Use this card to order copies of PDR® For Nonprescription Drugs

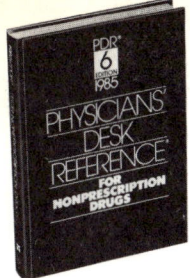

PDR For Nonprescription Drugs, 1985 is published in April, each year.

1. ☐ Send _____ copies of PDR For Nonprescription Drugs, 1985. My check is enclosed for $15.95 each.
2. ☐ Send _____ copies of PDR For Nonprescription Drugs, 1985. Bill me later for $17.95 each.

10% discount is granted for orders of 26 copies or more.

California and New Jersey residents add applicable sales tax.

Name _____

Institution _____

Street Address _____

MAIL THIS ORDER FORM, IN AN ENVELOPE, TO:
PDR For Nonprescription Drugs
Box 2019
Mahopac, New York 10541

City _____ State _____ Zip _____

Occupation _____

Signature _____

5R-AN-0

DETACH ALONG DOTTED LINE

Use this card to order copies of PDR® For Ophthalmology

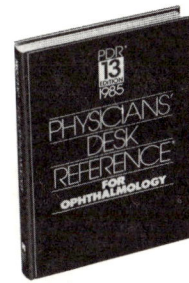

PDR For Ophthalmology 1985 was published in November, 1984.

1. ☐ Send _____ copies of PDR For Ophthalmology 1985. My check is enclosed for $21.95 each.
2. ☐ Send _____ copies of PDR For Ophthalmology 1985. Bill me later for $23.95 each.

10% discount is granted for orders of 26 copies or more.

California and New Jersey residents add applicable sales tax.

Name _____

Institution _____

Street Address _____

MAIL THIS ORDER FORM, IN AN ENVELOPE, TO:
PDR For Ophthalmology
Box 2017
Mahopac, New York 10541

City _____ State _____ Zip _____

Occupation _____

Signature _____

5R-AN-0

DETACH ALONG DOTTED LINE

Use this card to order extra copies of Physicians' Desk Reference®

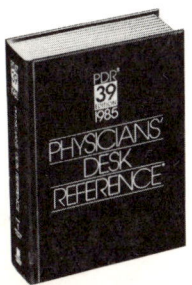

Physicians' Desk Reference is published in February, each year.

1. ☐ Send _____ copies of Physicians' Desk Reference, 1985. My check is enclosed for $25.95 each.
2. ☐ Send _____ copies of Physicians' Desk Reference, 1985. Bill me later for $27.95 each.
3. ☐ Send _____ copies of the 1985 PDR Supplements at $2.99 (Check must accompany order).

10% discount is granted for orders of 26 copies or more.

California and New Jersey residents add applicable sales tax.

Name _____

Institution _____

Street Address _____

MAIL THIS ORDER FORM, IN AN ENVELOPE, TO:
Physicians' Desk Reference
Box 2017
Mahopac, New York 10541

City _____ State _____ Zip _____

Occupation _____

Signature _____

5R-AN-0

Use this card to order copies of PDR® For Nonprescription Drugs

Use this card to order copies of PDR® For Ophthalmology

Use this card to order extra copies of Physicians' Desk Reference®

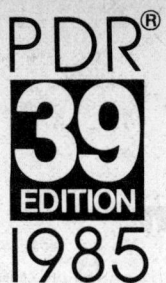

PHYSICIANS' DESK REFERENCE®

Publisher • EDWARD R. BARNHART

Director of Production
JEROME M. LEVINE

Managing Editor
BARBARA B. HUFF

Medical Consultant
IRVING M. LEVITAS, M.D.

Manager of Production Services
ELIZABETH H. CARUSO

Index Editor
ADELE L. DOWD

Editorial Assistants
F. EDYTHE PATERNITI
YVONNE HARLEY

Associate Editor
WILLIAM J. KNIPPING

Director of Printing
RALPH G. PELUSO

Circulation Director
THOMAS S. KRAEMER

Fulfillment Manager
JAMES SCIURBA

Research Director
CHARLOTTE E. SIBLEY

National Sales Manager
GARY J. GYSS

Account Managers
SALLY H. BERRIMAN
DAVID M. MJOLSNESS
PETER J. MURPHY

Design Director
JOHN NEWCOMB

Assistant Design Director
WILLIAM KUHN

Copyright © 1985 and published by Medical Economics Company Inc. at Oradell, N.J. 07649. All rights reserved. None of the content of this publication may be reproduced, stored in a retrieval system, or transmitted in any form or by any means (electronic, mechanical, photocopying, recording, or otherwise) without the prior written permission of the publisher. PHYSICIANS' DESK REFERENCE® and PDR® are trademarks of Medical Economics Company Inc., registered in the United States Patent and Trademark Office.

Officers of Medical Economics Company Inc.: Chairman and President, Charles P. Daly; Executive Vice President, Thomas J. McGill; Senior Vice Presidents: Theodore A. Maurer, Joseph M. Valenzano Jr.; Senior Vice President/Secretary, Stephen J. Sorkenn; Vice Presidents: Howard Clutterbuck, William J. Reynolds, Lewis A. Scaliti, Kathleen A. Starke.

ISBN 0-87489-878-1

Foreword to the thirty-ninth Edition

PHYSICIANS' DESK REFERENCE® is published annually by Medical Economics Company Inc. with the cooperation of the manufacturers whose products appear in the **Product Identification** (Gray Section), the **Product Information** (White Section), and the **Diagnostic Product Information** (Green Section). Intended primarily for physicans, PDR's purpose is to make available essential information on major pharmaceutical and diagnostic products. In addition to this volume, two other editions of PHYSICIANS' DESK REFERENCE will be published in 1985: PDR® For NONPRESCRIPTION DRUGS and PDR® For OPHTHALMOLOGY.

This edition of PHYSICIANS' DESK REFERENCE® includes the latest available information on over 2,500 products. During the year ahead as important new or revised information about these products becomes available to us, it will be published periodically in a PDR® Supplement. Retain the Supplement with PDR and before prescribing or administering any product described in PHYSICIANS' DESK REFERENCE, consult the latest PDR Supplement to determine if new information about the product has been published.

Special features in this edition include . . . Guide to the Management of Drug Overdose (inside back cover) . . . Poison Control Centers (page 446) . . . Educational Material (following manufacturer's product information) and Phonetic Spelling (below product name) in the Product Section.

The function of the Publisher is the compilation, organization, and distribution of this information. Product descriptions have been prepared by manufacturers, edited and approved by their medical department and/or medical consultant. Manufacturers suggest headings under which products should appear in the **Product Category Index** (Blue Section) and the **Generic and Chemical Name Index** (Yellow Section).

Under the federal Food, Drug, & Cosmetic [FD&C] Act, a drug approved for marketing may be labeled, promoted, and advertised by the manufacturer only for those uses for which the drug's safety and effectiveness have been established and which FDA has approved. The Code of Federal Regulations 201.100 (d)(i) pertaining to labeling for prescription products requires that for PDR content· "indications and usage, dosages, routes, methods and frequency and duration of administration, description, clinical pharmacology and supply and any relevant warnings, contraindications, adverse reactions, potential for drug abuse and dependence, overdosage and precautions" must be the *"same in language and emphasis"* as the approved labeling for the product. FDA regards the words *"same in language and emphasis"* as requiring VERBATIM use of the approved labeling providing such information. Furthermore, information in the approved labeling that is emphasized by the use of type set in a box or in capitals, bold face, or italics must also be given the same emphasis in PDR.

The FDA has also announced that the FD&C Act "does not, however, limit the manner in which a physician may use an approved drug. Once a product has been approved for marketing, a physician may prescribe it for uses or in treatment regimens or patient populations that are not included in approved labeling." Thus, the FDA states also that "accepted medical practice" often includes drug use that is not reflected in approved drug labeling.

For products which do not have official package circulars, the Publisher has emphasized to manufacturers the necessity of describing such products comprehensively so that physicians would have access to all information essential for intelligent and informed prescribing. In organizing and presenting the material in PHYSICIANS' DESK REFERENCE, the Publisher is providing all the information made available to PDR by manufacturers. Additional information on any product may be obtained from the manufacturer. In making this material available, the Publisher does not advocate the use of any described product.

EDWARD R. BARNHART
Publisher

Contents

MANUFACTURERS' INDEX 1
Section 1 (White) - Included are manufacturers who have provided prescribing information in this edition of PHYSICIANS' DESK REFERENCE®—their addresses, emergency phone numbers and a partial list of available products.

PRODUCT NAME INDEX AND DISCONTINUED PRODUCTS 101
Section 2 (Pink) - Part 1 - An alphabetical listing of products available from participating manufacturers. Where a page number is included, additional information can be found in other sections of this edition.
Part 2 - A list of products discontinued by manufacturers during the past year.

PRODUCT CATEGORY INDEX 201
Section 3 (Blue) - Products are listed according to the appropriate category, which has been determined by the Publisher in cooperation with each manufacturer. The opening pages contain the "Quick-Reference" to headings in this edition.

GENERIC AND CHEMICAL NAME INDEX 301
Section 4 (Yellow) - In this section products are listed under generic and chemical name headings according to the principal ingredient(s). The headings have been determined by the Publisher with the cooperation of the individual manufacturers.

PRODUCT IDENTIFICATION SECTION 401
Section 5 - Under company headings capsules and tablets are shown in color and actual size as an aid to identification. An index of participating manufacturers appears on page 402.

POISON CONTROL CENTERS 446
A list of centers and emergency telephone numbers.

PRODUCT INFORMATION SECTION 501
Section 6 (White) - An alphabetical arrangement by manufacturer of over 2,500 pharmaceuticals which are fully described as to indications and usage, dosage, administration, description, clinical pharmacology, supply, warnings, contraindications, adverse reactions, overdosage and precautions and other information concerning their use, including common names, generic compositions or chemical names. See inside back cover for information concerning overdosage.

DIAGNOSTIC PRODUCT INFORMATION 3001
Section 7 (Green) - Diagnostic product descriptions, listed alphabetically by manufacturer, to aid the physician in their use.

GUIDE TO MANAGEMENT OF DRUG OVERDOSE .... Inside Back Cover
Information concerning drug overdosage compiled by Eric G. Comstock, M.D., Director of the Institute of Clinical Toxicology.

SECTION 1
Manufacturers' Index

The manufacturers appearing in this index (white pages) have provided information concerning their pharmaceutical products in either the Product Information or Diagnostic Product Information Section. It is through their patronage that PHYSICIANS' DESK REFERENCE® is made available to you.

Included in this index are the names and addresses of manufacturers, individuals or departments to whom you may address inquiries, a partial list of products as well as emergency telephone numbers wherever available. The symbol ♦ indicates the product is shown in the Product Identification Section. The symbol •◘ indicates the product is described in PDR® FOR NONPRESCRIPTION DRUGS.

PAGE

ABBOTT LABORATORIES 403, 502
North Chicago, IL 60064
ABBOTT PHARMACEUTICALS, INC.
North Chicago, IL 60064
Address Medical Information Inquiries to:
Pharmaceutical Products Division
    (312) 937-7069
Hospital Products Division (312) 937-3806
Consumer Products Division (312) 937-3806
Distribution Centers
ATLANTA
  Stone Mountain, GA 30302
  P.O. Box 5049 (404) 493-8330
CHICAGO
  Abbott Park
  North Chicago, IL 60064
  P.O. Box 68 (312) 937-5153
DALLAS
  Dallas, TX 75265
  P.O. Box 225295 (214) 387-1350
LOS ANGELES
  Los Angeles, CA 90060
  60162 Terminal Annex (213) 582-6341
PHILADELPHIA
  King of Prussia, PA 19406
  920 Eighth Ave., East (215) 265-9100
Products Available
Abbokinase
Abbokinase Open-Cath
Abbo-Pac
Abbott Unit Dose Packages
  E.E.S. Granules
  Enduron Tablets
  Enduronyl Tablets
  Ery-Tab Tablets
  Erythrocin Stearate Filmtab
  Erythromycin Base Filmtab
  Fero-Grad-500 Filmtab
  Iberet-500 Filmtab
  K-Lor
  K-Tab Filmtab
  Nembutal Sodium Capsules
  Oretic Tablets
  Panwarfin Tablets
  Placidyl Capsules

PAGE

Surbex-T Filmtab
Tranxene Capsules
Acetic Acid Irrigation
Aerohalor
A-hydroCort
Alcohol, Absolute, Ampoules
5% Alcohol & 5% Dextrose Injection
A-methaPred
Aminophyllin 250 mg., 10 ml., Ampul & Vial
Aminophyllin 500 mg., 20 ml., Ampul & Vial
Aminosyn 3.5% M
Aminosyn 5%
Aminosyn 7%
Aminosyn 7% Kit
Aminosyn 7% with Electrolytes
Aminosyn 7% with Electrolytes TPN Kit
Aminosyn 8.5%
Aminosyn 8.5% TPN Kit
Aminosyn 8.5% with Electrolytes
Aminosyn 10%
Aminosyn 10% TPN Kit
Ammonium Chloride
Atropine 0.1 mg./ml., 5 ml., Abboject, Syringe
Atropine 0.1 mg./ml., 10 ml., Abboject, Syringe
Bupivacaine Hydrochloride Injection, USP, 0.5%
Butesin Picrate Ointment
Butyn Dental Ointment
Calcidrine Syrup
Calcium Chloride 10%, Abboject
Calcium Glucaptate Injection Ampoule & Abboject
Cecon Solution
♦ Cefol Filmtab
Cenolate Ampoules
♦ Chlorthalidone Tablets
Chromium 10 ml. (4 mg./ml.)
Colchicine Tablets
Copper 10 ml. (4 mg./ml.)
Covicone Cream
♦ Cylert Chewable Tablets
♦ Cylert Tablets
L-Cysteine Hydrochloride
Dayalets Filmtab

PAGE

Dayalets plus Iron Filmtab
♦ Depakene Capsules & Syrup
♦ Depakote Tablets
Desoxyn
♦ Desoxyn Gradumet Tablets
6% Dextran w/v & 5% Dextrose Injection
6% Dextran w/v & 0.9% Sodium Chloride Injection
2.5% Dextrose & ½ Str Lact Ringer's Injection
5% Dextrose & Lact Ringer's Injection
5% Dextrose & Ringer's Injection
2.5% Dextrose & 0.45% Sodium Chloride Injection
5% Dextrose & 0.225% Sodium Chloride Injection
5% Dextrose & 0.3% Sodium Chloride Injection
5% Dextrose & 0.45% Sodium Chloride Injection
5% Dextrose & 0.9% Sodium Chloride Injection
10% Dextrose & 0.9% Sodium Chloride Injection
2.5% Dextrose Injection
5% Dextrose Injection
5% Dextrose Injection (Partial fill)
10% Dextrose Injection
20% Dextrose Injection
50% Dextrose Injection
5% Dextrose & 0.075% Pot Chl Injection (10 mEq)
5% Dextrose & 0.15% Pot Chl Injection (20 mEq)
5% Dextrose & 0.224% Pot Chl Injection (30 mEq)
5% Dextrose & 0.3% Pot Chl Injection (40 mEq)
5% Dextrose & 0.225% Sodium Chloride with 0.075% Potassium Chloride Injection (10 mEq)

(♦ Shown in Product Identification Section)   (•◘ Described in PDR For Nonprescription Drugs)

Manufacturers' Index

5% Dextrose & 0.225% Sodium Chloride with 0.15% Potassium Chloride Injection (20 mEq)
5% Dextrose & 0.225% Sodium Chloride with 0.224% Potassium Chloride Injection (30 mEq)
5% Dextrose & 0.225% Sodium Chloride with 0.3% Potassium Chloride Injection (40 mEq)
5% Dextrose & 0.45% Sodium Chloride with 0.075% Potassium Chloride Injection (10 mEq)
5% Dextrose & 0.45% Sodium Chloride with 0.15% Potassium Chloride Injection (20 mEq)
5% Dextrose & 0.45% Sodium Chloride with 0.224% Potassium Chloride Injection (30 mEq)
5% Dextrose & 0.45% Sodium Chloride with 0.3% Potassium Chloride Injection (40 mEq)
10% Dextrose Injection
20% Dextrose Injection
30% Dextrose Injection
40% Dextrose Injection
50% Dextrose Injection
60% Dextrose Injection
70% Dextrose Injection
Dical-D Capsules & Wafers
Dical-D with Iron Capsules
Dical-D with Vitamin C Capsules
♦ Dicumarol Tablets
♦ E.E.S. Chewable Tablets
E.E.S. Drops
E.E.S. Granules
E.E.S. 200 Liquid
♦ E.E.S. 400 Filmtab
E.E.S. 400 Liquid
Empty Evacuated Container
Endrate Solution, Ampoules
♦ Enduron Tablets
♦ Enduronyl Forte Tablets
♦ Enduronyl Tablets
Ephedrine Sulfate, Injection
Epinephrine 1:10,000, 10 ml., Abboject
EryDerm
EryPed Granules
♦ Ery-Tab Tablets
Erythrocin Lactobionate-I.V.
Erythrocin Piggyback
Erythrocin Stearate Filmtab
Erythromycin Base Filmtab
♦ Eutonyl Filmtab
♦ Eutron Filmtab Tablets
♦ Fero-Folic-500 Filmtab
♦ Fero-Grad-500 Filmtab
Fero-Gradumet Filmtab
10% Fructose Injection
Gemonil Tablets
Gerilets Filmtab
Gerix Elixir
Glycine Solution, 1.5%, Irrigation/Aqualite
H-BIG
Halazone Tablets
Halothane
Harmonyl Tablets
Hydron Wound Dressing
Hydroxyzine HCl Injection, Abbojects, Ampuls, Vials, Syringes
Iberet Filmtab
♦ Iberet-500 Filmtab
Iberet-500 Liquid
♦ Iberet-Folic-500 Filmtab
Iberet Liquid
Iberol Filmtab
Iberol-F Filmtab
Inpersol & 1.5% Dextrose
Inpersol & 4.25% Dextrose
10% Invert Sugar Injection
Ionosol B & 5% Dextrose Injection
Ionosol B & 10% Invert Sugar Injection
Ionosol D & 10% Invert Sugar Injection
Ionosol D-CM & 5% Dextrose Injection
Ionosol G & 10% Dextrose Injection
Ionosol G & 10% Invert Sugar Injection
Ionosol MB & 5% Dextrose Injection
Ionosol T & 5% Dextrose Injection
Isoproterenol HCl 1:5,000 1 mg. Pintop
Isoproterenol HCl 1:5,000 2 mg. Pintop
Isoproterenol HCl 1:5,000 5 ml., Universal Add Syringe
Isoproterenol HCl 1:5,000 10 ml., Universal Add Syringe
Isoproterenol HCl 1:50,000, 10 ml., Abboject
♦ Janimine Filmtab
♦ K-Lor Powder
♦ K-Tab Filmtab
10% LMD w/v in 5% Dextrose Injection
10% LMD w/v with 0.9% Sodium Chloride Injection
LTA Kit, Preattached
LTA II Kit
LTA Pediatric Kit
Lactated Ringer's Injection
Lidocaine 0.2% in 5% Dextrose in water
Lidocaine 0.4% in 5% Dextrose in water
Lidocaine 1%, 5 ml., Abboject

Lidocaine 1%, 5 ml., Sterile Pack Abboject
Lidocaine 2%, 5 ml., Abboject
Lidocaine 2%, 5 ml., Sterile Pack Abboject
Lidocaine 20%, 5 ml., 1 gram-Pintop, U.A.S.
Lidocaine 20%, 10 ml., 2 gram-Pintop, U.A.S.
Lidocaine HCl, 5%, with 7.5% Dextrose
Lidocaine Hydrochloride Injection, U.S.P.
Liposyn 10%, 50, 100, 500, 200 ml.
Lubritine
Magnesium Sulfate 12.5%, 8 ml., Pintop
Magnesium Sulfate 50% w/v Ampoules & Abboject
Mammol Ointment
Manganese 10 ml. (1 mg./ml.)
5% Mannitol Injection
10% Mannitol Injection
15% Mannitol Injection
20% Mannitol Injection
25% Mannitol Injection
♦ Nembutal Sodium Capsules
Nembutal Sodium Solution
Nembutal Sodium Suppositories
Neut Abbo-Vial & Pintop
Niacin Tablets
Nitropress
Norisodrine Aerotrol
Norisodrine w/Calcium Iodide Syrup
Normosol-M 900 CAL
Normosol-M & 5% Dextrose Injection
Normosol-M & Surbex-T & 5% Dextrose Injection
Normosol-R & 5% Dextrose Injection
Normosol-R/K +& 5% Dextrose Injection
♦ Ogen Tablets
Ogen Vaginal Cream
Optilets-500 Filmtab
Optilets-M-500 Filmtab
♦ Oretic Tablets
Oreticyl Tablets
Oreticyl Forte Tablets
Panhematin
♦ Panwarfin Tablets
♦ Paradione Capsules & Oral Solution
Peganone Tablets
Penthrane
Pentothal Kit
Pentothal Rectal Suspension in Syringe
Pentothal Sodium Thiopental for Injection
Pentothal (Sterile Powder)
Pentothal Syringe
Phenobarbital Sodium Ampoules
Phenurone Tablets
Physiosol Irrigation/Aqualite
♦ Placidyl Capsules
Potassium Acetate 40 mEq Vial, Pintop & Fliptop
Potassium Chloride Injection Ampoules & Vials, Pintop & Universal Additive Syringe
Potassium Chloride 20 mEq. in D-5 W in Abbo-Vac
Potassium Phosphate 15 mM Vial, Pintop & Fliptop
Potassium Phosphate 45 mM Vial
Procaine Hydrochloride Injection 1% & 2% Vial
Quelicin (Succinylcholine Chloride Injection) Ampul & Vial, Pintop
Quelidrine Syrup
Ringer's Injection
Selsun Lotion
Selsun Suspension
Sodium Acetate 40 mEq Vial
5% Sodium Bicarbonate Injection
0.45% Sodium Chloride
5% Sodium Chloride
20% Sodium Chloride
0.9% Sodium Chloride Injection
Sorbital-Mannitol Irrigating Solution/Aqualite
Sterile Urea
Sulfadiazine Dulcet Tablets
Surbex Filmtab
Surbex w/C Filmtab
♦ Surbex-750 with Iron Filmtab
♦ Surbex-750 with Zinc Filmtab
♦ Surbex-T Filmtab
Surbex-T & 5% Dextrose Injection
TPN Electrolytes
Tham E
Tham Solution
Tral Filmtab
Tral Gradumet Tablets
♦ Tranxene Capsules & Tablets
♦ Tranxene-SD Half Strength Tablets
♦ Tranxene-SD Tablets
♦ Tridione Capsules
♦ Tridione Dulcet Tablets
Tridione Solution
Tronothane Hydrochloride Cream & Jelly
Tubocurarine Chloride Injection, USP
Ureaphil
Urological Solution G
Vercyte Tablets
Vita-Kaps Filmtab
Vita-Kaps M Filmtab
Vitamin C Filmtab

Water for Injection, Ampoules, Vial
Water for Injection Bacteriostatic 30 ml. Fliptop
Water for Injection, Sterile, Sterile Water
Water, for Irrigation, Sterile/Aqualite
Zinc 10 ml. (1 mg./1 ml.)

Gamma Counting Systems
Automatic and Manual
Auto-Logic 50
Auto-Logic 100
System Options
Logic 201
Logic 211
Logic 221

Hepatitis
Ausab Hepatitis B Surface Antigen [125I] (Human) Radioimmunoassay Diagnostic Kit
Ausab Hepatitis B Surface Antigen [125I] (Human) Radioimmunoassay Confirmatory Test
Auscell Antibody to Hepatitis B Surface Antigen (Guinea Pig) Reversed Passive Hemagglutination (RPHA) Diagnostic Kit
Auscell Antibody to Hepatitis B Surface Antigen (Human) Reversed Passive Hemagglutination (RPHA) Confirmatory Test Kit
Ausria II-125 Antibody to Hepatitis B Surface Antigen [125I] (Human) Radioimmunoassay Diagnostic Kit
Ausria II-125 Antibody to Hepatitis B Surface Antigen (Human) Radioimmunoassay Confirmatory Test
Aus-tect Test System, Rheophoresis Procedure

Thyroid
HTSH•RIA Diagnostic Kit
Prolactin RIA Diagnostic Kit
Quantisorb-125 T4N Diagnostic Kit
T3RIA (PEG) Diagnostic Kit
T4RIA (PEG) Diagnostic Kit
Thypinone (Protirelin) Synthetic TRH
Thyroscreen T4 Neonate
Triobead T3 Diagnostic Kit

Radiopharmaceuticals
Sensor [Radionuclide-Labeled ([125I]) Fibrinogen (Human)Glofil]

Diagnostics, General
Digoxin I 125 Imusay Diagnostic Kit
Reptilase-R (Bothrops atrox) (Lyophilized) Coagulation Test
Ruba-tect Rubella Diagnostic Test Systems (Kaolin or Heparin-Manganese Chloride)
Rubacell Rubella Screening Test
Strep-tect FA Group A Beta Hemolytic Streptococcus Fluorescent Antibody Detection System
UTI-tect Bacteriuria Diagnostic Test System

ABBOTT LABORATORIES   3002
DIAGNOSTICS DIVISION
Abbott Park
Abbott Park, IL 60064
Outside Illinois call toll free (800) 323-9100
In Illinois   1(800) 942-9117
Address inquiries to:
Marketing Services Dept. 49B
Products Available
Thypinone

ADRIA LABORATORIES   404, 571, 3003
INC.
Division of Erbamont Inc.
Administrative Offices:
5000 Post Road
Dublin, OH 43017
Mailing Address:
P. O. Box 16529
Columbus, OH 43216
Address inquiries to:
Medical Department   (614) 764-8100
Products Available
Adriamycin
Adrucil
Axotal
Chymex
efficin
Epsilan-M Capsules
Evac-Q-Kit
Evac-Q-Kwik
Fluidil
Folex for Injection
Ilopan Injection (Ampuls & Vials)
Ilopan Stat-Pak (Disposable Syringes)
Ilopan-Choline Tablets
Ilozyme Tablets
Kaochlor 10% Liquid
Kaochlor-Eff Tablets
Kaochlor S-F 10% Liquid
♦ Kaon Cl-10
Kaon Elixir, Grape Flavor
Kaon Elixir, Lemon-Lime Flavor
♦ Kaon Tablets
♦ Kaon-Cl
Kaon-Cl 20%
Magan Tablets
Modane Bulk
Modane Mild

(♦ Shown in Product Identification Section)   (▣ Described in PDR For Nonprescription Drugs)

Manufacturers' Index

Modane Mild Tablets
Modane Plus
Modane Soft
Modane Tablets
Myoflex Creme
Neosar for Injection
Pektamalt
Ratio Tablets
Taloin Ointment
Tympagesic Otic Solution
Tymtran Injection
W-T Lotion
Xylo-Pfan

ALCON LABORATORIES, INC. 588
Alcon Laboratories, Inc.
And its affiliates Inc.
Corporate Headquarters
P.O. Box 1959
6201 South Freeway
Fort Worth, TX 76134
Address inquiries to:
Sales Services (817) 293-0450
Products Available
A.I.D.S. (Alcon Instrument Delivery System)
Adsorbocarpine
Adsorbonac
Adsorbotear
Alcaine
Alcon Closure System, A.C.S.
Alcon Indirect Ophthalmoscope/Camera
Alcon Surgical System (Irrigation/Aspiration Kits; Phacoemulsification Kits)
BSS (15ml, 250ml, 500ml)
BSS Plus
BSS & BSS Plus Irrigation Solution Administration Set
Cetamide Ointment
Cetapred Ointment
Cryophake
Cyclogyl
Cyclomydril
Digilab Model 30D Pneuma-Tonometer
Digilab Model 30R Pneuma-Tonometer
Digilab Model 30R/T Pneuma-Tonometer-Tonographer
Duratears
Econochlor Solution & Ointment
Econopred
Econopred Plus
Enuclene
Epinal
Eye Pak
Eye Stream
Fluorescite
Glaucon
Gonioscopic Prism Solution
I-Knife
Ismotic
Isopto Atropine
Isopto Carbachol
Isopto Carpine
Isopto Cetamide
Isopto Cetapred
Isopto Homatropine
Isopto Hyoscine
Maxidex Suspension & Ointment
Maxitrol Suspension & Ointment
Microphake
Microsponge
Miostat
Mydfrin 2.5%
Mydriacyl
Naphcon
Naphcon-A
Naphcon Forte
Natacyn
Optemp
Osmoglyn
PTG
Steri-Units
Tears Naturale
Terry Keratometer
Tobrex Solution & Ointment
Zincfrin
Zolyse

ALCON (PUERTO RICO) INC. 588
P.O. Box 3000
Humacao, Puerto Rico 00661
Address inquiries to:
Medical Department
P.O. Box 1959
Fort Worth, TX 76101
(817) 293-0450
Products Available
Avitene

ALLERGAN PHARMACEUTICALS, INC. 589
2525 Dupont Drive
Irvine, CA 92715
Address inquiries to:
(714) 752-4500
(See also Herbert Laboratories)
Products Available
Albalon Liquifilm ophthalmic solution
Albalon-A Liquifilm ophthalmic solution
Allergan Hydrocare Cleaning & Disinfecting Solution
Allergan Hydrocare Preserved Saline Solution
Allergan Sorbi-Care Saline Solution
Atropine Sulfate ½% S.O.P. ophthalmic ointment
Atropine Sulfate 1.0% S.O.P. ophthalmic ointment
Atropine Sulfate ophthalmic solution 1%
Bleph-10 Liquifilm ophthalmic solution
Bleph-10 S.O.P. ophthalmic ointment
Blephamide Liquifilm ophthalmic suspension
Blephamide S.O.P. ophthalmic ointment
Blink-N-Clean hard contact lens solution
Chloroptic ophthalmic solution
Chloroptic S.O.P. ophthalmic ointment
Chloroptic-P S.O.P. ophthalmic ointment
Clean-N-Soak hard contact lens cleaning & soaking solution
Clean-N-Soakit hard contact lens storage case
Clean-N-Stow hard contact lens storage case
Epifrin ophthalmic solution
FML Liquifilm ophthalmic suspension
Genoptic S.O.P. ophthalmic ointment
Genoptic ophthalmic solution
HMS Liquifilm ophthalmic suspension
Herplex Liquifilm ophthalmic solution
LC-65 Daily Contact Lens Cleaner for Polycon & Paraperm O_2 gas permeable lenses & all hard & soft lenses
Lacril artificial tears
Lacri-Lube S.O.P. ophthalmic ointment
Lens Plus Daily Cleaner
Lens Plus Saline Solution
Lensrins preserved saline solution
Lens-Wet lubricating & rewetting solution
Liquifilm Forte enhanced artificial tears
Liquifilm Tears artificial tears
Liquifilm Wetting Solution hard contact lens solution
Ophthetic ophthalmic solution
P.V. Carpine Liquifilm ophthalmic solution
Poly-Pred Liquifilm ophthalmic suspension
Pred Forte ophthalmic suspension
Pred Mild ophthalmic suspension
Prefrin Liquifilm eye drops
Prefrin-A ophthalmic solution
Prefrin-Z Liquifilm ophthalmic solution
Propine ophthalmic solution
Soakare hard contact lens soaking solution
Soflens Enzymatic Contact Lens Cleaner
Tears Plus artificial tears
Total all-in-one hard contact lens solution
Wet-N-Soak wetting and soaking solution for hard contact lenses & Polycon & Paraperm O_2 gas permeable lenses

ALPHA THERAPEUTIC CORPORATION 589
5555 Valley Boulevard
Los Angeles, CA 90032
Address inquiries to:
2410 Lillyvale Avenue
Los Angeles, CA 90032
(213) 227-7470
For Medical Emergencies Contact:
Dr. Clyde McAuley (213) 227-7419
Products Available
Albutein 5%
Albutein 25%
Plasmatein 5%
Profilate
Profilate, Heat-Treated
Profilnine
Profilnine Heat-Treated

ALTO PHARMACEUTICALS, INC. 404, 589
15509 Casey Rd. Ext.
Tampa, FL 33624
Address inquiries to:
Professional Services
P.O. Box 271369
Tampa, FL 33688 (813) 961-1010
Products Available
Akne Drying Lotion
Akne Kaps
Akne pH Lotion
Alto-Pred Soluble Injection
Anabolin IM Injection
Anabolin LA-100 Injection
Cefinal II Tablets
D'Alpha-E Capsules
Dexamethasone Injection
◆ Efed II Capsules (Black)
◆ Efed II Capsules (Yellow)
Efed Tablets
Lotio-P Lotion
Methandrostenolone Tablets
Microcort Lotion
◆ Zinc-220 Capsules (Zinc Sulfate Capsules)

ALZA CORPORATION 404, 590
950 Page Mill Road
P.O. Box 10950
Palo Alto, California 94303-0802
Address inquiries to:
Marie E. Barry, Product Manager
(415) 494-5575
For Medical Emergencies Contact:
Virgil A. Place, Medical Director
(415) 494-5310
Products Available
Ocusert Ocular Therapeutic Systems
Pilo-20
Pilo-40
◆ Progestasert Intrauterine Contraceptive System

AMERICAN CRITICAL CARE 592
American Hospital Supply Corp.
McGaw Park, IL 60085
Address inquiries to:
Medical Director or in Emergency
Call: (312) 473-3000
Products Available
Bretylol Injection
Calciparine Injection
Hespan Injection
Intropin Injection
Inulin Solution, Purified
Tridil

AMERICAN DERMAL CORPORATION 599
12 Worlds Fair Drive
Somerset New Jersey 08873
Address Inquiries to:
Professional Services Department
(800) 526-0199
In New Jersey call: (201) 356-5544
Products Available
Drithocreme
Dritho-Scalp
Viranol

AMES DIVISION 3004
Miles Laboratories, Inc.
1127 Myrtle Street
P.O. Box 70
Elkhart, IN 46515
Order/Pricing Information:
(219) 264-8645
Customer Services
(800) 348-8100
Products Available
Ames Instruments
Clini-Tek Reflectance Photometer
Dextrometer Reflectance Colorimeter
Fluorostat Filter Fluorometer
Glucometer Reflectance Photometer
Optimate Alpha Automated Fluorometer/Photometer
Seralyzer Reflectance Photometer
Ames Tests
Ames Seralyzer Solid Phase Reagent Strips for: ALT/SGPT, AST/SGOT, Total Bilirubin, BUN, Cholesterol, Creatinine, CK, Glucose, Hemoglobin, LDH, Triglycerides, Uric Acid, Theophylline
Ames TDA Therapeutic Drug Assays-Fluorescent Immunoassays for Quantitative Determination of Therapeutic Drugs & Proteins in Serum on OPTIMATE Alpha
CHEK-STIX Urinalysis Control Strips
Dextrostix Reagent Strips
Diastix Reagent Strips
Hema-Chek Fecal Occult Blood Test with Control
Keto-Diastix Reagent Strips
Microcult-GC-Miniaturized Culture Test for Detection of *Neisseria gonorrhoeae*
Microstix-3 Reagent Strips
Microstix-Candida Miniaturized Culture Test
Microstix-Nitrite Kit
N-Multistix SG Reagent Strips
N-Uristix Reagent Strips
Visidex II Reagent Strips

ARCO PHARMACEUTICALS, INC. 600
105 Orville Drive
Bohemia, NY 11716
Address inquiries to:
Professional Service Dept. (516) 567-9500
Products Available
Arco-Cee Tablets
Arco-Lase Tablets
Arco-Lase Plus Tablets
Arcoret Tablets
Arcoret w/Iron Tablets
Arcotinic Liquid
Arcotinic Tablets
C-B Time Capsules
C-B Time 500 Tablets
C-B Time Liquid
⊞Codexin Capsules
Co-Gel Tablets
Mega-B
Megadose
Spantuss Liquid
Spantuss Tablets

AR-EX PRODUCTS CO. 600
1036 West Van Buren St.
Chicago, IL 60607
Address inquiries to:
Robert W. Francke (312) 226-5241
Products Available
Ar-Ex Hypo-Allergenic Cosmetics
Bath Oil - unscented
Body Lotion - unscented

(◆ Shown in Product Identification Section) (⊞ Described in PDR For Nonprescription Drugs)

Manufacturers' Index

Brush-On Complexion Coloring - unscented
Brush-On Eyeshadow - unscented
Chap Cream - scented & unscented
Cleansing Cream - scented & unscented
Cold Cream - scented & unscented
Compact Powder - unscented
Cream for Dry Skin - scented & unscented
Cream for Oily Skin - scented & unscented
Deodorant (Cream, Spray, Roll-On) - unscented
Disappear (Blemish Stick) - unscented
Eye Cream - unscented
Eye Makeup Remover Pads - unscented
Eye Pencil - unscented
Eye Shadow Stick - unscented
Face Powder - unscented
Foundation Cream - unscented
Lip Gloss & Sun Screen Stick - unscented
Moisture Cream - unscented
Moisture Lotion - scented & unscented
Night Cream - scented & unscented
Protein Hair Dressing & Conditioner - unscented
Roll-On Mascara - unscented
Shampoo - unscented
Special Formula Lipstick - unscented
Superfatted Soap - unscented
Safe Suds - unscented

**ARLO INTERAMERICAN CORPORATION 601
OF PUERTO RICO**
212 Mayaguez St.
Hato Rey, PR 00917
Address Inquiries to:
P.O. Box 1775
Hato Rey, PR 00919   (809) 767-2072
For Medical Emergencies Contact:
Professional Service Dept.
                          (809) 767-7281
Products Available
Apetigen Drops
Apetigen Elixir
Apetigen Plus Caps
Apetigen Plus Liquid
Arlon Forte
Dietex T.D.
Digestol Elixir
Duralgina Ampules
Duralgina Suppositories
Espasmotex Tablets
Fermolate Elixir
Forticon Liquid
Gumsol M.W. (mouthwash)
Gumsol Solution
Gumsol Spray
Hedal H-C Suppositories
Karbokoff Tablets
Oticol Sterile Ear Drops
Pasmex Drops
Pre-Protein Liquid
Pricort Cream
Pricort Lotion
Primotest Forte Tablets
Primotest Tablets
Primotest 225 Injection
Tocoferon 600 Tabs
Varisan Injection
Varisan Tabs
Vigoril 3 Tabs

**ARMOUR PHARMACEUTICAL 404, 601
COMPANY**
Executive Office
303 South Broadway
Tarrytown, NY 10591   (914) 631-8888
Eastern Distribution Center
P.O. Box 383
South Plainfield, NJ 07080 (201) 668-0110
Midwest Distribution Center
P.O. Box 511
Kankakee, IL 60901   (815) 932-6771
Western Distribution Center
P.O. Box 63249
Los Angeles, CA 90063   (213) 263-9359
Products Available
Acthar
◆ Aquasol A Capsules
Aquasol A Drops
Aquasol A Parenteral
◆ Aquasol E Capsules
Aquasol E Drops
Arm-a-char
Arm-a-Med
  Isoetharine Hychrochloride
  Isoproterenol Hydrochloride
Arm-a-Vial
  Sodium Chloride 0.45%
  Sodium Chloride 0.9%
  Sterile Water
Barotrast
Biozyme-C
C-B Vone Capsules
C.V.P. Capsules
Chrometrace
Clysodrast
Coppertrace
◆ Dialume
duo-C.V.P. Capsules

Esophotrast
HP Acthar Gel
Lufa Capsules
◆ M.V.I. (Multi-Vitamin Infusion)
M.V.I. Concentrate
M.V.I. Pediatric
M.V.I.-12 (Multi-Vitamin Infusion)
M.V.I.-12 Lyophilized (Multi-Vitamin Infusion)
Mangatrace
Methischol Capsules
Multitrace 5
Multitrace Pediatric
Multitrace Solution & Concentrate
Oratrast
Plasma Derivative Products
Albuminar-5, Normal Serum Albumin (Human) U.S.P. 5%
Albuminar-25, Normal Serum Albumin (Human) U.S.P. 25%
Factorate, Antihemophilic Factor (Human) Dried
Factorate, Generation II
Gammar, Immune Serum Globulin (Human) U.S.P.
Gamulin Rh
H.T. Factorate, Antihemophilic Factor (Human) Dried, Heat Treated
H.T. Factorate, Generation II
Mini-Gamulin Rh
Plasma Plex
Prothar, Factor IX Complex
Thrombinar
Selenitrace
Stimate Injection
Thrombinar
Thytropar
Trace Elements
  Chrometrace
  Coppertrace
  Mangatrace
  Multitrace 5
  Multitrace Pediatric
  Multitrace Solution & Concentrate
  Selenitrace
  Zinctrace
Vi-Aqua Capsules
Vi-Aqua Forte Capsules
Vi-Aquamin Forte Capsules
Zinctrace

ARTHER, INC. 614
Box 335
Mountain Lakes, NJ 07046
Address inquiries to:
A. Arthur Lowenthal, President
                          (800) 327-7914
                          (201) 263-2050
Products Available
Tryptacin

B. F. ASCHER & COMPANY, INC. 614
15501 W 109th St.
Lenexa, KS 66219
Address inquiries to:
Product Information Dept. (913) 888-1880
Products Available
Adipost Capsules
Anaspaz PB Tablets
Anaspaz Tablets
Ayr Saline Nasal Drops
Ayr Saline Nasal Mist
Converspaz Improved Capsules
Converzyme Improved Capsules
Dalca Tablets
Drize Capsules
Drotic Ear Drops
Ethaquin Tablets
Hycodaphen Tablets
Metronid Tablets
Mobidin Tablets
Mobigesic Tablets
Mobisyl Cream
Niloric Tablets
Soft 'N Soothe Creme
Tolfrinic Tablets
Unilax Tablets

**ASTRA PHARMACEUTICAL 615
PRODUCTS INC.**
50 Otis Street
Westboro, MA 01581-4428
Address inquiries to:
Professional Information Department
                          (617) 366-1100
Products Available
Citanest Solutions
Dopamine Solutions
Duranest Hydrochloride & Duranest Hydrochloride with Epinephrine 1:200,000
Dyclone, 0.5% & 1%
Nesacaine Solutions
Nesacaine-CE Solutions
Sensorcaine Hydrochloride & Sensorcaine Hydrochloride with Epinephrine 1:200,000
Xylocaine 2% Jelly
⊡ Xylocaine 2.5% Ointment
Xylocaine 5% Ointment

Xylocaine 10% Oral Spray
Xylocaine Hydrochloride, Xylocaine Hydrochloride with Epinephrine 1:100,000, & Xylocaine Hydrochloride with Epinephrine 1:200,000
Xylocaine Solution for Ventricular Arrhythmias-Intravenous Injection or Continuous Infusion; or Intramuscular Injection
Xylocaine 1.5% Solution with Dextrose 7.5%
Xylocaine 4% Sterile Solution
Xylocaine 5% Solution with Glucose 7.5%
Xylocaine 4% Topical Solution
Xylocaine 2% Viscous Solution
Yutopar Intravenous Injection
Yutopar Tablets

AYERST LABORATORIES 404, 634, 3007
Division of American Home Products Corp.
685 Third Ave.
New York, NY 10017
For Medical Information
Business hours only (9:00 a.m. to 5:00 p.m. EST), call   (212) 878-5900
For Medical Emergency Information After Hours or On Weekends, call
                          (212) 986-1000
                          (212) 878-5900
                          (212) 878-5000
Regional Sales Offices
Burlingame, CA 94010
  Suite 100
  840 Hinckley Road   (415) 692-4258
Chamblee, GA (Atlanta) 30341
  3600 American Drive   (404) 451-9578
Chicago, IL 60648
  7545 N. Natchez Ave.   (312) 647-8948
Lakewood, OH 44107
  Suite 440
  14701 Detroit Ave.   (216) 226-4128
Los Angeles, CA 90061
  12833 S. Spring St.
                         (213) 321-5550/1/2
Mesquite, TX (Dallas) 75149
  3601 Executive Blvd.   (214) 285-8741
Rockville, MD 20852
  6252 Montrose Rd.   (301) 984-9140
South Plainfield, NJ 07080
  4000 Hadley Rd.   (201) 754-6220 (NJ)
                         (212) 964-3903 (NY)
Distribution Centers
Chamblee—3600 American Drive
  Chamblee, GA 30341   (404) 457-2518
Chicago—7545 N. Natchez Ave.
  Chicago, IL 60648
                         (312) 763-0888 (Chicago)
                         (312) 647-8840 or 8841 (Niles)
Cleveland—15620 Industrial Parkway
  Cleveland, OH 44135   (216) 267-9090
Lenexa—10700 Pflumm Road
  Lenexa, KS 66210   (913) 888-4310
Los Angeles—12833 S. Spring St.
  Los Angeles, CA 90061
                         (213) 321-5550-1-2
Mesquite—3601 Executive Blvd.
  Mesquite, TX 75149   (214) 285-8741
Seattle—405 Baker Blvd., Andover Park
  Seattle, WA 98188   (206) 244-1921
South Plainfield—4000 Hadley Road
  South Plainfield, NJ 07080
                         (201) 754-6220 (NJ)
                         (212) 964-3903 (NY)
Products Available
A.P.L.
Almocarpine
◆ Anacin-3 with Codeine Tablets
◆ Antabuse
◆ Atromid-S
Auralgan Otic Solution
◆ Aygestin
◆ Beminal-500
Beminal Forte w/Vitamin C
◆ Beminal Stress Plus
Clusivol Capsules
Clusivol Syrup
Clusivol 130 Tablets
Cytoferin Hematinic Tablets
Dermoplast
◆ Diucardin
Enzactin Cream
Ayerst Epitrate
Estradurin
Estrogenic Substance (estrone) In Aqueous Suspension
◆ Factrel
Fluor-I-Strip Applicators
Fluor-I-Strip-A.T. Applicators
Fluothane
◆ Grisactin
◆ Grisactin Ultra
◆ Inderal
◆ Inderal LA Long Acting Capsules
◆ Inderide
Kerodex Cream (water-miscible)
Kerodex Cream (water-repellent)
Larylgan Throat Spray
◆ Mediatric Capsules
Mediatric Liquid

(◆ Shown in Product Identification Section)   (⊡ Described in PDR For Nonprescription Drugs)

Manufacturers' Index

◆ Mediatric Tablets
Mysoline Suspension
◆ Mysoline Tablets
Ophthalgan
◆ PMB 200 & PMB 400
Peptavlon
Phospholine Iodide
◆ Plegine
Premarin Intravenous
◆ Premarin Tablets
◆ Premarin Vaginal Cream
◆ Premarin w/Methyltestosterone
Protopam Chloride for Injection
Protopam Chloride Tablets
◆ Riopan Antacid Chew Tablets
◆ Riopan Antacid Chew Tablets in Rollpack
Riopan Antacid Suspension
◆ Riopan Antacid Swallow Tablets
◆ Riopan Plus Chew Tablets
Riopan Plus Chew Tablets in Rollpack
Riopan Plus Suspension
Sonacide
Thiosulfil Duo-Pak Package
◆ Thiosulfil Forte Tablets
◆ Thiosulfil Tablets
◆ Thiosulfil-A Forte Tablets
◆ Thiosulfil-A Tablets
Turgasept Aerosol

BAKER/CUMMINS 683
Dermatological Div. of Key Pharmaceuticals, Inc.
50 N.W. 176th Street
Miami, FL 33169
  In Florida (305) 652-2276
    (800) 327-9054
Products Available
Acno Lotion & Cleanser
Acticort Lotion 100
▣Complex 15 Lotion & Cream
▣P&S Liquid
▣P&S Plus Gel
▣P&S Shampoo
Panscol Lotion & Ointment
Phacid Shampoo
Ultra Derm Moisturizer
▣Ultra Mide 25 Lotion
▣Xseb Shampoo
▣Xseb-T Shampoo

BARNES-HIND, INC. 683
A Revlon Vision Care Company
895 Kifer Road
Sunnyvale, CA 94086
Address inquiries to:
Mr. James Tasker
Sales Services Dept. (408) 736-5462
    (800) 538-1562
Products Available
Barseb HC Scalp Lotion
Barseb Thera-Spray
HEB Cream Base
Komed Acne Lotion
Komed HC Lotion
Komex
Pro-Cort Cream
Pro-Cort M Cream
Tinver Lotion
The following Barium Products now sold by Armour Pharmaceuticals
Barotrast
Clysodrast
Esophotrast
Oratrast

BARRY LABORATORIES, INC. 685
461 N.E. 27th Street
P.O. Box 1967
Pompano Beach, FL 33061
In Florida call (1-305) 943-7722
Outside of Florida
Toll Free WATS Line (1-800) 327-1141
Address Inquiries to:
Special Services Department
Products Available
Allergenic Extracts, Diagnosis and/or Immunotherapy
  Dusts
  Epidermals
  Foods
  Fungi (molds & smuts)
  Inhalents
  Insects
  Poison Ivy, Oak, Sumac combined, (Rhus All Antigen)
  Pollens
  Stinging Insects (Stinging Insect Antigen) #108
Allergenic Extracts for Immunotherapy
Immunorex-Prescription allergy treatment sets
  Rhus All Antigen (Poison Ivy, Oak. Sumac combined)
  Stinging Insect Antigen #108
Diagnostic Allegenic Extracts
  Cutaneous
  Intracutaneous

Diagnostic Allergenic Test Sets
"50+" Includes a selection of perennial and seasonal allergens for each of 5 botanical zones
Sensi-Test Kit (Disposable Allergy Scarifier)
Merphene Germicidal Concentrate
Rhus All Antigen - Poison Ivy, Oak, Sumac Combined

A. J. BART, INC. 685
Gurabo Industrial Park
P.O. Box 813
Gurabo, Puerto Rico 00658
  (809) 737-8445
  (809) 737-8446
  (809) 737-8447
Address inquiries to:
Mr. Bob Bibars (809) 737-8445
Products Available
Alba-3 Ointment
Alba-3 Ophthalmic Ointment
Alba-3 Ophthalmic Solution
Alba-Ce Liquid, Drops, Tablets
Albacort Cream
Alba-Dex Injectable, Liquid & Tablets
Albaform-HC Cream
Albafort Injectable
Alba-Gyn Vaginal Cream
Alba-Lybe
Alba-Temp Suppositories, Liquid, Tablets & Drops
Albatussin (Sugar Free)
Alvimin
Asmex KI Liquid
Asmex Liquid
Benzotic Ear Drops
Dramatrol Injectable
Myoforte Tablets
Myophen Injectable
Pasmin Injectable, Liquid, Capsules
Sedaril
Tia-Doce Injectable Solution

BEACH PHARMACEUTICALS 405, 685
Division of Beach Products, Inc.
Executive Office
5220 S. Manhattan Ave.
Tampa, FL 33611 (813) 839-6565
Manufacturing and Distribution
Main St. at Perimeter Rd.
Conestee, SC 29605
  Toll Free 1-(800) 845-8210
Address inquiries to:
Richard Stephen Jenkins (813) 839-6565
Products Available
◆ Beelith Tablets
Citrolith Tablets
Fer-Bid Improved
◆ K-Phos M.F. (Modified Formula) Tablets
◆ K-Phos Neutral
◆ K-Phos No. 2 Tablets
◆ K-Phos Original Formula 'Sodium Free' Tablets
K-Phos w/S.A.P.
◆ Thiacide Tablets
◆ Uroqid-Acid
◆ Uroqid-Acid No. 2

BEECHAM PRODUCTS 687
Division of Beecham Inc.
P.O. Box 1467
Pittsburgh, PA 15230
Address inquiries to:
Professional Services Dept.
  800-BEECHAM
PA Residents: 800-242-1718
Products Available
Massengill Disposable Douche
Massengill Liquid Concentrate
Massengill Medicated Disposable Douche
Massengill Powder

BEECHAM LABORATORIES 405, 688
Division of Beecham, Inc.
Bristol, TN 37620
Address inquiries to:
Director, Professional Relations
Beecham Laboratories
501 Fifth Street
Bristol, TN 37620 (615) 764-5141
Products Available
Actol Expectorant Liquid
Actol Expectorant Tablets
◆ Amoxil Capsules, Oral Suspension & Chewable Tablets
Amoxil Pediatric Drops for Oral Suspension
Anexsia w/Codeine Tablets
Anexsia-D Tablets
◆ Augmentin Tablets & Powder for Oral Suspension
◆ Bactocill Capsules
Bactocill for Injection
Beepen-VK Oral Solution & Tablets
◆ Cloxapen Capsules
Conar Expectorant Syrup
Conar Suspension
Conar-A Suspension
Conar-A Tablets
Corrective Mixture w/Paregoric

Daricon
Daricon PB
Dasin Capsules
◆ Dycill Capsules
Enarax Tablets
◆ Fastin Capsules
Hybephen Tablets
Hycal Liquid
Klebcil for Injection
Livitamin Capsules
Livitamin Capsules w/Intrinsic Factor
Livitamin Chewable Tablets
Livitamin Liquid
Menest Tablets
Morphine & Atropine Injectable
Nallpen for Injection
◆ Nucofed Capsules
Nucofed Expectorant
Nucofed Pediatric Expectorant
Nucofed Syrup
Pyopen Injectable
Semets Troches
Theralax Suppositories
Ticar for Injection
◆ Tigan Capsules
Tigan Injectable
Tigan Suppositories
Totacillin Capsules
Totacillin For Oral Suspension
Totacillin-N Injectable

BERLEX LABORATORIES INC. 406, 699
Cedar Knolls, NJ 07927
Address inquiries to:
Professional Services
300 Fairfield Road
Wayne, NJ 07470 (201) 694-4100
For Medical Information
Medical Department
110 East Hanover Avenue
Cedar Knolls, NJ 07927 (201) 540-8700
Products Available
Anodynos DHC Tablets
Deconamine Elixir
◆ Deconamine SR Capsules
Deconamine Syrup
◆ Deconamine Tablets
◆ Elixicon Suspension
◆ Elixophyllin Capsules
Elixophyllin Elixir
◆ Elixophyllin SR Capsules
Elixophyllin-GG
Elixophyllin-KI Elixir
Kay Ciel Oral Solution 10%
Kay Ciel Powder
Pyocidin-Otic Solution
◆ Quinaglute Dura-Tabs
◆ Sus-Phrine Injection

BEUTLICH, INC. 705
7149 North Austin
Niles, IL 60048 (312) 262-7900
Products Available
Ceo-Two Rectal Suppositories
Hurricaine Liquid 1/4cc Unit Dose
Hurricaine Oral, Topical Anesthetic Gel
Hurricaine Oral, Topical Anesthetic Liquid
Hurricaine Spray Extension Tubes
Hurricaine Topical Anesthetic Spray
Hurricaine Topical Anesthetic Spray Kit
Mevanin-C Capsules
Peridin-C Tablets

BIOCRAFT LABORATORIES, INC. 705
92 Route 46
Elmwood Park, NJ 07407
Address Inquiries to:
  (201) 796-3434
Products Available
Amitriptyline HCl Tablets
Amoxicillin Capsules
Amoxicillin Suspension
Ampicillin Capsules
Ampicillin Suspension
Ampicillin-Probenecid Suspension
Chloroquine Phosphate Tablets
Cloxacillin Capsules
Cloxacillin Solution
Dicloxacillin Capsules
Imipramine HCl Tablets
Neomycin Sulfate Tablets
Oxacillin Capsules
Oxacillin Solution
Penicillin G Potassium Tablets
Penicillin V Potassium Solution
Penicillin V Potassium Tablets
Sulfamethoxazole & Trimethoprim Pediatric Suspension
Sulfamethoxazole and Trimethoprim Tablets
Trimethoprim Tablets

BOCK PHARMACAL COMPANY 705
5435 Highland Park Drive
St. Louis, MO 63110
Address inquiries to:
Professional Services Dept. (314) 535-4060
Products Available
Amobell Capsules
Broncholate Capsules

(◆ Shown in Product Identification Section)   (▣ Described in PDR For Nonprescription Drugs)

Manufacturers' Index

Broncholate Syrup
Demasone Injectable
Demasone-LA Injectable
Dolprn #3 Tablets
Hemaspan Tablets
Limit Tablets
Onset-5 Tablets
Onset-10 Tablets
Pavadyl Capsules
Poly-Histine Capsules
Poly-Histine Elixir
Poly-Histine Expectorant Plain
Poly-Histine Expectorant with Codeine
Poly-Histine-D Capsules
Poly-Histine-D Elixir
Poly-Histine-D Pediatric Capsules
Poly-Histine-DX Capsules
Prenate 90 Tablets
Theon Syrup
Vitamin B$_{12}$ Injectable
Zephrex Tablets
Zephrex-LA Tablets

BOEHRINGER INGELHEIM LTD.   406, 706
90 East Ridge
P.O. Box 368
Ridgefield, CT 06877
Address inquiries to:
Medical Services Dept.   (203) 438-0311
Products Available
Alupent Inhalent Solution 5% & Solution Unit Dose 0.6%
Alupent Metered Dose Inhaler
Alupent Syrup
◆ Alupent Tablets
◆ Catapres Tablets
◆ Combipres Tablets
◆ Dulcolax Suppositories
◆ Dulcolax Tablets
◆ Persantine Tablets
◆ Prelu-2 Capsules
Preludin Endurets
Preludin Tablets
◆ Respbid
Serentil Ampuls
Serentil Concentrate
◆ Serentil Tablets
◆ Thalitone Tablets
Torecan Ampuls
Torecan Suppositories
Torecan Tablets

**BOEHRINGER MANNHEIM   3009
DIAGNOSTICS, INC.**
Bio-Dynamics Division
9115 Hague Road
Indianapolis, IN 46250   (317) 845-2000
Products Available
Chemstrip bG Blood Glucose Test
Chemstrip Urine Testing System

BOOTS PHARMACEUTICALS, INC.   406, 717
6540 Line Avenue
Shreveport, LA 71106
Address inquiries to:
Medical Director   (318) 869-3551
Products Available
F-E-P Creme
◆ Lopurin Tablets
◆ Rufen Tablets
Ru-Tuss Expectorant
Ru-Tuss Plain
◆ Ru-Tuss Tablets
◆ Ru-Tuss II Capsules
Ru-Tuss with Hydrocodone
Twin-K Liquid
Twin-K-Cl Liquid
◆ Zorprin Tablets

BOYLE & COMPANY   726
13260 Moore St.
Cerritos, CA 90701
Address inquiries to:
Susan M. Boyle   (213) 926-8250
Products Available
Citra Forte Capsules
Citra Forte Syrup
Glytinic Tablets
Triva Combination
Triva Douche Powder
Triva Jel

BRAINTREE LABORATORIES, INC.   727
285 Washington Street
Braintree, MA 02184
Address inquiries to:
Mr. Vincent J. Heidenreich   (617) 843-2202
For Medical Emergencies Contact:
Geoffrey E. Clark, M.D.   (603) 749-2417
Products Available
GoLYTELY

BREON LABORATORIES, INC.
See WINTHROP-BREON LABORATORIES

BRISTOL LABORATORIES   407, 727
(Div. of Bristol-Myers Co.)
Thompson Rd., P.O. Box 4755
Syracuse, NY 13221   (315) 432-2000

Address medical inquiries to:
Dept. of Medical Services   (315) 432-2838
    or (315) 432-2000
Orders may be placed by calling the following toll free numbers:
Within New York State   1-(800) 962-7200
Continental U.S.   1-(800) 448-7700
Alaska - Hawaii   1-(800) 448-1100
Mail orders and all inquiries should be sent to:
Bristol Laboratories
Order Entry Department
P.O. Box 4755
Syracuse, NY 13221-4755
Products Available
Amikin
◆ Betapen-VK Tablets and Oral Solution
Bristoject Products
    Aminophyllin
    Atropine Sulfate
    Calcium Chloride
    Dexamethasone
    Dextrose
    Diphenhydromine HCl
    Dopamine HCl
    Ephedrine
    Epinephrine
    Lidocaine HCl
    Magnesium Sulfate
    Metaraminol Bitartrate
    Sodium Bicarbonate
Cefadyl for Intramuscular or Intravenous Injection
◆ Dynapen Capsules and Powder for Oral Suspension
◆ Kantrex Capsules
Kantrex Injection and Pediatric Injection
Nafcil
◆ Naldecon Syrup, Tablets, Pediatric Drops and Pediatric Syrup
⊞ Naldecon-CX Suspension
⊞ Naldecon-DX Pediatric Syrup
⊞ Naldecon-EX Pediatric Drops
◆ Naldegesic Tablets
◆ Polycillin Capsules, for Oral Suspension, and Pediatric Drops
Polycillin-N for Intramuscular or Injection
Polycillin-PRB (ampicillin-probenecid) for Oral Suspension
◆ Polymox Capsules, for Oral Suspension, and Pediatric Drops
Precef
◆ Prostaphlin Capsules, Oral Solution
Prostaphlin for Injection
◆ Saluron
◆ Salutensin/Salutensin-Demi
Stadol
Staphcillin Injection—Buffered
◆ Tegopen Capsules and For Oral Solution
◆ Ultracef Capsules, Tablets & Oral Suspension
Versapen Oral Suspension and Pediatric Drops
◆ Versapen-K Capsules

**BRISTOL-MYERS ONCOLOGY   407, 756
DIVISION**
(Bristol-Myers Company)
Thompson Road, P.O. Box 4755
Syracuse, NY 13221   (315) 432-2000
Address medical inquiries to:
Dept. of Medical Services
    (315) 432-9506
    or (315) 432-2000
Orders may be placed by calling the following toll free numbers:
Within New York State   1-(800) 962-7200
Continental US   1-(800) 448-7700
Alaska-Hawaii   1-(800) 448-1100
Mail orders and all inquiries should be sent to:
Bristol Laboratories
Order Entry Department
P.O. Box 4755
Syracuse, NY 13221-4755
Products Available
BiCNU
Blenoxane
◆ CeeNU
◆ Cytoxan
◆ Lysodren
◆ Megace Tablets
Mexate
Mutamycin
Platinol
VePesid Injection

BRISTOL-MYERS PRODUCTS   768
(Div. of Bristol-Myers Co.)
345 Park Avenue
New York, NY 10154
Address inquiries to:
Fredric B. Bauer M.D.
In Emergencies Call:
    (212) 546-2752 (9 AM-5 PM)
    (212) 546-4700 (other)
Products Available
Ammens medicated powder
Arthritis Strength Bufferin analgesic tablets

Aspirin Free Congespirin cold tablets
B.Q. cold tablets
Ban Basic antiperspirant
Ban cream antiperspirant
Ban roll-on antiperspirant
Ban Wide Ball antiperspirant
Body on Tap Shampoo and Conditioner
Bufferin analgesic tablets and capsules
Comtrex capsules
Comtrex liquid
Comtrex tablets
Congespirin aspirin-free chewable cold tablets for children
Congespirin cold tablets (aspirin formula)
Congespirin cough syrup
Congespirin liquid cold medicine
Excedrin Extra-Strength analgesic capsules
Excedrin Extra-Strength analgesic tablets
Excedrin P.M. analgesic tablets
Extra-Strength Bufferin capsules & tablets
Extra-Strength Datril capsules & tablets
4-Way cold tablets
4-Way long acting nasal spray
4-Way mentholated nasal spray
4-Way nasal spray
Minit-Rub analgesic balm
Mum cream deodorant
No Doz tablets
Nuprin ibuprofen/analgesic tablets
Pazo hemorrhoid ointment/suppositories
Score hair cream
Tickle antiperspirant
Ultra Ban Aerosol antiperspirant
Ultra Ban roll-on
Ultra Ban Solid antiperspirant/deodorant
Vitalis clear gel
Vitalis Dry Texture hair groom
Vitalis hair groom liquid
Vitalis Regular Hold hair spray
Vitalis Super Hold hair spray

**THE BROWN PHARMACEUTICAL   407, 771
COMPANY, INC.**
2500 West Sixth St.
P.O. Box 57925
Los Angeles, CA 90057
    (213) 389-1394/1395
Address inquiries to:
Professional Service Department
Products Available
◆ Android-5 Buccal
◆ Android-10 Tablets
◆ Android-25 Tablets
◆ Android-F Tablets
Brohembione
Calphosan B-12 I.M.
Calphosan I.M.
Lipo-Nicin/100 mg.
Lipo-Nicin/250 mg. Tablets
Lipo-Nicin/300 mg. Caps Timed
Vivikon I.M.

BURROUGHS WELLCOME CO.   407, 773
3030 Cornwallis Road
Research Triangle Park, NC 27709
    (919) 248-3000
Address inquiries to:
Public Affairs Dept.   (919) 248-4239
Branch Office
Burlingame, CA 94010
1760 Rollins Rd.   (415) 697-5630
Products Available
◆ A.P.C. with Codeine Nos. 3 & 4, Tabloid brand
◆ Actidil Tablets & Syrup
◆ Actifed Tablets & Syrup
Actifed with Codeine Cough Syrup
Aerosporin Powder
◆ Alkeran Tablets
Ammonia Aromatic, Vaporole
Amyl Nitrite, Vaporole
Anectine Flo-Pack
Anectine Injection
◆ Antepar Syrup & Tablets
Atropine Sulfate Injection, Wellcome
Borofax Ointment
◆ Cardilate Chewable Tablets
◆ Cardilate Oral/Sublingual Tablets
Cortisporin Cream
Cortisporin Ointment
Cortisporin Ophthalmic Ointment
Cortisporin Ophthalmic Suspension
Cortisporin Otic Solution
◆ Cortisporin Otic Suspension
◆ Daraprim Tablets
Digoxin (See Lanoxin)
◆ Empirin Aspirin Tablets
◆ Empirin w/Codeine Phosphate Nos. 2, 3 & 4
◆ Empracet with Codeine Phosphate Nos. 3 & 4
Erythrityl Tetranitrate (See Cardilate)
◆ Fedrazil Tablets
Imuran Injection
◆ Imuran Tablets
◆ Kemadrin Tablets
Lanoline, Wellcome
◆ Lanoxicaps
◆ Lanoxin—Tablets, Injection & Elixir Pediatric

(◆ Shown in Product Identification Section)   (⊞ Described in PDR For Nonprescription Drugs)

Manufacturers' Index

◆ Leukeran Tablets
Lubafax Surgical Lubricant, Sterile
Mantadil Cream
◆ Marezine Tablets & Injection
◆ Myleran Tablets
Neosporin Aerosol
Neosporin G.U. Irrigant
Neosporin Ointment
Neosporin Ophthalmic Ointment Sterile
Neosporin Ophthalmic Solution Sterile
Neosporin Topical Powder
Neosporin-G Cream
Polymyxin B Sulfate (see Aerosporin)
Polysporin Ointment
Polysporin Ophthalmic Ointment
◆ Proloprim Tablets
◆ Purinethol Tablets
Scopolamine Hydrobromide Injection, Wellcome
◆ Septra DS Tablets
Septra I.V. Infusion
Septra Suspension
◆ Septra Tablets
⊞ Sudafed Cough Syrup
◆ Sudafed Plus Syrup & Tablets
◆ Sudafed Pseudoephedrine Hydrochloride Syrup & Tablets
◆ Sudafed S.A. Capsules
◆ Tabloid Brand Thioguanine
Vasoxyl Injection
Vioptic Ophthalmic Solution
Wellcovorin Injection
◆ Wellcovorin Tablets
Zovirax Ointment 5%
Zovirax Sterile Powder
◆ Zyloprim Tablets

C & M PHARMACAL, INC.   **828**
1519 E. Eight Mile Rd.
Hazel Park, MI 48030-2696
Address Inquires to:
C & M Pharmacal, Inc.   (313) 548-7846
For Medical Emergencies Contact:
C & M Pharmacal, Inc.   (313) 548-7846
Or any Poison Control Center (All products have full ingredient disclosure)
Products Available
Acnotex
Aquaderm
Colladerm
Cortin 1% Cream
Drytergent
Drytex
Duplex
Duplex T
Finac
HI-COR 1.0
HI-COR 2.5
Hydropel
Pod-Ben-25
SLT Lotion
Schamberg's Lotion
Seale's Lotion Modified
Sofenol 5
Sulfoil
Therac
Theracort
Verr-Canth
Verrex
Verrusol

CAMPBELL LABORATORIES INC.   **829**
300 East 51st Street
New York, NY 10022   (212) 688-7684
Address inquiries to:
Richard C. Zahn, President
P.O. Box 812, FDR Station
New York, NY 10150
Products Available
Herpecin-L Cold Sore Lip Balm

THE CARLTON CORPORATION   **829**
See GLENWOOD, INC.

CARNRICK LABORATORIES, INC.   **408, 829**
65 Horse Hill Road
Cedar Knolls, NJ 07927   (201) 267-2670
Address inquiries to:
Medical Director   (201) 267-2670
Products Available
◆ Amen
◆ Bontril PDM
◆ Bontril Slow-Release
◆ Capital with Codeine Suspension
◆ Capital with Codeine Tablets
◆ Midrin
◆ Nolahist
◆ Nolamine
◆ Phrenilin
◆ Phrenilin Forte
◆ Phrenilin with Codeine No. 3
◆ Propagest & Propagest Syrup
◆ Sinulin
◆ Skelaxin

CENTER LABORATORIES   **835**
Division of EM Industries, Inc.
35 Channel Drive
Port Washington, NY 11050

Address Inquiries to:
Customer Services
    Call Toll Free (800) 645-6335
    In N.Y. (516) 767-1800
For Medical Emergencies Contact:
Technical Services   (516) 767-1800
Products Available
Center-Al—Allergenic Extracts Alum Precipitated
EpiPen—Epinephrine Auto-Injector
EpiPen Jr.

CENTRAL PHARMACEUTICALS, INC.   **409, 836**
120 East Third St.
Seymour, IN 47274
Address inquiries to:
Daniel J. Desmond   (812) 522-3915
Products Available
Analbalm, Liquid
Andronaq-50 Sterile Suspension
Andronaq-LA
Biotres Ointment
Cenocort A-40 Sterile Suspension
Cenocort Forte Sterile Suspension
Codiclear DH Syrup
Codimal DH Syrup
Codimal DM Syrup
Codimal Expectorant
Codimal PH Syrup
Codimal Tablets & Capsules
Codimal-A Injectable
◆ Codimal-L.A. Capsules
Co-Gesic Tablets
Co-Xan Syrup
Cyclocen Injectable
Dexacen LA-8 Sterile Suspension
Dexacen-4 Injectable
Dia-Eze
◆ Dia-Gesic
Diphenacen-10 and -50 Injectables
Dramocen Injectable
Estronol Aqueous Sterile Suspension
Estronol-LA Injectable
GG-Cen Syrup/Capsules
Hexalol Tablets
Hydroxacen Injectable
Lifolbex Injectable
◆ Mono-Gesic Tablets
Neocylate Tablets
Neocyten Injection
Neolax Tablets
Niferex Elixir
Niferex Forte Elixir
Niferex Tablets
Niferex w/Vitamin C Tablets
◆ Niferex-150 Capsules
◆ Niferex-150 Forte Capsules
◆ Niferex-PN Tablets
Pavacen Capsules
Phencen-50 Injectable
Prednicen-M Tablets
Prednisolone Acetate Sterile Suspension
Progestronaq-LA
Rep-Pred 40 Sterile Suspension
Rep-Pred 80 Sterile Suspension
Rubesol-1000 Injectable
Synophylate Elixir
Synophylate-GG Syrup
Synophylate-GG Tablets
◆ Theoclear L.A.-130 & -260 Capsules
Theoclear-80 Syrup

CETYLITE INDUSTRIES, INC.   **839**
P.O. Box CN6
9051 River Road
Pennsauken, NJ 08110
Address inquiries to:
Mr. Stanley L. Wachman, President
    (609) 665-6111
    (800) 257-7740
Products Available
Cetacaine Topical Anesthetic
Cetylcide Germicidal Concentrate
Protexin Oral Breath Spray
Protexin Oral Rinse Concentrate
Skin Screen Protective Skin Lotion

CHEMI-TECH LABS, INC.   **839**
74-80 Marine Street
Farmingdale, NY 11735
Address inquiries to:
Professional Services Dept.
    (516) 454-9282
Subsidiaries
DG Packaging, Inc.
Garden Pharmaceuticals, Inc.
Branch Offices
Dagoberto Rivera, Inc.
Salud 23 Int.
Station 6, Box 233
Ponce, Puerto Rico 00731
    (809) 842-6263
Products Available
HVS 1+2

CIBA PHARMACEUTICAL COMPANY   **409, 840**
Division of CIBA-GEIGY Corporation
Address inquiries to:
556 Morris Avenue
Summit, NJ 07901
    New Jersey (201) 277-5000
    New York (212) 267-6615
Division Offices
Warehouse Offices and Shipping Branches
Eastern
14 Henderson Drive
West Caldwell, NJ 07006   (201) 575-6510
Central
7530 No. Natchez Ave.
Niles, IL 60648   Niles (312) 647-9332
    Chicago (312) 763-8700
Western
12850 Moore St.
P.O. Box 6300
Cerritos, CA 90701
    Cerritos (213) 404-2651
Products Available
◆ Antrenyl Tablets
◆ Anturane Capsules
◆ Anturane Tablets
◆ Apresazide Capsules
◆ Apresoline Ampuls
◆ Apresoline Tablets
◆ Apresoline-Esidrix Tablets
Cibalith-S Syrup
Coramine Ampuls
Coramine Oral Solution
◆ Cytadren Tablets
Desferal Vials
◆ Esidrix Tablets
◆ Esimil Tablets
INH Tablets
◆ Ismelin Tablets
◆ Lithobid Tablets
◆ Ludiomil Tablets
◆ Metandren Linguets & Tablets
◆ Metopirone Tablets
Nupercainal Cream
Nupercainal Ointment
Nupercainal Suppositories
Nupercaine Ampuls 1:200
Nupercaine Ampuls 1:1500
Nupercaine (Heavy) Ampuls
Percorten Pellets
Percorten pivalate Multiple-dose Vials
Priscoline Multiple-dose Vials
Privine Nasal Solution
Privine Nasal Spray
Regitine
Regitine Hydrochloride Tablets
◆ Rimactane Capsules
Rimactane/INH Dual Pack
◆ Ritalin Tablets
◆ Ritalin-SR Tablets
◆ Ser-Ap-Es Tablets
Serpasil Parenteral Solution
◆ Serpasil Tablets
◆ Serpasil-Apresoline Tablets
◆ Serpasil-Esidrix Tablets
◆ Slow-K Tablets
◆ Transderm-Nitro Transdermal Therapeutic System
◆ Transderm Scōp Transdermal Therapeutic System
Vioform Cream
Vioform Ointment
Vioform-Hydrocortisone Cream
Vioform-Hydrocortisone Lotion
Vioform-Hydrocortisone Mild Cream
Vioform-Hydrocortisone Mild Ointment
Vioform-Hydrocortisone Ointment

CLINICAL NUTRITION DIVISION   **876**
SANDOZ NUTRITION CORPORATION
5320 West Twenty Third Street
P.O. Box 370
Minneapolis, MN 55440

Address inquiries to:
William Rush   (612) 925-2100
Products Available
Citrotein
Compleat Modified Formula
Compleat-B
Isotein HN
Meritene Liquid
Meritene Powder
Nutrisource Modular System
Stresstein

COLGATE-HOYT LABORATORIES   **410, 878**
Division of Colgate-Palmolive Company
575 University Avenue
Norwood MA 02062 USA
Address inquiries to:
Professional Services Dept. (800) 225-3756
Products Available
Luride Drops

(◆ Shown in Product Identification Section)   (⊞ Described in PDR For Nonprescription Drugs)

Manufacturers' Index

- ◆ Luride Lozi-Tabs Tablets
- ◆ Full-strength 1.0 mg F
- ◆ Luride-SF (no artificial flavor or color) 1.0 mg F
- ◆ Half-strength 0.5 mg F
- ◆ Quarter-strength 0.25 mg F

Orabase HCA Oral Paste
▣ Orabase Plain Oral Protective Paste
▣ Orabase with Benzocaine Analgesic Oral Protective Paste
▣ Peroxyl Mouthrinse
Phos-Flur Oral Rinse/Supplement
Point-Two Dental Rinse
PreviDent Brush-On Gel
Thera-Flur Topical Gel-Drops
Thera-Flur-N Topical Gel-Drops

CONSOLIDATED CHEMICAL, INC. 880
3224 S. Kingshighway Blvd.
St. Louis, MO 63139
Address inquiries to:
John C. Brereton (314) 772-4610
Products Available
CC-500
Consept
Consol Concentrate
Formula Magic
GCP Shampoo
New Consol 20
Perineal/Ostomy Spray Cleaner
Satin
Skin Magic
Staphoclean
Staphosan
Swirlsoft

COOK-WAITE LABORATORIES, INC. 881
90 Park Avenue
New York, NY 10016 (212) 907-2712
Products Available
Carbocaine Hydrochloride 3% Injection
Carbocaine Hydrochloride 2% with Neo-Cobefrin 1:20,000 Injection

COOPER DERMATOLOGY LABORATORIES, INC. 882
3145 Porter Drive
Palo Alto, CA 94304
Products Available
A-Fil Cream Neutral & Dark
Aveeno Bath Oilated
Aveeno Bath Regular
Aveenobar Medicated
Aveenobar Oilated
Aveenobar Regular
Benisone Gel/Cream/Lotion/Ointment
Maxafil Cream
Meted Shampoo
Nu-Flow Shampoo
Packer's Pine Tar Shampoo
Packer's Pine Tar Soap
Pentrax Tar Shampoo
sunDare Clear
sunDare Creamy
sunStick
Texacort Scalp Lotion

COOPERVISION PHARMACEUTICALS INC 883
San German, Puerto Rico 00753
Address inquiries to:
Professional Services
San German, Puerto Rico or call
(except California) (800) 227-8313
(California only) (800) 982-6194
For Medical or Contact Lens Solution Information
Write: Medical Department
P.O. Box 7264
Mountain View, CA 94039
Call: *(Business Hours Only)*
Joseph Krezanoski, Ph.D. (800) 227-8082
For Medical Emergency Information After Hours or on Weekends, call
Jerome F. Grattan (201) 821-8846
Products Available
Argyrol Stabilized Solution 10%
Atropisol Ophthalmic Solution 1%
Catarase 1:5,000 & 1:10,000

CooperVision Balanced Salt Solution
Cystex Tablets
Dacriose Ophthalmic Irrigating Solution
Dropperettes:
 Argyrol S.S. 20%
 Atropisol 0.5%, 1%, 2%
 Epinephrine 1:1000
 Fluorescein Sodium 2%
 Homatropine HBr 2%, 5%
 Phenylephrine HCl 10%
 Pilocar 1%, 2%, 4%
 Sulf-10 (Sodium Sulfacetamide 10%)
 Tetracaine HCl 0.5%
E-Pilo Ophthalmic Solutions 1, 2, 3, 4, 6
Eserine Sulfate Ophthalmic Ointment ¼ %
Funduscein-10 or -25 (Fluorescein sodium I.V.)
Gentacidin Ophthalmic Solution
Glucose-40 Ophthalmic Ointment 40%
Glyrol Solution
Goniosol Solution
Homatropine Hydrobromide Ophthalmic Solution 2%, 5%
Hypotears Lubricating Eye Drops
Inflamase Forte 1% Ophthalmic Solution
Inflamase Mild ⅛ % Ophthalmic Solution
Lens Care Products:
 Clerz
 Clerz 2
 Contactisol
 d-Film
 duo-Flow
 HGP Cleaner
 HGP Conditioning Solution
 Heat Case
 hy-Flow
 Lensine-5
 Lensine Extra Strength Cleaner
 Pliagel
 Unisol
 Unisol 4
Lipoflavonoid Vitamin Supplement (Capsule)
Lipotriad Vitamin Supplement (Capsule, Liquid)
Lydia Pinkham (Capsule, Liquid)
Miochol Intraocular
Phenylzin Ophthalmic Solution
Pilocar Ophthalmic Solutions 0.5%, 1%, 2%, 3%, 4%, 6%
Pilocar Ophthalmic Solutions Twin Pack 0.5%, 1%, 2%, 3%, 4%, 6%
Schirmer Tear Test
Sulf-10 Ophthalmic Solution
Tearisol Ophthalmic Solution
VasoClear Ophthalmic Decongestant Eye Drops
VasoClear A Decongestant Astrigent Lubricating Eye Drops
Vasocon Regular Ophthalmic Solution
Vasocon-A Ophthalmic Solution
Vasosulf Ophthalmic Solution

CUTTER BIOLOGICAL 883
Division of Miles Laboratories, Inc.
2200 Powell Street
Emeryville, CA 94662
Written inquiries to:
Professional Services Manager
Technical & Medical Inquiries:
(800) 227-1762 (outside CA)
(800) 227-3219 (within CA)
Branch Offices
To Order Call:
CHICAGO OFFICE
 725 Golf Lane
 Bensenville, IL 60106
 (800) 323-2549 (outside IL)
 (312) 595-3620 (in IL)
DALLAS TX 75240
 P.O. Box 400358
 (214) 661-5850 (Within AC 214)
 (800) 527-0382 (Outside TX)
 (800) 442-5701 (In TX, except AC 214)
LOS ANGELES OFFICE
 15320 East Salt Lake Avenue
 City of Industry, CA 91744
 (800) 423-9429 (outside CA)
 (800) 352-5495 (in CA)
NEW YORK OFFICE
 40 E. Cotters Lane
 East Brunswick, NJ 08816
 (800) 221-0831 (outside NJ)
 (201) 238-0140 (in NJ)
Products Available
Factor IX Complex (Human) (Factors II, VII, IX, and X) Konyne
Gamastan (Immune Serum Globulin-Human)
Gamimune (Immune Globulin Intravenous, 5% in 10% Maltose)
Hepatitis B Immune Globulin (Human) HyperHep
Hyperab (Rabies Immune Globulin-Human)
HyperHep (Hepatitis B Immune Globulin-Human)
Hyper-Tet (Tetanus Immune Globulin-Human)
HypRho-D (Rh₀-D Immune Globulin-Human)
HypRho-D Mini-Dose (Rh₀-D Immune Globulin-Human)
Immune Globulin Intravenous, 5% (In 10% Maltose) Gamimune
Immune Serum Globulin (Human) Gamastan
Koate-HT
Konyne (Factor IX Complex-Human) (Factors II, VII, IX and X)
Pertussis Immune Globulin (Human) Hypertussis
Plague Vaccine (Human)
Rh₀-D Immune Globulin (Human) HypRho-D
Rh₀-D Immune Globulin (Human) HypRho-D Mini-Dose
Rabies Immune Globulin (Human) Hyperab
Tetanus Immune Globulin (Human) Hyper-Tet

DALIN PHARMACEUTICALS, INC. 886
74-80 Marine Street
Farmingdale, NY 11735
Address inquiries to:
Professional Services Dept. (516) 454-9282
Subsidiaries
Chemi-Tech Labs, Inc.
DG Packaging, Inc.
Garden Pharmaceuticals, Inc.
Branch Offices
Dagoberto Rivera, Inc.
 Salud 23 Int.
 Station 6, Box 233
 Ponce, Puerto Rico 00731
 (809) 842-6263
Products Available
Audax Ear Drops
Ban Itch
Celluzyme Chewable Tablets
Cremesone
Dalex Lozenges
Dalex Pediatric Syrup
Dalex Syrup
Dalex Syrup Forte
Dalicote Lotion
Dalicreme
Daliderm Liquid
Dalidyne
Dalidyne Jel
Dalidyne Spray (Mouth and Throat)
Dalifort Tablets
Daligesic Liniment
Dalivim Forte Liquid & Tablets
Pentacort Cream
Phenagesic Capsules
Phenarex Syrup
Phenatuss Expectorant
Polysept Ointment
Sorbutuss

DANBURY PHARMACAL, INC. 887
131 West Street
P.O. Box 296
Danbury, CT 06810
Address Inquiries to:
Nessim Maleh
Ira Sacks
Milton Blitz (203) 744-7200
Products Available
Allopurinol Tablets
Bethanechol Chloride Tablets
Butalbital and Acetaminophen Tablets
Carisoprodol Compound Tablets
Carisoprodol Tablets
Chloroquine Phosphate Tablets
Chlorothiazide Tablets
Chlorpropamide Tablets
Chlorthalidone Tablets
Chlorzoxazone Tablets
Chlorzoxazone with APAP Tablets
Colchicine Tablets
Col-Probenecid Tablets
Cyproheptadine HCl Tablets
Dicyclomine HCl Capsules
Dicyclomine HCl Tablets
Diphenhydramine HCl Capsules
Dipyridamole Tablets
Disulfiram Tablets
Doxycycline Hyclate Capsules
Doxycycline Hyclate Tablets
Ergoloid Mesylates Oral Tablets
Ergoloid Mesylates Sublingual Tablets
Erythromycin Estolate Capsules
Folic Acid Tablets
Glutethimide Tablets
Glycopyrrolate Tablets
Hydralazine HCl Tablets
Hydrochlorothiazide, Hydralazine HCl, Reserpine Tablets
Hydrochlorothiazide/Reserpine Tablets
Hydrochlorothiazide Tablets
Hydrocortisone Tablets
Hydroxyzine Hydrochloride Tablets
Hydroxyzine Pamoate Capsules
Isoniazid Tablets
Isosorbide Dinitrate Oral Tablets
Isosorbide Dinitrate Sublingual Tablets
Isoxsuprine HCl Tablets
Meprobamate Tablets
Methocarbamol Tablets
Metronidazole Tablets
Nylidrin HCl Tablets
Papaverine HCl T.D. Capsules
Papaverine HCl Tablets
Phenobarbital Tablets
Phenylbutazone Tablets
Prednisolone Tablets
Prednisone Tablets
Primidone Tablets
Probenecid Tablets
Procainamide HCl Capsules
Propantheline Bromide Tablets
Pseudoephedrine HCl Tablets
Quindan Tablets
Quinidine Gluconate Sustained Action Tablets
Quinidine Sulfate Tablets
Spironolactone/Hydrochlorothiazide Tablets
Sulfamethoxazole with Trimethoprim Tablets
Sulfamethoxazole with Trimethoprim Tablets (Double Strength)
Sulfasalazine Tablets

(◆ Shown in Product Identification Section) (▣ Described in PDR For Nonprescription Drugs)

Manufacturers' Index

Sulfinpyrazone Tablets
Tetracycline HCl Capsules
Theofedral Tablets
Thioridazine HCl Tablets
Tolbutamide Tablets
Triamcinolone Tablets
Trihexyphenidyl HCl Tablets
Tripelennamine HCl Tablets
Tripodrine Tablets

DELMONT LABORATORIES, INC.   888
P.O. Box AA
Swarthmore, PA 19081
Address inquiries to:
(215) 543-3365
(215) 543-2747
Products Available
Staphage Lysate (SPL)

DERMIK LABORATORIES, INC.   888
500 Virginia Drive
Ft. Washington, PA 19034
Distribution Centers
Langhorne, PA 19047
  P.O. Box 247   (215) 752-1211
Oak Forest, IL 60452
  P.O. Box 280   (800) 323-4474
San Leandro, CA 94577
  1550 Factor Avenue   (415) 357-9471
Tucker, GA 30084
  4660 Hammermill Road   (800) 241-9120
Products Available
Anthra-Derm Ointment 1%, ½%, ¼%, 1/10%
5 Benzagel (5% benzoyl peroxide) & 10 Benzagel (10% benzoyl peroxide), Acne Gels, Microgel Formula
Comfortine Ointment
Drest Gel
Durrax Tablets 10mg, 25mg
Florone Cream 0.05%
Florone Ointment 0.05%
Hytone Cream 1%, 2 ½%
Hytone Lotion 1%, 2 ½%
Hytone Ointment ½%, 1%, 2 ½%
Jeri-Bath
Jeri-Lotion
Klaron Acne Lotion
Loroxide Acne Lotion
Rezamid Acne Lotion
Shepard's Cream Lotion
Shepard's Moisturizing Soap
Shepard's Skin Cream
Sulfacet-R Acne Lotion
Vanoxide Acne Lotion
Vanoxide-HC Acne Lotion
Vlemasque
Vytone Cream ½%, 1%
Zetar Emulsion
Zetar Shampoo

DISTA PRODUCTS COMPANY   410, 893
Division of Eli Lilly and Company
General Offices
307 East McCarty Street
Indianapolis, IN 46285
For Medical Information, Write:
Medical Department
307 East McCarty Street
Indianapolis, IN 46285   (317) 261-4000
Sales Offices
Aurora, CO 80014
  Suite 111, Cherry Creek Place I
  3131 South Vaughn Way (303) 695-7733
Bloomington, MN 55420
  Suite 1142, One Appletree Square
      (612) 854-0214
*Chicago, IL 60631
  Suite 270, O'Hare Plaza
  5735 East River Road   (312) 693-8360
Cincinnati, OH 45241
  Suite 413, 4055 Executive Park Drive
      (513) 563-7010
Cleveland, OH 44130
  Suite 395, Interstate Plaza
  16600 W. Sprague Road
      (216) 243-0047
Dallas, TX 75234
  4404 Beltwood Parkway, South
      (214) 661-5669
Dedham, MA 02026
  990 Washington Street   (617) 329-6858
Houston, TX 77042
  Suite 360, Richmond Plaza I
  9800 Richmond Ave.   (713) 975-6822
Indianapolis, IN 46268
  Suite 235, Northwest Plaza
  3901 West 86th St.   (317) 261-5770
      or (317) 261-4000
Jacksonville, FL 33216
  Suite 319-A, 7825 Baymeadows Way
      (904) 731-8530
Kansas City, MO 64114
  Suites 600, 610, 9200 Ward Parkway
      (816) 361-1020
Melville, NY 11747
  Suite 3S02
  One Huntington Quadrangle
      (516) 752-9839

Memphis, TN 38117
  Suite 224, 755 Crossover Lane
  Audubon Woods Business Campus
      (901) 767-3988
Metairie, LA 70002
  Suite 508, Security Homestead Bldg.
  4900 Veterans Memorial Boulevard
      (504) 455-0339
Morristown, NJ 07960
  Morristown Centre
  10 Madison Avenue   (201) 898-9507
Nashville, TN 37210
  Suite 310, 555 Marriott Drive
      (615) 885-2700
*Norcross, GA 30091
  5944 Peachtree Corners, East
      (404) 441-5404
*Pasadena, CA 91101
  Suite 916, Mutual Savings Bldg.
  301 East Colorado Blvd. (213) 792-3197
Pittsburgh, PA 15220
  Suite 602, Manor Oak Two
  1910 Cochran Road   (412) 561-5044
Raleigh, NC 27625
  Suite 103, 3109 Poplarwood Court
      (919) 872-5210
Redmond, WA 98052
  11811 Willows Road   (206) 881-6163
San Francisco, CA 94111
  Suite 1170, 100 California St.
      (415) 391-2767
Silver Spring, MD 20903
  Suite 111, Executive Court
  1734 Elton Road   (301) 439-1109
Southfield, MI 48075
  Suite 940, 3000 Town Center
      (313) 358-2278
St. Louis, MO 63131
  Suite 325, Corporate Hill II
  1633 Des Peres Rd.   (314) 821-0996
*Stamford, CT 06905
  Suite 301, 1600 Summer St.
      (203) 357-8872
Tampa, FL 33609
  Suite 630, Lincoln Center
  5401 West Kennedy Boulevard
      (813) 870-3086
Wynnewood, PA 19096
  Suite 202, Seven Wynnewood Road
      (215) 642-0420
*Regional Office
Products Available
Becotin Pulvules
Becotin with Vitamin C Pulvules
Becotin-T Tablets
◆ Cinobac Pulvules
Co-Pyronil 2, Pulvules, Pediatric Pulvules, and Suspension
Cordran Ointment & Lotion
Cordran SP Cream
Cordran Tape
Cordran-N Cream and Ointment
Ilosone Chewable Tablets
Ilosone, for Oral Suspension
Ilosone Liquids, Oral Suspensions
◆ Ilosone Pulvules & Tablets
Ilosone Ready-Mixed Drops
Ilotycin Gluceptate, IV, & Vials
Ilotycin Sterile Ophthalmic Ointment
Ilotycin Tablets
Keflex, for Oral Suspension
Keflex, for Pediatric Drops
◆ Keflex, Pulvules & Tablets
Mi-Cebrin Tablets
Mi-Cebrin T Tablets
◆ Nalfon Pulvules & Tablets
◆ Nalfon 200 Pulvules
Nebcin Vials & Hyporets
◆ Valmid Pulvules

DOAK PHARMACAL CO., INC.   908
128 Magnolia Avenue
Westbury, NY 11590
Address inquiries to:
Director of Physician Services
      1(800) 645-3191
      (516) 333-7222
Branch Offices
Obergfel Brothers
  2660 East 37th Street
  Vernon, CA 90058   (213) 583-8981
Products Available
Buro-Sol Antiseptic Powder
Diasporal Cream
Doak Oil & Doak Oil Forte
Doak Tar Lotion
Doak Tar Shampoo
Formula 405 Skin Care Products
  Body Smoothing Lotion
  Enriched Cream
  Eye Cream
  Le Pont Organic Nail Oil Treatment
  Light Textured Moisturizer
  Moisturizing Lotion
  Moisturizing Soap
  SPF 15+
  Skin Cleanser & Patented Buffing Mitt
  Solar Cream
  Therapeutic Bath Oil

Lavatar Tar Bath
Lotio Alsulfa
Normaderm Cream
Normaderm Lotion
Petro-Phylic Soap Cake
Tar Distillate "Doak"
Tarpaste
Tersaseptic Hygienic Skin Cleanser
Tersa-Tar
Unguentum Bossi

DORSEY LABORATORIES   908
Division of Sandoz, Inc.
P.O. Box 83288
Lincoln, NE 68501
Address Medical inquiries to:
Medical Department
Sandoz Pharmaceuticals
East Hanover, NJ 07936
      (201) 386-7500
Other Inquiries to:
Dorsey Laboratories   (402) 464-6311
Products Available
Acid Mantle Creme & Lotion
Cama Arthritis Pain Reliever
Chexit Tablets
Dorcol Children's Cough Syrup
Dorcol Children's Decongestant Liquid
Dorcol Children's Fever & Pain Reducer
Dorcol Children's Liquid Calcium Supplement
Dorcol Children's Liquid Cold Formula
Eclipse After Sun Moisturizer
Eclipse Lip and Face Protectant, SPF 15
Eclipse Partial Suntan Lotion, SPF 5
Eclipse Original Sunscreen Gel, SPF 10
Eclipse Original Sunscreen Moisturizing Lotion, SPF 10
Eclipse Total Sunscreen Cooling Alcohol Lotion, SPF 15
Eclipse Total Sunscreen Moisturizing Lotion, SPF 15
Kanulase Tablets
Metaprel Inhalant Solution 5%
Metaprel Metered Dose Inhaler
Metaprel Syrup
Metaprel Tablets, 10 mg
Metaprel Tablets, 20 mg
▣ Triaminic Allergy Tablets
▣ Triaminic Chewables
Triaminic Cold Syrup
Triaminic Cold Tablets
Triaminic Expectorant
Triaminic Expectorant DH
Triaminic Expectorant w/Codeine
Triaminic Juvelets
Triaminic Oral Infant Drops
Triaminic TR Tablets (Timed Release)
Triaminic-DM Cough Formula
Triaminic-12 Tablets
▣ Triaminicin Tablets
Triaminicol Multi-Symptom Cold Syrup
Triaminicol Multi-Symptom Cold Tablets
▣ Tussagesic Tablets & Suspension
▣ Ursinus Inlay-Tabs

DORSEY PHARMACEUTICALS
See SANDOZ, INC. PHARMACEUTICALS

DRUG INDUSTRIES CO., INC.   914
3237 Hilton Road
Ferndale, MI 48220
Address inquiries to:
John Hadd   (313) 547-3784
Products Available
Al-Vite
BC-Vite
Bilax
C-Caps 500
Calfer-Vite
Day-Vite
Di-Sosul
Di-Sosul Forte
E-Plus
Hemo-Vite
Hemo-Vite Liquid
Sinovan Timed
Trilax
Vanodonnal Timed
Vicef

DU PONT PHARMACEUTICALS   410, 915
E.I. du Pont de Nemours & Co. (Inc.)
Wilmington, Delaware 19898
Address inquiries to:
Director, Professional Services
      1 (800) 441-9861
  In Delaware (302) 992-3273
Distribution Centers
Garden City, NY 11530
  1000 Stewart Ave.
  New York State 1 (800) 645-3546
  Outside NY 1 (800) 645-3547
  In New York State call: (516) 832-2029
      (516) 832-2030
      (516) 832-2031

(◆ Shown in Product Identification Section)   (▣ Described in PDR For Nonprescription Drugs)

Manufacturers' Index

Chicago, IL 60641
    4956 W. Belmont Ave.   (312) 282-0440
Claremont, CA 91711
    1480 N. Claremont Blvd.
                           (714) 621-7986
                           (714) 621-7987

**DU PONT PHARMACEUTICALS   410, 915
CARIBE, INC.**
Subsidiary of E.I. du Pont de Nemours &
  Company (Inc.)
Post Office Box 12
Manati, Puerto Rico 00701
    Address inquiries to:
Du Pont Pharmaceuticals
E.I. du Pont de Nemours & Co. (Inc.)
Wilmington, Delaware 19898
Director, Professional Services
               1 (800) 441-9861
      In Delaware (302) 992-3273

**DU PONT PHARMACEUTICALS,   410, 915
INC.**
Subsidiary of E.I. du Pont de Nemours &
  Company (Inc.)
Post Office Box 363
Manati, Puerto Rico 00701
    Address Inquiries to:
Du Pont Pharmaceuticals
E.I. du Pont de Nemours & Co. (Inc.)
Wilmington, Delaware 19898
Director, Professional Services
               1 (800) 441-9861
      In Delaware (302) 992-3273
    Products Available
◆ Coumadin Injection & Tablets
  Endecon Tablets
  Endotussin-NN Pediatric Syrup
  Endotussin-NN Syrup
◆ Hycodan Syrup, Tablets
  Hycomine Compound Tablets
  Hycomine Pediatric Syrup
  Hycomine Syrup
  Hycotuss Expectorant Syrup
◆ Moban Tablets & Concentrate
◆ Narcan Injection
  Narcan Neonatal Injection
◆ Nubain Injection
  Numorphan Hydrochloride Injection,
    Suppositories
◆ Percocet Tablets
◆ Percodan Tablets
◆ Percodan-Demi Tablets
  Remsed Tablets
◆ Symmetrel Capsules & Syrup
◆ Tessalon Perles
  Valpin 50 Tablets

DURA PHARMACEUTICALS, INC   929
P.O. Box 28331
San Diego, CA 92128
    Address inquiries to:
Same as above   (619) 789-6840
   For Medical Emergencies Contact:
Craig Wheeler   (619) 789-6840
Tom Evangelisti
    Products Available
Dura Tap-PD
Dura-Vent
Dura-Vent/A
Dura-Vent/DA

ECOLOGICAL FORMULAS   929
Division of Cardiovascular Research, Ltd.
1061 Shary Circle
Concord, CA 94518
           Toll Free: 800-351-9429
                         415-827-2636
    Address Inquiries to:
Robert A. Da Prato, M.D., Medical Director
    Products Available
Caprystatin
Carnitine
Chondroitin-4-Sulphate
Glucostabil
Orithrush

ELDER PHARMACEUTICALS, INC.   411, 929
222 N. Vincent Ave.
Covina, CA 91722
    Address inquiries to:
222 N. Vincent Ave.
Covina, CA 91722
                    (800) 537-4294
                    (800) 423-8545
       In Ohio (800) 472-4588
    Products Available
Benoquin Cream 20%
Elaqua XX Cream
Eldecort Cream, 1%, 2.5%
Elder Psoralite
Eldopaque 2% Cream
Eldopaque Forte 4% Cream
Eldoquin 2% Cream
Eldoquin 2% Lotion
Eldoquin Forte 4% Cream
Fototar Cream 1.6%
Fototar Stik 5%
HQC Kit
◆ Oxsoralen Capsule

Oxsoralen Lotion 1%
Pabanol Lotion
Psoranide Cream 0.025%
RVP Ointment
RVPaba Lip Stick
RVPaque Ointment
Solaquin 2% Cream
Solaquin Forte 4% Cream
Solaquin Forte 4% Gel
◆ Trisoralen Tablets
Vitadye Lotion

ELKINS-SINN, INC.   938
A subsidiary of A.H. Robins Company
2 Esterbrook Lane
Cherry Hill, NJ 08034
                      (800) 257-8349
Address price and packaging inquiries to:
Marketing Department
Address scientific information inquiries to:
Professional Services Department
    Products Available
Aminocaproic Acid Injection
Aminophylline Injection
Atropine Sulfate Injection
Calcium Chloride Injection
Calcium Gluconate Injection
Chloramphenicol Sodium Succinate Injection
Chlorpromazine HCl Injection
Codeine Phosphate Injection
Cyanocobalamin (Vit. B$_{12}$) Injection
Dexamethasone Sodium Phosphate Injection
Dexpanthenol Injection (d-Pantothenyl
  Alcohol)
Dextrose Injection
Digoxin Injection
Diphenhydramine HCl Injection
Dopamine HCl Injection
Doxycycline Hyclate for Injection
Duramorph PF (Preservative-free morphine
  sulfate injection)
Epinephrine Injection
Fentanyl Citrate Injection
Furosemide Injection
Gentamicin Sulfate Injection
Heparin Sodium Injection
Hep-Lock (Heparin Lock Flush Solution)
Hep-Lock PF (Preservative-Free Heparin Lock
  Flush Solution)
Hydrocortisone Sodium Succinate for
  Injection
Hydromorphone HCl Injection
Hydroxyzine HCl Intramuscular Injection
Isoproterenol HCl Injection
Lidocaine HCl Injection
Lidocaine HCl Injection (Preservative-free)
Lidocaine Hydrochloride Injection for Cardiac
  Arrhythmias
Lidocaine HCl & Epinephrine Injection
Magnesium Sulfate Injection
Meperidine HCl Injection
Methylene Blue Injection
Methylprednisolone Sodium Succinate for
  Injection
Metronidazole Redi-Infusion
Mineral Oil, Sterile
Morphine Sulfate Injection
Neostigmine Methylsulfate Injection
Paraldehyde (Sterile)
Pentobarbital Sodium Injection
Phenobarbital Sodium Injection
Phenytoin Sodium Injection
Potassium Chloride Injection
Procaine HCl Injection
Prochlorperazine Edisylate Injection
Promethazine HCl Injection
Scopolamine Hydrobromide Injection
Sodium Chloride Injection (Preservative-free)
Sodium Chloride Injection, Bacteriostatic
Sodium Nitroprusside Injection
Sotradecol (Sodium Tetradecyl Sulfate
  Injection)
Thiamine HCl Injection
Vials, Sterile Empty
Water For Injection, Bacteriostatic
Water for Injection, Sterile

EVERETT LABORATORIES, INC.   941
76 Franklin Street
East Orange, NJ 07017
    Address inquiries to:
Professional Service Dept.   (201) 674-8455
    Products Available
Anafed Capsules & Syrup
Berovite Plus Tablets
Florvite Chewable Tablets 0.5 mg & 1 mg
Florvite Drops
Florvite + Iron Chewable Tablets 1 mg
Florvite + Iron Drops
Libidinal Capsules
Nicotym Capsules
Pavatym Capsules
Repan Tablets
Vitafol Tablets

FERNDALE LABORATORIES, INC.   942
780 W. Eight Mile Road
Ferndale, MI 48220

    Address inquiries to:
Professional Service Dept.   (313) 548-0900
    Products Available
Adphen Tablets
Aquaphyllin Syrup
Bellkatal Tablets
Benase Tablets
Betuline Liniment
Dapa Tablets
Dapacin Capsules
Dapex Capsules
Delaxin Tablets
Detachol Adhesive Remover
Doss 300 Capsule
Fastamine Tablets
Ferndex Tablets
Fernisolone-P-Tablets
Flavitab Tablets
Kronofed-A Jr. Kronocaps
Kronofed-A Kronocaps
Kronohist Kronocaps
Liqui-Doss
Lixaminol Elixir
Maigret Tablets
Mastisol Liquid Adhesive
Obestin-30 Capsules
Oxychinol Tablets
Phenobella Tablets
Pramosone Cream, Lotion & Ointment
Prax Cream & Lotion
Procute Cream & Lotion
Rhinocaps Capsules
Salatin Capsules
Strifon Forte Tablets
Synabrom Capsules
Tin-Ben Dispenser
Tin-Co-Ben Dispenser
Vio-Pramosone Cream
Vio-Pramosone Lotion

THE FIELDING COMPANY   942
2384 Centerline Industrial Drive
St. Louis, MO 63146
    Address inquiries to:
Professional Services Dept.
                      (314) 567-5462
   For Medical Emergencies Contact:
                      (314) 567-5462
    Products Available
Duracid
Gerimed
Irospan Capsules
Irospan Tablets
Metric 21 Tablets
Nestabs Tablets
Nestabs FA Tablets
Nestrex Tablets

FISONS CORPORATION   943
Pharmaceutical Division
Two Preston Court
Bedford, MA 01730
    Address inquiries to:
Professional Services Dept. (617) 275-1000
    Distribution Centers
ATLANTA
  James M. Hogan Co., Inc.
  5356 Ponce de Leon Ave.
  Stone Mountain, GA 30083
                      (404) 938-7901
BEDFORD
  Fisons Corporation
  2 Preston Court
  Bedford, MA 01730   (617) 275-1000
LOS ANGELES
  Obergfel Brothers
  2660 East 37th Street
  Vernon, CA 90058   (213) 583-8981
    Products Available
Bacid Capsules
Ergomar Sublingual Tablets
Intal
Intal Nebulizer Solution
Isoclor Timesule Capsules
Kondremul
Kondremul with Cascara
Kondremul with Phenolphthalein
Nasalcrom Nasal Solution
Neo-Cultol
Persistin
Proferdex
Somophyllin Oral Liquid
Somophyllin Rectal Solution
Somophyllin-CRT Capsules
Somophyllin-DF Liquid
Somophyllin-T Capsules
Vapo-Iso Solution
Vaponefrin Solution
Vitron-C
Vitron-C-Plus

C. B. FLEET CO., INC.   946, 3009
4615 Murray Pl.
Lynchburg, VA 24502-2235
    Address inquiries to:
Fred T. Wickis, Jr.   (804) 528-4000
    Products Available
Fleet Babylax
Fleet Bisacodyl Enema

(◆ Shown in Product Identification Section)   (⊞ Described in PDR For Nonprescription Drugs)

Manufacturers' Index

Fleet Detecatest
Fleet Enema
Fleet Enema Pediatric
Fleet Flavored Castor Oil Emulsion
Fleet Mineral Oil Enema
Fleet Phospho-Soda
Fleet Prep Kits
Fleet Relief
Summer's Eve Medicated Douche

FLEMING & COMPANY   948
1600 Fenpark Dr.
Fenton, MO 63026
Address inquiries to:
John J. Roth, M.D.   (314) 343-8200
Products Available
Aerolate Liquid
Aerolate III T.D. Capsules
Aerolate Jr. T.D. Capsules
Aerolate Sr. T.D. Capsules
Alumadrine Tablets
Congess Jr. T.D. Capsules
Congess Sr. T.D. Capsules
▣ Deter Jr. T.D. Capsules
▣ Deter Sr. T.D. Capsules
Ectasule Minus III T.D. Capsules
Ectasule Minus Jr. T.D. Capsules
Ectasule Minus Sr. T.D. Capsules
Ectasule III T.D. Capsules
Ectasule Jr. T.D. Capsules
Ectasule Sr. T.D. Capsules
Extendryl Chewable Tablets
Extendryl Sr. & Jr. T.D. Capsules
Extendryl Syrup
Impregon Concentrate
Magonate Tablets
▣ Marblen Suspension Peach/Apricot
▣ Marblen Suspension Unflavored
▣ Marblen Tablets
Nephrocaps
▣ Nephrox Suspension
Nicotinex Elixir
▣ Ocean Nasal Mist
Ocean-Plus Mist
Pima Syrup
▣ Purge Liquid
Rum-K Syrup
S-P-T "Liquid" Capsules

FLINT   411, 949
Division of Travenol Laboratories, Inc.
One Baxter Parkway
Deerfield, IL 60015   (312) 940-5224
Address inquiries to:
Product Management
Products Available
◆ Choloxin
◆ Flint SSD Cream
◆ Synthroid Injection
◆ Synthroid Tablets
◆ Travase Ointment

FLUORITAB CORPORATION   953
P.O. Box 381
Flint, MI 48501
Address inquiries to:
J. A. Vogt, Supervisor   (1-313) 239-9770
Products Available
Fluoritab Liquid
Fluoritab Tablets

FOREST LABORATORIES, INC.   953
919 Third Avenue
New York, NY 10022
Address inquiries to:
Professional Service Dept. (212) 421-7850
Products Available
Isochron Tablets

E. FOUGERA & COMPANY   953
Division of Altana, Inc.
60 Baylis Road
Melville, NY 11747
Address inquiries to:
Customer Service   (800) 645-9833
For Medical Emergencies Contact:
E. Fougera   (800) 645-9833
Products Available
Analgesic Balm
Analgesic Balm (Greaseless)
Atropine Sulfate Ophthalmic Ointment 1%
Bacitracin-Neomycin-Polymyxin Ointment
Bacitracin-Neomycin-Polymyxin Ophthalmic Ointment
Bacitracin Ointment
Bacitracin Ophthalmic Ointment
Bacitracin-Polymyxin Ointment
Betamethasone Valerate Cream, Lotion & Ointment 0.1%
Boric Acid Ointment
Boric Acid Ophthalmic Ointment 5%
Cold Cream
Dibucaine Ointment 1%
Efodine Ointment
Erythromycin Ophthalmic Ointment
Fluocinolone Acetonide Cream & Topical Solution 0.01%
Fluocinolone Acetonide Cream & Ointment 0.025%

Hydrocortisone Cream & Ointment 0.5%
Hydrocortisone Cream & Ointment 1%
Hydrophylic Ointment
Ichthammol Ointment 10% & 20%
Iodochlorhydroxyquin 3% with Hydrocortisone Cream
Lanolin & Lanolin Anhydrous
Lidocaine Ointment 5%
Nitroglycerin Ointment 2%
Nystatin Cream, Ointment & Vaginal Tablets
Nystatin-Neomycin-Gramicidin-Triamcinolone Cream & Ointment
Petrolatum (White) & Petrolatum (White) Ophthalmic Ointment
Polysorb Hydrate Cream
Sulfacetamide Sodium Ophthalmic Ointment
Surgilube Surgical Lubricant
Swim Ear
Triamcinolone Acetonide Cream 0.5%
Triamcinolone Acetonide Cream & Ointment 0.025% & 0.1%
Triple Sulfa Vaginal Cream
Vitamin A + Vitamin D Ointment
Whitfield's Ointment
Yellow Mercuric Oxide Ophthalmic Ointment 1% & 2%
Zinc Oxide Ointment

GEIGY PHARMACEUTICALS   411, 954
Division of CIBA-GEIGY Corporation
Ardsley, NY 10502
Address inquiries to:
Medical Services Dept.   (201) 277-5000
Products Available
Brethine Ampuls
◆ Brethine Tablets
◆ Butazolidin Capsules & Tablets
◆ Constant-T Tablets
◆ Lioresal Tablets
Lopressor Ampuls
◆ Lopressor Tablets
Otrivin Nasal Solution
Otrivin Nasal Spray
Otrivin Pediatric Solution
PBZ Elixir
PBZ Hydrochloride Cream
◆ PBZ Tablets
◆ PBZ-SR Tablets
◆ Tandearil
◆ Tegretol Chewable Tablets
◆ Tegretol Tablets
◆ Tofranil Ampuls
◆ Tofranil Tablets
◆ Tofranil-PM Capsules

GENEVA GENERICS   973
2599 W. Midway Blvd.
Broomfield, CO 80020
Address inquiries to:
Professional Services Department
                           (303) 466-2341
Products Available
APAP w/Codeine Tablets
APAP w/Codeine #3
APAP w/Codeine #4
Aminophylline Tablets
Amitriptyline HCl Tablets
Antibiotic Ear Drops
Aspirin w/Codeine Tablets
Azo-Sulfisoxazole Tablets
Bisacodyl Suppositories
Carisoprodol Tablets
Chloral Hydrate Capsules
Chlordiazepoxide Capsules
Chlorothiazide Tablets
Chlorothiazide w/Reserpine Tablets
Chlorpheniramine Maleate T.D. Capsules
Chlorpromazine Tablets & Concentrate Syrup
Chlorpropamide Tablets
Chlorzoxasone w/APAP Tablets
Conjugated Estrogens Tablets
Cyclandelate Capsules
Cyproheptadine HCl Tablets
Danthron Tablets
Deproist Expectorant w/Codeine
Diphenhydramine Capsules
Dipyridamole Tablets
Disobrom Tablets
Disulfiram Tablets
Doxycycline Hyclate Capsules & Tablets
Ergoloid Mesylates Tablets
Fluoxymesterone Tablets
Furosemide Tablets
Glutethimide Tablets
Hydralazine HCl Tablets
Hydralazine w/Hydrochlorothiazide Capsules
Hydrochlorothiazide Tablets
Hydrochlorothiazide w/Reserpine Tablets
Hydroflumethiazide with Reserpine
Hydroxyzine Hydrochloride Tablets
Hydroxyzine Tablets
Imipramine Tablets
Indomethacin
Isosorbide Dinitrate Tablets
Isosorbide Dinitrate T.D. Capsules & Tablets
Isoxsuprine Tablets
Lonox Tablets
Meclizine HCl Tablets

Meprobamate Tablets
Methocarbamol Tablets
Methocarbamol with Aspirin Tablets
Methyldopa Tablets
Metronidazole Tablets
Mygel Suspension
Nitroglycerin S.R. Capsules
Nylidrin Tablets
P.E.T.N. S.R. Tablets
Papaverine T.D. Capsules
Phenylbutazone Capsules
Phenylbutazone Tablets
Polyvite with Fluoride Drops
Potassium Chloride
Prednisolone Tablets
Prednisone Tablets
Primidone Tablets
Probenecid Tablets
Probenecid w/Colchicine Tablets
Procainamide Capsules
Prochlorperazine Tablets
Pro-Iso Capsules
Promethazine DM (Ped) Expectorant
Promethazine Expectorant Plain
Promethazine w/Codeine Expectorant
Promethazine VC Expectorant
Promethazine VC w/Codeine Expectorant
Propantheline Bromide Tablets
Propox 65 w/APAP Tablets
Propoxyphene-AC Capsules
Propoxyphene HCl Capsules
Pseudoephedrine Tablets
Quinidine Gluconate S.R. Tablets
Quinidine Sulfate Tablets
Quinine Sulfate Capsules
Quiphile Tablets
Resaid T.D. Tablets
Rescaps-D T.D. Capsules
Spironolactone Tablets
Spironolactone w/Hydrochlorothiazide Tablets
Sulfamethoxazole Tablets
Sulfamethoxazole w/Trimethoprim DS
Sulfamethoxazole w/Trimethoprim SS
Sulfasalazine Tablets
Sulfisoxazole Tablets
T.E.H. Tablets
T.E.P. Tablets
Tamine Elixir
Tamine S.R. Tablets
Theophylline Elixir
Theophylline S.R. Tablets
Thioridazine Tablets
Tolbutamide Tablets
Triamcinolone Tablets
Triamcinolone Acetonide Cream
Trichlormethiazide Tablets
Trifed Tablets & Syrup
Trifluoperazine Tablets
Triplevite w/Fluoride Drops
Uroblue Tablets

GERBER PRODUCTS COMPANY   974
Fremont, MI 49412   (616) 928-2000
Address inquiries to:
Professional Communications Department
Products Available
Gerber Bakery Products
Gerber Cereals
   Barley Cereal
   Cereals with Fruit
   High Protein Cereal
   Mixed Cereal
   Oatmeal Cereal
   Rice Cereal
Gerber Chunky Foods
Gerber High Meat Dinners (Strained & Junior)
Gerber Junior Foods
Gerber Junior Meats
Gerber Strained Egg Yolks
Gerber Strained Foods
Gerber Strained Juices (4.2 & 8 oz.)
Gerber Strained Meats
Gerber Toddler Meat Sticks (Chicken & Turkey)
MBF (Meat Base Formula) Liquid

GERIATRIC PHARMACEUTICAL CORP. 975
149 Covert Avenue
P.O. Box 1098
New Hyde Park, NY 11040 (516) 354-1121
Products Available
B-C-Bid Capsules (sustained release)
Bilezyme Tablets
Cal-Bio
Cal-Plus
Cevi-Bid Capsules (sustained release)
Cevi-Fer Capsules (sustained release)
Gaysal-S Tablets
Geritonic Liquid
Ger-O-Foam Aerosol
Gustalac Tablets
Gustase Tablets
Gustase-Plus Tablets
Iso-Bid Capsules (sustained release)

(◆ Shown in Product Identification Section)   (▣ Described in PDR For Nonprescription Drugs)

Manufacturers' Index

GILBERT LABORATORIES 411, 975
31 Fairmount Avenue
Chester NJ 07930
Address inquiries to:
Professional Service Dept. (201) 879-7374
Products Available
◆ Esgic Tablets & Capsules

GLAXO INC. 411, 976
Five Moore Drive
Research Triangle Park
North Carolina 27709 (919) 248-2100
Address inquiries to:
Professional Service Department
For Medical Emergencies Contact:
(919) 248-2100
(800) 334-0089
Products Available
Amesec Capsules
Atrocholin Tablets
BCG Vaccine
◆ Beclovent Oral Inhaler
◆ Beclovent Oral Inhaler Refill
◆ Beconase Nasal Inhaler
◆ Corticaine Cream
◆ Corticaine Suppositories
Ethatab Tablets
Seffin, Neutral
◆ Theobid Duracap Capsules
◆ Theobid Jr. Duracap Capsules
Trandate Injection
◆ Trandate Tablets
Tri-Cone Capsules
◆ Trinsicon/Trinsicon M Capsules
◆ Ventolin Inhaler
◆ Ventolin Inhaler Refill
◆ Ventolin Tablets
◆ Vicon Forte Capsules
◆ Vicon-C Capsules
◆ Vicon-Plus Capsules
◆ Vi-Zac Capsules
Zantac Injection
◆ Zantac Tablets
Zinacef

GLENBROOK LABORATORIES 412, 995
Division of Sterling Drug Inc.
90 Park Avenue
New York, NY 10016
Address inquiries to:
Medical Director (212) 972-4141
Products Available
◆ Arthritis Bayer Timed-Release Aspirin
◆ Bayer Aspirin
◆ Bayer Children's Chewable Aspirin
◆ Bayer Children's Cold Tablets
Bayer Cough Syrup for Children
◆ Children's Panadol Chewable Tablets, Liquid, Drops
Cope
Cosprin
Cosprin 650
Diaparene Line
◆ Fletcher's Castoria
◆ Infants Panadol Drops
◆ Maximum Bayer Aspirin
Maximum Strength Midol for Cramps
Maximum Strength Midol PMS
◆ Maximum Strength Panadol Capsules & Tablets
Midol-Original Formula
◆ Panadol Jr.
Phillips' Milk of Magnesia Liquid
Phillips' Milk of Magnesia Tablets
Vanquish

GLENWOOD, INC. 412, 998
83 North Summit Street
Tenafly, NJ 07670
Address inquiries to:
Professional Service Dept. (201) 569-0050
Products Available
Calphosan
Calphosan B-12
◆ Myotonachol
◆ Potaba
Primer Unna Boot
Pyridoxine HCl
◆ Renoquid
◆ Yodoxin
Zinc-Sulphate

GRAY PHARMACEUTICAL CO. 1000
Affiliate, The Purdue Frederick Company
100 Connecticut Avenue
Norwalk, CT 06854
Address inquiries to:
Medical Department (203) 853-0123
Products Available
X-Prep Bowel Evacuant Kit #1
X-Prep Bowel Evacuant Kit #2
X-Prep Liquid

GUARDIAN CHEMICAL 1000
A Division of United-Guardian, Inc.
230 Marcus Boulevard
P.O. Box 2500
Smithtown, NY 11787 (516) 273-0900
(800) 645-5566

Address inquiries to:
Director of Medical Research
Products Available
Clorpactin WCS-90
Clorpactin XCB
Lubrajel
Lubrajel HC
Lubraseptic Jelly
pHos-pHaid Tablets
Renacidin
Warexin

W. E. HAUCK, INC. 1001
P.O. Box 1065
Roswell, GA 30075
Address inquiries to:
Warren E. Hauck (404) 475-4758
Products Available
Anuject Injection
Besta Capsules
Butatran Tablets 30mg.
Cantri Vaginal Cream
Chlorafed H.S. Timecelles
Chlorafed Liquid
Chlorafed Timecelles
Diaqua Tablets
Dolacet Capsules
Entuss Expectorant
Entuss Tablets
Entuss-D Liquid & Tablets
G-1 Capsules
G-2 Capsules
G-3 Capsules
Geravite Elixir
Histor-D Syrup
Histor-D Timecelles
Isotrate Timecelles
Otic-HC Ear Drops
Otic-Plain Ear Drops
Palbar Tablets
Palmiron Tablets
Palmiron-C Tablets
Sinufed Timecelles
Vitormains
Wehless Capsules 35mg.
Wehless-105 Timecelles
Wehvert Tablets

HELENA LABORATORIES 3010
1530 Lindberg
P.O. Box 752
Beaumont, TX 77704
Address inquiries to:
(800) 231-5663
In TX (800) 392-3126
Products Available
ColoScreen/VPI

HERBERT LABORATORIES 1001
Dermatology Division of Allergan Pharmaceuticals, Inc.
2525 Dupont Drive
Irvine, CA 92715 (714) 752-4500
Products Available
Aeroseb-Dex Topical Aerosol Spray
Aeroseb-HC Topical Aerosol Spray
▣ Aquacare Dry Skin Cream & Lotion, 2% Urea Cream & Lotion
▣ Aquacare/HP Dry Skin Cream & Lotion, 10% Urea Cream & Lotion
▣ Bluboro Powder Astringent Soaking Solution
Clear By Design, Acne Skin Medication
▣ Danex Protein Enriched Dandruff Shampoo
Erymax Topical Solution
Exsel Lotion
Fluonid Ointment, Cream & Topical Solution
Fluoroplex Topical Solution & Cream
Gris-PEG Tablets, 125mg & 250mg
Maxiflor Cream
Maxiflor Ointment
Penecort Cream & Topical Solution 1%
Penecort Cream 2.5%
▣ Vanseb Cream Dandruff Shampoo
▣ Vanseb Lotion Dandruff Shampoo
▣ Vanseb-T Cream Tar Shampoo
▣ Vanseb-T Lotion Tar Shampoo

DOW B. HICKAM, INC. 1009
P.O. Box 2006
Sugar Land, TX 77487
Address inquiries to:
Professional Service Dept. (713) 240-1000
Products Available
Granulex
Proderm Topical Dressing

HIGH CHEMICAL COMPANY 1009
Div. Day & Frick, Inc.
1760 N. Howard St.
Philadelphia, PA 19122
Address inquiries to:
Professional Service Dept. (215) 634-2224
Products Available
Amo-Derm
Klorlyptus
Mus-L-Tone
Sarapin

HILL DERMACEUTICALS, INC. 1009
P.O. Box 19283
Orlando, FL 32814
Address inquiries to:
Mr. Jerry S. Roth, President
(305) 896-8280
Products Available
Burdeo
Derma Cas Gel
Derma-Smoothe/FS
Derma-Smoothe Oil
Derma-Sone Cream
Florida Foam Improved
Hill Cortac
Hill-Shade Lotion
R.S. Lotion No. 2

HOECHST-ROUSSEL PHARMACEUTICALS INC. 412, 1009
Route 202-206 North
Somerville, NJ 08876
Address inquiries to:
Medical Dept. (201) 231-2000
Products Available
◆ A/T/S
Claforan
◆ DiaBeta
◆ Doxidan
Doxinate
Doxinate Solution
Duadacin
◆ Festal II
◆ Festalan
◆ Lasix Oral Solution
◆ Lasix Tablets and Injection
◆ Loprox
Relefact TRH
Streptase
◆ Surfak
◆ Topicort Cream
◆ Topicort Gel
◆ Topicort LP
Topicort Ointment
◆ Trental

HOFFMANN-LA ROCHE INC.
See ROCHE LABORATORIES & ROCHE PRODUCTS INC.

HOLLAND-RANTOS COMPANY, INC. 1023
Post Office Box 385
865 Centennial Avenue
Piscataway, NJ 08854
See YOUNGS DRUG PRODUCTS CORPORATION

HOYT LABORATORIES 1023
See COLGATE-HOYT LABORATORIES

HYLAND THERAPEUTICS DIVISION 1023
Travenol Laboratories, Inc.
444 W. Glenoaks Blvd.
Glendale, CA 91202
Address inquiries to:
Product Management
(toll free) (800) 423-2862
For Medical Emergencies Contact:
Medical Director,
Hyland Therapeutics Div. (818) 956-3200
Branch Offices
Los Angeles, CA
4501 Colorado (800) 423-2862
(818) 240-5600
Coagulation Products Distributed By:
Hyland Therapeutics Division
Travenol Laboratories, Inc.
Glendale, CA 91202
(800) 423-2862
Plasma Extenders & Gamma Globulin
Products Distributed By:
Hyland Therapeutic Division
Travenol Laboratories, Inc.
Glendale, CA 91202 (818) 507-5472
Products Available
Autoplex, Anti-Inhibitor Coagulant Complex, Dried
Buminate 5%, Normal Serum Albumin (Human), U.S.P., 5% Solution
Buminate 25%, Normal Serum Albumin (Human), U.S.P., 25% Solution
Hemofil, Antihemophilic Factor (Human), Method Four, Dried
Hemofil T, Antihemophilic Factor (Human), Method Four, Dried, Heat-Treated
Hu-Tet, Tetanus Immune Globulin (Human), U.S.P.
Immune Serum Globulin (Human), U.S.P. Gamma Globulin
Proplex, Factor IX Complex (Human) (Factors II, VII, IX & X), Dried
Proplex SX, Factor IX Complex (Human)(Factors II, VII, IX & X), Dried
Proplex SX-T, Factor IX Complex (Human), Heat Treated
Protenate 5%, Plasma Protein Fraction (Human), U.S.P., 5% Solution

(◆ Shown in Product Identification Section) (▣ Described in PDR For Nonprescription Drugs)

Manufacturers' Index

HYNSON, WESTCOTT & DUNNING   1024
Division of Becton Dickinson and Co.
Charles & Chase Sts.
Baltimore, MD 21201   (301) 837-0890
Products Available
BAL in Oil Ampules
Cardio-Green Vials & Single Use Units
Indigo Carmine Ampules
▣ Lactinex Tablets & Granules
Phenolsulfonphthalein Solution Ampules
Thantis Lozenges

HYREX PHARMACEUTICALS   413, 1024
3494 Democrat Road
Memphis, TN 38118
Address inquiries to:
Professional Service Dept.   (901) 794-9050
Products Available
A-Spas
Atropine Sulfate Injection
Bronkotuss
C & T
Chorex
Cortisone Acetate Injection
Depogen
Depotest
Depotestogen
Dermarex Cream
Ear-Eze
Efedron Nasal Jelly
Everone
Glukor Injection
Hybolin Decanoate
Hydrate Injection
Hyplex Vari-Dose
Hyrex-105
Hytinic Capsules & Elixir
Hytinic Injection
◆ Hytuss Tablets
◆ Hytuss-2X Capsules
Hyzine-50 Injection
Kestrin Injection
Kestrone-5
Key-Pred
Key-Pred SP
Lipoderm Capsules
Lyopine Vari-Dose
Megaton Elixir
ND-Gesic Tablets
ND-Hist Capsules
ND-Stat Injection
Panzyme Tablets
Prorex Injection
Rexolate
Solurex Injection
◆ Trac Tablets 2X
Two-Dyne Capsules
Valergen
Valertest #2

ICN PHARMACEUTICALS, INC.   1025
222 N. Vincent Avenue
Covina, CA 91722
Address inquiries to:
Professional Service Dept.   (818) 967-5121
Products Available
Testred Capsules

IVES LABORATORIES INC.   413, 1026
685 Third Ave.
New York, NY 10017
Address medical inquiries to:
Medical Director
                            (Day) (212) 878-5164
Night Emergency   (212) 878-5273
General Information   (212) 878-5125
Branch Warehouses
Andover, MA 01810
   7 Lowell Junction Rd. Connector
                                (617) 475-7227
Atlanta, GA 30324
   221 Armour Dr., N.E.   (404) 875-8380
Baltimore, MD 21224
   101 Kane St.   (301) 633-4005
Buena Park, CA 90620
   6530 Altura Blvd.   (714) 523-5110
Dallas, TX 75238
   11240 Petal St.   (214) 341-1268
Denver, CO 80216
   4345 Oneida St.   (303) 377-0233
Honolulu, HI 96814
   1013 Kawaiahao St.   (808) 538-1988
N. Kansas City, MO 64116
   1340 Taney St.   (816) 842-3680
Memphis, TN 38127
   4171 Steele Road   (901) 353-5040
St. Paul, MN 55121
   935 Apollo Road
   Eagandale Center Indus. Pk.
                                (612) 454-1613
Kent, WA 98031
   19255 80th Ave. South (206) 872-8166
Skokie, IL 60187
   745 N. Gary Ave.   (312) 462-7400
Strongsville, OH 44136
   17647 Foltz Industrial Parkway
                                (216) 238-3820

Products Available
Cerose Compound Capsules
Cerose-DM
Cerubidine
Cetro-Cirose
◆ Cyclospasmol Capsules & Tablets
◆ Isordil Chewable
◆ Isordil Oral Titradose Tablets
◆ Isordil Sublingual Tablets
◆ Isordil Tembids Capsules
◆ Isordil Tembids Tablets
◆ Surmontil Capsules
◆ Synalgos-DC Capsules
Trecator-SC Tablets

JACOBUS PHARMACEUTICAL CO., INC.   1032
P.O. Box 5290
37, Cleveland Lane
Princeton, NJ 08540
Address inquiries to:
Professional Services   (609) 921-7447
For Medical Emergencies Contact:
Medical Department   (609) 921-7447
Products Available
Dapsone

JAMOL LABORATORIES INC.   1033
13 Ackerman Avenue
Emerson, NJ 07630
Address inquiries to:
                            (201) 262-6363
Products Available
Bahim Foot-Aide
Bahim Oil
Otide
Ponaris Nasal Mucosal Emollient
Prep-Aide
Roma-Nol Antiseptic

JANSSEN PHARMACEUTICA INC.   413, 1033
40 Kingsbridge Road
Piscataway, NJ 08854
                           (201) 524-9881
Products Available
Droperidol, See Inapsine
Fentanyl, See Sublimaze
◆ Imodium Capsules/Liquid
Inapsine Injection
Innovar Injection
Monistat I.V.
◆ Nizoral Tablets
◆ Sublimaze Injection
◆ Sufenta
◆ Sufentanil Citrate, See Sufenta
◆ Vermox Chewable Tablets

JOHNSON & JOHNSON PRODUCTS INC.   1044
A Johnson & Johnson Company
Patient Care Division
501 George Street
New Brunswick, NJ 08903
                          (201) 524-0400
Products Available
Debrisan Wound Cleaning Beads
Debrisan Wound Cleaning Paste
Surgicel Absorbable Hemostat

KENWOOD LABORATORIES, INC.   1046
490-A Main Street
New Rochelle, NY 10801   (914) 632-1002
Products Available
Apatate Liquid
Bonacal Plus Tablets
Glutofac Tablets
I.L.X. B_{12} Elixir
I.L.X. B_{12} Tablets
I.L.X. Elixir
Kenpectin
Kenpectin-P
Kenwood Therapeutic Liquid
Papavatral Tablets
Papavatral 20 Tablets
Posterisan Ointment
Posterisan Suppositories

KEY PHARMACEUTICALS, INC.   413, 1046
18425 N.W. 2nd Ave.
Miami, FL 33169
Address inquiries to:
Professional Service Dept.   (305) 652-2276
Products Available
AeroBid Inhaler System
Genapax
Guanidine HCl Tablets
InspirEase
Ipsatol Expectorant Syrup
Ircon Tablets
Ircon-FA Tablets
Nico-Span Capsules
◆ Nitro-Dur Transdermal Infusion System
Nitroglyn Tablets
Quinora Tablets
◆ Theo-Dur Sprinkle
◆ Theo-Dur Tablets
Tyzine Nasal Solution
Tyzine Pediatric Nasal Drops

KNOLL PHARMACEUTICAL COMPANY   414, 1056
30 North Jefferson Road
Whippany, NJ 07981   (201) 887-8300
Address inquiries to:
Professional Services Department
Products Available
Akineton Injection
◆ Akineton Tablets
Codeine Phosphate Injection
Codeine Sulfate Tablets
Dilaudid Cough Syrup
Dilaudid Injection
◆ Dilaudid-HP Injection
Dilaudid Multiple Dose Vials (Sterile Solution)
Dilaudid Powder
Dilaudid Rectal Suppositories
◆ Dilaudid Tablets
◆ Isoptin Ampules
◆ Isoptin for Intravenous Injection
◆ Isoptin Oral Tablets
Meperidine Hydrochloride Injection
Morphine Sulfate Injection
Promethazine Hydrochloride Injection
Quadrinal Suspension
◆ Quadrinal Tablets
Santyl Ointment
◆ Vicodin Tablets

KRAMER PHARMACAL, INC.   1069
8778 S.W. 8th Street
Miami, FL 33174
Address inquiries to:
8778 S.W. 8th Street
Miami, FL 33174   (305) 223-1287
For Medical Emergencies Contact:
Professional Director   (305) 223-1287
Branch Offices
Hato Rey, P.R. 00917
Arlo Laboratories
212 Mayaguez St.   (809) 767-7281
Products Available
Banquin Cream
Cortixin Otic Suspension
Fungi-Nail Tincture
Lysiplex Syrup
Otipyrin Otic Solution
Simetyl Elixir
Sulfadrin Nasal Drops
Uroseptic D-S Tablets
Vagisulf Cream
Vasoflex Tablets
Vasolin Drops
Yohimex Tablets
Yohimex P-Z (Dual Pack) Tablets
Zinckel-220 Tablets

KREMERS-URBAN COMPANY   1070
Please refer to WILLIAM H. RORER, INC. for product information.

LACTAID INC.   414, 1070
600 Fire Road, P.O. Box 111
Pleasantville, NJ 08232-0111
Address inquiries to:
Alan E. Kligerman   (609) 645-7500
Products Available
◆ LactAid brand lactase enzyme

LAFAYETTE PHARMACAL, INC.   1070
4200 South Hulen Street
Fort Worth, TX 76109
Address inquiries to:
Lafayette Pharmacal, Inc.
4200 South Hulen Street
Fort Worth, TX 76109   (817) 763-8011
Products Available
Konsyl
Konsyl-D (formerly L. A. Formula)

LAKESIDE PHARMACEUTICALS   421, 1358
Division of Merrell Dow Pharmaceuticals Inc.
P.O. Box 429553
Cincinnati, OH 45242-9553
Address inquiries to:
Professional Relations Manager
                            (513) 948-9111
These products currently listed under Merrell Dow in the Product Information Section will be listed under Lakeside in the next edition.
Products Available
◆ Bentyl 10 mg Capsules
Bentyl Injection
Bentyl Syrup
◆ Bentyl 20 mg Tablets
◆ Bricanyl Injection
◆ Bricanyl Tablets
▣ Novahistine Cough Formula
▣ Novahistine Cough & Cold Formula
◆ Novahistine DH
▣ Novahistine DMX
◆ Novahistine Elixir
◆ Novahistine Expectorant
◆ Singlet
◆ Tenuate Dospan Tablets
Tenuate Tablets

(◆ Shown in Product Identification Section)   (▣ Described in PDR For Nonprescription Drugs)

Manufacturers' Index

LAMBDA PHARMACAL CORPORATION 1071
Subsidiary of A. J. Bart, Inc.
P.O. Box 813
Gurabo, Puerto Rico 00658
Address inquiries to:
Mr. Bob Bibars
Gurabo Industrial Park, P.O. Box 813
Gurabo, Puerto Rico 00658
(809) 737-8445
Products Available
Dextrotussin Syrup
Migralam Capsules
Neuro B-12 Forte Injectable
Neuro B-12 Injectable
Vita-Numonyl Injectable

THE LANNETT COMPANY, INC. 1071
9000 State Road
Philadelphia, PA 19136
Address inquiries to:
Medical Service Dept. (215) 333-9000
Products Available
Acetazolamide Tablets
⊞Acnederm Lotion & Soap
Adalan Lanatabs
Alphamul Suspension
Amtren Tablets
Arithmin Tablets
Baroflave Powder
Bellafedrol AH Tablets
Bethanechol Chloride
Bisacodyl Suppositories & Tablets
Brompheniramine Maleate Tablets
Castaderm
Chlorpromazine Tablets
Chlorulan Tablets
Codalan
Dicalsonate Capsules
Diphenoxylate & Atropine Tablets
Disanthrol Capsules
Disolan Capsules
Disonate Capsules & Liquid
Efricon Expectorant
Glutethimide Tablets
Hydrochlorulan Tablets
Kaylixir
Lanacillin "400"
Lanahex Liquid
Lanamin Capsules
Lanatuss Expectorant
Lanorinal Capsules & Tablets
Lanvisone Cream
Lofene Tablets
Lycolan Elixir
⊞Magnatril Suspension & Tablets
Nitrofurantoin Tablets
Obalan Tablets
Orcophen Capsules
P-I-N Forte Tablets & Syrup
Paverolan Lanacaps
Potasalan Elixir
Primidone Tablets
Probenecid Tablets
Promethazine Expectorant
Promethazine Tablets
Pyrralan Expectorant DM
Rufolex Capsules
S-A-C Tablets
Salatar Cream
Sedragesic Tablets
Trichlorex Tablets
Trichlormethiazide Tablets
Veltane Tablets & Expectorant

LASALLE LABORATORIES, INC. 1071
Subsidiary of Mallard, Inc.
3021 Wabash Avenue
Detroit, MI 48216
Address inquiries to:
Mallard, Inc. (313) 964-3910
Products Available
Dytuss
Fetrin
Hyco-Pap
Orabex-TF Tablets
Pacaps
Protid Tablets, Improved Formula

LASER, INC. 1072
2000 N. Main Street,
P.O. Box 905, Crown Point, IN 46307
Address inquiries to:
Donald A. Laser (219) 663-1165
Products Available
Dallergy Capsules, Tablets, Syrup
Donatussin DC Syrup
Donatussin Drops
Fumatinic Capsules
Fumerin Tablets
Lactocal-F Tablets
Respaire-SR Capsules 60, 120
Theospan-SR Capsules 130 mg., 260 mg.
Theostat 80 Syrup
Trimstat Tablets

LEDERLE LABORATORIES 414, 1072, 3010
Division of American Cyanamid Co.
One Cyanamid Plaza

Wayne, NJ 07470
LEDERLE PARENTERALS, INC.
Carolina, Puerto Rico 00630
LEDERLE PIPERACILLIN, INC.
Carolina, Puerto Rico 00630
Address inquiries on medical matter to:
Professional Services Dept.
Lederle Laboratories
Pearl River, NY 10965 (914) 735-5000
Distribution Centers
ATLANTA
Bulk Address
Chamblee (Atlanta), GA 30341
5180 Peachtree Industrial Blvd.
Mail Address
Atlanta, GA 30302
P.O. Box 4272 (404) 455-0320
(All Other) (800) LEDERLE
CHICAGO
Bulk Address
Rosemont, IL 60018
10401 W. Touhy Ave.
Mail Address
Chicago, IL 60666
P.O. Box 66189 (312) 827-8871
(All Other) (800) LEDERLE
DALLAS
Bulk Address
Dallas, TX 75247
7611 Carpenter Freeway
Mail Address
Dallas, TX 75265
P.O. Box 225731 (214) 631-2130
(All Other) (800) LEDERLE
LOS ANGELES
Bulk Address
Los Angeles, CA 90040
2300 S. Eastern Ave.
Mail Address
Los Angeles, CA 90051
T.A. Box 2202 (213) 726-1016
(All Other) (800) LEDERLE
PHILADELPHIA
Fort Washington, PA 19034
185 Commerce Drive
(NY-NJ-MD-DE) (800) LEDERLE
(CT-VA-WV-DC) (800) LEDERLE
(Phila. Only) (215) 248-3900
(All Other) (215) 646-7000
Products Available
♦ Acetaminophen Capsules, Tablets, Elixir
Acetaminophen w/Codeine Tablets
Achromycin Intramuscular
Achromycin Intravenous
Achromycin Ophthalmic Ointment 1%
Achromycin Ophthalmic Suspension 1%
Achromycin 3% Ointment
♦ Achromycin V Capsules
Achromycin V Oral Suspension
Achrostatin V Capsules
♦ Amicar Intravenous, Syrup & Tablets
♦ Amitriptyline HCl Tablets
Amoxicillin Capsules, Suspension
♦ Ampicillin Trihydrate Capsules, Oral Suspension
♦ Aristocort A Topical Cream
♦ Aristocort A Topical Ointment
Aristocort Forte Parenteral
Aristocort Intralesional
Aristocort Syrup
♦ Aristocort Tablets
♦ Aristocort Topical Cream
♦ Aristocort Topical Ointment
Aristospan Suspension (Intraarticular)
Aristospan Suspension (Intralesional)
Artane Elixir
Artane Sequels
♦ Artane Tablets
Ascorbic Acid Tablets
♦ Asendin
Aureomycin Ointment 3%
Aureomycin Ointment (Ophthalmic) 1%
Brompheniramine Maleate, Phenylephrine & Phenylpropanolamine Sequels
⊞Caltrate 600
⊞Caltrate 600+Vitamin D
Caramiphen Edisylate & Phenylpropanolamine Sequels Sustained Release Tablets, Expectorant
♦ Centrum
⊞Centrum, Jr. (Childrens' Chewable)
Centrum, Jr. + C
Chlordiazepoxide HCl Capsules
Chlorothiazide Tablets
♦ Chlorpheniramine Maleate
Chlorpheniramine Maleate & Phenylpropanolamine Sequels, Tablets & Capsules
♦ Chlorpromazine HCl Tablets, Liquid Concentrate
Chlorpropamide Tablets
♦ Chlorthalidone Tablets
Chlorzoxazone Tablets
Cholera Vaccine (India Strains)
♦ Cloxacillin Capsules
♦ Cyclocort Cream
♦ Cyclocort Ointment
♦ Declomycin Capsules and Tablets

Diamox Parenteral
♦ Diamox Sequels, Tablets
Dicloxacillin Sodium Capsules
Dicyclomine HCl Capsules, Tablets
Diphenhydramine HCl Elixir, Cough Syrup
Diphenoxylate HCl Tablets
Diphtheria & Tetanus Toxoids, Adsorbed Purogenated
Diphtheria & Tetanus Toxoids & Pertussis Vaccine, Adsorbed
♦ Dipyridamole Tablets
♦ Docusate Sodium, USP (DSS) Capsules, Syrup
♦ Docusate Sodium, USP w/Casanthranol Capsules, Syrup
Dolene AP-65 Tablets
Dolene Capsules
♦ Doxycycline Hyclate Capsules, Tablets
♦ Ergoloid Mesylates Tablets
Erythromycin Estolate Oral Suspension
Erythromycin Ethylsuccinate Oral Suspension
♦ Erythromycin Stearate Tablets
♦ Ferro-Sequels
Ferrous Gluconate Iron Supplement Tablets
Ferrous Sulfate Tablets, Elixir
♦ Filibon F.A. Prenatal Vitamin Tablets
♦ Filibon Forte
♦ Filibon Prenatal Vitamin Tablets
♦ Folvite Parenteral & Tablets
⊞Footwork Athlete's Foot Remedy
♦ Furosemide Tablets
⊞Gevrabon Liquid
Gevral Protein Powder
♦ Gevral T Tablets
⊞Gevral Tablets
Gevrite Tablets
Guaifenesin Syrup
Guaifenesin w/D-Methorphan Hydrobromide Syrup
Hydralazine HCl Tablets
♦ Hydrochlorothiazide Tablets
♦ Hydromox R Tablets
♦ Hydromox Tablets
♦ Hydroxyzine HCl Tablets
♦ Imipramine HCl Tablets
⊞Incremin w/Iron Syrup
Indomethacin Capsules
Isosorbide Dinitrate Tablets
Isosorbide Dinitrate, Sublingual, Oral
Isosorbide Dinitrate T.D. Tablets
Isoxsuprine HCl Tablets
Ledercillin VK Oral Solution & Tablets
⊞Lederplex Capsules, Liquid & Tablets
♦ Leucovorin Calcium
Levoprome
Levothroxine Sodium Tablets
♦ Loxitane C Oral Concentrate
♦ Loxitane Capsules
♦ Loxitane IM
♦ Materna 1·60 Tablets
♦ Maxzide Tablets
♦ Meclizine HCl Tablets
Methenamine Mandelate Suspension
Methocarbamol Tablets
♦ Methotrexate Tablets & Parenteral
♦ Methyclothiazide Tablets
Methyldopa Tablets
♦ Metronidazole Tablets
♦ Minocin Capsules
Minocin Intravenous
♦ Minocin Oral Suspension
♦ Minocin Tablets
Myambutol Tablets
Neoloid Emulsified Castor Oil
Neomycin Sulfate Tablets
♦ Neptazane Tablets
Niacin
Nilstat for Preparation of Oral Suspension
Nilstat Oral Suspension
Nilstat Oral Tablets
Nilstat Topical Cream, Ointment
Nilstat Vaginal Tablets
♦ Nitroglycerin T.D. Capsules
Nylidrin HCl Tablets
Orimune Poliovirus Vaccine, Live, Oral, Trivalent
♦ Papaverine HCl Capsules
♦ Pathibamate Tablets
♦ Pathilon Tablets
Penicillin G Potassium Tablets
Penicillin V Potassium
Perihemin Capsules
⊞Peritinic Tablets
Phenobarbital Tablets
Pipracil
Pnu-Imune Pneumococcal Vaccine Polyvalent
Potassium Chloride Liquid
Potassium Gluconate Elixir
Prednisone Tablets
♦ Probenecid Tablets
♦ Probenecid with Colchicine Tablets
♦ Procainamide HCl Capsules
Promethazine HCl Expectorant, Plain
Promethazine HCl Expectorant V.C. Plain
Promethazine HCl Expectorant V.C. w/Codeine
Promethazine HCl Expectorant w/Codeine
Pronemia Capsules

(♦ Shown in Product Identification Section) (⊞ Described in PDR For Nonprescription Drugs)

Manufacturers' Index

Propantheline Bromide
Propoxyphene HCl
Propylthiouracil Tablets
Pseudoephedrine HCl Tablets & Syrup
◆ Pyrazinamide Tablets
Pyridoxine HCl Tablets
◆ Quinidine Gluconate Sustained Release Tablets
◆ Quinidine Sulfate Tablets
Quinine Sulfate Capsules
Reserpine, Hydrochlorothiazide & Hydralazine Tablets
▣ Spartus High Potency Vitamins & Minerals plus Electrolytes Tablets
▣ Spartus + Iron High Potency Vitamins & Minerals plus Electrolytes Tablets
◆ Spironolactone Tablets
◆ Spironolactone with Hydrochlorothiazide Tablets
▣ Stresscaps Capsules
▣ Stresstabs 600 Tablets, Advanced Formula
▣ Stresstabs 600 with Iron, Advanced Formula
▣ Stresstabs 600 with Zinc, Advanced Formula
Sulfadiazine-Sulfamerazine-Sulfamethazine
◆ Sulfamethoxazole & Trimethoprim Tablets and Pediatric Suspension
Sulfasalazine Tablets
Sulfisoxazole Tablets
Tetanus Toxoid, Adsorbed
Tetanus Toxoid Purogenated
Tetanus & Diphtheria Toxoids, Combined Purogenated
Thiamine HCl (Vitamin B-1) Tablets
◆ Thioridazine HCl Tablets
◆ Thiotepa Parenteral
Thyroid Tablets
Tolbutamide Tablets
◆ TriHemic 600 Tablets
Tri-Immunol
Triprolidine HCl with Pseudoephedrine Tablets, Syrup
Tuberculin, Old, Tine Test
Tuberculin Purified Protein Derivative Tine Test (PPD)
Vitamin A, Natural Capsules
Vitamin C Chewable Tablets
Vitamin E, Natural USP Capsules
Vitamin E USP Capsules
▣ Zincon Dandruff Shampoo, Improved Richer Formula

LEEMING DIVISION 1119
Pfizer Inc.
100 Jefferson Rd.
Parsippany, NJ 07054
Address inquiries to:
Research and Development Dept.
(201) 887-2100
Products Available
▣ Ben Gay External Analgesic Products
▣ Desitin Ointment
Rheaban Tablets
Unisom Nighttime Sleep-Aid
Visine A.C. Eye Drops
Visine Eye Drops

LEGERE PHARMACEUTICALS, INC. 1120
7326 E. Evans Road
Scottsdale, AZ 85260 (602) 991-4033
Address Inquiries to:
Customer Service & Product Information
Toll Free 1(800) 528-3144
Products Available
ACE + Z Tablets
Acetaco Tablets
Allerdryl 50
B-Complex 100
B-S-P
Brosema
Cee-500 (Ascorbic Acid)
Cee-1000 T.D. Tablets
Cinalone 40
Cinonide 40
Cobolin-M
Depo-Predate 40
Depo-Predate 80
Dexasone 4
Dexasone 10
Dexasone LA
Dexol T.D. Tablets
Dexol 300
Dextraron
Dieutrim Capsules
Di-Hydrotic
E-Cypionate
Estrone
Kabolin
KATO
Lidocaine 1% and 2%
Livolex
Megaplex I.M.
Menaval 20 & Menaval 40
Mersalyl-Theophylline
Natural Estrogenic Substance
Neucalm 50
O. B. Thera Tablets
PT 105 Capsules
Phenazine Tablets & Capsules

Predate 50
Predate S
Predate TBA
Probahist Capsules
Prodrox 250
Progesterone 50
Promet 50
Rodex
Rodex T.D. Capsules
Stemetic
T-Cypionate
Teramine Capsules
Testaval 90/4
Testosterone Suspension
Thera-Ron Tablets
Vagimide Cream
Vitabese Capsules

LEMMON COMPANY ETHICAL DIVISION 417, 1121
Post Office Box 630
Sellersville, PA 18960
Address inquiries to:
Toll Free (800) 523-6542
(215) 723-5544
Products Available
Acetaminophen Tablets and Capsules
Acetaminophen with Codeine Tablets and Capsules
◆ Adipex-P Tablets
Beta-Val Cream
Chlordiazepoxide Hydrochloride Capsules
Cotrim
Cotrim D.S.
Dexampex Tablets and Capsules
Donphen Tablets
Doxy-Lemmon Capsules
Glucamide Tablets
Indo-Lemmon Capsules
Methampex Tablets
Metryl and Metryl 500 Tablets
Myco-Triacet Cream and Ointment
Neothylline Tablets and Injection
Neothylline-GG Tablets
Nu'Leven Tablets
Nystatin Cream, Oral Tablets, and Vaginal Tablets
Otocort Sterile Ear Drops, Solution and Suspension
Phentermine HCl Capsules
Potage
Racet Cream
Racet LCD Cream
Racet-1% Cream
Rhinex D Lay Tablets
Rhus Tox Antigen Injection
S.B.P. Tablets
Statobex G Tablets
Triacet Cream
Triphed Tablets
Urinary #2 Tablets
Vagitrol Vaginal Cream

ELI LILLY AND COMPANY 417, 1122, 3012
For Medical Information, Write
Medical Department (317) 261-2000
307 E. McCarty St.
Indianapolis, IN 46285
Lilly Regional & District Offices
*Aurora, CO 80014
Suite 111, Cherry Creek Place I
3131 South Vaughn Way (303) 695-7730
Birmingham, AL 35223
Suite 309, Shades Brook Bldg.
3300 Cahaba Road (205) 879-2441
Bloomington, MN 55420
Suite 1142, One Appletree Square
(612) 854-3505
Charlotte, NC 28909
Suite 207, Park Seneca Bldg.
1515 Mockingbird Lane (704) 525-8905
*Chicago, IL 60631
Suite 270, O'Hare Plaza
5735 East River Road (312) 693-8740
Cincinnati, OH 45241
Suite 413, 4055 Executive Park Dr.
(513) 563-0720
*Dallas, TX 75234
4404 Beltwood Parkway, South
(214) 661-5620
Dedham, MA 02026
990 Washington St. (617) 329-4320
Enfield, CT 06082
150 Freshwater Boulevard
(203) 741-2055
Grand Rapids, MI 49506
Suite 170, 3040 Charlevoix Dr., S.E.
(616) 949-0876
Honolulu, HI 96825
6838 Niumalu Loop (808) 396-8444
Houston, TX 77042
Suite 360, Richmond Plaza I
9800 Richmond Ave. (713) 975-6766

Indianapolis, IN 46268
Suite 235, Northwest Plaza
3901 West 86th Street (317) 261-2512
Jacksonville, FL 32216
Suite 319-A, 7825 Baymeadows Way
(904) 731-7124
Kansas City, MO 64114
Suites 600, 610, 9200 Ward Parkway
(816) 361-6116
Louisville, KY 40223
Suite 150, Plainview Plaza II
10170 Linn Station Road
(502) 425-2372
Melville, NY 11747
Suite 3S02, One Huntington Quadrangle
(516) 752-9797
Memphis, TN 38117
Suite 224, 755 Crossover Lane
Audubon Woods Business Campus
(901) 767-0360
Metarie, LA 70002
Suite 508, Security Homestead Bldg.
4900 Veterans Memorial Blvd.
(504) 885-9645
Miami, FL 33156
Suite 412, Dadeland Square
7700 North Kendall Drive
(305) 596-6193
Middlebury Heights, OH 44130
Suite 395, Interstate Plaza
16600 W. Sprague Rd. (216) 243-3600
Morristown, NJ 07960
Morristown Centre
10 Madison Avenue (201) 898-9505
Nashville, TN 37210
Suite 310, 555 Marriott Drive
(615) 889-6010
*Norcross, GA 30091
5944 Peachtree Corners, East
(404) 441-5400
Oklahoma City, OK 73112
Suite 325, Grand Centre
5400 N.W. Grand Blvd. (405) 947-2482
Omaha, NE 68103
5600 South 42nd St. (402) 734-4635
*Pasadena, CA 91101
Suite 916, Mutual Savings Bldg.
301 E. Colorado Blvd. (213) 792-5121
Pittsburgh, PA 15220
Suite 602, Manor Oak Two
1910 Cochran Rd. (412) 922-9770
Portland, OR 97205
Suite 310, Morgan Bldg.
720 S.W. Washington St.
(503) 223-8298
Raleigh, NC 27625
Suite 103, 3109 Poplarwood Ct.
(919) 872-4836
Redmond, WA 98052
11811 Willows Road
(206) 881-5796
Richmond, VA 23229
Suite 105, Henrico Corporate Center
7798 Carousel Lane (804) 747-7160
St. Louis, MO 63131
Suite 325, Corporate Hill II
1633 Des Peres Road (314) 821-0190
Sacramento, CA 95814
Suite 715, 555 Capitol Mall
(916) 444-2173
San Antonio, TX 78216
GPM Life Bldg.
Suite 630 North Tower
800 N.W. Loop 410 (512) 341-2211
San Diego, CA 92103
Suite 618, Fifth Avenue Financial Center
2550 Fifth Ave. (619) 234-6664
San Francisco, CA 94111
Suite 1170, 100 California St.
(415) 362-0559
Silver Spring, MD 20903
Suite 111, Executive Court
1734 Elton Road (301) 439-7991
*Southfield, MI 48075
Suite 940, 3000 Town Center
(313) 358-2206
(313) 358-2207
(313) 358-2208
*Stamford, CT 06905
Suite 301, 1600 Summer St.
(203) 357-1422
Tampa, FL 33609
Suite 630, Lincoln Center
5401 W. Kennedy Blvd.
(813) 870-2036
Williamsville, NY 14221
Suite 204, 5820 Main St.
(716) 634-0178
Worthington, OH 43085
Suite 250, 300 E. Wilson Bridge Rd.
(614) 846-5090
Wynnewood, PA 19096
Suite 202, Seven Wynnewood Rd.
(215) 642-2649
(215) 477-8739
*Regional office also
Products Available
A.S.A. & Codeine Compound Pulvules & Tablets

(◆ Shown in Product Identification Section)   (▣ Described in PDR For Nonprescription Drugs)

Manufacturers' Index

A.S.A. Enseals, Pulvules, Suppositories & Tablets
Acidulin Pulvules
Aerolone Solution
Alphalin Gelseals
Amertan Jelly
Ammoniated Mercury Ointments
Ammonium Chloride Enseals
Amyl Nitrite, Aspirols
◆ Amytal Elixir & Tablets
Amytal Sodium Ampoules & Vials
◆ Amytal Sodium Pulvules
Analgesic Balm Ointment
Anhydron Tablets
Apomorphine Hydrochloride Soluble Tablets
Arnica Tincture
Aromatic Ammonia Aspirols & Spirit
Aromatic Elixir
Atropine Sulfate Vials, Sterile Ophthalmic Ointment, Tablets & Soluble Tablets
◆ Aventyl HCl Liquid & Pulvules
Bacitracin Ointment & Sterile Ophthalmic Ointment
Belladonna Extract Tablets
Belladonna Tincture
Benzoin Tincture
Betalin Complex Elixir
Betalin Compound Pulvules
Betalin S Ampoules, Vials, Elixir & Tablets
Betalin 12 Crystalline Vials
Bilron Pulvules
Boric Acid Ointment & Sterile Ophthalmic Ointments
Brevital Sodium Vials
Calcium Carbonate Tablets, Aromatic
Calcium Gluceptate, Ampoules
Calcium Gluconate Tablets
Calcium Gluconate w/Vitamin D Pulvules & Tablets
Calcium Hydroxide Powder
Calcium Lactate Tablets
Capastat Sulfate Vials
Capsules, Empty Gelatin
Carbarsone Capsules
Cascara, Aromatic, Fluid Extract
Cascara Compound Tablets
Cascara Sagrada Fluid Extract
Cascara Tablets
Castor Oil Elastic Filled Capsules
◆ Ceclor Pulvules & Suspension
Cevalin Ampoules & Tablets
Citrated Caffeine Tablets
Cocaine Hydrochloride Solvets
Codeine Phosphate Vials & Soluble Tablets
Codeine Sulfate Tablets & Soluble Tablets
Colchicine Ampoules & Tablets
Cold Cream, for Compounding Prescriptions, Ointment
Cologel Liquid
Compound Benzoin Tincture
Copavin, Pulvules
Crystodigin Ampoules
◆ Crystodigin Tablets
Cyanide Antidote Package
◆ Darvocet-N 50 Tablets
◆ Darvocet-N 100 Tablets
◆ Darvon Pulvules
◆ Darvon Compound Pulvules
◆ Darvon Compound-65 Pulvules
◆ Darvon with A.S.A. Pulvules
◆ Darvon-N Suspension & Tablets
◆ Darvon-N with A.S.A. Tablets
Deltalin Gelseals
Dibasic Calcium Phosphate Tablets
Dibasic Calcium Phosphate w/Vitamin D Pulvules
Diethylstilbestrol Enseals, Suppositories & Tablets
Digiglusin Tablets
Dobutrex Vials
Dolophine Hydrochloride Ampoules, Vials & Tablets
Drolban Vials
Duracillin A.S. Vials
◆ Dymelor Tablets
Emetine Hydrochloride Ampoules
En-Cebrin Pulvules
En-Cebrin F Pulvules
Ephedrine & Amytal Pulvules
Ephedrine Sulfate Ampoules, Pulvules, & Syrups
Eprolin Gelseals
Ergotrate Maleate Ampoules & Tablets
Extralin Pulvules
Ferrous Gluconate Pulvules
Ferrous Sulfate Enseals & Tablets
Folic Acid Tablets
Glucagon for Injection Vials
Green Soap Tincture
Haldrone Tablets
Heparin Sodium Vials
Hepicebrin Tablets
Hexa-Betalin Vials & Tablets
Histadyl and A.S.A. Pulvules
Histadyl E.C. Syrup
Histalog, Ampoules
Histamine Phosphate (For Gastric Test)

Histamine Phosphate (Histamine Test for Pheochromocytoma)
Homicebrin
Humulin N Vials
Humulin R Vials
Hydriodic Acid Syrup
Ichthammol Ointments
Lente Iletin I, 40 & 100 units
Regular Iletin I, 40 & 100 units
Regular Iletin II (Concentrated), 500 units
Semilente Iletin I, 40 & 100 units
Ultralente Iletin I, 40 & 100 units
NPH Iletin I, 40 & 100 units
Protamine, Zinc & Iletin I, 40 & 100 units
Beef Regular Iletin II, 100 units
Beef Lente Iletin II, 100 units
Beef NPH Iletin II, 100 units
Beef Protamine Zinc & Iletin II, 100 units
Pork Regular Iletin II, 100 units
Pork Lente Iletin II, 100 units
Pork NPH Iletin II, 100 units
Pork Protamine, Zinc & Iletin II, 100 units
Ipecac Syrup
Isoniazid Tablets
Isopropyl Alcohol, 91%
Keflin, Neutral, Vials & Faspak
Kefzol Vials & Faspak
Lactated Pepsin Elixir
Lextron Ferrous Pulvules
Lextron Pulvules
Liver Vials
Magnesium Sulfate Ampoules
Mandol Vials & Faspak
Mercuric Oxide, Yellow, Sterile Ophthalmic Ointments
Merthiolate, Aeropump, Glycerite, Solution & Tincture
◆ Methadone Hydrochloride Diskets
Methenamine & Sodium Biphosphate Tablets
Methyltestosterone Tablets
Metubine Iodide Vials
Milk of Bismuth
Morphine Sulfate Vials & Soluble Tablets
Moxam Vials
Multicebrin Tablets
Mumps Skin-Test Antigen
Myrrh Tincture
Neomycin Sulfate Ointment
Neomycin Sulfate Tablets
Neotrizine Suspension & Tablets
Niacin Tablets
Niacinamide Tablets
Nitroglycerin Sublingual Tablets
Oncovin Solution Vials
Opium (Deodorized) Tincture
Ox Bile Extract Enseals
Pancreatin Enseals & Tablets
Pantholin Tablets
Papaverine Hydrochloride, Ampoules, Powder, Tablets & Vials
Paregoric Tincture
Penicillin G Potassium Vials (Buffered)
Penicillin G Procaine Suspension, Sterile, Vials
Phenobarbital Elixir & Tablets
Phenobarbital Sodium Vials
Potassium Chloride Ampoules & Tablets
Potassium Iodide Enseals
Powder Papers
Progesterone Vials
Propylthiouracil Tablets
Protamine Sulfate Ampoules & Vials
Prunicodeine
Pyridoxine Hydrochloride Tablets
Quinidine Gluconate Vials
Quinidine Sulfate Pulvules & Tablets
Quinine Sulfate Pulvules & Tablets
Reserpine Tablets
Reticulex Pulvules
Reticulogen Vials
Reticulogen Fortified Vials
Riboflavin Tablets
Rose, Soluble, for Making Artificial Rose Water
Sandril, Vials
Scarlet Red Ointment
◆ Seconal Sodium Pulvules & Vials
Seconal Sodium Suppositories
Seromycin Pulvules
Silver Nitrate Wax Ampoules
Soda Mint Tablets
Sodium Bicarbonate Tablets
Sodium Chloride Vials, Enseals & Tablets
Sodium Iodide Ampoules
Sodium Salicylate Enseals
Streptomycin Sulfate Vials
Sulfadiazine Tablets
Sulfapyridine Tablets
Sulfur Ointment
Surfacaine Cream, Jelly & Ointment
Surfadil Cream & Lotion
Tapazole Tablets
Terpin Hydrate & Codeine Elixir
Terpin Hydrate Elixir
Tes-Tape
Testosterone Propionate Vials

Theracebrin Pulvules
Thiamine Hydrochloride Ampoules, Elixer, Tablets, & Vials
Thyroid Enseals & Tablets
Trikates Oral Solution
Tubocurarine Chloride Vials
◆ Tuinal Pulvules
Tycopan Pulvules
Tylosterone, Tablets
V-Cillin K for Oral Solution & Tablets
Valerian Tincture
Vancocin HCl, for Oral Solution
Vancocin HCl, Vials
Velban Vials
Vitamin A, Gelseals
Vitamin B Complex, Elixir & Pulvules
Vitamin C, Tablets
Vitamin D, Gelseals
Vitamin E, Gelseals
Whitfield's Ointment (Double Strength)
Wild Cherry Syrup
Zentinic Pulvules
Zentron Chewable Tablets
Zentron Liquid
Zinc Oxide Ointments
Zinc Oxide Paste Ointment
Zinc Sulfate Compound Powder

LYPHOMED, INC. 1181
2020 Ruby Street
Melrose Park, IL 60160
 (312) 345-6170
(except IL) (800) 621-3334
PENTAM Hotline (312) 34-LYPHO
Address medical or scientific inquiries to:
Manager, Professional Relations
Address other inquiries to:
Marketing Department
Distribution Centers
CHICAGO
Melrose Park, IL 60160
2020 Ruby Street
NEW YORK
Dayton, NJ 08810
P.O. Box 422
LOS ANGELES
Los Angeles, CA 90051
P.O. Box 4029
Products Available
Aminophylline Injection, USP, 25mg/ml
Calcium Chloride Injection, USP, 10%
Calcium Gluconate Injection, USP, 10%
Chloramphenicol Sodium Succinate for Injection, USP, 1 gm
Chorionic Gonadotropin for Injection, USP, 5,000/10,000/20,000 USP units
Chromic Chloride Injection, USP
Cupric Chloride Injection, USP
Dexamethasone Sodium Phosphate Injection, USP, 4 mg/ml
Doxy-100 & Doxy-200 (Doxycycline Hyclate for Injection, USP)
Furosemide Injection, USP, 10 mg/ml
Gentamicin Sulfate Injection, USP, 40 mg/ml
Glycopyrollate Injection, USP, 0.2 mg/ml
Heparin Lock Flush Solution, USP, 100 u/ml
Heparin Sodium Injection, USP, 1,000/5,000/10,000 units per ml
Heparin Sodium Injection, USP (Beef Lung Origin) 1,000 & 10,000 units per ml
HepFlush-10 (Heparin Lock Flush Solution, USP, 10 u/ml
Hydrocortisone Sodium Succinate for Injection, USP, 100, 250, 500 & 1,000 mg
Hydroxyzine Hydrochloride Injection, USP, 25 & 50 mg/ml
I.V. Transfer Spikes
Iodopen (Sodium Iodide Injection)
Kanamycin Sulfate Injection, USP, 75mg/2ml, 500mg/2ml, 1gm/3ml
LyphoLyte & LyphoLyte-II (Multielectrolyte Concentrate)
MTE-2
MTE-3
MTE-4 & MTE-4 Concentrated
MTE-5 & MTE-5 Concentrated
MTE-6 & MTE-6 Concentrated
MVC (Multivitamin Concentrate)
MVC 9+3 and MVC 9+3 VitaGard
Magnesium Sulfate Injection, USP, 10% & 50%
Manganese Sulfate Injection, USP
Maxifill Transfer Set
Methylprednisolone Sodium Succinate for Injection, USP, 40, 100, 125 & 500 mg
Molypen (Ammonium Molybdate Injection, USP)
NeoTrace-4
PTE-4
PedTrace-4
Pentam 300
Potassium Acetate Injection, USP
Potassium Chloride Injection, USP
Potassium Phosphates Injection, USP
Selepen (Selenious Acid Injection)
Sodium Acetate Injection, USP
Sodium Bicarbonate Additive Solution 4%

(◆ Shown in Product Identification Section)   (▣ Described in PDR For Nonprescription Drugs)

Manufacturers' Index

Sodium Bicarbonate Injection, USP, 7.5 & 8.4%
Sodium Chloride Injection, USP, 14.6 & 23.4%
Sodium Phosphates Injection, USP, 3mM/ml
TraceLyte & TraceLyte-II (Trace elements & electrolytes additive)
TraceLyte with Double Electrolytes & TraceLyte-II with Double Electrolytes
Transfer Needles, thin wall, 19 gauge

MACSIL, INC. 1181
1326 Frankford Avenue
Philadelphia, PA 19125 (215) 739-7300
Products Available
▣ Balmex Baby Powder
▣ Balmex Emollient Lotion
▣ Balmex Ointment

MALLARD INCORPORATED 1181
3021 Wabash Ave.
Detroit, MI 48216
Address inquiries to:
Sales Department (313) 964-3910

MARION LABORATORIES, INC. 417, 1181
Pharmaceutical Division
Marion Industrial Park
Marion Park Drive
Kansas City, MO 64137
Address inquiries to:
Product Surveillance Dept.
P.O. Box 9627
Kansas City, MO 64134 (816) 966-5000
Products Available
Ambenyl Cough Syrup
Ambenyl-D
♦ Carafate Tablets
♦ Cardizem 30-mg Tablets
♦ Cardizem 60-mg Tablets
Debrox Drops
Ditropan Syrup
♦ Ditropan Tablets
♦ Duotrate Plateau Caps
♦ Duotrate 45 Plateau Caps
Gaviscon Liquid
♦ Gaviscon Tablets
♦ Gaviscon-2 Tablets
Gly-Oxide Liquid
♦ Nico-400
Nitro-Bid IV
Nitro-Bid Ointment
♦ Nitro-Bid 2.5 Plateau Caps
♦ Nitro-Bid 6.5 Plateau Caps
♦ Nitro-Bid 9 Plateau Caps
♦ Os-Cal 250 Tablets
♦ Os-Cal 500 Tablets
♦ Os-Cal Forte Tablets
♦ Os-Cal Plus Tablets
♦ Os-Cal-Gesic Tablets
♦ Pavabid Capsules
♦ Pavabid HP Capsulets
Silvadene Cream
Throat Discs Throat Lozenges
♦ Thyroid Strong Tablets
♦ Thyroid Tablets

MARLYN COMPANY, INC. 1193
350 Pauma Place
Escondido, CA 92025
(714) 489-6115
Products Available
Albumin 500 Tablets
C Speridin Tablets, Sustained Release
Daily Nutritional Paks
..... Care-4
▣ ..... MARLYN PMS
..... Pro-Formance
Hep-Forte Capsules
Marbec Tablets
MARLYN Formula 50 Capsules
MARLYN Prolonged Release Vitamins
Balanced B 125
Clock E, 400 I.U.
Iron-L
Niacin, 400 mg.
Super One Daily
Super Citro Cee
Ultimate One
Vitamin B 12, 1000 mcg.
Vitamin C, 1000 mg.

MASON PHARMACEUTICALS, INC. 418, 1193
1201 Dove Street, Suite 520
Newport Beach, CA 92660 (714) 851-6860
Products Available
♦ Damacet-P
♦ Damason-P

MAYRAND, INC. 1196
P.O. Box 8869
4 Dundas Circle
Greensboro, NC 27419 (919) 292-5431
Products Available
Anamine Syrup
Anamine T.D. Caps
Anatuss Tablets & Syrup
Anatuss with Codeine Tablets & Syrup

Becomject-C
Benoject-10
Benoject-50
Buff-A Comp Caps
Buff-A Comp Tablets
Buff-A Comp No. 3 Tablets (with Codeine)
Corgonject-5
Cyanoject
Decaject
Decaject-L.A.
Depoject-40 & Depoject-80
Dramoject
Eldercaps
Eldertonic
Estroject
Estroject-LA
Flexoject
Glytuss Tabs
Histaject
Hydrotensin-50 Tablets
Hydro-Z-50 Tablets
Kenaject-40
Lidoject-1 & Lidoject-2
Lidoject-E-1 & Lidoject-E-2
Lifoject
Menoject-LA
Nu-Iron Elixir
Nu-Iron 150 Caps
Nu-Iron-Plus Elixir
Nu-Iron-V Tablets
Phenoject-50
Predaject-50
Progestaject-50
Sedapap-10 Tablets
Selestoject
Sorbide T.D. Caps
Spasmoject
Stera-Form Cream
Steramine Otic
Sterapred Uni-Pak
Sulfa-Gyn
Testoject-50
Testoject-100 L.A. & Testoject-200 L.A.
Tiject-20
Trimcaps
Trimtabs
Tristoject
Vistaject-25 & Vistaject-50

McGREGOR PHARMACEUTICALS 1197
32580 Grand River Avenue
Farmington, MI 48024
Address inquiries to:
Mr. Edward McGregor (313) 474-8727
Products Available
Rhindecon Capsules
Rhinolar Capsules
Rhinolar-EX Capsules
Rhinolar-EX 12 Capsules

McNEIL CONSUMER PRODUCTS CO. 418, 1197
McNEILAB, INC.
Fort Washington, PA 19034
Address inquiries to:
Professional Relations Department
Fort Washington, PA 19034
Manufacturing Divisions
Fort Washington, PA 19034
Southwest Manufacturing Plant
4001 N. I-35
Round Rock, TX 78664
Distribution Centers
Order Services
Fort Washington, PA 19034
Camp Hill Road
Local Area (215) 233-7000
Pennsylvania (800) 822-3978
Out of State (800) 523-3484
Arlington, TX 76010
3129 Pinewood Drive (817) 640-1167
Glendale, CA 91201
512 Paula Avenue (213) 245-1491
Montgomeryville, PA 18936
1390 Welsh Road (215) 641-1420
Products Available
♦ Children's CoTylenol Liquid Cold Formula
♦ Children's Tylenol acetaminophen Chewable Tablets, Elixir & Drops
♦ CoTylenol Cold Medication Tablets & Capsules
CoTylenol Liquid Cold Medication
Extra-Strength Sine-Aid Sinus Headache Capsules
♦ Extra-Strength Tylenol acetaminophen Capsules, Caplets, Tablets & Liquid
♦ Infants' Tylenol Drops
♦ Junior-Strength Tylenol
♦ Maximum-Strength Tylenol Sinus Medication Tablets & Capsules
♦ Regular Strength Tylenol acetaminophen Tablets & Capsules
Sine-Aid Sinus Headache Tablets

McNEIL PHARMACEUTICAL 418, 1201
McNEILAB, INC.
Spring House, PA 19477

Address inquiries to:
Professional Services Department
Spring House, PA 19477
(215) 628-5000
Manufacturing Affiliate
Dorado, Puerto Rico 00646
P.O. Box P
Fort Washington, PA 19034
Distribution Divisions
Burr Ridge, IL 60521
261 Shore Drive (312) 655-0366
Glendale, CA 91201
512 Paula Avenue (213) 245-0217
Montgomeryville PA 18936
Park Drive (215) 641-0250
Products Available
Butibel-Zyme Tablets
Carbinoxamine Maleate, see Clistin
Chlorzoxazone, see Paraflex
Clistin Tablets
Clistin-D Tablets
♦ Haldol Injection, Tablets & Concentrate
Haloperidol, see Haldol
Orap Tablets
♦ Pancrease
Paraflex Tablets
♦ Parafon Forte Tablets
Theophyl Chewable Tablets
Theophyl-SR
Theophyl-225 Elixir
Theophyl-225 Tablets
♦ Tolectin Tablets & DS Capsules
Tolmetin Sodium, see Tolectin Tablets
♦ Tylenol w/Codeine Capsules, Tablets & Elixir
♦ Tylox Capsules

MEAD JOHNSON LABORATORIES 419, 1216
Mead Johnson & Company
2404 West Pennsylvania St.
Evansville, IN 47721
(812) 426-6000
Address inquiries to:
Scientific Information Section
Medical Department
Products Available
♦ Estrace
♦ Estrace Vaginal Cream
♦ K-Lyte & K-Lyte DS
♦ K-Lyte/Cl & K-Lyte/Cl 50
♦ Natalins
♦ Natalins Rx
♦ Ovcon-35
♦ Ovcon-50
Questran
♦ Quibron & Quibron-300
♦ Quibron Plus
♦ Quibron-T & Quibron-T/SR

MEAD JOHNSON NUTRITIONAL DIVISION 1243
Mead Johnson & Company
2404 W. Pennsylvania St.
Evansville, IN 47721 (812) 426-6000
Address inquiries to:
Scientific Information Section
Medical Department
Products Available
▣ Casec
▣ Ce-Vi-Sol
▣ Criticare HN
▣ Enfamil
▣ Enfamil Nursette
▣ Enfamil Ready-To-Use
▣ Enfamil w/Iron
▣ Enfamil w/Iron Ready-To-Use
▣ Fer-In-Sol
▣ Isocal
Isocal HCN
▣ Lofenalac
▣ Lonalac
▣ Lytren
▣ MCT Oil
▣ Moducal
Naturacil
▣ Nutramigen
Poly-Vi-Flor 0.5 mg Vitamins w/Fluoride Chewable Tablets
Poly-Vi-Flor 1.0 mg Vitamins w/Fluoride Chewable Tablets
Poly-Vi-Flor 0.25 mg Vitamins w/Fluoride Drops
Poly-Vi-Flor 0.5 mg Vitamins w/Fluoride Drops
Poly-Vi-Flor 0.5 mg Vitamins w/Iron & Fluoride Chewable Tablets & Drops
Poly-Vi-Flor 1.0 Vitamins w/Iron & Fluoride Chewable Tablets
Poly-Vi-Flor 0.25 mg Vitamins w/Iron & Fluoride Drops
▣ Poly-Vi-Sol Vitamins Chewable Tablets & Drops
▣ Poly-Vi-Sol Vitamins with Iron & Zinc
▣ Poly-Vi-Sol Vitamins w/Iron Multivitamin & Iron Supplement Drops
▣ Portagen
▣ Pregestimil
▣ ProSobee

(♦ Shown in Product Identification Section) (▣ Described in PDR For Nonprescription Drugs)

Manufacturers' Index

⊞Sustacal
⊞Sustacal HC
⊞Sustagen
⊞Tempra
⊞Traumacal
⊞Trind
⊞Trind-DM
Tri-Vi-Flor 1.0 mg Vitamins w/Fluoride Chewable Tablets
Tri-Vi-Flor 0.25 mg Vitamins w/Fluoride Drops
Tri-Vi-Flor 0.5 mg Vitamins w/Fluoride Drops
Tri-Vi-Flor 0.25 mg Vitamins w/Iron & Fluoride Drops
⊞Tri-Vi-Sol Vitamins, Chewable Tablets & Drops
⊞Tri-Vi-Sol Vitamins w/Iron, Drops

MEAD JOHNSON 419, 1248
PHARMACEUTICAL DIVISION
Mead Johnson & Company
2404 W. Pennsylvania St.
Evansville, IN 47721 (812) 426-6000
Address inquiries to:
Scientific Information Section
Medical Department
Products Available
◆ Colace
◆ Deapril-ST
◆ Desyrel
◆ Duricef
◆ Klotrix
  Mucomyst
◆ Peri-Colace
◆ Vasodilan

MEDICAL PRODUCTS 1256
PANAMERICANA, INC.
Post Office Box 771
Coral Gables, FL 33134
Address inquiries to:
Professional Services Dept. (305) 545-6524
Branch and Distribution Division
San Juan, PR (809) 783-6736
Products Available
Aminobrain Capsules
Aminobrain Injection
Aminobrain Plus Capsules
Aminobrain Tablets
Atoximetin-B Capsules
Broncopectol Syrup
Digesplen Elixir
Digesplen-Plus Tablets
Ferlivit Capsules
Ferlivit Injection
Ferlivit Syrup
Medispray
Neurodep Injection Lyophilized
Novaflor Capsules
Rubroben-1000 Injection Lyophilized
Rutiplen-C
Tempotest 225
Trilycal-12
VG Capsules
Varidin Capsules

MEDICONE COMPANY 419, 1256
225 Varick St.
New York, NY 10014
Address inquiries to:
Professional Service Dept. (212) 924-5166
Products Available
⊞Derma Medicone Ointment
  Derma Medicone-HC
⊞Medicone Dressing Cream
⊞Mediconet
◆ Rectal Medicone Suppositories
⊞Rectal Medicone Unguent
◆ Rectal Medicone-HC Suppositories

MERCK SHARP & DOHME 420, 1256
Division of Merck & Co., Inc.
West Point, PA 19486 (215) 661-5000
For Medical or Drug Information
Write: Professional Information
Business hours only (8:30 a.m. to 4:45 p.m. EST), call (215) 661-7300
For Medical Emergency Information after hours or on weekends, call
  (215) 661-5000
Address other inquiries to:
Professional Service Department
West Point, PA 19486
Branch Offices
Arlington, TX 76011
  Great Southwest Industrial District
  925-111th Street (817) 261-7527
Atlanta Area:
  See Norcross, GA
Baltimore Area:
  see Columbia, MD
Boston Area:
  see Needham Heights, MA
Chicago Area:
  see Oak Brook, IL
Columbia, MD 21045
  9199 Red Branch Rd. (301) 730-8240
Columbus, OH 43228
  4242 Janitrol Road (614) 276-5308

Dallas/Ft. Worth Area:
  see Arlington, TX
Denver, CO 80216
  4900 Jackson Street (303) 355-1601
Kansas City Area:
  see Overland Park, KS
Kenner, LA 70062
  1431 E. Airline Highway (504) 464-0111
King of Prussia, PA 19406
  1045 First Avenue (215) 962-6900
Los Angeles, CA 90040
  6409 E. Gayhart Street (213) 723-9661
Memphis, TN 38106
  1980 Latham Street (901) 948-8501
Minneapolis, MN 55441
  12955 State Highway 55
    (612) 559-4445
Needham Heights, MA 02194
  40 A Street (617) 444-5510
New Orleans Area:
  see Kenner, LA
New York Area:
  see Teterboro, NJ
Oak Brook, IL 60521
  2010 Swift Drive (312) 920-2160
Norcross, GA 30071
  2825 Northwoods Parkway
    (404) 662-7200
Overland Park, KS 66215
  9001 Quivira Rd. (913) 888-1110
Philadelphia Area:
  see King of Prussia, PA
Portland, OR 97211
  717 N.E. Lombard St. (503) 285-2582
S. San Francisco, CA 94080
  340 Shaw Road (415) 583-4330
Teterboro, NJ 07608
  111 Central Avenue (201) 288-7710
Products Available
◆ Aldoclor Tablets
  Aldomet Ester HCl Injection
  Aldomet Oral Suspension
◆ Aldomet Tablets
◆ Aldoril Tablets
  alphaRedisol Injection
  Aminohippurate Sodium Injection
  Antivenin (Black Widow Spider)
  AquaMEPHYTON Injection
  Aramine Injection
  Attenuvax
◆ Benemid Tablets
  Biavax ₁₁
◆ Blocadren Tablets
◆ Clinoril Tablets
  Cogentin Tablets & Injection
◆ ColBENEMID Tablets
  Cortone Acetate Saline Suspension
  Cortone Acetate Tablets
  Cosmegen Injection
◆ Cuprimine Capsules
  Cyclaine Topical Solution
  Daranide Tablets
  Decaderm
  Decadron Elixir
  Decadron Phosphate Injection
  Decadron Phosphate Respihaler
  Decadron Phosphate Sterile Ophthalmic Ointment
  Decadron Phosphate Sterile Ophthalmic Solution
  Decadron Phosphate Topical Cream
  Decadron Phosphate Turbinaire
  Decadron Phosphate w/Xylocaine Injection
◆ Decadron Tablets
  Decadron-LA Suspension
  Decaspray Topical Aerosol
◆ Demser Capsules
  Diupres Tablets
  Diuril Intravenous Sodium
  Diuril Oral Suspension
◆ Diuril Tablets
◆ Dolobid Tablets
  Edecrin Sodium Intravenous
◆ Edecrin Tablets
  Elavil Injection
◆ Elavil Tablets
  Elspar
◆ Flexeril Tablets
  Floropryl Sterile Ophthalmic Ointment
  Hep-B-Gammagee
  Heptavax-B
  Humorsol Sterile Ophthalmic Solution
  Hydeltrasol Injection
  Hydeltra-T.B.A. Suspension
  Hydrocortone Acetate Saline Suspension
  Hydrocortone Acetate Sterile Ophthalmic Ointment and Ophthalmic Suspension
  Hydrocortone Phosphate Injection
  Hydrocortone Tablets
◆ HydroDIURIL Tablets
  Hydropres Tablets
◆ Indocin Capsules
◆ Indocin SR Capsules
◆ Indocin Suppositories
  Inversine Tablets
  Lacrisert Sterile Ophthalmic Insert
  M-M-R
  M-R-VAX ₁₁

Mefoxin
Mephyton Tablets
Meruvax ₁₁
◆ Midamor Tablets
◆ Mintezol Chewable Tablets
  Mintezol Suspension
◆ Moduretic Tablets
  Mumpsvax
  Mustargen
  Myochrysine Injection
  Neodecadron Sterile Ophthalmic Ointment
  Neodecadron Sterile Ophthalmic Solution
  Neodecadron Topical Cream
  Periactin Syrup
◆ Periactin Tablets
  Pneumovax 23
  Propadrine Capsules
  Redisol Injection
  Redisol Tablets
  Respihaler (see Decadron Phosphate Respihaler)
◆ Sinemet Tablets
◆ Timolide Tablets
  Timoptic Sterile Ophthalmic Solution
◆ Tonocard
◆ Triavil Tablets
  Turbinaire (see Decadron Phosphate Turbinaire)
  Urecholine Injection
◆ Urecholine Tablets
◆ Vivactil Tablets

MERICON INDUSTRIES, INC. 1358
8819 N. Pioneer Road
Peoria, IL 61615
Address inquiries to:
Thomas P. Morrissey (309) 693-2150
Products Available
⊞Orazinc Capsules
⊞Orazinc Lozenges

MERIEUX INSTITUTE, INC. 1358, 3013
P.O. Box 52-3980
Miami, FL 33152
Address inquiries to:
P.O. Box 52-3980
Miami, FL 33152 (305) 593-9577
For Medical Emergencies Contact:
Merieux Institute, Inc. (800) 327-2842
Alaska, FL, & HI, call Collect
  (305) 593-9577
Products Available
Imogam Rabies Immune Globulin (Human)
Imovax Rabies Vaccine
Mono-Vacc Test (O.T.)
Multitest CMI Skin Test Antigens for Cellular Hypersensitivity
Rabies Immune Globulin (Human), Imogam Rabies
Rabies Vaccine Human Diploid Cell, Imovax Rabies
Skin Test Antigens for Cellular Hypersensitivity, Multitest CMI
Tuberculin, Mono-Vacc Test (O.T.)

MERRELL DOW 421, 1358
PHARMACEUTICALS INC.
Subsidiary of The Dow Chemical Company
Cincinnati, OH 45242-9553
Address inquiries to:
Professional Relations Manager
  (513) 948-9111
Products Available
AVC Suppositories
AVC Vaginal Cream
AVC/Dienestrol Cream
AVC/Dienestrol Suppositories
Accurbron
◆ Bentyl 10 mg Capsules
  Bentyl Injection
  Bentyl Syrup
◆ Bentyl 20 mg Tablets
◆ Bricanyl Injection
◆ Bricanyl Tablets
◆ Cantil Tablets
⊞Cēpacol Anesthetic Lozenges (Troches)
⊞Cēpacol Mouthwash/Gargle
⊞Cēpacol Throat Lozenges
⊞CĒPASTAT Sore Throat Lozenges
⊞CĒPASTAT Sore Throat Lozenges, Cherry Flavor
◆ Cephulac Syrup
  Chloramphenicol Injection
◆ Chronulac Syrup
  Clomid Tablets
  DV Cream
  Delcid
  Dow-Isoniazid
  Hesper Bitabs
  Hesper Capsules
◆ Hiprex Tablets
  Imferon
⊞Kolantyl Gel
⊞Kolantyl Wafers
◆ Lorelco
◆ Metahydrin
◆ Metatensin
  Neo-Polycin Topical Antibiotic
◆ Nicorette

(◆ Shown in Product Identification Section) (⊞ Described in PDR For Nonprescription Drugs)

Manufacturers' Index

- ◆ Norpramin
- ◆ Novafed A Capsules
- Novafed A Liquid
- ◆ Novafed Capsules
- Novafed Liquid
- ▩ Novahistine Cough Formula
- ▩ Novahistine Cough & Cold Formula
- ◆ Novahistine DH
- ▩ Novahistine DMX
- ◆ Novahistine Elixir
- ◆ Novahistine Expectorant
- Orenzyme
- Orenzyme Bitabs
- Quide Tablets
- ◆ Quinamm Tablets
- ◆ Rifadin
- ◆ Rifamate
- ▩ Simron Capsules
- ▩ Simron Plus Capsules
- ◆ Singlet
- 2/G
- 2/G-DM
- ◆ TACE 12 mg Capsules
- ◆ TACE 25 mg Capsules
- ◆ TACE 72 mg Capsules
- ◆ Tenuate Dospan Tablets
- ◆ Tenuate Tablets
- Terpin Hydrate & Codeine Elixir
- ◆ Tussend Expectorant
- ◆ Tussend Liquid & Tablets

MILES LABORATORIES, INC. 1395
P.O. Box 340
Elkhart, IN 46515
Address inquiries to:
Medical Dept.   (219) 262-7886
Consumer Health Care Division only
Products Available
- Alka-Mints Chewable Antacid
- Alka-Seltzer Effervescent Antacid
- Alka-Seltzer Effervescent Pain Reliever and Antacid
- Alka-Seltzer Plus Cold Medicine
- ▩ Bactine Antiseptic-Anesthetic First Aid Spray
- ▩ Bactine Hydrocortisone Skin Care Cream
- Biocal Calcium Supplement Chewable Tablets
- Biocal Calcium Supplement Tablets
- ▩ Bugs Bunny Multivitamin Supplement
- ▩ Bugs Bunny Plus Iron Multivitamin Supplement
- ▩ Bugs Bunny Vitamins Plus Minerals (Sugar Free)
- ▩ Bugs Bunny With Extra C
- ▩ Flintstones Complete Multivitamin/Mineral Supplement
- ▩ Flintstones Multivitamin Supplement
- ▩ Flintstones Plus Iron Multivitamin Supplement
- ▩ Flintstones With Extra C
- Miles Nervine Nighttime Sleep-Aid
- One-A-Day Essential Multivitamin Supplement
- ▩ One-A-Day Maximum Formula (Multivitamin/Multimineral)
- ▩ One-A-Day Plus Extra C
- ▩ One-A-Day Stressgard Vitamins
- ▩ One-A-Day Within (Multivitamins Plus Iron & Calcium)

MILES PHARMACEUTICALS 421, 1396
Division of Miles Laboratories, Inc.
400 Morgan Lane
West Haven, CT 06516
Address Inquiries to:
Director, Medical Services   (203) 934-9221
Products Available
- Acne-Dome Lotion
- Acne-Dome Medicated Cleanser
- Azlin
- ◆ Biltricide
- Cort-Dome ⅛%, ¼%, ½%, and 1% Creme
- Cort-Dome ⅛%, ¼%, ½%, and 1% Lotion
- Cort-Dome High Potency Suppositories
- Cort-Dome Regular Potency Suppositories
- DTIC-Dome
- ◆ Decholin Tablets
- ◆ Domeboro Powder Packets, Effervescent Tablets
- Dome-Paste Bandage (Unna's Boot)
- Domol Bath & Shower Oil
- Lidaform-HC Creme
- ◆ Lithane Tablets
- Mezlin
- Mithracin
- ◆ Mycelex 1% Cream
- ◆ Mycelex 1% Solution
- ◆ Mycelex Troches
- Mycelex-G Vaginal Tablets
- Mycelex-G 1% Vaginal Cream
- Neo Cort-Dome Creme
- ◆ Niclocide Chewable Tablets
- Nystaform Ointment
- Otic Domeboro Solution
- Otic Tridesilon Solution 0.05%
- ◆ Stilphostrol Tablets and Ampuls
- Tridesilon Creme 0.05%
- Tridesilon Ointment 0.05%

MILEX PRODUCTS, INC. 1415
5915 Northwest Highway
Chicago, IL 60631   (312) 631-6484
Shipping Offices
Milex Western
  Post Office Box 46030
  Los Angeles, CA 90046   (213) 651-4301
Milex Central
  1873 Grove Street
  Glenview, IL 60025   (312) 729-5253
Milex Michigan
  Post Office Box 20264
  Ferndale, MI 48220   (313) 399-9223
Milex Puerto Rico
  GPO Box 554
  San Juan, PR 00936   (809) 791-3309
Milex Hawaii
  Box 6337
  Honolulu, HI 96818   (808) 422-9581
Milex Southeastern
  Post Office Drawer 4647
  Clearwater, FL 33518   (813) 461-1949
Milex Southern
  Post Office Drawer "M"
  Weatherford, TX 76086   (817) 594-6865
Milex Carolinas
  Post Office Box 23060
  Charlotte, NC 28212   (704) 545-4567
Milex Delaware Valley
  350 White Horse Pike
  Atco, NJ 08004   (609) 767-4818
Milex Delta
  Post Office Drawer 5684
  Shreveport, LA 71105   (318) 797-1554
Products Available
- Amino-Cerv
- Basal Thermometers
- Breast Self-Examination Kit
- Cannula Curette with Swivel Handle
- Dilateria
- Endometrial Suction Curettes
- Fertility Cannula
- Fertilo-Pak
- Laminaria Japonica
- Oligospermia Cups
- Pessaries
- Pro-Ception
- Seminal Pouches
- Shur-Seal Gel
- Spatula
- Tis-U-Trap
- Trimo-San
- Wide-Seal Diaphragm

MISSION PHARMACAL COMPANY 1415
1325 E. Durango
San Antonio, TX 78210
Address inquiries to:
Professional Service Dept.   (512) 533-7118
Post Office Box 1676
San Antonio, TX 78296
Products Available
- Calcet
- Calcet Plus
- Calcibind
- Compete
- Ferralet
- Fosfree
- Iromin-G
- Lithostat
- Mission Prenatal
- Mission Prenatal F.A.
- Mission Prenatal H.P.
- Mission Prenatal RX
- Mission Pre-Surgical
- Prulet
- Supac
- Therabid
- Thera-Gesic

MURO PHARMACEUTICAL, INC. 1420
890 East Street
Tewksbury, MA 01876-9987
Address inquiries to:
Professional Service Dept.
   1-(800) 225-0974
   (617) 851-5981
Products Available
- Bromfed Capsules (Timed Release)
- Bromfed-PD Capsules (Timed Release)
- Bromfed Tablets
- Duolube Ophthalmic Ointment
- Guaifed Capsules (Timed Release)
- Liquid Pred Syrup
- Muro 128 Ophthalmic Ointment
- Muro 128 Ophthalmic Solution
- Muro Tears Ophthalmic Solution
- Murocel - Ophthalmic Solution
- Murocoll-2 Ophthalmic Solution
- Muro's Opcon Ophthalmic Solution
- Muro's Opcon-A Ophthalmic Solution
- ▩ Salinex Nasal Mist and Drops
- Sulphrin Ophthalmic Suspension
- Sulten-10 Ophthalmic Solution

NATIONAL DERMACEUTICAL PRODUCTS, INC. 1421
8749 Surrey Place
Maineville, OH 45039

Address inquiries to:
Professional Service Dept.
   (513) 683-8855
Products Available
- Stimuzyme Plus
- Stimuzyme Topical Dressing

NEUTROGENA DERMATOLOGICS 1421
Division of Neutrogena Corp.
5755 West 96th Street
P.O. Box 45036
Los Angeles, CA 90045   (800) 421-6857
   In CA (213) 642-1150
Products Available
- Liquid Neutrogena
- Melanex 3% Topical Solution (Neutrogena)
- Neutrogena Acne Cleansing Formula Soap
- Neutrogena Acne-Drying Gel
- Neutrogena Acne Mask
- Neutrogena Baby Soap
- Neutrogena Body Lotion
- Neutrogena Dry Skin Formula Soap
- Neutrogena Moisture
- Neutrogena Norwegian Formula Hand Cream
- Neutrogena Original Formula Soap
- Neutrogena Rainbath Shower and Bath Gel
- Neutrogena Sesame Seed Body Oil
- Neutrogena Shampoo
- Neutrogena Solid Soap Shampoo
- Neutrogena T/Gel Therapeutic Shampoo
- T/Derm Tar Emollient
- T/Gel Scalp Solution (Neutrogena)
- Vehicle/N (Neutrogena)
- Vehicle/N Mild (Neutrogena)

NORCLIFF THAYER INC. 422, 1422
303 South Broadway
Tarrytown, NY 10591   (914) 631-0033
Products Available
- ◆ A-200 Pyrinate Pediculicide Shampoo, Liquid & Gel
- ▩ Esoterica Medicated Fade Cream
- ▩ Liquiprin Acetaminophen
- ▩ Nature's Remedy Laxative
- ▩ NoSalt Salt Alternative, Regular and Seasoned
- ▩ Oxy Clean Lathering Facial Scrub
- ▩ Oxy Clean Medicated Cleanser, Pads & Soap
- ▩ Oxy-5 Lotion with Sorboxyl
- ▩ Oxy-10 Lotion and Cover with Sorboxyl
- ▩ Oxy-10 Wash Antibacterial Skin Wash
- ▩ Tums Antacid Tablets, Regular & Extra Strength

NORDISK-USA 1422
6500 Rock Spring Drive
Suite 304
Bethesda, MD 20817
Address inquiries to:
Medical Director   (301) 897-9220
Products Available
- Insulatard NPH
- Mixtard
- Velosulin

NORGINE LABORATORIES, INC. 1424
2 Overhill Road
Scarsdale, NY 10583   (914) 472-3883
Products Available
- Bilamide Tablets
- Enzypan Tablets
- Movicol Granules
- Muripsin Tablets

NORWICH EATON 422, 1424
PHARMACEUTICALS, INC.
A Procter & Gamble Company
(formerly Eaton Laboratories,
Professional Products Group,
Norwich Products, or
Consumer Products Group)
13-27 Eaton Avenue
Norwich, NY 13815
Also see Procter & Gamble
Address medical inquiries to:
Medical Department
Norwich Eaton Pharmaceuticals, Inc.
Norwich, NY 13815   (607) 335-2565
Refer orders & other inquiries to:
Norwich Eaton Pharmaceuticals, Inc.
17 Eaton Avenue
Norwich, NY 13815-9989   (800) 448-4878
New York State customers only,
   (607) 335-2121
Products Available
- Alphaderm Cream
- ◆ Comhist LA Capsules
- Comhist Tablets
- Dantrium Capsules
- Dantrium Intravenous
- ◆ Didronel
- Dopar Capsules
- Duvoid Tablets
- Entex Capsules
- ◆ Entex LA Tablets
- Entex Liquid
- Furacin Preparations
  Furacin Soluble Dressing
  Furacin Topical Cream

(◆ Shown in Product Identification Section)   (▩ Described in PDR For Nonprescription Drugs)

Manufacturers' Index

Furadantin Oral Suspension
Furadantin Tablets
Furoxone Liquid Suspension
Furoxone Tablets
LABID 250 mg Tablets
◆ Macrodantin Capsules
Topicycline
Vivonex
   Standard Vivonex Diet
   High Nitrogen Vivonex Diet
   Vivonex T.E.N.
   Flavor Packets
   Devices
      Vivonex Acutrol Enteral Feeding System
      Vivonex Delivery System
      Vivonex Jejunostomy Kit
      Vivonex Moss Tube

NTRON INTERNATIONAL SALES CO.   **1443**
3833 Redwood Highway
P.O. Box 7000
San Rafael, CA 94912
Address inquiries to:
Customer Services   (415) 472-4600
For Medical Emergencies Contact:
Ken Levin, Biomedical Engineer
  (415) 472-4600
Products Available
NTRON TTS-2500 Transcutaneous Electrical Nerve Stimulator (TENS)

O'NEAL, JONES & FELDMAN   **422, 1443**
PHARMACEUTICALS
2510 Metro Blvd.
Maryland Heights, MO 63043
  (314) 569-3610
Products Available
A.C.T.H. "40" Injectable
A.C.T.H. "80" Injectable
Almora Tablets
Amonidrin Tablets
Anaids Tablets
Andro L.A. "200" Injectable
Andro "100" Injectable
Androgyn L.A. Injectable
Anergan "25" & "50" Injectable
Antilirium Injectable
Arbon Plus Injectable
Arbon Plus Tablets
Arbon Tablets
B-12 Plus Injectable
▣ Banalg Hospital Strength Arthritic Pain Reliever
▣ Banalg Liniment
Bancap Capsules
Bancap c̄ Codeine Capsules
◆ Bancap HC Capsules
Banesin Tablets
Banflex Injectable
Beesix Injectable
Belfer Tablets
Betaprone Liquid
Biamine Injectable
Calscorbate Tablets
Canz Tablets
Caquin Cream
Cebocap
Cetane Injection (w/o preservative)
Cetane Timed Capsules
Choron "10" Injectable Pak
Codroxomin Injectable
Conex DA Tablet
Conex Liquid
Conex Lozenges
Conex Plus Tablets
Conex c̄ Codeine Liquid
Cyomin Injectable
Dalalone Injectable
Dalalone D.P. Injectable
Dalalone L.A. Injectable
Dalcaine Injection
Dehist Capsules
Dehist Injectable
depAndro "100" & "200" Injectable
depAndrogyn Injectable
depGynogen Injectable
depMedalone "40" Injectable
depMedalone "80" Injectable
Diabismul Suspension
Diabismul Tablets
Disotate Injectable
Dommanate Injectable
Duradyne DHC Tablets
Duradyne Tablets
Dureze Drops
Eferol Ointment
Eferol Succinate Capsules
Enzymet Tablet
Feostat Drops
Feostat Injectable
Feostat Suspension
Feostat Tablets
G.B.S. Tablets
Gesterol "50" Injectable
Gesterol L.A. "250" Injectable
Glycate Tablets
Gynogen Injectable
Gynogen L.A. "10", "20" & "40" Injectable

Heparin Sodium w/o preservative Injectable
Hista-Derfule Capsules
Iodo-Niacin Tablets
KBP/O Capsules
Lidocaine 1% & 2% Injectable
Livroben Injectable
Magnesium Sulfate Injectable
Metra Tablets
N.B.P. Ointment
Nandrobolic Injectable
Nandrobolic L.A. Injectable
Neoquess Injectable
Neoquess Tablets
Niac Capsules
Obermine Capsules
Oxymycin Injectable
Panol Injectable
Panvitex Prenatal Tablets
Paral Injectable
Paral Liquid
◆ Pedameth Capsules
Pedameth Liquid
Petameth Capsules
Predalone 50 Injectable
Predalone T.B.A. Injectable
Proklar Tablets
Queltuss Tablets
Quiess Injectable
Rauverid Tablets
Rogenic Injectable
Rogenic Tablets
Solu-Eze Solvent
soluPredalone Injectable
Soniphen Tablets
Sulfaloid "500" Tablets
Sulfaloid Suspension
Tetracycline HCl Capsules
Tralmag Suspension
Triamolone "40" Injectable
Triamonide "40" Injectable
Urithol Tablets
Verazinc Capsules
Wolfina "50" & "100" Tablets

ORGANON PHARMACEUTICALS   **422, 1446**
375 Mount Pleasant Ave.
West Orange, NJ 07052   (201) 325-4500
Products Available
Accelerase
Bilogen
Cortrophin-Zinc
Cortrosyn
◆ Cotazym
Cotazym-B
◆ Cotazym-S
Deca-Durabolin
Doca Acetate
Durabolin
Heparin Sodium (from Beef Lung Sources)
Hexadrol Elixir
◆ Hexadrol Tablets
Hexadrol Phosphate Injection
Hexadrol Strip Packs
◆ Hexadrol Therapeutic Pack
Hydrocortisone USP
Liquaemin Sodium
◆ Liquamar Tablets
Maxibolin
Methylprednisolone Sodium Succinate
Norcuron (NC-45)
Pavulon
Pregnyl
Regonol
Succinylcholine
◆ Wigraine Tablets & Suppositories
◆ Wigraine-PB Suppositories
◆ Wigrettes

ORTHO DIAGNOSTIC SYSTEMS INC.   **1452**
Route 202
Raritan, NJ 08869
Address inquiries to:
Customer Service Div.   (201) 524-1732
  (201) 524-2374
Products Available
Fetaldex Quantitative Test for Fetal Red Blood Cells in the Maternal Blood Circulation
Fetalscreen Qualitative Screening Test for D(Rh$_o$) Positive Fetal Red Blood Cells in the Maternal Circulation
MICRhoGAM Rh$_o$(D) Immune Globulin (Human), Micro-Dose
RhoGAM Rh$_o$(D) Immune Globulin (Human)

ORTHO PHARMACEUTICAL   **422, 1453**
CORPORATION
Raritan, NJ 08869
For Medical Information Call:
  (201) 524-8895
  (201) 524-0504
For Product Information Call:
  (201) 524-2343
Products Available
Aci-Jel Therapeutic Vaginal Jelly
▣ Conceptrol Birth Control Cream
▣ Conceptrol Contraceptive Gel Disposable
▣ Delfen Contraceptive Foam
▣ Gynol II Contraceptive Jelly

Lippes Loop Intrauterine Double-S
▣ ◆ Massé Breast Cream
◆ Micronor Tablets
◆ Modicon 21 Tablets
Modicon 28 Tablets
Monistat 3 Vaginal Suppositories
◆ Monistat 7 Vaginal Cream
◆ Monistat 7 Vaginal Suppositories
Ortho Diaphragm Kit-All Flex
Ortho Diaphragm Kit-Coil Spring
Ortho Dienestrol Cream
▣ Ortho Disposable Applicator
▣ Ortho Personal Lubricant
▣ Ortho-Creme Contraceptive Cream
▣ Ortho-Gynol Contraceptive Jelly
◆ Ortho-Novum 1/35 ☐ 21
Ortho-Novum 1/35 ☐ 28
◆ Ortho-Novum 1/50 ☐ 21
Ortho-Novum 1/50 ☐ 28
◆ Ortho-Novum 1/80 ☐ 21
Ortho-Novum 1/80 ☐ 28
◆ Ortho-Novum 7/7/7 ☐.. 21 Tablets
Ortho-Novum 7/7/7 ☐.. 28 Tablets
◆ Ortho-Novum 10/11 ☐.. 21 Tablets
Ortho-Novum 10/11 ☐.. 28 Tablets
◆ Ortho-Novum Tablets 2 mg ☐ 21
Ortho-White Diaphragm Kit-Flat Spring
◆ Protostat Tablets
Sultrin Triple Sulfa Cream
Sultrin Triple Sulfa Vaginal Tablets

ORTHO PHARMACEUTICAL   **1472**
CORPORATION,
Dermatological Division
Route 202
Raritan, NJ 08869   (201) 524-0400
Products Available
Cloderm (clocortolone pivalate) Cream
Grifulvin V (griseofulvin microsize)
Meclan (meclocycline sulfosalicylate) Cream
Monistat-Derm (miconazole nitrate) Cream & Lotion
Persa-Gel (benzoyl peroxide)
Persa-Gel W (benzoyl peroxide)
▣ Purpose Dry Skin Cream
▣ Purpose Shampoo
▣ Purpose Soap
Retin-A (tretinoin)
Spectazole (econazole nitrate) Cream

PALISADES PHARMACEUTICALS, INC.   **1476**
219 County Road
Tenafly, NJ 07670
Address inquiries to:
Vice President   (201) 569-8502
For Medical Emergencies Contact:
Vice President   (201) 569-8502
Products Available
Yocon

PARKE-DAVIS   **423, 1477, 3014**
Division of Warner-Lambert Company
201 Tabor Road
Morris Plains, NJ 07950   (201) 540-2000
For Product Information call:
  1-(800) 223-0432
For Medical Information call:
  (201) 540-3950
Regional Sales Offices
Atlanta, GA 30328
  1140 Hammond Drive   (404) 396-4080
Baltimore (Hunt Valley), MD 21031
  11350 McCormick Road (301) 666-7810
Chicago (Schaumburg), IL 60195
  1111 Plaza Drive   (312) 884-6990
Dallas, TX 75234
  12200 Ford Road   (214) 484-5566
Detroit (Troy), MI 48084
  500 Stephenson Highway (313) 589-3292
Los Angeles (Tustin), CA 92680
  17822 East 17th Street (714) 731-3441
Memphis, TN 38119
  1355 Lynnfield Road   (901) 767-1921
New York (East Hartford, CT) 06108
  111 Founders Plaza   (203) 528-9601
Pittsburgh, PA 15220
  Manor Oak Two
  1910 Cochran Road   (412) 343-9855
Seattle (Bellevue), WA 98004
  301-116th Ave, Southeast
    (206) 451-1119
Products Available
ACTH Steri-Vial
Abdec Baby Vitamin Drops
Abdec with Fluoride Baby Vitamin Drops
Acetaminophen (Tapar)
Acetaminophen with Codeine Phosphate Tablets, No. 2
Acetaminophen with Codeine Phosphate Tablets, No. 3
Acetaminophen with Codeine Phosphate Tablets, No. 4
Adrenalin Chloride Solution 1:100 & 1:1,000
Agoral, Liquid Plain
Agoral, Marshmallow Flavor
Agoral, Raspberry Flavor
Alcohol, Rubbing (Lavacol)
Alophen Pills

(◆ Shown in Product Identification Section)   (▣ Described in PDR For Nonprescription Drugs)

Manufacturers' Index

- ◆ Amcill Capsules
- Amcill for Oral Suspension
- Amcill Pediatric Drops
- ◆ Amitriptyline Hydrochloride Tablets (Amitril)
- Amoxicillin for Oral Suspension
- ◆ Amoxicillin (Utimox) Capsules
- Antibiotics
- ◆ Amcill Products
- ◆ Amoxicillin Products
- ◆ Chloromycetin Products
- Coly-Mycin Products
- ◆ Erythromycin Stearate Tablets (Erypar)
- Humatin
- Penicillin Products
- Penicillin V Potassium Products (Penapar VK)
- ◆ Tetracycline Hydrochloride Capsules, (Cyclopar) (Cyclopar 500)
- Anusol Ointment
- ◆ Anusol Suppositories
- ◆ Anusol-HC Cream
- ◆ Anusol-HC Suppositories
- Aplisol (tuberculin PPD, diluted)
- Aplitest (tuberculin PPD, multiple-puncture device)
- Aspirin Tablets
- Aspirin with Codeine Phosphate Tablets, No. 2, No. 3 & No. 4
- ◆ Benadryl Capsules
- Benadryl Cream
- Benadryl Elixir
- ◆ Benadryl Kapseals
- Benadryl Steri-Vials, Ampoules, and Steri-Dose Syringe
- Benylin Cough Syrup
- ▣ Benylin DM Cough Syrup
- Brondecon Elixir
- ◆ Brondecon Tablets
- Caladryl Cream, Lotion
- Calcium Gluconate Injection
- Calcium Lactate Tablets
- ◆ Celontin (Half Strength) Kapseals
- ◆ Celontin Kapseals
- ◆ Centrax Capsules, Tablets
- Cherry Syrup
- Chloramphenicol (Chloromycetin)
- Chlordiazepoxide Hydrochloride Capsules
- Chloromycetin Cream, 1%
- Chloromycetin Hydrocortisone Ophthalmic
- ◆ Chloromycetin Kapseals
- Chloromycetin Ophthalmic
- Chloromycetin Ophthalmic Ointment, 1%
- ◆ Chloromycetin Ophthalmic Solution (Ophthochlor)
- Chloromycetin Otic
- Chloromycetin Palmitate, Oral Suspension
- Chloromycetin Sodium Succinate
- Chloromycetin-Polymyxin-Hydrocortisone Acetate Ophthalmic Ointment (Ophthocort)
- Chlorpromazine Hydrochloride Tablets (Promapar)
- Chlorthalidone Tablets, USP
- Choledyl Elixir
- Choledyl Pediatric Syrup
- ◆ Choledyl SA Tablets
- ◆ Choledyl Tablets
- Coly-Mycin M Parenteral
- Coly-Mycin S For Oral Suspension
- Coly-Mycin S Otic w/Neomycin & Hydrocortisone
- Corticotropin Injection (ACTH)
- Cyanocobalamin Injection (Sytobex)
- ◆ Cyclopar & Cyclopar 500 Capsules (tetracycline hydrochloride, USP)
- ◆ Dilantin Infatabs
- ◆ Dilantin Kapseals
- Dilantin, Parenteral
- ◆ Dilantin with Phenobarbital Kapseals
- Dilantin-30 Pediatric/Dilantin-125 Suspension
- ◆ Diphenhydramine Hydrochloride (Benadryl)
- Diphenoxylate Hydrochloride & Atropine Sulfate Tablets, USP
- Dispos-A-Med Flow Path Kit
- Dispos-A-Med, isoetharine hydrochloride; isoproterenol hydrochloride
- Dispos-A-Med Vials, Empty
- Dispos-A-Vial: Sterile Water, Normal Saline, Half Normal Saline
- Docusate Sodium Capsules (D-S-S Capsules)
- Docusate Sodium with Casanthranol Capsules (D-D-S Plus Capsules)
- Dopamine Hydrochloride Ampoules (Dopastat)
- ◆ Duraquin
- ◆ Easprin
- ◆ Elase
- Elase Ointment
- V-Applicator (for Elase Ointment)
- ◆ Elase-Chloromycetin Ointment
- ◆ Eldec Kapseals
- Epinephrine (Adrenalin)
- Ergostat
- ◆ ERYC
- ◆ Erythromycin Stearate Tablets (Erypar)
- ◆ Estrovis
- Ethosuximide (see Zarontin)
- ◆ Euthroid

- Ferrous Sulfate Filmseals
- Fluogen (influenza virus vaccine)
- Furosemide Injection, USP
- Furosemide Tablets, USP
- ◆ Gelusil Liquid & Tablets
- Gelusil-M Liquid & Tablets
- Gelusil-II Liquid & Tablets
- ◆ Geriplex-FS Kapseals
- Geriplex-FS Liquid
- Histoplasmin, Diluted
- ◆ Humatin Capsules
- Hydrochlorothiazide Tablets, USP (Thiuretic)
- Hydrogen Peroxide Solution
- ◆ Infatabs (Dilantin)
- Influenza Virus Vaccine (Fluogen)
- Ketalar
- Ketamine Hydrochloride Injection (Ketalar)
- Lavacol
- ◆ Loestrin ㉑ 1/20
- ◆ Loestrin Fe 1/20
- ◆ Loestrin ㉑ 1.5/30
- ◆ Loestrin Fe 1.5/30
- ◆ Lopid Capsules
- Mandelamine Granules
- Mandelamine Suspension
- Mandelamine Suspension Forte
- ◆ Mandelamine Tablets
- ◆ Meclomen
- Meprobamate Tablets
- ◆ Methsuximide (Celontin)
- Milontin Kapseals
- Myadec
- ◆ Nardil
- ◆ Natabec Kapseals
- ◆ Natabec Rx Kapseals
- ◆ Natabec with Fluoride Kapseals
- Natabec-FA Kapseals
- ◆ Natafort Filmseal
- Nema Worm Capsules
- ◆ Nitroglycerin Tablets (Nitrostat)
- Nitrostat Ointment 2%
- ◆ Nitrostat Tablets
- Nitrostat IV Ampoules
- Nitrostat IV Infusion Kit
- ◆ Nitrostat SR Capsules
- ◆ Norethindrone Acetate and Ethynyl Estradiol Tablets (Loestrin, Norlestrin)
- ◆ Norlestrin ㉑ 1/50
- ◆ Norlestrin ㉑ 2.5/50
- Norlestrin ㉘ 1/50
- ◆ Norlestrin Fe 1/50
- ◆ Norlestrin Fe 2.5/50
- ◆ Norlutate
- ◆ Norlutin
- Ophthochlor Ophthalmic Solution, 0.5%
- Ophthocort Ophthalmic Ointment
- Oxytocin Injection (Pitocin)
- ◆ Papase
- Paromomycin (Humatin)
- ◆ Parsidol
- Penicillin G Potassium for Injection
- Penicillin V Potassium for Oral Solution
- ◆ Penicillin V Potassium Tablets (Penapar VK)
- ◆ Peritrate Sustained Action
- ◆ Peritrate Tablets
- Peroxide, Hydrogen
- Phenobarbital Tablets
- ◆ Phensuximide (Milontin)
- Phenytoin Sodium (Dilantin)
- Pitocin Injection, Ampoules, Steri-Dose Syringes
- Pitressin Synthetic, Ampoules
- Pitressin Tannate in Oil Ampoules
- Pituitrin-S Ampoules
- Poison Ivy Extract
- ◆ Ponstel
- ◆ Povan Filmseals
- Prazepam Capsules
- ◆ Procan SR Tablets
- ◆ Proloid Tablets
- Propoxyphene Hydrochloride Capsules
- ◆ Pyridium
- ◆ Pyridium Plus
- ◆ Pyrvinium Pamoate (Povan)
- Quinidine Sulfate Tablets
- Quinine Sulfate Capsules
- Rubbing Alcohol (Lavacol)
- Siblin Granules
- ◆ Sinubid
- Spironolactone Tablets, USP
- Spironolactone w/Hydrochlorothiazide Tablets
- Surital Ampoules, Steri-Vials
- Sytobex (Cyanocobalamin Injection)
- ◆ Tabron Filmseal
- ◆ Tedral
- Tedral Elixir
- Tedral Expectorant
- ◆ Tedral SA
- Tedral Suspension
- ◆ Tedral Tablets
- Tedral-25 Tablets
- Terpin Hydrate & Codeine Elixir
- ◆ Tetracycline HCl Capsules (Cyclopar)
- ◆ Tetracycline HCl Capsules (Cyclopar 500)
- Theelin Aqueous Suspension
- ◆ Thera-Combex H-P Kapseals
- Thiamylal Sodium (Surital)

- Thiuretic (Hydrochlorothiazide Tablets)
- Thrombostat
- Tuberculin, Aplisol and Aplitest
- Tucks Cream
- Tucks Ointment
- Tucks Premoistened Pads
- Tucks Take-Alongs
- Unibase
- ◆ Uticort Cream, Gel, Lotion & Ointment
- V-Applicators for Elase Ointment
- Vasopressin Injection (Pitressin)
- Vira-A for Infusion
- ◆ Vira-A Ophthalmic Ointment, 3%
- ◆ Zarontin Capsules
- Zarontin Syrup
- Ziradryl Lotion

PEDINOL PHARMACAL INC.   1580
110 Bell Street
W. Babylon, NY 11704
Address inquiries to:
Director of Professional Services
(516) 293-9500
Products Available
- Alginate Styptic Gauze
- Breezee Mist Foot Powder
- Castellani Paint
- Fungoid Creme & Solution
- Fungoid Tincture
- G-myticin Creme and Ointment 0.1%
- Hydrisalic Gel
- Hydrisea Lotion
- Hydrisinol Creme & Lotion
- Osti-Derm Lotion
- PNS Unna Boot
- Pedi-Bath Salts
- Pedi-Boro Soak Paks
- Pedi-Cort V Creme
- Pedi-Dri Foot Powder
- Pedi-Pro Foot Powder
- Pedi-Vit A Creme
- Salactic Film
- Steri Unna Boot
- Ureacin Lotion & Creme

PENNWALT PRESCRIPTION DIVISION   426, 1581
Pennwalt Corporation
755 Jefferson Road
Rochester, NY 14623
Address inquiries to:
Director of Professional Relations
P.O. Box 1766
Rochester, NY 14603   (716) 475-9000
Products Available
- ◆ Adapin Capsules
- ◆ Biphetamine Capsules
- Cholan HMB
- Cholan-DH
- Corsym
- Delsym
- Emul-O-Balm
- ◆ Hylorel Tablets
- Infalyte
- ◆ Ionamin Capsules
- Kolyum Liquid and Powder
- Tussionex Capsules
- Tussionex Suspension
- Tussionex Tablets
- ◆ Zaroxolyn Tablets

PERSON & COVEY, INC.   1587
616 Allen Avenue
Glendale, CA 91201
Address inquiries to:
Lorne V. Person, President   (818) 240-1030
Products Available
- A.C.N. Tablets
- DHS Conditioning Rinse
- DHS Shampoo
- DHS Tar Shampoo
- DHS Zinc Dandruff Shampoo
- DOB Bath & Shower Oil (Formerly Tolakol)
- Drysol
- Enisyl Tablets
- Solbar PF
- Solbar Plus 15 Sun Protectant Cream
- Xerac
- Xerac AC
- Xerac BP5
- Xerac BP10
- Z-Pro-C Tablets

PERSONAL CARE PRODUCTS DIVISION   1588
Richardson-Vicks Inc.
10 Westport Road
Wilton, CT 06897
Address inquiries to:
Vicks Research Center   (203) 929-2500
For Medical Emergencies Contact
Medical Director
Vicks Research Center   (203) 929-2500
Products Available
- ▣ Clearasil Adult Care (Sulfur/Resorcinol)

(◆ Shown in Product Identification Section)   (▣ Described in PDR For Nonprescription Drugs)

Manufacturers' Index

▣ Clearasil 5% Benzoyl Peroxide Lotion Acne Treatment
▣ Clearasil Pore Deep Cleanser (Salicylic Acid 0.5%)
▣ Clearasil Super Strength Acne Treatment Cream (10% Benzoyl Peroxide)
▣ Denquel Sensitive Teeth Toothpaste
▣ Topex 10% Benzoyl Peroxide Lotion Buffered Acne Medication

PFIPHARMECS DIVISION 426, 1588
Pfizer Inc.
235 E. 42nd St.
New York, NY 10017
Address inquiries to:
Professional Services Dept. (212) 573-2323
Address Export inquiries to:
Pfizer International Inc. (212) 573-2323
Distribution Centers
Doraville, GA 30340
  4360 Northeast Expressway
    (404) 448-6666
Hoffman Estates, IL 60196
  2400 W. Central Road (312) 381-9500
Clifton, NJ 07012
  230 Brighton Rd. (201) 546-7700
Grand Prairie, TX 75050
  502 Fountain Parkway (817) 261-9131
Irvine, CA 92705
  16700 Red Hill Ave. (714) 540-9180
Products Available
◆ Antiminth Oral Suspension
Bacitracin Sterile
Bacitracin Topical Ointment
◆ Bonine Tablets
Cortril Topical Ointment
Coryban-D Capsules
Coryban-D Cough Syrup
Li-Ban Lice Control Spray
Permapen Isoject
Pfizerpen for Injection
Pfizerpen AS Aqueous Suspension
Polymixin B Sulfate Sterile
◆ RID Pediculicide
Streptomycin Sulfate Injection
Terra-Cortril Ophthalmic Suspension
◆ Terramycin Capsules
Terramycin Film-coated Tablets
Terramycin Intramuscular Solution
Terramycin Topical Ointment
Terramycin with Polymyxin B Sulfate Ophthalmic Ointment
Vansil Capsules
Vistaril Intramuscular Solution
◆ Wart-Off Wart Remover

PFIZER LABORATORIES 426, 1599
DIVISION
Pfizer Inc.
235 E. 42nd St.
New York, NY 10017
Address inquiries to:
Professional Services Dept. (212) 573-2422
Medical Emergency Calls
(Day or Night) (212) 573-2422
Address Export inquiries to:
Pfizer International Inc. (212) 573-2323
Distribution Centers
Doraville, GA 30340
  4360 Northeast Expressway
    (404) 448-6666
Hoffman Estates, IL 60196
  2400 W. Central Road (312) 381-9500
Clifton, NJ 07012
  230 Brighton Rd. (201) 546-7700
Grand Prairie, TX 75050
  502 Fountain Parkway (214) 647-0222
Irvine, CA 92714
  16700 Red Hill Ave. (714) 540-9180
Products Available
◆ Diabinese Tablets
◆ Feldene Capsules
◆ Minipress Capsules
◆ Minizide Capsules
◆ Moderil Tablets
◆ Procardia Capsules
◆ Renese Tablets
◆ Renese-R Tablets
Vibramycin Calcium Syrup
◆ Vibramycin Hyclate Capsules
Vibramycin Hyclate Intravenous
Vibramycin Monohydrate for Oral Suspension
◆ Vibra-Tabs Film Coated Tablets
◆ Vistaril Capsules
Vistaril Oral Suspension

PHARMACIA LABORATORIES 427, 1613
Division of Pharmacia Inc.
800 Centennial Ave.
Piscataway, NJ 08854
Address inquiries to:
Medical Director (201) 457-8000
Products Available
◆ Azulfidine Tablets, EN-tabs, Oral Suspension
Crescormon
Healon
Hyskon Hysteroscopy Fluid
Kabikinase
Macrodex

Rheomacrodex
Secretin-Kabi

PHARMACRAFT DIVISION 1616
Pennwalt Corporation
755 Jefferson Road
Rochester, NY 14623
Address inquiries to:
Professional Service Department
P.O. Box 1212
Rochester, NY 14603 (716) 475-9000
Products Available
▣ Allerest Tablets, Childrens Chewable Tablets, Headache Strength Tablets, Sinus Pain Formula Tablets, Eye Drops & Nasal Spray
▣ Allerest Timed Release Allergy Capsules
▣ CaldeCORT Hydrocortisone Multi-Purpose Anti-Itch Cream and Spray
▣ Caldesene Medicated Ointment
▣ Caldesene Medicated Baby Powder
▣ Cold Factor 12
▣ Cruex Antifungal Cream
▣ Cruex Antifungal Powder & Spray Powder
▣ Desenex Antifungal Cream, Ointment, Foam & Liquid
▣ Desenex Antifungal Powder & Spray Powder
▣ Sinarest Tablets, Extra Strength Tablets & Nasal Spray

PHARMADERM 1617
A division of Altana, Inc.
60 Baylis Road
Melville, NY 11747
Address inquiries to:
Customer Service Dept. (800) 645-9432
  (516) 454-8884
Betamethasone Dipropionate Cream & Ointment
Betamethasone Valerate Cream, Ointment & Lotion
Erythromycin Ophthalmic Ointment
Fluocinolone Acetonide Cream, Ointment & Topical Solution
Hydrocortisone Cream
Nystatin Cream, Ointment & Vaginal Tablets
Triamcinolone Acetonide Cream & Ointment
Triple Sulfa Vaginal Cream

PHARMAFAIR, INC. 1618
110 Kennedy Drive
Hauppauge, NY 11788
Address inquiries to:
Alfred Kahwaty 1-(800) 227-1427
or 1-(516) 231-0707
Products Available
Antipyrine & Benzocaine Otic Solution
Benzoyl Peroxide Gel
Borofair Otic
Cortifair Cream & Lotion ½ %
Cortifair Cream 1%
Fluocinolone Acetonide Topical Cream
Fluocinolone Acetonide Topical Ointment
Fluocinolone Acetonide Topical Solution
Gentafair Cream & Ointment
Iodo-Cortifair
Octicair Otic Solution & Suspension
Sterile Lubricating Jelly
Topisporin
Triamcinair Cream
Triprolidine HCl & Pseudoephedrine HCl Syrup

POYTHRESS LABORATORIES, INC. 1618
16 N. 22nd St.
Post Office Box 26946
Richmond, VA 23261 (804) 644-8591
Address inquiries to:
Special Services Department
Products Available
Antrocol Tablets, Capsules & Elixir
Bensulfoid
Bensulfoid Lotion
Lodrane Liquid-130 & 260
Mudrane GG Elixir
Mudrane GG Tablets
Mudrane GG-2 Tablets
Mudrane Tablets
Mudrane 2 Tablets
▣ Panalgesic
Solfoton Tablets & Capsules
Uro-Phosphate Tablets

PROCTER & GAMBLE 427, 1619
P.O. Box 171
Cincinnati, OH 45201
Also see Norwich Eaton Pharmaceuticals, Inc.
Address inquiries to:
Larry W. Farrell (513) 530-2154
For Medical Emergencies Contact:
W. S. Lainhart, M.D. (513) 627-7071
After Hours, call COLLECT (513) 751-5525
Products Available
Chloraseptic Preparations
  Children's Chloraseptic Lozenges
  Chloraseptic Liquid
  Chloraseptic Lozenges
◆ Encaprin
Head & Chest

▣ Head & Shoulders
Pepto-Bismol Liquid & Tablets

PROFESSIONAL HEALTH PRODUCTS, 1621
INC.
3496 Breakwater Court
Hayward, CA 94545
Address inquiries to:
Collect from CA, AK & HI (415) 783-5622
From outside of CA (800) 227-2224
For Medical Emergencies Contact:
Garry F. Gordon, M.D. (Same As Above)
Products Available
Added Protection III Multi-Vitamin & Multi-Mineral Supplement
Added Protection III Multi-Vitamin & Multi-Mineral Supplement without Copper
Added Protection III Multi-Vitamin & Multi-Mineral Supplement without Iron and Copper
Balance Gamma Linolenic Acid
Cardioguard Natural Lipotropic Dietary Supplement-Powder
Cardioguard Natural Lipotropic Dietary Supplement-Tablets
Hypoaller-C Hypoallergenic Vitamin C Powder (buffered)
MaxEPA Marine Lipid Concentrate
Protect! Natural Detoxification Formula

THE PURDUE FREDERICK 427, 1622
COMPANY
100 Connecticut Avenue
Norwalk, CT 06854 (203) 853-0123
Address inquiries to:
Medical Department
Products Available
Arthropan Liquid
Betadine Aerosol Spray
Betadine Antiseptic Gauze Pad
Betadine Antiseptic Gel
Betadine Antiseptic Lubricating Gel
Betadine Disposable Medicated Douche
Betadine Douche
Betadine Douche Kit
Betadine Helafoam Solution
Betadine Mouthwash/Gargle
Betadine Ointment
Betadine Perineal Wash Concentrate
Betadine Shampoo
Betadine Skin Cleanser
Betadine Skin Cleanser Foam
Betadine Solution
Betadine Solution Swab Aid
Betadine Solution Swabsticks
Betadine Surgical Scrub
Betadine Surgi-Prep Sponge-Brush
Betadine Viscous Formula Antiseptic Gauze Pad
Betadine Whirlpool Concentrate
◆ Cardioquin Tablets
Cerumenex Drops
◆ Fibermed Supplements
◆ MS Contin
Parelixir Liquid
Prioderm Lotion
Senokap DSS Capsules
Senokot Suppositories
Senokot Syrup
Senokot Tablets/Granules
Senokot Tablets Unit Strip Pack
Senokot-S Tablets
◆ Trilisate Tablets/Liquid
◆ Uniphyl 200 mg Tablets
◆ Uniphyl 400 mg Tablets

BLAIR LABORATORIES, INC.
Calamatum Lotion
Calamatum Ointment
Calamatum Spray
Fungacetin Ointment
Gentlax B Granules
Gentlax S Tablets
Isodine Antiseptic Solution
Isodine Mouthwash/Gargle
Kerid Ear Drops
Saratoga Ointment

SHIELD LABORATORIES, INC.
Central Venous Catheter Dressing Change Set

RAM LABORATORIES CORPORATION 1632
P. O. Box 559071
Miami, FL 33255
Address inquiries to:
In the United States (305) 264-6620
In Puerto Rico (809) 792-2002
Products Available
Algisin Capsules
Apetil Liquid
Digepepsin Tablets
Geroton Forte
Otisan Drops
Pasmol Tablets
Zincvit Capsules

(◆ Shown in Product Identification Section)   (▣ Described in PDR For Nonprescription Drugs)

Manufacturers' Index

REED & CARNRICK 427, 1632
1 New England Avenue
Piscataway, NJ 08854
Address inquiries to:
Professional Service Dept. (201) 981-0070
Products Available
Alphosyl Lotion, Cream
◆ Cortifoam
◆ Dilatrate-SR
◆ Epifoam
Kwell Cream
Kwell Lotion
Kwell Shampoo
Peptenzyme Elixir
◆ Phazyme
◆ Phazyme-95
◆ Phazyme-PB Tablets
◆ Proctofoam-HC
◆ proctoFoam/non-steroid
Proxigel
R&C Spray
Trichotine Liquid, Vaginal Douche
Trichotine Powder, Vaginal Douche

REID-PROVIDENT 427, 1637
LABORATORIES, INC.
Scientific Affairs and Manufacturing
25 Fifth Street, N.W.
Atlanta, GA 30308
Executive Offices
640 Tenth Street, N.W.
Atlanta, GA 30318 (404) 898-1000
Address inquiries to:
Medical Director
Products Available
Anduracaine Injection
Aquatag Tablets
Bacarate
Calinate-FA Tablets
◆ Compal Capsules
Crystimin-1000
◆ Curretab Tablets
Dentavite Chewable Tablets
Escot Capsules
Estraguard Vaginal Cream
◆ Estratab Tablets
◆ Estratest H.S. Tablets
◆ Estratest Tablets
Femguard Vaginal Cream
Fumatrin Forte
Histalet DM Syrup
◆ Histalet Forte Tablets
Histalet Syrup
Histalet X Syrup (New Formula)
◆ Histalet X Tablets (New Formula)
Melfiat Tablets
◆ Melfiat 105 Unicelles
Mity-Mycin Ointment
Mity-Quin Cream
Neotep Granucaps
Otoreid-HC Ear Drops
P-V-Tussin Syrup
◆ P-V-Tussin Tablets
Pavacap Unicelles
Proaqua Tablets
Proval #3 Capsules
Provigan Injection
Quinite Tablets
RP-Mycin Tablets
Reidamine Injection
Repen-VK Tablets
Retet-250 Capsules
Retet-500 Capsules
◆ Ru-Vert-M
Sumox Capsules
Sumox Oral Suspensions
Supen Capsules
Supen Oral Suspensions
Tranmep Tablets
Unifast Unicelles
◆ Unipres Tablets
Unproco Capsules
Vaso-80 Unicelles
◆ Zenate Tablets

REID-PROVIDENT LABORATORIES, INC.
DIRECT DIVISION
640 Tenth Street, N.W.
Atlanta GA 30318
Address inquiries to:
Professional Service Dept. (404) 898-1000
Products Available
Acetospan Injection
Alermine Tablets
Analone Injection
Appi-Plex Tablets
Aquatag Tablets
Bacarate Tablets
Baltron Injection
Bendylate Capsules
Bendylate Injection
C-BE Zinc Tablets
Cino-40 Injection
Codap Tablets
Dezone Injectable
Duoval P.A. Injection
E-Ionate P.A. Injection
Enoxa Tablets

Escot Capsules
Estraval 2X Injection
Estraval 4X Injection
Estraval-P.A. Injection
Fluoxymesterone Tablets
Ganphen Injection
Hyproval P.A. Injection
I.D. 50 Injection
Irolong II
L.A. Dezone Injection
Nandrolin Injection
Nautrol Injection
Neotep Granucaps
Nospaz Injection
P.S.P. IV (four) Injection
Pre-Dep 40 Injection
Pre-Dep 80 Injection
Prednisolone Acetate Injection
Pre-Enthus FA Capsules
Quinite Tablets
SPRX-1 Tablets
SPRX-3 Capsules
SPRX-105 Capsules
T.D. Alermine Granucaps
T.D. Therals Granucaps
T-E Ionate P.A. Injection
T-Ionate P.A. Injection
Tagatap Tablets
Testostroval P.A. Injection
Tora Tablets
Tora-30 Capsules
Trates Granucaps
Tuzon Tablets
Tuzyme Tablets
Unproco Capsules
Vernate Injection
X-Otag Injection
X-Otag S.R. Tablets
Zide Tablets

REXAR PHARMACAL CORP 1641
396 Rockaway Avenue
Valley Stream, NY 11581
Address inquiries to:
Rowena Melman (516) 561-7662
Products Available
Dextroamphetamine Sulfate, 5mg. & 10mg.
Methamphetamine Hydrochloride, 5mg. & 10mg.
Obetrol-10
Obetrol-20
Oby-Trim 30 Capsules
X-Trozine Capsules & Tablets
X-Trozine LA-105 Capsules

RIKER LABORATORIES, INC. 428, 1641
Subsidiary of 3M
225-1S-07 3M Center
St. Paul, MN 55144
For Medical Information
Write: Medical Services Department
Riker Laboratories, Inc.
225-1N-07 3M Center
St. Paul, MN 55144
Call: (612) 736-4930
For Medical Emergencies
Call: (612) 736-4930 (all hours)
Customer Service and other services:
Call: (800) 423-5197
or 423-5146 (Outside of CA only)
(818) 341-1300 (CA Residents)
Products Available
Alu-Cap Capsules
Alu-Tab Tablets
Calcium Disodium Versenate Injection
Cal-Sup
Circanol Tablets
◆ Disalcid Capsules
◆ Disalcid Tablets
Disipal Tablets
Duo-Medihaler Aerosol
Estomul-M Liquid & Tablets
Heparin Sodium Injection, Aqueous (Lipo-Hepin)
Lipo-Hepin (Heparin Sodium Injection USP)
◆ Medihaler Ergotamine Aerosol
Medihaler-Epi Aerosol
Medihaler-Iso Aerosol
◆ Norflex Injectable
◆ Norflex Tablets
◆ Norgesic Tablets
◆ Norgesic Forte Tablets
Rauwiloid Tablets
◆ Tepanil Tablets
◆ Tepanil Ten-tab Tablets
Theolair Liquid
◆ Theolair Tablets
◆ Theolair-Plus Tablets & Liquid
◆ Theolair-SR Tablets
◆ Urex Tablets

THE ROBERTSON/TAYLOR CO. 1645
A division of Intra-Medic Formulations, Inc.
1110 West Sunrise Boulevard
Fort Lauderdale, FL 33311

Address inquiries to:
Mitchell K. Friedlander (305) 763-5433
Products Available
Anorex-CCK
Intraderm-19 Emergency Acne Stick
Intraderm-19 Oral Acne Supplement
Intraderm-19 Overnight Acne Masque
Intraderm-19 Therapeutic Acne Scrub
Intraderm-19 Therapeutic Astringent Lotion
L-2000
Medi-Tec 90 New Therapeutic Overnight Concentrate
Medi-Tec 90 Therapeutic Conditioner with Strengthening Agents
Medi-Tec 90 Therapeutic Scalp Stimulant with Strengthening Agents
Medi-Tec 90 Therapeutic Shampoo & Scalp Conditioner with Strengthening Agents
Medi-Tec Vitamin-Mineral-Trace Mineral Supplement
Metabolite 2050
Revitalin-SL 90 Adult Supplement
Testorex-35 Adult Male Supplement

A. H. ROBINS COMPANY 428, 1647
Pharmaceutical Division
1407 Cummings Drive
Richmond, VA 23220
Address inquiries to:
The Medical Dept. (804) 257-2000
Medical Emergency calls (day or night) (804) 257-2000
If no answer, call answering service (804) 257-7788
Products Available
⊠ Allbee C-800 Plus Iron Tables
⊠ Allbee C-800 Tablets
⊠ Allbee w/C Capsules
Allbee-T Tablets
Arthralgen Tablets
Cough Calmers
◆ Dimacol Capsules
Dimacol Liquid
Dimetane-DC Cough Syrup
⊠ Dimetane Decongestant Elixir
⊠ Dimetane Decongestant Tablets
⊠ Dimetane Elixir
⊠ Dimetane Extentabs
⊠ Dimetane Tablets
Dimetane-Ten Injectable
Dimetapp Elixir
◆ Dimetapp Extentabs
Donnagel
Donnagel-PG
◆ Donnatal Capsules
Donnatal Elixir
◆ Donnatal Extentabs
◆ Donnatal No. 2 Tablets
◆ Donnatal Tablets
◆ Donnazyme Tablets
◆ Dopram Injectable
◆ Entozyme Tablets
◆ Exna Tablets
⊠ Extend 12 Liquid
◆ Micro-K Extencaps
◆ Micro-K 10 Extencaps
◆ Mitrolan Chewable Tablets
◆ Pabalate Tablets
◆ Pabalate-SF Tablets
◆ Phenaphen Capsules
◆ Phenaphen w/Codeine Capsules
◆ Phenaphen-650 with Codeine Tablets
◆ Pondimin Tablets
◆ Quinidex Extentabs
Reglan Injectable
Reglan Syrup
◆ Reglan Tablets
◆ Robaxin Injectable
◆ Robaxin Tablets
◆ Robaxin-750 Tablets
◆ Robaxisal Tablets
Robicillin VK Robitabs
Robimycin Robitabs
◆ Robinul Forte Tablets
◆ Robinul Injectable
◆ Robinul Tablets
Robitet '250' Hydrochloride Robicaps
Robitet '500' Hydrochloride Robicaps
⊠ Robitussin
Robitussin A-C
⊠ Robitussin-CF
Robitussin-DAC
⊠ Robitussin-DM
⊠ Robitussin Night Relief
⊠ Robitussin-PE
Silain Tablets
Silain-Gel Liquid
Viokase Powder
Viokase Tablets
⊠ Z-Bec Tablets

ROCHE LABORATORIES 429, 1665, 3015
Division of Hoffmann-La Roche Inc.
Nutley, NJ 07110 (201) 235-5000
For Medical Information
Write: Professional Services Department
Business hours only (8:30 a.m. to 5:00 p.m. EST), call (201) 235-2355

(◆ Shown in Product Identification Section)   (⊠ Described in PDR For Nonprescription Drugs)

Manufacturers' Index

For Medical Emergency Information only
after hours or on weekends, call
                                           (201) 235-2355

Branch Warehouses
Belvidere, NJ 07823
  Water Street   (201) 475-5337
Des Plaines, IL 60018
  105 E. Oakton St.   (312) 299-1106
  (Chicago)   (312) 775-0733

Products Available
- ◆ Accutane Capsules
- Alurate Elixir
- ◆ Ancobon Capsules
- Arfonad Ampuls
- ◆ Azo Gantanol Tablets
- ◆ Azo Gantrisin Tablets
- ◆ Bactrim DS Tablets
- Bactrim I.V. Infusion
- Bactrim Pediatric Suspension
- Bactrim Suspension
- ◆ Bactrim Tablets
- Berocca Parenteral Nutrition
- ◆ Berocca Plus Tablets
- ◆ Berocca Tablets
- Berocca-C & Berocca-C 500
- Bumex Injection
- ◆ Bumex Tablets
- ◆ Clonopin Tablets
- Efudex Cream
- Efudex Solution
- ◆ Emcyt Capsules
- FUDR Injectable
- ◆ Fansidar Tablets
- Fluorouracil Ampuls
- ◆ Gantanol DS Tablets
- Gantanol Suspension
- ◆ Gantanol Tablets
- ◆ Gantrisin Injectable
- Gantrisin Ophthalmic Ointment/Solution
- Gantrisin Pediatric Suspension
- Gantrisin Syrup
- ◆ Gantrisin Tablets
- Konakion Injectable
- ◆ Larobec Tablets
- ◆ Larodopa Capsules
- ◆ Larodopa Tablets
- Levo-Dromoran Injectable
- ◆ Levo-Dromoran Tablets
- Lipo Gantrisin
- Lorfan Injectable
- ◆ Marplan Tablets
- ◆ Matulane Capsules
- Mestinon Injectable
- Mestinon Syrup
- ◆ Mestinon Tablets
- ◆ Mestinon Timespan
- Nipride Injectable
- Nisentil Injectable
- ◆ Noludar Tablets
- ◆ Noludar 300 Capsules
- Pantopon Injectable
- Prostigmin Injectable
- ◆ Prostigmin Tablets
- ◆ Rocaltrol Capsules
- ◆ Solatene Capsules
- Synkayvite Injectable
- ◆ Synkayvite Tablets
- Taractan Concentrate
- Taractan Injectable
- ◆ Taractan Tablets
- ◆ Tel-E-Dose (unit dose) Products:
  - Bactrim Tablets
  - Bactrim DS Tablets
  - Bumex Tablets
  - Endep Tablets
  - Gantanol Tablets
  - Gantrisin Tablets
  - Trimpex Tablets
- Tensilon Injectable
- ◆ Trimpex Tablets
- ◆ Valrelease Capsules
- ◆ Vi-Penta F Chewables
- Vi-Penta F Infant Drops
- Vi-Penta F Multivitamin Drops
- Vi-Penta Infant Drops
- Vi-Penta Multivitamin Drops
- Vitamin K—see Synkayvite
- Vitamin K₁—see Konakion

ROCHE PRODUCTS INC.   **429, 1710**
Manati, Puerto Rico 00701
Address inquiries to:
Roche Laboratories   (see above)
Products Available
- ◆ Dalmane Capsules
- ◆ Endep Tablets
- ◆ Librax Capsules
- ◆ Libritabs Tablets
- ◆ Librium Capsules
- Librium Injectable
- ◆ Limbitrol Tablets
- ◆ Menrium Tablets
- ◆ Quarzan Capsules
- ◆ Tel-E-Dose (unit dose) Products:
  - Dalmane Capsules
  - Librax Capsules
  - Librium Capsules
  - Limbitrol Tablets

- Valium Tablets
- ◆ Valium Injectable
- ◆ Valium Tablets
- ◆ Valium Tel-E-Ject

ROERIG   **431, 1725**
A division of Pfizer Pharmaceuticals
235 E. 42nd St.
New York, NY 10017
Address inquiries to:
Medical Department   (212) 573-2187
Branch Offices
Doraville, GA 30340
  4360 N.E. Expressway
  (Southern Region)   (404) 448-6666
Hoffman Estates, IL 60196
  2400 W. Central Road (312) 381-9500
  (Midwestern & Great Lakes Regions)
Clifton, NJ 07012
  230 Brighton Road
  (Metro Region)   (201) 546-7700
Dallas, TX 75222
  P.O. Box 22249
  (Southwestern Region) (214) 647-0222
Irvine, CA 92705
  16700 Red Hill Ave.
  (Western Region)   (714) 540-9180
Products Available
- ◆ Antivert, Antivert/25 Tablets, Antivert/25 Chewable Tablets & Antivert/50 Tablets
- ◆ Atarax Tablets & Syrup
- Cefobid Intravenous/Intramuscular
- Emete-con Intramuscular/Intravenous
- ◆ Geocillin Tablets
- Geopen Intramuscular/Intravenous
- ◆ Glucotrol
- ◆ Heptuna Plus Capsules
- ◆ Marax Tablets & DF Syrup
- ◆ Navane Capsules and Concentrate
- Navane Intramuscular
- ◆ Sinequan Capsules
- Sinequan Oral Concentrate
- ◆ Spectrobid Tablets & Oral Suspension
- ◆ Sustaire Tablets
- ◆ Tao Capsules
- ◆ Urobiotic-250 Capsules

WILLIAM H. RORER, INC. **431, 1745**
500 Virginia Drive
Fort Washington, PA 19034
For Medical Emergencies Contact:
John F. A. Vance, M.D., Medical Director
                               (215) 628-6761
For Quality Matters Contact:
William E. Kinas, Vice President,
  Quality Assurance   (215) 628-6420
For Product Information Contact:
Ronald A. Amey, Marketing Services Manager
                               (215) 628-6492
Branch Offices
Langhorne, PA 19047
  2201 Cabot Blvd. West (215) 752-8555
Oak Forest, IL 60452
  P.O. Box 280
  4325 Frontage Rd.   (312) 687-7440
San Leandro, CA 94577
  P.O. Box 1569
  1550 Factor Avenue   (415) 357-9741
Tucker, GA 30084
  4660 Hammermill Road (404) 934-3091
Products Available
- Ananase Tablets
- ◆ Ascriptin Tablets
- ◆ Ascriptin A/D Tablets
- ◆ Ascriptin w/Codeine Tablets
- Azmacort Inhaler
- ◆ Calciferol Drops (Egocalciferol Oral Solution USP)
- ◆ Calciferol in Oil Injection (Egocalciferol USP)
- ◆ Calciferol Tablets (Ergocalciferol USP)
- ⬛ Camalox Suspension
- ◆ Camalox Tablets
- ◆ Chardonna-2 Tablets
- ⬛ Emetrol Solution
- Fedahist Expectorant
- ◆ Fedahist Gyrocaps
- Fedahist Syrup
- ◆ Fedahist Tablets
- ◆ Fermalox Tablets
- ◆ Gemnisyn Tablets
- ⬛ Kudrox Suspension (Double Strength)
- Kutapressin Injection
- ◆ Kutrase Capsules
- ◆ Ku-Zyme Capsules
- ◆ Ku-Zyme HP Capsules
- ◆ Lactrase Capsules
- ◆ Levsin Drops
- ◆ Levsin Elixir
- ◆ Levsin Injection
- ◆ Levsin Tablets
- Levsin-PB Drops
- Levsin/Phenobarbital Elixir
- Levsin/Phenobarbital Tablets
- ◆ Levsinex Timecaps
- Levsinex/Phenobarbital Timecaps
- ◆ Maalox No. 1 Tablets
- ◆ Maalox No. 2 Tablets
- ⬛ Maalox Plus Suspension

- ◆ Maalox Plus Tablets
- ⬛ Maalox TC Suspension
- ◆ Maalox TC Tablets
- ⬛ Milkinol
- ◆ Nitrol IV
- ◆ Nitrol Ointment
- Parepectolin Suspension
- ◆ Perdiem Granules
- ◆ Perdiem Plain Granules
- Pre-Pen
- Salimeph Forte
- ◆ Slo-bid Gyrocaps
- ◆ Slo-Phyllin Gyrocaps
- ◆ Slo-Phyllin Tablets
- ◆ Slo-Phyllin 80 Syrup
- ◆ Slo-Phyllin GG Capsules
- Slo-Phyllin GG Syrup

ROSS LABORATORIES   **432, 1761**
Div. Abbott Laboratories
Columbus, OH 43216
Address inquiries to:
Henry S. Sauls, M.D., Vice President,
  Medical Affairs   (614) 227-3333
Products Available
- Advance
- Clear Eyes Eye Drops
- Component Nipple System
- Ear Drops by Murine—See Murine Ear Wax Removal System
- Enrich
- Ensure
- Ensure HN
- Ensure Plus
- Ensure Plus HN
- Flexiflo Enteral Delivery System
  - Flexiflo Enteral Feeding Tube, 8 French
  - Flexiflo Enteral Feeding Tube, 8 French w/Stylet
  - Flexiflo Enteral Feeding Tube, 12 French
  - Flexiflo Enteral Nutrition Pump
  - Flexiflo Enteral Pump Set
  - Flexiflo Enteral Pump Set with Piercing Pin
  - Flexiflo-II Enteral Pump Set
  - Flexiflo-II Portable Enteral Nutrition Pump
  - Flexiflo-II Pump Set with Piercing Pin
  - Flexiflo-III Enteral Nutrition Pump
  - Flexiflo-III Enteral Pump Set
  - Flexiflo-III Pump Set with Piercing Pin
  - Flexiflo Gravity Gavage Set
  - Flexiflo Gravity Feeding Set with Piercing Pin
  - Flexitainer Enteral Nutrition Container
  - Flexitainer 500 Enteral Nutrition Container
- Forta Pudding
- Glucose Water 5% & 10%
- Isomil
- Isomil 20
- Isomil SF
- Isomil SF 20
- Murine Ear Wax Removal System/Murine Ear Drops
- Murine Eye Drops (Regular Formula)
- Murine Plus Eye Drops
- Osmolite
- Osmolite HN
- Pediaflor
- Pedialyte
- Pedialyte RS
- Pediamycin
- Pediazole
- Polycose
- ◆ Pramet FA
- ◆ Pramilet FA
- RCF
- Redi-Nurser System
- Rondec Oral Drops
- Rondec Syrup
- ◆ Rondec Tablet
- Rondec-DM Oral Drops
- Rondec-DM Syrup
- ◆ Rondec-TR Tablet
- Ross Hospital Formula System
- Ross SLD
- Selsun Blue Lotion
- Similac
- Similac PM 60/40
- Similac 13
- Similac 20
- Similac 24
- Similac 24 LBW
- Similac 27
- Similac Special Care 20
- Similac Special Care 24
- Similac With Iron
- Similac With Iron 13
- Similac With Iron 20
- Similac With Iron 24
- Similac With Whey + Iron
- Similac With Whey + Iron 20
- Sterilized Water
- Tronolane Anesthetic Hemorrhoidal Cream
- Tronolane Anesthetic Hemorrhoidal Suppositories
- TwoCal HN
- Vari-Flavors Flavor Pacs
- Vi-Daylin ADC Drops
- ◆ Vi-Daylin Chewable

(◆ Shown in Product Identification Section)   (⬛ Described in PDR For Nonprescription Drugs)

Manufacturers' Index

Vi-Daylin Drops
Vi-Daylin Liquid
Vi-Daylin Plus Iron ADC Drops
◆ Vi-Daylin + Iron Chewable
Vi-Daylin Plus Iron Drops
Vi-Daylin Plus Iron Liquid
Vi-Daylin/F ADC Drops
Vi-Daylin/F ADC + Iron Drops
◆ Vi-Daylin/F Chewable
Vi-Daylin/F Drops
◆ Vi-Daylin/F + Iron Chewable
Vi-Daylin/F + Iron Drops
Vital/High Nitrogen
Volu-Feed

ROWELL LABORATORIES, INC. 1786
210 Main Street, W.
Baudette, MN 56623
 Toll Free (800) 346-5040
 In Minn. Call (800) 542-5012
Address inquiries to:
Professional Service Dept.
Products Available
Balneol
C-Ron
C-Ron FA
C-Ron Forte
C-Ron Freckles
Chenix
Cin-Quin
Colrex Capsules
Colrex Compound Capsules
Colrex Compound Elixir
Colrex Decongestant
Colrex Expectorant
Colrex Syrup
Colrex Troches
Cortenema
Dermacort Cream
Dermacort Lotion-0.5%, 1%
Dexone 0.5, 0.75, 1.5, 4
Hydrocil Instant
Lithonate
Lithotabs
Multivitamins Rowell
Norlac
Norlac RX
Orasone 1, 5, 10, 20, 50
Perifoam
Prednisone Tablets
Proctocort
Quine Capsules
Quinidine Sulfate Capsules & Tablets
Ro-Bile
Vio-Bec
Vio-Bec Forte

ROXANE LABORATORIES, INC. 1788
330 Oak St., Columbus, OH 43216
Address inquiries to:
Professional Services Department
P.O. 16532
Columbus, OH 43216
 (Toll Free) (800) 848-0120
 (In Ohio call) (614) 228-5403
Products Available
Acetaminophen Elixir
Acetaminophen Elixir (Cherry)
Acetaminophen Suppositories
Acetaminophen Tablets
Acetaminophen with Codeine Phosphate Elixir
Acetaminophen with Codeine Phosphate Tablets
Aluminum Hydroxide Gel
Aluminum Hydroxide Gel-Concentrated
Aluminum Hydroxide Tablets
Aluminum & Magnesium Hydroxides with Simethicone I
Aluminum & Magnesium Hydroxides with Simethicone II
Aminophylline Tablets & Oral Solution
Amitriptyline Hydrochloride Tablets
Aromatic Cascara Fluidextract
Ascorbic Acid Tablets
Aspirin Suppositories
Bisacodyl Patient Pack
Bisacodyl Suppositories
Bisacodyl Tablets
Calcium Carbonate Tablets & Oral Suspension
Calcium Gluconate Tablets
Castor Oil
Castor Oil Flavored
Chloral Hydrate Capsules
Chloral Hydrate Syrup
Chlordiazepoxide Hydrochloride Capsules
Chlorpheniramine Maleate Tablets
Chlorpromazine Hydrochloride Tablets
Cocaine Hydrochloride Topical Solution
Codeine Phosphate Oral Solution
Codeine Sulfate Tablets
DHT (Dihydrotachysterol) Tablets, Oral Solution & Intensol
Dexamethasone Tablets, Oral Solution & Intensol
Diluent (Flavored) for Oral Use
Diphenhydramine Hydrochloride Capsules
Diphenhydramine Hydrochloride Elixir

Diphenoxylate Hydrochloride & Atropine Sulfate Tablets & Oral Solution
Docusate Sodium Capsules
Docusate Sodium Syrup
Docusate Sodium with Casanthranol Capsules
Ferrous Sulfate Liquid
Ferrous Sulfate Tablets
Gentz Wipes
Guaifenesin Syrup
Hydrochlorothiazide Tablets, Liquids, Intensol & Oral Solution
Imipramine Hydrochloride Tablets
Intensol Concentrated Oral Solutions (Package includes bottle & calibrated dropper)
  Chlorpromazine Hydrochloride Intensol
  DHT (Dihydrotachysterol) Intensol
  Dexamethasone Intensol
  Hydrochlorothiazine Intensol
  Roxanol (Morphine Sulfate Concentrated Oral Solution)
Ipecac Syrup
Isoetharine Hydrochloride Inhalation
Isoxsuprine Hydrochloride Tablets
Kaolin-Pectin-Concentrated
Kaolin-Pectin Suspension
Lithium Carbonate Capsules & Tablets
Lithium Citrate Syrup
Magnesia & Alumina Oral Suspension
Methadone Hydrochloride Oral Solution & Tablets
Methocarbamol Tablets
Milk of Magnesia
Milk of Magnesia-Concentrated
Milk of Magnesia-Cascara Suspension Concentrated
Milk of Magnesia-Mineral Oil Emulsion & Emulsion (Flavored)
Mineral Oil
Mineral Oil-Light Sterile
Morphine Sulfate Oral Solution
Morphine Sulfate Tablets
Neomycin Sulfate Tablets
Niacin Tablets
Oxycodone Hydrochloride Oral Solution
Oxycodone Hydrochloride Tablets
Oxycodone Hydrochloride USP Single Entity Tablets & Liquid
Oxycodone Hydrochloride & Acetaminophen Tablets
Oxycodone Hydrochloride, Oxycodone Terephthalate & Aspirin Tablets (Full Strength)
Papaverine Hydrochloride Capsules
Paregoric
Phenobarbital Elixir
Phenobarbital Tablets
Potassium Chloride for Oral Solution (Flavored)
Potassium Chloride Oral Solution
Potassium Chloride Powder Unflavored
Potassium Gluconate Elixir
Potassium Iodide Liquid
Potassium Iodide Oral Solution
Potassium Phosphates Oral Solution
Prednisolone Tablets
Prednisone Tablets
Propantheline Bromide Tablets
Propoxyphene Hydrochloride Capsules
Pseudoephedrine Syrup
Pseudoephedrine Hydrochloride Tablets
Quinidine Gluconate Sustained Release Tablets
Quinidine Sulfate Tablets
Roxanol (Morphine Sulfate Concentrated Oral Solution)
Saliva Substitute
Sodium Chloride Inhalation
Sodium Phosphates Oral Solution
Sodium Polystyrene Sulfonate Suspension
Sulfisoxazole Tablets
Terpin Hydrate & Codeine Elixir
Theophylline Oral Solution
Thioridazine Hydrochloride Tablets
Triprolidine Hydrochloride & Pseudoephedrine Hydrochloride Syrup
Triprolidine Hydrochloride & Pseudoephedrine Hydrochloride Tablets

RYDELLE LABORATORIES, INC. 1795
Subsidiary of S.C. Johnson & Son, Inc.
1525 Howe Street
Racine, Wisconsin 53403
Address inquiries to:
Carol Hansen, Consumer Affairs Director
 (414) 631-4000
For Medical Emergencies Contact:
Richard D. Stewart, M.D.
 (414) 631-3675
Products Available
Fiberall, Natural Flavor
Fiberall, Orange Flavor

RYSTAN COMPANY, INC. 1795
47 Center Avenue
P.O. Box 214
Little Falls, NJ 07424

Address inquiries to:
Professional Service Dept. (201) 256-3737
Products Available
Chloresium Dental Ointment
Chloresium Ointment
Chloresium Solution
Chloresium Tablets
Chloresium Toothpaste
Derifil Tablets & Powder
Panafil Ointment
Panafil-White Ointment
Prophyllin Wet Dressing Ointment & Powder

SANDOZ, INC. 432, 1796
Pharmaceuticals Division
Route 10, East Hanover, NJ 07936
Address inquiries to:
William F. Westlin, M.D. (201) 386-7500
New York City (212) 349-1212
Products Available
Asbron G Elixir
Asbron G Inlay-Tabs
◆ Belladenal Tablets
◆ Belladenal-S Tablets
Bellafoline Injection & Tablets
◆ Bellergal Tablets
◆ Bellergal-S Tablets
Cafergot Suppositories
◆ Cafergot Tablets
Cafergot P-B Suppositories
◆ Cafergot P-B Tablets
Cedilanid-D Injection
D.H.E. 45 Injection
Diapid Nasal Spray
◆ Fiogesic Tablets
◆ Fiorinal Capsules
◆ Fiorinal Tablets
◆ Fiorinal w/Codeine Capsules
◆ Hydergine Oral Tablets, Sublingual Tablets, & Liquid
◆ Hydergine LC Liquid Capsules
◆ Klorvess Effervescent Granules
◆ Klorvess Effervescent Tablets
Klorvess 10% Liquid
Mellaril Concentrate
Mellaril-S Suspension
◆ Mellaril Tablets
◆ Mesantoin Tablets
Methergine Injection
◆ Methergine Tablets
Neo-Calglucon Syrup
◆ Pamelor Capsules
Pamelor Solution
◆ Parlodel Capsules
◆ Parlodel Tablets
◆ Restoril Capsules
Sandimmune Ampuls
Sandimmune Oral Suspension
Sandoglobulin
◆ Sanorex Tablets
◆ Sansert Tablets
Syntocinon Injection
Syntocinon Nasal Spray
◆ Tavist Tablets
◆ Tavist-1 Tablets
◆ Tavist-D Tablets
◆ Visken

SAVAGE LABORATORIES 433, 1822
a division of Altana Inc.
60 Baylis Road
Post Office Box 2006
Melville, NY 11747 (516) 454-7677
Products Available
Alpha-Ruvite
Alphatrex Cream & Ointment
Aridose-R
Betatrex Cream, Ointment & Lotion
◆ Brexin Capsules
◆ Brexin L.A. Capsules
◆ Chromagen Capsules
Chromagen Injection
Chromagen OB
Cortigel-40
Cortigel-80
Dilor Elixir
◆ Dilor Injectable
◆ Dilor Tablets
◆ Dilor-400 Tablets
◆ Dilor-G Tablets & Liquid
Ditate
Ditate-DS
Estate
◆ Estrocon Tablets
Estrone
Ethiodol
Homo-Tet
Immuglobin
Libigen 10,000 & Diluent
Mepred-40
Mepred-80
Mytrex Cream & Ointment
Negatan
Nystex Cream & Ointment
Nystex Oral Suspension
Ruvite 1000
◆ Satric
Satric-500

(◆ Shown in Product Identification Section)   (■ Described in PDR For Nonprescription Drugs)

Manufacturers' Index

Savacort-50
Savacort-100
Savacort-D
Testate
Testosterone
Thiodyne
Tracilon
Trymex Cream & Ointment
Trysul

HENRY SCHEIN, INC.   **1828**
5 Harbor Park Drive
Port Washington, NY 11050
Address inquiries to:
Peter Schwartz   (516) 621-4300
Products Available
Acetazolamide Tablets
Allopurinol Tablets
Aminophylline Oral Liquid, Suppositories & Tabs
Amitriptyline HCl Tablets
Amoxicillin Trihydrate Capsules & Powder for Oral Suspension
Ampicillin Trihydrate Capsules & Powder for Oral Suspension
Antispasmodic Capsules, Elixir & Tablets
Apap 300 mg. with Codeine Capsules & Tabs
Apap with Codeine Elixir
Aspirin 325 mg. with Codeine Tabs
Azo-Sulfisoxazole Tablets
Benztropine Mesylate Tablets
Bromanyl Expectorant
Bromphen Compound Elixir - Sugar Free
Bromphen Compound Tablets
Bromphen DC Expectorant
Bromphen Expectorant
Butalbital Compound
Cafetrate-PB Suppositories
Cardec DM Drops & Syrup
Chloral Hydrate Capsules
Chloramphenicol Ophthalmic Solution 5%
Chlordiazepoxide HCl Capsules
Chloroserpine 250 & 500 Tablets
Chlorothiazide Tablets
Chlorpromazine HCl Tablets
Chlorthalidone Tablets
Chlorzone Forte Tablets
Clipoxide Capsules
Cloxacillin Sodium Capsules
Conjugated Estrogens Tablets - Coated
Cyclandelate Capsules
Cyproheptadine HCl Syrup & Tablets
Decongestant Elixir
Decongestant Expectorant
Decongestant-AT (Antitussive) Liquid
Detussin Expectorant
Detussin Liquid
Dexamethasone Tablets
Dexamycin Ophthalmic Ointment
Dexchlor Repeat Action Tablets
Dicloxacillin Sodium Capsules
Diethylpropion HCl Tablets & Timed Tablets
Dihydrocodeine Compound Tablets
Dioctocal Capsules - Docusate Calcium USP
Diphenhydramine HCl Caps
Diphenoxylate & Atropine HCl Liquid (DPXL) & Tabs
Dipyridamole Tablets
Disulfiram Tablets
Doxycycline Tablets
Doxycycline Hyclate Capsules
Effervescent Potassium Tablets
Erythromycin Estolate Capsules & Suspension
Erythromycin Ethylsuccinate Granules, Suspension & Tablets
Erythromycin Ophthalmic Ointment
Fluocinolone Acetonide Cream
Fluoxymesterone Tablets
Furosemide Tablets
Gentamicin Cream 0.1% & Ointment 0.1%
Gentamicin Ophthalmic Ointment & Solution
Glutethimide Tablets
Guiatuss Syrup
Guiatuss A-C Syrup
Guiatuss D-M Syrup
H-H-R Tablets
Hydralazine HCl Tablets
Hydralazine-Thiazide Capsules
Hydrochlorothiazide Tablets
Hydrocodone Syrup
Hydro-Ergoloid Oral & Sublingual Tablets
Hydroflumethiazide Tablets
Hydro-Fluserpine Tablets #1 & #2
Hydroserpine Tablets
Hydroxyzine HCl Syrup & Tablets
Hydroxyzine Pamoate
Imipramine HCl Tablets
Indomethacin Capsules
Iophen-C Liquid
Isoetharine Hydrochloride 1.0%
Isosorbide Dinitrate Tablets - Oral & Sublingual
Isosorbide Dinitrate Timed Capsules & Tablets
Isoxsuprine HCl Tablets
Kaolin, Pectin, Belladonna Mixture

Kaolin-Pectin Mixture
Kaolin-Pectin PG Mixture
Lidocaine HCl 2% Viscous Solution
Lindane Lotion & Shampoo
Liothyronine Sodium Tablets
Meclizine HCl MLT Tablets
Mepro Compound Tablets
Meprobamate Tablets
Methenamine Mandelate Forte Suspension & Tablets
Methocarbamol Tablets
Methocarbamol with Aspirin Tablets
Methyclothiazide Tablets
Methy-Deserpidine
Methylprednisolone Tablets
Metronidazole Oral Tablets
Nitrofurantoin Capsules & Tablets
Nitroglycerin Ointment 2%
Nitrolin Timed Capsules
Nylidrin HCl Tablets
Nystatin Cream, Oral & Vaginal Tablets
Nyst-olone Cream & Ointment
Oxacillin Sodium Capsules & Powder for Oral Suspension
Oxymeta-12 Nasal Spray
Oxytetracycline HCl Capsules
Papaverine HCl Timed Capsules
Penicillin VK Powder for Oral Solution & Tablets
Pentaerythritol Tetranitrate Tablets (PETN), Timed Capsules & Tablets
Phenobarbital Elixir & Tablets
Phentermine HCl Capsules & Tablets
Phenylbutazone Capsules & Tablets
Phenytoin Sodium Capsules-Prompt Action
Polyvitamin-Fluoride Drops & Tablets
Potassium Chloride Concentrate, Powder & Liquid
Potassium Gluconate Elixir
Prednisolone Tablets
Prednisone Tablets
Primidone Tablets
Probenecid Tablets
Probenecid with Colchicine Tablets
Procainamide HCl Capsules
Prochlor-Iso Timed Release Capsules
Propantheline Bromide Tablets
Propoxyphene & Apap Tablets 65/650
Propoxyphene Compound 65
Propoxyphene HCl Capsules
Pseudoephedrine HCl Tablets
Pyrinyl Liquid
Quadrahist Pediatric Syrup, Syrup & Timed Release Tablets
Quinidine Gluconate Tablets
Quinidine Sulfate Tablets
Quinine Sulfate Capsules & Tablets
Reserpine Tablets
Soprodol Tablets (Carisoprodol)
Spironazide Tablets
Spironolactone Tablets
Sulfasalazine Tablets
Sulfatrim & Sulfatrim D/S Tablets
Sulfinpyrazone Tablets
Sulfisoxazole Tablets
T-E-P Tablets
Tetracycline HCl Capsules & Syrup
Theophylline Anhydrous Tablets
Theophylline Elixir & KI Elixir
Theozine Syrup & Tablets - Dye-Free
Thioridazine Tablets
Thylline & Thylline-GG Tablets
L-Thyroxine Tablets
Tolbutamide Tablets
Triafed Syrup & Tablets
Triafed-C Expectorant
Triamcinolone Tablets
Triamcinolone Acetonide Cream
Trichlormethiazide Tablets
Trifluoperazine Tablets
Trimethobenzamide HCl Suppositories
Triple Sulfa Vaginal Cream
Tri-Thalmic Ophthalmic Solution
Tuss-Ade Timed Capsules
Vaginal Sulfa Suppositories
Warfarin Sodium Tablets

SCHERING CORPORATION   **433, 1831**
Galloping Hill Road
Kenilworth, NJ 07033   (201) 558-4000
Address inquiries to:
Professional Services Department
9:00 AM to 5:00 PM EST:
                       (201) 558-4908
After regular hours and on weekends:
                       (201) 558-4000
Branch Offices
Southeast Branch
5884 Peachtree Rd., N.E.
Chamblee, GA 30341   (404) 457-6315
Midwest Branch
7500 N. Natchez Ave.
Niles, IL 60648   (312) 647-9363

Southwest Branch
1921 Gateway Dr.
Irving, TX 75062   (214) 258-3545
West Coast Branch
14775 Wicks Blvd.
San Leandro, CA 94577   (415) 357-3125
Products Available
▣ A and D Hand Cream*
▣ A and D Ointment*
▣ Afrin Menthol Nasal Spray, 0.05%
▣ Afrin Nasal Spray 0.05%
▣ Afrin Nose Drops 0.05%
▣ Afrin Pediatric Nose Drops 0.025%
♦ Afrinol Repetabs Tablets Long-Acting Nasal Decongestant
Akrinol Cream
Celestone Cream
Celestone Phosphate Injection
Celestone 0.6 mg. Six-Day Pack
Celestone Soluspan Suspension
Celestone Syrup
♦ Celestone Tablets
▣ Chlor-Trimeton Allergy Syrup
♦ Chlor-Trimeton Allergy Tablets
♦ Chlor-Trimeton 12 mg Antihistamine Timed-Release Allergy Repetabs
♦ Chlor-Trimeton Decongestant Tablets
▣ Chlor-Trimeton Expectorant
Chlor-Trimeton Injection
♦ Chlor-Trimeton Long-Acting Allergy Repetabs Tablets
♦ Chlor-Trimeton Long-Acting Decongestant Repetabs Tablets
♦ Cod Liver Oil Concentrate Capsules*
♦ Cod Liver Oil Concentrate Tablets*
♦ Cod Liver Oil Concentrate Tablets w/Vitamin C*
▣ Coricidin Cough Syrup
♦ Coricidin "D" Decongestant Tablets
♦ Coricidin Decongestant Nasal Mist
♦ Coricidin Demilets Tablets For Children
♦ Coricidin Extra Strength Sinus Headache Tablets
♦ Coricidin Medilets Tablets For Children
♦ Coricidin Tablets
Corilin Infant Liquid
♦ Demazin Timed-Release Tablets
▣ Demazin Syrup
▣ Dermolate Anal-Itch Ointment
▣ Dermolate Anti-Itch Cream
▣ Dermolate Anti-Itch Spray
♦ Dermolate Scalp-Itch Lotion
Diprolene Ointment 0.05%
Diprosone Cream 0.05%
Diprosone Lotion 0.05% w/w
Diprosone Ointment 0.05%
Diprosone Topical Aerosol 0.1% w/w
♦ Disophrol Chronotab Sustained-Action Tablets*
♦ Disophrol Tablets*
♦ Drixoral Sustained-Action Tablets
▣ Emko Because Contraceptor Vaginal Contraceptive Foam
▣ Emko Pre-Fil Vaginal Contraceptive Foam
▣ Emko Vaginal Contraceptive Foam
♦ Estinyl Tablets
♦ Etrafon A Tablets (4-10)
♦ Etrafon 2-10 Tablets (2-10)
♦ Etrafon Tablets (2-25)
♦ Etrafon Forte Tablets (4-25)
♦ Fulvicin P/G Tablets
♦ Fulvicin P/G 165 & 330 Tablets
♦ Fulvicin-U/F Tablets
Garamycin Cream 0.1%
Garamycin Injectable
Garamycin Injectable Disposable Syringes
Garamycin Intrathecal Injection
Garamycin I.V. Piggyback Injection
Garamycin Ointment 0.1%
Garamycin Ophthalmic Ointment
Garamycin Ophthalmic Solution
Garamycin Pediatric Injectable
Gyne-Lotrimin Vaginal Cream 1%
♦ Gyne-Lotrimin Vaginal Tablets
Hyperstat I.V. Injection
Lotrimin Cream 1%
Lotrimin Lotion 1%
Lotrimin Solution 1%
Lotrisone Cream
♦ Meticorten Tablets
Meti-Derm Cream 0.5%
Metimyd Ophthalmic Ointment
Metimyd Ophthalmic Suspension
Metreton Ophthalmic/Otic Solution-Sterile
♦ Miradon Tablets
♦ Mol-Iron Chronosule Capsules*
♦ Mol-Iron Tablets*
♦ Mol-Iron w/Vitamin C Tablets
♦ Naqua Tablets
♦ Naquival Tablets
Netromycin Injection
Normodyne Injection
♦ Normodyne Tablets
♦ Optimine Tablets
Optimyd Ophthalmic Solution
Oreton Methyl Buccal Tablets
♦ Oreton Methyl Tablets
Otobiotic Otic Solution

(♦ Shown in Product Identification Section)   (▣ Described in PDR For Nonprescription Drugs)

Manufacturers' Index

◆ Paxipam Tablets
Permitil Oral Concentrate*
◆ Permitil Tablets*
◆ Polaramine Expectorant
◆ Polaramine Repetabs Tablets
Polaramine Syrup
◆ Polaramine Tablets
Proglycem Capsules
Proglycem Suspension
◆ Proventil Inhaler
◆ Proventil Tablets
◆ Rela Tablets
Sebizon Lotion
Sodium Sulamyd Ophthalmic Ointment 10%
Sodium Sulamyd Ophthalmic Solution 10%
Sodium Sulamyd Ophthalmic Solution 30%
Solganal Suspension
⊞ Sunril Premenstrual Capsules
◆ Theovent Long-Acting Capsules
⊞◆ Tinactin Cream 1%
⊞◆ Tinactin Jock Itch Cream 1%
⊞◆ Tinactin Jock Itch Spray Powder 1%
⊞◆ Tinactin Liquid 1% Aerosol
⊞◆ Tinactin Powder 1%
⊞◆ Tinactin Powder 1% Aerosol
⊞◆ Tinactin Solution 1%
Tindal Tablets
Trilafon Concentrate
Trilafon Injection
◆ Trilafon Repetabs Tablets
◆ Trilafon Tablets
◆ Trinalin Repetabs Tablets
Valisone Cream 0.1%
Valisone Lotion 0.1%
Valisone Ointment 0.1%
Valisone Reduced Strength Cream 0.01%
◆ Vancenase Nasal Inhaler
◆ Vanceril Inhaler
*Schering/White Product Line

SCHMID PRODUCTS COMPANY 1896
Division of Schmid Laboratories, Inc.
Route 46 West
Little Falls, NJ 07424
Address inquiries to:
Professional Service Dept. (201) 256-5500
Products Available
Ramses Bendex Flexible Cushioned Diaphragm
Ramses Contraceptive Vaginal Jelly
Ramses Flexible Cushioned Diaphragm
Vagisec Medicated Liquid Douche Concentrate
Vagisec Plus Suppositories

SCLAVO INC. 1897, 3017
5 Mansard Court
Wayne, NJ 07470
Address inquiries to:
Francis J. O'Grady (800) 526-5260
Products Available
Antirabies Serum (equine), Purified
Cholera Vaccine
Diphtheria Antitoxin (equine), Refined
Diphtheria & Tetanus Toxoids, Adsorbed (For Pediatric Use)
Diphtheria Toxoid, Adsorbed
SclavoTest-PPD, Tuberculin PPD Multiple Puncture Device
Tetanus Antitoxin (equine), Refined
Tetanus Toxoid, Adsorbed
Tetanus & Diphtheria Toxoids, Adsorbed (For Adult Use)

SCOT-TUSSIN PHARMACAL CO., INC. 1897
50 Clemence Street
Cranston, RI 02920-0217
Address inquiries to:
Professional Service Dept. (401) 942-8555
Products Available
Ferro-Bob Tablets
S-T Cort Lotion
S-T Decongest Sugar-Free & Dye-Free
S-T Febrol Tablets & Elixir
S-T Forte Sugar-Free
S-T Forte Syrup
Scot-Tussin DM Syrup
Scot-Tussin Sugar-Free Cough & Cold Medicine
Scot-Tussin Sugar-Free Expectorant, Dye-Free & Sodium-Free Cough Formula
Scot-Tussin Sugar-Free 5-Action Cold Formula
Scot-Tussin Syrup 5-Action Cold Formula
Tussirex Sugar-Free
Tussirex Syrup
Vita-Bob Capsules
Vita-Natal Capsules
Vita-Plus B 12, 10 ml. Vials, 1000 mcgm./ml.
Vita-Plus E Capsules Natural 400 I.U.
Vita-Plus G (geriatric) Capsules
Vita-Plus H (hematinic) Capsules
Vita-Plus H (hematinic) Sugar-Free, Liquid

SEAMLESS HOSPITAL PRODUCTS COMPANY 1897
Division of Dart Industries
P.O. Box 828
Barnes Industrial Park
Wallingford, CT 06492
Address inquiries to:
Medical Department (800) 243-3030
For Medical Emergencies Contact:
Patrick J. Lamb (800) 243-3030
Products Available
Anti-Sept

SEARLE PHARMACEUTICALS INC. 435, 1898
Box 5110
Chicago, IL 60680
Address medical inquiries to:
Medical Communications Department
G.D. Searle & Co.
4901 Searle Pkwy.
Skokie, IL 60077
Outside IL (800) 323-4204 (business hours)
Within IL (312) 982-7000 (at other times)
Products Available
Aminophyllin Injection
◆ Calan for IV Injection
◆ Cu-7
◆ Diulo
Dramamine Injection
Dramamine Liquid
◆ Dramamine Tablets
◆ Flagyl I.V.
◆ Flagyl I.V. RTU
◆ Nitrodisc
◆ Tatum-T

SEARLE CONSUMER PRODUCTS 1911
Division of G.D. Searle & Co.
Box 5110
Chicago, IL 60680
Address medical inquiries to:
Medical Communications Department
G.D. Searle & Co.
4901 Searle Pkwy.
Skokie, IL 60077
(312) 982-7000
Products Available
⊞ Dramamine Liquid
⊞ Dramamine Tablets
⊞ Equal
⊞ Icy Hot Balm
⊞ Icy Hot Rub
Metamucil, Instant Mix, Orange Flavor
Metamucil, Instant Mix, Regular Flavor
Metamucil, Powder, Orange Flavor
Metamucil, Powder, Regular Flavor
Metamucil, Powder, Strawberry Flavor
Metamucil, Powder, Sugar Free, Regular Flavor
Prompt

SEARLE & CO. 435, 1912
San Juan, Puerto Rico 00936
Address medical inquiries to:
Medical Communications Department
4901 Searle Pkwy.
Skokie, IL 60077
Products Available
◆ Aldactazide
◆ Aldactone
◆ Aminophyllin Tablets
◆ Anavar
◆ Banthine Tablets
◆ Calan Tablets
◆ Demulen 1/35-21
◆ Demulen 1/35-28
◆ Demulen 1/50-21
◆ Demulen 1/50-28
◆ Enovid 5 mg
◆ Enovid 10 mg
◆ Enovid-E 21
◆ Flagyl Tablets
Lomotil Liquid
◆ Lomotil Tablets
◆ Norpace Capsules
◆ Norpace CR Capsules
◆ Ovulen-21
◆ Ovulen-28
◆ Pro-Banthine Tablets
◆ Pro-Banthine w/Phenobarbital Tablets
◆ Theo-24

SERES LABORATORIES, INC. 1939
3331 Industrial Drive
Box 470
Santa Rosa, CA 95402
Address inquiries to:
Kathryn M. MacLeod, Ph.D. (707) 526-4526
Products Available
Cantharone
Cantharone Plus
Night Cast Formula R
Night Cast Formula S (Medicated Acne Mask)

SERONO LABORATORIES, INC. 1940
280 Pond Street
Randolph, MA 02368
Address inquiries to:
Medical Information Department
(outside MA) (800) 225-5185
(within MA) (617) 963-8154
For Medical Emergencies Contact 24 Hours:
Vice President, Research and Development
(outside MA) (800) 225-5185
(within MA) (617) 963-8154
Products Available
Asellacrin (somatropin)
Pergonal (menotropins USP)
Profasi HP (HCG)
Serophene (clomiphene citrate USP)

SMITH KLINE & FRENCH LABORATORIES 436, 1945
Division of SmithKline Beckman Corporation
1500 Spring Garden St.
P.O. Box 7929
Philadelphia, PA 19101
Address inquiries to:
Medical Dept. (215) 751-4000

SK&F CO. 436, 1945
Carolina, Puerto Rico 00630
Subsidiary of SmithKline Beckman Corporation
Address inquiries to:
Smith Kline & French Laboratories (see above)

SK&F LAB CO. 436, 1945
Carolina, Puerto Rico 00630
Subsidiary of SmithKline Beckman Corporation
Address inquiries to:
Smith Kline & French Laboratories (see above)

MENLEY & JAMES LABORATORIES 436, 1945
A SmithKline Beckman Company
P.O. Box 8082
Philadelphia, PA 19101
Address inquiries to
Medical Department (215) 751-5000
Products Available
Acnomel Cream*
Ancef Injection
◆ Anspor Capsules
Anspor for Oral Suspension
Benzedrex Inhaler*
Cefizox Injection
◆ Combid Spansule Capsules
Compazine Injection
◆ Compazine Spansule Capsules
◆ Compazine Suppositories
Compazine Syrup
◆ Compazine Tablets
◆ Cytomel Tablets
◆ Darbid Tablets
Dexedrine Elixir
◆ Dexedrine Spansule Capsules
◆ Dexedrine Tablets
◆ Dibenzyline Capsules
◆ Dyazide Capsules
◆ Dyrenium Capsules
Ecotrin Duentric Coated Aspirin*
Ecotrin, Maximum Strength Safety-Coated Aspirin Capsules*
Ecotrin, Maximum Strength Tablets*
Ecotrin, Regular Strength Safety-Coated Aspirin Capsules*
◆ Eskalith Capsules
◆ Eskalith Tablets
◆ Eskalith CR Controlled Release Tablets
Feosol Elixir
Feosol Plus Tablets*
Feosol Spansule Capsules*
Feosol Tablets*
◆ Hispril Spansule Capsules
Monocid Injection
Ornacol Capsules*
Ornacol Liquid*
◆ Ornade Spansule Capsules
Ornex Capsules*
Paredrine 1% w/Boric Acid, Ophthalmic Solution
◆ Parnate Tablets
⊞ Pragmatar w/Sulfur & Salicylic Acid Ointment*
SK-Amitriptyline Hydrochloride Tablets
SK-Ampicillin Capsules
SK-Ampicillin For Oral Suspension
SK-Ampicillin-N For Injection
SK-APAP with CODEINE Tablets
SK-Bamate Tablets
SK-Chloral Hydrate Capsules
SK-Chlorothiazide Tablets
SK-Dexamethasone Tablets
SK-Diphenoxylate Tablets
SK-Dipyridamole Tablets
SK-Erythromycin Tablets
SK-Furosemide Tablets
SK-Hydrochlorothiazide Tablets
SK-Lygen Capsules
SK-Metronidazole Tablets
SK-Oxycodone with Acetaminophen Tablets
SK-Oxycodone with Aspirin Tablets
SK-Penicillin G Tablets
SK-Penicillin VK For Oral Solution
SK-Penicillin VK Tablets
SK-Phenobarbital Tablets

(◆ Shown in Product Identification Section) (⊞ Described in PDR For Nonprescription Drugs)

Manufacturers' Index

SK-Potassium Chloride Oral Solution
SK-Pramine Tablets
SK-Prednisone Tablets
SK-Probenecid Tablets
SK-Propantheline Bromide Tablets
SK-Quinidine Sulfate Tablets
SK-Reserpine Tablets
SK-65 APAP Tablets
SK-65 Capsules
SK-65 Compound Capsules
SK-Soxazole Tablets
SK-Terpin Hydrate and Codeine Elixir
SK-Tetracycline Capsules
SK-Tetracycline Syrup
SK-Thioridazine Hydrochloride Tablets
SK-Tolbutamide Tablets
Spansule, sustained release capsules:
◆ 'Combid' Spansule Capsules
◆ 'Compazine' Spansule Capsules
◆ 'Dexedrine' Spansule Capsules
'Feosol' Spansule Capsules
◆ 'Hispril' Spansule Capsules
◆ 'Ornade' Spansule Capsules
◆ 'Temaril' Spansule Capsules
◆ 'Thorazine' Spansule Capsules
◆ 'Tuss-Ornade' Spansule Capsules
Stelazine Concentrate
Stelazine Injection
◆ Stelazine Tablets
Tagamet Injection
Tagamet Liquid
◆ Tagamet Tablets
Teldrin Multi-Symptom Allergy Reliever Capsules*
Teldrin Timed-Release Allergy Capsules*
◆ Temaril Spansule Capsules
Temaril Syrup
◆ Temaril Tablets
Thorazine Concentrate
Thorazine Injection
◆ Thorazine Spansule Capsules
◆ Thorazine Suppositories
Thorazine Syrup
◆ Thorazine Tablets
Troph-Iron Liquid & Tablets*
Trophite Liquid & Tablets*
Tuss-Ornade Liquid
◆ Tuss-Ornade Spansule Capsules
◆ Urispas Tablets
◆ Vontrol Tablets
*A product of Menley & James Laboratories, A SmithKline Beckman Company

SMITHKLINE DIAGNOSTICS, INC. 3017
A SmithKline Beckman Company
P.O. Box 61947
Sunnyvale, CA 94086
Ordering/Pricing/Technical Information:
Toll-free (800) 538-1581
Call Collect in California, Alaska and Hawaii
(408) 732-6000
Products Available
Gastroccult
Hemoccult
Isocult

SMITH LABORATORIES, INC. 437, 1983
2215 Sanders Road
Northbrook, IL 60062
Customer Service & Other Inquiries:
(800) 356-2225
For Medical Emergencies Contact:
Medical Department (312) 564-5700
Products Available
◆ Chymodiactin

SPRINGBOK PHARMACEUTICALS, INC. 1985
12502 South Garden Street
Houston, TX 77071
Address inquiries to:
Ralph Berson (713) 988-7373
For Medical Emergencies Contact:
Rocky Mountain Poison Center
(303) 893-7774
Products Available
E.N.T. Syrup
E.N.T. Tablets
Stopayne Capsules
Stopayne Syrup

E. R. SQUIBB & SONS INC. 437, 1985
General Offices
Post Office Box 4000
Princeton, NJ 08540 (609) 921-4000
Address inquiries to:
Squibb Professional Services Dept.
P.O. Box 4000
Princeton, NJ 08540 (609) 921-4006
Squibb Diagnostics
P.O. Box 191
New Brunswick, NJ 08903
(201) 545-1300
Distribution Centers
ATLANTA, GEORGIA
Post Office Box 16503
Atlanta, GA 30321

State of Ga. Customers Call (800) 282-9103
Customers in States of Ala., Fla., Miss., N.C., S.C., and Tenn. Call (800) 241-1744
All others call (800) 241-5364
For Radiopharmaceuticals (800) 241-8066
CHICAGO, ILLINOIS
Post Office Box 788
Arlington Heights, IL 60006
State of IL Customers Call (800) 942-0674
All others call (800) 323-0665
For Radiopharmaceuticals (800) 323-0831
DALLAS, TEXAS
Mail or telephone orders and customer service inquiries should be directed to Atlanta, GA (see above)
State of MS Customers Call (800) 241-1744
All others call (800) 241-5364
LOS ANGELES, CALIFORNIA
Post Office Box 428
La Mirada, CA 90638
State of CA Customers Call (800) 422-4254
State of HI Customers Call (714) 521-7050
All others call (800) 854-3050
SEATTLE, WASHINGTON
Mail or telephone orders and customer service inquiries should be directed to Los Angeles, CA (see above)
State of AK and MT Customers Call
(714) 521-7050
State of CA Customers Call
(800) 422-4254
All others call (800) 854-3050
NEW YORK AREA
E. R. Squibb & Sons, Inc.
Post Office Box 2013
New Brunswick, NJ 08903
State of ME Customers Call (201) 469-5400
State of NJ Customers Call (800) 352-4865
All others call (800) 631-5244
For Radiopharmaceuticals:
States of NJ and ME (201) 247-8100
All others call (800) 631-5245
For listing of standard and purified insulins, see SQUIBB-NOVO, INC.
Products Available
Aspirin Tablets USP
B Complex Vitamin Tablets
Brewer's Yeast Tablets
Broxodent Automatic-Action Toothbrush
Calcium, Phosphate and Vitamin D Tablets
◆ Capoten
Cardiografin
Castor Oil USP
Chlordiazepoxide Hydrochloride Capsules USP
Chlorothiazide Tablets USP
Cholografin Meglumine
Cholografin Meglumine for Infusion
Cod Liver Oil Capsules
Cod Liver Oil Plain & Mint Flavored
◆ Corgard
◆ Corzide
Crysticillin 300 A.S. & 600 A.S.
Cystografin
Cystografin Dilute
Deladumone
Deladumone OB
Delalutin
Delatestryl
Delestrogen
Diatrizoate Meglumine Injection USP 76%
◆ E.T. The Extra-Terrestrial Children's Chewable Vitamins
◆ E.T. The Extra-Terrestrial Children's Chewable Vitamins with Iron
Engran-HP Tablets
◆ Ethril '250' and Ethril '500' Tablets
Florinef Acetate Tablets
Follutein
Fungizone Cream, Lotion and Ointment
Fungizone for Tissue Culture
Fungizone Intravenous
Gastrografin
Halog Cream, Ointment & Solution
Halog-E Cream
◆ Hydrea Capsules
Iron and Vitamin C Tablets
Kenacort Diacetate Syrup
Kenacort Tablets
Kenalog Cream, Lotion, Ointment, Spray
Kenalog in Orabase
Kenalog-H Cream
Kenalog-10 Injection
Kenalog-40 Injection
Kinevac
Milk of Magnesia Liquid & Tablets
Mineral Oil
Mycolog Cream, Ointment
Mycostatin Cream, Ointment
Mycostatin Oral Suspension
◆ Mycostatin Oral Tablets
Mycostatin Powder (for laboratory use)
Mycostatin Topical Powder
◆ Mycostatin Vaginal Tablets
◆ Mysteclin-F Capsules
Mysteclin-F Syrup
Naturetin Tablets
Naturetin with K Tablets

Niacin Tablets USP
Nitrazine Paper
◆ Noctec Capsules
Noctec Syrup
Nuclear Medicine Products (Radiopharmaceuticals)
 A-C-D Solution Modified
 Albumotope I 131 Diagnostic Injection
 Chromalbin
 Chromitope Sodium Diagnostic Injection
 Cobatope-57 Reference Standard Solution
 Hipputope I 131 Diagnostic Injection
 Intrinsic Factor Concentrate Capsules
 Iodotope I 131 Diagnostic Capsules
 Iodotope I 131 Therapeutic Capsules
 Iodotope I 131 Therapeutic Oral Solution
 MDP-Squibb
 Macrotec
 Minitec
 Phosphotec
 Rubratope-57 Diagnostic Capsules
 Rubratope-57 Diagnostic Kit
 Sethotope
 Techneplex
 Tesuloid
Nydrazid Injection, Tablets
O-V Statin
Ophthaine Solution
Oragrafin Calcium Granules
Oragrafin Sodium Capsules
Ora-Testryl Tablets
Penicillin G Potassium for Injection USP
Penicillin G Sodium for Injection USP
Pentids for Syrup
Pentids '400' for Syrup
◆ Pentids '400' & '800' Tablets
Pentids Tablets
◆ Principen Capsules '250' & '500'
Principen for Oral Suspension '125' & '250'
Principen with Probenecid Capsules
Prolixin Decanoate
Prolixin Enanthate
Prolixin Elixir
Prolixin Injection
◆ Prolixin Tablets
◆ Pronestyl Capsules and Tablets
Pronestyl Injection
◆ Pronestyl-SR Tablets
◆ Raudixin Tablets
Rautrax Tablets
Rautrax-N Modified Tablets
Rautrax-N Tablets
◆ Rauzide Tablets
Renografin-60
Renografin-76
Reno-M-DIP
Reno-M-30
Reno-M-60
Renovist
Renovist II
Renovue-65
Renovue-DIP
Rubramin PC
Saccharin Tablets
Serenium Tablets
Sinografin
Spec-T Sore Throat Anesthetic Lozenges
Spec-T Sore Throat/Cough Suppressant Lozenges
Spec-T Sore Throat/Decongestant Lozenges
Spectrocin Ointment
Sucostrin Injection, High Potency
◆ Sumycin '250' & '500' Capsules
◆ Sumycin '250' and '500' Tablets
Sumycin Syrup
Suppositories, Glycerin, USP
Sweeta Liquid & Tablets
Terfonyl Tablets, Oral Suspension
Teslac Tablets
◆ Theragran Hematinic Tablets
Theragran Liquid
◆ Theragran Stress Formula
◆ Theragran Tablets
◆ Theragran-M Tablets
Trigesic Tablets
◆ Trimox '250' & '500' Capsules
Trimox '125' & '250' For Oral Suspension
Tubocurarine Chloride Injection USP
Valadol Tablets, Liquid
Veetids '125' & '250' for Oral Solution
◆ Veetids '250' & '500' Tablets
◆ Velosef '250' & '500' Capsules
Velosef for Infusion
Velosef for Injection
Velosef '125' & '250' for Oral Suspension
Vesprin Injection
Vesprin Tablets
Vigran plus Iron Tablets
Vigran Tablets
Vitamin A Capsules
Vitamin B₁ Tablets USP
Vitamin B₁₂ Capsules
Vitamin C Tablets
Vitamin E Capsules & Tablets
Yeast Tablets & Flavored Powder
Zinc Oxide Ointment USP

(◆ Shown in Product Identification Section) (⊛ Described in PDR For Nonprescription Drugs)

Manufacturers' Index

SQUIBB/CONNAUGHT, INC. 2033
330 Alexander Street
Princeton, NJ 08540
Address Inquiries and Medical Emergencies to:
Medical Director (609) 683-0400 (or)
 (800) V•A•C•C•I•N•E
Direct orders to:
E. R. Squibb and Sons, Inc.
 (Local Distribution Center)
Products Available
Diphtheria Antitoxin (Purified, Concentrated Globulin-Equine)
Diphtheria & Tetanus Toxoids Adsorbed USP
Diphtheria & Tetanus Toxoids & Pertussis Vaccine Adsorbed (for Pediatric Use)
Fluzone (Influenza Virus Vaccine), Whole Virion and Subvirion, Zonal Purified
Menomune (Meningococcal Polysaccharide Vaccine, Groups A,C,Y,W-135, Combined, and Groups A & C, Combined)
Poliomyelitis Vaccine (Purified) (For the Prevention of Poliomyelitis)
Tetanus Toxoid
Tetanus Toxoid Adsorbed
Tetanus & Diphtheria Toxoids Adsorbed (For Adult Use)
Tubersol (Tuberculin Purified Protein Derivative [Mantoux])
YF-VAX (Yellow Fever Vaccine)(Live, 17D Virus, Avian Leukosis-Free, Stabilized)

SQUIBB-NOVO, INC. 2033
120 Alexander Street
Princeton, NJ 08540
Address inquiries to:
Medical Communications (609) 921-8989
For Medical Emergencies Contact:
Medical Communications (609) 921-8989
Products Available
Lente
Lente Purified Pork Insulin Zinc Suspension
NPH
NPH Purified Pork Isophane Insulin Suspension
Novolin L
Novolin N
Novolin R
Regular Insulin
Regular Purified Pork Insulin
Semilente
Semilente Purified Pork Prompt Insulin Zinc Suspension
Ultralente
Ultralente Purified Beef Extended Insulin Zinc Suspension

STANDARD PROCESS LABORATORIES, INC. 2035
Home Office
2023 West Wisconsin Avenue
Milwaukee, WI 53233 (414) 933-2100
Branch Offices
Campbell, CA 95008
 501-C Vandell Way (408) 866-0707
(Los Angeles)
 City of Commerce, CA 90040
 2401 S. Atlantic Blvd. (213) 263-6133
Orlando, FL 32809
 7653 Currency Dr. (305) 851-6610
Seattle, WA 98101
 930 Terminal Sales Building
 (206) 622-6381
Watertown, MA 02172
 76 Coolidge Hill Road (617) 923-2330
Distributors
Cedar Hill, TX 75104
 1330 E. Wintergreen Road
 (214) 291-4258
Chilton, WI 53014
 253 East Main St. (414) 849-9014
Columbus, OH 43227
 5195 Ivyhurst Dr. (614) 866-5520
Fort Collins, CO 80526
 500 Apple Blossom Lane
 (303) 223-6262
Harrisburg, PA 17112
 5145 Jonestown Road (717) 545-9264
Kansas City, MO 64131
 8433 Passeo (816) 523-7600
Oklahoma City, OK 73112
 3419 N. Roff Ave. (405) 943-1056
Portland, OR 97220
 10704 N.E. Wygant St. (503) 252-2405
St. Joseph, MI 49085
 413 State Street (616) 983-3014
Products Available
Allorganic Trace Minerals-B12
Antronex
Betaine Hydrochloride
Biost Powder
Cal-Amo
Calcium Lactate (Fortified)
Cardio-Plus
Cardiotrophin (Heart)
Catalyn
Cataplex A-F & Betaris
Cataplex E-2

Cataplex F
Chlorophyll Complex Ointment (Fat Soluble)
Chlorophyll Complex Perles (Fat Soluble)
Choline
Comfrey, Pepsin—Formula E-3
Ferroplus
Inositol
Multizyme
Niacinamide B6
Ovex
Pneumotrophin (Lung)
Prost-X
Ribo-Nucleic Acid (RNA)
Thymex
Vasculin
Vitamin B-6 w/Niacinamide
Zypan Tablets

STAR PHARMACEUTICALS, INC. 2035
1990 N.W. 44th Street
R.R. 2, Box 904J
Pompano Beach, FL 33067-9802
Address inquiries to:
Scott L. Davidson, President
 (305) 971-9704
Stellar Pharmacal Corp.
A Star Pharmaceutical Co.,
1990 N.W. 44th St., R.R. 2
Pompano Beach, FL 33067
Address inquiries to:
Scott L. Davidson (305) 972-6060
Branch Office
Panamerican Pharmaceutical Distributors, Inc.
 Reparada Industrial Park
 Estacion #6
 Ponce, PR 00731 (809) 842-6263
Products Available
Prosed
Uro-KP-Neutral
Urolene Blue
Virilon

STELLAR PHARMACAL CORPORATION 2035
1990 N.W. 44th Street
R.R. 2, Box 904J
Pompano Beach, FL 33067-9802
Address inquiries to:
Scott L. Davidson, President
 (305) 971-9704
Branch Offices
Panamerican Pharmaceutical Distributors, Inc.
 Reparada Industrial Park
 Estacion #6
 Ponce, PR 00731 (809) 842-6263
Products Available
▣Star-Otic

STIEFEL LABORATORIES, INC. 2035
2801 Ponce de Leon Blvd.
Coral Gables, FL 33134
Address inquiries to:
Werner K. Stiefel (305) 443-3807
Branch Offices
CALIFORNIA
 P.O. Box 375
 Gardena, CA 90247 (213) 321-4006
GEORGIA
 Post Office Box 47789
 Doraville, GA 30362 (404) 455-1896
NEW YORK
 Route 145
 Oak Hill, NY 12460 (518) 239-6901
PUERTO RICO
 P.O. Box 387
 Mayaguez, PR 00708 (809) 832-1376
Products Available
Acne-Aid Cleansing Bar
Acne-Aid Cream
Acne-Aid Lotion
Benoxyl-5 Lotion
Benoxyl-10 Lotion
Brasivol Base
Brasivol Fine
Brasivol Medium
Brasivol Rough
Duofilm
Ichthyol Ointment
LactiCare Lotion
Lasan Creams, 0.1, 0.2, 0.4%
Lasan HP-1 Cream
Lasan Unguent
Oilatum Soap (Scented)
Oilatum Soap (Unscented)
PanOxyl 5, PanOxyl 10 Acne Gels
PanOxyl AQ 2½, 5 & 10 Acne Gels
PanOxyl Bar 5
PanOxyl Bar 10
Polytar Bath
Polytar Shampoo
Polytar Soap
Salicylic Acid Soap
Salicylic Acid & Sulfur Soap
Saligel
Sarna Lotion
SAStid (AL)

SAStid (Plain)
SAStid Soap
Scabene Lotion
Scabene Shampoo
Sulfoxyl Lotion Regular
Sulfoxyl Lotion Strong
Sulfur Soap
Surfol Bath Oil
Zeasorb Powder

STUART PHARMACEUTICALS 438, 2036
Div. of ICI Americas Inc.
Wilmington, DE 19897
Address inquiries to:
Yvonne Graham, Manager
 Professional Services (302) 575-2231
For Medical Emergencies Contact:
After Hours or On Weekends, call
 (302) 575-3000
Products Available
◆ ALternaGEL Liquid
◆ Bucladin-S Softab
◆ Dialose Capsules
◆ Dialose Plus Capsules
 Effersyllium Instant Mix
◆ Ferancee Tablets
◆ Ferancee-HP Tablets
◆ Hibiclens
◆ Hibiclens Sponge/Brush with Nail Cleaner
◆ Hibistat
◆ Kasof Capsules
◆ Kinesed Tablets
◆ Mulvidren-F Softab
◆ Mylanta Liquid
◆ Mylanta Tablets
◆ Mylanta-II Liquid
◆ Mylanta-II Tablets
 Mylicon Drops
◆ Mylicon Tablets
◆ Mylicon-80 Tablets
◆ Nolvadex Tablets
 Orexin Softab
◆ Probec-T Tablets
◆ Sorbitrate Chewable Tablets
◆ Sorbitrate Oral Tablets
◆ Sorbitrate Sublingual Tablets
◆ Sorbitrate Sustained Action Tablets
◆ The Stuart Formula (Tablets)
◆ Stuart Prenatal Tablets
◆ Stuartinic Tablets
◆ Stuartnatal 1 + 1 Tablets
◆ Tenoretic Tablets
◆ Tenormin Tablets

SWEEN CORPORATION 2047
Sween Building
P.O. Box 980
Lake Crystal, MN 56055 (507) 726-6200
Products Available
Fordustin'
Gentle Rain Shampoo
Methylbenzethonium Chloride
Micro-Guard
Peri-Care
Peri-Wash
Puri-Clens
Surgi-Kleen
Sween-A-Peel
Sween Cream
Sween Kind Touch
Sween Prep
Sween Soft Touch
Whirl-Sol
Xtracare II

SYNTEX (F.P.) INC. 440, 2049
Humacao, Puerto Rico 00661
Address inquiries to:
Syntex Laboratories, Inc. (see below)
Products Available
◆ Brevicon 21-Day Tablets
◆ Brevicon 28-Day Tablets
◆ Norinyl 1+35 21-Day Tablets
◆ Norinyl 1+35 28-Day Tablets
◆ Norinyl 1+50 21-Day Tablets
◆ Norinyl 1+50 28-Day Tablets
◆ Norinyl 1+80 21-Day Tablets
◆ Norinyl 1+80 28-Day Tablets
◆ Norinyl 2 mg. Tablets
◆ Nor-Q.D. Tablets
◆ Tri-Norinyl 21-Day Tablets
◆ Tri-Norinyl 28-Day Tablets
◆ Wallette Pill Dispenser

SYNTEX LABORATORIES, INC. 440, 2049
3401 Hillview Ave.
P.O. Box 10850
Palo Alto, CA 94303
Address Medical inquiries on marketed products to:
General Information (415) 855-5050
Medical Services Dept. (415) 855-5545
Report adverse reactions on marketed
 products to: (415) 852-1386
Products Available
◆ Anadrol-50 Tablets
 Carmol HC Cream
▣ Carmol 10 Lotion
▣ Carmol 20 Cream

(◆ Shown in Product Identification Section) (▣ Described in PDR For Nonprescription Drugs)

Manufacturers' Index

Lidex Cream, Gel, Ointment & Topical Solution
Lidex-E Cream
Nasalide Nasal Solution
Neo-Synalar Cream
Synacort Creams
Synalar Creams, Ointment and Topical Solution
Synalar-HP Cream
Synemol Cream
▩ Topic Gel

SYNTEX PUERTO RICO, INC. 440, 2049
Humacao, Puerto Rico 00661
Address Medical inquires to:
Syntex Laboratories, Inc. (see above)
Products Available
◆ Anaprox Tablets
◆ Naprosyn Tablets

THOMPSON MEDICAL COMPANY, INC. 2065
919 Third Avenue
New York, NY 10022
Address inquiries to:
Medical Services   (212) 688-4420
For Medical Emergencies Contact
Business Hours Only   (212) 688-4420
After Hours or on Weekends
     (212) 594-8855
Products Available
Appedrine, Maximum Strength
Aspercreme
Control Capsules, Maximum Strength
Dexatrim Capsules
Dexatrim Capsules, Extra Strength
Dexatrim Capsules, Extra Strength, Caffeine-Free
Dexatrim Capsules, Extra Strength, Plus Vitamins
Dexatrim • 15
Dexatrim • 15, Caffeine-Free
Prolamine Capsules, Maximum Strength

TRIMEN LABORATORIES, INC. 2067
80 - 26th Street
Pittsburgh, PA 15222
Address inquiries to:
Professional Service Dept. (412) 261-0339
Products Available
Allerid-D.C. Capsules
Allerid-O.D.-8 Capsules
Allerid-O.D.-12 Capsules
Amacodone Tablets
Amaphen Capsules
Amaphen with Codeine #3
Bellermine-O.D. Capsules
Deltamycin Capsules
Deltapen-VK Solution
Deltapen-VK Tablets
Deltavac Cream
Dilart Capsules
Dyrexan-OD Capsules
Fe-O.D. Tablets
Flexaphen Capsules
Hydrex Tablets
Korigesic Tablets
Laxatyl Tablets
Natacomp-FA Tablets
Neurate-400 Tablets
Sorate-5 Chewable Tablets
Sorate-10 Chewable Tablets
Titracid Tablets
Trimedine Expectorant
Viopan-T Tablets

TYSON and ASSOCIATES, INC. 2067
1661 Lincoln Blvd.
Santa Monica, CA 90404
Address Inquiries to:
Professional Services Dept. (213) 452-7844
Products Available
Amino B Plex Tablets
Amino Dox Tablets
Amino GTF Tablets
Amino K Tablets
Amino Lac Capsules
Aminolete
Amino Min D Tablets
Aminomine
Amino Opti C
Amino-Opti-E
Aminoplex Capsules & Powder
Aminosine
Aminostasis Capsules & Powder
Aminotate Capsules & Powder
Amino Vi Min Tablets
Aminoxin
Amino Zn Tablets
DL-Carnitine - Amino Acid Preparation
L-Carnitine
Endorphenyl
Iso-B Caps
Lyte-C
MVM Caps
Max-EPA
Maxovite Tablets
Nutrox Capsules
Optivite Tablets

Pantothenic Acid Capsules
Tyson Amino-ST
Tyson GABA
Tyson L-Alanine Capsules & Powder
Tyson L-Arginine Capsules & Powder
Tyson L-Aspartic Acid Capsules & Powder
Tyson L-Citrulline Capsules & Powder
Tyson L-Cysteine HCl Capsules & Powder
Tyson L-Cystine Capsules & Powder
Tyson L-Dopa
Tyson L-Glutamic Acid Capsules & Powder
Tyson L-Glutamine Caps & Powder
Tyson L-Glutathione
Tyson L-Glycine Capsules & Powder
Tyson L-Histidine Capsules & Powder
Tyson L-Isoleucine Capsules & Powder
Tyson L-Leucine Capsules & Powder
Tyson L-Lysine Powder & Caps
Tyson L-Methionine Powder & Caps
Tyson L-Phenylalanine Capsules & Powder
Tyson L-Proline Capsules & Powder
Tyson L-Serine Capsules & Powder
Tyson L-Threonine Powder & Caps
Tyson L-Tryptophan Capsules & Powder
Tyson L-Tyrosine Capsules & Powder
Tyson L-Valine Powder

UAD LABORATORIES, INC. 2069
6635 Highway 18 West
Jackson, MS 39209
Address inquiries to:
Professional Services Department
     (601) 372-7773
For Medical Emergencies Contact:
     (601) 372-7773
Products Available
AR-600
Adbeon
Adlone 40 and 80
Cezin & Cezin-S
Desone & Desone-LA
Dital
Endafed
Endal Plain
Eudal-SR
Lorcet
Lorcet-HD
Triad & Triad 650
UAD Cream & Cream Lotion
UAD Lotion Forte
UAD Pred
Zone-A Lotion 1%

U. S. ETHICALS INC.
37-02 48th Avenue
Long Island City, NY 11101
Address inquiries to:
Medical Director   (718) 786-8606
     (718) 786-8607
Products Available
Azlytal Tablets
Azmadrine Elixir & Tablets
Azmadrine S.A. Capsules
Bellastal Capsules
Bellastal Elixir & Tablets
Capa Tablets
Declofen SR Capsules
Eclabron Capsules
Eclabron Elixir (See Wharton Laboratories)
Eclabron-T/SR Capsules
Eclamide Capsules
Eclasufed Capsules
Eclasufed SR Capsules
Etnapa Elixir
Etnergan Syrup
Ferbetrin Tablets & Syrup
Gastrical Tablets
Geristone Capsules
Hepaferron Syrup
Histabs Tablets
Klavikordal Tablets
Natalac Capsules
Natalac Forte Capsules
Neocomplex Injection
Neodex Tablets & Syrup
Nicostrol Capsules
Niong Tablets
Nitromed
Nitronet Tablets
Nitrong Ointment (See Wharton Laboratories)
Nitrong Tablets (See Wharton Laboratories)
Nitrong SR Tablets (See Wharton Laboratories)
Supervim Drops, Tablets & Syrup
Ulcinal Tablets
Vitacoms Capsules

U.S. PHARMACEUTICAL CORPORATION 2070
2500 Park Central Blvd.
Decatur, GA 30030   (404) 987-4745
Mailing Address:
P.O. Box 1165
Decatur, GA 30030
Address inquiries to:
Marketing Director   (404) 987-4745
Products Available
Hemocyte Plus Tabules
Hemocyte Tablets

Hemocyte-F Tablets
Isovex Capsules
Magsal Tablets
Mediplex Tabules

USV LABORATORIES, DIVISION 440, 2070
USV PHARMACEUTICAL CORP.
303 South Broadway
Tarrytown, NY 10591
Address inquiries to:
Medical Department (914) 631-8500
Nights, Weekends and Holidays, call
     (914) 779-6300

USV LABORATORIES Inc. 440, 2070
Manati, Puerto Rico 00701
Address inquiries to:
USV Pharmaceutical Corp.   (see above)

USV (P.R.) DEVELOPMENT 440, 2070
CORP.
Manati, Puerto Rico 00701
Address inquiries to:
USV Pharmaceutical Corp.   (see above)
Products Available
◆ Arlidin Tablets
◆ Armour Thyroid Tablets
Azolid Capsules & Tablets
Bi-K
Biopar Forté
◆ Calcimar Solution
Cerespan Capsules
Chymoral
Chymoral-100
◆ DDAVP
◆ DDAVP Injection
◆ Demi-Regroton Tablets
Doriden Tablets
Histaspan-D Capsules
Histaspan-Plus Capsules
◆ Hygroton Tablets
◆ Levothroid for Injection
◆ Levothroid Tablets
◆ Lozol Tablets
◆ Nicobid
◆ Nicolar Tablets
◆ Nitrospan Capsules
Oxalid Tablets
Panthoderm Cream
Pentritol
◆ Pertofrane Capsules
◆ Regroton Tablets
Thyrar
◆ Thyrolar Tablets
Tussar DM
Tussar SF
Tussar-2

ULMER PHARMACAL COMPANY 2092
(A Krelitz Industries Company)
2440 Fernbrook Lane
Minneapolis, MN 55441
Address inquiries to:
Professional Service Dept. (612) 559-5887
In MN (800) 292-7918
In USA (800) 328-7157
Products Available
Aerosan
Andoin Ointment
Bi-Amine
Chloral Methylol Ointment
▩ Clinitar Cream
▩ Clinitar Shampoo
▩ Clinitar Stick
Gentle Shampoo
Kler-ro Liquid
Kler-ro Powder
Liquid Lather
▩ Lobana Bath Oil
▩ Lobana Body Lotion
▩ Lobana Body Powder
▩ Lobana Body Shampoo
▩ Lobana Conditioning Shampoo
▩ Lobana Derm-ADE Cream
▩ Lobana Liquid Hand Soap
▩ Lobana Peri-Gard
▩ Lobana Perineal Cleanse
M.O.M. - Suspension of Magnesium Hydroxide
Pheneen Solution
Reagent Alcohol
Surgel Liquid
Ta-Poff
Ta-Poff Aerosol
Ultracaine Injection
Versa-Quat
Verucid Gel
Vitamin A & D Ointment
▩ Vleminckx' Solution

THE UPJOHN COMPANY 440, 2092
7000 Portage Road
Kalamazoo, MI 49001
     (616) 323-4000
THE UPJOHN MANUFACTURING COMPANY
Barceloneta, Puerto Rico 00617
     (809) 846-4900

(◆ Shown in Product Identification Section)   (▩ Described in PDR For Nonprescription Drugs)

Manufacturers' Index

Emergency Medical Information
(616) 323-6615
Address inquiries to:
Medical Information
The Upjohn Company
Kalamazoo, MI 49001

Pharmaceutical Sales Areas and Distribution Centers

Atlanta (Chamblee), GA 30341	(404) 451-4822
Boca Raton, FL 33432	(305) 392-8500
Boston (Wellesley), MA 02181	(617) 431-7970
Buffalo (Cheektowaga), NY 14225	(716) 681-7160
Chicago (Oak Brook), IL 60521	(312) 654-3300
Cincinnati, OH 45237	(513) 242-4574
Dallas, TX 75204	(214) 824-3028
Denver, CO 80216	(303) 399-3113
Hartford (Enfield), CT 06082	(203) 741-3421
Honolulu, HI 96813	(808) 538-1181
Kalamazoo, MI 49001	(616) 323-7222
Kansas City, MO 64131	(816) 361-2291
Los Angeles, CA 90038	(213) 463-8101
Memphis, TN 38122	(901) 761-4170
Minneapolis, MN 55422	(612) 588-2786
New York (Garden City), NY 11530	(516) 294-3530
Orlando, FL 32809	(305) 859-4591
Philadelphia (Wayne), PA 19087	(215) 265-2100
Pittsburgh, (Bridgeville), PA 15017	(412) 257-0200
Portland, OR 97232	(503) 232-2133
St. Louis, MO 63146	(314) 872-8626
San Francisco (Palo Alto), CA 94306	(415) 493-8080
Washington, DC 20011	(202) 882-6163

Products Available
- ◆ Adeflor Chewable Tablets
- Adeflor Drops
- Adeflor M Tablets
- Albamycin Capsules
- Alkets Tablets
- Atgam Sterile Solution
- ▣ Baciguent Antibiotic Ointment
- Baciguent Ophthalmic Ointment
- Bacitracin, USP, Sterile Powder
- Berubigen Sterile Solution
- Calcium Chloride Injection, USP, Sterile Solution
- Calcium Gluconate Injection, USP, Sterile Solution
- Calcium Gluconate Tablets, USP
- Calcium Lactate Tablets, USP
- Calderol Capsules
- Cebenase Tablets
- Cheracol Cough Syrup
- ▣ Cheracol D Cough Syrup
- ▣ Cheracol Plus Head Cold/Cough Formula
- ▣ Citrocarbonate Antacid
- ◆ Cleocin HCl Capsules*
- Cleocin Pediatric Flavored Granules*
- ◆ Cleocin Phosphate Sterile Solution*
- ◆ Cleocin T Topical Solution*
- Clocream Skin Cream
- Colestid Granules
- ▣ Cortaid Cream
- ▣ Cortaid Lotion
- ▣ Cortaid Ointment
- ▣ Cortaid Spray
- Cortef Acetate Ointment
- Cortef Acetate Sterile Suspensiion
- ▣ Cortef Feminine Itch Cream
- Cortef Oral Suspension
- ▣ Cortef Rectal Itch Ointment
- Cortef Sterile Suspension IM
- Cortef Tablets
- Cortisone Acetate Tablets, USP
- Cytosar-U Sterile Powder
- Delta-Cortef Tablets
- ◆ Deltasone Tablets
- Depo-Estradiol Sterile Solution
- ◆ Depo-Medrol Sterile Aqueous Suspension
- Depo-Provera Sterile Aqueous Suspension
- Depo-Testadiol Sterile Solution
- Depo-Testosterone Sterile Solution
- ◆ Didrex Tablets
- Diostate D Tablets
- E-Mycin E Liquid
- ◆ E-Mycin Tablets
- ◆ Erythromycin Tablets (E-Mycin)
- Feminone Tablets
- Gelfilm Sterile Film
- Gelfilm Sterile Ophthalmic Film
- Gelfoam Dental Packs
- Gelfoam Packs
- Gelfoam Prostatectomy Cones
- Gelfoam Sterile Compressed Sponge
- Gelfoam Sterile Powder
- Gelfoam Sterile Sponge
- ◆ Halcion Tablets
- Halodrin Tablets
- ◆ Halotestin Tablets
- Heparin Sodium Injection, USP, Sterile Solution
- Hydrocortisone Acetate, U.S.P.; Micronized, Nonsterile Powder (For Prescription Compounding)
- Hydrocortisone, U.S.P. Micronized, Nonsterile Powder (For Prescription Compounding)
- ▣ Kaopectate Anti-Diarrhea Medicine
- Kaopectate Anti-Diarrhea Medicine (Bilingual) (English & Spanish labeling)
- ▣ Kaopectate Tablet Formula
- Lincocin Capsules
- Lincocin Pediatric Capsules
- Lincocin Sterile Solution
- Lipomul Oral Liquid
- ◆ Loniten Tablets
- ◆ Maolate Tablets
- Medrol ADT Pak Unit of Use
- Medrol Acetate Topical
- ◆ Medrol Dosepak Unit of Use
- Medrol Enpak Kit
- Medrol Enpak (Refill)
- ◆ Medrol Tablets
- Micronase Tablets
- ◆ Motrin Tablets*
- Mycifradin Oral Solution
- Mycifradin Sterile Powder
- Mycifradin Tablets
- ▣ Myciguent Antibiotic Cream & Ointment
- ▣ Mycitracin Antibiotic Ointment
- Neo-Cortef Cream
- Neo-Cortef Ointment
- Neo-Cortef Ophthalmic Suspension
- Neo-Delta-Cortef Ointment
- Neo-Delta-Cortef Ophthalmic Suspension
- Neo-Medrol Acetate Topical
- Orinase Diagnostic Sterile Powder
- ◆ Orinase Tablets
- Orthoxicol Cough Syrup
- P-A-C Revised Formula Analgesic Tablets
- Pamine Tablets
- Panmycin Capsules
- Phenolax Wafers
- Prostin VR Pediatric Sterile Solution
- Protamine Sulfate for Injection, USP, Sterile Powder
- ◆ Provera Tablets
- ▣ Pyrroxate Capsules
- Sigtab Tablets
- Sodium Chloride Injection, (Bacteriotstic) USP, Sterile Solution
- Solu-Cortef Sterile Powder
- ◆ Solu-Medrol Mix-O-Vial & Vials
- ◆ Solu-Medrol Sterile Powder
- Super D Perles
- ◆ Tolinase Tablets
- Trobicin Sterile Powder
- ▣ Unicap Capsules & Tablets
- ▣ Unicap Chewable Tablets
- ▣ Unicap M Tablets
- ▣ Unicap Plus Iron Tablets
- ▣ Unicap Senior Tablets
- ▣ Unicap T Tablets
- Upjohn Vitamin E Capsules, 200 I.U.
- Uracil Mustard Capsules
- Uticillin VK Tablets
- Water for Injection (Bacteriostatic), USP, Sterile Solution
- ◆ Xanax Tablets
- Zanosar Sterile Powder
- Zymacap Capsules

*Product of The Upjohn Manufacturing Company

UPSHER-SMITH LABORATORIES, INC.   2144
14905 23rd Avenue North
Minneapolis, MN 55441
Address inquiries to:
Professional Service Department
(612) 473-4412
For Medical Emergencies Contact:
Scientific Affairs Department
(612) 473-4412

Products Available
- Acetaminophen Uniserts Suppositories
- Aspirin Uniserts Suppositories
- Bisacodyl Tablets
- Bisacodyl Uniserts Suppositories
- Daily-M Tablets
- Docusate Sodium Capsules
- Docusate Sodium with Casanthranol Capsules
- Ferrous Gluconate Tablets
- Ferrous Sulfate Tablets
- Hemorrhoidal Uniserts Suppositories
- Hemorrhoidal-HC Uniserts Suppositories
- Hexavitamin Tablets
- Histatapp Elixir
- Histatapp T.D. Tablets
- Kerasol Therapeutic Bath Oil
- Klor-Con Powder
- Klor-Con/25 Powder
- Klor-Con 20% Solution
- Klor-10% Solution
- ▣ Lubrin Vaginal Lubricating Inserts
- Methocarbamol Tablets
- Papaverine Hydrochloride T.R. Capsules
- RMS Suppositories
- SSKI
- Sorbitol Solution
- Spironolactone Tablets
- Spironolactone w/Hydrochlorothiazide Tablets
- Stress-600 Tablets
- Stress-600 with Zinc
- Therapeutic B Complex with C Capsules
- Therapeutic Multivitamin Tablets
- Therapeutic Multivitamin & Mineral Tablets
- Trofan Tablets (L-Tryptophan)
- Zinc Sulfate Capsules

THE VALE CHEMICAL CO., INC.   2145
1201 Liberty St.
Allentown, PA 18102
Address inquiries to:
Elliot R. Davis   (215) 433-7579

Products Available
- Acedoval Tablets
- Acedyne Tablets
- Alkaline Aromatic Tablets
- Aluminum Hydroxide Gel, Tablets
- Aminophyllin Tablets
- Ammonium Chloride Tablets
- Antrin Tablets
- Aquabase (Beeler's) Hydrophyllic Ointment Base
- Ascorbic Acid Tablets
- Aspirin Tablets, 5 gr. & 10 gr.
- Aspir-10 Tablets
- Barbeloid Tablets
- Belexal Tablets
- Benzo-Menth Lozenges
- Biothesin Tablets
- Bipectol Wafers
- Bismapec Tablets
- Butalix
- Calcium Gluconate Tablets
- Calfos-D Tablets
- Dermaval Cream
- Double-Sal Tablets
- Dovacet Capsules
- Duphrene Syrup & Tablets
- Ephedrine & Sodium Phenobarbital Tablets
- Ephedrine Sulfate Capsules
- Extract of Ox Bile Tablets
- Ferate-C Tablets
- Flatulence Tablets
- Glucovite Tablets
- Glycofed
- ▣ Glycotuss Syrup & Tablets
- Glycotuss-dM Syrup & Tablets
- Guiosan Syrup
- Hydra-Mag Tablets
- Ironco-B Tablets
- Magmalin Tablets & Suspension
- Mandex Tablets
- Methenamine & Acid Sodium Phosphate Tablets
- Methiokap Capsules
- Neocet Tablets
- Neofed
- Neogesic Tablets
- Neo-Tab Tablets
- Nevrotose Capsutabs
- Niacin Tablets
- Nisaval Tablets
- Nyral Lozenges
- Obeval Tablets
- Oxynitral w/Veratrum Viride Tablets
- Pedric Elixir & Tablets
- Pedric Senior Tablets
- Phenobarbital Tablets
- Potassium Iodide Tablets
- Rauval Tablets
- Rhinogesic Tablets
- Rhinogesic-GG Tablets
- Serpate Tablets
- Sodium Butabarbital Tablets
- Sodium Salicylate Tablets
- Soothogel Cream
- Synthetar Cream
- Taurophyllin Tablets
- Taystron Tablets
- Terphan Elixir
- Thiamine Hydrochloride Tablets
- Thyroid Tablets
- Tono-B, Wafers
- Trioval Tablets
- Triple Sulfoid Tablets
- V-M Capsules
- Valacet Tablets
- Valax Tablets
- Valcaine Ointment
- Valcreme Lotion
- Valdeine Tablets
- Valdrene Expectorant Syrup
- Valdrene Tablets
- Val-Tep Tablets

VEREX LABORATORIES, INC.   442, 2145
8925 East Nichols Avenue
Englewood, CO 80112
(303) 799-4499
For Medical Emergencies Contact:
James M. Dunn, M.D.   (303) 799-4499

Products Available
- ◆ Help
- ◆ Verin

(◆ Shown in Product Identification Section)   (▣ Described in PDR For Nonprescription Drugs)

Manufacturers' Index

VICKS HEALTH CARE DIVISION   2146
Richardson-Vicks Inc.
10 Westport Road
Wilton, CT 06897
Address inquiries to:
Vicks Research Center   (203) 929-2500
For Medical Emergencies Contact
Medical Director
Vicks Research Center   (203) 929-2500
Products Available
▣ Daycare Daytime Colds Medicine-liquid
▣ Daycare Multi-Symptom Colds Medicine-capsules
▣ Formula 44 Cough Control Disc
▣ Formula 44 Cough Mixture
▣ Formula 44D Decongestant Cough Mixture
▣ Headway Capsules
▣ Headway Tablets
▣ Nyquil Nighttime Colds Medicine
▣ Oracin Cherry Flavor Cooling Throat Lozenges
▣ Oracin Cooling Throat Lozenges
▣ Sinex Decongestant Nasal Spray
▣ Sinex Long-Acting Decongestant Nasal Spray
▣ Tempo Antacid with Antigas Action
▣ Vaposteam
▣ Vatronol Nose Drops
▣ Vicks Cough Silencers Cough Drops
▣ Vicks Cough Syrup
▣ Vicks Inhaler
▣ Vicks Throat Lozenges
▣ Vicks Vaporub

VICKS PHARMACY PRODUCTS DIVISION   442, 2146
Richardson-Vicks Inc.
10 Westport Road
Wilton, CT 06897
Address inquiries to:
Vicks Research Center
                              (203) 929-2500
For Medical Emergencies Contact:
Medical Director, Vicks Research Center
                              (203) 929-2500
Products Available
◆ Cremacoat 1
◆ Cremacoat 2
◆ Cremacoat 3
◆ Cremacoat 4
◆ Percogesic Analgesic Tablets

VITALINE FORMULAS   2148
P.O. Box 6757
Incline Village, NV 89450
Address inquiries to:
Jed D. Meese,
Technical Director   (702) 831-5656
Products Available
Alka Aid (antacid)
B Complex 50 & 100
B Complex 50 & 100 (controlled time release)
Calcium (oyster shell)
Calcium (Vita Calcium)
Cal-Mag Aspartate (calcium/magnesium)
Chromium
Digestive Enzymes (chewable)
Digestive Supplement
E-Pherol (vitamin E succinate)
Enviro-Stress with Zinc & Selenium
Free Form Amino Acids
Fructose Wafers (orange, peanut, banana, strawberry & root beer)
Iron (Chelated Iron Plus)
L-Neuramine
Lipo Plus (lipotropics)
Magna Zinc (zinc 30 mg)
Magnesium (Cal-Mag Aspartate)
Magnesium (Vita-Mag)
Manganese
Multimineral Plus
NORx (appetite suppressant)
Oyster Shell Calcium
Pancreatin Tablets 2400 mg. N.F. (High Lipase)
Pantothenic Acid
Potassium Gluconate
Protein Powder
Protein Wafers (chewable)
S.O.D. (Superoxide Dismutase)
Selenium Tablets (200 mcg)
StimuLean (appetite suppressant)
Total Formula
Vitamin A (with beta carotene)
Vitamin B-6 200 mg
Vitamin B-6 200 mg (controlled time release)
Vitamin C 1000 mg (controlled time release)
Vitamin C 1000 mg with Bioflavonoids
Vitamin D-3 400 I.U.
Vitamin E 400 I.U. Capsules
Vitamin E 400 I.U. (E-Pherol)
Zinc 220 mg.

WALKER, CORP & CO., INC.   2148
Easthampton Pl. & N. Collingwood Ave.
Syracuse, NY 13201

Address inquiries to:
P.O. Box 1320
Syracuse, NY 13201   (315) 463-4511
Products Available
Evac-U-Gen

WALKER PHARMACAL COMPANY   2148
4200 Laclede Avenue
St. Louis, MO 63108
Address inquiries to:
Customer Service   (314) 533-9600
Products Available
Succus Cineraria Maritima

WALLACE LABORATORIES   442, 2149
P.O. Box 1
Cranbury, NJ 08512
Address inquiries to:
Professional Services   (609) 655-6000
Night and Weekend Emergencies
                           (609) 799-1167
Send all orders to:
Wallace Laboratories
Div. of Carter-Wallace, Inc.
Post Office Drawer 5
Cranbury, NJ 08512
Products Available
◆ Aquatensen Tablets
Avazyme/Avazyme-100 Tablets
Barbidonna Elixir & Tablets
Barbidonna No. 2 Tablets
Butibel Elixir & Tablets
Buticaps
◆ Butisol Sodium Elixir & Tablets
Covanamine Liquid
Covangesic Tablets
Dainite Tablets
Dainite-KI Tablets
Depen Titratable Tablets
Deprol Tablets
Diutensen Tablets
◆ Diutensen-R Tablets
Lufyllin Elixir
Lufyllin Injection
◆ Lufyllin & Lufyllin-400 Tablets
Lufyllin-EPG Elixir & Tablets
Lufyllin-GG Elixir & Tablets
▣ Maltsupex Liquid, Powder & Tablets
Meprospan Capsules
Micrainin
◆ Milpath Tablets
Milprem Tablets
◆ Miltown Tablets
◆ Miltown 600 Tablets
Miltrate Tablets
◆ Organidin Elixir, Solution & Tablets
◆ Rondomycin Capsules
▣ Ryna Liquid
▣ Ryna-C Liquid
▣ Ryna-CX Liquid
Rynatan Pediatric Suspension
◆ Rynatan Tablets
Rynatuss Pediatric Suspension
◆ Rynatuss Tablets
◆ Soma Tablets
◆ Soma Compound Tablets
◆ Soma Compound w/Codeine Tablets
Syllact Powder
Syllamalt Powder
◆ Theo-Organidin Elixir
◆ Tussi-Organidin DM Liquid
◆ Tussi-Organidin Liquid
◆ VōSol HC Otic Solution
◆ VōSol Otic Solution

WEBCON PHARMACEUTICALS   2171
Division of Alcon (Puerto Rico) Inc.
Post Office Box 3000
Humacao, Puerto Rico 00661
Address inquiries to:
Medical Department
Post Office Box 1959
Fort Worth, TX 76101   (817) 293-0450
Products Available
Alconefrin 12 Drops
Alconefrin 25 Drops
Alconefrin 50 Drops
Alconefrin 25 Spray
Anestacon Sterile Solution
Aquachloral
Azo-Standard Tablets
B & O No. 15A & No. 16A Supprettes
Cystospaz Tablets
Cystospaz-M Capsules
Neopap Supprettes
Urised Tablets
Urisedamine Tablets
WANS Children Supprettes
WANS No. 1 & No. 2 Supprettes

WESTWOOD PHARMACEUTICALS INC.   442, 2174
100 Forest Avenue
Buffalo, NY 14213
Address inquiries to:
Consumer Affairs Department
                           (716) 887-3773

Products Available
Alpha Keri Shower and Bath Oil
Alpha Keri Soap
Balnetar
Capitrol Cream Shampoo
Desquam-X 2.5 Gel
Desquam-X 5 Gel
Desquam-X 10 Gel
Desquam-X 5 Wash
Desquam-X 10 Wash
Estar Gel
Eurax Cream & Lotion
Fostex Medicated Cleansing Bar
Fostex Medicated Cleansing Cream
Fostex 5% Benzoyl Peroxide Gel
Fostex 10% Benzoyl Peroxide Cleansing Bar
Fostex 10% Benzoyl Peroxide Gel
Fostex 10% Benzoyl Peroxide Tinted Cream
Fostex 10% Benzoyl Peroxide Wash
Fostril
Halotex Cream & Solution
Keralyt Gel
Keri Creme
Keri Facial Soap
Keri Lotion
Lowila Cake
Moisturel
Pernox Lotion
Pernox Medicated Lathering Scrub
Pernox Shampoo
PreSun 4 Creamy Sunscreen
PreSun 8 Lotion, Creamy & Gel
PreSun 15 Creamy Sunscreen
PreSun 15 Sunscreen Lotion
Sebucare
Sebulex & Sebulex Cream Shampoo
Sebulex Shampoo with Conditioners
Sebulon Dandruff Shampoo
Sebutone & Sebutone Cream Shampoo
Staticin (erythromycin) 1.5% Topical Solution
T-Stat (erythromycin) 2.0% Topical Solution
◆ Tacaryl Chewable Tablets
◆ Tacaryl Syrup & Tablets
Transact
Westcort Cream
Westcort Ointment 0.2%

WHARTON LABORATORIES, INC.   2184
37-02 48th Ave.
Long Island City, NY 11101
Address inquiries to:
Medical Director   (718) 786-8606
                              (718) 786-8607
Products Available
Eclabron Elixir
Nitrong Ointment
Nitrong Ointment, Unit Dose
Nitrong 2.6 mg. Tablets
Nitrong 6.5 mg. Tablets
Nitrong 9 mg. Tablets
Nitrong SR 2.6 mg. Tablets
Nitrong SR 6.5 mg. Tablets

WHITEHALL LABORATORIES INC.   443, 2184
Division of American Home Products Corporation
685 Third Avenue
New York, NY 10017
Address Inquiries to:
Medical Department   (212) 878-5508
Products Available
◆ Advil Ibuprofen Tablets
◆ Anacin Analgesic Capsules
◆ Anacin Analgesic Tablets
◆ Anacin Maximum Strength Analgesic Capsules
◆ Anacin Maximum Strength Analgesic Tablets
◆ Anacin-3, Children's Acetaminophen Chewable Tablets, Elixir, Drops
◆ Anacin-3, Maximum Strength Acetaminophen Tablets and Capsules
◆ Anacin-3, Regular Strength Acetaminophen Tablets
◆ Anbesol Baby Teething Gel Antiseptic Anesthetic
◆ Anbesol Gel Antiseptic Anesthetic
◆ Anbesol Liquid Antiseptic Anesthetic
◆ Arthritis Pain Formula By the Makers of Anacin Analgesic Tablets
◆ Arthritis Pain Formula Aspirin-Free By the Makers of Anacin Analgesic Tablets
◆ Arthritis Pain Formula Safety-Coated by the Makers of Anacin Analgesic Tablets
Bisodol Antacid Powder
Bisodol Antacid Tablets
Bronitin Asthma Tablets
Bronitin Mist
Compound W Solution & Gel
Denalan Denture Cleanser

(◆ Shown in Product Identification Section)   (▣ Described in PDR For Nonprescription Drugs)

Manufacturers' Index

- ◆ Denorex Medicated Shampoo and Conditioner
- ◆ Denorex Medicated Shampoo, Regular & Mountain Fresh Herbal Scent
- ◆ Dristan, Advanced Formula Decongestant/Antihistamine/Analgesic Capsules
- ◆ Dristan, Advanced Formula Decongestant/Antihistamine/Analgesic Tablets
- Dristan Cough Formula
- Dristan Inhaler
- ◆ Dristan Long Lasting Nasal Spray, Regular & Menthol
- ◆ Dristan Nasal Spray, Regular & Menthol
- Dristan Room Vaporizer
- Dristan 12-Hour Nasal Decongestant Capsules
- ◆ Dristan Ultra Colds Formula Aspirin-Free Analgesic/Decongestant/Antihistamine/ Cough Suppressant Nighttime Liquid
- ◆ Dristan Ultra Colds Formula Aspirin-Free Analgesic/Decongestant/Antihistamine/ Cough Suppressant Tablets and Capsules
- Dristan-AF Decongestant/Antihistamine/ Analgesic Tablets
- Dry and Clear Acne Medication Lotion
- Dry and Clear Double Strength Cream
- Dry and Clear Medicated Acne Cleanser
- Freezone Solution
- Heather Feminine Deodorant Spray
- Heet Analgesic Liniment
- Heet Spray Analgesic
- InfraRub Analgesic Cream
- ◆ Medicated Cleansing Pads By the Makers of Preparation H Hemorrhoidal Remedies
- Momentum Muscular Backache Formula
- Neet Aerosol Depilatory
- Neet Depilatory Cream
- Neet Depilatory Lotion
- Outgro Solution
- Oxipor VHC Lotion for Psoriasis
- Predictor In-Home Early Pregnancy Test
- ◆ Preparation H Hemorrhoidal Ointment
- ◆ Preparation H Hemorrhoidal Suppositories
- Prepcort Hydrocortisone Cream 0.5%
- ◆ Primatene Mist
- Primatene Mist Suspension
- ◆ Primatene Tablets-M Formula
- ◆ Primatene Tablets-P Formula
- Quiet World Analgesic/Sleeping Aid
- ◆ Semicid Vaginal Contraceptive Suppositories
- Sleep-eze 3 Tablets
- Sudden Action Breath Freshener
- Sudden Beauty Country Air Mask
- Sudden Beauty Hair Spray
- Trendar Premenstrual Tablets
- Viro-Med Liquid
- Viro-Med Tablets

WILLEN DRUG COMPANY   2187
18 North High St.
Baltimore, MD 21202   (301) 752-1865
Products Available
- Bicitra—Sugar-Free
- Neutra-Phos Powder & Capsules
- Neutra-Phos-K Powder & Capsules
- Polycitra Syrup
- Polycitra-K Syrup
- Polycitra-LC—Sugar-Free

WINTHROP-BREON   443, 2189, 3018
LABORATORIES
90 Park Avenue
New York, NY 10016   (212) 907-2000
Professional Services Department
    (212) 907-2525
For INOCOR information:
Call toll-free   1-800-4INOCOR
Products Available
- Amipaque
- Anti-Rust Tablets
- Aralen Hydrochloride Injection
- ◆ Aralen Phosphate Tablets
- Aralen Phosphate w/Primaquine Phosphate
- Atabrine Hydrochloride Tablets
- Atropine & Demerol Carpuject
- ◆ Bilopaque Sodium
- Breonesin
- Bronkephrine Injection
- Bronkodyl
- Bronkolixir
- Bronkometer Aerosol
- Bronkosol
- Bronkotabs Tablets
- Carbocaine Hydrochloride Injection
- Codeine Phosphate Carpuject
- ◆ Danocrine
- ◆ Demerol APAP Tablets
- Demerol Carpuject
- Demerol Hydrochloride Injection
- Demerol Hydrochloride Syrup
- ◆ Demerol Hydrochloride Tablets
- Demerol Uni-Amp
- Dextrose Injection, 10%
- Drisdol 50,000 Unit Capsules
- Drisdol in Propylene Glycol
- Empty Sterile Carpuject
- ◆ Fergon Capsules
- Fergon Elixir
- Fergon Plus Caplets
- ◆ Fergon Tablets
- Heparin Lock Flush Solution Carpuject
- Heparin Sodium Carpuject
- HEP-PAK Convenience Package
- Hydromorphone Carpuject
- Hydroxyzine Carpuject
- Hypaque Meglumine 30%
- Hypaque Meglumine 60%
- Hypaque Sodium Oral Powder
- Hypaque Sodium Oral Solution
- Hypaque Sodium 20%
- Hypaque Sodium 25%
- Hypaque Sodium 50% Injection
- Hypaque-Cysto
- Hypaque-M, 75% Injection
- Hypaque-M, 90% Injection
- Hypaque-76 Injection
- Hytakerol Capsules & Liquid
- Inocor Lactate Injection
- Isuprel Hydrochloride Compound Elixir
- ◆ Isuprel Hydrochloride Glossets
- Isuprel Hydrochloride Injection 1:5000
- Isuprel Hydrochloride Mistometer
- Isuprel Hydrochloride Solution 1:200 & 1:100
- Kayexalate
- Levophed Bitartrate Injection
- Lotusate Caplets
- Luminal Ovoids
- Luminal Sodium Injection
- Marcaine Hydrochloride Injection
- Marcaine Hydrochloride with Epinephrine 1:200,000
- Marcaine Spinal
- Measurin Tablets
- ◆ Mebaral Tablets
- Morphine Sulfate Carpuject
- Mytelase Chloride Caplets
- ◆ NegGram Caplets
- NegGram Suspension
- Neo-Synephrine Hydrochloride 1% Carpuject
- Neo-Synephrine Hydrochloride 1% Injection
- Neo-Synephrine Hydrochloride (Ophthalmic)
- Novocain Hydrochloride for Spinal Anesthesia
- Novocain Hydrochloride Injection
- Pediacof Cough Syrup
- pHisoDerm
- pHisoHex
- pHisoScrub
- ◆ Plaquenil Sulfate Tablets
- Pontocaine Hydrochloride Eye Ointment
- Pontocaine Hydrochloride for Spinal Anesthesia
- Pontocaine Hydrochloride Topical Solution
- Primaquine Phosphate Tablets
- Sodium Chloride Carpuject
- Sulfamylon Acetate Cream
- ◆ Talacen
- Talwin Ampuls
- Talwin Carpuject
- Talwin Compound
- Talwin Injection
- ◆ Talwin Nx
- Telepaque Tablets
- ◆ Trancopal Caplets
- Vitamins
  - Vitamin D, USP
    - Drisdol 50,000 Unit Capsules
    - Drisdol in Propylene Glycol
- ◆ Winstrol Tablets
- Zephiran Chloride Aqueous Solution
- Zephiran Chloride Concentrate Solution
- Zephiran Chloride Spray
- Zephiran Chloride Tinted Tincture
- Zephiran Towelettes

WINTHROP CONSUMER PRODUCTS
- Astring-o-sol
- ▣ Bronkaid Mist
- ▣ Bronkaid Mist Suspension
- ▣ Bronkaid Tablets
- ▣ Campho-Phenique Lip Balm
- Caroid Laxative
- Caroid Tooth Powder
- Creamalin Tablets
- ▣ Haley's M-O, Regular & Flavored Mucilose Powder
- ▣ NTZ Long Acting Spray & Drops
- NāSal Saline Nasal Spray
- NāSal Saline Nose Drops
- Neocurtasal
- Neo-Synephrine Jelly
- ▣ Neo-Synephrine Nasal Spray (Mentholated)
- ▣ Neo-Synephrine Nasal Sprays
- ▣ Neo-Synephrine Nose Drops
- ▣ Neo-Synephrine 12 Hour Nasal Spray
- ▣ Neo-Synephrine 12 Hour Nose Drops (Adult & Children's Strengths)
- ▣ Neo-Synephrine 12 Hour Vapor Nasal Spray
- ▣ Neo-Synephrine II Long Acting Nasal Spray
- ▣ Neo-Synephrine II Long Acting Nose Drops (Adult & Children's Strengths)
- ▣ Neo-Synephrine II Long Acting Vapor Nasal Spray
- ▣ pHisoAc BP
- pHisoDan
- ▣ pHisoDerm Regular & Fresh Scent
- ▣ pHisoPUFF
- Soapure
- ▣ WinGel Liquid & Tablets

WYETH LABORATORIES   444, 2234
Division of American Home Products Corporation
P.O. Box 8299
Philadelphia, PA 19101
Address inquiries to:
Professional Service   (215) 341-2220
For Medical Emergency Information
Day or night call   (215) 688-4400
Wyeth Distribution Centers:
Andover, MA 01810
   P.O. Box 1776   (617) 475-9075
Atlanta, GA 30302
   P.O. Box 4365   (404) 873-1681
Baltimore, MD 21224
   101 Kane St.   (301) 633-4000
Boston Distribution Center,
   see under Andover, MA
Buena Park, CA 90622-5000
   P.O. Box 5000   (714) 523-5500
    (Los Angeles) (213) 627-5374
Chicago Distribution Center,
   see under Wheaton, IL
Cleveland, OH 44101
   P.O. Box 91549   (216) 238-9450
Dallas, TX 75238
   P.O. Box 38200   (214) 341-2299
Honolulu, HI 96814
   1013 Kawaiahao St.   (808) 538-1988
Kansas City Distribution Center, see under North Kansas City, MO
Kent, WA 98064-5609
   P.O. Box 5609   (206) 872-8790
Los Angeles Distribution Center, see under Buena Park, CA
Memphis, TN 38101
   P.O. Box 1698   (901) 353-4680
North Kansas City, MO 64116
   P.O. Box 7588   (816) 842-0680
Philadelphia Distribution Center
Paoli, PA 19301
   P.O. Box 61   (215) 644-8000
    Philadelphia (215) 878-9500
St. Paul, MN 55164
   P.O. Box 64034   (612) 454-6270
Seattle Distribution Center, see under Kent, WA
Wheaton, IL 60189-0140
   P.O. Box 140   (312) 462-7200
Products Available
- Alcohol Sponges
- ▣ Aludrox Suspension
- ▣ Aludrox Tablets
- Aminophylline Rectal Suppositories
- ▣ Amphojel Suspension
- ▣ Amphojel Suspension w/o Flavor
- ▣ Amphojel Tablets
- Antisnakebite Serum (see Antivenin)
- Antivenin (Crotalidae) Polyvalent
- Antivenin (Micrurus Fulvius)
- Aspirin Rectal Suppositories
- Aspirin Tablets, Redipak
- Ativan Injection
- ◆ Ativan Tablets
- Atropine Sulfate Injection
- Basaljel Capsules
- Basaljel Suspension
- Basaljel Suspension, Extra Strength
- Basaljel Swallow Tablets
- Benzathine Penicillin G (see Bicillin)
- Bicillin C-R Injection
- Bicillin C-R 900/300 Injection
- Bicillin Long-Acting Injection
- Bicillin Tablets
- Biologicals
- Bisacodyl Suppositories
- Chloral Hydrate Capsules, Redipak
- Chlorpromazine HCl Injection
- Cholera Vaccine
- Codeine Phosphate Injection
- Codeine Sulfate Tablets, Redipak
- ▣ Collyrium Eye Lotion
- ▣ Collyrium Z Eye Drops with Tetrahydrozoline
- Cyanocobalamin Injection
- Cyclapen-W for Oral Suspension
- ◆ Cyclapen-W Tablets
- Dexamethasone Sodium Phosphate Injection
- Digitoxin (see Purodigin)
- Digoxin Injection
- Dimenhydrinate Injection
- Diphenhydramine HCl Injection
- Diphtheria and Tetanus Toxoids Adsorbed (Adult Use) (see Tetanus and Diphtheria Toxoids Adsorbed)
- Diphtheria & Tetanus Toxoids Adsorbed, Pediatric
- Epinephrine Injection (1:1000)

(◆ Shown in Product Identification Section)   (▣ Described in PDR For Nonprescription Drugs)

Manufacturers' Index

- ◆ Equagesic Tablets
- ◆ Equanil Tablets
- ◆ Equanil Wyseals
- Erythromycin Ethylsuccinate Oral Suspension (See Wyamycin E Liquid)
- Erythromycin Stearate Tablets (see Wyamycin S Tablets)
- Furosemide Injection
- Heparin Lock Flush Solution
- Heparin Flush Kits
- Heparin Sodium Injection
- Hydromorphone HCl Injection
- Hydroxyzine HCl Injection
- Immune Serum Globulin (Human)
- Influenza Virus Vaccine Subvirion Type
- Largon Injection
- Lidocaine HCl Injection
- ◆ Lo/Ovral Tablets
- ◆ Lo/Ovral-28 Tablets
- ◆ Mazanor
- ◆ Mepergan Fortis Capsules
- Mepergan Injection
- Meperidine HCl Injection
- Meperidine HCl Tablets, Redipak
- Morphine Sulfate Injection
- ◆ Nordette-21 Tablets
- ◆ Nordette-28 Tablets
- ▣ Nursoy, Soy Protein Formula for Infants, Concentrated Liquid & Ready-to-Feed
- ◆ Omnipen Capsules
- Omnipen for Oral Suspension
- Omnipen Pediatric Drops
- Omnipen-N Injection
- Opium & Belladonna Rectal Suppositories
- ◆ Ovral Tablets
- ◆ Ovral-28 Tablets
- Ovrette Tablets
- Oxytocin Injection, Synthetic
- ◆ Pathocil Capsules
- Pathocil for Oral Suspension
- Pediatric Phenergan Expectorant w/Dextromethorphan
- Penicillin Preparations:
  - Bicillin Products
  - Penicillin G Potassium Tablets
  - Pen•Vee K Products
  - Wycillin Products
- Pentobarbital Sodium Injection
- Pen•Vee K for Oral Solution
- ◆ Pen•Vee K Tablets
- Petrogalar, Phenolphthalein
- Petrogalar, Plain
- ◆ Phenergan Compound Tablets
- Phenergan Injection
- Phenergan Syrup Fortis
- Phenergan Syrup Plain
- ◆ Phenergan Tablets & Rectal Suppositories
- Phenergan VC
- Phenergan VC with Codeine
- Phenergan with Codeine
- Phenergan with Dextromethorphan
- ◆ Phenergan-D Tablets
- Phenobarbital Sodium Injection
- Phenobarbital Tablets, Redipak
- Phosphaljel
- Polymagma Plain Tablets
- Potassium Penicillin G Tablets, Buffered
- Prochlorperazine Edisylate Injection
- Purodigin Tablets
- Redipak Unit Dose Medications (Strip Pack and/or Individually Wrapped) Products:
  - Aspirin Tablets
  - Ativan Tablets
  - Chloral Hydrate Capsules
  - Codeine Sulfate Tablets
- Equagesic Tablets
- Equanil Tablets
- Meperidine HCl Tablets
- Omnipen Capsules
- Pen•Vee K Tablets
- Phenergan Tablets
- Phenobarbital Tablets
- Serax Capsules
- Unipen Capsules
- Wygesic Tablets
- Redipak (Liquid Unit Dose) Products:
  - Omnipen Oral Suspension
  - Pen•Vee K Solution
- Redipak (Unit of Use Suppository Pack) Products:
  - Aminophylline Rectal Suppositories
  - Aspirin Rectal Suppositories
  - Phenergan Rectal Suppositories
- Redipak (Respiratory Therapy Unit) Products:
  - Sodium Chloride 0.9% and 0.45%
  - Sterile Distilled Water
- RediTemp-C, Disposable Cold Pack
- ▣ SMA Infant Formula, Liquid Concentrated
- ▣ SMA Infant Formula, Powder
- ▣ SMA Infant Formula, Ready-to-Feed
- Saline Solution (see Sodium Chloride Injection)
- Secobarbital Sodium Injection
- ◆ Serax Capsules
- ◆ Serax Tablets
- ▣ Simeco Suspension
- Snakebite Serum (see Antivenin)
- Sodium Chloride Injection, Bacteriostatic
- Sodium Chloride Solution, 0.9% & 0.45%
- Sopronol Ointment, Powder & Solution
- Sparine Concentrate
- Sparine Injection
- Sparine Syrup
- ◆ Sparine Tablets
- Tetanus & Diphtheria Toxoids Adsorbed (Adult)
- Tetanus & Diphtheria Toxoids Adsorbed (Pediatric) (see Diphtheria & Tetanus Toxoids Adsorbed)
- Tetanus Immune Globulin (Human)
- Tetanus Toxoid Adsorbed, Aluminum Phosphate
- Tetanus Toxoid Fluid, Purified
- ◆ Tetracycline HCl Capsules
- Thiamine HCl Injection
- ◆ Tubex Closed Injection System Products:
  - Ativan
  - Bicillin C-R
  - Bicillin C-R 900/300
  - Bicillin L-A
  - Chlorpromazine HCl
  - Codeine Phosphate
  - Cyanocobalamin (Vitamin B$_{12}$)
  - Dexamethasone Sodium Phosphate
  - Digoxin
  - Dimenhydrinate
  - Diphenhydramine HCl
  - Diphtheria & Tetanus Toxoids Adsorbed, Pediatric
  - Epinephrine
  - Furosemide
  - Heparin Lock Flush Solution
  - Heparin Sodium
  - Hydromorphone HCl
  - Hydroxyzine HCl
  - Immune Serum Globulin (Human)
  - Influenza Virus Vaccine, Trivalent, Purified, Subvirion
  - Largon
  - Lidocaine HCl
- Mepergan
- Meperidine HCl
- Morphine Sulfate
- Oxytocin, Synthetic
- Pentobarbital Sodium
- Phenergan
- Phenobarbital Sodium
- Prochlorperazine Edisylate
- Secobarbital Sodium
- Sodium Chloride, Bacteriostatic
- Sparine
- Tetanus & Diphtheria Toxoids Adsorbed (Adult)
- Tetanus Immune Globulin (Human)
- Tetanus Toxoid, Aluminum Phosphate Adsorbed
- Tetanus Toxoid Fluid, Purified
- Thiamine HCl
- Vitamin B$_{12}$ (Cyanocobalamin)
- Wyamine Sulfate
- Wycillin
- ◆ Tubex Hypodermic Syringe
- Tubex Sterile Cartridge-Needle Unit Empty
- Typhoid Vaccine
- ◆ Unipen Capsules
- Unipen Injection
- Unipen for Oral Solution
- ◆ Unipen Tablets
- Vitamin B$_{12}$ Injection (see Cyanocobalamin)
- Wyamine Sulfate Injection
- Wyamycin E Liquid
- ◆ Wyamycin S Tablets
- ◆ Wyanoids Hemorrhoidal Suppositories
- Wycillin Injection
- Wycillin Injection & Probenecid Tablets
- Wydase, Lyophilized
- Wydase, Stabilized Solution
- ◆ Wygesic Tablets
- ◆ Wymox Capsules
- Wymox for Oral Suspension
- Wyseals (see Equanil)
- ◆ Wytensin Tablets
- Wyvac Rabies Vaccine

YOUNGS DRUG PRODUCTS CORP.   2300
Post Office Box 385
865 Centennial Avenue
Piscataway, NJ 08854

Address inquiries to:
Mr. Phillip L. Frank or
Mr. Murray H. Glantz   (201) 885-5777
*Sole Distributor for products manufactured by
Holland-Rantos Company, Inc.
865 Centennial Avenue
Piscataway, NJ 08854

Products Available
- H-R Sterile Lubricating Jelly
- Koro-Flex Arcing Spring Diaphragm
- Koro-Flex Arcing Spring Diaphragm Compact Set
- Koro-Flex Fitting Rings, Set of
- Koromex Coil Spring Diaphragm
- Koromex Coil Spring Diaphragm Compact Set
- ▣ Koromex Contraceptive Cream
- ▣ Koromex Contraceptive Crystal Clear Gel
- ▣ Koromex Contraceptive Foam
- ▣ Koromex Contraceptive Jelly
- Koromex Diaphragm Introducer
- Koromex Fitting Rings, Set of
- Koromex Jelly/Cream Applicator
- Korostatin (Nystatin) Vaginal Tablets
- ▣ Nylmerate II Douche Concentrate
- Rantex Personal Cloth Wipes
- ▣ Transi-Lube
- ▣ Triple X

(◆ Shown in Product Identification Section)

(▣ Described in PDR For Nonprescription Drugs)

SECTION 2
Product Name Index

Part 1—In this section products are listed in alphabetical sequence by brand name or (if described) generic name. Only described products have page numbers to assist you in locating additional information. For additional information on other products, you may wish to contact the manufacturer directly.
The symbol ♦ indicates the product is shown in the Product Identification Section. The symbol ▣ indicates the product is described in PDR® FOR NONPRESCRIPTION DRUGS.

Part 2—A list of products that have been discontinued by manufacturers during the past year.

Part 1

A

▣ A and D Hand Cream (Schering)
▣ A and D Ointment (Schering)
ACE + Z Tablets (Legere) p 1120
A.C.N. Tablets (Person & Covey) p 1587
A.C.T.H. "40" Injectable (O'Neal, Jones & Feldman) p 1443
A.C.T.H. "80" Injectable (O'Neal, Jones & Feldman) p 1443
A-Fil Cream Neutral & Dark (Cooper Dermatology)
A.I.D.S. (Alcon Instrument Delivery System) (Alcon Labs.)
APAP w/Codeine Tablets (Geneva) p 973
APAP w/Codeine #3 (Geneva) p 973
APAP w/Codeine #4 (Geneva) p 973
♦ A.P.C. with Codeine Nos. 3 & 4, Tabloid brand (Burroughs Wellcome) p 407, 780
A.P.L. (Ayerst) p 636
AR-600 (UAD Labs.)
A.S.A. & Codeine Compound Pulvules & Tablets (Lilly)
A.S.A. Enseals, Pulvules, Suppositories & Tablets (Lilly)
A-Spas (Hyrex)
A/T/S (Hoechst-Roussel) p 412, 1009
♦ A-200 Pyrinate Pediculicide Shampoo, Liquid & Gel (Norcliff Thayer) p 422, 1422
AVC Cream (Merrell Dow) p 1358
AVC Suppositories (Merrell Dow) p 1358
AVC Vaginal Cream (Merrell Dow)
AVC/Dienestrol Cream (Merrell Dow)
AVC/Dienestrol Suppositories (Merrell Dow)
Abbokinase (Abbott) p 502
Abbokinase Open-Cath (Abbott) p 505
Abbo-Pac (Abbott) p 502
Abdec Baby Vitamin Drops (Parke-Davis)
Abdec with Fluoride Baby Vitamin Drops (Parke-Davis)
Accelerase (Organon)
Accurbron (Merrell Dow) p 1359
♦ Accutane Capsules (Roche) p 429, 1665
Acedoval Tablets (Vale)
Acedyne Tablets (Vale)
Acetaco Tablets (Legere) p 1120
♦ Acetaminophen Capsules, Tablets, Elixir (Lederle) p 416
Acetaminophen Elixir, Tablets, Suppositories (Roxane) p 1788
Acetaminophen Uniserts Suppositories (Upsher-Smith) p 2144
Acetaminophen with Codeine Tablets and Capsules (Lemmon) p 1122
Acetaminophen with Codeine Phosphate Tablets (Roxane) p 1788
Acetazolamide Tablets (Schein) p 1828

Acetospan Injection (Reid-Provident, Direct Div.)
Achromycin Intramuscular (Lederle) p 1074
Achromycin Intravenous (Lederle) p 1074
Achromycin Ophthalmic Ointment (Lederle) p 1077
Achromycin Ophthalmic Suspension 1% (Lederle) p 1075
Achromycin 3% Ointment (Lederle) p 1077
♦ Achromycin V Capsules (Lederle) p 414, 1076
Achromycin V Oral Suspension (Lederle) p 1076
Achrostatin V Capsules (Lederle)
Acid Mantle Creme & Lotion (Dorsey Laboratories) p 908
Acidulin (Lilly) p 1126
Aci-Jel Therapeutic Vaginal Jelly (Ortho Pharmaceutical) p 1453
Acne-Aid Cleansing Bar (Stiefel)
Acne-Aid Cream (Stiefel)
Acne-Aid Lotion (Stiefel)
▣ Acnederm Lotion & Soap (Lannett)
Acne-Dome Lotion (Miles Pharmaceuticals)
Acne-Dome Medicated Cleanser (Miles Pharmaceuticals)
Acno Lotion & Cleanser (Baker/Cummins)
Acnomel Cream (Smith Kline & French)
Acnotex (C & M)
Acthar (Armour) p 601
Acticort Lotion 100 (Baker/Cummins)
♦ Actidil Tablets & Syrup (Burroughs Wellcome) p 407
♦ Actifed Tablets & Syrup (Burroughs Wellcome) p 407
Actifed with Codeine Cough Syrup (Burroughs Wellcome) p 773
Actol Expectorant Liquid (Beecham Laboratories)
Actol Expectorant Tablets (Beecham Laboratories)
Adalan Lanatabs (Lannett)
♦ Adapin (Pennwalt) p 426, 1581
Adbeon (UAD Labs.)
Added Protection III Multi-Vitamin & Multi-Mineral Supplement (Professional Health) p 1621
Added Protection III Multi-Vitamin & Multi-Mineral Supplement without Copper (Professional Health)
Added Protection III Multi-Vitamin & Multi-Mineral Supplement without Iron and Copper (Professional Health)
♦ Adeflor Chewable Tablets (Upjohn) p 440, 2093
Adeflor Drops (Upjohn) p 2093
Adeflor M Tablets (Upjohn)
♦ Adipex-P Tablets (Lemmon) p 417, 1121
Adipost Capsules (Ascher)
Adlone 40 and 80 (UAD Labs.)

Adphen Tablets (Ferndale)
Adrenalin Chloride Solution, Injectable (Parke-Davis) p 1480
Adriamycin (Adria) p 571
Adrucil Injectable (Adria) p 573
Adsorbocarpine (Alcon Labs.)
Adsorbonac (Alcon Labs.)
Adsorbotear (Alcon Labs.)
Advance (Ross) p 1761
♦ Advil Ibuprofen Tablets (Whitehall) p 443, 2184
AeroBid Inhaler System (Key Pharmaceuticals) p 1046
Aerohalor (Abbott)
Aerolate Liquid (Fleming) p 948
Aerolate Sr. & Jr. & III Capsules (Fleming) p 948
Aerolone Solution (Lilly) p 1126
Aerosan (Ulmer)
Aeroseb-Dex Topical Aerosol Spray (Herbert) p 1001
Aeroseb-HC Topical Aerosol Spray (Herbert) p 1002
Aerosporin Powder (Burroughs Wellcome) p 775
▣ Afrin Menthol Nasal Spray, 0.05% (Schering)
▣ Afrin Nasal Spray 0.05% (Schering)
▣ Afrin Nose Drops 0.05% (Schering)
▣ Afrin Pediatric Nose Drops 0.025% (Schering)
♦ Afrinol Repetabs Tablets Long-Acting Nasal Decongestant (Schering) p 433
Agoral, Plain (Parke-Davis) p 1480
Agoral, Raspberry & Marshmallow Flavors (Parke-Davis) p 1480
A-hydroCort (Abbott) p 506
♦ Akineton (Knoll) p 414, 1056
Akne Drying Lotion (Alto)
Akne Kaps (Alto)
Akne pH Lotion (Alto)
Akrinol Cream (Schering)
Alba-3 Ointment (Bart)
Alba-3 Ophthalmic Ointment (Bart)
Alba-3 Ophthalmic Solution (Bart)
Alba-Ce Liquid, Drops, Tablets (Bart)
Albacort Cream (Bart)
Alba-Dex Injectable, Liquid & Tablets (Bart)
Albaform-HC Cream (Bart)
Albafort Injectable (Bart) p 685
Alba-Gyn Vaginal Cream (Bart)
Albalon Liquifilm ophthalmic solution (Allergan)
Albalon-A Liquifilm ophthalmic solution (Allergan)
Alba-Lybe (Bart) p 685
Albamycin Capsules (Upjohn)
Alba-Temp Suppositories, Liquid, Tablets & Drops (Bart)
Albatussin (Bart) p 685
Albumin 500 Tablets (Marlyn)

(♦ Shown in Product Identification Section)   (▣ Described in PDR For Nonprescription Drugs)   (Products without page numbers are not described)

Product Name Index

Albuminar-5, Normal Serum Albumin (Human) U.S.P. 5% (Armour) p 613
Albuminar-25, Normal Serum Albumin (Human) U.S.P. 25% (Armour) p 613
Albutein 5% (Alpha Theapeutic) p 589
Albutein 25% (Alpha Theapeutic) p 589
Alcaine (Alcon Labs.)
Alcon Closure System, A.C.S. (Alcon Labs.)
Alcon Indirect Ophthalmoscope/Camera (Alcon Labs.)
Alcon Surgical System (Irrigation/Aspiration Kits; Phacoemulsification Kits) (Alcon Labs.)
Alconefrin 12 Drops (Webcon)
Alconefrin 25 Drops (Webcon)
Alconefrin 50 Drops (Webcon)
Alconefrin 25 Spray (Webcon)
◆ Aldactazide (Searle & Co.) p 435, 1912
◆ Aldactone (Searle & Co.) p 435, 1914
◆ Aldoclor Tablets (Merck Sharp & Dohme) p 420, 1258
Aldomet Ester HCl Injection (Merck Sharp & Dohme) p 1261
Aldomet Oral Suspension (Merck Sharp & Dohme) p 1259
◆ Aldomet Tablets (Merck Sharp & Dohme) p 420, 1259
◆ Aldoril Tablets (Merck Sharp & Dohme) p 420, 1262
Alermine Tablets (Reid-Provident, Direct Div.)
Alginate Styptic Gauze (Pedinol)
Algisin Capsules (RAM Laboratories) p 1632
Alka Aid (antacid) (Vitaline)
Alkaline Aromatic Tablets (Vale)
Alka-Mints Chewable Antacid (Miles Laboratories)
Alka-Seltzer Effervescent Antacid (Miles Laboratories) p 1395
Alka-Seltzer Effervescent Pain Reliever and Antacid (Miles Laboratories) p 1395
Alka-Seltzer Plus Cold Medicine (Miles Laboratories) p 1395
◆ Alkeran (Burroughs Wellcome) p 407, 776
Alkets Tablets (Upjohn)
⊡ Allbee C-800 Plus Iron Tablets (Robins)
⊡ Allbee C-800 Tablets (Robins)
⊡ Allbee w/C Capsules (Robins)
Allbee-T Tablets (Robins)
Allerdryl 50 (Legere) p 1120
⊡ Allerest Tablets, Childrens Chewable Tablets, Headache Strength Tablets, Sinus Pain Formula Tablets, Eye Drops & Nasal Spray (Pharmacraft)
⊡ Allerest Timed Release Allergy Capsules (Pharmacraft)
Allergan Hydrocare Cleaning & Disinfecting Solution (Allergan)
Allergan Hydrocare Preserved Saline Solution (Allergan)
Allergan Sorbi-Care Saline Solution (Allergan)
Allergenic Extracts, Diagnosis and/or Immunotherapy (Barry) p 685
Allerid-D.C. Capsules (Trimen)
Allerid-O.D.-8 Capsules (Trimen)
Allerid-O.D.-12 Capsules (Trimen)
Allersone (Mallard) p 1181
Allopurinol Tablets (Danbury) p 887
Allopurinol Tablets (Schein) p 1828
Allorganic Trace Minerals-B12 (Standard Process)
Almocarpine (Ayerst)
Almora Tablets (O'Neal, Jones & Feldman)
Alophen Pills (Parke-Davis)
Alpha Keri Shower and Bath Oil (Westwood) p 2174
Alpha Keri Soap (Westwood) p 2175
Alphaderm (Norwich Eaton) p 1424
Alphalin Gelseals (Lilly)
Alphamul Suspension (Lannett)
alphaRedisol Injection (Merck Sharp & Dohme)
Alpha-Ruvite (Savage)
Alphatrex Cream & Ointment (Savage) p 1822
Alphosyl Lotion, Cream (Reed & Carnrick) p 1632
◆ ALternaGEL Liquid (Stuart) p 438, 2036
Alto-Pred Soluble Injection (Alto)
Alu-Cap Capsules (Riker) p 1641
⊡ Aludrox Oral Suspension (Wyeth) p 2235
Aludrox Tablets (Wyeth) p 2235
Alumadrine Tablets (Fleming)
Aluminum Hydroxide Gel (Roxane) p 1788
Aluminum Hydroxide Gel-Concentrated (Roxane) p 1788
Aluminum Hydroxide Tablets (Roxane) p 1788
Aluminum & Magnesium Hydroxides with Simethicone I (Roxane) p 1788
Aluminum & Magnesium Hydroxides with Simethicone II (Roxane) p 1788
Alupent Inhalent Solution 5% & Solution Unit Dose 0.6% (Boehringer Ingelheim) p 706
Alupent Metered Dose Inhaler (Boehringer Ingelheim) p 706
Alupent Syrup (Boehringer Ingelheim) p 706
◆ Alupent Tablets (Boehringer Ingelheim) p 406, 706
Alurate Elixir (Roche) p 1667
Alu-Tab Tablets (Riker) p 1641
Alvimin (Bart)
Al-Vite (Drug Industries) p 914
Amacodone Tablets (Trimen) p 2067

Amaphen Capsules (Trimen) p 2067
Amaphen with Codeine #3 (Trimen) p 2067
Ambenyl Cough Syrup (Marion) p 1181
Ambenyl-D Decongestant Cough Formula (Marion) p 1182
◆ Amcill Capsules (Parke-Davis) p 423, 1480
Amcill Oral Suspension (Parke-Davis) p 1480
Amcill Pediatric Drops (Parke-Davis)
◆ Amen (Carnrick) p 408, 829
Amertan Jelly (Lilly)
Ames TDA Therapeutic Drug Assays (Ames) p 3004
Amesec Capsules (Glaxo)
A-methaPred (Abbott) p 508
◆ Amicar (Lederle) p 414, 1077
Amikin (Bristol) p 727
Amino B Plex Tablets (Tyson)
Aminobrain Capsules (Medical Products)
Aminobrain Injection (Medical Products)
Aminobrain Plus Capsules (Medical Products)
Aminobrain Tablets (Medical Products)
Aminocaproic Acid Injection (Elkins-Sinn) p 938
Amino-Cerv (Milex) p 1415
Amino Dox Tablets (Tyson)
Amino GTF Tablets (Tyson)
Amino K Tablets (Tyson)
Amino Lac Capsules (Tyson)
Aminolete (Tyson) p 2067
Amino Min D Tablets (Tyson)
Aminomine (Tyson) p 2067
Amino Opti C (Tyson)
Amino-Opti-E (Tyson)
Aminophyllin Injection (Bristol) p 730
Aminophyllin Injection (Searle Pharmaceuticals) p 1898
◆ Aminophyllin Tablets (Searle & Co.) p 435, 1915
Aminophylline Injection (Elkins-Sinn) p 938
Aminophylline Oral Liquid, Suppositories & Tabs (Schein) p 1828
Aminophylline Tablets (Geneva) p 973
Aminophylline Tablets & Oral Solution (Roxane) p 1788
Aminoplex Capsules & Powder (Tyson) p 2068
Aminosine (Tyson) p 2068
Aminostasis Capsules & Powder (Tyson) p 2068
Aminotate Capsules & Powder (Tyson) p 2068
Amino Vi Min Tablets (Tyson)
Aminoxin (Tyson)
Amino Zn Tablets (Tyson)
Amipaque (Winthrop-Breon) p 3018
Amitriptyline HCl Tablets (Lederle) p 416
Amitriptyline HCl Tablets (Biocraft) p 705
Amitriptyline HCl Tablets (Geneva) p 973
Amitriptyline Hydrochloride Tablets (Roxane) p 1788
Amitriptyline HCl Tablets (Schein) p 1828
◆ Amitriptyline Hydrochloride Tablets (Parke-Davis) p 423, 1481
Ammens medicated powder (Bristol-Myers Products)
Ammonia Aromatic, Vaporole (Burroughs Wellcome)
Ammonium Chloride Enseals (Lilly)
Amobell Capsules (Bock)
Amo-Derm (High Chemical)
Amonidrin Tablets (O'Neal, Jones & Feldman)
◆ Amoxicillin Capsules (Parke-Davis) p 423, 1482
Amoxicillin for Oral Suspension (Parke-Davis) p 1482
Amoxicillin Suspension (Biocraft) p 705
Amoxicillin Trihydrate Capsules & Powder for Oral Suspension (Schein) p 1828
◆ Amoxil (Beecham Laboratories) p 405, 688
◆ Amphojel Suspension (Wyeth) p 2236
⊡ Amphojel Tablets (Wyeth) p 2236
Ampicillin Capsules (Biocraft) p 705
Ampicillin Suspension (Biocraft) p 705
◆ Ampicillin Trihydrate Capsules, Oral Suspension (Lederle) p 416
Ampicillin Trihydrate Capsules & Powder for Oral Suspension (Schein) p 1828
Ampicillin-Probenecid Suspension (Biocraft) p 705
Amtren Tablets (Lannett)
Amyl Nitrite, Aspirols (Lilly)
Amyl Nitrite, Vaporole (Burroughs Wellcome)
◆ Amytal (Lilly) p 417, 1127
Amytal Sodium Ampoules & Vials (Lilly) p 1127
◆ Amytal Sodium Pulvules (Lilly) p 417, 1128
Anabolin IM Injection (Alto)
Anabolin LA-100 Injection (Alto)
◆ Anacin Analgesic Capsules (Whitehall) p 443, 2184
◆ Anacin Analgesic Tablets (Whitehall) p 443, 2184
◆ Anacin Maximum Strength Analgesic Capsules (Whitehall) p 443
◆ Anacin Maximum Strength Analgesic Tablets (Whitehall) p 443
◆ Anacin-3, Children's Acetaminophen Chewable Tablets, Elixir, Drops (Whitehall) p 443, 2184
◆ Anacin-3, Maximum Strength Acetaminophen Tablets and Capsules (Whitehall) p 443, 2185
◆ Anacin-3, Regular Strength Acetaminophen Tablets (Whitehall) p 443

◆ Anacin-3 with Codeine Tablets (Ayerst) p 404, 634
◆ Anadrol-50 (Syntex) p 440, 2049
Anafed Capsules & Syrup (Everett) p 941
Anaids Tablets (O'Neal, Jones & Feldman)
Analbalm, Liquid (Central Pharmaceuticals)
Analgesic Balm (Fougera)
Analgesic Balm (Greaseless) (Fougera)
Analone Injection (Reid-Provident, Direct Div.)
Anamine Syrup (Mayrand) p 1196
Anamine T.D. Caps (Mayrand) p 1196
Ananase Tablets (Rorer)
◆ Anaprox Tablets (Syntex) p 440, 2050
Anaspaz PB Tablets (Ascher) p 614
Anaspaz Tablets (Ascher) p 614
Anatuss Tablets & Syrup (Mayrand)
Anatuss with Codeine Tablets & Syrup (Mayrand)
◆ Anavar (Searle & Co.) p 435, 1916
◆ Anbesol Baby Teething Gel Antiseptic Anesthetic (Whitehall) p 443, 2185
◆ Anbesol Gel Antiseptic Anesthetic (Whitehall) p 443, 2185
◆ Anbesol Liquid Antiseptic Anesthetic (Whitehall) p 443
Ancef (Smith Kline & French) p 1945
◆ Ancobon Capsules (Roche) p 429, 1669
Andoin Ointment (Ulmer)
Andro L.A. "200" Injectable (O'Neal, Jones & Feldman)
Andro "100" Injectable (O'Neal, Jones & Feldman)
Androgyn L.A. Injectable (O'Neal, Jones & Feldman)
◆ Android-5 Buccal (Brown) p 407, 771
◆ Android-10 (Brown) p 407, 771
◆ Android-25 (Brown) p 407, 771
◆ Android-F Tablets (Brown) p 407, 773
Andronaq-50 Sterile Suspension (Central Pharmaceuticals)
Andronaq-LA (Central Pharmaceuticals)
Anduracaine Injection (Reid-Provident Labs.)
Anectine (Burroughs Wellcome) p 778
Anectine Flo-Pack (Burroughs Wellcome)
Anergan "25" & "50" Injectable (O'Neal, Jones & Feldman)
Anestacon (Webcon) p 2171
Anexia w/Codeine Tablets (Beecham Laboratories)
Anexia-D Tablets (Beecham Laboratories)
Anhydron (Lilly) p 1129
Anodynos DHC Tablets (Berlex)
Anoquan (Mallard) p 1181
Anorex-CCK (Robertson/Taylor) p 1645
◆ Anspor (Smith Kline & French) p 436, 1948
◆ Antabuse (Ayerst) p 404, 635, 634
◆ Antepar (Burroughs Wellcome) p 407, 779
Anthra-Derm Ointment 1%, ½%, ¼%, 1/10% (Dermik) p 888
Antibiotic Ear Drops (Geneva)
Antilirium Injectable (O'Neal, Jones & Feldman) p 1443
◆ Antiminth Oral Suspension (Pfipharmecs) p 426, 1589
Antipyrine & Benzocaine Otic Solution (Pharmafair) p 1618
Antirabies Serum (equine), Purified (Sclavo) p 1897
Anti-Rust Tablets (Winthrop-Breon)
Anti-Sept (Seamless) p 1897
Antispasmodic Capsules, Elixir & Tablets (Schein) p 1828
Antivenin (Merck Sharp & Dohme) p 1264
Antivenin (Crotalidae) Polyvalent (equine origin) (Wyeth) p 2243
Antivenin (Micrurus Fulvius) (Wyeth) p 2245
◆ Antivert, Antivert/25 Tablets, Antivert/25 Chewable Tablets & Antivert/50 Tablets (Roerig) p 431, 1725
◆ Antrenyl bromide Tablets (CIBA) p 409, 841
Antrin Tablets (Vale)
Antrocol Tablets, Capsules & Elixir (Poythress) p 1618
Antronex (Standard Process)
◆ Anturane Tablets & Capsules (CIBA) p 409, 842
Anuject Injection (Hauck) p 1001
Anusol Ointment (Parke-Davis) p 1484
◆ Anusol Suppositories (Parke-Davis) p 423, 1484
◆ Anusol-HC (Parke-Davis) p 423, 1484
Apap 300 mg. with Codeine Capsules & Tabs (Schein) p 1828
Apap with Codeine Elixir (Schein) p 1828
Apatate Liquid (Kenwood)
Apetigen Drops (Arlo)
Apetigen Elixir (Arlo)
Apetigen Plus Caps (Arlo)
Apetigen Plus Liquid (Arlo)
Apetil Liquid (RAM Laboratories)
Aplisol (Parke-Davis) p 3014
Aplitest (Parke-Davis) p 3014
Apomorphine Hydrochloride Soluble Tablets (Lilly)
Appedrine, Maximum Strength (Thompson Medical) p 2065
Appi-Plex Tablets (Reid-Provident, Direct Div.)
◆ Apresazide (CIBA) p 409, 842
◆ Apresoline Hydrochloride (CIBA) p 409, 843
Apresoline Hydrochloride Parenteral (CIBA) p 844

(◆ Shown in Product Identification Section)   (⊡ Described in PDR For Nonprescription Drugs)   (Products without page numbers are not described)

Product Name Index

- Apresoline-Esidrix (CIBA) p 409, 844
  Aquabase (Beeler's) Hydrophyllic Ointment Base (Vale)
- Aquacare Dry Skin Cream & Lotion, 2% Urea Cream & Lotion (Herbert)
- Aquacare/HP Dry Skin Cream & Lotion, 10% Urea Cream & Lotion (Herbert)
  Aquachloral (Webcon)
  Aquaderm (C & M)
  AquaMEPHYTON Injection (Merck Sharp & Dohme) p 1265
  Aquaphyllin Syrup (Ferndale) p 942
- Aquasol A Capsules (Armour) p 404, 603
  Aquasol A Drops (Armour) p 604
  Aquasol A Parenteral (Armour)
- Aquasol E Capsules & Drops (Armour) p 404, 604
  Aquatag Tablets (Reid-Provident, Direct Div.)
  Aquatensen (Wallace) p 442, 2149
  Aralen Hydrochloride (Winthrop-Breon) p 2189
- Aralen Phosphate (Winthrop-Breon) p 443, 2190
  Aralen Phosphate w/Primaquine Phosphate (Winthrop-Breon) p 2191
  Aramine Injection (Merck Sharp & Dohme) p 1266
  Arbon Plus Injectable (O'Neal, Jones & Feldman)
  Arbon Plus Tablets (O'Neal, Jones & Feldman)
  Arbon Tablets (O'Neal, Jones & Feldman)
  Arco-Cee Tablets (Arco)
  Arco-Lase (Arco) p 600
  Arco-Lase Plus (Arco) p 600
  Arcoret Tablets (Arco)
  Arcoret w/Iron Tablets (Arco)
  Arcotinic Liquid (Arco)
  Arcotinic Tablets (Arco)
  Ar-Ex Hypo-Allergenic Cosmetics (Ar-Ex) p 600
    Protein Hair Dressing & Conditioner - unscented (Ar-Ex)
  Arfonad Ampuls (Roche) p 1670
  Argyrol S.S. 20% Dropperettes (CooperVision)
  Argyrol Stabilized Solution 10% (CooperVision)
  Aridose-R (Savage)
- Aristocort A Topical Cream & Ointment (Lederle) p 414, 415, 1084
  Aristocort Forte Parenteral (Lederle) p 1081
  Aristocort Intralesional (Lederle) p 1081
  Aristocort Syrup (Lederle) p 1078
- Aristocort Tablets (Lederle) p 414, 1078
- Aristocort Topical Products (Lederle) p 414, 415, 1080
  Aristospan Parenteral 20 mg./ml (Lederle) p 1085
  Aristospan Parenteral 5 mg./ml (Lederle) p 1085
  Arithmin Tablets (Lannett)
- Arlidin Tablets (USV Pharmaceutical) p 440, 2070
  Arlon Forte (Arlo)
  Arm-a-char (Armour) p 604
  Arm-a-Med (Armour)
    Isoetharine Hychrochloride (Armour)
    Isoproterenol Hydrochloride (Armour)
  Arm-a-Vial (Armour)
    Sodium Chloride 0.45% (Armour)
    Sodium Chloride 0.9% (Armour)
    Sterile Water (Armour)
- Armour Thyroid Tablets (USV Pharmaceutical) p 440, 2089
  Aromatic Cascara Fluidextract (Roxane) p 1788
  Artane Elixir (Lederle) p 1087
- Artane Sequels (Lederle) p 415, 1087
- Artane Tablets (Lederle) p 415, 1087
  Arthralgen Tablets (Robins)
- Arthritis Bayer Timed-Release Aspirin (Glenbrook) p 412, 995
- Arthritis Pain Formula By the Makers of Anacin Analgesic Tablets (Whitehall) p 443, 2185
- Arthritis Pain Formula Aspirin-Free By the Makers of Anacin Analgesic Tablets (Whitehall) p 443
- Arthritis Pain Formula Safety-Coated by the Makers of Anacin Analgesic Tablets (Whitehall) p 443, 2185
  Arthritis Strength Bufferin (Bristol-Myers Products) p 768
  Arthropan Liquid (Purdue Frederick)
  Asbron G Elixir (Sandoz Pharmaceutical Div.) p 1796
- Asbron G Inlay-Tabs (Sandoz Pharmaceutical Div.) p 432, 1796
  Ascorbic Acid Tablets (Roxane) p 1788
- Ascriptin Tablets (Rorer) p 431
- Ascriptin A/D Tablets (Rorer) p 431
- Ascriptin with Codeine (Rorer) p 431, 1745
  Asellacrin (somatropin) (Serono) p 1940
- Asendin (Lederle) p 415, 1088
  Asmex KI Liquid (Bart)
  Asmex Liquid (Bart)
  Aspercreme (Thompson Medical) p 2066
  Aspirin Free Congespirin cold tablets (Bristol-Myers Products)
  Aspirin Suppositories (Roxane) p 1788
  Aspirin w/Codeine Tablets (Geneva) p 973
  Aspirin 325 mg. with Codeine Tabs (Schein) p 1828
  Aspir-10 Tablets (Vale)
  Astring-o-sol (Winthrop Consumer Products)

  Atabrine Hydrochloride Tablets (Winthrop-Breon) p 2192
- Atarax Tablets & Syrup (Roerig) p 431, 1725
  Atgam Sterile Solution (Upjohn)
  Ativan in Tubex (Wyeth) p 2288
  Ativan Injection (Wyeth) p 2237
- Ativan Tablets (Wyeth) p 444, 2236
  Atoximetin-B Capsules (Medical Products)
  Atrocholin Tablets (Glaxo)
  Atromid-S (Ayerst) p 404, 636
  Atropine 0.1 mg./ml., 5 ml., Abboject, Syringe (Abbott)
  Atropine 0.1 mg./ml., 10 ml., Abboject, Syringe (Abbott)
  Atropine & Demerol Carpuject (Winthrop-Breon)
  Atropine Sulfate Injection (Bristol) p 730
  Atropine Sulfate Injection (Elkins-Sinn) p 938
  Atropine Sulfate Injection, Wellcome (Burroughs Wellcome)
  Atropine Sulfate Ophthalmic Ointment 1% (Fougera) p 953
  Atropisol 0.5%, 1%, 2% Dropperettes (CooperVision)
  Atropisol Ophthalmic Solution 1% (CooperVision)
  Attenuvax (Merck Sharp & Dohme) p 1267
  Audax Ear Drops (Dalin)
- Augmentin Tablets & Powder for Oral Suspension (Beecham Laboratories) p 405, 690
  Auralgan Otic Solution (Ayerst) p 638
  Aureomycin Ointment 3% (Lederle) p 1089
  Aureomycin Ointment (Ophthalmic) 1% (Lederle)
  Autoplex, Anti-Inhibitor Coagulant Complex, Dried (Hyland Therapeutics) p 1023
  Avazyme/Avazyme-100 Tablets (Wallace)
  Aveeno Bath Oilated (Cooper Dermatology) p 882
  Aveeno Bath Regular (Cooper Dermatology) p 882
  Aveenobar Medicated (Cooper Dermatology) p 882
  Aveenobar Oilated (Cooper Dermatology) p 882
  Aveenobar Regular (Cooper Dermatology) p 882
- Aventyl HCl (Lilly) p 417, 1130
  Avitene (Alcon P.R.) p 588
  Axotal (Adria) p 574
- Ayegestin (Ayerst) p 404, 638
  Ayr Saline Nasal Drops (Ascher)
  Ayr Saline Nasal Mist (Ascher)
  Azlin (Miles Pharmaceuticals) p 1396
  Azlytal Tablets (U.S. Ethicals)
  Azmacort Inhaler (Rorer) p 431, 1746
  Azmadrine Elixir & Tablets (U.S. Ethicals)
  Azmadrine S.A. Capsules (U.S. Ethicals)
  Azo Gantanol Tablets (Roche) p 429, 1670
  Azo Gantrisin Tablets (Roche) p 429, 1671
  Azolid Capsules & Tablets (USV Pharmaceutical) p 2070
  Azo-Standard Tablets (Webcon)
  Azo-Sulfisoxazole Tablets (Geneva) p 973
  Azo-Sulfisoxazole Tablets (Schein) p 1828
  Azulfidine Tablets, EN-tabs, Oral Suspension (Pharmacia) p 427, 1613

B

  B-12 Plus Injectable (O'Neal, Jones & Feldman)
  BCG Vaccine (Glaxo) p 976
  B-Complex 100 (Legere) p 1120
  B & O Supprettes No. 15A & No. 16A (Webcon) p 2172
  B-C-Bid Capsules (Geriatric) p 975
  BC-Vite (Drug Industries)
  B.Q. cold tablets (Bristol-Myers Products)
  B-S-P (Legere) p 1120
  BSS (15ml, 250ml, 500ml) (Alcon Labs.)
  BSS Plus (Alcon Labs.)
  BSS & BSS Plus Irrigation Solution Administration Set (Alcon Labs.)
  Bacarate Tablets (Reid-Provident, Direct Div.)
  Bacid Capsules (Fisons)
- Baciguent Antibiotic Ointment (Upjohn)
  Baciguent Ophthalmic Ointment (Upjohn)
  Bacitracin-Neomycin-Polymyxin Ointment (Fougera) p 953
  Bacitracin-Neomycin-Polymyxin Ophthalmic Ointment (Fougera) p 953
  Bacitracin Ointment (Fougera) p 953
  Bacitracin Ointment & Sterile Ophthalmic Ointment (Lilly)
  Bacitracin Ophthalmic Ointment (Fougera) p 953
  Bacitracin-Polymyxin Ointment (Fougera) p 953
  Bacitracin Topical Ointment (Pfipharmecs)
  Bacitracin, USP, Sterile Powder (Upjohn)
- Bactine Antiseptic-Anesthetic First Aid Spray (Miles Laboratories)
- Bactine Hydrocortisone Skin Care Cream (Miles Laboratories)
- Bactocill Capsules (Beecham Laboratories) p 406
  Bactocill for Injection (Beecham Laboratories)
  Bactrim DS Tablets (Roche) p 429, 1674
  Bactrim I.V. Infusion (Roche) p 1672
  Bactrim Pediatric Suspension (Roche) p 1674
  Bactrim Suspension (Roche) p 1674

- Bactrim Tablets (Roche) p 429, 1674
  Bahim Foot-Aide (Jamol)
  Bahim Oil (Jamol)
  BAL in Oil Ampules (Hynson, Westcott & Dunning) p 1024
  Balance Gamma Linolenic Acid (Professional Health)
  Balanced B 125 (Marlyn)
- Balmex Baby Powder (Macsil)
- Balmex Emollient Lotion (Macsil)
- Balmex Ointment (Macsil)
  Balneol (Rowell)
  Balnetar (Westwood) p 2175
  Baltron Injection (Reid-Provident, Direct Div.)
  Ban Basic antiperspirant (Bristol-Myers Products)
  Ban cream antiperspirant (Bristol-Myers Products)
  Ban Itch (Dalin)
  Ban roll-on antiperspirant (Bristol-Myers Products)
  Ban Wide Ball antiperspirant (Bristol-Myers Products)
- Banalg Hospital Strength Arthritic Pain Reliever (O'Neal, Jones & Feldman)
- Banalg Liniment (O'Neal, Jones & Feldman)
  Bancap Capsules (O'Neal, Jones & Feldman) p 1444
  Bancap c̄ Codeine Capsules (O'Neal, Jones & Feldman) p 1444
- Bancap HC Capsules (O'Neal, Jones & Feldman) p 422, 1444
  Banesin Tablets (O'Neal, Jones & Feldman)
  Banflex Injectable (O'Neal, Jones & Feldman)
  Banquin Cream (Kramer) p 1069
- Banthine Tablets (Searle & Co.) p 435
  Barbeloid Tablets (Vale)
  Barbidonna Elixir & Tablets (Wallace)
  Barbidonna No. 2 Tablets (Wallace)
  Baroflave Powder (Lannett)
  Barotrast (Armour)
  Barseb HC Scalp Lotion (Barnes-Hind) p 683
  Barseb Thera-Spray (Barnes-Hind) p 684
  Basaljel Capsules & Swallow Tablets (Wyeth) p 2239
  Basaljel Suspension & Suspension, Extra Strength (Wyeth) p 2239
  Basal Thermometers (Milex)
- Bayer Aspirin and Bayer Children's Chewable Aspirin (Glenbrook) p 412, 996
  Bayer Children's Cold Tablets (Glenbrook) p 996
  Bayer Cough Syrup for Children (Glenbrook) p 996
- Beclovent Oral Inhaler (Glaxo) p 411, 977
- Beclovent Oral Inhaler Refill (Glaxo) p 411
  Becomject-C (Mayrand)
- Beconase Nasal Inhaler (Glaxo) p 411, 978
  Becotin (Dista) p 893
  Becotin with Vitamin C (Dista) p 894
  Becotin-T (Dista) p 894
- Beelith Tablets (Beach) p 405, 685
- Beepen-VK Oral Solution & Tablets (Beecham Laboratories)
  Beesix Injectable (O'Neal, Jones & Feldman)
  Belexal Tablets (Vale)
  Belfer Tablets (O'Neal, Jones & Feldman)
- Belladenal Tablets (Sandoz Pharmaceutical Div.) p 432, 1798
- Belladenal-S Tablets (Sandoz Pharmaceutical Div.) p 432, 1798
  Bellafedrol AH Tablets (Lannett)
  Bellafoline Injection & Tablets (Sandoz Pharmaceutical Div.)
  Bellastal Capsules (U.S. Ethicals)
  Bellastal Elixir & Tablets (U.S. Ethicals)
- Bellergal Tablets (Sandoz Pharmaceutical Div.) p 432, 1798
- Bellergal-S Tablets (Sandoz Pharmaceutical Div.) p 432, 1798
  Bellermine-O.D. Capsules (Trimen)
  Bellkatal Tablets (Ferndale)
- Beminal-500 (Ayerst) p 404, 639
  Beminal Forte w/Vitamin C (Ayerst) p 639
- Beminal Stress Plus (Ayerst) p 404, 640
- Ben Gay External Analgesic Products (Leeming)
  Benadryl Cream (Parke-Davis)
  Benadryl Elixir (Parke-Davis) p 1485
- Benadryl Kapseals and Capsules (Parke-Davis) p 423, 1485
  Benadryl Parenteral (Parke-Davis) p 1485
  Benase Tablets (Ferndale)
  Bendylate Capsules (Reid-Provident, Direct Div.)
  Bendylate Injection (Reid-Provident, Direct Div.)
- Benemid Tablets (Merck Sharp & Dohme) p 420, 1268
  Benisone Gel/Cream/Lotion/Ointment (Cooper Dermatology)
  Benoject-10 (Mayrand)
  Benoject-50 (Mayrand)
  Benoquin Cream 20% (Elder) p 929
  Benoxyl-5 Lotion (Stiefel)
  Benoxyl-10 Lotion (Stiefel)
  Bensulfoid (Poythress)
  Bensulfoid Lotion (Poythress) p 1618
- Bentyl Capsules, Tablets, Syrup & Injection (Merrell Dow) p 421, 1359
  Benylin Cough Syrup (Parke-Davis) p 1486

(◆ Shown in Product Identification Section)   (❊ Described in PDR For Nonprescription Drugs)   (Products without page numbers are not described)

Product Name Index

⊞ Benylin DM Cough Syrup (Parke-Davis)
5 Benzagel (5% benzoyl peroxide) & 10 Benzagel (10% benzoyl peroxide), Acne Gels, Microgel Formula (Dermik) p 888
Benzedrex Inhaler (Smith Kline & French)
Benzo-Menth Lozenges (Vale)
Benzotic Ear Drops (Bart)
Benzoyl Peroxide Gel (Pharmafair) p 1618
Benztropine Mesylate Tablets (Schein) p 1828
Berocca Parenteral Nutrition (Roche) p 1676
◆ Berocca Plus Tablets (Roche) p 429, 1677
◆ Berocca Tablets (Roche) p 429, 1677
Berocca-C & Berocca-C 500 (Roche) p 1678
Berovite Plus Tablets (Everett) p 941
Berubigen Sterile Solution (Upjohn)
Besta Capsules (Hauck) p 1001
Betadine Aerosol Spray (Purdue Frederick) p 1622
Betadine Antiseptic Gauze Pad (Purdue Frederick)
Betadine Antiseptic Gel (Purdue Frederick) p 1622
Betadine Antiseptic Lubricating Gel (Purdue Frederick)
Betadine Disposable Medicated Douche (Purdue Frederick) p 1622
Betadine Douche (Purdue Frederick) p 1622
Betadine Douche Kit (Purdue Frederick)
Betadine Helafoam Solution (Purdue Frederick) p 1622
Betadine Mouthwash/Gargle (Purdue Frederick)
Betadine Ointment (Purdue Frederick) p 1622
Betadine Perineal Wash Concentrate (Purdue Frederick)
Betadine Shampoo (Purdue Frederick)
Betadine Skin Cleanser (Purdue Frederick) p 1622
Betadine Skin Cleanser Foam (Purdue Frederick)
Betadine Solution (Purdue Frederick) p 1622
Betadine Solution Swab Aid (Purdue Frederick)
Betadine Solution Swabsticks (Purdue Frederick)
Betadine Surgical Scrub (Purdue Frederick) p 1622
Betadine Surgi-Prep Sponge-Brush (Purdue Frederick)
Betadine Viscous Formula Antiseptic Gauze Pad (Purdue Frederick) p 1623
Betadine Whirlpool Concentrate (Purdue Frederick)
Betalin Complex Elixir (Lilly)
Betalin Compound Pulvules (Lilly)
Betalin S Ampoules, Vials, Elixir & Tablets (Lilly)
Betalin 12 Crystalline Vials (Lilly)
Betamethasone Dipropionate Cream & Ointment (Pharmaderm) p 1617
Betamethasone Valerate Cream, Lotion & Ointment 0.1% (Fougera) p 953
Betamethasone Valerate Cream, Ointment & Lotion (Pharmaderm) p 1617
◆ Betapen-VK (Bristol) p 407, 729
Betaprone Liquid (O'Neal, Jones & Feldman)
Betatrex Cream, Ointment & Lotion (Savage) p 1823
Beta-Val Cream 0.1% (Lemmon) p 1122
Bethanechol Chloride Tablets (Danbury) p 887
Betuline Liniment (Ferndale)
Biamine Injectable (O'Neal, Jones & Feldman)
Bi-Amine (Ulmer)
Biavax ॥ (Merck Sharp & Dohme) p 1269
Bicillin C-R Injection (Wyeth) p 2239
Bicillin C-R in Tubex (Wyeth) p 2288
Bicillin C-R 900/300 (Wyeth) p 2241
Bicillin C-R 900/300 in Tubex (Wyeth) p 2288
Bicillin L-A Injection (Wyeth) p 2242
Bicillin Tablets (Wyeth)
Bicitra—Sugar-Free (Willen) p 2187
BiCNU (Bristol-Myers Oncology) p 756
Bi-K (USV Pharmaceutical) p 2072
Bilamide Tablets (Norgine)
Bilax Capsules (Drug Industries) p 914
Bilezyme Tablets (Geriatric)
Bilogen (Organon) p 1446
◆ Bilopaque Sodium (Winthrop-Breon) p 443, 3023
Bilron Pulvules (Lilly)
◆ Biltricide (Miles Pharmaceuticals) p 421, 1399
Biocal Calcium Supplement Chewable Tablets (Miles Laboratories) p 1396
Biocal Calcium Supplement Tablets (Miles Laboratories) p 1396
Biopar Forté (USV Pharmaceutical)
Biost Powder (Standard Process)
Biothesin Tablets (Vale)
Biotres Ointment (Central Pharmaceuticals)
Biozyme-C Ointment (Armour) p 604
Bipectol Wafers (Vale)
◆ Biphetamine Capsules (Pennwalt) p 426
Bisacodyl Patient Pack, Suppositories, Tablets (Roxane) p 1788
Bisacodyl Suppositories (Geneva) p 973
Bisacodyl Suppositories (Wyeth)
Bismapec Tablets (Vale)
Bisodol Antacid Powder (Whitehall)
Bisodol Antacid Tablets (Whitehall)
Blenoxane (Bristol-Myers Oncology) p 757

Bleph-10 Liquifilm ophthalmic solution (Allergan)
Bleph-10 S.O.P. ophthalmic ointment (Allergan)
Blephamide Liquifilm ophthalmic suspension (Allergan)
Blephamide S.O.P. ophthalmic ointment (Allergan)
Blink-N-Clean hard contact lens solution (Allergan)
◆ Blocadren Tablets (Merck Sharp & Dohme) p 420, 1271
⊞ Bluboro Powder Astringent Soaking Solution (Herbert)
Body on Tap Shampoo and Conditioner (Bristol-Myers Products)
Bonacal Plus Tablets (Kenwood)
◆ Bonine Tablets (Pfipharmecs) p 426, 1589
◆ Bontril PDM (Carnrick) p 408, 830
◆ Bontril Slow-Release (Carnrick) p 408, 830
Boric Acid Ointment (Fougera) p 953
Boric Acid Ophthalmic Ointment 5% (Fougera) p 953
Borofair Otic (Pharmafair) p 1618
Borofax Ointment (Burroughs Wellcome)
Brasivol Base (Stiefel)
Brasivol Fine (Stiefel)
Brasivol Medium (Stiefel)
Brasivol Rough (Stiefel)
Breast Self-Examination Kit (Milex)
Breezee Mist Foot Powder (Pedinol) p 1580
Breonesin (Winthrop-Breon) p 2193
◆ Brethine (Geigy) p 411, 955
Brethine Ampuls (Geigy) p 956
Bretylol (American Critical Care) p 592
◆ Brevicon 21-Day Tablets (Syntex) p 440, 2052
◆ Brevicon 28-Day Tablets (Syntex) p 440, 2052
Brevital Sodium (Lilly) p 1131
◆ Brexin Capsules (Savage)
Brexin L.A. Capsules (Savage) p 433, 1824
◆ Bricanyl Injection (Merrell Dow) p 421, 1361
◆ Bricanyl Tablets (Merrell Dow) p 421, 1361
Bristoject Products (Bristol)
Brohembione (Brown)
Bromanyl Expectorant (Schein) p 1828
Bromfed Capsules (Timed Release) (Muro) p 1420
Bromfed-PD Capsules (Timed Release) (Muro) p 1420
Bromfed Tablets (Muro) p 1420
Bromphen Compound Elixir - Sugar Free (Schein) p 1828
Bromphen Compound Tablets (Schein) p 1828
Bromphen DC Expectorant (Schein) p 1828
Bromphen Expectorant (Schein) p 1828
Brompheniramine Maleate, Phenylephrine & Phenylpropanolamine Sequels (Lederle)
Broncholate Capsules (Bock)
Broncholate Syrup (Bock)
Broncopectol Syrup (Medical Products)
◆ Brondecon (Parke-Davis) p 423, 1486
Bronitin Asthma Tablets (Whitehall)
Bronitin Mist (Whitehall)
⊞ Bronkaid Mist (Winthrop Consumer Products)
⊞ Bronkaid Mist Suspension (Winthrop Consumer Products)
⊞ Bronkaid Tablets (Winthrop Consumer Products)
Bronkephrine Hydrochloride Injection (Winthrop-Breon) p 2193
Bronkodyl (Winthrop-Breon) p 2193
Bronkolixir (Winthrop-Breon) p 2193
Bronkometer (Winthrop-Breon) p 2193
Bronkosol (Winthrop-Breon) p 2193
Bronkotabs (Winthrop-Breon) p 2194
Bronkotuss (Hyrex) p 1024
Brosema (Legere) p 1120
Broxodent Automatic-Action Toothbrush (Squibb)
◆ Bucladin-S Softab Tablets (Stuart) p 439, 2036
Buff-A Comp Caps (Mayrand)
Buff-A Comp Tablets (Mayrand) p 1196
Buff-A Comp No. 3 Tablets (with Codeine) (Mayrand) p 1196
Bufferin (Bristol-Myers Products) p 769
⊞ Bugs Bunny Multivitamin Supplement (Miles Laboratories)
⊞ Bugs Bunny Plus Iron Multivitamin Supplement (Miles Laboratories)
⊞ Bugs Bunny Vitamins Plus Minerals (Sugar Free) (Miles Laboratories)
⊞ Bugs Bunny With Extra C (Miles Laboratories)
Bumex Injection (Roche) p 1678
◆ Bumex Tablets (Roche) p 429, 1678
Buminate 5%, Normal Serum Albumin (Human), U.S.P., 5% Solution (Hyland Therapeutics) p 1023
Buminate 25%, Normal Serum Albumin (Human), U.S.P., 25% Solution (Hyland Therapeutics) p 1023
Burdeo (Hill Dermaceuticals)
Buro-Sol Antiseptic Powder (Doak)
Butalbital and Acetaminophen Tablets (Danbury) p 887
Butalbital Compound (Schein) p 1828
Butalix (Vale)
Butatran Tablets 30mg. (Hauck)
◆ Butazolidin Capsules & Tablets (Geigy) p 411, 956
Butesin Picrate Ointment (Abbott) p 510

Butibel Elixir & Tablets (Wallace)
Butibel-Zyme Tablets (McNeil Pharmaceutical)
Buticaps (Wallace)
◆ Butisol Sodium Elixir & Tablets (Wallace) p 442, 2150

C

C & T (Hyrex)
C-B Time Capsules (Arco)
C-B Time 500 Tablets (Arco)
C-B Time Liquid (Arco)
C-B Vone Capsules (Armour)
C-BE Zinc Tablets (Reid-Provident, Direct Div.)
CC-500 (Consolidated Chemical)
C-Caps 500 (Drug Industries)
C-Ron (Rowell)
C-Ron FA (Rowell)
C-Ron Forte (Rowell)
C-Ron Freckles (Rowell)
C Speridin Tablets, Sustained Release (Marlyn)
C.V.P. Capsules (Armour)
◆ Cafergot (Sandoz Pharmaceutical Div.) p 432, 1799
◆ Cafergot P-B (Sandoz Pharmaceutical Div.) p 432, 1799
Cafetrate-PB Suppositories (Schein) p 1828
Caladryl (Parke-Davis) p 1486
Cal-Amo (Standard Process)
Calan for IV Injection (Searle Pharmaceuticals) p 435, 1900
◆ Calan Tablets (Searle & Co.) p 435, 1917
Cal-Bio (Geriatric)
Calcet (Mission) p 1415
Calcet Plus (Mission) p 1415
Calcibind (Mission) p 1416
Calcidrine Syrup (Abbott) p 510
◆ Calciferol Drops (Egocalciferol Oral Solution USP) (Rorer) p 431, 1748
◆ Calciferol in Oil Injection (Egocalciferol USP) (Rorer) p 431, 1748
◆ Calciferol Tablets (Ergocalciferol USP) (Rorer) p 431, 1748
◆ Calcimar Solution (USV Pharmaceutical) p 440, 2072
Calciparine Injection (American Critical Care) p 593
Calcium Carbonate Tablets & Oral Suspension (Roxane) p 1788
Calcium Chloride 10%, Abboject (Abbott)
Calcium Chloride Injection (Bristol) p 730
Calcium Chloride Injection (Elkins-Sinn) p 938
Calcium Disodium Versenate Injection (Riker) p 1641
Calcium Gluceptate Injection Ampoule & Abboject (Abbott)
Calcium Gluconate Injection (Elkins-Sinn) p 938
Calcium Gluconate Tablets (Roxane) p 1788
⊞ CaldeCORT Hydrocortisone Multi-Purpose Anti-Itch Cream and Spray (Pharmacraft)
Calderol Capsules (Upjohn) p 2093
Caldesene Medicated Ointment (Pharmacraft)
Caldesene Medicated Baby Powder (Pharmacraft)
Calfer-Vite (Drug Industries)
Calfos-D Tablets (Vale)
Calinate-FA Tablets (Reid-Provident Labs.)
Cal-Mag Aspartate (calcium/magnesium) (Vitaline)
Calphosan (Glenwood) p 998
Calphosan B-12 (Glenwood) p 998
Calphosan B-12 I.M. (Brown)
Calphosan I.M. (Brown)
Cal-Plus (Geriatric)
Calscorbate Tablets (O'Neal, Jones & Feldman)
Cal-Sup (Riker) p 1642
Caltrate 600 (Lederle)
Caltrate 600+Vitamin D (Lederle)
Cama Arthritis Pain Reliever (Dorsey Laboratories) p 908
⊞ Camalox Suspension (Rorer)
Camalox Tablets (Rorer) p 431
⊞ Campho-Phenique Lip Balm (Winthrop Consumer Products)
Cannula Curette with Swivel Handle (Milex)
Cantharone (Seres) p 1939
Cantharone Plus (Seres) p 1939
Cantil (Merrell Dow) p 421, 1362
Cantri Vaginal Cream (Hauck)
Canz Tablets (O'Neal, Jones & Feldman)
Capa Tablets (U.S. Ethicals)
Capastat Sulfate (Lilly) p 1132
◆ Capital with Codeine Suspension (Carnrick) p 408, 831
◆ Capital with Codeine Tablets (Carnrick) p 408, 831
Capitrol Cream Shampoo (Westwood) p 2175
Capoten (Squibb) p 437, 1986
Caprystatin (Ecological Formulas) p 929
Caquin Cream (O'Neal, Jones & Feldman)
◆ Carafate Tablets (Marion) p 417, 1182
Caramiphen Edisylate & Phenylpropanolamine Sequels Sustained Release Tablets, Expectorant (Lederle)
Carbarsone Capsules (Lilly)
Carbocaine Hydrochloride (Winthrop-Breon) p 2194

(◆ Shown in Product Identification Section)   (⊞ Described in PDR For Nonprescription Drugs)   (Products without page numbers are not described)

Product Name Index

Carbocaine Hydrochloride 3% Injection (Cook-Waite) p 881
Carbocaine Hydrochloride 2% with Neo-Cobefrin 1:20,000 Injection (Cook-Waite) p 881
Cardec DM Drops & Syrup (Schein) p 1828
◆ Cardilate Chewable Tablets (Burroughs Wellcome) p 407, 782
◆ Cardilate Oral/Sublingual Tablets (Burroughs Wellcome) p 407, 782
Cardiografin (Squibb)
Cardio-Green Vials & Single Use Units (Hynson, Westcott & Dunning)
Cardioguard Natural Lipotropic Dietary Supplement-Powder (Professional Health) p 1621
Cardioguard Natural Lipotropic Dietary Supplement-Tablets (Professional Health) p 1621
Cardio-Plus (Standard Process)
◆ Cardioquin Tablets (Purdue Frederick) p 427, 1623
◆ Cardizem (Marion) p 417, 1183
Care-4 (Marlyn)
Carisoprodol Compound Tablets (Danbury) p 887
Carisoprodol Tablets (Danbury) p 887
Carisoprodol Tablets (Geneva) p 973
Carmol HC Cream 1% (Syntex) p 2061
⊠ Carmol 10 Lotion (Syntex)
⊠ Carmol 20 Cream (Syntex)
Carnitine (Ecological Formulas)
DL-Carnitine - Amino Acid Preparation (Tyson) p 2068
L-Carnitine (Tyson) p 2068
Caroid Laxative (Winthrop Consumer Products)
Caroid Tooth Powder (Winthrop Consumer Products)
⊠ Casec (Mead Johnson Nutritional)
Castaderm (Lannett)
Castellani Paint (Pedinol) p 1580
Castor Oil, Castor Oil Favored (Roxane) p 1788
Catalyn (Standard Process)
Cataplex A-F & Betaris (Standard Process)
Cataplex E-2 (Standard Process)
Cataplex F (Standard Process)
◆ Catapres Tablets (Boehringer Ingelheim) p 406, 707
Catarase 1:5,000 & 1:10,000 (CooperVision)
Cebenase Tablets (Upjohn)
Cebocap (O'Neal, Jones & Feldman)
◆ Ceclor (Lilly) p 417, 1133
Cecon Solution (Abbott)
Cedilanid-D Injection (Sandoz Pharmaceutical Div.) p 1799
Cee-500 (Ascorbic Acid) (Legere) p 1120
Cee-1000 T.D. Tablets (Legere) p 1120
◆ CeeNU (Bristol-Myers Oncology) p 407, 758
Cefadyl (Bristol) p 731
Cefinal II Tablets (Alto)
Cefizox Injection (Smith Kline & French) p 1949
Cefobid Intravenous/Intramuscular (Roerig) p 1726
◆ Cefol Filmtab Tablets (Abbott) p 403, 510
Celestone Cream (Schering)
Celestone Phosphate Injection (Schering) p 1833
Celestone 0.6 mg. Six-Day Pack (Schering)
Celestone Soluspan Suspension (Schering) p 1835
◆ Celestone Syrup & Tablets (Schering) p 433, 1832
Celluzyme Chewable Tablets (Dalin) p 886
◆ Celontin (Half Strength) Kapseals (Parke-Davis) p 423, 1486
◆ Celontin Kapseals (Parke-Davis) p 423, 1486
Cenocort A-40 Sterile Suspension (Central Pharmaceuticals)
Cenocort Forte Sterile Suspension (Central Pharmaceuticals)
Cenolate Ampoules (Abbott)
Center-Al—Allergenic Extracts Alum Precipitated (Center)
◆ Centrax (Parke-Davis) p 423, 1487
⊠ Centrum (Lederle)
⊠ Centrum, Jr. (Childrens' Chewable) (Lederle)
Centrum, Jr. + C (Lederle)
Ceo-Two Suppositories (Beutlich) p 705
⊠ Cēpacol Anesthetic Lozenges (Troches) (Merrell Dow)
⊠ Cēpacol Mouthwash/Gargle (Merrell Dow)
⊠ Cēpacol Throat Lozenges (Merrell Dow)
⊠ CEPASTAT Sore Throat Lozenges (Merrell Dow)
⊠ CEPASTAT Sore Throat Lozenges, Cherry Flavor (Merrell Dow)
◆ Cephulac Syrup (Merrell Dow) p 421, 1362
Cerespan Capsules (USV Pharmaceutical) p 2074
Cerose Compound Capsules (Ives)
Cerose-DM (Ives)
Cerubidine (Ives) p 1026
Cerumenex Drops (Purdue Frederick) p 1624
Cetacaine Topical Anesthetic (Cetylite) p 839
Cetamide Ointment (Alcon Labs.)
Cetane Injection (w/o preservative) (O'Neal, Jones & Feldman)
Cetane Timed Capsules (O'Neal, Jones & Feldman)

Cetapred Ointment (Alcon Labs.)
Cetro-Cirose (Ives)
Cetylcide Solution (Cetylite) p 839
Cevalin Ampoules & Tablets (Lilly)
Cevi-Bid Capsules (Geriatric) p 975
Cevi-Fer Capsules (sustained release) (Geriatric) p 975
⊠ Ce-Vi-Sol (Mead Johnson Nutritional)
Cezin & Cezin-S (UAD Labs.)
◆ Chardonna-2 (Rorer) p 431, 1748
CHEK-STIX Urinalysis Control Strips (Ames) p 3004
Chemstrip bG Blood Glucose Test (Boehringer Mannheim) p 3009
Chemstrip Urine Testing System (Boehringer Mannheim) p 3009
Chenix (Rowell) p 1786
Cheracol Cough Syrup (Upjohn)
⊠ Cheracol D Cough Syrup (Upjohn)
⊠ Cheracol Plus Head Cold/Cough Formula (Upjohn)
Chexit Tablets (Dorsey Laboratories)
Children's Chloraseptic Lozenges (Procter & Gamble) p 1619
◆ Children's Panadol Chewable Tablets, Liquid, Drops (Glenbrook) p 412, 997
Chlorafed H.S. Timecelles (Hauck) p 1001
Chlorafed Liquid (Hauck) p 1001
Chlorafed Timecelles (Hauck) p 1001
Chloral Hydrate Capsules (Geneva) p 973
Chloral Hydrate Capsules, Syrup (Roxane) p 1788
Chloral Hydrate Capsules (Schein) p 1828
Chloral Methylol Ointment (Ulmer)
Chloramphenicol Ophthalmic Solution 5% (Schein) p 1828
Chloramphenicol Sodium Succinate Injection (Elkins-Sinn) p 938
Chloraseptic Liquid (Procter & Gamble) p 1619
Chloraseptic Lozenges (Procter & Gamble) p 1620
Chlordiazepoxide Capsules (Geneva) p 973
Chlordiazepoxide Hydrochloride Capsules (Roxane) p 1788
Chlordiazepoxide HCl Capsules (Schein) p 1828
Chloresium Dental Ointment (Rystan)
Chloresium Ointment (Rystan) p 1795
Chloresium Solution (Rystan) p 1795
Chloresium Tablets (Rystan)
Chloresium Toothpaste (Rystan)
Chloromycetin Cream, 1% (Parke-Davis) p 1487
Chloromycetin Hydrocortisone Ophthalmic (Parke-Davis) p 1488
◆ Chloromycetin Kapseals (Parke-Davis) p 423, 1489
Chloromycetin Ophthalmic (Parke-Davis)
Chloromycetin Ophthalmic Ointment, 1% (Parke-Davis) p 1491
◆ Chloromycetin Ophthalmic Solution (Ophthochlor) (Parke-Davis) p 425
Chloromycetin Otic (Parke-Davis) p 1491
Chloromycetin Palmitate (Parke-Davis) p 1491
Chloromycetin Sodium Succinate (Parke-Davis) p 1493
Chloromycetin-Polymyxin-Hydrocortisone Acetate Ophthalmic Ointment (Ophthocort) (Parke-Davis)
Chlorophyll Complex Ointment (Fat Soluble) (Standard Process)
Chlorophyll Complex Perles (Standard Process) p 2035
Chloroptic ophthalmic solution (Allergan)
Chloroptic S.O.P. ophthalmic ointment (Allergan)
Chloroptic-P S.O.P. ophthalmic ointment (Allergan)
Chloroquine Phosphate Tablets (Biocraft) p 705
Chloroquine Phosphate Tablets (Danbury) p 887
Chloroserpine 250 & 500 Tablets (Schein) p 1828
Chlorothiazide Tablets (Danbury) p 887
Chlorothiazide Tablets (Geneva) p 973
Chlorothiazide Tablets (Schein) p 1828
Chlorothiazide w/Reserpine Tablets (Geneva) p 973
◆ Chlorpheniramine Maleate (Lederle) p 416
Chlorpheniramine Maleate T.D. Capsules (Geneva) p 973
Chlorpheniramine Maleate Tablets (Roxane) p 1788
Chlorpheniramine Maleate & Phenylpropanolamine Sequels, Tablets & Capsules (Lederle)
Chlorpromazine HCl Injection (Elkins-Sinn) p 938
Chlorpromazine HCl Tablets (Schein) p 1828
Chlorpromazine HCl in Tubex (Wyeth) p 2288
Chlorpromazine Tablets & Concentrate Syrup (Geneva) p 973
◆ Chlorpromazine HCl Tablets, Liquid Concentrate (Lederle) p 416
Chlorpropamide Tablets (Danbury) p 887
Chlorpropamide Tablets (Geneva) p 973
◆ Chlorthalidone Tablets (Lederle) p 416
Chlorthalidone Tablets (Abbott) p 403, 510
Chlorthalidone Tablets (Danbury) p 887
Chlorthalidone Tablets (Schein) p 1828
Chlorthalidone Tablets, USP (Parke-Davis) p 1494

⊠ Chlor-Trimeton Allergy Syrup (Schering)
◆ Chlor-Trimeton Allergy Tablets (Schering) p 434
◆ Chlor-Trimeton 12 mg Antihistamine Timed-Release Allergy Tablets (Schering) p 434
◆ Chlor-Trimeton Decongestant Tablets (Schering) p 434
⊠ Chlor-Trimeton Expectorant (Schering)
Chlor-Trimeton Injection (Schering)
◆ Chlor-Trimeton Long-Acting Allergy Repetabs Tablets (Schering) p 434
◆ Chlor-Trimeton Long-Acting Decongestant Repetabs Tablets (Schering) p 434
Chlorulan Tablets (Lannett)
Chlorzone Forte Tablets (Schein) p 1828
Chlorzoxazone Tablets (Danbury) p 887
Chlorzoxazone with APAP Tablets (Danbury) p 887
Chlorzoxasone w/APAP Tablets (Geneva) p 973
Cholan HMB (Pennwalt)
Cholan-DH (Pennwalt)
◆ Choledyl (Parke-Davis) p 423, 1495
Choledyl Pediatric Syrup (Parke-Davis) p 1495
◆ Choledyl SA Tablets (Parke-Davis) p 423, 1497
Cholera Vaccine (Sclavo) p 1897
Cholera Vaccine (Wyeth) p 2245
Cholera Vaccine (India Strains) (Lederle) p 1089
Cholografin Meglumine (Squibb)
Cholografin Meglumine for Infusion (Squibb)
◆ Choloxin (Flint) p 411, 949
Chondroitin-4-Sulphate (Ecological Formulas)
Chorex (Hyrex)
Choron "10" Injectable Pak (O'Neal, Jones & Feldman)
◆ Chromagen Capsules (Savage) p 433, 1824
Chromagen Injection (Savage)
Chromagen OB (Savage) p 1824
Chrometrace (Armour) p 604
◆ Chronulac Syrup (Merrell Dow) p 421, 1363
Chymex (Adria) p 3003
◆ Chymodiactin (Smith) p 437, 1983
Chymoral (USV Pharmaceutical)
Chymoral-100 (USV Pharmaceutical)
Cibalith-S Syrup (CIBA) p 852
Cinalone 40 (Legere)
◆ Cinobac Pulvules (Dista) p 410, 894
Cino-40 Injection (Reid-Provident, Direct Div.)
Cinonide 40 (Legere) p 1120
Cin-Quin (Rowell)
Circanol (Riker) p 1642
Citanest Solutions (Astra)
Citra Forte Capsules (Boyle) p 726
Citra Forte Syrup (Boyle) p 726
⊠ Citrocarbonate Antacid (Upjohn)
Citrolith Tablets (Beach)
Citrotein (Clinical Nutrition) p 876
Claforan (Hoechst-Roussel) p 1010
Clean-N-Soak hard contact lens cleaning & soaking solution (Allergan)
Clean-N-Soakit hard contact lens storage case (Allergan)
Clean-N-Stow hard contact lens storage case (Allergan)
Clear By Design, Acne Skin Medication (Herbert)
Clear Eyes Eye Drops (Ross) p 1762
⊠ Clearasil Adult Care (Sulfur/Resorcinol) (Personal Care)
⊠ Clearasil 5% Benzoyl Peroxide Lotion Acne Treatment (Personal Care)
⊠ Clearasil Pore Deep Cleanser (Salicylic Acid 0.5%) (Personal Care)
⊠ Clearasil Super Strength Acne Treatment Cream (10% Benzoyl Peroxide) (Personal Care)
◆ Cleocin HCl Capsules* (Upjohn) p 441, 2094
Cleocin Pediatric Flavored Granules* (Upjohn) p 2096
◆ Cleocin Phosphate Sterile Solution* (Upjohn) p 440, 2097
◆ Cleocin T Topical Solution* (Upjohn) p 441, 2100
Clērz (CooperVision)
Clerz 2 (CooperVision)
⊠ Clinitar Cream (Ulmer)
⊠ Clinitar Shampoo (Ulmer)
⊠ Clinitar Stick (Ulmer)
Clini-Tek Reflectance Photometer (Ames)
◆ Clinoril Tablets (Merck Sharp & Dohme) p 420, 1274
Clipoxide Capsules (Schein) p 1828
Clistin Tablets (McNeil Pharmaceutical)
Clistin-D Tablets (McNeil Pharmaceutical)
Clock E, 400 I.U. (Marlyn)
Clocream Skin Cream (Upjohn)
Cloderm (Ortho Pharmaceutical (Dermatological Div.)) p 1472
Clomid (Merrell Dow) p 1364
◆ Clonopin Tablets (Roche) p 429, 1680
Clorpactin WCS-90 (Guardian) p 1000
Clorpactin XCB (Guardian)
◆ Cloxacillin Capsules (Lederle) p 416
Cloxacillin Capsules (Biocraft) p 705
Cloxacillin Sodium Capsules (Schein) p 1828
Cloxacillin Solution (Biocraft) p 705
◆ Cloxapen Capsules (Beecham Laboratories) p 406
Clusivol Capsules (Ayerst) p 640
Clusivol Syrup (Ayerst) p 640

(◆ Shown in Product Identification Section)   (⊠ Described in PDR For Nonprescription Drugs)   (Products without page numbers are not described)

Clusivol 130 Tablets (Ayerst) p 640
Clysodrast (Armour)
Cobolin-M (Legere) p 1120
Cocaine Hydrochloride Topical Solution (Roxane) p 1788
◆ Cod Liver Oil Concentrate Capsules (Schering) p 433
◆ Cod Liver Oil Concentrate Tablets* (Schering) p 433
◆ Cod Liver Oil Concentrate Tablets w/Vitamin C (Schering) p 433
Codalan (Lannett) p 1071
Codap Tablets (Reid-Provident, Direct Div.)
Codeine Phosphate Carpuject (Winthrop-Breon)
Codeine Phosphate Injection (Elkins-Sinn) p 938
Codeine Phosphate in Tubex (Wyeth) p 2288
Codeine Phosphate Oral Solution (Roxane) p 1788
Codeine Sulfate Tablets (Roxane) p 1788
⊛ Codexin Capsules (Arco)
Codiclear DH Syrup (Central Pharmaceuticals) p 836
Codimal DH (Central Pharmaceuticals) p 836
Codimal DM (Central Pharmaceuticals) p 836
Codimal Expectorant (Central Pharmaceuticals) p 836
Codimal PH (Central Pharmaceuticals) p 836
Codimal Tablets & Capsules (Central Pharmaceuticals)
Codimal-A Injectable (Central Pharmaceuticals)
◆ Codimal-L.A. Capsules (Central Pharmaceuticals) p 409, 836
Codroxomin Injectable (O'Neal, Jones & Feldman)
Co-Gel Tablets (Arco)
◆ Cogentin Tablets & Injection (Merck Sharp & Dohme) p 420, 1276
Co-Gesic Tablets (Central Pharmaceuticals) p 409, 836
◆ Colace (Mead Johnson Pharmaceutical) p 419, 1248
◆ ColBENEMID Tablets (Merck Sharp & Dohme) p 420, 1277
Colchicine Ampoules (Lilly) p 1134
Colchicine Tablets (Danbury) p 887
Colchicine Tablets (Lilly) p 1135
Cold Cream (Fougera)
⊛ Cold Factor 12 (Pharmacraft)
Colestid Granules (Upjohn) p 2100
Colladerm (C & M)
⊛ Collyrium Eye Lotion (Wyeth) p 2249
⊛ Collyrium 2 Eye Drops with Tetrahydrozoline (Wyeth) p 2249
Cologel Liquid (Lilly)
ColoScreen/VPI (Helena Labs.) p 3010
Col-Probenecid Tablets (Danbury) p 887
Colrex Capsules (Rowell)
Colrex Compound Capsules (Rowell)
Colrex Compound Elixir (Rowell)
Colrex Decongestant (Rowell)
Colrex Expectorant (Rowell)
Colrex Syrup (Rowell)
Colrex Troches (Rowell)
Coly-Mycin M Parenteral (Parke-Davis) p 1500
Coly-Mycin S Oral Suspension (Parke-Davis) p 1501
Coly-Mycin S Otic w/Neomycin & Hydrocortisone (Parke-Davis) p 1501
◆ Combid Spansule Capsules (Smith Kline & French) p 436, 1952
◆ Combipres Tablets (Boehringer Ingelheim) p 406, 708
Comfortine Ointment (Dermik)
Comfrey, Pepsin—Formula E-3 (Standard Process)
◆ Comhist LA Capsules (Norwich Eaton) p 422, 1425
Comhist Tablets (Norwich Eaton) p 1426
◆ Compal Capsules (Reid-Provident Labs.) p 427, 1637
◆ Compazine (Smith Kline & French) p 436, 1953
Compete (Mission) p 1416
Compleat Modified Formula (Clinical Nutrition) p 876
Compleat-B (Clinical Nutrition) p 877
⊛ Complex 15 Lotion & Cream (Baker/Cummins)
Component Nipple System (Ross) p 1777
Compound W Solution & Gel (Whitehall)
Comtrex (Bristol-Myers Products) p 769
Conar Expectorant Syrup (Beecham Laboratories)
Conar Suspension (Beecham Laboratories)
Conar-A Suspension (Beecham Laboratories)
Conar-A Tablets (Beecham Laboratories)
⊛ Conceptrol Birth Control Cream (Ortho Pharmaceutical)
⊛ Conceptrol Contraceptive Gel Disposable (Ortho Pharmaceutical)
Conex (O'Neal, Jones & Feldman) p 1445
Conex DA Tablet (O'Neal, Jones & Feldman)
Conex Lozenges (O'Neal, Jones & Feldman)
Conex Plus Tablets (O'Neal, Jones & Feldman)
Conex with Codeine (O'Neal, Jones & Feldman) p 1445
Congespirin Aspirin-Free Chewable Cold Tablets for Children (Bristol-Myers Products) p 769
Congespirin Cold Tablets (Aspirin Formula) (Bristol-Myers Products) p 769

Congespirin Cough Syrup (Bristol-Myers Products) p 770
Congespirin Liquid Cold Medicine (Bristol-Myers Products) p 770
Congess Jr. & Sr. T.D. Capsules (Fleming) p 948
Conjugated Estrogens Tablets (Geneva) p 973
Conjugated Estrogens Tablets - Coated (Schein) p 1828
Consept (Consolidated Chemical)
Consol Concentrate (Consolidated Chemical)
◆ Constant-T Tablets (Geigy) p 411, 958
Contactisol (CooperVision)
Control Capsules, Maximum Strength (Thompson Medical) p 2066
Converspaz Improved Capsules (Ascher)
Converzyme Improved Capsules (Ascher)
CooperVision Balanced Salt Solution (CooperVision)
Copavin, Pulvules (Lilly)
Cope (Glenbrook)
Coppertrace (Armour) p 605
Co-Pyronil 2 (Dista) p 895
Coramine (CIBA) p 846
Cordran Ointment & Lotion (Dista) p 895
Cordran SP Cream (Dista) p 895
Cordran Tape (Dista) p 897
Cordran-N (Dista) p 897
◆ Corgard (Squibb) p 437, 1989
Corgonject-5 (Mayrand)
◆ Coricidin Cough Syrup (Schering)
◆ Coricidin "D" Decongestant Tablets (Schering) p 434
⊛ Coricidin Decongestant Nasal Mist (Schering)
⊛ Coricidin Demilets Tablets For Children (Schering) p 434
⊛ Coricidin Extra Strength Sinus Headache Tablets (Schering) p 434
⊛ Coricidin Medilets Tablets For Children (Schering) p 434
⊛ Coricidin Tablets (Schering) p 434
Corilin Infant Liquid (Schering)
Corrective Mixture w/Paregoric (Beecham Laboratories)
Corsym (Pennwalt) p 1582
⊛ Cortaid Cream (Upjohn)
⊛ Cortaid Lotion (Upjohn)
⊛ Cortaid Ointment (Upjohn)
⊛ Cortaid Spray (Upjohn)
Cort-Dome ⅛%, ¼%, ½%, and 1% Creme (Miles Pharmaceuticals) p 1399
Cort-Dome ⅛%, ¼%, ½%, and 1% Lotion (Miles Pharmaceuticals) p 1400
Cort-Dome High Potency Suppositories (Miles Pharmaceuticals) p 1401
Cort-Dome Regular Potency Suppositories (Miles Pharmaceuticals) p 1401
Cortef Acetate Ointment (Upjohn)
Cortef Acetate Sterile Suspensiion (Upjohn)
⊛ Cortef Feminine Itch Cream (Upjohn)
Cortef Oral Suspension (Upjohn)
⊛ Cortef Rectal Itch Ointment (Upjohn)
Cortef Sterile Suspension IM (Upjohn)
Cortef Tablets (Upjohn)
Cortenema (Rowell)
◆ Corticaine Cream (Glaxo) p 412, 980
◆ Corticaine Suppositories (Glaxo) p 412, 980
◆ Cortifoam (Reed & Carnrick) p 427, 1632
Cortifair Cream & Lotion (Pharmafair) p 1618
Cortigel-40 (Savage)
Cortigel-80 (Savage)
Cortin 1% Cream (C & M)
Cortisone Acetate Tablets, USP (Upjohn)
Cortisporin Cream (Burroughs Wellcome) p 783
Cortisporin Ointment (Burroughs Wellcome) p 784
Cortisporin Ophthalmic Ointment (Burroughs Wellcome) p 784
Cortisporin Ophthalmic Suspension (Burroughs Wellcome) p 785
Cortisporin Otic Solution (Burroughs Wellcome) p 786
Cortisporin Otic Suspension (Burroughs Wellcome) p 786
Cortixin Otic Suspension (Kramer)
Cortone Acetate Saline Suspension (Merck Sharp & Dohme)
Cortone Acetate Tablets (Merck Sharp & Dohme)
Cortril Topical Ointment (Pfiphармecs) p 1589
Cortrophin-Zinc (Organon) p 1446
Cortrosyn (Organon) p 1446
Coryban-D Capsules (Pfipharmecs) p 1589
Coryban-D Cough Syrup (Pfipharmecs) p 1589
◆ Corzide (Squibb) p 437, 1990
Cosmegen Injection (Merck Sharp & Dohme) p 1278
Cosprin (Glenbrook) p 996
Cosprin 650 (Glenbrook) p 997
◆ Cotazym (Organon) p 422, 1446
Cotazym-B (Organon)
◆ Cotazym-S (Organon) p 422, 1446
Cotrim (Lemmon) p 1122
Cotrim D.S. (Lemmon) p 1122
◆ CoTylenol Cold Medication Tablets & Capsules (McNeil Consumer Products) p 418, 1197
CoTylenol Liquid Cold Medication (McNeil Consumer Products) p 1197

◆ CoTylenol Children's Liquid Cold Formula (McNeil Consumer Products) p 418, 1198
◆ Coumadin (Du Pont) p 410, 915
Covanamine Liquid (Wallace)
Covangesic Tablets (Wallace)
Covicone Cream (Abbott)
Co-Xan Syrup (Central Pharmaceuticals)
Creamalin Tablets (Winthrop Consumer Products)
◆ Cremacoat 1 (Vicks Pharmacy Products) p 442, 2146
◆ Cremacoat 2 (Vicks Pharmacy Products) p 442, 2147
◆ Cremacoat 3 (Vicks Pharmacy Products) p 442, 2147
◆ Cremacoat 4 (Vicks Pharmacy Products) p 442, 2147
Cremesone (Dalin)
Crescormon (Pharmacia) p 1616
⊛ Criticare HN (Mead Johnson Nutritional)
⊛ Cruex Antifungal Cream (Pharmacraft)
⊛ Cruex Antifungal Powder & Spray Powder (Pharmacraft)
Cryophake (Alcon Labs.)
Crysticillin 300 A.S. & Crysticillin 600 A.S. (Squibb) p 1992
Crystimin-1000 (Reid-Provident Labs.)
Crystodigin Ampoules (Lilly)
◆ Crystodigin Tablets (Lilly) p 417, 1135
◆ Cu-7 (Searle Pharmaceuticals) p 435, 1902
◆ Cuprimine Capsules (Merck Sharp & Dohme) p 420, 1280
Curretab Tablets (Reid-Provident Labs.) p 427, 1638
Cyanocobalamin in Tubex (Wyeth) p 445, 2288
Cyanocobalamin (Vit. B$_{12}$) Injection (Elkins-Sinn) p 938
Cyanoject (Mayrand)
Cyclaine Topical Solution (Merck Sharp & Dohme)
Cyclandelate Capsules (Geneva) p 973
Cyclandelate Capsules (Schein) p 1828
◆ Cyclapen-W (Wyeth) p 444, 2249
Cyclocen Injectable (Central Pharmaceuticals)
◆ Cyclocort Cream (Lederle) p 415, 1089
◆ Cyclocort Ointment (Lederle) p 415, 1089
Cyclogyl (Alcon Labs.)
Cyclomydril (Alcon Labs.)
◆ Cyclopar & Cyclopar 500 Capsules (tetracycline hydrochloride, USP) (Parke-Davis) p 426
◆ Cyclospasmol (Ives) p 413, 1028
◆ Cylert Chewable Tablets (Abbott) p 403
◆ Cylert Tablets (Abbott) p 403, 510
Cyomin Injectable (O'Neal, Jones & Feldman)
Cyproheptadine HCl Syrup & Tablets (Schein) p 1828
Cyproheptadine HCl Tablets (Danbury) p 887
Cyproheptadine HCl Tablets (Geneva) p 973
Cystex Tablets (CooperVision)
Cystografin (Squibb)
Cystografin Dilute (Squibb)
Cystospaz (Webcon) p 2172
Cystospaz-M (Webcon) p 2172
◆ Cytadren (CIBA) p 409, 846
Cytoferin Hematinic Tablets (Ayerst)
◆ Cytomel Tablets (Smith Kline & French) p 436, 1956
Cytosar-U Sterile Powder (Upjohn) p 2102
Cytoxan (Bristol-Myers Oncology) p 407, 759

D

D'Alpha-E Capsules (Alto)
◆ DDAVP (USV Pharmaceutical) p 440, 2074
◆ DDAVP Injection (USV Pharmaceutical) p 440, 2075
d-Film (CooperVision)
D.H.E. 45 (Sandoz Pharmaceutical Div.) p 1800
DHS Conditioning Rinse (Persön & Covey) p 1587
DHS Shampoo (Persön & Covey) p 1587
DHS Tar Shampoo (Persön & Covey) p 1587
DHS Zinc Dandruff Shampoo (Persön & Covey) p 1587
DHT (Dihydrotachysterol) Tablets, Oral Solution & Intensol (Roxane) p 1789
DOB Bath & Shower Oil (Formerly Tolakol) (Persön & Covey)
DTIC-Dome (Miles Pharmaceuticals) p 1402
DV Cream (Merrell Dow) p 1364
Dacriose Ophthalmic Irrigating Solution (CooperVision)
Daily-M Tablets (Upsher-Smith)
Daily Nutritional Paks (Marlyn)
Dainite Tablets (Wallace)
Dainite-KI Tablets (Wallace)
Dalalone Injectable (O'Neal, Jones & Feldman) p 1445
Dalalone D.P. Injectable (O'Neal, Jones & Feldman) p 1445
Dalalone L.A. Injectable (O'Neal, Jones & Feldman) p 1445
Dalca Tablets (Ascher)
Dalcaine Injection (O'Neal, Jones & Feldman) p 1445
Dalex Lozenges (Dalin)
Dalex Pediatric Syrup (Dalin)

(◆ Shown in Product Identification Section)   (⊛ Described in PDR For Nonprescription Drugs)   (Products without page numbers are not described)

Product Name Index

Dalex Syrup (Dalin)
Dalex Syrup Forte (Dalin)
Dalicote Lotion (Dalin)
Daliderm Liquid (Dalin)
Dalidyne (Dalin) p 886
Dalidyne Jel (Dalin)
Dalidyne Spray (Mouth and Throat) (Dalin)
Dalifort Tablets (Dalin)
Daligesic Liniment (Dalin)
Dalivim Forte Liquid & Tablets (Dalin)
Dallergy Capsules, Tablets, Syrup (Laser) p 1072
◆ Dalmane Capsules (Roche Products) p 429, 1710
◆ Damacet-P (Mason) p 418, 1193
◆ Damason-P (Mason) p 418, 1194
▥ Danex Protein Enriched Dandruff Shampoo (Herbert)
◆ Danocrine (Winthrop-Breon) p 443, 2195
Danthron Tablets (Geneva) p 973
Dantrium Capsules (Norwich Eaton) p 1426
Dantrium Intravenous (Norwich Eaton) p 1428
Dapa Tablets (Ferndale)
Dapacin Capsules (Ferndale)
Dapex Capsules (Ferndale)
Dapsone (Jacobus) p 1032
Daranide Tablets (Merck Sharp & Dohme)
Daraprim (Burroughs Wellcome) p 407, 787
◆ Darbid (Smith Kline & French) p 436, 1958
Daricon (Beecham Laboratories)
Daricon PB (Beecham Laboratories)
◆ Darvocet-N 50 (Lilly) p 417, 1136
◆ Darvocet-N 100 (Lilly) p 417, 1136
◆ Darvon (Lilly) p 417, 1139
◆ Darvon Compound (Lilly) p 417, 1139
◆ Darvon Compound-65 (Lilly) p 417, 1139
◆ Darvon with A.S.A. (Lilly) p 417, 1139
◆ Darvon-N (Lilly) p 417, 1136
◆ Darvon-N with A.S.A. (Lilly) p 417, 1136
Dasin Capsules (Beecham Laboratories)
Dayalets Filmtab (Abbott) p 511
Dayalets plus Iron Filmtab (Abbott) p 511
▥ Daycare Daytime Colds Medicine-liquid (Vicks Health Care)
▥ Daycare Multi-Symptom Colds Medicine-capsules (Vicks Health Care)
Day-Vite (Drug Industries)
◆ Deapril-ST (Mead Johnson Pharmaceutical) p 419, 1248
Debrisan Wound Cleaning Beads (Johnson & Johnson (Patient Care Div.)) p 1044
Debrisan Wound Cleaning Paste (Johnson & Johnson (Patient Care Div.)) p 1044
Debrox Drops (Marion) p 1184
Decaderm (Merck Sharp & Dohme)
Decadron Elixir (Merck Sharp & Dohme) p 1284
Decadron Phosphate Injection (Merck Sharp & Dohme) p 1288
Decadron Phosphate Respihaler (Merck Sharp & Dohme) p 1291
Decadron Phosphate Sterile Ophthalmic Ointment (Merck Sharp & Dohme) p 1290
Decadron Phosphate Sterile Ophthalmic Solution (Merck Sharp & Dohme) p 1291
Decadron Phosphate Topical Cream (Merck Sharp & Dohme)
Decadron Phosphate Turbinaire (Merck Sharp & Dohme) p 1293
Decadron Phosphate w/Xylocaine Injection (Merck Sharp & Dohme)
◆ Decadron Tablets (Merck Sharp & Dohme) p 420, 1286
Decadron-LA Suspension (Merck Sharp & Dohme) p 1294
Deca-Durabolin (Organon) p 1446
Decaject (Mayrand)
Decaject-L.A. (Mayrand)
Decaspray Topical Aerosol (Merck Sharp & Dohme) p 1296
Decholin Tablets (Miles Pharmaceuticals) p 421, 1402
Declofen SR Capsules (U.S. Ethicals)
◆ Declomycin Capsules and Tablets (Lederle) p 415, 1090
◆ Deconamine Tablets, Elixir, SR Capsules, Syrup (Berlex) p 406, 699
Decongestant Elixir (Schein) p 1828
Decongestant Expectorant (Schein) p 1828
Decongestant-AT (Antitussive) Liquid (Schein) p 1828
Dehist (O'Neal, Jones & Feldman) p 1445
Dehist Injectable (O'Neal, Jones & Feldman)
Deladumone (Squibb)
Deladumone OB (Squibb)
Delalutin (Squibb)
Delatestryl (Squibb)
Delaxin Tablets (Ferndale)
Delcid (Merrell Dow)
Delestrogen (Squibb)
▥ Delfen Contraceptive Foam (Ortho Pharmaceutical)
Delsym (Pennwalt) p 1582
Delta-Cortef Tablets (Upjohn) p 2107
Deltalin Gelseals (Lilly)
Deltamycin Capsules (Trimen)
Deltapen-VK Solution (Trimen)
Deltapen-VK Tablets (Trimen)
◆ Deltasone Tablets (Upjohn) p 441, 2107
Deltavac Cream (Trimen)

Demasone Injectable (Bock)
Demasone-LA Injectable (Bock)
◆ Demazin Timed-Release Tablets (Schering) p 434
▥ Demazin Syrup (Schering)
◆ Demerol APAP Tablets (Winthrop-Breon) p 443
Demerol Carpuject (Winthrop-Breon)
◆ Demerol Hydrochloride (Winthrop-Breon) p 443, 2197
◆ Demi-Regroton Tablets (USV Pharmaceutical) p 440, 2087
Demser Capsules (Merck Sharp & Dohme) p 420, 1297
◆ Demulen 1/35-21 (Searle & Co.) p 435, 1919
◆ Demulen 1/35-28 (Searle & Co.) p 435, 1919
◆ Demulen 1/50-21 (Searle & Co.) p 435, 1919
◆ Demulen 1/50-28 (Searle & Co.) p 435, 1919
Denalan Denture Cleanser (Whitehall)
◆ Denorex Medicated Shampoo and Conditioner (Whitehall) p 443, 2185
◆ Denorex Medicated Shampoo, Regular & Mountain Fresh Herbal Scent (Whitehall) p 443, 2185
▥ Denquel Sensitive Teeth Toothpaste (Personal Care)
Dentavite Chewable Tablets (Reid-Provident Labs.)
◆ Depakene Capsules & Syrup (Abbott) p 403, 512
◆ Depakote Tablets (Abbott) p 403, 513
depAndro "100" & "200" Injectable (O'Neal, Jones & Feldman)
depAndrogyn Injectable (O'Neal, Jones & Feldman)
Depen Titratable Tablets (Wallace) p 2152
depGynogen Injectable (O'Neal, Jones & Feldman)
depMedalone "40" Injectable (O'Neal, Jones & Feldman) p 1445
depMedalone "80" Injectable (O'Neal, Jones & Feldman) p 1445
Depo-Estradiol Sterile Solution (Upjohn)
Depoject-40 & Depoject-80 (Mayrand)
◆ Depo-Medrol (Upjohn) p 441, 2107
Depo-Predate 40 (Legere) p 1120
Depo-Predate 80 (Legere) p 1120
Depo-Provera (Upjohn) p 2109
Depotest (Hyrex)
Depo-Testadiol Sterile Solution (Upjohn)
Depotestogen (Hyrex)
Depo-Testosterone (Upjohn) p 2111
Deproist Expectorant w/Codeine (Geneva) p 973
Deprol (Wallace) p 2155
Derifil Tablets & Powder (Rystan) p 1796
Derma Cas Gel (Hill Dermaceuticals) p 1009
▥ Derma Medicone Ointment (Medicone)
Derma Medicone-HC Ointment (Medicone) p 1256
Dermacort Cream (Rowell)
Dermacort Lotion-0.5%, 1% (Rowell)
Dermarex Cream (Hyrex)
Derma-Smoothe/FS (Hill Dermaceuticals) p 1009
Derma-Smoothe Oil (Hill Dermaceuticals)
Derma-Sone Cream (Hill Dermaceuticals) p 1009
Dermaval Cream (Vale)
◆ Dermolate Anal-Itch Ointment (Schering)
▥ Dermolate Anti-Itch Cream (Schering)
▥ Dermolate Anti-Itch Spray (Schering)
▥ Dermolate Scalp-Itch Lotion (Schering)
Dermoplast Aerosol Spray (Ayerst) p 640
◆ Desenex Antifungal Cream, Ointment, Foam & Liquid (Pharmacraft)
◆ Desenex Antifungal Powder & Spray Powder (Pharmacraft)
Desferal mesylate (CIBA) p 847
▥ Desitin Ointment (Leeming)
Desone & Desone-LA (UAD Labs.)
Desoxyn (Abbott) p 515
◆ Desoxyn Graduмет Tablets (Abbott) p 403, 515
Desquam-X 2.5 Gel (Westwood) p 2175
Desquam-X 5 Gel (Westwood) p 2175
Desquam-X 10 Gel (Westwood) p 2175
Desquam-X 5 Wash (Westwood) p 2176
Desquam-X 10 Wash (Westwood) p 2176
◆ Desyrel (Mead Johnson Pharmaceutical) p 419, 1249
Detachol Adhesive Remover (Ferndale)
▥ Deter Jr. T.D. Capsules (Fleming)
Deter Sr. T.D. Capsules (Fleming)
Detussin Expectorant (Schein) p 1828
Detussin Liquid (Schein) p 1828
Dexacen LA-8 Sterile Suspension (Central Pharmaceuticals)
Dexacen-4 Injectable (Central Pharmaceuticals)
Dexamethasone Injection (Bristol) p 730
Dexamethasone Sodium Phosphate Injection (Elkins-Sinn) p 938
Dexamethasone Sodium Phosphate in Tubex (Wyeth) p 2288
Dexamethasone Tablets, Oral Solution & Intensol (Roxane) p 1788
Dexamethasone Tablets (Schein) p 1828
Dexampex Tablets and Capsules (Lemmon)
Dexamycin Ophthalmic Ointment (Schein) p 1828
Dexasone 4 (Legere) p 1120
Dexasone 10 (Legere) p 1120
Dexasone LA (Legere) p 1120
Dexatrim Capsules (Thompson Medical) p 2066

Dexatrim Capsules, Extra Strength (Thompson Medical) p 2066
Dexatrim Capsules, Extra Strength, Caffeine-Free (Thompson Medical) p 2066
Dexatrim Capsules, Extra Strength, Plus Vitamins (Thompson Medical) p 2066
Dexatrim • 15 (Thompson Medical) p 2066
Dexatrim • 15, Caffeine-Free (Thompson Medical) p 2066
Dexchlor Repeat Action Tablets (Schein) p 1828
◆ Dexedrine (Smith Kline & French) p 436, 1959
Dexol T.D. Tablets (Legere) p 1120
Dexol 300 (Legere) p 1120
Dexone (Rowell)
Dexpanthenol Injection (d-Pantothenyl Alcohol) (Elkins-Sinn) p 938
Dextraron (Legere) p 1120
Dextroamphetamine Sulfate, 5mg. & 10mg. (Rexar) p 1641
Dextrometer Reflectance Colorimeter (Ames) p 3006
Dextrose Injection (Bristol) p 730
Dextrose Injection (Elkins-Sinn) p 938
Dextrostix Reagent Strips (Ames) p 3005
Dextrotussin Syrup (Lambda)
Dezone Injectable (Reid-Provident, Direct Div.)
◆ DiaBeta (Hoechst-Roussel) p 412, 1012
◆ Diabinese (Pfizer) p 426, 1599
Diabismul Suspension (O'Neal, Jones & Feldman)
Diabismul Tablets (O'Neal, Jones & Feldman)
Dia-Eze (Central Pharmaceuticals)
Dia-Gesic (Central Pharmaceuticals) p 409, 837
Dialose Capsules (Stuart) p 439, 2036
Dialose Plus Capsules (Stuart) p 439, 2037
Dialume (Armour) p 404, 605
Diamox Parenteral (Lederle) p 1091
◆ Diamox Sequels, Tablets (Lederle) p 415, 1091
Diaparene Line (Glenbrook)
Diapid Nasal Spray (Sandoz Pharmaceutical Div.) p 1801
Diaqua Tablets (Hauck)
Diasporal Cream (Doak)
Diastix Reagent Strips (Ames) p 3004
Diatrizoate Meglumine Injection USP 76% (Squibb)
Dibasic Calcium Phosphate Tablets (Lilly)
Dibasic Calcium Phosphate w/Vitamin D Pulvules (Lilly)
◆ Dibenzyline Capsules (Smith Kline & French) p 436, 1960
Dibucaine Ointment 1% (Fougera) p 953
Dical-D Capsules & Wafers (Abbott) p 516
Dicalsonate Capsules (Lannett)
Dicloxacillin Capsules (Biocraft) p 705
Dicloxacillin Sodium Capsules (Schein) p 1828
◆ Dicumarol Tablets (Abbott) p 403, 517
Dicyclomine HCl Capsules (Danbury) p 887
Dicyclomine HCl Tablets (Danbury) p 887
◆ Didrex Tablets (Upjohn) p 441, 2111
◆ Didronel (Norwich Eaton) p 422, 1429
Dietex T.D. (Arlo)
◆ Diethylpropion HCl Tablets & Timed Tablets (Schein) p 1828
Diethylstilbestrol Enseals & Tablets (Lilly) p 1141
Diethylstilbestrol Suppositories (Lilly) p 1141
Dieutrim Capsules (Legere) p 1120
Digepepsin Tablets (RAM Laboratories) p 1632
Digesplen Elixir (Medical Products)
Digesplen-Plus Tablets (Medical Products)
Digestol Elixir (Arlo)
Digiglusin Tablets (Lilly)
Digilab Model 30D Pneuma-Tonometer (Alcon Labs.)
Digilab Model 30R Pneuma-Tonometer (Alcon Labs.)
Digilab Model 30R/T Pneuma-Tonometer-Tonographer (Alcon Labs.)
Digoxin Injection (Elkins-Sinn) p 938
Digoxin in Tubex (Wyeth) p 2288
Dihydrocodeine Compound Tablets (Schein) p 1828
Di-Hydrotic (Legere) p 1120
◆ Dilantin Infatabs (Parke-Davis) p 423, 1503
Dilantin Kapseals (Parke-Davis) p 423, 1502
Dilantin Parenteral (Parke-Davis) p 1505
◆ Dilantin with Phenobarbital (Parke-Davis) p 423, 1507
Dilantin-30 Pediatric/Dilantin-125 Suspension (Parke-Davis) p 1506
Dilart Capsules (Trimen)
Dilateria (Milex)
◆ Dilatrate-SR (Reed & Carnrick) p 427, 1632
Dilaudid Cough Syrup (Knoll) p 1058
◆ Dilaudid Hydrochloride (Knoll) p 414, 1057
◆ Dilaudid-HP Injection (Knoll) p 414, 1059
Dilor Elixir (Savage)
◆ Dilor Injectable (Savage) p 433
◆ Dilor Tablets (Savage) p 433, 1824
◆ Dilor-400 Tablets (Savage) p 433
◆ Dilor-G Tablets & Liquid (Savage) p 433, 1824
Diluent (Flavored) for Oral Use (Roxane) p 1788
▥ Dimacol Capsules (Robins)
Dimacol Liquid (Robins)
Dimenhydrinate in Tubex (Wyeth) p 2288
◆ Dimetane-DC Cough Syrup (Robins) p 1647

(◆ Shown in Product Identification Section)   (▥ Described in PDR For Nonprescription Drugs)   (Products without page numbers are not described)

Product Name Index

- ⊞ **Dimetane Decongestant Elixir** (Robins)
- ⊞ **Dimetane Decongestant Tablets** (Robins)
- ⊞ **Dimetane Elixir** (Robins)
- ⊞ **Dimetane Extentabs** (Robins)
- ⊞ **Dimetane Tablets** (Robins)
- **Dimetane-Ten Injectable** (Robins)
- **Dimetapp Elixir** (Robins) p 1648
- ◆ **Dimetapp Extentabs** (Robins) p 428, 1648
- **Dioctocal Capsules - Docusate Calcium USP** (Schein) p 1828
- **Diostate D Tablets** (Upjohn)
- **Diphenacen-10 and -50 Injectables** (Central Pharmaceuticals)
- **Diphenhydramine Capsules** (Geneva) p 973
- **Diphenhydramine HCl Caps** (Schein) p 1828
- **Diphenhydramine HCl Capsules** (Danbury) p 887
- **Diphenhydramine Hydrochloride Capsules, Elixir** (Roxane) p 1788
- **Diphenhydramine HCl Injection** (Bristol) p 730
- **Diphenhydramine HCl Injection** (Elkins-Sinn) p 938
- **Diphenhydramine HCl in Tubex** (Wyeth) p 2288
- **Diphenoxylate & Atropine Liquid (DPXL) & Tabs** (Schein) p 1828
- **Diphenoxylate Hydrochloride & Atropine Sulfate Tablets & Oral Solution** (Roxane) p 1788
- **Diphtheria Antitoxin (equine), Refined** (Sclavo) p 1897
- **Diphtheria Antitoxin (Purified, Concentrated Globulin-Equine)** (Squibb/Connaught) p 2033
- **Diphtheria & Tetanus Toxoids Adsorbed (Pediatric), Aluminum Phosphate Adsorbed, (Ultrafined)** (Wyeth) p 2245
- **Diphtheria & Tetanus Toxoids Adsorbed, Pediatric, in Tubex** (Wyeth) p 2288
- **Diphtheria & Tetanus Toxoids, Adsorbed (For Pediatric Use)** (Sclavo) p 1897
- **Diphtheria & Tetanus Toxoids, Adsorbed Purogenated** (Lederle) p 1093
- **Diphtheria & Tetanus Toxoids Adsorbed USP** (Squibb/Connaught) p 2033
- **Diphtheria & Tetanus Toxoids & Pertussis Vaccine, Adsorbed** (Lederle)
- **Diphtheria & Tetanus Toxoids & Pertussis Vaccine Adsorbed (for Pediatric Use)** (Squibb/Connaught) p 2033
- **Diphtheria Toxoid, Adsorbed** (Sclavo) p 1897
- **Diprolene Ointment 0.05%** (Schering) p 1837
- **Diprosone Cream 0.05%** (Schering) p 1838
- **Diprosone Lotion 0.05% w/w** (Schering) p 1838
- **Diprosone Ointment 0.05%** (Schering) p 1838
- **Diprosone Topical Aerosol 0.1% w/w** (Schering) p 1838
- ◆ **Dipyridamole Tablets** (Lederle) p 416
- **Dipyridamole Tablets** (Danbury) p 887
- **Dipyridamole Tablets** (Geneva) p 973
- **Dipyridamole Tablets** (Schein) p 1828
- ◆ **Disalcid** (Riker) p 428, 1642
- **Disanthrol Capsules** (Lannett)
- **Disipal Tablets** (Riker) p 1643
- **Disobrom Tablets** (Geneva) p 973
- **Disolan Capsules** (Lannett)
- **Disonate Capsules & Liquid** (Lannett) p 1071
- ◆ **Disophrol Chronotab Sustained-Action Tablets** (Schering) p 434
- **Disophrol Tablets** (Schering) p 434
- **Di-Sosul** (Drug Industries)
- **Di-Sosul Forte** (Drug Industries)
- **Disotate Injectable** (O'Neal, Jones & Feldman)
- **Dispenser Strip** (Lilly) p 1122
- **Dispos-A-Med Flow Path Kit** (Parke-Davis)
- **Dispos-A-Med, isoetharine hydrochloride; isoproterenol hydrochloride** (Parke-Davis)
- **Dispos-A-Med Vials, Empty** (Parke-Davis)
- **Dispos-A-Vial: Sterile Water, Normal Saline, Half Normal Saline** (Parke-Davis)
- **Disulfiram Tablets** (Danbury) p 887
- **Disulfiram Tablets** (Geneva) p 973
- **Disulfiram Tablets** (Schein) p 1828
- **Dital** (UAD Labs.)
- **Ditate** (Savage)
- **Ditate-DS** (Savage) p 1824
- **Ditropan Syrup** (Marion) p 1184
- ◆ **Ditropan Tablets** (Marion) p 417, 1184
- **Diucardin** (Ayerst) p 404, 640
- ◆ **Diulo** (Searle Pharmaceuticals) p 435, 1904
- ◆ **Diupres Tablets** (Merck Sharp & Dohme) p 420, 1298
- **Diuril Intravenous Sodium** (Merck Sharp & Dohme) p 1299
- ◆ **Diuril Tablets & Oral Suspension** (Merck Sharp & Dohme) p 420, 1301
- **Diutensen Tablets** (Wallace) p 2156
- ◆ **Diutensen-R Tablets** (Wallace) p 442, 2157
- **Doak Oil & Doak Oil Forte** (Doak)
- **Doak Tar Lotion** (Doak)
- **Doak Tar Shampoo** (Doak)
- **Dobutrex** (Lilly) p 1143
- **Doca Acetate** (Organon) p 1446
- **Docusate Sodium Capsules, Syrup** (Roxane) p 1788
- **Docusate Sodium with Casanthranol Capsules** (Roxane) p 1788
- ◆ **Docusate Sodium, USP (DSS) Capsules, Syrup** (Lederle) p 416

- **Docusate Sodium, USP w/Casanthranol Capsules, Syrup** (Lederle) p 416
- **Dolacet Capsules** (Hauck) p 1001
- **Dolene AP-65 Tablets** (Lederle)
- **Dolene Capsules** (Lederle)
- ◆ **Dolobid Tablets** (Merck Sharp & Dohme) p 420, 1302
- **Dolophine Hydrochloride Ampoules and Vials** (Lilly) p 1144
- **Dolophine Hydrochloride Tablets** (Lilly) p 1145
- **Dolprn #3 Tablets** (Bock) p 705
- ◆ **Domeboro Powder Packets & Tablets** (Miles Pharmaceuticals) p 422, 1402
- **Dome-Paste Bandage** (Miles Pharmaceuticals) p 1402
- **Dommanate Injectable** (O'Neal, Jones & Feldman)
- **Domol Bath & Shower Oil** (Miles Pharmaceuticals) p 1402
- **Donatussin DC Syrup** (Laser) p 1072
- **Donatussin Drops** (Laser) p 1072
- **Donnagel** (Robins)
- **Donnagel-PG** (Robins)
- ◆ **Donnatal Capsules** (Robins) p 428, 1648
- **Donnatal Elixir** (Robins) p 1648
- ◆ **Donnatal Extentabs** (Robins) p 428, 1649
- **Donnatal No. 2 Tablets** (Robins)
- ◆ **Donnatal Tablets** (Robins) p 428, 1648
- ◆ **Donnazyme Tablets** (Robins) p 428, 1650
- **Donphen Tablets** (Lemmon)
- **Dopamine Hydrochloride Ampoules (Dopastat)** (Parke-Davis) p 1510
- **Dopamine HCl Injection** (Bristol) p 730
- **Dopamine HCl Injection** (Elkins-Sinn) p 938
- **Dopamine Solutions** (Astra) p 615
- **Dopar Capsules** (Norwich Eaton)
- ◆ **Dopram Injectable** (Robins) p 428, 1650
- **Dorcol Children's Cough Syrup** (Dorsey Laboratories) p 909
- **Dorcol Children's Decongestant Liquid** (Dorsey Laboratories) p 909
- **Dorcol Children's Fever & Pain Reducer** (Dorsey Laboratories) p 909
- **Dorcol Children's Liquid Calcium Supplement** (Dorsey Laboratories) p 909
- **Dorcol Children's Liquid Cold Formula** (Dorsey Laboratories) p 909
- **Doriden Tablets** (USV Pharmaceutical) p 2076
- **Doss 300 Capsule** (Ferndale)
- **Double-Sal Tablets** (Vale)
- **Dovacet Capsules** (Vale)
- **Dow-Isoniazid** (Merrell Dow)
- ◆ **Doxidan** (Hoechst-Roussel) p 412, 1014
- **Doxinate** (Hoechst-Roussel)
- **Doxy-100 & Doxy-200 (Doxycycline Hyclate for Injection, USP)** (LyphoMed)
- **Doxycycline Hyclate Capsules** (Schein) p 1828
- **Doxycycline Hyclate Capsules** (Danbury) p 887
- **Doxycycline Hyclate Capsules & Tablets** (Geneva) p 973
- ◆ **Doxycycline Hyclate Capsules, Tablets** (Lederle) p 416
- **Doxycycline Hyclate Capsules** (Schein) p 1828
- **Doxycycline Hyclate for Injection** (Elkins-Sinn) p 938
- **Doxycycline Hyclate Tablets** (Danbury) p 887
- **Doxy-Lemmon Capsules** (Lemmon) p 1122
- **Dramamine Injection** (Searle Pharmaceuticals) p 1906
- **Dramamine Liquid** (Searle Pharmaceuticals) p 1906
- **Dramamine Tablets** (Searle Pharmaceuticals) p 435, 1906
- **Dramatrol Injectable** (Bart)
- **Dramocen Injectable** (Central Pharmaceuticals)
- **Dramoject** (Mayrand)
- **Drest Gel** (Dermik)
- **Drisdol 50,000 Unit Capsules** (Winthrop-Breon)
- **Drisdol in Propylene Glycol** (Winthrop-Breon)
- ◆ **Dristan, Advanced Formula Decongestant/Antihistamine/Analgesic Capsules** (Whitehall) p 443, 2186
- ◆ **Dristan, Advanced Formula Decongestant/Antihistamine/Analgesic Tablets** (Whitehall) p 443, 2186
- **Dristan Cough Formula** (Whitehall)
- **Dristan Inhaler** (Whitehall)
- ◆ **Dristan Long Lasting Nasal Spray, Regular & Menthol** (Whitehall) p 443, 2186
- ◆ **Dristan Nasal Spray, Regular & Menthol** (Whitehall) p 443, 2186
- **Dristan Room Vaporizer** (Whitehall)
- **Dristan 12-Hour Nasal Decongestant Capsules** (Whitehall)
- ◆ **Dristan Ultra Colds Formula Aspirin-Free Analgesic/Decongestant/Antihistamine/Cough Suppressant Nighttime Liquid** (Whitehall) p 443
- ◆ **Dristan Ultra Colds Formula Aspirin-Free Analgesic/Decongestant/Antihistamine/Cough Suppressant Tablets and Capsules** (Whitehall) p 443
- ◆ **Dristan-AF Decongestant/Antihistamine/Analgesic Tablets** (Whitehall)
- **Drithocreme** (American Dermal) p 599
- **Dritho-Scalp** (American Dermal) p 599
- ◆ **Drixoral Sustained-Action Tablets** (Schering) p 434
- **Drize Capsules** (Ascher)

- **Drolban Vials** (Lilly)
- **Droperidol, See Inapsine** (Janssen)
- **Drotic Ear Drops** (Ascher)
- **Dry and Clear Acne Medication Lotion** (Whitehall)
- **Dry and Clear Double Strength Cream** (Whitehall)
- **Dry and Clear Medicated Acne Cleanser** (Whitehall)
- **Drysol** (Person & Covey) p 1587
- **Drytergent** (C & M)
- **Drytex** (C & M)
- **Duadacin** (Hoechst-Roussel)
- ◆ **Dulcolax Suppositories** (Boehringer Ingelheim) p 406, 709
- ◆ **Dulcolax Tablets** (Boehringer Ingelheim) p 406, 709
- **duo-C.V.P. Capsules** (Armour)
- **Duofilm** (Stiefel) p 2035
- **duo-Flow** (CooperVision)
- **Duolube Ophthalmic Ointment** (Muro)
- **Duo-Medihaler** (Riker) p 1643
- ◆ **Duotrate Plateau Caps** (Marion) p 417, 1185
- ◆ **Duotrate 45 Plateau Caps** (Marion) p 418, 1185
- **Duoval P.A. Injection** (Reid-Provident, Direct Div.)
- **Duphrene Syrup & Tablets** (Vale)
- **Duplex** (C & M)
- **Duplex T** (C & M)
- **Durabolin** (Organon) p 1446
- **Duracid** (Fielding)
- **Duracillin A.S. Vials** (Lilly)
- **Duradyne DHC Tablets** (O'Neal, Jones & Feldman) p 1445
- **Duradyne Tablets** (O'Neal, Jones & Feldman)
- **Duralgina Ampules** (Arlo)
- **Duralgina Suppositories** (Arlo)
- **Duramorph PF (Preservative-free morphine sulfate injection)** (Elkins-Sinn) p 939
- **Duranest Hydrochloride & Duranest Hydrochloride with Epinephrine 1:200,000** (Astra) p 616
- ◆ **Duraquin** (Parke-Davis) p 423, 1511
- **Dura Tap-PD** (Dura) p 929
- **Duratears** (Alcon Labs.)
- **Dura-Vent** (Dura) p 929
- **Dura-Vent/A** (Dura) p 929
- **Dura-Vent/DA** (Dura) p 929
- **Dureze Drops** (O'Neal, Jones & Feldman)
- ◆ **Duricef** (Mead Johnson Pharmaceutical) p 419, 1250
- **Durrax Tablets 10mg, 25mg** (Dermik) p 888
- **Duvoid** (Norwich Eaton) p 1430
- ◆ **Dyazide** (Smith Kline & French) p 437, 1961
- ◆ **Dycill Capsules** (Beecham Laboratories) p 406
- **Dyclone, 0.5% & 1%** (Astra) p 618
- ◆ **Dymelor** (Lilly) p 417, 1146
- ◆ **Dynapen** (Bristol) p 407, 733
- ◆ **Dyrenium** (Smith Kline & French) p 436, 1963
- **Dyrexan-OD Capsules** (Trimen) p 2067
- **Dytuss** (LaSalle) p 1071

E

- **E-Cypionate** (Legere) p 1120
- ◆ **E.E.S. Chewable Tablets** (Abbott) p 403, 522
- **E.E.S. Drops** (Abbott) p 522
- **E.E.S. Granules** (Abbott) p 522
- **E.E.S. 200 Liquid** (Abbott) p 522
- ◆ **E.E.S. 400 Filmtab** (Abbott) p 403, 522
- **E.E.S. 400 Liquid** (Abbott) p 522
- **E-Ionate P.A. Injection** (Reid-Provident, Direct Div.)
- **E-Mycin E Liquid** (Upjohn) p 2113
- ◆ **E-Mycin Tablets** (Upjohn) p 441, 2112
- **E.N.T. Syrup** (Springbok) p 1985
- **E.N.T. Tablets** (Springbok) p 1985
- **E-Pherol (vitamin E succinate)** (Vitaline)
- **E-Pilo Ophthalmic Solutions 1, 2, 3, 4, 6** (CooperVision)
- **E-Plus** (Drug Industries)
- ◆ **E.T. The Extra-Terrestrial Children's Chewable Vitamins** (Squibb) p 438, 1994
- ◆ **E.T. The Extra-Terrestrial Children's Chewable Vitamins with Iron** (Squibb) p 438, 1994
- **Ear Drops by Murine—See Murine Ear Wax Removal System** (Ross) p 1762
- **Ear-Eze** (Hyrex)
- ◆ **Easprin** (Parke-Davis) p 424, 1512
- **Eclabron Capsules** (U.S. Ethicals)
- **Eclabron Elixir (See Wharton Laboratories)** (U.S. Ethicals)
- **Eclabron Elixir** (Wharton) p 2184
- **Eclabron-T/SR Capsules** (U.S. Ethicals)
- **Eclamide Capsules** (U.S. Ethicals)
- **Eclasufed Capsules** (U.S. Ethicals)
- **Eclasufed SR Capsules** (U.S. Ethicals)
- **Eclipse After Sun Moisturizer** (Dorsey Laboratories)
- **Eclipse Lip and Face Protectant, SPF 15** (Dorsey Laboratories)
- **Eclipse Partial Suntan Lotion, SPF 5** (Dorsey Laboratories)
- **Eclipse Original Sunscreen Gel, SPF 10** (Dorsey Laboratories)
- **Eclipse Original Sunscreen Moisturizing Lotion, SPF 10** (Dorsey Laboratories)

(◆ Shown in Product Identification Section)   (⊞ Described in PDR For Nonprescription Drugs)   (Products without page numbers are not described)

Product Name Index

Eclipse Total Sunscreen Cooling Alcohol Lotion, SPF 15 (Dorsey Laboratories) p 910
Eclipse Total Sunscreen Moisturizing Lotion, SPF 15 (Dorsey Laboratories) p 910
Econochlor Solution & Ointment (Alcon Labs.)
Econopred (Alcon Labs.)
Econopred Plus (Alcon Labs.)
Ecotrin Duentric Coated Aspirin (Smith Kline & French)
Ecotrin, Maximum Strength Safety-Coated Aspirin Capsules (Smith Kline & French)
Ecotrin, Maximum Strength Tablets (Smith Kline & French)
Ecotrin, Regular Strength Safety-Coated Aspirin Capsules (Smith Kline & French)
Ectasule Minus III T.D. Capsules (Fleming)
Ectasule Minus Jr. T.D. Capsules (Fleming)
Ectasule Minus Sr. T.D. Capsules (Fleming)
Ectasule III T.D. Capsules (Fleming)
Ectasule Jr. T.D. Capsules (Fleming)
Ectasule Sr. T.D. Capsules (Fleming)
Edecrin Sodium Intravenous (Merck Sharp & Dohme) p 1304
◆ Edecrin Tablets (Merck Sharp & Dohme) p 420, 1304
◆ Efed II Capsules (Black) (Alto) p 404, 589
◆ Efed II Capsules (Yellow) (Alto) p 404, 589
Efed Tablets (Alto)
Efedron Nasal Jelly (Hyrex)
Eferol Ointment (O'Neal, Jones & Feldman)
Eferol Succinate Capsules (O'Neal, Jones & Feldman)
Effersyllium (Stuart) p 2037
Effervescent Potassium Tablets (Schein) p 1828
efficin (Adria)
Efodine Ointment (Fougera) p 953
Efricon Expectorant (Lannett)
Efudex Topical Solutions and Cream (Roche) p 1681
Elaqua XX Cream (Elder) p 930
◆ Elase (Parke-Davis) p 424, 1513
◆ Elase Ointment (Parke-Davis) p 424, 1513
◆ Elase-Chloromycetin Ointment (Parke-Davis) p 424, 1513
◆ Elavil Tablets & Injection (Merck Sharp & Dohme) p 420, 1306
◆ Eldec Kapseals (Parke-Davis) p 424, 1514
Eldecort Cream, 1%, 2.5% (Elder) p 930
Elder Psoralite (Elder) p 930
Eldercaps (Mayrand) p 1196
Eldertonic (Mayrand) p 1196
Eldopaque 2% Cream (Elder) p 930
Eldopaque Forte 4% Cream (Elder) p 930
Eldoquin 2% Cream & 2% Lotion (Elder) p 930
Eldoquin Forte 4% Cream (Elder) p 930
Elixicon Suspension (Berlex) p 406, 699
◆ Elixophyllin Capsules (Berlex) p 406, 699
Elixophyllin Elixir (Berlex) p 699
◆ Elixophyllin SR Capsules (Berlex) p 406, 699
◆ Elixophyllin-GG (Berlex) p 406, 702
Elixophyllin-KI Elixir (Berlex)
Elspar (Merck Sharp & Dohme) p 1308
◆ Emcyt Capsules (Roche) p 429, 1681
Emete-con (Roerig) p 1729
⊞ Emetrol Solution (Rorer)
⊞ Emko Because Contraceptor Vaginal Contraceptive Foam (Schering)
⊞ Emko Pre-Fil Vaginal Contraceptive Foam (Schering)
⊞ Emko Vaginal Contraceptive Foam (Schering)
◆ Empirin Aspirin Tablets (Burroughs Wellcome) p 407
◆ Empirin with Codeine (Burroughs Wellcome) p 408, 787
◆ Empracet with Codeine Phosphate Nos. 3 & 4 (Burroughs Wellcome) p 408, 789
Empty Sterile Carpuject (Winthrop-Breon)
Emul-O-Balm (Pennwalt)
Enarax Tablets (Beecham Laboratories)
◆ Encaprin (Procter & Gamble) p 427, 1620
En-Cebrin Pulvules (Lilly)
En-Cebrin F Pulvules (Lilly)
Endafed (UAD Labs.)
Endal Plain (UAD Labs.)
Endecon Tablets (Du Pont)
◆ Endep Tablets (Roche Products) p 429, 1711
Endometrial Suction Curettes (Milex)
Endorphenyl (Tyson) p 2068
Endotussin-NN Pediatric Syrup (Du Pont)
Endotussin-NN Syrup (Du Pont)
Endrate Solution, Ampoules (Abbott)
◆ Enduron Tablets (Abbott) p 403, 517
◆ Enduronyl Forte Tablets (Abbott) p 403, 518
◆ Enduronyl Tablets (Abbott) p 403, 518
⊞ Enfamil (Mead Johnson Nutritional)
⊞ Enfamil Nursette (Mead Johnson Nutritional)
⊞ Enfamil Ready-To-Use (Mead Johnson Nutritional)
⊞ Enfamil w/Iron (Mead Johnson Nutritional)
⊞ Enfamil w/Iron Ready-To-Use (Mead Johnson Nutritional)
Engran-HP Tablets (Squibb)
Enisyl Tablets (Person & Covey) p 1588
◆ Enovid 5 mg (Searle & Co.) p 435, 1919
◆ Enovid 10 mg (Searle & Co.) p 435, 1919
◆ Enovid-E 21 (Searle & Co.) p 436, 1919
Enoxa Tablets (Reid-Provident, Direct Div.)
Enrich (Ross) p 1762
Ensure (Ross) p 1762

Ensure HN (Ross) p 1764
Ensure Plus (Ross) p 1764
Ensure Plus HN (Ross) p 1765
Entex Capsules (Norwich Eaton) p 1431
◆ Entex LA Tablets (Norwich Eaton) p 422, 1432
Entex Liquid (Norwich Eaton) p 1431
◆ Entozyme Tablets (Robins) p 428, 1652
Entuss Expectorant Tablets & Liquid (Hauck) p 1001
Entuss Tablets (Hauck)
Entuss-D Liquid & Tablets (Hauck) p 1001
Enuclene (Alcon Labs.)
Enviro-Stress with Zinc & Selenium (Vitaline) p 2148
Enzactin Cream (Ayerst) p 642
Enzobile Improved Formula (Mallard) p 1181
Enzymet Tablet (O'Neal, Jones & Feldman)
Enzypan (Norgine) p 1424
Ephedrine Injection (Bristol) p 730
Ephedrine & Amytal Pulvules (Lilly)
Ephedrine Sulfate Ampoules, Pulvules, & Syrups (Lilly)
◆ Epifoam (Reed & Carnrick) p 427, 1634
Epifrin ophthalmic solution (Allergan)
Epinal (Alcon Labs.)
Epinephrine 1:10,000, 10 ml., Abboject (Abbott)
Epinephrine Injection (Bristol) p 730
Epinephrine Injection (Elkins-Sinn) p 938
Epinephrine 1:1000 Dropperettes (CooperVision)
Epinephrine in Tubex (Wyeth) p 2288
EpiPen—Epinephrine Auto-Injector (Center) p 835
EpiPen Jr. (Center) p 835
Eprolin Gelseals (Lilly)
Epsilan-M Capsules (Adria)
◆ Equagesic (Wyeth) p 444, 2250
⊞ Equal (Searle Consumer Products)
◆ Equanil Tablets and Wyseals (Wyeth) p 444, 2252
Ergoloid Mesylates Oral Tablets (Danbury) p 887
Ergoloid Mesylates Sublingual Tablets (Danbury) p 887
Ergoloid Mesylates Tablets (Geneva) p 973
◆ Ergoloid Mesylates Tablets (Lederle) p 416
Ergomar Sublingual Tablets (Fisons) p 943
◆ Ergostat (Parke-Davis) p 424, 1515
Ergotrate Maleate Ampoules (Lilly) p 1146
Ergotrate Maleate Tablets (Lilly) p 1147
◆ ERYC (Parke-Davis) p 424, 1515
EryDerm (Abbott) p 519
Erymax Topical Solution (Herbert) p 1003
EryPed Granules (Abbott) p 520
◆ Ery-Tab Tablets (Abbott) p 403, 521
Erythrocin Lactobionate-I.V. (Abbott) p 523
◆ Erythrocin Piggyback (Abbott) p 403, 524
◆ Erythrocin Stearate Filmtab (Abbott) p 403, 525
◆ Erythromycin Base Filmtab (Abbott) p 403, 526
Erythromycin Estolate Capsules (Danbury) p 887
Erythromycin Estolate Capsules & Suspension (Schein) p 1828
Erythromycin Ethylsuccinate Granules, Suspension & Tablets (Schein) p 1828
Erythromycin Ophthalmic Ointment (Fougera) p 953
Erythromycin Ophthalmic Ointment (Pharmaderm) p 1617
Erythromycin Ophthalmic Ointment (Schein) p 1828
Erythromycin Stearate Tablets (Lederle) p 416
◆ Erythromycin Stearate Tablets, USP (Erypar) (Parke-Davis) p 424, 1516
Escot Capsules (Reid-Provident, Direct Div.)
◆ Esgic Tablets & Capsules (Gilbert) p 411, 975
◆ Esidrix (CIBA) p 409, 848
◆ Esimil (CIBA) p 409, 849
◆ Eskalith Capsules & Tablets (Smith Kline & French) p 437, 1964
◆ Eskalith CR Controlled Release Tablets (Smith Kline & French) p 437, 1964
Esophotrast (Armour)
⊞ Esotérica Medicated Fade Cream (Norcliff Thayer)
Espasmotex Tablets (Arlo)
Estar Gel (Westwood) p 2176
Estate (Savage)
◆ Estinyl Tablets (Schering) p 434, 1839
Estomul-M Liquid & Tablets (Riker)
◆ Estrace (Mead Johnson Laboratories) p 419, 1216
Estrace Vaginal Cream (Mead Johnson Laboratories) p 419, 1219
Estradurin (Ayerst) p 642
Estraguard Vaginal Cream (Reid-Provident Labs.)
◆ Estratab Tablets (Reid-Provident Labs.) p 427, 1638
◆ Estratest H.S. Tablets (Reid-Provident Labs.) p 427, 1638
◆ Estratest Tablets (Reid-Provident Labs.) p 427, 1638
Estraval 2X Injection (Reid-Provident, Direct Div.)
Estraval 4X Injection (Reid-Provident, Direct Div.)
Estraval-P.A. Injection (Reid-Provident, Direct Div.)

◆ Estrocon Tablets (Savage) p 433, 1824
Estroject-2 (Mayrand)
Estroject-LA (Mayrand)
Estrone (Legere) p 1120
Estrone (Savage)
Estronol Aqueous Sterile Suspension (Central Pharmaceuticals)
Estronol-LA Injectable (Central Pharmaceuticals)
◆ Estrovis (Parke-Davis) p 424, 1517
Ethaquin Tablets (Ascher)
Ethatab (Glaxo) p 980
Ethiodol (Savage)
◆ Ethril '250' and Ethril '500' Tablets (Squibb) p 438
Etnapa Elixir (U.S. Ethicals)
Etnergan Syrup (U.S. Ethicals)
Etrafon Tablets (Schering) p 434, 1841
Eudal-SR (UAD Labs.)
Eurax Cream & Lotion (Westwood) p 2177
◆ Euthroid (Parke-Davis) p 424, 1520
◆ Eutonyl Filmtab Tablets (Abbott) p 403, 528
◆ Eutron Filmtab Tablets (Abbott) p 403
Evac-Q-Kit (Adria) p 575
Evac-Q-Kwik (Adria) p 575
Evac-U-Gen (Walker, Corp) p 2148
Everone (Hyrex)
Excedrin Extra-Strength (Bristol-Myers Products) p 770
Excedrin P.M. (Bristol-Myers Products) p 770
◆ Exna Tablets (Robins) p 428, 1652
Exsel Lotion (Herbert) p 1003
⊞ Extend 12 Liquid (Robins)
Extendryl Chewable Tablets (Fleming) p 948
Extendryl Sr. & Jr. T.D. Capsules (Fleming) p 948
Extendryl Syrup (Fleming) p 948
Extra-Strength Bufferin capsules & tablets (Bristol-Myers Products) p 769
Extra-Strength Datril capsules & tablets (Bristol-Myers Products) p 770
Extra-Strength Sine-Aid Sinus Headache Capsules (McNeil Consumer Products) p 1199
Extralin Pulvules (Lilly)
Eye Pak (Alcon Labs.)
Eye Stream (Alcon Labs.)

F

F-E-P Creme (Boots) p 717
FML Liquifilm ophthalmic suspension (Allergan)
4-Way Cold Tablets (Bristol-Myers Products) p 770
4-Way Long Acting Nasal Spray (Bristol-Myers Products) p 771
4-Way Nasal Spray (Bristol-Myers Products) p 770
FUDR Injectable (Roche) p 1684
Factor IX Complex (Human) (Factors II, VII, IX, and X) Konyne (Cutter Biological) p 886
Factorate, Antihemophilic Factor (Human) Dried (Armour) p 613
Factorate, Generation II (Armour) p 613
◆ Factrel (Ayerst) p 404, 643, 3007
◆ Fansidar Tablets (Roche) p 429, 1682
◆ Fastin Capsules (Beecham Laboratories) p 406, 692
Fedahist Expectorant (Rorer) p 1749
◆ Fedahist Gyrocaps, Syrup & Tablets (Rorer) p 431, 1749
◆ Fedrazil Tablets (Burroughs Wellcome) p 408
◆ Feldene Capsules (Pfizer) p 426, 1601
Femguard Vaginal Cream (Reid-Provident Labs.)
Feminone Tablets (Upjohn)
Fentanyl, See Sublimaze (Janssen)
Fentanyl Citrate Injection (Elkins-Sinn)
Fe-O.D. Tablets (Trimen)
Feosol Elixir (Smith Kline & French)
Feosol Plus Capsules (Smith Kline & French)
Feosol Spansule Capsules (Smith Kline & French)
Feosol Tablets (Smith Kline & French)
Feostat Injectable (O'Neal, Jones & Feldman)
Feostat Tablets, Suspension & Drops (O'Neal, Jones & Feldman) p 1445
◆ Ferancee Chewable Tablets (Stuart) p 439, 2037
◆ Ferancee-HP Tablets (Stuart) p 439, 2037
Ferate-C Tablets (Vale)
Ferbetrin Tablets & Syrup (U.S. Ethicals)
Fer-Bid Improved (Beach)
◆ Fergon Capsules (Winthrop-Breon) p 443, 2198
Fergon Elixir (Winthrop-Breon) p 2198
Fergon Plus (Winthrop-Breon) p 2198
◆ Fergon Tablets (Winthrop-Breon) p 443, 2198
⊞ Fer-In-Sol (Mead Johnson Nutritional)
Ferlivit Capsules (Medical Products)
Ferlivit Injection (Medical Products)
Ferlivit Syrup (Medical Products)
Fermalox Tablets (Rorer) p 431
Fermolate Elixir (Arlo)
Ferndex Tablets (Ferndale)
Fernisolone-P-Tablets (Ferndale)
◆ Fero-Folic-500 (Abbott) p 403, 529
◆ Fero-Grad-500 (Abbott) p 403, 530
Fero-Gradumet (Abbott) p 530
Ferralet (Mission) p 1416

(◆ Shown in Product Identification Section)   (⊞ Described in PDR For Nonprescription Drugs)   (Products without page numbers are not described)

Product Name Index

Ferro-Bob Tablets (Scot-Tussin)
◆ Ferro-Sequels (Lederle) p 415, 1093
Ferrous Gluconate Pulvules (Lilly)
Ferrous Sulfate Enseals & Tablets (Lilly)
Ferrous Sulfate Filmseals (Parke-Davis)
Ferrous Sulfate Liquid, Tablets (Roxane) p 1788
Fertility Cannula (Milex)
Fertilo-Pak (Milex)
Festal II (Hoechst-Roussel) p 412, 1014
◆ Festalan (Hoechst-Roussel) p 413, 1014
Fetaldex Quantitative Test for Fetal Red Blood Cells in the Maternal Blood Circulation (Ortho Diagnostic Systems)
Fetalscreen Qualitative Screening Test for D(Rh₀) Positive Fetal Red Blood Cells in the Maternal Circulation (Ortho Diagnostic Systems)
Fetrin (LaSalle) p 1071
Fiberall, Natural Flavor (Rydelle) p 1795
Fiberall, Orange Flavor (Rydelle) p 1795
◆ Fibermed Supplements (Purdue Frederick) p 427, 1624
◆ Filibon (Lederle) p 415, 1093
◆ Filibon F.A. (Lederle) p 415, 1093
◆ Filibon Forte (Lederle) p 415, 1093
Finac (C & M)
◆ Fiogesic Tablets (Sandoz Pharmaceutical Div.) p 432, 1801
◆ Fiorinal (Sandoz Pharmaceutical Div.) p 433, 1801
◆ Fiorinal w/Codeine (Sandoz Pharmaceutical Div.) p 432, 1802
◆ Flagyl I.V. (Searle Pharmaceuticals) p 436, 1907
◆ Flagyl I.V. RTU (Searle Pharmaceuticals) p 436, 1907
◆ Flagyl Tablets (Searle & Co.) p 436, 1929
Flatulence Tablets (Vale)
Flavitab Tablets (Ferndale)
Fleet Babylax (Fleet) p 946
Fleet Bisacodyl Enema (Fleet) p 946
Fleet Detecatest (Fleet) p 3009
Fleet Enema (Fleet) p 946
Fleet Flavored Castor Oil Emulsion (Fleet) p 947
Fleet Mineral Oil Enema (Fleet) p 947
Fleet Phospho-Soda (Fleet) p 947
Fleet Prep Kits (Fleet) p 947
Fleet Relief (Fleet) p 947
Fletcher's Castoria (Glenbrook)
Flexaphen Capsules (Trimen)
◆ Flexeril Tablets (Merck Sharp & Dohme) p 420, 1310
Flexiflo Enteral Delivery System (Ross) p 1766
Flexiflo Enteral Feeding Tube, 8 French (Ross)
Flexiflo Enteral Feeding Tube, 8 French w/Stylet (Ross)
Flexiflo Enteral Feeding Tube, 12 French (Ross)
Flexiflo Enteral Nutrition Pump (Ross)
Flexiflo Enteral Pump Set (Ross)
Flexiflo Enteral Pump Set with Piercing Pin (Ross)
Flexiflo-II Enteral Pump Set (Ross)
Flexiflo-II Portable Enteral Nutrition Pump (Ross)
Flexiflo-II Pump Set with Piercing Pin (Ross)
Flexiflo-III Enteral Nutrition Pump (Ross)
Flexiflo-III Enteral Pump Set (Ross)
Flexiflo-III Pump Set with Piercing Pin (Ross)
Flexiflo Gravity Gavage Set (Ross)
Flexiflo Gravity Feeding Set with Piercing Pin (Ross)
Flexitainer Enteral Nutrition Container (Ross)
Flexitainer 500 Enteral Nutrition Container (Ross)
Flexoject (Mayrand)
◆ Flint SSD Cream (Flint) p 411, 950
⊡ Flintstones Complete Multivitamin/Mineral Supplement (Miles Laboratories)
⊡ Flintstones Multivitamin Supplement (Miles Laboratories)
⊡ Flintstones Plus Iron Multivitamin Supplement (Miles Laboratories)
⊡ Flintstones With Extra C (Miles Laboratories)
Florida Foam Improved (Hill Dermaceuticals)
Florinef Acetate Tablets (Squibb)
Florone Cream 0.05% (Dermik) p 889
Florone Ointment 0.05% (Dermik) p 889
Floropryl Sterile Ophthalmic Ointment (Merck Sharp & Dohme)
Florvite Chewable Tablets 0.5 mg & 1 mg (Everett) p 941
Florvite Drops (Everett) p 941
Florvite + Iron Chewable Tablets 1 mg (Everett) p 941
Florvite + Iron Drops (Everett) p 941
Fluidil (Adria) p 571
Fluocinolone Acetonide Cream (Schein) p 1828
Fluocinolone Acetonide Cream & Topical Solution 0.01% (Fougera) p 953
Fluocinolone Acetonide Cream & Ointment 0.025% (Fougera) p 953
Fluocinolone Acetonide Cream, Ointment & Topical Solution (Pharmaderm) p 1617
Fluocinolone Acetonide Topical Cream, Ointment & Solution (Pharmafair) p 1618
Fluogen (Parke-Davis) p 1522
Fluonid Ointment, Cream & Topical Solution (Herbert) p 1003

Fluorescein Sodium 2% Dropperettes (CooperVision)
Fluorescite (Alcon Labs.)
Fluor-I-Strip Applicators (Ayerst)
Fluor-I-Strip-A.T. Applicators (Ayerst)
Fluoritab Tablets & Fluoritab Liquid (Fluoritab) p 953
Fluoroplex Topical Solution & Cream (Herbert) p 1004
Fluorostat Filter Fluorometer (Ames) p 3006
Fluorouracil Ampuls (Roche) p 1683
Fluothane (Ayerst) p 645
Fluoxymesterone Tablets (Reid-Provident, Direct Div.)
Fluoxymesterone Tablets (Geneva) p 973
Fluoxymesterone Tablets (Schein) p 1828
Fluzone (Influenza Virus Vaccine), Whole Virion and Subvirion, Zonal Purified (Squibb/Connaught) p 2033
Folex for Injection (Adria) p 576
Folic Acid Tablets (Lilly) p 1147
Folic Acid Tablets (Danbury) p 887
Follutein (Squibb)
Folvite (Lederle) p 1093
⊡ Footwork Athlete's Foot Remedy (Lederle)
Fordustin' (Sween) p 2097
⊡ Formula 44 Cough Control Disc (Vicks Health Care)
⊡ Formula 44 Cough Mixture (Vicks Health Care)
⊡ Formula 44D Decongestant Cough Mixture (Vicks Health Care)
Formula 405 Skin Care Products (Doak)
 Body Smoothing Lotion (Doak)
 Enriched Cream (Doak)
 Eye Cream (Doak)
 Le Pont Organic Nail Oil Treatment (Doak)
 Light Textured Moisturizer (Doak)
 Moisturizing Lotion (Doak)
 Moisturizing Soap (Doak)
 SPF 15+ (Doak)
 Skin Cleanser & Patented Buffing Mitt (Doak)
 Solar Cream (Doak)
 Therapeutic Bath Oil (Doak)
Formula Magic (Consolidated Chemical) p 880
Forta Pudding (Ross) p 1767
Forticon Liquid (Arlo)
Fosfree (Mission) p 1416
Fostex Medicated Cleansing Bar (Westwood) p 2177
Fostex Medicated Cleansing Cream (Westwood) p 2177
Fostex 5% Benzoyl Peroxide Gel (Westwood) p 2177
Fostex 10% Benzoyl Peroxide Cleansing Bar (Westwood) p 2177
Fostex 10% Benzoyl Peroxide Gel (Westwood) p 2178
Fostex 10% Benzoyl Peroxide Tinted Cream (Westwood) p 2178
Fostex 10% Benzoyl Peroxide Wash (Westwood) p 2178
Fostril (Westwood) p 2178
Fototar Cream 1.6% (Elder) p 931
Fototar Stik 5% (Elder) p 931
Free Form Amino Acids (Vitaline)
Freezone Solution (Whitehall)
◆ Fulvicin P/G Tablets (Schering) p 434, 1843
◆ Fulvicin P/G 165 & 330 Tablets (Schering) p 434, 1844
◆ Fulvicin-U/F Tablets (Schering) p 434, 1845
Fumatinic Capsules (Laser)
Fumatrin Forte (Reid-Provident Labs.)
Fumerin Tablets (Laser)
Funduscein-10 or -25 (Fluorescein sodium I.V.) (CooperVision)
Fungi-Nail Tincture (Kramer) p 1069
Fungizone Cream/Lotion/Ointment (Squibb) p 1994
Fungizone for Tissue Culture (Squibb)
Fungizone Intravenous (Squibb) p 1994
Fungoid Creme & Solution (Pedinol) p 1580
Fungoid Tincture (Pedinol) p 1580
Furacin Preparations (Norwich Eaton) p 1433
Furacin Soluble Dressing (Norwich Eaton) p 1433
Furacin Topical Cream (Norwich Eaton) p 1434
Furadantin Oral Suspension (Norwich Eaton) p 1432
Furadantin Tablets (Norwich Eaton) p 1432
Furosemide Injection (Elkins-Sinn) p 938
Furosemide Injection, USP (Parke-Davis) p 1522
Furosemide Injection (Wyeth) p 2252
Furosemide Tablets (Geneva) p 973
◆ Furosemide Tablets (Lederle) p 416
Furosemide Tablets (Schein) p 1828
Furosemide Tablets, USP (Parke-Davis) p 1524
Furoxone Liquid Suspension (Norwich Eaton) p 1435
Furoxone Tablets (Norwich Eaton) p 1435

G

G-1 Capsules (Hauck) p 1001
G-2 Capsules (Hauck) p 1001
G-3 Capsules (Hauck) p 1001
G.B.S. Tablets (O'Neal, Jones & Feldman)
GCP Shampoo (Consolidated Chemical)

GG-Cen Syrup/Capsules (Central Pharmaceuticals)
G-myticin Creme and Ointment 0.1% (Pedinol) p 1580
Gamastan (Immune Serum Globulin-Human) (Cutter Biological)
Gamimune (Immune Globulin Intraveneous, 5% in 10% Maltose) (Cutter Biological)
Gammar, Immune Serum Globulin (Human) U.S.P. (Armour) p 613
Gamulin Rh (Armour) p 613
Ganphen Injection (Reid-Provident, Direct Div.)
◆ Gantanol DS Tablets (Roche) p 429, 1685
Gantanol Suspension (Roche) p 1685
◆ Gantanol Tablets (Roche) p 429, 1685
Gantrisin Injectable (Roche) p 1686
Gantrisin Ophthalmic Ointment/Solution (Roche) p 1685
Gantrisin Pediatric Suspension (Roche) p 1686
Gantrisin Syrup (Roche) p 1686
◆ Gantrisin Tablets (Roche) p 429, 1686
◆ Garamycin Cream 0.1% and Ointment 0.1% (Schering) p 1846
Garamycin Injectable (Schering) p 1846
Garamycin Intrathecal Injection (Schering) p 1854
Garamycin I.V. Piggyback Injection (Schering) p 1851
Garamycin Ophthalmic Ointment-Sterile (Schering) p 1846
Garamycin Ophthalmic Solution-Sterile (Schering) p 1846
Garamycin Pediatric Injectable (Schering) p 1849
Gastrical Tablets (U.S. Ethicals)
Gastroccult (SmithKline Diagnostics) p 3017
Gastrografin (Squibb)
◆ Gaviscon Antacid Tablets (Marion) p 418, 1185
Gaviscon Liquid Antacid (Marion) p 1186
◆ Gaviscon-2 Antacid Tablets (Marion) p 418, 1186
Gaysal-S Tablets (Geriatric)
Gelfilm Sterile Film (Upjohn)
Gelfilm Sterile Ophthalmic Film (Upjohn)
Gelfoam Sterile Powder (Upjohn) p 2114
Gelfoam Sterile Sponge (Upjohn) p 2113
◆ Gelusil (Parke-Davis) p 424, 1525
Gelusil-M (Parke-Davis) p 1525
◆ Gelusil-II (Parke-Davis) p 424, 1526
◆ Gemnisyn Tablets (Rorer) p 431
Gemonil (Abbott) p 531
Genapax (Key Pharmaceuticals)
Genoptic S.O.P. ophthalmic ointment (Allergan)
Genoptic ophthalmic solution (Allergan)
Gentacidin Ophthalmic Solution (CooperVision)
Gentafair Cream & Ointment (Pharmafair) p 1618
Gentamicin Cream 0.1% & Ointment 0.1% (Schein) p 1828
Gentamicin Ophthalmic Ointment & Solution (Schein) p 1828
Gentamicin Sulfate Injection (Elkins-Sinn) p 938
Gentle Rain Shampoo (Sween) p 2047
Gentle Shampoo (Ulmer)
Gentz Wipes (Roxane)
◆ Geocillin Tablets (Roerig) p 431, 1730
Geopen (Roerig) p 1731
Geravite Elixir (Hauck) p 1001
Gerber Bakery Products (Gerber)
Gerber Cereals (Gerber)
Gerber Chunky Foods (Gerber)
Gerber High Meat Dinners (Strained & Junior) (Gerber)
Gerber Junior Foods (Gerber)
Gerber Junior Meats (Gerber)
Gerber Strained Egg Yolks (Gerber)
Gerber Strained Foods (Gerber)
Gerber Strained Juices (4.2 & 8 oz.) (Gerber)
Gerber Strained Meats (Gerber)
Gerber Toddler Meat Sticks (Chicken & Turkey) (Gerber)
Gerilets Filmtab (Abbott)
Gerimed (Fielding)
◆ Geriplex-FS Kapseals (Parke-Davis) p 424, 1527
◆ Geriplex-FS Liquid (Parke-Davis) p 1527
Geristone Capsules (U.S. Ethicals)
Geritonic Liquid (Geriatric)
Gerix Elixir (Abbott)
Ger-O-Foam (Geriatric) p 975
Geroton Forte (RAM Laboratories)
Gesterol "50" Injectable (O'Neal, Jones & Feldman)
Gesterol L.A. "250" Injectable (O'Neal, Jones & Feldman)
⊡ Gevrabon Liquid (Lederle)
Gevral Protein Powder (Lederle)
⊡ Gevral T Tablets (Lederle)
⊡ Gevral Tablets (Lederle)
Gevrite Tablets (Lederle)
Glaucon (Alcon Labs.)
Glucagon for Injection Ampoules (Lilly) p 1147
Glucamide Tablets (Lemmon) p 1122
Glucometer (Ames) p 3006
Glucose Water 5% & 10% (Ross)
Glucostabil (Ecological Formulas)
◆ Glucotrol (Roerig) p 431, 1733
◆ Glucovite Tablets (Vale)

(◆ Shown in Product Identification Section) (⊡ Described in PDR For Nonprescription Drugs) (Products without page numbers are not described)

Product Name Index

Glukor Injection (Hyrex) p 1024
Glutethimide Tablets (Danbury) p 887
Glutethimide Tablets (Geneva) p 973
Glutethimide Tablets (Schein) p 1828
Glutofac Tablets (Kenwood) p 1046
Glycate Tablets (O'Neal, Jones & Feldman)
Glycofed (Vale)
Glycopyrrolate Tablets (Danbury) p 887
*▫ Glycotuss Syrup & Tablets (Vale)
Glycotuss-dM Syrup & Tablets (Vale)
Gly-Oxide Liquid (Marion) p 1186
Glyrol Solution (CooperVision)
Glytinic Tablets (Boyle) p 726
Glytuss Tabs (Mayrand)
GoLYTELY (Braintree) p 727
Gonioscopic Prism Solution (Alcon Labs.)
Goniosol Solution (CooperVision)
Granulex (Hickam) p 1009
Grifulvin V (Ortho Pharmaceutical (Dermatological Div.)) p 1473
◆ Grisactin (Ayerst) p 404, 646
◆ Grisactin Ultra (Ayerst) p 405, 646
Gris-PEG Tablets, 125mg & 250mg (Herbert) p 1005
Guaifed Capsules (Timed Release) (Muro) p 1421
Guaifenesin Syrup (Roxane) p 1788
Guanidine HCl Tablets (Key Pharmaceuticals)
Guiatuss Syrup (Schein) p 1828
Guiatuss A-C Syrup (Schein) p 1828
Guiatuss D-M Syrup (Schein) p 1828
Guiosan Syrup (Vale)
Gumsol (Arlo) p 601
Gustalac Tablets (Geriatric)
Gustase (Geriatric) p 975
Gustase-Plus Tablets (Geriatric)
Gyne-Lotrimin Vaginal Cream 1% (Schering) p 1856
◆ Gyne-Lotrimin Vaginal Tablets (Schering) p 434, 1856
Gynogen Injectable (O'Neal, Jones & Feldman)
Gynogen L.A. "10", "20" & "40" Injectable (O'Neal, Jones & Feldman)
*▫ Gynol II Contraceptive Jelly (Ortho Pharmaceutical)

H

H-BIG (Abbott) p 531
HEB Cream Base (Barnes-Hind)
H-H-R Tablets (Schein) p 1828
HMS Liquifilm ophthalmic suspension (Allergan)
HP Acthar Gel (Armour) p 601
HQC Kit (Elder)
H-R Sterile Lubricating Jelly (Youngs)
H.T. Factorate (Armour) p 613
H.T. Factorate, Generation II (Armour) p 613
HVS 1+2 (Chemi-Tech) p 839
Halazone Tablets (Abbott)
◆ Halcion Tablets (Upjohn) p 441, 2114
◆ Haldol Tablets, Concentrate, Injection (McNeil Pharmaceutical) p 418, 1201
Haldrone Tablets (Lilly)
*▫ Haley's M-O, Regular & Flavored (Winthrop Consumer Products)
Halodrin Tablets (Upjohn)
Halog Cream/Ointment/Solution (Squibb) p 1996
Halog-E Cream (Squibb) p 1996
◆ Halotestin Tablets (Upjohn) p 441, 2116
Halotex Cream & Solution (Westwood) p 2178
Harmonyl (Abbott) p 532
Head & Chest (Procter & Gamble) p 1620
◆ Head & Shoulders (Procter & Gamble)
*▫ Headway Capsules (Vicks Health Care)
*▫ Headway Tablets (Vicks Health Care)
Healon (Pharmacia) p 1615
Heather Feminine Deodorant Spray (Whitehall)
Hedal H-C Suppositories (Arlo)
Heet Analgesic Liniment (Whitehall)
Heet Spray Analgesic (Whitehall)
◆ Help (Verex) p 442, 2145
Hema-Chek Slide Test for Fecal Occult Blood Test with Control (Ames) p 3005
Hemaspan Tablets (Bock)
Hemoccult (SmithKline Diagnostics) p 3017
Hemocyte Plus Tabules (U.S. Pharmaceutical) p 2070
Hemocyte Tablets (U.S. Pharmaceutical) p 2070
Hemocyte-F Tablets (U.S. Pharmaceutical) p 2070
Hemofil, Antihemophilic Factor (Human), Method Four, Dried (Hyland Therapeutics) p 1023
Hemofil T, Antihemophilic Factor (Human), Method Four, Dried, Heat-Treated (Hyland Therapeutics) p 1024
Hemo-Vite (Drug Industries) p 914
Hemo-Vite Liquid (Drug Industries) p 914
Hepaferron Syrup (U.S. Ethicals)
Heparin Flush Kits (Wyeth)
Heparin Lock Flush Solution, USP, 100 u/ml (LyphoMed)
Heparin Lock Flush Solution Carpuject (Winthrop-Breon)
Heparin Lock Flush Solution in Tubex (Wyeth) p 2253

Heparin Sodium (Lilly) p 1149
Heparin Sodium (from Beef Lung Sources) (Organon) p 1446
Heparin Sodium Carpuject (Winthrop-Breon)
Heparin Sodium in Tubex (Wyeth) p 2288
Heparin Sodium Injection (Elkins-Sinn) p 938
Heparin Sodium Injection (Wyeth) p 2254
Heparin Sodium Injection, USP, Sterile Solution (Upjohn) p 2117
Heparin Sodium w/o preservative Injectable (O'Neal, Jones & Feldman) p 1445
Hepatitis B Immune Globulin (Human) HyperHep (Cutter Biological) p 884
Hep-B-Gammagee (Merck Sharp & Dohme) p 1311
HepFlush-10 (Heparin Lock Flush Solution, USP, 10 u/ml (LyphoMed)
Hep-Forte Capsules (Marlyn) p 1193
Hepicebrin Tablets (Lilly)
Hep-Lock (Heparin Lock Flush Solution) (Elkins-Sinn) p 938
Hep-Lock PF (Preservative-Free Heparin Lock Flush Solution) (Elkins-Sinn) p 938
HEP-PAK Convenience Package (Winthrop-Breon)
Heptavax-B (Merck Sharp & Dohme) p 1312
Heptuna Plus (Roerig) p 431, 1735
Herpecin-L Cold Sore Lip Balm (Campbell) p 829
Herplex Liquifilm ophthalmic solution (Allergan)
Hespan (American Critical Care) p 595
Hesper Bitabs (Merrell Dow)
Hesper Capsules (Merrell Dow)
Hexa-Betalin Vials & Tablets (Lilly)
Hexadrol Elixir (Organon) p 1446
Hexadrol Tablets (Organon) p 422, 1446
Hexadrol Phosphate Injection (Organon) p 1446
Hexadrol Strip Packs (Organon) p 1446
Hexadrol Therapeutic Pack (Organon) p 422, 1446
Hexalol Tablets (Central Pharmaceuticals)
◆ Hibiclens Antimicrobial Skin Cleanser (Stuart) p 439, 2037
◆ Hibiclens Sponge/Brush with Nail Cleaner (Stuart) p 439
◆ Hibistat Germicidal Hand Rinse (Stuart) p 439, 2038
HI-COR 1.0 (C & M)
HI-COR 2.5 (C & M)
Hill Cortac (Hill Dermaceuticals) p 1009
Hill-Shade Lotion (Hill Dermaceuticals) p 1009
◆ Hiprex (Merrell Dow) p 421, 1366
◆ Hispril Spansule Capsules (Smith Kline & French) p 437, 1965
Histabs Tablets (U.S. Ethicals)
Hista-Derfule Capsules (O'Neal, Jones & Feldman)
Histadyl and A.S.A. Pulvules (Lilly)
Histadyl E.C. Syrup (Lilly)
Histaject (Mayrand)
Histalet DM Syrup (Reid-Provident Labs.) p 1638
◆ Histalet Forte Tablets (Reid-Provident Labs.) p 428, 1638
Histalet Syrup (Reid-Provident Labs.) p 1638
Histalet X Syrup & Tablets (New Formula) (Reid-Provident Labs.) p 428, 1638
Histalog, Ampoules (Lilly)
Histamine Phosphate (For Gastric Test) (Lilly) p 3012
Histamine Phosphate (Histamine Test for Pheochromocytoma) (Lilly) p 3012
Histaspan-D Capsules (USV Pharmaceutical) p 2077
Histaspan-Plus Capsules (USV Pharmaceutical) p 2077
Histatapp Elixir (Upsher-Smith)
Histatapp T.D. Tablets (Upsher-Smith)
Histoplasmin, Diluted (Parke-Davis)
Histor-D Syrup (Hauck)
Histor-D Timecelles (Hauck) p 1001
Homatropine HBr 2%, 5% Dropperettes (CooperVision)
Homicebrin (Lilly)
Homo-Tet (Savage) p 1825
◆ Humatin Capsules (Parke-Davis) p 424, 1527
Humorsol Sterile Ophthalmic Solution (Merck Sharp & Dohme)
Humulin N Vials (Lilly) p 1150
Humulin R Vials (Lilly) p 1152
Hurricaine Liquid 1/4cc Unit Dose (Beutlich) p 705
Hurricaine Oral, Topical Anesthetic Gel, Liquid, Spray (Beutlich) p 705
Hurricaine Spray Extension Tubes (Beutlich)
Hurricaine Topical Anesthetic Spray Kit (Beutlich)
Hu-Tet, Tetanus Immune Globulin (Human), U.S.P. (Hyland Therapeutics) p 1024
Hybephen Tablets (Beecham Laboratories)
Hybolin Decanoate (Hyrex)
Hycal Liquid (Beecham Laboratories)
◆ Hycodan (Du Pont) p 410, 917
Hycodaphen Tablets (Ascher)
Hycomine Compound (Du Pont) p 919
Hycomine Pediatric Syrup (Du Pont) p 917
Hycomine Syrup (Du Pont) p 917
Hyco-Pap (LaSalle) p 1071
Hycotuss Expectorant (Du Pont) p 920
Hydeltrasol Injection (Merck Sharp & Dohme)

Hydeltra-T.B.A. Suspension (Merck Sharp & Dohme) p 1314
◆ Hydergine Oral Tablets, Sublingual Tablets, & Liquid (Sandoz Pharmaceutical Div.) p 433, 1802
◆ Hydergine LC Liquid Capsules (Sandoz Pharmaceutical Div.) p 433, 1802
Hydralazine HCl Tablets (Danbury) p 887
Hydralazine HCl Tablets (Geneva) p 973
Hydralazine HCl Tablets (Schein) p 1828
Hydralazine-Thiazide Capsules (Schein) p 1828
Hydralazine w/Hydrochlorothiazide Capsules (Geneva) p 973
Hydra-Mag Tablets (Vale)
Hydrate Injection (Hyrex)
◆ Hydrea Capsules (Squibb) p 438, 1997
Hydrex Tablets (Trimen) p 2067
Hydrisalic Gel (Pedinol) p 1580
Hydrisea Lotion (Pedinol) p 1580
Hydrisinol Creme & Lotion (Pedinol) p 1580
Hydrochlorothiazide, Hydralazine HCl, Reserpine Tablets (Danbury) p 887
Hydrochlorothiazide/Reserpine Tablets (Danbury) p 887
Hydrochlorothiazide Tablets (Danbury) p 887
Hydrochlorothiazide Tablets (Geneva) p 973
◆ Hydrochlorothiazide Tablets (Lederle) p 416
Hydrochlorothiazide Tablets, Liquids, Intensol & Oral Solution (Roxane) p 1788
Hydrochlorothiazide Tablets (Schein) p 1828
Hydrochlorothiazide Tablets, USP (Thiuretic) (Parke-Davis) p 1527
Hydrochlorothiazide w/Reserpine Tablets (Geneva) p 973
Hydrocil Instant (Rowell)
Hydrocodone Syrup (Schein) p 1828
Hydrocortisone USP (Organon) p 1446
Hydrocortisone Cream (Pharmaderm) p 1617
Hydrocortisone Cream & Ointment 0.5% (Fougera) p 953
Hydrocortisone Cream & Ointment 1% (Fougera) p 953
Hydrocortisone Sodium Succinate for Injection (Elkins-Sinn) p 938
Hydrocortisone Tablets (Danbury) p 887
Hydrocortisone Acetate Saline Suspension (Merck Sharp & Dohme)
Hydrocortone Acetate Sterile Ophthalmic Ointment and Ophthalmic Suspension (Merck Sharp & Dohme) p 1316
Hydrocortone Phosphate Injection (Merck Sharp & Dohme)
Hydrocortone Tablets (Merck Sharp & Dohme)
◆ HydroDIURIL Tablets (Merck Sharp & Dohme) p 420, 1316
Hydro-Ergoloid Oral & Sublingual Tablets (Schein) p 1828
Hydroflumethiazide Tablets (Schein) p 1828
Hydroflumethiazide with Reserpine (Geneva) p 973
Hydro-Fluserpine Tablets #1 & #2 (Schein) p 1828
Hydromorphone Carpuject (Winthrop-Breon)
Hydromorphone HCl Injection (Elkins-Sinn) p 938
Hydromorphone HCl in Tubex (Wyeth) p 2288
◆ Hydromox R Tablets (Lederle) p 415, 1094
◆ Hydromox Tablets (Lederle) p 415, 1094
Hydropel (Fougera)
Hydrophylic Ointment (Fougera)
◆ Hydropres Tablets (Merck Sharp & Dohme) p 420, 1317
Hydroserpine Tablets (Schein) p 1828
Hydrotensin-50 Tablets (Mayrand)
Hydroxacen Injectable (Central Pharmaceuticals)
Hydroxyzine Carpuject (Winthrop-Breon)
Hydroxyzine HCl Injection, Abbojects, Ampuls, Vials, Syringes (Abbott)
Hydroxyzine HCl Intramuscular Injection (Elkins-Sinn) p 938
Hydroxyzine HCl in Tubex (Wyeth) p 2288
Hydroxyzine HCl Syrup & Tablets (Schein) p 1828
Hydroxyzine Hydrochloride Tablets (Danbury) p 887
Hydroxyzine Hydrochloride Tablets (Geneva) p 973
◆ Hydroxyzine HCl Tablets (Lederle) p 416
Hydroxyzine Pamoate Capsules (Danbury) p 887
Hydroxyzine Pamoate (Schein) p 1828
Hydro-Z-50 Tablets (Mayrand)
hy-Flow (CooperVision)
◆ Hygroton Tablets (USV Pharmaceutical) p 440, 2078
◆ Hylorel Tablets (Pennwalt) p 426, 1582
Hypaque Meglumine 30% (Winthrop-Breon) p 3032
Hypaque Meglumine 60% (Winthrop-Breon) p 3039
Hypaque Sodium Oral Powder (Winthrop-Breon) p 3024
Hypaque Sodium Oral Solution (Winthrop-Breon) p 3025
Hypaque Sodium 20% (Winthrop-Breon) p 3026
Hypaque Sodium 25% (Winthrop-Breon) p 3028
Hypaque Sodium 50% (Winthrop-Breon) p 3034
Hypaque-Cysto (Winthrop-Breon) p 3030

(◆ Shown in Product Identification Section)   (*▫ Described in PDR For Nonprescription Drugs)   (Products without page numbers are not described)

Hypaque-M, 75% (Winthrop-Breon) p 3044
Hypaque-M, 90% (Winthrop-Breon) p 3053
Hypaque-76 Injection (Winthrop-Breon) p 3049
Hyperab (Rabies Immune Globulin-Human) (Cutter Biological)
HyperHep (Hepatitis B Immune Globulin-Human) (Cutter Biological)
Hyperstat I.V. Injection (Schering) p 1856
Hyper-Tet (Tetanus Immune Globulin-Human) (Cutter Biological)
Hyplex Vari-Dose (Hyrex)
Hypoaller-C Hypoallergenic Vitamin C Powder (buffered) (Professional Health)
Hypotears Lubricating Eye Drops (CooperVision)
HypRho-D (Rh₀-D Immune Globulin-Human) (Cutter Biological)
HypRho-D Mini-Dose (Rh₀-D Immune Globulin-Human) (Cutter Biological)
Hyproval P.A. Injection (Reid-Provident, Direct Div.)
Hyrex-105 (Hyrex) p 1024
Hyskon Hysteroscopy Fluid (Pharmacia) p 1616
Hysone (Mallard) p 1181
Hytakerol Capsules & Liquid (Winthrop-Breon)
Hytinic Capsules & Elixir (Hyrex) p 1024
Hytinic Injection (Hyrex)
Hytone Cream, Lotion & Ointment (Dermik) p 890
◆ Hytuss Tablets and Hytuss-2X Capsules (Hyrex) p 413, 1024
Hyzine-50 Injection (Hyrex)

I

I.D. 50 Injection (Reid-Provident, Direct Div.)
I-Knife (Alcon Labs.)
I.L.X. B₁₂ Elixir Crystalline (Kenwood) p 1046
I.L.X. B₁₂ Tablets (Kenwood) p 1046
I.L.X. Elixir (Kenwood)
INH Tablets (CIBA) p 850
I.V. Transfer Spikes (LyphoMed)
Iberet (Abbott) p 532
◆ Iberet-500 (Abbott) p 403, 532
Iberet-500 Liquid (Abbott) p 533
◆ Iberet-Folic-500 (Abbott) p 403, 529
Iberet Liquid (Abbott) p 533
Iberol Filmtab (Abbott)
Iberol-F Filmtab (Abbott)
Ichthammol Ointment 10% & 20% (Fougera) p 953
Ichthyol Ointment (Stiefel)
⊡ Icy Hot Balm (Searle Consumer Products)
⊡ Icy Hot Rub (Searle Consumer Products)
Identi-Dose (Lilly) p 1122
Iletin I, Lente (Lilly) p 1156
Iletin I, Regular (Lilly) p 1154
Iletin II, Regular (Concentrated), U-500 (Lilly) p 1155
Iletin I, Semilente (Lilly) p 1156
Iletin I, Ultralente (Lilly) p 1156
Ilopan Injection (Adria) p 578
Ilopan-Choline Tablets (Adria)
◆ Ilosone Oral Preparations (Dista) p 410, 897
Ilotycin Gluceptate (Dista) p 900
Ilotycin Sterile Ophthalmic Ointment (Dista) p 899
Ilotycin Tablets (Dista) p 899
Ilozyme Tablets (Adria)
Imferon (Merrell Dow) p 1367
◆ Imipramine HCl Tablets (Lederle) p 416
Imipramine HCl Tablets (Biocraft) p 705
Imipramine Hydrochloride Tablets (Roxane) p 1788
Imipramine HCl Tablets (Schein) p 1828
Imipramine Tablets (Geneva) p 973
Immuglobin (Savage) p 1825
Immune Globulin Intravenous, 5% (In 10% Maltose) Gamimune (Cutter Biological) p 883
Immune Serum Globulin (Human) (Wyeth) p 2245
Immune Serum Globulin (Human) in Tubex (Wyeth) p 2288
Immune Serum Globulin (Human), U.S.P. Gamma Globulin (Hyland Therapeutics) p 1024
Immune Serum Globulin (Human) Gamastan (Cutter Biological) p 883
◆ Imodium Capsules/Liquid (Janssen) p 413, 1033
Imogam Rabies Immune Globulin (Human) (Merieux) p 1358
Imovax Rabies Vaccine (Merieux) (Merieux) p 1358
Impregon Concentrate (Fleming)
Imuran Injection (Burroughs Wellcome)
◆ Imuran Tablets (Burroughs Wellcome) p 408, 790
Inapsine Injection (Janssen) p 1034
⊡ Incremin w/Iron Syrup (Lederle)
◆ Inderal Tablets & Injectable (Ayerst) p 405, 647
◆ Inderal LA Long Acting Capsules (Ayerst) p 405, 650
◆ Inderide (Ayerst) p 405, 651
◆ Indocin Capsules (Merck Sharp & Dohme) p 420, 1319
◆ Indocin SR Capsules (Merck Sharp & Dohme) p 420, 1319
◆ Indocin Suppositories (Merck Sharp & Dohme) p 420, 1319

Indo-Lemmon Capsules (Lemmon) p 1122
Indomethacin (Geneva) p 973
Indomethacin Capsules (Schein) p 1828
Infalyte (Pennwalt) p 1584
◆ Infants Panadol Drops (Glenbrook) p 412
◆ Infants' Tylenol Drops (McNeil Consumer Products) p 418
◆ Infatabs (Dilantin) (Parke-Davis) p 424
Inflamase Forte 1% Ophthalmic Solution (CooperVision)
Inflamase Mild ⅛% Ophthalmic Solution (CooperVision)
Influenza Virus Vaccine Subvirion Type (Wyeth) p 2246
Influenza Virus Vaccine Subvirion Type in Tubex (Wyeth) p 2288
InfraRub Analgesic Cream (Whitehall)
Innovar Injection (Janssen) p 1035
Inocor Lactate Injection (Winthrop-Breon) p 2199
Inpersol & 1.5% Dextrose (Abbott)
Inpersol & 4.25% Dextrose (Abbott)
InspirEase (Key Pharmaceuticals) p 1049
Insulatard NPH (Nordisk-USA) p 1422
Insulin Injection USP (Regular) (Squibb-Novo) p 2033
Intal (Fisons) p 943
Intal Nebulizer Solution (Fisons) p 943
Intensol Concentrated Oral Solutions (Package includes bottle & calibrated dropper) (Roxane)
   Chlorpromazine Hydrochloride Intensol (Roxane)
   DHT (Dihydrotachysterol) Intensol (Roxane)
   Dexamethasone Intensol (Roxane)
   Hydrochlorothiazine Intensol (Roxane)
   Roxanol (Morphine Sulfate Concentrated Oral Solution) (Roxane)
Intraderm-19 Emergency Acne Stick (Robertson/Taylor) p 1645
Intraderm-19 Oral Acne Supplement (Robertson/Taylor) p 1645
Intraderm-19 Overnight Acne Masque (Robertson/Taylor) p 1645
Intraderm-19 Therapeutic Acne Scrub (Robertson/Taylor) p 1645
Intraderm-19 Therapeutic Astringent Lotion (Robertson/Taylor) p 1646
Intropin (American Critical Care) p 596
Inversine Tablets (Merck Sharp & Dohme)
Iodochlorhydroxyquin 3% with Hydrocortisone Creams (Fougera) p 953
Iodo-Cortifair (Pharmafair) p 1618
Iodo-Niacin Tablets (O'Neal, Jones & Feldman) p 1445
Iodopen (Sodium Iodide Injection) (LyphoMed)
◆ Ionamin (Pennwalt) p 426, 1585
Ionosol B & 5% Dextrose Injection (Abbott)
Ionosol B & 10% Invert Sugar Injection (Abbott)
Ionosol D & 10% Invert Sugar Injection (Abbott)
Ionosol D-CM & 5% Dextrose Injection (Abbott)
Ionosol G & 10% Dextrose Injection (Abbott)
Ionosol G & 10% Invert Sugar Injection (Abbott)
Ionosol MB & 5% Dextrose Injection (Abbott)
Ionosol T & 5% Dextrose Injection (Abbott)
Iophen-C Liquid (Schein) p 1828
Ipecac (Lilly) p 1156
Ipecac Syrup (Roxane) p 1788
Ipsatol Expectorant Syrup (Key Pharmaceuticals)
Ircon Tablets (Key Pharmaceuticals)
Ircon-FA (Key Pharmaceuticals) p 1050
Irolong II (Reid-Provident, Direct Div.)
Iromin-G (Mission) p 1416
Iron (Chelated Iron Plus) (Vitaline)
Iron-L (Marlyn)
Ironco-B Tablets (Vale)
Irospan Capsules (Fielding) p 942
Irospan Tablets (Fielding) p 942
◆ Ismelin (CIBA) p 409, 851
Ismotic (Alcon Labs.)
Iso-B Caps (Tyson) p 2068
Iso-Bid Capsules (Geriatric) p 975
⊡ Isocal (Mead Johnson Nutritional)
Isocal HCN (Mead Johnson Nutritional)
Isochron Tablets (Forest) p 953
Isoclor Timesule Capsules (Fisons) p 944
Isocult (SmithKline Diagnostics) p 3018
Isoetharine Hydrochloride Inhalation (Roxane) p 1788
Isoetharine Hydrochloride 1.0% (Schein) p 1828
Isomil (Ross) p 1767
Isomil 20 (Ross)
Isomil SF (Ross) p 1768
Isomil SF 20 (Ross) p 1777
Isoniazid Tablets (Danbury) p 887
Isoniazid Tablets (Lilly)
Isopropyl Alcohol, 91% (Lilly)
Isoproterenol HCl Injection (Elkins-Sinn) p 938
Isoproterenol HCl 1:5,000 1 mg. Pintop (Abbott)
Isoproterenol HCl 1:5,000 2 mg. Pintop (Abbott)

Isoproterenol HCl 1:5,000 5 ml., Universal Add Syringe (Abbott)
Isoproterenol HCl 1:5,000 10 ml., Universal Add Syringe (Abbott)
Isoproterenol HCl 1:50,000, 10 ml., Abboject (Abbott)
◆ Isoptin Ampules (Knoll) p 414, 1061
◆ Isoptin for Intravenous Injection (Knoll) p 414, 1061
◆ Isoptin Oral Tablets (Knoll) p 414, 1063
Isopto Atropine (Alcon Labs.)
Isopto Carbachol (Alcon Labs.)
Isopto Carpine (Alcon Labs.)
Isopto Cetamide (Alcon Labs.)
Isopto Cetapred (Alcon Labs.)
Isopto Homatropine (Alcon Labs.)
Isopto Hyoscine (Alcon Labs.)
◆ Isordil Chewable (10 mg.) (Ives) p 413, 1028
◆ Isordil Oral Titradose (5 mg.) (Ives) p 413, 1028
◆ Isordil Oral Titradose (10 mg.) (Ives) p 413, 1028
◆ Isordil Oral Titradose (20 mg.) (Ives) p 413, 1028
◆ Isordil Oral Titradose (30 mg.) (Ives) p 413, 1028
◆ Isordil Oral Titradose (40 mg.) (Ives) p 413, 1028
◆ Isordil Sublingual 2.5 mg., 5 mg. & 10 mg. (Ives) p 413, 1028
◆ Isordil Tembids Capsules & Tablets (40 mg.) (Ives) p 413, 1028
Isosorbide Dinitrate Oral Tablets (Danbury) p 887
Isosorbide Dinitrate Sublingual Tablets (Danbury) p 887
Isosorbide Dinitrate Tablets (Geneva) p 973
Isosorbide Dinitrate Tablets - Oral & Sublingual (Schein) p 1828
Isosorbide Dinitrate T.D. Capsules & Tablets (Geneva) p 973
Isosorbide Dinitrate Timed Capsules & Tablets (Schein) p 1828
Isotein HN (Clinical Nutrition) p 877
Isotrate Timecelles (Hauck) p 1001
Isovex Capsules (U.S. Pharmaceutical) p 2070
Isoxsuprine Hydrochloride Tablets (Roxane) p 1788
Isoxsuprine HCl Tablets (Danbury) p 887
Isoxsuprine HCl Tablets (Schein) p 1828
Isoxsuprine Tablets (Geneva) p 973
Isuprel Hydrochloride Compound Elixir (Winthrop-Breon) p 2204
◆ Isuprel Hydrochloride Glossets (Winthrop-Breon) p 443, 2204
Isuprel Hydrochloride Injection 1:5000 (Winthrop-Breon) p 2201
Isuprel Hydrochloride Mistometer (Winthrop-Breon) p 2203
Isuprel Hydrochloride Solution 1:200 & 1:100 (Winthrop-Breon) p 2203

J

◆ Janimine Filmtab Tablets (Abbott) p 403, 533
Jeri-Bath (Dermik)
Jeri-Lotion (Dermik)

K

KBP/O Capsules (O'Neal, Jones & Feldman)
◆ K-Lor Powder (Abbott) p 403, 533
K-Lyte & K-Lyte DS (Mead Johnson Laboratories) p 419, 1222
K-Lyte/Cl & K-Lyte/Cl 50 (Mead Johnson Laboratories) p 419, 1222
K-Phos M.F. (Modified Formula) Tablets (Beach) p 405, 686
K-Phos Neutral Tablets (Beach) p 405, 686
K-Phos No. 2 Tablets (Beach) p 405, 686
K-Phos Original Formula 'Sodium Free' Tablets (Beach) p 405, 686
K-Phos w/S.A.P. (Beach)
◆ K-Tab (Abbott) p 403, 534
Kabikinase (Pharmacia) p 1616
Kabolin (Legere) p 1120
◆ Kantrex Capsules (Bristol) p 407, 734
Kantrex Injection (Bristol) p 735
Kantrex Pediatric Injection (Bristol) p 735
Kanulase (Dorsey Laboratories) p 910
Kaochlor 10% Liquid (Adria) p 579
Kaochlor-Eff Tablets (Adria)
Kaochlor S-F 10% Liquid (Sugar-free) (Adria) p 580
Kaolin, Pectin, Belladonna Mixture (Schein) p 1828
Kaolin-Pectin-Concentrated (Roxane) p 1788
Kaolin-Pectin Mixture (Schein) p 1828
Kaolin-Pectin PG Mixture (Schein) p 1828
Kaolin-Pectin Suspension (Roxane) p 1788
◆ Kaon Cl-10 (Adria) p 404, 582
Kaon Elixir, Grape Flavor (Adria) p 580
Kaon Elixir, Lemon-Lime Flavor (Adria)
◆ Kaon Tablets (Adria) p 404, 581
◆ Kaon-Cl Tabs (Adria) p 404, 581
◆ Kaon-Cl 20% (Adria) p 582
⊡ Kaopectate Anti-Diarrhea Medicine (Upjohn)
⊡ Kaopectate Anti-Diarrhea Medicine (Bilingual) (English & Spanish labeling) (Upjohn)
⊡ Kaopectate Tablet Formula (Upjohn)
Karbokoff Tablets (Arlo) p 601
Kasof Capsules (Stuart) p 439, 2038
KATO (Legere) p 1120

(◆ Shown in Product Identification Section)   (⊡ Described in PDR For Nonprescription Drugs)   (Products without page numbers are not described)

Product Name Index

Glukor Injection (Hyrex) p 1024
Glutethimide Tablets (Danbury) p 887
Glutethimide Tablets (Geneva) p 973
Glutethimide Tablets (Schein) p 1828
Glutofac Tablets (Kenwood) p 1046
Glycate Tablets (O'Neal, Jones & Feldman)
Glycofed (Vale)
Glycopyrrolate Tablets (Danbury) p 887
*❊ Glycotuss Syrup & Tablets (Vale)
Glycotuss-dM Syrup & Tablets (Vale)
Gly-Oxide Liquid (Marion) p 1186
Glyrol Solution (CooperVision)
Glytinic Tablets (Boyle) p 726
Glytuss Tabs (Mayrand)
GoLYTELY (Braintree) p 727
Gonioscopic Prism Solution (Alcon Labs.)
Goniosol Solution (CooperVision)
Granulex (Hickam) p 1009
Grifulvin V (Ortho Pharmaceutical (Dermatological Div.)) p 1473
◆ Grisactin (Ayerst) p 404, 646
◆ Grisactin Ultra (Ayerst) p 405, 646
Gris-PEG Tablets, 125mg & 250mg (Herbert) p 1005
Guaifed Capsules (Timed Release) (Muro) p 1421
Guaifenesin Syrup (Roxane) p 1788
Guanidine HCl Tablets (Key Pharmaceuticals)
Guiatuss Syrup (Schein) p 1828
Guiatuss A-C Syrup (Schein) p 1828
Guiatuss D-M Syrup (Schein) p 1828
Guiosan Syrup (Vale)
Gumsol (Arlo) p 601
Gustalac Tablets (Geriatric)
Gustase (Geriatric) p 975
Gustase-Plus Tablets (Geriatric)
Gyne-Lotrimin Vaginal Cream 1% (Schering) p 1856
◆ Gyne-Lotrimin Vaginal Tablets (Schering) p 434, 1856
Gynogen Injectable (O'Neal, Jones & Feldman)
Gynogen L.A. "10", "20" & "40" Injectable (O'Neal, Jones & Feldman)
*❊ Gynol II Contraceptive Jelly (Ortho Pharmaceutical)

H

H-BIG (Abbott) p 531
HEB Cream Base (Barnes-Hind)
H-H-R Tablets (Schein) p 1828
HMS Liquifilm ophthalmic suspension (Allergan)
HP Acthar Gel (Armour) p 601
HQC Kit (Elder)
H-R Sterile Lubricating Jelly (Youngs)
H.T. Factorate (Armour) p 613
H.T. Factorate, Generation II (Armour) p 613
HVS 1+2 (Chemi-Tech) p 839
Halazone Tablets (Abbott)
◆ Halcion Tablets (Upjohn) p 441, 2114
◆ Haldol Tablets, Concentrate, Injection (McNeil Pharmaceutical) p 418, 1201
Haldrone Tablets (Lilly)
*❊ Haley's M-O, Regular & Flavored (Winthrop Consumer Products)
Halodrin Tablets (Upjohn)
Halog Cream/Ointment/Solution (Squibb) p 1996
Halog-E Cream (Squibb) p 1996
◆ Halotestin Tablets (Upjohn) p 441, 2116
Halotex Cream & Solution (Westwood) p 2178
Harmonyl (Abbott) p 532
Head & Chest (Procter & Gamble) p 1620
◆ Head & Shoulders (Procter & Gamble)
*❊ Headway Capsules (Vicks Health Care)
*❊ Headway Tablets (Vicks Health Care)
Healon (Pharmacia) p 1615
Heather Feminine Deodorant Spray (Whitehall)
Hedal H-C Suppositories (Arlo)
Heet Analgesic Liniment (Whitehall)
Heet Spray Analgesic (Whitehall)
◆ Help (Verex) p 442, 2145
Hema-Chek Slide Test for Fecal Occult Blood Test with Control (Ames) p 3005
Hemaspan Tablets (Bock)
Hemoccult (SmithKline Diagnostics) p 3017
Hemocyte Plus Tabules (U.S. Pharmaceutical) p 2070
Hemocyte Tablets (U.S. Pharmaceutical) p 2070
Hemocyte-F Tablets (U.S. Pharmaceutical) p 2070
Hemofil, Antihemophilic Factor (Human), Method Four, Dried (Hyland Therapeutics) p 1023
Hemofil T, Antihemophilic Factor (Human), Method Four, Dried, Heat-Treated (Hyland Therapeutics) p 1024
Hemo-Vite (Drug Industries) p 914
Hemo-Vite Liquid (Drug Industries) p 914
Hepaferron Syrup (U.S. Ethicals)
Heparin Flush Kits (Wyeth)
Heparin Lock Flush Solution, USP, 100 u/ml (LyphoMed)
Heparin Lock Flush Solution Carpuject (Winthrop-Breon)
Heparin Lock Flush Solution in Tubex (Wyeth) p 2253

Heparin Sodium (Lilly) p 1149
Heparin Sodium (from Beef Lung Sources) (Organon) p 1446
Heparin Sodium Carpuject (Winthrop-Breon)
Heparin Sodium in Tubex (Wyeth) p 2288
Heparin Sodium Injection (Elkins-Sinn) p 938
Heparin Sodium Injection (Wyeth) p 2254
Heparin Sodium Injection, USP, Sterile Solution (Upjohn) p 2117
Heparin Sodium w/o preservative Injectable (O'Neal, Jones & Feldman) p 1445
Hepatitis B Immune Globulin (Human) HyperHep (Cutter Biological) p 884
Hep-B-Gammagee (Merck Sharp & Dohme) p 1311
HepFlush-10 (Heparin Lock Flush Solution, USP, 10 u/ml (LyphoMed)
Hep-Forte Capsules (Marlyn) p 1193
Hepicebrin Tablets (Lilly)
Hep-Lock (Heparin Lock Flush Solution) (Elkins-Sinn) p 938
Hep-Lock PF (Preservative-Free Heparin Lock Flush Solution) (Elkins-Sinn) p 938
HEP-PAK Convenience Package (Winthrop-Breon)
Heptavax-B (Merck Sharp & Dohme) p 1312
◆ Heptuna Plus (Roerig) p 431, 1735
Herpecin-L Cold Sore Lip Balm (Campbell) p 829
Herplex Liquifilm ophthalmic solution (Allergan)
Hespan (American Critical Care) p 595
Hesper Bitabs (Merrell Dow)
Hesper Capsules (Merrell Dow)
Hexa-Betalin Vials & Tablets (Lilly)
Hexadrol Elixir (Organon) p 1446
◆ Hexadrol Tablets (Organon) p 422, 1446
Hexadrol Phosphate Injection (Organon) p 1446
Hexadrol Strip Packs (Organon) p 1446
Hexadrol Therapeutic Pack (Organon) p 422, 1446
Hexalol Tablets (Central Pharmaceuticals)
◆ Hibiclens Antimicrobial Skin Cleanser (Stuart) p 439, 2037
◆ Hibiclens Sponge/Brush with Nail Cleaner (Stuart) p 439
◆ Hibistat Germicidal Hand Rinse (Stuart) p 439, 2038
HI-COR 1.0 (C & M)
HI-COR 2.5 (C & M)
Hill Cortac (Hill Dermaceuticals) p 1009
Hill-Shade Lotion (Hill Dermaceuticals) p 1009
◆ Hiprex (Merrell Dow) p 421, 1366
◆ Hispril Spansule Capsules (Smith Kline & French) p 437, 1965
Histabs Tablets (U.S. Ethicals)
Hista-Derfule Capsules (O'Neal, Jones & Feldman)
Histadyl and A.S.A. Pulvules (Lilly)
Histadyl E.C. Syrup (Lilly)
Histaject (Mayrand)
Histalet DM Syrup (Reid-Provident Labs.) p 1638
◆ Histalet Forte Tablets (Reid-Provident Labs.) p 428, 1638
Histalet Syrup (Reid-Provident Labs.) p 1638
Histalet X Syrup & Tablets (New Formula) (Reid-Provident Labs.) p 428, 1638
Histalog, Ampoules (Lilly)
Histamine Phosphate (For Gastric Test) (Lilly) p 3012
Histamine Phosphate (Histamine Test for Pheochromocytoma) (Lilly) p 3012
Histaspan-D Capsules (USV Pharmaceutical) p 2077
Histaspan-Plus Capsules (USV Pharmaceutical) p 2077
Histatapp Elixir (Upsher-Smith)
Histatapp T.D. Tablets (Upsher-Smith)
Histoplasmin, Diluted (Parke-Davis)
Histor-D Syrup (Hauck)
Histor-D Timecelles (Hauck) p 1001
Homatropine HBr 2%, 5% Dropperettes (CooperVision)
Homicebrin (Lilly)
Homo-Tet (Savage) p 1825
◆ Humatin Capsules (Parke-Davis) p 424, 1527
Humorsol Sterile Ophthalmic Solution (Merck Sharp & Dohme)
Humulin N Vials (Lilly) p 1150
Humulin R Vials (Lilly) p 1152
Hurricaine Liquid 1/4cc Unit Dose (Beutlich) p 705
Hurricaine Oral, Topical Anesthetic Gel, Liquid, Spray (Beutlich) p 705
Hurricaine Spray Extension Tubes (Beutlich)
Hurricaine Topical Anesthetic Spray Kit (Beutlich)
Hu-Tet, Tetanus Immune Globulin (Human), U.S.P. (Hyland Therapeutics) p 1024
Hybephen Tablets (Beecham Laboratories)
Hybolin Decanoate (Hyrex)
Hycal Liquid (Beecham Laboratories)
◆ Hycodan (Du Pont) p 410, 917
Hycodaphen Tablets (Ascher)
Hycomine Compound (Du Pont) p 919
Hycomine Pediatric Syrup (Du Pont) p 917
Hycomine Syrup (Du Pont) p 917
Hyco-Pap (LaSalle) p 1071
Hycotuss Expectorant (Du Pont) p 920
Hydeltrasol Injection (Merck Sharp & Dohme)

Hydeltra-T.B.A. Suspension (Merck Sharp & Dohme) p 1314
◆ Hydergine Oral Tablets, Sublingual Tablets, & Liquid (Sandoz Pharmaceutical Div.) p 433, 1802
◆ Hydergine LC Liquid Capsules (Sandoz Pharmaceutical Div.) p 433, 1802
Hydralazine HCl Tablets (Danbury) p 887
Hydralazine HCl Tablets (Geneva) p 973
Hydralazine HCl Tablets (Schein) p 1828
Hydralazine-Thiazide Capsules (Schein) p 1828
Hydralazine w/Hydrochlorothiazide Capsules (Geneva) p 973
Hydra-Mag Tablets (Vale)
Hydrate Injection (Hyrex)
◆ Hydrea Capsules (Squibb) p 438, 1997
Hydrex Tablets (Trimen) p 2067
Hydrisalic Gel (Pedinol) p 1580
Hydrisea Lotion (Pedinol) p 1580
Hydrisinol Creme & Lotion (Pedinol) p 1580
Hydrochlorothiazide, Hydralazine HCl, Reserpine Tablets (Danbury) p 887
Hydrochlorothiazide/Reserpine Tablets (Danbury) p 887
◆ Hydrochlorothiazide Tablets (Danbury) p 887
◆ Hydrochlorothiazide Tablets (Geneva) p 973
◆ Hydrochlorothiazide Tablets (Lederle) p 416
Hydrochlorothiazide Tablets, Liquids, Intensol & Oral Solution (Roxane) p 1788
Hydrochlorothiazide Tablets (Schein) p 1828
Hydrochlorothiazide Tablets, USP (Thiuretic) (Parke-Davis) p 1527
Hydrochlorothiazide w/Reserpine Tablets (Geneva) p 973
Hydrocil Instant (Rowell)
Hydrocodone Syrup (Schein) p 1828
Hydrocortisone USP (Organon) p 1446
Hydrocortisone Cream (Pharmaderm) p 1617
Hydrocortisone Cream & Ointment 0.5% (Fougera) p 953
Hydrocortisone Cream & Ointment 1% (Fougera) p 953
Hydrocortisone Sodium Succinate for Injection (Elkins-Sinn) p 938
Hydrocortisone Tablets (Danbury) p 887
Hydrocortone Acetate Saline Suspension (Merck Sharp & Dohme)
Hydrocortone Acetate Sterile Ophthalmic Ointment and Ophthalmic Suspension (Merck Sharp & Dohme) p 1316
Hydrocortone Phosphate Injection (Merck Sharp & Dohme)
Hydrocortone Tablets (Merck Sharp & Dohme)
◆ HydroDIURIL Tablets (Merck Sharp & Dohme) p 420, 1316
Hydro-Ergoloid Oral & Sublingual Tablets (Schein) p 1828
Hydroflumethiazide Tablets (Schein) p 1828
Hydroflumethiazide with Reserpine (Geneva) p 973
Hydro-Fluserpine Tablets #1 & #2 (Schein) p 1828
Hydromorphone Carpuject (Winthrop-Breon)
Hydromorphone HCl Injection (Elkins-Sinn) p 938
Hydromorphone HCl in Tubex (Wyeth) p 2288
◆ Hydromox R Tablets (Lederle) p 415, 1094
◆ Hydromox Tablets (Lederle) p 415, 1094
Hydropel (C & M)
Hydrophylic Ointment (Fougera)
◆ Hydropres Tablets (Merck Sharp & Dohme) p 420, 1317
Hydroserpine Tablets (Schein) p 1828
Hydrotensin-50 Tablets (Mayrand)
Hydroxacen Injectable (Central Pharmaceuticals)
Hydroxyzine Carpuject (Winthrop-Breon)
Hydroxyzine HCl Injection, Abbojects, Ampuls, Vials, Syringes (Abbott)
Hydroxyzine HCl Intramuscular Injection (Elkins-Sinn) p 938
Hydroxyzine HCl in Tubex (Wyeth) p 2288
Hydroxyzine HCl Syrup & Tablets (Schein) p 1828
Hydroxyzine Hydrochloride Tablets (Danbury) p 887
Hydroxyzine Hydrochloride Tablets (Geneva) p 973
◆ Hydroxyzine HCl Tablets (Lederle) p 416
Hydroxyzine Pamoate Capsules (Danbury) p 887
Hydroxyzine Pamoate (Schein) p 1828
Hydro-Z-50 Tablets (Mayrand)
hy-Flow (CooperVision)
◆ Hygroton Tablets (USV Pharmaceutical) p 440, 2078
◆ Hylorel Tablets (Pennwalt) p 426, 1582
Hypaque Meglumine 30% (Winthrop-Breon) p 3032
Hypaque Meglumine 60% (Winthrop-Breon) p 3039
Hypaque Sodium Oral Powder (Winthrop-Breon) p 3024
Hypaque Sodium Oral Solution (Winthrop-Breon) p 3025
Hypaque Sodium 20% (Winthrop-Breon) p 3026
Hypaque Sodium 25% (Winthrop-Breon) p 3028
Hypaque Sodium 50% (Winthrop-Breon) p 3034
Hypaque-Cysto (Winthrop-Breon) p 3030

(◆ Shown in Product Identification Section)   (*❊ Described in PDR For Nonprescription Drugs)   (Products without page numbers are not described)

Product Name Index

Hypaque-M, 75% (Winthrop-Breon) p 3044
Hypaque-M, 90% (Winthrop-Breon) p 3053
Hypaque-76 Injection (Winthrop-Breon) p 3049
Hyperab (Rabies Immune Globulin-Human) (Cutter Biological)
HyperHep (Hepatitis B Immune Globulin-Human) (Cutter Biological)
Hyperstat I.V. Injection (Schering) p 1856
Hyper-Tet (Tetanus Immune Globulin-Human) (Cutter Biological)
Hyplex Vari-Dose (Hyrex)
Hypoaller-C Hypoallergenic Vitamin C Powder (buffered) (Professional Health)
Hypotears Lubricating Eye Drops (CooperVision)
HypRho-D (Rh_o-D Immune Globulin-Human) (Cutter Biological)
HypRho-D Mini-Dose (Rh_o-D Immune Globulin-Human) (Cutter Biological)
Hyproval P.A. Injection (Reid-Provident, Direct Div.)
Hyrex-105 (Hyrex) p 1024
Hyskon Hysteroscopy Fluid (Pharmacia) p 1616
Hysone (Mallard) p 1181
Hytakerol Capsules & Liquid (Winthrop-Breon)
Hytinic Capsules & Elixir (Hyrex) p 1024
Hytinic Injection (Hyrex)
Hytone Cream, Lotion & Ointment (Dermik) p 890
◆ Hytuss Tablets and Hytuss-2X Capsules (Hyrex) p 413, 1024
Hyzine-50 Injection (Hyrex)

I

I.D. 50 Injection (Reid-Provident, Direct Div.)
I-Knife (Alcon Labs.)
I.L.X. B_{12} Elixir Crystalline (Kenwood) p 1046
I.L.X. B_{12} Tablets (Kenwood) p 1046
I.L.X. Elixir (Kenwood)
INH Tablets (CIBA) p 850
I.V. Transfer Spikes (LyphoMed)
Iberet (Abbott) p 532
◆ Iberet-500 (Abbott) p 403, 532
Iberet-500 Liquid (Abbott) p 533
◆ Iberet-Folic-500 (Abbott) p 403, 529
Iberet Liquid (Abbott) p 533
Iberol Filmtab (Abbott)
Iberol-F Filmtab (Abbott)
Ichthammol Ointment 10% & 20% (Fougera) p 953
Ichthyol Ointment (Stiefel)
⊡ Icy Hot Balm (Searle Consumer Products)
⊡ Icy Hot Rub (Searle Consumer Products)
Identi-Dose (Lilly) p 1122
Iletin I, Lente (Lilly) p 1156
Iletin I, Regular (Lilly) p 1154
Iletin I, Regular (Concentrated), U-500 (Lilly) p 1155
Iletin I, Semilente (Lilly) p 1156
Iletin I, Ultralente (Lilly) p 1156
Ilopan Injection (Adria) p 578
Ilopan-Choline Tablets (Adria)
◆ Ilosone Oral Preparations (Dista) p 410, 897
Ilotycin Glucoptate (Dista) p 900
Ilotycin Sterile Ophthalmic Ointment (Dista) p 899
Ilotycin Tablets (Dista) p 899
Ilozyme Tablets (Adria)
Imferon (Merrell Dow) p 1367
Imipramine HCl Tablets (Biocraft) p 705
◆ Imipramine HCl Tablets (Lederle) p 416
Imipramine Hydrochloride Tablets (Roxane) p 1788
Imipramine HCl Tablets (Schein) p 1828
Imipramine Tablets (Geneva) p 973
Immuglobin (Savage) p 1825
Immune Globulin Intravenous, 5% (In 10% Maltose) Gamimune (Cutter Biological) p 883
Immune Serum Globulin (Human) (Wyeth) p 2245
Immune Serum Globulin (Human) in Tubex (Wyeth) p 2288
Immune Serum Globulin (Human), U.S.P. Gamma Globulin (Hyland Therapeutics) p 1024
Immune Serum Globulin (Human) Gamastan (Cutter Biological) p 883
◆ Imodium Capsules/Liquid (Janssen) p 413, 1033
Imogam Rabies Immune Globulin (Human) (Merieux) p 1358
Imovax Rabies Vaccine (Merieux) (Merieux) p 1358
Impregon Concentrate (Fleming)
Imuran Injection (Burroughs Wellcome)
◆ Imuran Tablets (Burroughs Wellcome) p 408, 790
Inapsine Injection (Janssen) p 1034
⊡ Incremin w/Iron Syrup (Lederle)
◆ Inderal Tablets & Injectable (Ayerst) p 405, 647
◆ Inderal LA Long Acting Capsules (Ayerst) p 405, 650
Inderide (Ayerst) p 405, 651
Indocin Capsules (Merck Sharp & Dohme) p 420, 1319
◆ Indocin SR Capsules (Merck Sharp & Dohme) p 420, 1319
◆ Indocin Suppositories (Merck Sharp & Dohme) p 420, 1319

Indo-Lemmon Capsules (Lemmon) p 1122
Indomethacin (Geneva) p 973
Indomethacin Capsules (Schein) p 1828
Infalyte (Pennwalt) p 1584
◆ Infants Panadol Drops (Glenbrook) p 412
◆ Infants' Tylenol Drops (McNeil Consumer Products) p 418
◆ Infatabs (Dilantin) (Parke-Davis) p 424
Inflamase Forte 1% Ophthalmic Solution (CooperVision)
Inflamase Mild ⅛% Ophthalmic Solution (CooperVision)
Influenza Virus Vaccine Subvirion Type (Wyeth) p 2246
Influenza Virus Vaccine Subvirion Type in Tubex (Wyeth) p 2288
InfraRub Analgesic Cream (Whitehall)
Innovar Injection (Janssen) p 1035
Inocor Lactate Injection (Winthrop-Breon) p 2199
Inpersol & 1.5% Dextrose (Abbott)
Inpersol & 4.25% Dextrose (Abbott)
InspirEase (Key Pharmaceuticals) p 1049
Insulatard NPH (Nordisk-USA) p 1422
Insulin Injection USP (Regular) (Squibb-Novo) p 2033
Intal (Fisons) p 943
Intal Nebulizer Solution (Fisons) p 943
Intensol Concentrated Oral Solutions (Package includes bottle & calibrated dropper) (Roxane)
  Chlorpromazine Hydrochloride Intensol (Roxane)
  DHT (Dihydrotachysterol) Intensol (Roxane)
  Dexamethasone Intensol (Roxane)
  Hydrochlorothiazine Intensol (Roxane)
  Roxanol (Morphine Sulfate Concentrated Oral Solution) (Roxane)
Intraderm-19 Emergency Acne Stick (Robertson/Taylor) p 1645
Intraderm-19 Oral Acne Supplement (Robertson/Taylor) p 1645
Intraderm-19 Overnight Acne Masque (Robertson/Taylor) p 1645
Intraderm-19 Therapeutic Acne Scrub (Robertson/Taylor) p 1645
Intraderm-19 Therapeutic Astringent Lotion (Robertson/Taylor) p 1646
Intropin (American Critical Care) p 596
Inversine Tablets (Merck Sharp & Dohme)
Iodochlorhydroxyquin 3% with Hydrocortisone Creams (Fougera) p 953
Iodo-Cortifair (Pharmafair) p 1618
Iodo-Niacin Tablets (O'Neal, Jones & Feldman) p 1445
Iodopen (Sodium Iodide Injection) (LyphoMed)
◆ Ionamin (Pennwalt) p 426, 1585
Ionosol B & 5% Dextrose Injection (Abbott)
Ionosol B & 10% Invert Sugar Injection (Abbott)
Ionosol D & 10% Invert Sugar Injection (Abbott)
Ionosol D-CM & 5% Dextrose Injection (Abbott)
Ionosol G & 10% Dextrose Injection (Abbott)
Ionosol G & 10% Invert Sugar Injection (Abbott)
Ionosol MB & 5% Dextrose Injection (Abbott)
Ionosol T & 5% Dextrose Injection (Abbott)
Iophen-C Liquid (Schein) p 1828
Ipecac (Lilly) p 1156
Ipecac Syrup (Roxane) p 1788
Ipsatol Expectorant Syrup (Key Pharmaceuticals)
Ircon Tablets (Key Pharmaceuticals)
Ircon-FA (Key Pharmaceuticals) p 1050
Irolong II (Reid-Provident, Direct Div.)
Iromin-G (Mission) p 1416
Iron (Chelated Iron Plus) (Vitaline)
Iron-L (Marlyn)
Ironco-B Tablets (Vale)
Irospan Capsules (Fielding) p 942
Irospan Tablets (Fielding) p 942
◆ Ismelin (CIBA) p 409, 851
Ismotic (Alcon Labs.)
Iso-B Caps (Tyson) p 2068
Iso-Bid Capsules (Geriatric) p 975
⊡ Isocal (Mead Johnson Nutritional)
Isocal HCN (Mead Johnson Nutritional)
Isochron Tablets (Forest) p 953
Isoclor Timesule Capsules (Fisons) p 944
Isocult (SmithKline Diagnostics) p 3018
Isoetharine Hydrochloride Inhalation (Roxane) p 1788
Isoetharine Hydrochloride 1.0% (Schein) p 1828
Isomil (Ross) p 1767
Isomil SF (Ross) p 1768
Isomil SF 20 (Ross) p 1777
Isoniazid Tablets (Danbury) p 887
Isoniazid Tablets (Lilly)
Isopropyl Alcohol, 91% (Lilly)
Isoproterenol HCl Injection (Elkins-Sinn) p 938
Isoproterenol HCl 1:5,000 1 mg. Pintop (Abbott)
Isoproterenol HCl 1:5,000 2 mg. Pintop (Abbott)

Isoproterenol HCl 1:5,000 5 ml., Universal Add Syringe (Abbott)
Isoproterenol HCl 1:5,000 10 ml., Universal Add Syringe (Abbott)
Isoproterenol HCl 1:50,000, 10 ml., Abboject (Abbott)
◆ Isoptin Ampules (Knoll) p 414, 1061
◆ Isoptin for Intravenous Injection (Knoll) p 414, 1061
◆ Isoptin Oral Tablets (Knoll) p 414, 1063
Isopto Atropine (Alcon Labs.)
Isopto Carbachol (Alcon Labs.)
Isopto Carpine (Alcon Labs.)
Isopto Cetamide (Alcon Labs.)
Isopto Cetapred (Alcon Labs.)
Isopto Homatropine (Alcon Labs.)
Isopto Hyoscine (Alcon Labs.)
◆ Isordil Chewable (10 mg.) (Ives) p 413, 1028
◆ Isordil Oral Titradose (5 mg.) (Ives) p 413, 1028
◆ Isordil Oral Titradose (10 mg.) (Ives) p 413, 1028
◆ Isordil Oral Titradose (20 mg.) (Ives) p 413, 1028
◆ Isordil Oral Titradose (30 mg.) (Ives) p 413, 1028
◆ Isordil Oral Titradose (40 mg.) (Ives) p 413, 1028
◆ Isordil Sublingual 2.5 mg., 5 mg. & 10 mg. (Ives) p 413, 1028
◆ Isordil Tembids Capsules & Tablets (40 mg.) (Ives) p 413, 1028
Isosorbide Dinitrate Oral Tablets (Danbury) p 887
Isosorbide Dinitrate Sublingual Tablets (Danbury) p 887
Isosorbide Dinitrate Tablets (Geneva) p 973
Isosorbide Dinitrate Tablets - Oral & Sublingual (Schein) p 1828
Isosorbide Dinitrate T.D. Capsules & Tablets (Geneva) p 973
Isosorbide Dinitrate Timed Capsules & Tablets (Schein) p 1828
Isotein HN (Clinical Nutrition) p 877
Isotrate Timecelles (Hauck) p 1001
Isovex Capsules (U.S. Pharmaceutical) p 2070
Isoxsuprine Hydrochloride Tablets (Roxane) p 1788
Isoxsuprine HCl Tablets (Danbury) p 887
Isoxsuprine HCl Tablets (Schein) p 1828
Isoxsuprine Tablets (Geneva) p 973
Isuprel Hydrochloride Compound Elixir (Winthrop-Breon) p 2204
◆ Isuprel Hydrochloride Glossets (Winthrop-Breon) p 443, 2204
Isuprel Hydrochloride Injection 1:5000 (Winthrop-Breon) p 2201
Isuprel Hydrochloride Mistometer (Winthrop-Breon) p 2203
Isuprel Hydrochloride Solution 1:200 & 1:100 (Winthrop-Breon) p 2203

J

◆ Janimine Filmtab Tablets (Abbott) p 403, 533
Jeri-Bath (Dermik)
Jeri-Lotion (Dermik)

K

KBP/O Capsules (O'Neal, Jones & Feldman)
◆ K-Lor Powder (Abbott) p 403, 533
◆ K-Lyte & K-Lyte DS (Mead Johnson Laboratories) p 419, 1222
◆ K-Lyte/Cl & K-Lyte/Cl 50 (Mead Johnson Laboratories) p 419, 1222
◆ K-Phos M.F. (Modified Formula) Tablets (Beach) p 405, 686
◆ K-Phos Neutral Tablets (Beach) p 405, 686
◆ K-Phos No. 2 Tablets (Beach) p 405, 686
◆ K-Phos Original Formula 'Sodium Free' Tablets (Beach) p 405, 686
K-Phos w/S.A.P. (Beach)
◆ K-Tab (Abbott) p 403, 534
Kabikinase (Pharmacia) p 1616
Kabolin (Legere) p 1120
◆ Kantrex Capsules (Bristol) p 407, 734
Kantrex Injection (Bristol) p 735
Kantrex Pediatric Injection (Bristol) p 735
Kanulase (Dorsey Laboratories) p 910
Kaochlor 10% Liquid (Adria) p 579
Kaochlor-Eff Tablets (Adria)
Kaochlor S-F 10% Liquid (Sugar-free) (Adria) p 580
Kaolin, Pectin, Belladonna Mixture (Schein) p 1828
Kaolin-Pectin-Concentrated (Roxane) p 1788
Kaolin-Pectin Mixture (Schein) p 1828
Kaolin-Pectin PG Mixture (Schein) p 1828
Kaolin-Pectin Suspension (Roxane) p 1788
◆ Kaon Cl-10 (Adria) p 404, 582
Kaon Elixir, Grape Flavor (Adria) p 580
Kaon Elixir, Lemon-Lime Flavor (Adria)
◆ Kaon Tablets (Adria) p 404, 581
◆ Kaon-Cl Tabs (Adria) p 404, 581
◆ Kaon-Cl 20% (Adria) p 582
⊡ Kaopectate Anti-Diarrhea Medicine (Upjohn)
⊡ Kaopectate Anti-Diarrhea Medicine (Bilingual) (English & Spanish labeling) (Upjohn)
⊡ Kaopectate Tablet Formula (Upjohn)
Karbokoff Tablets (Arlo) p 601
◆ Kasof Capsules (Stuart) p 439, 2038
KATO (Legere) p 1120

(◆ Shown in Product Identification Section)   (⊡ Described in PDR For Nonprescription Drugs)   (Products without page numbers are not described)

Product Name Index

Kay Ciel Oral Solution 10% (Berlex) p 702
Kay Ciel Powder (Berlex) p 702
Kayexalate (Winthrop-Breon) p 2204
Kaylixir (Lannett)
◆ Keflex Oral Preparations (Dista) p 410, 901
Keflin, Neutral, Vials & Faspak (Lilly) p 1157
Kefzol (Lilly) p 1159
◆ Kemadrin (Burroughs Wellcome) p 408, 792
Kenacort Diacetate Syrup (Squibb)
Kenacort Tablets (Squibb)
Kenaject-40 (Mayrand)
Kenalog Cream/Lotion/Ointment (Squibb) p 1998
Kenalog in Orabase (Squibb) p 2003
Kenalog Spray (Squibb) p 1998
Kenalog-H Cream (Squibb)
Kenalog-10 Injection (Squibb) p 2001
Kenalog-40 Injection (Squibb) p 1999
Kenpectin (Kenwood)
Kenpectin-P (Kenwood)
Kenwood Therapeutic Liquid (Kenwood)
Keralyt Gel (Westwood) p 2179
Kerasol Therapeutic Bath Oil (Upsher-Smith)
Keri Creme (Westwood) p 2179
Keri Facial Soap (Westwood) p 2180
Keri Lotion (Westwood) p 2180
Kerodex (Ayerst) p 653
Kestrin Injection (Hyrex)
Kestrone-5 (Hyrex)
Ketalar (Parke-Davis) p 1528
Keto-Diastix Reagent Strips (Ames) p 3004
Key-Pred (Hyrex)
Key-Pred SP (Hyrex)
◆ Kinesed Tablets (Stuart) p 439, 2038
Kinevac (Squibb)
Klaron Acne Lotion (Dermik)
Klavikordal Tablets (U.S. Ethicals)
Klebcil for Injection (Beecham Laboratories)
Kler-ro Liquid (Ulmer)
Kler-ro Powder (Ulmer)
Klor-Con Powder (Upsher-Smith) p 2144
Klor-Con/25 Powder (Upsher-Smith) p 2144
Klor-Con 20% (Upsher-Smith) p 2144
Klorlyptus (High Chemical)
Klor-10% (Upsher-Smith) p 2144
Klorvess Effervescent Granules (Sandoz Pharmaceutical Div.) p 1803
Klorvess Effervescent Tablets (Sandoz Pharmaceutical Div.) p 433, 1803
Klorvess 10% Liquid (Sandoz Pharmaceutical Div.) p 1803
◆ Klotrix (Mead Johnson Pharmaceutical) p 419, 1251
Koate-HT (Cutter Biological) p 886
🅢🅓 Kolantyl Gel (Merrell Dow)
🅢🅓 Kolantyl Wafers (Merrell Dow)
Kolyum Liquid and Powder (Pennwalt)
Komed Acne Lotion (Barnes-Hind) p 684
Komed HC Lotion (Barnes-Hind) p 684
Komex (Barnes-Hind) p 684
Konakion Injectable (Roche) p 1687
Kondremul (Fisons)
Kondremul with Cascara (Fisons)
Kondremul with Phenolphthalein (Fisons)
Konsyl (Lafayette) p 1070
Konsyl-D (formerly L. A. Formula) (Lafayette) p 1070
Konÿne (Factor IX Complex-Human) (Factors II, VII, IX and X) (Cutter Biological)
Korigesic Tablets (Trimen) p 2067
Koro-Flex Arcing Spring Diaphragm (Youngs) p 2300
Koro-Flex Fitting Rings, Set of (Youngs)
Koromex Coil Spring Diaphragm (Youngs) p 2301
🅢🅓 Koromex Contraceptive Cream (Youngs)
🅢🅓 Koromex Contraceptive Crystal Clear Gel (Youngs)
🅢🅓 Koromex Contraceptive Foam (Youngs)
🅢🅓 Koromex Contraceptive Jelly (Youngs)
Koromex Diaphragm Introducer (Youngs)
Koromex Fitting Rings, Set of (Youngs)
Koromex Jelly/Cream Applicator (Youngs)
Korostatin Vaginal Tablets (Youngs) p 2301
Kronofed-A Jr. Kronocaps (Ferndale) p 942
Kronofed-A Kronocaps (Ferndale) p 942
Kronohist Kronocaps (Ferndale) p 942
🅢🅓 Kudrox Suspension (Double Strength) (Rorer)
Kutapressin Injection (Rorer)
◆ Kutrase Capsules (Rorer) p 431, 1750
◆ Ku-Zyme Capsules (Rorer) p 431, 1750
◆ Ku-Zyme HP Capsules (Rorer) p 431, 1751
Kwell Cream (Reed & Carnrick) p 1635
Kwell Lotion (Reed & Carnrick) p 1635
Kwell Shampoo (Reed & Carnrick) p 1635

L

L-2000 (Robertson/Taylor) p 1646
L.A. Dezone Injection (Reid-Provident, Direct Div.)
LC-65 Daily Contact Lens Cleaner for Polycon & Paraperm O₂ gas permeable lenses & all hard & soft lenses (Allergan)
L-Neuramine (Vitaline)
LTA Kit, Preattached (Abbott)
LTA II Kit (Abbott)
LTA Pediatric Kit (Abbott)

LABID 250 mg Tablets (Norwich Eaton) p 1436
Lacril artificial tears (Allergan)
Lacri-Lube S.O.P. ophthalmic ointment (Allergan)
Lacrisert Sterile Ophthalmic Insert (Merck Sharp & Dohme) p 1322
◆ LactAid (LactAid) p 414, 1070
LactiCare Lotion (Stiefel)
🅢🅓 Lactinex Tablets & Granules (Hynson, Westcott & Dunning)
Lactocal-F Tablets (Laser) p 1072
◆ Lactrase Capsules (Rorer) p 431
Laminaria Japonica (Milex)
Lanacillin "400" (Lannett)
Lanahex Liquid (Lannett)
Lanamin Capsules (Lannett)
Lanatuss Expectorant (Lannett)
Lanolin & Lanolin Anhydrous (Fougera) p 953
Lanoline, Wellcome (Burroughs Wellcome)
Lanorinal Capsules & Tablets (Lannett)
◆ Lanoxicaps (Burroughs Wellcome) p 408, 793
◆ Lanoxin (Burroughs Wellcome) p 408, 797
Lanvisone Cream (Lannett)
Largon in Tubex (Wyeth) p 2288
◆ Larobec Tablets (Roche) p 429, 1687
◆ Larodopa Capsules (Roche) p 429, 1688
◆ Larodopa Tablets (Roche) p 429, 1688
Larylgan Throat Spray (Ayerst) p 653
Lasan Creams, 0.1, 0.2, 0.4% (Stiefel)
Lasan HP-1 Cream (Stiefel)
Lasan Unguent (Stiefel)
◆ Lasix Oral Solution (Hoechst-Roussel) p 413, 1015
◆ Lasix Tablets and Injection (Hoechst-Roussel) p 413, 1015
Lavacol (Parke-Davis)
Lavatar Tar Bath (Doak)
Laxatyl Tablets (Trimen)
Ledercillin VK Oral Solution & Tablets (Lederle)
🅢🅓 Lederplex Capsules, Liquid & Tablets (Lederle)
Lens Plus Daily Cleaner (Allergan)
Lens Plus Saline Solution (Allergan)
Lensine-5 (CooperVision)
Lensine Extra Strength Cleaner (CooperVision)
Lensrins preserved saline solution (Allergan)
Lens-Wet lubricating & rewetting solution (Allergan)
Lente Insulin (Insulin Zinc Suspension USP) (Squibb-Novo) p 2033
Lente Purified Pork Insulin Zinc Suspension (Squibb-Novo) p 2034
◆ Leucovorin Calcium Injection (Lederle) p 415, 1096
◆ Leukeran (Burroughs Wellcome) p 408, 801
Levo-Dromoran Injectable (Roche) p 1689
◆ Levo-Dromoran Tablets (Roche) p 429, 1689
Levophed Bitartrate (Winthrop-Breon) p 2205
Levoprome (Lederle)
◆ Levothroid for Injection (USV Pharmaceutical) p 440, 2079
◆ Levothroid Tablets (USV Pharmaceutical) p 440, 2080
◆ Levsin Tablets, Injection, Elixir & Drops (Rorer) p 432, 1751
Levsin/Phenobarbital Tablets, Elixir & Drops (Rorer) p 1751
◆ Levsinex Timecaps (Rorer) p 432, 1751
Levsinex/Phenobarbital Timecaps (Rorer) p 1751
Lextron Ferrous Pulvules (Lilly)
Lextron Pulvules (Lilly)
Li-Ban Spray (Pfipharmecs) p 1589
Libidinal Capsules (Everett) p 942
Libigen 10,000 & Diluent (Savage)
◆ Librax Capsules (Roche Products) p 430, 1713
◆ Libritabs Tablets (Roche Products) p 430, 1714
◆ Librium Capsules (Roche Products) p 430, 1714
Librium Injectable (Roche Products) p 1715
Lidaform-HC Creme (Miles Pharmaceuticals)
Lidex Cream 0.05% (Syntex) p 2061
Lidex Gel 0.05% (Syntex) p 2061
Lidex Ointment 0.05% (Syntex) p 2061
Lidex Topical Solution 0.05% (Syntex) p 2061
Lidex-E Cream 0.05% (Syntex) p 2061
Lidocaine 1%, 5 ml., Abboject (Abbott)
Lidocaine 1%, 5 ml., Sterile Pack Abboject (Abbott)
Lidocaine 2%, 5 ml., Abboject (Abbott)
Lidocaine 2%, 5 ml., Sterile Pack Abboject (Abbott)
Lidocaine HCl Injection (Bristol) p 730
Lidocaine HCl Injection (Elkins-Sinn) p 938
Lidocaine HCl Injection (Preservative-free) (Elkins-Sinn) p 938
Lidocaine Hydrochloride Injection for Cardiac Arrhythmias (Elkins-Sinn) p 938
Lidocaine Hydrochloride Injection, U.S.P. (Abbott) p 535
Lidocaine HCl in Tubex (Wyeth) p 2288
Lidocaine HCl 2% Viscous Solution (Schein) p 1828
Lidocaine 1% and 2% (Legere) p 1120
Lidocaine Ointment 5% (Fougera) p 953
Lidoject-1 & Lidoject-2 (Mayrand)
Lidoject-E-1 & Lidoject-E-2 (Mayrand)
Lifoject (Mayrand)
Lifolbex Injectable (Central Pharmaceuticals)

◆ Limbitrol Tablets (Roche Products) p 430, 1716
Limit Tablets (Bock)
Lincocin (Upjohn) p 2119
Lindane Lotion & Shampoo (Schein) p 1828
◆ Lioresal Tablets (Geigy) p 411, 959
Liothyronine Sodium Tablets (Schein) p 1828
Lipo Gantrisin (Roche) p 1686
Lipo Plus (lipotropics) (Vitaline)
Lipoderm Capsules (Hyrex)
Lipoflavonoid Vitamin Supplement (Capsule) (CooperVision)
Lipo-Hepin (Heparin Sodium Injection USP) (Riker)
Lipomul Oral Liquid (Upjohn)
Lipo-Nicin (Brown) p 773
Lipotriad Vitamin Supplement (Capsule, Liquid) (CooperVision)
Lippes Loop Intrauterine Double-S (Ortho Pharmaceutical) p 1454
Liquaemin Sodium (Organon) p 1446
◆ Liquamar Tablets (Organon) p 422, 1447
Liqui-Doss (Ferndale) p 942
Liquid Lather (Ulmer)
Liquid Neutrogena (Neutrogena)
Liquid Pred Syrup (Muro) p 1421
Liquifilm Forte enhanced artificial tears (Allergan)
Liquifilm Tears artificial tears (Allergan)
Liquifilm Wetting Solution hard contact lens solution (Allergan)
🅢🅓 Liquiprin Acetaminophen (Norcliff Thayer)
◆ Lithane (Miles Pharmaceuticals) p 422, 1403
Lithium Carbonate Capsules & Tablets (Roxane) p 1789
Lithium Citrate Syrup (Roxane) p 1790
◆ Lithobid Tablets (CIBA) p 409, 852
Lithonate (Rowell)
Lithostat (Mission) p 1418
Lithotabs (Rowell)
🅢🅓 Livitamin Capsules (Beecham Laboratories)
Livitamin Capsules w/Intrinsic Factor (Beecham Laboratories)
🅢🅓 Livitamin Chewable Tablets (Beecham Laboratories)
🅢🅓 Livitamin Liquid (Beecham Laboratories)
Livolex (Legere) p 1120
Livroben Injectable (O'Neal, Jones & Feldman)
Lixaminol Elixir (Ferndale)
🅢🅓 Lobana Bath Oil (Ulmer)
🅢🅓 Lobana Body Lotion (Ulmer)
🅢🅓 Lobana Body Powder (Ulmer)
🅢🅓 Lobana Body Shampoo (Ulmer)
🅢🅓 Lobana Conditioning Shampoo (Ulmer)
🅢🅓 Lobana Derm-ADE Cream (Ulmer)
🅢🅓 Lobana Liquid Hand Soap (Ulmer)
🅢🅓 Lobana Peri-Gard (Ulmer)
🅢🅓 Lobana Perineal Cleanse (Ulmer)
Lodrane Capsules-130 & 260 (Poythress) p 1618
◆ Loestrin 21 1/20 (Parke-Davis) p 424, 1531
◆ Loestrin Fe 1/20 (Parke-Davis) p 424, 1531
◆ Loestrin 21 1.5/30 (Parke-Davis) p 424, 1531
◆ Loestrin Fe 1.5/30 (Parke-Davis) p 424, 1531
🅢🅓 Lofenalac (Mead Johnson Nutritional)
Lofene Tablets (Lannett)
Lomotil Liquid (Searle & Co.) p 1931
◆ Lomotil Tablets (Searle & Co.) p 436, 1931
🅢🅓 Lonalac (Mead Johnson Nutritional)
◆ Loniten Tablets (Upjohn) p 441, 2120
Lonox Tablets (Geneva) p 973
◆ Lo/Ovral Tablets (Wyeth) p 444, 2255
◆ Lo/Ovral-28 Tablets (Wyeth) p 444, 2263
◆ Lopid Capsules (Parke-Davis) p 424, 1539
Lopressor Ampuls (Geigy) p 960
◆ Lopressor Tablets (Geigy) p 411, 960
◆ Loprox Cream 1% (Hoechst-Roussel) p 413, 1017
Lopurin (Boots) p 406, 718
Lorcet (UAD Labs.) p 2069
Lorcet-HD (UAD Labs.) p 2069
◆ Lorelco (Merrell Dow) p 421, 1368
Lorfan Injectable (Roche) p 1689
Loroxide Acne Lotion (Dermik)
Lotio Alsulfa (Doak)
Lotio-P Lotion (Alto)
Lotrimin Cream 1% (Schering) p 1857
Lotrimin Lotion 1% (Schering) p 1857
Lotrimin Solution 1% (Schering) p 1857
Lotrisone Cream (Schering) p 1858
Lotusate Caplets (Winthrop-Breon) p 2206
Lowila Cake (Westwood) p 2180
◆ Loxitane C Oral Concentrate (Lederle) p 415, 1096
◆ Loxitane Capsules (Lederle) p 415, 1096
◆ Loxitane IM (Lederle) p 415, 1096
◆ Lozol Tablets (USV Pharmaceutical) p 440, 2081
Lubafax Surgical Lubricant, Sterile (Burroughs Wellcome)
Lubrajel (Guardian)
Lubrajel HC (Guardian)
Lubraseptic Jelly (Guardian) p 1000
🅢🅓 Lubrin Vaginal Lubricating Inserts (Upsher-Smith)
Lubritine (Guardian)
◆ Ludiomil (CIBA) p 409, 854
Lufa Capsules (Armour)
Lufyllin Elixir (Wallace) p 2158
Lufyllin Injection (Wallace) p 442, 2159
◆ Lufyllin & Lufyllin-400 Tablets (Wallace) p 442, 2160

(◆ Shown in Product Identification Section) (🅢🅓 Described in PDR For Nonprescription Drugs) (Products without page numbers are not described)

Product Name Index

Lufyllin-EPG Elixir & Tablets (Wallace)
◆ Lufyllin-GG (Wallace) p 442, 2161
Luminal Ovoids (Winthrop-Breon)
Luminal Sodium Injection (Winthrop-Breon)
Luride Drops (Colgate-Hoyt) p 878
◆ Luride Lozi-Tabs Tablets (Colgate-Hoyt) p 410, 878
◆ Full-strength 1.0 mg F (Colgate-Hoyt) p 410
Luride-SF (no artificial flavor or color) 1.0 mg F (Colgate-Hoyt) p 410
Half-strength 0.5 mg F (Colgate-Hoyt) p 410
Quarter-strength 0.25 mg F (Colgate-Hoyt) p 410
Lycolan Elixir (Lannett)
Lydia Pinkham (Capsule, Liquid) (CooperVision)
Lyopine Vari-Dose (Hyrex)
LyphoLyte & LyphoLyte-II (Multielectrolyte Concentrate) (LyphoMed)
Lysiplex Syrup (Kramer)
◆ Lysodren (Bristol-Myers Oncology) p 407, 760
Lyte-C (Tyson) p 2068
⊞ Lytren (Mead Johnson Nutritional)

M

MBF (Meat Base Formula) Liquid (Gerber) p 974
⊞ MCT Oil (Mead Johnson Nutritional)
M-M-R ∥ (Merck Sharp & Dohme) p 1323
M.O.M.- Suspension of Magnesium Hydroxide (Ulmer)
M-R-VAX ∥ (Merck Sharp & Dohme) p 1325
◆ MS Contin (Purdue Frederick) p 1625
MTE-2 (LyphoMed)
MTE-3 (LyphoMed)
MTE-4 & MTE-4 Concentrated (LyphoMed)
MTE-5 & MTE-5 Concentrated (LyphoMed)
MTE-6 & MTE-6 Concentrated (LyphoMed)
MVC (Multivitamin Concentrate) (LyphoMed)
MVC 9+3 and MVC 9+3 VitaGard (LyphoMed)
◆ M.V.I. (Armour) p 404, 605
M.V.I. Concentrate (Armour) p 605
M.V.I. Pediatric (Armour) p 607
M.V.I.-12 (Armour) p 606
M.V.I.-12 Lyophilized (Armour) p 606
MVM Caps (Tyson) p 2068
◆ Maalox No. 1 Tablets (Rorer) p 432
◆ Maalox No. 2 Tablets (Rorer) p 432
⊞ Maalox Plus Suspension (Rorer)
◆ Maalox Plus Tablets (Rorer) p 432
◆ Maalox TC Suspension (Rorer)
◆ Maalox TC Tablets (Rorer) p 432
◆ Macrodantin Capsules (Norwich Eaton) p 422, 1436
Macrodex (Pharmacia) p 1616
Magan (Adria) p 583
Magmalin Tablets & Suspension (Vale)
⊞ Magnatril Suspension & Tablets (Lannett)
Magnesia & Alumina Oral Suspension (Roxane) p 1788
Magnesium Sulfate 50% Injection (Bristol) p 730
Magnesium Sulfate 50% w/v Ampoules & Abboject (Abbott)
Magnesium Sulfate Injectable (O'Neal, Jones & Feldman) p 1445
Magnesium Sulfate Injection (Elkins-Sinn) p 938
Magonate Tablets (Fleming)
Magsal Tablets (U.S. Pharmaceutical) p 2070
Maigret Tablets (Ferndale)
⊞ Maltsupex Liquid, Powder & Tablets (Wallace)
Mammol Ointment (Abbott)
◆ Mandelamine (Parke-Davis) p 424, 1540
Mandex Tablets (Vale)
Mandol (Lilly) p 1161
Mangatrace (Armour) p 607
◆ Maolate Tablets (Upjohn) p 441, 2123
◆ Marax Tablets & DF Syrup (Roerig) p 431, 1737
Marbec Tablets (Marlyn)
⊞ Marblen Suspension Peach/Apricot (Fleming)
⊞ Marblen Suspension Unflavored (Fleming)
⊞ Marblen Tablets (Fleming)
Marcaine Hydrochloride (Winthrop-Breon) p 2206
Marcaine Hydrochloride with Epinephrine 1:200,000 (Winthrop-Breon) p 2206
Marcaine Spinal (Winthrop-Breon) p 2210
◆ Marezine (Burroughs Wellcome) p 408, 803
MARLYN Formula 50 (Marlyn) p 1193
⊞ MARLYN PMS (Marlyn)
MARLYN Prolonged Release Vitamins (Marlyn)
◆ Marplan Tablets (Roche) p 430, 1689
⊞ Massé Breast Cream (Ortho Pharmaceutical)
Massengill Disposable Douche (Beecham Products) p 687
Massengill Liquid Concentrate (Beecham Products) p 687
Massengill Medicated Disposable Douche (Beecham Products) p 688
Massengill Powder (Beecham Products) p 687
Mastisol Liquid Adhesive (Ferndale)
◆ Materna 1·60 Tablets (Lederle) p 415, 1098
◆ Matulane Capsules (Roche) p 430, 1691
Maxafil Cream (Cooper Dermatology)
Max-EPA (Tyson)

MaxEPA Marine Lipid Concentrate (Professional Health)
Maxibolin (Organon) p 1447
Maxidex Suspension & Ointment (Alcon Labs.)
Maxifill Transfer Set (LyphoMed)
Maxiflor Cream (Herbert) p 1006
Maxiflor Ointment (Herbert) p 1006
◆ Maximum Bayer Aspirin (Glenbrook) p 412, 996
Maximum Strength Midol for Cramps (Glenbrook) p 997
Maximum Strength Midol PMS (Glenbrook) p 997
◆ Maximum Strength Panadol Capsules & Tablets (Glenbrook) p 412, 997
Maxitrol Suspension & Ointment (Alcon Labs.)
Maxovite Tablets (Tyson) p 2068
◆ Maxzide Tablets (Lederle) p 415, 1098
Mazanor (Wyeth) p 444, 2263
Measurin Tablets (Winthrop-Breon)
◆ Mebaral (Winthrop-Breon) p 444, 2213
Meclan (Ortho Pharmaceutical (Dermatological Div.)) p 1474
Meclizine HCl MLT Tablets (Schein) p 1828
Meclizine HCl Tablets (Geneva) p 973
◆ Meclizine HCl Tablets (Lederle) p 416
◆ Meclomen (Parke-Davis) p 424, 1541
◆ Mediatric Capsules, Tablets & Liquid (Ayerst) p 405, 654
◆ Medicated Cleansing Pads By the Makers of Prepartion H Hemmorrhoidal Remedies (Whitehall) p 443
⊞ Medicone Dressing Cream (Medicone)
◆ Mediconet (Medicone)
◆ Medihaler Ergotamine Aerosol (Riker) p 428, 1643
Medihaler-Epi (Riker) p 1643
Medihaler-Iso (Riker) p 1644
Mediplex Tablets (U.S. Pharmaceutical) p 2070
Medispray (Medical Products)
Medi-Tec 90 New Therapeutic Overnight Concentrate (Robertson/Taylor) p 1646
Medi-Tec 90 Therapeutic Conditioner with Strengthening Agents (Robertson/Taylor) p 1646
Medi-Tec 90 Therapeutic Scalp Stimulant with Strengthening Agents (Robertson/Taylor) p 1646
Medi-Tec 90 Therapeutic Shampoo & Scalp Conditioner with Strengthening Agents (Robertson/Taylor) p 1646
Medi-Tec Vitamin-Mineral-Trace Mineral Supplement (Robertson/Taylor) p 1646
Medrol Acetate Topical (Upjohn) p 2124
Medrol Dosepak Unit of Use (Upjohn) p 441
Medrol Enpak Kit (Upjohn)
◆ Medrol Tablets (Upjohn) p 441, 2124
Mefoxin (Merck Sharp & Dohme) p 1326
Mega-B (Arco) p 600
◆ Megace Tablets (Bristol-Myers Oncology) p 407, 761
Megadose (Arco) p 600
Megaplex I.M. (Legere) p 1120
Megaton Elixir (Hyrex) p 1025
Melanex 3% Topical Solution (Neutrogena) (Neutrogena) p 1421
Melfiat Tablets (Reid-Provident Labs.) p 1639
◆ Melfiat 105 Unicelles (Reid-Provident Labs.) p 428, 1639
◆ Mellaril (Sandoz Pharmaceutical Div.) p 433, 1804
Mellaril-S (Sandoz Pharmaceutical Div.) p 1804
Menaval 20 & Menaval 40 (Legere) p 1120
Menest (Beecham Laboratories)
Menoject-LA (Mayrand)
Menomune (Meningococcal Polysaccharide Vaccine, Groups A,C,Y,W-135, Combined, and Groups A & C, Combined) (Squibb/Connaught) p 2033
◆ Menrium Tablets (Roche Products) p 430, 1717
◆ Mepergan Fortis Capsules (Wyeth) p 444
Mepergan Injection (Wyeth) p 2264
Mepergan in Tubex (Wyeth) p 2288
Meperidine HCl in Tubex (Wyeth) p 2288
Meperidine HCl Injection (Elkins-Sinn) p 938
Mephyton Tablets (Merck Sharp & Dohme)
Mepred-40 (Savage)
Mepred-80 (Savage)
Mepro Compound Tablets (Schein) p 1828
Meprobamate Tablets (Danbury) p 887
Meprobamate Tablets (Geneva) p 973
Meprobamate Tablets (Schein) p 1828
Meprospan (Wallace) p 2161
Meritene Liquid (Clinical Nutrition) p 877
Meritene Powder (Clinical Nutrition) p 877
Merphene Germicidal Concentrate (Barry)
Mersalyl-Theophylline (Legere) p 1120
Merthiolate, Aeropump, Glycerite, Solution & Tincture (Lilly)
Meruvax ∥ (Merck Sharp & Dohme) p 1329
◆ Mesantoin (Sandoz Pharmaceutical Div.) p 433, 1805
Mestinon Injectable (Roche) p 1692
Mestinon Syrup (Roche) p 1692
Mestinon Tablets (Roche) p 430, 1692
Mestinon Timespan Tablets (Roche) p 430, 1692
Metabolite 2050 (Robertson/Taylor) p 1646
Metahydrin (Merrell Dow) p 421, 1370
Metamucil, Instant Mix, Orange Flavor (Searle Consumer Products) p 1912

Metamucil, Instant Mix, Regular Flavor (Searle Consumer Products) p 1911
Metamucil, Powder, Orange Flavor (Searle Consumer Products) p 1911
Metamucil, Powder, Regular Flavor (Searle Consumer Products) p 1911
Metamucil, Powder, Strawberry Flavor (Searle Consumer Products) p 1911
Metamucil, Powder, Sugar Free, Regular Flavor (Searle Consumer Products) p 1911
◆ Metandren Linguets & Tablets (CIBA) p 409, 855
Metaprel Inhalant Solution, Metered Dose Inhaler, Syrup & Tablets (Dorsey Laboratories) p 910
Metaraminol Bitartrate Injection (Bristol) p 730
◆ Metatensin (Merrell Dow) p 421, 1370
Meted Shampoo (Cooper Dermatology)
◆ Methadone Hydrochloride Diskets (Lilly) p 417, 1164
Methadone Hydrochloride Oral Solution & Tablets (Roxane) p 1791
Methamphetamine Hydrochloride, 5mg. & 10mg. (Rexar) p 1641
Methandrostenolone Tablets (Alto)
Methenamine Mandelate Forte Suspension & Tablets (Schein) p 1828
◆ Methergine (Sandoz Pharmaceutical Div.) p 433, 1806
Methiokap Capsules (Vale)
Methischol Capsules (Armour)
Methocarbamol Tablets (Danbury) p 887
Methocarbamol Tablets (Geneva) p 973
Methocarbamol Tablets (Roxane) p 1788
Methocarbamol Tablets (Schein) p 1828
Methocarbamol with Aspirin Tablets (Schein) p 1828
◆ Methotrexate Tablets & Parenteral (Lederle) p 415, 1100
Methyclothiazide Tablets (Lederle) p 416
Methyclothiazide Tablets (Schein) p 1828
Methy-Deserpidine (Schein)
Methylbenzethonium Chloride (Sween) p 2047
Methyldopa Tablets (Geneva) p 973
Methylene Blue Injection (Elkins-Sinn) p 938
Methylprednisolone Tablets (Schein) p 1828
Methylprednisolone Sodium Succinate (Organon) p 1447
Methylprednisolone Sodium Succinate for Injection (Elkins-Sinn) p 938
◆ Meticorten Tablets (Schering) p 434
Meti-Derm Cream 0.5% (Schering)
Metimyd Ophthalmic Ointment - Sterile (Schering) p 1860
Metimyd Ophthalmic Suspension (Schering) p 1860
◆ Metopirone (CIBA) p 409, 856
Metra Tablets (O'Neal, Jones & Feldman)
Metreton Ophthalmic/Otic Solution-Sterile (Schering) p 1861
Metric 21 Tablets (Fielding) p 942
Metronid Tablets (Ascher)
Metronidazole Oral Tablets (Schein) p 1828
Metronidazole Redi-Infusion (Elkins-Sinn) p 938
Metronidazole Tablets (Danbury) p 887
Metronidazole Tablets (Geneva) p 973
◆ Metronidazole Tablets (Lederle) p 416
Metryl and Metryl 500 Tablets (Lemmon) p 1122
Metubine Iodide (Lilly) p 1165
Mevanin-C Capsules (Beutlich) p 705
Mexate (Bristol-Myers Oncology) p 762
Mezlin (Miles Pharmaceuticals) p 1404
Mi-Cebrin (Dista) p 903
Mi-Cebrin T (Dista) p 903
Micrainin (Wallace)
MICRhoGAM (Ortho Diagnostic Systems) p 1452
Microcort Lotion (Alto)
Microcult-GC (Ames) p 3005
Micro-Guard (Sween) p 2048
◆ Micro-K Extencaps (Robins) p 428, 1653
◆ Micro-K 10 Extencaps (Robins) p 1653
◆ Micronase Tablets (Upjohn) p 441, 2126
◆ Micronor Tablets (Ortho Pharmaceutical) p 423, 1461
Microphake (Alcon Labs.)
Microsponge (Alcon Labs.)
Microstix-Candida Miniaturized Culture Test (Ames) p 3006
Microstix-Nitrite Kit (Ames)
Microstix-3 Reagent Strips (Ames) p 3005
◆ Midamor Tablets (Merck Sharp & Dohme) p 420, 1331
Midol-Original Formula (Glenbrook) p 997
◆ Midrin Capsules (Carnrick) p 408, 832
Migralam Capsules (Lambda) p 1071
⊞ Miles Nervine Nighttime Sleep-Aid (Miles Laboratories)
Milk of Magnesia, Milk of Magnesia-Concentrated (Roxane) p 1788
Milk of Magnesia-Cascara Suspension Concentrated (Roxane) p 1788
Milk of Magnesia-Mineral Oil Emulsion & Emulsion (Flavored) (Roxane) p 1788
⊞ Milkinol (Rorer)
◆ Milontin Kapseals (Parke-Davis) p 424, 1543
◆ Milpath Tablets (Wallace) p 442
Milprem Tablets (Wallace)

(◆ Shown in Product Identification Section)   (⊞ Described in PDR For Nonprescription Drugs)   (Products without page numbers are not described)

Product Name Index

- ◆ Miltown (Wallace) p 442, 2162
- ◆ Miltown 600 (Wallace) p 442, 2162
- Miltrate Tablets (Wallace)
- Mineral Oil-Light Sterile, Mineral Oil (Roxane) p 1788
- Mini-Gamulin Rh (Armour) p 613
- ◆ Minipress (Pfizer) p 426, 1603
- Minit-Rub analgesic balm (Bristol-Myers Products)
- ◆ Minizide Capsules (Pfizer) p 426, 1604
- ◆ Minocin (Lederle) p 415, 1103
- Minocin Oral Suspension (Lederle) p 1104
- ◆ Mintezol Chewable Tablets & Suspension (Merck Sharp & Dohme) p 420, 1332
- Miochol Intraocular (CooperVision)
- Miostat (Alcon Labs.)
- ◆ Miradon Tablets (Schering) p 434
- Mission Prenatal (Mission) p 1419
- Mission Prenatal F.A. (Mission) p 1419
- Mission Prenatal H.P. (Mission) p 1419
- Mission Prenatal RX (Mission) p 1419
- Mission Pre-Surgical (Mission) p 1419
- Mithracin (Miles Pharmaceuticals) p 1407
- ◆ Mitrolan (Robins) p 428, 1654
- Mity-Mycin Ointment (Reid-Provident Labs.)
- Mity-Quin Cream (Reid-Provident Labs.)
- Mixtard (Nordisk-USA) p 1423
- ◆ Moban Tablets & Concentrate (Du Pont) p 410, 921
- Mobidin Tablets (Ascher)
- Mobigesic Tablets (Ascher)
- Mobisyl Creme (Ascher)
- Modane Bulk (Adria) p 584
- Modane Plus (Adria) p 585
- Modane Soft (Adria) p 584
- Modane, Tablets & Liquid (Adria) p 584
- ◆ Moderil (Pfizer) p 426, 1605
- ◆ Modicon 21 Tablets (Ortho Pharmaceutical) p 423, 1461
- Modicon 28 Tablets (Ortho Pharmaceutical) p 1461
- Moducal (Mead Johnson Nutritional)
- ◆ Moduretic Tablets (Merck Sharp & Dohme) p 420, 1333
- Moisturel (Westwood) p 2180
- ◆ Mol-Iron Chronosule Capsules (Schering) p 434
- ◆ Mol-Iron Tablets (Schering) p 434
- ◆ Mol-Iron w/Vitamin C Tablets (Schering) p 434
- Molypen (Ammonium Molybdate Injection, USP) (LyphoMed)
- Momentum Muscular Backache Formula (Whitehall)
- Monistat-Derm (miconazole nitrate) Cream & Lotion (Ortho Pharmaceutical (Dermatological Div.)) p 1474
- Monistat I.V. (Janssen) p 1037
- Monistat 3 Vaginal Suppositories (Ortho Pharmaceutical) p 1456
- ◆ Monistat 7 Vaginal Cream (Ortho Pharmaceutical) p 423, 1455
- ◆ Monistat 7 Vaginal Suppositories (Ortho Pharmaceutical) p 423, 1456
- Monocid Injection (Smith Kline & French) p 1966
- ◆ Mono-Gesic Tablets (Central Pharmaceuticals) p 409, 837
- Mono-Vacc Test (O.T.) (Merieux) p 1358
- Morphine Sulfate Carpuject (Winthrop-Breon)
- Morphine Sulfate Injection (Elkins-Sinn) p 938
- Morphine Sulfate Oral Solution (Roxane) p 1792
- Morphine Sulfate Tablets (Roxane) p 1792
- Morphine Sulfate in Tubex (Wyeth) p 2288
- ◆ Motrin Tablets* (Upjohn) p 441, 2128
- Movicol (Norgine) p 1424
- Moxam Vials (Lilly) p 1166
- Mucilose Powder (Winthrop Consumer Products)
- Mucomyst (Mead Johnson Pharmaceutical) p 1252
- Mudrane GG Elixir (Poythress) p 1619
- Mudrane GG Tablets (Poythress) p 1619
- Mudrane GG-2 Tablets (Poythress) p 1619
- Mudrane Tablets (Poythress) p 1618
- Mudrane-2 Tablets (Poythress) p 1619
- Multicebrin (Lilly) p 1169
- Multitest CMI Skin Test Antigens for Cellular Hypersensitivity (Merieux) p 1358, 3013
- Multitrace 5 (Armour) p 608
- Multitrace Pediatric (Armour) p 609
- Multitrace Solution & Concentrate (Armour) p 609
- Multivitamins Rowell (Rowell)
- Multizyme (Standard Process)
- Mulvidren-F Softab Tablets (Stuart) p 439, 2039
- Mum cream deodorant (Bristol-Myers Products)
- Mumpsvax (Merck Sharp & Dohme) p 1336
- Murine Ear Wax Removal System/Murine Ear Drops (Ross) p 1769
- Murine Eye Drops (Regular Formula) (Ross) p 1769
- Murine Plus Eye Drops (Ross) p 1769
- Muripsin (Norgine) p 1424
- Muro 128 Ophthalmic Ointment (Muro)
- Muro 128 Ophthalmic Solution (Muro)
- Muro Tears Ophthalmic Solution (Muro)
- Murocel - Ophthalmic Solution (Muro)
- Murocoll-2 Ophthalmic Solution (Muro)
- Muro's Opcon Ophthalmic Solution (Muro)
- Muro's Opcon-A Ophthalmic Solution (Muro)
- Mus-L-Tone (High Chemical)

- Mustargen (Merck Sharp & Dohme) p 1337
- Mutamycin (Bristol-Myers Oncology) p 764
- Myadec (Parke-Davis) p 1543
- Myambutol Tablets (Lederle) p 1106
- Mycelex 1% Cream (Miles Pharmaceuticals) p 1409
- Mycelex 1% Solution (Miles Pharmaceuticals) p 1409
- ◆ Mycelex Troches (Miles Pharmaceuticals) p 422, 1409
- ◆ Mycelex-G (Miles Pharmaceuticals) p 422, 1410
- Mycelex-G 1% Vaginal Cream (Miles Pharmaceuticals) p 1410
- Mycifradin Oral Solution (Upjohn)
- Mycifradin Sterile Powder (Upjohn)
- Mycifradin Tablets (Upjohn)
- ▣ Myciguent Antibiotic Cream & Ointment (Upjohn)
- Mycitracin Antibiotic Ointment (Upjohn)
- Mycolog Cream and Ointment (Squibb) p 2003
- Mycostatin Cream & Ointment (Squibb) p 2004
- Mycostatin Oral Suspension (Squibb) p 2004
- ◆ Mycostatin Oral Tablets (Squibb) p 438, 2005
- Mycostatin Powder (for laboratory use) (Squibb)
- Mycostatin Topical Powder (Squibb) p 2004
- ◆ Mycostatin Vaginal Tablets (Squibb) p 438, 2005
- Myco-Triacet Cream and Ointment (Lemmon) p 1122
- Mydfrin 2.5% (Alcon Labs.)
- Mydriacyl (Alcon Labs.)
- Mygel Suspension (Geneva) p 973
- ◆ Mylanta Liquid (Stuart) p 439, 2039
- ◆ Mylanta Tablets (Stuart) p 439, 2039
- ◆ Mylanta-II Liquid (Stuart) p 439, 2039
- ◆ Mylanta-II Tablets (Stuart) p 439, 2039
- Myleran (Burroughs Wellcome) p 408, 804
- Mylicon Drops (Stuart) p 2039
- Mylicon Tablets (Stuart) p 439, 2039
- ◆ Mylicon-80 Tablets (Stuart) p 439, 2040
- Myochrysine Injection (Merck Sharp & Dohme) p 1339
- Myoflex Creme (Topical Analgesic) (Adria) p 585
- Myoforte Tablets (Bart)
- Myophen Injectable (Bart)
- Myotonachol (Glenwood) p 412, 998
- Mysoline (Ayerst) p 405, 657
- ◆ Mysteclin-F Capsules (Squibb) p 438, 2005
- Mysteclin-F Syrup (Squibb) p 2005
- Mytelase Chloride Caplets (Winthrop-Breon)
- Mytrex Cream & Ointment (Savage) p 1825

N

- N.B.P. Ointment (O'Neal, Jones & Feldman)
- ND-Gesic Tablets (Hyrex)
- ND-Hist Capsules (Hyrex)
- ND-Stat Injection (Hyrex)
- N-Multistix SG Reagent Strips (Ames) p 3004
- NPH Insulin (Isophane Insulin Suspension USP) (Squibb-Novo) p 2034
- NPH Iletin I (Lilly) p 1156
- NPH Purified Pork Isophane Insulin Suspension (Squibb-Novo) p 2034
- NTRON TTS-2500 Transcutaneous Electrical Nerve Stimulator (TENS) (NTRON International) p 1443
- ▣ NTZ Long Acting Spray & Drops (Winthrop Consumer Products)
- N-Uristix Reagent Strips (Ames) p 3006
- Nafcil (Bristol) p 736
- ◆ Naldecon (Bristol) p 407, 738
- ▣ Naldecon-CX Suspension (Bristol) p 739
- ▣ Naldecon-DX Pediatric Syrup (Bristol) p 739
- ▣ Naldecon-EX Pediatric Drops (Bristol) p 740
- ◆ Naldegesic Tablets (Bristol) p 407
- ◆ Nalfon Pulvules & Tablets (Dista) p 410, 903
- ◆ Nalfon 200 Pulvules (Dista) p 410, 903
- Nallpen for Injection (Beecham Laboratories)
- Nandrobolic Injectable (O'Neal, Jones & Feldman)
- Nandrobolic L.A. Injectable (O'Neal, Jones & Feldman)
- Nandrolin Injection (Reid-Provident, Direct Div.)
- Naphcon (Alcon Labs.)
- Naphcon-A (Alcon Labs.)
- Naphcon Forte (Alcon Labs.)
- ◆ Naprosyn (Syntex) p 440, 2062
- ◆ Naqua Tablets (Schering) p 434, 1861
- ◆ Naturetil Tablets (Schering) p 434, 1862
- ◆ Narcan and Narcan Neonatal (Du Pont) p 410, 922
- ◆ Nardil (Parke-Davis) p 424, 1543
- NāSal Saline Nasal Spray (Winthrop Consumer Products)
- NāSal Saline Nose Drops (Winthrop Consumer Products)
- Nasalcrom Nasal Solution (Fisons) p 944
- Nasalide Nasal Solution 0.025% (Syntex) p 2064
- ◆ Natabec Kapseals (Parke-Davis) p 424, 1545
- ◆ Natabec Rx Kapseals (Parke-Davis) p 424, 1545
- ◆ Natabec with Fluoride Kapseals (Parke-Davis) p 424
- Natabec-FA Kapseals (Parke-Davis)
- Natacomp-FA Tablets (Trimen) p 2067
- Natacyn (Alcon Labs.)

- ◆ Natafort Filmseal (Parke-Davis) p 424, 1545
- Natalac Capsules (U.S. Ethicals)
- Natalac Forte Capsules (U.S. Ethicals)
- ◆ Natalins Rx (Mead Johnson Laboratories) p 419, 1224
- ◆ Natalins Tablets (Mead Johnson Laboratories) p 419, 1224
- Naturacil (Mead Johnson Nutritional) p 1243
- Natural Estrogenic Substance (Legere) p 1120
- ▣ Nature's Remedy Laxative (Norcliff Thayer)
- ◆ Naturetin Tablets (Squibb) p 438, 2006
- Naturetin with K Tablets (Squibb)
- Nautrol Injection (Reid-Provident, Direct Div.)
- ◆ Navane Capsules and Concentrate (Roerig) p 431, 1737
- Navane Intramuscular (Roerig) p 1739
- Nebcin (Dista) p 905
- Nebcin, Sterile (Dista) p 907
- Neet Aerosol Depilatory (Whitehall)
- Neet Depilatory Cream (Whitehall)
- Neet Depilatory Lotion (Whitehall)
- Negatan (Savage)
- ◆ NegGram Caplets (Winthrop-Breon) p 444, 2215
- NegGram Suspension (Winthrop-Breon) p 2215
- Nema Worm Capsules (Parke-Davis)
- ◆ Nembutal Sodium Capsules (Abbott) p 403, 538
- Nembutal Sodium Solution (Abbott) p 541
- Nembutal Sodium Suppositories (Abbott) p 543
- Neo-Calglucon Syrup (Sandoz Pharmaceutical Div.) p 1806
- Neocet Capsules (Vale)
- Neocomplex Injection (U.S. Ethicals)
- Neo Cort-Dome Creme (Miles Pharmaceuticals)
- Neo-Cortef Cream (Upjohn)
- Neo-Cortef Ointment (Upjohn)
- Neo-Cortef Ophthalmic Suspension (Upjohn)
- Neo-Cultol (Fisons)
- Neocurtasal (Winthrop Consumer Products)
- Neocylate Tablets (Central Pharmaceuticals)
- Neocyten Injection (Central Pharmaceuticals)
- Neodecadron Sterile Ophthalmic Ointment (Merck Sharp & Dohme) p 1340
- Neodecadron Sterile Ophthalmic Solution (Merck Sharp & Dohme) p 1341
- Neodecadron Topical Cream (Merck Sharp & Dohme)
- Neo-Delta-Cortef Ointment (Upjohn)
- Neo-Delta-Cortef Ophthalmic Suspension (Upjohn)
- Neodex Tablets & Syrup (U.S. Ethicals)
- Neofed (Vale)
- Neogesic Tablets (Vale)
- Neolax Tablets (Central Pharmaceuticals) p 838
- Neoloid (Lederle) p 1107
- Neo-Medrol Acetate Topical (Upjohn)
- Neomycin Sulfate Tablets (Biocraft) p 705
- Neomycin Sulfate Tablets (Roxane) p 1788
- Neopap Suppretes (Webcon)
- Neo-Polycin (Merrell Dow) p 1372
- Neoquess Injectable (O'Neal, Jones & Feldman)
- Neoquess Tablets (O'Neal, Jones & Feldman)
- Neosar for Injection (Adria) p 586
- Neosporin Aerosol (Burroughs Wellcome) p 806
- Neosporin G.U. Irrigant (Burroughs Wellcome) p 807
- Neosporin Ointment (Burroughs Wellcome) p 808
- Neosporin Ophthalmic Ointment Sterile (Burroughs Wellcome) p 808
- Neosporin Ophthalmic Solution Sterile (Burroughs Wellcome) p 809
- Neosporin Powder (Burroughs Wellcome) p 810
- Neosporin-G Cream (Burroughs Wellcome) p 807
- Neostigmine Methylsulfate Injection (Elkins-Sinn) p 938
- Neo-Synalar Cream (Syntex) p 2061
- Neo-Synephrine Hydrochloride 1% Carpuject (Winthrop-Breon)
- Neo-Synephrine Hydrochloride 1% Injection (Winthrop-Breon) p 2216
- Neo-Synephrine Hydrochloride (Ophthalmic) (Winthrop-Breon) p 2217
- Neo-Synephrine Jelly (Winthrop Consumer Products)
- ▣ Neo-Synephrine Nasal Spray (Mentholated) (Winthrop Consumer Products)
- ▣ Neo-Synephrine Nasal Sprays (Winthrop Consumer Products)
- ▣ Neo-Synephrine Nose Drops (Winthrop Consumer Products)
- ▣ Neo-Synephrine 12 Hour Nasal Spray (Winthrop Consumer Products)
- ▣ Neo-Synephrine 12 Hour Nose Drops (Adult & Children's Strengths) (Winthrop Consumer Products)
- ▣ Neo-Synephrine 12 Hour Vapor Nasal Spray (Winthrop Consumer Products)
- ▣ Neo-Synephrine II Long Acting Nasal Spray (Winthrop Consumer Products)
- ▣ Neo-Synephrine II Long Acting Nose Drops (Adult & Children's Strengths) (Winthrop Consumer Products)
- ▣ Neo-Synephrine II Long Acting Vapor Nasal Spray (Winthrop Consumer Products)
- Neo-Tab Tablets (Vale)
- Neotep Granucaps (Reid-Provident, Direct Div.)
- Neothylline Tablets and Injection (Lemmon)
- Neothylline-GG Tablets (Lemmon)
- NeoTrace-4 (LyphoMed)
- Neotrizine Suspension & Tablets (Lilly)

(◆ Shown in Product Identification Section)   (▣ Described in PDR For Nonprescription Drugs)   (Products without page numbers are not described)

Product Name Index

Nephrocaps (Fleming) p 948
▣ **Nephrox Suspension** (Fleming)
◆ **Neptazane Tablets** (Lederle) p 415, 1107
Nesacaine Solutions (Astra) p 618
Nesacaine-CE Solutions (Astra) p 618
Nestabs Tablets (Fielding)
Nestabs FA Tablets (Fielding) p 942
Nestrex Tablets (Fielding)
Netromycin Injection (Schering) p 1863
Neucalm 50 (Legere) p 1120
Neurate-400 Tablets (Trimen)
Neuro B-12 Forte Injectable (Lambda) p 1071
Neuro B-12 Injectable (Lambda) p 1071
Neurodep Injection Lyophilized (Medical Products)
Neut Abbo-Vial & Pintop (Abbott)
Neutra-Phos Powder & Capsules (Willen) p 2188
Neutra-Phos-K Powder & Capsules (Willen) p 2188
Neutrogena Acne Cleansing Formula Soap (Neutrogena)
Neutrogena Acne-Drying Gel (Neutrogena)
Neutrogena Acne Mask (Neutrogena)
Neutrogena Baby Soap (Neutrogena)
Neutrogena Body Lotion (Neutrogena)
Neutrogena Dry Skin Formula Soap (Neutrogena)
Neutrogena Moisture (Neutrogena)
Neutrogena Norwegian Formula Hand Cream (Neutrogena)
Neutrogena Original Formula Soap (Neutrogena)
Neutrogena Rainbath Shower and Bath Gel (Neutrogena)
Neutrogena Sesame Seed Body Oil (Neutrogena)
Neutrogena Shampoo (Neutrogena)
Neutrogena Solid Soap Shampoo (Neutrogena)
Neutrogena T/Gel Therapeutic Shampoo (Neutrogena)
Nevrotose Capsutabs (Vale)
New Consol 20 (Consolidated Chemical)
Niac Capsules (O'Neal, Jones & Feldman)
Niacin Tablets (Roxane) p 1788
◆ **Niclocide Chewable Tablets** (Miles Pharmaceuticals) p 422, 1411
◆ **Nicobid** (USV Pharmaceutical) p 440, 2083
Nico-400 (Marion) p 418, 1186
◆ **Nicolar Tablets** (USV Pharmaceutical) p 440, 2083
◆ **Nicorette** (Merrell Dow) p 421, 1372
Nico-Span Capsules (Key Pharmaceuticals)
Nicostrol Capsules (U.S. Ethicals)
▣ **Nicotinex Elixir** (Fleming)
Nicotym Capsules (Everett)
Niferex Forte Elixir (Central Pharmaceuticals) p 838
Niferex Tablets/Elixir (Central Pharmaceuticals) p 838
Niferex w/Vitamin C (Central Pharmaceuticals) p 838
◆ **Niferex-150 Capsules** (Central Pharmaceuticals) p 409, 838
◆ **Niferex-150 Forte Capsules** (Central Pharmaceuticals) p 409, 838
◆ **Niferex-PN** (Central Pharmaceuticals) p 409, 838
Night Cast Formula R (Seres) p 1939
Night Cast Formula S (Medicated Acne Mask) (Seres) p 1939
Niloric Tablets (Ascher)
Nilstat for Preparation of Oral Suspension (Lederle) p 1108
Nilstat Oral Suspension (Lederle) p 1108
Nilstat Oral Tablets (Lederle) p 1109
Nilstat Topical Cream & Ointment (Lederle) p 1109
Nilstat Vaginal Tablets (Lederle) p 1108
Niong Tablets (U.S. Ethicals)
Nipride Injectable (Roche) p 1693
Nisaval Tablets (Vale)
Nisentil Injectable (Roche) p 1694
Nitrazine Paper (Squibb)
Nitro-Bid IV (Marion) p 1187
Nitro-Bid Ointment (Marion) p 1188
◆ **Nitro-Bid 2.5 Plateau Caps** (Marion) p 418, 1186
◆ **Nitro-Bid 6.5 Plateau Caps** (Marion) p 418, 1186
◆ **Nitro-Bid 9 Plateau Caps** (Marion) p 418, 1186
◆ **Nitrodisc** (Searle Pharmaceuticals) p 436, 1909
◆ **Nitro-Dur Transdermal Infusion System** (Key Pharmaceuticals) p 413, 1050
Nitrofurantoin Capsules & Tablets (Schein) p 1828
Nitroglycerin Ointment 2% (Fougera) p 953
Nitroglycerin Ointment 2% (Schein) p 1828
Nitroglycerin S.R. Capsules (Geneva) p 973
◆ **Nitroglycerin Tablets (Nitrostat)** (Parke-Davis) p 424
◆ **Nitroglycerin T.D. Capsules** (Lederle) p 416
Nitroglyn (Key Pharmaceuticals) p 1051
◆ **Nitrol IV** (Rorer) p 432
◆ **Nitrol Ointment** (Rorer) p 432, 1752
Nitrolin Timed Capsules (Schein) p 1828
Nitromed (U.S. Ethicals)
Nitronet Tablets (Lemmon)
Nitrong Ointment (See Wharton Laboratories) (U.S. Ethicals)
Nitrong Ointment (Wharton) p 2184
Nitrong Ointment, Unit Dose (Wharton)

Nitrong Tablets (See Wharton Laboratories) (U.S. Ethicals)
Nitrong 2.6 mg. Tablets (Wharton) p 2184
Nitrong 6.5 mg. Tablets (Wharton) p 2184
Nitrong 9 mg. Tablets (Wharton) p 2184
Nitrong SR Tablets (See Wharton Laboratories) (U.S. Ethicals)
Nitrong SR 2.6 mg. Tablets (Wharton)
Nitrong SR 6.5 mg. Tablets (Wharton)
Nitropress (Abbott) p 546
◆ **Nitrospan Capsules** (USV Pharmaceutical) p 440, 2084
◆ **Nitrostat Ointment 2%** (Parke-Davis) p 425, 1545
◆ **Nitrostat Tablets** (Parke-Davis) p 424, 1546
◆ **Nitrostat IV** (Parke-Davis) p 424, 1546
◆ **Nitrostat SR Capsules** (Parke-Davis) p 425
◆ **Nizoral Tablets** (Janssen) p 413, 1038
No Doz (Bristol-Myers Products) p 771
◆ **Noctec Capsules & Syrup** (Squibb) p 438, 2007
◆ **Nolahist** (Carnrick) p 408, 832
◆ **Nolamine Tablets** (Carnrick) p 408, 833
◆ **Noludar & Noludar 300** (Roche) p 430, 1696
◆ **Nolvadex Tablets** (Stuart) p 439, 2040
Norcuron (NC-45) (Organon) p 1447
◆ **Nordette-21 Tablets** (Wyeth) p 444, 2266
◆ **Nordette-28 Tablets** (Wyeth) p 444, 2270
◆ **Norflex** (Riker) p 428, 1644
◆ **Norgesic & Norgesic Forte** (Riker) p 428, 1644
◆ **Norinyl 1+35 Tablets 21-Day** (Syntex) p 440, 2052
◆ **Norinyl 1+35 Tablets 28-Day** (Syntex) p 440, 2052
◆ **Norinyl 1+50 21-Day** (Syntex) p 440, 2052
◆ **Norinyl 1+50 28-Day** (Syntex) p 440, 2052
◆ **Norinyl 1+80 21-Day** (Syntex) p 440, 2052
◆ **Norinyl 1+80 28-Day** (Syntex) p 440, 2052
◆ **Norinyl 2 mg.** (Syntex) p 440, 2052
Norisodrine Aerotrol (Abbott) p 547
Norisodrine w/Calcium Iodide Syrup (Abbott) p 548
Norlac (Rowell)
Norlac RX (Rowell)
◆ **Norlestrin 21 1/50** (Parke-Davis) p 425, 1548
◆ **Norlestrin 21 2.5/50** (Parke-Davis) p 425, 1548
◆ **Norlestrin 28 1/50** (Parke-Davis) p 425, 1548
◆ **Norlestrin Fe 1/50** (Parke-Davis) p 425, 1548
◆ **Norlestrin Fe 2.5/50** (Parke-Davis) p 425, 1548
◆ **Norlutate** (Parke-Davis) p 425, 1556
◆ **Norlutin** (Parke-Davis) p 425, 1556
Normaderm Cream (Doak)
Normaderm Lotion (Doak)
Normodyne Injection (Schering) p 1867
◆ **Normodyne Tablets** (Schering) p 434, 1870
Normosol M 900 CAL (Abbott)
Normosol-M & 5% Dextrose Injection (Abbott)
Normosol-M & Surbex-T & 5% Dextrose Injection (Abbott)
Normosol-R & 5% Dextrose Injection (Abbott)
Normosol-R/K + & 5% Dextrose Injection (Abbott)
◆ **Norpace Capsules** (Searle & Co.) p 436, 1933
◆ **Norpace CR Capsules** (Searle & Co.) p 436, 1933
Norpramin (Merrell Dow) p 421, 1374
Nor-Q.D. (Syntex) p 440, 2052
NORx (appetite suppressant) (Vitaline)
◆ **NoSalt Salt Alternative, Regular and Seasoned** (Norcliff Thayer)
Nospaz Injection (Reid-Provident, Direct Div.)
◆ **Novafed A Capsules** (Merrell Dow) p 421, 1377
◆ **Novafed A Liquid** (Merrell Dow) p 1377
◆ **Novafed Capsules** (Merrell Dow) p 421, 1376
◆ **Novafed Liquid** (Merrell Dow) p 1376
Novaflor Capsules (Medical Products)
▣ **Novahistine Cough Formula** (Merrell Dow)
▣ **Novahistine Cough & Cold Formula** (Merrell Dow)
◆ **Novahistine DH** (Merrell Dow) p 421, 1378
◆ **Novahistine DMX** (Merrell Dow)
◆ **Novahistine Elixir** (Merrell Dow)
◆ **Novahistine Expectorant** (Merrell Dow) p 421, 1378
Novocain Hydrochloride (Winthrop-Breon) p 2219
Novocain Hydrochloride for Spinal Anesthesia (Winthrop-Breon) p 2220
Novolin L (Squibb-Novo) p 2034
Novolin N (Squibb-Novo) p 2034
Novolin R (Squibb-Novo) p 2034
◆ **Nubain** (Du Pont) p 410, 923
Nuclear Medicine Products (Radiopharmaceuticals) (Squibb)
◆ **Nucofed Capsules** (Beecham Laboratories) p 406, 692
Nucofed Expectorant (Beecham Laboratories) p 693
Nucofed Pediatric Expectorant (Beecham Laboratories) p 694
Nucofed Syrup (Beecham Laboratories) p 692
Nu-Flow Shampoo (Cooper Dermatology)
Nu-Iron Elixir (Mayrand) p 1196
Nu-Iron 150 Caps (Mayrand) p 1196
Nu-Iron-Plus Elixir (Mayrand) p 1196
Nu-Iron-V Tablets (Mayrand) p 1196
Nu'Leven Tablets (Lemmon)
Numorphan (Du Pont) p 924
Nupercainal Cream & Ointment (CIBA) p 856
Nupercainal Suppositories (CIBA) p 857
Nupercaine Heavy Solution (CIBA) p 860

Nupercaine hydrochloride 1:200 (CIBA) p 857
Nupercaine hydrochloride 1:1500 (CIBA) p 858
Nuprin (Bristol-Myers Products) p 771
▣ **Nursoy** (Wyeth) p 2271
▣ **Nutramigen** (Mead Johnson Nutritional)
Nutrisource Modular System (Clinical Nutrition) p 877
Nutrox Capsules (Tyson) p 2069
Nydrazid Injection, Tablets (Squibb)
Nylidrin Tablets (Geneva) p 973
Nylidrin HCl Tablets (Danbury) p 887
Nylidrin HCl Tablets (Schein) p 1828
▣ **Nylmerate II Douche Concentrate** (Youngs)
▣ **Nyquil Nighttime Colds Medicine** (Vicks Health Care)
Nyral Lozenges (Vale)
Nystaform Ointment (Miles Pharmaceuticals) p 1411
Nystatin Cream, Ointment & Vaginal Tablets (Fougera) p 953
Nystatin Cream, Ointment & Vaginal Tablets (Pharmaderm) p 1617
Nystatin Cream, Oral & Vaginal Tablets (Schein) p 1828
Nystatin Cream, Oral Tablets, and Vaginal Tablets (Lemmon) p 1122
Nystatin-Neomycin-Gramicidin-Triamcinolone Cream & Ointment (Fougera) p 953
Nystex Cream & Ointment (Savage) p 1825
Nystex Oral Suspension (Savage) p 1825
Nyst-olone Cream & Ointment (Schein) p 1828

O

O. B. Thera Tablets (Legere) p 1120
O-V Statin (Squibb) p 2008
Obalan Tablets (Lannett)
Obermine Capsules (O'Neal, Jones & Feldman)
Obestin-30 Capsules (Ferndale)
Obetrol-10 (Rexar) p 1641
Obetrol-20 (Rexar) p 1641
Obeval Tablets (Vale)
Oby-Trim 30 Capsules (Rexar) p 1641
▣ **Ocean Nasal Mist** (Fleming)
Ocean-Plus Mist (Fleming)
Octicair Otic Solution & Suspension (Pharmafair) p 1618
Ocusert Ocular Therapeutic Systems (Alza)
Pilo-20 (Alza)
Pilo-40 (Alza)
◆ **Ogen Tablets** (Abbott) p 403, 548
Ogen Vaginal Cream (Abbott) p 551
Oilatum Soap (Scented) (Stiefel)
Oilatum Soap (Unscented) (Stiefel)
Oligospermia Cups (Milex)
◆ **Omnipen Capsules** (Wyeth) p 444, 2271
Omnipen for Oral Suspension (Wyeth) p 2271
Omnipen Pediatric Drops (Wyeth) p 2271
Omnipen-N (Wyeth) p 2271
Oncovin (Lilly) p 1169
◆ **One-A-Day Essential Multivitamin Supplement** (Miles Laboratories)
▣ **One-A-Day Maximum Formula (Multivitamin/Multimineral)** (Miles Laboratories)
▣ **One-A-Day Plus Extra C** (Miles Laboratories)
▣ **One-A-Day Stressgard Vitamins** (Miles Laboratories)
▣ **One-A-Day Within (Multivitamins Plus Iron & Calcium)** (Miles Laboratories)
Onset-5 Tablets (Bock)
Onset-10 Tablets (Bock)
Ophthaine Solution (Squibb)
Ophthalgan (Ayerst)
Ophthalmic Products (Alcon Labs.) p 588
Ophthalmic Products (Allergan) p 589
Ophthalmic Products (CooperVision) p 883
Ophthetic ophthalmic solution (Allergan)
◆ **Ophthochlor, 0.5%** (Parke-Davis) p 425, 1557
Ophthocort (Parke-Davis) p 1558
Optemp (Alcon Labs.)
◆ **Optilets-500 Filmtab** (Abbott) p 403
◆ **Optilets-M-500 Filmtab** (Abbott) p 403
Optimate Alpha Automated Fluorometer/Photometer (Ames) p 3006
◆ **Optimine Tablets** (Schering) p 434, 1872
Optimyd Ophthalmic Solution (Schering)
Optivite Tablets (Tyson)
Orabase HCA (Colgate-Hoyt) p 879
▣ **Orabase Plain Oral Protective Paste** (Colgate-Hoyt)
▣ **Orabase with Benzocaine Analgesic Oral Protective Paste** (Colgate-Hoyt)
Orabex-TF (LaSalle) p 1071
▣ **Oracin Cherry Flavor Cooling Throat Lozenges** (Vicks Health Care)
▣ **Oracin Cooling Throat Lozenges** (Vicks Health Care)
Oragrafin Calcium Granules (Squibb)
Oragrafin Sodium Capsules (Squibb)
◆ **Orap Tablets** (McNeil Pharmaceutical) p 1203
Orasone (Rowell)
Ora-Testryl Tablets (Squibb)
Oratrast (Armour)
Orazinc Capsules (Mericon)
▣ **Orazinc Lozenges** (Mericon)
Orcophen Capsules (Lannett)
Orenzyme (Merrell Dow) p 1379

(◆ Shown in Product Identification Section) (▣ Described in PDR For Nonprescription Drugs) (Products without page numbers are not described)

Product Name Index

Orenzyme Bitabs (Merrell Dow) p 1379
◆ Oretic (Abbott) p 403, 554
Oreticyl (Abbott) p 555
Oreticyl Forte Tablets (Abbott)
◆ Oreton Methyl Tablets & Buccal Tablets (Schering) p 434, 1873
Orexin Softab Tablets (Stuart) p 2034
◆ Organidin (Wallace) p 442, 2163
Orimune Poliovirus Vaccine, Live, Oral, Trivalent (Lederle) p 1109
Orinase Diagnostic Sterile Powder (Upjohn)
◆ Orinase Tablets (Upjohn) p 441, 2130
Orithrush (Ecological Formulas)
Ornacol Capsules (Smith Kline & French)
Ornacol Liquid (Smith Kline & French)
◆ Ornade Spansule Capsules (Smith Kline & French) p 437, 1968
Ornex Capsules (Smith Kline & French)
Ortho Diaphragm Kit-All Flex (Ortho Pharmaceutical) p 1457
Ortho Diaphragm Kit-Coil Spring (Ortho Pharmaceutical) p 1457
Ortho Dienestrol Cream (Ortho Pharmaceutical) p 1457
⊠ Ortho Disposable Applicator (Ortho Pharmaceutical)
⊠ Ortho Personal Lubricant (Ortho Pharmaceutical)
⊠ Ortho-Creme Contraceptive Cream (Ortho Pharmaceutical)
⊠ Ortho-Gynol Contraceptive Jelly (Ortho Pharmaceutical)
◆ Ortho-Novum 1/35☐21 (Ortho Pharmaceutical) p 422, 1461
Ortho-Novum 1/35☐28 (Ortho Pharmaceutical) p 1461
◆ Ortho-Novum 1/50☐21 (Ortho Pharmaceutical) p 422, 1461
Ortho-Novum 1/50☐28 (Ortho Pharmaceutical) p 1461
◆ Ortho-Novum 1/80☐21 (Ortho Pharmaceutical) p 423, 1461
Ortho-Novum 1/80☐28 (Ortho Pharmaceutical) p 1461
◆ Ortho-Novum 7/7/7 ☐.. 21 Tablets (Ortho Pharmaceutical) p 422, 1461
Ortho-Novum 7/7/7 ☐.. 28 Tablets (Ortho Pharmaceutical) p 1461
◆ Ortho-Novum 10/11☐.. 21 Tablets (Ortho Pharmaceutical) p 422, 1461
Ortho-Novum 10/11☐.. 28 Tablets (Ortho Pharmaceutical) p 1461
Ortho-Novum Tablets 2 mg☐21 (Ortho Pharmaceutical) p 423, 1461
Ortho-White Diaphragm Kit-Flat Spring (Ortho Pharmaceutical) p 1457
Orthoxicol Cough Syrup (Upjohn)
◆ Os-Cal 250 Tablets (Marion) p 418, 1188
◆ Os-Cal 500 Tablets (Marion) p 418, 1188
◆ Os-Cal Forte Tablets (Marion) p 418, 1189
◆ Os-Cal Plus Tablets (Marion) p 418, 1189
◆ Os-Cal-Gesic Tablets (Marion) p 418, 1189
Osmoglyn (Alcon Labs.)
Osmolite (Ross) p 1769
Osmolite HN (Ross) p 1770
Osti-Derm Lotion (Pedinol) p 1580
Otic Domeboro Solution (Miles Pharmaceuticals) p 1411
Otic Tridesilon Solution 0.05% (Miles Pharmaceuticals) p 1414
Otic-HC Ear Drops (Hauck) p 1001
Otic-Plain Ear Drops (Hauck)
Oticol Sterile Ear Drops (Arlo) p 601
Otide (Jamol)
Otipyrin Otic Solution (Kramer) p 1069
Otisan Drops (RAM Laboratories)
Otobiotic Otic Solution (Schering) p 1875
Otocort Sterile Ear Drops, Solution and Suspension (Lemmon) p 1122
Otoreid-HC Ear Drops (Reid-Provident Labs.)
Otrivin (Geigy) p 963
Outgro Solution (Whitehall)
◆ Ovcon-35 (Mead Johnson Laboratories) p 419, 1224
◆ Ovcon-50 (Mead Johnson Laboratories) p 419, 1224
Ovex (Standard Process)
◆ Ovral Tablets (Wyeth) p 444, 2271
◆ Ovral-28 Tablets (Wyeth) p 444, 2272
◆ Ovrette Tablets (Wyeth) p 2272
◆ Ovulen-21 (Searle & Co.) p 436, 1919
◆ Ovulen-28 (Searle & Co.) p 436, 1919
Ox Bile Extract Enseals (Lilly)
Oxacillin Capsules (Biocraft) p 705
Oxacillin Solution (Biocraft) p 705
Oxacillin Sodium Capsules & Powder for Oral Suspension (Schein) p 1828
Oxalid Tablets (USV Pharmaceutical) p 2084
Oxipor VHC Lotion for Psoriasis (Whitehall)
◆ Oxsoralen Capsule (Elder) p 411, 932
Oxsoralen Lotion 1% (Elder) p 935
⊠ Oxy Clean Lathering Facial Scrub (Norcliff Thayer)
⊠ Oxy Clean Medicated Cleanser, Pads & Soap (Norcliff Thayer)
⊠ Oxy-5 Lotion with Sorboxyl (Norcliff Thayer)
⊠ Oxy-10 Lotion and Cover with Sorboxyl (Norcliff Thayer)

⊠ Oxy-10 Wash Antibacterial Skin Wash (Norcliff Thayer)
Oxychinol Tablets (Ferndale)
Oxycodone Hydrochloride Oral Solution & Tablets (Roxane) p 1792
Oxycodone Hydrochloride USP Single Entity Tablets & Liquid (Roxane) p 1788
Oxycodone Hydrochloride & Acetaminophen Tablets (Roxane) p 1788
Oxycodone Hydrochloride, Oxycodone Terephthalate & Aspirin Tablets (Full Strength) (Roxane) p 1788
Oxymeta-12 Nasal Spray (Schein) p 1828
Oxymycin Injectable (O'Neal, Jones & Feldman) p 1445
Oxynitral w/Veratrum Viride Tablets (Vale)
Oxytetracycline HCl Capsules (Schein) p 1828
Oxytocin Injection (Wyeth) p 2273
Oxytocin in Tubex (Wyeth) p 2288
Oyster Shell Calcium (Vitaline)

P

⊠ P&S Liquid (Baker/Cummins)
⊠ P&S Plus Gel (Baker/Cummins)
⊠ P&S Shampoo (Baker/Cummins)
P-A-C Revised Formula Analgesic Tablets (Upjohn)
PBZ Hydrochloride Cream (Geigy) p 964
◆ PBZ Tablets & Elixir (Geigy) p 411, 964
PBZ-SR Tablets (Geigy) p 411, 963
P.E.T.N. S.R. Tablets (Geneva) p 973
P-I-N Forte Tablets & Syrup (Lannett)
◆ PMB 200 & PMB 400 (Ayerst) p 405, 660
PNS Unna Boot (Pedinol)
P.S.P. IV (four) Injection (Reid-Provident, Direct Div.)
PT 105 Capsules (Legere) p 1120
PTE-4 (LyphoMed)
PTG (Alcon Labs.)
P.V. Carpine Liquifilm ophthalmic solution (Allergan)
P-V-Tussin Syrup (Reid-Provident Labs.) p 1640
◆ P-V-Tussin Tablets (Reid-Provident Labs.) p 428, 1640
◆ Pabalate Tablets (Robins) p 428, 1654
◆ Pabalate-SF Tablets (Robins) p 428, 1655
Pabanol Lotion (Elder)
Pacaps (LaSalle) p 1071
Packer's Pine Tar Shampoo (Cooper Dermatology)
Packer's Pine Tar Soap (Cooper Dermatology)
Palbar Tablets (Hauck)
Palmiron Tablets (Hauck)
Palmiron-C Tablets (Hauck)
◆ Pamelor (Sandoz Pharmaceutical Div.) p 433, 1807
Pamine Tablets (Upjohn) p 2132
◆ Panadol Jr. (Glenbrook) p 412
Panafil Ointment (Rystan) p 1796
Panafil-White Ointment (Rystan) p 1796
◆ Panalgesic (Poythress) p 1619
◆ Pancrease (McNeil Pharmaceutical) p 418, 1205
Pancreatin Enseals & Tablets (Lilly)
Pancreatin Tablets 2400 mg. N.F. (High Lipase) (Vitaline) p 2148
Panhematin (Abbott) p 557
Panol Injectable (O'Neal, Jones & Feldman)
Panmycin Capsules (Upjohn)
PanOxyl 5, PanOxyl 10 Acne Gels (Stiefel)
PanOxyl AQ 2½, 5 & 10 Acne Gels (Stiefel)
PanOxyl Bar 5 (Stiefel)
PanOxyl Bar 10 (Stiefel)
Panscol Lotion & Ointment (Baker/Cummins)
Panthoderm Cream (USV Pharmaceutical)
Pantholin Tablets (Lilly)
Pantopon Injectable (Roche) p 1697
Panvitex Prenatal Tablets (O'Neal, Jones & Feldman)
◆ Panwarfin (Abbott) p 403, 558
Panzyme Tablets (Hyrex)
◆ Papase (Parke-Davis) p 425, 1558
Papavatral Tablets (Kenwood)
Papavatral 20 Tablets (Kenwood)
Papaverine T.D. Capsules (Geneva) p 973
Papaverine HCl Capsules (Lederle) p 416
Papaverine Hydrochloride Capsules (Roxane) p 1788
Papaverine HCl T.D. Capsules (Danbury) p 887
Papaverine HCl Timed Capsules (Schein) p 1828
Papaverine HCl Tablets (Danbury) p 887
◆ Paradione (Abbott) p 403, 558
Paraflex Tablets (McNeil Pharmaceutical) p 1205
◆ Parafon Forte Tablets (McNeil Pharmaceutical) p 419, 1206
Paral Injectable (O'Neal, Jones & Feldman)
Paral Liquid (O'Neal, Jones & Feldman)
Paraldehyde (Sterile) (Elkins-Sinn) p 938
Paredrine 1% w/Boric Acid, Ophthalmic Solution (Smith Kline & French) p 1968
Paregoric (Roxane) p 1788
Parelixir Liquid (Purdue Frederick)
Parepectolin (Rorer) p 1752
◆ Parlodel Capsules & Tablets (Sandoz Pharmaceutical Div.) p 433, 1808
◆ Parnate (Smith Kline & French) p 437, 1969
◆ Parsidol (Parke-Davis) p 425, 1559
Pasmex Drops (Arlo)
Pasmin Injectable, Liquid, Capsules (Bart)

Pasmol Tablets (RAM Laboratories) p 1632
◆ Pathibamate (Lederle) p 415, 1110
◆ Pathilon (Lederle) p 415, 1112
Pathocil Capsules, for Oral Suspension (Wyeth) p 444, 2274
◆ Pavabid Capsules (Marion) p 418, 1189
◆ Pavabid HP Capsulets (Marion) p 418, 1189
Pavacap Unicelles (Reid-Provident Labs.)
Pavacen Capsules (Central Pharmaceuticals)
Pavadyl Capsules (Bock)
Pavatym Capsules (Everett) p 942
Paverolan Lanacaps (Lannett)
Pavulon (Organon) p 1449
◆ Paxipam Tablets (Schering) p 434, 1876
Pazo Hemorrhoid Ointment/Suppositories (Bristol-Myers Products)
◆ Pedameth Capsules (O'Neal, Jones & Feldman) p 422, 1445
Pedameth Liquid (O'Neal, Jones & Feldman) p 1445
Pediacof (Winthrop-Breon) p 2221
Pediaflor Drops (Ross) p 1771
Pedialyte (Ross) p 1771
Pedialyte RS (Ross) p 1772
Pediamycin (Ross) p 1772
Pediazole (Ross) p 1774
Pedi-Bath Salts (Pedinol) p 1581
Pedi-Boro Soak Paks (Pedinol) p 1581
Pedi-Cort V Creme (Pedinol) p 1581
Pedi-Dri Foot Powder (Pedinol) p 1581
Pedi-Pro Foot Powder (Pedinol) p 1581
Pedi-Vit A Creme (Pedinol) p 1581
Pedric Elixir & Tablets (Vale)
Pedric Senior Tablets (Vale)
PedTrace-4 (LyphoMed)
◆ Peganone (Abbott) p 403, 559
Pektamalt (Adria)
Penecort Cream & Topical Solution 1% (Herbert) p 1007
Penecort Cream 2.5% (Herbert) p 1008
Penicillin G Potassium for Injection USP (Squibb) p 2009
Penicillin G Potassium Tablets (Biocraft) p 705
Penicillin G Procaine Suspension, Sterile, Vials (Lilly) p 1170
Penicillin G Sodium for Injection USP (Squibb) p 2010
Penicillin V Potassium Solution (Biocraft) p 705
Penicillin V Potassium Tablets (Biocraft) p 705
◆ Penicillin V, Potassium (Penapar VK) (Parke-Davis) p 425, 1559
Penicillin VK Powder for Oral Solution & Tablets (Schein) p 1828
Pentacort Cream (Dalin)
Pentaerythritol Tetranitrate Tablets (PETN), Timed Capsules & Tablets (Schein) p 1828
Pentam 300 (LyphoMed) p 1181
Penthrane (Abbott) p 560
Pentids for Syrup (Squibb) p 2011
◆ Pentids Tablets, Pentids 400 & 800 Tablets (Squibb) p 438, 2011
Pentobarbital Sodium Injection (Elkins-Sinn) p 938
Pentobarbital Sodium in Tubex (Wyeth) p 2288
Pentothal (Abbott) p 562
Pentrax Tar Shampoo (Cooper Dermatology) p 882
Pentritol (USV Pharmaceutical) p 2086
◆ Pen•Vee K, for Oral Solution & Tablets (Wyeth) p 444, 2275
Peptavlon (Ayerst) p 657, 3008
Peptenzyme Elixir (Reed & Carnrick)
Pepto-Bismol Liquid & Tablets (Procter & Gamble) p 1620
◆ Percocet (Du Pont) p 410, 925
◆ Percodan & Percodan-Demi Tablets (Du Pont) p 410, 925
Percogesic Analgesic Tablets (Vicks Pharmacy Products) p 442, 2147
Percorten Pellets (CIBA) p 861
Percorten pivalate (CIBA) p 862
Perdiem Granules (Rorer) p 432
◆ Perdiem Plain Granules (Rorer) p 432
Pergonal (menotropins USP) (Serono) p 1941
◆ Periactin Syrup (Merck Sharp & Dohme) p 1342
◆ Periactin Tablets (Merck Sharp & Dohme) p 420, 1342
Peri-Care (Sween) p 2048
◆ Peri-Colace (Mead Johnson Pharmaceutical) p 419, 1255
Peridin-C (Beutlich) p 705
Perifoam (Rowell)
Perihemin (Lederle) p 1112
Perineal/Ostomy Spray Cleaner (Consolidated Chemical) p 881
◆ Peritinic Tablets (Lederle) p 1112
◆ Peritrate SA (Parke-Davis) p 425, 1560
◆ Peritrate Tablets 10 mg., 20 mg. and 40 mg. (Parke-Davis) p 425, 1560
Peri-Wash (Sween) p 2048
Permapen Isoject (Pfipharmecs) p 1590
Permitil Oral Concentrate (Schering) p 1877
◆ Permitil Tablets (Schering) p 434, 1877
Pernox Lotion (Westwood) p 2180
Pernox Medicated Lathering Scrub (Westwood) p 2180
Pernox Shampoo (Westwood) p 2180
◆ Peroxyl Mouthrinse (Colgate-Hoyt)

(◆ Shown in Product Identification Section)   (⊠ Described in PDR For Nonprescription Drugs)   (Products without page numbers are not described)

Product Name Index

Persa-Gel 5% & 10% (Ortho Pharmaceutical (Dermatological Div.)) p 1474
Persa-Gel W 5% & 10% (Ortho Pharmaceutical (Dermatological Div.)) p 1474
◆ Persantine Tablets (Boehringer Ingelheim) p 406, 710
Persistin (Fisons)
◆ Pertofrane Capsules (USV Pharmaceutical) p 440, 2086
Pertussis Immune Globulin (Human) Hypertussis (Cutter Biological) p 884
Pessaries (Milex)
Petameth Capsules (O'Neal, Jones & Feldman)
Petrogalar, Plain (Wyeth)
Petrolatum (White) & Petrolatum (White) Ophthalmic Ointment (Fougera) p 953
Petro-Phylic Soap Cake (Doak)
Pfizerpen for Injection (Pfipharmecs) p 1590
Pfizerpen-AS Aqueous Suspension (Pfipharmecs) p 1592
Phacid Shampoo (Baker/Cummins)
◆ Phazyme Tablets (Reed & Carnrick) p 427, 1636
◆ Phazyme-95 Tablets (Reed & Carnrick) p 427, 1636
◆ Phazyme-PB Tablets (Reed & Carnrick) p 427, 1636
Phenagesic Capsules (Dalin)
◆ Phenaphen Capsules (Robins) p 428
◆ Phenaphen w/Codeine Capsules (Robins) p 428, 1656
◆ Phenaphen-650 with Codeine Tablets (Robins) p 428, 1656
Phenarex Syrup (Dalin)
Phenate (Mallard) p 1181
Phenatuss Expectorant (Dalin)
Phenazine Tablets & Capsules (Legere) p 1120
Phencen-50 Injectable (Central Pharmaceuticals)
Pheneen Solution (Ulmer)
◆ Phenergan Compound Tablets (Wyeth) p 445
Phenergan Injection (Wyeth) p 2275
Phenergan in Tubex (Wyeth) p 2288
Phenergan Syrup Fortis (Wyeth) p 2276
Phenergan Syrup Plain (Wyeth) p 2276
◆ Phenergan Tablets & Rectal Suppositories (Wyeth) p 444,445, 2278
Phenergan VC (Wyeth) p 2282
Phenergan VC with Codeine (Wyeth) p 2284
Phenergan with Codeine (Wyeth) p 2278
Phenergan with Dextromethorphan (Wyeth) p 2280
◆ Phenergan-D Tablets (Wyeth) p 445
Phenobarbital Elixir, Tablets (Roxane) p 1788
Phenobarbital Elixir & Tablets (Schein) p 1828
Phenobarbital Sodium Injection (Elkins-Sinn) p 938
Phenobarbital Sodium in Tubex (Wyeth) p 2288
Phenobarbital Tablets (Danbury) p 887
Phenobella Tablets (Ferndale)
Phenoject-50 (Mayrand)
Phenolax Wafers (Upjohn)
Phentermine HCl Capsules & Tablets (Schein) p 1828
Phenurone (Abbott) p 564
Phenylbutazone Capsules (Geneva) p 973
Phenylbutazone Capsules & Tablets (Schein) p 1828
Phenylbutazone Tablets (Danbury) p 887
Phenylbutazone Tablets (Geneva) p 973
Phenylephrine HCl 10% Dropperettes (CooperVision)
Phenylzin Ophthalmic Solution (CooperVision)
Phenytoin Sodium Capsules-Prompt Action (Schein) p 1828
Phenytoin Sodium Injection (Elkins-Sinn) p 938
Phillips' Milk of Magnesia (Glenbrook) p 997
▣ pHisoAc BP (Winthrop Consumer Products)
pHisoDan (Winthrop Consumer Products)
pHisoDerm (Winthrop-Breon)
▣ pHisoDerm Regular & Fresh Scent (Winthrop Consumer Products)
pHisoHex (Winthrop-Breon) p 2222
▣ pHisoPUFF (Winthrop Consumer Products)
pHisoScrub (Winthrop-Breon)
Phos-Flur Oral Rinse/Supplement (Colgate-Hoyt) p 879
pHos-pHaid (Guardian) p 1000
Phosphaljel (Wyeth)
Phospholine Iodide (Ayerst) p 658
◆ Phrenilin Forte (Carnrick) p 408, 833
◆ Phrenilin Tablets (Carnrick) p 408, 833
◆ Phrenilin No. 3 with Codeine (Carnrick) p 409, 834
Physiosol Irrigation/Aqualite (Abbott)
Pilocar 1%, 2%, 4% Dropperettes (CooperVision)
Pilocar Ophthalmic Solutions 0.5%, 1%, 2%, 3%, 4%, 6% (CooperVision)
Pilocar Ophthalmic Solutions Twin Pack 0.5%, 1%, 2%, 3%, 4%, 6% (CooperVision)
Pima Syrup (Fleming) p 948
◆ Pipracil (Lederle) p 416, 1113
Pitocin Injection (Parke-Davis) p 1561
Pitressin (Parke-Davis) p 1562
Pitressin Tannate in Oil (Parke-Davis) p 1562
Pituitrin-S Ampoules (Parke-Davis)
◆ Placidyl (Abbott) p 403, 566
Plague Vaccine (Human) (Cutter Biological) p 886

◆ Plaquenil Sulfate (Winthrop-Breon) p 444, 2223
Plasma-Plex (Armour) p 613
Plasmatein 5% (Alpha Theapeutic) p 589
Platinol (Bristol-Myers Oncology) p 765
◆ Plegine (Ayerst) p 405, 659
Pliagel (CooperVision)
Pneumotrophin (Lung) (Standard Process)
Pneumovax 23 (Merck Sharp & Dohme) p 1343
Pnu-Imune (Lederle) p 1116
Pod-Ben-25 (C & M) p 828
Point-Two Dental Rinse (Colgate-Hoyt) p 880
Poison Ivy Extract (Parke-Davis)
Polaramine Expectorant (Schering)
◆ Polaramine Repetabs Tablets (Schering) p 434, 1879
Polaramine Syrup (Schering) p 1879
◆ Polaramine Tablets (Schering) p 434, 1879
Poliomyelitis Vaccine (Purified) (For the Prevention of Poliomyelitis) (Squibb/Connaught) p 2033
◆ Polycillin (Bristol) p 407, 740
Polycillin-N for Injection (Bristol) p 740
Polycillin-PRB (Bristol) p 741
Polycitra Syrup (Willen) p 2188
Polycitra-K Syrup (Willen) p 2189
Polycitra-LC—Sugar-Free (Willen) p 2188
Polycose (Ross) p 1775
Poly-Histine Capsules (Bock)
Poly-Histine Elixir (Bock)
Poly-Histine Expectorant Plain (Bock) p 705
Poly-Histine Expectorant with Codeine (Bock) p 705
Poly-Histine-D Capsules (Bock) p 705
Poly-Histine-D Elixir (Bock) p 705
Poly-Histine-D Pediatric Capsules (Bock) p 705
Poly-Histine-DX Capsules (Bock) p 706
Polymagma Plain Tablets (Wyeth)
◆ Polymox Capsules (Bristol) p 407, 742
Polymox For Oral Suspension (Bristol) p 742
Polymox Pediatric Drops (Bristol) p 742
Polymyxin B Sulfate (see Aerosporin) (Burroughs Wellcome) p 775
Poly-Pred Liquifilm ophthalmic suspension (Allergan)
Polysept Ointment (Dalin)
Polysorb Hydrate Cream (Fougera)
Polysporin Ointment (Burroughs Wellcome) p 810
Polysporin Ophthalmic Ointment (Burroughs Wellcome) p 810
Polytar Bath (Stiefel)
Polytar Shampoo (Stiefel)
Polytar Soap (Stiefel)
Poly-Vi-Flor 0.25 mg Vitamins w/Fluoride Drops (Mead Johnson Nutritional) p 1244
Poly-Vi-Flor 1.0 mg Vitamins w/Fluoride Chewable Tablets (Mead Johnson Nutritional) p 1243
Poly-Vi-Flor 0.5 mg Vitamins w/Fluoride Drops (Mead Johnson Nutritional) p 1244
Poly-Vi-Flor 0.5 mg Vitamins w/Iron & Fluoride Chewable Tablets (Mead Johnson Nutritional) p 1245
Poly-Vi-Flor 1.0 mg Vitamins w/Iron & Fluoride Chewable Tablets (Mead Johnson Nutritional) p 1245
Poly-Vi-Flor 0.25 mg Vitamins w/Fluoride Drops (Mead Johnson Nutritional) p 1244
Poly-Vi-Flor 0.25 mg Vitamins w/Iron & Fluoride Drops (Mead Johnson Nutritional) p 1245
Poly-Vi-Flor 0.5 mg Vitamins w/Iron & Fluoride Drops (Mead Johnson Nutritional) p 1245
▣ Poly-Vi-Sol Vitamins Chewable Tablets & Drops (Mead Johnson Nutritional)
▣ Poly-Vi-Sol Vitamins with Iron & Zinc (Mead Johnson Nutritional)
▣ Poly-Vi-Sol Vitamins w/Iron Multivitamin & Iron Supplement Drops (Mead Johnson Nutritional)
Polyvitamin-Fluoride Drops & Tablets (Schein) p 1828
Polyvite with Fluoride Drops (Geneva) p 973
Ponaris Nasal Mucosal Emollient (Jamol) p 1033
◆ Pondimin Tablets (Robins) p 428, 1657
◆ Ponstel (Parke-Davis) p 425, 1562
Pontocaine Hydrochloride Eye Ointment (Winthrop-Breon)
Pontocaine Hydrochloride for Spinal Anesthesia (Winthrop-Breon) p 2225
Pontocaine Hydrochloride Topical Solution (Winthrop-Breon)
▣ Portagen (Mead Johnson Nutritional)
Posterisan Ointment (Kenwood)
Posterisan Suppositories (Kenwood)
Potaba (Glenwood) p 412, 998
Potage (Lemmon) p 1122
Potasalan Elixir (Lannett)
Potassium Chloride Concentrate, Powder & Liquid (Schein) p 1828
Potassium Chloride (Geneva) p 973
Potassium Chloride for Oral Solution (Flavored), Oral Solution, Powder (Unflavored) (Roxane) p 1788
Potassium Chloride Injection (Elkins-Sinn) p 938

Potassium Chloride Oral Solution, Powder & for Oral Solution (Roxane) p 1793
Potassium Gluconate Elixir (Roxane) p 1788
Potassium Gluconate Elixir (Schein) p 1828
Potassium Iodide Liquid (Roxane) p 1788
Potassium Phosphates Oral Solution (Roxane) p 1788
◆ Povan Filmseals (Parke-Davis) p 425, 1563
▣ Pragmatar Ointment (Smith Kline & French)
◆ Pramet FA (Ross) p 432, 1775
◆ Pramilet FA (Ross) p 432, 1775
Pramosone Cream, Lotion & Ointment (Ferndale) p 942
Prax Cream & Lotion (Ferndale) p 942
Precef (Bristol) p 743
Pred Forte ophthalmic suspension (Allergan)
Pred Mild ophthalmic suspension (Allergan)
Predaject-50 (Mayrand)
Predalone 50 Injectable (O'Neal, Jones & Feldman)
Predalone T.B.A. Injectable (O'Neal, Jones & Feldman)
Predate 50 (Legere) p 1120
Predate S (Legere) p 1120
Predate TBA (Legere) p 1120
Pre-Dep 40 Injection (Reid-Provident, Direct Div.)
Pre-Dep 80 Injection (Reid-Provident, Direct Div.)
Predictor In-Home Early Pregnancy Test (Whitehall)
Prednicen-M Tablets (Central Pharmaceuticals)
Prednisolone Tablets (Danbury) p 887
Prednisolone Tablets (Geneva) p 973
Prednisolone Tablets (Roxane) p 1788
Prednisolone Tablets (Schein) p 1828
Prednisone Tablets (Danbury) p 887
Prednisone Tablets (Geneva) p 973
Prednisone Tablets (Roxane) p 1793
Prednisone Tablets (Schein) p 1828
Pre-Enthus FA Capsules (Reid-Provident, Direct Div.)
Prefrin Liquifilm eye drops (Allergan)
Prefrin-A ophthalmic solution (Allergan)
Prefrin-Z Liquifilm ophthalmic solution (Allergan)
▣ Pregestimil (Mead Johnson Nutritional)
Pregnyl (Organon) p 1450
◆ Prelu-2 Timed Release Capsules (Boehringer Ingelheim) p 406, 711
◆ Preludin Endurets (Boehringer Ingelheim) p 406, 710
Preludin Tablets (Boehringer Ingelheim) p 710
Premarin Intravenous (Ayerst) p 667
◆ Premarin Tablets (Ayerst) p 405, 664
◆ Premarin Vaginal Cream (Ayerst) p 405, 670
◆ Premarin w/Methyltestosterone (Ayerst) p 405, 674
Prenate 90 Tablets (Bock) p 706
Prep-Aide (Jamol)
◆ Preparation H Hemorrhoidal Ointment (Whitehall) p 443, 2186
◆ Preparation H Hemorrhoidal Suppositories (Whitehall) p 443, 2186
Prepcort Hydrocortisone Cream 0.5% (Whitehall)
Pre-Pen (Rorer) p 1753
Pre-Protein Liquid (Arlo) p 601
PreSun 4 Creamy Sunscreen (Westwood) p 2180
PreSun 8 Lotion, Creamy & Gel (Westwood) p 2180
PreSun 15 Creamy Sunscreen (Westwood) p 2181
PreSun 15 Sunscreen Lotion (Westwood) p 2181
PreviDent Brush-On Gel (Colgate-Hoyt) p 880
Pricort Cream (Arlo)
Pricort Lotion (Arlo)
Primaquine Phosphate Tablets (Winthrop-Breon)
◆ Primatene Mist (Whitehall) p 443, 2186
Primatene Mist Suspension (Whitehall) p 2187
◆ Primatene Tablets-M Formula (Whitehall) p 443, 2187
◆ Primatene Tablets-P Formula (Whitehall) p 443, 2187
Primer Unna Boot (Glenwood) p 999
Primidone Tablets (Danbury) p 887
Primidone Tablets (Geneva) p 973
Primidone Tablets (Schein) p 1828
Primotest Forte Tablets (Arlo)
Primotest Tablets (Arlo)
Primotest 225 Injection (Arlo)
◆ Principen Capsules (Squibb) p 438, 2012
Principen for Oral Suspension (Squibb) p 2012
Principen with Probenecid Capsules (Squibb) p 2013
Prioderm Lotion (Purdue Frederick) p 1626
Priscoline Hydrochloride Multiple-Dose Vials (CIBA) p 862
Privine Hydrochloride 0.05% Nasal Solution (CIBA) p 863
Privine Hydrochloride 0.05% Nasal Spray (CIBA) p 863
Proaqua Tablets (Reid-Provident Labs.)
Probahist Capsules (Legere) p 1120
◆ Pro-Banthine Tablets (Searle & Co.) p 436, 1936
◆ Pro-Banthine w/Phenobarbital (Searle & Co.) p 436, 1936

(◆ Shown in Product Identification Section)   (▣ Described in PDR For Nonprescription Drugs)   (Products without page numbers are not described)

Product Name Index

◆ Probec-T Tablets (Stuart) p 439, 2040
◆ Probenecid Tablets (Lederle) p 416
Probenecid Tablets (Danbury) p 887
Probenecid Tablets (Geneva) p 973
Probenecid Tablets (Schein) p 1828
Probenecid w/Colchicine Tablets (Geneva) p 973
◆ Probenecid with Colchicine Tablets (Lederle) p 416
Probenecid with Colchicine Tablets (Schein) p 1828
Procainamide Capsules (Geneva) p 973
◆ Procainamide HCl Capsules (Lederle) p 417
Procainamide HCl Capsules (Danbury) p 887
Procainamide HCl Capsules (Schein) p 1828
Procaine HCl Injection (Elkins-Sinn) p 938
◆ Procan SR (Parke-Davis) p 425, 1564
◆ Procardia Capsules (Pfizer) p 426, 1606
Pro-Ception (Milex) p 1415
Prochlor-Iso Timed Release Capsules (Schein) p 1828
Prochlorperazine Tablets (Geneva) p 973
Prochlorperazine Edisylate Injection (Elkins-Sinn) p 938
Prochlorperazine Edisylate in Tubex (Wyeth) p 2288
Pro-Cort Cream (Barnes-Hind) p 684
Pro-Cort M Cream (Barnes-Hind) p 684
Proctocort (Rowell)
◆ Proctofoam-HC (Reed & Carnrick) p 427, 1636
◆ proctoFoam/non-steroid (Reed & Carnrick) p 427, 1636
Procute Cream & Lotion (Ferndale)
Proderm Topical Dressing (Hickam)
Profasi HP (HCG) (Serono) p 1943
Proferdex (Fisons) p 943
Profilate (Alpha Theapeutic) p 589
Profilate, Heat-Treated (Alpha Theapeutic) p 589
Profilnine (Alpha Theapeutic) p 589
Profilnine Heat-Treated (Alpha Theapeutic) p 589
Pro-Formance (Marlyn)
Progestaject-50 (Mayrand)
◆ Progestasert Intrauterine Contraceptive System (Alza) p 404, 590
Progesterone 50 (Legere) p 1120
Progestronaq-LA (Central Pharmaceuticals)
Proglycem Capsules, Suspension (Schering) p 1880
Pro-Iso Capsules (Geneva) p 973
Proklar Tablets (O'Neal, Jones & Feldman)
Prolamine Capsules, Maximum Strength (Thompson Medical) p 2067
Prolixin Decanoate (Squibb) p 2015
Prolixin Enanthate (Squibb)
Prolixin Elixir & Injection (Squibb) p 2014
◆ Prolixin Tablets (Squibb) p 438, 2014
◆ Proloid Tablets (Parke-Davis) p 425, 1565
Proloprim (Burroughs Wellcome) p 408, 810
Promet 50 (Legere) p 1120
Promethazine DM (Ped) Expectorant (Geneva) p 973
Promethazine Expectorant Plain (Geneva) p 973
Promethazine HCl Injection (Elkins-Sinn) p 938
Promethazine w/Codeine Expectorant (Geneva) p 973
Promethazine VC Expectorant (Geneva) p 973
Promethazine VC w/Codeine Expectorant (Geneva) p 973
Prompt (Searle Consumer Products) p 1912
Pronemia Capsules (Lederle) p 1118
◆ Pronestyl Capsules and Tablets (Squibb) p 438, 2017
Pronestyl Injection (Squibb) p 2018
◆ Pronestyl-SR Tablets (Squibb) p 438, 2019
Propadrine Capsules (Merck Sharp & Dohme)
◆ Propagest & Propagest Syrup (Carnrick) p 408, 834
Propantheline Bromide Tablets (Danbury) p 887
Propantheline Bromide Tablets (Geneva) p 973
Propantheline Bromide Tablets (Roxane) p 1788
Propantheline Bromide Tablets (Schein) p 1828
Prophyllin (Rystan) p 1796
Propine ophthalmic solution (Allergan)
Proplex, Factor IX Complex (Human) (Factors II, VII, IX & X), Dried (Hyland Therapeutics) p 1024
Proplex SX, Factor IX Complex (Human)(Factors II, VII, IX & X), Dried (Hyland Therapeutics) p 1024
Proplex SX-T, Factor IX Complex (Human), Heat Treated (Hyland Therapeutics) p 1024
Propox 65 w/APAP Tablets (Geneva) p 973
Propoxyphene-AC Capsules (Geneva) p 973
Propoxyphene & Apap Tablets 65/650 (Schein) p 1828
Propoxyphene Compound 65 (Schein) p 1828
Propoxyphene HCl Capsules (Geneva) p 973
Propoxyphene Hydrochloride Capsules (Roxane) p 1788
Propoxyphene HCl Capsules (Schein) p 1828
Prorex Injection (Hyrex)
Prosed (Star)
*□ ProSobee (Mead Johnson Nutritional)
◆ Prostaphlin Capsules, Oral Solution (Bristol) p 407, 745
Prostaphlin for Injection (Bristol) p 745
Prostigmin Injectable (Roche) p 1698

◆ Prostigmin Tablets (Roche) p 430, 1699
Prostin VR Pediatric Sterile Solution (Upjohn) p 2132
Prost-X (Standard Process)
Protamine Sulfate (Lilly) p 1171
Protamine Sulfate for Injection, USP, Sterile Powder (Upjohn) p 2133
Protamine, Zinc & Iletin I (Lilly) p 1156
Protecti Natural Detoxification Formula (Professional Health)
Protein Powder (Vitaline)
Protein Wafers (chewable) (Vitaline)
Protenate 5%, Plasma Protein Fraction (Human), U.S.P., 5% Solution (Hyland Therapeutics) p 1024
Protexin Oral Breath Spray (Cetylite)
Protexin Oral Rinse Concentrate (Cetylite)
Prothar (Armour) p 613
Protid, Improved Formula (LaSalle) p 1071
Protopam Chloride (Ayerst) p 678
Protostat Tablets (Ortho Pharmaceutical) p 423, 1470
Proval #3 Capsules (Reid-Provident Labs.)
◆ Proventil Inhaler (Schering) p 435, 1882
◆ Proventil Tablets (Schering) p 435, 1883
◆ Provera Tablets (Upjohn) p 441, 2133
Provigan Injection (Reid-Provident Labs.)
Proxigel (Reed & Carnrick) p 1637
Prulet (Mission) p 1420
Prunicodeine (Lilly)
Pseudoephedrine Tablets (Geneva) p 973
Pseudoephedrine HCl Tablets (Danbury) p 887
Pseudoephedrine Hydrochloride Tablets (Roxane) p 1788
Pseudoephedrine HCl Tablets (Schein) p 1828
Psoranide Cream 0.025% (Elder) p 936
*□ Purge Liquid (Fleming)
Puri-Clens (Sween) p 2048
◆ Purinethol (Burroughs Wellcome) p 408, 811
Purodigin Tablets (Wyeth)
*□ Purpose Dry Skin Cream (Ortho Pharmaceutical (Dermatological Div.))
*□ Purpose Shampoo (Ortho Pharmaceutical (Dermatological Div.))
*□ Purpose Soap (Ortho Pharmaceutical (Dermatological Div.))
Pyocidin-Otic Solution (Berlex) p 702
Pyopen Injectable (Beecham Laboratories)
◆ Pyrazinamide Tablets (Lederle) p 417
◆ Pyridium (Parke-Davis) p 425, 1567
◆ Pyridium Plus (Parke-Davis) p 425, 1568
Pyrinyl Liquid (Schein) p 1828
Pyrralan Expectorant DM (Lannett)
*□ Pyrroxate Capsules (Upjohn)

Q

Quadrahist Pediatric Syrup, Syrup & Timed Release Tablets (Schein) p 1828
◆ Quadrinal Tablets & Suspension (Knoll) p 414, 1065
◆ Quarzan Capsules (Roche Products) p 430, 1721
Quelicin (Succinylcholine Chloride Injection) Ampul & Vial, Pintop (Abbott)
Quelidrine Syrup (Abbott) p 567
Queltuss Tablets (O'Neal, Jones & Feldman)
Questran (Mead Johnson Laboratories) p 1231
Quibron & Quibron-300 (Mead Johnson Laboratories) p 419, 1233
Quibron Plus (Mead Johnson Laboratories) p 419, 1236
Quibron-T & Quibron-T/SR (Mead Johnson Laboratories) p 419, 1236
Quide (Merrell Dow) p 1379
Quiess Injectable (O'Neal, Jones & Feldman)
Quiet World Analgesic/Sleeping Aid (Whitehall)
Quinaglute Dura-Tabs (Berlex) p 406, 702
Quinamm (Merrell Dow) p 421, 1380
Quindan Tablets (Danbury) p 887
Quine Capsules (Rowell)
◆ Quinidex Extentabs (Robins) p 428, 1659
Quinidine Gluconate Sustained Action Tablets (Danbury) p 887
Quinidine Gluconate S.R. Tablets (Geneva) p 973
Quinidine Gluconate Sustained Release Tablets (Lederle) p 417
Quinidine Gluconate Sustained Release Tablets (Roxane) p 1788
Quinidine Gluconate Tablets (Schein) p 1828
Quinidine Sulfate Tablets (Danbury) p 887
Quinidine Sulfate Tablets (Geneva) p 973
Quinidine Sulfate Tablets (Lederle) p 417
Quinidine Sulfate Tablets (Roxane) p 1788
Quinidine Sulfate Tablets (Schein) p 1828
Quinine Sulfate Capsules (Geneva) p 973
Quinine Sulfate Capsules & Tablets (Schein) p 1828
Quinora (Key Pharmaceuticals) p 1051
Quiphile Tablets (Geneva) p 973

R

R&C Spray (Reed & Carnrick) p 1637
RCF (Ross) p 1775
Rh₀-D Immune Globulin (Human) HypRho-D (Cutter Biological) p 885

Rh₀-D Immune Globulin (Human) HypRho-D Mini-Dose (Cutter Biological) p 884
◆ RID Liquid Pediculicide (Pfipharmecs) p 426, 1593
RMS Suppositories (Upsher-Smith) p 2144
RP-Mycin Tablets (Reid-Provident Labs.)
R.S. Lotion No. 2 (Hill Dermaceuticals)
RVP Ointment (Elder) p 936
RVPaba Lip Stick (Elder) p 936
RVPaque Ointment (Elder) p 936
Rabies Immune Globulin (Human) Hyperab (Cutter Biological) p 884
Rabies Immune Globulin (Human), Imogam Rabies (Merieux) p 1358
Rabies Vaccine Human Diploid Cell, Imovax Rabies (Merieux) p 1358
Racet Cream (Lemmon)
Racet LCD Cream (Lemmon)
Racet-1% Cream (Lemmon)
Ramses Bendex Flexible Cushioned Diaphragm (Schmid)
Ramses Contraceptive Vaginal Jelly (Schmid) p 1896
Ramses Flexible Cushioned Diaphragm (Schmid)
Rantex Personal Cloth Wipes (Youngs)
Ratio Tablets (Adria)
◆ Raudixin Tablets (Squibb) p 438, 2020
Rautrax Tablets (Squibb)
Rautrax-N Modified Tablets (Squibb)
Rautrax-N Tablets (Squibb)
Rauval Tablets (Vale)
Rauverid Tablets (O'Neal, Jones & Feldman)
Rauwiloid Tablets (Riker) p 1644
◆ Rauzide Tablets (Squibb) p 438, 2021
◆ Rectal Medicone Suppositories (Medicone) p 419, 1256
◆ Rectal Medicone Unguent (Medicone)
◆ Rectal Medicone-HC Suppositories (Medicone) p 419, 1256
Redi-Nurser System (Ross) p 1777
Redipak Unit Dose Medications (Wyeth)
Redisol Injection (Merck Sharp & Dohme)
RediTemp-C, Disposable Cold Pack (Wyeth)
Regitine (CIBA) p 863
Reglan Injectable (Robins) p 1659
Reglan Syrup (Robins) p 1659
◆ Reglan Tablets (Robins) p 428, 1659
Regonol (Organon) p 1450
◆ Regroton Tablets (USV Pharmaceutical) p 440, 2087
Regular Purified Pork Insulin (Squibb-Novo) p 2034
Reidamine Injection (Reid-Provident Labs.)
Rela Tablets (Schering) p 435
Relefact TRH (Hoechst-Roussel) p 1017
Remsed Tablets (Du Pont) p 926
Renacidin (Guardian) p 1000
◆ Renese (Pfizer) p 426, 1608
◆ Renese-R (Pfizer) p 426, 1608
Renografin-60 (Squibb)
Renografin-76 (Squibb)
Reno-M-DIP (Squibb)
Reno-M-30 (Squibb)
Reno-M-60 (Squibb)
Renoquid (Glenwood) p 412, 999
Renovist (Squibb)
Renovist II (Squibb)
Renovue-65 (Squibb)
Renovue-DIP (Squibb)
Repan Tablets (Everett) p 942
Repen-VK Tablets (Reid-Provident Labs.)
Rep-Pred 40 Sterile Suspension (Central Pharmaceuticals)
Rep-Pred 80 Sterile Suspension (Central Pharmaceuticals)
Resaid T.D. Capsules (Geneva) p 973
Rescaps-D T.D. Capsules (Geneva) p 973
Reserpine, Hydrochlorothiazide & Hydralazine Tablets (Lederle)
Reserpine Tablets (Schein) p 1828
Respaire-SR Capsules 60, 120 (Laser) p 1072
◆ Respbid (Boehringer Ingelheim) p 406, 712
Respihaler (see Decadron Phosphate Respihaler) (Merck Sharp & Dohme)
◆ Restoril Capsules (Sandoz Pharmaceutical Div.) p 433, 1810
Retet-250 Capsules (Reid-Provident Labs.)
Retet-500 Capsules (Reid-Provident Labs.)
Reticulex Pulvules (Lilly)
Reticulogen Vials (Lilly)
Reticulogen Fortified Vials (Lilly)
Retin-A (tretinoin) (Ortho Pharmaceutical (Dermatological Div.)) p 1475
Reverse-numbered Package (Lilly) p 1122
Revitalin-SL 90 Adult Supplement (Robertson/Taylor) p 1646
Rexolate (Hyrex)
Rezamid Acne Lotion (Dermik)
Rheaban Tablets (Leeming)
Rheomacrodex (Pharmacia) p 1616
Rhindecon Capsules (McGregor) p 1197
Rhinex D Lay Tablets (Lemmon)
Rhinocaps Capsules (Ferndale)
Rhinogesic Tablets (Vale)
Rhinogesic-GG Tablets (Vale)
Rhinolar Capsules (McGregor) p 1197
Rhinolar-EX Capsules (McGregor) p 1197
Rhinolar-EX 12 Capsules (McGregor) p 1197

(◆ Shown in Product Identification Section) (*□ Described in PDR For Nonprescription Drugs) (Products without page numbers are not described)

Product Name Index

RhoGAM (Ortho Diagnostic Systems) p 1453
Rhus All Antigen - Poison Ivy, Oak, Sumac Combined (Barry) p 685
Rhus Tox Antigen Injection (Lemmon) p 1122
◆ Rifadin (Merrell Dow) p 421, 1382
◆ Rifamate (Merrell Dow) p 421, 1383
◆ Rimactane Capsules (CIBA) p 409, 864
Rimactane/INH Dual Pack (CIBA)
◆ Riopan (Ayerst) p 405, 680
◆ Riopan Antacid Swallow Tablets (Ayerst) p 405
◆ Riopan Plus (Ayerst) p 405, 680
◆ Ritalin Hydrochloride Tablets (CIBA) p 409, 864
◆ Ritalin-SR Tablets (CIBA) p 409, 864
◆ Robaxin Injectable (Robins) p 429, 1661
◆ Robaxin Tablets (Robins) p 428, 1662
◆ Robaxin-750 Tablets (Robins) p 428, 1662
◆ Robaxisal Tablets (Robins) p 429, 1662
Robicillin VK Robitabs (Robins)
Ro-Bile (Rowell)
Robimycin Robitabs (Robins)
◆ Robinul Forte Tablets (Robins) p 429, 1662
◆ Robinul Injectable (Robins) p 429, 1663
◆ Robinul Tablets (Robins) p 429, 1662
Robitet '250' Hydrochloride Robicaps (Robins)
Robitet '500' Hydrochloride Robicaps (Robins)
⊞ Robitussin (Robins)
Robitussin A-C (Robins) p 1664
⊞ Robitussin-CF (Robins)
⊞ Robitussin-DAC (Robins) p 1665
⊞ Robitussin-DM (Robins)
Robitussin Night Relief (Robins)
⊞ Robitussin-PE (Robins)
◆ Rocaltrol Capsules (Roche) p 430, 1700
Rodex (Legere) p 1120
Rodex T.D. Capsules (Legere) p 1120
Rogenic Injectable (O'Neal, Jones & Feldman) p 1446
Rogenic Tablets (O'Neal, Jones & Feldman)
Roma-Nol Antiseptic (Jamol) p 1033
Rondec Oral Drops (Ross) p 1776
Rondec Syrup (Ross) p 1776
◆ Rondec Tablet (Ross) p 432, 1776
Rondec-DM Oral Drops (Ross) p 1777
Rondec-DM Syrup (Ross) p 1777
◆ Rondec-TR Tablet (Ross) p 432, 1776
◆ Rondomycin (Wallace) p 442, 2164
Rose, Soluble, for Making Artificial Rose Water (Lilly)
Ross Hospital Formula System (Ross)
Ross SLD (Ross) p 1778
Roxanol (Morphine Sulfate Concentrated Oral Solution) (Roxane) p 1793
Rubesol-1000 Injectable (Central Pharmaceuticals)
Rubramin PC (Squibb)
Rubroben-1000 Injection Lyophilized (Medical Products)
◆ Rufen Tablets (Boots) p 406, 720
Rufolex Capsules (Lannett)
Rum-K (Fleming) p 948
Rutiplen-C (Medical Products)
◆ Ru-Tuss Expectorant (Boots) p 722
Ru-Tuss Plain (Boots) p 723
◆ Ru-Tuss Tablets (Boots) p 406, 723
◆ Ru-Tuss II Capsules (Boots) p 406, 723
Ru-Tuss with Hydrocodone (Boots) p 722
◆ Ru-Vert-M (Reid-Provident Labs.) p 428, 1640
Ruvite 1000 (Savage)
⊞ Ryna Liquid (Wallace)
⊞ Ryna-C Liquid (Wallace)
⊞ Ryna-CX Liquid (Wallace)
◆ Rynatan Tablets & Pediatric Suspension (Wallace) p 442, 2165
◆ Rynatuss Tablets & Pediatric Suspension (Wallace) p 442, 2165

S

S-A-C Tablets (Lannett)
SK-Amitriptyline Hydrochloride Tablets (Smith Kline & French) p 1971
SK-Ampicillin Capsules & For Oral Suspension (Smith Kline & French) p 1971
SK-Ampicillin-N For Injection (Smith Kline & French) p 1971
SK-APAP with CODEINE Tablets (Smith Kline & French) p 1971
SK-Bamate Tablets (Smith Kline & French) p 1971
SK-Chloral Hydrate Capsules (Smith Kline & French) p 1971
SK-Chlorothiazide Tablets (Smith Kline & French) p 1971
SK-Dexamethasone Tablets (Smith Kline & French) p 1971
SK-Diphenoxylate Tablets (Smith Kline & French) p 1971
SK-Dipyridamole Tablets (Smith Kline & French) p 1971
SK-Erythromycin Tablets (Smith Kline & French) p 1971
SK-Furosemide Tablets (Smith Kline & French) p 1971
SK-Hydrochlorothiazide Tablets (Smith Kline & French) p 1971
SK-Lygen Capsules (Smith Kline & French) p 1971

SK-Metronidazole Tablets (Smith Kline & French) p 1971
SK-Oxycodone with Acetaminophen Tablets (Smith Kline & French) p 1971
SK-Oxycodone with Aspirin Tablets (Smith Kline & French) p 1971
SK-Penicillin G Tablets (Smith Kline & French) p 1971
SK-Penicillin VK For Oral Solution & Tablets (Smith Kline & French) p 1971
SK-Phenobarbital Tablets (Smith Kline & French) p 1971
SK-Pramine Tablets (Smith Kline & French) p 1971
SK-Prednisone Tablets (Smith Kline & French) p 1971
SK-Probenecid Tablets (Smith Kline & French) p 1971
SK-Propantheline Bromide Tablets (Smith Kline & French) p 1971
SK-Quinidine Sulfate Tablets (Smith Kline & French) p 1971
SK-Reserpine Tablets (Smith Kline & French) p 1971
SK-65 APAP Tablets (Smith Kline & French) p 1971
SK-65 Capsules (Smith Kline & French) p 1971
SK-65 Compound Capsules (Smith Kline & French) p 1971
SK-Soxazole Tablets (Smith Kline & French) p 1971
SK-Terpin Hydrate and Codeine Elixir (Smith Kline & French) p 1971
SK-Tetracycline Capsules (Smith Kline & French) p 1971
SK-Tetracycline Syrup (Smith Kline & French) p 1971
SK-Thioridazine Hydrochloride Tablets (Smith Kline & French) p 1971
SK-Tolbutamide Tablets (Smith Kline & French) p 1971
SLT Lotion (C & M)
⊞ SMA Infant Formula, Ready-to-Feed, Concentrated Liquid, Powder (Wyeth) p 2286
S.O.D. (Superoxide Dismutase) (Vitaline)
SPRX-1 Tablets (Reid-Provident, Direct Div.)
SPRX-3 Capsules (Reid-Provident, Direct Div.)
SPRX-105 Capsules (Reid-Provident, Direct Div.)
S-P-T (Fleming) p 949
SSKI (Upsher-Smith) p 2145
S-T Cort Lotion (Scot-Tussin)
S-T Decongest Sugar-Free & Dye-Free (Scot-Tussin) p 1897
S-T Febrol Tablets & Elixir (Scot-Tussin)
S-T Forte Syrup & Sugar-Free (Scot-Tussin) p 1897
Safe Suds (Ar-Ex) p 601
Salactic Film (Pedinol) p 1581
Salatar Cream (Lannett)
Salatin Capsules (Ferndale)
Saleto (Mallard) p 1181
Saligel (Stiefel)
Salimeph Forte (Rorer)
⊞ Salinex Nasal Mist and Drops (Muro)
Saliva Substitute (Roxane)
◆ Saluron (Bristol) p 407, 747
◆ Salutensin/Salutensin-Demi (Bristol) p 407, 748
Sandimmune Ampuls (Sandoz Pharmaceutical Div.) p 1811
Sandimmune Oral Suspension (Sandoz Pharmaceutical Div.) p 1811
Sandoglobulin (Sandoz Pharmaceutical Div.) p 1813
Sandril, Vials (Lilly)
◆ Sanorex (Sandoz Pharmaceutical Div.) p 433, 1815
◆ Sansert (Sandoz Pharmaceutical Div.) p 433, 1816
Santyl Ointment (Knoll) p 1067
Sarapin (High Chemical) p 1009
Sarna Lotion (Stiefel)
SAStid (AL) (Stiefel)
SAStid (Plain) (Stiefel)
SAStid Soap (Stiefel)
Satin (Consolidated Chemical) p 881
◆ Sātric (Savage) p 433, 1825
Sātric-500 (Savage)
Savacort-50 (Savage)
Savacort-100 (Savage)
Savacort-D (Savage)
Scabene Lotion (Stiefel) p 2035
Scabene Shampoo (Stiefel) p 2036
Scarlet Red Ointment (Lilly)
Schamberg's Lotion (C & M)
Schirmer Tear Test (CooperVision)
SclavoTest-PPD (Sclavo) p 3017
Scopolamine Hydrobromide Injection (Elkins-Sinn) p 938
Scopolamine Hydrobromide Injection, Wellcome (Burroughs Wellcome)
Score hair cream (Bristol-Myers Products)
Scot-Tussin DM Syrup (Scot-Tussin)
Scot-Tussin Sugar-Free Cough & Cold Medicine (Scot-Tussin)
Scot-Tussin Sugar-Free Expectorant (Scot-Tussin) p 1897
Scot-Tussin Sugar-Free 5-Action Cold Formula (Scot-Tussin) p 1897

Scot-Tussin Syrup 5-Action Cold Formula (Scot-Tussin)
Seale's Lotion Modified (C & M)
Sebizon Lotion (Schering)
Sebucare (Westwood) p 2181
Sebulex & Sebulex Cream Shampoo (Westwood) p 2181
Sebulex Shampoo with Conditioners (Westwood) p 2181
Sebulon Dandruff Shampoo (Westwood) p 2181
Sebutone & Sebutone Cream Shampoo (Westwood) p 2181
Secobarbital Sodium in Tubex (Wyeth) p 2288
◆ Seconal Sodium Pulvules & Vials (Lilly) p 417, 1172
Seconal Sodium Suppositories (Lilly)
Secretin-Kabi (Pharmacia) p 1616
Sedapap-10 Tablets (Mayrand) p 1196
Sedaril (Bart)
Sedragesic Tablets (Lannett)
Seffin, Neutral (Glaxo) p 980
Selenitrace (Armour) p 610
Selenium Tablets (200 mcg) (Vitaline) p 2148
Selepen (Selenious Acid Injection) (LyphoMed)
Selestoject (Mayrand)
Selsun Blue Lotion (Ross) p 1778
Selsun Lotion (Abbott) p 567
Semets Troches (Beecham Laboratories)
◆ Semicid Vaginal Contraceptive Suppositories (Whitehall) p 443, 2187
Semilente Insulin (Prompt Insulin Zinc Suspension USP) (Squibb-Novo) p 2033
Semilente Purified Pork Prompt Insulin Zinc Suspension (Squibb-Novo) p 2034
Seminal Pouches (Milex)
Senokap DSS Capsules (Purdue Frederick)
Senokot Suppositories (Purdue Frederick)
Senokot Syrup (Purdue Frederick) p 1626
Senokot Tablets/Granules (Purdue Frederick) p 1626
Senokot Tablets Unit Strip Pack (Purdue Frederick)
Senokot-S Tablets (Purdue Frederick) p 1627
Sensorcaine Hydrochloride & Sensorcaine Hydrochloride with Epinephrine 1:200,000 (Astra) p 619
◆ Septra DS Tablets (Burroughs Wellcome) p 408, 815
Septra I.V. Infusion (Burroughs Wellcome) p 813
Septra Suspension (Burroughs Wellcome) p 815
◆ Septra Tablets (Burroughs Wellcome) p 408, 815
Seralyzer Reflectance Photometer (Ames) p 3006
Seralyzer Solid Phase Reagent Strips (Ames)
◆ Ser-Ap-Es (CIBA) p 409, 866
◆ Serax Capsules, Tablets (Wyeth) p 445, 2287
Serenium Tablets (Squibb)
Serentil Ampuls (Boehringer Ingelheim) p 714
Serentil Concentrate (Boehringer Ingelheim) p 714
◆ Serentil Tablets (Boehringer Ingelheim) p 406, 714
Seromycin (Lilly) p 1174
Serophene (clomiphene citrate USP) (Serono) p 1943
Serpasil Parenteral Solution (CIBA) p 868
◆ Serpasil Tablets (CIBA) p 409, 867
◆ Serpasil-Apresoline (CIBA) p 409, 869
◆ Serpasil-Esidrix (CIBA) p 409, 870
Serpate Tablets (Vale)
Shepard's Cream Lotion (Dermik)
Shepard's Moisturizing Soap (Dermik)
Shepard's Skin Cream (Dermik)
Shur-Seal Gel (Milex)
Siblin Granules (Parke-Davis)
Sigtab Tablets (Upjohn) p 2135
Silain Tablets (Robins)
Silain-Gel Liquid (Robins)
Silvadene Cream (Marion) p 1189
Silver Nitrate (Lilly) p 1174
⊞ Simeco (Wyeth) p 2288
Simetyl Elixir (Kramer)
Similac (Ross) p 1778
Similac PM 60/40 (Ross) p 1779
Similac 13 (Ross) p 1777
Similac 20 (Ross) p 1777
Similac 24 (Ross) p 1777
Similac 24 LBW (Ross) p 1777
Similac 27 (Ross) p 1777
Similac Special Care 20 (Ross) p 1777
Similac Special Care 24 (Ross) p 1777
Similac With Iron (Ross) p 1779
Similac With Iron 13 (Ross) p 1777
Similac With Iron 20 (Ross) p 1777
Similac With Iron 24 (Ross) p 1777
Similac With Whey + Iron (Ross) p 1780
Similac With Whey + Iron 20 (Ross) p 1777
⊞ Simron Capsules (Merrell Dow)
⊞ Simron Plus Capsules (Merrell Dow)
⊞ Sinarest Tablets, Extra Strength Tablets & Nasal Spray (Pharmacraft)
Sine-Aid Extra-Strength Sinus Headache Capsules (McNeil Consumer Products) p 1199
Sine-Aid Sinus Headache Tablets (McNeil Consumer Products) p 1198
◆ Sinemet Tablets (Merck Sharp & Dohme) p 420, 1345
◆ Sinequan (Roerig) p 431, 1740

(◆ Shown in Product Identification Section) (⊞ Described in PDR For Nonprescription Drugs) (Products without page numbers are not described)

Product Name Index

- ℞ Sinex Decongestant Nasal Spray (Vicks Health Care)
- ℞ Sinex Long-Acting Decongestant Nasal Spray (Vicks Health Care)
- ◆ Singlet (Merrell Dow) p 421, 1385
- Sinografin (Squibb)
- Sinovan Timed (Drug Industries) p 915
- ◆ Sinubid (Parke-Davis) p 425, 1569
- Sinufed Timecelles (Hauck) p 1001
- ◆ Sinulin Tablets (Carnrick) p 409, 835
- ◆ Skelaxin (Carnrick) p 409, 835
- Skin Magic (Consolidated Chemical) p 881
- Skin Screen Protective Skin Lotion (Cetylite)
- Skin Test Antigens for Cellular Hypersensitivity, Multitest CMI (Merieux) p 1358, 3013
- Sleep-eze 3 Tablets (Whitehall)
- ◆ Slo-bid Gyrocaps (Rorer) p 432, 1754
- ◆ Slo-Phyllin Gyrocaps, Tablets (Rorer) p 432, 1756
- Slo-Phyllin 80 Syrup (Rorer) p 1756
- ◆ Slo-Phyllin GG Capsules, Syrup (Rorer) p 432, 1759
- ◆ Slow-K (CIBA) p 409, 872
- Snakebite Serum (see Antivenin) (Wyeth)
- Soakare hard contact lens soaking solution (Allergan)
- Soapure (Winthrop Consumer Products)
- Sodium Bicarbonate (Bristol) p 730
- Sodium Chloride, Bacteriostatic in Tubex (Wyeth) p 2288
- Sodium Chloride Carpuject (Winthrop-Breon)
- Sodium Chloride Inhalation (Roxane) p 1788
- Sodium Chloride Injection (Preservative-free) (Elkins-Sinn) p 938
- Sodium Chloride Injection, Bacteriostatic (Elkins-Sinn) p 938
- Sodium Nitroprusside Injection (Elkins-Sinn) p 938
- Sodium Phosphates Oral Solution (Roxane) p 1788
- Sodium Polystyrene Sulfonate Suspension (Roxane) p 1794
- Sodium Sulamyd Ophthalmic Solutions & Ointment-Sterile (Schering) p 1884
- Sofenol 5 (C & M)
- Soflens Enzymatic Contact Lens Cleaner (Allergan)
- Soft 'N Soothe Creme (Ascher)
- Solaquin 2% Cream (Elder) p 936
- Solaquin Forte 4% Cream (Elder) p 936
- Solaquin Forte 4% Gel (Elder) p 937
- ◆ Solatene Capsules (Roche) p 430, 1701
- Solbar PF (Persön & Covey) p 1588
- Solbar Plus 15 Sun Protectant Cream (Persön & Covey) p 1588
- Solfoton Tablets & Capsules (Poythress) p 1619
- Solganal Suspension (Schering) p 1884
- Solu-Cortef Plain & Mix-O-Vial (Upjohn) p 2135
- Solu-Eze Solvent (O'Neal, Jones & Feldman)
- ◆ Solu-Medrol Mix-O-Vial & Vials (Upjohn) p 441
- Solu-Medrol Sterile Powder (Upjohn) p 441, 2137
- soluPredalone Injectable (O'Neal, Jones & Feldman)
- Solurex Injection (Hyrex)
- ◆ Soma (Wallace) p 442, 2166
- ◆ Soma Compound (Wallace) p 442, 2166
- ◆ Soma Compound w/Codeine (Wallace) p 442, 2169
- Somophyllin & Somophyllin-DF Oral Liquids (Fisons) p 945
- Somophyllin Rectal Solution (Fisons) p 945
- Somophyllin-CRT Capsules (Fisons) p 945
- Somophyllin-T Capsules (Fisons) p 945
- Sonacide (Ayerst)
- Soniphen Tablets (O'Neal, Jones & Feldman)
- Soothogel Cream (Vale)
- Soprodol Tablets (Carisoprodol) (Schein) p 1828
- Sopronol Ointment, Powder & Solution (Wyeth)
- Sorate-5 Chewable Tablets (Trimen) p 2067
- Sorate-10 Chewable Tablets (Trimen) p 2067
- Sorbide (Mayrand) p 1196
- Sorbitol Solution (Upsher-Smith)
- Sorbitrate Tablets (Stuart) p 439, 2041
- Sorbutuss (Dalin) p 886
- Sotradecol Injection (Elkins-Sinn) p 941
- Spantuss Liquid (Arco)
- Spantuss Tablets (Arco)
- Sparine Concentrate (Wyeth)
- Sparine Injection (Wyeth)
- Sparine Injection in Tubex (Wyeth) p 2288
- Sparine Syrup (Wyeth)
- ◆ Sparine Tablets (Wyeth) p 445
- ℞ Spartus High Potency Vitamins & Minerals plus Electrolytes Tablets (Lederle)
- ℞ Spartus + Iron High Potency Vitamins & Minerals plus Electrolytes Tablets (Lederle)
- Spasmoject (Mayrand)
- Spatula (Milex)
- Spec-T Sore Throat Anesthetic Lozenges (Squibb)
- Spec-T Sore Throat/Cough Suppressant Lozenges (Squibb)
- Spec-T Sore Throat/Decongestant Lozenges (Squibb)

- Spectazole Cream (Ortho Pharmaceutical (Dermatological Div.)) p 1476
- ◆ Spectrobid Tablets & Oral Suspension (Roerig) p 431, 1741
- Spectrocin Ointment (Squibb)
- Spironazide Tablets (Schein) p 1828
- Spironolactone Tablets (Geneva) p 973
- ◆ Spironolactone Tablets (Lederle) p 417
- Spironolactone Tablets (Schein) p 1828
- Spironolactone Tablets, USP (Parke-Davis) p 1569
- Spironolactone/Hydrochlorothiazide Tablets (Danbury) p 887
- Spironolactone w/Hydrochlorothiazide Tablets (Geneva) p 973
- Spironolactone w/Hydrochlorothiazide Tablets (Parke-Davis) p 1570
- ◆ Spironolactone with Hydrochlorothiazide Tablets (Lederle) p 417
- Stadol (Bristol) p 750
- Staphage Lysate (SPL) (Delmont) p 888
- Staphcillin (Bristol) p 751
- Staphoclean (Consolidated Chemical)
- Staphosol (Consolidated Chemical)
- ℞ Star-Otic (Stellar)
- Staticin 1.5% Topical Solution (Westwood) p 2181
- Statobex G Tablets (Lemmon)
- ◆ Stelazine (Smith Kline & French) p 437, 1971
- Stemetic (Legere) p 1120
- Stera-Form Cream (Mayrand)
- Steramine Otic (Mayrand)
- Sterapred Uni-Pak (Mayrand) p 1196
- Steri-Units (Alcon Labs.)
- Steri Unna Boot (Pedinol)
- Sterile Lubricating Jelly (Pharmafair)
- Sterilized Water (Ross) p 1777
- ◆ Stilphostrol (Miles Pharmaceuticals) p 422, 1412
- Stimate Injection (Armour) p 611
- StimuLean (appetite suppressant) (Vitaline)
- Stimuzyme Plus (National Dermaceutical) p 1421
- Stimuzyme Topical Dressing (National Dermaceutical)
- Stopayne Capsules (Springbok) p 1985
- Stopayne Syrup (Springbok) p 1985
- Streptase (Hoechst-Roussel) p 1018
- Streptomycin Sulfate Injection (Pfipharmecs) p 1593
- Stress-600 Tablets (Upsher-Smith)
- Stress-600 with Zinc (Upsher-Smith)
- ℞ Stresscaps Capsules (Lederle)
- ℞ Stresstabs 600 Tablets, Advanced Formula (Lederle)
- ℞ Stresstabs 600 with Iron, Advanced Formula (Lederle)
- ℞ Stresstabs 600 with Zinc, Advanced Formula (Lederle)
- Stresstein (Clinical Nutrition) p 878
- Strifon Forte Tablets (Ferndale)
- ◆ The Stuart Formula Tablets (Stuart) p 439, 2042
- ◆ Stuart Prenatal Tablets (Stuart) p 439, 2034
- ◆ Stuartinic Tablets (Stuart) p 439, 2034
- ◆ Stuartnatal 1+1 Tablets (Stuart) p 439, 2043
- ◆ Sublimaze Injection (Janssen) p 413, 1039
- Succus Cineraria Maritima (Walker Pharmacal) p 2148
- Sucostrin Injection, High Potency (Squibb)
- ℞ Sudafed Cough Syrup (Burroughs Wellcome)
- ◆ Sudafed Plus Syrup & Tablets (Burroughs Wellcome) p 408
- ◆ Sudafed Pseudoephedrine Hydrochloride Syrup & Tablets (Burroughs Wellcome) p 408
- ◆ Sudafed S.A. Capsules (Burroughs Wellcome) p 408
- Sudden Action Breath Freshener (Whitehall)
- Sudden Beauty Country Air Mask (Whitehall)
- Sudden Beauty Hair Spray (Whitehall)
- ◆ Sufenta (Janssen) p 413, 1040
- Sulfacet-R Acne Lotion (Dermik) p 891
- Sulfacetamide Sodium Ophthalmic Ointment (Fougera) p 953
- Sulfadrin Nasal Drops (Kramer)
- Sulfa-Gyn (Mayrand)
- Sulfaloid "500" Tablets (O'Neal, Jones & Feldman)
- Sulfaloid Suspension (O'Neal, Jones & Feldman)
- Sulfamethoxazole Tablets (Geneva) p 973
- Sulfamethoxazole & Trimethoprim Pediatric Suspension (Biocraft) p 705
- Sulfamethoxazole and Trimethoprim Tablets (Biocraft) p 705
- ◆ Sulfamethoxazole & Trimethoprim Tablets and Pediatric Suspension (Lederle) p 417
- Sulfamethoxazole with Trimethoprim Tablets (Danbury) p 887
- Sulfamethoxazole with Trimethoprim Tablets (Double Strength) (Danbury) p 887
- Sulfamethoxazole w/Trimethoprim DS (Geneva) p 973
- Sulfamethoxazole w/Trimethoprim SS (Geneva) p 973
- Sulfamylon Acetate Cream (Winthrop-Breon) p 2226
- Sulfasalazine Tablets (Danbury) p 887
- Sulfasalazine Tablets (Geneva) p 973
- Sulfasalazine Tablets (Schein) p 1828
- Sulfatrim & Sulfatrim D/S Tablets (Schein) p 1828
- Sulfinpyrazone Tablets (Danbury) p 887

- Sulfinpyrazone Tablets (Schein) p 1828
- Sulfisoxazole Tablets (Geneva) p 973
- Sulfisoxazole Tablets (Schein) p 1828
- Sulfoil (C & M)
- Sulfoxyl Lotion Regular (Stiefel)
- Sulf-10 Ophthalmic Solution (CooperVision)
- Sulf-10 (Sodium Sulfacetamide 10% Dropperettes) (CooperVision)
- Sulphrin Ophthalmic Suspension (Muro)
- Sulten-10 Ophthalmic Solution (Muro)
- Sultrin Triple Sulfa Cream (Ortho Pharmaceutical) p 1472
- Sultrin Triple Sulfa Vaginal Tablets (Ortho Pharmaceutical) p 1472
- Summer's Eve Medicated Douche (Fleet) p 948
- Sumox Capsules (Reid-Provident Labs.)
- Sumox Oral Suspensions (Reid-Provident Labs.)
- ◆ Sumycin Capsules (Squibb) p 438, 2022
- ◆ Sumycin Tablets (Squibb) p 438, 2022
- Sumycin Syrup (Squibb) p 2022
- sunDare Clear (Cooper Dermatology)
- sunDare Creamy (Cooper Dermatology)
- ℞ Sunril Premenstrual Capsules (Schering)
- sunStick (Cooper Dermatology)
- Supac (Mission) p 1420
- Supen Capsules (Reid-Provident Labs.)
- Supen Oral Suspensions (Reid-Provident Labs.)
- Super Citro Cee (Marlyn)
- Super D Perles (Upjohn)
- Super One Daily (Marlyn)
- Supervim Drops, Tablets & Syrup (U.S. Ethicals)
- Surbex Filmtab (Abbott) p 567
- Surbex w/C Filmtab (Abbott) p 567
- ◆ Surbex-750 with Iron Filmtab (Abbott) p 404
- ◆ Surbex-750 with Zinc Filmtab (Abbott) p 404
- ◆ Surbex-T Filmtab (Abbott) p 404
- Surfacaine Cream, Jelly & Ointment (Lilly)
- Surfadil Cream & Lotion (Lilly)
- ◆ Surfak (Hoechst-Roussel) p 413, 1021
- Surfol Bath Oil (Stiefel)
- Surgel Liquid (Ulmer)
- Surgicel Absorbable Hemostat (Johnson & Johnson (Patient Care Div.)) p 1044
- Surgi-Kleen (Sween) p 2048
- Surgilube Surgical Lubricant (Fougera)
- Surital (Parke-Davis) p 1572
- ◆ Surmontil Capsules 25 mg, 50 mg, & 100 mg (Ives) p 413, 1029
- ◆ Sus-Phrine (Berlex) p 406, 704
- ℞ Sustacal (Mead Johnson Nutritional)
- ℞ Sustacal HC (Mead Johnson Nutritional)
- ℞ Sustagen (Mead Johnson Nutritional)
- ◆ Sustaire Tablets (Roerig) p 431, 1743
- Sween-A-Peel (Sween) p 2048
- Sween Cream (Sween) p 2049
- Sween Kind Touch (Sween) p 2047
- Sween Prep (Sween) p 2049
- Sween Soft Touch (Sween) p 2049
- Sweeta Liquid & Tablets (Squibb)
- Swim Ear (Fougera)
- Swirleoft (Consolidated Chemical)
- Syllact Powder (Wallace)
- Syllamalt Powder (Wallace)
- ◆ Symmetrel (Du Pont) p 410, 927
- Synabrom Capsules (Ferndale)
- Synacort Creams 1%, 2.5% (Syntex) p 2061
- Synalar Creams 0.025%, 0.01% (Syntex) p 2061
- Synalar Ointment 0.025% (Syntex) p 2061
- Synalar Topical Solution 0.01% (Syntex) p 2061
- Synalar-HP Cream 0.2% (Syntex) p 2061
- ◆ Synalgos-DC Capsules (Ives) p 413, 1031
- Synemol Cream 0.025% (Syntex) p 2061
- Synkayvite Injectable (Roche) p 1701
- ◆ Synkayvite Tablets (Roche) p 430, 1702
- Synophylate Elixir (Central Pharmaceuticals) p 839
- Synophylate-GG Tablets/Syrup (Central Pharmaceuticals) p 839
- Synthetar Cream (Vale)
- ◆ Synthroid (Flint) p 411, 951
- Syntocinon Injection (Sandoz Pharmaceutical Div.) p 1817
- Syntocinon Nasal Spray (Sandoz Pharmaceutical Div.) p 1818
- Sytobex (Cyanocobalamin Injection) (Parke-Davis)

T

- T-Cypionate (Legere) p 1120
- T/Derm Tar Emollient (Neutrogena)
- T.D. Alermine Granucaps (Reid-Provident, Direct Div.)
- T.D. Therals Granucaps (Reid-Provident, Direct Div.)
- T-E Ionate P.A. Injection (Reid-Provident, Direct Div.)
- T.E.H. Tablets (Geneva) p 973
- T-E-P Tablets (Schein) p 1828
- T.E.P. Tablets (Geneva) p 973
- T/Gel Scalp Solution (Neutrogena) (Neutrogena)
- T-Ionate P.A. Injection (Reid-Provident, Direct Div.)
- T-Stat 2.0% Topical Solution (Westwood) p 2181
- 2/G (Merrell Dow)

(◆ Shown in Product Identification Section)   (℞ Described in PDR For Nonprescription Drugs)   (Products without page numbers are not described)

Product Name Index

2/G-DM (Merrell Dow)
♦ Tabloid Brand Thioguanine (Burroughs Wellcome) p 408, 817
♦ Tabron Filmseal (Parke-Davis) p 425, 1572
♦ Tacaryl Chewable Tablets (Westwood) p 442, 2182
♦ Tacaryl Syrup & Tablets (Westwood) p 442, 2182
♦ TACE 12 mg Capsules (Merrell Dow) p 421, 1385
♦ TACE 25 mg Capsules (Merrell Dow) p 421, 1385
♦ TACE 72 mg Capsules (Merrell Dow) p 421, 1389
♦ Tagamet (Smith Kline & French) p 437, 1973
Tagatap Tablets (Reid-Provident, Direct Div.)
♦ Talacen (Winthrop-Breon) p 444, 2227
Taloin Ointment (Adria)
Talwin Ampuls (Winthrop-Breon)
Talwin Carpuject (Winthrop-Breon)
Talwin Compound (Winthrop-Breon) p 2229
Talwin Injection (Winthrop-Breon) p 2228
♦ Talwin Nx (Winthrop-Breon) p 444, 2230
Tamine Elixir (Geneva)
Tamine S.R. Tablets (Geneva) p 973
♦ Tandearil (Geigy) p 411, 964
♦ Tao Capsules (Roerig) p 431, 1744
Tapazole (Lilly) p 1175
Ta-Poff (Ulmer)
Ta-Poff Aerosol (Ulmer)
Tar Distillate "Doak" (Doak)
Taractan Concentrate (Roche) p 1703
Taractan Injectable (Roche) p 1703
Taractan Tablets (Roche) p 1703
Tarpaste (Doak)
♦ Tatum-T (Searle Pharmaceuticals) p 436, 1909
Taurophyllin Tablets (Vale)
♦ Tavist Tablets (Sandoz Pharmaceutical Div.) p 433, 1818
♦ Tavist-1 Tablets (Sandoz Pharmaceutical Div.) p 433, 1818
♦ Tavist-D Tablets (Sandoz Pharmaceutical Div.) p 433, 1819
Taystron Tablets (Vale)
Tearisol Ophthalmic Solution (CooperVision)
Tears Naturale (Alcon Labs.)
Tears Plus artificial tears (Allergan)
Tedral Elixir & Suspension (Parke-Davis) p 1573
Tedral Expectorant (Parke-Davis)
Tedral SA Tablets (Parke-Davis) p 425, 1573
Tedral Tablets (Parke-Davis) p 425
Tedral-25 Tablets (Parke-Davis) p 425
Tegopen (Bristol) p 407, 753
Tegretol Chewable Tablets (Geigy) p 411, 966
Tegretol Tablets (Geigy) p 411, 966
Teldrin Multi-Symptom Allergy Reliever Capsules (Smith Kline & French)
Teldrin Timed-Release Allergy Capsules (Smith Kline & French)
♦ Tel-E-Dose (Roche) p 430, 1705
♦ Telepaque (Winthrop-Breon) p 443, 3058
♦ Temaril (Smith Kline & French) p 437, 1976
▣ Tempo Antacid with Antigas Action (Vicks Health Care)
Tempotest 225 (Medical Products)
▣ Tempra (Mead Johnson Nutritional)
♦ Tenoretic Tablets (Stuart) p 439, 2043
♦ Tenormin Tablets (Stuart) p 439, 2045
Tensilon Injectable (Roche) p 1705, 3015
♦ Tenuate Dospan (Merrell Dow) p 421, 1393
♦ Tenuate 25 mg (Merrell Dow) p 421, 1393
♦ Tepanil (Riker) p 428, 1645
♦ Tepanil Ten-tab (Riker) p 428, 1645
Teramine Capsules (Legere) p 1120
Terfonyl Tablets, Oral Suspension (Squibb)
Terphan Elixir (Vale)
Terpin Hydrate & Codeine Elixir (Roxane) p 1788
Terra-Cortril Ophthalmic Suspension (Pfipharmecs) p 1594
♦ Terramycin Capsules (Pfipharmecs) p 426, 1595
Terramycin Film-coated Tablets (Pfipharmecs) p 1595
Terramycin Intramuscular Solution (Pfipharmecs) p 1596
Terramycin Ointment (Pfipharmecs) p 1598
Terramycin with Polymyxin B Sulfate Ophthalmic Ointment (Pfipharmecs) p 1598
Terry Keratometer (Alcon Labs.)
Tersaseptic Hygienic Skin Cleanser (Doak)
Tersa-Tar (Doak)
Teslac Tablets (Squibb) p 2023
♦ Tessalon (Du Pont) p 411, 928
Tes-Tape (Lilly) p 3013
Testate (Savage)
Testaval 90/4 (Legere) p 1120
Testoject-50 (Mayrand)
Testoject-100 L.A. & Testoject-200 L.A. (Mayrand)
Testorex-35 Adult Male Supplement (Robertson/Taylor) p 1646
Testosterone Suspension (Legere) p 1120
Testostroval P.A. Injection (Reid-Provident, Direct Div.)
Testred (ICN Pharmaceuticals) p 1025
Tetanus & Diphtheria Toxoids Adsorbed (Adult) (Wyeth) p 2246
Tetanus & Diphtheria Toxoids Adsorbed (Adult) in Tubex (Wyeth) p 2288

Tetanus Antitoxin (equine), Refined (Sclavo) p 1897
Tetanus Immune Globulin (Human) (Wyeth) p 2246
Tetanus Immune Globulin (Human) in Tubex (Wyeth) p 2288
Tetanus Immune Globulin (Human) Hyper-Tet (Cutter Biological) p 884
Tetanus Toxoid (Squibb/Connaught) p 2033
Tetanus Toxoid Adsorbed (Squibb/Connaught) p 2033
Tetanus Toxoid, Adsorbed (Sclavo) p 1897
Tetanus Toxoid Adsorbed, Aluminum Phosphate Adsorbed, Ultrafined (Wyeth) p 2246
Tetanus Toxoid Adsorbed, Aluminum Phosphate Adsorbed, Ultrafined in Tubex (Wyeth) p 2288
Tetanus Toxoid, Adsorbed Purogenated (Lederle) p 1118
Tetanus Toxoid Fluid, Purified, Ultrafined (Wyeth) p 2246
Tetanus Toxoid Fluid, Purified, Ultrafined in Tubex (Wyeth) p 2288
Tetanus Toxoid Purogenated (Lederle) p 1118
Tetanus & Diphtheria Toxoids, Adsorbed Purogenated (Lederle) p 1118
Tetanus & Diphtheria Toxoids Adsorbed (For Adult Use) (Squibb/Connaught) p 2033
Tetanus & Diphtheria Toxoids Adsorbed (For Adult Use) (Sclavo) p 1897
Tetracaine HCl 0.5% Dropperettes (CooperVision)
Tetracycline HCl Capsules (Danbury) p 887
Tetracycline HCl Capsules & Syrup (Schein) p 1828
♦ Tetracycline HCl Capsules (Wyeth) p 445
Tetracycline HCl Capsules (Cyclopar) (Parke-Davis) p 425, 1573
Tetracycline HCl Capsules (Cyclopar 500) (Parke-Davis) p 425, 1573
Texacort Scalp Lotion (Cooper Dermatology) p 882
♦ Thalitone Tablets (Boehringer Ingelheim) p 406, 715
Tham E (Abbott)
Tham Solution (Abbott)
Thantis Lozenges (Hynson, Westcott & Dunning)
Theelin Aqueous Suspension (Parke-Davis)
♦ Theo-24 (Searle & Co.) p 436, 1937
♦ Theobid, Theobid Jr. Duracap (Glaxo) p 412, 982
♦ Theoclear L.A.-130 & -260 Capsules (Central Pharmaceuticals) p 409, 839
Theoclear-80 Syrup (Central Pharmaceuticals) p 839
♦ Theo-Dur Sprinkle (Key Pharmaceuticals) p 414, 1053
♦ Theo-Dur Tablets (Key Pharmaceuticals) p 414, 1051
Theofedral Tablets (Danbury) p 887
♦ Theolair & Theolair-SR (Riker) p 428, 1645
♦ Theolair-Plus Tablets & Liquid (Riker) p 428, 1645
Theon Syrup (Bock) p 706
♦ Theo-Organidin Elixir (Wallace) p 442, 2170
Theophyl Chewable Tablets (McNeil Pharmaceutical) p 1207
Theophylline Anhydrous Tablets (Schein) p 1828
Theophylline Elixir (Geneva) p 973
Theophylline Elixir & KI Elixir (Schein) p 1828
Theophylline Oral Solution (Roxane) p 1788
Theophylline S.R. Tablets (Geneva) p 973
Theophyl-SR (McNeil Pharmaceutical) p 1208
Theophyl-225 Elixir (McNeil Pharmaceutical) p 1210
Theophyl-225 Tablets (McNeil Pharmaceutical) p 1210
Theospan-SR Capsules 130 mg., 260 mg. (Laser) p 1072
Theostat 80 Syrup (Laser) p 1072
♦ Theovent Long-Acting Capsules (Schering) p 435, 1886
Theozine Syrup & Tablets - Dye-Free (Schein) p 1828
Therabid (Mission) p 1420
Therac (C & M)
Theracebrin Pulvules (Lilly)
♦ Thera-Combex H-P (Parke-Davis) p 425, 1574
Theracort (C & M)
Thera-Flur Gel-Drops (Colgate-Hoyt) p 880
Thera-Flur-N Topical Gel-Drops (Colgate-Hoyt)
Thera-Gesic (Mission) p 1420
♦ Theragran Hematinic (Squibb) p 438, 2024
Theragran Liquid (Squibb) p 2024
♦ Theragran Stress Formula (Squibb) p 438, 2025
♦ Theragran Tablets (Squibb) p 438, 2025
♦ Theragran-M Tablets (Squibb) p 438, 2025
Theralax Suppositories (Beecham Laboratories)
Thera-Ron Tablets (Legere) p 1120
♦ Thiacide Tablets (Beach) p 405, 687
Thiamine HCl Injection (Elkins-Sinn) p 938
Thiamine HCl in Tubex (Wyeth) p 2288
Thiodyne (Savage)
Thioridazine Tablets (Geneva) p 973
Thioridazine Tablets (Schein) p 1828
Thioridazine HCl Tablets (Danbury) p 887
♦ Thioridazine HCl Tablets (Lederle) p 417

Thioridazine Hydrochloride Tablets (Roxane) p 1788
Thiosulfil Duo-Pak (Ayerst) p 682
♦ Thiosulfil Forte (Ayerst) p 405, 680
♦ Thiosulfil Tablets (Ayerst) p 405
♦ Thiosulfil-A Forte (Ayerst) p 405, 681
♦ Thiosulfil-A Tablets (Ayerst) p 405, 681
Thiotepa (Lederle) p 416, 1118
Thiuretic (Hydrochlorothiazide Tablets) (Parke-Davis)
♦ Thorazine (Smith Kline & French) p 437, 1977
Throat Discs Throat Lozenges (Marion) p 1190
Thrombinar (Armour) p 613
Thrombostat (Parke-Davis) p 1574
Thylline & Thylline-GG Tablets (Schein) p 1828
Thymex (Standard Process)
Thypinone (Abbott Diagnostics Div.) p 3002
Thyrar (USV Pharmaceutical)
♦ Thyroid Strong Tablets (Marion) p 418, 1190
Thyroid Tablets (Lederle)
♦ Thyroid Tablets (Marion) p 418, 1190
♦ Thyrolar Tablets (USV Pharmaceutical) p 440, 2091
L-Thyroxine Tablets (Schein) p 1828
Thytropar (Armour) p 612
Tia-Doce Injectable Solution (Bart) p 685
Ticar (Beecham Laboratories) p 695
Tickle antiperspirant (Bristol-Myers Products)
♦ Tigan (Beecham Laboratories) p 406, 698
Tiject-20 (Mayrand)
♦ Timolide Tablets (Merck Sharp & Dohme) p 420, 1346
Timoptic Sterile Ophthalmic Solution (Merck Sharp & Dohme) p 1349
▣ Tinactin Cream 1% (Schering)
▣ Tinactin Jock Itch Cream 1% (Schering)
▣ Tinactin Jock Itch Spray Powder 1% (Schering)
▣ Tinactin Liquid 1% Aerosol (Schering)
▣ Tinactin Powder 1% (Schering)
▣ Tinactin Powder 1% Aerosol (Schering)
▣ Tinactin Solution 1% (Schering)
Tin-Ben Dispenser (Ferndale)
Tin-Co-Ben Dispenser (Ferndale)
Tindal Tablets (Ayerst)
Tinver Lotion (Barnes-Hind) p 685
Tis-U-Trap (Milex)
Titracid Tablets (Trimen)
Tobrex Solution & Ointment (Alcon Labs.)
Tocoferon 600 Tabs (Arlo)
Tofranil Ampuls (Geigy) p 969
♦ Tofranil Tablets (Geigy) p 411, 969
♦ Tofranil-PM Capsules (Geigy) p 411, 971
Tolbutamide Tablets (Danbury) p 887
Tolbutamide Tablets (Geneva) p 973
Tolbutamide Tablets (Schein) p 1828
♦ Tolectin Tablets & DS Capsules (McNeil Pharmaceutical) p 419, 1212
Tolfrinic Tablets (Ascher)
♦ Tolinase Tablets (Upjohn) p 441, 2139
Tono-B, Wafers (Vale)
♦ Tonocard (Merck Sharp & Dohme) p 421, 1351
▣ Topex 10% Benzoyl Peroxide Lotion Buffered Acne Medication (Personal Care)
▣ Topic Gel (Syntex)
♦ Topicort Emollient Cream 0.25% (Hoechst-Roussel) p 413, 1021
♦ Topicort Gel 0.05% (Hoechst-Roussel) p 413, 1021
♦ Topicort LP Emollient Cream 0.05% (Hoechst-Roussel) p 413, 1021
Topicort Ointment 0.25% (Hoechst-Roussel) p 1021
Topicycline (Norwich Eaton) p 1438
Topisporin (Pharmafair) p 1618
Tora Tablets (Reid-Provident, Direct Div.)
Tora-30 Capsules (Reid-Provident, Direct Div.)
Torecan Injection (Ampuls) (Boehringer Ingelheim) p 716
Torecan Suppositories (Boehringer Ingelheim) p 716
♦ Torecan Tablets (Boehringer Ingelheim) p 406, 716
Totacillin Capsules (Beecham Laboratories)
Totacillin For Oral Suspension (Beecham Laboratories)
Totacillin-N Injectable (Beecham Laboratories)
Total all-in-one hard contact lens solution (Allergan)
Total Formula (Vitaline) p 2148
♦ Trac Tabs 2X (Hyrex) p 413, 1025
Trace Elements (Armour)
  Chrometrace (Armour)
  Coppertrace (Armour)
  Mangatrace (Armour)
  Multitrace 5 (Armour)
  Multitrace Pediatric (Armour)
  Multitrace Solution & Concentrate (Armour)
  Selenitrace (Armour)
  Zinctrace (Armour)
TraceLyte & TraceLyte-II (Trace elements & electrolytes additive) (LyphoMed)
TraceLyte with Double Electrolytes & TraceLyte-II with Double Electrolytes (LyphoMed)
Tracilon (Savage)
Tral Filmtab Tablets (Abbott) p 568
Tral Gradumet Tablets (Abbott)
Tralmag Suspension (O'Neal, Jones & Feldman)

(♦ Shown in Product Identification Section) (▣ Described in PDR For Nonprescription Drugs) (Products without page numbers are not described)

Product Name Index

◆ Trancopal (Winthrop-Breon) p 444, 2232
Trandate Injection (Glaxo) p 983
◆ Trandate Tablets (Glaxo) p 412, 983
Tranmep Tablets (Reid-Provident Labs.)
Transact (Westwood) p 2183
◆ Transderm-Nitro Transdermal Therapeutic System (CIBA) p 410, 873
◆ Transderm Scōp Transdermal Therapeutic System (CIBA) p 409, 874
Transfer Needles, thin wall, 19 gauge (LyphoMed)
⊞ Transi-Lube (Youngs)
◆ Tranxene Capsules & Tablets (Abbott) p 404, 568
◆ Tranxene-SD (Abbott) p 404, 568
◆ Tranxene-SD Half Strength (Abbott) p 404, 568
Trates Granucaps (Reid-Provident, Direct Div.)
Travase Ointment (Flint) p 411, 952
⊞ Traumacal (Mead Johnson Nutritional)
Trecator-SC (Ives) p 1031
Trendar Premenstrual Tablets (Whitehall)
◆ Trental (Hoechst-Roussel) p 413, 1022
Triacet Cream (Lemmon)
Triad & Triad 650 (UAD Labs.)
Triafed Syrup & Tablets (Schein) p 1828
Triafed-C Expectorant (Schein) p 1828
Triamcinair Cream (Pharmafair) p 1618
Triamcinolone Tablets (Danbury) p 887
Triamcinolone Tablets (Geneva) p 973
Triamcinolone Tablets (Schein) p 1828
Triamcinolone Acetonide Cream 0.5% (Fougera) p 953
Triamcinolone Acetonide Cream (Geneva) p 973
Triamcinolone Acetonide Cream (Schein) p 1828
Triamcinolone Acetonide Cream & Ointment 0.025% & 0.1% (Fougera) p 953
Triamcinolone Acetonide Cream & Ointment (Pharmaderm) p 1617
⊞ Triaminic Allergy Tablets (Dorsey Laboratories)
⊞ Triaminic Chewables (Dorsey Laboratories)
Triaminic Cold Syrup (Dorsey Laboratories) p 911
Triaminic Cold Tablets (Dorsey Laboratories) p 911
Triaminic Expectorant (Dorsey Laboratories) p 911
Triaminic Expectorant DH (Dorsey Laboratories)
Triaminic Expectorant w/Codeine (Dorsey Laboratories) p 911
Triaminic Juvelets (Dorsey Laboratories) p 912
Triaminic Oral Infant Drops (Dorsey Laboratories) p 912
Triaminic TR Tablets (Timed Release) (Dorsey Laboratories) p 912
Triaminic-DM Cough Formula (Dorsey Laboratories) p 913
Triaminic-12 Tablets (Dorsey Laboratories) p 913
⊞ Triaminicin Tablets (Dorsey Laboratories)
Triaminicol Multi-Symptom Cold Syrup (Dorsey Laboratories) p 913
Triaminicol Multi-Symptom Cold Tablets (Dorsey Laboratories) p 914
Triamolone "40" Injectable (O'Neal, Jones & Feldman)
Triamonide "40" Injectable (O'Neal, Jones & Feldman)
◆ Triavil Tablets (Merck Sharp & Dohme) p 420, 1354
Trichlorex Tablets (Lannett)
Trichlormethiazide Tablets (Geneva) p 973
Trichlormethiazide Tablets (Schein) p 1828
Trichotine Liquid, Vaginal Douche (Reed & Carnrick) p 1637
Trichotine Powder, Vaginal Douche (Reed & Carnrick) p 1637
Tri-Cone Capsules (Glaxo) p 986
Tridesilon Creme 0.05% (Miles Pharmaceuticals) p 1412
Tridesilon Ointment 0.05% (Miles Pharmaceuticals) p 1413
Tridil (American Critical Care) p 597
◆ Tridione (Abbott) p 404, 570
◆ Tridione Dulcet Tablets (Abbott) p 404
Trifed Tablets & Syrup (Geneva) p 973
Trifluoperazine Tablets (Geneva) p 973
Trifluoperazine Tablets (Schein) p 1828
Trigesic Tablets (Squibb)
◆ TriHemic 600 (Lederle) p 416, 1119
Trihexyphenidyl HCl Tablets (Danbury) p 887
Tri-Immunol (Lederle) p 1119
Trikates Oral Solution (Lilly)
◆ Trilafon Tablets, Repetabs Tablets, Concentrate & Injection (Schering) p 435, 1888
Trilax (Drug Industries) p 915
◆ Trilisate Tablets/Liquid (Purdue Frederick) p 427, 1627
Trilycal-12 (Medical Products)
Trimcaps (Mayrand) p 1196
Trimedine Expectorant (Trimen)
Trimethobenzamide HCl Suppositories (Schein) p 1828
Trimethoprim Tablets (Biocraft) p 705
Trimo-San (Milex)
◆ Trimox Capsules & for Oral Suspension (Squibb) p 438, 2025
◆ Trimpex Tablets (Roche) p 430, 1706
Trimstat Tablets (Laser) p 1072
Trimtabs (Mayrand) p 1197

◆ Trinalin Repetabs Tablets (Schering) p 435, 1890
⊞ Trind (Mead Johnson Nutritional)
Trind-DM (Mead Johnson Nutritional)
Tri-Norinyl 21-Day Tablets (Syntex) p 440, 2052
Tri-Norinyl 28-Day Tablets (Syntex) p 440, 2052
◆ Trinsicon/Trinsicon M Capsules (Glaxo) p 412, 986
Trioval Tablets (Vale)
Tripelennamine HCl Tablets (Danbury) p 887
Triphed Tablets (Lemmon)
Triple Sulfa Vaginal Cream (Fougera) p 953
Triple Sulfa Vaginal Cream (Pharmaderm)
Triple Sulfa Vaginal Cream (Schein) p 1828
Triple Sulfoid Tablets (Vale)
◆ Triple X (Youngs)
Triplevite w/Fluoride Drops (Geneva) p 973
Tripodrine Tablets (Danbury) p 887
Triprolidine HCl & Pseudoephedrine HCl Syrup (Pharmafair) p 1618
Triprolidine Hydrochloride & Pseudoephedrine Hydrochloride Syrup, Tablets (Roxane) p 1788
◆ Trisoralen Tablets (Elder) p 411, 937
Tristoject (Mayrand)
Tri-Thalmic Ophthalmic Solution (Schein) p 1828
Triva Combination (Boyle) p 726
Triva Douche Powder (Boyle) p 726
Triva Jel (Boyle) p 726
Tri-Vi-Flor 1.0 mg Vitamins w/Fluoride Chewable Tablets (Mead Johnson Nutritional) p 1246
Tri-Vi-Flor 0.25 mg Vitamins w/Fluoride Drops (Mead Johnson Nutritional) p 1247
Tri-Vi-Flor 0.5 mg Vitamins w/Fluoride Drops (Mead Johnson Nutritional) p 1247
Tri-Vi-Flor 0.25 mg Vitamins w/Iron & Fluoride Drops (Mead Johnson Nutritional) p 1248
⊞ Tri-Vi-Sol Vitamins, Chewable Tablets & Drops (Mead Johnson Nutritional)
⊞ Tri-Vi-Sol Vitamins w/Iron, Drops (Mead Johnson Nutritional)
Trobicin Sterile Powder (Upjohn) p 2141
Trofan Tablets (Upsher-Smith) p 2145
Tronolane Anesthetic Hemorrhoidal Cream (Ross) p 1781
Tronolane Anesthetic Hemorrhoidal Suppositories (Ross) p 1781
Tronothane Hydrochloride (Abbott) p 570
Troph-Iron Liquid & Tablets (Smith Kline & French)
Trophite Liquid & Tablets (Smith Kline & French)
Trymex Cream & Ointment (Savage) p 1827
Tryptacin (Arther) p 614
Trysul (Savage) p 1827
Tuberculin, Mono-Vacc Test (O.T.) (Merieux) p 3013
Tuberculin, Old, Tine Test (Rosenthal) (Lederle) p 3010
Tuberculin Purified Protein Derivative Tine Test (PPD) (Lederle) p 3011
Tubersol (Tuberculin Purified Protein Derivative [Mantoux]) (Squibb/Connaught) p 2033
◆ Tubex (Wyeth) p 445, 2288
◆ Tubex Hypodermic Syringe (Wyeth) p 445
Tubocurarine Chloride (Lilly) p 1175
Tucks Cream (Parke-Davis) p 1575
Tucks Ointment (Parke-Davis) p 1575
Tucks Premoistened Pads (Parke-Davis) p 1575
Tucks Take-Alongs (Parke-Davis)
Tuinal (Lilly) p 417, 1176
⊞ Tums Antacid Tablets, Regular & Extra Strength (Norcliff Thayer)
Turbinaire (see Decadron Phosphate Turbinaire) (Merck Sharp & Dohme)
Turgasept Aerosol (Ayerst)
Tuss-Ade Timed Capsules (Schein) p 1828
◆ Tussagesic Tablets & Suspension (Dorsey Laboratories)
Tussar DM (USV Pharmaceutical) p 2091
Tussar SF (USV Pharmaceutical) p 2092
Tussar-2 (USV Pharmaceutical) p 2092
◆ Tussend Expectorant (Merrell Dow) p 421, 1394
◆ Tussend Liquid & Tablets (Merrell Dow) p 421, 1393
Tussionex Tablets, Capsules & Suspension (Pennwalt) p 1585
◆ Tussi-Organidin (Wallace) p 442, 2171
◆ Tussi-Organidin DM (Wallace) p 442, 2171
Tussirex Sugar-Free (Scot-Tussin) p 1897
Tussirex Syrup (Scot-Tussin) p 1897
Tuss-Ornade Liquid (Smith Kline & French) p 1980
◆ Tuss-Ornade Spansule Capsules (Smith Kline & French) p 437, 1981
Tuzon Tablets (Reid-Provident, Direct Div.)
Tuzyme Tablets (Reid-Provident, Direct Div.)
Twin-K (Boots) p 724
Twin-K-Cl (Boots) p 725
TwoCal HN (Ross) p 1781
Two-Dyne Capsules (Hyrex) p 1025
Tycopan Pulvules (Lilly)
◆ Tylenol acetaminophen Children's Chewable Tablets, Elixir, Infants' Drops (McNeil Consumer Products) p 418, 1199

Tylenol, Extra-Strength, acetaminophen Liquid Pain Reliever (McNeil Consumer Products) p 1200
◆ Tylenol, Extra-Strength, acetaminophen Tablets, Capsules & Caplets (McNeil Consumer Products) p 418, 1200
◆ Tylenol, Junior-Strength, acetaminophen Swallowable Tablets (McNeil Consumer Products) p 418
◆ Tylenol, Maximum-Strength, Sinus Medication Tablets & Capsules (McNeil Consumer Products) p 418, 1201
◆ Tylenol, Regular Strength, acetaminophen Tablets & Capsules (McNeil Consumer Products) p 418, 1199
◆ Tylenol w/Codeine Elixir (McNeil Pharmaceutical) p 419, 1214
◆ Tylenol w/Codeine Tablets, Capsules (McNeil Pharmaceutical) p 419, 1214
Tylosterone, Tablets (Lilly)
◆ Tylox Capsules (McNeil Pharmaceutical) p 419, 1215
Tympagesic Otic Solution (Adria) p 587
Tymtran Injection (Adria)
Typhoid Vaccine (Wyeth) p 2246
Tyson Amino-ST (Tyson)
Tyson GABA (Tyson)
Tyson L-Alanine Capsules & Powder (Tyson)
Tyson L-Arginine Capsules & Powder (Tyson)
Tyson L-Aspartic Acid Capsules & Powder (Tyson)
Tyson L-Citrulline Capsules & Powder (Tyson)
Tyson L-Cysteine HCl Capsules & Powder (Tyson)
Tyson L-Cystine Capsules & Powder (Tyson)
Tyson L-Dopa (Tyson)
Tyson L-Glutamic Acid Capsules & Powder (Tyson)
Tyson L-Glutamine Caps & Powder (Tyson)
Tyson L-Glutathione (Tyson)
Tyson L-Glycine Capsules & Powder (Tyson)
Tyson L-Histidine Capsules & Powder (Tyson)
Tyson L-Isoleucine Capsules & Powder (Tyson)
Tyson L-Leucine Capsules & Powder (Tyson)
Tyson L-Lysine Powder & Caps (Tyson)
Tyson L-Methionine Powder & Caps (Tyson)
Tyson L-Phenylalanine Capsules & Powder (Tyson)
Tyson L-Proline Capsules & Powder (Tyson)
Tyson L-Serine Capsules & Powder (Tyson)
Tyson L-Threonine Powder & Caps (Tyson)
Tyson L-Tryptophan Capsules & Powder (Tyson)
Tyson L-Tyrosine Capsules & Powder (Tyson)
Tyson L-Valine Powder (Tyson)
Tyzine (Key Pharmaceuticals) p 1056
Tyzine Pediatric Nasal Drops (Key Pharmaceuticals)

U

UAD Cream & Cream Lotion (UAD Labs.)
UAD Lotion Forte (UAD Labs.)
UAD Pred (UAD Labs.)
Ulcinal Tablets (U.S. Ethicals)
Ultimate One (Marlyn)
Ultra Ban Aerosol antiperspirant (Bristol-Myers Products)
Ultra Ban roll-on (Bristol-Myers Products)
Ultra Ban Solid antiperspirant/deodorant (Bristol-Myers Products)
Ultracaine Injection (Ulmer)
◆ Ultracef Capsules, Tablets & Oral Suspension (Bristol) p 407, 754
Ultra Derm Moisturizer (Baker/Cummins)
Ultralente Insulin (Extended Insulin Zinc Suspension USP) (Squibb-Novo) p 2034
Ultralente Purified Beef Extended Insulin Zinc Suspension (Squibb-Novo) p 2034
⊞ Ultra Mide 25 Lotion (Baker/Cummins)
Unguentum Bossi (Doak)
Unibase (Parke-Davis)
⊞ Unicap Capsules & Tablets (Upjohn)
⊞ Unicap Chewable Tablets (Upjohn)
⊞ Unicap M Tablets (Upjohn)
⊞ Unicap Plus Iron Tablets (Upjohn)
⊞ Unicap Senior Tablets (Upjohn)
⊞ Unicap T Tablets (Upjohn)
Unifast Unicelles (Reid-Provident Labs.)
Unilax Tablets (Ascher)
◆ Unipen Injection, Capsules, Powder for Oral Solution, & Tablets (Wyeth) p 445, 2290
◆ Uniphyl 200 mg Tablets (Purdue Frederick) p 427, 1627
◆ Uniphyl 400 mg Tablets (Purdue Frederick) p 427, 1629
◆ Unipres Tablets (Reid-Provident Labs.) p 428, 1640
Unisol (CooperVision)
Unisol 4 (CooperVision)
Unisom Nighttime Sleep-Aid (Leeming) p 1119
Unproco Capsules (Reid-Provident, Direct Div.)
Upjohn Vitamin E Capsules, 200 I.U. (Upjohn)
Uracil Mustard Capsules (Upjohn)
Ureacin Lotion & Creme (Pedinol) p 1581
Ureaphil (Abbott)
◆ Urecholine Injection & Tablets (Merck Sharp & Dohme) p 421, 1356

(◆ Shown in Product Identification Section)   (⊞ Described in PDR For Nonprescription Drugs)   (Products without page numbers are not described)

Product Name Index

◆ Urex (Riker) p 428, 1645
Urinary #2 Tablets (Lemmon)
Urised Tablets (Webcon) p 2173
Urisedamine Tablets (Webcon)
◆ Urispas (Smith Kline & French) p 437, 1981
Urithol Tablets (O'Neal, Jones & Feldman)
◆ Urobiotic-250 (Roerig) p 431, 1744
Uroblue Tablets (Geneva) p 973
Uro-KP-Neutral (Star) p 2035
Urolene Blue (Star) p 2035
Uro-Phosphate Tablets (Poythress) p 1619
◆ Uroqid-Acid Tablets (Beach) p 405, 687
◆ Uroqid-Acid No. 2 Tablets (Beach) p 405, 687
Uroseptic D-S Tablets (Kramer)
▣ Ursinus Inlay-Tabs (Dorsey Laboratories)
Uticillin VK Tablets (Upjohn)
◆ Uticort Cream, Gel, Lotion & Ointment (Parke-Davis) p 426, 1575

V

V-Applicators for Elase Ointment (Parke-Davis)
V-Cillin K for Oral Solution & Tablets (Lilly) p 1178
VG Capsules (Medical Products) p 1256
V-M Capsules (Vale)
Vagimide Cream (Legere) p 1120
Vaginal Sulfa Suppositories (Schein) p 1828
Vagisec Medicated Liquid Douche Concentrate (Schmid) p 1896
Vagisec Plus Suppositories (Schmid) p 1896
Vagisulf Cream (Kramer)
Vagitrol Vaginal Cream (Lemmon)
Valacet Tablets (Vale)
Valadol Tablets, Liquid (Squibb)
Valax Tablets (Vale)
Valcaine Ointment (Vale)
Valcreme Lotion (Vale)
Valdeine Tablets (Vale)
Valdrene Expectorant Syrup (Vale)
Valdrene Tablets (Vale)
Valergen (Hyrex)
Valertest #2 (Hyrex)
Valisone Cream 0.1% (Schering) p 1892
Valisone Lotion 0.1% (Schering) p 1892
Valisone Ointment 0.1% (Schering) p 1892
Valisone Reduced Strength Cream 0.01% (Schering) p 1892
◆ Valium Injectable (Roche Products) p 430, 1721
◆ Valium Tablets (Roche Products) p 430, 1723
◆ Valium Tel-E-Ject (Roche Products) p 430
Valmid Pulvules (Dista) p 410, 908
Valpin 50 (Du Pont) p 928
Valrelease Capsules (Roche) p 430, 1707
Val-Tep Tablets (Vale)
Vancenase Nasal Inhaler (Schering) p 435, 1893
◆ Vanceril Inhaler (Schering) p 435, 1894
Vancocin HCl, for Oral Solution (Lilly) p 1178
Vancocin HCl, Vials (Lilly) p 1177
Vanodonnal Timed (Drug Industries)
Vanoxide Acne Lotion (Dermik)
Vanoxide-HC Acne Lotion (Dermik) p 891
Vanquish (Glenbrook) p 998
▣ Vanseb Cream Dandruff Shampoo (Herbert)
▣ Vanseb Lotion Dandruff Shampoo (Herbert)
▣ Vanseb-T Cream Tar Shampoo (Herbert)
▣ Vanseb-T Lotion Tar Shampoo (Herbert)
Vansil Capsules (Pfipharmecs)
Vapo-Iso Solution (Fisons) p 943
Vaponefrin Solution (Fisons) p 943
▣ Vaposteam (Vicks Health Care)
Varidin Capsules (Medical Products)
Vari-Flavors Flavor Pacs (Ross) p 1782
Varisan Injection (Arlo)
Varisan Tabs (Arlo)
Vasculin (Standard Process)
Vaso-80 Unicelles (Reid-Provident Labs.)
VasoClear Ophthalmic Decongestant Eye Drops (CooperVision)
VasoClear A Decongestant Astrigent Lubricating Eye Drops (CooperVision)
Vasocon Regular Ophthalmic Solution (CooperVision)
Vasocon-A Ophthalmic Solution (CooperVision)
◆ Vasodilan (Mead Johnson Pharmaceutical) p 419, 1255
Vasoflex Tablets (Kramer)
Vasolin Drops (Kramer)
Vasosulf Ophthalmic Solution (CooperVision)
Vasoxyl Injection (Burroughs Wellcome) p 819
▣ Vatronol Nose Drops (Vicks Health Care)
Veetids for Oral Solution (Squibb) p 2026
Veetids Tablets (Squibb) p 438, 2026
Vehicle/N (Neutrogena) (Neutrogena) p 1422
Vehicle/N Mild (Neutrogena) (Neutrogena) p 1422
Velban (Lilly) p 1179
◆ Velosef Capsules (Squibb) p 438, 2027
Velosef for Infusion (Sodium-Free) (Squibb) p 2029
Velosef for Injection (Squibb) p 2030
Velosef for Oral Suspension (Squibb) p 2027
Velosulin (Nordisk-USA) p 1423
Veltane Tablets & Expectorant (Lannett)
◆ Ventolin Inhaler (Glaxo) p 412, 987
◆ Ventolin Inhaler Refill (Glaxo) p 412
◆ Ventolin Tablets (Glaxo) p 412, 988
VePesid Injection (Bristol-Myers Oncology) p 767

Verazinc Capsules (O'Neal, Jones & Feldman)
Vercyte Tablets (Abbott)
◆ Verin (Verex) p 442, 2146
◆ Vermox Chewable Tablets (Janssen) p 413, 1043
Vernate Injection (Reid-Provident, Direct Div.)
Verr-Canth (C & M) p 828
Verrex (C & M) p 828
Verrusol (C & M) p 828
Versapen Oral Suspension (Bristol) p 755
Versapen Pediatric Drops (Bristol) p 755
◆ Versapen-K Capsules (Bristol) p 407, 755
Versa-Quat (Ulmer)
Verucid Gel (Ulmer)
Vesprin Injection (Squibb)
Vesprin Tablets (Squibb)
Vi-Aqua Capsules (Armour)
Vi-Aqua Forte Capsules (Armour)
Vi-Aquamin Forte Capsules (Armour)
Vibramycin Calcium Syrup (Pfizer) p 1610
◆ Vibramycin Hyclate Capsules (Pfizer) p 426, 1610
Vibramycin Hyclate Intravenous (Pfizer) p 1611
Vibramycin Monohydrate for Oral Suspension (Pfizer) p 1610
◆ Vibra-Tabs Film Coated Tablets (Pfizer) p 426, 1610
Vicef (Drug Industries)
▣ Vicks Cough Silencers Cough Drops (Vicks Health Care)
▣ Vicks Cough Syrup (Vicks Health Care)
▣ Vicks Inhaler (Vicks Health Care)
▣ Vicks Throat Lozenges (Vicks Health Care)
▣ Vicks Vaporub (Vicks Health Care)
◆ Vicodin (Knoll) p 414, 1068
◆ Vicon Forte Capsules (Glaxo) p 412, 989
◆ Vicon-C Capsules (Glaxo) p 412, 989
◆ Vicon-Plus Capsules (Glaxo) p 412, 989
◆ Vi-Daylin ADC Drops (Ross) p 1782
◆ Vi-Daylin Chewable (Ross) p 432, 1784
◆ Vi-Daylin Drops (Ross) p 1782
◆ Vi-Daylin Liquid (Ross) p 1784
◆ Vi-Daylin Plus Iron ADC Drops (Ross) p 1784
◆ Vi-Daylin + Iron Chewable (Ross) p 432, 1784
◆ Vi-Daylin Plus Iron Drops (Ross) p 1783
◆ Vi-Daylin Plus Iron Liquid (Ross) p 1784
◆ Vi-Daylin/F ADC Drops (Ross) p 1782
◆ Vi-Daylin/F ADC + Iron Drops (Ross) p 1782
◆ Vi-Daylin/F Chewable (Ross) p 432, 1784
◆ Vi-Daylin/F Drops (Ross) p 1783
◆ Vi-Daylin/F + Iron Chewable (Ross) p 432, 1783
◆ Vi-Daylin/F + Iron Drops (Ross) p 1783
Vigoril 3 Tabs (Arlo)
Vigran plus Iron Tablets (Squibb)
Vigran Tablets (Squibb)
Vio-Bec (Rowell)
Vio-Bec Forte (Rowell) p 1788
Vioform (CIBA) p 876
Vioform-Hydrocortisone (CIBA) p 876
Viokase Powder (Robins) p 1665
Viokase Tablets (Robins) p 1665
Viopan-T Tablets (Trimen) p 2067
Vio-Pramosone Cream (Ferndale)
Vio-Pramosone Lotion (Ferndale)
◆ Vi-Penta F Chewables (Roche) p 430, 1708
Vi-Penta F Infant Drops (Roche) p 1709
Vi-Penta F Multivitamin Drops (Roche) p 1709
Vi-Penta Infant Drops (Roche) p 1710
Vi-Penta Multivitamin Drops (Roche) p 1710
Vira-A for Infusion (Parke-Davis) p 1576
◆ Vira-A Ophthalmic Ointment, 3% (Parke-Davis) p 426, 1578
Viranol (American Dermal) p 600
Virilon (Star) p 2035
Viro-Med Liquid (Whitehall)
Viro-Med Tablets (Whitehall)
Vioptic Ophthalmic Solution (Burroughs Wellcome) p 820
Visidex II Reagent Strips (Ames) p 3006
Visine A.C. Eye Drops (Leeming)
Visine Eye Drops (Leeming)
Visken (Sandoz Pharmaceutical Div.) p 433, 1820
Vistaject-25 & Vistaject-50 (Mayrand)
◆ Vistaril Capsules and Oral Suspension (Pfizer) p 427, 1612
Vistaril Intramuscular Solution (Pfipharmecs) p 1598
Vitabese Capsules (Legere) p 1120
Vita-Bob Capsules (Scot-Tussin)
Vitacoms Capsules (U.S. Ethicals)
Vitadye Lotion (Elder) p 938
Vitafol Tablets (Everett) p 942
Vita-Kaps Filmtab (Abbott)
Vita-Kaps M Filmtab (Abbott)
Vital/High Nitrogen (Ross) p 1785
Vitalis clear gel (Bristol-Myers Products)
Vitalis Dry Texture hair groom (Bristol-Myers Products)
Vitalis hair groom liquid (Bristol-Myers Products)
Vitalis Regular Hold hair spray (Bristol-Myers Products)
Vitalis Super Hold hair spray (Bristol-Myers Products)
Vitamin A + Vitamin D Ointment (Fougera) p 953
Vita-Natal Capsules (Scot-Tussin)
Vita-Numonyl Injectable (Lambda) p 1071
Vita-Plus B 12, 10 ml. Vials, 1000 mcgm./ml. (Scot-Tussin)

Vita-Plus E Capsules Natural 400 I.U. (Scot-Tussin)
Vita-Plus G (geriatric) Capsules (Scot-Tussin)
Vita-Plus H (Scot-Tussin)
Vita-Plus H (hematinic) Sugar-Free, Liquid (Scot-Tussin)
Vitormains (Hauck)
Vitron-C (Fisons)
Vitron-C-Plus (Fisons)
◆ Vivactil Tablets (Merck Sharp & Dohme) p 421, 1357
Vivikon I.M. (Brown)
Vivonex Acutrol Enteral Feeding System (Norwich Eaton) p 1441
Vivonex Delivery System (Norwich Eaton) p 1441
Vivonex Flavor Packets (Norwich Eaton) p 1441
Vivonex High Nitrogen Diet (Norwich Eaton) p 1439
Vivonex Jejunostomy Kit (Norwich Eaton) p 1441
Vivonex Moss Tube (Norwich Eaton) p 1441
Vivonex Standard Diet (Norwich Eaton) p 1438
Vivonex T.E.N. (Norwich Eaton) p 1441
◆ Vi-Zac Capsules (Glaxo) p 412, 990
Vlemasque (Dermik) p 891
◆ Vleminckx' Solution (Ulmer)
Volu-Feed (Ross) p 1777
◆ Vontrol Tablets (Smith Kline & French) p 437, 1981
◆ VōSol HC Otic Solution (Wallace) p 442, 2171
◆ VōSol Otic Solution (Wallace) p 442, 2171
Vytone Cream (Dermik) p 891

W

W-T Lotion (Adria)
◆ Wallette Pill Dispenser (Syntex) p 440
WANS (Webcon Anti-Nausea Suppretes) (Webcon) p 2173
Warexin (Guardian)
Warfarin Sodium Tablets (Schein) p 1828
◆ Wart-Off (Pfipharmecs) p 426, 1599
Wehless Capsules 35mg. (Hauck)
Wehless-105 Timecelles (Hauck) p 1001
Wehvert Tablets (Hauck)
Wellcovorin Injection (Burroughs Wellcome) p 821
◆ Wellcovorin Tablets (Burroughs Wellcome) p 408, 821
Westcort Cream 0.2% (Westwood) p 2183
Westcort Ointment 0.2% (Westwood) p 2183
Wet-N-Soak wetting and soaking solution for hard contact lenses & Polycon & Paraperm O_2 gas permeable lenses (Allergan)
Whirl-Sol (Sween) p 2049
Whitfield's Ointment (Fougera) p 953
Wide-Seal Diaphragm (Milex)
◆ Wigraine Tablets & Suppositories (Organon) p 422, 1451
◆ Wigraine-PB Suppositories (Organon) p 422, 1451
◆ Wigrettes (Organon) p 422, 1451
▣ WinGel Liquid & Tablets (Winthrop Consumer Products)
◆ Winstrol (Winthrop-Breon) p 444, 2232
Wolfina "50" & "100" Tablets (O'Neal, Jones & Feldman)
Wyamine Sulfate in Tubex (Wyeth) p 2288
Wyamycin E Liquid (Wyeth) p 2292
◆ Wyamycin S Tablets (Wyeth) p 445, 2292
◆ Wyanoids Hemorrhoidal Suppositories (Wyeth) p 445, 2293
Wycillin (Wyeth) p 2293
Wycillin in Tubex (Wyeth) p 2288
◆ Wycillin & Probenecid Tablets & Injection (Wyeth) p 2295
Wydase Injection (Wyeth) p 2296
Wydase, Stabilized Solution (Wyeth)
◆ Wygesic Tablets (Wyeth) p 445, 2297
◆ Wymox Capsules & Oral Suspension (Wyeth) p 445, 2298
◆ Wytensin Tablets (Wyeth) p 445, 2299
Wyvac Rabies Vaccine (Wyeth) p 2246

X

X-Otag Injection (Reid-Provident, Direct Div.)
X-Otag S.R. Tablets (Reid-Provident, Direct Div.)
X-Prep Bowel Evacuant Kit #1 (Gray)
X-Prep Bowel Evacuant Kit #2 (Gray)
X-Prep Liquid (Gray) p 1000
▣ Xseb Shampoo (Baker/Cummins)
▣ Xseb-T Shampoo (Baker/Cummins)
Xtracare II (Sween) p 2049
X-Trozine Capsules & Tablets (Rexar) p 1641
X-Trozine LA-105 Capsules (Rexar) p 1641
◆ Xanax Tablets (Upjohn) p 441, 2142
Xerac (Persōn & Covey) p 1588
Xerac AC (Persōn & Covey) p 1588
Xerac BP5 & Xerac BP10 (Persōn & Covey) p 1588
◆ Xylocaine 2% Jelly (Astra) p 629
▣ Xylocaine 2.5% Ointment (Astra)
◆ Xylocaine 5% Ointment (Astra) p 629
◆ Xylocaine 10% Oral Spray (Astra) p 630

(◆ Shown in Product Identification Section)   (▣ Described in PDR For Nonprescription Drugs)   (Products without page numbers are not described)

Product Name Index

Xylocaine Hydrochloride, Xylocaine Hydrochloride with Epinephrine 1:100,000, & Xylocaine Hydrochloride with Epinephrine 1:200,000 (Astra) p 623
Xylocaine Solution for Ventricular Arrhythmias-Intravenous Injection or Continuous Infusion; or Intramuscular Injection (Astra) p 625
Xylocaine 1.5% Solution with Dextrose 7.5% (Astra) p 629
Xylocaine 4% Sterile Solution (Astra) p 627
Xylocaine 5% Solution with Glucose 7.5% (Astra) p 629
Xylocaine 4% Topical Solution (Astra) p 628
Xylocaine 2% Viscous Solution (Astra) p 630
Xylo-Pfan (Adria)

Y

YF-VAX (Yellow Fever Vaccine)(Live, 17D Virus, Avian Leukosis-Free, Stabilized) (Squibb/Connaught) p 2033
Yellow Mercuric Oxide Ophthalmic Ointment 1% & 2% (Fougera) p 953
Yocon (Palisades Pharm.) p 1476
◆ Yodoxin (Glenwood) p 412, 999
Yohimex Tablets (Kramer) p 1069
Yohimex P-Z (Dual Pack) Tablets (Kramer)
Yutopar Intravenous Injection (Astra) p 632
Yutopar Tablets (Astra) p 632

Z

⊞ Z-Bec Tablets (Robins)
Z-Pro-C Tablets (Person & Covey)
Zanosar Sterile Powder (Upjohn)
Zantac Injection (Glaxo) p 990
◆ Zantac Tablets (Glaxo) p 412, 991
◆ Zarontin Capsules (Parke-Davis) p 426, 1579
Zarontin Syrup (Parke-Davis) p 1579
◆ Zaroxolyn (Pennwalt) p 426, 1586
Zeasorb Powder (Stiefel)
◆ Zenate Tablets (Reid-Provident Labs.) p 428, 1640
Zentinic Pulvules (Lilly)
Zentron Chewable Tablets (Lilly)
Zentron Liquid (Lilly)
Zephiran Chloride 1:750 (Winthrop-Breon) p 2233
Zephiran Chloride Spray (Winthrop-Breon) p 2233
Zephiran Chloride Tinted Tincture (Winthrop-Breon) p 2233
Zephiran Towelettes (Winthrop-Breon)
Zephrex Tablets (Bock) p 706
Zephrex-LA Tablets (Bock) p 706
Zetar Emulsion (Dermik) p 892
Zetar Shampoo (Dermik) p 892
Zinacef (Glaxo) p 993
Zinc Oxide Ointment (Fougera) p 953
◆ Zinc-220 Capsules (Alto) p 404, 589
Zincfrin (Alcon Labs.)
Zinckel-220 Tablets (Kramer)
⊞ Zincon Dandruff Shampoo, Improved Richer Formula (Lederle)
Zinctrace (Armour) p 612
Zincvit Capsules (RAM Laboratories) p 1632
Ziradryl Lotion (Parke-Davis) p 1580
Zolyse (Alcon Labs.)
Zone-A Lotion 1% (UAD Labs.) p 2069
◆ Zorprin (Boots) p 406, 725
Zovirax Ointment 5% (Burroughs Wellcome) p 822
Zovirax Sterile Powder (Burroughs Wellcome) p 823
◆ Zyloprim (Burroughs Wellcome) p 408, 825
Zymacap Capsules (Upjohn)
Zypan Tablets (Standard Process) p 2035

(◆ Shown in Product Identification Section) (⊞ Described in PDR For Nonprescription Drugs) (Products without page numbers are not described)

Discontinued Products

Listed below are products discontinued by manufacturers this past year. Please check the Product Name Index to determine if marketing has been assumed by another manufacturer.

Part 2

Adria Laboratories Inc.
  Thi-Cine Capsules
Allergan Pharmaceuticals Inc.
  Pre-Sert
Arlo Interamerica Corp.
  Duralina Vial
  Fermolate Vial
  Tineasol Lotion
Beecham Laboratories
  C M w/Paregoric
  Celbenin for Injection
  Corrective Mixture
  Cotrol-D Tablets
  Dasikon Capsules
  Guaifenesin Syrup
  Livitamin Prenatal Tablets
  Thalfed Tablets
Berlex Laboratories, Inc.
  Aminodur Dura-Tabs
  Enuretrol Tablets
  L-Glutavite Capsules
  Stomaseptine Douche Powder
  Therapav Capsules
  Vi-Twel Injection
Beutlich, Inc.
  Mevatinic-C Tablets
  Pregent Tablets
Bio-Craft Laboratories, Inc.
  Penicillin G Potassium Solution
    250,000 u/5 ml., 400,000 u/5 ml.
Bock Pharmacal Company
  Hemaspan-FA Capsules
  Nisolone-40 Injectable
  Poly-Histine-DX Syrup
Boyle & Company
  Glytinic Liquid, 16 oz.
Burroughs-Wellcome
  A.P.C. w/Codeine Tablets TABLOID Brand
    15 mg., No. 2 Bottle of 100,1000
  ACTIFED-C Expectorant
    (now ACTIFED w/Codeine Cough Syrup)
  SEPTRA Tablets, Bottle of 1000
C & M Pharmacal, Inc.
  Neomark
  Sebisol
  Soltex
Dorsey Laboratories
  Pabirin Buffered Tablets
Everett Laboratories
  Folic Acid Tablets
Fisons Corporation
  Somophylline-CRT 50 mg.
  Somophylline-T 50 mg.

Geneva Generics
  Carisoprodol Compound Tablets
  Chlorpheniramine Maleate, 12 mg., T.D. Capsules
  Pseudoephedrine, 120 mg., S.R. Capsules
Geriatric Pharmaceutical Corp.
  Bilezyme-Plus Tablets
  Stimulax Capsules
Glaxo Inc.
  Renalgin Tablets
  Tri-Cone Plus
W.E. Hauck, Inc.
  Cydel Capsules, 200 mg.
  Dolacet Tablets (Tablets Only)
  Orapav Timecelles
  Palmiron-Forte Tablets
Ives Laboratories Inc.
  Isordil w/Phenobarbital
Kenwood Laboratories, Inc.
  Cebral Capsules
  Papavatral L.A. Capsules
  Papavatral L.A. w/Phenobarbital Capsules
Laser Inc.
  Theostat Tablets, 100 mg.,200 mg.
  Theospan-SR Capsules, 65 mg.
Lederle Laboratories
  Folvron folic acid and iron capsules
Lemmon Company
  Quaalude
McGregor Pharmaceuticals Inc.
  Rhinafed Capsules
  Rhinafed-Ex Capsules
  Rhindecon-G Capsules
  Unitinic Tablets
Mead Johnson Pharmaceutical Division
  Mucomyst w/Isoproterenol
Medical Products Panamericana, Inc.
  Flebomedic
  Folisplen B-12 Capsules, Injection
Medicone Company
  DioMedicone, 50's
Merieux Institute, Inc.
  Imovax Rabies I.D., Rabies Vaccine
Miles Laboratories, Inc.
  Alka-2
  One-A-Day Enriched B Complex
  One-A-Day Enriched C
  One-A-Day Enriched E
  One-A-Day Plus Iron
  Vitapace
Mission Pharmacal Company
  Dilax 100
Norwich Eaton Pharmaceuticals, Inc.
  Comhist Liquid
  Ivadantin

  Sarenin
  Vivonex Decompression Tube
  Vivonex Tungsten Tip Feeding Tube
  Vivonex Tungsten Tip Feeding Tube Stylet
Person & Covey Inc.
  Solbar
Reid-Provident Laboratories, Inc.
  Dentavite Drops
  Suladyne Tablets
  Vasotrate Tablets
A.H. Robins Company, Inc.
  Dimetane Expectorant
  Dimetane Expectorant-DC
  Robicillin VK for Oral Solution
Roche Laboratories
  Roniacol Elixir
  Roniacol Tablets
  Roniacol Timespan Tablets
Roerig
  Cartrax 10 mg., 20 mg.
  Tao Oral Suspension
Schering Corporation
  Chlor-Trimeton 100 mg/ml., Injection
  Coriforte Capsules
  Dismiss Douche
  Gitaligin Tablets
  Meticortelone Acetate Aqueous Suspension
  Mol-Iron Liquid
  My Own Towelettes
  Tremin Tablets
Scot-Tussin
  Vita-Plus D Capsules
Searle & Company
  Amodrine
Star Pharmaceuticals
  Microsul 0.5 gm., 1.0 gm.
  Nitrex 50 mg., 100 mg.
  Vesicholine 25 mg.
Stuart Pharmaceuticals
  Hibitane (Tincture, Tinted and Non-Tinted)
Thompson Medical Company, Inc.
  Dexatrim 18 hour
  Dexatrim 18 Hour, Caffeine Free
Tyson & Associates, Inc.
  Enteric Coated Enzymes
  Selenicel
  Vitaplex C (renamed Lyte C)
Upsher-Smith Laboratories, Inc.
  Chardose Powder
  Suhist Tablets
  Theobron SR Capsules

SECTION 3
Product Category Index

Products described in the Product Information (White) or Diagnostic Product Information (Green) Sections are listed according to their classifications. The headings and sub-headings have been determined by the Publisher with the cooperation of the individual manufacturers. In cases where there were differences of opinion or where the manufacturer had no opinion, the Publisher made the final decision. A QUICK-REFERENCE INDEX of headings and sub-headings can be found below.

Product Category Quick-Reference

A
ADRENAL CORTICAL STEROID INHIBITOR
AEROSOLS
ALLERGENS
AMINO ACID PREPARATIONS
ANALEPTIC AGENTS
ANALGESICS
  Acetaminophen & Combinations
  Aspirin
  Aspirin with Antacids
  Aspirin with Codeine
  Aspirin Combinations
  Codeine, Morphine & Opium Derivatives, Synthetics & Combinations
  Devices
    Transcutaneous Electrical Nerve Stimulator
  Ibuprofen
  Opium Derivative
  Other Salicylates & Combinations
  Potent Synthetics & Combinations
  Topical-Analgesic
  Topical-Counterirritant
  Other
ANESTHETICS
  Caudal
  Epidural
  Inhalation
  Injectable
  Local, Topical
  Rectal
  Spinal
ANOREXICS
  Amphetamines
  Non-Amphetamines
ANTACIDS
  Antacids
    with Antiflatulents
ANTIALCOHOL PREPARATIONS
ANTIARTHRITICS
  Antiarthritics
  Antigout
ANTIASTHMA
ANTIBACTERIALS & ANTISEPTICS
  Antibacterial
  Antifungal
  Parenteral
  Sulfonamide Combinations
  Sulfonamides
  Topical
  Urinary Antibacterial
  Urinary Antibacterial with Analgesics

ANTIBIOTICS
  Amebicides
  Antifungal
  Antituberculosis
  Antiviral
  Broad & Medium Spectrum
  Broad & Medium Spectrum with Antimonilial
  Penicillin
ANTICATECHOLAMINE SYNTHESIS
ANTICHOLINERGIC DRUG INHIBITOR
ANTICOAGULANT ANTAGONIST
ANTICOAGULANTS
ANTICONVULSANTS
ANTIDEPRESSANTS
ANTIDIABETIC AGENTS
  Intermediate Acting Insulins
  Long Acting Insulins
  Oral
  Rapid Acting Insulins
ANTIDIARRHEALS
ANTIDIURETICS
ANTIDOTES
  Anticholinesterase
  General
ANTIENURESIS
ANTIFIBRINOLYTIC AGENTS
ANTIFIBROTICS, SYSTEMIC
ANTIFLATULENTS & COMBINATIONS
ANTIFUNGAL AGENTS
  Systemic
  Topical
ANTIGONADOTROPIN
ANTIHERPES
ANTIHISTAMINES
ANTIHYPERAMMONIA
ANTI-INFLAMMATORY AGENTS
  Enzymes
  Hormones
  Phenylbutazones
  Salicylates
  Steroids & Combinations
  Sulfonamides
  Other
ANTILEPROSY
ANTIMETABOLITES
ANTIMIGRAINE PREPARATIONS
ANTIMOTION SICKNESS
ANTINAUSEANTS
ANTINEOPLASTICS
  Antibiotic Derivatives
  Antiestrogen
  Antimetabolites
  Cytotoxic Agents

  Hormones
  Nitrogen Mustard Derivatives
  Steroids & Combinations
  Other
ANTIPARASITICS
  Arthropods
    Lice
    Scabies
  Helminths
    Ascaris (roundworm)
    Enterobius (pinworm)
    Hookworm
    Taenia (tapeworm)
    Trichuris (whipworm)
  Protozoa
    Amebas, extraintestinal
    Amebas, intestinal
    Giardis
    Malaria
    Toxoplasma
    Trichomonas
ANTIPARKINSONISM DRUGS
ANTIPLATELET
ANTIPORPHYRIA AGENT
ANTIPRURITICS
ANTIPSYCHOTICS
ANTIPYRETICS
ANTISHOCK EMERGENCY KIT
ANTISPASMODICS & ANTICHOLINERGICS
  Gastrointestinal
  Urinary
  Other
ANTIVERTIGO AGENTS
ANTIVIRAL AGENTS

B
BIOLOGICALS
  Antigens
  Antiserum
  Antitoxin
  Rh$_0$ (D) Immune Globulin (Human)
  Serum
  Toxoids
  Vaccines
  Vaccines (Live)
  Other
BISMUTH PREPARATIONS
BONE METABOLISM REGULATOR
  Antiheterotopic Ossification Agent
  Antipagetic Agent
  Other
BOWEL EVACUANTS
BRONCHIAL DILATORS
  Beta Adrenergic Stimulator
  Iodides & Combinations

  Sympathomimetics
  Sympathomimetics & Combinations
  Xanthine Derivatives & Combinations

C
CALCIUM PREPARATIONS
  Calcium Binding Agents
  Calcium Regulator
  Calcium Supplements
CARDIOVASCULAR PREPARATIONS
  Alpha Receptor Blocking Agent
  Alpha and Beta Receptor Blocking Agent
  Angiotensin Converting Enzyme Inhibitors
  Antianginal Preparations
  Antiarrhythimcs
  Antihypertensives
  Antihypertensives with Diuretics
  Beta Blocking Agents
  Calcium Channel Blocker
  Digitalis
  Hemorheologic Agents
  Inotropic Agent
  Myocardial Infarction Prophylaxis
  Quinidine
  Vasodilators, Cerebral
  Vasodilators, Coronary
  Vasodilators, General
  Vasodilators, Peripheral
  Vasodilators & Combinations
  Vasopressors
  Other Cardiovasculars
CENTRAL NERVOUS SYSTEM STIMULANTS
CERUMENOLYTICS
CHELATING AGENTS
CHOLESTEROL REDUCERS & ANTIHYPERLIPEMICS
COLORIMETERS
CONTRACEPTIVES
  Devices
  Devices, copper containing
  Oral
  Topical
COSMETICS
COUGH & COLD PREPARATIONS
  Cold Preparations
    Non-Narcotic
    with Narcotics
  Cough Preparations
    Non-Narcotic
    with Narcotics
  Cough & Cold Preparations
    Non-Narcotic
    with Narcotics

Product Category Index

D

DECONGESTANTS
- Oral
- Topical, Nasal

DECONGESTANTS, EXPECTORANTS & COMBINATIONS

DENTAL PREPARATIONS

DEODORANTS
- Oral
- Topical

DERMATOLOGICALS
- Abradant
- Antiacne Preparations
- Antibacterial
- Antibacterial, Antifungal & Combinations
- Antidermatitis
- Antidermatitis Herpetiformis
- Antifungal & Combinations
- Antiherpes
- Anti-Inflammatory Agents
- Antilupus Erythematosus
- Antiperspiration
- Antipruritics, Topical
- Antipsoriasis Agents
- Antiseborrhea
- Astringents
- Coal Tar
- Coal Tar & Sulfur
- Deodorant
- Depigmenting Agent
- Detergents
- Emollients
- Fungicides
- General
- Keratolytics
- Moisturizer
- Pediculicides
- Photosensitizer
- Powders
- Scabicides
- Shampoos
- Skin Bleaches
- Skin Protectant
- Soaps & Cleansers
- Steroids & Combinations
- Sulfur & Salicylic Acid
- Sun Screens
- UVA Light Source
- UVB Light Source
- Vesicants
- Wart Therapeutic Agent
- Wet Dressings
- Wound Dressings
- Other

DIAGNOSTICS
- ACTH Test
- Adrenocortical Function
- Adult Peripheral Arteriography
- Allergy, Skin Tests
- Angiocardiography
- Angiography
- Aortography
- Arthrography
- Blood Glucose
- Central Venography
- Cerebral Angiography
- Cholangiography
- Cholecystography
- Cisternography-CT
- CT Scan Enhancement
- Culture Media
- Cystourethrography
- Direct Cholangiography
- Discography
- Excretory Urography
- Fecal Testing
- Fluorometer
- Gastric Acid Test
- Gastric Hydrochloric Acid Test
- Gastrointestinal Radiography
- Glucose in Whole Blood
- Hysterosalpingography
- Hysteroscopic Fluid
- Intravenous Digital Arteriography
- Intravenous Infusion for Urography
- Intravenous Venography
- Luteinizing Hormone Releasing Hormone (LH-RH)
- Myelography
- Myelography-CT
- Occult Blood in Feces
- Occult Blood in Gastric Samples
- Pancreatic Function Test
- Pediatric Angiocardiography
- Peripheral Angiography
- Peripheral Arteriography
- Pheochromocytoma Test
- Reflectance Photometer & Reagent Strips
- Renal Venography
- Retrograde Cystourethrography
- Retrograde Pyelography
- Selective Renal Arteriography
- Selective Visceral Arteriography
- Splenoportography
- Thyroid Function Test
  - Thyrotropin
- Thyroid Releasing Factor
- Tuberculin
  - Tuberculin, Old
  - Tuberculin, P.P.D.
- Urine Test
  - Bilirubin
  - Blood
  - Controls
  - Culture
  - Glucose
  - Ketones
  - Ketones & Glucose
  - Leukocytes
  - Nitrite
  - pH
  - Protein
  - Specific Gravity
  - Urobilinogen
- Urography
- Venography
- X-ray Contrast

DIETARY SUPPLEMENTS

DIURETICS
- Antihypertensive-Saluretic
- Carbonic Anhydrase Inhibitors
- Loop Diuretics
  - Bumetanide
  - Ethacrynic Acid Derivatives
  - Furosemide
- Monosulfamyl
- Potassium Sparing
- Thiazides and Combinations

DOPAMINE RECEPTOR AGONIST

DRUG DELIVERY SYSTEM

DUODENAL ULCER ADHERENT COMPLEX

E

ELECTROLYTES
- Alkalinizing Agents
- Fluid Replacement Therapy
- Potassium Preparations

EMETICS

ENZYMES & DIGESTANTS
- Collagenolytic
- Digestants
- Fibrinolytic & Proteolytic
- Hydrolytic
- Injectable Proteolytic
- Topical

ENZYME INHIBITORS

ERGOT PREPARATIONS
- Anti-Migraine
- Uterine Contractant

F

FERTILITY AGENTS

FIBER SUPPLEMENT

FLUORINE PREPARATIONS

FOODS
- Allergy Diet
- Carbohydrate
- Carbohydrate Free
- Complete Therapeutic
- Dietetic
- Enteral
- Enteral Hyperalimentation Kit
- High Nitrogen
- Infant
  - (see under INFANT FORMULAS)
- Lactose Free
- Low Fat
- Low Residue
- Low Sodium
- Medium Chain Triglycerides
- Tube Feeding System

G

GALACTO KINETIC

GALL STONE DISSOLUTION AGENT

GASTROINTESTINAL MOTILITY FACTOR

GERIATRICS

GERMICIDES

H

HEMATINICS
- Cyanocobalamin
- Folic Acid
- Hydrochloric Acid
- Iron & Combinations
- Liver
- Vitamin B$_{12}$

HEMORRHOIDAL PREPARATIONS

HEMOSTATICS

HISTAMINE H$_2$ RECEPTOR ANTAGONIST

HORMONES
- ACTH
- Anabolics
- Androgen & Estrogen Combinations
- Androgens
- Corticoids & Analgesics
- Corticoids & Antibiotics, Topical
- Estrogens
- Glucocorticoid
- Gonadotropin
- Human Growth Hormone
- Hypocalcemic
- Menotropins
- Mineralocorticoid
- Progestogen
- Progestogen & Estrogen Combinations
- Vasopressin
- Other

HYPERGLYCEMIC AGENTS

HYPNOTICS

I

IMMUNOSUPPRESSIVES

INFANT FORMULAS, REGULAR
- Liquid Concentrate
- Liquid Ready-to-feed
- Powder

INFANT FORMULAS, SPECIAL PURPOSE
- Hypo-Allergenic
  - Liquid Concentrate
  - Liquid Ready-to-feed
  - Powder
- Iron Supplement
  - Liquid Concentrate
  - Liquid Ready-to-feed
  - Powder
- Lactose Free
  - Liquid Concentrate
  - Liquid Ready-to-feed
- Medium Chain Triglycerides
  - Liquid Ready-to-feed
- Milk Free
  - Liquid Concentrate
  - Liquid Ready-to-feed
- Nutritional Beverage
  - Liquid Concentrate
  - Liquid Ready-to-feed
- Sucrose Free
  - Liquid Concentrate
  - Liquid Ready-to-feed
- With Whey
  - Liquid Concentrate
  - Liquid Ready-to-feed
  - Powder

INSECT STING EMERGENCY KIT

L

LAXATIVES
- Bulk
- Combinations
- Enemas
- Fecal Softeners
- Mineral Oil
- Saline
- Stimulant

LIP BALM

LIPOTROPICS

M

MINERALS

MOUTHWASHES

MUCOLYTICS

MUSCLE RELAXANTS
- Neuromuscular Blocking Agent
- Skeletal Muscle Relaxants
- Skeletal Muscle Relaxants with Analgesics
- Smooth Muscle Relaxants

N

NARCOTIC ANTAGONISTS

NARCOTIC DETOXIFICATION

NASAL PREPARATIONS

O

OPHTHALMOLOGICALS
- Antibacterial
- Antiglaucomatous Agent
- Antiviral
- Eye Washes
- Lubricants
- Moisturizing Agent
- Mydriatics and Cycloplegics
- Ocular Decongestants
- Steroids and Combinations
- Steroids & Combinations
- Surgical Adjunct
- Other

OPTIC OPACITIES
- Symptomatic Relief

OTIC PREPARATIONS

OXYTOCICS

P

PARASYMPATHOLYTICS

PARASYMPATHOMIMETICS

PENICILLIN ADJUVANT

PERISTOMAL COVERING

PHOSPHORUS PREPARATIONS

PLASMA EXTENDERS

PLASMA FRACTIONS, HUMAN
- Antihemophilic Factor
- Factor IX Complex
- Immune Serum Globulin (Human)
- Normal Serum Albumin (Human)
- Plasma Protein Fraction (Human)
- Rh$_0$ (D) Immune Globulin (Human)

PROSTAGLANDINS

PSYCHOSTIMULANTS

Q

QUINIDINES

R

RESINS, ION EXCHANGE

RESPIRATORY STIMULANTS

S

SCLEROSING AGENTS

SEDATIVES
- Barbiturates
- Non-Barbiturates

SMOKING CESSATION AID

SYMPATHOLYTICS

SYMPATHOMIMETICS & COMBINATIONS

T

THERAPEUTIC DRUG ASSAYS

THROAT LOZENGES

THROMBOLYTICS

THYROID PREPARATIONS
- Antithyroid
- Synthetic Thyroid Hormone
- Thyroid
- Thyrotropic Hormone
- Thyroxine Sodium

TONICS

TRACE MINERALS

TRANQUILIZERS
- Benzodiazepine
- Butyrophenones & Combinations
- Hydroxyzines
- Lithium Preparations
- Meprobamate & Combinations
- Phenothiazines & Combinations
- Rauwolfia Serpentina
- Reserpine
- Thioxanthenes
- Other

TUBERCULOSIS PREPARATIONS

U

UNIT DOSE SYSTEMS

UNNA BOOT

URICOSURIC AGENTS

URINARY ACIDIFIERS

URINARY ALKALINIZING AGENTS

URINARY TRACT ANALGESIC

UROLOGICAL IRRIGANTS

UTERINE CONTRACTANTS

UTERINE, MUSCLE CONTRACTION INHIBITOR

V

VAGINAL THERAPEUTICS
- Capsules, Tablets
- Creams
- Douches
- Inserts, Suppositories
- Jellies, Ointments
- Trichomonacides

VITAMINS
- Geriatric
- Multivitamins
- Multivitamins with Minerals
- Parenteral
- Pediatric
- Pediatric with Fluoride
- Prenatal
- Therapeutic

X

X-RAY CONTRAST MEDIA

Product Category Index

A

ADRENAL CORTICAL STEROID INHIBITOR
Cytadren (CIBA) p 409, 846

AEROSOLS
AeroBid Inhaler System (Key Pharmaceuticals) p 1046
Aeroseb-Dex Topical Aerosol Spray (Herbert) p 1001
Aeroseb-HC Topical Aerosol Spray (Herbert) p 1002
Beclovent Oral Inhaler (Glaxo) p 411, 977
Beconase Nasal Inhaler (Glaxo) p 411, 978
Betadine Aerosol Spray (Purdue Frederick) p 1622
Betadine Helafoam Solution (Purdue Frederick) p 1622
Breezee Mist Foot Powder (Pedinol) p 1580
Cortifoam (Reed & Carnrick) p 427, 1632
Decadron Phosphate Respihaler (Merck Sharp & Dohme) p 1291
Decadron Phosphate Turbinaire (Merck Sharp & Dohme) p 1293
Decaspray Topical Aerosol (Merck Sharp & Dohme) p 1296
Diprosone Topical Aerosol 0.1% w/w (Schering) p 1838
Epifoam (Reed & Carnrick) p 427, 1634
Kenalog Spray (Squibb) p 1998
Neosporin Aerosol (Burroughs Wellcome) p 806
Proctofoam-HC (Reed & Carnrick) p 427, 1636
proctoFoam/non-steroid (Reed & Carnrick) p 427, 1636
Proventil Inhaler (Schering) p 435, 1882
R&C Spray (Reed & Carnrick) p 1637
Vancenase Nasal Inhaler (Schering) p 435, 1893
Vanceril Inhaler (Schering) p 435, 1894
Ventolin Inhaler (Glaxo) p 412, 987

ALLERGENS
Allergenic Extracts, Diagnosis and/or Immunotherapy (Barry) p 685
Rhus All Antigen - Poison Ivy, Oak, Sumac Combined (Barry) p 685
Rhus Tox Antigen Injection (Lemmon) p 1122

AMEBICIDES & TRICHOMONACIDES
(see under ANTIPARASITICS)

AMINO ACID PREPARATIONS
Alba-Lybe (Bart) p 685
Amino-Cerv (Milex) p 1415
Aminolete (Tyson) p 2067
Aminomine (Tyson) p 2067
Aminoplex Capsules & Powder (Tyson) p 2068
Aminosine (Tyson) p 2068
Aminostasis Capsules & Powder (Tyson) p 2068
Aminotate Capsules & Powder (Tyson) p 2068
DL-Carnitine - Amino Acid Preparation (Tyson) p 2068
Endorphenyl (Tyson) p 2068
MARLYN Formula 50 (Marlyn) p 1193
Pedameth Capsules (O'Neal, Jones & Feldman) p 422, 1445
Pedameth Liquid (O'Neal, Jones & Feldman) p 1445
Tryptacin (Arther) p 614
Vivonex High Nitrogen Diet (Norwich Eaton) p 1439
Vivonex Standard Diet (Norwich Eaton) p 1438
Vivonex T.E.N. (Norwich Eaton) p 1441

ANALEPTIC AGENTS
L-2000 (Robertson/Taylor) p 1646

ANALGESICS

Acetaminophen & Combinations
Acetaminophen Uniserts Suppositories (Upsher-Smith) p 2144
Anacin-3, Children's Acetaminophen Chewable Tablets, Elixir, Drops (Whitehall) p 443, 2184
Anacin-3, Maximum Strength Acetaminophen Tablets and Capsules (Whitehall) p 443, 2185
Capital with Codeine Suspension (Carnrick) p 408, 831
Capital with Codeine Tablets (Carnrick) p 408, 831
Children's Panadol Chewable Tablets, Liquid, Drops (Glenbrook) p 412, 997
Co-Gesic Tablets (Central Pharmaceuticals) p 409, 836
Comtrex (Bristol-Myers Products) p 769
Congespirin Liquid Cold Medicine (Bristol-Myers Products) p 770
Dorcol Children's Fever & Pain Reducer (Dorsey Laboratories) p 909
Dristan, Advanced Formula Decongestant/Antihistamine/Analgesic Capsules (Whitehall) p 443, 2186
Dristan, Advanced Formula Decongestant/Antihistamine/Analgesic Tablets (Whitehall) p 443, 2186
Empracet with Codeine Phosphate Nos. 3 & 4 (Burroughs Wellcome) p 408, 789
Esgic Tablets & Capsules (Gilbert) p 411, 975
Excedrin P.M. (Bristol-Myers Products) p 770
Extra-Strength Datril capsules & tablets (Bristol-Myers Products) p 770
Extra-Strength Sine-Aid Sinus Headache Capsules (McNeil Consumer Products) p 1199
Maximum Strength Midol PMS (Glenbrook) p 997
Maximum Strength Panadol Capsules & Tablets (Glenbrook) p 412, 997
Midrin Capsules (Carnrick) p 408, 832
Migralam Capsules (Lambda) p 1071
Parafon Forte Tablets (McNeil Pharmaceutical) p 419, 1206
Percocet (Du Pont) p 410, 925
Percogesic Analgesic Tablets (Vicks Pharmacy Products) p 442, 2147
Phenaphen w/Codeine Capsules (Robins) p 428, 1656
Phenaphen-650 with Codeine Tablets (Robins) p 428, 1656
Phrenilin Tablets (Carnrick) p 408, 833
Phrenilin Forte (Carnrick) p 408, 834
Phrenilin with Codeine No. 3 (Carnrick) p 409, 834
Sedapap-10 Tablets (Mayrand) p 1196
Singlet (Merrell Dow) p 421, 1385
Sinubid (Parke-Davis) p 425, 1569
Sinulin Tablets (Carnrick) p 409, 835
Supac (Mission) p 1420
Talacen (Winthrop-Breon) p 444, 2227
Tylenol acetaminophen Children's Chewable Tablets, Elixir, Infants' Drops (McNeil Consumer Products) p 418, 1199
Tylenol, Extra-Strength, acetaminophen Liquid Pain Reliever (McNeil Consumer Products) p 1200
Tylenol, Extra-Strength, acetaminophen Tablets, Capsules & Caplets (McNeil Consumer Products) p 418, 1200
Tylenol, Junior-Strength, acetaminphen Swallowable Tablets (McNeil Consumer Products) p 418
Tylenol, Regular Strength, acetaminophen Tablets & Capsules (McNeil Consumer Products) p 418, 1199
Vicodin (Knoll) p 414, 1068
Wygesic Tablets (Wyeth) p 445, 2297

Aspirin
Arthritis Bayer Timed-Release Aspirin (Glenbrook) p 412, 995
Arthritis Pain Formula Safety-Coated by the Makers of Anacin Analgesic Tablets (Whitehall) p 443, 2185
Bayer Aspirin and Bayer Children's Chewable Aspirin (Glenbrook) p 412, 996
Cosprin (Glenbrook) p 996
Cosprin 650 (Glenbrook) p 997
Easprin (Parke-Davis) p 424, 1512
Encaprin (Procter & Gamble) p 427, 1620
Maximum Bayer Aspirin (Glenbrook) p 412, 996

Aspirin with Antacids
Alka-Seltzer Effervescent Pain Reliever and Antacid (Miles Laboratories) p 1395
Arthritis Strength Bufferin (Bristol-Myers Products) p 768
Buff-A Comp Tablets (Mayrand) p 1196
Bufferin (Bristol-Myers Products) p 769
Cama Arthritis Pain Reliever (Dorsey Laboratories) p 908
Extra-Strength Bufferin capsules & tablets (Bristol-Myers Products) p 769

Aspirin with Codeine
Empirin with Codeine (Burroughs Wellcome) p 408, 787

Aspirin Combinations
A.P.C. with Codeine Nos. 3 & 4, Tabloid brand (Burroughs Wellcome) p 407, 780
Alka-Seltzer Plus Cold Medicine (Miles Laboratories) p 1395
Anacin Analgesic Capsules (Whitehall) p 443, 2184
Anacin Analgesic Tablets (Whitehall) p 443, 2184
Arthritis Pain Formula By the Makers of Anacin Analgesic Tablets (Whitehall) p 443, 2185
Axotal (Adria) p 574
Bayer Children's Cold Tablets (Glenbrook) p 996
Buff-A Comp Tablets (Mayrand) p 1196
Congespirin Cold Tablets (Aspirin Formula) (Bristol-Myers Products) p 769
Dia-Gesic (Central Pharmaceuticals) p 409, 837
Equagesic (Wyeth) p 444, 2250
Excedrin Extra-Strength (Bristol-Myers Products) p 770
4-Way Cold Tablets (Bristol-Myers Products) p 770
Fiogesic Tablets (Sandoz Pharmaceutical Div.) p 432, 1801
Fiorinal (Sandoz Pharmaceutical Div.) p 433, 1801
Maximum Strength Midol for Cramps (Glenbrook) p 997
Midol-Original Formula (Glenbrook) p 997
Norgesic & Norgesic Forte (Riker) p 428, 1644
Supac (Mission) p 1420
Synalgos-DC Capsules (Ives) p 413, 1031
Talwin Compound (Winthrop-Breon) p 2229
Vanquish (Glenbrook) p 998
Verin (Verex) p 442, 2146

Codeine, Morphine & Opium Derivatives, Synthetics & Combinations
A.P.C. with Codeine Nos. 3 & 4, Tabloid brand (Burroughs Wellcome) p 407, 780
Anacin-3 with Codeine Tablets (Ayerst) p 404, 634
Ascriptin with Codeine (Rorer) p 431, 1745
B & O Supprettes No. 15A & No. 16A (Webcon) p 2172
Bancap HC Capsules (O'Neal, Jones & Feldman) p 422, 1444
Capital with Codeine Suspension (Carnrick) p 408, 831
Capital with Codeine Tablets (Carnrick) p 408, 831
Codalan (Lannett) p 1071
Codeine Phosphate in Tubex (Wyeth) p 2288
Co-Gesic Tablets (Central Pharmaceuticals) p 409, 836
Compal Capsules (Reid-Provident Labs.) p 427, 1637
Damacet-P (Mason) p 418, 1193
Damason-P (Mason) p 418, 1194
Demerol Hydrochloride (Winthrop-Breon) p 443, 2197
Dia-Gesic (Central Pharmaceuticals) p 409, 837
Dilaudid Hydrochloride (Knoll) p 414, 1057
Dilaudid-HP Injection (Knoll) p 414, 1059
Dolophine Hydrochloride Ampoules and Vials (Lilly) p 1144
Dolophine Hydrochloride Tablets (Lilly) p 1145
Duramorph PF (Preservative-free morphine sulfate injection) (Elkins-Sinn) p 939
Empracet with Codeine Phosphate Nos. 3 & 4 (Burroughs Wellcome) p 408, 789
Fiorinal w/Codeine (Sandoz Pharmaceutical Div.) p 432, 1802
Hydromorphone HCl in Tubex (Wyeth) p 2288
Innovar Injection (Janssen) p 1035

Product Category Index

Levo-Dromoran Injectable (Roche) p 1689
Levo-Dromoran Tab (Roche) p 429, 1689
MS Contin (Purdue Frederick) p 1625
Mepergan Injection (Wyeth) p 2264
Mepergan in Tubex (Wyeth) p 2288
Meperidine HCl in Tubex (Wyeth) p 2288
Morphine Sulfate Oral (Roxane) p 1792
Morphine Sulfate Tablets (Roxane) p 1792
Morphine Sulfate in Tubex (Wyeth) p 2288
Nisentil Injectable (Roche) p 1694
Numorphan (Du Pont) p 924
Pantopon Injectable (Roche) p 1697
Percocet (Du Pont) p 410, 925
Percodan & Percodan-Demi Tablets (Du Pont) p 410, 925
Phenaphen w/Codeine Capsules (Robins) p 428, 1656
Phenaphen-650 with Codeine Tablets (Robins) p 428, 1656
Phrenilin with Codeine No. 3 (Carnrick) p 409, 834
Roxanol (Morphine Sulfate Concentrated Oral Solution) (Roxane) p 1793
Sublimaze Injection (Janssen) p 413, 1039
Sufenta (Janssen) p 413, 1040
Synalgos-DC Capsules (Ives) p 413, 1031
Tylenol w/Codeine Elixir (McNeil Pharmaceutical) p 419, 1214
Tylenol w/Codeine Tablets, Capsules (McNeil Pharmaceutical) p 419, 1214
Tylox Capsules (McNeil Pharmaceutical) p 419, 1215
Vicodin (Knoll) p 414, 1068

Devices
Transcutaneous Electrical Nerve Stimulator
NTRON TTS-2500 (TENS) (NTRON International) p 1443

Ibuprofen
Advil Ibuprofen Tablets (Whitehall) p 443, 2184

Opium Derivative
Oxycodone Hydrochloride Oral Solution & Tablets (Roxane) p 1792
RMS Suppositories (Upsher-Smith) p 2144

Other Salicylates & Combinations
Ger-O-Foam (Geriatric) p 975
Mono-Gesic Tablets (Central Pharmaceuticals) p 409, 837
Os-Cal-Gesic Tablets (Marion) p 418, 1189

Potent Synthetics & Combinations
Darvocet-N 50 (Lilly) p 417, 1136
Darvocet-N 100 (Lilly) p 417, 1136
Darvon (Lilly) p 417, 1139
Darvon Compound (Lilly) p 417, 1139
Darvon Compound-65 (Lilly) p 417, 1139
Darvon with A.S.A. (Lilly) p 417, 1139
Darvon-N (Lilly) p 417, 1136
Darvon-N w/A.S.A. (Lilly) p 417, 1136
Methadone Hydrochloride Oral Solution & Tablets (Roxane) p 1791
Nubain (Du Pont) p 410, 923
Oxycodone Hydrochloride Oral Solution & Tablets (Roxane) p 1792
Ponstel (Parke-Davis) p 425, 1562
Stadol (Bristol) p 750
Synalgos-DC Capsules (Ives) p 413, 1031
Talwin Compound (Winthrop-Breon) p 2229
Talwin Injection (Winthrop-Breon) p 2228
Talwin Nx (Winthrop-Breon) p 444, 2230
Tegretol Chewable Tablets (Geigy) p 411, 966
Tegretol Tablets (Geigy) p 411, 966
Wygesic Tablets (Wyeth) p 445, 2297

Topical-Analgesic
Anbesol Gel Antiseptic Anesthetic (Whitehall) p 443, 2185
Aspercreme (Thompson Medical) p 2066
Larylgan Throat Spray (Ayerst) p 653
Myoflex Creme (Adria) p 585
Thera-Gesic (Mission) p 1420

Topical-Counterirritant
Thera-Gesic (Mission) p 1420

Other
Anaprox Tablets (Syntex) p 440, 2050
Dolobid Tablets (Merck Sharp & Dohme) p 420, 1302
Endorphenyl (Tyson) p 2068
Magan (Adria) p 583
Motrin Tablets* (Upjohn) p 441, 2128
Nalfon Pulvules & Tablets (Dista) p 410, 903
Nalfon 200 Pulvules (Dista) p 410, 903
Norflex (Riker) p 428, 1644
Nuprin (Bristol-Myers Products) p 771
Pabalate Tablets (Robins) p 428, 1654
Pabalate-SF Tablets (Robins) p 428, 1655
Rufen Tablets (Boots) p 406, 720
Sarapin (High Chemical) p 1009

ANESTHETICS

Caudal
Carbocaine Hydrochloride (Winthrop-Breon) p 2194
Duranest Hydrochloride & Duranest Hydrochloride with Epinephrine 1:200,000 (Astra) p 616
Lidocaine Hydrochloride Injection, U.S.P. (Abbott) p 535
Marcaine Hydrochloride (Winthrop-Breon) p 2206
Marcaine Hydrochloride with Epinephrine 1:200,000 (Winthrop-Breon) p 2206
Nesacaine-CE Solutions (Astra) p 618
Sensorcaine Hydrochloride & Sensorcaine Hydrochloride with Epinephrine 1:200,000 (Astra) p 619
Xylocaine Hydrochloride, Xylocaine Hydrochloride with Epinephrine 1:100,000, & Xylocaine Hydrochloride with Epinephrine 1:200,000 (Astra) p 623

Epidural
Duranest Hydrochloride & Duranest Hydrochloride with Epinephrine 1:200,000 (Astra) p 616
Marcaine Hydrochloride (Winthrop-Breon) p 2206
Marcaine Hydrochloride with Epinephrine 1:200,000 (Winthrop-Breon) p 2206
Nesacaine-CE Solutions (Astra) p 618
Sensorcaine Hydrochloride & Sensorcaine Hydrochloride with Epinephrine 1:200,000 (Astra) p 619
Xylocaine Hydrochloride, Xylocaine Hydrochloride with Epinephrine 1:100,000, & Xylocaine Hydrochloride with Epinephrine 1:200,000 (Astra) p 623

Inhalation
Fluothane (Ayerst) p 645
Penthrane (Abbott) p 560

Injectable
Brevital Sodium (Lilly) p 1131
Carbocaine Hydrochloride (Winthrop-Breon) p 2194
Carbocaine Hydrochloride 3% Injection (Cook-Waite) p 881
Carbocaine Hydrochloride 2% with Neo-Cobefrin 1:20,000 Injection (Cook-Waite) p 881
Duranest Hydrochloride & Duranest Hydrochloride with Epinephrine 1:200,000 (Astra) p 616
Ketalar (Parke-Davis) p 1528
Lidocaine Hydrochloride Injection, U.S.P. (Abbott) p 535
Lidocaine HCl in Tubex (Wyeth) p 2288
Marcaine Hydrochloride (Winthrop-Breon) p 2206
Marcaine Hydrochloride with Epinephrine 1:200,000 (Winthrop-Breon) p 2206
Nesacaine Solutions (Astra) p 618
Nesacaine-CE Solutions (Astra) p 618
Novocain Hydrochloride (Winthrop-Breon) p 2219
Pentothal (Abbott) p 562
Sarapin (High Chemical) p 1009
Sensorcaine Hydrochloride & Sensorcaine Hydrochloride with Epinephrine 1:200,000 (Astra) p 619
Surital (Parke-Davis) p 1572
Xylocaine Hydrochloride, Xylocaine Hydrochloride with Epinephrine 1:100,000, & Xylocaine Hydrochloride with Epinephrine 1:200,000 (Astra) p 623
Xylocaine 4% Sterile Solution (Astra) p 627

Local, Topical
Anbesol Baby Teething Gel Antiseptic Anesthetic (Whitehall) p 443, 2185
Anbesol Gel Antiseptic Anesthetic (Whitehall) p 443, 2185
Anestacon (Webcon) p 2171
Cetacaine Topical Anesthetic (Cetylite) p 839
Children's Chloraseptic Lozenges (Procter & Gamble) p 1619
Chloraseptic Liquid (Procter & Gamble) p 1619
Chloraseptic Lozenges (Procter & Gamble) p 1620
Corticaine Cream (Glaxo) p 412, 980
Dalidyne (Dalin) p 886
Derma Medicone-HC Ointment (Medicone) p 1256
Dermoplast Aerosol Spray (Ayerst) p 640
Dyclone, 0.5% & 1% (Astra) p 618
Epifoam (Reed & Carnrick) p 427, 1634
Ger-O-Foam (Geriatric) p 975
Gumsol (Arlo) p 601
Hurricane Liquid 1/4cc Unit Dose (Beutlich) p 705
Hurricane Oral, Topical Anesthetic Gel, Liquid, Spray (Beutlich) p 705
Lidocaine Hydrochloride Injection, U.S.P. (Abbott) p 535
Lidocaine HCl in Tubex (Wyeth) p 2288
Lubraseptic Jelly (Guardian) p 1000
Nupercainal Cream & Ointment (CIBA) p 856
Pramosone Cream, Lotion & Ointment (Ferndale) p 942
Proctofoam-HC (Reed & Carnrick) p 427, 1636
proctoFoam/non-steroid (Reed & Carnrick) p 427, 1636
Rectal Medicone-HC Suppositories (Medicone) p 419, 1256
Tronothane Hydrochloride (Abbott) p 570
Xylocaine 2% Jelly (Astra) p 629
Xylocaine 5% Ointment (Astra) p 629
Xylocaine 10% Oral Spray (Astra) p 630
Xylocaine 4% Sterile Solution (Astra) p 627
Xylocaine 4% Topical Solution (Astra) p 628
Xylocaine 2% Viscous Solution (Astra) p 630

Rectal
Nupercainal Cream & Ointment (CIBA) p 856

Spinal
Marcaine Spinal (Winthrop-Breon) p 2210
Novocain Hydrochloride for Spinal Anesthesia (Winthrop-Breon) p 2220
Nupercaine Heavy Solution (CIBA) p 860
Nupercaine hydrochloride 1:200 (CIBA) p 857
Nupercaine hydrochloride 1:1500 (CIBA) p 858
Pontocaine Hydrochloride for Spinal Anesthesia (Winthrop-Breon) p 2225
Xylocaine 1.5% Solution with Dextrose 7.5% (Astra) p 629
Xylocaine 5% Solution with Glucose 7.5% (Astra) p 629

ANOREXICS

Amphetamines
Desoxyn (Abbott) p 515
Desoxyn Gradumet Tablets (Abbott) p 403, 515
Dexedrine (Smith Kline & French) p 436, 1959
Didrex Tablets (Upjohn) p 441, 2111

Non-Amphetamines
Adipex-P Tablets (Lemmon) p 417, 1121
Anorex-CCK (Robertson/Taylor) p 1645
Appedrine, Maximum Strength (Thompson Medical) p 2065
Bontril PDM (Carnrick) p 408, 830
Bontril Slow-Release (Carnrick) p 408, 830
Control Capsules, Maximum Strength (Thompson Medical) p 2066
Dexatrim Capsules (Thompson Medical) p 2066
Dexatrim Capsules, Extra Strength (Thompson Medical) p 2066
Dexatrim Capsules, Extra Strength, Caffeine-Free (Thompson Medical) p 2066
Dexatrim Capsules, Extra Strength, Plus Vitamins (Thompson Medical) p 2066
Dexatrim • 15 (Thompson Medical) p 2066
Dexatrim • 15, Caffeine-Free (Thompson Medical) p 2066
Fastin Capsules (Beecham Laboratories) p 406, 692
Help (Verex) p 442, 2145
Ionamin (Pennwalt) p 426, 1585
Mazanor (Wyeth) p 444, 2263
Melfiat Tablets (Reid-Provident Labs.) p 1639
Melfiat 105 Unicelles (Reid-Provident Labs.) p 428, 1639
Plegine (Ayerst) p 405, 659
Pondimin Tablets (Robins) p 428, 1657
Prelu-2 Timed Release Capsules (Boehringer Ingelheim) p 406, 711
Preludin Endurets (Boehringer Ingelheim) p 406, 710
Preludin Tablets (Boehringer Ingelheim) p 710
Prolamine Capsules, Maximum Strength (Thompson Medical) p 2067
Sanorex (Sandoz Pharmaceutical Div.) p 433, 1815
Tenuate Dospan (Merrell Dow) p 421, 1393
Tenuate 25 mg (Merrell Dow) p 421, 1393
Tepanil (Riker) p 428, 1645
Tepanil Ten-tab (Riker) p 428, 1645

ANTACIDS

Antacids
Alka-Seltzer Effervescent Antacid (Miles Laboratories) p 1395
ALternaGEL Liquid (Stuart) p 438, 2036
Alu-Cap Capsules (Riker) p 1641
Aludrox Oral Suspension (Wyeth) p 2235
Aludrox Tablets (Wyeth) p 2235
Alu-Tab Tablets (Riker) p 1641
Amphojel Suspension (Wyeth) p 2236
Amphojel Tablets (Wyeth) p 2236
Basaljel Capsules & Swallow Tablets (Wyeth) p 2239
Basaljel Suspension & Suspension, Extra Strength (Wyeth) p 2239
Bicitra—Sugar-Free (Willen) p 2187
Dialume (Armour) p 404, 605
Gaviscon Antacid Tablets (Marion) p 418, 1185
Gaviscon Liquid Antacid (Marion) p 1186
Gaviscon-2 Antacid Tablets (Marion) p 418, 1186
Gelusil (Parke-Davis) p 424, 1525
Phillips' Milk of Magnesia (Glenbrook) p 997
Polycitra Syrup (Willen) p 2188

Product Category Index

Polycitra-LC—Sugar-Free (Willen) p 2188
Riopan (Ayerst) p 405, 680
Riopan Plus (Ayerst) p 405, 680
Simeco (Wyeth) p 2288
with Antiflatulents
Gelusil-M (Parke-Davis) p 1525
Gelusil-II (Parke-Davis) p 424, 1526
Mylanta Liquid (Stuart) p 439, 2039
Mylanta Tablets (Stuart) p 439, 2039
Mylanta-II Liquid (Stuart) p 439, 2039
Mylanta-II Tablets (Stuart) p 439, 2039
Riopan Plus (Ayerst) p 405, 680
Simeco (Wyeth) p 2288

ANTHELMINTICS
(see under ANTIPARASITICS)

ANTIALCOHOL PREPARATIONS
Antabuse (Ayerst) p 404, 635, 634

ANTIARTHRITICS
Antiarthritics
A.P.C. with Codeine Nos. 3 & 4, Tabloid brand (Burroughs Wellcome) p 407, 780
Aristospan Parenteral 20 mg./ml (Lederle) p 1085
Arthritis Bayer Timed-Release Aspirin (Glenbrook) p 412, 995
Azolid Capsules & Tablets (USV Pharmaceutical) p 2070
Butazolidin Capsules & Tablets (Geigy) p 411, 956
Cama Arthritis Pain Reliever (Dorsey Laboratories) p 908
Celestone Phosphate Injection (Schering) p 1833
Celestone Soluspan Suspension (Schering) p 1835
Celestone Syrup & Tablets (Schering) p 433, 1832
Clinoril Tablets (Merck Sharp & Dohme) p 420, 1274
Cosprin (Glenbrook) p 996
Cosprin 650 (Glenbrook) p 997
Cuprimine Capsules (Merck Sharp & Dohme) p 420, 1280
Decadron Elixir (Merck Sharp & Dohme) p 1284
Decadron Phosphate Injection (Merck Sharp & Dohme) p 1288
Decadron Tablets (Merck Sharp & Dohme) p 420, 1286
Decadron-LA Suspension (Merck Sharp & Dohme) p 1294
Depen Titratable Tablets (Wallace) p 2152
Depo-Medrol (Upjohn) p 441, 2107
Dolobid Tablets (Merck Sharp & Dohme) p 420, 1302
Empirin with Codeine (Burroughs Wellcome) p 408, 787
Feldene Capsules (Pfizer) p 426, 1601
Ger-O-Foam (Geriatric) p 975
Hydeltra-T.B.A. Suspension (Merck Sharp & Dohme) p 1314
Indocin Capsules (Merck Sharp & Dohme) p 420, 1319
Indocin SR Capsules (Merck Sharp & Dohme) p 420, 1319
Indocin Suppositories (Merck Sharp & Dohme) p 420, 1319
Kenalog-10 Injection (Squibb) p 2001
Kenalog-40 Injection (Squibb) p 1999
Magan (Adria) p 583
Maximum Bayer Aspirin (Glenbrook) p 412, 996
Meclomen (Parke-Davis) p 424, 1541
Medrol Tablets (Upjohn) p 441, 2124
Mono-Gesic Tablets (Central Pharmaceuticals) p 409, 837
Motrin Tablets* (Upjohn) p 441, 2128
Myochrysine Injection (Merck Sharp & Dohme) p 1339
Nalfon Pulvules & Tablets (Dista) p 410, 903
Naprosyn (Syntex) p 440, 2062
Os-Cal-Gesic Tablets (Marion) p 418, 1189
Oxalid Tablets (USV Pharmaceutical) p 2084
Pabalate Tablets (Robins) p 428, 1654
Pabalate-SF Tablets (Robins) p 428, 1655
Plaquenil Sulfate (Winthrop-Breon) p 444, 2223
Rufen Tablets (Boots) p 406, 720
Solganal Suspension (Schering) p 1884
Tandearil (Geigy) p 411, 964
Tolectin Tablets & DS Capsules (McNeil Pharmaceutical) p 419, 1212
Trilisate Tablets/Liquid (Purdue Frederick) p 427, 1627
Zorprin (Boots) p 406, 725
Antigout
Anturane Tablets & Capsules (CIBA) p 409, 842
Azolid Capsules & Tablets (USV Pharmaceutical) p 2070
Benemid Tablets (Merck Sharp & Dohme) p 420, 1268
Butazolidin Capsules & Tablets (Geigy) p 411, 956

Clinoril Tablets (Merck Sharp & Dohme) p 420, 1274
ColBENEMID Tablets (Merck Sharp & Dohme) p 420, 1277
Colchicine Ampoules (Lilly) p 1134
Colchicine Tablets (Lilly) p 1135
Indocin Capsules (Merck Sharp & Dohme) p 420, 1319
Indocin Suppositories (Merck Sharp & Dohme) p 420, 1319
Lopurin (Boots) p 406, 718
Oxalid Tablets (USV Pharmaceutical) p 2084
Tandearil (Geigy) p 411, 964
Zyloprim (Burroughs Wellcome) p 408, 825

ANTIASTHMA
Accurbron (Merrell Dow) p 1359
AeroBid Inhaler System (Key Pharmaceuticals) p 1046
Aminophyllin Tablets (Searle & Co.) p 435, 1915
Aquaphyllin Syrup (Ferndale) p 942
Beclovent Oral Inhaler (Glaxo) p 411, 977
Brethine (Geigy) p 411, 955
Brethine Ampuls (Geigy) p 956
Bricanyl Injection (Merrell Dow) p 421, 1361
Bricanyl Tablets (Merrell Dow) p 421, 1361
Bronkephrine Hydrochloride Injection (Winthrop-Breon) p 2193
Bronkometer (Winthrop-Breon) p 2193
Bronkosol (Winthrop-Breon) p 2193
Choledyl Pediatric Syrup (Parke-Davis) p 1495
Choledyl SA Tablets (Parke-Davis) p 423, 1497
Decadron Phosphate Respihaler (Merck Sharp & Dohme) p 1291
Efed II Capsules (Yellow) (Alto) p 404, 589
Elixicon Suspension (Berlex) p 406, 699
Elixophyllin Capsules (Berlex) p 406, 699
Elixophyllin Elixir (Berlex) p 699
Elixophyllin SR Capsules (Berlex) p 406, 699
Epinephrine in Tubex (Wyeth) p 2288
Intal Nebulizer Solution (Fisons) p 943
Isuprel Hydrochloride Mistometer (Winthrop-Breon) p 2203
LABID 250 mg Tablets (Norwich Eaton) p 1436
Lodrane Capsules-130 & 260 (Poythress) p 1618
Metaprel Inhalant Solution, Metered Dose Inhaler, Syrup & Tablets (Dorsey Laboratories) p 910
Mudrane GG Elixir (Poythress) p 1619
Mudrane GG Tablets (Poythress) p 1619
Mudrane Tablets (Poythress) p 1618
Norisodrine Aerotrol (Abbott) p 547
Primatene Mist (Whitehall) p 443, 2186
Primatene Mist Suspension (Whitehall) p 2187
Primatene Tablets-M Formula (Whitehall) p 443, 2187
Primatene Tablets-P Formula (Whitehall) p 443, 2187
Proventil Inhaler (Schering) p 435, 1882
Proventil Tablets (Schering) p 435, 1883
Slo-bid Gyrocaps (Rorer) p 432, 1754
Slo-Phyllin Gyrocaps, Tablets (Rorer) p 432, 1756
Slo-Phyllin 80 Syrup (Rorer) p 1756
Slo-Phyllin GG Capsules, Syrup (Rorer) p 432, 1759
Sus-Phrine (Berlex) p 406, 704
Synophylate Elixir (Central Pharmaceuticals) p 839
Synophylate-GG Tablets/Syrup (Central Pharmaceuticals) p 839
Theo-24 (Searle & Co.) p 436, 1937
Theobid, Theobid Jr. Duracap (Glaxo) p 412, 982
Theo-Dur Sprinkle (Key Pharmaceuticals) p 414, 1053
Theo-Dur Tablets (Key Pharmaceuticals) p 414, 1051
Theolair & Theolair-SR (Riker) p 428, 1645
Theophyl Chewable Tablets (McNeil Pharmaceutical) p 1207
Theophyl-SR (McNeil Pharmaceutical) p 1208
Theophyl-225 Elixir (McNeil Pharmaceutical) p 1210
Theophyl-225 Tablets (McNeil Pharmaceutical) p 1210
Theovent Long-Acting Capsules (Schering) p 435, 1886
Uniphyl 200 mg Tablets (Purdue Frederick) p 427, 1627
Uniphyl 400 mg Tablets (Purdue Frederick) p 427, 1629
Vanceril Inhaler (Schering) p 435, 1894
Ventolin Inhaler (Glaxo) p 412, 987
Ventolin Tablets (Glaxo) p 412, 988

ANTIBACTERIALS & ANTISEPTICS
Antibacterial
Anti-Sept (Seamless) p 1897
Bactrim DS Tablets (Roche) p 429, 1674
Bactrim I.V. Infusion (Roche) p 1672

Bactrim Pediatric Suspension (Roche) p 1674
Bactrim Suspension (Roche) p 1674
Bactrim Tablets (Roche) p 429, 1674
Cefobid Intravenous/Intramuscular (Roerig) p 1726
Flagyl I.V. (Searle Pharmaceuticals) p 436, 1907
Flagyl I.V. RTU (Searle Pharmaceuticals) p 436, 1907
Flagyl Tablets (Searle & Co.) p 436, 1929
Flint SSD Cream (Flint) p 411, 950
Furadantin Oral Suspension (Norwich Eaton) p 1432
Furadantin Tablets (Norwich Eaton) p 1432
Hibiclens Antimicrobial Skin Cleanser (Stuart) p 439, 2037
Hibistat Germicidal Hand Rinse (Stuart) p 439, 2038
Macrodantin Capsules (Norwich Eaton) p 422, 1436
Methylbenzethonium Chloride (Sween) p 2047
Micro-Guard (Sween) p 2048
Mycolog Cream and Ointment (Squibb) p 2003
Mysteclin-F Capsules (Squibb) p 438, 2005
Mysteclin-F Syrup (Squibb) p 2005
Neo-Polycin (Merrell Dow) p 1372
Penicillin G Potassium for Injection USP (Squibb) p 2009
Penicillin G Sodium for Injection USP (Squibb) p 2010
Pentids for Syrup (Squibb) p 2011
Pentids Tablets, Pentids 400 & 800 Tablets (Squibb) p 438, 2011
Principen Capsules (Squibb) p 438, 2012
Principen for Oral Suspension (Squibb) p 2012
Principen with Probenecid Capsules (Squibb) p 2013
Proloprim (Burroughs Wellcome) p 408, 810
Protostat Tablets (Ortho Pharmaceutical) p 423, 1470
Pyocidin-Otic Solution (Berlex) p 702
Roma-Nol Antiseptic (Jamol) p 1033
Seffin, Neutral (Glaxo) p 980
Septra DS Tablets (Burroughs Wellcome) p 408, 815
Septra I.V. Infusion (Burroughs Wellcome) p 813
Septra Suspension (Burroughs Wellcome) p 815
Septra Tablets (Burroughs Wellcome) p 408, 815
Spectrobid Tablets & Oral Suspension (Roerig) p 431, 1741
Sumycin Capsules (Squibb) p 438, 2022
Sumycin Tablets (Squibb) p 438, 2022
Sumycin Syrup (Squibb) p 2022
Trimox Capsules & for Oral Suspension (Squibb) p 438, 2025
Trimpex Tablets (Roche) p 430, 1706
Veetids Tablets (Squibb) p 438, 2026
Velosef Capsules (Squibb) p 438, 2027
Velosef for Oral Suspension (Squibb) p 2027
Zinacef (Glaxo) p 993
Antifungal
Betadine Viscous Formula Antiseptic Gauze Pad (Purdue Frederick) p 1623
Castellani Paint (Pedinol) p 1580
Flint SSD Cream (Flint) p 411, 950
Fungizone Cream/Lotion/Ointment (Squibb) p 1994
Fungoid Creme & Solution (Pedinol) p 1580
Fungoid Tincture (Pedinol) p 1580
Gyne-Lotrimin Vaginal Cream 1% (Schering) p 1856
Gyne-Lotrimin Vaginal Tablets (Schering) p 434, 1856
Hibiclens Antimicrobial Skin Cleanser (Stuart) p 439, 2037
Hibistat Germicidal Hand Rinse (Stuart) p 439, 2038
Lotrimin Cream 1% (Schering) p 1857
Lotrimin Lotion 1% (Schering) p 1857
Lotrimin Solution 1% (Schering) p 1857
Lotrisone Cream (Schering) p 1858
Micro-Guard (Sween) p 2048
Monistat-Derm (miconazole nitrate) Cream & Lotion (Ortho Pharmaceutical (Dermatological Div.)) p 1474
Mycelex Troches (Miles Pharmaceuticals) p 422, 1409
Mycolog Cream and Ointment (Squibb) p 2003
Mycostatin Cream & Ointment (Squibb) p 2004
Mycostatin Oral Suspension (Squibb) p 2004
Mycostatin Oral Tablets (Squibb) p 438, 2005
Mycostatin Topical Powder (Squibb) p 2004
Mycostatin Vaginal Tablets (Squibb) p 438, 2005
Mysteclin-F Capsules (Squibb) p 438, 2005
Mysteclin-F Syrup (Squibb) p 2005
O-V Statin (Squibb) p 2008

Product Category Index

Spectazole Cream (Ortho Pharmaceutical (Dermatological Div.)) p 1476
Triva Combination (Boyle) p 726
Triva Douche Powder (Boyle) p 726

Parenteral
Bactrim I.V. Infusion (Roche) p 1672
Cefobid Intravenous/Intramuscular (Roerig) p 1726
Crysticillin 300 A.S. & Crysticillin 600 A.S. (Squibb) p 1992
Gantrisin Injectable (Roche) p 1686
Garamycin Injectable (Schering) p 1846
Garamycin Intrathecal Injection (Schering) p 1854
Garamycin I.V. Piggyback Injection (Schering) p 1851
Garamycin Pediatric Injectable (Schering) p 1849
Geopen (Roerig) p 1731
Netromycin Injection (Schering) p 1863
Penicillin G Potassium for Injection USP (Squibb) p 2009
Penicillin G Sodium for Injection USP (Squibb) p 2010
Polymyxin B Sulfate (see Aerosporin) (Burroughs Wellcome) p 775
Seffin, Neutral (Glaxo) p 980
Septra I.V. Infusion (Burroughs Wellcome) p 813
Velosef for Infusion (Sodium-Free) (Squibb) p 2029
Velosef for Injection (Squibb) p 2030
Zinacef (Glaxo) p 993

Sulfonamide Combinations
Bactrim DS Tablets (Roche) p 429, 1674
Bactrim I.V. Infusion (Roche) p 1672
Bactrim Pediatric Suspension (Roche) p 1674
Bactrim Suspension (Roche) p 1674
Bactrim Tablets (Roche) p 429, 1674
Metimyd Ophthalmic Ointment - Sterile (Schering) p 1860
Metimyd Ophthalmic Suspension (Schering) p 1860
Septra DS Tablets (Burroughs Wellcome) p 408, 815
Septra Suspension (Burroughs Wellcome) p 815
Septra Tablets (Burroughs Wellcome) p 408, 815
Thiosulfil Duo-Pak (Ayerst) p 682
Thiosulfil-A Forte (Ayerst) p 405, 681
Thiosulfil-A Tablets (Ayerst) p 405, 681

Sulfonamides
Azulfidine Tablets, EN-tabs, Oral Suspension (Pharmacia) p 427, 1613
Gantanol DS Tablets (Roche) p 429, 1685
Gantanol Suspension (Roche) p 1685
Gantanol Tablets (Roche) p 429, 1685
Gantrisin Injectable (Roche) p 1686
Gantrisin Ophthalmic Ointment/Solution (Roche) p 1685
Gantrisin Pediatric Suspension (Roche) p 1686
Gantrisin Syrup (Roche) p 1686
Gantrisin Tablets (Roche) p 429, 1686
Lipo Gantrisin (Roche) p 1686
Septra I.V. Infusion (Burroughs Wellcome) p 813
Sulfamylon Acetate Cream (Winthrop-Breon) p 2226
Sween Prep (Sween) p 2049
Thiosulfil Forte (Ayerst) p 405, 680
Thiosulfil Tablets (Ayerst) p 405

Topical
Aerosporin Powder (Burroughs Wellcome) p 775
Anbesol Gel Antiseptic Anesthetic (Whitehall) p 443, 2185
Anti-Sept (Seamless) p 1897
Betadine Aerosol Spray (Purdue Frederick) p 1622
Betadine Antiseptic Gel (Purdue Frederick) p 1622
Betadine Disposable Medicated Douche (Purdue Frederick) p 1622
Betadine Douche (Purdue Frederick) p 1622
Betadine Helafoam Solution (Purdue Frederick) p 1622
Betadine Ointment (Purdue Frederick) p 1622
Betadine Skin Cleanser (Purdue Frederick) p 1622
Betadine Solution (Purdue Frederick) p 1622
Betadine Surgical Scrub (Purdue Frederick) p 1622
Betadine Viscous Formula Antiseptic Gauze Pad (Purdue Frederick) p 1623
Clorpactin WCS-90 (Guardian) p 1000
Cortisporin Cream (Burroughs Wellcome) p 783
Cortisporin Ointment (Burroughs Wellcome) p 784
Cortisporin Ophthalmic Ointment (Burroughs Wellcome) p 784
Cortisporin Ophthalmic Suspension (Burroughs Wellcome) p 785
Cortisporin Otic Solution (Burroughs Wellcome) p 786
Cortisporin Otic Suspension (Burroughs Wellcome) p 786
Dalidyne (Dalin) p 886
Derma Medicone-HC Ointment (Medicone) p 1256
Flint SSD Cream (Flint) p 411, 950
Furacin Preparations (Norwich Eaton) p 1433
Furacin Soluble Dressing (Norwich Eaton) p 1433
Furacin Topical Cream (Norwich Eaton) p 1434
Gantrisin Ophthalmic Ointment/Solution (Roche) p 1685
Garamycin Cream 0.1% and Ointment 0.1% (Schering) p 1846
Garamycin Ophthalmic Ointment-Sterile (Schering) p 1846
Garamycin Ophthalmic Solution-Sterile (Schering) p 1846
Gly-Oxide Liquid (Marion) p 1186
Gumsol (Arlo) p 601
Hibiclens Antimicrobial Skin Cleanser (Stuart) p 439, 2037
Hibistat Germicidal Hand Rinse (Stuart) p 439, 2038
Lubraseptic Jelly (Guardian) p 1000
Metimyd Ophthalmic Ointment - Sterile (Schering) p 1860
Metimyd Ophthalmic Suspension (Schering) p 1860
Mycelex Troches (Miles Pharmaceuticals) p 422, 1409
Neo-Polycin (Merrell Dow) p 1372
Neosporin Aerosol (Burroughs Wellcome) p 806
Neosporin Ointment (Burroughs Wellcome) p 808
Neosporin Ophthalmic Ointment Sterile (Burroughs Wellcome) p 808
Neosporin Ophthalmic Solution Sterile (Burroughs Wellcome) p 809
Neosporin Powder (Burroughs Wellcome) p 810
Neosporin-G Cream (Burroughs Wellcome) p 807
Polysporin Ointment (Burroughs Wellcome) p 810
Polysporin Ophthalmic Ointment (Burroughs Wellcome) p 810
Prophyllin (Rystan) p 1796
Pyocidin-Otic Solution (Berlex) p 702
Rectal Medicone-HC Suppositories (Medicone) p 419, 1256
Roma-Nol Antiseptic (Jamol) p 1033
Silvadene Cream (Marion) p 1189
Sodium Sulamyd Ophthalmic Solutions & Ointment-Sterile (Schering) p 1884
Sulfamylon Acetate Cream (Winthrop-Breon) p 2226
Triva Combination (Boyle) p 726
Triva Douche Powder (Boyle) p 726
Triva Jel (Boyle) p 726
Zephiran Chloride 1:750 (Winthrop-Breon) p 2233
Zephiran Chloride Spray (Winthrop-Breon) p 2233
Zephiran Chloride Tinted Tincture (Winthrop-Breon) p 2233

Urinary Antibacterial
Bactrim DS Tablets (Roche) p 429, 1674
Bactrim I.V. Infusion (Roche) p 1672
Bactrim Pediatric Suspension (Roche) p 1674
Bactrim Suspension (Roche) p 1674
Bactrim Tablets (Roche) p 429, 1674
Cinobac Pulvules (Dista) p 410, 894
Furadantin Oral Suspension (Norwich Eaton) p 1432
Furadantin Tablets (Norwich Eaton) p 1432
Gantanol DS Tablets (Roche) p 429, 1685
Gantanol Suspension (Roche) p 1685
Gantanol Tablets (Roche) p 429, 1685
Gantrisin Injectable (Roche) p 1686
Gantrisin Pediatric Suspension (Roche) p 1686
Gantrisin Syrup (Roche) p 1686
Gantrisin Tablets (Roche) p 429, 1686
Geocillin Tablets (Roerig) p 431, 1730
Hiprex (Merrell Dow) p 421, 1366
Lipo Gantrisin (Roche) p 1686
Macrodantin Capsules (Norwich Eaton) p 422, 1436
NegGram Caplets (Winthrop-Breon) p 444, 2215
NegGram Suspension (Winthrop-Breon) p 2215
Neosporin G.U. Irrigant (Burroughs Wellcome) p 807
Proloprim (Burroughs Wellcome) p 408, 810
Renoquid (Glenwood) p 412, 999
Septra DS Tablets (Burroughs Wellcome) p 408, 815
Septra I.V. Infusion (Burroughs Wellcome) p 813
Septra Suspension (Burroughs Wellcome) p 815
Septra Tablets (Burroughs Wellcome) p 408, 815
Thiacide Tablets (Beach) p 405, 687
Thiosulfil Forte (Ayerst) p 405, 680
Thiosulfil Tablets (Ayerst) p 405
Trimpex Tablets (Roche) p 430, 1706
Urised Tablets (Webcon) p 2173
Uro-Phosphate Tablets (Poythress) p 1619
Uroqid-Acid Tablets (Beach) p 405, 687
Uroqid-Acid No. 2 Tablets (Beach) p 405, 687

Urinary Antibacterial with Analgesics
Azo Gantanol Tablets (Roche) p 429, 1670
Azo Gantrisin Tablets (Roche) p 429, 1671
Mandelamine (Parke-Davis) p 424, 1540
Thiosulfil Duo-Pak (Ayerst) p 682
Thiosulfil-A Forte (Ayerst) p 405, 681
Thiosulfil-A Tablets (Ayerst) p 405, 681
Urobiotic-250 (Roerig) p 431, 1744

ANTIBIOTICS

Amebicides
Aralen Hydrochloride (Winthrop-Breon) p 2189
Aralen Phosphate (Winthrop-Breon) p 443, 2190
Flagyl Tablets (Searle & Co.) p 436, 1929
Humatin Capsules (Parke-Davis) p 424, 1527

Antifungal
Caprystatin (Ecological Formulas) p 929
Fulvicin P/G Tablets (Schering) p 434, 1843
Fulvicin P/G 165 & 330 Tablets (Schering) p 434, 1844
Fulvicin-U/F Tablets (Schering) p 434, 1845
Fungizone Cream/Lotion/Ointment (Squibb) p 1994
Fungizone Intravenous (Squibb) p 1994
Grisactin (Ayerst) p 404, 646
Grisactin Ultra (Ayerst) p 405, 646
Gris-PEG Tablets, 125mg & 250mg (Herbert) p 1005
Korostatin Vaginal Tablets (Youngs) p 2301
Lotrimin Cream 1% (Schering) p 1857
Lotrimin Lotion 1% (Schering) p 1857
Lotrimin Solution 1% (Schering) p 1857
Lotrisone Cream (Schering) p 1858
Monistat-Derm (miconazole nitrate) Cream & Lotion (Ortho Pharmaceutical (Dermatological Div.)) p 1474
Mycostatin Cream & Ointment (Squibb) p 2004
Mycostatin Oral Suspension (Squibb) p 2004
Mycostatin Oral Tablets (Squibb) p 438, 2005
Mycostatin Topical Powder (Squibb) p 2004
Mycostatin Vaginal Tablets (Squibb) p 438, 2005
Nilstat for Preparation of Oral Suspension (Lederle) p 1108
Nilstat Oral Suspension (Lederle) p 1108
Nilstat Oral Tablets (Lederle) p 1109
Nilstat Topical Cream & Ointment (Lederle) p 1109
Nilstat Vaginal Tablets (Lederle) p 1108
O-V Statin (Squibb) p 2008
Spectazole Cream (Ortho Pharmaceutical (Dermatological Div.)) p 1476

Antituberculosis
Capastat Sulfate (Lilly) p 1132
INH Tablets (CIBA) p 850
Rifadin (Merrell Dow) p 421, 1382
Rifamate (Merrell Dow) p 421, 1383
Rimactane Capsules (CIBA) p 409, 864
Seromycin (Lilly) p 1174
Streptomycin Sulfate Injection (Pfipharmecs) p 1593

Antiviral
Vira-A for Infusion (Parke-Davis) p 1576
Vira-A Ophthalmic Ointment, 3% (Parke-Davis) p 426, 1578

Broad & Medium Spectrum
A/T/S (Hoechst-Roussel) p 412, 1009
Achromycin Intramuscular (Lederle) p 1074
Achromycin Intravenous (Lederle) p 1074
Achromycin V Capsules (Lederle) p 414, 1076
Achromycin V Oral Suspension (Lederle) p 1076
Aerosporin Powder (Burroughs Wellcome) p 775
Amikin (Bristol) p 727
Amoxil (Beecham Laboratories) p 405, 688
Ancef (Smith Kline & French) p 1945
Anspor (Smith Kline & French) p 436, 1948
Azlin (Miles Pharmaceuticals) p 1396
Ceclor (Lilly) p 417, 1133
Cefadyl (Bristol) p 731
Cefizox Injection (Smith Kline & French) p 1949
Cefobid Intravenous/Intramuscular (Roerig) p 1726
Chloromycetin Cream, 1% (Parke-Davis) p 1487

Product Category Index

Chloromycetin Hydrocortisone Ophthalmic (Parke-Davis) p 1488
Chloromycetin Kapseals (Parke-Davis) p 423, 1489
Chloromycetin Ophthalmic Ointment, 1% (Parke-Davis) p 1491
Chloromycetin Otic (Parke-Davis) p 1491
Chloromycetin Palmitate (Parke-Davis) p 1491
Chloromycetin Sodium Succinate (Parke-Davis) p 1493
Claforan (Hoechst-Roussel) p 1010
Cleocin HCl Capsules* (Upjohn) p 441, 2094
Cleocin Pediatric Flavored Granules* (Upjohn) p 2096
Cleocin Phosphate Sterile Solution* (Upjohn) p 440, 2097
Cleocin T Topical Solution* (Upjohn) p 441, 2100
Coly-Mycin M Parenteral (Parke-Davis) p 1500
Cortisporin Cream (Burroughs Wellcome) p 783
Cortisporin Ointment (Burroughs Wellcome) p 784
Cortisporin Ophthalmic Ointment (Burroughs Wellcome) p 784
Cortisporin Ophthalmic Suspension (Burroughs Wellcome) p 785
Cortisporin Otic Solution (Burroughs Wellcome) p 786
Cortisporin Otic Suspension (Burroughs Wellcome) p 786
Cyclapen-W (Wyeth) p 444, 2249
Declomycin Capsules and Tablets (Lederle) p 415, 1090
Duricef (Mead Johnson Pharmaceutical) p 419, 1250
E.E.S. Chewable Tablets (Abbott) p 403, 522
E.E.S. Drops (Abbott) p 522
E.E.S. Granules (Abbott) p 522
E.E.S. 200 Liquid (Abbott) p 522
E.E.S. 400 Filmtab (Abbott) p 403, 522
E.E.S. 400 Liquid (Abbott) p 522
E-Mycin E Liquid (Upjohn) p 2113
E-Mycin Tablets (Upjohn) p 441, 2112
ERYC (Parke-Davis) p 424, 1515
EryDerm (Abbott) p 519
Erymax Topical Solution (Herbert) p 1003
EryPed Granules (Abbott) p 520
Ery-Tab Tablets (Abbott) p 403, 521
Erythrocin Lactobionate-I.V. (Abbott) p 523
Erythrocin Piggyback (Abbott) p 403, 524
Erythrocin Stearate Filmtab (Abbott) p 403, 525
Erythromycin Base Filmtab (Abbott) p 403, 526
Erythromycin Stearate Tablets, USP (Erypar) (Parke-Davis) p 424, 1516
Furoxone Liquid Suspension (Norwich Eaton) p 1435
Furoxone Tablets (Norwich Eaton) p 1435
G-myticin Creme and Ointment 0.1% (Pedinol) p 1580
Garamycin Cream 0.1% and Ointment 0.1% (Schering) p 1846
Garamycin Injectable (Schering) p 1846
Garamycin Intrathecal Injection (Schering) p 1854
Garamycin I.V. Piggyback Injection (Schering) p 1851
Garamycin Ophthalmic Ointment-Sterile (Schering) p 1846
Garamycin Ophthalmic Solution-Sterile (Schering) p 1846
Garamycin Pediatric Injectable (Schering) p 1849
Geocillin Tablets (Roerig) p 431, 1730
Geopen (Roerig) p 1731
Humatin Capsules (Parke-Davis) p 424, 1527
Ilosone Oral Preparations (Dista) p 410, 897
Ilotycin Gluceptate (Dista) p 900
Ilotycin Sterile Ophthalmic Ointment (Dista) p 899
Ilotycin Tablets (Dista) p 899
Kantrex Capsules (Bristol) p 407, 734
Kantrex Injection (Bristol) p 735
Kantrex Pediatric Injection (Bristol) p 735
Keflex Oral Preparations (Dista) p 410, 901
Keflin, Neutral, Vials & Faspak (Lilly) p 1157
Kefzol (Lilly) p 1159
Lincocin (Upjohn) p 2119
Mandol (Lilly) p 1161
Mefoxin (Merck Sharp & Dohme) p 1326
Mezlin (Miles Pharmaceuticals) p 1404
Minocin (Lederle) p 415, 1103
Minocin Oral Suspension (Lederle) p 1104
Monocid Injection (Smith Kline & French) p 1966
Moxam Vials (Lilly) p 1166
Nebcin (Dista) p 905
Nebcin, Sterile (Dista) p 907
Neosporin Ointment (Burroughs Wellcome) p 808
Netromycin Injection (Schering) p 1863
Omnipen Capsules (Wyeth) p 444, 2271

Omnipen for Oral Suspension (Wyeth) p 2271
Omnipen Pediatric Drops (Wyeth) p 2271
Omnipen-N (Wyeth) p 2271
Ophthochlor, 0.5% (Parke-Davis) p 425, 1557
Ophthocort (Parke-Davis) p 1558
Pediamycin (Ross) p 1772
Pediazole (Ross) p 1774
Penicillin V, Potassium (Penapar VK) (Parke-Davis) p 425, 1559
Pen•Vee K, for Oral Solution & Tablets (Wyeth) p 444, 2275
Permapen Isoject (Pfipharmecs) p 1590
Pfizerpen for Injection (Pfipharmecs) p 1590
Pfizerpen-AS Aqueous Suspension (Pfipharmecs) p 1592
Pipracil (Lederle) p 416, 1113
Polycillin (Bristol) p 407, 740
Polycillin-N for Injection (Bristol) p 740
Polycillin-PRB (Bristol) p 741
Polymox Capsules (Bristol) p 407, 742
Polymox For Oral Suspension (Bristol) p 742
Polymox Pediatric Drops (Bristol) p 742
Polymyxin B Sulfate (see Aerosporin) (Burroughs Wellcome) p 775
Polysporin Ointment (Burroughs Wellcome) p 810
Precef (Bristol) p 743
Principen Capsules (Squibb) p 438, 2012
Principen for Oral Suspension (Squibb) p 2012
Principen with Probenecid Capsules (Squibb) p 2013
Protostat Tablets (Ortho Pharmaceutical) p 423, 1470
Rondomycin (Wallace) p 442, 2164
Seffin, Neutral (Glaxo) p 980
Seromycin (Lilly) p 1174
Spectrobid Tablets & Oral Suspension (Roerig) p 431, 1741
Staticin 1.5% Topical Solution (Westwood) p 2181
Streptomycin Sulfate Injection (Pfipharmecs) p 1593
Sumycin Capsules (Squibb) p 438, 2022
Sumycin Tablets (Squibb) p 438, 2022
Sumycin Syrup (Squibb) p 2022
T-Stat 2.0% Topical Solution (Westwood) p 2181
Tao Capsules (Roerig) p 431, 1744
Terramycin Capsules (Pfipharmecs) p 426, 1595
Terramycin Film-coated Tablets (Pfipharmecs) p 1595
Terramycin Intramuscular Solution (Pfipharmecs) p 1596
Terramycin with Polymyxin B Sulfate Ophthalmic Ointment (Pfipharmecs) p 1598
Tetracycline HCl Capsules (Cyclopar) (Parke-Davis) p 425, 1573
Tetracycline HCl Capsules (Cyclopar 500) (Parke-Davis) p 425, 1573
Ticar (Beecham Laboratories) p 695
Topicycline (Norwich Eaton) p 1438
Trimox Capsules & for Oral Suspension (Squibb) p 438, 2025
Trobicin Sterile Powder (Upjohn) p 2141
Ultracef Capsules, Tablets & Oral Suspension (Bristol) p 407, 754
Urobiotic-250 (Roerig) p 431, 1744
Vancocin HCl, for Oral Solution (Lilly) p 1178
Vancocin HCl, Vials (Lilly) p 1177
Velosef Capsules (Squibb) p 438, 2027
Velosef for Infusion (Sodium-Free) (Squibb) p 2029
Velosef for Injection (Squibb) p 2030
Velosef for Oral Suspension (Squibb) p 2027
Versapen Oral Suspension (Bristol) p 755
Versapen Pediatric Drops (Bristol) p 755
Versapen-K Capsules (Bristol) p 407, 755
Vibramycin Calcium Syrup (Pfizer) p 1610
Vibramycin Hyclate Capsules (Pfizer) p 426, 1610
Vibramycin Hyclate Intravenous (Pfizer) p 1611
Vibramycin Monohydrate for Oral Suspension (Pfizer) p 1610
Vibra-Tabs Film Coated Tablets (Pfizer) p 426, 1610
Wyamycin E Liquid (Wyeth) p 2292
Wyamycin S Tablets (Wyeth) p 445, 2292
Wymox Capsules & Oral Suspension (Wyeth) p 445, 2298
Zinacef (Glaxo) p 993

Broad & Medium Spectrum with Antimonilial

Mysteclin-F Capsules (Squibb) p 438, 2005
Mysteclin-F Syrup (Squibb) p 2005

Penicillin

Amcill Capsules (Parke-Davis) p 423, 1480
Amcill Oral Suspension (Parke-Davis) p 1480
Amoxicillin Capsules (Parke-Davis) p 423, 1482
Amoxicillin for Oral Suspension (Parke-Davis) p 1482

Amoxil (Beecham Laboratories) p 405, 688
Augmentin Tablets & Powder for Oral Suspension (Beecham Laboratories) p 405, 690
Betapen-VK (Bristol) p 407, 729
Bicillin C-R Injection (Wyeth) p 2239
Bicillin C-R in Tubex (Wyeth) p 2288
Bicillin C-R 900/300 (Wyeth) p 2241
Bicillin C-R 900/300 in Tubex (Wyeth) p 2288
Bicillin L-A Injection (Wyeth) p 2242
Crysticillin 300 A.S. & Crysticillin 600 A.S. (Squibb) p 1992
Cyclapen-W (Wyeth) p 444, 2249
Dynapen (Bristol) p 407, 733
Geocillin Tablets (Roerig) p 431, 1730
Geopen (Roerig) p 1731
Mezlin (Miles Pharmaceuticals) p 1404
Nafcil (Bristol) p 736
Omnipen Capsules (Wyeth) p 444, 2271
Omnipen for Oral Suspension (Wyeth) p 2271
Omnipen Pediatric Drops (Wyeth) p 2271
Omnipen-N (Wyeth) p 2271
Pathocil Capsules, for Oral Suspension (Wyeth) p 444, 2274
Penicillin G Potassium for Injection USP (Squibb) p 2009
Penicillin G Procaine Suspension, Sterile, Vials (Lilly) p 1170
Penicillin G Sodium for Injection USP (Squibb) p 2010
Pentids for Syrup (Squibb) p 2011
Pentids Tablets, Pentids 400 & 800 Tablets (Squibb) p 438, 2011
Pen•Vee K, for Oral Solution & Tablets (Wyeth) p 444, 2275
Polycillin (Bristol) p 407, 740
Polycillin-N for Injection (Bristol) p 740
Polycillin-PRB (Bristol) p 741
Polymox Capsules (Bristol) p 407, 742
Polymox For Oral Suspension (Bristol) p 742
Polymox Pediatric Drops (Bristol) p 742
Principen Capsules (Squibb) p 438, 2012
Principen for Oral Suspension (Squibb) p 2012
Principen with Probenecid Capsules (Squibb) p 2013
Prostaphlin Capsules, Oral Solution (Bristol) p 407, 745
Prostaphlin for Injection (Bristol) p 745
Spectrobid Tablets & Oral Suspension (Roerig) p 431, 1741
Staphcillin (Bristol) p 751
Tegopen (Bristol) p 407, 753
Ticar (Beecham Laboratories) p 695
Unipen Injection, Capsules, Powder for Oral Solution, & Tablets (Wyeth) p 445, 2290
V-Cillin K for Oral Solution & Tablets (Lilly) p 1178
Veetids for Oral Solution (Squibb) p 2026
Veetids Tablets (Squibb) p 438, 2026
Versapen Oral Suspension (Bristol) p 755
Versapen Pediatric Drops (Bristol) p 755
Versapen-K Capsules (Bristol) p 407, 755
Wycillin (Wyeth) p 2293
Wycillin in Tubex (Wyeth) p 2288
Wycillin & Probenecid Tablets & Injection (Wyeth) p 2295
Wymox Capsules & Oral Suspension (Wyeth) p 445, 2298

ANTICANCER PREPARATIONS (see under ANTINEOPLASTICS)

ANTICATECHOLAMINE SYNTHESIS

Demser Capsules (Merck Sharp & Dohme) p 420, 1297

ANTICHOLINERGIC DRUG INHIBITOR

Antilirium Injectable (O'Neal, Jones & Feldman) p 1443

ANTICOAGULANT ANTAGONIST

AquaMEPHYTON Injection (Merck Sharp & Dohme) p 1265

ANTICOAGULANTS

Calciparine Injection (American Critical Care) p 593
Coumadin (Du Pont) p 410, 915
Heparin Lock Flush Solution in Tubex (Wyeth) p 2253
Heparin Sodium (Lilly) p 1149
Heparin Sodium in Tubex (Wyeth) p 2288
Heparin Sodium Injection (Wyeth) p 2254
Heparin Sodium Injection, USP, Sterile Solution (Upjohn) p 2117
Protamine Sulfate (Lilly) p 1171
Protamine Sulfate for Injection, USP, Sterile Powder (Upjohn) p 2133

ANTICONVULSANTS

Amytal Sodium Ampoules & Vials (Lilly) p 1127
Celontin (Half Strength) Kapseals (Parke-Davis) p 423, 1486

Product Category Index

Celontin Kapseals (Parke-Davis) p 423, 1486
Clonopin Tablets (Roche) p 429, 1680
Depakote Capsules & Syrup (Abbott) p 403, 512
Depakote Tablets (Abbott) p 403, 513
Dilantin Infatabs (Parke-Davis) p 423, 1503
Dilantin Kapseals (Parke-Davis) p 423, 1502
Dilantin Parenteral (Parke-Davis) p 1505
Dilantin with Phenobarbital (Parke-Davis) p 423, 1507
Dilantin-30 Pediatric/Dilantin-125 Suspension (Parke-Davis) p 1506
Gemonil (Abbott) p 531
Mebaral (Winthrop-Breon) p 444, 2213
Mesantoin (Sandoz Pharmaceutical Div.) p 433, 1805
Milontin Kapseals (Parke-Davis) p 424, 1543
Mysoline (Ayerst) p 405, 657
Paradione (Abbott) p 403, 558
Peganone (Abbott) p 403, 559
Phenurone (Abbott) p 564
Tegretol Chewable Tablets (Geigy) p 411, 966
Tegretol Tablets (Geigy) p 411, 966
Tridione (Abbott) p 404, 570
Valium Injectable (Roche Products) p 430, 1721
Valium Tablets (Roche Products) p 430, 1723
Valrelease Capsules (Roche) p 430, 1707
Zarontin Capsules (Parke-Davis) p 426, 1579
Zarontin Syrup (Parke-Davis) p 1579

ANTIDEPRESSANTS

Adapin (Pennwalt) p 426, 1581
Amitriptyline Hydrochloride Tablets (Parke-Davis) p 423, 1481
Asendin (Lederle) p 415, 1088
Aventyl HCl (Lilly) p 417, 1130
Deprol (Wallace) p 2157
Desyrel (Mead Johnson Pharmaceutical) p 419, 1249
Elavil Tablets & Injection (Merck Sharp & Dohme) p 420, 1306
Endep Tablets (Roche Products) p 429, 1711
Etrafon Tablets (Schering) p 434, 1841
Limbitrol Tablets (Roche Products) p 430, 1716
Ludiomil (CIBA) p 409, 854
Marplan Tablets (Roche) p 430, 1689
Nardil (Parke-Davis) p 424, 1543
Norpramin (Merrell Dow) p 421, 1374
Pamelor (Sandoz Pharmaceutical Div.) p 433, 1807
Parnate (Smith Kline & French) p 437, 1969
Pertofrane Capsules (USV Pharmaceutical) p 440, 2086
Sinequan (Roerig) p 431, 1740
Surmontil Capsules 25 mg, 50 mg, & 100 mg (Ives) p 413, 1029
Tofranil Ampuls (Geigy) p 969
Tofranil Tablets (Geigy) p 411, 969
Tofranil-PM Capsules (Geigy) p 411, 971
Triavil Tablets (Merck Sharp & Dohme) p 420, 1354
Vivactil Tablets (Merck Sharp & Dohme) p 421, 1357

ANTIDIABETIC AGENTS

Intermediate Acting Insulins
Humulin N Vials (Lilly) p 1150
Iletin I, Lente (Lilly) p 1156
Insulatard NPH (Nordisk-USA) p 1422
Lente Insulin (Insulin Zinc Suspension USP) (Squibb-Novo) p 2033
Lente Purified Pork Insulin Zinc Suspension (Squibb-Novo) p 2034
Mixtard (Nordisk-USA) p 1423
NPH Insulin (Isophane Insulin Suspension USP) (Squibb-Novo) p 2034
NPH Iletin I (Lilly) p 1156
NPH Purified Pork Isophane Insulin Suspension (Squibb-Novo) p 2034
Novolin L (Squibb-Novo) p 2034
Novolin N (Squibb-Novo) p 2034

Long Acting Insulins
Iletin I, Ultralente (Lilly) p 1156
Mixtard (Nordisk-USA) p 1423
Protamine, Zinc & Iletin I (Lilly) p 1156
Ultralente Insulin (Extended Insulin Zinc Suspension USP) (Squibb-Novo) p 2034
Ultralente Purified Beef Extended Insulin Zinc Suspension (Squibb-Novo) p 2034

Oral
DiaBeta (Hoechst-Roussel) p 412, 1012
Diabinese (Pfizer) p 426, 1599
Dymelor (Lilly) p 417, 1146
Glucotrol (Roerig) p 431, 1733
Micronase Tablets (Upjohn) p 441, 2126
Orinase Tablets (Upjohn) p 441, 2130
Tolinase Tablets (Upjohn) p 441, 2139

Rapid Acting Insulins
Humulin R Vials (Lilly) p 1152
Iletin I, Regular (Lilly) p 1154

Iletin II, Regular (Concentrated), U-500 (Lilly) p 1155
Iletin I, Semilente (Lilly) p 1156
Insulin Injection USP (Regular) (Squibb-Novo) p 2033
Novolin R (Squibb-Novo) p 2034
Regular Purified Pork Insulin (Squibb-Novo) p 2034
Semilente Insulin (Prompt Insulin Zinc Suspension USP) (Squibb-Novo) p 2033
Semilente Purified Pork Prompt Insulin Zinc Suspension (Squibb-Novo) p 2034
Velosulin (Nordisk-USA) p 1423

ANTIDIARRHEALS

Arco-Lase Plus (Arco) p 600
Coly-Mycin S Oral Suspension (Parke-Davis) p 1501
Furoxone Liquid Suspension (Norwich Eaton) p 1435
Furoxone Tablets (Norwich Eaton) p 1435
Imodium Capsules/Liquid (Janssen) p 413, 1033
Lomotil Liquid (Searle & Co.) p 1931
Lomotil Tablets (Searle & Co.) p 436, 1931
Mitrolan (Robins) p 428, 1654
Parepectolin (Rorer) p 1752
Pepto-Bismol Liquid & Tablets (Procter & Gamble) p 1620

ANTIDIURETICS

DDAVP (USV Pharmaceutical) p 440, 2074
DDAVP Injection (USV Pharmaceutical) p 440, 2075
Diapid Nasal Spray (Sandoz Pharmaceutical Div.) p 1801
Pitressin (Parke-Davis) p 1562
Pitressin Tannate in Oil (Parke-Davis) p 1562
Stimate Injection (Armour) p 611

ANTIDOTES

Anticholinesterase
Antilirium Injectable (O'Neal, Jones & Feldman) p 1443
Protopam Chloride (Ayerst) p 678

General
Arm-a-char (Armour) p 604

ANTIENURESIS

Tofranil Tablets (Geigy) p 411, 969

ANTIFIBRINOLYTIC AGENTS

Amicar (Lederle) p 414, 1077

ANTIFIBROTICS, SYSTEMIC

Potaba (Glenwood) p 412, 998

ANTIFLATULENTS & COMBINATIONS

Arco-Lase (Arco) p 600
Arco-Lase Plus (Arco) p 600
Celluzyme Chewable Tablets (Dalin) p 886
Festal II (Hoechst-Roussel) p 412, 1014
Festalan (Hoechst-Roussel) p 413, 1014
Gelusil (Parke-Davis) p 424, 1525
Ilopan Injection (Adria) p 578
Kanulase (Dorsey Laboratories) p 910
Karbokoff Tablets (Arlo) p 601
Kutrase Capsules (Rorer) p 431, 1750
Ku-Zyme Capsules (Rorer) p 431, 1750
Mylicon Drops (Stuart) p 2039
Mylicon Tablets (Stuart) p 439, 2039
Mylicon-80 Tablets (Stuart) p 439, 2040
Phazyme Tablets (Reed & Carnrick) p 427, 1636
Phazyme-95 Tablets (Reed & Carnrick) p 427, 1636
Phazyme-PB Tablets (Reed & Carnrick) p 427, 1636
Simeco (Wyeth) p 2288
Tri-Cone Capsules (Glaxo) p 986
Zypan Tablets (Standard Process) p 2035

ANTIFUNGAL AGENTS

Systemic
(see also under ANTIBIOTICS)
Ancobon Capsules (Roche) p 429, 1669
Fulvicin P/G Tablets (Schering) p 434, 1843
Fulvicin P/G 165 & 330 Tablets (Schering) p 434, 1844
Fulvicin-U/F Tablets (Schering) p 434, 1845
Fungizone Intravenous (Squibb) p 1994
Grifulvin V (Ortho Pharmaceutical (Dermatological Div.)) p 1473
Gris-PEG Tablets, 125mg & 250mg (Herbert) p 1005
Monistat I.V. (Janssen) p 1037
Mycostatin Oral Suspension (Squibb) p 2004
Mycostatin Oral Tablets (Squibb) p 438, 2005
Nilstat for Preparation of Oral Suspension (Lederle) p 1108
Nizoral Tablets (Janssen) p 413, 1038
Nystex Oral Suspension (Savage) p 1825

Topical
(see also under DERMATOLOGICALS)
Betadine Aerosol Spray (Purdue Frederick) p 1622
Betadine Helafoam Solution (Purdue Frederick) p 1622
Betadine Ointment (Purdue Frederick) p 1622
Betadine Skin Cleanser (Purdue Frederick) p 1622
Betadine Solution (Purdue Frederick) p 1622
Betadine Surgical Scrub (Purdue Frederick) p 1622
Betadine Viscous Formula Antiseptic Gauze Pad (Purdue Frederick) p 1623
Breezee Mist Foot Powder (Pedinol) p 1580
Castellani Paint (Pedinol) p 1580
Flint SSD Cream (Flint) p 411, 950
Fungi-Nail Tincture (Kramer) p 1069
Fungizone Cream/Lotion/Ointment (Squibb) p 1994
Fungoid Creme & Solution (Pedinol) p 1580
Fungoid Tincture (Pedinol) p 1580
Gyne-Lotrimin Vaginal Cream 1% (Schering) p 1856
Gyne-Lotrimin Vaginal Tablets (Schering) p 434, 1856
Loprox Cream 1% (Hoechst-Roussel) p 413, 1017
Lotrimin Cream 1% (Schering) p 1857
Lotrimin Lotion 1% (Schering) p 1857
Lotrimin Solution 1% (Schering) p 1857
Lotrisone Cream (Schering) p 1858
Monistat-Derm (miconazole nitrate) Cream & Lotion (Ortho Pharmaceutical (Dermatological Div.)) p 1474
Monistat 3 Vaginal Suppositories (Ortho Pharmaceutical) p 1456
Mycelex 1% Cream (Miles Pharmaceuticals) p 1409
Mycelex 1% Solution (Miles Pharmaceuticals) p 1409
Mycelex-G 1% Vaginal Cream (Miles Pharmaceuticals) p 1410
Mycostatin Cream & Ointment (Squibb) p 2004
Mycostatin Topical Powder (Squibb) p 2004
Nystex Cream & Ointment (Savage) p 1825
Osti-Derm Lotion (Pedinol) p 1580
Pedi-Dri Foot Powder (Pedinol) p 1581
Pedi-Pro Foot Powder (Pedinol) p 1581
Spectazole Cream (Ortho Pharmaceutical (Dermatological Div.)) p 1476

ANTIGONADOTROPIN

Danocrine (Winthrop-Breon) p 443, 2195

ANTIHERPES

Anbesol Gel Antiseptic Anesthetic (Whitehall) p 443, 2185
HVS 1+2 (Chemi-Tech) p 839
Zovirax Ointment 5% (Burroughs Wellcome) p 822

ANTIHISTAMINES

Actifed with Codeine Cough Syrup (Burroughs Wellcome) p 773
Albatussin (Bart) p 685
Alka-Seltzer Plus Cold Medicine (Miles Laboratories) p 1395
Ambenyl Cough Syrup (Marion) p 1181
Atarax Tablets & Syrup (Roerig) p 431, 1725
Benadryl Elixir (Parke-Davis) p 1485
Benadryl Kapseals and Capsules (Parke-Davis) p 423, 1485
Benadryl Parenteral (Parke-Davis) p 1485
Bromfed Capsules (Timed Release) (Muro) p 1420
Bromfed-PD Capsules (Timed Release) (Muro) p 1420
Bromfed Tablets (Muro) p 1420
Citra Forte Capsules (Boyle) p 726
Citra Forte Syrup (Boyle) p 726
Codimal DH (Central Pharmaceuticals) p 836
Codimal DM (Central Pharmaceuticals) p 836
Codimal PH (Central Pharmaceuticals) p 836
Comhist LA Capsules (Norwich Eaton) p 422, 1425
Comhist Tablets (Norwich Eaton) p 1426
Comtrex (Bristol-Myers Products) p 769
Co-Pyronil 2 (Dista) p 895
Deconamine Tablets, Elixir, SR Capsules, Syrup (Berlex) p 406, 699
Dimetane-DC Cough Syrup (Robins) p 1647
Dimetapp Elixir (Robins) p 1648
Dimetapp Extentabs (Robins) p 428, 1648
Diphenhydramine HCl in Tubex (Wyeth) p 2288
Dristan, Advanced Formula Decongestant/Antihistamine/Analgesic Capsules (Whitehall) p 443, 2186
Dristan, Advanced Formula Decongestant/Antihistamine/Analgesic Tablets (Whitehall) p 443, 2186
Dristan Nasal Spray, Regular & Menthol (Whitehall) p 443, 2186

Product Category Index

Durrax Tablets 10mg, 25mg (Dermik) p 888
Extendryl Chewable Tablets (Fleming) p 948
Extendryl Sr. & Jr. T.D. Capsules (Fleming) p 948
Extendryl Syrup (Fleming) p 948
4-Way Cold Tablets (Bristol-Myers Products) p 770
Fedahist Expectorant (Rorer) p 1749
Fedahist Gyrocaps, Syrup & Tablets (Rorer) p 431, 1749
Fiogesic Tablets (Sandoz Pharmaceutical Div.) p 432, 1801
Hispril Spansule Capsules (Smith Kline & French) p 437, 1965
Histaspan-D Capsules (USV Pharmaceutical) p 2077
Histaspan-Plus Capsules (USV Pharmaceutical) p 2077
Isoclor Timesule Capsules (Fisons) p 944
Nolahist (Carnrick) p 408, 832
Nolamine Tablets (Carnrick) p 408, 833
Optimine Tablets (Schering) p 434, 1872
PBZ Hydrochloride Cream (Geigy) p 964
PBZ Tablets & Elixir (Geigy) p 411, 964
PBZ-SR Tablets (Geigy) p 411, 963
Percogesic Analgesic Tablets (Vicks Pharmacy Products) p 442, 2147
Periactin Syrup (Merck Sharp & Dohme) p 1342
Periactin Tablets (Merck Sharp & Dohme) p 420, 1342
Phenergan Injection (Wyeth) p 2275
Phenergan in Tubex (Wyeth) p 2288
Phenergan Syrup Fortis (Wyeth) p 2276
Phenergan Syrup Plain (Wyeth) p 2276
Phenergan Tablets & Rectal Suppositories (Wyeth) p 444, 445, 2278
Phenergan VC (Wyeth) p 2282
Phenergan VC with Codeine (Wyeth) p 2284
Phenergan with Codeine (Wyeth) p 2278
Phenergan with Dextromethorphan (Wyeth) p 2280
Polaramine Repetabs Tablets (Schering) p 434, 1879
Polaramine Syrup (Schering) p 1879
Polaramine Tablets (Schering) p 434, 1879
Quelidrine Syrup (Abbott) p 567
Rondec Oral Drops (Ross) p 1776
Rondec Syrup (Ross) p 1776
Rondec Tablet (Ross) p 432, 1776
Rondec-TR Tablets (Ross) p 432, 1776
Ru-Tuss Expectorant (Boots) p 722
Ru-Tuss Plain (Boots) p 723
Ru-Tuss Tablets (Boots) p 406, 723
Ru-Tuss II Capsules (Boots) p 406, 723
Ru-Tuss with Hydrocodone (Boots) p 722
Rynatan Tablets & Pediatric Suspension (Wallace) p 442, 2165
Rynatuss Tablets & Pediatric Suspension (Wallace) p 442, 2165
Scot-Tussin Sugar-Free 5-Action Cold Formula (Scot-Tussin) p 1897
Sinovan Timed (Drug Industries) p 915
Sinulin Tablets (Carnrick) p 409, 835
Tacaryl Chewable Tablets (Westwood) p 442, 2182
Tacaryl Syrup & Tablets (Westwood) p 442, 2182
Tavist Tablets (Sandoz Pharmaceutical Div.) p 433, 1818
Tavist-1 Tablets (Sandoz Pharmaceutical Div.) p 433, 1818
Tavist-D Tablets (Sandoz Pharmaceutical Div.) p 433, 1819
Triaminic Cold Syrup (Dorsey Laboratories) p 911
Triaminic Cold Tablets (Dorsey Laboratories) p 911
Triaminic Juvelets (Dorsey Laboratories) p 912
Triaminic Oral Infant Drops (Dorsey Laboratories) p 912
Triaminic TR Tablets (Timed Release) (Dorsey Laboratories) p 912
Triaminic-12 Tablets (Dorsey Laboratories) p 913
Triaminicol Multi-Symptom Cold Syrup (Dorsey Laboratories) p 913
Triaminicol Multi-Symptom Cold Tablets (Dorsey Laboratories) p 914
Trinalin Repetabs Tablets (Schering) p 435, 1890
Vistaril Capsules and Oral Suspension (Pfizer) p 427, 1612

ANTIHYPERAMMONIA
Cephulac Syrup (Merrell Dow) p 421, 1362

ANTIHYPERTENSIVES
(see under CARDIOVASCULAR PREPARATIONS)

ANTI-INFLAMMATORY AGENTS
Enzymes
Orenzyme (Merrell Dow) p 1379
Orenzyme Bitabs (Merrell Dow) p 1379
Papase (Parke-Davis) p 425, 1558

Hormones
Aristocort Syrup (Lederle) p 1078
Aristocort Tablets (Lederle) p 414, 1078

Phenylbutazones
Azolid Capsules & Tablets (USV Pharmaceutical) p 2070
Butazolidin Capsules & Tablets (Geigy) p 411, 956
Oxalid Tablets (USV Pharmaceutical) p 2084
Tandearil (Geigy) p 411, 964

Salicylates
Arthritis Bayer Timed-Release Aspirin (Glenbrook) p 412, 995
Barseb HC Scalp Lotion (Barnes-Hind) p 683
Barseb Thera-Spray (Barnes-Hind) p 684
Bayer Aspirin and Bayer Children's Chewable Aspirin (Glenbrook) p 412, 996
Cosprin (Glenbrook) p 996
Cosprin 650 (Glenbrook) p 997
Dia-Gesic (Central Pharmaceuticals) p 409, 837
Disalcid (Riker) p 428, 1642
Encaprin (Procter & Gamble) p 427, 1620
Komed HC Lotion (Barnes-Hind) p 684
Maximum Bayer Aspirin (Glenbrook) p 412, 996
Mono-Gesic Tablets (Central Pharmaceuticals) p 409, 837
Myoflex Creme (Topical Analgesic) (Adria) p 585
Trilisate Tablets/Liquid (Purdue Frederick) p 427, 1627
Verin (Verex) p 442, 2146

Steroids & Combinations
AeroBid Inhaler System (Key Pharmaceuticals) p 1046
Aeroseb-Dex Topical Aerosol Spray (Herbert) p 1001
Aeroseb-HC Topical Aerosol Spray (Herbert) p 1002
Alphaderm (Norwich Eaton) p 1424
Aristocort A Topical Cream & Ointment (Lederle) p 414, 415, 1084
Aristocort Forte Parenteral (Lederle) p 1081
Aristocort Intralesional (Lederle) p 1081
Aristocort Topical Products (Lederle) p 414, 415, 1080
Azmacort Inhaler (Rorer) p 431, 1746
Barseb HC Scalp Lotion (Barnes-Hind) p 683
Barseb Thera-Spray (Barnes-Hind) p 684
Beclovent Oral Inhaler (Glaxo) p 411, 977
Beconase Nasal Inhaler (Glaxo) p 411, 978
Celestone Phosphate Injection (Schering) p 1833
Celestone Soluspan Suspension (Schering) p 1835
Celestone Syrup & Tablets (Schering) p 433, 1832
Cloderm (Ortho Pharmaceutical (Dermatological Div.)) p 1472
Cort-Dome High Potency Suppositories (Miles Pharmaceuticals) p 1401
Corticaine Cream (Glaxo) p 412, 980
Corticaine Suppositories (Glaxo) p 412, 980
Cortifoam (Reed & Carnrick) p 427, 1632
Cortisporin Cream (Burroughs Wellcome) p 783
Cortisporin Ointment (Burroughs Wellcome) p 784
Cortisporin Ophthalmic Ointment (Burroughs Wellcome) p 784
Cortisporin Ophthalmic Suspension (Burroughs Wellcome) p 785
Cortisporin Otic Solution (Burroughs Wellcome) p 786
Cortisporin Otic Suspension (Burroughs Wellcome) p 786
Decadron Elixir (Merck Sharp & Dohme) p 1284
Decadron Phosphate Injection (Merck Sharp & Dohme) p 1288
Decadron Phosphate Respihaler (Merck Sharp & Dohme) p 1291
Decadron Phosphate Sterile Ophthalmic Ointment (Merck Sharp & Dohme) p 1290
Decadron Phosphate Sterile Ophthalmic Solution (Merck Sharp & Dohme) p 1291
Decadron Phosphate Turbinaire (Merck Sharp & Dohme) p 1293
Decadron Tablets (Merck Sharp & Dohme) p 420, 1286
Decadron-LA Suspension (Merck Sharp & Dohme) p 1294
Decaspray Topical Aerosol (Merck Sharp & Dohme) p 1296
Depo-Medrol (Upjohn) p 441, 2107
Derma Medicone-HC Ointment (Medicone) p 1256
Dexamethasone Sodium Phosphate in Tubex (Wyeth) p 2288
Diprolene Ointment 0.05% (Schering) p 1837
Diprosone Cream 0.05% (Schering) p 1838
Diprosone Lotion 0.05% w/w (Schering) p 1838
Diprosone Ointment 0.05% (Schering) p 1838

Diprosone Topical Aerosol 0.1% w/w (Schering) p 1838
Epifoam (Reed & Carnrick) p 427, 1634
Florone Cream 0.05% (Dermik) p 889
Florone Ointment 0.05% (Dermik) p 889
Halog Cream/Ointment/Solution (Squibb) p 1996
Halog-E Cream (Squibb) p 1996
Hydeltra-T.B.A. Suspension (Merck Sharp & Dohme) p 1314
Hydrocortone Acetate Sterile Ophthalmic Ointment and Ophthalmic Suspension (Merck Sharp & Dohme) p 1316
Hytone Cream, Lotion & Ointment (Dermik) p 890
Kenalog Cream/Lotion/Ointment (Squibb) p 1998
Kenalog in Orabase (Squibb) p 2003
Kenalog Spray (Squibb) p 1998
Kenalog-10 Injection (Squibb) p 2001
Kenalog-40 Injection (Squibb) p 1999
Komed HC Lotion (Barnes-Hind) p 684
Lidex Cream 0.05% (Syntex) p 2061
Lidex Gel 0.05% (Syntex) p 2061
Lidex Ointment 0.05% (Syntex) p 2061
Lidex Topical Solution 0.05% (Syntex) p 2061
Lidex-E Cream 0.05% (Syntex) p 2061
Lotrisone Cream (Schering) p 1858
Mantadil Cream (Burroughs Wellcome) p 803
Medrol Tablets (Upjohn) p 441, 2124
Metimyd Ophthalmic Ointment - Sterile (Schering) p 1860
Metimyd Ophthalmic Suspension (Schering) p 1860
Metreton Ophthalmic/Otic Solution-Sterile (Schering) p 1861
Neodecadron Sterile Ophthalmic Ointment (Merck Sharp & Dohme) p 1340
Neodecadron Sterile Ophthalmic Solution (Merck Sharp & Dohme) p 1341
Neo-Synalar Cream (Syntex) p 2061
Ophthocort (Parke-Davis) p 1558
Otobiotic Otic Solution (Schering) p 1875
Pedi-Cort V Creme (Pedinol) p 1581
Penecort Cream & Topical Solution 1% (Herbert) p 1007
Penecort Cream 2.5% (Herbert) p 1008
Pramosone Cream, Lotion & Ointment (Ferndale) p 942
Proctofoam-HC (Reed & Carnrick) p 427, 1636
Pyocidin-Otic Solution (Berlex) p 702
Rectal Medicone-HC Suppositories (Medicone) p 419, 1256
Solu-Cortef Plain & Mix-O-Vial (Upjohn) p 2135
Solu-Medrol Sterile Powder (Upjohn) p 441, 2137
Synacort Creams 1%, 2.5% (Syntex) p 2061
Synalar Creams 0.025%, 0.01% (Syntex) p 2061
Synalar Ointment 0.025% (Syntex) p 2061
Synalar Topical Solution 0.01% (Syntex) p 2061
Synalar-HP Cream 0.2% (Syntex) p 2061
Synemol Cream 0.025% (Syntex) p 2061
Topicort Emollient Cream 0.25% (Hoechst-Roussel) p 413, 1021
Topicort Gel 0.05% (Hoechst-Roussel) p 413, 1021
Topicort LP Emollient Cream 0.05% (Hoechst-Roussel) p 413, 1021
Topicort Ointment 0.25% (Hoechst-Roussel) p 1021
Tridesilon Ointment 0.05% (Miles Pharmaceuticals) p 1413
Uticort Cream, Gel, Lotion & Ointment (Parke-Davis) p 426, 1575
Valisone Cream 0.1% (Schering) p 1892
Valisone Lotion 0.1% (Schering) p 1892
Valisone Ointment 0.1% (Schering) p 1892
Valisone Reduced Strength Cream 0.01% (Schering) p 1892
Vancenase Nasal Inhaler (Schering) p 435, 1893
Vanceril Inhaler (Schering) p 435, 1894
Vioform-Hydrocortisone (CIBA) p 876
VōSol HC Otic Solution (Wallace) p 442, 2171
Vytone Cream (Dermik) p 891
Westcort Cream 0.2% (Westwood) p 2183
Westcort Ointment 0.2% (Westwood) p 2183

Sulfonamides
Azulfidine Tablets, EN-tabs, Oral Suspension (Pharmacia) p 427, 1613
Metimyd Ophthalmic Ointment - Sterile (Schering) p 1860
Metimyd Ophthalmic Suspension (Schering) p 1860

Other
Acthar (Armour) p 601
Barseb HC Scalp Lotion (Barnes-Hind) p 683
Barseb Thera-Spray (Barnes-Hind) p 684
Carmol HC Cream 1% (Syntex) p 2061

Product Category Index

Clinoril Tablets (Merck Sharp & Dohme) p 420, 1274
Dolobid Tablets (Merck Sharp & Dohme) p 420, 1302
HP Acthar Gel (Armour) p 601
Herpecin-L Cold Sore Lip Balm (Campbell) p 829
Indocin Capsules (Merck Sharp & Dohme) p 420, 1319
Indocin SR Capsules (Merck Sharp & Dohme) p 420, 1319
Indocin Suppositories (Merck Sharp & Dohme) p 420, 1319
Komed HC Lotion (Barnes-Hind) p 684
Mantadil Cream (Burroughs Wellcome) p 803
Meclomen (Parke-Davis) p 424, 1541
Motrin Tablets* (Upjohn) p 441, 2128
Nalfon Pulvules & Tablets (Dista) p 410, 903
Naprosyn (Syntex) p 440, 2062
Orabase HCA (Colgate-Hoyt) p 879
Plaquenil Sulfate (Winthrop-Breon) p 444, 2223
Pramosone Cream, Lotion & Ointment (Ferndale) p 942
Rufen Tablets (Boots) p 406, 720
Tolectin Tablets & DS Capsules (McNeil Pharmaceutical) p 419, 1212
Tridesilon Creme 0.05% (Miles Pharmaceuticals) p 1412

ANTILEPROSY
Dapsone (Jacobus) p 1032

ANTIMALARIALS
(see under ANTIPARASITICS)

ANTIMETABOLITES
Imuran Tablets (Burroughs Wellcome) p 408, 790
Purinethol (Burroughs Wellcome) p 408, 811
Tabloid Brand Thioguanine (Burroughs Wellcome) p 408, 817

ANTIMETAL POISONING
(see under CHELATING AGENTS)

ANTIMIGRAINE PREPARATIONS
Cafergot (Sandoz Pharmaceutical Div.) p 432, 1799
Cafergot P-B (Sandoz Pharmaceutical Div.) p 432, 1799
D.H.E. 45 (Sandoz Pharmaceutical Div.) p 1800
Ergostat (Parke-Davis) p 424, 1514
Inderal Tablets & Injectable (Ayerst) p 405, 647
Inderal LA Long Acting Capsules (Ayerst) p 405, 650
Medihaler Ergotamine Aerosol (Riker) p 428, 1643
Midrin Capsules (Carnrick) p 408, 832
Migralam Capsules (Lambda) p 1071
Sansert (Sandoz Pharmaceutical Div.) p 433, 1816
Wigraine Tablets & Suppositories (Organon) p 422, 1451
Wigraine-PB Suppositories (Organon) p 422, 1451
Wigrettes (Organon) p 422, 1451

ANTIMOTION SICKNESS
(see also under ANTINAUSEANTS)
Bonine Tablets (Pfipharmecs) p 426, 1589
Dimenhydrinate in Tubex (Wyeth) p 2288
Dramamine Injection (Searle Pharmaceuticals) p 1906
Dramamine Liquid (Searle Pharmaceuticals) p 1906
Dramamine Tablets (Searle Pharmaceuticals) p 435, 1906
Marezine (Burroughs Wellcome) p 408, 803
Phenergan Injection (Wyeth) p 2275
Phenergan in Tubex (Wyeth) p 2288
Phenergan Tablets & Rectal Suppositories (Wyeth) p 444, 445, 2278
Transderm Scōp Transdermal Therapeutic System (CIBA) p 409, 874

ANTINAUSEANTS
Antivert, Antivert/25 Tablets, Antivert/25 Chewable Tablets & Antivert/50 Tablets (Roerig) p 431, 1725
Atarax Tablets & Syrup (Roerig) p 431, 1725
Bonine Tablets (Pfipharmecs) p 426, 1589
Bucladin-S Softab Tablets (Stuart) p 439, 2036
Compazine (Smith Kline & French) p 436, 1953
Dimenhydrinate in Tubex (Wyeth) p 2288
Dramamine Injection (Searle Pharmaceuticals) p 1906
Dramamine Liquid (Searle Pharmaceuticals) p 1906
Dramamine Tablets (Searle Pharmaceuticals) p 435, 1906
Emete-con (Roerig) p 1729
Marezine (Burroughs Wellcome) p 408, 803
Pepto-Bismol Liquid & Tablets (Procter & Gamble) p 1620
Phenergan Injection (Wyeth) p 2275
Phenergan in Tubex (Wyeth) p 2288
Phenergan Tablets & Rectal Suppositories (Wyeth) p 444, 445, 2278
Prochlorperazine Edisylate in Tubex (Wyeth) p 2288
Reglan Injectable (Robins) p 1659
Thorazine (Smith Kline & French) p 437, 1977
Tigan (Beecham Laboratories) p 406, 698
Torecan Injection (Ampuls) (Boehringer Ingelheim) p 716
Torecan Suppositories (Boehringer Ingelheim) p 716
Torecan Tablets (Boehringer Ingelheim) p 406, 716
Transderm Scōp Transdermal Therapeutic System (CIBA) p 409, 874
Trilafon Tablets, Repetabs Tablets, Concentrate & Injection (Schering) p 435, 1888
Vistaril Capsules and Oral Suspension (Pfizer) p 427, 1612
Vontrol Tablets (Smith Kline & French) p 437, 1981
WANS (Webcon Anti-Nausea Suppretes) (Webcon) p 2173

ANTINEOPLASTICS

Antibiotic Derivatives
Adriamycin (Adria) p 571
Blenoxane (Bristol-Myers Oncology) p 757
Cerubidine (Ives) p 1026
Cosmegen Injection (Merck Sharp & Dohme) p 1278

Antiestrogen
Nolvadex Tablets (Stuart) p 439, 2040

Antimetabolites
Adrucil Injectable (Adria) p 573
Cerubidine (Ives) p 1026
Efudex Topical Solutions and Cream (Roche) p 1681
FUDR Injectable (Roche) p 1684
Fluoroplex Topical Solution & Cream (Herbert) p 1004
Fluorouracil Ampuls (Roche) p 1683
Folex for Injection (Adria) p 576
Methotrexate Tablets & Parenteral (Lederle) p 415, 1100
Mexate (Bristol-Myers Oncology) p 762
Mithracin (Miles Pharmaceuticals) p 1407
Purinethol (Burroughs Wellcome) p 408, 811
Tabloid Brand Thioguanine (Burroughs Wellcome) p 408, 817

Cytotoxic Agents
Adriamycin (Adria) p 571
BiCNU (Bristol-Myers Oncology) p 756
CeeNU (Bristol-Myers Oncology) p 407, 758
Cerubidine (Ives) p 1026
Cytosar-U Sterile Powder (Upjohn) p 2102
Cytoxan (Bristol-Myers Oncology) p 407, 759
Emcyt Capsules (Roche) p 429, 1681
Fluoroplex Topical Solution & Cream (Herbert) p 1004
Hydrea Capsules (Squibb) p 438, 1997
Matulane Capsules (Roche) p 430, 1691
Mutamycin (Bristol-Myers Oncology) p 764
Myleran (Burroughs Wellcome) p 408, 804
Neosar for Injection (Adria) p 586
Platinol (Bristol-Myers Oncology) p 765

Hormones
Depo-Provera (Upjohn) p 2109
Estinyl Tablets (Schering) p 434, 1839
Estrace (Mead Johnson Laboratories) p 419, 1216
Estrace Vaginal Cream (Mead Johnson Laboratories) p 419, 1219
Megace Tablets (Bristol-Myers Oncology) p 407, 761
Oreton Methyl Tablets & Buccal Tablets (Schering) p 434, 1873
Stilphostrol (Miles Pharmaceuticals) p 422, 1412
TACE 12 mg Capsules (Merrell Dow) p 421, 1385
TACE 25 mg Capsules (Merrell Dow) p 421, 1385
Teslac Tablets (Squibb) p 2023

Nitrogen Mustard Derivatives
Alkeran (Burroughs Wellcome) p 407, 776
Emcyt Capsules (Roche) p 429, 1681
Leukeran (Burroughs Wellcome) p 408, 801
Mustargen (Merck Sharp & Dohme) p 1337
Thiotepa (Lederle) p 416, 1118

Steroids & Combinations
Celestone Phosphate Injection (Schering) p 1833
Celestone Soluspan Suspension (Schering) p 1835
Celestone Syrup & Tablets (Schering) p 433, 1832

Other
DTIC-Dome (Miles Pharmaceuticals) p 1402
Elspar (Merck Sharp & Dohme) p 1308
Lysodren (Bristol-Myers Oncology) p 407, 760
Oncovin (Lilly) p 1169
Velban (Lilly) p 1179
VePesid Injection (Bristol-Myers Oncology) p 767

ANTIOBESITY PREPARATIONS
(see under ANOREXICS)

ANTIPARASITICS

Arthropods

Lice
A-200 Pyrinate Pediculicide Shampoo, Liquid & Gel (Norcliff Thayer) p 422, 1422
Kwell Cream (Reed & Carnrick) p 1635
Kwell Lotion (Reed & Carnrick) p 1635
Kwell Shampoo (Reed & Carnrick) p 1635
Li-Ban Spray (Pfipharmecs) p 1589
Prioderm Lotion (Purdue Frederick) p 1626
R&C Spray (Reed & Carnrick) p 1637
RID Liquid Pediculicide (Pfipharmecs) p 426, 1593
Scabene Shampoo (Stiefel) p 2036

Scabies
Eurax Cream & Lotion (Westwood) p 2177
Kwell Cream (Reed & Carnrick) p 1635
Kwell Lotion (Reed & Carnrick) p 1635
Scabene Lotion (Stiefel) p 2035
Scabene Shampoo (Stiefel) p 2036

Helminths

Ascaris (roundworm)
Antepar (Burroughs Wellcome) p 407, 779
Antiminth Oral Suspension (Pfipharmecs) p 426, 1589
Mintezol Chewable Tablets & Suspension (Merck Sharp & Dohme) p 420, 1332
Vermox Chewable Tablets (Janssen) p 413, 1043

Enterobius (pinworm)
Antepar (Burroughs Wellcome) p 407, 779
Antiminth Oral Suspension (Pfipharmecs) p 426, 1589
Mintezol Chewable Tablets & Suspension (Merck Sharp & Dohme) p 420, 1332
Povan Filmseals (Parke-Davis) p 425, 1563
Vermox Chewable Tablets (Janssen) p 413, 1043

Hookworm
Mintezol Chewable Tablets & Suspension (Merck Sharp & Dohme) p 420, 1332
Vermox Chewable Tablets (Janssen) p 413, 1043

Taenia (tapeworm)
Niclocide Chewable Tablets (Miles Pharmaceuticals) p 422, 1411

Trematodes (Schistosomes)
Biltricide (Miles Pharmaceuticals) p 421, 1399

Trichuris (whipworm)
Mintezol Chewable Tablets & Suspension (Merck Sharp & Dohme) p 420, 1332
Vermox Chewable Tablets (Janssen) p 413, 1043

Protozoa

Amebas, extraintestinal
Aralen Hydrochloride (Winthrop-Breon) p 2189
Aralen Phosphate (Winthrop-Breon) p 443, 2190
Flagyl Tablets (Searle & Co.) p 436, 1929
Protostat Tablets (Ortho Pharmaceutical) p 423, 1470
Satric (Savage) p 433, 1825

Amebas, intestinal
Flagyl Tablets (Searle & Co.) p 436, 1929
Protostat Tablets (Ortho Pharmaceutical) p 423, 1470
Satric (Savage) p 433, 1825
Yodoxin (Glenwood) p 412, 999

Giardias
Flagyl Tablets (Searle & Co.) p 436, 1929

Malaria
Aralen Hydrochloride (Winthrop-Breon) p 2189
Aralen Phosphate (Winthrop-Breon) p 443, 2190
Aralen Phosphate w/Primaquine Phosphate (Winthrop-Breon) p 2191
Daraprim (Burroughs Wellcome) p 407, 787
Fansidar Tablets (Roche) p 429, 1682
Plaquenil Sulfate (Winthrop-Breon) p 444, 2223

Toxoplasma
Daraprim (Burroughs Wellcome) p 407, 787

Trichomonas
AVC Cream (Merrell Dow) p 1358

Product Category Index

AVC Suppositories (Merrell Dow) p 1358
Betadine Disposable Medicated Douche (Purdue Frederick) p 1622
Betadine Douche (Purdue Frederick) p 1622
Betadine Solution (Purdue Frederick) p 1622
Flagyl Tablets (Searle & Co.) p 436, 1929
Protostat Tablets (Ortho Pharmaceutical) p 423, 1470
Satric (Savage) p 433, 1825
Triva Combination (Boyle) p 726
Triva Douche Powder (Boyle) p 726
Triva Jel (Boyle) p 726
Vagisec Medicated Liquid Douche Concentrate (Schmid) p 1896
Vagisec Plus Suppositories (Schmid) p 1896

ANTIPARKINSONISM DRUGS

Akineton (Knoll) p 414, 1056
Artane Elixir (Lederle) p 1087
Artane Sequels (Lederle) p 415, 1087
Artane Tablets (Lederle) p 415, 1087
Cogentin Tablets & Injection (Merck Sharp & Dohme) p 420, 1276
Kemadrin (Burroughs Wellcome) p 408, 792
Larodopa Capsules (Roche) p 429, 1688
Larodopa Tablets (Roche) p 429, 1688
Levsin Tablets, Injection, Elixir & Drops (Rorer) p 432, 1751
Levsinex Timecaps (Rorer) p 432, 1751
Parsidol (Parke-Davis) p 425, 1559
Sinemet Tablets (Merck Sharp & Dohme) p 420, 1345
Symmetrel (Du Pont) p 410, 927

ANTIPLATELET

Bayer Aspirin and Bayer Children's Chewable Aspirin (Glenbrook) p 412, 996

ANTIPORPHYRIA AGENT

Panhematin (Abbott) p 557
Solatene Capsules (Roche) p 430, 1701

ANTIPRURITICS

Aeroseb-Dex Topical Aerosol Spray (Herbert) p 1001
Aeroseb-HC Topical Aerosol Spray (Herbert) p 1002
Alphaderm (Norwich Eaton) p 1424
Atarax Tablets & Syrup (Roerig) p 431, 1725
Carmol HC Cream 1% (Syntex) p 2061
Corticaine Cream (Glaxo) p 412, 980
Corticaine Suppositories (Glaxo) p 412, 980
Derma Medicone-HC Ointment (Medicone) p 1256
Diprolene Ointment 0.05% (Schering) p 1837
Diprosone Cream 0.05% (Schering) p 1838
Diprosone Lotion 0.05% w/w (Schering) p 1838
Diprosone Ointment 0.05% (Schering) p 1838
Diprosone Topical Aerosol 0.1% w/w (Schering) p 1838
Durrax Tablets 10mg, 25mg (Dermik) p 888
Epifoam (Reed & Carnrick) p 427, 1634
Eurax Cream & Lotion (Westwood) p 2177
Halog Cream/Ointment/Solution (Squibb) p 1996
Halog-E Cream (Squibb) p 1996
Hytone Cream, Lotion & Ointment (Dermik) p 890
Kenalog Cream/Lotion/Ointment (Squibb) p 1998
Kenalog in Orabase (Squibb) p 2003
Kenalog Spray (Squibb) p 1998
Lidex Topical Solution 0.05% (Syntex) p 2061
Lotrisone Cream (Schering) p 1858
Mantadil Cream (Burroughs Wellcome) p 803
Osti-Derm Lotion (Pedinol) p 1580
Penecort Cream & Topical Solution 1% (Herbert) p 1007
Penecort Cream 2.5% (Herbert) p 1008
Pramosone Cream, Lotion & Ointment (Ferndale) p 942
Proctofoam-HC (Reed & Carnrick) p 427, 1636
proctoFoam/non-steroid (Reed & Carnrick) p 427, 1636
Rectal Medicone-HC Suppositories (Medicone) p 419, 1256
Sebulex & Sebulex Cream Shampoo (Westwood) p 2181
Sebulex Shampoo with Conditioners (Westwood) p 2181
Sebulon Dandruff Shampoo (Westwood) p 2181
Sebutone & Sebutone Cream Shampoo (Westwood) p 2181
Tacaryl Chewable Tablets (Westwood) p 442, 2182
Tacaryl Syrup & Tablets (Westwood) p 442, 2182
Tavist Tablets (Sandoz Pharmaceutical Div.) p 433, 1818
Tavist-1 Tablets (Sandoz Pharmaceutical Div.) p 433, 1818

Temaril (Smith Kline & French) p 437, 1976
Topicort Emollient Cream 0.25% (Hoechst-Roussel) p 413, 1021
Topicort Gel 0.05% (Hoechst-Roussel) p 413, 1021
Topicort LP Emollient Cream 0.05% (Hoechst-Roussel) p 413, 1021
Topicort Ointment 0.25% (Hoechst-Roussel) p 1021
Tronothane Hydrochloride (Abbott) p 570
Uticort Cream, Gel, Lotion & Ointment (Parke-Davis) p 426, 1575
Valisone Cream 0.1% (Schering) p 1892
Valisone Lotion 0.1% (Schering) p 1892
Valisone Ointment 0.1% (Schering) p 1892
Valisone Reduced Strength Cream 0.01% (Schering) p 1892
Vioform-Hydrocortisone (CIBA) p 876
Vytone Cream (Dermik) p 891
Westcort Cream 0.2% (Westwood) p 2183
Westcort Ointment 0.2% (Westwood) p 2183
Zone-A Lotion 1% (UAD Labs.) p 2069

ANTIPSYCHOTICS

Cibalith-S Syrup (CIBA) p 852
Compazine (Smith Kline & French) p 436, 1953
Eskalith Capsules & Tablets (Smith Kline & French) p 437, 1964
Eskalith CR Controlled Release Tablets (Smith Kline & French) p 437, 1964
Haldol Tablets, Concentrate, Injection (McNeil Pharmaceutical) p 418, 1201
Lithane (Miles Pharmaceuticals) p 422, 1403
Lithium Carbonate Capsules & Tablets (Roxane) p 1789
Lithobid Tablets (CIBA) p 409, 852
Loxitane C Oral Concentrate (Lederle) p 415, 1096
Loxitane Capsules (Lederle) p 415, 1096
Loxitane IM (Lederle) p 415, 1096
Mellaril (Sandoz Pharmaceutical Div.) p 433, 1804
Moban Tablets & Concentrate (Du Pont) p 410, 921
Navane Capsules and Concentrate (Roerig) p 431, 1737
Navane Intramuscular (Roerig) p 1739
Orap Tablets (McNeil Pharmaceutical) p 1203
Prochlorperazine Edisylate in Tubex (Wyeth) p 2288
Prolixin Decanoate (Squibb) p 2015
Prolixin Elixir & Injection (Squibb) p 2014
Prolixin Tablets (Squibb) p 438, 2014
Quide (Merrell Dow) p 1379
Stelazine (Smith Kline & French) p 437, 1971
Taractan Concentrate (Roche) p 1703
Taractan Injectable (Roche) p 1703
Taractan Tablets (Roche) p 1703
Thorazine (Smith Kline & French) p 437, 1977
Triavil Tablets (Merck Sharp & Dohme) p 420, 1354

ANTIPYRETICS

A.P.C. with Codeine Nos. 3 & 4, Tabloid brand (Burroughs Wellcome) p 407, 780
Acetaminophen Uniserts Suppositories (Upsher-Smith) p 2144
Bayer Aspirin and Bayer Children's Chewable Aspirin (Glenbrook) p 412, 996
Bayer Children's Cold Tablets (Glenbrook) p 996
Buff-A Comp Tablets (Mayrand) p 1196
Dia-Gesic (Central Pharmaceuticals) p 409, 837
Dorcol Children's Fever & Pain Reducer (Dorsey Laboratories) p 909
Empirin with Codeine (Burroughs Wellcome) p 408, 787
Empracet with Codeine Phosphate Nos. 3 & 4 (Burroughs Wellcome) p 408, 789
Encaprin (Procter & Gamble) p 427, 1620
Sedapap-10 Tablets (Mayrand) p 1196
Tylenol acetaminophen Children's Chewable Tablets, Elixir, Infants' Drops (McNeil Consumer Products) p 418, 1199
Tylenol, Extra-Strength, acetaminophen Liquid Pain Reliever (McNeil Consumer Products) p 1200
Tylenol, Extra-Strength, acetaminophen Tablets, Capsules & Caplets (McNeil Consumer Products) p 418, 1200
Tylenol, Junior-Strength, acetaminophen Swallowable Tablets (McNeil Consumer Products) p 418
Tylenol, Regular Strength, acetaminophen Tablets & Capsules (McNeil Consumer Products) p 418, 1199
Vanquish (Glenbrook) p 998

ANTISHOCK EMERGENCY KIT

EpiPen—Epinephrine Auto-Injector (Center) p 835

ANTISPASMODICS & ANTICHOLINERGICS

Gastrointestinal

Anaspaz PB Tablets (Ascher) p 614
Anaspaz Tablets (Ascher) p 614
Antrenyl bromide Tablets (CIBA) p 409, 841
Arco-Lase Plus (Arco) p 600
Belladenal Tablets (Sandoz Pharmaceutical Div.) p 432, 1798
Belladenal-S Tablets (Sandoz Pharmaceutical Div.) p 432, 1798
Bentyl Capsules, Tablets, Syrup & Injection (Merrell Dow) p 421, 1359
Cantil (Merrell Dow) p 421, 1362
Chardonna-2 (Rorer) p 431, 1748
Combid Spansule Capsules (Smith Kline & French) p 436, 1952
Darbid (Smith Kline & French) p 436, 1958
Donnatal Capsules (Robins) p 428, 1648
Donnatal Elixir (Robins) p 1648
Donnatal Extentabs (Robins) p 428, 1649
Donnatal Tablets (Robins) p 428, 1648
Festalan (Hoechst-Roussel) p 413, 1014
Kinesed Tablets (Stuart) p 439, 2038
Kutrase Capsules (Rorer) p 431, 1750
Levsin Tablets, Injection, Elixir & Drops (Rorer) p 432, 1751
Levsin/Phenobarbital Tablets, Elixir & Drops (Rorer) p 1751
Levsinex Timecaps (Rorer) p 432, 1751
Levsinex/Phenobarbital Timecaps (Rorer) p 1751
Librax Capsules (Roche Products) p 430, 1713
Pathibamate (Lederle) p 415, 1110
Pathilon (Lederle) p 415, 1112
Pro-Banthīne Tablets (Searle & Co.) p 436, 1936
Pro-Banthīne w/Phenobarbital (Searle & Co.) p 436, 1936
Quarzan Capsules (Roche Products) p 430, 1721
Robinul Forte Tablets (Robins) p 429, 1662
Robinul Injectable (Robins) p 429, 1663
Robinul Tablets (Robins) p 429, 1662
Tral Filmtab Tablets (Abbott) p 568
Valpin 50 (Du Pont) p 928

Urinary

Cystospaz (Webcon) p 2172
Cystospaz-M (Webcon) p 2172
Ditropan Syrup (Marion) p 1184
Ditropan Tablets (Marion) p 417, 1184
Levsinex Timecaps (Rorer) p 432, 1751
Pyridium Plus (Parke-Davis) p 425, 1568
Urised Tablets (Webcon) p 2173
Urispas (Smith Kline & French) p 437, 1981

Other

Midol-Original Formula (Glenbrook) p 997

ANTITOXOPLASMOSIS
(see under ANTIPARASITICS)

ANTITUSSIVE
(see under COUGH & COLD PREPARATIONS)

ANTIVERTIGO AGENTS

Antivert, Antivert/25 Tablets, Antivert/25 Chewable Tablets & Antivert/50 Tablets (Roerig) p 431, 1725
Bucladin-S Softab Tablets (Stuart) p 439, 2036
Vontrol Tablets (Smith Kline & French) p 437, 1981

ANTIVIRAL AGENTS

Symmetrel (Du Pont) p 410, 927
Vira-A for Infusion (Parke-Davis) p 1576
Viroptic Ophthalmic Solution (Burroughs Wellcome) p 820
Zovirax Ointment 5% (Burroughs Wellcome) p 822
Zovirax Sterile Powder (Burroughs Wellcome) p 823

ATARACTICS
(see under TRANQUILIZERS)

B

BIOLOGICALS

Antigens

Rhus All Antigen - Poison Ivy, Oak, Sumac Combined (Barry) p 685
Rhus Tox Antigen Injection (Lemmon) p 1122
Staphage Lysate (SPL) (Delmont) p 888

Antiserum

Antirabies Serum (equine), Purified (Sclavo) p 1897
Antivenin (Merck Sharp & Dohme) p 1264
Antivenin (Crotalidae) Polyvalent (equine origin) (Wyeth) p 2243

Product Category Index

Antivenin (Micrurus Fulvius) (Wyeth) p 2245
H-BIG (Abbott) p 531
Hepatitis B Immune Globulin (Human) HyperHep (Cutter Biological) p 884
Hep-B-Gammagee (Merck Sharp & Dohme) p 1311
Homo-Tet (Savage) p 1825
Hu-Tet, Tetanus Immune Globulin (Human), U.S.P. (Hyland Therapeutics) p 1024
Immuglobin (Savage) p 1825
Immune Globulin Intravenous, 5% (In 10% Maltose) Gamimune (Cutter Biological) p 883
Immune Serum Globulin (Human), U.S.P. Gamma Globulin (Hyland Therapeutics) p 1024
Immune Serum Globulin (Human) Gamastan (Cutter Biological) p 883
Imogam Rabies Immune Globulin (Human) (Merieux) p 1358
Pertussis Immune Globulin (Human) Hypertussis (Cutter Biological) p 884
Rabies Immune Globulin (Human) Hyperab (Cutter Biological) p 884
Rabies Immune Globulin (Human), Imogam Rabies (Merieux) p 1358
Tetanus Immune Globulin (Human) (Wyeth) p 2246
Tetanus Immune Globulin (Human) in Tubex (Wyeth) p 2288
Tetanus Immune Globulin (Human) Hyper-Tet (Cutter Biological) p 884

Antitoxin
Diphtheria Antitoxin (equine), Refined (Sclavo) p 1897
Diphtheria Antitoxin (Purified, Concentrated Globulin-Equine) (Squibb/Connaught) p 2033
Tetanus Antitoxin (equine), Refined (Sclavo) p 1897

Rh$_o$ (D) Immune Globulin (Human)
Gamulin Rh (Armour) p 613
MICRhoGAM (Ortho Diagnostic Systems) p 1452
Mini-Gamulin Rh (Armour) p 613
Rh$_o$-D Immune Globulin (Human) HypRho-D (Cutter Biological) p 885
Rh$_o$-D Immune Globulin (Human) HypRho-D Mini-Dose (Cutter Biological) p 884
RhoGAM (Ortho Diagnostic Systems) p 1453

Serum
Albuminar-5, Normal Serum Albumin (Human) U.S.P. 5% (Armour) p 613
Albuminar-25, Normal Serum Albumin (Human) U.S.P. 25% (Armour) p 613
Autoplex, Anti-Inhibitor Coagulant Complex, Dried (Hyland Therapeutics) p 1023
Buminate 5%, Normal Serum Albumin (Human), U.S.P., 5% Solution (Hyland Therapeutics) p 1023
Buminate 25%, Normal Serum Albumin (Human), U.S.P., 25% Solution (Hyland Therapeutics) p 1023
Factor IX Complex (Human) (Factors II, VII, IX, and X) Konyne (Cutter Biological) p 886
Factorate, Antihemophilic Factor (Human) Dried (Armour) p 613
Factorate, Generation II (Armour) p 613
Gammar, Immune Serum Globulin (Human) U.S.P. (Armour) p 613
H.T. Factorate (Armour) p 613
H.T. Factorate, Generation II (Armour) p 613
Hemofil, Antihemophilic Factor (Human), Method Four, Dried (Hyland Therapeutics) p 1023
Hemofil T, Antihemophilic Factor (Human), Method Four, Dried, Heat-Treated (Hyland Therapeutics) p 1024
Immune Serum Globulin (Human) (Wyeth) p 2245
Immune Serum Globulin (Human) in Tubex (Wyeth) p 2288
Plasma-Plex (Armour) p 613
Proplex, Factor IX Complex (Human) (Factors II, VII, IX & X), Dried (Hyland Therapeutics) p 1024
Proplex SX, Factor IX Complex (Human)(Factors II, VII, IX & X), Dried (Hyland Therapeutics) p 1024
Protenate 5%, Plasma Protein Fraction (Human), U.S.P., 5% Solution (Hyland Therapeutics) p 1024
Prothar (Armour) p 613
Rh$_o$-D Immune Globulin (Human) HypRho-D (Cutter Biological) p 885
Rh$_o$-D Immune Globulin (Human) HypRho-D Mini-Dose (Cutter Biological) p 884

Toxoids
Diphtheria & Tetanus Toxoids Adsorbed (Pediatric), Aluminum Phosphate Adsorbed, (Ultrafined) (Wyeth) p 2245
Diphtheria & Tetanus Toxoids Adsorbed, Pediatric, in Tubex (Wyeth) p 2288
Diphtheria & Tetanus Toxoids, Adsorbed (For Pediatric Use) (Sclavo) p 1897
Diphtheria & Tetanus Toxoids, Adsorbed Purogenated (Lederle) p 1093
Diphtheria & Tetanus Toxoids Adsorbed USP (Squibb/Connaught) p 2033
Diphtheria & Tetanus Toxoids & Pertussis Vaccine Adsorbed (for Pediatric Use) (Squibb/Connaught) p 2033
Diphtheria Toxoid, Adsorbed (Sclavo) p 1897
Tetanus & Diphtheria Toxoids Adsorbed (Adult) (Wyeth) p 2246
Tetanus & Diphtheria Toxoids Adsorbed (Adult) in Tubex (Wyeth) p 2288
Tetanus Toxoid (Squibb/Connaught) p 2033
Tetanus Toxoid Adsorbed (Squibb/Connaught) p 2033
Tetanus Toxoid, Adsorbed (Sclavo) p 1897
Tetanus Toxoid Adsorbed, Aluminum Phosphate Adsorbed, Ultrafined (Wyeth) p 2246
Tetanus Toxoid Adsorbed, Aluminum Phosphate Adsorbed, Ultrafined in Tubex (Wyeth) p 2288
Tetanus Toxoid, Adsorbed Purogenated (Lederle) p 1118
Tetanus Toxoid Fluid, Purified, Ultrafined (Wyeth) p 2246
Tetanus Toxoid Fluid, Purified, Ultrafined in Tubex (Wyeth) p 2288
Tetanus Toxoid Purogenated (Lederle) p 1118
Tetanus & Diphtheria Toxoids, Adsorbed Purogenated (Lederle) p 1118
Tetanus & Diphtheria Toxoids Adsorbed (For Adult Use) (Squibb/Connaught) p 2033
Tetanus & Diphtheria Toxoids, Adsorbed (For Adult Use) (Sclavo) p 1897

Vaccines
Cholera Vaccine (Sclavo) p 1897
Cholera Vaccine (Wyeth) p 2245
Cholera Vaccine (India Strains) (Lederle) p 1089
Diphtheria & Tetanus Toxoids & Pertussis Vaccine Adsorbed (for Pediatric Use) (Squibb/Connaught) p 2033
Fluogen (Parke-Davis) p 1522
Fluzone (Influenza Virus Vaccine), Whole Virion and Subvirion, Zonal Purified (Squibb/Connaught) p 2033
Heptavax-B (Merck Sharp & Dohme) p 1312
Imovax Rabies Vaccine (Merieux) (Merieux) p 1358
Influenza Virus Vaccine Subvirion Type (Wyeth) p 2246
Influenza Virus Vaccine Subvirion Type in Tubex (Wyeth) p 2288
Menomune (Meningococcal Polysaccharide Vaccine, Groups A,C,Y,W-135, Combined, and Groups A & C, Combined) (Squibb/Connaught) p 2033
Plague Vaccine (Human) (Cutter Biological) p 886
Pneumovax 23 (Merck Sharp & Dohme) p 1343
Pnu-Imune (Lederle) p 1116
Poliomyelitis Vaccine (Purified) (For the Prevention of Poliomyelitis) (Squibb/Connaught) p 2033
Rabies Vaccine Human Diploid Cell, Imovax Rabies (Merieux) p 1358
Staphage Lysate (SPL) (Delmont) p 888
Tri-Immunol (Lederle) p 1119
Typhoid Vaccine (Wyeth) p 2246
Wyvac Rabies Vaccine (Wyeth) p 2246

Vaccines (Live)
Attenuvax (Merck Sharp & Dohme) p 1267
Biavax$_{II}$ (Merck Sharp & Dohme) p 1269
M-M-R$_{II}$ (Merck Sharp & Dohme) p 1323
M-R-VAX$_{II}$ (Merck Sharp & Dohme) p 1325
Meruvax$_{II}$ (Merck Sharp & Dohme) p 1329
Mumpsvax (Merck Sharp & Dohme) p 1336
Orimune Poliovirus Vaccine, Live, Oral, Trivalent (Lederle) p 1109
YF-VAX (Yellow Fever Vaccine)(Live, 17D Virus, Avian Leukosis-Free, Stabilized) (Squibb/Connaught) p 2033

Other
Autoplex, Anti-Inhibitor Coagulant Complex, Dried (Hyland Therapeutics) p 1023
Factor IX Complex (Human) (Factors II, VII, IX, and X) Konyne (Cutter Biological) p 886
Factorate, Antihemophilic Factor (Human) Dried (Armour) p 613
H.T. Factorate (Armour) p 613
Hemofil, Antihemophilic Factor (Human), Method Four, Dried (Hyland Therapeutics) p 1023
Hemofil T, Antihemophilic Factor (Human), Method Four, Dried, Heat-Treated (Hyland Therapeutics) p 1024
Multitest CMI Skin Test Antigens for Cellular Hypersensitivity (Merieux) p 1358, 3013
Proplex, Factor IX Complex (Human) (Factors II, VII, IX & X), Dried (Hyland Therapeutics) p 1024
Proplex SX, Factor IX Complex (Human)(Factors II, VII, IX & X), Dried (Hyland Therapeutics) p 1024
Skin Test Antigens for Cellular Hypersensitivity, Multitest CMI (Merieux) p 1358, 3013
Thrombinar (Armour) p 613

BISMUTH PREPARATIONS
Pepto-Bismol Liquid & Tablets (Procter & Gamble) p 1620

BONE METABOLISM REGULATOR
Antiheterotopic Ossification Agent
Didronel (Norwich Eaton) p 422, 1429
Antipagetic Agent
Calcimar Solution (USV Pharmaceutical) p 440, 2072
Didronel (Norwich Eaton) p 422, 1429
Other
Calderol Capsules (Upjohn) p 2093

BOWEL EVACUANTS
Bilax Capsules (Drug Industries) p 914
Ceo-Two Suppositories (Beutlich) p 705
Evac-Q-Kit (Adria) p 575
Evac-Q-Kwik (Adria) p 575
Fleet Babylax (Fleet) p 946
GoLYTELY (Braintree) p 727
Trilax (Drug Industries) p 915
X-Prep Liquid (Gray) p 1000

BRONCHIAL DILATORS
Beta Adrenergic Stimulator
Alupent Inhalent Solution 5% & Solution Unit Dose 0.6% (Boehringer Ingelheim) p 706
Alupent Metered Dose Inhaler (Boehringer Ingelheim) p 706
Alupent Syrup (Boehringer Ingelheim) p 706
Alupent Tablets (Boehringer Ingelheim) p 406, 706
Brethine (Geigy) p 411, 955
Bricanyl Injection (Merrell Dow) p 421, 1361
Bricanyl Tablets (Merrell Dow) p 421, 1361
Bronkometer (Winthrop-Breon) p 2193
Bronkosol (Winthrop-Breon) p 2193
Duo-Medihaler (Riker) p 1643
Isuprel Hydrochloride Mistometer (Winthrop-Breon) p 2203
Isuprel Hydrochloride Solution 1:200 & 1:100 (Winthrop-Breon) p 2203
Metaprel Inhalant Solution, Metered Dose Inhaler, Syrup & Tablets (Dorsey Laboratories) p 910
Proventil Inhaler (Schering) p 435, 1882
Proventil Tablets (Schering) p 435, 1883
Ventolin Inhaler (Glaxo) p 412, 987
Ventolin Tablets (Glaxo) p 412, 988

Iodides & Combinations
Quadrinal Tablets & Suspension (Knoll) p 414, 1065
Theo-Organidin Elixir (Wallace) p 442, 2170

Sympathomimetics
Brethine (Geigy) p 411, 955
Brethine Ampuls (Geigy) p 956
Bricanyl Injection (Merrell Dow) p 421, 1361
Bricanyl Tablets (Merrell Dow) p 421, 1361
Bronkephrine Hydrochloride Injection (Winthrop-Breon) p 2193
Congess Jr. & Sr. T.D. Capsules (Fleming) p 948
Efed II Capsules (Yellow) (Alto) p 404, 589
Epinephrine in Tubex (Wyeth) p 2288
Medihaler-Epi (Riker) p 1643
Medihaler-Iso (Riker) p 1644
Metaprel Inhalant Solution, Metered Dose Inhaler, Syrup & Tablets (Dorsey Laboratories) p 910
Norisodrine Aerotrol (Abbott) p 547
Primatene Mist (Whitehall) p 443, 2186
Primatene Mist Suspension (Whitehall) p 2187
Primatene Tablets-M Formula (Whitehall) p 443, 2187
Primatene Tablets-P Formula (Whitehall) p 443, 2187
Proventil Inhaler (Schering) p 435, 1882
Proventil Tablets (Schering) p 435, 1883
Quibron Plus (Mead Johnson Laboratories) p 419, 1236
Sus-Phrine (Berlex) p 406, 704
Ventolin Inhaler (Glaxo) p 412, 987

Sympathomimetics & Combinations
Actifed with Codeine Cough Syrup (Burroughs Wellcome) p 773
Duo-Medihaler (Riker) p 1643
Marax Tablets & DF Syrup (Roerig) p 431, 1737
Norisodrine w/Calcium Iodide Syrup (Abbott) p 548
Quadrinal Tablets & Suspension (Knoll) p 414, 1065
Rynatuss Tablets & Pediatric Suspension (Wallace) p 442, 2165
Tedral Elixir & Suspension (Parke-Davis) p 1573
Tedral SA Tablets (Parke-Davis) p 425, 1573

Product Category Index

Xanthine Derivatives & Combinations
Accurbron (Merrell Dow) p 1359
Aerolate Liquid (Fleming) p 948
Aerolate Sr. & Jr. & III Capsules (Fleming) p 948
Aminophyllin Injection (Searle Pharmaceuticals) p 1898
Aminophyllin Tablets (Searle & Co.) p 435, 1915
Aquaphyllin Syrup (Ferndale) p 942
Asbron G Elixir (Sandoz Pharmaceutical Div.) p 1796
Asbron G Inlay-Tabs (Sandoz Pharmaceutical Div.) p 432, 1796
Brondecon (Parke-Davis) p 423, 1486
Choledyl (Parke-Davis) p 423, 1495
Choledyl SA Tablets (Parke-Davis) p 423, 1497
Constant-T Tablets (Geigy) p 411, 958
Dilor Tablets (Savage) p 433, 1824
Dilor-G Tablets & Liquid (Savage) p 433, 1824
Elixicon Suspension (Berlex) p 406, 699
Elixophyllin Capsules (Berlex) p 406, 699
Elixophyllin Elixir (Berlex) p 699
Elixophyllin SR Capsules (Berlex) p 406, 699
Elixophyllin-GG (Berlex) p 406, 702
LABID 250 mg Tablets (Norwich Eaton) p 1436
Lodrane Capsules-130 & 260 (Poythress) p 1618
Lufyllin Elixir (Wallace) p 2158
Lufyllin Injection (Wallace) p 442, 2159
Lufyllin & Lufyllin-400 Tablets (Wallace) p 442, 2160
Lufyllin-GG (Wallace) p 442, 2161
Marax Tablets & DF Syrup (Roerig) p 431, 1737
Mudrane GG Elixir (Poythress) p 1619
Mudrane GG Tablets (Poythress) p 1619
Mudrane Tablets (Poythress) p 1618
Quadrinal Tablets & Suspension (Knoll) p 414, 1065
Quibron & Quibron-300 (Mead Johnson Laboratories) p 419, 1233
Quibron Plus (Mead Johnson Laboratories) p 419, 1236
Quibron-T & Quibron-T/SR (Mead Johnson Laboratories) p 419, 1236
Respbid (Boehringer Ingelheim) p 406, 712
Slo-bid Gyrocaps (Rorer) p 432, 1754
Slo-Phyllin Gyrocaps, Tablets (Rorer) p 432, 1756
Slo-Phyllin 80 Syrup (Rorer) p 1756
Slo-Phyllin GG Capsules, Syrup (Rorer) p 432, 1759
Somophyllin & Somophyllin-DF Oral Liquids (Fisons) p 945
Somophyllin Rectal Solution (Fisons) p 945
Somophyllin-CRT Capsules (Fisons) p 945
Somophyllin-T Capsules (Fisons) p 945
Sustaire Tablets (Roerig) p 431, 1743
Synophylate Elixir (Central Pharmaceuticals) p 839
Synophylate-GG Tablets/Syrup (Central Pharmaceuticals) p 839
Tedral Elixir & Suspension (Parke-Davis) p 1573
Tedral SA Tablets (Parke-Davis) p 425, 1573
Theo-24 (Searle & Co.) p 436, 1937
Theobid, Theobid Jr. Duracap (Glaxo) p 412, 982
Theo-Dur Sprinkle (Key Pharmaceuticals) p 414, 1053
Theo-Dur Tablets (Key Pharmaceuticals) p 414, 1051
Theolair & Theolair-SR (Riker) p 428, 1645
Theo-Organidin Elixir (Wallace) p 442, 2170
Theophyl Chewable Tablets (McNeil Pharmaceutical) p 1207
Theophyl-SR (McNeil Pharmaceutical) p 1208
Theophyl-225 Elixir (McNeil Pharmaceutical) p 1210
Theophyl-225 Tablets (McNeil Pharmaceutical) p 1210
Theovent Long-Acting Capsules (Schering) p 435, 1886
Uniphyl 200 mg Tablets (Purdue Frederick) p 427, 1627
Uniphyl 400 mg Tablets (Purdue Frederick) p 427, 1629

C

CALCIUM PREPARATIONS

Calcium Binding Agents
Calcibind (Mission) p 1416

Calcium Regulator
Calciferol Drops (Egocalciferol Oral Solution USP) (Rorer) p 431, 1748
Calciferol in Oil Injection (Egocalciferol USP) (Rorer) p 431, 1748
Calciferol Tablets (Ergocalciferol USP) (Rorer) p 431, 1748
DHT (Dihydrotachysterol) Tablets, Oral Solution & Intensol (Roxane) p 1789
Didronel (Norwich Eaton) p 422, 1429

Calcium Supplements
Biocal Calcium Supplement Chewable Tablets (Miles Laboratories) p 1396
Biocal Calcium Supplement Tablets (Miles Laboratories) p 1396
Calcet (Mission) p 1415
Calcet Plus (Mission) p 1415
Calphosan (Glenwood) p 998
Calphosan B-12 (Glenwood) p 998
Cal-Sup (Riker) p 1642
Dical-D Capsules & Wafers (Abbott) p 516
Dorcol Children's Liquid Calcium Supplement (Dorsey Laboratories) p 909
Fosfree (Mission) p 1416
Iromin-G (Mission) p 1416
Mission Prenatal (Mission) p 1419
Mission Prenatal F.A. (Mission) p 1419
Mission Prenatal H.P. (Mission) p 1419
Neo-Calglucon Syrup (Sandoz Pharmaceutical Div.) p 1806
Niferex-PN (Central Pharmaceuticals) p 409, 838
Os-Cal 250 Tablets (Marion) p 418, 1188
Os-Cal 500 Tablets (Marion) p 418, 1188
Os-Cal Forte Tablets (Marion) p 418, 1189
Os-Cal Plus Tablets (Marion) p 418, 1189

CARDIOVASCULAR PREPARATIONS

Alpha Receptor Blocking Agent
Yocon (Palisades Pharm.) p 1476

Alpha and Beta Receptor Blocking Agent
Normodyne Injection (Schering) p 1867
Normodyne Tablets (Schering) p 434, 1870
Trandate Tablets (Glaxo) p 412, 983

Angiotensin Converting Enzyme Inhibitors
Capoten (Squibb) p 437, 1986

Antianginal Preparations
Calan Tablets (Searle & Co.) p 435, 1917
Cardilate Chewable Tablets (Burroughs Wellcome) p 407, 782
Cardilate Oral/Sublingual Tablets (Burroughs Wellcome) p 407, 782
Cardizem (Marion) p 417, 1183
Corgard (Squibb) p 437, 1989
Dilatrate-SR (Reed & Carnrick) p 427, 1632
Duotrate Plateau Caps (Marion) p 417, 1185
Duotrate 45 Plateau Caps (Marion) p 418, 1185
Inderal Tablets & Injectable (Ayerst) p 405, 647
Inderal LA Long Acting Capsules (Ayerst) p 405, 650
Iso-Bid Capsules (Geriatric) p 975
Isochron Tablets (Forest) p 953
Isoptin Oral Tablets (Knoll) p 414, 1063
Isordil Chewable (10 mg.) (Ives) p 413, 1028
Isordil Oral Titradose (5 mg.) (Ives) p 413, 1028
Isordil Oral Titradose (10 mg.) (Ives) p 413, 1028
Isordil Oral Titradose (20 mg.) (Ives) p 413, 1028
Isordil Oral Titradose (30 mg.) (Ives) p 413, 1028
Isordil Oral Titradose (40 mg.) (Ives) p 413, 1028
Isordil Sublingual 2.5 mg., 5 mg. & 10 mg. (Ives) p 413, 1028
Isordil Tembids Capsules & Tablets (40 mg.) (Ives) p 413, 1028
Nitro-Bid Ointment (Marion) p 1188
Nitro-Bid 2.5 Plateau Caps (Marion) p 418, 1186
Nitro-Bid 6.5 Plateau Caps (Marion) p 418, 1186
Nitro-Bid 9 Plateau Caps (Marion) p 418, 1186
Nitrodisc (Searle Pharmaceuticals) p 436, 1909
Nitro-Dur Transdermal Infusion System (Key Pharmaceuticals) p 413, 1050
Nitroglyn (Key Pharmaceuticals) p 1051
Nitrol Ointment (Rorer) p 432, 1752
Nitrostat Ointment 2% (Parke-Davis) p 425, 1545
Nitrostat Tablets (Parke-Davis) p 424, 1546
Nitrostat IV (Parke-Davis) p 424, 1546
Peritrate SA (Parke-Davis) p 425, 1560
Peritrate Tablets 10 mg., 20 mg. and 40 mg. (Parke-Davis) p 425, 1560
Persantine Tablets (Boehringer Ingelheim) p 406, 710
Procardia Capsules (Pfizer) p 426, 1606
Sorbitrate Tablets (Stuart) p 439, 2041
Transderm-Nitro Transdermal Therapeutic System (CIBA) p 410, 873
Tridil (American Critical Care) p 597

Antiarrhythmics
Bretylol (American Critical Care) p 592
Calan for IV Injection (Searle Pharmaceuticals) p 435, 1900
Cardioquin Tablets (Purdue Frederick) p 427, 1623
Duraquin (Parke-Davis) p 423, 1511
Inderal Tablets & Injectable (Ayerst) p 405, 647
Isoptin Ampules (Knoll) p 414, 1061
Isoptin for Intravenous Injection (Knoll) p 414, 1061
Isuprel Hydrochloride Injection 1:5000 (Winthrop-Breon) p 2201
Lidocaine Hydrochloride Injection, U.S.P. (Abbott) p 535
Norpace Capsules (Searle & Co.) p 436, 1933
Norpace CR Capsules (Searle & Co.) p 436, 1933
Procan SR (Parke-Davis) p 425, 1564
Pronestyl Capsules and Tablets (Squibb) p 438, 2017
Pronestyl Injection (Squibb) p 2018
Pronestyl-SR Tablets (Squibb) p 438, 2019
Quinaglute Dura-Tabs (Berlex) p 406, 702
Quinora (Key Pharmaceuticals) p 1051
Tonocard (Merck Sharp & Dohme) p 421, 1351
Vasoxyl Injection (Burroughs Wellcome) p 819
Xylocaine Solution for Ventricular Arrhythmias-Intravenous Injection or Continuous Infusion; or Intramuscular Injection (Astra) p 625

Antihypertensives
Aldactazide (Searle & Co.) p 435, 1912
Aldactone (Searle & Co.) p 435, 1914
Aldomet Ester HCl Injection (Merck Sharp & Dohme) p 1261
Aldomet Oral Suspension (Merck Sharp & Dohme) p 1259
Aldomet Tablets (Merck Sharp & Dohme) p 420, 1259
Apresoline Hydrochloride (CIBA) p 409, 843
Apresoline Hydrochloride Parenteral (CIBA) p 844
Aquatensen (Wallace) p 442, 2149
Arfonad Ampuls (Roche) p 1670
Blocadren Tablets (Merck Sharp & Dohme) p 420, 1271
Capoten (Squibb) p 437, 1986
Catapres Tablets (Boehringer Ingelheim) p 406, 707
Corgard (Squibb) p 437, 1989
Demi-Regroton Tablets (USV Pharmaceutical) p 440, 2087
Diucardin (Ayerst) p 404, 640
Diulo (Searle Pharmaceuticals) p 435, 1904
Diuril Tablets & Oral Suspension (Merck Sharp & Dohme) p 420, 1301
Enduron Tablets (Abbott) p 403, 517
Esidrix (CIBA) p 409, 848
Eutonyl Filmtab Tablets (Abbott) p 403, 528
Harmonyl (Abbott) p 532
HydroDIURIL Tablets (Merck Sharp & Dohme) p 420, 1316
Hygroton Tablets (USV Pharmaceutical) p 440, 2078
Hylorel Tablets (Pennwalt) p 426, 1582
Hyperstat I.V. Injection (Schering) p 1856
Inderal Tablets & Injectable (Ayerst) p 405, 647
Inderal LA Long Acting Capsules (Ayerst) p 405, 650
Inderide (Ayerst) p 405, 651
Ismelin (CIBA) p 409, 851
Loniten Tablets (Upjohn) p 441, 2120
Lopressor Ampuls (Geigy) p 960
Lopressor Tablets (Geigy) p 411, 960
Lozol Tablets (USV Pharmaceutical) p 440, 2081
Metahydrin (Merrell Dow) p 421, 1370
Minipress (Pfizer) p 426, 1603
Minizide Capsules (Pfizer) p 426, 1604
Moderil (Pfizer) p 426, 1605
Moduretic Tablets (Merck Sharp & Dohme) p 420, 1333
Naqua Tablets (Schering) p 434, 1861
Naturetin Tablets (Squibb) p 438, 2006
Nipride Injectable (Roche) p 1693
Nitropress (Abbott) p 546
Normodyne Injection (Schering) p 1867
Normodyne Tablets (Schering) p 434, 1870
Oretic (Abbott) p 403, 554
Raudixin Tablets (Squibb) p 438, 2020
Regroton Tablets (USV Pharmaceutical) p 440, 2087
Renese (Pfizer) p 426, 1608
Saluron (Bristol) p 407, 747
Serpasil Parenteral Solution (CIBA) p 868
Serpasil Tablets (CIBA) p 409, 867
Serpasil-Apresoline (CIBA) p 409, 869
Tenormin Tablets (Stuart) p 439, 2045
Trandate Tablets (Glaxo) p 412, 983
Visken (Sandoz Pharmaceutical Div.) p 433, 1820
Wytensin Tablets (Wyeth) p 445, 2299
Zaroxolyn (Pennwalt) p 426, 1586

Antihypertensives with Diuretics
Aldactazide (Searle & Co.) p 435, 1912
Aldoclor Tablets (Merck Sharp & Dohme) p 420, 1258

Product Category Index

Aldoril Tablets (Merck Sharp & Dohme) p 420, 1262
Apresazide (CIBA) p 409, 842
Apresoline-Esidrix (CIBA) p 409, 844
Combipres Tablets (Boehringer Ingelheim) p 406, 708
Corzide (Squibb) p 437, 1990
Diupres Tablets (Merck Sharp & Dohme) p 420, 1298
Diutensen Tablets (Wallace) p 2156
Diutensen-R Tablets (Wallace) p 442, 2157
Dyazide (Smith Kline & French) p 437, 1961
Enduronyl Forte Tablets (Abbott) p 403, 518
Enduronyl Tablets (Abbott) p 403, 518
Esimil (CIBA) p 409, 849
Exna Tablets (Robins) p 428, 1652
Hydromox R Tablets (Lederle) p 415, 1094
Hydromox Tablets (Lederle) p 415, 1094
Hydropres Tablets (Merck Sharp & Dohme) p 420, 1317
Metatensin Tablets (Merrell Dow) p 421, 1370
Naquival Tablets (Schering) p 434, 1862
Oreticyl (Abbott) p 555
Rauzide Tablets (Squibb) p 438, 2021
Renese-R (Pfizer) p 426, 1608
Salutensin/Salutensin-Demi (Bristol) p 407, 748
Ser-Ap-Es (CIBA) p 409, 866
Serpasil-Esidrix (CIBA) p 409, 870
Tenoretic Tablets (Stuart) p 439, 2043
Timolide Tablets (Merck Sharp & Dohme) p 420, 1346

Beta Blocking Agents
Blocadren Tablets (Merck Sharp & Dohme) p 420, 1271
Corgard (Squibb) p 437, 1989
Corzide (Squibb) p 437, 1990
Inderal Tablets & Injectable (Ayerst) p 405, 647
Inderal LA Long Acting Capsules (Ayerst) p 405, 650
Inderide (Ayerst) p 405, 651
Lopressor Ampuls (Geigy) p 960
Lopressor Tablets (Geigy) p 411, 960
Tenoretic Tablets (Stuart) p 439, 2043
Tenormin Tablets (Stuart) p 439, 2045
Timolide Tablets (Merck Sharp & Dohme) p 420, 1346
Visken (Sandoz Pharmaceutical Div.) p 433, 1820

Calcium Channel Blocker
Calan for IV Injection (Searle Pharmaceuticals) p 435, 1900
Calan Tablets (Searle & Co.) p 435, 1917
Cardizem (Marion) p 417, 1183
Isoptin Ampules (Knoll) p 414, 1061
Isoptin for Intravenous Injection (Knoll) p 414, 1061
Isoptin Oral Tablets (Knoll) p 414, 1063
Procardia Capsules (Pfizer) p 426, 1606

Digitalis
Cedilanid-D Injection (Sandoz Pharmaceutical Div.) p 1799
Crystodigin Tablets (Lilly) p 417, 1135
Digoxin in Tubex (Wyeth) p 2288
Lanoxicaps (Burroughs Wellcome) p 408, 793
Lanoxin (Burroughs Wellcome) p 408, 797

Hemorheologic Agent
Trental (Hoechst-Roussel) p 413, 1022

Inotropic Agent
Dopamine Solutions (Astra) p 615
Inocor Lactate Injection (Winthrop-Breon) p 2199

Myocardial Infarction Prophylaxis
Blocadren Tablets (Merck Sharp & Dohme) p 420, 1271

Quinidine
Quinaglute Dura-Tabs (Berlex) p 406, 702
Quinidex Extentabs (Robins) p 428, 1659

Vasodilators, Cerebral
Cerespan Capsules (USV Pharmaceutical) p 2074
Cyclospasmol (Ives) p 413, 1028
Ethatab (Glaxo) p 980
Lipo-Nicin (Brown) p 773
Pavabid Capsules (Marion) p 418, 1189
Pavabid HP Capsulets (Marion) p 418, 1189
Theo-24 (Searle & Co.) p 436, 1937
Vasodilan (Mead Johnson Pharmaceutical) p 419, 1255

Vasodilators, Coronary
Aerolate Liquid (Fleming) p 948
Aerolate Sr. & Jr. & III Capsules (Fleming) p 948
Aminophyllin Injection (Searle Pharmaceuticals) p 1898
Aminophyllin Tablets (Searle & Co.) p 435, 1915
Cardilate Chewable Tablets (Burroughs Wellcome) p 407, 782
Cardilate Oral/Sublingual Tablets (Burroughs Wellcome) p 407, 782

Duotrate Plateau Caps (Marion) p 417, 1185
Duotrate 45 Plateau Caps (Marion) p 418, 1185
Iso-Bid Capsules (Geriatric) p 975
Isochron Tablets (Forest) p 953
Isordil Chewable (10 mg.) (Ives) p 413, 1028
Isordil Oral Titradose (5 mg.) (Ives) p 413, 1028
Isordil Oral Titradose (10 mg.) (Ives) p 413, 1028
Isordil Oral Titradose (20 mg.) (Ives) p 413, 1028
Isordil Oral Titradose (30 mg.) (Ives) p 413, 1028
Isordil Oral Titradose (40 mg.) (Ives) p 413, 1028
Isordil Sublingual 2.5 mg., 5 mg. & 10 mg. (Ives) p 413, 1028
Isordil Tembids Capsules & Tablets (40 mg.) (Ives) p 413, 1028
Nitro-Bid IV (Marion) p 1187
Nitro-Bid 2.5 Plateau Caps (Marion) p 418, 1186
Nitro-Bid 6.5 Plateau Caps (Marion) p 418, 1186
Nitro-Bid 9 Plateau Caps (Marion) p 418, 1186
Nitroglyn (Key Pharmaceuticals) p 1051
Nitrol Ointment (Rorer) p 432, 1752
Nitrospan Capsules (USV Pharmaceutical) p 440, 2084
Nitrostat Ointment 2% (Parke-Davis) p 425, 1545
Nitrostat Tablets (Parke-Davis) p 424, 1546
Nitrostat IV (Parke-Davis) p 424, 1546
Pavabid Capsules (Marion) p 418, 1189
Pavabid HP Capsulets (Marion) p 418, 1189
Pentritol (USV Pharmaceutical) p 2086
Peritrate SA (Parke-Davis) p 425, 1560
Peritrate Tablets 10 mg., 20 mg. and 40 mg. (Parke-Davis) p 425, 1560
Persantine Tablets (Boehringer Ingelheim) p 406, 710
Sorbitrate Tablets (Stuart) p 439, 2041
Tridil (American Critical Care) p 597

Vasodilators, General
Arlidin Tablets (USV Pharmaceutical) p 440, 2070
Cerespan Capsules (USV Pharmaceutical) p 2074
Ethatab (Glaxo) p 980
Nitro-Bid Ointment (Marion) p 1188
Nitrol Ointment (Rorer) p 432, 1752
Tridil (American Critical Care) p 597

Vasodilators, Peripheral
Apresoline Hydrochloride (CIBA) p 409, 843
Apresoline Hydrochloride Parenteral (CIBA) p 844
Apresoline-Esidrix (CIBA) p 409, 844
Arfonad Ampuls (Roche) p 1670
Arlidin Tablets (USV Pharmaceutical) p 440, 2070
Cyclospasmol (Ives) p 413, 1028
Dibenzyline Capsules (Smith Kline & French) p 436, 1960
Esimil (CIBA) p 409, 849
Ethatab (Glaxo) p 980
Hyperstat I.V. Injection (Schering) p 1856
Ismelin (CIBA) p 409, 851
Lipo-Nicin (Brown) p 773
Loniten Tablets (Upjohn) p 441, 2120
Nico-400 (Marion) p 418, 1186
Pavabid Capsules (Marion) p 418, 1189
Pavabid HP Capsulets (Marion) p 418, 1189
Priscoline Hydrochloride Multiple-Dose Vials (CIBA) p 862
Serpasil-Apresoline (CIBA) p 409, 869
Serpasil-Esidrix (CIBA) p 409, 870
Vasodilan (Mead Johnson Pharmaceutical) p 419, 1255

Vasodilators & Combinations
Lipo-Nicin (Brown) p 773

Vasopressors
Aramine Injection (Merck Sharp & Dohme) p 1266
Dopamine Hydrochloride Ampoules (Dopastat) (Parke-Davis) p 1510
Dopamine HCl Injection (Elkins-Sinn) p 938
Intropin (American Critical Care) p 596
Levophed Bitartrate (Winthrop-Breon) p 2205
Neo-Synephrine Hydrochloride 1% Injection (Winthrop-Breon) p 2216
Vasoxyl Injection (Burroughs Wellcome) p 819
Wyamine Sulfate in Tubex (Wyeth) p 2288

Other Cardiovasculars
Added Protection III Multi-Vitamin & Multi-Mineral Supplement (Professional Health) p 1621
Cardioguard Natural Lipotropic Dietary Supplement-Tablets (Professional Health) p 1621
Demser Capsules (Merck Sharp & Dohme) p 420, 1297

Diuril Intravenous Sodium (Merck Sharp & Dohme) p 1299
Dobutrex (Lilly) p 1143
Edecrin Sodium Intravenous (Merck Sharp & Dohme) p 1304
Edecrin Tablets (Merck Sharp & Dohme) p 420, 1304
Prostin VR Pediatric Sterile Solution (Upjohn) p 2132

CENTRAL NERVOUS SYSTEM STIMULANTS
Cylert Tablets (Abbott) p 403, 510
Desoxyn (Abbott) p 515
Desoxyn Gradumet Tablets (Abbott) p 403, 515
Efed II Capsules (Black) (Alto) p 404, 589
No Doz (Bristol-Myers Products) p 771

CERUMENOLYTICS
Cerumenex Drops (Purdue Frederick) p 1624

CHELATING AGENTS
BAL in Oil Ampules (Hynson, Westcott & Dunning) p 1024
Calcium Disodium Versenate Injection (Riker) p 1641
Cuprimine Capsules (Merck Sharp & Dohme) p 420, 1280
Depen Titratable Tablets (Wallace) p 2152
Desferal mesylate (CIBA) p 847

CHOLESTEROL REDUCERS & ANTIHYPERLIPEMICS
Atromid-S (Ayerst) p 404, 636
Choloxin (Flint) p 411, 949
Colestid Granules (Upjohn) p 2100
Lopid Capsules (Parke-Davis) p 424, 1539
Lorelco (Merrell Dow) p 421, 1368
Nicolar Tablets (USV Pharmaceutical) p 440, 2083
Questran (Mead Johnson Laboratories) p 1231
S-P-T (Fleming) p 949

COLORIMETERS
Dextrometer Reflectance Colorimeter (Ames) p 3006

CONTRACEPTIVES
Devices
Koro-Flex Arcing Spring Diaphragm (Youngs) p 2300
Koromex Coil Spring Diaphragm (Youngs) p 2301
Lippes Loop Intrauterine Double-S (Ortho Pharmaceutical) p 1454
Ortho Diaphragm Kit-All Flex (Ortho Pharmaceutical) p 1457
Ortho Diaphragm Kit-Coil Spring (Ortho Pharmaceutical) p 1457
Ortho-White Diaphragm Kit-Flat Spring (Ortho Pharmaceutical) p 1457
Progestasert Intrauterine Contraceptive System (Alza) p 404, 590

Devices, copper containing
Cu-7 (Searle Pharmaceuticals) p 435, 1902
Tatum-T (Searle Pharmaceuticals) p 436, 1909

Oral
Brevicon 21-Day Tablets (Syntex) p 440, 2052
Brevicon 28-Day Tablets (Syntex) p 440, 2052
Demulen 1/35-21 (Searle & Co.) p 435, 1919
Demulen 1/35-28 (Searle & Co.) p 435, 1919
Demulen 1/50-21 (Searle & Co.) p 435, 1919
Demulen 1/50-28 (Searle & Co.) p 435, 1919
Enovid 5 mg (Searle & Co.) p 435, 1919
Enovid 10 mg (Searle & Co.) p 435, 1919
Enovid-E 21 (Searle & Co.) p 436, 1919
Loestrin 21 1/20 (Parke-Davis) p 424, 1531
Loestrin Fe 1/20 (Parke-Davis) p 424, 1531
Loestrin 21 1.5/30 (Parke-Davis) p 424, 1531
Loestrin Fe 1.5/30 (Parke-Davis) p 424, 1531
Lo/Ovral Tablets (Wyeth) p 444, 2255
Lo/Ovral-28 Tablets (Wyeth) p 444, 2263
Micronor Tablets (Ortho Pharmaceutical) p 423, 1461
Modicon 21 Tablets (Ortho Pharmaceutical) p 423, 1461
Modicon 28 Tablets (Ortho Pharmaceutical) p 1461
Nordette-21 Tablets (Wyeth) p 444, 2266
Nordette-28 Tablets (Wyeth) p 444, 2270
Norinyl 1+35 Tablets 21-Day (Syntex) p 440, 2052
Norinyl 1+35 Tablets 28-Day (Syntex) p 440, 2052
Norinyl 1+50 21-Day (Syntex) p 440, 2052

Product Category Index

Norinyl 1+50 28-Day (Syntex) p 440, 2052
Norinyl 1+80 21-Day (Syntex) p 440, 2052
Norinyl 1+80 28-Day (Syntex) p 440, 2052
Norinyl 2 mg. (Syntex) p 440, 2052
Norlestrin 21 1/50 (Parke-Davis) p 425, 1548
Norlestrin 21 2.5/50 (Parke-Davis) p 425, 1548
Norlestrin 28 1/50 (Parke-Davis) p 1548
Norlestrin Fe 1/50 (Parke-Davis) p 425, 1548
Norlestrin Fe 2.5/50 (Parke-Davis) p 425, 1548
Nor-Q.D. (Syntex) p 440, 2052
Ortho-Novum 1/35□21 (Ortho Pharmaceutical) p 422, 1461
Ortho-Novum 1/35□28 (Ortho Pharmaceutical) p 1461
Ortho-Novum 1/50□21 (Ortho Pharmaceutical) p 422, 1461
Ortho-Novum 1/50□28 (Ortho Pharmaceutical) p 1461
Ortho-Novum 1/80□21 (Ortho Pharmaceutical) p 423, 1461
Ortho-Novum 1/80□28 (Ortho Pharmaceutical) p 1461
Ortho-Novum 7/7/7 □.. 21 Tablets (Ortho Pharmaceutical) p 422, 1461
Ortho-Novum 7/7/7 □.. 28 Tablets (Ortho Pharmaceutical) p 1461
Ortho-Novum 10/11□.. 21 Tablets (Ortho Pharmaceutical) p 422, 1461
Ortho-Novum 10/11□.. 28 Tablets (Ortho Pharmaceutical) p 1461
Ortho-Novum Tablets 2 mg□21 (Ortho Pharmaceutical) p 423, 1461
Ovcon-35 (Mead Johnson Laboratories) p 419, 1224
Ovcon-50 (Mead Johnson Laboratories) p 419, 1224
Ovral Tablets (Wyeth) p 444, 2271
Ovral-28 Tablets (Wyeth) p 444, 2272
Ovrette Tablets (Wyeth) p 2272
Ovulen-21 (Searle & Co.) p 436, 1919
Ovulen-28 (Searle & Co.) p 436, 1919
Tri-Norinyl 21-Day Tablets (Syntex) p 440, 2052
Tri-Norinyl 28-Day Tablets (Syntex) p 440, 2052

Topical

Ramses Contraceptive Vaginal Jelly (Schmid) p 1896
Semicid Vaginal Contraceptive Suppositories (Whitehall) p 443, 2187

COSMETICS

Ar-Ex Hypo-Allergenic Cosmetics (Ar-Ex) p 600
Formula Magic (Consolidated Chemical) p 880
Herpecin-L Cold Sore Lip Balm (Campbell) p 829
RVPaba Lip Stick (Elder) p 936
Skin Magic (Consolidated Chemical) p 881

COUGH & COLD PREPARATIONS

Cold Preparations

Non-Narcotic

Albatussin (Bart) p 685
Alka-Seltzer Plus Cold Medicine (Miles Laboratories) p 1395
Bromfed Capsules (Timed Release) (Muro) p 1420
Bromfed-PD Capsules (Timed Release) (Muro) p 1420
Bromfed Tablets (Muro) p 1420
Children's Chloraseptic Lozenges (Procter & Gamble) p 1619
Chloraseptic Liquid (Procter & Gamble) p 1619
Chloraseptic Lozenges (Procter & Gamble) p 1620
Comtrex (Bristol-Myers Products) p 769
Congespirin Cold Tablets (Aspirin Formula) (Bristol-Myers Products) p 769
Congespirin Liquid Cold Medicine (Bristol-Myers Products) p 770
Corsym (Pennwalt) p 1582
CoTylenol Cold Medication Tablets & Capsules (McNeil Consumer Products) p 418, 1197
CoTylenol Liquid Cold Medication (McNeil Consumer Products) p 1197
CoTylenol Children's Liquid Cold Formula (McNeil Consumer Products) p 418, 1198
Cremacoat 3 (Vicks Pharmacy Products) p 442, 2147
Cremacoat 4 (Vicks Pharmacy Products) p 442, 2147
Deconamine Tablets, Elixir, SR Capsules, Syrup (Berlex) p 406, 699
Dimetapp Elixir (Robins) p 1648
Dimetapp Extentabs (Robins) p 428, 1648
Dorcol Children's Liquid Cold Formula (Dorsey Laboratories) p 909

Dristan, Advanced Formula Decongestant/Antihistamine/Analgesic Capsules (Whitehall) p 443, 2186
Dristan, Advanced Formula Decongestant/Antihistamine/Analgesic Tablets (Whitehall) p 443, 2186
Dristan Long Lasting Nasal Spray, Regular & Menthol (Whitehall) p 443, 2186
Dristan Nasal Spray, Regular & Menthol (Whitehall) p 443, 2186
Extendryl Chewable Tablets (Fleming) p 948
Extendryl Sr. & Jr. T.D. Capsules (Fleming) p 948
Extendryl Syrup (Fleming) p 948
Extra-Strength Sine-Aid Sinus Headache Capsules (McNeil Consumer Products) p 1199
Fedahist Gyrocaps, Syrup & Tablets (Rorer) p 431, 1749
Head & Chest (Procter & Gamble) p 1620
Naldecon (Bristol) p 407, 738
Nolamine Tablets (Carnrick) p 408, 833
Novafed A Capsules (Merrell Dow) p 421, 1377
Novafed A Liquid (Merrell Dow) p 1377
Novafed Capsules (Merrell Dow) p 421, 1376
Novafed Liquid (Merrell Dow) p 1376
Ornade Spansule Capsules (Smith Kline & French) p 437, 1968
Ponaris Nasal Mucosal Emollient (Jamol) p 1033
Propagest & Propagest Syrup (Carnrick) p 408, 834
Rondec Oral Drops (Ross) p 1776
Rondec Syrup (Ross) p 1776
Rondec Tablet (Ross) p 432, 1776
Rondec-TR Tablet (Ross) p 432, 1776
Rynatan Tablets & Pediatric Suspension (Wallace) p 442, 2165
Sine-Aid Extra-Strength Sinus Headache Capsules (McNeil Consumer Products) p 1199
Sine-Aid Sinus Headache Tablets (McNeil Consumer Products) p 1198
Sinubid (Parke-Davis) p 425, 1569
Sinulin Tablets (Carnrick) p 409, 835
Tavist-D Tablets (Sandoz Pharmaceutical Div.) p 433, 1819
Triaminic Cold Syrup (Dorsey Laboratories) p 911
Triaminic Cold Tablets (Dorsey Laboratories) p 911
Triaminic Juvelets (Dorsey Laboratories) p 912
Triaminic Oral Infant Drops (Dorsey Laboratories) p 912
Triaminic TR Tablets (Timed Release) (Dorsey Laboratories) p 912
Triaminic-12 Tablets (Dorsey Laboratories) p 913
Tylenol, Maximum-Strength, Sinus Medication Tablets & Capsules (McNeil Consumer Products) p 418, 1201
Vita-Numonyl Injectable (Lambda) p 1071

Cough Preparations

Non-Narcotic

Benylin Cough Syrup (Parke-Davis) p 1486
Breonesin (Winthrop-Breon) p 2193
Codimal DM (Central Pharmaceuticals) p 836
Codimal Expectorant (Central Pharmaceuticals) p 836
Congespirin Cough Syrup (Bristol-Myers Products) p 770
Cremacoat 1 (Vicks Pharmacy Products) p 442, 2146
Cremacoat 2 (Vicks Pharmacy Products) p 442, 2147
Cremacoat 3 (Vicks Pharmacy Products) p 442, 2147
Cremacoat 4 (Vicks Pharmacy Products) p 442, 2147
Delsym (Pennwalt) p 1582
Dorcol Children's Cough Syrup (Dorsey Laboratories) p 909
Fedahist Expectorant (Rorer) p 1749
Hytuss Tablets and Hytuss-2X Capsules (Hyrex) p 413, 1024
Phenergan Syrup Fortis (Wyeth) p 2276
Phenergan Syrup Plain (Wyeth) p 2276
Phenergan VC (Wyeth) p 2282
Phenergan with Dextromethorphan (Wyeth) p 2280
Pima Syrup (Fleming) p 948
Polaramine Repetabs Tablets (Schering) p 434, 1879
Polaramine Syrup (Schering) p 1879
Polaramine Tablets (Schering) p 434, 1879
Quelidrine Syrup (Abbott) p 567
Sinovan Timed (Drug Industries) p 915
Sorbutuss (Dalin) p 886
Tessalon (Du Pont) p 411, 928
Triaminicol Multi-Symptom Cold Syrup (Dorsey Laboratories) p 913
Triaminicol Multi-Symptom Cold Tablets (Dorsey Laboratories) p 914
Tussi-Organidin DM (Wallace) p 442, 2171

with Narcotics

A.P.C. with Codeine Nos. 3 & 4, Tabloid brand (Burroughs Wellcome) p 407, 780
Actifed with Codeine Cough Syrup (Burroughs Wellcome) p 773
Ambenyl Cough Syrup (Marion) p 1181
Calcidrine Syrup (Abbott) p 510
Codiclear DH Syrup (Central Pharmaceuticals) p 836
Codimal DH (Central Pharmaceuticals) p 836
Codimal PH (Central Pharmaceuticals) p 836
Dilaudid Cough Syrup (Knoll) p 1058
Dimetane-DC Cough Syrup (Robins) p 1647
Hycodan (Du Pont) p 410, 917
Hycotuss Expectorant (Du Pont) p 920
Nucofed Expectorant (Beecham Laboratories) p 693
Nucofed Pediatric Expectorant (Beecham Laboratories) p 694
Pediacof (Winthrop-Breon) p 2221
Phenergan VC with Codeine (Wyeth) p 2284
Phenergan with Codeine (Wyeth) p 2278
Robitussin A-C (Robins) p 1664
Tussar SF (USV Pharmaceutical) p 2092
Tussar-2 (USV Pharmaceutical) p 2092
Tussend Expectorant (Merrell Dow) p 421, 1394
Tussionex Tablets, Capsules & Suspension (Pennwalt) p 1585
Tussi-Organidin (Wallace) p 442, 2171

Cough & Cold Preparations

Non-Narcotic

Albatussin (Bart) p 685
Ambenyl-D Decongestant Cough Formula (Marion) p 1182
Bayer Cough Syrup for Children (Glenbrook) p 996
Entex Capsules (Norwich Eaton) p 1431
Entex LA Tablets (Norwich Eaton) p 422, 1432
Entex Liquid (Norwich Eaton) p 1431
Guaifed Capsules (Timed Release) (Muro) p 1421
Head & Chest (Procter & Gamble) p 1620
Histalet DM Syrup (Reid-Provident Labs.) p 1638
Histalet Syrup (Reid-Provident Labs.) p 1638
Hytuss Tablets and Hytuss-2X Capsules (Hyrex) p 413, 1024
Isoclor Timesule Capsules (Fisons) p 944
Naldecon-DX Pediatric Syrup (Bristol) p 739
Naldecon-EX Pediatric Drops (Bristol) p 740
Rondec-DM Oral Drops (Ross) p 1777
Rondec-DM Syrup (Ross) p 1777
Rynatuss Tablets & Pediatric Suspension (Wallace) p 442, 2165
Scot-Tussin Sugar-Free 5-Action Cold Formula (Scot-Tussin) p 1897
Singlet (Merrell Dow) p 421, 1385
Triaminic Expectorant (Dorsey Laboratories) p 911
Triaminic-DM Cough Formula (Dorsey Laboratories) p 913
Tussar DM (USV Pharmaceutical) p 2091
Tuss-Ornade Liquid (Smith Kline & French) p 1980
Tuss-Ornade Spansule Capsules (Smith Kline & French) p 437, 1981

with Narcotics

Citra Forte Capsules (Boyle) p 726
Citra Forte Syrup (Boyle) p 726
Codiclear DH Syrup (Central Pharmaceuticals) p 836
Hycomine Compound (Du Pont) p 919
Hycomine Pediatric Syrup (Du Pont) p 917
Hycomine Syrup (Du Pont) p 917
Naldecon-CX Suspension (Bristol) p 739
Novahistine DH (Merrell Dow) p 421, 1378
Novahistine Expectorant (Merrell Dow) p 421, 1378
Nucofed Capsules (Beecham Laboratories) p 406, 692
Nucofed Syrup (Beecham Laboratories) p 692
P-V-Tussin Syrup (Reid-Provident Labs.) p 1640
P-V-Tussin Tablets (Reid-Provident Labs.) p 428, 1640
Robitussin-DAC (Robins) p 1665
Ru-Tuss Expectorant (Boots) p 722
Ru-Tuss with Hydrocodone (Boots) p 722
Triaminic Expectorant w/Codeine (Dorsey Laboratories) p 911
Tussend Liquid & Tablets (Merrell Dow) p 421, 1393

D

DECONGESTANTS

Oral

Alka-Seltzer Plus Cold Medicine (Miles Laboratories) p 1395
Bromfed Capsules (Timed Release) (Muro) p 1420
Bromfed-PD Capsules (Timed Release) (Muro) p 1420
Bromfed Tablets (Muro) p 1420

Product Category Index

Comhist LA Capsules (Norwich Eaton) p 422, 1425
Comhist Tablets (Norwich Eaton) p 1426
Comtrex (Bristol-Myers Products) p 769
Congespirin Aspirin-Free Chewable Cold Tablets for Children (Bristol-Myers Products) p 769
Congespirin Liquid Cold Medicine (Bristol-Myers Products) p 770
Corsym (Pennwalt) p 1582
Cremacoat 3 (Vicks Pharmacy Products) p 442, 2147
Cremacoat 4 (Vicks Pharmacy Products) p 442, 2147
Deconamine Tablets, Elixir, SR Capsules, Syrup (Berlex) p 406, 699
Dimetapp Elixir (Robins) p 1648
Dimetapp Extentabs (Robins) p 428, 1648
Dorcol Children's Cough Syrup (Dorsey Laboratories) p 909
Dorcol Children's Decongestant Liquid (Dorsey Laboratories) p 909
Dorcol Children's Liquid Cold Formula (Dorsey Laboratories) p 909
Dristan, Advanced Formula Decongestant/Antihistamine/Analgesic Capsules (Whitehall) p 443, 2186
Dristan, Advanced Formula Decongestant/Antihistamine/Analgesic Tablets (Whitehall) p 443, 2186
Efed II Capsules (Yellow) (Alto) p 404, 589
Extra-Strength Sine-Aid Sinus Headache Capsules (McNeil Consumer Products) p 1199
4-Way Cold Tablets (Bristol-Myers Products) p 770
Guaifed Capsules (Timed Release) (Muro) p 1421
Naldecon-CX Suspension (Bristol) p 739
Naldecon-DX Pediatric Syrup (Bristol) p 739
Novafed A Capsules (Merrell Dow) p 421, 1377
Novafed A Liquid (Merrell Dow) p 1377
Novafed Capsules (Merrell Dow) p 421, 1376
Novafed Liquid (Merrell Dow) p 1376
Phenergan VC (Wyeth) p 2282
Phenergan VC with Codeine (Wyeth) p 2284
Propagest & Propagest Syrup (Carnrick) p 408, 834
Rondec-DM Oral Drops (Ross) p 1777
Rondec-DM Syrup (Ross) p 1777
Ru-Tuss Expectorant (Boots) p 722
Ru-Tuss Plain (Boots) p 723
Ru-Tuss Tablets (Boots) p 406, 723
Ru-Tuss II Capsules (Boots) p 406, 723
Ru-Tuss with Hydrocodone (Boots) p 722
Sine-Aid Extra-Strength Sinus Headache Capsules (McNeil Consumer Products) p 1199
Sine-Aid Sinus Headache Tablets (McNeil Consumer Products) p 1198
Sinovan Timed (Drug Industries) p 915
Tavist-D Tablets (Sandoz Pharmaceutical Div.) p 433, 1819
Triaminic Cold Syrup (Dorsey Laboratories) p 911
Triaminic Cold Tablets (Dorsey Laboratories) p 911
Triaminic-DM Cough Formula (Dorsey Laboratories) p 913
Triaminic-12 Tablets (Dorsey Laboratories) p 913
Trinalin Repetabs Tablets (Schering) p 435, 1890
Tussar DM (USV Pharmaceutical) p 2091
Tussar SF (USV Pharmaceutical) p 2092
Tussar-2 (USV Pharmaceutical) p 2092
Tylenol, Maximum-Strength, Sinus Medication Tablets & Capsules (McNeil Consumer Products) p 418, 1201

Topical, Nasal

Beconase Nasal Inhaler (Glaxo) p 411, 978
Dristan Long Lasting Nasal Spray, Regular & Menthol (Whitehall) p 443, 2186
Dristan Nasal Spray, Regular & Menthol (Whitehall) p 443, 2186
4-Way Long Acting Nasal Spray (Bristol-Myers Products) p 771
4-Way Nasal Spray (Bristol-Myers Products) p 770
Otrivin (Geigy) p 963
Privine Hydrochloride 0.05% Nasal Solution (CIBA) p 863
Privine Hydrochloride 0.05% Nasal Spray (CIBA) p 863
Tyzine (Key Pharmaceuticals) p 1056

DECONGESTANTS, EXPECTORANTS & COMBINATIONS

Actifed with Codeine Cough Syrup (Burroughs Wellcome) p 773
Albatussin (Bart) p 685
Alka-Seltzer Plus Cold Medicine (Miles Laboratories) p 1395
Ambenyl Cough Syrup (Marion) p 1181
Ambenyl-D Decongestant Cough Formula (Marion) p 1182

Bayer Children's Cold Tablets (Glenbrook) p 996
Codiclear DH Syrup (Central Pharmaceuticals) p 836
Codimal DH (Central Pharmaceuticals) p 836
Codimal DM (Central Pharmaceuticals) p 836
Codimal Expectorant (Central Pharmaceuticals) p 836
Codimal PH (Central Pharmaceuticals) p 836
Congespirin Cold Tablets (Aspirin Formula) (Bristol-Myers Products) p 769
Congess Jr. & Sr. T.D. Capsules (Fleming) p 948
Dimetane-DC Cough Syrup (Robins) p 1647
Dorcol Children's Cough Syrup (Dorsey Laboratories) p 909
Dorcol Children's Liquid Cold Formula (Dorsey Laboratories) p 909
Entex Capsules (Norwich Eaton) p 1431
Entex LA Tablets (Norwich Eaton) p 422, 1432
Entex Liquid (Norwich Eaton) p 1431
Extendryl Chewable Tablets (Fleming) p 948
Extendryl Sr. & Jr. T.D. Capsules (Fleming) p 948
Extendryl Syrup (Fleming) p 948
Fedahist Expectorant (Rorer) p 1749
Fedahist Gyrocaps, Syrup & Tablets (Rorer) p 431, 1749
Fiogesic Tablets (Sandoz Pharmaceutical Div.) p 432, 1801
Head & Chest (Procter & Gamble) p 1620
Histalet Forte Tablets (Reid-Provident Labs.) p 428, 1638
Histalet X Syrup & Tablets (New Formula) (Reid-Provident Labs.) p 428, 1638
Histaspan-D Capsules (USV Pharmaceutical) p 2077
Histaspan-Plus Capsules (USV Pharmaceutical) p 2077
Hytuss Tablets and Hytuss-2X Capsules (Hyrex) p 413, 1024
Lufyllin-GG (Wallace) p 442, 2161
Mudrane GG Elixir (Poythress) p 1619
Mudrane GG Tablets (Poythress) p 1619
Mudrane Tablets (Poythress) p 1618
Naldecon (Bristol) p 407, 738
Naldecon-EX Pediatric Drops (Bristol) p 740
Nolamine Tablets (Carnrick) p 408, 833
Novahistine DH (Merrell Dow) p 421, 1378
Novahistine Expectorant (Merrell Dow) p 421, 1378
Nucofed Capsules (Beecham Laboratories) p 406, 692
Nucofed Syrup (Beecham Laboratories) p 692
Organidin (Wallace) p 442, 2163
Ornade Spansule Capsules (Smith Kline & French) p 437, 1968
Pediacof (Winthrop-Breon) p 2221
Quadrinal Tablets & Suspension (Knoll) p 414, 1065
Quibron & Quibron-300 (Mead Johnson Laboratories) p 419, 1233
Robitussin-DAC (Robins) p 1665
Rynatan Tablets & Pediatric Suspension (Wallace) p 442, 2165
SSKI (Upsher-Smith) p 2145
Singlet (Merrell Dow) p 421, 1385
Sinubid (Parke-Davis) p 425, 1569
Sinulin Tablets (Carnrick) p 409, 835
Theo-Organidin Elixir (Wallace) p 442, 2170
Triaminic Expectorant (Dorsey Laboratories) p 911
Triaminic Expectorant w/Codeine (Dorsey Laboratories) p 911
Triaminic Juvelets (Dorsey Laboratories) p 912
Triaminic Oral Infant Drops (Dorsey Laboratories) p 912
Triaminic TR Tablets (Timed Release) (Dorsey Laboratories) p 912
Triaminicol Multi-Symptom Cold Syrup (Dorsey Laboratories) p 913
Triaminicol Multi-Symptom Cold Tablets (Dorsey Laboratories) p 914
Trinalin Repetabs Tablets (Schering) p 435, 1890
Tussend Expectorant (Merrell Dow) p 421, 1394
Tussend Liquid & Tablets (Merrell Dow) p 421, 1393
Tussi-Organidin (Wallace) p 442, 2171
Tussi-Organidin DM (Wallace) p 442, 2171
Vita-Numonyl Injectable (Lambda) p 1071

DENTAL PREPARATIONS

Anbesol Gel Antiseptic Anesthetic (Whitehall) p 443, 2185
B-C-Bid Capsules (Geriatric) p 975
Cevi-Bid Capsules (Geriatric) p 975
Chloraseptic Liquid (Procter & Gamble) p 1619
Chloraseptic Lozenges (Procter & Gamble) p 1620
Dalidyne (Dalin) p 886

Fluoritab Tablets & Fluoritab Liquid (Fluoritab) p 953
Gly-Oxide Liquid (Marion) p 1186
Hurricaine Liquid 1/4cc Unit Dose (Beutlich) p 705
Hurricaine Oral, Topical Anesthetic Gel, Liquid, Spray (Beutlich) p 705
Kenalog in Orabase (Squibb) p 2003
Luride Drops (Colgate-Hoyt) p 878
Luride Lozi-Tabs Tablets (Colgate-Hoyt) p 410, 878
Mulvidren-F Softab Tablets (Stuart) p 439, 2039
Orabase HCA (Colgate-Hoyt) p 879
Phos-Flur Oral Rinse/Supplement (Colgate-Hoyt) p 879
Point-Two Dental Rinse (Colgate-Hoyt) p 880
PreviDent Brush-On Gel (Colgate-Hoyt) p 880
Proxigel (Reed & Carnrick) p 1637
Thera-Flur Gel-Drops (Colgate-Hoyt) p 880

DEODORANTS

Oral

Derifil Tablets & Powder (Rystan) p 1796

Topical

Chloresium Ointment (Rystan) p 1795
Chloresium Solution (Rystan) p 1795
Derifil Tablets & Powder (Rystan) p 1796
Panafil Ointment (Rystan) p 1796
Puri-Clens (Sween) p 2048

DERMATOLOGICALS

Abradant

Pernox Lotion (Westwood) p 2180
Pernox Medicated Lathering Scrub (Westwood) p 2180
Ureacin Lotion & Creme (Pedinol) p 1581

Antiacne Preparations

A/T/S (Hoechst-Roussel) p 412, 1009
Accutane Capsules (Roche) p 429, 1665
Aveenobar Medicated (Cooper Dermatology) p 882
5 Benzagel (5% benzoyl peroxide) & 10 Benzagel (10% benzoyl peroxide), Acne Gels, Microgel Formula (Dermik) p 888
Cleocin T Topical Solution* (Upjohn) p 441, 2100
Desquam-X 2.5 Gel (Westwood) p 2175
Desquam-X 5 Gel (Westwood) p 2175
Desquam-X 10 Gel (Westwood) p 2175
Desquam-X 5 Wash (Westwood) p 2176
Desquam-X 10 Wash (Westwood) p 2176
EryDerm (Abbott) p 519
Erymax Topical Solution (Herbert) p 1003
Fostex Medicated Cleansing Bar (Westwood) p 2177
Fostex Medicated Cleansing Cream (Westwood) p 2177
Fostex 5% Benzoyl Peroxide Gel (Westwood) p 2177
Fostex 10% Benzoyl Peroxide Cleansing Bar (Westwood) p 2177
Fostex 10% Benzoyl Peroxide Gel (Westwood) p 2178
Fostex 10% Benzoyl Peroxide Tinted Cream (Westwood) p 2178
Fostex 10% Benzoyl Peroxide Wash (Westwood) p 2178
Fostril (Westwood) p 2178
Hill Cortac (Hill Dermaceuticals) p 1009
Intraderm-19 Emergency Acne Stick (Robertson/Taylor) p 1645
Intraderm-19 Overnight Acne Masque (Robertson/Taylor) p 1645
Intraderm-19 Therapeutic Acne Scrub (Robertson/Taylor) p 1645
Intraderm-19 Therapeutic Astringent Lotion (Robertson/Taylor) p 1646
Komed Acne Lotion (Barnes-Hind) p 684
Komed HC Lotion (Barnes-Hind) p 684
Komex (Barnes-Hind) p 684
Meclan (Ortho Pharmaceutical (Dermatological Div.)) p 1474
Pernox Lotion (Westwood) p 2180
Pernox Medicated Lathering Scrub (Westwood) p 2180
Persa-Gel 5% & 10% (Ortho Pharmaceutical (Dermatological Div.) p 1474
Persa-Gel W 5% & 10% (Ortho Pharmaceutical (Dermatological Div.)) p 1474
Retin-A (tretinoin) (Ortho Pharmaceutical (Dermatological Div.)) p 1475
Staticin 1.5% Topical Solution (Westwood) p 2181
Sulfacet-R Acne Lotion (Dermik) p 891
T-Stat 2.0% Topical Solution (Westwood) p 2181
Topicycline (Norwich Eaton) p 1438
Transact (Westwood) p 2183
Vanoxide-HC Acne Lotion (Dermik) p 891
Vlemasque (Dermik) p 891
Xerac (Persōn & Covey) p 1588
Xerac BP5 & Xerac BP10 (Persōn & Covey) p 1588

Product Category Index

Antibacterial
Achromycin 3% Ointment (Lederle) p 1077
Anbesol Gel Antiseptic Anesthetic (Whitehall) p 443, 2185
Barseb HC Scalp Lotion (Barnes-Hind) p 683
Barseb Thera-Spray (Barnes-Hind) p 684
Chloromycetin Cream, 1% (Parke-Davis) p 1487
Cortisporin Ointment (Burroughs Wellcome) p 784
EryDerm (Abbott) p 519
Flint SSD Cream (Flint) p 411, 950
Formula Magic (Consolidated Chemical) p 880
Fungoid Creme & Solution (Pedinol) p 1580
Furacin Preparations (Norwich Eaton) p 1433
Furacin Soluble Dressing (Norwich Eaton) p 1433
Furacin Topical Cream (Norwich Eaton) p 1434
Garamycin Cream 0.1% and Ointment 0.1% (Schering) p 1846
Komed Acne Lotion (Barnes-Hind) p 684
Komed HC Lotion (Barnes-Hind) p 684
Mytrex Cream & Ointment (Savage) p 1825
Neo-Polycin (Merrell Dow) p 1372
Neosporin Aerosol (Burroughs Wellcome) p 806
Neosporin Ointment (Burroughs Wellcome) p 808
Neosporin-G Cream (Burroughs Wellcome) p 807
Osti-Derm Lotion (Pedinol) p 1580
pHisoHex (Winthrop-Breon) p 2222
Polysporin Ointment (Burroughs Wellcome) p 810
Satin (Consolidated Chemical) p 881
Skin Magic (Consolidated Chemical) p 881
Sulfacet-R Acne Lotion (Dermik) p 891
Sulfamylon Acetate Cream (Winthrop-Breon) p 2226

Antibacterial, Antifungal & Combinations
Anti-Sept (Seamless) p 1897
Betadine Ointment (Purdue Frederick) p 1622
Betadine Skin Cleanser (Purdue Frederick) p 1622
Flint SSD Cream (Flint) p 411, 950
Fungi-Nail Tincture (Kramer) p 1069
Micro-Guard (Sween) p 2048
Mycolog Cream and Ointment (Squibb) p 2003
Nystaform Ointment (Miles Pharmaceuticals) p 1411
Pedi-Cort V Creme (Pedinol) p 1581
Vioform (CIBA) p 876
Vioform-Hydrocortisone (CIBA) p 876
VōSol HC Otic Solution (Wallace) p 442, 2171
VōSol Otic Solution (Wallace) p 442, 2171
Vytone Cream (Dermik) p 891

Antidermatitis
Aeroseb-Dex Topical Aerosol Spray (Herbert) p 1001
Aeroseb-HC Topical Aerosol Spray (Herbert) p 1002
Aveeno Bath Oilated (Cooper Dermatology) p 882
Aveeno Bath Regular (Cooper Dermatology) p 882
Aveenobar Oilated (Cooper Dermatology) p 882
Aveenobar Regular (Cooper Dermatology) p 882
Caladryl (Parke-Davis) p 1486
Cyclocort Cream (Lederle) p 415, 1089
Cyclocort Ointment (Lederle) p 415, 1089
Decaspray Topical Aerosol (Merck Sharp & Dohme) p 1296
Florone Cream 0.05% (Dermik) p 889
Florone Ointment 0.05% (Dermik) p 889
Fluonid Ointment, Cream & Topical Solution (Herbert) p 1003
Hytone Cream, Lotion & Ointment (Dermik) p 890
Lidex Topical Solution 0.05% (Syntex) p 2061
Maxiflor Cream (Herbert) p 1006
Maxiflor Ointment (Herbert) p 1006
Osti-Derm Lotion (Pedinol) p 1580
Penecort Cream & Topical Solution 1% (Herbert) p 1007
Penecort Cream 2.5% (Herbert) p 1008
Pro-Cort Cream (Barnes-Hind) p 684
Pro-Cort M Cream (Barnes-Hind) p 684
Sween Cream (Sween) p 2049
Ziradryl Lotion (Parke-Davis) p 1580

Antidermatitis Herpetiformis
Dapsone (Jacobus) p 1032

Antifungal & Combinations
Breezee Mist Foot Powder (Pedinol) p 1580
Castellani Paint (Pedinol) p 1580
Derma Cas Gel (Hill Dermaceuticals) p 1009
Enzactin Cream (Ayerst) p 642
Fulvicin P/G Tablets (Schering) p 434, 1843
Fulvicin P/G 165 & 330 Tablets (Schering) p 434, 1844
Fulvicin-U/F Tablets (Schering) p 434, 1845
Fungizone Cream/Lotion/Ointment (Squibb) p 1994
Fungoid Creme & Solution (Pedinol) p 1580
Fungoid Tincture (Pedinol) p 1580
Grisactin (Ayerst) p 404, 646
Grisactin Ultra (Ayerst) p 405, 646
Halotex Cream & Solution (Westwood) p 2178
Loprox Cream 1% (Hoechst-Roussel) p 413, 1017
Lotrimin Cream 1% (Schering) p 1857
Lotrimin Lotion 1% (Schering) p 1857
Lotrimin Solution 1% (Schering) p 1857
Lotrisone Cream (Schering) p 1858
Monistat-Derm (miconazole nitrate) Cream & Lotion (Ortho Pharmaceutical (Dermatological Div.)) p 1474
Mycelex 1% Cream (Miles Pharmaceuticals) p 1409
Mycelex 1% Solution (Miles Pharmaceuticals) p 1409
Mycostatin Cream & Ointment (Squibb) p 2004
Mycostatin Topical Powder (Squibb) p 2004
Mytrex Cream & Ointment (Savage) p 1825
Nystex Cream & Ointment (Savage) p 1825
Pedi-Dri Foot Powder (Pedinol) p 1581
Pedi-Pro Foot Powder (Pedinol) p 1581
Spectazole Cream (Ortho Pharmaceutical (Dermatological Div.)) p 1476

Antiherpes
Anbesol Gel Antiseptic Anesthetic (Whitehall) p 443, 2185
Herpecin-L Cold Sore Lip Balm (Campbell) p 829
Zovirax Ointment 5% (Burroughs Wellcome) p 822
Zovirax Sterile Powder (Burroughs Wellcome) p 823

Anti-Inflammatory Agents
Alphatrex Cream & Ointment (Savage) p 1822
Betatrex Cream, Ointment & Lotion (Savage) p 1823
Chloresium Ointment (Rystan) p 1795
Chloresium Solution (Rystan) p 1795
Cloderm (Ortho Pharmaceutical (Dermatological Div.)) p 1472
F-E-P Creme (Boots) p 717
Lidex Topical Solution 0.05% (Syntex) p 2061
Texacort Scalp Lotion (Cooper Dermatology) p 882
Zone-A Lotion 1% (UAD Labs.) p 2069

Antilupus Erythematosus
Plaquenil Sulfate (Winthrop-Breon) p 444, 2223

Antiperspiration
Breezee Mist Foot Powder (Pedinol) p 1580
Drysol (Persōn & Covey) p 1587
Osti-Derm Lotion (Pedinol) p 1580
Pedi-Dri Foot Powder (Pedinol) p 1581
Pedi-Pro Foot Powder (Pedinol) p 1581
Xerac AC (Persōn & Covey) p 1588

Antipruritics, Antipruritus
Aeroseb-Dex Topical Aerosol Spray (Herbert) p 1001
Aeroseb-HC Topical Aerosol Spray (Herbert) p 1002
Alpha Keri Shower and Bath Oil (Westwood) p 2174
Alphaderm (Norwich Eaton) p 1424
Alphatrex Cream & Ointment (Savage) p 1822
Alphosyl Lotion, Cream (Reed & Carnrick) p 1632
Aveeno Bath Oilated (Cooper Dermatology) p 882
Aveeno Bath Regular (Cooper Dermatology) p 882
Aveenobar Oilated (Cooper Dermatology) p 882
Aveenobar Regular (Cooper Dermatology) p 882
Balnetar (Westwood) p 2175
Barseb HC Scalp Lotion (Barnes-Hind) p 683
Barseb Thera-Spray (Barnes-Hind) p 684
Betamethasone Valerate Cream, Ointment & Lotion (Pharmaderm) p 1617
Betatrex Cream, Ointment & Lotion (Savage) p 1823
Caladryl (Parke-Davis) p 1486
Carmol HC Cream 1% (Syntex) p 2061
Cort-Dome ⅛%, ¼%, ½%, and 1% Creme (Miles Pharmaceuticals) p 1399
Cort-Dome ⅛%, ¼%, ½%, and 1% Lotion (Miles Pharmaceuticals) p 1400
Corticaine Cream (Glaxo) p 412, 980
Decaspray Topical Aerosol (Merck Sharp & Dohme) p 1296
Denorex Medicated Shampoo and Conditioner (Whitehall) p 443, 2185
Denorex Medicated Shampoo, Regular & Mountain Fresh Herbal Scent (Whitehall) p 443, 2185
Derma Medicone-HC Ointment (Medicone) p 1256
Diprolene Cream 0.05% (Schering) p 1837
Diprosone Cream 0.05% (Schering) p 1838
Diprosone Lotion 0.05% w/w (Schering) p 1838
Diprosone Ointment 0.05% (Schering) p 1838
Diprosone Topical Aerosol 0.1% w/w (Schering) p 1838
Estar Gel (Westwood) p 2176
Eurax Cream & Lotion (Westwood) p 2177
F-E-P Creme (Boots) p 717
Florone Cream 0.05% (Dermik) p 889
Florone Ointment 0.05% (Dermik) p 889
Fluonid Ointment, Cream & Topical Solution (Herbert) p 1003
Fototar Cream 1.6% (Elder) p 931
Fototar Stik 5% (Elder) p 931
Hytone Cream, Lotion & Ointment (Dermik) p 890
Kenalog Cream/Lotion/Ointment (Squibb) p 1998
Kenalog Spray (Squibb) p 1998
Keri Creme (Westwood) p 2179
Keri Lotion (Westwood) p 2180
Komed Acne Lotion (Barnes-Hind) p 684
Komed HC Lotion (Barnes-Hind) p 684
Lidex Topical Solution 0.05% (Syntex) p 2061
Lotrisone Cream (Schering) p 1858
Mantadil Cream (Burroughs Wellcome) p 803
Maxiflor Cream (Herbert) p 1006
Maxiflor Ointment (Herbert) p 1006
Osti-Derm Lotion (Pedinol) p 1580
PBZ Hydrochloride Cream (Geigy) p 964
Pedi-Cort V Creme (Pedinol) p 1581
Penecort Cream & Topical Solution 1% (Herbert) p 1007
Penecort Cream 2.5% (Herbert) p 1008
Pentrax Tar Shampoo (Cooper Dermatology) p 882
Pramosone Cream, Lotion & Ointment (Ferndale) p 942
Pro-Cort Cream (Barnes-Hind) p 684
Pro-Cort M Cream (Barnes-Hind) p 684
Rectal Medicone-HC Suppositories (Medicone) p 419, 1256
Sebucare (Westwood) p 2181
Sebulex & Sebulex Cream Shampoo (Westwood) p 2181
Sebulex Shampoo with Conditioners (Westwood) p 2181
Sebulon Dandruff Shampoo (Westwood) p 2181
Sebutone & Sebutone Cream Shampoo (Westwood) p 2181
Sween Cream (Sween) p 2049
Texacort Scalp Lotion (Cooper Dermatology) p 882
Topicort Emollient Cream 0.25% (Hoechst-Roussel) p 413, 1021
Topicort Gel 0.05% (Hoechst-Roussel) p 413, 1021
Topicort LP Emollient Cream 0.05% (Hoechst-Roussel) p 413, 1021
Topicort Ointment 0.25% (Hoechst-Roussel) p 1021
Tridesilon Creme 0.05% (Miles Pharmaceuticals) p 1412
Tridesilon Ointment 0.05% (Miles Pharmaceuticals) p 1412
Tronothane Hydrochloride (Abbott) p 570
Tucks Cream (Parke-Davis) p 1575
Tucks Ointment (Parke-Davis) p 1575
Tucks Premoistened Pads (Parke-Davis) p 1575
Valisone Cream 0.1% (Schering) p 1892
Valisone Lotion 0.1% (Schering) p 1892
Valisone Ointment 0.1% (Schering) p 1892
Valisone Reduced Strength Cream 0.01% (Schering) p 1892
Vanoxide-HC Acne Lotion (Dermik) p 891
Vioform-Hydrocortisone (CIBA) p 876
Vytone Cream (Dermik) p 891
Westcort Cream 0.2% (Westwood) p 2183
Westcort Ointment 0.2% (Westwood) p 2183
Whirl-Sol (Sween) p 2049
Xtracare II (Sween) p 2049
Zetar Emulsion (Dermik) p 892
Zetar Shampoo (Dermik) p 892

Antipsoriasis Agents
Alphosyl Lotion, Cream (Reed & Carnrick) p 1632
Anthra-Derm Ointment 1%, ½%, ¼%, 1/10% (Dermik) p 888
Balnetar (Westwood) p 2175
Denorex Medicated Shampoo and Conditioner (Whitehall) p 443, 2185
Denorex Medicated Shampoo, Regular & Mountain Fresh Herbal Scent (Whitehall) p 443, 2185
Drithocreme (American Dermal) p 599

Product Category Index

Dritho-Scalp (American Dermal) p 599
Estar Gel (Westwood) p 2176
Fototar Cream 1.6% (Elder) p 931
Fototar Stik 5% (Elder) p 931
Hydrisea Lotion (Pedinol) p 1580
Oxsoralen Capsule (Elder) p 411, 932
Pentrax Tar Shampoo (Cooper Dermatology) p 882
Sebutone & Sebutone Cream Shampoo (Westwood) p 2181
Sween Cream (Sween) p 2049
Zetar Emulsion (Dermik) p 892
Zetar Shampoo (Dermik) p 892

Antiseborrhea
Capitrol Cream Shampoo (Westwood) p 2175
DHS Zinc Dandruff Shampoo (Persōn & Covey) p 1587
Denorex Medicated Shampoo and Conditioner (Whitehall) p 443, 2185
Denorex Medicated Shampoo, Regular & Mountain Fresh Herbal Scent (Whitehall) p 443, 2185
Fototar Cream 1.6% (Elder) p 931
Fototar Stik 5% (Elder) p 931
Pentrax Tar Shampoo (Cooper Dermatology) p 882
Sebucare (Westwood) p 2181
Sebulex & Sebulex Cream Shampoo (Westwood) p 2181
Sebulex Shampoo with Conditioners (Westwood) p 2181
Sebulon Dandruff Shampoo (Westwood) p 2181
Sebutone & Sebutone Cream Shampoo (Westwood) p 2181
Sulfacet-R Acne Lotion (Dermik) p 891
Zetar Emulsion (Dermik) p 892
Zetar Shampoo (Dermik) p 892

Astringents
Intraderm-19 Therapeutic Astringent Lotion (Robertson/Taylor) p 1646
Tucks Premoistened Pads (Parke-Davis) p 1575

Coal Tar
Denorex Medicated Shampoo and Conditioner (Whitehall) p 443, 2185
Denorex Medicated Shampoo, Regular & Mountain Fresh Herbal Scent (Whitehall) p 443, 2185
Estar Gel (Westwood) p 2176
Fototar Cream 1.6% (Elder) p 931
Fototar Stik 5% (Elder) p 931
Pentrax Tar Shampoo (Cooper Dermatology) p 882
Sebutone & Sebutone Cream Shampoo (Westwood) p 2181
Zetar Emulsion (Dermik) p 892
Zetar Shampoo (Dermik) p 892

Coal Tar & Sulfur
Alphosyl Lotion, Cream (Reed & Carnrick) p 1632
Sebutone & Sebutone Cream Shampoo (Westwood) p 2181

Deodorant
Chloresium Ointment (Rystan) p 1795
Chloresium Solution (Rystan) p 1795
Derifil Tablets & Powder (Rystan) p 1796
Panafil Ointment (Rystan) p 1796
Puri-Clens (Sween) p 2048

Depigmenting Agent
Benoquin Cream 20% (Elder) p 929
Eldopaque 2% Cream (Elder) p 930
Eldopaque Forte 4% Cream (Elder) p 930
Eldoquin 2% Cream & 2% Lotion (Elder) p 930
Eldoquin Forte 4% Cream (Elder) p 930
Melanex 3% Topical Solution (Neutrogena) (Neutrogena) p 1421
Solaquin Forte 4% Cream (Elder) p 936
Solaquin Forte 4% Gel (Elder) p 937

Detergents
Betadine Skin Cleanser (Purdue Frederick) p 1622
Fostex Medicated Cleansing Bar (Westwood) p 2177
Fostex Medicated Cleansing Cream (Westwood) p 2177
Komex (Barnes-Hind) p 684
Lowila Cake (Westwood) p 2180
Perineal/Ostomy Spray Cleaner (Consolidated Chemical) p 881
Peri-Wash (Sween) p 2048
Pernox Lotion (Westwood) p 2180
Pernox Medicated Lathering Scrub (Westwood) p 2180
pHisoHex (Winthrop-Breon) p 2222
Safe Suds (Ar-Ex) p 601
Satin (Consolidated Chemical) p 881
Surgi-Kleen (Sween) p 2048

Emollients
Acid Mantle Creme & Lotion (Dorsey Laboratories) p 908
Alpha Keri Shower and Bath Oil (Westwood) p 2174

Alphaderm (Norwich Eaton) p 1424
Balnetar (Westwood) p 2175
Domol Bath & Shower Oil (Miles Pharmaceuticals) p 1402
Herpecin-L Cold Sore Lip Balm (Campbell) p 829
Hydrisea Lotion (Pedinol) p 1580
Hydrisinol Creme & Lotion (Pedinol) p 1580
Keri Creme (Westwood) p 2179
Keri Lotion (Westwood) p 2180
Pro-Cort Cream (Barnes-Hind) p 684
Pro-Cort M Cream (Barnes-Hind) p 684
RVP Ointment (Elder) p 936
RVPaba Lip Stick (Elder) p 936
Rectal Medicone-HC Suppositories (Medicone) p 419, 1256
Skin Magic (Consolidated Chemical) p 881
Sween Cream (Sween) p 2049
Ureacin Lotion & Creme (Pedinol) p 1581
Whirl-Sol (Sween) p 2049
Xtracare II (Sween) p 2049

Fungicides
Breezee Mist Foot Powder (Pedinol) p 1580
Castellani Paint (Pedinol) p 1580
Fungizone Cream/Lotion/Ointment (Squibb) p 1994
Fungoid Creme & Solution (Pedinol) p 1580
Fungoid Tincture (Pedinol) p 1580
Halotex Cream & Solution (Westwood) p 2178
Loprox Cream 1% (Hoechst-Roussel) p 413, 1017
Lotrimin Cream 1% (Schering) p 1857
Lotrimin Lotion 1% (Schering) p 1857
Lotrimin Solution 1% (Schering) p 1857
Lotrisone Cream (Schering) p 1858
Monistat-Derm (miconazole nitrate) Cream & Lotion (Ortho Pharmaceutical (Dermatological Div.)) p 1474
Mycostatin Cream & Ointment (Squibb) p 2004
Mycostatin Topical Powder (Squibb) p 2004
Nilstat Topical Cream & Ointment (Lederle) p 1109
Osti-Derm Lotion (Pedinol) p 1580
Spectazole Cream (Ortho Pharmaceutical (Dermatological Div.)) p 1476
Tinver Lotion (Barnes-Hind) p 685

General
Acid Mantle Creme & Lotion (Dorsey Laboratories) p 908
Alphosyl Lotion, Cream (Reed & Carnrick) p 1632
Betadine Skin Cleanser (Purdue Frederick) p 1622
Corticaine Cream (Glaxo) p 412, 980
Domeboro Powder Packets & Tablets (Miles Pharmaceuticals) p 422, 1402
Dome-Paste Bandage (Miles Pharmaceuticals) p 1402
Fordustin' (Sween) p 2047
Hydrisea Lotion (Pedinol) p 1580
Hydrisinol Creme & Lotion (Pedinol) p 1580
Kerodex (Ayerst) p 653
Neosporin Aerosol (Burroughs Wellcome) p 806
Pedi-Boro Soak Paks (Pedinol) p 1581
pHisoHex (Winthrop-Breon) p 2222
RVP Ointment (Elder) p 936
Selsun Blue Lotion (Ross) p 1778
Selsun Lotion (Abbott) p 567
Sween-A-Peel (Sween) p 2048
Sween Cream (Sween) p 2049
Ureacin Lotion & Creme (Pedinol) p 1581

Keratolytics
Duofilm (Stiefel) p 2035
Hydrisalic Gel (Pedinol) p 1580
Keralyt Gel (Westwood) p 2179
Salactic Film (Pedinol) p 1581

Moisturizer
Moisturel (Westwood) p 2180

Pediculicides
Scabene Lotion (Stiefel) p 2035
Scabene Shampoo (Stiefel) p 2036

Photosensitizer
Fototar Cream 1.6% (Elder) p 931
Fototar Stik 5% (Elder) p 931
Oxsoralen Capsule (Elder) p 411, 932
Oxsoralen Lotion 1% (Elder) p 935
Trisoralen Tablets (Elder) p 411, 937

Powders
Breezee Mist Foot Powder (Pedinol) p 1580
Fordustin' (Sween) p 2047
Formula Magic (Consolidated Chemical) p 880
Mycostatin Topical Powder (Squibb) p 2004
Pedi-Dri Foot Powder (Pedinol) p 1581
Pedi-Pro Foot Powder (Pedinol) p 1581

Scabicides
Kwell Cream (Reed & Carnrick) p 1635
Kwell Lotion (Reed & Carnrick) p 1635
Kwell Shampoo (Reed & Carnrick) p 1635
Scabene Lotion (Stiefel) p 2035

Shampoos
Capitrol Cream Shampoo (Westwood) p 2175

DHS Shampoo (Persōn & Covey) p 1587
DHS Tar Shampoo (Persōn & Covey) p 1587
DHS Zinc Dandruff Shampoo (Persōn & Covey) p 1587
Denorex Medicated Shampoo and Conditioner (Whitehall) p 443, 2185
Denorex Medicated Shampoo, Regular & Mountain Fresh Herbal Scent (Whitehall) p 443, 2185
Exsel Lotion (Herbert) p 1003
Fostex Medicated Cleansing Cream (Westwood) p 2177
Gentle Rain Shampoo (Sween) p 2047
Medi-Tec 90 New Therapeutic Overnight Concentrate (Robertson/Taylor) p 1646
Medi-Tec 90 Therapeutic Conditioner with Strengthening Agents (Robertson/Taylor) p 1646
Medi-Tec 90 Therapeutic Scalp Stimulant with Strengthening Agents (Robertson/Taylor) p 1646
Medi-Tec 90 Therapeutic Shampoo & Scalp Conditioner with Strengthening Agents (Robertson/Taylor) p 1646
Pentrax Tar Shampoo (Cooper Dermatology) p 882
Pernox Shampoo (Westwood) p 2180
Satin (Consolidated Chemical) p 881
Sebulex & Sebulex Cream Shampoo (Westwood) p 2181
Sebulex Shampoo with Conditioners (Westwood) p 2181
Sebulon Dandruff Shampoo (Westwood) p 2181
Sebutone & Sebutone Cream Shampoo (Westwood) p 2181
Selsun Blue Lotion (Ross) p 1778
Selsun Lotion (Abbott) p 567
Surgi-Kleen (Sween) p 2048
Zetar Shampoo (Dermik) p 892

Skin Bleaches
Banquin Cream (Kramer) p 1069
Benoquin Cream 20% (Elder) p 929
Eldopaque 2% Cream (Elder) p 930
Eldopaque Forte 4% Cream (Elder) p 930
Eldoquin 2% Cream & 2% Lotion (Elder) p 930
Eldoquin Forte 4% Cream (Elder) p 930
Melanex 3% Topical Solution (Neutrogena) (Neutrogena) p 1421
Solaquin Forte 4% Cream (Elder) p 936
Solaquin Forte 4% Gel (Elder) p 937

Skin Protectant
Peri-Care (Sween) p 2048
Sween-A-Peel (Sween) p 2048

Soaps & Cleansers
Alpha Keri Soap (Westwood) p 2175
Anti-Sept (Seamless) p 1897
Gentle Rain Shampoo (Sween) p 2047
Intraderm-19 Therapeutic Acne Scrub (Robertson/Taylor) p 1645
Keri Facial Soap (Westwood) p 2180
Perineal/Ostomy Spray Cleaner (Consolidated Chemical) p 881
Peri-Wash (Sween) p 2048
Puri-Clens (Sween) p 2048
Satin (Consolidated Chemical) p 881
Surgi-Kleen (Sween) p 2048
Sween Kind Touch (Sween) p 2047
Sween Soft Touch (Sween) p 2049

Steroids & Combinations
Aeroseb-Dex Topical Aerosol Spray (Herbert) p 1001
Aeroseb-HC Topical Aerosol Spray (Herbert) p 1002
Alphaderm (Norwich Eaton) p 1424
Aristocort A Topical Cream & Ointment (Lederle) p 414, 415, 1084
Aristocort Topical Products (Lederle) p 414, 415, 1080
Aristospan Parenteral 5 mg./ml (Lederle) p 1085
Barseb HC Scalp Lotion (Barnes-Hind) p 683
Barseb Thera-Spray (Barnes-Hind) p 684
Carmol HC Cream 1% (Syntex) p 2061
Cordran Ointment & Lotion (Dista) p 895
Cordran SP Cream (Dista) p 895
Cordran Tape (Dista) p 897
Cordran-N (Dista) p 897
Cort-Dome ⅛%, ¼%, ½%, and 1% Creme (Miles Pharmaceuticals) p 1399
Cort-Dome ⅛%, ¼%, ½%, and 1% Lotion (Miles Pharmaceuticals) p 1400
Corticaine (Glaxo) p 412, 980
Cortisporin Ointment (Burroughs Wellcome) p 784
Cyclocort Cream (Lederle) p 415, 1089
Cyclocort Ointment (Lederle) p 415, 1089
Decaspray Topical Aerosol (Merck Sharp & Dohme) p 1296
Derma Medicone-HC Ointment (Medicone) p 1256
Diprolene Ointment 0.05% (Schering) p 1837
Diprosone Cream 0.05% (Schering) p 1838

Product Category Index

Diprosone Lotion 0.05% w/w (Schering) p 1838
Diprosone Ointment 0.05% (Schering) p 1838
Diprosone Topical Aerosol 0.1% w/w (Schering) p 1838
Florone Cream 0.05% (Dermik) p 889
Florone Ointment 0.05% (Dermik) p 889
Fluonid Ointment, Cream & Topical Solution (Herbert) p 1003
Halog Cream/Ointment/Solution (Squibb) p 1996
Halog-E Cream (Squibb) p 1996
Hytone Cream, Lotion & Ointment (Dermik) p 890
Kenalog Cream/Lotion/Ointment (Squibb) p 1998
Kenalog Spray (Squibb) p 1998
Komed HC Lotion (Barnes-Hind) p 684
Lidex Cream 0.05% (Syntex) p 2061
Lidex Gel 0.05% (Syntex) p 2061
Lidex Ointment 0.05% (Syntex) p 2061
Lidex Topical Solution 0.05% (Syntex) p 2061
Lidex-E Cream 0.05% (Syntex) p 2061
Lotrisone Cream (Schering) p 1858
Maxiflor Cream (Herbert) p 1006
Maxiflor Ointment (Herbert) p 1006
Mycolog Cream and Ointment (Squibb) p 2003
Mytrex Cream & Ointment (Savage) p 1825
Neo-Synalar Cream (Syntex) p 2061
Pedi-Cort V Creme (Pedinol) p 1581
Penecort Cream 2.5% (Herbert) p 1008
Pramosone Cream, Lotion & Ointment (Ferndale) p 942
Pro-Cort Cream (Barnes-Hind) p 684
Pro-Cort M Cream (Barnes-Hind) p 684
Synacort Creams 1%, 2.5% (Syntex) p 2061
Synalar Creams 0.025%, 0.01% (Syntex) p 2061
Synalar Ointment 0.025% (Syntex) p 2061
Synalar Topical Solution 0.01% (Syntex) p 2061
Synalar-HP Cream 0.2% (Syntex) p 2061
Synemol Cream 0.025% (Syntex) p 2061
Texacort Scalp Lotion (Cooper Dermatology) p 882
Topicort Emollient Cream 0.25% (Hoechst-Roussel) p 413, 1021
Topicort Gel 0.05% (Hoechst-Roussel) p 413, 1021
Topicort LP Emollient Cream 0.05% (Hoechst-Roussel) p 413, 1021
Topicort Ointment 0.25% (Hoechst-Roussel) p 1021
Tridesilon Creme 0.05% (Miles Pharmaceuticals) p 1412
Tridesilon Ointment 0.05% (Miles Pharmaceuticals) p 1413
Uticort Cream, Gel, Lotion & Ointment (Parke-Davis) p 426, 1575
Valisone Cream 0.1% (Schering) p 1892
Valisone Lotion 0.1% (Schering) p 1892
Valisone Ointment 0.1% (Schering) p 1892
Valisone Reduced Strength Cream 0.01% (Schering) p 1892
Vanoxide-HC Acne Lotion (Dermik) p 891
Vioform-Hydrocortisone (CIBA) p 876
VōSol HC Otic Solution (Wallace) p 442, 2171
Vytone Cream (Dermik) p 891
Westcort Cream 0.2% (Westwood) p 2183
Westcort Ointment 0.2% (Westwood) p 2183

Sulfur & Salicylic Acid
Fostril (Westwood) p 2178
Pernox Lotion (Westwood) p 2180
Pernox Medicated Lathering Scrub (Westwood) p 2180
Sebulex Shampoo with Conditioners (Westwood) p 2181

Sun Screens
Eclipse Total Sunscreen Cooling Alcohol Lotion, SPF 15 (Dorsey Laboratories) p 910
Eclipse Total Sunscreen Moisturizing Lotion, SPF 15 (Dorsey Laboratories) p 910
Herpecin-L Cold Sore Lip Balm (Campbell) p 829
PreSun 4 Creamy Sunscreen (Westwood) p 2180
PreSun 8 Lotion, Creamy & Gel (Westwood) p 2180
PreSun 15 Creamy Sunscreen (Westwood) p 2181
PreSun 15 Sunscreen Lotion (Westwood) p 2181
RVP Ointment (Elder) p 936
RVPaba Lip Stick (Elder) p 936
RVPaque Ointment (Elder) p 936
Solbar PF (Persōn & Covey) p 1588
Solbar Plus 15 Sun Protectant Cream (Persōn & Covey) p 1588

UVA Light Source
Elder Psoralite (Elder) p 930

UVB Light Source
Elder Psoralite (Elder) p 930

Vesicants
Cantharone (Seres) p 1939
Cantharone Plus (Seres) p 1939
Verr-Canth (C & M) p 828
Verrusol (C & M) p 828

Wart Therapeutic Agent
Cantharone (Seres) p 1939
Cantharone Plus (Seres) p 1939
Duofilm (Stiefel) p 2035
Pod-Ben-25 (C & M) p 828
Salactic Film (Pedinol) p 1581
Verr-Canth (C & M) p 828
Verrex (C & M) p 828
Verrusol (C & M) p 828
Viranol (American Dermal) p 600
Wart-Off (Pfipharmecs) p 426, 1599

Wet Dressings
Domeboro Powder Packets & Tablets (Miles Pharmaceuticals) p 422, 1402
Pedi-Boro Soak Paks (Pedinol) p 1581
Prophyllin (Rystan) p 1796
Tucks Premoistened Pads (Parke-Davis) p 1575

Wound Dressings
Betadine Aerosol Spray (Purdue Frederick) p 1622
Betadine Helafoam Solution (Purdue Frederick) p 1622
Betadine Ointment (Purdue Frederick) p 1622
Betadine Skin Cleanser (Purdue Frederick) p 1622
Betadine Solution (Purdue Frederick) p 1622
Betadine Viscous Formula Antiseptic Gauze Pad (Purdue Frederick) p 1623
Chloresium Ointment (Rystan) p 1795
Chloresium Solution (Rystan) p 1795
Debrisan Wound Cleaning Beads (Johnson & Johnson (Patient Care Div.)) p 1044
Debrisan Wound Cleaning Paste (Johnson & Johnson (Patient Care Div.)) p 1044
Flint SSD Cream (Flint) p 411, 950
Granulex (Hickam) p 1009
Panafil Ointment (Rystan) p 1796
Panafil-White Ointment (Rystan) p 1796
Puri-Clens (Sween) p 2048
Stimuzyme Plus (National Dermaceutical) p 1421

Other
Biozyme-C Ointment (Armour) p 604
Butesin Picrate Ointment (Abbott) p 510
Chloresium Ointment (Rystan) p 1795
Chloresium Solution (Rystan) p 1795
Cortisporin Ointment (Burroughs Wellcome) p 784
DHS Conditioning Rinse (Persōn & Covey) p 1587
Debrisan Wound Cleaning Beads (Johnson & Johnson (Patient Care Div.)) p 1044
Debrisan Wound Cleaning Paste (Johnson & Johnson (Patient Care Div.)) p 1044
Exsel Lotion (Herbert) p 1003
Fluoroplex Topical Solution & Cream (Herbert) p 1004
Fordustin' (Sween) p 2047
Gelfoam Sterile Powder (Upjohn) p 2114
Oxsoralen Capsule (Elder) p 411, 932
Oxsoralen Lotion 1% (Elder) p 935
Peri-Wash (Sween) p 2048
Plaquenil Sulfate (Winthrop-Breon) p 444, 2223
RVP Ointment (Elder) p 936
RVPaque Ointment (Elder) p 936
Santyl Ointment (Knoll) p 1067
Sebucare (Westwood) p 2181
Sebulex & Sebulex Cream Shampoo (Westwood) p 2181
Sebulex Shampoo with Conditioners (Westwood) p 2181
Sebulon Dandruff Shampoo (Westwood) p 2181
Sebutone & Sebutone Cream Shampoo (Westwood) p 2181
Sween Cream (Sween) p 2049
Sween Prep (Sween) p 2049
Temaril (Smith Kline & French) p 437, 1976
Trisoralen Tablets (Elder) p 411, 937
Vehicle/N (Neutrogena) (Neutrogena) p 1422
Vehicle/N Mild (Neutrogena) (Neutrogena) p 1422
Vitadye Lotion (Elder) p 938
Xtracare II (Sween) p 2049

DIAGNOSTICS

ACTH Test
Metopirone (CIBA) p 409, 856

Adrenocortical Function
Acthar (Armour) p 601
HP Acthar Gel (Armour) p 601

Adult Peripheral Arteriography
Amipaque (Winthrop-Breon) p 3018

Allergy, Skin Tests
Allergenic Extracts, Diagnosis and/or Immunotherapy (Barry) p 685
Multitest CMI Skin Test Antigens for Cellular Hypersensitivity (Merieux) p 1358, 3013
Pre-Pen (Rorer) p 1753
Skin Test Antigens for Cellular Hypersensitivity, Multitest CMI (Merieux) p 1358, 3013

Angiocardiography
Hypaque-M, 75% (Winthrop-Breon) p 3044
Hypaque-M, 90% (Winthrop-Breon) p 3053
Hypaque-76 Injection (Winthrop-Breon) p 3049

Angiography
Hypaque-M, 75% (Winthrop-Breon) p 3044
Hypaque-M, 90% (Winthrop-Breon) p 3053

Aortography
Hypaque Sodium 50% (Winthrop-Breon) p 3034
Hypaque-M, 75% (Winthrop-Breon) p 3044
Hypaque-M, 90% (Winthrop-Breon) p 3053
Hypaque-76 Injection (Winthrop-Breon) p 3049

Arthrography
Hypaque Meglumine 60% (Winthrop-Breon) p 3039

Blood Glucose
Chemstrip bG Blood Glucose Test (Boehringer Mannheim) p 3009
Dextrostix Reagent Strips (Ames) p 3005
Glucometer (Ames) p 3006

Central Venography
Hypaque-76 Injection (Winthrop-Breon) p 3049

Cerebral Angiography
Hypaque Meglumine 60% (Winthrop-Breon) p 3039
Hypaque Sodium 50% (Winthrop-Breon) p 3034

Cholangiography
Telepaque (Winthrop-Breon) p 443, 3058

Cholecystography
Bilopaque Sodium (Winthrop-Breon) p 443, 3023
Telepaque (Winthrop-Breon) p 443, 3058

Cisternography-CT
Amipaque (Winthrop-Breon) p 3018

CT Scan Enhancement
Hypaque Meglumine 30% (Winthrop-Breon) p 3032
Hypaque Sodium 25% (Winthrop-Breon) p 3028
Hypaque-76 Injection (Winthrop-Breon) p 3049

Culture Media

Bacteriuria
Isocult (SmithKline Diagnostics) p 3018
Microstix-Candida Miniaturized Culture Test (Ames) p 3006

Candida (Monilia)
Isocult (SmithKline Diagnostics) p 3018

Gonococcus (Neisseria)
Isocult (SmithKline Diagnostics) p 3018
Microcult-GC (Ames) p 3005

Pseudomonas aeruginosa
Isocult (SmithKline Diagnostics) p 3018

Staphylococcus aureus
Isocult (SmithKline Diagnostics) p 3018

Streptococci
Isocult (SmithKline Diagnostics) p 3018

Trichomonas vaginalis
Isocult (SmithKline Diagnostics) p 3018

Direct Cholangiography
Hypaque Meglumine 60% (Winthrop-Breon) p 3039
Hypaque Sodium 50% (Winthrop-Breon) p 3034

Discography
Hypaque Meglumine 60% (Winthrop-Breon) p 3039

Excretory Urography
Hypaque Meglumine 60% (Winthrop-Breon) p 3039
Hypaque Sodium 50% (Winthrop-Breon) p 3034
Hypaque-76 Injection (Winthrop-Breon) p 3049

Fluorometer
Fluorostat Filter Fluorometer (Ames) p 3006
Optimate Alpha Automated Fluorometer/Photometer (Ames) p 3006

Gastric Acid Test
Histamine Phosphate (For Gastric Test) (Lilly) p 3012
Peptavlon (Ayerst) p 657, 3008

Gastric Hydrochloric Acid Test
Histamine Phosphate (For Gastric Test) (Lilly) p 3012

Product Category Index

Gastrointestinal Radiography
Hypaque Sodium Oral Powder (Winthrop-Breon) p 3024
Hypaque Sodium Oral Solution (Winthrop-Breon) p 3025

Glucose in Whole Blood
Visidex II Reagent Strips (Ames) p 3006

Hysterosalpingography
Hypaque Sodium 50% (Winthrop-Breon) p 3034
Hypaque-M, 90% (Winthrop-Breon) p 3053

Hysteroscopic Fluid
Hyskon Hysteroscopy Fluid (Pharmacia) p 1616

Intravenous Digital Arteriography
Amipaque (Winthrop-Breon) p 3018
Hypaque-76 (Winthrop-Breon) p 3049

Intravenous Infusion for Urography
Hypaque Meglumine 30% (Winthrop-Breon) p 3032
Hypaque Sodium 25% (Winthrop-Breon) p 3028

Intravenous Venography
Hypaque Sodium 50% (Winthrop-Breon) p 3034

Luteinizing Hormone Releasing Hormone (LH-RH)
Factrel (Ayerst) p 404, 643, 3007

Myelography
Amipaque (Winthrop-Breon) p 3018

Myelography - CT
Amipaque (Winthrop-Breon) p 3018

Occult Blood in Feces
ColoScreen/VPI (Helena Labs.) p 3010
Fleet Detecatest (Fleet) p 3009
Hema-Chek Slide Test for Fecal Occult Blood Test with Control (Ames) p 3005
Hemoccult (SmithKline Diagnostics) p 3017

Occult Blood in Gastric Samples
Gastroccult (SmithKline Diagnostics) p 3017

Pancreatic Function Test
Chymex (Adria) p 3003
Secretin-Kabi (Pharmacia) p 1616

Pediatric Angiocardiography
Amipaque (Winthrop-Breon) p 3018

Peripheral Angiography
Hypaque Sodium 50% (Winthrop-Breon) p 3034
Hypaque-76 (Winthrop-Breon) p 3049

Peripheral Arteriography
Hypaque Meglumine 60% (Winthrop-Breon) p 3039

Pheochromocytoma Test
Histamine Phosphate (Histamine Test for Pheochromocytoma) (Lilly) p 3012
Regitine (CIBA) p 863

Reflectance Photometer & Reagent Strips
Seralyzer Reflectance Photometer (Ames) p 3006

Renal Venography
Hypaque-76 (Winthrop-Breon) p 3049

Retrograde Cystourethrography
Hypaque-Cysto (Winthrop-Breon) p 3030

Retrograde Pyelography
Hypaque Sodium 20% (Winthrop-Breon) p 3026

Selective Renal Arteriography
Hypaque-76 (Winthrop-Breon) p 3049

Selective Visceral Arteriography
Hypaque-76 (Winthrop-Breon) p 3049

Splenoportography
Hypaque Meglumine 60% (Winthrop-Breon) p 3039
Hypaque Sodium 50% (Winthrop-Breon) p 3034

Thyroid Function Test
Thyrotropin
Thytropar (Armour) p 612

Thyroid Releasing Factor
Relefact TRH (Hoechst-Roussel) p 1017
Thypinone (Abbott Diagnostics Div.) p 3002

Tuberculin
Tuberculin, Old
Mono-Vacc Test (O.T.) (Merieux) p 1358
Tuberculin, Mono-Vacc Test (O.T.) (Merieux) p 3013
Tuberculin, Old, Tine Test (Rosenthal) (Lederle) p 3010
Tuberculin Purified Protein Derivative Tine Test (PPD) (Lederle) p 3011

Tuberculin, P.P.D.
Aplisol (Parke-Davis) p 3014
Aplitest (Parke-Davis) p 3014
SclavoTest-PPD (Sclavo) p 3017
Tubersol (Tuberculin Purified Protein Derivative [Mantoux]) (Squibb/Connaught) p 2033

Urine Test
Bilirubin
Chemstrip Urine Testing System (Boehringer Mannheim) p 3009
N-Multistix SG Reagent Strips (Ames) p 3004

Blood
Chemstrip Urine Testing System (Boehringer Mannheim) p 3009
N-Multistix SG Reagent Strips (Ames) p 3004

Controls
CHEK-STIX Urinalysis Control Strips (Ames) p 3004

Culture
Microstix-3 Reagent Strips (Ames) p 3005

Glucose
Diastix Reagent Strips (Ames) p 3004
N-Multistix SG Reagent Strips (Ames) p 3004
N-Uristix Reagent Strips (Ames) p 3006
Tes-Tape (Lilly) p 3013

Ketones
N-Multistix SG Reagent Strips (Ames) p 3004

Ketones & Glucose
Chemstrip Urine Testing System (Boehringer Mannheim) p 3009
Keto-Diastix Reagent Strips (Ames) p 3004

Leukocytes
Chemstrip Urine Testing System (Boehringer Mannheim) p 3009

Nitrite
Chemstrip Urine Testing System (Boehringer Mannheim) p 3009
Microstix-3 Reagent Strips (Ames) p 3005
N-Multistix SG Reagent Strips (Ames) p 3004
N-Uristix Reagent Strips (Ames) p 3006

pH
Chemstrip Urine Testing System (Boehringer Mannheim) p 3009
N-Multistix SG Reagent Strips (Ames) p 3004

Protein
Chemstrip Urine Testing System (Boehringer Mannheim) p 3009
N-Multistix SG Reagent Strips (Ames) p 3004
N-Uristix Reagent Strips (Ames) p 3006

Specific Gravity
N-Multistix SG Reagent Strips (Ames) p 3004

Urobilinogen
Chemstrip Urine Testing System (Boehringer Mannheim) p 3009
N-Multistix SG Reagent Strips (Ames) p 3004

Urography
Hypaque-M, 75% (Winthrop-Breon) p 3044
Hypaque-M, 90% (Winthrop-Breon) p 3053
Hypaque-76 Injection (Winthrop-Breon) p 3049

Venography
Hypaque Meglumine 60% (Winthrop-Breon) p 3039

X-ray Contrast
Hypaque Meglumine 30% (Winthrop-Breon) p 3032
Hypaque Sodium 25% (Winthrop-Breon) p 3028
Hypaque-Cysto (Winthrop-Breon) p 3030
Hypaque-76 Injection (Winthrop-Breon) p 3049

DIETARY SUPPLEMENTS
Alba-Lybe (Bart) p 685
Aminoplex Capsules & Powder (Tyson) p 2068
Aminostasis Capsules & Powder (Tyson) p 2068
Aminotate Capsules & Powder (Tyson) p 2068
B-C-Bid Capsules (Geriatric) p 975
Beelith Tablets (Beach) p 405, 685
Cardioguard Natural Lipotropic Dietary Supplement-Powder (Professional Health) p 1621
Cardioguard Natural Lipotropic Dietary Supplement-Tablets (Professional Health) p 1621
Cevi-Fer Capsules (sustained release) (Geriatric) p 975
Chlorophyll Complex Perles (Standard Process) p 2035
Citrotein (Clinical Nutrition) p 876
Compleat-B (Clinical Nutrition) p 877
Dorcol Children's Liquid Calcium Supplement (Dorsey Laboratories) p 909
Eldercaps (Mayrand) p 1196
Endorphenyl (Tyson) p 2068
Enisyl Tablets (Persōn & Covey) p 1588
Fibermed Supplements (Purdue Frederick) p 427, 1624
Glutofac Tablets (Kenwood) p 1046
Iso-B Caps (Tyson) p 2068
MVM Caps (Tyson) p 2068
Maxovite Tablets (Tyson) p 2068
Mediatric Capsules, Tablets & Liquid (Ayerst) p 405, 654
Meritene Liquid (Clinical Nutrition) p 877
Meritene Powder (Clinical Nutrition) p 877
Metabolite 2050 (Robertson/Taylor) p 1646
Mevanin-C Capsules (Beutlich) p 705
Mission Pre-Surgical (Mission) p 1419
Neutra-Phos Powder & Capsules (Willen) p 2188
Neutra-Phos-K Powder & Capsules (Willen) p 2188
Niferex w/Vitamin C (Central Pharmaceuticals) p 838
Niferex-PN (Central Pharmaceuticals) p 409, 838
Nu-Iron Elixir (Mayrand) p 1196
Nu-Iron 150 Caps (Mayrand) p 1196
Nu-Iron-V Tablets (Mayrand) p 1196
Nutrox Capsules (Tyson) p 2069
Pre-Protein Liquid (Arlo) p 601
Selenium Tablets (200 mcg) (Vitaline) p 2148
Tri-Cone Capsules (Glaxo) p 986
Vicon Forte Capsules (Glaxo) p 412, 989
Vicon-C Capsules (Glaxo) p 412, 989
Vicon-Plus Capsules (Glaxo) p 412, 989
Vivonex Flavor Packets (Norwich Eaton) p 1441
Vivonex High Nitrogen Diet (Norwich Eaton) p 1439
Vivonex Standard Diet (Norwich Eaton) p 1438
Vivonex T.E.N. (Norwich Eaton) p 1441
Vi-Zac Capsules (Glaxo) p 412, 990
Zinc-220 Capsules (Alto) p 404, 589

DIURETICS
Antihypertensive-Saluretic
Diulo (Searle Pharmaceuticals) p 435, 1904
Hydromox R Tablets (Lederle) p 415, 1094
Hydromox Tablets (Lederle) p 415, 1094
Lozol Tablets (USV Pharmaceutical) p 440, 2081
Zaroxolyn (Pennwalt) p 426, 1586

Carbonic Anhydrase Inhibitors
Diamox Parenteral (Lederle) p 1091
Diamox Sequels, Tablets (Lederle) p 415, 1091

Loop Diuretics
Bumetanide
Bumex Injection (Roche) p 1678
Bumex Tablets (Roche) p 429, 1678
Ethracrynic Acid Derivatives
Edecrin Sodium Intravenous (Merck Sharp & Dohme) p 1304
Edecrin Tablets (Merck Sharp & Dohme) p 420, 1304
Furosemide
Furosemide Injection (Elkins-Sinn) p 938
Furosemide Injection, USP (Parke-Davis) p 1522
Furosemide Injection (Wyeth) p 2252
Furosemide Tablets, USP (Parke-Davis) p 1524
Lasix Oral Solution (Hoechst-Roussel) p 413, 1015
Lasix Tablets and Injection (Hoechst-Roussel) p 413, 1015
SK-Furosemide Tablets (Smith Kline & French) p 1971

Monosulfamyl
Chlorthalidone Tablets, USP (Parke-Davis) p 1494
Hygroton Tablets (USV Pharmaceutical) p 440, 2078
Thalitone Tablets (Boehringer Ingelheim) p 406, 715

Potassium Sparing
Aldactazide (Searle & Co.) p 435, 1912
Aldactone (Searle & Co.) p 435, 1914
Dyazide (Smith Kline & French) p 437, 1961
Dyrenium (Smith Kline & French) p 436, 1963
Maxzide Tablets (Lederle) p 415, 1098
Midamor Tablets (Merck Sharp & Dohme) p 420, 1331
Moduretic Tablets (Merck Sharp & Dohme) p 420, 1333
Spironolactone Tablets, USP (Parke-Davis) p 1569
Spironolactone w/Hydrochlorothiazide Tablets (Parke-Davis) p 1570

Thiazides & Combinations
Aldactazide (Searle & Co.) p 435, 1912
Anhydron (Lilly) p 1129
Aquatensen (Wallace) p 442, 2149
Corzide (Squibb) p 437, 1990
Diucardin (Ayerst) p 404, 640

Product Category Index

Diuril Intravenous Sodium (Merck Sharp & Dohme) p 1299
Diuril Tablets & Oral Suspension (Merck Sharp & Dohme) p 420, 1301
Diutensen Tablets (Wallace) p 2156
Diutensen-R Tablets (Wallace) p 442, 2157
Dyazide (Smith Kline & French) p 437, 1961
Enduron Tablets (Abbott) p 403, 517
Enduronyl Forte Tablets (Abbott) p 403, 518
Enduronyl Tablets (Abbott) p 403, 518
Esidrix (CIBA) p 409, 848
Exna Tablets (Robins) p 428, 1652
Hydrochlorothiazide Tablets, USP (Thiuretic) (Parke-Davis) p 1527
HydroDIURIL Tablets (Merck Sharp & Dohme) p 420, 1316
Maxzide Tablets (Lederle) p 415, 1098
Metahydrin (Merrell Dow) p 421, 1370
Metatensin (Merrell Dow) p 421, 1370
Minizide Capsules (Pfizer) p 426, 1604
Moduretic Tablets (Merck Sharp & Dohme) p 420, 1333
Naqua Tablets (Schering) p 434, 1861
Naquival Tablets (Schering) p 434, 1862
Naturetin Tablets (Squibb) p 438, 2006
Oretic (Abbott) p 403, 554
Oreticyl (Abbott) p 555
Rauzide Tablets (Squibb) p 438, 2021
Renese (Pfizer) p 426, 1608
Renese-R (Pfizer) p 426, 1608
Saluron (Bristol) p 407, 747
Spironolactone w/Hydrochlorothiazide Tablets (Parke-Davis) p 1570

DOPAMINE RECEPTOR AGONIST
Parlodel Capsules & Tablets (Sandoz Pharmaceutical Div.) p 433, 1808

DRUG DELIVERY SYSTEM
InspirEase (Key Pharmaceuticals) p 1049

DUODENAL ULCER ADHERENT COMPLEX
Carafate Tablets (Marion) p 417, 1182

E

ELECTROLYTES
Alkalinizing Agents
Bicitra—Sugar-Free (Willen) p 2187
Polycitra Syrup (Willen) p 2188
Polycitra-K Syrup (Willen) p 2189
Polycitra-LC—Sugar-Free (Willen) p 2188
Fluid Replacement Therapy
Infalyte (Pennwalt) p 1584
Pedialyte (Ross) p 1771
Pedialyte RS (Ross) p 1772
Potassium Preparations
Bi-K (USV Pharmaceutical) p 2072
K-Lor Powder (Abbott) p 403, 533
K-Lyte & K-Lyte DS (Mead Johnson Laboratories) p 419, 1222
K-Lyte/Cl & K-Lyte/Cl 50 (Mead Johnson Laboratories) p 419, 1222
K-Tab (Abbott) p 403, 534
Kaochlor 10% Liquid (Adria) p 579
Kaochlor S-F 10% Liquid (Sugar-free) (Adria) p 580
Kaon Cl-10 (Adria) p 404, 582
Kaon Elixir, Grape Flavor (Adria) p 580
Kaon Tablets (Adria) p 404, 581
Kaon-Cl Tabs (Adria) p 404, 581
Kaon-Cl 20% (Adria) p 582
KATO (Legere) p 1120
Kay Ciel Oral Solution 10% (Berlex) p 702
Kay Ciel Powder (Berlex) p 702
Klor-Con Powder (Upsher-Smith) p 2144
Klor-Con/25 Powder (Upsher-Smith) p 2144
Klorvess Effervescent Granules (Sandoz Pharmaceutical Div.) p 1803
Klorvess Effervescent Tablets (Sandoz Pharmaceutical Div.) p 433, 1803
Klorvess 10% Liquid (Sandoz Pharmaceutical Div.) p 1803
Klotrix (Mead Johnson Pharmaceutical) p 419, 1251
Micro-K Extencaps (Robins) p 428, 1653
Micro-K 10 Extencaps (Robins) p 1653
Potage (Lemmon) p 1122
Potassium Chloride Oral Solution, Powder & for Oral Solution (Roxane) p 1793
Rum-K (Fleming) p 948
Slow-K (CIBA) p 409, 872
Twin-K (Boots) p 724
Twin-K-Cl (Boots) p 725

EMETICS
Ipecac (Lilly) p 1156

ENZYMES & DIGESTANTS
Collagenolytic
Santyl Ointment (Knoll) p 1067
Digestants
Arco-Lase (Arco) p 600
Arco-Lase Plus (Arco) p 600
Celluzyme Chewable Tablets (Dalin) p 886
Cotazym (Organon) p 422, 1446
Cotazym-S (Organon) p 422, 1446
Donnazyme Tablets (Robins) p 428, 1650
Entozyme Tablets (Robins) p 428, 1652
Enzypan (Norgine) p 1424
Festal II (Hoechst-Roussel) p 412, 1014
Festalan (Hoechst-Roussel) p 413, 1014
Gustase (Geriatric) p 975
Kanulase (Dorsey Laboratories) p 910
Karbokoff Tablets (Arlo) p 601
Kutrase Capsules (Rorer) p 431, 1750
Ku-Zyme Capsules (Rorer) p 431, 1750
Ku-Zyme HP Capsules (Rorer) p 431, 1751
LactAid (LactAid) p 414, 1070
Muripsin (Norgine) p 1424
Pancrease (McNeil Pharmaceutical) p 418, 1205
Pancreatin Tablets 2400 mg. N.F. (High Lipase) (Vitaline) p 2148
Phazyme Tablets (Reed & Carnrick) p 427, 1636
Phazyme-95 Tablets (Reed & Carnrick) p 427, 1636
Phazyme-PB Tablets (Reed & Carnrick) p 427, 1636
Tri-Cone Capsules (Glaxo) p 986
Viokase Powder (Robins) p 1665
Viokase Tablets (Robins) p 1665
Zypan Tablets (Standard Process) p 2035
Fibrinolytic & Proteolytic
Biozyme-C Ointment (Armour) p 604
Elase (Parke-Davis) p 424, 1513
Elase Ointment (Parke-Davis) p 424, 1513
Elase-Chloromycetin Ointment (Parke-Davis) p 424, 1513
Granulex (Hickam) p 1009
Panafil Ointment (Rystan) p 1796
Panafil-White Ointment (Rystan) p 1796
Stimuzyme Plus (National Dermaceutical) p 1421
Travase Ointment (Flint) p 411, 952
Hydrolytic
Wydase Injection (Wyeth) p 2296
Injectable, Proteolytic
Chymodiactin (Smith) p 437, 1983
Topical
Panafil Ointment (Rystan) p 1796
Panafil-White Ointment (Rystan) p 1796
Santyl Ointment (Knoll) p 1067
Travase Ointment (Flint) p 411, 952

ENZYME INHIBITORS
Lithostat (Mission) p 1418

ERGOT PREPARATIONS
Antimigraine
Wigraine Tablets & Suppositories (Organon) p 422, 1451
Wigraine-PB Suppositories (Organon) p 422, 1451
Wigrettes (Organon) p 422, 1451
Uterine Contractant
Ergotrate Maleate Ampoules (Lilly) p 1146
Ergotrate Maleate Tablets (Lilly) p 1147
Methergine (Sandoz Pharmaceutical Div.) p 433, 1806

F

FERTILITY AGENTS
Pergonal (menotropins USP) (Serono) p 1941
Pro-Ception (Milex) p 1415
Profasi HP (HCG) (Serono) p 1943
Serophene (clomiphene citrate USP) (Serono) p 1943

FIBER SUPPLEMENT
Fibermed Supplements (Purdue Frederick) p 427, 1624

FLUORESCENT IMMUNOASSAYS
(see under THERAPEUTIC DRUG ASSAYS)

FLUORINE PREPARATIONS
Fluoritab Tablets & Fluoritab Liquid (Fluoritab) p 953
Luride Drops (Colgate-Hoyt) p 878
Luride Lozi-Tabs Tablets (Colgate-Hoyt) p 410, 878
Pediaflor Drops (Ross) p 1771

FOODS
Allergy Diet
MBF (Meat Base Formula) Liquid (Gerber) p 974
Vivonex Standard Diet (Norwich Eaton) p 1438
Carbohydrate
Polycose (Ross) p 1775
Carbohydrate Free
RCF (Ross) p 1775
Complete Therapeutic
Compleat Modified Formula (Clinical Nutrition) p 876
Compleat-B (Clinical Nutrition) p 877
Enrich (Ross) p 1762
Ensure (Ross) p 1762
Ensure HN (Ross) p 1764
Ensure Plus (Ross) p 1764
Ensure Plus HN (Ross) p 1765
Forta Pudding (Ross) p 1767
Isotein HN (Clinical Nutrition) p 877
Nutrisource Modular System (Clinical Nutrition) p 877
Osmolite (Ross) p 1769
Osmolite HN (Ross) p 1770
Stresstein (Clinical Nutrition) p 878
TwoCal HN (Ross) p 1781
Vari-Flavors Flavor Pacs (Ross) p 1782
Vital/High Nitrogen (Ross) p 1785
Vivonex Flavor Packets (Norwich Eaton) p 1441
Vivonex High Nitrogen Diet (Norwich Eaton) p 1439
Vivonex Standard Diet (Norwich Eaton) p 1438
Vivonex T.E.N. (Norwich Eaton) p 1441
Dietetic
Compleat Modified Formula (Clinical Nutrition) p 876
Compleat-B (Clinical Nutrition) p 877
Isotein HN (Clinical Nutrition) p 877
Stresstein (Clinical Nutrition) p 878
Enteral
Citrotein (Clinical Nutrition) p 876
Compleat Modified Formula (Clinical Nutrition) p 876
Compleat-B (Clinical Nutrition) p 877
Enrich (Ross) p 1762
Ensure (Ross) p 1762
Ensure HN (Ross) p 1764
Ensure Plus (Ross) p 1764
Ensure Plus HN (Ross) p 1765
Flexiflo Enteral Delivery System (Ross) p 1766
Isotein HN (Clinical Nutrition) p 877
Meritene Liquid (Clinical Nutrition) p 877
Meritene Powder (Clinical Nutrition) p 877
Osmolite (Ross) p 1769
Osmolite HN (Ross) p 1770
Polycose (Ross) p 1775
Ross SLD (Ross) p 1778
Stresstein (Clinical Nutrition) p 878
Vital/High Nitrogen (Ross) p 1785
Vivonex High Nitrogen Diet (Norwich Eaton) p 1439
Vivonex Standard Diet (Norwich Eaton) p 1438
Vivonex T.E.N. (Norwich Eaton) p 1441
Enteral Hyperalimentation Kit
Flexiflo Enteral Delivery System (Ross) p 1766
Vivonex Acutrol Enteral Feeding System (Norwich Eaton) p 1441
Vivonex Delivery System (Norwich Eaton) p 1441
High Nitrogen
Ensure HN (Ross) p 1764
Ensure Plus HN (Ross) p 1765
Isotein HN (Clinical Nutrition) p 877
Osmolite HN (Ross) p 1770
Ross SLD (Ross) p 1778
Stresstein (Clinical Nutrition) p 878
TwoCal HN (Ross) p 1781
Vital/High Nitrogen (Ross) p 1785
Vivonex Flavor Packets (Norwich Eaton) p 1441
Vivonex High Nitrogen Diet (Norwich Eaton) p 1439
Vivonex T.E.N. (Norwich Eaton) p 1441
Infant
(see under INFANT FORMULAS)
Lactose Free
Compleat Modified Formula (Clinical Nutrition) p 876
Enrich (Ross) p 1762
Ensure (Ross) p 1762
Ensure HN (Ross) p 1764
Ensure Plus (Ross) p 1764
Ensure Plus HN (Ross) p 1765
Isotein HN (Clinical Nutrition) p 877
Osmolite (Ross) p 1769
Osmolite HN (Ross) p 1770
Ross SLD (Ross) p 1778
TwoCal HN (Ross) p 1781
Vivonex High Nitrogen Diet (Norwich Eaton) p 1439
Vivonex Standard Diet (Norwich Eaton) p 1438
Vivonex T.E.N. (Norwich Eaton) p 1441
Low Fat
Compleat Modified Formula (Clinical Nutrition) p 876
Ross SLD (Ross) p 1778
Low Residue
Ensure (Ross) p 1762
Ensure HN (Ross) p 1764
Ensure Plus (Ross) p 1764
Ensure Plus HN (Ross) p 1765
Isotein HN (Clinical Nutrition) p 877

Product Category Index

Osmolite (Ross) p 1769
Osmolite HN (Ross) p 1770
Ross SLD (Ross) p 1778
Stresstein (Clinical Nutrition) p 878
Vital/High Nitrogen (Ross) p 1785
Vivonex High Nitrogen Diet (Norwich Eaton) p 1439
Vivonex Standard Diet (Norwich Eaton) p 1438
Vivonex T.E.N. (Norwich Eaton) p 1441

Low Sodium
Compleat Modified Formula (Clinical Nutrition) p 876
Isotein HN (Clinical Nutrition) p 877

Medium Chain Triglycerides
Isotein HN (Clinical Nutrition) p 877
Osmolite (Ross) p 1769
Osmolite HN (Ross) p 1770
Stresstein (Clinical Nutrition) p 878
Vital/High Nitrogen (Ross) p 1785

Tube Feeding System
Flexiflo Enteral Delivery System (Ross) p 1766
Vivonex Acutrol Enteral Feeding System (Norwich Eaton) p 1441
Vivonex Delivery System (Norwich Eaton) p 1441
Vivonex Jejunostomy Kit (Norwich Eaton) p 1441
Vivonex Moss Tube (Norwich Eaton) p 1441

FORMULAS
(see under INFANT FORMULAS)

G

GALACTOKINETIC
Syntocinon Nasal Spray (Sandoz Pharmaceutical Div.) p 1818

GALL STONE DISSOLUTION AGENT
Chenix (Rowell) p 1786

GASTROINTESTINAL MOTILITY FACTOR
Reglan Injectable (Robins) p 1659
Reglan Syrup (Robins) p 1659
Reglan Tablets (Robins) p 428, 1659

GERIATRICS
Circanol (Riker) p 1642
Deapril-ST (Mead Johnson Pharmaceutical) p 419, 1248
Enviro-Stress with Zinc & Selenium (Vitaline) p 2148
Glutofac Tablets (Kenwood) p 1046
Hydergine Oral Tablets, Sublingual Tablets, & Liquid (Sandoz Pharmaceutical Div.) p 433, 1802
Hydergine LC Liquid Capsules (Sandoz Pharmaceutical Div.) p 433, 1802
Total Formula (Vitaline) p 2148

GERMICIDES
Betadine Aerosol Spray (Purdue Frederick) p 1622
Betadine Antiseptic Gel (Purdue Frederick) p 1622
Betadine Disposable Medicated Douche (Purdue Frederick) p 1622
Betadine Douche (Purdue Frederick) p 1622
Betadine Helafoam Solution (Purdue Frederick) p 1622
Betadine Ointment (Purdue Frederick) p 1622
Betadine Skin Cleanser (Purdue Frederick) p 1622
Betadine Solution (Purdue Frederick) p 1622
Betadine Surgical Scrub (Purdue Frederick) p 1622
Betadine Viscous Formula Antiseptic Gauze Pad (Purdue Frederick) p 1623
Cetylcide Solution (Cetylite) p 839
Clorpactin WCS-90 (Guardian) p 1000

H

HEMATINICS

Cyanocobalamin
Albafort Injectable (Bart) p 685
Alba-Lybe (Bart) p 685
Cyanocobalamin in Tubex (Wyeth) p 445, 2288
Trinsicon/Trinsicon M Capsules (Glaxo) p 412, 986
Vicon Forte Capsules (Glaxo) p 412, 989

Folic Acid
Al-Vite (Drug Industries) p 914
Cevi-Fer Capsules (sustained release) (Geriatric) p 975
Eldercaps (Mayrand) p 1196
Fero-Folic-500 (Abbott) p 403, 529
Folic Acid Tablets (Lilly) p 1147
Hemo-Vite (Drug Industries) p 914
Hemo-Vite Liquid (Drug Industries) p 914
Iberet-Folic-500 (Abbott) p 403, 529
Ircon-FA (Key Pharmaceuticals) p 1050
Niferex-PN (Central Pharmaceuticals) p 409, 838
Nu-Iron-V Tablets (Mayrand) p 1196
Tabron Filmseal (Parke-Davis) p 425, 1572
Trinsicon/Trinsicon M Capsules (Glaxo) p 412, 986
Vicon Forte Capsules (Glaxo) p 412, 989

Hydrochloric Acid
Acidulin (Lilly) p 1126

Iron & Combinations
Albafort Injectable (Bart) p 685
Cevi-Fer Capsules (sustained release) (Geriatric) p 975
Chromagen Capsules (Savage) p 433, 1824
Ferancee Chewable Tablets (Stuart) p 439, 2037
Ferancee-HP Tablets (Stuart) p 439, 2037
Fergon Capsules (Winthrop-Breon) p 443, 2198
Fergon Elixir (Winthrop-Breon) p 2198
Fergon Plus (Winthrop-Breon) p 2198
Fergon Tablets (Winthrop-Breon) p 443, 2198
Fero-Folic-500 (Abbott) p 403, 529
Fero-Grad-500 (Abbott) p 403, 530
Fero-Gradumet (Abbott) p 530
Ferralet (Mission) p 1416
Ferro-Sequels (Lederle) p 415, 1093
Fosfree (Mission) p 1416
Glytinic Tablets (Boyle) p 726
Hemo-Vite (Drug Industries) p 914
Hemo-Vite Liquid (Drug Industries) p 914
Heptuna Plus (Roerig) p 431, 1735
Hytinic Capsules & Elixir (Hyrex) p 1024
I.L.X. B_{12} Elixir Crystalline (Kenwood) p 1046
I.L.X. B_{12} Tablets (Kenwood) p 1046
Iberet (Abbott) p 532
Iberet-500 (Abbott) p 403, 532
Iberet-500 Liquid (Abbott) p 533
Iberet-Folic-500 (Abbott) p 403, 529
Iberet Liquid (Abbott) p 533
Imferon (Merrell Dow) p 1367
Ircon-FA (Key Pharmaceuticals) p 1050
Iromin-G (Mission) p 1416
Irospan Capsules (Fielding) p 942
Irospan Tablets (Fielding) p 942
Mission Prenatal (Mission) p 1419
Mission Prenatal F.A. (Mission) p 1419
Mission Prenatal H.P. (Mission) p 1419
Mission Pre-Surgical (Mission) p 1419
Niferex Tablets/Elixir (Central Pharmaceuticals) p 838
Niferex w/Vitamin C (Central Pharmaceuticals) p 838
Niferex-150 Capsules (Central Pharmaceuticals) p 409, 838
Niferex-PN (Central Pharmaceuticals) p 409, 838
Nu-Iron Elixir (Mayrand) p 1196
Nu-Iron 150 Caps (Mayrand) p 1196
Nu-Iron-V Tablets (Mayrand) p 1196
Perihemin (Lederle) p 1112
Peritinic Tablets (Lederle) p 1112
Pramet FA (Ross) p 432, 1775
Pramilet FA (Ross) p 432, 1775
Pronemia Capsules (Lederle) p 1118
Stuartinic Tablets (Stuart) p 439, 2034
Tabron Filmseal (Parke-Davis) p 425, 1572
Theragran Hematinic (Squibb) p 438, 2024
TriHemic 600 (Lederle) p 416, 1119
Trinsicon/Trinsicon M Capsules (Glaxo) p 412, 986

Liver
Albafort Injectable (Bart) p 685
Hep-Forte Capsules (Marlyn) p 1193
Heptuna Plus (Roerig) p 431, 1735
Trinsicon/Trinsicon M Capsules (Glaxo) p 412, 986

Vitamin B_{12}
Albafort Injectable (Bart) p 685
Alba-Lybe (Bart) p 685
Al-Vite (Drug Industries) p 914
Hemo-Vite (Drug Industries) p 914
Hemo-Vite Liquid (Drug Industries) p 914
Heptuna Plus (Roerig) p 431, 1735
I.L.X. B_{12} Elixir Crystalline (Kenwood) p 1046
I.L.X. B_{12} Tablets (Kenwood) p 1046
Tia-Doce Injectable Solution (Bart) p 685
Trinsicon/Trinsicon M Capsules (Glaxo) p 412, 986

HEMORRHOIDAL PREPARATIONS
Anusol Ointment (Parke-Davis) p 1484
Anusol Suppositories (Parke-Davis) p 423, 1484
Anusol-HC (Parke-Davis) p 423, 1484
Cort-Dome High Potency Suppositories (Miles Pharmaceuticals) p 1401
Cort-Dome Regular Potency Suppositories (Miles Pharmaceuticals) p 1401
Corticaine Cream (Glaxo) p 412, 980
Corticaine Suppositories (Glaxo) p 412, 980
Fleet Relief (Fleet) p 947
Hurricaine Oral, Topical Anesthetic Gel, Liquid, Spray (Beutlich) p 705
Lubraseptic Jelly (Guardian) p 1000
Nupercainal Cream & Ointment (CIBA) p 856
Nupercainal Suppositories (CIBA) p 857
Preparation H Hemorrhoidal Ointment (Whitehall) p 443, 2186
Preparation H Hemorrhoidal Suppositories (Whitehall) p 443, 2186
Proctofoam-HC (Reed & Carnrick) p 427, 1636
proctoFoam/non-steroid (Reed & Carnrick) p 427, 1636
Rectal Medicone-HC Suppositories (Medicone) p 419, 1256
Tronolane Anesthetic Hemorrhoidal Cream (Ross) p 1781
Tronolane Anesthetic Hemorrhoidal Suppositories (Ross) p 1781
Tucks Cream (Parke-Davis) p 1575
Tucks Ointment (Parke-Davis) p 1575
Tucks Premoistened Pads (Parke-Davis) p 1575
Wyanoids Hemorrhoidal Suppositories (Wyeth) p 445, 2293

HEMOSTATICS
Amicar (Lederle) p 414, 1077
Avitene (Alcon P.R.) p 588
DDAVP Injection (USV Pharmaceutical) p 440, 2075
Gelfoam Sterile Powder (Upjohn) p 2114
Gelfoam Sterile Sponge (Upjohn) p 2113
Konakion Injectable (Roche) p 1687
Premarin Intravenous (Ayerst) p 667
Stimate Injection (Armour) p 611
Surgicel Absorbable Hemostat (Johnson & Johnson (Patient Care Div.)) p 1044
Thrombinar (Armour) p 613
Thrombostat (Parke-Davis) p 1574

HISTAMINE H_2 RECEPTOR ANTAGONIST
Tagamet (Smith Kline & French) p 437, 1973
Zantac Injection (Glaxo) p 990
Zantac Tablets (Glaxo) p 412, 991

HORMONES

ACTH
Acthar (Armour) p 601
HP Acthar Gel (Armour) p 601

Anabolics
Anavar (Searle & Co.) p 435, 1916
Teslac Tablets (Squibb) p 2023
Winstrol (Winthrop-Breon) p 444, 2232

Androgen & Estrogen Combinations
Mediatric Capsules, Tablets & Liquid (Ayerst) p 405, 654
Premarin w/Methyltestosterone (Ayerst) p 405, 674

Androgens
Anadrol-50 (Syntex) p 440, 2049
Android-5 Buccal (Brown) p 407, 771
Android-10 (Brown) p 407, 771
Android-25 (Brown) p 407, 771
Halotestin Tablets (Upjohn) p 441, 2116
Metandren Linguets & Tablets (CIBA) p 409, 855
Oreton Methyl Tablets & Buccal Tablets (Schering) p 434, 1873
Testred (ICN Pharmaceuticals) p 1025

Corticoids & Analgesics
Corticaine Cream (Glaxo) p 412, 980
Epifoam (Reed & Carnrick) p 427, 1634
Pramosone Cream, Lotion & Ointment (Ferndale) p 942
Proctofoam-HC (Reed & Carnrick) p 427, 1636

Corticoids & Antibiotics, Topical
Mycolog Cream and Ointment (Squibb) p 2003

Estrogens
Diethylstilbestrol Enseals & Tablets (Lilly) p 1141
Diethylstilbestrol Suppositories (Lilly) p 1141
Estinyl Tablets (Schering) p 434, 1839
Estrace (Mead Johnson Laboratories) p 419, 1216
Estrace Vaginal Cream (Mead Johnson Laboratories) p 419, 1219
Estradurin (Ayerst) p 642
Estrocon Tablets (Savage) p 433, 1824
Estrovis (Parke-Davis) p 424, 1517
Menrium Tablets (Roche Products) p 430, 1717
Ogen Tablets (Abbott) p 403, 548
Ogen Vaginal Cream (Abbott) p 551
PMB 200 & PMB 400 (Ayerst) p 405, 660
Premarin Tablets (Ayerst) p 405, 664
TACE 12 mg Capsules (Merrell Dow) p 421, 1385
TACE 25 mg Capsules (Merrell Dow) p 421, 1385
TACE 72 mg Capsules (Merrell Dow) p 421, 1389

Product Category Index

Glucocorticoid
A-hydroCort (Abbott) p 506
A-methaPred (Abbott) p 508
Aristocort Forte Parenteral (Lederle) p 1081
Aristocort Intralesional (Lederle) p 1081
Aristocort Syrup (Lederle) p 1078
Aristocort Tablets (Lederle) p 414, 1078
Aristospan Parenteral 20 mg./ml (Lederle) p 1085
Aristospan Parenteral 5 mg./ml (Lederle) p 1085
Beclovent Oral Inhaler (Glaxo) p 411, 977
Celestone Phosphate Injection (Schering) p 1833
Celestone Soluspan Suspension (Schering) p 1835
Celestone Syrup & Tablets (Schering) p 433, 1832
Cloderm (Ortho Pharmaceutical (Dermatological Div.)) p 1472
Corticaine Suppositories (Glaxo) p 412, 980
Cortifoam (Reed & Carnrick) p 427, 1632
Decadron Elixir (Merck Sharp & Dohme) p 1284
Decadron Phosphate Injection (Merck Sharp & Dohme) p 1288
Decadron Phosphate Respihaler (Merck Sharp & Dohme) p 1291
Decadron Phosphate Turbinaire (Merck Sharp & Dohme) p 1293
Decadron Tablets (Merck Sharp & Dohme) p 420, 1286
Decadron-LA Suspension (Merck Sharp & Dohme) p 1294
Decaspray Topical Aerosol (Merck Sharp & Dohme) p 1296
Depo-Medrol (Upjohn) p 441, 2107
Diprolene Ointment 0.05% (Schering) p 1837
Diprosone Cream 0.05% (Schering) p 1838
Diprosone Lotion 0.05% w/w (Schering) p 1838
Diprosone Ointment 0.05% (Schering) p 1838
Diprosone Topical Aerosol 0.1% w/w (Schering) p 1838
Halog Cream/Ointment/Solution (Squibb) p 1996
Halog-E Cream (Squibb) p 1996
Hydeltra-T.B.A. Suspension (Merck Sharp & Dohme) p 1314
Kenalog Cream/Lotion/Ointment (Squibb) p 1998
Kenalog in Orabase (Squibb) p 2003
Kenalog Spray (Squibb) p 1998
Kenalog-10 Injection (Squibb) p 2001
Kenalog-40 Injection (Squibb) p 1999
Lotrisone Cream (Schering) p 1858
Medrol Tablets (Upjohn) p 441, 2124
Pramosone Cream, Lotion & Ointment (Ferndale) p 942
Solu-Cortef Plain & Mix-O-Vial (Upjohn) p 2135
Solu-Medrol Sterile Powder (Upjohn) p 441, 2137
Tridesilon Creme 0.05% (Miles Pharmaceuticals) p 1412
Tridesilon Ointment 0.05% (Miles Pharmaceuticals) p 1413
Valisone Cream 0.1% (Schering) p 1892
Valisone Lotion 0.1% (Schering) p 1892
Valisone Ointment 0.1% (Schering) p 1892
Valisone Reduced Strength Cream 0.01% (Schering) p 1892
Westcort Cream 0.2% (Westwood) p 2183
Westcort Ointment 0.2% (Westwood) p 2183

Gonadotropin
A.P.L. (Ayerst) p 636
Pregnyl (Organon) p 1450
Profasi HP (HCG) (Serono) p 1943

Human Growth Hormone
Asellacrin (somatropin) (Serono) p 1940
Crescormon (Pharmacia) p 1616

Hypocalcemic
Calcimar Solution (USV Pharmaceutical) p 440, 2072

Menotropins
Pergonal (menotropins USP) (Serono) p 1941

Mineralocorticoid
Percorten Pellets (CIBA) p 861
Percorten pivalate (CIBA) p 862

Progestogen
Amen (Carnrick) p 408, 829
Aygestin (Ayerst) p 404, 638
Curretab Tablets (Reid-Provident Labs.) p 427, 1638
Depo-Provera (Upjohn) p 2109
Micronor Tablets (Ortho Pharmaceutical) p 423, 1461
Norlutate (Parke-Davis) p 425, 1556
Norlutin (Parke-Davis) p 425, 1556
Nor-Q.D. (Syntex) p 440, 2052
Ovrette Tablets (Wyeth) p 2272
Provera Tablets (Upjohn) p 441, 2133

Progestogen & Estrogen Combinations
Brevicon 21-Day Tablets (Syntex) p 440, 2052
Brevicon 28-Day Tablets (Syntex) p 440, 2052
Demulen 1/35-21 (Searle & Co.) p 435, 1919
Demulen 1/35-28 (Searle & Co.) p 435, 1919
Demulen 1/50-21 (Searle & Co.) p 435, 1919
Demulen 1/50-28 (Searle & Co.) p 435, 1919
Enovid 5 mg (Searle & Co.) p 435, 1919
Enovid 10 mg (Searle & Co.) p 435, 1919
Enovid-E 21 (Searle & Co.) p 436, 1919
Lo/Ovral Tablets (Wyeth) p 444, 2255
Lo/Ovral-28 Tablets (Wyeth) p 444, 2263
Modicon 21 Tablets (Ortho Pharmaceutical) p 423, 1461
Modicon 28 Tablets (Ortho Pharmaceutical) p 1461
Nordette-21 Tablets (Wyeth) p 444, 2266
Nordette-28 Tablets (Wyeth) p 444, 2270
Norinyl 1+35 Tablets 21-Day (Syntex) p 440, 2052
Norinyl 1+35 Tablets 28-Day (Syntex) p 440, 2052
Norinyl 1+50 21-Day (Syntex) p 440, 2052
Norinyl 1+50 28-Day (Syntex) p 440, 2052
Norinyl 1+80 21-Day (Syntex) p 440, 2052
Norinyl 1+80 28-Day (Syntex) p 440, 2052
Norinyl 2 mg. (Syntex) p 440, 2052
Ortho-Novum 1/35☐21 (Ortho Pharmaceutical) p 422, 1461
Ortho-Novum 1/35☐28 (Ortho Pharmaceutical) p 1461
Ortho-Novum 1/50☐21 (Ortho Pharmaceutical) p 422, 1461
Ortho-Novum 1/50☐28 (Ortho Pharmaceutical) p 1461
Ortho-Novum 1/80☐21 (Ortho Pharmaceutical) p 423, 1461
Ortho-Novum 1/80☐28 (Ortho Pharmaceutical) p 1461
Ortho-Novum 7/7/7 ☐.. 21 Tablets (Ortho Pharmaceutical) p 422, 1461
Ortho-Novum 7/7/7 ☐.. 28 Tablets (Ortho Pharmaceutical) p 1461
Ortho-Novum 10/11☐.. 21 Tablets (Ortho Pharmaceutical) p 422, 1461
Ortho-Novum 10/11☐.. 28 Tablets (Ortho Pharmaceutical) p 1461
Ortho-Novum Tablets 2 mg☐21 (Ortho Pharmaceutical) p 423, 1461
Ovcon-35 (Mead Johnson Laboratories) p 419, 1224
Ovcon-50 (Mead Johnson Laboratories) p 419, 1224
Ovral Tablets (Wyeth) p 444, 2271
Ovral-28 Tablets (Wyeth) p 444, 2272
Ovulen-21 (Searle & Co.) p 436, 1919
Ovulen-28 (Searle & Co.) p 436, 1919
Tri-Norinyl 21-Day Tablets (Syntex) p 440, 2052
Tri-Norinyl 28-Day Tablets (Syntex) p 440, 2052

Vasopressin
Pitressin (Parke-Davis) p 1562

Other
Rocaltrol Capsules (Roche) p 430, 1700

HYPERGLYCEMIC AGENTS
Glucagon for Injection Ampoules (Lilly) p 1147
Proglycem Capsules, Suspension (Schering) p 1880

HYPNOTICS
Alurate Elixir (Roche) p 1667
Dalmane Capsules (Roche Products) p 429, 1710
Doriden Tablets (USV Pharmaceutical) p 2076
Halcion Tablets (Upjohn) p 441, 2114
Nembutal Sodium Capsules (Abbott) p 403, 538
Nembutal Sodium Solution (Abbott) p 541
Nembutal Sodium Suppositories (Abbott) p 543
Noctec Capsules & Syrup (Squibb) p 438, 2007
Noludar & Noludar 300 (Roche) p 430, 1696
Placidyl (Abbott) p 403, 566
Restoril Capsules (Sandoz Pharmaceutical Div.) p 433, 1810
Valmid Pulvules (Dista) p 410, 908

I

IMMUNOSUPPRESSIVES
Imuran Tablets (Burroughs Wellcome) p 408, 790
MICRhoGAM (Ortho Diagnostic Systems) p 1452

Rh₀-D Immune Globulin (Human) HypRho-D (Cutter Biological) p 885
Rh₀-D Immune Globulin (Human) HypRho-D Mini-Dose (Cutter Biological) p 884
RhoGAM (Ortho Diagnostic Systems) p 1453
Sandimmune Ampuls (Sandoz Pharmaceutical Div.) p 1811
Sandimmune Oral Suspension (Sandoz Pharmaceutical Div.) p 1811
Sandoglobulin (Sandoz Pharmaceutical Div.) p 1813

INFANT FORMULAS, REGULAR
Liquid Concentrate
SMA Infant Formula, Ready-to-Feed, Concentrated Liquid, Powder (Wyeth) p 2286
Similac (Ross) p 1778

Liquid Ready-to-feed
SMA Infant Formula, Ready-to-Feed, Concentrated Liquid, Powder (Wyeth) p 2286
Similac (Ross) p 1778
Similac 13 (Ross) p 1777
Similac 20 (Ross) p 1777
Similac 24 (Ross) p 1777
Similac 27 (Ross) p 1777

Powder
SMA Infant Formula, Ready-to-Feed, Concentrated Liquid, Powder (Wyeth) p 2286
Similac (Ross) p 1778

INFANT FORMULAS, SPECIAL PURPOSE
Hypo-Allergenic
  Liquid Concentrate
  Isomil (Ross) p 1767
  Isomil SF (Ross) p 1768
  MBF (Meat Base Formula) Liquid (Gerber) p 974
  Nursoy (Wyeth) p 2271
  Liquid Ready-to-feed
  Isomil (Ross) p 1767
  Isomil SF (Ross) p 1768
  Isomil SF 20 (Ross) p 1777
  Nursoy (Wyeth) p 2271
  Powder
  Isomil (Ross) p 1767

Iron Supplement
  Liquid Concentrate
  Advance (Ross) p 1761
  Similac With Iron (Ross) p 1779
  Similac With Whey + Iron (Ross) p 1780
  Liquid Ready-to-feed
  Advance (Ross) p 1761
  Similac With Iron (Ross) p 1779
  Similac With Iron 13 (Ross) p 1777
  Similac With Iron 20 (Ross) p 1777
  Similac With Iron 24 (Ross) p 1777
  Similac With Whey + Iron (Ross) p 1780
  Similac With Whey + Iron 20 (Ross) p 1777
  Powder
  Similac With Iron (Ross) p 1779
  Similac With Whey + Iron (Ross) p 1780

Lactose Free
  Liquid Concentrate
  Isomil (Ross) p 1767
  Isomil SF (Ross) p 1768
  Nursoy (Wyeth) p 2271
  Liquid Ready-to-feed
  Isomil (Ross) p 1767
  Isomil SF (Ross) p 1768
  Isomil SF 20 (Ross) p 1777
  Nursoy (Wyeth) p 2271
  Powder
  Isomil (Ross) p 1767

Medium Chain Triglycerides
  Liquid Ready-to-feed
  Similac 24 LBW (Ross) p 1777
  Similac Special Care 20 (Ross) p 1777
  Similac Special Care 24 (Ross) p 1777

Milk Free
  Liquid Concentrate
  Nursoy (Wyeth) p 2271
  Liquid Ready-to-feed
  Nursoy (Wyeth) p 2271

Nutritional Beverage
  Liquid Concentrate
  Advance (Ross) p 1761
  Liquid Ready-to-feed
  Advance (Ross) p 1761

Sucrose Free
  Liquid Concentrate
  Isomil SF (Ross) p 1768
  Liquid Ready-to-feed
  Isomil SF (Ross) p 1768
  Isomil SF 20 (Ross) p 1777

Product Category Index

With Whey
Liquid Concentrate
Similac With Whey + Iron (Ross) p 1780
Liquid Ready-to-feed
Similac PM 60/40 (Ross) p 1779
Similac Special Care 20 (Ross) p 1777
Similac Special Care 24 (Ross) p 1777
Similac With Whey + Iron (Ross) p 1780
Similac With Whey + Iron 20 (Ross) p 1777
Powder
Similac PM 60/40 (Ross) p 1779
Similac With Whey + Iron (Ross) p 1780

INSECT STING EMERGENCY KIT
EpiPen—Epinephrine Auto-Injector (Center) p 835
EpiPen Jr. (Center) p 835

L

LAXATIVES
Bulk
Effersyllium (Stuart) p 2037
Fiberall, Natural Flavor (Rydelle) p 1795
Fiberall, Orange Flavor (Rydelle) p 1795
Konsyl (Lafayette) p 1070
Konsyl-D (formerly L. A. Formula) (Lafayette) p 1070
Metamucil, Instant Mix, Orange Flavor (Searle Consumer Products) p 1912
Metamucil, Instant Mix, Regular Flavor (Searle Consumer Products) p 1911
Metamucil, Powder, Orange Flavor (Searle Consumer Products) p 1911
Metamucil, Powder, Regular Flavor (Searle Consumer Products) p 1911
Metamucil, Powder, Strawberry Flavor (Searle Consumer Products) p 1911
Metamucil, Powder, Sugar Free, Regular Flavor (Searle Consumer Products) p 1911
Mitrolan (Robins) p 428, 1654
Modane Bulk (Adria) p 584
Movicol (Norgine) p 1424
Naturacil (Mead Johnson Nutritional) p 1243
Prompt (Searle Consumer Products) p 1912
Combinations
Bilax Capsules (Drug Industries) p 914
Dialose Plus Capsules (Stuart) p 439, 2037
Doxidan (Hoechst-Roussel) p 412, 1014
Evac-Q-Kit (Adria) p 575
Evac-Q-Kwik (Adria) p 575
Fleet Flavored Castor Oil Emulsion (Fleet) p 947
Modane Plus (Adria) p 585
Movicol (Norgine) p 1424
Neolax Tablets (Central Pharmaceuticals) p 838
Neoloid (Lederle) p 1107
Peri-Colace (Mead Johnson Pharmaceutical) p 419, 1255
Senokot-S Tablets (Purdue Frederick) p 1627
Trilax (Drug Industries) p 915
Enemas
Fleet Enema (Fleet) p 946
Fleet Mineral Oil Enema (Fleet) p 947
Fecal Softeners
Bilax Capsules (Drug Industries) p 914
Chronulac Syrup (Merrell Dow) p 421, 1363
Colace (Mead Johnson Pharmaceutical) p 419, 1248
Dialose Capsules (Stuart) p 439, 2036
Dialose Plus Capsules (Stuart) p 439, 2037
Disonate Capsules & Liquid (Lannett) p 1071
Geriplex-FS Kapseals (Parke-Davis) p 424, 1527
Geriplex-FS Liquid (Parke-Davis) p 1527
Kasof Capsules (Stuart) p 439, 2038
Modane Soft (Adria) p 584
Neolax Tablets (Central Pharmaceuticals) p 838
Prompt (Searle Consumer Products) p 1912
Surfak (Hoechst-Roussel) p 413, 1021
Trilax (Drug Industries) p 915
Mineral Oil
Agoral, Plain (Parke-Davis) p 1480
Fleet Mineral Oil Enema (Fleet) p 947
Saline
Fleet Phospho-Soda (Fleet) p 947
Phillips' Milk of Magnesia (Glenbrook) p 997
Stimulant
Agoral, Raspberry & Marshmallow Flavors (Parke-Davis) p 1480
Ceo-Two Suppositories (Beutlich) p 705
Decholin Tablets (Miles Pharmaceuticals) p 421, 1402
Dialose Plus Capsules (Stuart) p 439, 2037
Dulcolax Suppositories (Boehringer Ingelheim) p 406, 709
Dulcolax Tablets (Boehringer Ingelheim) p 406, 709
Evac-U-Gen (Walker, Corp) p 2148
Fleet Babylax (Fleet) p 946

Fleet Bisacodyl Enema (Fleet) p 946
Fleet Prep Kits (Fleet) p 947
Modane, Tablets & Liquid (Adria) p 584
Neolax Tablets (Central Pharmaceuticals) p 838
Prompt (Searle Consumer Products) p 1912
Prulet (Mission) p 1420
Senokot Syrup (Purdue Frederick) p 1626
Senokot Tablets/Granules (Purdue Frederick) p 1626
Trilax (Drug Industries) p 915

LIP BALM
Herpecin-L Cold Sore Lip Balm (Campbell) p 829
RVPaba Lip Stick (Elder) p 936

LIPOTROPICS
Cardioguard Natural Lipotropic Dietary Supplement-Powder (Professional Health) p 1621
Cardioguard Natural Lipotropic Dietary Supplement-Tablets (Professional Health) p 1621
DL-Carnitine - Amino Acid Preparation (Tyson) p 2068
Nicolar Tablets (USV Pharmaceutical) p 440, 2083

M

MINERALS
Beelith Tablets (Beach) p 405, 685
Enviro-Stress with Zinc & Selenium (Vitaline) p 2148
Glutofac Tablets (Kenwood) p 1046
Megadose (Arco) p 600
Selenium Tablets (200 mcg) (Vitaline) p 2148
Total Formula (Vitaline) p 2148
Vicon Forte Capsules (Glaxo) p 412, 989
Vicon-C Capsules (Glaxo) p 412, 989
Vicon-Plus Capsules (Glaxo) p 412, 989
Vi-Zac Capsules (Glaxo) p 412, 990
Zinc-220 Capsules (Alto) p 404, 589

MOUTHWASHES
Chloraseptic Liquid (Procter & Gamble) p 1619
Dalidyne (Dalin) p 886
Prophyllin (Rystan) p 1796

MUCOLYTICS
Entex Capsules (Norwich Eaton) p 1431
Entex LA Tablets (Norwich Eaton) p 422, 1432
Entex Liquid (Norwich Eaton) p 1431
Hytuss Tablets and Hytuss-2X Capsules (Hyrex) p 413, 1024
Mucomyst (Mead Johnson Pharmaceutical) p 1252
Mudrane GG Elixir (Poythress) p 1619
Mudrane GG Tablets (Poythress) p 1619
Mudrane Tablets (Poythress) p 1618
Pima Syrup (Fleming) p 948
Quadrinal Tablets & Suspension (Knoll) p 414, 1065
Theo-Organidin Elixir (Wallace) p 442, 2170
Trichotine Liquid, Vaginal Douche (Reed & Carnrick) p 1637
Trichotine Powder, Vaginal Douche (Reed & Carnrick) p 1637
Tussi-Organidin (Wallace) p 442, 2171
Tussi-Organidin DM (Wallace) p 442, 2171

MUSCLE RELAXANTS
Neuromuscular Blocking Agent
Norcuron (NC-45) (Organon) p 1447
Pavulon (Organon) p 1449
Skeletal Muscle Relaxants
Anectine (Burroughs Wellcome) p 778
Dantrium Capsules (Norwich Eaton) p 1426
Dantrium Intravenous (Norwich Eaton) p 1428
Flexeril Tablets (Merck Sharp & Dohme) p 420, 1310
Lioresal Tablets (Geigy) p 411, 959
Metubine Iodide (Lilly) p 1165
Paraflex Tablets (McNeil Pharmaceutical) p 1205
Quinamm (Merrell Dow) p 421, 1380
Robaxin Injectable (Robins) p 429, 1661
Robaxin Tablets (Robins) p 428, 1662
Robaxin-750 Tablets (Robins) p 428, 1662
Skelaxin (Carnrick) p 409, 835
Soma (Wallace) p 442, 2166
Tubocurarine Chloride (Lilly) p 1175
Valium Injectable (Roche Products) p 430, 1721
Valium Tablets (Roche Products) p 430, 1723
Valrelease Capsules (Roche) p 430, 1707
Skeletal Muscle Relaxants with Analgesics
Parafon Forte Tablets (McNeil Pharmaceutical) p 419, 1206
Robaxisal Tablets (Robins) p 429, 1662

Soma Compound (Wallace) p 442, 2166
Soma Compound w/Codeine (Wallace) p 442, 2169
Smooth Muscle Relaxants
Urispas (Smith Kline & French) p 437, 1981

N

NARCOTIC ANTAGONISTS
Lorfan Injectable (Roche) p 1689
Narcan and Narcan Neonatal (Du Pont) p 410, 922

NARCOTIC DETOXIFICATION
Methadone Hydrochloride Diskets (Lilly) p 417, 1164

NARCOTICS
(see under ANALGESICS)

NASAL PREPARATIONS
Beconase Nasal Inhaler (Glaxo) p 411, 978
Dristan Long Lasting Nasal Spray, Regular & Menthol (Whitehall) p 443, 2186
Dristan Nasal Spray, Regular & Menthol (Whitehall) p 443, 2186
Nasalcrom Nasal Solution (Fisons) p 944
Nasalide Nasal Solution 0.025% (Syntex) p 2064
Otrivin (Geigy) p 963
Ponaris Nasal Mucosal Emollient (Jamol) p 1033
Vancenase Nasal Inhaler (Schering) p 435, 1893

O

OPHTHALMOLOGICALS
Antibacterial
Achromycin Ophthalmic Ointment (Lederle) p 1077
Achromycin Ophthalmic Suspension 1% (Lederle) p 1075
Chloromycetin Hydrocortisone Ophthalmic (Parke-Davis) p 1488
Chloromycetin Ophthalmic Ointment, 1% (Parke-Davis) p 1491
Cortisporin Ophthalmic Ointment (Burroughs Wellcome) p 784
Cortisporin Ophthalmic Suspension (Burroughs Wellcome) p 785
Gantrisin Ophthalmic Ointment/Solution (Roche) p 1685
Garamycin Ophthalmic Ointment-Sterile (Schering) p 1846
Garamycin Ophthalmic Solution-Sterile (Schering) p 1846
Ilotycin Sterile Ophthalmic Ointment (Dista) p 899
Metimyd Ophthalmic Ointment - Sterile (Schering) p 1860
Metimyd Ophthalmic Suspension (Schering) p 1860
Neosporin Ophthalmic Ointment Sterile (Burroughs Wellcome) p 808
Neosporin Ophthalmic Solution Sterile (Burroughs Wellcome) p 809
Ophthochlor, 0.5% (Parke-Davis) p 425, 1557
Ophthocort (Parke-Davis) p 1558
Polysporin Ophthalmic Ointment (Burroughs Wellcome) p 810
Silver Nitrate (Lilly) p 1174
Sodium Sulamyd Ophthalmic Solutions & Ointment-Sterile (Schering) p 1884
Terra-Cortril Ophthalmic Suspension (Pfipharmecs) p 1594
Antiglaucomatous Agent
Ayerst Epitrate (Ayerst) p 642
Diamox Parenteral (Lederle) p 1091
Diamox Sequels, Tablets (Lederle) p 415, 1091
Neptazane Tablets (Lederle) p 415, 1107
Phospholine Iodide (Ayerst) p 658
Timoptic Sterile Ophthalmic Solution (Merck Sharp & Dohme) p 1349
Antiviral
Vira-A Ophthalmic Ointment, 3% (Parke-Davis) p 426, 1578
Viroptic Ophthalmic Solution (Burroughs Wellcome) p 820
Eye Washes
Collyrium Eye Lotion (Wyeth) p 2249
Murine Eye Drops (Regular Formula) (Ross) p 1769
Lubricants
Lacrisert Sterile Ophthalmic Insert (Merck Sharp & Dohme) p 1322
Moisturizing Agent
Murine Eye Drops (Regular Formula) (Ross) p 1769
Mydriatics
Paredrine 1% w/Boric Acid, Ophthalmic Solution (Smith Kline & French) p 1968

Product Category Index

Mydriatics & Cycloplegics
Neo-Synephrine Hydrochloride (Ophthalmic) (Winthrop-Breon) p 2217

Ocular Decongestants
Clear Eyes Eye Drops (Ross) p 1762
Collyrium 2 Eye Drops with Tetrahydrozoline (Wyeth) p 2249
Murine Plus Eye Drops (Ross) p 1769

Steroids & Combinations
Decadron Phosphate Sterile Ophthalmic Ointment (Merck Sharp & Dohme) p 1290
Decadron Phosphate Sterile Ophthalmic Solution (Merck Sharp & Dohme) p 1291
Hydrocortone Acetate Sterile Ophthalmic Ointment and Ophthalmic Suspension (Merck Sharp & Dohme) p 1316
Metimyd Ophthalmic Ointment - Sterile (Schering) p 1860
Metimyd Ophthalmic Suspension (Schering) p 1860
Metreton Ophthalmic/Otic Solution-Sterile (Schering) p 1861
Neodecadron Sterile Ophthalmic Ointment (Merck Sharp & Dohme) p 1340
Neodecadron Sterile Ophthalmic Solution (Merck Sharp & Dohme) p 1341
Ophthocort (Parke-Davis) p 1558

Surgical Adjunct
Healon (Pharmacia) p 1615

OPTIC OPACITIES
Symptomatic Relief
Succus Cineraria Maritima (Walker Pharmacal) p 2148

OTIC PREPARATIONS
Auralgan Otic Solution (Ayerst) p 638
Cerumenex Drops (Purdue Frederick) p 1624
Chloromycetin Otic (Parke-Davis) p 1491
Coly-Mycin S Otic w/Neomycin & Hydrocortisone (Parke-Davis) p 1501
Cortisporin Otic Solution (Burroughs Wellcome) p 786
Cortisporin Otic Suspension (Burroughs Wellcome) p 786
Debrox Drops (Marion) p 1184
Decadron Phosphate Sterile Ophthalmic Solution (Merck Sharp & Dohme) p 1291
Ear Drops by Murine—See Murine Ear Wax Removal System (Ross) p 1762
Hydrocortone Acetate Sterile Ophthalmic Ointment and Ophthalmic Suspension (Merck Sharp & Dohme) p 1316
Metreton Ophthalmic/Otic Solution-Sterile (Schering) p 1861
Murine Ear Wax Removal System/Murine Ear Drops (Ross) p 1769
Otic Domeboro Solution (Miles Pharmaceuticals) p 1411
Otic Tridesilon Solution 0.05% (Miles Pharmaceuticals) p 1414
Otic-HC Ear Drops (Hauck) p 1001
Oticol Sterile Ear Drops (Arlo) p 601
Otipyrin Otic Solution (Kramer) p 1069
Otobiotic Otic Solution (Schering) p 1875
Pyocidin-Otic Solution (Berlex) p 702
Tympagesic Otic Solution (Adria) p 587
VōSol HC Otic Solution (Wallace) p 442, 2171
VōSol Otic Solution (Wallace) p 442, 2171

OXYTOCICS
Ergotrate Maleate Ampoules (Lilly) p 1146
Ergotrate Maleate Tablets (Lilly) p 1147
Methergine (Sandoz Pharmaceutical Div.) p 433, 1806
Oxytocin Injection (Wyeth) p 2273
Pitocin Injection (Parke-Davis) p 1561
Syntocinon Injection (Sandoz Pharmaceutical Div.) p 1817

P

PARASYMPATHOLYTICS
Akineton (Knoll) p 414, 1056
Antrenyl bromide Tablets (CIBA) p 409, 841
Bellergal Tablets (Sandoz Pharmaceutical Div.) p 432, 1798
Bellergal-S Tablets (Sandoz Pharmaceutical Div.) p 432, 1798
Bentyl Capsules, Tablets, Syrup & Injection (Merrell Dow) p 421, 1359
Cantil (Merrell Dow) p 421, 1362
Combid Spansule Capsules (Smith Kline & French) p 436, 1952
Darbid (Smith Kline & French) p 436, 1958
Kinesed Tablets (Stuart) p 439, 2038
Levsin Tablets, Injection, Elixir & Drops (Rorer) p 432, 1751
Levsin/Phenobarbital Tablets, Elixir & Drops (Rorer) p 1751
Levsinex Timecaps (Rorer) p 432, 1751
Levsinex/Phenobarbital Timecaps (Rorer) p 1751
Robinul Forte Tablets (Robins) p 429, 1662
Robinul Injectable (Robins) p 429, 1663
Robinul Tablets (Robins) p 429, 1662
Tral Filmtab Tablets (Abbott) p 568
Yocon (Palisades Pharm.) p 1476

PARASYMPATHOMIMETICS
Duvoid (Norwich Eaton) p 1430
Mestinon Injectable (Roche) p 1692
Mestinon Syrup (Roche) p 1692
Mestinon Tablets (Roche) p 430, 1692
Mestinon Timespan Tablets (Roche) p 430, 1692
Myotonachol (Glenwood) p 412, 998
Prostigmin Injectable (Roche) p 1698
Prostigmin Tablets (Roche) p 430, 1699
Regonol (Organon) p 1450
Tensilon Injectable (Roche) p 1705, 3015
Urecholine Injection & Tablets (Merck Sharp & Dohme) p 421, 1356

PARENTERAL INJECTION SYSTEMS
(see under UNIT DOSE SYSTEMS)

PEDICULICIDES
(see under ANTIPARASITICS)

PENICILLIN ADJUVANT
Benemid Tablets (Merck Sharp & Dohme) p 420, 1268

PHOSPHORUS PREPARATIONS
K-Phos M.F. (Modified Formula) Tablets (Beach) p 405, 686
K-Phos Neutral Tablets (Beach) p 405, 686
K-Phos No. 2 Tablets (Beach) p 405, 686
K-Phos Original Formula 'Sodium Free' Tablets (Beach) p 405, 686
Neutra-Phos Powder & Capsules (Willen) p 2188
Neutra-Phos-K Powder & Capsules (Willen) p 2188
Thiacide Tablets (Beach) p 405, 687
Uroqid-Acid Tablets (Beach) p 405, 687
Uroqid-Acid No. 2 Tablets (Beach) p 405, 687

PLASMA EXTENDERS
Albutein 5% (Alpha Theapeutic) p 589
Albutein 25% (Alpha Theapeutic) p 589
Buminate 5%, Normal Serum Albumin (Human), U.S.P., 5% Solution (Hyland Therapeutics) p 1023
Buminate 25%, Normal Serum Albumin (Human), U.S.P., 25% Solution (Hyland Therapeutics) p 1023
Hespan (American Critical Care) p 595
Plasmatein 5% (Alpha Theapeutic) p 589
Protenate 5%, Plasma Protein Fraction (Human), U.S.P., 5% Solution (Hyland Therapeutics) p 1024

PLASMA FRACTIONS, HUMAN
Antihemophilic Factor
Autoplex, Anti-Inhibitor Coagulant Complex, Dried (Hyland Therapeutics) p 1023
Factor IX Complex (Human) (Factors II, VII, IX, and X) Konyne (Cutter Biological) p 886
Factorate, Antihemophilic Factor (Human) Dried (Armour) p 613
Factorate, Generation II (Armour) p 613
H.T. Factorate (Armour) p 613
H.T. Factorate, Generation II (Armour) p 613
Hemofil, Antihemophilic Factor (Human), Method Four, Dried (Hyland Therapeutics) p 1023
Hemofil T, Antihemophilic Factor (Human), Method Four, Dried, Heat-Treated (Hyland Therapeutics) p 1024
Koāte-HT (Cutter Biological) p 886
Profilate (Alpha Theapeutic) p 589
Profilate, Heat-Treated (Alpha Theapeutic) p 589
Profilnine (Alpha Theapeutic) p 589
Proplex, Factor IX Complex (Human) (Factors II, VII, IX & X), Dried (Hyland Therapeutics) p 1024
Proplex SX, Factor IX Complex (Human)(Factors II, VII, IX & X), Dried (Hyland Therapeutics) p 1024

Factor IX Complex
Prothar (Armour) p 613

Immune Serum Globulin (Human)
Gammar, Immune Serum Globulin (Human) U.S.P. (Armour) p 613
Gamulin Rh (Armour) p 613
Hepatitis B Immune Globulin (Human) HyperHep (Cutter Biological) p 884
Hu-Tet, Tetanus Immune Globulin (Human), U.S.P. (Hyland Therapeutics) p 1024
Immune Globulin Intravenous, 5% (In 10% Maltose) Gamimune (Cutter Biological) p 883
Immune Serum Globulin (Human), U.S.P. Gamma Globulin (Hyland Therapeutics) p 1024

Immune Serum Globulin (Human) Gamastan (Cutter Biological) p 883
Imogam Rabies Immune Globulin (Human) (Merieux) p 1358
Mini-Gamulin Rh (Armour) p 613
Pertussis Immune Globulin (Human) Hypertussis (Cutter Biological) p 884
Rabies Immune Globulin (Human) Hyperab (Cutter Biological) p 884
Rabies Immune Globulin (Human), Imogam Rabies (Merieux) p 1358
Tetanus Immune Globulin (Human) Hyper-Tet (Cutter Biological) p 884

Normal Serum Albumin (Human)
Albuminar-5, Normal Serum Albumin (Human) U.S.P. 5% (Armour) p 613
Albuminar-25, Normal Serum Albumin (Human) U.S.P. 25% (Armour) p 613
Albutein 5% (Alpha Theapeutic) p 589
Albutein 25% (Alpha Theapeutic) p 589
Buminate 5%, Normal Serum Albumin (Human), U.S.P., 5% Solution (Hyland Therapeutics) p 1023
Buminate 25%, Normal Serum Albumin (Human), U.S.P., 25% Solution (Hyland Therapeutics) p 1023

Plasma Protein Fraction (Human)
Plasma-Plex (Armour) p 613
Plasmatein 5% (Alpha Theapeutic) p 589
Protenate 5%, Plasma Protein Fraction (Human), U.S.P., 5% Solution (Hyland Therapeutics) p 1024

Rh₀ (D) Immune Globulin (Human)
MICRhoGAM (Ortho Diagnostic Systems) p 1452
Rh₀-D Immune Globulin (Human) HypRho-D (Cutter Biological) p 885
Rh₀-D Immune Globulin (Human) HypRho-D Mini-Dose (Cutter Biological) p 884
RhoGAM (Ortho Diagnostic Systems) p 1453

PROSTAGLANDINS
Prostin VR Pediatric Sterile Solution (Upjohn) p 2132

PSYCHOSTIMULANTS
Cardioguard Natural Lipotropic Dietary Supplement-Tablets (Professional Health) p 1621
Cylert Tablets (Abbott) p 403, 510
Desoxyn (Abbott) p 515
Desoxyn Gradumet Tablets (Abbott) p 403, 515
Efed II Capsules (Black) (Alto) p 404, 589
Parnate (Smith Kline & French) p 437, 1969
Pertofrane Capsules (USV Pharmaceutical) p 440, 2086
Ritalin Hydrochloride Tablets (CIBA) p 409, 864
Ritalin-SR Tablets (CIBA) p 409, 864
Tofranil Ampuls (Geigy) p 969
Tofranil Tablets (Geigy) p 411, 969
Tofranil-PM Capsules (Geigy) p 411, 971

Q

QUINIDINES
Cardioquin Tablets (Purdue Frederick) p 427, 1623
Quinaglute Dura-Tabs (Berlex) p 406, 702
Quinidex Extentabs (Robins) p 428, 1659

R

RESINS, ION EXCHANGE
Ionamin (Pennwalt) p 426, 1585
Kayexalate (Winthrop-Breon) p 2204
Questran (Mead Johnson Laboratories) p 1231
Sodium Polystyrene Sulfonate Suspension (Roxane) p 1794
Tussionex Tablets, Capsules & Suspension (Pennwalt) p 1585

RESPIRATORY STIMULANTS
Coramine (CIBA) p 846
Dopram Injectable (Robins) p 428, 1650

S

SCABICIDES
(see under ANTIPARASITICS)

SCLEROSING AGENTS
Sotradecol Injection (Elkins-Sinn) p 941

SEDATIVES
Barbiturates
Alurate Elixir (Roche) p 1667
Amytal (Lilly) p 417, 1127
Amytal Sodium Pulvules (Lilly) p 417, 1128
Buff-A Comp Tablets (Mayrand) p 1196
Butisol Sodium Elixir & Tablets (Wallace) p 442, 2150

Product Category Index

Levsin/Phenobarbital Tablets, Elixir & Drops (Rorer) p 1751
Levsinex/Phenobarbital Timecaps (Rorer) p 1751
Mebaral (Winthrop-Breon) p 444, 2213
Nembutal Sodium Capsules (Abbott) p 403, 538
Nembutal Sodium Solution (Abbott) p 541
Nembutal Sodium Suppositories (Abbott) p 543
Pentobarbital Sodium in Tubex (Wyeth) p 2288
Pentothal (Abbott) p 562
Phenobarbital Sodium in Tubex (Wyeth) p 2288
Secobarbital Sodium in Tubex (Wyeth) p 2288
Seconal Sodium Pulvules & Vials (Lilly) p 417, 1172
Sedapap-10 Tablets (Mayrand) p 1196
Solfoton Tablets & Capsules (Poythress) p 1619
Tuinal (Lilly) p 417, 1176

Non-Barbiturates
Ativan Injection (Wyeth) p 2237
Dalmane Capsules (Roche Products) p 429, 1710
Equanil Tablets and Wyseals (Wyeth) p 444, 2252
Hydroxyzine HCl in Tubex (Wyeth) p 2288
Largon in Tubex (Wyeth) p 2288
Mepergan Injection (Wyeth) p 2264
Mepergan in Tubex (Wyeth) p 2288
Noctec Capsules & Syrup (Squibb) p 438, 2007
Phenergan Injection (Wyeth) p 2275
Phenergan in Tubex (Wyeth) p 2288
Phenergan Tablets & Rectal Suppositories (Wyeth) p 444, 445, 2278
Remsed Injection (Du Pont) p 926
Unisom Nighttime Sleep-Aid (Leeming) p 1119

SMOKING CESSATION AID
Nicorette (Merrell Dow) p 421, 1372

SUPPLEMENTS
(see under DIETARY SUPPLEMENTS)

SYMPATHOLYTICS
Bellergal Tablets (Sandoz Pharmaceutical Div.) p 432, 1798
Bellergal-S Tablets (Sandoz Pharmaceutical Div.) p 432, 1798
Regitine (CIBA) p 863
Yocon (Palisades Pharm.) p 1476
Yohimex Tablets (Kramer) p 1069

SYMPATHOMIMETICS & COMBINATIONS
Actifed with Codeine Cough Syrup (Burroughs Wellcome) p 773
Adrenalin Chloride Solution, Injectable (Parke-Davis) p 1480
Aerolate Liquid (Fleming) p 948
Aerolate Sr. & Jr. & III Capsules (Fleming) p 948
Aerolone Solution (Lilly) p 1126
Arlidin Tablets (USV Pharmaceutical) p 440, 2070
Brethine (Geigy) p 411, 955
Brethine Ampuls (Geigy) p 956
Bricanyl Injection (Merrell Dow) p 421, 1361
Bricanyl Tablets (Merrell Dow) p 421, 1361
Bronkephrine Hydrochloride Injection (Winthrop-Breon) p 2193
Bronkometer (Winthrop-Breon) p 2193
Bronkosol (Winthrop-Breon) p 2193
Comhist LA Capsules (Norwich Eaton) p 422, 1425
Comhist Tablets (Norwich Eaton) p 1426
Desoxyn (Abbott) p 515
Desoxyn Gradumet Tablets (Abbott) p 403, 515
Dexedrine (Smith Kline & French) p 436, 1959
Didrex Tablets (Upjohn) p 441, 2111
Efed II Capsules (Yellow) (Alto) p 404, 589
Entex Capsules (Norwich Eaton) p 1431
Entex LA Tablets (Norwich Eaton) p 422, 1432
Entex Liquid (Norwich Eaton) p 1431
Extendryl Chewable Tablets (Fleming) p 948
Extendryl Sr. & Jr. T.D. Capsules (Fleming) p 948
Extendryl Syrup (Fleming) p 948
Intropin (American Critical Care) p 596
Isuprel Hydrochloride Injection 1:5000 (Winthrop-Breon) p 2201
Isuprel Hydrochloride Mistometer (Winthrop-Breon) p 2203
Levophed Bitartrate (Winthrop-Breon) p 2205
Neo-Synephrine Hydrochloride 1% Injection (Winthrop-Breon) p 2216
Nolamine Tablets (Carnrick) p 408, 833
Novafed A Capsules (Merrell Dow) p 421, 1377
Novafed A Liquid (Merrell Dow) p 1377
Novafed Capsules (Merrell Dow) p 421, 1376
Novafed Liquid (Merrell Dow) p 1376
Novahistine DH (Merrell Dow) p 421, 1378
Novahistine Expectorant (Merrell Dow) p 421, 1378
Otrivin (Geigy) p 963
Rondec Oral Drops (Ross) p 1776
Rondec Syrup (Ross) p 1776
Rondec Tablet (Ross) p 432, 1776
Rondec-TR Tablet (Ross) p 432, 1776
Singlet (Merrell Dow) p 421, 1385
Sus-Phrine (Berlex) p 406, 704
Triaminic Expectorant (Dorsey Laboratories) p 911
Triaminic Expectorant w/Codeine (Dorsey Laboratories) p 911
Triaminic Juvelets (Dorsey Laboratories) p 912
Triaminic Oral Infant Drops (Dorsey Laboratories) p 912
Triaminic TR Tablets (Timed Release) (Dorsey Laboratories) p 912
Triaminicol Multi-Symptom Cold Syrup (Dorsey Laboratories) p 913
Triaminicol Multi-Symptom Cold Tablets (Dorsey Laboratories) p 914
Tussend Expectorant (Merrell Dow) p 421, 1394
Tussend Liquid & Tablets (Merrell Dow) p 421, 1393
Ventolin Inhaler (Glaxo) p 412, 987

T

THERAPEUTIC DRUG ASSAYS
Ames TDA Therapeutic Drug Assays (Ames) p 3004

THROAT LOZENGES
Children's Chloraseptic Lozenges (Procter & Gamble) p 1619
Chloraseptic Lozenges (Procter & Gamble) p 1620
Throat Discs Throat Lozenges (Marion) p 1190

THROMBOLYTICS
Abbokinase (Abbott) p 502
Abbokinase Open-Cath (Abbott) p 505
Kabikinase (Pharmacia) p 1616
Streptase (Hoechst-Roussel) p 1018

THYROID PREPARATIONS
Antithyroid
Tapazole (Lilly) p 1175

Synthetic Thyroid Hormone
Levothroid for Injection (USV Pharmaceutical) p 440, 2079
Levothroid Tablets (USV Pharmaceutical) p 440, 2080
Synthroid (Flint) p 411, 951
Thyrolar Tablets (USV Pharmaceutical) p 440, 2091

Thyroid
Armour Thyroid Tablets (USV Pharmaceutical) p 440, 2089
Cytomel Tablets (Smith Kline & French) p 436, 1956
Euthroid (Parke-Davis) p 424, 1520
Levothroid for Injection (USV Pharmaceutical) p 440, 2079
Levothroid Tablets (USV Pharmaceutical) p 440, 2080
Proloid Tablets (Parke-Davis) p 425, 1565
S-P-T (Fleming) p 949
Synthroid (Flint) p 411, 951
Thyroid Strong Tablets (Marion) p 418, 1190
Thyroid Tablets (Marion) p 418, 1190
Thyrolar Tablets (USV Pharmaceutical) p 440, 2091

Thyrotropic Hormone
Thytropar (Armour) p 612

Thyroxine Sodium
Synthroid (Flint) p 411, 951

TONICS
Alba-Lybe (Bart) p 685
Enviro-Stress with Zinc & Selenium (Vitaline) p 2148
Hemo-Vite (Drug Industries) p 914
Hemo-Vite Liquid (Drug Industries) p 914
Hep-Forte Capsules (Marlyn) p 1193
Hytinic Capsules & Elixir (Hyrex) p 1024
I.L.X. B_{12} Elixir Crystalline (Kenwood) p 1046
I.L.X. B_{12} Tablets (Kenwood) p 1046
Megadose (Arco) p 600
Niferex Tablets/Elixir (Central Pharmaceuticals) p 838
Niferex w/Vitamin C (Central Pharmaceuticals) p 838
Nu-Iron Elixir (Mayrand) p 1196
Revitalin-SL 90 Adult Supplement (Robertson/Taylor) p 1646
Testorex-35 Adult Male Supplement (Robertson/Taylor) p 1646

TRACE MINERALS
Chrometrace (Armour) p 604
Coppertrace (Armour) p 605
Mangatrace (Armour) p 607
Multitrace 5 (Armour) p 608
Multitrace Pediatric (Armour) p 609
Selenitrace (Armour) p 610
Zinctrace (Armour) p 612

TRANQUILIZERS
Benzodiazepine
Ativan in Tubex (Wyeth) p 2288
Ativan Injection (Wyeth) p 2237
Ativan Tablets (Wyeth) p 444, 2236
Centrax (Parke-Davis) p 423, 1487
Libritabs Tablets (Roche Products) p 430, 1714
Librium Capsules (Roche Products) p 430, 1714
Librium Injectable (Roche Products) p 1715
Limbitrol Tablets (Roche Products) p 430, 1716
Menrium Tablets (Roche Products) p 430, 1717
Paxipam Tablets (Schering) p 434, 1876
Serax Capsules, Tablets (Wyeth) p 445, 2287
Tranxene Capsules & Tablets (Abbott) p 404, 568
Tranxene-SD (Abbott) p 404, 568
Tranxene-SD Half Strength (Abbott) p 404, 568
Valium Injectable (Roche Products) p 430, 1721
Valium Tablets (Roche Products) p 430, 1723
Valrelease Capsules (Roche) p 430, 1707
Xanax Tablets (Upjohn) p 441, 2142

Butyrophenones & Combinations
Haldol Tablets, Concentrate, Injection (McNeil Pharmaceutical) p 418, 1201
Inapsine Injection (Janssen) p 1034
Innovar Injection (Janssen) p 1035

Hydroxyzines
Atarax Tablets & Syrup (Roerig) p 431, 1725
Durrax Tablets 10mg, 25mg (Dermik) p 888
Hydroxyzine HCl in Tubex (Wyeth) p 2288
Vistaril Capsules and Oral Suspension (Pfizer) p 427, 1612
Vistaril Intramuscular Solution (Pfipharmecs) p 1598

Lithium Preparations
Eskalith Capsules & Tablets (Smith Kline & French) p 437, 1964
Eskalith CR Controlled Release Tablets (Smith Kline & French) p 437, 1964
Lithane (Miles Pharmaceuticals) p 422, 1403
Lithium Carbonate Capsules & Tablets (Roxane) p 1789
Lithium Citrate Syrup (Roxane) p 1790

Meprobamate & Combinations
Deprol (Wallace) p 2155
Equanil Tablets and Wyseals (Wyeth) p 444, 2252
Meprospan (Wallace) p 2161
Miltown (Wallace) p 442, 2162
Miltown 600 (Wallace) p 442, 2162
PMB 200 & PMB 400 (Ayerst) p 405, 660
Pathibamate (Lederle) p 415, 1110

Phenothiazines & Combinations
Chlorpromazine HCl in Tubex (Wyeth) p 2288
Compazine (Smith Kline & French) p 436, 1953
Etrafon Tablets (Schering) p 434, 1841
Mellaril (Sandoz Pharmaceutical Div.) p 433, 1804
Mellaril-S (Sandoz Pharmaceutical Div.) p 1804
Permitil Oral Concentrate (Schering) p 1877
Permitil Tablets (Schering) p 434, 1877
Prolixin Decanoate (Squibb) p 2015
Prolixin Elixir & Injection (Squibb) p 2014
Prolixin Tablets (Squibb) p 438, 2014
Quide (Merrell Dow) p 1379
Serentil Ampuls (Boehringer Ingelheim) p 714
Serentil Concentrate (Boehringer Ingelheim) p 714
Serentil Tablets (Boehringer Ingelheim) p 406, 714
Stelazine (Smith Kline & French) p 437, 1971
Thorazine (Smith Kline & French) p 437, 1977
Triavil Tablets (Merck Sharp & Dohme) p 420, 1354
Trilafon Tablets, Repetabs Tablets, Concentrate & Injection (Schering) p 435, 1888

Product Category Index

Rauwolfia Serpentina
Raudixin Tablets (Squibb) p 438, 2020
Reserpine
Serpasil Parenteral Solution (CIBA) p 868
Serpasil Tablets (CIBA) p 409, 867
Thioxanthenes
Navane Capsules and Concentrate (Roerig) p 431, 1737
Navane Intramuscular (Roerig) p 1739
Other
Loxitane C Oral Concentrate (Lederle) p 415, 1096
Loxitane Capsules (Lederle) p 415, 1096
Loxitane IM (Lederle) p 415, 1096
Moban Tablets & Concentrate (Du Pont) p 410, 921
Orap Tablets (McNeil Pharmaceutical) p 1203
Sinequan (Roerig) p 431, 1740
Trancopal (Winthrop-Breon) p 444, 2232

TUBERCULOSIS PREPARATIONS

BCG Vaccine (Glaxo) p 976
Capastat Sulfate (Lilly) p 1132
INH Tablets (CIBA) p 850
Myambutol Tablets (Lederle) p 1106
Rifadin (Merrell Dow) p 421, 1382
Rifamate (Merrell Dow) p 421, 1383
Rimactane Capsules (CIBA) p 409, 864
Seromycin (Lilly) p 1174
Trecator-SC (Ives) p 1031

U

UNIT DOSE SYSTEMS

A.P.C. with Codeine Nos. 3 & 4, Tabloid brand (Burroughs Wellcome) p 407, 780
Abbo-Pac (Abbott) p 502
Acetaminophen Elixir, Tablets, Suppositories (Roxane) p 1788
Acetaminophen with Codeine Phosphate Tablets (Roxane) p 1788
Aldactazide (Searle & Co.) p 435, 1912
Aldactone (Searle & Co.) p 435, 1914
Aluminum Hydroxide Gel (Roxane) p 1788
Aluminum Hydroxide Gel-Concentrated (Roxane) p 1788
Aluminum Hydroxide Tablets (Roxane) p 1788
Aluminum & Magnesium Hydroxides with Simethicone I (Roxane) p 1788
Aluminum & Magnesium Hydroxides with Simethicone II (Roxane) p 1788
Aminophyllin Tablets (Searle & Co.) p 435, 1915
Aminophylline Tablets & Oral Solution (Roxane) p 1788
Amitriptyline Hydrochloride Tablets (Roxane) p 1788
Antivert, Antivert/25 Tablets, Antivert/25 Chewable Tablets & Antivert/50 Tablets (Roerig) p 431, 1725
Aquaphyllin Syrup (Ferndale) p 942
Aromatic Cascara Fluidextract (Roxane) p 1788
Ascorbic Acid Tablets (Roxane) p 1788
Aspirin Suppositories (Roxane) p 1788
Atarax Tablets & Syrup (Roerig) p 431, 1725
Ativan in Tubex (Wyeth) p 2288
Azulfidine Tablets, EN-tabs, Oral Suspension (Pharmacia) p 427, 1613
Bactrim DS Tablets (Roche) p 429, 1674
Bactrim Tablets (Roche) p 429, 1674
Bicillin C-R in Tubex (Wyeth) p 2288
Bicillin C-R 900/300 in Tubex (Wyeth) p 2288
Bicitra—Sugar-Free (Willen) p 2187
Bisacodyl Patient Pack, Suppositories, Tablets (Roxane) p 1788
Brethine (Geigy) p 411, 955
Bumex Injection (Roche) p 1678
Bumex Tablets (Roche) p 429, 1678
Butazolidin Capsules & Tablets (Geigy) p 411, 956
Calan Tablets (Searle & Co.) p 435, 1917
Calcium Carbonate Tablets & Oral Suspension (Roxane) p 1788
Calcium Gluconate Tablets (Roxane) p 1788
Castor Oil, Castor Oil Favored (Roxane) p 1788
Chloral Hydrate Capsules, Syrup (Roxane) p 1788
Chlordiazepoxide Hydrochloride Capsules (BCG) (Roxane) p 1788
Chlorpheniramine Maleate Tablets (Roxane) p 1788
Chlorpromazine HCl in Tubex (Wyeth) p 2288
Cocaine Hydrochloride Topical Solution (Roxane) p 1788
Codeine Phosphate in Tubex (Wyeth) p 2288
Codeine Phosphate Oral Solution (Roxane) p 1788
Codeine Sulfate Tablets (Roxane) p 1788
Constant-T Tablets (Geigy) p 411, 958
Corgard (Squibb) p 437, 1989

Cyanocobalamin in Tubex (Wyeth) p 445, 2288
Cytoxan (Bristol-Myers Oncology) p 407, 759
DHT (Dihydrotachysterol) Tablets, Oral Solution & Intensol (Roxane) p 1789
Dalmane Capsules (Roche Products) p 429, 1710
Dayalets Filmtab (Abbott) p 511
Dexamethasone Sodium Phosphate in Tubex (Wyeth) p 2288
Dexamethasone Tablets, Oral Solution & Intensol (Roxane) p 1788
Digoxin in Tubex (Wyeth) p 2288
Diluent (Flavored) for Oral Use (Roxane) p 1788
Dimenhydrinate in Tubex (Wyeth) p 2288
Dimetapp Elixir (Robins) p 1648
Dimetapp Extentabs (Robins) p 428, 1648
Diphenhydramine Hydrochloride Capsules, Elixir (Roxane) p 1788
Diphenhydramine HCl in Tubex (Wyeth) p 2288
Diphenoxylate Hydrochloride & Atropine Sulfate Tablets & Oral Solution (Roxane) p 1788
Diphtheria & Tetanus Toxoids Adsorbed, Pediatric, in Tubex (Wyeth) p 2288
Dispenser Strip (Lilly) p 1122
Ditropan Tablets (Marion) p 417, 1184
Docusate Sodium Capsules, Syrup (Roxane) p 1788
Docusate Sodium with Casanthranol Capsules (Roxane) p 1788
Donnatal Elixir (Robins) p 1648
Donnatal Extentabs (Robins) p 428, 1649
Donnatal Tablets (Robins) p 428, 1648
Dramamine Tablets (Searle Pharmaceuticals) p 435, 1906
E.E.S. Chewable Tablets (Abbott) p 403, 522
E.E.S. Granules (Abbott) p 522
E.E.S. 400 Filmtab (Abbott) p 403, 522
Elixophyllin Capsules (Berlex) p 406, 699
Elixophyllin SR Capsules (Berlex) p 406, 699
Empirin with Codeine (Burroughs Wellcome) p 408, 787
Empracet with Codeine Phosphate Nos. 3 & 4 (Burroughs Wellcome) p 408, 789
Endep Tablets (Roche Products) p 429, 1711
Enduron Tablets (Abbott) p 403, 517
Enduronyl Forte Tablets (Abbott) p 403, 518
Enduronyl Tablets (Abbott) p 403, 518
Epinephrine in Tubex (Wyeth) p 2288
Erythrocin Piggyback (Abbott) p 403, 524
Erythrocin Stearate Filmtab (Abbott) p 403, 525
Erythromycin Base Filmtab (Abbott) p 403, 526
Ethatab (Glaxo) p 980
Evac-Q-Kit (Adria) p 575
Evac-Q-Kwik (Adria) p 575
Fero-Grad-500 (Abbott) p 403, 530
Ferrous Sulfate Liquid, Tablets (Roxane) p 1788
Flagyl Tablets (Searle & Co.) p 436, 1929
Fleet Bisacodyl Enema (Fleet) p 946
Fleet Enema (Fleet) p 946
Fleet Flavored Castor Oil Emulsion (Fleet) p 947
Fleet Mineral Oil Enema (Fleet) p 947
Fleet Phospho-Soda (Fleet) p 947
Fleet Prep Kits (Fleet) p 947
Furadantin Tablets (Norwich Eaton) p 1432
Furosemide Injection (Wyeth) p 2252
Gantanol Tablets (Roche) p 429, 1685
Gantrisin Tablets (Roche) p 429, 1686
Geocillin Tablets (Roerig) p 431, 1730
Guaifenesin Syrup (Roxane) p 1788
Haldol Tablets, Concentrate, Injection (McNeil Pharmaceutical) p 418, 1201
Heparin Lock Flush Solution in Tubex (Wyeth) p 2253
Heparin Sodium in Tubex (Wyeth) p 2288
Heparin Sodium Injection (Wyeth) p 2254
Hurricaine Liquid 1/4cc Unit Dose (Beutlich) p 705
Hydrochlorothiazide Tablets, Liquids, Intensol & Oral Solution (Roxane) p 1788
Hydromorphone HCl in Tubex (Wyeth) p 2288
Hydroxyzine HCl in Tubex (Wyeth) p 2288
Iberet-500 (Abbott) p 403, 532
Identi-Dose (Lilly) p 1122
Ilopan Injection (Adria) p 578
Imipramine Hydrochloride Tablets (Roxane) p 1788
Immune Serum Globulin (Human) in Tubex (Wyeth) p 2288
Influenza Virus Vaccine Subvirion Type in Tubex (Wyeth) p 2288
Ipecac Syrup (Roxane) p 1788
Isoetharine Hydrochloride Inhalation (Roxane) p 1788
Isoxsuprine Hydrochloride Tablets (Roxane) p 1788
K-Lor Powder (Abbott) p 403, 533
Kaochlor 10% Liquid (Adria) p 579

Kaochlor S-F 10% Liquid (Sugar-free) (Adria) p 580
Kaolin-Pectin-Concentrated (Roxane) p 1788
Kaolin-Pectin Suspension (Roxane) p 1788
Kaon Cl-10 (Adria) p 404, 582
Kaon Elixir, Grape Flavor (Adria) p 580
Kaon Tablets (Adria) p 404, 581
Kaon-Cl Tabs (Adria) p 404, 581
Kay Ciel Powder (Berlex) p 702
Lanoxin (Burroughs Wellcome) p 408, 797
Largon in Tubex (Wyeth) p 2288
Librax Capsules (Roche Products) p 430, 1713
Librium Capsules (Roche Products) p 430, 1714
Lidocaine HCl in Tubex (Wyeth) p 2288
Limbitrol Tablets (Roche Products) p 430, 1716
Lioresal Tablets (Geigy) p 411, 959
Lithium Carbonate Capsules & Tablets (Roxane) p 1789
Lomotil Tablets (Searle & Co.) p 436, 1931
Lopressor Tablets (Geigy) p 411, 960
Lopurin (Boots) p 406, 718
Macrodantin Capsules (Norwich Eaton) p 422, 1436
Magnesia & Alumina Oral Suspension (Roxane) p 1788
Mepergan in Tubex (Wyeth) p 2288
Meperidine HCl in Tubex (Wyeth) p 2288
Metamucil, Instant Mix, Regular Flavor (Searle Consumer Products) p 1911
Metamucil, Powder, Regular Flavor (Searle Consumer Products) p 1911
Metamucil, Powder, Sugar Free, Regular Flavor (Searle Consumer Products) p 1911
Methadone Hydrochloride Oral Solution & Tablets (Roxane) p 1791
Methocarbamol Tablets (Roxane) p 1788
Micro-K Extencaps (Robins) p 428, 1653
Micro-K 10 Extencaps (Robins) p 1653
Milk of Magnesia, Milk of Magnesia-Concentrated (Roxane) p 1788
Milk of Magnesia-Cascara Suspension Concentrated (Roxane) p 1788
Milk of Magnesia-Mineral Oil Emulsion & Emulsion (Flavored) (Roxane) p 1788
Mineral Oil-Light Sterile, Mineral Oil (Roxane) p 1788
Modane, Tablets & Liquid (Adria) p 584
Morphine Sulfate Oral Solution (Roxane) p 1792
Morphine Sulfate Tablets (Roxane) p 1792
Morphine Sulfate in Tubex (Wyeth) p 2288
Mycostatin Oral Suspension (Squibb) p 2004
Mycostatin Oral Tablets (Squibb) p 438, 2005
Mycostatin Vaginal Tablets (Squibb) p 438, 2005
Mysteclin-F Capsules (Squibb) p 438, 2005
Navane Capsules and Concentrate (Roerig) p 431, 1737
Nembutal Sodium Capsules (Abbott) p 403, 538
Neomycin Sulfate Tablets (Roxane) p 1788
Neosporin Ointment (Burroughs Wellcome) p 808
Niacin Tablets (Roxane) p 1788
Noctec Capsules & Syrup (Squibb) p 438, 2007
Norpace Capsules (Searle & Co.) p 436, 1933
Norpace CR Capsules (Searle & Co.) p 436, 1933
Oretic (Abbott) p 403, 554
Oxycodone Hydrochloride Oral Solution & Tablets (Roxane) p 1792
Oxycodone Hydrochloride USP Single Entity Tablets & Liquid (Roxane) p 1788
Oxycodone Hydrochloride & Acetaminophen Tablets (Roxane) p 1788
Oxycodone Hydrochloride, Oxycodone Terephthalate & Aspirin Tablets (Full Strength) (Roxane) p 1788
Oxytocin in Tubex (Wyeth) p 2288
Panwarfin (Abbott) p 403, 558
Papaverine Hydrochloride Capsules (Roxane) p 1788
Parafon Forte Tablets (McNeil Pharmaceutical) p 419, 1206
Paregoric (Roxane) p 1788
Pavabid Capsules (Marion) p 418, 1189
Pentids Tablets, Pentids 400 & 800 Tablets (Squibb) p 438, 2011
Pentobarbital Sodium in Tubex (Wyeth) p 2288
Peri-Colace (Mead Johnson Pharmaceutical) p 419, 1255
Phenaphen w/Codeine Capsules (Robins) p 428, 1656
Phenaphen-650 with Codeine Tablets (Robins) p 428, 1656
Phenergan in Tubex (Wyeth) p 2288
Phenobarbital Elixir, Tablets (Roxane) p 1788
Phenobarbital Sodium in Tubex (Wyeth) p 2288
Placidyl (Abbott) p 403, 566

Product Category Index

Polysporin Ointment (Burroughs Wellcome) p 810
Potassium Chloride for Oral Solution (Flavored), Oral Solution, Powder (Unflavored) (Roxane) p 1788
Potassium Chloride Oral Solution, Powder & for Oral Solution (Roxane) p 1793
Potassium Gluconate Elixir (Roxane) p 1788
Potassium Iodide Liquid (Roxane) p 1788
Potassium Phosphates Oral Solution (Roxane) p 1788
Prednisolone Tablets (Roxane) p 1788
Principen Capsules (Squibb) p 438, 2012
Principen for Oral Suspension (Squibb) p 2012
Pro-Banthine Tablets (Searle & Co.) p 436, 1936
Pro-Banthine w/Phenobarbital (Searle & Co.) p 436, 1936
Prochlorperazine Edisylate in Tubex (Wyeth) p 2288
Prolixin Decanoate (Squibb) p 2015
Prolixin Tablets (Squibb) p 438, 2014
Prompt (Searle Consumer Products) p 1912
Pronestyl Capsules and Tablets (Squibb) p 438, 2017
Pronestyl-SR Tablets (Squibb) p 438, 2019
Propantheline Bromide Tablets (Roxane) p 1788
Propoxyphene Hydrochloride Capsules (Roxane) p 1788
Pseudoephedrine Hydrochloride Tablets (Roxane) p 1788
Quinaglute Dura-Tabs (Berlex) p 406, 702
Quinidex Extentabs (Robins) p 428, 1659
Quinidine Gluconate Sustained Release Tablets (Roxane) p 1788
Quinidine Sulfate Tablets (Roxane) p 1788
Reglan Tablets (Robins) p 428, 1659
Reverse-numbered Package (Lilly) p 1122
Robaxin Tablets (Robins) p 428, 1662
Robaxin-750 Tablets (Robins) p 428, 1662
Robaxisal Tablets (Robins) p 429, 1662
Secobarbital Sodium in Tubex (Wyeth) p 2288
Septra DS Tablets (Burroughs Wellcome) p 408, 815
Septra Tablets (Burroughs Wellcome) p 408, 815
Sinequan (Roerig) p 431, 1740
Slo-bid Gyrocaps (Rorer) p 432, 1754
Slo-Phyllin Gyrocaps, Tablets (Rorer) p 432, 1756
Slo-Phyllin 80 Syrup (Rorer) p 1756
Slo-Phyllin GG Capsules, Syrup (Rorer) p 432, 1759
Sodium Chloride, Bacteriostatic in Tubex (Wyeth) p 2288
Sodium Chloride Inhalation (Roxane) p 1788
Sodium Phosphates Oral Solution (Roxane) p 1788
Sodium Polystyrene Sulfonate Suspension (Roxane) p 1794
Sparine Injection in Tubex (Wyeth) p 2288
Summer's Eve Medicated Douche (Fleet) p 948
Sumycin Capsules (Squibb) p 438, 2022
Sustaire Tablets (Roerig) p 431, 1743
Synthroid (Flint) p 411, 951
Tandearil (Geigy) p 411, 964
Tegretol Chewable Tablets (Geigy) p 411, 966
Tegretol Tablets (Geigy) p 411, 966
Tel-E-Dose (Roche) p 430, 1705
Terpin Hydrate & Codeine Elixir (Roxane) p 1788
Tetanus & Diphtheria Toxoids Adsorbed (Adult) in Tubex (Wyeth) p 2288
Tetanus Immune Globulin (Human) in Tubex (Wyeth) p 2288
Tetanus Toxoid Adsorbed, Aluminum Phosphate Adsorbed, Ultrafined in Tubex (Wyeth) p 2288
Tetanus Toxoid Fluid, Purified, Ultrafined in Tubex (Wyeth) p 2288
Theo-24 (Searle & Co.) p 436, 1937
Theobid, Theobid Jr. Duracap (Glaxo) p 412, 982
Theophylline Oral Solution (Roxane) p 1788
Theragran Tablets (Squibb) p 438, 2025
Theragran-M Tablets (Squibb) p 438, 2025
Thiamine HCl in Tubex (Wyeth) p 2288
Thioridazine Hydrochloride Tablets (Roxane) p 1788
Tofranil Tablets (Geigy) p 411, 969
Tofranil-PM Capsules (Geigy) p 411, 971
Tranxene Capsules & Tablets (Abbott) p 404, 568
Trimox Capsules & for Oral Suspension (Squibb) p 438, 2025
Triprolidine Hydrochloride & Pseudoephedrine Hydrochloride Syrup, Tablets (Roxane) p 1788
Tubex (Wyeth) p 445, 2288
Tylenol, Extra-Strength, acetaminophen Liquid Pain Reliever (McNeil Consumer Products) p 1200

Tylenol, Extra-Strength, acetaminophen Tablets, Capsules & Caplets (McNeil Consumer Products) p 418, 1200
Tylenol, Regular Strength, acetaminophen Tablets & Capsules (McNeil Consumer Products) p 418, 1199
Tylenol w/Codeine Tablets, Capsules (McNeil Pharmaceutical) p 419, 1214
Tylox Capsules (McNeil Pharmaceutical) p 419, 1215
Valium Injectable (Roche Products) p 430, 1721
Valium Tablets (Roche Products) p 430, 1723
Veetids Tablets (Squibb) p 438, 2026
Velosef Capsules (Squibb) p 438, 2027
Vicon Forte Capsules (Glaxo) p 412, 989
Vicon-C Capsules (Glaxo) p 412, 989
Wyamine Sulfate in Tubex (Wyeth) p 2288
Wycillin in Tubex (Wyeth) p 2288
Zyloprim (Burroughs Wellcome) p 408, 825

UNNA BOOT
Primer Unna Boot (Glenwood) p 999

URICOSURIC AGENTS
Anturane Tablets & Capsules (CIBA) p 409, 842
Benemid Tablets (Merck Sharp & Dohme) p 420, 1268
ColBENEMID Tablets (Merck Sharp & Dohme) p 420, 1277

URINARY ACIDIFIERS
K-Phos M.F. (Modified Formula) Tablets (Beach) p 405, 686
K-Phos No. 2 Tablets (Beach) p 405, 686
K-Phos Original Formula 'Sodium Free' Tablets (Beach) p 405, 686
Pedameth Capsules (O'Neal, Jones & Feldman) p 422, 1445
Pedameth Liquid (O'Neal, Jones & Feldman) p 1445
pHos-pHaid (Guardian) p 1000
Thiacide Tablets (Beach) p 405, 687
Uro-Phosphate Tablets (Poythress) p 1619
Uroqid-Acid Tablets (Beach) p 405, 687
Uroqid-Acid No. 2 Tablets (Beach) p 405, 687

URINARY ALKALINIZING AGENTS
Bicitra—Sugar-Free (Willen) p 2187
Polycitra Syrup (Willen) p 2188
Polycitra-K Syrup (Willen) p 2189
Polycitra-LC—Sugar-Free (Willen) p 2188

URINARY TRACT ANALGESIC
Azo Gantanol Tablets (Roche) p 429, 1670
Azo Gantrisin Tablets (Roche) p 429, 1671
Pyridium (Parke-Davis) p 425, 1567
Pyridium Plus (Parke-Davis) p 425, 1568
Renoquid (Glenwood) p 412, 999
Thiosulfil Duo-Pak (Ayerst) p 682
Thiosulfil-A Forte (Ayerst) p 405, 681
Thiosulfil-A Tablets (Ayerst) p 405, 681

UROLOGICAL IRRIGANTS
Renacidin (Guardian) p 1000

UTERINE CONTRACTANTS
Oxytocin in Tubex (Wyeth) p 2288

UTERINE, MUSCLE CONTRACTION INHIBITOR
Yutopar Intravenous Injection (Astra) p 632
Yutopar Tablets (Astra) p 632

V

VAGINAL THERAPEUTICS
Capsules, Tablets
Flagyl Tablets (Searle & Co.) p 436, 1929
Gyne-Lotrimin Vaginal Tablets (Schering) p 434, 1856
Metric 21 Tablets (Fielding) p 942
Mycelex-G (Miles Pharmaceuticals) p 422, 1410
Mycostatin Vaginal Tablets (Squibb) p 438, 2005
Nilstat Vaginal Tablets (Lederle) p 1108
O-V Statin (Squibb) p 2008
Sultrin Triple Sulfa Vaginal Tablets (Ortho Pharmaceutical) p 1472
Creams
AVC Cream (Merrell Dow) p 1358
Amino-Cerv (Milex) p 1415
DV Cream (Merrell Dow) p 1364
Gyne-Lotrimin Vaginal Cream 1% (Schering) p 1856
Monistat 7 Vaginal Cream (Ortho Pharmaceutical) p 423, 1455
Mycelex-G 1% Vaginal Cream (Miles Pharmaceuticals) p 1410
Ogen Vaginal Cream (Abbott) p 551
Ortho Dienestrol Cream (Ortho Pharmaceutical) p 1457

Premarin Vaginal Cream (Ayerst) p 405, 670
Sultrin Triple Sulfa Cream (Ortho Pharmaceutical) p 1472
Douches
Betadine Disposable Medicated Douche (Purdue Frederick) p 1622
Betadine Douche (Purdue Frederick) p 1622
Massengill Disposable Douche (Beecham Products) p 687
Massengill Liquid Concentrate (Beecham Products) p 687
Massengill Medicated Disposable Douche (Beecham Products) p 688
Massengill Powder (Beecham Products) p 687
Pro-Ception (Milex) p 1415
Prophyllin (Rystan) p 1796
Summer's Eve Medicated Douche (Fleet) p 948
Trichotine Liquid, Vaginal Douche (Reed & Carnrick) p 1637
Trichotine Powder, Vaginal Douche (Reed & Carnrick) p 1637
Triva Combination (Boyle) p 726
Triva Douche Powder (Boyle) p 726
Vagisec Medicated Liquid Douche Concentrate (Schmid) p 1896
Inserts, Suppositories
AVC Suppositories (Merrell Dow) p 1358
Korostatin Vaginal Tablets (Youngs) p 2301
Monistat 3 Vaginal Suppositories (Ortho Pharmaceutical) p 1456
Monistat 7 Vaginal Suppositories (Ortho Pharmaceutical) p 423, 1456
Mycostatin Vaginal Tablets (Squibb) p 438, 2005
O-V Statin (Squibb) p 2008
Vagisec Plus Suppositories (Schmid) p 1896
Jellies, Ointments
Aci-Jel Therapeutic Vaginal Jelly (Ortho Pharmaceutical) p 1453
Betadine Antiseptic Gel (Purdue Frederick) p 1622
Triva Combination (Boyle) p 726
Triva Jel (Boyle) p 726
Trichomonacides
AVC Cream (Merrell Dow) p 1358
AVC Suppositories (Merrell Dow) p 1358
Flagyl Tablets (Searle & Co.) p 436, 1929
Metric 21 Tablets (Fielding) p 942
Satric (Savage) p 433, 1825
Vagisec Medicated Liquid Douche Concentrate (Schmid) p 1896
Vagisec Plus Suppositories (Schmid) p 1896

VITAMINS
Geriatric
Al-Vite (Drug Industries) p 914
B-C-Bid Capsules (Geriatric) p 975
Berocca Parenteral Nutrition (Roche) p 1676
Berocca Plus Tablets (Roche) p 429, 1677
Berocca Tablets (Roche) p 429, 1677
Berocca-C & Berocca-C 500 (Roche) p 1678
Cevi-Bid Capsules (Geriatric) p 975
Cevi-Fer Capsules (sustained release) (Geriatric) p 975
Eldec Kapseals (Parke-Davis) p 424, 1514
Eldercaps (Mayrand) p 1196
Fosfree (Mission) p 1416
Geriplex-FS Kapseals (Parke-Davis) p 424, 1527
Geriplex-FS Liquid (Parke-Davis) p 1527
Hemo-Vite (Drug Industries) p 914
Hemo-Vite Liquid (Drug Industries) p 914
Iromin-G (Mission) p 1416
Mega-B (Arco) p 600
Megadose (Arco) p 600
Orexin Softab Tablets (Stuart) p 2034
Vicon Forte Capsules (Glaxo) p 412, 989
Vicon-C Capsules (Glaxo) p 412, 989
Vicon-Plus Capsules (Glaxo) p 412, 989
Vi-Zac Capsules (Glaxo) p 412, 990
Multivitamins
A.C.N. Tablets (Persōn & Covey) p 1587
Albafort Injectable (Bart) p 685
Alba-Lybe (Bart) p 685
Al-Vite (Drug Industries) p 914
B-C-Bid Capsules (Geriatric) p 975
Becotin (Dista) p 893
Becotin with Vitamin C (Dista) p 894
Beminal-500 (Ayerst) p 404, 639
Beminal Forte w/Vitamin C (Ayerst) p 639
Berocca Parenteral Nutrition (Roche) p 1676
Berocca Tablets (Roche) p 429, 1677
Berocca-C & Berocca-C 500 (Roche) p 1678
Dayalets Filmtab (Abbott) p 511
E.T. The Extra-Terrestrial Children's Chewable Vitamins (Squibb) p 438, 1994
Enviro-Stress with Zinc & Selenium (Vitaline) p 2148
Geriplex-FS Liquid (Parke-Davis) p 1527
Larobec Tablets (Roche) p 429, 1687
M.V.I. (Armour) p 404, 605
M.V.I. Concentrate (Armour) p 605
M.V.I. Pediatric (Armour) p 607
M.V.I.-12 (Armour) p 606

Product Category Index

M.V.I.-12 Lyophilized (Armour) p 606
Mega-B (Arco) p 600
Megadose (Arco) p 600
Multicebrin (Lilly) p 1169
Mulvidren-F Softab Tablets (Stuart) p 439, 2039
Nephrocaps (Fleming) p 948
Nu-Iron-V Tablets (Mayrand) p 1196
Probec-T Tablets (Stuart) p 439, 2040
Surbex Filmtab (Abbott) p 567
Surbex w/C Filmtab (Abbott) p 567
Therabid (Mission) p 1420
Thera-Combex H-P (Parke-Davis) p 425, 1574
Theragran Liquid (Squibb) p 2024
Theragran Tablets (Squibb) p 438, 2025
Tia-Doce Injectable Solution (Bart) p 685
Vicon Forte Capsules (Glaxo) p 412, 989
Vicon-C Capsules (Glaxo) p 412, 989
Vicon-Plus Capsules (Glaxo) p 412, 989
Vi-Daylin Chewable (Ross) p 432, 1784
Vi-Daylin Drops (Ross) p 1782
Vi-Daylin Liquid (Ross) p 1784
Vi-Daylin/F ADC + Iron Drops (Ross) p 1782
Vi-Daylin/F Drops (Ross) p 1783
Vi-Daylin/F + Iron Chewable (Ross) p 432, 1783
Vi-Daylin/F + Iron Drops (Ross) p 1783
Vio-Bec Forte (Rowell) p 1788
Vi-Penta Multivitamin Drops (Roche) p 1710
Vi-Zac Capsules (Glaxo) p 412, 990

Multivitamins with Minerals
Added Protection III Multi-Vitamin & Multi-Mineral Supplement (Professional Health) p 1621
Beminal Stress Plus (Ayerst) p 404, 640
Berocca Plus Tablets (Roche) p 429, 1677
Chromagen OB (Savage) p 1824
Clusivol Capsules (Ayerst) p 640
Clusivol Syrup (Ayerst) p 640
Clusivol 130 Tablets (Ayerst) p 640
Compete (Mission) p 1416
Dayalets plus Iron Filmtab (Abbott) p 511
E.T. The Extra-Terrestrial Children's Chewable Vitamins with Iron (Squibb) p 438, 1994
Eldercaps (Mayrand) p 1196
Fosfree (Mission) p 1416
Geriplex-FS Kapseals (Parke-Davis) p 424, 1527
Geriplex-FS Liquid (Parke-Davis) p 1527
Glutofac Tablets (Kenwood) p 1046
Hemo-Vite (Drug Industries) p 914
Hemo-Vite Liquid (Drug Industries) p 914
I.L.X. B_{12} Elixir Crystalline (Kenwood) p 1046
I.L.X. B_{12} Tablets (Kenwood) p 1046
Intraderm-19 Oral Acne Supplement (Robertson/Taylor) p 1645
Iromin-G (Mission) p 1416
Medi-Tec Vitamin-Mineral-Trace Mineral Supplement (Robertson/Taylor) p 1646
Megadose (Arco) p 600
Mevanin-C Capsules (Beutlich) p 705
Mi-Cebrin (Dista) p 903
Mi-Cebrin T (Dista) p 903
Mission Pre-Surgical (Mission) p 1419
Myadec (Parke-Davis) p 1543
Natabec Kapseals (Parke-Davis) p 424, 1545
Natabec Rx Kapseals (Parke-Davis) p 424, 1545
Poly-Vi-Flor 0.5 mg Vitamins w/Iron & Fluoride Chewable Tablets (Mead Johnson Nutritional) p 1245
Poly-Vi-Flor 1.0 mg Vitamins w/Iron & Fluoride Chewable Tablets (Mead Johnson Nutritional) p 1245
Poly-Vi-Flor 0.25 mg Vitamins w/Iron & Fluoride Drops (Mead Johnson Nutritional) p 1245
Poly-Vi-Flor 0.5 mg Vitamins w/Iron & Fluoride Drops (Mead Johnson Nutritional) p 1245
The Stuart Formula Tablets (Stuart) p 439, 2042
Stuart Prenatal Tablets (Stuart) p 439, 2034
Stuartnatal 1+1 Tablets (Stuart) p 439, 2043
Theragran Hematinic (Squibb) p 438, 2024
Theragran Stress Formula (Squibb) p 438, 2025
Theragran-M Tablets (Squibb) p 438, 2025
Total Formula (Vitaline) p 2148
Tri-Vi-Flor 0.25 mg Vitamins w/Iron & Fluoride Drops (Mead Johnson Nutritional) p 1248
VG Capsules (Medical Products) p 1256
Vicon Forte Capsules (Glaxo) p 412, 989
Vicon-C Capsules (Glaxo) p 412, 989
Vicon-Plus Capsules (Glaxo) p 412, 989
Vi-Daylin + Iron Chewable (Ross) p 432, 1784
Vi-Daylin Plus Iron Drops (Ross) p 1783
Vi-Daylin Plus Iron Liquid (Ross) p 1784
Vi-Zac Capsules (Glaxo) p 412, 990

Parenteral
Albafort Injectable (Bart) p 685
AquaMEPHYTON Injection (Merck Sharp & Dohme) p 1265
Berocca Parenteral Nutrition (Roche) p 1676
Berocca-C & Berocca-C 500 (Roche) p 1678
Cyanocobalamin in Tubex (Wyeth) p 445, 2288
Ilopan Injection (Adria) p 578
M.V.I. (Armour) p 404, 605
M.V.I. Concentrate (Armour) p 605
M.V.I. Pediatric (Armour) p 607
M.V.I.-12 (Armour) p 606
M.V.I.-12 Lyophilized (Armour) p 606
Synkayvite Injectable (Roche) p 1701
Thiamine HCl in Tubex (Wyeth) p 2288
Vita-Numonyl Injectable (Lambda) p 1071

Pediatric
Alba-Lybe (Bart) p 685
Cevi-Fer Capsules (sustained release) (Geriatric) p 975
E.T. The Extra-Terrestrial Children's Chewable Vitamins (Squibb) p 438, 1994
E.T. The Extra-Terrestrial Children's Chewable Vitamins with Iron (Squibb) p 438, 1994
Hemo-Vite (Drug Industries) p 914
Hemo-Vite Liquid (Drug Industries) p 914
Vi-Daylin ADC Drops (Ross) p 1782
Vi-Daylin Chewable (Ross) p 432, 1784
Vi-Daylin Drops (Ross) p 1782
Vi-Daylin Liquid (Ross) p 1784
Vi-Daylin Plus Iron ADC Drops (Ross) p 1784
Vi-Daylin + Iron Chewable (Ross) p 432, 1784
Vi-Daylin Plus Iron Drops (Ross) p 1783
Vi-Daylin Plus Iron Liquid (Ross) p 1784
Vi-Penta Infant Drops (Roche) p 1710
Vi-Penta Multivitamin Drops (Roche) p 1710

Pediatric with Fluoride
Mulvidren-F Softab Tablets (Stuart) p 439, 2039
Poly-Vi-Flor 0.25 mg Vitamins w/Fluoride Drops (Mead Johnson Nutritional) p 1244
Poly-Vi-Flor 1.0 mg Vitamins w/Fluoride Chewable Tablets (Mead Johnson Nutritional) p 1243
Poly-Vi-Flor 0.5 mg Vitamins w/Fluoride Drops (Mead Johnson Nutritional) p 1244
Poly-Vi-Flor 0.5 mg Vitamins w/Iron & Fluoride Chewable Tablets (Mead Johnson Nutritional) p 1245
Poly-Vi-Flor 1.0 mg Vitamins w/Iron & Fluoride Chewable Tablets (Mead Johnson Nutritional) p 1245
Poly-Vi-Flor 0.25 mg Vitamins w/Fluoride Drops (Mead Johnson Nutritional) p 1244
Poly-Vi-Flor 0.25 mg Vitamins w/Iron & Fluoride Drops (Mead Johnson Nutritional) p 1245
Poly-Vi-Flor 0.5 mg Vitamins w/Iron & Fluoride Drops (Mead Johnson Nutritional) p 1245
Tri-Vi-Flor 1.0 mg Vitamins w/Fluoride Chewable Tablets (Mead Johnson Nutritional) p 1246
Tri-Vi-Flor 0.25 mg Vitamins w/Fluoride Drops (Mead Johnson Nutritional) p 1247
Tri-Vi-Flor 0.5 mg Vitamins w/Fluoride Drops (Mead Johnson Nutritional) p 1247
Tri-Vi-Flor 0.25 mg Vitamins w/Iron & Fluoride Drops (Mead Johnson Nutritional) p 1248
Vi-Daylin/F ADC Drops (Ross) p 1782
Vi-Daylin/F Chewable (Ross) p 432, 1784
Vi-Daylin/F Drops (Ross) p 1783
Vi-Daylin/F + Iron Chewable (Ross) p 432, 1783
Vi-Daylin/F + Iron Drops (Ross) p 1783
Vi-Penta F Chewables (Roche) p 430, 1708
Vi-Penta F Infant Drops (Roche) p 1709
Vi-Penta F Multivitamin Drops (Roche) p 1709

Prenatal
Chromagen OB (Savage) p 1824
Filibon (Lederle) p 415, 1093
Filibon F.A. (Lederle) p 415, 1093
Filibon Forte (Lederle) p 415, 1093
Fosfree (Mission) p 1416
Hemo-Vite (Drug Industries) p 914
Hemo-Vite Liquid (Drug Industries) p 914
Iromin-G (Mission) p 1416
Materna 1•60 Tablets (Lederle) p 415, 1098
Mission Prenatal (Mission) p 1419
Mission Prenatal F.A. (Mission) p 1419
Mission Prenatal H.P. (Mission) p 1419
Mission Prenatal RX (Mission) p 1419
Natabec Kapseals (Parke-Davis) p 424, 1545
Natabec Rx Kapseals (Parke-Davis) p 424, 1545
Natafort Filmseal (Parke-Davis) p 424, 1545
Natalins Rx (Mead Johnson Laboratories) p 419, 1224
Natalins Tablets (Mead Johnson Laboratories) p 419, 1224
Nestabs FA Tablets (Fielding) p 942

Niferex-PN (Central Pharmaceuticals) p 409, 838
Nu-Iron-V Tablets (Mayrand) p 1196
Pramet FA (Ross) p 432, 1775
Pramilet FA (Ross) p 432, 1775
Stuart Prenatal Tablets (Stuart) p 439, 2034
Stuartnatal 1+1 Tablets (Stuart) p 439, 2043
Zenate Tablets (Reid-Provident Labs.) p 428, 1640

Therapeutic
Added Protection III Multi-Vitamin & Multi-Mineral Supplement (Professional Health) p 1621
Al-Vite (Drug Industries) p 914
B-C-Bid Capsules (Geriatric) p 975
Becotin-T (Dista) p 894
Berocca Parenteral Nutrition (Roche) p 1676
Berocca Plus Tablets (Roche) p 429, 1677
Berocca Tablets (Roche) p 429, 1677
Berocca-C & Berocca-C 500 (Roche) p 1678
Calciferol Drops (Egocalciferol Oral Solution USP) (Rorer) p 431, 1748
Calciferol in Oil Injection (Egocalciferol USP) (Rorer) p 431, 1748
Calciferol Tablets (Ergocalciferol USP) (Rorer) p 431, 1748
DL-Carnitine - Amino Acid Preparation (Tyson) p 2068
Cevi-Bid Capsules (Geriatric) p 975
DHT (Dihydrotachysterol) Tablets, Oral Solution & Intensol (Roxane) p 1789
Eldercaps (Mayrand) p 1196
Enviro-Stress with Zinc & Selenium (Vitaline) p 2148
Folic Acid Tablets (Lilly) p 1147
Hemo-Vite (Drug Industries) p 914
Hemo-Vite Liquid (Drug Industries) p 914
Hep-Forte Capsules (Marlyn) p 1193
Lyte-C (Tyson) p 2068
Mega-B (Arco) p 600
Megadose (Arco) p 600
Mi-Cebrin T (Dista) p 903
Nico-400 (Marion) p 418, 1186
Nicolar Tablets (USV Pharmaceutical) p 440, 2083
Therabid (Mission) p 1420
Theragran Hematinic (Squibb) p 438, 2024
Total Formula (Vitaline) p 2148
Vicon Forte Capsules (Glaxo) p 412, 989
Vicon-C Capsules (Glaxo) p 412, 989
Vicon-Plus Capsules (Glaxo) p 412, 989
Vio-Bec Forte (Rowell) p 1788
Vita-Numonyl Injectable (Lambda) p 1071
Vi-Zac Capsules (Glaxo) p 412, 990

Other
Aquasol A Capsules (Armour) p 404, 603
Aquasol A Drops (Armour) p 604
Aquasol E Capsules & Drops (Armour) p 404, 604
Beelith Tablets (Beach) p 405, 685
Calciferol Drops (Egocalciferol Oral Solution USP) (Rorer) p 431, 1748
Calciferol in Oil Injection (Egocalciferol USP) (Rorer) p 431, 1748
Calciferol Tablets (Ergocalciferol USP) (Rorer) p 431, 1748
Cefol Filmtab Tablets (Abbott) p 403, 510
Chlorophyll Complex Perles (Standard Process) p 2035
Folvite (Lederle) p 1093
Ilopan Injection (Adria) p 578
Leucovorin Calcium Injection (Lederle) p 415, 1096
Mega-B (Arco) p 600
Megadose (Arco) p 600
Nicobid (USV Pharmaceutical) p 440, 2083
Orexin Softab Tablets (Stuart) p 2034
Os-Cal Forte Tablets (Marion) p 418, 1189
Os-Cal Plus Tablets (Marion) p 418, 1189
Synkayvite Tablets (Roche) p 430, 1702
Vita-Numonyl Injectable (Lambda) p 1071
Wellcovorin Tablets (Burroughs Wellcome) p 408, 821
Zinc-220 Capsules (Alto) p 404, 589

X
X-RAY CONTRAST MEDIA
Amipaque (Winthrop-Breon) p 3018
Bilopaque Sodium (Winthrop-Breon) p 443, 3023
Hypaque Meglumine 60% (Winthrop-Breon) p 3039
Hypaque Sodium Oral Powder (Winthrop-Breon) p 3024
Hypaque Sodium Oral Solution (Winthrop-Breon) p 3025
Hypaque Sodium 20% (Winthrop-Breon) p 3026
Hypaque Sodium 25% (Winthrop-Breon) p 3028
Hypaque-Cysto (Winthrop-Breon) p 3030
Hypaque-M, 75% (Winthrop-Breon) p 3044
Hypaque-M, 90% (Winthrop-Breon) p 3053
Hypaque-76 Injection (Winthrop-Breon) p 3049
Telepaque (Winthrop-Breon) p 443, 3058

SECTION 4
Generic and Chemical Name Index

In this section the products described in the Product Information (White) and Diagnostic Product Information (Green) Sections are listed under generic and chemical name headings according to the principal ingredient(s). The headings under which products are listed have been determined by the Publisher with the cooperation of the individual manufacturers.

A

Acetaminophen
APAP w/Codeine Tablets (Geneva) p 973
APAP w/Codeine #3 (Geneva) p 973
APAP w/Codeine #4 (Geneva) p 973
Acetaco Tablets (Legere) p 1120
Acetaminophen Elixir, Tablets, Suppositories (Roxane) p 1788
Acetaminophen Uniserts Suppositories (Upsher-Smith) p 2144
Acetaminophen with Codeine Tablets and Capsules (Lemmon) p 1122
Acetaminophen with Codeine Phosphate Tablets (Roxane) p 1788
Algisin Capsules (RAM Laboratories) p 1632
Amacodone Tablets (Trimen) p 2067
Amaphen Capsules (Trimen) p 2067
Amaphen with Codeine #3 (Trimen) p 2067
Anacin-3, Children's Acetaminophen Chewable Tablets, Elixir, Drops (Whitehall) p 443, 2184
Anacin-3, Maximum Strength Acetaminophen Tablets and Capsules (Whitehall) p 443, 2185
Anacin-3 with Codeine Tablets (Ayerst) p 404, 634
Anoquan (Mallard) p 1181
Apap 300 mg. with Codeine Capsules & Tabs (Schein) p 1828
Apap with Codeine Elixir (Schein) p 1828
Bancap Capsules (O'Neal, Jones & Feldman) p 1444
Bancap c̄ Codeine Capsules (O'Neal, Jones & Feldman) p 1444
Bancap HC Capsules (O'Neal, Jones & Feldman) p 422, 1444
Butalbital and Acetaminophen Tablets (Danbury) p 887
Capital with Codeine Suspension (Carnrick) p 408, 831
Capital with Codeine Tablets (Carnrick) p 408, 831
Children's Panadol Chewable Tablets, Liquid, Drops (Glenbrook) p 412, 997
Chlorzone Forte Tablets (Schein) p 1828
Chlorzoxazone with APAP Tablets (Danbury) p 887
Chlorzoxasone w/APAP Tablets (Geneva) p 973
Codalan (Lannett) p 1071
Co-Gesic Tablets (Central Pharmaceuticals) p 409, 836
Compal Capsules (Reid-Provident Labs.) p 427, 1637
Comtrex (Bristol-Myers Products) p 769
Congespirin Aspirin-Free Chewable Cold Tablets for Children (Bristol-Myers Products) p 769
Congespirin Liquid Cold Medicine (Bristol-Myers Products) p 770
CoTylenol Cold Medication Tablets & Capsules (McNeil Consumer Products) p 418, 1197
CoTylenol Liquid Cold Medication (McNeil Consumer Products) p 1197
CoTylenol Children's Liquid Cold Formula (McNeil Consumer Products) p 418, 1198
Darvocet-N 50 (Lilly) p 417, 1136
Darvocet-N 100 (Lilly) p 417, 1136
Dia-Gesic (Central Pharmaceuticals) p 409, 837
Dolacet Capsules (Hauck) p 1001
Dolprn #3 Tablets (Bock) p 705
Dorcol Children's Fever & Pain Reducer (Dorsey Laboratories) p 909
Dristan, Advanced Formula Decongestant/Antihistamine/Analgesic Capsules (Whitehall) p 443, 2186
Dristan, Advanced Formula Decongestant/Antihistamine/Analgesic Tablets (Whitehall) p 443, 2186
Duradyne DHC Tablets (O'Neal, Jones & Feldman) p 1445
Empracet with Codeine Phosphate Nos. 3 & 4 (Burroughs Wellcome) p 408, 789
Esgic Tablets & Capsules (Gilbert) p 411, 975
Excedrin Extra-Strength (Bristol-Myers Products) p 770
Excedrin P.M. (Bristol-Myers Products) p 770
Extra-Strength Datril capsules & tablets (Bristol-Myers Products) p 770
Extra-Strength Sine-Aid Sinus Headache Capsules (McNeil Consumer Products) p 1199
G-1 Capsules (Hauck) p 1001
G-2 Capsules (Hauck) p 1001
G-3 Capsules (Hauck) p 1001
Hycomine Compound (Du Pont) p 919
Hyco-Pap (LaSalle) p 1071
Korigesic Tablets (Trimen) p 2067
Lorcet (UAD Labs.) p 2069
Lorcet-HD (UAD Labs.) p 2069
Maximum Strength Midol PMS (Glenbrook) p 997
Maximum Strength Panadol Capsules & Tablets (Glenbrook) p 412, 997
Midrin Capsules (Carnrick) p 408, 832
Migralam Capsules (Lambda) p 1071
Oxycodone Hydrochloride & Acetaminophen Tablets (Roxane) p 1788
Pacaps (LaSalle) p 1071
Parafon Forte Tablets (McNeil Pharmaceutical) p 419, 1206
Percocet (Du Pont) p 410, 925
Percogesic Analgesic Tablets (Vicks Pharmacy Products) p 442, 2147
Phenaphen w/Codeine Capsules (Robins) p 428, 1656
Phenaphen-650 with Codeine Tablets (Robins) p 428, 1656
Phenate (Mallard) p 1181
Phrenilin Tablets (Carnrick) p 408, 833
Phrenilin Forte (Carnrick) p 408, 833
Phrenilin with Codeine No. 3 (Carnrick) p 409, 834
Propoxyphene & Apap Tablets 65/650 (Schein) p 1828
Protid, Improved Formula (LaSalle) p 1071
Repan Tablets (Everett) p 942
SK-APAP with CODEINE Tablets (Smith Kline & French) p 1971
SK-Oxycodone with Acetaminophen Tablets (Smith Kline & French) p 1971
SK-65 APAP Tablets (Smith Kline & French) p 1971
Saleto (Mallard) p 1181
Sedapap-10 Tablets (Mayrand) p 1196
Sine-Aid Extra-Strength Sinus Headache Capsules (McNeil Consumer Products) p 1199
Sine-Aid Sinus Headache Tablets (McNeil Consumer Products) p 1198
Singlet (Merrell Dow) p 421, 1385
Sinubid (Parke-Davis) p 425, 1569
Sinulin Tablets (Carnrick) p 409, 835
Stopayne Capsules (Springbok) p 1985
Stopayne Syrup (Springbok) p 1985
Supac (Mission) p 1420
Talacen (Winthrop-Breon) p 444, 2227
Two-Dyne Capsules (Hyrex) p 1025
Tylenol acetaminophen Children's Chewable Tablets, Elixir, Infants' Drops (McNeil Consumer Products) p 418, 1199
Tylenol, Extra-Strength, acetaminophen Liquid Pain Reliever (McNeil Consumer Products) p 1200
Tylenol, Extra-Strength, acetaminophen Tablets, Capsules & Caplets (McNeil Consumer Products) p 418, 1200
Tylenol, Junior-Strength, acetaminiphen Swallowable Tablets (McNeil Consumer Products) p 418
Tylenol, Maximum-Strength, Sinus Medication Tablets & Capsules (McNeil Consumer Products) p 418, 1201

Generic and Chemical Name Index

Tylenol, Regular Strength, acetaminophen Tablets & Capsules (McNeil Consumer Products) p 418, 1199
Tylenol w/Codeine Elixir (McNeil Pharmaceutical) p 419, 1214
Tylenol w/Codeine Tablets, Capsules (McNeil Pharmaceutical) p 419, 1214
Tylox Capsules (McNeil Pharmaceutical) p 419, 1215
Vanquish (Glenbrook) p 998
Vicodin (Knoll) p 414, 1068
Wygesic Tablets (Wyeth) p 445, 2297

Acetazolamide
Acetazolamide Tablets (Schein) p 1828
Diamox Parenteral (Lederle) p 1091
Diamox Sequels, Tablets (Lederle) p 415, 1091

Acetic Acid
Aci-Jel Therapeutic Vaginal Jelly (Ortho Pharmaceutical) p 1453
Borofair Otic (Pharmafair) p 1618
Fungi-Nail Tincture (Kramer) p 1069
Otic Domeboro Solution (Miles Pharmaceuticals) p 1411
Otic Tridesilon Solution 0.05% (Miles Pharmaceuticals) p 1414
Otic-HC Ear Drops (Hauck) p 1001
Otipyrin Otic Solution (Kramer) p 1069
VōSol HC Otic Solution (Wallace) p 442, 2171
VōSol Otic Solution (Wallace) p 442, 2171

Acetohexamide
Dymelor (Lilly) p 417, 1146

Acetohydroxamic Acid
Lithostat (Mission) p 1418

Acetyl Sulfisoxazole
Gantrisin Pediatric Suspension (Roche) p 1686
Gantrisin Syrup (Roche) p 1686
Lipo Gantrisin (Roche) p 1686
Pediazole (Ross) p 1774

Acetylcysteine
Mucomyst (Mead Johnson Pharmaceutical) p 1252

ACTH
(see under Adrenocorticotropic Hormone)

Acyclovir
Zovirax Ointment 5% (Burroughs Wellcome) p 822

Acyclovir Sodium
Zovirax Sterile Powder (Burroughs Wellcome) p 823

Adrenocorticotropic Hormone
A.C.T.H. "40" Injectable (O'Neal, Jones & Feldman) p 1443
A.C.T.H. "80" Injectable (O'Neal, Jones & Feldman) p 1443
Acthar (Armour) p 601
Cortrophin-Zinc (Organon) p 1446
Cortrosyn (Organon) p 1446
HP Acthar Gel (Armour) p 601

Albumin, Normal Serum
Albuminar-5, Normal Serum Albumin (Human) U.S.P. 5% (Armour) p 613
Albuminar-25, Normal Serum Albumin (Human) U.S.P. 25% (Armour) p 613
Albutein 5% (Alpha Theapeutic) p 589
Albutein 25% (Alpha Theapeutic) p 589
Buminate 5%, Normal Serum Albumin (Human), U.S.P., 5% Solution (Hyland Therapeutics) p 1023
Buminate 25%, Normal Serum Albumin (Human), U.S.P., 25% Solution (Hyland Therapeutics) p 1023

Albuterol
Proventil Inhaler (Schering) p 435, 1882
Proventil Tablets (Schering) p 435, 1883
Ventolin Inhaler (Glaxo) p 412, 987
Ventolin Tablets (Glaxo) p 412, 988

Allantoin
Alphosyl Lotion, Cream (Reed & Carnrick) p 1632
Herpecin-L Cold Sore Lip Balm (Campbell) p 829
Vagimide Cream (Legere) p 1120
Vaginal Sulfa Suppositories (Schein) p 1828

Allergenic Extracts
Allergenic Extracts, Diagnosis and/or Immunotherapy (Barry) p 685

Allopurinol
Allopurinol Tablets (Danbury) p 887

Allopurinol Tablets (Schein) p 1828
Lopurin (Boots) p 406, 718
Zyloprim (Burroughs Wellcome) p 408, 825

Alpha Tocopheral Acetate
(see under Vitamin E)

Alphaprodine Hydrochloride
Nisentil Injectable (Roche) p 1694

Alprazolam
Xanax Tablets (Upjohn) p 441, 2142

Alprostadil
Prostin VR Pediatric Sterile Solution (Upjohn) p 2132

Alseroxylon
Rauwiloid Tablets (Riker) p 1644

Alumina (Fused)
Magnesia & Alumina Oral Suspension (Roxane) p 1788

Aluminum Acetate
Acid Mantle Creme & Lotion (Dorsey Laboratories) p 908
Osti-Derm Lotion (Pedinol) p 1580
Otic Domeboro Solution (Miles Pharmaceuticals) p 1411

Aluminum Carbonate Gel
Basaljel Capsules & Swallow Tablets (Wyeth) p 2239
Basaljel Suspension & Suspension, Extra Strength (Wyeth) p 2239

Aluminum Chlorhydroxide
Pedi-Dri Foot Powder (Pedinol) p 1581
Pedi-Pro Foot Powder (Pedinol) p 1581

Aluminum Chloride
Drysol (Persōn & Covey) p 1587
Xerac AC (Persōn & Covey) p 1588

Aluminum Chlorohydrate
Breezee Mist Foot Powder (Pedinol) p 1580

Aluminum Hydroxide
Aluminum & Magnesium Hydroxides with Simethicone I (Roxane) p 1788
Aluminum & Magnesium Hydroxides with Simethicone II (Roxane) p 1788
Dialume (Armour) p 404, 605
Gaviscon Liquid Antacid (Marion) p 1186
Gelusil (Parke-Davis) p 424, 1525
Gelusil-M (Parke-Davis) p 1525
Gelusil-II (Parke-Davis) p 424, 1526
Mygel Suspension (Geneva) p 973

Aluminum Hydroxide Gel
ALternaGEL Liquid (Stuart) p 438, 2036
Aludrox Oral Suspension (Wyeth) p 2235
Aluminum Hydroxide Gel (Roxane) p 1788
Aluminum Hydroxide Gel-Concentrated (Roxane) p 1788
Amphojel Suspension (Wyeth) p 2236
Arthritis Pain Formula By the Makers of Anacin Analgesic Tablets (Whitehall) p 443, 2185
Mylanta Liquid (Stuart) p 439, 2039
Mylanta-II Liquid (Stuart) p 439, 2039
Simeco (Wyeth) p 2288

Aluminum Hydroxide Gel, Dried
Alu-Cap Capsules (Riker) p 1641
Aludrox Tablets (Wyeth) p 2235
Aluminum Hydroxide Tablets (Roxane) p 1788
Alu-Tab Tablets (Riker) p 1641
Amphojel Tablets (Wyeth) p 2236
Cama Arthritis Pain Reliever (Dorsey Laboratories) p 908
Dolprn #3 Tablets (Bock) p 705
Gaviscon Antacid Tablets (Marion) p 418, 1185
Gaviscon-2 Antacid Tablets (Marion) p 418, 1186
Mylanta Tablets (Stuart) p 439, 2039
Mylanta-II Tablets (Stuart) p 439, 2039

Aluminum Sulfate
Domeboro Powder Packets & Tablets (Miles Pharmaceuticals) p 422, 1402
Pedi-Boro Soak Paks (Pedinol) p 1581

Amantadine Hydrochloride
Symmetrel (Du Pont) p 410, 927

Amcinonide
Cyclocort Cream (Lederle) p 415, 1089
Cyclocort Ointment (Lederle) p 415, 1089

Amikacin Sulfate
Amikin (Bristol) p 727

Amiloride Hydrochloride
Midamor Tablets (Merck Sharp & Dohme) p 420, 1331
Moduretic Tablets (Merck Sharp & Dohme) p 420, 1333

Aminacrine Hydrochloride
Vagimide Cream (Legere) p 1120

Aminacrine Preparations
AVC Cream (Merrell Dow) p 1358
AVC Suppositories (Merrell Dow) p 1358
Vaginal Sulfa Suppositories (Schein) p 1828

Amino Acid Preparations
Added Protection III Multi-Vitamin & Multi-Mineral Supplement (Professional Health) p 1621
Amino-Cerv (Milex) p 1415
Aminolete (Tyson) p 2067
Aminomine (Tyson) p 2067
Aminoplex Capsules & Powder (Tyson) p 2068
Aminosine (Tyson) p 2068
Aminostasis Capsules & Powder (Tyson) p 2068
Aminotate Capsules & Powder (Tyson) p 2068
DL-Carnitine - Amino Acid Preparation (Tyson) p 2068
Endorphenyl (Tyson) p 2068
Geravite Elixir (Hauck) p 1001
MARLYN Formula 50 (Marlyn) p 1193
Pre-Protein Liquid (Arlo) p 601
Stresstein (Clinical Nutrition) p 878
Vivonex High Nitrogen Diet (Norwich Eaton) p 1439
Vivonex Standard Diet (Norwich Eaton) p 1438
Vivonex T.E.N. (Norwich Eaton) p 1441

2-Amino-6-Mercaptopurine
Tabloid Brand Thioguanine (Burroughs Wellcome) p 408, 817

Aminoacetic Acid
Glytinic Tablets (Boyle) p 726

Aminobenzoate Potassium
Potaba (Glenwood) p 412, 998

Aminobenzoic Acid
Potaba (Glenwood) p 412, 998
PreSun 15 Sunscreen Lotion (Westwood) p 2181

Aminobenzoic Preparations
Cetacaine Topical Anesthetic (Cetylite) p 839
Pabalate Tablets (Robins) p 428, 1654
Pabalate-SF Tablets (Robins) p 428, 1655
Potaba (Glenwood) p 412, 998

Aminocaproic Acid
Amicar (Lederle) p 414, 1077
Aminocaproic Acid Injection (Elkins-Sinn) p 938

Aminoglutethamide
Cytadren (CIBA) p 409, 846

Aminophylline
Aminophyllin Injection (Bristol) p 730
Aminophyllin Injection (Searle Pharmaceuticals) p 1898
Aminophyllin Tablets (Searle & Co.) p 435, 1915
Aminophylline Injection (Elkins-Sinn) p 938
Aminophylline Oral Liquid, Suppositories & Tabs (Schein) p 1828
Aminophylline Tablets (Geneva) p 973
Aminophylline Tablets & Oral Solution (Roxane) p 1788
Mudrane GG Tablets (Poythress) p 1619
Mudrane GG-2 Tablets (Poythress) p 1619
Mudrane Tablets (Poythress) p 1618
Mudrane-2 Tablets (Poythress) p 1619
Somophyllin & Somophyllin-DF Oral Liquids (Fisons) p 945
Somophyllin Rectal Solution (Fisons) p 945

Amitriptyline
Amitriptyline HCl Tablets (Geneva) p 973
SK-Amitriptyline Hydrochloride Tablets (Smith Kline & French) p 1971

Amitriptyline Hydrochloride
Amitriptyline HCl Tablets (Biocraft) p 705
Amitriptyline Hydrochloride Tablets (Roxane) p 1788
Amitriptyline Hydrochloride Tablets (Schein) p 1828
Amitriptyline Hydrochloride Tablets (Parke-Davis) p 423, 1481
Elavil Tablets & Injection (Merck Sharp & Dohme) p 420, 1306
Endep Tablets (Roche Products) p 429, 1711

Generic and Chemical Name Index

Etrafon Tablets (Schering) p 434, 1841
Limbitrol Tablets (Roche Products) p 430, 1716
Triavil Tablets (Merck Sharp & Dohme) p 420, 1354

Ammonium Chloride
Bromanyl Expectorant (Schein) p 1828
P-V-Tussin Syrup (Reid-Provident Labs.) p 1640
Quelidrine Syrup (Abbott) p 567
Ru-Tuss Expectorant (Boots) p 722
Twin-K-Cl (Boots) p 725
Zypan Tablets (Standard Process) p 2035

Amobarbital
Amytal (Lilly) p 417, 1127

Amobarbital Sodium
Amytal Sodium Ampoules & Vials (Lilly) p 1127
Amytal Sodium Pulvules (Lilly) p 417, 1128
Tuinal (Lilly) p 417, 1176

Amoxapine
Asendin (Lederle) p 415, 1088

Amoxicillin
Amoxicillin Capsules (Biocraft) p 705
Amoxicillin Capsules (Parke-Davis) p 423, 1482
Amoxicillin for Oral Suspension (Parke-Davis) p 1482
Amoxicillin Suspension (Biocraft) p 705
Amoxicillin Trihydrate Capsules & Powder for Oral Suspension (Schein) p 1828
Amoxil (Beecham Laboratories) p 405, 688
Augmentin Tablets & Powder for Oral Suspension (Beecham Laboratories) p 405, 690
Polymox Capsules (Bristol) p 407, 742
Polymox For Oral Suspension (Bristol) p 742
Polymox Pediatric Drops (Bristol) p 742
Trimox Capsules & for Oral Suspension (Squibb) p 438, 2025
Wymox Capsules & Oral Suspension (Wyeth) p 445, 2298

Amphetamine Aspartate
Obetrol-10 (Rexar) p 1641
Obetrol-20 (Rexar) p 1641

Amphetamine Sulfate
Obetrol-10 (Rexar) p 1641
Obetrol-20 (Rexar) p 1641

Amphotericin B
Fungizone Cream/Lotion/Ointment (Squibb) p 1994
Fungizone Intravenous (Squibb) p 1994
Mysteclin-F Capsules (Squibb) p 438, 2005
Mysteclin-F Syrup (Squibb) p 2005

Ampicillin
Amcill Capsules (Parke-Davis) p 423, 1480
Amcill Oral Suspension (Parke-Davis) p 1480
Ampicillin Capsules (Biocraft) p 705
Ampicillin Suspension (Biocraft) p 705
Ampicillin-Probenecid Suspension (Biocraft) p 705
Omnipen Capsules (Wyeth) p 444, 2271
Omnipen for Oral Suspension (Wyeth) p 2271
Omnipen Pediatric Drops (Wyeth) p 2271
Polycillin (Bristol) p 407, 740
Polycillin-N for Injection (Bristol) p 740
Polycillin-PRB (Bristol) p 741
SK-Ampicillin Capsules & For Oral Suspension (Smith Kline & French) p 1971

Ampicillin Sodium
Omnipen-N (Wyeth) p 2271
Polycillin-N for Injection (Bristol) p 740
SK-Ampicillin-N For Injection (Smith Kline & French) p 1971

Ampicillin Trihydrate
Ampicillin Trihydrate Capsules & Powder for Oral Suspension (Schein) p 1828
Principen Capsules (Squibb) p 438, 2012
Principen for Oral Suspension (Squibb) p 2012
Principen with Probenecid Capsules (Squibb) p 2013

Amrinone Lactate
Inocor Lactate Injection (Winthrop-Breon) p 2199

Amylolytic Enzyme
Arco-Lase (Arco) p 600
Arco-Lase Plus (Arco) p 600
Cotazym (Organon) p 422, 1446
Cotazym-S (Organon) p 422, 1446
Festal II (Hoechst-Roussel) p 412, 1014
Festalan (Hoechst-Roussel) p 413, 1014

Gustase (Geriatric) p 975
Kutrase Capsules (Rorer) p 431, 1750
Ku-Zyme Capsules (Rorer) p 431, 1750
Ku-Zyme HP Capsules (Rorer) p 431, 1751
Pancreatin Tablets 2400 mg. N.F. (High Lipase) (Vitaline) p 2148
Tri-Cone Capsules (Glaxo) p 986

Anisotropine Methylbromide
Valpin 50 (Du Pont) p 928

Anterior Pituitary Hormones
Acthar (Armour) p 601
HP Acthar Gel (Armour) p 601
Thytropar (Armour) p 612

Anthralin Preparations
Anthra-Derm Ointment 1%, ½%, ¼%, 1/10% (Dermik) p 888
Drithocreme (American Dermal) p 599
Dritho-Scalp (American Dermal) p 599

Anthraquinone Preparations
Modane Plus (Adria) p 585
Modane, Tablets & Liquid (Adria) p 584

Antihemophilic Factor (Human)
Factorate, Antihemophilic Factor (Human) Dried (Armour) p 613
Factorate, Generation II (Armour) p 613
H.T. Factorate (Armour) p 613
H.T. Factorate, Generation II (Armour) p 613
Hemofil, Antihemophilic Factor (Human), Method Four, Dried (Hyland Therapeutics) p 1023
Hemofil T, Antihemophilic Factor (Human), Method Four, Dried, Heat-Treated (Hyland Therapeutics) p 1024

Antihemophilic Factor (Human), VIII, AHF, AHG
Koate-HT (Cutter Biological) p 886
Profilate (Alpha Theapeutic) p 589
Profilate, Heat-Treated (Alpha Theapeutic) p 589

Antihemophilic Factor (Human), IX Complex
Profilnine (Alpha Theapeutic) p 589

Anti-Inhibitor Coagulant Complex
Autoplex, Anti-Inhibitor Coagulant Complex, Dried (Hyland Therapeutics) p 1023

Antipyrine
Antipyrine & Benzocaine Otic Solution (Pharmafair) p 1618
Auralgan Otic Solution (Ayerst) p 638
Collyrium Eye Lotion (Wyeth) p 2249
Otipyrin Otic Solution (Kramer) p 1069
Tympagesic Otic Solution (Adria) p 587

Antivenin (Crotalidae) Polyvalent
Antivenin (Crotalidae) Polyvalent (equine origin) (Wyeth) p 2243

Antivenin (Micrurus Fulvius)
Antivenin (Micrurus Fulvius) (Wyeth) p 2245

Aprobarbital
Alurate Elixir (Roche) p 1667

Ara-A
Vira-A Ophthalmic Ointment, 3% (Parke-Davis) p 426, 1578

Ascorbic Acid
(see under Vitamin C)

Asparaginase
Elspar (Merck Sharp & Dohme) p 1308

Aspirin
A.P.C. with Codeine Nos. 3 & 4, Tabloid brand (Burroughs Wellcome) p 407, 780
Alka-Seltzer Effervescent Pain Reliever and Antacid (Miles Laboratories) p 1395
Alka-Seltzer Plus Cold Medicine (Miles Laboratories) p 1395
Anacin Analgesic Capsules (Whitehall) p 443, 2184
Anacin Analgesic Tablets (Whitehall) p 443, 2184
Arthritis Bayer Timed-Release Aspirin (Glenbrook) p 412, 995
Arthritis Pain Formula By the Makers of Anacin Analgesic Tablets (Whitehall) p 443, 2185
Arthritis Pain Formula Safety-Coated by the Makers of Anacin Analgesic Tablets (Whitehall) p 443, 2185
Arthritis Strength Bufferin (Bristol-Myers Products) p 768
Ascriptin with Codeine (Rorer) p 431, 1745
Aspirin Suppositories (Roxane) p 1788
Aspirin w/Codeine Tablets (Geneva) p 973

Aspirin 325 mg. with Codeine Tabs (Schein) p 1828
Axotal (Adria) p 574
Bayer Aspirin and Bayer Children's Chewable Aspirin (Glenbrook) p 412, 996
Bayer Children's Cold Tablets (Glenbrook) p 996
Buff-A Comp Tablets (Mayrand) p 1196
Buff-A Comp No. 3 Tablets (with Codeine) (Mayrand) p 1196
Bufferin (Bristol-Myers Products) p 769
Cama Arthritis Pain Reliever (Dorsey Laboratories) p 908
Congespirin Cold Tablets (Aspirin Formula) (Bristol-Myers Products) p 769
Cosprin (Glenbrook) p 996
Cosprin 650 (Glenbrook) p 997
Darvon with A.S.A. (Lilly) p 417, 1139
Darvon-N with A.S.A. (Lilly) p 417, 1136
Dia-Gesic (Central Pharmaceuticals) p 409, 837
Dihydrocodeine Compound Tablets (Schein) p 1828
Dolprn #3 Tablets (Bock) p 705
Easprin (Parke-Davis) p 424, 1512
Empirin with Codeine (Burroughs Wellcome) p 408, 787
Encaprin (Procter & Gamble) p 427, 1620
Equagesic (Wyeth) p 444, 2250
Excedrin Extra-Strength (Bristol-Myers Products) p 770
Extra-Strength Bufferin capsules & tablets (Bristol-Myers Products) p 769
4-Way Cold Tablets (Bristol-Myers Products) p 770
Fiorinal (Sandoz Pharmaceutical Div.) p 433, 1801
Fiorinal w/Codeine (Sandoz Pharmaceutical Div.) p 432, 1802
Hyco-Pap (LaSalle) p 1071
Maximum Bayer Aspirin (Glenbrook) p 412, 996
Maximum Strength Midol for Cramps (Glenbrook) p 997
Mepro Compound Tablets (Schein) p 1828
Methocarbamol with Aspirin Tablets (Schein) p 1828
Midol-Original Formula (Glenbrook) p 997
Norgesic & Norgesic Forte (Riker) p 428, 1644
Oxycodone Hydrochloride, Oxycodone Terephthalate & Aspirin Tablets (Full Strength) (Roxane) p 1788
Percodan & Percodan-Demi Tablets (Du Pont) p 410, 925
Propoxyphene Compound 65 (Schein) p 1828
Robaxisal Tablets (Robins) p 429, 1662
SK-Oxycodone with Aspirin Tablets (Smith Kline & French) p 1971
SK-65 Compound Capsules (Smith Kline & French) p 1971
Saleto (Mallard) p 1181
Soma Compound (Wallace) p 442, 2166
Soma Compound w/Codeine (Wallace) p 442, 2169
Supac (Mission) p 1420
Synalgos-DC Capsules (Ives) p 413, 1031
Talwin Compound (Winthrop-Breon) p 2229
Vanquish (Glenbrook) p 998
Verin (Verex) p 442, 2146
Zorprin (Boots) p 406, 725

Atenolol
Tenoretic Tablets (Stuart) p 439, 2043
Tenormin Tablets (Stuart) p 439, 2045

Atropine Derivatives
Antispasmodic Capsules, Elixir & Tablets (Schein) p 1828
Diphenoxylate & Atropine Liquid (DPXL) & Tabs (Schein) p 1828
Trac Tabs 2X (Hyrex) p 413, 1025

Atropine Nitrate, Methyl
Festalan (Hoechst-Roussel) p 413, 1014

Atropine Sulfate
Antrocol Tablets, Capsules & Elixir (Poythress) p 1618
Arco-Lase Plus (Arco) p 600
Atropine Sulfate Injection (Bristol) p 730
Atropine Sulfate Injection (Elkins-Sinn) p 938
Atropine Sulfate Ophthalmic Ointment 1% (Fougera) p 953
Comhist Tablets (Norwich Eaton) p 1426
Diphenoxylate Hydrochloride & Atropine Sulfate Tablets & Oral Solution (Roxane) p 1788
Ru-Tuss Tablets (Boots) p 406, 723
SK-Diphenoxylate Tablets (Smith Kline & French) p 1971
Trac Tabs 2X (Hyrex) p 413, 1025
Urised Tablets (Webcon) p 2173

Aurothioglucose
Solganal Suspension (Schering) p 1884

Generic and Chemical Name Index

Azatadine Maleate
  Optimine Tablets (Schering) p 434, 1872
  Trinalin Repetabs Tablets (Schering) p 435, 1890

Azathioprine
  Imuran Tablets (Burroughs Wellcome) p 408, 790

Azlocillin Sodium
  Azlin (Miles Pharmaceuticals) p 1396

Azosulfisoxazole
  Azo-Sulfisoxazole Tablets (Geneva) p 973
  Azo-Sulfisoxazole Tablets (Schein) p 1828

B

BCG Vaccine
  BCG Vaccine (Glaxo) p 976

Bacampicillin Hydrochloride
  Spectrobid Tablets & Oral Suspension (Roerig) p 431, 1741

Bacitracin
  Bacitracin-Neomycin-Polymyxin Ointment (Fougera) p 953
  Bacitracin-Neomycin-Polymyxin Ophthalmic Ointment (Fougera) p 953
  Bacitracin Ointment (Fougera) p 953
  Bacitracin Ophthalmic Ointment (Fougera) p 953
  Bacitracin-Polymyxin Ointment (Fougera) p 953

Bacitracin Zinc
  Cortisporin Ointment (Burroughs Wellcome) p 784
  Cortisporin Ophthalmic Ointment (Burroughs Wellcome) p 784
  Neo-Polycin (Merrell Dow) p 1372
  Neosporin Aerosol (Burroughs Wellcome) p 806
  Neosporin Ointment (Burroughs Wellcome) p 808
  Neosporin Ophthalmic Ointment Sterile (Burroughs Wellcome) p 808
  Neosporin Powder (Burroughs Wellcome) p 810
  Polysporin Ointment (Burroughs Wellcome) p 810
  Polysporin Ophthalmic Ointment (Burroughs Wellcome) p 810
  Topisporin (Pharmafair) p 1618

Baclofen
  Lioresal Tablets (Geigy) p 411, 959

BAL
  BAL in Oil Ampules (Hynson, Westcott & Dunning) p 1024

Balsam Peru
  Anusol Ointment (Parke-Davis) p 1484
  Anusol Suppositories (Parke-Davis) p 423, 1484
  Granulex (Hickam) p 1009
  Rectal Medicone-HC Suppositories (Medicone) p 419, 1256
  Stimuzyme Plus (National Dermaceutical) p 1421

Barbiturate Preparations
  Alurate Elixir (Roche) p 1667
  Buff-A Comp Tablets (Mayrand) p 1196
  Buff-A Comp No. 3 Tablets (with Codeine) (Mayrand) p 1196
  Donnatal Capsules (Robins) p 428, 1648
  Donnatal Elixir (Robins) p 1648
  Donnatal Extentabs (Robins) p 428, 1649
  Donnatal Tablets (Robins) p 428, 1648
  G-1 Capsules (Hauck) p 1001
  G-2 Capsules (Hauck) p 1001
  G-3 Capsules (Hauck) p 1001
  Kinesed Tablets (Stuart) p 439, 2038
  Levsin/Phenobarbital Tablets, Elixir & Drops (Rorer) p 1751
  Levsinex/Phenobarbital Timecaps (Rorer) p 1751
  Lotusate Caplets (Winthrop-Breon) p 2206
  Mebaral (Winthrop-Breon) p 444, 2213
  Nembutal Sodium Capsules (Abbott) p 403, 538
  Nembutal Sodium Solution (Abbott) p 541
  Nembutal Sodium Suppositories (Abbott) p 543
  Repan Tablets (Everett) p 942

Basic Fuchsin
  Castellani Paint (Pedinol) p 1580

Beclomethasone Dipropionate
  Beclovent Oral Inhaler (Glaxo) p 411, 977
  Beconase Nasal Inhaler (Glaxo) p 411, 978

  Vancenase Nasal Inhaler (Schering) p 435, 1893
  Vanceril Inhaler (Schering) p 435, 1894

Belladonna Ergotamine
  Bellergal Tablets (Sandoz Pharmaceutical Div.) p 432, 1798
  Bellergal-S Tablets (Sandoz Pharmaceutical Div.) p 432, 1798

Belladonna Extract
  Chardonna-2 (Rorer) p 431, 1748

Belladonna Preparations
  Belladenal Tablets (Sandoz Pharmaceutical Div.) p 432, 1798
  Belladenal-S Tablets (Sandoz Pharmaceutical Div.) p 432, 1798
  Chardonna-2 (Rorer) p 431, 1748
  Comhist LA Capsules (Norwich Eaton) p 422, 1425
  Donnatal Capsules (Robins) p 428, 1648
  Donnatal Elixir (Robins) p 1648
  Donnatal Extentabs (Robins) p 428, 1649
  Donnatal Tablets (Robins) p 428, 1648
  Donnazyme Tablets (Robins) p 428, 1650
  Kaolin, Pectin, Belladonna Mixture (Schein) p 1828
  Kinesed Tablets (Stuart) p 439, 2038
  Trac Tabs 2X (Hyrex) p 413, 1025
  Wigraine-PB Suppositories (Organon) p 422, 1451

Benactyzine Hydrochloride
  Deprol (Wallace) p 2155

Bendroflumethiazide
  Corzide (Squibb) p 437, 1990
  Naturetin Tablets (Squibb) p 438, 2006
  Rauzide Tablets (Squibb) p 438, 2021

Bentiromide
  Chymex (Adria) p 3003

Benzalkonium Chloride
  Amino-Cerv (Milex) p 1415
  Cetylcide Solution (Cetylite) p 839
  Zephiran Chloride 1:750 (Winthrop-Breon) p 2233
  Zephiran Chloride Spray (Winthrop-Breon) p 2233
  Zephiran Chloride Tinted Tincture (Winthrop-Breon) p 2233

Benzalkonium Chloride Complex
  HVS 1+2 (Chemi-Tech) p 839

Benzethonium Chloride
  Dalidyne (Dalin) p 886

Benzocaine
  Anbesol Baby Teething Gel Antiseptic Anesthetic (Whitehall) p 443, 2185
  Anbesol Gel Antiseptic Anesthetic (Whitehall) p 443, 2185
  Antipyrine & Benzocaine Otic Solution (Pharmafair) p 1618
  Auralgan Otic Solution (Ayerst) p 638
  Cetacaine Topical Anesthetic (Cetylite) p 839
  Children's Chloraseptic Lozenges (Procter & Gamble) p 1619
  Dalidyne (Dalin) p 886
  Derma Medicone-HC Ointment (Medicone) p 1256
  Dermoplast Aerosol Spray (Ayerst) p 640
  Dieutrim Capsules (Legere) p 1120
  Fungi-Nail Tincture (Kramer) p 1069
  Ger-O-Foam (Geriatric) p 975
  Gumsol (Arlo) p 601
  Hurricaine Liquid 1/4cc Unit Dose (Beutlich) p 705
  Hurricaine Oral, Topical Anesthetic Gel, Liquid, Spray (Beutlich) p 705
  Otipyrin Otic Solution (Kramer) p 1069
  Rectal Medicone-HC Suppositories (Medicone) p 419, 1256
  Tympagesic Otic Solution (Adria) p 587

Benzoic Acid
  Trac Tabs 2X (Hyrex) p 413, 1025
  Whitfield's Ointment (Fougera) p 953

Benzonatate
  Tessalon (Du Pont) p 411, 928

Benzoyl Peroxide
  5 Benzagel (5% benzoyl peroxide) & 10 Benzagel (10% benzoyl peroxide), Acne Gels, Microgel Formula (Dermik) p 888
  Benzoyl Peroxide Gel (Pharmafair) p 1618
  Desquam-X 2.5 Gel (Westwood) p 2175
  Desquam-X 5 Gel (Westwood) p 2175
  Desquam-X 10 Gel (Westwood) p 2175
  Desquam-X 5 Wash (Westwood) p 2176
  Desquam-X 10 Wash (Westwood) p 2176

  Fostex 5% Benzoyl Peroxide Gel (Westwood) p 2177
  Fostex 10% Benzoyl Peroxide Cleansing Bar (Westwood) p 2177
  Fostex 10% Benzoyl Peroxide Gel (Westwood) p 2178
  Fostex 10% Benzoyl Peroxide Tinted Cream (Westwood) p 2178
  Fostex 10% Benzoyl Peroxide Wash (Westwood) p 2178
  Intraderm-19 Overnight Acne Masque (Robertson/Taylor) p 1645
  Persa-Gel 5% & 10% (Ortho Pharmaceutical (Dermatological Div.)) p 1474
  Persa-Gel W 5% & 10% (Ortho Pharmaceutical (Dermatological Div.)) p 1474
  Vanoxide-HC Acne Lotion (Dermik) p 891
  Xerac BP5 & Xerac BP10 (Persön & Covey) p 1588

Benzphetamine Hydrochloride
  Didrex Tablets (Upjohn) p 441, 2111

Benzquinamide Hydrochloride
  Emete-con (Roerig) p 1729

Benzthiazide
  Exna Tablets (Robins) p 428, 1652
  Hydrex Tablets (Trimen) p 2067

Benztropine Mesylate
  Benztropine Mesylate Tablets (Schein) p 1828
  Cogentin Tablets & Injection (Merck Sharp & Dohme) p 420, 1276

Benzylpenicilloyl-Polylysine
  Pre-Pen (Rorer) p 1753

Beta-carotene
  Added Protection III Multi-Vitamin & Multi-Mineral Supplement (Professional Health) p 1621
  Solatene Capsules (Roche) p 430, 1701

Betaine Hydrochloride
  Zypan Tablets (Standard Process) p 2035

Betamethasone
  Celestone Syrup & Tablets (Schering) p 433, 1832

Betamethasone Acetate
  Celestone Soluspan Suspension (Schering) p 1835

Betamethasone Benzoate
  Uticort Cream, Gel, Lotion & Ointment (Parke-Davis) p 426, 1575

Betamethasone Dipropionate
  Alphatrex Cream & Ointment (Savage) p 1822
  Betamethasone Dipropionate Cream & Ointment (Pharmaderm) p 1617
  Diprolene Ointment 0.05% (Schering) p 1837
  Diprosone Cream 0.05% (Schering) p 1838
  Diprosone Lotion 0.05% w/w (Schering) p 1838
  Diprosone Ointment 0.05% (Schering) p 1838
  Diprosone Topical Aerosol 0.1% w/w (Schering) p 1838
  Lotrisone Cream (Schering) p 1858

Betamethasone Sodium Phosphate
  B-S-P (Legere) p 1120
  Celestone Phosphate Injection (Schering) p 1833
  Celestone Soluspan Suspension (Schering) p 1835

Betamethasone Valerate
  Betamethasone Valerate Cream, Lotion & Ointment 0.1% (Fougera) p 953
  Betamethasone Valerate Cream, Ointment & Lotion (Pharmaderm) p 1617
  Betatrex Cream, Ointment & Lotion (Savage) p 1823
  Beta-Val Cream 0.1% (Lemmon) p 1122
  Valisone Cream 0.1% (Schering) p 1892
  Valisone Lotion 0.1% (Schering) p 1892
  Valisone Ointment 0.1% (Schering) p 1892
  Valisone Reduced Strength Cream 0.01% (Schering) p 1892

Bethanechol Chloride
  Bethanechol Chloride Tablets (Danbury) p 887
  Duvoid (Norwich Eaton) p 1430
  Myotonachol (Glenwood) p 412, 998
  Urecholine Injection & Tablets (Merck Sharp & Dohme) p 421, 1356

Generic and Chemical Name Index

Bile Salts
  Digepepsin Tablets (RAM Laboratories) p 1632

Bioflavonoids
  Mevanin-C Capsules (Beutlich) p 705
  Peridin-C (Beutlich) p 705

Biotin
  Mega-B (Arco) p 600
  Megadose (Arco) p 600
  Theragran Stress Formula (Squibb) p 438, 2025

Biperiden
  Akineton (Knoll) p 414, 1056

Bisacodyl
  Bisacodyl Patient Pack, Suppositories, Tablets (Roxane) p 1788
  Bisacodyl Suppositories (Geneva) p 973
  Dulcolax Suppositories (Boehringer Ingelheim) p 406, 709
  Dulcolax Tablets (Boehringer Ingelheim) p 406, 709
  Evac-Q-Kwik (Adria) p 575
  Fleet Bisacodyl Enema (Fleet) p 946
  Fleet Prep Kits (Fleet) p 947

Bishydroxycoumarin
  (see under Dicumarol)

Bismuth Oxyiodide
  Wyanoids Hemorrhoidal Suppositories (Wyeth) p 445, 2293

Bismuth Subcarbonate
  Wyanoids Hemorrhoidal Suppositories (Wyeth) p 445, 2293

Bismuth Subgallate
  Anusol Suppositories (Parke-Davis) p 423, 1484
  Anusol-HC (Parke-Davis) p 423, 1484

Bismuth Subsalicylate
  Pepto-Bismol Liquid & Tablets (Procter & Gamble) p 1620

Black Widow Spider Antivenin (Equine)
  Antivenin (Merck Sharp & Dohme) p 1264

Bleomycin Sulfate
  Blenoxane (Bristol-Myers Oncology) p 757

Boric Acid
  Boric Acid Ointment (Fougera) p 953
  Boric Acid Ophthalmic Ointment 5% (Fougera) p 953
  Clear Eyes Eye Drops (Ross) p 1762
  Collyrium Eye Lotion (Wyeth) p 2249
  Collyrium 2 Eye Drops with Tetrahydrozoline (Wyeth) p 2249
  Murine Plus Eye Drops (Ross) p 1769
  Wyanoids Hemorrhoidal Suppositories (Wyeth) p 445, 2293

Bretylium Tosylate
  Bretylol (American Critical Care) p 592

Brewers Yeast
  Glutofac Tablets (Kenwood) p 1046

Bromocriptine Mesylate
  Parlodel Capsules & Tablets (Sandoz Pharmaceutical Div.) p 433, 1808

Bromodiphenhydramine Hydrochloride
  Ambenyl Cough Syrup (Marion) p 1181
  Bromanyl Expectorant (Schein) p 1828

Brompheniramine Maleate
  Bromfed Capsules (Timed Release) (Muro) p 1420
  Bromfed-PD Capsules (Timed Release) (Muro) p 1420
  Bromfed Tablets (Muro) p 1420
  Bromphen Compound Elixir - Sugar Free (Schein) p 1828
  Bromphen Compound Tablets (Schein) p 1828
  Bromphen DC Expectorant (Schein) p 1828
  Bromphen Expectorant (Schein) p 1828
  Dimetane-DC Cough Syrup (Robins) p 1647
  Dimetapp Elixir (Robins) p 1648
  Dimetapp Extentabs (Robins) p 428, 1648
  Dura Tap-PD (Dura) p 929
  E.N.T. Syrup (Springbok) p 1985
  Poly-Histine-DX Capsules (Bock) p 706
  S-T Decongest Sugar-Free & Dye-Free (Scot-Tussin) p 1897
  Tamine S.R. Tablets (Geneva) p 973

Buclizine Hydrochloride
  Bucladin-S Softab Tablets (Stuart) p 439, 2036

Bumetanide
  Bumex Injection (Roche) p 1678
  Bumex Tablets (Roche) p 429, 1678

Bupivacaine Hydrochloride
  Marcaine Hydrochloride (Winthrop-Breon) p 2206
  Marcaine Hydrochloride with Epinephrine 1:200,000 (Winthrop-Breon) p 2206
  Marcaine Spinal (Winthrop-Breon) p 2210
  Sensorcaine Hydrochloride & Sensorcaine Hydrochloride with Epinephrine 1:200,000 (Astra) p 619

Busulfan
  Myleran (Burroughs Wellcome) p 408, 804

Butabarbital
  Pyridium Plus (Parke-Davis) p 425, 1568
  Quibron Plus (Mead Johnson Laboratories) p 419, 1236

Butabarbital Sodium
  (see under Sodium Butabarbital)

Butalbital
  Amaphen Capsules (Trimen) p 2067
  Amaphen with Codeine #3 (Trimen) p 2067
  Anoquan (Mallard) p 1181
  Axotal (Adria) p 574
  Bancap Capsules (O'Neal, Jones & Feldman) p 1444
  Bancap c̄ Codeine Capsules (O'Neal, Jones & Feldman) p 1444
  Buff-A Comp Tablets (Mayrand) p 1196
  Buff-A Comp No. 3 Tablets (with Codeine) (Mayrand) p 1196
  Butalbital and Acetaminophen Tablets (Danbury) p 887
  Butalbital Compound (Schein) p 1828
  Esgic Tablets & Capsules (Gilbert) p 411, 975
  Fiorinal (Sandoz Pharmaceutical Div.) p 433, 1801
  Fiorinal w/Codeine (Sandoz Pharmaceutical Div.) p 432, 1802
  G-1 Capsules (Hauck) p 1001
  G-2 Capsules (Hauck) p 1001
  G-3 Capsules (Hauck) p 1001
  Pacaps (LaSalle) p 1071
  Phrenilin Tablets (Carnrick) p 408, 833
  Phrenilin Forte (Carnrick) p 408, 833
  Phrenilin with Codeine No. 3 (Carnrick) p 409, 834
  Repan Tablets (Everett) p 942
  Sedapap-10 Tablets (Mayrand) p 1196
  Two-Dyne Capsules (Hyrex) p 1025

Butamben
  Cetacaine Topical Anesthetic (Cetylite) p 839

Butamben Picrate
  Butesin Picrate Ointment (Abbott) p 510

Butorphanol Tartrate
  Stadol (Bristol) p 750

Butyrophenone
  Haldol Tablets, Concentrate, Injection (McNeil Pharmaceutical) p 418, 1201
  Inapsine Injection (Janssen) p 1034
  Innovar Injection (Janssen) p 1035

C

Caffeine
  A.P.C. with Codeine Nos. 3 & 4, Tabloid brand (Burroughs Wellcome) p 407, 780
  Amaphen Capsules (Trimen) p 2067
  Amaphen with Codeine #3 (Trimen) p 2067
  Anacin Analgesic Capsules (Whitehall) p 443, 2184
  Anacin Analgesic Tablets (Whitehall) p 443, 2184
  Anoquan (Mallard) p 1181
  Buff-A Comp Tablets (Mayrand) p 1196
  Buff-A Comp No. 3 Tablets (with Codeine) (Mayrand) p 1196
  Cafergot (Sandoz Pharmaceutical Div.) p 432, 1799
  Cafergot P-B (Sandoz Pharmaceutical Div.) p 432, 1799
  Cafetrate-PB Suppositories (Schein) p 1828
  Compal Capsules (Reid-Provident Labs.) p 427, 1637
  Dexatrim • 15 (Thompson Medical) p 2066
  Dia-Gesic (Central Pharmaceuticals) p 409, 837
  Dihydrocodeine Compound Tablets (Schein) p 1828
  Efed II Capsules (Black) (Alto) p 404, 589
  Esgic Tablets & Capsules (Gilbert) p 411, 975
  Excedrin Extra-Strength (Bristol-Myers Products) p 770
  Fiorinal (Sandoz Pharmaceutical Div.) p 433, 1801
  Fiorinal w/Codeine (Sandoz Pharmaceutical Div.) p 432, 1802
  G-1 Capsules (Hauck) p 1001
  Korigesic Tablets (Trimen) p 2067
  Maximum Strength Midol for Cramps (Glenbrook) p 997
  Migralam Capsules (Lambda) p 1071
  No Doz (Bristol-Myers Products) p 771
  Pacaps (LaSalle) p 1071
  Propoxyphene Compound 65 (Schein) p 1828
  SK-65 Compound Capsules (Smith Kline & French) p 1971
  Synalgos-DC Capsules (Ives) p 413, 1031
  Two-Dyne Capsules (Hyrex) p 1025
  Vanquish (Glenbrook) p 998
  Wigraine Tablets & Suppositories (Organon) p 422, 1451
  Wigraine-PB Suppositories (Organon) p 422, 1451

Caffeine Citrate
  Tussirex Sugar-Free (Scot-Tussin) p 1897
  Tussirex Syrup (Scot-Tussin) p 1897

Calamine
  Caladryl (Parke-Davis) p 1486
  Dome-Paste Bandage (Miles Pharmaceuticals) p 1402

Calcifediol
  Calderol Capsules (Upjohn) p 2093

Calciferol
  Calciferol Drops (Egocalciferol Oral Solution USP) (Rorer) p 431, 1748
  Calciferol in Oil Injection (Egocalciferol USP) (Rorer) p 431, 1748
  Calciferol Tablets (Ergocalciferol USP) (Rorer) p 431, 1748

Calcitonin, Synthetic
  Calcimar Solution (USV Pharmaceutical) p 440, 2072

Calcitriol
  Rocaltrol Capsules (Roche) p 430, 1700

Calcium Acetate
  Domeboro Powder Packets & Tablets (Miles Pharmaceuticals) p 422, 1402
  Pedi-Boro Soak Paks (Pedinol) p 1581

Calcium Carbaspirin
  Fiogesic Tablets (Sandoz Pharmaceutical Div.) p 432, 1801

Calcium Carbonate
  Biocal Calcium Supplement Chewable Tablets (Miles Laboratories) p 1396
  Biocal Calcium Supplement Tablets (Miles Laboratories) p 1396
  Calcet (Mission) p 1415
  Calcet Plus (Mission) p 1415
  Calcium Carbonate Tablets & Oral Suspension (Roxane) p 1788
  Cal-Sup (Riker) p 1642
  Fosfree (Mission) p 1416
  Iromin-G (Mission) p 1416
  Mission Prenatal (Mission) p 1419
  Mission Prenatal F.A. (Mission) p 1419
  Mission Prenatal H.P. (Mission) p 1419
  Natacomp-FA Tablets (Trimen) p 2067
  Natalins Rx (Mead Johnson Laboratories) p 419, 1224
  Natalins Tablets (Mead Johnson Laboratories) p 419, 1224
  Nu-Iron-V Tablets (Mayrand) p 1196
  Os-Cal 250 Tablets (Marion) p 418, 1188
  Os-Cal 500 Tablets (Marion) p 418, 1188
  Pramet FA (Ross) p 432, 1775
  Pramilet FA (Ross) p 432, 1775
  Prenate 90 Tablets (Bock) p 706
  Zenate Tablets (Reid-Provident Labs.) p 428, 1640

Calcium Chloride
  Calcium Chloride Injection (Bristol) p 730
  Calcium Chloride Injection (Elkins-Sinn) p 938

Calcium Disodium Edetate
  Calcium Disodium Versenate Injection (Riker) p 1641

Calcium Glubionate
  Dorcol Children's Liquid Calcium Supplement (Dorsey Laboratories) p 909
  Neo-Calglucon Syrup (Sandoz Pharmaceutical Div.) p 1806

Calcium Gluconate
  Calcet (Mission) p 1415
  Calcet Plus (Mission) p 1415

Generic and Chemical Name Index

Calcium Gluconate Injection (Elkins-Sinn) p 938
Calcium Gluconate Tablets (Roxane) p 1788
Fosfree (Mission) p 1416
Iromin-G (Mission) p 1416
Mission Prenatal (Mission) p 1419
Mission Prenatal F.A. (Mission) p 1419
Mission Prenatal H.P. (Mission) p 1419

Calcium Glycerophosphate
Calphosan (Glenwood) p 998
Calphosan B-12 (Glenwood) p 998

Calcium Iodide
Calcidrine Syrup (Abbott) p 510
Norisodrine w/Calcium Iodide Syrup (Abbott) p 548

Calcium Lactate
Calcet (Mission) p 1415
Calcet Plus (Mission) p 1415
Calphosan (Glenwood) p 998
Calphosan B-12 (Glenwood) p 998
Fosfree (Mission) p 1416
Iromin-G (Mission) p 1416
Mevanin-C Capsules (Beutlich) p 705
Mission Prenatal (Mission) p 1419
Mission Prenatal F.A. (Mission) p 1419
Mission Prenatal H.P. (Mission) p 1419

Calcium (Oyster Shell)
Os-Cal 250 Tablets (Marion) p 418, 1188
Os-Cal 500 Tablets (Marion) p 418, 1188
Os-Cal Forte Tablets (Marion) p 418, 1189
Os-Cal Plus Tablets (Marion) p 418, 1189
Os-Cal-Gesic Tablets (Marion) p 418, 1189

Calcium Pantothenate
Al-Vite (Drug Industries) p 914
B-C-Bid Capsules (Geriatric) p 975
Eldercaps (Mayrand) p 1196
Glutofac Tablets (Kenwood) p 1046
Hemo-Vite (Drug Industries) p 914
Megadose (Arco) p 600
Therabid (Mission) p 1420

Calcium & Calcium-Phosphorus Preparations
Calphosan (Glenwood) p 998
Calphosan B-12 (Glenwood) p 998
Dical-D Capsules & Wafers (Abbott) p 516

Calcium Polycarbophil
Mitrolan (Robins) p 428, 1654

Cantharidin
Cantharone (Seres) p 1939
Cantharone Plus (Seres) p 1939
Verr-Canth (C & M) p 828
Verrusol (C & M) p 828

Capreomycin Sulfate
Capastat Sulfate (Lilly) p 1132

Caprylic Acid
Caprystatin (Ecological Formulas) p 929

Captopril
Capoten (Squibb) p 437, 1986

Caramiphen Edisylate
Rescaps-D T.D. Capsules (Geneva) p 973
Tuss-Ade Timed Capsules (Schein) p 1828
Tuss-Ornade Liquid (Smith Kline & French) p 1980
Tuss-Ornade Spansule Capsules (Smith Kline & French) p 437, 1981

Carbamazepine
Tegretol Chewable Tablets (Geigy) p 411, 966
Tegretol Tablets (Geigy) p 411, 966

Carbamide Peroxide
Ear Drops by Murine—See Murine Ear Wax Removal System (Ross) p 1762
Murine Ear Wax Removal System/Murine Ear Drops (Ross) p 1769
Proxigel (Reed & Carnrick) p 1637

Carbamide Preparations
Carmol HC Cream 1% (Syntex) p 2061
Debrox Drops (Marion) p 1184
Gly-Oxide Liquid (Marion) p 1186

Carbenicillin Disodium
(see under Disodium Carbenicillin)

Carbenicillin Indanyl Sodium
Geocillin Tablets (Roerig) p 431, 1730

Carbetapentane Citrate
Tussar SF (USV Pharmaceutical) p 2092
Tussar-2 (USV Pharmaceutical) p 2092

Carbetapentane Tannate
Rynatuss Tablets & Pediatric Suspension (Wallace) p 442, 2165

Carbidopa
Sinemet Tablets (Merck Sharp & Dohme) p 420, 1345

Carbinoxamine Maleate
Cardec DM Drops & Syrup (Schein) p 1828
Rondec Oral Drops (Ross) p 1776
Rondec Syrup (Ross) p 1776
Rondec Tablet (Ross) p 432, 1776
Rondec-DM Oral Drops (Ross) p 1777
Rondec-DM Syrup (Ross) p 1777
Rondec-TR Tablet (Ross) p 432, 1776

Carbon Dioxide
Evac-Q-Kit (Adria) p 575

Carboxymethylcellulose Sodium
Dieutrim Capsules (Legere) p 1120

Carisoprodol
Carisoprodol Compound Tablets (Danbury) p 887
Carisoprodol Tablets (Danbury) p 887
Carisoprodol Tablets (Geneva) p 973
Soma (Wallace) p 442, 2166
Soma Compound (Wallace) p 442, 2166
Soma Compound w/Codeine (Wallace) p 442, 2169
Soprodol Tablets (Carisoprodol) (Schein) p 1828

Carmustine (BCNU)
BiCNU (Bristol-Myers Oncology) p 756

L. Carnitine
L-Carnitine (Tyson) p 2068

Casanthranol
Dialose Plus Capsules (Stuart) p 439, 2037
Docusate Sodium with Casanthranol Capsules (Roxane) p 1788
Peri-Colace (Mead Johnson Pharmaceutical) p 419, 1255

Cascara Sagrada
Aromatic Cascara Fluidextract (Roxane) p 1788
Milk of Magnesia-Cascara Suspension Concentrated (Roxane) p 1788
Peri-Colace (Mead Johnson Pharmaceutical) p 419, 1255

Castor Oil
Castor Oil, Castor Oil Favored (Roxane) p 1788
Fleet Flavored Castor Oil Emulsion (Fleet) p 947
Fleet Prep Kits (Fleet) p 947
Granulex (Hickam) p 1009
Hydrisinol Creme & Lotion (Pedinol) p 1580
Neoloid (Lederle) p 1107
Stimuzyme Plus (National Dermaceutical) p 1421

Cefaclor
Ceclor (Lilly) p 417, 1133

Cefadroxil Monohydrate
Duricef (Mead Johnson Pharmaceutical) p 419, 1250
Ultracef Capsules, Tablets & Oral Suspension (Bristol) p 407, 754

Cefamandole Nafate
Mandol (Lilly) p 1161

Cefazolin Sodium
Ancef (Smith Kline & French) p 1945
Kefzol (Lilly) p 1159

Cefonicid Sodium
Monocid Injection (Smith Kline & French) p 1966

Cefoperazone Sodium
Cefobid Intravenous/Intramuscular (Roerig) p 1726

Ceforanide
Precef (Bristol) p 743

Cefotaxime Sodium
Claforan (Hoechst-Roussel) p 1010

Cefoxitin Sodium
Mefoxin (Merck Sharp & Dohme) p 1326

Ceftizoxime Sodium
Cefizox Injection (Smith Kline & French) p 1949

Cefuroxime Sodium
Zinacef (Glaxo) p 993

Cellulase
Celluzyme Chewable Tablets (Dalin) p 886
Enzobile Improved Formula (Mallard) p 1181
Kanulase (Dorsey Laboratories) p 910

Cellulolytic Enzyme
Arco-Lase (Arco) p 600
Arco-Lase Plus (Arco) p 600
Celluzyme Chewable Tablets (Dalin) p 886
Festal II (Hoechst-Roussel) p 412, 1014
Festalan (Hoechst-Roussel) p 413, 1014
Gustase (Geriatric) p 975
Kutrase Capsules (Rorer) p 431, 1750
Ku-Zyme Capsules (Rorer) p 431, 1750

Cellulose Sodium Phosphate
Calcibind (Mission) p 1416

Cephalexin
Keflex Oral Preparations (Dista) p 410, 901

Cephalothin Sodium
Keflin, Neutral, Vials & Faspak (Lilly) p 1157
Seffin, Neutral (Glaxo) p 980

Cephapirin Sodium
Cefadyl (Bristol) p 731

Cephradine
Anspor (Smith Kline & French) p 436, 1948
Velosef Capsules (Squibb) p 438, 2027
Velosef for Infusion (Sodium-Free) (Squibb) p 2029
Velosef for Injection (Squibb) p 2030
Velosef for Oral Suspension (Squibb) p 2027

Cervical Caps (Rubber)
Koro-Flex Arcing Spring Diaphragm (Youngs) p 2300
Koromex Coil Spring Diaphragm (Youngs) p 2301

Cetyl Dimethyl Ethyl Ammonium Bromide
Cetylcide Solution (Cetylite) p 839

Cetyl Pyridinium Chloride
Fungoid Creme & Solution (Pedinol) p 1580
Fungoid Tincture (Pedinol) p 1580
Gumsol (Arlo) p 601

Charcoal, Activated
Arm-a-char (Armour) p 604
Karbokoff Tablets (Arlo) p 601

Chenodiol
Chenix (Rowell) p 1786

Chloral Hydrate
Chloral Hydrate Capsules (Geneva) p 973
Chloral Hydrate Capsules, Syrup (Roxane) p 1788
Chloral Hydrate Capsules (Schein) p 1828
Noctec Capsules & Syrup (Squibb) p 438, 2007
SK-Chloral Hydrate Capsules (Smith Kline & French) p 1971

Chlorambucil
Leukeran (Burroughs Wellcome) p 408, 801

Chloramphenicol
Chloramphenicol Ophthalmic Solution 5% (Schein) p 1828
Chloromycetin Cream, 1% (Parke-Davis) p 1487
Chloromycetin Hydrocortisone Ophthalmic (Parke-Davis) p 1486
Chloromycetin Kapseals (Parke-Davis) p 423, 1489
Chloromycetin Ophthalmic Ointment, 1% (Parke-Davis) p 1491
Chloromycetin Otic (Parke-Davis) p 1491
Ophthochlor, 0.5% (Parke-Davis) p 425, 1557
Ophthocort (Parke-Davis) p 1558

Chloramphenicol Palmitate
Chloromycetin Palmitate (Parke-Davis) p 1491

Chloramphenicol Sodium Succinate
Chloramphenicol Sodium Succinate Injection (Elkins-Sinn) p 938
Chloromycetin Sodium Succinate (Parke-Davis) p 1493

Chlorcyclizine Hydrochloride
Mantadil Cream (Burroughs Wellcome) p 803

Chlordiazepoxide
Libritabs Tablets (Roche Products) p 430, 1714

Generic and Chemical Name Index

Limbitrol Tablets (Roche Products) p 430, 1716
Menrium Tablets (Roche Products) p 430, 1717

Chlordiazepoxide Hydrochloride
Chlordiazepoxide Capsules (Geneva) p 973
Chlordiazepoxide Hydrochloride Capsules (Roxane) p 1788
Chlordiazepoxide HCl Capsules (Schein) p 1828
Clipoxide Capsules (Schein) p 1828
Librax Capsules (Roche Products) p 430, 1713
Librium Capsules (Roche Products) p 430, 1714
Librium Injectable (Roche Products) p 1715
SK-Lygen Capsules (Smith Kline & French) p 1971

Chlorhexidine Gluconate
Hibiclens Antimicrobial Skin Cleanser (Stuart) p 439, 2037
Hibistat Germicidal Hand Rinse (Stuart) p 439, 2038

Chlormezanone
Trancopal (Winthrop-Breon) p 444, 2232

Chlorophyll Preparations
Chloresium Ointment (Rystan) p 1795
Chloresium Solution (Rystan) p 1795
Chlorophyll Complex Perles (Standard Process) p 2035
Derifil Tablets & Powder (Rystan) p 1796
Panafil Ointment (Rystan) p 1796
Prophyllin (Rystan) p 1796

Chloroprocaine Hydrochloride
Nesacaine Solutions (Astra) p 618
Nesacaine-CE Solutions (Astra) p 618

Chloroquine Hydrochloride
Aralen Hydrochloride (Winthrop-Breon) p 2189

Chloroquine Phosphate
Aralen Phosphate (Winthrop-Breon) p 443, 2190
Aralen Phosphate w/Primaquine Phosphate (Winthrop-Breon) p 2191
Chloroquine Phosphate Tablets (Biocraft) p 705
Chloroquine Phosphate Tablets (Danbury) p 887

Chlorothiazide
Aldoclor Tablets (Merck Sharp & Dohme) p 420, 1258
Chloroserpine 250 & 500 Tablets (Schein) p 1828
Chlorothiazide Tablets (Danbury) p 887
Chlorothiazide Tablets (Geneva) p 973
Chlorothiazide Tablets (Schein) p 1828
Chlorothiazide w/Reserpine Tablets (Geneva) p 973
Diupres Tablets (Merck Sharp & Dohme) p 420, 1298
Diuril Tablets & Oral Suspension (Merck Sharp & Dohme) p 420, 1301
SK-Chlorothiazide Tablets (Smith Kline & French) p 1971

Chlorothiazide Sodium
Diuril Intravenous Sodium (Merck Sharp & Dohme) p 1299

Chlorotrianisene
TACE 12 mg Capsules (Merrell Dow) p 421, 1385
TACE 25 mg Capsules (Merrell Dow) p 421, 1385
TACE 72 mg Capsules (Merrell Dow) p 421, 1389

Chloroxine
Capitrol Cream Shampoo (Westwood) p 2175

Chloroxylenol
Anti-Sept (Seamless) p 1897
Fungoid Creme & Solution (Pedinol) p 1580
Fungoid Tincture (Pedinol) p 1580
Micro-Guard (Sween) p 2048
Pedi-Pro Foot Powder (Pedinol) p 1581
Sween Prep (Sween) p 2049
Sween Soft Touch (Sween) p 2049

Chlorphenesin Carbamate
Maolate Tablets (Upjohn) p 441, 2123

Chlorpheniramine
Dallergy Capsules, Tablets, Syrup (Laser) p 1072
Decongestant Elixir (Schein) p 1828
Donatussin Drops (Laser) p 1072

Probahist Capsules (Legere) p 1120
Quadrahist Pediatric Syrup, Syrup & Timed Release Tablets (Schein) p 1828

Chlorpheniramine Maleate
Alka-Seltzer Plus Cold Medicine (Miles Laboratories) p 1395
Anafed Capsules & Syrup (Everett) p 941
Anamine Syrup (Mayrand) p 1196
Anamine T.D. Caps (Mayrand) p 1196
Brexin L.A. Capsules (Savage) p 433, 1824
Bronkotuss (Hyrex) p 1024
Chlorafed H.S. Timecelles (Hauck) p 1001
Chlorafed Liquid (Hauck) p 1001
Chlorafed Timecelles (Hauck) p 1001
Chlorpheniramine Maleate T.D. Capsules (Geneva) p 973
Chlorpheniramine Maleate Tablets (Roxane) p 1788
Citra Forte Capsules (Boyle) p 726
Citra Forte Syrup (Boyle) p 726
Codimal-L.A. Capsules (Central Pharmaceuticals) p 409, 836
Comhist LA Capsules (Norwich Eaton) p 422, 1425
Comhist Tablets (Norwich Eaton) p 1426
Comtrex (Bristol-Myers Products) p 769
Co-Pyronil 2 (Dista) p 895
Coryban-D Capsules (Pfipharmecs) p 1589
CoTylenol Cold Medication Tablets & Capsules (McNeil Consumer Products) p 418, 1197
CoTylenol Liquid Cold Medication (McNeil Consumer Products) p 1197
CoTylenol Children's Liquid Cold Formula (McNeil Consumer Products) p 418, 1198
Deconamine Tablets, Elixir, SR Capsules, Syrup (Berlex) p 406, 699
Decongestant-AT (Antitussive) Liquid (Schein) p 1828
Dehist (O'Neal, Jones & Feldman) p 1445
Dorcol Children's Liquid Cold Formula (Dorsey Laboratories) p 909
Dristan, Advanced Formula Decongestant/Antihistamine/Analgesic Capsules (Whitehall) p 443, 2186
Dristan, Advanced Formula Decongestant/Antihistamine/Analgesic Tablets (Whitehall) p 443, 2186
Dura-Vent/A (Dura) p 929
Dura-Vent/DA (Dura) p 929
E.N.T. Tablets (Springbok) p 1985
Extendryl Chewable Tablets (Fleming) p 948
Extendryl Sr. & Jr. T.D. Capsules (Fleming) p 948
Extendryl Syrup (Fleming) p 948
4-Way Cold Tablets (Bristol-Myers Products) p 770
Fedahist Expectorant (Rorer) p 1749
Fedahist Gyrocaps, Syrup & Tablets (Rorer) p 431, 1749
Histalet DM Syrup (Reid-Provident Labs.) p 1638
Histalet Forte Tablets (Reid-Provident Labs.) p 428, 1638
Histalet Syrup (Reid-Provident Labs.) p 1638
Histaspan-D Capsules (USV Pharmaceutical) p 2077
Histaspan-Plus Capsules (USV Pharmaceutical) p 2077
Histor-D Timecelles (Hauck) p 1001
Hycomine Compound (Du Pont) p 919
Iophen-C Liquid (Schein) p 1828
Isoclor Timesule Capsules (Fisons) p 944
Korigesic Tablets (Trimen) p 2067
Kronofed-A Jr. Kronocaps (Ferndale) p 942
Kronofed-A Kronocaps (Ferndale) p 942
Kronohist Kronocaps (Ferndale) p 942
Naldecon (Bristol) p 407, 738
Nolamine Tablets (Carnrick) p 408, 833
Novafed A Capsules (Merrell Dow) p 421, 1377
Novafed A Liquid (Merrell Dow) p 1377
Novahistine DH (Merrell Dow) p 421, 1378
Ornade Spansule Capsules (Smith Kline & French) p 437, 1968
P-V-Tussin Syrup (Reid-Provident Labs.) p 1640
Pediacof (Winthrop-Breon) p 2221
Phenate (Mallard) p 1181
Protid, Improved Formula (LaSalle) p 1071
Quelidrine Syrup (Abbott) p 567
Resaid T.D. Capsules (Geneva) p 973
Rhinolar Capsules (McGregor) p 1197
Rhinolar-EX Capsules (McGregor) p 1197
Rhinolar-EX 12 Capsules (McGregor) p 1197
Ru-Tuss Tablets (Boots) p 406, 723
Ru-Tuss II Capsules (Boots) p 406, 723
Scot-Tussin Sugar-Free 5-Action Cold Formula (Scot-Tussin) p 1897
Singlet (Merrell Dow) p 421, 1385
Sinovan Timed (Drug Industries) p 915
Sinulin Tablets (Carnrick) p 409, 835
Triaminic Cold Syrup (Dorsey Laboratories) p 911
Triaminic Cold Tablets (Dorsey Laboratories) p 911

Triaminic-12 Tablets (Dorsey Laboratories) p 913
Triaminicol Multi-Symptom Cold Syrup (Dorsey Laboratories) p 913
Triaminicol Multi-Symptom Cold Tablets (Dorsey Laboratories) p 914
Tussar DM (USV Pharmaceutical) p 2091
Tussar SF (USV Pharmaceutical) p 2092
Tussar-2 (USV Pharmaceutical) p 2092

Chlorpheniramine Polistirex
Corsym (Pennwalt) p 1582

Chlorpheniramine Preparations
Deconamine Tablets, Elixir, SR Capsules, Syrup (Berlex) p 406, 699
Fedahist Expectorant (Rorer) p 1749
Fedahist Gyrocaps, Syrup & Tablets (Rorer) p 431, 1749

Chlorpheniramine Tannate
Rynatan Tablets & Pediatric Suspension (Wallace) p 442, 2165
Rynatuss Tablets & Pediatric Suspension (Wallace) p 442, 2165

Chlorpromazine
Chlorpromazine Tablets & Concentrate Syrup (Geneva) p 973
Thorazine (Smith Kline & French) p 437, 1977

Chlorpromazine Hydrochloride
Chlorpromazine HCl Injection (Elkins-Sinn) p 938
Chlorpromazine HCl Tablets (Schein) p 1828
Chlorpromazine HCl in Tubex (Wyeth) p 2288

Chlorpropamide
Chlorpropamide Tablets (Danbury) p 887
Chlorpropamide Tablets (Geneva) p 973
Diabinese (Pfizer) p 426, 1599
Glucamide Tablets (Lemmon) p 1122

Chlorprothixene
Taractan Tablets (Roche) p 1703

Chlorprothixene Hydrochloride
Taractan Concentrate (Roche) p 1703
Taractan Injectable (Roche) p 1703

Chlorprothixene Lactate
Taractan Concentrate (Roche) p 1703

Chlortetracycline Hydrochloride
Aureomycin Ointment 3% (Lederle) p 1089

Chlorthalidone
Chlorthalidone Tablets (Abbott) p 403, 510
Chlorthalidone Tablets (Danbury) p 887
Chlorthalidone Tablets (Schein) p 1828
Chlorthalidone Tablets, USP (Parke-Davis) p 1494
Combipres Tablets (Boehringer Ingelheim) p 406, 708
Demi-Regroton Tablets (USV Pharmaceutical) p 440, 2087
Hygroton Tablets (USV Pharmaceutical) p 440, 2078
Regroton Tablets (USV Pharmaceutical) p 440, 2087
Tenoretic Tablets (Stuart) p 439, 2043
Thalitone Tablets (Boehringer Ingelheim) p 406, 715

Chlorzoxazone
Algisin Capsules (RAM Laboratories) p 1632
Chlorzone Forte Tablets (Schein) p 1828
Chlorzoxazone Tablets (Danbury) p 887
Chlorzoxazone with APAP Tablets (Danbury) p 887
Chlorzoxasone w/APAP Tablets (Geneva) p 973
Paraflex Tablets (McNeil Pharmaceutical) p 1205
Parafon Forte Tablets (McNeil Pharmaceutical) p 419, 1206

Cholera Vaccine
Cholera Vaccine (Wyeth) p 2245
Cholera Vaccine (India Strains) (Lederle) p 1089

Cholestyramine
Questran (Mead Johnson Laboratories) p 1231

Choline
Cardioguard Natural Lipotropic Dietary Supplement-Powder (Professional Health) p 1621

Choline Bitartrate
Mega-B (Arco) p 600
Megadose (Arco) p 600

Generic and Chemical Name Index

Choline Magnesium Trisalicylate
 Trilisate Tablets/Liquid (Purdue Frederick) p 427, 1627

Chorionic Gonadotropin
 A.P.L. (Ayerst) p 636
 Glukor Injection (Hyrex) p 1024
 Pregnyl (Organon) p 1450
 Profasi HP (HCG) (Serono) p 1943

Chromic Chloride
 Chrometrace (Armour) p 604
 Multitrace 5 (Armour) p 608
 Multitrace Pediatric (Armour) p 609
 Multitrace Solution & Concentrate (Armour) p 609

Chromium
 Total Formula (Vitaline) p 2148

Chymopapain for Injection
 Chymodiactin (Smith) p 437, 1983

Chymotrypsin
 Orenzyme (Merrell Dow) p 1379
 Orenzyme Bitabs (Merrell Dow) p 1379

Ciclopirox Olamine
 Loprox Cream 1% (Hoechst-Roussel) p 413, 1017

Cimetidine
 Tagamet (Smith Kline & French) p 437, 1973

Cinnamedrine Hydrochloride
 Maximum Strength Midol for Cramps (Glenbrook) p 997
 Midol-Original Formula (Glenbrook) p 997

Cinoxacin
 Cinobac Pulvules (Dista) p 410, 894

Cisplatin
 Platinol (Bristol-Myers Oncology) p 765

Citric Acid
 Bicitra—Sugar-Free (Willen) p 2187
 Polycitra Syrup (Willen) p 2188
 Polycitra-K Syrup (Willen) p 2189
 Polycitra-LC—Sugar-Free (Willen) p 2188

Clemastine Fumarate
 Tavist Tablets (Sandoz Pharmaceutical Div.) p 433, 1818
 Tavist-1 Tablets (Sandoz Pharmaceutical Div.) p 433, 1818
 Tavist-D Tablets (Sandoz Pharmaceutical Div.) p 433, 1819

Clidinium Bromide
 Clipoxide Capsules (Schein) p 1828
 Librax Capsules (Roche Products) p 430, 1713
 Quarzan Capsules (Roche Products) p 430, 1721

Clindamycin Hydrochloride
 Cleocin HCl Capsules* (Upjohn) p 441, 2094

Clindamycin Palmitate Hydrochloride
 Cleocin Pediatric Flavored Granules* (Upjohn) p 2096

Clindamycin Phosphate
 Cleocin Phosphate Sterile Solution* (Upjohn) p 440, 2097
 Cleocin T Topical Solution* (Upjohn) p 441, 2100

Clocortolone Pivalate
 Cloderm (Ortho Pharmaceutical (Dermatological Div.)) p 1472

Clofibrate
 Atromid-S (Ayerst) p 404, 636

Clomiphene Citrate
 Clomid (Merrell Dow) p 1364
 Serophene (clomiphene citrate USP) (Serono) p 1943

Clonazepam
 Clonopin Tablets (Roche) p 429, 1680

Clonidine Hydrochloride
 Catapres Tablets (Boehringer Ingelheim) p 406, 707
 Combipres Tablets (Boehringer Ingelheim) p 406, 708

Clorazepate Dipotassium
 Tranxene Capsules & Tablets (Abbott) p 404, 568
 Tranxene-SD (Abbott) p 404, 568
 Tranxene-SD Half Strength (Abbott) p 404, 568

Clotrimazole
 Gyne-Lotrimin Vaginal Cream 1% (Schering) p 1856
 Gyne-Lotrimin Vaginal Tablets (Schering) p 434, 1856
 Lotrimin Cream 1% (Schering) p 1857
 Lotrimin Lotion 1% (Schering) p 1857
 Lotrimin Solution 1% (Schering) p 1857
 Lotrisone Cream (Schering) p 1858
 Mycelex 1% Cream (Miles Pharmaceuticals) p 1409
 Mycelex 1% Solution (Miles Pharmaceuticals) p 1409
 Mycelex Troches (Miles Pharmaceuticals) p 422, 1409
 Mycelex-G (Miles Pharmaceuticals) p 422, 1410
 Mycelex-G 1% Vaginal Cream (Miles Pharmaceuticals) p 1410

Cloxacillin
 Cloxacillin Capsules (Biocraft) p 705
 Cloxacillin Sodium Capsules (Schein) p 1828
 Cloxacillin Solution (Biocraft) p 705

Cloxacillin Sodium Monohydrate
 Tegopen (Bristol) p 407, 753

Coal Tar
 Denorex Medicated Shampoo and Conditioner (Whitehall) p 443, 2185
 Denorex Medicated Shampoo, Regular & Mountain Fresh Herbal Scent (Whitehall) p 443, 2185
 Fototar Cream 1.6% (Elder) p 931
 Fototar Stik 5% (Elder) p 931
 Pentrax Tar Shampoo (Cooper Dermatology) p 882
 Zetar Emulsion (Dermik) p 892
 Zetar Shampoo (Dermik) p 892

Cocaine Hydrochloride
 Cocaine Hydrochloride Topical Solution (Roxane) p 1788

Codeine
 APAP w/Codeine Tablets (Geneva) p 973
 APAP w/Codeine #3 (Geneva) p 973
 APAP w/Codeine #4 (Geneva) p 973
 Acetaminophen with Codeine Tablets and Capsules (Lemmon) p 1122
 Apap 300 mg. with Codeine Capsules & Tabs (Schein) p 1828
 Apap with Codeine Elixir (Schein) p 1828
 Aspirin 325 mg. with Codeine Tabs (Schein) p 1828
 Calcidrine Syrup (Abbott) p 510
 Empracet with Codeine Phosphate Nos. 3 & 4 (Burroughs Wellcome) p 408, 789
 Terpin Hydrate & Codeine Elixir (Roxane) p 1788

Codeine Phosphate
 A.P.C. with Codeine Nos. 3 & 4, Tabloid brand (Burroughs Wellcome) p 407, 780
 Acetaco Tablets (Legere) p 1120
 Acetaminophen with Codeine Phosphate Tablets (Roxane) p 1788
 Actifed with Codeine Cough Syrup (Burroughs Wellcome) p 773
 Amaphen with Codeine #3 (Trimen) p 2067
 Anacin-3 with Codeine Tablets (Ayerst) p 404, 634
 Ascriptin with Codeine (Rorer) p 431, 1745
 Bancap c̄ Codeine Capsules (O'Neal, Jones & Feldman) p 1444
 Bromanyl Expectorant (Schein) p 1828
 Bromphen DC Expectorant (Schein) p 1828
 Buff-A Comp No. 3 Tablets (with Codeine) (Mayrand) p 1196
 Capital with Codeine Suspension (Carnrick) p 408, 831
 Capital with Codeine Tablets (Carnrick) p 408, 831
 Codalan (Lannett) p 1071
 Codeine Phosphate Injection (Elkins-Sinn) p 938
 Codeine Phosphate in Tubex (Wyeth) p 2288
 Codeine Phosphate Oral Solution (Roxane) p 1788
 Codimal PH (Central Pharmaceuticals) p 836
 Conex with Codeine (O'Neal, Jones & Feldman) p 1445
 Decongestant Expectorant (Schein) p 1828
 Decongestant-AT (Antitussive) Liquid (Schein) p 1828
 Deproist Expectorant w/Codeine (Geneva) p 973
 Dimetane-DC Cough Syrup (Robins) p 1647
 Dolprn #3 Tablets (Bock) p 705
 Empirin with Codeine (Burroughs Wellcome) p 408, 787
 Fiorinal w/Codeine (Sandoz Pharmaceutical Div.) p 432, 1802
 G-2 Capsules (Hauck) p 1001
 G-3 Capsules (Hauck) p 1001
 Guiatuss A-C Syrup (Schein) p 1828
 Iophen-C Liquid (Schein) p 1828
 Naldecon-CX Suspension (Bristol) p 739
 Novahistine DH (Merrell Dow) p 421, 1378
 Novahistine Expectorant (Merrell Dow) p 421, 1378
 Nucofed Capsules (Beecham Laboratories) p 406, 692
 Nucofed Expectorant (Beecham Laboratories) p 693
 Nucofed Pediatric Expectorant (Beecham Laboratories) p 694
 Nucofed Syrup (Beecham Laboratories) p 692
 Pediacof (Winthrop-Breon) p 2221
 Phenaphen w/Codeine Capsules (Robins) p 428, 1656
 Phenaphen-650 with Codeine Tablets (Robins) p 428, 1656
 Phenergan VC with Codeine (Wyeth) p 2284
 Phenergan with Codeine (Wyeth) p 2278
 Phrenilin with Codeine No. 3 (Carnrick) p 409, 834
 Poly-Histine Expectorant with Codeine (Bock) p 705
 Robitussin A-C (Robins) p 1664
 Robitussin-DAC (Robins) p 1665
 Ru-Tuss Expectorant (Boots) p 722
 SK-APAP with CODEINE Tablets (Smith Kline & French) p 1971
 Soma Compound w/Codeine (Wallace) p 442, 2169
 Stopayne Syrup (Springbok) p 1985
 Triafed-C Expectorant (Schein) p 1828
 Triaminic Expectorant w/Codeine (Dorsey Laboratories) p 911
 Tussar SF (USV Pharmaceutical) p 2092
 Tussar-2 (USV Pharmaceutical) p 2092
 Tussi-Organidin (Wallace) p 442, 2171
 Tussirex Sugar-Free (Scot-Tussin) p 1897
 Tussirex Syrup (Scot-Tussin) p 1897
 Tylenol w/Codeine Elixir (McNeil Pharmaceutical) p 419, 1214
 Tylenol w/Codeine Tablets, Capsules (McNeil Pharmaceutical) p 419, 1214

Codeine Sulfate
 Ambenyl Cough Syrup (Marion) p 1181
 Aspirin w/Codeine Tablets (Geneva) p 973
 Codeine Sulfate Tablets (Roxane) p 1788

Colchicine
 ColBENEMID Tablets (Merck Sharp & Dohme) p 420, 1277
 Colchicine Ampoules (Lilly) p 1134
 Colchicine Tablets (Danbury) p 887
 Colchicine Tablets (Lilly) p 1135
 Col-Probenecid Tablets (Danbury) p 887
 Probenecid w/Colchicine Tablets (Geneva) p 973
 Probenecid with Colchicine Tablets (Schein) p 1828

Colestipol Hydrochloride
 Colestid Granules (Upjohn) p 2100

Colistimethate Sodium
 Coly-Mycin M Parenteral (Parke-Davis) p 1500

Colistin Sulfate
 Coly-Mycin S Oral Suspension (Parke-Davis) p 1501
 Coly-Mycin S Otic w/Neomycin & Hydrocortisone (Parke-Davis) p 1501

Collagenase
 Santyl Ointment (Knoll) p 1067

Colloidal Oatmeal
 Aveeno Bath Oilated (Cooper Dermatology) p 882
 Aveeno Bath Regular (Cooper Dermatology) p 882
 Aveenobar Oilated (Cooper Dermatology) p 882
 Aveenobar Regular (Cooper Dermatology) p 882

Copper
 Added Protection III Multi-Vitamin & Multi-Mineral Supplement (Professional Health) p 1621

Copper Sulfate
 Hemo-Vite (Drug Industries) p 914
 Vio-Bec Forte (Rowell) p 1788

Cortex Rhamni Frangulae
 Movicol (Norgine) p 1424

Generic and Chemical Name Index

Limbitrol Tablets (Roche Products) p 430, 1716
Menrium Tablets (Roche Products) p 430, 1717

Chlordiazepoxide Hydrochloride
Chlordiazepoxide Capsules (Geneva) p 973
Chlordiazepoxide Hydrochloride Capsules (Roxane) p 1788
Chlordiazepoxide HCl Capsules (Schein) p 1828
Clipoxide Capsules (Schein) p 1828
Librax Capsules (Roche Products) p 430, 1713
Librium Capsules (Roche Products) p 430, 1714
Librium Injectable (Roche Products) p 1715
SK-Lygen Capsules (Smith Kline & French) p 1971

Chlorhexidine Gluconate
Hibiclens Antimicrobial Skin Cleanser (Stuart) p 439, 2037
Hibistat Germicidal Hand Rinse (Stuart) p 439, 2038

Chlormezanone
Trancopal (Winthrop-Breon) p 444, 2232

Chlorophyll Preparations
Chloresium Ointment (Rystan) p 1795
Chloresium Solution (Rystan) p 1795
Chlorophyll Complex Perles (Standard Process) p 2035
Derifil Tablets & Powder (Rystan) p 1796
Panafil Ointment (Rystan) p 1796
Prophyllin (Rystan) p 1796

Chloroprocaine Hydrochloride
Nesacaine Solutions (Astra) p 618
Nesacaine-CE Solutions (Astra) p 618

Chloroquine Hydrochloride
Aralen Hydrochloride (Winthrop-Breon) p 2189

Chloroquine Phosphate
Aralen Phosphate (Winthrop-Breon) p 443, 2190
Aralen Phosphate w/Primaquine Phosphate (Winthrop-Breon) p 2191
Chloroquine Phosphate Tablets (Biocraft) p 705
Chloroquine Phosphate Tablets (Danbury) p 887

Chlorothiazide
Aldoclor Tablets (Merck Sharp & Dohme) p 420, 1258
Chloroserpine 250 & 500 Tablets (Schein) p 1828
Chlorothiazide Tablets (Danbury) p 887
Chlorothiazide Tablets (Geneva) p 973
Chlorothiazide Tablets (Schein) p 1828
Chlorothiazide w/Reserpine Tablets (Geneva) p 973
Diupres Tablets (Merck Sharp & Dohme) p 420, 1298
Diuril Tablets & Oral Suspension (Merck Sharp & Dohme) p 420, 1301
SK-Chlorothiazide Tablets (Smith Kline & French) p 1971

Chlorothiazide Sodium
Diuril Intravenous Sodium (Merck Sharp & Dohme) p 1299

Chlorotrianisene
TACE 12 mg Capsules (Merrell Dow) p 421, 1385
TACE 25 mg Capsules (Merrell Dow) p 421, 1385
TACE 72 mg Capsules (Merrell Dow) p 421, 1389

Chloroxine
Capitrol Cream Shampoo (Westwood) p 2175

Chloroxylenol
Anti-Sept (Seamless) p 1897
Fungoid Creme & Solution (Pedinol) p 1580
Fungoid Tincture (Pedinol) p 1580
Micro-Guard (Sween) p 2048
Pedi-Pro Foot Powder (Pedinol) p 1581
Sween Prep (Sween) p 2049
Sween Soft Touch (Sween) p 2049

Chlorphenesin Carbamate
Maolate Tablets (Upjohn) p 441, 2123

Chlorpheniramine
Dallergy Capsules, Tablets, Syrup (Laser) p 1072
Decongestant Elixir (Schein) p 1828
Donatussin Drops (Laser) p 1072
Probahist Capsules (Legere) p 1120
Quadrahist Pediatric Syrup, Syrup & Timed Release Tablets (Schein) p 1828

Chlorpheniramine Maleate
Alka-Seltzer Plus Cold Medicine (Miles Laboratories) p 1395
Anafed Capsules & Syrup (Everett) p 941
Anamine Syrup (Mayrand) p 1196
Anamine T.D. Caps (Mayrand) p 1196
Brexin L.A. Capsules (Savage) p 433, 1824
Bronkotuss (Hyrex) p 1024
Chlorafed H.S. Timecelles (Hauck) p 1001
Chlorafed Liquid (Hauck) p 1001
Chlorafed Timecelles (Hauck) p 1001
Chlorpheniramine Maleate T.D. Capsules (Geneva) p 973
Chlorpheniramine Maleate Tablets (Roxane) p 1788
Citra Forte Capsules (Boyle) p 726
Citra Forte Syrup (Boyle) p 726
Codimal-L.A. Capsules (Central Pharmaceuticals) p 409, 836
Comhist LA Capsules (Norwich Eaton) p 422, 1425
Comhist Tablets (Norwich Eaton) p 1426
Comtrex (Bristol-Myers Products) p 769
Co-Pyronil 2 (Dista) p 895
Coryban-D Capsules (Pfipharmecs) p 1589
CoTylenol Cold Medication Tablets & Capsules (McNeil Consumer Products) p 418, 1197
CoTylenol Liquid Cold Medication (McNeil Consumer Products) p 1197
CoTylenol Children's Liquid Cold Formula (McNeil Consumer Products) p 418, 1198
Deconamine Tablets, Elixir, SR Capsules, Syrup (Berlex) p 406, 699
Decongestant-AT (Antitussive) Liquid (Schein) p 1828
Dehist (O'Neal, Jones & Feldman) p 1445
Dorcol Children's Liquid Cold Formula (Dorsey Laboratories) p 909
Dristan, Advanced Formula Decongestant/Antihistamine/Analgesic Capsules (Whitehall) p 443, 2186
Dristan, Advanced Formula Decongestant/Antihistamine/Analgesic Tablets (Whitehall) p 443, 2186
Dura-Vent/A (Dura) p 929
Dura-Vent/DA (Dura) p 929
E.N.T. Tablets (Springbok) p 1985
Extendryl Chewable Tablets (Fleming) p 948
Extendryl Sr. & Jr. T.D. Capsules (Fleming) p 948
Extendryl Syrup (Fleming) p 948
4-Way Cold Tablets (Bristol-Myers Products) p 770
Fedahist Expectorant (Rorer) p 1749
Fedahist Gyrocaps, Syrup & Tablets (Rorer) p 431, 1749
Histalet DM Syrup (Reid-Provident Labs.) p 1638
Histalet Forte Tablets (Reid-Provident Labs.) p 428, 1638
Histalet Syrup (Reid-Provident Labs.) p 1638
Histaspan-D Capsules (USV Pharmaceutical) p 2077
Histaspan-Plus Capsules (USV Pharmaceutical) p 2077
Histor-D Timecelles (Hauck) p 1001
Hycomine Compound (Du Pont) p 919
Iophen-C Liquid (Schein) p 1828
Isoclor Timesule Capsules (Fisons) p 944
Korigesic Tablets (Trimen) p 2067
Kronofed-A Jr. Kronocaps (Ferndale) p 942
Kronofed-A Kronocaps (Ferndale) p 942
Kronohist Kronocaps (Ferndale) p 942
Naldecon (Bristol) p 407, 738
Nolamine Tablets (Carnrick) p 408, 833
Novafed A Capsules (Merrell Dow) p 421, 1377
Novafed A Liquid (Merrell Dow) p 1377
Novahistine DH (Merrell Dow) p 421, 1378
Ornade Spansule Capsules (Smith Kline & French) p 437, 1968
P-V-Tussin Syrup (Reid-Provident Labs.) p 1640
Pediacof (Winthrop-Breon) p 2221
Phenate (Mallard) p 1181
Protid, Improved Formula (LaSalle) p 1071
Quelidrine Syrup (Abbott) p 567
Resaid T.D. Capsules (Geneva) p 973
Rhinolar Capsules (McGregor) p 1197
Rhinolar-EX Capsules (McGregor) p 1197
Rhinolar-EX 12 Capsules (McGregor) p 1197
Ru-Tuss Tablets (Boots) p 406, 723
Ru-Tuss II Capsules (Boots) p 406, 723
Scot-Tussin Sugar-Free 5-Action Cold Formula (Scot-Tussin) p 1897
Singlet (Merrell Dow) p 421, 1385
Sinovan Timed (Drug Industries) p 915
Sinulin Tablets (Carnrick) p 409, 835
Triaminic Cold Syrup (Dorsey Laboratories) p 911
Triaminic Cold Tablets (Dorsey Laboratories) p 911
Triaminic-12 Tablets (Dorsey Laboratories) p 913
Triaminicol Multi-Symptom Cold Syrup (Dorsey Laboratories) p 913
Triaminicol Multi-Symptom Cold Tablets (Dorsey Laboratories) p 914
Tussar DM (USV Pharmaceutical) p 2091
Tussar SF (USV Pharmaceutical) p 2092
Tussar-2 (USV Pharmaceutical) p 2092

Chlorpheniramine Polistirex
Corsym (Pennwalt) p 1582

Chlorpheniramine Preparations
Deconamine Tablets, Elixir, SR Capsules, Syrup (Berlex) p 406, 699
Fedahist Expectorant (Rorer) p 1749
Fedahist Gyrocaps, Syrup & Tablets (Rorer) p 431, 1749

Chlorpheniramine Tannate
Rynatan Tablets & Pediatric Suspension (Wallace) p 442, 2165
Rynatuss Tablets & Pediatric Suspension (Wallace) p 442, 2165

Chlorpromazine
Chlorpromazine Tablets & Concentrate Syrup (Geneva) p 973
Thorazine (Smith Kline & French) p 437, 1977

Chlorpromazine Hydrochloride
Chlorpromazine HCl Injection (Elkins-Sinn) p 938
Chlorpromazine HCl Tablets (Schein) p 1828
Chlorpromazine HCl in Tubex (Wyeth) p 2288

Chlorpropamide
Chlorpropamide Tablets (Danbury) p 887
Chlorpropamide Tablets (Geneva) p 973
Diabinese (Pfizer) p 426, 1599
Glucamide Tablets (Lemmon) p 1122

Chlorprothixene
Taractan Tablets (Roche) p 1703

Chlorprothixene Hydrochloride
Taractan Concentrate (Roche) p 1703
Taractan Injectable (Roche) p 1703

Chlorprothixene Lactate
Taractan Concentrate (Roche) p 1703

Chlortetracycline Hydrochloride
Aureomycin Ointment 3% (Lederle) p 1089

Chlorthalidone
Chlorthalidone Tablets (Abbott) p 403, 510
Chlorthalidone Tablets (Danbury) p 887
Chlorthalidone Tablets (Schein) p 1828
Chlorthalidone Tablets, USP (Parke-Davis) p 1494
Combipres Tablets (Boehringer Ingelheim) p 406, 708
Demi-Regroton Tablets (USV Pharmaceutical) p 440, 2087
Hygroton Tablets (USV Pharmaceutical) p 440, 2078
Regroton Tablets (USV Pharmaceutical) p 440, 2087
Tenoretic Tablets (Stuart) p 439, 2043
Thalitone Tablets (Boehringer Ingelheim) p 406, 715

Chlorzoxazone
Algisin Capsules (RAM Laboratories) p 1632
Chlorzone Forte Tablets (Schein) p 1828
Chlorzoxazone Tablets (Danbury) p 887
Chlorzoxazone with APAP Tablets (Danbury) p 887
Chlorzoxasone w/APAP Tablets (Geneva) p 973
Paraflex Tablets (McNeil Pharmaceutical) p 1205
Parafon Forte Tablets (McNeil Pharmaceutical) p 419, 1206

Cholera Vaccine
Cholera Vaccine (Wyeth) p 2245
Cholera Vaccine (India Strains) (Lederle) p 1089

Cholestyramine
Questran (Mead Johnson Laboratories) p 1231

Choline
Cardioguard Natural Lipotropic Dietary Supplement-Powder (Professional Health) p 1621

Choline Bitartrate
Mega-B (Arco) p 600
Megadose (Arco) p 600

Generic and Chemical Name Index

Choline Magnesium Trisalicylate
Trilisate Tablets/Liquid (Purdue Frederick) p 427, 1627

Chorionic Gonadotropin
A.P.L. (Ayerst) p 636
Glukor Injection (Hyrex) p 1024
Pregnyl (Organon) p 1450
Profasi HP (HCG) (Serono) p 1943

Chromic Chloride
Chrometrace (Armour) p 604
Multitrace 5 (Armour) p 608
Multitrace Pediatric (Armour) p 609
Multitrace Solution & Concentrate (Armour) p 609

Chromium
Total Formula (Vitaline) p 2148

Chymopapain for Injection
Chymodiactin (Smith) p 437, 1983

Chymotrypsin
Orenzyme (Merrell Dow) p 1379
Orenzyme Bitabs (Merrell Dow) p 1379

Ciclopirox Olamine
Loprox Cream 1% (Hoechst-Roussel) p 413, 1017

Cimetidine
Tagamet (Smith Kline & French) p 437, 1973

Cinnamedrine Hydrochloride
Maximum Strength Midol for Cramps (Glenbrook) p 997
Midol-Original Formula (Glenbrook) p 997

Cinoxacin
Cinobac Pulvules (Dista) p 410, 894

Cisplatin
Platinol (Bristol-Myers Oncology) p 765

Citric Acid
Bicitra—Sugar-Free (Willen) p 2187
Polycitra Syrup (Willen) p 2188
Polycitra-K Syrup (Willen) p 2189
Polycitra-LC—Sugar-Free (Willen) p 2188

Clemastine Fumarate
Tavist Tablets (Sandoz Pharmaceutical Div.) p 433, 1818
Tavist-1 Tablets (Sandoz Pharmaceutical Div.) p 433, 1818
Tavist-D Tablets (Sandoz Pharmaceutical Div.) p 433, 1819

Clidinium Bromide
Clipoxide Capsules (Schein) p 1828
Librax Capsules (Roche Products) p 430, 1713
Quarzan Capsules (Roche Products) p 430, 1721

Clindamycin Hydrochloride
Cleocin HCl Capsules* (Upjohn) p 441, 2094

Clindamycin Palmitate Hydrochloride
Cleocin Pediatric Flavored Granules* (Upjohn) p 2096

Clindamycin Phosphate
Cleocin Phosphate Sterile Solution* (Upjohn) p 440, 2097
Cleocin T Topical Solution* (Upjohn) p 441, 2100

Clocortolone Pivalate
Cloderm (Ortho Pharmaceutical (Dermatological Div.)) p 1472

Clofibrate
Atromid-S (Ayerst) p 404, 636

Clomiphene Citrate
Clomid (Merrell Dow) p 1364
Serophene (clomiphene citrate USP) (Serono) p 1943

Clonazepam
Clonopin Tablets (Roche) p 429, 1680

Clonidine Hydrochloride
Catapres Tablets (Boehringer Ingelheim) p 406, 707
Combipres Tablets (Boehringer Ingelheim) p 406, 708

Clorazepate Dipotassium
Tranxene Capsules & Tablets (Abbott) p 404, 568
Tranxene-SD (Abbott) p 404, 568
Tranxene-SD Half Strength (Abbott) p 404, 568

Clotrimazole
Gyne-Lotrimin Vaginal Cream 1% (Schering) p 1856
Gyne-Lotrimin Vaginal Tablets (Schering) p 434, 1856
Lotrimin Cream 1% (Schering) p 1857
Lotrimin Lotion 1% (Schering) p 1857
Lotrimin Solution 1% (Schering) p 1857
Lotrisone Cream (Schering) p 1858
Mycelex 1% Cream (Miles Pharmaceuticals) p 1409
Mycelex 1% Solution (Miles Pharmaceuticals) p 1409
Mycelex Troches (Miles Pharmaceuticals) p 422, 1409
Mycelex-G (Miles Pharmaceuticals) p 422, 1410
Mycelex-G 1% Vaginal Cream (Miles Pharmaceuticals) p 1410

Cloxacillin
Cloxacillin Capsules (Biocraft) p 705
Cloxacillin Sodium Capsules (Schein) p 1828
Cloxacillin Solution (Biocraft) p 705

Cloxacillin Sodium Monohydrate
Tegopen (Bristol) p 407, 753

Coal Tar
Denorex Medicated Shampoo and Conditioner (Whitehall) p 443, 2185
Denorex Medicated Shampoo, Regular & Mountain Fresh Herbal Scent (Whitehall) p 443, 2185
Fototar Cream 1.6% (Elder) p 931
Fototar Stik 5% (Elder) p 931
Pentrax Tar Shampoo (Cooper Dermatology) p 882
Zetar Emulsion (Dermik) p 892
Zetar Shampoo (Dermik) p 892

Cocaine Hydrochloride
Cocaine Hydrochloride Topical Solution (Roxane) p 1788

Codeine
APAP w/Codeine Tablets (Geneva) p 973
APAP w/Codeine #3 (Geneva) p 973
APAP w/Codeine #4 (Geneva) p 973
Acetaminophen with Codeine Tablets and Capsules (Lemmon) p 1122
Apap 300 mg. with Codeine Capsules & Tabs (Schein) p 1828
Apap with Codeine Elixir (Schein) p 1828
Aspirin 325 mg. with Codeine Tabs (Schein) p 1828
Calcidrine Syrup (Abbott) p 510
Empracet with Codeine Phosphate Nos. 3 & 4 (Burroughs Wellcome) p 408, 789
Terpin Hydrate & Codeine Elixir (Roxane) p 1788

Codeine Phosphate
A.P.C. with Codeine Nos. 3 & 4, Tabloid brand (Burroughs Wellcome) p 407, 780
Acetaco Tablets (Legere) p 1120
Acetaminophen with Codeine Phosphate Tablets (Roxane) p 1788
Actifed with Codeine Cough Syrup (Burroughs Wellcome) p 773
Amaphen with Codeine #3 (Trimen) p 2067
Anacin-3 with Codeine Tablets (Ayerst) p 404, 634
Ascriptin with Codeine (Rorer) p 431, 1745
Bancap c̄ Codeine Capsules (O'Neal, Jones & Feldman) p 1444
Bromanyl Expectorant (Schein) p 1828
Bromphen DC Expectorant (Schein) p 1828
Buff-A Comp No. 3 Tablets (with Codeine) (Mayrand) p 1196
Capital with Codeine Suspension (Carnrick) p 408, 831
Capital with Codeine Tablets (Carnrick) p 408, 831
Codalan (Lannett) p 1071
Codeine Phosphate Injection (Elkins-Sinn) p 938
Codeine Phosphate in Tubex (Wyeth) p 2288
Codeine Phosphate Oral Solution (Roxane) p 1788
Codimal PH (Central Pharmaceuticals) p 836
Conex with Codeine (O'Neal, Jones & Feldman) p 1445
Decongestant Expectorant (Schein) p 1828
Decongestant-AT (Antitussive) Liquid (Schein) p 1828
Deproist Expectorant w/Codeine (Geneva) p 973
Dimetane-DC Cough Syrup (Robins) p 1647
Dolprn #3 Tablets (Bock) p 705
Empirin with Codeine (Burroughs Wellcome) p 408, 787
Fiorinal w/Codeine (Sandoz Pharmaceutical Div.) p 432, 1802
G-2 Capsules (Hauck) p 1001
G-3 Capsules (Hauck) p 1001
Guiatuss A-C Syrup (Schein) p 1828
Iophen-C Liquid (Schein) p 1828
Naldecon-CX Suspension (Bristol) p 739
Novahistine DH (Merrell Dow) p 421, 1378
Novahistine Expectorant (Merrell Dow) p 421, 1378
Nucofed Capsules (Beecham Laboratories) p 406, 692
Nucofed Expectorant (Beecham Laboratories) p 693
Nucofed Pediatric Expectorant (Beecham Laboratories) p 694
Nucofed Syrup (Beecham Laboratories) p 692
Pediacof (Winthrop-Breon) p 2221
Phenaphen w/Codeine Capsules (Robins) p 428, 1656
Phenaphen-650 with Codeine Tablets (Robins) p 428, 1656
Phenergan VC with Codeine (Wyeth) p 2284
Phenergan with Codeine (Wyeth) p 2278
Phrenilin with Codeine No. 3 (Carnrick) p 409, 834
Poly-Histine Expectorant with Codeine (Bock) p 705
Robitussin A-C (Robins) p 1664
Robitussin-DAC (Robins) p 1665
Ru-Tuss Expectorant (Boots) p 722
SK-APAP with CODEINE Tablets (Smith Kline & French) p 1971
Soma Compound w/Codeine (Wallace) p 442, 2169
Stopayne Syrup (Springbok) p 1985
Triafed-C Expectorant (Schein) p 1828
Triaminic Expectorant w/Codeine (Dorsey Laboratories) p 911
Tussar SF (USV Pharmaceutical) p 2092
Tussar-2 (USV Pharmaceutical) p 2092
Tussi-Organidin (Wallace) p 442, 2171
Tussirex Sugar-Free (Scot-Tussin) p 1897
Tussirex Syrup (Scot-Tussin) p 1897
Tylenol w/Codeine Elixir (McNeil Pharmaceutical) p 419, 1214
Tylenol w/Codeine Tablets, Capsules (McNeil Pharmaceutical) p 419, 1214

Codeine Sulfate
Ambenyl Cough Syrup (Marion) p 1181
Aspirin w/Codeine Tablets (Geneva) p 973
Codeine Sulfate Tablets (Roxane) p 1788

Colchicine
ColBENEMID Tablets (Merck Sharp & Dohme) p 420, 1277
Colchicine Ampoules (Lilly) p 1134
Colchicine Tablets (Danbury) p 887
Colchicine Tablets (Lilly) p 1135
Col-Probenecid Tablets (Danbury) p 887
Probenecid w/Colchicine Tablets (Geneva) p 973
Probenecid with Colchicine Tablets (Schein) p 1828

Colestipol Hydrochloride
Colestid Granules (Upjohn) p 2100

Colistimethate Sodium
Coly-Mycin M Parenteral (Parke-Davis) p 1500

Colistin Sulfate
Coly-Mycin S Oral Suspension (Parke-Davis) p 1501
Coly-Mycin S Otic w/Neomycin & Hydrocortisone (Parke-Davis) p 1501

Collagenase
Santyl Ointment (Knoll) p 1067

Colloidal Oatmeal
Aveeno Bath Oilated (Cooper Dermatology) p 882
Aveeno Bath Regular (Cooper Dermatology) p 882
Aveenobar Oilated (Cooper Dermatology) p 882
Aveenobar Regular (Cooper Dermatology) p 882

Copper
Added Protection III Multi-Vitamin & Multi-Mineral Supplement (Professional Health) p 1621

Copper Sulfate
Hemo-Vite (Drug Industries) p 914
Vio-Bec Forte (Rowell) p 1788

Cortex Rhamni Frangulae
Movicol (Norgine) p 1424

Generic and Chemical Name Index

Cortisol
(see under Hydrocortisone)

Coumarin Derivatives
Coumadin (Du Pont) p 410, 915
Dicumarol Tablets (Abbott) p 403, 517
Panwarfin (Abbott) p 403, 558

Cromolyn Sodium
Intal (Fisons) p 943
Intal Nebulizer Solution (Fisons) p 943
Nasalcrom Nasal Solution (Fisons) p 944

Cryptenamine Preparations
Diutensen Tablets (Wallace) p 2156

Cupric Chloride
Coppertrace (Armour) p 605
Multitrace 5 (Armour) p 608
Multitrace Pediatric (Armour) p 609
Multitrace Solution & Concentrate (Armour) p 609

Cyanocobalamin
Al-Vite (Drug Industries) p 914
B-C-Bid Capsules (Geriatric) p 975
Chromagen Capsules (Savage) p 433, 1824
Cyanocobalamin in Tubex (Wyeth) p 445, 2288
Cyanocobalamin (Vit. B_{12}) Injection (Elkins-Sinn) p 938
Eldertonic (Mayrand) p 1196
Hemo-Vite (Drug Industries) p 914
I.L.X. B_{12} Elixir Crystalline (Kenwood) p 1046
I.L.X. B_{12} Tablets (Kenwood) p 1046
Neuro B-12 Forte Injectable (Lambda) p 1071
Neuro B-12 Injectable (Lambda) p 1071
Niferex-150 Forte Capsules (Central Pharmaceuticals) p 409, 838
Nu-Iron-V Tablets (Mayrand) p 1196
Tia-Doce Injectable Solution (Bart) p 685
Trinsicon/Trinsicon M Capsules (Glaxo) p 412, 986
Vicon Forte Capsules (Glaxo) p 412, 989

Cyclacillin
Cyclapen-W (Wyeth) p 444, 2249

Cyclandelate
Cyclandelate Capsules (Geneva) p 973
Cyclandelate Capsules (Schein) p 1828
Cyclospasmol (Ives) p 413, 1028

Cyclizine Preparations
Marezine (Burroughs Wellcome) p 408, 803

Cyclobenzaprine Hydrochloride
Flexeril Tablets (Merck Sharp & Dohme) p 420, 1310

Cyclophosphamide
Cytoxan (Bristol-Myers Oncology) p 407, 759
Neosar for Injection (Adria) p 586

Cyclopropanecarboxylate
Li-Ban Spray (Pfipharmecs) p 1589

Cycloserine
Seromycin (Lilly) p 1174

Cyclothiazide
Anhydron (Lilly) p 1129
Fluidil (Adria) p 571

Cylosporine
Sandimmune Ampuls (Sandoz Pharmaceutical Div.) p 1811
Sandimmune Oral Suspension (Sandoz Pharmaceutical Div.) p 1811

Cyproheptadine Hydrochloride
Cyproheptadine HCl Syrup & Tablets (Schein) p 1828
Cyproheptadine HCl Tablets (Danbury) p 887
Cyproheptadine HCl Tablets (Geneva) p 973
Periactin Syrup (Merck Sharp & Dohme) p 1342
Periactin Tablets (Merck Sharp & Dohme) p 420, 1342

Cytarabine
Cytosar-U Sterile Powder (Upjohn) p 2102

Cytosine Arabinoside
Cytosar-U Sterile Powder (Upjohn) p 2102

D

Dacarbazine
DTIC-Dome (Miles Pharmaceuticals) p 1402

Dactinomycin
Cosmegen Injection (Merck Sharp & Dohme) p 1278

Danazol
Danocrine (Winthrop-Breon) p 443, 2195

Danthron
Danthron Tablets (Geneva) p 973
Doxidan (Hoechst-Roussel) p 412, 1014
Modane Plus (Adria) p 585
Modane, Tablets & Liquid (Adria) p 584

Dantrolene Sodium
Dantrium Capsules (Norwich Eaton) p 1426
Dantrium Intravenous (Norwich Eaton) p 1428

Dapsone
Dapsone (Jacobus) p 1032

Daunorubicin Hydrochloride
Cerubidine (Ives) p 1026

Dead Sea Salts
Hydrisea Lotion (Pedinol) p 1580

Deferoxamine Mesylate
Desferal mesylate (CIBA) p 847

Dehydrocholic Acid
Bilax Capsules (Drug Industries) p 914
Decholin Tablets (Miles Pharmaceuticals) p 421, 1402
Neolax Tablets (Central Pharmaceuticals) p 838
Trilax (Drug Industries) p 915

Demeclocycline
Declomycin Capsules and Tablets (Lederle) p 415, 1090

Deserpidine
Enduronyl Forte Tablets (Abbott) p 403, 518
Enduronyl Tablets (Abbott) p 403, 518
Harmonyl (Abbott) p 532
Oreticyl (Abbott) p 555

Desipramine Hydrochloride
Norpramin (Merrell Dow) p 421, 1374
Pertofrane Capsules (USV Pharmaceutical) p 440, 2086

Deslanoside
Cedilanid-D Injection (Sandoz Pharmaceutical Div.) p 1799

Desmopressin Acetate
DDAVP (USV Pharmaceutical) p 440, 2074
DDAVP Injection (USV Pharmaceutical) p 440, 2075
Stimate Injection (Armour) p 611

Desonide
Otic Tridesilon Solution 0.05% (Miles Pharmaceuticals) p 1414
Tridesilon Creme 0.05% (Miles Pharmaceuticals) p 1412
Tridesilon Ointment 0.05% (Miles Pharmaceuticals) p 1413

Desoximetasone
Topicort Emollient Cream 0.25% (Hoechst-Roussel) p 413, 1021
Topicort Gel 0.05% (Hoechst-Roussel) p 413, 1021
Topicort LP Emollient Cream 0.05% (Hoechst-Roussel) p 413, 1021
Topicort Ointment 0.25% (Hoechst-Roussel) p 1021

Desoxycorticosterone Acetate
Doca Acetate (Organon) p 1446
Percorten Pellets (CIBA) p 861

Desoxycorticosterone Pivalate
Percorten pivalate (CIBA) p 862

Desoxyribonuclease
Elase (Parke-Davis) p 424, 1513
Elase Ointment (Parke-Davis) p 424, 1513
Elase-Chloromycetin Ointment (Parke-Davis) p 424, 1513

Dexamethasone
Aeroseb-Dex Topical Aerosol Spray (Herbert) p 1001
Decadron Elixir (Merck Sharp & Dohme) p 1284
Decadron Tablets (Merck Sharp & Dohme) p 420, 1286
Decaspray Topical Aerosol (Merck Sharp & Dohme) p 1296
Dexamethasone Injection (Bristol) p 730
Dexamethasone Tablets, Oral Solution & Intensol (Roxane) p 1788
Dexamethasone Tablets (Schein) p 1828
Hexadrol Elixir (Organon) p 1446
Hexadrol Tablets (Organon) p 422, 1446
Hexadrol Strip Packs (Organon) p 1446
Hexadrol Therapeutic Pack (Organon) p 422, 1446
SK-Dexamethasone Tablets (Smith Kline & French) p 1971

Dexamethasone Acetate
Dalalone D.P. Injectable (O'Neal, Jones & Feldman) p 1445
Dalalone L.A. Injectable (O'Neal, Jones & Feldman) p 1445
Decadron-LA Suspension (Merck Sharp & Dohme) p 1294
Dexasone LA (Legere) p 1120

Dexamethasone Phosphate
Dexasone 4 (Legere) p 1120

Dexamethasone Sodium Phosphate
Decadron Phosphate Respihaler (Merck Sharp & Dohme) p 1291
Decadron Phosphate Sterile Ophthalmic Ointment (Merck Sharp & Dohme) p 1290
Decadron Phosphate Sterile Ophthalmic Solution (Merck Sharp & Dohme) p 1291
Decadron Phosphate Turbinaire (Merck Sharp & Dohme) p 1293
Dexasone 10 (Legere) p 1120
Neodecadron Sterile Ophthalmic Ointment (Merck Sharp & Dohme) p 1340
Neodecadron Sterile Ophthalmic Solution (Merck Sharp & Dohme) p 1341

Dexamethasone Sodium Phosphate Injection
Dalalone Injectable (O'Neal, Jones & Feldman) p 1445
Decadron Phosphate Injection (Merck Sharp & Dohme) p 1288
Dexamethasone Sodium Phosphate Injection (Elkins-Sinn) p 938
Dexamethasone Sodium Phosphate in Tubex (Wyeth) p 2288
Hexadrol Phosphate Injection (Organon) p 1446

Dexamycin Sodium Phosphate
Dexamycin Ophthalmic Ointment (Schein) p 1828

Dexbrompheniramine Maleate
Disobrom Tablets (Geneva) p 973

Dexchlorpheniramine Maleate
Dexchlor Repeat Action Tablets (Schein) p 1828
Polaramine Repetabs Tablets (Schering) p 434, 1879
Polaramine Syrup (Schering) p 1879
Polaramine Tablets (Schering) p 434, 1879

Dexpanthenol
Dexol 300 (Legere) p 1120
Dexpanthenol Injection (d-Pantothenyl Alcohol) (Elkins-Sinn) p 938
Ilopan Injection (Adria) p 578

Dextran-40
Rheomacrodex (Pharmacia) p 1616

Dextran-70
Hyskon Hysteroscopy Fluid (Pharmacia) p 1616
Macrodex (Pharmacia) p 1616

Dextrans (Low Molecular Weight)
Rheomacrodex (Pharmacia) p 1616

Dextroamphetamine Saccharate
Obetrol-10 (Rexar) p 1641
Obetrol-20 (Rexar) p 1641

Dextroamphetamine Sulfate
Dexedrine (Smith Kline & French) p 436, 1959
Dextroamphetamine Sulfate, 5mg. & 10mg. (Rexar) p 1641
Obetrol-10 (Rexar) p 1641
Obetrol-20 (Rexar) p 1641

Dextromethorphan
Guiatuss D-M Syrup (Schein) p 1828

Dextromethorphan Hydrobromide
Albatussin (Bart) p 685
Ambenyl-D Decongestant Cough Formula (Marion) p 1182
Bayer Cough Syrup for Children (Glenbrook) p 996
Cardec DM Drops & Syrup (Schein) p 1828
Codimal DM (Central Pharmaceuticals) p 836

Generic and Chemical Name Index

Comtrex (Bristol-Myers Products) p 769
Congespirin Cough Syrup (Bristol-Myers Products) p 770
Coryban-D Cough Syrup (Pfipharmecs) p 1589
CoTylenol Cold Medication Tablets & Capsules (McNeil Consumer Products) p 418, 1197
CoTylenol Liquid Cold Medication (McNeil Consumer Products) p 1197
Cremacoat 1 (Vicks Pharmacy Products) p 442, 2146
Cremacoat 3 (Vicks Pharmacy Products) p 442, 2147
Cremacoat 4 (Vicks Pharmacy Products) p 442, 2147
Dorcol Children's Cough Syrup (Dorsey Laboratories) p 909
Histalet DM Syrup (Reid-Provident Labs.) p 1638
Phenergan with Dextromethorphan (Wyeth) p 2280
Quelidrine Syrup (Abbott) p 567
Rondec-DM Oral Drops (Ross) p 1777
Rondec-DM Syrup (Ross) p 1777
Scot-Tussin Sugar-Free 5-Action Cold Formula (Scot-Tussin) p 1897
Sorbutuss (Dalin) p 886
Triaminic-DM Cough Formula (Dorsey Laboratories) p 913
Triaminicol Multi-Symptom Cold Syrup (Dorsey Laboratories) p 913
Triaminicol Multi-Symptom Cold Tablets (Dorsey Laboratories) p 914
Tussar DM (USV Pharmaceutical) p 2091
Tussi-Organidin DM (Wallace) p 442, 2171

Dextromethorphan Polistirex
Delsym (Pennwalt) p 1582

Dextrose
Dextrose Injection (Bristol) p 730
Dextrose Injection (Elkins-Sinn) p 938

Dextrothyroxine
Choloxin (Flint) p 411, 949

Diatrizoate Meglumine
Hypaque Meglumine 60% (Winthrop-Breon) p 3039
Hypaque-M, 75% (Winthrop-Breon) p 3044
Hypaque-M, 90% (Winthrop-Breon) p 3053
Hypaque-76 Injection (Winthrop-Breon) p 3049

Diatrizoate Preparations
Hypaque Meglumine 30% (Winthrop-Breon) p 3032
Hypaque Sodium 50% (Winthrop-Breon) p 3034
Hypaque-Cysto (Winthrop-Breon) p 3030
Hypaque-M, 75% (Winthrop-Breon) p 3044
Hypaque-M, 90% (Winthrop-Breon) p 3053
Hypaque-76 Injection (Winthrop-Breon) p 3049

Diatrizoate Sodium
Hypaque Sodium Oral Powder (Winthrop-Breon) p 3024
Hypaque Sodium Oral Solution (Winthrop-Breon) p 3025
Hypaque Sodium 20% (Winthrop-Breon) p 3026
Hypaque Sodium 25% (Winthrop-Breon) p 3028
Hypaque-M, 75% (Winthrop-Breon) p 3044
Hypaque-M, 90% (Winthrop-Breon) p 3053
Hypaque-76 Injection (Winthrop-Breon) p 3049

Diazepam
Valium Injectable (Roche Products) p 430, 1721
Valium Tablets (Roche Products) p 430, 1723
Valrelease Capsules (Roche) p 430, 1707

Diazoxide
Hyperstat I.V. Injection (Schering) p 1856
Proglycem Capsules, Suspension (Schering) p 1880

Dibucaine
Corticaine Cream (Glaxo) p 412, 980
Dibucaine Ointment 1% (Fougera) p 953
Nupercainal Cream & Ointment (CIBA) p 856

Dibucaine Hydrochloride
Nupercaine Heavy Solution (CIBA) p 860
Nupercaine hydrochloride 1:200 (CIBA) p 857
Nupercaine hydrochloride 1:1500 (CIBA) p 858

Dichloralphenazone
Midrin Capsules (Carnrick) p 408, 832

Dicloxacillin
Dicloxacillin Capsules (Biocraft) p 705

Dicloxacillin Sodium
Dicloxacillin Sodium Capsules (Schein) p 1828
Dynapen (Bristol) p 407, 733
Pathocil Capsules, for Oral Suspension (Wyeth) p 444, 2274

Dicumarol
Dicumarol Tablets (Abbott) p 403, 517

Dicyclomine Hydrochloride
Bentyl Capsules, Tablets, Syrup & Injection (Merrell Dow) p 421, 1359
Dicyclomine HCl Capsules (Danbury) p 887
Dicyclomine HCl Tablets (Danbury) p 887

Dienestrol
DV Cream (Merrell Dow) p 1364
Ortho Dienestrol Cream (Ortho Pharmaceutical) p 1457

Diethylpropion Hydrochloride
Diethylpropion HCl Tablets & Timed Tablets (Schein) p 1828
Tenuate Dospan (Merrell Dow) p 421, 1393
Tenuate 25 mg (Merrell Dow) p 421, 1393
Tepanil (Riker) p 428, 1645
Tepanil Ten-tab (Riker) p 428, 1645

Diethylstilbestrol
Diethylstilbestrol Enseals & Tablets (Lilly) p 1141
Diethylstilbestrol Suppositories (Lilly) p 1141

Diethylstilbestrol Diphosphate
Stilphostrol (Miles Pharmaceuticals) p 422, 1412

Diflorasone Diacetate
Florone Cream 0.05% (Dermik) p 889
Florone Ointment 0.05% (Dermik) p 889
Maxiflor Cream (Herbert) p 1006
Maxiflor Ointment (Herbert) p 1006

Diflunisal
Dolobid Tablets (Merck Sharp & Dohme) p 420, 1302

Digitalis Glycoside Preparations
Crystodigin Tablets (Lilly) p 417, 1135

Digoxin
Digoxin Injection (Elkins-Sinn) p 938
Digoxin in Tubex (Wyeth) p 2288
Lanoxicaps (Burroughs Wellcome) p 408, 793
Lanoxin (Burroughs Wellcome) p 408, 797

Dihydrocodeine Bitartrate
Compal Capsules (Reid-Provident Labs.) p 427, 1637
Synalgos-DC Capsules (Ives) p 413, 1031

Dihydrocodeinone Bitartrate
Dihydrocodeine Compound Tablets (Schein) p 1828

Dihydroergotamine Mesylate
D.H.E. 45 (Sandoz Pharmaceutical Div.) p 1800

Dihydromorphinone Hydrochloride (see also under Hydromorphone Hydrochloride)
Dilaudid Cough Syrup (Knoll) p 1058
Hydromorphone HCl Injection (Elkins-Sinn) p 938

Dihydrotachysterol
DHT (Dihydrotachysterol) Tablets, Oral Solution & Intensol (Roxane) p 1789

Diiodohydroxyquin (see under Iodoquinol)

Diisopropyl Sebacate
Domol Bath & Shower Oil (Miles Pharmaceuticals) p 1402

Diltiazem Hydrochloride
Cardizem (Marion) p 417, 1183

Dimenhydrinate
Dimenhydrinate in Tubex (Wyeth) p 2288
Dramamine Injection (Searle Pharmaceuticals) p 1906
Dramamine Liquid (Searle Pharmaceuticals) p 1906
Dramamine Tablets (Searle Pharmaceuticals) p 435, 1906

Dimercaprol
BAL in Oil Ampules (Hynson, Westcott & Dunning) p 1024

Dioctyl Sodium Sulfosuccinate (see under Docusate Sodium)

Dioxybenzone
Solbar PF (Persön & Covey) p 1588

Diphenhydramine
Caladryl (Parke-Davis) p 1486

Diphenhydramine Hydrochloride
Allerdryl 50 (Legere) p 1120
Benadryl Elixir (Parke-Davis) p 1485
Benadryl Kapseals and Capsules (Parke-Davis) p 423, 1485
Benadryl Parenteral (Parke-Davis) p 1485
Benylin Cough Syrup (Parke-Davis) p 1486
Bromanyl Expectorant (Schein) p 1828
Diphenhydramine Capsules (Geneva) p 973
Diphenhydramine HCl Caps (Schein) p 1828
Diphenhydramine HCl Capsules (Danbury) p 887
Diphenhydramine Hydrochloride Capsules, Elixir (Roxane) p 1788
Diphenhydramine HCl Injection (Bristol) p 730
Diphenhydramine HCl Injection (Elkins-Sinn) p 938
Diphenhydramine HCl in Tubex (Wyeth) p 2288
Dytuss (LaSalle) p 1071
Ziradryl Lotion (Parke-Davis) p 1580

Diphenidol
Vontrol Tablets (Smith Kline & French) p 437, 1981

Diphenoxylate
Diphenoxylate & Atropine Liquid (DPXL) & Tabs (Schein) p 1828
SK-Diphenoxylate Tablets (Smith Kline & French) p 1971

Diphenoxylate Hydrochloride
Diphenoxylate Hydrochloride & Atropine Sulfate Tablets & Oral Solution (Roxane) p 1788
Lomotil Liquid (Searle & Co.) p 1931
Lomotil Tablets (Searle & Co.) p 436, 1931
Lonox Tablets (Geneva) p 973

Diphenylhydantoin Sodium
Phenytoin Sodium Injection (Elkins-Sinn) p 938

Diphenylpyraline Hydrochloride
Hispril Spansule Capsules (Smith Kline & French) p 437, 1965

Diphtheria Antitoxin
Diphtheria Antitoxin (equine), Refined (Sclavo) p 1897
Diphtheria Antitoxin (Purified, Concentrated Globulin-Equine) (Squibb/Connaught) p 2033

Diphtheria & Tetanus Toxoids Adsorbed, (For Pediatric Use)
Diphtheria & Tetanus Toxoids, Adsorbed for Pediatric Use) (Sclavo) p 1897

Diphtheria & Tetanus Toxoids Combined, (For Pediatric Use)
Diphtheria & Tetanus Toxoids, Adsorbed Purogenated (Lederle) p 1093

Diphtheria & Tetanus Toxoids Combined, Pediatric, Aluminum Phosphate Adsorbed
Diphtheria & Tetanus Toxoids Adsorbed (Pediatric), Aluminum Phosphate Adsorbed, (Ultrafined) (Wyeth) p 2245
Diphtheria & Tetanus Toxoids Adsorbed, Pediatric, in Tubex (Wyeth) p 2288
Diphtheria & Tetanus Toxoids Adsorbed USP (Squibb/Connaught) p 2033

Diphtheria & Tetanus Toxoids w/Pertussis Vaccine Combined, Aluminum Phosphate Adsorbed
Tri-Immunol (Lederle) p 1119

Diphtheria & Tetanus Toxoids w/Pertussis Vaccine Combined, Aluminum Potassium Sulfate Adsorbed
Diphtheria & Tetanus Toxoids & Pertussis Vaccine Adsorbed (for Pediatric Use) (Squibb/Connaught) p 2033

Diphtheria Toxoid, Aluminum Hydroxide Adsorbed (For Pediatric Use)
Diphtheria Toxoid, Adsorbed (Sclavo) p 1897

Generic and Chemical Name Index

Diphylline
 Thylline & Thylline-GG Tablets (Schein) p 1828

Dipotassium Phosphate
 Uro-KP-Neutral (Star) p 2035

Dipyridamole
 Dipyridamole Tablets (Danbury) p 887
 Dipyridamole Tablets (Geneva) p 973
 Dipyridamole Tablets (Schein) p 1828
 Persantine Tablets (Boehringer Ingelheim) p 406, 710
 SK-Dipyridamole Tablets (Smith Kline & French) p 1971

Disodium Carbenicillin
 Geopen (Roerig) p 1731

Disodium Phosphate
 Uro-KP-Neutral (Star) p 2035

d-Isoephedrine Sulfate
 Fedahist Expectorant (Rorer) p 1749
 Fedahist Gyrocaps, Syrup & Tablets (Rorer) p 431, 1749

Disopyramide Phosphate
 Norpace Capsules (Searle & Co.) p 436, 1933
 Norpace CR Capsules (Searle & Co.) p 436, 1933

Disposable Injectable
 Tetanus Immune Globulin (Human) Hyper-Tet (Cutter Biological) p 884

Disulfiram
 Antabuse (Ayerst) p 404, 635, 634
 Disulfiram Tablets (Danbury) p 887
 Disulfiram Tablets (Geneva) p 973
 Disulfiram Tablets (Schein) p 1828

Divalproex Sodium
 Depakote Tablets (Abbott) p 403, 513

Dobutamine Hydrochloride
 Dobutrex (Lilly) p 1143

Docusate Calcium
 Dioctocal Capsules - Docusate Calcium USP (Schein) p 1828
 Doxidan (Hoechst-Roussel) p 412, 1014
 Surfak (Hoechst-Roussel) p 413, 1021

Docusate Potassium
 Dialose Capsules (Stuart) p 439, 2036
 Dialose Plus Capsules (Stuart) p 439, 2037
 Kasof Capsules (Stuart) p 439, 2038

Docusate Sodium
 Bilax Capsules (Drug Industries) p 914
 Colace (Mead Johnson Pharmaceutical) p 419, 1248
 Disonate Capsules & Liquid (Lannett) p 1071
 Docusate Sodium Capsules, Syrup (Roxane) p 1788
 Docusate Sodium with Casanthranol Capsules (Roxane) p 1788
 Ferro-Sequels (Lederle) p 415, 1093
 Geriplex-FS Kapseals (Parke-Davis) p 424, 1527
 Geriplex-FS Liquid (Parke-Davis) p 1527
 Liqui-Doss (Ferndale) p 942
 Modane Plus (Adria) p 585
 Modane Soft (Adria) p 584
 Neolax Tablets (Central Pharmaceuticals) p 838
 Peri-Colace (Mead Johnson Pharmaceutical) p 419, 1255
 Peritinic Tablets (Lederle) p 1112
 Prenate 90 Tablets (Bock) p 706
 Senokot-S Tablets (Purdue Frederick) p 1627
 Trilax (Drug Industries) p 915

Dopamine Hydrochloride
 Dopamine Hydrochloride Ampoules (Dopastat) (Parke-Davis) p 1510
 Dopamine HCl Injection (Bristol) p 730
 Dopamine HCl Injection (Elkins-Sinn) p 938
 Dopamine Solutions (Astra) p 615
 Intropin (American Critical Care) p 596

Doxapram Hydrochloride
 Dopram Injectable (Robins) p 428, 1650

Doxepin Hydrochloride
 Adapin (Pennwalt) p 426, 1581
 Sinequan (Roerig) p 431, 1740

Doxorubicin Hydrochloride
 Adriamycin (Adria) p 571

Doxycycline
 Doxycycline Tablets (Schein) p 1828

Doxycycline Calcium
 Vibramycin Calcium Syrup (Pfizer) p 1610

Doxycycline Hyclate
 Doxycycline Hyclate Capsules (Danbury) p 887
 Doxycycline Hyclate Capsules & Tablets (Geneva) p 973
 Doxycycline Hyclate Capsules (Schein) p 1828
 Doxycycline Hyclate for Injection (Elkins-Sinn) p 938
 Doxycycline Hyclate Tablets (Danbury) p 887
 Doxy-Lemmon Capsules (Lemmon) p 1122
 Vibramycin Hyclate Capsules (Pfizer) p 426, 1610
 Vibramycin Hyclate Intravenous (Pfizer) p 1611
 Vibra-Tabs Film Coated Tablets (Pfizer) p 426, 1610

Doxycycline Monohydrate
 Vibramycin Monohydrate for Oral Suspension (Pfizer) p 1610

Doxylamine Succinate
 Cremacoat 4 (Vicks Pharmacy Products) p 442, 2147
 Unisom Nighttime Sleep-Aid (Leeming) p 1119

Droperidol
 Inapsine Injection (Janssen) p 1034
 Innovar Injection (Janssen) p 1035

Dyclonine Hydrochloride
 Dyclone, 0.5% & 1% (Astra) p 618

Dyphylline
 Brosema (Legere) p 1120
 Dilor Tablets (Savage) p 433, 1824
 Dilor-G Tablets & Liquid (Savage) p 433, 1824
 Lufyllin Elixir (Wallace) p 2158
 Lufyllin Injection (Wallace) p 442, 2159
 Lufyllin & Lufyllin-400 Tablets (Wallace) p 442, 2160
 Lufyllin-GG (Wallace) p 442, 2161

E

Echothiophate Iodide
 Phospholine Iodide (Ayerst) p 658

Econazole Nitrate
 Spectazole Cream (Ortho Pharmaceutical (Dermatological Div.)) p 1476

Edrophonium Chloride
 Tensilon Injectable (Roche) p 1705, 3015

Endocrine
 S-P-T (Fleming) p 949
 Synthroid (Flint) p 411, 951

Entsufon Sodium
 pHisoHex (Winthrop-Breon) p 2222

Enzymes, Collagenolytic
 Santyl Ointment (Knoll) p 1067

Enzymes, Debridement
 Biozyme-C Ointment (Armour) p 604
 Elase (Parke-Davis) p 424, 1513
 Elase Ointment (Parke-Davis) p 424, 1513
 Elase-Chloromycetin Ointment (Parke-Davis) p 424, 1513
 Panafil Ointment (Rystan) p 1796
 Panafil-White Ointment (Rystan) p 1796
 Santyl Ointment (Knoll) p 1067
 Travase Ointment (Flint) p 411, 952

Enzymes, Digestant
 Kutrase Capsules (Rorer) p 431, 1750
 Ku-Zyme Capsules (Rorer) p 431, 1750
 Ku-Zyme HP Capsules (Rorer) p 431, 1751

Enzymes, Digestive
 Arco-Lase (Arco) p 600
 Arco-Lase Plus (Arco) p 600
 Zypan Tablets (Standard Process) p 2035

Enzymes, Fibrinolytic
 Elase (Parke-Davis) p 424, 1513
 Elase Ointment (Parke-Davis) p 424, 1513
 Elase-Chloromycetin Ointment (Parke-Davis) p 424, 1513

Enzymes, Proteolytic
 Panafil Ointment (Rystan) p 1796
 Panafil-White Ointment (Rystan) p 1796
 Papase (Parke-Davis) p 425, 1558
 Travase Ointment (Flint) p 411, 952
 Zypan Tablets (Standard Process) p 2035

Ephedrine
 Ephedrine Injection (Bristol) p 730
 Quibron Plus (Mead Johnson Laboratories) p 419, 1236
 T-E-P Tablets (Schein) p 1828

Ephedrine Hydrochloride
 Derma Medicone-HC Ointment (Medicone) p 1256
 Mudrane GG Elixir (Poythress) p 1619
 Mudrane GG Tablets (Poythress) p 1619
 Mudrane Tablets (Poythress) p 1618
 Primatene Tablets-M Formula (Whitehall) p 443, 2187
 Primatene Tablets-P Formula (Whitehall) p 443, 2187
 Quadrinal Tablets & Suspension (Knoll) p 414, 1065
 Quelidrine Syrup (Abbott) p 567
 T.E.P. Tablets (Geneva) p 973
 Tedral Elixir & Suspension (Parke-Davis) p 1573
 Tedral SA Tablets (Parke-Davis) p 425, 1573

Ephedrine Sulfate
 Bronkolixir (Winthrop-Breon) p 2193
 Bronkotabs (Winthrop-Breon) p 2194
 Bronkotuss (Hyrex) p 1024
 Efed II Capsules (Yellow) (Alto) p 404, 589
 Isuprel Hydrochloride Compound Elixir (Winthrop-Breon) p 2204
 Marax Tablets & DF Syrup (Roerig) p 431, 1737
 T.E.H. Tablets (Geneva) p 973
 Theofedral Tablets (Danbury) p 887
 Theozine Syrup & Tablets - Dye-Free (Schein) p 1828
 Wyanoids Hemorrhoidal Suppositories (Wyeth) p 445, 2293

Ephedrine Tannate
 Rynatuss Tablets & Pediatric Suspension (Wallace) p 442, 2165

Epinephrine
 Adrenalin Chloride Solution, Injectable (Parke-Davis) p 1480
 Epinephrine Injection (Bristol) p 730
 Epinephrine Injection (Elkins-Sinn) p 938
 Epinephrine in Tubex (Wyeth) p 2288
 EpiPen—Epinephrine Auto-Injector (Center) p 835
 EpiPen Jr. (Center) p 835
 Marcaine Hydrochloride with Epinephrine 1:200,000 (Winthrop-Breon) p 2206
 Primatene Mist (Whitehall) p 443, 2186
 Sus-Phrine (Berlex) p 406, 704

Epinephrine Bitartrate
 Ayerst Epitrate (Ayerst) p 642
 Medihaler-Epi (Riker) p 1643
 Primatene Mist Suspension (Whitehall) p 2187

Epinephrine, Racemic
 Vaponefrin Solution (Fisons) p 943

Epoxymethamine Bromide
 (see under Methscopolamine Bromide)

Ergocalciferol
 Calciferol Drops (Egocalciferol Oral Solution USP) (Rorer) p 431, 1748
 Calciferol in Oil Injection (Egocalciferol USP) (Rorer) p 431, 1748
 Calciferol Tablets (Ergocalciferol USP) (Rorer) p 431, 1748
 Os-Cal-Gesic Tablets (Marion) p 418, 1189
 Vi-Penta F Chewables (Roche) p 430, 1708
 Vi-Penta F Infant Drops (Roche) p 1709
 Vi-Penta F Multivitamin Drops (Roche) p 1709

Ergoloid Mesylates
 Circanol (Riker) p 1642
 Ergoloid Mesylates Oral Tablets (Danbury) p 887
 Ergoloid Mesylates Sublingual Tablets (Danbury) p 887
 Hydergine Oral Tablets, Sublingual Tablets, & Liquid (Sandoz Pharmaceutical Div.) p 433, 1802
 Hydergine LC Liquid Capsules (Sandoz Pharmaceutical Div.) p 433, 1802

Ergonovine Maleate
 Ergotrate Maleate Ampoules (Lilly) p 1146
 Ergotrate Maleate Tablets (Lilly) p 1147

Ergot Alkaloids (Hydrogenated)
 Deapril-ST (Mead Johnson Pharmaceutical) p 419, 1248
 Ergoloid Mesylates Tablets (Geneva) p 973

Generic and Chemical Name Index

Hydergine Oral Tablets, Sublingual Tablets, & Liquid (Sandoz Pharmaceutical Div.) p 433, 1802
Hydergine LC Liquid Capsules (Sandoz Pharmaceutical Div.) p 433, 1802
Hydro-Ergoloid Oral & Sublingual Tablets (Schein) p 1828

Ergotamine Tartrate
Bellergal Tablets (Sandoz Pharmaceutical Div.) p 432, 1798
Bellergal-S Tablets (Sandoz Pharmaceutical Div.) p 432, 1798
Cafergot (Sandoz Pharmaceutical Div.) p 432, 1799
Cafergot P-B (Sandoz Pharmaceutical Div.) p 432, 1799
Cafetrate-PB Suppositories (Schein) p 1828
Ergomar Sublingual Tablets (Fisons) p 943
Ergostat (Parke-Davis) p 1514
Medihaler Ergotamine Aerosol (Riker) p 428, 1643
Wigraine Tablets & Suppositories (Organon) p 422, 1451
Wigraine-PB Suppositories (Organon) p 422, 1451
Wigrettes (Organon) p 422, 1451

Erythrityl Tetranitrate
Cardilate Chewable Tablets (Burroughs Wellcome) p 407, 782
Cardilate Oral/Sublingual Tablets (Burroughs Wellcome) p 407, 782

Erythromycin
A/T/S (Hoechst-Roussel) p 412, 1009
ERYC (Parke-Davis) p 424, 1515
EryDerm (Abbott) p 519
Erymax Topical Solution (Herbert) p 1003
Ery-Tab Tablets (Abbott) p 403, 521
Erythromycin Base Filmtab (Abbott) p 403, 526
Erythromycin Ophthalmic Ointment (Fougera) p 953
Erythromycin Ophthalmic Ointment (Pharmaderm) p 1617
Erythromycin Ophthalmic Ointment (Schein) p 1828
Ilotycin Sterile Ophthalmic Ointment (Dista) p 899
Ilotycin Tablets (Dista) p 899
Pediamycin (Ross) p 1772
Pediazole (Ross) p 1774
Staticin 1.5% Topical Solution (Westwood) p 2181
T-Stat 2.0% Topical Solution (Westwood) p 2181

Erythromycin Enteric Coated Tablets
E-Mycin Tablets (Upjohn) p 441, 2112

Erythromycin Estolate
Erythromycin Estolate Capsules (Danbury) p 887
Erythromycin Estolate Capsules & Suspension (Schein) p 1828
Ilosone Oral Preparations (Dista) p 410, 897

Erythromycin Ethylsuccinate
E.E.S. Chewable Tablets (Abbott) p 403, 522
E.E.S. Drops (Abbott) p 522
E.E.S. Granules (Abbott) p 522
E.E.S. 200 Liquid (Abbott) p 522
E.E.S. 400 Filmtab (Abbott) p 403, 522
E.E.S. 400 Liquid (Abbott) p 522
E-Mycin E Liquid (Upjohn) p 2113
EryPed Granules (Abbott) p 520
Erythromycin Ethylsuccinate Granules, Suspension & Tablets (Schein) p 1828
Pediamycin (Ross) p 1772
Pediazole (Ross) p 1774
Wyamycin E Liquid (Wyeth) p 2292

Erythromycin Gluceptate
Ilotycin Gluceptate (Dista) p 900

Erythromycin Lactobionate
Erythrocin Lactobionate-I.V. (Abbott) p 523
Erythrocin Piggyback (Abbott) p 403, 524

Erythromycin Stearate
Erythromycin Stearate Filmtab (Abbott) p 403, 525
Erythromycin Stearate Tablets, USP (Erypar) (Parke-Davis) p 424, 1516
SK-Erythromycin Tablets (Smith Kline & French) p 1971
Wyamycin S Tablets (Wyeth) p 445, 2292

Estradiol
Estrace (Mead Johnson Laboratories) p 419, 1216
Estrace Vaginal Cream (Mead Johnson Laboratories) p 419, 1219

Estradiol Cypionate
E-Cypionate (Legere) p 1120

Estradiol Valerate
Ditate-DS (Savage) p 1824
Menaval 20 & Menaval 40 (Legere) p 1120
Testaval 90/4 (Legere) p 1120

Estramustine Phosphate Sodium
Emcyt Capsules (Roche) p 429, 1681

Estrogens, Conjugated
Conjugated Estrogens Tablets (Geneva) p 973
Conjugated Estrogens Tablets - Coated (Schein) p 1828
Estrocon Tablets (Savage) p 433, 1824
PMB 200 & PMB 400 (Ayerst) p 405, 660
Premarin Intravenous (Ayerst) p 667
Premarin Tablets (Ayerst) p 405, 664
Premarin Vaginal Cream (Ayerst) p 405, 670
Premarin w/Methyltestosterone (Ayerst) p 405, 674

Estrogens, Esterified
Estratab Tablets (Reid-Provident Labs.) p 427, 1638
Estratest H.S. Tablets (Reid-Provident Labs.) p 427, 1638
Estratest Tablets (Reid-Provident Labs.) p 427, 1638
Menrium Tablets (Roche Products) p 430, 1717

Estrone
Estrone (Legere) p 1120
Natural Estrogenic Substance (Legere) p 1120
Ogen Tablets (Abbott) p 403, 548
Ogen Vaginal Cream (Abbott) p 551

Estropipate
Ogen Tablets (Abbott) p 403, 548
Ogen Vaginal Cream (Abbott) p 551

Ethacrynate Sodium
Edecrin Sodium Intravenous (Merck Sharp & Dohme) p 1304

Ethacrynic Acid
Edecrin Tablets (Merck Sharp & Dohme) p 420, 1304

Ethambutol Hydrochloride
Myambutol Tablets (Lederle) p 1106

Ethaverine Hydrochloride
Ethatab (Glaxo) p 980
Isovex Capsules (U.S. Pharmaceutical) p 2070
Pasmol Tablets (RAM Laboratories) p 1632

Ethchlorvynol
Placidyl (Abbott) p 403, 566

Ethinamate
Valmid Pulvules (Dista) p 410, 908

Ethinyl Estradiol
Brevicon 21-Day Tablets (Syntex) p 440, 2052
Brevicon 28-Day Tablets (Syntex) p 440, 2052
Demulen 1/35-21 (Searle & Co.) p 435, 1919
Demulen 1/35-28 (Searle & Co.) p 435, 1919
Demulen 1/50-21 (Searle & Co.) p 435, 1919
Demulen 1/50-28 (Searle & Co.) p 435, 1919
Estinyl Tablets (Schering) p 434, 1839
Loestrin 21 1/20 (Parke-Davis) p 443, 1531
Loestrin Fe 1/20 (Parke-Davis) p 424, 1531
Loestrin 21 1.5/30 (Parke-Davis) p 424, 1531
Loestrin Fe 1.5/30 (Parke-Davis) p 424, 1531
Lo/Ovral Tablets (Wyeth) p 444, 2255
Lo/Ovral-28 Tablets (Wyeth) p 444, 2263
Modicon 21 Tablets (Ortho Pharmaceutical) p 423, 1461
Modicon 28 Tablets (Ortho Pharmaceutical) p 1461
Nordette-21 Tablets (Wyeth) p 444, 2266
Nordette-28 Tablets (Wyeth) p 444, 2270
Norinyl 1+35 Tablets 21-Day (Syntex) p 440, 2052
Norinyl 1+35 Tablets 28-Day (Syntex) p 440, 2052
Norlestrin 21 1/50 (Parke-Davis) p 425, 1548
Norlestrin 21 2.5/50 (Parke-Davis) p 425, 1548
Norlestrin 28 1/50 (Parke-Davis) p 1548
Norlestrin Fe 1/50 (Parke-Davis) p 425, 1548
Norlestrin Fe 2.5/50 (Parke-Davis) p 425, 1548
Ortho-Novum 1/35 21 (Ortho Pharmaceutical) p 422, 1461
Ortho-Novum 1/35 28 (Ortho Pharmaceutical) p 1461
Ortho-Novum 7/7/7 .. 21 Tablets (Ortho Pharmaceutical) p 422, 1461
Ortho-Novum 7/7/7 .. 28 Tablets (Ortho Pharmaceutical) p 1461
Ortho-Novum 10/11 .. 21 Tablets (Ortho Pharmaceutical) p 422, 1461
Ortho-Novum 10/11 .. 28 Tablets (Ortho Pharmaceutical) p 1461
Ovcon-35 (Mead Johnson Laboratories) p 419, 1224
Ovcon-50 (Mead Johnson Laboratories) p 419, 1224
Ovral Tablets (Wyeth) p 444, 2271
Ovral-28 Tablets (Wyeth) p 444, 2272
Tri-Norinyl 21-Day Tablets (Syntex) p 440, 2052
Tri-Norinyl 28-Day Tablets (Syntex) p 440, 2052

Ethionamide
Trecator-SC (Ives) p 1031

Ethoheptazine Citrate
Mepro Compound Tablets (Schein) p 1828

Ethopropazine Hydrochloride
Parsidol (Parke-Davis) p 425, 1559

Ethosuximide
Zarontin Capsules (Parke-Davis) p 426, 1579
Zarontin Syrup (Parke-Davis) p 1579

Ethotoin
Peganone (Abbott) p 403, 559

Ethyl Aminobenzoate
Derma Medicone-HC Ointment (Medicone) p 1256
Rectal Medicone-HC Suppositories (Medicone) p 419, 1256

Ethylestrenol
Maxibolin (Organon) p 1447

Ethylnorepinephrine Hydrochloride
Bronkephrine Hydrochloride Injection (Winthrop-Breon) p 2193

Ethylpapaverine Hydrochloride
(see under Ethaverine Hydrochloride)

Ethynodiol Diacetate
Demulen 1/35-21 (Searle & Co.) p 435, 1919
Demulen 1/35-28 (Searle & Co.) p 435, 1919
Demulen 1/50-21 (Searle & Co.) p 435, 1919
Demulen 1/50-28 (Searle & Co.) p 435, 1919
Ovulen-21 (Searle & Co.) p 436, 1919
Ovulen-28 (Searle & Co.) p 436, 1919

Etidocaine Hydrochloride
Duranest Hydrochloride & Duranest Hydrochloride with Epinephrine 1:200,000 (Astra) p 616

Etidronate Disodium (Diphosphonate)
Didronel (Norwich Eaton) p 422, 1429

Etoposide
VePesid Injection (Bristol-Myers Oncology) p 767

Eucalyptol
Ponaris Nasal Mucosal Emollient (Jamol) p 1033
Vita-Numonyl Injectable (Lambda) p 1071

F

Factor VIII (AHF, AHG)
Hemofil, Antihemophilic Factor (Human), Method Four, Dried (Hyland Therapeutics) p 1023
Hemofil T, Antihemophilic Factor (Human), Method Four, Dried, Heat-Treated (Hyland Therapeutics) p 1024

Factor IX Complex (Human)
Factor IX Complex (Human) (Factors II, VII, IX, and X) Konÿne (Cutter Biological) p 886
Profilnine Heat-Treated (Alpha Theapeutic) p 589
Proplex, Factor IX Complex (Human) (Factors II, VII, IX & X), Dried (Hyland Therapeutics) p 1024

Generic and Chemical Name Index

Proplex SX, Factor IX Complex (Human)(Factors II, VII, IX & X), Dried (Hyland Therapeutics) p 1024
Proplex SX-T, Factor IX Complex (Human), Heat Treated (Hyland Therapeutics) p 1024
Prothar (Armour) p 613

Fenfluramine Hydrochloride
Pondimin Tablets (Robins) p 428, 1657

Fenoprofen Calcium
Nalfon Pulvules & Tablets (Dista) p 410, 903
Nalfon 200 Pulvules (Dista) p 410, 903

Fentanyl
Innovar Injection (Janssen) p 1035
Sublimaze Injection (Janssen) p 413, 1039

Ferric Pyrophosphate
Hemo-Vite Liquid (Drug Industries) p 914

Ferrous Fumarate
Cevi-Fer Capsules (sustained release) (Geriatric) p 975
Chromagen Capsules (Savage) p 433, 1824
Feostat Tablets, Suspension & Drops (O'Neal, Jones & Feldman) p 1445
Ferancee Chewable Tablets (Stuart) p 439, 2037
Ferancee-HP Tablets (Stuart) p 439, 2037
Ferro-Sequels (Lederle) p 415, 1093
Fetrin (LaSalle) p 1071
Hemocyte Tablets (U.S. Pharmaceutical) p 2070
Hemocyte-F Tablets (U.S. Pharmaceutical) p 2070
Hemo-Vite (Drug Industries) p 914
Ircon-FA (Key Pharmaceuticals) p 1050
Natalins Rx (Mead Johnson Laboratories) p 419, 1224
Natalins Tablets (Mead Johnson Laboratories) p 419, 1224
Poly-Vi-Flor 1.0 mg Vitamins w/Iron & Fluoride Chewable Tablets (Mead Johnson Nutritional) p 1245
Pramilet FA (Ross) p 432, 1775
Prenate 90 Tablets (Bock) p 706
Stuartinic Tablets (Stuart) p 439, 2034
Trinsicon/Trinsicon M Capsules (Glaxo) p 412, 986
Zenate Tablets (Reid-Provident Labs.) p 428, 1640

Ferrous Gluconate
Albafort Injectable (Bart) p 685
Fergon Capsules (Winthrop-Breon) p 443, 2198
Fergon Elixir (Winthrop-Breon) p 2198
Fergon Plus (Winthrop-Breon) p 2198
Fergon Tablets (Winthrop-Breon) p 443, 2198
Ferralet (Mission) p 1416
Fosfree (Mission) p 1416
Glytinic Tablets (Boyle) p 726
I.L.X. B₁₂ Tablets (Kenwood) p 1046
Iromin-G (Mission) p 1416
Megadose (Arco) p 600
Mission Prenatal (Mission) p 1419
Mission Prenatal F.A. (Mission) p 1419
Mission Prenatal H.P. (Mission) p 1419
Mission Pre-Surgical (Mission) p 1419

Ferrous Sulfate
Dayalets plus Iron Filmtab (Abbott) p 511
Eldec Kapseals (Parke-Davis) p 424, 1514
Fero-Folic-500 (Abbott) p 403, 529
Fero-Grad-500 (Abbott) p 403, 530
Fero-Gradumet (Abbott) p 530
Ferrous Sulfate Liquid, Tablets (Roxane) p 1788
Heptuna Plus (Roerig) p 431, 1735
Iberet (Abbott) p 532
Iberet-500 (Abbott) p 403, 532
Iberet-500 Liquid (Abbott) p 533
Iberet-Folic-500 (Abbott) p 403, 529
Iberet Liquid (Abbott) p 533
Irospan Capsules (Fielding) p 942
Irospan Tablets (Fielding) p 942
Mevanin-C Capsules (Beutlich) p 705
Pramet FA (Ross) p 432, 1775

Fibrinolysin
Elase (Parke-Davis) p 424, 1513
Elase Ointment (Parke-Davis) p 424, 1513
Elase-Chloromycetin Ointment (Parke-Davis) p 424, 1513

Flavoxate Hydrochloride
Urispas (Smith Kline & French) p 437, 1981

Floxuridine
FUDR Injectable (Roche) p 1684

Flucytosine
Ancobon Capsules (Roche) p 429, 1669

Flunisolide
AeroBid Inhaler System (Key Pharmaceuticals) p 1046
Nasalide Nasal Solution 0.025% (Syntex) p 2064

Fluocinolone Acetonide
Derma-Smoothe/FS (Hill Dermaceuticals) p 1009
Fluocinolone Acetonide Cream (Schein) p 1828
Fluocinolone Acetonide Cream & Topical Solution 0.01% (Fougera) p 953
Fluocinolone Acetonide Cream & Ointment 0.025% (Fougera) p 953
Fluocinolone Acetonide Cream, Ointment & Topical Solution (Pharmaderm) p 1617
Fluocinolone Acetonide Topical Cream, Ointment & Solution (Pharmafair) p 1618
Fluonid Ointment, Cream & Topical Solution (Herbert) p 1003
Neo-Synalar Cream (Syntex) p 2061
Psoranide Cream 0.025% (Elder) p 936
Synalar Creams 0.025%, 0.01% (Syntex) p 2061
Synalar Ointment 0.025% (Syntex) p 2061
Synalar Topical Solution 0.01% (Syntex) p 2061
Synalar-HP Cream 0.2% (Syntex) p 2061
Synemol Cream 0.025% (Syntex) p 2061

Fluocinonide
Lidex Cream 0.05% (Syntex) p 2061
Lidex Gel 0.05% (Syntex) p 2061
Lidex Ointment 0.05% (Syntex) p 2061
Lidex Topical Solution 0.05% (Syntex) p 2061
Lidex-E Cream 0.05% (Syntex) p 2061

Fluorine & Fluoride Preparations
Adeflor Chewable Tablets (Upjohn) p 440, 2093
Adeflor Drops (Upjohn) p 2093
Fluoritab Tablets & Fluoritab Liquid (Fluoritab) p 953
Luride Drops (Colgate-Hoyt) p 878
Luride Lozi-Tabs Tablets (Colgate-Hoyt) p 410, 878
Mulvidren-F Softab Tablets (Stuart) p 439, 2039
Pediaflor Drops (Ross) p 1771
Phos-Flur Oral Rinse/Supplement (Colgate-Hoyt) p 879
Point-Two Dental Rinse (Colgate-Hoyt) p 880
Poly-Vi-Flor 1.0 mg Vitamins w/Fluoride Chewable Tablets (Mead Johnson Nutritional) p 1243
Poly-Vi-Flor 0.5 mg Vitamins w/Fluoride Drops (Mead Johnson Nutritional) p 1244
Poly-Vi-Flor 1.0 mg Vitamins w/Iron & Fluoride Chewable Tablets (Mead Johnson Nutritional) p 1245
Poly-Vi-Flor 0.5 mg Vitamins w/Iron & Fluoride Drops (Mead Johnson Nutritional) p 1245
PreviDent Brush-On Gel (Colgate-Hoyt) p 880
Thera-Flur Gel-Drops (Colgate-Hoyt) p 880
Tri-Vi-Flor 0.25 mg Vitamins w/Iron & Fluoride Drops (Mead Johnson Nutritional) p 1248
Vi-Daylin/F ADC Drops (Ross) p 1782
Vi-Daylin/F ADC + Iron Drops (Ross) p 1782
Vi-Daylin/F Chewable (Ross) p 432, 1784
Vi-Daylin/F Drops (Ross) p 1783
Vi-Daylin/F + Iron Chewable (Ross) p 432, 1783
Vi-Daylin/F + Iron Drops (Ross) p 1783
Vi-Penta F Chewables (Roche) p 430, 1708
Vi-Penta F Infant Drops (Roche) p 1709
Vi-Penta F Multivitamin Drops (Roche) p 1709

Fluorouracil
Adrucil Injectable (Adria) p 573
Efudex Topical Solutions and Cream (Roche) p 1681
Fluoroplex Topical Solution & Cream (Herbert) p 1004
Fluorouracil Ampuls (Roche) p 1683

Fluoxymesterone
Android-F Tablets (Brown) p 407, 773
Fluoxymesterone Tablets (Geneva) p 973
Fluoxymesterone Tablets (Schein) p 1828
Halotestin Tablets (Upjohn) p 441, 2116

Fluphenazine Decanoate
Prolixin Decanoate (Squibb) p 2015

Fluphenazine Hydrochloride
Permitil Oral Concentrate (Schering) p 1877
Permitil Tablets (Schering) p 434, 1877
Prolixin Elixir & Injection (Squibb) p 2014
Prolixin Tablets (Squibb) p 438, 2014

Flurandrenolide
Cordran Ointment & Lotion (Dista) p 895
Cordran SP Cream (Dista) p 895
Cordran Tape (Dista) p 897
Cordran-N (Dista) p 897

Flurazepam Hydrochloride
Dalmane Capsules (Roche Products) p 429, 1710

Folic Acid
Added Protection III Multi-Vitamin & Multi-Mineral Supplement (Professional Health) p 1621
Al-Vite (Drug Industries) p 914
Cefol Filmtab Tablets (Abbott) p 403, 510
Cevi-Fer Capsules (sustained release) (Geriatric) p 975
Dayalets Filmtab (Abbott) p 511
Dayalets plus Iron Filmtab (Abbott) p 511
Eldec Kapseals (Parke-Davis) p 424, 1514
Eldercaps (Mayrand) p 1196
Enviro-Stress with Zinc & Selenium (Vitaline) p 2148
Fero-Folic-500 (Abbott) p 403, 529
Filibon F.A. (Lederle) p 415, 1093
Filibon Forte (Lederle) p 415, 1093
Folic Acid Tablets (Lilly) p 1147
Folic Acid Tablets (Danbury) p 887
Folvite (Lederle) p 1093
Hemocyte-F Tablets (U.S. Pharmaceutical) p 2070
Hemo-Vite (Drug Industries) p 914
Hemo-Vite Liquid (Drug Industries) p 914
Iberet-Folic-500 (Abbott) p 403, 529
Ircon-FA (Key Pharmaceuticals) p 1050
Iromin-G (Mission) p 1416
Mega-B (Arco) p 600
Megadose (Arco) p 600
Mevanin-C Capsules (Beutlich) p 705
Niferex-150 Forte Capsules (Central Pharmaceuticals) p 409, 838
Nu-Iron-Plus Elixir (Mayrand) p 1196
Nu-Iron-V Tablets (Mayrand) p 1196
Orabex-TF (LaSalle) p 1071
Pramet FA (Ross) p 432, 1775
Pramilet FA (Ross) p 432, 1775
Prenate 90 Tablets (Bock) p 706
Pronemia Capsules (Lederle) p 1118
Stuartnatal 1+1 Tablets (Stuart) p 439, 2043
Trinsicon/Trinsicon M Capsules (Glaxo) p 412, 986
Vicon Forte Capsules (Glaxo) p 412, 989
Vio-Bec Forte (Rowell) p 1788
Vitafol Tablets (Everett) p 942
Zenate Tablets (Reid-Provident Labs.) p 428, 1640
Zincvit Capsules (RAM Laboratories) p 1632

Formaldehyde
Pedi-Dri Foot Powder (Pedinol) p 1581

Furazolidone
Furoxone Liquid Suspension (Norwich Eaton) p 1435
Furoxone Tablets (Norwich Eaton) p 1435

Furosemide
Furosemide Injection (Elkins-Sinn) p 938
Furosemide Injection, USP (Parke-Davis) p 1522
Furosemide Injection (Wyeth) p 2252
Furosemide Tablets (Geneva) p 973
Furosemide Tablets (Schein) p 1828
Furosemide Tablets, USP (Parke-Davis) p 1524
Lasix Oral Solution (Hoechst-Roussel) p 413, 1015
Lasix Tablets and Injection (Hoechst-Roussel) p 413, 1015
SK-Furosemide Tablets (Smith Kline & French) p 1971

G

Gamma Benzene Hexachloride
Kwell Cream (Reed & Carnrick) p 1635
Kwell Lotion (Reed & Carnrick) p 1635
Kwell Shampoo (Reed & Carnrick) p 1635
Scabene Lotion (Stiefel) p 2035
Scabene Shampoo (Stiefel) p 2036

Gamma Globulin
Gammar, Immune Serum Globulin (Human) U.S.P. (Armour) p 613
Hepatitis B Immune Globulin (Human) HyperHep (Cutter Biological) p 884
Hu-Tet, Tetanus Immune Globulin (Human), U.S.P. (Hyland Therapeutics) p 1024
Immuglobin (Savage) p 1825
Immune Globulin Intravenous, 5% (In 10% Maltose) Gamimune (Cutter Biological) p 883
Immune Serum Globulin (Human) (Wyeth) p 2245

Generic and Chemical Name Index

Immune Serum Globulin (Human) in Tubex (Wyeth) p 2288
Immune Serum Globulin (Human), U.S.P. Gamma Globulin (Hyland Therapeutics) p 1024
Immune Serum Globulin (Human) Gamastan (Cutter Biological) p 883
Imogam Rabies Immune Globulin (Human) (Merieux) p 1358
Pertussis Immune Globulin (Human) Hypertussis (Cutter Biological) p 884
Rabies Immune Globulin (Human) Hyperab (Cutter Biological) p 884
Rabies Immune Globulin (Human), Imogam Rabies (Merieux) p 1358
Tetanus Immune Globulin (Human) (Wyeth) p 2246
Tetanus Immune Globulin (Human) in Tubex (Wyeth) p 2288
Tetanus Immune Globulin (Human) Hyper-Tet (Cutter Biological) p 884

Gelatin Preparations
Dome-Paste Bandage (Miles Pharmaceuticals) p 1402
Gelfoam Sterile Powder (Upjohn) p 2114
Gelfoam Sterile Sponge (Upjohn) p 2113

Gemfibrozil
Lopid Capsules (Parke-Davis) p 424, 1539

Gentamicin
Gentamicin Ophthalmic Ointment & Solution (Schein) p 1828

Gentamicin Sulfate
G-myticin Creme and Ointment 0.1% (Pedinol) p 1580
Garamycin Cream 0.1% and Ointment 0.1% (Schering) p 1846
Garamycin Injectable (Schering) p 1846
Garamycin Intrathecal Injection (Schering) p 1854
Garamycin I.V. Piggyback Injection (Schering) p 1851
Garamycin Ophthalmic Ointment-Sterile (Schering) p 1846
Garamycin Ophthalmic Solution-Sterile (Schering) p 1846
Garamycin Pediatric Injectable (Schering) p 1849
Gentafair Cream & Ointment (Pharmafair) p 1618
Gentamicin Cream 0.1% & Ointment 0.1% (Schein) p 1828
Gentamicin Sulfate Injection (Elkins-Sinn) p 938

Glipizide
Glucotrol (Roerig) p 431, 1733

Globulin, Immune Serum (Human)
Gammar, Immune Serum Globulin (Human) U.S.P. (Armour) p 613
Hepatitis B Immune Globulin (Human) HyperHep (Cutter Biological) p 884
Immune Globulin Intravenous, 5% (In 10% Maltose) Gamimune (Cutter Biological) p 883
Immune Serum Globulin (Human) Gamastan (Cutter Biological) p 883
Tetanus Immune Globulin (Human) Hyper-Tet (Cutter Biological) p 884

Globulin, Poliomyelitis Immune (Human)
Gammar, Immune Serum Globulin (Human) U.S.P. (Armour) p 613

Glucagon
Glucagon for Injection Ampoules (Lilly) p 1147

Glucose
Infalyte (Pennwalt) p 1584

Glucose Polymers
Polycose (Ross) p 1775

Glutamic Acid Hydrochloride
Acidulin (Lilly) p 1126
Kanulase (Dorsey Laboratories) p 910
Muripsin (Norgine) p 1424

Glutethimide
Doriden Tablets (USV Pharmaceutical) p 2076
Glutethimide Tablets (Danbury) p 887
Glutethimide Tablets (Geneva) p 973
Glutethimide Tablets (Schein) p 1828

Glyburide
DiaBeta (Hoechst-Roussel) p 412, 1012
Micronase Tablets (Upjohn) p 441, 2126

Glycerin
Debrox Drops (Marion) p 1184
Dome-Paste Bandage (Miles Pharmaceuticals) p 1402
Fleet Babylax (Fleet) p 946
Gly-Oxide Liquid (Marion) p 1186
Otipyrin Otic Solution (Kramer) p 1069

Glycerin Dehydrated
Auralgan Otic Solution (Ayerst) p 638

Glyceryl Guaiacolate
(see under Guaifenesin)

Glyceryl Trinitrate
(see under Nitroglycerin)

Glycopyrrolate
Glycopyrrolate Tablets (Danbury) p 887
Robinul Forte Tablets (Robins) p 429, 1662
Robinul Injectable (Robins) p 429, 1663
Robinul Tablets (Robins) p 429, 1662

Gold Sodium Thiomalate
Myochrysine Injection (Merck Sharp & Dohme) p 1339

Gonadorelin Hydrochloride
Factrel (Ayerst) p 404, 643, 3007

Gonadotropins (Human Menopausal)
Pergonal (menotropins USP) (Serono) p 1941

Gramicidin
Mycolog Cream and Ointment (Squibb) p 2003
Myco-Triacet Cream and Ointment (Lemmon) p 1122
Mytrex Cream & Ointment (Savage) p 1825
Neosporin Ophthalmic Solution Sterile (Burroughs Wellcome) p 809
Neosporin-G Cream (Burroughs Wellcome) p 807
Nystatin-Neomycin-Gramicidin-Triamcinolone Cream & Ointment (Fougera) p 953
Nyst-olone Cream & Ointment (Schein) p 1828
Tri-Thalmic Ophthalmic Solution (Schein) p 1828

Griseofulvin
Fulvicin P/G Tablets (Schering) p 434, 1843
Fulvicin P/G 165 & 330 Tablets (Schering) p 434, 1844
Fulvicin-U/F Tablets (Schering) p 434, 1845
Grifulvin V (Ortho Pharmaceutical (Dermatological Div.)) p 1473
Grisactin (Ayerst) p 404, 646
Grisactin Ultra (Ayerst) p 405, 646
Gris-PEG Tablets, 125mg & 250mg (Herbert) p 1005

Guaiacolglycerylether
Eclabron Elixir (Wharton) p 2184

Guaifenesin
Ambenyl-D Decongestant Cough Formula (Marion) p 1182
Asbron G Elixir (Sandoz Pharmaceutical Div.) p 1796
Asbron G Inlay-Tabs (Sandoz Pharmaceutical Div.) p 432, 1796
Breonesin (Winthrop-Breon) p 2193
Bromphen DC Expectorant (Schein) p 1828
Bromphen Expectorant (Schein) p 1828
Brondecon (Parke-Davis) p 423, 1486
Bronkolixir (Winthrop-Breon) p 2193
Bronkotabs (Winthrop-Breon) p 2194
Bronkotuss (Hyrex) p 1024
Codimal Expectorant (Central Pharmaceuticals) p 836
Conex (O'Neal, Jones & Feldman) p 1445
Conex with Codeine (O'Neal, Jones & Feldman) p 1445
Congess Jr. & Sr. T.D. Capsules (Fleming) p 948
Coryban-D Cough Syrup (Pfipharmecs) p 1589
Cremacoat 2 (Vicks Pharmacy Products) p 442, 2147
Cremacoat 3 (Vicks Pharmacy Products) p 442, 2147
Decongestant Expectorant (Schein) p 1828
Deproist Expectorant w/Codeine (Geneva) p 973
Detussin Expectorant (Schein) p 1828
Dilaudid Cough Syrup (Knoll) p 1058
Dilor-G Tablets & Liquid (Savage) p 433, 1824
Donatussin DC Syrup (Laser) p 1072
Donatussin Drops (Laser) p 1072
Dorcol Children's Cough Syrup (Dorsey Laboratories) p 909
Dura-Vent (Dura) p 929
Elixophyllin-GG (Berlex) p 406, 702
Entex Capsules (Norwich Eaton) p 1431
Entex LA Tablets (Norwich Eaton) p 422, 1432
Entex Liquid (Norwich Eaton) p 1431
Entuss-D Liquid & Tablets (Hauck) p 1001
Fedahist Expectorant (Rorer) p 1749
Guaifed Capsules (Timed Release) (Muro) p 1421
Guaifenesin Syrup (Roxane) p 1788
Guiatuss Syrup (Schein) p 1828
Guiatuss A-C Syrup (Schein) p 1828
Guiatuss D-M Syrup (Schein) p 1828
Head & Chest (Procter & Gamble) p 1620
Histalet X Syrup & Tablets (New Formula) (Reid-Provident Labs.) p 428, 1638
Hycotuss Expectorant (Du Pont) p 920
Hytuss Tablets and Hytuss-2X Capsules (Hyrex) p 413, 1024
Lufyllin-GG (Wallace) p 442, 2161
Mudrane GG Elixir (Poythress) p 1619
Mudrane GG Tablets (Poythress) p 1619
Mudrane GG-2 Tablets (Poythress) p 1619
Naldecon-CX Suspension (Bristol) p 739
Naldecon-DX Pediatric Syrup (Bristol) p 739
Naldecon-EX Pediatric Drops (Bristol) p 740
Novahistine Expectorant (Merrell Dow) p 421, 1378
Nucofed Expectorant (Beecham Laboratories) p 693
Nucofed Pediatric Expectorant (Beecham Laboratories) p 694
P-V-Tussin Tablets (Reid-Provident Labs.) p 428, 1640
Poly-Histine Expectorant Plain (Bock) p 705
Poly-Histine Expectorant with Codeine (Bock) p 705
Quibron & Quibron-300 (Mead Johnson Laboratories) p 419, 1233
Quibron Plus (Mead Johnson Laboratories) p 419, 1236
Respaire-SR Capsules 60, 120 (Laser) p 1072
Robitussin A-C (Robins) p 1664
Robitussin-DAC (Robins) p 1665
S-T Forte Syrup & Sugar-Free (Scot-Tussin) p 1897
Scot-Tussin Sugar-Free Expectorant (Scot-Tussin) p 1897
Sinufed Timecelles (Hauck) p 1001
Slo-Phyllin GG Capsules, Syrup (Rorer) p 432, 1759
Sorbutuss (Dalin) p 886
Synophylate-GG Tablets/Syrup (Central Pharmaceuticals) p 839
Theolair-Plus Tablets & Liquid (Riker) p 428, 1645
Triafed-C Expectorant (Schein) p 1828
Triaminic Expectorant (Dorsey Laboratories) p 911
Triaminic Expectorant w/Codeine (Dorsey Laboratories) p 911
Tussar SF (USV Pharmaceutical) p 2092
Tussar-2 (USV Pharmaceutical) p 2092
Tussend Expectorant (Merrell Dow) p 421, 1394
Zephrex Tablets (Bock) p 706
Zephrex-LA Tablets (Bock) p 706

Guanabenz Acetate
Wytensin Tablets (Wyeth) p 445, 2299

Guanadrel Sulfate
Hylorel Tablets (Pennwalt) p 426, 1582

Guanethidine Monosulfate
Esimil (CIBA) p 409, 849

Guanethidine Sulfate
Ismelin (CIBA) p 409, 851

Gum Karaya
Movicol (Norgine) p 1424

H

Halazepam
Paxipam Tablets (Schering) p 434, 1876

Halcinonide
Halog Cream/Ointment/Solution (Squibb) p 1996
Halog-E Cream (Squibb) p 1996

Haloperidol
Haldol Tablets, Concentrate, Injection (McNeil Pharmaceutical) p 418, 1201

Haloprogin
Halotex Cream & Solution (Westwood) p 2178

Halothane
Fluothane (Ayerst) p 645

Hemin for Injection
Panhematin (Abbott) p 557

Heparin Calcium
Calciparine Injection (American Critical Care) p 593

Generic and Chemical Name Index

Heparin Sodium
  Heparin Lock Flush Solution in Tubex
    (Wyeth) p 2253
  Heparin Sodium (Lilly) p 1149
  Heparin Sodium (from Beef Lung Sources)
    (Organon) p 1446
  Heparin Sodium in Tubex (Wyeth) p 2288
  Heparin Sodium Injection (Elkins-Sinn) p 938
  Heparin Sodium Injection (Wyeth) p 2254
  Heparin Sodium Injection, USP, Sterile
    Solution (Upjohn) p 2117
  Heparin Sodium w/o preservative Injectable
    (O'Neal, Jones & Feldman) p 1445
  Hep-Lock (Heparin Lock Flush Solution)
    (Elkins-Sinn) p 938
  Hep-Lock PF (Preservative-Free Heparin Lock
    Flush Solution) (Elkins-Sinn) p 938
  Liquaemin Sodium (Organon) p 1446

Hepatitis B Immune Globulin (Human)
  H-BIG (Abbott) p 531
  Hep-B-Gammagee (Merck Sharp & Dohme)
    p 1311

Hepatitis B Vaccine
  Heptavax-B (Merck Sharp & Dohme) p 1312

Hesperidin Preparations
  Mevanin-C Capsules (Beutlich) p 705
  Peridin-C (Beutlich) p 705

Hetastarch
  Hespan (American Critical Care) p 595

Hexachlorophene
  pHisoHex (Winthrop-Breon) p 2222

Hexocyclium Methylsulfate
  Tral Filmtab Tablets (Abbott) p 568

Histamine Phosphate
  Histamine Phosphate (For Gastric Test)
    (Lilly) p 3012
  Histamine Phosphate (Histamine Test for
    Pheochromocytoma) (Lilly) p 3012

Homatropine Methylbromide
  Hydrocodone Syrup (Schein) p 1828
  Sinulin Tablets (Carnrick) p 409, 835

Hyaluronidase
  Wydase Injection (Wyeth) p 2296

Hydantoin Derivative
  Dilantin Infatabs (Parke-Davis) p 423, 1503
  Dilantin Kapseals (Parke-Davis) p 423, 1502
  Dilantin Parenteral (Parke-Davis) p 1505
  Dilantin with Phenobarbital (Parke-Davis)
    p 423, 1507
  Dilantin-30 Pediatric/Dilantin-125
    Suspension (Parke-Davis) p 1506

Hydralazine
  H-H-R Tablets (Schein) p 1828
  Hydralazine-Thiazide Capsules (Schein)
    p 1828
  Hydralazine w/Hydrochlorothiazide Capsules
    (Geneva) p 973

Hydralazine Hydrochloride
  Apresazide (CIBA) p 409, 842
  Apresoline Hydrochloride (CIBA) p 409, 843
  Apresoline Hydrochloride Parenteral (CIBA)
    p 844
  Apresoline-Esidrix (CIBA) p 409, 844
  Hydralazine HCl Tablets (Danbury) p 887
  Hydralazine HCl Tablets (Geneva) p 973
  Hydralazine HCl Tablets (Schein) p 1828
  Hydrochlorothiazide, Hydralazine HCl,
    Reserpine Tablets (Danbury) p 887
  Ser-Ap-Es (CIBA) p 409, 866
  Serpasil-Apresoline (CIBA) p 409, 869
  Unipres Tablets (Reid-Provident Labs.)
    p 428, 1640

Hydrochloric Acid Preparations
  Muripsin (Norgine) p 1424
  Zypan Tablets (Standard Process) p 2035

Hydrochlorothiazide
  Aldactazide (Searle & Co.) p 435, 1912
  Aldoril Tablets (Merck Sharp & Dohme)
    p 420, 1262
  Apresazide (CIBA) p 409, 842
  Apresoline-Esidrix (CIBA) p 409, 844
  Dyazide (Smith Kline & French) p 437, 1961
  Esidrix (CIBA) p 409, 848
  Esimil (CIBA) p 409, 849
  H-H-R Tablets (Schein) p 1828
  Hydralazine-Thiazide Capsules (Schein)
    p 1828
  Hydralazine w/Hydrochlorothiazide Capsules
    (Geneva) p 973
  Hydrochlorothiazide, Hydralazine HCl,
    Reserpine Tablets (Danbury) p 887
  Hydrochlorothiazide/Reserpine Tablets
    (Danbury) p 887
  Hydrochlorothiazide Tablets (Danbury) p 887
  Hydrochlorothiazide Tablets (Geneva) p 973
  Hydrochlorothiazide Tablets, Liquids, Intensol
    & Oral Solution (Roxane) p 1788
  Hydrochlorothiazide Tablets (Schein) p 1828
  Hydrochlorothiazide Tablets, USP (Thiuretic)
    (Parke-Davis) p 1527
  Hydrochlorothiazide w/Reserpine Tablets
    (Geneva) p 973
  HydroDIURIL Tablets (Merck Sharp &
    Dohme) p 420, 1316
  Hydropres Tablets (Merck Sharp & Dohme)
    p 420, 1317
  Hydroserpine Tablets (Schein) p 1828
  Inderide (Ayerst) p 405, 651
  Maxzide Tablets (Lederle) p 415, 1098
  Moduretic Tablets (Merck Sharp & Dohme)
    p 420, 1333
  Oretic (Abbott) p 403, 554
  Oreticyl (Abbott) p 555
  SK-Hydrochlorothiazide Tablets (Smith Kline
    & French) p 1971
  Ser-Ap-Es (CIBA) p 409, 866
  Serpasil-Esidrix (CIBA) p 409, 870
  Spironazide Tablets (Schein) p 1828
  Spironolactone/Hydrochlorothiazide Tablets
    (Danbury) p 887
  Spironolactone w/Hydrochlorothiazide
    Tablets (Geneva) p 973
  Spironolactone w/Hydrochlorothiazide
    Tablets (Parke-Davis) p 1570
  Timolide Tablets (Merck Sharp & Dohme)
    p 420, 1346
  Unipres Tablets (Reid-Provident Labs.)
    p 428, 1640

Hydrocodone Bitartrate
  Amacodone Tablets (Trimen) p 2067
  Bancap HC Capsules (O'Neal, Jones &
    Feldman) p 422, 1444
  Citra Forte Capsules (Boyle) p 726
  Citra Forte Syrup (Boyle) p 726
  Codiclear DH Syrup (Central
    Pharmaceuticals) p 836
  Codimal DH (Central Pharmaceuticals) p 836
  Co-Gesic Tablets (Central Pharmaceuticals)
    p 409, 836
  Damacet-P (Mason) p 418, 1193
  Damason-P (Mason) p 418, 1194
  Detussin Expectorant (Schein) p 1828
  Detussin Liquid (Schein) p 1828
  Dia-Gesic (Central Pharmaceuticals) p 409,
    837
  Dolacet Capsules (Hauck) p 1001
  Donatussin DC Syrup (Laser) p 1072
  Duradyne DHC Tablets (O'Neal, Jones &
    Feldman) p 1445
  Entuss Expectorant Tablets & Liquid (Hauck)
    p 1001
  Entuss-D Liquid & Tablets (Hauck) p 1001
  Hycodan (Du Pont) p 410, 917
  Hycomine Compound (Du Pont) p 919
  Hycomine Pediatric Syrup (Du Pont) p 917
  Hycomine Syrup (Du Pont) p 917
  Hyco-Pap (LaSalle) p 1071
  Hycotuss Expectorant (Du Pont) p 920
  Hydrocodone Syrup (Schein) p 1828
  Lorcet-HD (UAD Labs.) p 2069
  P-V-Tussin Syrup (Reid-Provident Labs.)
    p 1640
  P-V-Tussin Tablets (Reid-Provident Labs.)
    p 428, 1640
  Ru-Tuss with Hydrocodone (Boots) p 722
  S-T Forte Syrup & Sugar-Free (Scot-Tussin)
    p 1897
  Stopayne Capsules (Springbok) p 1985
  Tussend Expectorant (Merrell Dow) p 421,
    1394
  Tussend Liquid & Tablets (Merrell Dow)
    p 421, 1393
  Vicodin (Knoll) p 414, 1068

Hydrocodone Resin Complex
  Tussionex Tablets, Capsules & Suspension
    (Pennwalt) p 1585

Hydrocortisone
  Aeroseb-HC Topical Aerosol Spray (Herbert)
    p 1002
  Allersone (Mallard) p 1181
  Alphaderm (Norwich Eaton) p 1424
  Carmol HC Cream 1% (Syntex) p 2061
  Cort-Dome ⅛%, ¼%, ½%, and 1% Creme
    (Miles Pharmaceuticals) p 1399
  Cort-Dome ⅛%, ¼%, ½%, and 1% Lotion
    (Miles Pharmaceuticals) p 1400
  Corticaine Cream (Glaxo) p 412, 980
  Corticaine Suppositories (Glaxo) p 412, 980
  Cortifair Cream & Lotion (Pharmafair)
    p 1618
  Cortisporin Ophthalmic Ointment (Burroughs
    Wellcome) p 784
  Cortisporin Ophthalmic Suspension
    (Burroughs Wellcome) p 785
  Cortisporin Otic Solution (Burroughs
    Wellcome) p 786
  Cortisporin Otic Suspension (Burroughs
    Wellcome) p 786
  Cortril Topical Ointment (Pfipharmecs)
    p 1589
  Derma-Sone Cream (Hill Dermaceuticals)
    p 1009
  Di-Hydrotic (Legere) p 1120
  Eldecort Cream, 1%, 2.5% (Elder) p 930
  F-E-P Creme (Boots) p 717
  Hill Cortac (Hill Dermaceuticals) p 1009
  Hydrocortisone USP (Organon) p 1446
  Hydrocortisone Cream (Pharmaderm)
    p 1617
  Hydrocortisone Cream & Ointment 0.5%
    (Fougera) p 953
  Hydrocortisone Cream & Ointment 1%
    (Fougera) p 953
  Hydrocortisone Tablets (Danbury) p 887
  Hysone (Mallard) p 1181
  Hytone Cream, Lotion & Ointment (Dermik)
    p 890
  Iodochlorhydroxyquin 3% with
    Hydrocortisone Creams (Fougera) p 953
  Iodo-Cortifair (Pharmafair) p 1618
  Octicair Otic Solution & Suspension
    (Pharmafair) p 1618
  Otic-HC Ear Drops (Hauck) p 1001
  Oticol Sterile Ear Drops (Arlo) p 601
  Otobiotic Otic Solution (Schering) p 1875
  Otocort Sterile Ear Drops, Solution and
    Suspension (Lemmon) p 1122
  Pedi-Cort V Creme (Pedinol) p 1581
  Penecort Cream & Topical Solution 1%
    (Herbert) p 1007
  Penecort Cream 2.5% (Herbert) p 1008
  Pro-Cort Cream (Barnes-Hind) p 684
  Pro-Cort M Cream (Barnes-Hind) p 684
  Pyocidin-Otic Solution (Berlex) p 702
  Synacort Creams 1%, 2.5% (Syntex)
    p 2061
  Texacort Scalp Lotion (Cooper Dermatology)
    p 882
  Vanoxide-HC Acne Lotion (Dermik) p 891
  Vioform-Hydrocortisone (CIBA) p 876
  VōSol HC Otic Solution (Wallace) p 442,
    2171
  Vytone Cream (Dermik) p 891

Hydrocortisone Acetate
  Anusol-HC (Parke-Davis) p 423, 1484
  Carmol HC Cream 1% (Syntex) p 2061
  Coly-Mycin S Otic w/Neomycin &
    Hydrocortisone (Parke-Davis) p 1501
  Cort-Dome High Potency Suppositories (Miles
    Pharmaceuticals) p 1401
  Cort-Dome Regular Potency Suppositories
    (Miles Pharmaceuticals) p 1401
  Cortifoam (Reed & Carnrick) p 427, 1632
  Cortisporin Cream (Burroughs Wellcome)
    p 783
  Derma Medicone-HC Ointment (Medicone)
    p 1256
  Epifoam (Reed & Carnrick) p 427, 1634
  Hydrocortone Acetate Sterile Ophthalmic
    Ointment and Ophthalmic Suspension
    (Merck Sharp & Dohme) p 1316
  Komed HC Lotion (Barnes-Hind) p 684
  Mantadil Cream (Burroughs Wellcome) p 803
  Ophthocort (Parke-Davis) p 1558
  Orabase HCA (Colgate-Hoyt) p 879
  Pramosone Cream, Lotion & Ointment
    (Ferndale) p 942
  Proctofoam-HC (Reed & Carnrick) p 427,
    1636
  Rectal Medicone-HC Suppositories
    (Medicone) p 419, 1256
  Zone-A Lotion 1% (UAD Labs.) p 2069

Hydrocortisone (Alcohol)
  Barseb HC Scalp Lotion (Barnes-Hind) p 683
  Barseb Thera-Spray (Barnes-Hind) p 684
  Cortisporin Ointment (Burroughs Wellcome)
    p 784

Hydrocortisone Sodium Succinate
  A-hydroCort (Abbott) p 506
  Hydrocortisone Sodium Succinate for
    Injection (Elkins-Sinn) p 938
  Solu-Cortef Plain & Mix-O-Vial (Upjohn)
    p 2135

Hydrocortisone Valerate
  Westcort Cream 0.2% (Westwood) p 2183
  Westcort Ointment 0.2% (Westwood)
    p 2183

Hydroflumethiazide
  Diucardin (Ayerst) p 404, 640
  Hydroflumethiazide Tablets (Schein) p 1828
  Hydroflumethiazide with Reserpine (Geneva)
    p 973
  Hydro-Fluserpine Tablets #1 & #2 (Schein)
    p 1828
  Saluron (Bristol) p 407, 747
  Salutensin/Salutensin-Demi (Bristol) p 407,
    748

Generic and Chemical Name Index

Hydrogenated Vegetable Oil
Hydrisinol Creme & Lotion (Pedinol) p 1580

Hydromorphone
(see under Dihydromorphinone Hydrochloride)

Hydromorphone Hydrochloride
(see also under Dihydromorphinone Hydrochloride)
Dilaudid Cough Syrup (Knoll) p 1058
Dilaudid Hydrochloride (Knoll) p 414, 1057
Dilaudid-HP Injection (Knoll) p 414, 1059
Hydromorphone HCl Injection (Elkins-Sinn) p 938
Hydromorphone HCl in Tubex (Wyeth) p 2288

Hydroquinone
Banquin Cream (Kramer) p 1069
Eldopaque 2% Cream (Elder) p 930
Eldopaque Forte 4% Cream (Elder) p 930
Eldoquin 2% Cream & 2% Lotion (Elder) p 930
Eldoquin Forte 4% Cream (Elder) p 930
Melanex 4% Topical Solution (Neutrogena) (Neutrogena) p 1421
Solaquin Forte 4% Cream (Elder) p 936
Solaquin Forte 4% Gel (Elder) p 937

Hydroxyamphetamine Hydrobromide
Paredrine 1% w/Boric Acid, Ophthalmic Solution (Smith Kline & French) p 1968

Hydroxychloroquine Sulfate
Plaquenil Sulfate (Winthrop-Breon) p 444, 2223

Hydroxyprogesterone Caproate
Prodrox 250 (Legere) p 1120

Hydroxyquinoline Sulfate
Derma Medicone-HC Ointment (Medicone) p 1256
Rectal Medicone-HC Suppositories (Medicone) p 419, 1256

Hydroxyurea
Hydrea Capsules (Squibb) p 438, 1997

Hydroxyzine Hydrochloride
Atarax Tablets & Syrup (Roerig) p 431, 1725
Durrax Tablets 10mg, 25mg (Dermik) p 888
Hydroxyzine HCl Intramuscular Injection (Elkins-Sinn) p 938
Hydroxyzine HCl in Tubex (Wyeth) p 2288
Hydroxyzine HCl Syrup & Tablets (Schein) p 1828
Hydroxyzine Hydrochloride Tablets (Danbury) p 887
Hydroxyzine Hydrochloride Tablets (Geneva) p 973
Marax Tablets & DF Syrup (Roerig) p 431, 1737
Neucalm 50 (Legere) p 1120
T.E.H. Tablets (Geneva) p 973
Theozine Syrup & Tablets - Dye-Free (Schein) p 1828
Vistaril Intramuscular Solution (Pfipharmecs) p 1598

Hydroxyzine Pamoate
Hydroxyzine Pamoate Capsules (Danbury) p 887
Hydroxyzine Pamoate (Schein) p 1828
Vistaril Capsules and Oral Suspension (Pfizer) p 427, 1612

Hyoscine Hydrobromide
(see under Scopolamine Preparations)

Hyoscyamine
Antispasmodic Capsules, Elixir & Tablets (Schein) p 1828
Cystospaz (Webcon) p 2172

l-Hyoscyamine
Kutrase Capsules (Rorer) p 431, 1750
Levsin Tablets, Injection, Elixir & Drops (Rorer) p 432, 1751
Levsin/Phenobarbital Tablets, Elixir & Drops (Rorer) p 1751
Levsinex Timecaps (Rorer) p 432, 1751
Levsinex/Phenobarbital Timecaps (Rorer) p 1751
Urised Tablets (Webcon) p 2173

Hyoscyamine Hydrobromide
Pyridium Plus (Parke-Davis) p 425, 1568

Hyoscyamine Sulfate
Arco-Lase Plus (Arco) p 600
Cystospaz-M (Webcon) p 2172
Levsin Tablets, Injection, Elixir & Drops (Rorer) p 432, 1751
Levsin/Phenobarbital Tablets, Elixir & Drops (Rorer) p 1751
Levsinex Timecaps (Rorer) p 432, 1751
Levsinex/Phenobarbital Timecaps (Rorer) p 1751
Ru-Tuss Tablets (Boots) p 406, 723

l-Hyoscyamine Sulfate
Anaspaz PB Tablets (Ascher) p 614
Anaspaz Tablets (Ascher) p 614

Hyoscyamus Preparations
Trac Tabs 2X (Hyrex) p 413, 1025

I

Ibuprofen
Advil Ibuprofen Tablets (Whitehall) p 443, 2184
Motrin Tablets* (Upjohn) p 441, 2128
Nuprin (Bristol-Myers Products) p 771
Rufen Tablets (Boots) p 406, 720

Ichthammol
Derma Medicone-HC Ointment (Medicone) p 1256
Ichthammol Ointment 10% & 20% (Fougera) p 953

Imipramine Hydrochloride
Imipramine HCl Tablets (Biocraft) p 705
Imipramine Hydrochloride Tablets (Roxane) p 1788
Imipramine HCl Tablets (Schein) p 1828
Imipramine Tablets (Geneva) p 973
Janimine Filmtab Tablets (Abbott) p 403, 533
SK-Pramine Tablets (Smith Kline & French) p 1971
Tofranil Ampuls (Geigy) p 969
Tofranil Tablets (Geigy) p 411, 969

Imipramine Pamoate
Tofranil-PM Capsules (Geigy) p 411, 971

Immune Globulin Intravenous
Immune Globulin Intravenous, 5% (In 10% Maltose) Gamimune (Cutter Biological) p 883
Sandoglobulin (Sandoz Pharmaceutical Div.) p 1813

Immune Serum Globulin (Human)
Immuglobin (Savage) p 1825
Immune Globulin Intravenous, 5% (In 10% Maltose) Gamimune (Cutter Biological) p 883
Immune Serum Globulin (Human) (Wyeth) p 2245
Immune Serum Globulin (Human) in Tubex (Wyeth) p 2288
Immune Serum Globulin (Human), U.S.P. Gamma Globulin (Hyland Therapeutics) p 1024
Immune Serum Globulin (Human) Gamastan (Cutter Biological) p 883
MICRhoGAM (Ortho Diagnostic Systems) p 1452
RhoGAM (Ortho Diagnostic Systems) p 1453

Indapamide
Lozol Tablets (USV Pharmaceutical) p 440, 2081

Indomethacin
Indocin Capsules (Merck Sharp & Dohme) p 420, 1319
Indocin SR Capsules (Merck Sharp & Dohme) p 420, 1319
Indocin Suppositories (Merck Sharp & Dohme) p 420, 1319
Indo-Lemmon Capsules (Lemmon) p 1122
Indomethacin (Geneva) p 973
Indomethacin Capsules (Schein) p 1828

Influenza Virus Vaccine
Fluogen (Parke-Davis) p 1522
Fluzone (Influenza Virus Vaccine), Whole Virion and Subvirion, Zonal Purified (Squibb/Connaught) p 2033
Influenza Virus Vaccine Subvirion Type (Wyeth) p 2246
Influenza Virus Vaccine Subvirion Type in Tubex (Wyeth) p 2288

Inositol
Amino-Cerv (Milex) p 1415
Mega-B (Arco) p 600
Megadose (Arco) p 600

Insulin, Human
Humulin N Vials (Lilly) p 1150
Humulin R Vials (Lilly) p 1152
Novolin N (Squibb-Novo) p 2034
Novolin R (Squibb-Novo) p 2034

Insulin, Human, Zinc Suspension
Novolin L (Squibb-Novo) p 2034

Insulin, NPH
Insulatard NPH (Nordisk-USA) p 1422
Mixtard (Nordisk-USA) p 1423
NPH Iletin I (Lilly) p 1156
NPH Insulin (Isophane Insulin Suspension USP) (Squibb-Novo) p 2034
NPH Purified Pork Isophane Insulin Suspension (Squibb-Novo) p 2034
Novolin N (Squibb-Novo) p 2034

Insulin, Regular
Iletin I, Regular (Lilly) p 1154
Iletin II, Regular (Concentrated), U-500 (Lilly) p 1155
Insulin Injection USP (Regular) (Squibb-Novo) p 2033
Mixtard (Nordisk-USA) p 1423
Regular Purified Pork Insulin (Squibb-Novo) p 2034
Velosulin (Nordisk-USA) p 1423

Insulin, Zinc Crystals
NPH Iletin I (Lilly) p 1156

Insulin, Zinc Suspension
Iletin I, Lente (Lilly) p 1156
Iletin I, Semilente (Lilly) p 1156
Iletin I, Ultralente (Lilly) p 1156
Lente Insulin (Insulin Zinc Suspension USP) (Squibb-Novo) p 2033
Lente Purified Pork Insulin Zinc Suspension (Squibb-Novo) p 2034
Protamine, Zinc & Iletin I (Lilly) p 1156
Semilente Insulin (Prompt Insulin Zinc Suspension USP) (Squibb-Novo) p 2033
Semilente Purified Pork Prompt Insulin Zinc Suspension (Squibb-Novo) p 2034
Ultralente Insulin (Extended Insulin Zinc Suspension USP) (Squibb-Novo) p 2034
Ultralente Purified Beef Extended Insulin Zinc Suspension (Squibb-Novo) p 2034

Intrinsic Factor Concentrate
Al-Vite (Drug Industries) p 914
Fergon Plus (Winthrop-Breon) p 2198
Hemo-Vite (Drug Industries) p 914
Heptuna Plus (Roerig) p 431, 1735
Perihemin (Lederle) p 1112
Pronemia Capsules (Lederle) p 1118

Iodinated Glycerol
Iophen-C Liquid (Schein) p 1828
Organidin (Wallace) p 442, 2163
Theo-Organidin Elixir (Wallace) p 442, 2170
Tussi-Organidin (Wallace) p 442, 2171
Tussi-Organidin DM (Wallace) p 442, 2171

Iodine Preparations
Bronkotuss (Hyrex) p 1024
Calcidrine Syrup (Abbott) p 510
Pima Syrup (Fleming) p 948
Ponaris Nasal Mucosal Emollient (Jamol) p 1033
Prenate 90 Tablets (Bock) p 706
Roma-Nol Antiseptic (Jamol) p 1033

Iodochlorhydroxyquin
Hysone (Mallard) p 1181
Iodochlorhydroxyquin 3% with Hydrocortisone Creams (Fougera) p 953
Iodo-Cortifair (Pharmafair) p 1618
Nystaform Ointment (Miles Pharmaceuticals) p 1411
Pedi-Cort V Creme (Pedinol) p 1581
Vioform (CIBA) p 876
Vioform-Hydrocortisone (CIBA) p 876

Iodoquinol
Vytone Cream (Dermik) p 891
Yodoxin (Glenwood) p 412, 999

Iopanoic Acid
Telepaque (Winthrop-Breon) p 443, 3058

Ipecac Preparation
Ipecac (Lilly) p 1156
Ipecac Syrup (Roxane) p 1788

Iron & Ammonium Citrate
I.L.X. B$_{12}$ Elixir Crystalline (Kenwood) p 1046

Iron Dextran
Dextraron (Legere) p 1120
Imferon (Merrell Dow) p 1367
Proferdex (Fisons) p 943

Iron, Peptonized
Rogenic Injectable (O'Neal, Jones & Feldman) p 1446

Iron Polysaccharide Complex
Hytinic Capsules & Elixir (Hyrex) p 1024

Generic and Chemical Name Index

Niferex Forte Elixir (Central Pharmaceuticals) p 838
Niferex Tablets/Elixir (Central Pharmaceuticals) p 838
Niferex-150 Capsules (Central Pharmaceuticals) p 409, 838
Niferex-150 Forte Capsules (Central Pharmaceuticals) p 409, 838
Niferex-PN (Central Pharmaceuticals) p 409, 838
Nu-Iron Elixir (Mayrand) p 1196
Nu-Iron 150 Caps (Mayrand) p 1196
Nu-Iron-Plus Elixir (Mayrand) p 1196
Nu-Iron-V Tablets (Mayrand) p 1196

Iron Preparations
Added Protection III Multi-Vitamin & Multi-Mineral Supplement (Professional Health) p 1621
Advance (Ross) p 1761
Albafort Injectable (Bart) p 685
Beminal Stress Plus (Ayerst) p 404, 640
Ferancee Chewable Tablets (Stuart) p 439, 2037
Ferancee-HP Tablets (Stuart) p 439, 2037
Fergon Capsules (Winthrop-Breon) p 443, 2198
Fergon Elixir (Winthrop-Breon) p 2198
Fergon Plus (Winthrop-Breon) p 2198
Fergon Tablets (Winthrop-Breon) p 443, 2198
Fero-Folic-500 (Abbott) p 403, 529
Fero-Grad-500 (Abbott) p 403, 530
Fero-Gradumet (Abbott) p 530
Ferro-Sequels (Lederle) p 415, 1093
Florvite + Iron Chewable Tablets 1 mg (Everett) p 941
Florvite + Iron Drops (Everett) p 941
Fosfree (Mission) p 1416
Glytinic Tablets (Boyle) p 726
Hemocyte Plus Tabules (U.S. Pharmaceutical) p 2070
Hemocyte-F Tablets (U.S. Pharmaceutical) p 2070
Hemo-Vite (Drug Industries) p 914
Hemo-Vite Liquid (Drug Industries) p 914
Heptuna Plus (Roerig) p 431, 1735
Hytinic Capsules & Elixir (Hyrex) p 1024
I.L.X. B$_{12}$ Elixir Crystalline (Kenwood) p 1046
I.L.X. B$_{12}$ Tablets (Kenwood) p 1046
Iberet (Abbott) p 532
Iberet-500 (Abbott) p 403, 532
Iberet-500 Liquid (Abbott) p 533
Iberet-Folic-500 (Abbott) p 403, 529
Iberet Liquid (Abbott) p 533
Imferon (Merrell Dow) p 1367
Iromin-G (Mission) p 1416
Irospan Capsules (Fielding) p 942
Irospan Tablets (Fielding) p 942
Isomil (Ross) p 1767
Isomil SF (Ross) p 1768
Isomil SF 20 (Ross) p 1777
Megaton Elixir (Hyrex) p 1025
Mevanin-C Capsules (Beutlich) p 705
Niferex Forte Elixir (Central Pharmaceuticals) p 838
Niferex Tablets/Elixir (Central Pharmaceuticals) p 838
Niferex w/Vitamin C (Central Pharmaceuticals) p 838
Niferex-150 Capsules (Central Pharmaceuticals) p 409, 838
Niferex-150 Forte Capsules (Central Pharmaceuticals) p 409, 838
Niferex-PN (Central Pharmaceuticals) p 409, 838
Nu-Iron Elixir (Mayrand) p 1196
Nu-Iron 150 Caps (Mayrand) p 1196
Nu-Iron-Plus Elixir (Mayrand) p 1196
Nu-Iron-V Tablets (Mayrand) p 1196
Perihemin (Lederle) p 1112
Peritinic Tablets (Lederle) p 1112
Poly-Vi-Flor 1.0 mg Vitamins w/Iron & Fluoride Chewable Tablets (Mead Johnson Nutritional) p 1245
Poly-Vi-Flor 0.5 mg Vitamins w/Iron & Fluoride Drops (Mead Johnson Nutritional) p 1245
Prenate 90 Tablets (Bock) p 706
Pronemia Capsules (Lederle) p 1118
Similac With Iron (Ross) p 1779
Similac With Iron 13 (Ross) p 1777
Similac With Iron 20 (Ross) p 1777
Similac With Iron 24 (Ross) p 1777
Stuartinic Tablets (Stuart) p 439, 2034
Tabron Filmseal (Parke-Davis) p 425, 1572
TriHemic 600 (Lederle) p 416, 1119
Tri-Vi-Flor 0.25 mg Vitamins w/Iron & Fluoride Drops (Mead Johnson Nutritional) p 1248
Vi-Daylin Plus Iron ADC Drops (Ross) p 1784
Vi-Daylin + Iron Chewable (Ross) p 432, 1784
Vi-Daylin Plus Iron Drops (Ross) p 1783
Vi-Daylin Plus Iron Liquid (Ross) p 1784
Vi-Daylin/F ADC + Iron Drops (Ross) p 1782

Vi-Daylin/F + Iron Chewable (Ross) p 432, 1783
Vi-Daylin/F + Iron Drops (Ross) p 1783

Isocarboxazid
Marplan Tablets (Roche) p 430, 1689

d-Isoephedrine Hydrochloride
Isoetharine Hydrochloride Inhalation (Roxane) p 1788

Isoetharine
Bronkometer (Winthrop-Breon) p 2193
Bronkosol (Winthrop-Breon) p 2193
Isoetharine Hydrochloride 1.0% (Schein) p 1828

Isometheptene Mucate
Midrin Capsules (Carnrick) p 408, 832
Migralam Capsules (Lambda) p 1071

Isoniazid
INH Tablets (CIBA) p 850
Isoniazid Tablets (Danbury) p 887
Rifamate (Merrell Dow) p 421, 1383

Isopropamide Iodide
Combid Spansule Capsules (Smith Kline & French) p 436, 1952
Darbid (Smith Kline & French) p 436, 1958
Ornade Spansule Capsules (Smith Kline & French) p 437, 1968
Prochlor-Iso Timed Release Capsules (Schein) p 1828
Pro-Iso Capsules (Geneva) p 973

Isopropyl Alcohol
Cetylcide Solution (Cetylite) p 839
Komed Acne Lotion (Barnes-Hind) p 684
Komed HC Lotion (Barnes-Hind) p 684
Tinver Lotion (Barnes-Hind) p 685

Isopropyl Myristate
Domol Bath & Shower Oil (Miles Pharmaceuticals) p 1402

Isoproterenol Hydrochloride
Isoproterenol HCl Injection (Elkins-Sinn) p 938
Vapo-Iso Solution (Fisons) p 943

Isoproterenol Preparations
Aerolone Solution (Lilly) p 1126
Duo-Medihaler (Riker) p 1643
Isuprel Hydrochloride Compound Elixir (Winthrop-Breon) p 2204
Isuprel Hydrochloride Glossets (Winthrop-Breon) p 443, 2204
Isuprel Hydrochloride Injection 1:5000 (Winthrop-Breon) p 2201
Isuprel Hydrochloride Mistometer (Winthrop-Breon) p 2203
Isuprel Hydrochloride Solution 1:200 & 1:100 (Winthrop-Breon) p 2203
Medihaler-Iso (Riker) p 1644
Norisodrine Aerotrol (Abbott) p 547
Norisodrine w/Calcium Iodide Syrup (Abbott) p 548

Isosorbide Dinitrate
Dilatrate-SR (Reed & Carnrick) p 427, 1632
Iso-Bid Capsules (Geriatric) p 975
Isochron Tablets (Forest) p 953
Isordil Chewable (10 mg.) (Ives) p 413, 1028
Isordil Oral Titradose (5 mg.) (Ives) p 413, 1028
Isordil Oral Titradose (10 mg.) (Ives) p 413, 1028
Isordil Oral Titradose (20 mg.) (Ives) p 413, 1028
Isordil Oral Titradose (30 mg.) (Ives) p 413, 1028
Isordil Oral Titradose (40 mg.) (Ives) p 413, 1028
Isordil Sublingual 2.5 mg., 5 mg & 10 mg. (Ives) p 413, 1028
Isordil Tembids Capsules & Tablets (40 mg.) (Ives) p 413, 1028
Isosorbide Dinitrate Oral Tablets (Danbury) p 887
Isosorbide Dinitrate Sublingual Tablets (Danbury) p 887
Isosorbide Dinitrate Tablets (Geneva) p 973
Isosorbide Dinitrate Tablets - Oral & Sublingual (Schein) p 1828
Isosorbide Dinitrate T.D. Capsules & Tablets (Geneva) p 973
Isosorbide Dinitrate Timed Capsules & Tablets (Schein) p 1828
Isotrate Timecelles (Hauck) p 1001
Sorate-5 Chewable Tablets (Trimen) p 2067
Sorate-10 Chewable Tablets (Trimen) p 2067
Sorbide (Mayrand) p 1196
Sorbitrate Tablets (Stuart) p 439, 2041

Isotretinoin
Accutane Capsules (Roche) p 429, 1665

Isoxsuprine Hydrochloride
Isoxsuprine Hydrochloride Tablets (Roxane) p 1788
Isoxsuprine HCl Tablets (Danbury) p 887
Isoxsuprine HCl Tablets (Schein) p 1828
Isoxsuprine Tablets (Geneva) p 973
Vasodilan (Mead Johnson Pharmaceutical) p 419, 1255

K

Kanamycin Sulfate
Kantrex Capsules (Bristol) p 407, 734
Kantrex Injection (Bristol) p 735
Kantrex Pediatric Injection (Bristol) p 735

Kaolin
Kaolin, Pectin, Belladonna Mixture (Schein) p 1828
Kaolin-Pectin-Concentrated (Roxane) p 1788
Kaolin-Pectin Mixture (Schein) p 1828
Kaolin-Pectin PG Mixture (Schein) p 1828
Kaolin-Pectin Suspension (Roxane) p 1788
Parepectolin (Rorer) p 1752

Ketamine Hydrochloride
Ketalar (Parke-Davis) p 1528

Ketoconazole
Nizoral Tablets (Janssen) p 413, 1038

L

Labetalol Hydrochloride
Normodyne Injection (Schering) p 1867
Normodyne Tablets (Schering) p 434, 1870
Trandate Tablets (Glaxo) p 412, 983

Lactase (Beta-D-galactosidase)
LactAid (LactAid) p 414, 1070

Lactic Acid
Duofilm (Stiefel) p 2035
Salactic Film (Pedinol) p 1581
Viranol (American Dermal) p 600

Lactulose
Cephulac Syrup (Merrell Dow) p 421, 1362
Chronulac Syrup (Merrell Dow) p 421, 1363

Lanolin
Derma Medicone-HC Ointment (Medicone) p 1256
Lanolin & Lanolin Anhydrous (Fougera) p 953
pHisoHex (Winthrop-Breon) p 2222

Lecithin
Cardioguard Natural Lipotropic Dietary Supplement-Powder (Professional Health) p 1621

Leucovorin, Calcium
Leucovorin Calcium Injection (Lederle) p 415, 1096
Wellcovorin Injection (Burroughs Wellcome) p 821
Wellcovorin Tablets (Burroughs Wellcome) p 408, 821

Levallorphan Tartrate
Lorfan Injectable (Roche) p 1689

Levodopa
Larodopa Capsules (Roche) p 429, 1688
Larodopa Tablets (Roche) p 429, 1688
Sinemet Tablets (Merck Sharp & Dohme) p 420, 1345

Levonordefrin Injection
Carbocaine Hydrochloride 2% with Neo-Cobefrin 1:20,000 Injection (Cook-Waite) p 881

Levonorgestrel
Nordette-21 Tablets (Wyeth) p 444, 2266
Nordette-28 Tablets (Wyeth) p 444, 2270

Levorphanol Tartrate
Levo-Dromoran Injectable (Roche) p 1689
Levo-Dromoran Tablets (Roche) p 429, 1689

Lidocaine
Lidocaine Ointment 5% (Fougera) p 953
Xylocaine 10% Oral Spray (Astra) p 630

Lidocaine Base
Xylocaine 5% Ointment (Astra) p 629

Generic and Chemical Name Index

Lidocaine Hydrochloride
  Anestacon (Webcon) p 2171
  Dalcaine Injection (O'Neal, Jones & Feldman) p 1445
  Lidocaine HCl Injection (Bristol) p 730
  Lidocaine HCl Injection (Elkins-Sinn) p 938
  Lidocaine HCl Injection (Preservative-free) (Elkins-Sinn) p 938
  Lidocaine Hydrochloride Injection for Cardiac Arrhythmias (Elkins-Sinn) p 938
  Lidocaine Hydrochloride Injection, U.S.P. (Abbott) p 535
  Lidocaine HCl in Tubex (Wyeth) p 2288
  Lidocaine HCl 2% Viscous Solution (Schein) p 1828
  Lidocaine 1% and 2% (Legere) p 1120
  Xylocaine 2% Jelly (Astra) p 629
  Xylocaine Hydrochloride, Xylocaine Hydrochloride with Epinephrine 1:100,000, & Xylocaine Hydrochloride with Epinephrine 1:200,000 (Astra) p 623
  Xylocaine Solution for Ventricular Arrhythmias-Intravenous Injection or Continuous Infusion; or Intramuscular Injection (Astra) p 625
  Xylocaine 1.5% Solution with Dextrose 7.5% (Astra) p 629
  Xylocaine 4% Sterile Solution (Astra) p 627
  Xylocaine 5% Solution with Glucose 7.5% (Astra) p 629
  Xylocaine 4% Topical Solution (Astra) p 628
  Xylocaine 2% Viscous Solution (Astra) p 630

Lincomycin Hydrochloride Monohydrate
  Lincocin (Upjohn) p 2119

Lindane
  Kwell Cream (Reed & Carnrick) p 1635
  Kwell Lotion (Reed & Carnrick) p 1635
  Kwell Shampoo (Reed & Carnrick) p 1635
  Lindane Lotion & Shampoo (Schein) p 1828
  Scabene Lotion (Stiefel) p 2035
  Scabene Shampoo (Stiefel) p 2036

Liothyronine Sodium
  Cytomel Tablets (Smith Kline & French) p 436, 1956
  Liothyronine Sodium Tablets (Schein) p 1828

Liotrix
  Euthroid (Parke-Davis) p 424, 1520
  Thyrolar Tablets (USV Pharmaceutical) p 440, 2091

Lipolytic Enzyme
  Arco-Lase (Arco) p 600
  Arco-Lase Plus (Arco) p 600
  Celluzyme Chewable Tablets (Dalin) p 886
  Cotazym (Organon) p 422, 1446
  Cotazym-S (Organon) p 422, 1446
  Festal II (Hoechst-Roussel) p 412, 1014
  Festalan (Hoechst-Roussel) p 413, 1014
  Kutrase Capsules (Rorer) p 431, 1750
  Ku-Zyme Capsules (Rorer) p 431, 1750
  Ku-Zyme HP Capsules (Rorer) p 431, 1751
  Tri-Cone Capsules (Glaxo) p 986

Lipolytic Preparations
  Arco-Lase (Arco) p 600
  Arco-Lase Plus (Arco) p 600
  Cardioguard Natural Lipotropic Dietary Supplement-Tablets (Professional Health) p 1621
  Pancreatin Tablets 2400 mg. N.F. (High Lipase) (Vitaline) p 2148
  Tri-Cone Capsules (Glaxo) p 986

Lithium Carbonate
  Eskalith Capsules & Tablets (Smith Kline & French) p 437, 1964
  Eskalith CR Controlled Release Tablets (Smith Kline & French) p 437, 1964
  Lithane (Miles Pharmaceuticals) p 422, 1403
  Lithium Carbonate Capsules & Tablets (Roxane) p 1789
  Lithobid Tablets (CIBA) p 409, 852

Lithium Citrate
  Cibalith-S Syrup (CIBA) p 852
  Lithium Citrate Syrup (Roxane) p 1790

Liver, Desiccated
  Hep-Forte Capsules (Marlyn) p 1193
  Heptuna Plus (Roerig) p 431, 1735

Liver Preparations
  Albafort Injectable (Bart) p 685
  Hep-Forte Capsules (Marlyn) p 1193
  I.L.X. B$_{12}$ Elixir Crystalline (Kenwood) p 1046
  I.L.X. B$_{12}$ Tablets (Kenwood) p 1046
  Livolex (Legere) p 1120
  Trinsicon/Trinsicon M Capsules (Glaxo) p 412, 986

Lomustine (CCNU)
  CeeNU (Bristol-Myers Oncology) p 407, 758

Loperamide Hydrochloride
  Imodium Capsules/Liquid (Janssen) p 413, 1033

Lorazepam
  Ativan in Tubex (Wyeth) p 2288
  Ativan Injection (Wyeth) p 2237
  Ativan Tablets (Wyeth) p 444, 2236

Loxapine Hydrochloride
  Loxitane C Oral Concentrate (Lederle) p 415, 1096
  Loxitane IM (Lederle) p 415, 1096

Loxapine Succinate
  Loxitane Capsules (Lederle) p 415, 1096

Lypressin
  Diapid Nasal Spray (Sandoz Pharmaceutical Div.) p 1801

Lysine
  Alba-Lybe (Bart) p 685
  Geravite Elixir (Hauck) p 1001

l-Lysine
  Aminoplex Capsules & Powder (Tyson) p 2068

Lysine Monohydrochloride
  Enisyl Tablets (Persŏn & Covey) p 1588

M

Mafenide Acetate
  Sulfamylon Acetate Cream (Winthrop-Breon) p 2226

Magaldrate
  Riopan (Ayerst) p 405, 680
  Riopan Plus (Ayerst) p 405, 680

Magnesium
  Enviro-Stress with Zinc & Selenium (Vitaline) p 2148

Magnesium Carbonate
  Gaviscon Liquid Antacid (Marion) p 1186
  Osti-Derm Lotion (Pedinol) p 1580

Magnesium Citrate
  Evac-Q-Kit (Adria) p 575
  Evac-Q-Kwik (Adria) p 575

Magnesium Hydroxide
  Aludrox Oral Suspension (Wyeth) p 2235
  Aludrox Tablets (Wyeth) p 2235
  Aluminum & Magnesium Hydroxides with Simethicone I (Roxane) p 1788
  Aluminum & Magnesium Hydroxides with Simethicone II (Roxane) p 1788
  Arthritis Pain Formula By the Makers of Anacin Analgesic Tablets (Whitehall) p 443, 2185
  Dolprn #3 Tablets (Bock) p 705
  Gelusil (Parke-Davis) p 424, 1525
  Gelusil-M (Parke-Davis) p 1525
  Gelusil-II (Parke-Davis) p 424, 1526
  Magnesia & Alumina Oral Suspension (Roxane) p 1788
  Milk of Magnesia, Milk of Magnesia-Concentrated (Roxane) p 1788
  Milk of Magnesia-Cascara Suspension Concentrated (Roxane) p 1788
  Milk of Magnesia-Mineral Oil Emulsion & Emulsion (Flavored) (Roxane) p 1788
  Mygel Suspension (Geneva) p 973
  Mylanta Liquid (Stuart) p 439, 2039
  Mylanta Tablets (Stuart) p 439, 2039
  Mylanta-II Liquid (Stuart) p 439, 2039
  Mylanta-II Tablets (Stuart) p 439, 2039
  Phillips' Milk of Magnesia (Glenbrook) p 997
  Simeco (Wyeth) p 2288

Magnesium Oxide
  ACE + Z Tablets (Legere) p 1120
  Beelith Tablets (Beach) p 405, 685
  Cama Arthritis Pain Reliever (Dorsey Laboratories) p 908
  Prenate 90 Tablets (Bock) p 706

Magnesium Salicylate
  Magan (Adria) p 583
  Magsal Tablets (U.S. Pharmaceutical) p 2070
  Trilisate Tablets/Liquid (Purdue Frederick) p 427, 1627

Magnesium Sulfate
  Eldercaps (Mayrand) p 1196
  Eldertonic (Mayrand) p 1196
  Glutofac Tablets (Kenwood) p 1046

Magnesium Sulfate 50% Injection (Bristol) p 730
  Magnesium Sulfate Injectable (O'Neal, Jones & Feldman) p 1445
  Magnesium Sulfate Injection (Elkins-Sinn) p 938
  Pedi-Bath Salts (Pedinol) p 1581
  Vicon Forte Capsules (Glaxo) p 412, 989
  Vicon-C Capsules (Glaxo) p 412, 989
  Vicon-Plus Capsules (Glaxo) p 412, 989

Magnesium Trisilicate
  Gaviscon Antacid Tablets (Marion) p 418, 1185
  Gaviscon-2 Antacid Tablets (Marion) p 418, 1186

Malathion
  Prioderm Lotion (Purdue Frederick) p 1626

Manganese Chloride
  Mangatrace (Armour) p 607
  Multitrace 5 (Armour) p 608
  Multitrace Pediatric (Armour) p 609
  Multitrace Solution & Concentrate (Armour) p 609
  Vicon-Plus Capsules (Glaxo) p 412, 989

Manganese Sulfate
  Eldercaps (Mayrand) p 1196
  Eldertonic (Mayrand) p 1196
  Vicon Forte Capsules (Glaxo) p 412, 989

Maprotiline Hydrochloride
  Ludiomil (CIBA) p 409, 854

Mazindol
  Mazanor (Wyeth) p 444, 2263
  Sanorex (Sandoz Pharmaceutical Div.) p 433, 1815

Measles & Rubella Virus Vaccine, Live
  M-R-VAX II (Merck Sharp & Dohme) p 1325

Measles, Mumps & Rubella Virus Vaccine, Live
  M-M-R II (Merck Sharp & Dohme) p 1323

Measles Virus Vaccine, Live, Attenuated
  Attenuvax (Merck Sharp & Dohme) p 1267

Mebendazole
  Vermox Chewable Tablets (Janssen) p 413, 1043

Mechlorethamine Hydrochloride
  Mustargen (Merck Sharp & Dohme) p 1337

Meclizine Hydrochloride
  Antivert, Antivert/25 Tablets, Antivert/25 Chewable Tablets & Antivert/50 Tablets (Roerig) p 431, 1725
  Bonine Tablets (Pfipharmecs) p 426, 1589
  Meclizine HCl MLT Tablets (Schein) p 1828
  Meclizine HCl Tablets (Geneva) p 973
  Ru-Vert-M (Reid-Provident Labs.) p 428, 1640

Meclocycline Sulfosalicylate
  Meclan (Ortho Pharmaceutical (Dermatological Div.)) p 1474

Meclofenamate Sodium
  Meclomen (Parke-Davis) p 424, 1541

Medroxyprogesterone Acetate
  Amen (Carnrick) p 408, 829
  Curretab Tablets (Reid-Provident Labs.) p 427, 1638
  Depo-Provera (Upjohn) p 2109
  Provera Tablets (Upjohn) p 441, 2133

Mefenamic Acid
  Ponstel (Parke-Davis) p 425, 1562

Megestrol Acetate
  Megace Tablets (Bristol-Myers Oncology) p 407, 761

Melphalan
  Alkeran (Burroughs Wellcome) p 407, 776

Menadiol Diphosphate
  Synkayvite Injectable (Roche) p 1701
  Synkayvite Tablets (Roche) p 430, 1702

Meningococcal Polysaccharide Vaccine
  Menomune (Meningococcal Polysaccharide Vaccine, Groups A,C,Y,W-135, Combined, and Groups A & C, Combined) (Squibb/Connaught) p 2033

Menotropins
  Pergonal (menotropins USP) (Serono) p 1941

Generic and Chemical Name Index

Menthol
- Decongestant Elixir (Schein) p 1828
- Denorex Medicated Shampoo and Conditioner (Whitehall) p 443, 2185
- Denorex Medicated Shampoo, Regular & Mountain Fresh Herbal Scent (Whitehall) p 443, 2185
- Derma Medicone-HC Ointment (Medicone) p 1256
- Panalgesic (Poythress) p 1619
- Rectal Medicone-HC Suppositories (Medicone) p 419, 1256

Mepenzolate Bromide
- Cantil (Merrell Dow) p 421, 1362

Meperidine Hydrochloride
- Demerol Hydrochloride (Winthrop-Breon) p 443, 2197
- Mepergan Injection (Wyeth) p 2264
- Mepergan in Tubex (Wyeth) p 2288
- Meperidine HCl in Tubex (Wyeth) p 2288
- Meperidine HCl Injection (Elkins-Sinn) p 938

Mephentermine Sulfate
- Wyamine Sulfate in Tubex (Wyeth) p 2288

Mephenytoin
- Mesantoin (Sandoz Pharmaceutical Div.) p 433, 1805

Mephobarbital
- Mebaral (Winthrop-Breon) p 444, 2213

Mepivacaine Hydrochloride Injection
- Carbocaine Hydrochloride (Winthrop-Breon) p 2194
- Carbocaine Hydrochloride 3% Injection (Cook-Waite) p 881
- Carbocaine Hydrochloride 2% with Neo-Cobefrin 1:20,000 Injection (Cook-Waite) p 881

Meprobamate
- Deprol (Wallace) p 2155
- Equagesic (Wyeth) p 444, 2250
- Equanil Tablets and Wyseals (Wyeth) p 444, 2252
- Mepro Compound Tablets (Schein) p 1828
- Meprobamate Tablets (Danbury) p 887
- Meprobamate Tablets (Geneva) p 973
- Meprobamate Tablets (Schein) p 1828
- Meprospan (Wallace) p 2161
- Miltown (Wallace) p 442, 2162
- Miltown 600 (Wallace) p 442, 2162
- PMB 200 & PMB 400 (Ayerst) p 405, 660
- Pathibamate (Lederle) p 415, 1110
- SK-Bamate Tablets (Smith Kline & French) p 1971

Mercaptopurine
- Purinethol (Burroughs Wellcome) p 408, 811

Mesoridazine
- Serentil Ampuls (Boehringer Ingelheim) p 714
- Serentil Concentrate (Boehringer Ingelheim) p 714
- Serentil Tablets (Boehringer Ingelheim) p 406, 714

Mestranol Preparations
- Enovid 5 mg (Searle & Co.) p 435, 1919
- Enovid 10 mg (Searle & Co.) p 435, 1919
- Enovid-E 21 (Searle & Co.) p 436, 1919
- Norinyl 1+50 21-Day (Syntex) p 440, 2052
- Norinyl 1+50 28-Day (Syntex) p 440, 2052
- Norinyl 1+80 21-Day (Syntex) p 440, 2052
- Norinyl 1+80 28-Day (Syntex) p 440, 2052
- Norinyl 2 mg. (Syntex) p 440, 2052
- Ortho-Novum 1/50☐21 (Ortho Pharmaceutical) p 422, 1461
- Ortho-Novum 1/50☐28 (Ortho Pharmaceutical) p 1461
- Ortho-Novum 1/80☐21 (Ortho Pharmaceutical) p 423, 1461
- Ortho-Novum 1/80☐28 (Ortho Pharmaceutical) p 1461
- Ortho-Novum Tablets 2 mg☐21 (Ortho Pharmaceutical) p 423, 1461
- Ovulen-21 (Searle & Co.) p 436, 1919
- Ovulen-28 (Searle & Co.) p 436, 1919

Metaproterenol Sulfate
- Alupent Inhalent Solution 5% & Solution Unit Dose 0.6% (Boehringer Ingelheim) p 706
- Alupent Metered Dose Inhaler (Boehringer Ingelheim) p 706
- Alupent Syrup (Boehringer Ingelheim) p 706
- Alupent Tablets (Boehringer Ingelheim) p 406, 706
- Metaprel Inhalent Solution, Metered Dose Inhaler, Syrup & Tablets (Dorsey Laboratories) p 910

Metaraminol Bitartrate
- Aramine Injection (Merck Sharp & Dohme) p 1266
- Metaraminol Bitartrate Injection (Bristol) p 730

Metaxalone
- Skelaxin (Carnrick) p 409, 835

Methacycline Hydrochloride
- Rondomycin (Wallace) p 442, 2164

Methadone Hydrochloride
- Dolophine Hydrochloride Ampoules and Vials (Lilly) p 1144
- Dolophine Hydrochloride Tablets (Lilly) p 1145
- Methadone Hydrochloride Diskets (Lilly) p 417, 1164
- Methadone Hydrochloride Oral Solution & Tablets (Roxane) p 1791

Methamphetamine Hydrochloride
- Desoxyn (Abbott) p 515
- Desoxyn Gradumet Tablets (Abbott) p 403, 515
- Methamphetamine Hydrochloride, 5mg. & 10mg. (Rexar) p 1641

Metharbital
- Gemonil (Abbott) p 531

Methazolamide
- Neptazane Tablets (Lederle) p 415, 1107

Methdilazine
- Tacaryl Chewable Tablets (Westwood) p 442, 2182

Methdilazine Hydrochloride
- Tacaryl Syrup & Tablets (Westwood) p 442, 2182

Methenamine
- Trac Tabs 2X (Hyrex) p 413, 1025
- Urised Tablets (Webcon) p 2173
- Uroblue Tablets (Geneva) p 973
- Uro-Phosphate Tablets (Poythress) p 1619

Methenamine Hippurate
- Hiprex (Merrell Dow) p 421, 1366
- Urex (Riker) p 428, 1645

Methenamine Mandelate
- Mandelamine (Parke-Davis) p 424, 1540
- Methenamine Mandelate Forte Suspension & Tablets (Schein) p 1828
- Thiacide Tablets (Beach) p 405, 687
- Uroqid-Acid Tablets (Beach) p 405, 687
- Uroqid-Acid No. 2 Tablets (Beach) p 405, 687

Methicillin Sodium
- Staphcillin (Bristol) p 751

Methimazole
- Tapazole (Lilly) p 1175

Methionine
- Amino-Cerv (Milex) p 1415
- Aminoplex Capsules & Powder (Tyson) p 2068

Methocarbamol
- Methocarbamol Tablets (Danbury) p 887
- Methocarbamol Tablets (Geneva) p 973
- Methocarbamol Tablets (Roxane) p 1788
- Methocarbamol Tablets (Schein) p 1828
- Methocarbamol with Aspirin Tablets (Schein) p 1828
- Robaxin Injectable (Robins) p 429, 1661
- Robaxin Tablets (Robins) p 428, 1662
- Robaxin-750 Tablets (Robins) p 428, 1662
- Robaxisal Tablets (Robins) p 429, 1662

Methohexital Sodium
- Brevital Sodium (Lilly) p 1131

Methotrexate
- Methotrexate Tablets & Parenteral (Lederle) p 415, 1100

Methotrexate Sodium
- Folex for Injection (Adria) p 576
- Mexate (Bristol-Myers Oncology) p 762

Methoxamine Hydrochloride
- Vasoxyl Injection (Burroughs Wellcome) p 819

Methoxsalen
- Oxsoralen Capsule (Elder) p 411, 932
- Oxsoralen Lotion 1% (Elder) p 935

Methoxyflurane
- Penthrane (Abbott) p 560

Methscopolamine Bromide
- Pamine Tablets (Upjohn) p 2132

Methscopolamine Nitrate
- Dura-Vent/DA (Dura) p 929
- Extendryl Chewable Tablets (Fleming) p 948
- Extendryl Sr. & Jr. T.D. Capsules (Fleming) p 948
- Extendryl Syrup (Fleming) p 948
- Histaspan-D Capsules (USV Pharmaceutical) p 2077
- Histor-D Timecelles (Hauck) p 1001
- Rhinolar Capsules (McGregor) p 1197
- Sinovan Timed (Drug Industries) p 915

Methsuximide
- Celontin (Half Strength) Kapseals (Parke-Davis) p 423, 1486
- Celontin Kapseals (Parke-Davis) p 423, 1486

Methyclothiazide
- Aquatensen (Wallace) p 442, 2149
- Diutensen Tablets (Wallace) p 2156
- Diutensen-R Tablets (Wallace) p 442, 2157
- Enduron Tablets (Abbott) p 403, 517
- Enduronyl Forte Tablets (Abbott) p 403, 518
- Enduronyl Tablets (Abbott) p 403, 518
- Methyclothiazide Tablets (Schein) p 1828

Methyl Cellulose
- Anorex-CCK (Robertson/Taylor) p 1645

Methyl Salicylate
- Ger-O-Foam (Geriatric) p 975
- Panalgesic (Poythress) p 1619
- Thera-Gesic (Mission) p 1420

Methylbenzethonium Chloride
- Fordustin' (Sween) p 2047
- Methylbenzethonium Chloride (Sween) p 2047
- Peri-Care (Sween) p 2048
- Peri-Wash (Sween) p 2048
- Puri-Clens (Sween) p 2048
- Surgi-Kleen (Sween) p 2048
- Sween Cream (Sween) p 2049
- Xtracare II (Sween) p 2049

Methyldopa
- Aldoclor Tablets (Merck Sharp & Dohme) p 420, 1258
- Aldomet Oral Suspension (Merck Sharp & Dohme) p 1259
- Aldomet Tablets (Merck Sharp & Dohme) p 420, 1259
- Aldoril Tablets (Merck Sharp & Dohme) p 420, 1262
- Methyldopa Tablets (Geneva) p 973

Methyldopate Hydrochloride
- Aldomet Ester HCl Injection (Merck Sharp & Dohme) p 1261

Methylene Blue
- Methylene Blue Injection (Elkins-Sinn) p 938
- Trac Tabs 2X (Hyrex) p 413, 1025
- Urised Tablets (Webcon) p 2173
- Uroblue Tablets (Geneva) p 973
- Urolene Blue (Star) p 2035

Methylergonovine Maleate
- Methergine (Sandoz Pharmaceutical Div.) p 433, 1806

Methylphenidate Hydrochloride
- Ritalin Hydrochloride Tablets (CIBA) p 409, 864
- Ritalin-SR Tablets (CIBA) p 409, 864

Methylphenylsuccinimide
(see under Phensuximide)

Methylprednisolone
- Medrol Tablets (Upjohn) p 441, 2124
- Methylprednisolone Tablets (Schein) p 1828
- Methylprednisolone Sodium Succinate (Organon) p 1447

Methylprednisolone Acetate
- depMedalone "40" Injectable (O'Neal, Jones & Feldman) p 1445
- depMedalone "80" Injectable (O'Neal, Jones & Feldman) p 1445
- Depo-Medrol (Upjohn) p 441, 2107
- Depo-Predate 40 (Legere) p 1120
- Depo-Predate 80 (Legere) p 1120
- Medrol Acetate Topical (Upjohn) p 2124

Methylprednisolone Sodium Succinate
- A-methaPred (Abbott) p 508
- Methylprednisolone Sodium Succinate for Injection (Elkins-Sinn) p 938

Generic and Chemical Name Index

Solu-Medrol Sterile Powder (Upjohn) p 441, 2137

Methyltestosterone
Android-5 Buccal (Brown) p 407, 771
Android-10 (Brown) p 407, 771
Android-25 (Brown) p 407, 771
Estratest H.S. Tablets (Reid-Provident Labs.) p 427, 1638
Estratest Tablets (Reid-Provident Labs.) p 427, 1638
Metandren Linguets & Tablets (CIBA) p 409, 855
Oreton Methyl Tablets & Buccal Tablets (Schering) p 434, 1873
Premarin w/Methyltestosterone (Ayerst) p 405, 674
Testred (ICN Pharmaceuticals) p 1025
Virilon (Star) p 2035

Methyprylon
Noludar & Noludar 300 (Roche) p 430, 1696

Methysergide Maleate
Sansert (Sandoz Pharmaceutical Div.) p 433, 1816

Metoclopramide Hydrochloride
Reglan Injectable (Robins) p 1659
Reglan Syrup (Robins) p 1659
Reglan Tablets (Robins) p 428, 1659

Metocurine Iodide
Metubine Iodide (Lilly) p 1165

Metolazone
Diulo (Searle Pharmaceuticals) p 435, 1904
Zaroxolyn (Pennwalt) p 426, 1586

Metoprolol Tartrate
Lopressor Ampuls (Geigy) p 960
Lopressor Tablets (Geigy) p 411, 960

Metrizamide
Amipaque (Winthrop-Breon) p 3018

Metronidazole
Flagyl I.V. RTU (Searle Pharmaceuticals) p 436, 1907
Flagyl Tablets (Searle & Co.) p 436, 1929
Metric 21 Tablets (Fielding) p 942
Metronidazole Oral Tablets (Schein) p 1828
Metronidazole Redi-Infusion (Elkins-Sinn) p 938
Metronidazole Tablets (Danbury) p 887
Metronidazole Tablets (Geneva) p 973
Metryl and Metryl 500 Tablets (Lemmon) p 1122
Protostat Tablets (Ortho Pharmaceutical) p 423, 1470
SK-Metronidazole Tablets (Smith Kline & French) p 1971
Satric (Savage) p 433, 1825

Metronidazole Hydrochloride
Flagyl I.V. (Searle Pharmaceuticals) p 436, 1907

Metyrapone
Metopirone (CIBA) p 409, 856

Metyrosine
Demser Capsules (Merck Sharp & Dohme) p 420, 1297

Mezlocillin Sodium
Mezlin (Miles Pharmaceuticals) p 1404

Miconazole
Monistat I.V. (Janssen) p 1037

Miconazole Nitrate
Monistat-Derm (miconazole nitrate) Cream & Lotion (Ortho Pharmaceutical (Dermatological Div.)) p 1474
Monistat 3 Vaginal Suppositories (Ortho Pharmaceutical) p 1456
Monistat 7 Vaginal Cream (Ortho Pharmaceutical) p 423, 1455
Monistat 7 Vaginal Suppositories (Ortho Pharmaceutical) p 423, 1456

Microfibrillar Collagen
Avitene (Alcon P.R.) p 588

Mineral Oil
Agoral, Plain (Parke-Davis) p 1480
Agoral, Raspberry & Marshmallow Flavors (Parke-Davis) p 1480
Fleet Mineral Oil Enema (Fleet) p 947
Liqui-Doss (Ferndale) p 942
Milk of Magnesia-Mineral Oil Emulsion & Emulsion (Flavored) (Roxane) p 1788
Mineral Oil-Light Sterile, Mineral Oil (Roxane) p 1788

Whirl-Sol (Sween) p 2049

Minocycline Hydrochloride
Minocin (Lederle) p 415, 1103
Minocin Oral Suspension (Lederle) p 1104

Minoxidil
Loniten Tablets (Upjohn) p 441, 2120

Mitomycin (mitomycin-C)
Mutamycin (Bristol-Myers Oncology) p 764

Mitotane
Lysodren (Bristol-Myers Oncology) p 407, 760

Molindone Hydrochloride
Moban Tablets & Concentrate (Du Pont) p 410, 921

Molybdenum
Total Formula (Vitaline) p 2148

Monoamine-Oxidase Inhibitors
Eutonyl Filmtab Tablets (Abbott) p 403, 528
Nardil (Parke-Davis) p 424, 1543
Parnate (Smith Kline & French) p 437, 1969

Monobenzone
Benoquin Cream 20% (Elder) p 929

Morphine Sulfate
Duramorph PF (Preservative-free morphine sulfate injection) (Elkins-Sinn) p 939
MS Contin (Purdue Frederick) p 1625
Morphine Sulfate Injection (Elkins-Sinn) p 938
Morphine Sulfate Oral Solution (Roxane) p 1792
Morphine Sulfate Tablets (Roxane) p 1792
Morphine Sulfate in Tubex (Wyeth) p 2288
RMS Suppositories (Upsher-Smith) p 2144
Roxanol (Morphine Sulfate Concentrated Oral Solution) (Roxane) p 1793

Moxalactam Disodium
Moxam Vials (Lilly) p 1166

Mumps Virus Vaccine, Live
Mumpsvax (Merck Sharp & Dohme) p 1336

N

Nadolol
Corgard (Squibb) p 437, 1989
Corzide (Squibb) p 437, 1990

Nafcillin Sodium
Nafcil (Bristol) p 736
Unipen Injection, Capsules, Powder for Oral Solution, & Tablets (Wyeth) p 445, 2290

Nalbuphine Hydrochloride
Nubain (Du Pont) p 410, 923

Nalidixic Acid
NegGram Caplets (Winthrop-Breon) p 444, 2215
NegGram Suspension (Winthrop-Breon) p 2215

Naloxone Hydrochloride
Narcan and Narcan Neonatal (Du Pont) p 410, 922
Talwin Nx (Winthrop-Breon) p 444, 2230

Nandrolone Decanoate
Deca-Durabolin (Organon) p 1446
Kabolin (Legere) p 1120

Nandrolone Phenpropionate
Durabolin (Organon) p 1446

Naphazoline Hydrochloride
Clear Eyes Eye Drops (Ross) p 1762
4-Way Nasal Spray (Bristol-Myers Products) p 770
Privine Hydrochloride 0.05% Nasal Solution (CIBA) p 863
Privine Hydrochloride 0.05% Nasal Spray (CIBA) p 863

Naproxen
Naprosyn (Syntex) p 440, 2062

Naproxen Sodium
Anaprox Tablets (Syntex) p 440, 2050

Nebulizers
Norisodrine Aerotrol (Abbott) p 547

Neomycin Sulfate
Bacitracin-Neomycin-Polymyxin Ointment (Fougera) p 953

Bacitracin-Neomycin-Polymyxin Ophthalmic Ointment (Fougera) p 953
Coly-Mycin S Otic w/Neomycin & Hydrocortisone (Parke-Davis) p 1501
Cortisporin Cream (Burroughs Wellcome) p 783
Cortisporin Ointment (Burroughs Wellcome) p 784
Cortisporin Ophthalmic Ointment (Burroughs Wellcome) p 784
Cortisporin Ophthalmic Suspension (Burroughs Wellcome) p 785
Cortisporin Otic Solution (Burroughs Wellcome) p 786
Cortisporin Otic Suspension (Burroughs Wellcome) p 786
Mycolog Cream and Ointment (Squibb) p 2003
Myco-Triacet Cream and Ointment (Lemmon) p 1122
Mytrex Cream & Ointment (Savage) p 1825
Neodecadron Sterile Ophthalmic Ointment (Merck Sharp & Dohme) p 1340
Neodecadron Sterile Ophthalmic Solution (Merck Sharp & Dohme) p 1341
Neomycin Sulfate Tablets (Biocraft) p 705
Neomycin Sulfate Tablets (Roxane) p 1788
Neo-Polycin (Merrell Dow) p 1372
Neosporin Aerosol (Burroughs Wellcome) p 806
Neosporin G.U. Irrigant (Burroughs Wellcome) p 807
Neosporin Ointment (Burroughs Wellcome) p 808
Neosporin Ophthalmic Ointment Sterile (Burroughs Wellcome) p 808
Neosporin Ophthalmic Solution Sterile (Burroughs Wellcome) p 809
Neosporin Powder (Burroughs Wellcome) p 810
Neosporin-G Cream (Burroughs Wellcome) p 807
Neo-Synalar Cream (Syntex) p 2061
Nystatin-Neomycin-Gramicidin-Triamcinolone Cream & Ointment (Fougera) p 953
Nyst-olone Cream & Ointment (Schein) p 1828
Octicair Otic Solution & Suspension (Pharmafair) p 1618
Otocort Sterile Ear Drops, Solution and Suspension (Lemmon) p 1122
Topisporin (Pharmafair) p 1618
Tri-Thalmic Ophthalmic Solution (Schein) p 1828

Neostigmine Bromide
Prostigmin Tablets (Roche) p 430, 1699

Neostigmine Methylsulfate
Neostigmine Methylsulfate Injection (Elkins-Sinn) p 938
Prostigmin Injectable (Roche) p 1698

Netilmicin Sulfate
Netromycin Injection (Schering) p 1863

Niacin
Cardioguard Natural Lipotropic Dietary Supplement-Tablets (Professional Health) p 1621
Niacin Tablets (Roxane) p 1788
Nicobid (USV Pharmaceutical) p 440, 2083
Nicolar Tablets (USV Pharmaceutical) p 440, 2083

Niacinamide
A.C.N. Tablets (Persōn & Covey) p 1587
Albafort Injectable (Bart) p 685
Al-Vite (Drug Industries) p 914
B-C-Bid Capsules (Geriatric) p 975
Eldercaps (Mayrand) p 1196
Eldertonic (Mayrand) p 1196
Geravite Elixir (Hauck) p 1001
Glutofac Tablets (Kenwood) p 1046
Hemo-Vite (Drug Industries) p 914
Hemo-Vite Liquid (Drug Industries) p 914
Mega-B (Arco) p 600
Megadose (Arco) p 600
Natalins Rx (Mead Johnson Laboratories) p 419, 1224
Natalins Tablets (Mead Johnson Laboratories) p 419, 1224
Nu-Iron-V Tablets (Mayrand) p 1196
Prenate 90 Tablets (Bock) p 706
Therabid (Mission) p 1420

Niacinamide Hydroiodide
Iodo-Niacin Tablets (O'Neal, Jones & Feldman) p 1445

Niclosamide
Niclocide Chewable Tablets (Miles Pharmaceuticals) p 422, 1411

Nicotinamide
I.L.X. B$_{12}$ Elixir Crystalline (Kenwood) p 1046

Generic and Chemical Name Index

I.L.X. B₁₂ Tablets (Kenwood) p 1046

Nicotine Polacrilex
Nicorette (Merrell Dow) p 421, 1372

Nicotinic Acid
Lipo-Nicin (Brown) p 773
Nicobid (USV Pharmaceutical) p 440, 2083
Nico-400 (Marion) p 418, 1186
Nicolar Tablets (USV Pharmaceutical) p 440, 2083

Nifedipine
Procardia Capsules (Pfizer) p 426, 1606

Nikethamide
Coramine (CIBA) p 846

Nitrate & Nitrite Preparations
Cardilate Chewable Tablets (Burroughs Wellcome) p 407, 782
Cardilate Oral/Sublingual Tablets (Burroughs Wellcome) p 407, 782
Dilatrate-SR (Reed & Carnrick) p 427, 1632
Iso-Bid Capsules (Geriatric) p 975
Nitrol Ointment (Rorer) p 432, 1752
Pentritol (USV Pharmaceutical) p 2086
Peritrate SA (Parke-Davis) p 425, 1560
Peritrate Tablets 10 mg., 20 mg. and 40 mg. (Parke-Davis) p 425, 1560
Sorbide (Mayrand) p 1196

Nitrofurantoin
Furadantin Oral Suspension (Norwich Eaton) p 1432
Furadantin Tablets (Norwich Eaton) p 1432
Nitrofurantoin Capsules & Tablets (Schein) p 1828

Nitrofurantoin Macrocrystals
Macrodantin Capsules (Norwich Eaton) p 422, 1436

Nitrofurazone
Furacin Preparations (Norwich Eaton) p 1433
Furacin Soluble Dressing (Norwich Eaton) p 1433
Furacin Topical Cream (Norwich Eaton) p 1434

Nitroglycerin
Nitro-Bid IV (Marion) p 1187
Nitro-Bid Ointment (Marion) p 1188
Nitro-Bid 2.5 Plateau Caps (Marion) p 418, 1186
Nitro-Bid 6.5 Plateau Caps (Marion) p 418, 1186
Nitro-Bid 9 Plateau Caps (Marion) p 418, 1186
Nitrodisc (Searle Pharmaceuticals) p 436, 1909
Nitro-Dur Transdermal Infusion System (Key Pharmaceuticals) p 413, 1050
Nitroglycerin Ointment 2% (Fougera) p 953
Nitroglycerin Ointment 2% (Schein) p 1828
Nitroglycerin S.R. Capsules (Geneva) p 973
Nitroglyn (Key Pharmaceuticals) p 1051
Nitrol Ointment (Rorer) p 432, 1752
Nitrolin Timed Capsules (Schein) p 1828
Nitrong Ointment (Wharton) p 2184
Nitrong 2.6 mg. Tablets (Wharton) p 2184
Nitrong 6.5 mg. Tablets (Wharton) p 2184
Nitrong 9 mg. Tablets (Wharton) p 2184
Nitrospan Capsules (USV Pharmaceutical) p 440, 2084
Nitrostat Ointment 2% (Parke-Davis) p 425, 1545
Nitrostat Tablets (Parke-Davis) p 424, 1546
Nitrostat IV (Parke-Davis) p 424, 1546
Transderm-Nitro Transdermal Therapeutic System (CIBA) p 410, 873
Tridil (American Critical Care) p 597

Nonoxynol-9
Ramses Contraceptive Vaginal Jelly (Schmid) p 1896
Semicid Vaginal Contraceptive Suppositories (Whitehall) p 443, 2187

Norepinephrine Bitartrate
Levophed Bitartrate (Winthrop-Breon) p 2205

Norethindrone Acetate
Aygestin (Ayerst) p 404, 638
Norlutate (Parke-Davis) p 425, 1556

Norethindrone Preparations
Brevicon 21-Day Tablets (Syntex) p 440, 2052
Brevicon 28-Day Tablets (Syntex) p 440, 2052
Loestrin 21 1/20 (Parke-Davis) p 424, 1531
Loestrin Fe 1/20 (Parke-Davis) p 424, 1531

Loestrin 21 1.5/30 (Parke-Davis) p 424, 1531
Loestrin Fe 1.5/30 (Parke-Davis) p 424, 1531
Micronor Tablets (Ortho Pharmaceutical) p 423, 1461
Modicon 21 Tablets (Ortho Pharmaceutical) p 423, 1461
Modicon 28 Tablets (Ortho Pharmaceutical) p 1461
Norinyl 1+35 Tablets 21-Day (Syntex) p 440, 2052
Norinyl 1+35 Tablets 28-Day (Syntex) p 440, 2052
Norinyl 1+50 21-Day (Syntex) p 440, 2052
Norinyl 1+50 28-Day (Syntex) p 440, 2052
Norinyl 1+80 21-Day (Syntex) p 440, 2052
Norinyl 1+80 28-Day (Syntex) p 440, 2052
Norinyl 2 mg. (Syntex) p 440, 2052
Norlestrin 21 1/50 (Parke-Davis) p 425, 1548
Norlestrin 21 2.5/50 (Parke-Davis) p 425, 1548
Norlestrin 28 1/50 (Parke-Davis) p 1548
Norlestrin Fe 1/50 (Parke-Davis) p 425, 1548
Norlestrin Fe 2.5/50 (Parke-Davis) p 425, 1548
Norlutin (Parke-Davis) p 425, 1556
Nor-Q.D. (Syntex) p 440, 2052
Ortho-Novum 1/35☐21 (Ortho Pharmaceutical) p 422, 1461
Ortho-Novum 1/35☐28 (Ortho Pharmaceutical) p 1461
Ortho-Novum 1/50☐21 (Ortho Pharmaceutical) p 422, 1461
Ortho-Novum 1/50☐28 (Ortho Pharmaceutical) p 1461
Ortho-Novum 1/80☐21 (Ortho Pharmaceutical) p 423, 1461
Ortho-Novum 1/80☐28 (Ortho Pharmaceutical) p 1461
Ortho-Novum 7/7/7 ☐.. 21 Tablets (Ortho Pharmaceutical) p 422, 1461
Ortho-Novum 7/7/7 ☐.. 28 Tablets (Ortho Pharmaceutical) p 1461
Ortho-Novum 10/11☐.. 21 Tablets (Ortho Pharmaceutical) p 422, 1461
Ortho-Novum 10/11☐.. 28 Tablets (Ortho Pharmaceutical) p 1461
Ortho-Novum Tablets 2 mg☐21 (Ortho Pharmaceutical) p 423, 1461
Ovcon-35 (Mead Johnson Laboratories) p 419, 1224
Ovcon-50 (Mead Johnson Laboratories) p 419, 1224
Tri-Norinyl 21-Day Tablets (Syntex) p 440, 2052
Tri-Norinyl 28-Day Tablets (Syntex) p 440, 2052

Norethynodrel
Enovid 5 mg (Searle & Co.) p 435, 1919
Enovid 10 mg (Searle & Co.) p 435, 1919
Enovid-E 21 (Searle & Co.) p 436, 1919

Norgestrel
Lo/Ovral Tablets (Wyeth) p 444, 2255
Lo/Ovral-28 Tablets (Wyeth) p 444, 2263
Ovral Tablets (Wyeth) p 444, 2271
Ovral-28 Tablets (Wyeth) p 444, 2272
Ovrette Tablets (Wyeth) p 2272

Nortriptyline Hydrochloride
Aventyl HCl (Lilly) p 417, 1130
Pamelor (Sandoz Pharmaceutical Div.) p 433, 1807

Nylidrin
Arlidin Tablets (USV Pharmaceutical) p 440, 2070

Nylidrin Hydrochloride
Nylidrin Tablets (Geneva) p 973
Nylidrin HCl Tablets (Danbury) p 887
Nylidrin HCl Tablets (Schein) p 1828

Nystatin
Korostatin Vaginal Tablets (Youngs) p 2301
Mycolog Cream and Ointment (Squibb) p 2003
Mycostatin Cream & Ointment (Squibb) p 2004
Mycostatin Oral Suspension (Squibb) p 2004
Mycostatin Oral Tablets (Squibb) p 438, 2005
Mycostatin Topical Powder (Squibb) p 2004
Mycostatin Vaginal Tablets (Squibb) p 438, 2005
Myco-Triacet Cream and Ointment (Lemmon) p 1122
Mytrex Cream & Ointment (Savage) p 1825
Nilstat for Preparation of Oral Suspension (Lederle) p 1108
Nilstat Oral Suspension (Lederle) p 1108
Nilstat Oral Tablets (Lederle) p 1109
Nilstat Topical Cream & Ointment (Lederle) p 1109

Nilstat Vaginal Tablets (Lederle) p 1108
Nystaform Ointment (Miles Pharmaceuticals) p 1411
Nystatin Cream, Ointment & Vaginal Tablets (Fougera) p 953
Nystatin Cream, Ointment & Vaginal Tablets (Pharmaderm) p 1617
Nystatin Cream, Oral & Vaginal Tablets (Schein) p 1828
Nystatin Cream, Oral Tablets, and Vaginal Tablets (Lemmon) p 1122
Nystatin-Neomycin-Gramicidin-Triamcinolone Cream & Ointment (Fougera) p 953
Nystex Cream & Ointment (Savage) p 1825
Nystex Oral Suspension (Savage) p 1825
Nyst-olone Cream & Ointment (Schein) p 1828
O-V Statin (Squibb) p 2008

O

Opium Preparations
B & O Supprettes No. 15A & No. 16A (Webcon) p 2172
Pantopon Injectable (Roche) p 1697
Parepectolin (Rorer) p 1752

Opium, Tincture of
Parepectolin (Rorer) p 1752

Orphenadrine Citrate
Norflex (Riker) p 428, 1644
Norgesic & Norgesic Forte (Riker) p 428, 1644

Orphenadrine Hydrochloride
Disipal Tablets (Riker) p 1643

Ox Bile Extract
Bilogen (Organon) p 1446
Enzobile Improved Formula (Mallard) p 1181
Enzypan (Norgine) p 1424
Kanulase (Dorsey Laboratories) p 910
Karbokoff Tablets (Arlo) p 601

Oxacillin
Oxacillin Capsules (Biocraft) p 705
Oxacillin Solution (Biocraft) p 705

Oxacillin Sodium
Oxacillin Sodium Capsules & Powder for Oral Suspension (Schein) p 1828
Prostaphlin Capsules, Oral Solution (Bristol) p 407, 745
Prostaphlin for Injection (Bristol) p 745

Oxandrolone
Anavar (Searle & Co.) p 435, 1916

Oxazepam
Serax Capsules, Tablets (Wyeth) p 445, 2287

Oxidized Regenerated Cellulose
Surgicel Absorbable Hemostat (Johnson & Johnson (Patient Care Div.)) p 1044

Oxtriphylline
Brondecon (Parke-Davis) p 423, 1486
Choledyl (Parke-Davis) p 423, 1495
Choledyl Pediatric Syrup (Parke-Davis) p 1495
Choledyl SA Tablets (Parke-Davis) p 423, 1497

Oxybenzone
Eclipse Total Sunscreen Cooling Alcohol Lotion, SPF 15 (Dorsey Laboratories) p 910
Eclipse Total Sunscreen Moisturizing Lotion, SPF 15 (Dorsey Laboratories) p 910
PreSun 8 Lotion, Creamy & Gel (Westwood) p 2180
PreSun 15 Creamy Sunscreen (Westwood) p 2181
PreSun 15 Sunscreen Lotion (Westwood) p 2181
Solbar PF (Persōn & Covey) p 1588
Solbar Plus 15 Sun Protectant Cream (Persōn & Covey) p 1588

Oxybutynin Chloride
Ditropan Syrup (Marion) p 1184
Ditropan Tablets (Marion) p 417, 1184

Oxycodone Hydrochloride
Oxycodone Hydrochloride Oral Solution & Tablets (Roxane) p 1792
Oxycodone Hydrochloride USP Single Entity Tablets & Liquid (Roxane) p 1788
Oxycodone Hydrochloride & Acetaminophen Tablets (Roxane) p 1788
Oxycodone Hydrochloride, Oxycodone Terephthalate & Aspirin Tablets (Full Strength) (Roxane) p 1788
Percocet (Du Pont) p 410, 925

Generic and Chemical Name Index

Percodan & Percodan-Demi Tablets (Du Pont) p 410, 925
SK-Oxycodone with Acetaminophen Tablets (Smith Kline & French) p 1971
SK-Oxycodone with Aspirin Tablets (Smith Kline & French) p 1971
Tylox Capsules (McNeil Pharmaceutical) p 419, 1215

Oxycodone Terephthalate
Oxycodone Hydrochloride, Oxycodone Terephthalate & Aspirin Tablets (Full Strength) (Roxane) p 1788
SK-Oxycodone with Aspirin Tablets (Smith Kline & French) p 1971

Oxymetazoline Hydrochloride
Dristan Long Lasting Nasal Spray, Regular & Menthol (Whitehall) p 443, 2186
Oxymeta-12 Nasal Spray (Schein) p 1828

Oxymetholone
Anadrol-50 (Syntex) p 440, 2049

Oxymorphone Hydrochloride
Numorphan (Du Pont) p 924

Oxyphenbutazone
Oxalid Tablets (USV Pharmaceutical) p 2084
Tandearil (Geigy) p 411, 964

Oxyphenonium Bromide
Antrenyl bromide Tablets (CIBA) p 409, 841

Oxyquinoline Sulfate
Aci-Jel Therapeutic Vaginal Jelly (Ortho Pharmaceutical) p 1453
Otipyrin Otic Solution (Kramer) p 1069
Triva Combination (Boyle) p 726
Triva Douche Powder (Boyle) p 726
Triva Jel (Boyle) p 726

Oxytetracycline
Oxymycin Injectable (O'Neal, Jones & Feldman) p 1445
Terramycin Film-coated Tablets (Pfipharmecs) p 1595
Terramycin Intramuscular Solution (Pfipharmecs) p 1596
Terramycin Ointment (Pfipharmecs) p 1598
Urobiotic-250 (Roerig) p 431, 1744

Oxytetracycline Hydrochloride
Oxytetracycline HCl Capsules (Schein) p 1828
Terra-Cortril Ophthalmic Suspension (Pfipharmecs) p 1594
Terramycin Capsules (Pfipharmecs) p 426, 1595
Terramycin Intramuscular Solution (Pfipharmecs) p 1596
Terramycin Ointment (Pfipharmecs) p 1598
Terramycin with Polymyxin B Sulfate Ophthalmic Ointment (Pfipharmecs) p 1598

Oxytocin (Injection)
Oxytocin Injection (Wyeth) p 2273
Oxytocin in Tubex (Wyeth) p 2288
Pitocin Injection (Parke-Davis) p 1561
Syntocinon Injection (Sandoz Pharmaceutical Div.) p 1817

Oxytocin (Nasal Spray)
Syntocinon Nasal Spray (Sandoz Pharmaceutical Div.) p 1818

P

Padimate O (Octyl dimethyl PABA)
Banquin Cream (Kramer) p 1069
Eclipse Total Sunscreen Cooling Alcohol Lotion, SPF 15 (Dorsey Laboratories) p 910
Eclipse Total Sunscreen Moisturizing Lotion, SPF 15 (Dorsey Laboratories) p 910
Herpecin-L Cold Sore Lip Balm (Campbell) p 829
PreSun 4 Creamy Sunscreen (Westwood) p 2180
PreSun 8 Lotion, Creamy & Gel (Westwood) p 2180
PreSun 15 Creamy Sunscreen (Westwood) p 2181
PreSun 15 Sunscreen Lotion (Westwood) p 2181
Solbar Plus 15 Sun Protectant Cream (Persōn & Covey) p 1588

Pamabron
Maximum Strength Midol PMS (Glenbrook) p 997

Pancreatic Preparations
Arco-Lase (Arco) p 600
Arco-Lase Plus (Arco) p 600
Cotazym (Organon) p 422, 1446
Cotazym-S (Organon) p 422, 1446
Digepepsin Tablets (RAM Laboratories) p 1632

Donnazyme Tablets (Robins) p 428, 1650
Entozyme Tablets (Robins) p 428, 1652
Enzobile Improved Formula (Mallard) p 1181
Enzypan (Norgine) p 1424
Glucagon for Injection Ampoules (Lilly) p 1147
Kanulase (Dorsey Laboratories) p 910
Karbokoff Tablets (Arlo) p 601
Ku-Zyme HP Capsules (Rorer) p 431, 1751
Pancrease (McNeil Pharmaceutical) p 418, 1205
Pancreatin Tablets 2400 mg. N.F. (High Lipase) (Vitaline) p 2148
Phazyme Tablets (Reed & Carnrick) p 427, 1636
Phazyme-95 Tablets (Reed & Carnrick) p 427, 1636
Phazyme-PB Tablets (Reed & Carnrick) p 427, 1636
Viokase Powder (Robins) p 1665
Viokase Tablets (Robins) p 1665
Zypan Tablets (Standard Process) p 2035

Pancreatin
(see under Pancreatic Preparations)

Pancuronium Bromide Injection
Pavulon (Organon) p 1449

Panthenol
Albafort Injectable (Bart) p 685
Eldertonic (Mayrand) p 1196
Ilopan Injection (Adria) p 578

Pantothenate, Calcium
Mega-B (Arco) p 600
Natalins Rx (Mead Johnson Laboratories) p 419, 1224
Natalins Tablets (Mead Johnson Laboratories) p 419, 1224

Pantothenic Acid
Dexol T.D. Tablets (Legere) p 1120

Papain
Cardioguard Natural Lipotropic Dietary Supplement-Powder (Professional Health) p 1621
Cardioguard Natural Lipotropic Dietary Supplement-Tablets (Professional Health) p 1621
Panafil Ointment (Rystan) p 1796
Panafil-White Ointment (Rystan) p 1796

Papaverine
Papaverine T.D. Capsules (Geneva) p 973

Papaverine Hydrochloride
Cerespan Capsules (USV Pharmaceutical) p 2074
Papaverine Hydrochloride Capsules (Roxane) p 1788
Papaverine HCl T.D. Capsules (Danbury) p 887
Papaverine HCl Timed Capsules (Schein) p 1828
Papaverine HCl Tablets (Danbury) p 887
Pavabid Capsules (Marion) p 418, 1189
Pavabid HP Capsulets (Marion) p 418, 1189
Pavatym Capsules (Everett) p 942

Para-Aminobenzoate, Potassium
Potaba (Glenwood) p 412, 998

Para-Aminobenzoic Acid
Hill-Shade Lotion (Hill Dermaceuticals) p 1009
Mega-B (Arco) p 600
RVPaba Lip Stick (Elder) p 936

Parachlorometaxylenol
Fungi-Nail Tincture (Kramer) p 1069
Otic-HC Ear Drops (Hauck) p 1001
Oticol Sterile Ear Drops (Arlo) p 601

Paraldehyde
Paraldehyde (Sterile) (Elkins-Sinn) p 938

Paramethadione
Paradione (Abbott) p 403, 558

Paramomycin Sulfate
Humatin Capsules (Parke-Davis) p 424, 1527

Paregoric
Paregoric (Roxane) p 1788
Parepectolin (Rorer) p 1752

Pargyline Hydrochloride
Eutonyl Filmtab Tablets (Abbott) p 403, 528

Pectin
Kaolin, Pectin, Belladonna Mixture (Schein) p 1828
Kaolin-Pectin-Concentrated (Roxane) p 1788

Kaolin-Pectin Mixture (Schein) p 1828
Kaolin-Pectin PG Mixture (Schein) p 1828
Kaolin-Pectin Suspension (Roxane) p 1788
Parepectolin (Rorer) p 1752

Pemoline
Cylert Tablets (Abbott) p 403, 510

Penicillamine
Cuprimine Capsules (Merck Sharp & Dohme) p 420, 1280
Depen Titratable Tablets (Wallace) p 2152

Penicillin G, Benzathine
Bicillin C-R Injection (Wyeth) p 2239
Bicillin C-R in Tubex (Wyeth) p 2288
Bicillin C-R 900/300 (Wyeth) p 2241
Bicillin C-R 900/300 in Tubex (Wyeth) p 2288
Bicillin L-A Injection (Wyeth) p 2242
Permapen Isoject (Pfipharmecs) p 1590

Penicillin G, Dibenzylethyenediamine
(see under Penicillin G, Benzathine)

Penicillin G Potassium
Penicillin G Potassium for Injection USP (Squibb) p 2009
Penicillin G Potassium Tablets (Biocraft) p 705
Pentids for Syrup (Squibb) p 2011
Pentids Tablets, Pentids 400 & 800 Tablets (Squibb) p 438, 2011
Pfizerpen for Injection (Pfipharmecs) p 1590
SK-Penicillin G Tablets (Smith Kline & French) p 1971

Penicillin G Procaine
Bicillin C-R Injection (Wyeth) p 2239
Bicillin C-R in Tubex (Wyeth) p 2288
Bicillin C-R 900/300 (Wyeth) p 2241
Bicillin C-R 900/300 in Tubex (Wyeth) p 2288
Crysticillin 300 A.S. & Crysticillin 600 A.S. (Squibb) p 1992
Penicillin G Procaine Suspension, Sterile, Vials (Lilly) p 1170
Pfizerpen-AS Aqueous Suspension (Pfipharmecs) p 1592
Wycillin (Wyeth) p 2293
Wycillin in Tubex (Wyeth) p 2288
Wycillin & Probenecid Tablets & Injection (Wyeth) p 2295

Penicillin G Sodium
Penicillin G Sodium for Injection USP (Squibb) p 2010

Penicillin (Oral)
Cyclapen-W (Wyeth) p 444, 2249
Omnipen Capsules (Wyeth) p 444, 2271
Omnipen for Oral Suspension (Wyeth) p 2271
Omnipen Pediatric Drops (Wyeth) p 2271
Pathocil Capsules, for Oral Suspension (Wyeth) p 444, 2274
Pentids for Syrup (Squibb) p 2011
Pentids Tablets, Pentids 400 & 800 Tablets (Squibb) p 438, 2011
Pen•Vee K, for Oral Solution & Tablets (Wyeth) p 444, 2275
Principen Capsules (Squibb) p 438, 2012
Principen for Oral Suspension (Squibb) p 2012
Principen with Probenecid Capsules (Squibb) p 2013
Unipen Injection, Capsules, Powder for Oral Solution, & Tablets (Wyeth) p 445, 2290
Veetids for Oral Solution (Squibb) p 2026
Veetids Tablets (Squibb) p 438, 2026
Wymox Capsules & Oral Suspension (Wyeth) p 445, 2298

Penicillin, Potassium Phenoxymethyl
(see under Penicillin V Potassium)

Penicillin (Repository)
Bicillin C-R Injection (Wyeth) p 2239
Bicillin C-R in Tubex (Wyeth) p 2288
Bicillin C-R 900/300 (Wyeth) p 2241
Bicillin C-R 900/300 in Tubex (Wyeth) p 2288
Bicillin L-A Injection (Wyeth) p 2242

Penicillin V Potassium
Betapen-VK (Bristol) p 407, 729
Penicillin V Potassium Solution (Biocraft) p 705
Penicillin V Potassium Tablets (Biocraft) p 705
Penicillin V, Potassium (Penapar VK) (Parke-Davis) p 425, 1559
Penicillin VK Powder for Oral Solution & Tablets (Schein) p 1828
Pen•Vee K, for Oral Solution & Tablets (Wyeth) p 444, 2275

Generic and Chemical Name Index

SK-Penicillin VK For Oral Solution & Tablets (Smith Kline & French) p 1971
V-Cillin K for Oral Solution & Tablets (Lilly) p 1178
Veetids for Oral Solution (Squibb) p 2026
Veetids Tablets (Squibb) p 438, 2026

Pentaerythritol Tetranitrate
Duotrate Plateau Caps (Marion) p 417, 1185
Duotrate 45 Plateau Caps (Marion) p 418, 1185
P.E.T.N. S.R. Tablets (Geneva) p 973
Pentaerythritol Tetranitrate Tablets (PETN), Timed Capsules & Tablets (Schein) p 1828
Pentritol (USV Pharmaceutical) p 2086
Peritrate SA (Parke-Davis) p 425, 1560
Peritrate Tablets 10 mg., 20 mg. and 40 mg. (Parke-Davis) p 425, 1560

Pentagastrin
Peptavlon (Ayerst) p 657, 3008

Pentamidine Isethionate
Pentam 300 (LyphoMed) p 1181

Pentazocine Hydrochloride
Talacen (Winthrop-Breon) p 444, 2227
Talwin Compound (Winthrop-Breon) p 2229
Talwin Nx (Winthrop-Breon) p 444, 2230

Pentazocine Lactate
Talwin Injection (Winthrop-Breon) p 2228

Pentobarbital
Wigraine-PB Suppositories (Organon) p 422, 1451

Pentobarbital Sodium
(see under Sodium Pentobarbital)

Pentoxifylline
Trental (Hoechst-Roussel) p 413, 1022

Pepsin
Digepepsin Tablets (RAM Laboratories) p 1632
Donnazyme Tablets (Robins) p 428, 1650
Entozyme Tablets (Robins) p 428, 1652
Enzobile Improved Formula (Mallard) p 1181
Enzypan (Norgine) p 1424
Kanulase (Dorsey Laboratories) p 910
Muripsin (Norgine) p 1424
Zypan Tablets (Standard Process) p 2035

Peroxide Preparations
Debrox Drops (Marion) p 1184
Gly-Oxide Liquid (Marion) p 1186

Perphenazine
Etrafon Tablets (Schering) p 434, 1841
Triavil Tablets (Merck Sharp & Dohme) p 420, 1354
Trilafon Tablets, Repetabs Tablets, Concentrate & Injection (Schering) p 435, 1888

Pertussis Immune Globulin (Human)
Pertussis Immune Globulin (Human) Hypertussis (Cutter Biological) p 884

Petrolatum
Petrolatum (White) & Petrolatum (White) Ophthalmic Ointment (Fougera) p 953

Phenacemide
Phenurone (Abbott) p 564

Phenacetin
A.P.C. with Codeine Nos. 3 & 4, Tabloid brand (Burroughs Wellcome) p 407, 780
Propoxyphene Compound 65 (Schein) p 1828

Phenazopyridine
Urobiotic-250 (Roerig) p 431, 1744

Phenazopyridine Hydrochloride
Azo Gantanol Tablets (Roche) p 429, 1670
Azo Gantrisin Tablets (Roche) p 429, 1671
Pyridium (Parke-Davis) p 425, 1567
Pyridium Plus (Parke-Davis) p 425, 1568
Thiosulfil Duo-Pak (Ayerst) p 682
Thiosulfil-A (Ayerst) p 405, 681
Thiosulfil-A Tablets (Ayerst) p 405, 681

Phendimetrazine
PT 105 Capsules (Legere) p 1120
Phenazine Tablets & Capsules (Legere) p 1120

Phendimetrazine Tartrate
Bontril PDM (Carnrick) p 408, 830
Bontril Slow-Release (Carnrick) p 408, 830
Dyrexan-OD Capsules (Trimen) p 2067

Hyrex-105 (Hyrex) p 1024
Melfiat Tablets (Reid-Provident Labs.) p 1639
Melfiat 105 Unicelles (Reid-Provident Labs.) p 428, 1639
Plegine (Ayerst) p 405, 659
Prelu-2 Timed Release Capsules (Boehringer Ingelheim) p 406, 711
Trimcaps (Mayrand) p 1196
Trimstat Tablets (Laser) p 1072
Trimtabs (Mayrand) p 1197
Wehless-105 Timecelles (Hauck) p 1001
X-Trozine Capsules & Tablets (Rexar) p 1641
X-Trozine LA-105 Capsules (Rexar) p 1641

Phenelzine Sulfate
Nardil (Parke-Davis) p 424, 1543

Phenindamine Tartrate
Nolahist (Carnrick) p 408, 832
Nolamine Tablets (Carnrick) p 408, 833
P-V-Tussin Syrup (Reid-Provident Labs.) p 1640
P-V-Tussin Tablets (Reid-Provident Labs.) p 428, 1640

Pheniramine Maleate
Citra Forte Capsules (Boyle) p 726
Citra Forte Syrup (Boyle) p 726
Dristan Nasal Spray, Regular & Menthol (Whitehall) p 443, 2186
Fiogesic Tablets (Sandoz Pharmaceutical Div.) p 432, 1801
Poly-Histine-D Capsules (Bock) p 705
Poly-Histine-D Elixir (Bock) p 705
Poly-Histine-D Pediatric Capsules (Bock) p 705
Ru-Tuss Expectorant (Boots) p 722
Ru-Tuss Plain (Boots) p 723
Ru-Tuss with Hydrocodone (Boots) p 722
S-T Forte Syrup & Sugar-Free (Scot-Tussin) p 1897
Triaminic Juvelets (Dorsey Laboratories) p 912
Triaminic Oral Infant Drops (Dorsey Laboratories) p 912
Triaminic TR Tablets (Timed Release) (Dorsey Laboratories) p 912
Tussirex Sugar-Free (Scot-Tussin) p 1897
Tussirex Syrup (Scot-Tussin) p 1897

Phenmetrazine Hydrochloride
Preludin Endurets (Boehringer Ingelheim) p 406, 710
Preludin Tablets (Boehringer Ingelheim) p 710

Phenobarbital
Antispasmodic Capsules, Elixir & Tablets (Schein) p 1828
Antrocol Tablets, Capsules & Elixir (Poythress) p 1618
Arco-Lase Plus (Arco) p 600
Bronkolixir (Winthrop-Breon) p 2193
Bronkotabs (Winthrop-Breon) p 2194
Chardonna-2 (Rorer) p 431, 1748
Isuprel Hydrochloride Compound Elixir (Winthrop-Breon) p 2204
Levsin/Phenobarbital Tablets, Elixir & Drops (Rorer) p 1751
Levsinex/Phenobarbital Timecaps (Rorer) p 1751
Mudrane GG Elixir (Poythress) p 1619
Mudrane GG Tablets (Poythress) p 1619
Mudrane Tablets (Poythress) p 1618
Phazyme-PB Tablets (Reed & Carnrick) p 427, 1636
Phenobarbital Elixir, Tablets (Roxane) p 1788
Phenobarbital Elixir & Tablets (Schein) p 1828
Phenobarbital Tablets (Danbury) p 887
Primatene Tablets-P Formula (Whitehall) p 443, 2177
Pro-Banthine w/Phenobarbital (Searle & Co.) p 436, 1936
Quadrinal Tablets & Suspension (Knoll) p 414, 1065
SK-Phenobarbital Tablets (Smith Kline & French) p 1971
Solfoton Tablets & Capsules (Poythress) p 1619
T-E-P Tablets (Schein) p 1828
T.E.P. Tablets (Geneva) p 973
Theofedral Tablets (Danbury) p 887

Phenobarbital Sodium
Phenobarbital Sodium Injection (Elkins-Sinn) p 938
Phenobarbital Sodium in Tubex (Wyeth) p 2288

Phenol
Anbesol Gel Antiseptic Anesthetic (Whitehall) p 443, 2185
Castellani Paint (Pedinol) p 1580

Chloraseptic Liquid (Procter & Gamble) p 1619
Chloraseptic Lozenges (Procter & Gamble) p 1620
Derma Cas Gel (Hill Dermaceuticals) p 1009
Osti-Derm Lotion (Pedinol) p 1580

Phenolphthalein
Agoral, Raspberry & Marshmallow Flavors (Parke-Davis) p 1480
Evac-Q-Kit (Adria) p 575
Evac-Q-Kwik (Adria) p 575
Evac-U-Gen (Walker, Corp) p 2148
Prulet (Mission) p 1420
Trilax (Drug Industries) p 915

Phenothiazine Derivatives
Compazine (Smith Kline & French) p 436, 1953
Largon in Tubex (Wyeth) p 2288
Phenergan Injection (Wyeth) p 2275
Phenergan in Tubex (Wyeth) p 2288
Phenergan Syrup Fortis (Wyeth) p 2276
Phenergan Syrup Plain (Wyeth) p 2276
Phenergan Tablets & Rectal Suppositories (Wyeth) p 444,445, 2278
Phenergan VC (Wyeth) p 2282
Phenergan VC with Codeine (Wyeth) p 2284
Phenergan with Codeine (Wyeth) p 2278
Phenergan with Dextromethorphan (Wyeth) p 2280
Sparine Injection in Tubex (Wyeth) p 2288
Stelazine (Smith Kline & French) p 437, 1971
Temaril (Smith Kline & French) p 437, 1976
Thorazine (Smith Kline & French) p 437, 1977

Phenoxybenzamine Hydrochloride
Dibenzyline Capsules (Smith Kline & French) p 436, 1960

Phenprocoumon
Liquamar Tablets (Organon) p 422, 1447

Phensuximide
Milontin Kapseals (Parke-Davis) p 424, 1543

Phentermine Hydrochloride
Adipex-P Tablets (Lemmon) p 417, 1121
Fastin Capsules (Beecham Laboratories) p 406, 692
Oby-Trim 30 Capsules (Rexar) p 1641
Phentermine HCl Capsules & Tablets (Schein) p 1828
Teramine Capsules (Legere) p 1120

Phentermine Resin
Ionamin (Pennwalt) p 426, 1585

Phentolamine
Regitine (CIBA) p 863

Phenyl Salicylate
Trac Tabs 2X (Hyrex) p 413, 1025

D-Phenylalanine
Endorphenyl (Tyson) p 2068

Phenylazodiamino Pyridine Hydrochloride
(see under Phenazopyridine Hydrochloride)

Phenylbutazone
Azolid Capsules & Tablets (USV Pharmaceutical) p 2070
Butazolidin Capsules & Tablets (Geigy) p 411, 956
Phenylbutazone Capsules (Geneva) p 973
Phenylbutazone Capsules & Tablets (Schein) p 1828
Phenylbutazone Tablets (Danbury) p 887
Phenylbutazone Tablets (Geneva) p 973

Phenylephrine
Donatussin Drops (Laser) p 1072
Quadrahist Pediatric Syrup, Syrup & Timed Release Tablets (Schein) p 1828
Sinovan Timed (Drug Industries) p 915

Phenylephrine Bitartrate
Duo-Medihaler (Riker) p 1643

Phenylephrine Hydrobromide
Albatussin (Bart) p 685

Phenylephrine Hydrochloride
Bromphen Compound Elixir - Sugar Free (Schein) p 1828
Bromphen Compound Tablets (Schein) p 1828
Bromphen DC Expectorant (Schein) p 1828
Bromphen Expectorant (Schein) p 1828
Codimal DH (Central Pharmaceuticals) p 836
Codimal DM (Central Pharmaceuticals) p 836
Codimal PH (Central Pharmaceuticals) p 836

Generic and Chemical Name Index

Comhist LA Capsules (Norwich Eaton) p 422, 1425
Comhist Tablets (Norwich Eaton) p 1426
Congespirin Aspirin-Free Chewable Cold Tablets for Children (Bristol-Myers Products) p 769
Congespirin Cold Tablets (Aspirin Formula) (Bristol-Myers Products) p 769
Coryban-D Cough Syrup (Pfipharmecs) p 1589
Dallergy Capsules, Tablets, Syrup (Laser) p 1072
Dimetapp Elixir (Robins) p 1648
Dimetapp Extentabs (Robins) p 428, 1648
Donatussin DC Syrup (Laser) p 1072
Dristan, Advanced Formula Decongestant/Antihistamine/Analgesic Capsules (Whitehall) p 443, 2186
Dristan, Advanced Formula Decongestant/Antihistamine/Analgesic Tablets (Whitehall) p 443, 2186
Dristan Nasal Spray, Regular & Menthol (Whitehall) p 443, 2186
Dura Tap-PD (Dura) p 929
Dura-Vent/DA (Dura) p 929
E.N.T. Syrup (Springbok) p 1985
E.N.T. Tablets (Springbok) p 1985
Entex Capsules (Norwich Eaton) p 1431
Entex Liquid (Norwich Eaton) p 1431
Extendryl Chewable Tablets (Fleming) p 948
Extendryl Sr. & Jr. T.D. Capsules (Fleming) p 948
Extendryl Syrup (Fleming) p 948
4-Way Nasal Spray (Bristol-Myers Products) p 770
Histalet Forte Tablets (Reid-Provident Labs.) p 428, 1638
Histaspan-D Capsules (USV Pharmaceutical) p 2077
Histaspan-Plus Capsules (USV Pharmaceutical) p 2077
Histor-D Timecelles (Hauck) p 1001
Hycomine Compound (Du Pont) p 919
Korigesic Tablets (Trimen) p 2067
Naldecon (Bristol) p 407, 738
Neo-Synephrine Hydrochloride 1% Injection (Winthrop-Breon) p 2216
Neo-Synephrine Hydrochloride (Ophthalmic) (Winthrop-Breon) p 2217
P-V-Tussin Syrup (Reid-Provident Labs.) p 1640
Pediacof (Winthrop-Breon) p 2221
Phenergan VC (Wyeth) p 2282
Phenergan VC with Codeine (Wyeth) p 2284
Protid, Improved Formula (LaSalle) p 1071
Quelidrine Syrup (Abbott) p 567
Ru-Tuss Expectorant (Boots) p 722
Ru-Tuss Plain (Boots) p 723
Ru-Tuss Tablets (Boots) p 406, 723
Ru-Tuss with Hydrocodone (Boots) p 722
S-T Decongest Sugar-Free & Dye-Free (Scot-Tussin) p 1897
S-T Forte Syrup & Sugar-Free (Scot-Tussin) p 1897
Singlet (Merrell Dow) p 421, 1385
Tamine S.R. Tablets (Geneva) p 973
Tussar DM (USV Pharmaceutical) p 2091
Tussirex Sugar-Free (Scot-Tussin) p 1897
Tussirex Syrup (Scot-Tussin) p 1897
Tympagesic Otic Solution (Adria) p 587

Phenylephrine Tannate
Rynatan Tablets & Pediatric Suspension (Wallace) p 442, 2165
Rynatuss Tablets & Pediatric Suspension (Wallace) p 442, 2165

Phenylpropanolamine
Alka-Seltzer Plus Cold Medicine (Miles Laboratories) p 1395
Bromphen Compound Elixir - Sugar Free (Schein) p 1828
Bromphen DC Expectorant (Schein) p 1828
Bromphen Expectorant (Schein) p 1828
Decongestant Elixir (Schein) p 1828
Decongestant Expectorant (Schein) p 1828
Decongestant-AT (Antitussive) Liquid (Schein) p 1828
Dexatrim Capsules, Extra Strength, Plus Vitamins (Thompson Medical) p 2066
Dexatrim • 15 (Thompson Medical) p 2066
Dexatrim • 15, Caffeine-Free (Thompson Medical) p 2066
Quadrahist Pediatric Syrup, Syrup & Timed Release Tablets (Schein) p 1828
Tuss-Ade Timed Capsules (Schein) p 1828

Phenylpropanolamine Hydrochloride
Appedrine, Maximum Strength (Thompson Medical) p 2065
Bayer Children's Cold Tablets (Glenbrook) p 996
Bayer Cough Syrup for Children (Glenbrook) p 996
Bromphen Compound Tablets (Schein) p 1828
Codimal Expectorant (Central Pharmaceuticals) p 836
Comtrex (Bristol-Myers Products) p 769
Conex (O'Neal, Jones & Feldman) p 1445
Conex with Codeine (O'Neal, Jones & Feldman) p 1445
Congespirin Liquid Cold Medicine (Bristol-Myers Products) p 770
Control Capsules, Maximum Strength (Thompson Medical) p 2066
Coryban-D Capsules (Pfipharmecs) p 1589
CoTylenol Children's Liquid Cold Formula (McNeil Consumer Products) p 418, 1198
Cremacoat 3 (Vicks Pharmacy Products) p 442, 2147
Cremacoat 4 (Vicks Pharmacy Products) p 442, 2147
Dehist (O'Neal, Jones & Feldman) p 1445
Dexatrim Capsules (Thompson Medical) p 2066
Dexatrim Capsules, Extra Strength (Thompson Medical) p 2066
Dexatrim Capsules, Extra Strength, Caffeine-Free (Thompson Medical) p 2066
Dieutrim Capsules (Legere) p 1120
Dimetane-DC Cough Syrup (Robins) p 1647
Dimetapp Elixir (Robins) p 1648
Dimetapp Extentabs (Robins) p 428, 1648
Dura Tap-PD (Dura) p 929
Dura-Vent (Dura) p 929
Dura-Vent/A (Dura) p 929
E.N.T. Syrup (Springbok) p 1985
E.N.T. Tablets (Springbok) p 1985
Entex Capsules (Norwich Eaton) p 1431
Entex LA Tablets (Norwich Eaton) p 422, 1432
Entex Liquid (Norwich Eaton) p 1431
4-Way Cold Tablets (Bristol-Myers Products) p 770
Fiogesic Tablets (Sandoz Pharmaceutical Div.) p 432, 1801
Head & Chest (Procter & Gamble) p 1620
Help (Verex) p 442, 2145
Histalet Forte Tablets (Reid-Provident Labs.) p 428, 1638
Hycomine Pediatric Syrup (Du Pont) p 917
Hycomine Syrup (Du Pont) p 917
Korigesic Tablets (Trimen) p 2067
Kronohist Kronocaps (Ferndale) p 942
Naldecon (Bristol) p 407, 738
Naldecon-CX Suspension (Bristol) p 739
Naldecon-DX Pediatric Syrup (Bristol) p 739
Naldecon-EX Pediatric Drops (Bristol) p 740
Nolamine Tablets (Carnrick) p 408, 833
Ornade Spansule Capsules (Smith Kline & French) p 437, 1968
Phenate (Mallard) p 1181
Poly-Histine Expectorant Plain (Bock) p 705
Poly-Histine Expectorant with Codeine (Bock) p 705
Poly-Histine-D Capsules (Bock) p 705
Poly-Histine-D Elixir (Bock) p 705
Poly-Histine-D Pediatric Capsules (Bock) p 705
Prolamine Capsules, Maximum Strength (Thompson Medical) p 2067
Propagest & Propagest Syrup (Carnrick) p 408, 834
Resaid T.D. Capsules (Geneva) p 973
Rescaps-D T.D. Capsules (Geneva) p 973
Rhindecon Capsules (McGregor) p 1197
Rhinolar Capsules (McGregor) p 1197
Rhinolar-EX Capsules (McGregor) p 1197
Rhinolar-EX 12 Capsules (McGregor) p 1197
Ru-Tuss Expectorant (Boots) p 722
Ru-Tuss Plain (Boots) p 723
Ru-Tuss Tablets (Boots) p 406, 723
Ru-Tuss II Capsules (Boots) p 406, 723
Ru-Tuss with Hydrocodone (Boots) p 722
S-T Decongest Sugar-Free & Dye-Free (Scot-Tussin) p 1897
S-T Forte Syrup & Sugar-Free (Scot-Tussin) p 1897
Sinubid (Parke-Davis) p 425, 1569
Sinulin Tablets (Carnrick) p 409, 835
Tamine S.R. Tablets (Geneva) p 973
Tavist-D Tablets (Sandoz Pharmaceutical Div.) p 433, 1819
Triaminic Cold Syrup (Dorsey Laboratories) p 911
Triaminic Cold Tablets (Dorsey Laboratories) p 911
Triaminic Expectorant (Dorsey Laboratories) p 911
Triaminic Expectorant w/Codeine (Dorsey Laboratories) p 911
Triaminic Juvelets (Dorsey Laboratories) p 912
Triaminic Oral Infant Drops (Dorsey Laboratories) p 912
Triaminic TR Tablets (Timed Release) (Dorsey Laboratories) p 912
Triaminic-DM Cough Formula (Dorsey Laboratories) p 913
Triaminic-12 Tablets (Dorsey Laboratories) p 913
Triaminicol Multi-Symptom Cold Syrup (Dorsey Laboratories) p 913
Triaminicol Multi-Symptom Cold Tablets (Dorsey Laboratories) p 914
Tuss-Ornade Liquid (Smith Kline & French) p 1980
Tuss-Ornade Spansule Capsules (Smith Kline & French) p 437, 1981

Phenylpropanolamine Polistirex
Corsym (Pennwalt) p 1582

Phenyltoloxamine
Quadrahist Pediatric Syrup, Syrup & Timed Release Tablets (Schein) p 1828

Phenyltoloxamine Citrate
Comhist LA Capsules (Norwich Eaton) p 422, 1425
Comhist Tablets (Norwich Eaton) p 1426
Magsal Tablets (U.S. Pharmaceutical) p 2070
Naldecon (Bristol) p 407, 738
Percogesic Analgesic Tablets (Vicks Pharmacy Products) p 442, 2147
Poly-Histine-D Capsules (Bock) p 705
Poly-Histine-D Elixir (Bock) p 705
Poly-Histine-D Pediatric Capsules (Bock) p 705
Sinubid (Parke-Davis) p 425, 1569

Phenyltoloxamine Dihydrogen Citrate
Kutrase Capsules (Rorer) p 431, 1750

Phenyltoloxamine Resin Complex
Tussionex Tablets, Capsules & Suspension (Pennwalt) p 1585

Phenytoin
Dilantin Infatabs (Parke-Davis) p 423, 1503
Dilantin-30 Pediatric/Dilantin-125 Suspension (Parke-Davis) p 1506

Phenytoin Sodium
Dilantin Kapseals (Parke-Davis) p 423, 1502
Dilantin Parenteral (Parke-Davis) p 1505
Dilantin with Phenobarbital (Parke-Davis) p 423, 1507
Phenytoin Sodium Capsules-Prompt Action (Schein) p 1828
Phenytoin Sodium Injection (Elkins-Sinn) p 938

Phosphorus Preparations
K-Phos M.F. (Modified Formula) Tablets (Beach) p 405, 686
K-Phos Neutral Tablets (Beach) p 405, 686
K-Phos No. 2 Tablets (Beach) p 405, 686
K-Phos Original Formula 'Sodium Free' Tablets (Beach) p 405, 686
Neutra-Phos Powder & Capsules (Willen) p 2188
Neutra-Phos-K Powder & Capsules (Willen) p 2188
Phos-Flur Oral Rinse/Supplement (Colgate-Hoyt) p 879
Thera-Flur Gel-Drops (Colgate-Hoyt) p 880
Thiacide Tablets (Beach) p 405, 687
Uro-KP-Neutral (Star) p 2035
Uroqid-Acid Tablets (Beach) p 405, 687
Uroqid-Acid No. 2 Tablets (Beach) p 405, 687

Physostigmine Salicylate
Antilirium Injectable (O'Neal, Jones & Feldman) p 1443

Phytonadione
AquaMEPHYTON Injection (Merck Sharp & Dohme) p 1265
Konakion Injectable (Roche) p 1687

Pimozide
Orap Tablets (McNeil Pharmaceutical) p 1203

Pindolol
Visken (Sandoz Pharmaceutical Div.) p 433, 1820

Piperacetazine
Quide (Merrell Dow) p 1379

Piperacillin Sodium
Pipracil (Lederle) p 416, 1113

Piperazine Preparations
Antepar (Burroughs Wellcome) p 407, 779

Piperonyl Butoxide
A-200 Pyrinate Pediculicide Shampoo, Liquid & Gel (Norcliff Thayer) p 422, 1422
Pyrinyl Liquid (Schein) p 1828
RID Liquid Pediculicide (Pfipharmecs) p 426, 1593

Piroxicam
Feldene Capsules (Pfizer) p 426, 1601

Pitcher Plant Distillate
Sarapin (High Chemical) p 1009

Generic and Chemical Name Index

Pitressin Tannate
  Pitressin Tannate in Oil (Parke-Davis) p 1562

Plague Vaccine
  Plague Vaccine (Human) (Cutter Biological) p 886

Plantago Seed
  Konsyl (Lafayette) p 1070
  Konsyl-D (formerly L. A. Formula) (Lafayette) p 1070

Plasma Fractions, Human
  Albutein 5% (Alpha Theapeutic) p 589
  Albutein 25% (Alpha Theapeutic) p 589
  Autoplex, Anti-Inhibitor Coagulant Complex, Dried (Hyland Therapeutics) p 1023
  Buminate 5%, Normal Serum Albumin (Human), U.S.P., 5% Solution (Hyland Therapeutics) p 1023
  Buminate 25%, Normal Serum Albumin (Human), U.S.P., 25% Solution (Hyland Therapeutics) p 1023
  Factor IX Complex (Human) (Factors II, VII, IX, and X) Konÿne (Cutter Biological) p 886
  Hemofil, Antihemophilic Factor (Human), Method Four, Dried (Hyland Therapeutics) p 1023
  Hemofil T, Antihemophilic Factor (Human), Method Four, Dried, Heat-Treated (Hyland Therapeutics) p 1024
  Hepatitis B Immune Globulin (Human) HyperHep (Cutter Biological) p 884
  Hu-Tet, Tetanus Immune Globulin (Human), U.S.P. (Hyland Therapeutics) p 1024
  Immuglobin (Savage) p 1825
  Immune Globulin Intravenous, 5% (In 10% Maltose) Gamimune (Cutter Biological) p 883
  Immune Serum Globulin (Human), U.S.P. Gamma Globulin (Hyland Therapeutics) p 1024
  Immune Serum Globulin (Human) Gamastan (Cutter Biological) p 883
  Imogam Rabies Immune Globulin (Human) (Merieux) p 1358
  Pertussis Immune Globulin (Human) Hypertussis (Cutter Biological) p 884
  Plasma-Plex (Armour) p 613
  Plasmanin 5% (Alpha Theapeutic) p 589
  Profilate (Alpha Theapeutic) p 589
  Profilate, Heat-Treated (Alpha Theapeutic) p 589
  Profilnine (Alpha Theapeutic) p 589
  Proplex, Factor IX Complex (Human) (Factors II, VII, IX & X), Dried (Hyland Therapeutics) p 1024
  Proplex SX, Factor IX Complex (Human)(Factors II, VII, IX & X), Dried (Hyland Therapeutics) p 1024
  Protenate 5%, Plasma Protein Fraction (Human), U.S.P., 5% Solution (Hyland Therapeutics) p 1024
  Rh₀-D Immune Globulin (Human) HypRho-D (Cutter Biological) p 885
  Rh₀-D Immune Globulin (Human) HypRho-D Mini-Dose (Cutter Biological) p 884
  Rabies Immune Globulin (Human) Hyperab (Cutter Biological) p 884
  Rabies Immune Globulin (Human), Imogam Rabies (Merieux) p 1358
  Tetanus Immune Globulin (Human) Hyper-Tet (Cutter Biological) p 884

Plicamycin
  Mithracin (Miles Pharmaceuticals) p 1407

Pneumococcal Vaccine, Polyvalent
  Pneumovax 23 (Merck Sharp & Dohme) p 1343
  Pnu-Imune (Lederle) p 1116

Podophyllin
  Cantharone Plus (Seres) p 1939
  Pod-Ben-25 (C & M) p 828
  Verrex (C & M) p 828
  Verrusol (C & M) p 828

Poison Ivy Extract
  Rhus Tox Antigen Injection (Lemmon) p 1122

Poison Ivy, Oak, Sumac Extract Combined
  Rhus All Antigen - Poison Ivy, Oak, Sumac Combined (Barry) p 685

Poliomyelitis Vaccine Purified, Trivalent Types 1,2,3 (Salk)
  Poliomyelitis Vaccine (Purified) (For the Prevention of Poliomyelitis) (Squibb/Connaught) p 2033

Poliovirus Vaccine, Live, Oral, Trivalent, Types 1,2,3 (Sabin)
  Orimune Poliovirus Vaccine, Live, Oral, Trivalent (Lederle) p 1109

Polyestradiol Phosphate
  Estradurin (Ayerst) p 642

Polyethylene Glycol
  GoLYTELY (Braintree) p 727

Polymyxin B Sulfate
  Aerosporin Powder (Burroughs Wellcome) p 775
  Bacitracin-Neomycin-Polymyxin Ointment (Fougera) p 953
  Bacitracin-Neomycin-Polymyxin Ophthalmic Ointment (Fougera) p 953
  Bacitracin-Polymyxin Ointment (Fougera) p 953
  Cortisporin Cream (Burroughs Wellcome) p 783
  Cortisporin Ointment (Burroughs Wellcome) p 784
  Cortisporin Ophthalmic Ointment (Burroughs Wellcome) p 784
  Cortisporin Ophthalmic Suspension (Burroughs Wellcome) p 785
  Cortisporin Otic Solution (Burroughs Wellcome) p 786
  Cortisporin Otic Suspension (Burroughs Wellcome) p 786
  Neo-Polycin (Merrell Dow) p 1372
  Neosporin Aerosol (Burroughs Wellcome) p 806
  Neosporin G.U. Irrigant (Burroughs Wellcome) p 807
  Neosporin Ointment (Burroughs Wellcome) p 808
  Neosporin Ophthalmic Ointment Sterile (Burroughs Wellcome) p 808
  Neosporin Ophthalmic Solution Sterile (Burroughs Wellcome) p 809
  Neosporin Powder (Burroughs Wellcome) p 810
  Neosporin-G Cream (Burroughs Wellcome) p 807
  Octicair Otic Solution & Suspension (Pharmafair) p 1618
  Ophthocort (Parke-Davis) p 1558
  Otobiotic Otic Solution (Schering) p 1875
  Otocort Sterile Ear Drops, Solution and Suspension (Lemmon) p 1122
  Polymyxin B Sulfate (see Aerosporin) (Burroughs Wellcome) p 775
  Polysporin Ointment (Burroughs Wellcome) p 810
  Polysporin Ophthalmic Ointment (Burroughs Wellcome) p 810
  Pyocidin-Otic Solution (Berlex) p 702
  Terramycin Ointment (Pfipharmecs) p 1598
  Terramycin with Polymyxin B Sulfate Ophthalmic Ointment (Pfipharmecs) p 1598
  Topisporin (Pharmafair) p 1618
  Tri-Thalmic Ophthalmic Solution (Schein) p 1828

Polymyxin Preparations
  Neosporin G.U. Irrigant (Burroughs Wellcome) p 807
  Polysporin Ointment (Burroughs Wellcome) p 810
  Pyocidin-Otic Solution (Berlex) p 702

Polysaccharides
  Cardioguard Natural Lipotropic Dietary Supplement-Powder (Professional Health) p 1621

Polythiazide
  Minizide Capsules (Pfizer) p 426, 1604
  Renese (Pfizer) p 426, 1608
  Renese-R (Pfizer) p 426, 1608

Potassium Acid Phosphate
  K-Phos M.F. (Modified Formula) Tablets (Beach) p 405, 686
  K-Phos Neutral Tablets (Beach) p 405, 686
  K-Phos No. 2 Tablets (Beach) p 405, 686
  K-Phos Original Formula 'Sodium Free' Tablets (Beach) p 405, 686
  Thiacide Tablets (Beach) p 405, 687

Potassium Bicarbonate
  K-Lyte & K-Lyte DS (Mead Johnson Laboratories) p 419, 1222
  K-Lyte/Cl & K-Lyte/Cl 50 (Mead Johnson Laboratories) p 419, 1222
  Klorvess Effervescent Granules (Sandoz Pharmaceutical Div.) p 1803
  Klorvess Effervescent Tablets (Sandoz Pharmaceutical Div.) p 433, 1803

Potassium Bitartrate
  Ceo-Two Suppositories (Beutlich) p 705

Potassium Chloride
  Infalyte (Pennwalt) p 1584
  K-Lor Powder (Abbott) p 403, 533
  K-Lyte/Cl & K-Lyte/Cl 50 (Mead Johnson Laboratories) p 419, 1222
  K-Tab (Abbott) p 403, 534
  Kaochlor 10% Liquid (Adria) p 579
  Kaochlor S-F 10% Liquid (Sugar-free) (Adria) p 580
  Kaon Cl-10 (Adria) p 404, 582
  Kaon-Cl Tabs (Adria) p 404, 581
  Kaon-Cl 20% (Adria) p 582
  KATO (Legere) p 1120
  Kay Ciel Oral Solution 10% (Berlex) p 702
  Kay Ciel Powder (Berlex) p 702
  Klor-Con Powder (Upsher-Smith) p 2144
  Klor-Con/25 Powder (Upsher-Smith) p 2144
  Klor-Con 20% (Upsher-Smith) p 2144
  Klor-10% (Upsher-Smith) p 2144
  Klorvess Effervescent Granules (Sandoz Pharmaceutical Div.) p 1803
  Klorvess Effervescent Tablets (Sandoz Pharmaceutical Div.) p 433, 1803
  Klorvess 10% Liquid (Sandoz Pharmaceutical Div.) p 1803
  Klotrix (Mead Johnson Pharmaceutical) p 419, 1251
  Micro-K Extencaps (Robins) p 428, 1653
  Micro-K 10 Extencaps (Robins) p 1653
  Potage (Lemmon) p 1122
  Potassium Chloride Concentrate, Powder & Liquid (Schein) p 1828
  Potassium Chloride (Geneva) p 973
  Potassium Chloride for Oral Solution (Flavored), Oral Solution, Powder (Unflavored) (Roxane) p 1788
  Potassium Chloride Injection (Elkins-Sinn) p 938
  Potassium Chloride Oral Solution, Powder & for Oral Solution (Roxane) p 1793
  Rum-K (Fleming) p 948
  Slow-K (CIBA) p 409, 872

Potassium Citrate
  Alka-Seltzer Effervescent Antacid (Miles Laboratories) p 1395
  Bi-K (USV Pharmaceutical) p 2072
  K-Lyte & K-Lyte DS (Mead Johnson Laboratories) p 419, 1222
  K-Lyte/Cl & K-Lyte/Cl 50 (Mead Johnson Laboratories) p 419, 1222
  Polycitra Syrup (Willen) p 2188
  Polycitra-K Syrup (Willen) p 2189
  Polycitra-LC—Sugar-Free (Willen) p 2188
  Twin-K (Boots) p 724
  Twin-K-Cl (Boots) p 725

Potassium Clavulanate
  Augmentin Tablets & Powder for Oral Suspension (Beecham Laboratories) p 405, 690

Potassium Gluconate
  Bi-K (USV Pharmaceutical) p 2072
  Kaon Elixir, Grape Flavor (Adria) p 580
  Kaon Tablets (Adria) p 404, 581
  Potassium Gluconate Elixir (Roxane) p 1788
  Potassium Gluconate Elixir (Schein) p 1828
  Twin-K (Boots) p 724
  Twin-K-Cl (Boots) p 725

Potassium Guaiacolsulfonate
  Albatussin (Bart) p 685
  Bromanyl Expectorant (Schein) p 1828
  Codiclear DH Syrup (Central Pharmaceuticals) p 836
  Entuss Expectorant Tablets & Liquid (Hauck) p 1001

Potassium Hetacillin
  Versapen Oral Suspension (Bristol) p 755
  Versapen Pediatric Drops (Bristol) p 755
  Versapen-K Capsules (Bristol) p 407, 755

Potassium Iodide
  Iodo-Niacin Tablets (O'Neal, Jones & Feldman) p 1445
  Isuprel Hydrochloride Compound Elixir (Winthrop-Breon) p 2204
  Mudrane Tablets (Poythress) p 1618
  Mudrane-2 Tablets (Poythress) p 1619
  Pediacof (Winthrop-Breon) p 2221
  Pedi-Bath Salts (Pedinol) p 1581
  Pima Syrup (Fleming) p 948
  Potassium Iodide Liquid (Roxane) p 1788
  Quadrinal Tablets & Suspension (Knoll) p 414, 1065
  SSKI (Upsher-Smith) p 2145

Potassium Phosphate, Dibasic
  Neutra-Phos Powder & Capsules (Willen) p 2188
  Neutra-Phos-K Powder & Capsules (Willen) p 2188
  Potassium Phosphates Oral Solution (Roxane) p 1788

Generic and Chemical Name Index

Potassium Phosphate, Monobasic
- K-Phos M.F. (Modified Formula) Tablets (Beach) p 405, 686
- K-Phos Neutral Tablets (Beach) p 405, 686
- K-Phos Original Formula 'Sodium Free' Tablets (Beach) p 405, 686
- Neutra-Phos Powder & Capsules (Willen) p 2188
- Neutra-Phos-K Powder & Capsules (Willen) p 2188
- Potassium Phosphates Oral Solution (Roxane) p 1788
- Thiacide Tablets (Beach) p 405, 687

Potassium Preparations
- Effervescent Potassium Tablets (Schein) p 1828
- K-Lor Powder (Abbott) p 403, 533
- Kaochlor 10% Liquid (Adria) p 579
- Kaochlor S-F 10% Liquid (Sugar-free) (Adria) p 580
- Kaon Cl-10 (Adria) p 404, 582
- Kaon Elixir, Grape Flavor (Adria) p 580
- Kaon Tablets (Adria) p 404, 581
- Kaon-Cl Tabs (Adria) p 404, 581
- Kaon-Cl 20% (Adria) p 582
- Klorvess Effervescent Granules (Sandoz Pharmaceutical Div.) p 1803
- Klorvess Effervescent Tablets (Sandoz Pharmaceutical Div.) p 433, 1803
- Klorvess 10% Liquid (Sandoz Pharmaceutical Div.) p 1803
- Pima Syrup (Fleming) p 948

Potassium Salicylate
- Pabalate-SF Tablets (Robins) p 428, 1655

Povidone-Iodine
- Betadine Aerosol Spray (Purdue Frederick) p 1622
- Betadine Antiseptic Gel (Purdue Frederick) p 1622
- Betadine Disposable Medicated Douche (Purdue Frederick) p 1622
- Betadine Douche (Purdue Frederick) p 1622
- Betadine Helafoam Solution (Purdue Frederick) p 1622
- Betadine Ointment (Purdue Frederick) p 1622
- Betadine Skin Cleanser (Purdue Frederick) p 1622
- Betadine Solution (Purdue Frederick) p 1622
- Betadine Surgical Scrub (Purdue Frederick) p 1622
- Betadine Viscous Formula Antiseptic Gauze Pad (Purdue Frederick) p 1623
- Efodine Ointment (Fougera) p 953
- Summer's Eve Medicated Douche (Fleet) p 948

Pralidoxime Chloride
- Protopam Chloride (Ayerst) p 678

Pramoxine Hydrochloride
- Anusol Ointment (Parke-Davis) p 1484
- Anusol Suppositories (Parke-Davis) p 423, 1484
- Derma-Smoothe/FS (Hill Dermaceuticals) p 1009
- Derma-Sone Cream (Hill Dermaceuticals) p 1009
- F-E-P Creme (Boots) p 717
- Fleet Relief (Fleet) p 947
- Otic-HC Ear Drops (Hauck) p 1001
- Oticol Sterile Ear Drops (Arlo) p 601
- Pramosone Cream, Lotion & Ointment (Ferndale) p 942
- Prax Cream & Lotion (Ferndale) p 942
- proctoFoam/non-steroid (Reed & Carnrick) p 427, 1636
- Tronolane Anesthetic Hemorrhoidal Cream (Ross) p 1781
- Tronolane Anesthetic Hemorrhoidal Suppositories (Ross) p 1781
- Tronothane Hydrochloride (Abbott) p 570
- Zone-A Lotion 1% (UAD Labs.) p 2069

Prazepam
- Centrax (Parke-Davis) p 423, 1487

Praziquantel
- Biltricide (Miles Pharmaceuticals) p 421, 1399

Prazosin Hydrochloride
- Minipress (Pfizer) p 426, 1603
- Minizide Capsules (Pfizer) p 426, 1604

Prednisolone
- Delta-Cortef Tablets (Upjohn) p 2107
- Prednisolone Tablets (Danbury) p 887
- Prednisolone Tablets (Geneva) p 973
- Prednisolone Tablets (Roxane) p 1788
- Prednisolone Tablets (Schein) p 1828

Prednisolone Acetate
- Metimyd Ophthalmic Ointment - Sterile (Schering) p 1860
- Metimyd Ophthalmic Suspension (Schering) p 1860
- Predate 50 (Legere) p 1120

Prednisolone Sodium Phosphate
- Metreton Ophthalmic/Otic Solution-Sterile (Schering) p 1861
- Predate S (Legere) p 1120

Prednisolone Tebutate
- Hydeltra-T.B.A. Suspension (Merck Sharp & Dohme) p 1314
- Predate TBA (Legere) p 1120

Prednisone
- Deltasone Tablets (Upjohn) p 441, 2107
- Liquid Pred Syrup (Muro) p 1421
- Prednisone Tablets (Danbury) p 887
- Prednisone Tablets (Roxane) p 1793
- Prednisone Tablets (Geneva) p 973
- Prednisone Tablets (Schein) p 1828
- SK-Prednisone Tablets (Smith Kline & French) p 1971
- Sterapred Uni-Pak (Mayrand) p 1196

Primaquine Phosphate
- Aralen Phosphate w/Primaquine Phosphate (Winthrop-Breon) p 2191

Primidone
- Mysoline (Ayerst) p 405, 657
- Primidone Tablets (Danbury) p 887
- Primidone Tablets (Geneva) p 973
- Primidone Tablets (Schein) p 1828

Probenecid
- Ampicillin-Probenecid Suspension (Biocraft) p 705
- Benemid Tablets (Merck Sharp & Dohme) p 420, 1268
- ColBENEMID Tablets (Merck Sharp & Dohme) p 420, 1277
- Col-Probenecid Tablets (Danbury) p 887
- Polycillin-PRB (Bristol) p 741
- Principen with Probenecid Capsules (Squibb) p 2013
- Probenecid Tablets (Danbury) p 887
- Probenecid Tablets (Geneva) p 973
- Probenecid Tablets (Schein) p 1828
- Probenecid w/Colchicine Tablets (Geneva) p 973
- Probenecid with Colchicine Tablets (Schein) p 1828
- SK-Probenecid Tablets (Smith Kline & French) p 1971
- Wycillin & Probenecid Tablets & Injection (Wyeth) p 2295

Probucol
- Lorelco (Merrell Dow) p 421, 1368

Procainamide
- Procainamide Capsules (Geneva) p 973

Procainamide Hydrochloride
- Procainamide HCl Capsules (Danbury) p 887
- Procainamide HCl Capsules (Schein) p 1828
- Procan SR (Parke-Davis) p 425, 1564
- Pronestyl Capsules and Tablets (Squibb) p 438, 2017
- Pronestyl Injection (Squibb) p 2018
- Pronestyl-SR Tablets (Squibb) p 438, 2019

Procaine
- Anuject Injection (Hauck) p 1001

Procaine Hydrochloride
- Novocain Hydrochloride (Winthrop-Breon) p 2219
- Novocain Hydrochloride for Spinal Anesthesia (Winthrop-Breon) p 2220
- Procaine HCl Injection (Elkins-Sinn) p 938

Procarbazine Hydrochloride
- Matulane Capsules (Roche) p 430, 1691

Prochlorperazine
- Combid Spansule Capsules (Smith Kline & French) p 436, 1952
- Compazine (Smith Kline & French) p 436, 1953
- Prochlor-Iso Timed Release Capsules (Schein) p 1828
- Prochlorperazine Tablets (Geneva) p 973

Prochlorperazine Edisylate
- Prochlorperazine Edisylate Injection (Elkins-Sinn) p 938
- Prochlorperazine Edisylate in Tubex (Wyeth) p 2288

Prochlorperazine Maleate
- Pro-Iso Capsules (Geneva) p 973

Procyclidine Hydrochloride
- Kemadrin (Burroughs Wellcome) p 408, 792

Progesterone
- Progestasert Intrauterine Contraceptive System (Alza) p 404, 590
- Progesterone 50 (Legere) p 1120

Promazine Hydrochloride
- Sparine Injection in Tubex (Wyeth) p 2288

Promethazine
- Dihydrocodeine Compound Tablets (Schein) p 1828
- Promethazine DM (Ped) Expectorant (Geneva) p 973
- Promethazine Expectorant Plain (Geneva) p 973
- Promethazine w/Codeine Expectorant (Geneva) p 973
- Promethazine VC Expectorant (Geneva) p 973
- Promethazine VC w/Codeine Expectorant (Geneva) p 973

Promethazine Hydrochloride
- Mepergan Injection (Wyeth) p 2264
- Mepergan in Tubex (Wyeth) p 2288
- Phenergan Injection (Wyeth) p 2275
- Phenergan in Tubex (Wyeth) p 2288
- Phenergan Syrup Fortis (Wyeth) p 2276
- Phenergan Syrup Plain (Wyeth) p 2276
- Phenergan Tablets & Rectal Suppositories (Wyeth) p 444,445, 2278
- Phenergan VC (Wyeth) p 2282
- Phenergan VC with Codeine (Wyeth) p 2284
- Phenergan with Codeine (Wyeth) p 2278
- Phenergan with Dextromethorphan (Wyeth) p 2280
- Promet 50 (Legere) p 1120
- Promethazine HCl Injection (Elkins-Sinn) p 938
- Remsed Tablets (Du Pont) p 926

Propantheline Bromide
- Pro-Banthine Tablets (Searle & Co.) p 436, 1936
- Pro-Banthine w/Phenobarbital (Searle & Co.) p 436, 1936
- Propantheline Bromide Tablets (Danbury) p 887
- Propantheline Bromide Tablets (Geneva) p 973
- Propantheline Bromide Tablets (Roxane) p 1788
- Propantheline Bromide Tablets (Schein) p 1828
- SK-Propantheline Bromide Tablets (Smith Kline & French) p 1971

Propiomazine Hydrochloride Injection
- Largon in Tubex (Wyeth) p 2288

Propoxyphene Hydrochloride
- Darvon (Lilly) p 417, 1139
- Darvon Compound (Lilly) p 417, 1139
- Darvon Compound-65 (Lilly) p 417, 1139
- Darvon with A.S.A. (Lilly) p 417, 1139
- Lorcet (UAD Labs.) p 2069
- Propox 65 w/APAP Tablets (Geneva) p 973
- Propoxyphene-AC Capsules (Geneva) p 973
- Propoxyphene & Apap Tablets 65/650 (Schein) p 1828
- Propoxyphene Compound 65 (Schein) p 1828
- Propoxyphene HCl Capsules (Geneva) p 973
- Propoxyphene Hydrochloride Capsules (Roxane) p 1788
- Propoxyphene HCl Capsules (Schein) p 1828
- SK-65 APAP Tablets (Smith Kline & French) p 1971
- SK-65 Capsules (Smith Kline & French) p 1971
- SK-65 Compound Capsules (Smith Kline & French) p 1971
- Wygesic Tablets (Wyeth) p 445, 2297

Propoxyphene Napsylate
- Darvocet-N 50 (Lilly) p 417, 1136
- Darvocet-N 100 (Lilly) p 417, 1136
- Darvon-N (Lilly) p 417, 1136
- Darvon-N with A.S.A. (Lilly) p 417, 1136

Propranolol Hydrochloride
- Inderal Tablets & Injectable (Ayerst) p 405, 647
- Inderal LA Long Acting Capsules (Ayerst) p 405, 650
- Inderide (Ayerst) p 405, 651

Protamine Sulfate
- Protamine Sulfate (Lilly) p 1171
- Protamine Sulfate for Injection, USP, Sterile Powder (Upjohn) p 2133

Protein Preparations
- MARLYN Formula 50 (Marlyn) p 1193

Generic and Chemical Name Index

Plasmatein 5% (Alpha Theapeutic) p 589

Proteolytic Preparations
Arco-Lase (Arco) p 600
Arco-Lase Plus (Arco) p 600
Biozyme-C Ointment (Armour) p 604
Celluzyme Chewable Tablets (Dalin) p 886
Cotazym (Organon) p 422, 1446
Cotazym-S (Organon) p 422, 1446
Festal II (Hoechst-Roussel) p 412, 1014
Festalan (Hoechst-Roussel) p 413, 1014
Gustase (Geriatric) p 975
Kutrase Capsules (Rorer) p 431, 1750
Ku-Zyme Capsules (Rorer) p 431, 1750
Ku-Zyme HP Capsules (Rorer) p 431, 1751
Panafil Ointment (Rystan) p 1796
Panafil-White Ointment (Rystan) p 1796
Pancreatin Tablets 2400 mg. N.F. (High Lipase) (Vitaline) p 2148
Travase Ointment (Flint) p 411, 952
Tri-Cone Capsules (Glaxo) p 986

Protirelin
Relefact TRH (Hoechst-Roussel) p 1017
Thypinone (Abbott Diagnostics Div.) p 3002

Protriptyline Hydrochloride
Vivactil Tablets (Merck Sharp & Dohme) p 421, 1357

Pseudoephedrine Hydrochloride
Actifed with Codeine Cough Syrup (Burroughs Wellcome) p 773
Ambenyl-D Decongestant Cough Formula (Marion) p 1182
Anafed Capsules & Syrup (Everett) p 941
Anamine Syrup (Mayrand) p 1196
Anamine T.D. Caps (Mayrand) p 1196
Brexin L.A. Capsules (Savage) p 433, 1824
Bromfed Capsules (Timed Release) (Muro) p 1420
Bromfed-PD Capsules (Timed Release) (Muro) p 1420
Bromfed Tablets (Muro) p 1420
Cardec DM Drops & Syrup (Schein) p 1828
Chlorafed H.S. Timecelles (Hauck) p 1001
Chlorafed Liquid (Hauck) p 1001
Chlorafed Timecelles (Hauck) p 1001
Codimal-L.A. Capsules (Central Pharmaceuticals) p 409, 836
Congess Jr. & Sr. T.D. Capsules (Fleming) p 948
CoTylenol Cold Medication Tablets & Capsules (McNeil Consumer Products) p 418, 1197
CoTylenol Liquid Cold Medication (McNeil Consumer Products) p 1197
Deconamine Tablets, Elixir, SR Capsules, Syrup (Berlex) p 406, 699
Dorcol Children's Cough Syrup (Dorsey Laboratories) p 909
Dorcol Children's Decongestant Liquid (Dorsey Laboratories) p 909
Dorcol Children's Liquid Cold Formula (Dorsey Laboratories) p 909
Extra-Strength Sine-Aid Sinus Headache Capsules (McNeil Consumer Products) p 1199
Fedahist Expectorant (Rorer) p 1749
Fedahist Gyrocaps, Syrup & Tablets (Rorer) p 431, 1749
Guaifed Capsules (Timed Release) (Muro) p 1421
Histalet DM Syrup (Reid-Provident Labs.) p 1638
Histalet Syrup (Reid-Provident Labs.) p 1638
Histalet X Syrup & Tablets (New Formula) (Reid-Provident Labs.) p 428, 1638
Isoclor Timesule Capsules (Fisons) p 944
Kronofed-A Jr. Kronocaps (Ferndale) p 942
Kronofed-A Kronocaps (Ferndale) p 942
Novafed A Capsules (Merrell Dow) p 421, 1377
Novafed A Liquid (Merrell Dow) p 1377
Novafed Capsules (Merrell Dow) p 421, 1376
Novafed Liquid (Merrell Dow) p 1376
Novahistine DH (Merrell Dow) p 421, 1378
Novahistine Expectorant (Merrell Dow) p 421, 1378
Nucofed Capsules (Beecham Laboratories) p 406, 692
Nucofed Expectorant (Beecham Laboratories) p 693
Nucofed Pediatric Expectorant (Beecham Laboratories) p 694
Nucofed Syrup (Beecham Laboratories) p 692
Poly-Histine-DX Capsules (Bock) p 706
Pseudoephedrine HCl Tablets (Danbury) p 887
Pseudoephedrine Hydrochloride Tablets (Roxane) p 1788
Pseudoephedrine HCl Tablets (Schein) p 1828
Respaire-SR Capsules 60, 120 (Laser) p 1072
Robitussin-DAC (Robins) p 1665
Sine-Aid Extra-Strength Sinus Headache Capsules (McNeil Consumer Products) p 1199
Sine-Aid Sinus Headache Tablets (McNeil Consumer Products) p 1198
Triafed-C Expectorant (Schein) p 1828
Trifed Tablets & Syrup (Geneva) p 973
Tripodrine Tablets (Danbury) p 887
Triprolidine HCl & Pseudoephedrine HCl Syrup (Pharmafair) p 1618
Triprolidine Hydrochloride & Pseudoephedrine Hydrochloride Syrup, Tablets (Roxane) p 1788
Tussend Expectorant (Merrell Dow) p 421, 1394
Tussend Liquid & Tablets (Merrell Dow) p 421, 1393
Tylenol, Maximum-Strength, Sinus Medication Tablets & Capsules (McNeil Consumer Products) p 418, 1201
Zephrex Tablets (Bock) p 706
Zephrex-LA Tablets (Bock) p 706

Pseudoephedrine Sulfate
Trinalin Repetabs Tablets (Schering) p 435, 1890

Pseudoephedrine Preparations
Chlorafed H.S. Timecelles (Hauck) p 1001
Chlorafed Liquid (Hauck) p 1001
Chlorafed Timecelles (Hauck) p 1001
Co-Pyronil 2 (Dista) p 895
Deconamine Tablets, Elixir, SR Capsules, Syrup (Berlex) p 406, 699
Deproist Expectorant w/Codeine (Geneva) p 973
Detussin Expectorant (Schein) p 1828
Detussin Liquid (Schein) p 1828
Disobrom Tablets (Geneva) p 973
Entuss-D Liquid & Tablets (Hauck) p 1001
Fedahist Expectorant (Rorer) p 1749
Fedahist Gyrocaps, Syrup & Tablets (Rorer) p 431, 1749
Poly-Histine-DX Capsules (Bock) p 706
Probahist Capsules (Legere) p 1120
Pseudoephedrine Tablets (Geneva) p 973
Rondec Oral Drops (Ross) p 1776
Rondec Syrup (Ross) p 1776
Rondec Tablet (Ross) p 432, 1776
Rondec-DM Oral Drops (Ross) p 1777
Rondec-DM Syrup (Ross) p 1777
Rondec-TR Tablet (Ross) p 432, 1776
Sinufed Timecelles (Hauck) p 1001
Triafed Syrup & Tablets (Schein) p 1828

Psyllium Preparations
Effersyllium (Stuart) p 2037
Fiberall, Natural Flavor (Rydelle) p 1795
Fiberall, Orange Flavor (Rydelle) p 1795
Konsyl (Lafayette) p 1070
Konsyl-D (formerly L. A. Formula) (Lafayette) p 1070
Metamucil, Instant Mix, Orange Flavor (Searle Consumer Products) p 1912
Metamucil, Instant Mix, Regular Flavor (Searle Consumer Products) p 1911
Metamucil, Powder, Orange Flavor (Searle Consumer Products) p 1911
Metamucil, Powder, Regular Flavor (Searle Consumer Products) p 1911
Metamucil, Powder, Strawberry Flavor (Searle Consumer Products) p 1911
Metamucil, Powder, Sugar Free, Regular Flavor (Searle Consumer Products) p 1911
Modane Bulk (Adria) p 584
Naturacil (Mead Johnson Nutritional) p 1243
Prompt (Searle Consumer Products) p 1912

Pyrantel Pamoate
Antiminth Oral Suspension (Pfipharmecs) p 426, 1589

Pyrethrins
A-200 Pyrinate Pediculicide Shampoo, Liquid & Gel (Norcliff Thayer) p 422, 1422
Pyrinyl Liquid (Schein) p 1828
RID Liquid Pediculicide (Pfipharmecs) p 426, 1593

Pyrethroids
R&C Spray (Reed & Carnrick) p 1637

Pyridostigmine Bromide
Mestinon Injectable (Roche) p 1692
Mestinon Syrup (Roche) p 1692
Mestinon Tablets (Roche) p 430, 1692
Mestinon Timespan Tablets (Roche) p 430, 1692
Regonol (Organon) p 1450

Pyridoxine
Herpecin-L Cold Sore Lip Balm (Campbell) p 829
Rodex T.D. Capsules (Legere) p 1120

Pyridoxine Hydrochloride
Alba-Lybe (Bart) p 685
Al-Vite (Drug Industries) p 914
Beelith Tablets (Beach) p 405, 685
Eldertonic (Mayrand) p 1196
Glutofac Tablets (Kenwood) p 1046
Hemo-Vite (Drug Industries) p 914
Hemo-Vite Liquid (Drug Industries) p 914
Mega-B (Arco) p 600
Neuro B-12 Forte Injectable (Lambda) p 1071
Nu-Iron-V Tablets (Mayrand) p 1196
Rodex (Legere) p 1120
Vicon-C Capsules (Glaxo) p 412, 989
Vicon-Plus Capsules (Glaxo) p 412, 989

Pyrilamine Maleate
Albatussin (Bart) p 685
Citra Forte Capsules (Boyle) p 726
Citra Forte Syrup (Boyle) p 726
Codimal DH (Central Pharmaceuticals) p 836
Codimal DM (Central Pharmaceuticals) p 836
Codimal PH (Central Pharmaceuticals) p 836
Excedrin P.M. (Bristol-Myers Products) p 770
4-Way Nasal Spray (Bristol-Myers Products) p 770
Fiogesic Tablets (Sandoz Pharmaceutical Div.) p 432, 1801
Histalet Forte Tablets (Reid-Provident Labs.) p 428, 1638
Kronohist Kronocaps (Ferndale) p 942
Maximum Strength Midol PMS (Glenbrook) p 997
P-V-Tussin Syrup (Reid-Provident Labs.) p 1640
Poly-Histine-D Capsules (Bock) p 705
Poly-Histine-D Elixir (Bock) p 705
Poly-Histine-D Pediatric Capsules (Bock) p 705
Primatene Tablets-M Formula (Whitehall) p 443, 2187
Ru-Tuss Expectorant (Boots) p 722
Ru-Tuss Plain (Boots) p 723
Ru-Tuss with Hydrocodone (Boots) p 722
Triaminic Juvelets (Dorsey Laboratories) p 912
Triaminic Oral Infant Drops (Dorsey Laboratories) p 912
Triaminic TR Tablets (Timed Release) (Dorsey Laboratories) p 912
WANS (Webcon Anti-Nausea Suppretes) (Webcon) p 2173

Pyrilamine Tannate
Rynatan Tablets & Pediatric Suspension (Wallace) p 442, 2165

Pyrimethamine
Daraprim (Burroughs Wellcome) p 407, 787
Fansidar Tablets (Roche) p 429, 1682

Pyrvinium Pamoate
Povan Filmseals (Parke-Davis) p 425, 1563

Q

Quinacrine Hydrochloride
Atabrine Hydrochloride Tablets (Winthrop-Breon) p 2192

Quinestrol
Estrovis (Parke-Davis) p 424, 1517

Quinethazone
Hydromox R Tablets (Lederle) p 415, 1094
Hydromox Tablets (Lederle) p 415, 1094

Quinidine Gluconate
Duraquin (Parke-Davis) p 423, 1511
Quinaglute Dura-Tabs (Berlex) p 406, 702
Quinidine Gluconate Sustained Action Tablets (Danbury) p 887
Quinidine Gluconate S.R. Tablets (Geneva) p 973
Quinidine Gluconate Sustained Release Tablets (Roxane) p 1788
Quinidine Gluconate Tablets (Schein) p 1828

Quinidine Polygalacturonate
Cardioquin Tablets (Purdue Frederick) p 427, 1623

Quinidine Sulfate
Quinidex Extentabs (Robins) p 428, 1659
Quinidine Sulfate Tablets (Danbury) p 887
Quinidine Sulfate Tablets (Geneva) p 973
Quinidine Sulfate Tablets (Roxane) p 1788
Quinidine Sulfate Tablets (Schein) p 1828
Quinora (Key Pharmaceuticals) p 1051
SK-Quinidine Sulfate Tablets (Smith Kline & French) p 1971

Quinine Sulfate
Quinamm (Merrell Dow) p 421, 1380
Quindan Tablets (Danbury) p 887
Quinine Sulfate Capsules (Geneva) p 973

Generic and Chemical Name Index

Quinine Sulfate Capsules & Tablets (Schein) p 1828
Quiphile Tablets (Geneva) p 973

R

Rabies Antiserum
Antirabies Serum (equine), Purified (Sclavo) p 1897

Rabies Immune Globulin (Human)
Imogam Rabies Immune Globulin (Human) (Merieux) p 1358
Rabies Immune Globulin (Human) Hyperab (Cutter Biological) p 884
Rabies Immune Globulin (Human), Imogam Rabies (Merieux) p 1358

Rabies Vaccine
Imovax Rabies Vaccine (Merieux) (Merieux) p 1358
Rabies Vaccine Human Diploid Cell, Imovax Rabies (Merieux) p 1358
Wyvac Rabies Vaccine (Wyeth) p 2246

Racemethionine
Pedameth Capsules (O'Neal, Jones & Feldman) p 422, 1445
Pedameth Liquid (O'Neal, Jones & Feldman) p 1445

Ranitidine Hydrochloride
Zantac Injection (Glaxo) p 990
Zantac Tablets (Glaxo) p 412, 991

Rauwolfia Preparations
Harmonyl (Abbott) p 532
Raudixin Tablets (Squibb) p 438, 2020
Rauwiloid Tablets (Riker) p 1644

Rauwolfia Serpentina
Raudixin Tablets (Squibb) p 438, 2020
Rauzide Tablets (Squibb) p 438, 2021

Red Petrolatum
RVP Ointment (Elder) p 936
RVPaba Lip Stick (Elder) p 936
RVPaque Ointment (Elder) p 936

Rescinnamine
Moderil (Pfizer) p 426, 1605

Reserpine
Chloroserpine 250 & 500 Tablets (Schein) p 1828
Chlorothiazide w/Reserpine Tablets (Geneva) p 973
Demi-Regroton Tablets (USV Pharmaceutical) p 440, 2087
Diupres Tablets (Merck Sharp & Dohme) p 420, 1298
Diutensen-R Tablets (Wallace) p 442, 2157
H-H-R Tablets (Schein) p 1828
Hydrochlorothiazide, Hydralazine HCl, Reserpine Tablets (Danbury) p 887
Hydrochlorothiazide/Reserpine Tablets (Danbury) p 887
Hydrochlorothiazide w/Reserpine Tablets (Geneva) p 973
Hydroflumethiazide with Reserpine (Geneva) p 973
Hydro-Fluserpine Tablets #1 & #2 (Schein) p 1828
Hydromox R Tablets (Lederle) p 415, 1094
Hydropres Tablets (Merck Sharp & Dohme) p 420, 1317
Hydroserpine Tablets (Schein) p 1828
Metatensin (Merrell Dow) p 421, 1370
Naquival Tablets (Schering) p 434, 1862
Regroton Tablets (USV Pharmaceutical) p 440, 2087
Renese-R (Pfizer) p 426, 1608
Reserpine Tablets (Schein) p 1828
SK-Reserpine Tablets (Smith Kline & French) p 1971
Salutensin/Salutensin-Demi (Bristol) p 407, 748
Ser-Ap-Es (CIBA) p 409, 866
Serpasil Parenteral Solution (CIBA) p 868
Serpasil Tablets (CIBA) p 409, 867
Serpasil-Apresoline (CIBA) p 409, 869
Serpasil-Esidrix (CIBA) p 409, 870
Unipres Tablets (Reid-Provident Labs.) p 428, 1640

Resorcinol
Castellani Paint (Pedinol) p 1580
Derma Cas Gel (Hill Dermaceuticals) p 1009
Night Cast Formula R (Seres) p 1939

Rh₀ (D) Immune Globulin (Human)
Gamulin Rh (Armour) p 613
MICRhoGAM (Ortho Diagnostic Systems) p 1452
Mini-Gamulin Rh (Armour) p 613

Rh₀-D Immune Globulin (Human) HypRho-D (Cutter Biological) p 885
Rh₀-D Immune Globulin (Human) HypRho-D Mini-Dose (Cutter Biological) p 884
RhoGAM (Ortho Diagnostic Systems) p 1453

Riboflavin
(see under Vitamin B₂)

Ricinoleic Acid
Aci-Jel Therapeutic Vaginal Jelly (Ortho Pharmaceutical) p 1453

Rifampin
Rifadin (Merrell Dow) p 421, 1382
Rifamate (Merrell Dow) p 421, 1383
Rimactane Capsules (CIBA) p 409, 864

Ritodrine Hydrochloride
Yutopar Intravenous Injection (Astra) p 632
Yutopar Tablets (Astra) p 632

Rubella & Mumps Virus Vaccine, Live
Biavax ॥ (Merck Sharp & Dohme) p 1269

Rubella Virus Vaccine, Live
Meruvax ॥ (Merck Sharp & Dohme) p 1329

S

Salicylamide
Codalan (Lannett) p 1071
Korigesic Tablets (Trimen) p 2067
Os-Cal-Gesic Tablets (Marion) p 418, 1189
Saleto (Mallard) p 1181
Sinulin Tablets (Carnrick) p 409, 835

Salicylic Acid
Aveenobar Medicated (Cooper Dermatology) p 882
Barseb HC Scalp Lotion (Barnes-Hind) p 683
Barseb Thera-Spray (Barnes-Hind) p 684
Cantharone Plus (Seres) p 1939
Duofilm (Stiefel) p 2035
Fostex Medicated Cleansing Bar (Westwood) p 2177
Fostex Medicated Cleansing Cream (Westwood) p 2177
Fungi-Nail Tincture (Kramer) p 1069
Hydrisalic Gel (Pedinol) p 1580
Keralyt Gel (Westwood) p 2179
Komed Acne Lotion (Barnes-Hind) p 684
Komed HC Lotion (Barnes-Hind) p 684
Night Cast Formula S (Medicated Acne Mask) (Seres) p 1939
Pernox Lotion (Westwood) p 2180
Pernox Medicated Lathering Scrub (Westwood) p 2180
Salactic Film (Pedinol) p 1581
Sebucare (Westwood) p 2181
Sebulex & Sebulex Cream Shampoo (Westwood) p 2181
Sebulex Shampoo with Conditioners (Westwood) p 2181
Sebutone & Sebutone Cream Shampoo (Westwood) p 2181
Tinver Lotion (Barnes-Hind) p 685
Verrex (C & M) p 828
Verrusol (C & M) p 828
Viranol (American Dermal) p 600
Wart-Off (Pfipharmecs) p 426, 1599
Whitfield's Ointment (Fougera) p 953

Salicylsalicylic Acid
Disalcid (Riker) p 428, 1642
Mono-Gesic Tablets (Central Pharmaceuticals) p 409, 837

Scopolamine Hydrobromide
Ru-Tuss Tablets (Boots) p 406, 723
Scopolamine Hydrobromide Injection (Elkins-Sinn) p 938

Scopolamine Preparations
Dallergy Capsules, Tablets, Syrup (Laser) p 1072
Transderm Scōp Transdermal Therapeutic System (CIBA) p 409, 874

Secobarbital Sodium
Secobarbital Sodium in Tubex (Wyeth) p 2288
Seconal Sodium Pulvules & Vials (Lilly) p 417, 1172
Tuinal (Lilly) p 417, 1176

Secretin
Secretin-Kabi (Pharmacia) p 1616

Selenious Acid
Multitrace 5 (Armour) p 608
Selenitrace (Armour) p 610

Selenium
Added Protection III Multi-Vitamin & Multi-Mineral Supplement (Professional Health) p 1621
Enviro-Stress with Zinc & Selenium (Vitaline) p 2148
Selenium Tablets (200 mcg) (Vitaline) p 2148
Total Formula (Vitaline) p 2148

Selenium Sulfide
Exsel Lotion (Herbert) p 1003
Selsun Blue Lotion (Ross) p 1778
Selsun Lotion (Abbott) p 567

Senecio Cineraria Extracts
Succus Cineraria Maritima (Walker Pharmacal) p 2148

Senna
Senokot Syrup (Purdue Frederick) p 1626

Senna Concentrates
Senokot Tablets/Granules (Purdue Frederick) p 1626
Senokot-S Tablets (Purdue Frederick) p 1627
X-Prep Liquid (Gray) p 1000

Shark Liver Oil
Preparation H Hemorrhoidal Ointment (Whitehall) p 443, 2186
Preparation H Hemorrhoidal Suppositories (Whitehall) p 443, 2186

Silicon Dioxide
Cardioguard Natural Lipotropic Dietary Supplement-Powder (Professional Health) p 1621

Silver Nitrate
Silver Nitrate (Lilly) p 1174

Silver Sulfadiazine
Flint SSD Cream (Flint) p 411, 950
Silvadene Cream (Marion) p 1189

Simethicone
Aluminum & Magnesium Hydroxides with Simethicone I (Roxane) p 1788
Aluminum & Magnesium Hydroxides with Simethicone II (Roxane) p 1788
Celluzyme Chewable Tablets (Dalin) p 886
Gelusil-M (Parke-Davis) p 1525
Gelusil-II (Parke-Davis) p 424, 1526
Mygel Suspension (Geneva) p 973
Mylanta Liquid (Stuart) p 439, 2039
Mylanta Tablets (Stuart) p 439, 2039
Mylanta-II Liquid (Stuart) p 439, 2039
Mylanta-II Tablets (Stuart) p 439, 2039
Mylicon Drops (Stuart) p 2039
Mylicon Tablets (Stuart) p 439, 2039
Mylicon-80 Tablets (Stuart) p 439, 2040
Phazyme Tablets (Reed & Carnrick) p 427, 1636
Phazyme-95 Tablets (Reed & Carnrick) p 427, 1636
Phazyme-PB Tablets (Reed & Carnrick) p 427, 1636
Riopan Plus (Ayerst) p 405, 680
Simeco (Wyeth) p 2288
Tri-Cone Capsules (Glaxo) p 986

Skin Test Antigens
Multitest CMI Skin Test Antigens for Cellular Hypersensitivity (Merieux) p 1358, 3013
Skin Test Antigens for Cellular Hypersensitivity, Multitest CMI (Merieux) p 1358, 3013

Sodium Acid Phosphate
K-Phos No. 2 Tablets (Beach) p 405, 686
Uroqid-Acid Tablets (Beach) p 405, 687
Uroqid-Acid No. 2 Tablets (Beach) p 405, 687

Sodium Ampicillin
(see under Ampicillin Sodium)

Sodium Bicarbonate
Ceo-Two Suppositories (Beutlich) p 705
Infalyte (Pennwalt) p 1584
Pedi-Bath Salts (Pedinol) p 1581
Sodium Bicarbonate (Bristol) p 730

Sodium Biphosphate
Sodium Phosphates Oral Solution (Roxane) p 1788
Uro-Phosphate Tablets (Poythress) p 1619

Sodium Borate
Trichotine Liquid, Vaginal Douche (Reed & Carnrick) p 1637

Generic and Chemical Name Index

Sodium Butabarbital
- Butisol Sodium Elixir & Tablets (Wallace) p 442, 2150

Sodium Chloride
- Infalyte (Pennwalt) p 1584
- Pedi-Bath Salts (Pedinol) p 1581
- Sodium Chloride, Bacteriostatic in Tubex (Wyeth) p 2288
- Sodium Chloride Inhalation (Roxane) p 1788
- Sodium Chloride Injection (Preservative-free) (Elkins-Sinn) p 938
- Sodium Chloride Injection, Bacteriostatic (Elkins-Sinn) p 938
- Trichotine Powder, Vaginal Douche (Reed & Carnrick) p 1637

Sodium Citrate
- Alka-Seltzer Effervescent Antacid (Miles Laboratories) p 1395
- Alka-Seltzer Effervescent Pain Reliever and Antacid (Miles Laboratories) p 1395
- Bicitra—Sugar-Free (Willen) p 2187
- Polycitra Syrup (Willen) p 2188
- Polycitra-LC—Sugar-Free (Willen) p 2188
- Tussar SF (USV Pharmaceutical) p 2092
- Tussar-2 (USV Pharmaceutical) p 2092
- Tussirex Sugar-Free (Scot-Tussin) p 1897
- Tussirex Syrup (Scot-Tussin) p 1897

Sodium Cloxacillin Monohydrate (see under Cloxacillin Sodium Monohydrate)

Sodium Dextrothyroxine
- Choloxin (Flint) p 411, 949

Sodium Fluoride
- Fluoritab Tablets & Fluoritab Liquid (Fluoritab) p 953
- Luride Drops (Colgate-Hoyt) p 878
- Luride Lozi-Tabs Tablets (Colgate-Hoyt) p 410, 878
- Pediaflor Drops (Ross) p 1771
- Phos-Flur Oral Rinse/Supplement (Colgate-Hoyt) p 879
- Point-Two Dental Rinse (Colgate-Hoyt) p 880
- Poly-Vi-Flor 1.0 mg Vitamins w/Fluoride Chewable Tablets (Mead Johnson Nutritional) p 1243
- Poly-Vi-Flor 0.5 mg Vitamins w/Fluoride Drops (Mead Johnson Nutritional) p 1244
- Poly-Vi-Flor 1.0 mg Vitamins w/Iron & Fluoride Chewable Tablets (Mead Johnson Nutritional) p 1245
- Polyvitamin-Fluoride Drops & Tablets (Schein) p 1828
- PreviDent Brush-On Gel (Colgate-Hoyt) p 880
- Thera-Flur Gel-Drops (Colgate-Hoyt) p 880
- Tri-Vi-Flor 1.0 mg Vitamins w/Fluoride Chewable Tablets (Mead Johnson Nutritional) p 1246
- Tri-Vi-Flor 0.25 mg Vitamins w/Fluoride Drops (Mead Johnson Nutritional) p 1247
- Tri-Vi-Flor 0.5 mg Vitamins w/Fluoride Drops (Mead Johnson Nutritional) p 1247

Sodium Hyaluronate
- Healon (Pharmacia) p 1615

Sodium Lauryl Sulfate
- Peri-Wash (Sween) p 2048
- Surgi-Kleen (Sween) p 2048
- Trichotine Liquid, Vaginal Douche (Reed & Carnrick) p 1637
- Trichotine Powder, Vaginal Douche (Reed & Carnrick) p 1637

Sodium Levothyroxine
- Levothroid for Injection (USV Pharmaceutical) p 440, 2079
- Levothroid Tablets (USV Pharmaceutical) p 440, 2080
- Synthroid (Flint) p 411, 951
- Thyrolar Tablets (USV Pharmaceutical) p 440, 2091

Sodium Liothyronine
- Thyrolar Tablets (USV Pharmaceutical) p 440, 2091

Sodium Monobasic
- Uro-KP-Neutral (Star) p 2035

Sodium Nitroprusside
- Nipride Injectable (Roche) p 1693
- Nitropress (Abbott) p 546
- Sodium Nitroprusside Injection (Elkins-Sinn) p 938

Sodium Oxychlorosene
- Clorpactin WCS-90 (Guardian) p 1000

Sodium Pentobarbital
- Nembutal Sodium Capsules (Abbott) p 403, 538
- Nembutal Sodium Solution (Abbott) p 541
- Nembutal Sodium Suppositories (Abbott) p 543
- Pentobarbital Sodium Injection (Elkins-Sinn) p 938
- Pentobarbital Sodium in Tubex (Wyeth) p 2288
- WANS (Webcon Anti-Nausea Suppretes) (Webcon) p 2173

Sodium Perborate
- Trichotine Powder, Vaginal Douche (Reed & Carnrick) p 1637

Sodium Phosphate
- Fleet Enema (Fleet) p 946
- Fleet Phospho-Soda (Fleet) p 947
- Fleet Prep Kits (Fleet) p 947
- Sodium Phosphates Oral Solution (Roxane) p 1788

Sodium Phosphate, Dibasic
- Fleet Enema (Fleet) p 946
- Fleet Phospho-Soda (Fleet) p 947
- Fleet Prep Kits (Fleet) p 947
- K-Phos Neutral Tablets (Beach) p 405, 686
- Neutra-Phos Powder & Capsules (Willen) p 2188

Sodium Phosphate, Monobasic
- K-Phos M.F. (Modified Formula) Tablets (Beach) p 405, 686
- K-Phos Neutral Tablets (Beach) p 405, 686
- K-Phos No. 2 Tablets (Beach) p 405, 686
- Neutra-Phos Powder & Capsules (Willen) p 2188
- Uroqid-Acid Tablets (Beach) p 405, 687
- Uroqid-Acid No. 2 Tablets (Beach) p 405, 687

Sodium Polystyrene Sulfonate
- Kayexalate (Winthrop-Breon) p 2204
- Sodium Polystyrene Sulfonate Suspension (Roxane) p 1794

Sodium Propionate
- Amino-Cerv (Milex) p 1415

Sodium Salicylate
- Pabalate Tablets (Robins) p 428, 1654
- Tussirex Sugar-Free (Scot-Tussin) p 1897
- Tussirex Syrup (Scot-Tussin) p 1897

Sodium Sulfacetamide
- Metimyd Ophthalmic Ointment - Sterile (Schering) p 1860
- Metimyd Ophthalmic Suspension (Schering) p 1860
- Sulfacet-R Acne Lotion (Dermik) p 891

Sodium Sulfate
- GoLYTELY (Braintree) p 727
- Pedi-Bath Salts (Pedinol) p 1581

Sodium Tetradecyl Sulfate
- Sotradecol Injection (Elkins-Sinn) p 941

Sodium Thiopental
- Pentothal (Abbott) p 562

Sodium Thiosulfate
- Komed Acne Lotion (Barnes-Hind) p 684
- Komed HC Lotion (Barnes-Hind) p 684
- Tinver Lotion (Barnes-Hind) p 685

Somatropin
- Asellacrin (somatropin) (Serono) p 1940
- Crescormon (Pharmacia) p 1616

Soybean Preparations
- Isomil (Ross) p 1767
- Isomil SF (Ross) p 1768
- Isomil SF 20 (Ross) p 1777
- RCF (Ross) p 1775

Spectinomycin Hydrochloride
- Trobicin Sterile Powder (Upjohn) p 2141

Spironolactone
- Aldactazide (Searle & Co.) p 435, 1912
- Aldactone (Searle & Co.) p 435, 1914
- Spironazide Tablets (Schein) p 1828
- Spironolactone Tablets (Geneva) p 973
- Spironolactone Tablets (Schein) p 1828
- Spironolactone Tablets, USP (Parke-Davis) p 1569
- Spironolactone/Hydrochlorothiazide Tablets (Danbury) p 887
- Spironolactone w/Hydrochlorothiazide Tablets (Geneva) p 973
- Spironolactone w/Hydrochlorothiazide Tablets (Parke-Davis) p 1570

Stanozolol
- Winstrol (Winthrop-Breon) p 444, 2232

Staphylococcus Bacterial Antigen
- Staphage Lysate (SPL) (Delmont) p 888

Staphylococcus Vaccine
- Staphage Lysate (SPL) (Delmont) p 888

Streptokinase
- Kabikinase (Pharmacia) p 1616
- Streptase (Hoechst-Roussel) p 1018

Streptomycin Sulfate
- Streptomycin Sulfate Injection (Pfipharmecs) p 1593

Succinylcholine Chloride
- Anectine (Burroughs Wellcome) p 778

Sucralfate
- Carafate Tablets (Marion) p 417, 1182

Sufentanil Citrate
- Sufenta (Janssen) p 413, 1040

Sulfabenzamide
- Sultrin Triple Sulfa Cream (Ortho Pharmaceutical) p 1472
- Sultrin Triple Sulfa Vaginal Tablets (Ortho Pharmaceutical) p 1472
- Triple Sulfa Vaginal Cream (Fougera) p 953
- Triple Sulfa Vaginal Cream (Schein) p 1828
- Trysul (Savage) p 1827

Sulfacetamide
- Sultrin Triple Sulfa Cream (Ortho Pharmaceutical) p 1472
- Sultrin Triple Sulfa Vaginal Tablets (Ortho Pharmaceutical) p 1472
- Triple Sulfa Vaginal Cream (Fougera) p 953
- Triple Sulfa Vaginal Cream (Schein) p 1828
- Trysul (Savage) p 1827

Sulfacetamide Sodium
- Sodium Sulamyd Ophthalmic Solutions & Ointment-Sterile (Schering) p 1884
- Sulfacetamide Sodium Ophthalmic Ointment (Fougera) p 953

Sulfacytine
- Renoquid (Glenwood) p 412, 999

Sulfadoxine
- Fansidar Tablets (Roche) p 429, 1682

Sulfamethizole
- Thiosulfil Duo-Pak (Ayerst) p 682
- Thiosulfil Forte (Ayerst) p 405, 680
- Thiosulfil Tablets (Ayerst) p 405
- Thiosulfil-A Forte (Ayerst) p 405, 681
- Thiosulfil-A Tablets (Ayerst) p 405, 681
- Urobiotic-250 (Roerig) p 431, 1744

Sulfamethoxazole
- Azo Gantanol Tablets (Roche) p 429, 1670
- Bactrim DS Tablets (Roche) p 429, 1674
- Bactrim I.V. Infusion (Roche) p 1672
- Bactrim Pediatric Suspension (Roche) p 1674
- Bactrim Suspension (Roche) p 1674
- Bactrim Tablets (Roche) p 429, 1674
- Cotrim (Lemmon) p 1122
- Cotrim D.S. (Lemmon) p 1122
- Gantanol DS Tablets (Roche) p 429, 1685
- Gantanol Suspension (Roche) p 1685
- Gantanol Tablets (Roche) p 429, 1685
- Septra DS Tablets (Burroughs Wellcome) p 408, 815
- Septra I.V. Infusion (Burroughs Wellcome) p 813
- Septra Suspension (Burroughs Wellcome) p 815
- Septra Tablets (Burroughs Wellcome) p 408, 815
- Sulfamethoxazole Tablets (Geneva) p 973
- Sulfamethoxazole & Trimethoprim Pediatric Suspension (Biocraft) p 705
- Sulfamethoxazole and Trimethoprim Tablets (Biocraft) p 705
- Sulfamethoxazole with Trimethoprim Tablets (Danbury) p 887
- Sulfamethoxazole with Trimethoprim Tablets (Double Strength) (Danbury) p 887
- Sulfamethoxazole w/Trimethoprim DS (Geneva) p 973
- Sulfamethoxazole w/Trimethoprim SS (Geneva) p 973
- Sulfatrim & Sulfatrim D/S Tablets (Schein) p 1828

Sulfanilamide
- AVC Cream (Merrell Dow) p 1358
- AVC Suppositories (Merrell Dow) p 1358
- Vagimide Cream (Legere) p 1120
- Vaginal Sulfa Suppositories (Schein) p 1828

Generic and Chemical Name Index

Sulfasalazine
 Azulfidine Tablets, EN-tabs, Oral Suspension (Pharmacia) p 427, 1613
 Sulfasalazine Tablets (Danbury) p 887
 Sulfasalazine Tablets (Geneva) p 973
 Sulfasalazine Tablets (Schein) p 1828

Sulfathiazole
 Sultrin Triple Sulfa Cream (Ortho Pharmaceutical) p 1472
 Sultrin Triple Sulfa Vaginal Tablets (Ortho Pharmaceutical) p 1472
 Triple Sulfa Vaginal Cream (Fougera) p 953
 Triple Sulfa Vaginal Cream (Schein) p 1828
 Trysul (Savage) p 1827

Sulfinpyrazone
 Anturane Tablets & Capsules (CIBA) p 409, 842
 Sulfinpyrazone Tablets (Danbury) p 887
 Sulfinpyrazone Tablets (Schein) p 1828

Sulfisoxazole
 Azo Gantrisin Tablets (Roche) p 429, 1671
 Gantrisin Tablets (Roche) p 429, 1686
 Pediazole (Ross) p 1774
 SK-Soxazole Tablets (Smith Kline & French) p 1971
 Sulfisoxazole Tablets (Geneva) p 973
 Sulfisoxazole Tablets (Schein) p 1828

Sulfisoxazole Diolamine
 Gantrisin Injectable (Roche) p 1686
 Gantrisin Ophthalmic Ointment/Solution (Roche) p 1685

Sulfur
 Aveenobar Medicated (Cooper Dermatology) p 882
 Hill Cortac (Hill Dermaceuticals) p 1009
 Night Cast Formula R (Seres) p 1939
 Night Cast Formula S (Medicated Acne Mask) (Seres) p 1939
 Pedi-Bath Salts (Pedinol) p 1581
 Sulfacet-R Acne Lotion (Dermik) p 891
 Transact (Westwood) p 2183

Sulfur (Colloidal)
 Bensulfoid Lotion (Poythress) p 1618

Sulfur Preparations
 Fostex Medicated Cleansing Bar (Westwood) p 2177
 Fostex Medicated Cleansing Cream (Westwood) p 2177
 Fostril (Westwood) p 2178
 Intraderm-19 Emergency Acne Stick (Robertson/Taylor) p 1645
 Pernox Lotion (Westwood) p 2180
 Pernox Medicated Lathering Scrub (Westwood) p 2180
 Sebulex & Sebulex Cream Shampoo (Westwood) p 2181
 Sebulex Shampoo with Conditioners (Westwood) p 2181
 Sebutone & Sebutone Cream Shampoo (Westwood) p 2181
 Xerac (Persön & Covey) p 1588

Sulfurated Lime
 Vlemasque (Dermik) p 891

Sulindac
 Clinoril Tablets (Merck Sharp & Dohme) p 420, 1274

Sutilains
 Travase Ointment (Flint) p 411, 952

T

Talbutal
 Lotusate Caplets (Winthrop-Breon) p 2206

Tamoxifen Citrate
 Nolvadex Tablets (Stuart) p 439, 2040

Tannic Acid
 Dalidyne (Dalin) p 886
 Gumsol (Arlo) p 601

Tar Preparations
 Alphosyl Lotion, Cream (Reed & Carnrick) p 1632
 Balnetar (Westwood) p 2175
 DHS Tar Shampoo (Persön & Covey) p 1587
 Estar Gel (Westwood) p 2176
 Fototar Cream 1.6% (Elder) p 931
 Fototar Stik 5% (Elder) p 931
 Sebutone & Sebutone Cream Shampoo (Westwood) p 2181
 Zetar Emulsion (Dermik) p 892
 Zetar Shampoo (Dermik) p 892

Temazepam
 Restoril Capsules (Sandoz Pharmaceutical Div.) p 433, 1810

Terbutaline Sulfate
 Brethine (Geigy) p 411, 955
 Brethine Ampuls (Geigy) p 956
 Bricanyl Injection (Merrell Dow) p 421, 1361
 Bricanyl Tablets (Merrell Dow) p 421, 1361

Terpin Hydrate
 SK-Terpin Hydrate and Codeine Elixir (Smith Kline & French) p 1971
 Terpin Hydrate & Codeine Elixir (Roxane) p 1788

Testolactone
 Teslac Tablets (Squibb) p 2023

Testosterone
 Testosterone Suspension (Legere) p 1120

Testosterone Cypionate
 Depo-Testosterone (Upjohn) p 2111
 T-Cypionate (Legere) p 1120

Testosterone Enanthate
 Ditate-DS (Savage) p 1824
 Testaval 90/4 (Legere) p 1120

Tetanus Antitoxin
 Tetanus Antitoxin (equine), Refined (Sclavo) p 1897
 Tetanus Immune Globulin (Human) Hyper-Tet (Cutter Biological) p 884

Tetanus & Diphtheria Toxoids Adsorbed (For Adult Use)
 Tetanus & Diphtheria Toxoids, Adsorbed Purogenated (Lederle) p 1118
 Tetanus & Diphtheria Toxoids, Adsorbed (For Adult Use) (Sclavo) p 1897

Tetanus & Diphtheria Toxoids Combined, Aluminum Phosphate Adsorbed (For Adult Use)
 Tetanus & Diphtheria Toxoids Adsorbed (Adult) (Wyeth) p 2246
 Tetanus & Diphtheria Toxoids Adsorbed (Adult) in Tubex (Wyeth) p 2288

Tetanus & Diphtheria Toxoids Combined, Aluminum Potassium Sulfate Adsorbed (For Adult Use)
 Tetanus & Diphtheria Toxoids Adsorbed (For Adult Use) (Squibb/Connaught) p 2033

Tetanus Immune Globulin (Human)
 Homo-Tet (Savage) p 1825
 Tetanus Immune Globulin (Human) (Wyeth) p 2246
 Tetanus Immune Globulin (Human) in Tubex (Wyeth) p 2288
 Tetanus Immune Globulin (Human) Hyper-Tet (Cutter Biological) p 884

Tetanus Toxoid, Aluminum Hydroxide Adsorbed
 Tetanus Toxoid, Adsorbed (Sclavo) p 1897

Tetanus Toxoid, Aluminum Phosphate Adsorbed
 Tetanus Toxoid Adsorbed, Aluminum Phosphate Adsorbed, Ultrafined (Wyeth) p 2246
 Tetanus Toxoid Adsorbed, Aluminum Phosphate Adsorbed, Ultrafined in Tubex (Wyeth) p 2288

Tetanus Toxoid, Aluminum Potassium Sulfate Adsorbed
 Tetanus Toxoid Adsorbed (Squibb/Connaught) p 2033

Tetanus Toxoid, Fluid
 Tetanus Toxoid (Squibb/Connaught) p 2033
 Tetanus Toxoid Fluid, Purified, Ultrafined (Wyeth) p 2246
 Tetanus Toxoid Fluid, Purified, Ultrafined in Tubex (Wyeth) p 2288

Tetracaine Hydrochloride
 Cetacaine Topical Anesthetic (Cetylite) p 839
 Pontocaine Hydrochloride for Spinal Anesthesia (Winthrop-Breon) p 2225

Tetracycline
 Achromycin V Oral Suspension (Lederle) p 1076
 Mysteclin-F Capsules (Squibb) p 438, 2005
 Mysteclin-F Syrup (Squibb) p 2005
 SK-Tetracycline Syrup (Smith Kline & French) p 1971
 Sumycin Syrup (Squibb) p 2022

Tetracycline HCl Capsules (Cyclopar) (Parke-Davis) p 425, 1573
 Tetracycline HCl Capsules (Cyclopar 500) (Parke-Davis) p 425, 1573

Tetracycline Hydrochloride
 Achromycin Intramuscular (Lederle) p 1074
 Achromycin Intravenous (Lederle) p 1074
 Achromycin Ophthalmic Ointment (Lederle) p 1077
 Achromycin Ophthalmic Suspension 1% (Lederle) p 1075
 Achromycin 3% Ointment (Lederle) p 1077
 Achromycin V Capsules (Lederle) p 414, 1076
 Mysteclin-F Capsules (Squibb) p 438, 2005
 Mysteclin-F Syrup (Squibb) p 2005
 SK-Tetracycline Capsules (Smith Kline & French) p 1971
 Sumycin Capsules (Squibb) p 438, 2022
 Sumycin Tablets (Squibb) p 438, 2022
 Tetracycline HCl Capsules (Danbury) p 887
 Tetracycline HCl Capsules & Syrup (Schein) p 1828
 Topicycline (Norwich Eaton) p 1438

Tetrahydrozoline Hydrochloride
 Collyrium 2 Eye Drops with Tetrahydrozoline (Wyeth) p 2249
 Murine Plus Eye Drops (Ross) p 1769
 Tyzine (Key Pharmaceuticals) p 1056

Theophyllinate
 Eclabron Elixir (Wharton) p 2184

Theophylline
 Accurbron (Merrell Dow) p 1359
 Aerolate Liquid (Fleming) p 948
 Aerolate Sr. & Jr. & III Capsules (Fleming) p 948
 Aquaphyllin Syrup (Ferndale) p 942
 Bronkolixir (Winthrop-Breon) p 2193
 Bronkotabs (Winthrop-Breon) p 2194
 Constant-T Tablets (Geigy) p 411, 958
 Elixicon Suspension (Berlex) p 406, 699
 Elixophyllin Capsules (Berlex) p 406, 699
 Elixophyllin Elixir (Berlex) p 699
 Elixophyllin SR Capsules (Berlex) p 406, 699
 Elixophyllin-GG (Berlex) p 406, 702
 Isuprel Hydrochloride Compound Elixir (Winthrop-Breon) p 2204
 LABID 250 mg Tablets (Norwich Eaton) p 1436
 Lodrane Capsules-130 & 260 (Poythress) p 1618
 Marax Tablets & DF Syrup (Roerig) p 431, 1737
 Mersalyl-Theophylline (Legere) p 1120
 Mudrane GG Elixir (Poythress) p 1619
 Primatene Tablets-M Formula (Whitehall) p 443, 2187
 Primatene Tablets-P Formula (Whitehall) p 443, 2187
 Quibron & Quibron-300 (Mead Johnson Laboratories) p 419, 1233
 Quibron Plus (Mead Johnson Laboratories) p 419, 1236
 Quibron-T & Quibron-T/SR (Mead Johnson Laboratories) p 419, 1236
 Respbid (Boehringer Ingelheim) p 406, 712
 Slo-bid Gyrocaps (Rorer) p 432, 1754
 Slo-Phyllin Gyrocaps, Tablets (Rorer) p 432, 1756
 Slo-Phyllin 80 Syrup (Rorer) p 1756
 Slo-Phyllin GG Capsules, Syrup (Rorer) p 432, 1759
 Somophyllin-CRT Capsules (Fisons) p 945
 Somophyllin-T Capsules (Fisons) p 945
 Sustaire Tablets (Roerig) p 431, 1743
 Synophylate Elixir (Central Pharmaceuticals) p 839
 Synophylate-GG Tablets/Syrup (Central Pharmaceuticals) p 839
 T.E.H. Tablets (Geneva) p 973
 T-E-P Tablets (Schein) p 1828
 T.E.P. Tablets (Geneva) p 973
 Tedral Elixir & Suspension (Parke-Davis) p 1573
 Tedral SA Tablets (Parke-Davis) p 425, 1573
 Theobid, Theobid Jr. Duracap (Glaxo) p 412, 982
 Theoclear L.A.-130 & -260 Capsules (Central Pharmaceuticals) p 409, 839
 Theoclear-80 Syrup (Central Pharmaceuticals) p 839
 Theo-Dur Sprinkle (Key Pharmaceuticals) p 414, 1051
 Theo-Dur Tablets (Key Pharmaceuticals) p 414, 1051
 Theofedral Tablets (Danbury) p 887
 Theolair & Theolair-SR (Riker) p 428, 1645
 Theolair-Plus Tablets & Liquid (Riker) p 428, 1645
 Theon (Bock) p 706
 Theo-Organidin Elixir (Wallace) p 442, 2170
 Theophyl Chewable Tablets (McNeil Pharmaceutical) p 1207

Generic and Chemical Name Index

Theophylline Elixir (Geneva) p 973
Theophylline Elixir & KI Elixir (Schein) p 1828
Theophylline Oral Solution (Roxane) p 1788
Theophylline S.R. Tablets (Geneva) p 973
Theophyl-SR (McNeil Pharmaceutical) p 1208
Theophyl-225 Elixir (McNeil Pharmaceutical) p 1210
Theophyl-225 Tablets (McNeil Pharmaceutical) p 1210
Theospan-SR Capsules 130 mg., 260 mg. (Laser) p 1072
Theostat 80 Syrup (Laser) p 1072
Theozine Syrup & Tablets - Dye-Free (Schein) p 1828

Theophylline Anhydrous
Bronkodyl (Winthrop-Breon) p 2193
Theo-24 (Searle & Co.) p 436, 1937
Theophylline Anhydrous Tablets (Schein) p 1828
Theovent Long-Acting Capsules (Schering) p 435, 1886
Uniphyl 200 mg Tablets (Purdue Frederick) p 427, 1627
Uniphyl 400 mg Tablets (Purdue Frederick) p 427, 1629

Theophylline Calcium Salicylate
Quadrinal Tablets & Suspension (Knoll) p 414, 1065

Theophylline Dihydroxypropyl (Glyceryl)
(see under Dyphylline)

Theophylline Ethylenediamine
(see under Aminophylline)

Theophylline Sodium Glycinate
Asbron G Elixir (Sandoz Pharmaceutical Div.) p 1796
Asbron G Inlay-Tabs (Sandoz Pharmaceutical Div.) p 432, 1796
Synophylate Elixir (Central Pharmaceuticals) p 839
Synophylate-GG Tablets/Syrup (Central Pharmaceuticals) p 839

Thiabendazole
Mintezol Chewable Tablets & Suspension (Merck Sharp & Dohme) p 420, 1332

Thiamine Hydrochloride
Albafort Injectable (Bart) p 685
Alba-Lybe (Bart) p 685
Eldercaps (Mayrand) p 1196
Eldertonic (Mayrand) p 1196
Geravite Elixir (Hauck) p 1001
Glutofac Tablets (Kenwood) p 1046
I.L.X. B$_{12}$ Elixir Crystalline (Kenwood) p 1046
I.L.X. B$_{12}$ Tablets (Kenwood) p 1046
Neuro B-12 Forte Injectable (Lambda) p 1071
Neuro B-12 Injectable (Lambda) p 1071
Thiamine HCl Injection (Elkins-Sinn) p 938
Thiamine HCl in Tubex (Wyeth) p 2288
Tia-Doce Injectable Solution (Bart) p 685

Thiamine Mononitrate
Mega-B (Arco) p 600
Megadose (Arco) p 600
Nu-Iron-V Tablets (Mayrand) p 1196
Prenate 90 Tablets (Bock) p 706
Vicon-C Capsules (Glaxo) p 412, 989

Thiamylal Sodium
Surital (Parke-Davis) p 1572

Thiethylperazine
Torecan Injection (Ampuls) (Boehringer Ingelheim) p 716
Torecan Suppositories (Boehringer Ingelheim) p 716
Torecan Tablets (Boehringer Ingelheim) p 406, 716

Thioguanine
Tabloid Brand Thioguanine (Burroughs Wellcome) p 408, 817

Thioridazine
Mellaril (Sandoz Pharmaceutical Div.) p 433, 1804
Mellaril-S (Sandoz Pharmaceutical Div.) p 1804
Thioridazine Tablets (Geneva) p 973
Thioridazine Tablets (Schein) p 1828

Thioridazine Hydrochloride
SK-Thioridazine Hydrochloride Tablets (Smith Kline & French) p 1971
Thioridazine HCl Tablets (Danbury) p 887
Thioridazine Hydrochloride Tablets (Roxane) p 1788

Thiotepa
Thiotepa (Lederle) p 416, 1118

Thiothixene
Navane Capsules and Concentrate (Roerig) p 431, 1737
Navane Intramuscular (Roerig) p 1739

Thioxanthene Derivatives
Navane Capsules and Concentrate (Roerig) p 431, 1737
Navane Intramuscular (Roerig) p 1739

Thrombin
Thrombinar (Armour) p 613
Thrombostat (Parke-Davis) p 1574

Thymol
Bensulfoid Lotion (Poythress) p 1618

Thyroglobulin
Proloid Tablets (Parke-Davis) p 425, 1565

Thyroid
Armour Thyroid Tablets (USV Pharmaceutical) p 440, 2089
Cytomel Tablets (Smith Kline & French) p 436, 1956
Euthroid (Parke-Davis) p 424, 1520
Levothroid for Injection (USV Pharmaceutical) p 440, 2079
Levothroid Tablets (USV Pharmaceutical) p 440, 2080
Proloid Tablets (Parke-Davis) p 425, 1565
S-P-T (Fleming) p 949
Synthroid (Flint) p 411, 951
Thyroid Strong Tablets (Marion) p 418, 1190
Thyroid Tablets (Marion) p 418, 1190
Thyrolar Tablets (USV Pharmaceutical) p 440, 2091

Thyrotropic Hormone
Thytropar (Armour) p 612

Thyroxine
Choloxin (Flint) p 411, 949
Euthroid (Parke-Davis) p 424, 1520
Levothroid for Injection (USV Pharmaceutical) p 440, 2079
Levothroid Tablets (USV Pharmaceutical) p 440, 2080
Synthroid (Flint) p 411, 951
Thyrolar Tablets (USV Pharmaceutical) p 440, 2091
L-Thyroxine Tablets (Schein) p 1828

Thyroxine Sodium
Choloxin (Flint) p 411, 949
Synthroid (Flint) p 411, 951

Ticarcillin Disodium
Ticar (Beecham Laboratories) p 695

Timolol Maleate
Blocadren Tablets (Merck Sharp & Dohme) p 420, 1271
Timolide Tablets (Merck Sharp & Dohme) p 420, 1346
Timoptic Sterile Ophthalmic Solution (Merck Sharp & Dohme) p 1349

Titanium Dioxide
Intraderm-19 Emergency Acne Stick (Robertson/Taylor) p 1645

Tobramycin Sulfate
Nebcin (Dista) p 905
Nebcin, Sterile (Dista) p 907

Tocainide Hydrochloride
Tonocard (Merck Sharp & Dohme) p 421, 1351

Tolazamide
Tolinase Tablets (Upjohn) p 441, 2139

Tolazoline Hydrochloride
Priscoline Hydrochloride Multiple-Dose Vials (CIBA) p 862

Tolbutamide
Orinase Tablets (Upjohn) p 441, 2130
SK-Tolbutamide Tablets (Smith Kline & French) p 1971
Tolbutamide Tablets (Danbury) p 887
Tolbutamide Tablets (Geneva) p 973
Tolbutamide Tablets (Schein) p 1828

Tolmetin Sodium
Tolectin Tablets & DS Capsules (McNeil Pharmaceutical) p 419, 1212

Tranylcypromine Sulfate
Parnate (Smith Kline & French) p 437, 1969

Trazodone Hydrochloride
Desyrel (Mead Johnson Pharmaceutical) p 419, 1249

Tretinoin
Retin-A (tretinoin) (Ortho Pharmaceutical (Dermatological Div.)) p 1475

Triacetin
Enzactin Cream (Ayerst) p 642
Fungoid Creme & Solution (Pedinol) p 1580
Fungoid Tincture (Pedinol) p 1580

Triamcinolone
Aristocort Tablets (Lederle) p 414, 1078
Nystatin-Neomycin-Gramicidin-Triamcinolone Cream & Ointment (Fougera) p 953
Triamcinolone Tablets (Danbury) p 887
Triamcinolone Tablets (Geneva) p 973
Triamcinolone Tablets (Schein) p 1828

Triamcinolone Acetonide
Aristocort A Topical Cream & Ointment (Lederle) p 414, 415, 1084
Aristocort Topical Products (Lederle) p 414, 415, 1080
Azmacort Inhaler (Rorer) p 431, 1746
Cinonide 40 (Legere) p 1120
Kenalog Cream/Lotion/Ointment (Squibb) p 1998
Kenalog in Orabase (Squibb) p 2003
Kenalog Spray (Squibb) p 1998
Kenalog-10 Injection (Squibb) p 2001
Kenalog-40 Injection (Squibb) p 1999
Mycolog Cream and Ointment (Squibb) p 2003
Myco-Triacet Cream and Ointment (Lemmon) p 1122
Mytrex Cream & Ointment (Savage) p 1825
Nyst-olone Cream & Ointment (Schein) p 1828
Triamcinair Cream (Pharmafair) p 1618
Triamcinolone Acetonide Cream 0.5% (Fougera) p 953
Triamcinolone Acetonide Cream (Geneva) p 973
Triamcinolone Acetonide Cream (Schein) p 1828
Triamcinolone Acetonide Cream & Ointment 0.025% & 0.1% (Fougera) p 953
Triamcinolone Acetonide Cream & Ointment (Pharmaderm) p 1617
Trymex Cream & Ointment (Savage) p 1827

Triamcinolone Diacetate
Aristocort Forte Parenteral (Lederle) p 1081
Aristocort Intralesional (Lederle) p 1081
Aristocort Syrup (Lederle) p 1078
Cinalone 40 (Legere) p 1120

Triamcinolone Hexacetonide
Aristospan Parenteral 20 mg./ml (Lederle) p 1085
Aristospan Parenteral 5 mg./ml (Lederle) p 1085

Triamterene
Dyazide (Smith Kline & French) p 437, 1961
Dyrenium (Smith Kline & French) p 436, 1963
Maxzide Tablets (Lederle) p 415, 1098

Triazolam
Halcion Tablets (Upjohn) p 441, 2114

Trichlormethiazide
Metahydrin (Merrell Dow) p 421, 1370
Metatensin (Merrell Dow) p 421, 1370
Naqua Tablets (Schering) p 434, 1861
Naquival Tablets (Schering) p 434, 1862
Trichlormethiazide Tablets (Geneva) p 973
Trichlormethiazide Tablets (Schein) p 1828

Tridihexethyl Chloride
Pathibamate (Lederle) p 415, 1110
Pathilon (Lederle) p 415, 1112

Triethanolamine Polypeptide Oleate-Condensate
Cerumenex Drops (Purdue Frederick) p 1624

Triethanolamine Salicylate
Aspercreme (Thompson Medical) p 2066
Myoflex Creme (Topical Analgesic) (Adria) p 585

Triethylenethiophosphoramide
Thiotepa (Lederle) p 416, 1118

Trifluoperazine Hydrochloride
Stelazine (Smith Kline & French) p 437, 1971
Trifluoperazine Tablets (Geneva) p 973
Trifluoperazine Tablets (Schein) p 1828

Trifluorothymidine
(see under Trifluridine)

Trifluridine
Viroptic Ophthalmic Solution (Burroughs Wellcome) p 820

Generic and Chemical Name Index

Trihexyphenidyl Hydrochloride
  Trihexyphenidyl HCl Tablets (Danbury) p 887
Trihexyphenidyl Preparations
  Artane Elixir (Lederle) p 1087
  Artane Sequels (Lederle) p 415, 1087
  Artane Tablets (Lederle) p 415, 1087
Triiodothyronine
  Thyrolar Tablets (USV Pharmaceutical) p 440, 2091
Trimeprazine Tartrate
  Temaril (Smith Kline & French) p 437, 1976
Trimethadione
  Tridione (Abbott) p 404, 570
Trimethaphan Camsylate
  Arfonad Ampuls (Roche) p 1670
Trimethobenzamide Hydrochloride
  Stemetic (Legere) p 1120
  Tigan (Beecham Laboratories) p 406, 698
  Trimethobenzamide HCl Suppositories (Schein) p 1828
Trimethoprim
  Bactrim DS Tablets (Roche) p 429, 1674
  Bactrim I.V. Infusion (Roche) p 1672
  Bactrim Pediatric Suspension (Roche) p 1674
  Bactrim Suspension (Roche) p 1674
  Bactrim Tablets (Roche) p 429, 1674
  Cotrim (Lemmon) p 1122
  Cotrim D.S. (Lemmon) p 1122
  Proloprim (Burroughs Wellcome) p 408, 810
  Septra DS Tablets (Burroughs Wellcome) p 408, 815
  Septra I.V. Infusion (Burroughs Wellcome) p 813
  Septra Suspension (Burroughs Wellcome) p 815
  Septra Tablets (Burroughs Wellcome) p 408, 815
  Sulfamethoxazole & Trimethoprim Pediatric Suspension (Biocraft) p 705
  Sulfamethoxazole and Trimethoprim Tablets (Biocraft) p 705
  Sulfamethoxazole with Trimethoprim Tablets (Danbury) p 887
  Sulfamethoxazole with Trimethoprim Tablets (Double Strength) (Danbury) p 887
  Sulfamethoxazole w/Trimethoprim DS (Geneva) p 973
  Sulfamethoxazole w/Trimethoprim SS (Geneva) p 973
  Sulfatrim & Sulfatrim D/S Tablets (Schein) p 1828
  Trimethoprim Tablets (Biocraft) p 705
  Trimpex Tablets (Roche) p 430, 1706
Trimipramine Maleate
  Surmontil Capsules 25 mg, 50 mg, & 100 mg (Ives) p 413, 1029
Trioxsalen
  Trisoralen Tablets (Elder) p 411, 937
Tripelennamine Hydrochloride
  PBZ Hydrochloride Cream (Geigy) p 964
  PBZ-SR Tablets (Geigy) p 411, 963
  Tripelennamine HCl Tablets (Danbury) p 887
Tripelennamine Preparations
  PBZ Tablets & Elixir (Geigy) p 411, 964
Triprolidine Hydrochloride
  Actifed with Codeine Cough Syrup (Burroughs Wellcome) p 773
  Triafed-C Expectorant (Schein) p 1828
  Trifed Tablets & Syrup (Geneva) p 973
  Tripodrine Tablets (Danbury) p 887
  Triprolidine HCl & Pseudoephedrine HCl Syrup (Pharmafair) p 1618
  Triprolidine Hydrochloride & Pseudoephedrine Hydrochloride Syrup, Tablets (Roxane) p 1788
Triprolidine Preparations
  Triafed Syrup & Tablets (Schein) p 1828
Troleandomycin
  Tao Capsules (Roerig) p 431, 1744
Trypsin
  Granulex (Hickam) p 1009
  Orenzyme (Merrell Dow) p 1379
  Orenzyme Bitabs (Merrell Dow) p 1379
  Stimuzyme Plus (National Dermaceutical) p 1421
  Zypan Tablets (Standard Process) p 2035
L. Tryptophan
  Trofan Tablets (Upsher-Smith) p 2145
  Tryptacin (Arther) p 614
Tuberculin, Old
  Mono-Vacc Test (O.T.) (Merieux) p 1358
  Tuberculin, Mono-Vacc Test (O.T.) (Merieux) p 3013
  Tuberculin, Old, Tine Test (Rosenthal) (Lederle) p 3010

Tuberculin, Purified Protein Derivative, Multiple Puncture Device
  Aplitest (Parke-Davis) p 3014
  SclavoTest-PPD (Sclavo) p 3017
Tuberculin, Purified Protein Derivative for Mantoux Test
  Aplisol (Parke-Davis) p 3014
  Tubersol (Tuberculin Purified Protein Derivative [Mantoux]) (Squibb/Connaught) p 2033
Tubocurarine Chloride
  Tubocurarine Chloride (Lilly) p 1175
Typhoid Vaccine
  Typhoid Vaccine (Wyeth) p 2246
Tyropanoate Sodium
  Bilopaque Sodium (Winthrop-Breon) p 443, 3023

U—V

Undecylenic Acid
  Breezee Mist Foot Powder (Pedinol) p 1580
Urea Preparations
  Amino-Cerv (Milex) p 1415
  Carmol HC Cream 1% (Syntex) p 2061
  Debrox Drops (Marion) p 1184
  Elaqua XX Cream (Elder) p 930
  Gly-Oxide Liquid (Marion) p 1186
  Panafil Ointment (Rystan) p 1796
  Panafil-White Ointment (Rystan) p 1796
  Proxigel (Reed & Carnrick) p 1637
  Ureacin Lotion & Creme (Pedinol) p 1581
Urine Glucose Enzymatic Test Strip
  Tes-Tape (Lilly) p 3013
Urokinase
  Abbokinase (Abbott) p 502
  Abbokinase Open-Cath (Abbott) p 505
Vaccines (Live)
  Attenuvax (Merck Sharp & Dohme) p 1267
  Biavax II (Merck Sharp & Dohme) p 1269
  M-M-R II (Merck Sharp & Dohme) p 1323
  M-R-VAX II (Merck Sharp & Dohme) p 1325
  Meruvax II (Merck Sharp & Dohme) p 1329
  Mumpsvax (Merck Sharp & Dohme) p 1336
Vaginal Diaphragm & Apparatus
  Koro-Flex Arcing Spring Diaphragm (Youngs) p 2300
  Koromex Coil Spring Diaphragm (Youngs) p 2301
Valproic Acid
  Depakene Capsules & Syrup (Abbott) p 403, 512
Vanadium
  Total Formula (Vitaline) p 2148
Vancomycin
  Vancocin HCl, for Oral Solution (Lilly) p 1178
  Vancocin HCl, Vials (Lilly) p 1177
Vasopressin
  Pitressin (Parke-Davis) p 1562
Vecuronium Bromide
  Norcuron (NC-45) (Organon) p 1447
Verapamil Hydrochloride
  Calan for IV Injection (Searle Pharmaceuticals) p 435, 1900
  Calan Tablets (Searle & Co.) p 435, 1917
  Isoptin Ampules (Knoll) p 414, 1061
  Isoptin for Intravenous Injection (Knoll) p 414, 1061
  Isoptin Oral Tablets (Knoll) p 414, 1063
Versenate, Calcium Disodium
  Calcium Disodium Versenate Injection (Riker) p 1641
Vidarabine
  Vira-A Ophthalmic Ointment, 3% (Parke-Davis) p 426, 1578
Vidarabine Monohydrate
  Vira-A for Infusion (Parke-Davis) p 1576
Vinblastine Sulfate
  Velban (Lilly) p 1179
Vincristine Sulfate
  Oncovin (Lilly) p 1169
Vitamin A
  ACE + Z Tablets (Legere) p 1120
  Al-Vite (Drug Industries) p 914
  Aquasol A Parenteral (Armour) p 404, 603
  Aquasol A Drops (Armour) p 604
  Eldercaps (Mayrand) p 1196
  Iromin-G (Mission) p 1416
  Megadose (Arco) p 600
  Natacomp-FA Tablets (Trimen) p 2067
  Natalins Rx (Mead Johnson Laboratories) p 419, 1224

  Natalins Tablets (Mead Johnson Laboratories) p 419, 1224
  Pedi-Vit A Creme (Pedinol) p 1581
  Prenate 90 Tablets (Bock) p 706
  Therabid (Mission) p 1420
  Triplevite w/Fluoride Drops (Geneva) p 973
  Tri-Vi-Flor 1.0 mg Vitamins w/Fluoride Chewable Tablets (Mead Johnson Nutritional) p 1246
  Tri-Vi-Flor 0.25 mg Vitamins w/Fluoride Drops (Mead Johnson Nutritional) p 1247
  Tri-Vi-Flor 0.5 mg Vitamins w/Fluoride Drops (Mead Johnson Nutritional) p 1247
  Vicon Forte Capsules (Glaxo) p 412, 989
  Vicon-Plus Capsules (Glaxo) p 412, 989
  Vi-Daylin ADC Drops (Ross) p 1782
  Vi-Penta F Chewables (Roche) p 430, 1708
  Vi-Penta F Infant Drops (Roche) p 1709
  Vi-Penta F Multivitamin Drops (Roche) p 1709
  Vi-Penta Infant Drops (Roche) p 1710
  Vi-Penta Multivitamin Drops (Roche) p 1710
  Vitamin A + Vitamin D Ointment (Fougera) p 953
  Vita-Numonyl Injectable (Lambda) p 1071
  Vi-Zac Capsules (Glaxo) p 412, 990
Vitamins A & D
  Adeflor Chewable Tablets (Upjohn) p 440, 2093
  Adeflor Drops (Upjohn) p 2093
  Al-Vite (Drug Industries) p 914
  Dayalets Filmtab (Abbott) p 511
  Dayalets plus Iron Filmtab (Abbott) p 511
  Eldercaps (Mayrand) p 1196
  Iromin-G (Mission) p 1416
  M.V.I. (Armour) p 404, 605
  M.V.I. Concentrate (Armour) p 605
  M.V.I. Pediatric (Armour) p 607
  M.V.I.-12 (Armour) p 606
  M.V.I.-12 Lyophilized (Armour) p 606
  Megadose (Arco) p 600
  Natacomp-FA Tablets (Trimen) p 2067
  Nu-Iron-V Tablets (Mayrand) p 1196
  Sigtab Tablets (Upjohn) p 2135
  Vi-Daylin ADC Drops (Ross) p 1782
  Vi-Daylin Plus Iron ADC Drops (Ross) p 1784
  Vi-Daylin/F ADC Drops (Ross) p 1782
  Vi-Daylin/F ADC + Iron Drops (Ross) p 1782
  Viopan-T Tablets (Trimen) p 2067
Vitamin B$_1$
  Al-Vite (Drug Industries) p 914
  B-C-Bid Capsules (Geriatric) p 975
  Eldercaps (Mayrand) p 1196
  Eldertonic (Mayrand) p 1196
  Geravite Elixir (Hauck) p 1001
  Hemo-Vite (Drug Industries) p 914
  Mega-B (Arco) p 600
  Megadose (Arco) p 600
  Natacomp-FA Tablets (Trimen) p 2067
  Neuro B-12 Forte Injectable (Lambda) p 1071
  Neuro B-12 Injectable (Lambda) p 1071
  Nu-Iron-V Tablets (Mayrand) p 1196
  Orexin Softab Tablets (Stuart) p 2034
  Prenate 90 Tablets (Bock) p 706
  The Stuart Formula Tablets (Stuart) p 439, 2042
  Therabid (Mission) p 1420
  Viopan-T Tablets (Trimen) p 2067
Vitamin B$_2$
  Albafort Injectable (Bart) p 685
  Alba-Lybe (Bart) p 685
  Al-Vite (Drug Industries) p 914
  B-C-Bid Capsules (Geriatric) p 975
  Eldercaps (Mayrand) p 1196
  Eldertonic (Mayrand) p 1196
  Geravite Elixir (Hauck) p 1001
  Glutofac Tablets (Kenwood) p 1046
  Hemo-Vite (Drug Industries) p 914
  I.L.X. B$_{12}$ Elixir Crystalline (Kenwood) p 1046
  I.L.X. B$_{12}$ Tablets (Kenwood) p 1046
  Mega-B (Arco) p 600
  Megadose (Arco) p 600
  Natacomp-FA Tablets (Trimen) p 2067
  Nu-Iron-V Tablets (Mayrand) p 1196
  Prenate 90 Tablets (Bock) p 706
  The Stuart Formula Tablets (Stuart) p 439, 2042
  Therabid (Mission) p 1420
  Vicon-C Capsules (Glaxo) p 412, 989
Vitamin B$_6$
  Al-Vite (Drug Industries) p 914
  B-C-Bid Capsules (Geriatric) p 975
  Eldercaps (Mayrand) p 1196
  Eldertonic (Mayrand) p 1196
  Glutofac Tablets (Kenwood) p 1046
  Hemo-Vite (Drug Industries) p 914
  Hemo-Vite Liquid (Drug Industries) p 914
  Mega-B (Arco) p 600
  Megadose (Arco) p 600
  Natacomp-FA Tablets (Trimen) p 2067
  Neuro B-12 Forte Injectable (Lambda) p 1071

Generic and Chemical Name Index

Nu-Iron-V Tablets (Mayrand) p 1196
Orexin Softab Tablets (Stuart) p 2034
Prenate 90 Tablets (Bock) p 706
The Stuart Formula Tablets (Stuart) p 439, 2042
Therabid (Mission) p 1420
Viopan-T Tablets (Trimen) p 2067

Vitamin B$_{12}$

Albafort Injectable (Bart) p 685
Alba-Lybe (Bart) p 685
Al-Vite (Drug Industries) p 914
B-C-Bid Capsules (Geriatric) p 975
Cobolin-M (Legere) p 1120
Cyanocobalamin (Vit. B$_{12}$) Injection (Elkins-Sinn) p 938
Eldertonic (Mayrand) p 1196
Fergon Plus (Winthrop-Breon) p 2198
Fetrin (LaSalle) p 1071
Geravite Elixir (Hauck) p 1001
Hemo-Vite (Drug Industries) p 914
Hemo-Vite Liquid (Drug Industries) p 914
Heptuna Plus (Roerig) p 431, 1735
I.L.X. B$_{12}$ Elixir Crystalline (Kenwood) p 1046
I.L.X. B$_{12}$ Tablets (Kenwood) p 1046
Mega-B (Arco) p 600
Megadose (Arco) p 600
Natacomp-FA Tablets (Trimen) p 2067
Neuro B-12 Forte Injectable (Lambda) p 1071
Neuro B-12 Injectable (Lambda) p 1071
Nu-Iron-Plus Elixir (Mayrand) p 1196
Nu-Iron-V Tablets (Mayrand) p 1196
Orexin Softab Tablets (Stuart) p 2034
Perihemin (Lederle) p 1112
Prenate 90 Tablets (Bock) p 706
Pronemia Capsules (Lederle) p 1118
The Stuart Formula Tablets (Stuart) p 439, 2042
Therabid (Mission) p 1420
Tia-Doce Injectable Solution (Bart) p 685
Vicon Forte Capsules (Glaxo) p 412, 989
Viopan-T Tablets (Trimen) p 2067

Vitamin B Complex

Added Protection III (Professional Health) p 1621
B-Complex 100 (Legere) p 1120
Becotin (Dista) p 893
Cefol Filmtab Tablets (Abbott) p 403, 510
Dayalets Filmtab (Abbott) p 511
Dayalets plus Iron Filmtab (Abbott) p 511
Hemo-Vite (Drug Industries) p 914
Hemo-Vite Liquid (Drug Industries) p 914
Iberet-500 (Abbott) p 403, 532
Iromin-G (Mission) p 1416
Mega-B (Arco) p 600
Megadose (Arco) p 600
Natalins Rx (Mead Johnson Laboratories) p 419, 1224
Natalins Tablets (Mead Johnson Laboratories) p 419, 1224
Orexin Softab Tablets (Stuart) p 2034
Prenate 90 Tablets (Bock) p 706
Probec-T Tablets (Stuart) p 439, 2040
The Stuart Formula Tablets (Stuart) p 439, 2042
Vicon Forte Capsules (Glaxo) p 412, 989
Vicon-C Capsules (Glaxo) p 412, 989
Vicon-Plus Capsules (Glaxo) p 412, 989
Vi-Penta F Chewables (Roche) p 430, 1708
Vi-Penta F Multivitamin Drops (Roche) p 1709
Vi-Penta Multivitamin Drops (Roche) p 1710

Vitamin B Complex with Vitamin C

Added Protection III (Professional Health) p 1621
Adeflor Chewable Tablets (Upjohn) p 440, 2093
Al-Vite (Drug Industries) p 914
B-C-Bid Capsules (Geriatric) p 975
Becotin with Vitamin C (Dista) p 894
Becotin-T (Dista) p 894
Beminal-500 (Ayerst) p 404, 639
Beminal Forte w/Vitamin C (Ayerst) p 639
Beminal Stress Plus (Ayerst) p 404, 640
Berocca Tablets (Roche) p 429, 1677
Berocca-C & Berocca-C 500 (Roche) p 1678
Eldercaps (Mayrand) p 1196
Enviro-Stress with Zinc & Selenium (Vitaline) p 2148
Hemocyte Plus Tabules (U.S. Pharmaceutical) p 2070
Hemo-Vite (Drug Industries) p 914
Heptuna Plus (Roerig) p 431, 1735
Iberet (Abbott) p 532
Iberet-500 Liquid (Abbott) p 533
Iberet-Folic-500 (Abbott) p 403, 529
Iberet Liquid (Abbott) p 533
Iromin-G (Mission) p 1416
Larobec Tablets (Roche) p 429, 1687
M.V.I. (Armour) p 404, 605
M.V.I. Concentrate (Armour) p 605
M.V.I. Pediatric (Armour) p 607
M.V.I.-12 (Armour) p 606
M.V.I.-12 Lyophilized (Armour) p 606

Mediplex Tabules (U.S. Pharmaceutical) p 2070
Nu-Iron-V Tablets (Mayrand) p 1196
Orabex-TF (LaSalle) p 1071
Prenate 90 Tablets (Bock) p 706
Probec-T Tablets (Stuart) p 439, 2040
Sigtab Tablets (Upjohn) p 2135
Surbex Filmtab (Abbott) p 567
Surbex w/C Filmtab (Abbott) p 567
Tabron Filmseal (Parke-Davis) p 425, 1572
Thera-Combex H-P (Parke-Davis) p 425, 1574
Vicon Forte Capsules (Glaxo) p 412, 989
Vicon-C Capsules (Glaxo) p 412, 989
Vicon-Plus Capsules (Glaxo) p 412, 989
Vio-Bec Forte (Rowell) p 1788
Viopan-T Tablets (Trimen) p 2067

Vitamin C

ACE + Z Tablets (Legere) p 1120
Al-Vite (Drug Industries) p 914
Ascorbic Acid Tablets (Roxane) p 1788
B-C-Bid Capsules (Geriatric) p 975
Cee-500 (Ascorbic Acid) (Legere) p 1120
Cee-1000 T.D. Tablets (Legere) p 1120
Cefol Filmtab Tablets (Abbott) p 403, 510
Cevi-Bid Capsules (Geriatric) p 975
Cevi-Fer Capsules (sustained release) (Geriatric) p 975
Dayalets Filmtab (Abbott) p 511
Dayalets plus Iron Filmtab (Abbott) p 511
Eldercaps (Mayrand) p 1196
Enviro-Stress with Zinc & Selenium (Vitaline) p 2148
Ferancee Chewable Tablets (Stuart) p 439, 2037
Ferancee-HP Tablets (Stuart) p 439, 2037
Fergon Plus (Winthrop-Breon) p 2198
Fetrin (LaSalle) p 1071
Glutofac Tablets (Kenwood) p 1046
Hemo-Vite (Drug Industries) p 914
I.L.X. B$_{12}$ Tablets (Kenwood) p 1046
Iromin-G (Mission) p 1416
Lyte-C (Tyson) p 2068
Mevanin-C Capsules (Beutlich) p 705
Natacomp-FA Tablets (Trimen) p 2067
Natalins Rx (Mead Johnson Laboratories) p 419, 1224
Natalins Tablets (Mead Johnson Laboratories) p 419, 1224
Niferex w/Vitamin C (Central Pharmaceuticals) p 838
Nu-Iron-V Tablets (Mayrand) p 1196
Peridin-C (Beutlich) p 705
Prenate 90 Tablets (Bock) p 706
Probec-T Tablets (Stuart) p 439, 2040
The Stuart Formula Tablets (Stuart) p 439, 2042
Stuartinic Tablets (Stuart) p 439, 2034
Therabid (Mission) p 1420
Trinsicon/Trinsicon M Capsules (Glaxo) p 412, 986
Triplevite w/Fluoride Drops (Geneva) p 973
Tri-Vi-Flor 1.0 mg Vitamins w/Fluoride Chewable Tablets (Mead Johnson Nutritional) p 1246
Tri-Vi-Flor 0.25 mg Vitamins w/Fluoride Drops (Mead Johnson Nutritional) p 1247
Tri-Vi-Flor 0.5 mg Vitamins w/Fluoride Drops (Mead Johnson Nutritional) p 1247
Vicon Forte Capsules (Glaxo) p 412, 989
Vicon-C Capsules (Glaxo) p 412, 989
Vicon-Plus Capsules (Glaxo) p 412, 989
Vi-Daylin ADC Drops (Ross) p 1782
Vi-Daylin Plus Iron ADC Drops (Ross) p 1784
Vi-Daylin/F ADC Drops (Ross) p 1782
Vi-Daylin/F ADC + Iron Drops (Ross) p 1782
Viopan-T Tablets (Trimen) p 2067
Vi-Penta F Chewables (Roche) p 430, 1708
Vi-Penta F Infant Drops (Roche) p 1709
Vi-Penta F Multivitamin Drops (Roche) p 1709
Vi-Penta Infant Drops (Roche) p 1710
Vi-Penta Multivitamin Drops (Roche) p 1710
Vi-Zac Capsules (Glaxo) p 412, 990

Vitamin D

Al-Vite (Drug Industries) p 914
Iromin-G (Mission) p 1416
Megadose (Arco) p 600
Natalins Rx (Mead Johnson Laboratories) p 419, 1224
Natalins Tablets (Mead Johnson Laboratories) p 419, 1224
Prenate 90 Tablets (Bock) p 706
Triplevite w/Fluoride Drops (Geneva) p 973
Tri-Vi-Flor 1.0 mg Vitamins w/Fluoride Chewable Tablets (Mead Johnson Nutritional) p 1246
Tri-Vi-Flor 0.25 mg Vitamins w/Fluoride Drops (Mead Johnson Nutritional) p 1247
Tri-Vi-Flor 0.5 mg Vitamins w/Fluoride Drops (Mead Johnson Nutritional) p 1247
Vi-Daylin ADC Drops (Ross) p 1782
Vi-Penta Infant Drops (Roche) p 1710
Vi-Penta Multivitamin Drops (Roche) p 1710
Vitamin A + Vitamin D Ointment (Fougera) p 953

Vita-Numonyl Injectable (Lambda) p 1071

Vitamin D$_2$

Calcet (Mission) p 1415
Calciferol Drops (Egocalciferol Oral Solution USP) (Rorer) p 431, 1748
Calciferol in Oil Injection (Egocalciferol USP) (Rorer) p 431, 1748
Calciferol Tablets (Ergocalciferol USP) (Rorer) p 431, 1748
Dical-D Capsules & Wafers (Abbott) p 516
Eldercaps (Mayrand) p 1196
Therabid (Mission) p 1420

Vitamin D$_3$

Al-Vite (Drug Industries) p 914

Vitamin E

ACE + Z Tablets (Legere) p 1120
Al-Vite (Drug Industries) p 914
Aquasol E Capsules & Drops (Armour) p 404, 604
Cefol Filmtab Tablets (Abbott) p 403, 510
Dayalets Filmtab (Abbott) p 511
Dayalets plus Iron Filmtab (Abbott) p 511
Eldercaps (Mayrand) p 1196
Enviro-Stress with Zinc & Selenium (Vitaline) p 2148
Libidinal Capsules (Everett) p 942
M.V.I. (Armour) p 404, 605
M.V.I. Concentrate (Armour) p 605
M.V.I. Pediatric (Armour) p 607
M.V.I.-12 (Armour) p 606
M.V.I.-12 Lyophilized (Armour) p 606
Mediplex Tabules (U.S. Pharmaceutical) p 2070
Megadose (Arco) p 600
Natacomp-FA Tablets (Trimen) p 2067
Natalins Rx (Mead Johnson Laboratories) p 419, 1224
Natalins Tablets (Mead Johnson Laboratories) p 419, 1224
Prenate 90 Tablets (Bock) p 706
The Stuart Formula Tablets (Stuart) p 439, 2042
Therabid (Mission) p 1420
Vicon Forte Capsules (Glaxo) p 412, 989
Vicon-Plus Capsules (Glaxo) p 412, 989
Vi-Penta F Chewables (Roche) p 430, 1708
Vi-Penta F Infant Drops (Roche) p 1709
Vi-Penta F Multivitamin Drops (Roche) p 1709
Vi-Penta Infant Drops (Roche) p 1710
Vi-Penta Multivitamin Drops (Roche) p 1710
Vi-Zac Capsules (Glaxo) p 412, 990

Vitamin K

Chlorophyll Complex Perles (Standard Process) p 2035
Synkayvite Injectable (Roche) p 1701
Synkayvite Tablets (Roche) p 430, 1702

Vitamin K$_1$

AquaMEPHYTON Injection (Merck Sharp & Dohme) p 1265
Konakion Injectable (Roche) p 1687
M.V.I. Pediatric (Armour) p 607

Vitamin P

Mevanin-C Capsules (Beutlich) p 705
Peridin-C (Beutlich) p 705

Vitamin (Parenteral)

Berocca Parenteral Nutrition (Roche) p 1676

Vitamin (Therapeutic)

Added Protection III (Professional Health) p 1621
Al-Vite (Drug Industries) p 914
Berocca Parenteral Nutrition (Roche) p 1676
Cefol Filmtab Tablets (Abbott) p 403, 510
Hemo-Vite Liquid (Drug Industries) p 914
Hep-Forte Capsules (Marlyn) p 1193
Mega-B (Arco) p 600
Megadose (Arco) p 600
Megaplex I.M. (Legere) p 1120
Niferex-PN (Central Pharmaceuticals) p 409, 838
Peridin-C (Beutlich) p 705
Surbex Filmtab (Abbott) p 567
Surbex w/C Filmtab (Abbott) p 567
Theragran Hematinic (Squibb) p 438, 2024
Vicon Forte Capsules (Glaxo) p 412, 989
Vicon-C Capsules (Glaxo) p 412, 989
Vicon-Plus Capsules (Glaxo) p 412, 989
Viopan-T Tablets (Trimen) p 2067
Vi-Zac Capsules (Glaxo) p 412, 990

Vitamins, Supplement

A.C.N. Tablets (Persōn & Covey) p 1587
Added Protection III (Professional Health) p 1621
B-C-Bid Capsules (Geriatric) p 975
Berovite Plus Tablets (Everett) p 941
Dayalets Filmtab (Abbott) p 511
Dayalets plus Iron Filmtab (Abbott) p 511
Dexatrim Capsules, Extra Strength, Plus Vitamins (Thompson Medical) p 2066
E.T. The Extra-Terrestrial Children's Chewable Vitamins (Squibb) p 438, 1994

Hemo-Vite Liquid (Drug Industries) p 914
Iso-B Caps (Tyson) p 2068
Mevanin-C Capsules (Beutlich) p 705
Natabec Kapseals (Parke-Davis) p 424, 1545
Natabec Rx Kapseals (Parke-Davis) p 424, 1545
Natacomp-FA Tablets (Trimen) p 2067
Natafort Filmseal (Parke-Davis) p 424, 1545
Nephrocaps (Fleming) p 948
Niferex-PN (Central Pharmaceuticals) p 409, 838
Nutrox Capsules (Tyson) p 2069
O. B. Thera Tablets (Legere) p 1120
Peridin-C (Beutlich) p 705
Prenate 90 Tablets (Bock) p 706
Sigtab Tablets (Upjohn) p 2135
Theragran Liquid (Squibb) p 2024
Theragran Tablets (Squibb) p 438, 2025
Total Formula (Vitaline) p 2148
Vi-Daylin ADC Drops (Ross) p 1782
Vi-Daylin Chewable (Ross) p 432, 1784
Vi-Daylin Drops (Ross) p 1782
Vi-Daylin Liquid (Ross) p 1784
Vi-Daylin Plus Iron ADC Drops (Ross) p 1784
Vi-Daylin + Iron Chewable (Ross) p 432, 1784
Viopan-T Tablets (Trimen) p 2067

Vitamins with Fluoride
Florvite Chewable Tablets 0.5 mg & 1 mg (Everett) p 941
Florvite Drops (Everett) p 941
Florvite + Iron Chewable Tablets 1 mg (Everett) p 941
Florvite + Iron Drops (Everett) p 941
Poly-Vi-Flor 0.5 mg Vitamins w/Iron & Fluoride Chewable Tablets (Mead Johnson Nutritional) p 1245
Poly-Vi-Flor 0.25 mg Vitamins w/Iron & Fluoride Drops (Mead Johnson Nutritional) p 1245
Polyvitamin-Fluoride Drops & Tablets (Schein) p 1828
Polyvite with Fluoride Drops (Geneva) p 973
Triplevite w/Fluoride Drops (Geneva) p 973
Vi-Daylin/F ADC + Iron Drops (Ross) p 1782
Vi-Daylin/F Chewable (Ross) p 432, 1784
Vi-Penta F Chewables (Roche) p 430, 1708
Vi-Penta F Infant Drops (Roche) p 1709
Vi-Penta F Multivitamin Drops (Roche) p 1709

Vitamins with Iron
Added Protection III (Professional Health) p 1621
E.T. The Extra-Terrestrial Children's Chewable Vitamins with Iron (Squibb) p 438, 1994
Hemo-Vite Liquid (Drug Industries) p 914
Livolex (Legere) p 1120
Megaton Elixir (Hyrex) p 1025
Poly-Vi-Flor 0.5 mg Vitamins w/Iron & Fluoride Chewable Tablets (Mead Johnson Nutritional) p 1245
Poly-Vi-Flor 0.25 mg Vitamins w/Iron & Fluoride Drops (Mead Johnson Nutritional) p 1245
Prenate 90 Tablets (Bock) p 706
Theragran Stress Formula (Squibb) p 438, 2025

Vitamins with Minerals
Added Protection III (Professional Health) p 1621
Berocca Plus Tablets (Roche) p 429, 1677
Calcet Plus (Mission) p 1415
Chromagen OB (Savage) p 1824
Clusivol Capsules (Ayerst) p 640
Clusivol Syrup (Ayerst) p 640
Clusivol 130 Tablets (Ayerst) p 640
Compete (Mission) p 1416
Eldercaps (Mayrand) p 1196
Enviro-Stress with Zinc & Selenium (Vitaline) p 2148
Filibon (Lederle) p 415, 1093
Filibon F.A. (Lederle) p 415, 1093
Filibon Forte (Lederle) p 415, 1093
Intraderm-19 Oral Acne Supplement (Robertson/Taylor) p 1645
Lactocal-F Tablets (Laser) p 1072
MVM Caps (Tyson) p 2068
Materna 1•60 Tablets (Lederle) p 415, 1098
Maxovite Tablets (Tyson) p 2068
Medi-Tec Vitamin-Mineral-Trace Mineral Supplement (Robertson/Taylor) p 1646
Mi-Cebrin (Dista) p 903
Mission Prenatal (Mission) p 1419
Mission Prenatal F.A. (Mission) p 1419
Mission Prenatal H.P. (Mission) p 1419
Mission Prenatal RX (Mission) p 1419
Myadec (Parke-Davis) p 1543
Natabec Kapseals (Parke-Davis) p 424, 1545
Natabec Rx Kapseals (Parke-Davis) p 424, 1545

Natacomp-FA Tablets (Trimen) p 2067
Natafort Filmseal (Parke-Davis) p 424, 1545
Natalins Rx (Mead Johnson Laboratories) p 419, 1224
Natalins Tablets (Mead Johnson Laboratories) p 419, 1224
Nestabs FA Tablets (Fielding) p 942
Niferex-PN (Central Pharmaceuticals) p 409, 838
Nu-Iron-V Tablets (Mayrand) p 1196
Peritinic Tablets (Lederle) p 1112
Pramet FA (Ross) p 432, 1775
Pramilet FA (Ross) p 432, 1775
Prenate 90 Tablets (Bock) p 706
The Stuart Formula Tablets (Stuart) p 439, 2042
Stuart Prenatal Tablets (Stuart) p 439, 2034
Stuartinic Tablets (Stuart) p 439, 2034
Stuartnatal 1+1 Tablets (Stuart) p 439, 2043
Theragran-M Tablets (Squibb) p 438, 2025
Thera-Ron Tablets (Legere) p 1120
Total Formula (Vitaline) p 2148
VG Capsules (Medical Products) p 1256
Viopan-T Tablets (Trimen) p 2067
Vitafol Tablets (Everett) p 942
Zenate Tablets (Reid-Provident Labs.) p 428, 1640
Zincvit Capsules (RAM Laboratories) p 1632

Vitamins with Minerals, Therapeutic
Added Protection III Multi-Vitamin & Multi-Mineral Supplement (Professional Health) p 1621
Berovite Plus Tablets (Everett) p 941
Besta Capsules (Hauck) p 1001
Eldercaps (Mayrand) p 1196
Enviro-Stress with Zinc & Selenium (Vitaline) p 2148
Megadose (Arco) p 600
Mi-Cebrin T (Dista) p 903
Mission Pre-Surgical (Mission) p 1419
Niferex-PN (Central Pharmaceuticals) p 409, 838
Theragran Hematinic (Squibb) p 438, 2024
Total Formula (Vitaline) p 2148
Vicon Forte Capsules (Glaxo) p 412, 989
Vicon-C Capsules (Glaxo) p 412, 989
Vicon-Plus Capsules (Glaxo) p 412, 989
Viopan-T Tablets (Trimen) p 2067
Vitabese Capsules (Legere) p 1120
Vi-Zac Capsules (Glaxo) p 412, 990

W–Z

Warfarin Sodium
Coumadin (Du Pont) p 410, 915
Panwarfin (Abbott) p 403, 558
Warfarin Sodium Tablets (Schein) p 1828

Water-Soluble Vitamins
Berocca Tablets (Roche) p 429, 1677
Larobec Tablets (Roche) p 429, 1687
Mega-B (Arco) p 600

Witch Hazel
Tucks Cream (Parke-Davis) p 1575
Tucks Ointment (Parke-Davis) p 1575
Tucks Premoistened Pads (Parke-Davis) p 1575

Wound Cleaning Beads
Debrisan Wound Cleaning Beads (Johnson & Johnson (Patient Care Div.)) p 1044
Debrisan Wound Cleaning Paste (Johnson & Johnson (Patient Care Div.)) p 1044

Xanthine Oxidase Inhibitor
Zyloprim (Burroughs Wellcome) p 408, 825

Xanthine Preparations
Aerolate Liquid (Fleming) p 948
Aerolate Sr. & Jr. & III Capsules (Fleming) p 948
Aquaphyllin Syrup (Ferndale) p 942
Asbron G Elixir (Sandoz Pharmaceutical Div.) p 1796
Asbron G Inlay-Tabs (Sandoz Pharmaceutical Div.) p 432, 1796
Brondecon (Parke-Davis) p 423, 1486
Bronkolixir (Winthrop-Breon) p 2193
Bronkotabs (Winthrop-Breon) p 2194
Choledyl (Parke-Davis) p 423, 1495
Elixicon Suspension (Berlex) p 406, 699
Elixophyllin Capsules (Berlex) p 406, 699
Elixophyllin Elixir (Berlex) p 699
Elixophyllin SR Capsules (Berlex) p 406, 699
LABID 250 mg Tablets (Norwich Eaton) p 1436
Lufyllin-GG (Wallace) p 442, 2161
Slo-bid Gyrocaps (Rorer) p 432, 1754
Slo-Phyllin Gyrocaps, Tablets (Rorer) p 432, 1756
Slo-Phyllin 80 Syrup (Rorer) p 1756
Slo-Phyllin GG Capsules, Syrup (Rorer) p 432, 1759
Tedral Elixir & Suspension (Parke-Davis) p 1573
Tedral SA Tablets (Parke-Davis) p 425, 1573

Theobid, Theobid Jr. Duracap (Glaxo) p 412, 982
Theoclear L.A.-130 & -260 Capsules (Central Pharmaceuticals) p 409, 839
Theoclear-80 Syrup (Central Pharmaceuticals) p 839
Theolair & Theolair-SR (Riker) p 428, 1645
Theolair-Plus Tablets & Liquid (Riker) p 428, 1645

Xylometazoline Hydrochloride
4-Way Long Acting Nasal Spray (Bristol-Myers Products) p 771
Otrivin (Geigy) p 963

Yeast Cell Derivative
Preparation H Hemorrhoidal Ointment (Whitehall) p 443, 2186
Preparation H Hemorrhoidal Suppositories (Whitehall) p 443, 2186

Yellow Fever Vaccine
YF-VAX (Yellow Fever Vaccine)(Live, 17D Virus, Avian Leukosis-Free, Stabilized) (Squibb/Connaught) p 2033

Yellow Mercuric Oxide
Yellow Mercuric Oxide Ophthalmic Ointment 1% & 2% (Fougera) p 953

Yohimbine Hydrochloride
Yocon (Palisades Pharm.) p 1476
Yohimex Tablets (Kramer) p 1069

Zinc
Beminal Stress Plus (Ayerst) p 404, 640
Eldercaps (Mayrand) p 1196
Enviro-Stress with Zinc & Selenium (Vitaline) p 2148
Megadose (Arco) p 600
Prenate 90 Tablets (Bock) p 706
Total Formula (Vitaline) p 2148
Vicon Forte Capsules (Glaxo) p 412, 989
Vicon-C Capsules (Glaxo) p 412, 989
Vicon-Plus Capsules (Glaxo) p 412, 989
Vi-Zac Capsules (Glaxo) p 412, 990
Zinc-220 Capsules (Alto) p 404, 589
Zincvit Capsules (RAM Laboratories) p 1632

Zinc Chloride
Multitrace 5 (Armour) p 608
Multitrace Pediatric (Armour) p 609
Multitrace Solution & Concentrate (Armour) p 609
Zinctrace (Armour) p 612

Zinc Gluconate
Libidinal Capsules (Everett) p 942
Megadose (Arco) p 600

Zinc Oxide
Allersone (Mallard) p 1181
Anusol Ointment (Parke-Davis) p 1484
Anusol Suppositories (Parke-Davis) p 423, 1484
Anusol-HC (Parke-Davis) p 423, 1484
Bensulfoid Lotion (Poythress) p 1618
Derma Medicone-HC Ointment (Medicone) p 1256
Dome-Paste Bandage (Miles Pharmaceuticals) p 1402
Hill Cortac (Hill Dermaceuticals) p 1009
Intraderm-19 Emergency Acne Stick (Robertson/Taylor) p 1645
Osti-Derm Lotion (Pedinol) p 1580
Primer Unna Boot (Glenwood) p 999
RVPaque Ointment (Elder) p 936
Rectal Medicone-HC Suppositories (Medicone) p 419, 1256
Wyanoids Hemorrhoidal Suppositories (Wyeth) p 445, 2293
Zinc Oxide Ointment (Fougera) p 953
Ziradryl Lotion (Parke-Davis) p 1580

Zinc Phenosulfonate
Intraderm-19 Overnight Acne Masque (Robertson/Taylor) p 1645

Zinc Pyrithione
DHS Zinc Dandruff Shampoo (Persōn & Covey) p 1587
Sebulon Dandruff Shampoo (Westwood) p 2181

Zinc Sulfate
ACE + Z Tablets (Legere) p 1120
Eldercaps (Mayrand) p 1196
Eldertonic (Mayrand) p 1196
Glutofac Tablets (Kenwood) p 1046
Hemocyte Plus Tabules (U.S. Pharmaceutical) p 2070
Mediplex Tabules (U.S. Pharmaceutical) p 2070
Vicon Forte Capsules (Glaxo) p 412, 989
Vicon-C Capsules (Glaxo) p 412, 989
Vicon-Plus Capsules (Glaxo) p 412, 989
Vio-Bec Forte (Rowell) p 1788
Vi-Zac Capsules (Glaxo) p 412, 990
Zinc-220 Capsules (Alto) p 404, 589

Zinc Undecylenate
Pedi-Dri Foot Powder (Pedinol) p 1581
Pedi-Pro Foot Powder (Pedinol) p 1581

Product Identification Section

Designed to help you identify products, this section contains actual size, full-color reproductions selected for inclusion by participating manufacturers.

Because tablets and capsules, for the most part, are shown here, you should not infer that these are the only dosage forms. Where other dosage forms are available, the product name is preceded by the † symbol. Refer to the product's description in the PRODUCT INFORMATION (White Section) or check directly with manufacturer.

Letters and/or numbers followed by an asterisk (*) accompanying a product photograph designate the manufacturers' identification code.

While every effort has been made to reproduce products faithfully, this section should be considered only as a quick reference identification aid.

If overdosage is suspected, the user may wish to consult Guide to Management of Drug Overdose printed inside the back cover.

INDEX BY MANUFACTURER

This section is made possible through the courtesy of the manufacturers whose products appear on the following pages. Page numbers of individual products included can be found in the Product Name, Generic and Product Category Indices.

Abbott Laboratories—
   Abbott Pharmaceuticals, Inc. 403
Adria Laboratories, Inc. 404
Alto Pharmaceuticals, Inc. 404
Alza Corporation 404
Armour Pharmaceutical Company 404
Ayerst Laboratories 404

Beach Pharmaceuticals 405
Beecham Laboratories 405
Berlex Laboratories, Inc. 406
Boehringer Ingelheim Ltd. 406
Boots Pharmaceuticals, Inc. 406
Bristol Laboratories 407
Bristol-Myers Oncology Division 407
The Brown Pharmaceutical Co., Inc. 407
Burroughs Wellcome Company 407

Carnrick Laboratories, Inc. 408
Central Pharmaceuticals, Inc. 409
CIBA Pharmaceutical Company 409
Colgate-Hoyt Laboratories 410

Dista Products Company 410
Du Pont Pharmaceuticals 410

Elder Pharmaceuticals, Inc. 411

Flint 411

Geigy Pharmaceuticals 411
Gilbert Laboratories 411
Glaxo Inc. 411
Glenbrook Laboratories 412
Glenwood, Inc. 412

Hoechst-Roussel Pharmaceuticals Inc. 412
Hyrex Pharmaceuticals 413

Ives Laboratories Incorporated 413

Janssen Pharmaceutica Inc. 413

Key Pharmaceuticals, Inc. 413
Knoll Pharmaceutical Company 414

LactAid Inc. 414
Lederle Laboratories 414
Lemmon Company 417
Eli Lilly and Company 417

Marion Laboratories, Inc. 417
Mason Pharmaceuticals, Inc. 418
McNeil Consumer Products Co. 418

McNeil Pharmaceutical 418
Mead Johnson Laboratories 419
Mead Johnson Pharmaceutical Division 419
Medicone Company 419
Merck Sharp & Dohme 420
Merrell Dow Pharmaceuticals Inc. 421
Miles Pharmaceuticals 421

Norcliff Thayer Inc. 422
Norwich Eaton Pharmaceuticals, Inc. 422

O'Neal, Jones
   & Feldman Pharmaceuticals 422
Organon Pharmaceuticals 422
Ortho Pharmaceutical Corporation 422

Parke-Davis 423
Pennwalt Corporation 426
Pfipharmecs Division 426
Pfizer Laboratories Division 426
Pharmacia Laboratories 427
Procter & Gamble 427
The Purdue Frederick Company 427

Reed & Carnrick 427
Reid-Provident Laboratories, Inc. 427
Riker Laboratories, Inc. 428
A. H. Robins Company 428
Roche Laboratories 429
Roerig 431
William H. Rorer, Incorporated 431
Ross Laboratories 432

Sandoz, Inc. 432
Savage Laboratories 433
Schering Corporation 433
Searle Pharmaceuticals, Inc., Searle & Co. ... 435
Smith Kline & French Laboratories 436
Smith Laboratories, Inc. 437
E. R. Squibb & Sons, Inc. 437
Stuart Pharmaceuticals 438
Syntex Laboratories, Inc. 440

USV Laboratories, Division 440
The Upjohn Company 440

Verex Laboratories, Inc. 442
Vicks Pharmacy Products Division 442

Wallace Laboratories 442
Westwood Pharmaceuticals, Inc. 442
Whitehall Laboratories Inc. 443
Winthrop-Breon Laboratories 443
Wyeth Laboratories 444

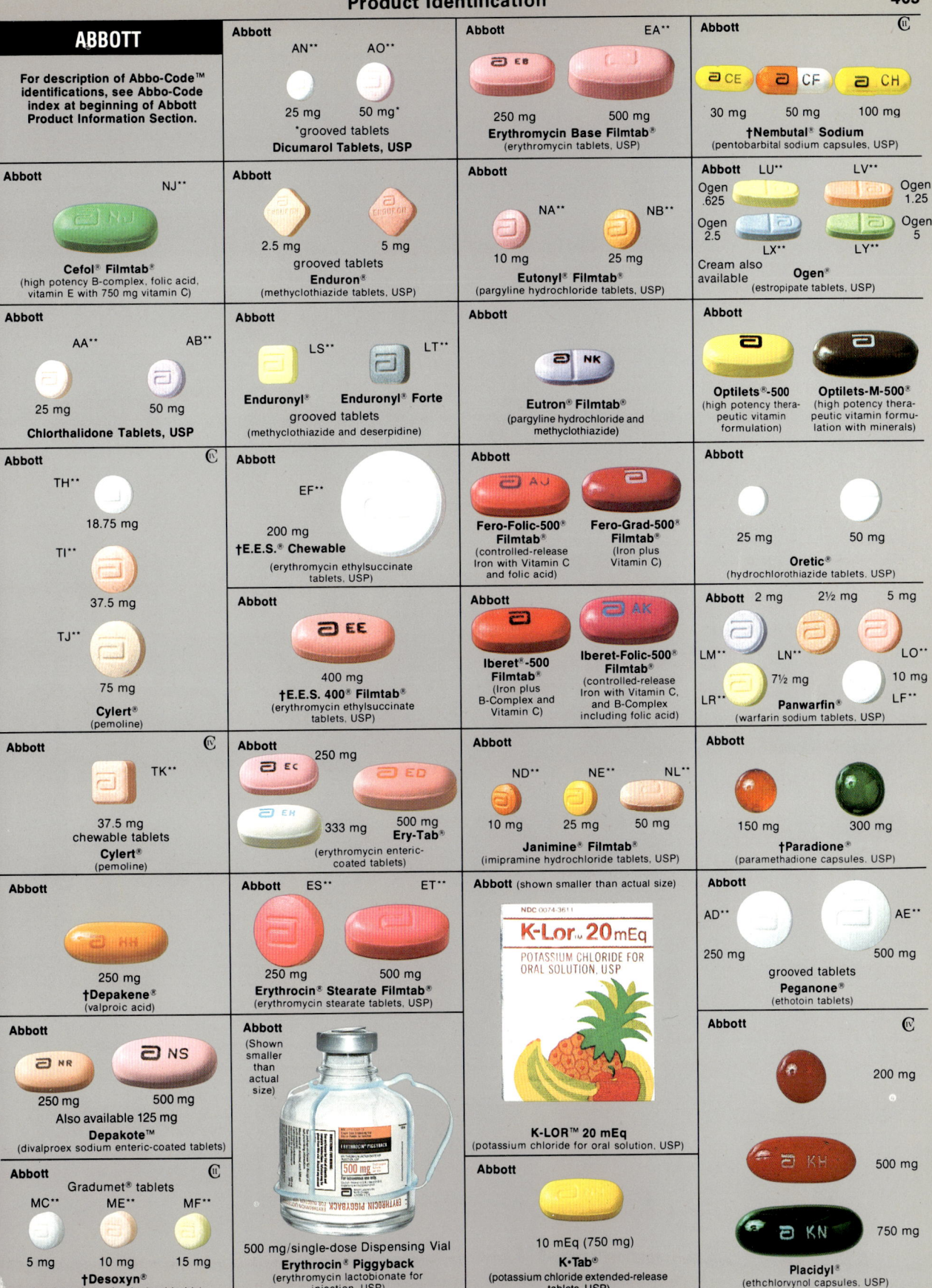

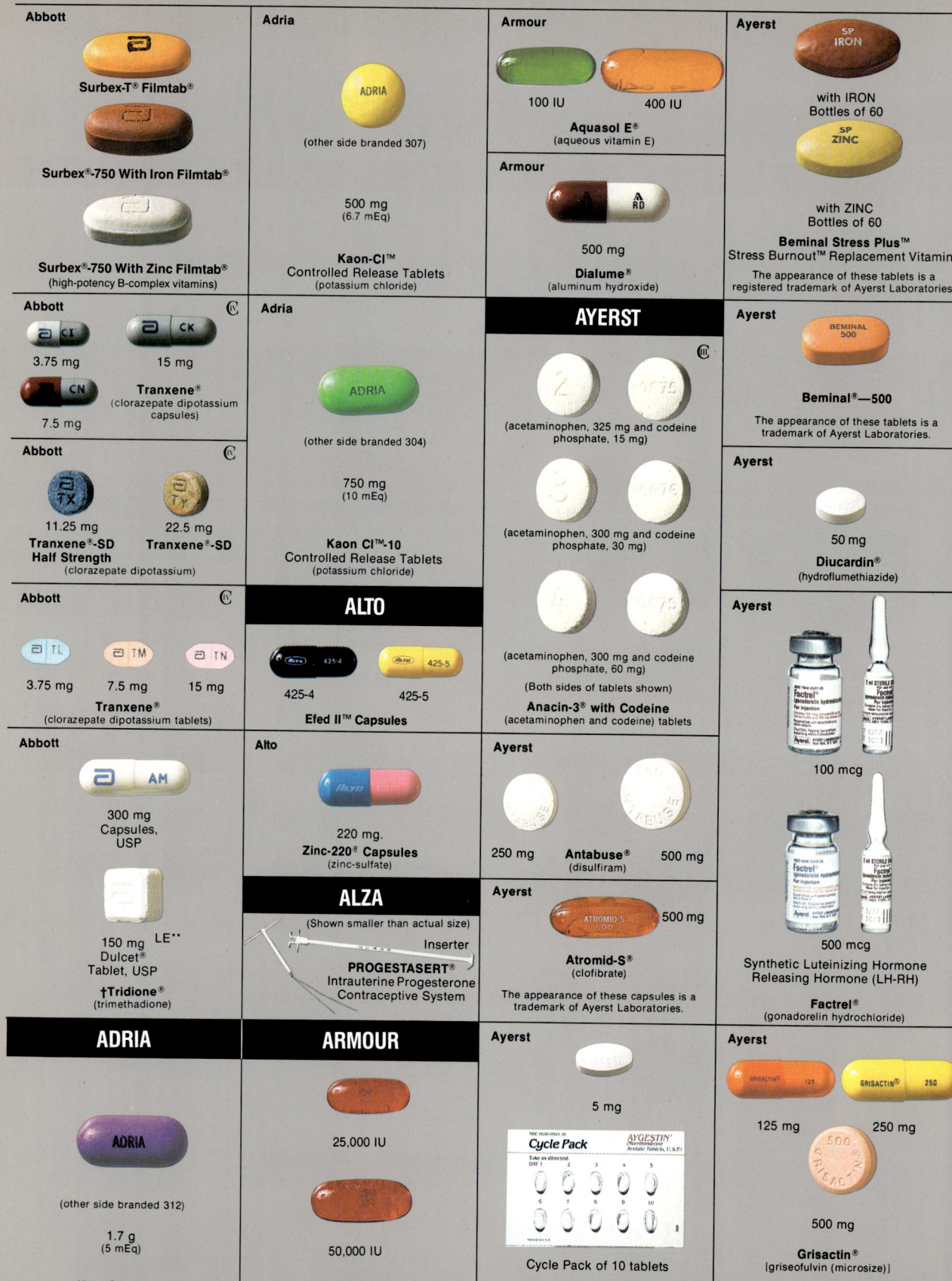

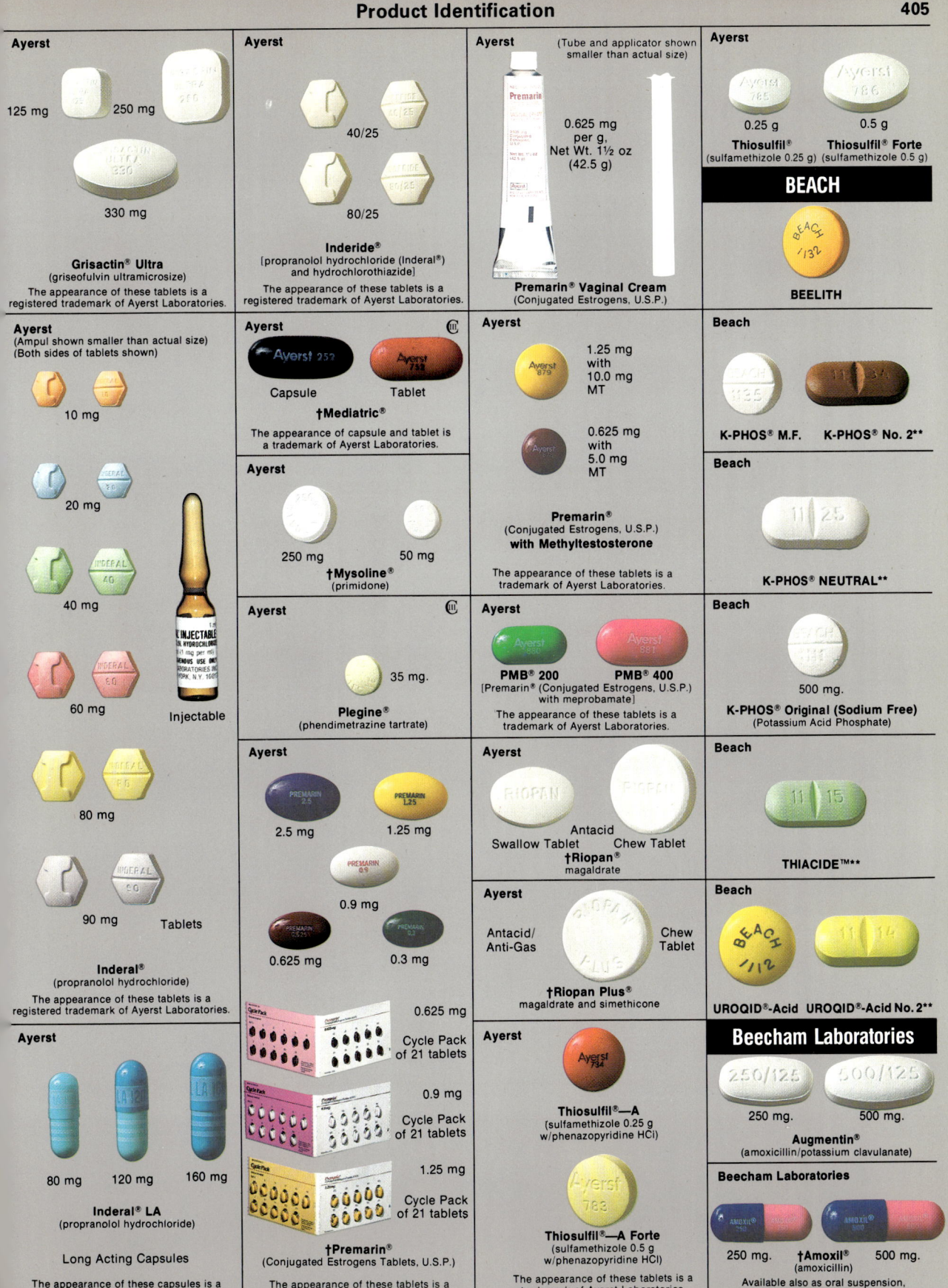

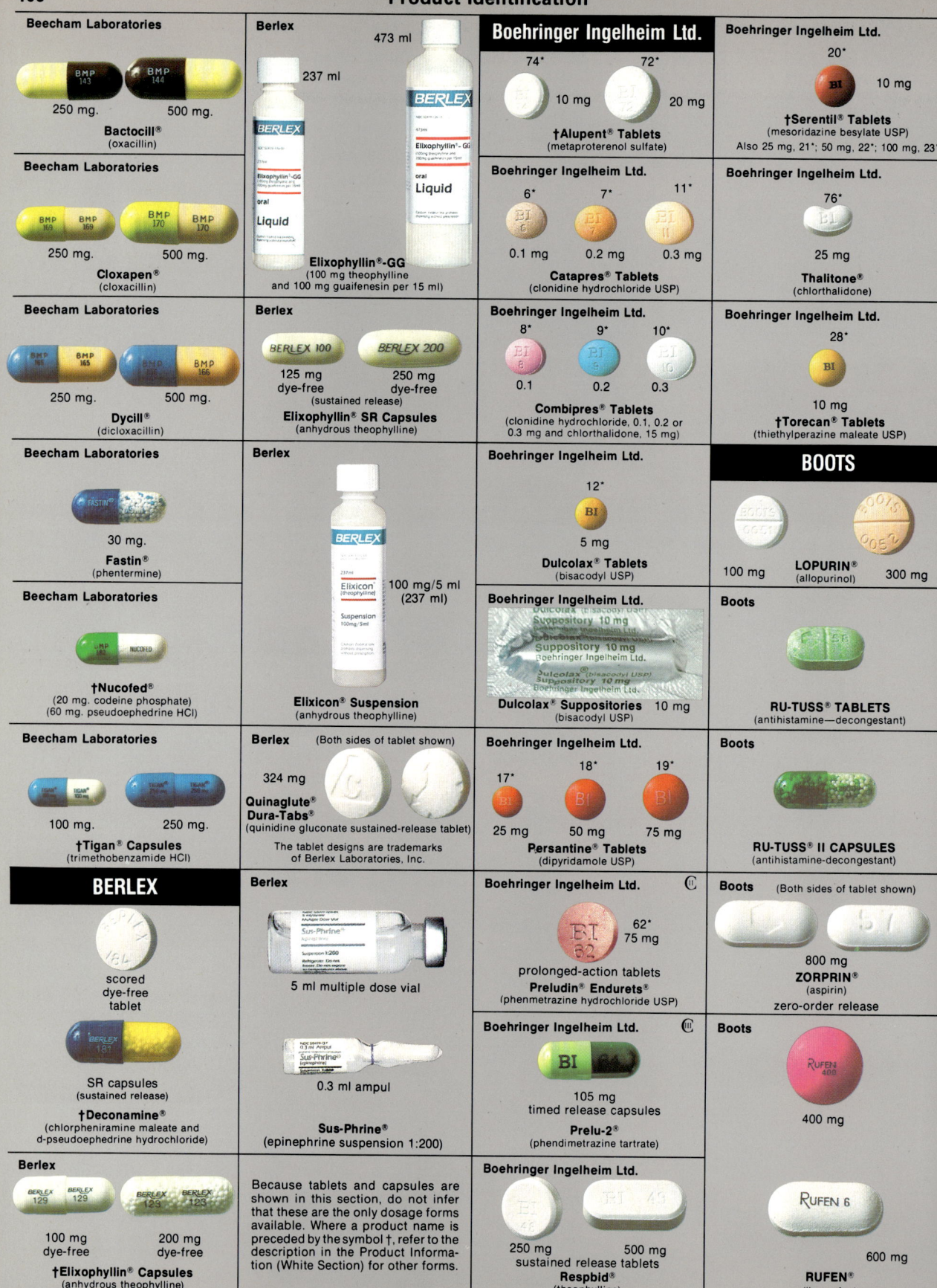

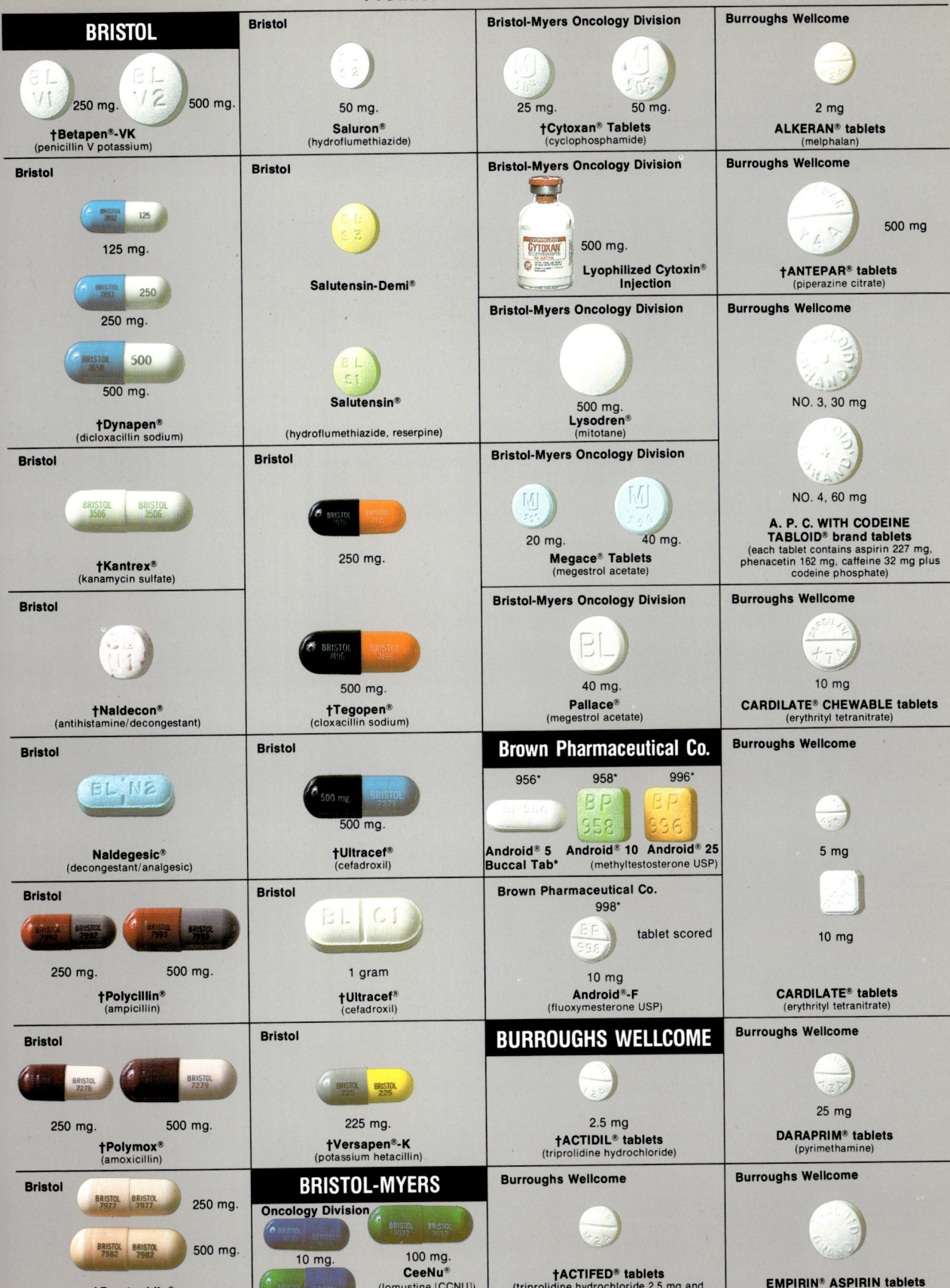

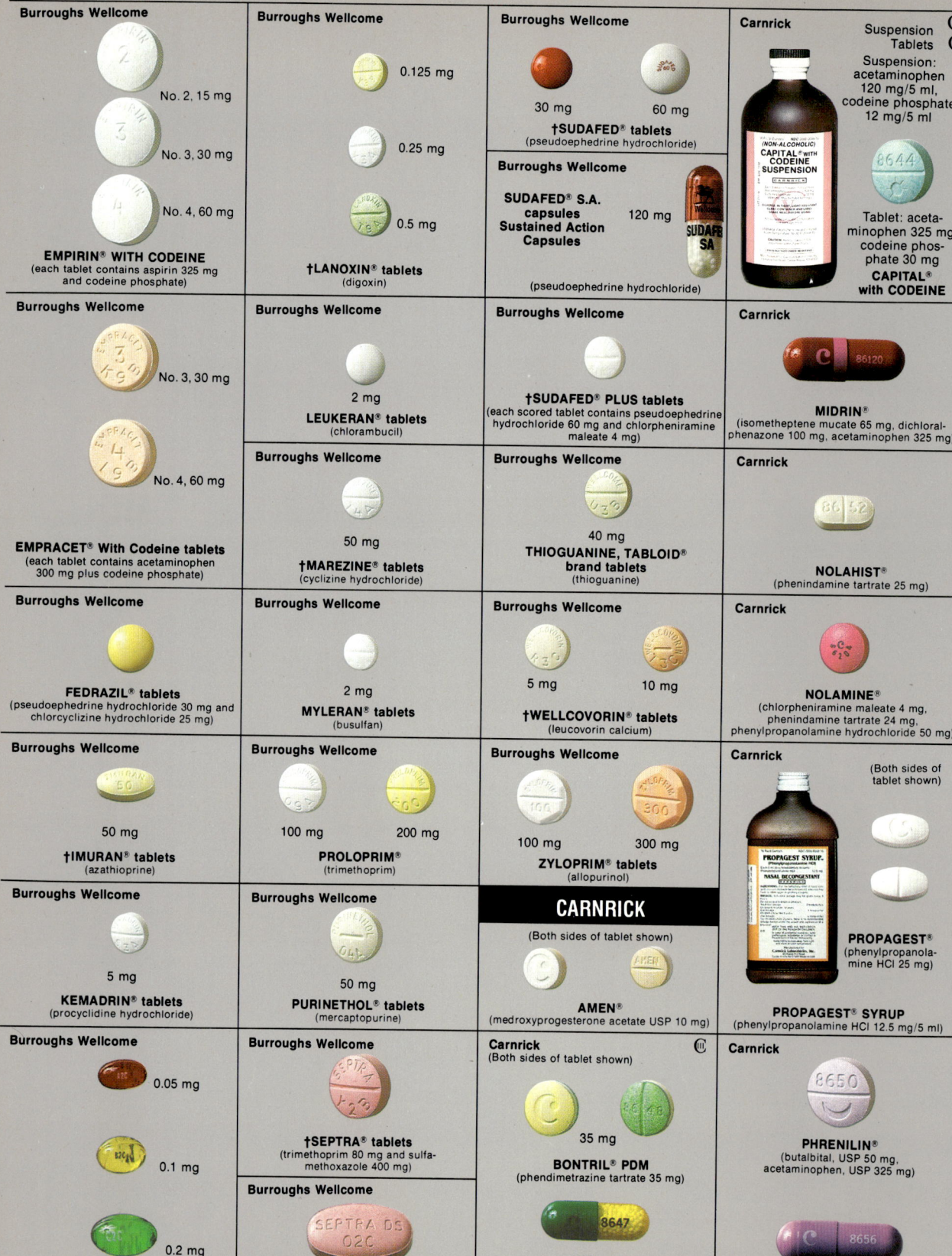

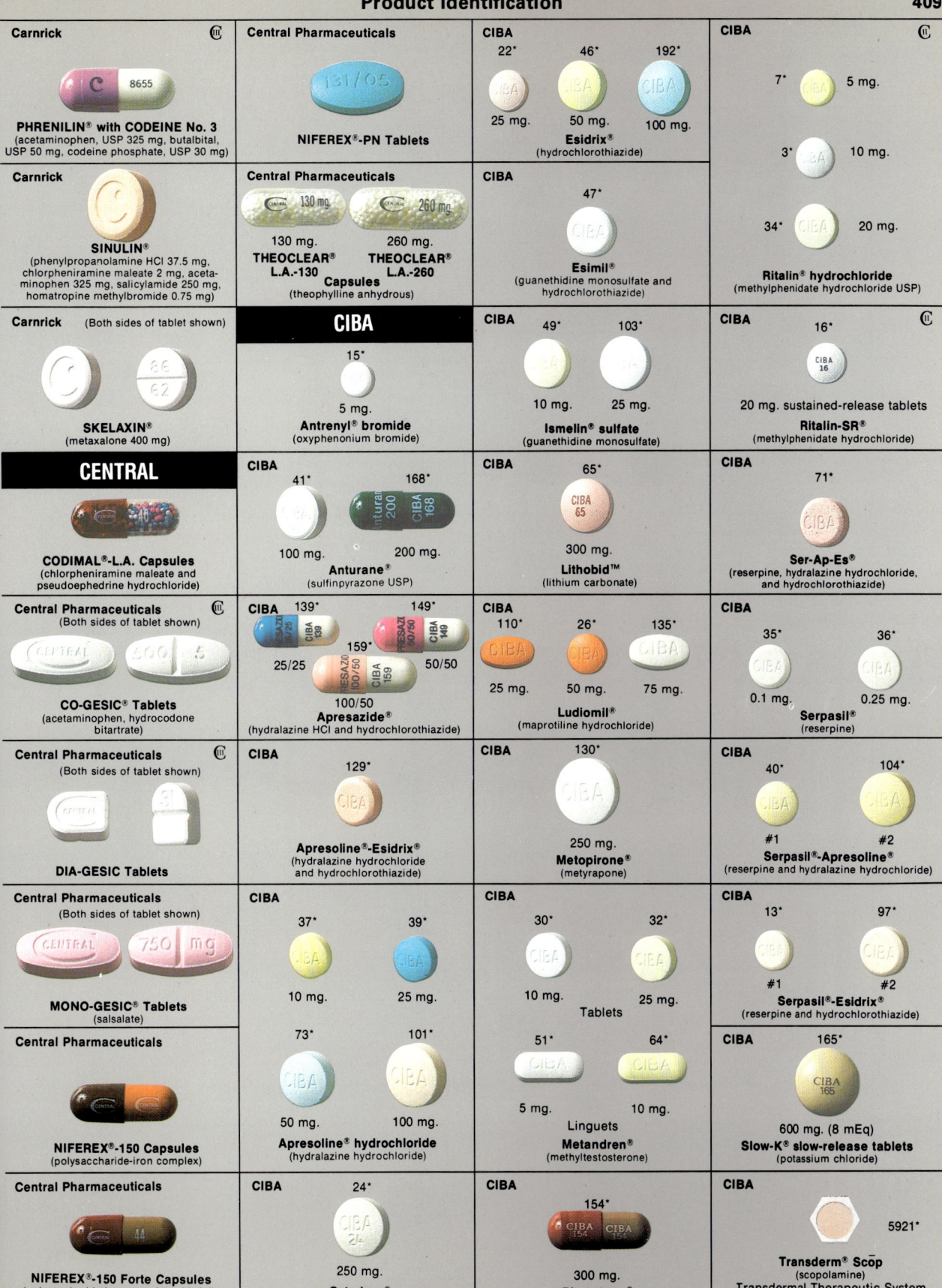

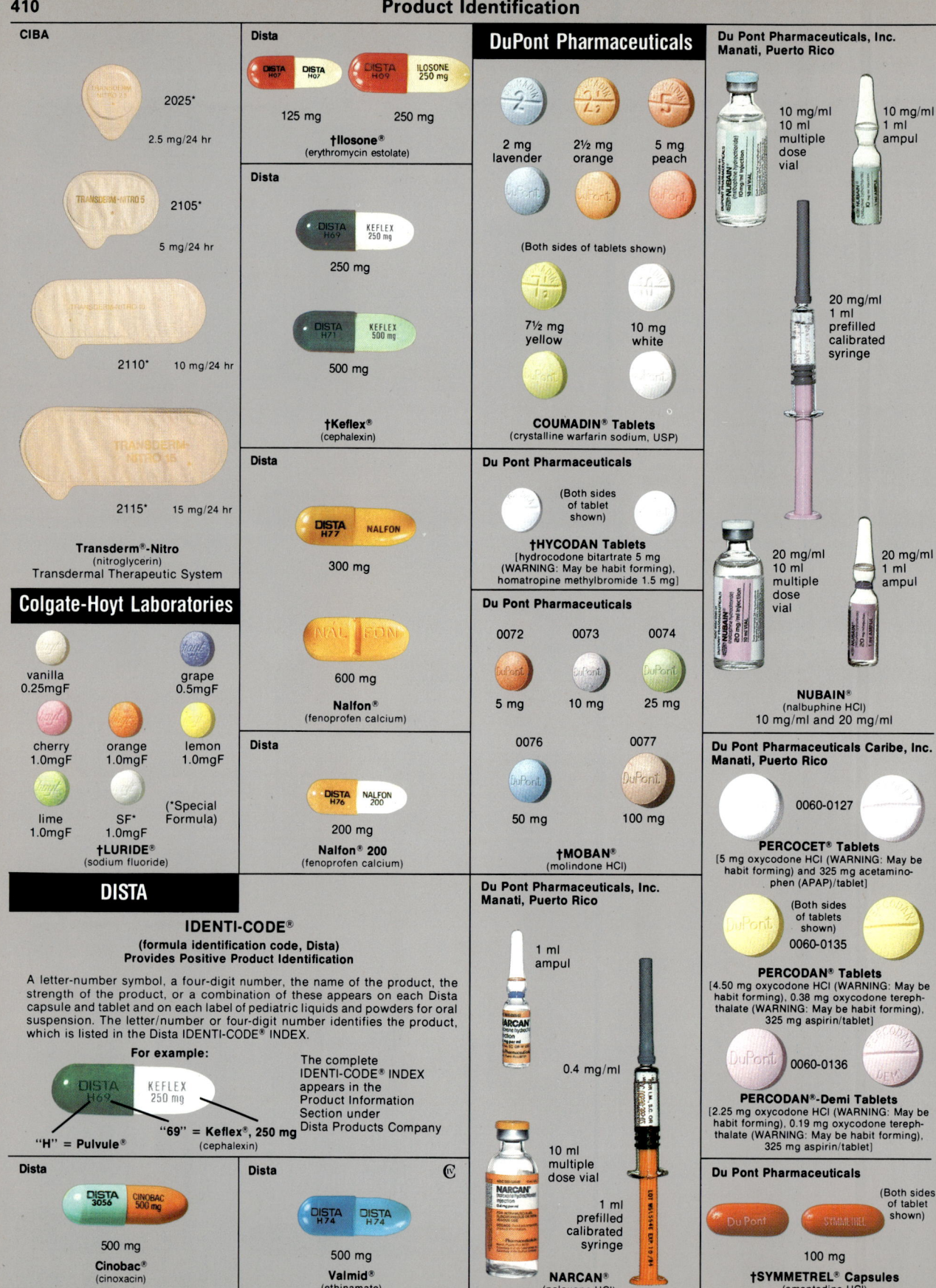

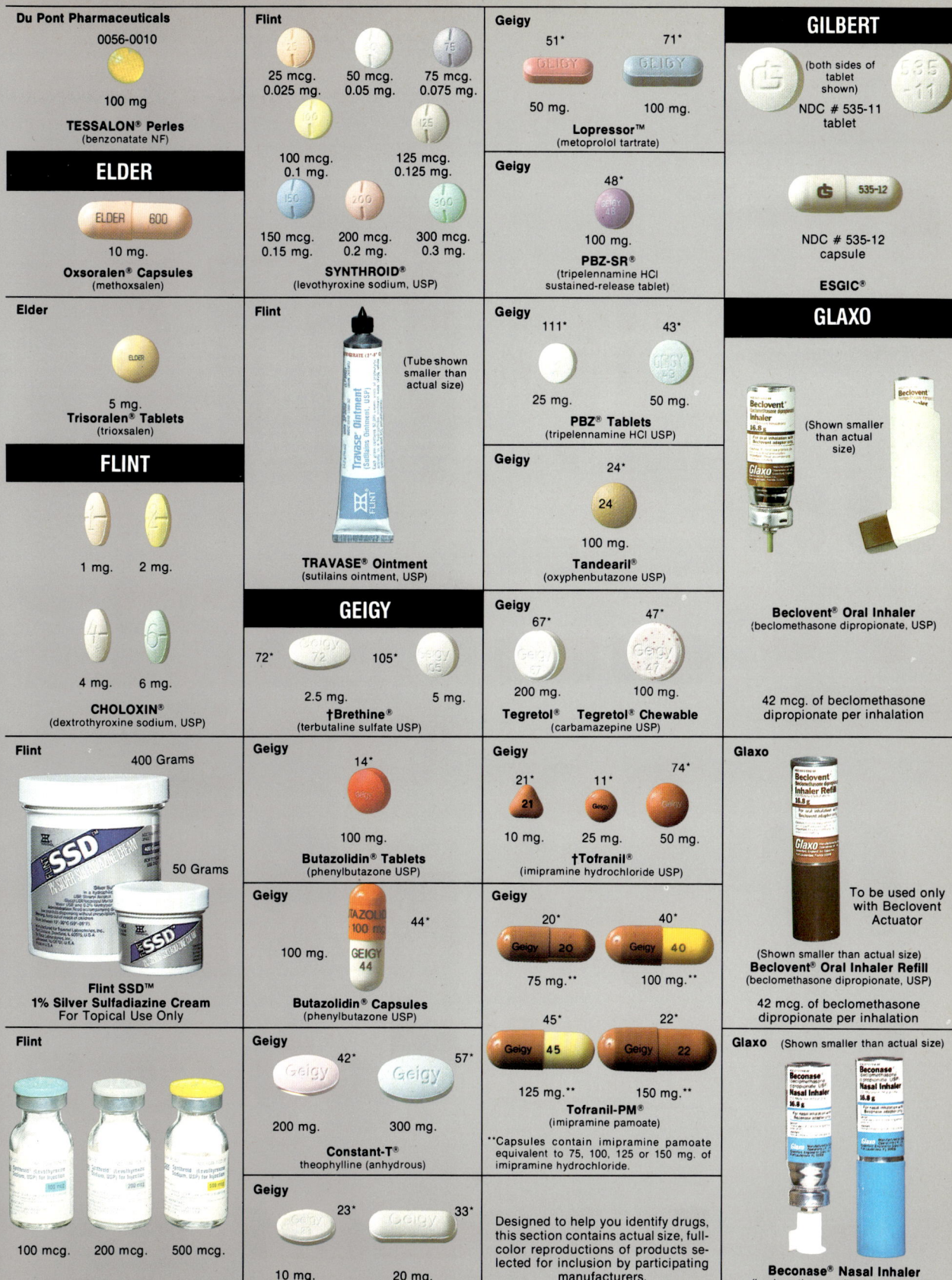

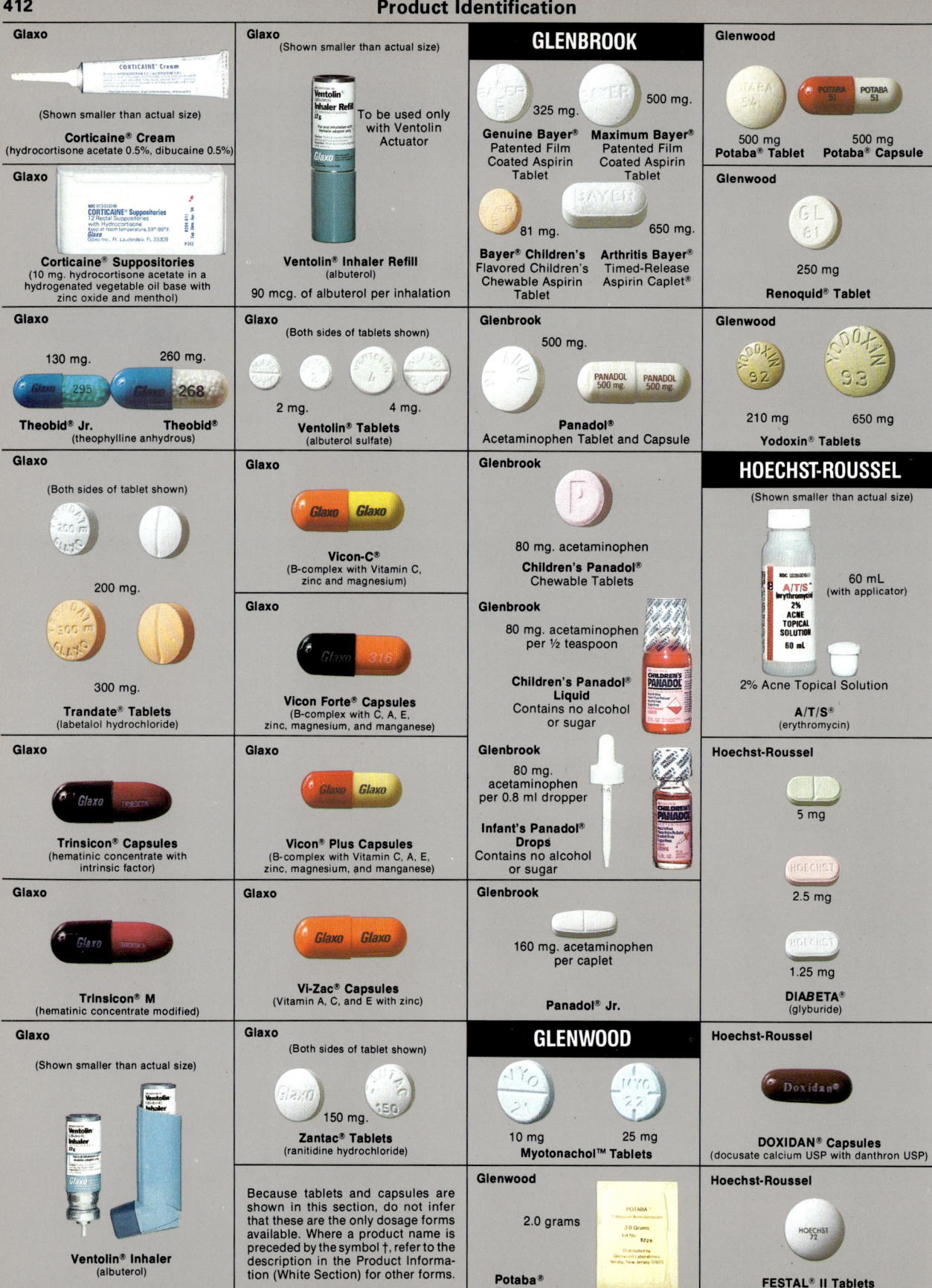

Product Identification

Hoechst-Roussel
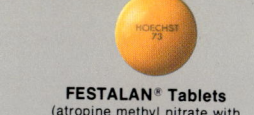
FESTALAN® Tablets
(atropine methyl nitrate with digestive enzymes)

Hoechst-Roussel
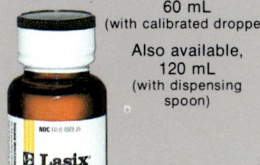
60 mL (with calibrated dropper)
Also available, 120 mL (with dispensing spoon)

LASIX® Oral Solution
(furosemide)

(Lasix Oral Solution shown smaller than actual size)

Hoechst-Roussel
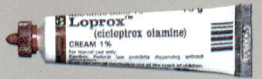
20 mg
40 mg
80 mg
LASIX® Tablets
(furosemide)

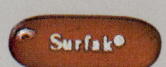 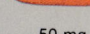

Ampuls 2, 4 and 10 mL (10 mg/mL)
LASIX® Injection
(furosemide)

2, 4 and 10 mL (10 mg/mL)
LASIX® Prefilled Syringe

(Ampul and syringe shown smaller than actual size)

Hoechst-Roussel
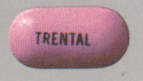
15 and 30 g tubes
LOPROX® Cream 1%
(ciclopirox olamine)

Hoechst-Roussel
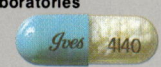
240 mg   50 mg
SURFAK® Capsules
(docusate calcium USP)

Hoechst-Roussel
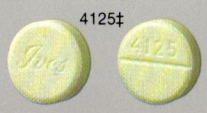
400 mg
Trental®
(pentoxifylline)

Hoechst-Roussel
(Tubes shown smaller than actual size)
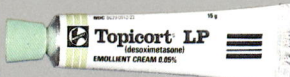
15 g, 60 g, and 4 oz. tubes
TOPICORT® Emollient Cream 0.25%
(desoximetasone)

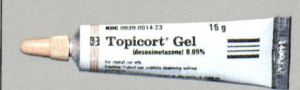
15 and 60 g tubes
TOPICORT® LP Emollient Cream 0.05%
(desoximetasone)

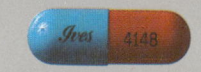
15 and 60 g tubes
TOPICORT® Gel 0.05%
(desoximetasone)

HYREX PHARMACEUTICALS
 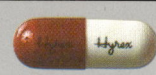
Sugar Free
100 mg.   200 mg.
HYTUSS™   **HYTUSS 2X™**
(guaifenesin USP)

Hyrex Pharmaceuticals

TRAC TABS 2X™

IVES LABORATORIES
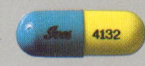
400 mg.

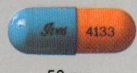
200 mg.   100 mg.
CYCLOSPASMOL®
(cyclandelate)

Ives Laboratories
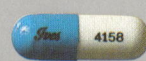
Tembids® Capsules

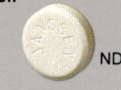
Tembids® Tablets
Sustained Action 40 mg.
The appearance of these capsules/tablets is a trademark of Ives Laboratories.
ISORDIL®
(isosorbide dinitrate)

Ives Laboratories
10 mg.   5 mg.   2.5 mg.
Sublingual   4164‡
Both sides of tablet shown
Chewable 10 mg.

Oral Titradose® Dosage Forms:
4152‡   4153‡
5 mg. Titradose®   10 mg. Titradose®
4154‡   4159‡
20 mg. Titradose®   30 mg. Titradose®
4192‡
40 mg. Titradose®
Both sides of Titradose tablets shown above
ISORDIL®
(isosorbide dinitrate)

Ives Laboratories
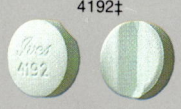
4132   4133
25 mg.   50 mg.
4158
100 mg.
SURMONTIL®
(trimipramine maleate)
The appearance of these capsules is a trademark of Ives Laboratories.

Ives Laboratories
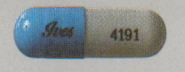
4191
SYNALGOS®-DC
The appearance of this capsule is a trademark of Ives Laboratories.

JANSSEN
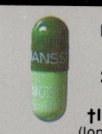
NDC 50458-400-50
2 mg capsules
†IMODIUM®
(loperamide HCl)

Janssen
NDC 50458-220-10
200 mg tablets
†NIZORAL®
(ketoconazole)

Janssen
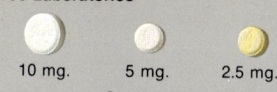
NDC 50458-110-30
100 mg tablet
VERMOX®
(mebendazole)

Janssen
NDC 50458-030-20
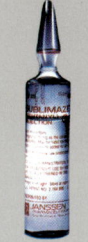 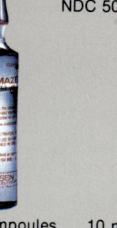
NDC 50458-030-10

20 ml ampoules   10 ml ampoules
†SUBLIMAZE® Injection
(fentanyl)

Janssen
NDC 50458-030-02
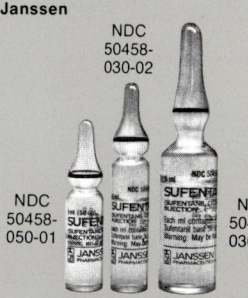
NDC 50458-030-05
NDC 50458-050-01

1 ml   2 ml   5 ml
ampoules
SUFENTA®
(sufentanil citrate)

Key Pharmaceuticals
(Shown smaller than actual size)
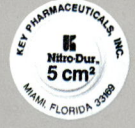
5 cm²

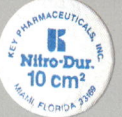
10 cm²

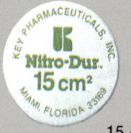
15 cm²

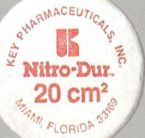
20 cm²

Nitro-Dur®
(nitroglycerin)
Transdermal Infusion System

413

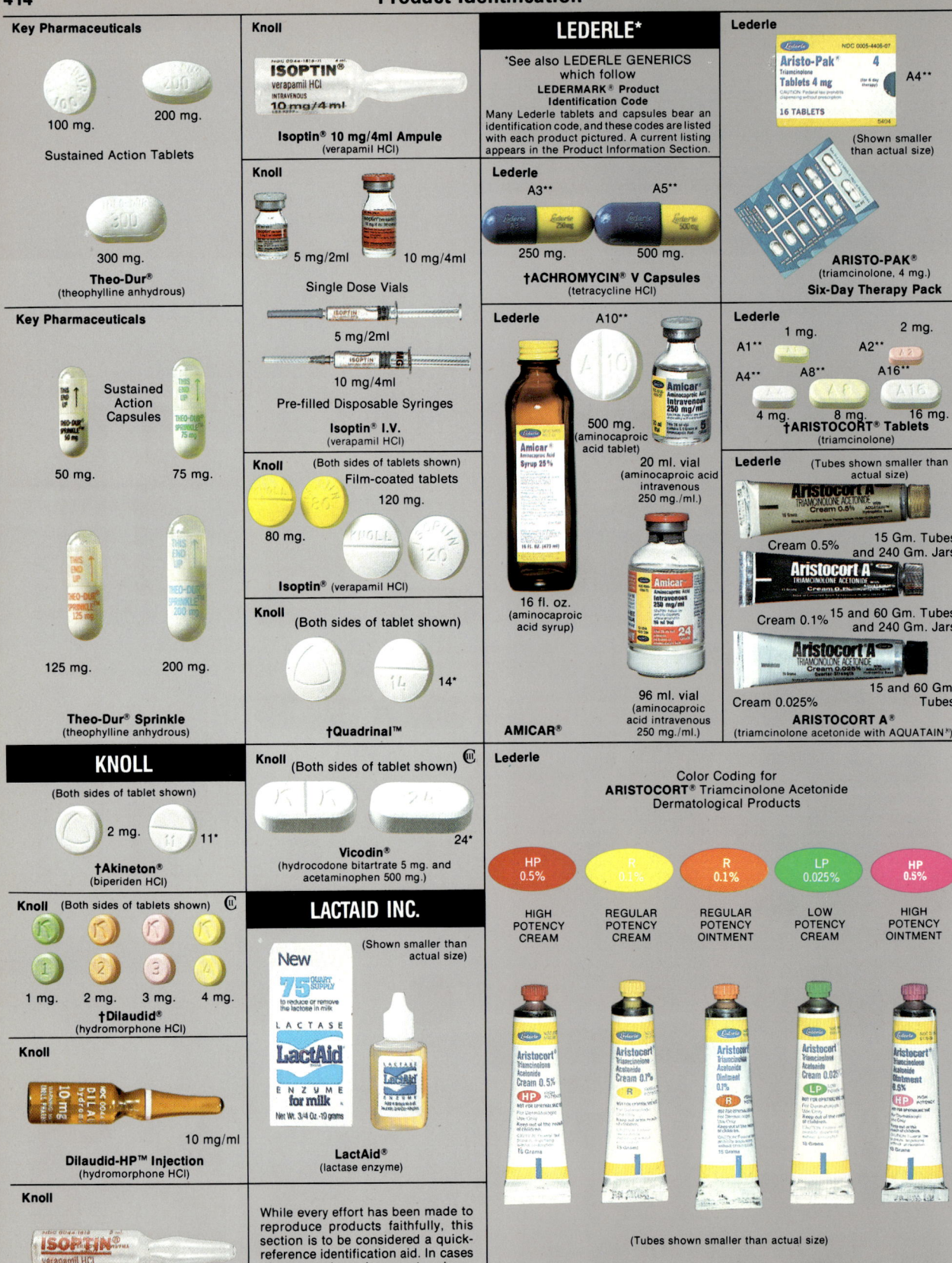

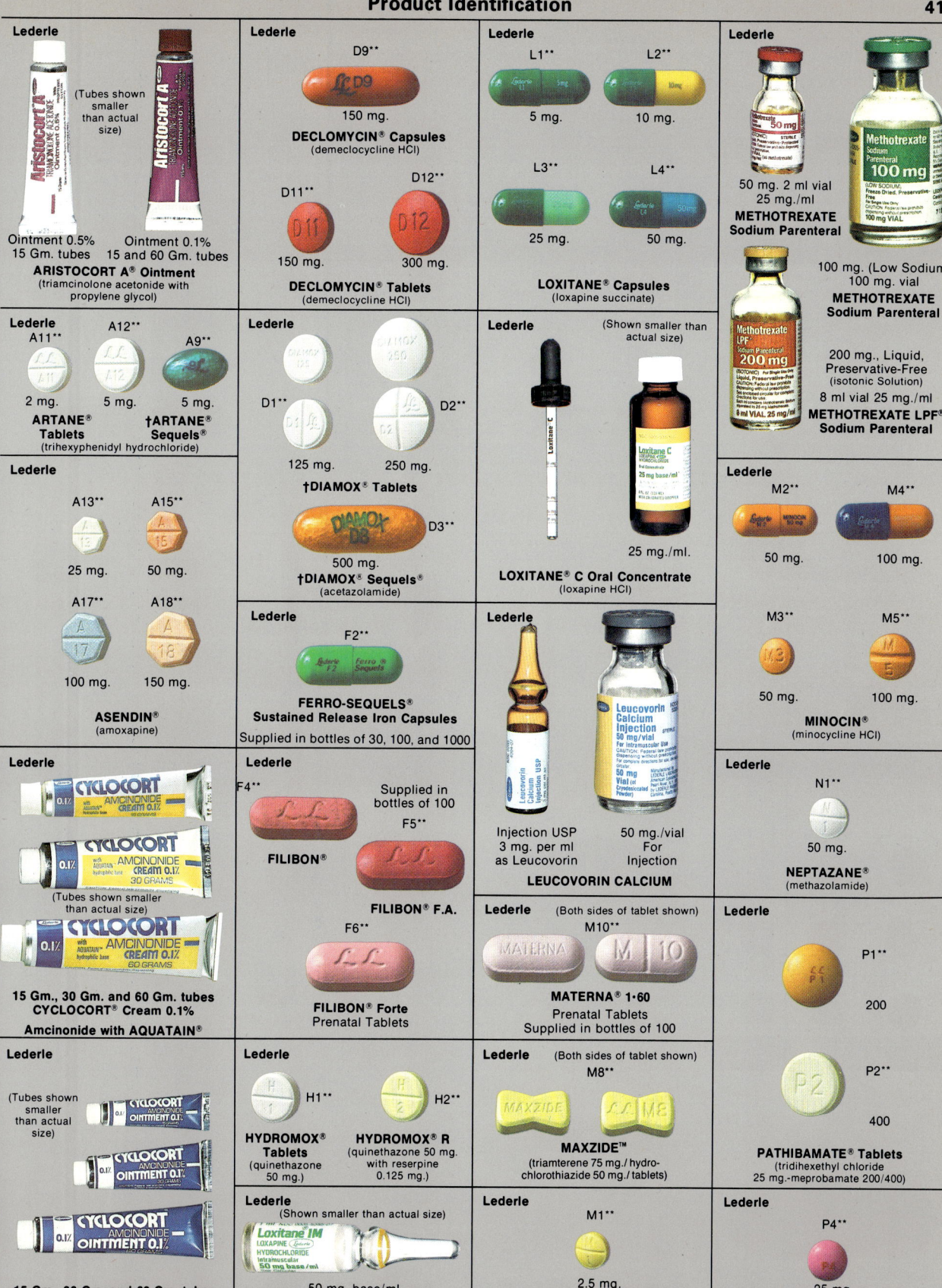

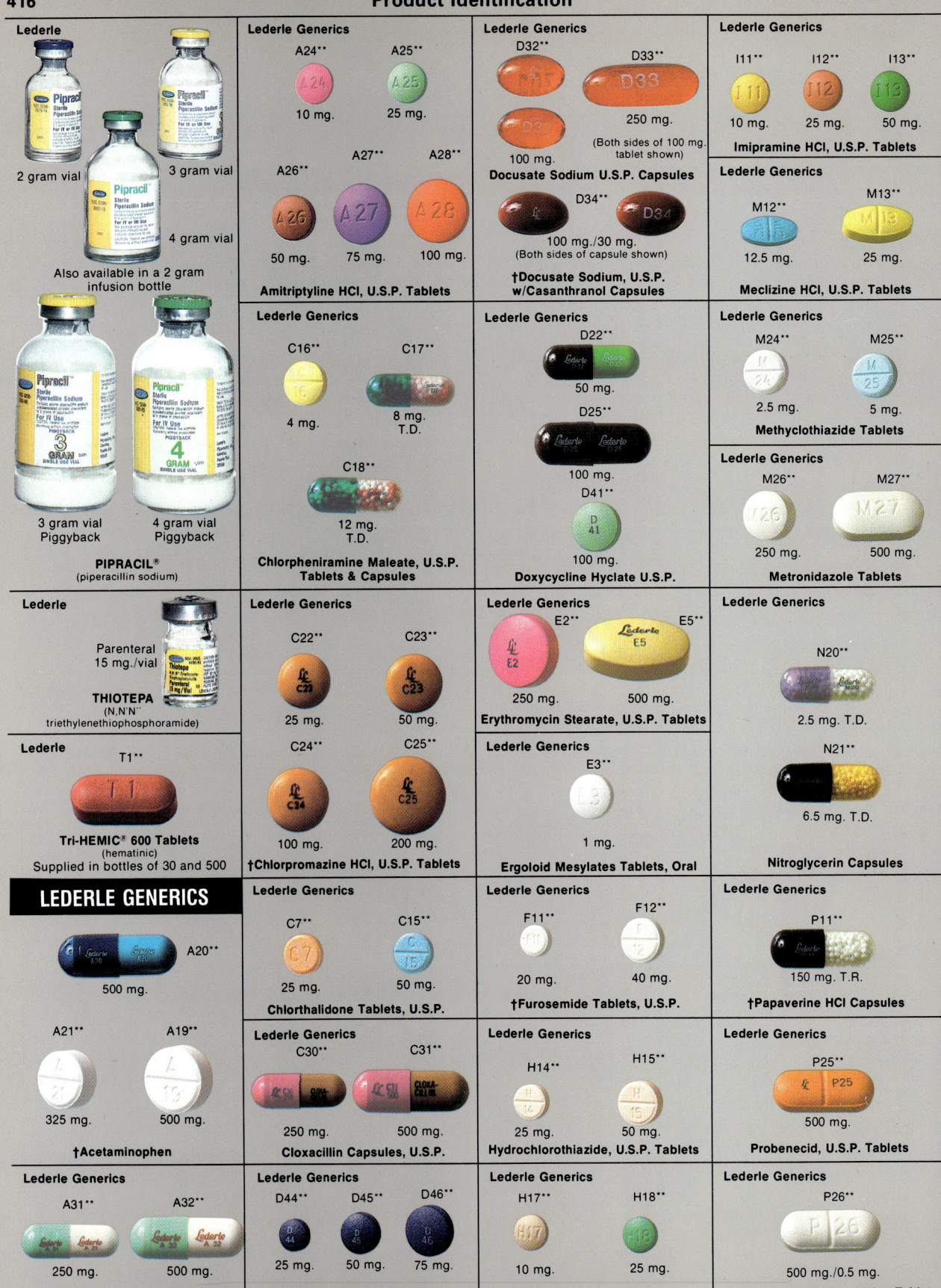

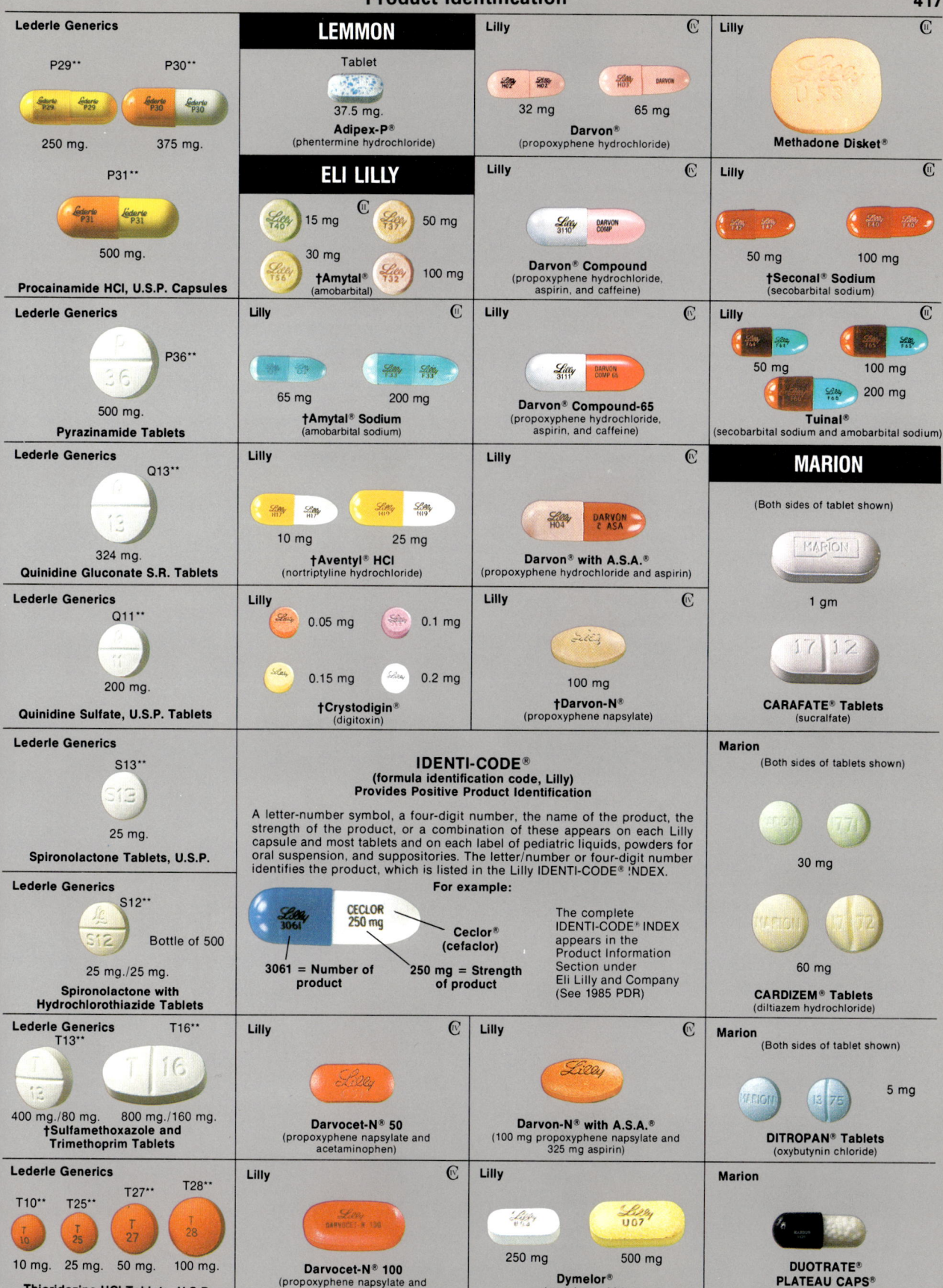

Product Identification

Marion

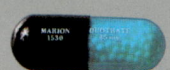
DUOTRATE® 45 PLATEAU CAPS®
(pentaerythritol tetranitrate)

Marion (Both sides of tablet shown)
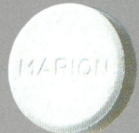
GAVISCON® Antacid Tablets

Marion (Both sides of tablet shown)
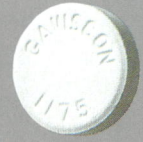
GAVISCON®-2 Antacid Tablets

Marion
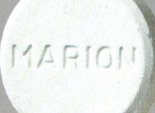
400 mg
NICO-400®
(nicotinic acid)

Marion
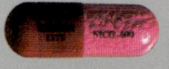
2.5 mg
NITRO-BID® 2.5 PLATEAU CAPS®
(nitroglycerin)

Marion
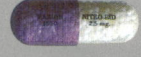
6.5 mg
NITRO-BID® 6.5 PLATEAU CAPS®
(nitroglycerin)

Marion
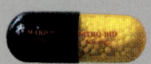
9 mg
NITRO-BID® 9 PLATEAU CAPS®
(nitroglycerin)

Marion

OS-CAL® 250 Tablets

OS-CAL® 500 Tablets

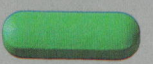
OS-CAL FORTE® Tablets

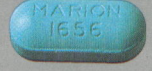
OS-CAL-GESIC® Tablets

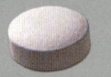
OS-CAL® PLUS Tablets

(oyster shell calcium family)

Marion
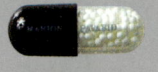
150 mg
PAVABID® PLATEAU CAPS®
(papaverine hydrochloride)

Marion (Both sides of tablet shown)
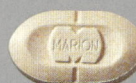 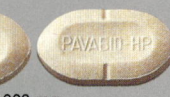
300 mg
PAVABID® HP Capsulets
(papaverine hydrochloride)

Marion

1 grain (60 mg)
(Also available in 2-grain tablets)
THYROID Tablets, USP

Marion

1 grain (60 mg), plain
(Also available in ½-grain and 2-grain plain tablets)

Marion

1 grain (60 mg), sugar-coated
(Also available in ½-grain, 2-grain and 3-grain sugar-coated tablets)
THYROID STRONG Tablets
(50% stronger than USP)

MASON PHARMACEUTICALS

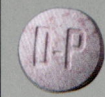 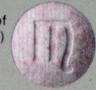
DAMACET-P®
(hydrocodone bitartrate 5 mg;
acetaminophen 500 mg)

Mason Pharmaceuticals (Both sides of tablet shown)
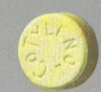 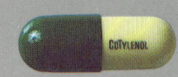
DAMASON-P®
(hydrocodone bitartrate 5 mg;
aspirin 224 mg; caffeine 32 mg)

McNeil Consumer Products

 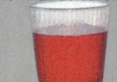
†CoTYLENOL® Cold Medication Tablets and Capsules

Also Available:
CoTYLENOL® Liquid Cold Medication

McNeil Consumer Products
(Dosage cup shown smaller than actual size)
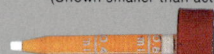
Children's CoTYLENOL® Chewable Cold Tablets and Liquid Cold Medication

McNeil Consumer Products
(Shown smaller than actual size)
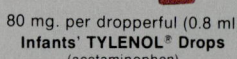
80 mg. per dropperful (0.8 ml)
Infants' TYLENOL® Drops
(acetaminophen)

McNeil Consumer Products
(Shown smaller than actual size)

80 mg. per ½ tsp.
Children's TYLENOL® Elixir
(acetaminophen)

McNeil Consumer Products
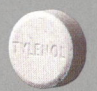
80 mg.
Children's TYLENOL® Chewable Tablets
(acetaminophen)

McNeil Consumer Products
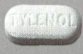
160 mg.
Junior Strength TYLENOL® Swallowable Tablets
(acetaminophen)

McNeil Consumer Products

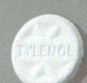 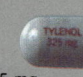
325 mg.
Regular Strength TYLENOL® Tablets and Capsules
(acetaminophen)

McNeil Consumer Products
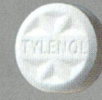
500 mg.
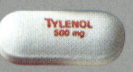
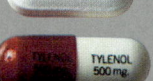
†Extra-Strength TYLENOL® Tablets, Caplets and Capsules
(acetaminophen)
Also Available: Extra-Strength TYLENOL® Adult Liquid

McNeil Consumer Products
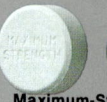 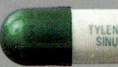
Maximum-Strength TYLENOL® Sinus Medication Tablets and Capsules

McNeil Pharmaceutical

Tablets
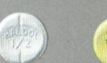 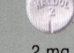
½ mg   1 mg   2 mg

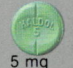 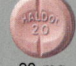
5 mg   10 mg   20 mg

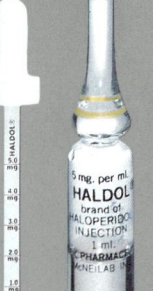

Concentrate 2 mg per ml | Injectable 5 mg per ml (1 ml/ampul) | Pre-filled Syringe 5 mg

HALDOL®
(haloperidol)

McNeil Pharmaceutical

Enteric Coated Microspheres 0095*
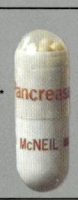
PANCREASE® Capsules
(brand of pancrelipase)
Bottles of 100 and 250

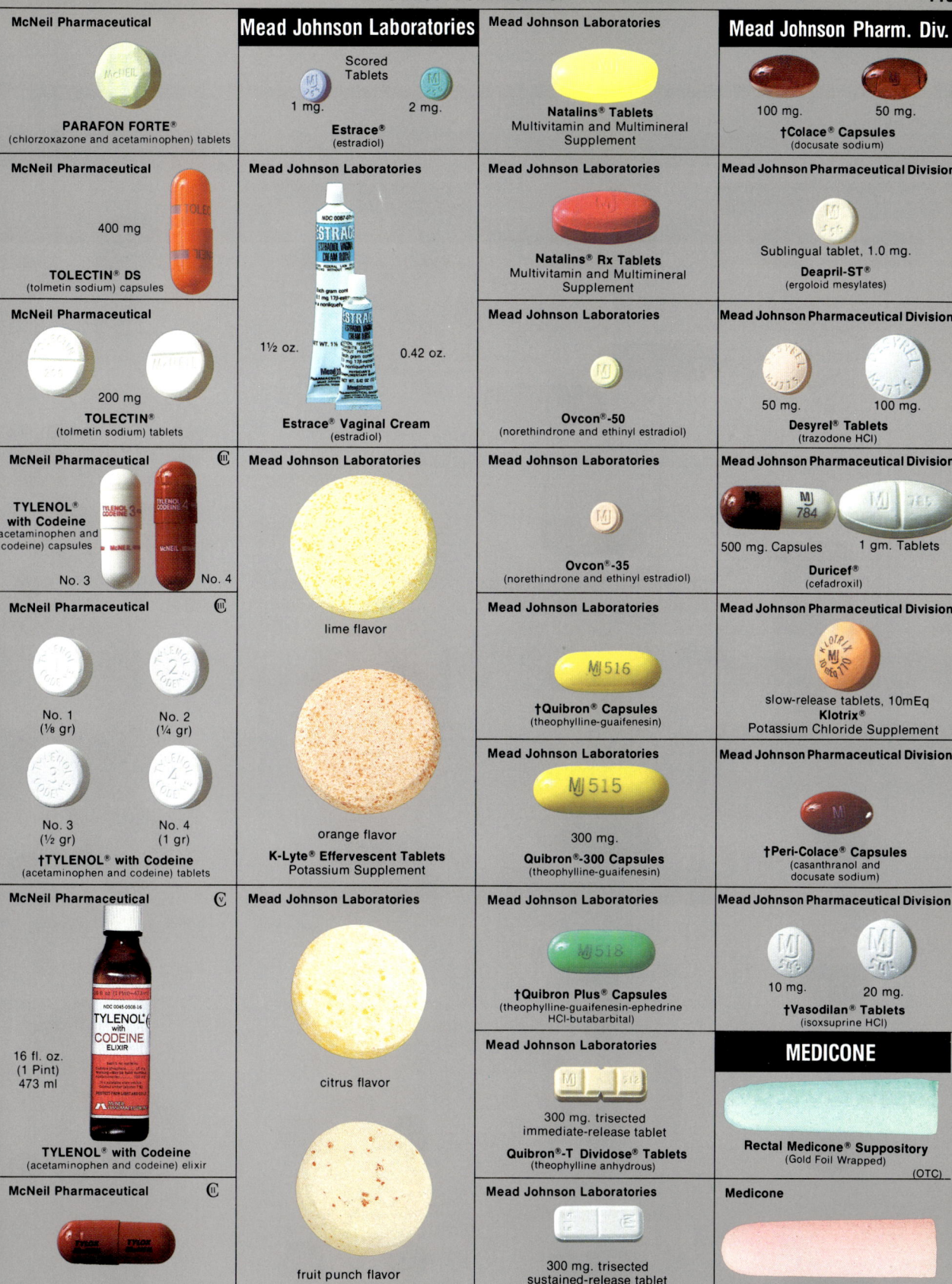

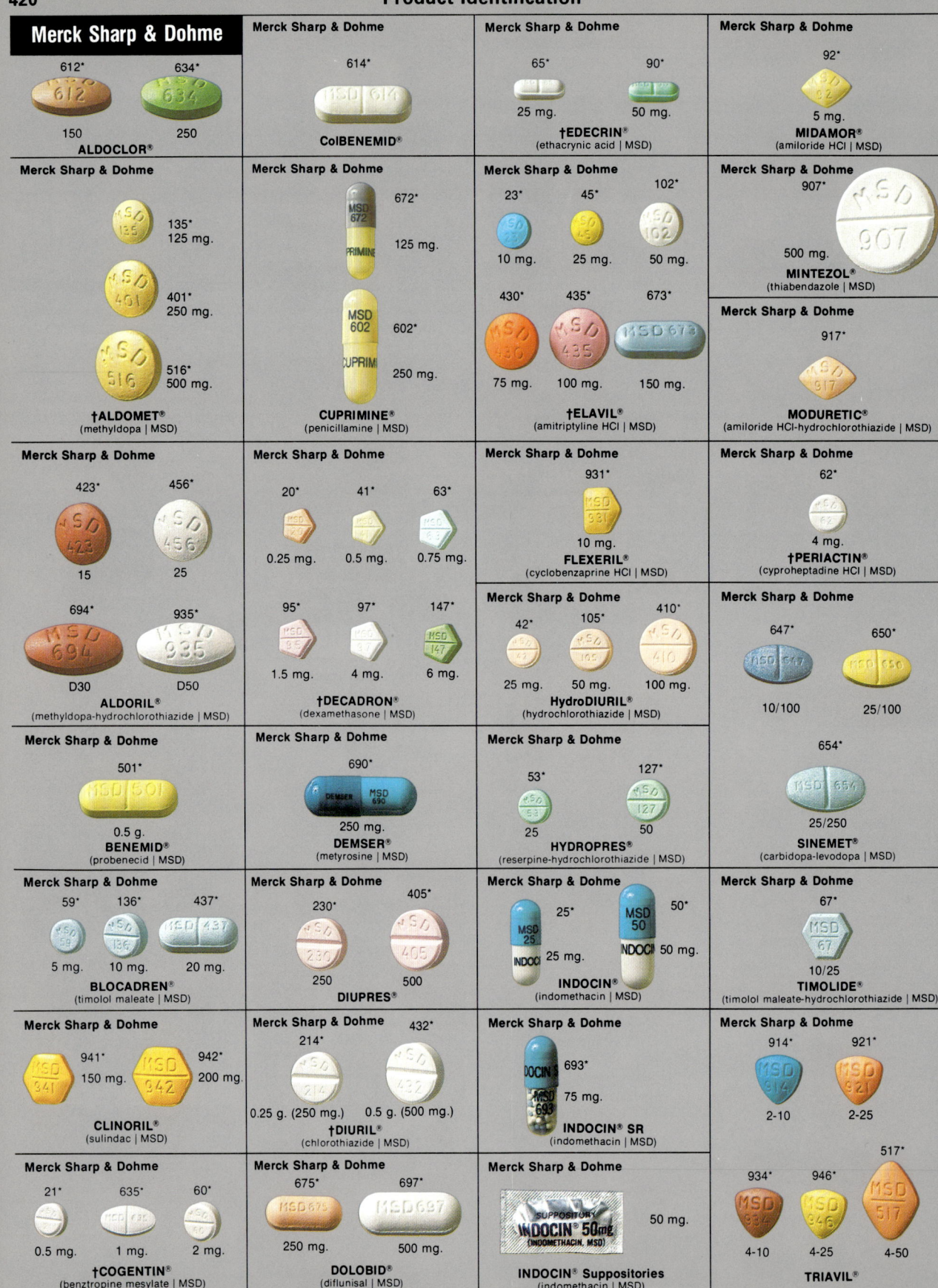

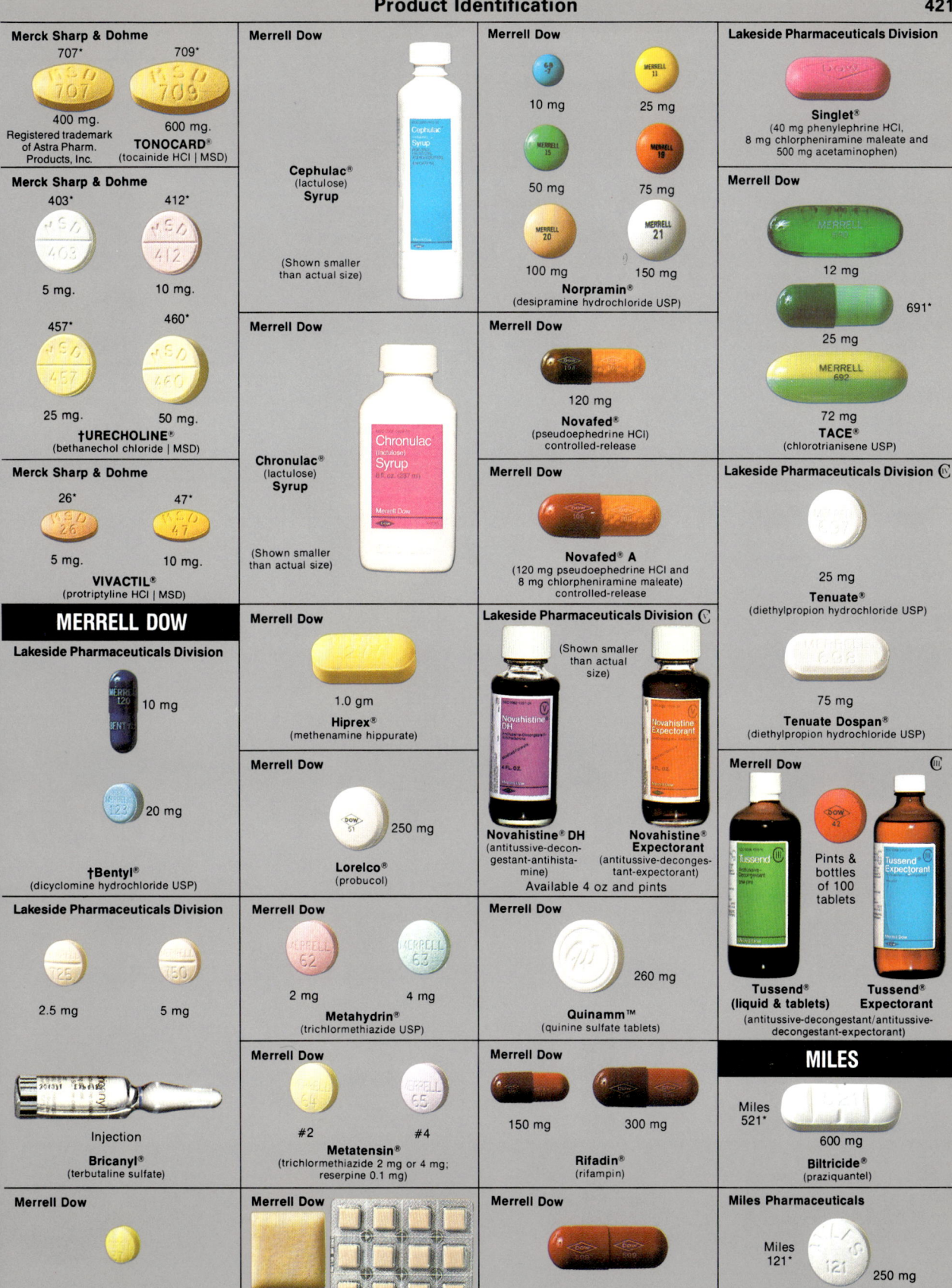

Product Identification

Miles Pharmaceuticals

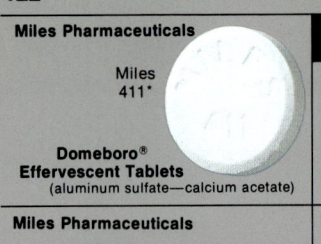
Miles 411*
Domeboro® Effervescent Tablets
(aluminum sulfate—calcium acetate)

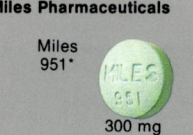
Miles 951*
300 mg
Lithane®
(lithium carbonate)

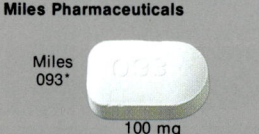
Miles 093*
100 mg
Mycelex®-G Vaginal Tablets
(clotrimazole)

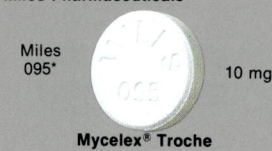
Miles 095*
10 mg
Mycelex® Troche
(clotrimazole)

Miles 721*
500 mg
Niclocide™ Chewable Tablets
(niclosamide)

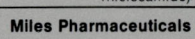
Miles 132*
50 mg
Stiphostrol®
(diethyl stilbestrol diphosphate)

NORCLIFF THAYER

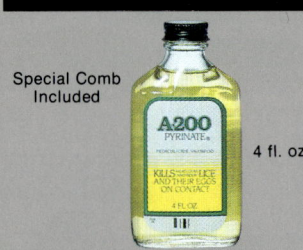
Special Comb Included
4 fl. oz.
A-200 Pyrinate® Pediculicide Shampoo
Also available:
A-200 Pyrinate Shampoo, 2 fl. oz.
A-200 Pyrinate Shampoo Gel, 1 oz.

Because tablets and capsules are shown in this section, do not infer that these are the only dosage forms available. Where a product name is preceded by the symbol †, refer to the description in the Product Information (White Section) for other forms.

NORWICH EATON

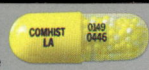
sustained release
Comhist® LA Capsules
(chlorpheniramine maleate 4 mg., phenyltoloxamine citrate 50 mg., phenylephrine HCl 20 mg.)

Norwich Eaton
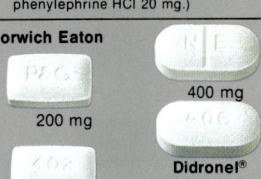
200 mg   400 mg
Didronel®
(etidronate disodium)

Norwich Eaton
sustained release
Entex® LA Tablets
(guaifenesin 400 mg., phenylpropanolamine HCl 75 mg.)

Eaton Laboratories Inc.
Manati, Puerto Rico

25 mg   50 mg

100 mg
Macrodantin® Capsules
(nitrofurantoin macrocrystals)

O'Neal, Jones & Feldman

OJF 610
Bancap HC®
(hydrocodone bitartrate, 5 mg and acetaminophen, 500 mg)

O'Neal, Jones & Feldman

†**Pedameth®** Capsules
(racemethionine, OJF)

ORGANON

388*
Cotazym-S™
enteric coated spheres
(pancrelipase, USP)

Organon
381*   386*
†**Cotazym®**   386
†**Cotazym®** Cherry Flavored
(pancrelipase capsules, USP)

Organon

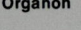
795*
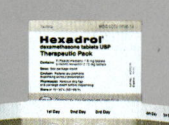
Hexadrol Therapeutic Pack

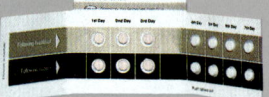
(pack shown smaller than actual size)
6 Hexadrol 1.5 mg. tablets and
8 Hexadrol 0.75 mg. tablets
Hexadrol® Therapeutic Pack
(dexamethasone tablets, USP)

Organon
792*   791*
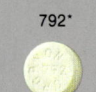 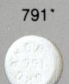
0.5 mg.   0.75 mg.

790*   798*
 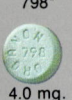
1.5 mg.   4.0 mg.
†**Hexadrol®**
(dexamethasone tablets, USP)

Organon
821*
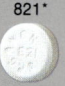
3 mg.
Liquamar®
(phenprocouman tablets, USP)

Organon
542*
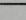
Wigraine®
(ergotamine tartrate and caffeine tablets, USP)

Organon
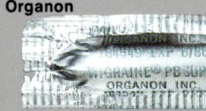
Wigraine®
(ergotamine tartrate and caffeine suppositories, USP)

Organon
Wigraine®-PB
(ergotamine tartrate, caffeine, belladonna alkaloids, pentobarbital suppositories, USP)

Organon
547*

Wigrettes®
(ergotamine tartrate sublingual tablets, USP)

ORTHO

Ortho compacts shown smaller than actual size

Also available in 28-day regimen containing 7 inert green tablets

ORTHO-NOVUM™
7/7/7□21 Day Regimen
(Each white tablet contains 0.5 mg of norethindrone and 0.035 mg of ethinyl estradiol)
(Each light peach tablet contains 0.75 mg of norethindrone and 0.035 mg of ethinyl estradiol)
(Each peach tablet contains 1 mg of norethindrone and 0.035 mg of ethinyl estradiol)

Ortho

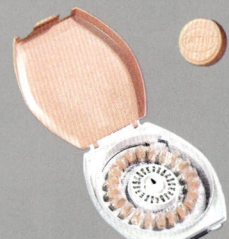

Also available in 28-day regimen containing 7 inert green tablets

ORTHO-NOVUM™
10/11□21 Day Regimen
(Each white tablet contains 0.5 mg of norethindrone with 0.035 mg of ethinyl estradiol)
(Each peach tablet contains 1 mg of norethindrone with 0.035 mg of ethinyl estradiol)

Ortho

ORTHO-NOVUM™
1/35□21 Day Regimen
(1 mg of norethindrone with 0.035 mg of ethinyl estradiol)
Also available in 28-day regimen containing 7 inert green tablets

Ortho

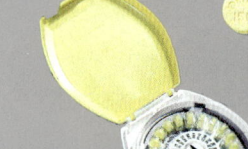

ORTHO-NOVUM™
1/50□21 Day Regimen
(1 mg of norethindrone with 0.05 mg of mestranol)
Also available in 28-day regimen containing 7 inert green tablets

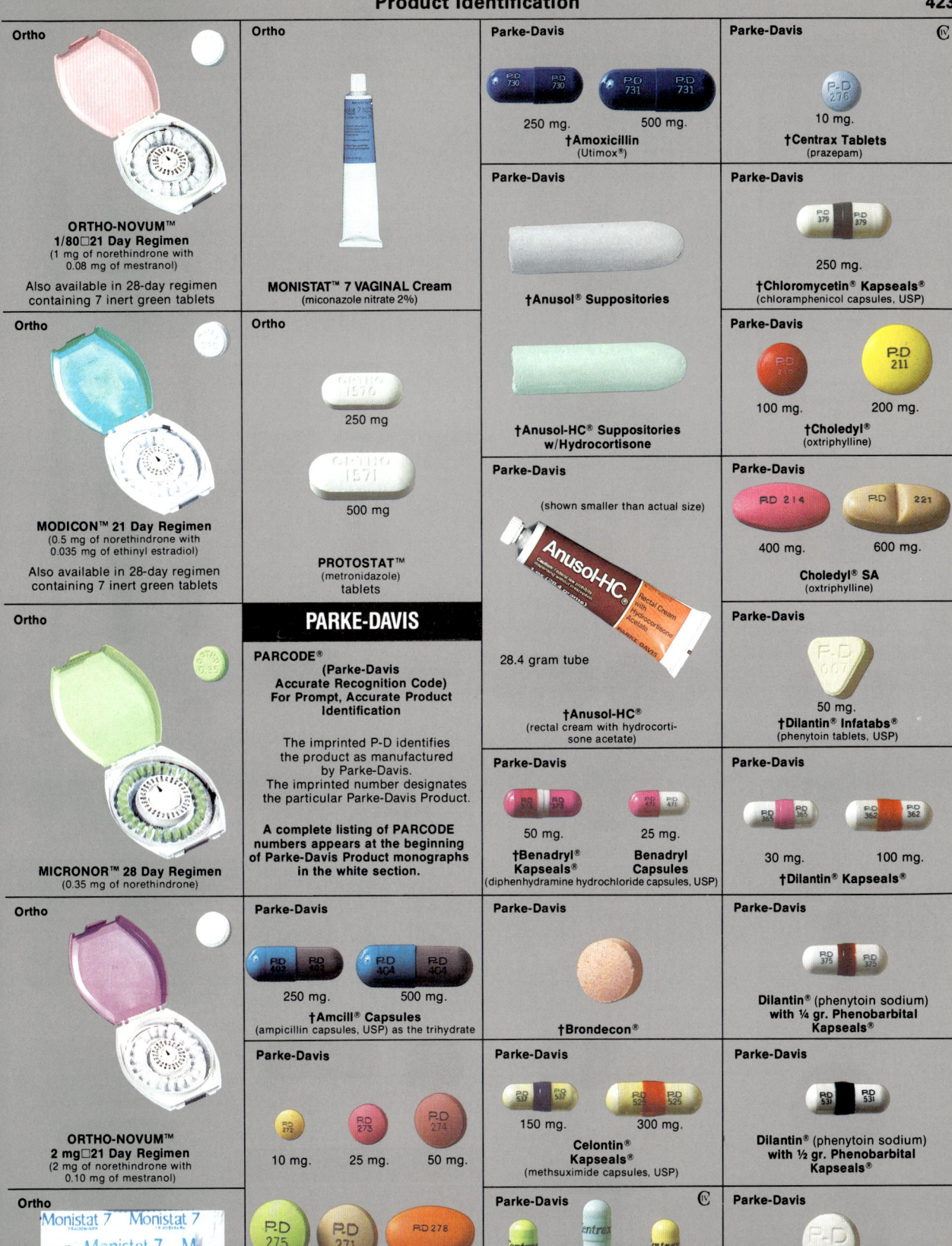

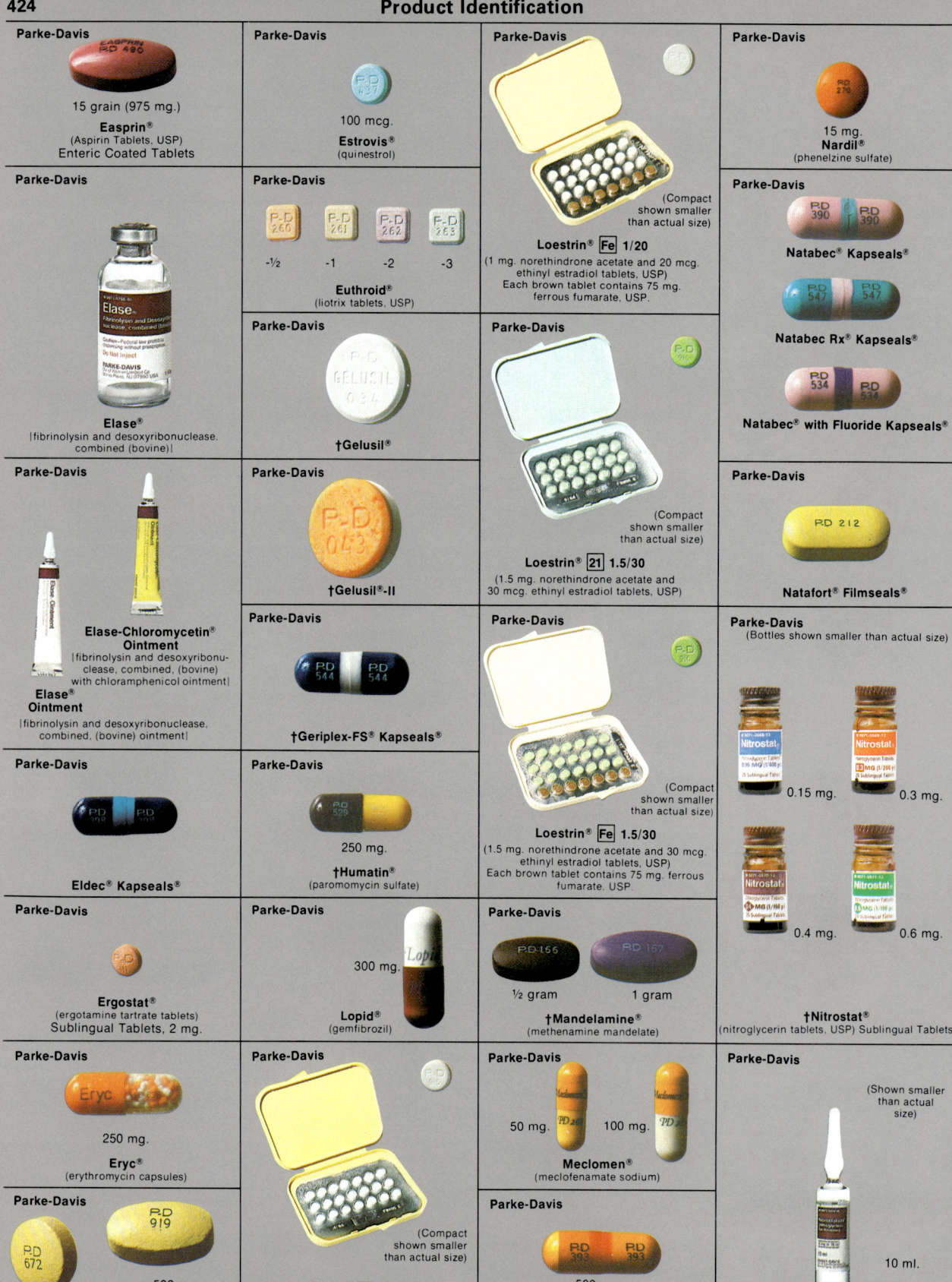

Product Identification

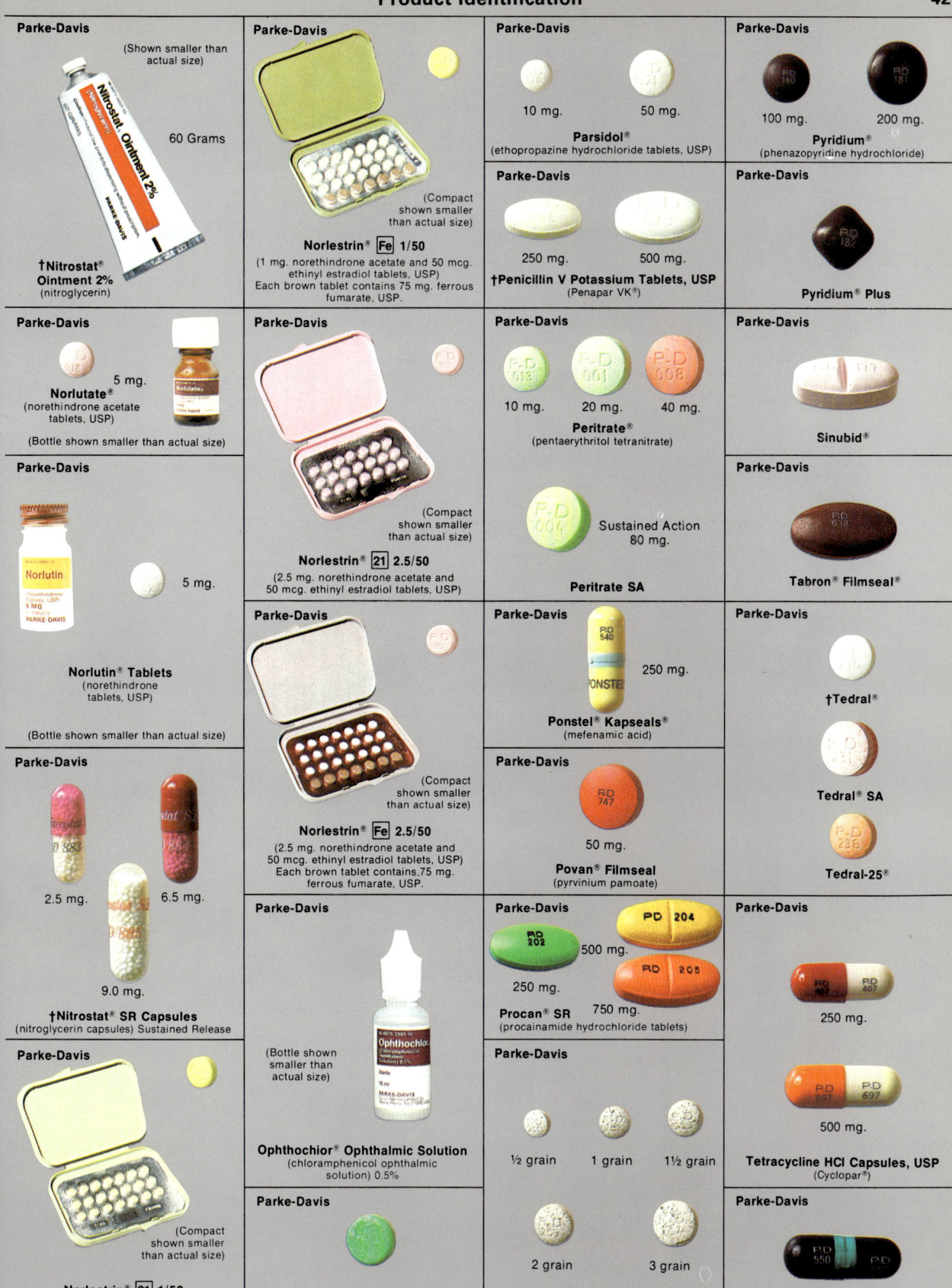

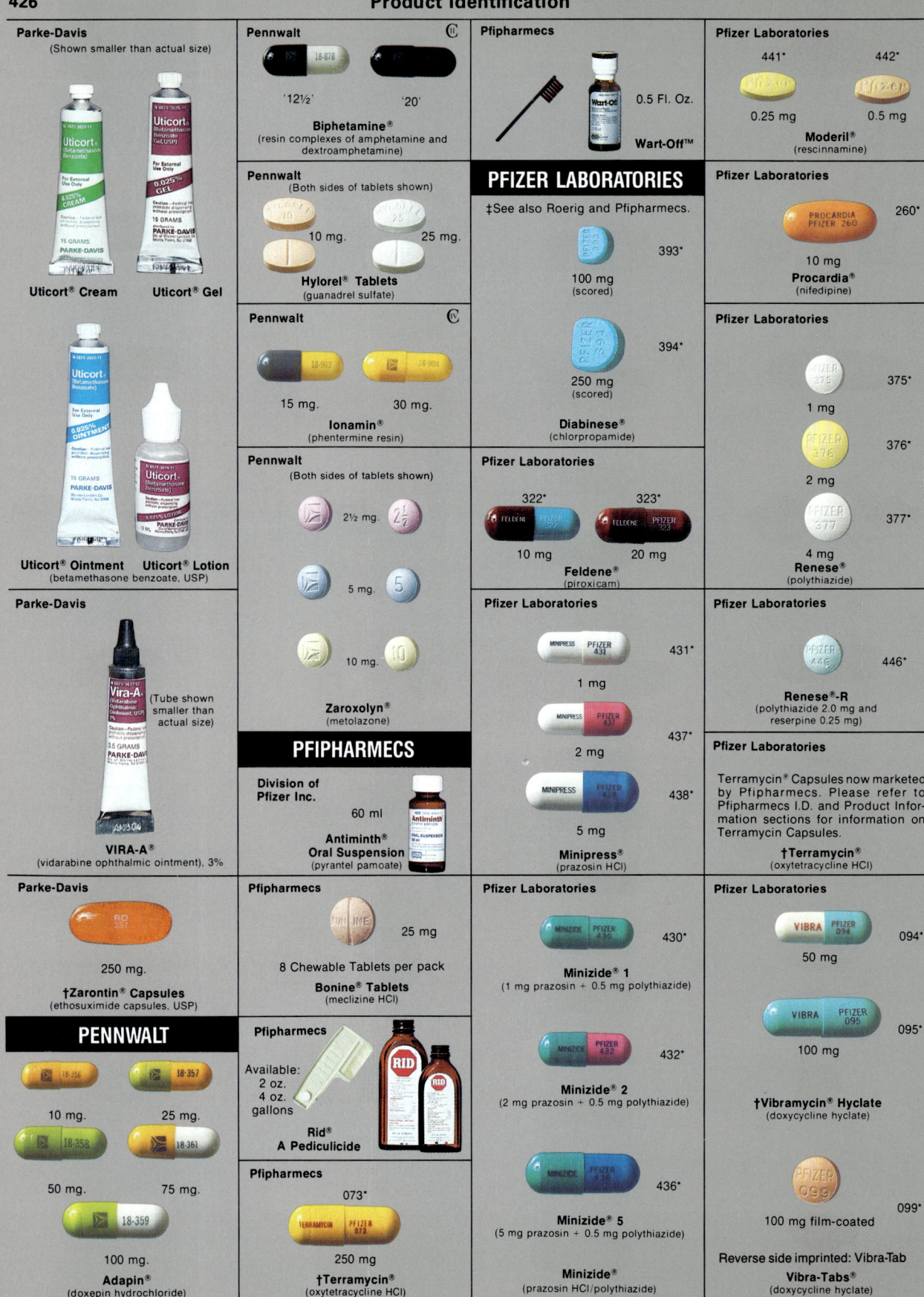

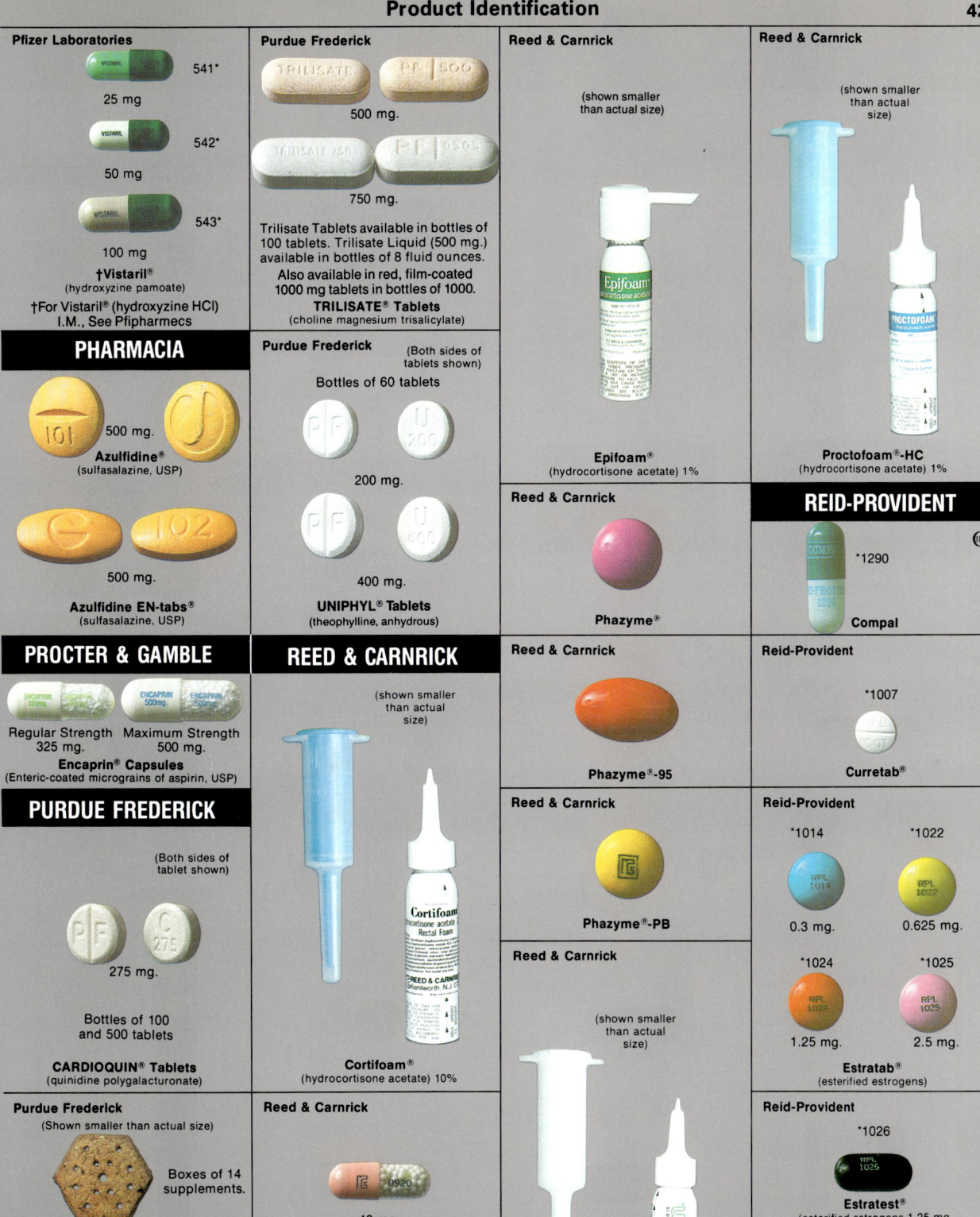

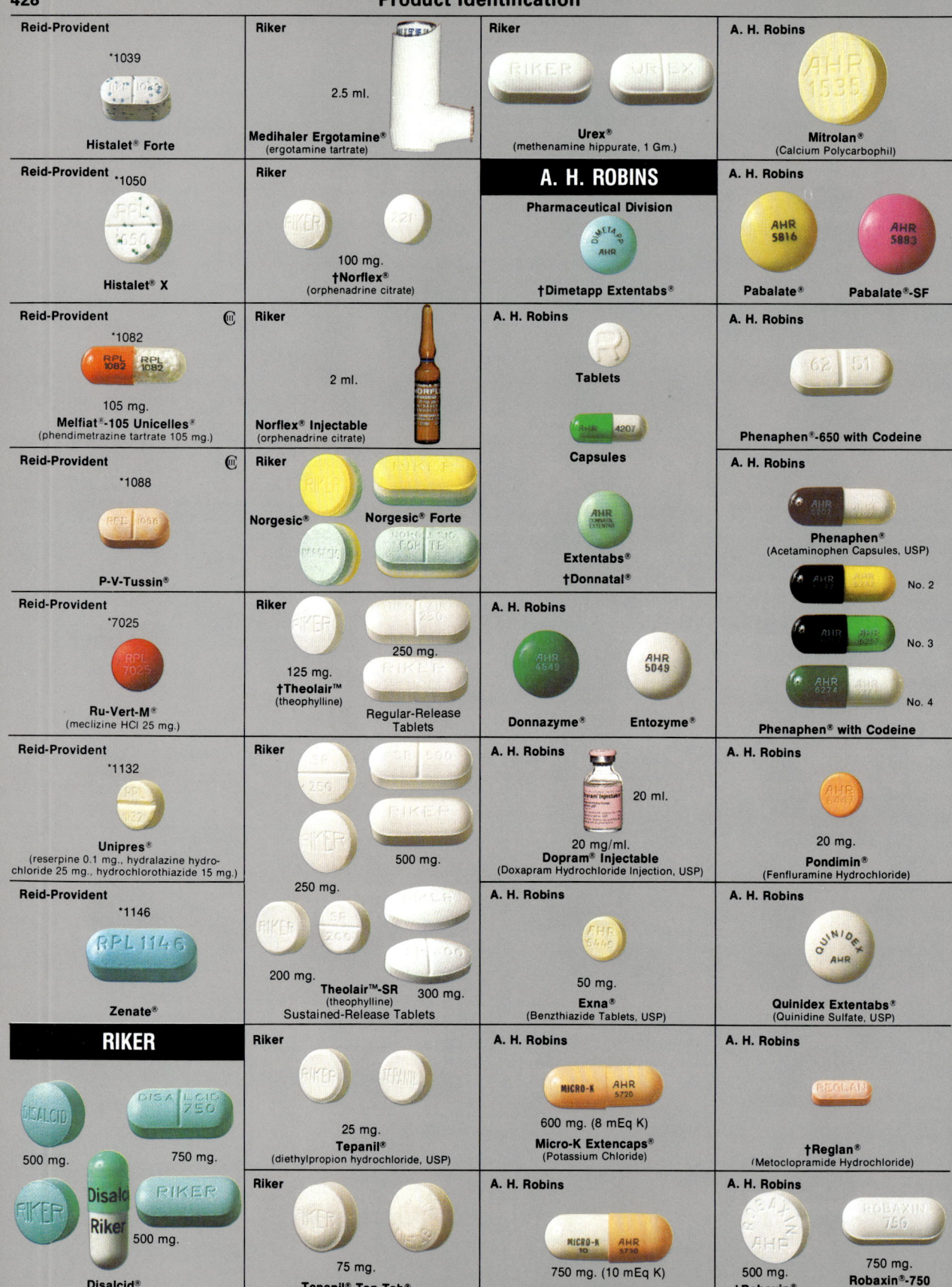

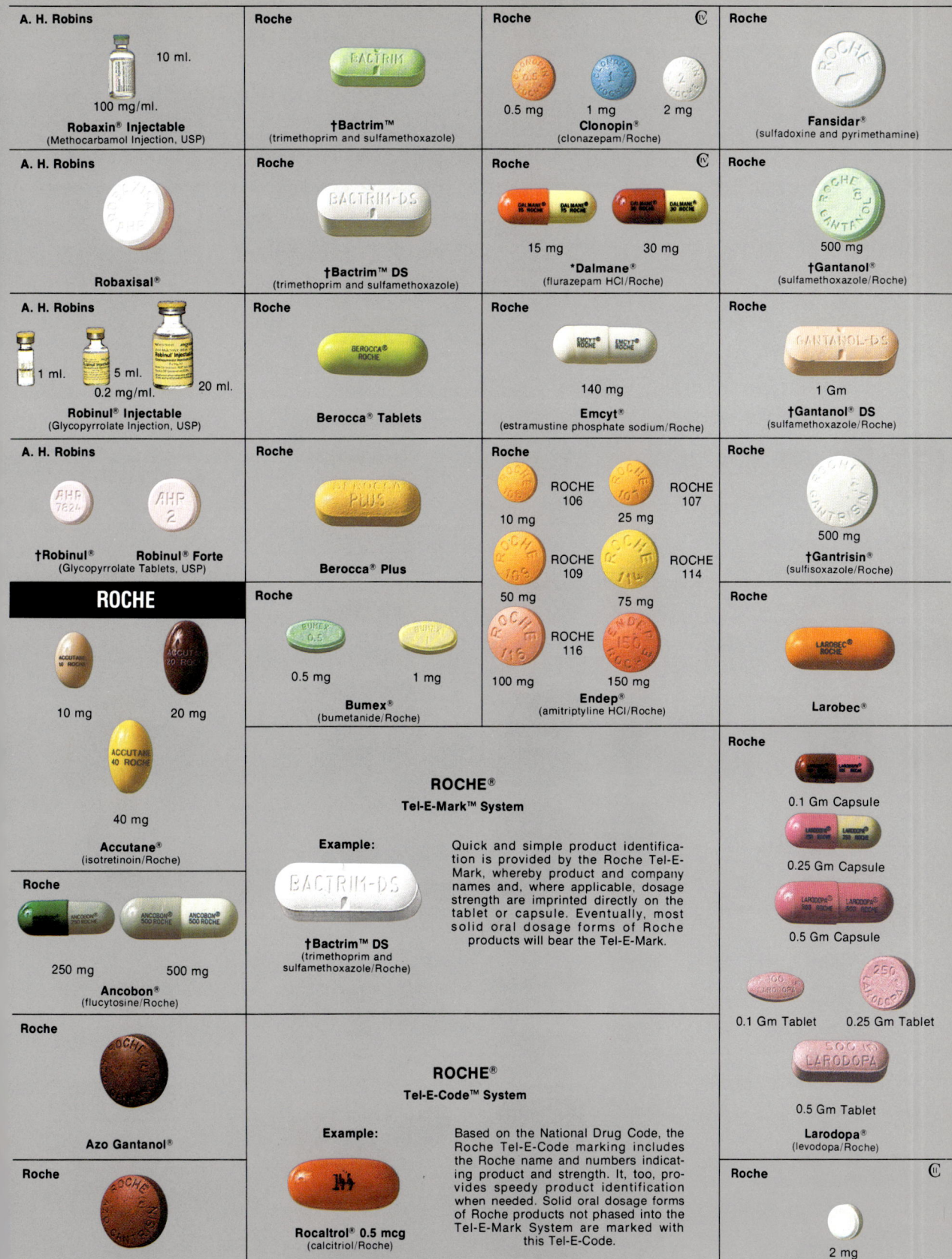

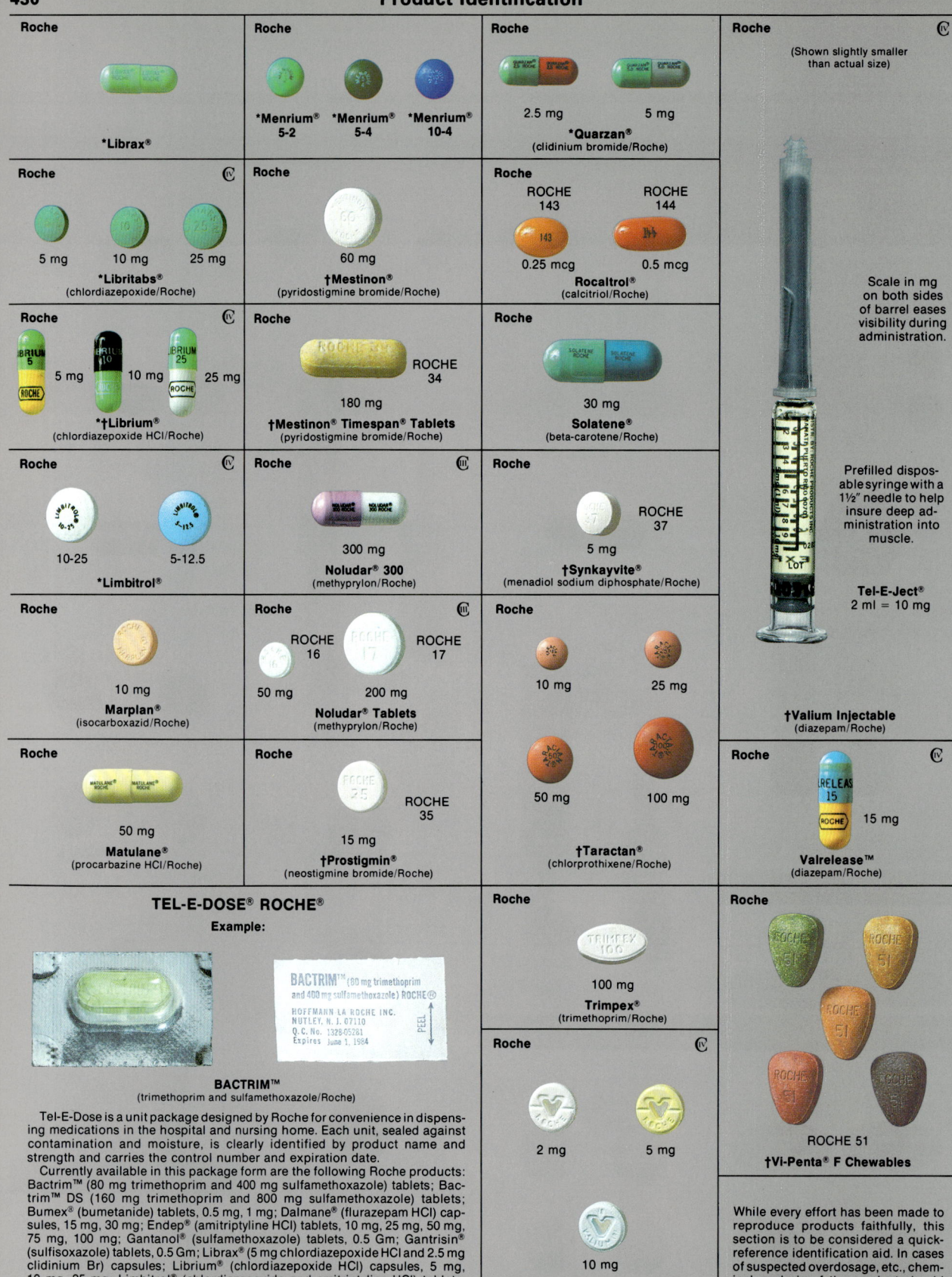

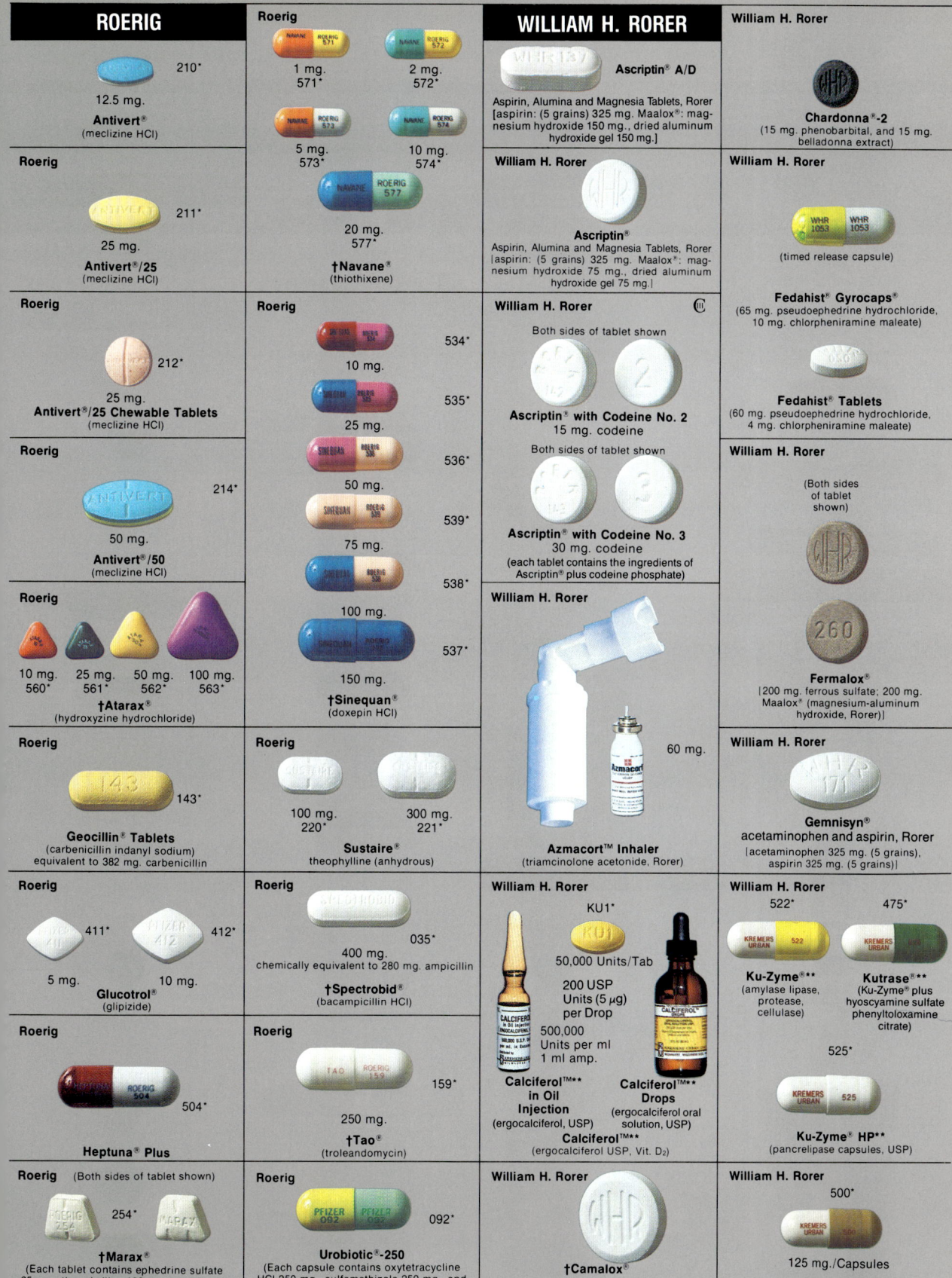

432 Product Identification

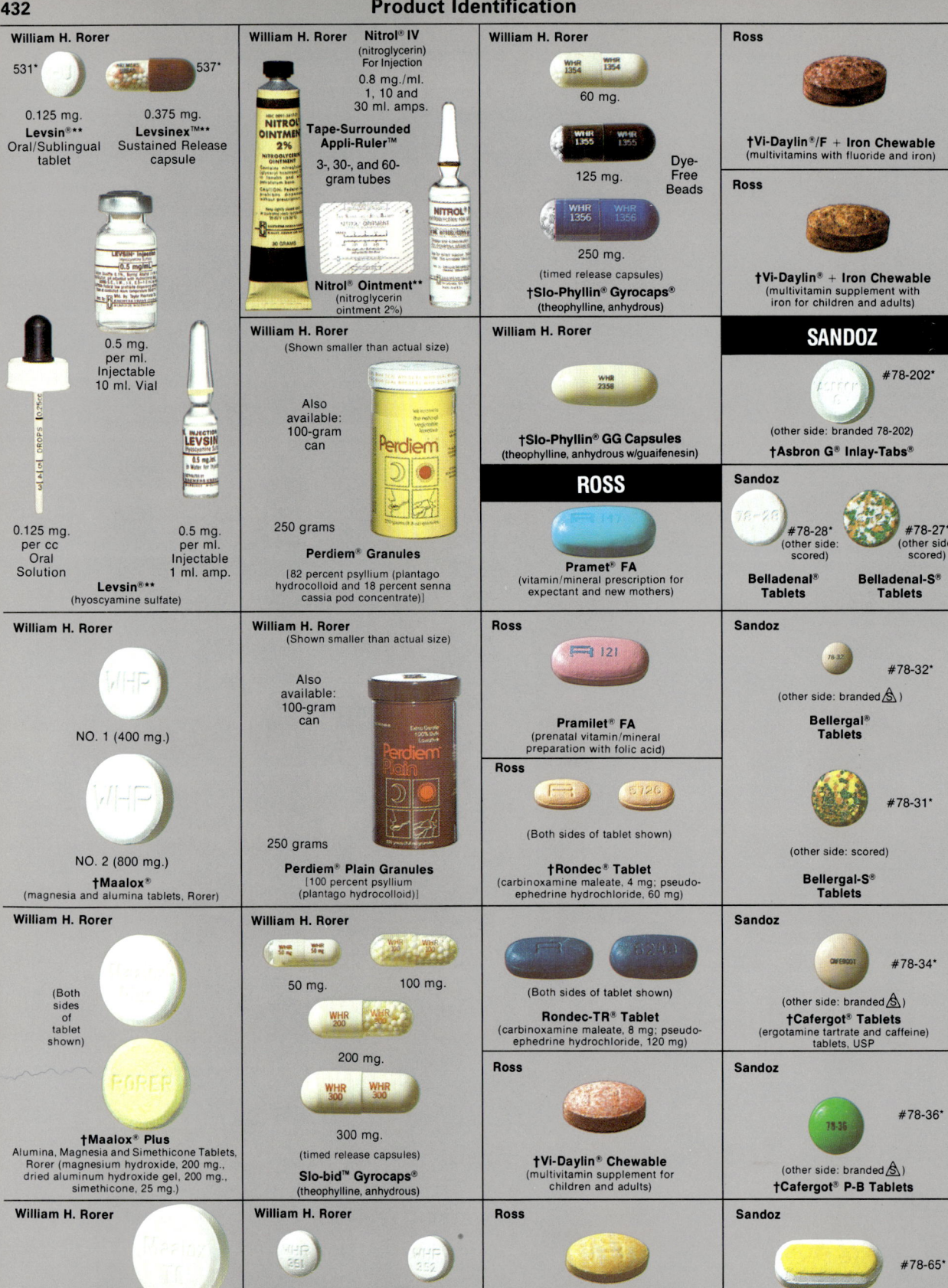

**During the next year, Rorer identification may appear on the products.

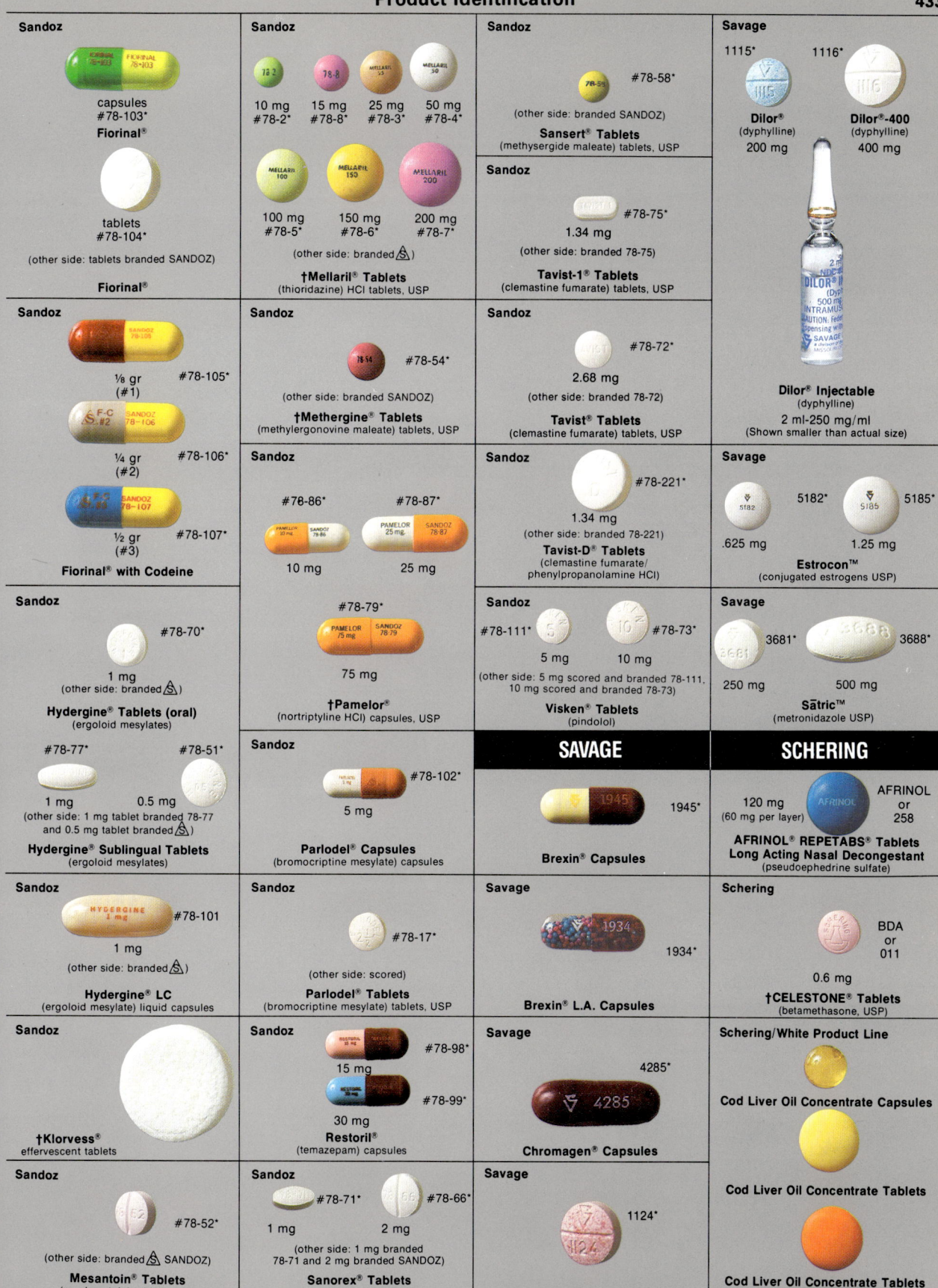

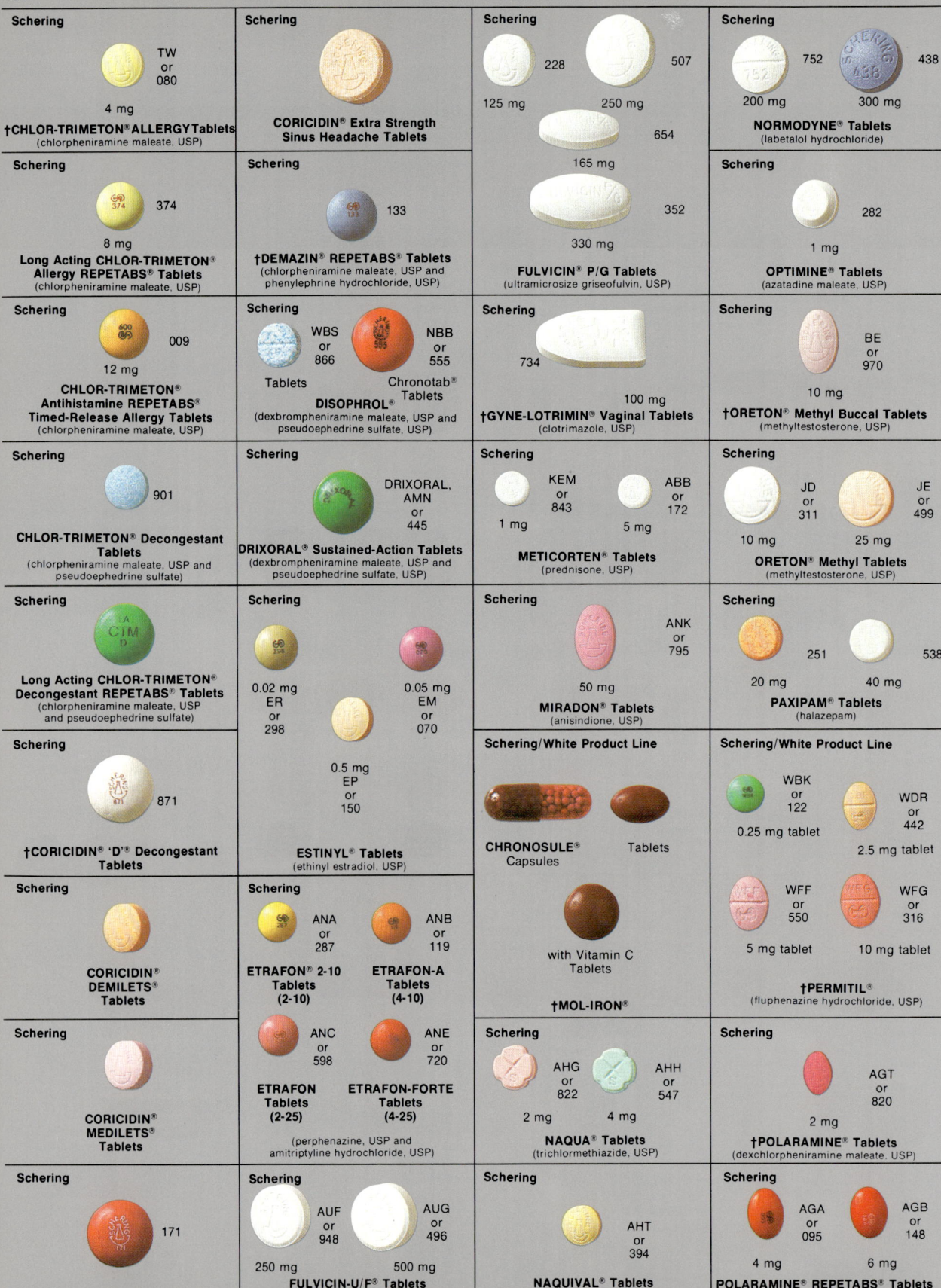

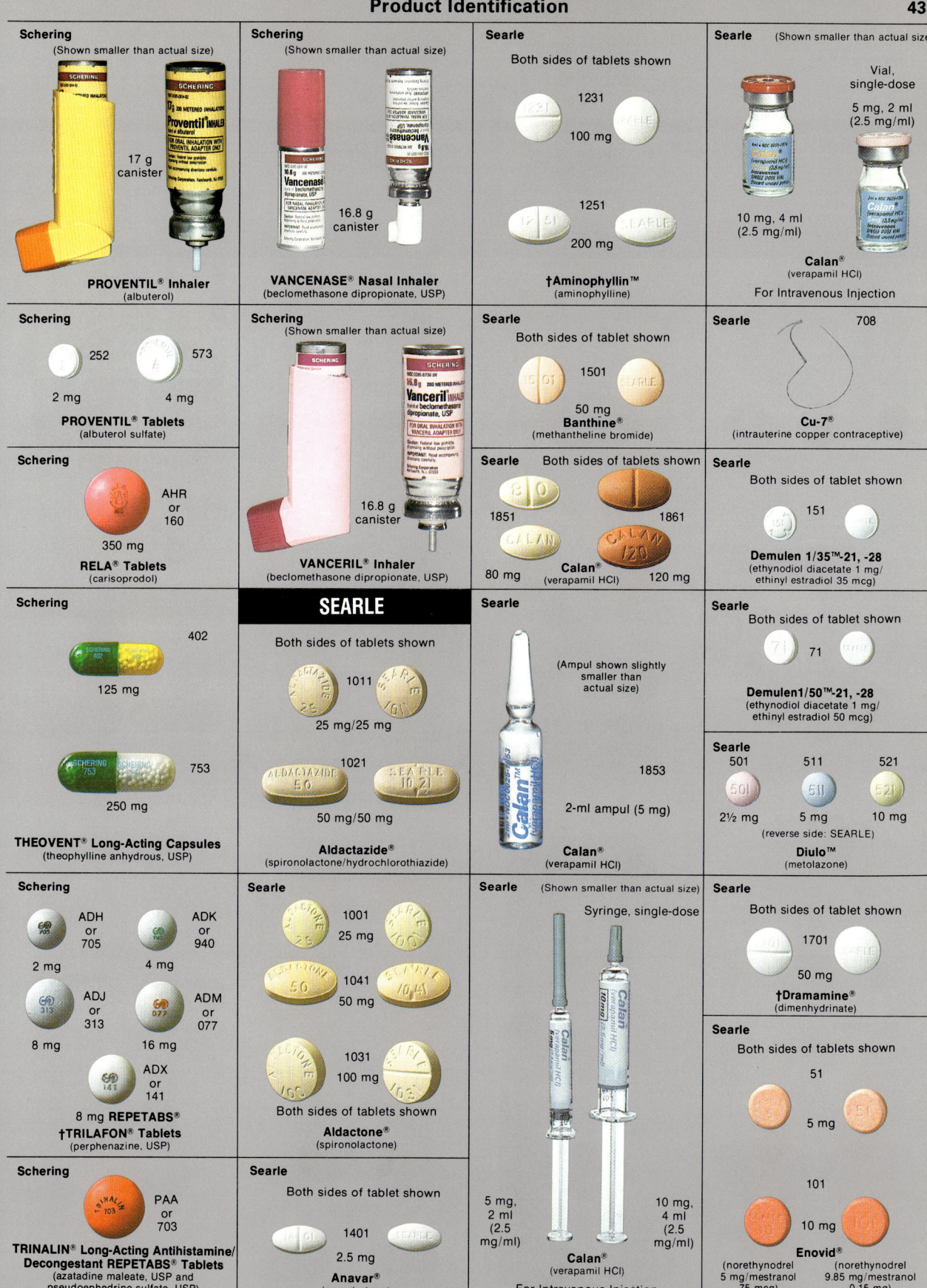

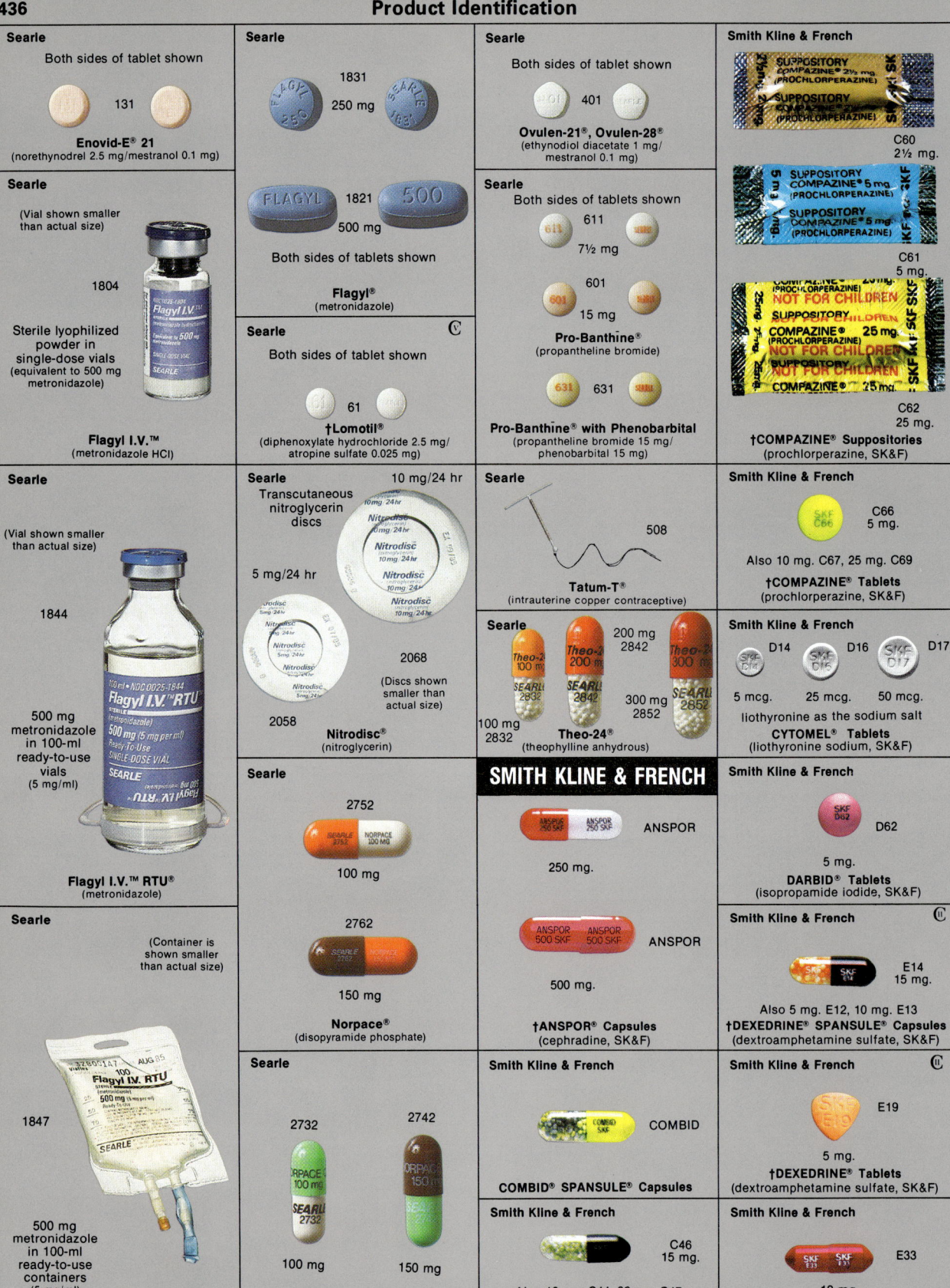

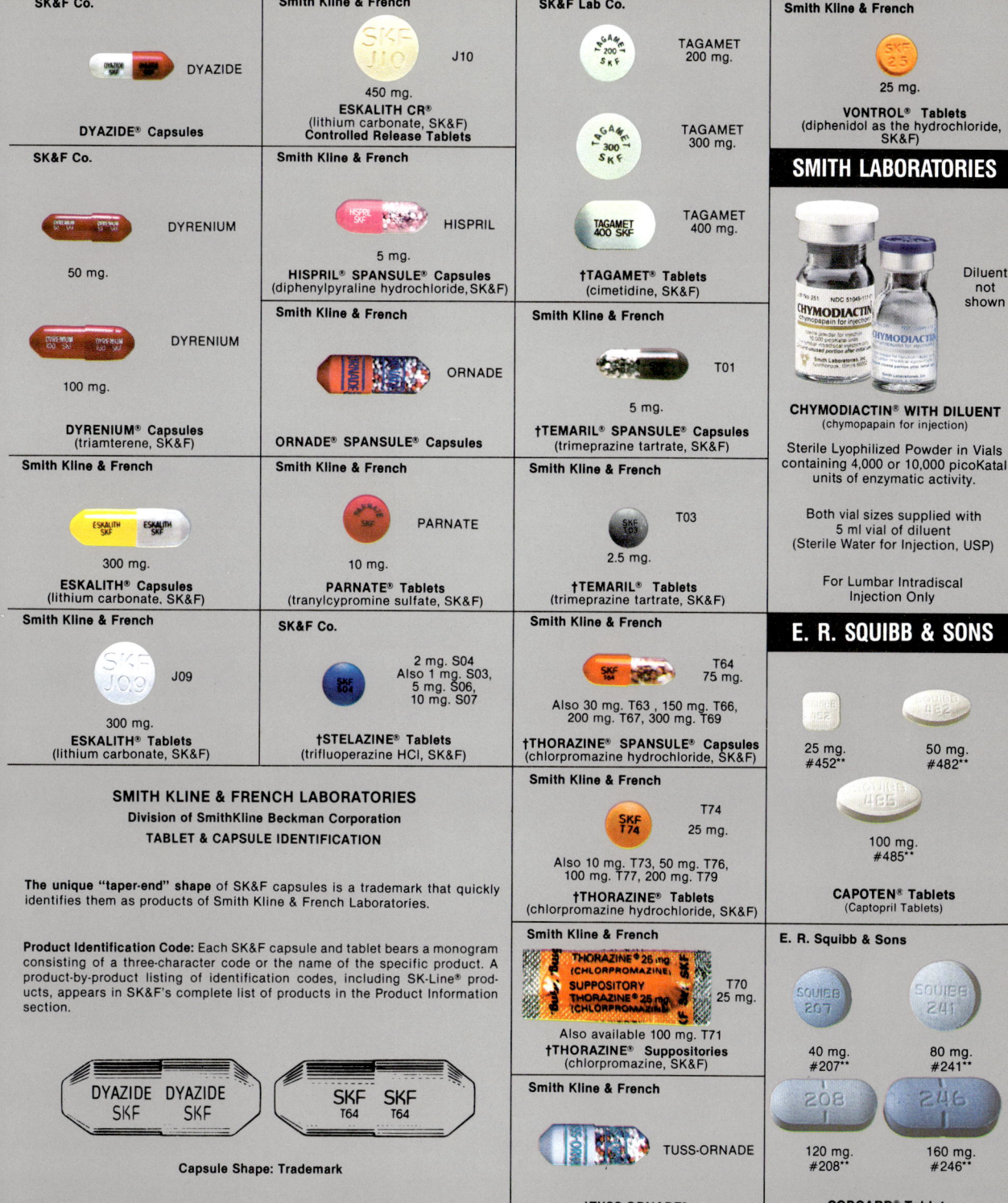

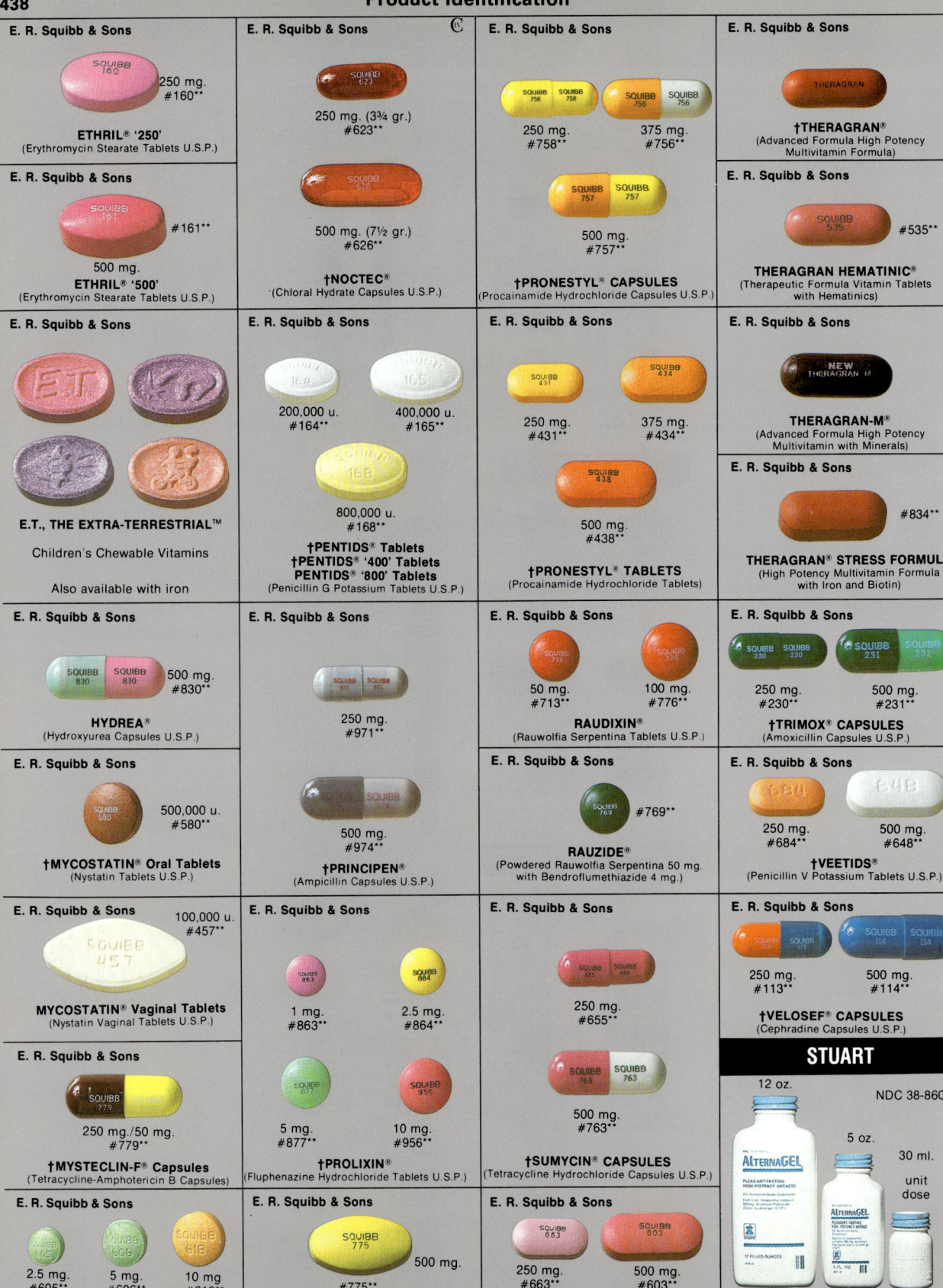

Product Identification

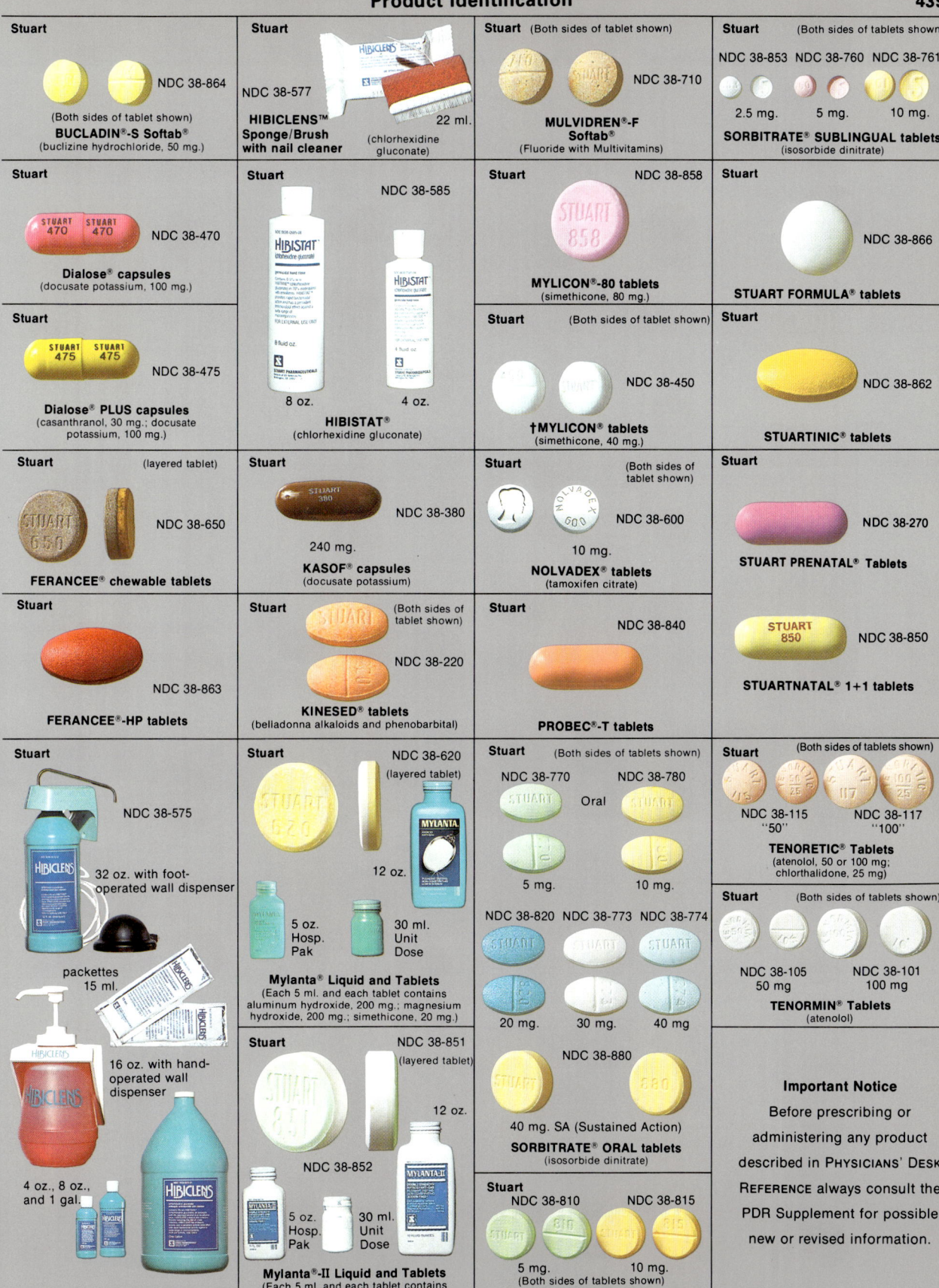

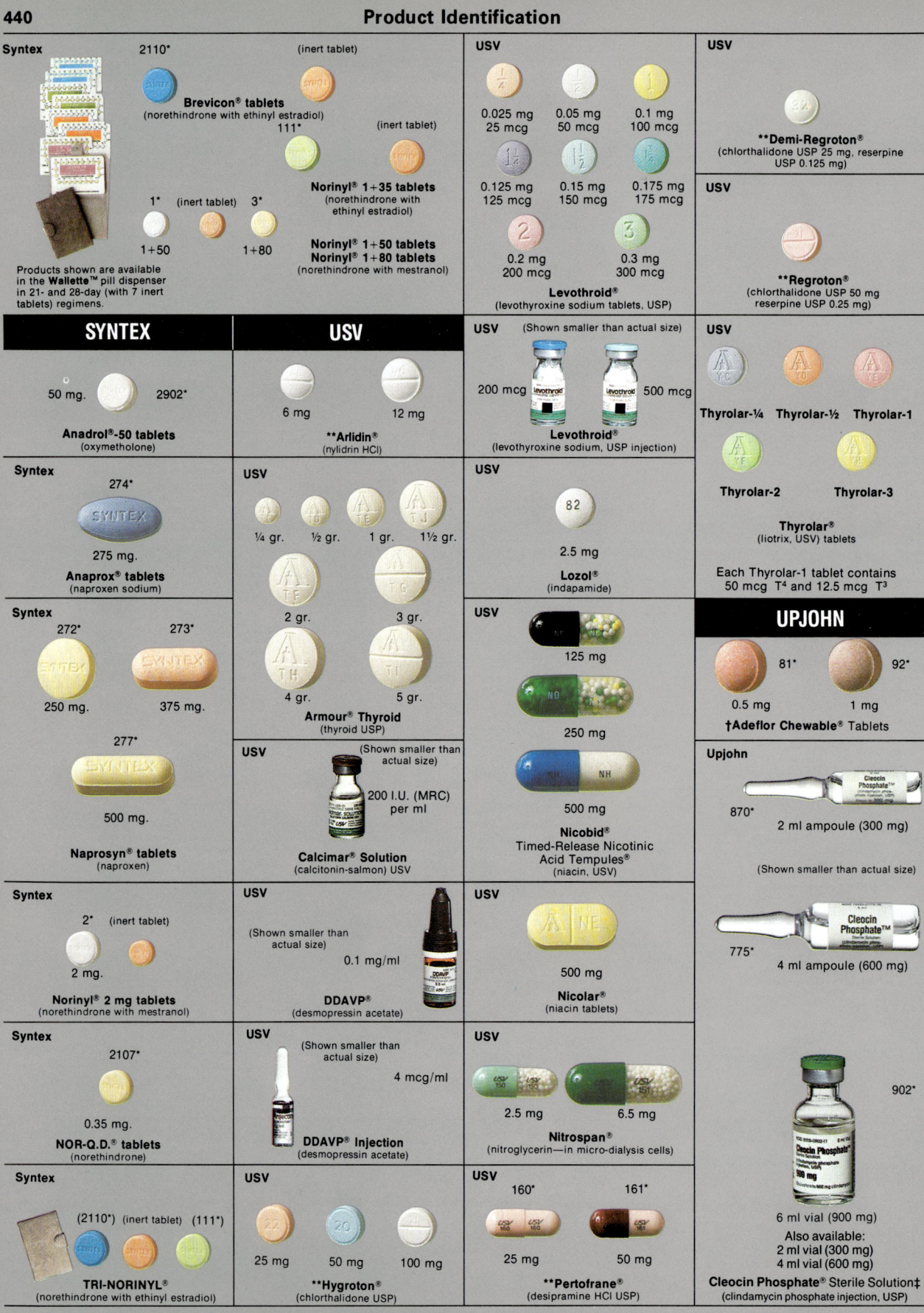

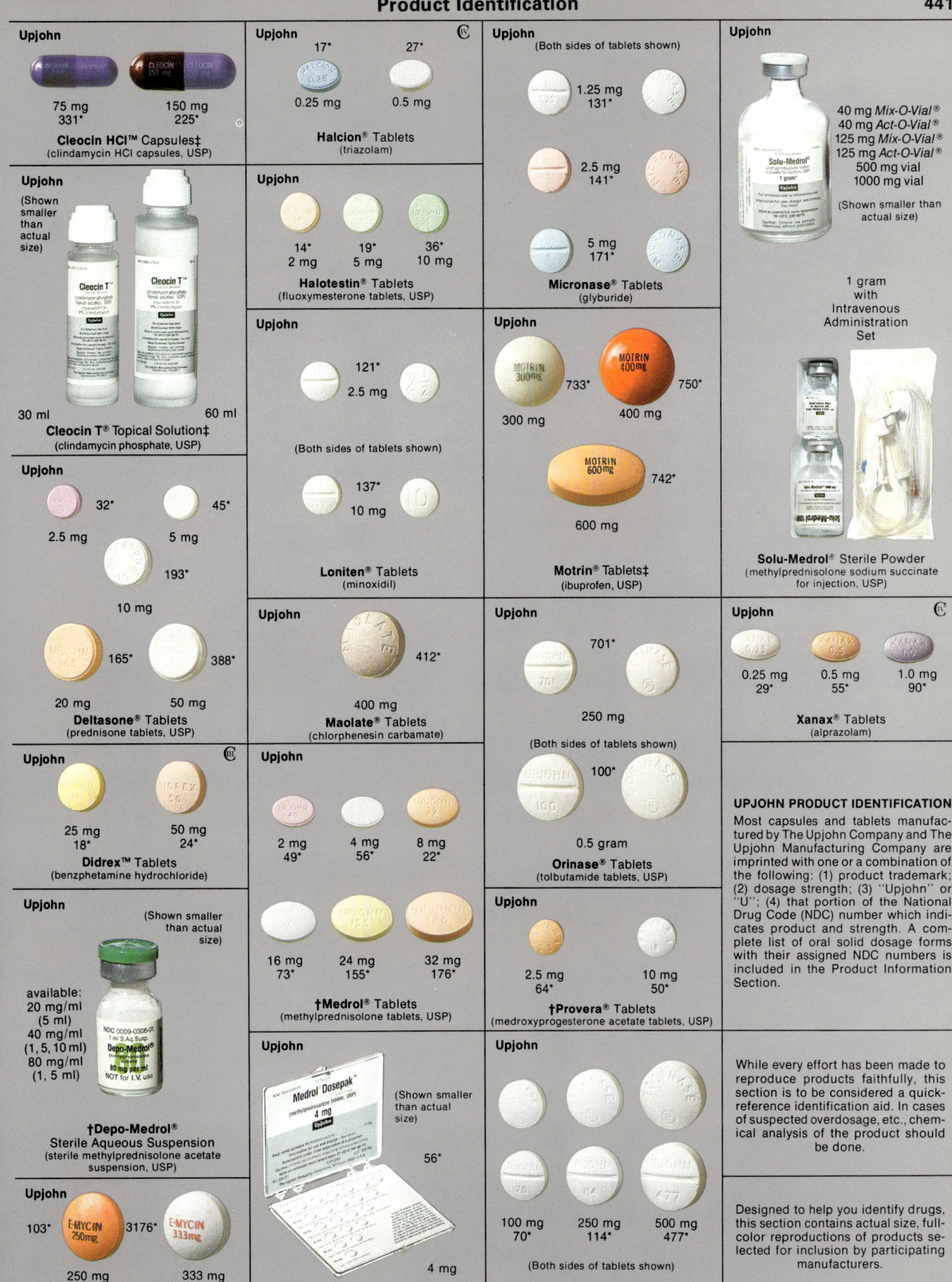

Product Identification

VEREX

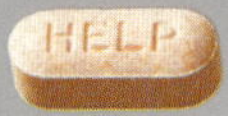

Help® 75 mg.
(constant release rate phenylpropanolamine)

Verex

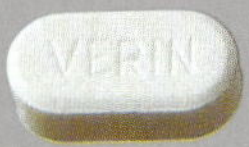

Verin® 650 mg.
(constant release rate aspirin)

VICKS PHARMACY

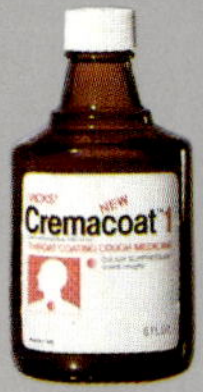

Cremacoat™ 1 dextromethorphan hydrobromide

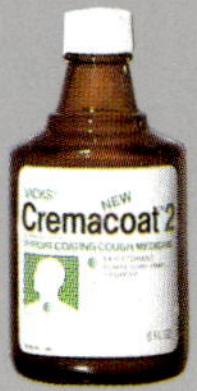

Cremacoat™ 2 guaifenesin (glyceryl guaiacolate)

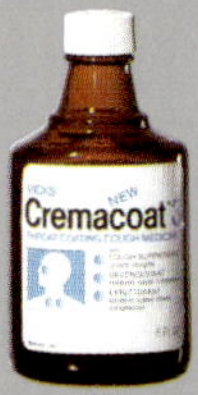

Cremacoat™ 3 dextromethorphan hydrobromide, phenyl-propanolamine hydrochloride, guaifenesin (glyceryl guaiacolate)

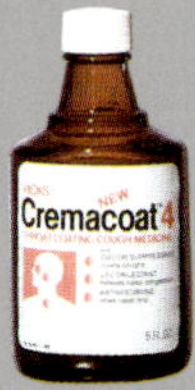

Cremacoat™ 4 dextromethorphan hydrobromide, phenylpropanolamine hydrochloride, doxylamine succinate

All available in 3 oz. and 6 oz. sizes

Vicks Pharmacy

Available in blister strip boxes of 24 tablets and bottles of 50 and 90.

Percogesic® acetaminophen, phenyltoloxamine citrate

WALLACE

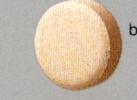

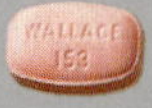

Aquatensen® (methylclothiazide 5 mg.)

Wallace

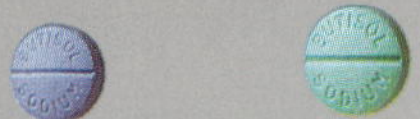

15 mg. / 30 mg.

†Butisol Sodium Tablets (butabarbital)

Wallace

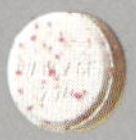

Diutensen®-R (methyclothiazide, 2.5 mg. and reserpine, 0.1 mg.)

Wallace

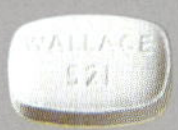

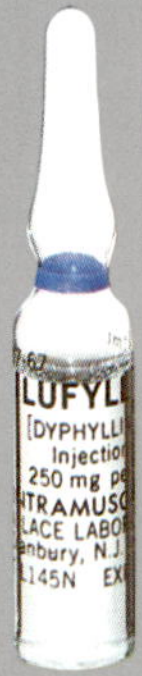

200 mg. **†Lufyllin®** (dyphylline)

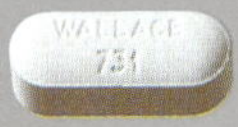

400 mg. **Lufyllin®-400** (dyphylline)

2 ml. (250 mg./ml.) **Lufyllin® Injection** (dyphylline) (ampul shown slightly smaller than actual size)

Wallace

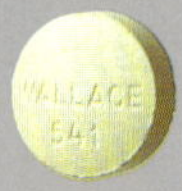

†Lufyllin®-GG (dyphylline, 200 mg. and guaifenesin, 200 mg.)

Wallace

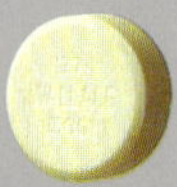

Milpath®—400

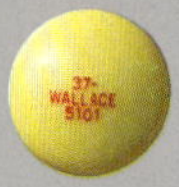

Milpath®—200 (meprobamate 400 mg. or 200 mg. + tridihexethyl chloride 25 mg.)

Wallace

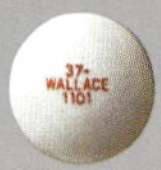

200 mg.

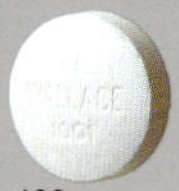

400 mg.

600 mg. **Miltown** (meprobamate)

Wallace

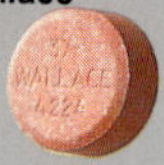

30 mg. **†Organidin®** (iodinated glycerol)

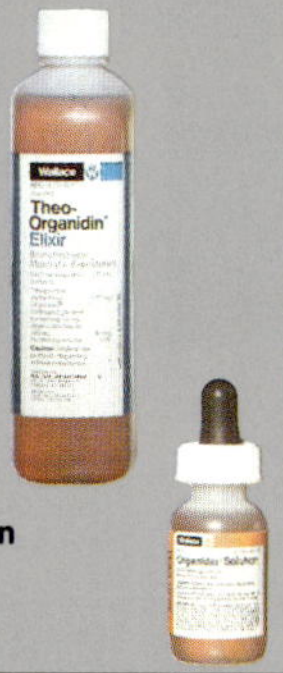

Organidin® Elixir (iodinated glycerol) per 5 mL-1.2%, 60 mg. Organidin

Organidin® Solution (iodinated glycerol) per mL-5%, 50 mg. Organidin

Wallace

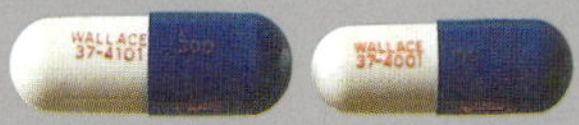

300 mg. / 150 mg. **†Rondomycin®** (methacycline HCl)

Wallace (Both sides of tablet shown)

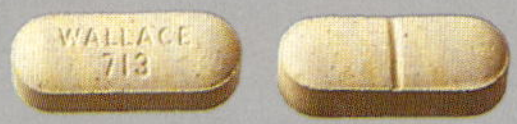

Rynatan® (phenylephrine tannate, 25 mg., chlorpheniramine tannate, 8 mg. and pyrilamine tannate, 25 mg.)

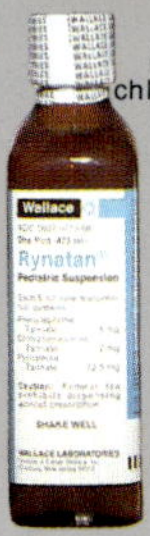

Rynatan® Pediatric Suspension (in 5 mL-phenylephrine tannate, 5 mg.; chlorpheniramine tannate, 2 mg.; pyrilamine tannate, 12.5 mg.)

Wallace

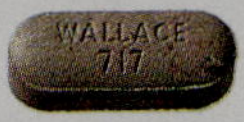

Rynatuss® (carbetapentane tannate, 60 mg., chlorpheniramine tannate, 5 mg., ephedrine tannate, 10 mg. and phenylephrine tannate, 10 mg.)

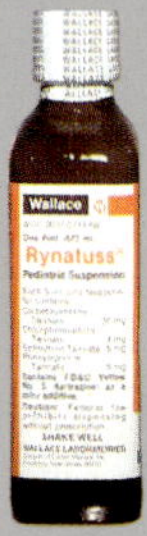

Rynatuss® Pediatric Suspension (in 5 mL-carbetapentane tannate, 30 mg.; chlorpheniramine tannate, 4 mg.; phenylephrine tannate, 5 mg.)

Wallace

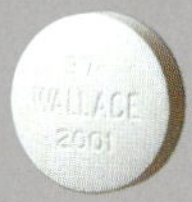

350 mg. **Soma®** (carisoprodol)

Wallace

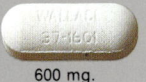

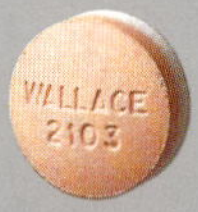

Soma® Compound (200 mg. carisoprodol + 325 mg. aspirin)

Wallace

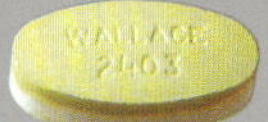

Soma® Compound with Codeine (200 mg. carisoprodol + 325 mg. aspirin + 16 mg. codeine phosphate)

Wallace

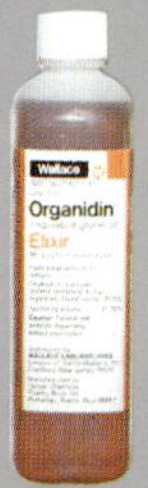

Theo-Organidin™ Elixir [15 mL contains: theophylline (anhydrous), 120 mg.; Organidin (iodinated glycerol containing 15 mg. organically bound iodine), 30 mg.; 15% alcohol by volume]

Wallace

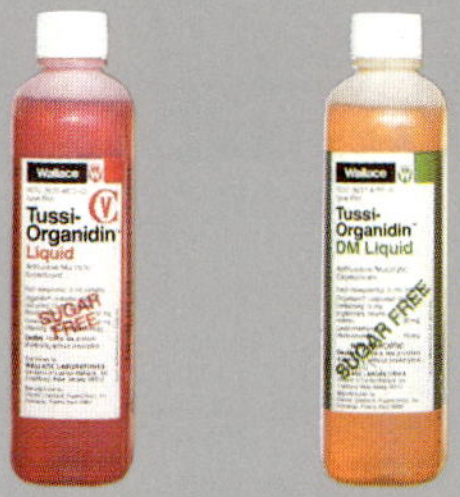

Tussi-Organidin® Liquid [(per 5 mL)-Organidin (iodinated glycerol) 30 mg.; codeine phosphate, 16 mg.]

Tussi-Organidin® DM Liquid [(per 5 mL)-Organidin (iodinated glycerol) 30 mg.; dextromethorphan hydrobromide, 10 mg.]

Wallace (shown smaller than actual size)

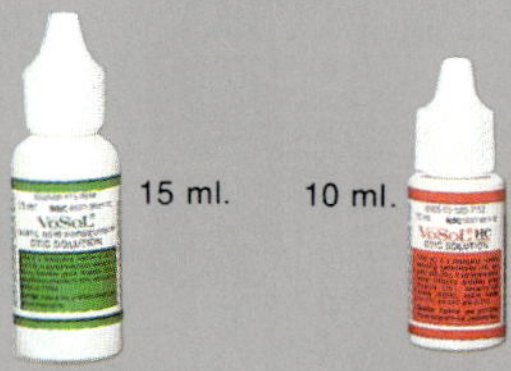

15 ml. / 10 ml.

VōSol (acetic acid-nonaqueous 2%)

VōSol HC (hydrocortisone 1% acetic acid-nonaqueous 2%)

30 ml.

VōSol (acetic acid-nonaqueous 2%)

WESTWOOD

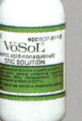

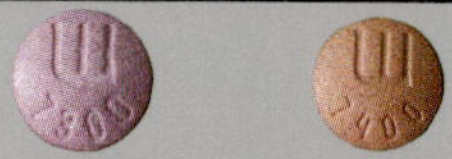

3.6 mg. / 8 mg.

†Tacaryl (methdilazine base and hydrochloride)

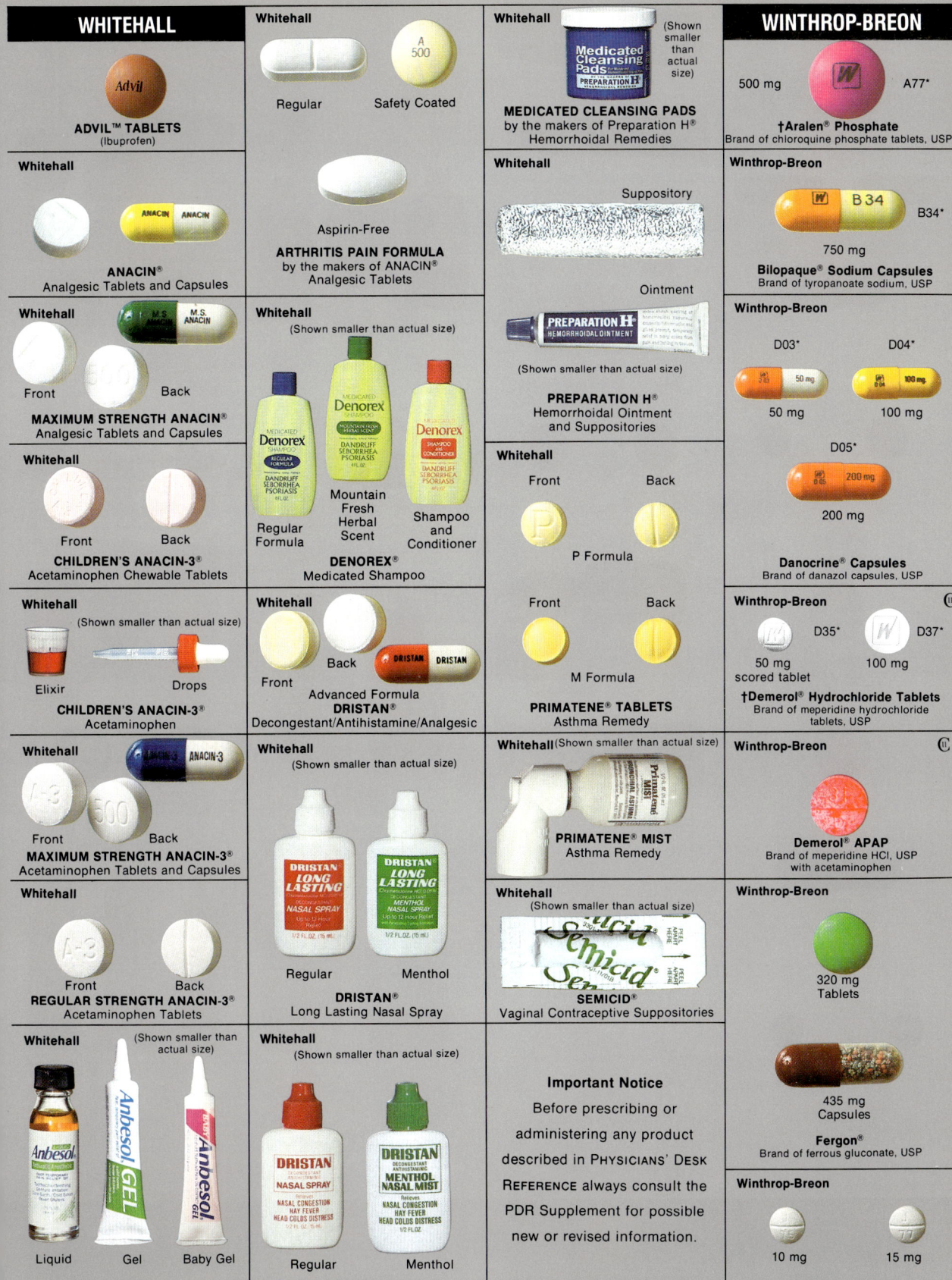

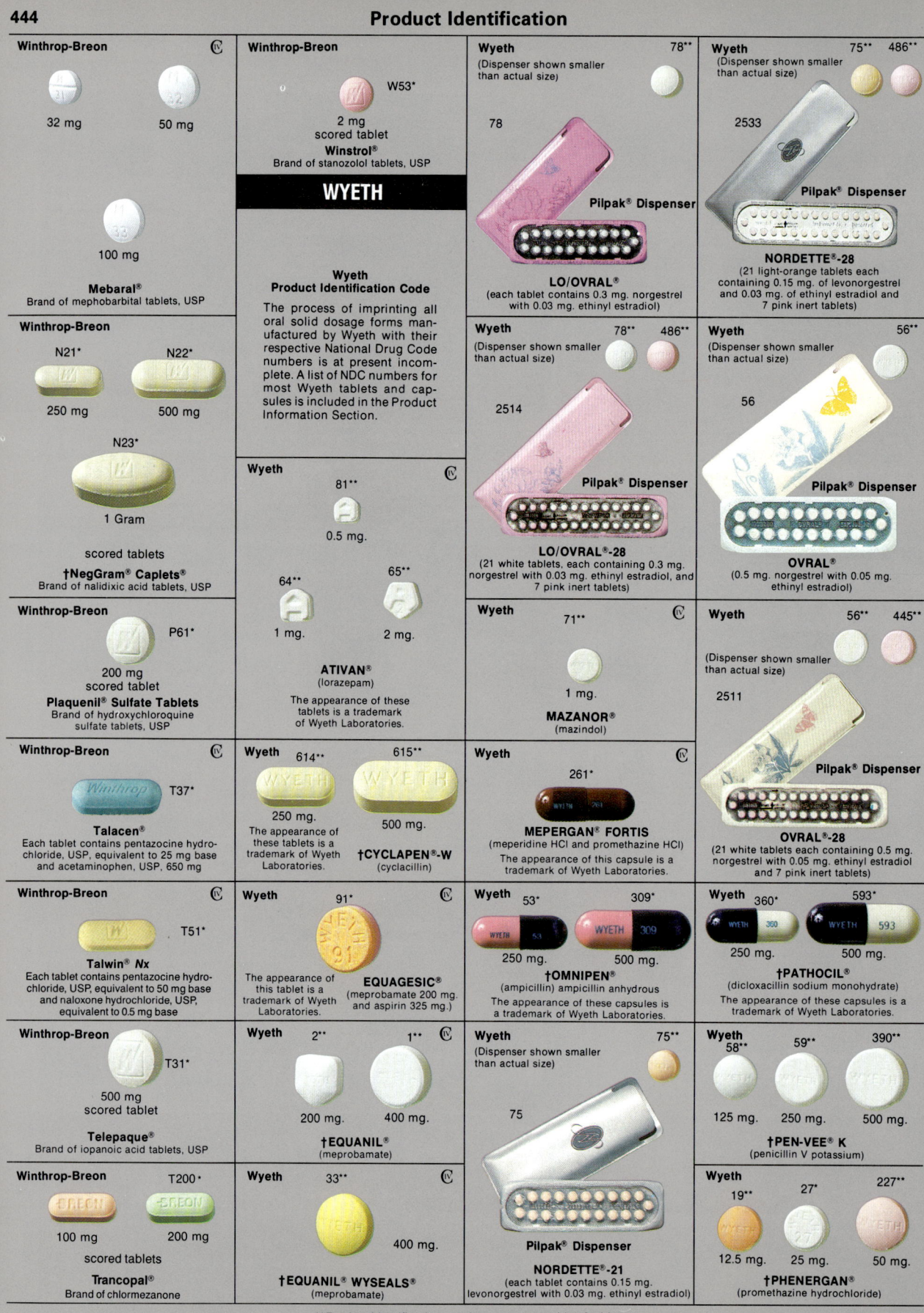

Product Identification

445

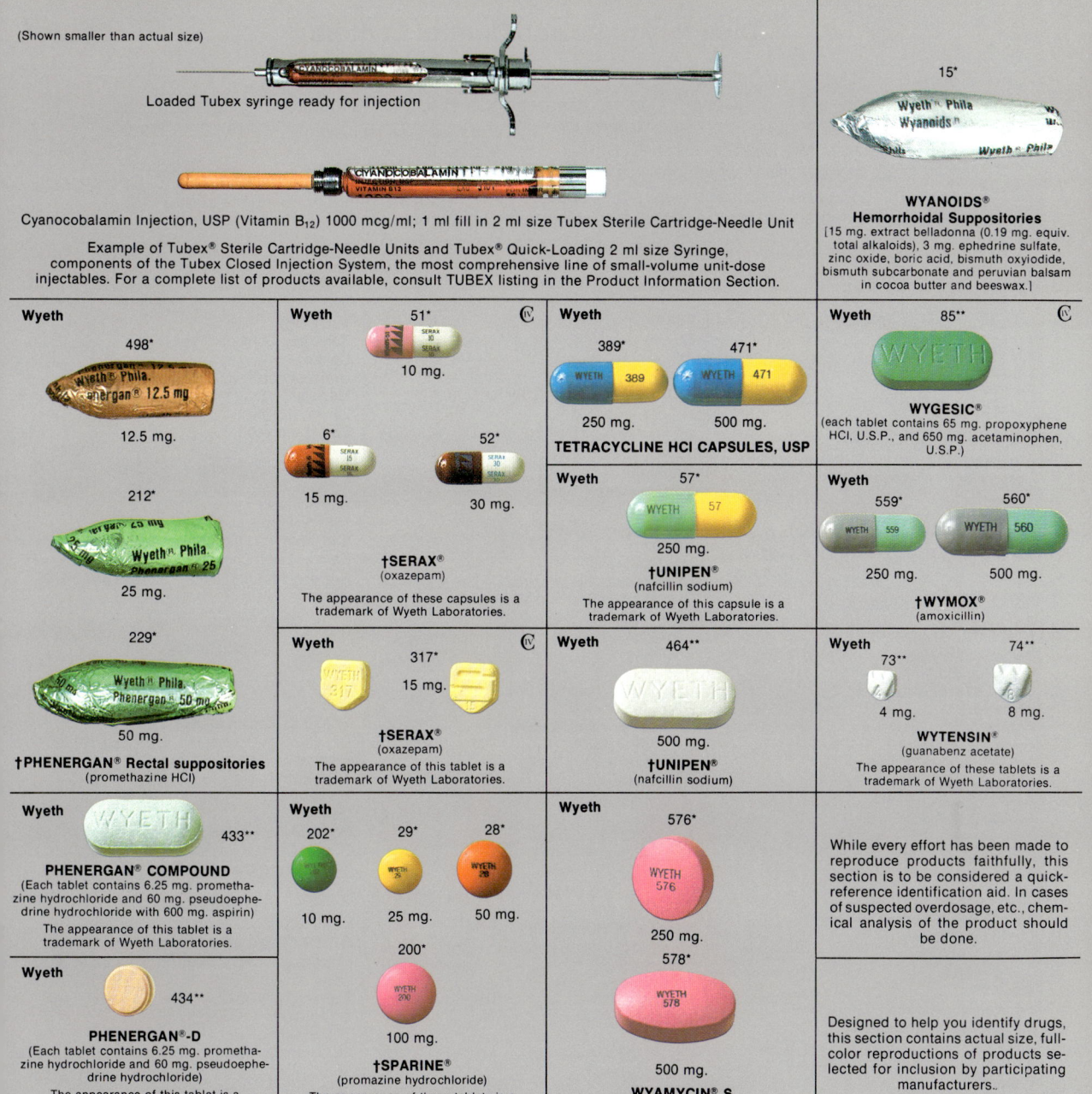

Directory of Poison Control Centers

The Directory of Poison Control Centers has been compiled from information furnished by the National Clearinghouse for Poison Control Centers, Bureau of Drugs, 5600 Fishers Lane, Room 1347, Rockville, Md. 20857.

It includes those facilities which provide for the medical profession, on a 24-hour basis, information concerning the prevention and treatment of accidents involving ingestion of poisonous and potentially poisonous substances. Unless otherwise noted, inquiries should be addressed to:
Poison Control Center

ALABAMA

STATE COORDINATOR
Department of Public Health (205) 832-3194
Montgomery 36117 832-3935
Birmingham
Children's Hospital 933-4050
of Birmingham 800/292-6678
1601 6th Ave., S. 35233 (Statewide)
Tuscaloosa
The Alabama Poison Control Center
Druid City Hospital (205) 345-0600
809 University Blvd., E. (800) 462-0800
(Statewide)

ALASKA

STATE COORDINATOR
Department of Health & (907) 465-3100
Social Services
Juneau 99811
Anchorage
Anchorage Poison Center 274-6535
Providence Hospital
3200 Providence Dr. 99504
Fairbanks
Fairbanks Poison Center (907) 456-7182
Fairbanks Memorial Hospital
1650 Cowles 99701

ARIZONA

STATE COORDINATOR
Arizona Poison Control System
College of Pharmacy (602) 626-6016
University of Arizona 800/362-0101
Tucson 85724 (Statewide)
Flagstaff
Flagstaff Hospital and 779-0555
Medical Center of Northern
Arizona
1215 N. Beaver St. 86001
Phoenix
St. Luke's Hospital and 253-3334
Medical Center
525 N. 18th St. 85006
Tucson
Arizona Poison and Drug 626-6016
Information Center (800) 362-0101
Arizona Hlth. Sciences Ctr. (Statewide)
University of Arizona
85724

ARKANSAS

STATE COORDINATOR
Division of Environmental (501) 661-2301
Health Protection
Little Rock 72201
El Dorado
Warner Brown Hospital 863-2266
Emergency Room
460 West Oak St. 71730

Fort Smith
St. Edward's Mercy Medical 452-5100
Center Ext. 2401
Emergency Room
7301 Rogers Avenue 72904
Emergency Room
Sparks Regional Med. Center 441-5011
1311 S. Eye St. 72902
Harrison
Boone County Hospital 741-6141
Emergency Room Ext. 275
620 N. Willow St. 72601
Helena
Helena Hospital 338-6411
Emergency Room Ext. 340
Hi-Way 49 By Pass 72342
Little Rock
U.A.M. Sc College of 1-800-428-8948
Pharmacy
SLOT 522
4301 W. Markham St. 72205
Osceola
Osceola Memorial Hospital 563-7182
Emergency Room 563-3174
611 Lee Ave. West 72370
Pine Bluff
Jefferson Regional Medical 541-7111
Center 541-7100
Emergency Department Ext. 5350
1515 W. 42nd Ave. 71601

CALIFORNIA

STATE COORDINATOR
Emergency Medical Services
Authority (916) 322-4336
1600 Ninth St.
Room 460
Sacramento 95814
Fresno
Central Valley Regional 445-1222
Poison Control Ctr.
Fresno Community Hospital and
Medical Center
Fresno & R Sts. 93715
Los Angeles
Los Angeles County 484-5151
Medical Association
Regional Poison Information Center
1925 Wilshire Blvd. 90057
Oakland
Children's Hosp. Medical 428-3248
Center of Northern California
51st & Grove St. 94609
Orange
University of California 634-5988
Irvine Medical Center
101 City Drive, Route 32 92688
Sacramento
Sacramento Medical Center 453-3692
Univ. of California, Davis 800/852-7221
2315 Stockton Blvd. 95817 (N. Cal.)

San Diego
San Diego Regional Poison 294-6000
Center
University Calif. at San Diego
Medical Center
225 W. Dickinson St. 92103
San Francisco
San Francisco Bay Area 666-2845
Regional Poison Center 800/792-0720
Room IE 86 (N. Cal.)
San Francisco General Hosp.
1001 Potrero Ave. 94110
San Jose
Central-Coast Counties 279-5112
Regional Poison Control (800) 662-9886
Center
Santa Clara Valley Medical
Center (Statewide)
751 S. Bascom Ave. 95128

COLORADO

STATE COORDINATOR
Department of Health (303) 320-8476
Emergency Medical Services Div
4210 E. 11th Ave.
Denver 80220
Denver
Rocky Mountain Poison Center 629-1123
Denver General Hospital 800/332-3073
W. 8th Ave. & Cherokee Sts. 80204

CONNECTICUT

STATE COORDINATOR
University of Connecticut (203) 674-3456
Health Center
Farmington 06032
Bridgeport
Bridgeport Hospital 384-3566
267 Grant St. 06602
St. Vincent's Medical Center 576-5178
2800 Main St. 06606
Danbury
Danbury Hospital 797-7300
95 Locust Ave. 06810
Farmington
Connecticut Poison Control 674-3456
Center
University of Connecticut
Health Center 06032
Middletown
Middlesex Memorial Hospital 344-6684
28 Crescent St. 06457
New Haven
The Hospital of St. Raphael 789-3464
1450 Chapel St. 06511
Dept. of Pediatrics
Yale-New Haven Hospital 785-2222
20 York St. 06504
Norwalk
Department of Emergency Medicine

Norwalk Hospital	852-2160
Maple St. 06856	

St. Mary's Hospital   574-6011
Emergency Room
56 Franklin St. 06702

DELAWARE

STATE COORDINATOR
Wilmington Medical Center   (302) 655-3389
Delaware Division
Wilmington 19801

Wilmington
Wilmington Medical Center   655-3389
Delaware Division
501 W. 14th St. 19899

DISTRICT OF COLUMBIA

STATE COORDINATOR
Washington, D.C.
National Capital Poison
Center
Georgetown University   625-3333
Hospital
3800 Reservoir Rd.
Washington, D.C. 20007

FLORIDA

STATE COORDINATOR
Department of Health and   (904) 487-1566
Rehabilitative Services Office of
Emergency Medical Services
Tallahassee 32301

Bradenton
Manatee Memorial Hospital   748-2121
206 2nd St. E. 33505

Daytona Beach
Halifax Hospital   258-1513
Emergency Department
P.O. Box 1990   32014

Ft. Lauderdale
Broward General Medical   463-3131
Center
Poison Control Center   Ext. 1955/6
1600 S. Andrews Ave. 33316

Fort Myers
Lee Memorial Hospital   334-5287
2776 Cleveland Ave.
P.O. Drawer 2218   33902

Ft. Walton Beach
General Hospital of   862-1111
Ft. Walton Beach   Ext. 106
1000 Mar-Walt Drive 32548

Gainesville
Shands Teaching Hosp.   392-3389
and Clinics
University of Florida 32610

Inverness
Citrus Memorial Hosp.   726-2800
502 Highland Blvd. 32650

Jacksonville
St. Vincent's Medical Center   387-7500
P.O. Box 2982 32203   387-7499

Lakeland
Lakeland Regional Medical   687-1137
Center
Lakeland General Hospital
Lakeland Hills Blvd.
Drawer 448   33802

Leesburg
Leesburg Regional Medical   787-9900
Center
600 E. Dixie 32748

Melbourne
James E. Holmes Regional   727-7000
Medical Center   Ext. 675
Emergency Department
1350 S. Hickory St. 32901

Naples
Naples Community Hospital   262-3131
350 7th St. N. 33940

Ocala
Munroe Regional Medical   351-7607
Center
131 S.W. 15th St.   Ext. 187
P.O. Box 6000   32670

Orlando
Orlando Reg. Med. Ctr.   841-5222
Orange Memorial Division
1414 S. Kuhl Ave. 32806

Pensacola
Gulf Region Poison Center   434-4611
Baptist Hospital   (800) 342-3222
P.O. Box 17500   32522   (Statewide)

Punta Gorda
Medical Center Hospital   637-2529
809 E. Marion Ave. 33950

Rockledge
Wuesthoff Memorial Hospital   636-4357
110 Longwood Ave. 32955

St. Petersburg
Bay Front Medical Center, Inc.   282-3171
701 6th St., S. 33701   (Statewide)

Sarasota
Memorial Hospital   953-1332
1901 Arlington St. 33579

Tallahassee
Tallahassee Memorial   681-5411
Regional Medical Center
1300 Miccosukee Road 32304

Tampa
Tampa Bay Regional Poison
Control Center   251-6995
Tampa General Hospital   (800) 282-3171
Davis Island 33606   (Statewide)

Titusville
Jess Parrish Mem. Hospital   268-6260
P.O. Drawer W
951 N. Washington Ave. 32780

West Palm Beach
Good Samaritan Hospital   655-5511
Palm Beach Lakes Blvd.   Ext. 4250
West Palm Beach 33402

Winter Haven
Poison Control Center
Winter Haven Hospital, Inc.   299-9701
200 Avenue F., N.E. 33880

GEORGIA

STATE COORDINATOR
Department of Human   (404) 894-5170
Resources
Emergency Health Section
Atlanta 30303

Albany
Phoebe Putney Memorial   888-4150
Hosp.
417 Third Avenue 31705

Athens
Athens General Hospital   543-5215
1199 Prince Ave. 30613

Atlanta
Georgia Poison Control   588-4400
Center   (800) 282-5846
Grady Memorial Hospital   (Statewide)
P.O. Box 26066   (Deaf) 404 525-3323
    80 Butler St., S.E. 30335

Augusta
University Hospital   724-5050
1350 Walton Way 30902

Columbus
The Medical Center   571-1080
710 Center Street 31902

Macon
Medical Center of Central Georgia   744-1427
Regional Poison Control Center
777 Hemlock St. 31201

Rome
Floyd Hospital   295-5500
Turner McCall Blvd. 31061

Savannah
Savannah Reg. EMS Poison Ctr.   355-5228
Depart. of Emergency Medicine
Memorial Medical Center
P.O. Box 23089   31403

Thomasville
John D. Archbold   226-4121
Memorial Hospital   Ext. 169
900 Gordon Ave. 31792

Valdosta
S. Georgia Medical Center   333-1110
P.O. Box 1727   31603

Waycross
Memorial Hospital   283-3030
410 Darling Ave. 31501

HAWAII

STATE COORDINATOR
Department of Health   (808) 531-7776
Honolulu 96801

Honolulu
Kapiolani-Childrens Medical   941-4411
Center
319 Punahou St. 96826   (808) 362-3585

IDAHO

STATE COORDINATOR
Department of Health   (208) 334-4245
and Welfare
Boise 83720

Boise
Idaho Emergency Medical   334-2241
Poison Center   (800) 632-8000
1055 N. Curtis Rd. 83706   (Statewide)

Idaho Falls
Consolidated Hospitals   522-3600
Emergency Department
900 Memorial Dr. 83401

Pocatello
Idaho Drug Information   234-0777
Service and Poison Control   Ext. 2019
Center   (800) 632-9490
Pocatello Regional Medical Center (Statewide)
777 Hospital Way 83202

ILLINOIS

STATE COORDINATOR
Division of Emergency   (217) 785-2080
Medical Services and
Highway Safety
Springfield 62761

Chicago
Rush-Presbyterian-St. Lukes   942-5969
Medical Center   800 942-5969
1753 W. Congress Parkway 60612

Peoria
Peoria Poison Center
St. Francis Hospital &   672-2334
Medical Center   800 322-5330
530 N.E. Glen Oak Avenue 61637

Springfield
Central & Southern Illinois
Poison Resource Center   753-3330
St. John's Hospital   (800) 252-2022
800 East Carpenter 62769   (Statewide)

INDIANA

STATE COORDINATOR
Indiana State Board   (317) 633-0332
of Health
Hazardous Products Section
and Division of Drug Control
P.O. Box 1964
Indianapolis 46206

Poison Control Centers

Anderson
Community Hospital 646-5143
1515 N. Madison Ave. 46012
St. John's Hickey 646-8222
Memorial Hospital
2015 Jackson St. 46014
Angola
Cameron Memorial Hospital 665-2141
416 East Maumee St. 46703 Ext. 146
Crown Point
St. Anthony Medical Ctr. 738-2100
Main at Franciscan Rd. 46307 Ext. 1311
Evansville
Deaconess Hospital 426-3333
600 Mary St. 47710

Welborn Memorial 426-8336
Baptist Hospital
401 S.E. 6th St. 47713
Fort Wayne
Lutheran Hospital 458-2211
Emergency Dept.
3024 Fairfield Ave. 46807

Indiana Poison Center 484-9711
2200 Randalia Dr. 46805

St. Joseph's Hospital 426-8280
700 Broadway 46802
Gary
Methodist Hospital of 886-4710
Gary, Inc.
600 Grant St. 46402
Hammond
St. Margaret's Hospital 931-4477
Poison Control Center
25 Douglas St. 46320
Indianapolis
Indiana Poison Center 630-7351
1001 West 10th St. 46202 800 382-9097
Kokomo
Howard Community Hospital 453-8444
3500 S. LaFountain St. 46901
Lafayette
Lafayette Home Hospital 447-6811
2400 South Street 47902

Poison Control Center
St. Elizabeth Hospital 423-6699
1501 Hartford St. 47904
Lebanon
Witham Memorial Hospital 482-2700
1124 N. Lebanon St. 46052 Ext. 241
Madison
King's Daughter's Hospital 265-5211
112 Presbyterian Ave. 47250 Ext. 131
Marion
Marion General Hospital 662-4693
Wabash & Euclid Ave. 46952
Muncie
Ball Memorial Hospital 747-4321
2401 University Ave. 47303
Richmond
Reid Memorial Hospital 983-3148
1401 Chester Blvd. 47374
Shelbyville
Wm. S. Major Hospital 392-3211
150 W. Washington St. 46176 Ext. 252
South Bend
St. Joseph's Medical Center 237-7264
811 E. Madison St. 46622
Terre Haute
Union Hospital, Inc. 238-7000
1606 N. 7th St. 47804 Ext. 7523
Valparaiso
Porter Memorial Hosp. 464-8611
814 LaPorte Ave. 46383 Ext. 301

Vincennes
The Good Samaritan 885-3348
Hospital
520 S. 7th St. 47591

IOWA

STATE COORDINATOR
Department of Health (515) 281-4964
Des Moines 50319
Des Moines
Variety Club Poison and 283-6254
Drug Information Center 800 362-2327
Iowa Methodist Medical (Statewide)
Center
1200 Pleasant St. 50308
Dubuque
Mercy Health Center 589-9099
Mercy Drive 52001
Fort Dodge
Trinity Regional Hospital 573-3101
Poison Information Center
Kenyon Rd. 50501
Iowa City
Univ. of Iowa Hospitals 356-2922
and Clinics 800 272-6477
Poison Control Center 52242 (Statewide)
Waterloo
Allen Memorial Hospital 235-3893
Emergency Department
1825 Logan Avenue 50703

KANSAS

STATE COORDINATOR
Department of Health & (913) 862-9360
Environment Ext. 541
Bureau of Food and Drug
Forbes Field Topeka 66620
Atchison
Atchison Hospital 367-2131
1301 N. 2nd St. 66002 Ext. 111
Dodge City
Dodge City Regional Hosp. 225-9050
Ross & Ave. "A" 67801 Ext. 381
Emporia
Newman Memorial Hospital 343-6800
12th & Chestnut Sts. 66801 Ext. 545
Fort Riley
Irwin Army Hospital 239-7776
Emergency Room 66442
Fort Scott
Mercy Hospital 223-2200
821 Burke St. 66701 Ext. 136
Great Bend
Central Kansas Medical 792-2511
Center Ext. 115
3515 Broadway 67530
Hays
Hadley Regional Medical 628-8251
Center
201 E. 7th St. 67601 Ext. 145
Kansas City
Mid-America Poison Center
University of Kansas 588-6633
Medical Center (800) 332-6633
39th & Rainbow Blvd. 66103 (Statewide)
Lawrence
Lawrence Memorial Hospital 843-3680
325 Maine St. 66044 Ext. 162
Salina
St. John's Hospital 827-3187
139 N. Penn St. 67401
Topeka
Stormont-Vail Regional Med. 354-6100
Ctr.
10th & Washburn Sts. 66606
Northeast Kansas Poison Center
St. Francis Hospital 295-8094
and Medical Center
1700 W. 7th St. 66606
Wichita
Wesley Medical Center 688-2277
550 N. Hillside Ave. 67214

KENTUCKY

STATE COORDINATOR
Department For Human (502) 564-3970
Resources
Frankfort 40601
Fort Thomas
St. Lukes Hospital 572-3215
85 N. Grand Ave. 41075 800 352-9900
Lexington
Central Baptist Hospital 278-3411
1740 S. Limestone St. 40503 Ext. 363
Drug Information Center 233-5320
University of Kentucky
Medical Center 40536
Louisville
Kentucky Regional Poison 589-8222
Center of Kosair-Children's 800 722-5725
Hospital
NKC, Inc.
P.O. Box 35070 40232
Murray
Murray-Calloway County 753-7588
Hospital
803 Popular 42071
Owensboro
Owensboro-Daviess County 926-3030
Hospital Ext. 180
811 Hospital Court 42301
Paducah
Western Baptist Hospital 444-5180
2501 Kentucky Ave. 42001
Prestonburg
Poison Control Center 886-8511
Highlands Regional Medical Ext. 132
Center 41653

LOUISIANA

STATE COORDINATOR
L.S.U. Poison Control and 425-1524
Drug Abuse Information
Center
Louisiana State University
Medical Center
P.O. Box 33932 71130
Alexandria
Rapides General Hospital 445-4665
Poison Control Center
P.O. Box 7146 71301
Lafayette
Our Lady of Lourdes Hosp. 234-7381
611 St. Landry St. 70501
Lake Charles
Lake Charles Memorial Hosp. 478-6800
P.O. Drawer M 70601
Monroe
Northeast Louisiana University 342-3008
School of Pharmacy
700 University Ave. 71209
St. Francis Hospital 325-6454
P.O. Box 1901 71301
New Orleans
Charity Hospital 568-5222
1532 Tulane Ave. 70140
Shreveport
Louisiana State University
Poison Control and Drug
Abuse Information Center
LSU Medical Center 425-1524
P.O. Box 33932 71130

MAINE

STATE COORDINATOR
Maine Poison (207) 871-2950
Control Center
Portland 04102

Listings Continued Following Product Information Section

Poison Control Centers

Portland
Maine Medical Center 871-2381
Emergency Division 800 442-6305
22 Bramhall St. 04102 (Statewide)

MARYLAND

STATE COORDINATOR
Maryland Poison Center
University of Maryland (301) 528-7604
School of Pharmacy (Statewide)
636 W. Lombard St.
Baltimore 21201
Baltimore
Maryland Poison Center 528-7701
University of Maryland (Statewide)
School of Pharmacy
636 W. Lombard St. 21201
Cumberland
Tri-State Poison Center
Sacred Heart Hospital 722-6677
900 Seton Drive 21502

MASSACHUSETTS

STATE COORDINATOR
Department of Public Health (617) 727-2700
Boston 02111
Boston
Massachusetts Poison Control 232-2120
System 800 682-9211
300 Longwood Ave. 02115 (Statewide)

MICHIGAN

STATE COORDINATOR
Department of Public Health (517) 373-1406
Emergency Medical Services
Lansing 48909
Adrian
Emma L. Bixby Hospital 263-2412
Poison Control Center
818 Riverside Ave. 49221
Ann Arbor
University Hospital 764-7667
Poison Control Center
1405 E. Ann St. 48104
Battle Creek
Community Hospital 963-5521
Pharmacy Dept.
183 West St. 49016
Bay City
Bay Medical Center 894-3131
1900 Columbus Ave. 48706
Coldwater
Community Health Center 278-7361
of Branch County
274 E. Chicago St. 49036
Detroit
Children's Hospital 494-5711
Poison Center (800) 572-1655
Children's Hospital (Statewide)
3901 Beaubien 48201
Flint
Poison Information Center
Hurley Medical Center 257-9111
One Hurley Plaza 48502 (800) 572-5396
Grand Rapids
Western Michigan Regional 774-7854
Poison Center (800) 632-2727
Blodgett Memorial Medical (Statewide)
Center
1840 Wealthy, S.E. 49506
Kalamazoo
Midwest Poison Center 383-7104
Borgess Medical Center (800) 632-4177
1521 Gull Rd. 49001 (Statewide)
Great Lakes Poison Center 383-6409
Bronson Methodist Hospital (Statewide)
252 E. Lovell St. 49006

Lansing
St. Lawrence Hospital 372-5112
1210 W. Saginaw St. 48914
Marquette
Upper Peninsula Regional
Poison Center
Marquette General Hospital 228-9440
420 W. Magnetic Dr.
49855 (800) 562-9781
Pontiac
St. Joseph Mercy Hospital 858-7373
900 S. Woodward Ave. 48053
Port Huron
Port Huron Hospital 987-5555
Poison Control Center
1001 Kearney St. 48060
Saginaw
Saginaw Region Poison Center
Saginaw General Hospital 755-1111
1447 N. Harrison 48602
Traverse City
Munson Medical Center 947-6140
Sixth and Madison Sts 49684 Ext. 303

MINNESOTA

STATE COORDINATOR
EMS Section
Minnesota Department
of Health (612) 623-5284
717 S.E. Delaware St.
Minneapolis 55404
Duluth
St. Luke's Hospital 726-5466
Poison Control Center
915 E. First St. 55805
St. Mary's Hospital 726-4500
407 E. 3rd St. 55805
Fridley
Unity Medical Center 786-2200
550 Osborne Rd. 55432 Ext. 6844
Mankato
Immanuel - St. Joseph's 625-4031
Hospital Ext. 2760
Poison Control Center
325 Garden Blvd. 56001
Minneapolis
Hennepin Poison Ctr. 347-3141
Hennepin County Medical Center
701 Park Ave. 55415
Morris
Stevens County Memorial 589-1313
Hospital 56267 Ext. 231
Rochester
Southeastern Minnesota 285-6162
Poison Control Ctr.
St. Mary's Hospital
1216 Second St., S.W. 55901
St. Cloud
St. Cloud Hospital 255-5617
1406 6th Avenue, N. 56301
St. Paul
St. John's Hospital 228-3132
403 Maria Ave. 55106
United and Children's 298-8402
Hospitals
333 N. Smith 55102
Minnesota Poison
Information Center
St. Paul-Ramsey 221-2113
Medical Center
640 Jackson St. 55101
Worthington
Worthington Regional Hosp. 372-2941
1016 6th Ave. 56187 Ext. 109

MISSISSIPPI

STATE COORDINATOR
State Board of Health (601) 354-7660
Jackson 39205

Biloxi
Gulf Coast Community Hospital 388-1919
4642 West Beach Blvd. 39531
USAF Hospital Keesler 377-6555
Keesler Air Force Base 39534
Brandon
Rankin General Hospital 825-2811
Emergency Department
350 Crossgates Blvd. 39042 Ext. 405
Columbia
Marion County General 736-6303
Hospital Ext. 1020
Sumrall Rd. 39429
Greenwood
Greenwood-LeFlore Hosp. 459-2790
River Road 38930
Hattiesburg
Forrest County General Hosp 264-4235
400 S. 28th Ave. 39401
Jackson
St. Dominic- 982-0121
Jackson Mem. Hosp
969 Lakeland Dr. Ext. 2345
39216
University Medical Center 354-7660
2500 N. State St. 39216
Laurel
Jones County 649-4000
Community Hospital Ext. 630
Jefferson St. at 13th Ave.
39440
Meridian
Meridian Regional Hosp. 483-6211
Highway 39, North 39301 Ext. 440
Pascagoula
Singing River Hospital 938-5162
Emergency Room
2609 Denny Ave. East 39567
University
University of Mississippi 234-1522
School of Pharmacy
Poison Information Center 38677

MISSOURI

STATE COORDINATOR
Bureau of EMS
Missouri Division of (314) 751-2713
Health
of Jefferson City 65102
Cape Girardeau
St. Francis Medical Ctr. 651-6235
St. Francis Drive 63701
Columbia
University of Missouri 882-8091
Hospital and Clinics
807 Stadium Blvd. 65212
Hannibal
St. Elizabeth Hospital, 221-0414
Pharmacy Dept. Ext. 264
109 Virginia St. 63401
Jefferson City
Charles E. Still 635-7141
Osteopathic Hospital Ext. 215
1125 Madison 65101
Joplin
St. John's Medical Center 781-2727
2727 McClelland Blvd. 64801 Ext. 2305
Kansas City
Children's Mercy Hospital 234-3000
24th & Gillham Rd. 64108
Kirksville
Kirksville Osteopathic Health 626-2266
Center
Box 949
1 Osteopathy Ave. 63501
Poplar Bluff
Lucy Lee Hospital 785-7721
2620 N. Westwood Blvd. 63901 Ext. 264
Rolla
Phelps County Regional 364-3100

Poison Control Centers

Medical Center.   Ext. 287
1000 W. 10th St. 65401
St. Joseph
Methodist   271-7580
Medical Center   232-8481
Seventh to Ninth on Faron Sts. 64501
St. Louis
Cardinal Glennon Memorial   772-5200
Hospital for Children
1465 S. Grand Ave. 63104

St. Louis Children's Hosp.   454-6099
500 S. Kingshighway 63110
Springfield
Ozark Poison Center   831-9746
Lester E. Cox Medical Center
1423 N. Jefferson St. 65802

MONTANA

STATE COORDINATOR
Department of Health and   (406) 449-3895
Environmental Sciences
Helena 59620
Helena
Montana Poison   442-2480
Control System   (800)-525-5042
Cogswell Bldg.
Helena 59620

NEBRASKA

STATE COORDINATOR
Department of Health   (402) 471-2122
Lincoln 68502
Omaha
Mid-Plains Regional   390-5400
Poison Center
Children's Memorial Hospital   800-642-9999
8301 Dodge 68114   (Statewide)
Nebraska   800-228-9515
   Surrounding States

NEVADA

STATE COORDINATOR
Department of Human   (702) 885-4750
Resources
Carson City 89710
Las Vegas
Southern Nevada Memorial   385-1277
Hosp.
1800 W. Charleston Blvd. 89102

Sunrise Hospital Med. Ctr.   732-4989
3186 South Maryland Parkway 89109
Reno
St. Mary's Hospital   789-3013
235 W. 6th 89520

Washoe Medical Center   785-4129
77 Pringle Way 89520

NEW HAMPSHIRE

STATE COORDINATOR
New Hampshire Poison Center (603) 646-5000
NH Dartmouth Hitchcock   (800) 562-8236
Medical Center   (Statewide)
2 Maynard St. 03756
Hanover
New Hampshire Poison Center (603) 646-5000
Mary Hitchcock Hospital   (800) 562-8236
2 Maynard St. 03756   (Statewide)

NEW JERSEY

STATE COORDINATOR
New Jersey Poison
Information and Education
System
201 Lyons Avenue
Newark, N.J. 07112
(201) 926-7443

Newark
New Jersey Poison
Control Center   800-962-1253 (NJ only)
926-8005 (out of state)
Medical Center
201 Lyons Ave. 07112

NEW MEXICO

STATE COORDINATOR
N.M. Poison, Drug   (505) 843-2551
Inf. & Med. Crisis   800-432-6866
Center
University of New Mexico
Albuquerque 87131

NEW YORK

STATE COORDINATOR
Department of Health   (518) 474-3785
Albany 12237
Binghampton
Southern Tier Poison Center
United Health Services
Binghampton General Hospital   723-8929
Mitchell Avenue 13903

Our Lady of Lourdes   798-5231
Memorial Hospital
169 Riverside Drive 13905
Buffalo
Western N.Y. Poison Control   878-7654
Center
Children's Hospital of Buffalo
219 Bryant St. 14222
Dunkirk
Brooks Memorial Hospital   366-1111
10 West 6th St. 14048   Ext. 414
East Meadow
Long Island Regional Poison   542-2323
Center
Nassau County Medical Ctr.   542-2324
2201 Hempstead Tpk. 11554
Elmira
Arnot Ogden Memorial Hosp.   737-4194
Roe Ave. & Grove St. 14901
St. Joseph's Hospital   734-2662
Health Center
555 E. Market St. 14901
Endicott
Ideal Hospital   754-7171
600 High St. 13760
Glens Falls
Glens Falls Hospital   761-5261
100 Park St. 12801   Ext. 456
Jamestown
W.C.A. Hospital   484-8648
207 Foote Ave. 14701
Johnson City
Wilson Memorial Hospital   773-6611
33 Harrison St. 13790
Kingston
Kingston Hospital   331-3313
396 Broadway 12401
New York
N.Y. City Poison Center   340-4494
Dept. of Health   764-7667
Bureau of Laboratories
455 First Ave. 10016
Nyack
Hudson Valley Poison Center   353-1000
Nyack Hospital (Pharmacy)
North Midland Ave. 10960
Rochester
Finger Lakes Poison   275-5151
Control Center   275-2700
Life Line, Univ. of
Rochester Medical Center 14642
Schenectady
Ellis Hospital Poison Control   382-4039
1101 Nott Street 12308   382-4121

Syracuse
Syracuse Poison Inf. Ctr.   476-7529
750 E. Adams St. 13210
Troy
St. Mary's Hospital   272-5792
Poison Control Center
1300 Massachusetts Ave. 12180
Utica
St. Luke's Memorial Hospital   798-6200
Center
P.O. Box 479   13502
Watertown
House of the Good   788-8700
Samaritan Hospital
Washington & Pratt Sts. 13602

NORTH CAROLINA

STATE COORDINATOR
Duke University Medical   (919)684-8111
Center   (800)672-1697
Durham 27710   (Statewide)
Asheville
Western N.C. Poison Control
Center   255-4490
Memorial Mission Hospital
509 Biltimore Ave. 28801
Charlotte
Mercy Hospital   379-5827
2001 Vail Ave. 28207
Durham
Duke University Medical   684-8111
Center
Poison Control Center
P.O. Box 3007 27710
Greensboro
Triad Poison Center
Moses H. Cone Memorial   379-4105
Hospital
1200 N. Elm St. 27401
Hendersonville
Margaret R. Pardee Memorial   693-6522
Hospital   Ext. 555
Fleming St. 28739
Hickory
Catawba Memorial Hospital   322-6649
Fairgrove-Church Rd. 28601
Jacksonville
Onslow Memorial Hospital   577-2555
Western Blvd. 28540
Wilmington
New Hanover Memorial Hosp.   343-7046
2131 S. 17th St. 28401
Winston-Salem
Wake Forest University
Medical Center   748-4991
North Carolina Baptist Hosp.
300 S. Hawthorne Rd. 27103

NORTH DAKOTA

STATE COORDINATOR
Department of Health   (701) 224-2388
Bismarck 58505
Bismarck
Bismarck Hospital   223-4357
300 N. 7th St. 58501
Fargo
St. Luke's Hosptal   280-5575
Fifth St. at Mills Ave. 58122
Grand Forks
United Hospital   780-5282
1200 S. Columbia Rd. 58201
Minot
St. Joseph's Hospital   857-2553
Third St. & Fourth Ave., S.E. 58701
Williston
Mercy Hospital   572-7661
1301 15th Ave. W. 58801

Poison Control Centers

OHIO

STATE COORDINATOR
Department of Health (614)466-5190
Columbus 43216

Akron
Children's Hospital 379-8562
Medical Center of Akron (800) 362-9922 (Ohio)
281 Locust St. 44308

Canton
Aultman Hospital 452-9911
2600 Sixth St., S.W. 44710 438-6203

Cincinnati
Drug & Poison Inf. Ctr.
Bridge Medical Science Bldg.
Univ. of Cincinnati 872-5111
Rm. 7701
231 Bethesda Ave. 45267

Cleveland
Greater Cleveland Poison Control Center
2119 Abington Rd. 44106 231-4455

Columbus
Central Ohio Poison Center 228-1323
Children's Hospital of Ohio
700 Children's Dr. 43205

Dayton
Children's Medical Center 222-2227
One Children's Plaza 45404 (800) 762-0727

Lorain
Lorain Community Hospital 282-2220
3700 Kolbe Rd. 44053

Mansfield
Mansfield General Hospital 522-3411
335 Glessner Ave. 44903 Ext. 2545

Springfield
Community Hospital 325-1255
2615 E. High St. 44505

Toledo
Medical College Hospital 381-3897
P.O. Box 6190 43679

Youngstown
Mahoning Valley Poison Control Center
St. Elizabeth Hospital & Med Ctr. 746-2222
1044 Belmont Ave. 44501 746-5510

Zanesville
Bethesda Hospital 454-4221
Bethesda Poison Control Center
2951 Maple Ave. 43701

OKLAHOMA

STATE COORDINATOR
Oklahoma Poison Control Ctr (405) 271-5454
Oklahoma Children's 800-522-4611
Memorial Hospital
P.O. Box 26307
Oklahoma City 73126

Ada
Valley View Hospital 332-2323
1300 E. 6th St. 74820 Ext. 200

Lawton
Comanche County Memorial 355-8620
Hospital Ext. 296
3401 Gore Blvd. 73501

McAlester
McAlester General Hospital, West 426-1800
P.O. Box 669 74501 Ext. 240

Oklahoma City
Oklahoma Children's 271-5454
Memorial Hospital 800-522-4611
P.O. Box 26307 73126 (Statewide)

Ponca City
St. Joseph Medical Center 765-0584
14th & Hartford 74601

Tulsa
Hillcrest Medical Center 560-5755
1120 S. Utica 74104

OREGON

Portland
Oregon Poison Control and
Drug Info. Center
University of Oregon (503) 225-8968
Health Sciences Center 97201 1-800-452-7165
(Statewide)

PENNSYLVANIA

STATE COORDINATOR
Director, Division of Drugs,
Devices and Cosmetics (717) 787-2307
Department of Health
P.O. Box 90
Harrisburg 17108

Allentown
Lehigh Valley Poison Center 433-2311
Allentown General Hospital
17th & Chew St. 18102

Altoona
Keystone Region Poison Center 946-3711
Mercy Hospital
2500 Seventh Ave. 16603

Bloomsburg
The Bloomsburg Hospital 784-4241
549 E. Fair St. 17815

Chester
Sacred Heart General Hosp. 494-4400
9th and Wilson St. 19013

Danville
Susquehanna Poison Center 275-6116
Geisinger Medical Center
North Academy Ave. 17821

Erie
Doctors Osteopathic Hospital 454-2120
252 W. 11th St. 16502
Hamot Medical Center 452-4242
201 State St. 16550
Millcreek Community Hospital 864-4031
5515 Peach St. 16509
St. Vincent's Health Center 452-3232
232 W. 25th St. 16544

Gettysburg
Annie M. Warner Hospital 334-9155
S. Washington St. 17325

Hanover
Hanover General Hospital 637-3711
300 Highland Ave. 17331

Hershey
Capital Area Poison Center 534-6111
Milton S. Hershey Medical Center
University Dr. 17033

Jersey Shore
Jersey Shore Hospital 398-0100
Thompson St. 17740

Johnstown
Conemaugh Valley Memorial 535-5351
1086 Franklin St. 15905
Laurel Highlands Poison Center 535-8255
320 Main St. 15901
Mercy Hospital 535-5353
1020 Franklin St. 15905

Lancaster
Lancaster General Hospital 295-8322
555 North Duke St. 17604
St. Joseph's Hospital 299-4546
250 College Ave. 17604

Lehighton
Gnaden-Huetten Memorial Hospital 377-1300
11th & Hamilton St. 18235

Lewistown
Lewistown Hospital 248-5411
Highland Ave. 17044

Nanticoke
Nanticoke State Hospital 735-5000
N. Washington St. 18634

Paoli
Paoli Memorial Hospital 19301 648-1043

Philadelphia
Philadelphia Poison 922-5523
Information 922-5524
321 University Ave. 19104

Philipsburg
Philipsburg State General Hospital 342-3320
Loch Lomond Rd. 16866

Pittsburgh
Pittsburgh Poison Center
Children's Hospital 681-6669
125 DeSoto St. 15214 647-5600

Reading
Community General Hospital 375-9115
145 N. 6th St. 19601

Sayre
The Robert Packer Hospital 888-6666
Guthrie Square 18840

Sellersville
Grandview Hospital 18960 257-3611

State College
Centre Community Hospital 238-4351
Orchard Rd. 16801

York
Memorial Osteopathic Hospital 843-8623
325 S. Belmont St. 17403 Ext. 123
York Hospital 771-2311
1001 S. George St. 17405

RHODE ISLAND

STATE COORDINATOR
Rhode Island Poison Control Center
Rhode Island Hospital (401) 277-5727
593 Eddy St. Providence 02902

Providence
Rhode Island Hospital 277-5727
Annex Bldg. 442
593 Eddy St. 02902

SOUTH CAROLINA

STATE COORDINATOR
Department of Health & (803) 758-5654
Environmental Control
Columbia 29201

Charleston
National Pesticide
Telecommunications Network 792-4201
Medical University of (800) 845-7633
South Carolina
171 Ashley Ave. 29403

Columbia
Palmetto Poison Center 765-7359
College of Pharmacy (800) 922-1117
University of S.C. 29208

SOUTH DAKOTA

STATE COORDINATOR
Department of Health (605) 773-3361
Pierre 57501

Aberdeen 225-1880
The Dakota Midland (800) 592-1889
1400 15th Ave., N.W. 57401

Rapid City
Rapid City Regional 341-3333
Poison Control P.O. Box 6000 800-742-8925
353 Fairmont Blvd. 57709

Sioux Falls
McKennan Hospital 336-3894
800 East 21st St. 57101 (800) 952-0123

TENNESSEE

STATE COORDINATOR
Department of Public Health (615) 741-2407
Division of Emergency Serices
Nashville 37216

Chattanooga
T.C. Thompson Children's Hospital 755-6100
910 Blackford St. 37403

Columbia
Maury County Hospital 778-4500
1224 Trotwood Ave. 38401 Ext. 110

Cookeville
Cookeville General Hospital 526-4818
142 W. 5th St. 38501

Jackson
Jackson-Madison General Hospital 424-0424
708 W. Forest 38301 Ext. 525

Poison Control Centers

Johnson City
Medical Center Hospital 461-6572
400 State of Franklin Rd. 37601
Knoxville
Memorial Research Center 971-3261
and Hospital
1924 Alcoa Highway 37920
Memphis
Southern Poison Center 528-6048
LeBonheur Children's Medical Center
848 Adams Ave. 38103
Nashville
Vanderbilt University Hospital 322-6435
21st & Garland 37232

TEXAS
STATE COORDINATOR
Texas Department of Health (512) 458-7254
Div. of Occupational Health
Austin 78756
Abilene
Hendrick Hospital 677-7762
19th & Hickory Sts. 79601
Amarillo
Amarillo Hospital District 376-4292
Amarillo Emergency Receiving Center
P.O. Box 1110
1501 Coulter Dr. 79175
Austin
Brackenridge Hospital 478-4490
14th & Sabine Sts. 78701
Beaumont
Baptist Hospital of Southeast Texas 833-7409
P.O. Box 1591
College & 11th St. 77701
Corpus Christi
Memorial Medical Center 881-4559
P.O. Box 5280
2606 Hospital Blvd. 78405
El Paso
El Paso Poison Control Center 533-1244
R.E. Thomason General Hospital
4815 Alameda Ave. 79905
Fort Worth
W.I. Cook Children's Hospital 336-6611
1212 W. Lancaster 76102
Galveston
Southeast Texas Poison 765-1420
Control Center
The University of Texas Medical Branch
8th & Mechanic Sts. 77550
Harlingen
Valley Baptist Hospital 421-1859
P.O. Box 2588
2101 S. Commerce St. 78550
Houston
Southeast Texas Poison 654-1701
Control Center
8th and Mechanic St.
Galveston, Tex. 77550
Laredo
Mercy Hospital 724-6247
1515 Logan St. 78040
Lubbock
Methodist Hospital 793-4366
3615 19th St. 79410
Odessa
Medical Center Hospital 333-1231
P.O. Box 7239 79760
Plainview
Central Plains Regional Hospital 296-9601
2601 Dimmitt Rd. 79072
San Angelo
Shannon West Texas 653-6741
Memorial Hospital Ext. 318
120 E. Harris 76901
San Antonio
Department of Pediatrics 223-6361
Univ. of Texas Health Ext. 473
Science Center at San Antonio
7703 Floyd Curl Dr. 78284

Tyler
Medical Center Hospital 597-0351
1000 S. Beckham St. 75701
Waco
Hillcrest Baptist Hosp. 753-1412
3000 Herring Ave. 76708
Wichita Falls
Wichita Falls General Hospital 322-6771
Emergency Room
1600 8th St. 76301

UTAH
STATE COORDINATOR
Utah Department of Health (801) 533-6161
Division Family Health Services
Salt Lake City 84113
Salt Lake City
Intermountain Regional 581-2151
Poison Control Center
50 N. Medical Drive 84132

VERMONT
STATE COORDINATOR
Department of Health (802) 862-5701
Burlington 05401
Burlington
Vermont Poison Control 658-3456
Medical Center Hospital 05401

VIRGINIA
STATE COORDINATOR
Division of Emergency (804) 786-5188
Medical Services
Room 1102, 109 Governor St.
Richmond 23219
Alexandria
Alexandria Hospital 379-3070
4320 Seminary Rd. 22314
Arlington
Arlington Hospital 558-6161
5129 N. 16th St. 22205
Blacksburg
Montgomery County 951-1111
Community Hospital Ext. 140
Rt. 460, S. 24060
Charlottesville
Blue Ridge Poison Center 924-5543
Univ. of Virginia Hospital 22903
(800) 446-9876 (Deaf Out-of-State)
(Statewide) (800) 552-3723
Falls Church
Fairfax Hospital 698-3600
3300 Gallows Rd. 22046
Hampton
Hampton General Hospital 722-1131
3120 Victoria Blvd. 23661
Harrisonburg
Rockingham Memorial Hospital 433-8311
235 Cantrell 22801
Lexington
Stonewall Jackson Hosp. 463-9141
22043 Ext. 219
Lynchburg
Gen. Marshall Lodge Hosp., Inc. 528-2066
Tate Springs Rd. 24504
Nassawadox
Northampton-Accomack 442-8700
Memorial Hospital 23413
Newport News
Riverside Hospital 599-2050
500 J. Clyde Morris Blvd. 23601
Norfolk
DePaul Hospital 489-5288
Granby St. at Kingsley Lane 23505
Portsmouth
U.S. Naval Hospital 23708 398-5898
Richmond
Central Virginia Poison Center 786-9123
Medical College of Virginia

Virginia Commonwealth University
Box 522 MCV Station 23298
Roanoke
Southwest Virginia Poison
Center
Roanoke Memorial Hospital 981-7336
Belleview at Jefferson St.
P.O. Box 13367 24033
Staunton
King's Daughters' Hospital 885-6848
P.O. Box 3000 24401
Waynesboro
Waynesboro Community Hospital 942-4096
501 Oak Ave. 22980
Williamsburg
Williamsburg Community Hosp. 253-6005
1238 Mt. Vernon Ave.
P.O. Drawer H 23185

WASHINGTON
STATE COORDINATOR
Department of Social & (206) 522-7478
Health Services
Emergency Medical Services
Olympia 98504
Seattle
Children's Orthopedic 634-5252
Hosp. & Med. Center (800) 732-6985
4800 Sandpoint Way, N.E. 98105
Spokane
Deaconess Hospital 747-1077
800 W. 5th Ave. 99210 (800) 572-5842
Tacoma
Mary Bridge Children's Hospital 272-1281
311 S. L St. 98405 (800) 542-6319
Yakima
Central Washington Poison Center
Yakima Valley Memorial 248-4400
Hospital (800) 572-9176
2811 Tieton Dr. 98902 (Statewide)

WEST VIRGINIA
STATE COORDINATOR
West Virginia University (800) 642-3625
3110 MacCorkle Ave. SE 348-4211
Charleston 25304

WISCONSIN
STATE COORDINATOR
Department of Health & Social (608) 267-7174
Services, Div. of Health
Madison 53701
Eau Claire
Luther Hospital 835-1515
1225 Whipple 54701
Green Bay
St. Vincent Hospital 433-8100
835 S. Van Buren St. 54305
LaCrosse
St. Francis Hospital 784-3971
700 West Ave. N 54601
Madison
University Hospital and Clinic 262-3702
600 Highland Ave. 53792
Milwaukee
Milwaukee Children's Hospital 931-4114
1700 W. Wisconsin 53233

WYOMING
STATE COORDINATOR
Office of Emergency Medical (307) 777-7955
Services
Department of Health & Social Services
Cheyenne 82002
Cheyenne
Wyoming Poison Center 635-9256
De Paul Hospital (800) 442-2704
2600 East 18th St. 82001

SECTION 6
Product Information Section

This section is made possible through the courtesy of the manufacturers whose products appear on the following pages. The information concerning each product has been prepared, edited and approved by the medical department, medical director, and/or medical counsel of each manufacturer.

Products described in PHYSICIANS' DESK REFERENCE® which have official package circulars must be in full compliance with Food & Drug Administration regulations pertaining to labeling for prescription drugs. These regulations require that for PDR copy, "indications and usage, dosages, routes, methods, and frequency and duration of administration, description, clinical pharmacology and supply and any relevant warnings, hazards, contraindications, adverse reactions, potential for drug abuse and dependence, overdosage and precautions" must be in the *"same language and emphasis"* as the approved labeling for the product. FDA regards the words *"same language and emphasis"* as requiring VERBATIM use of the approved labeling providing such information. Furthermore, the information in the approved labeling that is emphasized by the use of type set in a box or in capitals, bold face, or italics must be given the same emphasis in PDR. For products which do not have official package circulars, the Publisher has emphasized to manufacturers the necessity of describing such products comprehensively so that physicians would have access to all information essential for intelligent and informed prescribing. In organizing and presenting the material in PHYSICIANS' DESK REFERENCE, the Publisher is providing all the information made available to PDR by manufacturers.

This edition of PHYSICIANS' DESK REFERENCE contains the latest product information available at press-time. During the year, however, new and revised information about the products described herein may be furnished us. This information will be published in the PDR Supplement. Therefore, before prescribing or administering any product described in the following pages, you should first consult the PDR Supplement.

In presenting the following material to the medical profession, the Publisher is not necessarily advocating the use of any product listed.

Abbott Laboratories—Abbott Pharmaceuticals, Inc.
Pharmaceutical Products Division
NORTH CHICAGO, IL 60064

ABBO–CODE™ INDEX

The Abbo-Code identification system provides positive identification of a drug and dosage strength. The following Abbott products are imprinted or debossed with an Abbo-Code designation:

PRODUCT	ABBO-CODE
Cefol® Filmtab® Tablets B-complex vitamins with folic acid, vitamin E, and vitamin C	NJ
Chlorthalidone Tablets, USP	
25 mg	AA
50 mg	AB
Colchicine Tablets, USP	
0.6 mg	AF
Cylert® Tablets ℭ (pemoline)	
18.75 mg	TH
37.5 mg	TI
75 mg	TJ
37.5 mg Chewable	TK
Depakene® Capsules (valproic acid capsules)	
250 mg	HH
Depakote™ Tablets (divalproex sodium enteric-coated tablets)	
250 mg	NR
500 mg	NS
Desoxyn® ℭ (methamphetamine hydrochloride)	
5 mg Tablet	TE
5 mg Gradumet®	MC
10 mg Gradumet	ME
15 mg Gradumet	MF
Dicumarol Tablets, USP	
25 mg	AN
50 mg	AO
Ery-Tab® Tablets (erythromycin enteric-coated tablets)	
250 mg	EC
333 mg	EH
500 mg	ED
E.E.S.® Chewable Tablets (erythromycin ethylsuccinate, USP)	
200 mg erythromycin activity	EF
E.E.S. 400® Filmtab® Tablets (erythromycin ethylsuccinate, USP)	
400 mg erythromycin activity	EE
Enduron® Tablets (methyclothiazide tablets, USP)	
2.5 mg	ENDURON
5 mg	ENDURON
Enduronyl® Tablets 5 mg methyclothiazide and 0.25 mg deserpidine	LS
Enduronyl® Forte Tablets 5 mg methyclothiazide and 0.5 mg deserpidine	LT
Erythrocin® Stearate Filmtab® Tablets (erythromycin stearate tablets, USP)	
250 mg erythromycin activity	ES
500 mg erythromycin activity	ET
Erythromycin Base Filmtab® Tablets (erythromycin tablets, USP)	
250 mg	EB
500 mg	EA
Eutonyl® Filmtab® Tablets (pargyline hydrochloride tablets, USP)	
10 mg	NA
25 mg	NB
Eutron® Filmtab® Tablets 25 mg pargyline hydrochloride and 5 mg methyclothiazide	NK
Fero-Folic-500® Filmtab® Tablets controlled-release iron, folic acid, and vitamin C	AJ
Gemonil® Tablets ℭ (metharbital tablets, USP)	
100 mg	TF
Harmonyl® Tablets (deserpidine tablets)	
0.25 mg	LK
Iberet-Folic-500® Filmtab® Tablets controlled-release iron, B-complex vitamins with folic acid, and vitamin C	AK
Janimine® Filmtab® Tablets (imipramine hydrochloride tablets, USP)	
10 mg	ND
25 mg	NE
50 mg	NL
K · Tab® Filmtab® Tablets (potassium chloride extended-release tablets, USP)	
10 mEq (750 mg)	NM
Nembutal® Sodium Capsules ℭ (pentobarbital sodium capsules, USP)	
50 mg	CF
100 mg	CH
Ogen® Tablets (estropipate tablets, USP)	
0.625 tablet (0.75 mg estropipate)	LU
1.25 tablet (1.5 mg estropipate)	LV
2.5 tablet (3 mg estropipate)	LX
5 tablet (6 mg estropipate)	LY
Oretic® Tablets (hydrochlorothiazide tablets, USP)	
25 mg	ORETIC
50 mg	ORETIC
Oreticyl® 25 Tablets 25 mg hydrochlorothiazide and 0.125 mg deserpidine	AH
Oreticyl® 50 Tablets 50 mg hydrochlorothiazide and 0.125 mg deserpidine	AI
Oreticyl® Forte Tablets 25 mg hydrochlorothiazide and 0.25 mg deserpidine	LL
Panwarfin® Tablets (warfarin sodium tablets, USP)	
2 mg	LM
2.5 mg	LN
5 mg	LO
7.5 mg	LR
10 mg	LF
Peganone® Tablets (ethotoin tablets)	
250 mg	AD
500 mg	AE
Phenurone® Tablets (phenacemide tablets, USP)	
500 mg	II
Placidyl® Capsules ℭ (ethchlorvynol capsules, USP)	
500 mg	KH
750 mg	KN
Tral® Filmtab® Tablets (hexocyclium methylsulfate tablets)	
25 mg	NF
Tranxene® ℭ (clorazepate dipotassium)	
3.75 mg Capsule	CI
7.5 mg Capsule	CN
15 mg Capsule	CK
3.75 mg Tablet	TL
7.5 mg Tablet	TM
15 mg Tablet	TN
Tranxene®-SD ℭ Single Dose Tablets (clorazepate dipotassium)	
22.5 mg	TY
11.25 mg Half Strength	TX
Tridione® Dulcet® Tablets (trimethadione tablets, USP)	
150 mg	LE
Tridione® Capsules (trimethadione capsules, USP)	
300 mg	AM
Vercyte® Tablets (pipobroman tablets, USP)	
25 mg	AT

ABBO-PAC®
Unit Dose Packages

The Abbo-Pac unit dose system from Abbott Laboratories offers a wide range of drugs. Each individual dose is clearly identified by generic name, Abbott name, strength, NDC identification number, expiration date and lot number. Abbo-Pac unit dose containers are designed to accommodate virtually all hospital pharmacy storage racks and to provide maximum accessibility and ease of handling.

The following is a list of products which are now available:

PRODUCT	DOSAGE STRENGTH
Depakene® Capsules (valproic acid)	250 mg
Depakote™ Tablets (divalproex sodium enteric-coated tablets)	250 mg
Depakote Tablets	500 mg
Enduron® Tablets (methyclothiazide tablets, USP)	5 mg
Enduronyl® Tablets (methyclothiazide 5 mg and deserpidine 0.25 mg)	
E.E.S. 400® Filmtab (erythromycin ethylsuccinate tablets, USP)	400 mg
E.E.S.® Granules (erythromycin ethylsuccinate for oral suspension, USP)	200 mg/5 ml
EryPed® Granules (erythromycin ethylsuccinate for oral suspension, USP)	400 mg/5 ml
Ery-Tab® (erythromycin enteric-coated tablets)	250 mg
Ery-Tab	333 mg
Ery-Tab	500 mg
Erythrocin® Stearate Filmtab (erythromycin stearate tablets, USP)	250 mg
Erythromycin Base Filmtab® (erythromycin tablets, USP)	250 mg
Fero-Grad-500® Filmtab Controlled-Release Iron plus Vitamin C	
Iberet®-500 Filmtab Controlled-Release Iron plus B-Complex and Vitamin C	
K-Lor™ 20 mEq (potassium chloride for oral solution, USP)	20 mEq Potassium 20 mEq Chloride/Packet
K-Lor™ 15 mEq	15 mEq Potassium 15 mEq Chloride/Packet
K·Tab® Filmtab (potassium chloride extended-release tablets, USP)	10 mEq (750 mg)
Nembutal® Sodium Capsules ℭ (pentobarbital sodium capsules, USP)	100 mg
Oretic® Tablets (hydrochlorothiazide tablets, USP)	25 mg
Oretic® Tablets	50 mg
Panwarfin® Tablets (warfarin sodium tablets, USP)	2 mg
Panwarfin® Tablets	2.5 mg
Panwarfin® Tablets	5 mg
Panwarfin® Tablets	7.5 mg
Panwarfin® Tablets	10 mg
Placidyl® Capsules ℭ (ethchlorvynol capsules, USP)	500 mg
Surbex-T® Filmtab High-Potency B-Complex Vitamins with Vitamin C	
Tranxene® Capsules ℭ (clorazepate dipotassium)	3.75 mg
Tranxene® Capsules ℭ	7.5 mg
Tranxene® Capsules ℭ	15 mg

ABBOKINASE®
[ab-bo-kī'nāze]
Urokinase For Injection

ABBOKINASE (urokinase for injection) should be used in hospitals where the recommended diagnostic and monitoring techniques are available. Thrombolytic therapy should be considered in all situations where the benefits to be achieved outweigh the risk of potentially serious hemorrhage. When internal bleeding does occur, it may be more difficult to manage than that which occurs with conventional anticoagulant therapy.

Urokinase treatment should be instituted as soon as possible after onset of pulmonary embolism, preferably no later than seven days after onset. Any delay in instituting lytic therapy to evaluate the effect of heparin decreases the potential for optimal efficacy.[1]

When urokinase is used for treatment of coronary artery thrombosis associated with evolving transmural myocardial infarction, therapy should be instituted within six hours of symptom onset.

Description: Urokinase is an enzyme (protein) produced by the kidney, and found in the urine. There are two forms of urokinase differing in molecular weight but having similar clinical effects. ABBOKINASE (urokinase for injection) is a thrombolytic agent obtained from human kidney cells by tissue culture techniques and is primarily the low molecular weight form. It is supplied as a sterile lyophilized white powder containing mannitol (25 mg/vial) and sodium chloride (45 mg/vial).

Thin translucent filaments may occasionally occur in reconstituted ABBOKINASE vials, but do not indicate any decrease in potency of this product. No clinical problems have been associated with these filaments. See "Dosage and Administration" section.

Following reconstitution with 5.2 ml of Sterile Water for Injection, USP, it is a clear, practically colorless solution; each ml contains 50,000 IU of urokinase activity, 0.5% mannitol, and 0.9% sodium chloride. The pH is adjusted with sodium hydroxide and/or hydrochloric acid prior to lyophilization.

ABBOKINASE is for intravenous and intracoronary infusion only.

Clinical Pharmacology: Urokinase acts on the endogenous fibrinolytic system. It converts plasminogen to the enzyme plasmin. Plasmin degrades fibrin clots as well as fibrinogen and other plasma proteins.

Intravenous infusion of urokinase in doses recommended for lysis of pulmonary embolism is followed by increased fibrinolytic activity. This effect disappears within a few hours after discontinuation, but a decrease in plasma levels of fibrinogen and plasminogen and an increase in the amount of circulating fibrin (ogen) degradation products may persist for 12-24 hours.[3,4] There is a lack of correlation between embolus resolution and changes in coagulation and fibrinolytic assay results.

Information is incomplete about the pharmacokinetic properties in man. Urokinase administered by intravenous infusion is cleared rapidly by the liver. The serum half-life in man is 20 minutes or less. Patients with impaired liver function (e.g., cirrhosis) would be expected to show a prolongation in half-life. Small fractions of an administered dose are excreted in bile and urine.

Indications and Usage:
Pulmonary Embolism: ABBOKINASE (urokinase for injection) is indicated in adults:
— For the lysis of acute massive pulmonary emboli, defined as obstruction of blood flow to a lobe or multiple segments.
— For the lysis of pulmonary emboli accompanied by unstable hemodynamics, i.e., failure to maintain blood pressure without supportive measures.

The diagnosis should be confirmed by objective means, such as pulmonary angiography via an upper extremity vein, or non-invasive procedures such as lung scanning.

Angiographic and hemodynamic measurements demonstrate a more rapid improvement with lytic therapy than with heparin therapy.[5,6,7,8,9]

Coronary Artery Thrombosis: ABBOKINASE has been reported to lyse acute thrombi obstructing coronary arteries, associated with evolving transmural myocardial infarction.[2] The majority of patients who received ABBOKINASE by intracoronary infusion within six hours following onset of symptoms showed recanalization of the involved vessel.

IT HAS NOT BEEN ESTABLISHED THAT INTRACORONARY ADMINISTRATION OF ABBOKINASE DURING EVOLVING TRANSMURAL MYOCARDIAL INFARCTION RESULTS IN SALVAGE OF MYOCARDIAL TISSUE, NOR THAT IT REDUCES MORTALITY. THE PATIENTS WHO MIGHT BENEFIT FROM THIS THERAPY CANNOT BE DEFINED.

I.V. Catheter Clearance: ABBOKINASE is indicated for the restoration of patency to intravenous catheters, including central venous catheters, obstructed by clotted blood or fibrin.[10,11] (See separate section at end of insert concerning I.V. catheter clearance for information regarding warnings, precautions, adverse reactions, and dosage and administration.)

Contraindications: Because thrombolytic therapy increases the risk of bleeding, urokinase is contraindicated in the following situations: (See WARNINGS.)
— Active internal bleeding
— Recent (within two months) cerebrovascular accident, intracranial or intraspinal surgery
— Intracranial neoplasm

Warnings:
Bleeding: The aim of urokinase is the production of sufficient amounts of plasmin for lysis of intravascular deposits of fibrin; however, fibrin deposits which provide hemostasis, for example, at sites of needle puncture, will also lyse, and bleeding from such sites may occur.

Intramuscular injections and nonessential handling of the patient must be avoided during treatment with urokinase. Venipunctures should be performed carefully and as infrequently as possible.

Should an arterial puncture be necessary (except for intracoronary administration), upper extremity vessels are preferable. Pressure should be applied for at least 30 minutes, a pressure dressing applied, and the puncture site checked frequently for evidence of bleeding.

In the following conditions, the risks of therapy may be increased and should be weighed against the anticipated benefits:
— Recent (within 10 days) major surgery, obstetrical delivery, organ biopsy, previous puncture of non-compressible vessels
— Recent (within 10 days) serious gastrointestinal bleeding
— Recent trauma including cardiopulmonary resuscitation
— Severe uncontrolled arterial hypertension
— High likelihood of a left heart thrombus, e.g., mitral stenosis with atrial fibrillation
— Subacute bacterial endocarditis
— Hemostatic defects including those secondary to severe hepatic or renal disease
— Pregnancy
— Cerebrovascular disease
— Diabetic hemorrhagic retinopathy
— Any other condition in which bleeding might constitute a significant hazard or be particularly difficult to manage because of its location

Should serious spontaneous bleeding (not controllable by local pressure) occur, the infusion of urokinase should be terminated immediately, and treatment instituted as described under ADVERSE REACTIONS.

Use of Anticoagulants: Concurrent use of anticoagulants with intravenous administration of ABBOKINASE is not recommended. However, concurrent use of heparin may be required during intracoronary administraion of ABBOKINASE. A clinical study[2] with concurrent use of heparin and ABBOKINASE during intracoronary administration has demonstrated no tendency toward increased bleeding that would not be attributable to the procedure or ABBOKINASE alone. Nevertheless, careful monitoring for excessive bleeding is advised.

Arrhythmias: Rapid lysis of coronary thrombi has been reported occasionally to cause atrial or ventricular dysrhythmias as a result of reperfusion requiring immediate treatment. Careful monitoring for arrhythmias should be maintained during and immediately following intracoronary administration of ABBOKINASE.

Precautions:
Laboratory Tests: Before commencing thrombolytic therapy, obtain a hematocrit, platelet count, and a thrombin time (TT), activated partial thromboplastin time (APTT), or prothrombin time (PT). If heparin has been given, it should be discontinued unless it is to be used in conjunction with ABBOKINASE for intracoronary administration. TT or APTT should be less than twice the normal control value before thrombolytic therapy is started.

During the infusion, coagulation tests and/or measures of fibrinolytic activity may be performed if desired. Results do not, however, reliably predict either efficacy or a risk of bleeding. The clinical response should be observed frequently, and vital signs, i.e., pulse, temperature, respiratory rate and blood pressure, should be checked at least every four hours. The blood pressure should not be taken in the lower extremities to avoid dislodgment of possible deep vein thrombi.

Following the intravenous infusion, *before (re)instituting heparin*, the TT or APTT should be less than twice the upper limits of normal. Following intracoronary infusion of ABBOKINASE, blood coagulation parameters should be determined and heparin therapy continued as appropriate.

Drug Interactions: The interaction of urokinase with other drugs has not been studied. Drugs that alter platelet function should not be used. Common examples are: aspirin, indomethacin and phenylbutazone.

Although a bolus dose of heparin is recommended prior to intracoronary use of urokinase, oral anticoagulants or heparin should not be given concurrently with large doses of urokinase such as those used for pulmonary embolism. Concomitant use of intravenous urokinase and oral anticoagulants or heparin may increase the risk of hemorrhage. (See "WARNINGS" section.)

Carcinogenicity: Adequate data is not available on the long-term potential for carcinogenicity in animals or humans.

Pregnancy: Pregnancy category B. Reproduction studies have been performed in mice and rats at doses up to 1,000 times the human dose and have revealed no evidence of impaired fertility or harm to the fetus due to urokinase. There are, however, no adequate and well-controlled studies in pregnant women. Because animal reproduction studies are not always predictive of human response, this drug should be used during pregnancy only if clearly needed.

Nursing Mothers: It is not known whether this drug is excreted in human milk. Because many drugs are excreted in human milk, caution should be exercised when urokinase is administered to a nursing woman.

Pediatric Use: Safety and effectiveness in children have not been established.

Adverse Reactions: The following adverse reactions have been associated with intravenous therapy but may also occur with intracoronary artery infusion.

Bleeding: The type of bleeding associated with thrombolytic therapy can be placed into two broad categories:
— Superficial or surface bleeding, observed mainly at invaded or disturbed sites (e.g., venous cutdowns, arterial punctures, sites of recent surgical intervention, etc.).
— Internal bleeding, involving, e.g., the gastrointestinal tract, genitourinary tract, vagina, or intramuscular, retroperitoneal, or intracerebral sites.

Several fatalities due to cerebral or retroperitoneal hemorrhage have occurred during thrombolytic therapy.

Should serious bleeding occur, urokinase infusion should be discontinued and, if necessary, blood loss and reversal of the bleeding tendency can be effec-

Continued on next page

If desired, additional literature on any Abbott Product will be provided upon request to Abbott Laboratories.

Abbott—Cont.

tively managed with whole blood (fresh blood preferable), packed red blood cells and cryoprecipitate or fresh frozen plasma. Dextran should not be used. Although the use of aminocaproic acid (ACA, AMICAR®) in humans as an antidote for urokinase has not been documented, it may be considered in an emergency situation.

Allergic Reactions: *In vitro* tests with urokinase, as well as intradermal tests in humans, gave no evidence of induced antibody formation. Relatively mild allergic type reactions, e.g., bronchospasm and skin rash, have been reported rarely. When such reactions occur, they usually respond to conventional therapy.

Fever: Febrile episodes have occurred in approximately 2–3% of treated patients. A cause and effect relationship has not been established. Symptomatic treatment with acetaminophen is usually sufficient to alleviate discomfort. Aspirin is not recommended.

Dosage and Administration: ABBOKINASE IS INTENDED FOR INTRAVENOUS AND INTRACORONARY INFUSION ONLY.

A. Pulmonary Embolism:

Preparation: Reconstitute ABBOKINASE (urokinase for injection) by aseptically adding 5.2 ml of Sterile Water for Injection, USP, to the vial. (It is important that ABBOKINASE be reconstituted *only* with Sterile Water for Injection, USP, *without* preservatives. Bacteriostatic Water for Injection should not be used.) Each vial should be visually inspected for discoloration (practically colorless solution) and for the presence of particulate material. Highly colored solutions should not be used. Because ABBOKINASE contains no preservatives, it should not be reconstituted until immediately before using. Any unused portion of the reconstituted material should be discarded.

To minimize formation of filaments, avoid shaking the vial during reconstitution. Roll and tilt the vial to enhance reconstitution. The solution may be terminally filtered, e.g., through a 0.45 micron or smaller cellulose membrane filter. No other medication should be added to this solution.

Reconstituted ABBOKINASE is diluted with 0.9% Sodium Chloride Injection, USP or 5% Dextrose Injection, USP, prior to intravenous infusion. (See Table I, Dose Preparation.)

Administration: Administer ABBOKINASE (urokinase for injection) by means of a constant infusion pump that is capable of delivering a total volume of 195 ml. The following table may be used as an aid in the preparation of ABBOKINASE (urokinase for injection) for administration.

A priming dose of 2,000 IU/lb (4,400 IU/kg) of ABBOKINASE is given as the ABBOKINASE -0.9% Sodium Chloride Injection or 5% Dextrose Injection admixture at a rate of 90 ml/hour over a period of 10 minutes. This is followed by a continuous infusion of 2,000 IU/lb/hr (4,400 IU/kg/hr) of ABBOKINASE at a rate of 15 ml/hour for 12 hours. Since some ABBOKINASE admixture will remain in the tubing at the end of an infusion pump delivery cycle, the following flush procedure should be performed to insure that the total dose of ABBOKINASE is administered. A solution of 0.9% Sodium Chloride Injection or 5% Dextrose Injection approximately equal in amount to the volume of the tubing in the infusion set should be administered via the pump to flush the ABBOKINASE admixture from the entire length of the infusion set. The pump should be set to administer the flush solution at the continuous infusion rate of 15 ml/hour.

Anticoagulation After Terminating Urokinase Treatment: At the end of urokinase therapy, treatment with heparin by continuous intravenous infusion is recommended to prevent recurrent thrombosis. Heparin treatment, without a loading dose, should not begin until the thrombin time has decreased to *less than twice* the normal control value (approximately 3 to 4 hours after completion of the infusion). See manufacturer's prescribing information for proper use of heparin.

This should then be followed by oral anticoagulants in the conventional manner.

B. Lysis of Coronary Artery Thrombi:[2]

Preparation: Reconstitute three (3) 250,000 I.U. vials of ABBOKINASE by aseptically adding 5.2 ml of Sterile Water for Injection, USP, to the vial. (It is important that ABBOKINASE be reconstituted *only* with Sterile Water for Injection, USP, *without* preservatives. Bacteriostatic Water for Injection should *not* be used.) Each vial should be visually inspected for discoloration (practically colorless solution) and for the presence of particulate material. Highly colored solutions should not be used. Because ABBOKINASE contains no preservatives, it should not be reconstituted until immediately before using. Any unused portion of the reconstituted material should be discarded.

To minimize formation of filaments, avoid shaking the vial during reconstitution. Roll and tilt the vial to enhance reconstitution. The solution may be terminally filtered, e.g., through a 0.45 micron or smaller cellulose membrane filter.

Add the contents of the three (3) reconstituted ABBOKINASE vials to 500 ml of 5% Dextrose Injection, USP. The resulting solution admixture will have a concentration of approximately 1500 I.U. per ml. No other medication should be added to the solution.

The admixture should be administered immediately as described under Administration. Any solution remaining after administration should be discarded.

NOTE: Adsorption of drug from dilute protein solutions to various materials has been reported in the literature. Therefore, the directions for Preparation and Administration must be followed to assure that significant drug loss does not occur.

Administration: Prior to the infusion of ABBOKINASE, a bolus dose of heparin ranging from 2500 to 10,000 units should be administered intravenously. Prior heparin administration should be considered when calculating the heparin dose for this procedure. Following the bolus dose of heparin, the prepared ABBOKINASE solution should be infused into the occluded artery at a rate of 4 ml per minute (6000 I.U. per minute) for periods up to 2 hours. In a clinical study, the average total dose of ABBOKINASE utilized for lysis of coronary artery thrombi was 500,000 I.U.[2]

To determine response to ABBOKINASE therapy, periodic angiography during the infusion is recommended. It is suggested that the angiography be repeated at approximately 15 minute intervals. ABBOKINASE therapy should be continued until the artery is maximally opened, usually 15 to 30 minutes after the initial opening. Following the infusion, coagulation parameters should be determined. It is advisable to continue heparin therapy after the artery is opened by ABBOKINASE.

When ABBOKINASE was administered selectively into thrombosed coronary arteries via coronary catheter within 6 hours following onset of symptoms of acute transmural myocardial infarction, 60% of the occlusions were opened.[2]

I.V. Catheter Clearance:

Warnings: Excessive pressure should be avoided when ABBOKINASE is injected into the catheter. Such force could cause rupture of the catheter or expulsion of the clot into the circulation.

Precautions: Catheters may be occluded by substances other than blood products, such as drug precipitate. ABBOKINASE is not effective in such a case, and there is a possibility that the precipitate may be forced into the vascular system.

Adverse Reactions: Although there have been no adverse reactions reported as a result of using ABBOKINASE for the removal of clot obstruction from I.V. catheters, the possibility of reactions should nevertheless be considered.

Dosage and Administration:

Preparation: Reconstitute ABBOKINASE (urokinase for injection) by aseptically adding 5.2 ml of Sterile Water for Injection, USP, to the vial. (It is important that ABBOKINASE be reconstituted *only* with Sterile Water for Injection, USP, *without* preservatives. Bacteriostatic Water for Injection should *not* be used.) Add 1 ml of the reconstituted drug to 9.0 ml Sterile Water for Injection, USP, to make a final dilution equivalent to 5,000 IU/ml. One ml of this preparation is to be utilized for each catheter clearing procedure. BECAUSE ABBOKINASE CONTAINS NO PRESERVATIVES, IT SHOULD NOT BE RECONSTITUTED UNTIL IMMEDIATELY BEFORE USING.

Administration: NOTE: When the following procedure is used to clear a central venous catheter, the patient should be instructed to exhale and hold his breath any time the catheter is not connected to I.V. tubing or a syringe. This is to prevent air from entering the open catheter.

Aseptically disconnect the I.V. tubing connection at the catheter hub and attach a 10 ml syringe. Determine occlusion of the catheter by *gently* attempting to aspirate blood from the catheter with the 10 ml syringe. If aspiration is not possible, remove the 10 ml syringe and attach a 1 ml tuberculin syringe filled with prepared ABBOKINASE to the catheter. Slowly and gently inject an amount of ABBOKINASE equal to the volume of the catheter. Aseptically remove the tuberculin syringe and connect a 5 ml syringe to the catheter. Wait at least 5 minutes before attempting to aspirate the drug and residual clot with the 5 ml syringe. Repeat aspiration attempts every 5 minutes. If the catheter is not open within 30 minutes, the catheter may be capped allowing ABBOKINASE to remain in the catheter for 30 to 60 minutes before again attempting to aspirate. A second injection of ABBOKINASE may be necessary in resistant cases.

When patency is restored, aspirate 4 to 5 ml of blood to assure removal of all drug and clot residual. Remove the blood-filled syringe and replace it with a 10 ml syringe filled with 0.9% Sodium Chloride Injection, USP. The catheter should then be gently irrigated with this solution to assure patency of the catheter. After the catheter has been irrigated, remove the 10 ml syringe and aseptically reconnect sterile I.V. tubing to the catheter hub.

How Supplied: ABBOKINASE (urokinase for injection) is supplied as a sterile lyophilized preparation (**NDC** 0074-6109-05). Each vial contains 250,000 IU urokinase activity, 25 mg mannitol, and 45 mg sodium chloride. Store ABBOKINASE powder at 2° to 8°C.

[See table on next page].

References:

1. Sherry, S., *et al:* Thrombolytic Therapy in Thrombosis: A National Institutes of Health Consensus Development Conference. Ann. Intern. Med. *93*:141–144 (1980).
2. Tennant, S. N., Campbell, W.B., *et al:* Intracoronary Thrombolysis In Acute Myocardial Infarction: Comparison of the Efficacy of Urokinase to Streptokinase. Accepted for Publication, Circulation.
3. Bang, N. U.: Physiology and Biochemistry of Fibrinolysis in *Thrombosis and Bleeding Disorders* (Bang, N. U., Beller, F. K., Deutsch, E., Mammen, E. F., eds.). Academic Press (1971). pp. 292–327.
4. McNicol, G. P.: The Fibrinolytic Enzyme System. Postgrad. Med. J. (August Suppl. 5). *49*:10–12 (1973).
5. Sasahara, A. A., Hyers, T. M., Cole, C. M., *et al.:* The Urokinase Pulmonary Embolism Trial Circulation, (Suppl. II) *47*:1–108 (1973).
6. Urokinase pulmonary embolism trial study group: Urokinase-Streptokinase Embolism Trial. JAMA *229*:1606-1613 (1974).
7. Sasahara, A. A., Bell, W. R., Simon, T. L., Stengle, J. M. and Sherry, S.: The Phase II Urokinase-Streptokinase Pulmonary Embolism Trial. Thrombos. Diathes. Haemorrh. (Stuttg.) *33*:464–476 (1975).
8. Bell, W. R.: Thrombolytic Therapy: A Comparison Between Urokinase and Streptokinase. Sem. Thromb. Hemost. *2*:1–13 (1975).
9. Fratantoni, J. C., Ness, P., Simon, T. L.: Thrombolytic Therapy: Current Status. N. Eng. J. Med., *293*:1073–1078 (1975).
10. Lawson, M., *et al:* The Use of Urokinase to Restore the Patency of Occluded Central Venous Catheters. Am J. Intravenous Therapy and Clinical Nutrition, 9:29–32 (Oct. 1982).

11. Glynn, M.F.X., et al: Therapy for Thrombotic Occlusion of Long-term Intravenous Alimentation Catheters, Journal of Parenteral and Enteral Nutrition, 4(4):387–390 (July/Aug. 1980).

Abbott Laboratories
North Chicago, IL 60064
Ref. 01-2307-R6

ABBOKINASE® OPEN–CATH™ ℞
[ab-bō-kī¹ nāze open-cath]
Urokinase for Catheter Clearance

Description: Urokinase is an enzyme (protein) produced by the kidney and found in the urine. There are two forms of urokinase differing in molecular weight but having similar clinical effects. Urokinase is a thrombolytic agent obtained from human kidney cells by tissue culture techniques and is primarily the low molecular weight form. It is supplied as a sterile lyophilized white powder. Following reconstitution ABBOKINASE OPEN-CATH is a clear, practically colorless solution.

Each ml of reconstituted ABBOKINASE OPEN-CATH contains 5000 IU of urokinase activity, 5 mg gelatin, 15 mg mannitol, 1.7 mg sodium chloride and 4.6 mg monobasic sodium phosphate anhydrous. The pH of ABBOKINASE is adjusted with sodium hydroxide and/or hydrochloric acid prior to lyophilization.

Clinical Pharmacology: Urokinase acts on the endogenous fibrinolytic system. It converts plasminogen to the enzyme plasmin. Plasmin degrades fibrin clots as well as fibrinogen and other plasma proteins.

When used as directed for I.V. catheter clearance, only small amounts of urokinase may reach the circulation; therefore, therapeutic serum levels are not expected to be achieved. Nevertheless, one should be aware of the clinical pharmacology of urokinase.

Intravenous infusion of urokinase in doses recommended for lysis of pulmonary embolism is followed by increased fibrinolytic activity. This effect disappears within a few hours after discontinuation, but a decrease in plasma levels of fibrinogen and plasminogen and an increase in the amount of circulating fibrin (ogen) degradation products may persist for 12–24 hours.[1,2] There is a lack of correlation between embolus resolution and changes in coagulation and fibrinolytic assay results.

Information is incomplete about the pharmacokinetic properties in man. Urokinase administered by intravenous infusion is cleared rapidly by the liver. The serum half-life in man is 20 minutes or less. Patients with impaired liver function (e.g., cirrhosis) would be expected to show a prolongation in half-life. Small fractions of an administered dose are excreted in bile and urine.

Indications and Usage: ABBOKINASE OPEN-CATH (urokinase for catheter clearance) is indicated for the restoration of patency to intravenous catheters, including central venous catheters, obstructed by clotted blood or fibrin.[3,4,5]

Contraindications: Because thrombolytic therapy increases the risk of bleeding, urokinase is contraindicated in the following situations:
—Active internal bleeding
—Recent (within two months) cerebrovascular accident, intracranial or intraspinal surgery
—Intracranial neoplasm

There have been no reports, however, which would suggest a contraindication for the use of urokinase for I.V. catheter clearance.

Warnings: Excessive pressure should be avoided when ABBOKINASE is injected into the catheter. Such force could cause rupture of the catheter or expulsion of the clot into the circulation. During attempts to determine catheter occlusion, vigorous suction should not be applied due to possible damage to the vascular wall or collapse of soft-wall catheters.

Catheters may be occluded by substances other than fibrin clots, such as drug precipitates. ABBOKINASE is not effective in such cases and there is the possibility that the substances may be forced into the vascular system.

TABLE 1
Dose Preparation–Pulmonary Embolism

Weight (pounds)	Total Dose* Urokinase (IU)	Number Vials ABBOKINASE (urokinase for injection)	Volume of ABBOKINASE After Reconstitution (ml)**	+	Volume of Diluent (ml)	=	Final Volume (ml)
81–90	2,250,000	9	45		150		195
91–100	2,500,000	10	50		145		195
101–110	2,750,000	11	55		140		195
111–120	3,000,000	12	60		135		195
121–130	3,250,000	13	65		130		195
131–140	3,500,000	14	70		125		195
141–150	3,750,000	15	75		120		195
151–160	4,000,000	16	80		115		195
161–170	4,250,000	17	85		110		195
171–180	4,500,000	18	90		105		195
181–190	4,750,000	19	95		100		195
191–200	5,000,000	20	100		95		195
201–210	5,250,000	21	105		90		195
211–220	5,500,000	22	110		85		195
221–230	5,750,000	23	115		80		195
231–240	6,000,000	24	120		75		195
241–250	6,250,000	25	125		70		195

Infusion Rate:	Priming Dose	Dose for 12-Hour Period
	15 ml/10 min***	15 ml/hr for 12 hrs

*Priming dose + dose administered during 12-hour period.
**After addition of 5.2 ml of Sterile Water for Injection, USP, per vial (See Preparation.)
***Pump rate = 90 ml/hr

Precautions:
Carcinogenicity: Adequate data is not available on the long-term potential for carcinogenicity in animals or humans.
Pregnancy: Pregnancy category B. Reproduction studies have been performed in mice and rats at doses up to 1,000 times the human therapeutic dose and have revealed no evidence of impaired fertility or harm to the fetus due to urokinase. There are, however, no adequate and well-controlled studies in pregnant women. Because animal reproduction studies are not always predictive of human response, this drug should be used during pregnancy only if clearly needed.
Nursing Mothers: It is not known whether this drug is excreted in human milk. Because many drugs are excreted in human milk, caution should be exercised when urokinase is administered to a nursing woman.
Pediatric Use: Safety and effectiveness in children have not been established.
Adverse Reactions: Although there have been no adverse reactions reported as a result of using ABBOKINASE for the removal of clot obstruction from I.V. catheters, the possibility of reactions should nevertheless be considered. The following reactions have been associated with ABBOKINASE in doses recommended for lysis of pulmonary embolism.
Bleeding: The type of bleeding associated with thrombolytic therapy can be placed into two broad categories:
—Superficial or surface bleeding, observed mainly at invaded or disturbed sites (e.g., venous cutdowns, arterial punctures, sites of recent surgical intervention, etc.).
—Internal bleeding, involving, e.g., the gastrointestinal tract, genitourinary tract, vagina, or intramuscular, retroperitoneal, or intracerebral sites.

Several fatalities due to cerebral or retroperitoneal hemorrhage have occurred during thrombolytic therapy.

Should serious bleeding occur, urokinase infusion should be discontinued and, if necessary, blood loss and reversal of the bleeding tendency can be effectively managed with whole blood (fresh blood preferable), packed red blood cells and cryoprecipitate or fresh frozen plasma. Dextran should not be used. Although the use of aminocaproic acid (ACA, AMICAR®) in humans as an antidote for urokinase has not been documented, it may be considered in an emergency situation.

Allergic Reactions: In vitro tests with urokinase, as well as intradermal tests in humans, gave no evidence of induced antibody formation. Relatively mild allergic type reactions, e.g., bronchospasm and skin rash, have been reported rarely. When such reactions occur, they usually respond to conventional therapy.
Fever: Febrile episodes have occurred in approximately 2–3% of treated patients. A cause and effect relationship has not been established. Symptomatic treatment with acetaminophen is usually sufficient to alleviate discomfort. Aspirin is not recommended.
Dosage and Administration: USE IMMEDIATELY AFTER RECONSTITUTION
Preparation of Solution: *Univial:*
1. Remove protective cap. Turn plunger-stopper a quarter turn and press to force diluent into lower chamber.
2. Roll and tilt to effect solution. Use only a clear, colorless solution.
3. Sterilize top of stopper with a suitable germicide.
4. Insert needle through the center of stopper until tip is barely visible. Invert vial and withdraw dose.

It is recommended that vigorous shaking be avoided during reconstitution; roll and tilt to enhance reconstitution.

Parenteral drug products should be inspected visually for particulate matter and discoloration prior to administration, whenever solution and container permit.

Administration: When the following procedure is used to clear a central venous catheter, the patient should be instructed to exhale and hold his breath any time the catheter is not connected to I.V. tubing or a syringe. This is to prevent air from entering the open catheter.

Aseptically disconnect the I.V. tubing connection at the catheter hub and attach an empty 10 ml syringe. Determine occlusion of the catheter by *gently* attempting to aspirate blood from the catheter with the 10 ml syringe. If aspiration is not possible, remove the 10 ml syringe and attach a 1 ml tuberculin syringe filled with prepared ABBOKI-

Continued on next page

If desired, additional literature on any Abbott Product will be provided upon request to Abbott Laboratories.

Abbott—Cont.

NASE OPEN-CATH to the catheter. Slowly and gently inject an amount of ABBOKINASE equal to the volume of the catheter. Aseptically remove the tuberculin syringe and connect an empty syringe (e.g., 5 ml) to the catheter. Wait at least 5 minutes before attempting to aspirate the drug and residual clot with the empty syringe. Repeat aspiration attempts every 5 minutes. If the catheter is not open within 30 minutes, the catheter may be capped allowing ABBOKINASE to remain in the catheter for 30 to 60 minutes before again attempting to aspirate. A second injection of ABBOKINASE may be necessary in resistant cases.

When patency is restored, aspirate 4 to 5 ml of blood to assure removal of all drug and clot residual. Remove the blood-filled syringe and replace it with a 10 ml syringe filled with 0.9% Sodium Chloride Injection, USP. The catheter should then be gently irrigated with this solution to assure patency of the catheter. After the catheter has been irrigated, remove the 10 ml syringe and aseptically reconnect sterile I.V. tubing to the catheter hub.

How Supplied: ABBOKINASE OPEN-CATH (urokinase for catheter clearance) is supplied as a sterile lyophilized preparation in a 1-ml single dose Univial® package (**NDC** 0074-6111-01). Each Univial contains 5000 I.U. urokinase activity, 5 mg gelatin, 15 mg mannitol, 1.7 mg sodium chloride and 4.6 mg monobasic sodium phosphate anhydrous. Store powder at 2° to 8°C.

References:
1. Bang, N. U.: Physiology and Biochemistry of Fibrinolysis In *Thrombosis and Bleeding Disorders* (Bang, N. U., Beller, F. K., Deutsch, E., Mammen, E. F., eds.). Academic Press (1971). pp. 292–327.
2. McNicol, G. P.: The Fibrinolytic Enzyme System. Postgrad. Med. J. (August Suppl. 5). 49:10–12 (1973).
3. Hurtubise, Michel R., M.D., Bottino, Joseph C., M.D., Lawson, Millie, R.N., McCredie, Kenneth B., M.D.: Restoring Patency of Occluded Central Venous Catheters. Arch. Surg. 115:212–213 (1980).
4. Glynn, M. F. X., *et al:* Therapy for Thrombotic Occlusion of Long-term Intravenous Alimentation Catheters. Journal of Parenteral and Enteral Nutrition. 4(4):387–390 (July/Aug. 1980).
5. Lawson, M., Bottino, J. C., Hurtubise, M. R., McCredie, K. B.: The Use of Urokinase to Restore the Patency of Occluded Central Venous Catheters. Am. J. I.V. Ther. and Clin. Nutr., 9(9):29–30,32 (October, 1982).

Abbott Laboratories
North Chicago, IL 60064

A-HYDROCORT™   ℞
[*ā-hī'dro-cort"*]
(hydrocortisone sodium succinate for injection, USP)
For Intravenous or Intramuscular Use

Description: Hydrocortisone sodium succinate, USP, an adrenocortical-like steroid, is the sodium succinate ester of hydrocortisone.
It occurs as a white, or nearly white, odorless hygroscopic amorphous solid. Hydrocortisone sodium succinate is very soluble in water and in alcohol; it is insoluble in chloroform and is very slightly soluble in acetone.
Hydrocortisone sodium succinate is soluble in water and is especially well suited for intravenous use in situations in which high blood levels of hydrocortisone are required rapidly.
A-HYDROCORT (hydrocortisone sodium succinate for injection, USP) is available as:
100 mg Univial®—Each 2 ml (when mixed) contains hydrocortisone sodium succinate equivalent to 100 mg hydrocortisone; also 0.8 mg monobasic sodium phosphate anhydrous; 8.73 mg dibasic sodium phosphate anhydrous; and 18 mg of benzyl alcohol.
250 mg Univial—Each 2 ml (when mixed) contains hydrocortisone sodium succinate equivalent to 250 mg hydrocortisone; also 2 mg monobasic sodium phosphate anhydrous; 21.8 mg dibasic sodium phosphate anhydrous; and 18 mg of benzyl alcohol.
500 mg Univial—Each 4 ml (when mixed) contains hydrocortisone sodium succinate equivalent to 500 mg hydrocortisone; also 4 mg monobasic sodium phosphate anhydrous; 44 mg dibasic sodium phosphate anhydrous; and 36 mg benzyl alcohol.
1000 mg Univial—Each 8 ml (when mixed) contains hydrocortisone sodium succinate equivalent to 1000 mg hydrocortisone; also 8 mg monobasic sodium phosphate anhydrous; 88 mg dibasic sodium phosphate anhydrous; and 72 mg benzyl alcohol.
100 mg Vial with Diluent—Each 2 ml (when mixed) contains hydrocortisone sodium succinate equivalent to 100 mg hydrocortisone; also 0.8 mg monobasic sodium phosphate anhydrous; 8.73 mg dibasic sodium phosphate anhydrous; and 18 mg of benzyl alcohol.
The pH of each formula was adjusted with sodium hydroxide and/or hydrochloric acid.
Important: The solid contents of A-HYDROCORT should not be used with any diluent other than that provided. **Use within 3 days after mixing.**
When reconstituted as directed, the pH of the solutions ranges from 7–8 and the tonicities are: for the 100 mg per 2 ml solution, 0.36 osmolar; for the 250 mg per 2 ml, 500 mg per 4 ml, and 1000 mg per 8 ml solutions, 0.57 osmolar. [Isotonic saline (0.9% Sodium Chloride Injection, USP) = 0.28 osmolar.]
Clinical Pharmacology: Hydrocortisone sodium succinate has potent anti-inflammatory effects. Because it is an adrenocortical-like steroid, hydrocortisone sodium succinate may cause profound and varied metabolic effects in addition to modifying the body's immune response to diverse stimuli. When given parenterally and in equimolar quantities, hydrocortisone sodium succinate and hydrocortisone are equivalent in biologic activity.
Following intravenous injection of hydrocortisone sodium succinate, demonstrable effects are evident within one hour and persist for a variable period. Excretion of the administered dose is nearly complete within 12 hours. Thus, if constantly high blood levels are required, injections should be made every four to six hours.
This preparation is also rapidly absorbed when administered intramuscularly and is excreted in a pattern similar to that observed after intravenous injection.
Indications: Sterile A-HYDROCORT (hydrocortisone sodium succinate) is indicated in situations requiring a rapid and intense hormonal effect.
Intravenous administration of A-HYDROCORT is most appropriate for the following indications:
1. **Endocrine disorders:**
    a. Acute adrenocortical insufficiency (hydrocortisone or cortisone is the drug of choice; mineralocorticoid supplementation may be necessary, particularly when synthetic analogs are used).
    b. Preoperatively and in the event of serious trauma or illness, in patients with known adrenal insufficiency or when adrenocortical reserve is doubtful.
    c. Shock unresponsive to conventional therapy if adrenocortical insufficiency exists or is suspected.
2. **Collagen diseases**—During an exacerbation or as maintenance therapy in selected cases of:
    a. Acute rheumatic carditis.
3. **Allergic states**—Control of severe or incapacitating allergic conditions intractable to adequate trials of conventional treatment in:
    a. Bronchial asthma.
    b. Serum sickness.
    c. Drug hypersensitivity reactions.
    d. Urticarial transfusion reactions.
    e. Acute noninfectious laryngeal edema (epinephrine is the drug of first choice).
4. **Hematologic disorders:**
    a. Idiopathic thrombocytopenic purpura in adults (I.M. administration is contraindicated).

Intramuscular administration of A-HYDROCORT is appropriate for the following indications:
1. **Endocrine disorders:**
    a. Primary or secondary adrenocortical insufficiency (hydrocortisone or cortisone is the drug of choice; synthetic analogs may be used in conjunction with mineralocorticoids where applicable; in infancy, mineralocorticoid supplementation is of particular importance).
    b. Acute adrenocortical insufficiency (hydrocortisone or cortisone is the drug of choice; mineralocorticoid supplementation may be necessary, particularly when synthetic analogs are used).
    c. Preoperatively and in the event of serious trauma or illness, in patients with known adrenal insufficiency or when adrenocortical reserve is doubtful.
    d. Shock unresponsive to conventional therapy if adrenocortical insufficiency exists or is suspected.
    e. Congenital adrenal hyperplasia.
    f. Nonsuppurative thyroiditis.
    g. Hypercalcemia associated with cancer.
2. **Rheumatic disorders**—As adjunctive therapy for short-term administration (to tide the patient over an acute episode or exacerbation) in:
    a. Post-traumatic osteoarthritis.
    b. Synovitis of osteoarthritis.
    c. Rheumatoid arthritis, including juvenile rheumatoid arthritis (selected cases may require low-dose maintenance therapy).
    d. Acute and subacute bursitis.
    e. Epicondylitis.
    f. Acute nonspecific tenosynovitis.
    g. Acute gouty arthritis.
    h. Psoriatic arthritis.
    i. Ankylosing spondylitis.
3. **Collagen diseases**—During an exacerbation or as maintenance therapy in selected cases of:
    a. Systemic lupus erythematosus.
    b. Acute rheumatic carditis.
4. **Dermatologic diseases:**
    a. Severe erythema multiforme (Stevens-Johnson syndrome).
    b. Exfoliative dermatitis.
    c. Bullous dermatitis herpetiformis.
    d. Severe seborrheic dermatitis.
    e. Severe psoriasis.
    f. Pemphigus.
    g. Mycosis fungoides.
    h. Systemic dermatomyositis (polymyositis).
5. **Allergic states**—Control of severe or incapacitating allergic conditions intractable to adequate trials of conventional treatment in:
    a. Bronchial asthma.
    b. Contact dermatitis.
    c. Atopic dermatitis.
    d. Serum sickness.
    e. Seasonal or perennial allergic rhinitis.
    f. Drug hypersensitivity reactions.
    g. Urticarial transfusion reactions.
    h. Acute noninfectious laryngeal edema (epinephrine is the drug of first choice).
6. **Ophthalmic diseases**—Severe acute and chronic allergic and inflammatory processes involving the eye, such as:
    a. Herpes zoster ophthalmicus.
    b. Iritis, iridocyclitis.
    c. Chorioretinitis.
    d. Diffuse posterior uveitis and choroiditis.
    e. Optic neuritis.
    f. Sympathetic ophthalmia.
    g. Anterior segment inflammation.
    h. Allergic conjunctivitis.
    i. Allergic corneal marginal ulcers.
7. **Gastrointestinal diseases**—To tide the patient over a critical period of disease in:
    a. Ulcerative colitis—(Systemic therapy).
    b. Regional enteritis—(Systemic therapy).
8. **Respiratory diseases:**
    a. Symptomatic sarcoidosis.

b. Berylliosis.
   c. Fulminating or disseminated pulmonary tuberculosis when concurrently accompanied by appropriate antituberculous chemotherapy.
   d. Aspiration pneumonitis.
   e. Loeffler's syndrome not manageable by other means.
9. **Hematologic disorders:**
   a. Acquired (autoimmune) hemolytic anemia.
   b. Secondary thrombocytopenia in adults.
   c. Erythroblastopenia (RBC anemia).
   d. Congenital (erythroid) hypoplastic anemia.
10. **Neoplastic diseases**—For palliative management of:
    a. Leukemias and lymphomas in adults.
    b. Acute leukemia of childhood.
11. **Edematous state**—To induce diuresis or remission of proteinuria in the nephrotic syndrome, without uremia, of the idiopathic type or that due to lupus erythematosus.
12. **Nervous system**—Acute exacerbations of multiple sclerosis.
13. **Miscellaneous:**
    a. Tuberculous meningitis with subarachnoid block or impending block when used concurrently with appropriate antituberculous chemotherapy.
    b. Trichinosis with neurologic or myocardial involvement.

Contraindications: Systemic fungal infections.
Not for use in newborns. Benzyl alcohol, a preservative in the Bacteriostatic Water for Injection provided with these products, has been associated with toxicity in newborns. Data are unavailable on the toxicity of other preservatives in this age group.

Warnings: In patients on corticosteroid therapy subjected to any unusual stress, increased dosage of rapidly acting corticosteroids before, during, and after the stressful situation is indicated.

Corticosteroids may mask some signs of infection, and new infections may appear during their use. There may be decreased resistance and inability to localize infection when corticosteroids are used.

Prolonged use of corticosteroids may produce posterior subcapsular cataracts, glaucoma with possible damage to the optic nerves, and may enhance the establishment of secondary ocular infections due to fungi or viruses.

Average and large doses of cortisone or hydrocortisone can cause elevation of blood pressure, salt and water retention, and increased excretion of potassium. These effects are less likely to occur with the synthetic derivatives except when used in large doses. Dietary salt restriction and potassium supplementation may be necessary. All corticosteroids increase calcium excretion.

While on corticosteroid therapy patients should not be vaccinated against smallpox. Other immunization procedures should not be undertaken in patients who are on corticosteroids, especially on high dose, because of possible hazards of neurological complications and a lack of antibody response.

The use of A-HYDROCORT (hydrocortisone sodium succinate) in active tuberculosis should be restricted to those cases of fulminating or disseminated tuberculosis in which the corticosteroid is used for the management of the disease in conjunction with appropriate antituberculous regimen.

If corticosteroids are indicated in patients with latent tuberculosis or tuberculin reactivity, close observation is necessary as reactivation of the disease may occur. During prolonged corticosteroid therapy, these patients should receive chemoprophylaxis.

Because rare instances of anaphylactoid reactions have occurred in patients receiving parenteral corticosteroid therapy, appropriate precautionary measures should be taken prior to administration, especially when the patient has a history of allergy to any drug.

Usage in Pregnancy: Since adequate human reproduction studies have not been done with corticosteroids, the use of these drugs in pregnancy, nursing mothers, or women of childbearing potential requires that the possible benefits of the drug be weighed against the potential hazards to the mother and embryo or fetus. Infants born of mothers who have received substantial doses of corticosteroids during pregnancy should be carefully observed for signs of hypoadrenalism.

Precautions: Drug-induced secondary adrenocortical insufficiency may be minimized by gradual reduction of dosage. This type of relative insufficiency may persist for months after discontinuation of therapy; therefore, in any situation of stress occurring during that period, hormone therapy should be reinstituted. Since mineralocorticoid secretion may be impaired, salt and/or a mineralocorticoid should be administered concurrently.

There is an enhanced effect of corticosteroids on patients with hypothyroidism and in those with cirrhosis.

Corticosteroids should be used cautiously in patients with ocular herpes simplex because of possible corneal perforation.

The lowest possible dose of corticosteroid should be used to control the condition under treatment, and when reduction in dosage is possible, the reduction should be gradual.

Psychic derangements may appear when corticosteroids are used, ranging from euphoria, insomnia, mood swings, personality changes and severe depression, to frank psychotic manifestations. Also, existing emotional instability or psychotic tendencies may be aggravated by corticosteroids.

Aspirin should be used cautiously in conjunction with corticosteroids in hypoprothrombinemia.

Steroids should be used with caution in nonspecific ulcerative colitis, if there is a probability of impending perforation, abscess or other pyogenic infection; diverticulitis; fresh intestinal anastomoses; active or latent peptic ulcer; renal insufficiency; hypertension; osteoporosis; and myasthenia gravis.

Growth and development of infants and children on prolonged corticosteroid therapy should be carefully observed.

Although controlled clinical trials have shown corticosteroids to be effective in speeding the resolution of acute exacerbations of multiple sclerosis they do not show that they affect the ultimate outcome or natural history of the disease. The studies do show that relatively high doses of corticosteroids are necessary to demonstrate a significant effect. (See "Dosage and Administration"section).

Since complications of treatment with glucocorticoids are dependent on the size of the dose and the duration of treatment a risk/benefit decision must be made in each individual case as to dose and duration of treatment and as to whether daily or intermittent therapy should be used.

Adverse Reactions:
Fluid and Electrolyte Disturbances
   Sodium retention
   Fluid retention
   Congestive heart failure in susceptible patients
   Potassium loss
   Hypokalemic alkalosis
   Hypertension
Musculoskeletal
   Muscle weakness
   Steroid myopathy
   Loss of muscle mass
   Osteoporosis
   Vertebral compression fractures
   Aseptic necrosis of femoral and humeral heads
   Pathologic fracture of long bones
Gastrointestinal
   Peptic ulcer with possible perforation and hemorrhage
   Pancreatitis
   Abdominal distention
   Ulcerative esophagitis
Dermatologic
   Impaired wound healing
   Thin fragile skin
   Petechiae and ecchymoses
   Facial erythema
   Increased sweating
   May suppress reactions to skin tests
Neurological
   Increased intracranial pressure with papilledema (pseudo-tumor cerebri) usually after treatment
   Convulsions
   Vertigo
   Headache
Endocrine
   Development of Cushingoid state
   Suppression of growth in children
   Secondary adrenocortical and pituitary unresponsiveness, particularly in times of stress, as in trauma, surgery or illness
   Menstrual irregularities
   Decreased carbohydrate tolerance
   Manifestations of latent diabetes mellitus
   Increased requirements for insulin or oral hypoglycemic agents in diabetics
Ophthalmic
   Posterior subcapsular cataracts
   Increased intraocular pressure
   Glaucoma
   Exophthalmos
Metabolic
   Negative nitrogen balance due to protein catabolism

The following additional adverse reactions are related to parenteral corticosteroid therapy:
   Hyperpigmentation or hypopigmentation
   Subcutaneous and cutaneous atrophy
   Sterile abscess

Dosage and Administration: This preparation may be administered by intravenous injection, by intravenous infusion, or by intramuscular injection, the preferred method for initial emergency use being intravenous injection. Following the initial emergency period, consideration should be given to employing a longer acting injectable preparation or an oral preparation.

Therapy is initiated by administering hydrocortisone sodium succinate intravenously over a period of 30 seconds (e.g., 100 mg) to 10 minutes (e.g., 500 mg or more). In general, high dose corticosteroid therapy should be continued only until the patient's condition has stabilized—usually not beyond 48 to 72 hours. Although adverse effects associated with high dose, short-term corticoid therapy are uncommon, peptic ulceration may occur. Prophylactic antacid therapy may be indicated.

When high dose hydrocortisone therapy must be continued beyond 48 to 72 hours, hypernatremia may occur. Under such circumstances it may be desirable to replace hydrocortisone sodium succinate with a corticoid which causes little or no sodium retention.

The initial dose of hydrocortisone sodium succinate is 100 mg to 500 mg depending upon the severity of the condition. This dose may be repeated at intervals of 2, 4 or 6 hours as indicated by the patient's response and clinical condition. While the dose may be reduced for infants and children, it is governed more by the severity of the condition and response of the patient than by age or body weight but should not be less than 25 mg daily. Patients subjected to severe stress following corticosteroid therapy should be observed closely for signs and symptoms of adrenocortical insufficiency.

Corticoid therapy is an adjunct to, and not a replacement for, conventional therapy.

Multiple Sclerosis:
In the treatment of acute exacerbations of multiple sclerosis, daily doses of 200 mg of prednisolone for a week followed by 80 mg every other day for one month have been shown to be effective (20 mg of hydrocortisone is equivalent to 5 mg of prednisolone).

Continued on next page

If desired, additional literature on any Abbott Product will be provided upon request to Abbott Laboratories.

Abbott—Cont.

Preparation of Solutions:
Univial:
1. Remove protective cap, give the plunger-stopper a quarter turn and press to force diluent into lower compartment.
2. Gently agitate to effect solution. Use solution within 72 hours.
3. Sterilize top of plunger-stopper with a suitable germicide.
4. Insert needle squarely through center of plunger-stopper until tip is just visible. Invert vial and withdraw dose.

100 mg/2 ml Combination Package:
Prepare solution by aseptically adding 2 ml of Bacteriostatic Water for Injection to the vial.
Further dilution is not necessary for intravenous or intramuscular injection.
For Intravenous Infusion:
Prepare solution as described above. The 100 mg solution may then be added to 100 to 1000 ml (but not less than 100 ml) of 5% Dextrose Injection (or 0.9% Sodium Chloride Injection or 5% Dextrose and 0.9% Sodium Chloride Injection if patient is not on sodium restriction). The 250 mg solution may be added to 250 to 1000 ml (but not less than 250 ml), the 500 mg solution may be added to 500 to 1000 ml (but not less than 500 ml) and the 1000 mg solution to not less than 1000 ml of the same diluents.

How Supplied: Sterile A-HYDROCORT (hydrocortisone sodium succinate for injection, USP) is available in the following packages:
  100 mg/2 ml Univial **NDC** 0074-5671-02;
  250 mg/2 ml Univial **NDC** 0074-5672-02;
  500 mg/4 ml Univial **NDC** 0074-5673-04;
  1000 mg/8 ml Univial **NDC** 0074-5674-08;
  100 mg/2 ml Combination Package
  NDC 0074-5676-02.

Store unreconstituted products below 86°F. Protect from light and avoid freezing.
Abbott Laboratories
North Chicago, IL 60064

A-METHAPRED® ℞
[ā-meth′a-pred″]
(methylprednisolone sodium succinate for injection, USP)
For Intravenous or Intramuscular Use

Description: Methylprednisolone sodium succinate, USP, an adrenocortical-like steroid, is the sodium succinate ester of methylprednisolone.
It occurs as a white, or nearly white, odorless hygroscopic, amorphous solid.
Methylprednisolone sodium succinate is extremely soluble in water and is especially well suited for intravenous use in situations in which high blood levels of methylprednisolone are required rapidly.
A-METHAPRED (methylprednisolone sodium succinate for injection, USP) is available as:
40 mg Univial®—Each 1 ml (when mixed) contains methylprednisolone sodium succinate equivalent to 40 mg methylprednisolone; also 1.6 mg monobasic sodium phosphate anhydrous; 17.46 mg dibasic sodium phosphate anhydrous; 25 mg lactose anhydrous; and 9 mg of benzyl alcohol.
125 mg Univial—Each 2 ml (when mixed) contains methylprednisolone sodium succinate equivalent to 125 mg methylprednisolone; also 1.6 mg monobasic sodium phosphate anhydrous; 17.4 mg dibasic sodium phosphate anhydrous; and 18 mg of benzyl alcohol.
500 mg Univial—Each 4 ml (when mixed) contains methylprednisolone sodium succinate equivalent to 500 mg methylprednisolone; also 6.4 mg monobasic sodium phosphate anhydrous; 69.6 mg dibasic sodium phosphate anhydrous; and 36 mg of benzyl alcohol.
1000 mg Univial—Each 8 ml (when mixed) contains methylprednisolone sodium succinate equivalent to 1000 mg methylprednisolone; also 12.8 mg monobasic sodium phosphate anhydrous; 139.2 mg dibasic sodium phosphate anhydrous; and 72 mg of benzyl alcohol.

The pH of each formula was adjusted with sodium hydroxide and/or hydrochloric acid.
NOTE: The 40 mg and 125 mg Univial should be used within 48 hours after mixing. The 500 mg and 1000 mg Univial should be used within 72 hours after mixing.

Clinical Pharmacology: Methylprednisolone sodium succinate is a potent anti-inflammatory steroid. It has a greater anti-inflammatory potency than prednisolone and even less tendency than prednisolone to induce sodium and water retention. Like the adrenocortical steroids, methylprednisolone sodium succinate may cause profound and varied metabolic effects in addition to modifying the body's immune response to diverse stimuli.

When given parenterally and in equimolar quantities, methylprednisolone sodium succinate and methylprednisolone are equivalent in biologic activity.

The relative potency of methylprednisolone sodium succinate and hydrocortisone sodium succinate, as indicated by depression of eosinophil count, following intravenous administration, is at least four to one. This is in good agreement with the relative oral potency of methylprednisolone and hydrocortisone.

Indications: When oral therapy is not feasible, and the strength, dosage form and route of administration of the drug reasonably lend the preparation to the treatment of the condition, A-METHAPRED (methylprednisolone sodium succinate) is indicated for intravenous or intramuscular use in the following conditions:
1. **Endocrine disorders:**
   a. Primary or secondary adrenocortical insufficiency (hydrocortisone or cortisone is the drug of choice, synthetic analogs may be used in conjunction with mineralocorticoids where applicable; in infancy, mineralocorticoid supplementation is of particular importance).
   b. Acute adrenocortical insufficiency (hydrocortisone or cortisone is the drug of choice; mineralocorticoid supplementation may be necessary, particularly when synthetic analogs are used).
   c. Preoperatively and in the event of serious trauma or illness, in patients with known adrenal insufficiency or when adrenocortical reserve is doubtful.
   d. Shock unresponsive to conventional therapy if adrenocortical insufficiency exists or is suspected.
   e. Congenital adrenal hyperplasia.
   f. Hypercalcemia associated with cancer.
   g. Nonsuppurative thyroiditis.
2. **Rheumatic disorders**—As adjunctive therapy for short-term administration (to tide the patient over an acute episode or exacerbation) in:
   a. Post-traumatic osteoarthritis.
   b. Synovitis of osteoarthritis.
   c. Rheumatoid arthritis, including juvenile rheumatoid arthritis (selected cases may require low-dose maintenance therapy).
   d. Acute and subacute bursitis.
   e. Epicondylitis.
   f. Acute nonspecific tenosynovitis.
   g. Acute gouty arthritis.
   h. Psoriatic arthritis.
   i. Ankylosing spondylitis.
3. **Collagen diseases** — During an exacerbation or as maintenance therapy in selected cases of:
   a. Systemic lupus erythematosus.
   b. Acute rheumatic carditis.
   c. Systemic dermatomyositis (polymyositis).
4. **Dermatologic diseases:**
   a. Severe erythema multiforme (Stevens-Johnson syndrome).
   b. Exfoliative dermatitis.
   c. Bullous dermatitis herpetiformis.
   d. Severe seborrheic dermatitis.
   e. Severe psoriasis.
   f. Pemphigus.
   g. Mycosis fungoides.
5. **Allergic states** — Control of severe or incapacitating allergic conditions intractable to adequate trials of conventional treatment in:
   a. Bronchial asthma.
   b. Contact dermatitis.
   c. Atopic dermatitis.
   d. Serum sickness.
   e. Seasonal or perennial allergic rhinitis.
   f. Drug hypersensitivity reactions.
   g. Urticarial transfusion reactions.
   h. Acute noninfectious laryngeal edema (epinephrine is the drug of first choice).
6. **Ophthalmic diseases** — Severe acute and chronic allergic and inflammatory processes involving the eye, such as:
   a. Herpes zoster ophthalmicus.
   b. Iritis, iridocyclitis.
   c. Chorioretinitis.
   d. Diffuse posterior uveitis and choroiditis.
   e. Optic neuritis.
   f. Sympathetic ophthalmia.
   g. Anterior segment inflammation.
   h. Allergic conjunctivitis.
   i. Allergic corneal marginal ulcers.
   j. Keratitis.
7. **Gastrointestinal diseases** — To tide the patient over a critical period of disease in:
   a. Ulcerative colitis — (Systemic therapy).
   b. Regional enteritis — (Systemic therapy).
8. **Respiratory diseases:**
   a. Symptomatic sarcoidosis.
   b. Berylliosis.
   c. Fulminating or disseminated pulmonary tuberculosis when concurrently accompanied by appropriate antituberculous chemotherapy.
   d. Aspiration pneumonitis.
   e. Loeffler's syndrome not manageable by other means.
9. **Hematologic disorders:**
   a. Acquired (autoimmune) hemolytic anemia.
   b. Idiopathic thrombocytopenic purpura in adults (IV only; IM administration is contraindicated).
   c. Secondary thrombocytopenia in adults.
   d. Erythroblastopenia (RBC anemia).
   e. Congenital (erythroid) hypoplastic anemia.
10. **Neoplastic diseases** — For palliative management of:
    a. Leukemias and lymphomas in adults.
    b. Acute leukemia of childhood.
11. **Edematous state** — To induce diuresis or remission of proteinuria in the nephrotic syndrome, without uremia, of the idiopathic type or that due to lupus erythematosus.
12. **Nervous System:**
    a. Acute exacerbations of multiple sclerosis.
13. **Miscellaneous:**
    a. Tuberculous meningitis with subarachnoid block or impending block when used concurrently with appropriate antituberculous chemotherapy.
    b. Trichinosis with neurologic or myocardial involvement.

Contraindications: Systemic fungal infections.
Not for use in newborns. Benzyl alcohol, a preservative in the Bacteriostatic Water for Injection provided with these products, has been associated with toxicity in newborns. Data are unavailable on the toxicity of other preservatives in this age group.
Warnings: In patients on corticosteroid therapy subjected to any unusual stress, increased dosage of rapidly acting corticosteroids before, during, and after the stressful situation is indicated.
Corticosteroids may mask some signs of infection, and new infections may appear during their use. There may be decreased resistance and inability to localize infection when corticosteroids are used.
Prolonged use of corticosteroids may produce posterior subcapsular cataracts, glaucoma with possible damage to the optic nerves, and may enhance the establishment of secondary ocular infections due to fungi or viruses.
Average and large doses of cortisone or hydrocortisone can cause elevation of blood pressure, salt and water retention, and increased excretion of potassium. These effects are less likely to occur with the synthetic derivatives except when used in large doses. Dietary salt restriction and potassium sup-

plementation may be necessary. All corticosteroids increase calcium excretion.

While on corticosteroid therapy patients should not be vaccinated against smallpox. Other immunization procedures should not be undertaken in patients who are on corticosteroids, especially on high dose, because of possible hazards of neurological complications and a lack of antibody response.

The use of A-METHAPRED (methylprednisolone sodium succinate) in active tuberculosis should be restricted to those cases of fulminating or disseminated tuberculosis in which the corticosteroid is used for the management of the disease in conjunction with appropriate antituberculous regimen.

If corticosteroids are indicated in patients with latent tuberculosis or tuberculin reactivity, close observation is necessary as reactivation of the disease may occur. During prolonged corticosteroid therapy, these patients should receive chemoprophylaxis.

Because rare instances of anaphylactoid reactions have occurred in patients receiving parenteral corticosteroid therapy, appropriate precautionary measures should be taken prior to administration, especially when the patient has a history of allergy to any drug.

There are reports of cardiac arrhythmias and/or circulatory collapse and/or cardiac arrest following the rapid administration of large IV doses of methylprednisolone sodium succinate (greater than 0.5 gram administered over a period of less than 10 minutes).

Usage in Pregnancy: Since adequate human reproduction studies have not been done with corticosteroids, the use of these drugs in pregnancy, nursing mothers, or women of childbearing potential requires that the possible benefits of the drug be weighed against the potential hazards to the mother and embryo or fetus. Infants born of mothers who have received substantial doses of corticosteroids during pregnancy should be carefully observed for signs of hypoadrenalism.

Precautions: Drug-induced secondary adrenocortical insufficiency may be minimized by gradual reduction of dosage. This type of relative insufficiency may persist for months after discontinuation of therapy; therefore, in any situation of stress occurring during that period, hormone therapy should be reinstituted. Since mineralocorticoid secretion may be impaired, salt and/or a mineralocorticoid should be administered concurrently.

There is an enhanced effect of corticosteroids on patients with hypothyroidism and in those with cirrhosis.

Corticosteroids should be used cautiously in patients with ocular herpes simplex because of possible corneal perforation.

The lowest possible dose of corticosteroid should be used to control the condition under treatment, and when reduction in dosage is possible, the reduction should be gradual.

Psychic derangements may appear when corticosteroids are used, ranging from euphoria, insomnia, mood swings, personality changes and severe depression, to frank psychotic manifestations. Also, existing emotional instability or psychotic tendencies may be aggravated by corticosteroids. Aspirin should be used cautiously in conjunction with corticosteroids in hypoprothrombinemia.

Steroids should be used with caution in nonspecific ulcerative colitis, if there is a probability of impending perforation, abscess or other pyogenic infection; diverticulitis; fresh intestinal anastomoses; active or latent peptic ulcer; renal insufficiency; hypertension; osteoporosis, and myasthenia gravis.

Growth and development of infants and children on prolonged corticosteroid therapy should be carefully observed.

Although controlled clinical trials have shown corticosteroids to be effective in speeding the resolution of acute exacerbations of multiple sclerosis, they do not show that corticosteroids affect the ultimate outcome or natural history of the disease. The studies do show that relatively high doses of corticosteroids are necessary to demonstrate a significant effect. (See "Dosage and Administration" section).

Since complications of treatment with glucocorticoids are dependent on the size of the dose and the duration of treatment, a risk/benefit decision must be made in each individual case as to dose and duration of treatment and as to whether daily or intermittent therapy should be used.

Adverse Reactions:
Fluid and Electrolyte Disturbances
 Sodium retention
 Fluid retention
 Congestive heart failure in susceptible patients
 Potassium loss
 Hypokalemic alkalosis
 Hypertension
Musculoskeletal
 Muscle weakness
 Steroid myopathy
 Loss of muscle mass
 Severe arthralgia
 Osteoporosis
 Vertebral compression fractures
 Aseptic necrosis of femoral and humeral heads
 Pathologic fracture of long bones
Gastrointestinal
 Peptic ulcer with possible perforation and hemorrhage
 Pancreatitis
 Abdominal distention
 Ulcerative esophagitis
Dermatologic
 Impaired wound healing
 Thin fragile skin
 Petechiae and ecchymoses
 Facial erythema
 Increased sweating
 May suppress reactions to skin tests
Neurological
 Increased intracranial pressure with papilledema (pseudo-tumor cerebri) usually after treatment
 Convulsions
 Vertigo
 Headache
Endocrine
 Development of Cushingoid state
 Suppression of growth in children
 Secondary adrenocortical and pituitary unresponsiveness particularly in times of stress, as in trauma, surgery or illness
 Menstrual irregularities
 Decreased carbohydrate tolerance
 Manifestations of latent diabetes mellitus
 Increased requirements for insulin or oral hypoglycemic agents in diabetics
Ophthalmic
 Posterior subcapsular cataracts
 Increased intraocular pressure
 Glaucoma
 Exophthalmos
Metabolic
 Negative nitrogen balance due to protein catabolism

The following additional adverse reactions are related to parenteral corticosteroid therapy:
 Hyperpigmentation or hypopigmentation
 Subcutaneous and cutaneous atrophy
 Sterile abscess
 Anaphylactic reaction with or without circulatory collapse, cardiac arrest, bronchospasm
 Urticaria
 Nausea and vomiting
 Cardiac arrhythmias, hypotension or hypertension

Dosage and Administration: When high dose therapy is desired, the recommended dose of methylprednisolone as the sodium succinate is 30 mg/kg administered intravenously over a 10 to 20-minute period. This dose may be repeated every 4 to 6 hours. In general, high dose corticosteroid therapy should be continued only until the patient's condition has stabilized, usually not beyond 48 to 72 hours.

Although adverse effects associated with high dose short-term corticoid therapy are uncommon, peptic ulceration may occur. Prophylactic antacid therapy may be indicated.

In other indications initial dosage will vary from 10 to 40 mg of methylprednisolone depending on the clinical problem being treated. The larger doses may be required for short-term management of severe, acute conditions. The initial dose usually should be given intravenously over a period of one to several minutes. Subsequent doses may be given intravenously or intramuscularly at intervals dictated by the patient's response and clinical condition. Corticoid therapy is an adjunct to, and not replacement for conventional therapy.

Dosage may be reduced for infants and children but should be governed more by the severity of the condition and response of the patient than by age or size. It should not be less than 0.5 mg/kg every 24 hours.

Dosage must be decreased or discontinued gradually when the drug has been administered for more than a few days. If a period of spontaneous remission occurs in a chronic condition, treatment should be discontinued. Routine laboratory studies, such as urinalysis, two-hour postprandial blood sugar, determination of blood pressure and body weight, and a chest X-ray should be made at regular intervals during prolonged therapy. Upper GI X-rays are desirable in patients with an ulcer history or significant dyspepsia.

Methylprednisolone may be administered intravenously by direct push, or by intermittent or continuous infusion; or by intramuscular injection. The preferred method for initial emergency use is either direct I.V. push or intermittent infusion. To administer by intravenous (or intramuscular) injection, prepare solution as directed. The desired dose may be administered intravenously over a period of one to several minutes (for doses of 40 mg or less).

Multiple Sclerosis: In treatment of acute exacerbations of multiple sclerosis, daily doses of 200 mg of prednisolone for a week followed by 80 mg every other day for 1 month have been shown to be effective (4 mg of methylprednisolone is equivalent to 5 mg of prednisolone).

Preparation of Solutions:
1. Remove protective cap, give the plunger-stopper a quarter turn and press to force diluent into the lower compartment.
2. Gently agitate to effect solution. Use solution in 40 mg and 125 mg Univial within 48 hours. Use solution in 500 mg and 1000 mg Univial within 72 hours.
3. Sterilize top of plunger-stopper with a suitable germicide.
4. Insert needle squarely through center of plunger-stopper until tip is just visible. Invert vial and withdraw dose.

Storage: After mixing, store solution below 86°F; avoid freezing. Refrigeration not required.
For Intravenous Infusion:
To prepare solutions for intravenous infusion, first prepare the solution for injection as directed. This solution may then be added to indicated amounts of 5% Dextrose Injection, 0.9% Sodium Chloride Injection, USP or 5% Dextrose and 0.9% Sodium Chloride Injection, USP.

How Supplied: Sterile A-METHAPRED (methylprednisolone sodium succinate for injection, USP) is available in the following packages:
40 mg/ml Univial **NDC** 0074-5684-01;
125 mg/2 ml Univial **NDC** 0074-5685-02;
500 mg/4 ml Univial **NDC** 0074-5630-04;
1000 mg/8 ml Univial **NDC** 0074-5631-08.
Store unreconstituted products below 86°F. Protect from light and avoid freezing.

Continued on next page

If desired, additional literature on any Abbott Product will be provided upon request to Abbott Laboratories.

Abbott—Cont.

Abbott Laboratories
North Chicago, IL 60064
Ref. 01-2301-R1

BUTESIN® PICRATE Ointment
[bū'ti-sin pick'rate]
(butamben picrate)

Description: Butesin Picrate is an anesthetic ointment containing Butesin Picrate (Butamben Picrate), 1%.

Indication: For temporary relief of pain due to minor burns.

Warning: Certain persons, due to idiosyncrasy, are sensitive to this ointment and may develop a rash following its application. In such cases its use should be discontinued, and the ointment remaining on the skin removed with soap and water.

Precautions: Should not be applied repeatedly or to large areas except under a physician's instructions. As Butesin Picrate stains cannot be removed from animal fibers, contact with silk or wool fabrics and hair should be avoided.

Dosage and Administration: Spread thinly on painful or denuded lesions of the skin, if these are small. Apply a loose bandage to protect the clothing.

How Supplied: 1 oz tube (**NDC** 0074-4392-01).
Abbott Laboratories
North Chicago, IL 60064
Ref. 09-5413-2/R4

CALCIDRINE® SYRUP ℞ ©
[cal'si-drīne]

Description: Calcidrine is an oral antitussive, expectorant syrup. Each 5 ml (teaspoonful) contains Codeine, USP, 8.4 mg, (Warning —May be habit forming); Calcium Iodide, anhydrous 152 mg, in a palatable syrup. Alcohol 6%.
The chemical formula for calcium iodide is CaI_2. Codeine is methylmorphine, a natural alkaloid of opium. The chemical formula for codeine is $C_{18}H_{21}NO_3 \cdot H_2O$.

Clinical Pharmacology: The major effects of codeine in man are on the central nervous system. The antitussive effect is produced by depression of the cough reflex. Codeine is rapidly absorbed from the gastrointestinal tract and is metabolized in the liver.
Iodides are readily absorbed from the gastrointestinal tract and are distributed to extracellular fluid as well as gastric and salivary secretions. Iodides are accumulated by the thyroid gland. Excretion occurs mainly through the kidneys.

Indications and Usage: In adults and children as an expectorant, and for symptomatic relief of coughs.

Contraindications: Calcidrine should not be used in patients with a history of iodism, or with known hypersensitivity to iodides or codeine. Long-term use of iodide-containing preparations is contraindicated during pregnancy.

Warnings: Physiological dependence may develop with the use of codeine.

Usage During Pregnancy: Calcidrine Syrup can cause fetal harm when administered to a pregnant woman. Maternal ingestion of large amounts of iodides during pregnancy has been associated with development of fetal goiter and resultant acute respiratory distress of the neonate. If this drug is used during pregnancy, or if the patient becomes pregnant while taking this drug, the patient should be apprised of the potential hazard to the fetus.
Severe and occasionally fatal skin eruptions have been reported rarely in patients receiving prolonged administration of iodides.

Precautions: *Laboratory Tests:* Patients who must receive prolonged iodide therapy should be evaluated periodically for possible depression of thyroid function.

Drug Interactions: The concurrent administration of calcium iodide and lithium carbonate may enhance the hypothyroid and goitrogenic effects of either drug.

Laboratory Test Interactions: Elevated values may be obtained on thyroid function tests or protein-bound iodine tests when iodide-containing compounds have been ingested. False positive results may be obtained if iodides have been ingested prior to guaiac or benzidine testing.

Carcinogenesis: No data is available on long-term carcinogenicity in animals or humans.

Pregnancy: Pregnancy Category D. See "WARNINGS" section.

Nursing Mothers: Iodine is excreted in breast milk. Caution should be exercised when Calcidrine is administered to a nursing woman.

Adverse Reactions: In decreasing order of severity: severe and sometimes fatal skin eruptions (ioderma) occur rarely after the prolonged use of iodides. Iodism can occur. Symptoms of iodism include metallic taste, acneform skin lesions, mucous membrane irritation, salivary gland swelling, and gastric distress. These side effects subside quickly upon discontinuance of the iodide-containing drug.
Codeine may produce vomiting, nausea, and constipation.

Overdosage: Symptoms of acute codeine poisoning include respiratory and central nervous system depression, pinpoint pupils and coma. Blood pressure and body temperature may fall.
Acute iodide poisoning is associated with gastrointestinal irritation. Angioedema with laryngeal swelling may develop. Shock may also occur.
Treatment for overdose of Calcidrine is:
a. Establish a patent airway and ventilate if needed. b. Gastric evacuation. c. Treatment for shock. d. General supportive measures including replacement of fluids and electrolytes may be indicated. e. The use of naloxone to antagonize the narcotic depression of the central nervous system should be considered.

Dosage and Administration: Adults and children over ten years of age, usual dose, 1 to 2 teaspoonfuls every 4 hours. Children 6 to 10 years of age, ½ to 1 teaspoonful every 4 hours. Children 2 to 6 years of age, ½ teaspoonful every 4 hours.

How Supplied: Orange-colored syrup with a pleasant apricot-menthol flavor in 4 fl oz (**NDC** 0074-5763-04), pint (**NDC** 0074-5763-16), and gallon (**NDC** 0074-5763-11) bottles.
Calcidrine must be dispensed in USP tight, light-resistant glass containers.
Abbott Laboratories
North Chicago, IL 60064
Ref. 02-6039-2/R5

CEFOL® Filmtab® Tablets ℞
[c'full]
(B-Complex, folic acid, vitamin E with 750 mg vitamin C)

Description: Each oral Cefol Filmtab vitamin tablet provides:

Ascorbic Acid (C)	750 mg
Niacinamide	100 mg
Calcium Pantothenate	20 mg
Thiamine Mononitrate (B_1)	15 mg
Riboflavin (B_2)	10 mg
Pyridoxine Hydrochloride (B_6)	5 mg
Folic Acid	500 mcg
Cyanocobalamin (B_{12})	6 mcg
Vitamin E (as dl-alpha tocopheryl acetate)	30 IU

Clinical Pharmacology: The vitamin components of Cefol are absorbed by the active transport process. All but Vitamin E are rapidly eliminated and not stored in the body. Vitamin E is stored in body tissues.

Indications and Usage: Cefol is indicated in non-pregnant* adults for the treatment of Vitamin C deficiency states with an associated deficient intake or increased need for Vitamin B-Complex, Folic Acid, and Vitamin E.
*Pregnancy may require greater Folic Acid intake.

Contraindications: Rare hypersensitivity to Folic Acid.

Warnings: Folic Acid alone is improper treatment of pernicious anemia and other megaloblastic anemias where Vitamin B_{12} is deficient.

Precautions: Folic Acid above 0.1 mg daily may obscure pernicious anemia (hematologic remission may occur while neurological manifestations remain progressive).

Adverse Reactions: Allergic sensitization has been reported following oral and parenteral administration of Folic Acid.

Dosage: Usual adult dose is one tablet daily.

How Supplied: Cefol is supplied as green Filmtab tablets in bottles of 100 (**NDC** 0074-6089-13).
Filmtab—Film-sealed tablets, Abbott.
Shown in Product Identification Section, page 403
Abbott Pharmaceuticals, Inc.
North Chicago, IL 60064
Ref. 03-1080-9/R13

CHLORTHALIDONE Tablets, USP ℞
[clor-thal'i-dōne]

How Supplied: Abbott Chlorthalidone Tablets, USP are available as scored tablets in two dosage strengths:
25 mg, peach-colored:
Bottles of 100 (**NDC** 0074-4325-13).
50 mg, lavender-colored:
Bottles of 100 (**NDC** 0074-4338-13).
Bottles of 500 (**NDC** 0074-4338-53).
Shown in Product Identification Section, page 403

CYLERT® Tablets ℞ ©
[cī'lert]
(Pemoline)

Description: CYLERT (pemoline) is a central nervous system stimulant. Pemoline is structurally dissimilar to the amphetamines and methylphenidate.
It is an oxazolidine compound and is chemically identified as 2-amino-5-phenyl-2- oxazolin-4-one.
Pemoline is a white, tasteless, odorless powder, relatively insoluble (less than 1 mg/ml) in water, chloroform, ether, acetone, and benzene; its solubility in 95% ethyl alcohol is 2.2 mg/ml.
CYLERT (pemoline) is supplied as tablets containing 18.75 mg, 37.5 mg or 75 mg of pemoline for oral administration. CYLERT is also available as chewable tablets containing 37.5 mg of pemoline.

Clinical Pharmacology: CYLERT (pemoline) has a pharmacological activity similar to that of other known central nervous system stimulants; however, it has minimal sympathomimetic effects. Although studies indicate that pemoline may act in animals through dopaminergic mechanisms, the exact mechanism and site of action of the drug in man is not known.
There is neither specific evidence which clearly establishes the mechanism whereby CYLERT produces its mental and behavioral effects in children, nor conclusive evidence regarding how these effects relate to the condition of the central nervous system.
Pemoline is rapidly absorbed from the gastrointestinal tract. Approximately 50% is bound to plasma proteins. The serum half-life of pemoline is approximately 12 hours. Peak serum levels of the drug occur within 2 to 4 hours after ingestion of a single dose. Multiple dose studies in adults at several dose levels indicate that steady state is reached in approximately 2 to 3 days. In animals given radiolabeled pemoline, the drug was widely and uniformly distributed throughout the tissues, including the brain.
Pemoline is metabolized by the liver. Metabolites of pemoline include pemoline conjugate, pemoline dione, mandelic acid, and unidentified polar compounds. CYLERT is excreted primarily by the kidneys with approximately 50% excreted unchanged and only minor fractions present as metabolites. CYLERT (pemoline) has a gradual onset of action. Using the recommended schedule of dosage titration, significant clinical benefit may not be evident until the third or fourth week of drug administration.

Indications and Usage: CYLERT (pemoline) is indicated in Attention Deficit Disorder (ADD) with hyperactivity as an integral part of a total treatment program which typically includes other remedial measures (psychological, educational, social) for a stabilizing effect in children with a behavioral syndrome characterized by the following group of developmentally inappropriate symptoms: moderate to severe distractibility, short attention span, hyperactivity, emotional lability, and impulsivity. The diagnosis of this syndrome should not be made with finality when these symptoms are only of comparatively recent origin. Non-localizing (soft) neurological signs, learning disability, and abnormal EEG may or may not be present, and a diagnosis of central nervous system dysfunction may or may not be warranted.

Contraindications: CYLERT (pemoline) is contraindicated in patients with known hypersensitivity or idiosyncrasy to the drug. CYLERT should not be administered to patients with impaired hepatic function. (See "ADVERSE REACTIONS" section.)

Warnings: Decrements in the predicted growth (i.e., weight gain and/or height) rate have been reported with the long-term use of stimulants in children. Therefore, patients requiring long-term therapy should be carefully monitored.

Precautions:
General: Clinical experience suggests that in psychotic children, administration of CYLERT may exacerbate symptoms of behavior disturbance and thought disorder.

CYLERT should be administered with caution to patients with significantly impaired renal function.

Laboratory Tests: Liver function tests should be performed prior to and periodically during therapy with CYLERT. The drug should be discontinued if abnormalities are revealed and confirmed by follow-up tests. (See "ADVERSE REACTIONS" section regarding reports of abnormal liver function tests, hepatitis and jaundice.)

Drug Interactions: The interaction of CYLERT with other drugs has not been studied in humans. Patients who are receiving CYLERT concurrently with other drugs, especially drugs with CNS activity, should be monitored carefully.

Decreased seizure threshold has been reported in patients receiving CYLERT concomitantly with *antiepileptic* medications.

Carcinogenesis: Long-term studies have been conducted in rats with doses as high as 150 mg/kg/day for eighteen months. There was no significant difference in the incidence of any neoplasm between treated and control animals.

Mutagenesis: Data are not available concerning long-term effects on mutagenicity in animals or humans.

Impairment of Fertility: The results of studies in which rats were given 18.75 and 37.5 mg/kg/day indicated that pemoline did not affect fertility in males or females at those doses.

Pregnancy: Teratogenic effects: Pregnancy Category B. Reproduction studies have been performed in rats and rabbits at doses of 18.75 and 37.5 mg/kg/day and have revealed no evidence of impaired fertility or harm to the fetus. There are, however, no adequate and well-controlled studies in pregnant women. Because animal reproduction studies are not always predictive of human response, this drug should be used during pregnancy only if clearly needed.

Nonteratogenic effects: Studies in rats have shown an increased incidence of stillbirths and cannibalization when pemoline was administered at a dose of 37.5 mg/kg/day. Postnatal survival of off-spring was reduced at doses of 18.75 and 37.5 mg/kg/day.

Nursing Mothers: It is not known whether this drug is excreted in human milk. Because many drugs are excreted in human milk, caution should be exercised when CYLERT is administered to a nursing woman.

Pediatric Use: Safety and effectiveness in children below the age of 6 years have not been established.

Long-term effects of CYLERT in children have not been established (See "WARNINGS" section).

CNS stimulants, including pemoline, have been reported to precipitate motor and phonic tics and Tourette's syndrome. Therefore, clinical evaluation for tics and Tourette's syndrome in children and their families should precede use of stimulant medications.

Drug treatment is not indicated in all cases of ADD with hyperactivity and should be considered only in light of complete history and evaluation of the child. The decision to prescribe CYLERT should depend on the physician's assessment of the chronicity and severity of the child's symptoms and their appropriateness for his/her age. Prescription should not depend solely on the presence of one or more of the behavioral characteristics.

Adverse Reactions: The following are adverse reactions in decreasing order of severity within each category associated with CYLERT:

Hepatic: There have been reports of hepatic dysfunction including elevated liver enzymes, hepatitis and jaundice in patients taking CYLERT. The occurrence of elevated liver enzymes is not rare and these reactions appear to be reversible upon drug discontinuance. Most patients with elevated liver enzymes were asymptomatic. Although no causal relationship has been established, two hepatic-related fatalities have been reported involving patients taking CYLERT.

Central Nervous System: The following CNS effects have been reported with the use of CYLERT: convulsive seizures; literature reports indicate that CYLERT may precipitate attacks of Gilles de la Tourette syndrome; hallucinations; dyskinetic movements of the tongue, lips, face and extremities; abnormal oculomotor function including nystagmus and oculogyric crisis; mild depression; dizziness; increased irritability; headache; and drowsiness.

Insomnia is the most frequently reported side effect of CYLERT; it usually occurs early in therapy prior to an optimum therapeutic response. In the majority of cases it is transient in nature or responds to a reduction in dosage.

Gastrointestinal: Anorexia and weight loss may occur during the first weeks of therapy. In the majority of cases it is transient in nature; weight gain usually resumes within three to six months.

Nausea and stomach ache have also been reported.

Miscellaneous: Suppression of growth has been reported with the long-term use of stimulants in children. (See "WARNINGS" section.) Skin rash has been reported with CYLERT.

Mild adverse reactions appearing early during the course of treatment with CYLERT often remit with continuing therapy. If adverse reactions are of a significant or protracted nature, dosage should be reduced or the drug discontinued.

Drug Abuse and Dependence:
Controlled Substance: CYLERT is subject to control under DEA schedule IV.

Abuse: CYLERT failed to demonstrate a potential for self-administration in primates. However, the pharmacologic similarity of pemoline to other psychostimulants with known dependence liability suggests that psychological and/or physical dependence might also occur with CYLERT. There have been isolated reports of transient psychotic symptoms occurring in adults following the long-term misuse of excessive oral doses of pemoline. CYLERT should be given with caution to emotionally unstable patients who may increase the dosage on their own initiative.

Overdosage: Signs and symptoms of acute overdosage, resulting principally from overstimulation of the central nervous system and from excessive sympathomimetic effects, may include the following: vomiting, agitation, tremors, hyperreflexia, muscle twitching, convulsions (may be followed by coma), euphoria, confusion, hallucinations, delirium, sweating, flushing, headache, hyperpyrexia, tachycardia, hypertension and mydriasis. Treatment consists of appropriate supportive measures. The patient must be protected against self-injury and against external stimuli that would aggravate overstimulation already present. If signs and symptoms are not too severe and the patient is conscious, gastric contents may be evacuated. Chlorpromazine has been reported in the literature to be useful in decreasing CNS stimulation and sympathomimetic effects.

Efficacy of peritoneal dialysis or extracorporeal hemodialysis for CYLERT overdosage has not been established.

Dosage and Administration: CYLERT (pemoline) is administered as a single oral dose each morning. The recommended starting dose is 37.5 mg/day. This daily dose should be gradually increased by 18.75 mg at one week intervals until the desired clinical response is obtained. The effective daily dose for most patients will range from 56.25 to 75 mg. The maximum recommended daily dose of pemoline is 112.5 mg.

Clinical improvement with CYLERT is gradual. Using the recommended schedule of dosage titration, significant benefit may not be evident until the third or fourth week of drug administration. Where possible, drug administration should be interrupted occasionally to determine if there is a recurrence of behavioral symptoms sufficient to require continued therapy.

How Supplied: CYLERT (pemoline) is supplied as monogrammed, grooved tablets in three dosage strengths:

18.75 mg tablets (white) in bottles of 100 (**NDC** 0074-6025-13)

37.5 mg tablets (orange-colored) in bottles of 100 (**NDC** 0074-6057-13)

75 mg tablets (tan-colored) in bottles of 100 (**NDC** 0074-6073-13)

CYLERT Chewable is supplied as monogrammed, grooved tablets in one dosage strength:

37.5 mg tablets (orange-colored) in bottles of 100 (**NDC** 0074-6088-13)

Shown in Product Identification Section, page 403
Abbott Pharmaceuticals, Inc.
North Chicago, IL 60064

DAYALETS® Filmtab®
[dāy'a-lets]
Multivitamin Supplement for adults and children 4 or more years of age
DAYALETS® PLUS IRON Filmtab®
Multivitamin Supplement with Iron for adults and children 4 or more years of age

Description: Dayalets provide 100% of the recommended daily allowances of essential vitamins. Dayalets Plus Iron provides 100% of the recommended daily allowances of essential vitamins plus the mineral iron.

Daily dosage (one Dayalets tablet) provides:

VITAMINS		% U.S. RDA
Vitamin A........... (1.5 mg)......... 5000 IU		100%
Vitamin D........... (10 mcg)......... 400 IU		100%
Vitamin E............................... 30 IU		100%
Vitamin C............................... 60 mg		100%
Folic Acid .... 0.4 mg		100%
Thiamine (Vitamin B_1)............... 1.5 mg		100%
Riboflavin (Vitamin B_2)............... 1.7 mg		100%
Niacin .... 20 mg		100%
Vitamin B_6 .... 2 mg		100%
Vitamin B_{12} .... 6 mcg		100%

Ingredients: Ascorbic acid, cellulose, dl-alpha tocopheryl acetate, niacinamide, povidone, pyridoxine hydrochloride, riboflavin, thiamine hydrochloride, vitamin A acetate, vitamin A palmitate, folic acid, cholecalciferol, and cyanocobalamin in a film-coated tablet with vanillin flavoring and artificial coloring added.

Each Dayalets Plus Iron Filmtab® represents all the vitamins in the Dayalets formula in the same concentrations, plus the mineral iron 18 mg (100% U.S. R.D.A.), as ferrous sulfate. Dayalets Plus Iron contain the same ingredients as Dayalets.

These products contain no sugar and essentially no calories.

Continued on next page

If desired, additional literature on any Abbott Product will be provided upon request to Abbott Laboratories.

Abbott—Cont.

Indications: Dietary supplement and supplement with iron for adults and children 4 or more years of age.
Administration and Dosage: One Filmtab tablet daily.
How Supplied: Daylets® Filmtab® in bottles of 100 tablets (NDC 0074-3925-01).
Daylets®Plus Iron Filmtab in bottles of 100 tablets (NDC 0074-6667-01).
® Filmtab—Film-sealed tablets, Abbott.
Abbott Laboratories
North Chicago, IL 60064
Ref. 02-6438-7/R6, Ref. 02-6452-8/R7

DEPAKENE® Capsules and Syrup ℞
[dep'a-kāne]
(Valproic Acid)

> **Warning:** HEPATIC FAILURE RESULTING IN FATALITIES HAS OCCURRED IN PATIENTS RECEIVING DEPAKENE. THESE INCIDENTS USUALLY HAVE OCCURRED DURING THE FIRST SIX MONTHS OF TREATMENT WITH DEPAKENE. SERIOUS OR FATAL HEPATOTOXICITY MAY BE PRECEDED BY NONSPECIFIC SYMPTOMS SUCH AS LOSS OF SEIZURE CONTROL, MALAISE, WEAKNESS, LETHARGY, ANOREXIA AND VOMITING. LIVER FUNCTION TESTS SHOULD BE PERFORMED PRIOR TO THERAPY AND AT FREQUENT INTERVALS THEREAFTER, ESPECIALLY DURING THE FIRST SIX MONTHS.

Description: DEPAKENE (valproic acid) is a carboxylic acid designated as 2-propylpentanoic acid. It is also known as dipropylacetic acid.
Valproic acid (pKa 4.8) has a molecular weight of 144 and occurs as a colorless liquid with a characteristic odor. It is slightly soluble in water (1.3 mg/ml) and very soluble in organic solvents.
DEPAKENE is supplied as soft elastic capsules and syrup for oral administration. Each capsule contains 250 mg valproic acid. The syrup contains the equivalent of 250 mg valproic acid per 5 ml as the sodium salt.
Clinical Pharmacology: DEPAKENE is an antiepileptic agent which is chemically unrelated to other drugs used to treat seizure disorders. It has no nitrogen or aromatic moiety characteristic of other antiepileptic drugs. The mechanism by which DEPAKENE exerts its antiepileptic effects has not been established. It has been suggested that its activity is related to increased brain levels of gamma-aminobutyric acid (GABA). The effect on the neuronal membrane is unknown.
DEPAKENE is rapidly absorbed after oral administration. Peak serum levels of valproic acid occur approximately one to four hours after a single oral dose of DEPAKENE. The serum half-life of the parent compound is typically in the range of six to sixteen hours. Half-lives in the lower part of the above range are usually found in patients taking other antiepileptic drugs. A slight delay in absorption occurs when the drug is administered with meals but this does not affect the total absorption.
Valproic acid is rapidly distributed and at therapeutic drug concentrations, drug is highly bound (90%) to human plasma proteins. Increases in dose may result in decreases in the extent of protein binding and variable changes in valproate clearance and elimination.
Elimination of DEPAKENE and its metabolites occurs principally in the urine, with minor amounts in the feces and expired air. Very little unmetabolized parent drug is excreted in the urine. The drug is primarily metabolized in the liver and is excreted as the glucuronide conjugate. Other metabolites in the urine are products of beta omega-1, and omega oxidation (C-3, C-4, and C-5 positions). The major oxidative metabolite in the urine is 2-propyl-3-keto-pentanoic acid; minor metabolites are 2-propyl-glutaric acid, 2-propyl-5-hydroxypentanoic acid, 2-propyl-3-hydroxypentanoic acid and 2-propyl-4-hydroxypentanoic acid.

Indications: DEPAKENE (valproic acid) is indicated for use as sole and adjunctive therapy in the treatment of simple (petit mal) and complex absence seizures. DEPAKENE may also be used adjunctively in patients with multiple seizure types which include absence seizures.
In accordance with the International Classification of Seizures, simple absence is defined as very brief clouding of the sensorium or loss of consciousness (lasting usually 2–15 seconds), accompanied by certain generalized epileptic discharges without other detectable clinical signs. Complex absence is the term used when other signs are also present.
SEE "WARNINGS" SECTION FOR STATEMENT REGARDING FATAL HEPATIC DYSFUNCTION.
Contraindications: DEPAKENE (valproic acid) should not be administered to patients with hepatic disease or significant dysfunction.
DEPAKENE is contraindicated in patients with known hypersensitivity to the drug.
Warnings: **Hepatic failure resulting in fatalities has occurred in patients receiving DEPAKENE. These incidents usually have occurred during the first six months of treatment with DEPAKENE. Serious or fatal hepatotoxicity may be preceded by non-specific symptoms such as loss of seizure control, malaise, weakness, lethargy, anorexia and vomiting. Liver function tests should be performed prior to therapy and at frequent intervals thereafter, especially during the first six months. However, physicians should not rely totally on serum biochemistry since these tests may not be abnormal in all instances, but should also consider the results of careful interim medical history and physical examination. Caution should be observed when administering DEPAKENE to patients with a prior history of hepatic disease. Patients with various unusual congenital disorders, those with severe seizure disorders accompanied with mental retardation, and those with organic brain disease may be at particular risk.**
The drug should be discontinued immediately in the presence of significant hepatic dysfunction, suspected or apparent. In some cases, hepatic dysfunction has progressed in spite of discontinuation of drug. The frequency of adverse effects (particularly elevated liver enzymes) may be dose-related. The benefit of improved seizure control which may accompany the higher doses should therefore be weighed against the possibility of a greater incidence of adverse effects.
Usage in Pregnancy: ACCORDING TO RECENT REPORTS IN THE MEDICAL LITERATURE, DEPAKENE MAY PRODUCE TERATOGENICITY IN THE OFFSPRING OF HUMAN FEMALES RECEIVING THE DRUG DURING PREGNANCY. THE INCIDENCE OF NEURAL TUBE DEFECTS IN THE FETUS MAY BE INCREASED IN MOTHERS RECEIVING VALPROATE DURING THE FIRST TRIMESTER OF PREGNANCY. BASED UPON A SINGLE FRENCH REPORT[1], THE CENTERS FOR DISEASE CONTROL (CDC) HAS ESTIMATED THE RISK OF VALPROIC ACID EXPOSED WOMEN HAVING CHILDREN WITH SPINA BIFIDA TO BE APPROXIMATELY 1.2%.[2] THIS RISK IS SIMILAR TO THAT FOR NONEPILEPTIC WOMEN WHO HAVE HAD CHILDREN WITH NEURAL TUBE DEFECTS (ANENCEPHALY AND SPINA BIFIDA).
THERE ARE MULTIPLE REPORTS IN THE CLINICAL LITERATURE WHICH INDICATE THAT THE USE OF ANTIEPILEPTIC DRUGS DURING PREGNANCY RESULTS IN AN INCREASED INCIDENCE OF BIRTH DEFECTS IN THE OFFSPRING. ALTHOUGH DATA ARE MORE EXTENSIVE WITH RESPECT TO TRIMETHADIONE, PARAMETHADIONE, PHENYTOIN, AND PHENOBARBITAL, REPORTS INDICATE A POSSIBLE SIMILAR ASSOCIATION WITH THE USE OF OTHER ANTIEPILEPTIC DRUGS. THEREFORE, ANTIEPILEPTIC DRUGS SHOULD BE ADMINISTERED TO WOMEN OF CHILDBEARING POTENTIAL ONLY IF THEY ARE CLEARLY SHOWN TO BE ESSENTIAL IN THE MANAGEMENT OF THEIR SEIZURES.
ANIMAL STUDIES HAVE ALSO DEMONSTRATED DEPAKENE INDUCED TERATOGENICITY. Studies in rats and human females demonstrated placental transfer of the drug. Doses greater than 65 mg/kg/day given to pregnant rats and mice produced skeletal abnormalities in the offspring, primarily involving ribs and vertebrae; doses greater than 150 mg/kg/day given to pregnant rabbits produced fetal resorptions and (primarily) soft-tissue abnormalities in the offspring. In rats a dose-related delay in the onset of parturition was noted. Postnatal growth and survival of the progeny were adversely affected, particularly when drug administration spanned the entire gestation and early lactation period.
Antiepileptic drugs should not be discontinued in patients in whom the drug is administered to prevent major seizures because of the strong possibility of precipitating status epilepticus with attendant hypoxia and threat to life. In individual cases where the severity and frequency of the seizure disorder are such that the removal of medication does not pose a serious threat to the patient, discontinuation of the drug may be considered prior to and during pregnancy, although it cannot be said with any confidence that even minor seizures do not pose some hazard to the developing embryo or fetus.
The prescribing physician will wish to weigh these considerations in treating or counseling epileptic women of childbearing potential.
Precautions:
Hepatic dysfunction: See "Contraindications" and "Warnings" sections.
General: Because of reports of thrombocytopenia and inhibition of the secondary phase of platelet aggregation, platelet counts and bleeding time determination are recommended before initiating therapy and at periodic intervals. It is recommended that patients receiving DEPAKENE be monitored for platelet count prior to planned surgery. Clinical evidence of hemorrhage, bruising or a disorder of hemostasis/coagulation is an indication for reduction of DEPAKENE dosage or withdrawal of therapy pending investigation.
Hyperammonemia with or without lethargy or coma has been reported and may be present in the absence of abnormal liver function tests. If elevation occurs, DEPAKENE should be discontinued.
Since DEPAKENE (valproic acid) may interact with concurrently administered antiepileptic drugs, periodic serum level determinations of concomitant antiepileptic drugs are recommended during the early course of therapy. (See "Drug Interactions" section.)
DEPAKENE is partially eliminated in the urine as a keto-metabolite which may lead to a false interpretation of the urine ketone test.
Information for Patients: Since DEPAKENE may produce CNS depression, especially when combined with another CNS depressant (e.g., alcohol), patients should be advised not to engage in hazardous occupations, such as driving an automobile or operating dangerous machinery, until it is known that they do not become drowsy from the drug.
Drug Interactions: DEPAKENE may potentiate the CNS depressant activity of alcohol.
THERE IS EVIDENCE THAT DEPAKENE CAN CAUSE AN INCREASE IN SERUM PHENOBARBITAL LEVELS BY IMPAIRMENT OF NONRENAL CLEARANCE. THIS PHENOMENON CAN RESULT IN SEVERE CNS DEPRESSION. THE COMBINATION OF DEPAKENE AND PHENOBARBITAL HAS ALSO BEEN REPORTED TO PRODUCE CNS DEPRESSION WITHOUT SIGNIFICANT ELEVATIONS OF BARBITURATE OR VALPROATE SERUM LEVELS. ALL PATIENTS RECEIVING CONCOMITANT BARBITURATE THERAPY SHOULD BE CLOSELY MONITORED FOR NEUROLOGICAL TOXICITY. SERUM BARBITURATE LEVELS SHOULD BE OBTAINED, IF POSSIBLE, AND

THE BARBITURATE DOSAGE DECREASED, IF APPROPRIATE.

Primidone is metabolized into a barbiturate and, therefore, may also be involved in a similar or identical interaction.

THERE HAVE BEEN REPORTS OF BREAKTHROUGH SEIZURES OCCURRING WITH THE COMBINATION OF DEPAKENE AND PHENYTOIN. MOST REPORTS HAVE NOTED A DECREASE IN TOTAL PLASMA PHENYTOIN CONCENTRATION. HOWEVER, INCREASES IN TOTAL PHENYTOIN SERUM CONCENTRATION HAVE BEEN REPORTED. AN INITIAL FALL IN TOTAL PHENYTOIN LEVELS WITH SUBSEQUENT INCREASE IN PHENYTOIN LEVELS HAS ALSO BEEN REPORTED. IN ADDITION, A DECREASE IN TOTAL SERUM PHENYTOIN WITH AN INCREASE IN THE FREE VS. PROTEIN BOUND PHENYTOIN LEVELS HAS BEEN REPORTED. THE DOSAGE OF PHENYTOIN SHOULD BE ADJUSTED AS REQUIRED BY THE CLINICAL SITUATION.

THE CONCOMITANT USE OF VALPROIC ACID AND CLONAZEPAM MAY PRODUCE ABSENCE STATUS.

Caution is recommended when DEPAKENE (valproic acid) is administered with drugs affecting coagulation, e.g., aspirin and warfarin. (See "Adverse Reactions" section.)

There have been reports of altered thyroid function tests associated with DEPAKENE. The clinical significance of these is unknown.

Carcinogenesis: DEPAKENE was administered to Sprague Dawley rats and ICR (HA/ICR) mice at doses of 0, 80 and 170 mg/kg/day for two years. Although a variety of neoplasms were observed in both species, the chief findings were a statistically significant increase in the incidence of subcutaneous fibrosarcomas in high dose male rats receiving DEPAKENE and a statistically significant dose-related trend for benign pulmonary adenomas in male mice receiving DEPAKENE. The significance of these findings for man is unknown at present.

Mutagenesis: Studies on DEPAKENE have been performed using bacterial and mammalian systems. These studies have provided no evidence of a mutagenic potential for DEPAKENE.

Fertility: Chronic toxicity studies in juvenile and adult rats and dogs demonstrated reduced spermatogenesis and testicular atrophy at doses greater than 200 mg/kg/day in rats and greater than 90 mg/kg/day in dogs. Segment I fertility studies in rats have shown doses up to 350 mg/kg/day for 60 days to have no effect on fertility. THE EFFECT OF DEPAKENE (VALPROIC ACID) ON THE DEVELOPMENT OF THE TESTES AND ON SPERM PRODUCTION AND FERTILITY IN HUMANS IS UNKNOWN.

Pregnancy: See "WARNINGS" section.

Nursing Mothers: DEPAKENE is excreted in breast milk. Concentrations in breast milk have been reported to be 1-10% of serum concentrations. It is not known what effect this would have on a nursing infant. Caution should be exercised when DEPAKENE is administered to a nursing woman.

Adverse Reactions: Since DEPAKENE (valproic acid) has usually been used with other antiepileptic drugs, it is not possible, in most cases, to determine whether the following adverse reactions can be ascribed to DEPAKENE alone, or the combination of drugs.

Gastrointestinal: The most commonly reported side effects at the initiation of therapy are nausea, vomiting and indigestion. These effects are usually transient and rarely require discontinuation of therapy. Diarrhea, abdominal cramps and constipation have been reported. Both anorexia with some weight loss and increased appetite with weight gain have also been reported.

CNS Effects: Sedative effects have been noted in patients receiving valproic acid alone but are found most often in patients receiving combination therapy. Sedation usually disappears upon reduction of other antiepileptic medication. Ataxia, headache, nystagmus, diplopia, asterixis, "spots before eyes", tremor, dysarthria, dizziness, and incoordination have rarely been noted. Rare cases of coma have been noted in patients receiving valproic acid alone or in conjunction with phenobarbital.

Dermatologic: Transient increases in hair loss have been observed. Skin rash and petechiae have rarely been noted.

Psychiatric: Emotional upset, depression, psychosis, aggression, hyperactivity and behavioral deterioration have been reported.

Musculoskeletal: Weakness has been reported.

Hematopoietic: Thrombocytopenia has been reported. Valproic acid inhibits the secondary phase of platelet aggregation. (See "Drug Interactions" section.) This may be reflected in altered bleeding time. Bruising, hematoma formation and frank hemorrhage have been reported. Relative lymphocytosis and hypofibrinogenemia have been noted. Leukopenia and eosinophilia have also been reported. Anemia and bone marrow suppression have been reported.

Hepatic: Minor elevations of transaminases (e.g., SGOT and SGPT) and LDH are frequent and appear to be dose related. Occasionally, laboratory test results include, as well, increases in serum bilirubin and abnormal changes in other liver function tests. These results may reflect potentially serious hepatotoxicity. (See "Warnings" section.)

Endocrine: There have been reports of irregular menses and secondary amenorrhea occurring in patients receiving DEPAKENE.

Abnormal thyroid function tests have been reported. (see "Precautions" section.)

Pancreatic: There have been reports of acute pancreatitis occurring in patients receiving DEPAKENE.

Metabolic: Hyperammonemia. (See "Precautions" section.)

Hyperglycinemia has been reported and has been associated with a fatal outcome in a patient with preexistent nonketotic hyperglycinemia.

Overdosage: Overdosage with valproic acid may result in deep coma.

Since DEPAKENE is absorbed very rapidly, the value of gastric evacuation will vary with the time since ingestion. General supportive measures should be applied with particular attention being given to the maintenance of adequate urinary output.

Naloxone has been reported to reverse the CNS depressant effects of DEPAKENE overdosage. Because naloxone could theoretically also reverse the antiepileptic effects of DEPAKENE it should be used with caution.

Dosage and Administration: DEPAKENE (valproic acid) is administered orally. The recommended initial dose is 15 mg/kg/day, increasing at one week intervals by 5 to 10 mg/kg/day, until seizures are controlled or side effects preclude further increases. The maximum recommended dosage is 60 mg/kg/day. If the total daily dose exceeds 250 mg, it should be given in a divided regimen.

The following table is a guide for the initial daily dose of DEPAKENE (valproic acid) (15 mg/kg/day): [See table above]

The frequency of adverse effects (particularly elevated liver enzymes) may be dose-related. The benefit of improved seizure control which may accompany the higher doses should therefore be weighed against the possibility of a greater incidence of adverse reactions.

A good correlation has not been established between daily dose, serum level and therapeutic effect, however, therapeutic serum levels for most patients will range from 50 to 100 mcg/ml. Occasional patients may be controlled with serum levels lower or higher than this range.

As the DEPAKENE dosage is titrated upward, blood levels of phenobarbital and/or phenytoin may be affected. (See "Precautions" section.)

Patients who experience G.I. irritation may benefit from administration of the drug with food or by slowly building up the dose from an initial low level.

THE CAPSULES SHOULD BE SWALLOWED WITHOUT CHEWING TO AVOID LOCAL IRRITATION OF THE MOUTH AND THROAT.

How Supplied: DEPAKENE (valproic acid) is available as orange-colored soft gelatin capsules of 250 mg valproic acid in bottles of 100 capsules (NDC 0074-5681-13), in ABBO-PAC® unit dose packages of 100 capsules (NDC 0074-5681-11), and as a red syrup containing the equivalent of 250 mg valproic acid per 5 ml as the sodium salt in bottles of 16 ounces (NDC 0074-5682-16).

References:
1. Robert E., Guibaud, P., Maternal Valproic Acid and Congenital Neural Tube Defects, *The Lancet*, 2(8304):937, 1982.
2. Centers for Disease Control, Valproic Acid and Spina Bifida: A Preliminary Report—France, *Morbidity and Mortality Weekly Report*, 31(42): 565-566, 1982.

Shown in Product Identification Section, page 403
Abbott Laboratories
North Chicago, IL 60064
Ref. 01-2275-R11

DEPAKOTE™ B
[dep′ả-cōat]
(Divalproex Sodium)
Enteric-Coated Tablets

Warning: HEPATIC FAILURE RESULTING IN FATALITIES HAS OCCURRED IN PATIENTS RECEIVING VALPROIC ACID AND ITS DERIVATIVES. THESE INCIDENTS USUALLY HAVE OCCURRED DURING THE FIRST SIX MONTHS OF TREATMENT. SERIOUS OR FATAL HEPATOTOXICITY MAY BE PRECEDED BY NON-SPECIFIC SYMPTOMS SUCH AS LOSS OF SEIZURE CONTROL, MALAISE, WEAKNESS, LETHARGY, ANOREXIA AND VOMITING. LIVER FUNCTION TESTS SHOULD BE PERFORMED PRIOR TO THERAPY AND AT FREQUENT INTERVALS THEREAFTER, ESPECIALLY DURING THE FIRST SIX MONTHS.

Description: Divalproex sodium is a stable coordination compound comprised of sodium valproate and valproic acid in a 1:1 molar relationship and formed during the partial neutralization of valproic acid with 0.5 equivalent of sodium hydroxide. Chemically it is designated as sodium hydrogen bis (2-propylpentanoate).

Divalproex sodium has a molecular weight of 310.41 and occurs as a white powder with a characteristic odor.

Continued on next page

If desired, additional literature on any Abbott Product will be provided upon request to Abbott Laboratories.

Recommended Initial Dosages for DEPAKENE

Weight (kg)	Weight (lb)	Total Daily Dose (mg)	Dose 1	Dose 2	Dose 3
10—24.9	22— 54.9	250	0	0	1
25—39.9	55— 87.9	500	1	0	1
40—59.9	88—131.9	750	1	1	1
60—74.9	132—164.9	1,000	1	1	2
75—89.9	165—197.9	1,250	2	1	2

Number of Capsules or Teaspoonfuls of Syrup

Abbott—Cont.

DEPAKOTE is an oral antiepileptic supplied as enteric-coated tablets in three dosage strengths containing divalproex sodium equivalent to 125 mg, 250 mg or 500 mg of valproic acid.

Clinical Pharmacology: DEPAKOTE is an antiepileptic agent which is chemically related to valproic acid. It has no nitrogen or aromatic moiety characteristic of other antiepileptic drugs. The mechanism by which DEPAKOTE exerts its antiepileptic effects has not been established. It has been suggested that its activity is related to increased brain levels of gamma-aminobutyric acid (GABA). The effect on the neuronal membrane is unknown. DEPAKOTE dissociates into valproate in the gastrointestinal tract.

Because of the enteric coating of DEPAKOTE, absorption is delayed one hour following oral administration. Thereafter, DEPAKOTE is uniformly and reliably absorbed, as shown by studies in normal volunteers. Peak serum levels of valproate occur in 3 to 4 hours. Bioavailability of divalproex sodium tablets was found to be equivalent to that of DEPAKENE ® (valproic acid) capsules. Concomitant administration with food would be expected to slow absorption but not affect the extent of absorption. The serum half-life of valproate is typically in the range of six to sixteen hours. Half-lives in the lower part of the above range are usually found in patients taking other antiepileptic drugs capable of enzyme induction.

Valproate is rapidly distributed and at therapeutic drug concentrations, drug is highly bound (90%) to human plasma proteins. Increases in dose may result in decreases in the extent of protein binding and increased valproate clearance and elimination.

Elimination of DEPAKOTE and its metabolites occurs principally in the urine, with minor amounts in the feces and expired air. Very little unmetabolized parent drug is excreted in the urine. The drug is primarily metabolized in the liver and is excreted as the glucuronide conjugate. Other metabolites in the urine are products of beta, omega-1, and omega oxidation (C-3, C-4 and C-5 positions). The major oxidative metabolite in the urine is 2-propyl-3-keto-pentanoic acid; minor metabolites are 2-propyl-glutaric acid, 2-propyl-5-hydroxypentanoic acid, 2-propyl-3-hydroxypentanoic acid and 2-propyl-4-hydroxypentanoic acid.

Indications and Usage: DEPAKOTE (divalproex sodium) is indicated for use as sole and adjunctive therapy in the treatment of simple (petit mal) and complex absence seizures. DEPAKOTE may also be used adjunctively in patients with multiple seizure types which include absence seizures.

In accordance with the International Classification of Seizures, simple absence is defined as very brief clouding of the sensorium or loss of consciousness (lasting usually 2–15 seconds), accompanied by certain generalized epileptic discharges without other detectable clinical signs. Complex absence is the term used when other signs are also present.

SEE "WARNINGS" SECTION FOR STATEMENT REGARDING FATAL HEPATIC DYSFUNCTION.

Contraindications: DEPAKOTE (DIVALPROEX SODIUM) SHOULD NOT BE ADMINISTERED TO PATIENTS WITH HEPATIC DISEASE OR SIGNIFICANT DYSFUNCTION.

DEPAKOTE is contraindicated in patients with known hypersensitivity to the drug.

Warnings: Hepatic failure resulting in fatalities has occurred in patients receiving valproic acid. These incidents usually have occurred during the first six months of treatment. Serious or fatal hepatotoxicity may be preceded by nonspecific symptoms such as loss of seizure control, malaise, weakness, lethargy, anorexia and vomiting. Liver function tests should be performed prior to therapy and at frequent intervals thereafter, especially during the first six months. However, physicians should not rely totally on serum biochemistry since these tests may not be abnormal in all instances, but should also consider the results of careful interim medical history and physical examination. Caution should be observed when administering DEPAKOTE to patients with a prior history of hepatic disease. Patients with various unusual congenital disorders, those with severe seizure disorders accompanied by mental retardation, and those with organic brain disease may be at particular risk.

The drug should be discontinued immediately in the presence of significant hepatic dysfunction, suspected or apparent. In some cases, hepatic dysfunction has progressed in spite of discontinuation of drug. The frequency of adverse effects (particularly elevated liver enzymes) may be dose-related. The benefit of improved seizure control which may accompany the higher doses should therefore be weighed against the possibility of a greater incidence of adverse effects.

Usage in Pregnancy: ACCORDING TO RECENT REPORTS IN THE MEDICAL LITERATURE, VALPROIC ACID MAY PRODUCE TERATOGENICITY IN THE OFFSPRING OF HUMAN FEMALES RECEIVING THE DRUG DURING PREGNANCY. THE INCIDENCE OF NEURAL TUBE DEFECTS IN THE FETUS MAY BE INCREASED IN MOTHERS RECEIVING VALPROATE DURING THE FIRST TRIMESTER OF PREGNANCY. BASED UPON A SINGLE FRENCH REPORT,[1] THE CENTERS FOR DISEASE CONTROL (CDC) HAS ESTIMATED THE RISK OF VALPROIC ACID EXPOSED WOMEN HAVING CHILDREN WITH SPINA BIFIDA TO BE APPROXIMATELY 1.2%.[2] THIS RISK IS SIMILAR TO THAT FOR NONEPILEPTIC WOMEN WHO HAVE HAD CHILDREN WITH NEURAL TUBE DEFECTS (ANENCEPHALY AND SPINA BIFIDA).

THERE ARE MULTIPLE REPORTS IN THE CLINICAL LITERATURE WHICH INDICATE THAT THE USE OF ANTIEPILEPTIC DRUGS DURING PREGNANCY RESULTS IN AN INCREASED INCIDENCE OF BIRTH DEFECTS IN THE OFFSPRING. ALTHOUGH DATA ARE MORE EXTENSIVE WITH RESPECT TO TRIMETHADIONE, PARAMETHADIONE, PHENYTOIN, AND PHENOBARBITAL, REPORTS INDICATE A POSSIBLE SIMILAR ASSOCIATION WITH THE USE OF OTHER ANTIEPILEPTIC DRUGS. THEREFORE, ANTIEPILEPTIC DRUGS SHOULD BE ADMINISTERED TO WOMEN OF CHILDBEARING POTENTIAL ONLY IF THEY ARE CLEARLY SHOWN TO BE ESSENTIAL IN THE MANAGEMENT OF THEIR SEIZURES.

ANIMAL STUDIES HAVE ALSO DEMONSTRATED VALPROIC ACID INDUCED TERATOGENICITY. Studies in rats and human females demonstrated placental transfer of the drug. Doses greater than 65 mg/kg/day given to pregnant rats and mice produced skeletal abnormalities in the offspring, primarily involving ribs and vertebrae; doses greater than 150 mg/kg/day given to pregnant rabbits produced fetal resorptions and (primarily) soft-tissue abnormalities in the offspring. In rats a dose-related delay in the onset of parturition was noted. Postnatal growth and survival of the progeny were adversely affected, particularly when drug administration spanned the entire gestation and early lactation period.

Antiepileptic drugs should not be discontinued in patients in whom the drug is administered to prevent major seizures because of the strong possibility of precipitating status epilepticus with attendant hypoxia and threat to life. In individual cases where the severity and frequency of the seizure disorder are such that the removal of medication does not pose a serious threat to the patient, discontinuation of the drug may be considered prior to and during pregnancy, although it cannot be said with any confidence that even minor seizures do not pose some hazard to the developing embryo or fetus.

The prescribing physician will wish to weigh these considerations in treating or counseling epileptic women of childbearing potential.

Precautions: *Hepatic Dysfunction:* See "Contraindications" and "Warnings" sections.

General: Because of reports of thrombocytopenia and inhibition of the secondary phase of platelet aggregation, platelet counts and bleeding time determination are recommended before initiating therapy and at periodic intervals. It is recommended that patients receiving DEPAKOTE be monitored for platelet count prior to planned surgery. Clinical evidence of hemorrhage, bruising or a disorder of hemostasis/coagulation is an indication for reduction of DEPAKOTE dosage or withdrawal of therapy pending investigation.

Hyperammonemia with or without lethargy or coma has been reported and may be present in the absence of abnormal liver function tests. If elevation occurs, DEPAKOTE should be discontinued.

Since DEPAKOTE (divalproex sodium) may interact with concurrently administered antiepileptic drugs, periodic serum level determinations of concomitant antiepileptic drugs are recommended during the early course of therapy. (See "Drug Interactions" section).

Valproate is partially eliminated in the urine as a keto-metabolite which may lead to a false interpretation of the urine ketone test.

Information for Patients: Since DEPAKOTE may produce CNS depression, especially when combined with another CNS depressant (e.g., alcohol), patients should be advised not to engage in hazardous occupations, such as driving an automobile or operating dangerous machinery, until it is known that they do not become drowsy from the drug.

Drug Interactions: Valproic acid may potentiate the CNS depressant activity of alcohol.

THERE IS EVIDENCE THAT VALPROIC ACID CAN CAUSE AN INCREASE IN SERUM PHENOBARBITAL LEVELS BY IMPAIRMENT OF NONRENAL CLEARANCE. THIS PHENOMENON CAN RESULT IN SEVERE CNS DEPRESSION. THE COMBINATION OF VALPROIC ACID AND PHENOBARBITAL HAS ALSO BEEN REPORTED TO PRODUCE CNS DEPRESSION WITHOUT SIGNIFICANT ELEVATIONS OF BARBITURATE OR VALPROATE SERUM LEVELS. ALL PATIENTS RECEIVING CONCOMITANT BARBITURATE THERAPY SHOULD BE CLOSELY MONITORED FOR NEUROLOGICAL TOXICITY. SERUM BARBITURATE LEVELS SHOULD BE OBTAINED, IF POSSIBLE, AND THE BARBITURATE DOSAGE DECREASED, IF APPROPRIATE.

Primidone is metabolized into a barbiturate and, therefore, may also be involved in a similar or identical interaction.

THERE HAVE BEEN REPORTS OF BREAKTHROUGH SEIZURES OCCURRING WITH THE COMBINATION OF VALPROIC ACID AND PHENYTOIN. MOST REPORTS HAVE NOTED A DECREASE IN TOTAL PLASMA PHENYTOIN CONCENTRATION. HOWEVER, INCREASES IN TOTAL PHENYTOIN SERUM CONCENTRATION HAVE BEEN REPORTED. AN INITIAL FALL IN TOTAL PHENYTOIN LEVELS WITH SUBSEQUENT INCREASE IN PHENYTOIN LEVELS HAS ALSO BEEN REPORTED. IN ADDITION, A DECREASE IN TOTAL SERUM PHENYTOIN WITH AN INCREASE IN THE FREE VS. PROTEIN BOUND PHENYTOIN LEVELS HAS BEEN REPORTED. THE DOSAGE OF PHENYTOIN SHOULD BE ADJUSTED AS REQUIRED BY THE CLINICAL SITUATION.

THE CONCOMITANT USE OF VALPROIC ACID AND CLONAZEPAM MAY PRODUCE ABSENCE STATUS.

Caution is recommended when DEPAKOTE (divalproex sodium) is administered with drugs affecting coagulation, e.g., aspirin and warfarin. (See "Adverse Reactions" section).

There have been reports of altered thyroid function tests associated with valproate. The clinical significance of these is unknown.

Carcinogenesis: Valproic acid was administered to Sprague Dawley rats and ICR (HA /ICR) mice at doses of 0, 80 and 170 mg/kg/day for two years. Although a variety of neoplasms were observed in both species, the chief findings were a statistically significant increase in the incidence of subcutaneous fibrosarcomas in high dose male rats receiving

valproic acid and a statistically significant dose-related trend for benign pulmonary adenomas in male mice receiving valproic acid. The significance of these findings for man is unknown at present.
Mutagenesis: Studies on valproic acid have been performed using bacterial and mammalian systems. These studies have provided no evidence of a mutagenic potential for DEPAKOTE.
Fertility: Chronic toxicity studies in juvenile and adult rats and dogs demonstrated reduced spermatogenesis and testicular atrophy at doses greater than 200 mg/kg/day in rats and greater than 90 mg/kg/day in dogs. Segment I fertility studies in rats have shown doses up to 350 mg/kg/day for 60 days to have no effect on fertility. THE EFFECT OF DEPAKOTE (DIVALPROEX SODIUM) ON THE DEVELOPMENT OF THE TESTES AND ON SPERM PRODUCTION AND FERTILITY IN HUMANS IS UNKNOWN.
Pregnancy: Pregnancy Category D: See "Warnings" section.
Nursing Mothers: Valproate is excreted in breast milk. Concentrations in breast milk have been reported to be 1–10% of serum concentrations. It is not known what effect this would have on a nursing infant. Caution should be exercised when DEPAKOTE is administered to a nursing woman.
Adverse Reactions: Since valproic acid and its derivatives have usually been used with other antiepileptic drugs, it is not possible, in most cases, to determine whether the following adverse reactions can be ascribed to valproic acid alone, or the combination of drugs.
Gastrointestinal: The most commonly reported side effects at the initiation of therapy are nausea, vomiting and indigestion. These effects are usually transient and rarely require discontinuation of therapy. Diarrhea, abdominal cramps and constipation have been reported. Both anorexia with some weight loss and increased appetite with weight gain have also been reported.
CNS Effects: Sedative effects have been noted in patients receiving valproic acid alone but are found most often in patients receiving combination therapy. Sedation usually disappears upon reduction of other antiepileptic medication. Ataxia, headache, nystagmus, diplopia, asterixis, "spots before eyes," tremor, dysarthria, dizziness, and incoordination have rarely been noted. Rare cases of coma have been noted in patients receiving valproic acid alone or in conjunction with phenobarbital.
Dermatologic: Transient increases in hair loss have been observed. Skin rash and petechiae have rarely been noted.
Psychiatric: Emotional upset, depression, psychosis, aggression, hyperactivity and behavioral deterioration have been reported.
Musculoskeletal: Weakness has been reported.
Hematopoietic: Thrombocytopenia has been reported. Valproic acid inhibits the secondary phase of platelet aggregation. (See "Drug Interactions" section). This may be reflected in altered bleeding time. Bruising, hematoma formation and frank hemorrhage have been reported. Relative lymphocytosis and hypofibrinogenemia have been noted. Leukopenia and eosinophilia have also been reported. Anemia and bone marrow suppression have been reported.
Hepatic: Minor elevations of transaminases (e.g., SGOT and SGPT) and LDH are frequent and appear to be dose related. Occasionally, laboratory test results include, as well, increases in serum bilirubin and abnormal changes in other liver function tests. These results may reflect potentially serious hepatotoxicity. (See "Warnings" section).
Endocrine: There have been reports of irregular menses and secondary amenorrhea occurring in patients receiving valproic acid and its derivatives.
Abnormal thyroid function tests have been reported. (See "Precautions" section).
Pancreatic: There have been reports of acute pancreatitis occurring in patients receiving valproic acid and its derivatives.
Metabolic: Hyperammonemia. (See "Precautions" section).

Hyperglycinemia has been reported and has been associated with a fatal outcome in a patient with preexistent nonketotic hyperglycinemia.
Overdosage: Overdosage with valproic acid may result in deep coma.
Since DEPAKOTE tablets are enteric-coated, the benefit of gastric lavage or emesis will vary with the time since ingestion. General supportive measures should be applied with particular attention being given to the maintenance of adequate urinary output.
Naloxone has been reported to reverse the CNS depressant effects of valproate overdosage. Because naloxone could theoretically also reverse the antiepileptic effects of DEPAKOTE it should be used with caution.
Dosage and Administration: DEPAKOTE is administered orally. The recommended initial dose is 15 mg/kg/day, increasing at one week intervals by 5 to 10 mg/kg/day until seizures are controlled or side effects preclude further increases. The maximum recommended dosage is 60 mg/kg/day. If the total daily dose exceeds 250 mg, it should be given in a divided regimen. A twice-a-day dosage is suggested wherever feasible.
The frequency of adverse effects (particularly elevated liver enzymes) may be dose-related. The benefit of improved seizure control which may accompany higher doses should therefore be weighed against the possibility of a greater incidence of adverse reactions.
A good correlation has not been established between daily dose, serum level and therapeutic effect, however, therapeutic valproate serum levels for most patients will range from 50 to 100 mcg/ml. Occasional patients may be controlled with serum levels lower or higher than this range. As the DEPAKOTE dosage is titrated upward, blood levels of phenobarbital and/or phenytoin may be affected. (See "Precautions" section).
Patients who experience G. I. irritation may benefit from administration of the drug with food or by slowly building up the dose from an initial low level.
How Supplied: DEPAKOTE (divalproex sodium enteric-coated tablets) are supplied as:
125 mg salmon pink-colored tablets in bottles of 100 (**NDC** 0074-6212-13).
250 mg peach-colored tablets in bottles of 100 (**NDC** 0074-6214-13) and Abbo-Pac® unit dose packages of 100 (**NDC** 0074-6214-11).
500 mg lavender-colored tablets in bottles of 100 (**NDC** 0074-6215-13) and Abbo-Pac® unit dose packages of 100 (**NDC** 0074-6215-11).
References:
1. Robert E., Guibaud, P., Maternal Valproic Acid and Congenital Neural Tube Defects, *The Lancet*, 2(8304): 937, 1982.
2. Centers for Disease Control. Valproic Acid and Spina Bifida: A Preliminary Report— France, *Morbidity and Mortality Weekly Report*, 31(42): 565–566, 1982.
Abbott Laboratories
North Chicago, IL 60064
Ref. 01-2294-R4
Shown in Product Identification Section, page 403

DESOXYN® R ©
(methamphetamine hydrochloride)
Tablets—Gradumet® Tablets

METHAMPHETAMINE HAS A HIGH POTENTIAL FOR ABUSE. IT SHOULD THUS BE TRIED ONLY IN WEIGHT REDUCTION PROGRAMS FOR PATIENTS IN WHOM ALTERNATIVE THERAPY HAS BEEN INEFFECTIVE. ADMINISTRATION OF METHAMPHETAMINE FOR PROLONGED PERIODS OF TIME IN OBESITY MAY LEAD TO DRUG DEPENDENCE AND MUST BE AVOIDED. PARTICULAR ATTENTION SHOULD BE PAID TO THE POSSIBILITY OF SUBJECTS OBTAINING METHAMPHETAMINE FOR NON-THERAPEUTIC USE OR DISTRIBUTION TO OTH-

ERS, AND THE DRUG SHOULD BE PRESCRIBED OR DISPENSED SPARINGLY.

Description: DESOXYN (methamphetamine hydrochloride), chemically known as (S)-N, α-dimethylbenzeneethanamine hydrochloride, is a member of the amphetamine group of sympathomimetic amines.
DESOXYN is available as Gradumet sustained-release tablets containing 5 mg, 10 mg or 15 mg of methamphetamine hydrochloride and as conventional tablets containing 5 mg methamphetamine hydrochloride, for oral administration. The Gradumet is an inert, porous, plastic matrix, which is impregnated with DESOXYN. The drug is leached slowly from the Gradumet as it passes through the gastrointestinal tract. The expended matrix is not absorbed and is excreted in the stool.
Clinical Pharmacology: DESOXYN is a sympathomimetic amine with CNS stimulant activity. Peripheral actions include elevation of systolic and diastolic blood pressures and weak bronchodilator and respiratory stimulant action. Drugs of this class used in obesity are commonly known as "anorectics" or "anorexigenics." It has not been established, however, that the action of such drugs in treating obesity is primarily one of appetite suppression. Other central nervous system actions, or metabolic effects, may be involved, for example.
Adult obese subjects instructed in dietary management and treated with "anorectic" drugs, lose more weight on the average than those treated with placebo and diet, as determined in relatively short-term clinical trials.
The magnitude of increased weight loss of drug-treated patients over placebo-treated patients is only a fraction of a pound a week. The rate of weight loss is greatest in the first weeks of therapy for both drug and placebo subjects and tends to decrease in succeeding weeks. The origins of the increased weight loss due to the various possible drug effects are not established. The amount of weight loss associated with the use of an "anorectic" drug varies from trial to trial, and the increased weight loss appears to be related in part to variables other than the drug prescribed, such as the physician-investigator, the population treated, and the diet prescribed. Studies do not permit conclusions as to the relative importance of the drug and non-drug factors on weight loss.
The natural history of obesity is measured in years, whereas the studies cited are restricted to a few weeks duration; thus, the total impact of drug-induced weight loss over that of diet alone must be considered clinically limited.
The mechanism of action involved in producing the beneficial behavioral changes seen in hyperkinetic children receiving DESOXYN is unknown.
In humans, methamphetamine is rapidly absorbed from the gastrointestinal tract. The primary site of metabolism is in the liver by aromatic hydroxylation, N-dealkylation and deamination. At least seven metabolites have been identified in the urine. The biological half-life has been reported in the range of 4 to 5 hours. Excretion occurs primarily in the urine and is dependent on urine pH. Alkaline urine will significantly increase the drug half-life. Approximately 62% of an oral dose is eliminated in the urine within the first 24 hours with about one-third as intact drug and the remainder as metabolites.
Indications and Usage: *Attention Deficit Disorder with Hyperactivity*—DESOXYN is indicated as an integral part of a total treatment program which typically includes other remedial measures (psychological, educational, social) for a stabilizing effect in children over 6 years of age with a behavioral syndrome characterized by the following group of developmentally inappropriate symp-

Continued on next page

If desired, additional literature on any Abbott Product will be provided upon request to Abbott Laboratories.

Abbott—Cont.

toms: moderate to severe distractibility, short attention span, hyperactivity, emotional lability, and impulsivity. The diagnosis of this syndrome should not be made with finality when these symptoms are only of comparatively recent origin. Non-localizing (soft) neurological signs, learning disability, and abnormal EEG may or may not be present, and a diagnosis of central nervous system disfunction may or may not be warranted.

Exogenous Obesity—as a short-term (i.e., a few weeks) adjunct in a regimen of weight reduction based on caloric restriction, for patients in whom obesity is refractory to alternative therapy, e.g., repeated diets, group programs, and other drugs. The limited usefulness of DESOXYN (see "Clinical Pharmacology" section) should be weighed against possible risks inherent in use of the drug, such as those described below.

Contraindications: DESOXYN (methamphetamine hydrochloride) is contraindicated during or within 14 days following the administration of monoamine oxidase inhibitors; hypertensive crises may result. It is also contraindicated in patients with glaucoma, advanced arteriosclerosis, symptomatic cardiovascular disease, moderate to severe hypertension, hyperthyroidism or known hypersensitivity or idiosyncrasy to sympathomimetic amines. Methamphetamine should not be given to patients who are in an agitated state or who have a history of drug abuse.

Warnings: Tolerance to the anorectic effect usually develops within a few weeks. When this occurs, the recommended dose should not be exceeded in an attempt to increase the effect; rather, the drug should be discontinued (see "Drug Abuse and Dependence" section).

Decrements in the predicted growth (i.e., weight gain and/or height) rate have been reported with the long-term use of stimulants in children. Therefore, patients requiring long-term therapy should be carefully monitored.

Precautions:
General: DESOXYN (methamphetamine hydrochloride) should be used with caution in patients with even mild hypertension.

Methamphetamine should not be used to combat fatigue or to replace rest in normal persons.

Prescribing and dispensing of methamphetamine should be limited to the smallest amount that is feasible at one time in order to minimize the possibility of overdosage.

The 15 mg dosage strength of DESOXYN Gradumet tablets contains FD&C Yellow No. 5 (tartrazine) which may cause allergic-type reactions (including bronchial asthma) in certain susceptible individuals. Although the overall incidence of FD&C Yellow No. 5 (tartrazine) sensitivity in the general population is low, it is frequently seen in patients who also have aspirin hypersensitivity.

Information for Patients: The patient should be informed that methamphetamine may impair the ability to engage in potentially hazardous activities, such as, operating machinery or driving a motor vehicle.

The patient should be cautioned not to increase dosage, except on advice of the physician.

Drug Interactions: Insulin requirements in diabetes mellitus may be altered in association with the use of methamphetamine and concomitant dietary regimen.

Methamphetamine may decrease the hypotensive effect of *guanethidine*.

DESOXYN should not be used concurrently with *monoamine oxidase inhibitors* (see "Contraindications" section).

Concurrent administration of *tricyclic antidepressants* and indirect-acting sympathomimetic amines such as amphetamines, should be closely supervised and dosage carefully adjusted.

Phenothiazines are reported in the literature to antagonize the CNS stimulant action of the amphetamines.

Drug/Laboratory Test Interactions: Literature reports suggest that amphetamines may be associated with significant elevation of plasma corticosteroids. This should be considered if determination of plasma corticosteroid levels is desired in a person receiving amphetamines.

Carcinogensis, Mutagenesis, Impairment of Fertility: Data are not available on long-term potential for carcinogenicity, mutagenicity, or impairment of fertility.

Pregnancy: Teratogenic effects: Pregnancy Category C. Methamphetamine has been shown to have teratogenic and embryocidal effects in mammals given high multiples of the human dose. There are no adequate and well-controlled studies in pregnant women. DESOXYN should not be used during pregnancy unless the potential benefit justifies the potential risk to the fetus.

Nonteratogenic effects: Infants born to mothers dependent on amphetamines have an increased risk of premature delivery and low birth weight. Also, these infants may experience symptoms of withdrawal as demonstrated by dysphoria, including agitation and significant lassitude.

Nursing Mothers: It is not known whether this drug is excreted in human milk. Because many drugs are excreted in human milk, caution should be exercised when DESOXYN is administered to a nursing woman.

Pediatric Use: Safety and effectiveness for use as an anorectic agent in children below the age of 12 years have not been established.

Long-term effects of DESOXYN in children have not been established (see "Warnings" section).

Drug treatment is not indicated in all cases of the behavioral syndrome characterized by moderate to severe distractibility, short attention span, hyperactivity, emotional lability and impulsivity. It should be considered only in light of the complete history and evaluation of the child. The decision to prescribe DESOXYN should depend on the physician's assessment of the chronicity and severity of the child's symptoms and their appropriateness for his/her age. Prescription should not depend solely on the presence of one or more of the behavioral characteristics.

When these symptoms are associated with acute stress reaction, treatment with DESOXYN is usually not indicated.

Clinical experience suggests that in psychotic children, administration of DESOXYN may exacerbate symptoms of behavior disturbance and thought disorder.

Amphetamines have been reported to exacerbate motor and phonic tics and Tourette's syndrome. Therefore, clinical evaluation for tics and Tourette's syndrome in children and their families should precede use of stimulant medications.

Adverse Reactions: The following are adverse reactions in decreasing order of severity within each category that have been reported with DESOXYN:

Cardiovascular: Elevation of blood pressure, tachycardia and palpitation.

Central Nervous System: Psychotic episodes have been rarely reported at recommended doses. Dizziness, dysphoria, overstimulation, euphoria, insomnia, tremor, restlessness and headache. Exacerbation of motor and phonic tics and Tourette's syndrome.

Gastrointestinal: Diarrhea, constipation, dryness of mouth, unpleasant taste and other gastrointestinal disturbances.

Hypersensitivity: Urticaria.

Endocrine: Impotence and changes in libido.

Miscellaneous: Suppression of growth has been reported with the long-term use of stimulants in children (see "Warnings" section).

Drug Abuse and Dependence: *Controlled Substance:* DESOXYN (methamphetamine hydrochloride) is subject to control under DEA schedule II.

Abuse: DESOXYN has been extensively abused. Tolerance, extreme psychological dependence, and severe social disability have occurred. There are reports of patients who have increased the dosage to many times that recommended. Abrupt cessation following prolonged high dosage administration results in extreme fatigue and mental depression; changes are also noted on the sleep EEG. Manifestations of chronic intoxication with Desoxyn include severe dermatoses, marked insomnia, irritability, hyperactivity, and personality changes. The most severe manifestation of chronic intoxication is psychosis, often clinically indistinguishable from schizophrenia.

Overdosage: Manifestations of acute overdosage with methamphetamine include restlessness, tremor, hyperreflexia, rapid respiration, confusion, assaultiveness, hallucinations, and panic states. Fatigue and depression usually follow the central stimulation. Cardiovascular effects include arrhythmias, hypertension or hypotension, and circulatory collapse. Gastrointestinal symptoms include nausea, vomiting, diarrhea, and abdominal cramps. Fatal poisoning usually terminates in convulsions and coma.

Management of acute methamphetamine intoxication is largely symptomatic and includes gastric evacuation and sedation with a barbiturate. Experience with hemodialysis or peritoneal dialysis is inadequate to permit recommendations in this regard.

Acidification of urine increases methamphetamine excretion. Intravenous phentolamine (Regitine®) has been suggested for possible acute, severe hypertension, if this complicates methamphetamine overdosage. Usually a gradual drop in blood pressure will result when sufficient sedation has been achieved. Chlorpromazine has been reported to be useful in decreasing CNS stimulation and sympathomimetic effects.

Since the Gradumet tablet releases methamphetamine gradually, therapy should be directed at reversing the effects of the ingested drug and at supporting the patient until symptoms subside. Saline cathartics are useful for hastening the evacuation of the tablets that have not already released medication.

Dosage and Administration: DESOXYN (methamphetamine hydrochloride) is given orally.

Methamphetamine should be administered at the lowest effective dosage, and dosage should be individually adjusted. Late evening medication should be avoided because of the resulting insomnia.

Attention Deficit Disorder with Hyperactivity:

For treatment of children 6 years or older with a behavioral syndrome characterized by moderate to severe distractibility, short attention span, hyperactivity, emotional lability and impulsivity: an initial dose of 5 mg DESOXYN (methamphetamine hydrochloride) once or twice a day is recommended. Daily dosage may be raised in increments of 5 mg at weekly intervals until optimum clinical response is achieved. The usual effective dose is 20 to 25 mg daily. The total daily dose may be given as conventional tablets in two divided doses daily or once daily using the Gradumet tablet. The Gradumet form should not be utilized for initiation of dosage nor until the conventional titrated daily dosage is equal to or greater than the dosage provided in a Gradumet tablet.

Where possible, drug administration should be interrupted occasionally to determine if there is a recurrence of behavioral symptoms sufficient to require continued therapy.

For obesity: one Gradumet tablet, 10 or 15 mg, once a day in the morning. When the conventional tablet form is prescribed, 5 mg should be taken one-half hour before each meal. Treatment should not exceed a few weeks in duration. Methamphetamine is not recommended for use as an anorectic agent in children under 12 years of age.

How Supplied: DESOXYN (methamphetamine hydrochloride) is supplied as follows:

Gradumet Tablets, 5 mg, white, in bottles of 100 (**NDC 0074-6941-04**); 10 mg, orange, in bottles of 100 (**NDC 0074-6948-08**) and 500 (**NDC 0074-6948-09**); and 15 mg, yellow, in bottles of 100 (**NDC 0074-6959-07**) and 500 (**NDC 0074-6959-08**).

Tablets, 5 mg, white, in bottles of 100 (**NDC 0074-3377-04**).

Ref. 03-4260-R6

DICAL-D® CAPSULES—WAFERS
[dī′cal-d]
(Dibasic Calcium Phosphate with Vitamin D)

Description:
Capsules
Daily dosage (three capsules) provides:

Vitamin D............ 399 IU .... 99% USRDA*
                    (10 mcg)
Calcium................. 0.35 g............. 35% USRDA
Phosphorous........... 0.27 g............. 27% USRDA
Each gelatin capsule contains:
Dibasic Calcium Phosphate, hydrous
  (as anhydrous form).................................. 500 mg
Cholecalciferol............................ 3.33 mcg (133 IU)
Corn starch added.
Calcium to phosphorous ratio 1.3 to 1.
Wafers
Daily dosage (two wafers) provides:
Vitamin D............... 400 IU........... 100% USRDA
                    (10 mcg)
Calcium................. 0.464 g........... 46% USRDA
Phosphorous........... 0.36 g............. 36% USRDA
Each wafer contains:
Cholecalciferol.. 5 mcg (200 IU)
Dibasic Calcium Phosphate, hydrous............... 1 g
Added dextrose, sucrose, talc, stearic acid, mineral oil, salt, and natural and artificial flavorings.
Calcium to phosphorous ratio 1.29 to 1.
*% U.S. Recommended Daily Allowance for adults and children 4 or more years of age.
Indications: For those individuals who must restrict their intake of dairy products.
Dosage and Administration: Usual dose for adults and children 4 years and older:
Wafers—Chew 1 wafer twice daily with meals, or as directed by the physician or dentist.
Capsules—1 capsule 3 times daily with meals, or as directed by the physician or dentist.
How Supplied:
Dical-D Capsules in bottles of 100 (NDC 0074-3594-04) and 500 (NDC 0074-3594-02).
Dical-D Wafers in box of 51 (NDC 0074-3589-01).
Abbott Laboratories/
Abbott Pharmaceuticals, Inc.
North Chicago, IL 60064
Ref. 03-1160-5/R13 & 09-5876-5/R8

DICUMAROL Tablets, USP ℞
[dī-cū'ma-roll]

How Supplied: Dicumarol tablets are supplied as:
  25 mg tablets:
   bottles of 100 (**NDC** 0074-3794-01);
   bottles of 1000 (**NDC** 0074-3794-06).
  50 mg tablets:
   bottles of 100 (**NDC** 0074-3773-01);
   bottles of 1000 (**NDC** 0074-3773-02).
Shown in Product Identification Section, page 403
Abbott Pharmaceuticals, Inc.
North Chicago, IL 60064

ENDURON® ℞
[en'de-ron]
(methyclothiazide tablets, USP)

Description: ENDURON (methyclothiazide) is a member of the benzothiadiazine (thiazide) family of drugs. It is an analogue of hydrochlorothiazide. Clinically, ENDURON is an oral diuretic-antihypertensive agent.

Actions: The diuretic and saluretic effects of ENDURON result from a drug-induced inhibition of the renal tubular reabsorption of electrolytes. The excretion of sodium and chloride is greatly enhanced. Potassium excretion is also enhanced to a variable degree, as it is with the other thiazides. Although urinary excretion of bicarbonate is increased slightly, there is usually no significant change in urinary pH. Methyclothiazide has a per mg natriuretic activity approximately 100 times that of the prototype thiazide, chlorothiazide. At maximal therapeutic dosages, all thiazides are approximately equal in their diuretic/natriuretic effects.

There is significant natriuresis and diuresis within two hours after administration of a single dose of methyclothiazide. These effects reach a peak in about six hours and persist for 24 hours following oral administration of a single dose.

Like other benzothiadiazines, ENDURON also has antihypertensive properties, and may be used for this purpose either alone or to enhance the antihypertensive action of other drugs. The mechanism by which the benzothiadiazines, including methyclothiazide, produce a reduction of elevated blood pressure is not known. However, sodium depletion appears to be involved.

ENDURON is rapidly absorbed and slowly eliminated by the kidneys as both intact drug and as a metabolite showing no diuretic activity in a rat model.

Indications: ENDURON is indicated in the management of hypertension either as the sole therapeutic agent or to enhance the effect of other antihypertensive drugs in the more severe forms of hypertension.

ENDURON (methyclothiazide) is indicated as adjunctive therapy in edema associated with congestive heart failure, hepatic cirrhosis, and corticosteroid and estrogen therapy.

ENDURON has also been found useful in edema due to various forms of renal dysfunction such as the nephrotic syndrome, acute glomerulonephritis, and chronic renal failure.

Usage in Pregnancy: The routine use of diuretics in an otherwise healthy pregnant woman is inappropriate and exposes mother and fetus to unnecessary hazard. Diuretics do not prevent development of toxemia of pregnancy, and there is no satisfactory evidence that they are useful in the treatment of developed toxemia.

Edema during pregnancy may arise from pathological causes or from the physiological and mechanical consequences of pregnancy. Thiazides are indicated in pregnancy when edema is due to pathological causes, just as they are in the absence of pregnancy (however, see Warnings, below). Dependent edema in pregnancy, resulting from restriction of venous return by the expanded uterus, is properly treated through elevation of the lower extremities and use of support hose; use of diuretics to lower intravascular volume in this case is illogical and unnecessary. There is hypervolemia during normal pregnancy which is harmful to neither the fetus nor the mother (in the absence of cardiovascular disease), but which is associated with edema, including generalized edema, in the majority of pregnant women. If this edema produces discomfort, increased recumbency will often provide relief. In rare instances, this edema may cause extreme discomfort which is not relieved by rest. In these cases, a short course of diuretics may provide relief and may be appropriate.

Contraindications: Renal decompensation. Hypersensitivity to this or other sulfonamide-derived drugs.

Warnings: Methyclothiazide shares with other thiazides the propensity to deplete potassium reserves to an unpredictable degree.

Thiazides should be used with caution in patients with renal disease or significant impairment of renal function, since azotemia may be precipitated and cumulative drug effects may occur.

Thiazides should be used with caution in patients with impaired hepatic function or progressive liver disease, since minor alterations of fluid and electrolyte balance may precipitate hepatic coma.

Thiazides may be additive or potentiative of the action of other antihypertensive drugs. Potentiation occurs with ganglionic or peripheral adrenergic blocking drugs.

Sensitivity reactions may occur in patients with a history of allergy or bronchial asthma.

The possibility of exacerbation or activation of systemic lupus erythematosus has been reported.

Usage in Pregnancy: Thiazides cross the placental barrier and appear in cord blood. The use of thiazides in pregnant women requires that the anticipated benefit be weighed against possible hazards to the fetus. These hazards include fetal or neonatal jaundice, thrombocytopenia, and possible other adverse reactions that have occurred in the adult.

Nursing Mothers: Thiazides appear in breast milk. If use of the drug is deemed essential, the patient should stop nursing.

Precautions: Periodic determinations of serum electrolytes should be performed at appropriate intervals for the purpose of detecting possible electrolyte imbalances such as hyponatremia, hypochloremic alkalosis, and hypokalemia. Serum and urine electrolyte determinations are particularly important when a patient is vomiting excessively or receiving parenteral fluids. All patients should be observed for other clinical signs of electrolyte imbalances such as dryness of mouth, thirst, weakness, lethargy, drowsiness, restlessness, muscle pains or cramps, muscular fatigue, hypotension, oliguria, tachycardia, and gastrointestinal disturbances such as nausea and vomiting.

Hypokalemia may develop with thiazides as with any other potent diuretic, especially when brisk diuresis occurs, severe cirrhosis is present, or when corticosteroids or ACTH are given concomitantly. Interference with the adequate oral intake of electrolytes will also contribute to the possible development of hypokalemia. Potassium depletion, even of a mild degree, resulting from thiazide use, may sensitize a patient to the effects of cardiac glycosides such as digitalis.

Any chloride deficit is generally mild and usually does not require specific treatment except under extraordinary circumstances (as in liver disease or renal disease). Dilutional hyponatremia may occur in edematous patients in hot weather; appropriate therapy is water restriction rather than administration of salt, except in rare instances when the hyponatremia is life threatening.

In actual salt depletion, appropriate replacement is the therapy of choice.

Hyperuricemia may occur or frank gout may be precipitated in certain patients receiving thiazide therapy.

Insulin requirements in diabetic patients may be increased, decreased, or unchanged. Latent diabetes mellitus may become manifest during thiazide administration.

Thiazide drugs may increase the responsiveness to tubocurarine.

The antihypertensive effects of the drug may be enhanced in the postsympathectomy patient.

Thiazides may decrease arterial responsiveness to norepinephrine. This diminution is not sufficient to preclude effectiveness of the pressor agent for therapeutic use.

If progressive renal impairment becomes evident as indicated by a rising nonprotein nitrogen or blood urea nitrogen, a careful reappraisal of therapy is necessary with consideration given to withholding or discontinuing diuretic therapy.

Thiazides may decrease serum PBI levels without signs of thyroid disturbance.

Thiazides have been reported, on rare occasions, to have elevated serum calcium to hypercalcemic levels. The serum calcium levels have returned to normal when the medication has been stopped. This phenomenon may be related to the ability of the thiazide diuretics to lower the amount of calcium excreted in the urine.

Adverse Reactions: Gastrointestinal system reactions: Anorexia, gastric irritation, nausea, vomiting, cramping, diarrhea, constipation, jaundice (intrahepatic cholestatic jaundice), pancreatitis.

Central nervous system reactions: Dizziness, vertigo, paresthesias, headache, xanthopsia.

Hematologic reactions: Leukopenia, agranulocytosis, thrombocytopenia, aplastic anemia.

Dermatologic—hypersensitivity reactions: Purpura, photosensitivity, rash, urticaria, necrotizing angiitis (vasculitis) (cutaneous vasculitis).

Cardiovascular reaction: Orthostatic hypotension may occur and may be aggravated by alcohol, barbiturates, or narcotics.

Other: Hyperglycemia, glycosuria, hypercalcemia, hyperuricemia, muscle spasm, weakness, restlessness.

There have been isolated reports that certain nonedematous individuals developed severe fluid and electrolyte derangements after only brief exposure to normal doses of thiazide and non-thiazide diuretics. The condition is usually manifested

Continued on next page

If desired, additional literature on any Abbott Product will be provided upon request to Abbott Laboratories.

Abbott—Cont.

as severe dilutional hyponatremia, hypokalemia, and hypochloremia. It has been reported to be due to inappropriately increased ADH secretion and appears to be idiosyncratic. Potassium replacement is apparently the most important therapy in the treatment of this syndrome along with removal of the offending drug.

Whenever adverse reactions are severe, treatment should be discontinued.

Dosage and Administration: ENDURON (methyclothiazide) is administered orally. Therapy should be individualized according to patient response. This therapy should be titrated to gain maximal therapeutic response as well as the minimal dose possible to maintain that therapeutic response.

For edematous conditions: The usual adult dose ranges from 2.5 to 10 mg once daily. Maximum effective single dose is 10 mg; larger single doses do not accomplish greater diuresis, and are not recommended.

For the treatment of hypertension: The usual adult dose ranges from 2.5 to 5 mg once daily. If control of blood pressure is not satisfactory after 8 to 12 weeks of therapy with 5 mg once daily, another antihypertensive drug should be added. Increase of the dosage of ENDURON will usually not result in further lowering of blood pressure.

Methyclothiazide may be either employed alone for mild to moderate hypertension or concurrently with other antihypertensive drugs in the management of more severe forms of hypertension. Combined therapy may provide adequate control of hypertension with lower dosage of the component drugs and fewer or less severe side effects. An enhanced response frequently follows its concurrent administration with Harmonyl® (deserpidine) so that dosage of both drugs may be reduced. When other antihypertensive agents are to be added to the regimen, this should be accomplished gradually. Ganglionic blocking agents should be given at only half the usual dose since their effect is potentiated by pretreatment with ENDURON.

Overdosage: Symptoms of overdosage include electrolyte imbalance and signs of potassium deficiency such as confusion, dizziness, muscular weakness, and gastrointestinal disturbances. General supportive measures including replacement of fluids and electrolytes may be indicated in treatment of overdosage.

How Supplied: ENDURON (methyclothiazide tablets, USP) is provided in two dosage sizes as monogrammed, grooved, square-shaped tablets:

2.5 mg, orange-colored:
bottles of 100 (**NDC 0074-6827-01**),
bottles of 1000 (**NDC 0074-6827-02**).

5 mg, salmon-colored:
bottles of 100 (**NDC 0074-6812-01**),
bottles of 1000 (**NDC 0074-6812-02**),
bottles of 5000 (**NDC 0074-6812-03**),
Abbo-Pac® unit dose packages of 100 (**NDC 0074-6812-10**).

Shown in Product Identification Section, page 403
Abbott Pharmaceuticals, Inc.
North Chicago, IL 60064
Ref. 03-4235-R8

ENDURONYL® Tablets ℞
[en-du're-nol]
(methyclothiazide and deserpidine)

Oral thiazide-rauwolfia therapy for hypertension.

Warning:
This fixed combination drug is not indicated for initial therapy of hypertension. Hypertension requires therapy titrated to the individual patient. If the fixed combination represents the dosage so determined, its use may be more convenient in patient management. The treatment of hypertension is not static, but must be reevaluated as conditions in each patient warrant.

Description: ENDURONYL is an orally-administered combination of Enduron® (methyclothiazide) and Harmonyl® (deserpidine). Methyclothiazide is an oral diuretic-antihypertensive of the benzothiadiazine (thiazide) class. Deserpidine is a purified rauwolfia alkaloid, chemically identified as 11-desmethoxyreserpine, which produces antihypertensive effects.

Actions: The combined antihypertensive actions of methyclothiazide and deserpidine result in a total clinical antihypertensive effect which is greater than can ordinarily be achieved by either drug given individually.

The diuretic and saluretic effects of methyclothiazide result from a drug-induced inhibition of the renal tubular reabsorption of electrolytes. The excretion of sodium and chloride is greatly enhanced. Potassium excretion is also enhanced to a variable degree, as it is with the other thiazides. Although urinary excretion of bicarbonate is increased slightly, there is usually no significant change in urinary pH. Methyclothiazide has a per mg natriuretic activity approximately 100 times that of the prototype thiazide, chlorothiazide. At maximal therapeutic dosages, all thiazides are approximately equal in their diuretic/natriuretic effects.

There is significant natriuresis and diuresis within two hours after administration of a single dose of methyclothiazide. These effects reach a peak in about six hours and persist for 24 hours following oral administration of a single dose.

Like other benzothiadiazines, methyclothiazide also has antihypertensive properties, and may be used for this purpose either alone or to enhance the antihypertensive action of other drugs. The mechanism by which the benzothiadiazines, including methyclothiazide, produce a reduction of elevated blood pressure is not known. However, sodium depletion appears to be involved.

Methyclothiazide is rapidly absorbed and slowly eliminated by the kidney as both intact drug and as a metabolite showing no diuretic activity in a rat model.

The pharmacologic actions of Harmonyl (deserpidine) are essentially the same as those of other active rauwolfia alkaloids. Deserpidine probably produces its antihypertensive effects through depletion of tissue stores of catecholamines (epinephrine and norepinephrine) from peripheral sites. The antihypertensive effect is often accompanied by bradycardia. There is no significant alteration in cardiac output or renal blood flow. The carotid sinus reflex is inhibited, but postural hypotension is rarely seen with the use of conventional doses of Harmonyl alone.

Deserpidine, like other rauwolfia alkaloids, is characterized by slow onset of action and sustained effect which may persist following withdrawal of the drug.

Indications: ENDURONYL (methyclothiazide and deserpidine) is indicated in the treatment of mild to moderately severe hypertension (see boxed warning). In many cases ENDURONYL alone produces an adequate reduction of blood pressure. In resistant or unusually severe cases ENDURONYL also may be supplemented by more potent antihypertensive agents. When administered with ENDURONYL, more potent agents can be given at reduced dosage to minimize undesirable side effects.

Contraindications: Methyclothiazide is contraindicated in patients with renal decompensation and in those who are hypersensitive to this or other sulfonamide-derived drugs.

Deserpidine is contraindicated in patients with known hypersensitivity, mental depression especially with suicidal tendencies, active peptic ulcer, and ulcerative colitis. It is also contraindicated in patients receiving electroconvulsive therapy.

Warnings:
Methyclothiazide
Methyclothiazide shares with other thiazides the propensity to deplete potassium reserves to an unpredictable degree.

Thiazides should be used with caution in patients with renal disease or significant impairment of renal function, since azotemia may be precipitated and cumulative drug effects may occur.

Thiazides should be used with caution in patients with impaired hepatic function or progressive liver disease, since minor alterations of fluid and electrolyte balance may precipitate hepatic coma.
Thiazides may be additive or potentiative of the action of other antihypertensive drugs. Potentiation occurs with ganglionic or peripheral adrenergic blocking drugs.

Sensitivity reactions may occur in patients with a history of allergy or bronchial asthma.

The possibility of exacerbation or activation of systemic lupus erythematosus has been reported.

Deserpidine
Extreme caution should be exercised in treating patients with a history of mental depression. Discontinue the drug at the first sign of despondency, early morning insomnia, loss of appetite, impotence, or self-deprecation. Drug-induced depression may persist for several months after drug withdrawal and may be severe enough to result in suicide.

Usage in Pregnancy and Lactation:
Methyclothiazide
Thiazides cross the placental barrier and appear in cord blood. The use of thiazides in pregnant women requires that the anticipated benefit be weighed against possible hazards to the fetus. These hazards include fetal or neonatal jaundice, thrombocytopenia, and possible other adverse reactions that have occurred in the adult.

Thiazides appear in breast milk. If use of the drug is deemed essential, the patient should stop nursing.

Deserpidine
The safety of deserpidine for use during pregnancy or lactation has not been established; therefore, it should be used in pregnant women or in women of childbearing potential only when in the judgment of the physician its use is deemed essential to the welfare of the patient. Increased respiratory secretions, nasal congestion, cyanosis, and anorexia may occur in infants born to rauwolfia alkaloid-treated mothers, since these preparations are known to cross the placental barrier to enter the fetal circulation and appear in cord blood. They also are secreted by nursing mothers into breast milk.

Reproductive and teratology studies in rats reduced the mating index and neonatal survival indices; the no-effect dosage has not been established.

Precautions: Periodic determinations of serum electrolytes should be performed at appropriate intervals for the purpose of detecting possible electrolyte imbalances such as hyponatremia, hypochloremic alkalosis, and hypokalemia. Serum and urine electrolyte determinations are particularly important when a patient is vomiting excessively or receiving parenteral fluids. All patients should be observed for other clinical signs of electrolyte imbalances such as dryness of mouth, thirst, weakness, lethargy, drowsiness, restlessness, muscle pains or cramps, muscular fatigue, hypotension, oliguria, tachycardia, and gastrointestinal disturbances such as nausea and vomiting.

Hypokalemia may develop with thiazides as with any other potent diuretic, especially when brisk diuresis occurs, severe cirrhosis is present, or when corticosteroids or ACTH are given concomitantly. Interference with the adequate oral intake of electrolytes will also contribute to the possible development of hypokalemia. Potassium depletion, even of a mild degree, resulting from thiazide use, may sensitize a patient to the effects of cardiac glycosides such as digitalis.

Any chloride deficit is generally mild and usually does not require specific treatment except under extraordinary circumstances (as in liver disease or renal disease). Dilutional hyponatremia may occur in edematous patients in hot weather; appropriate therapy is water restriction rather than administration of salt, except in rare instances when the hyponatremia is life threatening.

In actual salt depletion, appropriate replacement is the therapy of choice.

Hyperuricemia may occur or frank gout may be precipitated in certain patients receiving thiazide therapy.

Insulin requirements in diabetic patients may be increased, decreased, or unchanged. Latent diabetes mellitus may become manifest during thiazide administration.

Thiazide drugs may increase the responsiveness to tubocurarine.

The antihypertensive effects of the drug may be enhanced in the postsympathectomy patient.

Thiazides may decrease arterial responsiveness to norepinephrine. This diminution is not sufficient to preclude effectiveness of the pressor agent for therapeutic use.

If progressive renal impairment becomes evident as indicated by a rising nonprotein nitrogen or blood urea nitrogen, a careful reappraisal of therapy is necessary with consideration given to withholding or discontinuing diuretic therapy.

Thiazides may decrease serum PBI levels without signs of thyroid disturbance.

Thiazides have been reported, on rare occasions, to have elevated serum calcium to hypercalcemic levels. The serum calcium levels have returned to normal when the medication has been stopped. This phenomenon may be related to the ability of the thiazide diuretics to lower the amount of calcium excreted in the urine.

Because rauwolfia preparations increase gastrointestinal motility and secretion, this drug should be used cautiously in patients with a history of peptic ulcer, ulcerative colitis, or gallstones, where biliary colic may be precipitated.

Caution should be exercised when treating hypertensive patients with renal insufficiency since they adjust poorly to lowered blood pressure levels.

Use deserpidine cautiously with digitalis and quinidine since cardiac arrhythmias have occurred with rauwolfia preparations.

Preoperative withdrawal of deserpidine does not assure that circulatory instability will not occur. It is important that the anesthesiologist be aware of the patient's drug intake and consider this in the overall management, since hypotension has occurred in patients receiving rauwolfia preparations. Anticholinergic and/or adrenergic drugs (metaraminol, norepinephrine) have been employed to treat adverse vagocirculatory effects.

Animal tumorigenicity: There are no studies demonstrating that deserpidine is an animal tumorigen, although it is a prolactin stimulator and structurally related to reserpine. Rodent studies with reserpine, however, have shown that reserpine is an animal tumorigen, causing an increased incidence of mammary fibroadenomas in female mice, malignant tumors of the seminal vesicles in male mice, and malignant adrenal medullary tumors in male rats. These findings arose in 2 year studies in which the drug was administered in the feed at concentrations of 5 to 10 ppm—about 100 to 300 times the usual human dose. The breast neoplasms are thought to be related to reserpine's prolactin-elevating effect. Several other prolactin-elevating drugs have also been associated with an increased incidence of mammary neoplasia in rodents.

The extent to which these findings indicate a risk to humans is uncertain. Tissue culture experiments show that about one-third of human breast tumors are prolactin-dependent *in vitro,* a factor of considerable importance if the use of the drug is contemplated in a patient with previously detected breast cancer. The possibility of an increased risk of breast cancer in reserpine users has been studied extensively; however, no firm conclusion has emerged. Although a few epidemiologic studies have suggested a slightly increased risk (less than twofold in all studies except one) in women who have used reserpine, other studies of generally similar design have not confirmed this. Epidemiologic studies conducted using other drugs (neuroleptic agents) that, like reserpine, increase prolactin levels and, therefore, would be considered rodent mammary carcinogens, have not shown an association between chronic administration of the drug and human mammary tumorigenesis. While long-term clinical observation has not suggested such an association, the available evidence is considered too limited to be conclusive at this time. An association of reserpine intake with pheochromocytoma or tumors of the seminal vesicles has not been explored.

Adverse Reactions:
Methyclothiazide
Gastrointestinal System Reactions: Anorexia, gastric irritation, nausea, vomiting, cramping, diarrhea, constipation, jaundice (intrahepatic cholestatic jaundice), pancreatitis.
Central Nervous System Reactions: Dizziness, vertigo, paresthesias, headache, xanthopsia.
Hematologic Reactions: Leukopenia, agranulocytosis, thrombocytopenia, aplastic anemia.
Dermatologic — Hypersensitivity Reactions: Purpura, photosensitivity, rash, urticaria, necrotizing angiitis (vasculitis) (cutaneous vasculitis).
Cardiovascular Reaction: Orthostatic hypotension may occur and may be aggravated by alcohol, barbiturates, or narcotics.
Other: Hyperglycemia, glycosuria, hypercalcemia, hyperuricemia, muscle spasm, weakness, restlessness.

There have been isolated reports that certain nonedematous individuals developed severe fluid and electrolyte derangements after only brief exposure to normal doses of thiazide and non-thiazide diuretics. The condition is usually manifested as severe dilutional hyponatremia, hypokalemia, and hypochloremia. It has been reported to be due to inappropriately increased ADH secretion and appears to be idiosyncratic. Potassium replacement is apparently the most important therapy in the treatment of this syndrome along with removal of the offending drug.

Whenever adverse reactions are severe, treatment should be discontinued.

Deserpidine
The following adverse reactions have been reported with rauwolfia preparations. These reactions are usually reversible and disappear when the drug is discontinued.
Gastrointestinal: Including hypersecretion, anorexia, diarrhea, nausea, and vomiting.
Cardiovascular: Including angina-like symptoms, arrhythmias (particularly when used concurrently with digitalis or quinidine), and bradycardia.
Central Nervous System: Including drowsiness, depression, nervousness, paradoxical anxiety, nightmares, extrapyramidal tract symptoms, CNS sensitization manifested by dull sensorium, and deafness.
Dermatologic—Hypersensitivity: Including pruritus, rash, and asthma in asthmatic patients.
Ophthalmologic: Including glaucoma, uveitis, optic atrophy, and conjunctival injection.
Hematologic: Thrombocytopenic purpura.
Miscellaneous: Nasal congestion, weight gain, impotence or decreased libido, dysuria, dyspnea, muscular aches, dryness of mouth, dizziness, and headache.

Dosage and Administration: Dosage should be determined by individual titration of ingredients (see boxed warning). Dosage of both components should be carefully adjusted to the needs of the individual patient. Since at least ten days to two weeks may elapse before the full effects of the drugs become manifest, the dosage of the drugs should not be adjusted more frequently.

Two tablet strengths, ENDURONYL (methyclothiazide 5 mg, deserpidine 0.25 mg) and ENDURONYL FORTE (methyclothiazide 5 mg, deserpidine 0.5 mg), each grooved, are provided to permit considerable latitude in meeting the dosage requirements of individual patients.*

The following table will help in determining which dose of ENDURONYL or ENDURONYL FORTE best represents the equivalent of the titrated dose.

Daily Dosage of ENDURONYL	methyclothiazide	deserpidine
½ tablet	2.5 mg	0.125 mg
1 tablet	5.0 mg	0.250 mg
1½ tablet	7.5 mg	0.375 mg
2 tablets	10.0 mg	0.500 mg

Daily Dosage of ENDURONYL FORTE	methyclothiazide	deserpidine
½ tablet	2.5 mg	0.250 mg
1 tablet	5.0 mg	0.500 mg
1½ tablet	7.5 mg	0.750 mg
2 tablets	10.0 mg	1.000 mg

The appropriate dose of ENDURONYL is administered orally, once daily. The usual adult dosage is one lower-strength ENDURONYL tablet daily.

There is no contraindication to combining the administration of ENDURONYL with other antihypertensive agents. When other antihypertensive agents are to be added to the regimen, this should be accomplished gradually. Ganglionic blocking agents should be given at only half the usual dose since their effect is potentiated by pretreatment with ENDURONYL.

Overdosage: Symptoms of thiazide overdosage include electrolyte imbalance and signs of potassium deficiency such as confusion, dizziness, muscular weakness, and gastrointestinal disturbances. General supportive measures including replacement of fluids and electrolytes may be indicated in treatment of overdosage.

An overdosage of deserpidine is characterized by flushing of the skin, conjunctival injection, and pupillary constriction. Sedation ranging from drowsiness to coma may occur. Hypotension, hypothermia, central respiratory depression and bradycardia may develop in cases of severe overdosage. Treatment consists of the careful evacuation of stomach contents followed by the usual procedures for the symptomatic management of CNS depressant overdosage. If severe hypotension occurs it should be treated with a direct acting vasopressor such as norepinephrine bitartrate injection.

How Supplied: ENDURONYL (methyclothiazide and deserpidine) is supplied as monogrammed, grooved, square-shaped tablets in the following dosage sizes and quantities:

ENDURONYL (5 mg of methyclothiazide and 0.25 mg of deserpidine) yellow tablets in bottles of 100 (NDC 0074-6838-01) and 1000 (NDC 0074-6838-02). Also available in ABBO-PAC® unit dose packages, 100 tablets (NDC 0074-6838-06), in strips of 10 tablets.

ENDURONYL FORTE (5 mg of methyclothiazide and 0.5 mg of deserpidine) gray-colored tablets in bottles of 100 (NDC 0074-6854-01) and 1000 (NDC 0074-6854-02).

*Each component is separately available as ENDURON (methyclothiazide) and HARMONYL (deserpidine).

Shown in Product Identification Section, page 403
Abbott Pharmaceuticals, Inc.
North Chicago, IL 60064
Ref. 03-4258/R5

ERYDERM® 2% ℞
[*e-ry′derm*]
erythromycin topical solution, USP

Description: Erythromycin is an antibiotic produced from a strain of *Streptomyces erythraeus.* It is basic and readily forms salts with acids. Each ml of ERYDERM 2% (erythromycin topical solution) contains 20 mg of erythromycin base in a vehicle consisting of polyethylene glycol, acetone, and alcohol 77%.

Actions: Although the mechanism by which ERYDERM acts in reducing inflammatory lesions of acne vulgaris is unknown, it is presumably due to its antibiotic action.

Indications: ERYDERM is indicated for the topical control of acne vulgaris.

Continued on next page

If desired, additional literature on any Abbott Product will be provided upon request to Abbott Laboratories.

Abbott—Cont.

Contraindications: ERYDERM is contraindicated in persons who have shown hypersensitivity to any of its ingredients.

Warnings: The safe use of ERYDERM during pregnancy or lactation has not been established.

Precautions: ERYDERM is for external use only and should be kept away from the eyes and mucous membranes including those of the nose and mouth. Do not allow solution to contact clothing and furniture. Concomitant topical acne therapy should be used with caution because a cumulative irritant effect may occur, especially with the use of peeling, desquamating, or abrasive agents.

The use of antimicrobial agents may be associated with the overgrowth of antibiotic resistant organisms. If this occurs, administration of this drug should be discontinued and appropriate measures taken.

Adverse Reactions: Adverse conditions experienced included dryness, pruritus, erythema, desquamation, and burning sensation.

Dosage and Administration: ERYDERM should be applied with applicator or pad to the affected area twice a day after the skin is thoroughly washed with warm water and soap. The solution should be applied with a dabbing action when the applicator is used. Use enough solution to cover the affected area lightly.

How Supplied: ERYDERM 2% (erythromycin topical solution, USP) is supplied in 60 ml bottles with applicator (**NDC** 0074-2698-02) and without an applicator. Store at temperatures below 86°F (30°C).

Abbott Laboratories
North Chicago, IL 60064
Ref. 09-5849-3/R1

ERYPED® ℞
[ere¹ ped]
(erythromycin ethylsuccinate for oral suspension, USP)

Description: Erythromycin is produced by a strain of *Streptomyces erythraeus* and belongs to the macrolide group of antibiotics. It is basic and readily forms salts with acids. The base, the stearate salt, and the esters are poorly soluble in water. Erythromycin ethylsuccinate is an ester of erythromycin suitable for oral administration. EryPed (erythromycin ethylsuccinate for oral suspension) is for reconstitution with water to form a suspension containing erythromycin ethylsuccinate equivalent to 400 mg of erythromycin per 5 ml (teaspoonful) with an appealing banana flavor. After mixing, EryPed must be stored below 77°F (25°C) and used within 35 days; refrigeration is not required. This product is intended primarily for pediatric use but can also be used in adults.

Actions:
Microbiology: Biochemical tests demonstrate that erythromycin inhibits protein synthesis of the pathogen without directly affecting nucleic acid synthesis. Antagonism has been demonstrated between clindamycin and erythromycin. NOTE: Many strains of *Hemophilus influenzae* are resistant to erythromycin alone, but are susceptible to erythromycin and sulfonamides together. Staphylococci resistant to erythromycin may emerge following a course of erythromycin therapy. Culture and susceptibility testing should be performed.

Disc Susceptibility Tests: Quantitative methods that require measurement of zone diameters give the most precise estimates of antibiotic susceptibility. One recommended procedure (21 CFR section 460.1) uses erythromycin class discs for testing susceptibility; interpretations correlate zone diameters of this disc test with MIC values for erythromycin. With this procedure, a report from the laboratory of "susceptible" indicates that the infecting organism is likely to respond to therapy. A report of "resistant" indicates, that the infective organism is not likely to respond to therapy. A report of "intermediate susceptibility" suggests that the organism would be susceptible if higher doses were used.

Clinical Pharmacology: Erythromycin binds to the 50 S ribosomal subunits of susceptible bacteria and suppresses protein synthesis.

Orally administered erythromycin ethylsuccinate suspension is readily and reliably absorbed under both fasting and nonfasting conditions.

Erythromycin diffuses readily into most body fluids. Only low concentrations are normally achieved in the spinal fluid, but passage of the drug across the blood-brain barrier increases in meningitis. In the presence of normal hepatic function, erythromycin is concentrated in the liver and excreted in the bile; the effect of hepatic dysfunction on excretion of erythromycin by the liver into the bile is not known. Less than 5 percent of the orally administered dose of erythromycin is excreted in active form in the urine.

Erythromycin crosses the placental barrier and is excreted in breast milk.

Indications: *Streptococcus pyogenes* (Group A beta-hemolytic streptococcus): Upper and lower respiratory tract, skin, and soft tissue infections of mild to moderate severity.

Injectable benzathine penicillin G is considered by the American Heart Association to be the drug of choice in the treatment and prevention of streptococcal pharyngitis and in long-term prophylaxis of rheumatic fever.

When oral medication is preferred for treatment of the above conditions, penicillin G, V, or erythromycin are alternate drugs of choice.

When oral medication is given, the importance of strict adherence by the patient to the prescribed dosage regimen must be stressed. A therapeutic dose should be administered for at least 10 days.

Alpha-hemolytic streptococci (viridans group): Although no controlled clinical efficacy trials have been conducted, oral erythromycin has been suggested by the American Heart Association and American Dental Association for use in a regimen for prophylaxis against bacterial endocarditis in patients hypersensitive to penicillin who have congenital heart disease, or rheumatic or other acquired valvular heart disease when they undergo dental procedures and surgical procedures of the upper respiratory tract.[1] Erythromycin is not suitable prior to genitourinary or gastrointestinal tract surgery. NOTE: When selecting antibiotics for the prevention of bacterial endocarditis the physician or dentist should read the full joint statement of the American Heart Association and the American Dental Association.[1]

Staphylococcus aureus: Acute infections of skin and soft tissue of mild to moderate severity. Resistant organisms may emerge during treatment.

Streptococcus pneumoniae (Diplococcus pneumoniae): Upper respiratory tract infections (e.g., otitis media, pharyngitis) and lower respiratory tract infections (e.g., pneumonia) of mild to moderate degree.

Mycoplasma pneumoniae (Eaton agent, PPLO): For respiratory infections due to this organism.

Hemophilus influenzae: For upper respiratory tract infections of mild to moderate severity when used concomitantly with adequate doses of sulfonamides. (See sulfonamide labeling for appropriate prescribing information). The concomitant use of the sulfonamides is necessary since not all strains of *Hemophilus influenzae* are susceptible to erythromycin at the concentrations of the antibiotic achieved with usual therapeutic doses.

Chlamydia trachomatis: For the treatment of urethritis in adult males due to *Chlamydia trachomatis*.

Ureaplasma urealyticum: For the treatment of urethritis in adult males due to *Ureaplasma urealyticum*.

Treponema pallidum: Erythromycin is an alternate choice of treatment for primary syphilis in patients allergic to the penicillins. In treatment of primary syphilis, spinal fluid examinations should be done before treatment and as part of follow-up after therapy.

Corynebacterium diphtheriae: As an adjunct to antitoxin, to prevent establishment of carriers, and to eradicate the organism in carriers.

Corynebacterium minutissimum: For the treatment of erythrasma.

Entamoeba histolytica: In the treatment of intestinal amebiasis only. Extraenteric amebiasis requires treatment with other agents.

Listeria monocytogenes: Infections due to this organism.

Bordetella pertussis: Erythromycin is effective in eliminating the organism from the nasopharynx of infected individuals, rendering them non-infectious. Some clinical studies suggest that erythromycin may be helpful in the prophylaxis of pertussis in exposed susceptible individuals.

Legionnaires' Disease: Although no controlled clinical efficacy studies have been conducted, *in vitro* and limited preliminary clinical data suggest that erythromycin may be effective in treating Legionnaires' Disease.

Contraindications: Erythromycin is contraindicated in patients with known hypersensitivity to this antibiotic.

Precautions: Erythromycin is principally excreted by the liver. Caution should be exercised in administering the antibiotic to patients with impaired hepatic function. There have been reports of hepatic dysfunction, with or without jaundice occurring in patients receiving oral erythromycin products.

Areas of localized infection may require surgical drainage in addition to antibiotic therapy.

Recent data from studies of erythromycin reveal that its use in patients who are receiving high doses of theophylline may be associated with an increase of serum theophylline levels and potential theophylline toxicity. In case of theophylline toxicity and/or elevated serum theophylline levels, the dose of theophylline should be reduced while the patient is receiving concomitant erythromycin therapy.

Usage during pregnancy and lactation: The safety of erythromycin for use during pregnancy has not been established.

Erythromycin crosses the placental barrier. Erythromycin also appears in breast milk.

Adverse Reactions: The most frequent side effects of erythromycin preparations are gastrointestinal, such as abdominal cramping and discomfort, and are dose related. Nausea, vomiting, and diarrhea occur infrequently with usual oral doses. During prolonged or repeated therapy, there is a possibility of overgrowth of nonsusceptible bacteria or fungi. If such infections occur, the drug should be discontinued and appropriate therapy instituted.

Allergic reactions ranging from urticaria and mild skin eruptions to anaphylaxis have occurred.

There have been isolated reports of reversible hearing loss occurring chiefly in patients with renal insufficiency and in patients receiving high doses of erythromycin.

Dosage and Administration: EryPed (erythromycin ethylsuccinate for oral suspension) may be administered without regard to meals.

Children: Age, weight, and severity of the infection are important factors in determining the proper dosage. In mild to moderate infections the usual dosage of erythromycin ethylsuccinate for children is 30 to 50 mg/kg/day in equally divided doses. For more severe infections this dosage may be doubled.

The following dosage schedule is suggested for mild to moderate infections:

Body Weight	Total Daily Dose
Under 10 lbs	30-50 mg/kg/day 15-25 mg/lb/day
10 to 15 lbs	200 mg
16 to 25 lbs	400 mg
26 to 50 lbs	800 mg
51 to 100 lbs	1200 mg
over 100 lbs	1600 mg

Adults: 400 mg erythromycin ethylsuccinate every 6 hours is the usual dose. Dosage may be increased up to 4 g per day according to the severity of the infection.

If twice-a-day dosage is desired in either adults or children, one-half of the total daily dose may be given every 12 hours. Doses may also be given three times daily if desired by administering one-third of the total daily dose every 8 hours.

In the treatment of streptococcal infections, a therapeutic dosage of erythromycin ethylsuccinate should be administered for at least 10 days. In continuous prophylaxis against recurrences of streptococcal infections in persons with a history of rheumatic heart disease, the usual dosage is 400 mg twice a day.

For prophylaxis against bacterial endocarditis[1] in patients with congenital heart disease, or rheumatic or other acquired valvular heart disease when undergoing dental procedures or surgical procedures of the upper respiratory tract, give 1.6 g (20 mg/kg for children) orally 1 $\frac{1}{2}$ to 2 hours before the procedure, and then, 800 mg (10 mg/kg for children) orally every 6 hours for 8 doses.

For treatment of urethritis due to *C. trachomatis* or *U. urealyticum*: 800 mg three times a day for 7 days.

For treatment of primary syphilis: Adults: 48 to 64 g given in divided doses over a period of 10 to 15 days.

For intestinal amebiasis: Adults: 400 mg four times daily for 10 to 14 days. Children: 30 to 50 mg/kg/day in divided doses for 10 to 14 days.

For use in pertussis: Although optimal dosage and duration have not been established, doses of erythromycin utilized in reported clinical studies were 40 to 50 mg/kg/day, given in divided doses for 5 to 14 days.

For treatment of Legionnaires' Disease: Although optimal doses have not been established, doses utilized in reported clinical data were 1.6 to 4 g daily in divided doses.

How Supplied: EryPed (erythromycin ethylsuccinate for oral suspension, USP), 400 mg per 5 ml, is supplied in 60-ml (NDC 0074-6305-60), 100-ml (**NDC 0074-6305-13**) and 200-ml (**NDC 0074-6305-53**) bottles, and 5-ml unit dose in ABBO-PAC® packages of 100 bottles (**NDC 0074-6305-05**). After reconstitution, EryPed must be stored below 77°F (25°C) and used within 35 days; refrigeration not required.

Reference: 1. American Heart Association. 1977. Prevention of bacterial endocarditis. Circulation 56:139A-143A.

Abbott Laboratories
North Chicago, IL 60064
Ref. 07-5295-R4

ERY-TAB® ℞
[ĕrē¹ tab]
(erythromycin enteric-coated tablets)

Description: Erythromycin is produced by a strain of *Streptomyces erythraeus* and belongs to the macrolide group of antibiotics. It is basic and readily forms salts with acids. The base is white to off-white crystals or powder slightly soluble in water, soluble in alcohol, in chloroform, and in ether. ERY-TAB (erythromycin enteric-coated tablets) is specially coated to protect the contents from the inactivating effects of gastric acidity and to permit efficient absorption of the antibiotic in the small intestine. ERY-TAB is available in three dosage strengths containing either 250 mg, 333 mg, or 500 mg of erythromycin as the free base.

Actions: The mode of action of erythromycin is inhibition of protein synthesis without affecting nucleic acid synthesis. Resistance to erythromycin of some strains of *Hemophilus influenzae* and staphylococci has been demonstrated. Culture and susceptibility testing should be done. If the Kirby-Bauer method of disc susceptibility is used, a 15 mcg erythromycin disc should give a zone diameter of at least 18 mm when tested against an erythromycin susceptible organism.

Bioavailability data are available from Abbott Laboratories, Dept. 498.

ERY-TAB is well absorbed and may be given without regard to meals.

After absorption, erythromycin diffuses readily into most body fluids. In the absence of meningeal inflammation, low concentrations are normally achieved in the spinal fluid but passage of the drug across the blood-brain barrier increases in meningitis. In the presence of normal hepatic function, erythromycin is concentrated in the liver and excreted in the bile; the effect of hepatic dysfunction on excretion of erythromycin by the liver into the bile is not known. After oral administration, less than 5 percent of the activity of the administered dose can be recovered in the urine.

Erythromycin crosses the placental barrier but fetal plasma levels are low.

Indications: *Streptococcus pyogenes* (Group A beta-hemolytic streptococcus): For upper and lower respiratory tract, skin, and soft tissue infections of mild to moderate severity.

Injectable benzathine penicillin G is considered by the American Heart Association to be the drug of choice in the treatment and prevention of streptococcal pharyngitis and in long-term prophylaxis of rheumatic fever.

When oral medication is preferred for treatment of the above conditions, penicillin G, V, or erythromycin are alternate drugs of choice.

When oral medication is given, the importance of strict adherence by the patient to the prescribed dosage regimen must be stressed. A therapeutic dose should be administered for at least 10 days.

Alpha-hemolytic streptococci (viridans group): Although no controlled clinical efficacy trials have been conducted, oral erythromycin has been suggested by the American Heart Association and American Dental Association for use in a regimen for prophylaxis against bacterial endocarditis in patients hypersensitive to penicillin who have congenital heart disease, or rheumatic or other acquired valvular heart disease when they undergo dental procedures and surgical procedures of the upper respiratory tract.[1] Erythromycin is not suitable prior to genitourinary or gastrointestinal tract surgery. NOTE: When selecting antibiotics for the prevention of bacterial endocarditis the physician or dentist should read the full joint statement of the American Heart Association and the American Dental Association.[1]

Staphylococcus aureus: For acute infections of skin and soft tissue of mild to moderate severity. Resistant organisms may emerge during treatment.

Streptococcus pneumoniae (Diplococcus pneumoniae): For upper respiratory tract infections (e.g., otitis media, pharyngitis) and lower respiratory tract infections (e.g., pneumonia) of mild to moderate degree.

Mycoplasma pneumoniae (Eaton agent, PPLO): For respiratory infections due to this organism.

Hemophilus influenzae: For upper respiratory tract infections of mild to moderate severity when used concomitantly with adequate doses of sulfonamides. Not all strains of this organism are susceptible at the erythromycin concentrations ordinarily achieved (see appropriate sulfonamide labeling for prescribing information).

Chlamydia trachomatis: Erythromycin is indicated for treatment of the following infections caused by *Chlamydia trachomatis:* conjunctivitis of the newborn, pneumonia of infancy and urogenital infections during pregnancy. When tetracyclines are contraindicated or not tolerated, erythromycin is indicated for the treatment of uncomplicated urethral, endocervical, or rectal infections in adults due to *Chlamydia trachomatis*.[2]

Treponema pallidum: Erythromycin is an alternate choice of treatment for primary syphilis in patients allergic to the penicillins. In treatment of primary syphilis, spinal fluid examinations should be done before treatment and as part of follow-up after therapy.

Corynebacterium diphtheriae and C. minutissimum: As an adjunct to antitoxin, to prevent establishment of carriers, and to eradicate the organism in carriers.

In the treatment of erythrasma.

Entamoeba histolytica: In the treatment of intestinal amebiasis only. Extra-enteric amebiasis requires treatment with other agents.

Listeria monocytogenes: Infections due to this organism.

Neisseria gonorrhoeae: Erythrocin® Lactobionate-I.V. (erythromycin lactobionate for injection, USP) in conjunction with erythromycin base orally, as an alternative drug in treatment of acute pelvic inflammatory disease caused by *N. gonorrhoeae* in female patients with a history of sensitivity to penicillin. Before treatment of gonorrhea, patients who are suspected of also having syphilis should have a microscopic examination for *T. pallidum* (by immunofluorescence or darkfield) before receiving erythromycin, and monthly serologic tests for a minimum of 4 months.

Bordetella pertussis: Erythromycin is effective in eliminating the organism from the nasopharynx of infected individuals, rendering them non-infectious. Some clinical studies suggest that erythromycin may be helpful in the prophylaxis of pertussis in exposed susceptible individuals.

Legionnaires' Disease: Although no controlled clinical efficacy studies have been conducted, *in vitro* and limited preliminary clinical data suggest that erythromycin can be effective in treating Legionnaires' Disease.

Contraindications: Erythromycin is contraindicated in patients with known hypersensitivity to this antibiotic.

Warning: *Usage in pregnancy:* Safety for use in pregnancy has not been established.

Precautions: Erythromycin is principally excreted by the liver. Caution should be exercised in administering the antibiotic to patients with impaired hepatic function.

There have been reports of hepatic dysfunction, with or without jaundice, occurring in patients receiving oral erythromycin products.

Recent data from studies of erythromycin reveal that its use in patients who are receiving high doses of theophylline may be associated with an increase of serum theophylline levels and potential theophylline toxicity. In cases of theophylline toxicity and/or elevated serum theophylline levels, the dose of theophylline should be reduced while the patient is receiving concomitant erythromycin therapy.

Surgical procedures should be performed when indicated.

Adverse Reactions: The most frequent side effects of erythromycin preparations are gastrointestinal, such as abdominal cramping and discomfort, and are dose-related. Nausea, vomiting, and diarrhea occur infrequently with usual oral doses. During prolonged or repeated therapy, there is a possibility of overgrowth of nonsusceptible bacteria or fungi. If such infections occur, the drug should be discontinued and appropriate therapy instituted.

Mild allergic reactions such as urticaria and other skin rashes have occurred. Serious allergic reactions, including anaphylaxis, have been reported. Allergic reactions should be handled in the usual manner.

There have been isolated reports of reversible hearing loss occurring chiefly in patients with renal insufficiency and in patients receiving high doses of erythromycin.

Dosage and Administration: ERY-TAB (erythromycin enteric-coated tablets) is well absorbed and may be given without regard to meals.

Adults: The usual dose is 250 mg four times daily in equally spaced doses. The 333 mg tablet is recommended if dosage is desired every 8 hours. If twice-a-day dosage is desired, the recommended dose is 500 mg every 12 hours.

Continued on next page

If desired, additional literature on any Abbott Product will be provided upon request to Abbott Laboratories.

Abbott—Cont.

Dosage may be increased up to 4 or more grams per day according to the severity of the infection. Twice-a-day dosing is not recommended when doses larger than 1 gram daily are administered. Children: Age, weight, and severity of the infection are important factors in determining the proper dosage. 30 to 50 mg/kg/day, in divided doses, is the usual dose. For more severe infections, this dose may be doubled.

In the treatment of streptococcal infections, a therapeutic dosage of erythromycin should be administered for at least 10 days. In continuous prophylaxis of streptococcal infections in persons with a history of rheumatic heart disease, the dose is 250 mg twice a day.

For prophylaxis against bacterial endocarditis[1] in patients with congenital heart disease, or rheumatic or other acquired valvular heart disease when undergoing dental procedures or surgical procedures of the upper respiratory tract, give 1 g (20 mg/kg for children) orally 1½ to 2 hours before the procedure, and then, 500 mg (10 mg/kg in children) orally every 6 hours for 8 doses.

For conjunctivitis of the newborn caused by *Chlamydia trachomatis:* Oral erythromycin suspension 50 mg/kg/day in 4 divided doses for at least 2 weeks.[2]

For pneumonia of infancy caused by *Chlamydia trachomatis:* Although the optimal duration of therapy has not been established, the recommended therapy is oral erythromycin suspension 50 mg/kg/day in 4 divided doses for at least 3 weeks.[2]

For urogenital infections during pregnancy due to *Chlamydia trachomatis:* Although the optimal dose and duration of therapy have not been established, the suggested treatment is erythromycin 500 mg, by mouth, 4 times a day for at least 7 days. For women who cannot tolerate this regimen, a decreased dose of 250 mg, by mouth, 4 times a day should be used for at least 14 days.[2]

For adults with uncomplicated urethral, endocervical, or rectal infections caused by *Chlamydia trachomatis* in whom tetracyclines are contraindicated or not tolerated: 500 mg, by mouth, 4 times a day for at least 7 days.[2]

For treatment of primary syphilis: 30 to 40 grams given in divided doses over a period of 10 to 15 days.

For treatment of acute pelvic inflammatory disease caused by *N. gonorrhoeae:* After initial treatment with Erythrocin® Lactobionate-I.V. (erythromycin lactobionate for injection, USP) 500 mg every 6 hours for 3 days, the oral dosage recommendation is 250 mg every 6 hours for 7 days.

For dysenteric amebiasis: 250 mg four times daily for 10 to 14 days, for adults; 30 to 50 mg/kg/day in divided doses for 10 to 14 days, for children.

For use in pertussis: Although optimal dosage and duration have not been established, doses of erythromycin utilized in reported clinical studies were 40 to 50 mg/kg/day, given in divided doses for 5 to 14 days.

For treatment of Legionnaires' Disease: Although optimal doses have not been established, doses utilized in reported clinical data were 1 to 4 grams erythromycin base daily in divided doses.

Overdosage: Gastrointestinal side effects of erythromycin are dose related. Some individuals may exhibit gastric intolerance to even therapeutic amounts.

Erythromycin serum levels are not appreciably affected by hemodialysis or peritoneal dialysis.

How Supplied: ERY-TAB (erythromycin enteric-coated tablets), 250 mg, is supplied as pink tablets in bottles of 100 (**NDC 0074-6304-13**), bottles of 500 (**NDC 0074-6304-53**), and Abbo-Pac® unit dose packages of 100 (**NDC 0074-6304-11**).

ERY-TAB, 333 mg, is supplied as white tablets in bottles of 100 (**NDC 0074-6320-13**), and Abbo-Pac® unit dose packages of 100 (**NDC 0074-6320-11**).

ERY-TAB, 500 mg, is supplied as pink tablets in bottles of 100 (**NDC 0074-6321-13**) and Abbo-Pac unit dose packages of 100 (**NDC 0074-6321-11**).

References: 1. American Heart Association. 1977. Prevention of bacterial endocarditis. Circulation 56:139A-143A.
2. CDC Sexually Transmitted Diseases Treatment Guidelines 1982.

U.S. Pat. No. 4,340,582.
Shown in Product Identification Section, page 403
Abbott Laboratories
North Chicago, IL 60064
Ref: 01-2320-R7

E.E.S.® R
[ē-ē-ś]
(erythromycin ethylsuccinate)

Description: Erythromycin is produced by a strain of *Streptomyces erythraeus* and belongs to the macrolide group of antibiotics. It is basic and readily forms salts with acids. The base, the stearate salt, and the esters are poorly soluble in water. Erythromycin ethylsuccinate is an ester of erythromycin suitable for oral administration.

The cherry-flavored, chewable tablets are easily ingested and are particularly acceptable for the administration of antibiotic medication to young children who are unable to swallow regular tablets or in whom persuasion of a pleasant taste insures cooperation. Each chewable tablet, providing the equivalent of 200 mg of erythromycin, is conveniently scored for division into half-dose (100 mg) portions.

The granules and drops are intended for reconstitution with water. When reconstituted, they are palatable cherry-flavored suspensions.

The pleasant tasting, fruit-flavored liquids are supplied ready for oral administration.

Granules, drops and ready-made suspensions are intended primarily for pediatric use but can also be used in adults.

The Filmtab® tablets are intended primarily for adults or older children.

Actions: Microbiology: Biochemical tests demonstrate that erythromycin inhibits protein synthesis of the pathogen without directly affecting nucleic acid synthesis. Antagonism has been demonstrated between clindamycin and erythromycin. NOTE: Many strains of *Hemophilus influenzae* are resistant to erythromycin alone, but are susceptible to erythromycin and sulfonamides together. Staphylococci resistant to erythromycin may emerge during a course of erythromycin therapy. Culture and susceptibility testing should be performed.

Disc Susceptibility Tests: Quantitative methods that require measurement of zone diameters give the most precise estimates of antibiotic susceptibility. One recommended procedure (21 CFR section 460.1) uses erythromycin class discs for testing susceptibility; interpretations correlate zone diameters of this disc test with MIC values for erythromycin. With this procedure, a report from the laboratory of "susceptible" indicates that the infecting organism is likely to respond to therapy. A report of "resistant" indicates that the infective organism is not likely to respond to therapy. A report of "intermediate susceptibility" suggests that the organism would be susceptible if higher doses were used.

Clinical Pharmacology: Erythromycin binds to the 50 S ribosomal subunits of susceptible bacteria and suppresses protein synthesis.

Orally administered erythromycin ethylsuccinate suspensions and Filmtab tablets are readily and reliably absorbed. Erythromycin ethylsuccinate chewable tablets are readily and reliably absorbed when chewed. Comparable serum levels of erythromycin are achieved in the fasting and nonfasting states.

Erythromycin diffuses readily into most body fluids. Only low concentrations are normally achieved in the spinal fluid, but passage of the drug across the blood-brain barrier increases in meningitis. In the presence of normal hepatic function, erythromycin is concentrated in the liver and excreted in the bile; the effect of hepatic dysfunction on excretion of erythromycin by the liver into the bile is not known. Less than 5 percent of the orally administered dose of erythromycin is excreted in active form in the urine.

Erythromycin crosses the placental barrier and is excreted in breast milk.

Indications: *Streptococcus pyogenes* (Group A beta-hemolytic streptococcus): Upper and lower respiratory tract, skin, and soft tissue infections of mild to moderate severity.

Injectable benzathine penicillin G is considered by the American Heart Association to be the drug of choice in the treatment and prevention of streptococcal pharyngitis and in long-term prophylaxis of rheumatic fever.

When oral medication is preferred for treatment of the above conditions, penicillin G, V, or erythromycin are alternate drugs of choice.

When oral medication is given, the importance of strict adherence by the patient to the prescribed dosage regimen must be stressed. A therapeutic dose should be administered for at least 10 days.

Alpha-hemolytic streptococci (viridans group): Although no controlled clinical efficacy trials have been conducted, oral erythromycin has been suggested by the American Heart Association and American Dental Association for use in a regimen for prophylaxis against bacterial endocarditis in patients hypersensitive to penicillin who have congenital heart disease, or rheumatic or other acquired valvular heart disease when they undergo dental procedures and surgical procedures of the upper respiratory tract.[1] Erythromycin is not suitable prior to genitourinary or gastrointestinal tract surgery. NOTE: When selecting antibiotics for the prevention of bacterial endocarditis the physician or dentist should read the full joint statement of the American Heart Association and the American Dental Association.[1]

Staphylococcus aureus: Acute infections of skin and soft tissue of mild to moderate severity. Resistant organisms may emerge during treatment.

Streptococcus pneumoniae (Diplococcus pneumoniae): Upper respiratory tract infections (e.g., otitis media, pharyngitis) and lower respiratory tract infections (e.g., pneumonia) of mild to moderate degree.

Mycoplasma pneumoniae (Eaton agent, PPLO): For respiratory infections due to this organism.

Hemophilus influenzae: For upper respiratory tract infections of mild to moderate severity when used concomitantly with adequate doses of sulfonamides. (See sulfonamide labeling for appropriate prescribing information). The concomitant use of the sulfonamides is necessary since not all strains of *Hemophilus influenzae* are susceptible to erythromycin at the concentrations of the antibiotic achieved with usual therapeutic doses.

Chlamydia trachomatis: For the treatment of urethritis in adult males due to *Chlamydia trachomatis.*

Ureaplasma urealyticum: For the treatment of urethritis in adult males due to *Ureaplasma urealyticum.*

Treponema pallidum: Erythromycin is an alternate choice of treatment for primary syphilis in patients allergic to the penicillins. In treatment of primary syphilis, spinal fluid examinations should be done before treatment and as part of follow-up after therapy.

Corynebacterium diphtheriae: As an adjunct to antitoxin, to prevent establishment of carriers, and to eradicate the organism in carriers.

Corynebacterium minutissimum: For the treatment of erythrasma.

Entamoeba histolytica: In the treatment of intestinal amebiasis only. Extraenteric amebiasis requires treatment with other agents.

Listeria monocytogenes: Infections due to this organism.

Bordetella pertussis: Erythromycin is effective in eliminating the organism from the nasopharynx of infected individuals, rendering them non-infectious. Some clinical studies suggest that erythromycin may be helpful in the prophylaxis of pertussis in exposed susceptible individuals.

Legionnaires' Disease: Although no controlled clinical efficacy studies have been conducted, *in vitro* and limited preliminary clinical data suggest that erythromycin may be effective in treating Legionnaires' Disease.

Contraindications: Erythromycin is contraindicated in patients with known hypersensitivity to this antibiotic.

Precautions: Erythromycin is principally excreted by the liver. Caution should be exercised in administering the antibiotic to patients with impaired hepatic function. There have been reports of hepatic dysfunction, with or without jaundice occurring in patients receiving oral erythromycin products.

Areas of localized infection may require surgical drainage in addition to antibiotic therapy.

Recent data from studies of erythromycin reveal that its use in patients who are receiving high doses of theophylline may be associated with an increase of serum theophylline levels and potential theophylline toxicity. In case of theophylline toxicity and/or elevated serum theophylline levels, the dose of theophylline should be reduced while the patient is receiving concomitant erythromycin therapy.

Usage during pregnancy and lactation: The safety of erythromycin for use during pregnancy has not been established.

Erythromycin crosses the placental barrier. Erythromycin also appears in breast milk.

Adverse Reactions: The most frequent side effects of erythromycin preparations are gastrointestinal, such as abdominal cramping and discomfort, and are dose related. Nausea, vomiting, and diarrhea occur infrequently with usual oral doses. During prolonged or repeated therapy, there is a possibility of overgrowth of nonsusceptible bacteria or fungi. If such infections occur, the drug should be discontinued and appropriate therapy instituted.

Allergic reactions ranging from urticaria and mild skin eruptions to anaphylaxis have occurred.

There have been isolated reports of reversible hearing loss occurring chiefly in patients with renal insufficiency and in patients receiving high doses of erythromycin.

Dosage and Administration: Erythromycin ethylsuccinate suspensions, Filmtab tablets and chewable tablets may be administered without regard to meals. For full therapeutic effect, the chewable tablets must be chewed.

Children: Age, weight, and severity of the infection are important factors in determining the proper dosage. In mild to moderate infections the usual dosage of erythromycin ethylsuccinate for children is 30 to 50 mg/kg/day in equally divided doses. For more severe infections this dosage may be doubled.

The following dosage schedule is suggested for mild to moderate infections:

Body Weight	Total Daily Dose
Under 10 lbs	30–50 mg/kg/day 15–25 mg/lb/day
10 to 15 lbs	200 mg
16 to 25 lbs	400 mg
26 to 50 lbs	800 mg
51 to 100 lbs	1200 mg
over 100 lbs	1600 mg

Adults: 400 mg erythromycin ethylsuccinate every 6 hours is the usual dose. Dosage may be increased up to 4 g per day according to the severity of the infection.

If twice-a-day dosage is desired in either adults or children, one-half of the total daily dose may be given every 12 hours. Doses may also be given three times daily if desired by administering one-third of the total daily dose every 8 hours.

In the treatment of streptococcal infections, a therapeutic dosage of erythromycin ethylsuccinate should be administered for at least 10 days. In continuous prophylaxis against recurrences of streptococcal infections in persons with a history of rheumatic heart disease, the usual dosage is 400 mg twice a day.

For prophylaxis against bacterial endocarditis[1] in patients with congenital heart disease, or rheumatic or other acquired valvular heart disease when undergoing dental procedures or surgical procedures of the upper respiratory tract, give 1.6 g (20 mg/kg for children) orally 1½ to 2 hours before the procedure, and then, 800 mg (10 mg/kg for children) orally every 6 hours for 8 doses.

For treatment of urethritis due to *C. trachomatis* or *U. urealyticum:* 800 mg three times a day for 7 days.

For treatment of primary syphilis: Adults: 48 to 64 g given in divided doses over a period of 10 to 15 days.

For intestinal amebiasis: Adults: 400 mg four times daily for 10 to 14 days. Children: 30 to 50 mg/kg/day in divided doses for 10 to 14 days.

For use in pertussis: Although optimal dosage and duration have not been established, doses of erythromycin utilized in reported clinical studies were 40 to 50 mg/kg/day, given in divided doses for 5 to 14 days.

For treatment of Legionnaires' Disease: Although optimal doses have not been established, doses utilized in reported clinical data were 1.6 to 4 g daily in divided doses.

How Supplied: E.E.S. 200 LIQUID (erythromycin ethylsuccinate oral suspension, USP) is supplied in 1 pint bottles (**NDC** 0074-6306-16) and in packages of six 100-ml bottles (**NDC** 0074-6306-13). Each 5-ml teaspoonful of fruit-flavored suspension contains activity equivalent to 200 mg of erythromycin.

E.E.S. 400® LIQUID (erythromycin ethylsuccinate oral suspension, USP) is supplied in 1 pint bottles (**NDC** 0074-6373-16) and in packages of six 100-ml bottles (**NDC** 0074-6373-13). Each 5-ml teaspoonful of orange, fruit-flavored suspension contains activity equivalent to 400 mg of erythromycin.

Both liquid products require refrigeration to preserve taste until dispensed. Refrigeration by patient is not required if used within 14 days.

E.E.S. GRANULES (erythromycin ethylsuccinate for oral suspension, USP) is supplied in 60-ml (**NDC** 0074-6369-01), 100-ml (**NDC** 0074-6369-02) and 200-ml (**NDC** 0074-6369-10) size bottles. Each 5-ml teaspoonful of reconstituted cherry-flavored suspension contains activity equivalent to 200 mg of erythromycin. E.E.S. GRANULES is also available in 5-ml bottles (when reconstituted) in the ABBO-PAC® unit dose packages of 100 bottles (**NDC** 0074-6369-05).

E.E.S. DROPS (erythromycin ethylsuccinate for oral suspension, USP) is supplied in 50-ml size bottles (**NDC** 0074-6360-50). Each 2.5-ml dropperful (½ teaspoonful) of reconstituted cherry-flavored suspension contains activity equivalent to 100 mg of erythromycin.

E.E.S. CHEWABLE (erythromycin ethylsuccinate tablets, USP) cherry-flavored wafers containing the equivalent of 200 mg of erythromycin are available in packages of 50 (**NDC** 0074-6371-50). Each wafer is individually sealed in a blister package.

E.E.S. 400 Filmtab tablets (erythromycin ethylsuccinate tablets, USP) 400 mg, are available in bottles of 100 (**NDC** 0074-5729-13) and 500 (**NDC** 0074-5729-53), and in ABBO-PAC® unit dose strip packages of 100 (**NDC** 0074-5729-11). Tablets are pink in color.

Reference: 1. American Heart Association. 1977. Prevention of bacterial endocarditis. Circulation 56: 139A-143A.

Filmtab—Film-sealed tablets, Abbott.
Shown in Product Identification Section, page 403
Abbott Laboratories
North Chicago, IL 60064
Ref. 07-5294-R10

ERYTHROCIN® LACTOBIONATE-I.V. ℞
[*e-rith'ro-sin lac-tō-bī'ō-nāte ĭ. v.*]
(erythromycin lactobionate for injection, USP)
For I.V. use only

Description: Erythromycin is produced by a strain of *Streptomyces erythraeus* and belongs to the macrolide group of antibiotics. It is basic and readily forms salts with acids.

ERYTHROCIN LACTOBIONATE is a soluble salt of erythromycin suitable for intravenous administration.

Actions: Microbiology: Biochemical tests demonstrate that erythromycin inhibits protein synthesis of the pathogen without directly affecting nucleic acid synthesis. Antagonism has been demonstrated between clindamycin and erythromycin.

NOTE: Many strains of *Hemophilus influenzae* are resistant to erythromycin alone, but are susceptible to erythromycin and sulfonamides together. Staphylococci resistant to erythromycin may emerge during a course of erythromycin therapy. Culture and susceptibility testing should be performed.

Disc Susceptibility Tests: Quantitative methods that require measurement of zone diameters give the most precise estimates of antibiotic susceptibility. One recommended procedure (21 CFR section 460.1) uses erythromycin class discs for testing susceptibility; interpretations correlate zone diameters of this disc test with MIC values for erythromycin. With this procedure, a report from the laboratory of "susceptible" indicates that the infecting organism is likely to respond to therapy. A report of "resistant" indicates that the infective organism is not likely to respond to therapy. A report of "intermediate susceptibility" suggests that the organism would be susceptible if higher doses were used.

Clinical Pharmacology: Erythromycin binds to the 50 S ribosomal subunits of susceptible bacteria and suppresses protein synthesis.

Intravenous infusion of 500 mg erythromycin lactobionate at a constant rate over 1 hour in fasting adults produced a mean serum erythromycin level of approximately 7 mcg/ml at 20 minutes, 10 mcg/ml at 1 hour, 2.6 mcg/ml at 2.5 hours, and 1 mcg/ml at 6 hours.

Erythromycin diffuses readily into most body fluids. Only low concentrations are normally achieved in the spinal fluid, but passage of the drug across the blood-brain barrier increases in meningitis. In the presence of normal hepatic function, erythromycin is concentrated in the liver and excreted in the bile; the effect of hepatic dysfunction on excretion of erythromycin by the liver into the bile is not known. From 12 to 15 percent of intravenously administered erythromycin is excreted in active form in the urine.

Erythromycin crosses the placental barrier and is excreted in breast milk.

Indications: ERYTHROCIN LACTOBIONATE is indicated in the treatment of patients where oral administration is not possible or where the severity of the infection requires immediate high serum levels of erythromycin. Intravenous therapy should be replaced by oral administration at the appropriate time.

Streptococcus pyogenes (Group A beta-hemolytic streptococcus): Upper and lower respiratory tract, skin, and soft tissue infections of mild to moderate severity.

Injectable benzathine penicillin G is considered by the American Heart Association to be the drug of choice in the treatment and prevention of streptococcal pharyngitis and in long-term prophylaxis of rheumatic fever.

When oral medication is preferred for treatment of the above conditions, penicillin G, V, or erythromycin are alternate drugs of choice.

Continued on next page

If desired, additional literature on any Abbott Product will be provided upon request to Abbott Laboratories.

Abbott—Cont.

Staphylococcus aureus: Acute infections of skin and soft tissue of mild to moderate severity. Resistant organisms may emerge during treatment.
Streptococcus pneumoniae (Diplococcus pneumoniae): For upper respiratory tract infections (e.g., otitis media, pharyngitis) and lower respiratory tract infections (e.g., pneumonia) of mild to moderate severity.
Mycoplasma pneumoniae (Eaton agent, PPLO): For respiratory infections due to this organism.
Hemophilus influenzae: For upper respiratory tract infections of mild to moderate severity when used concomitantly with adequate doses of sulfonamides. (See sulfonamide labeling for appropriate prescribing information). The concomitant use of the sulfonamides is necessary since not all strains of *Hemophilus influenzae* are susceptible to erythromycin at the concentrations of the antibiotic achieved with usual therapeutic doses.
Corynebacterium diphtheriae: As an adjunct to antitoxin, to prevent the establishment of carriers, and to eradicate the organism in carriers.
Corynebacterium minutissimum: In the treatment of erythrasma.
Listeria monocytogenes: Infections due to this organism.
Neisseria gonorrhoeae: ERYTHROCIN LACTOBIONATE-I.V. in conjunction with erythromycin stearate or base orally, as an alternative drug in treatment of acute pelvic inflammatory disease caused by *N. gonorrhoeae* in female patients with a history of sensitivity to penicillin. Before treatment of gonorrhea, patients who are suspected of also having syphilis should have a microscopic examination for *T. pallidum* (by immunofluorescence or darkfield) before receiving erythromycin, and monthly serologic tests for a minimum of 4 months.
Legionnaires' Disease: Although no controlled clinical efficacy studies have been conducted, *in vitro* and limited preliminary clinical data suggest that erythromycin may be effective in treating Legionnaires' Disease.
Contraindications: Erythromycin is contraindicated in patients with known hypersensitivity to this antibiotic.
Precautions: Since erythromycin is principally excreted by the liver, caution should be exercised when erythromycin is administered to patients with impaired hepatic function.
Prolonged or repeated use of erythromycin may result in an overgrowth of non-susceptible bacteria or fungi. If superinfection occurs, erythromycin should be discontinued and appropriate therapy instituted.
Areas of localized infection may require surgical drainage in addition to antibiotic therapy.
Recent data from studies of erythromycin reveal that its use in patients who are receiving high doses of theophylline may be associated with an increase of serum theophylline levels and potential theophylline toxicity. In case of theophylline toxicity and/or elevated serum theophylline levels, the dose of theophylline should be reduced while the patient is receiving concomitant erythromycin therapy.
Usage during pregnancy and lactation: The safety of erythromycin for use during pregnancy has not been established.
Erythromycin crosses the placental barrier. Erythromycin also appears in breast milk.
Adverse Reactions: Side effects following the use of intravenous erythromycin are rare. Occasional venous irritation has been encountered, but if the infusion is given slowly, in dilute solution, preferably by continuous intravenous infusion or intermittent infusion in no less than 20 to 60 minutes, pain and vessel trauma are minimized.
Allergic reactions, ranging from urticaria and mild skin eruptions to anaphylaxis, have occurred with intravenously administered erythromycin.
Reversible hearing loss associated with the intravenous infusion of 4 g or more per day of erythromycin lactobionate has been reported rarely.

Dosage and Administration: For the treatment of severe infections in adults and children, the recommended intravenous dose of erythromycin lactobionate is 15 to 20 mg/kg/day. Higher doses, up to 4 g/day, may be given for very severe infections. ERYTHROCIN LACTOBIONATE-I.V. must be administered by continuous or intermittent intravenous infusion only. Due to the irritative properties of erythromycin, I.V. push is an unacceptable route of administration.
Continuous infusion of erythromycin lactobionate is preferable due to the slower infusion rate and lower concentration of erythromycin; however, intermittent infusion at intervals not greater than every six hours is also effective. Intravenous erythromycin should be replaced by oral erythromycin as soon as possible.
For slow continuous infusion: The final diluted solution of erythromycin lactobionate is prepared to give a concentration of 1 g per liter (1 mg/ml).
For intermittent infusion: Administer one-fourth the total daily dose of erythromycin lactobionate by intravenous infusion in 20 to 60 minutes at intervals not greater than every six hours. The final diluted solution of erythromycin lactobionate is prepared to give a concentration of 1 to 5 mg/ml. No less than 100 ml of I.V. diluent should be used. Infusion should be sufficiently slow to minimize pain along the vein.
For treatment of acute pelvic inflammatory disease caused by *N. gonorrhoeae*, in female patients hypersensitive to penicillins, administer 500 mg erythromycin lactobionate every six hours for three days, followed by oral administration of 250 mg erythromycin stearate or base every six hours for seven days.
For treatment of Legionnaires' Disease: Although optimal doses have not been established, doses utilized in reported clinical data were 1 to 4 grams daily in divided doses.
Preparation of Solution:
1. **PREPARE THE INITIAL SOLUTION OF ERYTHROCIN® LACTOBIONATE-I.V. BY ADDING 10 ML OF STERILE WATER FOR INJECTION, USP, TO THE 500 MG VIAL OR 20 ML OF STERILE WATER FOR INJECTION, USP, TO THE 1 G VIAL. Use only Sterile Water for Injection, USP, as other diluents may cause precipitation during reconstitution. Do not use diluents containing preservatives or inorganic salts. Note: When the product is reconstituted as directed above, the resulting solution contains an effective microbial preservative.**
After reconstitution, each ml contains 50 mg of erythromycin activity. The initial solution is stable at refrigerator temperature for two weeks, or for 24 hours at room temperature.
2. ADD THE INITIAL DILUTION TO ONE OF THE FOLLOWING DILUENTS BEFORE ADMINISTRATION to give a concentration of 1 g of erythromycin activity per liter (1 mg/ml) for continuous infusion or 1 to 5 mg/ml for intermittent infusion:
0.9% SODIUM CHLORIDE INJECTION, USP
LACTATED RINGER'S INJECTION, USP
NORMOSOL®-R
3. THE FOLLOWING SOLUTIONS MAY ALSO BE USED PROVIDING THEY ARE FIRST BUFFERED WITH NEUT® (4% SODIUM BICARBONATE, ABBOTT) by adding 1 ml of Neut per 100 ml of solution:
5% DEXTROSE INJECTION, USP
5% DEXTROSE AND LACTATED RINGER'S INJECTION
5% DEXTROSE AND 0.9% SODIUM CHLORIDE INJECTION, USP
Neut® (4% sodium bicarbonate, Abbott) must be added to these solutions so that their pH is in the optimum range for erythromycin lactobionate stability. Acidic solutions of erythromycin lactobionate are unstable and lose their potency rapidly. A pH of at least 5.5 is desirable for the final diluted solution of erythromycin lactobionate.
No drug or chemical agent should be added to an erythromycin lactobionate-I.V. fluid admixture unless its effect on the chemical and physical stability of the solution has first been determined.

Stability: The final diluted solution of erythromycin lactobionate should be completely administered within 8 hours, since it is not suitable for storage.*
How Supplied: ERYTHROCIN LACTOBIONATE-I.V. (erythromycin lactobionate for injection, USP) is supplied as a sterile, lyophilized powder in packages of 5 vials (**NDC** 0074-6342-05), each vial containing the equivalent of 1 g of erythromycin with 180 mg benzyl alcohol added as preservative; and in packages of 5 vials (**NDC** 0074-6365-02), each vial containing the equivalent of 500 mg of erythromycin with 90 mg benzyl alcohol added as preservative.
*Contact Abbott Laboratories, Dept. 498 for additional stability data.
Abbott Laboratories
North Chicago, IL 60064
Ref. 01-2163-R13

ERYTHROCIN® PIGGYBACK ℞
[*e-rith'ro-sin pig'gy back*]
(erythromycin lactobionate for injection, USP)
Single Dose Dispensing Vial
For I.V. use only

Description: Erythromycin is produced by a strain of *Streptomyces erythraeus* and belongs to the macrolide group of antibiotics. It is basic and readily forms salts with acids.
Erythromycin lactobionate is a soluble salt of erythromycin. ERYTHROCIN PIGGYBACK is a dosage form suitable for intermittent intravenous administration.
Actions: Microbiology: Biochemical tests demonstrate that erythromycin inhibits protein synthesis of the pathogen without directly affecting nucleic acid synthesis. Antagonism has been demonstrated between clindamycin and erythromycin.
NOTE: Many strains of *Hemophilus influenzae* are resistant to erythromycin alone, but are susceptible to erythromycin and sulfonamides together. Staphylococci resistant to erythromycin may emerge during a course of erythromycin therapy. Culture and susceptibility testing should be performed.
Disc Susceptibility Tests: Quantitative methods that require measurement of zone diameters give the most precise estimates of antibiotic susceptibility. One recommended procedure (21 CFR section 460.1) uses erythromycin class discs for testing susceptibility; interpretations correlate zone diameters of this disc test with MIC values for erythromycin. With this procedure, a report from the laboratory of "susceptible" indicates that the infecting organism is likely to respond to therapy. A report of "resistant" indicates that the infective organism is not likely to respond to therapy. A report of "intermediate susceptibility" suggests that the organism would be susceptible if higher doses were used.
Clinical Pharmacology: Erythromycin binds to the 50 S ribosomal subunits of susceptible bacteria and suppresses protein synthesis.
Intravenous infusion of 500 mg erythromycin lactobionate at a constant rate over 1 hour in fasting adults produced a mean serum erythromycin level of approximately 7 mcg/ml at 20 minutes, 10 mcg/ml at 1 hour, 2.6 mcg/ml at 2.5 hours, and 1 mcg/ml at 6 hours.
Erythromycin diffuses readily into most body fluids. Only low concentrations are normally achieved in the spinal fluid, but passage of the drug across the blood-brain barrier increases in meningitis. In the presence of normal hepatic function, erythromycin is concentrated in the liver and excreted in the bile; the effect of hepatic dysfunction on excretion of erythromycin by the liver into the bile is not known. From 12 to 15 percent of intravenously administered erythromycin is excreted in active form in the urine.
Erythromycin crosses the placental barrier and is excreted in breast milk.
Indications: ERYTHROCIN PIGGYBACK is indicated in the treatment of patients where oral administration is not possible or where the severity of the infection requires immediate high serum levels of erythromycin. Intravenous therapy

should be replaced by oral administration at the appropriate time.

Steptococcus pyogenes (Group A beta-hemolytic streptococcus): Upper and lower respiratory tract, skin, and soft tissue infections of mild to moderate severity.

Injectable benzathine penicillin G is considered by the American Heart Association to be the drug of choice in the treatment and prevention of streptococcal pharyngitis and in long-term prophylaxis of rheumatic fever.

When oral medication is preferred for treatment of the above conditions, penicillin G, V, or erythromycin are alternate drugs of choice.

Staphylococcus aureus: Acute infections of skin and soft tissue of mild to moderate severity. Resistant organisms may emerge during treatment.

Streptococcus pneumoniae (Diplococcus pneumoniae): For upper respiratory tract infections (e.g., otitis media, pharyngitis) and lower respiratory tract infections (e.g., pneumonia) of mild to moderate severity.

Mycoplasma pneumoniae (Eaton agent, PPLO): For respiratory infections due to this organism.

Hemophilus influenzae: For upper respiratory tract infections of mild to moderate severity when used concomitantly with adequate doses of sulfonamides. (See sulfonamide labeling for appropriate prescribing information). The concomitant use of the sulfonamides is necessary since not all strains of *Hemophilus influenzae* are susceptible to erythromycin at the concentrations of the antibiotic achieved with usual therapeutic doses.

Corynebacterium diphtheriae: As an adjunct to antitoxin, to prevent the establishment of carriers, and to eradicate the organism in carriers.

Corynebacterium minutissimum: In the treatment of erythrasma.

Listeria monocytogenes: Infections due to this organism.

Neisseria gonorrhoeae: ERYTHROCIN PIGGYBACK in conjunction with erythromycin stearate or base orally, as an alternative drug in treatment of acute pelvic inflammatory disease caused by *N. gonorrhoeae* in female patients with a history of sensitivity to penicillin. Before treatment of gonorrhea, patients who are suspected of also having syphilis should have a microscopic examination for *T. pallidum* (by immunofluorescence or darkfield) before receiving erythromycin, and monthly serologic tests for a minimum of 4 months.

Legionnaires' Disease: Although no controlled clinical efficacy studies have been conducted, *in vitro* and limited preliminary clinical data suggest that erythromycin may be effective in treating Legionnaires' Disease.

Contraindications: Erythromycin is contraindicated in patients with known hypersensitivity to this antibiotic.

Precautions: Since erythromycin is principally excreted by the liver, caution should be exercised when erythromycin is administered to patients with impaired hepatic function.

Prolonged or repeated use of erythromycin may result in an overgrowth of nonsusceptible bacteria or fungi. If superinfection occurs, erythromycin should be discontinued and appropriate therapy instituted.

Areas of localized infection may require surgical drainage in addition to antibiotic therapy.

Recent data from studies of erythromycin reveal that its use in patients who are receiving high doses of theophylline may be associated with an increase of serum theophylline levels and potential theophylline toxicity. In case of theophylline toxicity and/or elevated serum theophylline levels, the dose of theophylline should be reduced while the patient is receiving concomitant erythromycin therapy.

Usage during pregnancy and lactation: The safety of erythromycin for use during pregnancy has not been established.

Erythromycin crosses the placental barrier. Erythromycin also appears in breast milk.

Adverse Reactions: Side effects following the use of intravenous erythromycin are rare. Occasional venous irritation has been encountered.

Allergic reactions, ranging from urticaria and mild skin eruptions to anaphylaxis, have occurred with intravenously administered erythromycin. Reversible hearing loss associated with the intravenous infusion of 4 g or more per day of erythromycin lactobionate has been reported rarely.

Dosage and Administration: For the treatment of severe infections in adults and children, the recommended intravenous dose of erythromycin lactobionate is 15 to 20 mg/kg/day. Higher doses, up to 4 g/day, may be given for very severe infections. ERYTHROCIN PIGGYBACK should be administered by intravenous infusion. Due to the high concentration of erythromycin, I.V. push is not an acceptable route of administration. Intravenous erythromycin should be replaced by oral erythromycin as soon as possible.

After reconstitution each ml of ERYTHROCIN PIGGYBACK solution contains 5 mg of erythromycin activity (500 mg in 100 ml). The drug may be administered directly from the vial. When this preparation is administered by intermittent infusion one-fourth the total daily dose of erythromycin lactobionate should be administered over a 20 to 60 minute period at intervals not greater than every 6 hours. The infusion should be sufficiently slow to minimize pain along the vein.

For treatment of acute pelvic inflammatory disease caused by *N. gonorrhoeae*, in female patients hypersensitive to penicillins, administer 500 mg erythromycin lactobionate every 6 hours for 3 days, followed by oral administration of 250 mg erythromycin stearate or base every 6 hours for 7 days.

For treatment of Legionnaires' Disease: Although optimal doses have not been established, doses utilized in reported clinical data were 1 to 4 grams daily in divided doses.

Preparation of Solution: Prepare the ERYTHROCIN PIGGYBACK solution by adding 100 ml of 0.9% Sodium Chloride Injection, USP, or Lactated Ringer's Injection, USP, or Normosol®-R Solution to the dispensing vial. Immediately after adding diluent, the product should be shaken well to aid dissolution. Lack of immediate agitation will greatly increase time required for complete dissolution. Reconstitution may also be made using 100 ml of the following solutions to which 1 ml of Neut® (4% sodium bicarbonate, Abbott) has first been added:

5% Dextrose Injection, USP
5% Dextrose and Lactated Ringer's Injection
5% Dextrose and 0.9% Sodium Chloride Injection, USP
Normosol®-M and 5% Dextrose Injection
Normosol®-R and 5% Dextrose Injection

Neut® (4% sodium bicarbonate, Abbott) must be added to these solutions so that their pH is in the optimum range for erythromycin lactobionate stability. Acidic solutions of erythromycin lactobionate are unstable and lose their potency rapidly. A pH of at least 5.5 is desirable.

No drug or chemical agent should be added to an erythromycin lactobionate-I.V. fluid admixture unless its effect on the chemical and physical stability of the solution has first been determined.

Stability: The solution should be used within 8 hours if stored at room temperature and 24 hours if stored in the refrigerator. If the solution is to be frozen, it should be frozen ($-10°C$ to $-20°C$) within 4 hours of preparation. Frozen solution may be stored for 30 days. Frozen solution should be thawed in the refrigerator and used within 8 hours after thawing is completed. THAWED SOLUTION MUST NOT BE REFROZEN.

How Supplied: ERYTHROCIN PIGGYBACK (erythromycin lactobionate for injection, USP) is supplied as a sterile, lyophilized powder in packages of 5 single dose dispensing vials (**NDC** 0074-6368-13). Each vial contains the equivalent of 500 mg of erythromycin with 90 mg of benzyl alcohol.

Shown in Product Identification Section, page 403
Abbott Laboratories
North Chicago, IL 60064
Ref. 01-2161-R4

ERYTHROCIN® STEARATE ℞
[e-ry' thrō-sin]
(erythromycin stearate tablets, USP)
Filmtab® Tablets

Description: Erythromycin is produced by a strain of *Streptomyces erythraeus* and belongs to the macrolide group of antibiotics. It is basic and readily forms salts with acids. The base, the stearate salt, and the esters are poorly soluble in water, and are suitable for oral administration.

ERYTHROCIN STEARATE Filmtab tablets contain the stearate salt of the antibiotic in a unique film coating.

Actions: Microbiology: Biochemical tests demonstrate that erythromycin inhibits protein synthesis of the pathogen without directly affecting nucleic acid synthesis. Antagonism has been demonstrated between clindamycin and erythromycin. NOTE: Many strains of *Hemophilus influenzae* are resistant to erythromycin alone, but are susceptible to erythromycin and sulfonamides together. Staphylococci resistant to erythromycin may emerge during a course of erythromycin therapy. Culture and susceptibility testing should be performed.

Disc Susceptibility Tests: Quantitative methods that require measurement of zone diameters give the most precise estimates of antibiotic susceptibility. One recommended procedure (21 CFR section 460.1) uses erythromycin class discs for testing susceptibility; interpretations correlate zone diameters of this disc test with MIC values for erythromycin. With this procedure, a report from the laboratory of "susceptible" indicates that the infecting organism is likely to respond to therapy. A report of "resistant" indicates that the infective organism is not likely to respond to therapy. A report of "intermediate susceptibility" suggests that the organism would be susceptible if higher doses were used.

Clinical Pharmacology: Erythromycin binds to the 50 S ribosomal subunits of susceptible bacteria and suppresses protein synthesis.

Orally administered ERYTHROCIN STEARATE tablets are readily and reliably absorbed. Optimal serum levels of erythromycin are reached when the drug is taken in the fasting state or immediately before meals.

Erythromycin diffuses readily into most body fluids. Only low concentrations are normally achieved in the spinal fluid, but passage of the drug across the blood-brain barrier increases in meningitis. In the presence of normal hepatic function, erythromycin is concentrated in the liver and excreted in the bile; the effect of hepatic dysfunction on excretion of erythromycin by the liver into the bile is not known. Less than 5 percent of the orally administered dose of erythromycin is excreted in active form in the urine.

Erythromycin crosses the placental barrier and is excreted in breast milk.

Indications: *Streptococcus pyogenes* (Group A beta-hemolytic streptococcus): Upper and lower respiratory tract, skin, and soft tissue infections of mild to moderate severity.

Injectable benzathine penicillin G is considered by the American Heart Association to be the drug of choice in the treatment and prevention of streptococcal pharyngitis and in long-term prophylaxis of rheumatic fever.

When oral medication is preferred for treatment of the above conditions, penicillin G, V, or erythromycin are alternate drugs of choice.

When oral medication is given, the importance of strict adherence by the patient to the prescribed dosage regimen must be stressed. A therapeutic dose should be administered for at least 10 days.

Alpha-hemolytic streptococci (viridans group): Although no controlled clinical efficacy trials have been conducted, oral erythromycin has been sug-

Continued on next page

If desired, additional literature on any Abbott Product will be provided upon request to Abbott Laboratories.

Abbott—Cont.

gested by the American Heart Association and American Dental Association for use in a regimen for prophylaxis against bacterial endocarditis in patients hypersensitive to penicillin who have congenital heart disease, or rheumatic or other acquired valvular heart disease when they undergo dental procedures and surgical procedures of the upper respiratory tract.[1] Erythromycin is not suitable prior to genitourinary or gastrointestinal tract surgery. NOTE: When selecting antibiotics for the prevention of bacterial endocarditis the physician or dentist should read the full joint statement of the American Heart Association and the American Dental Association.[1]

Staphylococcus aureus: Acute infections of skin and soft tissue of mild to moderate severity. Resistant organisms may emerge during treatment.

Streptococcus pneumoniae (Diplococcus pneumoniae): Upper respiratory tract infections (e.g., otitis media, pharyngitis) and lower respiratory tract infections (e.g., pneumonia) of mild to moderate degree.

Mycoplasma pneumoniae (Eaton agent, PPLO): For respiratory infections due to this organism.

Hemophilus influenzae: For upper respiratory tract infections of mild to moderate severity when used concomitantly with adequate doses of sulfonamides. (See sulfonamide labeling for appropriate prescribing information). The concomitant use of the sulfonamides is necessary since not all strains of *Hemophilus influenzae* are susceptible to erythromycin at the concentrations of the antibiotic achieved with usual therapeutic doses.

Chlamydia trachomatis: Erythromycin is indicated for treatment of the following infections caused by *Chlamydia trachomatis:* conjunctivitis of the newborn, pneumonia of infancy and urogenital infections during pregnancy. When tetracyclines are contraindicated or not tolerated, erythromycin is indicated for the treatment of uncomplicated urethral, endocervical, or rectal infections in adults due to *Chlamydia trachomatis.*[2]

Treponema pallidum: Erythromycin is an alternate choice of treatment for primary syphilis in patients allergic to the penicillins. In treatment of primary syphilis, spinal fluid examinations should be done before treatment and as part of follow-up after therapy.

Corynebacterium diphtheriae: As an adjunct to antitoxin, to prevent establishment of carriers, and to eradicate the organism in carriers.

Corynebacterium minutissimum: For the treatment of erythrasma.

Entamoeba histolytica: In the treatment of intestinal amebiasis only. Extra-enteric amebiasis requires treatment with other agents.

Listeria monocytogenes: Infections due to this organism.

Neisseria gonorrhoeae: Erythrocin Lactobionate-I.V. (erythromycin lactobionate for injection) in conjunction with erythromycin stearate orally, as an alternative drug in treatment of acute pelvic inflammatory disease caused by *N. gonorrhoeae* in female patients with a history of sensitivity to penicillin. Before treatment of gonorrhea, patients who are suspected of also having syphilis should have a microscopic examination for *T. pallidum* (by immunofluorescence or darkfield) before receiving erythromycin, and monthly serologic tests for a minimum of 4 months.

Bordetella pertussis: Erythromycin is effective in eliminating the organism from the nasopharynx of infected individuals, rendering them non-infectious. Some clinical studies suggest that erythromycin may be helpful in the prophylaxis of pertussis in exposed susceptible individuals.

Legionnaires' Disease: Although no controlled clinical efficacy studies have been conducted, *in vitro* and limited preliminary clinical data suggest that erythromycin may be effective in treating Legionnaires' Disease.

Contraindications: Erythromycin is contraindicated in patients with known hypersensitivity to this antibiotic.

Precautions: Erythromycin is principally excreted by the liver. Caution should be exercised in administering the antibiotic to patients with impaired hepatic function. There have been reports of hepatic dysfunction, with or without jaundice occurring in patients receiving oral erythromycin products.

Areas of localized infection may require surgical drainage in addition to antibiotic therapy.

Recent data from studies of erythromycin reveal that its use in patients who are receiving high doses of theophylline may be associated with an increase of serum theophylline levels and potential theophylline toxicity. In case of theophylline toxicity and/or elevated serum theophylline levels, the dose of theophylline should be reduced while the patient is receiving concomitant erythromycin therapy.

Usage during pregnancy and lactation: The safety of erythromycin for use during pregnancy has not been established.

Erythromycin crosses the placental barrier. Erythromycin also appears in breast milk.

Adverse Reactions: The most frequent side effects of oral erythromycin preparations are gastrointestinal, such as abdominal cramping and discomfort, and are dose-related. Nausea, vomiting, and diarrhea occur infrequently with usual oral doses.

During prolonged or repeated therapy, there is a possibility of overgrowth of nonsusceptible bacteria or fungi. If such infections occur, the drug should be discontinued and appropriate therapy instituted.

Allergic reactions ranging from urticaria and mild skin eruptions to anaphylaxis have occurred.

There have been isolated reports of reversible hearing loss occurring chiefly in patients with renal insufficiency and in patients receiving high doses of erythromycin.

Dosage and Administration: Optimal serum levels of erythromycin are reached when ERYTHROCIN STEARATE (erythromycin stearate) is taken in the fasting state or immediately before meals.

Adults: The usual dosage is 250 mg every 6 hours; or 500 mg every 12 hours, taken in the fasting state or immediately before meals. Up to 4 g per day may be administered, depending upon the severity of the infection.

Children: Age, weight, and severity of the infection are important factors in determining the proper dosage. For the treatment of mild to moderate infections, the usual dosage is 30 to 50 mg/kg/day in 3 or 4 divided doses. When dosage is desired on a twice-a-day schedule, one-half of the total daily dose may be taken every 12 hours in the fasting state or immediately before meals. For the treatment of more severe infections the total daily dose may be doubled.

In the treatment of streptococcal infections, a therapeutic dosage of erythromycin should be administered for at least 10 days. In continuous prophylaxis of streptococcal infections in persons with a history of rheumatic heart disease, the dose is 250 mg twice a day.

For prophylaxis against bacterial endocarditis[1] in patients with congenital heart disease, or rheumatic or other acquired valvular heart disease when undergoing dental procedures or surgical procedures of the upper respiratory tract, give 1 g (20 mg/kg for children) orally 1½ to 2 hours before the procedure, and then, 500 mg (10 mg/kg for children) orally every 6 hours for 8 doses.

For conjunctivitis of the newborn caused by *Chlamydia trachomatis:* Oral erythromycin suspension 50 mg/kg/day in 4 divided doses for at least 2 weeks.[2]

For pneumonia of infancy caused by *Chlamydia trachomatis:* Although the optimal duration of therapy has not been established, the recommended therapy is oral erythromycin suspension 50 mg/kg/day in 4 divided doses for at least 3 weeks.[2]

For urogenital infections during pregnancy due to *Chlamydia trachomatis:* Although the optimal dose and duration of therapy have not been established, the suggested treatment is erythromycin 500 mg, by mouth, 4 times a day on an empty stomach for at least 7 days. For women who cannot tolerate this regimen, a decreased dose of 250 mg, by mouth, 4 times a day should be used for at least 14 days.[2]

For adults with uncomplicated urethral, endocervical, or rectal infections caused by *Chlamydia trachomatis* in whom tetracyclines are contraindicated or not tolerated: 500 mg, by mouth, 4 times a day for at least 7 days.[2]

For treatment of primary syphilis: 30 to 40 g given in divided doses over a period of 10 to 15 days.

For treatment of acute pelvic inflammatory disease caused by *N. gonorrhoeae:* 500 mg Erythrocin Lactobionate-I.V. (erythromycin lactobionate for injection) every 6 hours for 3 days, followed by 250 mg ERYTHROCIN STEARATE every 6 hours for 7 days.

For intestinal amebiasis: Adults: 250 mg four times daily for 10 to 14 days. Children: 30 to 50 mg/kg/day in divided doses for 10 to 14 days.

For use in pertussis: Although optimal dosage and duration have not been established, doses of erythromycin utilized in reported clinical studies were 40 to 50 mg/kg/day, given in divided doses for 5 to 14 days.

For treatment of Legionnaires' Disease: Although optimal doses have not been established, doses utilized in reported clinical data were 1 to 4 g daily in divided doses.

How Supplied: ERYTHROCIN STEARATE Filmtab Tablets (erythromycin stearate tablets, USP) are supplied as:

Erythrocin Stearate Filmtab, 250 mg
Bottles of 20......................................(NDC 0074-6346-23)
Bottles of 100....................................(NDC 0074-6346-20)
Bottles of 500....................................(NDC 0074-6346-53)
ABBO-PAC® unit dose strip packages of
100 tablets..(NDC 0074-6346-38)

Erythrocin Stearate Filmtab, 500 mg
Bottles of 100....................................(NDC 0074-6316-13)

References: 1. American Heart Association. 1977. Prevention of bacterial endocarditis. Circulation 56: 139A-143A.
2. CDC Sexually Transmitted Diseases Treatment Guidelines 1982.

FILMTAB—Film-sealed tablets, Abbott
Shown in Product Identification Section, page 403
Abbott Laboratories
North Chicago, IL 60064
Ref: 07-5266-R7

ERYTHROMYCIN BASE FILMTAB® ℞
[*e-ri-thrō-mī' sin*]
(erythromycin tablets, USP)

Description: Erythromycin is produced by a strain of *Streptomyces erythraeus* and belongs to the macrolide group of antibiotics. It is basic and readily forms salts with acids. The base, the stearate salt, and the esters are poorly soluble in water, and are suitable for oral administration.

ERYTHROMYCIN BASE FILMTAB tablets contain erythromycin, USP, in a unique, nonenteric film coating.

Actions: Microbiology: Biochemical tests demonstrate that erythromycin inhibits protein synthesis of the pathogen without directly affecting nucleic acid synthesis. Antagonism has been demonstrated between clindamycin and erythromycin. NOTE: Many strains of *Hemophilus influenzae* are resistant to erythromycin alone, but are susceptible to erythromycin and sulfonamides together. Staphylococci resistant to erythromycin may emerge during a course of erythromycin therapy. Culture and susceptibility testing should be performed.

Disc Susceptibility Tests: Quantitative methods that require measurement of zone diameters give the most precise estimates of antibiotic susceptibility. One recommended procedure (21 CFR section 460.1) uses erythromycin class discs for testing susceptibility; interpretations correlate zone diameters of this disc test with MIC values for erythromycin. With this procedure, a report from the laboratory of "susceptible" indicates that the infecting organism is likely to respond to therapy. A report of "resistant" indicates that the infective organism is not likely to respond to therapy. A report of "intermediate susceptibility" suggests that the organism would be susceptible if higher doses were used.

Clinical Pharmacology: Erythromycin binds to the 50 S ribosomal subunits of susceptible bacteria and suppresses protein synthesis.

Orally administered erythromycin is readily absorbed by most patients, especially on an empty stomach, but patient variation is observed. Due to its formulation and nonenteric coating, this erythromycin tablet gives reliable blood levels in the average subject; however, the levels may vary with the individual.

Erythromycin diffuses readily into most body fluids. Only low concentrations are normally achieved in the spinal fluid, but passage of the drug across the blood-brain barrier increases in meningitis. In the presence of normal hepatic function, erythromycin is concentrated in the liver and excreted in the bile; the effect of hepatic dysfunction on excretion of erythromycin by the liver into the bile is not known. Less than 5 percent of the orally administered dose of erythromycin is excreted in active form in the urine.

Erythromycin crosses the placental barrier and is excreted in breast milk.

Indications: *Streptococcus pyogenes* (Group A beta-hemolytic streptococcus): Upper and lower respiratory tract, skin, and soft tissue infections of mild to moderate severity.

Injectable benzathine penicillin G is considered by the American Heart Association to be the drug of choice in the treatment and prevention of streptococcal pharyngitis and in long-term prophylaxis of rheumatic fever.

When oral medication is preferred for treatment of the above conditions, penicillin G, V, or erythromycin are alternate drugs of choice.

When oral medication is given, the importance of strict adherence by the patient to the prescribed dosage regimen must be stressed. A therapeutic dose should be administered for at least 10 days.

Alpha-hemolytic streptococci (viridans group): Although no controlled clinical efficacy trials have been conducted, oral erythromycin has been suggested by the American Heart Association and American Dental Association for use in a regimen for prophylaxis against bacterial endocarditis in patients hypersensitive to penicillin who have congenital heart disease, or rheumatic or other acquired valvular heart disease when they undergo dental procedures and surgical procedures of the upper respiratory tract.[1] Erythromycin is not suitable prior to genitourinary or gastrointestinal tract surgery. NOTE: When selecting antibiotics for the prevention of bacterial endocarditis the physician or dentist should read the full joint statement of the American Heart Association and the American Dental Association.[1]

Staphylococcus aureus: Acute infections of skin and soft tissue of mild to moderate severity. Resistant organisms may emerge during treatment.

Streptococcus pneumoniae (Diplococcus pneumoniae): Upper respiratory tract infections (e.g., otitis media, pharyngitis) and lower respiratory tract infections (e.g., pneumonia) of mild to moderate degree.

Mycoplasma pneumoniae (Eaton agent, PPLO): For respiratory infections due to this organism.

Hemophilus influenzae: For upper respiratory tract infections of mild to moderate severity when used concomitantly with adequate doses of sulfonamides. (See sulfonamide labeling for appropriate prescribing information). The concomitant use of the sulfonamides is necessary since not all strains of *Hemophilus influenzae* are susceptible to erythromycin at the concentrations of the antibiotic achieved with usual therapeutic doses.

Chlamydia trachomatis: Erythromycin is indicated for treatment of the following infections caused by *Chlamydia trachomatis:* conjunctivitis of the newborn, pneumonia of infancy and urogenital infections during pregnancy. When tetracyclines are contraindicated or not tolerated, erythromycin is indicated for the treatment of uncomplicated urethral, endocervical, or rectal infections in adults due to *Chlamydia trachomatis.*[2]

Treponema pallidum: Erythromycin is an alternate choice of treatment for primary syphilis in patients allergic to the penicillins. In treatment of primary syphilis, spinal fluid examinations should be done before treatment and as part of follow-up after therapy.

Corynebacterium diphtheriae: As an adjunct to antitoxin, to prevent establishment of carriers, and to eradicate the organism in carriers.

Corynebacterium minutissimum: For the treatment of erythrasma.

Entamoeba histolytica: In the treatment of intestinal amebiasis only. Extra-enteric amebiasis requires treatment with other agents.

Listeria monocytogenes: Infections due to this organism.

Neisseria gonorrhoeae: Erythrocin® Lactobionate-I.V. (erythromycin lactobionate for injection) in conjunction with erythromycin base orally, as an alternative drug in treatment of acute pelvic inflammatory disease caused by *N. gonorrhoeae* in female patients with a history of sensitivity to penicillin. Before treatment of gonorrhea, patients who are suspected of also having syphilis should have a microscopic examination for *T. pallidum* (by immunofluorescence or darkfield) before receiving erythromycin, and monthly serologic tests for a minimum of 4 months.

Bordetella pertussis: Erythromycin is effective in eliminating the organism from the nasopharynx of infected individuals, rendering them non-infectious. Some clinical studies suggest that erythromycin may be helpful in the prophylaxis of pertussis in exposed susceptible individuals.

Legionnaires' Disease: Although no controlled clinical efficacy studies have been conducted, *in vitro* and limited preliminary clinical data suggest that erythromycin may be effective in treating Legionnaires' Disease.

Contraindications: Erythromycin is contraindicated in patients with known hypersensitivity to this antibiotic.

Precautions: Erythromycin is principally excreted by the liver. Caution should be exercised in administering the antibiotic to patients with impaired hepatic function. There have been reports of hepatic dysfunction, with or without jaundice occurring in patients receiving oral erythromycin products.

Areas of localized infection may require surgical drainage in addition to antibiotic therapy.

Recent data from studies of erythromycin reveal that its use in patients who are receiving high doses of theophylline may be associated with an increase of serum theophylline levels and potential theophylline toxicity. In case of theophylline toxicity and/or elevated serum theophylline levels, the dose of theophylline should be reduced while the patient is receiving concomitant erythromycin therapy.

Usage during pregnancy and lactation: The safety of erythromycin for use during pregnancy has not been established.

Erythromycin crosses the placental barrier. Erythromycin also appears in breast milk.

Adverse Reactions: The most frequent side effects of oral erythromycin preparations are gastrointestinal, such as abdominal cramping and discomfort, and are dose-related. Nausea, vomiting, and diarrhea occur infrequently with usual oral doses.

During prolonged or repeated therapy, there is a possibility of overgrowth of nonsusceptible bacteria or fungi. If such infections occur, the drug should be discontinued and appropriate therapy instituted.

Allergic reactions ranging from urticaria and mild skin eruptions to anaphylaxis have occurred.

There have been isolated reports of reversible hearing loss occurring chiefly in patients with renal insufficiency and in patients receiving high doses of erythromycin.

Dosage and Administration: Optimum blood levels are obtained when doses are given on an empty stomach.

Adults: 250 mg every 6 hours is the usual dose; or 500 mg every 12 hours one hour before meals. Dosage may be increased up to 4 g per day according to the severity of the infection.

Children: Age, weight, and severity of the infection are important factors in determining the proper dosage. 30 to 50 mg/kg/day, in divided doses, is the usual dose. For more severe infections this dose may be doubled. If dosage is desired on a twice-a-day schedule, one-half of the total daily dose may be given every 12 hours, one hour before meals.

For the treatment of streptococcal infections: a therapeutic dosage should be administered for at least 10 days. In continuous prophylaxis of streptococcal infections in persons with rheumatic heart disease history, the dose is 250 mg twice a day.

For prophylaxis against bacterial endocarditis[1] in patients with congenital heart disease, or rheumatic or other acquired valvular heart disease when undergoing dental procedures or surgical procedures of the upper respiratory tract, give 1 g (20 mg/kg for children) orally 1½ to 2 hours before the procedure, and then, 500 mg (10 mg/kg for children) orally every 6 hours for 8 doses.

For conjunctivitis of the newborn caused by *Chlamydia trachomatis:* Oral erythromycin suspension 50 mg/kg/day in 4 divided doses for at least 2 weeks.[2]

For pneumonia of infancy caused by *Chlamydia trachomatis:* Although the optimal duration of therapy has not been established, the recommended therapy is oral erythromycin suspension 50 mg/kg/day in 4 divided doses for at least 3 weeks.[2]

For urogenital infections during pregnancy due to *Chlamydia trachomatis:* Although the optimal dose and duration of therapy have not been established, the suggested treatment is erythromycin 500 mg, by mouth, 4 times a day on an empty stomach for at least 7 days. For women who cannot tolerate this regimen, a decreased dose of 250 mg, by mouth 4 times a day should be used for at least 14 days.[2]

For adults with uncomplicated urethral, endocervical, or rectal infections caused by *Chlamydia trachomatis* in whom tetracyclines are contraindicated or not tolerated: 500 mg, by mouth, 4 times a day for at least 7 days.[2]

For treatment of primary syphilis: 30 to 40 g given in divided doses over a period of 10 to 15 days.

For treatment of acute pelvic inflammatory disease caused by *N. gonorrhoeae:* 500 mg Erythrocin Lactobionate-I.V. (erythromycin lactobionate for injection) every 6 hours for 3 days, followed by 250 mg erythromycin base every 6 hours for 7 days.

For intestinal amebiasis: Adults: 250 mg four times daily for 10 to 14 days. Children: 30 to 50 mg/kg/day in divided doses for 10 to 14 days.

For use in pertussis: Although optimal dosage and duration have not been established, doses of erythromycin utilized in reported clinical studies were 40 to 50 mg/kg/day, given in divided doses for 5 to 14 days.

For treatment of Legionnaires' Disease: Although optimal doses have not been established, doses utilized in reported clinical data were 1 to 4 g daily in divided doses.

How Supplied: ERYTHROMYCIN BASE FILMTAB tablets (erythromycin tablets, USP) are supplied as pink capsule-shaped tablets in two dosage strengths:

250 mg tablets:
Bottles of 100 ....(NDC 0074-6326-13)
ABBO-PAC® unit dose strip packages of
100 tablets................................(NDC 0074-6326-11)
500 mg tablets:
Bottles of 100 ....(NDC 0074-6227-13).
References: 1. American Heart Association. 1977. Prevention of bacterial endocarditis. Circulation. 56: 139A-143A.

Continued on next page

If desired, additional literature on any Abbott Product will be provided upon request to Abbott Laboratories.

Abbott—Cont.

2. CDC Sexually Transmitted Diseases Treatment Guidelines 1982.

FILMTAB—Film-sealed tablets, Abbott.
Shown in Product Identification Section, page 403
Abbott Laboratories
North Chicago, IL 60064
Ref: 01-2288-R8

EUTONYL® Filmtab® Tablets ℞
(pargyline hydrochloride tablets, USP)

Description: EUTONYL (pargyline hydrochloride) is a non-hydrazine monoamine oxidase (MAO) inhibitor with hypotensive activity and is chemically identified as N-methyl-N-2-propynylbenzylamine hydrochloride. Clinically, EUTONYL is an effective oral antihypertensive agent which is primarily useful in the treatment of moderate to severe hypertension. EUTONYL is available as Filmtab tablets in two strengths containing 10 mg or 25 mg of pargyline hydrochloride.

Clinical Pharmacology: EUTONYL is a MAO inhibitor which has a potent antihypertensive action. Its exact mode of action is uncertain. The antihypertensive effect of pargyline is greatest when the patient is in the standing position. In about half of the patients treated, reduction of blood pressure in the sitting and supine positions was nearly as great as in the standing position. An interval of four days to three weeks or more may elapse following initiation of therapy before the full therapeutic effects of a given dosage schedule become manifest. A similar interval may be required for effects to subside after withdrawal of the drug, because the termination of drug effect is dependent on the regeneration of inhibited enzymes.

Information is limited on human pharmacokinetics for pargyline hydrochloride. It is extensively metabolized in the liver. The metabolites N-methyl benzylamine and propioladehyde have been identified. Pargyline passes the blood-brain barrier in rats and has been found in most tissues. In humans less than one percent of a given dose is excreted unchanged in the urine. Studies in the dog indicate that metabolic products are extensively eliminated in the urine.

Indications and Usage: EUTONYL is indicated in the treatment of moderate to severe hypertension. *It is not recommended for use in patients with mild or labile hypertension.* EUTONYL does not interfere with or obviate the use of diuretic therapy in hypertensive patients who may have an associated edema.

EUTONYL may be used alone or concurrently with most other antihypertensive agents. It is often effective at reduced dosage when administered with one of the thiazides and/or rauwolfia alkaloids.

Contraindications: EUTONYL (pargyline hydrochloride) is contraindicated in patients with pheochromocytoma, paranoid schizophrenia, hyperthyroidism, and advanced renal failure.

EUTONYL should not be administered to those with malignant hypertension or to children under twelve years of age because significant clinical information concerning the use of the drug in these conditions is not available.

In general, the following drugs or agents are contraindicated in patients receiving EUTONYL due to the possibility of precipitating a sudden rise in blood pressure, including hypertensive crisis (see "Warnings" section):

Centrally acting sympathomimetic amines such as amphetamine and related compounds (includes most anorectic agents).

Peripherally acting sympathomimetic drugs such as ephedrine and its derivatives (also found in nasal decongestants, cold remedies, and hay fever preparations).

In some patients receiving pargyline, tyramine may precipitate an abrupt rise in blood pressure, including hypertensive crisis. Therefore, aged cheese (e.g., Cheddar, Camembert, and Stilton), processed cheese, beer and wine (especially, Chianti wine), and other foods require the action of bacteria or molds for their preparation or preservation because of the presence of pressor substances such as tyramine should be avoided. Other foods which should be avoided during pargyline therapy because of their high pressor amine content include chocolate, yeast extract, avocado, pickled herring, pods of broad beans, ripened bananas, papaya products (including certain meat tenderizers), and chicken livers. Cream cheese, ricotta, and cottage cheese can be allowed in the diet during pargyline therapy since tyramine content is inconsequential.

Parenteral reserpine or guanethidine. Parenteral use of these drugs in patients receiving monoamine oxidase inhibitors results in a sudden release of accumulated catecholamines which may cause a hypertensive reaction. Reserpine and guanethidine should not be given parenterally during, and for at least one week following, treatment with pargyline.

Imipramine, amitriptyline, desipramine, nortriptyline, protriptyline, doxepin, or their analogues. The use of these drugs with a monoamine oxidase inhibitor has been reported to cause vascular collapse and hyperthermia which may be fatal. A drug-free interval (about two weeks) should separate therapy bun with EUTONYL (pargyline hydrochloride) and use of these agents.

Other monoamine oxidase inhibitors. These may augment the effects of pargyline.

Methyldopa or dopamine. These drugs may cause hyperexcitability in patients receiving pargyline.

L-dopa. There have been several reports of potentiation of the pressor effects of this drug by various monoamine oxidase inhibitors. At least one month should elapse after the discontinuation of pargyline before L-dopa is given.

Warnings: The most serious reactions to EUTONYL involve changes in blood pressure.

Hypertensive Crises: The most important reaction associated with EUTONYL administration is the occurrence of hypertensive crises precipitated by its interaction with numerous drug and food substances (see "Contraindications" and "Precautions" sections). These reactions have sometimes been fatal.

These crises are characterized by some or all of the following symptoms: occipital headache which may radiate frontally, palpitation, neck stiffness or soreness, nausea, vomiting, sweating (sometimes with fever and sometimes with cold, clammy skin), dilated pupils, photophobia, visual disturbances, stertorous breathing and coma. Either tachycardia or bradycardia may be present and can be associated with constricting chest pain.

NOTE: Intracranial bleeding has been reported in association with the increase in blood pressure. Blood pressure should be observed frequently to detect evidence of any pressor response in all patients receiving EUTONYL. Therapy should be discontinued immediately upon the occurrence of palpitation or frequent headaches during therapy.

Recommended Treatment in Hypertensive Crisis: If a hypertensive crisis occurs, EUTONYL should be discontinued and therapy to lower blood pressure should be instituted immediately. Headache tends to abate as blood pressure is lowered. On the basis of present evidence, phentolamine is recommended. (The dosage reported for phentolamine is 5 mg. I.V.). Care should be taken to administer this drug slowly in order to avoid producing an excessive hypotensive effect. Fever should be managed by means of external cooling. Other symptomatic and supportive measures may be desirable in particular cases. Do not use parenteral reserpine.

Precautions:
General: All patients with impaired circulation to vital organs from any cause including those with angina pectoris, coronary artery disease, and cerebral arteriosclerosis should be closely observed for symptoms of orthostatic hypotension. If hypotension develops in these patients, EUTONYL (pargyline hydrochloride) dosage should be reduced or therapy discontinued since severe and/or prolonged hypotension may precipitate cerebral or coronary vessel thrombosis.

The hypotensive effect of EUTONYL may be augmented by febrile illnesses. It may be advisable to withdraw the drug during such diseases.

Care should be exercised in using EUTONYL in patients with impaired renal function. Since pargyline is excreted primarily in the urine, patients with impaired renal function may experience cumulative drug effects. Such patients should also be watched for elevations of blood urea nitrogen and other evidence of progressive renal failure. If such alterations should persist and progress, the drug should be discontinued.

EUTONYL should not be used in individuals with hyperactive or hyperexcitable personalities, as some of these patients show an undesirable increase in motor activity with restlessness, confusion, agitation, and disorientation. Clinical studies have shown that pargyline may unmask severe psychotic symptoms such as hallucinations or paranoid delusions in some patients with pre-existing serious emotional problems. This can usually be controlled by judicious administration of chlorpromazine intramuscularly, or other phenothiazines, the patient remaining supine for one hour after administration.

Pargyline should be used with caution in patients with Parkinsonism, as it may increase symptoms. In addition, great care is required if pargyline is administered in conjunction with anti-parkinsonian agents.

Documented cases of eye changes or optic atrophy have not been reported with the use of pargyline as they have with the use of certain other monoamine oxidase inhibitors. However, since nonspecific visual disturbances and aggravation of glaucoma have occurred occasionally, it is advisable that patients receiving EUTONYL be examined for changes in color perception, visual fields, fundi, and visual acuity.

The 25 mg dosage strength of EUTONYL tablets contains FD&C Yellow No. 5 (tartrazine) which may cause allergic-type reactions (including bronchial asthma) in certain susceptible individuals. Although the overall incidence of FD&C Yellow No. 5 (tartrazine) sensitivity in the general population is low, it is frequently seen in patients who also have aspirin hypersensitivity.

Information for Patients:
1. PATIENTS SHOULD BE WARNED AGAINST THE USE OF ANY OVER-THE-COUNTER PREPARATIONS, PARTICULARLY "COLD PREPARATIONS" AND ANTIHISTAMINES, OR PRESCRIPTION DRUGS WITHOUT THE KNOWLEDGE AND CONSENT OF THE PHYSICIAN.
2. PATIENTS SHOULD BE CAUTIONED ON THE USE OF CHEESE AND OTHER FOODS WITH HIGH TYRAMINE CONTENT (See "Contraindications" section) AND ALCOHOLIC BEVERAGES IN ANY FORM.
3. PATIENTS SHOULD BE WARNED ABOUT THE LIKELIHOOD OF THE OCCURRENCE OF ORTHOSTATIC HYPOTENSION.
4. PATIENTS SHOULD BE INSTRUCTED TO REPORT PROMPTLY THE OCCURRENCE OF SEVERE HEADACHE OR OTHER UNUSUAL SYMPTOMS.
5. PATIENTS WITH ANGINA PECTORIS OR CORONARY ARTERY DISEASE SHOULD BE ESPECIALLY WARNED NOT TO INCREASE THEIR PHYSICAL ACTIVITIES IN RESPONSE TO A DIMINUTION IN ANGINAL SYMPTOMS OR AN INCREASE IN WELL-BEING OCCURRING DURING TREATMENT WITH EUTONYL.

Laboratory Tests: There have been no substantiated reports of hepatotoxicity associated with pargyline therapy. However, since liver damage has resulted from use of certain other monoamine oxidase inhibitors, and since transient alterations in liver enzyme levels have occasionally occurred with pargyline, it is advisable that patients receiving EUTONYL (pargyline hydrochloride) have periodic liver function tests.

Drug Interactions: The therapeutic response to a variety of drugs may be changed or exaggerated in patients receiving a monoamine oxidase inhibitor such as pargyline hydrochloride. *Caffeine, alcohol, antihistamines, barbiturates, chloral hydrate* and other *hypnotics, sedatives, tranquilizers,* and *narcotics (meperidine* should not be used) should be used cautiously and at reduced dosage in patients who are taking pargyline. (See "Contraindications" section).

An increased response to *central depressants* may be manifested by acute hypotension and increased sedative effect. EUTONYL also may augment the hypotensive effects of anesthetic agents, and surgery. For this reason, the drug should be discontinued at least two weeks prior to surgery.

In the event of emergency surgery, ¼ to ⅕ of the usual dose of narcotics, sedatives, analgesics and other premedications should be used. If severe hypotension should occur, this can be controlled by small doses of a vasopressor agent such as norepinephrine.

EUTONYL may induce hypoglycemia. Therefore, EUTONYL should be given with caution to diabetics receiving *hypoglycemic agents* because severe hypoglycemia may occur. If it is necessary to administer EUTONYL to patients receiving insulin or other hypoglycemic agents, the dose of these agents should be reduced accordingly and the patient carefully monitored.

Clinical reports state that certain individuals receiving pargyline for a prolonged period of time are refractory to the nerve-blocking effects of *local anesthetics*, e.g., lidocaine.

Foods containing pressor substances, such as tyramine, should be avoided during pargyline therapy. (See "Contraindications" section).

Carcinogenesis, Mutagenesis, Impairment of Fertility: Adequate data are not available on long-term potential for carcinogenicity in animals or humans for pargyline hydrochloride.

The results of one study in which rats were injected with pargyline 15 mg/kg for ten days revealed seminiferous tubular degeneration with depletion of spermatogenic elements.

Pregnancy: Pregnancy Category C. Inadequate animal data is available to determine teratogenic potential for pargyline hydrochloride. However, limited studies reported in the literature indicate an embryocidal potential.

In one study, two groups of pregnant mice were given pargyline hydrochloride 2 mg/day subcutaneously during either early or late pregnancy. The results indicated that only three out of nineteen in the group treated during early pregnancy had normal litters. The remainder exhibited no signs of implantation. Four out of five litters in the group treated during late pregnancy were normal. In another study pregnant rats were injected intraamniotically with a single 2.8-4.6 mg/kg dose of pargyline hydrochloride during various stages of pregnancy. Fetal death was noted following pargyline injection during every stage of pregnancy.

One study has been reported in which the intraamniotic administration of 50 to 100 mg of EUTONYL produced abortion in 19 out of 20 pregnant human females during the tenth to twenty-fourth week of gestation.

There are no adequate and well-controlled studies of systemically administered EUTONYL in pregnant women. EUTONYL should be used during pregnancy only if the potential benefit justifies the potential risk to the fetus.

Nursing Mothers: It is not known whether this drug is excreted in human milk. Because many drugs are excreted in human milk and because of the potential for serious adverse reactions in nursing infants from EUTONYL, a decision should be made whether to discontinue nursing or to discontinue the drug, taking into account the importance of the drug to the mother.

Pediatric Use: Safety and effectiveness in children below the age of 12 years have not been established.

Adverse Reactions: Generally side effects are not severe or serious when the recommended dosages are used and necessary precautions are observed. If side effects are severe or persist the drug should be discontinued. See also "Warnings" and "Precautions" sections. The following adverse reactions are listed by order of decreasing severity within each category.

Cardiovascular: Hypertensive crisis has been precipitated by concurrent use of sympathomimetic drugs or foods containing tyramine. (See "Contraindications" and "Warnings" sections).

Congestive heart failure has been reported in patients with reduced cardiac reserve.

The most frequently occurring side effects are those associated with orthostatic hypotension (dizziness, weakness, palpitation, or fainting). These usually respond to a reduction of dosage. Patients should be warned against rising to a standing position too quickly, especially when getting out of bed. Severe and persistent orthostatic hypotension should be avoided by reduction in dosage or discontinuation of therapy.

Central Nervous System: Increased neuromuscular activity (muscle twitching) and other extrapyramidal symptoms have been reported. Hyperexcitability, insomnia and headache have also occurred.

Gastrointestinal: Vomiting, nausea, mild constipation, increased appetite and dry mouth.

Genitourinary: Difficulty in micturition, impotence and delayed ejaculation.

Dermatologic: Purpura, rash and sweating.

Miscellaneous: In some patients reduction of blood sugar has been noted. Although the significance of this has not been elucidated, the possibility of hypoglycemic effects should be borne in mind. Aggravation of glaucoma, blurred vision, fluid retention, arthralgia, drug fever (rare) and nightmares have been reported. Gain in weight may be due to either edema or increased appetite.

Overdosage: The characteristic symptoms that may be caused by overdosage are usually those described on the preceding pages.

However, an intensification of these symptoms and sometimes severe additional manifestations may be seen, depending on the degree of overdosage and on individual susceptibility. Some patients exhibit insomnia, restlessness and anxiety, progressing in severe cases to agitation, mental confusion and incoherence. Hypotension, dizziness, weakness and drowsiness may occur, progressing in severe cases to extreme dizziness and shock. A few patients have displayed hypertension with severe headache and other symptoms. Rare instances have been reported in which hypertension was accompanied by twitching or myoclonic fibrillation of skeletal muscles with hyperpyrexia, sometimes progressing to generalized rigidity and coma.

Gastric evacuation is helpful if performed early. Treatment should normally consist of general supportive measures, close observations of vital signs and steps to counteract specific symptoms as they occur, since MAO inhibition may persist. The management of hypertensive crises is described under Hypertensive Crises. (See "Warnings" section).

External cooling is recommended if hyperpyrexia occurs. Barbiturates have been reported to help relieve myoclonic reaction, but frequency of administration should be controlled carefully because EUTONYL (pargyline hydrochloride) may prolong barbiturate activity. When hypotension requires treatment, the standard measures for managing circulatory shock should be initiated. If pressor agents are used, the rate of infusion should be regulated by careful observation of the patient because an exaggerated pressor response sometimes occurs in the presence of MAO inhibition. Remember that the toxic effect of EUTONYL may be delayed or prolonged following the last dose of the drug. Therefore, the patient should be closely observed for at least a week.

Dosage and Administration: EUTONYL is orally administered as a single daily dose; there is no known advantage in prescribing the drug more frequently than once daily. Clinical response to the drug is not immediate. Four days to three weeks or more may be required to produce the full effects of a given daily dosage. *For this reason it is generally unwise to increase dosage more frequently than once a week.* Likewise the effects of the drug may persist following reduction of dosage or withdrawal. If therapy must be interrupted because of undesirable side-effects, the drug should be withheld until all such effects have disappeared. Therapy is then reinstituted at a lower dosage. Because the drug exerts an orthostatic effect on blood pressure, dosage adjustments should be based upon the blood pressure response *in the standing position.* The usual adult dosage for initiating therapy in hypertensive patients not receiving other antihypertensive agents is 25 mg once daily. This dosage may be increased once a week by 10 mg increments until the desired response is obtained. The total daily dose of pargyline should not exceed 200 mg if excessive side effects are to be avoided.

Patients over age 65, or those who have undergone sympathectomy may be unusually sensitive to the antihypertensive properties of the drug. In such patients the initial daily dosage should be 10 to 25 mg. When EUTONYL is added to an established antihypertensive regimen, the initial dose should not exceed 25 mg daily (less in sympathectomized or elderly patients).

EUTONYL should not be administered to children under 12 years of age because of limited experience with the drug in this group.

Reduction of blood pressure is often maintained in hypertensive patients with a daily dose of 25 to 50 mg of EUTONYL alone. Larger doses may be tried in resistant cases. In general, dosage should be kept at the minimum level required to maintain a desirable reduction in blood pressure without encountering undue side effects. A few patients may develop a relative tolerance to the antihypertensive effects of the drug. The administration of additional antihypertensive agents may be considered in cases not controlled by EUTONYL alone.

How Supplied: EUTONYL (pargyline hydrochloride tablets, USP) is available in Filmtab tablet strengths of 10 mg and 25 mg. The tablets are available in the following packages: 10 mg pink tablets in bottles of 100 (**NDC** 0074-6876-02) and 25 mg apricot-colored tablets in bottles of 100 (**NDC** 0074-6878-01).

Abbott Pharmaceuticals, Inc.
North Chicago, IL 60064

Shown in Product Identification Section, page 403

FERO–FOLIC–500® Filmtab® Tablets ℞
[fe'ro fo-lic]
Controlled-Release Iron with Folic Acid and Vitamin C

IBERET–FOLIC–500® Filmtab® ℞
Tablets
Controlled-Release Iron with Vitamin C, and B-Complex, including Folic Acid

Description: FERO-FOLIC-500 Filmtab is a hematinic for oral administration containing 525 mg of ferrous sulfate (equivalent to 105 mg of elemental iron) in a unique controlled-release vehicle, the Gradumet®. In addition, this product contains 800 mcg of folic acid and 500 mg of ascorbic acid present as sodium ascorbate.

IBERET-FOLIC-500 is an Abbott hematinic containing iron in the Gradumet® controlled-release vehicle; vitamin C for enhancement of iron absorption; and the B-Complex vitamins including folic acid. The IBERET-FOLIC-500 Filmtab is for oral use.

Each Filmtab tablet provides:
*Ferrous Sulfate ....525 mg
(equivalent to 105 mg of elemental iron)
Ascorbic Acid (present as
 sodium ascorbate) (C) ....500 mg
Niacinamide .... 30 mg
Calcium Pantothenate .... 10 mg
Thiamine Mononitrate (B_1) .... 6 mg
Riboflavin (B_2) .... 6 mg
Pyridoxine Hydrochloride (B_6) .... 5 mg
Folic Acid ....800 mcg

Continued on next page

If desired, additional literature on any Abbott Product will be provided upon request to Abbott Laboratories.

Abbott—Cont.

Cyanocobalamin (B$_{12}$) .... 25 mcg
*In controlled-release form (Gradumet)

Controlled-release of iron from the Gradumet protects against gastric side effects. The Gradumet is an inert, porous, plastic matrix which is impregnated with ferrous sulfate. Iron is leached from the Gradumet as it passes through the gastrointestinal tract, and the expended matrix is excreted harmlessly in the stool. Controlled-release iron is particularly helpful in patients who have demonstrated intolerance to oral iron preparations.

Clinical Pharmacology: Oral iron is absorbed most efficiently when it is administered between meals. Conventional iron preparations, however, frequently cause gastric irritation when taken on an empty stomach. Studies with iron in the Gradumet have indicated that relatively little of the iron is released in the stomach, gastric intolerance is seldom encountered, and hematologic response ranks with that obtained from plain ferrous sulfate.

Iron is found in the body principally as hemoglobin. Storage in the form of ferritin occurs in the liver, spleen, and bone marrow. Concentrations of plasma iron and the total iron-binding capacity of plasma vary greatly in different physiological conditions and disease states.

Large amounts of ascorbic acid administered orally with ferrous sulfate have been shown to enhance iron absorption. Apparently this is due to the ability of ascorbic acid to prevent the oxidation of ferrous iron to the less effectively absorbed ferric form.

Folic acid and iron are absorbed in the proximal small intestine, particularly the duodenum. Folic acid is absorbed maximally and rapidly at this site, and iron is absorbed in a descending gradient from the duodenum distally.

After absorption folic acid is rapidly converted into its metabolically active forms. Approximately two-thirds is bound to plasma protein. Half of the folic acid stored in the body is found in the liver. Folic acid is also concentrated in spinal fluid.

Except for the folates ingested in liver, yeast, and egg yolk, the percentage of absorption of food folates averages about 10%.

The B-complex vitamins in IBERET-FOLIC-500 are absorbed by the active transport process. B-complex vitamins are rapidly eliminated and therefore are not stored in the body.

Calcium pantothenate is absorbed readily from the gastrointestinal tract and distributed to all body tissues.

Indications and Usage: FERO-FOLIC-500 is indicated for the treatment of iron deficiency and prevention of concomitant folic acid deficiency in nonpregnant adults. FERO-FOLIC-500 is also indicated in pregnancy for the prevention and treatment of iron deficiency and to supply a maintenance dosage of folic acid.

IBERET-FOLIC-500 is indicated in non-pregnant adults for the treatment of iron deficiency and prevention of concomitant folic acid deficiency where there is an associated deficient intake or increased need for the B-complex vitamins. IBERET-FOLIC-500 is also indicated in pregnancy for the prevention and treatment of iron deficiency where there is a concomitant deficient intake or increased need for the B-complex vitamins (including folic acid).

Contraindications: FERO-FOLIC-500 and IBERET-FOLIC-500 are contraindicated in patients with pernicious anemia.

FERO-FOLIC-500 and IBERET-FOLIC-500 are also contraindicated in the rare instance of hypersensitivity to folic acid.

Warnings: Folic acid alone is improper therapy in the treatment of pernicious anemia and other megaloblastic anemias where vitamin B$_{12}$ is deficient.

Precautions: Where anemia exists, its nature should be established and underlying causes determined.

FERO-FOLIC-500 and IBERET-FOLIC-500 contain 800 mcg of folic acid per tablet. Folic acid especially in doses above 0.1 mg daily may obscure pernicious anemia, in that hematologic remission may occur while neurological manifestations remain progressive. Concomitant parenteral therapy with vitamin B$_{12}$ may be necessary in patients with deficiency of vitamin B$_{12}$. Pernicious anemia is rare in women of childbearing age, and the likelihood of its occurrence along with pregnancy is reduced by the impairment of fertility associated with vitamin B$_{12}$ deficiency.

Like other oral iron preparations, FERO-FOLIC-500 and IBERET-FOLIC-500 should be stored out of the reach of children to guard against accidental iron poisoning (see Overdosage).

Laboratory Tests: In older patients and those with conditions tending to lead to vitamin B$_{12}$ depletion, serum B$_{12}$ levels should be regularly assessed during treatment with FERO-FOLIC-500 or IBERET-FOLIC-500.

Drug Interactions: Absorption of iron is inhibited by *magnesium trisilicate* and *antacids containing carbonates*.

Ferrous sulfate may interfere with the absorption of *tetracyclines*.

The antiparkinsonism effects of *levodopa* may be reversed by pyridoxine.

Iron absorption is inhibited by the ingestion of eggs or milk.

Carcinogenesis: Adequate data is not available on long-term potential for carcinogenesis in animals or humans.

Pregnancy: Pregnancy Category A. Studies in pregnant women have not shown that FERO-FOLIC-500 or IBERET-FOLIC-500 increase the risk of fetal abnormalities if administered during pregnancy. If either of these drugs is used during pregnancy, the possibility of fetal harm appears remote. Because studies cannot rule out the possibility of harm, however, FERO-FOLIC-500 or IBERET-FOLIC-500 should be used during pregnancy only if clearly needed.

Nursing Mothers: Folic acid, ascorbic acid, and B-complex vitamins are excreted in breast milk.

Adverse Reactions: The likelihood of gastric intolerance to iron in the controlled-release Gradumet vehicle is remote. If such should occur, the tablet may be taken after a meal. Allergic sensitization has been reported following both oral and parenteral administration of folic acid.

Overdosage: Signs of serious toxicity may be delayed because the iron is in a controlled-release dose form. Increased capillary permeability, reduced plasma volume, increased cardiac output, and sudden cardiovascular collapse may occur in acute iron intoxication. In overdosage, efforts should be made to hasten the elimination of the Gradumet tablets ingested. An emetic should be administered as soon as possible, followed by gastric lavage if indicated. Immediately following emesis, a large dose of a saline cathartic should be used to speed passage through the intestinal tract. X-ray examination may then be considered to determine the position and number of Gradumet tablets remaining in the gastrointestinal tract.

Dosage and Administration: FERO-FOLIC-500 is administered orally and may be taken on an empty stomach.

Adults: For treatment of iron deficiency and prevention of folic acid deficiency, the recommended dose is one tablet daily.

Pregnant Adults: For prevention and treatment of iron deficiency and to supply a maintenance dosage of folic acid, the recommended dose is one tablet daily.

IBERET-FOLIC-500 is administered orally and may be taken on an empty stomach.

Adults: For the treatment of iron deficiency and prevention of concomitant folic acid deficiency where there is an associated deficient intake or increased need for the B-complex vitamins, the recommended dose is one tablet daily.

Pregnant Adults: For the prevention and treatment of iron deficiency where there is a concomitant deficient intake or increased need for the B-complex vitamins including folic acid, the recommended dose is one tablet daily.

How Supplied: FERO-FOLIC-500 is supplied as red Filmtab tablets in bottles of 100 (NDC 0074-7079-13) and 500 (NDC 0074-7079-53).

IBERET-FOLIC-500 is supplied as red Filmtab tablets in bottles of 60 (NDC 0074-7125-60).

Abbott Pharmaceuticals, Inc.
North Chicago, IL 60064
Ref. 03-4240-R3
Shown in Product Identification Section, page 403

FERO–GRAD–500® Filmtab® tablets
[fe′ro-grad]
IRON plus Vitamin C
Well-tolerated once-daily hematinic
with controlled-release iron.

FERO-GRADUMET® Filmtab® tablets
Hematinic supplying controlled-release dose of iron

Description: Each Fero-Gradumet and Fero-Grad-500 tablet contains the equivalent of 105 mg of elemental iron (525 mg of ferrous sulfate) in a unique controlled-release vehicle, the Gradumet®. In addition, each Fero-Grad-500 tablet contains 500 mg of vitamin C (as sodium ascorbate) to improve iron absorption.

The Gradumet, an inert, porous, plastic matrix, is impregnated with ferrous sulfate. Iron is leached from the Gradumet as it passes through the gastrointestinal tract, and the expended matrix is excreted harmlessly in the stool. Controlled-release iron is particularly helpful in patients who have demonstrated intolerance to other oral iron preparations.

Indications: Fero-Grad-500: For the treatment of iron deficiency or iron deficiency anemia. Fero-Gradumet: For the prevention and treatment of iron deficiency.

Precautions: Where anemia exists, its nature should be established and underlying cause determined.

Like other oral iron preparations Fero-Gradumet and Fero-Grad-500 should be stored out of the reach of children to protect against accidental iron poisoning. (see Overdosage).

Adverse Reactions: The likelihood of gastric intolerance to iron in the controlled-release Gradumet vehicle is slight. If it should occur, the tablet may be taken after a meal.

Dosage and Administration: Fero-Gradumet and Fero-Grad-500 are administered orally and may be taken on an empty stomach. The Gradumet controlled-release vehicle reduces the incidence of gastric side effects by delaying the release of almost all the iron until the tablet has passed the stomach.

Fero-Grad-500: Usual adult dose, including pregnant females: One tablet daily, or as directed by the physician.

Fero-Gradumet: Usual adult dose: Prevention: One tablet daily; Treatment: One tablet twice daily, or as directed by the physician. Pregnant females: Prevention: One tablet daily, or as directed by physician.

Overdosage: Signs of serious toxicity may be delayed because the iron is in a controlled-release dose form. Increased capillary permeability, reduced plasma volume, increased cardiac output, and sudden cardiovascular collapse may occur in acute iron intoxication. In overdosage, efforts should be made to hasten the elimination of the Gradumet tablets ingested. An emetic should be administered as soon as possible, followed by gastric lavage if indicated. Immediately following emesis, a large dose of a saline cathartic should be used to speed passage through the intestinal tract. X-ray examination may then be considered to determine the position and number of Gradumet tablets remaining in the gastrointestinal tract.

How Supplied: Fero-Gradumet is supplied as red tablets in bottles of 100 (NDC 0074-6852-02); Fero-Grad-500 is supplied as red tablets in bottles of 30 (NDC 0074-7238-30), 100 (NDC 0074-7238-01) and 500 (NDC 0074-7238-02). The ingredients of these products are listed in one or more of the Medicare designated compendia.

for possible revisions

Abbott Pharmaceuticals, Inc.
North Chicago, IL 60064
Shown in Product Identification Section, page 403

GEMONIL®
[ge'mō-nil]
(metharbital tablets, USP)

Description: GEMONIL (metharbital) is a synthetic, N-methylated derivative of barbital which is identified chemically as 5,5-diethyl-1-methylbarbituric acid.

Actions: GEMONIL produces anticonvulsant effects which are similar to those produced by phenobarbital and mephobarbital. In experimental animals the drug has been shown to be unusually effective against pentylenetetrazol-induced convulsions. GEMONIL is less effective against convulsions induced by electroshock. Toxicity studies in mice, rats, cats and dogs indicate that the drug is less toxic and has less sedative effect than phenobarbital.

GEMONIL is adequately absorbed from the gastrointestinal tract following oral administration. It is demethylated in the liver to barbital, and is excreted largely in this form by the kidneys.

Indications: GEMONIL is indicated for the control of grand mal, petit mal, myoclonic and mixed types of seizures.

Contraindications: GEMONIL is contraindicated in patients with known hypersensitivity to barbiturates, and in those with a history of manifest or latent porphyria.

Warnings: Metharbital may be habit forming.
USAGE DURING PREGNANCY AND LACTATION: THERE ARE MULTIPLE REPORTS IN THE CLINICAL LITERATURE WHICH INDICATE THAT THE USE OF ANTICONVULSANT DRUGS DURING PREGNANCY RESULTS IN AN INCREASED INCIDENCE OF BIRTH DEFECTS IN THE OFFSPRING. ALTHOUGH DATA ARE MORE EXTENSIVE WITH RESPECT TO TRIMETHADIONE, PARAMETHADIONE, PHENYTOIN, AND PHENOBARBITAL, REPORTS INDICATE A POSSIBLE SIMILAR ASSOCIATION WITH THE USE OF OTHER ANTICONVULSANT DRUGS. THEREFORE, ANTICONVULSANT DRUGS SHOULD BE ADMINISTERED TO WOMEN OF CHILDBEARING POTENTIAL ONLY IF THEY ARE CLEARLY SHOWN TO BE ESSENTIAL IN THE MANAGEMENT OF THEIR SEIZURES.

ANTICONVULSANT DRUGS SHOULD NOT BE DISCONTINUED IN PATIENTS IN WHOM THE DRUG IS ADMINISTERED TO PREVENT MAJOR SEIZURES BECAUSE OF THE STRONG POSSIBILITY OF PRECIPITATING STATUS EPILEPTICUS WITH ATTENDANT HYPOXIA AND RISK TO BOTH MOTHER AND THE UNBORN CHILD. CONSIDERATION SHOULD, HOWEVER, BE GIVEN TO DISCONTINUATION OF ANTICONVULSANTS PRIOR TO AND DURING PREGNANCY WHEN THE NATURE, FREQUENCY AND SEVERITY OF THE SEIZURES DO NOT POSE A SERIOUS THREAT TO THE PATIENT. IT IS NOT, HOWEVER, KNOWN WHETHER EVEN MINOR SEIZURES CONSTITUTE SOME RISK TO THE DEVELOPING EMBRYO OR FETUS.

REPORTS HAVE SUGGESTED THAT THE MATERNAL INGESTION OF ANTICONVULSANT DRUGS, PARTICULARLY BARBITURATES, IS ASSOCIATED WITH A NEONATAL COAGULATION DEFECT THAT MAY CAUSE BLEEDING DURING THE EARLY (USUALLY WITHIN 24 HOURS OF BIRTH) NEONATAL PERIOD. THE POSSIBILITY OF THE OCCURRENCE OF THIS DEFECT WITH THE USE OF GEMONIL SHOULD BE KEPT IN MIND. THE DEFECT IS CHARACTERIZED BY DECREASED LEVELS OF VITAMIN K-DEPENDENT CLOTTING FACTORS, AND PROLONGATION OF EITHER THE PROTHROMBIN TIME OR THE PARTIAL THROMBOPLASTIN TIME, OR BOTH. IT HAS BEEN SUGGESTED THAT VITAMIN K BE GIVEN PROPHYLACTICALLY TO THE MOTHER ONE MONTH PRIOR TO AND DURING DELIVERY, AND TO THE INFANT, INTRAVENOUSLY, IMMEDIATELY AFTER BIRTH.

THE SAFETY OF GEMONIL FOR USE DURING LACTATION HAS NOT BEEN ESTABLISHED. THE PHYSICIAN SHOULD WEIGH THESE CONSIDERATIONS IN TREATMENT AND COUNSELING OF EPILEPTIC WOMEN OF CHILDBEARING POTENTIAL.

Precautions: There is evidence that some barbiturates stimulate hepatic microsomal enzymes and therefore may increase the rate of metabolism of some drugs including the coumarin anticoagulants. Although metharbital has not been directly associated with such effect, caution is advised in patients receiving such anticoagulants.

Since metharbital is detoxified primarily in the liver, GEMONIL should be used with caution in patients with hepatic impairment.

In patients with convulsive disorders who have been taking regular daily doses, withdrawal of GEMONIL should be gradual since abrupt discontinuation of barbiturates given for the treatment of epilepsy may result in status epilepticus.

Adverse Reactions: GEMONIL (metharbital) has a low toxicity, and side effects are usually infrequent and mild. Gastric distress, dizziness, increased irritability, skin rash and drowsiness (large doses) may occur. If side effects become severe or cannot be controlled by dosage adjustment, the drug should be gradually withdrawn.

Dosage and Administration: GEMONIL is administered orally. As with all antiepileptic therapy, it is particularly important to adjust the dosage for each patient to obtain optimal effect. For adults, the usual starting dose is 100 mg, one to three times daily. The usual initial pediatric dose should be one-half of a 100 mg tablet, one to three times daily, depending on the age and weight of the patient. A dose of 5 to 15 mg/kg per day has been recommended for children. According to the patient's tolerance these dosages may be gradually increased to the level required to control seizures. In some cases very small doses may be effective, whereas in other instances as much as 600 to 800 mg daily are required for adequate control.

GEMONIL may be used alone or in conjunction with other antiepileptic drugs such as Tridione® (trimethadione), Paradione® (paramethadione), Phenurone® (phenacemide), Peganone® (ethotoin), phenytoin sodium, or mephenytoin. Frequently, more effective control of seizures can be achieved by a combination of drugs. When added to an established regimen to replace or supplement other anticonvulsant therapy, the dosage of other medication should be gradually reduced while increasing that of GEMONIL so as to avoid or minimize recurrence of seizures.

Overdosage: Symptoms of overdosage include drowsiness, irritability, dizziness, and gastric distress. Loss of consciousness and coma may occur following very high doses. Treatment is the same as that for barbiturate intoxication.

How Supplied: GEMONIL (metharbital tablets, USP) is supplied as grooved, 100 mg tablets in bottles of 100 (**NDC** 0074-6401-01).

This product is listed in USP, a Medicare designated compendium.

Abbott Laboratories
North Chicago, IL 60064
Ref. 01-2109-R3

H-BIG®
(Hepatitis B Immune Globulin [Human])

Description: Hepatitis B Immune Globulin (Human)—H-BIG®—is a sterile solution of immunoglobulin (10–18% protein) which is prepared by cold alcohol fractionation from pooled venous plasma of individuals with high titers of antibody to the hepatitis B suface antigen (anti-HBs). The product is stabilized with 0.3 M glycine and contains 1:10,000 Thimerosal (a mercury derivative) as a preservative. The solution has a pH of 6.8 ± 0.4 adjusted with sodium carbonate. Each vial contains anti-HBs antibody equivalent to or exceeding the potency of anti-HBs in a U.S. reference hepatitis B immune globulin (Office of Biologics Research and Review, FDA).

This product has been prepared from large pools of human venous plasma. Each individual unit of plasma has been found nonreactive for hepatitis B surface antigen (HBsAg) using a U.S. Federally approved test with third-generation sensitivity.

Clinical Pharmacology: Hepatitis B Immune Globulin (Human) provides passive immunization for individuals exposed to the hepatitis B virus (HBV) as evidenced by a reduction in the attack rate of hepatitis B following its use. The administration of the usual recommended dose of H-BIG® generally results in a detectable level of circulating anti-HBs which persists for approximately two months or longer. Cases of type B hepatitis are rarely seen following exposure to HBV in persons with pre-existing anti-HBs. No confirmed instance of transmission of hepatitis B has been associated with this product.

Indications and Usage: H-BIG® is indicated for post-exposure prophylaxis following either parenteral exposure, e.g., by accidental "needlestick," or direct mucous membrane contact (accidental splash), or oral ingestion (pipetting accident) involving HBsAg positive materials such as blood, plasma or serum.

H-BIG® is also indicated for prophylaxis of infants born to HBsAg positive mothers. Such infants are at risk of being infected with hepatitis B virus and becoming chronic carriers. The carrier state can be prevented in about 75% of such infections if newborns are given H-BIG® immediately after birth and in the early months of life.

Contraindications: None known.

Warnings: H-BIG® should be given with caution to patients with a history of prior systemic allergic reactions following the administration of human immune globulin preparations.

In patients who have severe thrombocytopenia or any coagulation disorder that would contraindicate intramuscular injections, Hepatitis B Immune Globulin (Human) should be given only if the expected benefits outweigh the risks.

Precautions:
General
Hepatitis B Immune Globulin (Human) should *not* be administered intravenously because of the potential for serious reactions. Injections should be made intramuscularly, and care should be taken to draw back on the plunger of the syringe before injection in order to be certain that the needle is not in a blood vessel. Although systemic reactions to immune globulin preparations are rare, epinephrine should be available.

Drug Interactions
Antibodies in the globulin preparation may interfere with the response to live viral vaccines such as measles, mumps, polio and rubella. Therefore, use of such vaccines should be deferred until approximately three months after H-BIG® administration.

No interactions with other products are known.

Pregnancy Category C
Animal reproduction studies have not been conducted with H-BIG®. It is also not known whether Hepatitis B Immune Globulin (Human) can cause fetal harm when administered to a pregnant woman or can affect reproduction capacity. H-BIG® should be given to a pregnant woman only if clearly needed.

Adverse Reactions: Local pain and tenderness at the injection site, and urticaria and angioedema may occur; anaphylactic reactions, although rare, have been reported following the injection of human immune globulin preparations.

Overdosage: Although no data are available, clinical experience with other immunoglobulin preparations suggests that the only manifestations would be pain and tenderness at the injection site.

Dosage and Administration: The recommended dose is 0.06 mL per kilogram of body

Continued on next page

If desired, additional literature on any Abbott Product will be provided upon request to Abbott Laboratories.

Abbott—Cont.

weight; the usual adult dose is 3 to 5 mL. The appropriate dose should be administered as soon after exposure as possible (preferably within 7 days) and repeated 28–30 days after the initial dose. H-BIG® is administered intramuscularly, preferably in the gluteal or deltoid region, in adults.

It is recommended that H-BIG® be given to infants born to HBsAg positive mothers. The recommended dose for at-risk newborns is 0.5 mL intramuscularly, as soon after birth as possible, preferably no later than 24 hours; the same dose (0.5 mL) should be repeated 3 months and 6 months after the initial dose.

Parenteral drug products should be inspected visually for particulate matter and discoloration prior to administration, whenever solution and container permit.

How Supplied: No. 8399—H-BIG®—is supplied in 1 mL, 4 mL and 5 mL vials.

Storage: Store at 2 to 8°C (35 to 46°F). Do not freeze. Do not use after expiration date.

HARMONYL® Tablets ℞
[har′mō-nil]
(deserpidine)

Description: Harmonyl (deserpidine) is a purified rauwolfia alkaloid chemically identified as 11-desmethoxyreserpine.

Actions: The pharmacologic actions of HARMONYL (deserpidine) are essentially the same as those of other active rauwolfia alkaloids. Deserpidine probably produces its antihypertensive effects through depletion of tissue stores of catecholamines (epinephrine and norepinephrine) from peripheral sites. By contrast, its sedative and tranquilizing properties are thought to be related to depletion of 5-hydroxytryptamine from the brain.

The antihypertensive effect is often accompanied by bradycardia. There is no significant alteration in cardiac output or renal blood flow. The carotid sinus reflex is inhibited, but postural hypotension is rarely seen with the use of conventional doses of HARMONYL alone.

Deserpidine, like other rauwolfia alkaloids, is characterized by slow onset of action and sustained effect which may persist following withdrawal of the drug.

Indications: HARMONYL (deserpidine) is indicated for the treatment of mild essential hypertension. It is also useful as adjunctive therapy with other antihypertensive agents in the more severe forms of hypertension.

The drug is also indicated for the relief of symptoms in agitated psychotic states, e.g., schizophrenia—primarily in those individuals unable to tolerate phenothiazine derivatives or those who also require antihypertensive medication.

Contraindications: HARMONYL (deserpidine) is contraindicated in patients with known hypersensitivity, mental depression especially with suicidal tendencies, active peptic ulcer, and ulcerative colitis. It is also contraindicated in patients receiving electroconvulsive therapy.

Warnings: Extreme caution should be exercised in treating patients with a history of mental depression. Discontinue the drug at the first sign of despondency, early morning insomnia, loss of appetite, impotence, or self-deprecation. Drug-induced depression may persist for several months after drug withdrawal and may be severe enough to result in suicide.

Usage in Pregnancy and Lactation
The safety of deserpidine for use during pregnancy or lactation has not been established; therefore, it should be used in pregnant women or in women of childbearing potential only when, in the judgment of the physician, its use is deemed essential to the welfare of the patient. Increased respiratory secretions, nasal congestion, cyanosis, and anorexia may occur in infants born to rauwolfia alkaloid-treated mothers since these preparations are known to cross the placental barrier to enter the fetal circulation and appear in cord blood. They also are secreted by nursing mothers into breast milk.

Reproductive and teratology studies in rats reduced the mating index and neonatal survival indices; the no-effect dosage has not been established.

Precautions: Because rauwolfia preparations increase gastrointestinal motility and secretion, this drug should be used cautiously in patients with a history of peptic ulcer, ulcerative colitis, or gallstones, where biliary colic may be precipitated. Caution should be exercised when treating hypertensive patients with renal insufficiency since they adjust poorly to lowered blood pressure levels.

Use HARMONYL (deserpidine) cautiously with digitalis and quinidine since cardiac arrhythmias have occurred with rauwolfia preparations.

Preoperative withdrawal of deserpidine does not assure that circulatory instability will not occur. It is important that the anesthesiologist be aware of the patient's drug intake and consider this in the overall management, since hypotension has occurred in patients receiving rauwolfia preparations. Anticholinergic and/or adrenergic drugs (metaraminol, norepinephrine) have been employed to treat adverse vagocirculatory effects.

The 0.1 mg dosage strength of HARMONYL contains FD&C Yellow No. 5 (tartrazine) which may cause allergic-type reactions (including bronchial asthma) in certain susceptible individuals. Although the overall incidence of FD&C Yellow No. 5 (tartrazine) sensitivity in the general population is low, it is frequently seen in patients who also have aspirin hypersensitivity.

Adverse Reactions: The following adverse reactions have been reported with rauwolfia preparations. These reactions are usually reversible and disappear when the drug is discontinued.
Gastrointestinal: Including hypersecretion, anorexia, diarrhea, nausea, and vomiting.
Cardiovascular: Including angina-like symptoms, arrhythmias (particularly when used concurrently with digitalis or quinidine), and bradycardia.
Central Nervous System: Including drowsiness, depression, nervousness, paradoxical anxiety, nightmares, extrapyramidal tract symptoms, CNS sensitization manifested by dull sensorium, and deafness.
Dermatologic-Hypersensitivity: Including pruritus, rash, and asthma in asthmatic patients.
Ophthalmologic: Including glaucoma, uveitis, optic atrophy, and conjunctival injection.
Hematologic: Thrombocytopenic purpura.
Miscellaneous: Nasal congestion, weight gain, impotence or decreased libido, dysuria, dyspnea, muscular aches, dryness of mouth, dizziness, and headache.

Water retention with edema in patients with hypertensive vascular disease may occur rarely, but the condition generally clears with cessation of therapy or with the administration of a diuretic agent.

Dosage and Administration: HARMONYL (deserpidine) is administered orally. For the management of mild essential hypertension in the average patient not receiving other antihypertensive agents, the usual initial adult dose is 0.75 to 1 mg daily. Because 10 to 14 days are required to produce the full effects of the drug, adjustments in dosage should not be made more frequently. If the therapeutic response is not adequate, it is generally advisable to add another antihypertensive agent to the regimen. For maintenance, dosage should be reduced. A single daily dose of 0.25 mg of deserpidine may suffice for some patients.

Concomitant use of deserpidine with ganglionic blocking agents, guanethidine, veratrum, hydralazine, methyldopa, chlorthalidone, or thiazides necessitates careful titration of dosage with each agent.

For psychiatric disorders: The average initial oral dose is 0.5 mg daily with a range of 0.1 to 1 mg. Adjust dosage upward or downward according to the patient's response.

Overdosage: An overdosage of deserpidine is characterized by flushing of the skin, conjunctival injection, and pupillary constriction. Sedation ranging from drowsiness to coma may occur. Hypotension, hypothermia, central respiratory depression and bradycardia may develop in cases of severe overdosage.

Treatment consists of the careful evacuation of stomach contents followed by the usual procedures for the symptomatic management of CNS depressant overdosage. If severe hypotension occurs, it should be treated with a direct acting vasopressor such as Levophed® (norepinephrine bitartrate injection, USP).

How Supplied: HARMONYL (deserpidine) Tablets, 0.1 mg, are yellow and supplied in bottles of 100 (NDC 0074-6901-01).
HARMONYL (deserpidine) Tablets (grooved), 0.25 mg, are salmon-pink and supplied in bottles of 100 (NDC 0074-6906-07).
Abbott Laboratories
North Chicago, IL 60064

IBERET®–500 Filmtab® tablets
[i′ be-ret]
IRON plus B-complex and Vitamin C
Well-tolerated once-daily hematinic with controlled-release iron.

IBERET® Filmtab® tablets
Hematinic Supplying Controlled-Release Iron, Vitamin C and Vitamin B-Complex

Description: Each Iberet-500 and Iberet Filmtab tablet contains 525 mg of ferrous sulfate (equivalent to 105 mg elemental iron) in the Gradumet® controlled-release vehicle. To enhance iron absorption, 500 mg of vitamin C has been added to each Iberet-500 Filmtab.

The Gradumet is an inert, porous, plastic matrix which is impregnated with ferrous sulfate. Iron is leached from the Gradumet as it passes through the gastrointestinal tract, and the expended matrix is excreted harmlessly in the stool. Controlled-release iron is particularly helpful in patients who have demonstrated intolerance to other oral iron preparations.

Each Iberet-500 Filmtab tablet contains:
Ferrous Sulfate ....525 mg
  (equivalent to 105 mg of elemental iron)
Vitamin C (as Sodium Ascorbate)...............500 mg
Niacinamide ....30 mg
Calcium Pantothenate..................................10 mg
Vitamin B$_1$ (Thiamine Mononitrate).............6 mg
Vitamin B$_2$ (Riboflavin).................................6 mg
Vitamin B$_6$ (Pyridoxine Hydrochloride)........5 mg
Vitamin B$_{12}$ (Cyanocobalamin)...................25 mcg

The formulation of Iberet differs from Iberet-500 only in that it contains a lesser amount of vitamin C, 150 mg per Filmtab tablet.

Indications: Iberet-500: For the treatment of iron deficiency or iron deficiency anemia where there is a deficient intake or increased need for B-complex vitamins.* Iberet: For conditions in which iron deficiency and vitamin C deficiency occur concomitantly with deficient intake or increased need for the B-complex vitamins.*
*Contains no folic acid.

Precautions: Where anemia exists, its nature should be established and underlying cause determined.

Like other oral iron preparations, Iberet-500 and Iberet should be stored out of the reach of children to protect against accidental iron poisoning (see Overdosage).

Adverse Reactions: The likelihood of gastric intolerance to iron in the controlled-release Gradumet vehicle is slight. If it should occur, the tablet may be taken after a meal.

Dosage and Administration: Iberet-500 and Iberet are administered orally and may be taken on an empty stomach. Iberet-500: Usual Adult Dose: One tablet daily, or as directed by the physician. Iberet: Usual Adult Dose, including pregnant females: One tablet daily, or as directed by the physician.

Overdosage: Signs of serious iron toxicity may be delayed because the iron is in a controlled-release dose form. Increased capillary permeability, reduced plasma volume, increased cardiac output, and sudden cardiovascular collapse may occur in acute iron intoxication. In overdosage, efforts should be made to hasten the elimination of the Gradumet tablets ingested. An emetic should be administered as soon as possible, followed by gastric lavage if indicated. Immediately following emesis, a saline cathartic should be administered to hasten passage through the intestinal tract. X-ray examination may then be considered to determine the position and number of Gradumet tablets remaining in the gastrointestinal tract.

How Supplied: Iberet-500 is supplied as red, oval shaped tablets in bottles of 30 (**NDC** 0074-7235-30), 60 (**NDC** 0074-7235-01) and 500 (**NDC** 0074-7235-03), and in Abbo-Pac® unit dose packages of 100 (**NDC** 0074-7235-11); Iberet is supplied as red, round tablets in bottles of 60 (**NDC** 0074-6863-01) and 500 (**NDC** 0074-6863-02).

Shown in Product Identification Section, page 403
Abbott Pharmaceuticals, Inc.
North Chicago, IL 60064

IBERET–FOLIC–500®   ℞
Controlled-Release Iron with Vitamin C, and B-Complex, including Folic Acid Filmtab® Tablets

See combined listing under FERO-FOLIC-500.

IBERET®–500 LIQUID
[ī′ bĕ-rĕt]
Hematinic Supplying Iron, Vitamin C and Vitamin B-Complex*

IBERET®–LIQUID
Hematinic Supplying Iron, Vitamin C and Vitamin B-Complex*

Description: Iberet-500 Liquid and Iberet-Liquid are hematinic preparations of ferrous sulfate, B-complex vitamins* and ascorbic acid. Each teaspoonful (5 ml) of Iberet-500 Liquid provides:
Elemental Iron (as ferrous sulfate) ....26.25 mg
Vitamin C (Ascorbic Acid) ....125 mg
Niacinamide ....7.5 mg
Dexpanthenol ....2.5 mg
Vitamin B$_1$ (Thiamine Hydrochloride) ....1.5 mg
Vitamin B$_2$ (Riboflavin) ....1.5 mg
Vitamin B$_6$ (Pyridoxine Hydrochloride) ..1.25 mg
Vitamin B$_{12}$ (Cyanocobalamin) ....6.25 mcg
In a citrus-flavored vehicle.

Iberet-Liquid has a raspberry-mint flavored vehicle, alcohol 1%; it has the same formula as Iberet-500 Liquid except for a smaller amount of ascorbic acid: 37.5 mg per teaspoonful.

Indications: Iberet-500 Liquid: For conditions in which iron deficiency occurs concomitantly with deficient intake or increased need for the B-complex vitamins.* Iberet-Liquid: For conditions in which iron deficiency and vitamin C deficiency occur concomitantly with deficient intake or increased need for the B-complex vitamins.*

* Contains no folic acid.

Precautions: Where anemia exists, its nature should be established and underlying cause determined. Iberet-500 Liquid and Iberet-Liquid should be stored out of the reach of children because of the possibility of iron intoxication from accidental overdosage.

Adverse Reactions: If gastrointestinal symptoms appear as a sign of iron intolerance, smaller individual doses may be given at more frequent intervals to provide the desired daily amount. Administering Iberet-500 Liquid or Iberet-Liquid after meals may also reduce such effects.

Like other liquid iron preparations, Iberet-500 Liquid or Iberet-Liquid may stain the teeth on continued use. Stains may be prevented to a large extent by taking the dose through a straw, first mixing it with water or fruit juice, and by following the dose with a drink of plain water or juice. Brushing the teeth with sodium bicarbonate or hydrogen peroxide will usually remove existing stains.

Dosage and Administration: Iberet-500 Liquid and Iberet-Liquid are administered orally, preferably after meals. Each has a fruit-flavored vehicle, and is suitable for pediatric patients who are unable to take tablets or capsules, and for patients who prefer or can better tolerate liquid medication. Iberet-500 Liquid and Iberet-Liquid may be administered by spoon or incorporated into infant formulas, water, or fruit juices. Iberet-500 Liquid: Usual dosage: Adults and children 4 years of age and older—2 teaspoonfuls (10 ml) twice daily, after meals; Children 1–3 years of age—1 teaspoonful (5 ml) twice daily, after meals. Otherwise as directed by the physician. Iberet-Liquid: Usual dosage: Adults and children 4 years of age and older—2 teaspoonfuls (10 ml) three times daily, after meals; Children 1–3 years of age—1 teaspoonful (5 ml) three times daily, after meals. Otherwise as directed by the physician.

How Supplied: Iberet-500 Liquid (**NDC** 0074-8422-02) and Iberet-Liquid (**NDC** 0074-7173-01) are supplied in 8 fl oz bottles.
Abbott Laboratories
North Chicago, IL 60064
Ref. 02-6289-3/R14, 02-6290-4/R12

JANIMINE® Filmtab® Tablets   ℞
[ja-ni-mīne]
(imipramine hydrochloride tablets, USP)

How Supplied: JANIMINE is provided in three dosage sizes as monogrammed tablets:
  10 mg, round-shaped, orange-colored, in bottles of 100 (**NDC** 0074-1897-13) and bottles of 1000 (**NDC** 0074-1897-19).
  25 mg, round-shaped, yellow, in bottles of 100 (**NDC** 0074-1898-13) and bottles of 1000 (**NDC** 0074-1898-19).
  50 mg, ovaloid-shaped, peach-colored, in bottles of 100 (**NDC** 0074-1899-13) and bottles of 1000 (**NDC** 0074-1899-19).

Shown in Product Identification Section, page 403
Abbott Laboratories
North Chicago, IL 60064

K–LOR™ Powder   ℞
[k′lor]
(potassium chloride for oral solution, USP)

Description: Natural fruit-flavored K-LOR (potassium chloride for oral solution, USP) is an oral potassium supplement offered as a powder for reconstitution in individual packets. Each packet of K-LOR 20 mEq contains potassium 20 mEq and chloride 20 mEq provided by potassium chloride 1.5 Gm. Each packet of K-LOR 15 mEq contains potassium 15 mEq and chloride 15 mEq provided by potassium chloride 1.125 Gm.

Clinical Pharmacology: Potassium ion is the principal intracellular cation of most body tissues. Potassium ions participate in a number of essential physiological processes, including the maintenance of intracellular tonicity, the transmission of nerve impulses, the contraction of cardiac, skeletal, and smooth muscle and the maintenance of normal renal function.

Potassium depletion may occur whenever the rate of potassium loss through renal excretion and/or loss from the gastrointestinal tract exceeds the rate of potassium intake. Such depletion usually develops slowly as a consequence of prolonged therapy with oral diuretics, primary or secondary hyperaldosteronism, diabetic ketoacidosis, severe diarrhea, or inadequate replacement of potassium in patients on prolonged parenteral nutrition. Potassium depletion due to these causes is usually accompanied by a concomitant deficiency of chloride and is manifested by hypokalemia and metabolic alkalosis. Potassium depletion may produce weakness, fatigue, disturbances of cardiac rhythm (primarily ectopic beats), prominent U-waves in the electrocardiogram, and in advanced cases flaccid paralysis and/or impaired ability to concentrate urine.

Potassium depletion associated with metabolic alkalosis is managed by correcting the fundamental causes of the deficiency whenever possible and administering supplemental potassium chloride, in the form of high potassium food or potassium chloride solution or tablets. In rare circumstances, (e.g., patients with renal tubular acidosis) potassium depletion may be associated with metabolic acidosis and hyperchloremia. In such patients potassium replacement should be accomplished with potassium salts other than the chloride, such as potassium bicarbonate, potassium citrate, potassium gluconate, or potassium acetate.

Indications and Usage:
1. For therapeutic use in patients with hypokalemia with or without metabolic alkalosis; in digitalis intoxication and in patients with hypokalemic familial periodic paralysis.
2. For prevention of potassium depletion when the dietary intake of potassium is inadequate in the following conditions: patients receiving digitalis and diuretics for congestive heart failure; hepatic cirrhosis with ascites; states of aldosterone excess with normal renal function; potassium-losing nephropathy, and certain diarrheal states.
3. The use of potassium salts in patients receiving diuretics for uncomplicated essential hypertension is often unnecessary when such patients have a normal dietary pattern. Serum potassium should be checked periodically, however, and, if hypokalemia occurs, dietary supplementation with potassium-containing foods may be adequate to control milder cases. In more severe cases supplementation with potassium salts may be indicated.

Contraindications: Potassium supplements are contraindicated in patients with hyperkalemia since a further increase in serum potassium concentration in such patients can produce cardiac arrest. Hyperkalemia may complicate any of the following conditions: chronic renal failure, systemic acidosis such as diabetic acidosis, acute dehydration, extensive tissue breakdown as in severe burns or adrenal insufficiency. Potassium supplements are contraindicated in patients receiving potassium-sparing diuretics (e.g., spironolactone, triamterene), since such use may produce severe hyperkalemia.

Potassium chloride supplements are contraindicated in hypokalemic patients with metabolic acidosis. These patients should be treated with an alkalinizing potassium salt such as potassium bicarbonate, potassium citrate, potassium gluconate, or potassium acetate.

Warnings: *Hyperkalemia:* In patients with impaired mechanisms for excreting potassium, the administration of potassium salts can produce hyperkalemia and cardiac arrest. This occurs most commonly in patients given potassium by the intravenous route but may also occur in patients given potassium orally. Potentially fatal hyperkalemia can develop rapidly and be asymptomatic.

Interaction with Potassium-Sparing Diuretics: Hypokalemia should not be treated by the concomitant administration of potassium salts and a potassium-sparing diuretic (e.g., spironolactone or triamterene), since the simultaneous administration of these agents can produce severe hyperkalemia.

Precautions: The diagnosis of potassium depletion is ordinarily made by demonstrating hypokalemia in a patient with a clinical history suggesting some cause for potassium depletion. In interpreting the serum potassium level, the physician should bear in mind that acute alkalosis *per se* can produce hypokalemia in the absence of a deficit in total body potassium, while acute acidosis *per se* can increase the serum potassium concentration into the normal range even in the presence of a reduced total body potassium. The treatment of potassium depletion, particularly in the presence of cardiac disease, renal disease, or acidosis, requires careful attention to acid-base balance and appropriate monitoring of serum electrolytes, the electrocardiogram, and the clinical status of the patient.

The use of potassium salts in patients with chronic renal disease, or any other condition which impairs potassium excretion, requires particularly

Continued on next page

If desired, additional literature on any Abbott Product will be provided upon request to Abbott Laboratories.

Abbott—Cont.

careful monitoring of the serum potassium concentration and appropriate dosage adjustment.

Carcinogenesis: No data are available on long-term potential for carcinogenicity in animals or humans.

Pregnancy: K-LOR is not expected to cause fetal harm when administered in dosages which will not result in hyperkalemia.

Nursing Mothers: Although no studies have been done, it is presumed that potassium chloride is excreted in human milk. Caution should be exercised when K-LOR is administered to a nursing woman.

Pediatric Use: Safety and effectiveness in children have not been established.

Adverse Reactions: One of the most severe adverse effects is hyperkalemia (see CONTRAINDICATIONS, WARNINGS and OVERDOSAGE). The most common adverse reactions to oral potassium salts are nausea, vomiting, abdominal discomfort, and diarrhea. These symptoms are due to irritation of the gastrointestinal tract and are best managed by diluting the preparation further, taking the dose with meals, or reducing the dose.

Skin rash has been reported rarely.

Overdosage: The administration of oral potassium salts to persons with normal excretory mechanisms for potassium rarely causes serious hyperkalemia. However, if excretory mechanisms are impaired or if potassium is administered too rapidly intravenously, potentially fatal hyperkalemia can result (see Contraindications and Warnings). It is important to recognize that hyperkalemia is usually asymptomatic and may be manifested only by an increased serum potassium concentration and characteristic electrocardiographic changes (peaking of T-waves, loss of P-waves, depression of S-T segments, and prolongation of QT intervals). Late manifestations include muscle paralysis and cardiovascular collapse from cardiac arrest.

Treatment measures for hyperkalemia include the following: (1) elimination of foods and medications containing potassium and of potassium-sparing diuretics; (2) intravenous administration of 300 to 500 ml/hr of dextrose injection (10–25%), containing 10 units of insulin/20 g dextrose; (3) correction of acidosis, if present, with intravenous sodium bicarbonate; (4) use of exchange resins, hemodialysis, or peritoneal dialysis. In treating hyperkalemia, it should be recalled that in patients who have been stabilized on digitalis, too rapid a lowering of the serum potassium concentration can produce digitalis toxicity.

Dosage and Administration: The dosage depends on the severity of the condition. The usual adult dose is 20 to 80 mEq of potassium per day (1 K-LOR 20 mEq packet 1 to 4 times daily after meals, or 1 K-LOR 15 mEq packet 2 to 5 times daily after meals).

Each 20 mEq (one K-LOR 20 mEq packet) of potassium should be dissolved in at least 4 oz (approximately ½ glassful) cold water or juice. Each 15 mEq (one K-LOR 15 mEq packet) of potassium should be dissolved in at least 3 oz (approximately ½ glassful) cold water or juice. These preparations, like other potassium supplements, must be properly diluted to avoid the possibility of gastrointestinal irritation.

How Supplied: K-LOR 20 mEq (potassium chloride for oral solution, USP) is supplied in cartons of 30 packets (NDC 0074-3611-01), and cartons of 100 packets (NDC 0074-3611-02). Each packet contains potassium, 20 mEq, and chloride, 20 mEq, provided by potassium chloride, 1.5 Gm.

K-LOR 15 mEq (potassium chloride for oral solution, USP) is supplied in cartons of 100 packets (NDC 0074-3633-11). Each packet contains potassium, 15 mEq, and chloride, 15 mEq, provided by potassium chloride, 1.125 Gm.

Abbott Laboratories
North Chicago, IL 60064
TM—Trademark
Shown in Product Identification Section, page 403
Ref. 01-2079-R8

K•Tab®
[k'tâb]
(Potassium Chloride Extended-Release Tablets, USP)

R

Description: K-TAB (potassium chloride extended-release tablets) is a film-coated (not enteric-coated) tablet containing 750 mg of potassium chloride (equivalent to 10 mEq) in an inert, porous, wax/polymer matrix. This oral potassium supplement formulation is intended to provide a controlled release of potassium from the matrix to minimize the likelihood of producing high localized concentrations of potassium within the gastrointestinal tract. The expended inert, porous, wax/polymer matrix is not absorbed and may be excreted intact in the stool.

Clinical Pharmacology: Potassium ion is the principal intracellular cation of most body tissues. Potassium ions participate in a number of essential physiological processes, including the maintenance of intracellular tonicity, the transmission of nerve impulses, the contraction of cardiac, skeletal, and smooth muscle and the maintenance of normal renal function.

Potassium depletion may occur whenever the rate of potassium loss through renal excretion and/or loss from the gastrointestinal tract exceeds the rate of potassium intake. Such depletion usually develops slowly as a consequence of prolonged therapy with oral diuretics, primary or secondary hyperaldosteronism, diabetic ketoacidosis, severe diarrhea, or inadequate replacement of potassium in patients on prolonged parenteral nutrition. Potassium depletion due to these causes is usually accompanied by a concomitant deficiency of chloride and is manifested by hypokalemia and metabolic alkalosis. Potassium depletion may produce weakness, fatigue, disturbances of cardiac rhythm (primarily ectopic beats), prominent U-waves in the electrocardiogram, and in advanced cases flaccid paralysis and/or impaired ability to concentrate urine.

Potassium depletion associated with metabolic alkalosis is managed by correcting the fundamental causes of the deficiency whenever possible and administering supplemental potassium chloride, in the form of high potassium food or potassium chloride solution or tablets. In rare circumstances, (e.g., patients with renal tubular acidosis) potassium depletion may be associated with metabolic acidosis and hyperchloremia. In such patients potassium replacement should be accomplished with potassium salts other than the chloride, such as potassium bicarbonate, potassium citrate, potassium gluconate, or potassium acetate.

Bioavailability: Studies of urinary potassium excretion in subjects with potassium balance controlled by dietary measures were used to determine bioavailability of K-TAB (potassium chloride extended-release tablets). There were no significant differences in the cumulative amount of potassium excreted over 48 hours between K-TAB and 10% potassium chloride liquid demonstrating the bioequivalence of K-TAB to the 10% liquid.

Indications and Usage: BECAUSE OF REPORTS OF INTESTINAL AND GASTRIC ULCERATION AND BLEEDING WITH EXTENDED-RELEASE POTASSIUM CHLORIDE PREPARATIONS, THESE DRUGS SHOULD BE RESERVED FOR THOSE PATIENTS WHO CANNOT TOLERATE OR REFUSE TO TAKE LIQUID OR EFFERVESCENT POTASSIUM PREPARATIONS OR FOR PATIENTS IN WHOM THERE IS A PROBLEM OF COMPLIANCE WITH THESE PREPARATIONS.

1. For therapeutic use in patients with hypokalemia with or without metabolic alkalosis; in digitalis intoxication and in patients with hypokalemic familial periodic paralysis.
2. For prevention of potassium depletion when the dietary intake of potassium is inadequate in the following conditions: patients receiving digitalis and diuretics for congestive heart failure; hepatic cirrhosis with ascites; states of aldosterone excess with normal renal function; potassium-losing nephropathy, and certain diarrheal states.
3. The use of potassium salts in patients receiving diuretics for uncomplicated essential hypertension is often unnecessary when such patients have a normal dietary pattern. Serum potassium should be checked periodically, however, and, if hypokalemia occurs, dietary supplementation with potassium-containing foods may be adequate to control milder cases. In more severe cases supplementation with potassium salts may be indicated.

Contraindications: Potassium supplements are contraindicated in patients with hyperkalemia since a further increase in serum potassium concentration in such patients can produce cardiac arrest. Hyperkalemia may complicate any of the following conditions: chronic renal failure, systemic acidosis such as diabetic acidosis, acute dehydration, extensive tissue breakdown as in severe burns, or adrenal insufficiency. Potassium supplements are contraindicated in patients receiving potassium-sparing diuretics (e.g., spironolactone, triamterene), since such use may produce severe hyperkalemia.

Wax matrix potassium chloride preparations have produced esophageal ulceration in certain cardiac patients with esophageal compression due to an enlarged left atrium. Their use in such patients is contraindicated.

All solid dosage forms of potassium supplements are contraindicated in any patient in whom there is cause for arrest or delay in tablet passage through the gastrointestinal tract. In these instances, potassium supplementation should be with a liquid preparation.

Potassium chloride supplements are contraindicated in hypokalemic patients with metabolic acidosis. These patients should be treated with an alkalinizing potassium salt such as potassium bicarbonate, potassium citrate, potassium gluconate, or potassium acetate.

Warnings: *Hyperkalemia:* In patients with impaired mechanisms for excreting potassium, the administration of potassium salts can produce hyperkalemia and cardiac arrest. This occurs most commonly in patients given potassium by the intravenous route but may also occur in patients given potassium orally. Potentially fatal hyperkalemia can develop rapidly and be asymptomatic.

Interaction with Potassium-Sparing Diuretics: Hypokalemia should not be treated by the concomitant administration of potassium salts and a potassium-sparing diuretic (e.g., spironolactone or triamterene), since the simultaneous administration of these agents can produce severe hyperkalemia.

Gastrointestinal lesions:
Potassium chloride tablets have produced stenotic and/or ulcerative lesions of the small bowel and deaths. These lesions are caused by a high localized concentration of potassium ion in the region of a rapidly dissolving tablet, which injures the bowel wall and thereby produces obstruction, hemorrhage, or perforation. K-TAB (potassium chloride extended-release tablets) is an inert, porous, wax/polymer matrix tablet formulated to provide a controlled rate of release of potassium chloride and thus to minimize the possibility of a high local concentration of potassium ion near the bowel wall. While the reported frequency of small-bowel lesions is much less with wax matrix tablets (less than one per 100,000 patient-years) than with enteric-coated potassium chloride tablets (40–50 per 100,000 patient-years), cases associated with wax matrix tablets have been reported both in foreign countries and in the United States. In addition, perhaps because the wax matrix tablet preparations are not enteric-coated and release potassium in the stomach, there have been reports of upper gastrointestinal bleeding associated with these products. The total number of gastrointestinal lesions remains less than one per 100,000 patient-years. Potassium chloride extended-release tablets should be discontinued immediately and the possibility of bowel obstruction or perforation considered if severe vomiting, abdominal pain, distention, or gastrointestinal bleeding occurs.

Precautions: The diagnosis of potassium depletion is ordinarily made by demonstrating hypokalemia in a patient with a clinical history suggesting some cause for potassium depletion. In interpreting the serum potassium level, the physician should bear in mind that acute alkalosis *per se* can produce hypokalemia in the absence of a deficit in total body potassium, while acute acidosis *per se* can increase the serum potassium concentration into the normal range even in the presence of a reduced total body potassium. The treatment of potassium depletion, particularly in the presence of cardiac disease, renal disease, or acidosis, requires careful attention to acid-base balance and appropriate monitoring of serum electrolytes, the electrocardiogram, and the clinical status of the patient.

The use of potassium salts in patients with chronic renal disease, or any other condition which impairs potassium excretion, requires particularly careful monitoring of the serum potassium concentration and appropriate dosage adjustment.

Carcinogenesis: No data are available on long-term potential for carcinogenicity in animals or humans.

Pregnancy: K-TAB tablets are not expected to cause fetal harm when administered in dosages which will not result in hyperkalemia.

Nursing Mothers: Although no studies have been done, it is presumed that potassium chloride is excreted in human milk. Caution should be exercised when K-TAB is administered to a nursing woman.

Pediatric use: Safety and effectiveness in children have not been established.

Adverse Reactions: One of the most severe adverse effects is hyperkalemia (see Contraindications, Warnings, and Overdosage). There also have been reports of upper and lower gastrointestinal conditions including obstruction, bleeding, ulceration, and perforation (see Contraindications and Warnings); other factors known to be associated with such conditions were present in many of these patients.

The most common adverse reactions to oral potassium salts are nausea, vomiting, abdominal discomfort, and diarrhea. These symptoms are due to irritation of the gastrointestinal tract and are best managed by diluting the preparation further, taking the dose with meals, or reducing the dose.

Skin rash has been reported rarely.

Overdosage: The administration of oral potassium salts to persons with normal excretory mechanisms for potassium rarely causes serious hyperkalemia. However, if excretory mechanisms are impaired or if potassium is administered too rapidly intravenously, potentially fatal hyperkalemia can result (see Contraindications and Warnings). It is important to recognize that hyperkalemia is usually asymptomatic and may be manifested only by an increased serum potassium concentration and characteristic electrocardiographic changes (peaking of T-waves, loss of P-waves, depression of S-T segments, and prolongation of QT intervals). Late manifestations include muscle paralysis and cardiovascular collapse from cardiac arrest.

Treatment measures for hyperkalemia include the following: (1) elimination of foods and medications containing potassium and of potassium-sparing diuretics; (2) intravenous administration of 300 to 500 ml/hr of dextrose injection (10–25%), containing 10 units of insulin/20 g dextrose; (3) correction of acidosis, if present, with intravenous sodium bicarbonate; (4) use of exchange resins, hemodialysis, or peritoneal dialysis. In treating hyperkalemia, it should be recalled that in patients who have been stabilized on digitalis, too rapid a lowering of the serum potassium concentration can produce digitalis toxicity.

Dosage and Administration: The usual dietary intake of potassium by the average adult is 40 to 80 mEq per day. Potassium depletion sufficient to cause hypokalemia usually requires the loss of 200 or more mEq of potassium from the total body store. Dosage must be adjusted to the individual needs of each patient but the usual adult dose is 20–80 mEq of potassium per day. One K-TAB tablet twice daily provides 20 mEq of potassium and 20 mEq of chloride.

NOTE: K-TAB IS TO BE SWALLOWED WHOLE AND NOT CRUSHED OR CHEWED.

How Supplied: K-TAB (potassium chloride extended-release tablets, USP) contains 750 mg of potassium chloride (equivalent to 10 mEq). K-TAB is provided as yellow, ovaloid, extended-release Filmtab® tablets in bottles of 100 (**NDC** 0074-7804-13) and 1000 (**NDC** 0074-7804-19) and in ABBO-PAC® unit dose packages of 100 (**NDC** 0074-7804-11).

Shown in Product Identification Section, page 403

Filmtab—Film-sealed tablets, Abbott
Abbott Pharmaceuticals, Inc.
North Chicago, IL 60064
Ref. 03-4236-R8

LIDOCAINE HYDROCHLORIDE INJECTION, USP ℞
[lie'dō-cāne]
AQUEOUS SOLUTIONS FOR ACUTE MANAGEMENT OF CARDIAC ARRHYTHMIAS OR FOR LOCAL ANESTHESIA.

Abboject® Unit of Use Syringe
Ampul
Fliptop Vial
Multiple-dose Fliptop Vial
Pintop Vial
Pressurized Pintop Vial
Universal Additive Syringe

Description: Lidocaine Hydrochloride Injection, USP is a sterile, nonpyrogenic solution of lidocaine hydrochloride in water for injection for parenteral administration in various concentrations with characteristics as follows:

Lidocaine HCl (anhydrous)

Conc.	0.5%	1%	1.5%	2%	4%	10%*	20%*
mg/ml (anhyd.)	5	10	15	20	40	100	200
pH (approx.)	6.5	6.5	6.5	6.5	6.5	5.7	5.7

*10% and 20% concentrations FOR DILUTION ONLY. **Must not be administered without proper dilution prior to injection.**

Multiple-dose vials contain 0.1% of methylparaben added as preservative. Single dose vials contain no preservative and unused portions must be discarded after use. May contain sodium hydroxide and hydrochloric acid for pH adjustment. May contain sodium chloride to adjust tonicity.

Lidocaine has cardiac antiarrhythmic properties and is a local anesthetic of the amide type.

Lidocaine Hydrochloride, USP is chemically designated 2-(diethylamino)-2',6'-acetoxylidide monohydrochloride monohydrate, a white powder freely soluble in water. It has the following structural formula:

$$CH_3\text{-}C_6H_3(CH_3)\text{-}NHCOCH_2N(C_2H_5)_2 \cdot HCl \cdot H_2O$$

FOR CARDIAC ARRHYTHMIAS

Clinical Pharmacology:
Mechanism of Action and Electrophysiology:
Studies of the effects of therapeutic concentrations of lidocaine on the electrophysiological properties of mammalian Purkinje fibers have shown that lidocaine attenuates phase 4 diastolic depolarization, decreases automaticity and causes a decrease or no change in excitability and membrane responsiveness. Action potential duration and effective refractory period of Purkinje fibers are decreased while the ratio of effective refractory period to action potential duration is increased. Action potential duration and effective refractory period of ventricular muscle are also decreased. Effective refractory period of the AV node may increase, decrease or remain unchanged and atrial effective refractory period is unchanged. Lidocaine raises the ventricular fibrillation threshold. No significant interactions between lidocaine and the autonomic nervous system have been described and consequently lidocaine has little or no effect on autonomic tone.

Clinical electrophysiological studies with lidocaine have demonstrated no change in sinus node recovery time or sinoatrial conduction time, AV nodal conduction time is unchanged or shortened and His-Purkinje conduction time is unchanged.

Hemodynamics:
At therapeutic doses, lidocaine has minimal hemodynamic effects in normal subjects and in patients with heart disease. Lidocaine has been shown to cause no, or minimal decrease in ventricular contractility, cardiac output, arterial pressure or heart rate.

Pharmacokinetics and Metabolism:
Lidocaine is rapidly metabolized by the liver and less than 10% of a dose is excreted unchanged in the urine. Oxidative N-dealkylation, a major pathway of metabolism, results in the metabolites monoethylglycinexylidide and glycinexylidide. The pharmacological/toxicological activities of these metabolites are similar to but less potent than lidocaine. The primary metabolite in urine is a conjugate of 4-hydroxy-2,6-dimethylaniline.

The elimination half-life of lidocaine following an intravenous bolus injection is typically 1.5 to 2.0 hours. There are data that indicate that the half-life may be 3 hours or longer following infusions of greater than 24 hours.

Because of the rapid rate at which lidocaine is metabolized, any condition that alters liver function, including changes in liver blood flow which could result from severe congestive heart failure or shock may alter lidocaine kinetics. The half-life may be two-fold or more greater in patients with liver dysfunction. Renal dysfunction does not affect lidocaine kinetics, but may increase the accumulation of metabolites.

Therapeutic effects of lidocaine are generally associated with plasma levels of 6 to 25 μmole/L (1.5 to 6 μg free base per ml). The blood to plasma distribution ratio is approximately 0.84. Objective adverse manifestations become increasingly apparent with increasing plasma levels above 6.0 μg free base per ml.

The plasma protein binding of lidocaine is dependent on drug concentration and the fraction bound decreases with increasing concentration. At concentrations of 1 to 4 μg free base per ml, 60 to 80 percent of lidocaine i protein bound. In addition to lidocaine concentration, the binding is dependent on the plasma concentration of the α-1-acid glycoprotein.

Lidocaine readily crosses the placental and blood-brain barriers. Dialysis has negligible effects on the kinetics of lidocaine.

Indications and Usage: Lidocaine hydrochloride administered intravenously, is specifically indicated in the acute management of ventricular arrhythmias such as those occurring in relation to acute myocardial infarction, or during cardiac manipulation, such as cardiac surgery.

Contraindications: Lidocaine hydrochloride is contraindicated in patients with a known history of hypersensitivity to local anesthetics of the amide type. Lidocaine hydrochloride should not be used in patients with Stokes-Adams syndrome, Wolff-Parkinson-White syndrome or with severe degrees of sinoatrial, atrioventricular or intraventricular block in the absence of an artificial pacemaker.

Continued on next page

If desired, additional literature on any Abbott Product will be provided upon request to Abbott Laboratories.

Abbott—Cont.

Warnings: IN ORDER TO MANAGE POSSIBLE ADVERSE REACTIONS, RESUSCITATIVE EQUIPMENT, OXYGEN AND OTHER RESUSCITATIVE DRUGS SHOULD BE IMMEDIATELY AVAILABLE WHEN LIDOCAINE HYDROCHLORIDE INJECTION IS USED.
THE 10% AND 20% CONCENTRATED SOLUTIONS MUST NOT BE INJECTED UNDILUTED. See DOSAGE AND ADMINISTRATION.

Systemic toxicity may result in manifestations of central nervous system depression (sedation) or irritability (twitching), which may progress to frank convulsions accompanied by respiratory depression and/or arrest. Early recognition of premonitory signs, assurance of adequate oxygenation and, where necessary, establishment of artificial airway with ventilatory support are essential to management of this problem. Should convulsions persist despite ventilatory therapy with oxygen, *small* increments of anticonvulsant drugs may be used intravenously. Examples of such agents include benzodiazepines (e.g., diazepam), ultrashort-acting barbiturates (e.g., thiopental or thiamylal) or a short-acting barbiturate (e.g., pentobarbital or secobarbital). If the patient is under anesthesia, a short-acting muscle relaxant (e.g., succinylcholine) may be used. Longer acting drugs should be used only when recurrent convulsions are evidenced.

Should circulatory depression occur, vasopressors may be used.

Constant electrocardiographic monitoring is essential to the proper administration of lidocaine hydrochloride. Signs of excessive depression of cardiac electrical activity such as sinus node dysfunction, prolongation of the P-R interval and QRS complex or the appearance or aggravation of arrhythmias, should be followed by flow adjustment and, if necessary, prompt cessation of the intravenous infusion of this agent. Ocasionally, acceleration of ventricular rate may occur when lidocaine hydrochloride is administered to patients with atrial flutter or fibrillation.

Precautions:
1. **General:** Caution should be employed in the use of lidocaine hydrochloride in patients with severe liver or kidney disease because accumulation of the drug or metabolites may occur. Lidocaine Hydrochloride Injection, USP should be used with caution in the treatment of patients with hypovolemia, severe congestive heart failure, shock and all forms of heart block. In patients with sinus bradycardia or incomplete heart block, the administration of lidocaine hydrochloride intravenously for the elimination of ventricular ectopic beats without prior acceleration in heart rate (e.g., by atropine, isoproterenol or electric pacing) may promote more frequent and serious ventricular arrhythmias or complete heart block. (See CONTRAINDICATIONS.)

Dosage should be reduced for children and for debilitated and/or elderly patients, commensurate with their age and physical status.

The safety of amide local anesthetic agents in patients with genetic predisposition of malignant hyperthermia has not been fully assessed; therefore, lidocaine should be used with caution in such patients.

In hospital environments where drugs known to be triggering agents for malignant hyperthermia (fulminant hypermetabolism) are administered, it is suggested that a standard protocol for management should be available.

It is not known whether lidocaine may trigger this reaction, however, large doses resulting in significant plasma concentrations, as may be achieved by intravenous infusion, pose potential risk to these individuals. Recognition of early unexplained signs of tachycardia, tachypnea, labile blood pressure and metabolic acidosis may precede temperature elevation. Successful outcome is dependent on early diagnosis, prompt discontinuance of the triggering agent and institution of treatment including oxygen therapy, supportive measures and dantrolene (for details see dantrolene package insert).

2. **Patient Information:** The patient should be advised of the possible occurrence of the experiences listed under ADVERSE REACTIONS.
3. **Laboratory Tests:** None known.
4. **Drug Interactions:** Lidocaine Hydrochloride Injection, USP should be used with caution in patients with digitalis toxicity accompanied by atrioventricular block. Concomitant use of beta-blocking agents may reduce hepatic blood flow and thereby reduce lidocaine clearance.
5. **Carcinogenesis, Mutagenesis, Impairment of Fertility:** Long term studies in animals to evaluate the carcinogenic and mutagenic potential or the effect on fertility of lidocaine HCl have not been conducted.
6. **Pregnancy:**
Teratogenic Effects: *Pregnancy Category B.* Reproduction studies have been performed in rats at doses up to 6.6 times the maximum human doses and have revealed no significant findings. There are, however, no adequate and well-controlled studies in pregnant women. Because animal reproduction studies are not always predictive of human response, this drug should be used during pregnancy only if clearly needed.
7. **Labor and Delivery:** The effects of lidocaine HCl on the mother and the fetus, when used in the managment of cardiac arrhythmias during labor and delivery are not known. Lidocaine readily crosses the placental barrier.
8. **Nursing Mothers:** It is not known whether this drug is excreted in human milk. Because many drugs are excreted in human milk, caution should be exercised when lidocaine is administered to a nursing woman.
9. **Pediatric Use:** Safety and effectiveness in children have not been established by controlled clinical studies. (See DOSAGE AND ADMINISTRATION).

Adverse Reactions: Adverse experiences following the administration of lidocaine are similar in nature to those observed with other amide local anesthetic agents. Adverse experiences may result from high plasma levels caused by excessive dosage or may result from a hypersensitivity, idiosyncrasy or diminished tolerance on the part of the patient. Serious adverse experiences are generally systemic in nature. The following types are those most commonly reported. The adverse experiences under Central Nervous System and Cardiovascular System are listed in general in a progression from mild to severe.

1. **Central Nervous System**
CNS reactions are excitatory and/or depressant and may be characterized by light-headedness, nervousness, apprehension, euphoria, confusion, dizziness, drowsiness, tinnitus, blurred or double vision, vomiting, sensations of heat, cold or numbness, twitching, tremors, convulsions, unconsciousness, respiratory depression and arrest. The excitatory reactions may be very brief or may not occur at all, in which case, the first manifestation of toxicity may be drowsiness, merging into unconsciousness and respiratory arrest.
2. **Cardiovascular System**
Cardiovascular reactions are usually depressant in nature and are characterized by bradycardia, hypotension and cardiovascular collapse, which may lead to cardiac arrest.
3. Allergic reactions as a result of sensitivity to lidocaine are extremely rare and, if they occur, should be managed by conventional means.

Drug Abuse and Dependence: Although specific studies have not been conducted, lidocaine HCl has been used clinically without evidence of abuse of this drug or of psychological or physical dependence as a result of its use.

Overdosage: Overdosage of lidocaine HCl usually results in signs of central nervous system or cardiovascular toxicity. See ADVERSE REACTIONS.

Should convulsions or signs of respiratory depression and arrest develop, the patency of the airway and adequacy of ventilation must be assured immediately. Should convulsions persist despite ventilatory therapy with oxygen, small increments of anticonvulsive agents may be given intravenously. Examples of such agents include a benzodiazepine (e.g., diazepam), an ultrashort-acting barbiturate (e.g., thiopental or thiamylal) or a short-acting barbiturate (e.g., pentobarbital or secobarbital). If the patient is under general anesthesia, a short-acting muscle relaxant (e.g., succinylcholine) may be administered.

Should circulatory depression occur, vasopressors may be used.

Dialysis is of negligible value in the treatment of acute overdosage from lidocaine HCl.

Dosage and Administration:

Adults

Single Direct Intravenous Injection (bolus): The usual dose is 50 to 100 mg of lidocaine hydrochloride (0.70 to 1.4 mg/kg; 0.32 to 0.63 mg/lb) administered intravenously under ECG monitoring. This dose may be administered at the rate of approximately 25 to 50 mg/min (0.35 to 0.70 mg/kg/min; 0.16 to 0.32 mg/lb/min). Sufficient time should be allowed to enable a slow circulation to carry the drug to the site of action. If the initial injection of 50 to 100 mg does not produce a desired response, a second dose may be injected after five minutes. NO MORE THAN 200 to 300 MG OF LIDOCAINE HYDROCHLORIDE SHOULD BE ADMINISTERED DURING A ONE HOUR PERIOD.

Continuous Intravenous Infusion: Following bolus administration, intravenous infusions of lidocaine hydrochloride may be initiated at the rate of 1 to 4 mg/min of lidocaine hydrochloride (0.014 to 0.057 mg/kg/min; 0.006 to 0.026 mg/lb/min). The rate of intravenous infusions should be reassessed as soon as the patient's basic cardiac rhythm appears to be stable or at the earliest signs of toxicity. It should rarely be necessary to continue intravenous infusions of lidocaine for prolonged periods.

Solutions for intravenous infusion may be prepared by the addition of one gram (or two grams) of lidocaine hydrochloride to one liter of 5% dextrose in water using aseptic technique. Approximately a 0.1% (or 0.2%) solution will result from this procedure; that is, each milliliter will contain approximately 1 (or 2 mg) of lidocaine hydrochloride. In those cases in which fluid restriction is medically appropriate, a more concentrated solution may be prepared.

The 20% concentration of lidocaine hydrochloride should be diluted with a suitable large volume parenteral as follows to achieve the above final concentrations for continuous infusion:

20% (200 mg/ml)	LVP Size	Final Conc.
1 g in 5 ml	1000 ml	0.1%
1 g in 5 ml	500 ml	0.2%
1 g in 5 ml	250 ml	0.4%
2 g in 10 ml	1000 ml	0.2%
2 g in 10 ml	500 ml	0.4%

The 10% concentration of lidocaine hydrochloride should be diluted with a suitable large volume parenteral as follows to achieve the above final concentrations for continuous infusion:

10% (100 mg/ml)	LVP Size	Final Conc.
1 g in 10 ml	1000 ml	0.1%
1 g in 1 ml	500 ml	0.2%
1 g in 10 ml	250 ml	0.4%

Lidocaine Hydrochloride Injection, USP has been found to be chemically stable for 24 hours after dilution in 5% dextrose in water. However, as with all intravenous admixtures, dilution of the solution should be made just prior to its administration.

When administering lidocaine hydrochloride (or any potent medication) by continuous intravenous infusion, it is advisable to use a precision volume control I.V. set.

Pediatric

Although controlled clinical studies to establish pediatric dosing schedules have not been conducted, the American Heart Association's *Standards and Guidelines* recommends a bolus dose of 1 mg/kg followed by an infusion rate of 3 µg/kg/min.

NOTE: Regarding Prolonged Infusions. There are data that indicate the half-life may be 3 hours or longer following infusions of greater than 24 hours in duration.

Parenteral drug products should be inspected visually for particulate matter and discoloration prior to administration, whenever solution and container permit.

FOR LOCAL ANESTHESIA

Clinical Pharmacology: Lidocaine stabilizes the neuronal membrane and prevents the initiation and conduction of nerve impulses, thereby effecting local anesthetic action.

Lidocaine is metabolized mainly in the liver and excreted via the kidneys. Approximately 90% of lidocaine administered is excreted in the form of various metabolites, while less than 10% is excreted unchanged.

Indications: Lidocaine Hydrochloride Injection, USP is indicated for production of local or regional anesthesia, by infiltration techniques, including percutaneous injection and intravenous regional anesthesia by peripheral nerve block techniques such as brachial plexus and intercostal blocks and by central neural techniques, including epidural and caudal blocks, when the accepted procedures for these techniques as described in standard textbooks are followed.

Contraindications: Lidocaine hydrochloride is contraindicated in patients with a known history of hypersensitivity either to local anesthetic agents of the amide type or to other components of the injectable formulations.

Warnings:
1. RESUSCITATIVE EQUIPMENT AND DRUGS, INCLUDING OXYGEN, SHOULD BE IMMEDIATELY AVAILABLE WHEN ANY LOCAL ANESTHETIC AGENT IS USED.
2. **Use in Pregnancy:** Reproductive studies have been performed in rats and rabbits without evidence of harm to the animal fetus. However, the safe use of lidocaine in humans has not been established with respect to possible adverse effects upon fetal development. Careful consideration should be given to this fact before administering this drug to women of childbearing potential, particularly during early pregnancy. This does not exclude the use of the drug at term for obstetrical analgesia. Lidocaine HCl has been used effectively for obstetrical analgesia. Adverse effect on the fetus, course of labor or delivery have rarely been observed when proper dosage and proper technique have been employed.
3. Local anesthetic procedures should be used with caution when there is inflammation and/or sepsis in the region of the proposed injection.
4. Vasopressor agents (administered for the treatment of hypotension related to caudal or other epidural blocks) should be used with caution in the presence of oxytocic drugs, as a severe persistent hypertension and even rupture of a cerebral blood vessel may occur.
5. The solutions which contain a vasoconstrictor should be used with extreme caution for patients whose medical history and physical evaluation suggest the existence of hypertension, arteriosclerotic heart disease, cerebral vascular insufficiency, heart block, thyrotoxicosis or diabetes, etc. The solutions which contain a vasoconstrictor should also be used with extreme caution in patients receiving drugs known to produce blood pressure alterations (e.g., MAO inhibitors, tricyclic antidepressants, phenothiazines, etc.) as either sustained hypotension or hypertension may occur.

Precautions: The safety and effectiveness of Lidocaine Hydrochloride Injection, USP depends on proper dosage, correct technique, adequate precautions and readiness for emergencies. Standard textbooks should be consulted for specific techniques and precautions for various regional anesthetic procedures.

The lowest dosage that results in effective anesthesia should be used. Injection of repeated doses of lidocaine HCl may cause significant increases in blood levels with each repeated dose due to slow accumulation of lidocaine or its metabolites. Tolerance varies with the status of the patient. Debilitated, elderly patients, acutely ill patients and children should be given reduced doses commensurate with their age and physical status. Lidocaine HCl should also be used with caution in patients with severe shock or heart block.

In using lidocaine HCl for infiltration or regional nerve block anesthesia, injection should always be made slowly and with frequent aspirations. Proper tourniquet technique is essential in the performance of intravenous regional anesthesia. Solutions containing epinephrine or other vasoconstrictors should not be used for this technique.

Epidural anesthesia and caudal anesthesia should be used with extreme caution in persons with the following conditions: Existing neurological disease, spinal deformities, septicemia, severe hypertension and extreme youth.

Fetal bradycardia frequently follows paracervical block and may be associated with fetal acidosis. Fetal heart rate should always be monitored during paracervical anesthesia. Added risk appears to be present in prematurity, postmaturity, toxemia of pregnancy, uteroplacental insufficiency and fetal distress. The physician should weigh the possible advantages against dangers when considering paracervical block in these conditions. When the recommended dose is exceeded, the incidence of fetal bradycardia increases. Short-term neonatal neurobehavioral alterations have been observed in association with some local anesthetics administered during labor and delivery. The short-term and long-term significance of these alterations is not known.

Solutions containing a vasoconstrictor should be used cautiously and in carefully circumscribed quantities in areas of the body supplied by end arteries or having otherwise compromised blood supply (e.g., digits, nose, external ear, penis, etc.). Serious cardiac arrhythmias may occur if preparations containing a vasoconstrictor are employed in patients during or following the administration of chloroform, halothane, cyclopropane, trichloroethylene or other related agents.

Lidocaine Hydrochloride Injection, USP should be used with caution in persons with known drug sensitivities. Patients allergic to para-aminobenzoic acid derivatives (procaine, tetracaine, benzocaine, etc.) have not shown cross sensitivity to lidocaine.

The safety of amid local anesthetics in patients with malignant hyperthermia has not been assessed, and therefore, these agents should be used with caution in such patients. Drowsiness following an injection of lidocaine HCl is usually an early indication of a high blood level of the drug and may occur following inadvertent intravascular administration or rapid absorption of lidocaine. Local anesthetics react with certain metals and cause the release of their respective ions which, if injected, may cause severe local irritation. Adequate precautions should be taken to avoid this type of interaction. (See STERILIZATION, STORAGE AND TECHNICAL PROCEDURES).

Adverse Reactions: Reactions to lidocaine HCl are similar in character to those observed with other local anesthetic agents. Adverse reactions may be due to high plasma levels as a result of excessive dosage, rapid absorption or inadvertent intravascular injection. Such reactions are systemic in nature and involve the central nervous system and/or the cardiovascular system.

Rarely, reactions may result from hypersensitivity, idiosyncrasy or diminished tolerance on the part of the patient.

CNS reactions are excitatory and/or depressant, and may be characterized by nervousness, dizziness, blurred vision and tremors, followed by drowsiness, convulsions, unconsciousness and, possibly, respiratory arrest. The excitatory reactions may be very brief or may not occur at all, in which case the first manifestations of toxicity may be drowsiness, merging into unconsciousness and respiratory arrest.

Hypotension and bradycardia may occur as normal physiological phenomena following sympathetic block with central neural blocks. Toxic cardiovascular reactions to local anesthetics are usually depressant in nature and are characterized by peripheral vasodilation, hypotension, myocardial depression, bradycardia and, possibly cardiac arrest.

Treatment of a patient with toxic manifestations consists of assuring and maintaining a patent airway, supporting ventilation with oxygen, and assisted or controlled ventilation (respiration) as required. This usually will be sufficient in the management of most reactions.

Should a convulsion persist despite ventilatory therapy with oxygen, small increments of anticonvulsive agents may be given intravenously. Examples of such agents include a benzodiazepine (e.g., diazepam), ultrashort-acting barbiturates (e.g., thiopental or thiamylal) or a short-acting barbiturate (e.g., pentobarbital or secobarbital). Cardiovascular depression may require circulatory assistance with intravenous fluids and/or vasopressors (e.g., ephedrine) as dictated by the clinical situation.

Allergic reactions may occur as a result of sensitivity either to local anesthetics or to the methylparaben used as a preservative in multiple-dose vials. Anaphylactoid type symptomatology and reactions, characterized by cutaneous lesions, urticaria, and edema should be managed by conventional means. The detection of potential sensitivity by skin testing is of limited value.

Dosage and Administration: Table I (Recommended Dosages) summarizes the recommended volumes and concentrations of Lidocaine Hydrochloride Injection, USP for various types of anesthetic procedures. The dosages suggested in this table are for normal healthy adults and refer to the use of epinephrine-free solutions. When larger dosages are required, only solutions containing epinephrine should be used except in those cases where vasopressor drugs may be contraindicated. These recommended doses serve only as a guide to the amount of anesthetic required for most routine procedures. The actual volume and concentrations to be used depend on a number of factors, such as type and extent of surgical procedure, degree of muscular relaxation required, duration of anesthesia required, the physical state of the patient, etc. In all cases the lowest concentration and smallest dose that will produce the desired result should be given. Dosages should be reduced for children and for elderly and debilitated patients. The onset of anesthesia, the duration of anesthesia and the degree of muscular relaxation are proportional to the volume and concentration of local anesthetic solution used. Thus, an increase in concentration and volume of lidocaine HCl administered will decrease the onset of anesthesia, prolong the duration of anesthesia, provide a greater degree of muscular relation and increase the segmental spread of anesthesia. However, increasing the concentration and volume of lidocaine HCl administered may result in a more profound fall in blood pressure when used in epidural anesthesia. Although the incidence of side effects with lidocaine HCl is quite low, caution should be exercised particularly when employing large volumes and concentrations of lidocaine HCl, since the incidence of side effects is directly related to the total dose of local anesthetic agent injected.

It is important that a single dose container be employed for epidural anesthesia and major peripheral nerve block.

Continued on next page

If desired, additional literature on any Abbott Product will be provided upon request to Abbott Laboratories.

Abbott—Cont.

FOR EPIDURAL OR SPINAL ANESTHESIA, USE ONLY SOLUTIONS WITHOUT PRESERVATIVES.

IMPORTANT: *A test dose of 2 to 5 ml should be administered at least 5 minutes prior to injecting the total required volume for central neural blocks (e.g., epidural or caudal anesthesia).*

Maximum Recommended Dosages
For normal healthy adults, the individual dose of lidocaine hydrochloride with epinephrine should be such that the dose of lidocaine hydrochloride is kept below 500 mg and, in any case, should not exceed 7 mg/kg (3.2 mg/lb) of body weight. When used without epinephrine, the amount of Lidocaine Hydrochloride Injection, USP administered should be such that the dose of lidocaine hydrochloride is kept below 300 mg, and in any case, should not exceed 4.5 mg/kg (2.0 mg/lb) of body weight. For continuous epidural or caudal anesthesia, the maximum recommended dosage should not be administered at intervals of less than 90 minutes. For paracervical block for obstetrical analgesia, (including abortion) the maximum recommended dosage (200 mg) should not be administered at intervals of less than 90 minutes. When paracervical block is used for non-obstetrical procedures, more drug may be administered if required to obtain adequate anesthesia. For intravenous regional anesthesia in adults (using lidocaine hydrochloride 0.5% solution without epinephrine), the dose administered should not exceed 4 mg/kg (1.8 mg/lb) of body weight.

Children:
It is difficult to recommend a maximum dose of any drug for children since this varies as a function of age and weight. For children of less than ten years who have a normal lean body mass and normal body development, the maximum dose may be determined by the application of one of the standard pediatric dose formulas (e.g., Clark's rule). For example, in a child of five years weighing 50 lbs. the dose of lidocaine hydrochloride should not exceed 75 to 100 mg when calculated according to Clark's rule. In any case, the maximum dose of lidocaine HCl with epinephrine should not exceed 7 mg/kg (3.2 mg/lb) of body weight. When used without epinephrine, the amount of lidocaine HCl administered should not exceed 4.5 mg/kg (2.0 mg/lb) of body weight. In order to minimize the possibility of toxic reactions, the use of lidocaine HCl 0.5% or 1.0% is recommended for most anesthetic procedures involving pediatric patients. The use of even more dilute solutions (e.g., 0.25% to 0.5%) and total dosages not to exceed 3 mg/kg (1.4 mg/lb) are recommended for induction of intravenous regional anesthesia in children.

Parenteral drug products should be inspected visually for particulate matter and discoloration prior to administration, whenever solution and container permit.
[See table below].

Sterilization, Storage and Technical Procedures: Disinfecting agents containing heavy metals, which cause release of respective ions (mercury, zinc, copper, etc.) should not be used for skin or mucous membrane disinfection as they have been related to incidence of swelling and edema. When chemical disinfection of multi-dose vials is desired, either isopropyl alcohol (91%) or 70% ethyl alcohol is recommended. Many commercially available brands of rubbing alcohol, as well as solutions of ethyl alcohol not of USP grade, contain denaturants which are injurious to rubber and, therefore, are not to be used. It is recommended that chemical disinfection be accomplished by wiping the vial or ampul thoroughly with cotton or gauze that has been moistened with the recommended alcohol just prior to use.

How Supplied: Lidocaine Hydrochloride Injection, USP is available in a variety of dosage strengths, containers and sizes. Consult Abbott Labortories for a current listing.
Exposure of pharmaceutical products to heat should be minimized. Avoid excessive heat. Protect from freezing. It is recommended that the product be stored at room temperature (25° C); however, brief exposure up to 40° C does not adversely affect the product.

Caution: Federal (USA) law prohibits dispensing without prescription.
06-3508 R16 Rev. Apr., 1984

Table I
Recommended Dosages of Lidocaine Hydrochloride Injection, USP for Various Anesthetic Procedures in Normal Healthy Adults

Procedure	Lidocaine Hydrochloride Injection, USP (without Epinephrine)		
	Conc. (%)	Vol. (ml)	Total Dose (mg)
Infiltration			
Percutaneous	0.5 or 1.0	1–60	5–300
Intravenous Regional	0.5	10–60	50–300
Peripheral Nerve Blocks, e.g.			
Brachial	1.5	15–20	225–300
Dental	2.0	1–5	20–100
Intercostal	1.0	3	30
Paravertebral	1.0	3–5	30–50
Pudendal (each side)	1.0	10	100
Paracervical			
Obstetrical Analgesia (each side)	1.0	10	100
Sympathetic Nerve Blocks, e.g.			
Cervical (stellate ganglion)	1.0	5	50
Lumbar	1.0	5–10	50–100
Central Neural Blocks			
Epidural*			
Thoracic	1.0	20–30	200–300
Lumbar			
Analgesia	1.0	25–30	250–300
Anesthesia	1.5	15–20	225–300
	2.0	10–15	200–300
Caudal			
Obstetrical Analgesia	1.0	20–30	200–300
Surgical Anesthesia	1.5	15–20	225–300

* Dose determined by number of dermatomes to be anesthetized (2 to 3 ml/dermatome).
THE ABOVE SUGGESTED CONCENTRATIONS AND VOLUMES SERVE ONLY AS A GUIDE. OTHER VOLUMES AND CONCENTRATIONS MAY BE USED PROVIDED THE TOTAL MAXIMUM RECOMMENDED DOSE IS NOT EXCEEDED.

NEMBUTAL® SODIUM CAPSULES
[nĕm-bū-tal sō-dĭ-um]
(pentobarbital sodium capsules, USP)

WARNING: MAY BE HABIT FORMING

Description: The barbiturates are nonselective central nervous system depressants which are primarily used as sedative hypnotics. The barbiturates and their sodium salts are subject to control under the Federal Controlled Substances Act (See "Drug Abuse and Dependence" section).
Barbiturates are substituted pyrimidine derivatives in which the basic structure common to these drugs is barbituric acid, a substance which has no central nervous system (CNS) activity. CNS activity is obtained by substituting alkyl, alkenyl, or aryl groups on the pyrimidine ring. Nembutal (pentobarbital sodium) is chemically represented by sodium 5-ethyl-5-(1-methylbutyl) barbiturate.
The sodium salt of pentobarbital occurs as a white, slightly bitter powder which is freely soluble in water and alcohol but practically insoluble in benzene and ether. Nembutal Sodium capsules for oral administration contain either 50 mg or 100 mg of pentobarbital sodium.

Clinical Pharmacology: Barbiturates are capable of producing all levels of CNS mood alteration from excitation to mild sedation, to hypnosis, and deep coma. Overdosage can produce death. In high enough therapeutic doses, barbiturates induce anesthesia.
Barbiturates depress the sensory cortex, decrease motor activity, alter cerebellar function, and produce drowsiness, sedation, and hypnosis.
Barbiturate-induced sleep differs from physiological sleep. Sleep laboratory studies have demonstrated that barbiturates reduce the amount of time spent in the rapid eye movement (REM) phase of sleep or dreaming stage. Also, Stages III and IV sleep are decreased. Following abrupt cessation of barbiturates used regularly, patients may experience markedly increased dreaming, nightmares, and/or insomnia. Therefore, withdrawal of a single therapeutic dose over 5 or 6 days has been recommended to lessen the REM rebound and disturbed sleep which contribute to drug withdrawal syndrome (for example, decrease the dose from 3 to 2 doses a day for 1 week).
In studies, secobarbital sodium and pentobarbital sodium have been found to lose most of their effectiveness for both inducing and maintaining sleep by the end of 2 weeks of continued drug administration at fixed doses. The short-, intermediate-, and, to a lesser degree, long-acting barbiturates have been widely prescribed for treating insomnia. Although the clinical literature abounds with claims that the short-acting barbiturates are superior for producing sleep while the intermediate-acting compounds are more effective in maintaining sleep, controlled studies have failed to demonstrate these differential effects. Therefore, as sleep medications, the barbiturates are of limited value beyond short-term use.
Barbiturates have little analgesic action at subanesthetic doses. Rather, in subanesthetic doses these drugs may increase the reaction to painful stimuli. All barbiturates exhibit anticonvulsant activity in anesthetic doses. However, of the drugs in this class, only phenobarbital, mephobarbital, and metharbital have been clinically demonstrated to be effective as oral anticonvulsants in subhypnotic doses.
Barbiturates are respiratory depressants. The degree of respiratory depression is dependent upon dose. With hypnotic doses, respiratory depression produced by barbiturates is similar to that which occurs during physiologic sleep with slight decrease in blood pressure and heart rate. Studies in laboratory animals have shown that barbiturates cause reduction in the tone and contractility of the uterus, ureters, and urinary bladder. However, concentrations of the drugs required to produce this effect in humans are not reached with sedative-hypnotic doses.
Barbiturates do not impair normal hepatic function, but have been shown to induce liver microsomal enzymes, thus increasing and/or altering

the metabolism of barbiturates and other drugs. (See "Precautions—*Drug Interactions*" section).

Pharmacokinetics: Barbiturates are absorbed in varying degrees following oral, rectal, or parenteral administration. The salts are more rapidly absorbed than are the acids. The rate of absorption is increased if the sodium salt is ingested as a dilute solution or taken on an empty stomach.

The onset of action for oral or rectal administration varies from 20 to 60 minutes.

Duration of action, which is related to the rate at which the barbiturates are redistributed throughout the body, varies among persons and in the same person from time to time. In Table 1, the barbiturates are classified according to their duration of action. This classification should not be used to predict the exact duration of effect, but the grouping of drugs should be used as a guide in the selection of barbiturates.

No studies have demonstrated that the different routes of administration are equivalent with respect to bioavailability.

[See Table 1.]

Barbiturates are weak acids that are absorbed and rapidly distributed to all tissues and fluids with high concentrations in the brain, liver, and kidneys. Lipid solubility of the barbiturates is the dominant factor in their distribution within the body. The more lipid soluble the barbiturate, the more rapidly it penetrates all tissues of the body. Barbiturates are bound to plasma and tissue proteins to a varying degree with the degree of binding increasing directly as a function of lipid solubility. The plasma half-life for pentobarbital in adults is 15 to 50 hours and appears to be dose dependent.

Barbiturates are metabolized primarily by the hepatic microsomal enzyme system, and the metabolic products are excreted in the urine, and less commonly, in the feces. Approximately 25 to 50 percent of a dose of aprobarbital or phenobarbital is eliminated unchanged in the urine, whereas the amount of other barbiturates excreted unchanged in the urine is negligible. The excretion of unmetabolized barbiturate is one feature that distinguishes the long-acting category from those belonging to other categories which are almost entirely metabolized. The inactive metabolites of the barbiturates are excreted as conjugates of glucuronic acid.

Indications and Usage: *Oral:*
a. Sedatives.
b. Hypnotics, for the short-term treatment of insomnia, since they appear to lose their effectiveness for sleep induction and sleep maintenance after 2 weeks (See "Clinical Pharmacology" section).
c. Preanesthetics.

Contraindications: Barbiturates are contraindicated in patients with known barbiturate sensitivity. Barbiturates are also contraindicated in patients with a history of manifest or latent porphyria.

Warnings:
1. *Habit forming:* Barbiturates may be habit forming. Tolerance, psychological and physical dependence may occur with continued use. (See "Drug Abuse and Dependence" and "Pharmacokinetics" sections). Patients who have psychological dependence on barbiturates may increase the dosage or decrease the dosage interval without consulting a physician and may subsequently develop a physical dependence on barbiturates. To minimize the possibility of overdosage or the development of dependence, the prescribing and dispensing of sedative-hypnotic barbiturates should be limited to the amount required for the interval until the next appointment. Abrupt cessation after prolonged use in the dependent person may result in withdrawal symptoms, including delirium, convulsions, and possibly death. Barbiturates should be withdrawn gradually from any patient known to be taking excessive dosage over long periods of time. (See "Drug Abuse and Dependence" section).

Table 1.—*Classification, Onset, and Duration of Action of Commonly used Barbiturates Taken Orally*

Classification	Onset of action	Duration of action
Long-acting Phenobarbital.	1 hour or longer	10 to 12 hours
Intermediate Amobarbital. Butabarbital.	¾ to 1 hour	6 to 8 hours
Short-acting Pentobarbital Secobarbital.	10 to 15 minutes	3 to 4 hours

2. *Acute or chronic pain:* Caution should be exercised when barbiturates are administered to patients with acute or chronic pain, because paradoxical excitement could be induced or important symptoms could be masked. However, the use of barbiturates as sedatives in the postoperative surgical period and as adjuncts to cancer chemotherapy is well established.

3. *Use in pregnancy:* Barbiturates can cause fetal damage when administered to a pregnant woman. Retrospective, case-controlled studies have suggested a connection between the maternal consumption of barbiturates and a higher than expected incidence of fetal abnormalities. Following oral or parenteral administration, barbiturates readily cross the placental barrier and are distributed throughout fetal tissues with highest concentrations found in the placenta, fetal liver, and brain.

Withdrawal symptoms occur in infants born to mothers who receive barbiturates throughout the last trimester of pregnancy. (See "Drug Abuse and Dependence" section). If this drug is used during pregnancy, or if the patient becomes pregnant while taking this drug, the patient should be apprised of the potential hazard to the fetus.

4. *Synergistic effects:* The concomitant use of alcohol or other CNS depressants may produce additive CNS depressant effects.

Precautions:

General: Barbiturates may be habit forming. Tolerance and psychological and physical dependence may occur with continuing use. (See "Drug Abuse and Dependence" section). Barbiturates should be administered with caution, if at all, to patients who are mentally depressed, have suicidal tendencies, or a history of drug abuse.

Elderly or debilitated patients may react to barbiturates with marked excitement, depression, and confusion. In some persons, barbiturates repeatedly produce excitement rather than depression.

In patients with hepatic damage, barbiturates should be administered with caution and initially in reduced doses. Barbiturates should not be administered to patients showing the premonitory signs of hepatic coma.

The 100 mg capsules of Nembutal Sodium contain FD&C Yellow No. 5 (tartrazine) which may cause allergic-type reactions (including bronchial asthma) in certain susceptible individuals. Although the overall incidence of FD&C Yellow No. 5 (tartrazine) sensitivity in the general population is low, it is frequently seen in patients who also have aspirin hypersensitivity.

Information for the patient: Practitioners should give the following information and instructions to patients receiving barbiturates.
1. The use of barbiturates carries with it an associated risk of psychological and/or physical dependence. The patient should be warned against increasing the dose of the drug without consulting a physician.
2. Barbiturates may impair mental and/or physical abilities required for the performance of potentially hazardous tasks (e.g., driving, operating machinery, etc.).
3. Alcohol should not be consumed while taking barbiturates. Concurrent use of the barbiturates with other CNS depressants (e.g., alcohol, narcotics, tranquilizers, and antihistamines) may result in additional CNS depressant effects.

Laboratory tests: Prolonged therapy with barbiturates should be accompanied by periodic laboratory evaluation of organ systems, including hematopoietic, renal, and hepatic systems. (See "Precautions—*General*" and "Adverse Reactions" sections).

Drug interactions: Most reports of clinically significant drug interactions occurring with the barbiturates have involved phenobarbital. However, the application of these data to other barbiturates appears valid and warrants serial blood level determinations of the relevant drugs when there are multiple therapies.

1. *Anticoagulants:* Phenobarbital lowers the plasma levels of dicumarol (name previously used: bishydroxycoumarin) and causes a decrease in anticoagulant activity as measured by the prothrombin time. Barbiturates can induce hepatic microsomal enzymes resulting in increased metabolism and decreased anticoagulant response of oral anticoagulants (e.g., warfarin, acenocoumarol, dicumarol, and phenprocoumon). Patients stabilized on anticoagulant therapy may require dosage adjustments if barbiturates are added to or withdrawn from their dosage regimen.

2. *Corticosteroids:* Barbiturates appear to enhance the metabolism of exogenous corticosteroids probably through the induction of hepatic microsomal enzymes. Patients stabilized on corticosteroid therapy may require dosage adjustments if barbiturates are added to or withdrawn from their dosage regimen.

3. *Griseofulvin:* Phenobarbital appears to interfere with the absorption of orally administered griseofulvin, thus decreasing its blood level. The effect of the resultant decreased blood levels of griseofulvin on therapeutic response has not been established. However, it would be preferable to avoid concomitant administration of these drugs.

4. *Doxycycline:* Phenobarbital has been shown to shorten the half-life of doxycycline for as long as 2 weeks after barbiturate therapy is discontinued.

This mechanism is probably through the induction of hepatic microsomal enzymes that metabolize the antibiotic. If phenobarbital and doxycycline are administered concurrently, the clinical response to doxycycline should be monitored closely.

5. *Phenytoin, sodium valproate, valproic acid:* The effect of barbiturates on the metabolism of phenytoin appears to be variable. Some investigators report an accelerating effect, while others report no effect. Because the effect of barbiturates on the metabolism of phenytoin is not predictable, phenytoin and barbiturate blood levels should be monitored more frequently if these drugs are given concurrently. Sodium valproate and valproic acid appear to decrease barbiturate metabolism; therefore, barbiturate blood levels should be monitored and appropriate dosage adjustments made as indicated.

6. *Central nervous system depressants:* The concomitant use of other central nervous system

Continued on next page

If desired, additional literature on any Abbott Product will be provided upon request to Abbott Laboratories.

Abbott—Cont.

depressants including other sedatives or hypnotics, antihistamines, tranquilizers, or alcohol, may produce additive depressant effects.

7. *Monoamine oxidase inhibitors (MAOI):* MAOI prolong the effects of barbiturates probably because metabolism of the barbiturate is inhibited.
8. *Estradiol, estrone, progesterone and other steroidal hormones:* Pretreatment with or concurrent administration of phenobarbital may decrease the effect of estradiol by increasing its metabolism. There have been reports of patients treated with antiepileptic drugs (e.g., phenobarbital) who became pregnant while taking oral contraceptives. An alternate contraceptive method might be suggested to women taking phenobarbital.

Carcinogenesis: Adequate data are not available on long-term potential for carcinogenicity in humans or animals for pentobarbital.

Data from one retrospective study of 235 children in which the types of barbiturates are not identified suggested an association between exposure to barbiturates prenatally and an increased incidence of brain tumor. (Gold, E., et al., "Increased Risk of Brain Tumors in Children Exposed to Barbiturates," Journal of National Cancer Institute, 61:1031–1034, 1978).

Pregnancy: 1. *Teratogenic effects.* Pregnancy Category D—See "Warnings—Use in Pregnancy" section.

2. *Nonteratogenic effects.* Reports of infants suffering from long-term barbiturate exposure in utero included the acute withdrawal syndrome of seizures and hyperirritability from birth to a delayed onset of up to 14 days. (See "Drug Abuse and Dependence" section).

Labor and delivery: Hypnotic doses of these barbiturates do not appear to significantly impair uterine activity during labor. Full anesthetic doses of barbiturates decrease the force and frequency of uterine contractions. Administration of sedative-hypnotic barbiturates to the mother during labor may result in respiratory depression in the newborn. Premature infants are particularly susceptible to the depressant effects of barbiturates. If barbiturates are used during labor and delivery, resuscitation equipment should be available.

Data are currently not available to evaluate the effect of these barbiturates when forceps delivery or other intervention is necessary. Also, data are not available to determine the effect of these barbiturates on the later growth, development, and functional maturation of the child.

Nursing mothers: Caution should be exercised when a barbiturate is administered to a nursing woman since small amounts of barbiturates are excreted in the milk.

Adverse Reactions: The following adverse reactions and their incidence were compiled from surveillance of thousands of hospitalized patients. Because such patients may be less aware of certain of the milder adverse effects of barbiturates, the incidence of these reactions may be somewhat higher in fully ambulatory patients.

More than 1 in 100 patients. The most common adverse reaction estimated to occur at a rate of 1 to 3 patients per 100 is: *Nervous System:* Somnolence.

Less than 1 in 100 patients. Adverse reactions estimated to occur at a rate of less than 1 in 100 patients listed below, grouped by organ system, and by decreasing order of occurrence are:

Nervous system: Agitation, confusion, hyperkinesia, ataxia, CNS depression, nightmares, nervousness, psychiatric disturbance, hallucinations, insomnia, anxiety, dizziness, thinking abnormality.
Respiratory system: Hypoventilation, apnea.
Cardiovascular system: Bradycardia, hypotension, syncope.
Digestive system: Nausea, vomiting, constipation.
Other reported reactions: Headache, injection site reactions, hypersensitivity reactions (angioedema, skin rashes, exfoliative dermatitis), fever, liver damage, megaloblastic anemia following chronic phenobarbital use.

Drug Abuse and Dependence: Pentobarbital sodium capsules are subject to control by the Federal Controlled Substances Act under DEA schedule II.

Barbiturates may be habit forming. Tolerance, psychological dependence, and physical dependence may occur especially following prolonged use of high doses of barbiturates. Daily administration in excess of 400 mg of pentobarbital or secobarbital for approximately 90 days is likely to produce some degree of physical dependence. A dosage of from 600 to 800 mg taken for at least 35 days is sufficient to produce withdrawal seizures. The average daily dose for the barbiturate addict is usually about 1.5 grams. As tolerance to barbiturates develops, the amount needed to maintain the same level of intoxication increases; tolerance to a fatal dosage, however, does not increase more than two-fold. As this occurs, the margin between an intoxicating dosage and fatal dosage becomes smaller.

Symptoms of acute intoxication with barbiturates include unsteady gait, slurred speech, and sustained nystagmus. Mental signs of chronic intoxication include confusion, poor judgment, irritability, insomnia, and somatic complaints.

Symptoms of barbiturate dependence are similar to those of chronic alcoholism. If an individual appears to be intoxicated with alcohol to a degree that is radically disproportionate to the amount of alcohol in his or her blood the use of barbiturates should be suspected. The lethal dose of a barbiturate is far less if alcohol is also ingested.

The symptoms of barbiturate withdrawal can be severe and may cause death. Minor withdrawal symptoms may appear 8 to 12 hours after the last dose of a barbiturate. These symptoms usually appear in the following order: anxiety, muscle twitching, tremor of hands and fingers, progressive weakness, dizziness, distortion in visual perception, nausea, vomiting, insomnia, and orthostatic hypotension. Major withdrawal symptoms (convulsions and delirium) may occur within 16 hours and last up to 5 days after abrupt cessation of these drugs. Intensity of withdrawal symptoms gradually declines over a period of approximately 15 days. Individuals susceptible to barbiturate abuse and dependence include alcoholics and opiate abusers, as well as other sedative-hypnotic and amphetamine abusers.

Drug dependence to barbiturates arises from repeated administration of a barbiturate or agent with barbiturate-like effect on a continuous basis, generally in amounts exceeding therapeutic dose levels. The characteristics of drug dependence to barbiturates include: (a) a strong desire or need to continue taking the drug; (b) a tendency to increase the dose; (c) a psychic dependence on the effects of the drug related to subjective and individual appreciation of those effects; and (d) a physical dependence on the effects of the drug requiring its presence for maintenance of homeostasis and resulting in a definite, characteristic, and self-limited abstinence syndrome when the drug is withdrawn.

Treatment of barbiturate dependence consists of cautious and gradual withdrawal of the drug. Barbiturate-dependent patients can be withdrawn by using a number of different withdrawal regimens. In all cases withdrawal takes an extended period of time. One method involves substituting a 30 mg dose of phenobarbital for each 100 to 200 mg dose of barbiturate that the patient has been taking. The total daily amount of phenobarbital is then administered in 3 to 4 divided doses, not to exceed 600 mg daily. Should signs of withdrawal occur on the first day of treatment, a loading dose of 100 to 200 mg of phenobarbital may be administered IM in addition to the oral dose. After stabilization on phenobarbital, the total daily dose is decreased by 30 mg a day as long as withdrawal is proceeding smoothly. A modification of this regimen involves initiating treatment at the patient's regular dosage level and decreasing the daily dosage by 10 percent if tolerated by the patient.

Infants physically dependent on barbiturates may be given phenobarbital 3 to 10 mg/kg/day. After withdrawal symptoms (hyperactivity, disturbed sleep, tremors, hyperreflexia) are relieved, the dosage of phenobarbital should be gradually decreased and completely withdrawn over a 2 week period.

Overdosage: The toxic dose of barbiturates varies considerably. In general, an oral dose of 1 g of most barbiturates produces serious poisoning in an adult. Death commonly occurs after 2 to 10 g of ingested barbiturate. Barbiturate intoxication may be confused with alcoholism, bromide intoxication, and with various neurological disorders. Acute overdosage with barbiturates is manifested by CNS and respiratory depression which may progress to Cheyne-Stokes respiration, areflexia, constriction of the pupils to a slight degree (though in severe poisoning they may show paralytic dilation), oliguria, tachycardia, hypotension, lowered body temperature, and coma. Typical shock syndrome (apnea, circulatory collapse, respiratory arrest, and death) may occur.

In extreme overdose, all electrical activity in the brain may cease, in which case a "flat" EEG normally equated with clinical death cannot be accepted. This effect is fully reversible unless hypoxic damage occurs. Consideration should be given to the possibility of barbiturate intoxication even in situations that appear to involve trauma. Complications such as pneumonia, pulmonary edema, cardiac arrhythmias, congestive heart failure, and renal failure may occur. Uremia may increase CNS sensitivity to barbiturates. Differential diagnosis should include hypoglycemia, head trauma, cerebrovascular accidents, convulsive states, and diabetic coma. Blood levels from acute overdosage for some barbiturates are listed in Table 2.

[See table on next page].

Treatment of overdosage is mainly supportive and consists of the following:

1. Maintenance of an adequate airway, with assisted respiration and oxygen administration as necessary.
2. Monitoring of vital signs and fluid balance.
3. If the patient is conscious and has not lost the gag reflex, emesis may be induced with ipecac. Care should be taken to prevent pulmonary aspiration of vomitus. After completion of vomiting, 30 g activated charcoal in a glass of water may be administered.
4. If emesis is contraindicated, gastric lavage may be performed with a cuffed endotracheal tube in place with the patient in the face down position. Activated charcoal may be left in the emptied stomach and a saline cathartic administered.
5. Fluid therapy and other standard treatment for shock, if needed.
6. If renal function is normal, forced diuresis may aid in the elimination of the barbiturate. Alkalinization of the urine increases renal excretion of some barbiturates, especially phenobarbital, also aprobarbital, and mephobarbital (which is metabolized to phenobarbital).
7. Although not recommended as a routine procedure, hemodialysis may be used in severe barbiturate intoxications or if the patient is anuric or in shock.
8. Patient should be rolled from side to side every 30 minutes.
9. Antibiotics should be given if pneumonia is suspected.
10. Appropriate nursing care to prevent hypostatic pneumonia, decubiti, aspiration, and other complications of patients with altered states of consciousness.

Dosage and Administration: *Adults:* Daytime sedation can ordinarily be provided by one 30 mg capsule of NEMBUTAL Sodium (pentobarbital sodium) taken 3 or 4 times per day.

The usual hypnotic dose consists of 100 mg.

Children: Daytime sedation can be provided by 2 to 6 mg/kg/24 hours (maximum 100 mg), depending on age, weight, and the desired degree of sedation.

The proper hypnotic dose for children must be judged on the basis of individual age and weight. Dosages of barbiturates must be individualized with full knowledge of their particular characteristics and recommended rate of administration. Factors of consideration are the patient's age, weight, and condition.

Special patient population: Dosage should be reduced in the elderly or debilitated because these patients may be more sensitive to barbiturates. Dosage should be reduced for patients with impaired renal function or hepatic disease.

How Supplied: NEMBUTAL Sodium Capsules (pentobarbital sodium capsules, USP) are supplied as follows:

50 mg transparent and orange-colored capsules in bottles of 100 (**NDC** 0074-3150-11);

100 mg yellow capsules in bottles of 100 (**NDC** 0074-3114-01), 500 (**NDC** 0074-3114-02), and in the Abbo-Pac® unit dose packages of 100 (**NDC** 0074-3114-21).

Abbott Pharmaceuticals, Inc.
North Chicago, IL 60064

Shown in Product Identification Section, page 403

Table 2.—*Concentration of Barbiturate in the Blood Versus Degree of CNS Depression*
Blood barbiturate level in ppm (μg/ml)

Barbiturate	Onset/duration	1	2	3	4	5
Pentobarbital	Fast/short	≤2	0.5 to 3	10 to 15	12 to 25	15 to 40
Secobarbital	Fast/short	≤2	0.5 to 5	10 to 15	15 to 25	15 to 40
Amobarbital	Intermediate/intermediate	≤3	2 to 10	30 to 40	30 to 60	40 to 80
Butabarbital	Intermediate/intermediate	≤5	3 to 25	40 to 60	50 to 80	60 to 100
Phenobarbital	Slow/long	≤10	5 to 40	50 to 80	70 to 120	100 to 200

Degree of depression in nontolerant persons*

* Categories of degree of depression in nontolerant persons.
1. Under the influence and appreciably impaired for purposes of driving a motor vehicle or performing tasks requiring alertness and unimpaired judgment and reaction time.
2. Sedated, therapeutic range, calm, relaxed, and easily aroused.
3. Comatose, difficult to arose, significant depression of respiration.
4. Compatible with death in aged or ill persons or in presence of obstructed airway, other toxic agents, or exposure to cold.
5. Usual lethal level, the upper end of the range includes those who received some supportive treatment.

NEMBUTAL® SODIUM SOLUTION ℞ ©
[nem'-bū-tal]
(pentobarbital sodium injection, USP)
Ampuls—Vials

WARNING: MAY BE HABIT FORMING. DO NOT USE IF MATERIAL HAS PRECIPITATED.

Description: The barbiturates are nonselective central nervous system depressants which are primarily used as sedative hypnotics and also anticonvulsants in subhypnotic doses. The barbiturates and their sodium salts are subject to control under the Federal Controlled Substances Act (See "Drug Abuse and Dependence" section).

The sodium salts of amobarbital, pentobarbital, phenobarbital, and secobarbital are available as sterile parenteral solutions.

Barbiturates are substituted pyrimidine derivatives in which the basic structure common to these drugs is barbituric acid, a substance which has no central nervous system (CNS) activity. CNS activity is obtained by substituting alkyl, alkenyl, or aryl groups on the pyrimidine ring.

NEMBUTAL Sodium Solution (pentobarbital sodium injection) is a sterile solution for intravenous or intramuscular injection. Each ml contains pentobarbital sodium 50 mg, in a vehicle of propylene glycol, 40%, alcohol, 10% and water for injection, to volume. The pH is adjusted to approximately 9.5 with hydrochloric acid and/or sodium hydroxide.

NEMBUTAL Sodium is a short-acting barbiturate, chemically designated as sodium 5-ethyl-5-(1-methylbutyl) barbiturate.

The sodium salt occurs as a white, slightly bitter powder which is freely soluble in water and alcohol but practically insoluble in benzene and ether.

Clinical Pharmacology: Barbiturates are capable of producing all levels of CNS mood alteration from excitation to mild sedation, to hypnosis, and deep coma. Overdosage can produce death. In high enough therapeutic doses, barbiturates induce anesthesia.

Barbiturates depress the sensory cortex, decrease motor activity, alter cerebellar function, and produce drowsiness, sedation, and hypnosis.

Barbiturate-induced sleep differs from physiological sleep. Sleep laboratory studies have demonstrated that barbiturates reduce the amount of time spent in the rapid eye movement (REM) phase of sleep or dreaming stage. Also, Stages III and IV sleep are decreased. Following abrupt cessation of barbiturates used regularly, patients may experience markedly increased dreaming, nightmares, and/or insomnia. Therefore, withdrawal of a single therapeutic dose over 5 or 6 days has been recommended to lessen the REM rebound and disturbed sleep which contribute to drug withdrawal syndrome (for example, decrease the dose from 3 to 2 doses a day for 1 week).

In studies, secobarbital sodium and pentobarbital sodium have been found to lose most of their effectiveness for both inducing and maintaining sleep by the end of 2 weeks of continued drug administration at fixed doses. The short-, intermediate-, and, to a lesser degree, long-acting barbiturates have been widely prescribed for treating insomnia. Although the clinical literature abounds with claims that the short-acting barbiturates are superior for producing sleep while the intermediate-acting compounds are more effective in maintaining sleep, controlled studies have failed to demonstrate these differential effects. Therefore, as sleep medications, the barbiturates are of limited value beyond short-term use.

Barbiturates have little analgesic action at subanesthetic doses. Rather, in subanesthetic doses these drugs may increase the reaction to painful stimuli. All barbiturates exhibit anticonvulsant activity in anesthetic doses. However, of the drugs in this class, only phenobarbital, mephobarbital, and metharbital have been clinically demonstrated to be effective as oral anticonvulsants in subhypnotic doses.

Barbiturates are respiratory depressants. The degree of respiratory depression is dependent upon dose. With hypnotic doses, respiratory depression produced by barbiturates is similar to that which occurs during physiologic sleep with slight decrease in blood pressure and heart rate. Studies in laboratory animals have shown that barbiturates cause reduction in the tone and contractility of the uterus, ureters, and urinary bladder. However, concentration of the drugs required to produce this effect in humans are not reached with sedative-hypnotic doses.

Barbiturates do not impair normal hepatic function, but have been shown to induce liver microsomal enzymes, thus increasing and/or altering the metabolism of barbiturates and other drugs. (See "Precautions—*Drug Interactions*" section).

Pharmacokinetics: Barbiturates are absorbed in varying degrees following oral, rectal, or parenteral administration. The salts are more rapidly absorbed than are the acids.

The onset of action for oral or rectal administration varies from 20 to 60 minutes. For IM administration, the onset of action is slightly faster. Following IV administration, the onset of action ranges from almost immediately for pentobarbital sodium to 5 minutes for phenobarbital sodium. Maximal CNS depression may not occur until 15 minutes or more after IV administration for phenobarbital sodium.

Duration of action, which is related to the rate at which the barbiturates are redistributed throughout the body, varies among persons and in the same person from time to time.

No studies have demonstrated that the different routes of administration are equivalent with respect to bioavailability.

Barbiturates are weak acids that are absorbed and rapidly distributed to all tissues and fluids with high concentration in the brain, liver, and kidneys. Lipid solubility of the barbiturates is the dominant factor in their distribution within the body. The more lipid soluble the barbiturate, the more rapidly it penetrates all tissues of the body. Barbiturates are bound to plasma and tissue proteins to a varying degree with the degree of binding increasing directly as a function of lipid solubility. The plasma half-life for pentobarbital in adults is 15 to 50 hours and appears to be dose-dependent. Barbiturates are metabolized primarily by the hepatic microsomal enzyme system, and the metabolic products are excreted in the urine, and less commonly, in the feces. Approximately 25 to 50 percent of a dose of aprobarbital or phenobarbital is eliminated unchanged in the urine, whereas the amount of other barbiturates excreted unchanged in the urine is negligible. The excretion of unmetabolized barbiturate is one feature that distinguishes the long-acting category from those belonging to other categories which are almost entirely metabolized. The inactive metabolites of the barbiturates are excreted as conjugates of glucuronic acid.

Indications and Usage:
Parenteral:
a. Sedatives.
b. Hypnotics, for the short-term treatment of insomnia, since they appear to lose their effectiveness for sleep induction and sleep maintenance after 2 weeks (See "Clinical Pharmacology" section).
c. Preanesthetics.
d. Anticonvulsant, in anesthetic doses, in the emergency control of certain acute convulsive episodes, e.g., those associated with status epilepticus, cholera, eclampsia, meningitis, tetanus, and toxic reactions to strychnine or local anesthetics.

Contraindications: Barbiturates are contraindicated in patients with known barbiturate sensitivity. Barbiturates are also contraindicated in patients with a history of manifest or latent porphyria.

Warnings: 1. *Habit forming:* Barbiturates may be habit forming. Tolerance, psychological and physical dependence may occur with continued use. (See "Drug Abuse and Dependence" and "Pharmacokinetics" sections). Patients who have psychological dependence on barbiturates may increase the dosage or decrease the dosage interval without consulting a physician and may subsequently develop a physical dependence on barbiturates. To minimize the possibility of overdosage or the development of dependence, the prescribing and dispensing of sedative-hypnotic barbiturates should be limited to the amount required for the interval until the

Continued on next page

If desired, additional literature on any Abbott Product will be provided upon request to Abbott Laboratories.

Abbott—Cont.

next appointment. Abrupt cessation after prolonged use in the dependent person may result in withdrawal symptoms, including delirium, convulsions, and possibly death. Barbiturates should be withdrawn gradually from any patient known to be taking excessive dosage over long periods of time. (See "Drug Abuse and Dependence" section).

2. *IV administration:* Too rapid administration may cause respiratory depression, apnea, laryngospasm, or vasodilation with fall in blood pressure.

3. *Acute or chronic pain:* Caution should be exercised when barbiturates are administered to patients with acute or chronic pain, because paradoxical excitement could be induced or important symptoms could be masked. However, the use of barbiturates as sedatives in the postoperative surgical period and as adjuncts to cancer chemotherapy is well established.

4. *Use in pregnancy:* Barbiturates can cause fetal damage when administered to a pregnant woman. Retrospective, case-controlled studies have suggested a connection between the maternal consumption of barbiturates and a higher than expected incidence of fetal abnormalities. Following oral or parenteral administration, barbiturates readily cross the placental barrier and are distributed throughout fetal tissues with highest concentrations found in the placenta, fetal liver, and brain. Fetal blood levels approach maternal blood levels following parenteral administration.

Withdrawal symptoms occur in infants born to mothers who receive barbiturates throughout the last trimester of pregnancy. (See "Drug Abuse and Dependence" section). If this drug is used during pregnancy, or if the patient becomes pregnant while taking this drug, the patient should be apprised of the potential hazard to the fetus.

5. *Synergistic effects:* The concomitant use of alcohol or other CNS depressants may produce additive CNS depressant effects.

Precautions: *General:* Barbiturates may be habit forming. Tolerance and psychological and physical dependence may occur with continuing use. (See "Drug Abuse and Dependence" section). Barbiturates should be administered with caution, if at all, to patients who are mentally depressed, have suicidal tendencies, or a history of drug abuse.

Elderly or debilitated patients may react to barbiturates with marked excitement, depression, and confusion. In some persons, barbiturates repeatedly produce excitement rather than depression.

In patients with hepatic damage, barbiturates should be administered with caution and initially in reduced doses. Barbiturates should not be administered to patients showing the premonitory signs of hepatic coma.

Parenteral solutions of barbiturates are highly alkaline. Therefore, extreme care should be taken to avoid perivascular extravasation or intra-arterial injection. Extravascular injection may cause local tissue damage with subsequent necrosis; consequences of intra-arterial injection may vary from transient pain to gangrene of the limb. Any complaint of pain in the limb warrants stopping the injection.

Information for the patient: Practitioners should give the following information and instructions to patients receiving barbiturates.

1. The use of barbiturates carries with it an associated risk of psychological and/or physical dependence. The patient should be warned against increasing the dose of the drug without consulting a physician.

2. Barbiturates may impair mental and/or physical abilities required for the performance of potentially hazardous tasks (e.g., driving, operating machinery, etc.).

3. Alcohol should not be consumed while taking barbiturates. Concurrent use of the barbiturates with other CNS depressants (e.g., alcohol, narcotics, tranquilizers, and antihistamines) may result in additional CNS depressant effects.

Laboratory tests: Prolonged therapy with barbiturates should be accompanied by periodic laboratory evaluation of organ systems, including hematopoietic, renal, and hepatic systems. (See "Precautions-*General*" and "Adverse Reactions" sections).

Drug interactions: Most reports of clinically significant drug interactions occurring with the barbiturates have involved phenobarbital. However, the application of these data to other barbiturates appears valid and warrants serial blood level determinations of the relevant drugs when there are multiple therapies.

1. *Anticoagulants:* Phenobarbital lowers the plasma levels of dicumarol (name previously used: bishydroxycoumarin) and causes a decrease in anticoagulant activity as measured by the prothrombin time. Barbiturates can induce hepatic microsomal enzymes resulting in increased metabolism and decreased anticoagulant response of oral anticoagulants (e.g., warfarin, acenocoumarol, dicumarol, and phenprocoumon). Patients stabilized on anticoagulant therapy may require dosage adjustments if barbiturates are added to or withdrawn from their dosage regimen.

2. *Corticosteroids:* Barbiturates appear to enhance the metabolism of exogenous corticosteroids probably through the induction of hepatic microsomal enzymes. Patients stabilized on corticosteroid therapy may require dosage adjustments if barbiturates are added to or withdrawn from their dosage regimen.

3. *Griseofulvin:* Phenobarbital appears to interfere with the absorption of orally administered griseofulvin, thus decreasing its blood level. The effect of the resultant decreased blood levels of griseofulvin on therapeutic response has not been established. However, it would be preferable to avoid concomitant administration of these drugs.

4. *Doxycycline:* Phenobarbital has been shown to shorten the half-life of doxycycline for as long as 2 weeks after barbiturate therapy is discontinued.

This mechanism is probably through the induction of hepatic microsomal enzymes that metabolize the antibiotic. If phenobarbital and doxycycline are administered concurrently, the clinical response to doxycycline should be monitored closely.

5. *Phenytoin, sodium valproate, valproic acid:* The effect of barbiturates on the metabolism of phenytoin appears to be variable. Some investigators report an accelerating effect, while others report no effect. Because the effect of barbiturates on the metabolism of phenytoin is not predictable, phenytoin and barbiturate blood levels should be monitored more frequently if these drugs are given concurrently. Sodium valproate and valproic acid appear to decrease barbiturate metabolism; therefore, barbiturate blood levels should be monitored and appropriate dosage adjustments made as indicated.

6. *Central nervous system depressants:* The concomitant use of other central nervous system depressants, including other sedatives or hypnotics, antihistamines, tranquilizers, or alcohol, may produce additive depressant effects.

7. *Monoamine oxidase inhibitors (MAOI):* MAOI prolong the effects of barbiturates probably because metabolism of the barbiturate is inhibited.

8. *Estradiol, estrone, progesterone and other steroidal hormones:* Pretreatment with or concurrent administration of phenobarbital may decrease the effect of estradiol by increasing its metabolism. There have been reports of patients treated with antiepileptic drugs (e.g., phenobarbital) who became pregnant while taking oral contraceptives. An alternate contraceptive method might be suggested to women taking phenobarbital.

Carcinogenesis: Adequate data are not available on long-term potential for carcinogenicity in humans or animals for pentobarbital.

Data from one retrospective study of 235 children in which the types of barbiturates are not identified suggested an association between exposure to barbiturates prenatally and an increased incidence of brain tumor. (Gold, E., et al., "Increased Risk of Brain Tumors in Children Exposed to Barbiturates," Journal of National Cancer Institute, 61:1031–1034, 1978).

Pregnancy: 1. *Teratogenic effects.* Pregnancy Category D—See "Warnings—Use in Pregnancy" section.

2. *Nonteratogenic effects.* Reports of infants suffering from long-term barbiturate exposure in utero included the acute withdrawal syndrome of seizures and hyperirritability from birth to a delayed onset of up to 14 days. (See "Drug Abuse and Dependence" section).

Labor and delivery: Hypnotic doses of these barbiturates do not appear to significantly impair uterine activity during labor. Full anesthetic doses of barbiturates decrease the force and frequency of uterine contractions. Administration of sedative-hypnotic barbiturates to the mother during labor may result in respiratory depression in the newborn. Premature infants are particularly susceptible to the depressant effects of barbiturates. If barbiturates are used during labor and delivery, resuscitation equipment should be available.

Data are currently not available to evaluate the effect of these barbiturates when forceps delivery or other intervention is necessary. Also, data are not available to determine the effect of these barbiturates on the later growth, development, and functional maturation of the child.

Nursing mothers: Caution should be exercised when a barbiturate is administered to a nursing woman since small amounts of barbiturates are excreted in the milk.

Adverse Reactions: The following adverse reactions and their incidence were compiled from surveillance of thousands of hospitalized patients. Because such patients may be less aware of certain of the milder adverse effects of barbiturates, the incidence of these reactions may be somewhat higher in fully ambulatory patients.

More than 1 in 100 patients. The most common adverse reaction estimated to occur at a rate of 1 to 3 patients per 100 is: *Nervous System:* Somnolence.

Less than 1 in 100 patients. Adverse reactions estimated to occur at a rate of less than 1 in 100 patients listed below, grouped by organ system, and by decreasing order of occurrence are:

Nervous system: Agitation, confusion, hyperkinesia, ataxia, CNS depression, nightmares, nervousness, psychiatric disturbance, hallucinations, insomnia, anxiety, dizziness, thinking abnormality.

Respiratory system: Hypoventilation, apnea.

Cardiovascular system: Bradycardia, hypotension, syncope.

Digestive system: Nausea, vomiting, constipation.

Other reported reactions: Headache, injection site reactions, hypersensitivity reactions (angioedema, skin rashes, exfoliative dermatitis), fever, liver damage, megaloblastic anemia following chronic phenobarbital use.

Drug Abuse and Dependence: Pentobarbital sodium injection is subject to control by the Federal Controlled Substances Act under DEA schedule II.

Barbiturates may be habit forming. Tolerance, psychological dependence, and physical dependence may occur especially following prolonged use of high doses of barbiturates. Daily administration in excess of 400 mg of pentobarbital or secobarbital for approximately 90 days is likely to produce some degree of physical dependence. A dosage of from 600 to 800 mg taken for at least 35 days is sufficient to produce withdrawal seizures. The average daily dose for the barbiturate addict is usually about 1.5 g. As tolerance to barbiturates develops, the amount needed to maintain the same level of intoxication increases; tolerance to a fatal dosage, however, does not increase more than two-fold. As this occurs, the margin between an intoxicating dosage and fatal dosage becomes smaller.

Symptoms of acute intoxication with barbiturates include unsteady gait, slurred speech, and sustained nystagmus. Mental signs of chronic intoxication include confusion, poor judgment, irritability, insomnia, and somatic complaints.

Symptoms of barbiturate dependence are similar to those of chronic alcoholism. If an individual appears to be intoxicated with alcohol to a degree that is radically disproportionate to the amount of alcohol in his or her blood the use of barbiturates should be suspected. The lethal dose of a barbiturate is far less if alcohol is also ingested.

The symptoms of barbiturate withdrawal can be severe and may cause death. Minor withdrawal symptoms may appear 8 to 12 hours after the last dose of a barbiturate. These symptoms usually appear in the following order: anxiety, muscle twitching, tremor of hands and fingers, progressive weakness, dizziness, distortion in visual perception, nausea, vomiting, insomnia, and orthostatic hypotension. Major withdrawal symptoms (convulsions and delirium) may occur within 16 hours and last up to 5 days after abrupt cessation of these drugs. Intensity of withdrawal symptoms gradually declines over a period of approximately 15 days. Individuals susceptible to barbiturate abuse and dependence include alcoholics and opiate abusers, as well as other sedative-hypnotic and amphetamine abusers.

Drug dependence to barbiturates arises from repeated administration of a barbiturate or agent with barbiturate-like effect on a continuous basis, generally in amounts exceeding therapeutic dose levels. The characteristics of drug dependence to barbiturates include: (a) a strong desire or need to continue taking the drug; (b) a tendency to increase the dose; (c) a psychic dependence on the effects of the drug related to subjective and individual appreciation of those effects; and (d) a physical dependence on the effects of the drug requiring its presence for maintenance of homeostasis and resulting in a definite, characteristic, and self-limited abstinence syndrome when the drug is withdrawn.

Treatment of barbiturate dependence consists of cautious and gradual withdrawal of the drug. Barbiturate-dependent patients can be withdrawn by using a number of different withdrawal regimens. In all cases withdrawal takes an extended period of time. One method involves substituting a 30 mg dose of phenobarbital for each 100 to 200 mg dose of barbiturate that the patient has been taking. The total daily amount of phenobarbital is then administered in 3 to 4 divided doses, not to exceed 600 mg daily. Should signs of withdrawal occur on the first day of treatment, a loading dose of 100 to 200 mg of phenobarbital may be administered IM in addition to the oral dose. After stabilization on phenobarbital, the total daily dose is decreased by 30 mg a day as long as withdrawal is proceeding smoothly. A modification of this regimen involves initiating treatment at the patient's regular dosage level and decreasing the daily dosage by 10 percent if tolerated by the patient.

Infants physically dependent on barbiturates may be given phenobarbital 3 to 10 mg/kg/day. After withdrawal symptoms (hyperactivity, disturbed sleep, tremors, hyperreflexia) are relieved, the dosage of phenobarbital should be gradually decreased and completely withdrawn over a 2-week period.

Overdosage: The toxic dose of barbiturates varies considerably. In general, an oral dose of 1 g of most barbiturates produces serious poisoning in an adult. Death commonly occurs after 2 to 10 g of ingested barbiturate. Barbiturate intoxication may be confused with alcoholism, bromide intoxication, and with various neurological disorders.

Acute overdosage with barbiturates is manifested by CNS and respiratory depression which may progress to Cheyne-Stokes respiration, areflexia, constriction of the pupils to a slight degree (though in severe poisoning they may show paralytic dilation), oliguria, tachycardia, hypotension, lowered body temperature, and coma. Typical shock syndrome (apnea, circulatory collapse, respiratory arrest, and death) may occur.

In extreme overdose, all electrical activity in the brain may cease, in which case a "flat" EEG normally equated with clinical death cannot be accepted. This effect is fully reversible unless hypoxic damage occurs. Consideration should be given to the possibility of barbiturate intoxication even in situations that appear to involve trauma.

Complications such as pneumonia, pulmonary edema, cardiac arrhythmias, congestive heart failure, and renal failure may occur. Uremia may increase CNS sensitivity to barbiturates. Differential diagnosis should include hypoglycemia, head trauma, cerebrovascular accidents, convulsive states, and diabetic coma. Blood levels from acute overdosage for some barbiturates are listed in Table 2. [See Table 2 in Nembutal Capsules prescribing information.]

Treatment of overdosage is mainly supportive and consists of the following:
1. Maintenance of an adequate airway, with assisted respiration and oxygen administration as necessary.
2. Monitoring of vital signs and fluid balance.
3. Fluid therapy and other standard treatment for shock, if needed.
4. If renal function is normal, forced diuresis may aid in the elimination of the barbiturate. Alkalinization of the urine increases renal excretion of some barbiturates, especially phenobarbital, also aprobarbital, and mephobarbital (which is metabolized to phenobarbital).
5. Although not recommended as a routine procedure, hemodialysis may be used in severe barbiturate intoxications or if the patient is anuric or in shock.
6. Patient should be rolled from side to side every 30 minutes.
7. Antibiotics should be given if pneumonia is suspected.
8. Appropriate nursing care to prevent hypostatic pneumonia, decubiti, aspiration, and other complications of patients with altered states of consciousness.

Dosage and Administration: Dosages of barbiturates must be individualized with full knowledge of their particular characteristics and recommended rate of administration. Factors of consideration are the patient's age, weight, and condition. Parenteral routes should be used only when oral administration is impossible or impractical.

Intramuscular Administration: IM injection of the sodium salts of barbiturates should be made deeply into a large muscle, and a volume of 5 ml should not be exceeded at any one site because of possible tissue irritation. After IM injection of a hypnotic dose, the patient's vital signs should be monitored. The usual adult dosage of NEMBUTAL Sodium Solution is 150 to 200 mg as a single IM injection; the recommended pediatric dosage ranges from 2 to 6 mg/kg as a single IM injection not to exceed 100 mg.

Intravenous Administration: IV injection is restricted to conditions in which other routes are not feasible, either because the patient is unconscious (as in cerebral hemorrhage, eclampsia, or status epilepticus, or because the patient resists (as in delirium), or because prompt action is imperative. Slow IV injection is essential and patients should be carefully observed during administration. This requires that blood pressure, respiration, and cardiac function be maintained, vital signs be recorded, and equipment for resuscitation and artificial ventilation be available. The rate of IV injection should not exceed 50 mg/min for pentobarbital sodium.

There is no average intravenous dose of NEMBUTAL Sodium Solution (pentobarbital sodium injection) that can be relied on to produce similar effects in different patients. The possibility of overdose and respiratory depression is remote when the drug is injected slowly in fractional doses.

A commonly used initial dose for the 70 kg adult is 100 mg. Proportional reduction in dosage should be made for pediatric or debilitated patients. At least one minute is necessary to determine the full effect of intravenous pentobarbital. If necessary, additional small increments of the drug may be given up to a total of from 200 to 500 mg for normal adults.

Anticonvulsant use: In convulsive states, dosage of NEMBUTAL Sodium Solution should be kept to a minimum to avoid compounding the depression which may follow convulsions. The injection must be made slowly with due regard to the time required for the drug to penetrate the blood-brain barrier.

Special patient population: Dosage should be reduced in the elderly or debilitated because these patients may be more sensitive to barbiturates. Dosage should be reduced for patients with impaired renal function or hepatic disease.

Inspection: Parenteral drug products should be inspected visually for particulate matter and discoloration prior to administration, whenever solution containers permit. Solutions for injection showing evidence of precipitation should not be used.

How Supplied: NEMBUTAL Sodium Solution (pentobarbital sodium injection, USP) is available in the following sizes:
2-ml ampul, 100 mg (1½ gr), in boxes of 25 (**NDC** 0074-6899-04); 20-ml multiple-dose vial, 1 g, in boxes of 5 (**NDC** 0074-3778-04); and 50-ml multiple-dose vial, 2.5 g, in boxes of 5 (**NDC** 0074-3778-05).
Each ml contains:
Pentobarbital Sodium,
derivative of barbituric acid ....50 mg (¾ gr)
Warning—May be habit forming.
Propylene glycol ....40% v/v
Alcohol 10%
Water for Injection ....qs
(pH adjusted to approximately 9.5 with hydrochloric acid and/or sodium hydroxide.)
Abbott Laboratories
North Chicago, IL 60064
Ref. 07-5165/R2

NEMBUTAL® SODIUM SUPPOSITORIES ℞
[nêm-bū' tal]
(pentobarbital sodium suppositories)

WARNING: MAY BE HABIT FORMING

Description: The barbiturates are nonselective central nervous system depressants which are primarily used as sedative hypnotics. The barbiturates and their sodium salts are subject to control under the Federal Controlled Substances Act (See "Drug Abuse and Dependence" section).

Barbiturates are substituted pyrimidine derivatives in which the basic structure common to these drugs is barbituric acid, a substance which has no central nervous system (CNS) activity. CNS activity is obtained by substituting alkyl, alkenyl, or aryl groups on the pyrimidine ring. Nembutal (pentobarbital sodium) is chemically represented by sodium 5-ethyl-5-(1-methylbutyl) barbiturate. The sodium salt of pentobarbital occurs as a white, slightly bitter powder which is freely soluble in water and alcohol but practically insoluble in benzene and ether. Each rectal suppository contains either 30 mg, 60 mg, 120 mg, or 200 mg of pentobarbital sodium.

Clinical Pharmacology: Barbiturates are capable of producing all levels of CNS mood alteration from excitation to mild sedation, to hypnosis, and deep coma. Overdosage can produce death. In high enough therapeutic doses, barbiturates induce anesthesia.

Barbiturates depress the sensory cortex, decrease motor activity, alter cerebellar function, and produce drowsiness, sedation, and hypnosis.

Barbiturate-induced sleep differs from physiological sleep. Sleep laboratory studies have demonstrated that barbiturates reduce the amount of time spent in the rapid eye movement (REM) phase of sleep or dreaming stage. Also, Stages III

Continued on next page

If desired, additional literature on any Abbott Product will be provided upon request to Abbott Laboratories.

Abbott—Cont.

and IV sleep are decreased. Following abrupt cessation of barbiturates used regularly, patients may experience markedly increased dreaming, nightmares, and/or insomnia. Therefore, withdrawal of a single therapeutic dose over 5 or 6 days has been recommended to lessen the REM rebound and disturbed sleep which contribute to drug withdrawal syndrome (for example, decrease the dose from 3 to 2 doses a day for 1 week).

In studies, secobarbital sodium and pentobarbital sodium have been found to lose most of their effectiveness for both inducing and maintaining sleep by the end of 2 weeks of continued drug administration at fixed doses. The short-, intermediate-, and, to a lesser degree, long-acting barbiturates have been widely prescribed for treating insomnia. Although the clinical literature abounds with claims that the short-acting barbiturates are superior for producing sleep while the intermediate-acting compounds are more effective in maintaining sleep, controlled studies have failed to demonstrate these differential effects. Therefore, as sleep medications, the barbiturates are of limited value beyond short-term use.

Barbiturates have little analgesic action at subanesthetic doses. Rather, in subanesthetic doses these drugs may increase the reaction to painful stimuli. All barbiturates exhibit anticonvulsant activity in anesthetic doses. However, of the drugs in this class, only phenobarbital, mephobarbital, and metharbital have been clinically demonstrated to be effective as oral anticonvulsants in subhypnotic doses.

Barbiturates are respiratory depressants. The degree of respiratory depression is dependent upon dose. With hypnotic doses, respiratory depression produced by barbiturates is similar to that which occurs during physiologic sleep with slight decrease in blood pressure and heart rate. Studies in laboratory animals have shown that barbiturates cause reduction in the tone and contractility of the uterus, ureters, and urinary bladder. However, concentrations of the drugs required to produce this effect in humans are not reached with sedative-hypnotic doses.

Barbiturates do not impair normal hepatic function, but have been shown to induce liver microsomal enzymes, thus increasing and/or altering the metabolism of barbiturates and other drugs. (See "Precautions—*Drug Interactions*" section).

Pharmacokinetics: Barbiturates are absorbed in varying degrees following oral, rectal, or parenteral administration.

The onset of action for oral or rectal administration varies from 20 to 60 minutes.

Duration of action, which is related to the rate at which the barbiturates are redistributed throughout the body, varies among persons and in the same person from time to time.

No studies have demonstrated that the different routes of administration are equivalent with respect to bioavailability.

Barbiturates are weak acids that are absorbed and rapidly distributed to all tissues and fluids with high concentrations in the brain, liver, and kidneys. Lipid solubility of the barbiturates is the dominant factor in their distribution within the body. The more lipid soluble the barbiturate, the more rapidly it penetrates all tissues of the body. Barbiturates are bound to plasma and tissue proteins to a varying degree with the degree of binding increasing directly as a function of lipid solubility. The plasma half-life for pentobarbital in adults is 15 to 50 hours and appears to be dose dependent. Barbiturates are metabolized primarily by the hepatic microsomal enzyme system, and the metabolic products are excreted in the urine, and less commonly, in the feces. Approximately 25 to 50 percent of a dose of aprobarbital or phenobarbital is eliminated unchanged in the urine, whereas the amount of other barbiturates excreted unchanged in the urine is negligible. The excretion of unmetabolized barbiturate is one feature that distinguishes the long-acting category from those belonging to other categories which are almost entirely metabolized. The inactive metabolites of the barbiturates are excreted as conjugates of glucuronic acid.

Indications and Usage: *Rectal:* Barbiturates administered rectally are absorbed from the colon and are used when oral or parenteral administration may be undesirable.
1. Sedative.
2. Hypnotic, for the short-term treatment of insomnia, since they appear to lose their effectiveness for sleep induction and sleep maintenance after 2 weeks (See "Clinical Pharmacology" section).

Contraindications: Barbiturates are contraindicated in patients with known barbiturate sensitivity. Barbiturates are also contraindicated in patients with a history of manifest or latent porphyria.

Warnings: 1. *Habit forming:* Barbiturates may be habit forming. Tolerance, psychological and physical dependence may occur with continued use. (See "Drug Abuse and Dependence" and "Pharmacokinetics" sections). Patients who have psychological dependence on barbiturates may increase the dosage or decrease the dosage interval without consulting a physician and may subsequently develop a physical dependence on barbiturates. To minimize the possibility of overdosage or the development of dependence, the prescribing and dispensing of sedative-hypnotic barbiturates should be limited to the amount required for the interval until the next appointment. Abrupt cessation after prolonged use in the dependent person may result in withdrawal symptoms, including delirium, convulsions, and possibly death. Barbiturates should be withdrawn gradually from any patient known to be taking excessive dosage over long periods of time. (See "Drug Abuse and Dependence" section).

2. *Acute or chronic pain:* Caution should be exercised when barbiturates are administered to patients with acute or chronic pain, because paradoxical excitement could be induced or important symptoms could be masked. However, the use of barbiturates as sedatives in the postoperative surgical period and as adjuncts to cancer chemotherapy is well established.

3. *Use in pregnancy:* Barbiturates can cause fetal damage when administered to a pregnant woman. Retrospective, case-controlled studies have suggested a connection between the maternal consumption of barbiturates and a higher than expected incidence of fetal abnormalities. Following oral or parenteral administration, barbiturates readily cross the placental barrier and are distributed throughout fetal tissues with highest concentrations found in the placenta, fetal liver, and brain. It is presumed that this effect will also be seen following rectal administration.

Withdrawal symptoms occur in infants born to mothers who receive barbiturates throughout the last trimester of pregnancy. (See "Drug Abuse and Dependence" section). If this drug is used during pregnancy, or if the patient becomes pregnant while taking this drug, the patient should be apprised of the potential hazard to the fetus.

4. *Synergistic effects:* The concomitant use of alcohol or other CNS depressants may produce additive CNS depressant effects.

Precautions: *General:* Barbiturates may be habit forming. Tolerance and psychological and physical dependence may occur with continuing use. (See "Drug Abuse and Dependence" section). Barbiturates should be administered with caution, if at all, to patients who are mentally depressed, have suicidal tendencies, or a history of drug abuse.

Elderly or debilitated patients may react to barbiturates with marked excitement, depression, and confusion. In some persons, barbiturates repeatedly produce excitement rather than depression.

In patients with hepatic damage, barbiturates should be administered with caution and initially in reduced doses. Barbiturates should not be administered to patients showing the premonitory signs of hepatic coma.

Information for the patient: Practitioners should give the following information and instructions to patients receiving barbiturates.
1. The use of barbiturates carries with it an associated risk of psychological and/or physical dependence. The patient should be warned against increasing the dose of the drug without consulting a physician.
2. Barbiturates may impair mental and/or physical abilities required for the performance of potentially hazardous tasks (e.g., driving, operating machinery, etc.).
3. Alcohol should not be consumed while taking barbiturates. Concurrent use of the barbiturates with other CNS depressants (e.g., alcohol, narcotics, tranquilizers, and antihistamines) may result in additional CNS depressant effects.

Laboratory tests: Prolonged therapy with barbiturates should be accompanied by periodic laboratory evaluation of organ systems, including hematopoietic, renal, and hepatic systems. (See "Precautions — *General*" and "Adverse Reactions" sections).

Drug interactions: Most reports of clinically significant drug interactions occurring with the barbiturates have involved phenobarbital. However, the application of these data to other barbiturates appears valid and warrants serial blood level determinations of the relevant drugs when there are multiple therapies.

1. *Anticoagulants:* Phenobarbital lowers the plasma levels of dicumarol (name previously used: bishydroxycoumarin) and causes a decrease in anticoagulant activity as measured by the prothrombin time. Barbiturates can induce hepatic microsomal enzymes resulting in increased metabolism and decreased anticoagulant response of oral anticoagulants (e.g., warfarin, acenocoumarol, dicumarol, and phenprocoumon). Patients stabilized on anticoagulant therapy may require dosage adjustments if barbiturates are added to or withdrawn from their dosage regimen.

2. *Corticosteroids:* Barbiturates appear to enhance the metabolism of exogenous corticosteroids probably through the induction of hepatic microsomal enzymes. Patients stabilized on corticosteroid therapy may require dosage adjustments if barbiturates are added to or withdrawn from their dosage regimen.

3. *Griseofulvin:* Phenobarbital appears to interfere with the absorption of orally administered griseofulvin, thus decreasing its blood level. The effect of the resultant decreased blood levels of griseofulvin on therapeutic response has not been established. However, it would be preferable to avoid concomitant administration of these drugs.

4. *Doxycycline:* Phenobarbital has been shown to shorten the half-life of doxycycline for as long as 2 weeks after barbiturate therapy is discontinued.

This mechanism is probably through the induction of hepatic microsomal enzymes that metabolize the antibiotic. If phenobarbital and doxycycline are administered concurrently, the clinical response to doxycycline should be monitored closely.

5. *Phenytoin, sodium valproate, valproic acid:* The effect of barbiturates on the metabolism of phenytoin appears to be variable. Some investigators report an accelerating effect, while others report no effect. Because the effect of barbiturates on the metabolism of phenytoin is not predictable, phenytoin and barbiturate blood levels should be monitored more frequently if these drugs are given concurrently. Sodium valproate and valproic acid appear to decrease barbiturate metabolism; therefore, barbiturate blood levels should be monitored and appropriate dosage adjustments made as indicated.

6. *Central nervous system depressants:* The concomitant use of other central nervous system depressants, including other sedatives or hypnotics, antihistamines, tranquilizers, or alcohol, may produce additive depressant effects.

7. *Monoamine oxidase inhibitors (MAOI):* MAOI prolong the effects of barbiturates probably because metabolism of the barbiturate is inhibited.
8. *Estradiol, estrone, progesterone and other steroidal hormones:* Pretreatment with or concurrent administration of phenobarbital may decrease the effect of estradiol by increasing its metabolism. There have been reports of patients treated with antiepileptic drugs (e.g., phenobarbital) who became pregnant while taking oral contraceptives. An alternate contraceptive method might be suggested to women taking phenobarbital.

Carcinogenesis: Adequate data are not available on long-term potential for carcinogenicity in humans or animals for pentobarbital.

Data from one retrospective study of 235 children in which the types of barbiturates are not identified suggested an association between exposure to barbiturates prenatally and an increased incidence of brain tumor. (Gold, E., et al, "Increased Risk of Brain Tumors in Children Exposed to Barbiturates," Journal of National Cancer Institute, 61:1031–1034, 1978).

Pregnancy: 1. *Teratogenic effects.* Pregnancy Category D — See "Warnings — Use in Pregnancy" section.
2. *Nonteratogenic effects.* Reports of infants suffering from long-term barbiturate exposure in utero included the acute withdrawal syndrome of seizures and hyperirritability from birth to a delayed onset of up to 14 days. (See "Drug Abuse and Dependence" section).

Labor and delivery: Hypnotic doses of these barbiturates do not appear to significantly impair uterine activity during labor. Full anesthetic doses of barbiturates decrease the force and frequency of uterine contractions. Administration of sedative-hypnotic barbiturates to the mother during labor may result in respiratory depression in the newborn. Premature infants are particularly susceptible to the depressant effects of barbiturates. If barbiturates are used during labor and delivery, resuscitation equipment should be available.

Data are currently not available to evaluate the effect of these barbiturates when forceps delivery or other intervention is necessary. Also, data are not available to determine the effect of these barbiturates on the later growth, development, and functional maturation of the child.

Nursing mothers: Caution should be exercised when a barbiturate is administered to a nursing woman since small amounts of barbiturates are excreted in the milk.

Adverse Reactions: The following adverse reactions and their incidence were compiled from surveillance of thousands of hospitalized patients. Because such patients may be less aware of certain of the milder adverse effects of barbiturates, the incidence of these reactions may be somewhat higher in fully ambulatory patients.

More than 1 in 100 patients. The most common adverse reaction estimated to occur at a rate of 1 to 3 patients per 100 is: *Nervous System:* Somnolence.

Less than 1 in 100 patients. Adverse reactions estimated to occur at a rate of less than 1 in 100 patients listed below, grouped by organ system, and by decreasing order of occurrence are:

Nervous system: Agitation, confusion, hyperkinesia, ataxia, CNS depression, nightmares, nervousness, psychiatric disturbance, hallucinations, insomnia, anxiety, dizziness, thinking abnormality.
Respiratory system: Hypoventilation, apnea.
Cardiovascular system: Bradycardia, hypotension, syncope.
Digestive system: Nausea, vomiting, constipation.
Other reported reactions: Headache, injection site reactions, hypersensitivity reactions (angioedema, skin rashes, exfoliative dermatitis), fever, liver damage, megaloblastic anemia following chronic phenobarbital use.

Drug Abuse and Dependence: Pentobarbital sodium suppositories are subject to control by the Federal Controlled Substances Act under DEA schedule III.

Barbiturates may be habit forming. Tolerance, psychological dependence, and physical dependence may occur especially following prolonged use of high doses of barbiturates. Daily administration in excess of 400 mg of pentobarbital or secobarbital for approximately 90 days is likely to produce some degree of physical dependence. A dosage of from 600 to 800 mg taken for at least 35 days is sufficient to produce withdrawal seizures. The average daily dose for the barbiturate addict is usually about 1.5 grams. As tolerance to barbiturates develops, the amount needed to maintain the same level of intoxication increases; tolerance to a fatal dosage, however, does not increase more than two-fold. As this occurs, the margin between an intoxicating dosage and fatal dosage becomes smaller.

Symptoms of acute intoxication with barbiturates include unsteady gait, slurred speech, and sustained nystagmus. Mental signs of chronic intoxication include confusion, poor judgment, irritability, insomnia, and somatic complaints.

Symptoms of barbiturate dependence are similar to those of chronic alcoholism. If an individual appears to be intoxicated with alcohol to a degree that is radically disproportionate to the amount of alcohol in his or her blood the use of barbiturates should be suspected. The lethal dose of a barbiturate is far less if alcohol is also ingested.

The symptoms of barbiturate withdrawal can be severe and may cause death. Minor withdrawal symptoms may appear 8 to 12 hours after the last dose of a barbiturate. These symptoms usually appear in the following order: anxiety, muscle twitching, tremor of hands and fingers, progressive weakness, dizziness, distortion in visual perception, nausea, vomiting, insomnia, and orthostatic hypotension. Major withdrawal symptoms (convulsions and delirium) may occur within 16 hours and last up to 5 days after abrupt cessation of these drugs. Intensity of withdrawal symptoms gradually declines over a period of approximately 15 days. Individuals susceptible to barbiturate abuse and dependence include alcoholics and opiate abusers, as well as other sedative-hypnotic and amphetamine abusers.

Drug dependence to barbiturates arises from repeated administration of a barbiturate or agent with barbiturate-like effect on a continuous basis, generally in amounts exceeding therapeutic dose levels. The characteristics of drug dependence to barbiturates include: (a) a strong desire or need to continue taking the drug; (b) a tendency to increase the dose; (c) a psychic dependence on the effects of the drug related to subjective and individual appreciation of those effects; and (d) a physical dependence on the effects of the drug requiring its presence for maintenance of homeostasis and resulting in a definite, characteristic, and self-limited abstinence syndrome when the drug is withdrawn.

Treatment of barbiturate dependence consists of cautious and gradual withdrawal of the drug. Barbiturate-dependent patients can be withdrawn by using a number of different withdrawal regimens. In all cases withdrawal takes an extended period of time. One method involves substituting a 30 mg dose of phenobarbital for each 100 to 200 mg dose of barbiturate that the patient has been taking. The total daily amount of phenobarbital is then administered in 3 to 4 divided doses, not to exceed 600 mg daily. Should signs of withdrawal occur on the first day of treatment, a loading dose of 100 to 200 mg of phenobarbital may be administered IM in addition to the oral dose. After stabilization on phenobarbital, the total daily dose is decreased by 30 mg a day as long as withdrawal is proceeding smoothly. A modification of this regimen involves initiating treatment at the patient's regular dosage level and decreasing the daily dosage by 10 percent if tolerated by the patient.

Infants physically dependent on barbiturates may be given phenobarbital 3 to 10 mg/kg/day. After withdrawal symptoms (hyperactivity, disturbed sleep, tremors, hyperreflexia) are relieved, the dosage of phenobarbital should be gradually decreased and completely withdrawn over a 2 week period.

Overdosage: The toxic dose of barbiturates varies considerably. In general, an oral dose of 1 g of most barbiturates produces serious poisoning in an adult. Death commonly occurs after 2 to 10 g of ingested barbiturate. Barbiturate intoxication may be confused with alcoholism, bromide intoxication, and with various neurological disorders. Acute overdosage with barbiturates is manifested by CNS and respiratory depression which may progress to Cheyne-Stokes respiration, areflexia, constriction of the pupils to a slight degree (though in severe poisoning they may show paralytic dilation), oliguria, tachycardia, hypotension, lowered body temperature, and coma. Typical shock syndrome (apnea, circulatory collapse, respiratory arrest, and death) may occur.

In extreme overdose, all electrical activity in the brain may cease, in which case a "flat" EEG normally equated with clinical death cannot be accepted. This effect is fully reversible unless hypoxic damage occurs. Consideration should be given to the possibility of barbiturate intoxication even in situations that appear to involve trauma.

Complications such as pneumonia, pulmonary edema, cardiac arrhythmias, congestive heart failure, and renal failure may occur. Uremia may increase CNS sensitivity to barbiturates. Differential diagnosis should include hypoglycemia, head trauma, cerebrovascular accidents, convulsive states, and diabetic coma. Blood levels from acute overdosage for some barbiturates are listed in Table 2. [See Table 2 shown in Nembutal Capsules prescribing information.]

Treatment of overdosage is mainly supportive and consists of the following:

1. Maintenance of an adequate airway, with assisted respiration and oxygen administration as necessary.
2. Monitoring of vital signs and fluid balance.
3. Fluid therapy and other standard treatment for shock, if needed.
4. If renal function is normal, forced diuresis may aid in the elimination of the barbiturate. Alkalinization of the urine increases renal excretion of some barbiturates, especially phenobarbital, also aprobarbital, and mephobarbital (which is metabolized to phenobarbital).
5. Although not recommended as a routine procedure, hemodialysis may be used in severe barbiturate intoxications or if the patient is anuric or in shock.
6. Patient should be rolled from side to side every 30 minutes.
7. Antibiotics should be given if pneumonia is suspected.
8. Appropriate nursing care to prevent hypostatic pneumonia, decubiti, aspiration, and other complications of patients with altered states of consciousness.

Dosage and Administration: Typical hypnotic doses for adults and children are given below. These are intended only as a guide, and administration should be adjusted to the individual needs of each patient. For sedation, in children 5–14 years and in adults, reduce dose appropriately. Adults (average to above average weight)— one 120 mg or one 200 mg suppository.

Children —

12–14 years ....one 60 mg or one	
(80–110 lbs)	120 mg suppository
5–12 years ....one 60 mg suppository	
(40–80 lbs)	
1–4 years ....one 30 mg or one	
(20–40 lbs)	60 mg suppository
2 months–1 year ....one 30 mg	
(10–20 lbs)	suppository

Suppositories should not be divided.

Dosages of barbiturates must be individualized with full knowledge of their particular characteristics and recommended rate of administration.

Continued on next page

If desired, additional literature on any Abbott Product will be provided upon request to Abbott Laboratories.

Abbott—Cont.

Factors of consideration are the patient's age, weight, and condition.
Special patient population: Dosage should be reduced in the elderly or debilitated because these patients may be more sensitive to barbiturates. Dosage should be reduced for patients with impaired renal function or hepatic disease.
How Supplied: NEMBUTAL Sodium Suppositories (pentobarbital sodium suppositories) are available as suppositories containing pentobarbital sodium in the amount of 30 mg (½ gr) (NDC 0074-3272-01); 60 mg (1 gr) (NDC 0074-3148-01); 120 mg (2 gr) (NDC 0074-3145-01) and 200 mg (3 gr) (NDC 0074-3164-01). Supplied in boxes of 12 suppositories.
Semi-synthetic glycerides provide the base for each suppository.
Store in a refrigerator (36°–46°F).
Abbott Laboratories
North Chicago, IL 60064
Ref. 07-5174-R9

NITROPRESS® ℞
[ni¹ tro-press]
(sterile sodium nitroprusside, USP)

> NITROPRESS is only to be used as an infusion with sterile 5% dextrose injection. Not for direct injection.
> NITROPRESS should be used only when the necessary facilities and equipment for continuous monitoring of blood pressure are available.
> If at infusion rates of up to 10 mcg/kg/minute, an adequate reduction of blood pressure is not obtained within ten minutes, administration of NITROPRESS should be stopped.
> The instructions included herein should be reviewed thoroughly before administration of NITROPRESS.

Description: This antihypertensive agent is for intravenous infusion only. When mixed, each 2 ml of NITROPRESS (sterile sodium nitroprusside, USP) in injectable form contains the equivalent of 50 mg of sodium nitroprusside dihydrate (sodium nitrosylpentacyanoferrate [III]) in sterile water for injection in an amber-colored, single dose Univial.®
Chemically, sodium nitroprusside is $Na_2[Fe(CN)_5NO] \cdot 2H_2O$. It is a reddish-brown powder which is soluble in water. In aqueous solution, it is photosensitive and should be protected from light.
Clinical Pharmacology: NITROPRESS is a potent, immediate acting, intravenous hypotensive agent. This action is probably due to the nitroso (NO) group. Its effect is almost immediate and ends when the IV infusion is stopped. Generally, NITROPRESS is rapidly metabolized to cyanide and subsequently converted to thiocyanate through the mediation of a hepatic enzyme, rhodanase. The rate of conversion from cyanide to thiocyanate is dependent on the availability of sulfur, usually thiosulfate. The hypotensive effect is augmented by ganglionic blocking agents, volatile liquid anesthetics (such as halothane and enflurane), and by most other circulatory depressants.
The hypotensive effects of NITROPRESS are caused by peripheral vasodilation as a result of a direct action on the blood vessels, independent of autonomic innervation. No relaxation is seen in the smooth muscle of the uterus or duodenum *in situ* in animals.
Sodium nitroprusside administered intravenously to hypertensive and normotensive patients produced a marked lowering of the arterial blood pressure, slight increase in heart rate, a mild decrease in cardiac output and a moderate diminution in calculated total peripheral vascular resistance.
The decrease in calculated total peripheral vascular resistance suggests arteriolar vasodilatation. The decreases in cardiac and stroke index noted may be due to the peripheral vascular pooling of blood.
In hypertensive patients, moderate depressor doses induce renal vasodilatation roughly equivalent to the decrease in pressure without an appreciable increase in renal blood flow or a decrease in glomerular filtration.
In normotensive subjects, acute reduction of mean arterial pressure to 60 to 75 mmHg by infusion of sodium nitroprusside caused a significant increase in renin activity of renal venous plasma in correlation with the degree of reduction in pressure. Renal response to reduction in pressure was more striking in renovascular hypertensive patients, with significant increase in renin release occurring from the involved kidney at mean arterial pressures ranging from 90 to 137 mmHg. Furthermore, the magnitude of renin release from the involved kidney was significantly greater when compared with that in normotensive subjects, while in the contralateral, uninvolved kidney, no significant release of renin was detected during the reduction of pressure.
Indications and Usage: NITROPRESS (sterile sodium nitroprusside) is indicated for the immediate reduction of blood pressure of patients in hypertensive crises. Concomitant oral antihypertensive medication should be started while the hypertensive emergency is being brought under control with NITROPRESS.
NITROPRESS is also indicated for producing controlled hypotension during anesthesia in order to reduce bleeding in surgical procedures where surgeon and anesthesiologist deem it appropriate.
Contraindications: NITROPRESS should not be used in the treatment of compensatory hypertension, *e.g.*, arteriovenous shunt or coarctation of the aorta.
The use of NITROPRESS to produce controlled hypotension during surgery is contraindicated in patients with known inadequate cerebral circulation. NITROPRESS is not intended for use during emergency surgery in moribund patients (A.S.A. Class 5E).
Warnings:

> If excessive amounts of NITROPRESS are used and/or sulfur—usually thiosulfate—supplies are depleted, cyanide toxicity can occur. (See Overdosage.)
> If sodium nitroprusside infusion is to be extended, particularly if renal impairment is present, close attention should be given to not exceeding the recommended maximum infusion rate of 10 mcg/kg/min. If in the course of therapy increased tolerance to the drug (as shown by the need for higher infusion rate) develops, it is essential to monitor blood acid-base balance, as metabolic acidosis is the earliest and most reliable evidence of cyanide toxicity. If signs of metabolic acidosis appear, NITROPRESS should be discontinued and an alternate drug administered.
> Serum thiocyanate levels do not reflect cyanide toxicity. However, serum thiocyanate levels should be monitored daily if treatment is to be extended, especially in patients with renal dysfunction. Thiocyanate accumulation and toxicity may manifest itself as tinnitus, blurred vision, delirium.

The following warnings apply to use of NITROPRESS for controlled hypotension during anesthesia:
1. Tolerance to blood loss, anemia and hypovolemia may be diminished. If possible, pre-existing anemia and hypovolemia should be corrected prior to employing controlled hypotension.
2. Hypotensive anesthetic techniques may alter pulmonary ventilation perfusion ratio. Patients intolerant of additional dead air space at ordinary oxygen partial pressure may benefit from higher oxygen partial pressure.
3. Extreme caution should be exercised in patients who are especially poor surgical risks (A.S.A. Class 4 and 4E).

NITROPRESS IS ONLY TO BE USED AS AN INFUSION WITH 5% DEXTROSE INJECTION. NOT FOR DIRECT INJECTION.
Infusion rates greater than 10 mcg/kg/minute are rarely required. If, at this rate, an adequate reduction in blood pressure is not obtained within 10 minutes, administration of NITROPRESS (sterile sodium nitroprusside) should be stopped.
Precautions:
General: Adequate facilities, equipment and personnel should be available for frequent and vigilant monitoring of blood pressure, since the hypotensive effect of NITROPRESS occurs rapidly.
When the infusion is slowed or stopped, blood pressure usually begins to rise immediately and returns to pretreatment levels within one to ten minutes. It should be used with caution and initially in low doses in elderly patients, since they may be more sensitive to the hypotensive effects of the drug. Young, vigorous males may require somewhat larger than ordinary doses of sodium nitroprusside for hypotensive anesthesia; however, the infusion rate of 10 mcg/kg/minute should not be exceeded. Deepening of anesthesia, if indicated, might permit satisfactory conditions to exist within the recommended dosage range.
Because of the rapid onset of action and potency of NITROPRESS, it should preferably be administered with the use of an infusion pump, micro-drip regulator, or any similar device that would allow precise measurement of the flow rate.
Since cyanide is converted into thiocyanate through the mediation of a hepatic enzyme, rhodanase, NITROPRESS should be used with caution in patients with hepatic insufficiency.
Since thiocyanate inhibits both the uptake and binding of iodine, caution should be exercised in using NITROPRESS in patients with hypothyroidism or severe renal impairment.
Hypertensive patients are more sensitive to the intravenous effect of sodium nitroprusside than are normotensive subjects. Patients who are receiving concomitant antihypertensive medications are more sensitive to the hypotensive effect of sodium nitroprusside and the dosage should be adjusted accordingly.
Once dissolved in solution, NITROPRESS tends to deteriorate in the presence of light. Therefore, it must be protected from light by covering the container of the prepared solution with the light-protective sleeve supplied with the product, or aluminum foil, or other opaque materials. If properly protected from light, the freshly reconstituted and diluted solution is stable for 24 hours.
NITROPRESS in aqueous solution yields the nitroprusside ion which reacts with even minute quantities of a wide variety of inorganic and organic substances to form usually highly colored reaction products (blue, green or dark red). If this occurs, the infusion should be replaced.
Drug Interactions: The hypotensive effect of sodium nitroprusside is augmented by *ganglionic blocking agents. Volatile liquid anesthetics* (such as halothane and enflurane) also augment the hypotensive effect. Most other *circulatory depressants* will augment the hypotensive effect of sodium nitroprusside.
Carcinogenesis: No data are available on long-term potential for carcinogenicity in animals or humans for sodium nitroprusside.
Usage During Pregnancy: Pregnancy Category C. Animal reproduction studies have not been conducted with NITROPRESS. It is also not known whether NITROPRESS (sterile sodium nitroprusside) can cause fetal harm when administered to a pregnant woman or can affect reproduction capacity. NITROPRESS should be given to a pregnant woman only if clearly needed.
Nursing Mothers: It is not known whether this drug is excreted in human milk. Because many drugs are excreted in human milk, caution should be exercised when NITROPRESS is administered to a nursing woman.
Adverse Reactions: Nausea, retching, diaphoresis, apprehension, headache, restlessness, muscle twitching, retrosternal discomfort, palpitations, dizziness and abdominal pain have been noted with too rapid reduction in blood pressure,

but these symptoms rapidly disappeared with slowing of the rate of the infusion or temporary discontinuation of infusion and did not reappear with continued slower rate of administration. Irritation at the infusion site may occur.

One case of hypothyroidism following prolonged therapy with intravenous sodium nitroprusside has been reported. A patient with severe hypertension with uremia received 3900 mg of sodium nitroprusside intravenously over a period of 21 days. This is one of the longest reported intravenous uses of this agent. There was no tachyphylaxis, but the patient developed evidence of hypothyroidism, together with retention of thiocyanate (9.5 mg/100 ml). With peritoneal dialysis the thiocyanate level diminished and the signs of hypothyroidism subsided.

Overdosage: The first signs of sodium nitroprusside overdosage are those of profound hypotension. As with instances of depletion of thiosulfate supplies, overdosage may lead to cyanide toxicity. Metabolic acidosis and increasing tolerance to the drug are early indications of overdosage. These may be associated with or followed by dyspnea, headache, vomiting, dizziness, ataxia and loss of consciousness. Sodium nitroprusside should then be immediately discontinued. Other signs of cyanide poisoning are coma, imperceptible pulse, absent reflexes, widely dilated pupils, pink color, distant heart sounds, and shallow breathing. Oxygen alone will not provide relief. Nitrites should be administered to induce methemoglobin formation. Methemoglobin, in turn, combines with cyanide bound to cytochrome oxidase to liberate cytochrome oxidase and form a non-toxic complex, cyanmethemoglobin. Cyanide then gradually dissociates from the latter and is converted by administration of thiosulfate to sodium thiocyanate in the presence of rhodanase.

Treatment: In cases of massive overdosage when signs of cyanide toxicity are present use the following regimen:

1. Discontinue administration of NITROPRESS.
2. Administer amyl nitrite inhalations for 15 to 30 seconds each minute until 3% sodium nitrite solution can be prepared for I.V. administration.
3. Sodium nitrite 3% solution should be injected intravenously at a rate not exceeding 2.5 to 5 ml/minute up to a total dose of 10 to 15 ml with careful monitoring of the blood pressure.
4. Following the above steps, inject sodium thiosulfate intravenously, 12.5 g in 50 ml of 5% dextrose injection over a ten-minute period.
5. Since signs of overdosage may reappear, the patient must be observed for several hours.
6. If signs of overdosage reappear, sodium nitrite and sodium thiosulfate injections are repeated in one-half of the above doses.
7. During the administration of nitrites and later when thiocyanate formation is taking place, blood pressure may drop but can be corrected with vasopressor agents.

Dosage and Administration:
Reconstitution Directions for Univial:
1. Remove protective cap.
Turn plunger-stopper a quarter turn and press to force sterile water for injection into lower chamber.
2. Shake gently to effect solution.
Use only a clear solution.
3. Sterilize top of stopper with a suitable germicide.
4. Insert needle through the center of stopper until tip is barely visible. Withdraw dose.

Depending on the desired concentration, all of the reconstituted Univial solution should be diluted in 250 to 1000 ml of 5% dextrose injection and promptly covered with light-protective sleeve supplied with the product, or aluminum foil, or other opaque materials to protect from light. *If properly protected from light, the freshly reconstituted and diluted solution is stable for 24 hours.* The freshly prepared solution for infusion has a very faint brownish tint. If it is highly colored, it should be discarded (see Precautions). *The infusion fluid used for the administration of NITROPRESS should not be employed as a vehicle for simultaneous administration of any other drug.*

In patients who are not receiving antihypertensive drugs, the average dose of NITROPRESS (sterile sodium nitroprusside) for both adults and children is 3 mcg/kg/minute (range of 0.5 to 10 mcg/kg/minute). Usually, at 3 mcg/kg/minute, blood pressure can be lowered by about 30 to 40% below the pretreatment diastolic levels and maintained. In hypertensive patients receiving concomitant antihypertensive medications, smaller doses are required. In order to avoid excessive levels of thiocyanate and lessen the possibility of a precipitous drop in blood pressure, infusion rates greater than 10 mcg/kg/minute should rarely be used. If, at this rate, an adequate reduction of blood pressure is not obtained within 10 minutes, administration of NITROPRESS should be stopped.

One Univial (50 mg) NITROPRESS in 1000 ml 5% dextrose injection provides a concentration of 50 mcg/ml.

One Univial (50 mg) NITROPRESS in 500 ml 5% dextrose injection provides a concentration of 100 mcg/ml.

One Univial (50 mg) NITROPRESS in 250 ml 5% dextrose injection provides a concentration of 200 mcg/ml.

Dose	mcg/kg/min.
Average	3
Range	0.5 to 10

The intravenous infusion of NITROPRESS should be administered by an infusion pump, micro-drip regulator or any similar device that will allow precise measurement of the flow rate. Care should be taken to avoid extravasation. The rate of administration should be adjusted to maintain the desired antihypertensive or hypotensive effect, as determined by frequent blood pressure determinations. It is recommended that the blood pressure should not be allowed to drop at a too rapid rate and the systolic pressure not be lowered below 60 mmHg. In hypertensive emergencies NITROPRESS infusion may be continued until the patient can safely be treated with oral antihypertensive medications.

How Supplied: NITROPRESS (sterile sodium nitroprusside, USP) is supplied in an amber-colored, single dose Univial (**NDC** 0074-3019-02), each 2 ml (when mixed) containing the equivalent of 50 mg sodium nitroprusside dihydrate in sterile water for injection. Exposure of pharmaceutical products to heat should be minimized. Avoid excessive heat. Protect from freezing. It is recommended that unreconstituted product be stored below 86°F (30°C); however, brief exposure up to 104°F (40°C) does not adversely affect the product. Protect from light—store in carton until use.

Univial®—Sterile two-compartment vial, Abbott.
Abbott Laboratories
North Chicago, IL 60064
Ref. 01-2313-R4

NORISODRINE® AEROTROL®   R
[no-ris'o-drene air'ō-trol]
(isoproterenol hydrochloride inhalation aerosol, USP)
In a Controlled-Dose Nebulizer
Description: Isoproterenol HCl 0.25% w/w (=2.8 mg/ml) in inert chlorofluorohydrocarbon propellants; alcohol 33%; ascorbic acid 0.1% as preservative; and artificial and natural flavors. Each depression of the valve delivers approximately 0.12 mg to the patient.
Actions: Isoproterenol is a short-acting sympathomimetic drug. It produces pharmacologic response in the cardiovascular system and on the smooth muscles of the bronchial tree. The drug will prevent or overcome histamine-induced asthma in both experimental animals and man, and is effective when used prophylactically. It is one of the most potent bronchodilators known and can be used in patients who do not respond to the bronchodilating action of epinephrine. Isoproterenol has a cardio-accelerating effect, but its vasoconstricting action is less pronounced than that of epinephrine. Therapeutic doses may produce a slight increase in systolic blood pressure, but a slight decrease in diastolic. Larger doses may cause peripheral vasodilatation in the renal, mesenteric and femoral beds and some patients respond with a decrease in diastolic, but no change in systolic pressure. Such effects are usually of very short duration.

Indications: For the treatment of bronchospasm associated with acute and chronic bronchial asthma, pulmonary emphysema, bronchitis, and bronchiectasis.

Contraindications: Use of isoproterenol in patients with pre-existing cardiac arrhythmias associated with tachycardia is contraindicated because the cardiac stimulant effects of the drug may aggravate such disorders.

Warnings: Excessive use of an adrenergic aerosol should be discouraged, as it may lose its effectiveness. Occasional patients have been reported to develop severe paradoxical airway resistance with repeated excessive use of isoproterenol inhalation preparations. The cause of this refractory state is unknown. It is advisable that in such instances the use of this preparation be discontinued immediately and alternative therapy instituted, since in the reported cases the patients did not respond to other forms of therapy until the drug was withdrawn.

Deaths have been reported following excessive use of isoproterenol inhalation preparations and the exact cause is unknown. Cardiac arrest was noted in several instances.

Precautions: Isoproterenol and epinephrine may be used interchangeably if the patient becomes unresponsive to one or the other but should not be used concurrently. If desired, these drugs may be alternated, provided an interval of at least four hours has elapsed.

As with all sympathomimetic drugs, isoproterenol should be used with great caution in the presence of cardiovascular disorders, including coronary insufficiency, hypertension, hyperthyroidism and diabetes, or when there is a sensitivity to sympathomimetic amines.

Although there has been no evidence of teratogenic effects with this drug, use of any drug in pregnancy, lactation, or in women of childbearing age requires that the potential benefit of the drug be weighed against its possible hazard to the mother and child.

Adverse Reactions: Only a small percentage of patients experience any side effects following oral inhalation of aerosolized isoproterenol. Overdosage may produce tachycardia with resultant coronary insufficiency, palpitations, vertigo, nausea, tremors, headache, insomnia, central excitation, and blood pressure changes. These reactions are similar to those produced by other sympathomimetic agents.

Dosage and Administration: The usual dose for the relief of dyspnea in the acute episode is 1 to 2 inhalations. Start with one inhalation. If no relief is evident after 2 to 5 minutes, a second inhalation may be taken. For daily maintenance, use 1 to 2 inhalations 4 to 6 times daily, or as directed by the physician. The physician should be careful to instruct the patient in the proper technique of administration so that the number of inhalations per treatment and the frequency of treatment may be titrated to the patient's response.

No more than two inhalations should be taken at any one time, or more than 6 inhalations in any hour during a 24-hour period, unless advised by physician.

Directions for Use: Before each use, remove cap and assemble.
1. Breathe out fully. Place mouthpiece well into the mouth, aimed at the back of the throat.
2. As you begin to breathe in deeply, press the vial firmly down into the adapter. This releases one dose. Continue to breathe in until your lungs are completely filled.

Continued on next page

If desired, additional literature on any Abbott Product will be provided upon request to Abbott Laboratories.

Abbott—Cont.

3. Remove from mouth. Hold your breath for several seconds, then breathe out slowly.

Warning: Do not exceed the dose prescribed by your physician. If difficulty in breathing persists, contact your physician immediately.

How Supplied: NORISODRINE AEROTROL (isoproterenol hydrochloride inhalation aerosol, USP), 0.25% w/w, is supplied in a 15 ml controlled-dose nebulizer (NDC 0074-6869-03).

Manufactured for
Abbott Laboratories
North Chicago, IL 60064
Ref. 01-2149-R3

NORISODRINE® WITH CALCIUM IODIDE SYRUP ℞
[nō-rī′sō-drēen]
(isoproterenol sulfate and calcium iodide)

How Supplied: Each teaspoonful of NORISODRINE WITH CALCIUM IODIDE SYRUP contains 3 mg of isoproterenol sulfate, 150 mg of anhydrous calcium iodide and 6% alcohol in a palatable syrup. Norisodrine with Calcium Iodide Syrup is supplied in pint (NDC 0074-6953-01) bottles.

Abbott Laboratories
North Chicago, IL 60064

OGEN® ℞
[ō′gĕn]
(estropiate tablets, USP)

WARNING:
1. ESTROGENS HAVE BEEN REPORTED TO INCREASE THE RISK OF ENDOMETRIAL CARCINOMA.

Three independent case control studies have shown an increased risk of endometrial cancer in postmenopausal women exposed to exogenous estrogens for prolonged periods.[1-3] This risk was independent of the other known risk factors for endometrial cancer. These studies are further supported by the finding that incidence rates of endometrial cancer have increased sharply since 1969 in eight different areas of the United States with population-based cancer reporting systems, an increase which may be related to the rapidly expanding use of estrogens during the last decade.[4]

The three case control studies reported that the risk of endometrial cancer in estrogen users was about 4.5 to 13.9 times greater than in nonusers. The risk appears to depend on both duration of treatment[1] and on estrogen dose.[3] In view of these findings, when estrogens are used for the treatment of menopausal symptoms, the lowest dose that will control symptoms should be utilized and medication should be discontinued as soon as possible. When prolonged treatment is medically indicated, the patient should be reassessed on at least a semiannual basis to determine the need for continued therapy. Although the evidence must be considered preliminary, one study suggests that cyclic administration of low doses of estrogen may carry less risk than continuous administration;[3] it therefore appears prudent to utilize such a regimen.

Close clinical surveillance of all women taking estrogens is important. In all cases of undiagnosed persistent or recurring abnormal vaginal bleeding, adequate diagnostic measures should be undertaken to rule out malignancy.

There is no evidence at present that "natural" estrogens are more or less hazardous than "synthetic" estrogens at equiestrogenic doses.

2. OGEN SHOULD NOT BE USED DURING PREGNANCY.

According to some investigators, the use of female sex hormones, both estrogens and progestogens, during early pregnancy may seriously damage the offspring. Studies have reported that females exposed in utero to diethylstilbestrol, a non-steroidal estrogen, have an increased risk of developing in later life a form of vaginal or cervical cancer that is ordinarily extremely rare.[5,6] In one of these studies, this risk was estimated as not greater than 4 per 1000 exposures.[7] Furthermore, there are reports that a high percentage of such exposed women (from 30 to 90 percent) have been found to have vaginal adenosis,[8-12] epithelial changes of the vagina and cervix. Although these reported changes are histologically benign, the investigators have not determined whether they are precursors of adenocarcinoma.

Several reports suggest an association between intrauterine exposure to female sex hormones and congenital anomalies in the offspring, including heart defects and limb reduction defects.[13-16] One case control study[16] estimated a 4.7 fold increased risk of limb reduction defects in infants exposed in utero to sex hormones (oral contraceptives, hormone withdrawal tests for pregnancy, or attempted treatment for threatened abortion). Some of these exposures were very short and involved only a few days of treatment. The data suggest that the risk of limb reduction defects in exposed fetuses is somewhat less than 1 per 1000.

In the past, female sex hormones have been used during pregnancy in an attempt to treat threatened or habitual abortion. OGEN has not been studied for these uses, and therefore should not be used during pregnancy. There is no evidence from well controlled studies that progestogens are effective for these uses.

If OGEN (estropipate tablets) is used during pregnancy, or if the patient becomes pregnant while taking this drug, she should be apprised of the potential risks to the fetus, and the question of continuation of the pregnancy should be addressed.

Description: OGEN (estropipate tablets), (formerly piperazine estrone sulfate), is a natural estrogenic substance prepared from purified crystalline estrone, solubilized as the sulfate and stabilized with piperazine. It is appreciably soluble in water and has almost no odor or taste—properties which are ideally suited for oral administration. The amount of piperazine in OGEN is not sufficient to exert a pharmacological action. Its addition ensures solubility, stability, and uniform potency of the estrone sulfate. Chemically estropipate is represented by estra-1,3,5(10)-trien-17-one, 3-(sulfooxy)-, compound with piperazine (1:1).

OGEN is available as tablets for oral administration containing either 0.75 mg (OGEN .625), 1.5 mg (OGEN 1.25), 3 mg (OGEN 2.5) or 6 mg (OGEN 5) estropipate.

Clinical Pharmacology: Estrogens are important in the development and maintenance of the female reproductive system and secondary sex characteristics. They promote growth and development of the vagina, uterus, and fallopian tubes, and enlargement of the breasts. Indirectly, they contribute to the shaping of the skeleton, maintenance of tone and elasticity of urogenital structures, changes in the epiphyses of the long bones that allow for the pubertal growth spurt and its termination, growth of axillary and pubic hair, and pigmentation of the nipples and genitals. Along with other hormones such as progesterone, estrogens are intricately involved in the process of menstruation. Estrogens also affect the release of pituitary gonadotropins.

Estropipate owes its therapeutic action to estrone, one of the three principal estrogenic steroid hormones of man: estradiol, estrone, and estriol. Estradiol is rapidly hydrolyzed in the body to estrone, which in turn may be hydrated to the less active estriol. These transformations occur readily, mainly in the liver, where there is also free interconversion between estrone and estradiol.

Gastrointestinal absorption of orally administered estrogens is usually prompt and complete. Inactivation of estrogens in the body occurs mainly in the liver. During cyclic passage through the liver, estrogens are degraded to less active estrogenic compounds and conjugated with sulfuric and glucuronic acids. Estrone is 50–80% bound to protein as it circulates in the blood, primarily as a conjugate with sulfate.

Indications and Usage: The cyclic administration of OGEN (estropipate tablets) is indicated for the treatment of estrogen deficiency associated with (See "DOSAGE AND ADMINISTRATION" section):

1. Moderate to severe *vasomotor* symptoms of menopause. (There is no evidence that estrogens are effective for nervous symptoms or depression which might occur during menopause, and they should not be used to treat these conditions.)
2. Atrophic vaginitis.
3. Kraurosis vulvae.
4. Female hypogonadism.
5. Female castration.
6. Primary ovarian failure.

OGEN (estropipate tablets) HAS NOT BEEN TESTED FOR EFFICACY FOR ANY PURPOSE DURING PREGNANCY. SINCE ITS EFFECT UPON THE FETUS IS UNKNOWN, IT CANNOT BE RECOMMENDED FOR ANY CONDITION DURING PREGNANCY (SEE BOXED WARNING).

Contraindications: OGEN should not be used in women with any of the following conditions:

1. Known or suspected cancer of the breast.
2. Known or suspected estrogen dependent neoplasia.
3. OGEN may cause fetal harm when administered to a pregnant woman. OGEN is contraindicated in women who are or may become pregnant (See Box Warning).
4. Undiagnosed abnormal genital bleeding.
5. Active thrombophlebitis or thromboembolic disorders.
6. A past history of thrombophlebitis, thrombosis, or thromboembolic disorders associated with previous estrogen use.

Warnings:

1. *Induction of malignant neoplasms.* Long-term continuous administration of natural and synthetic estrogens in certain animal species has been reported by some investigators to increase the frequency of carcinomas of the breast, cervix, vagina, and liver. There is now evidence that estrogens increase the risk of carcinoma of the endometrium in humans. (See Boxed Warning.)

At the present time there is no conclusive evidence that estrogens given to postmenopausal women increase the risk of cancer of the breast.[17,40,41] There are, however, a few retrospective studies which suggest a small but statistically significant increase in the risk factor for breast cancer among these women.[18,42-44] Therefore, caution should be exercised when administering estrogens to women with a strong family history of breast cancer or who have breast nodules, fibrocystic disease, or abnormal mammograms. Careful breast examinations should be performed periodically.

2. *Gallbladder disease.* A recent study has reported a 2 to 3 fold increase in the risk of surgically confirmed gallbladder disease in women receiving postmenopausal estrogens,[17] similar to the 2-fold increase previously noted in users of oral contraceptives.[19,22] In the case of oral contraceptives, the increased risk appeared after two years of use.[22]

3. *Effects similar to those caused by estrogen-progestogen oral contraceptives.* There are several serious adverse effects of oral contraceptives, most of which have not, up to now, been documented as consequences of postmenopausal estrogen therapy. This may reflect the comparatively low doses of estrogen used in postmenopausal women. It would be expected that the larger doses of estrogen used to treat postpartum breast engorgement would be more likely to result in these adverse effects, and, in fact, it has been shown that there is an increased risk of thrombosis in women receiving estrogens for postpartum breast engorgement.[20,21]

a. *Thromboembolic disease.* It is now well established that users of oral contraceptives have an increased risk of various thromboembolic and thrombotic vascular diseases, such as thrombophlebitis, pulmonary embolism, stroke, and myocardial infarction.[22-29] Cases of retinal thrombosis, mesenteric thrombosis, and optic neuritis have been reported in oral contraceptive users. There is evidence that the risk of several of these adverse reactions is related to the dose of the drug.[30,31] An increased risk of post-surgery thromboembolic complications has also been reported in users of oral contraceptives.[32,33] If feasible, estrogen should be discontinued at least 4 weeks before surgery of the type associated with an increased risk of thromboembolism; it should also be discontinued during periods of prolonged immobilization. While an increased rate of thromboembolic and thrombotic disease in postmenopausal users of estrogens has not been found[17,34] this does not rule out the possibility that such an increase may be present or that subgroups of women who have underlying risk factors or who are receiving relatively large doses of estrogens may have increased risk. Therefore, estrogens should not be used in persons with active thrombophlebitis or thromboembolic disorders, and they should not be used in persons with a history of such disorders in association with estrogen use. They should be used with caution in patients with cerebral vascular or coronary artery disease and only for those in whom estrogens are clearly needed.

Large doses of estrogen (5 mg conjugated estrogens per day), comparable to those used to treat cancer of the prostate and breast, have been shown in a large prospective clinical trial in men[35] to increase the risk of nonfatal myocardial infarction, pulmonary embolism and thrombophlebitis. When estrogen doses of this size are used, any of the thromboembolic and thrombotic adverse effects associated with oral contraceptive use should be considered a clear risk.

b. *Hepatic adenoma.* Benign hepatic adenomas appear to be associated with the use of oral contraceptives.[36-38] Although benign, and rare, these may rupture and cause death through intraabdominal hemorrhage. Such lesions have not yet been reported in association with other estrogen or progestogen preparations but should be considered in estrogen users having abdominal pain and tenderness, abdominal mass, or hypovolemic shock. Hepatocellular carcinoma has also been reported in women taking estrogen-containing oral contraceptives.[37] The relationship of this malignancy to these drugs is not known at this time.

c. *Elevated blood pressure.* Increased blood pressure is not uncommon in women using oral contraceptives. There is now a report that this may occur with use of estrogens in the menopause[39] and blood pressure should be monitored with estrogen use, especially if high doses are used.

d. *Glucose tolerance.* A worsening of glucose tolerance has been observed in a significant percentage of patients on estrogen-containing oral contraceptives. For this reason, diabetic patients should be carefully observed while receiving estrogen.

4. *Hypercalcemia.* Administration of estrogens may lead to severe hypercalcemia in patients with breast cancer and bone metastases. If this occurs, the drug should be stopped and appropriate measures taken to reduce the serum calcium level.

Precautions:
A. General Precautions.
1. A complete medical and family history should be taken prior to the initiation of any estrogen therapy. The pretreatment and periodic physical examinations should include special reference to blood pressure, breasts, abdomen, and pelvic organs, and should include a Papanicolau smear. As a general rule, estrogen should not be prescribed for longer than one year without another physical examination being performed.
2. Fluid retention—Estrogens may cause some degree of fluid retention. Therefore, patients with conditions such as epilepsy, migraine, and cardiac or renal dysfunction, which might be influenced by this factor, require careful observation.

3. Certain patients may develop undesirable manifestations of excessive estrogenic stimulation, such as abnormal or excessive uterine bleeding, mastodynia, etc.
4. Oral contraceptives appear to be associated with an increased incidence of mental depression.[22] Although it is not clear whether this is due to the estrogenic or progestogenic component of the contraceptive, patients with a history of depression should be carefully observed.
5. Preexisting uterine leiomyomata may increase in size during estrogen use.
6. The pathologist should be advised of the patient's use of estrogen therapy when relevant specimens are submitted.
7. Patients with a past history of jaundice during pregnancy have an increased risk of recurrence of jaundice while receiving estrogen containing oral contraceptive therapy. If jaundice develops in any patient receiving estrogen, the medication should be discontinued while the cause is investigated.
8. Estrogens may be poorly metabolized in patients with impaired liver function and they should be administered with caution in such patients.
9. Because estrogens influence the metabolism of calcium and phosphorus, they should be used with caution in patients with metabolic bone diseases that are associated with hypercalcemia or in patients with renal insufficiency.

B. Information for the Patient. See text of Patient Package Insert which appears after PHYSICIAN REFERENCES.

C. Drug Interactions. The concomitant use of any drugs which can induce hepatic microsomal enzymes with estrogens may produce estrogen levels which are lower than would be expected from the dose of estrogen administered.

The use of *broad spectrum antibiotics* which profoundly effect intestinal flora may influence the absorption of steroidal compounds including the estrogens.

Diabetics receiving *insulin* may have increased insulin requirements when receiving estrogens.

Laboratory Test Interference. Certain endocrine and liver function tests may be affected by estrogen-containing oral contraceptives. The following similar changes may be expected with larger doses of estrogen:
a. Increased sulfobromophthalein retention.
b. Increased prothrombin and factors VII, VIII, IX, and X; decreased antithrombin 3; increased norepinephrine-induced platelet aggregability.
c. Increased thyroid binding globulin (TBG) leading to increased circulating total thyroid hormone, as measured by PBI, T4 by column, or T4 by radioimmunoassay. Free T3 resin uptake is decreased, reflecting the elevated TBG; free T4 concentration is unaltered.
d. Abnormal glucose tolerance test results.
e. Decreased pregnanediol excretion.
f. Reduced response to metyrapone test.
g. Reduced serum folate concentration.
h. Increased serum triglyceride and phospholipid concentration.

D. Carcinogenesis. Studies have shown an increased risk of endometrial cancer in postmenopausal women exposed to exogenous estrogens for prolonged periods (see Boxed Warning). At the present time there is no conclusive evidence that estrogens given to postmenopausal women increase the risk of cancer of the breast.[17,40,41] There are, however, a few retrospective studies which suggest a small, but statistically significant increase in the risk factor for breast cancer among these women.[18,42,44] (See "WARNINGS" section.)

E. Pregnancy. Pregnancy Category X. See "CONTRAINDICATIONS" section and Boxed Warning.

F. Nursing Mothers. Estrogens have been reported to be excreted in human breast milk. Caution should be exercised when OGEN is administered to a nursing woman.

G. Pediatric Use. Because of the effects of estrogens on epiphyseal closure, they should be used judiciously in young patients in whom bone growth is not complete.

Adverse Reactions: (See Warnings regarding reports of possible induction of neoplasia, unknown effects upon the fetus, increased incidence of gall bladder disease, and adverse effects similar to those of oral contraceptives, including thromboembolism.) The following additional adverse reactions in decreasing order of severity within each category have been reported with estrogenic therapy, including oral contraceptives:

1. *Genitourinary system.*
Increase in size of uterine fibromyomata.
Vaginal candidiasis.
Cystitis-like syndrome.
Dysmenorrhea.
Amenorrhea during and after treatment.
Change in cervical eversion and in degree of cervical secretion.
Breakthrough bleeding, spotting, change in menstrual flow.
Premenstrual-like syndrome.
2. *Breast.*
Tenderness, enlargement, secretion.
3. *Gastrointestinal.*
Cholestatic jaundice.
Vomiting, nausea.
Abdominal cramps, bloating.
4. *Skin.*
Hemorrhagic eruption.
Erythema nodosum.
Erythema multiforme.
Hirsutism.
Chloasma or melasma which may persist when drug is discontinued.
Loss of scalp hair.
5. *Eyes.*
Steepening of corneal curvature.
Intolerance to contact lenses.
6. *CNS.*
Chorea.
Mental depression
Migraine, dizziness, headache.
7. *Miscellaneous.*
Aggravation of porphyria.
Edema.
Reduced carbohydrate tolerance.
Increase or decrease in weight.
Changes in libido.

Overdosage: Numerous reports of ingestion of large doses of estrogen-containing oral contraceptives by young children indicate that serious ill effects do not occur. Overdosage of oral estrogen may cause nausea and withdrawal bleeding may occur in females.

Dosage and Administration:
1. *Given cyclically for short-term use:*
For treatment of moderate to severe *vasomotor* symptoms, atrophic vaginitis, or kraurosis vulvae associated with the menopause.
The lowest dose that will control symptoms should be chosen and medication should be discontinued as promptly as possible.
Administration should be cyclic (e.g., 3 weeks on and 1 week off).
Attempts to discontinue or taper medication should be made at 3 to 6 month intervals.
Usual dosage ranges:

Vasomotor symptoms—One OGEN .625 (estropipate) Tablet to one OGEN 5 Tablet per day. The lowest dose that will control symptoms should be chosen. If the patient has not menstruated within the last two months or more, cyclic administration is started arbitrarily. If the patient is menstruating, cyclic administration is started on day 5 of bleeding.

Atrophic vaginitis and kraurosis vulvae—One OGEN .625 Tablet to one OGEN 5 Tablet daily, depending upon the tissue response of the individual patient. The lowest dose that will control symptoms should be chosen. Administer cyclically.

2. *Given cyclically.*
Female hypogonadism; Female castration; primary ovarian failure.

Continued on next page

If desired, additional literature on any Abbott Product will be provided upon request to Abbott Laboratories.

Abbott—Cont.

Usual dosage ranges:
Female hypogonadism—A daily dose of one OGEN 1.25 Tablet to three OGEN 2.5 Tablets may be given for the first three weeks of a theoretical cycle, followed by a rest period of eight to ten days. The lowest dose that will control symptoms should be chosen. If bleeding does not occur by the end of this period, the same dosage schedule is repeated. The number of courses of estrogen therapy necessary to produce bleeding may vary depending on the responsiveness of the endometrium. If satisfactory withdrawal bleeding does not occur, an oral progestogen may be given in addition to estrogen during the third week of the cycle.

Female castration and primary ovarian failure—A daily dose of one OGEN 1.25 Tablet to three OGEN 2.5 Tablets may be given for the first three weeks of a theoretical cycle, followed by a rest period of eight to ten days. Adjust dosage upward or downward according to severity of symptoms and response of the patient. For maintenance, adjust dosage to lowest level that will provide effective control.

Treated patients with an intact uterus should be monitored closely for signs of endometrial cancer and appropriate diagnostic measures should be taken to rule out malignancy in the event of persistent or recurring abnormal vaginal bleeding.

How Supplied: OGEN (estropipate tablets, USP) is supplied as OGEN .625 (0.75 mg estropipate), yellow tablets, **NDC** 0074-3943-04; OGEN 1.25 (1.5 mg estropipate), peach-colored tablets, **NDC** 0074-3946-04; OGEN 2.5 (3 mg estropipate), blue tablets, **NDC** 0074-3951-04; and OGEN 5 (6 mg estropipate), light green tablets, **NDC** 0074-3958-13. Tablets of all four dosage levels are standardized to provide uniform estrone activity and are grooved (Divide-Tab®) to provide dosage flexibility. All tablet sizes of OGEN are available in bottles of 100.

Shown in Product Identification Section, page 403

Physician References:
[1] Ziel, H. K., Finkel, W. D., "Increased Risk of Endometrial Carcinoma Among Users of Conjugated Estrogens," *New England Journal of Medicine*, 293:1167-1170, 1975.
[2] Smith, D. C., Prentic, R., Thompson, D. J., et al., "Association of Exogenous Estrogen and Endometrial Carcinoma," *New England Journal of Medicine*, 293:1164-1167, 1975.
[3] Mack, T. M., Pike, M. C., Henderson, B.E., et al., "Estrogens and Endometrial Cancer in a Retirement Community," *New England Journal of Medicine*, 294:1262-1267, 1976.
[4] Weiss, N. S., Szekely, D. R., Austin, D. F., "Increasing Incidence of Endometrial Cancer in the United States," *New England Journal of Medicine*, 294:1259-1262, 1976.
[5] Herbst, A. L., Ulfelder, H., Poskanzer, D. C., "Adenocarcinoma of Vagina," *New England Journal of Medicine*, 284:878-881, 1971.
[6] Greenwald, P., Barlow, J., Nasca, P., et al., "Vaginal Cancer after Maternal Treatment with Synthetic Estrogens," *New England Journal of Medicine*, 285:390-392, 1971.
[7] Lanier, A., Noller, K., Decker, D., et al., "Cancer and Stilbestrol A Follow Up of 1719 Persons Exposed to Estrogens In Utero and Born 1943-1959," *Mayo Clinic Proceedings*, 48:793-799, 1973.
[8] Herbst, A., Kurman, R., Scully, R., "Vaginal and Cervical Abnormalities After Exposure to Stilbestrol In Utero," *Obstetrics and Gynecology*, 40:287-298, 1972.
[9] Herbst, A., Robboy, S., Macdonald, G., et al., "The Effects of Local Progesterone on Stilbestrol Associated Vaginal Adenosis," *American Journal of Obstetrics and Gynecology*, 118:607-615, 1974.
[10] Herbst, A., Poskanzer, D., Robboy, S., et al., "Prenatal Exposure to Stilbestrol, A Prospective Comparison of Exposed Female Offspring with Unexposed Controls," *New England Journal of Medicine*, 292:334-339, 1975.
[11] Stafl, A., Mattingly, R., Foley, D., et al., "Clinical Diagnosis of Vaginal Adenosis," *Obstetrics and Gynecology*, 43:118-128, 1974.
[12] Sherman, A. I., Goldrath, M., Berlin, A., et al., "Cervical-Vaginal Adenosis After *In Utero* Exposure to Synthetic Estrogens," *Obstetrics and Gynecology*, 44:531-545, 1974.
[13] Gal, I., Kirman, B., Stern, J., "Hormone Pregnancy Tests and Congenital Malformation," *Nature*, 216:83, 1967.
[14] Levy, E. P., Cohen, A., Fraser, F. C., "Hormone Treatment During Pregnancy and Congenital Heart Defects," *Lancet*, 1:611, 1973.
[15] Nora, J., Nora, A., "Birth Defects and Oral Contraceptives," *Lancet*, 1:941-942, 1973.
[16] Janerich, D. T., Piper, J. M., Clebatis, D.M., "Oral Contraceptives and Congenital Limb-Reduction Defects," *New England Journal of Medicine*, 291:697-700, 1974.
[17] Boston Collaborative Drug Surveillance Program "Surgically Confirmed Gall Bladder Disease, Venous Thromboembolism and Breast Tumors in Relation to Post-Menopausal Estrogen Therapy," *New England Journal of Medicine*, 290:15-19, 1974.
[18] Brinton, L. A., Hoover, R. N., Szklo, M., et al., "Menopausal Estrogen Use and Risk of Breast Cancer," *Cancer*, 47(10):2517-2522, 1981.
[19] Boston Collaborative Drug Surveillance Program, "Oral Contraceptives and Venous Thromboembolic Disease, Surgically Confirmed Gall Bladder Disease and Breast Tumors," *Lancet*, 1:1399-1404, 1973.
[20] Daniel, D.G., Campbell, H., Turnbull, A. C., "Puerperal Thromboembolism and Suppression of Lactation," *Lancet*, 2:287-289, 1967.
[21] Bailar, J. C., "Thromboembolism and Oestrogen Therapy," *Lancet*, 2:560, 1967.
[22] Royal College of General Practitioners, "Oral Contraception and Thromboembolic Disease," *Journal of the Royal College of General Practitioners*, 13:267-279, 1967.
[23] Inman, W. H. W., Vessey, M. P., "Investigation of Deaths from Pulmonary, Coronary, and Cerebral Thrombosis and Embolism in Women of Child Bearing Age," *British Medical Journal*, 2:193-199, 1968.
[24] Vessey, M. P., Doll, R., "Investigation of Relation Between Use of Oral Contraceptives and Thromboembolic Disease. A Further Report," *British Medical Journal*, 2:651-657, 1969.
[25] Sartwell, P. E., Masi, A. T., Arthes, F. G., et al. "Thromboembolism and Oral Contraceptives: An Epidemiological Case Control Study," *American Journal of Epidemiology*, 90:365-380, 1969.
[26] Collaborative Group for the Study of Stroke in Young Women, "Oral Contraception and Increased Risk of Cerebral Ischemia or Thrombosis," *New England Journal of Medicine*, 288:871-878, 1973.
[27] Collaborative Group for the Study of Stroke in Young Women, "Oral Contraceptives and Stroke in Young Women: Associated Risk Factors," *Journal of American Medical Association*, 231:718-722, 1975.
[28] Mann, J. I., Inman, W. H. W., "Oral Contraceptives and Death from Myocardial Infarction," *British Medical Journal*, 2:245-248, 1975.
[29] Mann, J. I., Vessey, M. P., Thorogood, M., et al., "Myocardial Infarction in Young Women with Special Reference to Oral Contraceptives Practice," *British Medical Journal*, 2:241-245, 1975.
[30] Inman, W. H. W., Vessey, M. P., Westerholm, B., et al., "Thromboembolic Disease and the Steroidal Content of Oral Contraceptives," *British Medical Journal*, 2:203-209, 1970.
[31] Stolley, P. D., Tonascia, J. A., Tockman, M. S., et al., "Thrombosis with Low-Estrogen Oral Contraceptives," *American Journal of Epidemiology*, 102:197-208, 1975.
[32] Vessey, M. P., Doll, R., Fairbairn, A. S., et al., "Post Operative Thromboembolism and the Use of the Oral Contraceptives," *British Medical Journal*, 3:123-126, 1970.
[33] Greene, G. R., Sartwell, P. E., "Oral Contraceptive Use in Patients with Thromboembolism Following Surgery, Trauma or Infection," *American Journal of Public Health*, 62:680-685, 1972.
[34] Rosenberg, L., Armstrong, M. B., Jick, H., "Myocardial Infarction and Estrogen Therapy in Postmenopausal Women," *New England Journal of Medicine*, 294:1256-1259, 1976.
[35] Coronary Drug Project Research Group, "The Coronary Drug Project: Initial Findings Leading to Modifications of Its Research Protocol," *Journal of the American Medical Association*, 214:1303-1313, 1970.
[36] Baum, J., Holtz, F., Bookstein, J.J., et al., "Possible Association Between Benign Hepatomas and Oral Contraceptives," *Lancet*, 2:926-928, 1973.
[37] Mays, E. T., Christopherson, W. M., Mahr, M. M., et al., "Hepatic Changes in Young Women Ingesting Contraceptive Steroids, Hepatic Hemorrhage and Primary Hepatic Tumors," *Journal of the American Medical Association*, 235:730-782, 1976.
[38] Edmondson, H. A., Henderson, B., Benton, B., "Liver Cell Adenomas Associated with the Use of Oral Contraceptives," *New England Journal of Medicine*, 294:470-472, 1976.
[39] Pfeffer, R. I., Van Den Noort, S., "Estrogen Use and Stroke Risk in Postmenopausal Women," *American Journal of Epidemiology*, 103:445-456, 1976.
[40] Gambrell, R. D., Massey, F. M., Castaneda, T. A., et al., "Estrogen Therapy and Breast Cancer in Postmenopausal Women," *Journal of the American Geriatrics Society*, 28(6):251-257, 1980.
[41] Kelsey, J. L., Fischer, D. B., Holford, T. R., et al., "Exogenous Estrogens and Other Factors in the Epidemiology of Breast Cancer," *Journal of the National Cancer Institute*, 57(2):327-333, 1981.
[42] Ross, R. K., Paganini-Hill, A., Gerkins, V., et al., "A Case-Control Study of Menopausal Estrogen Therapy and Breast Cancer," *Journal of the American Medical Association*, 243(16):1635-1639, 1980.
[43] Hoover, R., Glass, A., Finkel, W. D., et al., "Conjugated Estrogens and Breast Cancer Risk in Women," *Journal of the National Cancer Institute*, 67(4):815-820, 1981.
[44] Lawson, D. H., Jick, H., Hunter, J. R., et al., "Exogenous Estrogens and Breast Cancer," *American Journal of Epidemiology*, 114(5):710, 1981.

INFORMATION FOR PATIENTS
OGEN®
(estropipate tablets, USP)
WHAT YOU SHOULD KNOW ABOUT ESTROGENS

Estrogens are female hormones produced by the ovaries. The ovaries make several different kinds of estrogens. In addition, scientists have been able to make a variety of synthetic estrogens. As far as we know, all these estrogens have similar properties and therefore much the same usefulness, side effects, and risks. This leaflet is intended to help you understand what estrogens are used for, the risks involved in their use, and how to use them as safely as possible.

This leaflet includes the most important information about estrogens, but not all the information. If you want to know more, you can ask your doctor or pharmacist to let you read the package insert prepared for the doctor.

Uses of Estrogen: Estrogens are prescribed by doctors for a number of purposes, including:
1. To provide estrogen during a period of adjustment when a woman's ovaries no longer produce it, in order to prevent certain uncomfortable symptoms of estrogen deficiency. (All women normally stop producing estrogens, generally between the ages of 45 and 55; this is called the menopause.)
2. To prevent symptoms of estrogen deficiency when a woman's ovaries have been removed surgically before the natural menopause.
3. To prevent pregnancy. (Estrogens are given along with a progestogen, another female hormone; these combinations are called oral contraceptives or birth control pills. Patient labeling is available to women taking oral contraceptives and they will not be discussed in this leaflet.)

THERE IS NO PROPER USE OF OGEN (ESTROPIPATE) IN A PREGNANT WOMAN.

Estrogens in the Menopause: In the natural course of their lives, all women eventually experience a decrease in estrogen production. This usually occurs between ages 45 and 55 but may occur earlier or later. Sometimes the ovaries may need to be removed before natural menopause by an operation, producing a "surgical menopause."

When the amount of estrogen in the blood begins to decrease, many women may develop typical symptoms: Feelings of warmth in the face, neck, and chest or sudden intense episodes of heat or sweating throughout the body (called "hot flashes" or "hot flushes"). These symptoms are sometimes very uncomfortable. A few women eventually develop changes in the vagina (called "atrophic vaginitis") which cause discomfort, especially during and after intercourse.

Estrogens can be prescribed to treat these symptoms of the menopause. It is estimated that considerably more than half of all women undergoing the menopause have only mild symptoms or no symptoms at all and therefore do not need estrogens. Other women may need estrogens for a few months, while their bodies adjust to lower estrogen levels. Sometimes the need will be for periods longer than six months. In an attempt to avoid overstimulation of the uterus (womb), oral estrogens are usually given cyclically during each month of use, that is three weeks of pills followed by one week without pills.

Sometimes women experience nervous symptoms or depression during menopause. There is no evidence that estrogens are effective for such symptoms and they should not be used to treat them, although other treatment may be needed.

You may have heard that taking estrogens for long periods (years) after the menopause will keep your skin soft and supple and keep you feeling young. There is no evidence that this is so, however, and such long-term treatment carries important risks.

The Dangers of Estrogens:

1. *Cancer of uterus.* If estrogens are used in the postmenopausal period for more than a year, there is an increased risk of *endometrial cancer* (cancer of the uterus). Women taking estrogens have roughly 5 to 10 times as great a chance of getting this cancer as women who take no estrogens. To put this another way, while a postmenopausal woman not taking estrogens has 1 chance in 1,000 each year of getting cancer of the uterus, a woman taking estrogens has 5 to 10 chances in 1,000 each year. For this reason *it is important to take estrogens only when you really need them.*

The risk of this cancer is greater the longer estrogens are used and also seems to be greater when larger doses are taken. For this reason *it is important to take the lowest dose of estrogen that will control symptoms and to take it only as long as it is needed.* If estrogens are needed for longer periods of time, your doctor will want to reevaluate your need for estrogens at least every six months.

Women using estrogens should report any irregular vaginal bleeding to their doctors; such bleeding may be of no importance, but it can be an early warning of cancer of the uterus. If you have undiagnosed vaginal bleeding, you should not use estrogens until a diagnosis is made and you are certain there is no cancer of the uterus.

If you have had your uterus completely removed (total hysterectomy), there is no danger of developing cancer of the uterus.

2. *Other possible cancers.* Estrogens can cause development of other tumors in animals, such as tumors of the breast, cervix, vagina, or liver, when given for a long time. At present there is no good evidence that women using estrogen in the menopause have an increased risk of such tumors, but there is no way yet to be sure they do not; and one study raises the possibility that use of estrogens in the menopause may increase the risk of breast cancer many years later. This is a further reason to use estrogens only when clearly needed. While you are taking estrogens, it is important that you go to your doctor at least once a year for a physical examination. Also, if members of your family have had breast cancer or if you have breast nodules or abnormal mammograms (breast x-rays), your doctor may wish to carry out more frequent examinations of your breasts.

3. *Gallbladder disease.* Women who use estrogens after menopause are more likely to develop gallbladder disease needing surgery than women who do not use estrogens. Birth control pills have a similar effect.

4. *Abnormal blood clotting.* Oral contraceptives increase the risk of blood clotting in various parts of the body. This can result in a stroke (if the clot is in the brain), a heart attack (clot in a blood vessel of the heart), or a pulmonary embolus (a clot which forms in the legs or pelvis, then breaks off and travels to the lungs). Any of these can be fatal. At this time use of estrogens in the menopause is not known to cause such blood clotting, but this has not been fully studied and there could still prove to be such a risk. It is recommended that if you have had clotting in the legs or lungs or a heart attack or stroke while you were using estrogens or birth control pills, you should not use estrogens. If you have had a stroke or heart attack or if you have angina pectoris, estrogens should be used with great caution and only if clearly needed (for example, if you have severe symptoms of the menopause.)

Special Warning About Pregnancy: You should not receive OGEN (estropipate) if you are pregnant. Some scientists have reported that, if estrogens are used during pregnancy, there may be a greater than usual chance that the developing baby will be born with a birth defect, although the risk remains small. In addition, other scientists have reported that there is an association between another estrogen-type product (diethylstilbestrol) and appearance of a particular cancer of the vagina or cervix (adenocarcinoma) in young women whose mothers took that drug in pregnancy. Every effort should be made to avoid exposure to OGEN in pregnancy. If exposure occurs, see your doctor.

Other Effects of Estrogens: In addition to the serious known risks of estrogens described above, estrogens have the following side effects and potential risks:

1. *Nausea and vomiting.* The most common side effect of estrogen therapy is nausea. Vomiting is less common.

2. *Effects on breasts.* Estrogens may cause breast tenderness or enlargement and may cause the breasts to secrete a liquid. These effects are not dangerous.

3. *Effects on the uterus.* Estrogens may cause benign fibroid tumors of the uterus to get larger. Some women will have menstrual bleeding when estrogens are stopped. But if the bleeding occurs on days you are still taking estrogens you should report this to your doctor.

4. *Effects on liver.* Women taking oral contraceptives develop on rare occasions a tumor of the liver which can rupture and bleed into the abdomen. So far, these tumors have not been reported in women using estrogens in the menopause, but you should report any swelling or unusual pain or tenderness in the abdomen to your doctor immediately.

Women with a past history of jaundice (yellowing of the skin and white parts of the eyes) may get jaundice again during estrogen use. If this occurs, stop taking estrogens and see your doctor.

5. *Other effects.* Estrogens may cause excess fluid to be retained in the body. This may make some conditions worse, such as epilepsy, migraine, heart disease, or kidney disease.

Summary: Estrogens have important uses, but they have serious risks as well. You must decide, with your doctor, whether the risks are acceptable to you in view of the benefits of treatment. You should not use OGEN (estropipate tablets) if you have cancer of the breast or uterus, are pregnant, have undiagnosed abnormal vaginal bleeding, clotting in the legs or lungs, or have had a stroke, heart attack or angina, or clotting in the legs or lungs in the past while you were taking estrogens. You can use estrogens as safely as possible by understanding that your doctor will require regular physical examinations while you are taking them and will try to discontinue the drug as soon as possible and use the smallest dose possible. Be alert for signs of trouble including:

1. Abnormal bleeding from the vagina.
2. Pains in the calves or chest or sudden shortness of breath, or coughing blood (indicating possible clots in the legs, heart, or lungs).
3. Severe headache, dizziness, faintness, or changes in vision (indicating possible developing clots in the brain or eye).
4. Breast lumps (you should ask your doctor how to examine your own breasts).
5. Jaundice (yellowing of the skin).
6. Mental depression.

Based on his or her assessment of your medical needs, your doctor has prescribed this drug for you. Do not give the drug to anyone else.

Abbott Pharmaceuticals, Inc.
North Chicago, IL 60064

OGEN® VAGINAL CREAM ℞
[*o'gĕn*]
(estropipate vaginal cream, USP)

WARNING:

1. ESTROGENS HAVE BEEN REPORTED TO INCREASE THE RISK OF ENDOMETRIAL CARCINOMA.

Three independent case control studies have shown an increased risk of endometrial cancer in postmenopausal women exposed to exogenous estrogens for prolonged periods.[1-3] This risk was independent of the other known risk factors for endometrial cancer. These studies are further supported by the finding that incidence rates of endometrial cancer have increased sharply since 1969 in eight different areas of the United States with population-based cancer reporting systems, an increase which may be related to the rapidly expanding use of estrogens during the last decade.[4]

The three case control studies reported that the risk of endometrial cancer in estrogen users was about 4.5 to 13.9 times greater than in nonusers. The risk appears to depend on both duration of treatment[1] and on estrogen dose.[3] In view of these findings, when estrogens are used for the treatment of menopausal symptoms, the lowest dose that will control symptoms should be utilized and medication should be discontinued as soon as possible. When prolonged treatment is medically indicated, the patient should be reassessed on at least a semiannual basis to determine the need for continued therapy. Although the evidence must be considered preliminary, one study suggests that cyclic administration of low doses of estrogen may carry less risk than continuous administration;[3] it therefore appears prudent to utilize such a regimen.

Close clinical surveillance of all women taking estrogens is important. In all cases of undiagnosed persistent or recurring abnormal vaginal bleeding, adequate diagnostic measures should be undertaken to rule out malignancy.

There is no evidence at present that "natural" estrogens are more or less hazardous than "synthetic" estrogens at equiestrogenic doses.

2. OGEN VAGINAL CREAM SHOULD NOT BE USED DURING PREGNANCY.

According to some investigators, the use of female sex hormones, both estrogens and progestogens, during early pregnancy may seriously damage the offspring. Studies have reported that females exposed in utero to diethylstilbestrol, a non-steroidal estrogen, have an increased risk of developing in later life a form of vaginal or cervical cancer that is ordinarily extremely rare.[5,6] In one of these studies, this risk was estimated as not greater than 4 per 1000 exposures.[7] Furthermore, there are reports that a high percentage of such exposed women (from 30 to 90 percent)

Continued on next page

If desired, additional literature on any Abbott Product will be provided upon request to Abbott Laboratories.

Abbott—Cont.

have been found to have vaginal adenosis,[8-12] epithelial changes of the vagina and cervix. Although these reported changes are histologically benign, the investigators have not determined whether they are precursors of adenocarcinoma.

Several reports suggest an association between intra-uterine exposure to female sex hormones and congenital anomalies in the offspring, including heart defects and limb reduction defects.[13-16] One case control study[16] estimated a 4.7 fold increased risk of limb reduction defects in infants exposed in utero to sex hormones (oral contraceptives, hormone withdrawal tests for pregnancy, or attempted treatment for threatened abortion). Some of these exposures were very short and involved only a few days of treatment. The data suggest that the risk of limb reduction defects in exposed fetuses is somewhat less than 1 per 1000.

In the past, female sex hormones have been used during pregnancy, in an attempt to treat threatened or habitual abortion. OGEN Vaginal Cream is not intended for these uses, nor has it been studied for these uses, and therefore should not be used during pregnancy. There is no evidence from well controlled studies that progestogens are effective for these uses.

If OGEN Vaginal Cream (estropipate) is used during pregnancy, or if the patient becomes pregnant while using this drug, she should be apprised of the potential risks to the fetus, and the question of continuation of the pregnancy should be addressed.

Description: OGEN (estropipate), (formerly piperazine estrone sulfate), is a natural estrogenic substance prepared from purified crystalline estrone, solubilized as the sulfate and stabilized with piperazine. It is appreciably soluble in water and has almost no odor or taste. The amount of piperazine in OGEN is not sufficient to exert a pharmacological action. Its addition ensures solubility, stability, and uniform potency of the estrone sulfate. Chemically estropipate is represented by estra-1,3,5(10)-trien-17-one,3-(sulfooxy)-, compound with piperazine (1:1).

Each gram of OGEN Vaginal Cream contains 1.5 mg estropipate in a base composed of the following ingredients: glycerin, mineral oil, glyceryl monostearate, polyethylene glycol ether complex of higher fatty alcohols, cetyl alcohol, anhydrous lanolin, sodium biphosphate, cis-N-(3-chloroallyl) hexaminium chloride, propylparaben, methylparaben, piperazine hexahydrate, citric acid and water.

Clinical Pharmacology: Estrogens are important in the development and maintenance of the female reproductive system and secondary sex characteristics. They promote growth and development of the vagina, uterus, and fallopian tubes, and enlargement of the breasts. Indirectly, they contribute to the shaping of the skeleton, maintenance of tone and elasticity of urogenital structures, changes in the epiphyses of the long bones that allow for the pubertal growth spurt and its termination, growth of axillary and pubic hair, and pigmentation of the nipples and genitals. Along with other hormones such as progesterone, estrogens are intricately involved in the process of menstruation. Estrogens also affect the release of pituitary gonadotropins.

OGEN (estropipate) Vaginal Cream owes its therapeutic action to estrone, one of the three principal estrogenic steroidal hormones of man: estradiol, estrone, and estriol. Estradiol is rapidly hydrolyzed in the body to estrone, which in turn may be hydrated to the less active estriol. These transformations occur readily, mainly in the liver, where there is also free interconversion between estrone and estradiol.

A depletion of endogenous estrogens occurs postmenopausally as a result of a decline in ovarian function, and may cause symptomatic vulvovaginal epithelial atrophy. The signs and symptoms of these atrophic changes in the vaginal and vulval epithelia may be alleviated by the topical application of an estrogenic hormone such as OGEN.

OGEN Vaginal Cream may be absorbed transmucosally and may produce systemic estrogenic effects. Inactivation of estrogens in the body occurs mainly in the liver. During cyclic passage through the liver, estrogens are degraded to less active estrogenic compounds and conjugated with sulfuric and glucuronic acids. Estrone is 50–80% bound to proteins as it circulates in the blood, principally as a conjugate with sulfate.

Indications and Usage: The cyclic administration of OGEN Vaginal Cream is indicated for the treatment of atrophic vaginitis or kraurosis vulvae. (See "DOSAGE AND ADMINISTRATION" section.)

OGEN VAGINAL CREAM HAS NOT BEEN TESTED FOR EFFICACY FOR ANY PURPOSE DURING PREGNANCY. SINCE ITS EFFECT UPON THE FETUS IS UNKNOWN, IT CANNOT BE RECOMMENDED FOR ANY CONDITION DURING PREGNANCY (SEE BOXED WARNING).

Contraindications: OGEN Vaginal Cream should not be used in women with any of the following conditions:
1. Known or suspected cancer of the breast.
2. Known or suspected estrogen-dependent neoplasia.
3. OGEN may cause fetal harm when administered to a pregnant women. OGEN is contraindicated in women who are or may become pregnant (See Boxed Warning).
4. Undiagnosed abnormal genital bleeding.
5. Active thrombophlebitis, thrombosis, or thromboembolic disorders.
6. A past history of thrombophlebitis, thrombosis, or thromboembolic disorders associated with previous estrogen use.

OGEN Vaginal Cream (estropipate) is contraindicated in patients hypersensitive to its ingredients.

Warnings: 1. *Induction of malignant neoplasms.* Long-term continuous administration of natural and synthetic estrogens in certain animal species has been reported by some investigators to increase the frequency of carcinomas of the breast, cervix, vagina, and liver. There is now evidence that estrogens increase the risk of carcinoma of the endometrium in humans. (See Boxed Warning).

At the present time there is no conclusive evidence that estrogens given to postmenopausal women increase the risk of cancer of the breast,[17,40,41] There are, however, a few retrospective studies which suggest a small but statistically significant increase in the risk factor for breast cancer among these women.[18,42-44] Therefore, caution should be exercised when administering estrogens to women with a strong family history of breast cancer or who have breast nodules, fibrocystic disease, or abnormal mammograms. Careful breast examinations should be performed periodically.

2. *Gall bladder disease.* A recent study has reported a 2 to 3-fold increase in the risk of surgically confirmed gall bladder disease in women receiving postmenopausal estrogens,[17] similar to the 2-fold increase previously noted in users of oral contraceptives.[19,22] In the case of oral contraceptives, the increased risk appeared after two years of use.[22]

3. *Effects similar to those caused by estrogen-progestogen oral contraceptives.* There are several serious adverse effects of oral contraceptives, most of which have not, up to now, been documented as consequences of postmenopausal estrogen therapy. This may reflect the comparatively low doses of estrogen used in postmenopausal women. It would be expected that the larger doses of estrogen used to treat postpartum breast engorgement would be more likely to result in these adverse effects, and, in fact, it has been shown that there is an increased risk of thrombosis in women receiving estrogens for postpartum breast engorgement.[20,21]

a. *Thromboembolic disease.* It is now well established that users of oral contraceptives have an increased risk of various thromboembolic and thrombotic vascular diseases, such as thrombophlebitis, pulmonary embolism, stroke, and myocardial infarction.[22-29] Cases of retinal thrombosis, mesenteric thrombosis, and optic neuritis have been reported in oral contraceptive users. There is evidence that the risk of several of these adverse reactions is related to the dose of the drug.[30,31] An increased risk of post-surgery thromboembolic complications has also been reported in users of oral contraceptives.[32,33] If feasible, estrogen should be discontinued at least 4 weeks before surgery of the type associated with an increased risk of thromboembolism; it should also be discontinued during periods of prolonged immobilization. While an increased rate of thromboembolic and thrombotic disease in postmenopausal users of estrogens has not been found[17,34] this does not rule out the possibility that such an increase may be present or that subgroups of women who have underlying risk factors or who are receiving relatively large doses of estrogens may have increased risk. Therefore estrogens should not be used in persons with active thrombophlebitis or thromboembolic disorders, and they should not be used in persons with a history of such disorders in association with estrogen use. They should be used with caution in patients with cerebral vascular or coronary artery disease and only for those in whom estrogens are clearly needed.

Large doses of estrogen (5 mg conjugated estrogens per day), comparable to those used to treat cancer of the prostate and breast, have been shown in a large prospective clinical trial in men[35] to increase the risk of nonfatal myocardial infarction, pulmonary embolism and thrombophlebitis. When estrogen doses of this size are used, any of the thromboembolic and thrombotic adverse effects associated with oral contraceptive use should be considered a clear risk.

b. *Hepatic adenoma.* Benign hepatic adenomas appear to be associated with the use of oral contraceptives.[36-38] Although benign, and rare, these may rupture and cause death through intraabdominal hemorrhage. Such lesions have not yet been reported in association with other estrogen or progestogen preparations but should be considered in estrogen users having abdominal pain and tenderness, abdominal mass, or hypovolemic shock. Hepatocellular carcinoma has also been reported in women taking estrogen-containing oral contraceptives.[37] The relationship of this malignancy to these drugs is not known at this time.

c. *Elevated blood pressure.* Increased blood pressure is not uncommon in women using oral contraceptives. There is now a report that this may occur with use of estrogens in the menopause[39] and blood pressure should be monitored with estrogen use, especially if high doses are used.

d. *Glucose tolerance.* A worsening of glucose tolerance has been observed in a significant percentage of patients on estrogen-containing oral contraceptives. For this reason, diabetic patients should be carefully observed while receiving estrogen.

4. *Hypercalcemia.* Administration of estrogens may lead to severe hypercalcemia in patients with breast cancer and bone metastases. If this occurs, the drug should be stopped and appropriate measures taken to reduce the serum calcium level.

Precautions: A. General.
1. A complete medical and family history should be taken prior to the initiation of any estrogen therapy. The pretreatment and periodic physical examinations should include special reference to blood pressure, breasts, abdomen, and pelvic organs, and should include a Papanicolau smear. As a general rule, estrogen should not be prescribed for longer than one year without another physical examination being performed.
2. Diagnostic measures should be taken to rule out gonorrhea or neoplasia before prescribing OGEN Vaginal Cream. Trichomonal, monilial, or bacterial infection should be treated by appropriate anti-microbial therapy.

3. Fluid retention—Estrogens may cause some degree of fluid retention. Therefore, patients with conditions such as epilepsy, migraine, and cardiac or renal dysfunction, which might be influenced by this factor, require careful observation.
4. Certain patients may develop undesirable manifestations of excessive estrogenic stimulation, such as abnormal or excessive uterine bleeding, mastodynia, etc.
5. Oral contraceptives appear to be associated with an increased incidence of mental depression.[22] Although it is not clear whether this is due to the estrogenic or progestogenic component of the contraceptive, patients with a history of depression should be carefully observed.
6. Preexisting uterine leiomyomata may increase in size during estrogen use.
7. The pathologist should be advised of the patient's use of estrogen therapy when relevant specimens are submitted.
8. Patients with a past history of jaundice during pregnancy have an increased risk of recurrence of jaundice while receiving estrogen-containing oral contraceptive therapy. If jaundice develops in any patient receiving estrogen, the medication should be discontinued while the cause is investigated.
9. Estrogens may be poorly metabolized in patients with impaired liver function and they should be administered with caution in such patients.
10. Because estrogens influence the metabolism of calcium and phosphorus, they should be used with caution in patients with metabolic bone diseases that are associated with hypercalcemia or in patients with renal insufficiency.

B. Information for the Patient. See text of Patient Package Insert which appears after PHYSICIAN REFERENCES.

C. Drug Interactions. The concomitant use of any drugs which can induce hepatic microsomal enzymes with estrogens may produce estrogen levels which are lower than would be expected from the dose of estrogen administered.

Diabetics receiving *insulin* may have increased insulin requirements when receiving estrogens.
Laboratory Test Interference. Certain endocrine and liver function tests may be affected by estrogen-containing oral contraceptives. The following similar changes may be expected with larger doses of estrogen:
a. Increased sulfobromophthalein retention.
b. Increased prothrombin and factors VII, VIII, IX, and X; decreased antithrombin 3; increased norepinephrine-induced platelet aggregability.
c. Increased thyroid binding globulin (TBG) leading to increased circulating total thyroid hormone, as measured by PBI, T4 by column, or T4 by radioimmunoassay. Free T3 resin uptake is decreased, reflecting the elevated TBG; free T4 concentration is unaltered.
d. Abnormal glucose tolerance test results.
e. Decreased pregnanediol excretion.
f. Reduced response to metyrapone test.
g. Reduced serum folate concentration.
h. Increased serum triglyceride and phospholipid concentration.

D. Carcinogenesis. Studies have shown an increased risk of endometrial cancer in postmenopausal women exposed to exogenous estrogens for prolonged periods (see Boxed Warning). At the present time there is no conclusive evidence that estrogens given to postmenopausal women increase the risk of cancer of the breast.[17,40,41] There are, however, a few retrospective studies which suggest a small but statistically significant increase in the risk factor for breast cancer among these women.[18,42-44] (See "WARNINGS" section.)

E. Pregnancy. Pregnancy Category X. See "CONTRAINDICATIONS" section and Boxed Warning.

F. Nursing Mothers. Estrogens have been reported to be excreted in human breast milk. Caution should be exercised when OGEN is administered to a nursing woman.

G. Pediatric Use. Because of the effects of estrogens on epiphyseal closure, they should be used judiciously in young patients to whom bone growth is not complete.

Adverse Reactions: Hypersensitivity reactions, systemic effects such as breast tenderness, and rarely, withdrawal bleeding, have occurred with the use of topical estrogens. Local irritation (especially when prior inflammation is present) has occurred at initiation of therapy.

The following additional adverse reactions in decreasing order of severity within each category have been reported with estrogenic therapy, including oral contraceptives (See WARNINGS regarding reports of possible induction of neoplasia, unknown effects upon the fetus, increased incidence of gall bladder disease, and adverse effects similar to those of oral contraceptives, including thromboembolism.):

1. *Genitourinary system.*
Increase in size of uterine fibromyomata.
Vaginal candidiasis.
Cystitis-like syndrome.
Dysmenorrhea.
Amenorrhea during and after treatment.
Change in cervical eversion and in degree of cervical secretion.
Breakthrough bleeding, spotting, change in menstrual flow.
Premenstrual-like syndrome.
2. *Breast.*
Tenderness, enlargement, secretion.
3. *Gastrointestinal.*
Cholestatic jaundice.
Vomiting, nausea.
Abdominal cramps, bloating.
4. *Skin.*
Hemorrhagic eruption.
Erythema nodosum.
Erythema multiforme.
Hirsutism.
Chloasma or melasma which may persist when drug is discontinued.
Loss of scalp hair.
5. *Eyes.*
Steepening of corneal curvature.
Intolerance to contact lenses.
6. *CNS.*
Chorea.
Mental depression.
Migraine, dizziness, headache.
7. *Miscellaneous.*
Aggravation of porphyria.
Edema.
Reduced carbohydrate tolerance.
Increase or decrease in weight.
Changes in libido.

Dosage and Administration: *To be administered cyclically for short-term use only:*
For treatment of atrophic vaginitis or kraurosis vulvae.
The lowest dose that will control symptoms should be chosen and medication should be discontinued as promptly as possible.
Administration should be cyclic (e.g., three weeks on and one week off).
Attempts to discontinue or taper medication should be made at three to six-month intervals.
Treated patients with an intact uterus should be monitored closely for signs of endometrial cancer and appropriate diagnostic measures should be taken to rule out malignancy in the event of persistent or recurring abnormal vaginal bleeding.
Usual dosage: Intravaginally, 2 to 4 grams of OGEN Vaginal Cream daily, depending upon the severity of the condition.
The following instructions for use are intended for the patient and are printed on the carton label for OGEN Vaginal Cream (estropipate):
1. Remove cap from tube.
2. Make sure plunger of applicator is all the way into the barrel.
3. Screw nozzle end of applicator onto the tube.
4. Squeeze tube to force sufficient cream into applicator so that number on plunger indicating prescribed dose is level with top of barrel.
5. Unscrew applicator from tube and replace cap on tube.
6. To deliver medication, insert end of applicator into vagina and push plunger all the way down.
Between uses, pull plunger out of barrel and wash applicator in warm, soapy water. DO NOT PUT APPLICATOR IN HOT OR BOILING WATER.

How Supplied: OGEN (estropipate vaginal cream, USP), 1.5 mg estropipate per gram, is available in packages containing a 1½ oz (42.5 Gm) tube with one plastic applicator calibrated at 2, 3 and 4 Gm levels. (NDC 0074-2467-42).

Physician References: [1]Ziel, H. K., Finkle, W. D., "Increased Risk of Endometrial Carcinoma Among Users of Conjugated Estrogens," *New England Journal of Medicine*, 293:1167–1170, 1975.
[2]Smith, D. C., Prentic, R., Thompson, D. J., et al., "Association of Exogenous Estrogen and Endometrial Carcinoma," *New England Journal of Medicine*, 293:1164–1167, 1975.
[3]Mack, T. M., Pike, M. C., Henderson, B. E., et al., "Estrogens and Endometrial Cancer in a Retirement Community," *New England Journal of Medicine*, 294:1262–1267, 1976.
[4]Weiss, N. S., Szekely, D. R., Austin, D. F., "Increasing Incidence of Endometrial Cancer in the United States," *New England Journal of Medicine*, 294:1259–1262, 1976.
[5]Herbst, A., Ulfelder, H., Poskanzer, D. C., "Adenocarcinoma of Vagina," *New England Journal of Medicine*, 284: 878–881, 1971.
[6]Greenwald, P., Barlow, J., Nasca, P., et al., "Vaginal Cancer after Maternal Treatment with Synthetic Estrogens," *New England Journal of Medicine*, 285:390–392, 1971.
[7]Lanier, A., Noller, K., Decker, D., et al., "Cancer and Stilbestrol. A Follow-up of 1719 Persons Exposed to Estrogens In Utero and Born 1943-1959," *Mayo Clinic Proceedings*, 48:793–799, 1973.
[8]Herbst, A., Kurman, R., Scully, R., "Vaginal and Cervical Abnormalities After Exposure to Stilbestrol in Utero," *Obstetrics and Gynecology*, 40:287–298, 1972.
[9]Herbst, A., Robboy, S., Macdonald, G., et al., "The Effects of Local Progesterone on Stilbestrol-Associated Vaginal Adenosis," *Journal of Obstetrics and Gynecology*, 118:607–615, 1974.
[10]Herbst, A., Poskanzer, D., Robboy, S., et al., "Prenatal Exposure to Stilbestrol, A Prospective Comparison of Exposed Female Offspring with Unexposed Controls," *New England Journal of Medicine*, 292:334–339, 1975.
[11]Stafl, A., Mattingly, R., Foley, D., et al., "Clinical Diagnosis of Vaginal Adenosis," *Obstetrics and Gynecology*, 43:118–128, 1974.
[12]Sherman, A. I., Goldrath, M., Berlin, A., et al., "Cervical-Vaginal Adenosis After *In Utero* Exposure to Synthetic Estrogens," *Obstetrics and Gynecology*, 44:531–545, 1974.
[13]Gal, I., Kirman, B., Stern, J., "Hormone Pregnancy Tests and Congenital Malformation," *Nature*, 216:83, 1967.
[14]Levy, E. P., Cohen, A., Fraser, F. C., "Hormone Treatment During Pregnancy and Congenital Heart Defects," *Lancet*, 1:611, 1973.
[15]Nora, J., Nora, A., "Birth Defects and Oral Contraceptives," *Lancet*, 1:941–942, 1973.
[16]Janerich, D. T., Piper, J. M., Glebatis, D. M., "Oral Contraceptives and Congenital Limb-Reduction Defects," *New England Journal of Medicine*, 291:697–700, 1974.
[17]Boston Collaborative Drug Surveillance Program "Surgically Confirmed Gall Bladder Disease, Venous Thromboembolism and Breast Tumors in Relation to Postmenopausal Estrogen Therapy," *New England Journal of Medicine*, 290:15–19, 1974.
[18]Brinton, L. A., Hoover, R. N., Szklo, M., et al., "Menopausal Estrogen Use and Risk of Breast Cancer," *Cancer*, 47(10):2517–2522, 1981.
[19]Boston Collaborative Drug Surveillance Program, "Oral Contraceptives and Venous Thromboembolic Disease, Surgically Confirmed Gall Blad-

Continued on next page

If desired, additional literature on any Abbott Product will be provided upon request to Abbott Laboratories.

Abbott—Cont.

der Disease and Breast Tumors," *Lancet* 1:1399–1404, 1973.
[20]Daniel, D. G., Campbell, H., Turnbull, A. C., "Puerperal Thromboembolism and Suppression of Lactation," *Lancet*, 2:287–289, 1967.
[21]Bailar, J. C., "Thromboembolism and Oestrogen Therapy," *Lancet*, 2:560, 1967.
[22]Royal College of General Practitioners, "Oral Contraception and Thromboembolic Disease," *Journal of the Royal College of General Practitioners*, 13:267–279, 1967.
[23]Inman, W. H. W., Vessey, M. P., "Investigation of Deaths from Pulmonary, Coronary, and Cerebral Thrombosis and Embolism in Women of Child-Bearing Age," *British Medical Journal*, 2:193–199, 1968.
[24]Vessey, M. P., Doll, R., "Investigation of Relation Between Use of Oral Contraceptives and Thromboembolic Disease. A Further Report," *British Medical Journal*, 2:651–657, 1969.
[25]Sartwell, P. E., Masi, A. T., Arthes, F. G., et al., "Thromboembolism and Oral Contraceptives: An Epidemiological Case Control Study," *American Journal of Epidemiology*, 90:365–380, 1969.
[26]Collaborative Group for the Study of Stroke in Young Women, "Oral Contraception and Increased Risk of Cerebral Ischemia or Thrombosis," *New England Journal of Medicine*, 288:871–878, 1973.
[27]Collaborative Group for the Study of Stroke in Young Women, "Oral Contraceptives and Stroke in Young Women: Associated Risk Factors," *Journal of the American Medical Association*, 231:718–722, 1975.
[28]Mann, J. I., Inman, W. H. W., "Oral Contraceptives and Death from Myocardial Infarction," *British Medical Journal*, 2:245–248, 1975.
[29]Mann, J. I., Vessey, M. P., Thorogood, M., et al. "Myocardial Infarction in Young Women with Special Reference to Oral Contraceptive Practice," *British Medical Journal*, 2:241–245, 1975.
[30]Inman, W. H. W., Vessey, M. P., Westerholm, B., et al., "Thromboembolic Disease and the Steroidal Content of Oral Contraceptives," *British Medical Journal*, 20:203–209, 1970.
[31]Stolley, P. D., Tonascia, J. A., Tockman, M. S., et al., "Thrombosis with Low-Estrogen Oral Contraceptives," *American Journal of Epidemiology*, 102:197–208, 1975.
[32]Vessey, M. P., Doll. R., Fairbairn, A. S., et al., "Post-Operative Thromboembolism and the Use of the Oral Contraceptives," *British Medical Journal*, 3:123–126, 1970.
[33]Greene, G. R., Sartwell, P. E., "Oral Contraceptive Use in Patients with Thromboembolism Following Surgery, Trauma or Infection," *American Journal of Public Health*, 62:680–685, 1972.
[34]Rosenberg, L., Armstrong, M. B., Jick, H., "Myocardial Infarction and Estrogen Therapy in Postmenopausal Women," *New England Journal of Medicine*, 294:1256–1259, 1976.
[35]Coronary Drug Project Research Group, "The Coronary Drug Project: Initial Findings Leading to Modifications of Its Research Protocol," *Journal of the American Medical Association*, 214:1303–1313, 1970.
[36]Baum, J., Holtz, F., Bookstein, J. J., et al., "Possible Association Between Benign Hepatomas and Oral Contraceptives," *Lancet*, 2:926–928, 1973.
[37]Mays, E. T., Christophersen, W. M., Mahr, M. M., et al., "Hepatic Changes in Young Women Ingesting Contraceptive Steroids, Hepatic Hemorrhage and Primary Hepatic Tumors," *Journal of the American Medical Association*, 235:730–782, 1976.
[38]Edmondson, H. A., Henderson, B., Benton B., "Liver Cell Adenomas Associated with the Use of Oral Contraceptives," *New England Journal of Medicine*, 294:470–472, 1976.
[39]Pfeffer, R. I., Van Den Noort, S., "Estrogen Use and Stroke Risk in Postmenopausal Women," *American Journal of Epidemiology*, 103:445–456, 1976.
[40]Gambrell, R. D., Massey, F. M., Castaneda, T. A., et al., "Estrogen Therapy and Breast Cancer in Postmenopausal Women," *Journal of the American Geriatrics Society*, 28(6):251–257, 1980.
[41]Kelsey, J. L. Fischer, D. B., Holford, T. R., et al., "Exogenous Estrogens and Other Factors in the Epidemiology of Breast Cancer," *Journal of the National Cancer Institute*, 57(2):237–333, 1981.
[42]Ross, R. K., Paganini-Hill, A., Gerkins, V., et al., "A Case-Control Study of Menopausal Estrogen Therapy and Breast Cancer," *Journal of the American Medical Association*, 243(16):1635–1639, 1980.
[43]Hoover, R., Glass, A., Finkle, W. D., et al., "Conjugated Estrogens and Breast Cancer Risk in Women," *Journal of the National Cancer Institute*, 67(4):815–820, 1981.
[44]Lawson, D. H., Jick, H., Hunter, J. R., et al., "Exogenous Estrogens and Breast Cancer," *American Journal of Epidemiology*, 114(5):710, 1981.

INFORMATION FOR PATIENTS
OGEN® VAGINAL CREAM
(estropipate vaginal cream, USP)

You have been given an estrogen cream that is used for the local treatment of certain symptoms of estrogen deficiency: the soreness and itching of the vagina and vulva caused by drying and thinning (atrophy) of these tissues.
The discussion in the Ogen (estropipate tablets) patient labeling is about estrogens that are taken internally for the treatment of symptoms of estrogen deficiency. Some or all of the information on the systemic use of estrogens may also apply to the estrogen cream prescribed for you.
Abbott Laboratories
North Chicago IL 60064, U.S.A.
Ref. 01-2305-R3

OPTILETS®-500
[ŏp′ ti-lets]
High potency multivitamin for use in treatment of multivitamin deficiency.
OPTILETS-M-500®
High potency multivitamin for use in treatment of multivitamin deficiency. Mineral supplementation added.

(See PDR For Nonprescription Drugs)
Shown in Product Identification Section, page 403

ORETIC® ℞
[ō-re′ tic]
(hydrochlorothiazide tablets, USP)

Description: ORETIC (hydrochlorothiazide) is a member of the benzothiadiazine (thiazide) family of drugs. It is closely related to chlorothiazide. Clinically, ORETIC is an orally active diuretic-antihypertensive agent.
Actions: The diuretic and saluretic effects of ORETIC result from a drug-induced inhibition of the renal tubular reabsorption of electrolytes. The excretion of sodium and chloride is greatly enhanced. Potassium excretion is also enhanced to a variable degree, as it is with the other thiazides. Although urinary excretion of bicarbonate is increased slightly, there is usually no significant change in urinary pH. Hydrochlorothiazide has a per mg natriuretic activity approximately 10 times that of the prototype thiazide, chlorothiazide. At maximal therapeutic dosages, all thiazides are approximately equal in their diuretic/natriuretic effects.
There is significant natriuresis and diuresis within two hours after administration of a single oral dose of hydrochlorothiazide. These effects reach a peak in about six hours and persist for about 12 hours following oral administration of a single dose.
Like other benzothiadiazines, ORETIC also has antihypertensive properties, and may be used for this purpose either alone or to enhance the antihypertensive action of other drugs. The mechanism by which the benzothiadiazines, including hydrochlorothiazide, produce a reduction of elevated blood pressure is not known. However, sodium depletion appears to be involved.
ORETIC (hydrochlorothiazide) is readily absorbed from the gastrointestinal tract and is excreted unchanged by the kidneys.
Indications: ORETIC is indicated in the management of hypertension either as the sole therapeutic agent or to enhance the effect of other antihypertensive drugs in the more severe forms of hypertension.
ORETIC is indicated as adjunctive therapy in edema associated with congestive heart failure, hepatic cirrhosis, and corticosteroid and estrogen therapy.
ORETIC has also been found useful in edema due to various forms of renal dysfunction such as the nephrotic syndrome, acute glomerulonephritis and chronic renal failure.
Usage in Pregnancy: The routine use of diuretics in an otherwise healthy pregnant woman is inappropriate and exposes mother and fetus to unnecessary hazard. Diuretics do not prevent development of toxemia of pregnancy, and there is no satisfactory evidence that they are useful in the treatment of developed toxemia.
Edema during pregnancy may arise from pathological causes or from the physiological and mechanical consequences of pregnancy. Thiazides are indicated in pregnancy when edema is due to pathological causes, just as they are in the absence of pregnancy (however, see Warnings, below). Dependent edema in pregnancy, resulting from restriction of venous return by the expanded uterus, is properly treated through elevation of the lower extremities and use of support hose; use of diuretics to lower intravascular volume in this case is illogical and unnecessary. There is hypervolemia during normal pregnancy which is harmful to neither the fetus nor the mother (in the absence of cardiovascular disease), but which is associated with edema, including generalized edema, in the majority of pregnant women. If this edema produces discomfort, increased recumbency will often provide relief. In rare instances, this edema may cause extreme discomfort which is not relieved by rest. In these cases, a short course of diuretics may provide relief and may be appropriate.
Contraindications: Renal decompensation. Hypersensitivity to this or other sulfonamide-derived drugs.
Warnings: Hydrochlorothiazide shares with other thiazides the propensity to deplete potassium reserves to an unpredictable degree.
Thiazides should be used with caution in patients with renal disease or significant impairment of renal function, since azotemia may be precipitated and cumulative drug effects may occur.
Thiazides should be used with caution in patients with impaired hepatic function or progressive liver disease, since minor alterations of fluid and electrolyte balance may precipitate hepatic coma.
Thiazides may be additive to potentiative of the action of other antihypertensive drugs. Potentiation occurs with ganglionic or peripheral adrenergic blocking drugs.
Sensitivity reactions may occur in patients with a history of allergy or bronchial asthma.
The possibility of exacerbation or activation of systemic lupus erythematosus has been reported.
Usage in Pregnancy: Thiazides cross the placental barrier and appear in cord blood. The use of thiazides in pregnant women requires that the anticipated benefit be weighed against possible hazards to the fetus. These hazards include fetal or neonatal jaundice, thrombocytopenia, and possible other adverse reactions that have occurred in the adult.
Nursing Mothers: Thiazides appear in breast milk. If use of the drug is deemed essential, the patient should stop nursing.
Precautions: Periodic determinations of serum electrolytes should be performed at appropriate intervals for the purpose of detecting possible electrolyte imbalances such as hyponatremia, hypochloremic alkalosis, and hypokalemia. Serum and urine electrolyte determinations are particularly important when a patient is vomiting excessively or receiving parenteral fluids. All patients should be observed for other clinical signs of electrolyte imbalances such as dryness of mouth, thirst, weakness, lethargy, drowsiness, restlessness, muscle

pains or cramps, muscular fatigue, hypotension, oliguria, tachycardia, and gastrointestinal disturbances such as nausea and vomiting.

Hypokalemia may develop with thiazides as with any other potent diuretic, especially when brisk diuresis occurs, severe cirrhosis is present, or when corticosteroids or ACTH are given concomitantly. Interference with the adequate oral intake of electrolytes will also contribute to the possible development of hypokalemia. Potassium depletion, even of a mild degree, resulting from thiazide use, may sensitize a patient to the effects of cardiac glycosides such as digitalis.

Any chloride deficit is generally mild and usually does not require specific treatment except under extraordinary circumstances (as in liver disease or renal disease). Dilutional hyponatremia may occur in edematous patients in hot weather; appropriate therapy is water restriction rather than administration of salt, except in rare instances when the hyponatremia is life threatening.

In actual salt depletion, appropriate replacement is the therapy of choice.

Hyperuricemia may occur or frank gout may be precipitated in certain patients receiving thiazide therapy.

Insulin requirements in diabetic patients may be increased, decreased, or unchanged. Latent diabetes mellitus may become manifest during thiazide administration.

Thiazide drugs may increase the responsiveness to tubocurarine.

The antihypertensive effects of the drug may be enhanced in the postsympathectomy patient.

Thiazides may decrease arterial responsiveness to norepinephrine. This diminution is not sufficient to preclude effectiveness of the pressor agent for therapeutic use.

If progressive renal impairment becomes evident as indicated by a rising-nonprotein nitrogen or blood urea nitrogen, a careful reappraisal of therapy is necessary with consideration given to withholding or discontinuing diuretic therapy.

Thiazides may decrease serum PBI levels without signs of thyroid disturbance.

Thiazides have been reported, on rare occasions, to have elevated serum calcium to hypercalcemic levels. The serum calcium levels have returned to normal when the medication has been stopped. This phenomenon may be related to the ability of the thiazide diuretics to lower the amount of calcium excreted in the urine.

Adverse Reactions: Gastrointestinal system reactions: Anorexia, gastric irritation, nausea, vomiting, cramping, diarrhea, constipation, jaundice (intrahepatic cholestatic jaundice), pancreatitis.

Central nervous system reactions: Dizziness, vertigo, paresthesias, headache, xanthopsia.

Hematologic reactions: Leukopenia, agranulocytosis, thrombocytopenia, aplastic anemia.

Dermatologic — hypersensitivity reactions: Purpura, photosensitivity, rash, urticaria, necrotizing angiitis (vasculitis) (cutaneous vasculitis).

Cardiovascular reaction: Orthostatic hypotension may occur and may be aggravated by alcohol, barbiturates, or narcotics.

Other: Hyperglycemia, glycosuria, hypercalcemia, hyperuricemia, muscle spasm, weakness, restlessness.

There have been isolated reports that certain nonedematous individuals developed severe fluid and electrolyte derangements after only brief exposure to normal doses of thiazide and non-thiazide diuretics. The condition is usually manifested as severe dilutional hyponatremia, hypokalemia, and hypochloremia. It has been reported to be due to inappropriately increased ADH secretion and appears to be idiosyncratic. Potassium replacement is apparently the most important therapy in the treatment of this syndrome along with removal of the offending drug.

Whenever adverse reactions are severe, treatment should be discontinued.

Dosage and Administration: ORETIC (hydrochlorothiazide) is administered orally. Therapy should be individualized according to patient response. This therapy should be titrated to gain maximal therapeutic response as well as the minimal dose possible to maintain that therapeutic response.

For the management of edema the adult dosage ranges from 25 to 200 mg daily and may be given in single or divided doses. Usually 75 to 100 mg will produce the desired diuretic effect.

For the management of hypertension the usual initial adult dosage is 25 to 50 mg two times daily. The dosage may be increased if necessary to a maximum of 100 mg twice daily.

When therapy is prolonged or large doses are used, particular attention should be given to the patient's electrolyte status. Supplemental potassium may be required.

In the treatment of hypertension hydrochlorothiazide may be either employed alone or concurrently with other antihypertensive drugs. Combined therapy may provide adequate control of hypertension with lower dosage of the component drugs and fewer or less severe side effects. An enhanced response frequently follows its concurrent administration with Harmonyl® (deserpidine) so that dosage of both drugs may be reduced.

For treatment of moderately severe or severe hypertension, supplemental use of other more potent antihypertensive agents such as Eutonyl® (pargyline hydrochloride) may be indicated.

When other antihypertensive agents are to be added to the regimen, this should be accomplished gradually. Additional potent antihypertensive agents should be given at only half the usual dose since their effect is potentiated by pretreatment with ORETIC.

Overdosage: Symptoms of overdosage include electrolyte imbalance and signs of potassium deficiency such as confusion, dizziness, muscular weakness, and gastrointestinal disturbances. General supportive measures including replacement of fluids and electrolytes may be indicated in treatment of overdosage.

How Supplied: ORETIC (hydrochlorothiazide tablets, USP) is provided in two dosage sizes as white tablets:
25 mg tablets:
bottles of 100 (**NDC** 0074-6978-01),
bottles of 1000 (**NDC** 0074-6978-02),
Abbo-Pac® unit dose packages, 100 tablets (**NDC** 0074-6978-05).
50 mg tablets:
bottles of 100 (**NDC** 0074-6985-01),
bottles of 1000 (**NDC** 0074-6985-02),
Abbo-Pac unit dose packages, 100 tablets (**NDC** 0074-6985-06).

Shown in Product Identification Section, page 403
Abbott Laboratories
North Chicago, IL 60064
Ref. 01-2131-R3

ORETICYL®   ℞
[ō-re'ti-sill]
(hydrochlorothiazide and deserpidine tablets)

Oral thiazide-rauwolfia therapy for hypertension.

> **Warning:**
> This fixed combination drug is not indicated for initial therapy of hypertension. Hypertension requires therapy titrated to the individual patient. If the fixed combination represents the dosage so determined, its use may be more convenient in patient management. The treatment of hypertension is not static, but must be reevaluated as conditions in each patient warrant.

Description: ORETICYL is an orally administered combination of Oretic® (hydrochlorothiazide) and Harmonyl® (deserpidine). Hydrochlorothiazide is a diuretic-antihypertensive agent of the benzothiadiazine (thiazide) class. Deserpidine is a purified rauwolfia alkaloid, chemically identified as 11-desmethoxyreserpine, which produces antihypertensive effects.

Actions: The combined antihypertensive actions of hydrochlorothiazide and deserpidine result in a total clinical antihypertensive effect which is greater than can ordinarily be achieved by either drug given individually.

The diuretic and saluretic effects of hydrochlorothiazide result from a drug-induced inhibition of the renal tubular reabsorption of electrolytes. The excretion of sodium and chloride is greatly enhanced. Potassium excretion is also enhanced to a variable degree, as it is with the other thiazides. Although urinary excretion of bicarbonate is increased slightly, there is usually no significant change in urinary pH. Hydrochlorothiazide has a per mg natriuretic activity approximately 10 times that of the prototype thiazide, chlorothiazide. At maximal therapeutic dosages, all thiazides are approximately equal in their diuretic/natriuretic effects.

There is significant natriuresis and diuresis within two hours after administration of a single oral dose of hydrochlorothiazide. These effects reach a peak in about six hours and persist for about 12 hours following oral administration of a single dose.

Like other benzothiadiazines, hydrochlorothiazide also has antihypertensive properties, and may be used for this purpose either alone or to enhance the antihypertensive action of other drugs. The mechanism by which the benzothiadiazines, including hydrochlorothiazide, produce a reduction of elevated blood pressure is not known. However, sodium depletion appears to be involved.

Hydrochlorothiazide is readily absorbed from the gastrointestinal tract and is excreted unchanged by the kidneys.

The pharmacologic actions of Harmonyl (deserpidine) are essentially the same as those of other active rauwolfia alkaloids. Deserpidine probably produces its antihypertensive effects through depletion of tissue stores of catecholamines (epinephrine and norepinephrine) from peripheral sites. The antihypertensive effect is often accompanied by bradycardia. There is no significant alteration in cardiac output or renal blood flow. The carotid sinus reflex is inhibited, but postural hypotension is rarely seen with the use of conventional doses of Harmonyl alone.

Deserpidine, like other rauwolfia alkaloids, is characterized by slow onset of action and sustained effect which may persist following withdrawal of the drug.

Indications: ORETICYL (hydrochlorothiazide and deserpidine) is indicated in the treatment of patients with mild to moderately severe hypertension (see boxed warning). It may be used alone for this purpose or added to other antihypertensive agents for the management of more severe hypertension. When administered with ORETICYL, more potent agents can be given at reduced dosage to minimize undesirable side effects.

Contraindications: Hydrochlorothiazide is contraindicated in patients with renal decompensation and in those who are hypersensitive to this or other sulfonamide-derived drugs.

Deserpidine is contraindicated in patients with known hypersensitivity, mental depression especially with suicidal tendencies, active peptic ulcer, and ulcerative colitis. It is also contraindicated in patients receiving electroconvulsive therapy.

Warnings:
Hydrochlorothiazide
Hydrochlorothiazide shares with other thiazides the propensity to deplete potassium reserves to an unpredictable degree.

Thiazides should be used with caution in patients with renal disease or significant impairment of renal function, since azotemia may be precipitated and cumulative drug effects may occur.

Thiazides should be used with caution in patients with impaired hepatic function or progressive

Continued on next page

If desired, additional literature on any Abbott Product will be provided upon request to Abbott Laboratories.

Abbott—Cont.

liver disease, since minor alterations of fluid and electrolyte balance may precipitate hepatic coma. Thiazides may be additive or potentiative of the action of other antihypertensive drugs. Potentiation occurs with ganglionic or peripheral adrenergic blocking drugs.

Sensitivity reactions may occur in patients with a history of allergy or bronchial asthma.

The possibility of exacerbation or activation of systemic lupus erythematosus has been reported.

Deserpidine

Extreme caution should be exercised in treating patients with a history of mental depression. Discontinue the drug at the first sign, of despondency, early morning insomnia, loss of appetite, impotence, or self-deprecation. Drug-induced depression may persist for several months after drug withdrawal and may be severe enough to result in suicide.

Usage in Pregnancy and Lactation:

Hydrochlorothiazide

Thiazides cross the placental barrier and appear in cord blood. The use of thiazides in pregnant women requires that the anticipated benefit be weighed against possible hazards to the fetus. These hazards include fetal or neonatal jaundice, thrombocytopenia, and possible other adverse reactions that have occurred in the adult.

Thiazides appear in breast milk. If use of the drug is deemed essential, the patient should stop nursing.

Deserpidine

The safety of deserpidine for use during pregnancy or lactation has not been established; therefore, it should be used in pregnant women or in women of childbearing potential only when in the judgment of the physician its use is deemed essential to the welfare of the patient. Increased respiratory secretions, nasal congestion, cyanosis, and anorexia may occur in infants born to rauwolfia alkaloid-treated mothers, since these preparations are known to cross the placental barrier to enter the fetal circulation and appear in cord blood. They also are secreted by nursing mothers into breast milk.

Reproductive and teratology studies in rats reduced the mating index and neonatal survival indices. The no-effect dosage has not been established.

Precautions: Periodic determinations of serum electrolytes should be performed at appropriate intervals for the purpose of detecting possible electrolyte imbalances such as hyponatremia, hypochloremic alkalosis, and hypokalemia. Serum and urine electrolyte determinations are particularly important when a patient is vomiting excessively or receiving parenteral fluids. All patients should be observed for other clinical signs of electrolyte imbalances such as dryness of mouth, thirst, weakness, lethargy, drowsiness, restlessness, muscle pains or cramps, muscular fatigue, hypotension, oliguria, tachycardia, and gastrointestinal disturbances such as nausea and vomiting.

Hypokalemia may develop with thiazides as with any other potent diuretic, especially when brisk diuresis occurs, severe cirrhosis is present, or when corticosteroids or ACTH are given concomitantly. Interference with the adequate oral intake of electrolytes will also contribute to the possible development of hypokalemia. Potassium depletion, even of a mild degree, resulting from thiazide use, may sensitize a patient to the effects of cardiac glycosides such as digitalis.

Any chloride deficit is generally mild and usually does not require specific treatment except under extraordinary circumstances (as in liver disease or renal disease). Dilutional hyponatremia may occur in edematous patients in hot weather; appropriate therapy is water restriction rather than administration of salt, except in rare instances when the hyponatremia is life threatening.

In actual salt depletion, appropriate replacement is the therapy of choice.

Hyperuricemia may occur or frank gout may be precipitated in certain patients receiving thiazide therapy.

Insulin requirements in diabetic patients may be increased, decreased, or unchanged. Latent diabetes mellitus may become manifest during thiazide administration.

Thiazide drugs may increase the responsiveness to tubocurarine.

The antihypertensive effects of the drug may be enhanced in the postsympathectomy patient.

Thiazides may decrease arterial responsiveness to norepinephrine. This diminution is not sufficient to preclude effectiveness of the pressor agent for therapeutic use.

If progressive renal impairment becomes evident as indicated by a rising-nonprotein nitrogen or blood urea nitrogen, a careful reappraisal of therapy is necessary with consideration given to withholding or discontinuing diuretic therapy.

Thiazides may decrease serum PBI levels without signs of thyroid disturbance.

Thiazides have been reported, on rare occasions, to have elevated serum calcium to hypercalcemic levels. The serum calcium levels have returned to normal when the medication has been stopped. This phenomenon may be related to the ability of the thiazide diuretics to lower the amount of calcium excreted in the urine.

Because rauwolfia preparations increase gastrointestinal motility and secretion, this drug should be used cautiously in patients with a history of peptic ulcer, ulcerative colitis, or gallstones, where biliary colic may be precipitated.

Caution should be exercised when treating hypertensive patients with renal insufficiency since they adjust poorly to lowered blood pressure levels.

Use deserpidine cautiously with digitalis and quinidine since cardiac arrhythmias have occurred with rauwolfia preparations.

Preoperative withdrawal of deserpidine does not assure that circulatory instability will not occur. It is important that the anesthesiologist be aware of the patient's drug intake and consider this in the overall management, since hypotension has occurred in patients receiving rauwolfia preparations. Anticholinergic and/ or adrenergic drugs (metaraminol, norepinephrine) have been employed to treat adverse vagocirculatory effects.

Animal tumorigenicity: There are no studies demonstrating that deserpidine is an animal tumorigen, although it is a prolactin stimulator and structurally related to reserpine. Rodent studies with reserpine, however, have shown that reserpine is an animal tumorigen, causing an increased incidence of mammary fibroadenomas in female mice, malignant tumors of the seminal vesicles in male mice, and malignant adrenal medullary tumors in male rats. These findings arose in 2 year studies in which the drug was administered in the feed at concentrations of 5 and 10 ppm—about 100 to 300 times the usual human dose. The breast neoplasms are though to be related to reserpine's prolactin-elevating effect. Several other prolactin-elevating drugs have also been associated with an increased incidence of mammary neoplasia in rodents.

The extent to which these findings indicate a risk to humans is uncertain. Tissue culture experiments show that about one-third of human breast tumors are prolactin-dependent *in vitro*, a factor of considerable importance if the use of the drug is contemplated in a patient with previously detected breast cancer. The possibility of an increased risk of breast cancer in reserpine users has been studied extensively; however, no firm conclusion has emerged. Although a few epidemiologic studies have suggested a slightly increased risk (less than twofold in all studies except one) in women who have used reserpine, other studies of generally similar design have not confirmed this. Epidemiologic studies conducted using other drugs (neuroleptic agents) that, like reserpine, increase prolactin levels and, therefore, would be considered rodent mammary carcinogens, have not shown an association between chronic administration of the drug and human mammary tumorigenesis. While long-term clinical observation has not suggested such an association, the available evidence is considered too limited to be conclusive at this time. An association of reserpine intake with pheochromocytoma or tumors of the seminal vesicles has not been explored.

Adverse Reactions:

Hydrochlorothiazide

Gastrointestinal System Reactions: Anorexia, gastric irritation, nausea, vomiting, cramping, diarrhea, constipation, jaundice (intrahepatic cholestatic jaundice), pancreatitis.

Central Nervous System Reactions: Dizziness, vertigo, paresthesias, headache, xanthopsia.

Hematologic Reactions: Leukopenia, agranulocytosis, thrombocytopenia, aplastic anemia.

Dermatologic — Hypersensitivity Reactions: Purpura, photosensitivity, rash, urticaria, necrotizing angitis (vasculitis) (cutaneous vasculitis).

Cardiovascular Reaction: Orthostatic hypotension may occur and may be aggravated by alcohol, barbiturates, or narcotics.

Other: Hyperglycemia, glycosuria, hypercalcemia, hyperuricemia, muscle spasm, weakness, restlessness.

There have been isolated reports that certain nonedematous individuals developed severe fluid and electrolyte derangements after only brief exposure to normal doses of thiazide and non-thiazide diuretics. The condition is usually manifested as severe dilutional hyponatremia, hypokalemia, and hypochloremia. It has been reported to be due to inappropriately increased ADH secretion and appears to be idiosyncratic. Potassium replacement is apparently the most important therapy in the treatment of this syndrome along with the removal of the offending drug.

Whenever adverse reactions are severe, treatment should be discontinued.

Deserpidine

The following adverse reactions have been reported with rauwolfia preparations. These reactions are usually reversible and disappear when the drug is discontinued.

Gastrointestinal: Including hypersecretion, anorexia, diarrhea, nausea, and vomiting.

Cardiovascular: Including angina-like symptoms, arrhythmias (particularly when used concurrently with digitalis or quinidine), and bradycardia.

Central Nervous System: Including drowsiness, depression, nervousness, paradoxical anxiety, nightmares, extrapyramidal tract symptoms, CNS sensitization manifested by dull sensorium, and deafness.

Dermatologic—Hypersensitivity: Including pruritus, rash, and asthma in asthmatic patients.

Ophthalmologic: Including glaucoma, uveitis, optic atrophy, and conjunctival injection.

Hematologic: Thrombocytopenic purpura.

Miscellaneous: Nasal congestion, weight gain, impotence or decreased libido, dysuria, dyspnea, muscular aches, dryness of mouth, dizziness and headache.

Dosage and Administration: Dosage should be determined by individual titration of ingredients (see boxed warning). Dosage of both components should be carefully adjusted to the needs of the individual patient. Since at least ten days to two weeks may elapse before the full effects of the drugs become manifest, the dosage should not be adjusted more frequently.

Three tablet strengths, ORETICYL 25 (hydrochlorothiazide 25 mg, deserpidine 0.125 mg); ORETICYL 50 (hydrochlorothiazide 50 mg, deserpidine 0.125 mg); and ORETICYL FORTE (hydrochlorothiazide 25 mg, deserpidine 0.25 mg), all grooved, are provided to permit considerable latitude in meeting the dosage requirements of individual patients.

The table below will help in determining which dose of ORETICYL 25, ORETICYL 50, or ORETICYL FORTE best represents the equivalent of the titrated dose.

ORETICYL 25	hydro-chlorothiazide	deserpidine
1 tablet bid	25.0 mg bid	0.125 mg bid

1½ tablet bid	37.5 mg bid	0.188 mg bid
2 tablets bid	50.0 mg bid	0.250 mg bid
ORETICYL 50	hydro-chlorothiazide	deserpidine
1 tablet bid	50 mg bid	0.125 mg bid
1½ tablet bid	75 mg bid	0.188 mg bid
2 tablets bid	100 mg bid	0.250 mg bid
ORETICYL FORTE	hydro-chlorothiazide	deserpidine
1 tablet bid	25.0 mg bid	0.250 mg bid
1½ tablet bid	37.5 mg bid	0.375 mg bid
2 tablets bid	50.0 mg bid	0.500 mg bid

The usual adult dosage is one ORETICYL 50 two times daily.

When other antihypertensive agents are to be added to the regimen, this should be accomplished gradually. Ganglionic blocking agents should be given at only half the usual dose since their effect is potentiated by pretreatment with ORETICYL (hydrochlorothiazide and deserpidine).

Overdosage: Symptoms of thiazide overdosage include electrolyte imbalance and signs of potassium deficiency such as confusion, dizziness, muscular weakness, and gastrointestinal disturbances. General supportive measures including replacement of fluids and electrolytes may be indicated in treatment of overdosage.

An overdosage of deserpidine is characterized by flushing of the skin, conjunctival injection, and pupillary constriction. Sedation ranging from drowsiness to coma may occur. Hypotension, hypothermia, central respiratory depression and bradycardia may develop in cases of severe overdosage. Treatment consists of the careful evacuation of stomach contents followed by the usual procedures for the symptomatic management of CNS depressant overdosage. If severe hypotension occurs it should be treated with a direct acting vasopressor such as norepinephrine bitartrate injection.

How Supplied: ORETICYL is supplied as grooved tablets in the following dosage sizes:

Rose-colored ORETICYL 25, contains hydrochlorothiazide 25 mg, deserpidine 0.125 mg, in bottles of 100 (**NDC** 0074-6922-01).

Rose-colored ORETICYL 50, contains hydrochlorothiazide 50 mg, deserpidine 0.125 mg, in bottles of 100 (**NDC** 0074-6931-01).

Gray-colored ORETICYL FORTE, contains hydrochlorothiazide 25 mg, deserpidine 0.25 mg, in bottles of 100 (**NDC** 0074-6927-01).

Abbott Laboratories
North Chicago, IL 60064
Ref. 01-2316-R5

PANHEMATIN™ ℞
[pan-he'ma-tin]
(hemin for injection)
For I.V. Use Only

> PANHEMATIN (hemin for injection) should only be used by physicians experienced in the management of porphyrias in hospitals where the recommended clinical and laboratory diagnostic and monitoring techniques are available.
> PANHEMATIN therapy should be considered after an appropriate period of alternate therapy (i.e., 400 g glucose/day for 1 to 2 days). (See "WARNINGS", "PRECAUTIONS" and "DOSAGE AND ADMINISTRATION" sections.)

Description: PANHEMATIN (hemin for injection) is an enzyme inhibitor derived from processed red blood cells. Hemin for injection was known previously as hematin. The term hematin has been used to describe the chemical reaction product of hemin and sodium carbonate solution. Hemin is an iron containing metalloporphyrin. Chemically hemin is represented as chloro[7,12-diethenyl-3,8,13,17-tetramethyl-21H,23H-porphine-2,18-dipropanoato(2-)-$N^{21},N^{22},N^{23},N^{24}$] iron.

PANHEMATIN is a sterile, lyophilized powder suitable for intravenous administration after reconstitution. Each dispensing vial of PANHEMATIN contains the equivalent of 313 mg hemin, 215 mg sodium carbonate and 300 mg of sorbitol. The pH may have been adjusted with hydrochloric acid; the product contains no preservatives. When mixed as directed with 43 ml Sterile Water for Injection, USP, hemin 313 mg/43 ml is approximately equivalent to hematin 7 mg/ml.

Clinical Pharmacology: Heme acts to limit the hepatic and/or marrow synthesis of porphyrin. This action is likely due to the inhibition of delta-aminolevulinic acid synthetase, the enzyme which limits the rate of the porphyrin/heme biosynthetic pathway. The exact mechanism by which hematin produces symptomatic improvement in patients with acute episodes of the hepatic porphyrias has not been elucidated.[1,9]

Following intravenous administration of hematin in non-jaundiced human patients, an increase in fecal urobilinogen can be observed which is roughly proportional to the amount of hematin administered. This suggests an enterohepatic pathway as at least one route of elimination. Bilirubin metabolites are also excreted in the urine following hematin injections.[2]

PANHEMATIN (hemin for injection) therapy for the acute porphyrias is not curative. After discontinuation of PANHEMATIN treatment, symptoms generally return although in some cases remission is prolonged. Some neurological symptoms have improved weeks to months after therapy although little or no response was noted at the time of treatment.

Other aspects of human pharmacokinetics have not been defined.

Indications and Usage: PANHEMATIN (hemin for injection) is indicated for the amelioration of recurrent attacks of acute intermittent porphyria temporally related to the menstrual cycle in susceptible women.

Manifestations such as pain, hypertension, tachycardia, abnormal mental status and mild to progressive neurologic signs may be controlled in selected patients with this disorder.

Similar findings have been reported in other patients with acute intermittent porphyria, porphyria variegata and hereditary coproporphyria. PANHEMATIN is not indicated in porphyria cutanea tarda.

Contraindications: Hemin for injection is contraindicated in patients with known hypersensitivity to this drug.

Warnings: PANHEMATIN (hemin for injection) therapy is intended to limit the rate of porphyria/heme biosynthesis possibly by inhibiting the enzyme delta-aminolevulinic acid synthetase. For this reason, drugs such as estrogens, barbituric acid derivatives and steroid metabolites which increase the activity of delta-aminolevulinic acid synthetase should be avoided.

Also, because PANHEMATIN has exhibited transient, mild anticoagulant effects during clinical studies, concurrent anticoagulant therapy should be avoided.[9] The extent and duration of the hypocoagulable state induced by PANHEMATIN has not been established.

Precautions: *General:*
Clinical benefit from PANHEMATIN depends on prompt administration. Attacks of porphyria may progress to a point where irreversible neuronal damage has occurred. PANHEMATIN therapy is intended to prevent an attack from reaching the critical stage of neuronal degeneration. PANHEMATIN is not effective in repairing neuronal damage.[9] Recommended dosage guidelines should be strictly followed. Reversible renal shutdown has been observed in a case where an excessive hematin dose (12.2 mg/kg) was administered in a single infusion. Oliguria and increased nitrogen retention occurred although the patient remained asymptomatic.[4] No worsening of renal function has been seen with administration of recommended dosages of hematin.[9]

A large arm vein or a central venous catheter should be utilized for the administration of hemin for injection to avoid the possibility of phlebitis.

Since reconstituted PANHEMATIN is not transparent, any undissolved particulate matter is difficult to see when inspected visually. Therefore, terminal filtration through a sterile 0.45 micron or smaller filter is recommended.

Tests for Diagnosis and Monitoring of Therapy: Before PANHEMATIN therapy is begun, the presence of acute porphyria must be diagnosed using the following criteria:[9]
a. Presence of clinical symptoms.
b. Positive Watson-Schwartz or Hoesch test. (A negative Watson-Schwartz or Hoesch test indicates a porphyric attack is highly unlikely. When in doubt quantitative measures of delta-aminolevulinic acid and porphobilinogen in serum or urine may aid in diagnosis.)

Urinary concentrations of the following compounds may be *monitored* during PANHEMATIN therapy. Drug effect will be demonstrated by a decrease in one or more of the following compounds:[3-6] ALA—delta-aminolevulinic acid, UPG—uroporphyrinogen, PBG—porphobilinogen or coproporphyrin.

Carcinogenesis, Mutagenesis, Impairment of Fertility: No data are available on potential for carcinogenicity, mutagenicity or impairment of fertility in animals or humans.

Pregnancy: Teratogenic effects: Pregnancy Category C. Animal reproduction studies have not been conducted with hematin. It is also not known whether hematin can cause fetal harm when administered to a pregnant woman or can affect reproduction capacity. For this reason hemin for injection should not be given to a pregnant woman unless the expected benefits are sufficiently important to the health and welfare of the patient to outweigh the unknown hazard to the fetus.

Nursing Mothers: It is not known whether this drug is excreted in human milk. Because many drugs are excreted in human milk, caution should be exercised when hemin for injection is administered to a nursing woman.

Pediatric Use: Safety and effectiveness in children have not been established.

Adverse Reactions: Reversible renal shutdown has occurred with administration of excessive doses (See "PRECAUTIONS" section).

Phlebitis with or without leucocytosis and with or without mild pyrexia has occurred after administration of hematin through small arm veins.

There has been one report in the literature[8] of coagulopathy occurring in a patient receiving hematin therapy. This patient exhibited prolonged prothrombin time and partial thromboplastin time, thrombocytopenia, mild hypofibrinogenemia, mild elevation of fibrin split products and a 10% fall in hematocrit.

Overdosage: Reversible renal shutdown has been observed in a case where an excessive hematin dose (12.2 mg/kg) was administered in a single infusion. Treatment of this case consisted of ethacrynic acid and mannitol.[7]

Dosage and Administration: Before administering hemin for injection, an appropriate period of alternate therapy (i.e., 400 g glucose/day for 1 to 2 days) must be considered. If improvement is unsatisfactory for the treatment of acute attacks of porphyria, an intravenous infusion of PANHEMATIN containing a dose of 1 to 4 mg/kg/day of hematin should be given over a period of 10 to 15 minutes for 3 to 14 days based on the clinical signs. In more severe cases this dose may be repeated no earlier than every 12 hours. No more than 6 mg/kg of hematin should be given in any 24-hour period.

After reconstitution each ml of PANHEMATIN contains the equivalent of approximately 7 mg of hematin (313 mg hemin/43 ml), 5 mg sodium carbonate (215 mg/43 ml) and 7 mg sorbitol. The drug may be administered directly from the vial.

Continued on next page

If desired, additional literature on any Abbott Product will be provided upon request to Abbott Laboratories.

Abbott—Cont.

Dosage Calculation Table

1 mg hematin equivalent = 0.14 ml PANHEMATIN
2 mg hematin equivalent = 0.28 ml PANHEMATIN
3 mg hematin equivalent = 0.42 ml PANHEMATIN
4 mg hematin equivalent = 0.56 ml PANHEMATIN

Since reconstituted PANHEMATIN is not transparent, any undissolved particulate matter is difficult to see when inspected visually. Therefore, terminal filtration through a sterile 0.45 micron or smaller filter is recommended.

Preparation of Solution: Reconstitute PANHEMATIN by aseptically adding 43 ml of Sterile Water for Injection, USP, to the dispensing vial. Immediately after adding diluent, the product should be shaken well for a period of 2 to 3 minutes to aid dissolution. **NOTE:** Because PANHEMATIN contains no preservative and because PANHEMATIN undergoes rapid chemical decomposition in solution, it should not be reconstituted until immediately before use. After the first withdrawal from the vial, any solution remaining must be discarded.

No drug or chemical agent should be added to a PANHEMATIN fluid admixture unless its effect on the chemical and physical stability has first been determined.

How Supplied: PANHEMATIN (hemin for injection) is supplied as a sterile, lyophilized black powder in single dose dispensing vials (**NDC** 0074-2000-43). Each dispensing vial contains the equivalent of 313 mg hemin, 215 mg sodium carbonate and 300 mg sorbitol (43 ml when mixed as directed). The pH may have been adjusted with hydrochloric acid; the product contains no preservatives. Hemin 313 mg/43 ml is approximately equivalent to 7 mg hematin/ml. Store lyophilized powder frozen until time of use.

References:
1. Bickers, D., Treatment of the Porphyrias: Mechanisms of Action, *J Invest Dermatol* 77(1):107–113, 1981.
2. Watson, C. J., Hematin and Porphyria, editorial, *N Engl J Med* 293(12):605–607, September 18, 1975.
3. Lamon, J. M., Hematin Therapy for Acute Porphyria, *Medicine* 58(3):252–269, 1979.
4. Dhar, G. J., et al., Effects of Hematin in Hepatic Porphyria, *Ann Intern Med* 83:20–30, 1975.
5. Watson, C. J., et al., Use of Hematin in the Acute Attack of the "Inducible" Hepatic Porphyrias, *Adv Intern Med* 23:265–286, 1978.
6. McColl, K. E., et al., Treatment with Haematin in Acute Hepatic Porphyria, *Q J Med*, New Series L (198):161–174, Spring, 1981.
7. Dhar, G. J., et al., Transitory Renal Failure Following Rapid Administration of a Relatively Large Amount of Hematin in a Patient with Acute Intermittent Porphyria in Clinical Remission, *Acta Med Scand* 203:437–443, 1978.
8. Morris, D. L., et al., Coagulopathy Associated with Hematin Treatment for Acute Intermittent Porphyria, *Ann Intern Med* 95:700–701, 1981.
9. Pierach, C. A., Hematin Therapy for the Porphyric Attack, *Semin Liver Dis* 2(2):125–131, May, 1982.

Abbott Laboratories
North Chicago, IL 60064
Ref. 01-2296-R2

PANWARFIN® ℞
[pǎn-wăr′fin]
(warfarin sodium tablets, USP)

How Supplied: PANWARFIN (warfarin sodium tablets, USP) for oral administration, grooved and bearing dosage strength numerals are available as follows:

2 mg, lavender-colored: bottles of 100 (**NDC** 0074-6626-03), and ABBO-PAC® unit dose packages of 100 tablets (**NDC** 0074-6626-07).

2½ mg, orange-colored: bottles of 100 (**NDC** 0074-7202-01), and ABBO-PAC unit dose packages of 100 tablets (**NDC** 0074-7202-05).

5 mg, peach-colored: bottles of 100 (**NDC** 0074-7210-01), 500 (**NDC** 0074-7210-09), and ABBO-PAC unit dose packages of 100 tablets (**NDC** 0074-7210-05).

7½ mg, yellow: bottles of 100 (**NDC** 0074-6638-03), and ABBO-PAC unit dose packages of 100 tablets (**NDC** 0074-6638-07).

10 mg, white: bottles of 100 (**NDC** 0074-7218-01), and ABBO-PAC unit dose packages of 100 tablets (**NDC** 0074-7218-05).

Shown in Product Identification Section, page 403
Abbott Pharmaceuticals, Inc.
North Chicago, IL 60064

PARADIONE® ℞
[pă-rǎ-dī′own]
(paramethadione)
Capsules and Oral Solution

> BECAUSE OF ITS POTENTIAL TO PRODUCE FETAL MALFORMATIONS AND SERIOUS SIDE EFFECTS, PARADIONE (paramethadione) SHOULD ONLY BE UTILIZED WHEN OTHER LESS TOXIC DRUGS HAVE BEEN FOUND INEFFECTIVE IN CONTROLLING ABSENCE (PETIT MAL) SEIZURES.

Description: PARADIONE (paramethadione) is an antiepileptic agent. An oxazolidinedione compound, it is chemically identified as 5-Ethyl-3,5-dimethyl-2,4-oxazolidinedione. PARADIONE is a synthetic, oily, slightly water-soluble liquid. It is supplied in capsular and liquid forms for oral use only. The capsules are available in two dosage strengths. One strength contains 150 mg the other 300 mg of paramethadione per capsule. Each ml of the liquid contains 300 mg of paramethadione; alcohol 65%.

Clinical Pharmacology: PARADIONE has been shown to prevent pentylenetetrazol-induced and thujone-induced seizures in experimental animals; the drug has a less marked effect on seizures induced by picrotoxin, procaine, cocaine, or strychnine. Unlike the hydantoins and antiepileptic barbiturates, PARADIONE does not modify the maximal seizure pattern in patients undergoing electroconvulsive therapy. PARADIONE has a sedative effect that may increase to the point of ataxia when excessive doses are used. A toxic dose of the drug in animals (approximately 1 Gm/kg) produced sleep, unconsciousness, and respiratory depression.

Paramethadione is rapidly absorbed from the gastrointestinal tract. It is demethylated by liver microsomes to an active N-demethylated metabolite, and is excreted slowly in this form by the kidney; almost no unmetabolized PARADIONE is excreted.

Indications and Usage: PARADIONE (paramethadione) is indicated for the control of absence (petit mal) seizures that are refractory to treatment with other drugs.

Contraindications: PARADIONE is contraindicated in patients with a known hypersensitivity to the drug.

Warnings: PARADIONE may cause serious side effects. Strict medical supervision of the patient is mandatory, especially during the initial year of therapy.

USAGE DURING PREGNANCY: THERE ARE MULTIPLE REPORTS IN THE CLINICAL LITERATURE WHICH INDICATE THAT THE USE OF ANTIEPILEPTIC DRUGS DURING PREGNANCY RESULTS IN AN INCREASED INCIDENCE OF BIRTH DEFECTS IN THE OFFSPRING. DATA ARE MORE EXTENSIVE WITH RESPECT TO TRIMETHADIONE, PARAMETHADIONE, PHENYTOIN AND PHENOBARBITAL THAN WITH OTHER ANTIEPILEPTIC DRUGS.

THEREFORE, ANTIEPILEPTIC DRUGS SUCH AS PARADIONE (PARAMETHADIONE) SHOULD BE ADMINISTERED TO WOMEN OF CHILDBEARING POTENTIAL ONLY IF THEY ARE CLEARLY SHOWN TO BE ESSENTIAL IN THE MANAGEMENT OF THEIR SEIZURES. EFFECTIVE MEANS OF CONTRACEPTION SHOULD ACCOMPANY THE USE OF PARADIONE IN SUCH PATIENTS. IF A PATIENT BECOMES PREGNANT WHILE TAKING PARADIONE, TERMINATION OF THE PREGNANCY SHOULD BE CONSIDERED. A PATIENT WHO REQUIRES THERAPY WITH PARADIONE AND WHO WISHES TO BECOME PREGNANT SHOULD BE ADVISED OF THE RISKS.

REPORTS HAVE SUGGESTED THAT THE MATERNAL INGESTION OF ANTIEPILEPTIC DRUGS, PARTICULARLY BARBITURATES, IS ASSOCIATED WITH A NEONATAL COAGULATION DEFECT THAT MAY CAUSE BLEEDING DURING THE EARLY (USUALLY WITHIN 24 HOURS OF BIRTH) NEONATAL PERIOD. THE POSSIBILITY OF THE OCCURRENCE OF THIS DEFECT WITH THE USE OF PARADIONE SHOULD BE KEPT IN MIND. THE DEFECT IS CHARACTERIZED BY DECREASED LEVELS OF VITAMIN K-DEPENDENT CLOTTING FACTORS, AND PROLONGATION OF EITHER THE PROTHROMBIN TIME OR THE PARTIAL THROMBOPLASTIN TIME, OR BOTH. IT HAS BEEN SUGGESTED THAT PROPHYLACTIC VITAMIN K BE GIVEN TO THE MOTHER ONE MONTH PRIOR TO, AND DURING DELIVERY, AND TO THE INFANT, INTRAVENOUSLY, IMMEDIATELY AFTER BIRTH.

Precautions: *General:* Abrupt discontinuation of PARADIONE may precipitate absence (petit mal) status. PARADIONE (paramethadione) should always be withdrawn gradually unless serious adverse effects dictate otherwise. In the latter case, another antiepileptic may be substituted to protect the patient.

PARADIONE (paramethadione) should be withdrawn promptly if skin rash appears, because of the grave possibility of the occurrence of exfoliative dermatitis or severe forms of erythema multiforme. Even a minor acneiform or morbilliform rash should be allowed to clear completely before treatment with PARADIONE is resumed; reinstitute therapy cautiously.

PARADIONE should ordinarily not be used in patients with severe blood dyscrasias.

Hepatitis has been associated rarely with the use of oxazolidinediones. Jaundice or other signs of liver dysfunction are an indication for withdrawal of PARADIONE. PARADIONE should ordinarily not be used in patients with severe hepatic impairment. Fatal nephrosis has been reported with the use of oxazolidinediones. Persistent or increasing albuminuria, or the development of any other significant renal abnormality, is an indication for withdrawal of the drug. PARADIONE should ordinarily not be used in patients with severe renal dysfunction.

Hemeralopia has occurred with the use of oxazolidinedione compounds; this appears to be an effect of the drugs on the neural layers of the retina, and usually can be reversed by a reduction in dosage. Scotomata are an indication for withdrawal of the drug. Caution should be observed when treating patients who have diseases of the retina or optic nerve.

Manifestations of systemic lupus erythematosus have been associated with the use of the oxazolidinediones, as they have with the use of certain other antiepileptics. Lymphadenopathies simulating malignant lymphoma have also occurred. Lupus-like manifestations or lymph node enlargement are indications for withdrawal of PARADIONE. Signs and symptoms may disappear after discontinuation of therapy, and specific treatment may be unnecessary.

A myasthenia gravis-like syndrome has been associated with the chronic use of the oxazolidinediones. Symptoms suggestive of this condition are indications for withdrawal of PARADIONE.

The 300 mg capsule of PARADIONE contains FD&C Yellow No. 5 (tartrazine) which may cause allergic-type reactions (including bronchial asthma) in certain susceptible individuals. Although the overall incidence of FD&C Yellow No. 5 (tartrazine) sensitivity in the general population is low, it is frequently seen in patients who also have aspirin hypersensitivity.

Information for Patients: Patients should be advised to report immediately such signs and symptoms as sore throat, fever, malaise, easy-bruising, petechiae, or epistaxis, or others that may be indicative of an infection or bleeding tendency.

Laboratory Tests: A complete blood count should be done prior to initiating therapy with PARADIONE, and at monthly intervals thereafter. A marked depression of the blood count is an indication for withdrawal of the drug. If no abnormality appears within 12 months, the interval between blood counts may be extended. A moderate degree of neutropenia with or without a corresponding drop in the leukocyte count is not uncommon. Therapy need not be withdrawn unless the neutrophil count is 2500 or less; more frequent blood examinations should be done when the count is less than 3,000. Other blood dyscrasias, including leukopenia, eosinophilia, thrombocytopenia, pancytopenia, agranulocytosis, hypoplastic anemia, and fatal aplastic anemia, have occurred with the use of oxazolidinediones.

Liver function tests should be done prior to initiating therapy with PARADIONE, and at monthly intervals thereafter.

A urinalysis should be done prior to initiating therapy with PARADIONE and at monthly intervals thereafter.

Drug Interactions: Drugs known to cause toxic effects similar to those of the oxazolidinediones should be avoided or used only with extreme caution during therapy with PARADIONE.

Carcinogenesis: No data are available on long-term potential for carcinogenicity in animals or humans.

Pregnancy: Pregnancy Category D. See "Warnings" section.

Nursing Mothers: It is not known whether this drug is excreted in human milk. Because many drugs are excreted in human milk and because of the potential for serious adverse reactions in nursing infants from PARADIONE, a decision should be made whether to discontinue nursing or to discontinue the drug, taking into account the importance of the drug to the mother.

Adverse Reactions: The following side effects, in decreasing order of severity, have been associated with the use of oxazolidinedione compounds. Although not all of them have been reported with the use of PARADIONE, the possibility of their occurrence should be kept in mind when the drug is prescribed.

Renal: Fatal nephrosis has occurred. Albuminuria.

Hematologic: Fatal aplastic anemia, hypoplastic anemia, pancytopenia, agranulocytosis, leukopenia, neutropenia, thrombocytopenia, eosinophilia, retinal and petechial hemorrhages, vaginal bleeding, epistaxis, and bleeding gums.

Hepatic: Hepatitis has been reported rarely.

Dermatologic: Acneiform or morbilliform skin rash that may progress to severe forms of erythema multiforme or to exfoliative dermatitis. Hair loss.

CNS/Neurologic: A myasthenia gravis-like syndrome has been reported. Precipitation of tonic-clonic (grand mal) seizures, vertigo, personality changes, increased irritability, drowsiness, headache, paresthesias, fatigue, malaise, and insomnia. Drowsiness usually subsides with continued therapy. If it persists, a reduction in dosage is indicated.

Ophthalmologic: Diplopia, hemeralopia, and photophobia.

Cardiovascular: Changes in blood pressure.

Gastrointestinal: Vomiting, abdominal pain, gastric distress, nausea, anorexia, weight loss, and hiccups.

Other: Lupus erythematosus, and lymphadenopathies simulating malignant lymphoma, have been reported. Pruritus associated with lymphadenopathy and hepatosplenomegaly has occurred in hypersensitive individuals.

Overdosage: Symptoms of acute PARADIONE overdosage include drowsiness, nausea, dizziness, ataxia, visual disturbances. Coma may follow massive overdosage.

Gastric evacuation, either by induced emesis, or by lavage, or both, should be done immediately. General supportive care, including frequent monitoring of the vital signs and close observation of the patient, are required.

It has been reported that alkalinization of the urine may be expected to increase the excretion of the N-demethylated metabolite of PARADIONE.

A blood count and a careful evaluation of hepatic and renal function should be done following recovery.

Dosage and Administration: PARADIONE is administered orally.

Because PARADIONE Oral Solution contains alcohol 65%, it may be desirable to dilute the preparation with water before administering it to small children.

Usual Adult Dosage: 0.9–2.4 Gm daily in 3 or 4 equally divided doses (i.e., 300–600 mg 3 or 4 times daily).

Initially, give 0.9 Gm daily; increase this dose by 300 mg at weekly intervals until therapeutic results are seen or until toxic symptoms appear. Maintenance dosage should be the least amount of drug required to maintain control.

Children's Dosage: Usually 0.3–0.9 Gm daily in 3 or 4 equally divided doses.

How Supplied: PARADIONE Capsules (paramethadione capsules, USP) are round capsules supplied as 150 mg (orange color) (**NDC** 0074-3976-01), and 300 mg (green color) (**NDC** 0074-3838-01) in bottles of 100.

Shown in Product Identification Section, page 403

PARADIONE Solution (paramethadione oral solution, USP), 300 mg per ml, is supplied in 50-ml bottles (**NDC** 0074-3860-01). A dropper is provided with each bottle, which is marked to permit easy measurement of 0.5 ml and 1 ml doses. The solution is clear and colorless.

Abbott Laboratories
North Chicago, IL 60064
Ref. 01-2200/R5

PEGANONE® ℞
[pĕg′ă-noon]
(ethotoin tablets)

Description: PEGANONE (ethotoin) is an oral antiepileptic of the hydantoin series and is chemically identified as 3-ethyl-5-phenyl-2, 4-imidazolidinedione. PEGANONE tablets are available in two dosage strengths of 250 mg and 500 mg respectively.

Clinical Pharmacology: PEGANONE (ethotoin) exerts an antiepileptic effect without causing general central nervous system depression. The mechanism of action is probably very similar to that of phenytoin. The latter drug appears to stabilize rather than to raise the normal seizure threshold, and to prevent the spread of seizure activity rather than to abolish the primary focus of seizure discharges.

In laboratory animals, the drug was found effective against electroshock convulsions, and to a lesser extent, against complex partial (psychomotor) and pentylenetetrazol-induced seizures.

In mice, the duration of antiepileptic activity was prolonged by hepatic injury but not by bilateral nephrectomy; the drug is apparently biotransformed by the liver.

Ethotoin is fairly rapidly absorbed; the extent of oral absorption is not known. The drug exhibits saturable metabolism with respect to the formation of N-deethyl and p-hydroxyl-ethotoin, the major metabolites. Where plasma concentrations are below about 8 mg/l, the elimination half-life of ethotoin is in the range of 3 to 9 hours. Above this concentration, the dose-dependent, nonlinear kinetics of the drug preclude definition of any conventional half-life. Experience suggests that therapeutic plasma concentrations fall in the range of 15 to 50 mg/l; however, this range is not as extensively documented as those quoted for other antiepileptics.

Indications and Usage: PEGANONE (ethotoin) is indicated for the control of tonic-clonic (grand mal) and complex partial (psychomotor) seizures.

Contraindications: PEGANONE (ethotoin) is contraindicated in patients with hepatic abnormalities or hematologic disorders.

Warnings: USAGE DURING PREGNANCY—THERE ARE MULTIPLE REPORTS IN THE CLINICAL LITERATURE WHICH INDICATE THAT THE USE OF ANTIEPILEPTIC DRUGS DURING PREGNANCY RESULTS IN AN INCREASED INCIDENCE OF BIRTH DEFECTS IN THE OFFSPRING. ALTHOUGH DATA ARE MORE EXTENSIVE WITH RESPECT TO TRIMETHADIONE, PARAMETHADIONE, PHENYTOIN, AND PHENOBARBITAL, REPORTS INDICATE A POSSIBLE SIMILAR ASSOCIATION WITH THE USE OF OTHER ANTIEPILEPTIC DRUGS.

THEREFORE, ANTIEPILEPTIC DRUGS SHOULD BE ADMINISTERED TO WOMEN OF CHILDBEARING POTENTIAL ONLY IF THEY ARE CLEARLY SHOWN TO BE ESSENTIAL IN THE MANAGEMENT OF THEIR SEIZURES. ANTIEPILEPTIC DRUGS SHOULD NOT BE DISCONTINUED IN PATIENTS IN WHOM THE DRUG IS ADMINISTERED TO PREVENT MAJOR SEIZURES BECAUSE OF THE STRONG POSSIBILITY OF PRECIPITATING STATUS EPILEPTICUS WITH ATTENDANT HYPOXIA AND RISK TO BOTH MOTHER AND THE UNBORN CHILD. CONSIDERATION SHOULD, HOWEVER, BE GIVEN TO DISCONTINUATION OF ANTIEPILEPTICS PRIOR TO AND DURING PREGNANCY WHEN THE NATURE, FREQUENCY AND SEVERITY OF THE SEIZURES DO NOT POSE A SERIOUS THREAT TO THE PATIENT. IT IS NOT, HOWEVER, KNOWN WHETHER EVEN MINOR SEIZURES CONSTITUTE SOME RISK TO THE DEVELOPING EMBRYO OR FETUS.

REPORTS HAVE SUGGESTED THAT THE MATERNAL INGESTION OF ANTIEPILEPTIC DRUGS, PARTICULARLY BARBITURATES, IS ASSOCIATED WITH A NEONATAL COAGULATION DEFECT THAT MAY CAUSE BLEEDING DURING THE EARLY (USUALLY WITHIN 24 HOURS OF BIRTH) NEONATAL PERIOD. THE POSSIBILITY OF THE OCCURRENCE OF THIS DEFECT WITH THE USE OF PEGANONE SHOULD BE KEPT IN MIND. THE DEFECT IS CHARACTERIZED BY DECREASED LEVELS OF VITAMIN K-DEPENDENT CLOTTING FACTORS, AND PROLONGATION OF EITHER THE PROTHROMBIN TIME OR THE PARTIAL THROMBOPLASTIN TIME, OR BOTH. IT HAS BEEN SUGGESTED THAT VITAMIN K BE GIVEN PROPHYLACTICALLY TO THE MOTHER ONE MONTH PRIOR TO, AND DURING DELIVERY, AND TO THE INFANT, INTRAVENOUSLY, IMMEDIATELY AFTER BIRTH.

THE PHYSICIAN SHOULD WEIGH THESE CONSIDERATIONS IN TREATMENT AND COUNSELING OF EPILEPTIC WOMEN OF CHILDBEARING POTENTIAL.

Precautions: *General:* Blood dyscrasias have been reported in patients receiving PEGANONE. Although the etiologic role of PEGANONE has not been definitely established, physicians should be alert for general malaise, sore throat and other symptoms indicative of possible blood dyscrasia. There is some evidence suggesting that hydantoin-like compounds may interfere with folic acid metabolism, precipitating a megaloblastic anemia. If this should occur during gestation, folic acid therapy should be considered.

Information for Patients: Patients should be advised to report immediately such signs and symptoms as sore throat, fever, malaise, easy bruising, petechiae, epistaxis, or others that may be indicative of an infection or bleeding tendency.

Continued on next page

If desired, additional literature on any Abbott Product will be provided upon request to Abbott Laboratories.

Abbott—Cont.

Laboratory Tests: Liver function tests should be performed if clinical evidence suggests the possibility of hepatic dysfunction. Signs of liver damage are indication for withdrawal of the drug.

It is recommended that blood counts and urinalyses be performed when therapy is begun and at monthly intervals for several months thereafter. As in patients receiving other hydantoin compounds and other antiepileptic drugs, blood dyscrasias have been reported in patients receiving PEGANONE (ethotoin). Marked depression of the blood count is indication for withdrawal of the drug.

Drug Interactions: PEGANONE used in combination with other drugs known to adversely affect the hematopoietic system should be avoided if possible.

Considerable caution should be exercised if PEGANONE is administered concurrently with *Phenurone (phenacemide)* since paranoid symptoms have been reported during therapy with this combination.

A two-way interaction between the hydantoin antiepileptic, *phenytoin*, and the *coumarin anticoagulants* has been suggested. Presumably, phenytoin acts as a stimulator of coumarin metabolism and has been reported to cause decreased serum levels of the coumarin anticoagulants and increased prothrombin-proconvertin concentrations. Conversely, the coumarin anticoagulants have been reported to increase the serum levels and prolong the serum half-life of phenytoin by inhibiting its metabolism. Although there is no documentation of such, a similar interaction between ethotoin and the coumarin anticoagulants may occur. Caution is therefore advised when administering PEGANONE to patients receiving coumarin anticoagulants.

Carcinogenesis: No data are available on long-term potential for carcinogenicity in animals or humans.

Pregnancy: Pregnancy Category C. See "Warnings" section.

Nursing Mothers: Ethotoin is excreted in breast milk. Because of the potential for serious adverse reactions in nursing infants from ethotoin, a decision should be made whether to discontinue nursing or to discontinue the drug, taking into account the importance of the drug to the mother.

Adverse Reactions: Adverse reactions associated with PEGANONE, in decreasing order of severity, are:

Isolated cases of lymphadenopathy and systemic lupus erythematosus have been reported in patients taking hydantoin compounds, and lymphadenopathy has occurred with PEGANONE. Withdrawal of therapy has resulted in remission of the clinical and pathological findings. Therefore, if a lymphoma-like syndrome develops, the drug should be withdrawn and the patient should be closely observed for regression of signs and symptoms before treatment is resumed.

Ataxia and gum hypertrophy have occurred only rarely—usually only in patients receiving an additional hydantoin derivative. It is of interest to note that ataxia and gum hypertrophy have subsided in patients receiving other hydantoins when PEGANONE was given as a substitute antiepileptic.

Occasionally, vomiting or nausea after ingestion of PEGANONE has been reported, but if the drug is administered after meals, the incidence of gastric distress is reduced. Other side effects have included chest pain, nystagmus, diplopia, fever, dizziness, diarrhea, headache, insomnia, fatigue, numbness and skin rash.

Overdosage: Symptoms of acute overdosage include drowsiness, visual disturbance, nausea and ataxia. Coma is possible at very high dosage. Treatment should be begun by inducing emesis; gastric lavage may be considered as an alternative. General supportive measures will be necessary. A careful evaluation of blood-forming organs should be made following recovery.

Dosage and Administration: PEGANONE is administered orally in 4 to 6 divided doses daily. The drug should be taken after food, and doses should be spaced as evenly as practicable. Initial dosage should be conservative. For adults, the initial daily dose should be 1 g or less, with subsequent gradual dosage increases over a period of several days. The optimum dosage must be determined on the basis of individual response. The usual adult maintenance dose is 2 to 3 g daily. Less than 2 g daily has been found ineffective in most adults.

Pediatric dosage depends upon the age and weight of the patient. The initial dose should not exceed 750 mg daily. The usual maintenance dose in children ranges from 500 mg to 1 g daily, although occasionally 2 or (rarely) 3 g daily may be necessary.

If a patient is receiving another antiepileptic drug, it should not be discontinued when PEGANONE therapy is begun. The dosage of the other drug should be reduced gradually as that of PEGANONE is increased. PEGANONE may eventually replace the other drug or the optimal dosage of both antiepileptics may be established.

PEGANONE is compatible with all commonly employed antiepileptic medications with the possible exception of Phenurone® (phenacemide). In tonic-clonic (grand mal) seizures, use of the drug with Gemonil® (metharbital) or phenobarbital may be beneficial. PEGANONE may be used in combination with drugs such as Tridione® (trimethadione) or Paradione® (paramethadione), as an adjunct in those patients with absence (petit mal) associated with tonic-clonic (grand mal).

How Supplied: PEGANONE (ethotoin) grooved, white tablets are supplied in two dosage strengths: 250 mg, bottles of 100 (**NDC** 0074-6902-01); 500 mg, bottles of 100 (**NDC** 0074-6905-04).

This product is listed in N.D., a Medicare designated compendium.

Abbott Laboratories
North Chicago, IL 60064

Shown in Product Identification Section, page 403
Ref. 01-2206-R4

PENTHRANE® ℞
[pen'thrāne]
(methoxyflurane, USP)

Description: PENTHRANE® (Methoxyflurane, USP), a volatile liquid, is intended only for vaporization at suitable concentrations for administration by inhalation with appropriate anesthesia equipment or devices.

PENTHRANE is an inhalation anesthetic/analgesic which belongs to the fluorinated hydrocarbon group of volatile anesthetics. It is chemically designated 2,2 - dichloro -1, 1 - difluoroethyl methyl ether and has the following structural formula:

$$CHCl_2CF_2-O-CH_3$$

PENTHRANE has a mildly pungent odor.
Some of the physical constants are:

Molecular weight	164.97
Boiling point at 760 mm Hg	104.6°C
Partition coefficients at 37°C	
Water/gas	4.5
Blood/gas (mean range)	10.20 to 14.06
Oil/gas	825
Vapor Pressure 17.7°C	20 mm Hg
Flash points	
in air	62.8°C
in oxygen (closed system)	32.8°C
in nitrous oxide 50% with 50% oxygen	28.2°C
Lower limits of flammability of vapor concentration	
in air	7.0%
in oxygen	5.4%
in N_2O 50%	4.6%

PENTHRANE (Methoxyflurane, USP) is stable and does not decompose in contact with soda lime. An antioxidant, butylated hydroxytoluene 0.01% w/w is added to insure stability on standing. This slowly oxidizes to a yellow pigment that progressively turns to brown, and which may accumulate on the vaporizer wick. The colored matter may be removed by rinsing the wick with diethyl ether. The wick must be dried after cleaning to avoid introducing diethyl ether into the system.

Polyvinyl chloride plastics are extracted by PENTHRANE, therefore, contact should be avoided. PENTHRANE does not extract polyethylene plastics, polypropylene plastics, fluorinated hydrocarbon plastics or nylon. It is very soluble in rubber and soda lime. Disposable conductive plastic circuits should be discarded after a single use to avoid cross contamination and because PENTHRANE may reduce conductivity of such materials below safe limits for subsequent administration of a flammable anesthetic.

The vapor concentration of PENTHRANE is limited by its vapor pressure at room temperature to a maximum of about 3.5% at 23°C. In practice, this concentration is not easily reached due to the cooling effect of vaporization. PENTHRANE is not flammable except at vapor concentrations well above those recommended for its use. Recommended concentrations are nonflammable and nonexplosive in air, oxygen and nitrous oxide mixtures at ordinary room temperature.

Clinical Pharmacology: PENTHRANE provides anesthesia and/or analgesia.

After surgical anesthesia with PENTHRANE, analgesia and drowsiness may persist after consciousness has returned. This may obviate or reduce the need for narcotics in the immediate postoperative period.

When used alone in safe concentration, PENTHRANE (Methoxyflurane, USP) will not produce appreciable skeletal muscle relaxation. A muscle relaxing agent, e.g., succinylcholine chloride (Quelicin®) or tubocurarine chloride should be used as an adjunct.

Bronchiolar constriction or laryngeal spasm is not ordinarily provoked by PENTHRANE.

During PENTHRANE anesthesia, the cardiac rhythm is usually regular. The myocardium is only minimally sensitized by PENTHRANE to epinephrine. Some decrease in blood pressure often accompanies light planes of anesthesia. This may be accompanied by bradycardia. The hypotension noted is accompanied by reduced cardiac contractile force and reduced cardiac output.

When used for obstetrical delivery, light planes of PENTHRANE anesthesia have little effect on uterine contractions. There are no known contraindications to the concomitant use of PENTHRANE and oxytocic agents.

Biotransformation of PENTHRANE occurs in man. Approximately 20% of PENTHRANE uptake is recovered in the exhaled air, while urinary excretion of organic fluorine, fluoride and oxalic acid accounts for about 30% of the PENTHRANE uptake.

Studies have shown that higher peak blood fluoride levels are obtained earlier in obese patients than in non-obese.

Indications and Usage:
1. PENTHRANE is indicated usually in combination with oxygen and nitrous oxide to provide anesthesia for surgical procedures in which total duration of PENTHRANE administration is anticipated to be 4 hours or less, and in which PENTHRANE is not to be used in concentrations that will provide skeletal muscle relaxation; see WARNINGS regarding time and dose relationships.
2. PENTHRANE (Methoxyflurane, USP) may be used alone with hand held inhalers or in combination with oxygen and nitrous oxide for analgesia in obstetrics and in minor surgical procedures.

Contraindications: See WARNINGS.
Warnings: SEQUENTIAL ANESTHESIA WITH PENTHRANE AND HALOTHANE, OR HALOTHANE AND PENTHRANE, IN EITHER ORDER, HAS BEEN FOLLOWED BY JAUNDICE IN A FEW RARE CASES. WHEN A PREVIOUS EXPOSURE TO PENTHRANE (METHOXYFLURANE, USP) OR HALOTHANE HAS BEEN

FOLLOWED BY UNEXPLAINED HEPATIC DYSFUNCTION AND/OR JAUNDICE, CONSIDERATION SHOULD BE GIVEN TO THE USE OF OTHER AGENTS.
THE NEPHROTOXICITY ASSOCIATED WITH PENTHRANE ADMINISTRATION APPEARS TO BE RELATED TO THE TOTAL DOSE (TIME AND CONCENTRATION). SEE PARAGRAPH 5. THE MANIFESTATIONS RANGE IN SEVERITY FROM REVERSIBLE ALTERATIONS IN LABORATORY FINDINGS TO POLYURIC OR OLIGURIC RENAL FAILURE, SOMETIMES FATAL. POLYURIC RENAL FAILURE IS CHARACTERIZED BY THE DEVELOPMENT, EARLY IN THE POSTOPERATIVE PERIOD, OF THE FOLLOWING:
WEIGHT LOSS
URINE: LOW SPECIFIC GRAVITY, LARGE VOLUME EQUAL TO OR IN EXCESS OF FLUID INTAKE, DECREASED OSMOLALITY.
SERUM/BLOOD: ELEVATION OF SODIUM, CHLORIDE, URIC ACID, BUN, CREATININE.
THIS SYNDROME IS BELIEVED TO BE RELATED TO RELEASE OF THE FLUORIDE ION, A METABOLIC PRODUCT OF PENTHRANE AND TO BE RELATED TO THE TOTAL DOSAGE ADMINISTERED. THEREFORE, THE LOWEST EFFECTIVE DOSAGE SHOULD BE ADMINISTERED, ESPECIALLY IN AGED OR OBESE PATIENTS AND IN SURGICAL PROCEDURES OF LONG DURATION, BEARING IN MIND THAT THE TOTAL DOSE DELIVERED TO THE PATIENT IS A FACTOR OF DURATION OF ADMINISTRATION AND CONCENTRATION OF VAPOR.
OXALATE CRYSTALS AND/OR ACUTE TUBULAR NECROSIS HAVE BEEN NOTED AT AUTOPSY.
The guiding principles in minimizing the possibility of renal injury are:
1. AVOID USING PENTHRANE (METHOXYFLURANE, USP) AS THE SOLE OR PRINCIPLE AGENT TO ACHIEVE MUSCULAR RELAXATION.
2. PATIENTS WITH PRE-EXISTING RENAL DISEASE, IMPAIRMENT OF RENAL FUNCTION, TOXEMIA OF PREGNANCY, AND PATIENTS UNDERGOING VASCULAR SURGERY AT OR NEAR THE RENAL VESSELS SHOULD NOT RECEIVE PENTHRANE UNLESS IN THE JUDGMENT OF THE PHYSICIAN THE BENEFITS OUTWEIGH THE INCREASED RISK OF NEPHROTOXIC EFFECT.
3. URINARY OUTPUT SHOULD BE MONITORED IN ALL PATIENTS IF EXCESSIVE URINE OUTPUT OCCURS, APPROPRIATE LABORATORY STUDIES SHOULD BE DONE TO ASSESS RENAL FUNCTION. IN HIGH RISK PATIENTS (SEE 2, ABOVE) SERIAL TESTS OF RENAL FUNCTION AND MEASUREMENTS OF FLUID AND ELECTROLYTE BALANCE ARE IMPERATIVE. ALL FLUID AND ELECTROLYTE LOSSES SHOULD BE PROMPTLY REPLACED.
4. THE CONCURRENT USE OF TETRACYCLINE AND PENTHRANE HAS BEEN REPORTED TO RESULT IN FATAL RENAL TOXICITY. THE POSSIBILITY EXISTS THAT PENTHRANE MAY ENHANCE THE ADVERSE RENAL EFFECTS OF OTHER DRUGS INCLUDING CERTAIN ANTIBIOTICS OF KNOWN NEPHROTOXIC POTENTIAL SUCH AS GENTAMICIN, KANAMYCIN, COLISTIN, POLYMYXIN B, CEPHALORIDINE AND AMPHOTERICIN B. THIS SHOULD BE CAREFULLY CONSIDERED WHEN PRESCRIBING SUCH DRUGS DURING THE PREOPERATIVE, OPERATIVE AND POSTOPERATIVE PERIODS.
5. BECAUSE OF THE DOSE-RELATED NEPHROTOXICITY POTENTIAL OF PENTHRANE (METHOXYFLURANE, USP), IT IS SUGGESTED THAT THE TOTAL DURATION OF LIGHT ANESTHETIC DEPTH WITH PENTHRANE NOT EXCEED APPROXIMATELY 4 HOURS AT A SINGLE ADMINISTRATION.

Precautions: Diabetic patients may have an increased likelihood of developing nephropathy if they have impaired renal function or polyuria, are obese, or are not optimally controlled.
Caution should be exercised in using PENTHRANE in patients under treatment with enzyme inducing drugs (e.g., barbiturates) as such agents may enhance the metabolism of PENTHRANE, resulting in increased fluoride levels. Ventilation should be assessed carefully and, if depressed, should be augmented to insure adequate oxygenation and carbon dioxide removal. Parenteral anesthetic adjuncts (e.g., barbiturates, narcotics and neuromuscular blocking agents) may also cause depression of respiration requiring assisted or controlled ventilation. A sufficient reduction in respiratory minute volume occurs during deep anesthesia to produce a significant respiratory acidosis if ventilation is not adequately assisted. PENTHRANE causes a slight metabolic acidosis.
PENTHRANE augments the effect of nondepolarizing muscle relaxants so that their usual dosage should be reduced by approximately one-half.
Epinephrine or levarterenol (norepinephrine) should be employed cautiously during PENTHRANE anesthesia.
When PENTHRANE is used under the conditions of dosage and administration shown below, in surgery or obstetrics, inorganic fluoride levels may infrequently reach those at which changes in renal laboratory values have been seen.
General anesthesia, including general anesthesia with PENTHRANE (Methoxyflurane, USP), has been associated in susceptible individuals with the acute onset of fulminant hypermetabolism of skeletal muscle known as *malignant hyperthermic crisis*. This syndrome is characterized by the acute onset of skeletal muscle overactivity and resulting high oxygen demand which usually exceeds supply. TACHYCARDIA and TACHYPNEA are the most important early signs; these may be associated with increased utilization of anesthesia circuit carbon dioxide absorber, arrhythmias, cyanosis, skin mottling, profuse sweating, unstable blood pressure, rapidly rising body temperature (usually appearing sometime after the first signs, when noted) and other indications of markedly increased oxygen demand. Laboratory tests usually confirm the excessive oxygen demand and resulting metabolic acidosis (blood gases); hyperkalemia and myoglobinemia are also frequently noted. Hypoglobinuria and renal failure may develop later. When these signs suggests a diagnosis of malignant hyperthermic crisis, it is important to terminate the anesthetic, cancel the surgery when possible, confirm the diagnosis and initiate management of the condition.
Dantrolene sodium intravenous is indicated, along with supportive measures, in the management of malignant hyperthermic crisis. These necessary supportive measures must be individualized, but will usually involve discontinuance of the suspect triggering agents, attendance to increased oxygen requirements and carbon dioxide production, management of metabolic acidosis, assurance of adequate urinary output, management of electrolyte imbalance and institution of measures to control rising temperature, when indicated. Consult literature references and the prescribing information for dantrolene sodium intravenous for additional information about the management of malignant hyperthermic crisis.
Information for patients:
When appropriate, as in some cases where discharge is anticipated soon after methoxyflurane anesthesia, patients should be cautioned not to drive an automobile, operate hazardous machinery or engage in hazardous sports for 24 hours or more (depending upon total dosage of methoxyflurane, condition of the patient and consideration given to other drugs administered) after anesthesia.
Carcinogenesis, mutagenesis, impairment of fertility:
A 15 month transplacental inhalation study of methoxyflurane at a subanesthetic concentration of 0.13% in the mouse revealed no evidence of anesthetic-related carcinogenesis. This concentration is equivalent to 36 hours of 0.2% methoxyflurane.
Mutagenesis testing of methoxyflurane was negative. Tests included: Ames bacterial assay, mouse sperm morphology assay and sister chromated exchange in Chinese hamster ovary cells.
Studies of the effect on fertility have not been reported.
Pregnancy Category C: Methoxyflurane has been shown to cause fetal growth retardation in the rat at levels equivalent to 67 hours exposure of 0.2% methoxyflurane. There are no adequate and well-controlled studies in pregnant women. Methoxyflurane should be used during pregnancy only if the potential benefit justifies the potential risk to the fetus.
Nursing Mothers: Caution should be exercised when PENTHRANE (Methoxyflurane, USP) is administered to a nursing mother.
Labor and Delivery: In obstetrics attention should be given to the directions for Dosage and Administration shown below. Fluoride levels in cord blood are usually less than, but may equal those of the mother at delivery. The effect of inorganic fluoride on the infant is not known. However, clinical experience has demonstrated that cases of high output renal failure in either mother or child must be considered unlikely.
Pediatric Use: Safety and effectiveness of PENTHRANE (Methoxyflurane, USP) in children have not been established.
Adverse Reactions: Renal dysfunction: See WARNINGS.
Hepatic dysfunction, jaundice, and fatal hepatic necrosis have occurred following PENTHRANE anesthesia. Also as with other anesthetics, transient alterations in liver function tests may follow PENTHRANE administration. Hepatic complications rarely have involved reported cross reactions between PENTHRANE and Halothane.
Some patients exhibity pallor during recovery from PENTHRANE anesthesia.
Other adverse reactions which have been reported include cardiac arrest, malignant hyperpyrexia, prolonged postoperative somnolence, respiratory depression laryngospasm, bronchospasm, nausea, vomiting postoperative headache, hypotension and emergence delirium.
Overdosage: Patients should be closely observed for signs of excessive dosage during administration of PENTHRANE. PENTHRANE overdosage is characterized by decrease in tidal and minute volume; decrease in blood pressure, pallor, cyanosis and muscle relaxation. If the above signs are observed, turn off vaporizer and increase ventilation. If anesthesia exceeds light levels, vapor concentration should be reduced promptly. Prolonged administration (beyond four hours) and/or excessive vapor concentration beyond the equivalent of four hours of 0.25% delivered methoxyflurane may cause nephrotoxic effects attributable to metabolic release of free fluoride ion. See WARNINGS, PRECAUTIONS and DOSAGE AND ADMINISTRATION.
In the event of postoperative excessive urine output, fluid and electrolyte losses should be promptly replaced.
Dosage and Administration: THE LOWEST EFFECTIVE DOSAGE OF PENTHRANE (METHOXYFLURANE, USP) SHOULD BE USED IN ORDER TO MINIMIZE THE POSSIBILITY OF NEPHROPATHY AND TO ALLOW FOR OPTIMAL RECOVERY TIME. IN CASES OF UNUSUALLY HIGH MAINTENANCE REQUIREMENTS, THE USE OF ANESTHETIC ADJUNCTS OR ANOTHER AGENT MAY BE INDICATED. THE ABSENCE OF HYPOTENSION CANNOT BE RELIED UPON AS EVIDENCE

Continued on next page

If desired, additional literature on any Abbott Product will be provided upon request to Abbott Laboratories.

Abbott—Cont.

THAT DOSAGE HAS NOT BEEN EXCESSIVE DURING MAINTENANCE.

Analgesia
For analgesia, intermittent inhalation of vapor concentrations in the range of 0.3 to 0.8% are recommended. PENTHRANE may be self administered by hand held inhalers (e.g., Analgizer, Cyprane) if the patient is kept under close observation.

For intermittent administration from the hand-held inhaler, dosage for each patient is limited to not more than a single 15 ml charge of liquid PENTHRANE. Such analgesia in labor should not be instituted before relief becomes necessary. Use of the hand-held inhaler does not preclude transfer of the patient to a conventional anesthesia machine for inhalation anesthesia, but concentrations should be kept at the lowest effective dosage. Total time for anesthesia combined with analgesia should be as short as possible, bearing in mind the recommended duration for continuous anesthesia (four hours).

Anesthesia
A light level of anesthesia should be used. The use of deeper levels to achieve muscle relaxation should be avoided.

Apparatus: PENTHRANE should be vaporized by calibrated, temperature compensated, out of circle vaporizers (e.g., Pentec II, Pentomatic) or other methods which provide accurate delivered vapor concentration. Anesthetic uptake by rubber tubing, bags and soda lime which may prolong induction and recovery time can be reduced by the use of nonabsorptive plastic circuit material (not polyvinyl chloride) and fresh moist Baralyme. The fresh gas inlet should be located downstream of the CO_2 absorber in order to avoid excessive anesthetic absorption, and the rebreathing bag and pop-off valve should be located on the expiratory side.

Premedication: The usual preanesthetic medications may be administered prior to PENTHRANE (Methoxyflurane, USP) anesthesia, see PRECAUTIONS.

Induction: Use of a parenteral induction agent (such as an ultra-short acting barbiturate) is recommended unless contraindicated in an individual patient.

Carrier Gases: For general surgery, PENTHRANE should usually be administered with a carrier gas flow consisting of oxygen and at least 50% nitrous oxide in order to minimize the total PENTHRANE dose unless nitrous oxide is contraindicated.

Muscle Relaxation: PENTHRANE should not be administered at levels required to achieve muscle relaxation. Adequate relaxation should be obtained from adjunctive use of a muscle relaxant, e.g., succinylcholine chloride (Quelicin®) or tubocurarine chloride. The usual dosage of nondepolarizing muscle relaxants should be reduced by approximately one-half.

Vapor Concentrations: Initially PENTHRANE concentrations may be increased as tolerated to a maximum of approximately 2.0%. This concentration should only be continued for about two to five minutes, or until patient signs of light anesthesia are evident. The concentration of PENTHRANE should then be reduced by frequent decrements to the lowest possible levels consistent with the maintenance of adequate anesthesia. For example, in a 70 kg patient, the following sequential reduction in the delivered vapor concentration of PENTHRANE (Methoxyflurane, USP) may be appropriate:

Elapsed Minutes				
0 to 5	5 to 20	20 to 60	60 to 120	120 to 240

Vapor Conc.*				
2.0%	0.6%	0.4%	0.2%	0.1%

* Concentrations are approximate and subject to adjustment according to patient signs of anesthesia. Based on 5 liters per minute gas flow and ventilation rate throughout procedure, 50/50 N_2O and oxygen.

Concentration may be increased or decreased according to the requirements of the individual patient. Four hours of 0.25% delivered methoxyflurane should not be exceeded in normal adult patients unless, in the opinion of the clinician, the anticipated benefits outweigh the increased risk of dose related nephrotoxicity. The product of these two factors (four hours of 0.25% delivered methoxyflurane) may be used to estimate other combinations of time and dose: Thus two hours of 0.5%, for example, should not ordinarily be exceeded. In sufficiently long cases, PENTHRANE should be discontinued 30 to 40 minutes before the end of surgery. Rapid flushing will not remove PENTHRANE absorbed by rubber circuit components.

Patient signs and levels: The PENTHRANE level of conscious analgesia is suited for pain relief, as in labor and uncomplicated vaginal deliveries. The level of unconscious analgesia is suitable for many minor surgical procedures. The level of light anesthesia is recommended for general surgical use. Deep anesthesia with PENTHRANE (Methoxyflurane, USP) is not recommended.

Appropriate patient signs of PENTHRANE anesthesia should be observed closely as a guide to proper depth. A blood pressure decrease of about 22 mm Hg may be seen during induction. A greater decrease may occur in hypertensive patients. Blood pressure usually recovers as a level of light anesthesia is reached. The absence of hypotension cannot be relied upon as evidence that dosage has not been excessive during maintenance.

How Supplied: PENTHRANE (Methoxyflurane, USP) is supplied in 125 and 15 ml bottles, List 6864.

Preserve in tight, light-resistant containers and avoid exposure to excessive heat.

Protect from light. Protect from freezing and extreme heat.

Caution: Federal (USA) law prohibits dispensing without prescription.
06-3179-R26-3/82
Marketed by
Abbott Laboratories

PENTOTHAL®
[pen'tō-thal]
(thiopental sodium for injection, USP)

WARNING: MAY BE HABIT FORMING.

Description: Pentothal (Thiopental Sodium for Injection, USP) is a thiobarbiturate, the sulfur analogue of sodium pentobarbital.

The drug is prepared as a sterile powder and after reconstitution with an appropriate diluent is administered by the intravenous route.

Pentothal is chemically designated sodium 5-ethyl-5-(1-methylbutyl)-2-thiobarbiturate and has the following structural formula:

The drug is a yellowish, hygroscopic powder, stabilized with anhydrous sodium carbonate as a buffer (60 mg/g of thiopental sodium).

Clinical Pharmacology: Pentothal (Thiopental Sodium for Injection, USP) is an ultrashort-acting depressant of the central nervous system which induces hypnosis and anesthesia, but not analgesia. It produces hypnosis within 30 to 40 seconds of intravenous injection. Recovery after a small dose is rapid, with some somnolence and retrograde amnesia. Repeated intravenous doses lead to prolonged anesthesia because fatty tissues act as a reservoir; they accumulate Pentothal in concentrations 6 to 12 times greater than the plasma concentration, and then release the drug slowly to cause prolonged anesthesia.

The half-life of the elimination phase after a single intravenous dose is three to eight hours.

The distribution and fate of Pentothal (as with other barbiturates) is influenced chiefly by its lipid solubility (partition coefficient), protein binding and extent of ionization. Pentothal has a partition coefficient of 580.

Approximately 80% of the drug in the blood is bound to plasma protein. Pentothal is largely degraded in the liver and to a smaller extent in other tissues, especially the kidney and brain. It has a pk_a of 7.4.

Concentration in spinal fluid is slightly less than in the plasma.

Biotransformation products of thiopental are pharmacologically inactive and mostly excreted in the urine.

Indications and Usage: Pentothal (Thiopental Sodium for Injection, USP) is indicated (1) as the sole anesthetic agent for brief (15 minute) procedures, (2) for induction of anesthesia prior to administration of other anesthetic agents, (3) to supplement regional anesthesia, (4) to provide hypnosis during balanced anesthesia with other agents for analgesia or muscle relaxation, (5) for the control of convulsive states during or following inhalation anesthesia, local anesthesia, or other causes, (6) in neurosurgical patients with increased intracranial pressure, if adequate ventilation is provided, and (7) for narcoanalysis and narcosynthesis in psychiatric disorders.

Contraindications:

Absolute Contraindications:
(1) Absence of suitable veins for intravenous administration,
(2) hypersensitivity (allergy) to barbiturates, (3) status asthmaticus, and (4) latent or manifest porphyria.

Relative Contraindications:
(1) Severe cardiovascular disease, (2) hypotension or shock, (3) conditions in which the hypnotic effect may be prolonged or potentiated — excessive premedication, Addison's disease, hepatic or renal dysfunction, myxedema, increased blood urea, severe anemia, asthma and myasthenia gravis.

Warnings: KEEP RESUSCITATIVE AND ENDOTRACHEAL INTUBATION EQUIPMENT AND OXYGEN READILY AVAILABLE. MAINTAIN PATENCY OF THE AIRWAY AT ALL TIMES.

This drug should be administered only by persons qualified in the use of intravenous anesthetics.

Avoid extravasation or intra-arterial injection.

WARNING: MAY BE HABIT FORMING.

Precautions: Observe aseptic precautions at all times in preparation and handling of Pentothal (Thiopental Sodium for Injection, USP) solutions. If used in conditions involving relative contraindications, reduce dosage and administer slowly.

Care should be taken in administering the drug to patients with advanced cardiac disease, increased intracranial pressure, asthma, myasthenia gravis and endocrine insufficiency (pituitary, thyroid, adrenal, pancreas).

Nursing Mothers: Thiopental sodium readily crosses the placental barrier and small amounts may appear in the milk of nursing mothers following administration of large doses.

Pregnancy Category C. Animal reproduction studies have not been conducted with Pentothal. It is also not known whether Pentothal can cause fetal harm when administered to a pregnant woman or can affect reproduction capacity. Pentothal should be given to a pregnant woman only if clearly needed.

Adverse Reactions: Adverse reactions include respiratory depression, myocardial depression, cardiac arrhythmias, prolonged somnolence and recovery, sneezing, coughing, bronchospasm, laryngospasm and shivering. Hypersensitivity reactions to barbiturates, including Pentothal (Thiopental Sodium for Injection, USP), have been reported.

Drug Abuse and Dependence:
WARNING: MAY BE HABIT FORMING. Thiopental sodium is classified as a Schedule III controlled substance.

Overdosage: Overdosage may occur from too rapid or repeated injections. Too rapid injection may be followed by an alarming fall in blood pressure even to shock levels. Apnea, occasional laryngospasm, coughing and other respiratory difficulties with excessive or too rapid injections may occur. In the event of suspected or apparent overdosage, the drug should be discontinued, a patent airway established (intubate if necessary) or maintained, and oxygen should be administered, with assisted ventilation if necessary. The lethal dose of barbiturates varies and cannot be stated with certainty. Lethal blood levels may be as low as 1 mg/100 ml for short-acting barbiturates; less if other depressant drugs or alcohol are also present.

Dosage and Administration: Pentothal (Thiopental Sodium for Injection, USP) is administered by the intravenous route only. Individual response to the drug is so varied that there can be no fixed dosage. The drug should be titrated against patient requirements as governed by age, sex and body weight. Younger patients require relatively larger doses than middle-aged and elderly persons; the latter metabolize the drug more slowly. Prepuberty requirements are the same for both sexes, but adult females require less than adult-males. Dose is usually proportional to body weight and obese patients require a larger dose than relatively lean persons of the same weight.

Premedication
Premedication usually consists of atropine or scopolamine to suppress vagal reflexes and inhibit secretions. In addition, a barbiturate or an opiate is often given. Sodium pentobarbital injection (Nembutal®) is suggested because it provides a preliminary indication of how the patient will react to barbiturate anesthesia. Ideally, the peak effect of these medications should be reached shortly before the time of induction.

Test Dose
It is advisable to inject a small "test" dose of 25 to 75 mg (1 to 3 ml of a 2.5% solution) of Pentothal (Thiopental Sodium for Injection, USP) to assess tolerance or unusual sensitivity to Pentothal, and pausing to observe patient reaction for at least 60 seconds. If unexpectedly deep anesthesia develops or if respiratory depression occurs, consider these possibilities: (1) the patient may be unusually sensitive to Pentothal, (2) the solution may be more concentrated than had been assumed, or (3) the patient may have received too much premedication.

Use in Anesthesia
Moderately slow induction can usually be accomplished in the "average" adult by injection of 50 to 75 mg (2 to 3 ml of a 2.5% solution) at intervals of 20 to 40 seconds, depending on the reaction of the patient. Once anesthesia is established, additional injections of 25 to 50 mg can be given whenever the patient moves.

Slow injection is recommended to minimize respiratory depression and the possibility of overdosage. The smallest dose consistent with attaining the surgical objective is the desired goal. Momentary apnea following each injection is typical, and progressive decrease in the amplitude of respiration appears with increasing dosage. Pulse remains normal or increases slightly and returns to normal. Blood pressure usually falls slightly but returns toward normal. Muscles usually relax about 30 seconds after unconsciousness is attained, but this may be masked if a skeletal muscle relaxant is used. The tone of jaw muscles is a fairly reliable index. The pupils may dilate but later contract; sensitivity to light is not usually lost until a level of anesthesia deep enough to permit surgery is attained. Nystagmus and divergent strabismus are characteristic during early stages, but at the level of surgical anesthesia, the eyes are central and fixed. Corneal and conjunctival reflexes disappear during surgical anesthesia.

When Pentothal (Thiopental Sodium for Injection, USP) is used for induction in balanced anesthesia with a skeletal muscle relaxant and an inhalation agent, the total dose of Pentothal can be estimated and then injected in two to four fractional doses. With this technique, brief periods of apnea may occur which may require assisted or controlled pulmonary ventilation. As an initial dose, 210 to 280 mg (3 to 4 mg/kg) of Pentothal is usually required for rapid induction in the average adult (70 kg).

When Pentothal (Thiopental Sodium for Injection, USP) is used as the sole anesthetic agent, the desired level of anesthesia can be maintained by injection of small repeated doses as needed or by using a continuous intravenous drip in a 0.2% or 0.4% concentration. (Sterile water should not be used as the diluent in these concentrations, since hemolysis will occur). With continuous drip, the depth of anesthesia is controlled by adjusting the rate of infusion.

Use in Convulsive States
For the control of convulsive states following anesthesia (inhalation or local) or other causes, 75 to 125 mg (3 to 5 ml of a 2.5% solution) should be given as soon as possible after the convulsion begins. Convulsions following the use of a local anesthetic may require 125 to 250 mg of Pentothal (Thiopental Sodium for Injection), given over a ten minute period. If the convulsion is caused by a local anesthetic, the required dose of Pentothal will depend upon the amount of local anesthetic given and its convulsant properties.

Use in Neurosurgical Patients with Increased Intracranial Pressure
In neurosurgical patients, intermittent bolus injections of 1.5 to 3.5 mg/kg of body weight may be given to reduce intraoperative elevations of intracranial pressure, if adequate ventilation is provided.

Use in Psychiatric Disorders
For narcoanalysis and narcosynthesis in psychiatric disorders, premedication with an anticholinergic agent may precede administration of Pentothal. After a test dose, Pentothal is injected at a slow rate of 100 mg/min (4 ml/min of a 2.5% solution) with the patient counting backwards from 100. Shortly after counting becomes confused but before actual sleep is produced, the injection is discontinued. Allow the patient to return to a semidrowsy state where conversation is coherent. Alternatively, Pentothal (Thiopental Sodium for Injection, USP) may be administered by rapid I.V. drip using a 0.2% concentration in 5% dextrose and water. At this concentration, the rate of administration should not exceed 50 ml/min.

Management of Some Complications: *Respiratory depression* (hypoventilation, apnea), which may result from either unusual responsiveness to Pentothal (Thiopental Sodium for Injection, USP) or overdosage, is managed as stated above. Pentothal should be considered to have the same potential for producing respiratory depression as an inhalation agent, and patency of the airway must be protected at all times.

Laryngospasm may occur with light Pentothal narcosis at intubation, or in the absence of intubation if foreign matter or secretions in the respiratory tract create irritation. Laryngeal and bronchial vagal reflexes can be suppressed, and secretions minimized by giving atropine or scopolamine premedication and a barbiturate or opiate. Use of a skeletal muscle relaxant or positive pressure oxygen will usually relieve laryngospasm. Tracheostomy may be indicated in difficult cases.

Myocardial depression, proportioned to the amount of drug in direct contact with the heart, can occur and may cause hypotension, particularly in patients with an unhealthy myocardium. Arrhythmias may appear if P_{CO_2} is elevated, but they are uncommon with adequate ventilation. Management of myocardial depression is the same as for overdosage. Pentothal (Thiopental Sodium for Injection, USP) does not sensitize the heart to epinephrine or other sympathomimetic amines.

Extravascular infiltration should be avoided. Care should be taken to insure that the needle is within the lumen of the vein before injection of Pentothal. Extravascular injection may cause chemical irritation of the tissues varying from slight tenderness to venospasm, extensive necrosis and sloughing. This is due primarily to the high alkaline pH (10 to 11) of clinical concentrations of the drug. If extravasation occurs, the local irritant effects can be reduced by injection of 1% procaine locally to relieve pain and enhance vasodilatation. Local application of heat also may help to increase local circulation and removal of the infiltrate.

Intra-arterial injection can occur inadvertently, especially if an aberrant superficial artery is present at the medial aspect of the antecubital fossa. The area selected for intravenous injection of the drug should be palpated for detection of an underlying pulsating vessel. Accidental intra-arterial injection can cause arteriospasm and severe pain along the course of the artery with blanching of the arm and fingers. Appropriate corrective measures should be instituted promptly to avoid possible development of gangrene. Any patient complaint of pain warrants stopping the injection. Methods suggested for dealing with this complication vary with the severity of symptoms. The following have been suggested:

1. Dilute the injected Pentothal (Thiopental Sodium for Injection, USP) by removing the tourniquet and any restrictive garments.
2. Leave the needle in place, if possible.
3. Inject the artery with a dilute solution of papaverine, 40 to 80 mg, or 10 ml of 1% procaine, to inhibit smooth muscle spasm.
4. If necessary, perform sympathetic block of the brachial plexus and/or stellate ganglion to relieve pain and assist in opening collateral circulation. Papaverine can be injected into the subclavian artery, if desired.
5. Unless otherwise contraindicated, institute immediate heparinization to prevent thrombus formation.
6. Consider local infiltration of an alpha-adrenergic blocking agent such as phentolamine into the vasospastic area.
7. Provide additional symptomatic treatment as required.

Shivering after Pentothal anesthesia, manifested by twitching face muscles and occasional progression to tremors of the arms, head, shoulder and body, is a thermal reaction due to increased sensitivity to cold. Shivering appears if the room environment is cold and if a large ventilatory heat loss has been sustained with balanced inhalation anesthesia employing nitrous oxide. Treatment consists of warming the patient with blankets, maintaining room temperature near 22° C (72°F), and administration of chlorpromazine or methylphenidate.

Preparation of Solutions: Pentothal (Thiopental Sodium for Injection, USP) is supplied as a yellowish, hygroscopic powder in a variety of different containers. Solutions should be prepared aseptically with one of the three following diluents. Sterile Water for Injection, USP, Sodium Chloride Injection, USP or 5% Dextrose Injection, USP. Clinical concentrations used for intermittent intravenous administration vary between 2.0% and 5.0%. A 2.0% or 2.5% solution is most commonly used. A 3.4% concentraton in sterile water for injection is isotonic; concentrations less than 2.0% in this diluent are not used because they cause hemolysis. For continuous intravenous drip administration, concentrations of 0.2% or 0.4% are used. Solutions may be prepared by adding Pentothal to 5% Dextrose Injection, USP, Sodium Chloride Injection, USP or Normosol® R pH 7.4. Since Pentothal (Thiopental Sodium for Injection, USP) contains no added bacteriostatic agent, extreme care in preparation and handling should be exercised at all times to prevent the introduction of microbial contaminants. Solutions should be freshly prepared and used promptly; when reconstituted for administration to several patients, unused portions should be discarded after 24

Continued on next page

If desired, additional literature on any Abbott Product will be provided upon request to Abbott Laboratories.

Abbott—Cont.

hours. Sterilization by heating should not be attempted.

Warning: The 2.5 g and larger sizes contain adequate medication for several patients.

Compatibility: Any solution of Pentothal (Thiopental Sodium for Injection, USP) with a visible precipitate should not be administered. The stability of Pentothal solutions depends upon several factors, including the diluent, temperature of storage and the amount of carbon dioxide from room air that gains access to the solution. Any factor or condition which tends to lower pH (increase acidity) of Pentothal solutions will increase the likelihood of precipitation of thiopental acid. Such factors include the use of diluents which are too acid and the absorption of carbon dioxide which can combine with water to form carbonic acid.

Solutions of succinylcholine, tubocurarine or other drugs which have an acid pH should not be mixed with Pentothal solutions. The most stable solutions are those reconstituted in water or isotonic saline, kept under refrigeration and tightly stoppered. The presence or absence of a visible precipitate offers a practical guide to the physical compatibility of prepared solutions of Pentothal (Thiopental Sodium for Injection, USP).

Calculations for Various Concentrations:

Concentration Desired Percent	mg/ml	Amounts to Use Pentothal g	Diluent ml
0.2	2	1	500
0.4	4	1	250
		2	500
2.0	20	5	250
		10	500
2.5	25	1	40
		5	200
5	50	1	20
		5	100

Reconstituted solutions of Pentothal should be inspected visually for particulate matter and discoloration, whenever solution and container permit.

How Supplied: Pentothal (Thiopental Sodium for Injection, USP) is available in a variety of sizes and containers in combination packages with diluent as shown at the end of this insert.

Diluents in Pentothal® Kits
READY-TO-MIX SYRINGES AND VIALS
(For preparing solutions of Thiopental Sodium for Injection, USP)

Description: The following diluents in various container, syringe and vial sizes are provded in Pentothal Kits, Pentothal Ready-to-Mix Syringes and Vials for preparing solutions of Pentothal (Thiopental Sodium for Injection, USP) for clinical use:

Sterile Water for Injection, USP is sterile, nonpyrogenic preparation of water for injection which contains no bacteriostat, antimicrobial agents or added buffers. The pH is 5.7 (approximate).

Sterile Water for Injection, USP is a pharmaceutic aid (solvent) for intravenous administration only after addition of a solute.

Water is chemically designated H_2O.

0.9% Sodium Chloride Injection, USP is a sterile, nonpyrogenic, isotonic solution of sodium chloride and water for injection. Each ml contains sodium chloride 9 mg (308 mOsm/liter calc). It contains no bacteriostat, antimicrobial agents or added buffers except for pH adjustment. May contain hydrochloric acid or sodium hydroxide for pH adjustment. Approximate pH 5.7.

0.9% Sodium Chloride Injection, USP is an isotonic vehicle fo intravenous administration of another solute.

Sodium chloride is chemically designated NaCl, a white crystalline compound freely soluble in water.

The semi-rigid vial contained in List Nos. 3329 and 6435 is fabricated from a specially formulated polyolefin. It is a copolymer of ethylene and propylene. The safety of the plastic has been confirmed by tests in animals according to USP biological standards for plastic containers. The container requires no vapor barrier to maintain the proper labeled volume.

Clinical Pharmacology: Sterile Water for Injection, USP serves only as a pharmaceutic aid for diluting or dissolving drugs prior to administration.

Water is an essential constituent of all body tissues and accounts for approximately 70% of total body weight. Average normal adult daily requirement ranges from two to three liters (1.0 to 1.5 liters each for insensible water loss by perspiration and urine excretion).

Water balance is maintained by various regulatory mechanisms. Water distribution depends primarily on the concentration of dissociated electrolytes in the body compartments and sodium (Na+) plays a major role in maintaining a physiologic equilibrium between fluid intake and output. 0.9% Sodium Chloride Injection, USP serves only as an isotonic vehicle for drugs prior to administration.

Sodium chloride in water is an electrolyte solution of sodium (Na+) and chloride (Cl−) ions. These ions are normal constituents of the body fluids (principally extracellular) and are essential for maintaining electrolyte balance.

The distribution and excretion of sodium (Na+) and chloride (Cl−) are largely under the control of the kidney which maintains a balance between intake and output of these ions.

The small volumes of fluid and amounts of sodium chloride provided by 0.9% Sodium Chloride Injection in Ready-to-Mix Syringes are unlikely to produce a significant effect on fluid or electrolyte balance.

Indications and Usage: These products are indicated only for preparing Pentothal (Thiopental Sodium for Injection, USP) solutions for clinical use.

Contraindications: Do not use unless the diluent is clear and the bottle or vial seal or syringe package is undamaged.

Diluents in Pentothal Kits, Ready-to-Mix Syringes or Vials should not be used for fluid or sodium chloride replacement.

Warnings: Intravenous administration of Sterile Water for Injection, USP without a solute may result in hemolysis.

Protect Kits, Ready-to-Mix Syringes and Vials from freezing and extreme heat or temperatures above 38° C (100° F).

Use aseptic technique for preparing Pentothal (Thiopental Sodium for Injection, USP) solutions when using Pentothal Kits, Syringes or Vials and during withdrawal from reconstituted single or multiple use containers.

Administer only clear reconstituted solutions.

Avoid storing reconstituted solutions at extreme temperatures and use within 24 hours after preparation. Discard unused portions.

Precautions: Inspect reconstituted (mixed) solutions of Pentothal (Thiopental Sodium for Injection, USP) for clarity and freedom from precipitation or discoloration prior to administration.

Use Transfer Label in each Pentothal Kit and affix to container of reconstituted solution to show concentration and time of preparation.

Pregnancy Category C. Animal reproduction studies have not been conducted with sodium chloride. It is also not known whether sodium chloride can cause fetal harm when administered to a pregnant woman or can affect reproduction capacity. Sodium chloride should be given a pregnant woman only if clearly needed.

Adverse Reactions: Reactions which may occur because of the diluents, technique of preparation or mixing, or administration of reconstituted solutions of Pentothal (Thiopental Sodium for Injection, USP) include febrile response or infection at the site of injection, venous thrombosis or phlebitis extending from the site of injection and extravasation.

If an adverse reaction does occur, discontinue the injection, evaluate the patient, institute appropriate therapeutic countermeasures and save the remainder of unused solution (or the used container or syringe) for examination if deemed necessary.

Drug Abuse and Dependence: None known.

Overdosage: Used as diluents for preparing solutions of Pentothal (Thiopental Sodium for Injection, USP) the small volumes of administered fluid (from Sterile Water for Injection in bottles and vials) and amounts of sodium chloride (from 0.9% Sodium Chloride Injection in Ready-to-Mix Syringes) are unlikely to pose a threat of fluid or sodium chloride overload.

Dosage and Administration: Pentothal (Thiopental Sodium for Injection, USP) solutions should be administered only by intravenous injection and by individuals experienced in the conduct of intravenous anesthesia.

The volume of choice of diluent for preparing Pentothal (Thiopental Sodium for Injection, USP) solutions for clinical use depends on the concentration and vehicle desired. Pentothal Kits provide only Sterile Water for Injection as the diluent for individual or multi-patient use; Pentothal Ready-to-Mix Syringes provide only 0.9% Sodium Chloride Injection, USP as the diluent for individual patient use; vials provide only Sterile Water for Injection, USP as the diluent for individual patient use.

Parenteral drug products should be inspected visually for particulate matter and discoloration prior to administration, whenever solution and container permit. See PRECAUTIONS.

How Supplied: The diluent in Pentothal Kits is supplied in various size partial-fill glass containers with various dosage sizes of Pentothal (Thiopental Sodium for Injection, USP). Kits include all items needed for aseptic transfer of Pentothal powder from a squeeze bottle into the diluent partial-fill container.

The diluent in Pentothal Ready-to-Mix Syringes is supplied in a separate vial injector to permit intrasyringe mixing with the Pentothal in a powder vial which is then removed to permit immediate intravenous injection of reconstituted solution into a vein or attachment to a standard stopcock assembly.

Vials are supplied in cartons with different dosage sizes of Pentothal (Thiopental Sodium for Injection, USP) for preparing 2.0% or 2.5% concentrations by using a separate syringe (not supplied) for mixing.

See attached table for list of sizes available.
[See table on next page].

Exposure of pharmaceutical products to heat should be minimized. Avoid excessive heat. Protect from freezing. It is recommended that the product be stored at room temperature (25° C); however, brief exposure up to 40° C does not adversely affect the product.

Keep reconstituted solution in a cool place.

Caution: Federal (USA) law prohibits dispensing without prescription.
06-3485-R2-2/84

PHENURONE® ℞
[fĕn´ū-rōne]
(phenacemide tablets, USP)

Description: PHENURONE (phenacemide) is a valuable antiepileptic drug for use in selected patients with epilepsy. Since therapy with PHENURONE involves certain risks, *physicians should thoroughly familiarize themselves with the undesirable side effects which may occur and the precautions to be observed.* PHENURONE (phenacemide) is a substituted acetylurea derivative. Chemically PHENURONE is identified as N-(aminocarbonyl)-benzeneacetamide. PHENURONE tablets contain 500 mg phenacemide for oral administration.

Clinical Pharmacology: In experimental animals, PHENURONE in doses well below those causing neurological signs, elevates the threshold for minimal electroshock convulsions and abolishes the tonic phase of maximal electroshock seizures. The drug prevents or modifies seizures induced by pentylenetetrazol or other convulsants. In comparative tests, PHENURONE was found to be equal or more effective than other commonly used antiepileptics against complex partial (psychomotor) seizures which were induced in mice by low frequency stimulation of the cerebral cortex. Studies in mice have shown that PHENURONE exerts a synergistic antiepileptic effect with mephenytoin, phenobarbital, or trimethadione.

Given orally to laboratory animals, PHENURONE has a low acute toxicity. In mice, slight ataxia appears at 400 mg/kg and light sleep occurs at 800 mg/kg. In high doses the drug causes marked ataxia and coma, the fatal dose being in the range of 3 to 5 g/kg for mice, rats, and cats.

PHENURONE is metabolized by the liver, however, further definition of human pharmacokinetics has not been determined.

Indications and Usage: PHENURONE (phenacemide) is indicated for the control of severe epilepsy, particularly mixed forms of complex partial (psychomotor) seizures, refractory to other drugs.

Contraindications: PHENURONE should not be administered unless other available antiepileptics have been found to be ineffective in satisfactorily controlling seizures.

Warnings: PHENURONE (phenacemide) can produce serious side effects as well as direct organ toxicity. As a consequence its use entails the assumption of certain risks which must be weighed against the benefit to the patient. *Ordinarily* PHENURONE *should not be administered unless other available antiepileptics have been found to be ineffective in controlling seizures.*

Death attributable to liver damage during therapy with PHENURONE has been reported. PHENURONE should be used with caution in patients with a history of previous liver dysfunction. If jaundice or other signs of hepatitis appear, the drug should be discontinued.

Aplastic anemia has occurred in association with PHENURONE therapy and death from this condition has been reported. PHENURONE should ordinarily not be used in patients with severe blood dyscrasias. Marked depression of the blood count is an indication for withdrawal of the drug.

Usage During Pregnancy: PHENURONE can cause fetal harm when administered to a pregnant woman. There are multiple reports in the clinical literature which indicate that the use of antiepileptic drugs during pregnancy results in an increased incidence of birth defects in the offspring. Reports have also suggested that the maternal ingestion of antiepileptic drugs, particularly barbiturates, is associated with a neonatal coagulation defect that may cause bleeding during the early (usually within 24 hours of birth) neonatal period. The possibility of the occurrence of this defect with the use of PHENURONE should be kept in mind. The defect is characterized by decreased levels of vitamin K-dependent clotting factors, and prolongation of either the prothrombin time or the partial thromboplastin time, or both. It has been suggested that vitamin K be given prophylactically to the mother one month prior to and during delivery, and to the infant, intravenously, immediately after birth. If this drug is used during pregnancy, or if the patient becomes pregnant while taking this drug, the patient should be apprised of the potential hazard to the fetus.

Precautions: *General:* Extreme caution must be exercised in treating patients who previously have shown personality disorders. It may be advisable to hospitalize such patients during the first week of treatment. Personality changes, including attempts at suicide and the occurrence of psychoses requiring hospitalization, have been reported during therapy with PHENURONE (phenacemide). Severe or exacerbated personality changes are an indication for withdrawal of the drug.

PHENURONE (phenacemide) should be used with caution in patients with a history of previous liver dysfunction.

PHENURONE should be administered with caution to patients with a history of allergy, particularly in association with the administration of other antiepileptics. The drug should be discontinued at the first sign of a skin rash or other allergic manifestation.

Pentothal® and Diluent in Kits, Ready-to-Mix Syringes and Vials

List No.	Pentothal	Pentothal Container	Diluent (ml)	Diluent Container	Reconstituted Conc. (%)
6259	2.5 g	Squeeze Bottle	W (125)	PF Bottle	2.0
6108	5.0 g	Squeeze Bottle	W (250)	PF Bottle	2.0
6244	1.0 g	Squeeze Bottle	W (40)	PF Bottle	2.5
6260	2.5 g	Squeeze Bottle	W (100)	PF Bottle	2.5
6504	5.0 g	Squeeze Bottle	W (200)	PF Bottle	2.5
6435	1.0 g	Vial	W (50)	Plastic Vial	2.0
3329	500 mg	Vial	W (20)	Plastic Vial	2.5
6246	400 mg	Syringe	S (20)	Syringe	2.0
6241	250 mg	Syringe	S (10)	Syringe	2.5
6243	500 mg	Syringe	S (20)	Syringe	2.5

PF — denotes Partial Fill
W — denotes Sterile Water for Injection, USP
S — denotes 0.9% Sodium Chloride Injection, USP

Information for Patients: The patient and his family should be aware of the possibility of personality changes so the family can watch for changes in the behavior of the patient such as decreased interest in surroundings, depression, or aggressiveness.

The patient should be told to report immediately any symptoms indicative of a developing blood dyscrasia such as malaise, sore throat, or fever.

Laboratory Tests: Liver function tests should be performed before and during therapy. Death attributable to liver damage during therapy with PHENURONE has been reported. If jaundice or other signs of hepatitis appear, the drug should be discontinued.

Complete blood counts should be made before instituting PHENURONE, and at monthly intervals thereafter. If no abnormality appears within 12 months, the interval between blood counts may be extended. Blood changes have been reported with leukopenia (leukocyte count of 4,000 or less per cubic millimeter of blood) as the most commonly observed effect. However, aplastic anemia has occurred in association with PHENURONE therapy, and death from this condition has been reported. *The total number of each cellular element per cubic millimeter is a better index of possible blood dyscrasia than the percentage of cells.* Marked depression of the blood count is an indication for withdrawal of the drug.

Similarly, as nephritis has occasionally occurred in patients on PHENURONE, the urine should be examined at regular intervals. Abnormal urinary findings are an indication for discontinuance of therapy.

Drug Interactions: Extreme caution is essential if PHENURONE is administered with any other antiepileptic which is known to cause similar toxic effects.

Considerable caution should be exercised if PHENURONE (phenacemide) is administered concurrently with *Peganone (ethotoin)* since paranoid symptoms have been reported during therapy with this combination.

Carcinogenesis: No data are available on long-term potential for carcinogenicity in animals or humans.

Pregnancy: Pregnancy Category D. See "Warnings" section.

Nursing Mothers: It is not known whether this drug is excreted in human milk. Because many drugs are excreted in human milk and because of the potential for serious adverse reactions in nursing infants from PHENURONE, a decision should be made whether to discontinue nursing or to discontinue the drug, taking into account the importance of the drug to the mother.

Pediatric Use: Safety and effectiveness in children below the age of 5 years have not been established.

Adverse Reactions: The following adverse effects associated with PHENURONE are listed by decreasing order of frequency based on data from one large clinical study.[1]

Psychiatric: Psychic changes (17 in 100 patients).
Gastrointestinal: Gastrointestinal disturbances (8 in 100 patients), including anorexia (5 in 100 patients) and weight loss (less than 1 in 100 patients).
Dermatologic: Skin rash (5 in 100 patients).
CNS: Drowsiness (4 in 100 patients), headache (2 in 100 patients), insomnia (1 in 100 patients), dizziness and paresthesias (less than 1 in 100 patients).
Hematopoietic: Blood dyscrasias (primarily leukopenia), including fatal aplastic anemia (2 in 100 patients).
Hepatic: Hepatitis, including fatalities (2 in 100 patients).
Renal: Abnormal urinary findings, including a rise in serum creatinine[2], and nephritis (1 in 100 patients or less).
Other: Fatigue, fever, muscle pain and palpitation (less than 1 in 100 patients).

Overdosage: Symptoms of acute overdosage include excitement or mania, followed by drowsiness, ataxia and coma. In one case of acute overdosage, dizziness was followed by coma which lasted nearly 24 hours. Treatment should be started by inducing emesis; gastric lavage may be considered as an alternative or adjunct. General supportive measures will be necessary. A careful evaluation of liver and kidney function, mental state, and the blood-forming organs should be made following recovery.

Dosage and Administration: PHENURONE is administered orally.

Since PHENURONE may produce serious toxic effects, it is strongly recommended that the dosage be held to the minimum amount necessary to achieve an adequate therapeutic effect.

For adults the usual starting dose is 1.5 g daily, administered in three divided doses of 500 mg each. After the first week, if seizures are not controlled and the drug is well tolerated, an additional 500 mg tablet may be taken upon arising. In the third week, if necessary, the dosage may be further increased by another 500 mg at bedtime. Satisfactory results have been noted in some patients on an initial dose of 250 mg three times per day. The effective total daily dose for adults usually ranges from 2 to 3 g, although some patients have required as much as 5 g daily.

For the pediatric patient from 5 to 10 years of age, approximately one-half the adult dose is recommended. It should be given at the same intervals as for adults.

PHENURONE may be administered alone or in conjunction with other antiepileptics. However, extreme caution must be exercised if other antiepileptics cause toxic effects similar to PHENURONE. When PHENURONE is to replace other antiepileptic medication, the latter should be withdrawn gradually as the dosage of PHENURONE is increased to maintain seizure control.

How Supplied: PHENURONE (Phenacemide Tablets, USP), grooved, white, 500 mg are supplied in bottles of 100 (**NDC 0074-3971-05**).

Continued on next page

If desired, additional literature on any Abbott Product will be provided upon request to Abbott Laboratories.

Abbott—Cont.

References:
1. Tyler, M. W., King, E. Q.: Phenacemide in Treatment of Epilepsy. JAMA 147: 17-21 (1951).
2. Richards, R.K., Bjornsson, T. D., Waterbury, L. D.: Rise in Serum and Urine Creatinine After Phenacemide. Clin. Pharmacol. Ther. 23: 430-437 (1978).

Abbott Laboratories
North Chicago, IL 60064
Ref. 01-2238-R7

PLACIDYL® ℞ ©
[pla'ci-dil]
(ethchlorvynol capsules, USP)
Oral hypnotic

Description: PLACIDYL (ethchlorvynol) is a tertiary carbinol. It is chemically designated as 1-chloro-3-ethyl-1-penten-4-yn-3-ol. Ethchlorvynol occurs as a liquid which is immiscible with water and miscible with most organic solvents. PLACIDYL is an oral hypnotic available in capsule form containing either 100 mg, 200 mg, 500 mg or 750 mg of ethchlorvynol.

Clinical Pharmacology: The usual hypnotic dose of PLACIDYL induces sleep within 15 minutes to one hour. The duration of the hypnotic effect is about five hours. The mechanism of action is unknown. PLACIDYL is rapidly absorbed from the gastrointestinal tract with peak plasma concentrations usually occurring within two hours after a single oral fasting dose. Plasma concentrations required for hypnotic effects are unknown. The plasma half-life (t½, β) of the parent compound is approximately ten to twenty hours. Studies with ^{14}C-PLACIDYL have demonstrated that within 24 hours, 33% of a single 500 mg dose is excreted in the urine mostly as metabolites. The major plasma and urinary metabolite is the secondary alcohol of PLACIDYL. The free and conjugated forms of this metabolite in the urine account for about 40% of the dose. Other minor metabolites have been identified as the primary alcohol and a secondary alcohol with an altered acetylene group. Studies with ^{14}C-PLACIDYL in animals indicate that the parent compound and its metabolites undergo extensive enterohepatic recirculation.

Distribution studies indicate that there is extensive tissue localization of ethchlorvynol, particularly in adipose tissue. Ethchlorvynol and/or its metabolites have also been detected in liver, kidneys, spleen, brain, bile and cerebrospinal fluid.

Indications and Usage: PLACIDYL is indicated as short-term hypnotic therapy for periods up to one week in duration for the management of insomnia. If retreatment becomes necessary, after drug-free intervals of one or more weeks, it should only be undertaken upon further evaluation of the patient.

Contraindications: PLACIDYL is contraindicated in patients with known hypersensitivity to the drug and in patients with porphyria.

Warnings: PLACIDYL SHOULD BE ADMINISTERED WITH CAUTION IN MENTALLY DEPRESSED PATIENTS WITH OR WITHOUT SUICIDAL TENDENCIES. IT SHOULD ALSO BE ADMINISTERED WITH CAUTION TO THOSE WHO HAVE A PSYCHOLOGICAL POTENTIAL FOR DRUG DEPENDENCE. THE LEAST AMOUNT OF DRUG THAT IS FEASIBLE SHOULD BE PRESCRIBED FOR THESE PATIENTS.

Psychological and Physical Dependence: PROLONGED USE OF PLACIDYL MAY RESULT IN TOLERANCE AND PSYCHOLOGICAL AND PHYSICAL DEPENDENCE. PROLONGED ADMINISTRATION OF THE DRUG IS NOT RECOMMENDED. (See "Drug Abuse and Dependence" section.)

Precautions: *General:* Elderly or debilitated patients should receive the smallest effective amount of PLACIDYL (ethchlorvynol).

Caution should be exercised when treating patients with impaired hepatic or renal function. Patients who exhibit unpredictable behavior, or paradoxical restlessness or excitement in response to barbiturates or alcohol may react in this manner to PLACIDYL.

PLACIDYL should not be used for the management of insomnia in the presence of pain unless insomnia persists after pain is controlled with analgesics.

The 750 mg dosage strength of PLACIDYL contains FD&C Yellow No. 5 (tartrazine) which may cause allergic-type reactions (including bronchial asthma) in certain susceptible individuals. Although the overall incidence of FD&C Yellow No. 5 (tartrazine) sensitivity in the general population is low, it is frequently seen in patients who also have aspirin hypersensitivity.

Information for Patients: The use of ethchlorvynol carries with it an associated risk of psychological and/or physical dependence. The patient should be warned against increasing the dose of the drug without consulting a physician.

Patients should be advised that, for the duration of the effect of PLACIDYL, mental and/or physical abilities required for the performance of potentially hazardous tasks such as the operation of dangerous machinery including motor vehicles, may be impaired.

Patients should be cautioned to avoid the concomitant use of PLACIDYL with alcohol, barbiturates, other CNS depressants, MAO inhibitors.

Drug Interactions: The concomitant use of PLACIDYL with alcohol, barbiturates, other CNS depressants, or MAO inhibitors may produce exaggerated depressant effects.

Ethchlorvynol may cause a decreased prothrombin time response to coumarin anticoagulants; therefore, the dosage of these drugs may require adjustment when therapy with ethchlorvynol is initiated and after it is discontinued.

Transient delirium has been reported with the concomitant use of PLACIDYL and amitriptyline; therefore, PLACIDYL should be administered with caution to patients receiving tricyclic antidepressants.

Carcinogenesis: A study in mice receiving oral doses of PLACIDYL up to 7 times the maximum human daily dose for 22 to 24 months produced equivocal results. When compared to controls, a statistically significant increase in total lung tumors was found in female mice given the high dose of PLACIDYL. However, the 48% incidence is not substantially higher than the high value (39%) reported for the historical laboratory controls.

No evidence of carcinogenic potential was observed in rats given PLACIDYL at 5 to 15 times the maximum human daily dose for up to 2 years.

Usage During Pregnancy: 1. Teratogenic—Pregnancy Category C. Ethchlorvynol has been associated with a higher percentage of stillbirths and a lower survival rate of progeny among rats given 40 mg/kg/day. There are no adequate and well-controlled studies in pregnant women. Therefore, ethchlorvynol is not recommended for use during the first and second trimesters of pregnancy. Ethchlorvynol should be used during pregnancy only if the potential benefit justifies the potential risk to the fetus.

2. Non-teratogenic—Clinical experience has indicated that ethchlorvynol taken during the third trimester of pregnancy may produce CNS depression and transient withdrawal symptoms in the newborn. These symptoms resemble congenital narcotic withdrawal symptoms (See "Drug Abuse and Dependence" section).

Nursing Mothers: It is not known whether this drug is excreted in breast milk. Because many drugs are excreted in human milk and because of the potential for serious adverse reactions in nursing infants from PLACIDYL, a decision should be made whether to discontinue nursing or to discontinue the drug, taking into account the importance of the drug to the mother.

Pediatric Use: PLACIDYL is not recommended for use in children since its safety and effectiveness in the pediatric age group has not been determined.

Adverse Reactions: Adverse effects in decreasing order of severity within each of the following categories are:

Hypersensitivity: cholestatic jaundice, urticaria and rash.
Hematologic: thrombocytopenia—one case of fatal immune thrombocytopenia due to ethchlorvynol has been reported.
Gastrointestinal: vomiting, gastric upset, nausea and aftertaste.
Neurologic: dizziness and facial numbness.
Miscellaneous: blurred vision, hypotension and mild "hangover".

The following idiosyncratic responses have been reported occasionally: syncope without marked hypotension, profound muscular weakness, hysteria, marked excitement, prolonged hypnosis and mild stimulation.

Transient ataxia and giddiness have occurred in patients in whom absorption of the drug is especially rapid. These effects can sometimes be controlled by giving PLACIDYL with food.

(See "Drug Abuse and Dependence" section for the signs and symptoms of chronic intoxication).

Drug Abuse and Dependence: PLACIDYL is subject to control by the Federal Controlled Substances Act under DEA schedule IV.

Abuse: Pulmonary edema of rapid onset has resulted from the I.V. abuse of PLACIDYL (ethchlorvynol).

Dependence: Signs and symptoms of intoxication have been reported with the prolonged use of doses as low as 1 g/day. Signs and symptoms of chronic intoxication may include incoordination, tremors, ataxia, confusion, slurred speech, hyperreflexia, diplopia, and generalized muscle weakness. Toxic amblyopia, scotoma, nystagmus, and peripheral neuropathy have also been reported with prolonged use of ethchlorvynol; these symptoms are usually reversible.

Severe withdrawal symptoms similar to those seen during barbiturate and alcohol withdrawal have been reported following abrupt discontinuance of prolonged use of PLACIDYL. These symptoms may appear as late as nine days after sudden withdrawal of the drug. Signs and symptoms of PLACIDYL withdrawal may include convulsions, delirium, schizoid reaction, perceptual distortions, memory loss, ataxia, insomnia, slurring of speech, unusual anxiety, irritability, agitation, and tremors. Other signs and symptoms may include anorexia, nausea, vomiting, weakness, dizziness, sweating, muscle twitching, and weight loss.

Management of a patient who manifests withdrawal symptoms from PLACIDYL involves readministration of the drug to approximately the same level of chronic intoxication which existed before the abrupt discontinuance. (Phenobarbital may be substituted for PLACIDYL.) A gradual, stepwise reduction of dosage may then be made over a period of days or weeks. A phenothiazine compound may be used in addition to this regimen for those patients who exhibit psychotic symptoms during the withdrawal period. The patient undergoing withdrawal from PLACIDYL must be hospitalized or closely observed, and given general supportive care as indicated.

In one report an infant born to a mother who received 500 mg PLACIDYL at bedtime daily throughout the third trimester, exhibited withdrawal symptoms on the second day of life. The symptoms included episodic jitteriness, hyperactivity, restlessness, irritability, disturbed sleep and hunger. The neonate responded to a single oral dose of phenobarbital (3 mg/kg). The withdrawal symptoms gradually decreased and completely disappeared by the tenth day of life.

Overdosage: Acute intoxication is characterized by prolonged deep coma, severe respiratory depression, hypothermia, hypotension, and relative bradycardia. Nystagmus and pancytopenia resulting from acute PLACIDYL overdose have been reported.

Although death has occurred following the ingestion of 6 g of PLACIDYL, there have been reports of patients who have survived overdoses of 50 g and more with intensive care. Fatal blood concentrations usually range from 20 to 50 μg/ml.[1] Because large amounts of ethchlorvynol are taken up by adipose tissue, the blood concentration is an unreliable indicator of the magnitude of overdose.

Management of acute PLACIDYL intoxication is similar to that of acute barbiturate intoxication.[2] Gastric evacuation should be performed immediately. (In the unconscious patient, gastric lavage should be preceded by tracheal intubation with a cuffed tube.) Supportive care (assisted ventilation, frequent and careful monitoring of vital signs, control of blood pressure) is essential. Emphasis should be placed on pulmonary care and monitoring of blood gases. Hemoperfusion utilizing the Amberlite column technique has been reported in the literature to be the most effective method in the management of acute PLACIDYL overdose.[3] In addition, hemodialysis and peritoneal dialysis have each been reported to be of some value. (Aqueous and oil dialysates have been used. Forced diuresis with maintenance of a high urinary output has also been reported of some value.)

(See "Drug Abuse and Dependence" section for the signs and symptoms of chronic intoxication.)

Dosage and Administration: The usual adult hypnotic dose of PLACIDYL (ethchlorvynol) is 500 mg taken orally at bedtime. A dose of 750 mg may be required for patients whose sleep response to a 500 mg capsule is inadequate, or for patients being changed from barbiturates or other nonbarbiturate hypnotics. Up to 1000 mg may be given as a single bedtime dose when insomnia is unusually severe. A single supplemental dose of 100 to 200 mg may be given to reinstitute sleep in patients who may awaken after the original bedtime dose of 500 or 750 mg.

For patients whose insomnia is characterized only by untimely awakening during the early morning hours, a single dose of 100 to 200 mg taken upon awakening may be adequate for relief.

The smallest effective dose of PLACIDYL should be given to elderly or debilitated patients.

PLACIDYL should not be prescribed for periods exceeding one week. (See "Drug Abuse and Dependence" section.)

How Supplied: PLACIDYL (ethchlorvynol capsules, USP) is supplied as:
100 mg red capsules:
Bottles of 100 ....(NDC 0074-6649-04)
200 mg red capsules:
Bottles of 100 ....(NDC 0074-6661-08)
500 mg red capsules:
Bottles of 100 ....(NDC 0074-6685-15)
Bottles of 500 ....(NDC 0074-6685-02)
ABBO-PAC® unit dose strip packages of
100..(NDC 0074-6685-10)
750 mg green capsules:
Bottles of 100 ....(NDC 0074-6630-01)
ABBO-PAC unit dose strip packages of
100..(NDC 0074-6630-10)

References:
1. AMA Dept. of Drugs. *AMA Drug Evaluations*, Massachusetts: Publishing Sciences Group, Inc., 1980.
2. Khantzian, E. J., McKenna, G. J., Acute Toxic and Withdrawal Reactions Associated with Drug Abuse, *Annals of Internal Medicine*, 90:361–372, 1979.
3. Lynn, R.I., et al. Resin Hemoperfusion for Treatment of Ethchlorvynol Overdose, *Annals of Internal Medicine*, 91:549–553, 1979.

Shown in Product Identification Section, page 403
Abbott Laboratories
North Chicago, IL 60064
Ref. 01-2318-R5

QUELIDRINE® SYRUP
[*quel'i-drēen*]
(non-narcotic, antihistaminic cough suppressant)

Composition: Each teaspoonful (5 ml) contains:
Dextromethorphan Hydrobromide ....10 mg
Chlorpheniramine Maleate ....2 mg
Ephedrine Hydrochloride ....5 mg
Phenylephrine Hydrochloride ....5 mg
Ammonium Chloride ....40 mg
Ipecac Fluidextract ....0.005 ml
Alcohol 2%
in a palatable, aromatic syrup.

Action and Indications: Quelidrine is designed as an aid in the management of cough associated with acute or subacute simple respiratory infections. Quelidrine provides a wide range of therapeutic action against the cough complex—without the risk of addiction or the production of undue central depression.

Warnings: As with any drug, if you are pregnant or nursing a baby, seek the advice of a health professional before using this product. Keep this and all medicines out of the reach of children.

Precautions: Quelidrine should be administered with caution to patients with hypertension, serious organic heart disease, angina pectoris, diabetes, thyroid disease, or to persons receiving digitalis. When cough persists or accompanies a high fever, the underlying cause and need for other medication should be reevaluated.

Side Effects: Quelidrine is safe for patients of all ages, but professional supervision of dosage for young patients is essential. Side effects are infrequent. Drowsiness, nausea, vomiting, nervousness, palpitation, blurred vision and insomnia may occur in susceptible patients. Constipation is seldom a problem. If side effects are encountered, dosage should be reduced or medication withdrawn.

Dosage and Administration: *Adults*—1 teaspoonful, one to four times daily. Children 6 years of age or older, ½ teaspoonful, one to four times daily. Children 2 to 6 years old, ¼ teaspoonful one to four times daily. Under 2, as directed by physician. Quelidrine may be diluted with Syrup, NF in order to facilitate pediatric administration.

How Supplied: Quelidrine Syrup is supplied in bottles of 4 fluid ounces (NDC 0074-6883-04), with or without a prescription.
Store below 77°F (25°C).
Abbott Laboratories
North Chicago, IL 60064
Ref. 07-5233-4/R19

SELSUN® ℞
[*sel'sun*]
(selenium sulfide lotion, USP)

Description: SELSUN (selenium sulfide lotion) is a liquid antiseborrheic, antifungal preparation for topical application, containing selenium sulfide 2 ½% w/v in aqueous suspension; also contains: bentonite, lauric diethanolamide, ethylene glycol monostearate, titanium dioxide, amphoteric-2, sodium lauryl sulfate, sodium phosphate (monobasic), glyceryl monoricinoleate, citric acid, captan, and perfume.

Clinical Pharmacology: Selenium sulfide appears to have a cytostatic effect on cells of the epidermis and follicular epithelium, thus reducing corneocyte production.

Indications and Usage: For the treatment of dandruff and seborrheic dermatitis of the scalp. For treatment of tinea versicolor.

Contraindications: SELSUN should not be used by patients allergic to any of its components.

Precautions: *General:* Should not be used when acute inflammation or exudation is present as increased absorption may occur.

Information for Patients: Application to skin or scalp may produce skin irritation or sensitization. If sensitivity reactions occur, use should be discontinued. May be irritating to mucous membranes of the eyes and contact with this area should be avoided. When applied to the body for treatment of tinea versicolor, SELSUN may produce skin irritation especially in the genital area and where skin folds occur. These areas should be thoroughly rinsed after application.

Carcinogenesis: Studies in mice using dermal application of 25% and 50% solutions of 2.5% selenium sulfide lotion over an 88 week period, indicated no carcinogenic effects.

Pregnancy: WHEN USED ON BODY SURFACES FOR THE TREATMENT OF TINEA VERSICOLOR, SELSUN IS CLASSIFIED AS PREGNANCY CATEGORY C. Animal reproduction studies have not been conducted with SELSUN. It is also not known whether SELSUN can cause fetal harm when applied to body surfaces of a pregnant woman or can affect reproduction capacity. Under ordinary circumstances SELSUN should not be used for the treatment of tinea versicolor in pregnant women.

Pediatric Use: Safety and effectiveness in infants have not been established.

Adverse Reactions: In decreasing order of severity: skin irritation; occasional reports of increase in amount of normal hair loss; discoloration of hair (can be avoided or minimized by thorough rinsing of hair after treatment). As with other shampoos, oiliness or dryness of hair and scalp may occur.

Overdosage: Accidental Oral Ingestion:
Selsun is intended for external use only. There have been no documented reports of serious toxicity in humans resulting from acute ingestion of SELSUN, however, acute toxicity studies in animals suggest that ingestion of large amounts could result in potential human toxicity. For this reason, evacuation of the stomach contents should be considered in cases of acute oral ingestion.

Dosage and Administration: *For treatment of dandruff and seborrheic dermatitis:*
1. Massage about 1 or 2 teaspoonfuls of shampoo into wet scalp.
2. Allow to remain on the scalp for 2 to 3 minutes.
3. Rinse scalp thoroughly.
4. Repeat application and rinse thoroughly.
5. After treatment, wash hands well.

For the usual case, two applications each week for two weeks will afford control. After this, the lotion may be used at less frequent intervals—weekly, every two weeks, or even every 3 or 4 weeks in some cases. The preparation should not be applied more frequently than required to maintain control.

For treatment of tinea versicolor: Apply to affected areas and lather with a small amount of water. Allow product to remain on skin for 10 minutes, then rinse the body thoroughly. Repeat this procedure once a day for 7 days. The product may damage jewelry; jewelry should be removed before use.

How Supplied: SELSUN (selenium sulfide lotion, USP) is supplied in 4-fluidounce nonbreakable plastic bottles (NDC 0074-2660-04). SELSUN is to be dispensed only on the prescription of a physician.
Abbott Laboratories
North Chicago, IL 60064

SURBEX®
[*sir'bex*]
Vitamin B-Complex*
SURBEX® with C
Vitamin B-Complex* with Vitamin C

Description: Each Surbex Filmtab tablet provides:
Niacinamide ....30 mg
Calcium Pantothenate ....10 mg
Vitamin B_1 (thiamine mononitrate) ....6 mg
Vitamin$_2$ (riboflavin)...6 mg
Vitamin B_6
(pyridoxine hydrochloride).......................2.5 mg
Vitamin B_{12} (cyanocobalamin)......................5 mcg
Each Surbex with C Filmtab tablet provides the same ingredients as Surbex, plus 250 mg Vitamin C (as sodium ascorbate).

Indications: Surbex is indicated for treatment of Vitamin B-Complex* deficiency.
Surbex with C is indicated for use in treatment of Vitamin B-Complex* with Vitamin C deficiency.
*Contains no folic acid; not for treatment of folate deficiency.

Dosage and Administration: Usual adult dosage is one tablet twice daily or as directed by physician.

How Supplied: Surbex is supplied as bright orange-colored tablets in bottles of 100 (NDC 0074-4876-13).

Continued on next page

If desired, additional literature on any Abbott Product will be provided upon request to Abbott Laboratories.

Abbott—Cont.

Surbex with C is supplied as yellow-colored tablets in bottles of 100 (NDC 0074-4877-13) and 500 (NDC 0074-4877-53).
Abbott Pharmaceuticals, Inc.
North Chicago, IL 60064
Ref. 03-1070-3/R8, 03-1071-3/R7

SURBEX-T®
[sir′bex-t]
High-Potency Vitamin B-Complex with 500 mg of Vitamin C

(See PDR For Nonprescription Drugs)
Shown in Product Identification Section, page 404

SURBEX®-750 with IRON
[sir′bex ī-ron]
High-potency B-complex with iron, vitamin E and 750 mg vitamin C

(See PDR For Nonprescription Drugs)
Shown in Product Identification Section, page 404

SURBEX®-750 with ZINC
[sir′bex zinc]
High-potency B-complex with zinc, vitamin E and 750 mg vitamin C

(See PDR For Nonprescription Drugs)
Shown in Product Identification Section, page 404

TRAL® Filmtab® Tablets   ℞
[trāl]
(hexocyclium methylsulfate)

Description: TRAL (hexocyclium methylsulfate) is a quaternary ammonium salt. Chemically, it is designated as N-(beta-cyclohexyl-beta-hydroxy-beta-phenylethyl)-N′-methylpiperazine methosulfate. Physically, TRAL is a white powder soluble in water or physiological saline yielding a stable solution.

Actions: Clinically, TRAL is an effective anticholinergic agent which inhibits gastric secretion and gastrointestinal motility.

The drug has an antimuscarinic action similar to that of other quaternary ammonium compounds which produce anticholinergic effects. In experimental animals the drug has been shown to decrease gastric secretion, prevent gastric ulceration, decrease gastrointestinal motility, dilate the pupils, inhibit salivation, increase the heart rate, and counteract the peripheral muscarinic effect of choline esters. With massive overdosage the drug also may produce a peripheral curare-like neuromuscular block and ganglionic blockade. In studies with human subjects, TRAL produced a decrease in gastric acidity, and a decrease in the volume of gastric secretion.

TRAL is absorbed from the gastrointestinal tract but the degree of absorption varies. Following oral administration of a single dose of the drug in conventional tablet form, its effects persist for 3 to 4 hours. The metabolic fate and route of excretion are unknown.

Indications: TRAL is indicated as adjunctive therapy in the treatment of peptic ulcer. IT SHOULD BE NOTED AT THIS POINT IN TIME THAT THERE IS A LACK OF CONCURRENCE AS TO THE VALUE OF ANTICHOLINERGICS IN THE TREATMENT OF GASTRIC ULCER. IT HAS NOT BEEN SHOWN WHETHER ANTICHOLINERGIC DRUGS AID IN THE HEALING OF A PEPTIC ULCER, DECREASE THE RATE OF RECURRENCES OR PREVENT COMPLICATION. To be effective the dosage must be titrated to the individual patient's needs.

Contraindications: TRAL is contraindicated in patients with glaucoma; obstructive uropathy (for example, bladder neck obstruction due to prostatic hypertrophy); obstructive disease of the gastrointestinal tract (as in achalasia, paralytic ileus, pyloroduodenal stenosis, etc.); intestinal atony of the elderly or debilitated patient; unstable cardiovascular status; in acute hemorrhage; severe ulcerative colitis; toxic megacolon complicating ulcerative colitis; myasthenia gravis.

Warnings: In the presence of a high environmental temperature, heat prostration can occur with drug use (fever and heat stroke due to decreased sweating).

TRAL may produce drowsiness or blurred vision. In this event, the patient should be warned not to engage in activities requiring mental alertness such as operating a motor vehicle or other machinery, or perform hazardous work while taking this drug.

Usage in Pregnancy and Lactation: The safety of TRAL for use during pregnancy or lactation has not been established.

When given to pregnant rabbits at daily oral doses of 2.5 and 40 mg/kg/day, which are 1.2 and 20 times the human dose, TRAL increased the rate of abortion and fetal resorption.

As with all anticholinergic drugs, an inhibitory effect on lactation may occur.

Precautions: TRAL should be used with caution in patients with:

- Autonomic neuropathy.
- Hepatic or renal disease.
- Ulcerative colitis—large doses may suppress intestinal motility to the point of producing a paralytic ileus and the use of this drug may precipitate or aggravate the serious complication of toxic megacolon.
- Hyperthyroidism, coronary heart disease, congestive heart failure, cardiac arrhythmias, hypertension and non-obstructing prostatic hypertrophy.
- Hiatal hernia associated with reflux esophagitis since anticholinergic drugs may aggravate this condition.

It should be noted that the use of anticholinergic drugs in the treatment of gastric ulcer may produce a delay in gastric emptying time and may complicate such therapy (antral stasis).

Investigate any tachycardia before giving anticholinergic (atropine-like) drugs since they may increase the heart rate.

With overdosage, a curare-like action may occur. This product contains FD&C Yellow No. 5 (tartrazine) which may cause allergic-type reactions (including bronchial asthma) in certain susceptible individuals. Although the overall incidence of FD&C Yellow No. 5 (tartrazine) sensitivity in the general population is low, it is frequently seen in patients who also have aspirin hypersensitivity.

Adverse Reactions: Adverse reactions may include xerostomia, urinary hesitancy and retention, blurred vision, mydriasis, cycloplegia, increased intra-ocular tension, tachycardia, palpitations, headaches, nervousness, drowsiness, weakness, dizziness, insomnia, nausea, vomiting, impotency, dysphagia, altered taste perception, heartburn, bloated feeling, constipation, paralytic ileus, flushing, decreased sweating, urticaria and other dermal manifestations, severe allergic reaction or drug idiosyncrasies, and some degree of mental confusion and/or excitement especially in elderly persons.

When side effects are severe and cannot be controlled by reduction of dosage, the medication should be withdrawn.

Dosage and Administration: TRAL is administered orally. The usual recommended adult dose of TRAL is one 25 mg Filmtab tablet four times daily, taken before meals and at bedtime.

For optimal therapeutic effect, dosage should be adjusted to the patient's response.

TRAL is not for use in children.

Overdosage: The first sign of overdosage may be indicated by an atropine-like flush, particularly in the blush areas. Other manifestations of overdosage are revealed by the appearance or an increase in intensity of dryness of the mouth or other side effects.

With unusually large doses the quaternary ammonium type of anticholinergic agent may produce a curare-like action and ganglionic blockade manifested by respiratory paralysis and circulatory collapse. This is unlikely to occur with therapeutic doses. Neostigmine methylsulfate at a dose of 0.5 to 2 mg given by slow intravenous injection and repeated as required may be administered as an antidote. Only in exceptional cases should the total dose of neostigmine methylsulfate exceed 5 mg. Artificial respiration and other supportive measures should be applied if needed.

How Supplied: TRAL (hexocyclium methylsulfate) Filmtab tablets, 25 mg, green, (NDC 0074-6698-02) are supplied in bottles of 100.
Abbott Laboratories
North Chicago, IL 60064
Ref. 01-2061-R5

TRANXENE®   ℞ ©
[tran′zēen]
(clorazepate dipotassium)
Capsules
Tablets

TRANXENE®-SD & TRANXENE-SD HALF STRENGTH
(clorazepate dipotassium)
Tablets

Description: Chemically, TRANXENE (clorazepate dipotassium) is a benzodiazepine. The empirical formula is $C_{16}H_{11}ClK_2N_2O_4$; the molecular weight is 408.92.

The compound occurs as a fine, light yellow, practically odorless powder. It is insoluble in the common organic solvents, but very soluble in water. Aqueous solutions are unstable, clear, light yellow, and alkaline.

Actions: Pharmacologically, clorazepate dipotassium has the characteristics of the benzodiazepines. It has depressant effects on the central nervous system. The primary metabolite, nordiazepam, quickly appears in the blood stream. The serum half-life is about 2 days. The drug is metabolized in the liver and excreted primarily in the urine. (See ANIMAL AND CLINICAL PHARMACOLOGY section).

Indications: TRANXENE is indicated for the management of anxiety disorders or for the short-term relief of the symptoms of anxiety. Anxiety or tension associated with the stress of everyday life usually does not require treatment with an anxiolytic.

TRANXENE is indicated as adjunctive therapy in the management of partial seizures.

The effectiveness of TRANXENE in long-term management of anxiety, that is, more than 4 months, has not been assessed by systematic clinical studies. Long-term studies in epileptic patients, however, have shown continued therapeutic activity. The physician should reassess periodically the usefulness of the drug for the individual patient.

TRANXENE is indicated for the symptomatic relief of acute alcohol withdrawal.

Contraindications: TRANXENE is contraindicated in patients with a known hypersensitivity to the drug, and in those with acute narrow angle glaucoma.

Warnings: TRANXENE is not recommended for use in depressive neuroses or in psychotic reactions.

Patients on TRANXENE should be cautioned against engaging in hazardous occupations requiring mental alertness, such as operating dangerous machinery including motor vehicles.

Since TRANXENE has a central nervous system depressant effect, patients should be advised against the simultaneous use of other CNS-depressant drugs, and cautioned that the effects of alcohol may be increased.

Because of the lack of sufficient clinical experience, TRANXENE is not recommended for use in patients less than 9 years of age.

Physical and Psychological Dependence: Withdrawal symptoms (similar in character to those noted with barbiturates and alcohol) have occurred following abrupt discontinuance of clorazepate. Symptoms of nervousness, insomnia, irritability, diarrhea, muscle aches and memory impairment have followed abrupt withdrawal after long-term use of high dosage. Withdrawal symptoms have also been reported following abrupt discontinuance of benzodiazepines taken continuously at therapeutic levels for several months.

Caution should be observed in patients who are considered to have a psychological potential for drug dependence.

Evidence of drug dependence has been observed in dogs and rabbits which was characterized by convulsive seizures when the drug was abruptly withdrawn or the dose was reduced; the syndrome in dogs could be abolished by administration of clorazepate.

Usage in Pregnancy: An increased risk of congenital malformations associated with the use of minor tranquilizers (chlordiazepoxide, diazepam, and meprobamate) during the first trimester of pregnancy has been suggested in several studies. TRANXENE, a benzodiazepine derivative, has not been studied adequately to determine whether it, too, may be associated with an increased risk of fetal abnormality. Because use of these drugs is rarely a matter of urgency, their use during this period should almost always be avoided. The possibility that a woman of childbearing potential may be pregnant at the time of institution of therapy should be considered. Patients should be advised that if they become pregnant during therapy or intend to become pregnant they should communicate with their physician about the desirability of discontinuing the drug.

Usage during Lactation: TRANXENE should not be given to nursing mothers since it has been reported that nordiazepam is excreted in human breast milk.

Precautions: In those patients in which a degree of depression accompanies the anxiety, suicidal tendencies may be present and protective measures may be required. The least amount of drug that is feasible should be available to the patient.

Patients on TRANXENE for prolonged periods should have blood counts and liver function tests periodically. The usual precautions in treating patients with impaired renal or hepatic function should also be observed.

In elderly or debilitated patients, the initial dose should be small, and increments should be made gradually, in accordance with the response of the patient, to preclude ataxia or excessive sedation.

Adverse Reactions: The side effect most frequently reported was drowsiness. Less commonly reported (in descending order of occurrence) were: dizziness, various gastrointestinal complaints, nervousness, blurred vision, dry mouth, headache, and mental confusion. Other side effects included insomnia, transient skin rashes, fatigue, ataxia, genitourinary complaints, irritability, diplopia, depression and slurred speech.

There have been reports of abnormal liver and kidney function tests and of decrease in hematocrit.

Decrease in systolic blood pressure has been observed.

Dosage and Administration: *For the symptomatic relief of anxiety:* TRANXENE capsules and tablets are administered orally in divided doses. The usual daily dose is 30 mg. The dose should be adjusted gradually within the range of 15 to 60 mg daily in accordance with the response of the patient. In elderly or debilitated patients it is advisable to initiate treatment at a daily dose of 7.5 or 15 mg.

TRANXENE capsules and tablets may also be administered in a single dose daily at bedtime; the recommended initial dose is 15 mg. After the initial dose, the response of the patient may require adjustment of subsequent dosage. Lower doses may be indicated in the elderly patient. Drowsiness may occur at the initiation of treatment and with dosage increment.

TRANXENE-SD (22.5 mg tablets) may be administered as a single dose every 24 hours. This tablet is intended as an alternate dosage form for the convenience of patients stabilized on a dose of 7.5 mg capsules or tablets three times a day. TRANXENE-SD should not be used to initiate therapy.

TRANXENE-SD HALF STRENGTH (11.25 mg tablets) may be administered as a single dose every 24 hours.

For the symptomatic relief of acute alcohol withdrawal:
The following dosage schedule is recommended:

1st 24 hours (Day 1)	30 mg Tranxene, initially; followed by 30 to 60 mg in divided doses
2nd 24 hours (Day 2)	45 to 90 mg in divided doses
3rd 24 hours (Day 3)	22.5 to 45 mg in divided doses
Day 4	15 to 30 mg in divided doses

Thereafter, gradually reduce the daily dose to 7.5 to 15 mg. Discontinue drug therapy as soon as patient's condition is stable.

The maximum recommended total daily dose is 90 mg. Avoid excessive reductions in the total amount of drug administered on successive days.

As an Adjunct to Antiepileptic Drugs:
In order to minimize drowsiness, the recommended initial dosages and dosage increments should not be exceeded.

Adults: The maximum recommended initial dose in patients over 12 years old is 7.5 mg three times a day. Dosage should be increased by no more than 7.5 mg every week and should not exceed 90 mg/day.

Children (9-12 years): The maximum recommended initial dose is 7.5 mg two times a day. Dosage should be increased by no more than 7.5 mg every week and should not exceed 60 mg/day.

Drug Interactions: If TRANXENE is to be combined with other drugs acting on the central nervous system, careful consideration should be given to the pharmacology of the agents to be employed. Animal experience indicates that TRANXENE prolongs the sleeping time after hexobarbital or after ethyl alcohol, increases the inhibitory effects of chlorpromazine, but does not exhibit monoamine oxidase inhibition. Clinical studies have shown increased sedation with concurrent hypnotic medications. The actions of the benzodiazepines may be potentiated by barbiturates, narcotics, phenothiazines, monoamine oxidase inhibitors or other antidepressants.

If TRANXENE is used to treat anxiety associated with somatic disease states, careful attention must be paid to possible drug interaction with concomitant medication.

In bioavailability studies with normal subjects, the concurrent administration of antacids at therapeutic levels did not significantly influence the bioavailability of TRANXENE.

Management of Overdosage: Overdosage is usually manifested by varying degrees of CNS depression ranging from slight sedation to coma. As in the management of overdosage with any drug, it should be borne in mind that multiple agents may have been taken.

There are no specific antidotes for the benzodiazepines. The treatment of overdosage should consist of the general measures employed in the management of overdosage of any CNS depressant. Gastric evacuation either by the induction of emesis, lavage, or both, should be performed immediately. General supportive care, including frequent monitoring of the vital signs and close observation of the patient, is indicated. Hypotension, though rarely reported, may occur with large overdoses. In such cases the use of agents such as Levophed® Bitartrate (norepinephrine bitartrate injection, USP) or Aramine® Injection (metaraminol bitartrate injection, USP) should be considered.

While reports indicate that individuals have survived overdoses of TRANXENE as high as 450 to 675 mg, these doses are not necessarily an accurate indication of the amount of drug absorbed since the time interval between ingestion and the institution of treatment was not always known. Sedation in varying degrees was the most common physiological manifestation of TRANXENE overdosage. Deep coma when it occurred was usually associated with the ingestion of other drugs in addition to TRANXENE.

Animal and Clinical Pharmacology: Studies in rats and monkeys have shown a substantial difference between doses producing tranquilizing, sedative and toxic effects. In rats, conditioned avoidance response was inhibited at an oral dose of 10 mg/kg; sedation was induced at 32 mg/kg; the LD_{50} was 1320 mg/kg. In monkeys aggressive behavior was reduced at an oral dose of 0.25 mg/kg; sedation (ataxia) was induced at 7.5 mg/kg; the LD_{50} could not be determined because of the emetic effect of large doses, but the LD_{50} exceeds 1600 mg/kg.

Twenty-four dogs were given TRANXENE orally in a 22-month toxicity study; doses up to 75 mg/kg were given. Drug-related changes occurred in the liver; weight was increased and cholestasis with minimal hepatocellular damage was found, but lobular architecture remained well preserved.

Eighteen rhesus monkeys were given oral doses of TRANXENE from 3 to 36 mg/kg daily for 52 weeks. All treated animals remained similar to control animals. Although total leucocyte count remained within normal limits it tended to fall in the female animals on the highest doses.

Examination of all organs revealed no alterations attributable to TRANXENE. There was no damage to liver function or structure.

Reproduction Studies: Standard fertility, reproduction, and teratology studies were conducted in rats and rabbits. Oral doses in rats up to 150 mg/kg and in rabbits up to 15 mg/kg produced no abnormalities in the fetuses. TRANXENE (clorazepate dipotassium) did not alter the fertility indices or reproductive capacity of adult animals. As expected, the sedative effect of high doses interfered with care of the young by their mothers (see Usage in Pregnancy).

Clinical Pharmacology: Studies in healthy men have shown that TRANXENE has depressant effects on the central nervous system. Prolonged administration of single daily doses as high as 120 mg was without toxic effects. Abrupt cessation of high doses was followed in some patients by nervousness, insomnia, irritability, diarrhea, muscle aches, or memory impairment.

Absorption—Excretion: After oral administration of TRANXENE there is essentially no circulating parent drug. Nordiazepam, its primary metabolite, quickly appears in the blood stream. In 2 volunteers given 15 mg (50 μC) of ^{14}C-Tranxene, about 80% was recovered in the urine and feces within 10 days. Excretion was primarily in the urine with about 1% excreted per day on day 10.

How Supplied: TRANXENE (clorazepate dipotassium) is supplied as:
3.75 mg gray and white capsules:
Bottles of 100 ....(NDC 0074-3417-13)
Bottles of 500 ....(NDC 0074-3417-53)
ABBO-PAC® unit dose packages:
100 ....(NDC 0074-3417-11)
7.5 mg gray and maroon capsules:
Bottles of 100 ....(NDC 0074-3418-13)
Bottles of 500 ....(NDC 0074-3418-53)
ABBO-PAC unit dose packages:
100 ....(NDC 0074-3418-11)
4 cartons of 25
(reverse-numbered) ....(NDC 0074-3418-25)
15 mg gray capsules:
Bottles of 100 ....(NDC 0074-3419-13)
Bottles of 500 ....(NDC 0074-3419-53)
ABBO-PAC unit dose packages:
100 ....(NDC 0074-3419-11)
3.75 mg blue-colored, scored tablets:
Bottles of 100 ....(NDC 0074-4389-13)
7.5 mg peach-colored, scored tablets:
Bottles of 100 ....(NDC 0074-4390-13)
15 mg lavender-colored, scored tablets:
Bottles of 100 ....(NDC 0074-4391-13)
TRANXENE-SD 22.5 mg tan-colored, single dose tablets:
Bottles of 100 ....(NDC 0074-2997-13)
TRANXENE-SD HALF STRENGTH 11.25 mg blue-colored, single dose tablets:
Bottles of 100 ....(NDC 0074-2699-13)

Shown in Product Identification Section, page 404
Abbott Pharmaceuticals, Inc.
North Chicago, IL 60064
Ref. 03-4224-R14

Continued on next page

Abbott—Cont.

TRIDIONE® ℞
[try'dē-own]
(trimethadione)
Tablets, Capsules, and Oral Solution

BECAUSE OF ITS POTENTIAL TO PRODUCE FETAL MALFORMATIONS AND SERIOUS SIDE EFFECTS, TRIDIONE (trimethadione) SHOULD ONLY BE UTILIZED WHEN OTHER LESS TOXIC DRUGS HAVE BEEN FOUND INEFFECTIVE IN CONTROLLING PETIT MAL SEIZURES.

Description: TRIDIONE (trimethadione) is an antiepileptic agent. An oxazolidinedione compound, it is chemically identified as 3,5,5-trimethyloxozolidine-2,4-dione.
TRIDIONE is a synthetic, water-soluble, white, crystalline powder. It is supplied in capsular, tablet, and liquid forms for oral use only.

Clinical Pharmacology: TRIDIONE has been shown to prevent pentylenetetrazol-induced and thujone-induced seizures in experimental animals; the drug has a less marked effect on seizures induced by picrotoxin, procaine, cocaine, or strychnine. Unlike the hydantoins and antiepileptic barbiturates, TRIDIONE does not modify the maximal seizure pattern in patients undergoing electroconvulsive therapy.
TRIDIONE has a sedative effect that may increase to the point of ataxia when excessive doses are used. A toxic dose of the drug in animals (approximately 2 Gm/kg) produced sleep, unconsciousness, and respiratory depression.
Trimethadione is rapidly absorbed from the gastrointestinal tract. It is demethylated by liver microsomes to the active metabolite, dimethadione. Approximately 3% of a daily dose of TRIDIONE is recovered in the urine as unchanged drug. The majority of trimethadione is excreted slowly by the kidney in the form of dimethadione.

Indications: TRIDIONE (trimethadione) is indicated for the control of petit mal seizures that are refractory to treatment with other drugs.

Contraindications: TRIDIONE is contraindicated in patients with a known hypersensitivity to the drug.

Warnings: TRIDIONE may cause serious side effects. Strict medical supervision of the patient is mandatory, especially during the initial year of therapy.
TRIDIONE (trimethadione) should be withdrawn promptly if skin rash appears, because of the grave possibility of the occurrence of exfoliative dermatitis or severe forms of erythema multiforme. Even a minor acneiform or morbilliform rash should be allowed to clear completely before treatment with TRIDIONE is resumed; reinstitute therapy cautiously.
A complete blood count should be done prior to intiating therapy with TRIDIONE, and at monthly intervals thereafter. A marked depression of the blood count is an indication for withdrawal of the drug. If no abnormality appears within 12 months, the interval between blood counts may be extended. A moderate degree of neutropenia with or without a corresponding drop in the leukocyte count is not uncommon. Therapy need not be withdrawn unless the neutrophil count is 2500 or less; more frequent blood examinations should be done when the count is less than 3,000. Other blood dyscrasias, including leukopenia, eosinophilia, thrombocytopenia, pancytopenia, agranulocytosis, hypoplastic anemia, and fatal aplastic anemia, have occurred. Patients should be advised to report immediately such signs and symptoms as sore throat, fever, malaise, easy bruising, petechiae, or epistaxis, or others that may be indicative of an infection or bleeding tendency. TRIDIONE should ordinarily not be used in patients with severe blood dyscrasias.
Liver function tests should be done prior to initiating therapy with TRIDIONE, and at monthly intervals thereafter. Hepatitis has been reported rarely. Jaundice or other signs of liver dysfunction are an indication for withdrawal of the drug. TRIDIONE should ordinarily not be used in patients with severe hepatic impairment.
A urinalysis should be done prior to initiating therapy with TRIDIONE and at monthly intervals thereafter. Fatal nephrosis has been reported. Persistent or increasing albuminuria, or the development of any other significant renal abnormality, is an indication for withdrawal of the drug. TRIDIONE should ordinarily not be used in patients with severe renal dysfunction.
Hemeralopia has occurred; this appears to be an effect of TRIDIONE on the neural layers of the retina, and usually can be reversed by a reduction in dosage. Scotomata are an indication for withdrawal of the drug. Caution should be observed when treating patients who have diseases of the retina or optic nerve.
Manifestations of systemic lupus erythematosus have been associated with the use of TRIDIONE, as they have with the use of certain other anticonvulsants. Lymphadenopathies simulating malignant lymphoma have occurred. Lupus-like manifestations or lymph node enlargement are indications for withdrawal of the drug. Signs and symptoms may disappear after discontinuation of therapy, and specific treatment may be unnecessary.
A myasthenia gravis-like syndrome has been associated with the chronic use of trimethadione. Symptoms suggestive of this condition are indications for withdrawal of the drug.
Drugs known to cause toxic effects similar to those of TRIDIONE should be avoided or used only with extreme caution during therapy with TRIDIONE.

USAGE DURING PREGNANCY AND LACTATION:
THERE ARE MULTIPLE REPORTS IN THE CLINICAL LITERATURE WHICH INDICATE THAT THE USE OF ANTICONVULSANT DRUGS DURING PREGNANCY RESULTS IN AN INCREASED INCIDENCE OF BIRTH DEFECTS IN THE OFFSPRING. DATA ARE MORE EXTENSIVE WITH RESPECT TO TRIMETHADIONE, PARAMETHADIONE, PHENYTOIN AND PHENOBARBITAL THAN WITH OTHER ANTICONVULSANT DRUGS.
THEREFORE, ANTICONVULSANT DRUGS SUCH AS TRIDIONE (TRIMETHADIONE) SHOULD BE ADMINISTERED TO WOMEN OF CHILDBEARING POTENTIAL ONLY IF THEY ARE CLEARLY SHOWN TO BE ESSENTIAL IN THE MANAGEMENT OF THEIR SEIZURES. EFFECTIVE MEANS OF CONTRACEPTION SHOULD ACCOMPANY THE USE OF TRIDIONE IN SUCH PATIENTS. IF A PATIENT BECOMES PREGNANT WHILE TAKING TRIDIONE, TERMINATION OF THE PREGNANCY SHOULD BE CONSIDERED. A PATIENT WHO REQUIRES THERAPY WITH TRIDIONE AND WHO WISHES TO BECOME PREGNANT SHOULD BE ADVISED OF THE RISKS.
REPORTS HAVE SUGGESTED THAT THE MATERNAL INGESTION OF ANTICONVULSANT DRUGS, PARTICULARLY BARBITURATES, IS ASSOCIATED WITH A NEONATAL COAGULATION DEFECT THAT MAY CAUSE BLEEDING DURING THE EARLY (USUALLY WITHIN 24 HOURS OF BIRTH) NEONATAL PERIOD. THE POSSIBILITY OF THE OCCURRENCE OF THIS DEFECT WITH THE USE OF TRIDIONE SHOULD BE KEPT IN MIND. THE DEFECT IS CHARACTERIZED BY DECREASED LEVELS OF VITAMIN K-DEPENDENT CLOTTING FACTORS, AND PROLONGATION OF EITHER THE PROTHROMBIN TIME OR THE PARTIAL THROMBOPLASTIN TIME, OR BOTH. IT HAS BEEN SUGGESTED THAT PROPHYLACTIC VITAMIN K BE GIVEN TO THE MOTHER ONE MONTH PRIOR TO, AND DURING DELIVERY, AND TO THE INFANT, INTRAVENOUSLY, IMMEDIATELY AFTER BIRTH.
THE SAFETY OF TRIDIONE FOR USE DURING LACTATION HAS NOT BEEN ESTABLISHED.

Precautions: Abrupt discontinuation of TRIDIONE may precipitate petit mal status. TRIDIONE should always be withdrawn gradually unless serious adverse effects dictate otherwise. In the latter case, another anticonvulsant may be substituted to protect the patient.

Usage during Pregnancy and Lactation: See WARNINGS.

Adverse Reactions: The following side effects, some of them serious, have been associated with the use of TRIDIONE.
Gastrointestinal: nausea, vomiting, abdominal pain, gastric distress.
CNS/Neurologic: drowsiness, fatigue, malaise, insomnia, vertigo, headache, paresthesias, precipitation of grand mal seizures, increased irritability, personality changes.
Drowsiness usually subsides with continued therapy. If it persists, a reduction in dosage is indicated.
Hematologic: bleeding gums, epistaxis, retinal and petechial hemorrhages, vaginal bleeding; neutropenia, leukopenia, eosinophilia, thrombocytopenia, pancytopenia, agranulocytosis, hypoplastic anemia, and fatal aplastic anemia.
Dermatologic: acneiform or morbilliform skin rash that may progress to exfoliative dermatitis or to severe forms of erythema multiforme.
Other: hiccups, anorexia, weight loss, hair loss, changes in blood pressure, albuminuria, hemeralopia, photophobia, diplopia.
Fatal nephrosis has occurred.
Hepatitis has been reported rarely.
Lupus erythematosus, and lymphadenopathies simulating malignant lymphoma, have been reported.
Pruritus associated with lymphadenopathy and hepatosplenomegaly has occurred in hypersensitive individuals.
A myasthenia gravis-like syndrome has been reported.

Overdosage: Symptoms of acute TRIDIONE overdosage include drowsiness, nausea, dizziness, ataxia, visual disturbances. Coma may follow massive overdosage.
Gastric evacuation, either by induced emesis, or by lavage, or both, should be done immediately. General supportive care, including frequent monitoring of the vital signs and close observation of the patient, are required.
Alkalinization of the urine has been reported to enhance the renal excretion of dimethadione, the active metabolite of TRIDIONE.
A blood count and a careful evaluation of hepatic and renal function should be done following recovery.

Dosage and Administration: TRIDIONE is administered orally.
Usual Adult Dosage: 0.9–2.4 Gm daily in 3 or 4 equally divided doses (i.e. 300–600 mg 3 or 4 times daily).
Initially, give 0.9 Gm daily; increase this dose by 300 mg at weekly intervals until therapeutic results are seen or until toxic symptoms appear.
Maintenance dosage should be the least amount of drug required to maintain control.
Children's Dosage: Usually 0.3–0.9 Gm daily in 3 or 4 equally divided doses.

How Supplied: TRIDIONE Capsules (trimethadione capsules, USP), 300 mg (white) are supplied in bottles of 100 (NDC 0074-3709-01).
TRIDIONE Dulcet® Tablets (trimethadione tablets, USP), 150 mg (white) chewable tablets are supplied in bottles of 100 (NDC 0074-3753-01).
Shown in Product Identification Section, page 404
TRIDIONE Solution (trimethadione oral solution, USP), 1.2 Gm per fluidounce (40 mg per ml), is supplied in pint bottles (NDC 0074-3721-01).
Abbott Laboratories/
Abbott Pharmaceuticals, Inc.
North Chicago, IL 60064
®Dulcet—Sweetened tablets, Abbott.
Ref. 03-4194/R3

TRONOTHANE® HYDROCHLORIDE
[tro'nō-thāne hy-drō-clō'rīde]
(pramoxine hydrochloride)
Cream

Description: Tronothane Hydrochloride (pramoxine hydrochloride) is a surface anesthetic agent, chemically unrelated to the benzoate esters of the "caine" type. It is chemically designated as 4-n-butoxyphenyl gammamorpholinopropyl ether

Caution should be observed in patients who are considered to have a psychological potential for drug dependence.

Evidence of drug dependence has been observed in dogs and rabbits which was characterized by convulsive seizures when the drug was abruptly withdrawn or the dose was reduced; the syndrome in dogs could be abolished by administration of clorazepate.

Usage in Pregnancy: **An increased risk of congenital malformations associated with the use of minor tranquilizers (chlordiazepoxide, diazepam, and meprobamate) during the first trimester of pregnancy has been suggested in several studies. TRANXENE, a benzodiazepine derivative, has not been studied adequately to determine whether it, too, may be associated with an increased risk of fetal abnormality. Because use of these drugs is rarely a matter of urgency, their use during this period should almost always be avoided. The possibility that a woman of childbearing potential may be pregnant at the time of institution of therapy should be considered. Patients should be advised that if they become pregnant during therapy or intend to become pregnant they should communicate with their physician about the desirability of discontinuing the drug.**

Usage during Lactation: TRANXENE should not be given to nursing mothers since it has been reported that nordiazepam is excreted in human breast milk.

Precautions: In those patients in which a degree of depression accompanies the anxiety, suicidal tendencies may be present and protective measures may be required. The least amount of drug that is feasible should be available to the patient.

Patients on TRANXENE for prolonged periods should have blood counts and liver function tests periodically. The usual precautions in treating patients with impaired renal or hepatic function should also be observed.

In elderly or debilitated patients, the initial dose should be small, and increments should be made gradually, in accordance with the response of the patient, to preclude ataxia or excessive sedation.

Adverse Reactions: The side effect most frequently reported was drowsiness. Less commonly reported (in descending order of occurrence) were: dizziness, various gastrointestinal complaints, nervousness, blurred vision, dry mouth, headache, and mental confusion. Other side effects included insomnia, transient skin rashes, fatigue, ataxia, genitourinary complaints, irritability, diplopia, depression and slurred speech.

There have been reports of abnormal liver and kidney function tests and of decrease in hematocrit.

Decrease in systolic blood pressure has been observed.

Dosage and Administration: *For the symptomatic relief of anxiety:* TRANXENE capsules and tablets are administered orally in divided doses. The usual daily dose is 30 mg. The dose should be adjusted gradually within the range of 15 to 60 mg daily in accordance with the response of the patient. In elderly or debilitated patients it is advisable to initiate treatment at a daily dose of 7.5 to 15 mg.

TRANXENE capsules and tablets may also be administered in a single dose daily at bedtime; the recommended initial dose is 15 mg. After the initial dose, the response of the patient may require adjustment of subsequent dosage. Lower doses may be indicated in the elderly patient. Drowsiness may occur at the initiation of treatment and with dosage increment.

TRANXENE-SD (22.5 mg tablets) may be administered as a single dose every 24 hours. This tablet is intended as an alternate dosage form for the convenience of patients stabilized on a dose of 7.5 mg capsules or tablets three times a day. TRANXENE-SD should not be used to initiate therapy.

TRANXENE-SD HALF STRENGTH (11.25 mg tablets) may be administered as a single dose every 24 hours.

For the symptomatic relief of acute alcohol withdrawal:

The following dosage schedule is recommended:

1st 24 hours (Day 1)	30 mg Tranxene, initially; followed by 30 to 60 mg in divided doses
2nd 24 hours (Day 2)	45 to 90 mg in divided doses
3rd 24 hours (Day 3)	22.5 to 45 mg in divided doses
Day 4	15 to 30 mg in divided doses

Thereafter, gradually reduce the daily dose to 7.5 to 15 mg. Discontinue drug therapy as soon as patient's condition is stable.

The maximum recommended total daily dose is 90 mg. Avoid excessive reductions in the total amount of drug administered on successive days.

As an Adjunct to Antiepileptic Drugs:
In order to minimize drowsiness, the recommended initial dosages and dosage increments should not be exceeded.

Adults: The maximum recommended initial dose in patients over 12 years old is 7.5 mg three times a day. Dosage should be increased by no more than 7.5 mg every week and should not exceed 90 mg/day.

Children (9-12 years): The maximum recommended initial dose is 7.5 mg two times a day. Dosage should be increased by no more than 7.5 mg every week and should not exceed 60 mg/day.

Drug Interactions: If TRANXENE is to be combined with other drugs acting on the central nervous system, careful consideration should be given to the pharmacology of the agents to be employed. Animal experience indicates that TRANXENE prolongs the sleeping time after hexobarbital or after ethyl alcohol, increases the inhibitory effects of chlorpromazine, but does not exhibit monoamine oxidase inhibition. Clinical studies have shown increased sedation with concurrent hypnotic medications. The actions of the benzodiazepines may be potentiated by barbiturates, narcotics, phenothiazines, monoamine oxidase inhibitors or other antidepressants.

If TRANXENE is used to treat anxiety associated with somatic disease states, careful attention must be paid to possible drug interaction with concomitant medication.

In bioavailability studies with normal subjects, the concurrent administration of antacids at therapeutic levels did not significantly influence the bioavailability of TRANXENE.

Management of Overdosage: Overdosage is usually manifested by varying degrees of CNS depression ranging from slight sedation to coma. As in the management of overdosage with any drug, it should be borne in mind that multiple agents may have been taken.

There are no specific antidotes for the benzodiazepines. The treatment of overdosage should consist of the general measures employed in the management of overdosage of any CNS depressant. Gastric evacuation either by the induction of emesis, lavage, or both, should be performed immediately. General supportive care, including frequent monitoring of the vital signs and close observation of the patient, is indicated. Hypotension, though rarely reported, may occur with large overdoses. In such cases the use of agents such as Levophed® Bitartrate (norepinephrine bitartrate injection, USP) or Aramine® Injection (metaraminol bitartrate injection, USP) should be considered.

While reports indicate that individuals have survived overdoses of TRANXENE as high as 450 to 675 mg, these doses are not necessarily an accurate indication of the amount of drug absorbed since the time interval between ingestion and the institution of treatment was not always known. Sedation in varying degrees was the most common physiological manifestation of TRANXENE overdosage. Deep coma when it occurred was usually associated with the ingestion of other drugs in addition to TRANXENE.

Animal and Clinical Pharmacology: Studies in rats and monkeys have shown a substantial difference between doses producing tranquilizing, sedative and toxic effects. In rats, conditioned avoidance response was inhibited at an oral dose of 10 mg/kg; sedation was induced at 32 mg/kg; the LD_{50} was 1320 mg/kg. In monkeys aggressive behavior was reduced at an oral dose of 0.25 mg/kg; sedation (ataxia) was induced at 7.5 mg/kg; the LD_{50} could not be determined because of the emetic effect of large doses, but the LD_{50} exceeds 1600 mg/kg.

Twenty-four dogs were given TRANXENE orally in a 22-month toxicity study; doses up to 75 mg/kg were given. Drug-related changes occurred in the liver; weight was increased and cholestasis with minimal hepatocellular damage was found, but lobular architecture remained well preserved.

Eighteen rhesus monkeys were given oral doses of TRANXENE from 3 to 36 mg/kg daily for 52 weeks. All treated animals remained similar to control animals. Although total leucocyte count remained within normal limits it tended to fall in the female animals on the highest doses.

Examination of all organs revealed no alterations attributable to TRANXENE. There was no damage to liver function or structure.

Reproduction Studies: Standard fertility, reproduction, and teratology studies were conducted in rats and rabbits. Oral doses in rats up to 150 mg/kg and in rabbits up to 15 mg/kg produced no abnormalities in the fetuses. TRANXENE (clorazepate dipotassium) did not alter the fertility indices or reproductive capacity of adult animals. As expected, the sedative effect of high doses interfered with care of the young by their mothers (see Usage in Pregnancy).

Clinical Pharmacology: Studies in healthy men have shown that TRANXENE has depressant effects on the central nervous system. Prolonged administration of single daily doses as high as 120 mg was without toxic effects. Abrupt cessation of high doses was followed in some patients by nervousness, insomnia, irritability, diarrhea, muscle aches, or memory impairment.

Absorption—Excretion: After oral administration of TRANXENE there is essentially no circulating parent drug. Nordiazepam, its primary metabolite, quickly appears in the blood stream. In 2 volunteers given 15 mg (50 μC) of ^{14}C-Tranxene, about 80% was recovered in the urine and feces within 10 days. Excretion was primarily in the urine with about 1% excreted per day on day 10.

How Supplied: TRANXENE (clorazepate dipotassium) is supplied as:

3.75 mg gray and white capsules:
Bottles of 100 ....(NDC 0074-3417-13)
Bottles of 500 ....(NDC 0074-3417-53)
ABBO-PAC® unit dose packages:
100 ....(NDC 0074-3417-11).
7.5 mg gray and maroon capsules:
Bottles of 100 ....(NDC 0074-3418-13)
Bottles of 500 ....(NDC 0074-3418-53)
ABBO-PAC unit dose packages:
100 ....(NDC 0074-3418-11)
4 cartons of 25
(reverse-numbered) ....(NDC 0074-3418-25).
15 mg gray capsules:
Bottles of 100 ....(NDC 0074-3419-13)
Bottles of 500 ....(NDC 0074-3419-53)
ABBO-PAC unit dose packages:
100 ....(NDC 0074-3419-11).
3.75 mg blue-colored, scored tablets:
Bottles of 100 ....(NDC 0074-4389-13).
7.5 mg peach-colored, scored tablets:
Bottles of 100 ....(NDC 0074-4390-13).
15 mg lavender-colored, scored tablets:
Bottles of 100 ....(NDC 0074-4391-13).
TRANXENE-SD 22.5 mg tan-colored, single dose tablets:
Bottles of 100 ....(NDC 0074-2997-13).
TRANXENE-SD HALF STRENGTH 11.25 mg blue-colored, single dose tablets:
Bottles of 100 ....(NDC 0074-2699-13).

Shown in Product Identification Section, page 404
Abbott Pharmaceuticals, Inc.
North Chicago, IL 60064
Ref. 03-4224-R14

Continued on next page

Abbott—Cont.

TRIDIONE®
[try'dē-own]
(trimethadione)
Tablets, Capsules, and Oral Solution

BECAUSE OF ITS POTENTIAL TO PRODUCE FETAL MALFORMATIONS AND SERIOUS SIDE EFFECTS, TRIDIONE (trimethadione) SHOULD ONLY BE UTILIZED WHEN OTHER LESS TOXIC DRUGS HAVE BEEN FOUND INEFFECTIVE IN CONTROLLING PETIT MAL SEIZURES.

Description: TRIDIONE (trimethadione) is an antiepileptic agent. An oxazolidinedione compound, it is chemically identified as 3,5,5-trimethyloxozolidine-2,4-dione.
TRIDIONE is a synthetic, water-soluble, white, crystalline powder. It is supplied in capsular, tablet, and liquid forms for oral use only.

Clinical Pharmacology: TRIDIONE has been shown to prevent pentylenetetrazol-induced and thujone-induced seizures in experimental animals; the drug has a less marked effect on seizures induced by picrotoxin, procaine, cocaine, or strychnine. Unlike the hydantoins and antiepileptic barbiturates, TRIDIONE does not modify the maximal seizure pattern in patients undergoing electroconvulsive therapy.
TRIDIONE has a sedative effect that may increase to the point of ataxia when excessive doses are used.
A toxic dose of the drug in animals (approximately 2 mg/kg) produced sleep, unconsciousness, and respiratory depression.
Trimethadione is rapidly absorbed from the gastrointestinal tract. It is demethylated by liver microsomes to the active metabolite, dimethadione. Approximately 3% of a daily dose of TRIDIONE is recovered in the urine as unchanged drug. The majority of trimethadione is excreted slowly by the kidney in the form of dimethadione.

Indications: TRIDIONE (trimethadione) is indicated for the control of petit mal seizures that are refractory to treatment with other drugs.

Contraindications: TRIDIONE is contraindicated in patients with a known hypersensitivity to the drug.

Warnings: TRIDIONE may cause serious side effects. Strict medical supervision of the patient is mandatory, especially during the initial year of therapy.
TRIDIONE (trimethadione) should be withdrawn promptly if skin rash appears, because of the grave possibility of the occurrence of exfoliative dermatitis or severe forms of erythema multiforme. Even a minor acneiform or morbilliform rash should be allowed to clear completely before treatment with TRIDIONE is resumed; reinstitute therapy cautiously.
A complete blood count should be done prior to intiating therapy with TRIDIONE, and at monthly intervals thereafter. A marked depression of the blood count is an indication for withdrawal of the drug. If no abnormality appears within 12 months, the interval between blood counts may be extended. A moderate degree of neutropenia with or without a corresponding drop in the leukocyte count is not uncommon. Therapy need not be withdrawn unless the neutrophil count is 2500 or less; more frequent blood examinations should be done when the count is less than 3,000. Other blood dyscrasias, including leukopenia, eosinophilia, thrombocytopenia, pancytopenia, agranulocytosis, hypoplastic anemia, and fatal aplastic anemia, have occurred. Patients should be advised to report immediately such signs and symptoms as sore throat, fever, malaise, easy bruising, petechiae, or epistaxis, or others that may be indicative of an infection or bleeding tendency. TRIDIONE should ordinarily not be used in patients with severe blood dyscrasias.
Liver function tests should be done prior to initiating therapy with TRIDIONE, and at monthly intervals thereafter. Hepatitis has been reported rarely. Jaundice or other signs of liver dysfunction are an indication for withdrawal of the drug. TRIDIONE should ordinarily not be used in patients with severe hepatic impairment.
A urinalysis should be done prior to initiating therapy with TRIDIONE and at monthly intervals thereafter. Fatal nephrosis has been reported. Persistent or increasing albuminuria, or the development of any other significant renal abnormality, is an indication for withdrawal of the drug. TRIDIONE should ordinarily not be used in patients with severe renal dysfunction.
Hemeralopia has occurred; this appears to be an effect of TRIDIONE on the neural layers of the retina, and usually can be reversed by a reduction in dosage. Scotomata are an indication for withdrawal of the drug. Caution should be observed when treating patients who have diseases of the retina or optic nerve.
Manifestations of systemic lupus erythematosus have been associated with the use of TRIDIONE, as they have with the use of certain other anticonvulsants. Lymphadenopathies simulating malignant lymphoma have occurred. Lupus-like manifestations or lymph node enlargement are indications for withdrawal of the drug. Signs and symptoms may disappear after discontinuation of therapy, and specific treatment may be unnecessary.
A myasthenia gravis-like syndrome has been associated with the chronic use of trimethadione. Symptoms suggestive of this condition are indications for withdrawal of the drug.
Drugs known to cause toxic effects similar to those of TRIDIONE should be avoided or used only with extreme caution during therapy with TRIDIONE.

USAGE DURING PREGNANCY AND LACTATION:
THERE ARE MULTIPLE REPORTS IN THE CLINICAL LITERATURE WHICH INDICATE THAT THE USE OF ANTICONVULSANT DRUGS DURING PREGNANCY RESULTS IN AN INCREASED INCIDENCE OF BIRTH DEFECTS IN THE OFFSPRING. DATA ARE MORE EXTENSIVE WITH RESPECT TO TRIMETHADIONE, PARAMETHADIONE, PHENYTOIN AND PHENOBARBITAL THAN WITH OTHER ANTICONVULSANT DRUGS.
THEREFORE, ANTICONVULSANT DRUGS SUCH AS TRIDIONE (TRIMETHADIONE) SHOULD BE ADMINISTERED TO WOMEN OF CHILDBEARING POTENTIAL ONLY IF THEY ARE CLEARLY SHOWN TO BE ESSENTIAL IN THE MANAGEMENT OF THEIR SEIZURES. EFFECTIVE MEANS OF CONTRACEPTION SHOULD ACCOMPANY THE USE OF TRIDIONE IN SUCH PATIENTS. IF A PATIENT BECOMES PREGNANT WHILE TAKING TRIDIONE, TERMINATION OF THE PREGNANCY SHOULD BE CONSIDERED. A PATIENT WHO REQUIRES THERAPY WITH TRIDIONE AND WHO WISHES TO BECOME PREGNANT SHOULD BE ADVISED OF THE RISKS.
REPORTS HAVE SUGGESTED THAT THE MATERNAL INGESTION OF ANTICONVULSANT DRUGS, PARTICULARLY BARBITURATES, IS ASSOCIATED WITH A NEONATAL COAGULATION DEFECT THAT MAY CAUSE BLEEDING DURING THE EARLY (USUALLY WITHIN 24 HOURS OF BIRTH) NEONATAL PERIOD. THE POSSIBILITY OF THE OCCURRENCE OF THIS DEFECT WITH THE USE OF TRIDIONE SHOULD BE KEPT IN MIND. THE DEFECT IS CHARACTERIZED BY DECREASED LEVELS OF VITAMIN K-DEPENDENT CLOTTING FACTORS, AND PROLONGATION OF EITHER THE PROTHROMBIN TIME OR THE PARTIAL THROMBOPLASTIN TIME, OR BOTH. IT HAS BEEN SUGGESTED THAT PROPHYLACTIC VITAMIN K BE GIVEN TO THE MOTHER ONE MONTH PRIOR TO, AND DURING DELIVERY, AND TO THE INFANT, INTRAVENOUSLY, IMMEDIATELY AFTER BIRTH.
THE SAFETY OF TRIDIONE FOR USE DURING LACTATION HAS NOT BEEN ESTABLISHED.

Precautions: Abrupt discontinuation of TRIDIONE may precipitate petit mal status. TRIDIONE should always be withdrawn gradually unless serious adverse effects dictate otherwise. In the latter case, another anticonvulsant may be substituted to protect the patient.
Usage during Pregnancy and Lactation: See WARNINGS.

Adverse Reactions: The following side effects, some of them serious, have been associated with the use of TRIDIONE.
Gastrointestinal: nausea, vomiting, abdominal pain, gastric distress.
CNS/Neurologic: drowsiness, fatigue, malaise, insomnia, vertigo, headache, paresthesias, precipitation of grand mal seizures, increased irritability, personality changes.
Drowsiness usually subsides with continued therapy. If it persists, a reduction in dosage is indicated.
Hematologic: bleeding gums, epistaxis, retinal and petechial hemorrhages, vaginal bleeding; neutropenia, leukopenia, eosinophilia, thrombocytopenia, pancytopenia, agranulocytosis, hypoplastic anemia, and fatal aplastic anemia.
Dermatologic: acneiform or morbilliform skin rash that may progress to exfoliative dermatitis or to severe forms of erythema multiforme.
Other: hiccups, anorexia, weight loss, hair loss, changes in blood pressure, albuminuria, hemeralopia, photophobia, diplopia.
Fatal nephrosis has occurred.
Hepatitis has been reported rarely.
Lupus erythematosus, and lymphadenopathies simulating malignant lymphoma, have been reported.
Pruritus associated with lymphadenopathy and hepatosplenomegaly has occurred in hypersensitive individuals.
A myasthenia gravis-like syndrome has been reported.

Overdosage: Symptoms of acute TRIDIONE overdosage include drowsiness, nausea, dizziness, ataxia, visual disturbances. Coma may follow massive overdosage.
Gastric evacuation, either by induced emesis, or by lavage, or both, should be done immediately. General supportive care, including frequent monitoring of the vital signs and close observation of the patient, are required.
Alkalinization of the urine has been reported to enhance the renal excretion of dimethadione, the active metabolite of TRIDIONE.
A blood count and a careful evaluation of hepatic and renal function should be done following recovery.

Dosage and Administration: TRIDIONE is administered orally.
Usual Adult Dosage: 0.9–2.4 Gm daily in 3 or 4 equally divided doses (i.e. 300–600 mg 3 or 4 times daily).
Initially, give 0.9 Gm daily; increase this dose by 300 mg at weekly intervals until therapeutic results are seen or until toxic symptoms appear. Maintenance dosage should be the least amount of drug required to maintain control.
Children's Dosage: Usually 0.3–0.9 Gm daily in 3 or 4 equally divided doses.

How Supplied: TRIDIONE Capsules (trimethadione capsules, USP), 300 mg (white) are supplied in bottles of 100 (NDC 0074-3709-01).
TRIDIONE Dulcet® Tablets (trimethadione tablets, USP), 150 mg (white) chewable tablets are supplied in bottles of 100 (NDC 0074-3753-01).
Shown in Product Identification Section, page 404
TRIDIONE Solution (trimethadione oral solution, USP), 1.2 Gm per fluidounce (40 mg per ml), is supplied in pint bottles (NDC 0074-3721-01).
Abbott Laboratories/
Abbott Pharmaceuticals, Inc.
North Chicago, IL 60064
®Dulcet—Sweetened tablets, Abbott.
Ref. 03-4194/R3

TRONOTHANE® HYDROCHLORIDE
[tro'nō-thāne hy-drō-clō'rīde]
(pramoxine hydrochloride)
Cream

Description: Tronothane Hydrochloride (pramoxine hydrochloride) is a surface anesthetic agent, chemically unrelated to the benzoate esters of the "caine" type. It is chemically designated as 4-n-butoxyphenyl gammamorpholinopropyl ether hydrochloride.

Indications: Tronothane Hydrochloride is indicated for temporary relief of pain and itching due to minor burns, sunburn, minor cuts, abrasions, insect bites, minor skin irritations, hemorrhoids and other anorectal disorders.

Contraindications: Tronothane Hydrochloride is not suitable for and should not be injected into the tissues. It should not be used for bronchoscopy or gastroscopy, or in patients who are hypersensitive to the drug.

Warnings: Tronothane Hydrochloride is not intended for prolonged use. Do not apply to large areas of the body. Do not use in the eyes or nose. If condition worsens, or persists for 7 days, consult physician. If bleeding or increased pain occurs when using the product in the rectum, consult physician promptly.

For topical use in children under 2 years or anorectal use in children under 12 years, use only as directed by physician. Keep out of reach of children.

Adverse Reactions: Local skin reactions, e.g. stinging and burning. Discontinue use if redness, irritation, swelling or pain occur.

Dosage and Administration: *Topical*—Adults and children 2 years of age or older: Apply to affected area 3 to 4 times daily, or as directed by a physician.

Anorectal—When practical, wash the area with soap and warm water, and rinse off all soap before application. Adults and children 12 years of age or older: Apply up to 5 times daily, especially morning, night and after bowel movements, or as directed by a physician.

External—Apply liberally to affected area.

Intrarectal—Remove cap from tube and attach clean applicator. Squeeze tube to fill and lubricate applicator. Gently insert applicator into rectum and squeeze tube. Thoroughly cleanse applicator with soap and warm water after use.

How Supplied: Tronothane Hydrochloride 1% Cream (pramoxine hydrochloride cream, USP), pramoxine hydrochloride 1% in a water miscible base containing cetyl alcohol, cetyl esters wax, glycerin, sodium lauryl sulfate, methylparaben, and propylparaben, is supplied in a 1-oz tube with rectal applicator (**NDC** 0074-6645-01).

These products are listed in USP, a Medicare designated compendium.

Abbott Laboratories
North Chicago, IL 60064

If desired, additional literature on any Abbott Product will be provided upon request to Abbott Laboratories.

Adria Laboratories
Division of Erbamont Inc.
5000 POST ROAD
DUBLIN, OH 43017

PRODUCT IDENTIFICATION CODES

To provide quick and positive identification of Adria Laboratories Inc. products, we have imprinted the product identification number on one side of all tablets and capsules. The other side of the tablet displays the name "ADRIA".

In order that you may quickly identify a product by its code number, we have compiled below a numerical list of code numbers of prescription products with their corresponding product names:

PRODUCT IDENTIFICATION CODE	NUMERICAL PRODUCT INDEX

130 Axotal (butalbital, USP, 50 mg and aspirin, USP, 650 mg. Warning: May be habit forming)
200 Ilozyme® (pancrelipase, USP) Tablets
231 Ilopan-Choline® Tablets (dexpanthenol 50 mg./choline bitartrate 25 mg)
304 Kaon CL™-10 (potassium chloride Controlled Release Tablets, 750 mg. (10 mEq)
305 Kaochlor-Eff® Tablets (potassium and chloride) 20 mEq.
307 Kaon-CL™ (potassium chloride) Controlled Release Tablets, 500 mg (6.7 mEq)
312 Kaon® (potassium gluconate) Tablets, 1.7 g (5 mEq)
412 Magan® (magnesium salicylate) Tablets, 545 mg.
648 Fluidil™ (cyclothiazide, USP) 2 mg.

ADRIAMYCIN™ ℞
[a′dreeah-mi″sin]
(doxorubicin hydrochloride)
for injection
FOR INTRAVENOUS USE ONLY

WARNINGS
1. Severe local tissue necrosis will occur if there is extravasation during administration. (See Dosage and Administration.) ADRIAMYCIN must not be given by the intramuscular or subcutaneous route.
2. Serious irreversible myocardial toxicity with delayed congestive failure often unresponsive to any cardiac supportive therapy may be encountered as total dosage approaches 550 mg/m². This toxicity may occur at lower cumulative doses in patients with prior mediastinal irradiation or on concurrent cyclophosphamide therapy.
3. Dosage should be reduced in patients with impaired hepatic function.
4. Severe myelosuppression may occur.
5. ADRIAMYCIN should be administered only under the supervision of a physician who is experienced in the use of cancer chemotherapeutic agents.

Description: Doxorubicin is a cytotoxic anthracycline antibiotic isolated from cultures of *Streptomyces peucetius* var. *caesius*. Doxorubicin consists of a naphthacenequinone nucleus linked through a glycosidic bond at ring atom 7 to an amino sugar, daunosamine. The structural formula is as follows:

Doxorubicin binds to nucleic acids, presumably by specific intercalation of the planar anthracycline nucleus with the DNA double helix. The anthracycline ring is lipophilic but the saturated end of the ring system contains abundant hydroxyl groups adjacent to the amino sugar, producing a hydrophilic center. The molecule is amphoteric, containing acidic functions in the ring phenolic groups and a basic function in the sugar amino group. It binds to cell membranes as well as plasma proteins. It is supplied in the hydrochloride form as a freeze-dried powder containing lactose.

Clinical Pharmacology: Though not completely elucidated, the mechanism of action of doxorubicin is related to its ability to bind to DNA and inhibit nucleic acid synthesis. Cell culture studies have demonstrated rapid cell penetration and perinucleolar chromatin binding, rapid inhibition of mitotic activity and nucleic acid synthesis, mutagenesis and chromosomal aberrations. Animal studies have shown activity in a spectrum of experimental tumors, immunosuppression, carcinogenic properties in rodents, induction of a variety of toxic effects, including delayed and progressive cardiac toxicity, myelosuppression in all species and atrophy to testes in rats and dogs.

Pharmacokinetic studies show the intravenous administration of normal or radiolabeled ADRIAMYCIN (doxorubicin hydrochloride) for Injection is followed by rapid plasma clearance and significant tissue binding. Urinary excretion, as determined by fluorimetric methods, accounts for approximately 4-5% of the administered dose in five days. Biliary excretion represents the major excretion route, 40-50% of the administered dose being recovered in the bile or the feces in seven days. Impairment of liver function results in slower excretion, and consequently, increased retention and accumulation in plasma and tissues. ADRIAMYCIN does not cross the blood brain barrier.

Indications and Usage: ADRIAMYCIN has been used successfully to produce regression in disseminated neoplastic conditions such as acute lymphoblastic leukemia, acute myeloblastic leukemia, Wilms' tumor, neuroblastoma, soft tissue and bone sarcomas, breast carcinoma, ovarian carcinoma, transitional cell bladder carcinoma, thryoid carcinoma, lymphomas of both Hodgkin and non-Hodgkin types, bronchogenic carcinoma in which the small cell histologic type is the most responsive compared to other cell types and gastric carcinoma.

A number of other solid tumors have also shown some responsiveness but in numbers too limited to justify specific recommendation. Studies to date have shown malignant melanoma, kidney carcinoma, large bowel carcinoma, brain tumors and metastases to the central nervous system not to be significantly responsive to ADRIAMYCIN therapy.

Contraindications: ADRIAMYCIN therapy should not be started in patients who have marked myelosuppression induced by previous treatment with other antitumor agents or by radiotherapy. Conclusive data are not available on pre-existing heart disease as a co-factor of increased risk of ADRIAMYCIN induced cardiac toxicity. Preliminary data suggest that in such cases cardiac toxicity may occur at doses lower than the recommended cumulative limit. It is therefore not recommended to start ADRIAMYCIN in such cases. ADRIAMYCIN treatment is contraindicated in patients who received previous treatment with complete cumulative doses of ADRIAMYCIN and/or daunorubicin.

Warnings: Special attention must be given to the cardiac toxicity exhibited by ADRIAMYCIN. Although uncommon, acute left ventricular failure has occurred, particularly in patients who have received total dosage of the drug exceeding the currently recommended limit of 550 mg/m². This limit appears to be lower (400 mg/m²) in patients who received radiotherapy to the mediastinal area or concomitant therapy with other potentially cardiotoxic agents such as cyclophosphamide. The total dose of ADRIAMYCIN administered to the individual patient should also take into account a previous or concomitant therapy with related compounds such as daunorubicin. Congestive heart failure and/or cardiomyopathy may be encountered several weeks after discontinuation of ADRIAMYCIN therapy.

Cardiac failure is often not favorably affected by presently known medical or physical therapy for cardiac support. Early clinical diagnosis of drug induced heart failure appears to be essential for successful treatment with digitalis, diuretics, low salt diet and bed rest. Severe cardiac toxicity may occur precipitously without antecedent EKG changes. A baseline EKG and EKGs performed prior to each dose or course after 300 mg/m² cumulative dose has been given is suggested. Transient EKG changes consisting of T-wave flattening, S-T depression and arrhythmias lasting for up to two weeks after a dose or course of ADRIAMYCIN are presently not considered indications for suspension of ADRIAMYCIN therapy. ADRIAMYCIN cardiomyopathy has been reported to be associated with a persistent reduction in the voltage of the QRS wave, a prolongation of the systolic time interval and a reduction of the ejection fraction as determined by echocardiography or radionuclide angiography. None of these tests have yet been confirmed to consistently identify those individual patients that are approaching their maximally tolerated cumulative dose of ADRIAMYCIN. If test results indicate change in cardiac function

Continued on next page

Adria—Cont.

associated with ADRIAMYCIN the benefit of continued therapy must be carefully evaluated against the risk of producing irreversible cardiac damage.

Acute life-threatening arrhythmias have been reported to occur during or within a few hours after ADRIAMYCIN adminstration.

There is a high incidence of bone marrow depression, primarily of leukocytes, requiring careful hematologic monitoring. With the recommended dosage schedule, leukopenia is usually transient, reaching its nadir at 10–14 days after treatment with recovery usually occurring by the 21st day. White blood cell counts as low as 1000 mm^3 are to be expected during treatment with appropriate doses of ADRIAMYCIN. Red blood cell and platelet levels should also be monitored since they may also be depressed. Hematologic toxicity may require dose reduction or suspension or delay of ADRIAMYCIN therapy. Persistent severe myelosuppression may result in superinfection or hemorrhage.

ADRIAMYCIN may potentiate the toxicity of other anticancer therapies. Exacerbation of cyclophosphamide induced hemorrhagic cystitis and enhancement of the hepatotoxicity of 6-mercaptopurine have been reported. Radiation induced toxicity to the myocardium, mucosae, skin and liver have been reported to be increased by the administration of ADRIAMYCIN.

Toxicity to recommended doses of ADRIAMYCIN is enhanced by hepatic impairment, therefore, prior to the individual dosing, evaluation of hepatic function is recommended using conventional clinical laboratory tests such as SGOT, SGPT, alkaline phosphatase and bilirubin. (See Dosage and Administration).

Necrotizing colitis manifested by typhlitis (cecal inflammation), bloody stools and severe and sometimes fatal infections have been associated with a combination of ADRIAMYCIN given by i.v. push daily for 3 days and cytarabine given by continuous infusion daily for 7 or more days.

On intravenous administration of ADRIAMYCIN extravasation may occur with or without an accompanying stinging or burning sensation and even if blood returns well on aspiration of the infusion needle (See Dosage and Administration). If any signs or symptoms of extravasation have occurred the injection or infusion should be immediately terminated and restarted in another vein.

ADRIAMYCIN and related compounds have also been shown to have mutagenic and carcinogenic properties when tested in experimental models.

Usage in Pregnancy—Safe use of ADRIAMYCIN in pregnancy has not been established. ADRIAMYCIN is embryotoxic and teratogenic in rats and embryotoxic and abortifacient in rabbits. Therefore, the benefits to the pregnant patient should be carefully weighed against the potential toxicity to fetus and embryo. The possible adverse effects on fertility in males and females in humans or experimental animals have not been adequately evaluated.

Precautions: Initial treatment with ADRIAMYCIN requires close observation of the patient and extensive laboratory monitoring. It is recommended, therefore, that patients be hospitalized at least during the first phase of the treatment.

Like other cytotoxic drugs, ADRIAMYCIN may induce hyperuricemia secondary to rapid lysis of neoplastic cells. The clinician should monitor the patient's blood uric acid level and be prepared to use such supportive and pharmacologic measures as might be necessary to control this problem.

ADRIAMYCIN imparts a red coloration to the urine for 1–2 days after administration and patients should be advised to expect this during active therapy.

ADRIAMYCIN is not an anti-microbial agent.

Adverse Reactions: Dose limiting toxicities of therapy are myelosuppression and cardiotoxicity (See Warnings). Other reactions reported are:

Cutaneous—Reversible complete alopecia occurs in most cases. Hyperpigmentation of nailbeds and dermal creases, primarily in children, have been reported in a few cases. Recall of skin reaction due to prior radiotherapy has occurred with ADRIAMYCIN administration.

Gastrointestinal—Acute nausea and vomiting occurs frequently and may be severe. This may be alleviated by antiemetic therapy. Mucositis (stomatitis and esophagitis) may occur 5–10 days after administration. The effect may be severe leading to ulceration and represents a site of origin for severe infections. The dose regimen consisting of administration of ADRIAMYCIN on three successive days results in the greater incidence and severity of mucositis. Ulceration and necrosis of the colon, especially the cecum, may occur leading to bleeding or severe infections which can be fatal. This reaction has been reported in patients with acute non-lymphocytic leukemia treated with a 3-day course of ADRIAMYCIN combined with cytarabine. Anorexia and diarrhea have been occasionally reported.

Vascular—Phlebosclerosis has been reported especially when small veins are used or a single vein is used for repeated administration. Facial flushing may occur if the injection is given too rapidly.

Local—Severe cellulitis, vesication and tissue necrosis will occur if ADRIAMYCIN is extravasated during administration. Erythematous streaking along the vein proximal to the site of the injection has been reported (See Dosage and Administration).

Hypersensitivity—Fever, chills and urticaria have been reported occasionally. Anaphylaxis may occur. A case of apparent cross sensitivity to lincomycin has been reported.

Other—Conjunctivitis and lacrimation occur rarely.

Overdosage: Acute overdosage with ADRIAMYCIN enhances the toxic effects of mucositis, leukopenia and thrombopenia. Treatment of acute overdosage consists of treatment of the severely myelosuppressed patient with hospitalization, antibiotics, platelet and granulocyte transfusions and symptomatic treatment of mucositis.

Chronic overdosage with cumulative doses exceeding 550 mg/m^2 increases the risk of cardiomyopathy and resultant congestive heart failure. Treatment consists of vigorous management of congestive heart failure with digitalis preparations and diuretics. The use of peripheral vasodilators has been recommended.

Dosage and Administration: Care in the administration of ADRIAMYCIN will reduce the chance of perivenous infiltration. It may also decrease the chance of local reactions such as urticaria and erythematous streaking. On intravenous administration of ADRIAMYCIN, extravasation may occur with or without an accompanying stinging or burning sensation and even if blood returns well on aspiration of the infusion needle. If any signs or symptoms of extravasation have occurred, the injection or infusion should be immediately terminated and restarted in another vein. If it is known or suspected that subcutaneous extravasation has occurred, local infiltration with an injectable corticosteroid and flooding the site with normal saline has been reported to lessen the local reaction. Because of the progressive nature of extravasation reactions, the area of injection should be frequently examined and plastic surgery consultation obtained. If ulceration begins, early wide excision of the involved area should be considered.[1]

The most commonly used dosage schedule is 60–75 mg/m^2 as a single intravenous injection administered at 21-day intervals. The lower dose should be given to patients with inadequate marrow reserves due to old age, or prior therapy, or neoplastic marrow infiltration. An alternative dose schedule is weekly doses of 20 mg/m^2 which has been reported to produce a lower incidence of congestive heart failure. Thirty mg/m^2 on each of three successive days repeated every 4 weeks has also been used. ADRIAMYCIN dosage must be reduced if the bilirubin is elevated as follows: Serum Bilirubin 1.2–3.0 mg/dl—give ½ normal dose, > 3 mg/dl—give ¼ normal dose.

Preparation of Solution: ADRIAMYCIN 10 mg vials and 50 mg vials should be reconstituted with 5 ml and 25 ml respectively of Sodium Chloride injection USP (0.9%) or Sterile Water for Injection USP to give a final concentration of 2 mg/ml of doxorubicin hydrochloride. If Sterile Water for Injection USP is used for reconstitution, the resulting solution must be brought towards isotonicity before injection by adding 2 to 3 times the volume of 0.9% Sodium Chloride Injection USP to the aqueous solution. An approriate volume of air should be withdrawn from the vial during reconstitution to avoid excessive pressure build-up. Bacteriostatic diluents are not recommended.

Skin reactions associated with ADRIAMYCIN have been reported. Caution in the handling and preparation of the powder and solution must be exercised and the use of gloves is recommended. If ADRIAMYCIN powder or solution contacts the skin or mucosae, immediately wash thoroughly with soap and water.

After adding the diluent, the vial should be shaken and the contents allowed to dissolve. The reconstituted solution is stable for 24 hours at room temperature and 48 hours under refrigeration (4–10°C). It should be protected from exposure to sunlight and any unused solution should be discarded. It is recommended that ADRIAMYCIN be slowly administered into the tubing of a freely running intravenous infusion of Sodium Chloride Injection USP or 5% Dextrose Injection USP. The tubing should be attached to a Butterfly® needle inserted preferably into a large vein. If possible, avoid veins over joints or in extremities with compromised venous or lymphatic drainage. The rate of administration is dependent on the size of the vein and the dosage. However the dose should be administered in not less than 3 to 5 minutes. Local erythematous streaking along the vein as well as facial flushing may be indicative of too rapid an administration. A burning or stinging sensation may be indicative of perivenous infiltration and the infusion should be immediately terminated and restarted in another vein. Perivenous infiltration may occur painlessly.

ADRIAMYCIN should not be mixed with heparin or 5-fluorouracil since it has been reported that these drugs are incompatible to the extent that a precipitate may form. Until specific compatibility data are available, it is not recommended that ADRIAMYCIN be mixed with other drugs.

ADRIAMYCIN has been used concurrently with other approved chemotherapeutic agents. Evidence is available that in some types of neoplastic disease combination chemotherapy is superior to single agents. The benefits and risks of such therapy continue to be elucidated; listed in CLINICAL STUDIES are combinations that have been reported to be clinically superior to any agent in the combination used alone.

How Supplied: ADRIAMYCIN™ (doxorubicin hydrochloride) for Injection is available in two sizes:

10 mg—Each vial contains 10 mg of doxorubicin HCl and 50 mg of lactose USP as a sterile red-orange lyophilized powder. Packaged and supplied in 10-vial cartons NDC 0013-1006-91.

50 mg—Each vial contains 50 mg of doxorubicin HCl and 250 mg of lactose USP as a sterile red-orange lyophilized powder. Packaged and supplied in a single vial carton NDC 0013-1016-79.

Clinical Studies: Clinical studies support the efficacy of ADRIAMYCIN used concurrently with other chemotherapeutic agents. Listed below are tumor types and drugs used concurrently with ADRIAMYCIN:

Acute lymphocytic leukemia in adults. ADRIAMYCIN with vincristine and prednisone[2,3] or with cytosine arabinoside, vincristine and prednisone[8].
Acute lymphocytic leukemia in children. ADRIAMYCIN with vincristine and prednisone[4,5].
Acute non-lymphocytic leukemia. ADRIAMYCIN with arabinosyl cytosine[6] or with arabinosyl cytosine, vincristine and prednisone[7,8].
Carcinoma of the breast. ADRIAMYCIN with 5-fluorouracil and/or cyclophosphamide[9,10] or with vincristine with or without cyclophosphamide[11].
Bronchogenic carcinoma, non-small cell: ADRIAMYCIN with cyclophosphamide, methotrexate and procarbazine[12] or with cyclophosphamide and

cisplatin[13]. Bronchogenic carcinoma, small cell: ADRIAMYCIN with vincristine and cyclophosphamide[14,15,16]

Hodgkin disease: ADRIAMYCIN with bleomycin, vincristine and dacarbazine[17,18].

Non-Hodgkin lymphoma: ADRIAMYCIN with cyclophosphamide, vincristine and prednisone[19], or bleomycin, cyclophosphamide, vincristine and prednisone[20].

Carcinoma of the ovary. ADRIAMYCIN with cisplatin[21,22].

Soft tissue sarcoma: ADRIAMYCIN with dacarbazine or with dacarbazine, cyclophosphamide and vincristine[23,24].

Carcinoma of the bladder. ADRIAMYCIN with cisplatin and cyclophosphamide[25] or with 5-flourouracil[26].

Carcinoma of the stomach. ADRIAMYCIN with 5-flourouracil and mitomycin-C[27,28]

References:

1. Rudolph R et al: Skin Ulcers Due to ADRIAMYCIN. Cancer 38: 1087–1094, Sept. 1976.
2. Muriel FS, Pavlovsky S, Penalver JA et al: Evaluation of Induction of Remission, Intensification, and Central Nervous System Prophylactic Treatment in Acute Lymphoblastic Leukemia. Cancer 34:418–426, 1974.
3. Shaw MT, Raab SO: ADRIAMYCIN in Combination Chemotherapy of Adult Acute Lymphoblastic Leukemia: A Southwest Oncology Group Study. Med Pediatr Oncol 3:261–266, 1977.
4. Sallan SE, Camitta BM, Cassady JR et al: Intermittent Combination Chemotherapy with ADRIAMYCIN for Childhood Acute Lymphoblastic Leukemia: Clinical Results. Blood 51:425–433, 1978.
5. Rivera G, Aur RJA, Dahl GV: Second Cessation of Therapy in Childhood Lymphocytic Leukemia. Blood 53:1114–1120, 1979.
6. Preisler HD, Rustum Y, Henderson ES, et al: Treatment of Acute Non-Lymphocytic Leukemia: Use of Anthracycline-Cytosine Arabinoside Induction Therapy and Comparision of Two Maintenance Regimens. Blood 53:455–464, 1979.
7. Weinstein HJ, Mayer RJ, Rosenthal DS: Treatment of Acute Myelogenous Leukemia in Children and Adults. N Engl J Med 303:473–478, 1980.
8. McCredie KB, Bodey GP, Freireich EJ, et al: Chemoimmunotherapy of Adult Acute Leukemia. Cancer 47:1256–1261, 1981.
9. Bull JM, Tormey DC, Li S-H, et al: A Randomized Comparative Trial of ADRIAMYCIN Versus Methotrexate in Combination Drug Therapy. Cancer 41:1649–1657, 1978.
10. Smalley RV, Bartolucci AA: Variations in Responsiveness and Survival of Clinical Subsets of patients with Metastatic Breast Cancer to Two Chemotherapy Combinations. Eur J Cancer (Suppl 1) 141–146, 1980.
11. Brambilla C, Valagussa P, Bonadonna G: Sequential combination Chemotherapy in Advanced Breast Cancer. Cancer Chemother Pharmacol 1:35–39, 1978.
12. Bitran JD, Desser RK, DeMeester TR, et al: Cyclophosphamide, ADRIAMYCIN, Methotrexate and Procarbazine (CAMP)-Effective Four-Drug Combination Chemotherapy for Metastatic Non-Oat Cell Bronchogenic Carcinoma. Cancer Treat Rep 60:1225–1230, 1976.
13. Eagan, RT, Frytak S, Creagan ET: Phase II Study of Cyclophosphamide, ADRIAMYCIN and Cis-dichlorodiammineplatinum II by Infusion in Patients with Adenocarcinoma and Large Cell Carcinoma of the Lung. Cancer Treat Rep 63:1589–1591, 1979.
14. Livingston RB, Moore TN, Heilbrun L, et al: Small Cell Carcinoma of the Lung: Combined Chemotherapy and Radiation. Ann Intern Med 88: 194–199, 1978.
15. Lyman GH, Hartmann RC, Hussain IS, et al: Combination Chemotherapy and Radiation Therapy of Undifferentiated Small Cell Bronchogenic Carcinoma. South Med J 71:519–524, 1978.
16. Greco FA, Richardson RL, Snell JD, et al: Small Cell Lung Cancer, Am J Med 66:625–630, 1979.
17. Bonadonna G, DeLena M, Monfardini S, et al: Combination Usage of ADRIAMYCIN (NSC 123127) in Malignant Lymphomas, Cancer Chemother Rep Part 3, Vol 6:381–388, 1975.
18. Case DC, Young CW, Nisce L, et al: Eight-Drug Combination Chemotherapy (MOPP and ABVD) and Local Radiotherapy for Advanced Hodgkin's Disease. Cancer Treat Rep 60:1217–1223, 1976.
19. McKelvey EM, Gottlieb JA, Wilson HE, et al: Hydroxyldaunomycin (ADRIAMYCIN) Combination Chemotherapy in Malignant Lymphoma. Cancer 38:1484–1493, 1976.
20. Schein PS, DeVita VT, Hubbard S, et al: Bleomycin, ADRIAMYCIN, Cyclophosphamide, Vincristine, and Prednisone (BACOP) Combination Chemotherapy in the Treatment of Advanced Diffuse Histocytic Lymphoma. Ann Intern Med 85:417–422, 1976.
21. Briscoe KE, Pasmantier MW, Ohnuma T, Kennedy BJ: Cis-Dichlorodiammine platinum (II) and ADRIAMYCIN Treatment of Advanced Ovarian Cancer. Cancer Treat Rep 62:2027–2030, 1978.
22. Bruckner HW, Cohen CJ, Goldberg JD, et al: Improved chemotherapy in Ovarian Cancer with Cis-diamminedichloroplatinum and ADRIAMYCIN, Cancer 47:2288–2294, May 1, 1981.
23. Gottlieb JA, Baker LH, O'Bryan RM, et al: ADRIAMYCIN (NSC-123127) Used Alone and in Combination for Soft Tissue and Bony Sarcoma. Cancer Chemother Rep Part 3 Vol 6:271–282, 1975.
24. Yap BS, Baker LH, Sinkovics JG, et al: Cyclophosphamide, Vincristine, ADRIAMYCIN and DTIC (CYVADIC) Combination Chemotherapy for the Treatment of Advanced Sarcomas. Cancer Treat Rep 64:93–98, 1980.
25. Kedia KR, Gibbons C, Persky L: The Management of Advanced Bladder Carcinoma. J Urol 125:655–658, 1981.
26. Martino S, Samal B, Al-Sarraf M: Phase II Study of 5-Fluorouracil and ADRIAMYCIN In Transitional Cell Carcinoma of the Urinary Tract. Cancer Treat Rep 64:161–163, 1980.
27. Macdonald JS, Schein PS, Woolley PV, et al: 5-Fluorouracil, Doxorubicin and Mitomycin (FAM) Combination Chemotherapy for Advanced Gastric Cancer. Ann Intern Med 93:533–536, 1980.
28. Panettiere FJ, Heilbran L: Experiences with two treatment Schedules in the Combination Chemotherapy of Advanced Gastric Carcinoma. In: Mitomycin C. Current Status and New Developments. Schein PS ed., New York, Academic Press 1979 pp. 145–157.

Distributed by: Adria Laboratories Inc., Columbus, Ohio 43215. Manufactured by: Farmitalia Carlo Erba S.p.A., Milan, Italy.

ADRUCIL® R
[a'drew-sill"]
(fluorouracil)
INJECTABLE, USP
FOR INTRAVENOUS USE ONLY

WARNINGS

Adrucil should be administered only by or under the supervision of a qualified physician who is experienced in cancer chemotherapy and the use of potent antimetabolites. Because severe toxic reactions may occur, it is recommended that patients be hospitalized during the initial course of therapy. Before administering Adrucil, the contents of this insert should be thoroughly reviewed.

Description: Fluorouracil is a fluorinated pyrimidine belonging to the category of antimetabolites. Fluorouracil resembles the natural uracil molecule except it has been fluorinated in the 5 position; it has the following structural formula:

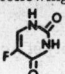

Molecular formula: $C_4H_3FN_2O_2$
Molecular Weight: 130.08

It is sparingly soluble in water (12.2 mg/ml) at pH 7 and has pK's of 8.0 and 13.0.

Adrucil (Fluorouracil) Injectable, USP is supplied as a sterile aqueous solution for intravenous injection. It has a pH of 8.6 to 9.0. The ampules are filled with a 5% excess to permit withdrawal and administration of the labeled volume.

A precipitate may form as a result of exposure to low temperatures. Redissolve by heating to 140°F (60°C) with vigorous shaking, and allow to cool to body temperature prior to use.

Actions: The mechanism of action of fluorouracil is mainly related to competitive inhibition of thymidylate synthetase, the enzyme catalyzing the methylation of deoxyuridylic acid to thymidylic acid. The consequent thymidine deficiency results in inhibition of deoxyribonucleic acid (DNA) synthesis, thus inducing cell death. Also, moderate inhibition of ribonucleic acid (RNA) and incorporation of fluorouracil into RNA have been observed, but these effects do not appear to play a significant role in the determination of the antitumor action of fluorouracil.

The effects of DNA and RNA deprivation are most marked on those cells which grow rapidly and which take up fluorouracil at more rapid pace. Inactive degradation products (e.g., CO_2, urea, α-fluoro-β-alanine) result from the extensive catabolic metabolism of fluorouracil. Following intravenous injection, no intact drug can be detected in the plasma after 3 hours and 60 to 80% of the dose is excreted as respiratory CO_2 in 8 to 12 hours. Within 6 hours approximately 15% of the total drug administered is excreted unchanged in the urine with over 90% of this excretion occurring in the first hour.

Indications: Adrucil is effective in the palliative management of carcinoma of the colon, rectum, breast, stomach and pancreas in patients who are considered incurable by surgery or other means.

Contraindications: Adrucil therapy should not be started in patients with a poor nutritional state, depressed bone marrow function, or potentially serious infections.

Warnings: THE DAILY DOSE OF ADRUCIL IS NOT TO EXCEED 800 MG AND IT IS RECOMMENDED THAT PATIENTS BE HOSPITALIZED DURING THEIR FIRST COURSE OF TREATMENT.

Adrucil (Fluorouracil) Injectable, USP should be used with extreme caution in poor risk patients with a history of high-dose pelvic irradiation, previous use of alkylating agents, or who have a widespread involvement of bone marrow by metastatic tumors, or impaired hepatic or renal function. The drug is not intended as an adjuvant to surgery. Although severe toxicity and fatalities are more likely to occur in poor risk patients, these effects have occasionally been encountered in patients in relatively good condition. Severe hematologic toxicity, gastrointestinal hemorrhage, and even death may result from use of Adrucil (Fluorouracil) Injectable, USP despite meticulous selection of patients and careful adjustment of dosage.

Usage in Pregnancy: Safe use of Adrucil (Fluorouracil) Injectable, USP has not been established with respect to adverse effects on fetal development. Therefore, this drug should not be used during pregnancy, particularly in the first trimester, unless in the judgement of the physician the potential benefits to the patient outweigh the hazards.

Because the risk of mutagenesis has not been evaluated, such possible effects on males and females must be considered.

Combination Therapy: Any form of therapy which adds to the stress of the patient, interferes with nutrition or depresses bone marrow function

Continued on next page

Adria—Cont.

will increase the toxicity of Adrucil (Fluorouracil) Injectable, USP.

Precautions: Adrucil® (Fluorouracil) Injectable, USP is a highly toxic drug with a narrow margin of safety. Special attention must be given to the toxicity exhibited by fluorouracil. Patients should be carefully supervised since it must be recognized that therapeutic response is unlikely to occur without some evidence of toxicity. Patients should be advised of expected toxic effects, especially oral manifestations. White blood counts with differential are recommended before each dose. Knowledge of WBC nadir is necessary for eventual subsequent dosage adjustments.

Administration of Adrucil (Fluorouracil) Injectable, USP is to be discontinued promptly when one of the following signs appear:

1. Stomatitis or esophagopharyngitis (at first visible sign)
2. Leukopenia (WBC < 3500 mm^3) or rapidly falling white blood count
3. Vomiting (intractable)
4. Diarrhea (frequent bowel movements or watery stools)
5. Gastrointestinal ulceration and bleeding
6. Thrombocytopenia (platelets < 100,000 mm^3)
7. Hemorrhage (from any site)

Adverse Reactions: Stomatitis and esophagopharyngitis (which may lead to sloughing and ulceration), diarrhea, anorexia, nausea and emesis are common.

Myelosuppression almost uniformly accompanies a course of adequate therapy with fluorouracil. Low WBC counts are usually first observed between the 9th and 14th day after the first course of treatment with nadir occurring during the third week, although at times delayed for as long as 25 days. By the 30th day the count is usually within the normal range. Thrombocytopenia also may occur.

Alopecia and dermatitis are seen in a substantial number of cases and patients should be advised of this consequence of treatment. The alopecia is reported to be reversible. The dermatitis is often a pruritic maculopapular rash generally appearing on the extremities and less frequently on the trunk. It is usually reversible and responsive to symptomatic treatment. Dry skin and fissuring have also been noted.

Photosensitivity, as manifested by erythema or increased pigmentation of the skin, may occasionally occur. Also reported were photophobia, lacrimation, epistaxis, euphoria, acute cerebellar syndrome (which may persist following discontinuation of treatment) and nail changes including loss of nails. Myocardial ischemia has also been reported.

Dosage and Administration:

Note:

The recommended route of administration of Adrucil is only by intravenous injection, using care to avoid extravasation. No dilution of Adrucil is required.

It is recommended that all dosages be based on the patient's actual weight. However, if the patient is obese or if there has been a spurious weight gain due to edema, ascites, or other forms of abnormal fluid retention, then the estimated lean body mass (dry weight) should be used.

Prior to treatment, it is recommended that each patient be carefully evaluated to accurately estimate the optimum initial dosage of Adrucil.

Initial Therapy (See Contraindications, Warnings and Precautions before prescribing):

I. A dose of 12 mg/kg is given intravenously once daily for 4 successive days. The daily dose should not be more than 800 mg. If no toxicity is observed at any time during the course of therapy, 6 mg/kg are given on the 6th, 8th, 10th and 12th days. No therapy is given on the 5th, 7th, 9th or 11th days. Therapy is to be discontinued at the end of the 12th day, even if no toxicity has become apparent.

II. In poor risk patients or those who are not in an adequate nutritional state, a dose level of 6 mg/kg/day for 3 days is recommended. If no toxicity is observed at any time during the treatment, 3 mg/kg may be given on the 5th, 7th and 9th days. No therapy is given on the 4th, 6th or 8th days. The daily dose should not exceed 400 mg.

A sequence of injections on either schedule constitutes a "course of therapy."

Therapy should be discontinued promptly when any of the signs of toxicity listed under PRECAUTIONS appears.

Maintenance Therapy: When toxicity has not been a problem, or after the toxic signs from the initial course of therapy have subsided, therapy should be continued using either of the following schedules:

A. Repeat dosage of the first course, beginning 30 days after the last day of the previous course of treatment.
B. Administer a maintenance dosage of 10 to 15 mg/kg/week. Do not exceed 1 gram per week. Reduced doses should be used for poor risk patients.

The dosage of drug to be used should take into account the patient's reaction to the previous course of therapy and be adjusted accordingly. Some patients have received from 9 to 45 courses of treatment during periods which ranged from 12 to 60 months.

Adrucil (Fluorouracil) Injectable, USP should not be mixed with IV additives or chemotherapeutic agents.

How Supplied: Adrucil (Fluorouracil) Injectable, USP is available in 10 ml ampules, as a colorless to faint yellow aqueous solution containing 500 mg of fluorouracil and pH adjusted with sodium hydroxide to 8.6 to 9.0. Packaged and supplied in individual cartons, there are 10 ampules per shelf container NDC 0013-1026-91.

NOTE: Although Adrucil ampule solution may discolor slightly during storage, the potency and safety are not adversely affected. Store at room temperature 59–86°F (15–30°C) and protect from light. If a precipitate occurs due to exposure to low temperatures, re-solubilize by heating to 140°F (60°C) with vigorous shaking; allow to cool to body temperature before using.

Distributed by: Adria Laboratories Inc., Columbus, Ohio 43215

Manufactured by: Taylor Pharmacal Co., Decatur, Illinois 62525

Reformulated
AXOTAL®   ℞
[ax'ō-tall"]
(Butalbital and Aspirin)

Warning: May be habit forming.

Description: Each AXOTAL tablet for oral administration contains: butalbital, USP, 50 mg (Warning: May be habit forming) and aspirin, USP, 650 mg.

Butalbital, 5-allyl-5-isobutyl barbituric acid, a white odorless crystalline powder, is a short to intermediate-acting barbiturate. Its molecular formula is $C_{11}H_{16}N_2O_3$ and molecular weight 224.26. The chemical structure of butalbital is:

Actions: Pharmacologically, AXOTAL combines the analgesic properties of aspirin with the anxiolytic and muscle relaxant properties of butalbital.

Indications: AXOTAL is indicated for the relief of the symptom complex of tension (or muscle contraction) headaches.

Contraindications: Hypersensitivity to aspirin or barbiturates. Patients with porphyria.

Precautions: *General*—AXOTAL should be used with caution in patients with certain medical problems, including those with a history of asthma, allergies and nasal polyps. Also, the drug must be prescribed carefully for patients with hemophilia or other bleeding problems, peptic ulcer, renal impairment, or a history of drug abuse or dependence.

Information for patients—AXOTAL may impair the mental and/or physical abilities required for the performance of potentially hazardous tasks, such as driving a car or operating machinery. The patient should be cautioned accordingly.

Drug Interactions—Patients receiving narcotic analgesics, antipsychotics, antianxiety agents, or other CNS depressants (including alcohol) concomitantly with AXOTAL may exhibit additive CNS depressant effects. When combined therapy is contemplated, the dose of one or both agents should be reduced.

Drugs	Effect
Aspirin with anti-inflammatory agents	Increased ulcerogenic effects
Butalbital with coumarin anticoagulants	Decreased effect of anticoagulant because of increased metabolism resulting from enzyme induction.
Butalbital with tricyclic anti-depressants	Decreased blood levels of anti-depressant

Usage in Pregnancy—Adequate studies have not been performed in animals to determine whether this drug affects fertility in males or females, has teratogenic potential or has other adverse effects on the fetus. Although there is no clearly defined risk, experience cannot exclude the possibility of infrequent or subtle damage to the human fetus. AXOTAL should be used in pregnant women only when clearly needed.

Nursing Mothers—The effects of AXOTAL on infants of nursing mothers are not known. Salicylates and barbiturates are excreted in the breast milk of nursing mothers. The serum levels in infants are believed to be insignificant with therapeutic doses.

Pediatric Use—Safety and effectiveness in children below the age of 12 have not been established.

Adverse Reactions: The most frequent adverse reactions are drowsiness and dizziness. Less frequent adverse reactions are lightheadness and gastrointestinal disturbances including nausea, vomiting and flatulence. Mental confusion or depression can occur due to intolerance or overdosage of butalbital.

Drug Abuse and Dependence: Prolonged use of barbiturates can produce drug dependence, characterized by psychic dependence, and less frequently, physical dependence, and tolerance. The abuse liability of AXOTAL is similar to that of other barbiturate-containing drug combinations. Caution should be exercised when prescribing medication for patients with a known propensity for taking excessive quantities of drugs which is not uncommon in patients with chronic tension headaches.

Overdosage: The toxic effects of acute overdosage of AXOTAL are attributable mainly to its barbiturate component and, to a lesser extent, aspirin. Symptoms attributable to acute *barbiturate poisoning* include drowsiness, confusion and coma, respiratory depression, hypertension and shock. Symptoms of *salicylate overdosage* include central nausea and vomiting, tinnitus and deafness, vertigo and headaches, mental dullness and confusion, diaphoresis, rapid pulse and increased respiration leading to respiratory alkalosis. Treatment consists primarily of management of barbiturate intoxication and the correction of acid-base imbalance due to salicylism. Vomiting should be induced mechanically or with emetics, such as ipecac syrup, in the conscious patient. Gastric lavage may be used if the pharyngeal and laryngeal reflexes are present and if less than 4 hours have elapsed since ingestion. A cuffed endotracheal tube should be inserted before gastric lavage of the unconscious patient and when necessary to provide assisted respiration. Gastric lavage followed by activated charcoal is recommended regardless of time since ingestion. Diuresis, alkalinization of the urine, and correction of electrolyte disturbances should be accomplished through administration of intravenous fluids such as 1% sodium bicarbonate in 5% dextrose in water. Meticulous attention should be given to maintaining adequate pulmonary ventilation. Exchange transfusion is most feasible for a small infant while intermittent peritoneal dialysis is useful for cases of moderate severity in adults. Hemodialysis with the artifical kidney is the most effective means of removing salicylate and is indicated for the very severe cases of salicylate intoxication. Hypoprothrombinemia should be treated with intravenous Vitamin K (phytonadione). Methemoglobinemia over 30% should be treated with methylene blue administered slowly intravenously.

In all cases of suspected overdose, immediately call your regional poison center for assistance.

Dosage and Administration: One tablet every four hours as needed. Do not exceed 6 tablets per day.

Medication should be taken with food or a full glass of water or milk to lessen gastric irritation caused by aspirin.

How Supplied: Each AXOTAL tablet contains butalbital USP, 50 mg, and aspirin 650 mg.

AXOTAL is available for oral administration as uncoated, white, capsule-shaped tablets coded ADRIA, 130.

Tablets are supplied as follows:
NDC 0013-1301-17 in bottles of 100
NDC 0013-1301-18 STAT-PAK® (unit dose) box of 100 tablets.
NDC 0013-1301-21 in bottles of 500

Store in a tight container below 30°C (86°F). Protect from moisture.

EVAC-Q-KIT®
[ē-vak'cue-kit]

Description: Each EVAC-Q-KIT® contains:
1. EVAC-Q-MAG®—10 fl. oz. Sugar-Free. Ingredients: Magnesium citrate, citric acid and potassium citrate in cherry flavored base. Carbonated.
2. EVAC-Q-TABS® — 2 tablets. Ingredients: Each tablet contains 2 grains (130 mg) of Phenolphthalein.
3. EVAC-Q-SERT®—2 suppositories. Ingredients: Potassium bitartrate and sodium bicarbonate in polyethylene glycol base.
4. 1 Instruction Sheet (In English and Spanish)

Actions: Bowel Evacuant.

Indications: Preparations of the colon for single and multiple radiology examinations requiring a clean colon.

Contraindications: EVAC-Q-MAG is contraindicated in the presence of severe renal insufficiency.

Warnings: Do not use any of these preparations when abdominal pain, nausea, or vomiting are present. Frequent and continued use may cause dependence upon laxatives. Rectal bleeding or failure to respond may indicate a serious condition. Consult physician. As with any drug, if you are pregnant or nursing a baby, seek the advice of a health professional before using this product. KEEP OUT OF REACH OF CHILDREN.

Precautions: If skin rash appears, do not use this or any other preparation containing phenolphthalein.

Dosage and Administration:
Instructions for Patients—early schedule* Your physician is preparing you for an X-ray examination that requires thorough clearing of the intestinal tract. He is using this EVAC-Q-KIT® routine to make this procedure more comfortable for you. BE SURE TO FOLLOW EACH STEP AND COMPLETE ALL INSTRUCTIONS OR ENTIRE X-RAY EXAMINATION MAY HAVE TO BE REPEATED.

DAY BEFORE EXAMINATION
IMPORTANT: A high fluid intake is essential to the success of this regimen. You MUST take a large glass (8 oz.) of fluid at specified times. ▯ =8 oz. fluid.) Drink only black coffee, plain tea, strained fruit juice, soft drinks or water at the times indicated. NO MILK OR CREAM.

☐ **Noon.** Light lunch. Clear soup, two hard-boiled eggs, plain Jell-O, fluid.
☐ **12:30 P.M.** (or ½ hr. after lunch) Drink entire contents—EVAC-Q-MAG® (#1 in your kit), over Ice.
☐ **1:00 P.M.** + ▯.
☐ **3:00 P.M.** Take two (2) EVAC-Q-TABS® laxative tablets (#2 in your kit) with large glass of water.
☐ **4:00 P.M.** + ▯.
☐ **5:00 P.M.** Liquid dinner. Clear Soup, plain Jell-O + ▯.
☐ **6:00 P.M.** + ▯.
☐ **9:00 P.M.** + ▯.
☐ **10:00 P.M.** Remove cover from EVAC-Q-SERT® suppository (#3 in your kit). Moisten the suppository in tap water. Insert suppository into rectum. Wait at least 10–15 minutes before evacuating, even if urge is strong.
☐ **BEDTIME:** + ▯.

DAY OF TEST. No breakfast.
☐ **6:00 A.M.** (must be at least 2 hours before test).
Use remaining EVAC-Q-SERT® suppository (#4 in your kit). Follow same directions as 10:00 P.M. night before.

BE SURE TO DRINK ALL THE FLUID SPECIFIED.

NOTE: This product information is for professional use only.

How Supplied: Each EVAC-Q-KIT NDC 0013-2199 contains:
1. One 10 fl. oz. EVAC-Q-MAG
2. Two tablets—EVAC-Q-TABS
3. Two suppositories—EVAC-Q-SERT
4. 1 Instruction Sheet
Shipping Unit: 12 EVAC-Q-KIT units per carton.

*Late schedule also available. See Instruction Sheet in EVAC-Q-KIT. (Instruction sheet printed in both English and Spanish.)

EVAC-Q-KWIK®
[ē-vak'cue-kwik]
Bowel Evacuant System

Description: EVAC-Q-KWIK is a bowel evacuant system comprised of three separate products that are intended to be administered sequentially at intervals intended to minimize the overlap of pharmacological activity. These three products are augmented by the sequential administration of liquids in a manner to promote the flushing of the G.I. tract. Together, the products and the liquids comprise the bowel evacuant system.
1. EVAC-Q-MAG®—Each bottle contains 10 fl. oz., magnesium citrate oral solution, USP, in a cherry flavored base, sugar-free, carbonated base. It contains sodium 0.84 mEq, potassium 2.1 mEq, magnesium 250 mg and 66.7 calories.
2. EVAC-Q-TABS®—2 tablets. Each tablet contains phenolphthalein 130 mg.
3. EVAC-Q-KWIK SUPPOSITORY—bisacodyl 10 mg.
4. Illustrated bilingual instruction sheet.

Magnesium citrate is a saline laxative and has a mild purgative action. It is chemically 2-hydroxy-1,2,3-propanetricarboxylic acid, magnesium salt and has the following structure:

$$\left[\begin{array}{c} CH_2COO- \\ HO-C-COO- \\ CH_2COO- \end{array} \right]_2 \cdot Mg_3$$

Magnesium citrate occurs as white crystalline powder or granules, slightly soluble in water, soluble in dilute acids. Its molecular weight citrate is 451.12.

Phenolphthalein, a contact laxative, is a diphenylmethane derivative. It is chemically 3,3-bis(4-hydroxyphenyl)-1(3H)-isobenzofuranone and has the following structure:

It occurs as a white, or yellowish-white, crystalline powder and is practically insoluble in water, soluble in alcohol and dilute alkali solutions. Its molecular weight is 318.33.

Bisacodyl, a contact laxative, is also a diphenylmethane derivative. It is chemically 4,4'-(2-pyridylmethylene) diphenol diacetate and has the following structure:

Bisacodyl occurs as a white or off-white crystalline powder, practically insoluble in water, sparingly soluble in alcohol and soluble in chloroform. Its molecular weight is 361.40.

Clinical Pharmacology: Magnesium citrate is a saline laxative. It acts mainly on the small intestine by drawing water into the gut thus increasing intraluminal pressure and intestinal motility, resulting in evacuation of the bowel usually in 3–6 hours or less. Substantial fluid intake is required for this purpose. Approximately 15–30% of the magnesium present in its salts may be absorbed. The magnesium and potassium ions are excreted primarily by the kidney and may accumulate in patients with impaired renal function, in the newborn and in the elderly.

Phenolphthalein, a contact laxative, acts primarily on the large intestine to produce a semifluid stool usually in 4–8 hours. It is dissolved by bile salts and alkaline intestinal secretions and may impart a red color to alkaline feces and urine. Up to 15% of the dose may be absorbed and excreted mainly by the kidney in the conjugated glucuronide form.

Bisacodyl is also a contact laxative which acts on the large intestine to produce brief and strong peristaltic movements resulting in evacuation usually within 15–60 minutes after rectal administration. It is minimally (about 5%) absorbed and excreted mainly in the feces and partly in the urine as the glucuronide.

Indications and Usage: EVAC-Q-KWIK is indicated for use as a bowel evacuant in the preparation of the colon for single or multiple radiological examination requiring a clean colon.

Contraindications: The EVAC-Q-MAG component is contraindicated in patients with severe renal insufficiency.

Warnings: Do not use any laxative preparations when abdominal pain, nausea or vomiting are present. Frequent and continued use may cause dependence upon laxatives. Rectal bleeding or failure to respond may indicate a serious underlying condition and require a physician's consultation. KEEP THIS PRODUCT OUT OF REACH OF CHILDREN.

As with any drug, if the patient is pregnant or nursing a baby, she should consult a health professional before using. (See Precautions: Pregnancy, Nursing Mothers.)

Precautions:
General—If skin rash appears, do not use EVAC-Q-TABS or any other preparation containing phenolphthalein. The EVAC-Q-KWIK SUPPOSITORY should be used with caution in patients with rectal fissures or ulcerated hemorrhoids.
Phenolphthalein, the active ingredient of EVAC-Q-TABS, may color alkaline feces and urine red.
Laboratory Test Interactions—Phenolphthalein in EVAC-Q-TABS may interfere with the ACE-TEST® and KETOSTIX® urine tests for ketones to produce a pink color. It may also give false-positive test results for urinary urobilinogen and for estrogens measured by the Kober procedure.
Carcinogenesis, Mutagenesis, Impairment of Fertility—There have been no studies in animals or humans to evaluate the carcinogenesis, mutagenesis or impairment of fertility potential of the EVAC-Q-KWIK.
Pregnancy—Category C. Animal reproduction studies have not been conducted with any of the components of EVAC-Q-KWIK. It is also not known whether the EVAC-Q-KWIK can cause fetal harm when administered to a pregnant

Continued on next page

Adria—Cont.

woman or can affect reproduction capacity. EVAC-Q-KWIK should be given to a pregnant woman only if clearly needed.

Nursing Mothers—Small amounts of magnesium are excreted in the milk and saliva. Phenolphthalein and bisacodyl are also excreted in human milk. Therefore, caution should be exercised when EVAC-Q-KWIK is administered to a nursing woman.

Pediatric Use—Safety and effectiveness in children below the age of 12 has not been established.

Adverse Reactions: Excessive bowel activity, usually diarrhea or abdominal discomfort, nausea, vomiting, cramps, weakness, dizziness, palpitations, sweating and fainting may follow the administration of an evacuant. Diarrhea may lead to fluid and electrolyte deficits. Allergic reactions, mainly skin rashes attributed to phenolphthalein, have been reported. Bisacodyl in the EVAC-Q-KWIK SUPPOSITORY may cause irritation or a sensation of burning of the rectal mucosa.

Overdosage: Accidental or intentional overdosage may lead to severe diarrhea and excessive loss of body fluids and electrolytes, muscle weakness and tremor, gastrointestinal disturbances and fainting. Depressed deep tendon reflexes, sedation, EKG changes or heart block and respiratory paralysis may occur with high plasma magnesium levels.

The excretion of magnesium may be increased by the administration of a diuretic. Only small amounts of phenolphthalein or bisacodyl are absorbed. If ingestion is recent or food is present in the stomach, induction of emesis with ipecac syrup, gastric emptying and lavage and introduction of activated charcoal may be recommended. Fluid and electrolyte administration is also recommended to correct dehydration and electrolyte imbalance.

Dosage and Administration: A high fluid intake and a low residue diet are essential for a successful colon preparation. Recommended liquids are black coffee, plain tea, strained fruit juice, soft drinks or water and NO MILK OR CREAM. The directions provided in the Instruction Sheet and the following schedule should be adhered to closely.

Time Schedule:
NOON	Light lunch: clear soup, plain gelatin, fluid.
4:00 P.M.	Drink entire contents of EVAC-Q-MAG (#1 in the kit), over ice.
5:00 P.M.	8 oz. of fluid.
6:00 P.M.	Liquid dinner. Clear soup, plain gelatin, 8 oz. of fluid.
7:00 P.M.	Take two (2) EVAC-Q-TABS laxative tablets (#2 in the kit) with a large glass of water.
8:00 P.M.	8 oz. of fluid.
9:00 P.M.	8 oz. of fluid.
10:00 P.M.	Insert one EVAC-Q-KWIK SUPPOSITORY (#3 in the kit) into rectum as far as possible, retain as long as comfort will permit—usually 10–15 minutes—before defecating. Nothing by mouth, after 10:00 P.M. until x-ray examination. Prescription medications can be taken as scheduled with a glass of water.

DRINK ALL THE FLUID SPECIFIED.

Alternate Schedule:
(For patients admitted in the afternoon on the day before examination.)
6:00 P.M.	Liquid dinner. Clear soup, plain gelatin, 8 oz. of fluid.
7:00 P.M.	Drink entire contents of EVAC-Q-MAG (#1 in the kit), over ice.
8:00 P.M.	8 oz. of fluid.
9:00 P.M.	8 oz. of fluid.
10:00 P.M.	Take two (2) EVAC-Q-TABS laxative tablets (#2 in the kit) with a large glass of water. Nothing by mouth, after 10:00 p.m. until x-ray examination. Prescription medications can be taken as scheduled with a glass of water.
6:00 A.M.	Insert one EVAC-Q-KWIK SUPPOSITORY (#3 in the kit) into rectum as far as possible, retain as long as comfort will permit—usually 10–15 minutes—before defecating.

DRINK ALL THE FLUID SPECIFIED.
See also: Illustrated Multilingual Instruction Sheet.
NOTE: This product information is for professional use only.

How Supplied: Each EVAC-Q-KWIK, NDC 0013-2189, contains:
1. One 10 fl. oz. EVAC-Q-MAG
2. Two tablets EVAC-Q-TABS
3. One EVAC-Q-KWIK SUPPOSITORY
4. Instruction Sheet

Store at controlled room temperature (15–30°C, 59–86°F).
Avoid freezing.

EVAC-Q-MAG
Manufactured by:
NATIONAL MAGNESIA CO., INC.
GLENDALE, NEW YORK 11385

EVAC-Q-KWIK SUPPOSITORY
Manufactured by:
G & W LABORATORIES, INC.
SOUTH PLAINFIELD, NJ 07050

Distributed by:
ADRIA LABORATORIES INC.
COLUMBUS, OHIO 43215

FOLEX® FOR INJECTION B
[fō¹ lĕx]
(methotrexate sodium)

> **WARNINGS**
> METHOTREXATE MUST BE USED ONLY BY PHYSICIANS EXPERIENCED IN ANTIMETABOLITE CHEMOTHERAPY.
> BECAUSE OF THE POSSIBILITY OF FATAL OR SEVERE TOXIC REACTIONS THE PATIENT SHOULD BE FULLY INFORMED BY THE PHYSICIAN OF THE RISKS INVOLVED AND SHOULD BE UNDER HIS CONSTANT SUPERVISION.
> DEATHS HAVE BEEN REPORTED WITH THE USE OF METHOTREXATE IN THE TREATMENT OF PSORIASIS. IN THE TREATMENT OF PSORIASIS METHOTREXATE SHOULD BE RESTRICTED TO SEVERE, RECALCITRANT, DISABLING PSORIASIS WHICH IS NOT ADEQUATELY RESPONSIVE TO OTHER FORMS OF THERAPY, BUT ONLY WHEN THE DIAGNOSIS HAS BEEN ESTABLISHED AS BY BIOPSY AND/OR AFTER DERMATOLOGIC CONSULTATION.
> 1. Methotrexate may produce marked depression of bone marrow, anemia, leukopenia, thrombocytopenia and bleeding.
> 2. Methotrexate may be hepatotoxic, particularly at high dosage or with prolonged therapy. Liver atrophy, necrosis, cirrhosis, fatty changes, and periportal fibrosis have been reported. Since changes may occur without previous signs of gastrointestinal or hematologic toxicity, it is imperative that hepatic function be determined prior to initiation of treatment and monitored regularly throughout therapy. Special caution is indicated in the presence of preexisting liver damage or impaired hepatic function. Concomitant use of other drugs with hepatotoxic potential (including alcohol) should be avoided.
> 3. Methotrexate has caused fetal death and/or congenital anomalies, therefore, it is not recommended in women of childbearing potential unless there is appropriate medical evidence that the benefits can be expected to outweigh the considered risks. Pregnant psoriatic patients should not receive methotrexate. If methotrexate is used during pregnancy or if the patient becomes pregnant while taking the drug, the patient should be apprised of the potential hazard to the fetus.
> 4. Impaired renal function is usually a contraindication.
> 5. Diarrhea and ulcerative stomatitis are frequent toxic effects and require interruption of therapy, otherwise hemorrhagic enteritis and death from intestinal perforation may occur.

Description: FOLEX FOR INJECTION (methotrexate sodium) is an antimetabolite used in the treatment of certain neoplastic diseases.

4-amino-N^{10}-methylpteroylglutamic acid

FOLEX FOR INJECTION is available in 25, 50, and 100 mg strengths, each available as sterile lyophilized powder in vials, containing no preservatives, for single use only.

Each 25 mg vial contains methotrexate USP, 25 mg, prepared as the sodium salt; sodium hydroxide to adjust pH to about 8.5.

Each 50 mg vial contains methotrexate USP, 50 mg, prepared as the sodium salt; sodium hydroxide to adjust pH to about 8.5.

Each 100 mg vial contains methotrexate USP, 100 mg, prepared as the sodium salt; sodium hydroxide to adjust pH to about 8.5.

Clinical Pharmacology: Methotrexate has as its principal mechanism of action the competitive inhibition of the enzyme dihydrofolate reductase. Folic acid must be reduced to tetrahydrofolic acid by this enzyme in the process of DNA synthesis and cellular replication. Methotrexate binds almost irreversibly to dihydrofolate reductase and inhibits the formation of tetrahydrofolates necessary for the metabolic transfer of one-carbon units in a variety of intracellular biochemical processes. The conversion of deoxyuridylate to thymidylate by one-carbon transfer is required for DNA synthesis. One-carbon transfer is also necessary for purine, RNA, amino acid and protein synthesis, thus methotrexate can disrupt several biological processes involved in cell growth.

Actively proliferating tissues such as malignant cells, bone marrow, fetal cells, dermal epithelium, buccal and intestinal mucosa and cells of the urinary bladder are in general more sensitive to this effect of methotrexate than slowly proliferating tissues. Cellular proliferation in malignant tissue is greater than in most normal tissue and thus methotrexate may impair malignant growth without causing irreversible damage to normal tissues. After parenteral injection, peak serum levels are seen in about 30 to 60 minutes. Orally administered methotrexate is absorbed rapidly in most, but not all patients, and reaches peak serum levels in 1-2 hours. The mean plasma half life of methotrexate is about 2 hours. After injection approximately one half the methotrexate is reversibly bound to serum protein, but exchanges with body fluids easily and diffuses into the body tissue cells. Metabolism of methotrexate in man does not seem to occur to a significant degree.

Excretion of single daily doses occurs through the kidneys in amounts from 55% to 88% or higher within 24 hours. Repeated doses daily result in more sustained serum levels and some retention of methotrexate over each 24-hour period which may result in accumulation of the drug within the tissues. The liver cells appear to retain certain amounts of the drug for prolonged periods even after a single therapeutic dose. Methotrexate is retained in the presence of impaired renal function and may increase rapidly in the serum and in the tissue cells under such conditions. Methotrexate does not penetrate the blood cerebrospinal fluid barrier in therapeutic amounts when given parenterally. High concentrations of the drug when needed may be attained by direct intrathecal administration.

In psoriasis, the rate of production of epithelial cells in the skin is greatly increased over normal skin. This differential in reproductive rates is the basis for use of methotrexate to control the psoriatic process.

Indications and Usage:
Anti-neoplastic Chemotherapy—FOLEX is indicated for the treatment of gestational choriocarcinoma, and in patients with chorioadenoma destruens and hydatidiform mole.

FOLEX is indicated for the palliation of acute lymphocytic leukemia. It is also indicated in the treatment and prophylaxis of meningeal leukemia. In combination with other anticancer drugs or suitable agents, FOLEX may be used for induction of remission, but it is most commonly used, as described in the literature, in the maintenance of induced remissions.

FOLEX is also effective in the treatment of the advanced stages (III and IV, Ann Arbor Staging System) of malignant lymphoma, particularly in those cases in children; and in advanced cases of mycosis fungoides.

Psoriasis Chemotherapy—(See box warnings.) Because of high risk attending its use, FOLEX is only indicated in the symptomatic control of severe, recalcitrant, disabling psoriasis which is not adequately responsive to other forms of therapy, *but only when the diagnosis has been established, as by biopsy and/or after dermatologic consultation.*

Contraindications:
Pregnant psoriatic patients should not receive FOLEX. Psoriatic patients with severe renal or hepatic disorders should not receive FOLEX. Psoriatic patients with preexisting blood dyscrasias, such as bone marrow hypoplasia, leukopenia, thrombocytopenia or anemia, should not receive FOLEX.

Warnings:
See box warnings.

Precautions:
Methotrexate has a high potential toxicity, usually dose-related. The physician should be familiar with the various characteristics of the drug and its established clinical usage. Patients undergoing therapy should be subject to appropriate supervision so the signs or symptoms of possible toxic effects or adverse reactions may be detected and evaluated with minimal delay. Pretreatment and periodic hematologic studies are essential to the use of methotrexate in chemotherapy because of its common effect of hematopoetic suppression. This may occur abruptly and on apparent safe dosage, and any profound drop in bloodcell count indicates immediate stopping of the drug and appropriate therapy. In patients with malignant disease who have preexisting bone marrow aplasia, leukopenia, thrombocytopenia or anemia, the drug should be used with caution, if at all.

Methotrexate is excreted principally by the kidneys. Its use in the presence of impaired renal function may result in accumulation of toxic amounts or even additional renal damage. The patient's renal status should be determined prior to and during methotrexate therapy and proper caution exercised should significant renal impairment be disclosed. Drug dosage should be reduced or discontinued until renal function is improved or restored.

In general, the following laboratory tests are recommended as part of essential clinical evaluation and appropriate monitoring of patients chosen for or receiving methotrexate therapy: complete hemogram, hematocrit, urinalysis, renal function tests, and liver function tests. A chest x-ray is also recommended. The purpose is to determine any existing organ dysfunction or system impairment. The tests should be performed prior to therapy, at appropriate periods during therapy and after termination of therapy. It may be useful or important to perform liver biopsy or bone marrow aspiration studies where high dose or long-term therapy is being followed.

Methotrexate is bound in part to serum albumin after absorption, and toxicity may be increased because of displacement by certain drugs such as salicylates, sulfonamides, diphenylhydantoin, phenylbutazone, and some antibacterials such as tetracycline, chloramphenicol and para-aminobenzoic acid. These drugs, especially salicylates, phenylbutazone, and sulfonamides, whether antibacterial, hypoglycemic or diuretic, should not be given concurrently until the significance of these findings is established.

Vitamin preparations containing folic acid or its derivatives may alter responses to methotrexate. Methotrexate should be used with extreme caution in the presence of infection, peptic ulcer, ulcerative colitis, debility and in extreme youth or old age.

If profound leukopenia occurs during therapy, bacterial infection may occur or become a threat. Cessation of the drug and appropriate antibiotic therapy is usually indicated. In severe bone marrow depression, blood or platelet transfusions may be necessary.

Since it is reported that methotrexate may have an immunosuppressive action, this factor must be taken into consideration in evaluating the use of the drug where immune responses in a patient may be important or essential.

In all instances where the use of methotrexate is considered for chemotherapy, the physician must evaluate the need and usefulness of the drug against the risks of toxic effects or adverse reaction. Most such adverse reactions are reversible if detected early. When such effects or reactions do occur, the drug should be reduced in dosage or discontinued and appropriate corrective measures should be taken, according to the clinical judgment of the physician. Reinstitution of methotrexate therapy should be carried out with caution, with adequate consideration of further need for the drug and alertness as to possible recurrence of toxicity. Tests were negative for carcinogenesis in the Ames test and by sister chromatid exchange in lymphocyte cultures of patients receiving methotrexate. Weak carcinogenesis was reported in one animal study and no carcinogenesis in another.

Usage in Pregnancy—Category D. (See box warnings.) Defective oogenesis or spermatogenesis caused by methotrexate has been reported.

Methotrexate is excreted in breast milk and although no problems in humans have been documented, caution should be exercised when methotrexate is administered to a nursing woman.

Adverse Reactions:
The most common adverse reactions include ulcerative stomatitis, leukopenia, nausea and abdominal distress. Others reported are malaise, undue fatigue, chills and fever, dizziness and decreased resistance to infection. In general, the incidence and severity of side effects are considered to be dose-related. Adverse reactions as reported for the various systems are as follows:

Skin—erythematous rashes, pruritus, urticaria, photosensitivity depigmentation, alopecia, ecchymosis, telangiectasia, acne, furunculosis. Lesions of psoriasis may be aggravated by concomitant exposure to ultraviolet radiation.

Blood—bone marrow depression, leukopenia, thrombocytopenia, anemia, hypogammaglobulinemia, hemorrhage from various sites, septicemia.

Pulmonary System—an acute reversible pneumonitis may develop characterized by fever, cough, shortness of breath, peripheral eosinophilia and patchy pulmonary infiltrates.

Alimentary System—gingivitis, pharyngitis, stomatitis, anorexia, vomiting, diarrhea, hematemesis, melena, gastrointestinal ulceration and bleeding, enteritis, hepatic toxicity resulting in acute liver atrophy, necrosis, fatty metamorphosis, periportal fibrosis, or hepatic cirrhosis.

Urogenital System—renal failure azotemia, cystitis, hematuria; defective oogenesis or spermatogenesis, transient oligospermia, menstrual dysfunction; infertility, abortion, fetal defects, severe nephropathy.

Central Nervous System—headaches, drowsiness, blurred vision. Aphasia, hemiparesis, paresis and convulsions have also occurred following administration of methotrexate.

There have been reports of leucoencephalopathy following intravenous administration of methotrexate to patients who have had craniospinal irradiation.

After the intrathecal use of methotrexate, the central nervous system toxicity which may occur can be classified as follows: (1) chemical arachnoiditis manifested by such symptoms as headache, back pain, nuchal rigidity, and fever; (2) paresis, usually transient, manifested by paraplegia associated with involvement of one or more spinal nerve roots; (3) leucoencephalopathy manifested by confusion, irritability, somnolence, ataxia, dementia, and occasionally major convulsions.

Other reactions related to or attributed to the use of methotrexate such as metabolic changes, precipitating diabetes, osteoporotic effects, abnormal tissue cell changes, and even sudden death have been reported.

Overdosage:
Overdosage may lead to severe toxicity, especially of the hematopoetic and gastrointestinal systems and death may result. Leucovorin (citrovorum factor) is a potent agent for neutralizing the immediate toxic effects of methotrexate. Where large doses or overdoses are given, calcium leucovorin may be administered by intravenous infusion in doses up to 75 mg within 12 hours, followed by 12 mg intramuscularly every 6 hours for 4 doses. Where average doses of methotrexate appear to have an adverse effect, 2 to 4 ml (6 to 12 mg) of calcium leucovorin may be given intramuscularly every 6 hours for 4 doses. In general, where over-dosage is suspected, the dose of leucovorin should be equal to or higher than the offending dose of methotrexate and should best be administered within the first hour. Use of calcium leucovorin after an hour delay is much less effective.

Dosage and Administration:
Anti-neoplastic chemotherapy—FOLEX FOR INJECTION may be given by intramuscular, intravenous, intraarterial or intrathecal routes. Initial treatment is usually undertaken with the patient under hospital care. For conversion of mg/kg body weight to mg/m^2 of body surface area or the reverse, a ratio of 1:30 is given as a guideline. The conversion factor varies between 1:20 and 1:40 depending on age and body build.

Choriocarcinoma and similar trophoblastic diseases—FOLEX is administered intramuscularly in doses of 15 to 30 mg daily for a 5 day course. Such courses are usually repeated for 3 to 5 times as required, with rest periods of one or more weeks interposed between courses, until any manifesting toxic symptoms subside. The effectiveness of therapy is ordinarily evaluated by quantitative analysis of the beta subunit of the serum human chorionic gonadotropin (hCG), which should return to less than 5 mlU/ml usually after the 3rd or 4th course and should usually be followed by a complete resolution of measurable lesions in 4 to 6 weeks. One to two courses of methotrexate after normalization of hCG is usually recommended. Before each course of the drug careful clinical assessment is essential. Cyclic combination therapy of methotrexate with other antitumor drugs has been reported as being useful.

Since hydatidiform mole may precede or be followed by choriocarcinoma, prophylactic chemotherapy with methotrexate has been recommended. Chorioadenoma destruens is considered to be an invasive form of hydatidiform mole. Methotrexate is administered in these disease states in doses similar to those recommended for choriocarcinoma.

Leukemia—Acute lymphatic (lymphoblastic) leukemia in children and young adolescents is the most responsive to present day chemotherapy. In young adults and older patients, clinical remission is more difficult to obtain and early relapse is more common. In chronic lymphatic leukemia, the prognosis for adequate response is less encouraging. Methotrexate alone or in combination with steroids was used initially for induction of remission of lymphoblastic leukemias. More recently corticosteroid therapy in combination with other antileukemic drugs or in cyclic combinations with methotrexate included appears to produce rapid and effective remissions. When remission is achieved and supportive care has produced general clinical improvement, maintenance therapy is initiated as follows: FOLEX is administered 2

Continued on next page

Adria—Cont.

times weekly intramuscularly in doses of 30 mg/m^2. It has also been given in doses of 2.5 mg/kg intravenously every 14 days if and when relapse does occur, reinduction of remission can again usually be obtained by repeating the initial induction regimen. Various experts have recently introduced a variety of dosage schedules for both induction and maintenance of remission with various combinations of alkylating and antifolic agents. Multiple drug therapy with several agents, including methotrexate, given concomitantly is gaining increasing support in both the acute and chronic forms of leukemia. The physician should familiarize himself with the new advances in antileukemic therapy.

Acute granulocytic leukemia is rare in children but common in adults. This form of leukemia responds poorly to chemotherapy and remissions are short with relapses common, and resistance to therapy develops rapidly.

Meningeal leukemia—Patients with leukemia are subject to leukemic invasion of the central nervous system. This may manifest characteristic signs or symptoms or may remain silent and be diagnosed only by examination of the cerebrospinal fluid which contains leukemic cells in such cases. Therefore, the CSF should be examined in all leukemic patients. Since passage of methotrexate from blood serum to the cerebrospinal fluid is minimal, for adequate therapy the drug is administered intrathecally. It is now common practice because of the noted increased frequency of meningeal leukemia to administer methotrexate intrathecally as prophylaxis in all cases of lymphocytic leukemia.

By intrathecal injection, the FOLEX FOR INJECTION is administered in solution in doses of 12 mg per square meter of body surface or in an empirical dose of 15 mg. The solution is made in a strength of 1 mg per ml with an appropriate, sterile, preservative-free medium such as 0.9% Sodium Chloride Injection, U.S.P.

For the treatment of meningeal leukemia, methotrexate is given at intervals of 2 to 5 days. Methotrexate is administered until the cell count of the cerebrospinal fluid returns to normal. At this point one additional dose is advisable.

For prophylaxis against meningeal leukemia, the dosage is the same as for treatment except for the intervals of administration. On this subject, it is advisable for the physician to consult the medical literature.

Large doses may cause convulsions. Untoward side effects may occur with any given intrathecal injection and are commonly neurological in character. Methotrexate given by the intrathecal route appears significantly in the systemic circulation and may cause systemic methotrexate toxicity. Therefore systemic antileukemic therapy with the drug should be appropriately adjusted, reduced or discontinued. Focal leukemic involvement of the central nervous system may not respond to intrathecal chemotherapy and is best treated with radiotherapy.

Lymphomas—In Burkitt's Tumor, Stages I-II, methotrexate has produced prolonged remissions in some cases. In Stage III methotrexate is commonly given concomitantly with other antitumor agents. Treatment in all stages usually consists of several courses of the drug interposed with 7 to 10 day rest periods. Malignant lymphomas in Stage III may respond to combined drug therapy with methotrexate given in doses of 0.625 mg to 2.5 mg/kg daily.

Mycosis fungoides—Therapy with methotrexate appears to produce clinical remissions in about one half of the cases treated. Dosage is usually daily by mouth for weeks or months. Dose levels of drug and adjustment of dose regimen by reduction or cessation of drug are guided by patient response and hematologic monitoring. Methotrexate has also been given intramuscularly in doses of 50 mg once weekly or 25 mg 2 times weekly.

Psoriasis Chemotherapy—The patient should be fully informed of the risks involved and should be under constant supervision of the physician. Assessment of renal function, liver function, and blood elements should be made by history, physical examination, and laboratory tests (such as CBC, urinalysis, serum creatinine, liver function studies, and liver biopsy if indicated) periodically and before reinstituting methotrexate therapy after a rest period. Blood counts should be taken weekly during treatment. Appropriate steps should be taken to avoid conception during and for at least eight weeks following methotrexate therapy.

There are three commonly used general types of dosage schedules:
1. weekly oral or parenteral intermittent large doses
2. divided dose intermittent oral schedule over a 36-hour period
3. daily oral with a rest period

All schedules should be continually tailored to the individual patient. Dose schedules cited below pertain to an average 70 kg adult. An initial test dose one week prior to initiation of therapy is recommended to detect any idiosyncrasy. A suggested dose range is 5 to 10 mg parenterally.

Recommended starting dose schedule:
1. Weekly single, IM or IV dose schedule: 10 to 25 mg per week until adequate response is achieved. With this dosage schedule, 50 mg per week should ordinarily not be exceeded.
2. Divided daily oral doses for one or four days each week.

Special Note—Available data suggest that the four days per week schedule may carry an increased risk of serious liver pathology.

Dosages may be gradually adjusted to achieve optimal clinical response, but not to exceed the maximum stated in the schedule.

Once an optimal clinical response has been achieved, the dosage schedule should be reduced to the lowest possible amount of drug and to the longest possible rest period. The use of methotrexate may permit the return to conventional topical therapy, which should be encouraged.

Caution: *Pharmacist*—Because of its potential to cause severe toxicity, methotrexate therapy requires close supervision of the patient by the physician. Pharmacists should dispense no more than a seven (7) day supply of the drug at one time. Refill of such prescriptions should be by direct order (written or oral) of the physician only.

Directions for Use: Reconstitute FOLEX FOR INJECTION (methotrexate sodium) immediately prior to use with 2 to 10 ml depending on the route of administration, of an appropriate preservative-free medium such as 0.9% Sodium Chloride Injection, USP. FOLEX FOR INJECTION does not contain an antimicrobial agent and care must be taken to ensure the sterility of prepared solutions. The sterile reconstituted solution has been shown to be stable for 24 hours at room temperature.

How Supplied:
FOLEX FOR INJECTION (methotrexate sodium)
NDC 0013-2226-86 25 mg vial
NDC 0013-2236-86 50 mg vial
NDC 0013-2246-86 100 mg vial

Store products at room temperature and protect from light.

Manufactured by:
BEN VENUE LABORATORIES
BEDFORD, OHIO 44146
for:
ADRIA LABORATORIES INC.
COLUMBUS, OHIO 43215

ILOPAN® INJECTION ℞
[ī′ lō-pan]
(dexpanthenol)

Description: ILOPAN® INJECTION (dexpanthenol) is a derivative of pantothenic acid, a member of the B complex of vitamins. ILOPAN INJECTION is a sterile aqueous solution indicated for use as a gastrointestinal stimulant. The chemical name is D-(+)-2, 4-dihydroxy-N-(3-hydroxypropyl)-3,3-dimethylbutyramide. The structural formula is

$$HOCH_2-\underset{\underset{CH_3}{|}}{\overset{\overset{CH_3}{|}}{C}}-\underset{\underset{H}{|}}{\overset{\overset{OH}{|}}{C}}-CONHCH_2CH_2CH_2OH$$

The empirical formula is $C_9H_{19}NO_4$.

Each ml contains dexpanthenol 250 mg in distilled water for injection.

Clinical Pharmacology: Pantothenic acid is a precursor of coenzyme A, which serves as a cofactor for a variety of enzyme-catalyzed reactions involving transfer of acetyl groups. The final step in the synthesis of acetylcholine consists of the choline acetylase transfer of an acetyl group from acetylcoenzyme A to choline. Acetylcholine is the neurohumoral transmitter in the parasympathetic system and as such maintains the normal functions of the intestine. Decrease in acetylcholine content would result in decreased peristalsis and in extreme cases adynamic ileus. The pharmacological mode of action of the drug is unknown. Pharmacokinetic data in humans are unavailable.

Indications and Usage: Prophylactic use immediately after major abdominal surgery to minimize the possibility of paralytic ileus. Intestinal atony causing abdominal distention; postoperative or postpartum retention of flatus, or postoperative delay in resumption of intestinal motility; paralytic ileus.

Contraindications: There are no known contraindications to the use of ILOPAN INJECTION.

Warnings: There have been rare instances of allergic reactions of unknown cause during the concomitant use of ILOPAN INJECTION with drugs such as antibiotics, narcotics and barbiturates.

Administration of ILOPAN INJECTION directly into the vein is not advised (See Dosage and Administration).

ILOPAN INJECTION should not be administered within one hour of succinylcholine.

Precautions:
General—If any signs of a hypersensitivity reaction appear, ILOPAN INJECTION should be discontinued. If ileus is a secondary consequence of mechanical obstruction, primary attention should be directed to the obstruction.

The management of adynamic ileus includes the correction of any fluid and electrolyte imbalance (especially hypokalemia), anemia and hypoproteinemia, treatment of infection, avoidance where possible of drugs which are known to decrease gastrointestinal motility and decompression of the gastrointestinal tract when considerably distended by nasogastric suction or use of a long intestinal tube.

Drug Interactions—The effects of succinylcholine appeared to have been prolonged in a woman administered dexpanthenol.

Carcinogenicity, Mutagenicity, and Impairment of Fertility—There have been no studies in animals to evaluate the carcinogenic, mutagenic, or impairment of fertility potential of dexpanthenol.

Pregnancy—Category C. Animal reproduction studies have not been conducted with ILOPAN INJECTION. It is also not known whether ILOPAN INJECTION can cause fetal harm when administered to a pregnant woman or can affect reproduction capacity. ILOPAN INJECTION should be given to a pregnant woman only if clearly needed.

Nursing Mothers—It is not known whether this drug is excreted in human milk. Because many drugs are excreted in human milk, caution should be exercised when ILOPAN INJECTION is administered to a nursing woman.

Pediatric Use—Safety and effectiveness in children have not been established.

Adverse Reactions: There have been a few reports of allergic reactions and single reports of several other adverse events in association with the administration of dexpanthenol. A causal relationship is uncertain. One patient experienced itching, tingling, difficulty in breathing. Another patient had red patches of skin. Two patients had generalized dermatitis and one patient urticaria. One patient experienced temporary respiratory difficulty following administration of ILOPAN INJECTION 5 minutes after succinylcholine was discontinued.

One patient experienced a noticeable but slight drop in blood pressure after administration of dexpanthenol while in the recovery room.

One patient experienced intestinal colic one-half hour after the drug was administered.

Two patients vomited following administration and two patients had diarrhea 10 days post-surgery and after ILOPAN INJECTION.

One elderly patient became agitated after administration of the drug.

Dosage and Administration: Prevention of post-operative adynamic ileus: 250 mg (1 ml) or 500 mg (2 ml) intramuscularly. Repeat in 2 hours and then every 6 hours until all danger of adynamic ileus has passed.

Treatment of adynamic ileus: 500 mg (2 ml) intramuscularly. Repeat in 2 hours and then every 6 hours as needed.

Intravenous administration: ILOPAN INJECTION 2 ml (500 mg) may be mixed with bulk I.V. solutions such as glucose or lactate-Ringer's and slowly infused intravenously.

Parenteral drug products should be inspected visually for particulate matter and discoloration prior to administration, whenever solution and container permit.

How Supplied: Each milliliter of ILOPAN INJECTION contains dexpanthenol, 250 mg in Water for Injection. ILOPAN INJECTION is available as follows:
ILOPAN INJECTION
  NDC 0013-2356-93 2 ml Ampuls, Box of 12
  NDC 0013-2356-95 2 ml Ampuls, Box of 25
  NDC 0013-2356-97 2 ml Ampuls, Box of 100
Ampules maufactured by:
TAYLOR PHARMACAL CO.
DECATUR, ILLINOIS 62525
ILOPAN INJECTION
  NDC 0013-2356-86 10 ml Vial
ILOPAN INJECTION STAT-PAK® (unit dose)
  NDC 0013-2366-95 Disposable Syringe 2 ml, Box of 25
Protect from freezing or excessive heat.

KAOCHLOR® ℞
[ka'ō-kloor]
(Potassium Chloride)
10% Liquid
Contains Sugar

Description: Each 15 ml (tablespoonful) of KAOCHLOR 10% Liquid supplies 20 mEq each of potassium and chloride (as potassium chloride, 1.5 g) with sugar, saccharin, flavoring, and alcohol 5%. Contains FD&C Yellow No. 5 (tartrazine) as a color additive. The chemical name of the drug is potassium chloride.

Clinical Pharmacology: Potassium ion is the principal intracellular cation of most body tissues. Potassium ions participate in a number of essential physiological processes including the maintenance of intracellular tonicity, the transmission of nerve impulses, the contraction of cardiac, skeletal and smooth muscle and the maintenance of normal renal function.

Potassium depletion may occur whenever the rate of potassium loss through renal excretion and/or loss from the gastrointestinal tract exceeds the rate of potassium intake. Such depletion usually develops slowly as a consequence of prolonged therapy with oral diuretics, primary or secondary hyperaldosteronism, diabetic ketoacidosis, or inadequate replacement of potassium in patients on prolonged parenteral nutrition. Such depletion can develop rapidly with severe diarrhea, especially if associated with vomiting. Potassium depletion due to these causes is usually accompanied by a concomitant loss of chloride and is manifested by hypokalemia and metabolic alkalosis. Potassium depletion may produce weakness, fatigue, disturbances of cardiac rhythm (primarily ectopic beats), prominent U-waves in the electrocardiogram, and in advanced cases, flaccid paralysis and/or impaired ability to concentrate urine.

Potassium depletion associated with metabolic alkalosis is managed by correcting the fundamental cause of the deficiency whenever possible and administering supplemental potassium chloride, in the form of high potassium food or potassium chloride solution or tablets.

In rare circumstances (e.g., patients with renal tubular acidosis) potassium depletion may be associated with metabolic acidosis and hyperchloremia. In such patients potassium replacement should be accomplished with potassium salts other than the chloride, such as potassium bicarbonate, potassium citrate, potassium acetate, or potassium gluconate.

Indications and Usage:
1. For therapeutic use in patients with hypokalemia with or without metabolic alkalosis, in digitalis intoxication and in patients with hypokalemic familial periodic paralysis.
2. For the prevention of potassium depletion when the dietary intake is inadequate in the following conditions: Patients receiving digitalis and diuretics for congestive heart failure, hepatic cirrhosis with ascites, states of aldosterone excess with normal renal function, potassium-losing nephropathy, and with certain diarrheal states.
3. The use of potassium salts in patients receiving diuretics for uncomplicated essential hypertension is often unnecessary when such patients have a normal dietary pattern. Serum potassium should be checked periodically, however, and if hypokalemia occurs, dietary supplementation with potassium-containing foods may be adequate to control milder cases. In more severe cases supplementation with potassium salts may be indicated.

Contraindications: Potassium supplements are contraindicated in patients with hyperkalemia since a further increase in serum potassium concentration in such patients can produce cardiac arrest. Hyperkalemia may complicate any of the following conditions: Chronic renal failure, systemic acidosis such as diabetic acidosis, acute dehydration, extensive tissue breakdown as in severe burns, adrenal insufficiency, or the administration of a potassium-sparing diuretic (e.g., spironolactone, triamterene).

Warnings: Do not administer full strength. KAOCHLOR 10% Liquid will cause gastrointestinal irritation if administered undiluted. For details regarding adequate dilution, see Dosage and Administration.

Hyperkalemia—In patients with impaired mechanisms for excreting potassium, the administration of potassium salts can produce hyperkalemia and cardiac arrest. This occurs most commonly in patients given potassium by the intravenous route but may also occur in patients given potassium orally. Potentially fatal hyperkalemia can develop rapidly and be asymptomatic. The use of potassium salts in patients with chronic renal disease, or any other condition which impairs potassium excretion, requires particularly careful monitoring of the serum potassium concentration and appropriate dosage adjustment.

Interaction with Potassium Sparing Diuretics—Hypokalemia should not be treated by the concomitant administration of potassium salts and a potassium-sparing diuretic (e.g., spironolactone or triamterene) since the simultaneous administration of these agents can produce severe hyperkalemia.

Metabolic Acidosis—Hypokalemia in patients with metabolic acidosis should be treated with an alkalinizing potassium salt such as potassium bicarbonate, potassium citrate, potassium acetate or potassium gluconate.

Precautions:
General—The diagnosis of potassium depletion is ordinarily made by demonstrating hypokalemia in a patient with a clinical history suggesting some cause for potassium depletion.

This product contains FD&C Yellow No. 5 (tartrazine) which may cause allergic-type reactions (including bronchial asthma) in certain susceptible individuals. Although the overall incidence of FD&C Yellow No. 5 (tartrazine) sensitivity in the general population is low, it is frequently seen in patients who also have aspirin hypersensitivity.

Laboratory Tests—In interpreting the serum potassium level, the physician should bear in mind that acute alkalosis *per se* can produce hypokalemia in the absence of a deficit in total body potassium while acute acidosis *per se* can increase the serum potassium concentration into the normal range even in the presence of a reduced total body potassium. The treatment of potassium depletion, particularly in the presence of cardiac disease, renal disease, or acidosis, requires careful attention to acid-base balance and appropriate monitoring of serum electrolytes, the electrocardiogram, and the clinical status of the patient.

It is important to recognize that hyperkalemia is usually asymptomatic and may be manifested only by an increased serum potassium concentration and characteristic electrocardiographic changes (peaking of T-waves, loss of P-wave, depression of S-T segment, and prolongation of the QT interval). (See Contraindications, Warnings and Overdosage.)

The use of potassium salts in patients with chronic renal disease, or any other condition which impairs potassium excretion, requires particularly careful monitoring of the serum potassium concentration and appropriate dosage adjustment.

When blood is drawn for analysis of plasma potassium levels, it is important to recognize that artifactual elevations do occur after repeated fist clenching to make veins more prominent during application of a tourniquet.

Carcinogenesis, Mutagenesis, Impairment of Fertility—There have been no studies in animals or humans to evaluate the carcinogenesis, mutagenesis or impairment of fertility for potassium.

Pregnancy—Category C. Animal reproduction studies have not been conducted with KAOCHLOR 10% Liquid. It is also not known whether KAOCHLOR 10% Liquid can cause fetal harm when administered to a pregnant woman or can affect reproduction capacity. KAOCHLOR 10% Liquid should be given to a pregnant woman only if clearly needed.

Nursing Mothers—It is not known whether this drug is excreted in human milk. Because many drugs are excreted in human milk, caution should be exercised when KAOCHLOR 10% Liquid is administered to a nursing woman.

Pediatric Use—Safety and effectiveness in children have not been established.

Adverse Reactions: The most severe effect is hyperkalemia (see Contraindications, Warnings and Overdosage).

The most common adverse reactions to oral potassium salts are nausea, vomiting, abdominal discomfort, and diarrhea. These symptoms are due to irritation of the gastrointestinal tract and are best managed by diluting the preparation further, taking the dose with meals, or reducing the dose.

Overdosage: The administration of oral potassium salts to persons with normal excretory mechanisms for potassium rarely causes serious hyperkalemia. However, if excretory mechanisms are impaired or if potassium is administered too rapidly intravenously, potentially fatal hyperkalemia can result (see Contraindications and Warnings). It is important to recognize that hyperkalemia is usually asymptomatic and may be manifested only by an increased serum potassium concentration and characteristic electrocardiographic changes (peaking of T-waves, loss of P-wave, depression of S-T segment, and prolongation of the QT interval). Late manifestations include muscle-paralysis and cardiovascular collapse from cardiac arrest.

Treatment for hyperkalemia includes the following:
1. Elimination of foods and medications containing potassium and potassium-sparing diuretics.
2. Intravenous administration of 300 to 500 ml/hr of 10% dextrose solution containing 10-20 units of crystalline insulin per 1,000 ml.

Continued on next page

Adria—Cont.

3. Correction of acidosis, if present, with intravenous sodium bicarbonate.
4. Use of exchange resins, hemodialysis, or peritoneal dialysis.

In treating hyperkalemia, it should be recalled that in patients who have been stabilized on digitalis, too rapid a lowering of the serum potassium concentration can produce digitalis toxicity.

Dosage and Administration: The usual dietary intake of potassium by the average adult is 40 to 80 mEq per day. Potassium depletion sufficient to cause hypokalemia usually requires the loss of 200 or more mEq of potassium from the total body store.

Dosage must be adjusted to the individual needs of each patient but is typically in the range of 20 mEq per day for the prevention of hypokalemia to 40-100 mEq per day or more for the treatment of potassium depletion.

To minimize gastrointestinal irritation, patients must follow directions regarding dilution. Each tablespoonful (15 ml) should be diluted with three (3) fluid ounces or more of water or other liquid. One (1) tablespoonful (15 ml) twice daily (after morning and evening meals) supplies 40 mEq of potassium. Deviations from this recommendation may be indicated, since no average total daily dose can be defined but must be governed by close observation for clinical effects. However, potassium intoxication may result from any therapeutic dosage. See "Overdosage" and "Precautions".

How Supplied:
KAOCHLOR 10% Liquid supplies 20 mEq each of potassium and chloride per tablespoonful (15 ml).
NDC 0013-3103-51 Pint
NDC 0013-3103-53 Gallon
NDC 0013-3103-56 Bottle of 4 Fl. oz. (36's only)
NDC 0013-3103-58 Bottle of 15 ml, Stat-Pak® (Unit Dose), 100's only.
Storage Conditions—Protect from cold.

KAOCHLOR® S-F ℞
[ka'ō-kloor s-f]
(Potassium Chloride)
10% Liquid
Sugar-Free

Description: Each 15 ml (tablespoonful) of KAOCHLOR S-F 10% Liquid supplies 20 mEq each of potassium and chloride (as potassium chloride, 1.5g) with saccharin, flavoring, and alcohol 5%. The chemical name of the drug is potassium chloride.
Clinical Pharmacology: See KAOCHLOR 10% LIQUID
Indications and Usage: See KAOCHLOR 10% LIQUID
Contraindications: See KAOCHLOR 10% LIQUID
Warnings: See KAOCHLOR 10% LIQUID
Precautions:
General—The diagnosis of potassium depletion is ordinarily made by demonstrating hypokalemia in patients with a clinical history suggesting some cause for potassium depletion.
Laboratory Tests—See KAOCHLOR 10% LIQUID
Carcinogenesis, Mutagenesis, Impairment of Fertility—See KAOCHLOR 10% LIQUID
Pregnancy—See KAOCHLOR 10% LIQUID
Nursing Mothers—See KAOCHLOR 10% LIQUID
Pediatric Use—See KAOCHLOR 10% LIQUID
Adverse Reactions: See KAOCHLOR 10% LIQUID
Overdosage: See KAOCHLOR 10% LIQUID
Dosage and Administration: See KAOCHLOR 10% LIQUID
How Supplied: KAOCHLOR S-F 10% Liquid supplies 20 mEq each of potassium and chloride per tablespoonful (15 ml).
NDC 0013-3093-51 Pint
NDC 0013-3093-53 Gallon
NDC 0013-3093-56 Bottle of 4 Fl. Oz. (36's only)
NDC 0013-3093-58 Bottle of 15 ml Stat-Pak® (Unit Dose) 100's only.
Storage Conditions—Protect from cold.

KAON® ELIXIR ℞
[kā'ŏn]
(Potassium Gluconate)
Grape Flavor
Sugar-Free

Description: Each 15 ml (tablespoonful) supplies 20 mEq of potassium (as potassium gluconate, 4.68 g) with saccharin and aromatics and alcohol 5%. The chemical name of the drug is gluconic acid potassium salt. The structural formula is:

$$HOCH_2-\underset{\underset{H}{|}}{\overset{\overset{H}{|}}{C}}-\underset{\underset{OH}{|}}{\overset{\overset{H}{|}}{C}}-\underset{\underset{H}{|}}{\overset{\overset{OH}{|}}{C}}-\underset{\underset{OH}{|}}{\overset{\overset{H}{|}}{C}}-COOK$$

Clinical Pharmacology: Potassium ion is the principal intracellular cation of most body tissues. Potassium ions participate in a number of essential physiological processes including the maintenance of intracellular tonicity, the transmission of nerve impulses, the contraction of cardiac, skeletal and smooth muscle and the maintenance of a normal renal function.

Potassium depletion may occur whenever the rate of potassium loss through renal excretion and/or loss from the gastrointestinal tract exceeds the rate of potassium intake. Potassium depletion sufficient to cause hypokalemia usually requires the loss of 200 or more mEq of potassium from the total body store. Such depletion usually develops slowly as a consequence of prolonged therapy with oral diuretics, primary or secondary hyperaldosteronism, diabetic ketoacidosis, or inadequate replacement of potassium in patients on prolonged parenteral nutrition. Such depletion can develop rapidly with severe diarrhea, especially if associated with vomiting. Potassium depletion may produce weakness, fatigue, disturbances of cardiac rhythm (primarily ectopic beats), prominent U-waves in the electrocardiogram, and in advanced cases, flaccid paralysis and/or impaired ability to concentrate urine.

Indications and Usage:
1. For therapeutic use in patients with hypokalemia with or without metabolic alkalosis, in digitalis intoxication and in patients with hypokalemic familial periodic paralysis.
2. For the prevention of potassium depletion when the dietary intake is inadequate in the following conditions: Patients receiving digitalis and diuretics for congestive heart failure; hepatic cirrhosis with ascites, states of aldosterone excess with normal renal function, potassium-losing nephropathy, and with certain diarrheal states.
3. The use of potassium salts in patients receiving diuretics for uncomplicated essential hypertension is often unnecessary when such patients have a normal dietary pattern. Serum potassium should be checked periodically, however, and if hypokalemia occurs, dietary supplementation with potassium-containing foods may be adequate to control milder cases. In more severe cases supplementation with potassium salts may be indicated.
4. Hypokalemia in patients with metabolic acidosis should be treated with an alkalinizing potassium salt such as potassium gluconate.

Contraindications: Potassium supplements are contraindicated in patients with hyperkalemia since a further increase in serum potassium concentration in such patients can produce cardiac arrest. Hyperkalemia may complicate any of the following conditions: Chronic renal failure, systemic acidosis such as diabetic acidosis, acute dehydration, extensive tissue breakdown as in severe burns, adrenal insufficiency, or the administration of a potassium-sparing diuretic (e.g., spironolactone, triamterene).

Warnings: Do not administer full strength. KAON ELIXIR may cause gastrointestinal irritation if administered undiluted. For details regarding adequate dilution, see Dosage and Administration.

Hyperkalemia—In patients with impaired mechanisms for excreting potassium, the administration of potassium salts can produce hyperkalemia and cardiac arrest. This occurs most commonly in patients given potassium by the intravenous route but may also occur in patients given potassium orally. Potentially fatal hyperkalemia can develop rapidly and be asymptomatic. The use of potassium salts in patients with chronic renal disease, or any other condition which impairs potassium excretion, requires particularly careful monitoring of the serum potassium concentration and appropriate dosage adjustment.

Interaction with Potassium Sparing Diuretics —Hypokalemia should not be treated by the concomitant administration of potassium salts and a potassium-sparing diuretic (e.g., spironolactone or triamterene) since the simultaneous administration of these agents can produce severe hyperkalemia.

Precautions:
General—The diagnosis of potassium depletion is ordinarily made by demonstrating hypokalemia in a patient with a clinical history suggesting some cause for potassium depletion.

In hypokalemic states, especially in patients on a low-salt diet, hypochloremic alkalosis is a possibility that may require chloride as well as potassium supplementation. In these circumstances, potassium replacement with potassium chloride may be more advantageous than with other potassium salts.

However, KAON ELIXIR can be supplemented with chloride. Ammonium chloride is an excellent source of chloride ion (18.7 mEq per gram) but it should not be used in patients with hepatic cirrhosis where ammonium salts are contraindicated.

Laboratory Tests—In interpreting the serum potassium level, the physician should bear in mind that acute alkalosis *per se* can produce hypokalemia in the absence of a deficit in total body potassium while acute acidosis *per se* can increase the serum potassium concentration into the normal range even in the presence of a reduced total body potassium. The treatment of potassium depletion, particularly in the presence of cardiac disease, renal disease, or acidosis, requires careful attention to acid-base balance and appropriate monitoring of serum electrolytes, the electrocardiogram, and the clinical status of the patient.

It is important to recognize that hyperkalemia is usually asymptomatic and may be manifested only by an increased serum potassium concentration and characteristic electrocardiographic changes (peaking of T-waves, loss of P-wave, depression of S-T segment, and prolongation of the QT interval). (See Contraindications, Warnings, and Overdosage.)

The use of potassium salts in patients with chronic renal disease, or any other condition which impairs potassium excretion, requires particularly careful monitoring of the serum potassium concentration and appropriate dosage adjustment.

When blood is drawn for analysis of plasma potassium levels, it is important to recognize that artifactual elevations do occur after repeated fist clenching to make veins more prominent during application of a tourniquet.

Carcinogenesis, Mutagenesis, Impairment of Fertility—There have been no studies in animals or humans to evaluate the carcinogenesis, mutagenesis or impairment of fertility for potassium.

Pregnancy—Category C. Animal reproduction studies have not been conducted with KAON ELIXIR. It is also not known whether KAON ELIXIR can cause fetal harm when administered to a pregnant woman or can affect reproduction capacity. KAON ELIXIR should be given to a pregnant woman only if clearly needed.

Nursing Mothers—It is not known whether this drug is excreted in human milk. Because many drugs are excreted in human milk, caution should be exercised when KAON ELIXIR is administered to a nursing woman.

Pediatric Use—Safety and effectiveness in children have not been established.

Adverse Reactions: The most severe adverse effect is hyperkalemia (see Contraindications, Warnings and Overdosage).

The most common adverse reactions to oral potassium salts are nausea, vomiting, abdominal discomfort, and diarrhea. These symptoms are due to irritation of the gastrointestinal tract and are best managed by diluting the preparation further, taking the dose with meals, or reducing the dose.

Overdosage: The administration of oral potassium salts to persons with normal excretory mechanisms for potassium rarely causes serious hyperkalemia. However, if excretory mechanisms are impaired or if potassium is administered too rapidly intravenously, potentially fatal hyperkalemia can result (see Contraindications and Warnings). It is important to recognize that hyperkalemia is usually asymptomatic and may be manifested only by an increased serum potassium concentration and characteristic electrocardiographic changes (peaking of T-waves, loss of P-wave, depression of S-T segment, and prolongation of the QT interval). Late manifestations include muscle-paralysis and cardiovascular collapse from cardiac arrest.

Treatment for hyperkalemia includes the following:
1. Elimination of foods and medications containing potassium and potassium-sparing diuretics.
2. Intravenous administration of 300 to 500 ml/hr of 10% dextrose solution containing 10–20 units of crystalline insulin per 1,000 ml.
3. Correction of acidosis, if present, with intravenous sodium bicarbonate.
4. Use of exchange resins, hemodialysis, or peritoneal dialysis.

In treating hyperkalemia, it should be recalled that in patients who have been stabilized on digitalis, too rapid a lowering of the serum potassium concentration can produce digitalis toxicity.

Dosage and Administration: The usual dietary intake of potassium by the average adult is 40 to 80 mEq per day. Potassium depletion sufficient to cause hypokalemia usually requires the loss of 200 or more mEq of potassium from the total body store.

Dosage must be adjusted to the individual needs of each patient but is typically in the range of 20 mEq per day for the prevention of hypokalemia to 40–100 mEq per day or more for the treatment of potassium depletion.

To minimize gastrointestinal irritation, patients must follow directions regarding dilution. Each tablespoonful (15 ml) should be diluted with one fluid ounce or more of water or other liquid.

One tablespoonful twice daily (after morning and evening meals) supplies 40 mEq of potassium. Deviations from this recommendation may be indicated, since no average total daily dose can be defined but must be governed by close observation for clinical effects. However, potassium intoxications may result from any therapeutic dosage. See "Overdosage" and "Precautions".

How Supplied: KAON ELIXIR (potassium gluconate), Grape, supplies 20 mEq of potassium (as potassium gluconate, 4.68g) per tablespoonful (15 ml).
NDC 0013-3203-51 Pint
NDC 0013-3203-53 Gallon
NDC 0013-3203-56 Bottle of 4 Fl. Oz. (36's only).
NDC 0013-3203-58 Bottle of 15 ml, Stat-Pak® (Unit Dose) 100's only.

Storage Conditions: Protect from cold.

KAON® TABLETS
[kā'ŏn]
(Potassium Gluconate)

Description: Each sugar coated tablet supplies 5 mEq of elemental potassium (as potassium gluconate 1.17 g). KAON Tablets are sugar coated, not enteric coated, which favors dissolution in the stomach and absorption before reaching the small intestine where the lesions with enteric potassium chloride have occurred. The sugar coating merely adds to palatability and ease of swallowing, not to delay absorption as does the enteric coating.

Indications: Oral potassium therapy for the prevention and treatment of hypokalemia which may occur secondary to diuretic or corticosteroid administration. It may be used in the treatment of cardiac arrhythmias due to digitalis intoxication.

Contraindications: Severe renal impairment with oliguria or azotemia, untreated Addison's disease, adynamia episodica hereditaria, acute dehydration, heat cramps and hyperkalemia from any cause.

Warning: There have been several reports, published and unpublished, concerning nonspecific small-bowel lesions consisting of stenosis, with or without ulceration, associated with the administration of enteric-coated thiazides with potassium salts. These lesions may occur with enteric-coated potassium tablets alone or when they are used with nonenteric-coated thiazides or certain other oral diuretics. These small bowel lesions have caused obstruction, hemorrhage and perforation. Surgery was frequently required and deaths have occurred. Available information tends to implicate enteric-coated potassium salts, although lesions of this type also occur spontaneously. Therefore, coated potassium-containing formulations should be administered only when indicated and should be discontinued immediately if abdominal pain, distention, nausea, vomiting, or gastrointestinal bleeding occur. Coated potassium tablets should be used only when adequate dietary supplementation is not practical.

Precautions: In response to a rise in the concentration of body potassium, renal excretion of the ion is increased. With normal kidney function, it is difficult, therefore, to produce potassium intoxication by oral adminstration. However, potassium supplements must be administered with caution, since the amount of the deficiency or daily dosage is not accurately known. Frequent checks of the clinical status of the patient, and periodic ECG and/or serum potassium levels should be made. High serum concentrations of potassium ion may cause death through cardiac depression, arrhythmias or arrest. This drug should be used with caution in the presence of cardiac disease. In hypokalemic states, especially in patients on a salt-free diet, hypochloremic alkalosis is a possibility that may require chloride as well as potassium supplementation. In these circumstances, KAON (potassium gluconate) should be supplemented with chloride. Ammonium chloride is an excellent source of chloride ion (18.7 mEq per Gram), but it should not be used in patients with hepatic cirrhosis where ammonium salts are contraindicated. Other sources for chloride are sodium chloride and Diluted Hydrochloric Acid, NF. It should also be kept in mind that ammonium cycle cation exchange resin, sometimes used to treat hyperkalemia, should not be administered to patients with hepatic cirrhosis.

Adverse Reactions: Nausea, vomiting, diarrhea and abdominal discomfort have been reported. The symptoms and signs of potassium intoxication include paresthesias of the extremities, flaccid paralysis, listlessness, mental confusion, weakness and heaviness of the legs, fall in blood pressure, cardiac arrhythmias and heart block. Hyperkalemia may exhibit the following electrocardiographic abnormalities: disappearance of the P wave, widening and slurring of QRS complex, changes of the S-T segment, tall peaked T waves, etc.

Dosage and Adminstration: The usual adult dosage is 2 tablets four times daily (after meals and at bedtime). This supplies 40 mEq of elemental potassium, the approximate minimum adult daily requirement for potassium. Deviations from this recommendation may be indicated, since no average total daily dose can be defined but must be governed by close observation for clinical effects. However, potassium intoxication may result from any therapeutic dosage. See "Overdosage" and "Precautions."

Overdosage: Potassium intoxication may result from overdosage of potassium or from therapeutic dosage in conditions stated under "Contraindications." Hyperkalemia, when detected, must be treated immediately because lethal levels can be reached in a few hours.

Treatment of Hyperkalemia:
1. Dextrose solution, 10 or 25% containing 10 units of crystalline insulin per 20 g dextrose, given I.V. in a dose of 300 to 500 ml in an hour.
2. Adsorption and exchange of potassium using sodium or ammonium cycle cation exchange resin, orally and as retention enema. See "Precautions."
3. Hemodialysis and peritoneal dialysis.
4. The use of potassium-containing foods or medicaments must be eliminated.

In cases of digitalization too rapid a lowering of plasma potassium concentration can cause digitalis toxicity.

How Supplied:
NDC 0013-3121-17 Bottle of 100 Tablets
NDC 0013-3121-21 Bottle of 500 Tablets
NDC 0013-3121-18 Stat-Pak® (Unit Dose) 100's only

Shown in Product Identification Section, page 404

KAON–CL™
[kā'ŏn sēē-ĕl"]
(Potassium Chloride)
CONTROLLED RELEASE TABLETS

Description: KAON-CL 6.7 mEq is a sugar coated (not enteric-coated) tablet containing 500 mg potassium chloride (equivalent to 6.7 mEq potassium chloride) in a wax matrix. Contains color additives including FD&C Yellow No. 5 (tartrazine). This formulation is intended to provide a controlled release of potassium from the matrix to minimize the likelihood of producing high localized concentrations of potassium within the gastrointestinal tract.

Actions: Potassium ion is the principal intracellular cation of most body tissues. Potassium ions participate in a number of essential physiological processes including the maintenance of intracellular tonicity, the transmission of nerve impulses, the contraction of cardiac, skeletal and smooth muscle and the maintenance of normal renal function.

Potassium depletion may occur whenever the rate of potassium loss through renal excretion and/or loss from the gastrointestinal tract exceeds the rate of potassium intake. Such depletion usually develops slowly as a consequence of prolonged therapy with oral diuretics, primary or secondary hyperaldosteronism, diabetic ketoacidosis, severe diarrhea, or inadequate replacement of potassium in patients on prolonged parenteral nutrition. Potassium depletion due to these causes is usually accompanied by a concomitant deficiency of chloride and is manifested by hypokalemia and metabolic alkalosis. Potassium depletion may produce weakness, fatigue, disturbances of cardiac rhythm (primarily ectopic beats), prominent U-waves in the electrocardiogram, and in advanced cases, flaccid paralysis and/or impaired ability to concentrate urine.

Potassium depletion associated with metabolic alkalosis is managed by correcting the fundamental cause of the deficiency whenever possible and administering supplemental potassium chloride, in the form of high potassium food or potassium chloride solution or tablets. In rare circumstances (e.g., patients with renal tubular acidosis) potassium depletion may be associated with metabolic acidosis and hyperchloremia. In such patients potassium replacement should be accomplished with potassium salts other than the chloride, such as potassium bicarbonate, potassium citrate, potassium acetate, or potassium gluconate.

Indications:

BECAUSE OF REPORTS OF INTESTINAL AND GASTRIC ULCERATION AND BLEEDING WITH SLOW RELEASE POTASSIUM CHLORIDE PREPARATIONS, THESE DRUGS SHOULD BE RESERVED FOR THOSE PATIENTS WHO CANNOT TOLERATE OR REFUSE TO TAKE LIQUIDS OR EFFERVESCENT POTASSIUM PREPARATIONS OR FOR PATIENTS IN WHOM THERE IS A PROBLEM OF COMPLIANCE WITH THESE PREPARATIONS.

1. For therapeutic use in patients with hypokalemia with or without metabolic alkalosis, in digitalis intoxication and in patients with hypokalemic familial periodic paralysis.

Continued on next page

Adria—Cont.

2. For the prevention of potassium depletion when the dietary intake is inadequate in the following conditions: Patients receiving digitalis and diuretics for congestive heart failure, hepatic cirrhosis with ascites, states of aldosterone excess with normal renal function, potassium-losing nephropathy, and with certain diarrheal states.
3. The use of potassium salts in patients receiving diuretics for uncomplicated essential hypertension is often unnecessary when such patients have a normal dietary pattern. Serum potassium should be checked periodically, however, and if hypokalemia occurs, dietary supplementation with potassium-containing foods may be adequate to control milder cases. In more severe cases supplementation with potassium salts may be indicated.

Contraindications: Potassium supplements are contraindicated in patients with hyperkalemia since a further increase in serum potassium concentration in such patients can produce cardiac arrest. Hyperkalemia may complicate any of the following conditions: Chronic renal failure, systemic acidosis such as diabetic acidosis, acute dehydration, extensive tissue breakdown as in severe burns, adrenal insufficiency, or the administration of a potassium-sparing diuretic (e.g., spironolactone, triamterene).

Wax-matrix potassium chloride preparations have produced esophageal ulceration in certain cardiac patients with esophageal compression due to enlarged left atrium. Potassium supplementation, when indicated in such patients, should be with a liquid preparation.

All solid dosage forms of potassium chloride supplements are contraindicated in any patient in whom there is cause for arrest or delay in tablet passage through the gastrointestinal tract. In these instances, potassium supplementation should be with a liquid preparation.

Warnings:
Hyperkalemia—In patients with impaired mechanisms for excreting potassium, the administration of potassium salts can produce hyperkalemia and cardiac arrest. This occurs most commonly in patients given potassium by the intravenous route but may also occur in patients given potassium orally. Potentially fatal hyperkalemia can develop rapidly and be asymptomatic. The use of potassium salts in patients with chronic renal disease, or any other condition which impairs potassium excretion, requires particularly careful monitoring of the serum potassium concentration and appropriate dosage adjustment.

Interaction with Potassium Sparing Diuretics—Hypokalemia should not be treated by the concomitant administration of potassium salts and a potassium-sparing diuretic (e.g., spironolactone or triamterene) since the simultaneous administration of these agents can produce severe hyperkalemia.

Gastrointestinal Lesions—Potassium chloride tablets have produced stenotic and/or ulcerative lesions of the small bowel and deaths. These lesions are caused by a high localized concentration of potassium ion in the region of a rapidly dissolving tablet, which injures the bowel wall and thereby produces obstruction, hemorrhage or perforation. KAON-CL 6.7 mEq (potassium chloride) is a wax-matrix tablet formulated to provide a controlled rate of release of potassium chloride and thus to minimize the possibility of a high local concentration of potassium ion near the bowel wall. While the reported frequency of small bowel lesions is much less with wax-matrix tablets (less than one per 100,000 patient years) than with enteric-coated potassium chloride tablets (40-50 per 100,000 patient years) cases associated with wax-matrix tablets have been reported both in foreign countries and in the United States. In addition, perhaps because the wax-matrix preparations are not enteric-coated and release potassium in the stomach, there have been reports of upper gastrointestinal bleeding associated with these products. The total number of gastrointestinal lesions remains less than one per 100,000 patient years. KAON-CL 6.7 mEq should be discontinued immediately and the possibility of bowel obstruction or perforation considered if severe vomiting, abdominal pain, distention, or gastrointestinal bleeding occurs.

Metabolic Acidosis—Hypokalemia in patients with metabolic acidosis should be treated with an alkalinizing potassium salt such as potassium bicarbonate, potassium citrate, potassium acetate, or potassium gluconate.

Precautions: The diagnosis of potassium depletion is ordinarily made by demonstrating hypokalemia in a patient with a clinical history suggesting some cause for potassium depletion. In interpreting the serum potassium level, the physician should bear in mind that acute alkalosis *per se* can produce hypokalemia in the absence of a deficit in total body potassium while acute acidosis *per se* can increase the serum potassium concentration into the normal range even in the presence of a reduced total body potassium. The treatment of potassium depletion, particularly in the presence of cardiac arrest, renal disease, or acidosis requires careful attention to acid-base balance and appropriate monitoring of serum electrolytes, the electrocardiogram, and the clinical status of the patient.

This product contains FD&C Yellow No. 5 (tartrazine) which may cause allergic-type reactions (including bronchial asthma) in certain susceptible individuals. Although the overall incidence of FD&C Yellow No. 5 (tartrazine) sensitivity in the general population is low, it is frequently seen in patients who also have aspirin hypersensitivity.

Adverse Reactions: The most common adverse reactions to oral potassium salts are nausea, vomiting, abdominal discomfort and diarrhea. These symptoms are due to irritation of the gastrointestinal tract and are best managed by diluting the preparation further, taking the dose with meals, or reducing the dose. The most severe adverse effects are hyperkalemia (see Contraindications, Warnings and Overdosage) and gastrointestinal obstruction, bleeding or perforation (see Warnings).

Overdosage: The administration of oral potassium salts to persons with normal excretory mechanisms for potassium rarely causes serious hyperkalemia. However, if excretory mechanisms are impaired or if potassium is administered too rapidly intravenously, potentially fatal hyperkalemia can result (see Contraindications and Warnings). It is important to recognize that hyperkalemia is usually asymptomatic and may be manifested only by an increased serum potassium concentration and characteristic electrocardiographic changes (peaking of T-waves, loss of P-wave, depression of S-T segment, and prolongation of the QT interval). Late manifestations include muscle-paralysis and cardiovascular collapse from cardiac arrest.

Treatment measures for hyperkalemia include the following:
1. Elimination of foods and medications containing potassium and of potassium-sparing diuretics.
2. Intravenous administration of 300 to 500 ml/hr of 10% dextrose solution containing 10–20 units of crystalline insulin per 1,000 ml.
3. Correction of acidosis, if present, with intravenous sodium bicarbonate.
4. Use of exchange resins, hemodialysis, or peritoneal dialysis.

In treating hyperkalemia, it should be recalled that in patients who have been stabilized on digitalis, too rapid a lowering of the serum potassium concentration can produce digitalis toxicity.

Dosage and Administration: The usual dietary intake of potassium by the average adult is 40 to 80 mEq per day. Potassium depletion sufficient to cause hypokalemia usually requires the loss of 200 or more mEq of potassium from the total body store.

Dosage must be adjusted to the individual needs of each patient but is typically in the range of 20 mEq per day for the prevention of hypokalemia to 40–100 mEq per day or more for the treatment of potassium depletion.

One KAON-CL 6.7 mEq three times daily provides 20 mEq of potassium chloride. Two KAON-CL 6.7 mEq three times daily provides 40 mEq of potassium chloride.

Tablets should be taken with a glass of water or other liquid.

How Supplied:
NDC 0013-3071-17 Bottle of 100 Tablets.
NDC 0013-3071-19 Bottle of 250 Tablets.
NDC 0013-3071-23 Bottle of 1000 Tablets.
NDC 0013-3071-18 Stat-Pak® Unit Dose Box of 100 Tablets

Shown in Product Identification Section, page 404

KAON CL™-10 ℞
[kā'ŏn see-el" ten]
(Potassium Chloride)
CONTROLLED RELEASE TABLETS

Description: KAON CL-10 mEq is a sugar coated (not enteric-coated) tablet containing 750 mg potassium chloride (equivalent to 10 mEq potassium chloride) in a wax matrix. This formulation is intended to provide a controlled release of potassium from the matrix to minimize the likelihood of producing high localized concentrations of potassium within the gastrointestinal tract.

Actions: See KAON-CL™ TABLETS
Indications: See KAON-CL TABLETS
Contraindications: See KAON-CL TABLETS
Warnings: See KAON-CL TABLETS
Precautions: The diagnosis of potassium depletion is ordinarily made by demonstrating hypokalemia in a patient with a clinical history suggesting some cause for potassium depletion. In interpreting the serum potassium level, the physician should bear in mind that acute alkalosis *per se* can produce hypokalemia in the absence of a deficit in total body potassium while acute acidosis *per se* can increase the serum potassium concentration into the normal range even in the presence of a reduced total body potassium. The treatment of potassium depletion, particularly in the presence of cardiac disease, renal disease, or acidosis requires careful attention to acid-base balance and appropriate monitoring of serum electrolytes, the electrocardiogram, and the clinical status of the patient.

Adverse Reactions: See KAON-CL TABLETS
Overdosage: See KAON-CL TABLETS
Dosage and Administration: The usual dietary intake of potassium by the average adult is 40 to 80 mEq per day. Potassium depletion sufficient to cause hypokalemia usually requires the loss of 200 or more mEq of potassium from the total body store.

Dosage must be adjusted to the individual needs of each patient but is typically in the range of 20 mEq per day for the prevention of hypokalemia to 40–100 mEq per day or more for the treatment of potassium depletion.

One KAON CL-10 mEq two times daily provides 20 mEq of potassium chloride. Two KAON CL-10 mEq two times daily provides 40 mEq of potassium chloride.

Tablets should be taken with a glass of water or other liquid.

Caution: Federal law prohibits dispensing without prescription.

How Supplied:
NDC 0013-3041-17 Bottles of 100 Tablets
NDC 0013-3041-21 Bottle of 500 Tablets
NDC 0013-3041-18 Stat-Pak® (Unit Dose) Box of 100 Tablets

Shown in Product Identification Section, page 404

KAON-CL 20% ℞
[kā'ŏn-see-el" 20%]
(Potassium Chloride)
Sugar-Free

Description: Each 15 ml (tablespoonful) of KAON-CL 20% supplies 40 mEq each of potassium and chloride (as potassium chloride, 3g) with saccharin, flavoring, and alcohol 5%. The chemical name of the drug is potassium chloride.

Clinical Pharmacology: See KAOCHLOR 10% LIQUID
Indications and Usage: See KAOCHLOR 10% LIQUID
Contraindications: See KAOCHLOR 10% LIQUID
Warnings: See KAOCHLOR 10% LIQUID
Precautions:
General: The diagnosis of potassium depletion is ordinarily made by demonstrating hypokalemia in a patient with a clinical history suggesting some cause for potassium depletion.
Laboratory Tests—See KAOCHLOR 10% LIQUID
Carcinogenesis, Mutagenesis, Impairment of Fertility—See KAOCHLOR 10% LIQUID
Pregnancy—See KAOCHLOR 10% LIQUID
Nursing Mothers:—See KAOCHLOR 10% LIQUID
Pediatric Use:—See KAOCHLOR 10% LIQUID
Adverse Reactions: See KAOCHLOR 10% LIQUID
Overdosage: See KAOCHLOR 10% LIQUID
Dosage and Administration: The usual dietary intake of potassium by the average adult is 40 to 80 mEq per day. Potassium depletion sufficient to cause hypokalemia usually requires the loss of 200 or more mEq of potassium from the total body store.
Dosage must be adjusted to the individual needs of each patient but is typically in the range of 20 mEq per day for the prevention of hypokalemia to 40-100 mEq per day or more for the treatment of potassium depletion.
To minimize gastrointestinal irritation, patients must follow directions regarding dilution. Each tablespoonful (15 ml) should be diluted with six (6) fluid ounces or more of water or other liquid.
One (1) tablespoonful (15 ml) per day (after the morning meal) supplies 40 mEq of potassium. One tablespoonful twice a day, in six (6) or more fluid ounces of water or other fluid, provides 80 mEq potassium chloride. Deviations from these recommendations may be indicated, since no average total daily dose can be defined but must be governed by close observation for clinical effects. However, potassium intoxication may result from any therapeutic dosage. See "Overdosage" and "Precautions".
How Supplied: KAON-CL 20% supplies 40 mEq each of potassium and chloride per tablespoonful (15 ml).
NDC 0013-3113-51 Pint
NDC 0013-3113-53 Gallon
NDC 0013-3113-56 Bottles of 4 Fl. Oz. (36's only).
Storage Conditions: Protect from cold or excessive heat.

MAGAN® ℞
[mā-găn¹]
(Magnesium Salicylate)

Description: Each MAGAN uncoated, pink, capsule-shaped tablet for oral administration contains 545 mg of magnesium salicylate equivalent to 500 mg of salicylate. Magnesium salicylate is a non-steroidal, antiinflammatory agent with antipyretic and analgesic properties. Its molecular weight is 298.54. It has the following structural formula:

Magnesium salicylate is a white, odorless, crystalline powder with a sweet taste. It is soluble in water and alcohol.
Clinical Pharmacology: Salicylic acid is the active moiety released into the plasma by MAGAN (magnesium salicylate). Salicylic acid is enzymatically biotransformed through two pathways to salicyluric acid and salicylphenolic glucuronide and eliminated in the urine.
Oral salicylates are absorbed rapidly, partly from the stomach but mostly from the upper intestine. Salicylic acid is rapidly distributed throughout all body tissues and most transcellular fluids, mainly by pH-dependent passive processes. It can be detected in synovial, spinal and peritoneal fluid, in saliva and milk. It readily crosses the placental barrier. From 50% to 90% of salicylic acid is bound to plasma proteins, especially albumin.
Following the ingestion of a single dose of 524 mg of magnesium salicylate, a peak concentration of 3.6 mg/dl salicylic acid is reached in 1.5 hours with a T ½ of 2 hours. The major biotransformation paths for the elimination of salicylic acid from the plasma become saturated by low doses of salicylic acid. As a result, repeated doses of MAGAN increase the plasma concentration and markedly prolong the plasma half-time. The plasma concentration of salicylic acid is increased by conditions that reduce the glomerular filtration rate or tubular secretion such as renal disease or the presence of inhibitors that compete for the transport system such as probenecid.
Therapeutic plasma concentrations of salicylic acid for an adequate antiinflammatory effect needed for the treatment of rheumatoid arthritis range between 20–30 mg/dl. Effective analgesia is achieved at lower concentrations. Salicylates relieve pain by both a peripheral and a CNS effect. Salicylates inhibit the synthesis of prostaglandins; the importance of this mechanism in analgesia and antiinflammation has not been fully elucidated. Salicylates have a antipyretic effect in febrile patients but little in subjects with normal temperatures. This appears to be due to the inhibition of the synthesis of prostaglandins which are powerful pyrogens that affect the hypothalamus. Higher therapeutic concentrations cause reversible tinnitus and high tone hearing loss. Full therapeutic doses of salicylates increase oxygen consumption and CO_2 production. They cause an extracellular and intracellular respiratory alkalosis which is rapidly compensated. Salicylates irritate the gastric mucosa and frequently lead to blood loss in the stool; this effect is more pronounced with aspirin than magnesium salicylate. Salicylates in large doses (over 6 g/day) reduce the plasma prothrombin level. In contrast to aspirin, magnesium salicylate does not affect platelets. Salicylic acid increases the urinary excretion of urates at higher doses but may decrease excretion at lower doses.
Indications and Usage: MAGAN is indicated for the relief of the signs and symptoms of rheumatoid arthritis, osteoarthritis, bursitis and other musculoskeletal disorders.
Contraindications: MAGAN is contraindicated in patients with advanced chronic renal insufficiency. It may counteract the effect of uricosuric agents and should not be prescribed for patients on such drugs.
Warnings: As with all salicylates, MAGAN should be avoided or administered with caution to patients with liver damage, pre-existing hypoprothrombinemia, vitamin K deficiency and before surgery.
Precautions:
General—Appropriate precautions should be taken in prescribing MAGAN for persons known to be sensitive to salicylates and in patients with erosive gastritis or peptic ulcer. If a reaction develops, the drug should be discontinued. MAGAN should be used with caution, if at all, concomitantly with anticoagulants. Appropriate precautions should be taken in administering MAGAN to patients with any impairment of renal function including discontinuing other drugs containing magnesium and monitoring serum magnesium levels if dosage levels of MAGAN are high.
Drug Interactions—Even small doses of MAGAN should not be given with uricosuric agents such as probenecid that decrease tubular reabsorption because it counteracts their effect. Large doses of MAGAN cause hypoprothrombinemia. Lower doses enhance the effects of anticoagulants such as coumadin and must be used with caution in patients receiving anticoagulants that affect the prothrombin time. Caution should also be exercised in patients concurrently treated with a sulfonylurea hypoglycemic agent or methotrexate because of the drug's capability of displacing them from the plasma protein binding sites, resulting in enhanced action of these agents. A similar displacement of barbiturates and diphenylhydantoin may occur; diphenylhydantoin intoxication has been precipitated by the consumption of aspirin. Salicylates inhibit the diuretic action of spironolactone.
Carcinogenesis, Mutagenesis, Impairment of Fertility—There have been no studies in animals or humans to evaluate the carcinogenesis, mutagenesis or impairment of fertility for magnesium salicylate. Aspirin causes testicular atrophy and inhibition of spermatogenesis in animals.
Pregnancy—Category C.
1. *Teratogenic effects*—Aspirin has been shown to be teratogenic in animals and to increase the incidence of still births and neonatal deaths in women. There are no adequate or well-controlled studies of MAGAN in pregnant women. MAGAN should be used during pregnancy only if the potential benefit justifies the potential risk to the fetus.
2. *Non-Teratogenic effects*—Chronic, high dose salicylate therapy of pregnant women increases the length of gestation and the frequency of post maturity and prolongs spontaneous labor. It is recommended MAGAN be taken during the last three months of pregnancy only under the close supervision of a physician.
Nursing Mothers—Since salicylates are excreted in human milk, caution should be exercised when MAGAN is administered to a nursing woman.
Pediatric Use—Safety and effectiveness of MAGAN in children have not been established.
Adverse Reactions: Magnesium salicylate in large doses has a hypoprothrombinemic effect and should be given with caution in patients receiving anticoagulant drugs, patients with liver damage, pre-existing hypoprothrombinemia, vitamin K deficiency or before surgery.
Salicylates given in overdose produce stimulation (often manifested as tinnitus) followed by depression of the central nervous system. The dosage should be lowered at the onset of tinnitus.
Salicylates may cause gastric mucosal irritation and bleeding. However, fecal blood loss in patients taking MAGAN is significantly less than in those taking aspirin.
MAGAN should not be given to patients with severe renal damage because of the possibility of hypermagnesemia.
In moderate to high doses, salicylates lower the blood glucose in diabetics. Aspirin-induced hypoglycemia has been described in adults undergoing hemodialysis.
Unlike aspirin, magnesium salicylate is not known to affect the platelet adhesiveness involved in the clotting mechanism; and therefore, does not prolong bleeding time. MAGAN has not been associated with reactions causing asthmatic attacks in susceptible people.
Overdosage: Acute overdosage results in salicylate toxicity. Early signs and symptoms from repeated larger doses as well as a large single dose consist of headache, dizziness, tinnitus (which may be absent in children or the elderly), difficulty in hearing, dimness of vision, mental confusion, lassitude, drowsiness, sweating, thirst, hyperventilation, nausea, vomiting and occasionally diarrhea. More severe salicylate poisoning is manifested by CNS disturbances including EEG abnormalities. Hyperventilation occurs producing initial respiratory alkalosis. This is followed by severe metabolic acidosis with dehydration and loss of potassium. Restlessness, garrulity, incoherent speech, apprehension, vertigo, tremor, diplopia, maniacal delirium, hallucinations, generalized convulsions and coma may occur. Toxic symptoms may occur at serum levels greater than 20 mg/dl in patients over 60 years of age. Hyperventilation may occur at plasma salicylate levels over 35 mg/dl. Death may result from salicylate levels between 45–75 mg/dl. As with other salicylates, 10 to 30 g of the drug may be fatal. Renal or hepatic insufficiency and fever and dehydration in children enhance the acute toxicity of salicylate overdoses. Treatment of

Continued on next page

Adria—Cont.

acute poisoning is a medical emergency and should be undertaken in a hospital. Serum Na, K, Cl, CO_2 levels, pH, BUN, blood glucose and urine pH and specific gravity should be obtained. Emesis should be induced or gastric lavage performed. Activated charcoal may be administered. Hyperthermia should be controlled with tepid water sponging. Dehydration should be treated and acid-base imbalance corrected. A high concentration of salicylic acid in the brain may be fatal. Correction of acidosis shifts salicylate from the brain to the plasma. A bicarbonate solution should be infused to maintain an alkaline diuresis. Care should be taken to avoid pulmonary edema. The blood pH, plasma pCO_2 and plasma glucose level should be monitored frequently. Ketosis and hypoglycemia may be corrected by glucose infusions and hypokalemia by potassium chloride added to the intravenous infusate. Avoid respiratory depressants. Shock may be combatted by plasma infusions. Hemorrhagic phenomena may necessitate whole blood transfusions or vitamin K_1. In severe intoxication, exchange transfusion, peritoneal dialysis, hemodialysis or hemoperfusion should be performed to remove plasma salicylic acid. Dialysis should be seriously considered if the patient's condition is worsening despite appropriate therapy.

Dosage and Administration: The dosage for MAGAN in the treatment of musculoskeletal disorders such as arthritis should be adjusted according to individual patient's needs. The recommended initial regimen is two tablets three times per day. Dosage may be increased, if necessary, to achieve the desired therapeutic effect. In adjusting the dosage, the physician should monitor the dose limiting parameters such as tinnitus and/or serum salicylate over 30 mg/dl.

How Supplied: Each MAGAN tablet contains 545 mg of magnesium salicylate equivalent to 500 mg salicylate. MAGAN is available for oral administration as uncoated, pink, capsule-shaped tablets coded Adria 412. They are supplied as follows:
NDC 0013-4121-17 in bottles of 100
NDC 0013-4121-21 in bottles of 500
Store at room temperature and protect from light.

MODANE® BULK
[mō′dāne bulk]
(psyllium and dextrose)

Description: MODANE BULK is a powdered mixture of equal parts of psyllium, a bulking agent, and dextrose, as a dispersing agent. Psyllium is a highly efficient dietary fiber derived from the husk of the seed of *Plantago ovata*. Each rounded teaspoonful contains approximately 3.5 g psyllium, 3.5 g dextrose, 2 mg sodium and 37 mg potassium, and provides 14 calories.

Clinical Pharmacology: Psyllium absorbs water and expands. When taken with adequate amounts of water, it increases the water content and bulk volume of the stool. The initial response usually occurs in 12 to 24 hours but, in patients who have used laxatives chronically, up to three days may elapse before the initial response.

Indications and Usage: MODANE BULK is indicated in the treatment of constipation resulting from a diet low in residue. It is used also as adjunctive therapy in patients with diverticular disease, spastic or irritable colon, hemorrhoids, in pregnancy, and in convalescent and senile patients.

Contraindications: Intestinal obstruction, fecal impaction.

Precautions *General*—Impaction or obstruction may occur if the bulk-forming agent is temporarily arrested in its passage through parts of the alimentary canal. In this case, water is absorbed and the bolus may become inspissated. Use of this product in patients with narrowing of the intestinal lumen may be hazardous. Inspissation should not occur in a normal gastrointestinal tract if the product is taken with one or more glasses of water.

Drug Interactions—Psyllium may combine with certain other drugs. Products containing psyllium should not be taken with salicylates, digitalis and other cardiac glycosides, or nitrofurantoin.

Adverse Reactions: Adverse reactions are uncommon, and most often have resulted from inadequate intake of water or from underlying organic disease. Esophageal, gastric, small intestinal and rectal obstruction have resulted from the accumulation of the mucilaginous components of psyllium.

Dosage and Administration: Adults and children over 12 years of age—ONE ROUNDED TEASPOONFUL ONE TO THREE TIMES DAILY STIRRED INTO AN 8 OUNCE GLASS OF WATER, JUICE OR OTHER SUITABLE LIQUID AND PREFERABLY FOLLOWED BY A SECOND GLASSFUL OF LIQUID. Children 6 to 12 years of age —one-half the adult dose in 8 ounces of liquid.

How Supplied: Each rounded teaspoonful of MODANE BULK powder contains approximately 3.5 g psyllium.
NDC 0013-5025-72 14 oz. container.
Store at room temperature.

MODANE® SOFT
[mō′dāne soft]
(docusate sodium)
Capsules

Description: Each MODANE SOFT capsule contains docusate sodium 100 mg. in a soft gelatin capsule. Docusate sodium is classified as a stool softener. Chemically, docusate sodium is sulfobutanedioic acid 1,4-bis (2-ethylhexyl) ester sodium salt. The chemical structure is:

$$\begin{array}{c} C_2H_5 \\ | \\ COOCH_2CH(CH_2)_3CH_3 \\ | \\ CH_2 \\ | \\ CH-SO_3Na \\ | \\ COOCH_2CH(CH_2)_3CH_3 \\ | \\ C_2H_5 \end{array}$$

docusate sodium

The empirical formula is $C_{20}H_{37}O_7SNa$ and the molecular weight is 444.56. At 25°C the solubility of docusate sodium in water is 15 g/l.

Clinical Pharmacology: Hydration of the stool has been attributed to the drug's surfactant effect on the intestinal contents which was assumed to facilitate penetration of the fecal mass by water and lipids. Although this emollient effect may exist, there is evidence that mucosal permeability is increased and water absorption is inhibited in the jejunum. Similar concentrations inhibit colonic absorption and/or increase intraluminal water and electrolytes. In these respects, it is similar to bile salts and in this manner, may also be considered as a stimulant laxative.

Docusate sodium is absorbed to some extent in the duodenum and proximal jejunum. It appears in the bile.

Indications and Usage: MODANE SOFT is indicated for the management of functional constipation associated with dry hard stools. It is especially useful when it is desirable to lessen the strain of defecation (e.g. in persons with painful rectal lesions, hernia or cardiovascular disease). The effect on the stools may not be apparent until 1-3 days after the first dose.

Contraindications: Mineral oil administration or when abdominal pain, nausea, vomiting, or other signs and/or symptoms of appendicitis are present.

Precautions: *Drug Interactions*—MODANE SOFT may increase the intestinal absorption of mineral oil and may increase the intestinal absorption and/or hepatic uptake of other drugs administered concurrently.

Carcinogenesis, Mutagenesis, Impairment of Fertility—There have been no long term studies of docusate to evaluate carcinogenic potential. There have been no studies to evaluate mutagenic potential or to determine whether docusate has the potential to impair fertility.

Teratogenic Effects—Pregnancy Category C. Animal reproduction studies have not been conducted with docusate. It is also not known whether MODANE SOFT can cause fetal harm when administered to a pregnant woman or can affect reproductive capacity. MODANE SOFT should be given to a pregnant woman only if clearly needed.

Nursing Mothers—It is not known whether this drug is excreted in human milk. Caution should be exercised when MODANE SOFT is administered to a nursing woman.

Pediatric Use—Because of its dosage size, MODANE SOFT is not recommended for use by children less than 6 years of age.

Adverse Reactions: Adverse reactions are uncommon. Diarrhea, cramping pains and rash have been reported.

Overdosage: Docusates have a low potential for toxicity. Single doses as large as 50 mg/kg have not produced adverse effects in children. Anorexia, vomiting and diarrhea may result from overdosage.

Dosage and Administration: Adults and children over 12 years of age—1 to 3 capsules daily. Children 6–12 years of age—one capsule daily.

How Supplied: Each MODANE SOFT green, soft gelatin capsule contains docusate sodium 100 mg coded 13 503.
NDC 0013-5031-13 Package of 30 Capsules
Store at controlled room temperature (59°– 86°F, 15°–30°C).

MODANE®
[mō′dāne]
(danthron)
Tablets and Liquid

Description: MODANE® Tablets (yellow)—Each tablet contains danthron 75 mg.
MODANE® MILD Tablets—Each tablet contains danthron 37.5 mg.
MODANE® Liquid—Each 5 ml (teaspoonful) contains danthron 37.5 mg and alcohol 5%.
Danthron is classified as a stimulant laxative and is chemically 1,8-dihydroxyanthraquinone. Its chemical structure is:

danthron

The empirical formula is $C_{14}H_8O_4$ and the molecular weight is 240.21. It is practically insoluble in water.

Clinical Pharmacology: Stimulant cathartics act on the intestinal mucosa and have effects both on the net absorption of electrolytes and water and on motility. This group includes danthron, the docusates, castor oil, and bile acids. Despite similarity of their mechanism of action, there are differences among these drugs which are due, for the most part, to dosage and the major site of action, i.e. small intestine or colon.

Anthraquinone cathartics vary in their effects depending upon their anthraquinone content and the ease of liberation of the active constituents from their inactive precursor glycosides. Danthron, although a free anthraquinone, is similar to the pro-drug glycosides in its pharmacological properties. A soft or semifluid stool is passed 6 to 8 hours after administration of an anthraquinone glycoside cathartic such as danthron.

Danthron is absorbed from the small intestine to a limited extent, circulated through the portal system and into the general circulation and excreted in the bile, urine, saliva, colonic mucosa and milk.

Indications and Usage: MODANE is indicated for the management of constipation. It may be useful in the management of constipation in geriatric, cardiac, surgical and postpartum patients.

MODANE may be useful in the management of constipation which may occur with or during the concomitant use of antihypertensive agents, ganglionic blocking agents, antihistamines, tranquilizers, sympathomimetics and anticholinergics. A soft or semifluid stool is passed 6 to 8 hours after administration.

Adequate bulk should be provided in the diet and, if the diet does not provide sufficient bulk, by hydrophilic bulking agents. Poor bowel habits should be corrected.

Contraindications: Should not be used when abdominal pain, nausea, vomiting or other signs and/or symptoms of appendicitis are present.

Precautions: *General*—MODANE may cause harmless pink discoloration of urine (the urine may be pink-red, red-violet or red-brown if alkaline).

As with all laxatives, frequent or prolonged use may result in dependence.

Drug Interactions—The absorption of danthron from the gastrointestinal tract and/or its uptake by hepatic cells may be increased by the co-administration of docusate.

Carcinogenesis, Mutagenesis, Impairment of Fertility—There have been no long term studies of MODANE to evaluate carcinogenic potential. There have been no studies to evaluate mutagenic potential or whether MODANE has the potential to impair fertility.

Teratogenic Effects—Pregnancy Category C. Animal reproduction studies have not been conducted with danthron. It is also not known whether danthron can cause fetal harm when administered to a pregnant woman or can affect reproductive capacity. MODANE should be given to a pregnant woman only if clearly needed.

Nursing Mothers—Danthron is excreted in human milk and has been reported to increase bowel activity in infants nursed by women taking it. Caution should be exercised when MODANE is administered to a nursing woman.

Pediatric Use—In general stimulant cathartics should seldom be used in children.

Adverse Reactions: Adverse reactions are uncommon. These are in order of frequency: excessive bowel activity (griping, diarrhea, nausea, vomiting), peri-anal irritation, weakness, dizziness, palpitations and sweating. Temporary brownish mucosal staining has occurred with prolonged use. There has also been reported a suspected allergic reaction with facial swelling, redness and discomfort.

Overdosage: The lowest reported lethal dose in mice and rats is 500 mg/kg. Overdosage may be expected to result in excessive bowel activity. Treatment is symptomatic when the duration of effects is prolonged.

Dosage and Administration: MODANE Tablet (yellow)–Adults—1 tablet with evening meal. MODANE MILD Tablets (half-strength, pink)–Adults—1 or 2 tablets with the evening meal. For adults who have previously responded with excessive bowel activity to a mild laxative or who are diet-restricted or who are bedfast and for children 6-12 years of age—1 tablet with the evening meal. MODANE Liquid–Adults—1 to 2 teaspoonfuls with the evening meal. For adults who have previously responded with excessive bowel activity to a mild laxative or who are diet-restricted or who are bedfast and children who are 6-12 years of age—1 teaspoonful with the evening meal.

How Supplied:
Each MODANE Tablet contains danthron 75 mg in a yellow, round, sugar coated tablet, coded 13 501.
NDC 0013-5011-17 Bottle of 100 Tablets
NDC 0013-5011-23 Bottle of 1000 Tablets
NDC 0013-5011-18 STAT-PAK® (unit dose) 100 Tablets
NDC 0013-5011-07 Package of 10 Tablets
NDC 0013-5011-13 Package of 30 Tablets
Store at room temperature.
Each MODANE MILD Tablet contains danthron 37.5 mg in a pink, round, sugar coated tablet, coded 13 502.
NDC 0013-5021-17 Bottle of 100 Tablets
NDC 0013-5021-23 Bottle of 1000 Tablets
Store at room temperature.
Each 5 ml (teaspoonful) of MODANE Liquid contains danthron 37.5 mg in a red liquid.
NDC 0013-5033-51 Pint Bottles
Protect from cold.

MODANE® PLUS
[mō'dāne plŭs]
(danthron and docusate sodium) Tablets

Description: Each MODANE PLUS tablet contains danthron 50 mg and docusate sodium 100 mg. Danthron is classified as a stimulant cathartic and docusate sodium is a stool softener. Chemically docusate sodium is sulfobutanedioic acid 1,4-bis (2-ethylhexyl) ester sodium salt and danthron is 1,8-dihydroxyanthraquinone. The empirical formula of docusate sodium is $C_{20}H_{37}O_7SNa$ and its molecular weight is 444.56. The empirical formula of danthron is $C_{14}H_8O_4$ and its molecular weight is 240.21.

danthron   docusate sodium

Danthron is practically insoluble in water. At 25°C the solubility of docusate sodium in water is 15 g/1.

Clinical Pharmacology: Contact cathartics act on the intestinal mucosa and have effects both on the net absorption of electrolytes and water and on motility. This group includes danthron, the docusates, castor oil, and bile acids. Despite similarity of their mechanism of action, there are differences among these drugs which are due, for the most part, to dosage and the major site of action, i.e. small intestine or colon.

Anthraquinone cathartics vary in their effects depending upon their anthraquinone content and the ease of liberation of the active constituents from their precursor glycosides. Danthron, although a free anthraquinone, is similar to the pro-drug glycosides in its pharmacological properties. A soft or semifluid stool is passed 6 to 8 hours after administration of an anthraquinone glycoside cathartic or danthron.

Hydration of the stool has been attributed to docusate sodium's surfactant effect on the intestinal contents which was assumed to facilitate penetration of the fecal mass by water and lipids. Although this emollient effect may exist, there is evidence that mucosal permeability is increased and water absorption is inhibited in the jejunum. Similar concentrations inhibit colonic absorption and/or increase intraluminal water and electrolytes. In these respects docusate sodium is similar to bile salts and in this manner may also be considered as a stimulant laxative.

Danthron is absorbed from the small intestine to a limited extent, circulated through the portal system and into the general circulation and excreted in the bile, urine, saliva, colonic mucosa and milk. Docusate sodium is absorbed to some extent in the duodenum and proximal jejunum. It appears in the bile.

Indications and Usage: MODANE PLUS is indicated for the management of constipation where a combination of a stimulant plus a stool softener is needed. It may be useful in geriatric or inactive patients, following surgery, and in patients refractory to other laxatives (see MODANE, MODANE SOFT and MODANE BULK). Adequate bulk should be provided in the diet and, if the diet does not provide sufficient bulk, by hydrophilic bulking agents (MODANE BULK). Poor bowel habits should be corrected.

Contraindications: Mineral oil administration, or when abdominal pain, nausea, vomiting or other signs and/or symptoms of appendicitis are present.

Precautions: *General*—It may cause harmless discoloration of urine (the urine may be pink-red, red-violet or red-brown if alkaline).

As with all laxatives, frequent or prolonged use may result in dependence.

Drug Interactions—Docusate sodium may increase the intestinal absorption and/or hepatic uptake of other drugs administered concurrently.

Carcinogenesis, Mutagenesis, Impairment of Fertility—There have been no long term studies of MODANE PLUS to evaluate carcinogenic potential. There have been no studies to evaluate mutagenic potential or to determine whether MODANE PLUS has the potential to impair fertility.

Teratogenic Effects—Pregnancy Category C. Animal reproduction studies have not been conducted with danthron and docusate sodium. It is also not known whether MODANE PLUS can cause fetal harm when administered to a pregnant woman or can affect reproductive capacity. MODANE PLUS should be given to a pregnant woman only if clearly needed.

Nursing Mothers—Danthron is excreted in human milk and has been reported to increase bowel activity in infants nursed by women taking it. Caution should be exercised when MODANE PLUS is administered to a nursing woman.

Pediatric Use—Because of its dosage size, MODANE PLUS is not recommended for use by children less than 12 years.

Adverse Reactions: Adverse reactions are uncommon. These are in order of frequency: Excessive bowel activity (griping, diarrhea, nausea, vomiting), peri-anal irritation, weakness, dizziness, palpitations and sweating. Temporary brownish mucosal staining has occurred with prolonged use. There have also been reports of rash and a report of facial swelling, redness and discomfort.

Overdosage: Docusates and danthron have low potential for toxicity. The oral LD_{50} values of danthron, docusate sodium and danthron— docusate sodium combination in mice were greater than 7 g/kg, 2.64 g/kg and 3.44 g/kg, respectively. The lowest reported lethal dose of danthron in mice and rats is 500 mg/kg. Single doses of docusate sodium, as large as 50 mg/kg, have not produced adverse effects in children. Overdosage may be expected to result in anorexia, vomiting and diarrhea. Treatment is symptomatic when the duration of effects is prolonged.

Dosage and Administration: Adults and children over 12 years of age—1 tablet daily with evening meal.

How Supplied Each MODANE PLUS tablet contains a combination of danthron 50 mg and docusate sodium 100 mg in a brown, round, sugar coated tablet coded 13 504.
NDC 0013-5041-13   30 Tablet Package
NDC 0013-5041-17   Bottle of 100 Tablets
Store at room temperature
AHFS 56:12

MYOFLEX® CREME
[mī'ō-flex]
(Trolamine Salicylate)

Description: Trolamine (formerly Triethanolamine) salicylate 10% in a nongreasy base is a nonirritating, nonburning, odorless, stainless, readily absorbed cream. Trolamine salicylate is a topical analgesic. The empirical formula of trolamine salicylate is $C_6H_{15}NO_3 \cdot C_7H_6O_3$, molecular weight 287.31. Its chemical structure is:

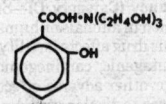

Continued on next page

Adria—Cont.

Trolamine salicylate is a light reddish viscous liquid with a faint odor. It is miscible in all proportions with water, glycerin, propylene glycol, and ethyl alcohol.

Clinical Pharmacology: Salicylic acid is the active moiety of MYOFLEX. Salicylic acid is enzymatically biotransformed to salicyluric acid and salicylphenolic glucuronide and eliminated in the urine. Salicylic acid is rapidly distributed throughout all body tissues, mainly by pH-dependent passive processes. It can be detected in synovial, spinal and peritoneal fluids, in saliva and in milk. It readily crosses the placental barrier. About 50% to 90% of salicylic acid is bound to plasma proteins, mainly to albumin.

The urinary excretion of salicylic acid equivalents was studied in 12 normal, healthy male subjects after MYOFLEX application. Salicylic acid was absorbed from MYOFLEX in 11 of 12 normal subjects over the 24-hour period post-application with a mean salicylic acid excretion of 13.5%.

Trolamine salicylate does not block neuronal membranes as do topical anesthetics. Some degree of percutaneous absorption occurs through the skin and blood levels have been demonstrated following topical application in animals and humans. Trolamine salicylate is not a counterirritant analgesic.

Indications: MYOFLEX is indicated as a topical analgesic for the temporary relief of minor aches and pains of muscles and joints due to muscle strains, sprains and bruises or overexertion. It is a useful topical adjunct in arthritis and rheumatism as a cream for patients with minor rheumatic stiffness or sore hands and feet.

Contraindications: MYOFLEX is contraindicated in patients sensitive to its ingredients and patients with advanced chronic renal insufficiency.

Warnings: For external use only. Avoid contact with eyes or mucous membranes. Keep out of the reach of children.

If condition worsens, or if symptoms persist for more than 7 days, or clear up and occur again within a few days, discontinue use and consult a doctor.

As with any drug, if you are pregnant or nursing a baby, seek the advice of a health professional before using this product.

As with all salicylates, MYOFLEX should be avoided or used with caution in patients with liver damage, pre-existing hypoprothrombinemia, vitamin K deficiency and before surgery.

Precautions: General—Apply to affected parts only. Do not apply to broken or irritated skin. Appropriate precautions should be taken by persons known to be sensitive to salicylates or with impairment of renal function. If a reaction develops, the drug should be discontinued.

Drug Interactions—There are no known drug interactions with MYOFLEX. However, salicylates may counteract the effects of uricosuric agents such as probenecid and enhance the effects of oral anticoagulants such as coumadin. Therefore, they must be used with caution in patients on anticoagulants that affect the prothrombin time. Caution should also be exercised in patients concurrently treated with a sulfonylurea hypoglycemic agent, methotrexate, barbiturates and diphenylhydantoin, because these drugs may be displaced from plasma protein binding sites by salicylate resulting in an enhanced effect. Diphenylhydantoin intoxication has been precipitated by concomitant use of aspirin. The diuretic action of spironolactone is inhibited by salicylates.

Usage in Pregnancy (Category C)—Studies have not been performed in animals or humans to determine whether this drug affects fertility in males or females, has mutagenic, carcinogenic or teratogenic potential or other adverse effects on the fetus. Aspirin causes testicular atrophy and inhibition of spermatogenesis in animals and has been shown to be teratogenic in animals and to increase the incidence of still births and neonatal deaths in pregnant women. As with other salicylates, MYOFLEX should be used during pregnancy only if the potential benefit justifies the potential risk to the fetus.

Chronic, high dose salicylate therapy of pregnant women increases the length of gestation and the frequency of post-maturity and prolongs spontaneous labor. It is, therefore, recommended that MYOFLEX be taken during the last three months of pregnancy only under the close supervision of a physician.

Nursing Mothers—Salicylates are excreted in the breast milk of nursing mothers. Caution should be therefore exercised when MYOFLEX is administered to a nursing woman.

Pediatric Use—Safety and effectiveness of MYOFLEX in children have not been established.

Adverse Reactions: If applied to large skin areas, the absorbed salicylate may cause typical salicylate side effects such as tinnitus, nausea, or vomiting.

Overdosage: Acute overdosage with MYOFLEX is unlikely. A 2 oz. MYOFLEX tube contains the salicylate equivalent of about 56 grains of aspirin. Early signs and symptoms from repeated large doses consist of headache, dizziness, tinnitus (which may be absent in children or the elderly), difficulty in hearing, dimness of vision, mental confusion, lassitude, drowsiness, sweating, thirst, hyperventilation, nausea, vomiting and occasionally diarrhea. Treatment of acute salicylate poisoning is a medical emergency and should be undertaken in a hospital.

Dosage and Administration: Adults—Rub into painful or sore area two or three times daily. Wrists, elbows, knees or ankles may be wrapped loosely with 2″ or 3″ elastic bandage after application.

How Supplied:
NDC 0013-5404-61 Tubes, 2 oz.
NDC 0013-5404-60 Tubes, 4 oz.
NDC 0013-5404-65 Jars, 8 oz.
NDC 0013-5404-74 Jars, 1 lb.
Store at controlled room temperature (15–30°C, 59–86°F) (jars).
Protect from freezing or excessive heat (tubes).

NEOSAR® FOR INJECTION ℞
[nē′ ō-sär]
(cyclophosphamide USP)

Description: NEOSAR® FOR INJECTION (cyclophosphamide USP) is supplied as a sterile powder, containing sufficient sodium chloride to produce an isotonic solution for parenteral use when reconstituted as directed with Sterile Water for Injection USP. NEOSAR is cyclophosphamide, a member of the nitrogen mustard class of antineoplastic drugs. It is a white crystalline powder which is soluble in water, physiological saline, or alcohol. Cyclophosphamide is 2-[Bis(2-chloroethyl)-amino] tetrahydro-2H-1,3,2-oxazaphosphorine 2-oxide monohydrate. The structural formula is:

$$\text{structural formula: } N(CH_2CH_2Cl)_2 \cdot H_2O$$

Clinical Pharmacology: Cyclophosphamide is first hydroxylated by hepatic mixed function oxidases to the intermediate metabolites 4-hydroxycyclophosphamide and aldophosphamide. These are enzymatically oxidized to several inactive metabolites and to the active antineoplastic alkylating compounds nor-nitrogen mustard and phosphoramide mustard. Acrolein is also formed. The mechanism of action of the active metabolites is alkylation, principally of DNA, which interferes with growth of susceptible neoplasms and to some extent, normal tissues. Acrolein has no antineoplastic activity but is considered responsible for irritation of the bladder mucosa. The $t\frac{1}{2}$ of cyclophosphamide ranges from 6 to 12 hours with a volume (Vc) of the central compartment of 0.2 to 0.6 L/kg. The $t\frac{1}{2}$ is shortened by barbiturate and previous cyclophosphamide administration. It is not known whether the rate of activation and metabolism of cyclophosphamide has any clinical significance. Cyclophosphamide or its metabolites do not readily cross the blood brain barrier. Cyclophosphamide is excreted in breast milk. It, or its active metabolites cross the placenta. Cyclophosphamide and its metabolites are excreted by the kidneys.

Indications: Cyclophosphamide, though effective alone in susceptible malignancies, is more frequently used concurrently or sequentially with other antineoplastic drugs. The following malignancies are often susceptible to cyclophosphamide treatment:

1. Malignant lymphomas (Stages III and IV, Ann Arbor Staging System).
   a. Hodgkin's disease
   b. Lymphoma (nodular or diffuse)
   c. Mixed-cell type lymphoma
   d. Histiocytic lymphoma
   e. Burkitt's lymphoma.
2. Multiple myeloma.
3. Leukemias:
   a. Chronic lymphocytic leukemia.
   b. Chronic granulocytic leukemia (it is ineffective in acute blastic crises).
   c. Acute myelogenous and monocytic leukemia.
   d. Acute lymphoblastic (stem-cell) leukemia in children (cyclophosphamide given during remission is effective in prolonging its duration).
4. Mycosis fungoides (advanced disease).
5. Neuroblastoma.
6. Adenocarcinoma of the ovary.
7. Retinoblastoma.
8. Carcinoma of the breast.

Contraindications: None known.

Warnings: Since cyclophosphamide has been reported to be more toxic in adrenalectomized dogs, adjustment of the doses of both replacement steroids and cyclophosphamide may be necessary for the adrenalectomized patient.

The rate of metabolism and the leukopenic activity of cyclophosphamide reportedly are increased by chronic administration of high doses of phenobarbital. The physician should be alert for possible combined drug actions, desirable or undesirable, involving cyclophosphamide even though cyclophosphamide has been used successfully concurrently with other drugs, including other cytotoxic drugs.

Cyclophosphamide may interfere with normal wound healing.

Precautions: Cyclophosphamide should be given cautiously to patients with any of the following conditions:
1. Leukopenia
2. Thrombocytopenia
3. Tumor cell infiltration of bone marrow
4. Previous X-ray therapy
5. Previous therapy with other cytotoxic agents
6. Impaired hepatic function
7. Impaired renal function

Because cyclophosphamide may exert a suppressive action on immune mechanisms, interruption or modification of dosage should be considered for patients who develop bacterial, fungal or viral infections. This is especially true for patients receiving concomitant steroid therapy and perhaps those with a recent history of steroid therapy, since infections in some of these patients have been fatal. Varicella zoster infections appear to be particularly dangerous under these circumstances.

Patients should be instructed to increase their fluid intake for 24 hours before, during, and for at least 24 hours after receiving cyclophosphamide. They should also be instructed to void frequently for 24 hours after receiving cyclophosphamide. Patients should be informed of the possibility of hair loss.

A white blood cell count should be obtained regularly while treating patients with cyclophosphamide.

Secondary Neoplasia: Secondary malignancies have developed in some patients treated with cyclophosphamide alone or in association with other antineoplastic drugs and/or modalities. These malignancies most frequently have been urinary bladder, myeloproliferative, and lymphoproliferative malignancies. Secondary malignancies most frequently have developed in the cyclophosphamide-treated patients with primary myeloproliferative and lymphoproliferative malignancies and primary non-malignant diseases in which immune processes are believed to be involved pathologically. In some cases, the secondary malignancy was detected up to several years after cyclophosphamide treatment was discontinued. The secondary urinary bladder malignancies generally have occurred in patients who previously developed hemorrhagic cystitis (see Genitourinary under Adverse Reactions). Although no cause-effect relationship has been established between cyclophosphamide and the development of malignancy in humans, the possibility of secondary malignancy, based on available data, should be considered in any benefit-to-risk assessment for the use of the drug.

Pregnancy Category C. Cyclophosphamide has been shown to be teratogenic and embryotoxic in mice, rats, rabbits, and monkeys when given respectively, in doses 0.02, 0.08, 0.5 and 0.07 times the human dose.

There are no adequate and well-controlled studies in pregnant women. Cyclophosphamide should not be used in pregnancy, particularly in early pregnancy, unless in the judgment of the physician the potential benefits outweigh the possible risks. Cyclophosphamide is excreted in breast milk and breast feeding should be terminated prior to institution of cyclophosphamide therapy.

Patients, male or female, capable of conception ordinarily should be advised of the mutagenic potential of cyclophosphamide. Adequate methods of contraception appear desirable for such patients receiving cyclophosphamide.

Adverse Reactions:
Hematopoietic: Leukopenia is an expected effect and ordinarily is used as a guide to therapy. Thrombocytopenia or anemia may occur in a few patients. These effects are almost always reversible when therapy is interrupted.
Gastrointestinal: Anorexia, nausea, or vomiting are common and related to dose as well as individual susceptibility. There are isolated reports of hemorrhagic colitis, oral mucosal ulceration and jaundice occurring during therapy.
Genitourinary: Sterile hemorrhagic cystitis can result from the administration of cyclophosphamide. THIS CAN BE SEVERE, EVEN FATAL, and is probably due to metabolites in the urine. Nonhemorrhagic cystitis and/or fibrosis of the bladder also have been reported to result from cyclophosphamide administration. Atypical epithelial cells may be found in the urinary sediment. **Ample fluid intake and frequent voiding help to prevent the development of cystitis,** but when it occurs it is ordinarily necessary to interrupt cyclophosphamide therapy. Hematuria usually resolves spontaneously within a few days after cyclophosphamide therapy is discontinued, but may persist for several months. In severe cases replacement of blood loss may be required. The application of electrocautery to telangiectatic areas of the bladder and diversion of urine flow have been successful methods used in treatment of protracted cases. Cryosurgery has also been used. (See also Secondary Neoplasia under Precautions.) Nephrotoxicity, including hemorrhage and clot formation in the renal pelvis, have been reported.
Gonadal suppression, resulting in amenorrhea or azoospermia, has been reported in a number of patients treated with cyclophosphamide and appears to be related to dosage and duration of therapy. This side effect, possibly irreversible, should be anticipated in patients treated with cyclophosphamide. It is not known to what extent cyclophosphamide may affect prepuberal gonads. Fibrosis of the ovary following cyclophosphamide therapy has been reported also.
Integument: It is ordinarily advisable to inform patients in advance of possible alopecia, a frequent complication of cyclophosphamide therapy. Regrowth of hair can be expected although occasionally the new hair may be of a different color or texture. The skin and fingernails may become darker during therapy. Non-specific dermatitis has been reported to occur with cyclophosphamide.
Pulmonary: Interstitial pulmonary fibrosis has been reported in patients receiving high doses of cyclophosphamide over a prolonged period.

Overdosage: No reports of cyclophosphamide overdosage have been published and no reports of overdosage from NEOSAR have been received. It is expected that acute overdosage of cyclophosphamide will cause severe leukopenia and thrombocytopenia. Cardiac damage, manifested by heart failure has been reported to occur within 15 days of the initial dose of 4 to 10 day courses of cyclophosphamide at total doses per course greater than 140 mg/kg (5.2 g/m^2). Impairment of water excretion with hyponatremia, weight gain and inappropriately concentrated urine has been reported after cyclophosphamide doses greater than 50 mg/kg (2 g/m^2). Patients in whom overdosage is known or suspected should be hospitalized for supportive therapy. No specific antidote is known. Cyclophosphamide is theoretically dialyzable but no studies have been performed to confirm the efficacy of dialysis in a clinical situation.

Dosage and Administration: Chemotherapy with NEOSAR, as with other drugs used in cancer chemotherapy, is potentially hazardous and fatal complications can occur. It is recommended that it be administered only by physicians aware of the associated risks. Therapy may be aimed at either induction or maintenance of remission.
Induction Therapy: The usual initial intravenous loading dose for patients with no hematologic deficiency is 40–50 mg/kg (1500–1800 mg/m^2). This total initial intravenous loading dose usually is given in divided doses over a period of two to five days.
Patients with any previous treatment that may have compromised the functional capacity of the bone marrow, such as X-ray or cytotoxic drugs, and patients with tumor infiltration of the bone marrow may require reduction of the initial loading dose by $\frac{1}{3}$ to $\frac{1}{2}$.
A marked leukopenia is usually associated with the above doses, but recovery usually begins after 7–10 days. The white blood cell count should be monitored closely during induction therapy.
Maintenance Therapy: It is frequently necessary to maintain chemotherapy in order to suppress or retard neoplastic growth. A variety of schedules has been used:
1. 10–15 mg/kg (350–550 mg/m^2) i.v. every 7–10 days
2. 3–5 mg/kg (110–185 mg/m^2) i.v. twice weekly

Unless the disease is unusually sensitive to NEOSAR, it is advisable to give the largest maintenance dose that can be reasonably tolerated by the patient. The total leukocyte count is a good objective guide for regulating the maintenance dose. Ordinarily a leukopenia of 3000–4000 cells/mm^3 can be maintained without undue risk of serious infection or other complications.
Preparation and Handling of Solutions: NEOSAR should be prepared for parenteral use by adding **Sterile Water for Injection USP or Bacteriostatic Water for Injection USP (paraben preserved only)** to the vial and shaking to dissolve. Use 5 ml for the 100 mg vial, 10 ml for the 200 mg vial, 25 ml for the 500 mg vial, or 50 ml for the 1 g vial. Solutions of NEOSAR may be injected intravenously, intramuscularly, intraperitoneally or intrapleurally or they may be infused intravenously in Dextrose Injection USP (5% dextrose) or Dextrose and Sodium Chloride Injection USP (5% dextrose and 0.9% sodium chloride). These solutions should be used within 24 hours if stored at room temperature or within 6 days if stored under refrigeration (2–8°C; 36–46°F). NEOSAR does not contain an antimicrobial agent and **care must be taken to insure the sterility of prepared solutions.**
Parenteral drug products should be inspected visually for particulate matter and discoloration prior to administration whenever solution and container permit.

How Supplied: NEOSAR FOR INJECTION (cyclophosphamide USP) is available as follows:

NDC 0013-5606-93 100 mg vials, cartons of 12
NDC 0013-5616-93 200 mg vials, cartons of 12
NDC 0013-5626-93 500 mg vials, cartons of 12
NDC 0013-5636-93 1 g vial, individual carton

Store at a temperature not exceeding 86°F (30°C) and preferably below 77°F (25°C).
References on selected topics and a physician's brochure are available by writing to: Medical Oncology Section, Adria Laboratories, P.O. Box 16529, Columbus, OH 43216.
Manufactured by:
ASTA-WERKE A.G.
BIELEFELD, GERMANY
for:
ADRIA LABORATORIES INC.
COLUMBUS, OHIO 43215

TYMPAGESIC® ℞
[*tim″pah-jē′sik*]
Otic Solution

Analgesic-Decongestant Ear Drops

Description: TYMPAGESIC Otic Solution, analgesic-decongestant ear drops, contains phenylephrine hydrochloride USP 0.25%, antipyrine USP 5% and benzocaine USP 5% v/v in propylene glycol USP.

Phenylephrine hydrochloride is a sympathomimetic amine with local vasoconstriction or decongestant action. It is chemically (R)-3-hydroxy-α-[(methylamino)methyl] benzenemethanol hydrochloride and has the following structure:

It occurs as white crystals, has bitter taste and is freely soluble in water and alcohol. Its molecular weight is 203.67.

Antipyrine is an analgesic with local anesthetic action. It is chemically 2:3-dimethyl-1-phenyl-3-pyrazolin-5-one and has the following structure:

Antipyrine occurs as colorless crystals or white powder, has a slightly bitter taste and is soluble in water and alcohol. Its molecular weight is 188.23.
Benzocaine is a local anesthetic. It is chemically ethyl p-aminobenzoate and has the following structure:

It occurs as white crystals or white crystalline powder and is slightly soluble in water and soluble in organic solvents. Its molecular weight is 165.19.

Clinical Pharmacology: Topical application of phenylephrine produces vasoconstriction mainly by a direct effect on α-adrenergic receptors. The effects of phenylephrine are similar to those of epinephrine. However, phenylephrine is considered less CNS and cardiostimulatory than epinephrine. Phenylephrine, after its absorption, is metabolized in the liver and the intestine by the enzyme monoamine oxidase (MAO). The type, route and rate of excretion of metabolites have not been defined.

Like other local anesthetics, benzocaine acts by blocking nerve conduction first in autonomic, then in sensory and finally in motor nerve fibers. Its

Continued on next page

Adria—Cont.

effect appears to be due to decreased nerve cell membrane permeability to sodium ions or competition with calcium ions for membrane binding sites. A vasoconstrictor, such as phenylephrine, is added to decrease the rate of absorption and prolong the duration of action of the anesthetic. Ester-type anesthetics, which include benzocaine, after absorption are comparatively rapidly degraded by esterases mainly in the liver and excreted in the urine as metabolites and in small amounts as the unchanged drug.

Antipyrine is believed to have analgesic and local anesthetic effects on the nerve endings. After absorption, it is slowly metabolized in the liver by oxidation and conjugation with glucuronic acid and is excreted in the urine mainly in the conjugated form.

Indications and Usage: TYMPAGESIC Otic Solution may be used as a topical anesthetic in the external auditory canal to relieve ear pain.

It may be used concomitantly with systemic antibiotics as in the treatment of acute otitis media.

Contraindications: TYMPAGESIC is contraindicated in the presence of a perforated tympanic membrane or ear discharge and in individuals with a history of hypersensitivity to any of its ingredients.

Warnings: As with all drugs containing a sympathomimetic or an anesthetic, systemic reactions may occur after local application. Phenylephrine may cause blanching and a feeling of coolness in the skin. Allergic and idiosyncratic reactions to local anesthetics have been observed infrequently. Such reactions are unlikely because absorption from the skin of the ear drum or the external ear canal is minimal.

Cross-sensitivity reactions between members of the *caine* group of local anesthetics have been reported.

Precautions:

General—Drugs containing a sympathomimetic should be used with caution in the elderly and in patients with hypertension, increased intraocular pressure, diabetes mellitus, ischemic heart disease, hyperthyroidism and prostatic hypertrophy. High plasma levels of benzocaine and antipyrine may cause CNS stimulation with nausea and vomiting. Such levels, however, are unlikely to be attained following local application in the external ear.

Drug Interactions—MAO inhibitors and β-adrenergic blockers enhance the effects of sympathomimetics. Benzocaine is hydrolyzed in the body to p-aminobenzoic acid which competes with the antibacterial action of sulfonamides. However, these are unlikely to occur because of limited absorption from the external ear canal.

Carcinogenesis, Mutagenesis, Impairment of Fertility—There have been no studies in animals or humans to evaluate the carcinogenesis, mutagenesis or impairment of fertility for Tympagesic.

Pregancy—Category C. Animal reproduction studies have not been conducted with TYMPAGESIC. It is also not known whether TYMPAGESIC can cause fetal harm when administered to a pregnant woman or can effect reproduction capacity. Tympagesic should be given to a pregnant woman only if clearly needed.

Nursing Mothers—It is not known whether this drug is excreted in human milk. Because many drugs are excreted in human milk, caution should be exercised when TYMPAGESIC is administered to a nursing woman.

Pediatric Use—Safety and effectiveness in children below the age of 12 has not been established.

Adverse Reactions: Following its absorption, phenylephrine may produce a pressor response or cause restlessness, anxiety, nervousness, weakness, pallor, headache and dizziness. Absorption of benzocaine and antipyrine in the plasma may cause chills, nausea, vomiting, tinnitus and agranulocytosis. Such reactions are unlikely following application of TYMPAGESIC on the external ear canal.

Benzocaine can cause a hypersensitivity reaction consisting of rash, urticaria and edema. Individuals frequently exposed to ester-type local anesthetics can develop contact dermatitis characterized by erythema and pruritus which may progress to vesiculation and oozing.

Overdosage: It is more likely to be associated with accidental or deliberate ingestion rather than cutaneous absorption. Phenylephrine present in a bottle (13 ml) of TYMPAGESIC, if absorbed, may cause hypertension, headache, vomiting and palpitations. Effects of benzocaine overdosage may include yawning, restlessness, excitement, nausea and vomiting. Antipyrine overdosage may cause giddiness, tremor, sweating and skin eruptions. Treatment is symptomatic. If ingestion of the contents of a bottle or more of TYMPAGESIC is recent or food is present in the stomach, induction of emesis with ipecac syrup, gastric emptying and lavage and introduction of activated charcoal may be recommended.

Dosage and Administration: Using the dropper, instill TYMPAGESIC Otic Solution in the external ear canal allowing the solution to run into the canal until filled. Insert a cotton pledget into the meatus after moistening with the otic solution. Repeat every 2 to 4 hours, if necessary, until pain is relieved.

Replace dropper in bottle without rinsing.

How Supplied: TYMPAGESIC Otic Solution is supplied in 13 ml amber glass dropper bottles (NDC 0013-7363-39).

Store at 15–30°C (59–86°F).

Alcon Laboratories, Inc.
and its affiliates
CORPORATE HEADQUARTERS:
PO BOX 1959
6201 SOUTH FREEWAY
FORT WORTH, TX 76134

OPHTHALMIC PRODUCTS

For information on Alcon ophthalmic products, consult the PDR for Ophthalmology. See a complete listing of products in the Manufacturer's Index Section of this book. For information, literature, samples or service items contact Alcon Sales Services.

Alcon (Puerto Rico) Inc.
P.O. BOX 3000
HUMACAO, PUERTO RICO 00661

AVITENE®
[ăv'itēne]
(Microfibrillar Collagen Hemostat)

Description: Avitene® (Microfibrillar Collagen Hemostat, or MCH), is an absorbable topical hemostatic agent prepared as a dry, sterile, fibrous, water insoluble partial hydrochloric acid salt of purified bovine corium collagen. It is prepared in a loose fibrous form and in a compacted "non-woven" web form. In its manufacture, swelling of the native collagen fibrils is controlled by ethyl alcohol to permit non-covalent attachment of hydrochloric acid to amine groups on the collagen molecule and preservation of the essential morphology of native collagen molecules. Dry heat sterilization causes some cross-linking which is evidenced by reduction of hydrating properties, and a decrease of molecular weight which implies some degradation of collagen molecules. However, the characteristics of collagen which are essential to its effect on the blood coagulation mechanisms are preserved.

Actions: Avitene (MCH), in contact with a bleeding surface, attracts platelets which adhere to the fibrils and undergo the release phenomenon to trigger aggregation of platelets into thrombi in the interstices of the fibrous mass. The effect on platelet adhesion and aggregation is not inhibited by heparin *in vitro*. It has been found effective in heparinized dogs and in eight of nine fully heparinized human subjects. Platelets of patients with clinical thrombasthenia do not adhere to MCH *in vitro*. However, in clinical trials it was effective in 50 of 68 patients receiving aspirin. MCH cannot control bleeding due to systemic coagulation disorders. Appropriate therapy to correct the underlying coagulopathy should be instituted prior to use of the product. MCH is tenaciously adherent to surfaces wet with blood but excess material not involved in the hemostatic clot may be removed by teasing or irrigation, usually without causing rebleeding. In animal and human studies, it has been shown to stimulate a mild, chronic cellular inflammatory response. When implanted in animal tissues, it is absorbed in less than 84 days. In human studies of hemostasis in osteotomy cuts, it has been shown not to interfere with bone regeneration or healing. In animal studies, it has been demonstrated that MCH does not predispose to stenosis at vascular anastomotic sites. These findings have not been confirmed in human use. Studies have been performed using MCH (fibrous form) in experimental wounds contaminated with hemolytic *Staphylococcus aureus*. The presence of MCH does not enhance or initiate staphylococcus wound infections to a greater or lesser extent than control agents employed for the same purpose. The effects of MCH (fibrous form) on experimental wounds contaminated with a gram-negative aerobic rod and an anaerobic non-spore forming bacteria are currently under investigation.

Indications: Avitene (MCH) is used in surgical procedures as an adjunct to hemostasis when control of bleeding by ligature or conventional procedures is ineffective or impractical.

Contraindications: Avitene (MCH) should not be used in the closure of skin incisions as it may interfere with the healing of the skin edges. This is due to simple mechanical interposition of dry collagen and not to any intrinsic interference with wound healing. By filling porosities of cancellous bone, MCH may significantly reduce the bond strength of methylmethacrylate adhesives. MCH should not, therefore, be employed on bone surfaces to which prosthetic materials are to be attached with methylmethacrylate adhesives.

Warnings: Avitene (MCH) is inactivated by autoclaving. Ethylene oxide reacts with bound hydrochloric acid to form ethylene chlorohydrin. This product should not be resterilized. It is not for injection. Moistening MCH or wetting with saline or thrombin impairs its hemostatic efficacy. It should be used dry. Discard any unused portion. As with any foreign substance, use in contaminated wounds may enhance infection.

Precautions: Only that amount of Avitene (MCH) necessary to produce hemostasis should be used. After several minutes, excess material should be removed; this is usually possible without the re-initiation of active bleeding. Failure to remove excess MCH may result in bowel adhesion or mechanical pressure sufficient to compromise the ureter. In otolaryngological surgery, precautions against aspiration should include removal of all excess dry material and thorough irrigation of the pharynx. MCH contains a low, but detectable, level of intercalated bovine serum protein which reacts immunologically as does beef serum albumin. Increases in anti-BSA titer have been observed following treatment with MCH. About two-thirds of individuals exhibit antibody titers because of ingestion of food products of bovine origin. Intradermal skin tests have occasionally shown a weak positive reaction to BSA or MCH but these have not been correlated with IgG titers to BSA. Tests have failed to demonstrate clinically significant elicitation of antibodies of the IgE class against BSA following MCH therapy. Care should be exercised to avoid spillage on nonbleeding surfaces, particularly in abdominal or thoracic viscera. Teratology studies in rats and rabbits have revealed no harm to the animal fetus. There are no well-controlled studies in pregnant women; therefore, MCH should be used in pregnant women only when clearly needed.

Adverse Reactions: The most serious adverse reactions reported which may be related to the use of Avitene (MCH) are potentiation of infection including abscess formation, hematoma, wound dehiscence and mediastinitis. Other reported adverse reactions possibly related are adhesion formation, allergic reaction, foreign body reaction and subgaleal seroma (report of a single case). The use of MCH in dental extraction sockets has been reported to increase the incidence of alveolalgia. Transient laryngospasm due to aspiration of dry material has been reported following use of MCH in tonsillectomy.

Dosage and Administration: Avitene (MCH) must be applied directly to the source of bleeding. Because of its adhesiveness, it may seal over the exit site of deeper hemorrhage and conceal an underlying hematoma as in penetrating liver wounds. Surfaces to be treated should be compressed with dry sponges immediately prior to application of the dry MCH. It is then necessary to apply pressure over the MCH with a dry sponge for a period of time which varies with the force and severity of bleeding. A minute may suffice for capillary bleeding (e.g., skin graft donor sites, dermatologic curettage) but three to five or more minutes may be required for brisk bleeding (e.g., splenic tears) or high pressure leaks in major artery suture holes. For control of oozing from cancellous bone, it should be firmly packed into the spongy bone surface. After five to ten minutes, excess MCH should be teased away (see **Precautions**); this can usually be accomplished with blunt forceps and is facilitated by wetting with sterile 0.9% saline solution and irrigation. If breakthrough bleeding occurs in areas of thin application, additional MCH may be applied. The amount required depends, again, on the severity of bleeding. In capillary bleeding, one gram will usually be sufficient for a 50 cm^2 area. Thicker coverage will be required for more brisk bleeding. MCH will adhere to wet gloves, instruments, or tissue surfaces. To facilitate handling, dry smooth forceps should be used. Gloved fingers should not be used to apply pressure. In neurosurgical and other procedures the non-woven web may conveniently be used by applying small squares to bleeding areas and then covering the sites with moist cottonoid "patties". To prevent wetting of the MCH, and to apply needed pressure, a suction tip should be held against the cottonoid for one to several minutes, depending on the briskness of bleeding. After five to ten minutes excess MCH may be removed by teasing and irrigation.

How Supplied: Fibrous Form; in 1 g and 5 g sterile jars of sterile microfibrillar collagen hemostat all contained in a sealed can. Sterility of the jar exterior cannot be guaranteed if can seal is broken. Content of jar is sterile until opened. Non-woven Web form; as 70 mm × 70 mm × 1 mm (2.75" × 2.75" × .04") and 70 mm × 35 mm × 1 mm (2.75" × 1.4" × .04") sheets, each contained in a sterile blister pack within a foil pouch. Sterility of the blister pack cannot be guaranteed after the pouch is opened. Content of the blister pack is sterile until adhesive backing is removed.

"Avitene" is a registered trademark of Alcon (Puerto Rico) Inc.

Important Notice
Before prescribing or administering any product described in PHYSICIANS' DESK REFERENCE always consult the PDR Supplement for possible new or revised information

---

Allergan Pharmaceuticals, Inc.
2525 DUPONT DRIVE
IRVINE, CA 92715

OPHTHALMIC PRODUCTS

For information on Allergan prescription and OTC ophthalmic products, consult the Physicians' Desk Reference For Ophthalmology. For literature, service items or sample material, contact Allergan directly. See a complete listing of products in the Manufacturers' Index section of this book.

Alpha Therapeutic Corporation
5555 VALLEY BOULEVARD
LOS ANGELES, CA 90032

ALBUTEIN® 5% ℞
Normal Serum Albumin (Human), USP, 5% Solution

How Supplied: A 5% solution in 250 ml and 500 ml bottles. For use with intravenous administration set.

ALBUTEIN® 25% ℞
Normal Serum Albumin (Human), USP, 25% Solution

How Supplied: A 25% solution in 20 ml, 50 ml, and 100 ml vials. For use with intravenous administration set.

PLASMATEIN® 5% ℞
Plasma Protein Fraction (Human), USP, 5% Solution

How Supplied: A 5% solution in 250 ml and 500 ml bottles. For use with intravenous administration set.

PROFILATE® dried ℞
Antihemophilic Factor (Human), Factor VIII, AHF

How Supplied: In single dose 10 ml and 25 ml size (AHF activity is stated on label of each vial) with sterile diluent and micron filter spike for withdrawal.

PROFILATE® HEAT-TREATED dried ℞
Antihemophilic Factor (Human), factor VIII, AHF, heat-treated

How Supplied: In single dose 10 ml and 25 ml size (AHF activity is stated on label of each vial) with sterile diluent and micron filter spike for withdrawal.

PROFILNINE® HEAT-TREATED dried ℞
Factor IX Complex (Human)

How Supplied: In single dose 10 ml and 25 ml size (Factor IX activity is stated on label of each vial) with sterile diluent and micron filter spike for withdrawal.

IDENTIFICATION PROBLEM?
Consult PDR's
Product Identification Section
where you'll find over 1200 products pictured actual size and in full color.

Alto Pharmaceuticals, Inc.
PO BOX 271369
TAMPA, FL 33688

EFED II™ CAPSULES (Black)
[e'fed]

Description: Each Efed II Black capsule contains: Theionized® caffeine 200 mg.
Indications: Efed II capsules are safe, effective, and non-habit forming. Efed II fast acting ingredient give immediate relief from fatigue, drowsiness and stuffiness. Use as a stimulant to aid in mental alertness.
Warnings: Keep this and all medications out of the reach of small children. Do not exceed recommended dosage. Reduce dosage if nervousness, or restlessness, or sleeplessness occurs. As with any drug, if you are pregnant or nursing a baby, seek the advice of a health professional before using this product.
Caution: If under medical care do not take without consulting a pharmacist or physician. Do not take as a substitute for normal sleep. May interfere with sleep if taken within four (4) hours of bedtime.
Adult Dosage: One capsule every four hours, not to exceed four (4) capsules in a 24 hour period. Not recommended for children under 12 years of age.
How Supplied: Packages of 24 capsules and bottles of 100.
Shown in Product Identification Section, page 404

EFED II™ CAPSULES (Yellow)
[e'fed]

Active Ingredient: Each Efed II Yellow capsule contains Theionized ephedrine sulfate 25 mg.
Indications: Efed II fast acting ingredient give immediate relief from stuffiness. Use for the symptomatic relief of nasal and sinus congestion, allergic conditions such as hay fever and bronchial asthma.
Caution: If under medical care do not take without consulting a physician or pharmacist. Individuals with high blood pressure, heart disease, diabetes or thyroid disease should use only as directed by a physician.
Warning: Do not exceed recommended dosage. Reduce dosage if nervousness or restlessness or sleeplessness occurs. Because of the ephedrine component, this medicine should be used with caution by elderly males or those with prostatic hypertrophy. This product should not be used by pregnant or lactating women.
Adult Dosage: One capsule every four hours, not to exceed 4 capsules in a 24 hour period. Not recommended for children under 12 years of age.
How Supplied: Package of 24 capsules and bottles of 100.
Shown in Product Identification Section, page 404

ZINC-220® CAPSULES
[zĭnk]
(zinc sulfate 220 mg.)

Composition: Each opaque blue and pink capsule contains zinc sulfate 220 mg. delivering 55 mg. of elemental zinc. Zinc-220 Capsules do not contain dextrose or glucose.
Action and Uses: Zinc-220 Capsules are indicated as a dietary supplement. Normal growth and tissue repair are directly dependent upon an adequate supply of zinc in the diet. Zinc functions as an integral part of a number of enzymes important to protein and carbohydrate metabolism. Zinc-220 Capsules are recommended for deficiencies or the prevention of deficiencies of zinc.
Warnings: Zinc-220 if administered in stat dosages of 2 grams (9 capsules) will cause an emetic effect. This product should not be used by pregnant or lactating women.
Precaution: It is recommended that Zinc-220 Capsules be taken with meals or milk to avoid gastric distress.

Continued on next page

Alto—Cont.

Dosage: One capsule daily with milk or meals. One capsule daily provides approximately 5.3 times the recommended adult requirement for zinc.

How Supplied: Bottles of 100 and 1000 capsules and Unit Dose Strips boxes of 100 capsules. (NDC 0731-0401)

Shown in Product Identification Section, page 404

Alza Corporation
950 PAGE MILL ROAD
P.O. BOX 10950
PALO ALTO, CA 94303-0802

PROGESTASERT® ℞
[prō-jes-ta-sert]
Intrauterine Progesterone Contraceptive System
Release rated 65 μg/day progesterone for one year

Description: The PROGESTASERT® Intrauterine Progesterone Contraceptive System is a white, T-shaped unit constructed of ethylene/vinyl acetate copolymer (EVA) containing titanium dioxide. The 36-mm tubular vertical stem of the T contains a reservoir of 38 mg of progesterone, USP, together with barium sulfate, USP, for radiopacity; both are dispersed in medical grade silicone fluid. The 32-mm horizontal crossarms are solid EVA. Two monofilament nylon indicator/retrieval threads are fastened to the base of the T stem.

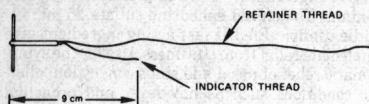

One tip of the shorter indicator thread is 9 cm from the top or leading end of the system and is used to ascertain correct placement at insertion. The long thread extends the length of the inserter where it is anchored by a plug and retains the system in the inserter. This thread is cut to length after insertion.

The PROGESTASERT® system is packaged sterile within its curved, malleable inserter. Progesterone is released from the system at an average rate of 65 μg/day for one year by membrane-controlled diffusion from the reservoir. None of the inert ingredients of the reservoir or membrane—barium sulfate, silicone fluid, titanium dioxide, or EVA—is released from the system.

Action: Available data indicate that the contraceptive effectiveness of the PROGESTASERT® system is enhanced by its continuous release of progesterone at an average rate of 65 μg/day for one year into the uterine cavity. The mechanism by which progesterone enhances the contraceptive effectiveness of the T is local, not systemic. The concentrations of luteinizing hormone, estradiol, and progesterone in systemic venous plasma follow regular cyclic patterns indicative of ovulation during use of the PROGESTASERT® system. Blood chemistry studies related to liver, kidney, and thyroid function also reveal no changes.

During use of the system the endometrium shows progestational influence. Progesterone from the system suppresses proliferation of the endometrial tissue (an anti-estrogenic effect). Following removal of the system, the endometrium rapidly returns to its normal cyclic pattern and can support pregnancy. The local mechanism by which continuously released progesterone enhances the contraceptive effectiveness of the T has not been conclusively demonstrated. The hypotheses that have been offered are: progesteone-induced inhibition of sperm capacitation or survival; and alteration of the uterine milieu so as to prevent nidation.

Indications and Usage: The PROGESTASERT® system is indicated for contraception in parous and nulliparous women.

Contraindications: The PROGESTASERT® system should not be inserted when the following conditions exist:
1. Pregnancy or suspicion of pregnancy.
2. Previous ectopic pregnancy.
3. Presence of, or a history of one or more episodes of, pelvic inflammatory disease.
4. Presence of, or a history of one or more episodes of, venereal disease, including gonorrhea, syphilis, or chlamydial infection of the genital tract.
5. Previous pelvic surgery.
6. Presence of, or a history of one or more episodes of, postpartum endometritis or infected abortion.
7. Abnormalities of the uterus which have resulted in distortion of the uterine cavity.
8. Known or suspected uterine or cervical malignancy including, but not limited to, an unresolved, abnormal "Pap" smear.
9. Genital bleeding of unknown etiology.
10. Acute cervicitis, unless and until infection has been completely controlled and has been shown to be nongonococcal.

Warnings:
1. Pregnancy
   a. *Long term effects.* Long term effects on the offspring when pregnancy occurs with the PROGESTASERT® system in place are unknown.
   b. *Septic Abortion.* Reports have indicated an increased incidence of septic abortion associated in some instances with septicemia, septic shock and death in patients becoming pregnant with an intrauterine device (IUD) in place. Most of these reports have been associated with the mid-trimester of pregnancy. In some cases, the initial symptoms have been insidious and not easily recognized. If pregnancy should occur with a PROGESTASERT® system *in situ*, it should be removed if the thread is visible or, if removal proves to be or would be difficult, termination of the pregnancy should be considered and offered the patient as an option, bearing in mind that the risks associated with an elective abortion increase with gestational age.
   c. *Continuation of pregnancy.* If the patient chooses to continue the pregnancy, she must be warned of the increased risk of spontaneous abortion and of the increased risk of sepsis, including death if the pregnancy continues with the system in place. The patient must be closely observed and she must be advised to report all abnormal symptoms, such as flu-like syndrome, fever, abdominal cramping and pain, bleeding, or vaginal discharge immediately because generalized symptoms of septicemia may be insidious.
2. Ectopic Pregnancy
   a. A pregnancy that occurs while a patient is wearing an IUD is much more likely to be ectopic than a pregnancy occurring without an IUD in place. Accordingly, patients in whom pregnancy occurs while wearing the system should be carefully evaluated for the possibility of an ectopic pregnancy.
   b. Special attention should be directed toward determining whether ectopic pregnancy has occurred in patients with delayed menses, slight metrorrhagia and/or unilateral pelvic pain, especially when associated with a falling or low hematocrit, and in patients who wish to terminate an unplanned pregnancy.
   c. Women who have previously had acute salpingitis (pelvic inflammatory disease) subsequently have an 8- to 10-fold greater than normal risk of ectopic pregnancy. Data provided to the FDA indicate an estimated incidence of ectopic pregnancy in women previously having had salpingitis of 2.7 per 100 woman years, compared with an estimated risk in normal women of 0.1 to 0.3 per 100 woman years. Since IUD use has little or no effect in preventing ectopic pregnancy, patients considering IUD use should be carefully evaluated for evidence of previous pelvic inflammatory disease. Previous pelvic surgery that has involved the reproductive tract, endometritis, and retrograde menstruation have also been recognized as risk factors for ectopic pregnancy, but the increased degree of risk with respect to each of these factors has not yet been quantified.
   d. There are no comparable clinical trial data on the incidence of ectopic pregnancy during use of unmedicated, copper, and progesterone IUDs. Data gathered from separate studies and presented to the FDA, however, indicated that the incidence of ectopic pregnancy was greater in the studies with the PROGESTASERT® system than in studies with other IUDs. These data on uterine and extrauterine pregnancies for the PROGESTASERT® system, unmedicated IUDs, and copper IUDs, given as rates per 100 woman years, are listed below.

[See table below].

Factors responsible for the differences in extrauterine pregnancies could include the increased incidence of salpingitis, the selection of patients, the criteria for diagnosing ectopic pregnancies, or other yet unexplained factors.

3. Pelvic infection. An increased risk of pelvic inflammatory disease associated with the use of IUDs has been reported. This risk is greatest for young women who are nulliparous and/or who have a multiplicity of sexual partners. Salpingitis can result in tubal damage and occlusion, thereby threatening future fertility, and/or can predispose to ectopic pregnancy as described above. It is recommended that patients be taught to recognize the symptoms of pelvic inflammatory disease and ectopic pregnancy. The decision to use an IUD in a particular case must be made by the physician and patient with the consideration of a possible deleterious effect on future fertility.

Pelvic infection may occur with PROGESTASERT® system *in situ*, and at times result in the development of tubo-ovarian abscesses or general peritonitis. The symptoms of pelvic infection include new development of menstrual disorders (prolonged or heavy bleeding), abnormal vaginal discharge, abdominal or pelvic pain or tenderness, dyspareunia, fever. The symptoms are especially significant if they occur following the first two or three cycles after insertion. Appropriate aerobic and anaerobic bacteriologic studies should be done and antibiotic therapy initiated promptly. The PROGESTASERT® system should be removed and the continuing treatment assessed on the basis of the results of culture and sensitivity tests.

4. Embedment. Partial penetration or lodging of an IUD in the endometrium can result in difficult removals.

5. Perforation. Partial or total perforation of the uterine wall or cervix may occur with the use of IUDs. The possiblity of perforation must be kept in mind during insertion and at the time of any subsequent examination. If perforation occurs, the system should be removed. Adhesions, foreign body reactions, and intestinal obstruction may result if an IUD is left in the peritoneal cavity.

6. Congenital anomalies. Systemically administered sex steroids, including progestational agents, have been associated with an increased risk of congenital anomalies. It is not known whether there is an increased or decreased risk of such anomalies when pregnancy is continued with a PROGESTASERT® system in place.

Precautions:
1. Patient Counseling. Prior to insertion the physician, nurse, or other trained health professional should provide the patient with the Patient Information Leaflet. The patient should be given the

	Woman Months	Intrauterine Pregnancy	Extrauterine Pregnancy
PROGESTASERT® System	126,800	1.7	0.4
Unmedicated IUD	343,365	2.7	0.12
Copper T-200	132,432	3.1	0.05
Cu-7	157,625	2.3	0.04

Product Information

opportunity to read the leaflet and discuss fully any questions she may have concerning the PROGESTASERT® system as well as other methods of contraception.

2. Patient Evaluation and Clinical Considerations.

a. A complete medical history should be obtained to determine conditions that might influence the selection of an IUD. Special attention must be given during the history to ascertain if the woman is at a high risk to ectopic pregnancy by virtue of previous pelvic inflammatory disease. Physical examination should include a pelvic examination, a "Pap" smear, gonorrhea culture, and, if indicated, appropriate tests for other forms of venereal disease.

b. The uterus should be carefully sounded prior to insertion to determine the degree of patency of the endocervical canal and the internal os, and the direction and depth of the uterine cavity. In occasional cases, severe cervical stenosis may be encountered. Do not use excessive force to overcome this resistance.

c. The uterus should sound to a depth of 6 to 10 centimeters (cm). Insertion of a PROGESTASERT® system into a uterine cavity measuring less than 6 cm by sounding may increase the incidence of expulsion, bleeding, and pain.

d. The possibility of insertion in the presence of an existing undetermined pregnancy is reduced if insertion is performed during or shortly following a menstrual period. The system should not be inserted postpartum or postabortion until involution of the uterus is completed. The incidence of perforation and expulsion is greater if involution is not completed.

e. IUDs should still be used with caution in those patients who have an anemia or a history of menorrhagia or hypermenorrhea. Patients experiencing menorrhagia and/or metrorrhagia following IUD insertion may be at risk for the development of hypochromic microcytic anemia. Also, IUDs should be used with caution in patients receiving anticoagulants or having a coagulopathy.

f. Syncope, bradycardia or other neurovascular episodes may occur during insertion or removal of IUDs, especially in patients with a previous disposition to these conditions.

g. Patients with valvular or congenital heart disease are more prone to develop subacute bacterial endocarditis than patients who do not have valvular or congenital heart disease. Use of an IUD in these patients may represent a potential source of septic emboli.

h. Use of an IUD in those patients with acute cervicitis should be postponed until proper treatment has cleared up the infection.

i. Since an IUD may be expelled or displaced, patients should be reexamined and evaluated shortly after the first postinsertion menses, but definitely within 3 months after insertion. Thereafter annual examination with appropriate medical and laboratory examination should be carried out. The PROGESTASERT® system should be replaced each year, since the level of contraceptive efficacy of the system after this time has yet to be established.

j. The patient should be told that some bleeding and cramps may occur during the first few weeks after insertion, but if her symptoms continue or are severe she should report them to her physician. She should be instructed on how to check after each menstrual period to make certain that the threads still protrude from the cervix, and she should be cautioned that there is no contraceptive protection if the system is expelled. She should be cautioned not to pull on the threads thus displacing the system. If partial expulsion occurs, removal is indicated and a new system may be inserted. The patient should be told to return in one year for replacement of the system.

Adverse Reactions: These adverse reactions are not listed in any order of frequency or severity. Reported adverse reactions of IUD use include: endometritis, spontaneous abortion, septic abortion, septicemia, perforation of uterus and cervix, pelvic infection, cervical erosion, vaginitis, leukorrhea, pregnancy, ectopic pregnancy, uterine embedment, difficult removal, complete or partial expulsion, intermenstrual spotting, prolongation of menstrual flow, anemia, amenorrhea or delayed menses, pain and cramping, dysmenorrhea, backaches, dyspareunia, neuro-vascular episodes including bradycardia, and syncope secondary to insertion. Perforation into the abdomen followed by abdominal adhesions, intestinal penetration, intestinal obstruction, and cystic masses in the pelvis has been reported in general IUD use, but these have not been reported with PROGESTASERT® system perforations to date.

Directions For Use: A single PROGESTASERT® system is to be inserted into the uterine cavity (see Precautions section). Present information indicates that the contraceptive effectiveness of the system is retained for one year, and must be replaced one year after insertion.

Insertion Instructions:

NOTE: Physicians are cautioned to become thoroughly familiar with the insertion instructions before attempting placement with the PROGESTASERT® system.

Description of Inserter: The inserter is a malleable, curved tube designed to conform to the anatomical configuration of most cervical-uterine cavities. The horizontal arms of the T are positioned outside of the inserter and are folded by an arm-cocker attachment immediately prior to insertion.

■ DO NOT REMOVE ANY COMPONENT FROM THE INSERTER BEFORE INSERTION OF THE SYSTEM INTO THE UTERUS.

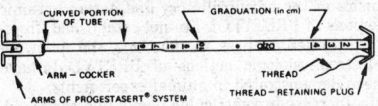

The PROGESTASERT® system inserter is designed to permit determination of the depth of uterine placement of the PROGESTASERT® system. The curvature of the inserter conforms with the usual orientation of the uterus; however, in cases of extreme flexion, the malleable inserter can be shaped gently to the desired curvature.

Preliminary Preparation and Precautions:

1. The completion of a medical history, a cervical Papanicolaou smear, gonorrhea culture, and pelvic examination is recommended prior to insertion of the PROGESTASERT® system.
2. Use of aseptic technique during insertion is essential.
3. Refer to the package insert for CONTRAINDICATIONS, WARNINGS, and PRECAUTIONS.
4. The system should preferably be inserted during or shortly after menstruation to ensure a nonpregnant state. (This approach may not be practical in certain clinical situations.)
5. The endocervix should be cleansed with an antiseptic solution and a tenaculum applied to the cervix with downward traction for correction of the angulation of the cervix and stabilization of the cervix.
6. Prior to insertion, it is desirable to ascertain the depth and position of the uterus and the patency of the cervical canal by uterine sounding. Insertion is not recommended into a uterus which sounds under 6 cm. or more than 10 cm.
7. THE PROGESTASERT® SYSTEM MUST BE USED ONLY WITH ITS SPECIALLY DESIGNED, PLUNGER-FREE INSERTER. This inserter will facilitate fundal placement and is designed to decrease the possibility of uterine perforation. No component should be removed from the inserter before insertion of the system into the uterus.

NOTE: Any intrauterine procedure can result in severe pain, bradycardia and syncope.

System Insertion:

1. Open the PROGESTASERT® system pouch by removing the clear cover.

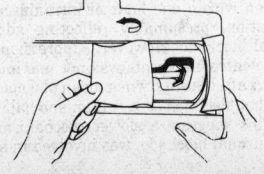

Remove the system and inserter by lifting the handle of the inserter. DO NOT CONTAMINATE THE END CONTAINING THE SYSTEM.

2. IMMEDIATELY PRIOR TO INSERTION, cock the arms of the PROGESTASERT® system by pressing straight down on the inserter onto the tray or other sterile field as shown. This will cause the arms to fold against the side of the inserter.

NOTE: To avoid alteration of system shape, do not leave the system in the folded position for more than a few minutes.

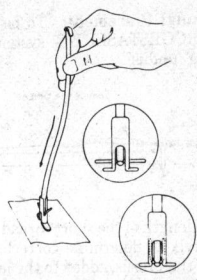

3. Examine the curvature of the inserter. If necessary, it can be easily reshaped to fit the flexion of the uterus. After aligning the curvature of the inserter with the direction of uterine flexion, introduce the inserter into the cervical canal. Be certain the thread-retaining plug is still secure in the end of the inserter. The arm-cocker will slide along the inserter shaft as the inserter moves through the cervical canal.

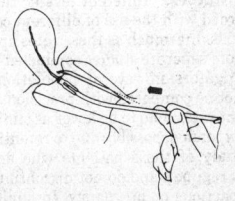

4. Sound steadily but gently with the inserter until the fundus is reached. While the inserter is in this position, note the number seen on the shaft at the base of the arm-cocker. This number approximates the depth in centimeters of the uterus.

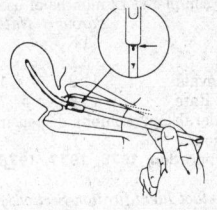

5. With the inserter still at the fundus, release the retaining thread by squeezing the wings of and removing the thread-retaining plug.

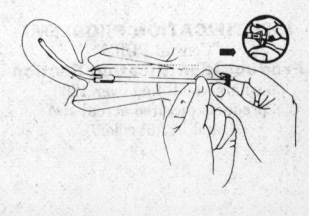

Continued on next page

Alza—Cont.

6. Slowly withdraw the inserter. The PROGESTASERT® system is released as the inserter is withdrawn.

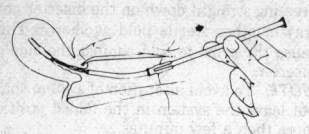

Correct Fundal Placement: To be fully effective, the PROGESTASERT® system must be placed at the fundus.

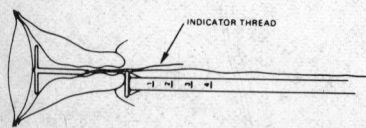

Estimate the length of the short thread protruding from the cervix to determine correct placement. The depth of the uterus, added to the length of the shorter "indicator" thread protruding from the cervix should approximate 9 cm. For example, with a uterine depth of 6 cm, you should see a 3 cm protrusion of the short "indicator" thread.
Trim the long thread to a standard 3 cm length from the cervix. This measurement is used for future reference in determining continued fundal placement.

How Supplied: Available in cartons containing six sterile systems (PROGESTASERT® system with an inserter).

Clinical Studies: Different event rates have been recorded with the use of different contraceptive methods. Inasmuch as these rates are usually derived from separate studies conducted by different investigators in several population groups, they cannot be compared with precision. Furthermore, event rates tend to be lower as clinical experience is expanded, possibly due to retention in the clinical study of those patients who accept the treatment regimen and do not discontinue due to adverse reactions or pregnancy. In clinical trials conducted by ALZA and the World Health Organization with the PROGESTASERT® system, use-effectiveness was determined as follows for parous and nulliparous women by the life table method. (Rates are expressed as events per 100 women through 12 months of use.) This experience is based on 68,780 woman-months of use with 7,614 women, of whom about 25% were nulliparous; 4,724 women completed 12 months of use.

	Parous	Nulliparous
Pregnancy	1.8	2.6
Expulsion	3.1	7.4
Medical Removals	11.2	15.1
Continuation Rate	79.8	71.8

Caution: Federal law prohibits dispensing without prescription.

© ALZA Corporation, 1975, 1977, 1978, 1980, 1984

Shown in Product Identification Section, page 404

IDENTIFICATION PROBLEM?
Consult PDR's
Product Identification Section
where you'll find over 1200
products pictured actual size
and in full color.

American Critical Care
American Hospital Supply
Corporation
McGAW PARK, IL 60085

BRETYLOL®
[bre'ti-lol"]
(bretylium tosylate)
INJECTION

For Intramuscular or Intravenous Use

Description: BRETYLOL (bretylium tosylate) is o-Bromobenzyl ethyl-dimethylammonium p-toluene sulfonate.
BRETYLOL is a white, crystalline powder with an extremely bitter taste. It is freely soluble in water and alcohol. Each ml of sterile, non-pyrogenic solution contains 50 mg bretylium tosylate in Water for Injection, USP. The pH is adjusted when necessary, with dilute hydrochloric acid or sodium hydroxide. BRETYLOL contains no preservative.

Clinical Pharmacology: BRETYLOL (bretylium tosylate) is a bromobenzyl quaternary ammonium compound which selectively accumulates in sympathetic ganglia and their postganglionic adrenergic neurons where it inhibits norepinephrine release by depressing adrenergic nerve terminal excitability.
BRETYLOL also suppresses ventricular fibrillation and ventricular arrhythmias. The mechanisms of the antifibrillatory and antiarrhythmic actions of BRETYLOL are not established. In efforts to define these mechanisms, the following electrophysiologic actions of BRETYLOL have been demonstrated in animal experiments:
1. Increase in ventricular fibrillation threshold.
2. Increase in action potential duration and effective refractory period without changes in heart rate.
3. Little effect on the rate of rise or amplitude of the cardiac action potential (Phase 0) or in resting membrane potential (Phase 4) in normal myocardium. However, when cell injury slows the rate of rise, decreases amplitude, and lowers resting membrane potential, BRETYLOL transiently restores these parameters toward normal.
4. In canine hearts with infarcted areas BRETYLOL decreases the disparity in action potential duration between normal and infarcted regions.
5. Increase in impulse formation and spontaneous firing rate of pacemaker tissue as well as increased ventricular conduction velocity.

The restoration of injured myocardial cell electrophysiology toward normal, as well as the increase of the action potential duration and effective refractory period without changing their ratio to each other, may be important factors in suppressing re-entry of aberrant impulses and decreasing induced dispersion of local excitable states.
BRETYLOL induces a chemical sympathectomy-like state which resembles a surgical sympathectomy. Catecholamine stores are not depleted by BRETYLOL, but catecholamine effects on the myocardium and on peripheral vascular resistance are often seen shortly after administration because BRETYLOL causes an early release of norepinephrine from the adrenergic postganglionic nerve terminals. Subsequently, BRETYLOL blocks the release of norepinephrine in response to neuron stimulation. Peripheral adrenergic blockade regularly causes orthostatic hypotension but has less effect on supine blood pressure. The relationship of adrenergic blockade to the antifibrillatory and antiarrhythmic actions of BRETYLOL is not clear. In a study in patients with frequent ventricular premature beats, peak plasma concentration of BRETYLOL and peak hypotensive effects were seen within one hour of intramuscular administration, presumably reflecting adrenergic neuronal blockade. However, suppression of premature ventricular beats was not maximal until 6-9 hours after dosing, when mean plasma concentration had declined to less than one-half of peak level. This suggests a slower mechanism, other than neuronal blockade, was involved in suppression of the arrhythmia. On the other hand, antifibrillatory effect can be seen within minutes of an intravenous injection, suggesting that the effect on the myocardium may occur quite rapidly.

BRETYLOL has a positive inotropic effect on the myocardium, but it is not yet certain whether this effect is direct or is mediated by catecholamine release.

BRETYLOL is eliminated intact by the kidneys. No metabolites have been identified following administration of BRETYLOL in man and laboratory animals. In man, approximately 70 to 80% of a ^{14}C-labelled intramuscular dose is excreted in the urine during the first 24 hours, with an additional 10% excreted over the next three days. The terminal half-life in four normal volunteers averaged 7.8 ± 0.6 hrs (range 6.9–8.1). In one patient with a creatinine clearance of 21.0 ml/min x 1.73 m^2, the half-life was 16 hours. In one patient with a creatinine clearance of 1.0 ml/min x 1.73 m^2 the half-life was 31.5 hours. During hemodialysis, this patient's arterial and venous BRETYLOL concentrations declined rapidly, resulting in a half-life of 13 hours. During dialysis there was a two-fold increase in total BRETYLOL clearance.

Effect on Heart Rate: There is sometimes an initial small increase in heart rate when BRETYLOL is administered, but this is an inconsistent and transient occurrence.

Hemodynamic Effects: Following intravenous administration of 5 mg/kg of BRETYLOL to patients with acute myocardial infarction, there was a mild increase in arterial pressure, followed by a modest decrease, remaining within normal limits throughout. Pulmonary artery pressures, pulmonary capillary wedge pressure, right atrial pressure, cardiac index, stroke volume index, and stroke work index were not significantly changed. These hemodynamic effects were not correlated with antiarrhythmic activity.

Onset of Action: Suppression of ventricular fibrillation is rapid, usually occurring within minutes following intravenous administration. Suppression of ventricular tachycardia and other ventricular arrhythmias develops more slowly, usually 20 minutes to 2 hours after parenteral administration.

Indications: BRETYLOL is indicated in the prophylaxis and therapy of ventricular fibrillation.

BRETYLOL is also indicated in the treatment of life-threatening ventricular arrhythmias, such as ventricular tachycardia, that have failed to respond to adequate doses of a first-line antiarrhythmic agent, such as lidocaine.

Use of BRETYLOL should be limited to intensive care units, coronary care units or other facilities where equipment and personnel for constant monitoring of cardiac arrhythmias and blood pressure are available.

Following injection of BRETYLOL there may be a delay of 20 minutes to 2 hours in the onset of antiarrhythmic action, although it appears to act within minutes in ventricular fibrillation. The delay in effect appears to be longer after intramuscular than after intravenous injection.

Contraindications: There are no contraindications to use in treatment of ventricular fibrillation or life-threatening refractory ventricular arrhythmias.

Warnings:
1. Hypotension
   Administration of BRETYLOL regularly results in postural hypotension, subjectively recognized by dizziness, light-headedness, vertigo or faintness. Some degree of hypotension is present in about 50% of patients while they are supine. Hypotension may occur at doses lower than those needed to suppress arrhythmias.

Patients should be kept in the supine position until tolerance to the hypotensive effect of BRETYLOL develops. Tolerance occurs unpredictably but may be present after several days.

Hypotension with supine systolic pressure greater than 75 mm Hg need not be treated unless there are associated symptoms. If supine systolic pressure falls below 75 mm Hg, an infusion of dopamine or norepinephrine may be used to raise blood pressure. When catecholamines are administered, a dilute solution should be employed and blood pressure monitored closely because the pressor effects of the catecholamines are enhanced by BRETYLOL. Volume expansion with blood or plasma and correction of dehydration should be carried out where appropriate.

2. **Transient Hypertension and Increased Frequency of Arrhythmias**
Due to the initial release of norepinephrine from adrenergic postganglionic nerve terminals by BRETYLOL, transient hypertension or increased frequency of premature ventricular contractions and other arrhythmias may occur in some patients.

3. **Caution During Use with Digitalis Glycosides**
The initial release of norepinephrine caused by BRETYLOL may aggravate digitalis toxicity. When a life-threatening cardiac arrhythmia occurs in a digitalized patient, BRETYLOL should be used only if the etiology of the arrhythmia does not appear to be digitalis toxicity and other antiarrhythmic drugs are not effective. Simultaneous initiation of therapy with digitalis glycosides and BRETYLOL (bretylium tosylate) should be avoided.

4. **Patients with Fixed Cardiac Output**
In patients with fixed cardiac output (i.e., severe aortic stenosis or severe pulmonary hypertension) BRETYLOL should be avoided since severe hypotension may result from a fall in peripheral resistance without a compensatory increase in cardiac output. If survival is threatened by the arrhythmia, BRETYLOL may be used but vasoconstrictive catecholamines should be given promptly if severe hypotension occurs.

Use in Pregnancy: The safety of BRETYLOL in human pregnancy has not been established. However, as the drug is intended for use only in life-threatening situations, it may be used in pregnant women when its benefits outweigh the potential risk to the fetus.

Use in Children: The safety and efficacy of this drug in children has not been established. BRETYLOL has been administered to a limited number of pediatric patients, but such use has been inadequate to define fully proper dosage and limitations for use.

Precautions:

1. **Dilution for Intravenous Use**
BRETYLOL should be diluted (one part BRETYLOL with four parts of Dextrose Injection, USP or Sodium Chloride Injection, USP) prior to intravenous use. Rapid intravenous administration may cause severe nausea and vomiting. Therefore, the diluted solution should be infused over a period greater than 8 minutes. In treating existing ventricular fibrillation BRETYLOL should be given as rapidly as possible and may be given without dilution.

2. **Use Various Sites for Intramuscular Injection**
When injected intramuscularly, not more than 5 ml should be given in a site, and injection sites should be varied since repeated intramuscular injection into the same site may cause atrophy and necrosis of muscle tissue, fibrosis, vascular degeneration and inflammatory changes.

3. **Reduce Dosage in Impaired Renal Function**
Since BRETYLOL is excreted principally via the kidney, the dosage interval should be increased in patients with impaired renal function. See 'Clinical Pharmacology' section for information on the effect of reduced renal function on half-life.

Adverse Reactions: Hypotension and postural hypotension have been the most frequently reported adverse reactions (see Warnings section). Nausea and vomiting occurred in about three percent of patients, primarily when BRETYLOL was administered rapidly by the intravenous route (see Precautions section). Vertigo, dizziness, lightheadedness and syncope, which sometimes accompanied postural hypotension, were reported in about 7 patients in 1000.

Bradycardia, increased frequency of premature ventricular contractions, transitory hypertension, initial increase in arrhythmias (see Warnings section), precipitation of anginal attacks, and sensation of substernal pressure have also been reported in a small number of patients, i.e., approximately 1–2 patients in 1000.

Renal dysfunction, diarrhea, abdominal pain, hiccups, erythematous macular rash, flushing, hyperthermia, confusion, paranoid psychosis, emotional lability, lethargy, generalized tenderness, anxiety, shortness of breath, diaphoresis, nasal stuffiness and mild conjunctivitis, have been reported in about 1 patient in 1000. The relationship of BRETYLOL administration to these reactions has not been clearly established.

Dosage and Administration: BRETYLOL is to be used clinically only for treatment of life-threatening ventricular arrhythmias under constant electrocardiographic monitoring. The clinical use of BRETYLOL is for short-term use only. Patients should either be kept supine during the course of BRETYLOL therapy or be closely observed for postural hypotension. The optimal dose schedule for parenteral administration of BRETYLOL has not been determined. There is comparatively little experience with dosages greater than 40 mg/kg/day, although such doses have been used without apparent adverse effects. The following schedule is suggested.

A. **For immediately Life-threatening Ventricular Arrhythmias such as Ventricular Fibrillation or Hemodynamically Unstable Ventricular Tachycardia:**
Administer undiluted BRETYLOL at a dosage of 5 mg/kg of body weight by rapid intravenous injection. Other usual cardiopulmonary resuscitative procedures, including electrical cardioversion, should be employed prior to and following the injection in accordance with good medical practice. If ventricular fibrillation persists, the dosage may be increased to 10 mg/kg and repeated as necessary.

For continuous suppression, dilute contents of one BRETYLOL ampul (10 ml containing 500 mg bretylium tosylate) to a minimum of 50 ml with Dextrose (5%) Injection, USP, or Sodium Chloride Injection, USP, and administer the diluted solution as a constant infusion of 1 to 2 mg BRETYLOL per minute. An alternative maintenance schedule is to infuse the diluted solution at a dosage of 5 to 10 mg BRETYLOL per kg body weight, over a period greater than 8 minutes, every 6 hours. More rapid infusion may cause nausea and vomiting.

B. **Other Ventricular Arrhythmias:**
1. Intravenous Use: **BRETYLOL must be diluted as described above before intravenous use.**
Administer the diluted solution at a dosage of 5 to 10 mg BRETYLOL per kg of body weight by intravenous infusion over a period greater than 8 minutes. More rapid infusion may cause nausea and vomiting. Subsequent doses may be given at 1 to 2 hour intervals if the arrhythmia persists.

For maintenance therapy, the same dosage may be administered every 6 hours, or a constant infusion of 1 to 2 mg BRETYLOL per minute may be given.

2. For intramuscular Injection: **Do not dilute BRETYLOL prior to intramuscular injection.** Inject 5 to 10 mg BRETYLOL per kg of body weight. Subsequent doses may be given at 1 to 2 hour intervals if the arrhythmia persists. Thereafter maintain the same dosage every 6 to 8 hours.

Intramuscular injection should not be made directly into or near a major nerve, and the site of injection should be varied on repeated injection.

As soon as possible, and when indicated, patients should be changed to an oral antiarrhythmic agent for maintenance therapy.

How Supplied: NDC 0094-0012-10: 10 ml ampul containing 500 mg bretylium tosylate in Water for Injection, USP. pH adjusted, when necessary, with dilute hydrochloric acid or sodium hydroxide. Sterile, non-pyrogenic.

Re. Pat. No. 29,618

CALCIPARINE® ℞
[cal-ci′ pū-rin]
(heparin calcium)
INJECTION

For Subcutaneous and IV Use

Description: Calciparine (heparin calcium injection) is a sterile solution of heparin calcium derived from porcine intestinal mucosa, standardized for use as an anticoagulant, in water for injection. The pH of the solution is adjusted to approximately 7 with calcium hydroxide or hydrochloric acid. The potency is determined by a biological assay using a USP reference standard based upon units of heparin activity per milligram.

Actions: Heparin inhibits reactions which lead to the clotting of blood and the formation of fibrin clots both *in vitro* and *in vivo*. Heparin acts at multiple sites in the normal coagulation system. Small amounts of heparin in combination with antithrombin III (heparin co-factor) can prevent the development of a hypercoagulable state by inactivating activated Factor X, preventing the conversion of prothrombin to thrombin. Once a hypercoagulable state exists, larger amounts of heparin in combination with antithrombin III can inhibit the coagulation process by inactivating thrombin and earlier clotting intermediates, thus preventing the conversion of fibrinogen to fibrin. Heparin also prevents the formation of a stable fibrin clot by inhibiting the activation of the fibrin stabilizing factor.

Bleeding time is usually unaffected by heparin. Clotting time is prolonged by full therapeutic doses of heparin; in most cases it is not measurably affected by low doses of heparin.

Heparin does not have fibrinolytic activity; therefore, it will not lyse existing clots.

Indications: Calciparine is indicated for anticoagulant therapy in prophylaxis and treatment of venous thrombosis and its extension; in low-dose regimen for prevention of postoperative deep venous thrombosis and pulmonary embolism in patients undergoing major abdominothoracic surgery who are at risk of developing thromboembolic disease (see DOSAGE AND ADMINISTRATION); for prophylaxis and treatment of pulmonary embolism; in atrial fibrillation with embolization; for diagnosis and treatment of acute and chronic consumptive coagulopathies (disseminated intravascular coagulation); for prevention of clotting in arterial and cardiac surgery; and for prevention of cerebral thrombosis in evolving stroke.

Heparin is indicated as an adjunct in treatment of coronary occlusion with acute myocardial infarction, and in prophylaxis and treatment of peripheral arterial embolism.

Heparin may also be employed as an anticoagulant in blood transfusion, extracorporeal circulation, dialysis procedures, and in blood samples for laboratory purposes.

Contraindications: Hypersensitivity to heparin.

Inability to perform suitable blood coagulation tests, e.g., the whole blood clotting time, partial thromboplastin time, etc., at required intervals. There is usually no need to monitor the effect of low-dose heparin in patients with normal coagulation parameters.

Continued on next page

American Critical—Cont.

Uncontrollable bleeding.

Warnings:

> Calciparine should be used with extreme caution in disease states in which there is an increased danger of hemorrhage.

Administration of Calciparine, when used in therapeutic dosage, should be regulated by frequent blood coagulation tests. If these are unduly prolonged or if hemorrhage occurs, Calciparine should be promptly discontinued. See OVERDOSAGE.

Some of the conditions in which increased danger of hemorrhage exists are:

Cardiovascular	subacute bacterial endocarditis; arterial sclerosis; increased capillary permeability; during and immediately following a) spinal tap or spinal anesthesia, b) major surgery, especially involving the brain, spinal cord, or eye.
Hematologic	conditions associated with increased bleeding tendencies such as hemophilia, some purpuras, and thrombocytopenia.
Gastrointestinal	inaccessible ulcerative lesions, and continuous tube drainage of the stomach or small intestine.

Calciparine may prolong the one-stage prothrombin time. Accordingly, when Calciparine is given with dicumarol or warfarin sodium, a period of at least 5 hours after the last intravenous dose and 24 hours after the last subcutaneous (intrafat) dose of Calciparine should elapse before blood is drawn, if a valid prothrombin time is to be obtained.

Drugs (such as acetylsalicylic acid, dextran, phenylbutazone, ibuprofen, indomethacin, dipyridamole, and hydroxychloroquine) which interfere with platelet aggregation reactions (the main hemostatic defense of heparinized patients) may induce bleeding and should be used with caution in patients on heparin therapy.

While there is experimental evidence that heparin may antagonize the action of ACTH, insulin, or corticoids, this effect has not been clearly defined. There is also evidence in animal experiments that heparin may modify or inhibit allergic reactions. However, the application of these findings to human patients has not been fully defined.

Larger doses of heparin may be necessary in the febrile state.

The use of digitalis, tetracyclines, nicotine, or antihistamines may partially counteract the anticoagulant action of heparin. An increased resistance to heparin is frequently encountered in cases of thrombosis, thrombophlebitis, infections with thrombosing tendency, myocardial infarction, cancer, and in the postoperative patient.

Usage in Pregnancy: Calciparine should be used with caution during pregnancy, especially during the last trimester and in the immediate postpartum period.

There is no adequate information as to whether heparin may affect human fertility, or have a teratogenic potential or other adverse effects on the fetus.

Heparin does not cross the placental barrier; it is not excreted in human milk.

Precautions: Because Calciparine is derived from animal tissue, it should be used with caution in patients with a history of allergy. Before a therapeutic dose is given to such a patient, a trial dose of 1,000 units may be advisable.

Calciparine should also be used with caution in the presence of hepatic or renal disease, hypertension, during menstruation, or in patients with indwelling catheters.

A higher incidence of bleeding may be seen in women over 60 years of age.

Caution should be exercised when administering ACD-converted blood (i.e., blood collected in Calciparine and later converted to ACD blood), since the anticoagulant activity of its heparin calcium content persists without loss for 22 days. ACD-converted blood may alter the coagulation system of the recipient, especially if it is given in multiple transfusions.

Adverse Reactions: Hemorrhage is the chief complication that may result from heparin therapy. An overly prolonged clotting time or minor bleeding during therapy can usually be controlled by withdrawing the drug. See OVERDOSAGE.

The occurrence of significant gastrointestinal or urinary tract bleeding during anticoagulant therapy may indicate the presence of an underlying occult lesion.

Adrenal hemorrhage with resultant acute adrenal insufficiency has occurred during anticoagulant therapy. Therefore such treatment should be discontinued in patients who develop signs and symptoms compatible with acute adrenal hemorrhage and insufficiency. Plasma cortisol levels should be measured immediately, and vigorous therapy with intravenous corticosteroids should be instituted promptly. Initiation of therapy should not depend upon laboratory confirmation of the diagnosis, since any delay in an acute situation may result in the patient's death.

Intramuscular injection of heparin frequently causes local irritation, mild pain, or hematoma, and for these reasons should be avoided. These effects are less often seen following deep subcutaneous (intrafat) injection. Histamin-like reactions have also been observed at the site of injection.

Hypersensitivity reactions have been reported with chills, fever, and urticaria as the most usual manifestations. Asthma, rhinitis, lacrimation, and anaphylactoid reactions have also been reported.

Vasospastic reactions may develop independent of the origin of heparin, 6 to 10 days after the initiation of therapy and last for 4 to 6 hours. The affected limb is painful, ischemic and cyanosed. An artery to this limb may have been recently catheterized. After repeat injections, the reaction may gradually increase, to include generalized vasospasm, with cyanosis, tachypnea, feeling of oppression, and headache. Protamine sulfate treatment has no marked therapeutic effect. Itching and burning, especially on the plantar side of the feet, is possibly based on a similar allergic vasospastic reaction. Chest pain, elevated blood pressure, arthralgias, and/or headache have also been reported in the absence of definite peripheral vasospasm. Anaphylactic shock has been reported rarely following the intravenous administration of heparin.

Acute reversible thrombocytopenia following the intravenous administration of heparin has been reported. Osteoporosis and suppression of renal function following long-term, high-dose administration, suppression of aldosterone synthesis, delayed transient alopecia, priapism, and rebound hyperlipemia following discontinuation of heparin have also been reported.

Dosage and Administration: Calciparine is not effective by oral administration and should be given by deep subcutaneous (intrafat, i.e., above iliac crest or into the abdominal fat layer) injection, by intermittent intravenous injection, or intravenous infusion. The intramuscular route of administration should be avoided because of the frequent occurrence of hematoma at the injection site.

The dosage of Calciparine should be adjusted according to the patient's coagulation test results, which during the first days of treatment should be determined just prior to each injection. There is usually no need to monitor the effect of low-dose heparin in patients with normal coagulation parameters. Dosage is considered adequate when the whole blood clotting time is elevated approximately 2.5 to 3 times the control value.

When Calciparine is administered by continuous intravenous infusion, coagulation tests should be performed approximately every 4 hours during the early stages of therapy. When it is administered intermittently by intravenous, or deep subcutaneous (intrafat) injection, coagulation tests should be performed before each injection during the early stages of treatment, and daily thereafter. When an oral anticoagulant of the coumadin or similar type is administered with Calciparine, coagulation tests and prothrombin activity should be determined at the start of therapy. For immediate anticoagulant effect, administer Calciparine in the usual therapeutic dosage. When the results of the initial prothrombin determination are known, administer the first dose of an oral anticoagulant in the usual initial amount. Thereafter, perform a coagulation test and determine the prothrombin activity at appropriate intervals. A period at least 5 hours after the last intravenous dose and 24 hours after the last subcutaneous (intrafat) dose of Calciparine should elapse before blood is drawn, if a valid prothrombin time is to be obtained. When the oral anticoagulant shows full effect and prothrombin activity is in the desired therapeutic range, Calciparine may be discontinued and therapy continued with the oral anticoagulant.

Therapeutic Anticoagulant Effect with Full-Dose Calciparine

Although dosage must be adjusted for the individual patient according to the results of suitable laboratory tests, the following dosage schedules may be used as guidelines:
[See table left].

1. *By deep subcutaneous (intrafat) injection.* After an initial I.V. injection of 5,000 units, inject 10,000 to 20,000 units of a concentrated Calciparine solution subcutaneously, followed by 8,000 to 10,000 units of a concentrated solution subcutaneously every 8 hours, or 15,000 to 20,000 units of a concentrated solution every 12 hours. A different site should be used for each injection to prevent the development of a massive hematoma.

2. *By intermittent intravenous injection.* 10,000 units initially, then 5,000 to 10,000 units every 4 to 6 hours. These amounts may be given either undiluted or diluted with 50 to 100 ml of isotonic sodium chloride injection.

METHOD OF ADMINISTRATION	FREQUENCY	RECOMMENDED DOSE based on 150 lb (68 kg) patient
Deep Subcutaneous (Intrafat) Injection	Initial Dose	5,000 units by I.V. injection followed by 10,000–20,000 units of a concentrated solution, subcutaneously
	Every 8 hours	8,000–10,000 units of a concentrated solution
	(or) Every 12 hours	15,000–20,000 units of a concentrated solution
Intermittent Intravenous Injection	Initial Dose	10,000 units, either undiluted or in 50–100 ml isotonic sodium chloride injection
	Every 4 to 6 hours	5,000–10,000 units, either undiluted or in 50–100 ml isotonic sodium chloride injection
Intravenous Infusion	Initial Dose	5,000 units by I.V. injection
	Continuous	20,000–40,000 units in 1,000 ml of isotonic sodium chloride solution for infusion/day

3. *By continuous intravenous infusion.* After an initial I.V. injection of 5,000 units of Calciparine add 20,000 to 40,000 units to 1,000 ml of isotonic sodium chloride solution for infusion. For most patients, the rate of flow should be adjusted to deliver approximately 20,000 to 40,000 units in 24 hours.

Surgery of the Heart and Blood Vessels: Patients undergoing total body perfusion for open heart surgery should receive an initial dose of not less than 150 units of Calciparine per kilogram of body weight. Frequently a dose of 300 units of Calciparine per kilogram of body weight is used for procedures estimated to last less than 60 minutes; or 400 units per kilgram for those estimated to last longer than 60 minutes.

Low-Dose Prophylaxis of Postoperative Thromboembolism: A number of well-controlled clinical trials have demonstrated that low-dose heparin prophylaxis, given just prior to and after surgery, will reduce the incidence of postoperative deep vein thrombosis in the legs, as measured by the I-125 fibrinogen technique and venography, and of clinical pulmonary embolism. The most widely used dosage has been 5,000 units 2 hours before surgery and 5,000 units every 8 to 12 hours thereafter for 7 days or until the patient is fully ambulatory, whichever is longer. The heparin is given by deep subcutaneous injection in the arm or abdomen with a fine needle (25–26 gauge) to minimize tissue trauma. A concentrated solution of Calciparine is recommended. Such prophylaxis should be reserved for patients over 40 undergoing major surgery. Patients with bleeding disorders, those having neurosurgery, spinal anesthesia, eye surgery, or potentially sanguinous operations should be excluded, as well as patients receiving oral anticoagulants or platelet-active drugs (see WARNINGS). The value of such prophylaxis in hip surgery has not been established. The possibility of increased bleeding during surgery or postoperatively should be borne in mind. If such bleeding occurs, discontinuance of Calciparine and neutralization with protamine sulfate is advisable. If clinical evidence of thromboembolism develops despite low-dose prophylaxis, full therapeutic doses of anticoagulants should be given unless contraindicated. All patients should be screened prior to heparinization to rule out bleeding disorders, and monitoring should be performed with appropriate coagulation tests just prior to surgery. Coagulation test values should be normal or only slightly elevated. There is usually no need for daily monitoring of the effect of low-dose Calciparine in patients with normal coagulation parameters.

Extracorporeal Dialysis Use: Follow equipment manufacturer's operating directions carefully.

Blood Transfusion: Addition of 400 to 600 units of Calciparine per 100 ml of whole blood. Usually, 7,500 units of Calciparine are added to 100 ml of sterile sodium chloride injection (or 75,000 units per 1,000 ml of sterile sodium chloride injection) and mixed, and from this sterile solution, 6 to 8 ml is added per 100 ml of whole blood. Leukocyte counts should be performed on heparinized blood within 2 hours after addition of Calciparine. Heparinized blood should not be used for isoagglutinin, complement, erythrocyte fragility tests, or platelet counts.

Laboratory Samples: Addition of 70 to 150 units of Calciparine per 10 to 20 ml sample of whole blood is usually employed to prevent coagulation of the sample. See comments under *Blood Transfusion.*

Overdosage: Protamine sulfate (1% solution) by slow infusion will neutralize heparin. No more than 50 mg should be given very slowly, in any 10-minute period. Each mg of protamine sulfate neutralizes approximately 100 units of heparin (or 1.0 to 1.5 mg neutralizes approximately 1.0 mg of heparin). Heparins derived from various animal sources require different amounts of protamine sulfate for neutralization. This fact is of most importance during procedures of regional heparinization, including dialysis.

Decreasing amounts of protamine are required as time from last heparin injection increases. Thirty minutes after a dose of heparin, approximately 0.5 mg of protamine sulfate is sufficient to neutralize each 100 units of administered heparin. Blood or plasma transfusions may be necessary; these dilute but do not neutralize heparin.

How Supplied: Calciparine (heparin calcium injection) is available as follows:
Calciparine 5,000 USP heparin units, 0.2 ml prefilled disposable syringe, carton of 10, NDC 0094-0030-02.
Calciparine 12,500 USP heparin units, 0.5 ml ampule with sterile syringe and attached 25-gauge ⅝″ needle, carton of 10, NDC 0094-0030-05.
Calciparine 20,000 USP heparin units, 0.8 ml ampule with sterile syringe and attached 25-gauge ⅝″ needle, carton of 10, NDC 0094-0030-08.

HESPAN® ℞
[hes′pan]
6% Hetastarch in
0.9% Sodium Chloride Injection

Description:
Composition per 100 ml:
Hetastarch .... 6.0 g
Sodium Chloride USP .... 0.90 g
Water for Injection USP .... qs
pH adjusted with Sodium Hydroxide
Concentration of Electrolytes (mEq/liter): Sodium 154, Chloride 154
pH: Approx. 5.5
Calculated Osmolarity: Approximately 310 mOsm/liter

Hetastarch is an artificial colloid derived from a waxy starch composed almost entirely of amylopectin. Hydroxyethyl ether groups are introduced into the glucose units of the starch and the resultant material is hydrolyzed to yield a product with a molecular weight suitable for use as a plasma expander. Clinical Hetastarch is characterized by its molecular weight and its degree of substitution. The weight average molecular weight is approximately 450,000 with 90% of the polymer units falling within the range of 10,000 to 1,000,000. The degree of substitution is 0.7 which means Hetastarch has 7 hydroxyethyl groups for every 10 glucose units. The polymerized glucose units in Hetastarch are joined primarily by 1–4 linkages with hydroxyethyl groups being attached primarily at the No. 2 position. The polymer closely resembles glycogen.

The Hespan dosage form is a clear, pale yellow to amber solution. Exposure to prolonged adverse storage conditions (temperatures above 40°C or below freezing) may result in a change to a turbid deep brown or the formation of a crystalline precipitate. Do not use the solution if these conditions are evident.

Actions: The colloidal properties of 6% Hetastarch approximate those of human albumin. Intravenous infusion of Hetastarch results in expansion of plasma volume slightly in excess of the volume infused which decreases from this maximum over the succeeding 24 to 36 hours. This expansion of plasma volume may improve the hemodynamic status for 24 hours and longer. Hetastarch molecules below 50,000 molecular weight are rapidly eliminated by renal excretion with approximately 40% of a given total dose appearing in the urine in 24 hours. This is a variable process but generally results in an intravascular Hetastarch concentration of less than 1% of the total dose injected by two weeks. The hydroxyethyl group is not cleaved by the body, but remains intact and attached to glucose units when excreted.

The addition of Hetastarch to whole blood increases the erythrocyte sedimentation rate. Therefore, Hetastarch is used to improve the efficiency of granulocyte collection by centrifugal means.

Indications: Hetastarch is indicated when plasma volume expansion is desired as an adjunct in the treatment of shock due to hemorrhage, burns, surgery, sepsis or other trauma. It is not a substitute for blood or plasma.

The adjunctive use of Hetastarch in leukapheresis has also been shown to be safe and efficacious in improving the harvesting and increasing the yield of granulocytes by centrifugal means.

Contraindications: Hetastarch is contraindicated in patients with severe bleeding disorders or with severe congestive cardiac and renal failure with oliguria or anuria.

Warnings: Large volumes may alter the coagulation mechanism. Thus, administration of Hetastarch may result in transient prolongation of prothrombin, partial thromboplastin and clotting times. With administration of large doses, the physician should also be alert to the possibility of transient prolongation of bleeding time.

Hematocrit may be decreased and plasma proteins diluted excessively by administration of large volumes of Hetastarch.

Usage of Leukapheresis: Significant declines in platelet counts and hemoglobin levels have been observed in donors undergoing repeated leukapheresis procedures due to the volume expanding effects of Hetastarch. Hemoglobin levels usually return to normal within 24 hours. Hemodilution by Hetastarch and saline may also result in 24 hour declines of total protein, albumin, calcium and fibrinogen values.

Usage in Pregnancy: Reproduction studies have been done in mice with no evidence of fetal damage. Relevance to humans is not known since Hetastarch has not been given to pregnant women. Therefore, it should not be used in pregnant women, particularly during early pregnancy, unless in the judgment of the physician the potential benefits outweigh the potential hazards.

Usage in Children: No data are available pertaining to use in children.
The safety and compatibility of additives have not been established.

Precautions: The possibility of circulatory overload should be kept in mind. Special care should be exercised in patients who have impaired renal clearance since this is the principal way in which Hetastarch is eliminated. Caution should be used when the risk of pulmonary edema and/or congestive heart failure is increased. Indirect bilirubin levels of 0.83 mg % (normal 0.0–0.7 mg %) have been reported in 2 out of 20 normal subjects who received multiple Hetastarch infusions. Total bilirubin was within normal limits at all times; indirect bilirubin returned to normal by 96 hours following the final infusion. The significance, if any, of these elevations is not known; however, caution should be observed before administering Hetastarch to patients with a history of liver disease.

Regular and frequent clinical evaluation and laboratory determinations are necessary for proper monitoring of Hetastarch use during leukapheresis. Studies should include CBC, total leukocyte and platelet counts, leukocyte differential count, hemoglobin, hematocrit, prothrombin time (PT), and partial thromboplastin time (PTT).

Hetastarch is nonantigenic. However, allergic or sensitivity reactions have been reported (see **Adverse Reactions**). If such reactions occur, they are readily controlled by discontinuation of the drug and, if necessary, administration of an antihistaminic agent.

Adverse Reactions: The following have been reported: vomiting, mild temperature elevation, chills, itching, submaxillary and parotid glandular enlargement, mild influenza-like symptoms, headaches, muscle pains, peripheral edema of the lower extremities, and anaphylactoid reactions consisting of periorbital edema, urticaria, and wheezing.

Dosage and Administration: Dosage in Plasma Volume Expansion: Hetastarch is administered by intravenous infusion only. Total dosage and rate of infusion depend upon the amount of blood lost and the resultant hemoconcentration. In adults, the amount usually administered is 500 to 1000 ml. Total dosage does not usually exceed 1500 ml per day or approximately 20 ml per kg of body weight for the typical 70 kg patient. In acute hemorrhagic shock, an administration rate approaching 20 ml per kg per hour may be used; in burn or septic shock it is usually administered at slower rates.

Dosage in Leukapheresis: In continuous-flow centrifugation (CFC) procedures, 250 to 700 ml

Continued on next page

American Critical—Cont.

Hetastarch is typically infused at a constant fixed ratio, usually 1:8, to venous whole blood.
Multiple CFC procedures using Hetastarch of up to 2 per week and a total of 7 to 10 have been reported to be safe and effective. Adequate data are not available to establish the safety of more frequent or a greater number of procedures.
How Supplied: NDC 0094-0037-05-Hespan® (6% Hetastarch in 0.9% Sodium Chloride Injection) is supplied sterile and nonpyrogenic in 500 ml intravenous infusion bottles.

INTROPIN® ℞
[in-trō'pin]
(dopamine HCl injection, USP) 5 ml VIAL and RAP-ADD® Syringe—
200 mg, 400 mg and 800 mg
5 ml AMPUL—200 mg

Description: INTROPIN (dopamine HCl injection, USP) is a clear, practically colorless, aqueous, additive solution for intravenous infusion after dilution. Each ml contains either 40 mg, 80 mg or 160 mg dopamine hydrochloride, USP (equivalent to 32.3 mg, 64.6 mg and 129.2 mg dopamine base, respectively) in Water for Injection, USP containing 1% sodium bisulfite as an antioxidant. Hydrochloric acid or sodium hydroxide added to adjust pH when necessary. The solution is sterile and non-pyrogenic. The pH is 2.5-4.5. INTROPIN, a naturally-occurring catecholamine, is an inotropic vasopressor agent. Its chemical name is 3,4 dihydroxyphenethylamine hydrochloride.
INTROPIN is sensitive to alkalis, iron salts and oxidizing agents. **It must be diluted in an appropriate, sterile parenteral solution** (see Dosage and Administration section) **before intravenous administration.**
Actions: INTROPIN exerts an inotropic effect on the myocardium resulting in an increased cardiac output. INTROPIN produces less increase in myocardial oxygen consumption than isoproterenol and its use is usually not associated with a tachyarrhythmia. Clinical studies indicate that INTROPIN usually increases systolic and pulse pressure with either no effect or a slight increase in diastolic pressure. Total peripheral resistance at low and intermediate therapeutic doses is usually unchanged. Blood flow to peripheral vascular beds may decrease while mesenteric flow increases. INTROPIN has also been reported to dilate the renal vasculature presumptively by activation of a "dopaminergic" receptor. This action is accompanied by increases in glomerular filtration rate, renal blood flow, and sodium excretion. An increase in urinary output produced by dopamine is usually not associated with a decrease in osmolality of the urine.
Indications: INTROPIN is indicated for the correction of hemodynamic imbalances present in the shock syndrome due to myocardial infarctions, trauma, endotoxic septicemia, open heart surgery, renal failure, and chronic cardiac decompensation as in congestive failure.
Where appropriate, restoration of blood volume with a suitable plasma expander or whole blood should be instituted or completed prior to administration of INTROPIN.
Patients most likely to respond adequately to INTROPIN are those in whom physiological parameters, such as urine flow, myocardial function, and blood pressure, have not undergone profound deterioration. Multiclinic trials indicate that the shorter the time interval between onset of signs and symptoms and initiation of therapy with volume correction and INTROPIN, the better the prognosis.
Poor Perfusion of Vital Organs—Urine flow appears to be one of the better diagnostic signs by which adequacy of vital organ perfusion can be monitored. Nevertheless, the physician should also observe the patient for signs of reversal of confusion or comatose condition. Loss of pallor, increase in toe temperature, and/or adequacy of nail bed capillary filling may also be used as indices of adequate dosage. Clinical studies have shown that when INTROPIN is administered before urine flow has diminished to levels approximately 0.3 ml/minute, prognosis is more favorable. Nevertheless, in a number of oliguric or anuric patients, administration of INTROPIN has resulted in an increase in urine flow which in some cases reached normal levels. INTROPIN may also increase urine flow in patients whose output is within normal limits and thus may be of value in reducing the degree of pre-existing fluid accumulation. It should be noted that at doses above those optimal for the individual patient, urine flow may decrease, necessitating reduction of dosage. Concurrent administration of INTROPIN and diuretic agents may produce an additive or potentiating effect.
Low Cardiac Output—Increased cardiac output is related to INTROPIN's direct inotropic effect on the myocardium. Increased cardiac output at low or moderate doses appears to be related to a favorable prognosis. Increase in cardiac output has been associated with either static or decreased systemic vascular resistance (SVR). Static or decreased SVR associated with low or moderate increments in cardiac output is believed to be a reflection of differential effects on specific vascular beds with increased resistance in peripheral beds (e.g. femoral) and concomitant decreases in mesenteric and renal vascular beds. Redistribution of blood flow parallels these changes so that an increase in cardiac output is accompanied by an increase in mesenteric and renal blood flow. In many instances the renal fraction of the total cardiac output has been found to increase. Increase in cardiac output produced by INTROPIN is not associated with substantial decreases in systemic vascular resistance as may occur with isoproterenol.
Hypotension—Hypotension due to inadequate cardiac output can be managed by administration of low to moderate doses of INTROPIN, which have little effect on SVR. At high therapeutic doses, INTROPIN's alpha adrenergic activity becomes more prominent and thus may correct hypotension due to diminished SVR. As in the case of other circulatory decompensation states, prognosis is better in patients whose blood pressure and urine flow have not undergone profound deterioration. Therefore, it is suggested that the physician administer INTROPIN as soon as a definite trend toward decreased systolic and diastolic pressure becomes evident.
Contraindications: INTROPIN should not be used in patients with pheochromocytoma.
Warnings: INTROPIN should not be administered in the presence of uncorrected tachyarrhythmias or ventricular fibrillation.
Do **NOT** add INTROPIN to any alkaline diluent solution, since the drug is inactivated in alkaline solution.
Patients who have been treated with monoamine oxidase (MAO) inhibitors prior to the administration of INTROPIN will require substantially reduced dosage. Dopamine is metabolized by MAO, and inhibition of this enzyme prolongs and potentiates the effect of INTROPIN. The starting dose in such patients should be reduced to at least one-tenth ($1/10$) of the usual dose.
Usage in Pregnancy—Animal studies have revealed no evidence of teratogenic effects from INTROPIN. In one study, administration of INTROPIN to pregnant rats resulted in a decreased survival rate of the newborn and a potential for cataract formation in the survivors. The drug may be used in pregnant women when, in the judgment of the physician, the expected benefits outweigh the potential risk to the fetus.
Usage in Children—The safety and efficacy of this drug in children has not been established. INTROPIN has been used in a limited number of pediatric patients, but such use has been inadequate to fully define proper dosage and limitations for use. Further studies are in progress.
Precautions: Avoid Hypovolemia—Prior to treatment with INTROPIN, hypovolemia should be fully corrected, if possible, with either whole blood or plasma as indicated.

Decreased Pulse Pressure—If a disproportionate rise in the diastolic pressure (i.e., a marked decrease in the pulse pressure) is observed in patients receiving INTROPIN, the infusion rate should be decreased and the patient observed carefully for further evidence of predominant vasoconstrictor activity, unless such an effect is desired.
Extravasation—INTROPIN should be infused into a large vein whenever possible to prevent the possibility of extravasation into tissue adjacent to the infusion site. Extravasation may cause necrosis and sloughing of surrounding tissue. Large veins of the antecubital fossa are preferred to veins in the dorsum of the hand or ankle. Less suitable infusion sites should be used only if the patient's condition requires immediate attention. The physician should switch to more suitable sites as rapidly as possible. The infusion site should be continuously monitored for free flow.
Occlusive Vascular Disease—Patients with a history of occlusive vascular disease (for example, atherosclerosis, arterial embolism, Raynaud's disease, cold injury, diabetic endarteritis, and Buerger's disease) should be closely monitored for any changes in color or temperature of the skin in the extremities. If a change in skin color or temperature occurs and is thought to be the result of compromised circulation to the extremities, the benefits of continued INTROPIN infusion should be weighed against the risk of possible necrosis. This condition may be reversed by either decreasing or discontinuing the rate of infusion.

IMPORTANT—Antidote for Peripheral Ischemia: To prevent sloughing and necrosis in ischemic areas, the area should be infiltrated as soon as possible with 10 to 15 ml. of saline solution containing from 5 to 10 mg. of Regitine® (brand of phentolamine), an adrenergic blocking agent. A syringe with a fine hypodermic needle should be used, and the solution liberally infiltrated throughout the ischemic area. Sympathetic blockade with phentolamine causes immediate and conspicuous local hyperemic changes if the area is infiltrated within 12 hours. Therefore, phentolamine should be given as soon as possible after the extravasation is noted.

Avoid Cyclopropane or Halogenated Hydrocarbon Anesthetics—Cyclopropane or halogenated hydrocarbon anesthetics increase cardiac autonomic irritability and therefore may sensitize the myocardium to the action of certain intravenously administered catecholamines. This interaction appears to be related both to pressor activity and to beta adrenergic stimulating properties of these catecholamines. Therefore, as with certain other catecholamines, and because of the theoretical arrhythmogenic potential, INTROPIN should be used with EXTREME CAUTION in patients inhaling cyclopropane or halogenated hydrocarbon anesthetics.
Careful Monitoring Required—Close monitoring of the following indices—urine flow, cardiac output and blood pressure—during INTROPIN infusion is necessary as in the case of any adrenergic agent.
Adverse Reactions: The most frequent adverse reactions observed in clinical evaluation of INTROPIN included ectopic beats, nausea, vomiting, tachycardia, anginal pain, palpitation, dyspnea, headache, hypotension, and vasoconstriction. Other adverse reactions which have been reported infrequently were aberrant conduction, bradycardia, piloerection, widened QRS complex, azotemia, and elevated blood pressure.
Dosage and Administration:
WARNING: This is a potent drug: It must be diluted before administration to patient.
Suggested Dilution—Transfer contents of one or more ampuls, vials or additive syringes by aseptic technique to either a 250 ml or 500 ml bottle of one of the following sterile intravenous solutions:
1) Sodium Chloride Injection, USP
2) Dextrose (5%) Injection, USP
3) Dextrose (5%) and Sodium Chloride (0.9%) Injection, USP

4) Dextrose (5%) in Sodium Chloride (0.45%) Solution
5) Dextrose (5%) in Lactated Ringer's Solution
6) Sodium Lactate (1/6 Molar) Injection, USP
7) Lactated Ringer's Injection, USP

INTROPIN has been found to be stable for a minimum of 24 hours after dilution in the sterile intravenous solutions listed above. However, as with all intravenous admixtures, dilution should be made just prior to administration.

Do **NOT** add INTROPIN to 5% Sodium Bicarbonate or other alkaline intravenous solutions, since the drug is inactivated in alkaline solution.

Rate of Administration—INTROPIN, after dilution, is administered intravenously through a suitable intravenous catheter or needle. An i.v. drip chamber or other suitable metering device is essential for controlling the rate of flow in drops/minute. Each patient must be individually titrated to the desired hemodynamic and/or renal response with INTROPIN. In titrating to the desired increase in systolic blood pressure, the optimum dosage rate for renal response may be exceeded, thus necessitating a reduction in rate after the hemodynamic condition is stablized.

Administration at rates greater than 50 mcg/kg/min has safely been used in advanced circulatory decompensation states. If unnecessary fluid expansion is of concern, adjustment of drug concentration may be preferred over increasing the flow rate of a less concentrated dilution.

Suggested Regimen:
1. When appropriate, increase blood volume with whole blood or plasma until central venous pressure is 10 to 15 cm H_2O or pulmonary wedge pressure is 14–18 mm Hg.
2. Begin administration of diluted solution at doses of 2–5 mcg/kg/minute INTROPIN in patients who are likely to respond to modest increments of heart force and renal perfusion. In more seriously ill patients, begin administration of diluted solution at doses of 5 mcg/kg/minute INTROPIN and increase gradually using 5 to 10 mcg/kg/minute increments up to 20 to 50 mcg/kg/minute as needed. If doses of INTROPIN in excess of 50 mcg/kg/minute are required, it is suggested that urine output be checked frequently. Should urine flow begin to decrease in the absence of hypotension, reduction of INTROPIN dosage should be considered. Multiclinic trials have shown that more than 50% of the patients were satisfactorily maintained on doses of INTROPIN less than 20 mcg/kg/minute. In patients who do not respond to these doses with adequate arterial pressures or urine flow, additional increments of INTROPIN may be employed in an effort to produce an appropriate arterial pressure and central perfusion.
3. Treatment of all patients requires constant evaluation of therapy in terms of the blood volume, augmentation of myocardial contractility, and distribution of peripheral perfusion. Dosage of INTROPIN should be adjusted according to the patient's response, with particular attention to diminution of established urine flow rate, increasing tachycardia or development of new dysrhythmias as indices for decreasing or temporarily suspending the dosage.
4. As with all potent intravenously administered drugs, care should be taken to control the rate of administration so as to avoid inadvertent administration of a bolus of drug.

Overdosage: In case of accidental overdosage, as evidenced by excessive blood pressure elevation, reduce rate of administration or temporarily discontinue INTROPIN until patient's condition stabilizes. Since INTROPIN's duration of action is quite short, no additional remedial measures are usually necessary. If these measures fail to stabilize the patient's condition, use of the short-acting alpha adrenergic blocking agent, phentolamine, should be considered.

How Supplied:
—200 mg (5 ml containing 40 mg dopamine HCl, USP per ml)
5 ml Ampul
5 ml Single-dose vial (color coded white)
5 ml RAP-ADD® Additive Syringe (color coded white)
—400 mg (5 ml containing 80 mg dopamine HCl, USP per ml)
5 ml Single-dose vial (color coded green)
5 ml RAP-ADD® Additive Syringe (color coded green)
—800 mg (5 ml containing 160 mg dopamine HCl, USP per ml)
5 ml Single-dose vial (color coded yellow)
5 ml RAP-ADD® Additive Syringe (color coded yellow)

Warning: NOT FOR DIRECT INTRAVENOUS INJECTION. MUST BE DILUTED BEFORE USE.

TRIDIL®
[tri′dil]
(nitroglycerin)

FOR INTRAVENOUS USE ONLY. NOT FOR DIRECT INTRAVENOUS INJECTION. TRIDIL® MUST BE DILUTED IN DEXTROSE (5%) INJECTION, USP OR SODIUM CHLORIDE (0.9%) INJECTION, USP PRIOR TO ITS INFUSION (SEE DOSAGE AND ADMINISTRATION SECTION). THE ADMINISTRATION SET USED FOR INFUSION WILL AFFECT THE AMOUNT OF TRIDIL DELIVERED TO THE PATIENT. (SEE WARNINGS, AND DOSAGE AND ADMINISTRATION SECTIONS).

Caution SEVERAL PREPARATIONS OF NITROGLYCERIN FOR INJECTION ARE AVAILABLE. THEY DIFFER IN CONCENTRATION AND/OR VOLUME PER VIAL. WHEN SWITCHING FROM ONE PRODUCT TO ANOTHER ATTENTION MUST BE PAID TO THE DILUTION AND DOSAGE AND ADMINISTRATION INSTRUCTIONS.

Description: TRIDIL (nitroglycerin) is a clear, practically colorless additive solution for intravenous infusion after dilution. Each ml of TRIDIL 5 mg contains 0.5 mg Nitroglycerin with 4.5 mg Lactose, USP; 10% Alcohol, USP; and 13.8 mg Monobasic Sodium Phosphate, USP as a buffer in Water for Injection, USP. Each ml of TRIDIL 25 mg or TRIDIL 50 mg contains 5 mg Nitroglycerin in 30% Alcohol, USP; 30% Propylene Glycol, USP; and Water for Injection, USP.

The solution is sterile, nonpyrogenic, and nonexplosive. TRIDIL, an organic nitrate, is a vasodilator. The chemical name for nitroglycerin is 1,2,3 propanetriol, trinitrate and its chemical structure is:

$$CH_2-ONO_2$$
$$|$$
$$CH-ONO_2$$
$$|$$
$$CH_2-ONO_2$$

$C_3H_5N_3O_9$ MOL. WT. 227.09

Clinical Pharmacology: Relaxation of vascular smooth muscle is the principal pharmacologic action of TRIDIL (nitroglycerin). Although venous effects predominate, nitroglycerin produces, in a dose-related manner, dilation of both arterial and venous beds. Dilation of the post-capillary vessels, including large veins, promotes peripheral pooling of blood and decreases venous return to the heart, reducing left ventricular end-diastolic pressure (pre-load). Arteriolar relaxation reduces systemic vascular resistance and arterial pressure (afterload). Myocardial oxygen consumption or demand (as measured by the pressure-rate product, tension-time index and stroke work index) is decreased by both the arterial and venous effects of nitroglycerin, and a more favorable supply-demand ratio can be achieved. Therapeutic doses of intravenous nitroglycerin reduce systolic, diastolic and mean arterial blood pressure. Effective coronary perfusion pressure is usually maintained, but can be compromised if blood pressure falls excessively or increased heart rate decreases diastolic filling time.

Elevated central venous and pulmonary capillary wedge pressures, pulmonary vascular resistance and systemic vascular resistance are also reduced by nitroglycerin therapy. Heart rate is usually slightly increased, presumably a reflex response to the fall in blood pressure. Cardiac index may be increased, decreased, or unchanged. Patients with elevated left ventricular filling pressure and systemic vascular resistance values in conjunction with a depressed cardiac index are likely to experience an improvement in cardiac index. On the other hand, when filling pressures and cardiac index are normal, cardiac index may be slightly reduced by intravenous nitroglycerin.

Nitroglycerin is widely distributed in the body with an apparent volume of distribution of approximately 200 liters in adult male subjects, and is rapidly metabolized to dinitrates and mononitrates, with a short half-life estimated at 1–4 minutes. This results in a low plasma concentration after intravenous infusion. At plasma concentrations of between 50 and 500 ng/ml, the binding of nitroglycerin to plasma proteins is approximately 60%, while that of 1,2 dinitroglycerin and 1,3 dinitroglycerin is 60% and 30% respectively. The activity and half-life of the dinitroglycerin metabolites are not well characterized. The mononitrate is not active.

Indications and Usage: TRIDIL is indicated for:
1. **Control of blood pressure in perioperative hypertension**, i.e., hypertension associated with surgical procedures, especially cardiovascular procedures, such as the hypertension seen during intratracheal intubation, anesthesia, skin incision, sternotomy, cardiac bypass, and in the immediate postsurgical period.
2. **Congestive Heart Failure Associated with Acute Myocardial Infarction.**
3. **Treatment of Angina Pectoris** in patients who have not responded to recommended doses of organic nitrates and/or a beta blocker.
4. **Production of controlled hypotension during surgical procedures.**

Contraindications: TRIDIL should not be administered to individuals with:
1. A known hypersensitivity to nitroglycerin or a known idiosyncratic reaction to organic nitrates.
2. Hypotension or uncorrected hypovolemia, as the use of TRIDIL in such states could produce severe hypotension or shock.
3. Increased intracranial pressure (e.g., head trauma or cerebral hemorrhage).
4. Constrictive pericarditis and pericardial tamponade.

Warnings:
1. Nitroglycerin readily migrates into many plastics. To avoid absorption of nitroglycerin into plastic parenteral solution containers, the dilution and storage of TRIDIL for intravenous infusion should be made only in *glass* parenteral solution bottles.
2. Some filters absorb nitroglycerin; they should be avoided.
3. Forty to 80% of the total amount of nitroglycerin in the final diluted solution for infusion is absorbed by the polyvinyl chloride (PVC) tubing of the intravenous administration sets currently in general use. The higher rates of absorption occur when flow rates are low, nitroglycerin concentrations are high, and the administration set is long. Although the rate of loss is highest during the early phase of infusion (when flow rates are lowest) the loss is neither constant nor self-limiting; consequently no simple calculation or correction can be performed to convert the theoretical infusion rate (based on the concentration of the infusion solution) to the actual delivery rate.

Because of this problem, American Critical Care has developed TRIDILSET® i.v. administration set and TRIDILSET V.I.P.® volumetric infusion pump connector set in which loss of TRIDIL is minimal. TRIDILSET or TRIDILSET V.I.P. are recommended for infusions of TRIDIL (see DOSAGE AND ADMINISTRATION).

Continued on next page

American Critical—Cont.

DOSING INSTRUCTIONS MUST BE FOLLOWED WITH CARE. IT SHOULD BE NOTED THAT WHEN TRIDILSET/TRIDILSET V.I.P. IS USED, THE CALCULATED DOSE WILL BE DELIVERED TO THE PATIENT BECAUSE THE LOSS OF TRIDIL DUE TO ABSORPTION IN STANDARD PVC TUBING WILL BE KEPT TO A MINIMUM. NOTE THAT THE DOSAGES COMMONLY USED IN PUBLISHED STUDIES UTILIZED GENERAL-USE PVC ADMINISTRATION SETS AND RECOMMENDED DOSES BASED ON THIS EXPERIENCE ARE TOO HIGH WHEN TRIDILSET/TRIDILSET V.I.P. IS USED.

Precautions: TRIDIL (nitroglycerin) should be used with caution in patients with severe liver or renal disease. Safety of intracoronary injection of this preparation has not been shown.

Excessive hypotension, especially for prolonged periods of time, must be avoided because of possible deleterious effects on the brain, heart, liver, and kidney from poor perfusion and the attendant risk of ischemia, thrombosis, and altered function of these organs. Paradoxical bradycardia and increased angina pectoris may accompany nitroglycerin-induced hypotension. Patients with normal or low pulmonary capillary wedge pressure are especially sensitive to the hypotensive effects of TRIDIL. If pulmonary capillary wedge pressure is being monitored, it will be noted that a fall in wedge pressure precedes the onset of arterial hypotension, and the pulmonary capillary wedge pressure is thus a useful guide to safe titration of the drug.

Carcinogenesis, mutagenesis, impairment of fertility
No long-term studies in animals were performed to evaluate carcinogenic potential of TRIDIL.

Pregnancy
Category C. Animal reproduction studies have not been conducted with TRIDIL. It is also not known whether TRIDIL can cause fetal harm when administered to a pregnant woman or can affect reproduction capacity. TRIDIL should be given to a pregnant woman only if clearly needed.

Nursing Mothers
It is not known whether nitroglycerin is excreted in human milk. Because many drugs are excreted in human milk, caution should be exercised when TRIDIL is administered to a nursing woman.

Pediatric Use
The safety and effectiveness of TRIDIL in children have not been established.

Adverse Reactions: The most frequent adverse reaction in patients treated with TRIDIL is headache, which occurs in approximately 2% of patients. Other adverse reactions occuring in less than 1% of patients are the following: tachycardia, nausea, vomiting, apprehension, restlessness, muscle twitching, retrosternal discomfort, palpitations, dizziness and abdominal pain.

The following additional adverse reactions have been reported with the oral and/or topical use of nitroglycerin: cutaneous flushing, weakness and occasionally drug rash or exfoliative dermatitis.

Overdosage: Accidental overdosage of TRIDIL may result in severe hypotension and reflex tachycardia which can be treated by elevating the legs and decreasing or temporarily terminating the infusion until the patient's condition stabilizes. Since the duration of the hemodynamic effects following TRIDIL administration is quite short, additional corrective measures are usually not required. However, if further therapy is indicated, administration of an intravenous alpha adrenergic agonist (e.g. methoxamine or phenylephrine) should be considered.

Dosage and Administration:
NOT FOR DIRECT INTRAVENOUS INJECTION
TRIDIL IS A CONCENTRATED, POTENT DRUG WHICH MUST BE DILUTED IN DEXTROSE (5%) INJECTION, USP OR SODIUM CHLORIDE (0.9%) INJECTION, USP PRIOR TO ITS INFUSION. TRIDIL SHOULD NOT BE ADMIXED WITH OTHER DRUGS.

1. Initial Dilution:
Aseptically transfer the contents of one TRIDIL ampul or vial (containing 25 or 50 mg of nitroglycerin) into a 500 ml *glass* bottle of either Dextrose (5%) Injection, USP or Sodium Chloride Injection (0.9%), USP. This yields a final concentration of 50 or 100 mcg/ml. Diluting 5 mg TRIDIL into 100 ml will also yield a final concentration of 50 mcg/ml.

2. Maintenance Dilution:
It is important to consider the fluid requirements of the patient as well as the expected duration of infusion in selecting the appropriate dilution of TRIDIL.

After the initial dosage titration, the concentration of the admixture solution may be increased, if necessary, to limit fluids given to the patient. The TRIDIL concentration should not exceed 400 mcg/ml. See chart.

Note: If the concentration is adjusted, it is imperative to flush TRIDILSET®/TRIDILSET VIP® before a new concentration is utilized. The deadspace of the set is approximately 15 ml, and depending on the flow rate it could take from 10 minutes to 3 hours for the new concentration to reach the patient if the set were not flushed. Invert the glass parenteral bottle several times following admixture to assure uniform dilution of TRIDIL. When stored in *glass* containers, the diluted solution is physically and chemically stable for up to 48 hours at room temperature, and up to seven days under refrigeration.

Dosage is affected by the type of container and administration set used. See WARNINGS.

Although the usual starting adult dose range reported in clinical studies was 25 mcg/min or more, these studies used PVC ADMINISTRATION SETS. THE USE OF NON-ABSORBING TUBING WILL RESULT IN THE NEED FOR REDUCED DOSES.

If a peristaltic action infusion pump is used, a TRIDILSET i.v. administration set should be selected. As the TRIDILSET drip chamber delivers approximately 60 microdrops/ml, the TRIDIL DILUTION AND ADMINISTRATION TABLE below may be used to calculate TRIDIL dilution and admixture flow rate in microdrops/minute to achieve the desired TRIDIL administration rate. If a volumetric infusion pump is used, a TRIDILSET V.I.P. volumetric infusion pump connector set should be selected. The TRIDIL DILUTION AND ADMINISTRATION TABLE below may still be used; however, admixture flow rate will be determined directly by the infusion pump and is independent of the drop size of the TRIDILSET V.I.P. drip chamber, which is approximately 15 drops/ml. Thus, the reference to "MICRODROPS/MIN" is not applicable and the corresponding flow rate in ML/HR should be used to determine pump settings. NOTE: the TRIDILSET V.I.P. is not intended for use as an i.v. administration set independent of a volumetric infusion pump.

The dosage for TRIDILSET/TRIDILSET VIP should initially be 5 mcg/min delivered through an infusion pump capable of exact and constant delivery of the drug. Subsequent titration must be adjusted to the clinical situation, with dose increments becoming more cautious as partial response is seen. Initial titration should be in 5 mcg/min increments with increases every 3–5 minutes until some response is noted. If no response is seen at 20 mcg/min, increments of 10 and later 20 mcg/min can be used. Once a partial blood pressure response is observed, the dose increase should be reduced and the interval between increases should be lengthened. Some patients with normal or low left ventricular filling pressures or pulmonary capillary wedge pressure (e.g. angina patients without other complications) may be hypersensitive to the effects of TRIDIL and may respond fully to doses as small as 5 mcg/min. These patients require especially careful titration and monitoring.

There is no fixed optimum dose of TRIDIL. Due to variations in the responsiveness of individual patients to the drug, each patient must be titrated to the desired level of hemodynamic function. Therefore, continuous monitoring of physiologic parameters (e.g. blood pressure and heart rate in all patients, other measurement such as pulmonary capillary wedge pressure, as appropriate MUST BE PERFORMED to achieve the correct dose. Adequate systemic blood pressure and coronary perfusion pressure must be maintained.

How Supplied:
NDC 0094-0073-10, 5 mg-10 ml ampul.
NDC 0094-0085-05, 25 mg-5 ml ampul.
NDC 0094-0085-86, 25 mg-5 ml single use vial.
NDC 0094-0090-10, 50 mg-10 ml ampul.
NDC 0094-0090-66, 50 mg-10 ml single use vial.
Protect from freezing.

[See table below].

TRIDIL DILUTION AND ADMINISTRATION TABLE

TRIDILSET ADMIXTURE FLOW RATE MICRO DROPS/ MIN = ML/HR	DILUTE 5 MG TRIDIL IN 100 ML OR 25 MG TRIDIL IN 500 ML	5 MG TRIDIL IN 50 ML OR 25 MG TRIDIL IN 250 ML OR 50 MG TRIDIL IN 500 ML	10 MG TRIDIL IN 50 ML OR 50 MG TRIDIL IN 250 ML OR 100 MG TRIDIL IN 500 ML	100 MG TRIDIL IN 250 ML OR 200 MG TRIDIL IN 500 ML
	TO YIELD			
	50 MCG/ML	100 MCG/ML	200 MCG/ML	400 MCG/ML
	TRIDIL ADMINISTRATION RATE MCG I.V. NITROGLYCERIN/MIN			
3	—		5	10	20
6	5	10	20	40
12	10	20	40	80
24	20	40	80	160
48	40	80	160	320
72	60	120	240	480
96	80	160	320	640

American Dermal Corporation
12 WORLDS FAIR DRIVE
SOMERSET, NJ 08873

DRITHOCREME® ℞
(anthralin) 0.1%, 0.25%, 0.5%, 1.0% (HP)

Description: Drithocreme is a pale yellow topical cream containing 0.1%, 0.25%, 0.5% or 1.0% anthralin USP in a base of white petrolatum, sodium lauryl sulfate, cetostearyl alcohol, ascorbic acid, salicylic acid, chlorocresol and purified water.
The chemical name of anthralin is 1,8,dihydroxy-9-anthrone or 1,8,9-trihydroxyanthracene.

Clinical Pharmacology: Although the precise mechanism of anthralin's anti-psoriatic action is not fully understood, in vitro evidence suggests that its antimitotic effect results from inhibition of DNA synthesis. Additionally, the chemically reducing properties of anthralin may upset oxidative metabolic processes, providing a further slowing down of epidermal mitosis.
Absorption in man has not been finally determined, but in a limited clinical study of Drithocreme, no traces of anthraquinone metabolites were detected in the urine of subjects treated.

Indications and Usage: An aid in the topical treatment of quiescent or chronic psoriasis. Treatment should be continued until the skin is entirely clear i.e. when there is nothing to feel with the fingers and the texture is normal.

Contraindications: In patients with acute psoriatic eruptions or a history or hypersensitivity to any of the ingredients.

Warnings: Avoid contact with the eyes or mucous membranes. Exercise care when applying Drithocreme to the face or intertriginous skin areas. Discontinue use if a sensitivity reaction occurs or if excessive irritation develops on uninvolved skin areas.

Precautions: For external use only. Keep out of the reach of children. To prevent the possibility of staining clothing or bed linen while gaining experience in using Drithocreme, it may be advisable to use protective dressings. To prevent the possibility of discoloration of the bath/shower, particularly where Drithocreme HP (1.0%) has been used, always rinse the bath/shower with hot water immediately after washing/showering and then use a household cleanser to remove any deposit on the surface of the bath or shower. Always wash hands thoroughly after use. Long-term studies in animals have not been performed to evaluate the carcinogenic potential of the drug. Although anthralin has been found to have tumor-promoting properties on mouse skin, there have been no reports to suggest carcinogenic effects in humans after many years of clinical use.

Pregnancy: Pregnancy Category C. Animal reproduction studies have not been conducted with Drithocreme. It is also not known whether Drithocreme can cause fetal harm when administered to a pregnant woman or can effect reproduction capacity. Drithocreme should be given to a pregnant woman only if clearly needed.

Nursing Mothers: It is not known whether this drug is excreted in human milk. Because many drugs are excreted in milk and because of the potential for tumorigenicity shown for anthralin in animal studies, a decision should be made whether to discontinue nursing or to discontinue the drug, taking into account the importance of the drug to the mother.

Pediatric Use: Safety in children has not been specifically established.

Adverse Reactions: Very few instances of contact allergic reactions to anthralin have been reported. However, transient primary irritation of uninvolved skin surrounding the treated lesions is more frequently seen. If the initial treatment produces excessive soreness or if the lesions spread, reduce frequency of application and, in extreme cases, discontinue use and consult physician. Some temporary discoloration of hair and fingernails may arise during the period of treatment but should be minimized by careful application.

Dosage and Administration: Generally, it is recommended that Drithocreme be applied once a day. The irritant potential of anthralin is directly related to the strength being used and each patient's individual tolerance. Therefore, where the response to anthralin treatment has not previously been established, always commence treatment for at least one week using 0.1% Drithocreme. Increase to the 0.25%, 0.5% or 1.0% (HP) strengths if appropriate.
Drithocreme should normally be applied once daily and removed by washing or showering. The optimal period of contact will vary according to the strength used and the patient's response to treatment.

For The Skin: Apply sparingly only to the psoriatic lesions and rub gently and carefully into the skin until absorbed. It is most important to avoid applying an excessive quantity which may cause unnecessary soiling and staining of the clothing and/or bed linen. At the end of each period of treatment, a bath or shower should be taken to remove any surplus cream which may have become red/brown in color. The margins of the lesions may gradually become stained purple/brown as treatment progresses, but this will disappear after cessation of treatment.

For The Scalp: Shampoo to remove scalar debris and any previous application. Dry the hair and, after suitably parting, rub the cream well into the lesions. Care should be taken to avoid application of the cream to uninvolved scalp margins. Remove any unintended residue which may be deposited behind the ears.
Keep tightly capped when not in use.
Store in a cool place (46°–59°F)

How Supplied: 50g tubes
Drithocreme 0.1%   NDC 51201-0029-1
Drithocreme 0.25%   NDC 51201-0028-1
Drithocreme 0.5%   NDC 51201-0027-1
Drithocreme HP 1.0% NDC 51201-0026-1

Caution: Federal law prohibits dispensing without prescription.

Revised 5/84
AMERICAN DERMAL CORPORATION
Somerset, New Jersey 08873

DRITHO-SCALP™ ℞
(anthralin) 0.25%, 0.5%

Description: Dritho-Scalp is a pale yellow topical cream containing 0.25% or 0.5% anthralin USP in a base of white petrolatum, mineral oil, sodium lauryl sulfate, cetostearyl alcohol, ascorbic acid, salicylic acid, chlorocresol and purified water.
The chemical name of anthralin is 1,8,dihydroxy-9-anthrone.
The structural formula is:

Clinical Pharmacology: Although the precise mechanism of anthralin's anti-psoriatic action is not fully understood, in vitro evidence suggests that its antimitotic effect results from inhibition of DNA synthesis. Additionally, the chemically reducing properties of anthralin may upset oxidative metabolic processes, providing a further slowing down of epidermal mitosis.
Absorption in man has not been finally determined.

Indications and Usage: An aid in the topical treatment of quiescent or chronic psoriasis of the scalp. Treatment should be continued until the skin is entirely clear i.e. when there is nothing to feel with the fingers and the texture is normal.

Contraindications: In patients with acute eruptions or a history of hypersensitivity to any of the ingredients.

Warnings: Avoid contact with the eyes or mucous membranes. Discontinue use if a sensitivity reaction occurs or if excessive irritation develops on uninvolved skin areas.

Precautions: For external use only. Keep out of the reach of children. Dritho-Scalp may stain the hair and should be applied sparingly and carefully to psoriasis lesions only. Contact with fabrics, plastics and other materials may cause staining and should be avoided. To prevent the possibility of discoloration, always rinse the bath/shower with hot water immediately after washing/showering and then use a suitable cleanser to remove any deposit on the surface of the bath or shower. Always wash hands thoroughly after use. Long-term studies in animals have not been performed to evaluate the carcinogenic potential of the drug. Although anthralin has been found to have tumor-promoting properties on mouse skin, there have been no reports to suggest carcinogenic effects in humans after many years of clinical use.

Pregnancy: Pregnancy Category C. Animal reproduction studies have not been conducted with Dritho-Scalp. It is also not known whether Dritho-Scalp can cause fetal harm when administered to a pregnant woman or can affect reproduction capacity. Dritho-Scalp should be given to a pregnant woman only if clearly needed.

Nursing Mothers: It is not known whether this drug is excreted in human milk. Because many drugs are excreted in milk and because of the potential for tumorigenicity shown for anthralin in animal studies, a decision should be made whether to discontinue nursing or to discontinue the drug, taking into account the importance of the drug to the mother.

Pediatric Use: Safety in children has not been specifically established.

Adverse Reactions: Very few instances of contact allergic reactions to anthralin have been reported. However, transient primary irritation of uninvolved skin surrounding the treated lesions is more frequently seen. If the initial treatment produces excessive soreness or if the lesions spread, reduce frequency of application and, in extreme cases, discontinue use and consult physician. Some temporary discoloration of hair and fingernails may arise during the period of treatment but should be minimized by careful application.

Dosage and Administration: Before initial use, the tube membrane should be pierced by inverting the white cap, which should then be discarded. The black applicator should then be screwed firmly onto the tube. This applicator includes a black cap which should always be replaced between treatments (see illustration). Generally, it is recommended that Dritho-Scalp be applied once a day. The irritant potential of anthralin is directly related to the strength being used and each patient's individual tolerance. Therefore, where the response to anthralin treatment has not previously been established, always commence treatment for at least one week using 0.25% Dritho-Scalp. Increase to the 0.5% strength only if appropriate.

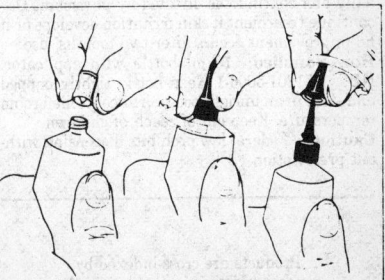

Dritho-Scalp should normally be applied once daily and removed by washing or showering. The optimal period of contact will vary according to the

Continued on next page

American Dermal—Cont.

strength used and the patient's response to treatment.

Comb the hair to remove scalar debris and, after suitably parting, apply Dritho-Scalp only to the lesions and rub in well, taking care to prevent the cream spreading onto the forehead. **Keep Dritho-Scalp well away from the eyes.** Avoid application of the cream to uninvolved scalp margins. Remove any unintended residue which may be deposited behind the ears. At the end of each period of contact, wash the hair and scalp to remove any surplus cream (which may have become red/brown in color). **Always wash hands thoroughly after use.** Store in a cool place (46°—59°F)
How Supplied: 50g tube with special applicator
Dritho-Scalp 0.25% NDC 51201-0024-1
Dritho-Scalp 0.5% NDC 51201-0023-1
Caution: Federal law prohibits dispensing without prescription.
Printed 9/84
Distributed by:
AMERICAN DERMAL CORPORATION
Somerset, New Jersey 08873

VIRANOL™

Description: Viranol™ is a solution for topical application containing 16.7% Salicylic Acid U.S.P., and 16.7% Lactic Acid U.S.P. in a vehicle of Flexible Collodion U.S.P.
Action: The active ingredients, Salicylic Acid and Lactic Acid are believed to exert a keratolytic action which effects the removal of wart epidermal cells infected by deoxyribonucleic acid viruses.
Indications: Viranol™ is indicated as an aid in the treatment and removal of plantar warts and other common warts.
Contraindications: Viranol™ should not be used by diabetics or individuals with impaired blood circulation.
Warnings: Viranol™ should not be applied to moles, birthmarks, unusual warts with protruding hair, genital warts, or warts on the face.
Precautions: Viranol™ is for external use only. Discontinue use if excessive irritation occurs on normal skin areas. Avoid contact with eyes or on mucous membranes. If contact with eyes or mucous membranes should occur, flush with water to remove Collodion film and continue rinsing for an additional 15 minutes. Viranol™ is highly flammable and should not be used or stored near fire or flame. Avoid inhaling vapors.
Adverse Reactions: Viranol™ may cause local irritation on normal skin. Care should be used to avoid contact with normal surrounding skin areas while applying Viranol™ directly to wart.
Dosage and Administration: Wash affected area and soak wart in hot water for 5 minutes. Dry thoroughly, then gently remove softened area of the wart by rubbing with a pumice stone, emery board or washcloth. Using the special applicator provided, apply 2 to 4 drops to the wart only. Keep Viranol™ away from surrounding skin (preferably by encircling the wart with a ring of petrolatum). Allow to dry before covering with a waterproof bandage. Repeat the above procedure once daily and continue as directed by physician. Discontinue treatment if skin irritation develops or if no improvement occurs after two months' use.
How Supplied: 10 ml bottle with applicator. NDC #51201-5006-1 Keep bottle tightly capped and store in an upright position at controlled room temperature. Keep out of reach of children.
Caution: Federal law prohibits dispensing without prescription.

Products are cross-indexed by generic and chemical names in the **YELLOW SECTION**

Arco Pharmaceuticals, Inc.
**105 ORVILLE DRIVE
BOHEMIA, NY 11716**

ARCO-LASE®
(broad pH spectrum digestant)

Composition: Each soft, mint flavored tablet contains Trizyme*, 38 mg., and Lipase, 25 mg.
*Contains the following standardized enzymes: amylolytic 30 mg.; proteolytic 6 mg.; cellulolytic 2 mg.
Action and Uses: Indicated for most gastrointestinal disorders due to poor digestion. Flatulence, gas and bloating, dyspepsia, distention, fullness, heartburn, or in any condition where normal digestion is impaired by digestive insufficiencies. Arcolase provides the highest standardized enzymatic activity, plus the protective action of the widest pH range. Thus it is effective throughout the entire G.I. tract. Requiring no enteric coating, there is assurance of a positive breakdown of its factors. This is advantageous, because quite often patients with digestive disorders cannot digest their food properly, let alone hard, or enteric coated capsules or tablets.
Side Effects: None.
Administration and Dosage: One tablet with or immediately following meals. Tablet may be swallowed or chewed.
Supplied: Bottles of 50's. NDC 275-4040.

ARCO–LASE® PLUS

Composition: Same as Arco-Lase, plus the addition of Hyoscyamine sulfate 0.10 mg., atropine sulfate 0.02 mg. and phenobarbital 1/8 gr. (Warning: may be habit forming.)
Action and Uses: Gastrointestinal disturbances, such as cramps, bloating, spasms, diarrhea, nausea, vomiting and peptic ulcer. The enzymes correct the digestive insufficiencies.
The antispasmodic and phenobarbital contribute to the symptomatic relief of hypermotility and nervous tension, which usually accompanies functional disturbances of the bowel.
Administration and Dosage: One tablet following meals.
Side Effects: May cause rapid pulse, dryness of mouth and blurred vision.
Contraindications: This product is contraindicated in the presence of glaucoma or prostatic hypertrophy.
Supplied: Bottles of 50's. NDC 275-45-45.
Literature Available: Yes.

CODEXIN™ Capsules
(See PDR For Nonprescription Drugs)

MEGA-B®
(super potency vitamin B complex, sugar & starch free)

Composition: Each Mega-B Tablet contains the following Mega Vitamins:

B₁ (Thiamine Mononitrate)	100 mg.
B₂ (Riboflavin)	100 mg.
B₆ (Pyridoxine Hydrochloride)	100 mg.
B₁₂ (Cyanocobalamin)	100 mcg.
Choline Bitartrate	100 mg.
Inositol	100 mg.
Niacinamide	100 mg.
Folic Acid	100 mcg.
Pantothenic Acid	100 mg.
d-Biotin	100 mcg.
Para-Aminobenzoic Acid (PABA)	100 mg.

In a base of yeast to provide the identified and unidentified B-Complex Factors.
Advantages: Each Mega-B capsule-shaped tablet provides the highest vitamin B complex available in a single dose.
Mega-B was designed for those patients who require truly Mega vitamin potencies with the convenience of minimum dosage.
Indications: Mega-B is indicated in conditions characterized by depletions or increased demand of the water-soluble B-complex vitamins. It may be useful in the nutritional management of patients during prolonged convalescence associated with major surgery. It is also indicated for stress conditions, as an adjunct to antibiotics and diuretic therapy, pre and post operative cases, liver conditions, gastro-intestinal disorders interffering with intake or absorbtion of water-soluble vitamins, prolonged or wasting diseases, diabetes, burns, fractures, severe infections, and some psychological disorders.
Warning: NOT INTENDED FOR TREATMENT OF PERNICIOUS ANEMIA, OR OTHER PRIMARY OR SECONDARY ANEMIAS.
Dosage: Usual dosage is one Mega-B tablet daily, or varied, depending on clinical needs.
Supplied: Yellow capsule shaped tablets in bottles of 30, 100 and 500.

MEGADOSE™
(multiple mega-vitamin formula with minerals, sugar and starch free)

Composition:

Vitamin A	25,000 USP Units
Vitamin D	1,000 USP Units
Vitamin C w/Rose Hips	250 mg.
Vitamin E	100 IU
Folic Acid	400 mcg.
Vitamin B₁	80 mg.
Vitamin B₂	80 mg.
Niacinamide	80 mg.
Vitamin B₆	80 mg.
Vitamin B₁₂	80 mcg.
Biotin	80 mcg.
Pantothenic Acid	80 mg.
Choline Bitartrate	80 mg.
Inositol	80 mg.
Para-Aminobenzoic Acid	80 mg.
Rutin	30 mg.
Citrus Bioflavonoids	30 mg.
Betaine Hydrochloride	30 mg.
Glutamic Acid	30 mg.
Hesperidin Complex	5 mg.
Iodine (from Kelp)	0.15 mg.
Calcium Gluconate*	50 mg.
Zinc Gluconate*	25 mg.
Potassium Gluconate*	10 mg.
Ferrous Gluconate*	10 mg.
Magnesium Gluconate*	7 mg.
Manganese Gluconate*	6 mg.
Copper Gluconate*	0.5 mg.

*Natural mineral chelates in a base containing natural ingredients.
Dosage: One tablet daily.
Supplied: Capsule shaped tablets in bottles of 30, 100 and 250.

Ar-Ex Products Co.
**1036 WEST VAN BUREN STREET
CHICAGO, IL 60607**

AR-EX HYPO–ALLERGENIC COSMETICS

Composition: Formulated so you can prescribe cosmetics as you prescribe medications or other therapeutic regimen in dermatological, respiratory, gastrointestinal and other allergies where usual cosmetics are contraindicated.
Action and Uses: To provide safe beauty aids and eliminate a whole field of potential irritants and sensitizers that may aggravate or precipitate allergic conditions, as: skin irritations and erythema, contact dermatitis, photosensitivity, dry, chapped skin, lipstick cheilitis, eyelid dermatitis, chronic coryza, chronic vasomotor rhinitis, chronic conjunctivitis, asthma, urticaria, colitis and other G-I symptoms, also other conditions where cosmetics may be prime or contributing offenders.
Unscented Cosmetics: Perfumes, natural or synthetic, and essential oils are known to be capable of irritating the skin, causing Berloque derma-

titis (photosensitivity), and causing or aggravating respiratory symptoms simulating asthma and hay fever. For these persons, all AR-EX Cosmetics are available Unscented, and contain absolutely no perfume, natural or synthetic.

A Complete Line: Following is a list of AR-EX Cosmetics, together with a partial list of potential irritants and allergens which they do NOT contain. When these substances are suspected etiological agents, you can rule them out of your diagnoses when you prescribe AR-EX Cosmetics *by brand name.*

Creams and Lotions: Contain no soap, almond oil, oil of orris, coconut oil, bergamot or other citrus oils, lanolin, cocoa butter, karaya gum, gum arabic, tragacanth, rose water or phenol. Unscented.

Deodorants: Cream, Spray and Roll-On. Contain no aluminum chloride, aluminum chlorhydroxide, aluminum acetate, aluminum sulfate, alum, salicylic acid, formaldehyde, alcohol or hexachlorophene.

Eye Makeup: Contain no lanolin, indelible or aniline dyes, perfume, turpentine, bergamot or other photosensitizers, chromium or nickel compounds, or pharaphenylenediamine.

Hair Preparations: Contain no soap, lanolin, sulfonated oil, palm or coconut oil, gum karaya, gum arabic, tragacanth, resin, lacquer, shellac. Unscented.

Powders: Contain no orris root, oil of orris, bergamot or other citrus oils, corn starch, rice starch, wheat starch, powdered gums or lanolin.

Soap: Low in excess alkali, superfatted. Contains no lanolin, perfumes, essential oils.

Foundation Lotion: Liquid makeup. Contains no gum acacia, karaya or tragacanth, lanolin, corn oil or other vegetable oils, oil of orris, perfumes or essential oils.

AR-EX Special Formula Lipstick: Contains no indelible dyes, eosin, mono-di-tri-or-tetra-bromfluorescein compounds, but achieves shades through use of lake pigments. Contains no perfumes or essential oils, lanolin, almond oil or cocoa butter.

Literature Available: For precise prescription of hypo-allergenic cosmetics in indicated conditions, refer to the AR-EX Professional Formulary. Sent on request.

SAFE SUDS

Composition: Hypo-allergenic, all-purpose detergent for patients whose hands or respiratory membranes are irritated by soaps or detergents. For dishes, laundry, floors, rugs, upholstery, etc. Suds in hard or soft water, with pH approximately 6.8. Contains no enzymes, phosphates, lanolin, fillers or bleaches. Biodegradable. NOT scented.

Arlo Interamerican Corp. of P.R.
**212 MAYAQUEZ STREET
HATO REY, P.R. 00917**

GUMSOL™   OTC
[gem' sol]
**Solution & Spray
Effective Treatment for the Oral Cavity**

Composition: Each 30 ml contains: Cetyl Pyridinium chloride (1: 1500 soln) 20mg; Benzocaine 600mg; Thymol 25mg; Menthol 23mg; Oil Peppermint 0.3ml; Glycerin 3 ml; Alcohol 65%; Tannic Acid 300mg.

Action and Uses: A cooling, soothing, quickdrying solution having germicidal, fungicidal, anesthethic, astringent and healing properties used in the treatment of: Teething Pain-Gingivitis- Trench Mouth- Herpes Simplex- Aphthous Stomatitis- Thrush- Denture Irritations- and Throat Irritations (as mouth wash or gargle).

Warnings: Do not use near the eyes. Keep this and all medications out of the reach of children.

Administration and Dosage: Solution: Topical Administration: Dry area and apply several times a day with cotton applicator. As Gargle or Mouth Wash: Dilute a 1/2 teaspoonful in 1/2 glass of warm water several times a day. Spray: Dry affected area with absorbent cotton, spray Gumsol three or four times a day.

How Supplied: Gumsol Solution is supplied in 1 fl oz. glass bottle (NDC 11475-703-01) and in 1 fl oz. bottle with spray applicator (NDC 11475-704-01).

KARBOKOFF™ Tablets   ℞
[kar-bō' koff]

Composition: Each tablet contains: Pancreatin 150mg; Ox Bile Salts 100mg; Activated Charcoal 150mg.

Actions: Pancreatin has three components: trypsin, amylase and lipase. Trypsin breaks down larger protein fractions into peptides; amylase converts starch into maltose; lipase splits fats into fatty acids and glycerin. Bile salts not only enhance the fat splitting action of lipase but also aids in the emulsification of fats and the absorbtion of fatty acids. The activated charcoal eliminates flatulence or belching associated with gastrointestinal disturbances.

Indications and Usage: Karbokoff is indicated as a digestive aid for the relief of flatulence and belching associated with incomplete digestion of food due to a deficiency of digestive enzymes.

Contraindications: Biliary tract obstruction. Hypersensitivity to any of its ingredients.

Adverse Reactions: Rash may occur in patients hypersensitive to any of its ingredients.

Dosage and Administration: Two tablets after meals or as directed by physician.

How Supplied: Karbokoff Tablets is supplied in bottles of 60 (NDC 11475-192-60).

OTICOL™   ℞
[o-ti' kōl]
Sterile Ear Drops

Composition: Each ml. contains; Hydrocortisone 0.5%; Pramoxine HCl 1.0%; Domiphen Bromide 0.1%; Parachlorometaxilenol 0.05% in a vehicle containing Propylene Glycol and Distilled Water.

Actions: Oticol is effective due to Hydrocortisone: Anti-inflammatory hormone; Pramoxine HCl: Potent topical anesthetic; Domiphen Bromide: Quaternary ammonium compound having bactericidal activity against a variety of gram positive and gram negative organisms; having also anti-fungal activity. (Blood and pus reduce its activity and its incompatible with soap.) Parachlorometaxilenol: Topical antiseptic.

Indications: An anti-inflammatory, antimicrobial preparation for use in the treatment of otitis externa caused by susceptible organisms.

Contraindications: Oticol is contraindicated in tuberculous and viral lesions and in persons who have shown sensitivity to any of its components.

Precautions: Oticol should be used with caution in the presence of perforated ear drums and long-standing otitis media because of the danger of ototoxicity. Care should be exercised to avoid contamination of the material during its use. Prolonged use may result in overgrowth of non-susceptible organisms.

Dosage: For topical use only. The external ear canal should be cleansed as thoroughly as possible, then dried. Apply 2-3 drops directly into the canal with sterile cotton that has been moistened with the solution. For the first few days, the cleansing application should be carried out three or four times daily. Thereafter, 2 or 4 drops in the affected ear, 2 or 3 times daily. Severe or chronic infections should be supplemented by systemic therapy.

How Supplied: Oticol Sterile ear drops is supplied in 5 ml plastic bottle with dropper tip (NDC 11475-911-11).

PRE-PROTEIN™   OTC
[pre' pro-tēn]
Liquid Predigested Proteins

Composition: Each 30 ml supplies (approximately) the following amino acids: Arginine 1180-1350mg; Lysine 585-780mg; Threonine 270-390mg; Leucine 420-525mg; Isoleucine 195-270mg; Phenylalanine 165-390mg; Methionine 105-130mg; Valine 315-510mg; Histidine 315-510 mg. Supplemented with Tryptophane 65mg. Each serving provides protein 15gm; calories 90; carbohydrates 0. The protein content is 23% of the US RDA.

Actions: Pre-Protein is a liquid predigested protein; a dietary supplement of proteins providing all essential amino acids. This products contains no sugar, fats, nor carbohydrates.

Indications: Pre-Protein is indicated as a dietary supplement of proteins in persons where the protein intake is reduced or where the protein requirements are increased.

Advantages: The protein used in this product is a predigested protein and is therefore utilized 100%. Prepared by hydrolyzing the animal protein collagen.

Warnings: Do not use for weight reduction or maintenance without medical supervision. Do not use without medical advise if you are taking prescription medications. Not for use by infants, children, pregnant or nursing mothers."

Dosage: Two tablespoonfuls daily as a dietary supplement to provide 15 gm of protein. Shake well before using.

How Supplied: Pre-Protein is supplied in 8 oz. bottles. (NDC 11475-533-08) and in 16 oz bottles (NDC 11475-533-16).

Armour Pharmaceutical Company
**303 SOUTH BROADWAY
TARRYTOWN, NY 10591**

H.P. ACTHAR® GEL*   ℞
[ăch pē ăk' thär jěl]
(repository corticotropin injection)
and
ACTHAR®   ℞
(corticotropin for injection)

Description: H.P. ACTHAR® GEL (Repository Corticotropin Injection) is a highly purified sterile preparation of the adrenocorticotropic hormone in 16% gelatin to provide a prolonged release after intramuscular or subcutaneous injection.
ACTHAR® (Corticotropin for Injection) is a sterile lyophilized ACTH which in dry form is stable at room temperature. Each vial contains 25 or 40 Units of Corticotropin U.S.P. and approximately 9 and 14 milligrams of hydrolyzed gelatin respectively. After reconstitution, this product is administered in the intravenous, intramuscular, or subcutaneous route.

Clinical Pharmacology: ACTH stimulates the adrenal cortex to secrete cortisol, corticosterone, aldosterone, and a number of weakly androgenic substances. Although ACTH does stimulate secretion of aldosterone, the rate is relatively independent. Prolonged administration of large doses of ACTH induces hyperplasia and hypertrophy of the adrenal cortex and continuous high output of cortisol, corticosterone, and weak androgens. The release of ACTH is under the influence of the nervous system via the corticotropin regulatory hormone released from the hypothalamus and by a negative corticosteroid feedback mechanism. Elevated plasma cortisol suppresses ACTH release. The trophic effects of ACTH on the adrenal cortex are not understood beyond the fact that they appear to be mediated by cyclic AMP.
ACTH rapidly disappears from the circulation following its intravenous administration; in man the plasma half-life is about 15 minutes.
The maximal effects of a trophic hormone on a target organ are achieved when optimal amounts of hormone are acting continuously. Thus, a fixed dose of ACTH will demonstrate a linear increase in adrenocortical secretion with increasing duration of the infusion.

Continued on next page

Armour—Cont.

Indications and Usage: ACTHAR® (Corticotropin for Injection) and H.P. ACTHAR® GEL (Repository Corticotropin Injection) are indicated for diagnostic testing of adrenocortical function.
ACTHAR® (Corticotropin for Injection) and H.P. ACTHAR® GEL (Repository Corticotropin Injection) have limited therapeutic value in those conditions responsive to corticosteroid therapy; in such case, corticosteroid therapy is considered to be the treatment of choice. ACTHAR® (Corticotropin for Injection) and H.P. ACTHAR® GEL (Repository Corticotropin Injection) may be employed in the following disorders:

ENDOCRINE DISORDERS: Nonsuppurative thyroiditis; Hypercalcemia associated with cancer.

NERVOUS SYSTEM DISEASES: Acute exacerbations of multiple sclerosis.

RHEUMATIC DISORDERS: As adjunctive therapy for short-term administration (to tide the patient over an acute episode or exacerbation) in:
Psoriatic arthritis; Rheumatoid arthritis, including juvenile rheumatoid arthritis (selected cases may require low-dose maintenance therapy); Ankylosing spondylitis; Acute and subacute bursitis; Acute nonspecific tenosynovitis; Acute gouty arthritis; Post-traumatic arthritis; Synovitis of osteoarthritis; Epicondylitis.

COLLAGEN DISEASES: During an exacerbation or as maintenance therapy in selected cases of: Systemic lupus erythematosus; Systemic dermatomyositis (polymyositis); Acute rheumatic carditis.

DERMATOLOGIC DISEASES: Pemphigus; Bullous dermatitis herpetiformis; Severe erythema multiforme (Stevens-Johnson syndrome); Exfoliative dermatitis; Severe psoriasis; Severe seborrheic dermatitis; Mycosis fungoides.

ALLERGIC STATES: Control of severe or incapacitating allergic conditions intractable to adequate trials of conventional treatment—
Seasonal or perennial allergic rhinitis; Bronchial asthma; Contact dermatitis; Atopic dermatitis; Serum sickness.

OPHTHALMIC DISEASES: Severe acute and chronic allergic and inflammatory processes involving the eye and its adnexa such as:
Allergic conjunctivitis; Keratitis; Herpes zoster ophthalmicus; Iritis and iridocyclitis; Diffuse posterior uveitis and choroiditis; Optic neuritis; Sympathetic ophthalmia; Chorioretinitis; Anterior segment inflammation; Allergic corneal marginal ulcers.

RESPIRATORY DISEASES: Symptomatic sarcoidosis; Loeffler's syndrome not manageable by other means; Berylliosis; Fulminating or disseminated pulmonary tuberculosis when used concurrently with antituberculous chemotherapy; Aspiration pneumonitis.

HEMATOLOGIC DISORDERS: Acquired (autoimmune) hemolytic anemia; Secondary thrombocytopenia in adults; Erythroblastopenia (RBC anemia); Congenital (erythroid) hypoplastic anemia.

NEOPLASTIC DISEASES: For palliative management of:
Leukemias and lymphomas in adults; Acute leukemia of childhood.

EDEMATOUS STATE: To induce a diuresis or a remission of proteinuria in the nephrotic syndrome without uremia of the idiopathic type or that due to lupus erythematosus.

GASTROINTESTINAL DISEASES: To tide the patient over a critical period of the disease in: Ulcerative colitis; Regional enteritis.

MISCELLANEOUS: Tuberculous meningitis with subarachnoid block or impending block when used concurrently with appropriate anti-tuberculous chemotherapy; Trichinosis with neurologic or myocardial involvement.

Contraindications: Corticotropin is contraindicated in patients with scleroderma, osteoporosis, systemic fungal infections, ocular herpes simplex, recent surgery, history of or the presence of a peptic ulcer, congestive heart failure, hypertension, or sensitivity to proteins of porcine origin.

Treatment of conditions listed within the indication section (see above) is contraindicated when they are accompanied by primary adrenocortical insufficiency or adrenocortical hyperfunction.

Intravenous administration of corticotropin is contraindicated for treatment of conditions listed within the indications section, but Acthar is used intravenously for diagnostic purposes (see DOSAGE AND ADMINISTRATION).

Warnings: Chronic administration of corticotropin may lead to adverse effects which are not reversible. Corticotropin may only suppress symptoms and signs of chronic diseases without altering the natural course of the disease. Neither H.P. ACTHAR® GEL (Repository Corticotropin Injection) nor ACTHAR® (Corticotropin for Injection) should be administered for treatment until adrenal responsiveness has been verified with the route of administration which will be utilized during treatment, intramuscularly or subcutaneously. A rise in urinary and plasma corticosteroid values provides direct evidence of a stimulatory effect. Prolonged administration of corticotropin increases the risk of hypersensitivity reactions. Although the action of corticotropin is similar to that of exogenous adrenocortical steroids the quantity of adrenocorticoid may be variable. In patients who receive prolonged corticotropin therapy the additional use of rapidly acting corticosteroids before, during, and after an unusual stressful situation is indicated.

Prolonged use of corticotropin may produce posterior subcapsular cataracts and glaucoma with possible damage to the optic nerves.

Corticotropin may mask some signs of infection, and new infections including those of the eye due to fungi or viruses may appear during its use. There may be decreased resistance and inability to localize infection when corticotropin is used.

Corticotropin can cause elevation of blood pressure, salt and water retention, and increased excretion of potassium. Dietary salt restriction and potassium supplementation may be necessary. Corticotropin increases calcium excretion.

While on corticotropin therapy, patients should not be vaccinated against smallpox. Other immunization procedures should be undertaken with caution in patients who are receiving corticotropin, especially when high doses are administered because of the possible hazards of neurological complications and lack of antibody response.

Precautions:
1. General
Corticotropin injection should be used in the lowest dose for the shortest period of time to accomplish the therapeutic goal. Corticotropin should be used for treatment only when the disease is intractable to non-steroid treatment.
There is an enhanced effect in patients with hypothyroidism and in those with cirrhosis of the liver. Sensitivity to porcine protein should be considered before starting therapy and during the course of treatment should symptoms arise.
When an infection is present, appropriate antibiotic therapy should be given. Patients with latent tuberculosis should be observed closely and if therapy is prolonged, chemoprophylaxis should be instituted.
Psychic symptoms may appear with use of corticotropin or pre-existing symptoms may be enhanced. These may range from mood alteration to a psychotic state.
Patients with a secondary disease may have that disease worsened. Caution should be used when prescribing corticotropin in patients with diabetes, renal insufficiency, diverticulitis, and myasthenia gravis.
Corticotropin often acts by suppressing symptoms without altering the course of the underlying disease. Since complications with corticotropin use are dependent on the dose and duration of treatment, a risk/benefit decision must be made in each case.

Suppression of the pituitary adrenal axis occurs following prolonged therapy which may be slow in returning to normal. Patients should be protected from the stress of trauma or surgery by the use of corticosteroids during the period of stress.

Since maximal corticotropin stimulation of the adrenals may be limited during the first few days of treatment, other drugs should be administered when an immediate therapeutic effect is desirable.

Although controlled clinical trials have shown ACTH to be effective in speeding the resolution of acute exacerbations of multiple sclerosis they do not show that it affects the ultimate outcome or natural history of the disease. The studies do show that relatively high doses of ACTH are necessary to demonstrate a significant effect. (See DOSAGE AND ADMINISTRATION section.)

Treatment of acute gouty arthritis should be limited to a few days. Since rebound attacks may occur when corticotropin is discontinued, conventional concomitant therapy should be administered during corticotropin treatment and for several days after it is stopped.

Aspirin should be used cautiously in conjunction with corticotropin in hypoprothrombinemia.

2. Drug Interactions
Corticotropin may accentuate the electrolyte loss associated with diuretic therapy.

3. Carcinogenesis, Mutagenesis, Impairment of Fetility
Adequate and well controlled studies have not been done in animals. Human use has not been associated with an increase in malignant disease. See Pregnancy warning below.

4. Pregnancy
Pregnancy Class C. Corticortropin has been shown to have an embryocidal effect. There are no adequate and well-controlled studies in pregnant women. Corticotropin should be used during pregnancy only if the potential benefit justifies the potential risk to the fetus.

5. Nursing Mothers
It is not known whether this drug is excreted in human milk. Because many drugs are excreted in human milk and because of the potential for serious adverse reactions in nursing infants from corticotropin, a decision should be made whether to discontinue nursing or to discontinue the drug, taking into account the importance of the drug to the mother.

6. Pediatric Use
Prolonged use of corticotropin in children will inhibit skeletal growth. If use is necessary, it should be given intermittently and the child carefully observed.

Adverse Reactions:
Fluid and electrolyte disturbances:
Sodium retention; fluid retention; potassium loss; hypokalemic alkalosis; calcium loss.

Musculoskeletal:
Muscle weakness; steroid myopathy; loss of muscle mass; osteoporosis; vertebral compression fractures; aseptic necrosis of femoral and humeral heads; pathologic fracture of long bones.

Gastrointestinal:
Peptic ulcer with possible perforation and hemorrhage; pancreatitis; abdominal distention; ulcerative esophagitis.

Dermatologic:
Impaired wound healing; thin fragile skin; petechiae and ecchymoses; facial erythema; increased sweating; suppression of skin test reactions; acne; hyperpigmentation.

Cardiovascular:
Hypertension, necrotizing angiitis; congestive heart failure.

Neurological:
Convulsions; increased intracranial pressure with papilledema, (pseudo-tumor cerebri) usually after treatment; headache, vertigo.

Endocrine:
Menstrual irregularities; development of Cushingoid state; suppression of growth in children; secondary adrenocortical pituitary unre-

sponsiveness, particularly in times of stress, as in trauma, surgery or illness; decreased carbohydrate tolerance; manifestations of latent diabetes mellitus; increased requirements for insulin or oral hypoglycemic agents in diabetics; hirsutism.

Ophthalmic:
Posterior subcapsular cataracts; increased intraocular pressure; glaucoma with possible damage to optic nerve; exophthalmos.

Metabolic:
Negative nitrogen balance due to protein catabolism.

Allergic reactions:
Especially in patients with allergic responses to proteins manifesting as dizziness, nausea and vomiting, shock, skin reactions.

Miscellaneous:
Abscess: prolonged use of ACTH may result in antibodies to it and resulting loss of stimulatory effect.

Drug Abuse and Dependence:
Although drug dependence does not occur, sudden withdrawal of corticotropin after prolonged use may lead to recurrent symptoms which make it difficult to stop. It may be necessary to taper the dose and increase the injection interval to gradually discontinue the medication.

Overdosage: An acute overdose would present no different adverse reactions.

Dosage and Administration: Standard tests for verification of adrenal responsiveness to corticotropin may utilize as much as 80 units as a single injection or one or more injections of a lesser dosage. Verification tests should be performed prior to treatment with corticotropins. The test should utilize the route(s) of administration proposed for treatment. Following verification, dosage should be individualized according to the disease under treatment and the general medical condition of each patient. Frequency and dose of the drug should be determined by considering severity of the disease, plasma and urine corticosteroid levels and the initial response of the patient. Only gradual change in dosage schedules should be attempted, after full drug effects have become apparent.

The chronic administration of more than 40 units daily may be associated with uncontrollable adverse effects.

When reduction in dosage is indicated this should be done gradually by either reducing the amount of each injection, or administering injections at longer intervals, or by a combination of both of the above. During reduction of dosage careful consideration should be given to the disease being treated, the general medical conditions of the patient and the duration over which corticotropin was administered.

Acthar must be reconstituted at the time of use by dissolving in a convenient volume of Sterile Water for Injection or Sodium Chloride Injection in such a manner that the individual dose will be contained in 1-2 ml. of solution. The reconstituted solution should be refrigerated and used within 24 hours.

H.P. ACTHAR® GEL (Repository Corticotropin Injection) and ACTHAR® (Corticotropin for Injection) may be administered intramuscularly or subcutaneously.

H.P. ACTHAR® GEL (Repository Corticotropin Injection) is given intramuscularly or subcutaneously every 24-72 hours in doses of 40-80 units. The usual intramuscular or subcutaneous dose for ACTHAR® (Corticotropin for Injection) is 20 units four times a day.

In the treatment of acute exacerbations of multiple sclerosis daily intramuscular doses of 80-120 units for 2-3 weeks may be administered.

For diagnostic purposes, ACTHAR® (Corticotropin for Injection) may be given intravenously in doses of 10-25 units dissolved in 500 ml. of 5% glucose infused over an 8-hour period.

How Supplied: H.P. ACTHAR® GEL (Repository Corticotropin Injection) is supplied in 5 milliliter multiple dose vials in strengths of 40 and 80 U.S.P. Units per milliliter and 1 milliliter vials containing 40 and 80 U.S.P. Units per milliliter.

ACTHAR® (Corticotropin for Injection) is supplied as a lyophilized powder in vials containing 25 and 40 U.S.P. Units per vial.

H.P. ACTHAR® GEL (Repository Corticotropin Injection) is stable for the period indicated on the label when stored under refrigeration between 2°-8°C (36°-46°F).

ACTHAR® (Corticotropin For Injection) is stable for the period indicated on the label when stored at controlled room temperature between 15°-30°C (59°-86°F).

*U.S. PAT. NO. 2,992,165
Revised: January 1983

AQUASOL A® ℞
[ăk'we-sŏl"ā]
water-miscible vitamin A
50,000 USP Units (15 mg)
vitamin A per capsule
25,000 USP Units (7.5 mg)
vitamin A per capsule

Description: AQUASOL A (water-miscible vitamin A) Capsules provide 50,000 USP Units (15 mg) or 25,000 USP Units (7.5 mg) of vitamin A per capsule as retinol in the form of vitamin A alcohol, a light yellow to amber oil. One USP Unit is equivalent to one international unit (IU) and to 0.3 mcg of retinol or 0.6 mcg of beta-carotene. One molecule of beta-carotene yields two molecules of retinol, which is known as provitamin A.

Vitamin A, one of the fat-soluble vitamins, includes vitamin A itself as well as its precursors, alpha, beta, and gamma-carotene and cryptoxanthin. Of the precursors, beta-carotene predominates in nature and is the most active; on splitting, it forms two molecules of vitamin A, whereas the other precursors form only one molecule of vitamin A.

Ordinarily fat-soluble, the vitamin A in this product has been water solubilized by special processing* to enable better absorption and utilization particularly in conditions in which absorption or utilization of fats and fat-soluble substances is impaired.

*Oil-soluble vitamin A water solubilized with polysorbate 80.

Clinical Pharmacology: Retinol combines with opsin, the rod pigment in the retina, to form rhodopsin, which is necessary for visual adaptation to darkness.

Vitamin A prevents retardation of growth and preserves the integrity of the epithelial cells.

Vitamin A deficiency is characterized by nyctalopia, keratomalacia, keratinization and drying of the skin, lowered resistance to infection, retardation of growth, thickening of bone, diminished production of cortical steroids, and fetal malformations. Vitamin A absorption requires bile salts, pancreatic lipase, and dietary fat. The vitamin is stored (primarily as the palmitate) in the Kupffer cells of the liver. The minimum daily requirement is approximately 20 units of vitamin A or 40 units of beta-carotene per kg of body weight. The daily Recommended Dietary Allowances (RDA) established by the National Academy of Sciences for selected categories of population are as follows: children 4-10 years of age, 2,500-3,000 units; adult males, 5,000 units; adult females, 4,000 units; pregnant women, 5,000 units; lactating women, 6,000 units.

The fat-soluble vitamins (A, D, E, and K) are absorbed by complex processes that parallel the absorption of fat. Thus, any condition that causes malabsorption of fat (e.g., celiac disease, tropical sprue, regional enteritis) may result in deficiency of one or all of these vitamins. Fat-soluble vitamins affect permeability or transport in various cell membranes and act as oxidation-reduction agents, coenzymes, or enzyme inhibitors. They are stored principally in the liver and excreted in the feces. Because these vitamins are metabolized very slowly, overdosage may produce toxic effects. Dietary fat is necessary for effective absorption of carotene, and protein is required for absorption of retinols. Protein and, possibly, zinc may be required to mobilize vitamin A reserves in the liver.

Vitamin A is more rapidly absorbed than carotene. Absorption of vitamin A from an aqueous vehicle is appreciably greater than when the drug is given in an oily solution.

Carotene is converted to vitamin A in the intestinal wall and in the liver. Vitamin A itself is found only in animal sources; it occurs in high concentrations in the liver of the cod, halibut, tuna, and shark. It is also prepared synthetically. Carotene is found only in plants.

Indications and Usage: AQUASOL A (water-miscible vitamin A) Capsules are effective for the treatment of vitamin A deficiency. Unlike fat-soluble vitamin A products, AQUASOL A Capsules are not contraindicated in the malabsorption syndrome, because of the water-solubilizing process.

Contraindications: Hypervitaminosis A. Sensitivity to any of the ingredients of this preparation.

Warnings: Avoid overdosage. Keep out of the reach of children.

Use in Pregnancy: Safety of amounts exceeding 5,000 units of vitamin A daily during pregnancy has not been established at this time. Therefore, for the protection of the fetus, the use of vitamin A in excess of the recommended dietary allowance should be avoided during normal pregnancy. Animal reproduction studies have shown fetal abnormalities associated with overdosage in several species. Malformations of the central nervous system, eye, palate, and genitourinary tract have been recorded.

Precautions: General: Protect from light. Vitamin A ingestion from fortified foods, dietary supplements, self-administered drugs and prescription drug sources should be evaluated. Prolonged daily dose administration over 25,000 units vitamin A should be under close supervision. Blood level assays are not a direct measure of liver storage. Liver storage should be adequate before discontinuing therapy. Single vitamin A deficiency is rare. Multiple vitamin deficiency is expected in any dietary deficiency.

Drug Interactions: Women receiving oral contraceptives have shown a significant increase in plasma vitamin A levels.

Pregnancy Category C: See Warnings section.
Nursing Mothers: The U.S. Recommended Dietary Allowance of vitamin A (6,000 units) is recommended for nursing mothers. Human milk supplies sufficient vitamin A for infants unless the maternal diet is grossly inadequate.

Adverse Reactions: See Overdosage section.

Overdosage: The following amounts have been found to be toxic orally. Toxicity manifestations depend on the age, dosage units, and duration of administration.

Acute toxicity—single dose (25,000 units/kg body weight)
Infant: 350,000 units
Adult: Over 2 million units

Chronic toxicity (4,000 units/kg body weight for 6 to 15 months)
Infants 3 to 6 months old: 18,500 units (water dispersed) per day for one to three months
Adult: 1 million units daily for three days, or 50,000 units daily for longer than 18 months, or 500,000 units daily for two months

Hypervitaminosis A Syndrome:
1. *General manifestations:* Fatigue, malaise, lethargy, abdominal discomfort, anorexia, and vomiting.
2. *Specific manifestations:*
   a. Skeletal: slow growth, hard tender cortical thickening over the radius and tibia, migratory arthralgia, and premature closure of the epiphysis:
   b. Central Nervous System: irritability, headache, and increased intracranial pressure as manifested by bulging fontanels, papilledema, and exophthalmos.
   c. Dermatologic: fissures of the lips, drying and cracking of the skin, alopecia, scaling, massive desquamation, and increased pigmentation.

Continued on next page

Armour—Cont.

d. Systemic: hypomenorrhea, hepatosplenomegaly, jaundice, leukopenia, vitamin A plasma level over 1,200 units.

The treatment of hypervitaminosis A consists of immediate withdrawal of the vitamin along with symptomatic and supportive treatment.

Dosage and Administration: For adults and children over eight years of age:
1. Severe deficiency with xerophthalmia: 500,000 units daily for three days, followed by 50,000 units daily for two weeks.
2. Severe deficiency: 100,000 units daily for three days followed by 50,000 units daily for two weeks.
3. Follow-up therapy: 10,000 to 20,000 units daily for two months.

Poor dietary habits should be corrected and an abundant and well-balanced dietary intake should be prescribed.

How Supplied: AQUASOL A Capsules (water-miscible vitamin A) 50,000 USP Units vitamin A, bottles of 100 (NDC 0053-0104-00) and 500 (NDC 0053-0104-05); 25,000 USP Units vitamin A, bottles of 100 (NDC 0053-0103-00). These products are dark red, soft gelatin capsules.

These products are manufactured for Armour Pharmaceutical Company, Kankakee, Illinois 60901 by R. P. Scherer Corp., Clearwater, FL 33518.

Shown in Product Identification Section, page 404
Issued: 12/82

AQUASOL A® DROPS
[ăk'we-sŏl"ā]

Composition: Oil-soluble vitamin A water solubilized with polysorbate 20 for faster, better absorption and utilization. Drops provide 5,000 IU vitamin A per 0.1 ml.

Actions: There is evidence that aqueous vitamin A produces a more rapid increase in the blood concentration and higher blood levels than the oily form of the vitamin.

Administration and Dosage: As a dietary supplement 0.1 ml (3 drops) daily for adults and children 4 or more years of age provides 100% of the U.S. RDA; 2 drops daily for children under 4, 133%.

How Supplied: Drops: 5,000 IU per 0.1 ml, bottles of 30 ml, with dropper.
Issued 12/82

AQUASOL E®
[ăk'we-sŏl ē]
(Aqueous Vitamin E Supplements, Oral)

Composition: Capsules, 100 IU or 400 IU vitamin E; Drops, 15 IU vitamin E per 0.3 ml. Oil-soluble vitamin E water solubilized with polysorbate 80 for more rapid and more complete absorption.

How Supplied: 100 IU capsules, bottles of 100; 400 IU capsules, bottles of 30. Drops, 12 ml and 30 ml.

Shown in Product Identification Section, page 404
Issued 12/82

ARM-A-CHAR™   OTC
[arm'a-char"]
Activated Charcoal, USP

ARM-A-CHAR™ (activated charcoal, USP) is supplied in bottles containing 30 grams of activated charcoal, USP suspended in 4 ounces of water.
Revised 10/83

BIOZYME®–C Ointment   ℞
[bī'ō-zim-sē"]
Collagenase

Description: BIOZYME®-C OINTMENT is a sterile enzymatic debriding ointment which contains 250 collagenase units per gram of white petrolatum USP. The enzyme collagenase is derived from the fermentation by *Clostridium histolyticum*. It possesses the unique ability to digest native and denatured collagen in necrotic tissue.

Clinical Pharmacology: Since collagen accounts for 75% of the dry weight of skin tissue, the ability of collagenase to digest collagen in the physiological pH range and temperature makes it particularly effective in the removal of detritus. Collagenase thus contributes towards the formation of granulation tissue and subsequent epithelization of dermal ulcers and severely burned areas. Collagen in healthy tissue or in newly formed granulation tissue is not attacked.

Indications: BIOZYME®-C OINTMENT is indicated for debriding chronic dermal ulcers and severely burned areas.

Contraindications: BIOZYME®-C OINTMENT is contraindicated in patients who have shown local or systemic hypersensitivity to collagenase.

Precautions: The optimal pH range of collagenase is 6 to 8. Higher or lower pH conditions will decrease the enzyme's activity and appropriate precautions should be taken. The enzymatic activity is also adversely affected by detergents, hexachlorophene and heavy metal ions such as mercury and silver which are used in some antiseptics. When it is suspected such materials have been used, the site should be carefully cleansed by repeated washings with normal saline before BIOZYME®-C OINTMENT is applied. Soaks containing metal ions or acidic solutions such as Burow's solution should be avoided because of the metal ion and low pH. Cleansing materials such as hydrogen peroxide, Dakin's solution, and sterile saline are compatible with BIOZYME®-C OINTMENT.

Debilitated patients should be closely monitored for systemic bacterial infections because of the theoretical possibility that debriding enzymes may increase the risk of bacteremia.

A slight transient erythema has been noted occasionally in the surrounding tissue, particularly when BIOZYME®-C OINTMENT was not confined to the lesion. Therefore, the ointment should be applied carefully within the area of the lesion.

Adverse Reactions: No allergic sensitivity or toxic reactions have been noted in the recorded clinical investigations. However, one case of systemic manifestations of hypersensitivity to collagenase in a patient treated for more than one year with a combination of collagenase and cortisone has been reported to us.

Overdosage: Action of the enzyme may be stopped, should this be desired, by the application of Burow's solution USP (pH 3.6-4.4) to the lesion.

Dosage and Administration: BIOZYME®-C OINTMENT should be applied once daily (or more frequently if the dressing becomes soiled, as from incontinence) in the following manner:

(1) Prior to application the lesion should be cleansed of debris and digested material by gently rubbing with a gauze pad saturated with hydrogen peroxide or Dakin's solution followed by sterile normal saline.
(2) Whenever infection is present it is desirable to use an appropriate topical antibacterial agent. Neomycin-Bacitracin-Polymyxin B (Neosporin) powder has been found to be compatible with BIOZYME®-C OINTMENT. The antibiotic should be applied to the lesion prior to the application of BIOZYME®-C OINTMENT. Should the infection not respond, therapy with BIOZYME®-C OINTMENT should be discontinued until remission of the infection.
(3) BIOZYME®-C OINTMENT should be applied directly from the tube. For shallow lesions, BIOZYME®-C OINTMENT may be applied to a sterile gauze pad which is then applied to the wound and properly secured.
(4) Crosshatching thick eschar with a #10 blade allows collagenase more surface contact with necrotic debris. It is also desirable to remove, with forceps and scissors, as much loosened detritus as can be done readily.
(5) All excess ointment should be removed each time dressing is changed.
(6) Use of BIOZYME®-C OINTMENT should be terminated when debridement of necrotic tissue is complete and granulation tissue is well established.

How Supplied: BIOZYME®-C OINTMENT contains 250 units of collagenase enzyme per gram of white petrolatum USP. The potency assay of collagenase is based on the digestion of undenatured collagen (from bovine Achilles tendon) at pH 7.2 and 37°C for 24 hours. The number of peptide bonds cleaved are measured by reaction with ninhydrin. Amino groups released by a trypsin digestion control are subtracted. One net collagenase unit will solubilize ninhydrin reactive material equivalent to 4 micromoles of leucine.
Manufactured by:
Advance Biofactures Corporation
35 Wilbur Street
Lynbrook, New York 11563
U.S. Gov't. License #383
Distributed by:
Armour Pharmaceutical Company
Kankakee, IL 60901
Revised: August, 1981

For dilution in intravenous infusions only
CHROMETRACE™   ℞
[krōm'trās]
Chromic Chloride Injection USP

4 mcg/ml

Chromic Chloride in Sodium Chloride Solution

Description: Chrometrace (Chromic Chloride Injection USP) (4 mcg chromium/ml) is a sterile, nonpyrogenic solution intended for use as an additive to intravenous solutions for total parenteral nutrition (TPN). Each ml of solution provides:

chromic chloride ....12.18 mcg
sodium ....3.34 mg
chloride ....5.29 mg

(not including ions for pH adjustment)
The pH is approximately 2.0, adjusted with hydrochloric acid and may be adjusted with sodium hydroxide. The solution is adjusted to isotonicity with sodium chloride. The osmolarity is approximately 0.300 mOsm/ml. The solution contains no bacteriostat, antimicrobial agent, or added buffer. Chromic chloride is chemically designated $CrCl_3$, a cystalline compound soluble in water. Sodium chloride USP is chemically designated NaCl, a white, crystalline compound freely soluble in water.

Clinical Pharmacology: Trivalent chromium is part of glucose tolerance factor, an essential activator of insulin-mediated reactions. Chromium helps to maintain normal glucose metabolism and peripheral nerve function.

Providing chromium during TPN helps prevent deficiency symptoms including impaired glucose tolerance, ataxia, peripheral neuropathy, and a confusional state similar to mild/moderate hepatic encephalopathy.

Serum chromium is bound to transferrin (siderophilin) in the beta-globulin fraction. Typical blood levels for chromium range from 1 to 5 mcg/liter, but blood levels are not considered a meaningful index of tissue stores. Administration of chromium supplements to chromium-deficient patients can result in normalization of the glucose tolerance curve from the diabetic-like curve typical of chromium deficiency. This response is viewed as a more meaningful indicator of chromium nutriture than serum chromium levels.

Excretion of chromium is via the kidneys, ranging from 3 to 50 mcg/day. Biliary excretion via the small intestine may be an ancillary route, but it is believed that only small amounts of chromium are excreted in this manner.

Indications and Usage: Chrometrace is indicated for use as a supplement to intravenous solutions given for total parenteral nutrition (TPN). Administration helps to maintain chromium serum levels and to prevent depletion of endogenous stores and subsequent deficiency symptoms.

Contraindications: Direct intramuscular or intravenous injection of Chrometrace is contraindicated, as the acidic pH of the solution (2.0) may cause considerable tissue irritation.

Warnings: None known.

Precautions: Do not use unless solution is clear and the seal is intact.

Chrometrace (Chromic Chloride Injection USP) should be used only in conjunction with a pharmacy-directed admixture program using aseptic technique in a laminar flow environment. The solution contains no preservatives; discard unused portion within 24 hours after opening.

In assessing the contribution of chromium supplements to maintenance of glucose homeostasis, consideration should be given to the possibility that the patient may be diabetic.

Pregnancy Category C. Animal reproduction studies have not been conducted with chromic chloride. It is also not known whether chromic chloride can cause fetal harm when administered to a pregnant woman or can affect reproductive capacity. Chromic chloride should be given to a pregnant woman only if clearly indicated.

Adverse Reactions: None known.
Drug Abuse and Dependence: None known.
Overdosage: Trivalent chromium administered intravenously to TPN patients has been shown to be nontoxic when given at dosage levels of up to 250 mcg/day for two consecutive weeks.

Reported toxic reactions to chromium include nausea, vomiting, ulcers of the gastrointestinal tract, renal and hepatic damage, convulsions, and coma. The acute LD_{50} for intravenous trivalent chromium in rats was reported as 10 to 18 mg/kg.

Dosage and Administration: Chrometrace contains 4 mcg chromium/ml and is administered intravenously only after dilution.

Adult: For the adult receiving TPN, the suggested additive dosage is 10 to 15 mcg chromium/day. The metabolically stable adult with intestinal fluid loss may require 20 mcg chromium/day, with frequent monitoring of blood levels as a guideline for subsequent administration.

Pediatric: For pediatric patients, the suggested additive dosage is 0.14 to 0.20 mcg/kg/day.

Parenteral drug products should be inspected visually for particulate matter and discoloration prior to administration, whenever solution and container permit. See Precautions section.

How Supplied:
Chrometrace 10-ml vials (NDC-0053-0830-22), boxes of 25.
Store at controlled room temperature—15°–30°C (59°–86°F); avoid excessive heat.
Revised: 1/84

For dilution in intravenous infusions only
COPPERTRACE™ ℞
[kŏp′er-trās″]
Cupric Chloride Injection USP
0.4 mg/ml
Cupric Chloride in Sodium Chloride Solution

Description: Coppertrace (Cupric Chloride Injection USP) (0.4 mg copper/ml) is a sterile nonpyrogenic solution intended for use as an additive to intravenous solutions for total parenteral nutrition (TPN). Each ml of solution provides:
cupric chloride .... 0.85 mg
sodium .... 3.19 mg
chloride .... 5.36 mg
(not including ions for pH adjustment).

The pH is approximately 2.0, adjusted with hydrochloric acid, and may be adjusted with sodium hydroxide. The solution is adjusted to isotonicity with sodium chloride. The osmolarity is approximately 0.300 mOsm/ml. The solution contains no bacteriostat, antimicrobial agent, or added buffer.

Cupric chloride is chemically designated $CuCl_2$, a crystalline compound freely soluble in water. Sodium chloride USP is chemically designated NaCl, a white crystalline compound freely soluble in water.

Clinical Pharmacology: Copper is an essential nutrient that serves as a cofactor for serum ceruloplasmin, an oxidase necessary for proper formation of the iron carrier protein, transferrin. Copper also helps maintain normal rates of red and white blood cell formation.

Providing copper during TPN helps prevent development of the following deficiency symptoms: Leukopenia, neutropenia, anemia, depressed ceruloplasmin levels, impaired transferrin formation, and secondary iron deficiency.

Normal serum copper values range from 80 to 163 mcg/dl (mean, approximately 110 mcg/dl). The serum copper level at which deficiency symptoms appear is not precisely defined. The daily turnover of copper through ceruloplasmin is approximately 0.5 mg. Excretion of copper is through the bile (80%), directly through the intestinal wall (16%), and in urine (4%).

Indications and Usage: Coppertrace is indicated for use as a supplement to intravenous solutions given for total parenteral nutrition (TPN). Administration helps to maintain copper serum levels and to prevent depletion of endogenous stores and subsequent deficiency symptoms.

Contraindications: Direct intramuscular or intravenous injection of Coppertrace is contraindicated, as the acidic pH of the solution (2.0) may cause considerable tissue irritation.

Warnings: Copper is eliminated via the bile. In patients with severe liver dysfunction and/or biliary tract obstruction, decreasing or omitting copper supplements entirely may be necessary.

Precautions: Do not use unless the solution is clear and the seal is intact.

Coppertrace should be used only in conjunction with a pharmacy-directed admixture program using aseptic technique in a laminar flow environment. The solution contains no preservatives; discard unused portion within 24 hours after opening. Twice monthly serum assays for copper and/or ceruloplasmin are suggested for monitoring copper concentrations in long-term TPN patients. As ceruloplasmin is a cuproenzyme, ceruloplasmin assays may be depressed secondary to copper deficiency.

Pregnancy Catergory C. Animal reproduction studies have not been conducted with cupric chloride. It is also not known whether cupric chloride can cause fetal harm when administered to a pregnant woman or can affect reproductive capacity. Cupric chloride should be given to a pregnant woman only if clearly indicated.

Adverse Reactions: None known.
Drug Abuse and Dependence: None known.
Overdosage: Copper toxicity can produce prostration, behavior change, diarrhea, progressive marasmus, hypotonia, photophobia and peripheral edema. Such symptoms have been reported with a serum copper level of 286 mcg/dl. D-penicillamine has been reported effective as an antidote.

Dosage and Administration: Coppertrace (Cupric Chloride Injection USP) contains 0.4 mg copper/ml and is administered intravenously only after dilution.

Adult: For the adult receiving TPN, the suggested additive dosage is 0.5 to 1.5 mg copper/day.

Pediatric: For pediatric patients, the suggested additive dosage is 20 mcg copper/kg/ day.

Parenteral drug products should be inspected visually for particulate matter and discoloration prior to administration, whenever solution and container permit. See Precautions section.

How Supplied: Coppertrace 10-ml vials (NDC 0053-0831-22), boxes of 25.
Store at controlled room temperature—15°–30°C (59°–86°F); avoid excessive heat.
Revised 12/82

DIALUME® OTC
[di-a-loom]
(Aluminum Hydroxide Capsules)

Composition: Each capsule contains:
Aluminum Hydroxide Powder .... 500 mg
Sodium Content Not More Than .... 1.2 mg
Magnesium Content Not More Than .... 1.0 mg
Calcium Content Not More Than .... 40 mg
Acid Neutralizing Capacity Per Capsule .10 mEq
Indications: For the relief of heartburn, sour stomach, or acid indigestion.
Drug Interaction Precaution: Do not take this product if you are presently taking a prescription antibiotic drug containing any form of tetracycline.

Warnings: Do not take more than six capsules daily for more than 2 weeks, except under the advice and supervision of a physician.
May cause constipation.
Directions: One or two capsules three times daily or as directed by a physician.
How Supplied: In bottles containing 100 capsules and 500 capsules.
Store and dispense in a tight container as defined in the U.S.P. at controlled room temperature between 15°–30°C (59°–86°F).
Revised 4/83

M.V.I.® ℞
[ĕm-vē-ī]
Multi-Vitamin Infusion

Composition: Each 10 ml ampul† or 5 ml Concentrate vial†† provides:
ascorbic acid (vitamin C) .... 500 mg
vitamin A* (retinol) .... 3 mg (a)
ergocalciferol* (vitamin D) .... 25 mcg (b)
thiamine (vitamin B_1)
  (as the hydrochloride) .... 50 mg
riboflavin (vitamin B_2)†† .... 10 mg
pyridoxine HCl (vitamin B_6) .... 15 mg
niacinamide .... 100 mg
dexpanthenol (d-pantothenyl
  alcohol) .... 25 mg
vitamin E* (dl-alpha
  tocopheryl acetate) .... 5 mg (c)
† with polysorbate 20 1%, sodium hydroxide for pH adjustment, butylated hydroxytoluene 0.003%, butylated hydroxyanisole 0.0008%; and gentisic acid ethanolamide 2.4% as preservative.
†† with propylene glycol 30% and gentisic acid ethanolamide 2% as stabilizers and preservatives, sodium hydroxide for pH adjustment, polysorbate 20 1.7%, butylated hydroxytoluene 0.006%, butylated hydroxyanisole 0.0015%; in Concentrate as riboflavin-5-phosphate sodium.
*Oil-soluble vitamins A, D and E water solubilized with polysorbate 20.
(a) 3 mg vitamin A equals 10,000 USP units.
(b) 25 mcg ergocalciferol equals 1,000 USP units.
(c) 5 mg vitamin E equals 5 USP units.

ORIGINAL "AQUEOUS" MULTIVITAMIN FORMULA FOR INTRAVENOUS INFUSION:
M.V.I. (Multi-Vitamin Infusion) makes available a combination of important oil-soluble and water-soluble vitamins in an aqueous solution, formulated specially for incorporation in intravenous infusions. Through special processing techniques, the liposoluble vitamins A, D and E have been solubilized in an aqueous medium, permitting intravenous administration of these vitamins.

Indications: *In Emergency Feedings*
Surgery, extensive burns, fractures and other trauma, severe infectious diseases, comatose states, etc. may provoke a "stress" situation with profound alterations in the body's metabolic demands and consequent tissue depletion of nutrients. As a result, wound healing may be impaired, enzyme activity disturbed, hematopoietic tissues affected; hypoproteinemia and edema may appear; convalescence is thus prolonged.

In such patients M.V.I. (administered in intravenous fluids under proper dilution) contributes optimum vitamin intake toward maintaining the body's normal resistance and repair processes.

Directions for Use: M.V.I. is ready for immediate use when added to intravenous infusion fluids. For intravenous feeding, one daily dose of 10 ml of M.V.I. or 5 ml of M.V.I. Concentrate added directly to not less than 500 ml, preferably 1,000 ml, of intravenous dextrose, saline or similar infusion solutions . . . plasma, protein hydrolysates, etc.

Precaution: Allergic reaction has been known to occur following intravenous administration of solutions containing thiamine.

Caution: Not to be given as a direct undiluted intravenous injection as it may give rise to dizziness, faintness, etc.

Therapeutic Note: Intravenous use should be discontinued as early as practical in favor of an

Continued on next page

Armour—Cont.

intramuscular or an oral vitamin preparation, if needed.

How Supplied: M.V.I.—10 ml ampuls, boxes of 25 and 100. M.V.I. CONCENTRATE—5 ml vials, boxes of 25. Available in 100s only.

PLEASE NOTE: M.V.I. ampuls contain a supersaturated solution of riboflavin, which may occasionally, due to climatic changes, crystallize out in yellow to dark green clusters. If this should occur, do not use.

STORE AT 2°-8°C (36°-46°F)
Revised: 12/82

For dilution in intravenous infusions only
M.V.I.®-12 ℞
[ĕm-vē-ī-twĕlv]
Multi-Vitamin Infusion

Description: This is a sterile product consisting of two vials, labeled Vial 1 and Vial 2.

Each 5 ml Vial 1† provides:
ascorbic acid (vitamin C) .... 100 mg
vitamin A* (retinol) .... 1 mg (a)
ergocalciferol* (vitamin D) .... 5 mcg (b)
thiamine (vitamin B$_1$)
 (as the hydrochloride) .... 3 mg
riboflavin (vitamin B$_2$) (as riboflavin-5-phosphate sodium) .... 3.6 mg
pyridoxine HCl (vitamin B$_6$) .... 4 mg
niacinamide .... 40 mg
dexpathenol (d-pantothenyl
 alcohol) .... 15 mg
vitamin E* (dl-alpha
 tocopheryl acetate) .... 10 mg (c)

† with propylene glycol 30% and gentisic acid ethanolamide 2% as stabilizers and preservatives, sodium hydroxide for pH adjustment, polysorbate 80 1.6%, polysorbate 20 0.028%, butylated hydroxytoluene 0.002%, butylated hydroxyanisole 0.0005%.

* Oil-soluble vitamins A, D and E water solubilized with polysorbate 80.

(a) 1 mg vitamin A equals 3,300 USP units.
(b) 5 mcg ergocalciferol equals 200 USP units.
(c) 10 mg vitamin E equals 10 USP units.

Each 5 ml Vial 2 provides:
biotin .... 60 mcg
folic acid .... 400 mcg
cyanocobalamin (vitamin B$_{12}$) .... 5 mcg
with propylene glycol 30%; and citric acid, sodium citrate, and sodium hydroxide for pH adjustment.

"Aqueous" multivitamin formula for intravenous infusion:

M.V.I.-12 (Multi-Vitamin Infusion) makes available a combination of important oil-soluble and water-soluble vitamins in an aqueous solution, formulated specially for incorporation into intravenous infusions. Through special processing techniques, the liposoluble vitamins A, D and E have been solubilized in an aqueous medium, permitting intravenous administration of these vitamins.

Indications and Usage: This formulation is indicated as daily multivitamin maintenance dosage for adults and children aged 11 and above receiving parenteral nutrition.

It is also indicated in other situations where administration by the intravenous route is required. Such situations include surgery, extensive burns, fractures and other trauma, severe infectious diseases, and comatose states, which may provoke a "stress" situation with profound alterations in the body's metabolic demands and consequent tissue depletion of nutrients.

The physician should not await the development of clinical signs of vitamin deficiency before initiating vitamin therapy. The use of a multivitamin product obviates the need to speculate on the status of individual vitamin nutriture.

M.V.I.-12 (administered in intravenous fluids under proper dilution) contributes intake of these necessary vitamins toward maintaining the body's normal resistance and repair processes.

Patients with multiple vitamin deficiencies or with markedly increased requirements may be given multiples of the daily dosage for two or more days as indicated by the clinical status.

M.V.I.-12 does not contain vitamin K, which may have to be administered separately.

Contraindications: Known hypersensitivity to any of the vitamins in this product or a pre-existing hypervitaminosis.

Precautions:

Drug Interactions: M.V.I.-12 (Multi-Vitamin Infusion) is not physically compatible with DIAMOX® (acetazolamide) 500 mg, DIURIL® Intravenous Sodium (chlorothiazide sodium) 500 mg, or moderately alkaline solutions. ACHROMYCIN® (tetracycline HCl) 500 mg may not be physically compatible with M.V.I.-12. It has been reported that folic acid is unstable in the presence of calcium salts such as calcium gluconate. Some of the vitamins in M.V.I.-12 may react with vitamin K bisulfite. Direct addition of M.V.I.-12 to intravenous fat emulsions is not recommended.

Carcinogenicity: Carcinogenicity studies have not been performed.

Pregnancy: Pregnant women should follow the U.S. Recommended Daily Allowance for their condition, because their vitamin requirements may exceed those of nonpregnant women.

Nursing Mothers: Lactating women should follow the U.S. Recommended Daily Allowance for their condition, because their vitamin requirements may exceed those of nonlactating women.

Pediatric Use: Safety and effectiveness in children below the age of 11 have not been established.

Overdosage: The possibility of hypervitaminosis A or D should be borne in mind.

Adverse Reactions: Allergic reaction has been known to occur following intravenous administration of thiamine. This risk, however, is negligible if the thiamine is administered with other vitamins of the B group.

Dosage and Administration: M.V.I.-12 (Multi-Vitamin Infusion) is ready for immediate use in adults and children aged 11 and above when added to intravenous infusion fluids.

M.V.I.-12 should not be given as a direct, undiluted intravenous injection as it may give rise to dizziness, faintness, and possible tissue irritation. For intravenous feeding, one daily dose of M.V.I.-12 (5 ml of Vial 1 plus 5 ml of Vial 2) added directly to not less than 500 ml, preferably 1,000 ml, of intravenous dextrose, saline or similar infusion solutions.

Parenteral drug products should be inspected visually for particulate matter and discoloration prior to administration, whenever solution and container permit.

After M.V.I.-12 is diluted in an intravenous infusion, the resulting solution should be refrigerated unless it is to be administered immediately, and in any event should be administered within 48 hours. Some of the vitamins in this product, particularly vitamins A and D, and riboflavin, are light sensitive, and exposure to light should be minimized.

STORE AT 2°-8°C (36°-46°F).

How Supplied: Boxes of 25 and cartons of 100. Each box contains two vials—Vial 1 (5 ml) and Vial 2 (5 ml), both vials to be used for a single dose.
Revised: 10/83

For dilution in intravenous infusions only
M.V.I.®-12 ℞
[ĕm-vē-ī-twĕlv li-ŏ'fĭl-īzd"]
Lyophilized
Multi-Vitamins for Infusion

Description: M.V.I.-12 Lyophilized is a sterile powder intended for reconstitution and dilution in intravenous infusions.

Each vial provides:
ascorbic acid (vitamin C) .... 100 mg
vitamin A† (retinol) .... 1.0 mg (a)
ergocalciferol† (vitamin D) .... 5 mcg (b)
thiamine (vitamin B$_1$)
 (as the base) .... 3.0 mg
riboflavin (vitamin B$_2$) (as riboflavin-5-phosphate sodium) .... 3.6 mg
pyridoxine (vitamin B$_6$)
 (as the base) .... 4.0 mg
niacinamide .... 40.0 mg
dexpanthenol (d-pantothenyl
 alcohol) .... 15.0 mg
vitamin E† (dl-alpha
 tocopheryl acetate) .... 10.0 mg (c)
biotin .... 60 mcg
folic acid .... 400 mcg
cyanocobalamin (vitamin B$_{12}$) .... 5 mcg
with mannitol 375 mg, sodium hydroxide for pH adjustment, polysorbate 80 80 mg, polysorbate 20 1.1 mg, butylated hydroxytoluene 82.5 mcg, butylated hydroxyanisole 20.6 mcg.

(a) 1 mg of vitamin A equals 3,300 USP units.
(b) 5 mcg ergocalciferol equals 200 USP units.
(c) 10 mg vitamin E equals 10 USP units.
† Oil soluble vitamins A, D and E water solubilized with polysorbate 80.

Multivitamin formula for intravenous infusion:
M.V.I.-12 Lyophilized (Multi-Vitamins for Infusion) provides a combination of important oil-soluble and water-soluble vitamins, formulated especially for incorporation into intravenous infusions after reconstitution. Through special processing techniques, the liposoluble vitamins A, D and E have been water solubilized with polysorbate 80, permitting intravenous administration of these vitamins.

Indications and Usage: This formulation is indicated as daily multivitamin maintenance dosage for adults and children aged 11 and above receiving parenteral nutrition.

It is also indicated in other situations where administration by the intravenous route is required. Such situations include surgery, extensive burns, fractures and other trauma, severe infectious diseases, and comatose states which may provoke a "stress" situation with profound alterations in the body's metabolic demands and consequent tissue depletion of nutrients.

The physician should not await the development of clinical signs of vitamin deficiency before initiating vitamin therapy. The use of a multivitamin product obviates the need to speculate on the status of individual vitamin nutriture.

M.V.I.-12 Lyophilized (reconstituted and administered in intravenous fluids under proper dilution) contributes intake of these necessary vitamins toward maintaining the body's normal resistance and repair processes.

Patients with multiple vitamin deficiencies or with markedly increased requirements may be given multiples of the daily dosage for two or more days as indicated by the clinical status.

M.V.I.-12 Lyophilized does not contain vitamin K, which may have to be administered separately.

Contraindications: Known hypersensitivity to any of the vitamins in this product or a pre-existing hypervitaminosis.

Precautions:

Drug Interactions: M.V.I.®-12 (Multi-Vitamins for Infusion) Lyophilized is not physically compatible with DIAMOX® (acetazolamide) 500 mg, DIURIL® Intravenous Sodium (chlorothiazide sodium) 500 mg, or moderately alkaline solutions. ACHROMYCIN® (tetracycline HCl) 500 mg may not be physically compatible with M.V.I.-12 Lyophilized. It has been reported that folic acid is unstable in the presence of calcium salts such as calcium gluconate. Some of the vitamins in M.V.I.-12 Lyophilized may react with vitamin K bisulfite. Direct addition of reconstituted M.V.I.-12 Lyophilized to intravenous fat emulsions is not recommended.

Carcinogenicity: Carcinogenicity studies have not been performed.

Pregnancy: Pregnant women should follow the U.S. Recommended Daily Allowance for their condition, because their vitamin requirements may exceed those of nonpregnant women.

Nursing Mothers: Lactating women should follow the U.S. Recommended Daily Allowance for their condition, because their vitamin requirements may exceed those of nonlactating women.

Pediatric Use: Safety and effectiveness in children below the age of 11 have not been established.

Adverse Reactions: Allergic reaction has been known to occur following intravenous administration of thiamine. This risk, however, is negligible if the thiamine is administered with other vitamins of the B group.

Overdosage: The possibility of hypervitaminosis A or D should be borne in mind.

Dosage and Administration: M.V.I.–12 Lyophilized is reconstituted by adding 5 ml of Sterile Water for Injection USP to the 10 ml vial. The vial may be swirled gently after the addition of the water to hasten reconstitution. The reconstituted solution is ready within five minutes for immediate use. The entire contents of the vial should be added to appropriate intravenous infusion fluids. The reconstituted M.V.I.–12 Lyophilized should not be given as a direct undiluted intravenous injection as it may give rise to dizziness, faintness and possible tissue irritation.

For intravenous feeding, administer one daily dose of reconstituted M.V.I.–12 Lyophilized added directly to not less than 500 ml, preferably 1,000 ml, of intravenous dextrose, saline or similar infusion solutions.

Parenteral drug products should be inspected visually for particulate matter and discoloration prior to administration, whenever solution and container permit.

After M.V.I.–12 Lyophilized is reconstituted and diluted in an intravenous infusion, the resulting solution should be refrigerated unless it is to be administered immediately, and in any event should be administered within 24 hours. Some of the vitamins in this product, particularly vitamins A and D, and riboflavin, are light sensitive, and exposure to light should be minimized.

How Supplied: Boxes of 25 vials (NDC 0053-1829-35) and cartons of 100 vials (NDC 0053-1829-37).

Revised: 7/83

For dilution in intravenous infusions only
M.V.I.® Pediatric   ℞
[ĕm-vē-i pē″dē-ăt′rĭk]
Multi-Vitamins for Infusion

Description: M.V.I.® Pediatric is a lyophilized, sterile powder intended for reconstitution and dilution in intravenous infusions.

Each vial provides:
ascorbic acid (vitamin C) .... 80 mg
vitamin A† (retinol) .... 0.7 mg (a)
ergocalciferol† (vitamin D) .... 10 mcg (b)
thiamine (vitamin B₁)
 (as the hydrochloride) .... 1.2 mg
riboflavin (vitamin B₂) (as ribo-
 flavin-5-phosphate sodium) .... 1.4 mg
pyridoxine (vitamin B₆)
 (as the hydrochloride) .... 1.0 mg
niacinamide .... 17.0 mg
dexpanthenol (d-pantothenyl
 alcohol) .... 5.0 mg
vitamin E† (dl-alpha
 tocopheryl acetate) .... 7 mg (c)
biotin .... 20 mcg
folic acid .... 140 mcg
cyanocobalamin (vitamin B₁₂) .... 1 mcg
phytonadione (vitamin K₁) .... 200 mcg
with mannitol 375 mg, sodium hydroxide for pH adjustment, polysorbate 80 50 mg, polysorbate 20 0.8 mg, butylated hydroxytoluene 58 mcg, butylated hydroxyanisole 14 mcg.

† Oil-soluble vitamins A, D and E water solubilized with polysorbate 80.

(a) 0.7 mg vitamin A equals 2,300 USP units.
(b) 10 mcg ergocalciferol equals 400 USP units.
(c) 7 mg vitamin E equals 7 USP units.

Multivitamin formula for intravenous infusion:
M.V.I.® Pediatric (Multi-Vitamins for Infusion) provides a combination of important oil-soluble and water-soluble vitamins, formulated especially for incorporation into intravenous infusions after reconstitution. Through special processing techniques, the liposoluble vitamins A, D and E have been water solubilized with polysorbate 80, permitting intravenous administration of these vitamins.

Indications and Usage: This formulation is indicated as daily multivitamin maintenance dosage for infants and children up to 11 years of age receiving parenteral nutrition.

It is also indicated in other situations where administration by the intravenous route is required. Such situations include surgery, extensive burns, fractures and other trauma, severe infectious diseases, and comatose states, which may provoke a "stress" situation with profound alterations in the body's metabolic demands and consequent tissue depletion of nutrients.

The physician should not await the development of clinical signs of vitamin deficiency before initiating vitamin therapy. The use of a multivitamin product obviates the need to speculate on the status of individual vitamin nutriture.

M.V.I.® Pediatric (reconstituted and administered in intravenous fluids under proper dilution) contributes intake of these necessary vitamins toward maintaining the body's normal resistance and repair processes.

Patients with multiple vitamin deficiencies or with markedly increased requirements may be given multiples of the daily dosage for two or more days as indicated by the clinical status.

Contraindications: Known hypersensitivity to any of the vitamins in this product or a pre-existing hypervitaminosis.

Precautions:
General: Unlike the adult formulation, M.V.I.®–12, this product contains phytonadione (vitamin K₁).

Drug Interactions: M.V.I.® Pediatric is not physically compatible with DIAMOX® (acetazolamide) 500 mg, DIURIL® Intravenous Sodium (chlorothiazide sodium) 500 mg, aminophylline 125 mg, ampicillin 500 mg, or moderately alkaline solutions. ACHROMYCIN® (tetracycline HCl) 500 mg may not be physically compatible with M.V.I.® Pediatric. It has been reported that folic acid is unstable in the presence of calcium salts such as calcium gluconate. Direct addition of M.V.I.® Pediatric to intravenous fat emulsions is not recommended.

Carcinogenicity: Carcinogenicity studies have not been performed.

Adverse Reactions: Allergic reaction has been known to occur following intravenous administration of thiamine. This risk, however, is negligible if the thiamine is administered with other vitamins of the B group.

Overdosage: The possibility of hypervitaminosis A or D should be borne in mind.

Dosage and Administration: M.V.I.® Pediatric is reconstituted by adding 5 ml of Sterile Water for Injection USP, Dextrose Injection USP 5%, or Sodium Chloride Injection to the 10 ml vial. The vial may be swirled gently after the addition of the water to hasten reconstitution. The reconstituted solution is ready within three minutes for immediate use. The amount to be administered should be added to appropriate intravenous infusion fluids (see below).

The reconstituted M.V.I.® Pediatric should not be given as a direct, undiluted intravenous injection as it may give rise to dizziness, faintness and possible tissue irritation.

For intravenous feeding, reconstituted M.V.I.® Pediatric should be added directly to not less than 100 ml of intravenous dextrose, saline or similar infusion solutions.

Infants weighing less than 3 kg: The daily dose is 65% of the contents of the vial.

Infants and children weighing 3 kg or more up to 11 years of age: The daily dose is the contents of one vial unless there is clinical or laboratory evidence for increasing or decreasing the dosage. Discard any unused portion.

Parenteral drug products should be inspected visually for particulate matter and discoloration prior to administration, whenever solution and container permit.

After M.V.I.® Pediatric is reconstituted and diluted in an intravenous infusion, the resulting solution should be refrigerated unless it is to be administered immediately, and in any event should be administered within 24 hours. Some of the vitamins in this product, particularly vitamins A and D, and riboflavin, are light sensitive, and exposure to light should be minimized.

How Supplied: Boxes of 25 vials (NDC 0053-0815-35) and cartons of 100 vials (NDC 0053-0815-37).

Revised: 5/83

For dilution in intravenous infusions only
MANGATRACE™   ℞
[măng′ga-trās]
Manganese Chloride Injection USP

0.1 mg/ml

Manganese Chloride in Sodium Chloride Solution

Description: Mangatrace, Manganese Chloride Injection USP (0.1 mg manganese/ml), is a sterile nonpyrogenic solution intended for use as an additive to intravenous solutions for total parenteral nutrition (TPN). Each ml of solution provides:
manganese chloride .... 0.23 mg
sodium .... 3.34 mg
chloride .... 5.29 mg
(not including ions for pH adjustment).

The pH is approximately 2.0, adjusted with hydrochloric acid, and may be adjusted with sodium hydroxide. The solution is adjusted to isotonicity with sodium chloride. The osmolarity is approximately 0.300 mOsm/ml. The solution contains no bacteriostat, antimicrobial agent, or added buffer. Manganese chloride is chemically designated $MnCl_2$, a deliquescent, crystalline compound soluble in water. Sodium chloride USP is chemically designated NaCl, a white crystalline compound freely soluble in water.

Clinical Pharmacology: Manganese is an essential nutrient that serves as an activator for enzymes such as polysaccharide polymerase, liver arginase, cholinesterase, and pyruvate carboxylase.

Providing manganese during TPN helps prevent development of deficiency symptoms such as nausea and vomiting, weight loss, dermatitis, and changes in growth and color of hair.

Under conditions of minimal intake, 20 mcg manganese/day is retained. Manganese is bound to a specific transport protein, transmanganin, a beta-1-globulin. Manganese is widely distributed but concentrates in the mitochondria-rich tissues such as brain, kidney, pancreas, and liver. Assays for manganese in whole blood result in concentrations ranging from 6 to 12 mcg/manganese/liter.

Excretion of manganese occurs mainly through the bile, but in the event of obstruction, ancillary excretion routes include pancreatic juice, or return into the lumen of the duodenum, jejunum, or ileum. Urinary excretion of manganese is negligible.

Indications and Usage: Mangatrace is indicated for use as a supplement to intravenous solutions given for total parenteral nutrition (TPN). Administration helps to maintain manganese serum levels and to prevent depletion of endogenous stores and subsequent deficiency symptoms.

Contraindications: Direct intramuscular or intravenous injection of Mangatrace is contraindicated, as the acidic pH of the solution (2.0) may cause considerable tissue irritation.

Warnings: **Manganese is eliminated via the bile. In patients with severe liver dysfunction and/or biliary tract obstruction, decreasing or omitting manganese supplements entirely may be necessary.**

Precautions: Do not use unless the solution is clear and the seal is intact.

Mangatrace should be used only in conjunction with a pharmacy-directed admixture program using aseptic technique in a laminar flow environment. The solution contains no preservatives; discard unused portion within 24 hours after opening.

Pregnancy Category C. Animal reproduction studies have not been conducted with manganese chloride. It is also not known whether manganese chloride can cause fetal harm when administered to a pregnant woman or can affect reproductive capacity. Manganese chloride should be given to a pregnant woman only if clearly indicated.

Continued on next page

Armour—Cont.

Adverse Reactions: None known.
Drug Abuse and Dependence: None known.
Overdosage: Manganese toxicity in TPN patients has not been reported.
Dosage and Administration: Mangatrace, Manganese Chloride Injection, contains 0.1 mg manganese/ml and is administered intravenously only after dilution.
Adult: For the adult receiving TPN, the suggested additive dosage for manganese is 0.15 to 0.8 mg/day.
Pediatric: For pediatric patients, a dosage of 2 to 10 mcg manganese/kg/day is recommended.
Periodic monitoring of manganese plasma levels is suggested as a guideline for subsequent administration.
Parenteral products should be inspected visually for particulate matter and discoloration prior to administration, whenever solution and container permit. See Precautions sections.
How Supplied: Mangatrace 10-ml vials (NDC 0053-0832-22), boxes of 25.
Store at controlled room temperature—15°–30°C (59°–86°F); avoid excessive heat.
Revised: 12/82

MULTITRACE™ 5   ℞
[mŭl' tē-trās]
Trace Element Mixture

Description: Multitrace™ 5, Trace Element Mixture, is a sterile, nonpyrogenic solution containing zinc, copper, manganese, chromium, and selenium for use as an additive to intravenous solutions for total parenteral nutrition (TPN).
Each ml of Multitrace™ 5 contains:
Zinc Chloride*...................................2.08 mg
Copper Chloride dihydrate**.....................1.07 mg
Manganese Chloride tetrahydrate***........0.36 mg
Chromium Chloride hexahydrate****.....20.5 mcg
Selenious Acid*****...................................32.7 mcg
Water for Injection...............................q.s.
*Equivalent to 1.0 mg Zn
**Equivalent to 0.4 mg Cu
***Equivalent to 0.1 mg Mn
****Equivalent to 4.0 mcg Cr
*****Equivalent to 20 mcg Se
pH adjusted with Hydrochloric Acid and/or Sodium Hydroxide
Zinc Chloride, USP is chemically designated $ZnCl_2$, a white crystalline compound freely soluble in water. Cupric Chloride is chemically designated $CuCl_2$, a crystalline compound freely soluble in water. Manganese Chloride is chemically designated $MnCl_2$, a deliquescent, crystalline compound soluble in water. Chromic Chloride is chemically designated $CrCl_3$, a crystalline compound soluble in water. Selenious Acid is chemically designated H_2Se, white or colorless crystals soluble in water or alcohol.
Clinical Pharmacology: Zinc is an essential nutritional requirement that serves as a cofactor for more than 70 different enzymes including carbonic anhydrase, alkaline phosphatase, lactic dehydrogenase, and both RNA and DNA polymerase. Zinc facilitates wound healing, helps maintain normal growth rates, normal skin hydration, and the senses of taste and smell. Providing zinc during TPN helps prevent development of deficiency symptoms and signs such as: Parakeratosis, hypogeusia, anorexia, dysosmia, geophagia, hypogonadism, growth retardation and hepatosplenomegaly. At plasma levels below 20 mcg zinc/dl, dermatitis followed by alopecia has been reported.
Copper is an essential nutrient that serves as a cofactor for serum ceruloplasmin, an oxidase necessary for proper formation of the iron carrier protein, transferrin. Copper also helps maintain normal rates of red and white blood cell formation. Providing copper during TPN helps prevent development of the following deficiency symptoms and signs: Leukopenia, neutropenia, anemia, depressed ceruloplasmin levels, impaired transferrin formation, and secondary iron deficiency. Normal serum copper values range from 80 to 163 mcg/dl.

Manganese is an essential nutrient that serves as an activator for enzymes such as polysaccharide polymerase, liver arginase, cholinesterase, and pyruvate carboxylase. Providing manganese during TPN helps prevent deficiency symptoms and signs such as nausea and vomiting, weight loss, dermatitis, and changes in growth and color of hair. Assays for manganese in whole blood result in concentrations ranging from 6 to 12 mcg manganese/liter.
Trivalent chromium is part of glucose tolerance factor, an essential activator of insulin-mediated reactions. Chromium helps maintain normal glucose metabolism and peripheral nerve function. Providing chromium during TPN helps prevent deficiency symptoms and signs including impaired glucose tolerance, ataxia, peripheral neuropathy, and a confusional state similar to mild/moderate hepatic encephalopathy. Typical blood levels for chromium range from 1 to 5 mcg/liter, but blood levels are not considered a meaningful index of tissue stores. A normalization of the glucose tolerance curve from the diabetic-like curve typical of chromium deficiency is viewed as a more meaningful indicator of chromium nutriture than serum chromium levels.
Selenium is an essential nutritional requirement that is part of glutathione peroxidase which protects cell components from oxidative damage resulting from peroxidase produced in cellular metabolism. Providing selenium during TPN helps prevent development of deficiency symptoms which include muscle pain and tenderness. Deficiency symptoms in humans have been reported with plasma selenium levels of 0.3 to 0.9 mcg/dl.
Indications and Usage: Multitrace 5 is indicated for use as a supplement to intravenous solutions given for total parenteral nutrition (TPN). Administration helps maintain zinc, copper, manganese, chromium, and selenium blood levels and prevents depletion of endogenous stores and subsequent deficiency states.
Contraindications: Direct intramuscular or intravenous injection of Multitrace 5, Trace Element Mixture, is contraindicated as the acidic pH of the solution (approximately 2.0) may cause considerable tissue irritation.
Warnings: Copper and manganese are eliminated via the bile. In patients with severe liver dysfunction and/or biliary tract obstruction, decreasing or omitting copper and manganese supplements entirely may be necessary.
Precautions: Do not use unless the solution is clear and the seal is intact. Multitrace 5, Trace Element Mixture, should be used only in conjunction with a pharmacy-directed admixture program using aseptic technique in a laminar flow environment. Multitrace 5 contains no preservative. Unused portions should be discarded within 24 hours after opening.
Frequent determination of serum levels of the various trace elements is suggested as a guideline for administering Multitrace 5. Zinc is eliminated via the kidneys and the possibility of retention should be considered in patients with renal dysfunction. Copper and manganese are eliminated via the bile and the possibility of retention should be considered in patients with biliary obstruction. In assessing the contribution of chromium supplements to maintenance of glucose homeostasis, consideration should be given to the possibility the patient may be diabetic. The primary route of elimination of selenium is in the urine, but significant losses also occur through feces. Selenium plasma level determinations are suggested as a guideline to adjust, reduce or omit selenium supplements in renal dysfunction and/or gastrointestinal malfunction.
Pregnancy Category C: Animal reproduction studies have not been conducted with Multitrace 5, Trace Element Mixture. It is also not known whether Multitrace 5 can cause fetal harm when administered to a pregnant woman or can affect reproductive capacity. Multitrace 5 should be given to a pregnant woman only if clearly indicated.

Adverse Reactions: None known.
Drug Abuse and Dependency: None known.
Overdosage: Single intravenous doses of 1 to 2 mg zinc/kg body weight have been given to adult leukemic patients without toxic manifestations. However, acute toxicity was reported in an adult when 10 mg zinc was infused over a period of one hour on each of four consecutive days. Symptoms included hypotension, pulmonary edema, diarrhea, vomiting, jaundice, oliguria, blurred vision, tachycardia, decreased level of consciousness, profuse sweating, and hypothermia. Death resulted from an overdose in which 1683 mg zinc was delivered intravenously over the course of 60 hours to a 72-year-old patient. Calcium supplements may confer a protective effect against zinc toxicity.
Copper toxicity can produce prostration, behavior change, diarrhea, progressive marasmus, hypotonia, photophobia, and peripheral edema. Such symptoms have been reported with a serum copper level of 286 mcg/dl. D-penicillamine has been reported effective as an antidote.
Manganese toxicity in TPN patients has not been reported.
Trivalent chromium administered intravenously to TPN patients has been shown to be nontoxic when given at dosage levels of up to 250 mcg/day for two consecutive weeks. Reported toxic reactions to chromium include nausea, vomiting, ulcers of the gastrointestinal tract, renal and hepatic damage, convulsions, and coma.
Exposure to selenium in industrial environments, intake of foods grown in seleniferous soils, application of selenium containing cosmetics, and use of selenium contaminated water have been reported to cause chronic toxicity in humans. Selenium toxicity symptoms include weakened nails, dental defects, hair loss, dermatitis, nervousness, gastrointestinal disorders, mental depression, metallic taste, vomiting and garlic odor of breath and sweat. Death resulted from ingestion of large amounts of selenium compounds. The histopathological changes included fulminating peripheral vascular collapse, internal vascular congestion, diffusely hemorrhagic congested and edematous lungs, and brick-red color gastric mucosa. Coma preceded death. There is no known effective antidote to selenium poisoning in humans.
Dosage and Administration: Each ml of Multitrace 5, Trace Element Mixture contains 1.0 mg Zn, 0.4 mg Cu, 0.1 mg Mn, 4.0 mcg Cr and 20 mcg Se and is administered intravenously only after dilution to a minimum of 1:200.
The following are suggested dosage ranges for the five trace elements.
Zinc: For the metabolically stable adult receiving TPN, the suggested intravenous dosage is 2.5 to 4 mg zinc/day. An additional 2 mg zinc/day is suggested for acute catabolic states. For the stable adult with fluid loss from the small bowel, an additional 12.2 mg zinc/liter of small bowel fluid lost, or an additional 17.1 mg zinc/kg of stool or ileostomy output is recommended. Frequent monitoring of zinc blood levels is suggested for patients receiving more than the usual maintenance dosage level of zinc.
For full term infants and children up to 5 years of age, 100 mcg zinc/kg/day is recommended. For premature infants (birth weight less than 1500 grams) up to 3 kg in body weight, 300 mcg/kg/day is suggested.
Copper: For the adult receiving TPN, the suggested additive dosage is 0.5 to 1.5 mg copper/day.
For pediatric patients, the suggested additive dosage is 20 mcg copper/day.
Manganese: For the adult receiving TPN, the suggested additive dosage for manganese is 0.15 to 0.8 mg/day.
For pediatric patients, a dosage of 2 to 10 manganese/kg/day is recommended.
Chromium: For the adult receiving TPN, the suggested additive dosage is 10 to 15 mcg chromium/day. The metabolically stable adult with intestinal fluid loss may require 20 mcg chromium/day with frequent monitoring of blood levels as a guideline for subsequent administration.
For pediatric patients, the suggested additive dosage is 0.14 to 0.20 mcg chromium/kg/day.

Selenium: For the metabolically stable adult receiving TPN, the suggested intravenous dosage level is 20 to 40 mcg selenium/day. In adults with selenium deficiency states resulting from long-term TPN support, selenious acid administered intravenously at 100 mcg/day for a period of 24 and 31 days, respectively, has been reported to reverse deficiency symptoms without toxicity.
Frequent monitoring of selenium blood levels is suggested for patients receiving more than the usual maintenance dose. The normal whole blood range for selenium is approximately 10–37 mcg/dl.
Pediatric: For children the suggested dosage level is 3 mcg/kg/day.
Parenteral drug products should be inspected visually for particulate matter and discoloration prior to administration, whenever solution and container permit.
How Supplied: Multitrace™ 5, Trace Element Mixture, in 10 ml Unit Dose vials in boxes of 25 (NDC 0053-1457-35).
Store at controlled room temperature between 15°–30°C (59°–86°F); avoid excessive heat.
Revised: March, 1984

MULTITRACE™ PEDIATRIC
[mŭl' tē-trās'']
Trace Element Mixture

Description: Multitrace™ Pediatric, Trace Element Mixture, is a sterile, nonpyrogenic solution containing zinc, copper, manganese and molybdenum for use as an additive to intravenous solutions for total parenteral nutrition (TPN).
Each ml of Multitrace™ Pediatric contains:
Zinc chloride .... 2.08 mg
Copper chloride dihydrate .... 0.27 mg
Manganese chloride tetrahydrate .... 0.09 mg
Chromium chloride hexahydrate ..... 5.12 mcg
Water for Injection .... q.s.
Equivalent to:
Zn .... 1.0 mg
Cu .... 0.1 mg
Mn .... 25.0 mcg
Cr .... 1.0 mcg
pH adjusted with sodium hydroxide and/or hydrochloric acid.
Zinc Chloride, USP is chemically designated $ZnCl_2$, a white crystalline compound freely soluble in water. Cupric Chloride is chemically designated $CuCl_2$, a crystalline compound freely soluble in water. Manganese Chloride is chemically designated $MnCl_2$, a deliquescent, crystalline compound soluble in water. Chromic Chloride is chemically designated $CrCl_3$, a crystalline compound soluble in water.
Clinical Pharmacology: Zinc is an essential nutritional requirement that serves as a cofactor for more than 70 different enzymes including carbonic anhydrase, alkaline phosphatase, lactic dehydrogenase, and both RNA and DNA polymerase. Zinc facilitates wound healing, helps maintain normal growth rates, normal skin hydration, and the senses of taste and smell. Providing zinc during TPN helps prevent development of deficiency symptoms and signs such as: Parakeratosis, hypogeusia, anorexia, dysosmia, geophagia, hypogonadism, growth retardation and hepatosplenomegaly. At plasma levels below 20 mcg zinc/dl, dermatitis followed by alopecia has been reported in adults.
Copper is an essential nutrient that serves as a cofactor for serum ceruloplasmin, an oxidase necessary for proper formation of the iron carrier protein, transferrin. Copper also helps maintain normal rates of red and white bood cell formation. Providing copper during TPN helps prevent development of the following deficiency symptoms and signs: Leukopenia, neutropenia, anemia, depressed ceruloplasmin levels, impaired transferrin formation, and secondary iron deficiency. Normal serum copper values range from 80 to 163 mcg/dl in adults.
Manganese is an essential nutrient that serves as an activator for enzymes such as polysaccharide polymerase, liver arginase, cholinesterase, and pyruvate carboxylase. Providing manganese during TPN helps prevent deficiency symptoms and signs such as nausea and vomiting, weight loss, dermatitis, and changes in growth and color of hair. Assays for manganese in whole blood result in concentrations ranging from 6 to 12 mcg manganese/liter in adults.
Trivalent chromium is part of glucose tolerance factor, an essential activator of insulin-mediated reactions. Chromium helps maintain normal glucose metabolism and peripheral nerve function. Providing chromium during TPN helps prevent deficiency symptoms and signs including impaired glucose tolerance, ataxia, peripheral neuropathy, and a confusional state similar to mild/moderate hepatic encephalopathy. Typical blood levels for chromium range from 1 to 5 mcg/liter in adults, but blood levels are not considered a meaningful index of tissue stores. A normalization of the glucose tolerance curve from the diabetic-like curve typical of chromium deficiency is viewed as a more meaningful indicator of chromium nutriture than serum chromium levels.
Indications and Usage: Multitrace™ Pediatric is indicated for use as a supplement to intravenous solutions given for total parenteral nutrition (TPN) for infants and children up to 11 years of age. Administration helps maintain zinc, copper, manganese, and chromium blood levels and prevents depletion of endogenous stores and subsequential deficiency states.
Contraindications: Direct intramuscular or intravenous injection of Multitrace™ Pediatric, Trace Element Mixture, is contraindicated as the acidic pH of the solution (approximately 2.0) may cause considerable tissue irritation.
Warnings: Copper and manganese are eliminated via the bile. In patients with severe liver dysfunction and/or biliary tract obstruction, decreasing or omitting copper and manganese supplements entirely may be necessary.
Precautions: Do not use unless the solution is clear and the seal is intact. Multitrace™ Pediatric, Trace Element Mixture, should be used only in conjunction with a pharmacy-directed admixture program using aseptic technique in a laminar flow environment. Single dose vials contain no preservative; unused portions should be discarded within 24 hours after opening.
Frequent determination of serum levels of the various trace elements is suggested as a guideline for administering Multitrace™ Pediatric. Zinc is eliminated via the kidneys and the possibility of retention should be considered in patients with renal dysfunction. Copper and manganese are eliminated via the bile and the possibility of retention should be considered in patients with biliary obstruction. In assessing the contribution of chromium supplements to maintenance of glucose homeostasis, consideration should be given to the possibility the patent may be diabetic.
Adverse Reactions: None known.
Drug Abuse and Dependency: None known.
Overdosage: Zinc toxicity signs and symptoms include hypotension, pulmonary edema, diarrhea, vomiting, jaundice, oliguria, blurred vision, tachycardia, decreased level of consciousness, profuse sweating, and hypothermia.
Copper toxicity can produce prostration, behavior change, diarrhea, progressive marasmus, hypotonia, photophobia, and peripheral edema. Such symptoms have been reported with a serum copper level of 286 mcg/dl. D-penicillamine has been reported effective as an antidote.
Manganese toxicity in TPN patients has not been reported.
Trivalent chromium administered intravenously to TPN patients has been shown to be nontoxic when given at dosage levels of up to 250 mcg/day for two consecutive weeks. Reported toxic reactions to chromium include nausea, vomiting, ulcers of the gastrointestinal tract, renal and hepatic damage, convulsions, and coma.
Dosage and Administration: Each ml of Multitrace™ Pediatric contains 1.0 mg Zn, 0.1 mg Cu, 25.0 mcg Mn, and 1.0 mcg Cr and is administered intravenously only after dilution to a minimum of 1:200. The following are suggested dosage ranges for the four trace elements.
Zinc: For full-term infants and children, 100 mcg zinc/kg/day is recommended. For premature infants (birth weight less than 1500 grams) up to 3 kg in body weight, 300 mcg/kg/day is suggested.
Copper: For pediatric patients, the suggested additive dosage is 20 mcg copper/kg/day.
Manganese: For pediatric patients, a dosage of 2 to 10 mcg manganese/kg/day is recommended.
Chromium: For pediatric patients, the suggested additive dosage is 0.14 to 0.20 mcg chromium/kg/day.
Parenteral drug products should be inspected visually for particulate matter and discoloration prior to administration whenever solution and container permit. See Precautions section.
How Supplied: Multitrace™ Pediatric, Trace Element Mixture, is supplied in 3 ml single-dose vials in boxes of 25.
Store at controlled room temperature between 15°–30°C (59°–86°F); avoid excessive heat.
Revised: February, 1984

MULTITRACE™ SOLUTION and CONCENTRATE
[mŭl' tē-trās'']
Trace Element Mixture

Description: Multitrace, Trace Element Mixture, is a sterile non-pyrogenic, isotonic solution containing zinc, copper, manganese and chromium for use as an additive to intravenous solutions for total parenteral nutrition (TPN).
Each ml of Multitrace Solution Contains:
Zinc Chloride* .... 2.085 mg
Copper Chloride dihydrate** .... 1,073 mg
Manganese Chloride tetrahydrate*** ..... 0.36 mg
Chromium Chloride hexahydrate**** .... 20.5 mcg
Sodium Chloride .... 6.35 mg
Water for Injection .... q.s.
*Equivalent to 1.0 mg Zn
**Equivalent to 0.4 mg Cu
***Equivalent to 0.1 mg Mn
****Equivalent to 4.0 mcg Cr
pH adjusted with Hydrochloric Acid
Multiple dose vials contain 0.9% Benzyl Alcohol as a preservative.
Each ml of Multitrace Concentrate Contains:
Zinc Chloride* .... 10.42 mg
Copper Chloride dihydrate** .... 2.68 mg
Manganese Chloride tetrahydrate*** ..... 1.80 mg
Chromium Chloride hexahydrate**** .... 51.2 mcg
Sodium Chloride .... 0.50 mg
Water for Injection .... q.s.
*Equivalent to 5.0 mg Zn
**Equivalent to 1.0 mg Cu
***Equivalent to 0.5 mg Mn
****Equivalent to 10.0 mcg Cr
pH adjusted with Hydrochloric Acid
Multiple dose vials contain 0.9% Benzyl Alcohol as a preservative.
Zinc Chloride, USP is chemically designated $ZnCl_2$, a white crystalline compound freely soluble in water. Cupric Chloride is chemically designated $CuCl_2$, a crystalline compound freely soluble in water. Manganese Chloride is chemically designated $MnCl_2$, a deliquescent, crystalline compound soluble in water. Chromic Chloride is chemically designated $CrCl_3$, a crystalline compound soluble in water. Sodium Chloride, USP is chemically designated NaCl, a white crystalline compound freely soluble in water.
Clinical Pharmacology: Zinc is an essential nutritional requirement that serves as a cofactor for more than 70 different enzymes including carbonic anhydrase, alkaline phosphatase, lactic dehydrogenase, and both RNA and DNA polymerase. Zinc facilitates wound healing, helps maintain normal growth rates, normal skin hydration, and the senses of taste and smell. Providing zinc during TPN helps prevent development of deficiency symptoms and signs such as: Parakeratosis, hypogeusia, anorexia, dysosmia, geophagia, hypogonadism, growth retardation and hepatosplenomeg-

Continued on next page

Armour—Cont.

aly. At plasma levels below 20 mcg zinc/dl, dermatitis followed by alopecia has been reported.
Copper is an essential nutrient that serves as a cofactor for serum ceruloplasmin, an oxidase necessary for proper formation of the iron carrier protein, transferrin. Copper also helps maintain normal rates of red and white blood cell formation. Providing copper during TPN helps prevent development of the following deficiency symptoms and signs: Leukopenia, neutropenia, anemia, depressed ceruloplasmin levels, impaired transferrin formation, and secondary iron deficiency. Normal serum copper values range from 80 to 163 mcg/dl.
Manganese is an essential nutrient that serves as an activator for enzymes such as polysaccharide polymerase, liver arginase, cholinesterase, and pyruvate carboxylase. Providing manganese during TPN helps prevent deficiency symptoms and signs such as nausea and vomiting, weight loss, dermatitis, and changes in growth and color of hair. Assays for manganese in whole blood result in concentrations ranging from 6 to 12 mcg manganese/liter.
Trivalent chromium is part of glucose tolerance factor, an essential activator of insulin-mediated reactions. Chromium helps maintain normal glucose metabolism and peripheral nerve function. Providing chromium during TPN helps prevent deficiency symptoms and signs including impaired glucose tolerance, ataxia, peripheral neuropathy, and a confusional state similar to mild/moderate hepatic encephalopathy. Typical blood levels for chromium range from 1 to 5 mcg/liter, but blood levels are not considered a meaningful index of tissue stores. A normalization of the glucose tolerance curve from the diabetic-like curve typical of chromium deficiency is viewed as a more meaningful indicator of chromium nutriture than serum chromium levels.

Indications and Usage: Multitrace is indicated for use as a supplement to intravenous solutions given for total parenteral nutrition (TPN). Administration helps maintain zinc, copper, manganese, and chromium blood levels and prevents depletion of endogenous stores and subsequential deficiency states.

Contraindications: Direct intramuscular or intravenous injection of Multitrace, Trace Element Mixture, is contraindicated as the acidic pH of the solution (2.0) may cause considerable tissue irritation.

Warnings: Copper and manganese are eliminated via the bile. In patients with severe liver dysfunction and/or biliary tract obstruction, decreasing or omitting copper and manganese supplements entirely may be necessary.

Precautions: Do not use unless the solution is clear and the seal is intact. Multitrace, Trace Element Mixture, should be used only in conjunction with a pharmacy-directed admixture program using aseptic technique in a laminar flow environment. Single dose vials contain no preservative; unused portions should be discarded within 24 hours after opening.
Frequent determination of serum levels of the various trace elements is suggested as a guideline for administering Multitrace. Zinc is eliminated via the kidneys and the possibility of retention should be considered in patients with renal dysfunction. Copper and manganese are eliminated via the bile and the possibility of retention should be considered in patients with biliary obstruction. In assessing the contribution of chromium supplements to maintenance of glucose homeostasis, consideration should be given to the possibility the patient may be diabetic.
Parenteral solutions which contain benzyl alcohol used for flushing intravascular catheters have been reported to cause a fatal toxic syndrome in neonates or in infants weighing less than 2500 grams. This product, as well as other parenteral micronutrient products, in multiple dose vials, contains benzyl alcohol and therefore should be used with caution in such patients.

Pregnancy Category C: Animal reproduction studies have not been conducted with Multitrace, Trace Element Mixture. It is also not known whether Multitrace can cause fetal harm when administered to a pregnant woman or can affect reproductive capacity. Multitrace should be given to a pregnant woman only if clearly indicated.

Adverse Reactions: None known.

Drug Abuse and Dependency: None known.

Overdosage: Single intravenous doses of 1 to 2 mg zinc/kg body weight have been given to adult leukemic patients without toxic manifestations. However, acute toxicity was reported in an adult when 10 mg zinc was infused over a period of one hour on each of four consecutive days. Symptoms included hypotension, pulmonary edema, diarrhea, vomiting, jaundice, oliguria, blurred vision, tachycardia, decreased level of consciousness, profuse sweating, and hypothermia. Death resulted from an overdose in which 1683 mg zinc was delivered intravenously over the course of 60 hours to a 72-year-old patient. Calcium supplements may confer a protective effect against zinc toxicity.
Copper toxicity can produce prostration, behavior change, diarrhea, progressive marasmus, hypotonia, photophobia, and peripheral edema. Such symptoms have been reported with a serum copper level of 286 mcg/dl. D-pencillamine has been reported effective as an antidote.
Manganese toxicity in TPN patients has not been reported.
Trivalent chromium administered intravenously to TPN patients has been shown to be nontoxic when given at dosage levels of up to 250 mcg/day for two consecutive weeks. Reported toxic reactions to chromium include nausea, vomiting, ulcers of the gastrointestinal tract, renal and hepatic damage, convulsions, and coma.

Dosage and Administration: Each ml of Multitrace Solution, Trace Element Mixture, contains 1.0 mg Zn, 0.4 mg Cu, 0.1 mg Mn and 4.0 mcg Cr and is administered intravenously only after dilution to a minimum of 1:200.
Each ml Multitrace Concentrate, Trace Element Mixture, contains 5.0 mg Zn, 1.0 mg Cu, 0.5 mg Mn, and 10.0 mcg Cr and is administered intravenously only after dilution to a minimum of 1:200. The following are suggested dosage ranges for the four trace elements.
Zinc: For the metabolically stable adult receiving TPN, the suggested intravenous dosage is 2.5 to 4 mg zinc/day. An additional 2 mg zinc/day is suggested for acute catabolic states. For the stable adult with fluid loss from the small bowel, an additional 12.2 mg zinc/liter of small bowel fluid lost, or an additional 17.1 mg zinc/kg of stool or ileostomy output is recommended. Frequent monitoring of zinc blood levels is suggested for patients receiving more than the usual maintenance dosage level of zinc.
For full-term infants and children up to 5 years of age, 100 mcg zinc/kg/day is recommended. For premature infants (birth weight less than 1500 grams) up to 3 kg in body weight, 300 mcg/kg/day is suggested.
Copper: For the adult receiving TPN, the suggested additive dosage is 0.5 to 1.5 mg copper/day. For pediatric patients, the suggested additive dosage is 20 mcg copper/kg/day.
Manganese: For the adult receiving TPN, the suggested additive dosage for manganese is 0.15 to 0.8 mg/day.
For pediatric patients, a dosage of 2 to 10 mcg manganese/kg/day is recommended.
Chromium: For the adult receiving TPN, the suggested additive dosage is 10 to 15 mcg chromium/day. The metabolically stable adult with intestinal fluid loss may require 20 mcg chromium/day with frequent monitoring of blood levels as a guideline for subsequent administration.
For pediatric patients, the suggested additive dosage is 0.14 to 0.20 mcg chromium/kg/day.
Parenteral drug products should be inspected visually for particulate matter and discoloration prior to administration whenever solution and container permit. See Precautions section.

How Supplied: Multitrace Solution, Trace Element Mixture in 10 ml, single dose vials in boxes of 25 and 30 ml multiple dose vials in boxes of 10. Multitrace Concentrate, Trace Element Mixture in 1 ml, single dose vials in boxes of 25 and 5 ml multiple dose vials in boxes of 10.
Store at controlled room temperature between 15°–30°C (59°–86°F); avoid excessive heat.
Revised: 1/84

SELENITRACE™ ℞
[sĕ-lĕ′ nē-trās″]
Selenious Acid Injection

Description: Selenitrace, Selenious Acid Injection (40 mcg selenium/ml) is a sterile nonpyrogenic solution intended for use as additive to intravenous solutions for total parenteral nutrition (TPN).
Each ml of solution provides:
Selenious Acid .... 65.34 mcg
Water for Injection .... q.s.
pH adjusted to approximately 2.0 with nitric acid
The solution contains no bacteriostat, antimicrobial agent, or added buffer.
Selenious acid is chemically designated H_2Se, white or colorless crystals soluble in water or alcohol.

Clinical Pharmacology: Selenium is an essential nutritional requirement that is part of glutathione peroxidase which protects cell components from oxidative damage resulting from peroxidase produced in cellular metabolism.
Providing selenium during TPN helps prevent development of deficiency symptoms which include muscle pain and tenderness.
In different human populations, normal blood levels of selenium have been found to vary and depend on the selenium content of the food consumed.
Deficiency symptoms in humans have been reported with plasma selenium levels of 0.3 and 0.9 mcg/dl.
The primary route of elimination of selenium is in the urine, but significant losses also occur through feces. The chemical form of the selenium used in supplementation affects the rate of excretion and the relative importance of the two routes. The lungs and skin are ancillary routes of elimination.

Indications and Usage: Selenitrace is indicated for use as a supplement to intravenous solutions given for TPN. Administration helps to maintain selenium serum levels and to prevent depletion of endogenous stores and subsequent deficiency symptoms.

Contraindications: Direct intramuscular or intravenous injection of Selenitrace is contraindicated as the acidic pH of the solution (2.0) may cause considerable tissue irritation.

Warnings: None known.

Precautions: Do not use unless the solution is clear and the seal is intact.
Selenitrace should be used only in conjunction with a pharmacy-directed admixture program using aseptic technique in a laminar flow environment. The solution contains no preservatives; discard unused portion within 24 hours after opening. Frequent selenium plasma level determinations are suggested as a guideline to adjust, reduce or omit selenium supplements in renal dysfunction and/or gastrointestinal malfunction.

Pregnancy Category C. Selenium at high dosage levels (15-30 mcg/egg) has been reported to have adverse embryological effects among chickens. There are no adequate and well-controlled studies in pregnant women. Selenitrace™ should be used during pregnancy only if the potential benefit justifies the potential risk to the fetus. The presence of selenium in placenta and umbilical cord has been reported.

Adverse Reactions: None known.

Drug Abuse and Dependence: None known.

Overdosage: Exposure to selenium in industrial environments, intake of foods grown in seleniferous soils, application of selenium-containing cosmetics, and use of selenium contaminated water have been reported to cause chronic toxicity in humans. Selenium toxicity symptoms include weakened nails, dental defects, hair loss, dermatitis, nervousness, gastrointestinal disorders, mental depression, metallic taste, vomiting and garlic odor of breath and sweat. Death resulted from ingestion of large amounts of selenium compounds. The histopathological changes included fulminating peripheral vascular collapse, internal vascular congestion, diffusely hemorrhagic congested and edematous lungs, and brick-red color gastric mucosa. Coma preceded death. There is no known effective antidote to selenium poisoning in humans.

Dosage and Administration: Selenitrace, Selenious Acid Injection, contains 40 mcg selenium/ml and is administered intravenously only after dilution to a minimum of 1:200.

Adult: For the metabolically stable adult receiving TPN, the suggested intravenous dosage level is 20 to 40 mcg selenium/day. In adults with selenium deficiency states resulting from long-term TPN support, selenious acid administered intravenously at 100 mcg/day for a period of 24 and 31 days, respectively, has been reported to reverse deficiency symptoms without toxicity.

Frequent monitoring of selenium blood levels is suggested for patients receiving more than the usual maintenance dose. The normal whole blood range for selenium is approximately 10-37 mcg/dl.

Pediatric: For children the suggested dosage level is 3 mcg/kg/day.

Parenteral drug products should be inspected visually for particulate matter and discoloration prior to administration, whenever solution and container permit.

How Supplied: Selenitrace 10 ml vials (NDC 0053-1449-35), boxes of 25.

Store at controlled room temperature 15°-30°C (59°-86°F).

Revised: 5/84

STIMATE™ ℞
[stĭm'āt]
(desmopressin acetate) INJECTION

Description: Desmopressin acetate is an antidiuretic hormone affecting renal water conservation and is a synthetic analogue of 8-arginine vasopressin. It is chemically defined as follows:
Mol. Wt. 1183.2
Empirical Formula: $C_{48}H_{74}N_{14}O_{17}S_2$
SCH$_2$CH$_2$CO-Tyr-Phe-Gln-Asn-Cys-Pro-D-Arg-
Gly-NH$_2 \cdot$ C$_2$H$_4$O$_2 \cdot$ 3H$_2$O

1-(3-mercaptopropionic acid)-8-D-arginine vasopressin mono-acetate (salt) trihydrate.

Stimate™ (desmopressin acetate) is provided as a sterile, aqueous solution for injection.

Each ml provides: Desmopressin acetate 4.0 mcg Chlorobutanol 5.0 mg Sodium chloride 9.0 mg Hydrochloric acid to adjust pH to 3.5.

Clinical Pharmacology: Stimate™ contains as active substance, 1-(3-mercaptopropionic acid)-8-D-arginine vasopressin, a synthetic analogue of the natural hormone arginine vasopressin. One ml (4 mcg) of Stimate™ has an antidiuretic activity of about 16 IU; 1 mcg of desmopressin acetate is equivalent to 4 IU.

Desmopressin acetate has been shown to be more potent than arginine vasopressin in increasing plasma levels of factor VIII activity in patients with hemophilia A and von Willebrand's disease Type 1.

Dose-response studies were performed in healthy persons, using doses of 0.1 to 0.4 mcg/kg body weight, infused over a 10-minute period. Maximal dose response occurred at 0.3 to 0.4 mcg/kg. The response to desmopressin acetate of factor VIII activity and plasminogen activator is dose-related, with maximal plasma levels of 300 to 400 percent of initial concentrations obtained after infusion of 0.4 mcg/kg body weight. The increase is rapid and evident within 30 minutes reaching a maximum at a point ranging from 90 minutes to two hours. The factor VIII-related antigen and ristocetin cofactor activity were also increased to a smaller degree, but still dose-dependent.

1. The biphasic half-lives of desmopressin acetate were 7.8 and 75.5 minutes for the fast and slow phases, respectively, compared with 2.5 and 14.5 minutes for lysine vasopressin, another form of the hormone. As a result, desmopressin acetate provides a prompt onset of antidiuretic action with a long duration after each administration.

2. The change in structure of arginine vasopressin to desmopressin acetate has resulted in a decreased vasopressor action and decreased actions on visceral smooth muscle relative to the enhanced antidiuretic activity, so that clinically effective antidiuretic doses are usually below threshold levels for effects on vascular or visceral smooth muscle.

3. When administered by injection, desmopressin acetate has an antidiuretic effect about ten times that of an equivalent dose administered intranasally.

4. The percentage increase of factor VIII levels in patients with mild hemophilia A and von Willebrand's disease was not significantly different from that observed in normal healthy individuals when treated with 0.3 mcg/kg of desmopressin acetate infused over 10 minutes. One hemophilia A patient treated with intravenous desmopressin acetate was shown to have a response that reached as much as five times the baseline value, and that occurred at 4½ hours after infusion.

5. Plasminogen activator activity increases rapidly after desmopressin acetate infusion, but there has been no clinically significant fibrinolysis in patients treated with desmopressin acetate.

6. The effect of repeated administration of desmopressin acetate when doses were given every 12 to 24 hours has generally shown a gradual diminution of the factor VIII activity increase noted with a single dose. The initial response is reproducible in any particular patient if there are 2 or 3 days between administration.

Indications and Usage: Hemophilia A
Stimate™ (desmopressin acetate) is indicated for patients with hemophilia A with factor VIII levels greater than 5%.

Stimate™ will often maintain hemostasis in patients with hemophilia A during surgical procedures and postoperatively when administered 30 minutes prior to scheduled procedure.

Stimate™ will also stop bleeding in hemophilia A patients with episodes of spontaneous or trauma-induced injuries such as hemarthroses, intramuscular hematomas or mucosal bleeding.

Stimate™ is not indicated for the treatment of hemophilia A with factor VIII levels equal to or less than 5%, or for the treatment of hemophilia B, or in patients who have factor VIII antibodies.

In certain clinical situations, it may be justified to try Stimate™ in patients with factor VIII levels between 2–5%; however these patients should be carefully monitored.

Von Willebrand's Disease (Type I)
Stimate™ is indicated for patients with mild to moderate classic von Willebrand's disease (Type I) with factor VIII levels greater than 5%. Stimate™ will often maintain hemostasis in patients with mild to moderate von Willebrand's disease during surgical procedures and postoperatively when administered 30 minutes prior to the scheduled procedure.

Stimate™ will usually stop bleeding in mild to moderate von Willebrand's patients with episodes of spontaneous or trauma-induced injuries such as hemarthroses, intramuscular hematomas or mucosal bleeding.

Those von Willebrand's disease patients who are least likely to respond are those with severe homozygous von Willebrand's disease with factor VIII coagulant activity, factor VIII antigen and von Willebrand's factor (ristocetin cofactor) activities less than 1%. Other patients may respond in a variable fashion depending on the type of molecular defect they have. Bleeding time and factor VIII coagulant activity, factor VIII antigen and von Willebrand's factor activities should be checked during administration of Stimate™ to ensure that adequate levels are being achieved.

Stimate™ is not indicated for the treatment of severe classic von Willebrand's disease (Type I) and when there is evidence of an abnormal molecular form of factor VIII antigen. See Warning.

Diabetes Insipidus
Stimate™ is indicated as antidiuretic replacement therapy in the management of central (cranial) diabetes insipidus and for the management of the temporary polyuria and polydipsia following head trauma or surgery in the pituitary region. Stimate™ is ineffective for the treatment of nephrogenic diabetes insipidus.

Desmopressin acetate is also available as an intranasal preparation, DDAVP.® However, this means of delivery can be compromised by a variety of factors that can make nasal insufflation ineffective or inappropriate. These include poor intranasal absorption, nasal congestion and blockage, nasal discharge, atrophy of nasal mucosa, and severe atrophic rhinitis. Intranasal delivery may be inappropriate where there is an impaired level of consciousness. In addition, cranial surgical procedures, such as transphenoidal hypophysectomy, create situations where an alternative route of administration is needed as in cases of nasal packing or recovery from surgery.

Contraindications: Known hypersensitivity to Stimate™ (desmopressin acetate).

Warning: Patients who do not have need of antidiuretic hormone for its antidiuretic effect, in particular those who are young or elderly, should be cautioned to ingest only enough fluid to satisfy thirst, in order to decrease the potential occurrence of water intoxication and hyponatremia.

Stimate™ (desmopressin acetate) should not be used to treat patients with Type IIB von Willebrand's disease since platelet aggregation may be induced.

Precautions:
GENERAL: For injection use only.

Desmopressin acetate has infrequently produced a slight elevation of blood pressure, which disappeared with a reduction in dosage. The drug should be used with caution in patients with coronary artery insufficiency and/or hypertensive cardiovascular disease, because of possible rise in blood pressure.

Severe allergic reactions have not been reported with desmopressin acetate. It is not known whether antibodies to desmopressin acetate are produced after repeated injections.

Hemophilia A
Laboratory tests for assessing patient status include levels of factor VIII coagulant, factor VIII antigen and factor VIII ristocetin cofactor (von Willebrand factor) as well as activated partial thromboplastin time. Factor VIII coagulant activity should be determined before giving desmopressin acetate for hemostasis. If factor VIII coagulant activity is present at less than 5% of normal, desmopressin acetate should not be relied on.

Von Willebrand's Disease
Laboratory tests for assessing patient status include levels of factor VIII coagulant, factor VIII antigen and factor VIII ristocetin cofactor (von Willebrand factor). The skin bleeding time may be helpful in following these patients.

Diabetes Insipidus
Laboratory tests for monitoring the patient include urine volume and osmolality. In some cases, plasma osmolality may be required.

DRUG INTERACTIONS: Although the pressor activity of desmopressin acetate is very low compared with the antidiuretic activity, use of doses as large as 0.3 mcg/kg of desmopressin acetate with other pressor agents should be done only with careful patient monitoring.

Desmopressin acetate has been used with epsilon aminocaproic acid without adverse effects.

CARCINOGENICITY, MUTAGENICITY, IMPAIRMENT OF FERTILITY: Teratology studies in rats have shown no abnormalities. No further data are available.

PREGNANCY CATEGORY B: Reproduction studies performed in rats and rabbits with subcutaneous doses up to 12.5 times the human dose when used for factor VIII stimulation and 125 times the human dose when used in diabetes insipidus have revealed no evidence of harm to the fe-

Continued on next page

Armour—Cont.

tus due to desmopressin acetate. There are several publications of management of diabetes insipidus in pregnant women with no harm to the fetus reported; however, there are no adequate and well-controlled studies in pregnant women. Published reports stress that, as opposed to preparations containing the natural hormones, desmopressin acetate in antidiuretic doses has no uterotonic action, but the physician will have to weigh possible therapeutic advantages against possible danger in each case.

NURSING MOTHERS: It is not known whether this drug is excreted in human milk. Because many drugs are excreted in human milk, caution should be exercised when desmopressin acetate is administered to a nursing woman.

PEDIATRIC USE: Use in infants and children will require careful fluid intake restriction to prevent possible hyponatremia and water intoxication. Stimate™ should not be used in infants younger than three months in the treatment of hemophilia A or von Willebrand's disease; safety and effectiveness in children under 12 years of age with diabetes insipidus have not been established.

Adverse Reactions: Infrequently, desmopressin acetate has produced transient headache, nausea, mild abdominal cramps and vulval pain. These symptoms disappeared with reduction in dosage. Occasionally, injection of desmopressin acetate has produced local erythema, swelling or burning pain. Occasional facial flushing has been reported with the administration of desmopressin acetate.

Desmopressin acetate has infrequently produced a slight elevation of blood pressure, which disappeared with a reduction in dosage.

See WARNING for the possibility of water intoxication and hyponatremia.

Overdosage: See ADVERSE REACTIONS above. In case of overdosage, the dosage should be reduced, frequency of administration decreased, or the drug withdrawn according to the severity of the condition.

There is no known specific antidote for desmopressin acetate. If considerable fluid retention causes concern, a saluretic may induce a diuresis.

An oral LD_{50} has not been established. An intravenous dose of 2 mg/kg in mice demonstrated no effect.

Dosage and Administration: Hemophilia A and von Willebrand's Disease (Type I)

Stimate™ is administered as an intravenous infusion at a dose of 0.3 mcg desmopressin acetate/kg body weight diluted in sterile physiological saline and infused slowly over 15 to 30 minutes. In adults and children weighing more than 10 kg, 50 ml of diluent is used; in children weighing 10 kg or less, 10 ml of diluent is used. Blood pressure and pulse should be monitored during infusion. If Stimate™ is used preoperatively, it should be administered 30 minutes prior to the scheduled procedure.

The necessity for repeat administration of Stimate™ or use of any blood products for hemostasis should be determined by laboratory response as well as the clinical condition of the patient. The tendency toward tachyphylaxis (lessening of response) with repeated administration given more frequently than every 48 hours should be considered in treating each patient.

Diabetes Insipidus

This formulation is administered subcutaneously or by direct intravenous injection. Stimate™ (desmopressin acetate) Injection dosage must be determined for each patient and adjusted according to the pattern of response. Response should be estimated by two parameters: adequate duration of sleep and adequate, not excessive, water turnover.

The usual dosage range in adults is 0.5 ml (2.0 mcg) to 1 ml (4.0 mcg) daily, administered intravenously or subcutaneously, usually in two divided doses. The morning and evening doses should be separately adjusted for an adequate diurnal rhythm of water turnover. For patients who have been controlled on intranasal desmopressin acetate and who must be switched to the injection form, either because of poor intranasal absorption or because of the need for surgery, the comparable antidiuretic dose of the injection is about one-tenth the intranasal dose.

Parenteral drug products should be inspected visually for particulate matter and discoloration prior to administration whenever solution and container permit.

How Supplied: Stimate™ (desmopressin acetate) Injection is available as a sterile solution in 10 ml multiple-dose vials, (NDC 0053-2451-02) each containing 4.0 mcg desmopressin acetate per ml. Keep refrigerated at about 4°C.

Manufactured for
Amour Pharmaceutical Company
Kankakee, Illinois 60901, U.S.A.
By Ferring Pharmaceuticals, Malmö, Sweden
Revised: February, 1984

THYTROPAR®
[thī' trō-pär']
(thyrotropin for injection)
U.S. PAT. No. 2,871,159

Description:
THYTROPAR® (Thyrotropin for Injection) is a highly purified and lyophilized thyrotropic or thyroid stimulating hormone (TSH) isolated from bovine anterior pituitary. The potency of THYTROPAR® is designated in terms of International Thyrotropin units and is free of significant amounts of adrenocorticotropic, gonadotropic, somatotropic and posterior pituitary hormones. It is soluble throughout a wide pH range and is stable at room temperature when kept in the dry state. It dissolves readily in physiologic saline and will retain its potency when in solution for at least two weeks if refrigerated.

THYTROPAR® Diluent (Sodium Chloride Injection) contains in each ml 9 mg of Sodium Chloride, Water for Injection, q.s.

It is a sterile preparation for intramuscular or subcutaneous use only. It is a glyco-protein with a molecular weight in the range of 28,000–30,000.

Clinical Pharmacology: The action of THYTROPAR® produces increased uptake of iodine by the thyroid, increased formation of thyroid hormone, increased release of thyroid hormone, and cellular hyperplasia of the thyroid on prolonged stimulation.

After injection, the effect on the thyroid in normal individuals is evident within 8 hours reaching a maximum in 24-48 hours.

Indications and Usage: THYTROPAR® is indicated for use as a diagnostic agent. It is used to differentiate thyroid failure from pituitary failure and to establish a diagnosis of decreased thyroid reserve.

Contraindications:
1. Hypersensitivity to thyrotropin.
2. Coronary thrombosis.
3. Untreated Addison's disease.

Warnings: Anaphylactic reactions have been reported on repeated administration.

Precautions:
General—Since THYTROPAR® can stimulate thyroid secretion, caution must be observed when using in patients with cardiac disease who are unable to tolerate additional stress.

Drug Interactions—THYTROPAR® (Thyrotropin for Injection) can be used with PBI or I^{131} uptake determinations.

Pregnancy Category C—Animal reproduction studies have not been conducted with THYTROPAR®. It is also not known whether THYTROPAR® can cause fetal harm when administered to a pregnant woman or can affect reproduction capacity. THYTROPAR® should be given to a pregnant woman only if clearly needed.

Nursing Mothers—It is not known whether this drug is excreted in human milk. Because many drugs are excreted in human milk, caution should be exercised when THYTROPAR® is administered to a nursing woman.

Pediatric Use—Safety and effectiveness in children have not been established.

Adverse Reactions:
Nausea, vomiting, headache, and urticaria are the most commonly seen reactions. Also seen and probably related to a sensitivity type reaction is transitory hypotension and tachycardia. Anaphylactic reactions with patient collapse have been reported.

Thyroid gland swelling has been reported particularly with larger doses (>10u).

Drug Abuse and Dependence: Drug abuse and dependence have not been reported.

Overdosage:
SYMPTOMS—Headache, irritability, nervousness, sweating, tachycardia, increased bowel motility, menstrual irregularities. Angina pectoris or congestive heart failure may be induced or aggravated. Shock may also develop. Excessive doses may result in symptoms resembling thyroid storm. Chronic excessive dosage will produce the signs and symptoms of hyperthyroidism.

TREATMENT—in shock, supportive measures and treatment of unrecognized adrenal insufficiency should be considered. Thyrotropin should be discontinued.

Dosage and Administration: THYTROPAR® is injected intramuscularly or subcutaneously in a dose of 10 I.U. for 1–3 days followed by a radioiodine uptake study 24 hours after the last injection. In thyroid failure, no response will be seen, in pituitary failure a substantial response should be seen. THYTROPAR® should be stored at controlled room temperature between 15°–30°C (59°–86°F.) After reconstitution store between 2°–8°C (36°–46°F), for not longer than two weeks.

Parenteral drug products should be inspected visually for particulate matter and discoloration prior to administration whenever solution and container permit.

How Supplied:
THYTROPAR® is supplied as a sterile lyophilized powder containing 10 International Units of Thyrotropic activity. Each package contains one vial of THYTROPAR® (Thyrotropin for Injection) and one vial of THYTROPAR® Diluent (Sodium Chloride Injection).

Revised: May, 1984

TRACE ELEMENTS See under:

Chrometrace™ (Chromic Chloride Injection USP)
Coppertrace™ (Cupric Chloride Injection USP)
Mangatrace™ (Manganese Chloride Injection USP)
Zinctrace™ (Zinc Chloride Injection USP)
Selenitrace™ (Selenious Acid Injection)

For dilution in intravenous infusions only
ZINCTRACE™
[zĭngk' trăs]
Zinc Chloride Injection USP

1 mg/ml

Zinc Chloride in Sodium Chloride Solution

Description: Zinctrace, Zinc Chloride Injection USP (1 mg zinc/ml), is a sterile, nonpyrogenic solution intended for use as an additive to intravenous solutions for total parenteral nutrition (TPN). Each ml of solution provides:

zinc chloride .... 2.09 mg
sodium .... 3.07 mg
chloride .... 5.82 mg
(not including ions for pH adjustment).

The pH is approximately 2.0, adjusted with hydrochloric acid, and may be adjusted with sodium hydroxide. The solution is adjusted to isotonicity with sodium chloride. The osmolarity is approximately 0.300 mOsm/ml. The solution contains no bacteriostat, antimicrobial agent, or added buffer. Zinc chloride USP is chemically designated $ZnCl_2$, a white crystalline compound freely soluble in water. Sodium chloride USP is chemically designated NaCl, a white crystalline compound freely soluble in water.

Clinical Pharmacology: Zinc is an essential nutritional requirement that serves as a cofactor for more than 70 different enzymes including carbonic anhydrase, alkaline phosphatase, lactic dehydrogenase, and both RNA and DNA polymerase. Zinc facilitates wound healing, helps maintain normal growth rates, normal skin hydration, and the senses of taste and smell.

Zinc resides in muscle, bone, skin, kidney, liver, pancreas, retina, prostate, and particularly in the red and white blood cells. Zinc binds to plasma albumin, Cl$_2$-macroglobulin, and some plasma amino acids including histidine, cysteine, threonine, glycine, and asparagine. Ingested zinc is excreted mainly in the stool (approximately 90%), and to a lesser extent in the urine and in perspiration.

Providing zinc during TPN helps prevent development of deficiency symptoms such as: Parakeratosis, hypogeusia, anorexia, dysosmia, geophagia, hypogonadism, growth retardation and hepatosplenomegaly.

The initial manifestations of hypozincemia in TPN are diarrhea, apathy, and depression. At plasma levels below 20 mcg zinc/dl, dermatitis followed by alopecia has been reported for TPN patients. Normal zinc plasma levels are 100 ± 12 mcg/dl.

Indications and Usage: Zinctrace is indicated for use as a supplement to intravenous solutions given for TPN. Administration helps to maintain zinc serum levels and to prevent depletion of endogenous stores and subsequent deficiency symptoms.

Contraindications: Direct intramuscular or intravenous injection of Zinctrace, is contraindicated as the acidic pH of the solution (2.0) may cause considerable tissue irritation.

Warnings: None known.

Precautions: Do not use unless the solution is clear and the seal is intact.

Zinctrace should be used only in conjunction with a pharmacy-directed admixture program using aseptic technique in a laminar flow environment. The solution contains no preservatives; discard unused portion within 24 hours after opening.

Zinctrace should not be given undiluted by direct injection into a peripheral vein because of the likelihood of infusion phlebitis and the potential for increased excretory loss of zinc from a bolus injection. Administration of zinc in the absence of copper may cause a decrease in serum copper levels. Periodic determinations of serum copper as well as zinc are suggested as a guideline for subsequent zinc administration.

Pregnancy Category C. Animal reproduction studies have not been conducted with zinc chloride. It is also not known whether zinc chloride can cause fetal harm when administered to a pregnant woman or can affect reproductive capacity. Zinc chloride should be given to a pregnant woman only if clearly needed.

Adverse Reactions: None known.

Drug Abuse and Dependence: None known.

Overdosage: Single intravenous doses of 1 to 2 mg zinc/kg body weight have been given to adult leukemic patients without toxic manifestations. However, acute toxicity was reported in an adult when 10 mg zinc was infused over a period of one hour on each of four consecutive days. Profuse sweating, decreased level of consciousness, blurred vision, tachycardia (140/min.), and marked hypothermia (94.2°F) on the fourth day were accompanied by a serum zinc concentration of 207 mcg/dl. Symptoms abated within three hours.

Hyperamylasemia may be a sign of impending zinc overdosage; patients receiving an inadvertent overdose (25 mg zinc/liter of TPN solution, equivalent to 50 to 70 mg zinc/day) developed hyperamylasemia (557 to 1850 Klein units; normal; 130 to 310).

Death resulted from an overdose in which 1683 mg zinc was delivered intravenously over the course of 60 hours to a 72-year-old patient.

Symptoms of zinc toxicity included hypotension (80/40 mm Hg), pulmonary edema, diarrhea, vomiting, jaundice, and oliguria, with a serum zinc level of 4184 mcg/dl.

Calcium supplements may confer a protective effect against zinc toxicity.

Dosage and Administration: Zinctrace, Zinc Chloride Injection USP, contains 1 mg zinc/ml and is administered intravenously only after dilution.

Adult: For the metabolically stable adult receiving TPN, the suggested intravenous dosage is 2.5 to 4 mg zinc/day. An additional 2 mg zinc/day is suggested for acute catabolic states. For the stable adult with fluid loss from the small bowel, an additional 12.2 mg zinc/liter of small bowel fluid lost, or an additional 17.1 mg zinc/kg of stool or ileostomy output is recommended. Frequent monitoring of zinc blood levels is suggested for patients receiving more than the usual maintenance dosage level of zinc.

Pediatric: For full-term infants and children up to 5 years of age, 100 mcg zinc/kg/day is recommended. For premature infants (birth weight less than 1500 grams) up to 3 kg in body weight, 300 mcg zinc/kg/day is suggested.

Parenteral drug products should be inspected visually for particulate matter and discoloration prior to administration, whenever solution and container permit. See Precautions section.

How Supplied: Zinctrace 10-ml vials (NDC 0053-0833-22), boxes of 25.

Store at controlled room temperature—15°-30°C (59°-86°F); avoid excessive heat.

Revised: 12/82

PLASMA DERIVATIVE PRODUCTS

ALBUMINAR®-5 ℞
[al-byōō'mĭn-är]
Normal Serum Albumin (Human) U.S.P. 5%

ALBUMINAR®-5 Normal Serum Albumin (Human) is supplied as a 5% solution in:
  50 ml. bottles containing 2.5 grams of albumin
  250 ml. bottles containing 12.5 grams of albumin
  500 ml. bottles containing 25.0 grams of albumin
  1000 ml. bottles containing 50 grams of albumin
For use with intravenous administration set. See directions on set supplied.

ALBUMINAR®-25 ℞
[ăl-byōō'mĭn-är']
Normal Serum Albumin (Human) U.S.P. 25%

ALBUMINAR®-25 Normal Serum Albumin (Human), is supplied as a 25% solution in:
  20 ml. vials containing 5.0 grams of albumin
  50 ml. vials containing 12.5 grams of albumin
  100 ml. vials containing 25.0 grams of albumin
For use with intravenous administration set. See directions on set supplied.

FACTORATE® ℞
[făk'tôr-āt'']
Antihemophilic Factor (Human) U.S.P. Dried

FACTORATE® Antihemophilic Factor (Human) Dried is supplied in single dose vials (I.U. activity is stated on label of each vial) with sterile diluent and needles for reconstitution and withdrawal.

FACTORATE® GENERATION II™ ℞
[făk'tôr-āt'']
Antihemophilic Factor (Human) Dried

FACTORATE® GENERATION II™ Antihemophilic Factor (Human) Dried is supplied in single dose vials (I.U. activity, total protein per vial and specific activity [I.U. per mg protein] are stated on carton label of each vial) with sterile diluent and needles for reconstitution and withdrawal.

GAMMAR® ℞
[găm'är]
Immune Serum Globulin (Human) U.S.P.

GAMMAR® Immune Serum Globulin (Human) U.S.P. is supplied in 2 ml. and 10 ml. vials.

GAMULIN® Rh ℞
[găm'yōō-lĭn'']
Rh$_o$ (D) Immune Globulin (Human)

A sterile Immune Globulin Solution containing Rh$_o$ (D) antibodies. Supplied in individual package containing a single dose vial of Gamulin Rh, patient identification card, directions for use, and patient information brochure and cartons containing 25 single dose vials of Gamulin Rh, 25 patient identification cards, 10 sets of directions for use, and 25 patient information brochures.

H.T. FACTORATE™ ℞
[făk'tôr-āt'']
Antihemophilic Factor (Human) Dried, Heat-Treated

H.T. Factorate™ Antihemophilic Factor (Human), Heat-Treated is supplied in single dose vials (I.U. activity is stated on label of each vial) with sterile diluent and needles for reconstitution and withdrawal.

H.T. FACTORATE™ GENERATION II™ ℞
[făk'tôr-āt'']
Antihemophilic Factor (Human) Dried, Heat-Treated

H.T. Factorate™ Generation II™ Antihemophilic Factor (Human), Heat-Treated is supplied in single dose vials (I.U. activity, total protein, and specific activity [I.U. per mg protein] are stated on carton label of each vial) with sterile diluent and needles for reconstitution and withdrawal.

MINI-GAMULIN™ Rh ℞
[mĭ-nē'' găm'yoo-lĭn]
Rh$_o$ (D) Immune Globulin (Human)

A sterile Immune Globulin Solution containing Rh$_o$ (D) antibodies. Mini-Gamulin Rh contains one-sixth the quantity of Rh$_o$ (D) antibody contained in a standard dose of Rh$_o$ (D) Immune Globulin (Human).

PLASMA-PLEX® ℞
[plăz'ma-plĕks]
Plasma Protein Fraction (Human) U.S.P.

As a 5% Solution in:
50 ml bottles containing 2.5 g of selected plasma proteins
250 ml bottles containing 12.5 g of selected plasma proteins
500 ml bottles containing 25.0 g of selected plasma proteins.
For use with intravenous administration set. See directions on set supplied.

PROTHAR™ ℞
[prō'thär]
Factor IX Complex (Human)

Prothar™ Factor IX Complex (Human) is supplied in single dose vials (Factor IX activity is stated on label of each vial) with sterile diluent and needles for reconstitution and withdrawal.

THROMBINAR™ ℞
[thrŏm'bĭn-är]
THROMBIN, TOPICAL (BOVINE), U.S.P.

Thrombin, Topical (Bovine), U.S.P. Thrombinar™ must not be injected! It is for topical use only.

Description: Thrombinar™ Thrombin, Topical (Bovine), U.S.P. is a protein product produced through activation of prothrombin of bovine origin by tissue thromboplastin in the presence of calcium chloride. It is supplied as a sterile powder that has been freeze-dried in the final container. Also contained in this preparation are 50% mannitol and 45% sodium chloride. Mannitol is included to make the dried product friable and more readily soluble. The material contains no preservative. This product is prepared under rigid assay control against U.S. Standard Thrombin.

Continued on next page

Armour—Cont.

Clinical Pharmacology: Thrombinar™ requires no intermediate physiological agent for its action. It clots the fibrinogen of the blood directly. Failure to clot blood occurs in the rare case where the primary clotting defect is the absence of fibrinogen itself. The speed with which thrombin clots blood is dependent upon its concentration.

Indications and Usage: Thrombinar™ Thrombin, Topical (Bovine) U.S.P., is indicated as an aid in hemostasis whenever oozing blood and minor bleeding from capillaries and small venules is accessible.

In various types of surgery solutions of thrombin may be used in conjunction with absorbable gelatin sponge, USP for hemostasis.

Contraindications: Thrombinar™ is contraindicated in persons known to be sensitive to any of its components and/or to material of bovine origin.

WARNING

Because of its action in the clotting mechanism, Thrombinar™ must not be injected or otherwise allowed to enter large blood vessels. Extensive intravascular clotting and even death may result.

Precautions: General—Consult the absorbable gelatin sponge product labeling for use prior to utilizing a thrombin saturated-sponge procedure. Pregnancy—Category C—Animal reproduction studies have not been conducted with Thrombin, Topical (Bovine) U.S.P. It is also not known whether Thrombin, Topical (Bovine), U.S.P. can cause fetal harm when administered to a pregnant woman or can affect reproduction capacity. Thrombin, Topical (Bovine), U.S.P. should be given to a pregnant woman only if clearly indicated. Pediatric Use—Safety and effectiveness in children have not been established.

Adverse Reactions: Allergic reactions may be encountered in persons known to be sensitive to bovine materials.

Dosage and Administration: Solutions of Thrombinar™ Thrombin, Topical (Bovine), U.S.P. may be prepared in Sterile Water for Injection, USP or isotonic saline. Sterile Water for Injection is recommended for reconstitution for 1000 units per ml or greater, isotonic saline for more dilute solutions. The intended use determines the strength of the solution to prepare. For general use such as plastic surgery, skin grafting, neurosurgery, solutions containing approximately 100 units per ml are frequently used. For this, 10 ml of diluent added to the 1000 unit vial is suitable. Where bleeding is profuse, concentrations as high as 1000 to 2000 units per ml may be required. For this, the 5,000 unit, 10,000 unit, or 20,000 unit vials dissolved in the appropriate amount of diluent supplied in each package is convenient. Other potencies to suit the needs of the case may be prepared by selecting the proper strength package and dissolving the contents in an appropriate volume of diluent. In many situations, it may be advantageous to use Thrombinar™ in dry form on oozing surfaces.

Caution: Product contains no preservative. Solution should be used immediately upon reconstitution. However, if several hours are to elapse before use, the solution should be refrigerated at approximately 5°C. Do not use after 48 hours.

The following techniques are suggested for the topical application of thrombin:

1. The recipient surface should be sponged (not wiped) free of blood before thrombin is applied.
2. A spray may be used or the surface may be flooded using a sterile syringe and small gauge needle. The most effective hemostasis results when the thrombin mixes freely with the blood as soon as it reaches the surface.
3. In instances where thrombin in dry form is needed, the vial is opened by removing the metal ring by grasping the edge where it is scored and tearing, using sterile pliers. The rubber-diaphragm cap may be easily removed and the dried thrombin is then broken up into a powder by means of sterile glass rod or other suitable sterile instrument.
4. Sponging of treated surfaces should be avoided in order that the clot remain securely in place. Thrombin, Topical (Bovine), U.S.P. may be used in conjunction with absorbable gelatin sponge, USP as follows:
   1. Prepare thrombin solution of the desired strength.
   2. Immerse sponge strips of the desired size in the thrombin solution. Knead the sponge strips vigorously with moistened fingers to remove trapped air, thereby facilitating saturation of the sponge.
   3. Apply saturated sponge to bleeding area. Hold in place for 10 to 15 seconds with a pledget of cotton or a small gauze sponge.

How Supplied: Thrombinar™ Thrombin, Topical (Bovine), U.S.P. is supplied in 1,000 U.S. Standard unit vials, 5,000 U.S. Standard unit vials, 10,000 U.S. Standard unit vials, 20,000 U.S. Standard unit vials, and 50,000 U.S. Standard unit vials of Thrombin, Topical. The 5,000 U.S. Standard unit vial is supplied with one 10 ml vial of Sterile Water for Injection, U.S.P. The 10,000 U.S. Standard unit vial and 20,000 U.S. Standard unit vial are each supplied with one 20 ml vial of Sterile Water for Injection U.S.P.

Storage: Store vials at 2°–8°C (36°–46°F).
Revised: May, 1984

EDUCATIONAL MATERIAL

Albuminar
"The Clinical Uses of normal serum Albumin (human)" (CME—Rutgers) cassette and accompanying brochure.
Available to physicians and pharmacists—contact your local Armour Sales Representative.

Factorate
Hemophilia booklets
—Management of hemophilia
—Boys with hemophilia
—Employment issues in hemophilia
—Employee with hemophilia
—Professional services in hemophilia
—Fluid Management—its a whole new ballgame
Available to physicians, pharmacists and patients—contact your local Armour Sales Representative or Armour Corporate Headquarters.

Gamulin
"Confidence Factor" booklets
—in Rh negative women
—in abortion
—in antepartum prophylaxis
—in prenatal diagnostic testing
The above literature is available to physicians, pharmacists and patients.
Monograph Series—"The Prevention of Rh Isoimmunization"
#1—Amniocentesis and Rh Isoimmunization
#2—Antenatal Rh Immune Globulin Use in an Uneventful Pregnancy
#3—Management of the High-Risk Pregnancy
#4—Massive Transplacental Hemorrhage, the Laboratory and the Blood Bank
Film—"Hemolytic disease of the newborn"
The Monograph Series and film are available to physicians and pharmacists—contact your local Armour Sales Representative or Armour Corporate Headquarters.

M.V.I. Product Line
"Establishing a Nutritional Support Team" —audiovisual presentation and accompanying brochure
Quarterly newsletter—"The Nutritional Support Team"
Available to physicians and pharmacists—contact your local Armour Sales Representative or Armour Corporate Headquarters.

Stimate
Booklets
—Questions and answers
—Mild hemophilia
Available to physicians and pharmacists—contact your local Armour Sales Representative or Armour Corporate Headquarters.

Thrombinar
Surgical casebook series
#1—Banded gastroplasty
#2—Abdominal aortic aneurysm inlay anastomosis
#3—Cholecystectomy
#4—Surgical intervention due to chemical peritonitis
#5—Repair of laceration of inferior vena cava
#6—The Whipple Procedure in chronic pancreatitis
Available to physicians and pharmacists—contact your local Armour Sales Representative or Armour Corporate Headquarters.

Arther, Inc.
(Formerly OLC Laboratories, Inc.)
BOX 335
MOUNTAIN LAKES, NJ 07046

TRYPTACIN™
(brand of l-tryptophan)

Description: TRYPTACIN - Chemically, l-tryptophan, aminoindole-3-propionic acid is white to slightly yellowish white crystals or crystalline powder, taste slightly bitter. When dried, contains not less than 98.5% and not more than 100.5% of l-tryptophan($C_{11}H_{12}N_2O_2$).

Action and Uses: For amino acid therapy. Claimed in latest research to be used as an antidepressant and to induce sleep.

Administration and Dosage: AS A DIETARY SUPPLEMENT. 125 mg.—1 to 2 tablets 4 times a day; 500 mg.—2 to 4 tablets after evening meal or one half hour before bedtime.

How Supplied: Scored tablets, 125 mg. bottles of 100 (NDC 48558-005-10). 500 mg. bottles of 100 (NDC 48558-001-10) and 250 (NDC 48558-001-25).

References:
Archives of Gen. Psych. Vol. 31-Sept., 1974
Diseases of the Nervous System, Jan., 1974
American Journal Psych. 134:4 April, 1977
ibid: 134:11, Nov., 1977
New England Journal of Med. Jan. 13, 1977
Journal Neurosurg., 53:44, July, 1980
Archives of Gen. Psych. 38:619, June, 1981

B.F. Ascher & Company, Inc.
15501 WEST 109TH STREET
LENEXA, KS 66219

ANASPAZ® Tablets   R
[an'ah-spāz]
(l-hyoscyamine sulfate)

Description: Each ANASPAZ tablet contains l-hyoscyamine sulfate 0.125 mg. ANASPAZ tablets are compressed, light yellow and scored with the Ascher logo on one side and 225/295 on the other.

Clinical Pharmacology: ANASPAZ is chemically pure l-hyoscyamine sulfate, one of the principal anticholinergic/antispasmodic components of belladonna alkaloids. ANASPAZ inhibits specifically the actions of acetylcholine on structures innervated by postganglionic cholinergic nerves and on smooth muscles that respond to acetylcholine but lack cholinergic innervation. These peripheral cholinergic receptors are present in the autonomic effector cells of smooth muscle, cardiac muscle, the sino-atrial node, the atrioventricular node and exocrine glands. It is completely devoid of any action in the autonomic ganglia. ANASPAZ inhibits gastrointestinal propulsive motility and decreases gastric acid secretion. ANASPAZ also controls excessive pharyngeal, tracheal and bronchial secretions. ANASPAZ is absorbed totally and completely by sublingual administration as well as oral administration. Once absorbed, ANASPAZ disappears rapidly from the blood and is distributed throughout the entire body. The half-life of ANASPAZ is 3.5 hours and the majority of drug is excreted in the urine unchanged within the first 12 hours. Only traces of this drug are found in breast milk.

Indications and Usage: ANASPAZ is effective as adjunctive therapy in the treatment of peptic ulcer and irritable bowel syndrome (irritable colon, spastic colon, mucous colitis), acute enterocolitis and other functional gastrointestinal disorders. It can also be used to control gastric secretion, visceral spasm and hypermotility in cystitis, pylorospasm and associated abdominal cramps. May be used in functional intestinal disorders to reduce symptoms such as those seen in mild dysenteries and diverticulitis. ANASPAZ is indicated (along with appropriate analgesics) in symptomatic relief of biliary and renal colic and as a drying agent in the relief of symptoms of acute rhinitis.

Contraindications: Glaucoma, obstructive uropathy (for example, bladder neck obstruction due to prostatic hypertrophy); obstructive disease of the gastrointestinal tract (as in achalasia, pyloroduodenal stenosis); paralytic ileus; intestinal atony of elderly or debilitated patients; unstable cardiovascular status; severe ulcerative colitis; toxic megacolon; myasthenia gravis; myocardial ischemia.

Warnings: In the presence of high environmental temperature, heat prostration can occur with drug use (fever and heat stroke due to decreased sweating). Diarrhea may be an early symptom of incomplete intestinal obstruction, especially in patients with ileostomy or colostomy. In this instance, treatment with this drug would be inappropriate and possibly harmful. Like other anticholinergic agents, ANASPAZ may produce drowsiness or blurred vision. In this event, the patient should be warned not to engage in activities requiring mental alertness such as operating a motor vehicle or other machinery or to perform hazardous work while taking this drug.

Precautions: Use with caution and only when clearly indicated in patients with autonomic neuropathy, hyperthyroidism, coronary heart disease, congestive heart failure and cardiac arrhythmias. Investigate any tachycardia before giving any anticholinergic drugs since they may increase the heart rate. Use with caution in patients with hiatal hernia associated with reflux esophagitis.

Adverse Reactions: Adverse reactions may include dryness of the mouth, urinary hesitancy, urinary retention, blurred vision, mydriasis, cycloplegia, tachycardia, palpitations, increased intraocular pressure, headache, nervousness, drowsiness, weakness, and decreased sweating. Allergic reactions or drug idiosyncrasies such as urticaria and other dermal manifestations may also occur.

Overdosage: The signs and symptoms of overdosage include dry mouth, blurred vision, tachycardia, arrhythmias, dry skin, fever, difficulty in swallowing, excitation, lethargy, stupor, coma, respiratory depression, and paralysis (with large overdoses). General measures such as emesis or gastric lavage and administration of activated charcoal should be undertaken immediately. Supportive therapy is given as needed, including artificial respiration if required. Physostigmine may be given by intravenous injection to reverse severe anticholinergic symptoms.

Dosage and Administration: One or two tablets three or four times a day, according to condition and severity of symptoms. ANASPAZ may be taken orally or sublingually. The dosage of ANASPAZ should be adjusted to the needs of the individual patient to assure symptomatic control with a minimum of adverse effects.

How Supplied: ANASPAZ is available as a compressed, yellow, scored tablet, imprinted with the Ascher logo and 225/295 in bottles of 100 tablets (NDC 0225-0295-15) and 500 tablets (NDC 0225-0295-20).

Also available:
ANASPAZ® PB tablets   ℞
l-hyoscyamine sulfate   0.125 mg
phenobarbital   15.0 mg.
(WARNING: May be habit forming)
Caution: Federal law prohibits dispensing without prescription.
Manufactured for B.F. Ascher & Co., Inc.
Lenexa, Kansas 66219

Astra Pharmaceutical Products, Inc.
50 OTIS STREET
WESTBORO, MA 01581-4428

DOPAMINE HCl   ℞
[*dó-pa-mean*]
Solution

Description: Dopamine hydrochloride is 3,4-dihydroxyphenethylamine hydrochloride, a naturally-occurring biochemical catecholamine precursor of norepinephrine. The chemical structure is:

Dopamine hydrochloride is a white, odorless crystalline powder, freely soluble in water and soluble in alcohol. It is sensitive to light, alkalis, iron salts and oxidizing agents.

Each ml of sterile, non-pyrogenic solution contains 40 mg of dopamine hydrochloride (equivalent to 32.3 mg of dopamine base), and 1% sodium bisulfite as an antioxidant. The pH of the solution may be adjusted with sodium hydroxide or hydrochloric acid to 2.5–4.5.

DOPAMINE HCl MUST BE DILUTED IN AN APPROPRIATE STERILE PARENTERAL SOLUTION BEFORE INTRAVENOUS ADMINISTRATION.

Actions: Dopamine hydrochloride exerts an inotropic effect on the myocardium resulting in an increased cardiac output. Dopamine hydrochloride produces less increase in myocardial oxygen consumption than isoproterenol and its use is usually not associated with a tachyarrhythmia. Clinical studies indicate that dopamine hydrochloride usually increases systolic and pulse pressure with either no effect or a slight increase in diastolic pressure. Total peripheral resistance at low and intermediate therapeutic doses is usually unchanged. Blood flow to peripheral vascular beds may decrease while mesenteric flow increases.

Dopamine hydrochloride has also been reported to dilate the renal vasculature presumptively by activation of a "dopaminergic" receptor. This action is accompanied by increases in glomerular filtration rate, renal blood flow, and sodium excretion. An increase in urinary output produced by dopamine is usually not associated with a decrease in osmolality of the urine.

Indications: Dopamine hydrochloride is indicated for the correction of hemodynamic imbalances present in the shock syndrome due to myocardial infarction, trauma, endotoxic septicemia, open heart surgery, renal failure, and chronic cardiac decompensation, as in congestive failure.

Where appropriate, restoration of blood volume with a suitable plasma expander or whole blood should be instituted or completed prior to administration of dopamine hydrochloride.

Patients most likely to respond adequately to dopamine hydrochloride are those in whom physiological parameters, such as urine flow, myocardial function, and blood pressure, have not undergone profound deterioration. Multiclinic trials indicate that the shorter the time interval between onset of signs and symptoms and initiation of therapy with volume correction and dopamine hydrochloride, the better the prognosis.

Poor Perfusion of Vital Organs—Urine flow appears to be one of the better diagnostic signs by which adequacy of vital organ perfusion can be monitored. Nevertheless, the physician should also observe the patient for signs of reversal of confusion or comatose condition. Loss of pallor, increase in toe temperature, and/or adequacy of nail bed capillary filling may also be used as indices of adequate dosage.

Clinical studies have shown that when dopamine hydrochloride is administered before urine flow has diminished to levels of approximately 0.3 ml/minute, prognosis is more favorable. Nevertheless, in a number of oliguric or anuric patients, administration of dopamine hydrochloride has resulted in an increase in urine flow, which in some cases reached normal levels. Dopamine hydrochloride may also increase urine flow in patients whose output is within normal limits and, thus, may be of value in reducing the degree of preexisting fluid accumulation. It should be noted that at doses above those optimal for the individual patient, urine flow may decrease, necessitating reduction of dosage.

Concurrent administration of dopamine hydrochloride and diuretic agents may produce an additive or potentiating effect.

Low Cardiac Output—Increased cardiac output is related to the direct inotropic effect of dopamine hydrochloride on the myocardium. Increased cardiac output at low or moderate doses appears to be related to a favorable prognosis. Increase in cardiac output has been associated with either static or decreased systemic vascular resistance (SVR). Static or decreased SVR associated with low or moderate increments in cardiac output is believed to be a reflection of differential effects on specific vascular beds with increased resistance in peripheral beds (e.g., femoral) and concomitant decreases in mesenteric and renal vascular beds.

Redistribution of blood flow parallels these changes, so that an increase in cardiac output is accompanied by an increase in mesenteric and renal blood flow. In many instances the renal fraction of the total cardiac output has been found to increase. Increase in cardiac output produced by dopamine hydrochloride is not associated with substantial decreases in systemic vascular resistance as may occur with isoproterenol.

Hypotension—Hypotension due to inadequate cardiac output can be managed by administration of low to moderate doses of dopamine hydrochloride, which have little effect on SVR. At high therapeutic doses, the alpha adrenergic activity of dopamine hydrochloride becomes more prominent and, thus, may correct hypotension due to diminished SVR. As in the case of other circulatory decompensation states, prognosis is better in patients whose blood pressure and urine flow has not undergone profound deterioration. Therefore, it is suggested that the physician administer dopamine hydrochloride as soon as a definite trend toward decreased systolic and diastolic pressure becomes evident.

Contraindications: Dopamine hydrochloride should not be used in patients with pheochromocytoma.

Warnings: Dopamine hydrochloride should not be administered in the presence of ventricular fibrillation or uncorrected tachyarrhythmias.

Do NOT add dopamine hydrochloride to any alkaline diluent solution, since the drug is inactivated in alkaline solution.

Patients who have been treated with monamine oxidase (MAO) inhibitors prior to the administration of dopamine hydrochloride will require substantially reduced dosage of dopamine hydrochloride. Dopamine is metabolized by MAO, and inhibition of this enzyme prolongs and potentiates the effect of dopamine hydrochloride. The initial dose in such patients should be reduced to no more than one-tenth (1/10) of the usual dose.

Continued on next page

Astra—Cont.

Usage in Pregnancy—Animal studies have revealed no evidence of teratogenic effects from dopamine hydrochloride. In one study, administration of dopamine hydrochloride to pregnant rats resulted in a decreased survival rate of the newborn and a potential for cataract formation in the survivors. The drug may be used in pregnant women when, in the judgment of the physician, the expected benefits outweigh the potential risk to the fetus.

Usage in Children—The safety and efficacy of this drug in children has not been established. Dopamine hydrochloride has been used in a limited number of pediatric patients, but such use has been inadequate to fully define proper dosage and limitations for use.

Precautions:

Avoid Hypovolemia—Prior to treatment with dopamine hydrochloride, hypovolemia should be fully corrected, if possible, with either whole blood or plasma as indicated.

Decreased Pulse Pressure—If a disporportionate rise in the diastolic pressure (i.e., a marked decrease in the pulse pressure) is observed in patients receiving dopamine hydrochloride, the infusion rate should be decreased and the patient observed carefully for further evidence of predominant vasoconstrictor activity, unless such an effect is desired.

Extravasation—Dopamine hydrochloride should be infused into a large vein whenever possible to prevent the possibility of extravasation into tissue adjacent to the infusion site. Extravasation may cause necrosis and sloughing of surrounding tissue.

Large veins of the antecubital fossa are preferred to veins in the dorsum of the hand or ankle. Less suitable infusion sites should be used only if the patient's condition requires immediate attention. The physician should switch to more suitable sites as rapidly as possible. The infusion site should be continuously monitored for free flow.

Occlusive Vascular Disease—Patients with a history of occlusive vascular disease (for example, atherosclerosis, arterial embolism, Raynaud's disease, cold injury, diabetic endarteritis, and Buerger's disease) should be closely monitored for any changes in color or temperature of the skin in the extremities. If a change in skin color or temperature occurs and is thought to be the result of compromised circulation to the extremities, the benefits of continued dopamine hydrochloride infusion should be weighed against the risk of possible necrosis. This condition may be reversed by either decreasing or discontinuing the rate of infusion.

IMPORTANT

Antidote for Peripheral Ischemia: To prevent sloughing and necrosis in ischemic areas, the area should be infiltrated as soon as possible with 10 to 15 ml of saline solution containing from 5 to 10 mg of phentolamine, an adrenergic blocking agent. A syringe with a fine hypodermic needle should be used, and the solution liberally infiltrated throughout the ischemic area. Sympathetic blockade with phentolamine causes immediate and conspicuous local hyperemic changes if the area is infiltrated within 12 hours. Therefore, _phentolamine should be given as soon as possible_ after the extravasation is noted.

Avoid Cyclopropane or Halogenated Hydrocarbon Anesthetics—Cyclopropane or halogenated hydrocarbon anesthetics increase cardiac autonomic irritability and therefore may sensitize the myocardium to the action of certain intravenously administered catecholamines. This interaction appears to be related botn to pressor activity and to the beta adrenergic stimulating properties of these catecholamines. Therefore, as with certain other catecholamines, and because of the theoretical arrhythmogenic potential, dopamine hydrochloride should be used with EXTREME CAUTION in patients inhaling cyclopropane or halogenated hydrocarbon anesthetics.

Careful Monitoring Required—As with any adrenergic agent close monitoring of the following indices—urine flow, cardiac output and blood pressure—during dopamine hydrochloride therapy is necessary as in the case of any adrenergic agent.

Adverse Reactions: The most frequent adverse reactions observed in clinical evaluation of dopamine hydrochloride included ectopic beats, nausea, vomiting, tachycardia, anginal pain, palpitation, dyspnea, headache, hypotension, and vasoconstriction. Other adverse reactions which have been reported infrequently were aberrant conduction, bradycardia, piloerection, widened QRS complex, azotemia, and elevated blood pressure.

Dosage and Administration:
WARNING: This is a potent drug: It must be diluted before administration to patient.

Suggested Dilution—Transfer contents of one or more ampules or additive syringes of dopamine hydrochloride by aseptic technique to either a 250 ml, 500 ml, or 1000 ml container of one of the following sterile intravenous solutions:
1. Sodium Chloride Injection, USP
2. Dextrose 5% Injection, USP
3. Dextrose (5%) and Sodium Chloride (0.9%) Injection, USP
4. 5% Dextrose in 0.45% Sodium Chloride Solution
5. Dextrose (5%) in Lactated Ringer's Solution
6. Sodium Lactate (1/6 Molar) Injection, USP
7. Lactated Ringer's Injection, USP

Dopamine hydrochloride has been found to be stable for a minimum of 24 hours after dilution in the sterile intravenous solutions listed above.

However, as with all intravenous admixtures, dilution should be made just prior to administration. Do NOT add dopamine hydrochloride solution to 5% sodium bicarbonate or other alkaline intravenous solutions, since the drug is inactivated in alkaline solution.

Rate of Administration—Dopamine hydrochloride, after dilution, is administered intravenously through a suitable intravenous catheter or needle. An i.v. drip chamber or other suitable metering device is essential for controlling the rate of flow in drops/minute. Each patient must be individually titrated to the desired hemodynamic and/or renal response with dopamine hydrochoride. In titrating to the desired increase in systolic blood pressure, the optimum dosage rate for renal response may be exceeded, thus necessitating a reduction in rate after the hemodynamic condition is stabilized. Administration at rates greater than 50 mcg/kg/min have been used safely in advanced circulatory decompensation states. If unnecessary fluid expansion is of concern, adjustment of drug concentration may be preferred over increasing the flow rate of a less concentrated dilution.

Suggested Regimen:
1. When appropriate, increase blood volume with whole blood or plasma until central venous pressure is 10 to 15 cm H$_2$O or pulmonary wedge pressure is 14–18 mm Hg.
2. Begin administration of diluted solution at doses of 2–5 mcg/kg/minute dopamine hydrochloride in patients who are likely to respond to modest increments of heart force and renal perfusion.
  In more seriously ill patients, begin administration of diluted solution at doses of 5 mcg/kg/minute dopamine hydrochloride and increase gradually using 5 to 10 mcg/kg/minute increments up to 20 to 50 mcg/kg/minute as needed. If doses in excess of 50 mcg/kg/minute are required, it is suggested that urine output be checked frequently. Should urine flow begin to decrease in the absence of hypotension, reduction of dosage should be considered. Multiclinic trials have shown that more than 50% of the patients were satisfactorily maintained on doses of dopamine hydrochloride less than 20 mcg/kg/minute. In patients who do not respond to these doses with adequate arterial pressures or urine flow, additional increments of dopamine hydrochloride may be employed in an effort to produce an appropriate arterial pressure and central perfusion.
3. Treatment of all patients requires constant evaluation of therapy in terms of the blood volume, augmentation of myocardial contractility, and distribution of peripheral perfusion. Dosage of dopamine hydrochloride should be adjusted according to the patient's response, with particular attention to diminution of established urine flow rate, increasing tachycardia or development of new dysrhythmias as indices for decreasing or temporarily suspending the dosage.
4. As with all potent intravenously administered drugs, care should be taken to control the rate of administration so as to avoid inadvertent administration of a bolus of drug.

Overdosage: In case of accidental overdosage, as evidenced by excessive blood pressure elevation, reduce rate of administration or temporarily discontinue dopamine hydrochloride until patient's condition stabilizes. Since duration of action is quite short, no additional remedial measures are usually necessary. If these measures fail to stabilize the patient's condition, use of the short-acting alpha adrenergic blocking agent, phentolamine, should be considered.

How Supplied: 5 ml (200 mg) ampule in packages of 10 (NDC 0186-1050-03), 5 ml (200 mg) additive syringe in packages of 10 (NDC 0186-0638-01), 10 ml (400 mg) ampule in packages of 5 (NDC 0186-1055-03), 10 ml (400 mg) additive syringe in packages of 10 (NDC 0186-0639-01).

WARNING: NOT FOR DIRECT INTRAVENOUS INJECTION, MUST BE DILUTED BEFORE USE.
021848-00   Iss. 5/83

DURANEST® (etidocaine hydrochloride) ℞
[_dur′a-nest_]
SOLUTION
STERILE AQUEOUS SOLUTION
Local anesthetic for
infiltration and nerve block

Description: Duranest (etidocaine hydrochloride) Solution is a local anesthetic of the amide type, chemically related to lidocaine. Its chemical name is (±)-2-(N-ethylpropylamino)-2′,6′-butyroxylidide monohydrochloride.

The pKa of etidocaine (7.74) is similar to that of lidocaine (7.86). However, etidocaine possesses a greater degree of lipid solubility (partition coefficient of 141 in heptane/7.4 phosphate buffer system) and protein binding capacity (94%) as compared to lidocaine (partition coefficient = 3.6, protein binding = 55%).

Duranest Solutions are sterile, and except for the 1.5% concentration, are available with or without epinephrine 1:200,000. Duranest solutions without epinephrine may be reautoclaved if necessary.

Please refer to Table 1 for the composition of available solutions.

[See table on next page].

Actions: Etidocaine stabilizes the neuronal membrane and prevents the initiation and conduction of nerve impulses, thereby effecting local anesthetic action. _In vivo_ animal studies have shown that Duranest (etidocaine hydrochloride) Solution has a rapid onset (3–5 minutes) and a prolonged duration of action (5–10 hours). Based on comparative clinical studies of lidocaine and etidocaine, the anesthetic properties of etidocaine in man may be characterized as follows: Initial onset of sensory analgesia and motor blockade is rapid (usually 3–5 minutes) and similar to that produced by lidocaine. Duration of sensory analgesia is 1.5 to 2 times longer than that of lidocaine, by the peridural route. The difference in analgesic duration between etidocaine and lidocaine may be even greater following peripheral nerve blockade than following central neural block. Duration of analgesia in excess of 9 hours is not infrequent when etidocaine is used for peripheral nerve blocks such as brachial plexus blockade. Etidocaine produces a profound degree of motor blockade and abdominal muscle relaxation when used for peridural analgesia.

Following absorption from the site of injection, etidocaine redistributes rapidly and demonstrates a larger volume of distribution than that seen with comparable local anesthetic drugs due to its high tissue solubility.

The rate of metabolism is similar to that of lidocaine. Etidocaine is metabolized in the liver and its metabolites are excreted via the kidneys. Little unchanged drug is recovered in the urine. Animal studies to date indicate that no single metabolite will account for more than 10% of the administered dose.

Clinical trials to date demonstrate that etidocaine does not produce methemoglobinemia or tissue irritation.

Indications: Duranest Solution is indicated for percutaneous infiltration anesthesia, peripheral nerve blocks, and central neural blocks, i.e., caudal or epidural blocks.

Contraindications: Duranest Solution is contraindicated in patients with a known history of hypersensitivity to local anesthetic agents of the amide type.

Warnings:
1. RESUSCITATIVE EQUIPMENT AND DRUGS, INCLUDING OXYGEN, SHOULD BE IMMEDIATELY AVAILABLE WHEN ANY LOCAL ANESTHETIC AGENT IS USED.
2. *Use in Pregnancy:* Reproductive studies have been performed in rats and rabbits without evidence of harm to the animal fetus. However, the safe use of Duranest Solution in humans has not been established with respect to adverse effects upon fetal development. Careful consideration should be given to this fact before administering this drug to women of childbearing potential, particularly during early pregnancy. This does not exclude the use of the drug at term for obstetrical analgesia. Duranest Solution has been used for obstetrical analgesia by the peridural route without evidence of adverse effects on the fetus. The use of Duranest Solution by the paracervical route have *not* been investigated for effects on the fetus.
3. Local anesthetic procedures should be used with caution when there is inflammation and/or sepsis in the region of the proposed injection.
4. Solutions which contain epinephrine or other vasoconstrictor agents should be used with extreme caution in patients receiving drugs known to produce blood pressure alterations (i.e., MAO inhibitors, tricyclic antidepressants, phenothiazines, etc.) as either severe sustained hypertension or hypotension may occur.
5. Vasopressor agents (administered for the treatment of hypotension related to caudal or other epidural blocks) should be used with extreme caution in the presence of oxytocic drugs as they are known to interact and may produce severe persistent hypertension and/or rupture of cerebral blood vessels.
6. The use of Duranest Solution has not been investigated in children under 14 years of age.

Precautions: The safety and effectiveness of Duranest Solutions depend on proper dosage, correct technique, adequate precautions, and readiness for emergencies. Consult standard textbooks for specific techniques and precautions for various regional anesthetic procedures.

The lowest dosage that results in effective anesthesia should be used to avoid high plasma levels and possible adverse effects. Tolerance varies with the status of the patient. For example, debilitated, elderly or acutely ill patients should be given reduced doses commensurate with their physical status. Duranest Solutions should also be used with caution in patients with severe shock or heart block.

INJECTIONS SHOULD ALWAYS BE MADE SLOWLY AND WITH FREQUENT ASPIRATIONS TO AVOID INADVERTENT RAPID INTRAVASCULAR ADMINISTRATION WHICH CAN PRODUCE SYSTEMIC TOXICITY.

Duranest Solution

TABLE 1. COMPOSITION OF AVAILABLE SOLUTIONS

Product Identification		Formula		
		Single Dose Vials		
Duranest (etidocaine) HCl Concentration	Epinephrine (as the bitartrate) Dilution	Sodium chloride (mg/ml)	Sodium metabisulfite (mg/ml)	Citric Acid (mg/ml)
1.0	None	7.1	None	—
1.0	1:200,000	7.1	0.5	0.2
1.5	1:200,000	6.2	0.5	0.2

NOTE: pH of all solutions adjusted with sodium hydroxide and/or hydrochloric acid. Duranest Solutions with epinephrine are adjusted to pH 3–4.5. Duranest Solutions without epinephrine are adjusted to pH 4.5.

Occasionally, duration of motor block may appear to exceed that of sensory block (see ACTIONS). Consideration should be given to the profound motor block and its effect on the need for voluntary expulsive muscles when using Duranest Solutions for epidural block in obstetrics.

Epidural anesthesia and caudal anesthesia should be used with extreme caution in persons with the following conditions: existing neurological disease, septicemia, severe hypertension, or spinal deformities which may affect the quality of the block. Solutions which contain a vasoconstrictor agent should be used with caution in the presence of diseases which may adversely affect the patient's cardiovascular system. Serious cardiac arrhythmias may occur if preparations containing a vasoconstrictor drug are employed in patients during or following the administration of chloroform, halothane, cyclopropane, trichlorethylene, or other related agents. Solutions containing epinephrine should be used cautiously in areas with limited blood supply.

Duranest Solutions should be used with caution in persons with known drug sensitivities. Patients allergic to paraaminobenzoic acid derivatives (procaine, tetracaine, benzocaine, etc.) have not shown cross sensitivity to agents of the amide type such as etidocaine. Since etidocaine is metabolized in the liver and excreted via the kidneys, it should be used cautiously in patients with liver and renal disease.

Consideration should be given to the long duration of peripheral nerve block (8–10 hours) when using this drug for ambulatory patients.

Adverse Reactions: Reactions to etidocaine are similar in character to those observed with other local anesthetic agents such as lidocaine. Adverse reactions may result from high plasma levels due to excessive dosage, rapid absorption or inadvertent intravascular injection. Such reactions are systemic in nature and involve the central nervous system and/or the cardiovascular system.

A small number of reactions may result from hypersensitivity, idiosyncrasy or diminished tolerance on the part of the patient.

CNS reactions are excitatory and/or depressant, and are usually characterized by nervousness, dizziness, blurred vision and tremors, followed by drowsiness, convulsions, unconsciousness and possibly respiratory arrest. Excitatory CNS effects commonly represent the initial signs of local anesthetic systemic toxicity. However, these reactions may be very brief or absent in some patients in which case the first manifestations of toxicity may be drowsiness, merging into unconsciousness and respiratory arrest.

Hypotension and bradycardia may occur as normal physiological phenomena following sympathetic block with central neural blocks. Toxic cardiovascular reactions to local anesthetics are usually depressant in nature and are characterized by peripheral vasodilation, hypotension, myocardial depression, bradycardia, and possibly cardiac arrest. However, direct cardiovascular depressant effects have not been seen with etidocaine in the absence of central nervous system toxicity.

Treatment of a patient wth toxic manifestations consists of assuring and maintaining a patent airway and supporting ventilation with oxygen and assisted or controlled respiration as required. This usually will be sufficient in the management of most reactions. Should a convulsion persist despite ventilatory therapy with oxygen, small increments of anticonvulsive agents may be given intravenously such as a benzodiazepine (e.g., diazepam), an ultra-short acting barbiturate (e.g., thiopental or thiamylal) or a short-acting barbiturate (e.g., pentobarbital or secobarbital). Cardiovascular depression may require circulatory assistance with intravenous fluids and/or vasopressor agents as dictated by the clinical situation. Allergic reactions may occur as a result of sensitivity to the local anesthetic or methylparaben used as a preservative (in multiple dose vials) and are characterized by cutaneous lesions, urticaria, edema or anaphylactoid type symtomatology. True allergic reactions should be managed by conventional means. The detection of potential sensitivity by skin testing is of limited value.

Dosage and Administration: As with all local anesthetic agents the dose of Duranest Solution to be employed will depend on the area to be anesthetized, the vascularity of the tissues, the number of neuronal segments to be blocked, the type of regional anesthetic technique and the status and tolerance of the individual patient. The maximum dose of Duranest Solution to be employed as a single injection should be determined on the basis of the status of the patient and the type of regional anesthetic technique to be performed. Although single injections of 450 mg have been employed for regional anesthesia without adverse effects, at present it is strongly recommended that the maximal dose of Duranest Solution as a single injection should not exceed 400 mg (approximately 5.5 mg/kg or 2.7 mg/lb) with epinephrine 1:200,000 and 300 mg (approximately 4 mg/kg or 2 mg/lb) without epinephrine. Because etidocaine has been shown to disappear quite rapidly from blood, toxicity is influenced by rapidity of administration, and therefore slow injection in vascular areas is highly recommended. Incremental doses of Duranest Solution may be repeated at 2–3 hour intervals. The following dosage recommendations are intended as guides for the use of Duranest Solution in the average adult patient. As indicated previously, the dosage should be reduced for elderly or debilitated patients or patients with severe renal disease.

No information is available on appropriate pediatric doses.

021569-00   Iss. 6/82

[See table on next page].

Continued on next page

Astra—Cont.

TABLE 2. Recommended Doses of Duranest Solutions For Various Anesthetic Procedures In Normal Healthy Adults

PROCEDURE	Duranest HCl with epinephrine 1:200,000		
	Conc. (%)	Vol. (ml)	Total Dose (mg)
Percutaneous Infiltration	0.5	1–80	5–400
Peripheral Nerve Block	{ 0.5 or 1.0	5–80 5–40	25–400 50–400
Central Neural Block			
Lumbar Peridural			
Intraabdominal or Pelvic Surgery Lower Limb Surgery Caesarean Section	{ 1.0 or 1.5	10–30 10–20	100–300 150–300
Vaginal Obstetrical and Gynecologic Procedures	{ 0.5 or 1.0	10–30 5–20	50–150 50–200
Caudal	{ 0.5 or 1.0	10–30 10–30	50–150 100–300

How Supplied:

Dosage Form and Volume	Duranest Solution Concentration	Epinephrine (as the bitartrate) Dilution
Single Dose Vials		
30 ml	1.0%	None
	1.0%	1:200,000
20 ml	1.5%	1:200,000

0.5% DYCLONE® ℞
[die-clone]
(dyclonine hydrochloride topical solution USP)
Topical Anesthetic
NOT FOR INJECTION OR OPHTHALMOLOGY

Full prescribing information is contained in the package insert.
For additional information, contact Astra's Professional Information Department.

How Supplied: Sterile, in one fluid ounce bottles (NDC 0186-3001-67).

1% DYCLONE® ℞
[die-clone]
(dyclonine hydrochloride topical solution USP)
Topical Anesthetic
NOT FOR INJECTION OR OPHTHALMOLOGY

Full prescribing information is contained in the package insert.
For additional information, contact Astra's Professional Information Department.

How Supplied: Sterile, in one fluid ounce bottles (NDC 0186-3002-67).

NESACAINE® ℞
[nés-a-caine]
(chloroprocaine hydrochloride)
with preservative, 1% and 2% solution
30 ml multiple-dose vial

NESACAINE®-CE ℞
(chloroprocaine hydrochloride)
without preservative, 2% and 3% solution
30 ml single-dose vial

Description: The active ingredient in Nesacaine and Nesacaine-CE is chloroprocaine hydrochloride (β-diethyl-aminoethyl-2-chloro-4-aminobenzoate hydrochloride) which is represented by the following structural formula:

$$H_2N-\text{C}_6H_3(Cl)-CO\cdot O\cdot CH_2\cdot CH_2\cdot N(CH_2CH_3)_2 \cdot HCl$$

It is incompatible with caustic alkalis and their carbonates, soaps, silver salts, iodine, and iodides.
Nesacaine, supplied in multidose vials, contains methylparaben as a preservative and should not be used for caudal or epidural anesthesia.
Nesacaine-CE, is supplied in single-dose vials. It contains no preservative, hence, any unused portion should be discarded.
While Nesacaine and Nesacaine-CE are sterile solutions, the vials may be autoclaved for terminal sterilization, with no significant decrease in potency. Sterilization of vials with ethylene oxide is not recommended, since absorption through the closure may occur.
As with other anesthetics having a free aromatic amino group, Nesacaine and Nesacaine-CE solutions are slightly photosensitive and may become discolored after prolonged exposure to light. It is recommended that these vials be stored in the original outer containers, protected from direct sunlight. Discolored solution should not be administered. If exposed to low temperatures, Nesacaine (chloroprocaine hydrochloride) and Nesacaine-CE may deposit crystals of chloroprocaine hydrochloride, which will redissolve with shaking when returned to room temperature. The product should not be used if it contains undissolved material.
Clinical Pharmacology: The parenteral administration of Nesacaine and Nesacaine-CE stabilizes the neuronal membrane and prevents the initiation and transmission of nerve impulses, thereby effecting local anesthetic action. The onset of action is rapid (usually within 6 to 12 minutes) and the duration of anesthesia is up to 60 minutes depending upon the amount used, and the route of administration.
Chloroprocaine is rapidly hydrolyzed in plasma by pseudocholinesterase. The hydrolysis of chloroprocaine results in the production of 2-chloro-4-aminobenzoic acid and β-diethylaminoethanol. Solutions of Nesacaine and Nesacaine-CE do not injure nervous tissue and are not irritating to the other tissues in the concentrations recommended.
Indications: Nesacaine, in multidose vials with preservative is indicated for the production of local anesthesia by infiltration and regional nerve block. It is not to be used for caudal or epidural anesthesia.
Nesacaine-CE, in single dose vials without preservative, is indicated for the production of local anesthesia by infiltration and regional nerve block, including caudal and epidural blocks.
Contraindications: Nesacaine and Nesacaine-CE are contraindicated in patients hypersensitive (allergic) to drugs of the PABA ester group.
Although central nervous system disease is generally considered a contraindication to caudal or epidural nerve block, it is not a contraindication to peripheral nerve block. Pathologic changes of the vertebral column may make epidural puncture impossible or inadvisable.
Warnings: RESUSCITATIVE EQUIPMENT AND DRUGS SHOULD BE IMMEDIATELY AVAILABLE WHEN ANY LOCAL ANESTHETIC IS USED.
NESACAINE (Chloroprocaine Hydrochloride) INJECTION contains a preservative and should not be used for caudal or epidural anesthesia. As NESACAINE-CE contains no preservative, discard unused drug remaining in vial after initial use. Equipment and drugs necessary for the treatment of inadvertent intravascular injection, intrathecal injection, or excessive dosage should be immediately available.
Usage in Pregnancy: Safe use of chloroprocaine hydrochloride has not been established with respect to adverse effects upon fetal development. This fact should be carefully considered before administering this drug to women of childbearing potential, particularly during early pregnancy. This does not preclude the use of the drug at term for obstetrical analgesia. Adverse effects on the fetus, course of labor, or delivery have rarely been observed when proper dosage and proper technique have been employed.
There are no data concerning use of chloroprocaine for obstetrical paracervical block when toxemia of pregnancy is present or when fetal distress or prematurity is anticipated in advance of the block; such use is, therefore, not recommended.
The following information should be considered by clinicians who select chloroprocaine for obstetrical paracervical block anesthesia: 1. Fetal bradycardia (generally a heart rate of less than 120 per minute for more than 2 minutes) has been noted by electronic monitoring in about 5% to 10% of the cases (various studies) where initial total doses of 120 mg to 400 mg of chloroprocaine were employed. The incidence of bradycardia, within this dose range, might not be dose related. 2. Fetal acidosis has not been demonstrated by blood gas monitoring around the time of bradycardia or afterwards. These data are limited and are generally restricted to non-toxemic cases where fetal distress or prematurity was not anticipated in advance of the block. 3. No intact chloroprocaine, and only trace quantities of a hydrolysis product. 2-chloro-4-aminobenzoic acid, have been demonstrated in umbilical cord arterial or venous plasma following properly administered paracervical block with chloroprocaine. 4. The role of drug factors and non-drug factors associated with fetal bradycardia following paracervical block are unexplained at this time.
In obstetrics, if vasoconstrictor drugs are used either to correct hypotension or are added to the local anesthetic solution, the obstetrician should be warned that some oxytocic drugs may cause severe persistent hypertension, and even rupture of a cerebral blood vessel may occur during the postpartum period.
Solutions containing vasoconstrictors, particularly epinephrine and norepinephrine, should be used with extreme caution in patients receiving certain antidepressants, such as MAO inhibitors and tricyclic compounds, since severe prolonged hypertension may occur.
Precautions: The safety and effectiveness of chloroprocaine hydrochloride injections depend upon proper dosage, correct technique, adequate precautions and readiness for emergencies.
The lowest dosage that results in effective anesthesia should be used to avoid high plasma levels and serious undesirable systemic side effects. Tolerance varies with the status of the patient. Debilitated patients, elderly patients, acutely ill pa-

tients, and children should be given reduced doses commensurate with their age and physical status. Solutions containing vasoconstrictors should be used cautiously in the presence of disease which may adversely affect the patient's cardiovascular system.

INJECTIONS SHOULD ALWAYS BE MADE SLOWLY AND WITH FREQUENT ASPIRATIONS TO AVOID INADVERTENT RAPID INTRAVASCULAR ADMINISTRATION WHICH CAN PRODUCE SYSTEMIC TOXICITY.

Chloroprocaine hydrochloride should be employed cautiously in persons with known drug allergies or sensitivities.

The decision whether or not to use local anesthesia in the following conditions depends on the physician's appraisal of the advantages as opposed to the risk:

Injection of solutions containing epinephrine in areas where the blood supply is limited (i.e. ears, nose, digits, etc.) or when peripheral vascular disease is present.

Serious cardiac arrhythmias may occur if preparations containing a vasopressor are employed in patients during or following the administration of chloroform, halothane, cyclopropane, trichloroethylene, or other related agents.

Adverse Reactions
Systemic: Systemic adverse reactions result from high plasma levels due to rapid absorption, inadvertent intravascular injection or excessive dosage. Hypersensitivity, idiosyncrasy, or diminished tolerance (as in patients with plasma cholinesterase deficiency) are other causes of reactions. Reactions due to overdosage (high plasma levels) are systemic and involve the central nervous system and the cardiovascular system.

Central nervous system reactions: These are characterized by excitation and/or depression. Restlessness, anxiety, dizziness, blurred vision or tremors may occur, possibly proceeding to convulsions. However, excitement may be transient or absent, with depression the first manifestation of an adverse reaction. This may quickly be followed by drowsiness merging into unconsciousness and respiratory arrest.

Cardiovascular system reactions: High systemic doses cause depression of the myocardium manifested by an initial episode of hypotension and bradycardia, and even cardiac arrest.

Treatment of systemic reactions: Treatment of a patient with toxic manifestations consists of assuring and maintaining a patent airway and supporting ventilation with oxygen and assisted or controlled ventilation (respiration) as required. This usually will be sufficient in the management of most reactions. Should a convulsion persist despite ventilatory therapy, small increments of anticonvulsive agents may be given intravenously, such as a benzodiazepine (e.g. diazepam), or ultra-short acting barbiturate (e.g. thiopental or thiamylal) or a short-acting barbiturate (e.g. pentobarbital or secobarbital). Cardiovascular depression may require circulatory assistance with intravenous fluids and/or vasopressors (e.g. ephedrine) as dictated by the clinical situation. Allergic reactions are rare and may occur as a result of sensitivity to chloroprocaine or to methylparaben used as a preservative and are characterized by cutaneous lesions, urticaria, edema and anaphylactoid type symptomatology. These allergic reactions should be managed by conventional means. The detection of potential sensitivity by skin testing is of limited value.

Neurologic: In the practice of epidural block, occasional inadvertent penetration of the subarachnoid space by the catheter may occur. The subsequent reactions depend on the amount of drug administered subdurally and may include, among others, spinal block of varying magnitude, loss of bowel and bladder control, loss of perineal sensation and sexual function. Persistent neurological deficit of some lower spinal segments with slow recovery (several months) has been reported in rare instances. (See DOSAGE AND ADMINISTRATION, CAUDAL AND EPIDURAL BLOCK)

Dosage and Administration: The lowest dose needed to provide effective anesthesia should be administered. As with all local anesthetics, the dosage depends upon the area to be anesthetized, vascularity of the tissues, number of neuronal segments to be blocked, individual tolerance and the technique employed. For specific techniques and procedures, refer to standard textbooks.

The maximum single recommended doses of chloroprocaine hydrochloride are: without epinephrine, 800 mg; with epinephrine (1:200,000), 1000 mg. The recommended dosage is based on requirements for the average adult and should be reduced for elderly or debilitated patients and children.

Preparation of Epinephrine Solutions—To prepare a 1 to 200,000 epinephrine-chloroprocaine hydrochloride solution add 0.15 ml of a 1 to 1,000 epinephrine injection U.S.P. to 30 ml of Nesacaine-CE.

As a guide for some routine procedures, suggested doses are given below:

1. Infiltration and Nerve Block: Nesacaine or Nesacaine-CE (Chloroprocaine Hydrochloride) INJECTION

Local Infiltration: Quantity depends on the concentration of the solution, the site to be infiltrated, and the discretion of the operator.

Nerve Blocks	Volume	Concentration
Mandibular	2–3 ml	2%
Infraorbital	0.5–1 ml	2%
Brachial Plexus	30–40 ml	2%
Digital (without epinephrine)	3–4 ml	1%

Obstetrical	Volume	Concentration
Pudendal Block	10 ml each side	2%
Paracervical Block (see WARNINGS section)	3 ml per each of 4 sites	1%

2. CAUDAL AND EPIDURAL BLOCK: NESACAINE-CE (Chloroprocaine Hydrochloride) INJECTION: *For caudal anesthesia* the initial dose is 15 to 25 ml of a 2% or 3% solution. Repeated doses may be given at 40 to 60 minute intervals.

For epidural anesthesia in the lumbar and sacral regions 2.0 to 2.5 ml per segment of a 2% or 3% solution can be used. The usual total volume of Nesacaine-CE is from 15 to 25 ml. Repeated doses 2 to 6 ml less than the original dose may be given at 40 to 50 minute intervals.

In order to guard against possible adverse reactions resulting from inadvertent penetration of the subarachnoid space, the following procedures are recommended:

1. Use of an adequate (in the case of Nesacaine-CE, approximately 3 ml of 3% or 5 ml of 2%) test dose prior to induction of complete block. This test dose should be repeated if the patient is moved in such a fashion as to have displaced the epidural catheter. At least 5 minutes should elapse after each test dose prior to proceeding further.

2. Injection of a large, single therapeutic dose through a catheter should be avoided; instead, repeated fractional doses are advocated.

3. In the event of the known injection of a large volume of Nesacaine-CE into the subarachnoid space, an appropriate amount of cerebrospinal fluid (such as 10 ml) should be withdrawn through the catheter or by separate lumbar puncture.

How Supplied: NESACAINE (Chloroprocaine Hydrochloride) INJECTION is supplied as follows:
1% solution in 30 ml multiple dose vials, 12 vials per package.
Each ml contains 10 mg of Chloroprocaine Hydrochloride, 0.6% sodium chloride and 0.2% sodium bisulfite in water for injection, with methylparaben 0.1% added as preservative and hydrochloric acid to adjust pH.
2% solution in 30 ml multiple dose vials, 12 vials per package.
Each ml contains 20 mg of Chloroprocaine Hydrochloride, 0.4% sodium chloride and 0.2% sodium bisulfite in water for injection, with methylparaben 0.1% added as preservative and hydrochloric acid to adjust pH.
NESACAINE-CE (Chloroprocaine Hydrochloride) INJECTION is supplied as follows:
2% solution in 30 ml single dose vials, packaged 12 vials per package.
Each ml contains 20 mg of Chloroprocaine Hydrochloride, 0.4% sodium chloride, and 0.2% sodium bisulfite in water for injection, and hydrochloric acid to adjust pH.
3% solution in 30 ml single dose vials, packaged 12 vials per package.
Each ml contains 30 mg of Chloroprocaine Hydrochloride, 0.2% sodium chloride and 0.2% sodium bisulfite in water for injection, and hydrochloric acid to adjust pH.

Manufactured by
Astra Pharmaceutical Products, Inc.
by Taylor Pharmacal Co., Decatur, Illinois
021849-00   11-82

SENSORCAINE™ ℞
[sén-sor-caine]
(bupivacaine HCl)
Solutions for Infiltration and Nerve Block

Description: Sensorcaine™ (bupivacaine HCl) solutions are sterile isotonic solutions that contain a local anesthetic agent with and without epinephrine (as bitartrate) 1:200,000 and are administered parenterally by injection. See INDICATIONS AND USAGE for specific uses. The quantitative composition of each available solution is shown in Table 1. Solutions of bupivacaine HCl may be autoclaved if they do not contain epinephrine.

Sensorcaine™ solutions contain bupivacaine HCl which is chemically designated as 2-piperidinecarboxamide, 1-butyl-N-(2,6-dimethylphenyl)-monohydrochloride, monohydrate and has the following structure:

Epinephrine is (-)-3,4-Dihydroxy-α-[(methylamino)methyl] benzyl alcohol. It has the following structural formula:

The pKa of bupivacaine (8.1) is similar to that of lidocaine (7.86). However, bupivacaine possesses a greater degree of lipid solubility and is protein bound to a greater extent than lidocaine.

Bupivacaine is related chemically and pharmacologically to the aminoacyl local anesthetics. It is a homologue of mepivacaine and is chemically related to lidocaine. All three of these anesthetics contain an amide linkage between the aromatic nucleus and the amino or piperidine group. They differ in this respect from the procaine-type local anesthetics, which have an ester linkage.

[See table on next page.]

Clinical Pharmacology: Local anesthetics block the generation and the conduction of nerve impulses, presumably by increasing the threshold for electrical excitation in the nerve, by slowing the propagation of the nerve impulse, and by reducing the rate of rise of the action potential. In general, the progression of anesthesia is related to the diameter, myelination and conduction velocity of affected nerve fibers. Clinically, the order of loss of nerve function is as follows: (1) pain, (2) temperature, (3) touch, (4) proprioception, and (5) skeletal muscle tone.

Systemic absorption of local anesthetics produces effects on the cardiovascular and central nervous systems. At blood concentrations achieved with therapeutic doses, changes in cardiac conduction, excitability, refractoriness, contractility, and peripheral vascular resistance are minimal. However, toxic blood concentrations depress cardiac

Continued on next page

Astra—Cont.

conduction and excitability, which may lead to atrioventricular block, ventricular arrhythmias and to cardiac arrest. In addition, myocardial contractility is depressed and peripheral vasodilation occurs, leading to decreased cardiac output and arterial blood pressure.

Recent clinical reports and animal research suggest that these cardiovascular changes are more likely to occur with bupivacaine.

Following systemic absorption, local anesthetics can produce central nervous system stimulation, depression or both. Apparent central stimulation is usually manifested as restlessness, tremors and shivering, progressing to convulsions, followed by depression and coma, progressing ultimately to respiratory arrest. However, the local anesthetics have a primary depressant effect on the medulla and on higher centers. The depressed stage may occur without a prior excited stage.

Pharmacokinetics: The rate of systemic absorption of local anesthetics is dependent upon the total dose and concentration of drug administered, the route of administration, the vascularity of the administration site, and the presence or absence of epinephrine in the anesthetic solution. A dilute concentration of epinephrine (1:200,000 or 5 µg/ml) usually reduces the rate of absorption and peak plasma concentration of bupivacaine, permitting the use of moderately larger total doses and sometimes prolonging the duration of action. The onset of action with bupivacaine is rapid and anesthesia is long-lasting. It has also been noted that there is a period of analgesia that persists after the return of sensation, during which time the need for potent analgesics is reduced.

Local anesthetics are bound to plasma proteins in varying degrees. Generally, the lower the plasma concentration of drug, the higher the percentage of drug bound to plasma proteins.

Local anesthetics appear to cross the placenta by passive diffusion. The rate and degree of diffusion is governed by: (1) the degree of plasma protein binding, (2) the degree of ionization, and (3) the degree of lipid solubility. Fetal/maternal ratios of local anesthetics appear to be inversely related to the degree of plasma protein binding, because only the free, unbound drug is available for placental transfer. Bupivacaine, with a high protein binding capacity (95%), has a low fetal/maternal ratio (0.2–0.4). The extent of placental transfer is also determined by the degree of ionization and lipid solubility of the drug. Lipid soluble, nonionized drugs readily enter the fetal blood from the maternal circulation.

Depending upon the route of adminstration, local anesthetics are distributed to some extent to all body tissues, with high concentrations found in highly perfused organs such as the liver, lungs, heart and brain.

Pharmacokinetic studies on the plasma profile of bupivacaine after direct intravenous injection suggest a three-compartment open model. The first compartment is represented by the rapid intravascular distribution of the drug. The second compartment represents the equilibration of the drug throughout the highly perfused organs such as the brain, myocardium, lungs, kidneys and liver. The third compartment represents an equilibration of the drug with poorly perfused tissues, such as muscle and fat. The elimination of drug from tissue depends largely upon the ability of binding sites in the circulation to carry it to the liver where is is metabolized.

After injection of Sensorcaine™ (bupivacaine HCl) solution for caudal, epidural or peripheral nerve block in man, peak levels of bupivacaine in the blood are reached in 30 to 45 minutes, followed by a decline to insignificant levels during the next 3 to 6 hours.

Various pharmacokinetic parameters of the local anesthetics can be significantly altered by the presence of hepatic or renal disease, addition of epinephrine, factors affecting urinary pH, renal blood flow, the route of drug administration, and the age of the patient. The half-life of bupivacaine in adults is 3.5 ± 2.0 hours and in neonates 8.1 hours.

Amide-type local anesthetics such as bupivacaine are metabolized primarily in the liver via conjugation with glucuronic acid.

Patients with hepatic disease, especially those with severe hepatic disease, may be more susceptible to the potential toxicities of the amide-type local anesthetics. The major metabolite of bupivacaine is 2,6-pipecoloxylidine.

The kidney is the main excretory organ for most local anesthetics and their metabolities. Urinary excretion is affected by renal perfusion and factors affecting urinary pH. Only 5% of bupivacaine is excreted unchanged in the urine.

When administered in recommended doses and concentrations, Sensorcaine™ (bupivacaine HCl) solution does not ordinarily produce irritation or tissue damage and does not cause methemoglobinemia.

Indications and Usage: Sensorcaine™ (bupivacaine HCl) solution is indicated for the production of local or regional anesthesia or analgesia for surgery, for diagnostic and therapeutic procedures and for obstetrical procedures. Only the 0.25% and 0.5% concentrations are indicated for obstetrical anesthesia. (See WARNINGS.)

Experience with non-obstetrical surgical procedures in pregnant patients is not sufficient to recommend use of the 0.75% concentration in these patients. Sensorcaine™ (bupivacaine HCl) solution is not recommended for intravenous regional anesthesia (Bier Block). See WARNINGS.

The routes of administration and indicated Sensorcaine™ (bupivacaine HCl) concentrations are:

local infiltration	0.25%
peripheral nerve block	0.25%, 0.5%
retrobulbar block	0.75%
sympathetic block	0.25%
lumbar epidural	0.25%, 0.5% and 0.75% (non-obstetrical)
caudal	0.25%, 0.5%

(See DOSAGE AND ADMINISTRATION for additional information.) Standard textbooks should be consulted to deteminie the accepted procedures and techniques for the administration of Sensorcaine™ (bupivacaine HCl).

Contraindications: Sensorcaine™ (bupivacaine HCl) solution is contraindicated in obstetrical paracervical block anesthesia. Its use by this technique has resulted in fetal bradycardia and death.

Sensorcaine™ (bupivacaine HCl) is contraindicated in patients with a known hypersensitivity to it or to any local anesthetic agent of the amide type or to other components of bupivacaine solutions.

Warnings

> THE 0.75% CONCENTRATION OF SENSORCAINE™ (BUPIVACAINE HYDROCHLORIDE) SOLUTION IS NOT RECOMMENDED FOR OBSTETRICAL ANESTHESIA. THERE HAVE BEEN REPORTS OF CARDIAC ARREST WITH DIFFICULT RESUSCITATION OR DEATH DURING USE OF BUPIVACAINE FOR EPIDURAL ANESTHESIA IN OBSTETRICAL PATIENTS. IN MOST CASES, THIS HAS FOLLOWED USE OF THE 0.75% CONCENTRATION. RESUSCITATION HAS BEEN DIFFICULT OR IMPOSSIBLE DESPITE APPARENTLY ADEQUATE PREPARATION AND APPROPRIATE MANAGEMENT. CARDIAC ARREST HAS OCCURRED AFTER CONVULSIONS RESULTING FROM SYSTEMIC TOXICITY, PRESUMABLY FOLLOWING UNINTENTIONAL INTRAVASCULAR INJECTION. THE 0.75% CONCENTRATION SHOULD BE RESERVED FOR SURGICAL PROCEDURES WHERE A HIGH DEGREE OF MUSCLE RELAXATION AND PROLONGED EFFECT ARE NECESSARY.

LOCAL ANESTHETICS SHOULD ONLY BE EMPLOYED BY CLINICIANS WHO ARE WELL VERSED IN DIAGNOSIS AND MANAGEMENT OF DOSE-RELATED TOXICITY AND OTHER ACUTE EMERGENCIES WHICH MIGHT ARISE FROM THE BLOCK TO BE EMPLOYED, AND THEN ONLY AFTER ENSURING THE *IMMEDIATE* AVAILABILITY OF OXYGEN, OTHER RESUSCITATIVE DRUGS, CARDIOPULMONARY RESUSCITATIVE EQUIPMENT, AND THE PERSONNEL RESOURCES NEEDED FOR PROPER MANAGEMENT OF TOXIC REACTIONS AND RELATED EMERGENCIES. (See also ADVERSE REACTIONS and PRECAUTIONS.) DELAY IN PROPER MANAGEMENT OF DOSE-RELATED TOXICITY, UNDERVENTILATION FROM ANY CAUSE AND/OR ALTERED SENSITIVITY MAY LEAD TO THE DEVELOPMENT OF ACIDOSIS, CARDIAC ARREST AND, POSSIBLY, DEATH.

Local anesthetic solutions containing antimicrobial preservatives, i.e. those supplied in multiple dose vials, should not be used for epidural or caudal anesthesia because safety has not been established with regard to intrathecal injection, either intentional or unintentional, of such preservatives.

It is essential that aspiration for blood or cerebrospinal fluid (where applicable) be done prior to injecting any local anesthetic, both the original dose and all subsequent doses, to avoid intravascular or subarachnoid injection. However, a negative aspiration does *not* ensure against an intravascular or subarachnoid injection.

Bupivacaine HCl with epinephrine 1:200,000 or other vasopressors should not be used concomitantly with ergot-type oxytocic drugs, because a severe persistent hypertension may occur. Like-

TABLE 1. COMPOSITION OF AVAILABLE SOLUTIONS*

		Multiple Dose Vials				Ampules and Single Dose Vials		
Bupivacaine HCl Concentration %	Epinephrine (as bitratrate) Dilution	Sodium Chloride (mg/ml)	Citric Acid (mg/ml)	Sodium Metabisulfite (mg/ml)	Methylparaben (mg/ml)	Sodium Chloride (mg/ml)	Citric Acid (mg/ml)	Sodium Metabisulfite (mg/ml)
0.25	None	8.0	None	None	1.0	8.0	None	None
0.50	None	8.0	None	None	1.0	8.0	None	None
0.50	1:200,000	.... Not available				8.0	0.2	0.5
0.75	None	.... Not available				8.0	None	None
0.75	1:200,000	.... Not available				8.0	0.2	0.5

*pH of all solutions adjusted to 4.5–6.5 (plain solutions) or to 3.3–5.5 (epinephrine-containing solutions) with sodium hydroxide and/or hydrochloric acid.

wise, solutions of bupivacaine containing a vasoconstrictor, such as epinephrine, should be used with extreme caution in patients receiving monoamine oxidase (MAO) inhibitors or antidepressants of the triptyline or imipramine types, because severe prolonged hypertension may result. Until further experience is gained in children younger than 12 years, administration of bupivacaine in this age group is not recommended.

Reports of cardiac arrest and death have occurred with the use of bupivacaine for intravenous regional anesthesia (Bier Block). Information on safe dosages or techniques of administration of this product are lacking; therefore bupivacaine is not recommended for use by this technique.

Prior use of chloroprocaine may interfere with the subsequent use of bupivacaine. Because of this, and because safety of intercurrent use of bupivacaine and chloroprocaine has not been established, such use is not recommended.

Precautions:

General: The safety and effectiveness of local anesthetics depend on proper dosage, correct technique, adequate precautions and readiness for emergencies. Resuscitative equipment, oxygen and other resuscitative drugs should be available for immediate use. (See WARNINGS and ADVERSE REACTIONS.) During major regional nerve blocks, the patient should have I.V. fluids running via an indwelling catheter to assure a functioning intravenous pathway. The lowest dosage of local anesthetic that results in effective anesthesia should be used to avoid high plasma levels and serious adverse effects. Injections should be made slowly, with frequent aspirations before and during the injection to avoid intravascular injection.

Epidural Anesthesia: During epidural administration of bupivacaine, concentrated solutions (0.5–0.75%) should be administered in incremental doses of 3 to 5 ml with sufficient time between doses to detect toxic manifestations of unintentional intravascular or intrathecal injection. Syringe aspirations should also be performed before and during each supplemental injection in continuous (intermittent) catheter techniques. An intravascular injection is still possible even if aspirations for blood are negative.

During the administration of epidural anesthethesia, it is recommended that a test dose be administered initially and the effects monitored before the full dose is given. When using a "continuous" catheter technique, test doses should be given prior to both the original and all reinforcing doses, because plastic tubing in the epidural space can migrate into a blood vessel or through the dura. When clinical conditions permit, the test dose should contain epinephrine (10 to 15 μg have been suggested) to serve as a warning of unintentional intravascular injection. If injected into a blood vessel, this amount of epinephrine is likely to produce a transient "epinephrine response" within 45 seconds, consisting of an increase in heart rate and systolic blood pressure, circumoral pallor, palpitations and nervousness in the unsedated patient. The sedated patient may exhibit only a pulse rate increase of 20 or more beats per minute for 15 or more seconds. Therefore, following the test dose, the heart rate should be monitored for a heart rate increase. The test dose should also contain 10 to 15 mg of Sensorcaine™ (bupivacaine HCl) solution or an equivalent dose of a short-acting amide anesthetic such as 30 to 40 mg of lidocaine, to detect an unintentional intrathecal administration. This will be manifested with a few minutes by signs of spinal block (e.g. decreased sensation of the buttocks, paresis of the legs, or, in the sedated patient, absent knee jerk). Patients on beta-blockers may not manifest changes in heart rate, but blood pressure monitoring can detect an evanescent rise in systolic blood pressure.

Injection of repeated doses of local anesthetics may cause significant increases in plasma levels with each repeated dose due to slow accumulation of the drug or its metabolites or to slow metabolic degradation. Tolerance to elevated blood levels varies with the physical condition of the patient. Debilitated, elderly patients and acutely ill patients should be given reduced doses commensurate with their age and physical condition. Local anesthetics should also be used with caution in patients with hypotension or heart block.

Careful and constant monitoring of cardiovascular and respiratory vital signs (adequacy of ventilation) and the patient's state of consciousness should be performed after each local anesthetic injection. It should be kept in mind at such times that restlessness, anxiety, incoherent speech, light-headedness, numbness and tingling of the mouth and lips, metallic taste, tinnitus, dizziness, blurred vision, tremors, twitching, depression, or drowsiness may be early warning signs of central nervous system toxicity.

Local anesthetic solutions containing a vasoconstrictor should be used cautiously and in carefully restricted quantities in areas of the body supplied by end arteries or having otherwise compromised blood supply such as digits, nose, external ear, penis, etc. Patients with hypertensive vascular disease may exhibit exaggerated vasoconstrictor response. Ischemic injury or necrosis may result. Because amide-type local anesthetics such as bupivacaine are metabolized by the liver, these drugs, especially repeat doses, should be used cautiously in patients with hepatic disease. Patients with severe hepatic disease, because of their inability to metabolize local anesthetics normally, are at a greater risk of developing toxic plasma concentrations. Local anesthetics should also be used with caution in patients with impaired cardiovascular function because they may be less able to compensate for functional changes associated with the prolongation of A-V conduction produced by these drugs.

Serious dose-related cardiac arrythmias may occur if preparations containing a vasoconstrictor such as epinephrine are employed in patients during or following the administration of potent inhalation anesthetics. In deciding whether to use these products concurrently in the same patients, the combined action of both agents upon the myocardium, the concentration and volume of vasoconstrictor used, and the time since injection, when applicable, should be taken into account.

Many drugs used during the conduct of anesthesia are considered potential triggering agents for familial malignant hyperthermia. Because it is not known whether amide-type local anesthetics may trigger this reaction and because the need for supplemental general anesthesia cannot be predicted in advance, it is suggested that a standard protocol for management should be available. Early unexplained signs of tachycardia, tachypnea, labile blood pressure and metabolic acidosis may precede temperature elevation. Successful outcome is dependent on early diagnosis, prompt discontinuance of the suspect triggering agent(s) and prompt treatment, including oxygen therapy, dantrolene (consult dantrolene sodium intravenous package insert before using) and other supportive measures.

Use in Head and Neck Area: Small doses of local anesthetics injected into the head and neck area, including retrobulbar, dental and stellate ganglion blocks, may produce adverse reactions similar to systemic toxicity seen with unintentional intravascular injections of larger doses. Confusion, convulsions, respiratory depression and/or respiratory arrest, and cardiovascular stimulation or depression have been reported. These reactions may be due to intraarterial injection of the local anesthetic with retrograde flow to the cerebral circulation. Patients receiving these blocks should have their circulation and respiration monitored and be constantly observed. Resuscitative equipment and personnel for treating adverse reactions should be immediately available. Dosage recommendations should not be exceeded. (See DOSAGE AND ADMINISTRATION.)

Use in Ophthalmic Surgery: When Sensorcaine™ (bupivacaine HCl) 0.75% solution is used for retrobulbar block, complete corneal anesthesia usually precedes onset of clinically acceptable external ocular muscle akinesia. Therefore, the presence of akinesia rather than anesthesia alone should determine readiness of the patient for surgery.

Information for Patients: When appropriate, patients should be informed in advance that they may experience temporary loss of sensation and motor activity, usually in the lower half of the body following proper administration of caudal or lumbar epidural anesthesia. Also, when appropriate, the physician should discuss other information including adverse reactions in the Sensorcaine™ (bupivacaine HCl) package insert.

Clinically Significant Drug Interactions: The administration of local anesthetic solutions containing epinephrine or norepinephrine to patients receiving monoamine oxidase inhibitors or tricyclic antidepressants may produce severe, prolonged hypertension. Concurrent use of these agents should generally be avoided. In situations in which concurrent therapy is necessary, careful patient monitoring is essential.

Concurrent administration of vasopressor drugs and of ergot-type oxytocic drugs may cause severe, persistent hypertension or cerebrovascular accidents.

Phenothiazines and butyrophenones may reduce or reverse the pressor effect of epinephrine.

Carcinogenesis, Mutagenesis, and Impairment of Fertility: Long-term studies in animals of most local anesthetics, including bupivacaine, to evaluate the carcinogenic potential have not been conducted. Mutagenic potential or the effect on fertility have not been determined. There is no evidence from human data that bupivacaine may be carcinogenic or mutagenic or that it impairs fertility.

Pregnancy Category C: Decreased pup survival in rats and embryocidal effect in rabbits have been observed when bupivacaine HCl was administered to these species in doses comparable to nine and five times, respectively, the maximum recommended daily human dose (400 mg). There are no adequate and well-controlled studies in pregnant women of the effect of bupivacaine on the developing fetus. Sensorcaine™ (bupivacaine HCl) solution should be used during pregnancy only if the potential benefit justifies the potential risk to the fetus. This does not exclude the use of Sensorcaine™ (bupivacaine HCl) solution (0.25% and 0.5% concentrations) at term for obstetrical anesthesia or analgesia. (See LABOR AND DELIVERY.)

Labor and Delivery: See Box WARNING regarding obstetrical use of 0.75% concentration.

Sensorcaine™ (bupivacaine HCl) solution is contraindicated in obstetrical paracervical block anesthesia.

Local anesthetics rapidly cross the placenta, and when used for epidural, caudal or pudendal block anesthesia, can cause varying degrees of maternal, fetal and neonatal toxicity. (See CLINICAL PHARMACOLOGY.) The incidence and degree of toxicity depend upon the procedure performed, the type and amount of drug used, and the technique of drug administration. Adverse reactions in the parturient, fetus and neonate involve alterations of the central nervous system, peripheral vascular tone and cardiac function.

Maternal hypotension has resulted from regional anesthesia. Local anesthetics produce vasodilation by blocking sympathetic nerves. Elevating the patient's legs and positioning her on her left side will help prevent decreases in blood pressure. The fetal heart rate also should be monitored continuously, and electronic fetal monitoring is highly advisable.

Epidural, caudal, or pudendal anesthesia may alter the forces of parturition through changes in uterine contractility or maternal expulsive efforts. Epidural anesthesia has been reported to prolong the second stage of labor by removing the parturient's reflex urge to bear down or by interfering with motor function. The use of obstetrical anesthesia may increase the need for forceps assistance.

The use of some local anesthetic drug products during labor and delivery may be followed by di-

Continued on next page

Astra—Cont.

minished muscle strength and tone for the first day or two of life. This has not been reported with Sensorcaine™ (bupivacaine HCl) solution.

It is extremely important to avoid aortocaval compression by the gravid uterus during administration of regional block to parturients. To do this, the patient must be maintained in the left lateral decubitus position or a blanket roll or sandbag may be placed beneath the right hip and the gravid uterus displaced to the left.

Nursing Mothers: It is not known whether local anesthetic drugs are excreted in human milk. Because many drugs are excreted in human milk, caution should be exercised when local anesthetics are administered to a nursing mother.

Pediatric Use: Until further experience is gained in children younger than 12 years, administration of Sensorcaine™ (bupivacaine HCl) solution in this age group is not recommended.

Adverse Reactions: Reactions to bupivacaine are characteristic of those associated with other amide-type local anesthetics. A major cause of adverse reactions to this group of drugs may be associated with excessive plasma levels, which may be due to overdosage, unintentional intravascular injection or slow metabolic degradation.

Systemic: The most commonly encountered acute adverse experiences that demand immediate countermeasures are related to the central nervous system and the cardiovascular system. These adverse experiences are generally dose related and due to high plasma levels which may result from overdosage, rapid absorption from the injection site, diminished tolerance or from unintentional intravascular injection of the local anesthetic solution. In addition to systemic dose-related toxicity, unintentional subarachnoid injection of drug during the intended performance of caudal or lumbar epidural block or nerve blocks near the vertebral column (especially in the head and neck region) may result in underventilation or apnea ("Total or High Spinal"). Also, hypotension due to loss of sympathetic tone and respiratory paralysis or underventilation due to cephalad extension of the motor level of anesthesia may occur. This may lead to secondary cardiac arrest if untreated. Factors influencing plasma protein binding, such as acidosis, systemic diseases that alter protein production or competition with other drugs for protein binding sites, may diminish individual tolerance.

Central Nervous System Reactions: These are characterized by excitation and/or depression. Restlessness, anxiety, dizziness, tinnitus, blurred vision or tremors may occur, possibly proceeding to convulsions. However, excitement may be transient or absent, with depression being the first manifestation of an adverse reaction. This may quickly be followed by drowsiness merging into unconsciousness and respiratory arrest. Other central nervous system effects may be nausea, vomiting, chills, and constriction of the pupils.

The incidence of convulsions associated with the use of local anesthetics varies with the procedure used and the total dose administered. In a survey of studies of epidural anesthesia, overt toxicity progressing to convulsions occurred in approximately 0.1 percent of local anesthetic administrations.

Cardiovascular System Reactions: High doses or unintentional intravascular injection may lead to high plasma levels and related depression of the myocardium, decreased cardiac output, heart block, hypotension, bradycardia, ventricular arrhythmias, including ventricular tachycardia and ventricular fibrillation, and cardiac arrest. (See WARNINGS, PRECAUTIONS, and OVERDOSAGE sections).

Allergic: Allergic type reactions are rare and may occur as a result of sensitivity to the local anesthetic or to other formulation ingredients, such as the antimicrobial preservative methylparaben contained in multiple dose vials or sulfites in epinephrine-containing solutions. These reactions are characterized by signs such as urticaria, pruritis, erythema, angioneurotic edema (including laryngeal edema), tachycardia, sneezing, nausea, vomiting, dizziness, syncope, excessive sweating, elevated temperature, and possibly, anaphylactoid symptomatology (including severe hypotension). Cross sensitivity among members of the amide-type local anesthetic group has been reported. The usefulness of screening for sensitivity has not been definitely established.

Neurologic: The incidence of adverse neurologic reactions associated with the use of local anesthetics may be related to the total dose of local anesthetic administered and are also dependent upon the particular drug used, the route of administraion and the physical status of the patient. Many of these effects may be related to local anesthetic techniques, with or without a contribution from the drug.

In the practice of caudal or lumbar epidural block, occasional unintentional penetration of the subarachnoid space by the catheter or needle may occur. Subsequent adverse effects may depend partially on the amount of drug administered intrathecally and the physiological and physical effects of a dural puncture. A high spinal is characterized by paralysis of the legs, loss of consciousness, respiratory paralysis and bradycardia.

Neurologic effects following unintentional subarachnoid administration during epidural or caudal anesthesia may include spinal block by varying magnitude (including high or total spinal block); hypotension secondary to spinal block; urinary retention; fecal and urinary incontinence; loss of perineal sensation and sexual function; persistent anesthesia, paresthesia, weakness, paralysis of the lower extremities and loss of sphincter control, all of which may have slow, incomplete or no recovery; headache; backache; septic meningitis; meningismus; slowing of labor; increased incidence of forceps delivery; or cranial nerve palsies due to traction on nerves from loss of cerebrospinal fluid.

Overdosage: Acute emergencies from local anesthetics are generally related to high plasma levels encountered during therapeutic use of local anesthetics or to unintended subarachnoid injection of local anesthetic solution. (See ADVERSE REACTIONS, WARNINGS, and PRECAUTIONS).

Management of Local Anesthetic Emergencies: The first consideration is prevention, best accomplished by careful and constant monitoring of cardiovascular and respiratory vital signs and the patient's state of consciousness after each local anesthetic injection. At the first sign of change, oxygen should be administered.

The first step in the management of systemic toxic reactions, as well as underventilation or apnea due to unintentional subarachnoid injection of drug solution, consists of immediate attention to the establishment and maintenance of a patent airway and effective assisted or controlled ventilation with 100% oxygen with a delivery system capable of permitting immediate positive airway pressure by mask. This may prevent convulsions if they have not already occurred.

If necessary, use drugs to control the convulsions. A 50 to 100 mg bolus I.V. injection of succinylcholine will paralyze the patient without depressing the central nervous or cardiovascular systems and facilitate ventilation. A bolus I.V. dose of 5 to 10 mg of diazepam or 50 to 100 mg of thiopental will permit ventilation and counteract central nervous system stimulation, but these drugs also depress the central nervous system, respiratory and cardiac function, add to postictal depression, and may result in apnea. Intravenous barbiturates, anticonsulsant agents, or muscle relaxants should only be administered by those familiar with their use. Immediately after the institution of these ventilatory measures, the adequacy of the circulation should be evaluated. Supportive treatment of circulatory depression may require administration of intravenous fluids, and, when appropriate, a vasopressor dictated by the clinical situation (such as ephedrine or epinephrine to enhance myocardial contractile force).

If difficulty is encountered in the maintenance of a patent airway or if prolonged ventilatory support (assisted or controlled) is indicated, endotracheal intubation, employing drugs and techniques familiar to the clinician, may be indicated after initial administration of oxygen by mask.

Recent clinical data from patients experiencing local anesthetic induced convulsions demonstrated rapid development of hypoxia, hypercarbia and acidosis wih bupivacaine within a minute of the onset of convulsions. These observations suggest the oxygen consumption and carbon dioxide production are greatly increased during local anesthetic convulsions and emphasize the importance of immediate and effective ventilation with oxygen which may avoid cardiac arrest.

If not treated immediately, convulsions with simultaneous hypoxia, hypercarbia and acidosis, plus myocardial depression from the direct effects of the local anesthetic may result in cardiac arrhythmias, bradycardia, asystole, ventricular fibrillation, or cardiac arrest. Respiratory abnormalities, includng apnea, may occur. Underventilation or apnea due to unintentional subarachnoid injection of local anesthetic solution may produce these same signs and also lead to cardiac arrest if ventilatory support is not instituted. *If cardiac arrest should occur, a successful outcome may require prolonged resuscitative efforts.*

The supine position is dangerous in pregnant women at term because of aortocaval compression by the gravid uterus. Therefore, during treatment of systemic toxicity, maternal hypotension or fetal bradycardia following regional block, the parturient should be maintained in the left lateral decubitus position if possible, or manual displacement of the uterus off the great vessels be accomplished. The mean seizure dosage of bupivacaine in rhesus monkeys was found to be 4.4 mg/kg with mean arterial plasma concentration of 4.5 mcg/ml. The intravenous and subcutaneous LD50s in mice are 6 to 8mg/kg and 38 to 54mg/kg respectively.

Dosage and Administration: The dosage varies and depends upon the area to be anesthetized, the vascularity of the tissues, the number of neuronal segments to be blocked, individual tolerance, and the technique of anesthesia. The lowest dosage needed to provide effective anesthesia should be administered. The rapid injection of a large volume of local anesthetic solution should be avoided and fractional doses should be used when feasible. For specific techniques and procedures, refer to standard textbooks.

For most indications, the duration of anesthesia with Sensorcaine™ (bupivacaine HCl) solution is such that a single dose is sufficient.

In each case, the maximum dosage limit must be determined by evaluating the size and physical status of the patient and considering the usual rate of systemic absorption from a specific injection site. Most experience to date is with single doses up to 175 mg of bupivacaine HCl without epinephrine or 225 mg with epinephrine 1:200,000. More or less drug may be used depending on the physical condition of each case. The dose may be repeated as often as every 3 hours. In studies to date, total daily doses up to 400 mg have been reported. Until further experience is gained, this dose should not be exceeded in 24 hours. The dosages in the following table are recommended as a guide for use in the average adult. For young, elderly or debilitated patients, these dosages should be reduced. Until further experience is gained, Sensorcaine™ solution is not recommended for children younger than 12 years. Sensorcaine™ (bupivacaine HCl) is contraindicated in obstetrical paracervial block and is not recommended for use in intravenous regional anesthesia (Bier Block).

Use in Epidural Anesthesia: During epidural administration, Sensorcaine™ (bupivacaine HCl) 0.5% and 0.75% solutions should be administered in incremental doses of 3 to 5 ml, with sufficient time between doses to detect toxic manifestations of unintentional intravascular or intrathecal injection. In obstetrics, only the 0.5% and 0.25% concentrations should be used; incremental doses of 3 to 5 ml of the 0.5% solution, not exceeding 50–100 mg at any dosing interval, are recommended. Repeat doses should be preceded by a test dose containing epinephrine if the vasoconstrictor is not contraindicated.

UNUSED PORTIONS OF SOLUTIONS IN SINGLE DOSE CONTAINERS SHOULD BE DISCARDED, SINCE THIS PRODUCT FORM CONTAINS NO PRESERVATIVES.
[See table right].

NOTE: Parenteral drug products should be inspected visually for particulate matter and discoloration prior to administration whenever the solution and container permit. Solutions that are discolored and/or contain particulate matter should not be used.

How Supplied: SOLUTIONS OF SENSORCAINE™ (BUPIVACAINE HYDROCHLORIDE) SHOULD NOT BE USED FOR THE PRODUCTION OF SPINAL ANESTHESIA (SUBARACHNOID BLOCK) BECAUSE OF INSUFFICIENT DATA TO SUPPORT SUCH USE.
[See table below].

Disinfecting agents containing heavy metals, which cause release of respective ions (mercury, zinc, copper, etc.), should not be used for skin or mucous membrane disinfection since they have been related to incidents of swelling and edema. When chemical disinfection of the container surface is desired, either pure undiluted isopropyl alcohol (91%) or ethyl alcohol (70%) USP is recommended. It is recommended that chemical disinfection be accomplished by wiping the ampule or vial stopper thoroughly with cotton or gauze that has been moistened with the recommended alcohol just prior to use.

Solutions should be stored at controlled room temperature 15° to 30° C (59°–86°F).
Solutions containing epinephrine should be protected from light.

Product Information as of November, 1983
021851R06   1/84

TABLE 2. DOSAGE RECOMMENDATIONS—SENSORCAINE™ (bupivacaine HCl) SOLUTIONS WITHOUT EPINEPHRINE

Type of Block	conc.(%)	Each Dose ml.	mg.	Motor Block*
Local infiltration	0.25	up to 70	up to 175	—
Epidural	0.75**	10–20	75–150	Complete
	0.50	10–20	50–100	Moderate to complete
	0.25	10–20	25–50	Partial to moderate
Caudal	0.50	15–30	75–150	Moderate to complete
	0.25	15–30	37.5–75	Moderate
Peripheral	0.50	5–35	25–175	Moderate to complete
	0.25	5–70	12.5–175	Moderate to complete
Retrobulbar†	0.75	2–4	15–30	Complete
Sympathetic†	0.25	20–50	50–125	—

*With continuous techniques, repeat doses increase the degree of motor block. The first repeat dose of 0.5% may produce complete motor block. Intercostal nerve block with 0.25% may also produce complete motor block for intra-abdominal surgery.
**For single dose; not for continuous techniques; not for use in obstetrics.
†See PRECAUTIONS.

XYLOCAINE® (lidocaine hydrochloride) ℞
[zī'lo-caine]
STERILE AQUEOUS SOLUTIONS
Local anesthetic for infiltration and nerve block

Description: Xylocaine® (lidocaine hydrochloride) Solutions are sterile aqueous solutions prepared from lidocaine hydrochloride and water. Lidocaine hydrochloride is a local anesthetic chemically designated as 2-(diethylamino)-N-(2,6-dimethylphenyl)-acetamide monohydrochloride.

Xylocaine Solutions are available with or without epinephrine. Xylocaine Solutions without epinephrine may be reautoclaved if necessary
Please refer to Table I for the exact composition of available Xylocaine Solutions.
[See table on next page].

Clinical Pharmacology: Lidocaine stabilizes the neuronal membrane and prevents the initiation and conduction of nerve impulses, thereby effecting local anesthetic action.

Lidocaine is metabolized mainly in the liver and excreted via the kidneys. Approximately 90% of lidocaine administered is excreted in the form of various metabolites, while less than 10% is excreted unchanged.

Indications: Xylocaine Solutions are indicated for production of local or regional anesthesia, by infiltration techniques, including percutaneous injection and intravenous regional anesthesia, by peripheral nerve block techniques such as brachial plexus and intercostal blocks and by central neural techniques, including epidural and caudal blocks, when the accepted procedures for these techniques as described in standard textbooks are followed.

Contraindications: Xylocaine (lidocaine hydrochloride) Solutions are containdicated in patients with a known history of hypersensitivity either to local anesthetic agents of the amide type or to other components of the injectable formulations.

Warnings:
(1) RESUSCITATIVE EQUIPMENT AND DRUGS, INCLUDING OXYGEN, SHOULD BE IMMEDIATELY AVAILABLE WHEN ANY LOCAL ANESTHETIC AGENT IS USED.
(2) USE IN PREGNANCY: Reproductive studies have been performed in rats and rabbits without evidence of harm to the animal fetus. However, the safe use of lidocaine in humans has not been established with respect to possible adverse effects upon fetal development. Careful consideration should be given to this fact before administering this drug to women of childbearing potential, particularly during early pregnancy.
This does not exclude the use of the drug at term for obstetrical analgesia. Xylocaine Solution has been used effectively for obstetrical analgesia. Adverse effects on the fetus, course of labor or delivery have rarely been observed when proper dosage and proper technique have been employed.
(3) Local anesthetic procedures should be used with caution when there is inflammation and/or sepsis in the region of the proposed injection.
(4) Vasopressor agents (administered for the treatment of hypotension related to caudal or other epidural blocks) should be used with caution in the presence of oxytocic drugs, as a severe persistent hypertension and even rupture of cerebral blood vessels may occur.
(5) The solutions which contain a vasoconstrictor should be used with extreme caution for patients whose medical history and physical evaluation suggest the existence of hypertension, arteriosclerotic heart disease, cerebral vascular insufficiency, heart block, thyrotoxicosis or diabetes, etc. The solutions which contain a vasoconstrictor should also be used with extreme caution in patients receiving drugs known to produce blood pressure alterations (e.g., MAO inhibitors, tricyclic antidepressants, phenothiazines, etc.) as either sustained hypotension or hypertension may occur.

Precautions: The safety and effectiveness of Xylocaine Solution depends on proper dosage, correct technique, adequate precautions and readiness for emergencies. Standard textbooks should be consulted for specific techniques and precautions for various regional anesthetic procedures.

The lowest dosage that results in effective anesthesia should be used. Injection of repeated doses of Xylocaine Solution may cause significant increases in blood levels with each repeated dose due to slow accumulation of lidocaine or its metabolites. Tolerance varies with the status of the patient. Debilitated, elderly patients, acutely ill patients, and children should be given reduced doses commensurate with their age and physical status. Xylocaine Solution should also be used with caution in patients with severe shock or heart block. In using Xylocaine Solution for infiltration or regional block anesthesia, injection should always be made slowly and with frequent aspirations. Proper tourniquet technique is essential in the performance of intravenous regional anesthesia. Solutions containing epinephrine or other vasoconstrictors should not be used for this technique. Epidural anesthesia and caudal anesthesia should be used with extreme caution in persons with the following conditions: existing neurological disease, spinal deformities, septicemia, severe hypertension, and extreme youth.

Fetal bradycardia frequently follows paracervical block and may be associated with fetal acidosis. Fetal heart rate should always be monitored during paracervical anesthesia. Added risk appears to be present in prematurity, postmaturity, toxemia of pregnancy, uteroplacental insufficiency and fetal distress. The physician should weigh the possible advantages against dangers when considering paracervical block in these conditions. When the recommended dose is exceeded, the incidence of fetal bradycardia increases.

Short term neonatal neurobehavioral alterations have been observed in association with some local anesthetics administered during labor and delivery. The short term and long term significance of these alterations is not known.

Sensorcaine™ (bupivacaine HCl) solutions

Dosage Form	Concentrate	Astra Sterile-Pak™
Single Dose Vials, 30 ml	0.25% and 0.5% without epinephrine	x
	0.5% and 0.75% with epinephrine 1:200,000	x
Multiple dose Vials, 50 ml	0.25% and 0.5% without epinephrine	
Single Dose Ampules, 30 ml	0.25%, 0.5%, 0.75% without epinephrine	x
	0.5% and 0.75% with epinephrine 1:200,000	x
Single Dose Ampules, 5 ml	0.5% with epinephrine 1:200,000	

x–Package forms—also available in Astra Sterile-Pak™ Pre-sterilized vials or ampules in a Convenient Dispenser Carton.

Continued on next page

Astra—Cont.

Solutions containing a vasoconstrictor should be used cautiously and in carefully circumscribed quantities in areas of the body supplied by end arteries or having otherwise compromised blood supply (e.g., digits, nose, external ear, penis, etc.). Serious cardiac arrhythmias may occur if preparations containing a vasoconstrictor are employed in patients during or following the administration of chloroform, halothane, cyclopropane, trichlorethylene, or other related agents.

Xylocaine Solution should be used with caution in persons with known drug sensitivities. Patients allergic to para-aminobenzoic acid derivatives (procaine, tetracaine, benzocaine, etc.) have not shown cross sensitivity to lidocaine.

The safety of amide local anesthetics in patients with malignant hyperthermia has not been assessed, and therefore, these agents should be used with caution in such patients.

Drowsiness following an injection of Xylocaine Solution is usually an early indication of a high blood level of the drug and may occur following an inadvertent intravascular administration or rapid absorption of lidocaine.

Local anesthetics react with certain metals and cause the release of their respective ions which, if injected, may cause severe local irritation. Adequate precautions should be taken to avoid this type of interaction (see STERILIZATION, STORAGE AND TECHNICAL PROCEDURES).

Adverse Reactions: Reactions to Xylocaine Solutions are similar in character to those observed with other local anesthetic agents. Adverse reactions may be due to high plasma levels as a result of excessive dosage, rapid absorption or inadvertent intravascular injection. Such reactions are systemic in nature and involve the central nervous system and/or the cardiovascular system. Rarely reactions may result from hypersensitivity, idiosyncrasy or diminished tolerance on the part of the patient.

CNS reactions are excitatory and/or depressant, and may be characterized by nervousness, dizziness, blurred vision and tremors, followed by drowsiness, convulsions, unconsciousness and, possibly, respiratory arrest. The excitatory reactions may be very brief or may not occur at all, in which case the first manifestations of toxicity may be drowsiness, merging into unconsciousness and respiratory arrest.

Hypotension and bradycardia may occur as normal physiological phenomena following sympathetic block with central neural blocks. Toxic cardiovascular reactions to local anesthetics are usually depressant in nature and are characterized by peripheral vasodilation, hypotension, myocardial depression, bradycardia and, possibly cardiac arrest.

Treatment of a patient with toxic manifestations consists of assuring and maintaining a patent airway, supporting ventilation with oxygen, and assisted or controlled ventilation (respiration) as required. This usually will be sufficient in the management of most reactions.

Should a convulsion persist despite ventilatory therapy with oxygen, small increments of anticonvulsive agents may be given intravenously. Examples of such agents include a benzodiazepine (e.g. diazepam), ultra-short acting barbiturates (e.g., thiopental or thiamylal) or a short acting barbiturate (e.g. pentobarbital or secobarbital). Cardiovascular depression may require circulatory assistance with intravenous fluids and/or vasopressors (e.g., ephedrine) as dictated by the clinical situation.

Allergic reactions may occur as a result of sensitivity either to local anesthetics or to the methylparaben used as a preservative in multiple dose vials. Anaphylactoid type symptomatology and reactions, characterized by cutaneous lesions, urticaria, and edema, should be managed by conventional means. The detection of potential sensitivity by skin testing is of limited value.

Dosage and Administration: Table II (Recommended Dosages) summarizes the recommended volumes and concentrations of Xylocaine (lidocaine hydrochloride) Solutions for various types of anesthetic procedures. The dosages suggested in this table are for normal healthy adults and refer to the use of epinephrine-free solutions. When larger dosages are required, only solutions containing epinephrine should be used except in those cases where vasopressor drugs may be contraindicated.

[See table on top next page].

These recommended doses serve only as a guide to the amount of anesthetic required for most routine procedures. The actual volume and concentrations to be used depend on a number of factors, such as type and extent of surgical procedure, degree of muscular relaxation required, duration of anesthesia required, the physical state of the patient, etc. In all cases the lowest concentration and smallest dose that will produce the desired result should be given. Dosages should be reduced for children and for elderly and debilitated patients. The onset of anesthesia, the duration of anesthesia and the degree of muscular relaxation are proportional to the volume and concentration of local anesthetic solution used. Thus, an increase in concentration and volume of Xylocaine Solution administered will decrease the onset of anesthesia, prolong the duration of anesthesia, provide a greater degree of muscular relaxation and increase the segmental spread of anesthesia. However, increasing the concentration and volume of Xylocaine Solution administered may result in a more profound fall in blood pressure when used in epidural anesthesia. Although the incidence of side effects with Xylocaine Solution is quite low, caution should be exercised particularly when employing large volumes and concentrations of Xylocaine Solutions, since the incidence of side effects is directly related to the total dose of local anesthetic agent injected.

It is important that a single dose container be employed for epidural anesthesia and major peripheral nerve block. For intravenous regional anesthesia, only the single dose containers designated for intravenous regional anesthesia should be used.

Epidural Anesthesia

For epidural anesthesia, only the following dosage forms of Xylocaine Solution are recommended:

1% without epinephrine..................30 ml ampules
30 ml single dose vials

1% with epinephrine
1:200,000 ....30 ml ampules
30 ml single dose vials

1.5% without
epinephrine ....20 ml ampules
20 ml single dose vials

1.5% with epinephrine
1:200,000 ....30 ml ampules
30 ml single dose vials

2% without
epinephrine ....10 ml ampules
10 ml single dose vials

2% with epinephrine
1:200,000 ....20 ml ampules
20 ml single dose vials

Although these solutions are intended specifically for epidural anesthesia, they may also be used for infiltration and peripheral nerve block provided they are employed as single dose units. These solutions contain no bacteriostatic agent.

In epidural anesthesia, the dosage varies with the number of dermatomes to be anesthetized (generally 2-3 ml of the indicated concentration per dermatome).

IMPORTANT: *A test dose of 2-5 ml should be administered at least 5 minutes prior to injecting the total required volume for central neural blocks (e.g., epidural or caudal anesthesia).*

Maximum Recommended Dosages

For normal healthy adults, the individual dose of Xylocaine Solution with epinephrine should be such that the dose of lidocaine hydrochloride is kept below 500 mg and, in any case should not exceed 7 mg/kg (3.2 mg/lb) of body weight. When used without epinephrine, the amount of Xylocaine Solution administered should be such that the dose of lidocaine hydrochloride is kept below 300 mg and in any case should not exceed 4.5 mg/kg (2.0 mg per lb) of body weight. For continuous epidural or caudal anesthesia, the maximum

Xylocaine Sterile Aqueous Solutions
TABLE I COMPOSITION OF AVAILABLE SOLUTIONS

PRODUCT IDENTIFICATION		SINGLE DOSE VIALS AND AMPULES			FORMULA MULTIPLE DOSE VIALS			
Xylocaine (lidocaine hydrochloride) Solution (Percent)	Epinephrine (dilution)	Sodium Chloride (mg/ml)	Sodium Metabisulfite (mg/ml)	Citric Acid (mg/ml)	Sodium Chloride (mg/ml)	Sodium Metabisulfite (mg/ml)	Citric Acid (mg/ml)	Methyl-Paraben (mg/ml)
0.5	None	8.0	None	None	8.0	None	None	1.0
0.5	1:200,000	N.S.	N.S.	N.S.	8.0	0.5	0.2	1.0
1.0	None	7.0	None	None	7.0	None	None	1.0
1.0	1:200,000	7.0	0.5	0.2	N.S.	N.S.	N.S.	N.S.
1.0	1:100,000	N.S.	N.S.	N.S.	7.0	0.5	0.2	1.0
1.5	None	6.5	None	None	N.S.	N.S.	N.S.	N.S.
1.5	1:200,000	6.5	0.5	0.2	N.S.	N.S.	N.S.	N.S.
2.0	None	6.0	None	None	6.0	None	None	1.0
2.0	1:200,000	6.0	0.5	0.2	N.S.	N.S.	N.S.	N.S.
2.0	1:100,000	N.S.	N.S.	N.S.	6.0	0.5	0.2	1.0

N.S. Not Supplied
NOTE: pH of all solutions is adjusted to USP limits with sodium hydroxide and/or hydrochloric acid.

recommended dosage should not be administered at intervals of less than 90 minutes.
For paracervical block for obstetrical analgesia, (including abortion) the maximum recommended dosage (200 mg) should not be administered at intervals of less than 90 minutes. When paracervical block is used for non-obstetrical procedures, more drug may be administered if required to obtain adequate anesthesia. For intravenous regional anesthesia in adults (using Xylocaine 0.5% solution without epinephrine), the dose administered should not exceed 4 mg/kg (1.8 mg/lb) of body weight.

Children:
It is difficult to recommend a maximum dose of any drug for children since this varies as a function of age and weight. For children of less than ten years who have a normal lean body mass and normal body development, the maximum dose may be determined by the application of one of the standard pediatric drug formulas (e.g., Clark's rule). For example, in a child of five years weighing 50 lbs., the dose of lidocaine hydrochloride should not exceed 75–100 mg when calculated according to Clark's rule. In any case, the maximum dose of Xylocaine Solution with epinephrine should not exceed 7 mg/kg (3.2 mg/lb) of body weight. When used without epinephrine, the amount of Xylocaine Solution administered should not exceed 4.5 mg/kg (2.0 mg/lb) of body weight.

In order to minimize the possibility of toxic reactions, the use of Xylocaine 0.5% or 1.0% Solution is recommended for most anesthetic procedures involving pediatric patients. The use of even more dilute solutions (i.e., 0.25–0.5%) and total dosages not to exceed 3 mg/kg (1.4 mg/lb) are recommended for induction of intravenous regional anesthesia in children.

Sterilization, Storage and Technical Procedures:
Disinfecting agents containing heavy metals, which cause release of respective ions (mercury, zinc, copper, etc.) should not be used for skin or mucous membrane disinfection as they have been related to incidence of swelling and edema. When chemical disinfection of multi-dose vials is desired, either pure undiluted isoprophyl alcohol (91%) or 70% ethyl alcohol U.S.P. is recommended. Many commercially available brands of rubbing alcohol, as well as solutions of ethyl alcohol not of U.S.P. grade, contain denaturants which are injurious to rubber and, therefore, are not to be used.

It is recommended that chemical disinfection be accomplished by wiping the vial or ampule thoroughly with cotton or gauze that has been moistened with the recommended alcohol just prior to use.

021563-01   Rev. 10/83

How Supplied:
[See table below].

XYLOCAINE® SOLUTION
[zī' lo-caine]
(lidocaine hydrochloride)
FOR VENTRICULAR ARRHYTHMIAS

Description: Xylocaine (lidocaine hydrochloride) Solution is a sterile solution of an antiarrhythmic agent administered intravenously by either direct injection or continuous infusion, or intramuscularly by injection. The specific quantitative for each available solution appears in Table 1.
(See table next page)

Xylocaine Solutions are composed of aqueous solutions of lidocaine hydrochloride. Lidocaine hydrochloride is chemically designated acetamide, 2-(diethylamino)-N-(2, 6 dimethylphenyl)-, monohydrochloride and is represented by the following structural formula:

Clinical Pharmacology:
Mechanism of action and electrophysiology:
Studies of the effects of therapeutic concentrations of lidocaine on the electrophysiological properties of mammalian Purkinje fibers have shown that lidocaine attenuates phase 4 diastolic depolarization, decreases automaticity, and causes a decrease or no change in excitability and membrane responsiveness. Action potential duration and effective refractory period of Purkinje fibers are decreased, while the ratio of effective refractory period to action potential duration is increased. Action potential duration and effective refractory period of ventricular muscle are also decreased. Effective refractory period of the AV node may increase, decrease or remain unchanged, and atrial effective refractory period is unchanged. Lidocaine raises the ventricular fibrillation threshold. No significant interactions between lidocaine and the autonomic nervous system have been described and consequently, lidocaine has little or no effect on autonomic tone.

Clinical electrophysiological studies with lidocaine have demonstrated no change in sinus node recovery time or sinoatrial conduction time. AV nodal conduction time is unchanged or shortened, and His-Purkinje conduction time is unchanged.

Hemodynamics:
At therapeutic doses, lidocaine has minimal hemodynamic effects in normal subjects and in patients with heart disease. Lidocaine has been shown to cause no, or minimal, decrease in ventricular contractility, cardiac output, arterial pressure or heart rate.

Pharmacokinetics and metabolism:
Lidocaine is rapidly metabolized by the liver, and less than 10% of a dose is excreted unchanged in the urine. Oxidative N-dealkylation, a major pathway of metabolism, results in the metabolites monoethylglycinexylidide and glycinexylidide. The pharmacological/toxicological activities of these metabolites are similar to, but less potent than, lidocaine. The primary metabolite in urine is a conjugate of 4-hydroxy-2,6-dimethylaniline.

The elimination half-life of lidocaine following an intravenous bolus injection is typically 1.5 to 2.0 hours. There are data that indicate that the half-life may be 3 hours or longer following infusions of greater than 24 hours.

Because of the rapid rate at which lidocaine is metabolized, any condition that alters liver function, including changes in liver blood flow, which could result from severe congestive heart failure or shock, may alter lidocaine kinetics. The half-life

---

TABLE II Recommended dosages of Xylocaine (lidocaine hydrochloride) For Various Anesthetic Procedures In Normal Healthy Adults.

PROCEDURE	Xylocaine (lidocaine hydrochloride) Solution (without epinephrine)		
	Conc. (%)	Vol. (ml)	Total Dose (mg)
Infiltration			
Percutaneous	0.5 or 1.0	1–60	5–300
Intravenous regional	0.5	10–60	50–300
Peripheral Nerve Blocks, e.g.			
Brachial	1.5	15–20	225–300
Dental	2.0	1–5	20–100
Intercostal	1.0	3	30
Paravertebral	1.0	3–5	30–50
Pudendal (each side)	1.0	10	100
Paracervical			
Obstetrical analgesia (each side)	1.0	10	100
Sympathetic Nerve Blocks, e.g.			
Cervical (stellate ganglion)	1.0	5	50
Lumbar	1.0	5–10	50–100
Central Neural Blocks			
Epidural*			
Thoracic	1.0	20–30	200–300
Lumbar			
Analgesia	1.0	25–30	250–300
Anesthesia	1.5	15–20	225–300
	2.0	10–15	200–300
Caudal			
Obstetrical analgesia	1.0	20–30	200–300
Surgical anesthesia	1.5	15–20	225–300

*Dose determined by number of dermatomes to be anesthetized (2–3 ml/dermatome).

THE ABOVE SUGGESTED CONCENTRATIONS AND VOLUMES SERVE ONLY AS A GUIDE. OTHER VOLUMES AND CONCENTRATIONS MAY BE USED PROVIDED THE TOTAL MAXIMUM RECOMMENDED DOSE IS NOT EXCEEDED.

Xylocaine (lidocaine HCl) Concentration	/Epinephrine Dilution (if present)	Ampules (ml) 2	5	10	20	30	Single Dose Vials (ml) 20	30	50	Multiple Dose Vials (ml) 20	50
0.5%									X		X
0.5%	/1:200,000										X
1%		X	X.		X		X			X	X
1%	/1:100,000									X	X
1%	/1:200,000				X	X	X				
1.5%						X		X			
1.5%	/1:200,000					X		X			
2%		X	X							X	X
2%	/1:100,000									X	X
2%	/1:200,000				X		X	X			

All solutions should be stored at controlled room temperature 15°–30°C (59°–86°F).

Continued on next page

Astra—Cont.

may be two-fold or more greater in patients with liver dysfunction. Renal dysfunction does not affect lidocaine kinetics, but may increase the accumulation of metabolites.

Therapeutic effects of lidocaine are generally associated with plasma levels of 6 to 25 μmole/L (1.5 to 6μg free base per ml). The blood to plasma distribution ratio is approximately 0.84. Objective adverse manifestations become increasingly apparent with increasing plasma levels above 6.0 μg free base per ml.

The plasma protein binding of lidocaine is dependent on drug concentration, and the fraction bound decreases with increasing concentration. At concentrations of 1 to 4 μg free base per ml, 60 to 80 percent of lidocaine is protein bound. In addition to lidocaine concentration, the binding is dependent on the plasma concentration of the α-1-acid glycoprotein.

Lidocaine readily crosses the placental and blood-brain barriers. Dialysis has negligible effects on the kinetics of lidocaine.

When an appropriate dose of Xylocaine Solution is administered intramuscularly into the deltoid muscle, effective antiarrhythmic blood levels are usually obtained within 5 to 15 minutes and usually persist for 60 to 90 minutes. Absorption from other intramuscular sites such as the vastus lateralis and gluteus maximus is slower, resulting in significantly lower blood levels during the first hour.

Indications and Usage: Xylocaine Solution, administered intravenously or intramuscularly, is specifically indicated in the acute management of ventricular arrhythmias such as those occurring in relation to acute myocardial infarction, or during cardiac manipulation, such as cardiac surgery.

Contraindications: Xylocaine Solution is contraindicated in patients with a known history of hypersensitivity to local anesthetics of the amide type. Xylocaine Solution should not be used in patients with Stokes-Adams syndrome, Wolff-Parkinson-White syndrome, or with severe degrees of sinoatrial, atrioventricular, or intraventricular block in the absence of an artificial pacemaker.

Warnings: IN ORDER TO MANAGE POSSIBLE ADVERSE REACTIONS, RESUSCITATIVE EQUIPMENT, OXYGEN AND OTHER RESUSCITATIVE DRUGS SHOULD BE IMMEDIATELY AVAILABLE WHEN XYLOCAINE (LIDOCAINE HYDROCHLORIDE) SOLUTION IS USED.

Systemic toxicity may result in manifestations of central nervous sytem depression (sedation) or irritability (twitching), which may progress to frank convulsions accompanied by respiratory depression and/or arrest. Early recognition of premonitory signs, assurance of adequate oxygenation and, where necessary, establishment of artificial airway with ventilatory support are essential to management of this problem. Should convulsions persist despite ventilatory therapy with oxygen, *small* increments of anticonvulsant drugs may be used intravenously. Examples of such agents include benzodiazepines (e.g., diazepam), ultra short-acting barbiturates (e.g., thiopental or thiamylal), or a short-acting barbiturate (e.g., pentobarbital or secobarbital). If the patient is under anesthesia, a short-acting muscle relaxant (e.g., succinylcholine) may be used. Longer acting drugs should be used only when recurrent convulsions are evidenced.

Should circulatory depression occur, vasopressors may be used.

Constant electrocardiographic monitoring is essential to the proper administration of Xylocaine Solutions. Signs of excessive depression of cardiac electrical activity such as sinus node dysfunction, prolongation of the P-R interval and QRS complex or the appearance or aggravation of arrhythmias, should be followed by flow adjustment and, if necessary, prompt cessation of the intravenous infusion of this agent. Occasionally, acceleration of ventricular rate may occur when Xylocaine Solution is administered to patients with atrial flutter or fibrillation.

Precautions:
1. **General:** Caution should be employed in the use of Xylocaine Solution in patients with severe liver or kidney disease because accumulation of the drug or metabolites may occur.

Xylocaine Solution should be used with caution in the treatment of patients with hypovolemia, severe congestive heart failure, shock, and all forms of heart block. In patients with sinus bradycardia or incomplete heart block, the administration of Xylocaine Solution intravenously for the elimination of ventricular ectopic beats, without prior acceleration in heart rate (e.g., by atropine, isoproterenol or electric pacing), may promote more frequent and serious ventricular arrhythmia or complete heart block (see CONTRAINDICATIONS).

Dosage should be reduced for children and for debilitated and/or elderly patients, commensurate with their age and physical status.

The safety of amide local anesthetic agents in patients with genetic predispositon to malignant hyperthermia has not been fully assessed; therefore, lidocaine should be used with caution in such patients.

In hospital environments where drugs known to be triggering agents for malignant hyperthermia (fulminant hypermetabolism) are administered, it is suggested that a standard protocol for management should be available.

It is not known whether lidocaine may trigger this reaction; however, large doses resulting in significant plasma concentrations, as may be achieved by intravenous infusion, pose potential risk to these individuals. Recognition of early unexplained signs of tachycardia, tachypnea, labile blood pressure and metabolic acidosis may precede temperature elevation. Successful outcome is dependent on early diagnosis, prompt discontinuance of the triggering agent and institution of treatment including oxygen therapy, supportive measures and dantrolene (for details see dantrolene package insert).
2. **Patient information:** The patient should be advised of the possible occurrence of the experiences listed under ADVERSE REACTIONS.
3. **Laboratory tests:** None known.
4. a. **Drug interactions:** Xylocaine Solutions should be used with caution in patients with digitalis toxicity accompanied by atrioventricular block. Concomitant use of beta-blocking agents or cimetidine may reduce hepatic blood flow and thereby reduce lidocaine clearance.
   b. **Drug/Laboratory test interactions:** The intramuscular use of Xylocaine Solution may result in an increase in creatine phosphokinase levels. Thus, the use of this enzyme determination, without isoenzyme separation, as a diagnostic test for the presence of acute myocardial infarction may be compromised by the use of intramuscular Xylocaine Solution.
5. **Carcinogenesis, mutagenesis, impairment of fertility:** Long term studies in animals to evaluate the carcinogenic and mutagenic potential or the effect on fertility of Xylocaine Solution have not been conducted.
6. **Pregnancy:**
   a. **Teratogenic effects:** Pregnancy Category B. Reproduction studies have been performed in rats at doses up to 6.6 times the maximum human doses and have revealed no significant findings. There are, however, no adequate and well-controlled studies in pregnant women. Because animal reproduction studies ar not always predictive of human response, this drug should be used during pregnancy only if clearly needed.
7. **Labor and delivery:** The effects of Xylocaine Solution on the mother and the fetus, when used in the management of cardiac arrhythmias during labor and delivery, are not known. Lidocaine readily crosses the placental barrier.
8. **Nursing mothers:** It is not known whether this drug is excreted in human milk. Because many drugs are excreted in human milk, caution should be exercised when lidocaine is administered to a nursing woman.
9. **Pediatric use:** Safety and effectiveness in children have not been established by controlled clinical studies. (See DOSAGE AND ADMINISTRATION).

Adverse Reactions: Adverse experiences following the administration of lidocaine are similar in nature to those observed with other amide local anesthetic agents. Adverse experiences may result from high plasma levels caused by excessive dosage or may result from a hypersensitivity, idiosyncrasy or diminished tolerance on the part of the patient. Serious adverse experiences are generally systemic in nature. The following types are those most commonly reported. The adverse experiences under Central Nervous System and Cardiovascular System are listed, in general, in a progression from mild to severe.
1. **Central Nervous System:**
   CNS reactions are excitatory and/or depressant, and may be characterized by light-headedness, nervousness, apprehension, euphoria, confusion, dizziness, drowsiness, tinnitus, blurred or double vision, vomiting, sensations of heat, cold or numbness, twitching, tremors, convulsions, unconsciousness, respiratory depression and arrest. The excitatory reactions may be very brief or may not occur at all, in which case, the first manifestation of toxicity may be drowsiness, merging into unconsciousness and respiratory arrest.
2. **Cardiovascular System:**
   Cardiovascular reactions are usually depressant in nature and are characterized by bradycardia, hypotension, and cardiovascular collapse, which may lead to cardiac arrest.
3. Allergic reactions as a result of sensitivity to lidocaine are extremely rare and, if they occur, should be managed by conventional means.

TABLE 1 Composition of available solutions:

Dosage Form		Composition* lidocaine hydrochloride (mg per ml)	sodium chloride (mg per ml)
For Direct Intravenous Injection	5 ml (100 mg) prefilled syringe	20	6
	5 ml (100 mg) ampule	20	6
For Preparation of Intravenous Infusion Solutions	25 ml (One Gram) single use vial	40	None
	50 ml (Two Grams) single use vial	40	None
	5 ml (One Gram) additive syringe	200	None
	10 ml (Two Grams) additive syringe	200	None
For Intramuscular Injection	5 ml (500 mg) ampule	100	None

*pH of all solutions adjusted to 5.0-7.0 with sodium hydroxide and/or hydrochloric acid. All containers are for single use: solutions do not contain preservatives.

Drug Abuse and Dependence: Although specific studies have not been conducted, Xylocaine Solution has been used clinically without evidence of abuse of this drug or of psychological or physical dependence as a result of its use.

Overdosage: Overdosage of Xylocaine (lidocaine hydrochloride) Solution usually results in signs of central nervous system or cardiovascular toxicity. See ADVERSE REACTIONS.

Should convulsions or signs of respiratory depression and arrest develop, the patency of the airway and adequacy of ventilation must be assured immediately. Should convulsions persist despite ventilatory therapy with oxygen, small increments of anticonvulsive agents may be given intravenously. Examples of such agents include a benzodiazepine (e.g., diazepam), an ultrashort-acting barbiturate (e.g., thiopental or thiamylal), or a short-acting barbiturate (e.g., pentobarbital or secobarbital). If the patient is under general anesthesia, a short-acting muscle relaxant (e.g., succinylcholine) may be administered.

Should circulatory depression occur, vasopressors may be used. Should cardiac arrest occur, standard CPR procedures should be instituted.

Dialysis is of negligible value in the treatment of acute overdosage from Xylocaine Solution.

Dosage and Administration:
Adults
Single Direct Intravenous Injection (bolus):
ONLY THE 5 ML, 100 MG DOSAGE SIZE (20 MG/ML) should be used for direct intravenous injection. The usual dose is 50 to 100 mg of lidocaine hydrochloride (0.70 to 1.4 mg/kg: 0.32 to 0.63 mg/lb) administered intravenously under ECG monitoring. This dose may be administered at the rate of approximately 25 to 50 mg/min (0.35 to 0.70 mg/kg/min; 0.16 to 0.32 mg/lb/min). Sufficient time should be allowed to enable a slow circulation to carry the drug to the site of action. If the initial injection of 50 to 100 mg does not produce a desired response, a second dose may be injected after 5 minutes. The syringe should be activated immediately prior to the injection. (See illustrated instructions for use on produce package.) NO MORE THAN 200 TO 300 MG OF LIDOCAINE HYDROCHLORIDE SHOULD BE ADMINISTERED DURING A ONE HOUR PERIOD.

Continuous Intravenous Infusion:
Following bolus administration, intravenous infusions of Xylocaine Solution may be initiated at the rate of 1 to 4 mg/min of lidocaine hydrochloride (0.014 to 0.057 mg/kg/min; 0.006 to 0.026 mg/lb/min). The rate of intravenous infusions should be reassessed as soon as the patient's basic cardiac rhythm appears to be stable or at the earliest signs of toxicity. It should rarely be necessary to continue intravenous infusions of lidocaine for prolonged periods.

Solutions for intravenous infusion may be prepared by the addition of one gram (or two grams) of lidocaine hydrochloride to one liter of 5% dextrose in water using aseptic technique. Approximately a 0.1% (or 0.2%) solution will result from this procedure; that is, each milliliter will contain approximately 1 (or 2 mg) of lidocaine hydrochloride. In those cases in which fluid restriction is medically appropriate, a more concentrated solution may be prepared.

Xylocaine Solution has been found to be chemically stable for 24 hours after dilution in 5% dextrose in water. However, as with all intravenous admixtures, dilution of the solution should be made just prior to its administration.

Parenteral drug products should be inspected visually for particulate matter and discoloration prior to administration whenever the solution and container permit.

Intramuscular Injection:
The recommended dose of lidocaine hydrochloride by the intramuscular route is 300 mg (approximately 4.3 mg/kg or 20 mg/lb). The deltoid muscle is recommended as the preferred site of injection, since therapeutic blood levels of lidocaine occur faster and the peak blood level is significantly higher following deltoid administration as compared to injections into the lateral thigh or gluteus. Injections should be made with frequent aspiration to avoid possible inadvertent intravascular injection.

As soon as possible, and when indicated, patients should be changed to an intravenous infusion of Xylocaine Solution. However, if necessary, an additional intramuscular injection may be made after an interval of 60-90 minutes.

Pediatric
Although controlled clinical studies to establish pediatric dosing schedules have not been conducted, the American Heart Association's *Standards and Guidelines* recommends a bolus dose of 1 mg/kg followed by an infusion rate of 3 µg/kg/min.

Note regarding prolonged infusions: There are data that indicate the half-life may be 3 hours or longer following infusions of greater than 24 hours in duration.

How Supplied: For direct intravenous injection, Xylocaine (lidocaine hydrochloride) Solution without preservatives is supplied in 5 ml, 100 mg ampules (20 mg/ml) and in 5 ml, 100 mg prefilled syringes.

For intramuscular injection, Xylocaine Solution without preservatives is supplied in 5 ml, 500 mg ampules (100 mg/ml).

For preparing solutions for intravenous infusions, Xylocaine Solution without sodium chloride or preservatives is supplied in one and two gram additive syringes and in one and two gram single use vials. Vials are available with or without pre-sterilized transfer unit manufactured by the West Company.

021834-00   Iss. 1/83

XYLOCAINE® (lidocaine hydrochloride) ℞
[zī' lo-caine]
4% STERILE SOLUTION
For transtracheal use,
retrobulbar injection,
and for topical application

Description: Xylocaine® (lidocaine hydrochloride) 4% Sterile Solution, is a sterile aqueous solution prepared from lidocaine hydrochloride and water. Lidocaine hydrochloride is a local anesthetic chemically designated as 2-(diethylamino)-N-(2,6-dimethylphenyl)-acetamide monohydrochloride.

Xylocaine 4% Sterile Solution in 5 ml ampules may be autoclaved repeatedly, if necessary.

Composition of Xylocaine 4% Sterile Solution
Each ml contains:
Lidocaine hydrochloride..............................40 mg
Sodium hydroxide and/or hydrochloric acid to adjust pH to 5.0–7.0.

Actions: Lidocaine stabilizes the neuronal membrane and prevents the initiation and conduction of nerve impulses, thereby effecting local anesthetic action.

Lidocaine is metabolized mainly in the liver and excreted via the kidneys. Approximately 90% of lidocaine administered is excreted in the form of various metabolites; while less than 10% is excreted unchanged.

The onset of action is rapid. For retrobulbar injection, 4 ml of Xylocaine 4% Sterile Solution provides an average duration of action of 1 to 1½ hours. This duration may be extended for ophthalmic surgery by the addition of epinephrine, the usual recommended dilution being 1:50,000 to 1:100,000.

Indications: Xylocaine 4% Sterile Solution is indicated for the production of topical anesthesia of the mucous membranes of the respiratory tract or the genito-urinary tract. It may be injected trans-tracheally to anesthetize the larynx and trachea. It may be administered by retrobulbar injection to provide anesthesia for ophthalmic surgery.

Contraindications: Xylocaine 4% sterile solution is contraindicated in patients with a known history of hypersensitivity either to local anesthetics of the amide type or to other components of the sterile solution.

Warnings:
(1) RESUSCITATIVE EQUIPMENT AND DRUGS, INCLUDING OXYGEN, SHOULD BE IMMEDIATELY AVAILABLE WHEN ANY LOCAL ANESTHETIC IS USED.
(2) *Usage in Pregnancy:* Reproductive studies have been performed in rats and rabbits without evidence of harm to the animal fetus. However, the safe use of lidocaine has not been established with respect to adverse effects upon fetal development. Careful consideration should be given to this fact before administering this drug to women of childbearing potential, particularly during early pregnancy.
(3) Local anesthetic procedures should be used with caution when there is inflammation and/or sepsis in the region of the proposed injection.
(4) If a vasoconstrictor has been added to the solution, it should be used with extreme caution for patients whose medical history and physical evaluation suggest the existence of hypertension, arteriosclerotic heart disease, cerebral vascular insufficiency, heart block, thyrotoxicosis or diabetes, etc. The solutions which contain a vasoconstrictor should also be used with extreme caution in patients receiving drugs known to produce blood pressure alterations (e.g., MAO inhibitors, tricyclic antidepressants, phenothiazines, etc.) as either sustained hypotension or hypertension may occur.

Precautions: The safety and effectiveness of Xylocaine 4% Sterile Solution depend on proper dosage, correct technique, adequate precautions, and readiness for emergencies. Standard textbooks should be consulted for specific techniques and precautions for various anesthetic procedures. The lowest dosage that results in effective anesthesia should be used. Injection of repeated doses of Xylocaine 4% Sterile Solution may cause significant increases in blood levels with each repeated dose due to slow accumulation of the drug or its metabolites. Tolerance varies with the status of the patient. Debilitated, elderly patients, acutely ill patients, and children should be given reduced doses commensurate with their age and physical status. Xylocaine 4% Sterile Solution should also be used with caution in patients with severe shock or heart block.

As with all injections of local anesthetics, retrobulbar injection should always be made slowly and with frequent aspirations.

Solutions to which a vasoconstrictor has been added should be used with caution in the presence of diseases which may adversely affect the patient's cardiovascular system. Serious cardiac arrhythmias may occur if preparations containing a vasoconstrictor are employed in patients during or following the administration of chloroform, halothane, cyclopropane, trichlorethylene, or other related agents.

Xylocaine 4% Sterile Solution should be used with caution in persons with known drug sensitivities. Patients allergic to para-aminobenzoic acid derivatives (procaine, tetracaine, benzocaine, etc.) have not shown cross sensitivity to lidocaine HCl.

Local anesthetics react with certain metals and cause the release of their respective ions which, if injected, may cause severe local irritation. Adequate precaution should be taken to avoid this type of interaction.

The safety of amide local anesthetics in patients with malignant hyperthermia has not been assessed, and therefore lidocaine should be used with caution in such patients.

Drowsiness following an injection of Xylocaine 4% Sterile Solution is *usually* an early indication of a high blood level of the drug and may occur following inadvertent intravascular administration or *rapid absorption* of lidocaine.

Adverse Reactions: Reactions to Xylocaine 4% Sterile Solution are similar in nature to those observed with other local anesthetic agents.

Adverse reactions may result from high plasma levels due to excessive dosage, rapid absorption or inadvertent intravascular injection. Such reactions are systemic in nature and involve the central nervous system and/or the cardiovascular

Continued on next page

Astra—Cont.

system. A small number of reactions may result from a hypersensitivity, idiosyncrasy or diminished tolerance on the part of the patient.

CNS reactions are excitatory and/or depressant, and may be characterized by nervousness, dizziness, blurred vision and tremors, followed by drowsiness, convulsions, unconsciousness and possibly respiratory arrest. The excitatory reactions may be very brief or may not occur at all, in which case the first manifestations of toxicity may be drowsiness, merging into unconsciousness and respiratory arrest.

Toxic cardiovascular reactions to local anesthetics are usually depressant in nature and are characterized by hypotension, myocardial depression, bradycardia and possibly cardiac arrest.

Treatment of a patient with toxic manifestations consists of assuring and maintaining a patent airway, supporting ventilation with oxygen, and assisted or controlled ventilation (respiration) as required. This usually will be sufficient in the management of most reactions. Should a convulsion persist despite ventilatory therapy, small increments of anticonvulsive agents may be given intravenously. Examples of such agents include benzodiazepine (e.g., diazepam), ultrashort acting barbiturates (e.g., thiopental or thiamylal) or a short acting barbiturate (e.g., pentobarbital or secobarbital). Cardiovascular depression may require circulatory assistance with intravenous fluids and/or vasopressors (e.g., ephedrine) as dictated by the clinical situation.

Allergic reactions may occur as a result of sensitivity either to local anesthetics or to other components of the sterile solution. Anaphylactoid type symptomatology and reactions, characterized by cutaneous lesions, urticaria, and edema, should be managed by conventional means. The detection of potential sensitivity by skin testing is of limited value.

Dosage and Administration: The dosage varies and depends upon the area to be anesthetized, vascularity of the tissues, individual tolerance and the technique of anesthesia. The lowest dosage needed to provide effective anesthesia should be administered. Dosages should be reduced for children and for elderly and debilitated patients commensurate with their body weights and physical condition. Although the incidence of adverse effects with Xylocaine 4% Sterile Solution is quite low, caution should be exercised, particularly when employing large volumes of Xylocaine 4% Sterile Solution since the incidence of adverse effects is directly proportional to the total dose of local anesthetic agent administered.

For specific techniques and procedures refer to standard textbooks.

The dosages recommended below are for a normal, healthy 70 kg adult:

RETROBULBAR INJECTION: The suggested dose is 3–5 ml (120–200 mg of lidocaine hydrochloride), i.e. 1.7–3 mg/kg or 0.8–1.3 mg/lb body weight. A portion of this is injected retrobulbarly and the rest may be used to block the facial nerve.

TRANSTRACHEAL INJECTION: For local anesthesia by the transtracheal route 2–3 ml should be injected through a large enough needle so that the injection can be made rapidly. By injecting during inspiration some of the drug will be carried into the bronchi and the resulting cough will distribute the rest of the drug over the vocal cords and the epiglottis. Occasionally it may be necessary to spray the pharynx by oropharyngeal spray to achieve complete analgesia. For the combination of the injection and spray, it should rarely be necessary to utilize more than 5 ml (200 mg of lidocaine hydrochloride) i.e., 3 mg/kg or 1.3 mg/lb body weight.

TOPICAL APPLICATION: For laryngoscopy, bronchoscopy and endotracheal intubation, the pharynx and larynx may be sprayed with 1–5 ml (40–200 mg of lidocaine hydrochloride), i.e. 0.6–3 mg/kg or 0.3–1.3 mg/lb body weight.

Maximum Recommended Dosages:

Normal healthy adults:

The maximum recommended dose of Xylocaine 4% Sterile Solution should be such that the dose of lidocaine hydrochloride is kept below 300 mg and in any case should not exceed 4.3 mg/kg (2 mg/lb) body weight.

Children:

It is difficult to recommend a maximum dose of any drug for children since this varies as a function of age and weight. For children of less than ten years who have a normal lean body mass and normal body development, the maximum dose may be determined by the application of one of the standard pediatric drug formulas (e.g. Clark's rule). For example, in a child of five years weighing 50 lbs., the dose of lidocaine hydrochloride should not exceed 75–100 mg when calculated according to Clark's rule.

How Supplied: Xylocaine (lidocaine hydrochloride) 4% Sterile Solution: 5 ml ampule, package of 10; 5 ml prefilled sterile disposable syringe.

021562-03   Rev. 9/81

XYLOCAINE® R
[zi′ lo-caine]
(lidocaine hydrochloride) 4% TOPICAL SOLUTION
For topical application

Description: Lidocaine is a local anesthetic chemically designated as 2-(diethylamino)-N-(2,6-dimethylphenyl)-acetamide.

The 50 ml screw-cap bottle should not be autoclaved because the closure employed cannot withstand autoclaving temperatures and pressures.

Composition of Xylocaine 4% (lidocaine hydrochloride) Topical Solution

50 ml screw-cap bottle:

Each ml contains:

2-(diethylamino)-N-(2, 6-dimethylphenyl)-acetamide (lidocaine) hydrochloride .... 40 mg

methylparaben .... 1 mg

sodium hydroxide...

to adjust pH to 6.0–7.0

An aqueous solution. NOT FOR INJECTION.

Actions: Lidocaine stabilizes the neuronal membrane and prevents the initiation and conduction of nerve impulses, thereby effecting local anesthetic action.

Lidocaine is metabolized mainly in the liver and excreted via the kidneys. Approximately 90% of lidocaine administered is excreted in the form of various metabolites, while less than 10% is excreted unchanged.

Indications: Xylocaine 4% (lidocaine hydrochloride) Topical Solution is indicated for the production of topical anesthesia of accessible mucous membranes of the oral and nasal cavities and proximal portions of the digestive tract.

Contraindications: Lidocaine hydrochloride is contraindicated in patients with a known history of hypersensitivity either to local anesthetics of the amide type or to the components of the topical solution.

Local anesthetic agents should not be used in patients with severe shock or heart block. Xylocaine 4% Topical Solution should not be used to anesthetize mucous membranes of the tracheobronchial tree and urinary tract, nor should it be used for ophthalmologic procedures.

Warnings:
1. RESUSCITATIVE EQUIPMENT AND DRUGS SHOULD BE IMMEDIATELY AVAILABLE WHEN ANY LOCAL ANESTHETIC IS USED.
2. *Usage in Pregnancy:* Reproductive studies have been performed in rats and rabbits without evidence of harm to the fetus. However, safe use of lidocaine hydrochloride topical solution has not been established with respect to adverse effects upon fetal development. Careful consideration should be given to this fact before administering this drug to women of childbearing potential, particularly during early pregnancy.

Precautions: The safety and effectiveness of lidocaine hydrochloride topical solution depends on proper dosage, correct technique, adequate precautions, and readiness for emergencies. Standard textbooks should be consulted for specific techniques and precautions for various anesthetic procedures.

The lowest dosage that results in effective anesthesia should be used to avoid high plasma levels and serious adverse effects. Debilitated, elderly patients, acutely ill patients, and children should be given reduced doses commensurate with their age and physical status.

Lidocaine hydrochloride topical solution should be used with caution in patients with severely traumatized mucosa and sepsis in the region of the proposed application.

Lidocaine hydrochloride topical solution should be used with caution in persons with known drug sensitivities. Patients allergic to para-aminobenzoic acid derivatives (procaine, tetracaine, benzocaine, etc.) have not shown cross sensitivity to lidocaine.

Adverse Reactions: Reactions to lidocaine hydrochloride are similar in character to those observed with other local anesthetic agents. Adverse reactions may be due to high plasma levels as a result of excessive dosage, rapid absorption or inadvertent intravascular injection. Such reactions are systemic in nature and involve the central nervous system and/or the cardiovascular system. A small number of reactions may result from hypersensitivity, idiosyncrasy or diminished tolerance on the part of the patient.

CNS reactions are excitatory and/or depressant, and may be characterized by nervousness, dizziness, blurred vision and tremors, followed by drowsiness, convulsions, unconsciousness and possibly respiratory arrest. The excitatory reactions may be very brief or may not occur at all, in which case the first manifestations of toxicity may be drowsiness, merging into unconsciousness and respiratory arrest.

Toxic cardiovascular reactions to local anesthetics are usually depressant in nature and may be characterized by hypotension, myocardial depression, bradycardia and possibly cardiac arrest.

Treatment of a patient with toxic manifestations consists of assuring and maintaining a patent airway, supporting ventilation with oxygen, and assisted or controlled ventilation (respiration) as required. This usually will be sufficient in the management of most reactions. Should a convulsion persist despite ventilatory therapy, small increments of anticonvulsive agents may be given intravenously. Examples of such agents include benzodiazepine (e.g., diazepam), ultrashort acting barbiturates (e.g., thiopental or thiamylal) or a short acting barbiturate (e.g., pentobarbital or secobarbital). Cardiovascular depression may require circulatory assistance with intravenous fluids and/or vasopressors (e.g., ephedrine) as dictated by the clinical situation.

Allergic reactions may occur as a result of sensitivity either to local anesthetics or to other components of the topical solution. Anaphylactoid type symptomatology and reactions, characterized by cutaneous lesions, urticaria, and edema, should be managed by conventional means. The detection of potential sensitivity skin testing is of limited value.

Dosage and Administration: The dosage varies and depends upon the area to be anesthetized, vascularity of the tissues, individual tolerance and the technique of anesthesia. The lowest dosage needed to provide effective anesthesia should be administered. Dosages should be reduced for children and for elderly and debilitated patients. The maximum dose should not exceed 7 mg/kg (3.17 mg/lb) of body weight. Although the incidence of adverse effects with Xylocaine 4% (lidocaine hydrochloride) Topical Solution is quite low, caution should be exercised particularly when employing large volumes since the incidence of adverse effects is proportional to the total dose of local anesthetic agent administered.

The dosages recommended below are for normal, healthy adults:

When used as a spray, or when applied by means of cotton applicators or packs, as well as when instilled into a cavity, the suggested dosage of Xylocaine 4% Topical Solution is 1–5 ml (40–200 mg of lidocaine hydrochloride), i.e., 0.6–3.0 mg/kg or 0.3–1.5 mg/lb body weight.

NOTE: The solution may be applied from a sterile swab which should be discarded after use and never reused under any circumstances. When spraying, transfer the solution from the original container to an atomizer.

Maximum recommended dosages

Normal healthy adults:

The maximum recommended dose of Xylocaine 4% (lidocaine hydrochloride) Topical Solution should be such that the dose of lidocaine hydrochloride is kept below 300 mg and in any case should not exceed 4.5 mg/kg (2 mg/lb) body weight.

Children:

It is difficult to recommend a maximum dose of any drug for children since this varies as a function of age and weight. For childen of less than ten years who have a normal lean body mass and normal body development, the maximum dose may be determined by the application of one of the standard pediatric drug formulas (e.g., Clark's rule or Young's rule). For example, in a child of five years weighing 50 lbs., the dose of lidocaine should not exceed 75–100 mg when calculated according to Clark's rule or Young's rule.

How Supplied: Xylocaine 4% (lidocaine hydrochloride) Topical Solution 50 ml screw-cap bottle, cartoned. NOT FOR INJECTION.

021802-00   3/79

XYLOCAINE® (lidocaine) ℞
[zī' lo-caine]
HYDROCHLORIDE 1.5% WITH DEXTROSE 7.5%
Sterile Aqueous Solution Only
for Spinal Anesthesia
in Obstetrics

(For details of indications, dosage and administration, precautions, and adverse reactions, see circular in package.)

How Supplied: Xylocaine® (lidocaine) Hydrochloride 1.5% solution with Dextrose 7.5% is supplied in 2 ml ampules.

XYLOCAINE® (lidocaine hydrochloride) ℞
[zī' lo-cain]
5% SOLUTION WITH GLUCOSE 7.5%
Sterile Aqueous Solution
for Spinal Anesthesia

(For details of indications, dosage and administration, precautions, and adverse reactions, see circular in package.)

How Supplied: Xylocaine® (lidocaine hydrochloride) 5% solution with Glucose 7.5% is supplied in 2 ml ampules in packages of 10 and 100.

XYLOCAINE® 2% (lidocaine HCl) ℞
[zī' lo-caine]
JELLY
A Topical Anesthetic
for Urological Procedures
and Lubrication
of Endotracheal Tubes

Description: Lidocaine is a local anesthetic chemically designated as 2 - (Diethylamino) - N - (2,6 - Dimethylphenyl) - Acetamide. Xylocaine® (lidocaine hydrochloride) 2% Jelly is a sterile, aqueous solution thickened to a suitable viscosity, of the following composition:

Each ml contains:
Lidocaine hydrochloride 20mg
Methyl-p-hydroxybenzoate 0.7mg
Propyl-p-hydroxybenzoate 0.3mg
Sodium Hydroxide .... to adjust pH
Sodium Carboxymethylcellulose, to adjust to a suitable consistency.

Actions: Lidocaine stabilizes the neuronal membrane and prevents the initiation and conduction of nerve impulses, thereby effecting local anesthetic action.

Xylocaine (lidocaine hydrochloride) 2% Jelly effects local, topical anesthesia. The onset of action is 3–5 minutes. It is ineffective when applied to intact skin.

Lidocaine is metabolized mainly in the liver and excreted via the kidneys. Approximately 90% of lidocaine administered is excreted in the form of various metabolites, while less than 10% is excreted unchanged.

Indications: Xylocaine® (lidocaine hydrochloride) 2% Jelly is indicated for prevention and control of pain in procedures involving the male and female urethra and for topical treatment of painful urethritis.

It is also useful as an anesthetic lubricant for endotracheal intubation.

Contraindications: Xylocaine® (lidocaine hydrochloride) 2% Jelly is contraindicated in patients with a known history of hypersensitivity to local anesthetics of the amide type, or to other components of the jelly formulation.

USE IN PREGNANCY: Reproductive studies have been performed in rats and rabbits without evidence of harm to the animal fetus. However, the safe use of lidocaine in humans has not been established with respect to possible adverse effects upon fetal development. Careful consideration should be given to this fact before administering this drug to women of childbearing potential, particularly during early pregnancy.

Precautions: The safety and effectiveness of lidocaine depends on proper dosage, correct technique, adequate precautions and readiness for emergencies. The lowest dose that results in effective anesthesia should be used to avoid high plasma levels and serious adverse effects. Debilitated, elderly patients, acutely ill patients and children should be given reduced doses commensurate with their age and physical status. Standard textbooks should be consulted for specific technique and precautions. Xylocaine® (lidocaine hydrochloride) 2% Jelly should be used with caution in patients with severely traumatized mucosa and/or sepsis in the region of the proposed application.

Xylocaine 2% Jelly should be used with caution in persons with known drug sensitivities. Patients with allergic sensitivity to para-aminobenzoic acid derivatives (procaine, tetracaine, benzocaine, etc.) have not shown cross sensitivity to lidocaine.

Adverse Reactions: Systemic adverse reactions are extremely rare with Xylocaine® (lidocaine hydrochloride) 2% Jelly. However, as with any local anesthetic, adverse reactions may result from high plasma levels due to excessive dosage, or rapid absorption, or may result from a hypersensitivity, idiosyncrasy or diminished tolerance.

CNS reactions are excitatory and/or depressant, and may be characterized by nervousness, dizziness, blurred vision and tremors, followed by drowsiness, convulsions, unconsciousness and possibly respiratory arrest. The excitatory reactions may be very brief or may not occur at all, in which case the first manifestations of toxicity may be drowsiness, merging into unconsciousness and respiratory arrest.

Cardiovascular reactions are depressant, and may be characterized by hypotension, myocardial depression, bradycardia and possibly, cardiac arrest. Treatment of a patient with toxic manifestations consists of assuring and maintaining a patent airway, supporting ventilation with oxygen, and as-sisted or controlled ventilation (respiration) as required. This usually will be sufficient in the management of most reactions. Should a convulsion persist despite ventilatory therapy, small increments of anticonvulsive agents may be given intravenously. Examples of such agents include benzodiazepine (e.g. diazepam), ultra-short acting barbiturates (e.g. thiopental or thiamylal) or a short acting barbiturate (e.g. pentobarbital or secobarbital). Cardiovascular depression may require circulatory assistance with intravenous fluids and/or vasopressor (e.g. ephedrine) as dictated by the clinical situation.

Allergic reactions may occur as a result of sensitivity to local anesthetics or other components of the jelly formulation. Anaphylactoid type symptomatology and reactions, characterized by cutaneous lesions, urticaria, and edema, should be managed by conventional means. The detection of potential sensitivity by skin testing is of limited value.

Dosage and Administration:

For surface anesthesia of the male urethra: The outer orifice is washed and cleansed with a disinfectant. The plastic cone is sterilized for 5 minutes in boiling water, cooled, and attached to the tube. The cone may be gas sterilized or cold sterilized, if preferred. The tube key is attached. The jelly is instilled slowly into the urethra by turning the tube key until the patient has a feeling of tension or until almost half the tube (15 ml; 300 mg) is emptied. A penile clamp is then applied for several minutes at the corona and then the remaining contents of the tube are instilled.

Prior to sounding or cystoscopy, a penile clamp should be applied for 5 to 10 minutes to obtain adequate anesthesia. The contents of one tube (30 ml; 600 mg) are usually required to fill and dilate the male urethra.

Prior to catheterization, smaller volumes (5-10 ml; 100-200 mg) are usually adequate.

For surface anesthesia of the female urethra: The outer orifice is washed and cleansed with a disinfectant. The plastic cone is sterilized for 5 minutes in boiling water, cooled, and attached to the tube. The cone may be gas sterilized or cold sterilized, if preferred. The tube key is attached. Three to five ml of the jelly is instilled slowly into the urethra by turning the tube key (approximately 1½ - 2 full turns). If desired, some jelly may be deposited on a cotton swab and introduced into the urethra. In order to obtain adequate anesthesia, several minutes should be allowed prior to performing urological procedures.

For endotracheal intubation: Apply to the catheter, as needed, prior to intubation.

Maximum Dosage: No more than one tube should be given in any 12 hour period.

How Supplied: Collapsible tubes which deliver 30 ml. A detachable applicator cone and a key for expressing contents are included in each package.

021704-06   Rev. 5/79

XYLOCAINE® (lidocaine) ℞
[zī' lo-caine]
5% OINTMENT
A Water-Soluble Topical
Anesthetic Ointment

Description: Lidocaine is a local anesthetic chemically designated as 2-(Diethylamino-N-(2,6 Dimethylphenyl)-Acetamide.

Composition of Xylocaine 5% (lidocaine) Ointment: 2- (Diethylamino) - N - (2, 6 Dimethylphenyl)-Acetamide 5% in a water miscible ointment vehicle consisting of polyethylene glycols and propylene glycol.

Actions: Lidocaine stabilizes the neuronal membrane and prevents the initiation and conduction of nerve impulses, thereby effecting local anesthetic action. Xylocaine 5% (lidocaine) Ointment effects local, topical anesthesia. The onset of action is 3-5 minutes. It is ineffective when applied to intact skin.

Lidocaine is metabolized mainly in the liver and excreted via the kidneys. Approximately 90% of lidocaine administered is excreted in the form of various metabolites, while less than 10% is excreted unchanged.

Indications: Xylocaine 5% (lidocaine) Ointment is indicated for production of anesthesia of accessible mucous membranes of the oropharynx.

It is also useful as an anesthetic lubricant for endotracheal intubation, and for the temporary relief of pain associated with minor burns and abrasions of the skin.

Contraindications: Xylocaine 5% (lidocaine) Ointment is contraindicated in patients with a known history of hypersensitivity to local anesthetics of the amide type, or to other components of the ointment.

Warnings: USE IN PREGNANCY: Reproductive studies have been performed in rats and rabbits without evidence of harm to the animal fetus. However, the safe use of lidocaine in humans has

Continued on next page

Astra—Cont.

not been established with respect to possible adverse effects upon fetal development. Careful consideration should be given to this fact before administering this drug to women of childbearing potential, particularly during early pregnancy.

Precautions: The safety and effectiveness of lidocaine depends on proper dosage, correct technique, adequate precautions and readiness for emergencies. The lowest dose that results in effective anesthesia should be used to avoid high plasma levels and serious adverse effects. Debilitated, elderly patients, acutely ill patients and children should be given reduced doses commensurate with their age and physical status. Standard textbooks should be consulted for specific techniques and precautions.

Xylocaine 5% (lidocaine) Ointment should be used with caution in patients with severely traumatized mucosa and/or sepsis in the region of the proposed application.

Xylocaine 5% (lidocaine) Ointment should be used with caution in persons with known drug sensitivities. Patients with allergic sensitivity to para-aminobenzoic acid derivatives (procaine, tetracaine, benzocaine, etc.) have not shown cross sensitivity to lidocaine.

Adverse Reactions: Systemic adverse reactions are extremely rare with Xylocaine 5% (lidocaine) Ointment. However, as with any local anesthetic, adverse reactions may result from high plasma levels due to excessive dosage, or rapid absorption, or may result from hypersensitivity, idiosyncrasy, or diminished tolerance.

CNS reactions are excitatory, and/or depressant, and may be characterized by nervousness, dizziness, blurred vision and tremors, followed by drowsiness, convulsions, unconsciousness, and, possibly, respiratory arrest. The excitatory reactions may be very brief or may not occur at all, in which case the first manifestations of toxicity may be drowsiness, merging into unconsciousness and respiratory arrest.

Cardiovascular reactions are depressant, and may be characterized by hypotension, myocardial depression, bradycardia, and, possibly, cardiac arrest.

Treatment of a patient with toxic manifestations consists of assuring and maintaining a patent airway, supporting ventilation with oxygen, and assisted or controlled ventilation (respiration) as required. This usually will be sufficient in the management of most reactions. Should a convulsion persist despite ventilatory therapy, small increments of anticonvulsive agents may be given intravenously. Examples of such agents include benzodiazepine (e.g., diazepam), ultrashort acting barbiturates (e.g., thiopental or thiamylal) or a short acting barbiturate (e.g., pentobarbital or secobarbital). Cardiovascular depression may require circulatory assistance with intravenous fluids and/or vasopressors (e.g., ephedrine) as dictated by the clinical situation.

Allergic reactions may occur as a result of sensitivity to local anesthetics. Anaphylactoid type symptomatology and reactions, characterized by cutaneous lesions, urticaria, and edema, should be managed by conventional means. The detection of potential sensitivity by skin testing is of limited value.

Dosage and Administration: Apply topically for adequate control of symptoms. The use of a sterile gauze pad is suggested for application to broken skin tissue. Apply to the catheter prior to endotracheal intubation.

In dentistry, apply to previously dried oral mucosa. Subsequent removal of excess saliva with cotton rolls or saliva ejector minimizes dilution of the ointment and permits maximum penetration. Avoid cross-contamination between patients by aseptically transferring from its container to a separate plate or small dish the estimated amount of ointment required for each patient. Discard any unused portion. For use in connection with the insertion of new dentures, apply to all denture surfaces contacting mucosa.

IMPORTANT: Patients should consult dentist at intervals not exceeding 36 hours throughout the fitting period.

NOTE: No more than 35 grams should be administered in any one day.

How Supplied: Xylocaine 5% (lidocaine) Ointment is available in 35-gram tubes.

Xylocaine 5% (lidocaine) Ointment Flavored, for application within the oral cavity, is dispensed in 3.5-gram tubes, 10 tubes per carton, and in 35-gram jars.

KEEP CONTAINER TIGHTLY CLOSED AT ALL TIMES WHEN NOT IN USE.

021709-07 Rev. 8/79

XYLOCAINE® (lidocaine)
[zī' lo-cain]
2.5% OINTMENT

(See PDR For Nonprescription Drugs)

XYLOCAINE® (lidocaine) ℞
[zī' lo-caine]
10% Oral Spray
Flavored Topical Anesthetic
For Use In The Oral Cavity

WARNING—CONTENTS UNDER PRESSURE.
Read carefully other warnings included in insert.

Name of Drug: Xylocaine 10% (lidocaine) Oral Spray.

Description: Lidocaine is a local anesthetic, chemically designated as diethylaminoacet-2,6-xylidide. It has the following structural formula:

Composition of Xylocaine 10% Oral Spray:
Each actuation of the metered dose (0.1 ml) valve delivers:

Lidocaine	10.0 mg
absolute alcohol	4.92 mg
cetylpyridinium chloride	0.01 mg
saccharin	0.39 mg
flavor	3.27 mg
polyethylene glycol	20.79 mg

And as propellents: trichlorofluoromethane/dichlorodifluoromethane (65%/35%)

Actions: Xylocaine 10% Oral Spray acts on intact mucous membranes to produce local anesthesia. Anesthesia occurs usually within 1-2 minutes and persists for approximately 10–15 minutes.

Approximately 90% of an administered dose of Xylocaine is metabolized in the liver. The remainder (10%) of the drug is excreted unchanged via the kidneys.

Indications: Xylocaine 10% Oral Spray is indicated for the production of topical anesthesia of the gingival and oral mucous membranes.

Contraindications: Xylocaine is contraindicated in patients with a known history of hypersensitivity to local anesthetics of the amide type.

Warnings: RESUSCITATIVE EQUIPMENT AND DRUGS SHOULD BE IMMEDIATELY AVAILABLE WHEN ANY LOCAL ANESTHETIC IS USED.

Avoid contact with the eyes. Inhalation and swallowing should be avoided. The recommended dosage should not be exceeded because of the possibility of toxicity or side effects. Contents under pressure. Therefore, do not puncture or incinerate container and do not expose to heat or store at temperatures above 120°F. Keep out of the reach of children.

Precautions: The lowest dosage that results in effective anesthesia should be used to avoid high plasma levels and serious undesirable systemic side effects. Tolerance varies with the status of the patient. The debilitated, elderly, and acutely ill patients should be given reduced doses commensurate with their age and physical status.

The safety and effectiveness of Xylocaine depends upon proper dosage, correct technique, adequate precautions, and readiness for emergencies. Xylocaine should be used cautiously in patients with known drug allergies or sensitivities. Patients allergic to para-aminobenzoic acid derivatives (procaine, tetracaine, benzocaine, etc.) have not shown similar sensitivity to Xylocaine.

Adverse Reactions: Adverse reactions result from high plasma levels due to excessive dosage or rapid absorption. Hypersensitivity, idiosyncrasy or diminished tolerance may also be the cause of reactions. Reactions due to overdosage (high plasma levels) are systemic and involve the central nervous system and the cardiovascular system. Reactions involving the central nervous system are characterized by excitation and/or depression. Nervousness, dizziness, blurred vision or tremors may occur followed by convulsions, drowsiness, unconsciousness and possibly respiratory arrest. Excitement may be transient or absent and the first manifestations may be drowsiness merging into unconsciouness and respiratory arrest.

Reactions involving the cardiovascular system include depression of the myocardium, hypotension, bradycardia, and even cardiac arrest.

The treatment of a patient with toxic manifestations consists of assuring and maintaining a patent airway and supporting ventilation using oxygen and assisted or controlled respiration as required. This will be sufficient in the management of most reactions. Should circulatory depression occur, vasopressors such as ephedrine or metaraminol, and intravenous fluids may be used. Should a convulsion persist despite oxygen therapy small increments of an ultra-short acting barbiturate (thiopental or thiamylal) or a short acting barbiturate (pentobarbital or secobarbital) may be given intravenously.

Allergic reactions are characterized by cutaneous lesions, urticaria, edema, or anaphylactoid reactions. The detection of sensitivity by skin testing is of doubtful value.

Dosage and Administration: Two metered doses are recommended as the upper limit and under no circumstances, should one exceed three metered doses per quadrant of gingiva and oral mucosa over a one-half hour period to produce the desired anesthetic effect. Experience in children is inadequate to recommend a pediatric dose at this time. *Note:* Each actuation of the metered dose valve delivers 10 mg Xylocaine base. It is unnecessary to dry the site prior to application.

How Supplied: An 82.5 gm (60 ml) aerosol container equipped with a metered dose valve.

021731-03 Rev. 6/81

XYLOCAINE® 2% (lidocaine ℞
[zī' lo-caine]
hydrochloride) **VISCOUS SOLUTION**
A Topical Anesthetic
for the Mucous Membranes
of the Mouth and Pharynx

Description: Xylocaine (lidocaine HCl) 2% Viscous Solution contains a local anesthetic agent and is administered topically. Xylocaine 2% Viscous Solution contains lidocaine HCl, which is chemically designated as acetamide, 2-(diethylamino)-N-(2,6-dimethylphenyl)-, monohydrochloride.

The molecular formula of lidocaine is $C_{14}H_{22}N_2O$. The molecular weight is 234.34.

Composition of Solution: Each ml contains 20 mg of lidocaine HCl, flavoring, sodium saccharin, methylparaben, propylparaben and sodium carboxymethylcellulose in purified water. The pH is adjusted to 6.0–7.0 by means of sodium hydroxide and/or hydrochloric acid.

Clinical Pharmacology:

Mechanism of action: Lidocaine stabilizes the neuronal membrane by inhibiting the ionic fluxes required for the initiation and conduction of impulses, thereby effecting local anesthetic action.

Hemodynamics: Excessive blood levels may cause changes in cardiac output, total peripheral resistance, and mean arterial pressure. These changes may be attributable to a direct depressant effect of the local anesthetic agent on various components of the cardiovascular system. The net effect is normally a modest hypotension when the recommended dosages are not exceeded.

Pharmacokinetics and metabolism: Lidocaine is absorbed following topical administration to mucous membranes, its rate and extent of absorption being dependent upon concentration and total dose administered, the specific site of application, and duration of exposure. In general, the rate of absorption of local anesthetic agents following topical application occurs most rapidly after intratracheal administration. Lidocaine is also well-absorbed from the gastro-intestinal tract, but little intact drug appears in the circulation because of biotransformation in the liver.

The plasma binding of lidocaine is dependent on drug concentration, and the fraction bound decreases with increasing concentration. At concentrations of 1 to 4 ug of free base per ml, 60 to 80 percent of lidocaine is protein bound. Binding is also dependent on the plasma concentration of the alpha-1-acid glycoprotein.

Lidocaine crosses the blood-brain and placental barriers, presumably by passive diffusion.

Lidocaine is metabolized rapidly by the liver, and metabolites and unchanged drug are excreted by the kidneys. Biotransformation includes oxidative N-dealkylation, ring hydroxylation, cleavage of the amide linkage, and conjugation. N-dealkylation, a major pathway of biotransformation, yields the metabolites monoethylglycinexylidide and glycinexylidide. The pharmacological/toxicological actions of these metabolites are similar to, but less potent than, those of lidocaine. Approximately 90% of lidocaine administered is excreted in the form of various metabolites, and less than 10% is excreted unchanged. The primary metabolite in urine is a conjugate of 4-hydroxy-2, 6-dimethylaniline.

The elimination half-life of lidocaine following an intravenous bolus injection is typically 1.5 to 2.0 hours. Because of the rapid rate at which lidocaine is metabolized, any condition that affects liver function may alter lidocaine kinetics. The half-life may be prolonged two-fold or more in patients with liver dysfunction. Renal dysfunction does not affect lidocaine kinetics but may increase the accumulation of metabolites.

Factors such as acidosis and the use of CNS stimulants and depressants affect the CNS levels of lidocaine required to produce overt systemic effects. Objective adverse manifestations become increasingly apparent with increasing venous plasma levels above 6.0 ug free base per ml. In the rhesus monkey arterial blood levels of 18–21 ug/ml have been shown to be threshold for convulsive activity.

Indications and Usage: Xylocaine (lidocaine HCl)2% Viscous Solution is indicated for the production of topical anesthesia of irritated or inflamed mucous membranes of the mouth and pharynx. It is also useful for reducing gagging during the taking of X-ray pictures and dental impressions.

Contraindications: Lidocaine is contraindicated in patients with a known history of hypersensitivity to local anesthetics of the amide type, or to other components of the solution.

Warnings: EXCESSIVE DOSAGE, OR SHORT INTERVALS BETWEEN DOSES, CAN RESULT IN HIGH PLASMA LEVELS AND SERIOUS ADVERSE EFFECTS. PATIENTS SHOULD BE INSTRUCTED TO STRICTLY ADHERE TO THE RECOMMENDED DOSAGE AND ADMINISTRATION GUIDELINES AS SET FORTH IN THIS PACKAGE INSERT.

THE MANAGEMENT OF SERIOUS ADVERSE REACTIONS MAY REQUIRE THE USE OF RESUSCITATIVE EQUIPMENT, OXYGEN, AND OTHER RESUSCITATIVE DRUGS.

Xylocaine 2% Viscous Solution should be used with extreme caution if the mucosa in the area of application has been traumatized, since under such conditions there is the potential for rapid systemic absorption.

Precautions:
General: The safety and effectiveness of lidocaine depend on proper dosage, correct technique, adequate precautions, and readiness for emergencies (See WARNINGS and ADVERSE REACTIONS). The lowest dosage that results in effective anethesia should be used to avoid high plasma levels and serious adverse effects. Repeated doses of lidocaine may cause significant increases in blood levels with each repeated dose because of slow accumulation of the drug and/or its metabolites. Tolerance varies with the status of the patient. Debilitated, elderly patients, acutely ill patients, and children should be given reduced doses commensurate with their age, weight and physical condition. Lidocaine should also be used with caution in patients with severe shock or heart block. Xylocaine 2% Viscous Solution should be used with caution in persons with known drug sensitivities. Patients allergic to para-aminobenzoic acid derivatives (procaine, tetracaine, benzocaine, etc.) have not shown cross sensitivity to lidocaine.

Information for Patients: When topical anesthetics are used in the mouth or throat, the patient should be aware that the production of topical anesthesia may impair swallowing and thus enhance the danger of aspiration. For this reason, food should not be ingested for 60 minutes following use of local anesthetic preparations in the mouth or throat area. This is particularly important in children because of their frequency of eating.

Numbness of the tongue or buccal mucosa may increase the danger of biting trauma. For this reason food and/or chewing gum should not be used while the mouth or throat area is anesthetized. PATIENTS SHOULD BE INSTRUCTED TO STRICTLY ADHERE TO DOSING INSTRUCTIONS, AND TO KEEP THE SUPPLY OF MEDICATION OUT OF REACH OF CHILDREN.

Carcinogenesis, mutagenesis, impairment of fertility: Studies of lidocaine in animals to evaluate the carcinogenic and mutagenic potential or the effect on fertility have not been conducted.

Pregnancy: Teratogenic Effects. Pregnancy Category B. Reproduction studies have been performed in rats at doses up to 6.6 times the human dose and have revealed no evidence of harm to the fetus caused by lidocaine. There are, however, no adequate and well-controlled studies in pregnant women. Because animal reproduction studies are not always predictive of human response, this drug should be used in pregnancy only if clearly needed.

Nursing mothers: It is not known whether this drug is excreted in human milk. Because many drugs are excreted in human milk, caution should be exercised when lidocaine is administered to nursing women.

Pediatric use: Dosages in children should be reduced, commensurate with age, body weight and physical condition. See DOSAGE AND ADMINISTRATION.

Adverse Reactions: Adverse experiences following the adminstration of lidocaine are similar in nature to those observed with other amide local anesthetic agents. These adverse experiences are, in general, dose-related and may result from high plasma levels caused by excessive dosage or rapid absorption, or may result from a hupersensitivity, idiosyncrasy or diminshed tolerance on the part of the patient. Serious adverse experiences are generally systemic in nature. The following types are those most commonly reported.

Central nervous system: CNS manifestations are excitatory and/or depressant and may be characterized by lightheadedness, nervousness, apprehension, euphoria, confusion, dizziness, drowsiness, tinnitus, blurred or double vision, vomiting, sensations of heat, cold or numbness, twitching, tremors, convulsions, unconsciousness, respiratory depression and arrest. The excitatory manifestations may be very brief or may not occur at all, in which case the first manifestation of toxicity may be drowsiness merging into unconsciousness and respiratory arrest.

Drowsiness following the administration of lidocaine is usually an early sign of a high blood level of the drug and may occur as a consequence of rapid absorption.

Cariovascular system: Cardiovascular manifestations are usually depressant and are characterized by bradycardia, hypotension, and cardiovascular collapse, which may lead to cardiac arrest.

Allergic: Allergic reactions are characterized by cutaneous lesions, urticaria, edema or anaphylactoid reactions. Allergic reactions may occur as a result of sensitivity either to the local anesthetic agent or to the methylparaben and/or propylparaben used in this formulation. Allergic reactions as a result of sensitivity to lidocaine are extremely rare and, if they occur, should be managed by conventional means. The detection of sensitivity by skin testing is of doubtful value.

Overdosage: Acute emergencies from local anesthetics are generally related to high plasma levels encountered during therapeutic use of local anesthetics (see ADVERSE REACTIONS, WARNINGS, and PRECAUTIONS).

Management of local anesthetic emergencies: The first consideration is prevention, best accomplished by careful and constant monitoring of cardiovascular and respiratory vital signs and the patient's state of consciousness after each local anesthetic administration.

The first step in the management of convulsions consists of immediate attention to the maintenance of a patent airway and assisted or controlled ventilation with oxygen. In situations where trained personnel are readily available, ventilation should be maintained and oxygen should be delivered by a delivery system capable of permitting immediate positive airway pressure by mask. Immediately after the institution of these ventilatory measures, the adequacy of the circulation should be evaluated, keeping in mind that drugs used to treat convulsions sometimes depress the circulation when administered intravenously. Should convulsions persist despite adequate respiratory support, and if the status of the circulation permits, small increments of an ultra-short acting barbiturate (such as thiopental or thiamylal) or a benzodiazepine (such as diazepam) may be administered intravenously. The clinician should be familiar, prior to use of local anesthetics, with these anticonvulsant drugs. Supportive treatment of circulatory depression may require administration of intravenous fluids and, when appropriate, a vasopressor as indicated by the clinical situation (e.g., ephedrine).

If not treated immediately, both convulsions and cardiovascular depression can result in hypoxia, acidosis, bradycardia, arrhythmias and cardiac arrest. If cardiac arrest should occur, standard cardiopulmonary resuscitative measures should be instituted.

Dialysis is of negligible value in the treatment of acute overdosage with lidocaine.

The oral LD_{50} of lidocaine in non-fasted female rats is 459 (346–773) mg/kg (as the salt) and 214 (159–324) mg/kg (as the salt) in fasted female rats.

Dosage and Administration:
Adult
The maximum recommended single dose of Xylocaine (lidocaine HCl) 2% Viscous Solution for healthy adults should be such that the dose of lidocaine HCl does not exceed 4.5 mg/kg or 2 mg/lb body weight and does not in any case exceed a total of 300 mg.

For symptomatic treatment of irritated or inflamed mucous membranes of the mouth and pharynx, the usual adult dose is one 15 ml tablespoonful undiluted. For use in the mouth, the solution should be swished around in the mouth and spit out. For use on the pharynx, the undiluted solution should be gargled and may be swallowed. This dose should not be administered at intervals of less than three hours, and not more than eight doses should be given in a 24-hour period.

The dosage should be adjusted commensurate with the patient's age, weight and physical condition (see PRECAUTIONS).

Continued on next page

Astra—Cont.

Pediatric
It is difficult to recommend a maximum dose of any drug for children since this varies as function of age and weight. For children over 3 years of age who have a normal lean body mass and normal body development, the maximum dose is determined by the childs weight or age. For example, in a child of 5 years weighing 50 lbs. the dose of lidocaine hydrochloride should not exceed 75–100 mg ($^3/_4$ to 1 teaspoonful).
For infants and in children under 3 years of age, $^1/_4$ teaspoon of the solution should be accurately measured and applied to the immediate area with a cotton-tipped applicator. This dose should not be administered at intervals of less than three hours. Not more than four doses should be given in a 12-hour period.

How Supplied: Xylocaine 2% (lidocaine HCl) Viscous Solution is available in 100 ml (NDC 0186-0360-01) and 450 ml (NDC 0186-0360-11) polyethylene squeeze bottles and in unit of use (adult dose) packages of 25 (20 ml) polyethylene bottles (NDC 0186-0361-78).
The solutions should be stored at controlled room temperature 15°–30°C (59°–86°F).
021833-00   1/83

YUTOPAR® ℞
[yoū′ tow-par]
(ritodrine hydrochloride)
(Sterile Solution and Tablets)

CAUTION: Federal law prohibits dispensing without prescription.

Description: Yutopar, which contains the betamimetic (beta sympathomimetic amine) ritodrine hydrochloride, is available in two dosage forms. Yutopar for parenteral (intravenous) use is a clear, colorless, sterile, aqueous solution; each milliliter contains 10 mg. of ritodrine hydrochloride, 0.44% (w/v) of acetic acid, 0.24% (w/v) of sodium hydroxide, 0.1% (w/v) of sodium metabisulfite, and 0.29% (w/v) of sodium chloride in water for injection USP. Hydrochloric acid or additional sodium hydroxide is used to adjust pH. **FOR INTRAVENOUS USE ONLY. MUST BE DILUTED BEFORE USE. FOR DOSAGE AND ADMINISTRATION INSTRUCTIONS, SEE PRODUCT INFORMATION BELOW. DO NOT USE IF SOLUTION IS DISCOLORED OR CONTAINS A PRECIPITATE.**
Each Yutopar tablet contains 10 mg. of ritodrine hydrochloride.
Ritodrine hydrochloride is a white, odorless crystalline powder, freely soluble in water, with a melting point between 196° and 205° C. The chemical name of ritodrine hydrochloride is erythro-p-hydroxy-α-[1[(p-hydroxyphenethyl)-amino]ethyl]benzyl alcohol hydrochloride and has the chemical structure:

[Chemical structure diagram]

Clinical Pharmacology: Yutopar (ritodrine hydrochloride) is a beta-receptor agonist, which has been shown by *in vitro* and *in vivo* pharmacologic studies in animals to exert a preferential effect on the β_2 adrenergic receptors such as those in the uterine smooth muscle. Stimulation of the β_2 receptors inhibits contractility of the uterine smooth muscle.
In humans, intravenous infusions of 0.05 to 0.30 mg./min. or single oral doses of 10 to 20 mg. decreased the intensity and frequency of uterine contractions. These effects were antagonized by beta-blocking compounds. Intravenous administration induced an immediate dose-related elevation of heart rate with maximum mean increases between 19 and 40 beats per minute. Widening of the pulse pressure was also observed; the average increase in systolic blood pressure was 4.0 mm. Hg, and the average decrease in diastolic pressure was 12.3 mm. Hg. With oral intake, the increase in heart rate was mild and delayed.
During intravenous infusion in humans, transient elevations of blood glucose, insulin, and free fatty acids have been observed. Decreased serum potassium has also been found, but effects on other electrolytes have not been reported.
Serum kinetics in humans (non-pregnant females) of an intravenous infusion of 60 minutes duration were determined by measuring serum ritodrine levels by a radioimmunoassay technique. Three half-lives were calculated: the first of 6 to 9 minutes dominated the ascending phase of the serum drug-level curve; the second phase of 1.7 to 2.6 hours dominated the descending curve; and finally, a third phase, with a half-life of more than 10 hours, was discernible. In a study of serum kinetics after oral ingestion (male subjects), the decline of serum drug levels could be described in terms of a two-phase decay with an initial half-life of 1.3 hours and a final half-life of 12 hours. With either route of administration, 90% of the excretion was completed within 24 hours after the dose. Comparison of ritodrine serum levels after intravenous administration with those after oral dosage indicates the oral bioavailability is about 30%. Intravenous infusion at a rate of 0.15 mg./min. for 1 hour yielded maximum serum levels ranging between 32 and 52 ng./ml. in a group of 6 non-pregnant female volunteers; maximum serum levels following single and repeated (4 × 10 mg./24 hr.) 10 mg. oral doses ranged between 5 and 15 ng./ml. and were obtained within 30 to 60 minutes after ingestion.
Placental transfer was confirmed by measurement of drug concentrations in cord blood showing that ritodrine and its conjugates reach the fetal circulation.

Indications And Usage: Yutopar is indicated for the management of preterm labor in suitable patients.
Administered intravenously, the drug will decrease uterine activity and thus prolong gestation in the majority of such patients. After intravenous Yutopar has arrested the acute episode, oral administration may help to avert relapse. Additional acute episodes may be treated by repeating the intravenous infusion. The incidence of neonatal mortality and respiratory distress syndrome increases when the normal gestation period is shortened.
Since successful inhibition of labor is more likely with early treatment, therapy with Yutopar should be instituted as soon as the diagnosis of preterm labor is established and contraindications ruled out in pregnancies of 20 or more weeks' gestation. The efficacy and safety of Yutopar in advanced labor, that is, when cervical dilatation is more than 4 cm. or effacement is more than 80%, have not been established.

Contraindications: Yutopar is contraindicated before the 20th week of pregnancy.
Yutopar is also contraindicated in those conditions of the mother or fetus in which continuation of pregnancy is hazardous; specific contraindications include:
1. Antepartum hemorrhage which demands immediate delivery
2. Eclampsia and severe preeclampsia
3. Intrauterine fetal death
4. Chorioamnionitis
5. Maternal cardiac disease
6. Pulmonary hypertension
7. Maternal hyperthyroidism
8. Uncontrolled maternal diabetes mellitus (See PRECAUTIONS.)
9. Pre-existing maternal medical conditions that would be seriously affected by the known pharmacologic properties of a betamimetic drug; such as: hypovolemia, cardiac arrhythmias associated with tachycardia or digitalis intoxication, uncontrolled hypertension, pheochromocytoma, bronchial asthma already treated by betamimetics and/or steroids
10. Known hypersensitivity to any component of the product

Warnings:

Maternal pulmonary edema has been reported in patients treated with Yutopar, sometimes after delivery. It has occurred more often when patients were treated concomitantly with corticosteroids. Maternal death from this condition has been reported with or without corticosteroids given concomitantly with drugs of this class.
Patients so treated must be closely monitored in the hospital. The patient's state of hydration should be carefully monitored; fluid overload must be avoided. (See DOSAGE AND ADMINISTRATION.) Intravenous fluid loading may be aggravated by the use of betamimetics with or without corticosteroids and may turn into manifest circulatory overloading with subsequent pulmonary edema. If pulmonary edema develops during administration, the drug should be discontinueed. Edema should be managed by conventional means.

Intravenous administration of Yutopar should be supervised by persons having knowledge of the pharmacology of the drug and who are qualified to identify and manage complications of drug administration and pregnancy. *Because cardiovascular responses are common and more pronounced during intravenous administration of Yutopar, cardiovascular effects, including maternal pulse rate and blood pressure and fetal heart rate, should be closely monitored.* Care should be exercised for maternal signs and symptoms of pulmonary edema. A persistent high tachycardia (over 140 beats per minute) may be one of the signs of impending pulmonary edema with drugs of this class. Occult cardiac disease may be unmasked with the use of Yutopar. If the patient complains of chest pain or tightness of chest, the drug should be temporarily discontinued and an ECG should be done as soon as possible.
The drug should not be administered to patients with mild to moderate preeclampsia, hypertension, or diabetes unless the attending physician considers that the benefits clearly outweigh the risks.

Precautions: When Yutopar is used for the management of preterm labor in a patient with premature rupture of the membranes, the benefits of delaying delivery should be balanced against the potential risks of development of chorioamnionitis.
Among low birth weight infants, approximately 9% may be growth retarded for gestational age. Therefore, Intra-Uterine Growth Retardation (IUGR) should be considered in the differential diagnosis of preterm labor; this is especially important when the gestational age is in doubt. The decision to continue or reinitiate the administration of Yutopar will depend on an assessment of fetal maturity. In addition to clinical parameters, other studies, such as sonography or amniocentesis, may be helpful in establishing the state of fetal maturity if it is in doubt.
Baseline EKG
This should be done to rule out occult maternal heart disease.
Laboratory Tests
Because intravenous administration of Yutopar has been shown to elevate plasma insulin and glucose and to decrease plasma potassium concentrations, monitoring of glucose and electrolyte levels is recommended during protracted infusions. Decrease of plasma potassium concentrations is usually transient, returning to normal within 24 hours. Special attention should be paid to biochemical variables when treating diabetic patients or those receiving potassium-depleting diuretics.
Serial hemograms may be helpful as an index of state of hydration.
Drug Interactions
Corticosteroids used concomitantly may lead to pulmonary edema. (See Warnings.)
Cardiovascular effects of Yutopar solution (especially cardiac arrhythmia or hypotension) may be potentiated by concomitant use of the following drugs.
1. magnesium sulfate
2. diazoxide
3. meperidine
4. potent general anesthetic agents
Systemic hypertension may be exaggerated in the presence of parasympatholytic agents such as atropine.
The effects of other sympathomimetic amines may be potentiated when concurrently administered and these effects may be additive. A sufficient time

interval should elapse prior to administration of another sympathomimetic drug. With either oral or intravenous administration, 90% of the excretion of Yutopar is completed within 24 hours after the dose.
(See CLINICAL PHARMACOLOGY.)
Beta-adrenergic blocking drugs inhibit the action of Yutopar; coadministration of these drugs should, therefore, be avoided.
With anesthetics used in surgery, the possibility that hypotensive effects may be potentiated should be considered.
Migraine Headache
Transient cerebral ischemia associated with beta sympathomimetic therapy has been reported in two patients with migraine headache.
Carcinogenesis, Mutagenesis, Impairment of Fertility
In rats given oral doses of 1, 10 and 150 mg./kg./day of ritodrine hydrochloride for 82 weeks, benign and malignant tumors were found in the various dosage groups. Since there were no important differences between untreated controls and treated groups and no dose-related trends, it was concluded that there was no evidence of tumorigenicity. The incidence (2–4%) of tumors of the type found in this study is not unusual in this species.
Reproduction studies in rats and rabbits have revealed no evidence of impaired fertility due to ritodrine hydrochloride.
Pregnancy
Teratogenic Effects
(Pregnancy Category B)
Reproduction studies were performed in rats and rabbits. The doses employed intravenously were 1/9 (1 mg./kg.), 1/3 (3 mg./kg.), and 1 (9 mg./kg.) times the maximum human daily intravenous dose (but given to the animals as a bolus rather than by infusion). The oral doses, 10 and 100 mg./kg. represented 5 and 50 times the maximum human daily oral maintenance dose. The results of these studies have revealed no evidence of impaired fertility or harm to the fetus due to ritodrine hydrochloride.
No adverse fetal effects were encountered when single intravenous doses of 1, 3, and 9 mg./kg./day or oral doses of 10 and 100 mg./kg./day were given to rats and rabbits on Days 6 through 15 and 6 through 18 of gestation, respectively. Intravenous doses of 1 and 8 mg./kg./day or oral doses of 10 and 100 mg./kg./day administered to the mother from Day 15 of pregnancy to Day 21 postpartum did not affect perinatal or postnatal development in rats. A slight increase in fetal weight in the rat was observed. Oral administration to both sexes did not impair fertility or reproductive performance. Lethal doses to pregnant rats did not cause immediate fetal demise. There are no adequate and well-controlled studies of Yutopar effects in pregnant women before 20 weeks' gestation; therefore, *this drug should not be used before the 20th week of pregnancy.* Studies of Yutopar administered to pregnant women from the 20th week of gestation have not shown increased risk of fetal abnormalities. Follow-up of selected variables in a small number of children for up to 2 years has not revealed harmful effects on growth, developmental or functional maturation. Nonetheless, although clinical studies did not demonstrate a risk of permanent adverse fetal effects from Yutopar, the possibility cannot be excluded; therefore, Yutopar should be used only when clearly indicated.
Some studies indicate that infants born before 36 weeks' gestation make up less than 10% of all births but account for as many as 75% of perinatal deaths and one-half of all neurologically handicapped infants. There are data available indicating that infants born at any time prior to full term may manifest a higher incidence of neurologic or other handicaps than occurs in the total population of infants born at or after full term. In delaying or preventing preterm labor, the use of Yutopar should result in an overall increase in neonatal survival. Handicapped infants who might not have otherwise survived may survive.
Adverse Reactions: The unwanted effects of Yutopar are related to its betamimetic activity and usually are controlled by suitable dosage adjustments.
Effects Associated with Intravenous Administration
Usual effects (80–100% of patients)
Intravenous infusion of Yutopar leads almost invariably to dose-related alterations in maternal and fetal heart rates and in maternal blood pressure. During clinical studies in which the maximum infusion rate was limited to 0.35 mg./min. (one patient received 0.40 mg./min.), the maximum maternal and fetal heart rates averaged, respectively, 130 (range 60 to 180) and 164 (range 130 to 200) beats per minute. The maximum maternal systolic blood pressures averaged 128 mm. Hg (range 96 to 162 mm. Hg), an average increase of 12 mm. Hg from pretreatment levels. The minimum maternal diastolic blood pressures averaged 48 mm. Hg (range 0 to 76 mm. Hg), an average decrease of 23 mm. Hg from pretreatment levels. While the more severe effects were usually managed effectively by dosage adjustments, in less than 1% of patients, persistent maternal tachycardia or decreased diastolic blood pressure required withdrawal of the drug. A persistent high tachycardia (over 140 beats per minute) may be one of the signs of impending pulmonary edema. (See WARNINGS.)
Yutopar infusion is associated with transient elevation of blood glucose and insulin, which decreases toward normal values after 48 to 72 hours despite continuous infusion. Elevation of free fatty acids and cAMP has been reported. Reduction of potassium levels should be expected; other biochemical effects have not been reported.
Frequent effects (10–50% of patients)
Intravenous Yutopar, in about one-third of the patients, was associated with palpitation. Tremor, nausea, vomiting, headache, or erythema was observed in 10 to 15% of patients.
Occasional effects (5–10% of patients)
Nervousness, jitteriness, restlessness, emotional upset, or anxiety was reported in 5 to 6% of patients and malaise in similar numbers.
Infrequent effects (1–3% of patients)
Cardiac symptoms including chest pain or tightness (rarely associated with abnormalities of ECG) and arrhythmia were reported in 1 to 2% of patients. (See Warnings.)
Other infrequently reported maternal effects included: anaphylactic shock, rash, heart murmur, epigastric distress, ileus, bloating, constipation, diarrhea, dyspnea, hyperventilation, hemolytic icterus, glycosuria, lactic acidosis, sweating, chills, drowsiness, and weakness.
Neonatal Effects
Infrequently reported neonatal symptoms include hypoglycemia and ileus. In addition, hypocalcemia and hypotension have been reported in neonates whose mothers were treated with other betamimetic agents.
Effects Associated with Oral Administration
Frequent effects (< 50% of patients)
Oral ritodrine in clinical studies was often associated with small increases in maternal heart rate, but little or no effect upon either maternal systolic or diastolic blood pressure or upon fetal heart rate was found.
Oral ritodrine in 10 to 15% of patients was associated with palpitation or tremor. Nausea and jitteriness were less frequent (5 to 8%), while rash was observed in some patients (3 to 4%), and arrhythmia was infrequent (about 1%).
Overdosage: The symptoms of overdosage are those of excessive beta-adrenergic stimulation including exaggeration of the known pharmacologic effects, the most prominent being tachycardia (maternal and fetal), palpitation, cardiac arrhythmia, hypotension, dyspnea, nervousness, tremor, nausea, and vomiting. If an excess of ritodrine tablets is ingested, gastric lavage or induction of emesis should be carried out followed by administration of activated charcoal. When symptoms of overdose occur as a result of intravenous administration, ritodrine should be discontinued; an appropriate beta-blocking agent may be used as an antidote. Ritodrine hydrochloride is dialyzable.
Acute intravenous toxicity was studied in rats and rabbits and acute oral toxicity in mice, rats, guinea pigs, and dogs. The LD50 values in the most sensitive of the species used were 64 mg./kg. intravenously in the nonpregnant rabbit and 540 mg./kg. orally in the nonpregnant mouse. The intravenous LD50 value in the pregnant rat was 85 mg./kg. The amount of drug required to produce symptoms of overdose in humans is individually variable. No reports of human mortality due to overdose have been received.
Dosage And Administration: In the management of preterm labor, the initial intravenous treatment should usually be followed by oral administration. The optimum dose of Yutopar is determined by a clinical balance of uterine response and unwanted effects.
Intravenous Therapy
Do not use intravenous Yutopar if the solution is discolored or contains any precipitate or particulate matter. Yutopar solution should be used promptly after preparation, but in no case after 48 hours of preparation.
Method of Administration: To minimize the risks of hypotension, the patient should be maintained in the left lateral position throughout infusion and careful attention given to her state of hydration, but fluid overload must be avoided.
For appropriate control and dose titration, a controlled infusion device is recommended to adjust the rate of flow in drops/minute. An i.v. microdrip chamber (60 drops/ml.) can provide a convenient range of infusion rates within the recommended dose range for Yutopar.
Recommended Dilution: 150 mg. ritodrine hydrochloride (3 ampuls) in 500 ml. fluid yielding a final concentration of 0.3 mg./ml. Ritodrine for intravenous infusion should be diluted with 5% w/v dextrose solution. Because of the increased probability of pulmonary edema, saline diluents such as:
—0.9% w/v sodium chloride solution,
—compound sodium chloride solution (Ringer's solution)
—and Hartmann's solution, should be reserved for cases where dextrose solution is medically undesirable e.g. diabetes mellitus.
In those cases where fluid restriction is medically desirable, a more concentrated solution may be prepared.
Intravenous therapy should be started as soon as possible after diagnosis. The usual initial dose is 0.1 mg./minute (0.33 ml./min., 20 drops/min. using a microdrip chamber at the recommended dilution), to be gradually increased according to the results by 0.05 mg./minute (0.17 ml./min., 10 drops/min. using a microdrip chamber at the recommended dilution) every 10 minutes until the desired result is attained. The effective dosage usually lies between 0.15 and 0.35 mg./minute (0.50 to 1.17 ml./min., 30–70 drops/min. using a microdrip chamber at the recommended dilution). Frequent monitoring of maternal uterine contractions, heart rate, and blood pressure, and of fetal heart rate is required, with patients individually titrated according to response. If other drugs need to be given intravenously, the use of "piggyback" or other site of intravenous administration permits the continued independent control of the rate of infusion of the Yutopar.
The infusion should generally be continued for at least 12 hours after uterine contractions cease. With the recommended dilution, the maximum volume of fluid that might be administered after 12 hours at the highest dose (0.35 mg./min.) will be approximately 840 ml.
The amount of i.v. fluids administered and the rate of administration should be monitored to avoid circulatory fluid overload (over-hydration) or inadequate hydration. (See PRECAUTIONS, *Laboratory Tests.*)
Oral Maintenance
One tablet (10 mg.) may be given approximately 30 minutes before the termination of intravenous therapy. The usual dosage schedule for the first 24 hours of oral administration is 1 tablet (10 mg.) every two hours. Thereafter, the usual maintenance is 1 or 2 tablets (10 to 20 mg.) every four to six hours, the dose depending on uterine activity and unwanted effects. The total daily dose of oral

Continued on next page

Astra—Cont.

ritodrine should not exceed 120 mg. The treatment may be continued as long as the physician considers it desirable to prolong pregnancy.
Recurrence of unwanted preterm labor may be treated with repeated infusion of Yutopar.

How Supplied:
NDC 0186-0599-03: 5 ml. ampuls in boxes of 10. Each ampul contains 50 mg. (10 mg./ml.) of ritodrine hydrochloride.
NDC 0186-0595-60: 10 mg. tablets in bottles of 60. Each round, yellow tablet contains 10 mg. ritodrine hydrochloride and is inscribed YUTOPAR on one side and scored on the other.
NDC 0186-0595-78: 10 mg unit dose tablets in boxes of 100. Each round, yellow tablet contains 10 mg. ritodrine hydrochloride and is inscribed YUTOPAR on one side and scored on the other.
NDC 0186-0597-12: 10 ml vial in boxes of 6. Each vial contains 150 mg (15 mg/ml) of ritodrine hydrochloride.

Both the tablet and intravenous dosage forms should be stored at room temperature, preferably below 86°F. (30°C). Protect from excessive heat.
Oral dosage form manufactured by Merrell Dow Pharmaceuticals Inc.
Subsidiary of The Dow Chemical Company
Cincinnati, Ohio 45215, U.S.A. for
ASTRA®
Astra Pharmaceuticals Products, Inc.
Westborough MA 01581
Yutopar® licensed by Duphar B. V. Amsterdam, Holland
021829R03   5/84

For information on Astra products, write to:
Professional Information Dept.
Astra Pharmaceutical Products, Inc.
50 Otis Street
Westborough Massachusetts 01581-4428

Ayerst Laboratories
Division of American Home
Products Corporation
685 THIRD AVE.
NEW YORK, NY 10017

ANACIN-3® (acetaminophen)
[ăn'a-sĭn]
with Codeine
TABLETS

Description: Each Tablet Contains:
Acetaminophen, 325 mg, and Codeine Phosphate*, 15 mg
Acetaminophen, 300 mg, and Codeine Phosphate*, 30 mg
Acetaminophen, 300 mg, and Codeine Phosphate*, 60 mg

*WARNING: May be habit forming.
Acetaminophen occurs as a white, odorless crystalline powder, possessing a slightly bitter taste. Codeine is an alkaloid, obtained from opium or prepared from morphine by methylation. Codeine occurs as colorless or white crystals, effloresces slowly in dry air and is affected by light.

Actions: Acetaminophen is a nonopiate, nonsalicylate analgesic and antipyretic. Codeine is an opiate analgesic and antitussive. Codeine retains at least one-half of its analgesic activity when administered orally.

Indications: For the relief of mild to moderately severe pain.

Contraindications: Hypersensitivity to acetaminophen or codeine.

Warnings:
Drug Dependence: Codeine can produce drug dependence of the morphine type, and therefore, has the potential for being abused. Psychic dependence, physical dependence and tolerance may develop upon repeated administration of this drug and it should be prescribed and administered with the same degree of caution appropriate to the use of other oral narcotic medications.
This acetaminophen and codeine dosage form is subject to the Federal Controlled Substances Act (Schedule III).

Precautions:
1. **General:**
Head injury and increased intracranial pressure: The respiratory depressant effects of narcotics and their capacity to elevate cerebrospinal fluid pressure may be markedly exaggerated in the presence of head injury, other intracranial lesions or a pre-existing increase in intracranial pressure. Furthermore, narcotics produce adverse reactions which may obscure the clinical course of patients with head injuries.
Acute abdominal conditions: The administration of products containing codeine or other narcotics may obscure the diagnosis or clinical course in patients with acute abdominal conditions.
Special risk patients: Acetaminophen with codeine should be given with caution to certain patients such as the elderly or debilitated, and those with severe impairment of hepatic or renal function, hypothyroidism, Addison's disease, and prostatic hypertrophy or urethral stricture.

2. **Information for Patients:**
Codeine may impair the mental and/or physical abilities required for the performance of potentially hazardous tasks such as driving a car or operating machinery. The patient taking this drug should be cautioned accordingly.

3. **Drug-Interactions:**
Patients receiving other narcotic analgesics, antipsychotics, antianxiety, or other CNS depressants (including alcohol) concomitantly with acetaminophen and codeine may exhibit additive CNS depression due to the codeine component. When such therapy is contemplated, the dose of one or both agents should be reduced.
The use of MAO inhibitors or tricyclic antidepressants with codeine preparations may increase the effect of either the antidepressant or codeine.
The concurrent use of anticholinergics with codeine may produce paralytic ileus.

4. **Usage in Pregnancy:**
Safe use in pregnancy has not been established relative to possible adverse effects on fetal development. Therefore, acetaminophen and codeine should not be used in pregnant women unless, in the judgment of the physician, the potential benefits outweigh the possible hazards.

5. **Nursing Mothers:**
It is not known whether the components of this drug are excreted in human milk. Because many drugs are excreted in human milk, caution should be exercised when acetaminophen and codeine is administered to a nursing woman.

Adverse Reactions: The most frequently observed adverse reactions include light headedness, dizziness, sedation, shortness of breath, nausea and vomiting. These effects seem to be more prominent in ambulatory than in non-ambulatory patients, and some of these adverse reactions may be alleviated if the patient lies down.
Other adverse reactions include euphoria, dysphoria, constipation and pruritus. At higher doses codeine has most of the disadvantages of morphine including respiratory depression.

Overdosage:
Acetaminophen:
Signs and Symptoms: Acetaminophen in massive overdosage may cause hepatic toxicity in some patients. In all cases of suspected overdose, immediately call your regional poison center or the Rocky Mountain Poison Center's toll-free number (800-525-6115) for assistance in diagnosis and for directions in the use of N-acetylcysteine as an antidote, a use currently restricted to investigational status.
In adults, hepatic toxicity has rarely been reported with acute overdoses of less than 10 grams and fatalities with less than 15 grams. Importantly, young children seem to be more resistant than adults to the hepatotoxic effect of an acetaminophen overdose. Despite this, the measures outlined below should be initiated in any adult or child suspected of having ingested an acetaminophen overdose.
Early symptoms following a potentially hepatotoxic overdose may include: nausea, vomiting, diaphoresis and general malaise. Clinical and laboratory evidence of hepatic toxicity may not be apparent until 48 to 72 hours postingestion.
Treatment: The stomach should be emptied promptly by lavage or by induction of emesis with syrup of ipecac. Patients' estimates of the quantity of a drug ingested are notoriously unreliable. Therefore, if an acetaminophen overdose is suspected, a serum acetaminophen assay should be obtained as early as possible, but no sooner than four hours following ingestion. Liver function studies should be obtained initially and repeated at 24-hour intervals.
The antidote, N-acetylcysteine, should be administered as early as possible, and within 16 hours of the overdose ingestion for optimal results. Following recovery, there are no residual, structural or functional hepatic abnormalities.

Codeine:
Signs and Symptoms: Serious overdose with codeine is characterized by respiratory depression (a decrease in respiratory rate and/or tidal volume, Cheyne-Stokes respiration, cyanosis), extreme somnolence progressing to stupor or coma, skeletal muscle flaccidity, cold and clammy skin, and sometimes bradycardia and hypotension. In severe overdosage, apnea, circulatory collapse, cardiac arrest and death may occur.
Treatment: Primary attention should be given to the reestablishment of adequate respiratory exchange through provision of a patent airway and the institution of assisted or controlled ventilation. The narcotic antagonist naloxone is a specific antidote against respiratory depression which may result from overdosage or unusual sensitivity to narcotics, including codeine. Therefore, an appropriate dose of naloxone (see package insert) should be administered, preferably by the intravenous route, and simultaneously with efforts at respiratory resuscitation. Since the duration of action of codeine may exceed that of the antagonist, the patient should be kept under continued surveillance and repeated doses of the antagonist should be administered as needed to maintain adequate respiration.
An antagonist should not be administered in the absence of clinically significant respiratory or cardiovascular depression. Oxygen, intravenous fluids, vasopressors and other supportive measures should be employed as indicated.
Gastric emptying may be useful in removing unabsorbed drug.

Dosage and Administration: Dosage should be adjusted according to severity of pain and response of the patient. However, it should be kept in mind that tolerance to codeine can develop with continued use and that the incidence of untoward effects is dose related. This product is inappropriate even in high doses for severe or intractable pain. Adult doses of codeine higher than 60 mg fail to give commensurate relief of pain but merely prolong analgesia and are associated with an appreciably increased incidence of undesirable side effects. Equivalently high doses in children would have similar effects.

Adults: **Codeine**—15–30 mg (for mild to moderate pain) 60 mg (for moderate to moderately severe pain)
         Acetaminophen—300–600 mg
Children: **Codeine**—500 mcg/kg
Doses can be repeated up to every 4 hours.

How Supplied: White compressed tablets. Acetaminophen, 325 mg, and Codeine Phosphate, 15 mg—in bottles of 100 (NDC 0046-0250-81) and bottles of 500 (NDC 0046-0250-85).
Acetaminophen, 300 mg, and Codeine Phosphate, 30 mg—in bottles of 100 (NDC 0046-0251-81), bottles of 500 (NDC 0046-0251-85) and bottles of 1,000 (NDC 0046-0251-91).
Acetaminophen, 300 mg, and Codeine Phosphate, 60 mg—in bottles of 100 (NDC 0046-0254-81) and bottles of 500 (NDC 0046-0254-85).

CAUTION: Federal law prohibits dispensing without prescription.

Shown in Product Identification Section, page 404

ANTABUSE® ℞
[an'tah-būse]
**Brand of disulfiram
In Alcoholism**

CAUTION: Federal law prohibits dispensing without prescription.

> **Warning**
> ANTABUSE should never be administered to a patient when he is in a state of alcohol intoxication or without his full knowledge.
> The physician should instruct relatives accordingly.

Description: CHEMICAL NAME: bis(diethylthiocarbamoyl) disulfide STRUCTURAL FORMULA:

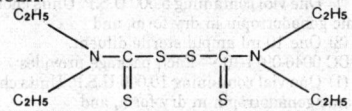

ANTABUSE occurs as a white to off-white, odorless, and almost tasteless powder, soluble in water to the extent of about 20 mg in 100 ml, and in alcohol to the extent of about 3.8 g in 100 ml.

Action: ANTABUSE produces a sensitivity to alcohol which results in a highly unpleasant reaction when the patient under treatment ingests even small amounts of alcohol.

ANTABUSE blocks the oxidation of alcohol at the acetaldehyde stage. During alcohol metabolism after ANTABUSE intake, the concentration of acetaldehyde occurring in the blood may be 5 to 10 times higher than that found during metabolism of the same amount of alcohol alone.

Accumulation of acetaldehyde in the blood produces the complex of highly unpleasant symptoms referred to hereinafter as the ANTABUSE-alcohol reaction. This reaction, which is proportional to the dosage of both ANTABUSE (disulfiram) and alcohol, will persist as long as alcohol is being metabolized. ANTABUSE does not appear to influence the rate of alcohol elimination from the body. ANTABUSE is slowly absorbed from the gastrointestinal tract and is slowly eliminated from the body. One (or even two) weeks after a patient has taken his last dose of ANTABUSE, ingestion of alcohol may produce unpleasant symptoms.

Prolonged administration of ANTABUSE does not produce tolerance; the longer a patient remains on therapy, the more exquisitely sensitive he becomes to alcohol.

Indication: ANTABUSE (disulfiram) is an aid in the management of selected chronic alcoholic patients who want to remain in a state of enforced sobriety so that supportive and psychotherapeutic treatment may be applied to best advantage. (Used alone, without proper motivation and without supportive therapy, ANTABUSE is not a cure for alcoholism, and it is unlikely that it will have more than a brief effect on the drinking pattern of the chronic alcoholic.)

Contraindications: Patients who are receiving or have recently received metronidazole, paraldehyde, alcohol, or alcohol-containing preparations, e.g. cough syrups, tonics and the like, should not be given ANTABUSE.

ANTABUSE is contraindicated in the presence of severe myocardial disease or coronary occlusion, psychoses, and hypersensitivity to disulfiram or to other thiuram derivatives used in pesticides and rubber vulcanization.

Warnings:

> ANTABUSE (disulfiram) should never be administered to a patient when he is in a state of alcohol intoxication or without his full knowledge.
> The physician should instruct relatives accordingly.

The patient must be fully informed of the ANTABUSE-alcohol reaction. He must be strongly cautioned against surreptitious drinking while taking the drug and he must be fully aware of possible consequences. He should be warned to avoid alcohol in disguised form, i.e. in sauces, vinegars, cough mixtures, and even aftershave lotions and back rubs. He should also be warned that reactions may occur with alcohol up to 14 days after ingesting ANTABUSE.

The ANTABUSE-ALCOHOL REACTION: ANTABUSE plus alcohol, even small amounts, produces flushing, throbbing in head and neck, throbbing headache, respiratory difficulty, nausea, copious vomiting, sweating, thirst, chest pain, palpitation, dyspnea, hyperventilation, tachycardia, hypotension, syncope, marked uneasiness, weakness, vertigo, blurred vision, and confusion. In severe reactions there may be respiratory depression, cardiovascular collapse, arrhythmias, myocardial infarction, acute congestive heart failure, unconsciousness, convulsions, and death.

The intensity of the reaction varies with each individual, but is generally proportional to the amounts of ANTABUSE and alcohol ingested. Mild reactions may occur in the sensitive individual when the blood alcohol concentration is increased to as little as 5 to 10 mg per 100 ml. Symptoms are fully developed at 50 mg per 100 ml and unconsciousness usually results when the blood alcohol level reaches 125 to 150 mg.

The duration of the reaction varies from 30 to 60 minutes to several hours in the more severe cases, or as long as there is alcohol in the blood.

DRUG INTERACTIONS: Disulfiram appears to decrease the rate at which certain drugs are metabolized and so may increase the blood levels and the possibility of clinical toxicity of drugs given concomitantly.

DISULFIRAM SHOULD BE USED WITH CAUTION IN THOSE PATIENTS RECEIVING PHENYTOIN AND ITS CONGENERS, SINCE THE CONCOMITANT ADMINISTRATION OF THESE TWO DRUGS CAN LEAD TO PHENYTOIN INTOXICATION. PRIOR TO ADMINISTERING DISULFIRAM TO A PATIENT ON PHENYTOIN THERAPY, A BASELINE PHENYTOIN SERUM LEVEL SHOULD BE OBTAINED. SUBSEQUENT TO INITIATION OF DISULFIRAM THERAPY, SERUM LEVELS ON PHENYTOIN SHOULD BE DETERMINED ON DIFFERENT DAYS FOR EVIDENCE OF AN INCREASE OR FOR A CONTINUING RISE IN LEVELS. INCREASED PHENYTOIN LEVELS SHOULD BE TREATED WITH APPROPRIATE DOSAGE ADJUSTMENT.

It may be necessary to adjust the dosage of oral anticoagulants upon beginning or stopping disulfiram, since disulfiram may prolong prothrombin time.

Patients taking isoniazid when disulfiram is given should be observed for the appearance of unsteady gait or marked changes in mental status and the disulfiram discontinued if such signs appear.

In rats, simultaneous ingestion of disulfiram and nitrite in the diet for 78 weeks has been reported to cause tumors, and it has been suggested that disulfiram may react with nitrites in the rat stomach to form a nitrosamine which is tumorigenic. Disulfiram alone in the diet of rats did not lead to such tumors. The relevance of this finding to humans is not known at this time.

CONCOMITANT CONDITIONS: Because of the possibility of an accidental ANTABUSE-alcohol reaction, ANTABUSE (disulfiram) should be used with extreme caution in patients with any of the following conditions: diabetes mellitus, hypothyroidism, epilepsy, cerebral damage, chronic and acute nephritis, hepatic cirrhosis or insufficiency.

USAGE IN PREGNANCY: The safe use of this drug in pregnancy has not been established. Therefore, ANTABUSE should be used during pregnancy only when, in the judgment of the physician, the probable benefits outweigh the possible risks.

Precautions: Patients with a history of rubber contact dermatitis should be evaluated for hypersensitivity to thiuram derivatives before receiving ANTABUSE (See Contraindications).

It is suggested that every patient under treatment carry an Identification Card, stating that he is receiving ANTABUSE and describing the symptoms most likely to occur as a result of the ANTABUSE-alcohol reaction. In addition, this card should indicate the physician or institution to be contacted in emergency. (Cards may be obtained from Ayerst Laboratories upon request.)

Alcoholism may accompany or be followed by dependence on narcotics or sedatives. Barbiturates have been administered concurrently with ANTABUSE without untoward effects, but the possibility of initiating a new abuse should be considered. Baseline and follow-up transaminase tests (10–14 days) are suggested to detect any hepatic dysfunction that may result with ANTABUSE therapy. In addition, a complete blood count and a sequential multiple analysis-12 (SMA-12) test should be made every six months.

Patients taking ANTABUSE Tablets should not be exposed to ethylene dibromide or its vapors. This precaution is based on preliminary results of animal research currently in progress which suggests a toxic interaction between inhaled ethylene dibromide and ingested disulfiram resulting in a higher incidence of tumors and mortality in rats. Correlation of this finding to humans, however, has not been demonstrated.

Adverse Reactions: (See Contraindications, Warnings, and Precautions.)
OPTIC NEURITIS, PERIPHERAL NEURITIS AND POLYNEURITIS MAY OCCUR FOLLOWING ADMINISTRATION OF ANTABUSE.

Occasional skin eruptions are, as a rule, readily controlled by concomitant administration of an antihistaminic drug.

In a small number of patients, a transient mild drowsiness, fatigability, impotence, headache, acneform eruptions, allergic dermatitis, or a metallic or garlic-like aftertaste may be experienced during the first two weeks of therapy. These complaints usually disappear spontaneously with the continuation of therapy or with reduced dosage. Psychotic reactions have been noted, attributable in most cases to high dosage, combined toxicity (with metronidazole or isoniazid), or to the unmasking of underlying psychoses in patients stressed by the withdrawal of alcohol.

One case of cholestatic hepatitis has been reported, but its relationship to ANTABUSE has not been unequivocally established.

One case of fulminant hepatitis temporally associated with administration of ANTABUSE has been reported.

Dosage and Administration: ANTABUSE (disulfiram) should never be administered until the patient has abstained from alcohol for at least 12 hours.

INITIAL DOSAGE SCHEDULE: In the first phase of treatment, a maximum of 500 mg daily is given in a single dose for one to two weeks. Although usually taken in the morning, ANTABUSE may be taken on retiring by patients who experience a sedative effect. Alternatively, to minimize, or eliminate, the sedative effect, dosage may be adjusted downward.

MAINTENANCE REGIMEN: The average maintenance dose is 250 mg daily (range, 125 to 500 mg); it should not exceed 500 mg daily.

NOTE: Occasional patients, while seemingly on adequate maintenance doses of ANTABUSE, report that they are able to drink alcoholic beverages with impunity and without any symptomatology. All appearances to the contrary, such patients must be presumed to be disposing of their tablets in some manner without actually taking them. Until such patients have been observed reliably taking their daily ANTABUSE tablets (preferably crushed and well mixed with liquid), it cannot be concluded that ANTABUSE is ineffective.

DURATION OF THERAPY: The daily, uninterrupted administration of ANTABUSE (disulfiram) must be continued until the patient is fully recovered socially and a basis for permanent self-control is established. Depending on the individual patient, maintenance therapy may be required for months or even years.

TRIAL WITH ALCOHOL: During early experience with ANTABUSE, it was thought advisable for each patient to have at least one supervised

Continued on next page

Ayerst—Cont.

alcohol-drug reaction. More recently, the test reaction has been largely abandoned. Furthermore, such a test reaction should never be administered to a patient over 50 years of age. A clear, detailed, and convincing description of the reaction is felt to be sufficient in most cases.

However, where a test reaction is deemed necessary, the suggested procedure is as follows:

After the first one to two weeks' therapy with 500 mg daily, a drink of 15 ml (½ oz) of 100 proof whiskey or equivalent is taken slowly. This test dose of alcoholic beverage may be repeated once only so that the total dose does not exceed 30 ml (1 oz) of whiskey. Once a reaction develops, no more alcohol should be consumed. Such tests should be carried out only when the patient is hospitalized, or comparable supervision and facilities, including oxygen, are available.

MANAGEMENT OF ANTABUSE-ALCOHOL REACTION: In severe reactions, whether caused by an excessive test dose or by the patient's unsupervised ingestion of alcohol, supportive measures to restore blood pressure and treat shock should be instituted. Other recommendations include: oxygen, carbogen (95 per cent oxygen and 5 per cent carbon dioxide), vitamin C intravenously in massive doses (1 g), and ephedrine sulfate. Antihistamines have also been used intravenously. Potassium levels should be monitored particularly in patients on digitalis since hypokalemia has been reported.

How Supplied: ANTABUSE—Each tablet (scored) contains 250 mg disulfiram, in bottles of 100 (NDC 0046-0809-81)—Each tablet (scored) contains 500 mg disulfiram, in bottles of 50 (NDC 0046-0810-50) and 1,000 (NDC 0046-0810-91).

Shown in Product Identification Section, page 404

A.P.L.® ℞
Brand of chorionic gonadotropin for injection, U.S.P.
For Intramuscular Injection Only

CAUTION: Federal law prohibits dispensing without prescription.

Description: Human chorionic gonadotropin (HCG), a polypeptide hormone produced by the human placenta, is composed of an alpha and a beta subunit. The alpha subunit is essentially identical to the alpha subunits of the human pituitary gonadotropins, luteinizing hormone (LH) and follicle-stimulating hormone (FSH), as well as to the alpha subunit of human thyroid stimulating hormone (TSH). The beta subunits of these hormones differ in amino acid sequence.

A.P.L. (chorionic gonadotropin, U.S.P.) is a gonad-stimulating principle obtained from the urine of pregnant women. It is an amorphous powder prepared by cryodesiccation, and is freely soluble in water.

Actions: The action of HCG is virtually identical to that of pituitary LH, although HCG appears to have a small degree of FSH activity as well. It stimulates production of gonadal steroid hormones by stimulating the interstitial cells (Leydig cells) of the testis to produce androgens and the corpus luteum of the ovary to produce progesterone. Androgen stimulation in the male leads to the development of secondary sex characteristics and may stimulate testicular descent when no anatomical impediment to descent is present. This descent is usually reversible when HCG is discontinued. During the normal menstrual cycle, LH participates with FSH in the development and maturation of the normal ovarian follicle, and the midcycle LH surge triggers ovulation. HCG can substitute for LH in this function.

During a normal pregnancy, HCG secreted by the placenta maintains the corpus luteum after LH secretion decreases, supporting continued secretion of estrogen and progesterone, and preventing menstruation. HCG HAS NO KNOWN EFFECT ON FAT MOBILIZATION, APPETITE OR SENSE OF HUNGER, OR BODY FAT DISTRIBUTION.

Indications: HCG HAS NOT BEEN DEMONSTRATED TO BE EFFECTIVE ADJUNCTIVE THERAPY IN THE TREATMENT OF OBESITY. THERE IS NO SUBSTANTIAL EVIDENCE THAT IT INCREASES WEIGHT LOSS BEYOND THAT RESULTING FROM CALORIC RESTRICTION, THAT IT CAUSES A MORE ATTRACTIVE OR "NORMAL" DISTRIBUTION OF FAT, OR THAT IT DECREASES THE HUNGER AND DISCOMFORT ASSOCIATED WITH CALORIE RESTRICTED DIETS.

1. Cryptorchidism not due to anatomic obstruction. In general, A.P.L. (Chorionic Gonadotropin for Injection, U.S.P.) is thought to induce testicular descent in situations when descent would have occurred at puberty. A.P.L. thus may help to predict whether or not orchiopexy will be needed in the future. Although, in some cases, descent following A.P.L. administration is permanent, in most cases the response is temporary. Therapy is usually instituted between the ages of 4 and 9.
2. Selected cases of male hypogonadism secondary to pituitary failure.
3. Induction of ovulation and pregnancy in the anovulatory, infertile woman in whom the cause of anovulation is secondary and not due to ovarian failure, and who has been appropriately pretreated with human menotropins.

Contraindications: Precocious puberty, prostatic carcinoma or other androgen-dependent neoplasia, prior allergic reaction to chorionic gonadotropin.

Warnings: HCG should be used in conjunction with human menopausal gonadotropins only by physicians experienced with infertility problems who are familiar with the criteria for patient selection, contraindications, warnings, precautions, and adverse reactions described in the package insert for menotropins. The principal serious adverse reactions during this use are: (1) ovarian enlargement, ascites with or without pain, and/or pleural effusion, (2) rupture of ovarian cysts with resultant hemoperitoneum, (3) multiple births, and (4) arterial thromboembolism.

Precautions: Induction of androgen secretion by chorionic gonadotropin may induce precocious puberty in patients treated for cryptorchidism. If signs of precocious puberty occur, therapy should be discontinued.

Since androgens may cause fluid retention, chorionic gonadotropin should be used with caution in patients with epilepsy, migraine, asthma, cardiac or renal disease.

Adverse Reactions:
Headache
Irritability
Restlessness
Depression
Tiredness
Edema
Precocious puberty
Gynecomastia
Pain at site of injection

Dosage and Administration: There is a marked variance of opinion concerning the dosage regimens to be used. Therefore the regimen employed in any particular case will depend upon the indication for use, the age and weight of the patient, and the physician's preference. The following regimens have been advocated by various authorities.

Cryptorchidism: (Therapy is usually instituted between the ages of 4 and 9.)

(1) 4,000 U.S.P. Units three times weekly for three weeks.

(2) 5,000 U.S.P. Units every second day for four injections.

(3) 15 injections of 500 to 1,000 U.S.P. Units over a period of six weeks.

(4) 500 U.S.P. Units three times weekly for four to six weeks. If this course of treatment is not successful, another is begun one month later, giving 1,000 U.S.P. Units per injection.

Selected cases of male hypogonadism secondary to pituitary failure:

(1) 500 to 1,000 U.S.P. Units three times a week for three weeks, followed by the same dose twice a week for three weeks.

(2) 1,000 to 2,000 U.S.P. Units three times weekly.

(3) 4,000 U.S.P. Units three times weekly for six to nine months, following which the dosage may be reduced to 2,000 U.S.P. Units three times weekly for an additional three months.

Induction of ovulation and pregnancy in the anovulatory, infertile woman in whom the cause of anovulation is secondary:

5,000 to 10,000 U.S.P. Units one day following the last dose of menotropins.

How Supplied: A.P.L. (Chorionic Gonadotropin for Injection, U.S.P.)

NDC 0046-0970-10 — Each package provides:
(1) One vial containing 5,000 U.S.P. Units chorionic gonadotropin in dry form, and
(2) One 10 ml ampul sterile diluent.

NDC 0046-0971-10 — Each package provides:
(1) One vial containing 10,000 U.S.P. Units chorionic gonadotropin in dry form, and
(2) One 10 ml ampul sterile diluent.

NDC 0046-0972-10 — Each package provides:
(1) One vial containing 20,000 U.S.P. Units chorionic gonadotropin in dry form, and
(2) One 10 ml ampul sterile diluent.

When reconstituted with 10 ml of accompanying sterile diluent, the resulting solutions also contain 2.0% benzyl alcohol, not more than 0.2% phenol, and the following concentrations of lactose: No. 970, 0.9%; No. 971, 1.8%; No. 972, 3.6%. The pH is adjusted with sodium hydroxide or hydrochloric acid.

MAY BE STORED FOR 90 DAYS IN A REFRIGERATOR AFTER RECONSTITUTION.

ATROMID-S® ℞
[ă' trō-mid]
Brand of clofibrate
Antilipidemic agent for reduction of elevated serum lipids

Actions: ATROMID-S is an antilipidemic agent. It acts to lower elevated serum lipids by reducing the very low density lipoprotein fraction ($S_f 20-400$) rich in triglycerides. Serum cholesterol, especially the low density lipoprotein fraction ($S_f 0-20$), is also decreased, particularly in those whose cholesterol levels are elevated at the outset.

The mechanism of action has not been established definitively. In man, clofibrate reduces cholesterol formation early in the biosynthetic chain. In addition, clofibrate has been shown to cause increased excretion of neutral sterols.

Animal studies suggest that clofibrate interrupts cholesterol biosynthesis prior to mevalonate formation.

Indications: Drug therapy should not be used for the routine treatment of elevated blood lipids for the prevention of coronary heart disease. Dietary therapy specific for the type of hyperlipidemia is the initial treatment of choice.[1] Excess body weight and alcoholic intake may be important factors in hypertriglyceridemia and should be addressed prior to any drug therapy. Physical exercise can be an important ancillary measure. Contributory diseases such as hypothyroidism or diabetes mellitus should be looked for and adequately treated. The use of drugs should be considered only when reasonable attempts have been made to obtain satisfactory results with non-drug methods. If the decision ultimately is to use drugs, the patient should be instructed that this does not reduce the importance of adhering to diet.

Because ATROMID-S (clofibrate) is associated with certain serious adverse findings reported in two large clinical trials (see WARNINGS), agents other than clofibrate may be more suitable for a particular patient.

ATROMID-S is indicated for Primary Dysbetalipoproteinemia (Type III hyperlipidemia) that does not respond adequately to diet.

ATROMID-S may be considered for the treatment of adult patients with very high serum triglyceride levels (Types IV and V hyperlipidemia) who present a risk of abdominal pain and pancreatitis and who do not respond adequately to a determined dietary effort to control them. Patients with triglyceride levels in excess of 750 mg per deciliter are likely to present such risk.

ATROMID-S has little effect on the elevated cholesterol levels of most subjects with hypercholesterolemia. A minority of subjects show a more pronounced response. However, it must be understood that there is no evidence that use of any lipid-altering agent will be beneficial in preventing death from coronary heart disease (See Warnings). Therefore, the physician should be very selective and confine clofibrate treatment to patients with clearly defined risk due to severe hypercholesterolemia (e.g. individuals with familial hypercholesterolemia starting in childhood) who inadequately respond to appropriate diet and more effective cholesterol-lowering drugs.

ATROMID-S is not useful for the hypertriglyceridemia of Type I hyperlipidemia.

The biochemical response to ATROMID-S (clofibrate) is variable, and it is not always possible to predict from the lipoprotein type or other factors which patients will obtain favorable results. It is essential that lipid levels be assessed and that the drug be discontinued in any patient in whom lipids do not show significant improvement.

Contraindications: Clofibrate is contraindicated in pregnant women. While teratogenic studies have not demonstrated any effect attributable to clofibrate, it is known that serum of the rabbit fetus accumulates a higher concentration of clofibrate than that found in maternal serum, and it is possible that the fetus may not have developed the enzyme system required for the excretion of clofibrate.

It is contraindicated in lactating women since it is not known if clofibrate is secreted in the milk.

It is contraindicated in patients with clinically significant hepatic or renal dysfunction.

It is contraindicated in patients with primary biliary cirrhosis since it may raise the already elevated cholesterol in these cases.

Warnings

In a large prospective study involving 5,000 patients in a clofibrate-treated group and 5,000 in a placebo-treated group followed for an average of five years on drug or placebo and one year beyond (the WHO study), there was a statistically significant 36% higher mortality due to noncardiovascular causes in the clofibrate-treated group than in a comparable placebo group. Half of this difference was due to malignancy; other causes of death included postcholecystectomy complications and pancreatitis.[2] In another prospective study involving 1,000 clofibrate- and 3,000 placebo-treated patients followed for an average of six years on drug or placebo (the Coronary Drug Project study), the noncardiovascular mortality rate, including that of malignancy, was not significantly different in the clofibrate- and placebo-treated groups.[3] This should not be interpreted to mean that clofibrate is not associated with an increased risk of noncardiovascular death because the patients in the Coronary Drug Project were much older than those in the WHO study and they all had had a previous myocardial infarction so that the deaths in the Coronary Drug Project were overwhelmingly due to cardiovascular causes and it would have been very difficult to discern a clofibrate-associated risk of death due to noncardiovascular causes if it existed. Both studies demonstrated that clofibrate users have twice the risk of developing cholelithiasis and cholecystitis requiring surgery as do nonusers.

A potential benefit of clofibrate was, however, reported in the WHO study which involved patients with hypercholesterolemia and no history of myocardial infarction or angina pectoris. In this study, there was noted a statistically significant 25% decrease in subsequent nonfatal myocardial infarctions in the clofibrate-treated group when compared with the placebo group. There was no difference in incidence of fatal myocardial infarction in the two groups. If the study had been continued longer, had included diet, had been restricted to patients who had both hyperlipidemia and increased risk factors *and* who obtained significant clofibrate-induced reduction in serum lipids, it is possible that it may have shown a decrease in fatal myocardial infarctions. In the Coronary Drug Project study, which involved patients with or without hypercholesterolemia and/or hypertriglyceridemia and with a history of previous myocardial infarction, there was no significant difference in incidence of either nonfatal or fatal myocardial infarction between the clofibrate- and placebo-treated groups.[2]

As a result of these and other studies, the following can be stated:

1. Clofibrate, in general, causes a relatively modest reduction of serum cholesterol and a somewhat greater reduction of serum triglycerides. In Type III hyperlipidemia, however, substantial reductions of both cholesterol and triglycerides can occur with use of clofibrate.
2. No study to date has shown a convincing reduction in incidence of *fatal* myocardial infarction.
3. A significantly increased incidence of cholelithiasis has been demonstrated consistently in clofibrate-treated groups, and an increase in morbidity from this complication and mortality from cholecystectomy must be anticipated during clofibrate treatment.
4. Several types of other undesirable events have been associated in a statistically significant way with clofibrate administration in the WHO or the Coronary Drug Project studies. There was an increase in incidence of noncardiovascular deaths reported in the WHO study. There was an increase in cardiac arrhythmias and intermittent claudication and in definite or suspected thromboembolic events and angina reported in the Coronary Drug Project, which was not, however, reported in the WHO study.
5. Administration of clofibrate to mice and rats in long-term studies at eight times the human dose, and to rats at five times the human dose, resulted in a higher incidence of benign and malignant liver tumors than in controls. Lower doses were not included in these studies.

BECAUSE OF THE HEPATIC TUMORIGENICITY OF CLOFIBRATE IN RODENTS AND THE POSSIBLE INCREASED RISK OF MALIGNANCY ASSOCIATED WITH CLOFIBRATE IN THE HUMAN, AS WELL AS THE INCREASED RISK OF CHOLELITHIASIS, AND BECAUSE THERE IS NOT, TO DATE, SUBSTANTIAL EVIDENCE OF A BENEFICIAL EFFECT ON CARDIOVASCULAR MORTALITY FROM CLOFIBRATE, THIS DRUG SHOULD BE UTILIZED ONLY FOR THOSE PATIENTS DESCRIBED IN THE INDICATIONS SECTION, AND SHOULD BE DISCONTINUED IF SIGNIFICANT LIPID RESPONSE IS NOT OBTAINED.

Concomitant Anticoagulants
CAUTION SHOULD BE EXERCISED WHEN ANTICOAGULANTS ARE GIVEN IN CONJUNCTION WITH ATROMID-S (CLOFIBRATE). THE DOSAGE OF THE ANTICOAGULANT SHOULD BE REDUCED USUALLY BY ONE-HALF (DEPENDING ON THE INDIVIDUAL CASE) TO MAINTAIN THE PROTHROMBIN TIME AT THE DESIRED LEVEL TO PREVENT BLEEDING COMPLICATIONS. FREQUENT PROTHROMBIN DETERMINATIONS ARE ADVISABLE UNTIL IT HAS BEEN DEFINITELY DETERMINED THAT THE PROTHROMBIN LEVEL HAS BEEN STABILIZED.

Avoidance of Pregnancy
Strict birth control procedures must be exercised by women of childbearing potential. In patients who plan to become pregnant, clofibrate should be withdrawn several months before conception. Because of the possibility of pregnancy occurring despite birth control precautions in patients taking clofibrate, the possible benefits of the drug to the patient must be weighed against possible hazards to the fetus.

Precautions: Before instituting therapy with clofibrate, attempts should be made to control serum lipids with appropriate dietary regimens, weight loss in obese patients, control of diabetes mellitus, etc.

Because of the long-term administration of a drug of this nature, adequate baseline studies should be performed to determine that the patient has significantly elevated serum lipid levels. Frequent determinations of serum lipids should be obtained during the first few months of ATROMID-S (clofibrate) administration, and periodic determinations thereafter. The drug should be withdrawn after three months if response is inadequate. However, in the case of xanthoma tuberosum, the drug should be employed for longer periods (even up to one year) provided that there is a reduction in the size and/or number of the xanthomata.

Subsequent serum lipid determinations should be done to detect a paradoxical rise in serum cholesterol or triglyceride levels. Clofibrate will not alter the seasonal variations of serum cholesterol peak elevations in midwinter and late summer and decreases in fall and spring. If the drug is discontinued, the patient should be continued on an appropriate hypolipidemic diet, and his serum lipids should be monitored until stabilized, as a rise in these values to or above the original baseline may occur.

During clofibrate therapy, frequent serum transaminase determinations and other liver function tests should be performed since the drug may produce abnormalities in these parameters. These effects are usually reversible when the drug is discontinued. Hepatic biopsies are usually within normal limits. If the hepatic function tests steadily rise or show excessive abnormalities, the drug should be withdrawn. Therefore use with caution in those patients with a past history of jaundice or hepatic disease.

Since cholelithiasis is a possible side effect of clofibrate therapy, appropriate diagnostic procedures should be performed if signs and symptoms related to disease of the biliary system should occur.

Clofibrate may produce "flu like" symptoms (muscular aching, soreness, cramping). The physician should differentiate this from actual viral and/or bacterial disease.

Use with caution in patients with peptic ulcer since reactivation has been reported. Whether this is drug-related is unknown.

Complete blood counts should be done periodically since anemia, and more frequently, leukopenia have been reported in patients who have been taking clofibrate.

Various cardiac arrhythmias have been reported with the use of clofibrate.

Several investigators have observed in their studies that clofibrate may produce a decrease in cholesterol linoleate but an increase in palmitoleate and oleate, the latter being considered atherogenic in experimental animals. The significance of this finding is unknown at this time.

Adverse Reactions: Of the pertinent reactions, the most common is nausea. Less frequently encountered gastrointestinal reactions are vomiting, loose stools, dyspepsia, flatulence, and abdominal distress. Reactions reported less often than gastrointestinal ones are headache, dizziness, and fatigue; muscle cramping, aching, and weakness; skin rash, urticaria, and pruritus; dry brittle hair, and alopecia.

Continued on next page

Ayerst—Cont.

The following reported adverse reactions are listed alphabetically by systems:
Cardiovascular
  Increased or decreased angina
  Cardiac arrhythmias
  Both swelling and phlebitis at site of xanthomas
Dermatologic
  Skin rash
  Alopecia
  Allergic reaction including urticaria
  Dry skin and dry brittle hair
  Puritus
Gastrointestinal
  Nausea
  Diarrhea
  Gastrointestinal upset (bloating, flatulence, abdominal distress)
  Hepatomegaly (not associated with hepatotoxicity)
  Gallstones
  Vomiting
  Stomatitis and gastritis
Genitourinary
  Impotence and decreased libido
  Findings consistent with renal dysfunction as evidenced by dysuria, hematuria, proteinuria, decreased urine output, One patient's renal biopsy suggested "allergic reaction."
Hematologic
  Leukopenia
  Potentiation of anticoagulant effect
  Anemia
  Eosinophilia
Musculoskeletal
  Myalgia (muscle cramping, aching, weakness)
  "Flu like" symptoms
  Arthralgia
Neurologic
  Fatigue, weakness, drowsiness
  Dizziness
  Headache
Miscellaneous
  Weight gain
  Polyphagia
Laboratory Findings
  Abnormal liver function tests as evidenced by increased transaminase (SGOT and SGPT), BSP retention, and increased thymol turbidity
  Proteinuria
  Increased creatine phosphokinase

Reported adverse reactions whose direct relationship with the drug has not been established: peptic ulcer, gastrointestinal hemorrhage, rheumatoid arthritis, tremors, increased perspiration, systemic lupus erythematosus, blurred vision, gynecomastia, thrombocytopenic purpura.

Dosage and Administration:
Initial: The recommended dosage for adults is 2 g daily in divided doses. Some patients may respond to a lower dosage.
Maintenance: Same as for initial dosage.
Note: In children, insufficient studies have been done to show safety and efficacy.

Drug Interactions: Caution should be exercised when anticoagulants are given in conjunction with ATROMID-S (clofibrate). The dosage of the anticoagulant should be reduced usually by one-half (depending on the individual case) to maintain the prothrombin time at the desired level to prevent bleeding complications. Frequent prothrombin determinations are advisable until it has been definitely determined that the prothrombin level has been stabilized.

Management of Overdosage: While there has been no reported case of overdosage, should it occur, symptomatic supportive measures should be taken.

How Supplied: ATROMID-S—Each capsule contains 500 mg clofibrate, in bottles of 100 (NDC 0046-0243-81).

References:
1. Coronary Risk Handbook (1973), American Heart Association.
2. Report from the Committee of Principal Investigators: A cooperative trial in the primary prevention of ischaemic heart disease using clofibrate, Br. Heart J. *40:*1069, 1978.
3. The Coronary Drug Project Research Group: Clofibrate and niacin in coronary heart disease, J.A.M.A. *231:*360, 1975.

Shown in Product Identification Section, page 404

AURALGAN® Otic Solution ℞
[aw-răl'gan]

Each ml contains:
  Antipyrine .... 54.0 mg
  Benzocaine .... 14.0 mg
  Glycerin dehydrated q.s. to .... 1.0 ml
  (contains not more than 0.6% moisture)
  (also contains oxyquinoline sulfate)

TOPICAL DECONGESTANT AND ANALGESIC
AURALGAN is an otic solution containing antipyrine, benzocaine, and dehydrated glycerin. The solution congeals at 0° C (32° F), but returns to normal consistency, unchanged, at room temperature.

Clinical Pharmacology: AURALGAN combines the hygroscopic property of dehydrated glycerin with the analgesic action of antipyrine and benzocaine to relieve pressure, reduce inflammation and congestion, and alleviate pain and discomfort in acute otitis media.
AURALGAN does not blanch the tympanic membrane or mask the landmarks and, therefore, does not distort the otoscopic picture.

Indications and Usage: *Acute otitis media of various etiologies*
  — prompt relief of pain and reduction of inflammation in the congestive and serous stages
  — adjuvant therapy during systemic antibiotic administration for resolution of the infection
Because of the close anatomical relationship of the eustachian tube to the nasal cavity, otitis media is a frequent problem, especially in children in whom the tube is shorter, wider, and more horizontal than in adults.
Removal of cerumen
  —facilitates the removal of excessive or impacted cerumen.

Contraindications: Hypersensitivity to any of the components or substances related to them.
In the presence of spontaneous perforation or discharge.

Precautions: *Carcinogenesis, Mutagenesis, Impairment of Fertility:* No long-term studies in animals or humans have been conducted. *Pregnancy Category C:* Animal reproduction studies have not been conducted with AURALGAN. It is also not known whether AURALGAN can cause fetal harm when administered to a pregnant woman, or can affect reproduction capacity. AURALGAN should be given to a pregnant woman only if clearly needed.
Nursing Mothers: It is not known whether this drug is excreted in human milk. Because many drugs are excreted in human milk, caution should be exercised when AURALGAN is administered to a nursing woman.

Dosage and Administration: *Acute otitis media:* Instill AURALGAN, permitting the solution to run along the wall of the canal until it is filled. Avoid touching the ear with dropper. Then moisten a cotton pledget with AURALGAN and insert into meatus. Repeat every one to two hours until pain and congestion are relieved.
Removal of cerumen
Before: Instill AURALGAN three times daily for two or three days to help detach cerumen from wall of canal and facilitate removal.
After: AURALGAN is useful for drying out the canal or relieving discomfort.
Before and after removal of cerumen, a cotton pledget moistened with AURALGAN should be inserted into the meatus following instillation.
NOTE: Do not rinse dropper after use. Replace in bottle and screw cap tightly.

How Supplied: AURALGAN® Otic Solution, in package containing 15 ml (½ fl oz) bottle with separate dropper-screw cap attachment (NDC 0046-1000-15).

AYGESTIN® ℞
[ā-jĕs'tĭn]
Brand of norethindrone acetate tablets, U.S.P.

WARNING:
THE USE OF PROGESTATIONAL AGENTS DURING THE FIRST FOUR MONTHS OF PREGNANCY IS NOT RECOMMENDED. Progestational agents have been used beginning with the first trimester of pregnancy in an attempt to prevent habitual abortion or treat threatened abortion. There is no adequate evidence that such use is effective and there is evidence of potential harm to the fetus when such drugs are given during the first four months of pregnancy. Furthermore, in the vast majority of women, the cause of abortion is a defective ovum, which progestational agents could not be expected to influence. In addition, the use of progestational agents with their uterine-relaxant properties, in patients with fertilized defective ova may cause a delay in spontaneous abortion. Therefore, the use of such drugs during the first four months of pregnancy is not recommended. Several reports suggest an association between intrauterine exposure to female sex hormones and congenital anomalies, including congenital heart defects and limb reduction defects.[1-5] One study[4] estimated a 4.7-fold increased risk of limb reduction defects in infants exposed in utero to sex hormones (oral contraceptives, hormone withdrawal tests for pregnancy, or attempted treatment for threatened abortion). Some of these exposures were very short and involved only a few days of treatment. The data suggest that the risk of limb reduction defects in exposed fetuses is somewhat less than 1 in 1,000 if the patient is exposed to AYGESTIN® (norethindrone acetate tablets, U.S.P.) during the first four months of pregnancy or if she becomes pregnant while taking this drug, she should be apprised of the potential risks to the fetus.

Description:
AYGESTIN®
(norethindrone acetate tablets, U.S.P.)—
5 mg oral tablets.
AYGESTIN, (17-hydroxy-19-nor-17α-pregn-4-en-20-yn-3-one acetate), a synthetic, orally active progestin, is the acetic acid ester of norethindrone. On a weight basis it is twice as potent as norethindrone. It is a white, or creamy white, crystalline powder.

Actions: Norethindrone acetate induces secretory changes in an estrogen-primed endometrium. It acts to inhibit the secretion of pituitary gonadotropins which, in turn, prevent follicular maturation and ovulation.

Indications: AYGESTIN is indicated for the treatment of secondary amenorrhea, endometriosis, and abnormal uterine bleeding due to hormonal imbalance in the absence of organic pathology such as submucous fibroids or uterine cancer.

Contraindications: Thrombophlebitis, thromboembolic disorders, cerebral apoplexy, or a past history of these conditions. Markedly impaired liver function or liver disease.
Known or suspected carcinoma of the breast
Undiagnosed vaginal bleeding
Missed abortion

As a diagnostic test for pregnancy

Warnings:
1. Discontinue medication pending examination if there is a sudden partial or complete loss of vision, or if there is sudden onset of proptosis, diplopia, or migraine. If examination reveals papilledema or retinal vascular lesions, medication should be withdrawn.
2. Detectable amounts of progestogens have been identified in the milk of mothers receiving them. The effect of this on the nursing infant has not been determined.
3. Because of the occasional occurrence of thrombophlebitis and pulmonary embolism in patients taking progestogens, the physician should be alert to the earliest manifestations of the disease.
4. Masculinization of the female fetus has occurred when progestogens have been used in pregnant women.
5. Some beagle dogs treated with medroxy-progesterone acetate developed mammary nodules. Although nodules occasionally appeared in control animals, they were intermittent in nature, whereas nodules in treated animals were larger and more numerous, and persisted. There is no general agreement as to whether the nodules are benign or malignant. Their significance with respect to humans has not been established.

Precautions:
A. General Precautions
1. The pretreatment physical examination should include special reference to breasts and pelvic organs, as well as a Papanicolaou smear.
2. Because this drug may cause some degree of fluid retention, conditions which might be influenced by this factor, such as epilepsy, migraine, asthma, cardiac or renal dysfunctions, require careful observation.
3. In cases of breakthrough bleeding, as in all cases of irregular bleeding per vaginam, nonfunctional causes should be borne in mind. In cases of undiagnosed vaginal bleeding, adequate diagnostic measures are indicated.
4. Patients who have a history of psychic depression should be carefully observed and the drug discontinued if the depression recurs to a serious degree.
5. Any possible influence of prolonged progestogen therapy on pituitary, ovarian, adrenal, hepatic, or uterine functions awaits further study.
6. A decrease in glucose tolerance has been observed in a small percentage of patients on estrogen-progestogen combination drugs. The mechanism of this decrease is obscure. For this reason, diabetic patients should be carefully observed while receiving progestogen therapy.
7. The age of the patient constitutes no absolute limiting factor, although treatment with progestogens may mask the onset of the climacteric.
8. The pathologist should be advised of progestogen therapy when relevant specimens are submitted.
B. Information for the Patient. See text which appears after REFERENCES.

Adverse Reactions: The following adverse reactions have been observed in women taking progestins:
breakthrough bleeding
spotting
change in menstrual flow
amenorrhea
edema
changes in weight (decreases, increases)
changes in cervical erosion and cervical secretions
cholestatic jaundice
rash (allergic) with and without pruritus
melasma or chloasma
mental depression

Progestins may alter the result of pregnanediol determinations. The following laboratory results may be altered by the concomitant use of estrogens with progestins:
hepatic function
coagulation tests—increase in prothrombin, factors VII, VIII, IX, and X
increase in PBI, BEI, and a decrease in T^3 uptake
metyrapone test

A statistically significant association has been demonstrated between use of estrogen-progestogen combination drugs and the following serious adverse reactions: thrombophlebitis, pulmonary embolism, and cerebral thrombosis and embolism. For this reason, patients on progestogen therapy should be carefully observed. Although available evidence is suggestive of an association, such a relationship has been neither confirmed nor refuted for the following serious adverse reactions: Neuro-ocular lesions, *e.g.*, retinal thrombosis and optic neuritis.

The following adverse reactions have been observed in patients receiving estrogen-progestogen combination drugs.
1. Rise in blood pressure in susceptible individuals
2. Premenstrual-like syndrome
3. Changes in libido
4. Changes in appetite
5. Cystitis-like syndrome
6. Headache
7. Nervousness
8. Dizziness
9. Fatigue
10. Backache
11. Hirsutism
12. Loss of scalp hair
13. Erythema multiforme
14. Erythema nodosum
15. Hemorrhagic eruption
16. Itching

In view of these observations, patients on progestogen therapy should be carefully observed.

Dosage and Administration: *Therapy with AYGESTIN® must be adapted to the specific indications and therapeutic response of the individual patient.* This dosage schedule assumes the interval between menses to be 28 days.

Secondary amenorrhea, abnormal uterine bleeding due to hormonal imbalance in the absence of organic pathology: 2.5 to 10 mg AYGESTIN may be given daily for from 5 to 10 days during the second half of the theoretical menstrual cycle to produce an optimum secretory transformation of an endometrium that has been adequately primed with either endogenous or exogenous estrogen.

Progestin withdrawal bleeding usually occurs within three to seven days after discontinuing AYGESTIN therapy. Patients with a past history of recurrent episodes of abnormal uterine bleeding may benefit from planned menstrual cycling with AYGESTIN.

Endometriosis:
Initial daily dosage of 5 mg AYGESTIN for two weeks. Dosage should be increased by 2.5 mg per day every two weeks until 15 mg per day of AYGESTIN is reached. Therapy may be held at this level for six to nine months or until annoying breakthrough bleeding demands temporary termination.

How Supplied: Each scored AYGESTIN tablet contains 5 mg norethindrone acetate, U.S.P., in bottles of 50 (NDC 0046-0894-50). Also available in Cycle Packs of 10 (0046-0894-10).

Physician References:
1. Gal I, Kirman B, Stern J: Hormonal pregnancy tests and congenital malformation. Nature 216:83, 1967.
2. Levy EP, Cohen A, Fraser FC: Hormone treatment during pregnancy and congenital heart defects. Lancet 1:611, 1973.
3. Nora JJ, Nora AH: Birth defects and oral contraceptives. Lancet 1:941-942, 1973.
4. Janerich DT, Piper JM, Glebatis DM: Oral contraceptives and congenital limb-reduction defects. N Engl J Med 291:697-700, 1974.
5. Hernonen OP, Stone D, Monson RR, et al: Cardiovascular birth defects and antenatal exposure to female sex hormones. N Engl J Med 296:67-70, 1977.

Information for the Patient: Your doctor has prescribed AYGESTIN® (norethindrone acetate tablets, U.S.P.), a progestin, for you. AYGESTIN is similar to the progesterone hormones naturally produced by the body. Progestins are used to treat menstrual disorders and to test if the body is producing certain hormones.

Warning: There is an increased risk of birth defects in children whose mothers take this drug during the first four months of pregnancy.

Progestins have been used as a test for pregnancy but such use is no longer considered safe because of possible damage to a developing baby. Also, more rapid methods for testing for pregnancy are now available.

These drugs have also been used to prevent miscarriage in the first few months of pregnancy. No adequate evidence is available to show that they are effective for this purpose and there is evidence of an increased risk of birth defects, such as heart or limb defects, if these drugs are taken during the first four months of pregnancy. Furthermore, most cases of early miscarriage are due to causes which could not be helped by these drugs.

The exact risk of taking these drugs early in pregnancy and having a baby with a birth defect is not known. However, one study found that babies born to women who had taken sex hormones (such as progesterone-like drugs) during the first three months of pregnancy were 4 to 5 times more likely to have abnormalities of the arms or legs than if their mothers had not taken such drugs. Some of these women had taken these drugs for only a few days. The chance that an infant whose mother had taken this drug will have this type of defect is about 1 in 1,000. If you take AYGESTIN (norethindrone acetate tablets, U.S.P.) and later find you were pregnant when you took it, be sure to discuss this with your doctor as soon as possible.

How Supplied: AYGESTIN® (norethindrone acetate tablets, U.S.P.)—scored 5 mg tablets, in bottles of 50, for oral administration. Also available in Cycle Packs of 10.

Shown in Product Identification Section, page 404

BEMINAL® 500
[bē'min-awl]
High potency vitamin supplement
vitamin B complex with 500 mg vitamin C

Each tablet contains:		% US RDA*
Thiamine mononitrate (Vit. B_1)	25.0 mg	1717%
Riboflavin (Vit. B_2)	12.5 mg	735%
Niacinamide (Vit. B_3) as niacinamide ascorbate	100.0 mg	500%
Pyridoxine hydrochloride (Vit. B_6)	10.0 mg	500%
Calcium pantothenate	20.0 mg	92%
Ascorbic acid (Vit. C) as ascorbic acid and niacinamide ascorbate	500.0 mg	833%
Cyanocobalamin (Vit. B_{12})	5.0 mcg	83%

Does not contain saccharin or other sweeteners.
*US Recommended Daily Allowance

Dosage: 12-year-olds and over, one tablet daily.
How Supplied: BEMINAL-500 Tablets, in bottles of 100 (NDC 0046-0830-81).

Shown in Product Identification Section, page 404

BEMINAL® FORTE
[bē'min-awl]
with VITAMIN C
High potency vitamin supplement
vitamin B complex with vitamin C

Each capsule contains:		% US RDA*
Thiamine mononitrate (Vit. B_1)	25.0 mg	1717%
Riboflavin (Vit. B_2)	12.5 mg	735%
Niacinamide (Vit. B_3) as niacinamide ascorbate	50.0 mg	250%
Pyridoxine HCl (Vit. B_6)	3.0 mg	150%
Calcium pantothenate	10.0 mg	46%
Ascorbic acid (Vit. C) as ascorbic acid and niacinamide ascorbate	250.0 mg	417%
Cyanocobalamin (Vit. B_{12})	2.5 mcg	42%

*U.S. Recommended Daily Allowance

Continued on next page

Ayerst—Cont.

Dosage: 12-year-olds and over, 1 capsule daily.
How Supplied: BEMINAL Forte with Vitamin C Capsules, in bottles of 100 (NDC 0046-0817-81).

BEMINAL STRESS PLUS™
[bē' mĭn-awl]
Stress potency replacement vitamins

BEMINAL STRESS PLUS™ with IRON

Each tablet contains:	% U.S. RDA*
Vitamin B1 as thiamine mononitrate, U.S.P., 25.0 mg	1717%
Vitamin B2 as riboflavin, U.S.P., 12.5 mg	735%
Vitamin B3 as niacinamide, 100.0 mg	504%
Vitamin B5 as calcium pantothenate, U.S.P., 20.0 mg	184%
Vitamin B6 as pyridoxine hydrochloride, U.S.P., 10.0 mg	411%
Vitamin B12 as cyanocobalamin, 25.0 mcg	417%
Vitamin Bc as folic acid, U.S.P., 400.0 mcg	100%
Vitamin C as sodium ascorbate, U.S.P., 787.0 mg	1166%
Vitamin E as dl-a-tocopheryl acetate, 45.0 I.U.	150%
Iron as ferrous fumarate, U.S.P., 82.2 mg	150%

*percentage of U.S. recommended daily allowance

BEMINAL STRESS PLUS™ with ZINC

Each tablet contains:	% U.S. RDA*
Vitamin B1 as thiamine mononitrate, U.S.P., 25.0 mg	1717%
Vitamin B2 as riboflavin, U.S.P., 12.5 mg	735%
Vitamin B3 as niacinamide, 100.0 mg	504%
Vitamin B5 as calcium pantothenate, U.S.P., 20.0 mg	184%
Vitamin B6 as pyridoxine hydrochloride, U.S.P., 10.0 mg	411%
Vitamin B12 as cyanocobalamin, 25.0 mcg	417%
Vitamin C as sodium ascorbate, U.S.P., 787.0 mg	1166%
Vitamin E as dl-a-tocopheryl acetate, 45.0 I.U.	150%
Zinc as zinc sulfate, 111.1 mg	300%

*percentage of U.S. recommended daily allowance
Indication: Dietary supplement.
Action and Uses: The BEMINAL STRESS PLUS formulas can help replenish the vitamins and minerals depleted by the stress of sickness, infections, and surgery. BEMINAL STRESS PLUS formulas may also be used where the demand on the body's store of vitamins and minerals may be increased by dieting, lack of sleep, the use of alcohol or cigarettes, jogging and other strenuous physical exercise.
Recommended Intake: *Adults,* one tablet daily.
How Supplied: BEMINAL STRESS PLUS with Iron—bottles of 60 tablets. BEMINAL STRESS PLUS with Zinc—bottles of 60 tablets.
Shown in Product Identification Section, page 404

CLUSIVOL® SYRUP
[klū'sĭ-vawl]
Vitamin supplement with minerals
Syrup for children and adults

Each 5 ml (1 teaspoonful) contains:	Percent US RDA*
Vitamin A (as palmitate)...2,500 U.S.P. Units	50
Cholecalciferol (Vit. D3)... 400 U.S.P. Units	100
Ascorbic acid (Vit. C)...... 15.0 mg	25
Cyanocobalamin (Vit. B12)...... 2.0 mcg	33
Thiamine HCl (Vit. B1)...... 1.0 mg	67
Riboflavin (Vit. B2)...... 1.0 mg	59
Niacinamide (Vit. B3)...... 5.0 mg	25
d-Panthenol...... 3.0 mg	32
Pyridoxine HCl (Vit. B6)...... 0.6 mg	30
Manganese†...... 0.5 mg	***
Zinc†...... 0.5 mg	3.3
Magnesium†...... 3.0 mg	**

†Supplied as the gluconates of manganese and magnesium, and zinc lactate.
*US Recommended Daily Allowance.
**Contains less than 2% US RDA.
*** US RDA not established.

A comprehensive nutritional formula incorporating essential fat- and water-soluble vitamins together with important minerals. Presented in a candy-flavored syrup base; particularly appealing to children, but also enjoyed by older individuals who prefer a liquid preparation.
Action and Uses: A vitamin and mineral supplement for better health for the entire family.
Dosage: *Children and Adults:* One teaspoonful (5 ml) daily.
How Supplied: CLUSIVOL Syrup, in bottles of 8 fl oz (½ pint) (NDC 0046-0920-08), and 16 fl oz (1 pint) (NDC 0046-0920-16).

CLUSIVOL® Tablet/Capsule
[klū'sĭ-vawl]
High potency vitamin supplement with minerals
Tablets for 12-year-olds and older

Each tablet contains:	% US RDA*
Vitamin A...... 10,000 U.S.P. Units (as palmitate)	200
Ergocalciferol... 400 U.S.P. Units (Vit. D2)	100
Ascorbic acid(Vit.C) 150.0 mg (as sodium ascorbate)	250
Thiamine mononitrate (Vit. B1)... 10.0 mg	687
Riboflavin (Vit. B2)... 5.0 mg	294
Pyridoxine HCl (Vit. B6)... 0.5 mg	25
d-Panthenol...... 1.0 mg	10.7
Cyanocobalamin (Vit. B12)... 2.5 mcg	42
Niacinamide...... 50.0 mg	250
Vitamin E†...... 0.5 I.U.	**
Iron†...... 15.0 mg	83
Calcium†...... 120.0 mg	12
Manganese†...... 0.5 mg	***
Zinc†...... 0.6 mg	4
Magnesium†...... 3.0 mg	**

†Supplied as dl-a-tocopheryl acetate, ferrous fumarate, calcium carbonate, manganese gluconate, zinc oxide, and magnesium oxide.
*US Recommended Daily Allowance
**Contains less than 2% US RDA
***US RDA not established

CLUSIVOL® Capsules
High potency vitamin supplement with minerals
Capsules for 12-year-olds and older

Each capsule contains:	% US RDA*
Vitamin A...... 10,000 U.S.P. Units (as palmitate)	200
Ergocalciferol......400 U.S.P. Units (Vit. D2)	100
Ascorbic acid(Vit.C) 150.0 mg (as sodium ascorbate)	250
Thiamine mononitrate (Vit. B1)... 10.0 mg	687
Riboflavin (Vit. B2)... 5.0 mg	294
Pyridoxine HCl (Vit. B6)... 0.5 mg	25
d-Panthenol...... 1.0 mg	10.7
Cyanocobalamin (Vit. B12)... 2.5 mcg	42
Niacinamide...... 50.0 mg	250
Vitamin E†...... 0.5 I.U.	**
Iron†...... 15.0 mg	83
Calcium†...... 120.0 mg	12
Manganese†...... 0.5 mg	***
Zinc†...... 0.6 mg	4
Magnesium†...... 3.0 mg	**

†Supplied as d-a-tocopheryl acetate concentrate, ferrous sulfate, calcium carbonate, manganous sulfate, zinc sulfate, and magnesium sulfate.
*US Recommended Daily Allowance
**Contains less than 2% US RDA
***US RDA not established.

Dosage and Administration: One tablet (capsule) daily.
How Supplied: CLUSIVOL 130, bottle of 130 tablets (NDC 0046-0270-81). CLUSIVOL Capsules, bottle of 100 (NDC 0046-0293-81).

DERMOPLAST® Aerosol Spray
[der' mō-plăst]
Topical anesthetic and antipruritic

Contains (exclusive of propellants) 20% benzocaine and 0.5% menthol in a water-dispersible base of TWEEN® 85 and polyethylene glycol 400 monolaurate with methylparaben as a preservative.
A topical anesthetic and antipruritic spray providing soothing, temporary relief of skin pain, itching, and discomfort due to episiotomy, pruritus vulvae, postpartum hemorrhoids, sunburn, abrasions, minor cuts, burns, and insect bites. May be applied without touching sensitive affected areas.
Warnings: FOR EXTERNAL USE ONLY. Avoid spraying in eyes. Contents under pressure. Do not puncture or incinerate. Do not expose to heat or temperatures above 120° F. Do not use near open flame. Use only as directed. Intentional misuse by deliberately concentrating and inhaling the contents can be harmful or fatal.
Do not take orally. Not for prolonged use. If the condition for which this preparation is used persists or if a rash or irritation develops, discontinue use and consult physician.
Directions for Use: Hold can in a comfortable position 6-12 inches away from affected area. Point spray nozzle and press button. To apply to face, spray in palm of hand. May be administered three or four times daily, or as directed by physician.
How Supplied: DERMOPLAST Aerosol Spray, in Net Wt 3 oz (85 g)—NDC 0046-1008-03; and in Net Wt 6 oz (170 g)—NDC 0046-1008-06.

DIUCARDIN® ℞
[dī"ū-car'din]
Brand of hydroflumethiazide
A diuretic-antihypertensive agent

CAUTION: Federal law prohibits dispensing without prescription.
Description: DIUCARDIN® (hydroflumethiazide) is an oral thiazide (benzothiadiazide) diuretic-antihypertensive agent.
DIUCARDIN is available in 50 mg tablets.
Chemical name: 3,4-Dihydro-6-(trifluoromethyl)-2H-1,2,4-benzothiadiazine-7-sulfonamide 1,1-dioxide.
Structural formula:

Hydroflumethiazide is an odorless white to cream colored, finely divided, crystalline powder. It has a melting point between 270° and 275° C. Hydroflumethiazide is freely soluble in acetone, soluble in alcohol, and slightly soluble in water.
Clinical Pharmacology: DIUCARDIN is a thiazide diuretic and antihypertensive. DIUCARDIN affects the renal tubular mechanism of electrolyte reabsorption. At maximal therapeutic dosage all thiazides are approximately equal in their diuretic potency.

DIUCARDIN increases excretion of sodium and chloride in approximately equivalent amounts. Natriuresis causes a secondary loss of potassium and bicarbonate.

The mechanism of the antihypertensive effect of DIUCARDIN is unknown. DIUCARDIN does not affect normal blood pressure.

Onset of action of DIUCARDIN occurs in two hours and the peak effect at about four hours. Its action persists for approximately 6 to 12 hours. Thiazides are eliminated rapidly by the kidney.

Indications and Usage: DIUCARDIN is indicated as adjunctive therapy in edema associated with congestive heart failure, hepatic cirrhosis and corticosteroid and estrogen therapy.

DIUCARDIN has also been found useful in edema due to various forms of renal dysfunction as: nephrotic syndrome; acute glomerulonephritis; and chronic renal failure.

DIUCARDIN is indicated in the management of hypertension either as the sole therapeutic agent or to enhance the effect of other antihypertensive drugs in the more severe forms of hypertension.

Usage in Pregnancy: The routine use of diuretics in an otherwise healthy woman is inappropriate and exposes mother and fetus to unnecessary hazard. Diuretics do not prevent development of toxemia of pregnancy, and there is no satisfactory evidence that they are useful in the treatment of developed toxemia.

Edema during pregnancy may arise from pathological causes or from the physiologic and mechanical consequences of pregnancy. Thiazides are indicated in pregnancy when edema is due to pathologic causes just as they are in the absence of pregnancy (however, see Warnings, below). Dependent edema in pregnancy, resulting from restriction of venous return by the expanded uterus, is properly treated through elevation of the lower extremities and use of support hose. Use of diuretics to lower intravascular volume in this case is illogical and unnecessary. There is hypervolemia during normal pregnancy which is harmful to neither the fetus nor the mother (in absence of cardiovascular disease), but which is associated with edema, including generalized edema, in the majority of pregnant women. If this edema produces discomfort, increased recumbency will often provide relief. In rare instances, this edema may cause extreme discomfort which is not relieved by rest. In these cases, a short course of diuretics may provide relief and may be appropriate.

Contraindications: Anuria.

Hypersensitivity to this or other sulfonamide-derived drugs.

Warnings: Thiazides should be used with caution in severe renal disease. In patients with renal disease, thiazides may precipitate azotemia. Cumulative effects of the drug may develop in patients with impaired renal function.

Thiazides should be used with caution in patients with impaired hepatic function or progressive liver disease, since minor alterations of fluid and electrolyte balance may precipitate hepatic coma.

Thiazides may add to or potentiate the action of other antihypertensive drugs. Potentiation occurs with ganglionic or peripheral adrenergic blocking drugs.

Sensitivity reactions may occur in patients with or without a history of allergy or bronchial asthma. The possibility of exacerbation or activation of systemic lupus erythematosus has been reported.

DIUCARDIN (hydroflumethiazide) can cause fetal harm when administered to a pregnant woman. Thiazides cross the placental barrier and appear in cord blood. Hazards to the fetus include fetal or neonatal jaundice, thrombocytopenia, and possibly other adverse reactions which have occurred in the adult. If this drug is used during pregnancy, or if the patient becomes pregnant while taking this drug, the patient should be apprised of the potential hazard to the fetus.

Lithium generally should not be given with diuretics because they reduce its renal clearance and add a high risk of lithium toxicity. Refer to the package insert on lithium before use of such concomitant therapy.

Precautions:
General:
Periodic determination of serum electrolytes to detect possible electrolyte imbalance should be performed at appropriate intervals.

All patients receiving thiazide therapy should be observed for clinical signs of fluid or electrolyte imbalance: namely, hyponatremia, hypochloremic alkalosis, and hypokalemia. Serum and urine electrolyte determinations are particularly important when the patient is vomiting excessively or receiving parenteral fluids. Medication such as digitalis may also influence serum electrolytes. Warning signs, irrespective of cause are: dryness of mouth, thirst, weakness, lethargy, drowsiness, restlessness, muscle pains or cramps, muscular fatigue, hypotension, oliguria, tachycardia, and gastrointestinal disturbances such as nausea and vomiting.

Hypokalemia may develop, especially with brisk diuresis, when severe cirrhosis is present, or during concomitant use of corticosteroids or ACTH. Interference with adequate oral electrolyte intake will also contribute to hypokalemia. Hypokalemia can sensitize or exaggerate the response of the heart to the toxic effects of digitalis (*e.g.*, increased ventricular irritability). Concurrent administration of a potassium sparing diuretic or potassium supplements may be indicated in these patients.

Any chloride deficit is generally mild and usually does not require specific treatment except under extraordinary circumstances (as in liver disease or renal disease). Dilutional hyponatremia may occur in edematous patients in hot weather; appropriate therapy is water restriction, rather than administration of salt, except in rare instances when the hyponatremia is life-threatening. In actual salt depletion, appropriate replacement is the therapy of choice.

Hyperuricemia may occur or frank gout may be precipitated in certain patients receiving thiazide therapy.

Diabetes mellitus which has been latent may become manifest during thiazide administration.

The antihypertensive effects of the drug may be enhanced in the postsympathectomy patient.

If progressive renal impairment becomes evident, consider withholding or discontinuing diuretic therapy.

Drug Interactions: Insulin requirements in diabetic patients may be increased, decreased or unchanged.

Thiazide drugs may increase the responsiveness to tubocurarine.

Thiazides may decrease aterial responsiveness to nonepinephrine. This diminution is not sufficient to preclude effectiveness of the pressor agent for therapeutic use.

Drug/laboratory test
Interactions: Thiazides may decrease serum PBI levels without signs of thyroid disturbance.

Calcium excretion is decreased by thiazides. Pathological changes in the parathyroid gland with hypercalcemia and hypophosphatemia have been observed in a few patients on prolonged thiazide therapy. The common complications of hyperparathyroidism such as renal lithiasis, bone resorption, and peptic ulceration have not been seen. Thiazides should be discontinued before carrying out tests for parathyroid function.

Carcinogenesis, mutagenesis, impairment of fertility: No long-term reproductive studies have been performed.

Pregnancy: *Teratogenic effects:* Pregnancy category D. See WARNINGS section.

Nonteratogenic effects: See WARNINGS section.

Nursing mothers: Thiazides appear in breast milk. If use of the drug is deemed essential, the patient should stop nursing.

Pediatric use: Safety and effectiveness in children have not been established.

Adverse Reactions:
Gastrointestinal System: anorexia, gastric irritation, nausea, vomiting, cramping, diarrhea, constipation, jaundice (intrahepatic cholestatic jaundice), pancreatitis, sialadenitis

Central Nervous System: dizziness, vertigo, paresthesias, headache, xanthopsia

Hematologic: leukopenia, agranulocytosis, thrombocytopenia, aplastic anemia, hemolytic anemia

Cardiovascular: orthostatic hypotension (may be aggravated by alcohol, barbiturates, or narcotics)

Hypersensitivity: purpura, photosensitivity, rash, urticaria, necrotizing angiitis (vasculitis, cutaneous vasculitis), fever, respiratory distress including pneumonitis, anaphylactic reactions

Other: hyperglycemia, glycosuria, hyperuricemia, muscle spasm, weakness, restlessness, transient blurred vision

Whenever adverse reactions are moderate or severe, thiazide dosage should be reduced or therapy withdrawn.

Overdosage: The following information is provided to serve as guidelines in treating overdosage.
HYDROFLUMETHIAZIDE
Signs and Symptoms:
Diuresis is to be expected; lethargy of varying degree may appear and may progress to coma within a few hours, with minimal depression of respiration and cardiovascular function, and without significant serum electrolyte changes or dehydration. The mechanism of CNS depression with thiazide overdosage is unknown.

G.I. irritation and hypermotility may occur; temporary elevation of BUN has been reported and serum electrolyte changes could occur, especially in patients with impairment of renal function.

Treatment:
Evacuate gastric contents but take care to prevent aspiration, especially in the stuporous or comatose patient. G.I. effects are usually of short duration, but may require symptomatic treatment.

Monitor serum electrolyte levels and renal function; institute supportive measures as required individually to maintain hydration, electrolyte balance, respiration, and cardiovascular-renal function.

DIUCARDIN (hydroflumethiazide) is slowly dialyzable.

Dosage and Administration: Therapy should be individualized according to patient response. Use the smallest dosage necessary to maintain the required response.

The usual daily dosages for antihypertensive and diuretic effect are:

Diuretic	Antihypertensive
Adult: 25 to 200 mg	50 to 100 mg

Dosage regimens using 25 mg DIUCARDIN may be adequate in some cases.

Dosage should not exceed 200 mg per day.

For Diuresis in the Adult:
Initial recommended dose is 50 mg once or twice a day. Daily maintenance dose may be as little as 25 mg or as much as 200 mg, depending on patient's response. With dosages in excess of 100 mg daily, it is generally preferable to administer DIUCARDIN in divided doses.

Many patients with edema respond to intermittent therapy, i.e., administration on alternate days or on three to five days each week. With an intermittent schedule, excessive response and the resulting undesirable electrolyte imbalance are less likely to occur.

For Control of Hypertension in the Adult:
Usual starting dose is 50 mg twice daily. Dosage is increased or decreased according to the blood pressure response of the patient. Usual maintenance dose is 50 mg to 100 mg per day. Dosage should not exceed 200 mg per day.

Careful observations for changes in blood pressure must be made when this compound is used with other antihypertensive drugs, especially during initial therapy. The dosage of other agents must be reduced by at least 50 percent as soon as it is added to the regimen to prevent excessive drop in blood pressure. As the blood pressure falls under the potentiating effect of this agent, a further reduc-

Continued on next page

Ayerst—Cont.

tion in dosage, or even discontinuation, of other antihypertensive drugs may be necessary.
How Supplied: DIUCARDIN—Each scored, white oval compressed tablet, inscribed "DIUCARDIN®50," contains 50 mg hydroflumethiazide, in bottles of 100 (NDC 0046-0702-81).
Store at room temperature (approximately 25° C).
Shown in Product Identification Section, page 404

ENZACTIN® Cream
[en-zăc'tin]
Brand of triacetin

Action: For prevention and treatment of athlete's foot and other superficial fungus infections. The "self-regulating" action of ENZACTIN (triacetin) releases a constant effective level of *free* fatty acid at the site of infection, in a concentration that is nonirritating.
"*Self-regulating*" *action*—At a neutral or higher pH of infected skin and in the presence of the enzyme esterase (found abundantly in skin, serum, and fungi), glycerol and free fatty acid (acetic) are rapidly liberated from triacetin. At this point, the growth of fungi is inhibited by the free acid.
With an accumulation of free acid, the pH drops and esterase activity decreases. Then, as the acid in the skin diffuses or becomes neutralized, the pH rises and esterase is reactivated, to release more free acid for fungistatic control.
Relieves itching and soreness promptly. Helps prevent spread of infection. Nonirritating. Odorless and stainless.
Indications: Athlete's foot and other superficial fungus infections.
Administration: Thoroughly cleanse affected and adjacent areas with dilute alcohol or a mild soap and warm water. Pat dry. Apply cream liberally twice daily, preferably morning and evening.
Note: Rayon fabrics should not come in contact with ENZACTIN (triacetin) Cream. For protection, cover treated areas with clean cotton cloth or bandage. If infection persists, consult a physician.
How Supplied: ENZACTIN *Cream*—250 mg triacetin per gram (in emollient base), in 1 oz (28.35 g) collapsible tubes (NDC 0046-0201-01).

Ayerst
EPITRATE® R
[ĕp'ĭ-trāt]
Brand of epinephrine bitartrate ophthalmic solution

Description: EPITRATE (epinephrine bitartrate) Ophthalmic Solution is a sterile aqueous solution of levorotatory epinephrine bitartrate, 2% (equivalent to 1.1% base). Inactive ingredients include chlorobutanol (chloral derivative) 0.55%, sodium bisulfite, sodium chloride, polyoxypropylene-polyoxyethylene-diol, and disodium edetate. Epinephrine bitartrate is an adrenergic agent with the chemical name (-)-3,4,-Dihydroxy-α-[(methylamino) methyl] benzyl alcohol (+) tartrate (1:1) salt. It has a low surface tension.
Clinical Pharmacology: EPITRATE lowers intraocular pressure by reducing the rate of aqueous formation. Improvement in outflow facility is also observed in certain cases following prolonged therapy.
Indications and Usage: Useful in management of chronic simple (open-angle) glaucoma, either alone or in combination with miotics. In selected cases, it may also be used with carbonic anhydrase inhibitors.
Contraindications: Prior to peripheral iridectomy, an epinephrine preparation is contraindicated in eyes that are capable of angle closure since its relatively weak mydriatic action may, nevertheless, precipitate angle block. Gonioscopy should be carried out on all patients before initiating therapy.
Warnings: Topical use of epinephrine in any form should be interrupted prior to general anesthesia with certain anesthetics such as cyclopropane or halothane which sensitize the myocardium to sympathomimetics.
Precautions: EPITRATE (epinephrine bitartrate) should be used with caution in the presence of hypertension, diabetes, hyperthyroidism, heart disease, and cerebral arteriosclerosis because of the possibility of systemic action.
Do not use the solution if it is brown or contains a precipitate.
Drug Interactions: See Warnings.
Carcinogenesis, Mutagenesis, Impairment of Fertility: No long-term studies in animals or humans have been conducted.
Pregnancy Category C: Animal reproduction studies have not been conducted with EPITRATE. It is also not known whether EPITRATE can cause fetal harm when administered to a pregnant woman or can affect reproduction capacity. EPITRATE should be given to a pregnant woman only if clearly needed.
Nursing Mothers: It is not known whether this drug is excreted in human milk. Because many drugs are excreted in human milk, caution should be exercised when EPITRATE is administered to a nursing woman.
Pediatric Use: Safety and effectiveness in children have not been established.
Adverse Reactions: As with other epinephrine solutions, transitory stinging on initial instillation may be expected. Headache or browache frequently occur on beginning EPITRATE therapy, but usually diminish as treatment is continued. Conjunctival allergy occurs occasionally. Pigmentary deposits in the lids, conjunctiva or cornea may occur after prolonged use of epinephrine eyedrops. In rare cases, maculopathy with a central scotoma may result from the use of topical epinephrine in aphakic patients; prompt reversal generally follows discontinuance of the drug. Systemic effects have occasionally been reported, such as: palpitation, tachycardia, extrasystoles, hypertension, trembling, sweating, and pallor.
Dosage and Administration: One drop, with frequency of instillation being individualized, from every two or three days to twice daily. More frequent instillation than one drop four times daily does not usually elicit any further improvement in therapeutic response.
How Supplied: EPITRATE—ophthalmic solution of epinephrine bitartrate 2% (equivalent to 1.1% base). Package containing 7.5 ml bottle with separate dropper-screw cap attachment (NDC 0046-1015-07).

ESTRADURIN® R
[ĕs" tra-dū' rin]
Brand of polyestradiol phosphate
For Intramuscular Injection Only

Description: ESTRADURIN (polyestradiol phosphate) is a water-soluble, high molecular weight polyester of phosphoric acid and 17β-estradiol. It is provided in a SECULE® containing 40 mg polyestradiol phosphate, 0.022 mg phenylmercuric nitrate, and 5.2 mg sodium phosphate. As solubilizing agents for the active ingredient, 25 mg niacinamide and 4 mg propylene glycol are also present. The pH is adjusted with sodium hydroxide.
One 2 ml ampul of sterile diluent is also provided.
Clinical Pharmacology: Estrogens are important in the development and maintenance of the female reproductive system. In responsive tissues estrogens enter the cell and are transported into the nucleus.
In the male patient with androgenic hormone-dependent conditions such as metastatic carcinoma of the prostate gland, estrogens counter the androgenic influence by competing for the receptor sites. As a result of treatment with estrogens, metastatic lesions in the bone may also show improvement.
Biologically active estradiol units are gradually split off from the large parent molecule, thus providing a continuous level of active estrogen over a prolonged period. The liberated estradiol is metabolized by the body in the same manner as the endogenous hormone. There is no depot effect at the site of injection—90 percent of injected dose leaves the bloodstream within 24 hours. Passive storage occurs in the reticuloendothelial system. As circulating levels of estradiol drop, more returns to the bloodstream from the site of storage for an even, continuous therapeutic effect. Increasing the dose acts to prolong the duration of pharmacologic action rather than to increase blood levels.
Metabolism and inactivation occur primarily in the liver. Some estrogens are excreted into the bile; however they are reabsorbed from the intestine and returned to the liver through the portal venous system. Water-soluble estrogen conjugates are strongly acidic and are ionized in body fluids, which favor excretion through the kidneys since tubular reabsorption is minimal.
Indication: ESTRADURIN (polyestradiol phosphate) is indicated in the treatment of prostatic carcinoma—palliative therapy of advanced disease.
Contraindications: Estrogens should not be used in men with any of the following conditions:
1. Known or suspected cancer of the breast except in appropriately selected patients being treated for metastatic disease.
2. Known or suspected estrogen-dependent neoplasia.
3. Active thrombophlebitis or thromboembolic disorders.
Warnings:
1. *Induction of malignant neoplasms.* Long term continuous administration of natural and synthetic estrogens in certain animal species increases the frequency of carcinomas of the breast, cervix, vagina, and liver.
2. *Gallbladder disease.* A recent study has reported a 2 to 3-fold increase in the risk of surgically confirmed gallbladder disease in women receiving postmenopausal estrogens,[1] similar to the 2-fold increase previously noted in users of oral contraceptives.[2,7a]
3. *Effects similar to those caused by estrogen-progestogen oral contraceptives.* There are several serious adverse effects of oral contraceptives. It has been shown that there is an increased risk of thrombosis in men receiving estrogens for prostatic cancer and women for postpartum breast engorgement.[3-6]
a. *Thromboembolic disease.* It is now well established that users of oral contraceptives have an increased risk of various thromboembolic and thrombotic vascular diseases, such as thrombophlebitis, pulmonary embolism, stroke, and myocardial infarction.[7-14] Cases of retinal thrombosis, mesenteric thrombosis, and optic neuritis have been reported in oral contraceptive users. There is evidence that the risk of several of these adverse reactions is related to the dose of the drug.[15,16] An increased risk of postsurgery thromboembolic complications has also been reported in users of oral contraceptives.[17,18] If feasible, estrogen should be discontinued at least 4 weeks before surgery of the type associated with an increased risk of thromboembolism, or during periods of prolonged immobilization.
Estrogens should not be used in persons with active thrombophlebitis or thromboembolic disorders. They should be used with caution in patients with cerebral vascular or coronary artery disease and only for those in whom estrogens are clearly indicated.
Large doses of estrogen (5 mg conjugated estrogens per day), comparable to those used to treat cancer of the prostate, have been shown in a large prospective clinical trial in men[19] to increase the risk of nonfatal myocardial infarction, pulmonary embolism and thrombophlebitis. When estrogen doses of this size are used, any of the thromboembolic and thrombotic adverse effects associated with oral contraceptive use should be considered a clear risk.
b. *Hepatic adenoma.* Benign hepatic adenomas appear to be associated with the use of oral contraceptives.[20-22] Although benign, and rare, these may rupture and may cause death through intra-abdominal hemorrhage. Such lesions have not yet been reported in association with other estrogen or

progestogen preparations but should be considered in estrogen users having abdominal pain and tenderness, abdominal mass, or hypovolemic shock. Hepatocellular carcinoma has also been reported in women taking estrogen-containing oral contraceptives.[21] The relationship of this malignancy to these drugs is not known at this time.

c. *Elevated blood pressure.* Women using oral contraceptives sometimes experience increased blood pressure which, in most cases, returns to normal on discontinuing the drug. There is now a report that this may occur with use of estrogens in the menopause[23] and blood pressure should be monitored with estrogen use, especially if high doses are used.

d. *Glucose tolerance.* A worsening of glucose tolerance has been observed in a significant percentage of patients on estrogen-containing oral contraceptives. For this reason, diabetic patients should be carefully observed while receiving estrogen.

4. *Hypercalcemia.* Administration of estrogens may lead to severe hypercalcemia in patients with breast cancer and bone metastases. If this occurs, the drug should be stopped and appropriate measures taken to reduce the serum calcium level.

Precautions:
1. A complete medical and family history should be taken prior to the initiation of any estrogen therapy. The pretreatment and periodic physical examinations should include special reference to blood pressure, breasts, abdomen, and pelvic organs. As a general rule, estrogen should not be prescribed for longer than one year without another physical examination being performed.
2. Fluid retention—Because estrogens may cause some degree of fluid retention, conditions which might be influenced by this factor such as asthma, epilepsy, migraine, and cardiac or renal dysfunction, require careful observation.
3. Certain patients may develop undesirable manifestations of excessive estrogenic stimulation, such as gynecomastia.
4. Oral contraceptives appear to be associated with an increased incidence of mental depression.[7a] Although it is not clear whether this is due to the estrogenic or progestogenic component of the contraceptive, patients with a history of depression should be carefully observed.
5. The pathologist should be advised of estrogen therapy when relevant specimens are submitted.
6. If jaundice develops in any patient receiving estrogen, the medication should be discontinued while the cause is investigated.
7. Estrogens may be poorly metabolized in patients with impaired liver function and they should be administered with caution in such patients.
8. Because estrogens influence the metabolism of calcium and phosphorus, they should be used with caution in patients with metabolic bone diseases that are associated with hypercalcemia or in patients with renal insufficiency.
9. Because of the effects of estrogens on epiphyseal closure, they should be used judiciously in young patients in whom bone growth is not complete.
10. Certain endocrine and liver function tests may be affected by estrogen-containing oral contraceptives. The following similar changes may be expected with larger doses of estrogen:
a. Increased sulfobromophthalein retention.
b. Increased prothrombin and factors VII, VIII, IX, and X; decreased antithrombin 3; increased norepinephrine-induced platelet aggregability.
c. Increased thyroid binding globulin (TBG) leading to increased circulating total thyroid hormone, as measured by PBI, T4 by column, or T4 by radioimmunoassay. Free T3 resin uptake is decreased, reflecting the elevated TBG; free T4 concentration is unaltered.
d. Impaired glucose tolerance.
e. Reduced response to metyrapone test.
f. Reduced serum folate concentration.
g. Increased serum triglyceride and phospholipid concentration.

Adverse Reactions: (See Warnings regarding induction of neoplasia, increased incidence of gallbladder disease, and adverse effects similar to those of oral contraceptives, including thromboembolism.) The following additional adverse reactions have been reported with estrogenic therapy, including oral contraceptives:
1. *Breasts:* Tenderness, enlargement, secretion.
2. *Gastrointestinal:* Nausea, vomiting; abdominal cramps, bloating; cholestatic jaundice.
3. *Skin:* Chloasma or melasma which may persist when drug is discontinued; erythema multiforme; erythema nodosum; hemorrhagic eruption; loss of scalp hair; hirsutism.
4. *Eyes:* Steepening of corneal curvature; intolerance to contact lenses.
5. *CNS:* Headache, migraine, dizziness; mental depression; chorea.
6. *Miscellaneous:* Increase or decrease in weight; reduced carbohydrate tolerance; aggravation of porphyria; edema; changes in libido.

Acute Overdosage: Numerous reports of ingestion of large doses of estrogen-containing oral contraceptives by young children indicate that acute serious ill effects do not occur. Overdosage of estrogen may cause nausea, and withdrawal bleeding may occur in females.

Dosage and Administration: Inoperable progressing prostatic cancer—40 mg intramuscularly every two to four weeks or less frequently, depending on clinical response of the patient. If the response is not satisfactory doses up to 80 mg may be used. Experimental evidence indicates that increasing the dose primarily prolongs the duration of action, but the amount of estrogen available at any one time is not significantly increased. The dosage should be adjusted as indicated by careful observation of the patient.

Deep intramuscular injection only is recommended. (Initially, some patients may experience a burning sensation at site of injection. This is transitory, and it may not recur with subsequent injections, or may be obviated by concomitant administration of a local anesthetic.)

If a response to estrogen therapy is going to occur, it will be apparent within three months of the beginning of therapy. If it does occur, the hormone should be continued until the disease is again progressive. The hormone should then be stopped, and the patient may obtain another period of improvement known as "rebound regression." This occurs in 30% of the patients who show objective improvement on estrogens.

DIRECTIONS FOR USE
Reconstitution for use:
1. Introduce sterile diluent into SECULE, preferably with a 20 gauge needle affixed to a 5 ml syringe.
2. Swirl gently until a solution is effected. (DO NOT AGITATE VIOLENTLY.)

Stability: After reconstitution, if storage is desired, the solution should be kept at room temperature and away from direct light. Under these conditions the solution is stable for about 10 days, so long as cloudiness or evidence of a precipitate has not occurred.

How Supplied: NDC 0046-0451-02—Each package provides:
1. One SECULE® containing 40 mg polyestradiol phosphate, 0.022 mg phenylmercuric nitrate, and 5.2 mg sodium phosphate. As solubilizing agents for the active ingredient, 25 mg niacinamide and 4 mg propylene glycol are also present. The pH is adjusted with sodium hydroxide.
2. One 2 ml ampul of sterile diluent.

ESTRADURIN (polyestradiol phosphate) is prepared by cryodesiccation.

Physician References:
1. Boston Collaborative Drug Surveillance Program: N. Engl. J. Med. *290*:15–19, 1974.
2. Boston Collaborative Drug Surveillance Program: Lancet *1*:1399–1404, 1973.
3. Daniel, D. G., *et al*: Lancet *2*:287–289, 1967.
4. The Veterans Administration Cooperative Urological Research Group: J. Urol. *98*:516–522, 1967.
5. Bailar, J. C.: Lancet *2*:560, 1967.
6. Blackard, C., *et al*: Cancer *26*:249–256, 1970.
7. Royal College of General Practitioners: J. R. Coll. Gen. Pract. *13*:267–279, 1967.
7a. Royal College of General Practitioners: Oral Contraceptives and Health, New York, Pitman Corp., 1974.
8. Inman, W. H. W., *et al*: Br. Med. J. *2*:193–199, 1968.
9. Vessey, M. P., *et al*: Br. Med. J. *2*:651–657, 1969.
10. Sartwell, P. E., *et al*: Am. J. Epidemiol. *90*:365–380, 1969.
11. Collaborative Group for the Study of Stroke in Young Women: N. Engl. J. Med. *288*:871–878, 1973.
12. Collaborative Group for the Study of Stroke in Young Women: J.A.M.A. *231*:718–722, 1975.
13. Mann, J. I., *et al*: Br. Med. J. *2*:245–248, 1975.
14. Mann, J. I., *et al*: Br. Med. J. *2*:241–245, 1975.
15. Inman, W. H. W., *et al*: Br. Med. J. *2*:203–209, 1970.
16. Stolley, P. D., *et al*: Am. J. Epidemiol. *102*:197–208, 1975.
17. Vessey, M. P., *et al*: Br. Med. J. *3*:123–126, 1970.
18. Greene, G. R., *et al*: Am. J. Public Health *62*:680–685, 1972.
19. Coronary Drug Project Research Group: J.A.M.A. *214*:1303–1313, 1970.
20. Baum, J., *et al*: Lancet *2*:926–928, 1973.
21. Mays, E. T., *et al*: J.A.M.A. *235*:730–732, 1976.
22. Edmondson, H. A., *et al*: N. Engl. J. Med. *294*:470–472, 1976.
23. Pfeffer, R. I., *et al*: Am. J. Epidemiol. *103*:445–456, 1976.

SECULE®—Trademark to designate a special vial containing an injectable preparation in dry form.

FACTREL® ℞
[făc-trĕl']
(gonadorelin hydrochloride)
Synthetic Luteinizing Hormone Releasing Hormone (LH-RH)
DIAGNOSTIC USE ONLY

Caution: Federal law prohibits dispensing without prescription.

Description: An agent for use in evaluating hypothalamic-pituitary gonadotropic function. FACTREL (gonadorelin hydrochloride) injectable is available as a sterile lyophilized powder for reconstitution and administration by subcutaneous or intravenous routes.

Chemical Name: 5-oxo-L-prolyl-L-histidyl-L-tryptophyl-L-seryl-L-tyrosyl-glycyl-L-leucyl-L-arginyl-L-prolyl glycinamide hydrochloride
[See table on next page].

FACTREL is $C_{55}H_{75}N_{17}O_{13}HCl$, as the mono- or dihydrochloride, or their mixture. The gonadorelin base has a molecular weight of 1182.33. It is a white powder, soluble in alcohol and water, hygroscopic and moisture-sensitive, and stable at room temperature. The synthetic decapeptide, FACTREL, has a chemical composition and structure identical to the natural hormone, identified from porcine or ovine hypothalami.

Each vial of FACTREL contains 100 or 500 mcg gonadorelin as the hydrochloride, with 100 mg lactose, U.S.P. Each ampul of sterile diluent contains 2% benzyl alcohol and Water for Injection, U.S.P.

Clinical Pharmacology: FACTREL has been shown to have gonadotropin-releasing effects upon the anterior pituitary. The range for normal baseline LH levels, as determined from the literature, is 5-25 mIU/ml in postpubertal males, and postpubertal and premenopausal females. The standard used is the Second International Reference Preparation—HMC. This range may not correspond in each laboratory performing the assay since the concentration of LH in normal individuals varies with different assay methods. The normal responses to FACTREL analyzed from the results of clinical studies included:
(1) LH peak (mIU/ml)
  (highest LH value post-FACTREL administration)

Continued on next page

Ayerst—Cont.

(2) Maximum LH increase (mIU/ml)
(peak LH value—LH baseline value)
(3) LH percent response
$$\frac{\text{peak LH} - \text{baseline LH}}{\text{baseline LH}} \times 100\%$$
(4) Time to peak (minutes)
(time required to reach LH peak value)

Normal adult subjects were shown to have these LH responses following FACTREL administration by subcutaneous or intravenous routes.

I. MALE ADULTS:
A) Subcutaneous Administration
The results are based on 18 tests in males between the ages of 18–42 years, inclusive:
(1) LH peak: mean 60.3 ± 26.2 mIU/ml
$100\% \geq 24.0$ mIU/ml
$90\% \geq 32.8$ mIU/ml
(2) Maximum LH increase: mean 46.7 ± 20.8 mIU/ml
$100\% \geq 12.3$ mIU/ml
$90\% \geq 20.9$ mIU/ml
(3) LH percent response: mean $437 \pm 243\%$
range: 66–1853%
$90\% \geq 188\%$

B) Intravenous Administration
The results are based on 26 tests in males between the ages of 19–58 years, inclusive:
(1) LH peak: mean 63.8 ± 40.3 mIU/ml
$100\% \geq 12.6$ mIU/ml
$90\% \geq 26.0$ mIU/ml
(2) Maximum LH increase: mean 51.3 ± 35.2 mIU/ml
$100\% \geq 7.4$ mIU/ml
$90\% \geq 14.8$ mIU/ml
(3) LH percent response: mean $481 \pm 184\%$
range: 67–2139%
$90\% \geq 142\%$
(4) Time to peak: mean 27 ± 14 min.

In males older than 50 years, the LH baseline and peak levels tend to be higher; however, the maximum LH increases do not differ in regard to age.

II. FEMALE ADULTS:
A) Subcutaneous Administration
The results are based on 38 tests in females between the ages of 19–36 years, inclusive:
(1) LH peak: mean 67.9 ± 27.5 mIU/ml
$100\% \geq 12.5$ mIU/ml
$90\% \geq 39.0$ mIU/ml
(2) Maximum LH increase: mean 52.8 ± 26.4 mIU/ml
$100\% \geq 7.5$ mIU/ml
$90\% \geq 23.8$ mIU/ml
(3) LH percent response: mean $374 \pm 221\%$
range: 108–981%
$90\% \geq 185\%$
(4) Time to peak: mean 71.5 ± 49.6 min.

B) Intravenous Administration
The results are based on 31 tests in females between the ages of 20–35 years inclusive:
(1) LH peak: mean 57.6 ± 36.7 mIU/ml
$100\% \geq 20.0$ mIU/ml
$90\% \geq 24.6$ mIU/ml
(2) Maximum LH increase: mean 44.5 ± 31.8 mIU/ml

$100\% \geq 7.5$ mIU/ml
$90\% \geq 16.2$ mIU/ml
(3) LH percent response: mean $356 \pm 282\%$
range: 60–1300%
$90\% \geq 142\%$
(4) Time to peak: mean 36 ± 24 min.

The FACTREL (gonadorelin hydrochloride) tests on which the normal female responses are based were performed in the early follicular phase of the menstrual cycle (Days 1–7).

In menopausal and postmenopausal females, the baseline LH levels are elevated and the maximum LH increases are exaggerated when compared with the premenopausal levels.

Patients with clinically diagnosed or suspected pituitary and/or hypothalamic dysfunction were often shown to have subnormal or no LH responses following FACTREL administration. For example, in clinical tests of 6 patients with known postpubertal panhypopituitarism, and 11 patients with Prader-Willi Syndrome, 100% showed subnormal responses or no rise in LH. Subnormal responses to the FACTREL test also were observed in 21 (95%) of 22 patients with prepubertal panhypopituitarism. In 19 patients with Sheehan Syndrome, 16 (84%) had a subnormal response. In the FACTREL test in 44 patients with Kallmann Syndrome, 33 (77%) had subnormal LH responses.

Indications and Usage: FACTREL as a single injection is indicated for evaluating the functional capacity and response of the gonadotropes of the anterior pituitary. This single injection test does not measure pituitary gonadotropic reserve for which more prolonged or repeated administration may be required. The LH response is useful in testing patients with suspected gonadotropin deficiency, whether due to the hypothalamus alone or in combination with anterior pituitary failure. FACTREL is also indicated for evaluating residual gonadotropic function of the pituitary following removal of a pituitary tumor by surgery and/or irradiation. In clinical studies to date, however, the single injection test has not been useful in differentiating pituitary disorders from hypothalamic disorders. The FACTREL test can be performed concomitantly with other post-treatment evaluations.

The results of the FACTREL test complement the clinical examination and other laboratory tests used to confirm or substantiate hypogonadotropic hypogonadism.

In cases where there is a normal response, it indicates the presence of functional pituitary gonadotropes. The single injection test does not measure pituitary gonadotropic reserve.

Contraindications: Hypersensitivity to gonadorelin hydrochloride or any of the components.

Precautions: Although allergic and hypersensitivity reactions have been observed with other polypeptide hormones, to date no such reactions have been encountered following the administration of a single 100 mcg dose of FACTREL. Antibody formulation has been rarely reported after chronic administration of large doses of FACTREL.

The FACTREL test should be conducted in the absence of other drugs which directly affect the pituitary secretion of the gonadotropins. These would include a variety of preparations which contain androgens, estrogens, progestins, or glucocorticoids. The gonadotropin levels may be transiently elevated by spironolactone, minimally elevated by levodopa, and suppressed by oral contraceptives and digoxin. The response to FACTREL may be blunted by phenothiazines and dopamine antagonists which cause a rise in prolactin.

Pregnancy Category B. Reproduction studies have been performed in mice, rats, and rabbits at doses up to 50 times the human dose, and have revealed no evidence of harm to the fetus due to FACTREL. There are, however, no adequate and well-controlled studies in pregnant women. Because animal reproduction studies are not always predictive of human response, this drug should be used during pregnancy only if clearly needed.

Appropriate precautions should be taken because the effects of LH-RH on the fetus and developing offspring have not been adequately evaluated. Repetitive, high doses of FACTREL may cause luteolysis and inhibition of spermatogenesis.

Adverse Reactions: Systemic complaints such as headaches, nausea, lightheadedness, abdominal discomfort, and flushing have been reported rarely following administration of 100 mcg of FACTREL. Local swelling, occasionally with pain and pruritus, at the injection site may occur if FACTREL is administered subcutaneously. Local and generalized skin rash have been noted after chronic subcutaneous administration.

Overdosage: FACTREL (gonadorelin hydrochloride) has been administered parenterally in doses up to 3 mg BID for 28 days without any signs or symptoms of overdosage. In case of overdosage or idiosyncrasy, symptomatic treatment should be administered as required.

Dosage and Administration: Adults: 100 mcg dose, subcutaneously or intravenously. In females for whom the phase of the menstrual cycle can be established, the test should be performed in the early follicular phase (Days 1–7).

Test Methodology: To determine the status of the gonadotropin secretory capacity of the anterior pituitary, a test procedure requiring seven venous blood samples for LH is recommended.

PROCEDURE:
1. Venous blood samples should be drawn at -15 minutes and immediately prior to FACTREL administration. The LH baseline is obtained by averaging the LH values of the two samples.
2. Administer a bolus of 100 mcg of FACTREL subcutaneously or intravenously.
3. Draw venous blood samples at 15, 30, 45, 60, and 120 minutes after administration.
4. Blood samples should be handled as recommended by the laboratory that will determine the LH content. It must be emphasized that the reliability of the test is directly related to the inter-assay and intra-assay reliability of the laboratory performing the assay.

Interpretation of Test Results: Interpretation of the LH response to FACTREL requires an understanding of the hypothalamic-pituitary physiology, knowledge of the clinical status of the individual patient, and familiarity with the normal ranges and the standards used in the laboratory performing the LH assays.

Figures 1 through 4 represent the LH response curves after FACTREL administration in normal subjects. The normal LH response curves were established between the 10th percentile (B line) and 90th percentile (A line) of all LH responses in normal subjects analyzed from the results of clinical studies. LH values are reported in units of mIU/ml and time is displayed in minutes. Individual patient responses should be plotted on the appropriate curve. A subnormal response in patients is defined as three or more LH values which fall below the B line of the normal LH response curve. In cases where there is a blunted or borderline response, the FACTREL (gonadorelin hydrochloride) test should be repeated.

Structural Formula:

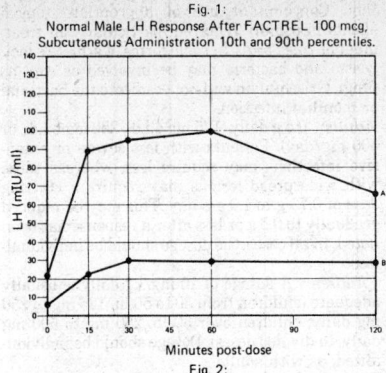

Fig. 1:
Normal Male LH Response After FACTREL 100 mcg, Subcutaneous Administration 10th and 90th percentiles.

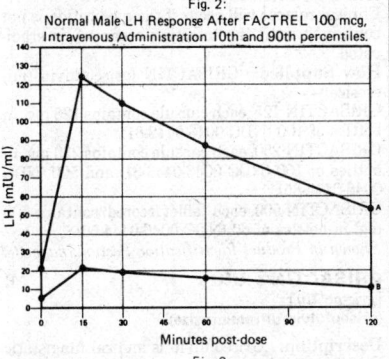

Fig. 2:
Normal Male LH Response After FACTREL 100 mcg, Intravenous Administration 10th and 90th percentiles.

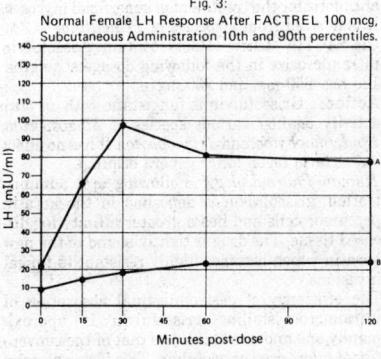

Fig. 3:
Normal Female LH Response After FACTREL 100 mcg, Subcutaneous Administration 10th and 90th percentiles.

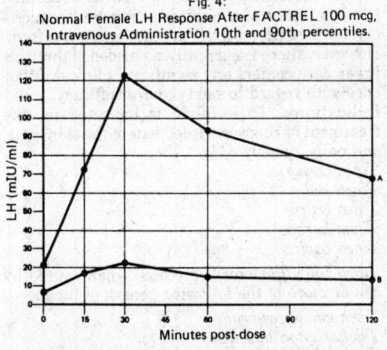

Fig. 4:
Normal Female LH Response After FACTREL 100 mcg, Intravenous Administration 10th and 90th percentiles.

The FACTREL (gonadorelin hydrochloride) test complements the clinical assessment of patients with a variety of endocrine disorders involving the hypothalamic-pituitary axis. In cases where there is a normal response, it indicates the presence of functional pituitary gonadotropes. The single injection test does not determine the pathophysiological cause for the subnormal response and does not measure pituitary gonadotropic reserve.

How Supplied: LYOPHILIZED POWDER in single-dose vials containing 100 mcg (NDC 0046-0507-05) and 500 mcg (NDC 0046-0509-05) gonadorelin as the hydrochloride with 100 mg lactose, U.S.P. Each vial is accompanied by one ampul containing 2 ml sterile diluent of 2% benzyl alcohol in Water for Injection, U.S.P.

Directions: Store at room temperature (approximately 25°C).
Reconstitute 100 mcg vial with 1.0 ml of the accompanying sterile diluent.
Reconstitute 500 mcg vial with 2.0 ml of the accompanying sterile diluent.
Prepare solution immediately before use.
After reconstitution, store at room temperature and use within 1 day.
Discard unused reconstituted solution and diluent.
Diagnostic Method of Use Patent 3,947,569
Shown in Product Identification Section, page 404

FLUOTHANE® ℞
[flū'o-thān]
Brand of halothane, U.S.P.

Description: FLUOTHANE, brand of halothane, U.S.P., is an inhalation anesthetic. It is 2-bromo-2-chloro-1,1,1-trifluoroethane.
The specific gravity is 1.872-1.877 at 20° C, and the boiling point (range) is 49° C-51° C at 760 mm Hg. The vapor pressure is 243 mm Hg at 20° C. The blood/gas coefficient is 2.5 at 37° C, and the olive oil/water coefficient is 220 at 37° C. Vapor concentrations within anesthetic range are nonirritating and have a pleasant odor. FLUOTHANE is nonflammable, and its vapors mixed with oxygen in proportions from 0.5 to 50 per cent (v/v) are not explosive.
FLUOTHANE does not decompose in contact with warm soda lime. When moisture is present, the vapor attacks aluminum, brass, and lead, but not copper. Rubber, some plastics, and similar materials are soluble in FLUOTHANE; such materials will deteriorate rapidly in contact with FLUOTHANE vapor or liquid. Stability of FLUOTHANE is maintained by the addition of 0.01 per cent thymol (w/w), up to 0.00025% ammonia (w/w), and storage is in amber colored bottles.
FLUOTHANE should not be kept indefinitely in vaporizer bottles not specifically designed for its use. Thymol does not volatilize along with FLUOTHANE, and therefore accumulates in the vaporizer, and may, in time, impart a yellow color to the remaining liquid or to wicks in vaporizers. The development of such discoloration may be used as an indicator that the vaporizer should be drained and cleaned, and the discolored FLUOTHANE (halothane, U.S.P.) discarded. Accumulation of thymol may be removed by washing with diethyl ether. After cleaning a wick or vaporizer, make certain all the diethyl ether has been removed before reusing the equipment to avoid introducing ether into the system.

Actions: FLUOTHANE is an inhalation anesthetic. Induction and recovery are rapid and depth of anesthesia can be rapidly altered. FLUOTHANE progressively depresses respiration. There may be tachypnea with reduced tidal volume and alveolar ventilation. FLUOTHANE is not an irritant to the respiratory tract, and no increase in salivary or bronchial secretions ordinarily occurs. Pharyngeal and laryngeal reflexes are rapidly obtunded. It causes bronchodilation. Hypoxia, acidosis, or apnea may develop during deep anesthesia.
FLUOTHANE reduces the blood pressure, and frequently decreases the pulse rate. The greater the concentration of the drug, the more evident these changes become. Atropine may reverse the bradycardia. FLUOTHANE does not cause the release of catecholamines from adrenergic stores. FLUOTHANE also causes dilation of the vessels of the skin and skeletal muscles.
Cardiac arrhythmias may occur during FLUOTHANE anesthesia. These include nodal rhythm, AV dissociation, ventricular extrasystoles and asystole. FLUOTHANE sensitizes the myocardial conduction system to the action of epinephrine and norepinephrine, and the combination may cause serious cardiac arrhythmias. FLUOTHANE increases cerebral spinal fluid pressure. FLUOTHANE produces moderate muscular relaxation. Muscle relaxants are used as adjuncts in order to maintain lighter levels of anesthesia. FLUOTHANE augments the action of nondepolarizing relaxants and ganglionic blocking agents. FLUOTHANE is a potent uterine relaxant.

Indications: FLUOTHANE (halothane, U.S.P.) is indicated for the induction and maintenance of general anesthesia.

Contraindications: FLUOTHANE is not recommended for obstetrical anesthesia except when uterine relaxation is required.

Warnings: When previous exposure to FLUOTHANE was followed by unexplained jaundice, consideration should be given to the use of other agents.
FLUOTHANE should be used in vaporizers that permit a reasonable approximation of output, and preferably of the calibrated type. The vaporizer should be placed out of circuit in closed circuit rebreathing systems; otherwise overdosage is difficult to avoid. The patient should be closely observed for signs of overdosage, *i.e.*, depression of blood pressure, pulse rate, and ventilation, particularly during assisted or controlled ventilation.
Usage in Pregnancy. Safe use of FLUOTHANE has not been established with respect to possible adverse effects upon fetal development. Therefore, FLUOTHANE should not be used in women where pregnancy is possible and particularly during early pregnancy, unless, in the judgment of the physician, the potential benefits outweigh the unknown hazards to the fetus.

Precautions: The uterine relaxation obtained with FLUOTHANE (halothane, U.S.P.) unless carefully controlled, may fail to respond to ergot derivatives and oxytocic posterior pituitary extract.
FLUOTHANE increases cerebrospinal fluid pressure. Therefore, in patients with markedly raised intracranial pressure, if FLUOTHANE is indicated, administration should be preceded by measures ordinarily used to reduce cerebrospinal fluid pressure. Ventilation should be carefully assessed, and it may be necessary to assist or control ventilation to insure adequate oxygenation and carbon dioxide removal.
Epinephrine or norepinephrine should be employed cautiously, if at all, during FLUOTHANE (halothane, U.S.P.) anesthesia since their simultaneous use may induce ventricular tachycardia or fibrillation.
Nondepolarizing relaxants and ganglionic blocking agents should be administered cautiously, since their actions are augmented by FLUOTHANE.
It has been reported that in genetically susceptible individuals, the use of general anesthetics and the muscle relaxant, succinylcholine, may trigger a syndrome known as malignant hyperthermic crisis. Monitoring temperature during surgery will aid in early recognition of this syndrome. Dantrolene sodium and supportive measures are generally indicated in the management of malignant hyperthermia.

Adverse Reactions: The following adverse reactions have been reported: mild, moderate and severe hepatic dysfunction (including hepatic necrosis), cardiac arrest, hypotension, respiratory arrest, cardiac arrhythmias, hyperpyrexia, shivering, nausea, and emesis.

Dosage and Administration: FLUOTHANE may be administered by the nonrebreathing technic, partial rebreathing, or closed technic. The induction dose varies from patient to patient. The maintenance dose varies from 0.5 per cent to 1.5 per cent.
FLUOTHANE may be administered with either oxygen or a mixture of oxygen and nitrous oxide.

How Supplied: Unit packages of 125 ml (NDC 0046-3125-81) and 250 ml (NDC 0046-3125-82) of halothane, U.S.P., stabilized with 0.01% thymol (w/w) and up to 0.00025% ammonia (w/w).

Continued on next page

Ayerst—Cont.

GRISACTIN®
[grĭz-ăc' tĭn]
brand of griseofulvin (microsize)

CAUTION: Federal law prohibits dispensing without prescription.

Description: Griseofulvin is an oral fungistatic antibiotic for the treatment of superficial mycoses. It is derived from a species of *Penicillium*. GRISACTIN is produced by a special process that fractures griseofulvin particles into minute crystals of irregular shape offering a greater and more effective surface area for increased gastrointestinal absorption.

Action: Griseofulvin is fungistatic with *in vitro* activity against various species of *Microsporum*, *Epidermophyton*, and *Trichophyton*. It has no effect on bacteria or on other genera of fungi.

Griseofulvin is deposited in the keratin precursor cells and has a greater affinity for diseased tissue. The drug is tightly bound to the new keratin which becomes highly resistant to fungal invasions.

Griseofulin absorption from the gastrointestinal tract varies considerably among individuals mainly because of insolubility of the drug in aqueous media of the upper G.I. tract. The peak serum level found in fasting adults given 0.5 g occurs at about four hours and ranges between 0.5 to 2.0 mcg/ml. The serum level may be increased by giving the drug with a meal with a high fat content.

Indications: Griseofulvin is indicated for the treatment of ringworm infections of the skin, hair, and nails, namely:

Tinea corporis
Tinea pedis
Tinea cruris
Tinea barbae
Tinea capitis

Tinea unguium (onychomycosis) when caused by one or more of the following genera of fungi:

Trichophyton rubrum
Trichophyton tonsurans
Trichophyton mentagrophytes
Trichophyton interdigitalis
Trichophyton verrucosum
Trichophyton megnini
Trichophyton gallinae
Trichophyton crateriform
Trichophyton sulphureum
Trichophyton schoenleini
Microsporum audouini
Microsporum canis
Microsporum gypseum
Epidermophyton floccosum

NOTE: Prior to therapy, the type of fungi responsible for the infection should be identified.

The use of this drug is not justified in minor or trivial infections which will respond to topical agents alone.

Griseofulvin is *not* effective in the following:
Bacterial infections
Candidiasis (Moniliasis)
Histoplasmosis
Actinomycosis
Sporotrichosis
Chromoblastomycosis
Coccidioidomycosis
North American Blastomycosis
Cryptococcosis (Torulosis)
Tinea versicolor
nocardiosis

Contraindications: This drug is contraindicated in patients with porphyria, hepatocellular failure, and in individuals with a history of hypersensitivity to griseofulvin.

Warnings:
Prophylactic Usage Safety and efficacy of griseofulvin for prophylaxis of fungal infections has not been established.

Animal Toxicology Chronic feeding of griseofulvin, at levels ranging from 0.5-2.5% of the diet, resulted in the development of liver tumors in several strains of mice, particularly males. Smaller particle sizes result in an enhanced effect. Lower oral dosage levels have not been tested. Subcutaneous administration of relatively small doses of griseofulvin, once a week, during the first three weeks of life has also been reported to induce hepatomata in mice. Although studies in other animal species have not yielded evidence of tumorigenicity, these studies were not of adequate design to form a basis for conclusions in this regard.

In subacute toxicity studies, orally administered griseofulvin produced hepatocellular necrosis in mice, but this has not been seen in other species. Disturbances in porphyrin metabolism have been reported in griseofulvin-treated laboratory animals. Griseofulvin has been reported to have a colchicine-like effect on mitosis and cocarcinogenicity with methylcholanthrene in cutaneous tumor induction in laboratory animals.

Usage in Pregnancy The safety of this drug during pregnancy has not been established.

Animal Reproduction Studies It has been reported in the literature that griseofulvin was found to be embryotoxic and teratogenic on oral administration to pregnant rats. Pups with abnormalities have been reported in the litters of a few bitches treated with griseofulvin. Additional animal reproduction studies are in progress.

Suppression of spermatogenesis has been reported to occur in rats, but investigation in man failed to confirm this.

Precautions: Patients on prolonged therapy with any potent medication should be under close observation. Periodic monitoring of organ system function, including renal, hepatic, and hematopoietic, should be done.

Since griseofulvin is derived from species of *Penicillium*, the possibility of cross-sensitivity with penicillin exists; however, known penicillin-sensitive patients have been treated without difficulty. Since a photosensitivity reaction is occasionally associated with griseofulvin therapy, patients should be warned to avoid exposure to intense natural or artificial sunlight. Should a photosensitivity reaction occur, lupus erythematosus may be aggravated.

Griseofulvin decreases the activity of warfarin-type anticoagulants so that patients receiving these drugs concomitantly may require dosage adjustment of the anticoagulant during and after griseofulvin therapy.

Barbiturates usually depress griseofulvin activity and concomitant administration may require a dosage adjustment of the antifungal agent.

Griseofulvin may augment or potentiate the effects of alcohol.

Adverse Reactions: When adverse reactions occur, they are most commonly of the hypersensitivity type such as skin rashes, urticaria, and rarely, angioneurotic edema, and may necessitate withdrawal of therapy and appropriate countermeasures. Paresthesias of the hands and feet have been reported rarely after extended therapy. Other side effects reported occasionally are oral thrush, nausea, vomiting, epigastric distress, diarrhea, headache, fatigue, dizziness, insomnia, mental confusion, and impairment of performance of routine activities.

Proteinuria and leukopenia have been reported rarely. Administration of the drug should be discontinued if granulocytopenia occurs.

When rare, serious reactions occur with griseofulvin, they are usually associated with high dosages, long periods of therapy, or both.

Dosage and Administration: Accurate diagnosis of the infecting organism is essential. Identification should be made either by direct microscopic examination of a mounting of infected tissue in a solution of potassium hydroxide or by culture on an appropriate medium.

Medication must be continued until the infecting organism is completely eradicated as indicated by appropriate clinical or laboratory examination. Representative treatment periods are—*tinea capitis*, 4 to 6 weeks; *tinea corporis*, 2 to 4 weeks; *tinea pedis*, 4 to 8 weeks; *tinea unguium*—depending on rate of growth—fingernails, at least 4 months: toenails, at least 6 months.

General measures in regard to hygiene should be observed to control sources of infection or reinfection. Concomitant use of appropriate topical agents is usually required, particularly in treatment of *tinea pedis*. In some forms of athlete's foot, yeasts and bacteria may be involved as well as fungi. Griseofulvin will not eradicate the bacterial or monilial infection.

Adults: 0.5 g daily (125 mg q.i.d., 250 mg b.i.d., or 500 mg/day). Patients with less severe or extensive infections may require less, whereas those with widespread lesions may require a starting dose of 0.75 g to 1.0 g a day. This may be reduced gradually to 0.5 g or less after a response has been noted. In all cases, the dosage should be individualized.

Children: A dosage of 10 mg/kg daily is usually adequate (children from 30 to 50 lb, 125 mg to 250 mg daily; children over 50 lb, 250 mg to 500 mg daily, in divided doses). Dosage should be individualized, as with adults.

Clinical relapse will occur if the medication is not continued until the infecting organism is eradicated.

How Supplied: GRISACTIN [griseofulvin (microsize)]—
GRISACTIN 125, each capsule contains 125 mg, in bottles of 100 (NDC 0046-0442-81).
GRISACTIN 250, each capsule contains 250 mg, in bottles of 100 (NDC 0046-0443-81) and 500 (NDC 0046-0443-85).
GRISACTIN 500, each tablet (scored) contains 500 mg, in bottles of 60 (NDC 0046-0444-60).

Shown in Product Identification Section, page 404

GRISACTIN® Ultra
[grĭz-ăc' tĭn]
(griseofulvin ultramicrosize)

Description: Griseofulvin is an oral fungistatic antibiotic for the treatment of superficial mycoses. It is derived from a species of *Penicillium*.
GRISACTIN Ultra tablets contain griseofulvin ultramicrosize in the following dosage strengths: 125 mg, 250 mg, and 330 mg.

Action: Griseofulvin is fungistatic with *in vitro* activity against various species of *Microsporum*, *Epidermophyton*, and *Trichophyton*. It has no effect on bacteria or on other genera of fungi.

Human Pharmacology: Following oral administration, griseofulvin is deposited in the keratin precursor cells and has a greater affinity for diseased tissue. The drug is tightly bound to the new keratin which becomes highly resistant to fungal invasions.

The efficiency of gastrointestinal absorption of ultramicrocrystalline griseofulvin is approximately one and one-half times that of the conventional microsized griseofulvin. This factor permits the oral intake of two-thirds as much ultramicrocrystalline griseofulvin as the microsize form. However, there is currently no evidence that this lower dose confers any significant clinical difference with regard to safety and/or efficacy.

Indications: Griseofulvin is indicated for the treatment of ringworm infections of the skin, hair, and nails, namely:

Tinea corporis
Tinea pedis
Tinea cruris
Tinea barbae
Tinea capitis

Tinea unguium (onychomycosis) when caused by one or more of the following genera of fungi:

Trichophyton rubrum
Trichophyton tonsurans
Trichophyton mentagrophytes
Trichophyton interdigitalis
Trichophyton verrucosum
Trichophyton megnini
Trichophyton gallinae
Trichophyton crateriform
Trichophyton sulphureum
Trichophyton schoenleini
Microsporum audouini
Microsporum canis
Microsporum gypseum
Epidermophyton floccosum

NOTE: Prior to therapy, the type of fungi responsible for the infection should be identified.

The use of this drug is not justified in minor or trivial infections which will respond to topical agents alone.

Griseofulvin is *not* effective in the following:

Bacterial infections
Candidiasis (Moniliasis)
Histoplasmosis
Actinomycosis
Sporotrichosis
Chromoblastomycosis
Coccidioidomycosis
North American Blastomycosis
Cryptococcosis (Torulosis)
Tinea versicolor
Nocardiosis

Contraindications: This drug is contraindicated in patients with porphyria, hepatocellular failure, and in individuals with a history of hypersensitivity to griseofulvin.

Warnings:
Prophylactic Usage
Safety and efficacy of griseofulvin for prophylaxis of fungal infections has not been established.
Animal Toxicology
Chronic feeding of griseofulvin, at levels ranging from 0.5-2.5% of the diet, resulted in the development of liver tumors in several strains of mice, particularly males. Smaller particle sizes result in an enhanced effect. Lower oral dosage levels have not been tested. Subcutaneous administration of relatively small doses of griseofulvin, once a week, during the first three weeks of life has also been reported to induce hepatomata in mice. Although studies in other animal species have not yielded evidence of tumorigenicity, these studies were not of adequate design to form a basis for conclusions in this regard.

In subacute toxicity studies, orally administered griseofulvin produced hepatocellular necrosis in mice, but this has not been seen in other species. Disturbances in porphyrin metabolism have been reported in griseofulvin-treated laboratory animals. Griseofulvin has been reported to have a colchicine-like effect on mitosis and cocarcinogenicity with methylcholanthrene in cutaneous tumor induction in laboratory animals.
Usage in Pregnancy
The safety of this drug during pregnancy has not been established.
Animal Reproduction Studies
It has been reported in the literature that griseofulvin was found to be embryotoxic and teratogenic on oral administration to pregnant rats. Pups with abnormalities have been reported in the litters of a few bitches treated with griseofulvin. Additional animal reproduction studies are in progress.

Suppression of spermatogenesis has been reported to occur in rats, but investigation in man failed to confirm this.

Precautions: Patients on prolonged therapy with any potent medication should be under close observation. Periodic monitoring of organ system function, including renal, hepatic, and hematopoietic, should be done.

Since griseofulvin is derived from species of *Penicillium*, the possibility of cross-sensitivity with penicillin exists; however, known penicillin-sensitive patients have been treated without difficulty. Since a photosensitivity reaction is occasionally associated with griseofulvin therapy, patients should be warned to avoid exposure to intense natural or artificial sunlight.

Lupus erythematosus or lupus-like syndromes have been reported in patients receiving griseofulvin.

Griseofulvin decreases the activity of warfarin-type anticoagulants so that patients receiving these drugs concomitantly may require dosage adjustment of the anticoagulant during and after griseofulvin therapy.

Barbiturates usually depress griseofulvin activity and concomitant administration may require a dosage adjustment of the antifungal agent.

The effect of alcohol may be potentiated by griseofulvin, producing such effects as tachycardia and flush.

Adverse Reactions: When adverse reactions occur, they are most commonly of the hypersensitivity type such as skin rashes, urticaria, and rarely, angioneurotic edema, and may necessitate withdrawal of therapy and appropriate countermeasures. Paresthesias of the hands and feet have been reported rarely after extended therapy. Other side effects reported occasionally are oral thrush, nausea, vomiting, epigastric distress, diarrhea, headache, fatigue, dizziness, insomnia, mental confusion, and impairment of performance of routine activities.

Proteinuria and leukopenia have been reported rarely. Administration of the drug should be discontinued if granulocytopenia occurs.

When rare, serious reactions occur with griseofulvin, they are usually associated with high dosages, long periods of therapy, or both.

Dosage and Administration: Accurate diagnosis of the infecting organism is essential. Identification should be made either by direct microscopic examination of a mounting of infected tissue in a solution of potassium hydroxide or by culture on an appropriate medium.

Medication must be continued until the infecting organism is completely eradicated as indicated by appropriate clinical or laboratory examination. Representative treatment periods are—*tinea capitis*, 4 to 6 weeks; *tinea corporis*, 2 to 4 weeks; *tinea pedis*, 4 to 8 weeks; *tinea unguium*—depending on rate of growth—fingernails, at least 4 months; toenails, at least 6 months.

General measures in regard to hygiene should be observed to control sources of infection or reinfection. Concomitant use of appropriate topical agents is usually required, particularly in treatment of *tinea pedis*. In some forms of athlete's foot, yeasts and bacteria may be involved as well as fungi. Griseofulvin will not eradicate the bacterial or monilial infection.

Adults: Daily administration of 330 mg (as a single dose or in divided doses) will give a satisfactory response in most patients with tinea corporis, tinea cruris, and tinea capitis. For those fungal infections more difficult to eradicate such as tinea pedis and tinea unguium, a divided dose of 660 mg is recommended.

Children: Approximately 3.3 mg per pound of body weight per day of ultra microsize griseofulvin is an effective dose for most children. On this basis the following dosage schedules are suggested:

Children weighing 35 to 50 lbs: 125 mg to 165 mg
Children weighing 50 to 75 lbs: 165 to 250 mg
Children weighing 75 lbs and over: 250 to 330 mg
Children 2 years of age and younger: dosage has not been established.

Clinical experience with griseofulvin in children with tinea capitis indicates that a single daily dose is effective. Clinical relapse will occur if the medication is not continued until the infecting organism is eradicated.

How Supplied: GRISACTIN® Ultra tablets, 125 mg: white, square shaped, compressed tablets impressed with the trade name and dosage strength, in bottles of 100 (NDC 0046-0434-81).
GRISACTIN® Ultra tablets, 250 mg: white, square shaped compressed tablets impressed with the trade name and dosage strength, in bottles of 100 (NDC 0046-0435-81).
GRISACTIN® Ultra tablets, 330 mg: scored, white, wide-oval shaped, compressed tablets impressed with the trade name and dosage strength, in bottles of 100 (NDC 0046-0437-81).
Store at room temperature (approximately 25°C).
Shown in Product Identification Section, page 405

INDERAL® ℞
[in'der-al]
Brand of propranolol hydrochloride

Description: INDERAL (propranolol hydrochloride) is a synthetic beta-adrenergic receptor blocking agent chemically described as 1-(Isopropylamino)-3-(1-naphthyloxy)-2-propanol hydrochloride. Its structural formula is

$$OCH_2CHOHCH_2NHCH(CH_3)_2 \cdot HCl$$

INDERAL is a stable, white, crystalline solid which is readily soluble in water and ethanol. Its molecular weight is 295.81.

INDERAL is available as 10 mg, 20 mg, 40 mg, 60 mg, 80 mg, and 90 mg tablets for oral administration and as a sterile injectable solution for intravenous administration.

Clinical Pharmacology: INDERAL is a nonselective beta-adrenergic receptor blocking agent possessing no other autonomic nervous system activity. Its specifically competes with beta-adrenergic receptor stimulating agents for available receptor sites. When access to beta-receptor sites is blocked by INDERAL, the chronotropic, inotropic, and vasodilator responses to beta-adrenergic stimulation are decreased proportionately.

Propranolol is almost completely absorbed from the gastrointestinal tract, but a portion is immediately bound by the liver. Peak effect occurs in one to one and one-half hours. The biologic half-life is approximately four hours.

There is no simple correlation between dose or plasma level and therapeutic effect, and the dose-sensitivity range as observed in clinical practice is wide. The principal reason for this is that sympathetic tone varies widely between individuals. Since there is no reliable test to estimate sympathetic tone or to determine whether total beta blockade has been achieved, proper dosage requires titration.

The mechanism of the antihypertensive effect of INDERAL has not been established. Among the factors that may be involved in contributing to the antihypertensive action are (1) decreased cardiac output, (2) inhibition of renin release by the kidneys, and (3) diminution of tonic sympathetic nerve outflow from vasomotor centers in the brain. Although total peripheral resistance may increase initially, it readjusts to or below the pretreatment level with chronic use. Effects on plasma volume appear to be minor and somewhat variable. INDERAL has been shown to cause a small increase in serum potassium concentration when used in the treatment of hypertensive patients.

In angina pectoris, propranolol generally reduces the oxygen requirement of the heart at any given level of effort by blocking the catecholamine-induced increases in the heart rate, systolic blood pressure, and the velocity and extent of myocardial contraction. Propranolol may increase oxygen requirements by increasing left ventricular fiber length, end diastolic pressure and systolic ejection period.

The net physiologic effect of beta adrenergic blockade is usually advantageous and is manifested during exercise by delayed onset of pain and increased work capacity.

Propranolol exerts its antiarrhythmic effects in concentrations associated with beta adrenergic blockade and this appears to be its principal antiarrhythmic mechanism of action. In dosages greater than required for beta blockade, INDERAL also exerts a quinidine-like or anesthetic-like membrane action which affects the cardiac action potential. The significance of the membrane action in the treatment of arrhythmias is uncertain.

The mechanism of the antimigraine effect of propranolol has not been established. Beta-adrenergic receptors have been demonstrated in the pial vessels of the brain.

Beta receptor blockage can be useful in conditions in which, because of pathologic or functional changes, sympathetic activity is detrimental to the patient. But there are also situations in which sympathetic stimulation is vital. For example, in patients with severely damaged hearts, adequate ventricular function is maintained by virtue of

Continued on next page

Ayerst—Cont.

sympathetic drive which should be preserved. In the presence of AV block greater than first degree, beta blockade may prevent the necessary facilitating effect of sympathetic activity on conduction. Beta blockade results in bronchial constriction by interfering with adrenergic bronchodilator activity which should be preserved in patients subject to bronchospasm.

Propranolol is not significantly dialyzable.

The Beta-Blocker Heart Attack Trial (BHAT) was a National Heart, Lung and Blood Institute-sponsored multicenter, randomized, double-blind placebo-controlled trial conducted in 31 U.S. centers (plus one in Canada) in 3,837 persons without history of severe congestive heart failure or presence of recent heart failure; certain conduction defects; angina since infarction, who had survived the acute phase of myocardial infarction. Propranolol was administered at either 60 or 80 mg t.i.d. based on blood levels achieved during an initial trial of 40 mg t.i.d. Therapy with INDERAL, begun 5–21 days following infarction, was shown to reduce overall mortality up to 39 months, the longest period of follow-up. This was primarily attributable to a reduction in cardiovascular mortality. The protective effect of INDERAL was consistent regardless of age, sex or site of infarction. Compared to placebo, total mortality was reduced 39% at 12 months and 26% over an average follow-up period of 25 months. The Norwegian Multicenter Trial in which propranolol was administered at 40 mg q.i.d. gave overall results which support the finings in the BHAT.

Although the clinical trials used either t.i.d. or q.i.d. dosing, clinical, pharmacologic and pharmacokinetic data provide a reasonable basis for concluding that b.i.d. dosing with propranolol should be adequate in the treatment of post-infarction patients.

CLINICAL: In the BHAT, patients on INDERAL were prescribed either 180 mg/day (82% of patients) or 240 mg/day (18% of patients). Patients were instructed to take the medication 3 times a day at mealtimes. This dosing schedule would result in an overnight dosing interval of 12 to 14 hours which is similar to the dosing interval for a b.i.d. regimen. In addition, blood samples were drawn at various times and analyzed for propranolol. When the patients were grouped into tertiles based on the blood levels observed and the mortality in the upper and lower tertiles were compared, there was no evidence that blood levels affected mortality.

PHARMACOLOGIC: Studies in normal volunteers have shown that a 90 mg b.i.d. regimen maintains beta-blockade at, or above, the minimum for 60 mg t.i.d. dosing for 24 hours even though differences occurred at two time intervals. At 10–12 hours after the first dose of the day, t.i.d. dosing gave more beta blockade than b.i.d. dosing, at 20–24 hours the trend of the relationship was reversed. These relationships were similar in direction to those observed for plasma propranolol levels (see Pharmacokinetic).

PHARMACOKINETIC: A bioavailability study in normal volunteers showed that the blood levels produced by 180 mg/day given b.i.d. are below those provided by the same daily dosage given t.i.d. at 10–12 hours after the first dose of the day but above those of a t.i.d. regimen at 20–24 hours. However, the blood levels produced by b.i.d. dosing were always equivalent to or above the minimum for t.i.d. dosing throughout the 24 hours. In addition, the mean AUC on the fourth day for the b.i.d. regimen was about 17% greater than for the t.i.d. regimen (1,194 vs. 1,024 ng/ml·hr).

Indications and Usage:
Hypertension
INDERAL is indicated in the management of hypertension. It may be used alone or used in combination with other antihypertensive agents, particularly a thiazide diuretic. INDERAL is not indicated in the management of hypertensive emergencies.

Angina Pectoris Due to Coronary Atherosclerosis
INDERAL is indicated for the long-term management of patients with angina pectoris.

Cardiac Arrhythmias
1.) Supraventricular arrhythmias
   a) Paroxysmal atrial tachycardias, particularly those arrhythmias induced by catecholamines or digitalis or associated with the Wolff-Parkinson-White syndrome. (See W-P-W under WARNINGS.)
   b) Persistent sinus tachycardia which is noncompensatory and impairs the well-being of the patient.
   c) Tachycardias and arrhythmias due to thyrotoxicosis when causing distress or increased hazard and when immediate effect is necessary as adjunctive, short term (2–4 weeks) therapy.
   May be used with, but not in place of, specific therapy. (See Thyrotoxicosis under WARNINGS.)
   d) Persistent atrial extrasystoles which impair the well-being of the patient and do not respond to conventional measures.
   e) Atrial flutter and fibrillation when ventricular rate cannot be controlled by digitalis alone, or when digitalis is contraindicated.
2.) Ventricular tachycardias
Ventricular arrhythmias do not respond to propranolol as predictably as do the supraventricular arrhythmias.
   a) Ventricular tachycardias
   With the exception of those induced by catecholamines or digitalis, INDERAL is not the drug of first choice. In critical situations when cardioversion technics or other drugs are not indicated or are not effective, INDERAL may be considered. If, after consideration of the risks involved, INDERAL is used, it should be given intravenously in low dosage and very slowly. (See DOSAGE AND ADMINISTRATION.) *Care in the administration of INDERAL with constant electrocardiographic monitoring is essential as the failing heart requires some sympathetic drive for maintenance of myocardial tone.*
   b) Persistent premature ventricular extrasystoles which do not respond to conventional measures and impair the well-being of the patient.
3.) Tachyarrhythmias of digitalis intoxication
If digitalis-induced tachyarrhythmias persist following discontinuance of digitalis and correction of electrolyte abnormalities, they are usually reversible with *oral* INDERAL. Severe bradycardia may occur (See OVERDOSAGE.) Intravenous propranolol hydrochloride is reserved for life-threatening arrhythmias. Temporary maintenance with oral therapy may be indicated. (See DOSAGE AND ADMINISTRATION.)
4.) Resistant tachyarrhythmias due to excessive catecholamine action during anesthesia
Tachyarrhythmias due to excessive catecholamine action during anesthesia may sometimes arise because of release of endogenous catecholamines or administration of catecholamines. When usual measures fail in such arrhythmias, INDERAL may be given intravenously to abolish them. All general inhalation anesthetics produce some degree of myocardial depression. Therefore, when INDERAL is used to treat arrhythmias during anesthesia, it should be used with extreme caution and constant ECG and central venous pressure monitoring. (See WARNINGS.)

Myocardial Infarction
INDERAL is indicated to reduce cardiovascular mortality in patients who have survived the acute phase of myocardial infarction and are clinically stable.

Migraine
INDERAL is indicated for the prophylaxis of common migraine headache. The efficacy of propranolol in the treatment of a migraine attack that has started has not been established and propranolol is not indicated for such use.

Hypertrophic Subsortic Stenosis
INDERAL is useful in the management of hypertrophic subaortic stenosis, especially for treatment of exertional or other stress-induced angina, palpitations, and syncope. INDERAL also improves exercise performance. The effectiveness of propranolol hydrochloride in this disease appears to be due to a reduction of the elevated outflow pressure gradient which is exacerbated by beta receptor stimulation. Clinical improvement may be temporary.

Pheochromocytoma
After primary treatment with an alpha-adrenergic blocking agent has been instituted, INDERAL may be useful as *adjunctive* therapy if the control of tachycardia becomes necessary before or during surgery.

It is hazardous to use INDERAL unless alpha-adrenergic blocking drugs are already in use, since this would predispose to serious blood pressure elevation. Blocking only the peripheral dilator (beta) action of epinephrine leaves its constrictor (alpha) action unopposed.

In the event of hemorrhage or shock, there is a disadvantage in having both beta and alpha blockade since the combination prevents the increase in heart rate and peripheral vasoconstriction needed to maintain blood pressure.

With inoperable or metastatic pheochromocytoma, INDERAL may be useful as an adjunct to the management of symtoms due to excessive beta receptor stimulation.

Contraindications: INDERAL is contraindicated in 1) cardiogenic shock, 2) sinus bradycardia and greater than first degree block, 3) bronchial asthma, 4) congestive heart failure (see WARNINGS) unless the failure is secondary to a tachyarrhythmia treatable with INDERAL.

Warnings: CARDIAC FAILURE: Sympathetic stimulation may be a vital component supporting circulatory function in patients with congestive heart failure, and its inhibition by beta blockade may precipitate more severe failure. Although beta blockers should be avoided in overt congestive heart failure, if necessary they can be used with close follow-up in patients with a history of failure who are well compensated and are receiving digitalis and diuretics. Beta-adrenergic blocking agents do not abolish the inotropic action of digitalis on heart muscle.

IN PATIENTS WITHOUT A HISTORY OF HEART FAILURE, continued use of beta blockers can, in some cases, lead to cardiac failure. Therefore, at the first sign or symptom of heart failure, the patient should be digitalized and/or treated with diuretics, and the response observed closely, or INDERAL should be discontinued (gradually, if possible).

IN PATIENTS WITH ANGINA PECTORIS, there have been reports of exacerbation of angina and, in some cases, myocardial infarction, following abrupt discontinuance of INDERAL therapy. Therefore, when discontinuance of INDERAL is planned the dosage should be gradually reduced over at least a few weeks and the patient should be cautioned against interruption or cessation of therapy without the physician's advice. If INDERAL therapy is interrupted and exacerbation of angina occurs, it usually is advisable to reinstitute INDERAL therapy and take other measures appropriate for the management of unstable angina pectoris. Since coronary artery disease may be unrecognized, it may be prudent to follow the above advice in patients considered at risk of having occult atherosclerotic heart disease who are given propranolol for other indications.

Nonallergic Bronchospasm (e.g., chronic bronchitis, emphysema)—PATIENTS WITH BRONCHOSPASTIC DISEASES SHOULD IN GENERAL NOT RECEIVE BETA BLOCKERS. INDERAL should be administered with caution since it may block bronchodilation produced by endogenous and exogenous catecholamine stimulation of beta receptors.

MAJOR SURGERY: The necessity or desirability of withdrawal of beta-blocking therapy prior to major surgery is controversial. It should be noted, however, that the impaired ability of the heart to respond to reflex adrenergic stimuli may augment the risks of general anesthesia and surgical procedures.

INDERAL, like other beta blockers, is a competitive inhibitor of beta-receptor agonists and its effects can be reversed by administration of such agents, e.g., dobutamine or isoproterenol. However, such patients may be subject to protracted severe hypotension. Difficulty in starting and maintaining the heartbeat has also been reported with beta blockers.

DIABETES AND HYPOGLYCEMIA: Beta-adrenergic blockade may prevent the appearance of certain premonitory signs and symptoms (pulse rate and pressure changes) of acute hypoglycemia in labile insulin-dependent diabetes. In these patients, it may be more difficult to adjust the dosage of insulin.

THYROTOXICOSIS: Beta blockade may mask certain clinical signs of hyperthyroidism. Therefore, abrupt withdrawal of propranolol may be followed by an exacerbation of symptoms of hyperthyroidism, including thyroid storm. Propranolol does not distort thyroid function tests.

IN PATIENTS WITH WOLFF-PARKINSON-WHITE SYNDROME, several cases have been reported in which, after propranolol, the tachycardia was replaced by a severe bradycardia requiring a demand pacemaker. In one case this resulted after an initial dose of 5 mg propranolol.

Precautions: General: Propranolol should be used with caution in patients with impaired hepatic or renal function. INDERAL is not indicated for the treatment of hypertensive emergencies.

Beta adrenoreceptor blockade can cause reduction of intraocular pressure. Patients should be told that INDERAL may interfere with the glaucoma screening test. Withdrawal may lead to a return of increased intraocular pressure.

Clinical Laboratory Tests: Elevated blood urea levels in patients with severe heart disease, elevated serum transaminase, alkaline phosphatase, lactate dehydrogenase.

DRUG INTERACTIONS: Patients receiving catecholamine-depleting drugs such as reserpine should be closely observed if INDERAL is administered. The added catecholamine-blocking action may produce an excessive reduction of resting sympathetic nervous activity which may result in hypotension, marked bradycardia, vertigo, syncopal attacks, or orthostatic hypotension.

Carcinogenesis, Mutagenesis, Impairment of Fertility: Long-term studies in animals have been conducted to evaluate toxic effects and carcinogenic potential. In 18-month studies in both rats and mice, employing doses up to 150 mg/kg/day, there was no evidence of significant drug-induced toxicity. There were no drug-related tumorigenic effects at any of the dosage levels. Reproductive studies in animals did not show any impairment of fertility that was attributable to the drug.

Pregnancy: Pregnancy Category C. INDERAL has been shown to be embryotoxic in animal studies at doses about 10 times greater than the maximum recommended human dose.

There are no adequate and well-controlled studies in pregnant women. INDERAL should be used during pregnancy only if the potential benefit justifies the potential risk to the fetus.

Nursing Mothers: INDERAL is excreted in human milk. Caution should be exercised when INDERAL is administered to a nursing woman.

Pediatric Use: Safety and effectiveness in children have not been established.

Adverse Reactions: Most adverse effects have been mild and transient and have rarely required the withdrawal of therapy.

Cardiovascular: bradycardia; congestive heart failure; intensification of AV block; hypotension; paresthesia of hands; thrombocytopenic purpura; arterial insufficiency, usually of the Raynaud type.

Central Nervous System: Lightheadedness; mental depression manifested by insomnia, lassitude, weakness, fatigue; reversible mental depression progressing to catatonia; visual disturbances; hallucinations; an acute reversible syndrome characterized by disorientation for time and place, short-term memory loss, emotional lability, slightly clouded sensorium, and decreased performance on neuropsychometrics.

Gastrointestinal: nausea, vomiting, epigastric distress, abdominal cramping, diarrhea, constipation, mesenteric arterial thrombosis, ischemic colitis.

Allergic: pharyngitis and agranulocytosis, erythematous rash, fever combined with aching and sore throat, laryngospasm and respiratory distress.

Respiratory: bronchospasm.

Hematologic: agranulocytosis, nonthrombocytopenic purpura, thrombocytopenic purpura.

Auto-Immune: In extremely rare instances, systemic lupus erythematosus has been reported.

Miscellaneous: alopecia, LE-like reactions, psoriasiform rashes, dry eyes, male impotence, and Peyronie's disease have been reported rarely. Oculomucocutaneous reactions involving the skin, serous membranes and conjunctivae reported for a beta blocker (practolol) have not been associated with propranolol.

Dosage and Administration:
The dosage range for INDERAL is different for each indication.

ORAL

HYPERTENSION—*Dosage must be individualized.*

The usual initial dosage is 40 mg INDERAL twice daily, whether used alone or added to a diuretic. Dosage may be increased gradually until adequate blood pressure control is achieved. The usual maintenance dosage is 120 to 240 mg per day. In some instances a dosage of 640 mg a day may be required. The time needed for full hypertensive response to a given dosage is variable and may range from a few days to several weeks.

While twice-daily dosing is effective and can maintain a reduction in blood pressure throughout the day, some patients, especially when lower doses are used, may experience a modest rise in blood pressure toward the end of the 12 hour dosing interval. This can be evaluated by measuring blood pressure near the end of the dosing interval to determine whether satisfactory control is being maintained throughout the day. If control is not adequate, a larger dose, or 3-times-daily therapy may achieve better control.

ANGINA PECTORIS—*Dosage must be individualized.*

Starting with 10–20 mg three or four times daily, before meals and at bedtime, dosage should be gradually increased at three to seven day intervals until optimum response is obtained. Although individual patients may respond at any dosage level, the average optimum dosage appears to be 160 mg per day. In angina pectoris, the value and safety of dosage exceeding 320 mg per day have not been established.

If treatment is to be discontinued, reduce dosage gradually over a period of several weeks. (See WARNINGS.)

ARRHYTHMIAS—10–30 mg three or four times daily before meals and at bedtime.

MYOCARDIAL INFARCTION

The recommended daily dosage is 180–240 mg per day in divided doses. Although a t.i.d. regimen was used in the Beta Blocker Heart Attack Trial and a q.i.d. regimen in the Norwegian Multicenter Trial, there is a reasonable basis for the use of either a t.i.d. or b.i.d. regimen (see Clinical Pharmacology). The effectiveness and safety of daily dosages greater than 240 mg for prevention of cardiac mortality have not been established. However, higher dosages may be needed to effectively treat coexisting disseases such as angina or hypertension (see above).

MIGRAINE—*Dosage must be individualized.*

The initial oral dose is 80 mg INDERAL daily in divided doses. The usual effective dose range is 160–240 mg per day. The dosage may be increased gradually to achieve optimum migraine prophylaxis.

If a satisfactory response is not obtained within four to six weeks after reaching the maximum dose, INDERAL therapy should be discontinued. It may be advisable to withdraw the drug gradually over a period of several weeks.

HYPERTROPHIC SUBAORTIC STENOSIS—20–40 mg three or four times daily, before meals and at bedtime.

PHEOCHROMOCYTOMA—*Preoperatively* — 60 mg daily in divided doses for three days prior to surgery, concomitantly with an alpha-adrenergic blocking agent.

—*Management of inoperable tumor*—30 mg daily in divided doses.

PEDIATRIC DOSAGE

At this time the data on the use of the drug in this age group are too limited to permit adequate directions for use.

INTRAVENOUS

Intravenous administration is reserved for life-threatening arrhythmias or those occurring under anesthesia. The usual dose is from 1 to 3 mg administered under careful monitoring, e.g., electrocardiographic, central venous pressure. The rate of administration should not exceed 1 mg (1 ml) per minute to diminish the possibility of lowering blood pressure and causing cardiac standstill. Sufficient time should be allowed for the drug to reach the site of action even when a slow circulation is present. If necessary, a second dose may be given after two minutes. Thereafter, additional drug should not be given in less than four hours. Additional INDERAL should not be given when the desired alteration in rate and/or rhythm is achieved.

Transference to oral therapy should be made as soon as possible.

The intravenous administration of INDERAL has not been evaluated adequately in the management of hypertensive emergencies.

OVERDOSAGE

INDERAL is not significantly dialyzable. In the event of overdosage or exaggerated response, the following measures should be employed.

General—If ingestion is or may have been recent, evacuate gastric contents, taking care to prevent pulmonary aspiration.

BRADYCARDIA—ADMINISTER ATROPINE (0.25 to 1.0 mg); IF THERE IS NO RESPONSE TO VAGAL BLOCKADE, ADMINISTER ISOPROTERENOL CAUTIOUSLY.

CARDIAC FAILURE—DIGITALIZATION AND DIURETICS.

HYPOTENSION—VASOPRESSORS, e.g. LEVARTERENOL OR EPINEPHRINE (THERE IS EVIDENCE THAT EPINEPHRINE IS THE DRUG OF CHOICE).

BRONCHOSPASM—ADMINISTER ISOPROTERENOL AND AMINOPHYLLINE.

How Supplied:

INDERAL
(propranolol hydrochloride)

TABLETS

INDERAL 10—Each hexagonal-shaped, orange, scored tablet is embossed with an "I" and imprinted with INDERAL 10, contains 10 mg propranolol hydrochloride, in bttles of 100 (NDC 0046-0421-81); 1,000 (NDC 0046-0421-91); and 5,000 (NDC 0046-0421-95). Also in unit dose packages of 100 (NDC 0046-0421-99).

INDERAL 20—Each hexagonal shaped, blue, scored tablet is embossed with an "I" and imprinted with "INDERAL 20," contains 20 mg propranolol hydrochloride, in bottles of 100 (NDC 0046-0422-81); 1,000 (NDC 0046-0422-91); and 5,000 (NDC 0046-0422-95). Also in unit dose packages of 100 (NDC 0046-0422-99).

INDERAL 40—Each hexagonal-shaped, green, scored tablet is embossed with an "I" and imprinted with "INDERAL 40," contains 40 mg propranolol hydrochloride, in bottles of 100 (NDC 0046-0424-81); 1,000 (NDC 0046-0424-91);

Continued on next page

Ayerst—Cont.

and 5,000 (NDC 0046-0424-95). Also in unit dose packages of 100 (NDC 0046-0424-99).

INDERAL 60—Each hexagonal-shaped, pink, scored tablet is embossed with an "I" and imprinted with "INDERAL 60," contains 60 mg propranolol hydrochloride, in bottles of 100 (NDC 0046-0426-81) and 1,000 (NDC 0046-0426-91). Also in unit dose packages of 100 (NDC 0046-0426-99).

INDERAL 80—Each hexagonal-shaped, yellow, scored tablet is embossed with an "I" and imprinted with "INDERAL 80," contains 80 mg propranolol hydrochloride, in bottles of 100 (NDC 0046-0428-81); 1,000 (NDC 0046-0428-91); and 5,000 (NDC 0046-0428-95). Also in unit dose packages of 100 (NDC 0046-0428-99).

INDERAL 90—Each hexagonal-shaped, lavender, scored tablet is embossed with an "I" and imprinted with "INDERAL 90," contains 90 mg propranolol hydrochloride, in bottles of 100 (NDC 0046-0439-81) and 1,000 (NDC 0046-0439-91). Also in unit dose packages of 100 (NDC 0046-0439-99).

The appearance of these tablets is a registered trademark of Ayerst Laboratories.

Store at room temperature (approximately 25°C).

INJECTABLE

—Each ml contains 1 mg of propranolol hydrochloride in Water for Injection. The pH is adjusted with citric acid. Supplied as: 1 ml ampuls in boxes of 10 (NDC 0046-3265-10).

Store at room temperature (approximately 25°C).

© 1983 AYERST LABORATORIES

Shown in Product Identification Section, page 405

INDERAL® LA ℞
[in'der-al]
Brand of propranolol hydrochloride
(Long Acting Capsules)

Description: INDERAL (propranolol hydrochloride) is a synthetic beta-adrenergic receptor blocking agent chemically described as 1-(Isopropylamino)-3-(1-naphthyloxy)-2-propanol hydrochloride. Its structural formula is

$$O-CH_2CHOHCH_2NHCH(CH_3)_2 \cdot HCl$$

INDERAL is a stable, white, crystalline solid which is readily soluble in water and ethanol. Its molecular weight is 295.81.

Inderal LA is formulated to provide a sustained release of propranolol hydrochloride. Inderal LA is available as 80 mg, 120 mg, and 160 mg capsules.

Clinical Pharmacology: INDERAL is a nonselective beta-adrenergic receptor blocking agent possessing no other autonomic nervous system activity. It specifically competes with beta-adrenergic receptor stimulating agents for available receptor sites. When access to beta-receptor sites is blocked by INDERAL, the chronotropic, inotropic, and vasodilator responses to beta-adrenergic stimulation are decreased proportionately.

INDERAL LA Capsules (80, 120, and 160 mg) release propranolol HCl at a controlled and predictable rate. Peak blood levels following dosing with INDERAL LA occur at about 6 hours and the apparent plasma half-life is about 10 hours. When measured at steady state over a 24-hour period the areas under the propranolol plasma concentration-time curve (AUCs) for the capsules are approximately 60% to 65% of the AUCs for a comparable divided daily dose of INDERAL tablets. The lower AUCs for the capsules are due to greater hepatic metabolism of propranolol, resulting from the slower rate of absorption of propranolol. Over a twenty-four (24) hour period, blood levels are fairly constant for about twelve (12) hours then decline exponentially.

INDERAL LA should not be considered a simple mg for mg substitute for conventional propranolol and the blood levels achieved do not match (are lower than) those of two to four times daily dosing with the same dose. When changing to INDERAL LA from conventional propranolol, a possible need for retitration upwards should be considered especially to maintain effectiveness at the end of the dosing interval. In most clinical settings, however, such as hypertension or angina where there is little correlation between plasma levels and clinical effect, INDERAL LA has been therapeutically equivalent to the same mg dose of conventional INDERAL as assessed by 24-hour effects on blood pressure and on 24-hour exercise responses of heart rate, systolic pressure and rate pressure product. INDERAL LA can provide effective beta blockade for a 24-hour period.

The mechanism of the antihypertensive effect of INDERAL has not been established. Among the factors that may be involved in contributing to the antihypertensive action are (1) decreased cardiac output, (2) inhibition of renin release by the kidneys, and (3) diminution of tonic sympathetic nerve outflow from vasomotor centers in the brain. Although total peripheral resistance may increase initially, it readjusts to or below the pretreatment level with chronic use. Effects on plasma volume appear to be minor and somewhat variable. INDERAL has been shown to cause a small increase in serum potassium concentration when used in the treatment of hypertensive patients.

In angina pectoris, propranolol generally reduces the oxygen requirement of the heart at any given level of effort by blocking the catecholamine-induced increases in the heart rate, systolic blood pressure, and the velocity and extent of myocardial contraction. Propranolol may increase oxygen requirements by increasing left ventricular fiber length, end diastolic pressure and systolic ejection period. The net physiologic effect of beta-adrenergic blockade is usually advantageous and is manifested during exercise by delayed onset of pain and increased work capacity.

In dosages greater than required for beta-blockade, INDERAL also exerts a quinidine-like or anesthetic-like membrane action which affects the cardiac action potential. The significance of the membrane action in the treatment of arrhythmias is uncertain.

The mechanism of the antimigraine effect of propranolol has not been established. Beta-adrenergic receptors have been demonstrated in the pial vessels of the brain.

Beta receptor blockade can be useful in conditions in which, because of pathologic or functional changes, sympathetic activity is detrimental to the patient. But there are also situations in which sympathetic stimulation is vital. For example, in patients with severely damaged hearts, adequate ventricular function is maintained by virtue of sympathetic drive which should be preserved. In the presence of AV block, greater than first degree, beta blockade may prevent the necessary facilitating effect of sympathetic activity on conduction. Beta blockade results in bronchial constriction by interfering with adrenergic bronchodilator activity which should be preserved in patients subject to bronchospasm.

Propranolol is not significantly dialyzable.

Indications and Usage:

Hypertension

INDERAL LA is indicated in the management of hypertension; it may be used alone or used in combination with other antihypertensive agents, particularly a thiazide diuretic. INDERAL LA is not indicated in the management of hypertensive emergencies.

Angina Pectoris Due to Coronary Atherosclerosis

INDERAL LA is indicated for the long-term management of patients with angina pectoris.

Migraine

INDERAL LA is indicated for the prophylaxis of common migraine headache. The efficacy of propranolol in the treatment of a migraine attack that has started has not been established and propranolol is not indicated for such use.

Hypertrophic Subaortic Stenosis

INDERAL LA is useful in the management of hypertrophic subaortic stenosis, especially for treatment of exertional or other stress-induced angina, palpitations, and syncope. INDERAL LA also improves exercise performance. The effectiveness of propranolol hydrochloride in this disease appears to be due to a reduction of the elevated outflow pressure gradient which is exacerbated by beta-receptor stimulation. Clinical improvement may be temporary.

Contraindications: INDERAL is contraindicated in 1) cardiogenic shock; 2) sinus bradycardia and greater than first degree block; 3) bronchial asthma; 4) congestive heart failure (see WARNINGS) unless the failure is secondary to a tachyarrhythmia treatable with INDERAL (propranolol hydrochloride).

Warnings:

CARDIAC FAILURE: Sympathetic stimulation may be a vital component supporting circulatory function in patients with congestive heart failure, and its inhibition by beta blockade may precipitate more severe failure. Although beta blockers should be avoided in overt congestive heart failure, if necessary, they can be used with close follow-up in patients with a history of failure who are well compensated and are receiving digitalis and diuretics. Beta-adrenergic blocking agents do not abolish the inotropic action of digitalis on heart muscle.

IN PATIENTS WITHOUT A HISTORY OF HEART FAILURE, continued use of beta blockers can, in some cases, lead to cardiac failure. Therefore, at the first sign or symptom of heart failure, the patient should be digitalized and/or treated with diuretics, and the response observed closely, or INDERAL should be discontinued (gradually, if possible).

IN PATIENTS WITH ANGINA PECTORIS, there have been reports of exacerbation of angina and, in some cases, myocardial infarction, following abrupt discontinuance of INDERAL therapy. Therefore, when discontinuance of INDERAL is planned the dosage should be gradually reduced over at least a few weeks, and the patient should be cautioned against interruption or cessation of therapy without the physician's advice. If INDERAL therapy is interrupted and exacerbation of angina occurs, it usually is advisable to reinstitute INDERAL therapy and take other measures appropriate for the management of unstable angina pectoris. Since coronary artery disease may be unrecognized, it may be prudent to follow the above advice in patients considered at risk of having occult atherosclerotic heart disease who are given propranolol for other indications.

Nonallergic Bronchospasm (e.g., chronic bronchitis, emphysema)—PATIENTS WITH BRONCHOSPASTIC DISEASES SHOULD IN GENERAL NOT RECEIVE BETA BLOCKERS. INDERAL should be administered with caution since it may block bronchodilation produced by endogenous and exogenous catecholamine stimulation of beta receptors.

MAJOR SURGERY: The necessity or desirability of withdrawal of beta-blocking therapy prior to major surgery is controversial. It should be noted, however, that the impaired ability of the heart to respond to reflex adrenergic stimuli may augment the risks of general anesthesia and surgical procedures.

INDERAL, like other beta blockers, is a competitive inhibitor of beta-receptor agonists and its effects can be reversed by administration of such agents, e.g., dobutamine or isoproterenol. However, such patients may be subject to protracted severe hypotension. Difficulty in starting and maintaining the heartbeat has also been reported with beta blockers.

DIABETES AND HYPOGLYCEMIA: Beta-adrenergic blockade may prevent the appearance of certain premonitory signs and symptoms (pulse rate and pressure changes) of acute hypoglycemia in labile insulin-dependent diabetes. In these patients, it may be more difficult to adjust the dosage of insulin.

THYROTOXICOSIS: Beta blockade may mask certain clinical signs of hyperthyroidism. Therefore, abrupt withdrawal of propranolol may be followed by an exacerbation of symptoms of hyperthyroidism, including thyroid storm. Propranolol does not distort thyroid function tests.

IN PATIENTS WITH WOLFF-PARKINSON-WHITE SYNDROME, several cases have been reported in which, after propranolol, the tachycardia was replaced by a severe bradycardia requiring a demand pacemaker. In one case this resulted after an initial dose of 5 mg propranolol.

Precautions: General: Propranolol should be used with caution in patients with impaired hepatic or renal function. INDERAL (propranolol hydrochloride) is not indicated for the treatment of hypertensive emergencies.

Beta adrenoreceptor blockade can cause reduction of intraocular pressure. Patients should be told that INDERAL may interfere with the glaucoma screening test. Withdrawal may lead to a return of increased intraocular pressure.

Clinical Laboratory Tests: Elevated blood urea levels in patients with severe heart disease, elevated serum transaminase, alkaline phosphatase, lactate dehydrogenase.

DRUG INTERACTIONS: Patients receiving catecholamine-depleting drugs such as reserpine should be closely observed if INDERAL is administered. The added catecholamine-blocking action may produce an excessive reduction of resting sympathetic nervous activity which may result in hypotension, marked bradycardia, vertigo, syncopal attacks, or orthostatic hypotension.

Carcinogenesis, Mutagenesis, Impairment of Fertility: Long-term studies in animals have been conducted to evaluate toxic effects and carcinogenic potential. In 18-month studies in both rats and mice, employing doses up to 150 mg/kg/day, there was no evidence of significant drug-induced toxicity. There were no drug-related tumorigenic effects at any of the dosage levels. Reproductive studies in animals did not show any impairment of fertility that was attributable to the drug.

Pregnancy: Pregnancy Category C. INDERAL has been shown to be embryotoxic in animal studies at doses about 10 times greater than the maximum recommended human dose.

There are no adequate and well-controlled studies in pregnant women. INDERAL should be used during pregnancy only if the potential benefit justifies the potential risk to the fetus.

Nursing Mothers: INDERAL is excreted in human milk. Caution should be exercised when INDERAL is administered to a nursing woman.

Pediatric Use: Safety and effectiveness in children have not been established.

Adverse Reactions: Most adverse effects have been mild and transient and have rarely required the withdrawal of therapy.

Cardiovascular: bradycardia; congestive heart failure; intensification of AV block; hypotension; paresthesia of hands; thrombocytopenic purpura; arterial insufficiency, usually of the Raynaud type.

Central Nervous System: Lightheadedness, mental depression manifested by insomnia, lassitude, weakness, fatigue, reversible mental depression progressing to catatonia; visual disturbances; hallucinations; an acute reversible syndrome characterized by disorientation for time and place, short-term memory loss, emotional lability, slightly clouded sensorium, and decreased performance on neuropsychometrics.

Gastrointestinal: nausea, vomiting, epigastric distress, abdominal cramping, diarrhea, constipation, mesenteric arterial thrombosis, ischemic colitis.

Allergic: pharyngitis and agranulocytosis, erythematous rash, fever combined with aching and sore throat, laryngospasm and respiratory distress.

Respiratory: bronchospasm.
Hematologic: agranulocytosis, nonthrombocytopenic purpura, thrombocytopenic purpura.
Auto-Immune: In extremely rare instances, systemic lupus erythematosus has been reported.
Miscellaneous: alopecia, LE-like reactions, psoriasiform rashes, dry eyes, male impotence, and Peyronie's disease have been reported rarely. Oculomucocutaneous reactions involving the skin, serous membranes and conjunctivae reported for a beta blocker (practolol) have not been associated with propranolol.

Dosage and Administration: INDERAL LA provides propranolol hydrochloride in a sustained-release capsule for administration once daily. If patients are switched from INDERAL tablets to INDERAL LA capsules, care should be taken to assure that the desired therapeutic effect is maintained. INDERAL LA should not be considered a simple mg for mg substitute for INDERAL. INDERAL LA has different kinetics and produces lower blood levels. Retitration may be necessary especially to maintain effectiveness at the end of the 24-hour dosing interval.

HYPERTENSION—*Dosage must be individualized.* The usual initial dosage is 80 mg INDERAL LA once daily, whether used alone or added to a diuretic. The dosage may be increased to 120 mg once daily or higher until adequate blood-pressure control is achieved. The usual maintenance dosage is 120 to 160 mg once daily. In some instances a dosage of 640 mg may be required. The time needed for full hypertensive response to a given dosage is variable and may range from a few days to several weeks.

ANGINA PECTORIS—*Dosage must be individualized.* Starting with 80 mg INDERAL LA once daily, dosage should be gradually increased at three to seven day intervals until optimum response is obtained. Although individual patients may respond at any dosage level, the average optimum dosage appears to be 160 mg once daily. In angina pectoris, the value and safety of dosage exceeding 320 mg per day have not been established.

If treatment is to be discontinued, reduce dosage gradually over a period of a few weeks (see WARNINGS).

MIGRAINE—*Dosage must be individualized.* The initial oral dose is 80 mg INDERAL LA once daily. The usual effective dose range is 160-240 mg once daily. The dosage may be increased gradually to achieve optimum migraine prophylaxis. If a satisfactory response is not obtained within four to six weeks after reaching the maximum dose, INDERAL LA therapy should be discontinued. It may be advisable to withdraw the drug gradually over a period of several weeks.

HYPERTROPHIC SUBAORTIC STENOSIS—80-160 mg INDERAL LA once daily.

PEDIATRIC DOSAGE

At this time the data on the use of the drug in this age group are too limited to permit adequate directions for use.

OVERDOSAGE

Inderal is not significantly dialyzable. In the event of overdosage or exaggerated response, the following measures should be employed:

General—If ingestion is or may have been recent, evacuate gastric contents, taking care to prevent pulmonary aspiration.

BRADYCARDIA—ADMINISTER ATROPINE (0.25 to 1.0 mg); IF THERE IS NO RESPONSE TO VAGAL BLOCKADE, ADMINISTER ISOPROTERENOL CAUTIOUSLY.

CARDIAC FAILURE—DIGITALIZATION AND DIURETICS.

HYPOTENSION—VASOPRESSORS, e.g. LEVARTERENOL OR EPINEPHRINE (THERE IS EVIDENCE THAT EPINEPHRINE IS THE DRUG OF CHOICE).

BRONCHOSPASM—ADMINISTER ISOPROTERENOL AND AMINOPHYLLINE.

How Supplied:

INDERAL LA CAPSULES
(propranolol hydrochloride)

—Each light-blue capsule, identified by 3 narrow bands and 1 wide band and "INDERAL LA 80,"

contains 80 mg of propranolol hydrochloride in bottles of 100 (NDC 0046-0471-81) and 1,000 (NDC 0046-0471-91). Also available in a unit dose package of 100 (NDC 0046-0471-99).

—Each light-blue/dark-blue capsule, identified by 3 narrow bands and 1 wide band and "INDERAL LA 120," contains 120 mg of propranolol hydrochloride in bottles of 100 (NDC 0046-0473-81) and 1,000 (NDC 0046-0473-91). Also available in a unit dose package of 100 (NDC 0046-0473-99).

—Each dark-blue capsule, identified by 3 narrow bands and 1 wide band and "INDERAL LA 160," contains 160 mg of propranolol hydrochloride in bottles of 100 (NDC 0046-0479-81) and 1,000 (NDC 0046-0479-91). Also available in a unit dose package of 100 (NDC 0046-0479-99).

The appearance of these capsules is a registered trademark of Ayerst Laboratories.

Store at room temperature (approximately 25°C).

© 1983 AYERST LABORATORIES

Shown in Product Identification Section, page 405

INDERIDE®   ℞
[in'de-ride]
Brand of propranolol hydrochloride (INDERAL®) and hydrochlorothiazide

No. 484—Each INDERIDE®-40/25 tablet contains:
Propranolol hydrochloride
 (Inderal®) ....40 mg
Hydrochlorothiazide ....25 mg
No. 488—Each INDERIDE®-80/25 tablet contains:
Propranolol hydrochloride
 (INDERAL®) ....80 mg
Hydrochlorothiazide ....25 mg

Warning

This fixed combination drug is not indicated for initial therapy of hypertension. Hypertension requires therapy titrated to the individual patient. If the fixed combination represents the dosage so determined, its use may be more convenient in patient management. The treatment of hypertension is not static, but must be reevaluated as conditions in each patient warrant.

Description: INDERIDE combines two antihypertensive agents: INDERAL (propranolol hydrochloride), a beta-adrenergic blocking agent, and hydrochlorothiazide, a thiazide diuretic-antihypertensive.

Propranolol hydrochloride is a stable, white to off-white, crystalline powder with a melting point of about 164°C. It is odorless and has a bitter taste. It is readily soluble in water and ethanol, and insoluble in non-polar solvents. Its chemical name is 1-(Isopropylamino)-3-(1-naphthyloxy)-2-propanol hydrochloride.

Hydrochlorothiazide is a white, or practically white, practically odorless, crystalline powder. It is slightly soluble in water, freely soluble in sodium hydroxide solution, sparingly soluble in methanol; insoluble in ether, chloroform, benzene, and dilute mineral acids. Its chemical name is 6-Chloro-3,4-dihydro-2H-1,2,4-benzothiadiazine-7-sulfonamide 1,1-dioxide.

Clinical Pharmacology:
Propranolol hydrochloride (INDERAL®):
Propranolol hydrochloride is a beta-adrenergic receptor blocking drug, possessing no other autonomic nervous system activity. It specifically competes with beta-adrenergic receptor stimulating agents for available beta-receptor sites. When access to beta-receptor sites is blocked by propranolol, the chronotropic, inotropic, and vasodilator responses to beta-adrenergic stimulation are decreased proportionately.

Propranolol is almost completely absorbed from the gastrointestinal tract, but a portion is immediately bound by the liver. Peak effect occurs in one to one and one-half hours. The biologic half-life is

Continued on next page

Ayerst—Cont.

approximately two to three hours. Propranolol is not significantly dialyzable. There is no simple correlation between dose or plasma level and therapeutic effect, and the dose-sensitivity range as observed in clinical practice is wide. The principal reason for this is that sympathetic tone varies widely between individuals. Since there is no reliable test to estimate sympathetic tone or to determine whether total beta blockade has been achieved, proper dosage requires titration.

The mechanism of the antihypertensive effects of propranolol has not been established. Among the factors that may be involved are (1) decreased cardiac output, (2) inhibition of renin release by the kidneys, and (3) diminution of tonic sympathetic nerve outflow from vasomotor centers in the brain.

Propranolol hydrochloride decreases heart rate, cardiac output, and blood pressure. Although total peripheral vascular resistance may increase initially, it readjusts to the pretreatment level or lower with chronic usage. Earlier studies indicate that plasma volume remains unchanged or may decrease. However, there are certain more recent studies suggesting that in the absence of sodium restriction, plasma volume may increase.

Beta-receptor blockade is useful in conditions in which, because of pathologic or functional changes, sympathetic activity is excessive or inappropriate, and detrimental to the patient. But there are also situations in which sympathetic stimulation is vital. For example, in patients with severely damaged hearts, adequate ventricular function is maintained by virtue of sympathetic drive which should be preserved. In the presence of AV block, beta blockade may prevent the necessary facilitating effect of sympathetic activity on conduction. Beta blockade results in bronchial constriction by interfering with adrenergic bronchodilator activity which should be preserved in patients subject to bronchospasm.

The proper objective of beta-blockade therapy is to decrease adverse sympathetic stimulation, but not to the degree that may impair necessary sympathetic support.

Hydrochlorothiazide:

Hydrochlorothiazide is a benzothiadiazine (thiazide) diuretic closely related to chlorothiazide. The mechanism of the antihypertensive effect of the thiazides is unknown. Thiazides do not affect normal blood pressure.

Thiazides affect the renal tubular mechanism of electrolyte reabsorption. At maximal therapeutic dosage, all thiazides are approximately equal in their diuretic potency.

Thiazides increase excretion of sodium and chloride in approximately equivalent amounts. Natriuresis causes a secondary loss of potassium and bicarbonate.

Onset of diuretic action of thiazides occurs in two hours, and the peak effect in about four hours. Its action persists for approximately six to 12 hours. Thiazides are eliminated rapidly by the kidney.

Indication: INDERIDE [propranolol HCl (INDERAL®) and hydrochlorothiazide] is indicated in the management of hypertension. (See boxed warning.)

Contraindications:

Propranolol hydrochloride (INDERAL®):
Propranolol hydrochloride is contraindicated in: 1) bronchial asthma; 2) allergic rhinitis during the pollen season; 3) sinus bradycardia and greater than first degree block; 4) cardiogenic shock; 5) right ventricular failure secondary to pulmonary hypertension; 6) congestive heart failure (see WARNINGS) unless the failure is secondary to a tachyarrhythmia treatable with propranolol; 7) in patients on adrenergic-augmenting psychotropic drugs (including MAO inhibitors), and during the two week withdrawal period from such drugs.

Hydrochlorothiazide:

Hydrochlorothiazide is contraindicated in patients with anuria or hypersensitivity to this or other sulfonamide-derived drugs.

Warnings:

Propranolol hydrochloride (INDERAL®):
CARDIAC FAILURE: Sympathetic stimulation is a vital component supporting circulatory function in congestive heart failure, and inhibition with beta blockade always carries the potential hazard of further depressing myocardial contractility and precipitating cardiac failure. Propranolol acts selectively without abolishing the inotropic action of digitalis on the heart muscle (*i.e.* that of supporting the strength of myocardial contractions). In patients already receiving digitalis, the positive inotropic action of digitalis may be reduced by propranolol's negative inotropic effect. The effects of propranolol and digitalis are additive in depressing AV conduction.

IN PATIENTS WITHOUT A HISTORY OF CARDIAC FAILURE, continued depression of the myocardium over a period of time can, in some cases, lead to cardiac failure. In rare instances, this has been observed during propranolol therapy. Therefore, at the first sign or symptom of impending cardiac failure, patients should be fully digitalized and/or given a diuretic, and the response observed closely: a) if cardiac failure continues, despite adequate digitalization and diuretic therapy, propranolol therapy should be immediately withdrawn; b) if tachyarrhythmia is being controlled, patients should be maintained on combined therapy and the patient closely followed until threat of cardiac failure is over.

IN PATIENTS WITH ANGINA PECTORIS, there have been reports of exacerbation of angina and, in some cases, myocardial infarction, following *abrupt* discontinuation of propranolol therapy. Therefore, when discontinuance of propranolol is planned the dosage should be gradually reduced and the patient carefully monitored. In addition, when propranolol is prescribed for angina pectoris, the patient should be cautioned against interruption or cessation of therapy without the physician's advice. If propranolol therapy is interrupted and exacerbation of angina occurs, it usually is advisable to reinstitute propranolol therapy and take other measures appropriate for the management of unstable angina pectoris. Since coronary artery disease may be unrecognized, it may be prudent to follow the above advice in patients considered at risk of having occult atherosclerotic heart disease, who are given propranolol for other indications.

IN PATIENTS WITH THYROTOXICOSIS, possible deleterious effects from long-term use have not been adequately appraised. Special consideration should be given to propranolol's potential for aggravating congestive heart failure. Propranolol may mask the clinical signs of developing or continuing hyperthyroidism or complications and give a false impression of improvement. Therefore, abrupt withdrawal of propranolol may be followed by an exacerbation of symptoms of hyperthyroidism, including thyroid storm. This is another reason for withdrawing propranolol slowly. Propranolol does not distort thyroid function tests.
IN PATIENTS WITH WOLFF-PARKINSON-WHITE SYNDROME, several cases have been reported in which, after propranolol, the tachycardia was replaced by a severe bradycardia requiring a demand pacemaker. In one case this resulted after an initial dose of 5 mg propranolol.
IN PATIENTS UNDERGOING MAJOR SURGERY, beta blockade impairs the ability of the heart to respond to reflex stimuli. For this reason, with the exception of pheochromocytoma, propranolol should be withdrawn 48 hours prior to surgery, at which time all chemical and physiologic effects are gone according to available evidence. However, in case of emergency surgery, since propranolol is a competitive inhibitor of beta-receptor agonists, its effects can be reversed by administration of such agents, *e.g.* isoproterenol or levarterenol. However, such patients may be subject to protracted severe hypotension. Difficulty in restarting and maintaining the heart beat has also been reported.
IN PATIENTS PRONE TO NONALLERGIC BRONCHOSPASM (*e.g.*, CHRONIC BRONCHITIS, EMPHYSEMA), propranolol should be administered with caution since it may block bronchodilation produced by endogenous and exogenous catecholamine stimulation of beta receptors.
DIABETICS AND PATIENTS SUBJECT TO HYPOGLYCEMIA: Because of its beta-adrenergic blocking activity, propranolol may prevent the appearance of premonitory signs and symptoms (pulse rate and pressure changes) of acute hypoglycemia. This is especially important to keep in mind in patients with labile diabetes. Hypoglycemic attacks may be accompanied by a precipitous elevation of blood pressure.

Hydrochlorothiazide:

Thiazides should be used with caution in severe renal disease. In patients with renal disease, thiazides may precipitate azotemia. In patients with impaired renal function, cumulative effects of the drug may develop.

Thiazides should also be used with caution in patients with impaired hepatic function or progressive liver disease, since minor alterations of fluid and electrolyte balance may precipitate hepatic coma.

Thiazides may add to or potentiate the action of other antihypertensive drugs. Potentiation occurs with ganglionic or peripheral adrenergic blocking drugs.

Sensitivity reactions may occur in patients with a history of allergy or bronchial asthma.

The possibility of exacerbation or activation of systemic lupus erythematosus has been reported.

USE IN PREGNANCY:

Propranolol hydrochloride (INDERAL®):
The safe use of propranolol in human pregnancy has not been established. Use of any drug in pregnancy or women of childbearing potential requires that the possible risk to mother and/or fetus be weighed against the expected therapeutic benefit. Embryotoxic effects have been seen in animal studies at doses about 10 times the maximum recommended human dose.

Hydrochlorothiazide:

Thiazides cross the placental barrier and appear in cord blood. The use of thiazides in pregnant women requires that the anticipated benefit be weighed against possible hazards to the fetus. These hazards include fetal or neonatal jaundice, thrombocytopenia, and possibly other adverse reactions which have occurred in the adult.
Nursing Mothers: Thiazides appear in breast milk. If the use of the drug is deemed essential, the patient should stop nursing.

Precautions:

Propranolol hydrochloride (INDERAL®):
Patients receiving catecholamine-depleting drugs such as reserpine should be closely observed if propranolol is administered. The added catecholamine blocking action of this drug may then produce an excessive reduction of the resting sympathetic nervous activity. Occasionally, the pharmacologic activity of propranolol may produce hypotension and/or marked bradycardia resulting in vertigo, syncopal attacks, or orthostatic hypotension.
As with any new drug given over prolonged periods, laboratory parameters should be observed at regular intervals. The drug should be used with caution in patients with impaired renal or hepatic function.

Hydrochlorothiazide:

Periodic determination of serum electrolytes to detect possible electrolyte imbalance should be performed at appropriate intervals.
All patients receiving thiazide therapy should be observed for clinical signs of fluid or electrolyte imbalance, namely: hyponatremia, hypochloremic alkalosis, and hypokalemia. Serum and urine electrolyte determinations are particularly important when the patient is vomiting excessively or receiving parenteral fluids. Medication such as digitalis may also influence serum electrolytes. Warning signs, irrespective of cause are: dryness of mouth, thirst, weakness, lethargy, drowsiness, restless-

ness, muscle pains or cramps, muscular fatigue, hypotension, oliguria, tachycardia, and gastrointestinal disturbances such as nausea and vomiting.

Hypokalemia may develop, especially with brisk diuresis, when severe cirrhosis is present or during concomitant use of corticosteroids or ACTH. Interference with adequate oral electrolyte intake will also contribute to hypokalemia. Hypokalemia can sensitize or exaggerate the response of the heart to the toxic effects of digitalis (*e.g.*, increased ventricular irritability). Hypokalemia may be avoided or treated by use of potassium supplements such as foods with a high potassium content.

Any chloride deficit is generally mild, and usually does not require specific treatment except under extraordinary circumstances (as in liver or renal disease). Dilutional hyponatremia may occur in edematous patients in hot weather; appropriate therapy is water restriction, rather than administration of salt, except in rare instances when the hyponatremia is life-threatening. In actual salt depletion, appropriate replacement is the therapy of choice.

Hyperuricemia may occur or frank gout may be precipitated in certain patients receiving thiazide therapy.

Insulin requirements in diabetic patients may be increased, decreased, or unchanged. Diabetes mellitus which has been latent may become manifest during thiazide administration.

Thiazide drugs may increase the responsiveness to tubocurarine.

The antihypertensive effects of the drug may be enhanced in the postsympathectomy patient. Thiazides may decrease arterial responsiveness to norepinephrine. This diminution is not sufficient to preclude effectiveness of the pressor agent for therapeutic use.

If progressive renal impairment becomes evident, consider withholding or discontinuing diuretic therapy.

Thiazides may decrease serum PBI levels without signs of thyroid disturbance.

Calcium excretion is decreased by thiazides. Pathologic changes in the parathyroid gland with hypercalcemia and hypophosphatemia have been observed in a few patients on prolonged thiazide therapy. The common complications of hyperparathyroidism such as renal lithiasis, bone resorption, and peptic ulceration, have not been seen. Thiazides should be discontinued before carrying out tests for parathyroid function.

Adverse Reactions:
Propranolol hydrochloride (INDERAL®):
Cardiovascular: bradycardia; congestive heart failure; intensification of AV block; hypotension; paresthesia of hands; arterial insufficiency, usually of the Raynaud type; thrombocytopenic purpura.
Central Nervous System: lightheadedness; mental depression manifested by insomnia, lassitude, weakness, fatigue, reversible mental depression progressing to catatonia; visual disturbances; hallucinations; an acute reversible syndrome characterized by disorientation for time and place, short term memory loss, emotional lability, slightly clouded sensorium, and decreased performance on neuropsychometrics.
Gastrointestinal: nausea, vomiting, epigastric distress, abdominal cramping, diarrhea, constipation, mesenteric arterial thrombosis, ischemic colitis.
Allergic: pharyngitis and agranulocytosis, erythematous rash, fever combined with aching and sore throat, laryngospasm and respiratory distress.
Respiratory: bronchospasm.
Hematologic: agranulocytosis, nonthrombocytopenic purpura, thrombocytopenic purpura.
Miscellaneous: reversible alopecia. Oculomucocutaneous reactions involving the skin, serous membranes and conjunctivae reported for a beta blocker (practolol) have not been conclusively associated with propranolol.
Clinical Laboratory Test Findings: Elevated blood urea levels in patients with severe heart disease,

elevated serum transaminase, alkaline phosphatase, lactate dehydrogenase.
Hydrochlorothiazide:
Gastrointestinal: anorexia, gastric irritation, nausea, vomiting, cramping, diarrhea, constipation, jaundice (intrahepatic cholestatic jaundice), pancreatitis, sialadenitis.
Central Nervous System: dizziness, vertigo, paresthesias, headache, xanthopsia.
Hematologic: leukopenia, agranulocytosis, thrombocytopenia, aplastic anemia.
Cardiovascular: orthostatic hypotension (may be aggravated by alcohol, barbiturates, or narcotics).
Hypersensitivity: purpura, photosensitivity, rash, urticaria, necrotizing angiitis (vasculitis, cutaneous vasculitis), fever, respiratory distress including pneumonitis, anaphylactic reactions.
Other: hyperglycemia, glycosuria, hyperuricemia, muscle spasm, weakness, restlessness, transient blurred vision.
Whenever adverse reactions are moderate or severe, thiazide dosage should be reduced or therapy withdrawn.

Dosage and Administration:
The dosage must be determined by individual titration (see boxed warning).
Hydrochlorothiazide is usually given at a dose of 50 to 100 mg per day. The initial dose of propranolol is 40 mg twice daily and it may be increased gradually until optimum blood pressure control is achieved. The usual effective dose is 160 to 480 mg per day.
One to two INDERIDE [propranolol HCl (INDERAL®) and hydrochlorothiazide] tablets twice daily can be used to administer up to 320 mg of propranolol and 100 mg of hydrochlorothiazide. For doses of propranolol greater than 320 mg, the combination products are not appropriate because their use would lead to an excessive dose of the thiazide component.
When necessary, another antihypertensive agent may be added gradually beginning with 50 percent of the usual recommended starting dose to avoid an excessive fall in blood pressure.

Overdosage or Exaggerated Response:
The propranolol hydrochloride (INDERAL) component may cause bradycardia, cardiac failure, hypotension, or bronchospasm.
The hydrochlorothiazide component can be expected to cause diuresis. Lethargy of varying degree may appear and may progress to coma within a few hours, with minimal depression of respiration and cardiovascular function, and in the absence of significant serum electrolyte changes or dehydration. The mechanism of central nervous system depression with thiazide overdosage is unknown. Gastrointestinal irritation and hypermotility can occur; temporary elevation of BUN has been reported, and serum electrolyte changes could occur, especially in patients with impairment of renal function.

TREATMENT
The following measures should be employed:
GENERAL—If ingestion is, or may have been, recent, induce gastric contents taking care to prevent pulmonary aspiration.
BRADYCARDIA—Administer atropine (0.25 to 1.0 mg). If there is no response to vagal blockade, administer isoproterenol cautiously.
CARDIAC FAILURE—Digitalization and diuretics.
HYPOTENSION—Vasopressors, *e.g.*, levarterenol or epinephrine.
BRONCHOSPASM—Administer isoproterenol and aminophylline.
STUPOR OR COMA—Administer supportive therapy as clinically warranted.
GASTROINTESTINAL EFFECTS—Though usually of short duration, these may require symptomatic treatment.
ABNORMALITIES IN BUN AND/OR SERUM ELECTROLYTES—Monitor serum electrolyte levels and renal function; institute supportive measures as required individually to maintain hydration, electrolyte balance, respiration, and cardiovascular-renal function.

How Supplied:
—Each hexagonal-shaped, off-white, scored INDERIDE 40/25 tablet is embossed with an "I" and imprinted with "INDERIDE 40/25," contains 40 mg propranolol hydrochloride (INDERAL®) and 25 mg hydrochlorothiazide, in bottles of 100 (NDC 0046-0484-81) and 1,000 (NDC 0046-0484-91). Also in unit dose package of 100 (NDC 0046-0484-99).
—Each hexagonal-shaped, off-white, scored INDERIDE 80/25 tablet is embossed with an "I" and imprinted with "INDERIDE 80/25," contains 80 mg propranolol hydrochloride (INDERAL®) and 25 mg hydrochlorothiazide, in bottles of 100 (NDC 0046-0488-81) and 1,000 (NDC 0046-0488-91). Also in unit dose package of 100 (NDC 0046-0488-99).
The appearance of these tablets is a registered trademark of Ayerst Laboratories.
Store at room temperature (approximately 25°C).
Shown in Product Identification Section, page 405

KERODEX®
[kĕr'o-dĕx]
Skin Barrier Cream

Action and Uses: A specially formulated barrier cream to help protect against potentially irritating chemicals, compounds, and solutions in common use. When applied and used as directed, KERODEX provides a barrier film that helps to block contact with skin irritants. KERODEX No. 71 (water-repellent) is for use in handling or working with *wet* materials; No. 51 is for *dry* or *oily* work. KERODEX is greaseless and stainless.
Application: 1. Wash hands clean and dry *thoroughly*. 2. Squeeze out ½ inch of cream into palm of one hand. Rub hands together with a washing motion until cream is *lightly* and *evenly* distributed, leaving no excess. Make sure cream reaches under nails, around cuticles, between fingers, across wrists and backs of hands (forearms, if necessary). 3. A second application is recommended.
NOTE: After applying KERODEX 71, "set" by holding hands under cold running water. Pat dry. After applying KERODEX 51, avoid contact with water. If hands become wet during work, reapply.
How Supplied: KERODEX (water-repellent cream for wet work), in 4 oz (113 g) tubes (NDC 0046-0071-04) and 1 lb. jars (NDC 0046-0071-01). KERODEX (water-miscible cream for dry or oily work), in 4 oz (113 g) tubes (NDC 0046-0051-04) and 1 lb. jars (NDC 0046-0051-01).

LARYLGAN® Throat Spray
[lăr'al-gan]

An aqueous solution containing:
Antipyrine 0.30%
Pyrilamine maleate 0.05%
Sodium caprylate 0.50%
Also contains menthol, gentian violet, methyl salicylate, methylparaben, propylparaben, peppermint oil, spearmint oil, anise oil, cinnamon oil, isobornyl acetate, benzyl alcohol 0.05%, ethyl alcohol 1.00%, glycerin, sodium saccharin, and other aromatics.

Action: The analgesic-like effect of LARYLGAN helps to allay pain of irritated mucosa. The glycerin dehydrated vehicle provides maximum spreading and penetrating properties to help the medication reach the affected areas. It is non-narcotic.
Indications: A soothing and refreshing spray for dry throat and for minor sore throat due to irritants such as smoking and postnasal drip.
Warning: Severe and persistent sore throat or sore throat accompanied by high fever, headache, nausea, and vomiting may be serious. Consult physician promptly. Do not use more than two days or administer to children under 3 years of age unless directed by physician.
Administration: *Instructions for Use:* Adults and children 3 years of age or older. Remove cap. Hold close to mouth. Spray as needed. If throat condition persists, consult a physician.

Continued on next page

Ayerst—Cont.

How Supplied: LARYLGAN Throat Spray, in 0.94 fl oz (28 ml) bottles (NDC 0046-1005-01).

MEDIATRIC®
[mē″dē-ăt′rik]

Each capsule or tablet contains:
Premarin®
 (Conjugated Estrogens, U.S.P.) ..... 0.25 mg
Methyltestosterone .... 2.5 mg
Ascorbic acid (Vit. C)* .... 100.0 mg
Cyanocobalamin .... 2.5 mcg
Thiamine mononitrate .... 10.0 mg
Riboflavin .... 5.0 mg
Niacinamide .... 50.0 mg
Pyridoxine HCl .... 3.0 mg
Calc. pantothenate .... 20.0 mg
Dried ferrous sulfate .... 30.0 mg
Methamphetamine HCl .... 1.0 mg

*For Capsules, provided as ascorbic acid, 70 mg, and as sodium ascorbate, 30 mg.

Also available: MEDIATRIC Liquid
Each 15 ml (3 teaspoonfuls) contains:
Premarin®
 (Conjugated Estrogens, U.S.P.) ..... 0.25 mg
Methyltestosterone .... 2.5 mg
Thiamine HCl .... 5.0 mg
Cyanocobalamin .... 1.5 mcg
Methamphetamine HCl .... 1.0 mg

Contains 15% alcohol—some loss unavoidable.

---

1. ESTROGENS HAVE BEEN REPORTED TO INCREASE THE RISK OF ENDOMETRIAL CARCINOMA.
Three independent case control studies have reported an increased risk of endometrial cancer in postmenopausal women exposed to exogenous estrogens for more than one year.[1-3] This risk was independent of the other known risk factors for endometrial cancer. These studies are further supported by the finding that incidence rates of endometrial cancer have increased sharply since 1969 in eight different areas of the United States with population-based cancer reporting systems, an increase which may be related to the rapidly expanding use of estrogens during the last decade.[4]
The three case control studies reported that the risk of endometrial cancer in estrogen users was about 4.5 to 13.9 times greater than in nonusers. The risk appears to depend on both duration of treatment[1] and on estrogen dose.[3] In view of these findings, when estrogens are used for the treatment of menopausal symptoms, the lowest dose that will control symptoms should be utilized and medication should be discontinued as soon as possible. When prolonged treatment is medically indicated, the patient should be reassessed on at least a semiannual basis to determine the need for continued therapy. Although the evidence must be considered preliminary, one study suggests that cyclic administration of low doses of estrogen may carry less risk than continuous administration;[3] it therefore appears prudent to utilize such a regimen.
Close clinical surveillance of all women taking estrogens is important. In all cases of undiagnosed persistent or recurring abnormal vaginal bleeding, adequate diagnostic measures should be undertaken to rule out malignancy.
There is no evidence at present that "natural" estrogens are more or less hazardous than "synthetic" estrogens at equiestrogenic doses.

2. ESTROGENS SHOULD NOT BE USED DURING PREGNANCY.
The use of female sex hormones, both estrogens and progestogens, during early pregnancy may seriously damage the offspring. It has been shown that females exposed in utero to diethylstilbestrol, a non-steroidal estrogen, have an increased risk of developing in later life a form of vaginal or cervical cancer that is ordinarily extremely rare.[5,6] This risk has been estimated as not greater than 4 per 1000 exposures.[7] Furthermore, a high percentage of such exposed women (from 30 to 90 percent) have been found to have vaginal adenosis,[8-12] epithelial changes of the vagina and cervix. Although these changes are histologically benign, it is not known whether they are precursors of malignancy. Although similar data are not available with the use of other estrogens, it cannot be presumed they would not induce similar changes.
Several reports suggest an association between intrauterine exposure to female sex hormones and congenital anomalies, including congenital heart defects and limb reduction defects.[13-16] One case control study[16] estimated a 4.7-fold increased risk of limb reduction defects in infants exposed in utero to sex hormones (oral contraceptives, hormone withdrawal tests for pregnancy, or attempted treatment for threatened abortion). Some of these exposures were very short and involved only a few days of treatment. The data suggest that the risk of limb reduction defects in exposed fetuses is somewhat less than 1 per 1000.
In the past, female sex hormones have been used during pregnancy in an attempt to treat threatened or habitual abortion. There is considerable evidence that estrogens are ineffective for these indications, and there is no evidence from well controlled studies that progestogens are effective for these uses.
If MEDIATRIC is used during pregnancy, or if the patient becomes pregnant while taking this drug, she should be apprised of the potential risks to the fetus, and the advisability of pregnancy continuation.

Description: MEDIATRIC provides estrogen and androgen in small doses, nutritional supplements, together with a mild antidepressant.
Action: MEDIATRIC provides (1) *steroids* to help counteract declining gonadal hormone secretion, and as important regulators of metabolic processes; (2) *nutritional supplements* specially selected to meet the needs of the aged and aging patient, and to act as necessary catalysts for the maintenance of efficient enzyme systems; and (3) *a mild antidepressant* to impart a gentle emotional uplift.
Indication: For use in aging patients of both sexes.
MEDIATRIC HAS NOT BEEN SHOWN TO BE EFFECTIVE FOR ANY PURPOSE DURING PREGNANCY AND ITS USE MAY CAUSE SEVERE HARM TO THE FETUS (SEE BOXED WARNING).
Contraindications: Estrogens should not be used in women (or men) with any of the following conditions:
1. Known or suspected cancer of the breast except in appropriately selected patients being treated for metastatic disease.
2. Known or suspected estrogen-dependent neoplasia.
3. Known or suspected pregnancy (See Boxed Warning).
4. Undiagnosed abnormal genital bleeding.
5. Active thrombophlebitis or thromboembolic disorders.
6. A past history of thrombophlebitis, thrombosis, or thromboembolic disorders associated with previous estrogen use (except when used in treatment of breast or prostatic malignancy).
Methyltestosterone should not be used in persons with any of the following conditions:
1. Known or suspected carcinoma of the prostate and in carcinoma of the male breast.
2. Severe liver damage.
3. Pregnancy or in breast-feeding mothers because of the possibility of masculinization of the female fetus or breast-fed infant.

Warnings:
Associated with Estrogens
1. *Induction of malignant neoplasms.* Long term continuous administration of natural and synthetic estrogens in certain animal species increases the frequency of carcinomas of the breast, cervix, vagina, and liver. There are now reports that estrogens increase the risk of carcinoma of the endometrium in humans. (See Boxed Warning.)
At the present time there is no satisfactory evidence that estrogens given to postmenopausal women increase the risk of cancer of the breast,[17] although a recent long-term followup of a single physician's practice has raised this possibility.[18] Because of the animal data, there is a need for caution in prescribing estrogens for women with a strong family history of breast cancer or who have breast nodules, fibrocystic disease, or abnormal mammograms.
2. *Gallbladder disease.* A recent study has reported a 2 to 3-fold increase in the risk of surgically confirmed gallbladder disease in women receiving postmenopausal estrogens,[17] similar to the 2-fold increase previously noted in users of oral contraceptives.[19,24a]
3. *Effects similar to those caused by estrogen-progestogen oral contraceptives.* There are several serious adverse effects of oral contraceptives, most of which have not, up to now, been documented as consequences of postmenopausal estrogen therapy. This may reflect the comparatively low doses of estrogen used in postmenopausal women. It would be expected that the larger doses of estrogen used to treat prostatic or breast cancer or postpartum breast engorgement are more likely to result in these adverse effects, and, in fact, it has been shown that there is an increased risk of thrombosis in men receiving estrogens for prostatic cancer and women for postpartum breast engorgement.[20-23]
a. *Thromboembolic disease.* It is now well established that users of oral contraceptives have an increased risk of various thromboembolic and thrombotic vascular diseases, such as thrombophlebitis, pulmonary embolism, stroke, and myocardial infarction.[24-31] Cases of retinal thrombosis, mesenteric thrombosis, and optic neuritis have been reported in oral contraceptive users. There is evidence that the risk of several of these adverse reactions is related to the dose of the drug.[32,33] An increased risk of postsurgery thromboembolic complications has also been reported in users of oral contraceptives.[34,35] If feasible, estrogen should be discontinued at least 4 weeks before surgery of the type associated with an increased risk of thromboembolism, or during periods of prolonged immobilization.
While an increased rate of thromboembolic and thrombotic disease in postmenopausal users of estrogens has not been found,[17-24,25-36] this does not rule out the possibility that such an increase may be present or that subgroups of women who have underlying risk factors or who are receiving relatively large doses of estrogens may have increased risk. Therefore estrogens should not be used in persons with active thrombophlebitis or thromboembolic disorders, and they should not be used (except in treatment of malignancy) in persons with a history of such disorders in association with estrogen use. They should be used with caution in patients with cerebral vascular or coronary artery disease and only for those in whom estrogens are clearly needed.
Large doses of estrogen (5 mg conjugated estrogens per day), comparable to those used to treat cancer of the prostate and breast, have been shown in a large prospective clinical trial in men[37] to increase the risk of nonfatal myocardial infarction, pulmonary embolism and thrombophlebitis. When estrogen doses of this size are used, any of the thromboembolic and thrombotic adverse effects associated with oral contraceptive use should be considered a clear risk.
b. *Hepatic adenoma.* Benign hepatic adenomas appear to be associated with the use of oral contraceptives.[38-40] Although benign, and rare, these may rupture and may cause death through intra-

abdominal hemorrhage. Such lesions have not yet been reported in association with other estrogen or progestogen preparations but should be considered in estrogen users having abdominal pain and tenderness, abdominal mass, or hypovolemic shock. Hepatocellular carcinoma has also been reported in women taking estrogen-containing oral contraceptives.[39] The relationship of this malignancy to these drugs is not known at this time.

c. *Elevated blood pressure.* Women using oral contraceptives sometimes experience increased blood pressure which, in most cases, returns to normal on discontinuing the drug. There is now a report that this may occur with use of estrogens in the menopause[41] and blood pressure should be monitored with estrogen use, especially if high doses are used.

d. *Glucose tolerance.* A worsening of glucose tolerance has been observed in a significant percentage of patients on estrogen-containing oral contraceptives. For this reason, diabetic patients should be carefully observed while receiving estrogen.

4. *Hypercalcemia.* Administration of estrogens may lead to severe hypercalcemia in patients with breast cancer and bone metastases. If this occurs, the drug should be stopped and appropriate measures taken to reduce the serum calcium level.

Associated with Methyltestosterone

1. Female patients should be watched carefully for symptoms or signs of virilization such as hoarseness or deepening of the voice, oily skin, acne, hirsutism, enlarged clitoris, stimulation of libido, and menstrual irregularities. At the dosage necessary to achieve a tumor response, androgens will cause masculinization of a female, but occasionally a sensitive female may exhibit one or more of these signs on smaller doses. Some of these changes, such as voice changes may be irreversible even after drug is stopped.

2. Cholestatic hepatitis with jaundice and altered liver function tests, such as increased BSP retention and rises in SGOT levels, have been reported with methyltestosterone. These changes appear to be related to dosage of the drug. Therefore, in the presence of any changes in liver function tests, the drug should be discontinued.

Precautions:
Associated with Estrogens
A. General Precautions.

1. A complete medical and family history should be taken prior to the initiation of any estrogen therapy. The pretreatment and periodic physical examinations should include special reference to blood pressure, breasts, abdomen, and pelvic organs, and should include a Papanicolau smear. As a general rule, estrogen should not be prescribed for longer than one year without another physical examination being performed.

2. Fluid retention—Because estrogens may cause some degree of fluid retention, conditions which might be influenced by this factor such as asthma, epilepsy, migraine, and cardiac or renal dysfunction, require careful observation.

3. Certain patients may develop undesirable manifestations of excessive estrogenic stimulation, such as abnormal or excessive uterine bleeding, mastodynia, etc.

4. Oral contraceptives appear to be associated with an increased incidence of mental depression.[24a] Although it is not clear whether this is due to the estrogenic or progestogenic component of the contraceptive, patients with a history of depression should be carefully observed.

5. Preexisting uterine leiomyomata may increase in size during estrogen use.

6. The pathologist should be advised of estrogen therapy when relevant specimens are submitted.

7. Patients with a past history of jaundice during pregnancy have an increased risk of recurrence of jaundice while receiving estrogen-containing oral contraceptive therapy. If jaundice develops in any patient receiving estrogen, the medication should be discontinued while the cause is investigated.

8. Estrogens may be poorly metabolized in patients with impaired liver function and they should be administered with caution in such patients.

9. Because estrogens influence the metabolism of calcium and phosphorus, they should be used with caution in patients with metabolic bone diseases that are associated with hypercalcemia or in patients with renal insufficiency.

10. Because of the effects of estrogens on epiphyseal closure, they should be used judiciously in young patients in whom bone growth is not complete.

11. Certain endocrine and liver function tests may be affected by estrogen-containing oral contraceptives. The following similar changes may be expected with larger doses of estrogen:

a. Increased sulfobromophthalein retention.

b. Increased prothrombin and factors VII, VIII, IX, and X; decreased antithrombin 3; increased norepinephrine-induced platelet aggregability.

c. Increased thyroid binding globulin (TBG) leading to increased circulating total thyroid hormone, as measured by PBI, T4 by column, or T4 by radioimmunoassay. Free T3 resin uptake is decreased, reflecting the elevated TBG; free T4 concentration is unaltered.

d. Impaired glucose tolerance.

e. Decreased pregnanediol excretion.

f. Reduced response to metyrapone test.

g. Reduced serum folate concentration.

h. Increased serum triglyceride and phospholipid concentration.

B. Information for the Patient. See text which appears after the PHYSICIAN REFERENCES.

C. Pregnancy Category X. See CONTRAINDICATIONS and Boxed Warning.

D. Nursing Mothers. As a general principle, the administration of any drug to nursing mothers should be done only when clearly necessary since many drugs are excreted in human milk.

Associated with Methyltestosterone

A. Prolonged dosage of androgen may result in sodium and fluid retention. This may present a problem, especially in patients with compromised cardiac reserve or renal disease.

B. If priapism or other signs of excessive sexual stimulation develop, discontinue therapy.

C. In the male, prolonged administration or excessive dosage may cause inhibition of testicular function, with resultant oligospermia and decrease in ejaculatory volume. Use cautiously in young boys to avoid possible premature epiphyseal closure or precocious sexual development.

D. Hypersensitivity and gynecomastia may occur rarely.

E. PBI may be decreased in patients taking androgens.

F. Hypercalcemia may occur. If this does occur, the drug should be discontinued.

Adverse Reactions:
Associated with Estrogens

(See Warnings regarding induction of neoplasia, adverse effects on the fetus, increased incidence of gallbladder disease, and adverse effects similar to those of oral contraceptives, including thromboembolism.) The following additional adverse reactions have been reported with estrogenic therapy, including oral contraceptives:

1. *Genitourinary system:* Breakthrough bleeding, spotting, change in menstrual flow; dysmenorrhea; premenstrual-like syndrome; amenorrhea during and after treatment; increase in size of uterine fibromyomata; vaginal candidiasis; change in cervical erosion and in degree of cervical secretion; cystitis-like syndrome.

2. *Breasts:* Tenderness, enlargement, secretion.

3. *Gastrointestinal:* Nausea, vomiting; abdominal cramps, bloating; cholestatic jaundice.

4. *Skin:* Chloasma or melasma which may persist when drug is discontinued; erythema multiforme; erythema nodosum; hemorrhagic eruption; loss of scalp hair; hirsutism.

5. *Eyes:* Steepening of corneal curvature; intolerance to contact lenses.

6. *CNS:* Headache, migraine, dizziness; mental depression; chorea.

7. *Miscellaneous:* Increase or decrease in weight; reduced carbohydrate tolerance; aggravation of porphyria; edema; changes in libido.

Associated with Methyltestosterone
Cholestatic jaundice
Hypercalcemia, particularly in patients with metastatic breast carcinoma. This usually indicates progression of bone metastases.
Sodium and water retention
Priapism
Virilization in female patients
Hypersensitivity and gynecomastia

Acute Overdosage: Numerous reports of ingestion of large doses of estrogen-containing oral contraceptives by young children indicate that acute serious ill effects do not occur. Overdosage of estrogen may cause nausea, and withdrawal bleeding may occur in females.

Dosage and Administration: *Male and female*—1 MEDIATRIC Capsule or Tablet daily. (MEDIATRIC Liquid, 3 teaspoonfuls daily.)

In the female: To avoid continuous stimulation of breast and uterus, cyclic therapy is recommended (3 week regimen with 1 week rest period—Withdrawal bleeding may occur during this 1 week rest period).

Treated patients with an intact uterus should be monitored closely for signs of endometrial cancer and appropriate diagnostic measures should be taken to rule out malignancy in the event of persistent or recurring abnormal vaginal bleeding.

In the male: A careful check should be made on the status of the prostate gland when therapy is given for protracted intervals.

How Supplied:
MEDIATRIC Capsules, in bottles of 100 (NDC 0046-0252-81).
MEDIATRIC Tablets, in bottles of 100 (NDC 0046-0752-81).
MEDIATRIC Liquid, in bottles of 16 fluidounces (NDC 0046-0910-16).

Physician References:

1. Ziel, H. K., *et al:* N. Engl. J. Med. *293:*1167–1170, 1975.
2. Smith, D. C., *et al:* N. Engl. J. Med. *293:*1164–1167, 1975.
3. Mack, T. M., *et al:* N. Engl. J. Med. *294:*1262–1267, 1976.
4. Weiss, N. S., *et al:* N. Engl. J. Med. *294:*1259–1262, 1976.
5. Herbst, A. L., *et al:* N. Engl. J. Med. *284:*878–881, 1971.
6. Greenwald, P., *et al:* N. Engl. J. Med. *285:*390–392, 1971.
7. Lanier, A., *et al:* Mayo Clin. Proc. *48:*793–799, 1973.
8. Herbst, A., *et al:* Obstet. Gynecol. *40:*287–298, 1972.
9. Herbst, A., *et al:* Am. J. Obstet. Gynecol. *118:*607–615, 1974.
10. Herbst, A., *et al:* N. Engl. J. Med. *292:*334–339, 1975.
11. Stafl, A., *et al:* Obstet. Gynecol. *43:*118–128, 1974.
12. Sherman, A. I., *et al:* Obstet. Gynecol. *44:*531–545, 1974.
13. Gal, I., *et al:* Nature *216:*83, 1967.
14. Levy, E. P., *et al:* Lancet *1:*611, 1973.
15. Nora, J., *et al:* Lancet *1:*941–942, 1973.
16. Janerich, D. T., *et al:* N. Engl. J. Med. *291:*697–700, 1974.
17. Boston Collaborative Drug Surveillance Program: N. Engl. J. Med. *290:*15–19, 1974.
18. Hoover, R., *et al:* N. Engl. J. Med. *295:*401–405, 1976.
19. Boston Collaborative Drug Surveillance Program: Lancet *1:*1399–1404, 1973.
20. Daniel, D. G., *et al:* Lancet *2:*287–289, 1967.
21. The Veterans Administration Cooperative Urological Research Group: J. Urol. *98:*516–522, 1967.
22. Bailar, J. C.: Lancet *2:*560, 1967.
23. Blackard, C., *et al:* Cancer *26:*249–256, 1970.
24. Royal College of General Practitioners: J. R. Coll. Gen. Pract. *13:*267–279, 1967.
24a. Royal College of General Practitioners: Oral Contraceptives and Health, New York, Pitman Corp., 1974.

Continued on next page

Ayerst—Cont.

25. Inman, W. H. W., et al: Br. Med. J. 2:193–199, 1968.
26. Vessey, M. P., et al: Br. Med. J. 2:651–657, 1969.
27. Sartwell, P. E., et al: Am. J. Epidemiol. 90:365–380, 1969.
28. Collaborative Group for the Study of Stroke in Young Women: N. Engl. J. Med. 288:871–878, 1973.
29. Collaborative Group for the Study of Stroke in Young Women: J.A.M.A. 231:718–722, 1975.
30. Mann, J. I., et al: Br. Med. J. 2:245–248, 1975.
31. Mann, J. I., et al: Br. Med. J. 2:241–245, 1975.
32. Inman, W. H. W., et al: Br. Med. J. 2:203–209, 1970.
33. Stolley, P. D., et al: Am. J. Epidemiol. 102:197–208, 1975.
34. Vessey, M. P., et al: Br. Med. J. 3:123–126, 1970.
35. Greene, G. R., et al: Am. J. Public Health 62:680–685, 1972.
36. Rosenberg, L., et al: N. Engl. J. Med. 294:1256–1259, 1976.
37. Coronary Drug Project Research Group: J.A.M.A. 214:1303–1313, 1970.
38. Baum, J., et al: Lancet 2:926–928, 1973.
39. Mays, E. T., et al: J.A.M.A. 235:730–732, 1976.
40. Edmondson, H. A., et al: N. Engl. J. Med. 294:470–472, 1976.
41. Pfeffer, R. I., et al: Am. J. Epidemiol. 103:445–456, 1976.

INFORMATION FOR THE PATIENT

What You Should Know about Estrogens:
Estrogens are female hormones produced by the ovaries. The ovaries make several different kinds of estrogens. In addition, scientists have been able to make a variety of synthetic estrogens. As far as we know, all these estrogens have similar properties and therefore much the same usefulness, side effects, and risks. This leaflet is intended to help you understand what estrogens are used for, the risks involved in their use, and how to use them as safely as possible.

This leaflet includes the most important information about estrogens, but not all the information. If you want to know more, you should ask your doctor for more information or you can ask your doctor or pharmacist to let you read the package insert prepared for the doctor.

Uses of Estrogen: THERE IS NO PROPER USE OF ESTROGENS IN A PREGNANT WOMAN. Estrogens are prescribed by doctors for a number of purposes, including:
1. To provide estrogen during a period of adjustment when a woman's ovaries stop producing a majority of her estrogens, in order to prevent certain uncomfortable symptoms of estrogen deficiency. (With the menopause, which generally occurs between the ages of 45 and 55, women produce a much smaller amount of estrogens.)
2. To prevent symptoms of estrogen deficiency when a woman's ovaries have been removed surgically before the natural menopause.
3. To prevent pregnancy. (Estrogens are given along with a progestogen, another female hormone; these combinations are called oral contraceptives or birth control pills. Patient labeling is available to women taking oral contraceptives and they will not be discussed in this leaflet.)
4. To treat certain cancers in women and men.
5. To prevent painful swelling of the breasts after pregnancy in women who choose not to nurse their babies.

Estrogens in the Menopause: In the natural course of their lives, all women eventually experience a decrease in estrogen production. This usually occurs between ages 45 and 55 but may occur earlier or later. Sometimes the ovaries may need to be removed before natural menopause by an operation, producing a "surgical menopause." When the amount of estrogen in the blood begins to decrease, many women may develop typical symptoms: feelings of warmth in the face, neck, and chest or sudden intense episodes of heat and sweating throughout the body (called "hot flashes" or "hot flushes"). These symptoms are sometimes very uncomfortable. Some women may also develop changes in the vagina (called "atrophic vaginitis") which cause discomfort, especially during and after intercourse.

Estrogens can be prescribed to treat these symptoms of the menopause. It is estimated that considerably more than half of all women undergoing the menopause have only mild symptoms or no symptoms at all and therefore do not need estrogens. Other women may need estrogens for a few months, while their bodies adjust to lower estrogen levels. Sometimes the need will be for periods longer than six months. In an attempt to avoid overstimulation of the uterus (womb), estrogens are usually given cyclically during each month of use, such as three weeks of pills followed by one week without pills.

Sometimes women experience nervous symptoms or depression during menopause. There is no evidence that estrogens are effective for such symptoms without associated vasomotor symptoms. In the absence of vasomotor symptoms, estrogens should not be used to treat nervous symptoms, although other treatment may be needed.

You may have heard that taking estrogens for long periods (years) after the menopause will keep your skin soft and supple and keep you feeling young. There is no evidence that this is so, however, and such long-term treatment carries important risks.

Estrogens to Prevent Swelling of the Breasts after Pregnancy: If you do not breast-feed your baby after delivery, your breasts may fill up with milk and become painful and engorged. This usually begins about 3 to 4 days after delivery and may last for a few days to up to a week or more. Sometimes the discomfort is severe, but usually it is not and can be controlled by pain-relieving drugs such as aspirin and by binding the breasts up tightly. Estrogens can be used to try to prevent the breasts from filling up. While this treatment is sometimes successful, in many cases the breasts fill up to some degree in spite of treatment. The dose of estrogens needed to prevent pain and swelling of the breasts is much larger than the dose needed to treat symptoms of the menopause and this may increase your chances of developing blood clots in the legs or lungs (see below). Therefore, it is important that you discuss the benefits and the risks of estrogen use with your doctor if you have decided not to breast-feed your baby.

The Dangers of Estrogens:
1. *Endometrial cancer.* There are reports that if estrogens are used in the postmenopausal period for more than a year, there is an increased risk of *endometrial cancer* (cancer of the lining of the uterus). Women taking estrogens have roughly 5 to 10 times as great a chance of getting this cancer as women who take no estrogens. To put this another way, while a postmenopausal woman not taking estrogens has 1 chance in 1,000 each year of getting endometrial cancer, a woman taking estrogens has 5 to 10 chances in 1,000 each year. For this reason *it is important to take estrogens only when they are really needed.*

The risk of this cancer is greater the longer estrogens are used and when larger doses are taken. Therefore you should not take more estrogen than your doctor prescribes. *It is important to take the lowest dose of estrogen that will control symptoms and to take it only as long as is needed.* If estrogens are needed for longer periods of time, your doctor will want to reevaluate your need for estrogens at least every six months.

Women using estrogens should report any vaginal bleeding to their doctors; such bleeding may be of no importance, but it can be an early warning of endometrial cancer. If you have undiagnosed vaginal bleeding, you should not use estrogens until a diagnosis is made and you are certain there is no endometrial cancer.

NOTE: If you have had your uterus removed (total hysterectomy), there is no danger of developing endometrial cancer.

2. *Other possible cancers.* Estrogens can cause development of other tumors in animals, such as tumors of the breast, cervix, vagina, or liver, when given for a long time. At present there is no good evidence that women using estrogen in the menopause have an increased risk of such tumors, but there is no way yet to be sure they do not; and one study raises the possibility that use of estrogens in the menopause may increase the risk of breast cancer many years later. This is a further reason to use estrogens only when clearly needed. While you are taking estrogens, it is important that you go to your doctor at least once a year for a physical examination. Also, if members of your family have had breast cancer or if you have breast nodules or abnormal mammograms (breast x-rays), your doctor may wish to carry out more frequent examinations of your breasts.

3. *Gallbladder disease.* Women who use estrogens after menopause are more likely to develop gallbladder disease needing surgery than women who do not use estrogens. Birth control pills have a similar effect.

4. *Abnormal blood clotting.* Oral contraceptives increase the risk of blood clotting in various parts of the body. This can result in a stroke (if the clot is in the brain), a heart attack (clot in a blood vessel of the heart), or a pulmonary embolus (a clot which forms in the legs or pelvis, then breaks off and travels to the lungs). Any of these can be fatal.
At this time use of estrogens in the menopause is not known to cause such blood clotting, but this has not been fully studied and there could still prove to be such a risk. It is recommended that if you have had clotting in the legs or lungs or a heart attack or stroke while you were using estrogens or birth control pills, you should not use estrogens (unless they are being used to treat cancer of the breast or prostate). If you have had a stroke or heart attack or if you have angina pectoris, estrogens should be used with great caution and only if clearly needed (for example, if you have severe symptoms of the menopause).

The larger doses of estrogen used to prevent swelling of the breasts after pregnancy have been reported to cause clotting in the legs and lungs.

Special Warning about Pregnancy: You should not receive estrogen if you are pregnant. If this should occur, there is a greater than usual chance that the developing child will be born with a birth defect, although the possibility remains fairly small. A female child may have an increased risk of developing cancer of the vagina or cervix later in life (in the teens or twenties). Every possible effort should be made to avoid exposure to estrogens during pregnancy. If exposure occurs, see your doctor.

Other Effects of Estrogens: In addition to the serious known risks of estrogens described above, estrogens have the following side effects and potential risks:
1. *Nausea and vomiting.* The most common side effect of estrogen therapy is nausea. Vomiting is less common.
2. *Effects on breasts.* Estrogens may cause breast tenderness or enlargement and may cause the breasts to secrete a liquid. These effects are not dangerous.
3. *Effects on the uterus.* Estrogens may cause benign fibroid tumors of the uterus to get larger.
4. *Effects on liver.* Women taking oral contraceptives develop on rare occasions a tumor of the liver which can rupture and bleed into the abdomen and may cause death. So far, these tumors have not been reported in women using estrogens in the menopause, but you should report any swelling or unusual pain or tenderness in the abdomen to your doctor immediately.

Women with a past history of jaundice (yellowing of the skin and white parts of the eyes) may get jaundice again during estrogen use. If this occurs, stop taking estrogens and see your doctor.

5. *Other effects.* Estrogens may cause excess fluid to be retained in the body. This may make some conditions worse, such as asthma, epilepsy, migraine, heart disease, or kidney disease.

Summary: Estrogens have important uses, but they have serious risks as well. You must decide,

for possible revisions — **Product Information** — 657

with your doctor, whether the risks are acceptable to you in view of the benefits of treatment. Except where your doctor has prescribed estrogens for use in special cases of cancer of the breast or prostate, you should not use estrogens if you have cancer of the breast or uterus, are pregnant, have undiagnosed abnormal vaginal bleeding, clotting in the legs or lungs, or have had a stroke, heart attack or angina, or clotting in the legs or lungs in the past while you were taking estrogens.

You can use estrogens as safely as possible by understanding that your doctor will require regular physical examinations while you are taking them and will try to discontinue the drug as soon as possible and use the smallest dose possible. Be alert for signs of trouble including:
1. Abnormal bleeding from the vagina.
2. Pains in the calves or chest or sudden shortness of breath, or coughing blood.
3. Severe headache, dizziness, faintness, or changes in vision.
4. Breast lumps (you should ask your doctor how to examine your own breasts).
5. Jaundice (yellowing of the skin).
6. Mental depression.

Your doctor has prescribed this drug for you and you alone. Do not give the drug to anyone else.

How Supplied:
MEDIATRIC®—provides estrogen and androgen in small doses, nutritional supplements, and a mild antidepressant. It is supplied as capsules, tablets, and liquid.

Shown in Product Identification Section, page 405

MYSOLINE® ℞
[mī'sō-lēn]
Brand of primidone
Anticonvulsant

Actions: MYSOLINE raises electro- or chemoshock seizure thresholds or alters seizure patterns in experimental animals. The mechanism(s) of primidone's antiepileptic action is not known. Primidone *per se* has anticonvulsant activity as do its two metabolites, phenobarbital and phenylethylmalonamide (PEMA). In addition to its anticonvulsant activity, PEMA potentiates that of phenobarbital in experimental animals.

Indications: MYSOLINE, either alone or used concomitantly with other anticonvulsants, is indicated in the control of grand mal, psychomotor, and focal epileptic seizures. It may control grand mal seizures refractory to other anticonvulsant therapy.

Contraindications: Primidone is contraindicated in: 1) patients with porphyria and 2) patients who are hypersensitive to phenobarbital (see ACTIONS).

Warnings: The abrupt withdrawal of antiepileptic medication may precipitate status epilepticus. The therapeutic efficacy of a dosage regimen takes several weeks before it can be assessed.

Usage in pregnancy: The effects of MYSOLINE (primidone) in human pregnancy and nursing infants are unknown.

Recent reports suggest an association between the use of anticonvulsant drugs by women with epilepsy and an elevated incidence of birth defects in children born to these women. Data are more extensive with respect to diphenylhydantoin and phenobarbital, but these are also the most commonly prescribed anticonvulsants; less systematic or anecdotal reports suggest a possible similar association with the use of all known anticonvulsant drugs.

The reports suggesting an elevated incidence of birth defects in children of drug-treated epileptic women cannot be regarded as adequate to prove a definite cause and effect relationship. There are intrinsic methodologic problems in obtaining adequate data on drug teratogenicity in humans; the possibility also exists that other factors, *e.g.*, genetic factors or the epileptic condition itself, may be more important than drug therapy in leading to birth defects. The great majority of mothers on anticonvulsant medication deliver normal infants. It is important to note that anticonvulsant drugs should not be discontinued in patients in whom the drug is administered to prevent major seizures because of the strong possibility of precipitating status epilepticus with attendant hypoxia and threat to life. In individual cases where the severity and frequency of the seizure disorder are such that the removal of medication does not pose a serious threat to the patient, discontinuation of the drug may be considered prior to and during pregnancy, although it cannot be said with any confidence that even minor seizures do not pose some hazard to the developing embryo or fetus. The prescribing physician will wish to weigh these considerations in treating or counseling epileptic women of childbearing potential.

Neonatal hemorrhage, with a coagulation defect resembling vitamin K deficiency, has been described in newborns whose mothers were taking primidone and other anticonvulsants. Pregnant women under anticonvulsant therapy should receive prophylactic vitamin K_1 therapy for one month prior to, and during, delivery.

Precautions: The total daily dosage should not exceed 2 g. Since MYSOLINE (primidone) therapy generally extends over prolonged periods, a complete blood count and a sequential multiple analysis-12 (SMA-12) test should be made every six months.

In nursing mothers: There is evidence that in mothers treated with primidone, the drug appears in the milk in substantial quantities. Since tests for the presence of primidone in biological fluids are too complex to be carried out in the average clinical laboratory, it is suggested that the presence of undue somnolence and drowsiness in nursing newborns of MYSOLINE-treated mothers be taken as an indication that nursing should be discontinued.

Adverse Reactions: The most frequently occurring early side effects are ataxia and vertigo. These tend to disappear with continued therapy, or with reduction of initial dosage. Occasionally, the following have been reported: nausea, anorexia, vomiting, fatigue, hyperirritability, emotional disturbances, sexual impotency, diplopia, nystagmus, drowsiness, and morbilliform skin eruptions. Occasionally, persistent or severe side effects may necessitate withdrawal of the drug. Megaloblastic anemia may occur as a rare idiosyncrasy to MYSOLINE and to other anticonvulsants. The anemia responds to folic acid without necessity of discontinuing medication.

Dosage and Administration: *Adult Dosage:* Patients 8 years of age and older who have received no previous treatment may be started on MYSOLINE (primidone) according to the following regimen using either 50 mg or scored 250 mg MYSOLINE tablets.

Days 1–3: 100 to 125 mg at bedtime
Days 4–6: 100 to 125 mg b.i.d.
Days 7–9: 100 to 125 mg t.i.d.
Day 10-maintenance: 250 mg t.i.d.

For most adults and children 8 years of age and over, the usual maintenance dosage is three to four 250 mg MYSOLINE tablets daily in divided doses (250 mg t.i.d. or q.i.d.). If required, an increase to five or six 250 mg tablets daily may be made but daily doses should not exceed 500 mg q.i.d.

INITIAL: ADULTS AND CHILDREN OVER 8

KEY: · = 50 mg tablet;   ● = 250 mg tablet

DAY	1	2	3	4	5	6
AM				·	·	·
NOON						·
PM	·	·	·	·	·	·

DAY	7	8	9	10	11	12
AM	·	·	·	●		
NOON	·	·	·		Adjust to	
PM	·	·	·	●	Maintenance	

Dosage should be individualized to provide maximum benefit. In some cases, serum blood level determinations of primidone may be necessary for optimal dosage adjustment. The clinically effective serum level for primidone is between 5–12 µg/ml.

In patients already receiving other anticonvulsants: MYSOLINE should be started at 100 to 125 mg at bedtime and gradually increased to maintenance level as the other drug is gradually decreased. This regimen should be continued until satisfactory dosage level is achieved for the combination, or the other medication is completely withdrawn. When therapy with MYSOLINE (primidone) alone is the objective, the transition from concomitant therapy should not be completed in less than two weeks.

Pediatric Dosage: For children under 8 years of age, the following regimen may be used:
Days 1–3: 50 mg at bedtime
Days 4–6: 50 mg b.i.d.
Days 7–9: 100 mg b.i.d.
Day 10-maintenance: 125 mg t.i.d. to 250 mg t.i.d.

For children under 8 years of age, the usual maintenance dosage is 125 to 250 mg three times daily, or 10–25 mg/kg/day in divided doses.

How Supplied:
MYSOLINE (primidone) Tablets
Each tablet contains 250 mg of primidone (scored), in bottles of 100 (NDC 0046-0430-81) and 1,000 (NDC 0046-0430-91).
Also in unit dose package of 100 (NDC 0046-0430-99).
Each tablet contains 50 mg of primidone (scored), in bottles of 100 (NDC 0046-0431-81) and 500 (NDC 0046-0431-85).
MYSOLINE Suspension
Each 5 ml (teaspoonful) contains 250 mg of primidone, in bottles of 8 fluidounces (NDC 0046-3850-08).

Shown in Product Identification Section, page 405

PEPTAVLON® ℞
[pĕp-tăv'lon]
Brand of
pentagastrin
A diagnostic agent for
evaluation of gastric acid
secretory function.

CAUTION: Federal law prohibits dispensing without prescription.

Description:
Chemical name: N-t-butyloxycarbonyl-B-alanyl-L-tryptophyl-L-methionyl- L-aspartyl- L-phenylalanyl amide.
Structural formula:

Pentagastrin is a synthetic pentapeptide containing the carboxyl terminal tetrapeptide, the active portion found in all natural gastrins. Pentagastrin is a colorless crystalline solid. It is soluble in dimethylformamide and dimethylsulfoxide; it is almost insoluble in water, ethanol, ether, benzene, chloroform, and ethyl acetate.

Actions: PEPTAVLON (pentagastrin) contains the C-terminal tetrapeptide responsible for the actions of the natural gastrins and, therefore, acts as a physiologic gastric acid secretagogue. The recommended dose of 6 mcg/kg subcutaneously produces a peak acid output which is reproducible when used in the same individual.

PEPTAVLON stimulates gastric acid secretion approximately ten minutes after subcutaneous injection, with peak responses occurring in most cases twenty to thirty minutes after administration.

Continued on next page

Ayerst—Cont.

Duration of activity is usually between sixty and eighty minutes.

Indications: PEPTAVLON (pentagastrin) is used as a diagnostic agent to evaluate gastric acid secretory function. It is useful in testing for:

Anacidity:—as a diagnostic aid in patients with suspected pernicious anemia, atrophic gastritis, or gastric carcinoma.

Hypersecretion:—as a diagnostic aid in patients with suspected duodenal ulcer or postoperative stomal ulcer, and for the diagnosis of Zollinger-Ellison tumor.

PEPTAVLON (pentagastrin) is also useful in determining the adequacy of acid-reducing operations for peptic ulcer.

Contraindications: Hypersensitivity or idio- syncrasy to pentagastrin.

Warnings: *Use in Pregnancy*—The use of pentagastrin in pregnancy has NOT been studied, and the benefit of administration of the drug must be weighed against any possible risk to the mother and/or fetus.

Use in Children—There are insufficient data to recommend the use of, or establish a dosage, in children.

****

In amounts in excess of the recommended dose, pentagastrin may cause inhibition of gastric acid secretion.

Precautions: Use with caution in patients with pancreatic, hepatic, or biliary disease. Like gastrin, pentagastrin could, in some cases, have the physiologic effect of stimulating pancreatic enzyme and bicarbonate secretion, as well as biliary flow.

Adverse Reactions: Pentagastrin causes fewer and less severe cardiovascular and other adverse reactions than histamine or betazole. The majority of reactions to pentagastrin are related to the gastrointestinal tract.

The following reactions associated with the use of pentagastrin have been reported.

Gastrointestinal: abdominal pain, desire to defecate, nausea, vomiting, borborygmi, blood-tinged mucus

Cardiovascular: flushing, tachycardia

Central Nervous System: dizziness, faintness or lightheadedness, drowsiness, sinking feeling, transient blurring of vision, tiredness, headache

Allergic and Hypersensitivity Reactions: May occur in some patients.

Miscellaneous: shortness of breath, heavy sensation in arms and legs, tingling in fingers, chills, sweating, generalized burning sensation, warmth, pain at site of injection, bile in collected specimens

Dosage and Administration: *Adults:* 6 mcg/kg subcutaneously. Effect begins in about ten minutes; peak response usually occurs in twenty to thirty minutes. (For discussion of the test and explicit directions, consult Baron, J.H.: Gastric Function Tests, in Wastell, C.: Chronic Duodenal Ulcer, New York, Appleton-Century-Crofts, 1972, pp. 82–114.)

Note: Data are inadequate to recommend the use of, or establish a dosage, in children.

Overdosage: In case of overdosage or idiosyncrasy, symptomatic treatment should be administered as required.

How Supplied: PEPTAVLON—In 2 ml ampuls. Each ml contains 0.25 mg (250 mcg) pentagastrin. Also contains 0.88% sodium chloride, and Water for Injection U.S.P. The pH is adjusted with ammonium hydroxide and/or hydrochloric acid . Cartons of 10 (NDC 0046-3290-10).

Clinical Studies:

Gastric Acid Secretion: Peak gastric output in mEq/hr caused by subcutaneous injection of 6 mcg/kg pentagastrin does not differ significantly from that caused by the standard subcutaneous injection of the histamine acid phosphate dose used in the augmented histamine test (40 mcg/kg). For example, in 25 normal volunteers, pentagastrin produced an average peak acid output of 28.4 mEq/hr compared with 24.7 mEq/hr by histamine. In 45 patients with duodenal ulcer, or suspected duodenal ulcer, pentagastrin produced an average peak gastric acid output of 39.7 mEq/hr compared with 33.7 mEq/hr by histamine. In 18 patients with gastric ulcer, or suspected gastric ulcer, pentagastrin produced an average peak output of 17.4 mEq/hr compared with 19.4 mEq/hr by histamine. The overall mean for peak acid secretion by pentagastrin was 24.8 mEq/hr compared with 22.6 mEq/hr by histamine. No biochemical abnormality which might indicate specific organ toxicity has been encountered following the administration of pentagastrin.

PHOSPHOLINE IODIDE®   R

[fŏs′ fo-lĭn ī′ o-dīd]
(echothiophate iodide for ophthalmic solution)

Description: PHOSPHOLINE IODIDE occurs as a white, crystalline, water-soluble, hygroscopic solid having a slight mercaptan-like odor. When freeze-dried in the presence of potassium acetate, the mixture appears as a white amorphous deposit on the walls of the bottle.

Each package contains materials for dispensing 5 ml of eyedrops: (1) bottle containing PHOSPHOLINE IODIDE in one of four potencies [1.5 mg (0.03%), 3.0 mg (0.06%), 6.25 mg (0.125%), or 12.5 mg (0.25%)] as indicated on the label, with 40 mg potassium acetate in each case. Sodium hydroxide or acetic acid may have been incorporated to adjust pH during manufacturing. (2) a 5 ml bottle of diluent containing chlorobutanol (chloral derivative), 0.5%; mannitol, 1.2%; boric acid, 0.06%; and exsiccated sodium phosphate, 0.026% (3) sterilized dropper.

Actions: PHOSPHOLINE IODIDE is a long-acting cholinesterase inhibitor for topical use which enhances the effect of endogenously liberated acetylcholine in iris, ciliary muscle, and other parasympathetically innervated structures of the eye. It thereby causes miosis, increase in facility of outflow of aqueous humor, fall in intraocular pressure, and potentiation of accommodation.

PHOSPHOLINE IODIDE (echothiophate iodide) will depress both plasma and erythrocyte cholinesterase levels in most patients after a few weeks of eyedrop therapy.

Indications: GLAUCOMA—Chronic open-angle glaucoma. Subacute or chronic angle-closure glaucoma after iridectomy or where surgery is refused or contraindicated. Certain non-uveitic secondary types of glaucoma, especially glaucoma following cataract surgery.

ACCOMMODATIVE ESOTROPIA—Concomitant esotropias with a significant accommodative component.

Contraindications:
1. Active uveal inflammation.
2. Most cases of angle-closure glaucoma, due to the possibility of increasing angle block.
3. Hypersensitivity to the active or inactive ingredients.

Warnings:
1. *Use in Pregnancy:* Safe use of anticholinesterase medications during pregnancy has not been established, nor has the absence of adverse effects on the fetus or on the respiration of the neonate.
2. Succinylcholine should be administered only with great caution, if at all, prior to or during general anesthesia to patients receiving anticholinesterase medication because of possible respiratory or cardiovascular collapse.
3. Caution should be observed in treating glaucoma with PHOSPHOLINE IODIDE (echothiophate iodide) in patients who are at the same time undergoing treatment with systemic anticholinesterase medications for myasthenia gravis, because of possible adverse additive effects.

Precautions:
1. Gonioscopy is recommended prior to initiation of therapy.
2. Where there is a quiescent uveitis or a history of this condition, anticholinesterase therapy should be avoided or used cautiously because of the intense and persistent miosis and ciliary muscle contraction that may occur.
3. While systemic effects are infrequent, proper use of the drug requires digital compression of the nasolacrimal ducts for a minute or two following instillation to minimize drainage into the nasal chamber with its extensive absorption area. The hands should be washed immediately following instillation.
4. Temporary discontinuance of medication is necessary if salivation, urinary incontinence, diarrhea, profuse sweating, muscle weakness, respiratory difficulties, or cardiac irregularities occur.
5. Patients receiving PHOSPHOLINE IODIDE who are exposed to carbamate or organophosphate type insecticides and pesticides (professional gardeners, farmers, workers in plants manufacturing or formulating such products, etc.) should be warned of the additive systemic effects possible from absorption of the pesticide through the respiratory tract or skin. During periods of exposure to such pesticides, the wearing of respiratory masks, and frequent washing and clothing changes may be advisable.
6. Anticholinesterase drugs should be used with extreme caution, if at all, in patients with marked vagotonia, bronchial asthma, spastic gastrointestinal disturbances, peptic ulcer, pronounced bradycardia and hypotension, recent myocardial infarction, epilepsy, parkinsonism, and other disorders that may respond adversely to vagotonic effects.
7. Anticholinesterase drugs should be employed prior to ophthalmic surgery only as a considered risk because of the possible occurrence of hyphema.
8. PHOSPHOLINE IODIDE (echothiophate iodide) should be used with great caution, if at all, where there is a prior history of retinal detachment.

Adverse Reactions:
1. Although the relationship, if any, of retinal detachment to the administration of PHOSPHOLINE IODIDE has not been established, retinal detachment has been reported in a few cases during the use of PHOSPHOLINE IODIDE in adult patients without a previous history of this disorder.
2. Stinging, burning, lacrimation, lid muscle twitching, conjunctival and ciliary redness, browache, induced myopia with visual blurring may occur.
3. Activation of latent iritis or uveitis may occur.
4. Iris cysts may form, and if treatment is continued, may enlarge and obscure vision. This occurrence is more frequent in children. The cysts usually shrink upon discontinuance of the medication, reduction in strength of the drops or frequency of instillation. Rarely, they may rupture or break free into the aqueous. Regular examinations are advisable when the drug is being prescribed for the treatment of accommodative esotropia.
5. Prolonged use may cause conjunctival thickening, obstruction of nasolacrimal canals.
6. Lens opacities occurring in patients under treatment for glaucoma with PHOSPHOLINE IODIDE have been reported and similar changes have been produced experimentally in normal monkeys. Routine examinations should accompany clinical use of the drug.
7. Paradoxical increase in intraocular pressure may follow anticholinesterase instillation. This may be alleviated by prescribing a sympathomimetic mydriatic such as phenylephrine.

Dosage and Administration:

GLAUCOMA—

Selection of Therapy: The *medication prescribed* should be that which will control the intraocular pressure around-the-clock with the least risk of side effects or adverse reactions. "Tonometric glaucoma" (ocular hypertension without other evidence of the disease) is frequently not treated with any medication, and PHOSPHOLINE IODIDE (echothiophate iodide) is certainly not recommended for this condition. In early chronic simple glaucoma with field loss or disc changes, pilocarpine is generally used for initial therapy and can be recommended so long as control is thereby maintained over the 24 hours of the day. When this is not the case, PHOSPHOLINE IODIDE 0.03% may be effective and probably has no greater potential for side effects. If this dosage is inadequate, epinephrine and a carbonic anhydrase inhibitor may be added to the regimen. When still more effective medication is required, the higher strengths of PHOSPHOLINE IODIDE may be prescribed with the recognition that the control of the intraocular pressure should have priority regardless of potential side effects. In secondary glaucoma following cataract surgery, the higher strengths of the drug are frequently needed and are ordinarily very well tolerated.

The *dosage regimen* prescribed should call for the lowest concentration that will control the intraocular pressure around-the-clock. Where tonometry around-the-clock is not feasible, it is suggested that appointments for tension-taking be made at different times of the day so that inadequate control may be more readily detected. Two doses a day are preferred to one in order to maintain as smooth a diurnal tension curve as possible, although a single dose per day or every other day has been used with satisfactory results. Because of the long duration of action of the drug, it is never necessary or desirable to exceed a schedule of twice a day. The daily dose or one of the two daily doses should always be instilled just before retiring to avoid inconvenience due to the miosis.

Early Chronic Simple Glaucoma: PHOSPHOLINE IODIDE (echothiophate iodide) 0.03% instilled twice a day, just before retiring and in the morning, may be prescribed advantageously for cases of early chronic simple glaucoma that are not controlled around-the-clock with pilocarpine. Because of prolonged action, control during the night and early morning hours may then sometimes be obtained. A change in therapy is indicated if, at any time, the tension fails to remain at an acceptable level on this regimen.

Advanced Chronic Simple Glaucoma and Glaucoma Secondary to Cataract Surgery: These cases may respond satisfactorily to PHOSPHOLINE IODIDE 0.03% twice a day as above. When the patient is being transferred to PHOSPHOLINE IODIDE (echothiophate iodide) because of unsatisfactory control with pilocarpine, carbachol, epinephrine, etc., one of the higher strengths, 0.06%, 0.125%, or 0.25% will usually be needed. In this case, a brief trial with the 0.03% eyedrops will be advantageous in that the higher strengths will then be more easily tolerated.

Concomitant Therapy: PHOSPHOLINE IODIDE may be used concomitantly with epinephrine, a carbonic anhydrase inhibitor, or both.

Technic: Good technic in the administration of PHOSPHOLINE IODIDE requires that finger pressure at the inner canthus should be exerted for a minute or two following instillation of the eyedrops, to minimize drainage into the nose and throat. Excess solution around the eye should be removed with tissue and any medication on the hands should be rinsed off.

ACCOMMODATIVE ESOTROPIA—

In Diagnosis: One drop of 0.125% may be instilled once a day in both eyes on retiring, for a period of two or three weeks. If the esotropia is accommodative, a favorable response will usually be noted which may begin within a few hours.

In Treatment: PHOSPHOLINE IODIDE (echothiophate iodide) is prescribed at the lowest concentration and frequency which gives satisfactory results. After the initial period of treatment for diagnostic purposes, the schedule may be reduced to 0.125% every other day or 0.06% every day. These dosages can often be gradually lowered as treatment progresses. The 0.03% strength has proven to be effective in some cases. The maximum usually recommended dosage is 0.125% once a day, although more intensive therapy has been used for short periods.

Technic: See Dosage and Administration, Section on Glaucoma.

Duration of Treatment

In diagnosis, only a short period is required and little time will be lost in instituting other procedures if the esotropia proves to be unresponsive. In therapy, there is no definite limit so long as the drug is well tolerated. However, if the eyedrops, with or without eyeglasses, are gradually withdrawn after about a year or two and deviation recurs, surgery should be considered. As with other miotics, tolerance may occasionally develop after prolonged use. In such cases, a rest period will restore the original activity of the drug.

Overdosage: Antidotes are atropine, 2 mg parenterally; PROTOPAM® CHLORIDE (pralidoxime chloride), 25 mg per kg intravenously; artificial respiration should be given if necessary.

Directions for Preparing Eyedrops
1. Use aseptic technic.
2. Tear off aluminum seals, and remove and discard rubber plugs from both drug and diluent containers.
3. Pour diluent into drug container.
4. Remove dropper assembly from its sterile wrapping. Holding dropper assembly by the screw cap and, WITHOUT COMPRESSING RUBBER BULB, insert into drug container and screw down tightly.
5. Shake for several seconds to ensure mixing.
6. Do not cover nor obliterate instructions to patient regarding storage of eyedrops.

Storage and Stability of Eyedrops

Keep eyedrops in refrigerator to obtain maximum useful life of six months. Room temperature is acceptable if drops will be used up within a month.

How Supplied: Each package contains PHOSPHOLINE IODIDE (echothiophate iodide), diluent, and dropper for dispensing 5 ml eyedrops of the strength indicated on the label. Four potencies are available:

NDC 0046-1062-05 .... 1.5 mg package for 0.03%
NDC 0046-1064-05 .... 3.0 mg package for 0.06%
NDC 0046-1065-05 .... 6.25 mg package for 0.125%
NDC 0046-1066-05 .... 12.5 mg package for 0.25%

PLEGINE® Tablets
[plĕj-ēn']
Brand of phendimetrazine tartrate
Anorexiant

CAUTION: Federal law prohibits dispensing without prescription.
Description:
Chemical name: (+)-3,4-Dimethyl-2-phenylmorpholine Tartrate
Structural formula:

PLEGINE is the dextro isomer of phendimetrazine tartrate. Phendimetrazine tartrate is a white, odorless powder with a bitter taste. It is soluble in water, methanol, and ethanol.

Actions: PLEGINE is a phenylalkylamine sympathomimetic with pharmacologic activity similar to the prototype drugs of this class used in obesity, the amphetamines. Actions include central nervous system stimulation and elevation of blood pressure. Tachyphylaxis and tolerance have been demonstrated with all drugs of this class in which these phenomena have been looked for.

Drugs of this class used in obesity are commonly known as "anorectics" or "anorexigenics." It has not been established, however, that the action of such drugs in treating obesity is primarily one of appetite suppression. Other central nervous system actions, or metabolic effects, may be involved, for example.

Adult obese subjects instructed in dietary management and treated with "anorectic" drugs, lose more weight on the average than those treated with placebo and diet, as determined in relatively short term clinical trials.

The magnitude of increased weight loss of drug-treated patients over placebo-treated patients is only a fraction of a pound a week. The rate of weight loss is greatest in the first weeks of therapy for both drug and placebo subjects and tends to decrease in succeeding weeks. The possible origins of the increased weight loss due to the various drug effects are not established. The amount of weight loss associated with the use of an "anorectic" drug varies from trial to trial, and the increased weight loss appears to be related in part to variables other than the drug prescribed, such as the physician-investigator, the population treated, and the diet prescribed. Studies do not permit conclusions as to the relative importance of the drug and non-drug factors on weight loss.

The natural history of obesity is measured in years, whereas the studies cited are restricted to a few weeks' duration; thus, the total impact of drug-induced weight loss over that of diet alone must be considered clinically limited.

Indications: PLEGINE (phendimetrazine tartrate) is indicated in the management of exogenous obesity as a short term adjunct (a few weeks) in a regimen of weight reduction based on caloric restriction. The limited usefulness of agents of this class should be measured against possible risk factors inherent in their use (see **Actions**).

Contraindications: Known hypersensitivity or idiosyncratic reactions to sympathomimetics.

Advanced arteriosclerosis, symptomatic cardiovascular disease, moderate and severe hypertension, hyperthyroidism

Highly nervous or agitated patients

Patients with a history of drug abuse

Patients taking other CNS stimulants, including monamine oxidase inhibitors

Warnings: DRUG DEPENDENCE: PLEGINE is related chemically and pharmacologically to the amphetamines. Amphetamines and related stimulant drugs have been extensively abused, and the possibility of abuse of PLEGINE should be kept in mind when evaluating the desirability of including a drug as part of a weight reduction program. Abuse of amphetamines and related drugs may be associated with intense psychological dependence and severe social dysfunction. There are reports of patients who have increased the dosage to many times that recommended. Abrupt cessation following prolonged high dosage administration results in extreme fatigue and mental depression; changes are also noted on the sleep EEG. Manifestations of chronic intoxication with anorectic drugs include severe dermatoses, marked insomnia, irritability, hyperactivity, and personality changes. The most severe manifestation of chronic intoxications is psychosis, often clinically indistinguishable from schizophrenia.

Tolerance to the anorectic effect of PLEGINE (phendimetrazine tartrate) develops within a few weeks. When this occurs, its use should be discontinued; the maximum recommended dose should not be exceeded.

Use of PLEGINE (phendimetrazine tartrate) within 14 days following the administration of monamine oxidase inhibitors may result in a hypertensive crisis.

Abrupt cessation of administration following prolonged high dosage results in extreme fatigue and depression. Because of the effect on the central nervous system, PLEGINE may impair the ability of the patient to engage in potentially hazardous activities such as operating machinery or driving a motor vehicle; the patient should therefore be cautioned accordingly.

Usage in Pregnancy: Safe use in pregnancy has not been established. Until more information is available, phendimetrazine tartrate should not be taken by women who are or may become pregnant

Continued on next page

Ayerst—Cont.

unless, in the opinion of the physician, the potential benefits outweigh the possible hazards.
Usage in Children: PLEGINE is not recommended for use in children under 12 years of age.
Precautions: Caution is to be exercised in prescribing PLEGINE for patients with even mild hypertension.
Insulin requirements in diabetes mellitus may be altered in association with the use of PLEGINE and the concomitant dietary regimen.
PLEGINE may decrease the hypotensive effect of guanethidine.
The least amount feasible should be prescribed or dispensed at one time in order to minimize the possibility of overdosage.
Adverse Reactions: Central Nervous System: Overstimulation, restlessness, insomnia, agitation, flushing, tremor, sweating, dizziness, headache, psychotic states, blurring of vision
Cardiovascular: Palpitation, tachycardia, elevated blood pressure
Gastrointestinal: Mouth dryness, nausea, diarrhea, constipation, stomach pain
Genitourinary: Urinary frequency, dysuria, changes in libido
Dosage and Administration: *Usual adult dosage:* 1 tablet (35 mg.) b.i.d. or t.i.d., one hour before meals.
Dosage should be individualized to obtain an adequate response with the lowest effective dosage. In some cases, ½ tablet per dose may be adequate; dosage should not exceed 2 tablets t.i.d.
Overdosage: Acute overdosage of phendimetrazine tartrate may manifest itself by the following signs and symptoms: unusual restlessness, confusion, belligerence, hallucinations, and panic states. Fatigue and depression usually follow the central stimulation. Cardiovascular effects include arrhythmias, hypertension, or hypotension and circulatory collapse. Gastrointestinal symptoms include nausea, vomiting, diarrhea, and abdominal cramps. Poisoning may result in convulsions, coma, and death.
The management of overdosage is largely symptomatic. It includes sedation with a barbiturate. If hypertension is marked, the use of a nitrate or rapid-acting alpha receptor-blocking agent should be considered. Experience with hemodialysis or peritoneal dialysis is inadequate to permit recommendations for its use.
How Supplied: PLEGINE—Each scored tablet contains 35 mg phendimetrazine tartrate, in bottles of 100 (NDC 0046-0755-81) and 1,000 (NDC 0046-0755-91).
Shown in Product Identification Section, page 405

PMB® 200 ℞

Each tablet contains:
Premarin® (Conjugated
 Estrogens, U.S.P.) ....0.45 mg
Meprobamate ....200.0 mg

PMB® 400

Each tablet contains:
Premarin® (Conjugated
 Estrogens, U.S.P.) ....0.45 mg
Meprobamate ....400.0 mg
CAUTION: Federal law prohibits dispensing without perscription.

> **1. ESTROGENS HAVE BEEN REPORTED TO INCREASE THE RISK OF ENDOMETRIAL CARCINOMA.**
> Three independent case control studies have reported an increased risk of endometrial cancer in postmenopausal women exposed to exogenous estrogens for more than one year.[1-3] This risk was independent of the other known risk factors for endometrial cancer. These studies are further supported by the finding that incidence rates of endometrial cancer have increased sharply since 1969 in eight different areas of the United States with population-based cancer reporting systems, an increase which may be related to the rapidly expanding use of estrogens during the last decade.[4]
> The three case control studies reported that the risk of endometrial cancer in estrogen users was about 4.5 to 13.9 times greater than in nonusers. The risk appears to depend on both duration of treatment[1] and on estrogen dose.[3] In view of these findings, when estrogens are used for the treatment of menopausal symptoms, the lowest dose that will control symptoms should be utilized and medication should be discontinued as soon as possible. When prolonged treatment is medically indicated, the patient should be reassessed on at least a semiannual basis to determine the need for continued therapy. Although the evidence must be considered preliminary, one study suggests that cyclic administration of low doses of estrogen may carry less risk than continuous administration;[3] it therefore appears prudent to utilize such a regimen.
> Close clinical surveillance of all women taking estrogens is important. In all cases of undiagnosed persistent or recurring abnormal vaginal bleeding, adequate diagnostic measures should be undertaken to rule out malignancy.
> There is no evidence at present that "natural" estrogens are more or less hazardous than "synthetic" estrogens at equiestrogenic doses.
>
> **2. ESTROGENS SHOULD NOT BE USED DURING PREGNANCY.**
> The use of female sex hormones, both estrogens and progestogens, during early pregnancy may seriously damage the offspring. It has been shown that females exposed in utero to diethylstilbestrol, a non-steroidal estrogen, have an increased risk of developing in later life a form of vaginal or cervical cancer that is ordinarily extremely rare.[5,6] This risk has been estimated as not greater than 4 per 1000 exposures.[7] Furthermore, a high percentage of such exposed women (from 30 to 90 percent) have been found to have vaginal adenosis,[8-12] epithelial changes of the vagina and cervix. Although these changes are histologically benign, it is not known whether they are precursors of malignancy. Although similar data are not available with the use of other estrogens, it cannot be presumed they would not induce similar changes.
> Several reports suggest an association between intrauterine exposure to female sex hormones and congenital anomalies, including congenital heart defects and limb reduction defects.[13-16] One case control study[16] estimated a 4.7-fold increased risk of limb reduction defects in infants exposed in utero to sex hormones (oral contraceptives, hormone withdrawal tests for pregnancy, or attempted treatment for threatened abortion). Some of these exposures were very short and involved only a few days of treatment. The data suggest that the risk of limb reduction defects in exposed fetuses is somewhat less than 1 per 1000.
> In the past, female sex hormones have been used during pregnancy in an attempt to treat threatened or habitual abortion. There is considerable evidence that estrogens are ineffective for these indications, and there is no evidence from well controlled studies that progestogens are effective for these uses.
> If PMB is used during pregnancy, or if the patient becomes pregnant while taking this drug, she should be apprised of the potential risks to the fetus, and the advisability of pregnancy continuation.
>
> **3. THIS FIXED COMBINATION DRUG IS NOT INDICATED FOR INITIAL THERAPY.**
> In cases where estrogen given alone has not alleviated anxiety and tension existing as part of the menopausal symptom complex, therapy may then consist of separate administration of estrogen and meprobamate in order to determine the appropriate dosage of each drug for the patient. If this fixed combination represents the dosage so determined, its use may be more convenient in patient management. The treatment of such patients is not static, but must be reevaluated as conditions in each patient warrant.

Description: PMB is a combination of PREMARIN® (Conjugated Estrogens, U.S.P.) and meprobamate, a tranquilizing agent, in tablet form for oral administration.
PREMARIN (Conjugated Estrogens, U.S.P.) is a mixture of estrogens, obtained exclusively from natural sources, occurring as the sodium salts of water-soluble estrogen sulfates blended to represent the average composition of material derived from pregnant mares' urine. It contains estrone, equilin, and 17α-dihydroequilin, together with smaller amounts of 17α-estradiol, equilenin, and 17 α-dihydroequilenin as salts of their sulfate esters.
Meprobamate is the dicarbamic acid ester of 2-methyl-2-*n*-propyl-1,3-propanediol.
Clinical Pharmacology: Estrogens are important in the development and maintenance of the female reproductive system and secondary sex characteristics. They promote growth and development of the vagina, uterus, and fallopian tubes, and enlargement of the breasts. Indirectly, they contribute to the shaping of the skeleton, maintenance of tone and elasticity of urogenital structures, changes in the epiphyses of the long bones that allow for the pubertal growth spurt and its termination, growth of axillary and pubic hair, and pigmentation of the nipples and genitals. Decline of estrogenic activity at the end of the menstrual cycle can bring on menstruation, although the cessation of progesterone secretion is the most important factor in the mature ovulatory cycle. However, in the preovulatory or nonovulatory cycle, estrogen is the primary determinant in the onset of menstruation. Estrogens also affect the release of pituitary gonadotropins.
The pharmacologic effects of conjugated estrogens are similar to those of endogenous estrogens. They are soluble in water and are well absorbed from the gastrointestinal tract.
In responsive tissues (female genital organs, breasts, hypothalamus, pituitary) estrogens enter the cell and are transported into the nucleus. As a result of estrogen action, specific RNA and protein synthesis occurs.
Metabolism and inactivation occur primarily in the liver. Some estrogens are excreted into the bile; however they are reabsorbed from the intestine and returned to the liver through the portal venous system. Water soluble estrogen conjugates are strongly acidic and are ionized in body fluids, which favor excretion through the kidneys since tubular reabsorption is minimal.
Meprobamate is used clinically for the reduction of anxiety and tension. The precise mechanism(s) of its action is not known. It is well-absorbed from the gastrointestinal tract and has a physiological half-life of about 10 hours. It is excreted in the urine primarily as hydroxymeprobamate and as a glucuronide.
The combination of PREMARIN with meprobamate as provided in PMB relieves the underlying estrogen deficiency and affords tranquilizing activity to ameliorate the anxiety and tension not due to estrogen deficiency.
Indication: For the treatment of moderate to severe vasomotor symptoms of the menopause when anxiety and tension are part of the symptom complex and only in those cases in which the use of estrogens alone has not resulted in alleviation of such symptoms.
PMB HAS NOT BEEN SHOWN TO BE EFFECTIVE FOR ANY PURPOSE DURING PREGNANCY AND ITS USE MAY CAUSE SEVERE HARM TO THE FETUS (SEE BOXED WARNING).

Contraindications: Estrogens should not be used in women with any of the following conditions:
1. Known or suspected cancer of the breast.
2. Known or suspected estrogen-dependent neoplasia.
3. Known or suspected pregnancy (See Boxed Warning).
4. Undiagnosed abnormal genital bleeding.
5. Active thrombophlebitis or thromboembolic disorders.
6. A past history of thrombophlebitis, thrombosis, or thromboembolic disorders associated with previous estrogen use.

Meprobamate should not be used in patients with the following conditions:
1. A history of allergic or idiosyncratic reactions to meprobamate or related compounds such as carisoprodol, mebutamate, tybamate, or carbromal.
2. Acute intermittent porphyria.

Warnings:
USAGE IN PREGNANCY AND LACTATION. An increased risk of congenital malformations associated with the use of minor tranquilizers (meprobamate, chlordiazepoxide, and diazepam) during the first trimester of pregnancy has been suggested in several studies. Because use of these drugs is rarely a matter of urgency, their use during this period should almost always be avoided. The possibility that a woman of childbearing potential may be pregnant at the time of institution of therapy should be considered. Patients should be advised that if they become pregnant during therapy or intend to become pregnant they should communicate with their physicians about the desirability of discontinuing the drug.

Meprobamate passes the placental barrier. It is present both in umbilical cord blood at or near maternal plasma levels and in breast milk of lactating mothers at concentrations two to four times that of maternal plasma. When use of meprobamate is contemplated in breast-feeding patients, the drug's higher concentrations in breast milk as compared to maternal plasma levels should be considered.

Usage in Children—PMB is not intended for use in children.

Associated with Estrogen Administration:
1. *Induction of malignant neoplasms.* Long term continuous administration of natural and synthetic estrogens in certain animal species increases the frequency of carcinomas of the breast, cervix, vagina, and liver. There are now reports that estrogens increase the risk of carcinoma of the endometrium in humans. (See Boxed Warning.)

At the present time there is no satisfactory evidence that estrogens given to postmenopausal women increase the risk of cancer of the breast,[17] although a recent long-term followup of a single physician's practice has raised this possibility.[18] Because of the animal data, there is a need for caution in prescribing estrogens for women with a strong family history of breast cancer or who have breast nodules, fibrocystic disease, or abnormal mammograms.

2. *Gallbladder disease.* A recent study has reported a 2 to 3-fold increase in the risk of surgically confirmed gallbladder disease in women receiving postmenopausal estrogens,[17] similar to the 2-fold increase previously noted in users of oral contraceptives.[19,24a]

3. *Effects similar to those caused by estrogen-progestogen oral contraceptives.* There are several serious adverse effects of oral contraceptives, most of which have not, up to now, been documented as consequences of postmenopausal estrogen therapy. This may reflect the comparatively low doses of estrogen used in postmenopausal women. It would be expected that the larger doses of estrogen used to treat prostatic or breast cancer or postpartum breast engorgement are more likely to result in these adverse effects, and, in fact, it has been shown that there is an increased risk of thrombosis in men receiving estrogens for prostatic cancer and women for postpartum breast engorgement.[20-23]

a. *Thromboembolic disease.* It is now well established that users of oral contraceptives have an increased risk of various thromboembolic and thrombotic vascular diseases, such as thrombophlebitis, pulmonary embolism, stroke, and myocardial infarction.[24-31] Cases of retinal thrombosis, mesenteric thrombosis, and optic neuritis have been reported in oral contraceptive users. There is evidence that the risk of several of these adverse reactions is related to the dose of the drug.[32,33] An increased risk of postsurgery thromboembolic complications has also been reported in users of oral contraceptives.[34,35] If feasible, estrogen should be discontinued at least 4 weeks before surgery of the type associated with an increased risk of thromboembolism, or during periods of prolonged immobilization.

While an increased rate of thromboembolic and thrombotic disease in postmenopausal users of estrogens has not been found,[17-24,25-36] this does not rule out the possibility that such an increase may be present or that subgroups of women who have underlying risk factors or who are receiving relatively large doses of estrogens may have increased risk. Therefore estrogens should not be used in persons with active thrombophlebitis or thromboembolic disorders, and they should not be used (except in treatment of malignancy) in persons with a history of such disorders in association with estrogen use. They should be used with caution in patients with cerebral vascular or coronary artery disease and only for those in whom estrogens are clearly needed.

Large doses of estrogen (5 mg conjugated estrogens per day), comparable to those used to treat cancer of the prostate and breast, have been shown in a large prospective clinical trial in men[37] to increase the risk of nonfatal myocardial infarction, pulmonary embolism and thrombophlebitis. When estrogen doses of this size are used, any of the thromboembolic and thrombotic adverse effects associated with oral contraceptive use should be considered a clear risk.

b. *Hepatic adenoma.* Benign hepatic adenomas appear to be associated with the use of oral contraceptives.[38-40] Although benign, and rare, these may rupture and may cause death through intraabdominal hemorrhage. Such lesions have not yet been reported in association with other estrogen or progestogen preparations but should be considered in estrogen users having abdominal pain and tenderness, abdominal mass, or hypovolemic shock. Hepatocellular carcinoma has also been reported in women taking estrogen-containing oral contraceptives.[39] The relationship of this malignancy to these drugs is not known at this time.

c. *Elevated blood pressure.* Women using oral contraceptives sometimes experience increased blood pressure which, in most cases, returns to normal on discontinuing the drug. There is now a report that this may occur with use of estrogens in the menopause[41] and blood pressure should be monitored with estrogen use, especially if high doses are used.

d. *Glucose tolerance.* A worsening of glucose tolerance has been observed in a significant percentage of patients on estrogen-containing oral contraceptives. For this reason, diabetic patients should be carefully observed while receiving estrogen.

4. *Hypercalcemia.* Administration of estrogens may lead to severe hypercalcemia in patients with breast cancer and bone metastases. If this occurs, the drug should be stopped and appropriate measures taken to reduce the serum calcium level.

Associated with Meprobamate Administration:
1. *Drug Dependence*—Physical dependence, psychological dependence, and abuse have occurred. When chronic intoxication from prolonged use occurs, it usually involves ingestion of greater than recommended doses and is manifested by ataxia, slurred speech, and vertigo. Therefore, careful supervision of dose and amounts prescribed is advised, as well as avoidance of prolonged administration, especially for alcoholics and other patients with a known propensity for taking excessive quantities of drugs.

Sudden withdrawal of the drug after prolonged and excessive use may precipitate recurrence of preexisting symptoms, such as anxiety, anorexia, or insomnia, or withdrawal reactions, such as vomiting, ataxia, tremors, muscle twitching, confusional states, hallucinosis, and, rarely, convulsive seizures. Such seizures are more likely to occur in persons with central nervous system damage or preexistent or latent convulsive disorders. Onset of withdrawal symptoms occurs usually within 12 to 48 hours after discontinuation of meprobamate; symptoms usually cease within the next 12 to 48 hours.

When excessive dosage has continued for weeks or months, dosage should be reduced gradually over a period of one or two weeks rather than abruptly stopped. Alternatively, a short-acting barbiturate may be substituted, then gradually withdrawn.

2. *Potentially Hazardous Tasks*—Patients should be warned that this drug may impair the mental and/or physical abilities required for the performance of potentially hazardous tasks such as driving a motor vehicle or operating machinery.

3. *Additive Effects*—Since the effects of meprobamate and alcohol or meprobamate and other CNS depressants or psychotropic drugs may be additive, appropriate caution should be exercised with patients who take more than one of these agents simultaneously.

Precautions:
Associated with Estrogen
A. General Precautions.
1. A complete medical and family history should be taken prior to the initiation of any estrogen therapy. The pretreatment and periodic physical examinations should include special reference to blood pressure, breasts, abdomen, and pelvic organs, and should include a Papanicolau smear. As a general rule, estrogen should not be prescribed for longer than one year without another physical examination being performed.

2. *Fluid retention*—Because estrogens may cause some degree of fluid retention, conditions which might be influenced by this factor such as asthma, epilepsy, migraine, and cardiac or renal dysfunction, require careful observation.

3. Certain patients may develop undesirable manifestations of excessive estrogenic stimulation, such as abnormal or excessive uterine bleeding, mastodynia, etc.

4. Oral contraceptives appear to be associated with an increased incidence of mental depression.[24a] Although it is not clear whether this is due to the estrogenic or progestogenic component of the contraceptive, patients with a history of depression should be carefully observed.

5. Preexisting uterine leiomyomata may increase in size during estrogen use.

6. The pathologist should be advised of estrogen therapy when relevant specimens are submitted.

7. Patients with a past history of jaundice during pregnancy have an increased risk of recurrence of jaundice while receiving estrogen-containing oral contraceptive therapy. If jaundice develops in any patient receiving estrogen, the medication should be discontinued while the cause is investigated.

8. Estrogens may be poorly metabolized in patients with impaired liver function and they should be administered with caution in such patients.

9. Because estrogens influence the metabolism of calcium and phosphorus, they should be used with caution in patients with metabolic bone diseases that are associated with hypercalcemia or in patients with renal insufficiency.

10. Because of the effects of estrogens on epiphyseal closure, they should be used judiciously in young patients in whom bone growth is not complete.

11. Certain endocrine and liver function tests may be affected by estrogen-containing oral contraceptives. The following similar changes may be expected with larger doses of estrogen:

Continued on next page

Ayerst—Cont.

a. Increased sulfobromophthalein retention.
b. Increased prothrombin and factors VII, VIII, IX, and X; decreased antithrombin 3; increased norepinephrine-induced platelet aggregability.
c. Increased thyroid binding globulin (TBG) leading to increased circulating total thyroid hormone, as measured by PBI, T4 by column, or T4 by radioimmunoassay. Free T3 resin uptake is decreased, reflecting the elevated TBG; free T4 concentration is unaltered.
d. Impaired glucose tolerance.
e. Decreased pregnanediol excretion.
f. Reduced response to metyrapone test.
g. Reduced serum folate concentration.
h. Increased serum triglyceride and phospholipid concentration.

B. Information for the Patient. See text which appears after the PHYSICIAN REFERENCES.
C. Pregnancy Category X. See CONTRAINDICATIONS and Boxed Warning.
D. Nursing Mothers. As a general principle, the administration of any drug to nursing mothers should be done only when clearly necessary since many drugs are excreted in human milk.

Associated with Meprobamate
A. The lowest effective dose should be administered, particularly to debilitated patients, in order to preclude oversedation.
B. The possibility of suicide attempts should be considered and the least amount of drug feasible should be dispensed at any one time.
C. Meprobamate is metabolized in the liver and excreted by the kidney; to avoid its excess accumulation, caution should be exercised in administration to patients with compromised liver or kidney function.
D. Meprobamate occasionally may precipitate seizures in epileptic patients.

Adverse Reactions:
Associated with Estrogen Administration
(See Warnings regarding induction of neoplasia, adverse effects on the fetus, increased incidence of gallbladder disease, and adverse effects similar to those of oral contraceptives, including thromboembolism.) The following additional adverse reactions have been reported with estrogenic therapy, including oral contraceptives:
1. *Genitourinary system:* Breakthrough bleeding, spotting, change in menstrual flow; dysmenorrhea; premenstrual-like syndrome; amenorrhea during and after treatment; increase in size of uterine fibromyomata; vaginal candidiasis; change in cervical erosion and in degree of cervical secretion; cystitis-like syndrome.
2. *Breasts:* Tenderness, enlargement, secretion.
3. *Gastrointestinal:* Nausea, vomiting; abdominal cramps, bloating; cholestatic jaundice.
4. *Skin:* Chloasma or melasma which may persist when drug is discontinued; erythema multiforme; erythema nodosum; hemorrhagic eruption; loss of scalp hair; hirsutism.
5. *Eyes:* Steepening of corneal curvature; intolerance to contact lenses.
6. *CNS:* Headache, migraine, dizziness; mental depression; chorea.
7. *Miscellaneous:* Increase or decrease in weight; reduced carbohydrate tolerance; aggravation of porphyria; edema; changes in libido.

The following have been reported with meprobamate therapy:
1. *Central Nervous System*—Drowsiness, ataxia, dizziness, slurred speech, headache, vertigo, weakness, paresthesias, impairment of visual accommodation, euphoria, overstimulation, paradoxical excitement, fast EEG activity.
2. *Gastrointestinal*—Nausea, vomiting, diarrhea.
3. *Cardiovascular*—Palpitations, tachycardia, various forms of arrhythmia, transient ECG changes, syncope; also, hypotensive crises (including one fatal case).
4. *Allergic or Idiosyncratic*—Allergic or idiosyncratic reactions are usually seen within the period of the first to fourth dose in patients having had no previous contact with the drug. Milder reactions are characterized by an itchy, urticarial, or erythematous maculopapular rash which may be generalized or confined to the groin. Other reactions have included leukopenia, acute nonthrombocytopenic purpura, petechiae, ecchymoses, eosinophilia, peripheral edema, adenopathy, fever, fixed drug eruption with cross reaction to carisoprodol, and cross sensitivity between meprobamate/mebutamate and meprobamate/carbromal.
More severe hypersensitivity reactions, rarely reported, include hyperpyrexia, chills, angioneurotic edema, bronchospasm, oliguria, and anuria. Also, anaphylaxis, erythema multiforme, exfoliative dermatitis, stomatitis, proctitis, Stevens-Johnson syndrome, and bullous dermatitis, including one fatal case of the latter, following administration of meprobamate in combination with prednisolone.
In case of allergic or idiosyncratic reactions to meprobamate, discontinue the drug and initiate appropriate symptomatic therapy, which may include epinephrine, antihistamines, and in severe cases corticosteroids. In evaluating possible allergic reactions, also consider allergy to excipients (information on excipients is available to physicians on request).
5. *Hematologic* (See also *Allergic or Idiosyncratic*).—Agranulocytosis and aplastic anemia have been reported, although no causal relationship has been established. These cases rarely were fatal. Rare cases of thrombocytopenic purpura have been reported.
6. *Other*—Exacerbation of porphyric symptoms.

Overdosage:
Acute overdosage (estrogen alone):
Numerous reports of ingestion of large doses of estrogen-containing oral contraceptives by young children indicate that acute serious ill effects do not occur. Overdosage of estrogen may cause nausea, and withdrawal bleeding may occur in females.
Acute simple overdosage (meprobamate alone): Death has been reported with ingestion of as little as 12 grams meprobamate and survival with as much as 40 grams.
Blood levels: 0.5–2.0 mg% represents the usual blood level range of meprobamate after therapeutic doses. The level may occasionally be as high as 3.0 mg%.
3—10 mg% usually corresponds to findings of mild to moderate symptoms of overdosage, such as stupor or light coma.
10—20 mg% usually corresponds to deeper coma, requiring more intensive treatment. Some fatalities occur.
At levels greater than 20 mg%, more fatalities than survivals can be expected.
Acute combined (alcohol or other CNS depressants or psychotropic drugs) **overdosage:** Since effects can be additive, a history of ingestion of a low dose of meprobamate plus any of these compounds (or of a relatively low blood or tissue level) cannot be used as a prognostic indicator.
In cases where excessive doses have been taken, sleep ensues rapidly and blood pressure, pulse, and respiratory rates are reduced to basal levels. Any drug remaining in the stomach should be removed and symptomatic therapy given. Should respiration or blood pressure become compromised, respiratory assistance, central nervous system stimulants, and pressor agents should be administered cautiously as indicated. Meprobamate is metabolized in the liver and excreted by the kidney. Diuresis, osmotic (mannitol) diuresis, peritoneal dialysis, and hemodialysis have been used successfully. Careful monitoring of urinary output is necessary and caution should be taken to avoid overhydration. Relapse and death, after initial recovery, have been attributed to incomplete gastric emptying and delayed absorption. Meprobamate can be measured in biological fluids by two methods: colorimetric[42] and gas chromatographic.[43]

Dosage and Administration:
Given cyclically for short term use only:
For the treatment of moderate to severe vasomotor symptoms of the menopause when anxiety and tension are part of the symptom complex and only in those cases in which the use of estrogens alone has not resulted in alleviation of such symptoms. The lowest dose that will control symptoms should be chosen and medication should be discontinued as promptly as possible. The usual dosage of conjugated estrogen is 1.25 milligrams daily. The usual dosage of meprobamate is 1,200 to 1,600 milligrams daily.
Administration should be cyclic (e.g., three weeks on and one week off).
Attempts to discontinue or taper medication should be made at three to six month intervals.

PMB® 200 & PMB® 400: The usual dosage is one tablet of either strength three times daily administered cyclically. Use of meprobamate during the rest period should be considered for those patients who may require continuing medication with tranquilizer. After the first few cycles of therapy, the patient's need for continuing the use of the meprobamate component should be reevaluated. Daily dosage should be adjusted to individual requirements. The daily dosage should not exceed 6 tablets of PMB 200 per day or 4 tablets of PMB 400 per day.
Treated patients with an intact uterus should be monitored closely for signs of endometrial cancer and appropriate diagnostic measures should be taken to rule out malignancy in the event of persistent or recurring abnormal vaginal bleeding.

How Supplied:
PMB® 200, in bottles of 60 (NDC 0046-0880-60).
PMB® 400, in bottles of 60 (NDC 0046-0881-60).

Physician References:
1. Ziel, H. K., *et al:* N. Engl. J. Med. 293:1167–1170, 1975.
2. Smith, D. C., *et al:* N. Engl. J. Med. 293:1164–1167, 1975.
3. Mack, T. M., *et al:* N. Engl. J. Med. 294:1262–1267, 1976.
4. Weiss, N. S., *et al:* N. Engl. J. Med. 294:1259–1262, 1976.
5. Herbst, A. L., *et al:* N. Engl. J. Med. 284:878–881, 1971.
6. Greenwald, P., *et al:* N. Engl. J. Med. 285:390–392, 1971.
7. Lanier, A., *et al:* Mayo Clin. Proc. 48:793–799, 1973.
8. Herbst, A., *et al:* Obstet. Gynecol. 40:287–298, 1972.
9. Herbst, A., *et al:* Am. J. Obstet. Gynecol. 118:607–615, 1974.
10. Herbst, A., *et al:* N. Engl. J. Med. 292:334–339, 1975.
11. Stafl, A., *et al:* Obstet. Gynecol. 43:118–128, 1974.
12. Sherman, A. I., *et al:* Obstet. Gynecol. 44:531–545, 1974.
13. Gal, I., *et al:* Nature 216:83, 1967.
14. Levy, E. P., *et al:* Lancet 1:611, 1973.
15. Nora, J., *et al:* Lancet 1:941–942, 1973.
16. Janerich, D. T., *et al:* N. Engl. J. Med. 291:697–700, 1974.
17. Boston Collaborative Drug Surveillance Program: N. Engl. J. Med. 290:15–19, 1974.
18. Hoover, R., *et al:* N. Engl. J. Med. 295:401–405, 1976.
19. Boston Collaborative Drug Surveillance Program: Lancet 1:1399–1404, 1973.
20. Daniel, D. G., *et al:* Lancet 2:287–289, 1967.
21. The Veterans Administration Cooperative Urological Research Group: J. Urol. 98:516–522, 1967.
22. Bailar, J. C.: Lancet 2:560, 1967.
23. Blackard, C., *et al:* Cancer 26:249–256, 1970.
24. Royal College of General Practitioners: J. R. Coll. Gen. Pract. 13:267–279, 1967.
24a. Royal College of General Practitioners: Oral Contraceptives and Health, New York, Pitman Corp., 1974.
25. Inman, W. H. W., *et al:* Br. Med. J. 2:193–199, 1968.
26. Vessey, M. P., *et al:* Br. Med. J. 2:651–657, 1969.
27. Sartwell, P. E., *et al:* Am. J. Epidemiol. 90:365–380, 1969.

28. Collaborative Group for the Study of Stroke in Young Women: N. Engl. J. Med. 288:871–878, 1973.
29. Collaborative Group for the Study of Stroke in Young Women: J.A.M.A. 231:718–722, 1975.
30. Mann, J. I., et al: Br. Med. J. 2:245–248, 1975.
31. Mann, J. I., et al: Br. Med. J. 2:241–245, 1975.
32. Inman, W. H. W., et al: Br. Med. J. 2:203–209, 1970.
33. Stolley, P. D., et al: Am. J. Epidemiol. 102:197–208, 1975.
34. Vessey, M. P., et al: Br. Med. J. 3:123–126, 1970.
35. Greene, G. R., et al: Am. J. Public Health 62:680–685, 1972.
36. Rosenberg, L., et al: N. Engl. J. Med. 294:1256–1259, 1976.
37. Coronary Drug Project Research Group: J.A.M.A. 214:1303–1313, 1970.
38. Baum, J., et al: Lancet 2:926–928, 1973.
39. Mays, E. T., et al: J.A.M.A. 235:730–732, 1976.
40. Edmondson, H. A., et al: N. Engl. J. Med. 294:470–472, 1976.
41. Pfeffer, R. I., et al: Am. J. Epidemiol. 103:445–456, 1976.
42. Hoffman, A. J., et al: J. Am. Pharm. Assoc. 48:740, 1959.
43. Douglas, J. F., et al: Anal. Chem. 39:956, 1967.

INFORMATION FOR THE PATIENT
What You Should Know About Estrogens

Estrogens are female hormones produced by the ovaries. The ovaries make several different kinds of estrogens. In addition, scientists have been able to make a variety of synthetic estrogens. As far as we know, all these estrogens have similar properties and therefore much the same usefulness, side effects, and risks. This leaflet is intended to help you understand what estrogens are used for, the risks involved in their use, and how to use them as safely as possible.

This leaflet includes the most important information about estrogens, but not all the information. If you want to know more, you should ask your doctor for more information or you can ask your doctor or pharmacist to let you read the package insert prepared for the doctor.

Uses of Estrogen
THERE IS NO PROPER USE OF ESTROGENS IN A PREGNANT WOMAN

Estrogens are prescribed by doctors for a number of purposes, including:

1. To provide estrogen during a period of adjustment when a woman's ovaries stop producing a majority of her estrogens, in order to prevent certain uncomfortable symptoms of estrogen deficiency. (With the menopause, which generally occurs between the ages of 45 and 55, women produce a much smaller amount of estrogens.)
2. To prevent symptoms of estrogen deficiency when a woman's ovaries have been removed surgically before the natural menopause.
3. To prevent pregnancy. (Estrogens are given along with a progestogen, another female hormone; these combinations are called oral contraceptives or birth control pills. Patient labeling is available to women taking oral contraceptives and they will not be discussed in this leaflet).
4. To treat certain cancers in women and men.
5. To prevent painful swelling of the breasts after pregnancy in women who choose not to nurse their babies.

Estrogens in the Menopause:
In the natural course of their lives, all women eventually experience a decrease in estrogen production. This usually occurs between ages 45 and 55 but may occur earlier or later. Sometimes the ovaries may need to be removed before natural menopause by an operation, producing a "surgical menopause."

When the amount of estrogen in the blood begins to decrease, many women may develop typical symptoms: feelings of warmth in the face, neck, and chest or sudden intense episodes of heat and sweating throughout the body (called "hot flashes" or "hot flushes"). These symptoms are sometimes very uncomfortable. Some women may also develop changes in the vagina (called "atrophic vagnitis") which cause discomfort, especially during and after intercourse.

Estrogens can be prescribed to treat these symptoms of the menopause. It is estimated that considerably more than half of all women undergoing the menopause have only mild symptoms or no symptoms at all and therefore do not need estrogens. Other women may need estrogens for a few months, while their bodies adjust to lower estrogen levels. Sometimes the need will be for periods longer than six months. In an attempt to avoid overstimulation of the uterus (womb), estrogens are usually given cyclically during each month of use, such as three weeks of pills followed by one week without pills.

Sometimes women experience nervous symptoms or depression during menopause. There is no evidence that estrogens are effective for such symptoms without associated vasomotor symptoms. In the absence of vasomotor symptoms, estrogens should not be used to treat nervous symptoms, although other treatment may be needed.

You may have heard that taking estrogens for long periods (years) after the menopause will keep your skin soft and supple and keep you feeling young. There is no evidence that this is so, however, and such long-term treatment carries important risks.

Estrogens to Prevent Swelling of the Breasts After Pregnancy
If you do not breast-feed your baby after delivery, your breasts may fill up with milk and become painful and engorged. This usually begins about 3 to 4 days after delivery and may last for a few days to up to a week or more. Sometimes the discomfort is severe, but usually it is not and can be controlled by pain-relieving drugs such as aspirin and by binding the breasts up tightly. Estrogens can be used to try to prevent the breasts from filling up. While this treatment is sometimes successful, in many cases the breasts fill up to some degree in spite of treatment. The dose of estrogens needed to prevent pain and swelling of the breasts is much larger than the dose needed to treat symptoms of the menopause and this may increase your chances of developing blood clots in the legs or lungs (see below). Therefore, it is important that you discuss the benefits and the risks of estrogen use with your doctor if you have decided not to breast-feed your baby.

The Dangers of Estrogens:
1. *Endometrial cancer.* There are reports that if estrogens are used in the postmenopausal period for more than a year there is an increased risk of *endometrial cancer* (cancer of the lining of the uterus). Women taking estrogens have roughly 5 to 10 times as great a chance of getting this cancer as women who take no estrogens. To put this another way, while a postmenopausal woman not taking estrogens has a 1 chance in 1,000 each year of getting endometrial cancer, a woman taking estrogens has 5 to 10 chances in 1,000 each year. For this reason *it is important to take estrogens only when they are really needed.*

The risk of this cancer is greater the longer estrogens are used and when larger doses are taken. Therefore you should not take more estrogen than your doctor prescribes. *It is important to take the lowest dose of estrogen that will control symptoms and to take it only as long as it is needed.* If estrogens are needed for longer periods of time, your doctor will want to reevaluate your need for estrogens at least every six months.

Women using estrogens should report any vaginal bleeding to their doctors; such bleeding may be of no importance, but it can be an early warning of endometrial cancer. If you have undiagnosed vaginal bleeding, you should not use estrogens until a diagnosis is made and you are certain there is no endometrial cancer.

NOTE: If you have had your uterus removed (total hysterectomy), there is no danger of developing endometrial cancer.

2. *Other possible cancers.* Estrogens can cause development of other tumors in animals, such as tumors of the breast, cervix, vagina, or liver, when given for a long time. At present there is no good evidence that women using estrogen in the menopause have an increased risk of such tumors, but there is no way yet to be sure they do not; and one study raises the possibility that use of estrogens in the menopause may increase the risk of breast cancer many years later. This is a further reason to use estrogens only when clearly needed. While you are taking estrogens, it is important that you go to your doctor at least once a year for a physical examination. Also, if members of your family have had breast cancer or if you have breast nodules or abnormal mammograms (breast x-rays), your doctor may wish to carry out more frequent examinations of your breasts.

3. *Gallbladder disease.* Women who use estrogens after menopause are more likely to develop gallbladder disease needing surgery then women who do not use estrogens. Birth control pills have a similar effect.

4. *Abnormal blood clotting.* Oral contraceptives increase the risk of blood clotting in various parts of the body. This can result in a stroke (if the clot is in the brain), a heart attack (clot in a blood vessel of the heart), or a pulmonary embolus (a clot which forms in the legs or pelvis, then breaks off and travels to the lungs). Any of these can be fatal. At this time use of estrogens in the menopause is not known to cause such blood clotting, but this has not been fully studied and there could still prove to be such a risk. It is recommended that if you have had clotting in the legs or lungs or a heart attack or stroke while you were using estrogens or birth control pills, you should not use estrogens (unless they are being used to treat cancer of the breast or prostrate). If you have had a stroke or heart attack or if you have angina pectoris, estrogens should be used with great caution and only if clearly needed (for example, if you have severe symptoms of the menopause).

The larger doses of estrogen used to prevent swelling of the breasts after pregnancy have been reported to cause clotting in the legs and lungs.

Special Warning About Pregnancy: You should not receive estrogen if you are pregnant. If this should occur, there is a greater than usual chance that the developing child will be born with a birth defect, although the possibility remains fairly small. A female child may have an increased risk of developing cancer of the vagina or cervix later in life (in the teens or twenties). Every possible effort should be made to avoid exposure to estrogens during pregnancy. If exposure occurs, see your doctor.

Other Effects of Estrogens: In addition to the serious known risks of estrogens described above, estrogens have the following side effects and potential risks:

1. *Nausea and vomiting.* The most common side effect of estrogen therapy is nausea. Vomiting is less common.
2. *Effects on breasts.* Estrogens may cause breast tenderness or enlargement and may cause the breasts to secrete a liquid. These effects are not dangerous.
3. *Effects on the uterus.* Estrogens may cause benign fibroid tumors of the uterus to get larger.
4. *Effects on liver.* Women taking oral contraceptives develop on rare occasions a tumor of the liver which can rupture and bleed into the abdomen and may cause death. So far, these tumors have not been reported in women using estrogens in the menopause, but you should report any swelling or unusual pain or tenderness in the abdomen to your doctor immediately.

Women with a past history of jaundice (yellowing of the skin and white parts of the eyes) may get jaundice again during estrogen use. If this occurs, stop taking estrogens and see your doctor.

5. *Other effects.* Estrogens may cause excess fluids to be retained in the body. This may make some conditions worse, such as asthma, epilepsy, migraine, heart disease, or kidney disease.

Summary: Estrogens have important uses, but they have serious risks as well. You must decide, with your doctor, whether the risks are acceptable

Continued on next page

Ayerst—Cont.

to you in view of the benefits of treatment. Except where your doctor has prescribed estrogens for use in special cases of cancer of the breast or prostate, you should not use estrogens if you have cancer of the breast or prostate, you should not use estrogens if you have cancer of the breast or uterus, are pregnant, have undiagnosed abnormal vaginal bleeding, clotting in the legs or lungs, or have had a stroke, heart attack or angina, or clotting in the legs or lungs in the past while you were taking estrogens.

You can use estrogens as safely as possible by understanding that your doctor will require regular physical examinations while you are taking them and will try to discontinue the drug as soon as possible and use the smallest dose possible. Be alert for signs of trouble including:
1. Abnormal bleeding from the vagina.
2. Pains in the calves or chest or sudden shortness of breath, or coughing blood.
3. Severe headache, dizziness, faintness, or changes in vision.
4. Breast lumps (you should ask your doctor how to examine your own breasts).
5. Jaundice (yellowing of the skin).
6. Mental depression.

Your doctor has prescribed this drug for you and you alone. Do not give the drug to anyone else.

How Supplied: PREMARIN® (Conjugated Estrogens Tablets, U.S.P.)—tablets for oral administration.

PREMARIN® VAGINAL CREAM—PREMARIN® in a nonliquefying base, designed for vaginal use.

PREMARIN® with METHYLTESTOSTERONE—a combination of PREMARIN and methyltestosterone (an androgen) in tablet form for oral administration.

PMB® 200, 400—a combination of PREMARIN® and meprobamate (a tranquilizing agent) in tablet form for oral administration.

PREMARIN® INTRAVENOUS—PREMARIN® specially prepared for intravenous and intramuscular use.

ESTROGENIC SUBSTANCE (Estrone) in Aqueous Suspension—a sterile aqueous suspension of estrone, a short-acting estrogen, for intramuscular injection only.

Shown in Product Identification Section, page 405

PREMARIN® ℞
[prĕm'a-rĭn]
Brand of Conjugated Estrogens Tablets, U.S.P.

1. ESTROGENS HAVE BEEN REPORTED TO INCREASE THE RISK OF ENDOMETRIAL CARCINOMA.

Three independent case control studies have reported an increased risk of endometrial cancer in postmenopausal women exposed to exogenous estrogens for more than one year.[1-3] This risk was independent of the other known risk factors for endometrial cancer. These studies are further supported by the finding that incidence rates of endometrial cancer have increased sharply since 1969 in eight different areas of the United States with population-based cancer reporting systems, an increase which may be related to the rapidly expanding use of estrogens during the last decade.[4]

The three case control studies reported that the risk of endometrial cancer in estrogen users was about 4.5 to 13.9 times greater than in nonusers. The risk appears to depend on both duration of treatment[1] and on estrogen dose.[3] In view of these findings, when estrogens are used for the treatment of menopausal symptoms, the lowest dose that will control symptoms should be utilized and medication should be discontinued as soon as possible. When prolonged treatment is medically indicated, the patient should be reassessed on at least a semiannual basis to determine the need for continued therapy. Although the evidence must be considered preliminary, one study suggests that cyclic administration of low doses of estrogen may carry less risk than continuous administration;[3] it therefore appears prudent to utilize such a regimen.

Close clinical surveillance of all women taking estrogens is important. In all cases of undiagnosed persistent or recurring abnormal vaginal bleeding, adequate diagnostic measures should be undertaken to rule out malignancy.

There is no evidence at present that "natural" estrogens are more or less hazardous than "synthetic" estrogens at equiestrogenic doses.

2. ESTROGENS SHOULD NOT BE USED DURING PREGNANCY.

The use of female sex hormones, both estrogens and progestogens, during early pregnancy may seriously damage the offspring. It has been shown that females exposed in utero to diethylstilbestrol, a non-steroidal estrogen, have an increased risk of developing in later life a form of vaginal or cervical cancer that is ordinarily extremely rare.[5,6] This risk has been estimated as not greater than 4 per 1000 exposures.[7] Furthermore, a high percentage of such exposed women (from 30 to 90 percent) have been found to have vaginal adenosis,[8-12] epithelial changes of the vagina and cervix. Although these changes are histologically benign, it is not known whether they are precursors of malignancy. Although similar data are not available with the use of other estrogens, it cannot be presumed they would not induce similar changes.

Several reports suggest an association between intrauterine exposure to female sex hormones and congenital anomalies, including congenital heart defects and limb reduction defects.[13-16] One case control study[16] estimated a 4.7-fold increased risk of limb reduction defects in infants exposed in utero to sex hormones (oral contraceptives, hormone withdrawal tests for pregnancy, or attempted treatment for threatened abortion). Some of these exposures were very short and involved only a few days of treatment. The data suggest that the risk of limb reduction defects in exposed fetuses is somewhat less than 1 per 1000.

In the past, female sex hormones have been used during pregnancy in an attempt to treat threatened or habitual abortion. There is considerable evidence that estrogens are ineffective for these indications, and there is no evidence from well controlled studies that progestogens are effective for these uses.

If PREMARIN is used during pregnancy, or if the patient becomes pregnant while taking this drug, she should be apprised of the potential risks to the fetus, and the advisability of pregnancy continuation.

Description: PREMARIN (Conjugated Estrogens Tablets, U.S.P.) for oral administration contains a mixture of estrogens, obtained exclusively from natural sources, occurring as the sodium salts of water-soluble estrogen sulfates blended to represent the average composition of material derived from pregnant mares' urine. It contains estrone, equilin, and 17 α-dihydroequilin, together with smaller amounts of 17 α-estradiol, equilenin, and 17 α-dihydroequilenin as salts of their sulfate esters.

Clinical Pharmacology: Estrogens are important in the development and maintenance of the female reproductive system and secondary sex characteristics. They promote growth and development of the vagina, uterus, and fallopian tubes, and enlargement of the breasts. Indirectly, they contribute to the shaping of the skeleton, maintenance of tone and elasticity of urogenital structures, changes in the epiphyses of the long bones that allow for the pubertal growth spurt and its termination, growth of axillary and pubic hair, and pigmentation of the nipples and genitals. Decline of estrogenic activity at the end of the menstrual cycle can bring on menstruation, although the cessation of progesterone secretion is the most important factor in the mature ovulatory cycle. However, in the preovulatory or nonovulatory cycle, estrogen is the primary determinant in the onset of menstruation. Estrogens also affect the release of pituitary gonadotropins.

The pharmacologic effects of conjugated estrogens are similar to those of endogenous estrogens. They are soluble in water and are well absorbed from the gastrointestinal tract.

In responsive tissues (female genital organs, breasts, hypothalamus, pituitary) estrogens enter the cell and are transported into the nucleus. As a result of estrogen action, specific RNA and protein synthesis occurs.

Metabolism and inactivation occur primarily in the liver. Some estrogens are excreted into the bile; however they are reabsorbed from the intestine and returned to the liver through the portal venous system. Water soluble estrogen conjugates are strongly acidic and are ionized in body fluids, which favor excretion through the kidneys since tubular reabsorption is minimal.

Indications: Based on a review of PREMARIN Tablets by the National Academy of Sciences—National Research Council and/or other information, FDA has classified the indications for use as follows:

Effective: 1. Moderate to severe *vasomotor* symptoms associated with the menopause. (There is no evidence that estrogens are effective for nervous symptoms or depression without associated vasomotor symptoms, and they should not be used to treat such conditions.)
2. Atrophic vaginitis.
3. Kraurosis vulvae.
4. Female hypogonadism.
5. Female castration.
6. Primary ovarian failure.
7. Breast cancer (for palliation only) in appropriately selected women and men with metastatic disease.
8. Prostatic carcinoma—palliative therapy of advanced disease.
9. Postpartum breast engorgement—Although estrogens have been widely used for the prevention of postpartum breast engorgement, controlled studies have demonstrated that the incidence of significant painful engorgement in patients not receiving such hormonal therapy is low and usually responsive to appropriate analgesic or other supportive therapy. Consequently, the benefit to be derived from estrogen therapy for this indication must be carefully weighed against the potential increased risk of puerperal thromboembolism associated with the use of large doses of estrogens.[20]

PREMARIN (Conjugated Estrogens Tablets, U.S.P.) HAS NOT BEEN SHOWN TO BE EFFECTIVE FOR ANY PURPOSE DURING PREGNANCY AND ITS USE MAY CAUSE SEVERE HARM TO THE FETUS (SEE BOXED WARNING).

"Probably" effective: For estrogen deficiency-induced osteoporosis, and only when used in conjunction with other important therapeutic measures such as diet, calcium, physiotherapy, and good general health-promoting measures. Final classification of this indication requires further investigation.

Contraindications: Estrogens should not be used in women (or men) with any of the following conditions:
1. Known or suspected cancer of the breast except in appropriately selected patients being treated for metastatic disease.
2. Known or suspected estrogen-dependent neoplasia.
3. Known or suspected pregnancy (See Boxed Warning).

4. Undiagnosed abnormal genital bleeding.
5. Active thrombophlebitis or thromboembolic disorders.
6. A past history of thrombophlebitis, thrombosis, or thromboembolic disorders associated with previous estrogen use (except when used in treatment of breast or prostatic malignancy).

Warnings:
1. *Induction of malignant neoplasms.* Long term continuous administration of natural and synthetic estrogens in certain animal species increases the frequency of carcinomas of the breast, cervix, vagina, and liver. There are now reports that estrogens increase the risk of carcinoma of the endometrium in humans. (See Boxed Warning.)

At the present time there is no satisfactory evidence that estrogens given to postmenopausal women increase the risk of cancer of the breast,[17] although a recent long-term followup of a single physician's practice has raised this possibility.[18] Because of the animal data, there is a need for caution in prescribing estrogens for women with a strong family history of breast cancer or who have breast nodules, fibrocystic disease, or abnormal mammograms.

2. *Gallbladder disease.* A recent study has reported a 2 to 3-fold increase in the risk of surgically confirmed gallbladder disease in women receiving postmenopausal estrogens,[17] similar to the 2-fold increase previously noted in users of oral contraceptives.[19,24a]

3. *Effects similar to those caused by estrogen-progestogen oral contraceptives.* There are several serious adverse effects of oral contraceptives, most of which have not, up to now, been documented as consequences of postmenopausal estrogen therapy. This may reflect the comparatively low doses of estrogen used in postmenopausal women. It would be expected that the larger doses of estrogen used to treat prostatic or breast cancer or postpartum breast engorgement are more likely to result in these adverse effects, and, in fact, it has been shown that there is an increased risk of thrombosis in men receiving estrogens for prostatic cancer and women for postpartum breast engorgement.[20-23]

a. *Thromboembolic disease.* It is now well established that users of oral contraceptives have an increased risk of various thromboembolic and thrombotic vascular diseases, such as thrombophlebitis, pulmonary embolism, stroke, and myocardial infarction.[24-31] Cases of retinal thrombosis, mesenteric thrombosis, and optic neuritis have been reported in oral contraceptive users. There is evidence that the risk of several of these adverse reactions is related to the dose of the drug.[32,33] An increased risk of postsurgery thromboembolic complications has also been reported in users of oral contraceptives.[34,35] If feasible, estrogen should be discontinued at least 4 weeks before surgery of the type associated with an increased risk of thromboembolism, or during periods of prolonged immobilization.

While an increased rate of thromboembolic and thrombotic disease in postmenopausal users of estrogens has not been found,[17-24,25-36] this does not rule out the possibility that such an increase may be present or that subgroups of women who have underlying risk factors or who are receiving relatively large doses of estrogens may have increased risk. Therefore estrogens should not be used in persons with active thrombophlebitis or thromboembolic disorders, and they should not be used (except in treatment of malignancy) in persons with a history of such disorders in association with estrogen use. They should be used with caution in patients with cerebral vascular or coronary artery disease and only for those in whom estrogens are clearly needed.

Large doses of estrogen (5 mg conjugated estrogens per day), comparable to those used to treat cancer of the prostate and breast, have been shown in a large prospective clinical trial in men[37] to increase the risk of nonfatal myocardial infarction, pulmonary embolism and thrombophlebitis. When estrogen doses of this size are used, any of the thromboembolic and thrombotic adverse effects associated with oral contraceptive use should be considered a clear risk.

b. *Hepatic adenoma.* Benign hepatic adenomas appear to be associated with the use of oral contraceptives.[38-40] Although benign, and rare, these may rupture and may cause death through intra-abdominal hemorrhage. Such lesions have not yet been reported in association with other estrogen or progestogen preparations but should be considered in estrogen users having abdominal pain and tenderness, abdominal mass, or hypovolemic shock. Hepatocellular carcinoma has also been reported in women taking estrogen-containing oral contraceptives.[39] The relationship of this malignancy to these drugs is not known at this time.

c. *Elevated blood pressure.* Women using oral contraceptives sometimes experience increased blood pressure which, in most cases, returns to normal on discontinuing the drug. There is now a report that this may occur with use of estrogens in the menopause[41] and blood pressure should be monitored with estrogen use, especially if high doses are used.

d. *Glucose tolerance.* A worsening of glucose tolerance has been observed in a significant percentage of patients on estrogen-containing oral contraceptives. For this reason, diabetic patients should be carefully observed while receiving estrogen.

4. *Hypercalcemia.* Administration of estrogens may lead to severe hypercalcemia in patients with breast cancer and bone metastases. If this occurs, the drug should be stopped and appropriate measures taken to reduce the serum calcium level.

Precautions:
A. General Precautions.
1. A complete medical and family history should be taken prior to the initiation of any estrogen therapy. The pretreatment and periodic physical examinations should include special reference to blood pressure, breasts, abdomen, and pelvic organs, and should include a Papanicolau smear. As a general rule, estrogen should not be prescribed for longer than one year without another physical examination being performed.
2. Fluid retention—Because estrogens may cause some degree of fluid retention, conditions which might be influenced by this factor such as asthma, epilepsy, migraine, and cardiac or renal dysfunction, require careful observation.
3. Certain patients may develop undesirable manifestations of excessive estrogenic stimulation, such as abnormal or excessive uterine bleeding, mastodynia, etc.
4. Prolonged administration of unopposed estrogen therapy has been reported to increase the risk of endometrial hyperplasia in some patients.
5. Oral contraceptives appear to be associated with an increased incidence of mental depression.[24a] Although it is not clear whether this is due to the estrogenic or progestogenic component of the contraceptive, patients with a history of depression should be carefully observed.
6. Preexisting uterine leiomyomata may increase in size during estrogen use.
7. The pathologist should be advised of estrogen therapy when relevant specimens are submitted.
8. Patients with a past history of jaundice during pregnancy have an increased risk of recurrence of jaundice while receiving estrogen-containing oral contraceptive therapy. If jaundice develops in any patient receiving estrogen, the medication should be discontinued while the cause is investigated.
9. Estrogens may be poorly metabolized in patients with impaired liver function and they should be administered with caution in such patients.
10. Because estrogens influence the metabolism of calcium and phosphorus, they should be used with caution in patients with metabolic bone diseases that are associated with hypercalcemia or in patients with renal insufficiency.
11. Because of the effects of estrogens on epiphyseal closure, they should be used judiciously in young patients in whom bone growth is not complete.
12. Certain endocrine and liver function tests may be affected by estrogen-containing oral contraceptives. The following similar changes may be expected with larger doses of estrogen:
a. Increased sulfobromophthalein retention.
b. Increased prothrombin and factors VII, VIII, IX, and X; decreased antithrombin 3; increased norepinephrine-induced platelet aggregability.
c. Increased thyroid binding globulin (TBG) leading to increased circulating total thyroid hormone, as measured by PBI, T4 by column, or T4 by radioimmunoassay. Free T3 resin uptake is decreased, reflecting the elevated TBG; free T4 concentration is unaltered.
d. Impaired glucose tolerance.
e. Decreased pregnanediol excretion.
f. Reduced response to metyrapone test.
g. Reduced serum folate concentration.
h. Increased serum triglyceride and phospholipid concentration.

B. **Information for the Patient.** See text which appears after the PHYSICIAN REFERENCES.
C. **Pregnancy Category X.** See CONTRAINDICATIONS and Boxed Warning.
D. **Nursing Mothers.** As a general principle, the administration of any drug to nursing mothers should be done only when clearly necessary since many drugs are excreted in human milk.

Adverse Reactions: (See Warnings regarding induction of neoplasia, adverse effects on the fetus, increased incidence of gallbladder disease, and adverse effects similar to those of oral contraceptives, including thromboembolism.) The following additional adverse reactions have been reported with estrogenic therapy, including oral contraceptives:
1. *Genitourinary system:* Breakthrough bleeding, spotting, change in menstrual flow; dysmenorrhea; premenstrual-like syndrome; amenorrhea during and after treatment; increase in size of uterine fibromyomata; vaginal candidiasis; change in cervical erosion and in degree of cervical secretion; cystitis-like syndrome.
2. *Breasts:* Tenderness, enlargement, secretion.
3. *Gastrointestinal:* Nausea, vomiting; abdominal cramps, bloating; cholestatic jaundice.
4. *Skin:* Chloasma or melasma which may persist when drug is discontinued; erythema multiforme; erythema nodosum; hemorrhagic eruption; loss of scalp hair; hirsutism.
5. *Eyes:* Steepening of corneal curvature; intolerance to contact lenses.
6. *CNS:* Headache, migraine, dizziness; mental depression; chorea.
7. *Miscellaneous:* Increase or decrease in weight; reduced carbohydrate tolerance; aggravation of porphyria; edema; changes in libido.

Acute Overdosage: Numerous reports of ingestion of large doses of estrogen-containing oral contraceptives by young children indicate that acute serious ill effects do not occur. Overdosage of estrogen may cause nausea, and withdrawal bleeding may occur in females.

Dosage and Administration:
1. *Given cyclically for short term use only:*
For treatment of moderate to severe *vasomotor* symptoms, atrophic vaginitis, or kraurosis vulvae associated with the menopause.
The lowest dose that will control symptoms should be chosen and medication should be discontinued as promptly as possible.
Administration should be cyclic (e.g., three weeks on and one week off).
Attempts to discontinue or taper medication should be made at three to six month intervals.
Usual dosage ranges:
Vasomotor symptoms—1.25 mg daily. If the patient has not menstruated within the last two months or more, cyclic administration is started arbitrarily. If the patient is menstruating, cyclic administration is started on day 5 of bleeding.
Atrophic vaginitis and kraurosis vulvae—0.3 mg to 1.25 mg or more daily, depending upon the tissue response of the individual patient. Administer cyclically.

Continued on next page

Ayerst—Cont.

2. *Given cyclically:* Female hypogonadism; female castration; primary ovarian failure; osteoporosis.
Usual dosage ranges:
Female hypogonadism—2.5 to 7.5 mg daily, in divided doses for 20 days, followed by a rest period of 10 days' duration. If bleeding does not occur by the end of this period, the same dosage schedule is repeated. The number of courses of estrogen therapy necessary to produce bleeding may vary depending on the responsiveness of the endometrium.
If bleeding occurs before the end of the 10 day period, begin a 20 day estrogen-progestin cyclic regimen with PREMARIN (Conjugated Estrogens Tablets, U.S.P.), 2.5 to 7.5 mg daily in divided doses, for 20 days. During the last five days of estrogen therapy, give an oral progestin. If bleeding occurs before this regimen is concluded, therapy is discontinued and may be resumed on the fifth day of bleeding.
Female castration and primary ovarian failure—1.25 mg daily, cyclically. Adjust dosage upward or downward according to severity of symptoms and response of the patient. For maintenance, adjust dosage to lowest level that will provide effective control.
Osteoporosis (to retard progression)—1.25 mg daily, cyclically.
3. *Given for a few days:* Prevention of postpartum breast engorgement—3.75 mg every four hours for five doses, or 1.25 mg every four hours for five days.
4. *Given chronically:* Inoperable progressing prostatic cancer—1.25 to 2.5 mg three times daily. The effectiveness of therapy can be judged by phosphatase determinations as well as by symptomatic improvement of the patient.
Inoperable progressing breast cancer in appropriately selected men and postmenopausal women. (See INDICATIONS)—Suggested dosage is 10 mg three times daily for a period of at least three months.
Treated patients with an intact uterus should be monitored closely for signs of endometrial cancer and appropriate diagnostic measures should be taken to rule out malignancy in the event of persistent or recurring abnormal vaginal bleeding.
How Supplied: PREMARIN (Conjugated Estrogens Tablets, U.S.P.)
—Each oval *purple* tablet contains 2.5 mg, in bottles of 100 (NDC 0046-0865-81) and 1,000 (NDC 0046-0865-91).
—Each oval *yellow* tablet contains 1.25 mg, in bottles of 100 (NDC 0046-0866-81) and 1,000 (NDC 0046-0866-91); and unit dose package of 100 (NDC 0046-0866-99). Also in Cycle Pack of 21 (NDC 0046-0866-21).
—Each oval *white* tablet contains 0.9 mg, in bottles of 100 (NDC 0046-0864-81). Also in Cycle Pack of 21 (NDC 0046-0864-21).
—Each oval *maroon* tablet contains 0.625 mg, in bottles of 100 (NDC 0046-0867-81), 1,000 (NDC 0046-0867-91); and unit dose package of 100 (NDC 0046-0867-99). Also in Cycle Pack of 21 (NDC 0046-0867-21).
—Each oval *green* tablet contains 0.3 mg, in bottles of 100 (NDC 0046-0868-81) and 1,000 (NDC 0046-0868-91).
The appearance of these tablets is a trademark of Ayerst Laboratories.
Physician References:
1. Ziel, H. K., *et al:* N. Engl. J. Med. 293:1167-1170, 1975.
2. Smith, D. C., *et al:* N. Engl. J. Med. 293:1164-1167, 1975.
3. Mack, T. M., *et al:* N. Engl. J. Med. 294:1262-1267, 1976.
4. Weiss, N. S., *et al:* N. Engl. J. Med. 294:1259-1262, 1976.
5. Herbst, A. L., *et al:* N. Engl. J. Med. 284:878-881, 1971.
6. Greenwald, P., *et al:* N. Engl. J. Med. 285:390-392, 1971.
7. Lanier, A., *et al:* Mayo Clin. Proc. 48:793-799, 1973.
8. Herbst, A., *et al:* Obstet. Gynecol. 40:287-298, 1972.
9. Herbst, A., *et al:* Am. J. Obstet. Gynecol. 118:607-615, 1974.
10. Herbst, A., *et al:* N. Engl. J. Med. 292:334-339, 1975.
11. Stafl, A., *et al:* Obstet. Gynecol. 43:118-128, 1974.
12. Sherman, A. I., *et al:* Obstet. Gynecol. 44:531-545, 1974.
13. Gal, I., *et al:* Nature 216:83, 1967.
14. Levy, E. P., *et al:* Lancet 1:611, 1973.
15. Nora, J., *et al:* Lancet 1:941-942, 1973.
16. Janerich, D. T., *et al:* N. Engl. J. Med. 291:697-700, 1974.
17. Boston Collaborative Drug Surveillance Program: N. Engl. J. Med. 290:15-19, 1974.
18. Hoover, R., *et al:* N. Engl. J. Med. 295:401-405, 1976.
19. Boston Collaborative Drug Surveillance Program: Lancet 1:1399-1404, 1973.
20. Daniel, D. G., *et al:* Lancet 2:287-289, 1967.
21. The Veterans Administration Cooperative Urological Research Group: J. Urol. 98:516-522, 1967.
22. Bailar, J. C.: Lancet 2:560, 1967.
23. Blackard, C., *et al:* Cancer 26:249-256, 1970.
24. Royal College of General Practitioners: J. R. Coll. Gen. Pract. 13:267-279, 1967.
24a. Royal College of General Practitioners: Oral Contraceptives and Health, New York, Pitman Corp., 1974.
25. Inman, W. H. W., *et al:* Br. Med. J. 2:193-199, 1968.
26. Vessey, M. P., *et al:* Br. Med. J. 2:651-657, 1969.
27. Sartwell, P. E., *et al:* Am. J. Epidemiol. 90:365-380, 1969.
28. Collaborative Group for the Study of Stroke in Young Women: N. Engl. J. Med. 288:871-878, 1973.
29. Collaborative Group for the Study of Stroke in Young Women: J.A.M.A. 231:718-722, 1975.
30. Mann, J. I., *et al:* Br. Med. J. 2:245-248, 1975.
31. Mann, J. I., *et al:* Br. Med. J. 2:241-245, 1975.
32. Inman, W. H. W., *et al:* Br. Med. J. 2:203-209, 1970.
33. Stolley, P. D., *et al:* Am. J. Epidemiol. 102:197-208, 1975.
34. Vessey, M. P., *et al:* Br. Med. J. 3:123-126, 1970.
35. Greene, G. R., *et al:* Am. J. Public Health 62:680-685, 1972.
36. Rosenberg, L., *et al:* N. Engl. J. Med. 294:1256-1259, 1976.
37. Coronary Drug Project Research Group: J.A.M.A. 214:1303-1313, 1970.
38. Baum, J., *et al:* Lancet 2: 926-928, 1973.
39. Mays, E. T., *et al:* J.A.M.A. 235:730-732, 1976.
40. Edmondson, H. A., *et al:* N. Engl. J. Med. 294:470-472, 1976.
41. Pfeffer, R. I., *et al:* Am. J. Epidemiol. 103:445-456, 1976.

INFORMATION FOR THE PATIENT

What You Should Know about Estrogens: Estrogens are female hormones produced by the ovaries. The ovaries make several different kinds of estrogens. In addition, scientists have been able to make a variety of synthetic estrogens. As far as we know, all these estrogens have similar properties and therefore much the same usefulness, side effects, and risks. This leaflet is intended to help you understand what estrogens are used for, the risks involved in their use, and how to use them as safely as possible.
This leaflet includes the most important information about estrogens, but not all the information. If you want to know more, you should ask your doctor for more information or you can ask your doctor or pharmacist to let you read the package insert prepared for the doctor.
Uses of Estrogen: THERE IS NO PROPER USE OF ESTROGENS IN A PREGNANT WOMAN.
Estrogens are prescribed by doctors for a number of purposes, including:
1. To provide estrogen during a period of adjustment when a woman's ovaries stop producing a majority of her estrogens, in order to prevent certain uncomfortable symptoms of estrogen deficiency. (With the menopause, which generally occurs between the ages of 45 and 55, women produce a much smaller amount of estrogens.)
2. To prevent symptoms of estrogen deficiency when a woman's ovaries have been removed surgically before the natural menopause.
3. To prevent pregnancy. (Estrogens are given along with a progestogen, another female hormone; these combinations are called oral contraceptives or birth control pills. Patient labeling is available to women taking oral contraceptives and they will not be discussed in this leaflet.)
4. To treat certain cancers in women and men.
5. To prevent painful swelling of the breasts after pregnancy in women who choose not to nurse their babies.
Estrogens in the Menopause: In the natural course of their lives, all women eventually experience a decrease in estrogen production. This usually occurs between ages 45 and 55 but may occur earlier or later. Sometimes the ovaries may need to be removed before natural menopause by an operation, producing a "surgical menopause."
When the amount of estrogen in the blood begins to decrease, many women may develop typical symptoms: feelings of warmth in the face, neck, and chest or sudden intense episodes of heat and sweating throughout the body (called "hot flashes" or "hot flushes"). These symptoms are sometimes very uncomfortable. Some women may also develop changes in the vagina (called "atrophic vaginitis") which cause discomfort, especially during and after intercourse.
Estrogens can be prescribed to treat these symptoms of the menopause. It is estimated that considerably more than half of all women undergoing the menopause have only mild symptoms or no symptoms at all and therefore do not need estrogens. Other women may need estrogens for a few months, while their bodies adjust to lower estrogen levels. Sometimes the need will be for periods longer than six months. In an attempt to avoid overstimulation of the uterus (womb), estrogens are usually given cyclically during each month of use, such as three weeks of pills followed by one week without pills.
Sometimes women experience nervous symptoms or depression during menopause. There is no evidence that estrogens are effective for such symptoms without associated vasomotor symptoms. In the absence of vasomotor symptoms, estrogens should not be used to treat nervous symptoms, although other treatment may be needed.
You may have heard that taking estrogens for long periods (years) after the menopause will keep your skin soft and supple and keep you feeling young. There is no evidence that this is so, however, and such long-term treatment carries important risks.
Estrogens to Prevent Swelling of the Breasts after Pregnancy: If you do not breast-feed your baby after delivery, your breasts may fill up with milk and become painful and engorged. This usually begins about 3 to 4 days after delivery and may last for a few days to up to a week or more. Sometimes the discomfort is severe, but usually it is not and can be controlled by pain-relieving drugs such as aspirin and by binding the breasts up tightly. Estrogens can be used to try to prevent the breasts from filling up. While this treatment is sometimes successful, in many cases the breasts fill up to some degree in spite of treatment. The dose of estrogens needed to prevent pain and swelling of the breasts is much larger than the dose needed to treat symptoms of the menopause and this may increase your chances of developing blood clots in the legs or lungs (see below). Therefore, it is important that you discuss the benefits and the risks of estrogen use with your doctor if you have decided not to breast-feed your baby.
The Dangers of Estrogens:
1. *Endometrial cancer.* There are reports that if

estrogens are used in the postmenopausal period for more than a year, there is an increased risk of *endometrial cancer* (cancer of the lining of the uterus). Women taking estrogens have roughly 5 to 10 times as great a chance of getting this cancer as women who take no estrogens. To put this another way, while a postmenopausal woman not taking estrogens has 1 chance in 1,000 each year of getting endometrial cancer, a woman taking estrogens has 5 to 10 chances in 1,000 each year. For this reason *it is important to take estrogens only when they are really needed.*

The risk of this cancer is greater the longer estrogens are used and when larger doses are taken. Therefore you should not take more estrogen than your doctor prescribes. *It is important to take the lowest dose of estrogen that will control symptoms and to take it only as long as it is needed.* If estrogens are needed for longer periods of time, your doctor will want to reevaluate your need for estrogens at least every six months.

Women using estrogens should report any vaginal bleeding to their doctors; such bleeding may be of no importance, but it can be an early warning of endometrial cancer. If you have undiagnosed vaginal bleeding, you should not use estrogens until a diagnosis is made and you are certain there is no endometrial cancer.

NOTE: If you have had your uterus removed (total hysterectomy), there is no danger of developing endometrial cancer.

2. *Other possible cancers.* Estrogens can cause development of other tumors in animals, such as tumors of the breast, cervix, vagina, or liver, when given for a long time. At present there is no good evidence that women using estrogen in the menopause have an increased risk of such tumors, but there is no way yet to be sure they do not; and one study raises the possibility that use of estrogens in the menopause may increase the risk of breast cancer many years later. This is a further reason to use estrogens only when clearly needed. While you are taking estrogens, it is important that you go to your doctor at least once a year for a physical examination. Also, if members of your family have had breast cancer or if you have breast nodules or abnormal mammograms (breast x-rays), your doctor may wish to carry out more frequent examinations of your breasts.

3. *Gallbladder disease.* Women who use estrogens after menopause are more likely to develop gallbladder disease needing surgery than women who do not use estrogens. Birth control pills have a similar effect.

4. *Abnormal blood clotting.* Oral contraceptives increase the risk of blood clotting in various parts of the body. This can result in a stroke (if the clot is in the brain), a heart attack (clot in a blood vessel of the heart), or a pulmonary embolus (a clot which forms in the legs or pelvis, then breaks off and travels to the lungs). Any of these can be fatal. At this time use of estrogens in the menopause is not known to cause such blood clotting, but this has not been fully studied and there could still prove to be such a risk. It is recommended that if you have had clotting in the legs or lungs or a heart attack or stroke while you were using estrogens or birth control pills, you should not use estrogens (unless they are being used to treat cancer of the breast or prostate). If you have had a stroke or heart attack or if you have angina pectoris, estrogens should be used with great caution and only if clearly needed (for example, if you have severe symptoms of the menopause).

The larger doses of estrogen used to prevent swelling of the breasts after pregnancy have been reported to cause clotting in the legs and lungs.

Special Warning about Pregnancy: You should not receive estrogen if you are pregnant. If this should occur, there is a greater than usual chance that the developing child will be born with a birth defect, although the possibility remains fairly small. A female child may have an increased risk of developing cancer of the vagina or cervix later in life (in the teens or twenties). Every possible effort should be made to avoid exposure to estrogens during pregnancy. If exposure occurs, see your doctor.

Other Effects of Estrogens: In addition to the serious known risks of estrogens described above, estrogens have the following side effects and potential risks:

1. *Nausea and vomiting.* The most common side effect of estrogen therapy is nausea. Vomiting is less common.
2. *Effects on breasts.* Estrogens may cause breast tenderness or enlargement and may cause the breasts to secrete a liquid. These effects are not dangerous.
3. *Effects on the uterus.* Estrogens may cause benign fibroid tumors of the uterus to get larger.
4. *Effects on liver.* Women taking oral contraceptives develop on rare occasions a tumor of the liver which can rupture and bleed into the abdomen and may cause death. So far, these tumors have not been reported in women using estrogens in the menopause, but you should report any swelling or unusual pain or tenderness in the abdomen to your doctor immediately.

Women with a past history of jaundice (yellowing of the skin and white parts of the eyes) may get jaundice again during estrogen use. If this occurs, stop taking estrogens and see your doctor.

5. *Other effects.* Estrogens may cause excess fluid to be retained in the body. This may make some conditions worse, such as asthma, epilepsy, migraine, heart disease, or kidney disease.

Summary: Estrogens have important uses, but they have serious risks as well. You must decide, with your doctor, whether the risks are acceptable to you in view of the benefits of treatment. Except where your doctor has prescribed estrogens for use in special cases of cancer of the breast or prostate, you should not use estrogens if you have cancer of the breast or uterus, are pregnant, have undiagnosed abnormal vaginal bleeding, clotting in the legs or lungs, or have had a stroke, heart attack or angina, or clotting in the legs or lungs in the past while you were taking estrogens.

You can use estrogens as safely as possible by understanding that your doctor will require regular physical examinations while you are taking them and will try to discontinue the drug as soon as possible and use the smallest dose possible. Be alert for signs of trouble including:

1. Abnormal bleeding from the vagina.
2. Pains in the calves or chest or sudden shortness of breath, or coughing blood.
3. Severe headache, dizziness, faintness, or changes in vision.
4. Breast lumps (you should ask your doctor how to examine your own breasts).
5. Jaundice (yellowing of the skin).
6. Mental depression.

Your doctor has prescribed this drug for you and you alone. Do not give the drug to anyone else.

How Supplied:
PREMARIN® (Conjugated Estrogens Tablets, U.S.P.)—tablets for oral administration.
Each oval *purple* tablet contains 2.5 mg
Each oval *yellow* tablet contains 1.25 mg
Each oval *white* tablet contains 0.9 mg
Each oval *maroon* tablet contains 0.625 mg
Each oval *green* tablet contains 0.3 mg
PREMARIN® with METHYLTESTOSTERONE—a combination of PREMARIN and methyltestosterone (an androgen) in tablet form for oral administration.
Each round *yellow* tablet contains 1.25 mg PREMARIN and 10 mg methyltestosterone
Each round *maroon* tablet contains 0.625 mg PREMARIN and 5 mg methyltestosterone
PMB® 200, 400—a combination of PREMARIN® and meprobamate (a tranquilizing agent) in tablet form for oral administration.
Each oblong *green* tablet contains 0.45 mg PREMARIN and 200 mg meprobamate
Each oblong *pink* tablet contains 0.45 mg PREMARIN and 400 mg meprobamate
The appearance of these tablets is a trademark of Ayerst Laboratories.
PREMARIN® VAGINAL CREAM—PREMARIN® in a nonliquefying base, designed for vaginal use.
PREMARIN® INTRAVENOUS—PREMARIN® specially prepared for intravenous and intramuscular use.
ESTROGENIC SUBSTANCE (Estrone) in Aqueous Suspension—a sterile aqueous suspension of estrone, a short-acting estrogen, for intramuscular injection only.
Shown in Product Identification Section, page 405

PREMARIN® INTRAVENOUS ℞
[prĕm'a-rĭn]
Brand of Conjugated Estrogens, U.S.P.,
for Injection
Specially prepared for Intravenous &
Intramuscular use

CAUTION: Federal law prohibits dispensing without prescription.

1. ESTROGENS HAVE BEEN REPORTED TO INCREASE THE RISK OF ENDOMETRIAL CARCINOMA.
Three independent case control studies have reported an increased risk of endometrial cancer in postmenopausal women exposed to exogenous estrogens for more than one year.[1-3] This risk was independent of the other known risk factors for endometrial cancer. These studies are further supported by the finding that incidence rates of endometrial cancer have increased sharply since 1969 in eight different areas of the United States with population-based cancer reporting systems, an increase which may be related to the rapidly expanding use of estrogens during the last decade.[4]

The three case control studies reported that the risk of endometrial cancer in estrogen users was about 4.5 to 13.9 times greater than in nonusers. The risk appears to depend on both duration of treatment[1] and on estrogen dose.[3] In view of these findings, when estrogens are used for the treatment of menopausal symptoms, the lowest dose that will control symptoms should be utilized and medication should be discontinued as soon as possible. When prolonged treatment is medically indicated, the patient should be reassessed on at least a semiannual basis to determine the need for continued therapy. Although the evidence must be considered preliminary, one study suggests that cyclic administration of low doses of estrogen may carry less risk than continuous administration;[3] it therefore appears prudent to utilize such a regimen.

Close clinical surveillance of all women taking estrogens is important. In all cases of undiagnosed persistent or recurring abnormal vaginal bleeding, adequate diagnostic measures should be undertaken to rule out malignancy.

There is no evidence at present that "natural" estrogens are more or less hazardous than "synthetic" estrogens at equiestrogenic doses.

2. ESTROGENS SHOULD NOT BE USED DURING PREGNANCY.
The use of female sex hormones, both estrogens and progestogens, during early pregnancy may seriously damage the offspring. It has been shown that females exposed in utero to diethylstilbestrol, a non-steroidal estrogen, have an increased risk of developing in later life a form of vaginal or cervical cancer that is ordinarily extremely rare.[5,6] This risk has been estimated as not greater than 4 per 1000 exposures.[7] Furthermore, a high percentage of such exposed women (from 30 to 90 percent) have been found to have vaginal adenosis,[8-12] epithelial changes of the vagina and cervix. Although these changes are histologically benign, it is not known whether they are precursors of malignancy. Although similar data are not available with the use of other estrogens, it cannot be presumed they would not induce similar changes.

Continued on next page

Ayerst—Cont.

Several reports suggest an association between intrauterine exposure to female sex hormones and congenital anomalies, including congenital heart defects and limb reduction defects.[13-16] One case control study[16] estimated a 4.7-fold increased risk of limb reduction defects in infants exposed in utero to sex hormones (oral contraceptives, hormone withdrawal tests for pregnancy, or attempted treatment for threatened abortion). Some of these exposures were very short and involved only a few days of treatment. The data suggest that the risk of limb reduction defects in exposed fetuses is somewhat less than 1 per 1000.

In the past, female sex hormones have been used during pregnancy in an attempt to treat threatened or habitual abortion. There is considerable evidence that estrogens are ineffective for these indications, and there is no evidence from well controlled studies that progestogens are effective for these uses.

If PREMARIN Intravenous (Conjugated Estrogens, U.S.P., for Injection) is used during pregnancy, or if the patient becomes pregnant while taking this drug, she should be apprised of the potential risks to the fetus, and the advisability of pregnancy continuation.

Description: Each Secule® contains 25 mg of Conjugated Estrogens, U.S.P. in a sterile lyophilized cake which also contains lactose 200 mg, sodium citrate 12.5 mg and simethicone 0.2 mg. The pH is adjusted with sodium hydroxide or hydrochloric acid. A sterile diluent (5 ml) containing 2% benzyl alcohol and Water for Injection, U.S.P. is provided for reconstitution. The reconstituted solution is suitable for intravenous or intramuscular injection.

PREMARIN (Conjugated Estrogens, U.S.P.) is a mixture of estrogens obtained exclusively from natural sources, occurring as the sodium salts of water-soluble estrogen sulfates blended to represent the average composition of material derived from pregnant mares' urine. It contains estrone, equilin, and 17 α-dihydroequilin, together with smaller amounts of 17 α-estradiol, equilenin, and 17 α-dihydroequilenin as salts of their sulfate esters.

Clinical Pharmacology: Estrogens are important in the development and maintenance of the female reproductive system and secondary sex characteristics. They promote growth and development of the vagina, uterus, and fallopian tubes, and enlargement of the breasts. Indirectly, they contribute to the shaping of the skeleton, maintenance of tone and elasticity of urogenital structures, changes in the epiphyses of the long bones that allow for the pubertal growth spurt and its termination, growth of axillary and pubic hair, and pigmentation of the nipples and genitals. Decline of estrogenic activity at the end of the menstrual cycle can bring on menstruation, although the cessation of progesterone secretion is the most important factor in the mature ovulatory cycle. However, in the preovulatory or nonovulatory cycle, estrogen is the primary determinant in the onset of menstruation. Estrogens also affect the release of pituitary gonadotropins.

The pharmacologic effects of conjugated estrogens are similar to those of endogenous estrogens. They are soluble in water and may be administered by intravenous or intramuscular injection.

In responsive tissues (female genital organs, breasts, hypothalamus, pituitary) estrogens enter the cell and are transported into the nucleus. As a result of estrogen action, specific RNA and protein synthesis occurs.

Metabolism and inactivation occur primarily in the liver. Some estrogens are excreted into the bile; however they are reabsorbed from the intestine and returned to the liver through the portal venous system. Water-soluble estrogen conjugates are strongly acidic and are ionized in body fluids, which favor excretion through the kidneys since tubular reabsorption is minimal.

Indication: PREMARIN Intravenous (Conjugated Estrogens, U.S.P., for Injection) is indicated in the treatment of abnormal uterine bleeding due to hormonal imbalance in the absence of organic pathology.

Contraindications: Estrogens should not be used in women with any of the following conditions:
1. Known or suspected cancer of the breast except in appropriately selected patients being treated for metastatic disease.
2. Known or suspected estrogen-dependent neoplasia.
3. Known or suspected pregnancy (See Boxed Warning).
4. Undiagnosed abnormal genital bleeding.
5. Active thrombophlebitis or thromboembolic disorders.
6. A past history of thrombophlebitis, thrombosis, or thromboembolic disorders associated with previous estrogen use (except when used in treatment of breast malignancy).

Warnings:
1. *Induction of malignant neoplasms.* Long term continuous administration of natural and synthetic estrogens in certain animal species increases the frequency of carcinomas of the breast, cervix, vagina, and liver. There are now reports that estrogens increase the risk of carcinoma of the endometrium in humans. (See Boxed Warning.)

At the present time there is no satisfactory evidence that estrogens given to postmenopausal women increase the risk of cancer of the breast,[17] although a recent long-term followup of a single physician's practice has raised this possibility.[18] Because of the animal data, there is a need for caution in prescribing estrogens for women with a strong family history of breast cancer or who have breast nodules, fibrocystic disease, or abnormal mammograms.

2. *Gallbladder disease.* A recent study has reported a 2 to 3-fold increase in the risk of surgically confirmed gallbladder disease in women receiving postmenopausal estrogens,[17] similar to the 2-fold increase previously noted in users of oral contraceptives.[19,24a]

3. *Effects similar to those caused by estrogen-progestogen oral contraceptives.* There are several serious adverse effects of oral contraceptives, most of which have not, up to now, been documented as consequences of postmenopausal estrogen therapy. This may reflect the comparatively low doses of estrogen used in postmenopausal women. It would be expected that the larger doses of estrogen used to treat prostatic or breast cancer or postpartum breast engorgement are more likely to result in these adverse effects, and, in fact, it has been shown that there is an increased risk of thrombosis in men receiving estrogens for prostatic cancer and women for postpartum breast engorgement.[20-23]

a. *Thromboembolic disease.* It is now well established that users of oral contraceptives have an increased risk of various thromboembolic and thrombotic vascular diseases, such as thrombophlebitis, pulmonary embolism, stroke, and myocardial infarction.[24-31] Cases of retinal thrombosis, mesenteric thrombosis, and optic neuritis have been reported in oral contraceptive users. There is evidence that the risk of several of these adverse reactions is related to the dose of the drug.[32,33] An increased risk of postsurgery thromboembolic complications has also been reported in users of oral contraceptives.[34,35] If feasible, estrogen should be discontinued at least 4 weeks before surgery of the type associated with an increased risk of thromboembolism, or during periods of prolonged immobilization.

While an increased rate of thromboembolic and thrombotic disease in postmenopausal users of estrogens has not been found,[17-24, 25-36] this does not rule out the possibility that such an increase may be present or that subgroups of women who have underlying risk factors or who are receiving relatively large doses of estrogens may have increased risk. Therefore estrogens should not be used in persons with active thrombophlebitis or thromboembolic disorders, and they should not be used (except in treatment of malignancy) in persons with a history of such disorders in association with estrogen use. They should be used with caution in patients with cerebral vascular or coronary artery disease and only for those in whom estrogens are clearly needed.

Large doses of estrogen (5 mg conjugated estrogens per day), comparable to those used to treat cancer of the prostate and breast, have been shown in a large prospective clinical trial in men[37] to increase the risk of nonfatal myocardial infarction, pulmonary embolism and thrombophlebitis. When estrogen doses of this size are used, any of the thromboembolic and thrombotic adverse effects associated with oral contraceptive use should be considered a clear risk.

b. *Hepatic adenoma.* Benign hepatic adenomas appear to be associated with the use of oral contraceptives.[38-40] Although benign, and rare, these may rupture and may cause death through intra-abdominal hemorrhage. Such lesions have not yet been reported in association with other estrogen or progestogen preparations but should be considered in estrogen users having abdominal pain and tenderness, abdominal mass, or hypovolemic shock. Hepatocellular carcinoma has also been reported in women taking estrogen-containing oral contraceptives.[39] The relationship of this malignancy to these drugs is not known at this time.

c. *Elevated blood pressure.* Women using oral contraceptives sometimes experience increased blood pressure which, in most cases, returns to normal on discontinuing the drug. There is now a report that this may occur with use of estrogens in the menopause[41] and blood pressure should be monitored with estrogen use, especially if high doses are used.

d. *Glucose tolerance.* A worsening of glucose tolerance has been observed in a significant percentage of patients on estrogen-containing oral contraceptives. For this reason, diabetic patients should be carefully observed while receiving estrogen.

4. *Hypercalcemia.* Administration of estrogens may lead to severe hypercalcemia in patients with breast cancer and bone metastases. If this occurs, the drug should be stopped and appropriate measures taken to reduce the serum calcium level.

Precautions:

A. General Precautions.
1. A complete medical and family history should be taken prior to the initiation of any estrogen therapy. The pretreatment and periodic physical examinations should include special reference to blood pressure, breasts, abdomen, and pelvic organs, and should include a Papanicolau smear. As a general rule, estrogen should not be prescribed for longer than one year without another physical examination being performed.
2. Fluid retention—Because estrogens may cause some degree of fluid retention, conditions which might be influenced by this factor such as asthma, epilepsy, migraine, and cardiac or renal dysfunction, require careful observation.
3. Certain patients may develop undesirable manifestations of excessive estrogenic stimulation, such as abnormal or excessive uterine bleeding, mastodynia, etc.
4. Oral contraceptives appear to be associated with an increased incidence of mental depression.[24a] Although it is not clear whether this is due to the estrogenic or progestogenic component of the contraceptive, patients with a history of depression should be carefully observed.
5. Preexisting uterine leiomyomata may increase in size during estrogen use.
6. The pathologist should be advised of estrogen therapy when relevant specimens are submitted.
7. Patients with a past history of jaundice during pregnancy have an increased risk of recurrence of jaundice while receiving estrogen-containing oral contraceptive therapy. If jaundice develops in any patient receiving estrogen, the medication should be discontinued while the cause is investigated.

8. Estrogens may be poorly metabolized in patients with impaired liver function and they should be administered with caution in such patients.
9. Because estrogens influence the metabolism of calcium and phosphorus, they should be used with caution in patients with metabolic bone diseases that are associated with hypercalcemia or in patients with renal insufficiency.
10. Because of the effects of estrogens on epiphyseal closure, they should be used judiciously in young patients in whom bone growth is not complete.
11. Certain endocrine and liver function tests may be affected by estrogen-containing oral contraceptives. The following similar changes may be expected with larger doses of estrogen:
a. Increased sulfobromophthalein retention.
b. Increased prothrombin and factors VII, VIII, IX, and X; decreased antithrombin 3; increased norepinephrine-induced platelet aggregability.
c. Increased thyroid binding globulin (TBG) leading to increased circulating total thyroid hormone, as measured by PBI, T4 by column, or T4 by radioimmunoassay. Free T3 resin uptake is decreased, reflecting the elevated TBG; free T4 concentration is unaltered.
d. Impaired glucose tolerance.
e. Decreased pregnanediol excretion.
f. Reduced response to metyrapone test.
g. Reduced serum folate concentration.
h. Increased serum triglyceride and phospholipid concentration.
B. **Information for the Patient.** See text which appears after the PHYSICIAN REFERENCES.
C. **Pregnancy Category X.** See CONTRAINDICATIONS and Boxed Warning.
D. **Nursing Mothers.** As a general principle, the administration of any drug to nursing mothers should be done only when clearly necessary since many drugs are excreted in human milk.

Adverse Reactions: (See Warnings regarding induction of neoplasia, adverse effects on the fetus, increased incidence of gallbladder disease, and adverse effects similar to those of oral contraceptives, including thromboembolism.) The following additional adverse reactions have been reported with estrogenic therapy, including oral contraceptives:
1. *Genitourinary system:* Breakthrough bleeding, spotting, change in menstrual flow; dysmenorrhea; premenstrual-like syndrome; amenorrhea during and after treatment; increase in size of uterine fibromyomata; vaginal candidiasis; change in cervical erosion and in degree of cervical secretion; cystitis-like syndrome.
2. *Breasts:* Tenderness, enlargement, secretion.
3. *Gastrointestinal:* Nausea, vomiting; abdominal cramps, bloating; cholestatic jaundice.
4. *Skin:* Chloasma or melasma which may persist when drug is discontinued; erythema multiforme; erythema nodosum; hemorrhagic eruption; loss of scalp hair; hirsutism.
5. *Eyes:* Steepening of corneal curvature; intolerance to contact lenses.
6. *CNS:* Headache, migraine, dizziness; mental depression; chorea.
7. *Miscellaneous:* Increase or decrease in weight; reduced carbohydrate tolerance; aggravation of porphyria; edema; changes in libido.

Acute Overdosage: Numerous reports of ingestion of large doses of estrogen-containing oral contraceptives by young children indicate that acute serious ill effects do not occur. Overdosage of estrogen may cause nausea, and withdrawal bleeding may occur in females.

Dosage and Administration: *Abnormal uterine bleeding due to hormonal imbalance:* One 25 mg injection, intravenously or intramuscularly. Intravenous use is preferred since more rapid response can be expected from this mode of administration.
Repeat in 6 to 12 hours if necessary. The use of PREMARIN Intravenous (Conjugated Estrogens, U.S.P., for Injection) does not preclude the advisability of other appropriate measures.

The usual precautionary measures governing intravenous administration should be adhered to. Injection should be made SLOWLY to obviate the occurrence of flushes.
Infusion of PREMARIN Intravenous (Conjugated Estrogens, U.S.P., for Injection) with other agents is not generally recommended. In emergencies, however, when an infusion has already been started, it may be expedient to make the injection into the tubing just distal to the infusion needle. If so used, compatibility of solutions must be considered.
Compatibility of solutions: PREMARIN Intravenous is compatible with normal saline, dextrose, and invert sugar solutions. IT IS NOT COMPATIBLE WITH PROTEIN HYDROLYSATE, ASCORBIC ACID, OR ANY SOLUTION WITH AN ACID pH.
Treated patients with an intact uterus should be monitored closely for signs of endometrial cancer and appropriate diagnostic measures should be taken to rule out malignancy in the event of persistent or recurring abnormal vaginal bleeding.

Directions for Storage and Reconstitution:
Storage before reconstitution: Store package in refrigerator, 2–8°C (36–46°F).
To reconstitute: First withdraw air from SECULE so as to facilitate introduction of sterile diluent. Then, flow the sterile diluent slowly against side of SECULE and agitate gently. DO NOT SHAKE VIOLENTLY.
Storage after reconstitution: It is common practice to utilize the reconstituted solution within a few hours. If it is necessary to keep the reconstituted solution for more than a few hours, store the reconstituted solution under refrigeration (2–8°C). Under these conditions, the solution is stable for 60 days, and is suitable for use unless darkening or precipitation occurs.
How Supplied: NDC 0046-0552-05-Each package provides: (1) One SECULE® containing 25 mg of Conjugated Estrogens, U.S.P., for Injection (also lactose 200 mg, sodium citrate 12.5 mg, and simethicone 0.2 mg). The pH is adjusted with sodium hydroxide or hydrochloric acid. (2)One 5 ml ampul sterile diluent with benzyl alcohol 2%, and Water for Injection, U.S.P.
PREMARIN Intravenous (Conjugated Estrogens, U.S.P., for Injection) is prepared by cryodesiccation.

Physician References:
1. Ziel, H. K., *et al:* N. Engl. J. Med. 293:1167–1170, 1975.
2. Smith, D. C., *et al:* N. Engl. J. Med. 293:1164–1167, 1975.
3. Mack, T. M., *et al:* N. Engl. J. Med. 294:1262–1267, 1976.
4. Weiss, N. S., *et al:* N. Engl. J. Med. 294:1259–1262, 1976.
5. Herbst, A. L., *et al:* N. Engl. J. Med. 284:878–881, 1971.
6. Greenwald, P., *et al:* N. Engl. J. Med. 285:390–392, 1971.
7. Lanier, A., *et al:* Mayo Clin. Proc. 48:793–799, 1973.
8. Herbst, A., *et al:* Obstet. Gynecol. 40:287–298, 1972.
9. Herbst, A., *et al:* Am. J. Obstet. Gynecol. 118:607–615, 1974.
10. Herbst, A., *et al:* N. Engl. J. Med. 292:334–339, 1975.
11. Stafl, A., *et al:* Obstet. Gynecol. 43:118–128, 1974.
12. Sherman, A. I., *et al:* Obstet. Gynecol. 44:531–545, 1974.
13. Gal, I., *et al:* Nature 216:83, 1967.
14. Levy, E. P., *et al:* Lancet 1:611, 1973.
15. Nora, J., *et al:* Lancet 1:941–942, 1973.
16. Janerich, D. T., *et al:* N. Engl. J. Med. 291:697–700, 1974.
17. Boston Collaborative Drug Surveillance Program: N. Engl. J. Med. 290:15–19, 1974.
18. Hoover, R., *et al:* N. Engl. J. Med. 295:401–405, 1976.
19. Boston Collaborative Drug Surveillance Program: Lancet 1:1399–1404, 1973.
20. Daniel, D. G., *et al:* Lancet 2:287–289, 1967.
21. The Veterans Administration Cooperative Urological Research Group: J. Urol. 98:516–522, 1967.
22. Bailar, J. C.: Lancet 2:560, 1967.
23. Blackard, C., *et al:* Cancer 26:249–256, 1970.
24. Royal College of General Practitioners: J. R. Coll. Gen. Pract. 13:267–279, 1967.
24a. Royal College of General Practitioners: Oral Contraceptives and Health, New York, Pitman Corp., 1974.
25. Inman, W. H. W., *et al:* Br. Med. J. 2:193–199, 1968.
26. Vessey, M. P., *et al:* Br. Med. J. 2:651–657, 1969.
27. Sartwell, P. E., *et al:* Am. J. Epidemiol. 90:365–380, 1969.
28. Collaborative Group for the Study of Stroke in Young Women: N. Engl. J. Med. 288:871–878, 1973.
29. Collaborative Group for the Study of Stroke in Young Women: J.A.M.A. 231:718–722, 1975.
30. Mann, J. I., *et al:* Br. Med. J. 2:245–248, 1975.
31. Mann, J. I., *et al:* Br. Med. J. 2:241–245, 1975.
32. Inman, W. H. W., *et al:* Br. Med. J. 2:203–209, 1970.
33. Stolley, P. D., *et al:* Am. J. Epidemiol. 102:197–208, 1975.
34. Vessey, M. P., *et al:* Br. Med. J. 3:123–126, 1970.
35. Greene, G. R., *et al:* Am. J. Public Health 62:680–685, 1972.
36. Rosenberg, L., *et al:* N. Engl. J. Med. 294:1256–1259, 1976.
37. Coronary Drug Project Research Group: J.A.M.A. 214:1303–1313, 1970.
38. Baum, J., *et al:* Lancet 2:926–928, 1973.
39. Mays, E. T., *et al:* J.A.M.A. 235:730–732, 1976.
40. Edmondson, H. A., *et al:* N. Engl. J. Med. 294:470–472, 1976.
41. Pfeffer, R. I., *et al:* Am. J. Epidemiol. 103:445–456, 1976.

INFORMATION FOR THE PATIENT
What you should know about estrogens
Estrogens are female hormones produced by the ovaries. The ovaries make several different kinds of estrogens. In addition, scientists have been able to make a variety of synthetic estrogens. As far as we know, all these estrogens have similar properties and therefore much the same usefulness, side effects, and risks. This leaflet is intended to help you understand what estrogens are used for, the risks involved in their use, and how to use them as safely as possible.
This leaflet includes the most important information about estrogens, but not all the information. If you want to know more, you should ask your doctor for more information or you can ask your doctor or pharmacist to let you read the package insert prepared for the doctor.

Uses of Estrogen:
THERE IS NO PROPER USE OF ESTROGENS IN A PREGNANT WOMAN.
Estrogens are prescribed by doctors for a number of purposes, including:
1. To provide estrogen during a period of adjustment when a woman's ovaries stop producing a majority of her estrogens, in order to prevent certain uncomfortable symptoms of estrogen deficiency. (With the menopause, which generally occurs between the ages of 45 and 55, women produce a much smaller amount of estrogens.)
2. To prevent symptoms of estrogen deficiency when a woman's ovaries have been removed surgically before the natural menopause.
3. To prevent pregnancy. (Estrogens are given along with a progestogen, another female hormone; these combinations are called oral contraceptives or birth control pills. Patient labeling is available to women taking oral contraceptives and they will not be discussed in this leaflet.)
4. To treat certain cancers in women and men.
5. To prevent painful swelling of the breasts after

Continued on next page

Ayerst—Cont.

pregnancy in women who choose not to nurse their babies.

Estrogens in the Menopause: In the natural course of their lives, all women eventually experience a decrease in estrogen production. This usually occurs between ages 45 and 55 but may occur earlier or later. Sometimes the ovaries may need to be removed before natural menopause by an operation, producing a "surgical menopause."

When the amount of estrogen in the blood begins to decrease, many women may develop typical symptoms: feelings of warmth in the face, neck, and chest or sudden intense episodes of heat and sweating throughout the body (called "hot flashes" or "hot flushes"). These symptoms are sometimes very uncomfortable. Some women may also develop changes in the vagina (called "atrophic vaginitis") which cause discomfort, especially during and after intercourse.

Estrogens can be prescribed to treat these symptoms of the menopause. It is estimated that considerably more than half of all women undergoing the menopause have only mild symptoms or no symptoms at all and therefore do not need estrogens. Other women may need estrogens for a few months, while their bodies adjust to lower estrogen levels. Sometimes the need will be for periods longer than six months. In an attempt to avoid overstimulation of the uterus (womb), estrogens are usually given cyclically during each month of use, such as three weeks of pills followed by one week without pills.

Sometimes women experience nervous symptoms or depression during menopause. There is no evidence that estrogens are effective for such symptoms without associated vasomotor symptoms. In the absence of vasomotor symptoms, estrogens should not be used to treat nervous symptoms, although other treatment may be needed.

You may have heard that taking estrogens for long periods (years) after the menopause will keep your skin soft and supple and keep you feeling young. There is no evidence that this is so, however, and such long-term treatment carries important risks.

Estrogens to Prevent Swelling of the Breasts After Pregnancy:

If you do not breast-feed your baby after delivery, your breasts may fill up with milk and become painful and engorged. This usually begins about 3 to 4 days after delivery and may last for a few days to up to a week or more. Sometimes the discomfort is severe, but usually it is not and can be controlled by pain-relieving drugs such as aspirin and by binding the breasts up tightly. Estrogens can be used to try to prevent the breasts from filling up. While this treatment is sometimes successful, in many cases the breasts fill up to some degree in spite of treatment. The dose of estrogens needed to prevent pain and swelling of the breasts is much larger than the dose needed to treat symptoms of the menopause and this may increase your chances of developing blood clots in the legs or lungs (see below). Therefore, it is important that you discuss the benefits and the risks of estrogen use with your doctor if you have decided not to breast-feed your baby.

The Dangers of Estrogens:

1. *Endometrial cancer.* There are reports that if estrogens are used in the postmenopausal period for more than a year, there is an increased risk of *endometrial cancer* (cancer of the lining of the uterus). Women taking estrogens have roughly 5 to 10 times as great a chance of getting this cancer as women who take no estrogens. To put this another way, while a postmenopausal woman not taking estrogens has 1 chance in 1,000 each year of getting endometrial cancer, a woman taking estrogens has 5 to 10 chances in 1,000 each year. For this reason *it is important to take estrogens only when they are really needed*.

The risk of this cancer is greater the longer estrogens are used and when larger doses are taken. Therefore you should not take more estrogen than your doctor prescribes. *It is important to take the lowest dose of estrogen that will control symptoms and to take it only as long as it is needed.* If estrogens are needed for longer periods of time, your doctor will want to reevaluate your need for estrogens at least every six months.

Women using estrogens should report any vaginal bleeding to their doctors; such bleeding may be of no importance, but it can be an early warning of endometrial cancer. If you have undiagnosed vaginal bleeding, you should not use estrogens until a diagnosis is made and you are certain there is no endometrial cancer.

NOTE: If you have had your uterus removed (total hysterectomy), there is no danger of developing endometrial cancer.

2. *Other possible cancers.* Estrogens can cause development of other tumors in animals, such as tumors of the breast, cervix, vagina, or liver, when given for a long time. At present there is no good evidence that women using estrogen in the menopause have an increased risk of such tumors, but there is no way yet to be sure they do not; and one study raises the possibility that use of estrogens in the menopause may increase the risk of breast cancer many years later. This is a further reason to use estrogens only when clearly needed. While you are taking estrogens, it is important that you go to your doctor at least once a year for a physical examination. Also, if members of your family have had breast cancer or if you have breast nodules or abnormal mammograms (breast x-rays), your doctor may wish to carry our more frequent examinations of your breasts.

3. *Gallbladder disease.* Women who use estrogens after menopause are more likely to develop gallbladder disease needing surgery than women who do not use estrogens. Birth control pills have a similar effect.

4. *Abnormal blood clotting.* Oral contraceptives increase the risk of blood clotting in various parts of the body. This can result in a stroke (if the clot is in the brain), a heart attack (clot in a blood vessel of the heart), or a pulmonary embolus (a clot which forms in the legs or pelvis, then breaks off and travels to the lungs). Any of these can be fatal. At this time use of estrogens in the menopause is not known to cause such blood clotting, but this has not been fully studied and there could still prove to be such a risk. It is recommended that if you had had clotting in the legs or lungs or a heart attack or stroke while you were using estrogens or birth control pills, you should not use estrogens (unless they are being used to treat cancer of the breast or prostate). If you have had a stroke or heart attack or if you have angina pectoris, estrogens should be used with great caution and only if clearly needed (for example, if you have severe symptoms of the menopause).

The larger doses of estrogen used to prevent swelling of the breasts after pregnancy have been reported to cause clotting in the legs and lungs.

Special Warning About Pregnancy: You should not receive estrogen if you are pregnant. If this should occur, there is a greater than usual chance that the developing child will be born with a birth defect, although the possibility remains fairly small. A female child may have an increased risk of developing cancer of the vagina or cervix later in life (in the teens or twenties). Every possible effort should be made to avoid exposure to estrogen during pregnancy. If exposure occurs, see your doctor.

Other Effects of Estrogens: In addition to the serious known risks of estrogens described above, estrogens have the following side effects and potential risks:

1. *Nausea and vomiting.* The most common side effect of estrogen therapy is nausea. Vomiting is less common.
2. *Effects on breasts.* Estrogens may cause breast tenderness or enlargement and may cause the breasts to secrete a liquid. These effects are not dangerous.
3. *Effects on the uterus.* Estrogens may cause benign fibroid tumors of the uterus to get larger.
4. *Effects on liver.* Women taking oral contraceptives develop on rare occasions a tumor of the liver which can rupture and bleed into the abdomen and may cause death. So far, these tumors have not been reported in women using estrogens in the menopause, but you should report any swelling or unusual pain or tenderness in the abdomen to your doctor immediately.

Women with a past history of jaundice (yellowing of the skin and white parts of the eyes) may get jaundice again during estrogen use. If this occurs, stop taking estrogens and see your doctor.

5. *Other effects.* Estrogens may cause excess fluid to be retained in the body. This may make some conditions worse, such as asthma, epilepsy, migraine, heart disease, or kidney disease.

Summary: Estrogens have important uses, but they have serious risks as well. You must decide, with your doctor, whether the risks are acceptable to you in view of the benefits of treatment. Except where your doctor has prescribed estrogens for use in special cases of cancer of the breast or prostate, you should not use estrogens if you have cancer of the breast or uterus, are pregnant, have undiagnosed abnormal vaginal bleeding, clotting in the legs or lungs, or have had a stroke, heart attack or angina, or clotting in the legs or lungs in the past while you were taking estrogens.

You can use estrogens as safely as possible by understanding that your doctor will require regular physical examinations while you are taking them and will try to discontinue the drug as soon as possible and use the smallest dose possible. Be alert for signs of trouble including:

1. Abnormal bleeding from the vagina.
2. Pains in the calves or chest or sudden shortness of breath, or coughing blood.
3. Severe headache, dizziness, faintness, or changes in vision.
4. Breast lumps (you should ask your doctor how to examine your own breasts).
5. Jaundice (yellowing of the skin).
6. Mental depression.

Your doctor has prescribed this drug for you and you alone. Do not give the drug to anyone else.

How Supplied: PREMARIN® (Conjugated Estrogens Tablets, U.S.P.)—tablets for oral administration.

PREMARIN® VAGINAL CREAM—PREMARIN® in a nonliquefying base, designed for vaginal use.

PREMARIN® with METHYLTESTOSTERONE—a combination of PREMARIN and methyltestosterone (an androgen) in tablet form for oral administration.

PMB® 200, 400—a combination of PREMARIN® and meprobamate (a tranquilizing agent) in tablet form for oral administration.

PREMARIN® INTRAVENOUS—PREMARIN® specially prepared for intravenous and intramuscular use.

ESTROGENIC SUBSTANCE (Estrone) in Aqueous Suspension—a sterile aqueous suspension of estrone, a short-acting estrogen, for intramuscular injection only.

PREMARIN® ℞
[prĕm'a-rin]
(CONJUGATED ESTROGENS, U.S.P.)
VAGINAL CREAM
in a nonliquefying base

CAUTION: Federal law prohibits dispensing without prescription.

---

1. ESTROGENS HAVE BEEN REPORTED TO INCREASE THE RISK OF ENDOMETRIAL CARCINOMA.

Three independent case control studies have reported an increased risk of endometrial cancer in postmenopausal women exposed to exogenous estrogens for more than one year.[1-3] This risk was independent of the other known risk factors for endometrial cancer. These studies are further supported by the finding that incidence rates of endometrial cancer have increased sharply since 1969 in eight different areas of the United States with population-based cancer reporting systems, an increase which may be related to the rapidly expanding use of estrogens during the last decade.[4]

The three case control studies reported that the risk of endometrial cancer in estrogen users was about 4.5 to 13.9 times greater than in non-users. The risk appears to depend on both duration of treatment[1] and on estrogen dose.[3] In view of these findings, when estrogens are used for the treatment of menopausal symptoms, the lowest dose that will control symptoms should be utilized and medication should be discontinued as soon as possible. When prolonged treatment is medically indicated, the patient should be reassessed on at least a semiannual basis to determine the need for continued therapy. Although the evidence must be considered preliminary, one study suggests that cyclic administration of low doses of estrogen may carry less risk than continuous administration;[3] it therefore appears prudent to utilize such a regimen.

Close clinical surveillance of all women taking estrogens is important. In all cases of undiagnosed persistent or recurring abnormal vaginal bleeding, adequate diagnostic measures should be undertaken to rule out malignancy.

There is no evidence at present that "natural" estrogens are more or less hazardous than "synthetic" estrogens at equiestrogenic doses.

2. ESTROGENS SHOULD NOT BE USED DURING PREGNANCY.

The use of female sex hormones, both estrogens and progestogens, during early pregnancy may seriously damage the offspring. It has been shown that females exposed in utero to diethylstilbestrol, a non-steroidal estrogen, have an increased risk of developing in later life a form of vaginal or cervical cancer that is ordinarily extremely rare.[5,6] This risk has been estimated as not greater than 4 per 1000 exposures.[7] Furthermore, a high percentage of such exposed women (from 30 to 90 percent) have been found to have vaginal adenosis,[8-12] epithelial changes of the vagina and cervix. Although these changes are histologically benign, it is not known whether they are precursors of malignancy. Although similar data are not available with the use of other estrogens, it cannot be presumed they would not induce similar changes.

Several reports suggest an association between intrauterine exposure to female sex hormones and congenital anomalies, including congenital heart defects and limb reduction defects.[13-16] One case control study[16] estimated a 4.7-fold increased risk of limb reduction defects in infants exposed in utero to sex hormones (oral contraceptives, hormone withdrawal tests for pregnancy, or attempted treatment for threatened abortion). Some of these exposures were very short and involved only a few days of treatment. The data suggest that the risk of limb reduction defects in exposed fetuses is somewhat less than 1 per 1000.

In the past, female sex hormones have been used during pregnancy in an attempt to treat threatened or habitual abortion. There is considerable evidence that estrogens are ineffective for these indications, and there is no evidence from well controlled studies that progestogens are effective for these uses.

If PREMARIN (Conjugated Estrogens, U.S.P.) Vaginal Cream is used during pregnancy, or if the patient becomes pregnant while taking this drug, she should be apprised of the potential risks to the fetus, and the advisability of pregnancy continuation.

Description: Each gram contains 0.625 mg Conjugated Estrogens, U.S.P., in a nonliquefying base containing cetyl esters wax, cetyl alcohol, white wax, glyceryl monostearate, propylene glycol monostearate, methyl stearate, phenylethyl alcohol, sodium lauryl sulfate, glycerin, and mineral oil.
PREMARIN (Conjugated Estrogens, U.S.P.) is a mixture of estrogens, obtained exclusively from natural sources, occurring as the sodium salts of water-soluble estrogen sulfates blended to represent the average composition of material derived from pregnant mares' urine. It contains estrone, equilin, and 17 α-dihydroequilin, together with smaller amounts of 17 α-estradiol, equilenin, and 17 α-dihydroequilenin as salts of their sulfate esters.

Clinical Pharmacology: Estrogens are important in the development and maintenance of the female reproductive system and secondary sex characteristics. They promote growth and development of the vagina, uterus, and fallopian tubes, and enlargement of the breasts. Indirectly, they contribute to the shaping of the skeleton, maintenance of tone and elasticity of urogenital structures, changes in the epiphyses of the long bones that allow for the pubertal growth spurt and its termination, growth of axillary and pubic hair, and pigmentation of the nipples and genitals. Decline of estrogenic activity at the end of the menstrual cycle can bring on menstruation, although the cessation of progesterone secretion is the most important factor in the mature ovulatory cycle. However, in the preovulatory or nonovulatory cycle, estrogen is the primary determinant in the onset of menstruation. Estrogens also affect the release of pituitary gonadotropins.

The pharmacologic effects of conjugated estrogens are similar to those of endogenous estrogens. They are soluble in water and may be absorbed from mucosal surfaces after local administration.

In responsive tissues (female genital organs, breasts, hypothalamus, pituitary) estrogens enter the cell and are transported into the nucleus. As a result of estrogen action, specific RNA and protein synthesis occurs.

Metabolism and inactivation occur primarily in the liver. Some estrogens are excreted into the bile; however they are reabsorbed from the intestine and returned to the liver through the portal venous system. Water-soluble estrogen conjugates are strongly acidic and are ionized in body fluids, which favor excretion through the kidneys since tubular reabsorption is minimal.

Indications: PREMARIN (Conjugated Estrogens, U.S.P.) Vaginal Cream is indicated in the treatment of atrophic vaginitis and kraurosis vulvae.

PREMARIN Vaginal Cream HAS NOT BEEN SHOWN TO BE EFFECTIVE FOR ANY PURPOSE DURING PREGNANCY AND ITS USE MAY CAUSE SEVERE HARM TO THE FETUS (SEE BOXED WARNING).

Contraindications: Estrogens should not be used in women with any of the following conditions:
1. Known or suspected cancer of the breast except in appropriately selected patients being treated for metastatic disease.
2. Known or suspected estrogen-dependent neoplasia.
3. Known or suspected pregnancy (See Boxed Warning).
4. Undiagnosed abnormal genital bleeding.
5. Active thrombophlebitis or thromboembolic disorders.
6. A past history of thrombophlebitis, thrombosis, or thromboembolic disorders with previous estrogen use (except when used in treatment of breast malignancy).

PREMARIN Vaginal Cream should not be used in patients hypersensitive to its ingredients.

Warnings:
1. *Induction of malignant neoplasms.* Long term continuous administration of natural and synthetic estrogens in certain animal species increases the frequency of carcinomas of the breast, cervix, vagina, and liver. There are now reports that estrogens increase the risk of carcinoma of the endometrium in humans. (See Boxed Warning.)

At the present time there is no satisfactory evidence that estrogens given to postmenopausal women increase the risk of cancer of the breast,[17] although a recent long-term follow-up of a single physician's practice has raised this possibility.[18] Because of the animal data, there is a need for caution in prescribing estrogens for women with a strong family history of breast cancer or who have breast nodules, fibrocystic disease, or abnormal mammograms.

2. *Gallbladder disease.* A recent study has reported a 2 to 3-fold increase in the risk of surgically confirmed gallbladder disease in women receiving postmenopausal estrogens,[17] similar to the 2-fold increase previously noted in users of oral contraceptives.[19,24a]

3. *Effects similar to those caused by estrogen-progestogen oral contraceptives.* There are several serious adverse effects of oral contraceptives, most of which have not, up to now, been documented as consequences of postmenopausal estrogen therapy. This may reflect the comparatively low doses of estrogen used in postmenopausal women. It would be expected that the larger doses of estrogen used to treat breast cancer or postpartum breast engorgement are more likely to result in these adverse effects, and, in fact, it has been shown that there is an increased risk of thrombosis in men receiving estrogens for prostatic cancer and women for postpartum breast engorgement.[20-23]

a. *Thromboembolic disease.* It is now well established that users of oral contraceptives have an increased risk of various thromboembolic and thrombotic vascular diseases, such as thrombophlebitis, pulmonary embolism, stroke, and myocardial infarction.[24-31] Cases of retinal thrombosis, mesenteric thrombosis, and optic neuritis have been reported in oral contraceptive users. There is evidence that the risk of several of these adverse reactions is related to the dose of the drug.[32,33] An increased risk of postsurgery thromboembolic complications has also been reported in users of oral contraceptives.[34,35] If feasible, estrogen should be discontinued at least 4 weeks before surgery of the type associated with an increased risk of thromboembolism, or during periods of prolonged immobilization.

While an increased rate of thromboembolic and thrombotic disease in postmenopausal users of estrogens has not been found,[17-24,25-36] this does not rule out the possibility that such an increase may be present or that subgroups of women who have underlying risk factors or who are receiving relatively large doses of estrogens may have increased risk. Therefore estrogens should not be used in persons with active thrombophlebitis or thromboembolic disorders, and they should not be used (except in treatment of malignancy) in persons with a history of such disorders in association with estrogen use. They should be used with caution in patients with cerebral vascular or coronary artery disease and only for those in whom estrogens are clearly needed.

Large doses of estrogen (5 mg conjugated estrogens per day), comparable to those used to treat cancer of the prostate and breast, have been shown in a large prospective clinical trial in men[37] to increase the risk of nonfatal myocardial infarction, pulmonary embolism and thrombophlebitis. When estrogen doses of this size are used, any of the thromboembolic and thrombotic adverse effects associated with oral contraceptive use should be considered a clear risk.

b. *Hepatic adenoma.* Benign hepatic adenomas appear to be associated with the use of oral contraceptives.[38-40] Although benign, and rare, these may rupture and may cause death through intraabdominal hemorrhage. Such lesions have not yet been reported in association with other estrogen or progestogen preparations but should be considered in estrogen users having abdominal pain and tenderness, abdominal mass, or hypovolemic shock. Hepatocellular carcinoma has also been reported in women taking estrogen-containing oral contraceptives.[39] The relationship of this malignancy to these drugs is not known at this time.

Continued on next page

Ayerst—Cont.

c. *Elevated blood pressure.* Women using oral contraceptives sometimes experience increased blood pressure which, in most cases, returns to normal on discontinuing the drug. There is now a report that this may occur with use of estrogens in the menopause[41] and blood pressure should be monitored with estrogen use, especially if high doses are used.

d. *Glucose tolerance.* A worsening of glucose tolerance has been observed in a significant percentage of patients on estrogen-containing oral contraceptives. For this reason, diabetic patients should be carefully observed while receiving estrogen.

4. *Hypercalcemia.* Administration of estrogens may lead to severe hypercalcemia in patients with breast cancer and bone metastases. If this occurs, the drug should be stopped and appropriate measures taken to reduce the serum calcium level.

Precautions:

A. General Precautions.

1. A complete medical and family history should be taken prior to the initiation of any estrogen therapy. The pretreatment and periodic physical examinations should include special reference to blood pressure, breasts, abdomen, and pelvic organs, and should include a Papanicolau smear. As a general rule, estrogen should not be prescribed for longer than one year without another physical examination being performed.

2. Fluid retention—Because estrogens may cause some degree of fluid retention, conditions which might be influenced by this factor such as asthma, epilepsy, migraine, and cardiac or renal dysfunction, require careful observation.

3. Certain patients may develop undesirable manifestations of excessive estrogenic stimulation, such as abnormal or excessive uterine bleeding, mastodynia, etc.

4. Prolonged administration of unopposed estrogen therapy has been reported to increase the risk of endometrial hyperplasia in some patients.

5. Oral contraceptives appear to be associated with an increased incidence of mental depression.[24a] Although it is not clear whether this is due to the estrogenic or progestogenic component of the contraceptive, patients with a history of depression should be carefully observed.

6. Preexisting uterine leiomyomata may increase in size during estrogen use.

7. The pathologist should be advised of estrogen therapy when relevant specimens are submitted.

8. Patients with a past history of jaundice during pregnancy have an increased risk of recurrence of jaundice while receiving estrogen-containing oral contraceptive therapy. If jaundice develops in any patient receiving estrogen, the medication should be discontinued while the cause is investigated.

9. Estrogens may be poorly metabolized in patients with impaired liver function and they should be administered with caution in such patients.

10. Because estrogens influence the metabolism of calcium and phosphorus, they should be used with caution in patients with metabolic bone diseases that are associated with hypercalcemia or in patients with renal insufficiency.

11. Because of the effects of estrogens on epiphyseal closure, they should be used judiciously in young patients in whom bone growth is not complete.

12. Certain endocrine and liver function tests may be affected by estrogen-containing oral contraceptives. The following similar changes may be expected with larger doses of estrogen:

a. Increased sulfobromophthalein retention.

b. Increased prothrombin and factors VII, VIII, IX, and X; decreased antithrombin 3; increased norepinephrine-induced platelet aggregability.

c. Increased thyroid binding globulin (TBG) leading to increased circulating total thyroid hormone, as measured by PBI, T4 by column, or T4 by radioimmunoassay. Free T3 resin uptake is decreased, reflecting the elevated TBG; free T4 concentration is unaltered.

d. Impaired glucose tolerance.

e. Decreased pregnanediol excretion.

f. Reduced response to metyrapone test.

g. Reduced serum folate concentration.

h. Increased serum triglyceride and phospholipid concentration.

B. Information for the Patient. See text which appears after the PHYSICIAN REFERENCES.

C. Pregnancy Category X. See CONTRAINDICATIONS and Boxed Warning.

D. Nursing Mothers. As a general principle, the administration of any drug to nursing mothers should be done only when clearly necessary since many drugs are excreted in human milk.

Adverse Reactions: (See Warnings regarding induction of neoplasia, adverse effects on the fetus, increased incidence of gallbladder disease, and adverse effects similar to those of oral contraceptives, including thromboembolism.) The following additional adverse reactions have been reported with estrogenic therapy, including oral contraceptives.

1. *Genitourinary system:* Breakthrough bleeding, spotting, change in menstrual flow; dysmenorrhea; premenstrual-like syndrome; amenorrhea during and after treatment; increase in size of uterine fibromyomata; vaginal candidiasis; change in cervical erosion and in degree of cervical secretion; cystitis-like syndrome.

2. *Breasts:* Tenderness, enlargement, secretion.

3. *Gastrointestinal:* Nausea, vomiting; abdominal cramps, bloating; cholestatic jaundice.

4. *Skin:* Chloasma or melasma which may persist when drug is discontinued; erythema multiforme; erythema nodosum; hemorrhagic eruption; loss of scalp hair; hirsutism.

5. *Eyes:* Steepening of corneal curvature; intolerance to contact lenses.

6. *CNS:* Headache, migraine, dizziness; mental depression; chorea.

7. *Miscellaneous:* Increase or decrease in weight; reduced carbohydrate tolerance; aggravation of porphyria; edema; changes in libido.

Acute Overdosage: Numerous reports of ingestion of large doses of estrogen-containing oral contraceptives by young children indicate that acute serious ill effects do not occur. Overdosage of estrogen may cause nausea, and withdrawal bleeding may occur in females.

Dosage and Administration:

Given cyclically for short-term use only:

For treatment of atrophic vaginitis, or kraurosis vulvae.

The lowest dose that will control symptoms should be chosen and medication should be discontinued as promptly as possible.

Administration should be cyclic (e.g., three weeks on and one week off).

Attempts to discontinue or taper medication should be made at three to six month intervals.

Usual dosage range: 2 to 4 g (½ applicatorful to 1 applicatorful) daily, intravaginally or topically, depending on the severity of the condition.

Treated patients with an intact uterus should be monitored closely for signs of endometrial cancer and appropriate diagnostic measures should be taken to rule out malignancy in the event of persistent or recurring abnormal vaginal bleeding.

How Supplied: PREMARIN (Conjugated Estrogens, U.S.P.) Vaginal Cream—Each gram contains 0.625 mg Conjugated Estrogens, U.S.P. (Also contains cetyl esters wax, cetyl alcohol, white wax, glyceryl monostearate, propylene glycol monostearate, methyl stearate, phenylethyl alcohol, sodium lauryl sulfate, glycerin, and mineral oil.)

Combination package: Each contains Net Wt. 1½ oz (42.5 g) tube with one plastic applicator calibrated in 1 g increments to a maximum of 4 g (NDC 0046-0872-93).

Also Available—Refill package: Each contains Net Wt. 1½ oz (42.5 g) tube (NDC 0046-0872-01).

Physician References:

1. Ziel, H. K., *et al:* N. Engl. J. Med. 293:1167–1170, 1975.
2. Smith, D. C., *et al:* N. Engl. J. Med. 293:1164–1167, 1975.
3. Mack, T. M., *et al:* N. Engl. J. Med. 294:1262–1267, 1976.
4. Weiss, N. S., *et al:* N. Engl. J. Med. 294:1259–1262, 1976.
5. Herbst, A. L., *et al:* N. Engl. J. Med. 284:878–881, 1971.
6. Greenwald, P., *et al:* N. Engl. J. Med. 285:390–392, 1971.
7. Lanier, A., *et al:* Mayo Clin. Proc. 48:793–799, 1973.
8. Herbst, A., *et al:* Obstet. Gynecol. 40:287–298, 1972.
9. Herbst, A., *et al:* Am. J. Obstet. Gynecol. 118:607–615, 1974.
10. Herbst, A., *et al:* N. Engl. J. Med. 292:334–339, 1975.
11. Stafl, A., *et al:* Obstet. Gynecol. 43:118–128, 1974.
12. Sherman, A. I., *et al:* Obstet. Gynecol. 44:531–545, 1974.
13. Gal, I., *et al:* Nature 216:83, 1967.
14. Levy, E. P., *et al:* Lancet 1:611, 1973.
15. Nora, J., *et al:* Lancet 1:941–942, 1973.
16. Janerich, D. T., *et al:* N. Engl. J. Med. 291:697–700, 1974.
17. Boston Collaborative Drug Surveillance Program: N. Engl. J. Med. 290:15–19, 1974.
18. Hoover, R., *et al:* N. Engl. J. Med. 295:401–405, 1976.
19. Boston Collaborative Drug Surveillance Program: Lancet 1:1399–1404, 1973.
20. Daniel, D. G., *et al:* Lancet 2:287–289, 1967.
21. The Veterans Administration Cooperative Urological Research Group: J. Urol. 98:516–522, 1967.
22. Bailar, J. C.: Lancet 2:560, 1967.
23. Blackard, C., *et al:* Cancer 26:249–256, 1970.
24. Royal College of General Practitioners: J. R. Coll. Gen. Pract. 13:267–279, 1967.
24a. Royal College of General Practitioners: Oral Contraceptives and Health, New York, Pitman Corp., 1974.
25. Inman, W. H. W., *et al:* Br. Med. J. 2:193–199, 1968.
26. Vessey, M. P., *et al:* Br. Med. J. 2:651–657, 1969.
27. Sartwell, P. E., *et al:* Am. J. Epidemiol. 90:365–380, 1969.
28. Collaborative Group for the Study of Stroke in Young Women: N. Engl. J. Med. 288:871–878, 1973.
29. Collaborative Group for the Study of Stroke in Young Women: J.A.M.A. 231:718–722, 1975.
30. Mann, J. I., *et al:* Br. Med. J. 2:245–248, 1975.
31. Mann, J. I., *et al:* Br. Med. J. 2:241–245, 1975.
32. Inman, W. H. W., *et al:* Br. Med. J. 2:203–209, 1970.
33. Stolley, P. D., *et al:* Am. J. Epidemiol. 102:197–208, 1975.
34. Vessey, M. P., *et al:* Br. Med. J. 3:123–126, 1970.
35. Greene, G. R., *et al:* Am. J. Public Health 62:680–685, 1972.
36. Rosenberg, L., *et al:* N. Engl. J. Med. 294:1256–1259, 1976.
37. Coronary Drug Project Research Group: J.A.M.A. 214:1303–1313, 1970.
38. Baum, J., *et al:* Lancet 2:926–928, 1973.
39. Mays, E. T., *et al:* J.A.M.A. 235:730–732, 1976.
40. Edmondson, H. A., *et al:* N. Engl. J. Med. 294:470–472, 1976.
41. Pfeffer, R. I., *et al:* Am. J. Epidemiol. 103:445–456, 1976.

INFORMATION FOR THE PATIENT

What You Should Know About Estrogens

Estrogens are female hormones produced by the ovaries. The ovaries make several different kinds of estrogens. In addition, scientists have been able to make a variety of synthetic estrogens. As far as we know, all these estrogens have similar properties and therefore much the same usefulness, side effects, and risks. This leaflet is intended to help you understand what estrogens are used for, the risks involved in their use, and how to use them as safely as possible.

This leaflet includes the most important information about estrogens, but not all the information. If you want to know more, you should ask your doctor for more information or you can ask your doctor or pharmacist to let you read the package insert prepared for the doctor.

Uses of Estrogen:

THERE IS NO PROPER USE OF ESTROGENS IN A PREGNANT WOMAN

Estrogens are prescribed by doctors for a number of purposes, including:

1. To provide estrogen during a period of adjustment when a woman's ovaries stop producing a majority of her estrogens, in order to prevent certain uncomfortable symptoms of estrogen deficiency. (With the menopause which generally occurs between the ages of 45 and 55, women produce a much smaller amount of estrogens.)
2. To prevent symptoms of estrogen deficiency when a woman's ovaries have been removed surgically before the natural menopause.
3. To prevent pregnancy. (Estrogens are given along with a progestogen, another female hormone; these combinations are called oral contraceptives or birth control pills. Patient labeling is available to women taking oral contraceptives and they will not be discussed in this leaflet.)
4. To treat certain cancers in women and men.
5. To prevent painful swelling of the breasts after pregnancy in women who choose not to nurse their babies.

Estrogens in the Menopause: In the natural course of their lives, all women eventually experience a decrease in estrogen production. This usually occurs between ages 45 and 55 but may occur earlier or later. Sometimes the ovaries may need to be removed before natural menopause by an operation, producing a "surgical menopause".

When the amount of estrogen in the blood begins to decrease, many women may develop typical symptoms: feelings of warmth in the face, neck, and chest or sudden intense episodes of heat and sweating throughout the body (called "hot flashes" or "hot flushes"). These symptoms are sometimes very uncomfortable. Some women may also develop changes in the vagina (called "atrophic vaginitis") which cause discomfort, especially during and after intercourse.

Estrogens can be prescribed to treat these symptoms of the menopause. It is estimated that considerably more than half of all women undergoing the menopause have only mild symptoms or no symptoms at all and therefore do not need estrogens. Other women may need estrogens for a few months, while their bodies adjust to lower estrogen levels. Sometimes the need will be for periods longer than six months. In an attempt to avoid overstimulation of the uterus (womb), estrogens are usually given cyclically during each month of use, such as three weeks of pills followed by one week without pills. Sometimes women experience nervous symptoms or depression during menopause. There is no evidence that estrogens are effective for such sumptoms without associated vasomotor symptoms. In the absence of vasomotor symptoms, estrogens should not be used to treat nervous symptoms, although other treatment may be needed. You may have heard that taking estrogens for long periods (years) after the menopause will keep your skin soft and supple and keep you feeling young. There is no evidence that this is so, however, and such long-term treatment carries important risks.

Estrogens to Prevent Swelling of the Breasts After Pregnancy

If you do not breast feed your baby after delivery, your breasts may fill up with milk and become painful and engorged. This usually begins about 3 to 4 days after delivery and may last for a few days to up to a week or more. Sometimes the discomfort is severe, but usually it is not and can be controlled by pain-relieving drugs such as aspirin and by binding the breasts up tightly. Estrogens can be used to try to prevent the breasts from filling up. While this treatment is sometimes successful, in many cases the breasts fill up to some degree in spite of treatment. The dose of estrogens needed to prevent pain and swelling of the breasts is much larger than the dose needed to treat symptoms of the menopause and this may increase your chances of developing blood clots in the legs or lungs (see below). Therefore, it is important that you discuss the benefits and the risks of estrogen use with your doctor if you have decided not to breast-feed your baby.

The Dangers of Estrogens: 1. *Endometrial cancer.* There are reports that if estrogens are used in the postmenopausal period for more than a year, there is an increased risk of *endometrial cancer* (cancer of the lining of the uterus). Women taking estrogens have roughly 5 to 10 times as great a chance of getting this cancer as women who take no estrogens. To put this another way, while a postmenopausal woman not taking estrogens has 1 chance in 1,000 each year of getting endometrial cancer, a woman taking estrogens has 5 to 10 chances in 1,000 each year. For this reason, *it is important to take estrogens only when they are really needed.*

The risk of this cancer is greater the longer estrogens are used and when larger doses are taken. Therefore you should not take more estrogen than your doctor prescribes. *It is important to take the lowest dose of estrogen that will control symptoms and to use only as long as it is needed.* If estrogens are needed for longer periods of time, your doctor will want to reevaluate your need for estrogens at least every six months.

Women using estrogens should report any vaginal bleeding to their doctors; such bleeding may be of no importance, but it can be an early warning of endometrial cancer. If you have undiagnosed vaginal bleeding, you should not use estrogens until a diagnosis is made and you are certain there is no endometrial cancer.

NOTE: If you have had your uterus removed (total hysterectomy), there is no danger of developing endometrial cancer.

2. *Other possible cancers.* Estrogens can cause development of other tumors in animals, such as tumors of the breast, cervix, vagina, or liver, when given for a long time. At present there is no good evidence that women using estrogen in the menopause have an increased risk of such tumors, but there is no way yet to be sure they do not; and one study raises the possibility that use of estrogens in the menopause may increase the risk of breast cancer many years later. This is a further reason to use estrogens only when clearly needed. While you are taking estrogens, it is important that you go to your doctor at least once a year for a physical examination. Also, if members of your family have had breast cancer or if you have breast nodules or abnormal mammograms (breast x-rays), your doctor may wish to carry out more frequent examinations of your breasts.

3. *Gallbladder disease.* Women who use estrogens after menopause are more likely to develop gallbladder disease needing surgery than women who do not use estrogens. Birth control pills have a similar effect.

4. *Abnormal blood clotting.* Oral contraceptives increase the risk of blood clotting in various parts of the body. This can result in a stroke (if the clot is in the brain), a heart attack (clot in a blood vessel of the heart), or a pulmonary embolus (a clot which forms in the legs or pelvis, then breaks off and travels to the lungs). Any of these can be fatal. At this time use of estrogens in the menopause is not known to cause such blood clotting, but this has not been fully studied and there could still prove to be such a risk. It is recommended that if you have had clotting in the legs or lungs or a heart attack or stroke while you were using estrogens or birth control pills, you should not use estrogens (unless they are being used to treat cancer of the breast or prostate). If you have had a stroke or heart attack or if you have angina pectoris, estrogens should be used with great caution and only if clearly needed (for example, if you have severe symptoms of the menopause).

The larger doses of estrogen used to prevent swelling of the breasts after pregnancy have been reported to cause clotting in the legs and lungs.

Special Warning About Pregnancy: You should not receive estrogen if you are pregnant. If this should occur, there is a greater than usual chance that the developing child will be born with a birth defect, although the possibility remains fairly small. A female child may have an increased risk of developing cancer of the vagina or cervix later in life (in the teens or twenties). Every possible effort should be made to avoid exposure to estrogens during pregnancy. If exposure occurs, see your doctor.

Other Effects of Estrogens: In additon to the serious known risks of estrogens described above, estrogens have the following side effects and potential risks:

1. *Nausea and vomiting.* The most common side effect of estrogen therapy is nausea. Vomiting is less common.
2. *Effects on breasts.* Estrogens may cause breast tenderness or enlargement and may cause the breasts to secrete a liquid. These effects are not dangerous.
3. *Effects on the uterus.* Estrogens may cause benign fibroid tumors of the uterus to get larger.
4. *Effects on liver.* Women taking oral contraceptives develop on rare occasions a tumor of the liver which can rupture and bleed into the abdomen and may cause death. So far, these tumors have not been reported in women using estrogens in the menopause, but you should report any swelling or unusual pain or tenderness in the abdomen to your doctor immediately.

Women with a past history of jaundice (yellowing of the skin and white parts of the eyes) may get jaundice again during estrogen use. If this occurs, stop taking estrogens and see your doctor.

5. *Other effects.* Estrogens may cause excess fluid to be retained in the body. This may make some conditions worse, such as asthma, epilepsy, migraine, heart disease, or kidney disease.

Summary: Estrogens have important uses, but they have serious risks as well. You must decide, with your doctor, whether the risks are acceptable to you in view of the benefits of treatment. Except where your doctor has prescribed estrogens for use in special cases of cancer of the breast or prostate, you should not use estrogens if you have cancer of the breast or uterus, are pregnant, have undiagnosed abnormal vaginal bleeding, clotting in the legs or lungs, or have had a stroke, heart attack or angina, or clotting in the legs or lungs in the past while you were taking estrogens.

You can use estrogens as safely as possible by understanding that your doctor will require regular physical examinations while you are taking them and will try to discontinue the drug as soon as possible and use the smallest dose possible. Be alert for signs of trouble including:

1. Abnormal bleeding from the vagina.
2. Pains in the calves or chest or sudden shortness of breath, or coughing blood.
3. Severe headache, dizziness, faintness, or changes in vision.
4. Breast lumps (you should ask your doctor how to examine your own breasts).
5. Jaundice (yellowing of the skin).
6. Mental depression.

Your doctor has prescribed this drug for you and you alone. Do not give the drug to anyone else.

How Supplied: PREMARIN® (Conjugated Estrogens Tablets, U.S.P.)—tablets for oral administration.

Each oval *purple* tablet contains 2.5 mg
Each oval *yellow* tablet contains 1.25 mg
Each oval *white* tablet contains 0.9 mg
Each oval *maroon* tablet contains 0.625 mg
Each oral *green* tablet contains 0.3 mg

PREMARIN® with METHYLTESTOSTERONE—a combination of PREMARIN and methyltestosterone (an androgen) in tablet form for oral administration.

Each round *yellow* tablet contains 1.25 mg PREMARIN and 10 mg methyltestosterone
Each round *maroon* tablet contains 0.625 mg PREMARIN and 5 mg methyltestosterone

Continued on next page

Ayerst—Cont.

PMB® 200, 400—a combination of PREMARIN® and meprobamate (a tranquilizing agent) in tablet form for oral administration.
    Each oblong *green* tablet contains 0.45 mg PREMARIN and 200 mg meprobamate
    Each oblong *pink* tablet contains 0.45 mg PREMARIN and 400 mg meprobamate
The appearance of these tablets is a trademark of Ayerst Laboratories.
PREMARIN® VAGINAL CREAM—PREMARIN® in a nonliquefying base, designed for vaginal use.
PREMARIN® INTRAVENOUS—PREMARIN® specially prepared for intravenous and intramuscular use.
ESTROGENIC SUBSTANCE (Estrone) in Aqueous Suspension—a sterile aqueous suspension of estrone, a short-acting estrogen, for intramuscular injection only.
Shown in Product Identification Section, page 405

PREMARIN® ℞
[prem'a-rin with meth"yl-tĕs-tŏs'ta-rŏn]
(Conjugated Estrogens, U.S.P.)
with METHYLTESTOSTERONE

No. 879—Each **yellow** tablet contains:
Premarin® (Conjugated
  Estrogens, U.S.P.) ....1.25 mg
Methyltestosterone ....10.0 mg
No. 878—Each **maroon** tablet contains:
Premarin® (Conjugated
  Estrogens, U.S.P.) ....0.625 mg
Methyltestosterone ....5.0 mg
CAUTION: Federal law prohibits dispensing without prescription.

1. ESTROGENS HAVE BEEN REPORTED TO INCREASE THE RISK OF ENDOMETRIAL CARCINOMA.

Three independent case control studies have reported an increased risk of endometrial cancer in postmenopausal women exposed to exogenous estrogens for more than one year.[1-3] This risk was independent of the other known risk factors for endometrial cancer. These studies are further supported by the finding that incidence rates of endometrial cancer have increased sharply since 1969 in eight different areas of the United States with population-based cancer reporting systems, an increase which may be related to the rapidly expanding use of estrogens during the last decade.[4]
The three case control studies reported that the risk of endometrial cancer in estrogen users was about 4.5 to 13.9 times greater than in nonusers. The risk appears to depend on both duration of treatment[1] and on estrogen dose.[3] In view of these findings, when estrogens are used for the treatment of menopausal symptoms, the lowest dose that will control symptoms should be utilized and medication should be discontinued as soon as possible. When prolonged treatment is medically indicated, the patient should be reassessed on at least a semiannual basis to determine the need for continued therapy. Although the evidence must be considered preliminary, one study suggests that cyclic administration of low doses of estrogen may carry less risk than continuous administration;[3] it therefore appears prudent to utilize such a regimen.
Close clinical surveillance of all women taking estrogens is important. In all cases of undiagnosed persistent or recurring abnormal vaginal bleeding, adequate diagnostic measures should be undertaken to rule out malignancy.
There is no evidence at present that "natural" estrogens are more or less hazardous than "synthetic" estrogens at equiestrogenic doses.

2. ESTROGENS SHOULD NOT BE USED DURING PREGNANCY.

The use of female sex hormones, both estrogens and progestogens, during early pregnancy may seriously damage the offspring. It has been shown that females exposed in utero to diethylstilbestrol, a non-steroidal estrogen, have an increased risk of developing in later life a form of vaginal or cervical cancer that is ordinarily extremely rare.[5,6] This risk has been estimated as not greater than 4 per 1000 exposures.[7] Furthermore, a high percentage of such exposed women (from 30 to 90 percent) have been found to have vaginal adenosis,[8-12] epithelial changes of the vagina and cervix. Although these changes are histologically benign, it is not known whether they are precursors of malignancy. Although similar data are not available with the use of other estrogens, it cannot be presumed they would not induce similar changes.
Several reports suggest an association between intrauterine exposure to female sex hormones and congenital anomalies, including congenital heart defects and limb reduction defects.[13-16] One case control study[16] estimated a 4.7-fold increased risk of limb reduction defects in infants exposed in utero to sex hormones (oral contraceptives, hormone withdrawal tests for pregnancy, or attempted treatment for threatened abortion). Some of these exposures were very short and involved only a few days of treatment. The data suggest that the risk of limb reduction defects in exposed fetuses is somewhat less than 1 per 1000.
In the past, female sex hormones have been used during pregnancy in an attempt to treat threatened or habitual abortion. There is considerable evidence that estrogens are ineffective for these indications, and there is no evidence from well controlled studies that progestogens are effective for these uses.
If PREMARIN with METHYLTESTOSTERONE is used during pregnancy, or if the patient becomes pregnant while taking this drug, she should be apprised of the potential risks to the fetus, and the advisability of pregnancy continuation.

Description: PREMARIN with METHYLTESTOSTERONE is provided in tablets for oral administration.
PREMARIN (Conjugated Estrogens, U.S.P.) is a mixture of estrogens, obtained exclusively from natural sources, occurring as the sodium salts of water-soluble estrogen sulfates blended to represent the average composition of material derived from pregnant mares' urine. It contains estrone, equilin, and 17 α-dihydroequilin, together with smaller amounts of 17 α-estradiol, equilenin, and 17 α-dihydroequilenin as salts of their sulfate esters.
Methyltestosterone is an androgen.
Androgens are derivatives of cyclopentano-perhydrophenanthrene. Endogenous androgens are C-19 steroids with a side chain at C-17, and with two angular methyl groups. Testosterone is the primary endogenous androgen. Fluoxymesterone and methyltestosterone are synthetic derivatives of testosterone.
Methylestosterone is a white to light yellow crystalline substance that is virtually insoluble in water but soluble in organic solvents. It is stable in air but decomposes in light.

Clinical Pharmacology:
Estrogens Estrogens are important in the development and maintenance of the female reproductive system and secondary sex characteristics. They promote growth and development of the vagina, uterus, and fallopian tubes, and enlargement of the breasts. Indirectly, they contribute to the shaping of the skeleton, maintenance of tone and elasticity of urogenital structures, changes in the epiphyses of the long bones that allow for the pubertal growth spurt and its termination, growth of axillary and pubic hair, and pigmentation of the nipples and genitals. Decline of estrogenic activity at the end of the menstrual cycle can bring on menstruation, although the cessation of progesterone secretion is the most important factor in the mature ovulatory cycle. However, in the preovulatory or nonovulatory cycle, estrogen is the primary determinant in the onset of menstruation. Estrogens also affect the release of pituitary gonadotropins.
The pharmacologic effects of conjugated estrogens are similar to those of endogenous estrogens. They are soluble in water and are well absorbed from the gastrointestinal tract.
In responsive tissues (female genital organs, breasts, hypothalamus, pituitary) estrogens enter the cell and are transported into the nucleus. As a result of estrogen action, specific RNA and protein synthesis occurs.
Estrogen Pharmacokinetics
Metabolism and inactivation occur primarily in the liver. Some estrogens are excreted into the bile; however they are reabsorbed from the intestine and returned to the liver through the portal venous system. Water soluble estrogen conjugates are strongly acidic and are ionized in body fluids, which favor excretion through the kidneys since tubular reabsorption is minimal.
Androgens Endogenous androgens are responsible for the normal growth and development of the male sex organs and for maintenance of secondary sex characteristics. These effects include the growth and maturation of prostate, seminal vesicles, penis, and scrotum; the development of male hair distribution, such as beard, pubic, chest, and axillary hair, laryngeal enlargement, vocal chord thickening, alterations in body musculature, and fat distribution. Drugs in this class also cause retention of nitrogen, sodium, potassium, phosphorus, and decreased urinary excretion of calcium. Androgens have been reported to increase protein anabolism and decrease protein catabolism. Nitrogen balance is improved only when there is sufficient intake of calories and protein.
Androgens are responsible for the growth spurt of adolescence and for the eventual termination of linear growth which is brought about by fusion of the epiphyseal growth centers. In children, exogenous androgens accelerate linear growth rates, but may cause a disproportionate advancement in bone maturation. Use over long periods may result in fusion of the eiphyseal growth centers and termination of growth process. Androgens have been reported to stimulate the production of red blood cells by enhancing the production of erythropoietic stimulating factor.
Androgen Pharmacokinetics
Testosterone given orally is metabolized by the gut and 44 percent is cleared by the liver in the first pass. Oral doses as high as 400 mg per day are needed to achieve clinically effective blood levels for full replacement therapy. The synthetic androgens (methyltestosterone and fluoxymesterone) are less extensively metabolized by the liver and have longer half-lives. They are more suitable than testosterone for oral administration.
Testosterone in plasma is 98 percent bound to a specific testosterone-estradiol binding globulin, and about 2 percent is free. Generally, the amount of this sex-hormone binding globulin in the plasma will determine the distribution of testosterone between free and bound forms, and the free testosterone concentration will determine its half-life. About 90 percent of a dose of testosterone is excreted in the urine as glucuronic and sulfuric acid conjugates of testosterone and its metabolites; about 6 percent of a dose is excreted in the feces, mostly in the unconjugated form. Inactivation of testosterone occurs primarily in the liver. Testosterone is metabolized to various 17-keto steroids through two different pathways. There are considerable variations of the half-life of testosterone as reported in the literature, ranging from 10 to 100 minutes.
In many tissues the activity of testosterone appears to depend on reduction to dihydrotestosterone, which binds to cytosol receptor proteins. The steroid-receptor complex is transported to the nu-

cleus where it initiates transcription events and cellular changes related to androgen action.

Indications: PREMARIN (Conjugated Estrogens, U.S.P.) with Methyltestosterone is indicated in the treatment of:

Moderate to severe *vasomotor* symptoms associated with the menopause in those patients not improved by estrogens alone. (There is no evidence that estrogens are effective for nervous symptoms or depression without associated vasomotor symptoms, and they should not be used to treat such conditions.)

PREMARIN with METHYLTESTOSTERONE HAS NOT BEEN SHOWN TO BE EFFECTIVE FOR ANY PURPOSE DURING PREGNANCY AND ITS USE MAY CAUSE SEVERE HARM TO THE FETUS (SEE BOXED WARNING).

Contraindications: Estrogens should not be used in women with any of the following conditions:

1. Known or suspected cancer of the breast except in appropriately selected patients being treated for metastatic disease.
2. Known or suspected estrogen-dependent neoplasia.
3. Known or suspected pregnancy (See Boxed Warning).
4. Undiagnosed abnormal genital bleeding.
5. Active thrombophlebitis or thromboembolic disorders.
6. A past history of thrombophlebitis, thrombosis, or thromboembolic disorders associated with previous estrogen use (except when used in treatment of breast malignancy).

Methyltestosterone should not be used in:
1. The presence of severe liver damage.
2. Pregnancy and in breast-feeding mothers because of the possibility of masculinization of the female fetus or breast-fed infant.

Warnings:
Associated with Estrogens
1. *Induction of malignant neoplasms.* Long term continuous administration of natural and synthetic estrogens in certain animal species increases the frequency of carcinomas of the breast, cervix, vagina, and liver. There are now reports that estrogens increase the risk of carcinoma of the endometrium in humans. (See Boxed Warning.)

At the present time there is no satisfactory evidence that estrogens given to postmenopausal women increase the risk of cancer of the breast,[17] although a recent long-term followup of a single physician's practice has raised this possibility.[18] Because of the animal data, there is a need for caution in prescribing estrogens for women with a strong family history of breast cancer or who have breast nodules, fibrocystic disease, or abnormal mammograms.

2. *Gallbladder disease.* A recent study has reported a 2 to 3-fold increase in the risk of surgically confirmed gallbladder disease in women receiving postmenopausal estrogens,[17] similar to the 2-fold increase previously noted in users of oral contraceptives.[19,24a]

3. *Effects similar to those caused by estrogen-progestogen oral contraceptives.* There are several serious adverse effects of oral contraceptives, most of which have not, up to now, been documented as consequences of postmenopausal estrogen therapy. This may reflect the comparatively low doses of estrogen used in postmenopausal women. It would be expected that the larger doses of estrogen used to treat prostatic or breast cancer or postpartum breast engorgement are more likely to result in these adverse effects, and, in fact, it has been shown that there is an increased risk of thrombosis in men receiving estrogens for prostatic cancer and women for postpartum breast engorgement.[20-23]

a. *Thromboembolic disease.* It is now well established that users of oral contraceptives have an increased risk of various thromboembolic and thrombotic vascular diseases, such as thrombophlebitis, pulmonary embolism, stroke, and myocardial infarction.[24-31] Cases of retinal thrombosis, mesenteric thrombosis, and optic neuritis have been reported in oral contraceptive users. There is evidence that the risk of several of these adverse reactions is related to the dose of the drug.[32,33] An increased risk of postsurgery thromboembolic complications has also been reported in users of oral contraceptives.[34,35] If feasible, estrogen should be discontinued at least 4 weeks before surgery of the type associated with an increased risk of thromboembolism, or during periods of prolonged immobilization.

While an increased rate of thromboembolic and thrombotic disease in postmenopausal users of estrogens has not been found,[17-24,25-36] this does not rule out the possibility that such an increase may be present or that subgroups of women who have underlying risk factors or who are receiving relatively large doses of estrogens may have increased risk. Therefore estrogens should not be used in persons with active thrombophlebitis or thromboembolic disorders, and they should not be used (except in treatment of malignancy) in persons with a history of such disorders in association with estrogen use. They should be used with caution in patients with cerebral vascular or coronary artery disease and only for those in whom estrogens are clearly needed.

Large doses of estrogen (5 mg conjugated estrogens per day), comparable to those used to treat cancer of the prostate and breast, have been shown in a large prospective clinical trial in men[37] to increase the risk of nonfatal myocardial infarction, pulmonary embolism and thrombophlebitis. When estrogen doses of this size are used, any of the thromboembolic and thrombotic adverse effects associated with oral contraceptive use should be considered a clear risk.

b. *Hepatic adenoma.* Benign hepatic adenomas appear to be associated with the use of oral contraceptives.[38-40] Although benign, and rare, these may rupture and may cause death through intra-abdominal hemorrhage. Such lesions have not yet been reported in association with other estrogen or progestogen preparations but should be considered in estrogen users having abdominal pain and tenderness, abdominal mass, or hypovolemic shock. Hepatocellular carcinoma has also been reported in women taking estrogen-containing oral contraceptives.[39] The relationship of this malignancy to these drugs is not known at this time.

c. *Elevated blood pressure.* Women using oral contraceptives sometimes experience increased blood pressure which, in most cases, returns to normal on discontinuing the drug. There is now a report that this may occur with use of estrogens in the menopause[41] and blood pressure should be monitored with estrogen use, especially if high doses are used.

d. *Glucose tolerance.* A worsening of glucose tolerance has been observed in a significant percentage of patients on estrogen-containing oral contraceptives. For this reason, diabetic patients should be carefully observed while receiving estrogen.

4. *Hypercalcemia.* Administration of estrogens may lead to severe hypercalcemia in patients with breast cancer and bone metastases. If this occurs, the drug should be stopped and appropriate measures taken to reduce the serum calcium level.

Associated with Methyltestosterone
In patients with breast cancer, androgen therapy may cause hypercalcemia by stimulating osteolysis. In this case, the drug should be discontinued. Prolonged use of high doses of androgens has been associated with the development of peliosis hepatis and hepatic neoplasms including hepatocellular carcinoma. (See PRECAUTIONS—*Carcinogensis*). Peliosis hepatis can be a life-threatening or fatal complication.

Cholestatic hepatitis and jaundice occur with 17-alpha-alkylandrogens at a relatively low dose. If cholestatic hepatitis with jaundice appears or if liver function tests become abnormal, the androgen should be discontinued and the etiology should be determined. Drug-induced jaundice is reversible when the medication is discontinued.

Edema with or without heart failure may be a serious complication in patients with preexisting cardiac, renal, or hepatic disease. In addition to discontinuation of the drug, diuretic therapy may be required.

Precautions:
Associated with Estrogens
A. General Precautions.

1. A complete medical and family history should be taken prior to the initiation of any estrogen therapy. The pretreatment and periodic physical examinations should include special reference to blood pressure, breasts, abdomen, and pelvic organs, and should include a Papanicolau smear. As a general rule, estrogen should not be prescribed for longer than one year without another physical examination being performed.

2. Fluid retention—Because estrogens may cause some degree of fluid retention, conditions which might be influenced by this factor such as asthma, epilepsy, migraine, and cardiac or renal dysfunction, require careful observation.

3. Certain patients may develop undesirable manifestations of excessive estrogenic stimulation, such as abnormal or excessive uterine bleeding, mastodynia, etc.

4. Prolonged administration of unopposed estrogen therapy has been reported to increase the risk of endometrial hyperplasia in some patients.

5. Oral contraceptives appear to be associated with an increased incidence of mental depression.[24a] Although it is not clear whether this is due to the estrogenic or progestogenic component of the contraceptive, patients with a history of depression should be carefully observed.

6. Preexisting uterine leiomyomata may increase in size during estrogen use.

7. The pathologist should be advised of estrogen therapy when relevant specimens are submitted.

8. Patients with a past history of jaundice during pregnancy have an increased risk of recurrence of jaundice while receiving estrogen-containing oral contraceptive therapy. If jaundice develops in any patient receiving estrogen, the medication should be discontinued while the cause is investigated.

9. Estrogens may be poorly metabolized in patients with impaired liver function and they should be administered with caution in such patients.

10. Because estrogens influence the metabolism of calcium and phosphorus, they should be used with caution in patients with metabolic bone diseases that are associated with hypercalcemia or in patients with renal insufficiency.

11. Because of the effects of estrogens on epiphyseal closure, they should be used judiciously in young patients in whom bone growth is not complete.

12. Certain endocrine and liver function tests may be affected by estrogen-containing oral contraceptives. The following similar changes may be expected with larger doses of estrogen.
a. Increased sulfobromophthalein retention.
b. Increased prothrombin and factors VII, VIII, IX, and X; decreased antithrombin 3; increased norepinephrine-induced platelet aggregability.
c. Increased thyroid binding globulin (TBG) leading to increased circulating total thyroid hormone, as measured by PBI, T4 by column, or T4 by radioimmunoassay. Free T3 resin uptake is decreased, reflecting the elevated TBG; free T4 concentration is unaltered.
d. Impaired glucose tolerance.
e. Decreased pregnanediol excretion.
f. Reduced response to metyrapone test.
g. Reduced serum folate concentration.
h. Increased serum triglyceride and phospholipid concentration.

B. Information for the Patient. See text which appears after the PHYSICIAN REFERENCES.

C. Pregnancy Category X. See CONTRAINDICATIONS and Boxed Warning.

D. Nursing Mothers. As a general principle, the administration of any drug to nursing mothers should be done only when clearly necessary since many drugs are excreted in human milk.

Continued on next page

Ayerst—Cont.

Associated with Methyltestosterone
A. General Precautions
1. Women should be observed for signs of virilization (deepening of the voice, hirsutism, acne, clitoromegaly, and menstrual irregularities). Discontinuation of drug therapy at the time of evidence of mild virilism is necessary to prevent irreversible virilization. Such virilization is usual following androgen use at high doses.
2. Prolonged dosage of androgen may result in sodium and fluid retention. This may present a problem, especially in patients with compromised cardiac reserve or renal disease.
3. Hypersensitivity may occur rarely.
4. PBI may be decreased in patients taking androgens.
D. Hypercalcemia may occur. If this does occur, the drug should be discontinued.

B. Information for the Patient
The physician should instruct patients to report any of the following side effects of androgens:
Women: Hoarseness, acne, changes in menstrual periods, or more hair on the face.
All Patients: Any nausea, vomiting, changes in skin color or ankle swelling.

C. Laboratory Tests
1. Women with disseminated breast carcinoma should have frequent determination of urine and serum calcium levels during the course of androgen therapy (See WARNINGS).
2. Because of the hepatotoxicity associated with the use of 17-alpha-alkylated androgens, liver function tests should be obtained periodically.
3. Hemoglobin and hematocrit should be checked periodically for polycythemia in patients who are receiving high doses of androgens.

D. Drug Interactions
1. *Anticoagulants* C-17 substituted derivatives of testosterone, such as methandrostenolone, have been reported to decrease the anticoagulant requirements of patients receiving oral anticoagulants. Patients receiving oral anticoagulant therapy require close monitoring, especially when androgens are started or stopped.
2. *Oxyphenbutazone.* Concurrent administration of oxyphenbutazone and androgens may result in elevated serum levels of oxyphenbutazone.
3. *Insulin.* In diabetic patients the metabolic effects of androgens may decrease blood glucose and insulin requirements.

E. Drug/Laboratory Test Interferences
Androgens may decrease levels of thyroxine-binding globulin, resulting in decreased T_4 serum levels and increased resin uptake of T_3 and T_4. Free thyroid hormone levels remain unchanged, however, and there is no clinical evidence of thyroid dysfunction.

F. Carcinogenesis
Animal Data. Testosterone has been tested by subcutaneous injection and implantation in mice and rats. The implant induced cervical-uterine tumors in mice, which metastasized in some cases. There is suggestive evidence that injection of testosterone into some strains of female mice increases their susceptibility to hepatoma. Testosterone is also known to increase the number of tumors and decrease the degree of differentiation of chemically induced carcinomas of the liver in rats.
Human Data. There are rare reports of hepatocellular carcinoma in patients receiving long-term therapy with androgens in high doses. Withdrawal of the drugs did not lead to regression of the tumors in all cases.
Geriatric patients treated with androgens may be at an increased risk for the development of prostatic hypertrophy and prostatic carcinoma.

G. Pregnancy
Teratogenic Effects. Pregnancy Category X (see CONTRAINDICATIONS).

H. Nursing Mothers
It is not known whether androgens are excreted in human milk. Because many drugs are excreted in human milk and because of the potential for serious adverse reactions in nursing infants from androgens, a decision should be made whether to discontinue nursing or to discontinue the drug, taking into account the importance of the drug to the mother.

Adverse Reactions:
Associated with Estrogens
(See Warnings regarding induction of neoplasia, adverse effects on the fetus, increased incidence of gallbladder disease, and adverse effects similar to those of oral contraceptives, including thromboembolism.) The following additional adverse reactions have been reported with estrogenic therapy, including oral contraceptives.
1. *Genitourinary system:* Breakthrough bleeding, spotting, change in menstrual flow; dysmenorrhea; premenstrual-like syndrome; amenorrhea during and after treatment; increase in size of uterine fibromyomata; vaginal candidiasis; change in cervical erosion and in degree of cervical secretion; cystitis-like syndrome.
2. *Breasts:* Tenderness, enlargement, secretion.
3. *Gastrointestinal:* Nausea, vomiting; abdominal cramps, bloating; cholestatic jaundice.
4. *Skin:* Chloasma or melasma which may persist when drug is discontinued; erythema multiforme; erythema nodosum; hemorrhagic eruption; loss of scalp hair; hirsutism.
5. *Eyes:* Steepening of corneal curvature; intolerance to contact lenses.
6. *CNS:* Headache, migraine, dizziness; mental depression; chorea.
7. *Miscellaneous:* Increase or decrease in weight; reduced carbohydrate tolerance; aggravation of porphyria; edema; changes in libido.

Associated with Methyltestosterone
A. Endocrine and Urogenital
1. *Female:* The most common side effects of androgen therapy are amenorrhea and other menstrual irregularities, inhibition of gonadotropin secretion, and virilization, including deepening of the voice and clitoral enlargement. The latter usually is not reversible after androgens are discontinued. When administered to a pregnant woman androgens cause virilization of external genitalia of the female fetus.
2. *Skin and Appendages:* Hirsutism, male pattern of baldness, and acne.
3. *Fluid and Electrolyte Disturbances:* Retention of sodium, chloride, water, potassium, calcium, and inorganic phosphates.
4. *Gastrointestinal:* Nausea, cholestatic jaundice, alterations in liver function test, rarely hepatocellular neoplasms, and peliosis hepatis (see WARNINGS).
5. *Hematologic:* Suppression of clotting factors II, V, VII, and X, bleeding in patients on concomitant anticoagulant therapy, and polycythemia.
6. *Nervous System:* Increased or decreased libido, headache, anxiety, depression, and generalized paresthesia.
7. *Metabolic:* Increased serum cholesterol.
8. *Miscellaneous:* Inflammation and pain at the site of intramuscular injection or subcutaneous implantation of testosterone containing pellets, stomatitis with buccal preparations, and rarely anaphylactoid reactions.

Acute Overdosage: Numerous reports of ingestion of large doses of estrogen-containing oral contraceptives by young children indicate that acute serious ill effects do not occur. Overdosage of estrogen may cause nausea, and withdrawal bleeding may occur in females.
There have been no reports of acute overdosage with the androgens.

Dosage and Administration: *Given cyclically for short-term use only:*
For treatment of moderate to severe *vasomotor* symptoms associated with the menopause in patients not improved by estrogen alone.
The lowest dose that will control symptoms should be chosen and medication should be discontinued as promptly as possible.
Administration should be cyclic (e.g., three weeks on and one week off).
Attempts to discontinue or taper medication should be made at three to six month intervals.

Usual dosage range:
1.25 mg Conjugated Estrogens, U.S.P. and 10.0 mg Methyltestosterone (1 yellow tablet, No. 879, or 2 maroon tablets, No. 878) daily and cyclically.
Treated patients with an intact uterus should be monitored closely for signs of endometrial cancer and appropriate diagnostic measures should be taken to rule out malignancy in the event of persistent or recurring abnormal vaginal bleeding.

How Supplied: PREMARIN (Conjugated Estrogens, U.S.P.) with Methyltestosterone Tablets
—Each round *yellow* tablet contains 1.25 mg PREMARIN and 10.0 mg Methyltestosterone, in bottles of 100 (NDC 0046-0879-81) and 1,000 (NDC 0046-0879-91).
—Each round *maroon* tablet contains 0.625 mg PREMARIN and 5.0 mg Methyltestosterone, in bottles of 100 (NDC 0046-0878-81) and 1,000 (NDC 0046-0878-91).
The appearance of these tablets is a trademark of Ayerst Laboratories.
Store at room temperature (approximately 25°C).

Physician References:
1. Ziel, H. K., *et al:* N. Engl. J. Med. 293:1167–1170, 1975.
2. Smith, D. C., *et al:* N. Engl. J. Med. 293:1164–1167, 1975.
3. Mack, T. M., *et al:* N. Engl. J. Med. 294:1262–1267, 1976.
4. Weiss, N. S., *et al:* N. Engl. J. Med. 294:1259–1262, 1976.
5. Herbst, A. L., *et al:* N. Engl. J. Med. 284:878–881, 1971.
6. Greenwald, P., *et al:* N. Engl. J. Med. 285:390–392, 1971.
7. Lanier, A., *et al:* Mayo Clin. Proc. 48:793–799, 1973.
8. Herbst, A., *et al:* Obstet. Gynecol. 40:287–298, 1972.
9. Herbst, A., *et al:* Am. J. Obstet. Gynecol. 118:607–615, 1974.
10. Herbst, A., *et al:* N. Engl. J. Med. 292:334–339, 1975.
11. Stafl, A., *et al:* Obstet. Gynecol. 43:118–128, 1974.
12. Sherman, A. I., *et al:* Obstet. Gynecol. 44:531–545, 1974.
13. Gal, I., *et al:* Nature 216:83, 1967.
14. Levy, E. P., *et al:* Lancet 1:611, 1973.
15. Nora, J., *et al:* Lancet 1:941–942, 1973.
16. Janerich, D. T., *et al:* N. Engl. J. Med. 291:697–700, 1974.
17. Boston Collaborative Drug Surveillance Program: N. Engl. J. Med. 290:15–19, 1974.
18. Hoover, R., *et al:* N. Engl. J. Med. 295:401–405, 1976.
19. Boston Collaborative Drug Surveillance Program: Lancet 1:1399–1404, 1973.
20. Daniel, D. G., *et al:* Lancet 2:287–289, 1967.
21. The Veterans Administration Cooperative Urological Research Group: J. Urol. 98:516–522, 1967.
22. Bailar, J. C.: Lancet 2:560, 1967.
23. Blackard, C., *et al:* Cancer 26:249–256, 1970.
24. Royal College of General Practitioners: J. R. Coll. Gen. Pract. 13:267–279, 1967.
24a. Royal College of General Practitioners: Oral Contraceptives and Health, New York, Pitman Corp., 1974.
25. Inman, W. H. W., *et al:* Br. Med. J. 2:193–199, 1968.
26. Vessey, M. P., *et al:* Br. Med. J. 2:651–657, 1969.
27. Sartwell, P. E., *et al:* Am. J. Epidemiol. 90:365–380, 1969.
28. Collaborative Group for the Study of Stroke in Young Women: N. Engl. J. Med. 288:871–878, 1973.
29. Collaborative Group for the Study of Stroke in Young Women: J.A.M.A. 231:718–722, 1975.
30. Mann, J. I., *et al:* Br. Med. J. 2:245–248, 1975.
31. Mann, J. I., *et al:* Br. Med. J. 2:241–245, 1975.
32. Inman, W. H. W., *et al:* Br. Med. J. 2:203–209, 1970.
33. Stolley, P. D., *et al:* Am. J. Epidemiol. 102:197–208, 1975.

34. Vessey, M. P., et al.: Br. Med. J. 3:123–126, 1970.
35. Greene, G. R., et al.: Am. J. Public Health 62:680–685, 1972.
36. Rosenberg, L., et al.: N. Engl. J. Med. 294:1256–1259, 1976.
37. Coronary Drug Project Research Group: J.A.M.A. 214:1303–1313, 1970.
38. Baum, J., et al.: Lancet 2:926–928, 1973.
39. Mays, E. T., et al.: J.A.M.A. 235:730–732, 1976.
40. Edmondson, H. A., et al.: N. Engl. J. Med. 294:470–472, 1976.
41. Pfeffer, R. I., et al.: Am. J. Epidemiol. 103:445–456, 1976.

Androgen references available upon request.

INFORMATION FOR THE PATIENT
What You Should Know About Estrogens

Estrogens are female hormones produced by the ovaries. The ovaries make several different kinds of estrogens. In addition, scientists have been able to make a variety of synthetic estrogens. As far as we know, all these estrogens have similar properties and therefore much the same usefulness, side effects, and risks. This leaflet is intended to help you understand what estrogens are used for, the risks involved in their use, and how to use them as safely as possible.

This leaflet includes the most important information about estrogens, but not all the information. If you want to know more, you should ask your doctor for more information or you can ask your doctor or pharmacist to let you read the package insert prepared for the doctor.

Uses of Estrogen:
THERE IS NO PROPER USE OF ESTROGENS IN A PREGNANT WOMAN.

Estrogens are prescribed by doctors for a number of purposes, including:
1. To provide estrogen during a period of adjustment when a woman's ovaries stop producing a majority of her estrogens, in order to prevent certain uncomfortable symptoms of estrogen deficiency. (With the menopause, which generally occurs between the ages of 45 and 55, women produce a much smaller amount of estrogens.)
2. To prevent symptoms of estrogen deficiency when a woman's ovaries have been removed surgically before the natural menopause.
3. To prevent pregnancy. (Estrogens are given along with a progestogen, another female hormone; these combinations are called oral contraceptives or birth control pills. Patient labeling is available to women taking oral contraceptives and they will not be discussed in this leaflet.)
4. To treat certain cancers in women and men.
5. To prevent painful swelling of the breasts after pregnancy in women who choose not to nurse their babies.

Estrogens in the Menopause: In the natural course of their lives, all women eventually experience a decrease in estrogen production. This usually occurs between ages 45 and 55 but may occur earlier or later. Sometimes the ovaries may need to be removed before natural menopause by an operation, producing a "surgical menopause."

When the amount of estrogen in the blood begins to decrease, many women may develop typical symptoms: feeling of warmth in the face, neck, and chest or sudden intense episodes of heat and sweating throughout the body (called "hot flashes" or "hot flushes"). These symptoms are sometimes very uncomfortable. Some women may also develop changes in the vagina (called "atrophic vaginitis") which cause discomfort, especially during and after intercourse.

Estrogens can be prescribed to treat these symptoms of the menopause. It is estimated that considerably more than half of all women undergoing the menopause have only mild symptoms or no symptoms at all and therefore do not need estrogens. Other women may need estrogens for a few months, while their bodies adjust to lower estrogen levels. Sometimes the need will be for periods longer than six months. In an attempt to avoid overstimulation of the uterus (womb), estrogens are usually given cyclically during each month of use, such as three weeks of pills followed by one week without pills.

Sometimes women experience nervous symptoms or depression during menopause. There is no evidence that estrogens are effective for such symptoms without associated vasomotor symptoms. In the absence of vasomotor symptoms, estrogens should not be used to treat nervous symptoms, although other treatment may be needed.

You may have heard that taking estrogens for long periods (years) after the menopause will keep your skin soft and supple and keep you feeling young. There is no evidence that this is so, however, and such long-term treatment carries important risks.

Estrogens to Prevent Swelling of the Breasts After Pregnancy: If you do not breast-feed your baby after delivery, your breasts may fill up with milk and become painful and engorged. This usually begins about 3 to 4 days after delivery and may last for a few days to up to a week or more. Sometimes the discomfort is severe, but usually it is not and can be controlled by pain-relieving drugs such as aspirin and by binding the breasts up tightly. Estrogens can be used to try to prevent the breasts from filling up. While this treatment is sometimes successful, in many cases the breasts fill up to some degree in spite of treatment. The dose of estrogens needed to prevent pain and swelling of the breasts is much larger than the dose needed to treat symptoms of the menopause and this may increase your chances of developing blood clots in the legs or lungs (see below). Therefore, it is important that you discuss the benefits and the risks of estrogen use with your doctor if you have decided not to breast-feed your baby.

The Dangers of Estrogens:

1. *Endometrial cancer.* There are reports that if estrogens are used in the postmenopausal period for more than a year, there is an increased risk of *endometrial cancer* (cancer of the lining of the uterus). Women taking estrogens have roughly 5 to 10 times as great a chance of getting this cancer as women who take no estrogens. To put this another way, while a postmenopausal woman not taking estrogens has a 1 chance in 1,000 each year of getting endometrial cancer, a woman taking estrogens has 5 to 10 chances in 1,000 each year. For this reason *it is important to take estrogens only when they are really needed.*

The risk of this cancer is greater the longer estrogens are used and when larger doses are taken. Therefore you should not take more estrogen than your doctor prescribes. *It is important to take the lowest dose of estrogen that will control symptoms and to take it only as long as it is needed.* If estrogens are needed for longer periods of time, your doctor will want to reevaluate your need for estrogens at least every six months.

Women using estrogens should report any vaginal bleeding to their doctors; such bleeding may be of no importance, but it can be an early warning of endometrical cancer. If you have undiagnosed vaginal bleeding, you should not use estrogens until a diagnosis is made and you are certain there is no endometrial cancer.

NOTE: If you have had your uterus removed (total hysterectomy), there is no danger of developing endometrial cancer.

2. *Other possible cancers.* Estrogens can cause development of other tumors in animals, such as tumors of the breast, cervix, vagina, or liver, when given for a long time. At present there is no good evidence that women using estrogen in the menopause have an increased risk of such tumors, but there is no way yet to be sure they do not; and one study raises the possibility that use of estrogens in the menopause may increase the risk of breast cancer many years later. This is a further reason to use estrogens only when clearly needed. While you are taking estrogens, it is important that you go to your doctor at least once a year for a physical examination. Also, if members of your family have had breast cancer or if you have breast nodules or abnormal mammograms (breast x-rays), your doctor may wish to carry out more frequent examinations of your breasts.

3. *Gallbladder disease.* Women who use estrogens after menopause are more likely to develop gallbladder disease needing surgery than women who do not use estrogens. Birth control pills have a similar effect.

4. *Abnormal blood clotting.* Oral contraceptives increase the risk of blood clotting in various parts of the body. This can result in a stroke (if the clot is in the brain), a heart attack (clot in a blood vessel of the heart), or a pulmonary embolus (a clot which forms in the legs or pelvis, then breaks off and travels to the lungs). Any of these can be fatal.

At this time use of estrogens in the menopause is not known to cause such blood clotting, but this has not been fully studied and there could still prove to be such a risk. It is recommended that if you have had clotting in the legs or lungs or a heart attack or stroke while you were using estrogens or birth control pills, you should not use estrogens (unless they are being used to treat cancer of the breast or prostate). If you have had a stroke or heart attack or if you have angina pectoris, estrogens should be used with great caution and only if clearly needed (for example, if you have severe symptoms of the menopause).

The larger doses of estrogen used to prevent swelling of the breasts after pregnancy have been reported to cause clotting in the legs and lungs.

Special Warning About Pregnancy: You should not receive estrogen if you are pregnant. If this should occur, there is a greater than usual chance that the developing child will be born with a birth defect, although the possibility remains fairly small. A female child may have an increased risk of developing cancer of the vagina or cervix later in life (in the teens or twenties). Every possible effort should be made to avoid exposure to estrogens during pregnancy. If exposure occurs, see your doctor.

Other Effects of Estrogens: In addition to the serious known risks of estrogens described above, estrogens have the following side effects and potential risks:

1. *Nausea and vomiting.* The most common side effect of estrogen therapy is nausea. Vomiting is less common.
2. *Effects on breasts.* Estrogens may cause breast tenderness or enlargement and may cause the breasts to secrete a liquid. These effects are not dangerous.
3. *Effects on the uterus.* Estrogens may cause benign fibroid tumors of the uterus to get larger.
4. *Effects on liver.* Women taking oral contraceptives develop on rare occasions a tumor of the liver which can rupture and bleed into the abdomen and may cause death. So far, these tumors have not been reported in women using estrogens in the menopause, but you should report any swelling or unusual pain or tenderness in the abdomen to your doctor immediately.

Women with a past history of jaundice (yellowing of the skin and white parts of the eyes) may get jaundice again during estrogen use. If this occurs, stop taking estrogens and see your doctor.

5. *Other effects.* Estrogens may cause excess fluid to be retained in the body. This may make some conditions worse, such as asthma, epilepsy, migraine, heart disease, or kidney disease.

Summary: Estrogens have important uses, but they have serious risks as well. You must decide, with your doctor, whether the risks are acceptable to you in view of the benefits of treatment. Except where your doctor has prescribed estrogens for use in special cases of cancer of the breast or prostrate, you should not use estrogens if you have cancer of the breast or uterus, are pregnant, have undiagnosed abnormal vaginal bleeding, clotting in the legs or lungs, or have had a stroke, heart attack or angina, or clotting in the legs or lungs in the past while you were taking estrogens.

You can use estrogens as safely as possible by understanding that your doctor will require physical examinations while you are taking them and will try to discontinue the drug as soon as possible and use the smallest dose possible. Be alert for signs of trouble including:

Continued on next page

Ayerst—Cont.

1. Abnormal bleeding from the vagina.
2. Pains in the calves or chest or sudden shortness of breath, or coughing blood.
3. Severe headache, dizziness, faintness, or changes in vision.
4. Breast lumps (you should ask your doctor how to examine your own breasts).
5. Jaundice (yellowing of the skin).
6. Mental depression.

Your doctor has prescribed this drug for you and you alone. Do not give the drug to anyone else.

How Supplied: PREMARIN® (Conjugated Estrogens Tablets, U.S.P.)—tablets for oral administration.
  Each oval *purple* tablet contains 2.5 mg
  Each oval *yellow* tablet contains 1.25 mg
  Each oval *white* tablet contains 0.9 mg
  Each oval *maroon* tablet contains 0.625 mg
  Each oval *green* tablet contains 0.3 mg

PREMARIN® with METHYLTESTOSTERONE—a combination of PREMARIN and methyltestosterone (an androgen) in tablet form for oral administration.
  Each round *yellow* tablet contains 1.25 mg PREMARIN and 10 mg methyltestosterone
  Each round *maroon* tablet contains 0.625 mg PREMARIN and 5 mg methyltestosterone

PMB® 200, 400—a combination of PREMARIN® and meprobamate (a tranquilizing agent) in tablet form for oral administration.
  Each oblong *green* tablet contains 0.45 mg PREMARIN and 200 mg meprobamate
  Each oblong *pink* tablet contains 0.45 mg PREMARIN and 400 mg meprobamate

The appearance of these tablets is a trademark of Ayerst Laboratories.

PREMARIN® VAGINAL CREAM—PREMARIN® in a nonliquefying base, designed for vaginal use.

PREMARIN® INTRAVENOUS—PREMARIN® specially prepared for intravenous and intramuscular use.

ESTROGENIC SUBSTANCE (Estrone) in Aqueous Suspension—a sterile aqueous suspension of estrone, a short-acting estroge, for intramuscular injection only.

Shown in Product Identification Section, page 405

PROTOPAM® CHLORIDE ℞
[prō″ tō-pam klaw′ rīde]
Brand of pralidoxime chloride

Caution: Federal law prohibits dispensing without prescription.

Description: PROTOPAM CHLORIDE (pralidoxime chloride) is a cholinesterase reactivator. Chemically, it is 2-formyl-1-methylpyridinium chloride oxime (pyridine-2-aldoxime methochloride), and has the generic name pralidoxime chloride. It has also been referred to as 2-PAM Chloride.

The chemical structure is:

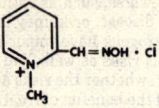

PROTOPAM CHLORIDE occurs as a white, nonhygroscopic, crystalline powder which is soluble in water to the extent of 1 g in less than 1 ml.

The specific activity of the drug resides in the 2-formyl-1-methylpyridinium ion and is independent of the particular salt employed.

Actions: The principal action of PROTOPAM (pralidoxime) is to reactivate cholinesterase (mainly outside of the central nervous system) which has been inactivated by phosphorylation due to an organophosphate pesticide or related compound. The destruction of accumulated acetylcholine can then proceed and neuromuscular junctions will again function normally. PROTOPAM also slows the process of "aging" of phosphorylated cholinesterase to a non-reactivatable form, and detoxifies certain organophosphates by direct chemical reaction. The drug has its most critical effect in relieving paralysis of the muscles of respiration. Because PROTOPAM is less effective in relieving depression of the respiratory center, atropine is always required concomitantly to block the effect of accumulated acetylcholine at this site. PROTOPAM relieves muscarinic signs and symptoms, salivation, bronchospasm, etc., but this action is relatively unimportant since atropine is adequate for this purpose.

PROTOPAM antagonizes the effects on the neuromuscular junction of the carbamate anticholinesterases, neostigmine, pyridostigmine and ambenonium, used in the treatment of myasthenia gravis. However, it is not nearly as effective as an antidote to these drugs as it is to the organophosphates.

PROTOPAM (pralidoxime) is distributed throughout the extracellular water; it is not bound to plasma protein. The drug is rapidly excreted in the urine partly unchanged, and partly as a metabolite produced by the liver. Consequently, PROTOPAM is relatively short acting and repeated doses may be needed, especially where there is any evidence of continuing absorption of the poison.

Indications: PROTOPAM is indicated as an antidote: (1) in the treatment of poisoning due to those pesticides and chemicals of the organophosphate class which have anticholinesterase activity, and (2) in the control of overdosage by anticholinesterase drugs used in the treatment of myasthenia gravis.

Warnings: Use of PROTOPAM should always be under supervision of the subject's personal physician or of the medical department of his employer. PROTOPAM is not effective in the treatment of poisoning due to phosphorus, inorganic phosphates or organophosphates not having anticholinesterase activity.

Until further information is available, no recommendation is made as to the use of PROTOPAM in intoxication by pesticides of the carbamate class.

Precautions: PROTOPAM (pralidoxime) has been very well tolerated in most cases, but it must be remembered that the desperate condition of the organophosphate-poisoned patient will generally mask such minor signs and symptoms as have been noted in normal subjects.

Intravenous administration of PROTOPAM should be carried out slowly and, preferably, by infusion, since certain side effects, such as tachycardia, laryngospasm, and muscle rigidity, have been attributed in a few cases to a too rapid rate of injection. (See Dosage and Administration.)

Because PROTOPAM is excreted in the urine, a decrease in renal function will result in increased blood levels of the drug. Thus, the dosage of PROTOPAM should be reduced in the presence of renal insufficiency.

PROTOPAM should be used with great caution in treating organophosphate overdosage in cases of myasthenia gravis since it may precipitate a myasthenic crisis.

The following precautions should be kept in mind in the treatment of anticholinesterase poisoning, although they do not bear directly on the use of PROTOPAM (pralidoxime): since barbiturates are potentiated by the anticholinesterases, they should be used cautiously in the treatment of convulsions; morphine, theophylline, aminophylline, succinylcholine, reserpine, and phenothiazine-type tranquilizers should be avoided in patients with organophosphate poisoning.

Adverse Reactions: Dizziness, blurred vision, diplopia and impaired accommodation, headache, drowsiness, nausea, tachycardia, hyperventilation, and muscular weakness have been reported after the use of PROTOPAM, but it is very difficult to differentiate the toxic effects produced by atropine or the organophosphate compounds from those of the drug. When atropine and PROTOPAM are used together, the signs of atropinization may occur earlier than might be expected when atropine is used alone. This is especially true if the total dose of atropine has been large and the administration of PROTOPAM has been delayed. Excitement and manic behavior immediately following recovery of consciousness have been reported in several cases. However, similar behavior has occurred in cases of organophosphate poisoning that were not treated with PROTOPAM.

Dosage and Administration:
Organophosphate poisoning

Initial measures should include removal of secretions, maintenance of a patent airway and, if necessary, artificial ventilation.

In the absence of cyanosis, atropine should be given intravenously in doses of 2 to 4 mg; where cyanosis is present, this dose of atropine should be given intramuscularly while simultaneously initiating measures for improving ventilation. Atropine administration should be repeated at 5 to 10 minute intervals until signs of atropine toxicity appear. Some degree of atropinization should be maintained for at least 48 hours.

PROTOPAM (pralidoxime) administration should be started at the same time as atropine.

In adults, inject an initial dose of 1 to 2 g of PROTOPAM (pralidoxime), preferably as an infusion in 100 ml of saline, over a 15 to 30 minute period. If this is not practicable or if pulmonary edema is present, the dose should be given slowly by intravenous injection as a 5 percent solution in water over not less than five minutes. After about an hour, a second dose of 1 to 2 g will be indicated if muscle weakness has not been relieved. Additional doses may be given cautiously if muscle weakness persists. If intravenous administration is not feasible, intramuscular or subcutaneous injection should be used.

In children, the dose should be 20 to 40 mg per kg. Treatment will be most effective if given within a few hours after poisoning has occurred. Usually, little will be accomplished if the drug is first administered more than 48 hours after exposure, but in severe poisoning, it is, nevertheless, indicated since occasionally patients have responded after such an interval.

In severe cases, especially after ingestion of the poison, it may be desirable to monitor the effect of therapy electrocardiographically because of the possibility of heart block due to the anticholinesterase. Where the poison has been ingested, it is particularly important to take into account the likelihood of continuing absorption from the lower bowel since this constitutes new exposure. In such cases, additional doses of PROTOPAM (pralidoxime) may be needed every three to eight hours. In effect, the patient should be "titrated" with PROTOPAM as long as signs of poisoning recur.

In the absence of severe gastrointestinal symptoms, resulting from the anticholinesterase intoxication, PROTOPAM (pralidoxime) may be administered orally in doses of 1 to 3 g (2 to 6 tablets) every five hours. As in all cases of organophosphate poisoning, care should be taken to keep the patient under observation for at least 24 hours.

If convulsions interfere with respiration, sodium thiopental (2.5 percent solution) may be given intravenously with care.

Anticholinesterase overdosage

As an antagonist to such anticholinesterases as neostigmine, pyridostigmine, and ambenonium, which are used in the treatment of myasthenia gravis, PROTOPAM may be given in a dosage of 1 to 2 g intravenously followed by increments of 250 mg every five minutes.

Overdosage: Artificial respiration and other supportive therapy should be administered as needed.

How Supplied: NDC 0046-0375-98—*Emergency Kit:* This contains one 20 ml vial of 1 g of sterile PROTOPAM CHLORIDE (pralidoxime chloride) white to off white porous cake*; one 20 ml ampul of Sterile Water for Injection, U.S.P. without preservative to be used as diluent; sterile, disposable 20 ml syringe; needle; alcohol swab. This is a single dose kit for intravenous administration. Intramuscular or subcutaneous injection may be used when intravenous injection is not feasible.

NDC 0046-0374-06—*Hospital Package:* This contains six 20 ml vials of 1 g each of sterile PROTOPAM CHLORIDE (pralidoxime chloride) white to off white porous cake*, without diluent or syringe. Solution may be prepared by adding 20 ml of Sterile Water for Injection, U.S.P. These are single dose vials for intravenous injection or for intravenous infusion after further dilution with physiologic saline. Intramuscular or subcutaneous injection may be used when intravenous injection is not feasible.

*When necessary, sodium hydroxide is added during processing to adjust the pH.

PROTOPAM CHLORIDE for Injection is prepared by cryodesiccation.
NDC 0046-0376-81—*Tablets:* Each tablet contains 500 mg of pralidoxime chloride, in bottles of 100.

A FULL DISCUSSION OF THE ACTIONS AND USES OF PROTOPAM (PRALIDOXIME) IS GIVEN IN A PROFESSIONAL BROCHURE WHICH IS AVAILABLE FROM AYERST LABORATORIES ON REQUEST.

Animal Pharmacology and Toxicology:
The following table lists chemical and trade or generic names of pesticides, chemicals, and drugs against which PROTOPAM (usually administered in conjunction with atropine) has been found to have antidotal activity on the basis of animal experiments. All compounds listed are organophosphates having anticholinesterase activity. A great many additional substances are in industrial use but have been omitted because of lack of specific information. The use of PROTOPAM should, nevertheless, be considered in any life-threatening situation resulting from poisoning by these compounds, since the limited and arbitrary conditions of pharmacologic screening do not always accurately reflect the usefulness of PROTOPAM (pralidoxime) in the clinical situation.

AAT—see PARATHION

AFLIX®—see FORMOTHION

ALKRON®—see PARATHION

AMERICAN CYANAMID 3422—see PARATHION

AMITON—diethyl -S- (2-diethyl-aminoethyl) phosphorothiolate

ANTHIO®—see FORMOTHION

APHAMITE—see PARATHION

ARMIN—ethyl-4-nitrophenyl-ethylphosphonate

AZINPHOS-METHYL—dimethyl-S- (4-oxo-1, 2, 3, -benzotriazin-3 (4 H) -ylmethyl) phosphorodithioate

AZODRIN—dimethyl phosphate of 3-hydroxy-N-methyl-cis-crotonamide

BAYER 16259—see ETHYL GUTHION

BAYER 19639—see DISULFOTON

BAYER 25141 — diethyl-4-methyl-sulfinyl- phenylphosphorothionate

BAYER 29493—see FENTHION

BAYER L13/59—see TRICHLOROFON

BAYER E605—see PARATHION

BAYTEX®—see FENTHION

CHIPMAN R6199—see AMITON

COMPOUND 3422—see PARATHION

COMPOUND 4049—see MALATHION

COMPOUND 4072—2-chloro-1-(2,4-dichloro- phenyl) vinyl diethyl-phosphate

CO-RAL®—see COUMAPHOS

COROTHION—see PARATHION

COUMAPHOS—3-chloro-4-methyl coumarin-7-yl-diethyl-phosphorothionate

DBD —see AZINPHOS-METHYL

DDVP—see DICHLORVOS

DELNAV—see DIOXATHION

DEMETON—Mixture of SYSTOX® and ISOSYSTOX®

DEMETON-S—see ISOSYSTOX®

DFP—see ISOFLUROPHATE

DIAZINON—diethyl- (2- isopropyl -4- methyl -6- pyrimidyl) phosphorothionate

DICHLORVOS—dimethyl-2, 2-dichloro vinyl phosphate

DIETHYL-p-NITROPHENYL-PHOSPHOROTHIONATE—see PARATHION

DIETHYL -p- NITROPHENYL - THIONO- PHOSPHATE—see PARATHION

DIOXATHION—2, 3-p-dioxanedithio-S, S-bis (0, 0-diethyl phosphorodithioate)

DIPTEREX®—see TRICHLOROFON

DISULFOTON—diethyl -S- (2-ethylthioethyl) phosphorodiothiate

DISYSTON®—see DISULFOTON

DITHIOSYSTOX—see DISULFOTON

DNTP—see PARATHION

DPP—see PARATHION

DSDP—see AMITON

DYFLOS—see DFP

DYLOX®—see TRICHLOROFON

E 600—see PARAOXON

E 601—see METHYL PARATHION

E 605—see PARATHION

E 1059—see SYSTOX

ECHOTHIOPHATE IODIDE—diethoxyphosphinylthio-choline iodide

EKATIN®—see MORPHOTHION

ENDOTHION—2- (dimethoxyphosphinylthiomethyl)-5-methoxy-4-pyrone

ENT 15108—see PARATHION

ENTEX®—see FENTHION

EPN—ethyl -4- nitrophenyl - phenylphosphonothionate

ETHION—0,0,0',0'-tetraethyl-S,S'-methylene-bis-phosphoro dithioate

ETHYL GUSATHION—see ETHYL GUTHION

ETHYL GUTHION®—diethyl-S-(4-oxo-1,2,3,-benzotriazinyl-3-methyl) phosphorodithioate

ETILON—see PARATHION

FENTHION—dimethyl-(4-methylthio-3-tolyl) phosphorothionate

FLOROPRYL®—see DFP

FOLIDOL®—see PARATHION

FORMOTHION—dimethyl -S- (N-formyl -N- methylcarbamyl-methyl) phosphorodithioate

G 24480—see DIAZINON

GB—see SARIN

GENITHION—see PARATHION

GUSATHION®—see AZINPHOSMETHYL

GUTHION®—see AZINPHOSMETHYL

HETP—see TEPP

I-ARMIN—isopropyl -4- nitro-phenyl methyl-phosphonate

ISOFLUROPHATE—diisopropyl - phosphorofluoridate

ISOSYSTOX®— diethyl-S-(2-ethylmercapto-ethyl)-phosphorothiolate

LEBACYD®—see FENTHION

MACKOTHION—see PARATHION

MALATHION—dimethyl -S- (1, 2-dicarbeth- oxyethyl) -phosphorodithioate

MALATHON—see MALATHION

M-ARMIN—ethyl-4-nitrophenyl methylphosphonate

MECARBAM—0, 0-dimethyl -S- (N-ethoxycarbonyl-N-methyl carbamoylmethyl) phosphorodithioate

METACIDE—see METHYL PARATHION

METASYSTOX®—see METHYL DEMETON

METASYSTOX I®—dimethyl -2- ethyl-mercapto-ethylphos-phorothiolate

METASYSTOX R®— see OXYDEMETON-METHYL

METHYL DEMETON—mixture of dimethyl(2-ethylmercapto-ethyl) phosphorothionate and di-methyl-S-(2-ethylmercapto-ethyl) phosphorothiolate

METHYL PARATHION—dimethyl - (4-ni- trophenyl) phosphorothionate

MEVINPHOS—1- carbomethoxy-1- propen-2- yl-dimethylphosphate

MINTACOL®—see PARAOXON

ML 97—see PHOSPHAMIDON

MORPHOTHION—dimethyl -S- 2-keto-2- (N-morpholyl ethyl-phosphorodithioate

NEGUVON®—see TRICHLOROFON

NIRAN®—see PARATHION

NITROSTIGMINE—see PARATHION

0, 0-DIETHYL -O- p-NITRO-PHENYL PHOSPHOROTHIOATE—see PARATHION

Continued on next page

Ayerst—Cont.

0, 0-DIETHYL -O- p-NITRO-PHENYLTHIO-PHOSPHATE —see PARATHION

OR 1191—see PHOSPHAMIDON

OS 1836—see VINYLPHOS

OXYDEMETONMETHYL—dimethyl -S- 2- (ethylsulfinyl) ethyl phosphorothiolate

PARAOXON—diethyl (4 - nitro - phenyl) phosphate.

PARATHION—diethyl (4-nitro-phenyl) phosphorothionate

PENPHOS—see PARATHION

PHENCAPTON—diethyl -S- (2, 5-dichloro- phenylmercaptomethyl) phosphorodithioate

PHOSDRIN®—see MEVINPHOS

PHOS-KIL—see PARATHION

PHOSPHAMIDON—1-chloro -1- diethylcar- bamoyl -1- propen -2- yl-dimethylphosphate

PHOSPHOLINE IODIDE®—see echothiophate iodide

PHOSPHOROTHIOIC ACID, 0,0-DIETHYL-0-p-NITRO-PHENYL ESTER—see PARATHION

PLANTHION—see PARATHION

QUELETOX—see FENTHION

RHODIATOX®—see PARATHION

RUELENE®— 4- tert-butyl -2- chlorophenylmethyl-N-methyl-phosphoroamidate

SARIN— isopropyl - methylphos - phonofluo- ridate

SHELL OS 1836—see VINYLPHOS

SHELL 2046—see MEVINPHOS

SNP—see PARATHION

SOMAN—pinacolyl - methyl - phosphonofluoridate

SYSTOX®—diethyl - (2-ethyl-mercaptoethyl) phosphorothionate

TEP—see TEPP

TEPP—tetraethylpyro phosphate

THIOPHOS®—see PARATHION

TIGUVON—see FENTHION

TRICHLOROFON—dimethyl -1- hydroxy-2, 2, 2-trichloro ethylphosphonate

VAPONA®— see DICHLORVOS

VAPOPHOS—see PARATHION

VINYLPHOS—diethyl -2- chloro - vinylphosphate

PROTOPAM appears to be ineffective, or marginally effective, against poisoning by:
CIODRIN® (alpha-methylbenzyl-3-[dimeth- oxyphosphinyloxy]-cis-crotonate)
DIMEFOX (tetramethylphosphorodiamidic fluoride)
DIMETHOATE (dimethyl-S-[N-methylcarbamoylmethyl]phosphorodithioate)
METHYL DIAZINON (dimethyl-[2-isopropyl-4-methylpyrimidyl]-phosphorothionate)
METHYL PHENCAPTON (dimethyl-S- [2, 5-dichlorophenylmercaptomethyl] phosphorodithioate)
PHORATE (diethyl-S-ethylmercaptomethyl- phosphorodithioate)
SCHRADAN (octamethylpyrophosphoramide)
WEPSYN® (5-amino-1-[bis-(dimethylamino)phosphinyl]-3-phenyl-1,2,4-triazole)

Clinical Studies: The use of PROTOPAM (pralidoxime) has been reported in the treatment of human cases of poisoning by the following substances:
    Azodrin
    Diazinon
    Dichlorvos (DDVP) with chlordane
    Disulfoton
    EPN
    Isoflurophate
    Malathion
    Metasystox I® and Fenthion
    Methyl demeton
    Methyl parathion
    Mevinphos
    Parathion
    Parathion and Mevinphos
    Phosphamidon
    Sarin
    Systox®
    TEPP

Of these cases, over 100 were due to parathion, about a dozen each to malathion, diazinon, and mevinphos, and a few to each of the other compounds.

RIOPAN®
[rī′opan]
magaldrate
Antacid

RIOPAN is a chemical entity (not a physical mixture), providing the advantages of a true buffer-antacid (not simply a neutralizing agent): (1) rapid action; (2) uniform buffering action; (3) high acid-consuming capacity; (4) no alkalinization or acid rebound.

Each teaspoonful (5 ml) of Suspension contains:
Magaldrate ....540 mg.
Each Chew Tablet contains:
Magaldrate ....480 mg.
Each Swallow Tablet contains:
Magaldrate ....480 mg.

Low Sodium Content: Not more than 0.1 mg (0.004 mEq) of sodium—per teaspoonful (5 ml) suspension—per chew tablet—per swallow tablet.
Acid-neutralizing Capacity—15.0 mEq/5 ml. 13.5 mEq per tablet.
Indications: For the relief of heartburn, sour stomach, acid indigestion and upset stomach associated with these symptoms. For symptomatic relief of hyperacidity associated with the diagnosis of peptic ulcer, gastritis, peptic esophagitis, gastric hyperacidity, and hiatal hernia.
Directions: RIOPAN (magaldrate) Antacid *Suspension*—Recommended dosage, one or two teaspoonfuls, between meals and at bedtime, or as directed by the physician. RIOPAN Antacid *Chew Tablets*—Recommended dosage, one or two tablets, between meals and at bedtime, or as directed by the physician. Chew before swallowing. RIOPAN Antacid *Swallow Tablets*—Recommended dosage, one or two tablets, between meals and at bedtime, or as directed by the physician. Take with enough water to swallow promptly.
Drug Interaction Precaution: Do not use in patients taking a prescription antibiotic drug containing any form of tetracycline.
Warnings: Patients should not take more than 18 teaspoonfuls or 20 tablets in a 24-hour period or use this maximum dosage for more than two weeks, except under the advice and supervision of a physician. If you have kidney disease, do not use this product except under the advice and supervision of a physician.
How Supplied: RIOPAN Antacid *Suspension* in 12 fl oz (355 ml) plastic bottles (NDC 0046-0765-12). Individual Cups, 1 fl oz (30 ml) ea., tray of 10—10 trays per packer (NDC 0046-0765-99). RIOPAN Antacid *Chew Tablets*—in bottles of 60 (NDC 0046-0928-59) and 100 (NDC 0046-0928-80) boxes of 60 (NDC 0046-0928-60) and 100 (NDC 0046-0928-81) in individual film strips (10 × 6 and 10 × 10, respectively). Also, single rollpacks of 12 tablets (NDC 0046-0941-12) and 3-roll rollpacks of 36 tablets (NDC 0046-0941-36). RIOPAN Antacid *Swallow Tablets*—Boxes of 60 (NDC 0046-0927-60) and 100 (NDC 0046-0927-81) in individual film strips (6 × 10 and 10 × 10, respectively).
Shown in Product Identification Section, page 405

RIOPAN PLUS®
[rī′opan]
magaldrate and SIMETHICONE
Antacid/Anti-Gas

Each teaspoonful (5 ml) of Suspension contains:
Magaldrate ....540 mg
Simethicone ....20 mg
Each Chew Tablet contains:
Magaldrate ....480 mg
Simethicone ....20 mg
Low Sodium Content: Not more than 0.1 mg (0.004 mEq) per teaspoonful (5 ml) or Chew Tablet.
Acid-neutralizing Capacity—15.0 mEq/5 ml. 13.5 mEq per tablet.
Indications: For the relief of heartburn, sour stomach, acid indigestion and upset stomach associated with these symptoms, accompanied by the symptoms of gas. For a symptomatic relief of hyperacidity associated with the diagnosis of peptic ulcer, gastritis, peptic esophagitis, gastric hyperacidity, and hiatal hernia. For postoperative gas pain or for use in endoscopic examinations.
Directions: RIOPAN PLUS (magaldrate and SIMETHICONE) Antacid/Anti-Gas *Suspension*—Recommended dosage, one or two teaspoonfuls between meals and at bedtime, or as directed by the physician.
RIOPAN PLUS Antacid/Anti-Gas *Chew Tablets*—Recommended dosage, one or two tablets, between meals and at bedtime, or as directed by the physician. Chew before swallowing.
Drug Interaction Precaution: Do not use in patients taking a prescription antibiotic drug containing any form of tetracycline.
Warnings: Patients should not take more than 18 teaspoonfuls or 20 tablets in a 24-hour period or use this maximum dosage for more than two weeks, except under the advice and supervision of a physician. If you have kidney disease, do not use this product except under the advice and supervision of a physician.
How Supplied: RIOPAN PLUS Antacid/Anti-Gas *Suspension*—in 12 fl oz (355 ml) plastic bottles (NDC 0046-0768-12) and 6 fl oz (176 ml) plastic bottles (NDC 0046-0768-06). Individual Cups, 1 fl oz (30 ml) ea., tray of 10—10 trays per packer (NDC 0046-0768-99).
RIOPAN PLUS Antacid *Chew Tablets*—in bottles of 60 (NDC 0046-0930-60) and 100 (NDC 0046-0930-80). Also single rollpacks of 12 Antacid tablets (NDC 0046-0930-12) and 3-roll rollpacks of 36 tablets (NDC 0046-0930-36).
Shown in Product Identification Section, page 405

THIOSULFIL® FORTE ℞
[thī′′o-sul′fil]
(sulfamethizole 500 mg with phenazopyridine HCl)
THIOSULFIL®
(sulfamethizole 250 with phenazopyridine HCl)
Bacteriostatic agent for use in Urinary Tract Infection (due to susceptible organisms)

Description: Chemical name: N′-(5-Methyl-1,3,4-thiadiazol-2-yl) sulfanilamide.
Structural formula:

$$H_2N-\underset{}{\underset{}{\bigcirc}}-SO_2-NH-\underset{S}{\overset{N-N}{C}}-CH_3$$

Sulfamethizole is a 5-membered heterocyclic sulfanilamide, occurring as a white or light buff-colored crystalline powder. Solubility in water is dependent upon the pH (1 g/5 ml at pH 7.5; 1 g/4000 ml at pH 6.5). It is soluble in alcohol, and practically insoluble in benzene.

Actions:
Mechanism of sulfonamide bacteriostatic action: The primary mechanism of bacteriostatic action by THIOSULFIL (sulfamethizole) is the same as that of most sulfonamides. By competing with the precursor para-aminobenzoic acid, sulfonamides inhibit bacterial synthesis of folic (pteroylglutamic) acid which is required for bacterial growth. Resistant strains are capable of utilizing folic acid precursors or preformed folic acid.

Antibacterial spectrum: The antibacterial spectrum of all sulfonamides is similar. *In vitro* sensitivity of bacteria to sulfonamides does not always reflect *in vivo* sensitivity. Therefore, efficacy must be carefully evaluated with bacteriologic and clinical responses in the individual patient. (See Warnings)

Factors determining efficacy: Efficacy of antimicrobial therapy is dependent upon a number of factors including the *in vivo* sensitivity of the involved organisms, the concentration of the drug required for bacteriostasis, and the achievable concentration of the sulfonamide at the desired site of action.

Because of the very rapid renal clearance of sulfamethizole, the blood levels attained are low, and accumulation of the drug in tissues outside the urinary tract is very limited. Therefore, sulfamethizole is not appropriate for treatment of systemic infections such as nocardiosis or for local lesions outside the urinary tract such as chancroid and trachoma. However, its low degree of acetylation and its rapid renal clearance permit high concentrations of active sulfamethizole to occur in the urinary tract, making it especially applicable for the treatment of infections of this tract. In addition, the possibility of crystalluria is minimized because of the high solubility of the drug in urine. Approximately 95 per cent of a given dose of sulfamethizole is not metabolized; less than 5 per cent is acetylated. As a consequence, almost all of a given dose of THIOSULFIL (sulfamethizole) is present in its active form in the body.

Approximately 80 per cent of an administered dose is recoverable within eight hours; approximately 98 per cent is cleared within 15 to 24 hours. Sulfamethizole is cleared by the kidney at a rate only 10 to 20 per cent lower than that for creatinine.

Indications: THIOSULFIL (sulfamethizole) is indicated in the treatment of urinary tract infections (primarily pyelonephritis, pyelitis, and cystitis) in the absence of obstructive uropathy or foreign bodies, when these infections are caused by susceptible strains of the following organisms: *Escherichia coli, Klebsiella-Enterobacter, Staphylococcus aureus, Proteus mirabilis,* and *Proteus vulgaris.*

Important note, *In vitro* sulfonamide sensitivity tests are not always reliable. The test must be carefully coordinated with bacteriologic and clinical reponse. When the patient is already taking sulfonamides, follow-up cultures should have aminobenzoic acid added to the culture media.

Currently, the increasing frequency of resistant organisms is a limitation of the usefulness of antibacterial agents, including the sulfonamides, especially in the treatment of recurrent and complicated urinary tract infections.

Wide variation in blood levels may result with identical doses. Blood levels should be measured in patients receiving sulfonamides for serious infections. Free sulfonamide blood levels of 5–15 mg per 100 ml may be considered therapeutically effective for most infections, with blood levels of 12–15 mg per 100 ml optimal for serious infections; 20 mg per 100 ml should be the maximum total sulfonamide level, as adverse reactions occur more frequently above this level.

Contraindications: Sulfonamides should not be used in patients hypersensitive to sulfa drugs. They should not be used in infants less than two months of age, in pregnancy at term, and during the nursing period because sulfonamides pass the placenta and are excreted in the milk and may cause kernicterus.

Warnings: Sulfonamides should not be used to treat group A streptococci infections or their sequelae. The occurrence of sore throat, fever, pallor, purpura, or jaundice during sulfonamide administration may be an early indication of serious blood dyscrasias.

Deaths associated with the administration of sulfonamides have been reported from hypersensitivity reactions, agranulocytosis, aplastic anemia, and other blood dyscrasias.

Frequent blood counts and renal function tests should be carried out during sulfonamide treatment, especially during prolonged administration. Microscopic urinalyses should be done once a week when a patient is treated for longer than two weeks. Urine cultures should be made to confirm eradication of bacteriuria.

Usage in Pregnancy: The safe use of sulfonamides in pregnancy has not been established. The teratogenicity potential of most sulfonamides has not been thoroughly investigated in either animals or humans. However, a significant increase in the incidence of cleft palate and other bony abnormalities of offspring has been observed when certain sulfonamides of the short-, intermediate-, and long-acting types were given to pregnant rats and mice at high oral doses (7 to 25 times the human dose).

Precautions: The usual precautions used in sulfonamide therapy should be observed, including the maintenance of an adequate fluid intake. Sulfonamides should be used with caution in patients with severe allergy or bronchial asthma, severe impairment of hepatic or renal function, and in patients with glucose-6-phosphate dehydrogenase deficiency since sulfas may cause hemolysis in this latter group.

Adverse Reactions: *Blood dyscrasias.* Agranulocytosis, aplastic anemia, thrombocytopenia, leukopenia, hemolytic anemia, purpura, hypoprothrombinemia, and methemoglobinemia.

Allergic reactions. Erythema multiforme (Stevens-Johnson Syndrome), generalized skin eruptions, epidermal necrolysis, urticaria, serum sickness, pruritus, exfoliative dermatitis, anaphylactoid reactions, periorbital edema, conjunctival and scleral injection, photosensitization, arthralgia, and allergic myocarditis.

Gastrointestinal reactions. Nausea, emesis, abdominal pains, hepatitis, diarrhea, anorexia, pancreatitis, and stomatitis.

C.N.S. reactions. Headache, peripheral neuritis, mental depression, convulsions, ataxia, hallucinations, tinnitus, vertigo, and insomnia.

Miscellaneous reactions. Drug fever, chills, and toxic nephrosis with oliguria and anuria. Periarteritis nodosum and L.E. phenomenon have occurred.

The sulfonamides bear certain chemical similarities to some goitrogens, diuretics (acetazolamide and the thiazides), and oral hypoglycemic agents. Goiter production, diuresis, and hypoglycemia have occurred rarely in patients receiving sulfonamides. Cross-sensitivity may exist with these agents.

Rats appear to be especially susceptible to the goitrogenic effects of sulfonamides, and long term administration has produced thyroid malignancies in the species.

Dosage and Administration: Usual dosage: *Adults:* 0.5 to 1.0 g three or four times daily.
Children and infants (over 2 months of age): 30 to 45 mg/kg/24 hours, divided into 4 doses.

How Supplied: THIOSULFIL Forte—Each tablet contains sulfamethizole 0.5 g (scored), in bottles of 100 (NDC 0046-0786-81).
Also in unit dose package of 100 (NDC 0046-0786-99).

Shown in Product Identification Section, page 405

THIOSULFIL®-A Forte ℞
[thi″o-sul′fil a fawrta]
(sulfamethizole 500 mg with phenazopyridine HCl)

Each tablet contains:
Sulfamethizole ....500 mg
Phenazopyridine HCl...........................50 mg

&

THIOSULFIL®-A
(sulfamethizole 250 mg with phenazopyridine HCl)

Each tablet contains:
Sulfamethizole ....250 mg
Phenazopyridine HCl...........................50 mg

Where pain is part of the problem in Urinary Tract Infection (due to susceptible organisms)

CAUTION: Federal law prohibits dispensing without prescription.

Description:
Sulfamethizole [N′-(5-Methyl-1,3,4-thiadiazol-2-yl) sulfanilamide] is a 5-membered heterocyclic sulfanilamide, occurring as a white or light buff-colored crystalline powder. Solubility in water is dependent upon the pH (1 g/5 ml at pH 7.5; 1 g/4000 ml at pH 6.5). It is soluble in alcohol, and practically insoluble in benzene.

Phenazopyridine HCl [2,6-Diamino-3-phenylazopyridine hydrochloride] occurs as brick-red microcrystals with a slight violet luster. It is soluble in boiling water, ethylene and propylene glycols, slightly soluble in alcohol and cold water, and insoluble in acetone and benzene.

Clinical Pharmacology: The combination of sulfamethizole and phenazopyridine HCl acts to eradicate urinary tract infections caused by susceptible organisms and to relieve associated pain and discomfort.

PHENAZOPYRIDINE HCl: Phenazopyridine HCl is an analgesic that acts on the mucosa of the urinary tract providing relief of pain and discomfort caused by inflammation associated with urinary tract infection.

SULFAMETHIZOLE: MECHANISM OF SULFONAMIDE BACTERIOSTATIC ACTION: The primary mechanism of bacteriostatic action by THIOSULFIL is the same as that of most sulfonamides. By competing with the precursor para-aminobenzoic acid, sulfonamides inhibit bacterial synthesis of folic (pteroylglutamic) acid which is required for bacterial growth. Resistant strains are capable of utilizing folic acid precursors or preformed folic acid.

SULFONAMIDE ANTIBACTERIAL SPECTRUM: The antibacterial spectrum of all sulfonamides is similar. *In vitro* sensitivity of bacteria to sulfonamides does not always reflect *in vivo* sensitivity. Therefore, efficacy must be carefully evaluated with bacteriologic and clinical responses in the individual patient. (See Warnings)

FACTORS DETERMINING ANTIBACTERIAL EFFICACY: Efficacy of antimicrobial therapy is dependent upon a number of factors including the *in vivo* sensitivity of the involved organisms, the concentration of the drug required for bacteriostasis, and the achievable concentration of the sulfonamide at the desired site of action.

Because of the very rapid renal clearance of sulfamethizole, the blood levels attained are low, and accumulation of the drug in tissues outside the urinary tract is very limited. Therefore, sulfamethizole is not appropriate for treatment of sys-

Continued on next page

Ayerst—Cont.

temic infections such as nocardiosis or for local lesions outside the urinary tract such as chancroid and trachoma. However, its low degree of acetylation and its rapid renal clearance permit high concentrations of active sulfamethizole to occur in the urinary tract, making it especially applicable for the treatment of infections of this tract. In addition, the possibility of crystalluria is minimized because of the high solubility of the drug in urine. Approximately 95 per cent of a given dose of sulfamethizole is not metabolized; less than 5 per cent is acetylated. As a consequence, almost all of a given dose of THIOSULFIL is present in its active form in the body.

Approximately 80 per cent of an administered dose is recoverable within eight hours; approximately 98 per cent is cleared within 15 to 24 hours. Sulfamethizole is cleared by the kidney at a rate only 10 to 20 per cent lower than that for creatinine.

Indications and Usage: For the initial treatment of uncomplicated urinary tract infections caused by susceptible strains of the following microorganisms: *Escherichia coli*, *Klebsiella* species, *Enterobacter* species, *Proteus mirabilis*, *Proteus vulgaris*, and *Staphylococcus aureus* when relief of symptoms of pain, burning or urgency is needed during the first 2 days of therapy. Treatment with THIOSULFIL-A Forte (sulfamethizole 500 mg with phenazopyridine HCl) or THIOSULFIL-A (sulfamethizole 250 mg with phenazopyridine HCl) should not exceed 2 days. There is a lack of evidence that the combination of sulfamethizole and phenazopyridine hydrochloride provide greater benefit than sulfamethizole alone after 2 days. Treatment beyond 2 days should only be continued with sulfamethizole. (See DOSAGE AND ADMINISTRATION section.)

Important note. *In vitro* sulfonamide sensitivity tests are not always reliable. The test must be carefully coordinated with bacteriologic and clinical reponse. When the patient is already taking sulfonamides, follow-up cultures should have aminobenzoic acid added to the culture media.

Currently, the increasing frequency of resistant organisms is a limitation of the usefulness of antibacterial agents, including the sulfonamides, especially in the treatment of recurrent and complicated urinary tract infections.

Wide variation in blood levels may result with identical doses. Blood levels should be measured in patients receiving sulfonamides for serious infections. Free sulfonamide blood levels of 5–15 mg per 100 ml may be considered therapeutically effective for most infections, with blood levels of 12–15 mg per 100 ml optimal for serious infections; 20 mg per 100 ml should be the maximum total sulfonamide level, as adverse reactions occur more frequently above this level.

Contraindications: Sulfonamides should not be used in patients hypersensitive to sulfa drugs. They should not be used in infants less than two months of age, in pregnancy at term, and during the nursing period because sulfonamides pass the placenta and are excreted in the milk and may cause kernicterus.

Phenazopyridine HCl is contraindicated in renal or hepatic failure, glomerulonephritis, and pyelonephritis of pregnancy with gastrointestinal disturbances.

Warnings: Sulfonamides should not be used to treat group A streptococci infections or their sequelae. The occurrence of sore throat, fever, pallor, purpura, or jaundice during sulfonamide administration may be an early indication of serious blood dyscrasias.

Deaths associated with the administration of sulfonamides have been reported from hypersensitivity reactions, agranulocytosis, aplastic anemia, and other blood dyscrasias.

Frequent blood counts and renal function tests should be carried out during sulfonamide treatment, especially during prolonged administration.

Microscopic urinalyses should be done once a week when a patient is treated for longer than two weeks. Urine cultures should be made to confirm eradication of bacteriuria.

Precautions: To allay any possible apprehension, patients should be told that this medication may color the urine orange or red.

The usual precautions used in sulfonamide therapy should be observed, including the maintenance of an adequate fluid intake. Sulfonamides should be used with caution in patients with severe allergy or bronchial asthma, severe impairment of hepatic or renal function, and in patients with glucose-6-phosphate dehydrogenase deficiency since sulfas may cause hemolysis in this latter group.

Carcinogenesis: THIOSULFIL-A Forte (sulfamethizole 500 mg with phenazopyridine HCl) and THIOSULFIL-A (sulfamethizole 250 mg with phenazopyridine HCl) have not undergone adequate trials relating to carcinogenicity; each component, however, has been evaluated separately. Rats appear to be especially susceptible to the goitrogenic effects of sulfonamides, and long-term administration of sulfonamides has resulted in thyroid malignancies in this species. Long-term administration of phenazopyridine hydrochloride has induced neoplasia in rats (large intestine) and mice (liver). Although no association between phenazopyridine hydrochloride and human neoplasia has been reported, adequate epidemiological studies have not been conducted.

Mutagenesis or Impairment of Fertility: No long-term studies in animals or humans have been conducted.

Pregnancy Category C: Certain sulfonamides of the short-, intermediate-, and long-acting types, when given to rats and mice in doses 7 to 25 times the human dose, have been associated with a significant increase in the incidence of cleft palate and other bony abnormalities of the offspring. There are no adequate and well-controlled studies in pregnant women. THIOSULFIL-A and THIOSULFIL-A Forte should be used during pregnancy only if the potential benefit justifies the potential risk to the fetus.

Nursing Mothers: See Contraindications.

Adverse Reactions:

Blood dyscrasias. Agranulocytosis, aplastic anemia, thrombocytopenia, leukopenia, hemolytic anemia, purpura, hypoprothrombinemia, and methemoglobinemia.

Allergic reactions. Erythema multiforme (Stevens-Johnson Syndrome), generalized skin eruptions, epidermal necrolysis, urticaria, serum sickness, pruritus, exfoliative dermatitis, anaphylactoid reactions, periorbital edema, conjunctival and scleral injection, photosensitization, arthralgia, and allergic myocarditis.

Gastrointestinal reactions. Nausea, emesis, abdominal pains, hepatitis, diarrhea, anorexia, pancreatitis, and stomatitis.

C.N.S. reactions. Headache, peripheral neuritis, mental depression, convulsions, ataxia, hallucinations, tinnitus, vertigo, and insomnia.

Miscellaneous reactions. Drug fever, chills, and toxic nephrosis with oliguria and anuria. Periarteritis nodosum and L.E. phenomenon have occurred.

The sulfonamides bear certain chemical similarities to some goitrogens, diuretics (acetazolamide and the thiazides), and oral hypoglycemic agents. Goiter production, diuresis, and hypoglycemia have occurred rarely in patients receiving sulfonamides. Cross-sensitivity may exist with these agents.

Dosage and Administration: Usual dosage in adults (based on sulfamethizole content):

THIOSULFIL-A Forte (sulfamethizole 500 mg with phenazopyridine HCl):
2 tablets three or four times daily for 2 days.
THIOSULFIL-A (sulfamethizole 250 mg with phenazopyridine HCl):
2–4 tablets three or four times daily for 2 days. Treatment with THIOSULFIL-A Forte or THIOSULFIL-A should not exceed 2 days. Treatment beyond 2 days should only be continued with sulfamethizole.

If pain persists, other causes for the discomfort should be investigated.

How Supplied: THIOSULFIL-A Forte (sulfamethizole 500 mg, phenazopyridine HCl 50 mg) Tablets, in bottles of 100 (NDC 0046-0783-81).
THIOSULFIL-A (sulfamethizole 250 mg, phenazopyridine HCl 50 mg) Tablets, in bottles of 100 (NDC 0046-0784-81).

Shown in Product Identification Section, page 405

THIOSULFIL® ℞
[thī″o″sul-fil′fĭl]
(sulfamethizole)
DUO-PAK®
Package

CAUTION: Federal law prohibits dispensing without prescription.

Description: This package contains 2 products:

Bottle No. 1—16 Tablets (*yellow*)

THIOSULFIL®-A Forte
(sulfamethizole 500 mg with phenazopyridine HCl)
Each tablet contains:
 Sulfamethizole .... 500 mg
 Phenazopyridine HCl .... 50 mg

Bottle No. 2—40 Tablets (*white*)

THIOSULFIL® Forte
(sulfamethizole 500 mg)
Each tablet contains:
 Sulfamethizole .... 500 mg

Sulfamethizole [N′-(5-Methyl-1,3,4-thiadiazol-2-yl) sulfanilamide] is a 5-membered heterocyclic sulfanilamide occurring as a white or light buff-colored crystalline powder. Solubility in water is dependent upon the pH (1 g 5 ml at pH 7.5; 1 g/4000 ml at pH 6.5). It is soluble in alcohol, and practically insoluble in benzene.

Phenazopyridine HCl [2,6-Diamino-3-phenylazopyridine hydrochloride] occurs as brick-red microcrystals with a slight violet luster. It is soluble in boiling water, ethylene and propylene glycols, slightly soluble in alcohol and cold water, and insoluble in acetone and benzene.

Clinical Pharmacology: The combination of sulfamethizole and phenazopyridine in THIOSULFIL-A Forte acts to eradicate urinary tract infections due to susceptible organisms, and relieve pain and discomfort associated with infection. Following relief of pain, THIOSULFIL Forte (sulfamethizole), containing only sulfamethizole, provides continuing antibacterial therapy.

PHENAZOPYRIDINE HCl: Phenazopyridine HCl is an analgesic that acts on the mucosa of the urinary tract to provide relief of pain and discomfort caused by inflammation associated with urinary tract infection.

SULFAMETHIZOLE:

Mechanism of sulfonamide bacteriostatic action: The primary mechanism of bacteriostatic action by THIOSULFIL (sulfamethizole) is the same as that of most sulfonamides. By competing with the precursor para-aminobenzoic acid, sulfonamides inhibit bacterial synthesis of folic (pteroylglutamic) acid which is required for bacterial growth. Resistant strains are capable of utilizing folic acid precursors of preformed folic acid.

Sulfonamide antibacterial spectrum: The antibacterial spectrum of all sulfonamides is similar. *In vitro* sensitivity of bacteria to sulfonamides does not always reflect *in vivo* sensitivity. Therefore, efficacy must be carefully evaluated with bacteriologic and clinical responses in the individual patient. (See Warnings)

Factors determining antibacterial efficacy: Efficacy of antimicrobial therapy is dependent upon a number of factors including the *in vivo* sensitivity of the involved organisms, the concentration of the drug required for bacteriostasis, and the achievable concentration of the sulfonamide at the desired site of action.

Because of the very rapid renal clearance of sulfamethizole, the blood levels attained are low, and accumulation of the drug in tissues outside the urinary tract is very limited. Therefore, sulfamethizole is not appropriate for treatment of systemic infections such as nocardiosis or for local lesions outside the urinary tract such as chancroid and trachoma. However, its low degree of acetylation and its rapid renal clearance permit high concentrations of active sulfamethizole to occur in the urinary tract, making it especially applicable for the treatment of infections of this tract. In addition, the possibility of crystalluria is minimized because of the high solubility of the drug in urine. Approximately 95 percent of a given dose of sulfamethizole is not metabolized; less than 5 percent is acetylated. As a consequence, almost all of a given dose of THIOSULFIL is present in its active form in the body.

Approximately 80 percent of an administered dose is recoverable within eight hours; approximately 98 percent is cleared within 15 to 24 hours. Sulfamethizole is cleared by the kidney at a rate only 10 to 20 percent lower than that for creatinine.

Indications and Usage: THIOSULFIL-A Forte (sulfamethizole 500 mg with phenazopyridine HCl)—Bottle No. 1—is indicated for the initial treatment of uncomplicated urinary tract infections caused by susceptible strains of the following microorganisms. *Escherichia coli, Klebsiella* species; *Enterobacter* species, *Proteus mirabilis, Proteus vulgaris,* and *Staphylococcus aureus* when relief of symptoms of pain, burning, or urgency is needed during the first 2 days of therapy. Treatment with THIOSULFIL-A Forte should not exceed 2 days. There is a lack of evidence that the combination of sulfamethizole and phenazopyridine hydrochloride provides greater benefit than sulfamethizole alone after 2 days. Treatment beyond 2 days should only be continued with sulfamethizole. (See DOSAGE AND ADMINISTRATION section.)

THIOSULFIL Forte (sulfamethizole)—Bottle No. 2—is indicated for continuing antibacterial therapy after pain and discomfort have been relieved.

Important note. *In vitro* sulfonamide sensitivity tests are not always reliable. The test must be carefully coordinated with bacteriologic and clinical response. When the patient is already taking sulfonamides, follow-up cultures should have aminobenzoic acid added to the culture media.

Currently the increasing frequency of resistant organisms is a limitation of the usefulness of antibacterial agents, including the sulfonamides, especially in the treatment of recurrent and complicated urinary tract infections.

Wide variation in blood levels may result with identical doses. Blood levels should be measured in patients receiving sulfonamides for serious infections. Free sulfonamide blood levels of 5-15 mg per 100 ml may be considered therapeutically effective for most infections, with blood levels of 12-15 mg per 100 ml optimal for serious infections; 20 mg per 100 ml should be the maximum total sulfonamide level, as adverse reactions occur more frequently above this level.

Contraindications: Sulfonamides should not be used in patients hypersensitive to sulfa drugs. They should not be used in infants less than two months of age, in pregnancy at term, and during the nursing period because sulfonamides pass the placenta and are excreted in the milk and may cause kernicterus.

Phenazopyridine HCl is contraindicated in renal or hepatic failure, glomerulonephritis, and pyelonephritis of pregnancy with gastrointestinal disturbances.

Warnings: Sulfonamides should not be used to treat group A streptococci infections or their sequelae. The occurrence of sore throat, fever, pallor, purpura, or jaundice during sulfonamide administration may be an early indication of serious blood dyscrasias.

Deaths associated with the administration of sulfonamides have been reported from hypersensitivity reactions, agranulocytosis, aplastic anemia, and other blood dyscrasias.

Frequent blood counts and renal function tests should be carried out during sulfonamide treatment, especially during prolonged administration. Microscopic urinalyses should be done once a week when a patient is treated for longer than two weeks. Urine cultures should be made to confirm eradication of bacteriuria.

Precautions: To allay any possible apprehension, patients should be told that this medication may color the urine orange or red.

The usual precautions used in sulfonamide therapy should be observed, including the maintenance of an adequate fluid intake. Sulfonamides should be used with caution in patients with severe allergy or bronchial asthma, severe impairment of hepatic or renal function, and in patients with glucose-6-phosphate dehydrogenase deficiency since sulfas may cause hemolysis in this latter group.

Carcinogenesis: THIOSULFIL-A Forte and THIOSULFIL Forte have not undergone adequate trials relating to carcinogenicity; each component, however, has been evaluated separately. Rats appear to be especially susceptible to the goitrogenic effects of sulfonamides, and long-term administration of sulfonamides has resulted in thyroid malignancies in this species. Long-term administration of phenazopyridine hydrochloride has induced neoplasia in rats (large intestine) and mice (liver). Although no association between phenazopyridine hydrochloride and human neoplasia has been reported, adequate epidemiological studies have not been conducted.

Mutagenesis or Impairment of Fertility: No long-term studies in animals or humans have been conducted.

Pregnancy Category C: Certain sulfonamides of the short, intermediate, and long-acting types, when given to rats and mice in doses 7 to 25 times the human dose, have been associated with a significant increase in the incidence of cleft palate and other bony abnormalities of the offspring. There are no adequate and well-controlled studies in pregnant women. THIOSULFIL®-Forte and THIOSULFIL®-A Forte should be used during pregnancy only if the potential benefit justifies the potential risk to the fetus.

Nursing Mothers: See Contraindications.

Adverse Reactions: *Blood dyscrasias.* Agranulocytosis, aplastic anemia, thrombocytopenia, leukopenia, hemolytic anemia, purpura, hypoprothrombinemia, and methemoglobinemia.

Allergic reactions. Erythema multiforme (Stevens-Johnson Syndrome), generalized skin eruptions, epidermal necrolysis, urticaria, serum sickness, pruritus, exfoliative dermatitis, anaphylactoid reactions, periorbital edema, conjunctival and scleral injection, photosensitization, arthralgia, and allergic myocarditis.

Gastrointestinal reactions. Nausea, emesis, abdominal pains, hepatitis, diarrhea, anorexia, pancreatitis, and stomatitis.

C.N.S. reactions. Headache, peripheral neuritis, mental depression, convulsions, ataxia, hallucinations, tinnitus, vertigo, and insomnia.

Miscellaneous reactions. Drug fever, chills, and toxic nephrosis with oliguria and anuria. Periarteritis nodosum and L.E. phenomenon have occurred.

The sulfonamides bear certain chemical similarities to some goitrogens, diuretics (acetazolamide and the thiazides), and oral hypoglycemic agents. Goiter production, diuresis, and hypoglycemia have occurred rarely in patients receiving sulfonamides. Cross-sensitivity may exist with these agents.

Dosage and Administration: *Adult dosage regimen:*

Start—Bottle No. 1 THIOSULFIL-A Forte (sulfamethizole 500 mg with phenazopyridine HCl)—2 *yellow* tablets three or four times daily for 2 days.

Continue—Bottle No. 2 THIOSULFIL Forte (sulfamethizole 500 mg)—2 *white* tablets four times daily for 5 days. Continue medication as recommended by physician.

Treatment with THIOSULFIL-A Forte or THIOSULFIL-A should not exceed 2 days. Treatment beyond 2 days should only be continued with sulfamethizole.

If pain persists, other causes for the discomfort should be investigated.

How Supplied: THIOSULFIL® (sulfamethizole) DUO-PAK® NDC 0046-0780-98.

Bottle No. 1—THIOSULFIL®-A Forte: 16 tablets (yellow).

Bottle No. 2—THIOSULFIL® Forte: 40 tablets (white).

Shown in Product Identification Section, page 405

Baker/Cummins
Dermatological Div. of
Key Pharmaceuticals, Inc.
50 N.W. 176TH STREET
MIAMI, FLORIDA 33169

COMPLEX 15™
Phospholipid Moisturizer
(See PDR For Nonprescription Drugs)

P&S® LIQUID
(See PDR For Nonprescription Drugs)

P&S® PLUS
GEL
(See PDR For Nonprescription Drugs)

P&S® SHAMPOO
Antiseborrheic Shampoo
(See PDR For Nonprescription Drugs)

ULTRA MIDE 25™ LOTION
(See PDR For Nonprescription Drugs)

XSEB® SHAMPOO
(See PDR For Nonprescription Drugs)

XSEB®-T SHAMPOO
(See PDR For Nonprescription Drugs)

Barnes-Hind, Inc.
A Revlon Vision Care Company
895 KIFER ROAD
SUNNYVALE, CA 94086

BARSEB® HC ℞
[*bar-sĕb hc*]
SCALP LOTION

Description: Contains hydrocortisone 1%, salicylic acid 0.5%, isopropyl alcohol 45%, propylene glycol, isopropyl myristate, ascorbic acid, and citric acid.

Actions: BARSEB® HC Scalp Lotion is primarily effective because of the anti-inflammatory, antipruritic, and vaso-constrictive actions of hydrocortisone, and salicylic acid aids in loosening and removing adherent sebum, crust, and epithelial debris.

Indications: For the relief of the inflammatory manifestations of corticosteroid-responsive dermatoses of the scalp.

Contraindications: Topical steroids are contraindicated in those patients with a history of hypersensitivity to any of the components of the preparations.

Precautions: If irritation develops, the product should be discontinued and appropriate therapy instituted.

In the presence of an infection, use of an appropriate antifungal or antibacterial agent should be instituted. If a favorable response does not occur promptly, the corticosteroid should be discontinued until the infection has been adequately controlled.

If extensive areas are treated or if the occlusive technique is used, there will be increased systemic

Continued on next page

Barnes-Hind—Cont.

absorption of the corticosteroid and suitable precautions should be taken, particularly in children and infants.

Although topical steroids have not been reported to have an adverse effect on human pregnancy, the safety of their use in pregnant women has not absolutely been established. In laboratory animals, increases in incidence of fetal abnormalities have been associated with exposure of gestating females to topical corticosteroids. Therefore, drugs of this class should not be used extensively on pregnant patients, in large amounts, or for prolonged periods of time.

Not for Ophthalmic Use or Use Around the Eyes.
Adverse Reactions: The following local adverse reactions have been reported with topical corticosteroids especially under occlusive dressings: burning, itching, irritation, dryness, folliculitis, hypertrichosis, acneform eruptions, hypopigmentation, perioral dermatitis, allergic contact dermatitis, maceration of the skin, secondary infection, skin atrophy, striae, and miliaria. Transient discomfort may occur when first applied to an inflamed scalp.
Dosage and Administration: Part hair, apply once or twice a day with gentle rubbing. Use sparingly. When a favorable response is obtained, reduce dosage as necessary.
Caution: Federal (U.S.A.) law prohibits dispensing without prescription.
For dermatologic use only.
How Supplied: BARSEB® HC is supplied in 1.75 fl. oz. (52 ml) plastic squeeze bottles.
Store at room temperature; avoid excessive heat (104°F.).

BARSEB® THERA=SPRAY® ℞
[bar-sĕb thĕr-a sprā]
Topical Aerosol

Description: Each bottle (84 g) contains 360 mg hydrocortisone, 288 mg salicylic acid, 14 mg benzalkonium chloride, 46 g alcohol with propylene glycol, isopropyl myristate, and butane as propellant.
After evaporation of the propellant, the vehicle contains 0.6% hydrocortisone, 0.48% salicylic acid, and 0.024% benzalkonium chloride.
Actions: BARSEB THERA-SPRAY is primarily effective because of the anti-inflammatory, antipruritic, and vasoconstrictive actions of hydrocortisone, and salicylic acid aids in loosening and removing adherent sebum, crusts, and epithelial debris.
Indications: BARSEB THERA-SPRAY is indicated for the relief of the inflammatory manifestations of corticosteroid-responsive dermatoses of the scalp.
Contraindications: Contraindicated in those patients with a history of hypersensitivity to any of the components of the aerosol.
Precautions: If irritation develops, discontinue use and institute appropriate therapy.
In the presence of an infection, use of an appropriate antifungal or antibacterial agent should be instituted. If a favorable response does not occur promptly, application of Barseb should be discontinued until the infection has been adequately controlled.
If extensive areas are treated or if the occlusive technique is used, there will be increased systemic absorption of the corticosteroid and suitable precautions should be taken, particularly with children and infants.
Avoid inhalation, ingestion or contact with the eyes or nose. If spray accidentally gets into eyes, flush with copious amounts of water.
Although topical steroids have not been reported to have an adverse effect on human pregnancy, the safety of their use in pregnant women has not absolutely been established. In laboratory animals, increases in incidence of fetal abnormalities have been associated with exposure of gestating females to topical corticosteroids, in some cases at rather low dosage levels. Therefore, drugs of this class should not be used extensively on pregnant patients, in large amounts, or for prolonged periods of time.
This product is not for ophthalmic use.
Adverse Reactions: The following local adverse reactions have been reported with topical corticosteroids, especially under occlusive dressings: burning, itching, irritation, dryness, folliculitis, hypertrichosis, acneform eruptions, hypopigmentation, perioral dermatitis, allergic contract dermatitis, maceration of the skin, secondary infection, skin atrophy, striae, and miliaria.
Transient discomfort may occur when first applied to an inflamed scalp.
Dosage and Administration: BARSEB THERA-SPRAY should be applied once daily during the acute phase or as directed by a physician. A maintenance schedule may be adjusted to the patient's response to therapy.
Directions For Use: Shake well. Hold the bottle upright (being careful not to spray forehead or eyes); insert applicator tube through hair to scalp at front hairline. Then start spraying and moving applicator tube slowly toward the back of the head. Repeat this procedure until all affected areas of the scalp are treated. Because of the spreading and penetrating properties of BARSEB THERA-SPRAY, it is not necessary to rub or massage medication into the scalp. Assembly directions are provided on the aerosol bottles.
How Supplied: BARSEB THERA-SPRAY is supplied in 84 g aerosol bottles with applicator tube.

KOMED® Acne Lotion OTC
[kō-mĕd]

Sodium thiosulfate	8%
Salicylic acid	2%
Isopropyl alcohol	25%

The above product also contains menthol, camphor, colloidal alumina, edetate disodium, and purified water.
Indications: Primarily indicated for the treatment of acne associated with oily skin. KOMED Acne Lotion is indicated in more severe conditions or where stronger keratolytic effect is desired. Komed Lotion features a thixotropic gel of colloidal alumina. It is greaseless and dries to an almost invisible film, forming a medicated base over which non-oily cosmetics may be applied.
Precautions: Do not use Komed Lotion on or near the eyes.
Dosage and Administration: Wash affected areas thoroughly. Shake lotion well and apply a thin film twice a day.
How Supplied: 1¾ fl. oz. (52.5 ml.) plastic squeeze bottles.

KOMED® HC Lotion ℞
[kō-mĕd hc]
(hydrocortisone)

Description: Contains hydrocortisone acetate 0.5%, sodium thiosulfate 8%, salicylic acid 2%, isopropyl alcohol 25%, menthol, camphor, colloidal alumina, edetate disodium, and purified water.
Indications: KOMED HC Acne Lotion is indicated for topical treatment of acne conditions when accompanied by inflammation. KOMED HC features a thixotropic gel of colloidal alumina. The lotion is greaseless and dries to an almost invisible film, forming a medicated base over which non-oily cosmetics may be applied.
Contraindications: Topical steroids are contraindicated in those patients with a history of hypersensitivity to any of the components of the preparation.
Precautions: If irritation develops, the product should be discontinued and appropriate therapy instituted.
In the presence of an infection, the use of an appropriate antifungal or antibacterial agent should be instituted. If a favorable response does not occur promptly, the corticosteroid should be discontinued until the infection has been adequately controlled.
If extensive areas are treated or if the occlusive technique is used, there will be increased systemic absorption of the corticosteroid and suitable precautions should be taken, particularly in children and infants.
Although topical steroids have not been reported to have an adverse effect on human pregnancy, the safety of their use in pregnant women has not been absolutely established. In laboratory animals, increases in incidence of fetal abnormalities have been associated with exposure of gestating females to topical corticosteroids. Therefore, drugs of this class should not be used extensively on pregnant patients, in large amounts, or for prolonged periods of time.
Not for Ophthalmic Use or Use Around the Eyes.
Adverse Reactions: The following local adverse reactions have been reported with topical corticosteroids especially under occlusive dressings: burning, itching, irritation, dryness, folliculitis, hypertrichosis, acneform eruptions, hypopigmentation, perioral dermatitis, allergic contact dermatitis, maceration of the skin, secondary infection, skin atrophy, striae, and miliaria.
Dosage and Administration: Wash affected areas thoroughly. Shake lotion well and apply a thin film twice a day, or as directed.
How Supplied: 1¾ fl. oz. (52.5 ml.) plastic squeeze bottles. Store at room temperature, avoid excessive heat.

KOMEX® OTC
[kō-mĕx]
(Scrub for Oily Skin and Make-up Removal)

Description: KOMEX® is a dissolving cleanser useful as an aid in reducing oily skin conditions associated with acne.
Contents: SCRUBULES, Barnes-Hind brand of dissolving particles (sodium tetraborate decahydrate), in a preserved base containing a unique combination of surface active soapless cleaning agents, and skin conditioners.
Directions: Use Komex in place of your usual soap or cleanser.
Skin Cleansing: Wet the face with warm water. Squeeze Komex onto your fingertips, and gently massage into the face. Continue scrubbing and adding water until Scrubules are completely dissolved (about one minute). Rinse thoroughly and dry. Use once or twice daily.
Caution: Avoid contact with eyes. If granules get into the eyes, flush thoroughly with water and avoid rubbing eyes. If skin irritation or excessive dryness develops, or increases, discontinue use. For external use only. Keep out of reach of children. Not to be used on infants. Do not use on inflamed skin.
How Supplied: 2.65 oz. (75 g.) plastic squeeze tube in unit carton.

PRO–CORT™ OTC
[prō-kort]
(Hydrocortisone ½% Cream–Unscented)

PRO–CORT M™ OTC
(Hydrocortisone ½% Cream–Scented)

Description: Pro-Cort and Pro-Cort M medication, with hydrocortisone ½%, is blended with a cooling, soothing emollient skin cream base (scented or unscented).
Indications: Pro-Cort's cooling, soothing and anti-itching properties offer effective, temporary relief of minor skin irritations, itching and rashes due to eczema, dermatitis, insect bites, poison ivy, poison sumac, soaps, detergents, cosmetics, and jewelry and for itchy genital and anal areas.
Directions for Use: For adults and children 2 years of age and older—apply to affected area not more than 3 to 4 times daily. For children under 2 years of age, there is no recommended dosage except under the advice and supervision of a physician.
Warnings: For external use only. Avoid contact with the eyes. Keep out of the reach of children.
How Supplied: Pro-Cort ½% is supplied in ½ oz. (15 g) tube or 1 oz. (30 g) tube in unit carton. Pro-

Cort M ½% is supplied in 1 oz. (30 g) tube in unit carton.

TINVER® LOTION ℞
[tin-ver]

Description: Sodium thiosulfate 25%, salicylic acid 1%, isopropyl alcohol 10%, propylene glycol, menthol, edetate disodium, colloidal alumina, purified water.
Indications: For topical use in treatment of tinea versicolor infections.
Precautions: Discontinue use if irritation or sensitivity develops. Do not use on or about the eyes.
Dosage and Administration: Thoroughly wash, rinse, and dry affected and susceptible areas before application. Apply thin film of TINVER twice a day. Although diagnostic evidence of the disease may disappear in a few days, it is advisable to continue treatment for a much longer period. Clothing should be boiled to prevent reinfection.
How Supplied: 4 fl. oz. (180 ml.) plastic squeeze bottles. Store at room temperature, avoid excessive heat.

Barry Laboratories, Inc.
461 N. E. 27th STREET
P. O. BOX 1967
POMPANO BEACH, FL 33061

ALLERGENIC EXTRACTS, DIAGNOSIS AND/OR IMMUNOTHERAPY ℞

Composition: Fluid allergens are available from the following categories: pollens, foods, dusts, epidermals, insects, fungi (molds & smuts), stinging insects, yeasts, and others.
Action and Uses: For diagnosis and immunotherapy of specific offenders in allergy.
Precautions: Usual precautions used in testing or treating hypersentive individuals. See product information circulars accompanying each product.
How Supplied: Diagnostic materials are availabe in liquid form for cutaneous or intracutaneous testing.
Diagnostic Test Sets: The "50 Plus"—includes a comprehensive selection of perennial and seasonal allergens for each of 5 botanical zones.
Immunorex®—Prescription Allergy Treatment Sets—Individualized, four vial treatment sets are prepared from the physician's instructions, based on the patients's skin test reactions and history. Refills of any dilution are available.
Literature Available: Send for free descriptive literature, report and case history forms.

RHUS ALL® ANTIGEN (Barry) ℞
Poison Ivy, Oak and Sumac Combined

Composition: A triple antigen of the active principles (urushiol) of poison ivy, oak and sumac in an oil vehicle.
Indications: Prophylactic for hyposensitization of Rhus Dermatitis.
Contraindications: Not recommended for treatment of active Rhus Dermatitis.
Administration and Dosage: Usual adult dosage: 1 ml. intramuscular injection a week, for two to three weeks prior to patient's exposure.
How Supplied: 5 ml. multiple dose vial.
Literature Available: Write for free Rhus All Antigen pamphlet.

Products are cross-indexed by generic and chemical names in the
YELLOW SECTION

A. J. Bart, Inc.
GURABO INDUSTRIAL PARK
POST OFFICE BOX 813
GURABO, PUERTO RICO 00658

ALBAFORT® INJECTABLE ℞
(Iron and B Complex)

Composition: Each ml of Albafort (Iron and B Complex) Injection contains: Iron as ferrous gluconate 50 mg; Vit. B_{12} 100 mcg; 20% Liver Extract N.F., (Vit. B_{12} eq. 10 mcq/ml); Thiamine HCl 12.5 mg; Riboflavin 0.5 mg; Pyridoxine HCl 2.0 mg, Panthenol 1.0 mg; Niacinamide 12.5 mg, with phenol 0.5% and Benzyl alcohol 1.5% as preservatives, water for injection q.s.
Actions: Albafort (Iron and B Complex) provides a combination of the hematinic effect of iron and the hematopoietic effect of liver.
Indications: Albafort (Iron and B Complex) is indicated in the treatment of hypochromic and macrocytic anemias, pernicious anemia and sprue that responds to B_{12} therapy. Hypochromic anemias are mostly due to prolonged loss of blood of the gastrointestinal tract, urinary tract and uterus. In addition, iron requirements must be increased at certain times of life such as, infancy and childhood, puberty (especially in females), during pregnancy and menopause. Albafort offers a balanced and stable formula for the treatment of hypochromic anemias.
Advantages: Iron in Albafort does not stain the skin. A Z-track technique need not be used nor deep needle injection in the gluteal area. No soft-tissue sarcomas have developed at site of injection as with iron dextran; no iron bound permanently to muscle and no fibromyositis. Due to the presence of 20% liver (ferritin present in liver) an excellent iron binding capacity occurs so there is more stimulation of the bone marrow to produce more erythrocites and greater levels of hemoglobin are obtained.
Warnings: As with other iron compounds toxic symptoms may occur at injection. The immediate reactions most frequently found are vomiting, nausea, lowering of blood pressure and pallor. These reactions are transitory and not frequent with ferrous gluconate. Some patients are sensitive to liver. Keep in a dark place at low temperature. DO NOT USE IF SEDIMENTATION OR PRECIPITATION SHOWS.
Contraindication: Individuals who have shown hypersensitivity to any of its components.
Dosage: Children—½ to 1 ml once or twice a week. Adults—1 to 2 ml once or twice a week or as the physician thinks necessary. For intramuscular use only.
How Supplied: 10 ml multidose vials (NDC 10023-100-10).

ALBA-LYBE® ℞

Composition: Each 5 cc contains: Lysine Monohydrochloride 275 mg., Vit. B_{12} Crystalline 10 mcq., Thiamine HCl 5 mg., Riboflavin 4 mg., Pyridoxine HCl 1 mg., Niacinamide 35 mg., Calcium Pantothenate 7 mg., Sorbitol q.s. (imitation sherry wine flavor).
Actions: Alba-Lybe provides lysine as an appetite stimulant and sorbitol q.s. to provide greater absorption of B_{12} and lysine.
Indications: As dietetic supplement of all ages, especially in states of anorexia and convalescence.
Advantages: Alba-Lybe can be administered to patients including the diabetic patient since it contains sorbitol. Sorbitol q.s. base has the advantage over the alcohol base since sorbitol is absorbed much more rapidly than alcohol, as well as the fact that the molecules of lysine and B_{12} adhere to sorbitol. This results in greater appetite and fixing of proteins producing weight increase and better anabolic results.
Dosage: Children—½ to 1 teaspoonful three times a day. Adults—1 tablespoonful three times a day.
How Supplied: 6 oz. bottle (NDC 10023-101-06).

ALBATUSSIN® ℞
(Antitussive, Expectorant, Sugar Free)

Composition: Each 5 cc contains: Dextromethorphan HBr 10 mg., pyrilamine maleate 8.33 mg., potassium guaiacolsulfonate 75 mg., phenylephrine HBr 5 mg., sodium citrate 215 mg., citric acid 50 mg., alcohol 4% with menthol, thymol and tolu in a sugar free base.
Actions: Albatussin suppresses coughing, helps in nasal decongestion, sneezing and expectoration.
Indications: For coughing relief due to colds or allergy, as well as an expectorant.
Advantages: Albatussin has a nice, pleasing flavor and can be given to diabetic patients and children of all ages as well as adults.
Dosage: Adults and older children—1 or 2 teaspoonfuls; Children six to twelve years—1 teaspoonful; four to six years—½ to 1 teaspoonful; one to four years—½ teaspoonful; under one year—¼ to ½ teaspoonful. These dosages should be given every four hours.
How Supplied: 4 oz bottle (NDC 10023-104-04).

TIA-DOCE® INJECTABLE SOLUTION ℞
(B_{12}—B_1)

Composition: Each ml. in Tia-Doce contains: Cyanocobalamin (Vit. B 12) 1000 mcg., Thiamine HCL (Vit. B 1) 100 mg. Benzyl Alcohol 1.5% and Sodium Chloride for injection q.s.
Action and Indications: Tia Doce Solution is indicated for the prevention and treatment of a variety of disorders associated with Vitamin B deficiency as well as for the management of certain sensory neuropathies responding to massive doses of Vitamin B 12. Specifically Vitamin B1 is indicated in the prevention and treatment of beriberi and in the correction of anorexia of dietary origin.
Warning: Contraindicated in persons who are hypersensitive to any of its components.
DO NOT USE IF PRECIPITATION OCCURS-PROTECT FROM LIGHT-REFRIGERATE.
Dosage: Tia Doce Solution is administered 0.5 to 1 cc intramusculary daily or as needed.
How Supplied: Tia Doce Solution is supplied in 10 ml. vials. (NDC 10023-185-10).

Beach Pharmaceuticals
Division of BEACH PRODUCTS, INC.
5220 SOUTH MANHATTAN AVE.
TAMPA, FL 33611

BEELITH Tablets OTC

Description: Each tablet contains magnesium oxide 600 mg and pyridoxine hydrochloride (Vitamin B_6) 25 mg equivalent to B_6 20 mg.
Inert Ingredients: caster oil, hydroxypropyl methylcellulose, magnesium stearate, microcrystalline cellulose, polyethylene glycol NF, propylene glycol USP, sodium starch glycolate. Also, D & C yellow #10, FDC yellow #6, titanium dioxide.
Warning: Keep this and all drugs out of the reach of children. In case of accidental overdose seek professional assistance or contact a Poison Control Center immediately. As with any drug, if you are pregnant or nursing a baby, seek the advice of a health professional before using this product.
Actions and Uses: BEELITH is a dietary supplement for patients deficient in magnesium and /or pyridoxine. Each tablet yields approximately 362 mg of elemental magnesium & supplies 1000% of the Adult U.S. Recommended Daily Allowance (RDA) for Vitamin B_6 and 90% of the RDA for magnesium.
Dosage: The usual adult dose is one or two tablets daily.
Precaution: Excessive dosage might cause laxation.
Caution: Use only under the supervision of a physician. Use with caution in renal insufficiency.

Continued on next page

Beach—Cont.

Drug Interaction Precautions: Do not take this product if you are presently taking a prescription antibiotic drug containing any form of tetracycline.
Storage: Keep tightly closed. Store at controlled room temperature 15°C–30°C (59°F–86°F).
How Supplied: Film coated tablet in bottles of 100 (NDC 0486-1132-01) and bottles of 500 (NDC 0486-1132-05) tablets.
Shown in Product Identification Section, page 406

K-PHOS® M.F. ℞
K-PHOS® No. 2 ℞
Phosphate Urinary Acidifiers

Description: K-PHOS® M.F.: Each tablet contains potassium acid phosphate 155 mg and sodium acid phosphate, anhydrous 350 mg. Each tablet yields approximately 125.6 mg of phosphorus, 44.5 mg of potassium or 1.1 mEq and 67 mg of sodium or 2.9 mEq. K-PHOS® No. 2: Each tablet contains potassium acid phosphate 305 mg and sodium acid phosphate, anhydrous 700 mg. Each tablet yields approximately 250 mg of phosphorus, 88 mg of potassium or 2.3 mEq and 134 mg of sodium or 5.8 mEq.
Actions: These products are highly effective urinary acidifiers.
Indications: For use in patients with elevated urinary pH. These products help keep calcium soluble and reduce odor and rash caused by ammoniacal urine. Also, by acidifying the urine they increase the antibacterial activity of methenamine mandelate and methenamine hippurate.
Precautions:
Pregnancy/Breast-feeding: Problems in humans have not been documented; however, risk/benefit must be considered.
Drug Interactions: Use of antacids containing magnesium or aluminum in conjunction with phosphate preparations may bind the phosphate and prevent is absorption. Concurrent use of antihypertensives, especially diazoxide, guanethidine, hydralazine, methyldopa or rauwolfia alkaloids; or corticosteroids, especially mineralocorticoids or corticotropin, with sodium phosphate may result in hypernatremia. Calcium preparations or vitamin D may antagonize the effects of phosphates in the treatment of hypercalcemia. Potassium-containing medications or potassium-sparing diuretics may cause hyperkalemia when used with potassium phosphates. Patients should have serum potassium level determinations at periodic intervals. Plasma levels of salicylates may be increased since salicylate excretion is decreased in acidified urine; addition of monobasic phosphates to patients stabilized on salicylates may lead to toxic salicylate levels.
Medical Problems—General: Use of this medication should be carefully considered when the following medical problems exist: Cardiac disease (particularly in digitalized patients), Addison's disease, acute dehydration, severe renal insufficiency, renal function impairment or chronic renal disease, extensive tissue breakdown, myotonia congenita, cardiac failure, cirrhosis of the liver or severe hepatic disease, peripheral and pulmonary edema, hypernatremia, hypertension, toxemia of pregnancy, hypoparathyroidism, osteomalacia, acute pancreatitis, and rickets.
The following procedures may be especially important in patient monitoring (other tests may be warranted in some patients, depending on condition); renal function determinations, serum calcium concentration, serum phosphorus concentration, serum potassium concentration, and serum sodium concentration determinations. (Checks may be required at periodic intervals during therapy; high phosphate levels increase the incidence of extraskeletal calcification.)
Side Effects: The following adverse effects have been reported: headaches; dizziness; mental confusion; seizures; weakness of legs; general fatigue or weakness; muscle cramps; numbness of or tingling of hands, lips, or feet; fast or irregular heartbeat; shortness of breath; swelling of feet or legs; unusual weight gain; low urine output; thirst; nausea; vomiting; stomach pain; diarrhea.
Dosage and Administration: K-PHOS® M.F.: Two tablets four times daily with a full glass of water. K-PHOS® No. 2: One tablet four times daily with a full glass of water. When the urine is difficult to acidify administer one tablet every two hours not to exceed eight tablets in a 24 hour period.
Caution: Federal law prohibits dispensing without prescription.
Storage: Keep tightly closed. Store at controlled room temperature, 15°C–30°C (59°F–86°F).
How Supplied: K-PHOS® M.F.: White scored tablet with the name BEACH and the number 1135 embossed on each tablet. Bottles of 100 (NDC 0486-1135-01) and bottles of 500 (NDC 0486-1135-05) tablets. K-PHOS® No. 2: Brown capsule shaped tablet with the name BEACH and the number 1134 embossed on each tablet. Bottles of 100 (NDC 0486-1134-01) and bottles of 500 (NDC 0486-1134-05) tablets. Form KMF-2 R8/84

K-PHOS® NEUTRAL ℞
Supplies 250 mg of phosphorus per tablet.

Description: Each tablet contains sodium phosphate dibasic, anhydrous 852 mg, potassium phosphate, monobasic 155 mg and sodium phosphate, monobasic 130 mg. Each tablet yields approximately 250 mg of phosphorus, 298 mg of sodium (13.0 mEq) and 45 mg of potassium (1.1 mEq).
Actions and Uses: K-PHOS® NEUTRAL lowers urinary calcium levels and increases phosphate and pyrophosphate. As a phosphorous supplement, each tablet supplies 25% of the U.S. Recommended Daily Allowance (U.S. RDA) of phosphorus for adults.
Precautions:
Pregnancy/Breast-feeding: Problems in humans have not been documented; however, risk/benefit must be considered.
Drug Interactions: Use of antacids containing magnesium or aluminum in conjunction with phosphate preparations may bind the phosphate and prevent its absorption. Concurrent use of antihypertensives, especially diazoxide, guanethidine, hydralazine, methyldopa or rauwolfia alkaloids; or corticosteroids, especially mineralocorticoids or corticotropin, with sodium phosphate may result in hypernatremia. Calcium preparations or vitamin D may antagonize the effects of phosphates in the treatment of hypercalcemia. Potassium-containing medications or potassium-sparing diuretics may cause hyperkalemia when used with potassium phosphates. Patients should have serum potassium level determinations at periodic intervals.
Medical Problems—General: Use of this medication should be carefully considered when the following medical problems exist: Cardiac disease (particularly in digitalized patients), Addison's disease, acute dehydration, severe renal insufficiency, renal function impairment or chronic renal disease, extensive tissue breakdown, myotonia congenita, cardiac failure, cirrhosis of the liver or severe hepatic disease, peripheral and pulmonary edema, hypernatremia, hypertension, toxemia of pregnancy, hypoparathyroidism, osteomalacia, acute pancreatitis, and rickets.
The following procedures may be especially important in patient monitoring (other tests may be warranted in some patients, depending on condition): renal function determinations, serum calcium concentration, serum phosphorus concentration, serum potassium concentration, and serum sodium concentration determinations. (Checks may be required at periodic intervals during therapy; high phosphate levels increase the incidence of extraskeletal calcification.)
Side Effects: The following adverse effects have been reported: headaches; dizziness; mental confusion; seizures; weakness of legs; general fatigue or weakness; muscle cramps; numbness of or tingling of hands, lips, or feet; fast or irregular heartbeat; shortness of breath; swelling of feet or legs; unusual weight gain; low urine output; thirst; nausea; vomiting; stomach pain; diarrhea.
Administration and Dosage: Adults; One or two tablets four times a day with a full glass of water.
Caution: Federal law prohibits dispensing without prescription.
Storage: Keep tightly closed. Store at controlled room temperature, 15°C–30°C (59°–86°F).
How Supplied: White, film coated, capsule shaped tablet with the name BEACH and the number 1125 embossed on each tablet. Bottles of 100 (NDC 0486-1125-01) and 500 (NDC 0486-1125-05) tablets.

K-PHOS® ORIGINAL (Sodium Free) ℞
(Potassium Acid Phosphate)
Urinary Acidifier
Supplies 114 mg of phosphorus per tablet.

Description: Each tablet contains potassium acid phosphate 500 mg. Each tablet yields approximately 114 mg of phosphorus and 144 mg of potassium or 3.7 mEq.
Actions: K-PHOS ORIGINAL (Sodium Free) is a highly effective urinary acidifier.
Indications: For use in patients with elevated urinary pH. Helps keep calcium soluble and reduces odor and rash caused by ammoniacal urine. Also, by acidifying the urine it increases the antibacterial activity of methenamine mandelate and methenamine hippurate.
Precautions:
Pregnancy/Breast-feeding: Problems in humans have not been documented; however, risk/benefit must be considered.
Drug Interactions: Use of antacids containing magnesium or aluminum in conjunction with phosphate preparations may bind the phosphate and prevent its absorption. Calcium preparations or vitamin D may antagonize the effects of phosphates in the treatment of hypercalcemia. Potassium-containing medications or potassium-sparing diuretics may should have serum potassium level determinations at periodic intervals. Plasma levels of salicylates may be increased since salicylate excretion is decreased in acidified urine; addition of monobasic potassium phosphate to patients stabilized on salicylates may lead to toxic salicylate levels.
Medical Problems—General: Use of this medication should be carefully considered when the following medical problems exist: Cardiac disease (particularly in digitalized patients), Addison's disease, acute dehydration, severe renal insufficiency, chronic renal disease, extensive tissue breakdown, myotonia congenita, cirrhosis of the liver or severe hepatic disease, hypoparathyroidism, osteomalacia, acute pancreatitis, and rickets. The following procedures may be especially important in patient monitoring (other tests may be warranted in some patients, depending on condition); renal function determinations, serum calcium concentration, serum phosphorus concentration, and serum potassium concentration. (Checks may be required at periodic intervals during therapy; high phosphate levels increase the incidence of extraskeletal calcification.)
Side Effects: The following adverse effects have been reported: bone and joint pain (possible phosphate induced osteomalacia); fast or irregular heartbreak; mental confusion; numbness or tingling of lips, hands, or feet; general fatigue or weakness; weakness of legs; muscle cramps; shortness of breath; diarrhea; nausea; stomach pain; vomiting.
Warning: There have been several reports, published and unpublished, concerning non-specific small-bowel lesions consisting of stenosis, with or without ulceration, associated with the administration of enteric-coated thiazides with potassium salts. These lesions may occur with enteric-coated potassium tablets alone or when they are used with nonenteric coated thiazides or certain other oral diuretics. These small-bowel lesions have caused obstruction, hemorrhage, and perforation. Surgery was frequently required and deaths have occurred. Based on a large survey of physicians

and hospitals, both United States and foreign, the incidence of these lesions is low, and a casual relationship in man has not been definitely established. Available information tends to implicate enteric-coated potassium salts, although lesions of this type also occur spontaneously. Therefore, coated potassium-containing formulations should be administered only when indicated and should be discontinued immediately if abdominal pain, distension, nausea, vomiting or gastrointestinal bleeding occur. Coated potassium tablets should be used only when adequate dietary supplementation is not practical.

Dosage: Two tablets dissolved in 6–8 oz. of water 4 times daily with meals and at bedtime. For best results let the tablets soak in water for 2 to 5 minutes, or more if necessary, and stir. If any tablet particles remain undissolved they may be crushed and stirred vigorously to speed dissolution.

Caution: Federal law prohibits dispensing without prescription.

Storage: Keep tightly closed. Store at controlled room temperature, 15°C–30°C (59°F–86°F).

How Supplied: White scored tablet with the name BEACH and the number 1111 embossed on each tablet. Bottles of 100 (NDC 0486-1111-01) and bottles of 500 (NDC 0486-1111-05) tablets.

UROQID-Acid®   R
UROQID-Acid® No. 2   R
THIACIDE™   R
(Sodium Free)
Methenamine mandelate with phosphate acidifiers

Description: Each UROQID-Acid® tablet contains methenamine mandelate 350 mg and sodium acid phosphate and monohydrate 200 mg. Each UROQID-Acid® No. 2 tablet contains methenamine mandelate 500 mg and sodium acid phosphate, monohydrate 500 mg.

Each THIACIDE tablet contains methenamine mandelate 500 mg and potassium acid phosphate 250 mg.

Clinical Pharmacology: Methenamine mandelate is rapidly absorbed and excreted in the urine. Formaldehyde is released by acid hydrolysis from methenamine with bactericidal levels rapidly reached at pH 5.0–5.5. Proportionally less formaldehyde is released as urinary pH approaches 6.0 and insufficient quantities are released above this level for therapeutic response. In acid urine, mandelic acid exerts its antibacterial action and also contributes to the acidification of the urine. Mandelic acid is excreted by both glomerular filtration and tubular excretion. In acid urine, there is equally effective antibacterial activity against both gram-positive and gram-negative organisms, since the antibacterial action of mandelic acid and formaldehyde is nonspecific. With Proteus vulgaris and urea splitting strains of Pseudomonas and Aerobacter results may be discouraging and particular attention is required in monitoring urinary pH and overall management.

Long-Term Prophylactic Use: For prevention of reinfection of a sterile urine by converting the urine into an antibacterial medium. Particular suitable for long-term therapy because of safety and because resistance to the nonspecific bactericidal action of formaldehyde does not develop. There is a growing body of evidence that long-term administration can prevent the recurrence of bacteriuria in patients with chronic pyelonephritis.

General Indications: Particularly useful in those infections which are often incurable because of stone or other obstruction, inlying catheter drainage or residual urine in the bladder in neurological disorders. Specifically recommended for the management of chronic urinary tract infection including pyelitis, pyelonephritis, cystitis and infection accompanying neurogenic bladder. Not recommended for acute infection with parenchymal involvement. A thorough diagnostic investigation as a part of the overall management of the urinary tract infection should accompany the use of this product.

Rationale: Methenamine mandelate should not be used unless urinary pH below 6.0 can be maintained. Sodium acid phosphate is a safe, dependable urinary acidifier. The concomitant use of sodium acid phosphate with methenamine mandelate is recommendd when the urinary pH is above 6.0 (See U.S. Dispensatory, 1960 Ed., pp 846–847.)

Contraindications: Renal insufficiency, severe hepatic disease and in patients who have exhibited hypersensitivity to this drug.

Precautions: Urine must be kept acid (on the average below 6.0) or therapy should be discontinued as methenamine mandelate is not effective at higher pH. Frequent urine pH tests are essential. This drug is a urine acidifier and can cause metabolic acidosis. Allergic reactions to Methenamine mandelate have been reported. Each UROQID-Acid® tablet contains approximately 33 mg of sodium and each UROQID-Acid®No. 2 tablet contains approximately 83 mg of sodium; therefore, caution is advised for patients on sodium restriction.

Each THIACIDE tablet contains approximately 72 mg of potassium and is sodium free.

"THIACIDE contains FD&C Yellow No. 5 (tartrazine) which may cause allergic-type reactions (including bronchial asthma) in certain susceptible individuals. Although the overall incidence of FD&C Yellow No. 5 (tartrazine) sensitivity in the general population is low, it is frequently seen in patients who also have aspirin hypersensitivity."

Drug Interactions: Formaldehyde and sulfamethizole form an insoluble precipitate in acid urine; therefore, do not administer concurrently with sulfamethizole.

Drug/Laboratory Test Interactions: Formaldehyde interferes with fluorometric procedures for determination of urinary catecholamines and vanilmandelic acid (VMA) causing erroneously high results. Formaldehyde also causes falsely decreased urine estriol levels by reacting with estriol when acid hydrolysis techniques are used; estriol determinations which use enzymatic hydrolysis are unaffected by folmaldehyde. Formaldehyde causes falsely elevated 17-hydroxy-corticosteroid levels when the Porter-Silber method is used and falsely decreased 5-hydroxy-indoleacetic acid (5HIAA) levels by inhibiting color development when nitrosonaphthol methods are used.

Pregnancy Category C: Animal reproduction studies have not been conducted. It is also not known whether fetal harm can be caused when administered to a pregnant woman or whether reproduction capacity can be affected. Administer to pregnant women only if clearly needed.

There have been no reports, in the literature, of increased risk of fetal abnormalities from use during pregnancy.

Side Effects: A mild laxative effect may be noted in an occasional patient. Methenamine mandelate may cause gastrointestinal upset and/or dysuria. An occasional patient may develop a generalized skin rash. Microscopic and rarely gross hematuria have been described.

Administration and Dosage: UROQID-Acid®; Initially, 3 tablets 4 times daily. For maintenance, 1 or 2 tablets, 4 times daily. UROQID-Acid® No. 2; Initially, 2 tablets 4 times daily. For maintenance, 2 to 4 tablets daily, in divided doses.

THIACIDE: One tablet every 2 to 4 hours with a glass of water not to exceed 8 tablets in 24 hours.

How Supplied: UROQID-Acid® is a yellow, sugar coated, tablet with the name BEACH and the number 1112 printed on each tablet. Packaged in bottles of 100 (NDC 0486-1112-01) and 500 (NDC 0486-1112-05) tablets. UROQID-Acid®No. 2 is a yellow, film coated, capsule shaped tablet with the name BEACH and the number 1114 embossed on each tablet. Packaged in bottles of 100 (NDC 0486-1114-01) and 500 (NDC 0486-1114-05) tablets.

THIACIDE is a light green, film coated, capsule shaped tablet with the name BEACH and the number 1115 embossed on each tablet. Packaged in bottles of 100 (NDC 0486-1115-01) tablets.

Storage: Keep tightly closed. Store at controlled room temperature (15°–30°C) (59°–86°F).

Caution: Federal law prohibits dispensing without prescription.

Supplied by: BEACH PHARMACEUTICALS, Div. Beach Products, Inc. Tampa, FL 33611

Rev. 8/84

Beecham Products
DIVISION OF BEECHAM INC.
POST OFFICE BOX 1467
PITTSBURGH, PA 15230

MASSENGILL®
[mas'sen-gil]
Disposable Douches
MASSENGILL®
Liquid Concentrate
MASSENGILL® Powder

Ingredients:
DISPOSABLES: Vinegar and Water—Water and Vinegar.

Belle-Mai—Water, SD Alcohol 40, Lactic Acid, Sodium Lactate, Octoxynol-9, Cetylpyridinium Chloride, Imidazolidinyl Urea, Disodium EDTA, Fragrance, FD&C Blue No. 1.

Country Flowers—Water, SD Alcohol 40, Lactic Acid, Sodium Lactate, Octoxynol-9, Cetylpyridinium Chloride, Imidazolidinyl Urea, Disodium EDTA, Fragrance, D&C Red No. 28, FD&C Blue No. 1.

Mountain Herbs—Water, SD Alcohol 40, Imidazolidinyl Urea, Lactic Acid, Sodium Lactate, Octoxynol-9, Cetylpyridinium Chloride, Fragrance, Disodium EDTA, D&C Yellow No. 10, FD&C Blue No. 1.

LIQUID CONCENTRATE: Water, SD Alcohol 40, Lactic Acid, Sodium Bicarbonate, Octoxynol-9, Fragrance, D&C Yellow No. 10, FD&C Yellow No. 6.

POWDER: Sodium Chloride, Ammonium alum, PEG-8, Phenol, Methyl Salicylate, Eucalyptus Oil, Menthol, Thymol, D&C Yellow No. 10, FD&C Yellow No. 6.

FLORAL POWDER: Sodium Chloride, Ammonium alum, Octoxynol-9, SD Alcohol 23-A, Fragrance, and FD&C Yellow No. 6.

Indications: Recommended for routine cleansing at the end of menstruation, after use of contraceptive creams or jellies (check the contraceptive package instructions first) or to rinse out the residue of prescribed vaginal medication (as directed by physician).

Actions: The buffered acid solutions of Massengill Douches are valuable adjuncts to specific vaginal therapy following the prescribed use of vaginal medication or contraceptives and in feminine hygiene.

Directions:
DISPOSABLES: Twist off flat, wing-shaped tab from bottle containing premixed solution, attach nozzle supplied and use. The unit is completely disposable.

LIQUID CONCENTRATE: Fill cap ¾ full, to measuring line, and pour contents into douche bag containing 1 quart of warm water. Mix thoroughly.

POWDER: Dissolve two rounded teaspoonfuls in a douche bag containing 1 quart of warm water. Mix thoroughly.

Warning: Vaginal cleansing douches should not be used more than twice weekly except on the advice of a physician. If irritation occurs, discontinue use. Keep out of reach of children. In case of accidental ingestion, seek professional assistance by contacting your physician, the local poison control center, or the Rocky Mt. Poison Control Center at 303-592-1710 (Collect), 24 hours a day.

How Supplied: Disposable—6 oz. disposable plastic bottle.

Liquid Concentrate—4 oz., 8 oz., plastic bottles.
Powder—4 oz., 8 oz., 16 oz., 22 oz., Packettes—10's, 12's.

Continued on next page

Beecham Products—Cont.

MASSENGILL® Medicated
[mas'sen-gil]
Disposable Douche

Active Ingredient: Ceptcin™ (0.23% povidone-iodine).

Indications: For symptomatic relief of minor irritation and itching associated with vaginitis due to Candida albicans, Trichomonas vaginalis and Gardnerella vaginalis.

Action: Povidone-iodine is widely recognized as an effective broad spectrum microbicide against both gram negative and gram positive bacteria, fungi, yeasts and protozoa. While remaining active in the presence of blood, serum or bodily secretions, it possesses virtually none of the irritating properties of iodine.

Warnings: If symptoms persist after seven days of use, or if redness, swelling or pain develop during treatment, consult a physician. Women with iodine-sensitivity should not use this product. Women may douche during menstruation if they douche gently. Do not douche during pregnancy unless directed by a physician. Douching does not prevent pregnancy. Keep out of reach of children. In case of accidental ingestion, seek professional assistance by contacting your physician, the local poison control center, or the Rocky Mt. Poison Control Center at 303-592-1710 (Collect), 24 hours a day.

Dosage and Administration: Dosage is provided as a single unit concentrate to be added to 6 oz. of sanitized water supplied in a disposable bottle. A specially designed nozzle is provided. After use, the unit is discarded. Use one bottle a day for seven days. Even if symptoms are relieved earlier, treatment should be continued for the full seven days.

How Supplied: 6 oz. bottle of sanitized water with 0.17 oz. vial of povidone-iodine and nozzle.

EDUCATIONAL MATERIAL

Booklet:
"A Personal Guide to Feminine Freshness"
A 16 page illustrated booklet on vaginal infections, feminine hygiene and douching. Free to physicians, pharmacists and patients in limited quantities by writing Beecham or calling 800-BEECHAM. (PA residents 800-242-1718)

Film, Video:
"Feminine Hygiene and You"
This 14 minute color film begins with a simple explanation of how a woman's body works (reproductive system, menstrual cycle, and vaginal secretions) then explains douching. Free loan to physicians, pharmacists and clinics. Available in 16mm, 3/4" video, Beta and VHS by writing Beecham or calling 800-BEECHAM. (PA residents 800-242-1718)

Important Notice

Before prescribing or administering
any product described in
PHYSICIANS' DESK REFERENCE
always consult the PDR Supplement for
possible new or revised information

Beecham Laboratories
DIV. OF BEECHAM INC.,
501 FIFTH STREET
BRISTOL, TN 37620

PRODUCT IDENTIFICATION CODES

To provide quick and positive identification of Beecham Laboratories' products, we have imprinted a code number or brand name on tablet and capsule products. In order that you may identify a product by its code and number, we have compiled below a numerical list of code numbers with their corresponding product names. The code number as it appears on tablets and capsules bears the letters BMP plus the numerical code. Amoxil® and Fastin® capsules, and Amoxil® Chewable Tablets bear the brand name only.

BMP Code No.   Product

105	ANEXSIA® w/Codeine Tablets
106	ANEXSIA®-D Tablets
107	CONAR®-A Tablets
112	DASIN® Capsules
119	HYBEPHEN® Tablets
121	LIVITAMIN® Capsules
122	LIVITAMIN® w/INTRINSIC FACTOR Capsules
123	LIVITAMIN® CHEWABLE Tablets
125	MENEST™ (Esterified Estrogens, U.S.P.) Tablets 0.3 mg.
126	MENEST™ (Esterified Estrogens, U.S.P.) Tablets 0.625 mg.
127	MENEST™ (Esterified Estrogens, U.S.P.) Tablets 1.25 mg.
128	MENEST™ (Esterified Estrogens, U.S.P.) Tablets 2.5 mg.
135	SEMETS®
140	TOTACILLIN® (Ampicillin) Capsules 250 mg.
141	TOTACILLIN® (Ampicillin) Capsules 500 mg.
143	BACTOCILL® (Oxacillin Sodium) Capsules 250 mg.
144	BACTOCILL® (Oxacillin Sodium) Capsules 500 mg.
145	DARICON® (Oxyphencyclimine HCl) Tablets 10 mg.
146	DARICON®-PB (Oxyphencyclimine HCl, 5 mg. and Phenobarbital, 15 mg.) Tablets
156	TIGAN® (Trimethobenzamide HCl) Capsules 100 mg.
157	TIGAN® (Trimethobenzamide HCl) Capsules 250 mg.
165	DYCILL® (Dicloxacillin Sodium) Capsules 250 mg.
166	DYCILL® (Dicloxacillin Sodium) Capsules 500 mg.
167	ACTOL EXPECTORANT® Tablets
169	CLOXAPEN® (Cloxacillin Sodium) Capsules 250 mg.
170	CLOXAPEN® (Cloxacillin Sodium) Capsules 500 mg.
182	NUCOFED® Capsules
185	BEEPEN–VK® (Penicillin V Potassium) Tablets 250 mg.
186	BEEPEN–VK® (Penicillin V Potassium) Tablets 500 mg.
194	ENARAX®5 (Oxphencyclimine HCl, 5 mg. and Hydroxyzine HCl, 25 mg.) Tablets
195	ENARAX®10 (Oxphencyclimine HCl, 10 mg, and Hydroxyzine HCl, 25 mg.) Tablets

AMOXIL®   B
[ă-mŏx'ĭl]
(amoxicillin)
capsules, for oral suspension and chewable tablets

Description: AMOXIL (Amoxicillin) is a semisynthetic antibiotic, an analog of ampicillin, with a broad spectrum of bactericidal activity against many Gram-positive and Gram-negative microorganisms. Chemically it is D- (-)-α -amino-p-hydroxybenzyl penicillin trihydrate.

Actions:

PHARMACOLOGY

Amoxicillin is stable in the presence of gastric acid and may be given without regard to meals. It is rapidly absorbed after oral administration. It diffuses readily into most body tissues and fluids, with the exception of brain and spinal fluid, except when meninges are inflamed. The half-life of amoxicillin is 61.3 minutes. Most of the amoxicillin is excreted unchanged in the urine; its excretion can be delayed by concurrent administration of probenecid. Amoxicillin is not highly protein-bound. In blood serum, Amoxicillin is approximately 20% protein-bound as compared to 60% for penicillin G.

Orally administered doses of 250 mg and 500 mg Amoxicillin capsules result in average peak blood levels one to two hours after administration in the range of 3.5 mcg/ml to 5.0 mcg/ml and 5.5 mcg/ml to 7.5 mcg/ml respectively.

Orally administered doses of Amoxicillin suspension 125 mg/5 ml and 250 mg/5 ml result in average peak blood levels one to two hours after administration in the range of 1.5 mcg/ml to 3.0 mcg/ml and 3.5 mcg/ml to 5.0 mcg/ml respectively. Amoxicillin chewable tablets, 125 mg and 250 mg, produced blood levels similar to those achieved with the corresponding doses of Amoxicillin oral suspensions.

Detectable serum levels are observed up to 8 hours after an orally administered dose of Amoxicillin. Following a 1 Gm dose and utilizing a special skin window technique to determine levels of the antibiotic, it was noted that therapeutic levels were found in the interstitial fluid. Approximately 60 percent of an orally administered dose of Amoxicillin is excreted in the urine within six to eight hours.

MICROBIOLOGY:

AMOXIL (Amoxicillin) is similar to ampicillin in its bactericidal action against susceptible organisms during the stage of active multiplication. It acts through the inhibition of biosynthesis of cell wall mucopeptide. *In vitro* studies have demonstrated the susceptibility of most strains of the following Gram-positive bacteria: alpha- and beta-hemolytic streptococci, *Diplococcus pneumoniae*, nonpenicillinase-producing staphylococci, and *Streptococcus faecalis*. It is active *in vitro* against many strains of *Haemophilus influenzae*, *Neisseria gonorrhoeae*, *Escherichia coli* and *Proteus mirabilis*. Because it does not resist destruction by penicillinase, it is not effective against penicillinase-producing bacteria, particularly resistant staphylococci. All strains of Pseudomonas and most strains of Klebsiella and Enterobacter are resistant.

DISC SUSCEPTIBILITY TESTS: Quantitative methods that require measurement of zone diameters give the most precise estimates of antibiotic susceptibility. One such procedure* has been recommended for use with discs for testing susceptibility to ampicillin-class antibiotics. Interpretations correlate diameters of the disc test with MIC values for Amoxicillin. With this procedure, a report from the laboratory of "susceptible" indicates that the infecting organism is likely to respond to therapy. A report of "resistant" indicates that the infecting organism is not likely to respond to therapy. A report of "intermediate susceptibility" suggests that the organism would be susceptible if high dosage is used, or if the infection is confined to tissues and fluids (e.g., urine), in which high antibiotic levels are attained.

*Bauer, A. W., Kirby, W. M. M., Sherris, J. C., and Turck, M.: Antibiotic Testing by a Standardized Single Disc Method, Am. J. Clin. Pathol., 45:493, 1966. Standardized Disc Susceptibility Test, FEDERAL REGISTER 37:20527-29, 1972.

Indications: AMOXIL (Amoxicillin) is indicated in the treatment of infections due to susceptible strains of the following:

Gram-negative organisms—*H. influenzae, E. coli, P. mirabilis* and *N. gonorrhoeae.*

Gram-positive organisms—Streptococci (including *Streptococcus faecalis*), *D. pneumoniae* and nonpenicillinase-producing staphylococci.

Therapy may be instituted prior to obtaining results from bacteriological and susceptibility studies to determine the causative organisms and their susceptibility to Amoxicillin. Indicated surgical procedures should be performed.

Contraindications: A history of allergic reaction to any of the penicillins is a contraindication.

Warnings: SERIOUS AND OCCASIONALLY FATAL HYPERSENSITIVITY (ANAPHYLACTOID) REACTIONS HAVE BEEN REPORTED IN PATIENTS ON PENICILLIN THERAPY. ALTHOUGH ANAPHYLAXIS IS MORE FREQUENT FOLLOWING PARENTERAL THERAPY, IT HAS OCCURRED IN PATIENTS ON ORAL PENICILLINS. THESE REACTIONS ARE MORE LIKELY TO OCCUR IN INDIVIDUALS WITH A HISTORY OF SENSITIVITY TO MULTIPLE ALLERGENS. THERE HAVE BEEN REPORTS OF INDIVIDUALS WITH A HISTORY OF PENICILLIN HYPERSENSITIVITY WHO HAVE EXPERIENCED SEVERE REACTIONS WHEN TREATED WITH CEPHALOSPORINS. BEFORE THERAPY WITH ANY PENICILLIN, CAREFUL INQUIRY SHOULD BE MADE CONCERNING PREVIOUS HYPERSENSITIVITY REACTIONS TO PENICILLINS, CEPHALOSPORINS, OR OTHER ALLERGENS. IF AN ALLERGIC REACTION OCCURS, APPROPRIATE THERAPY SHOULD BE INSTITUTED AND DISCONTINUANCE OF AMOXICILLIN THERAPY CONSIDERED. SERIOUS ANAPHYLACTOID REACTIONS REQUIRE IMMEDIATE EMERGENCY TREATMENT WITH EPINEPHRINE. OXYGEN, INTRAVENOUS STEROIDS, AND AIRWAY MANAGEMENT, INCLUDING INTUBATION, SHOULD ALSO BE ADMINISTERED AS INDICATED.

USAGE IN PREGNANCY
Safety for use in pregnancy has not been established.

Precautions: As with any potent drug, periodic assessment of renal, hepatic and hematopoietic function should be made during prolonged therapy.

The possibility of superinfections with mycotic or bacterial pathogens should be kept in mind during therapy. If superinfections occur (usually involving Enterobacter, Pseudomonas or Candida), the drug should be discontinued and/or appropriate therapy instituted.

Adverse Reactions: As with other penicillins, it may be expected that untoward reactions will be essentially limited to sensitivity phenomena. They are more likely to occur in individuals who have previously demonstrated hypersensitivity to penicillins and in those with a history of allergy, asthma, hay fever or urticaria. The following adverse reactions have been reported as associated with the use of the penicillins:

Gastrointestinal: Nausea, vomiting and diarrhea.

Hypersensitivity Reactions: Erythematous maculopapular rashes and urticaria have been reported.

NOTE: Urticaria, other skin rashes and serum sickness-like reactions may be controlled with antihistamines and, if necessary, systemic corticosteroids. Whenever such reactions occur, Amoxicillin should be discontinued unless, in the opinion of the physician, the condition being treated is life-threatening and amenable only to Amoxicillin therapy.

Liver: A moderate rise in serum glutamic oxaloacetic transaminase (SGOT) has been noted, but the significance of this finding is unknown.

Hemic and Lymphatic Systems: Anemia, thrombocytopenia, thrombocytopenic purpura, eosinophilia, leukopenia and agranulocytosis have been reported during therapy with the penicillins. These reactions are usually reversible on discontinuation of therapy and are believed to be hypersensitivity phenomena.

Dosage and Administration:
Infections of the ear, nose and throat due to streptococci, pneumococci, nonpenicillinase-producing staphylococci and *H. influenzae;*

Infections of the genitourinary tract due to *E. coli, Proteus mirabilis* and *Streptococcus faecalis;*

Infections of the skin and soft-tissues due to streptococci, susceptible staphylococci and *E. coli.*

USUAL DOSAGE:
Adults: 250 mg every 8 hours.
Children: 20 mg/kg/day in divided doses every 8 hours.
Children weighing 20 kg or more should be dosed according to the adult recommendations.

In severe infections or those caused by less susceptible organisms:
500 mg every 8 hours for adults, and 40 mg/kg/day in divided doses every 8 hours for children may be needed.

Infections of the lower respiratory tract due to streptococci, pneumococci, nonpenicillinase-producing staphylococci and *H. influenzae:*

USUAL DOSAGE:
Adults: 500 mg every 8 hours.
Children: 40 mg/kg/day in divided doses every 8 hours.
Children weighing 20 kg or more should be dosed according to the adult recommendations.

Gonorrhea, acute uncomplicated ano-genital and urethral infections due to *N. gonorrhoeae* (males and females):

USUAL DOSAGE:
Adults: 3 grams as a single oral dose.
Prepubertal children: 50 mg/kg amoxicillin combined with 25 mg/kg probenecid as a single dose.

NOTE: SINCE PROBENECID IS CONTRAINDICATED IN CHILDREN UNDER 2 YEARS, THIS REGIMEN SHOULD NOT BE USED IN THESE CASES.

Cases of gonorrhea with a suspected lesion of syphilis should have dark-field examinations before receiving Amoxicillin, and monthly serological tests for a minimum of four months. Larger doses may be required for stubborn or severe infections. The children's dosage is intended for individuals whose weight will not cause a dosage to be calculated greater than that recommended for adults. It should be recognized that in the treatment of chronic urinary tract infections, frequent bacteriological and clinical appraisals are necessary. Smaller doses than those recommended above should not be used. Even higher doses may be needed at times. In stubborn infections, therapy may be required for several weeks. It may be necessary to continue clinical and/or bacteriological follow-up for several months after cessation of therapy. Except for gonorrhea, treatment should be continued for a minimum of 48 to 72 hours beyond the time that the patient becomes asymptomatic or evidence of bacterial eradication has been obtained. It is recommended that there be at least 10 days' treatment for any infection caused by hemolytic streptococci to prevent the occurrence of acute rheumatic fever or glomerulonephritis.

Dosage and Administration of Pediatric Drops:

Usual dosage for all indications except infections of the lower respiratory tract:
Under 6 kg (13 lbs): 0.75 ml every 8 hours.
6—7 kg (13—15 lbs): 1.0 ml every 8 hours.
8 kg (16—18 lbs): 1.25 ml every 8 hours.
Infections of the lower respiratory tract:
Under 6 kg (13 lbs): 1.25 ml every 8 hours.
6—7 kg (13—15 lbs): 1.75 ml every 8 hours.
8 kg (16—18 lbs): 2.25 ml every 8 hours.

Children weighing more than 8 kg (18 lbs) should receive the appropriate dose of the Oral Suspension 125 mg or 250 mg/5 ml.

After reconstitution, the required amount of suspension should be placed directly on the child's tongue for swallowing. Alternate means of administration are to add the required amount of suspension to formula, milk, fruit juice, water, ginger ale or cold drinks. These preparations should then be taken immediately. To be certain the child is receiving full dosage, such preparations should be consumed in entirety.

Directions For Mixing Oral Suspension:
Prepare suspension at time of dispensing as follows: Tap bottle until all powder flows freely. Add approximately 1/3 of the total amount of water for reconstitution (see table below) and shake vigorously to wet powder. Add remainder of the water and again shake vigorously.

125 mg per 5 ml

Bottle Size	Amount of Water Required for Reconstitution
80 ml	62 ml
100 ml	78 ml
150 ml	116 ml

Each teaspoonful (5 ml) will contain 125 mg Amoxicillin.

| 125 mg unit dose | 5 ml |

250 mg per 5 ml

Bottle Size	Amount of Water Required for Reconstitution
80 ml	59 ml
100 ml	74 ml
150 ml	111 ml

Each teaspoonful (5 ml) will contain 250 mg Amoxicillin.

| 250 mg unit dose | 5 ml |
| 3 Gm single dose | 40 ml |

Directions For Mixing Pediatric Drops:
Prepare pediatric drops at time of dispensing as follows: Add the required amount of water (see table below) to the bottle and shake vigorously. Each ml of suspension will then contain Amoxicillin Trihydrate equivalent to 50 mg Amoxicillin.

Bottle Size	Amount of Water Required for Reconstitution
15 ml	12 ml
30 ml	23 ml

NOTE: SHAKE BOTH ORAL SUSPENSION AND PEDIATRIC DROPS WELL BEFORE USING. Keep bottle tightly closed. Any unused portion of the reconstituted suspension must be discarded after 14 days. Refrigeration preferable, but not required.

How Supplied:
AMOXIL (Amoxicillin) Capsules. Each capsule contains 250 mg or 500 mg Amoxicillin as the trihydrate.

250 mg/Capsule

NDC 0029-6006-24 ....bottles of 15
NDC 0029-6006-30 ....bottles of 100
NDC 0029-6006-32 ....bottles of 500
NDC 0029-6006-31 ....unit dose carton of 100

500 mg/Capsule

NDC 0029-6007-24 ....bottles of 15
NDC 0029-6007-29 ....bottles of 50
NDC 0029-6007-30 ....bottles of 100
NDC 0029-6007-32 ....bottles of 500
NDC 0029-6007-31 ....unit dose cartons of 100

Shown in Product Identification Section, page 000

Therapy Pack:
NDC 0029-6007-79 ....6 × 500 mg Capsules
(3 packs per carton)

AMOXIL (Amoxicillin) Chewable Tablets. Each scored tablet contains 125 mg or 250 mg Amoxicillin as the trihydrate.

Continued on next page

Beecham Laboratories—Cont.

125 mg/Tablet
NDC 0029-6004-39 ....bottles of 60
250 mg/Tablet
NDC 0029-6005-39 ....bottles of 60
NDC 0029-6005-30 ....bottles of 100
AMOXIL (Amoxicillin) for Oral Suspension.
125 mg/5 ml
NDC 0029-6008-21 ....80 ml bottle
NDC 0029-6008-23 ....100 ml bottle
NDC 0029-6008-22 ....150 ml bottle
250 mg/5 ml
NDC 0029-6009-21 ....80 ml bottle
NDC 0029-6009-23 ....100 ml bottle
NDC 0029-6009-22 ....150 ml bottle
Each 5 ml of reconstituted suspension contains 125 mg or 250 mg Amoxicillin as the trihydrate.
NDC 0029-6008-18 ....125 mg unit dose bottle
NDC 0029-6009-18 ....250 mg unit dose bottle
3 Gm for Oral Suspension:
NDC 0029-6037-28 ....single dose bottle
Each single dose bottle contains 3 grams Amoxicillin as the trihydrate.
AMOXIL (Amoxicillin) **Pediatric Drops for Oral Suspension.**
Each ml of reconstituted suspension contains 50 mg Amoxicillin as the trihydrate.
NDC 0029-6035-20 ....15 ml bottle
NDC 0029-6038-39 ....30 ml bottle
Rev. Aug., 1982

AUGMENTIN® ℞
(amoxicillin/potassium clavulanate)
Tablets and Powder for Oral Suspension

Description: AUGMENTIN is an oral antibacterial combination consisting of the semisynthetic antibiotic amoxicillin and the β-lactamase inhibitor, potassium clavulanate (the potassium salt of clavulanic acid. Amoxicillin is an analog of ampicillin, derived from the basic penicillin nucleus, 6-aminopenicillanic acid. Chemically, amoxicillin is D-(-)-α-amino-p-hydroxybenzyl-penicillin trihydrate and may be represented structurally as:

Clavulanic acid is produced by the fermentation of *Streptomyces clavuligerus*. It is a β-lactam structurally related to the penicillins and possesses the ability to inactivate a wide variety of β-lactamases by blocking the active sites of these enzymes. Clavulanic acid is particularly active against the clinically important plasmid mediated β-lactamases frequently responsible for transferred drug resistance to penicillins and cephalosporins. Chemically potassium clavulanate is potassium Z-(3R, 5R)-2-(β-hydroxyethylidene) clavam-3-carboxylate and may be represented structurally as:

AUGMENTIN is available in '250' and '500' white filmcoated tablets and '125' and '250' fruit flavored oral suspensions. Each AUGMENTIN '250' and '500' tablet contains 250 mg and 500 mg amoxicillin as the trihydrate, respectively, together with 125 mg clavulanic acid as the potassium salt. Following reconstitution, each teaspoonful (5 ml) of AUGMENTIN '125' oral suspension contains 125 mg amoxicillin and 31.25 mg clavulanic acid as the potassium salt while each 5 ml of AUGMENTIN '250' oral suspension contains 250 mg amoxicillin and 62.5 mg clavulanic acid as the potassium salt.
Each AUGMENTIN tablet contains 0.63 mEq potassium. Each 5 ml of reconstituted AUGMENTIN '125' and '250' oral suspension contains 0.16 mEq and 0.32 mEq potassium respectively.

Clinical Pharmacology: Amoxicillin and potassium clavulanate are well absorbed from the gastrointestinal tract after oral administration of AUGMENTIN. AUGMENTIN is stable in the presence of gastric acid and may be given without regard to meals.
Oral administration of one AUGMENTIN '250' or AUGMENTIN '500' tablet provides average peak serum concentrations one to two hours after dosing of 4.4 mcg/ml and 7.6 mcg/ml, respectively, for amoxicillin and 2.3 mcg/ml for clavulanic acid. The areas under the serum concentration curves obtained during the first 6 hours after dosing were 11.4 mcg/ml.hr and 20.2 mcg/ml.hr for amoxicillin, respectively, when one AUGMENTIN '250' or '500' tablet was administered to adult volunteers. The corresponding area under the serum concentration curve for calvulanic acid was 5 mcg/ml.hr.
Oral administration of 5 ml of AUGMENTIN '250' suspension or the equivalent dose of 10 ml of AUGMENTIN '125' suspension provides average peak serum concentrations approximately one hour after dosing of 6.9 mcg/ml for amoxicillin and 1.6 mcg/ml for clavulanic acid. The areas under the serum concentration curves obtained during the first 6 hours after dosing were 12.6 mcg/ml.hr for amoxicillin and 2.9 mcg/ml.hr for clavulanic acid when 5 ml of AUGMENTIN '250' suspension or the equivalent dose of 10 ml of AUGMENTIN '125' suspension was administered to adult volunteers.
Amoxicillin serum concentrations achieved with AUGMENTIN are similar to those produced by the oral administration of equivalent doses of amoxicillin alone. The half life of amoxicillin after the oral administration of AUGMENTIN is 1.3 hours and that of clavulanic acid is 1.0 hour.
Approximately 50-70% of the amoxicillin and approximately 25-40% of the clavulanic acid are excreted unchanged in urine during the first six hours after administration of a single AUGMENTIN '250' or '500' tablet or 10 ml of AUGMENTIN '250' suspension.
Concurrent administration of probenecid delays amoxicillin excretion but does not delay renal excretion of clavulanic acid.
Neither component in AUGMENTIN is highly protein-bound; clavulanic acid has been found to be approximately 30% bound to human serum and amoxicillin approximately 20% bound.
Amoxicillin diffuses readily into most body tissues and fluids with the exception of the brain and spinal fluids. The results of experiments involving the administration of clavulanic acid to animals suggest that this compound, like amoxicillin, is well distributed in body tissues.
Two hours after oral administration of a single 35 mg/kg dose of AUGMENTIN suspension to fasting children, average concentrations of 3.0 mcg/ml of amoxicillin and 0.5 mcg/ml of clavulanic acid were detected in middle ear effusions.
Microbiology: Amoxicillin is a semisynthetic antibiotic with a broad spectrum of bactericidal activity against many Gram-positive and Gram-negative microorganisms. Amoxicillin is, however, susceptible to degradation by β-lactamases and therefore the spectrum of activity does not include organisms which produce these enzymes.
Clavulanic acid is a β-lactam, structurally related to the penicillins, which possesses the ability to inactivate a wide range of β-lactamase enzymes commonly found in microorganisms resistant to penicillins and cephalosporins. In particular, it has good activity against the clinically important plasmid mediated β-lactamases frequently responsible for transferred drug resistance.
The formulation of amoxicillin with clavulanic acid in AUGMENTIN protects amoxicillin from degradation by β-lactamase enzymes and effectively extends the antibiotic spectrum of amoxicillin to include many bacteria normally resistant to amoxicillin and other β-lactam antibiotics. Thus AUGMENTIN possesses the distinctive properties of a broad spectrum antibiotic and a β-lactamase inhibitor.
While *in vitro* studies have demonstrated the susceptibility of most strains of the following organisms, clinical efficacy for infections other than those included in the Indications and Usage section has not been documented:

GRAM-POSITIVE BACTERIA: *Staphylococcus aureus* (β-lactamase and non-β-lactamase producing), *Staphylococcus epidermidis* (β-lactamase and non-β-lactamase producing), *Staphylococcus saprophyticus* (β-lactamase and non-β-lactamase producing), *Streptococcus faecalis** (Enterococcus), *Streptococcus pneumoniae**(D. pneumoniae), *Streptococcus pyogenes**, *Streptococcus viridans**
ANAEROBES: *Clostridium* species*, *Peptococcus* species*, *Peptostreptococcus* species*
*These are non-β-lactamase producing strains and therefore are susceptible to amoxicillin alone.
GRAM NEGATIVE BACTERIA: *Hemophilus influenzae* (β-lactamase and non-B-lactamase producing), *Branhamella catarrhalis (Neisseria catarrhalis)* (β-lactamase and non-β-lactamase producing); *Escherichia coli* (β-lactamase and non-β-lactamase producing), *Klebsiella* species (All known strains are β-lactamase producing), *Enterobacter* species (Although most strains of *Enterobacter* species are resistant *in vitro*, clinical efficacy has been demonstrated with AUGMENTIN in urinary tract infections caused by these organisms.), *Proteus mirabilis* (β-lactamase and non-β-lactamase producing), *Proteus vulgaris* (β-lactamase and non-β-lactamase producing), *Neisseria gonorrhoeae* (β-lactamase and non-β-lactamase producing), *Legionella* species (β-lactamase and non-β-lactamase producing)
ANAEROBES: *Bacteroides* species, including *B. fragilis* (β-lactamase and non-β-lactamase producing).

SUSCEPTIBILITY TESTING
Diffusion Technique: For Kirby-Bauer method of susceptibility testing, a 30 mcg AUGMENTIN (20 mcg amoxicillin + 10 mcg clavulanic acid) diffusion disk should be used. With this procedure, a report from the laboratory of "Susceptible" indicates that the infecting organism is likely to respond to AUGMENTIN therapy and a report of "Resistant" indicates that the infecting organism is not likely to respond to therapy. An "intermediate susceptibility" report suggests that the infecting organism would be susceptible to AUGMENTIN if the higher dosage is used or if the infection is confined to tissues or fluids (e.g. urine) in which high antibiotic levels are attained.
Dilution Techniques: Broth or agar dilution methods may be used to determine the minimal inhibitory concentration (MIC) value for susceptibility of bacterial isolates to AUGMENTIN. Tubes should be inoculated to contain 10^4 to 10^5 organisms/ml or plates "spotted" with 10^3 to 10^4 organisms.
The recommended dilution method employs a constant amoxicillin/clavulanic acid ratio of 2 to 1 in all tubes with increasing concentrations of amoxicillin. MIC's are reported in terms of amoxicillin concentration in the presence of clavulanic acid at a constant 2 parts amoxicillin to 1 part clavulanic acid.
[See table on next page].
[1] The non-β-lactamase-producing organisms which are normally susceptible to ampicillin, such as *Streptococci*, will have similar zone sizes as for ampicillin disks.
[2] The quality control cultures should have the following assigned daily ranges for AUGMENTIN:

		Disks	Mode MIC (mcg/ml)
E. coli	(ATCC 25922)	19-25 mm	4/2-8/4
S. aureus	(ATCC 25923)	28-36 mm	0.25/0.2-0.5/0.25
E. coli	(ATCC 35218)	18-22 mm	4/2-8/4

[3] Expressed as concentration of amoxicillin/clavulanic acid
[4] Organisms which show susceptibility to AUGMENTIN but are resistant to methicillin/oxacillin should be considered resistant.

Indications and Usage: AUGMENTIN is indicated in the treatment of infections caused by susceptible strains of the designated organisms in the conditions listed below:

Lower Respiratory Infections—caused by β-lactamase producing strains of *Hemophilus influenzae*.

Otitis Media—caused by β-lactamase producing strains of *Hemophilus influenzae* and *Branhamella catarrhalis*.

Sinusitis—caused by β-lactamase producing strains of *Hemophilus influenzae* and *Branhamella catarrhalis*.

Skin and Skin Structure Infections—caused by β-lactamase producing strains of *Staphylococcus aureus*, *Escherichia coli*, and *Klebsiella* spp.

Urinary Tract Infections—caused by β-lactamase producing strains of *Escherichia coli*, *Klebsiella* spp. and *Enterobacter* spp.

While AUGMENTIN is indicated only for the conditions listed above, infections caused by ampicillin susceptible organisms are also amenable to AUGMENTIN treatment due to its amoxicillin content. Therefore, mixed infections caused by ampicillin susceptible organisms and β-lactamase producing organisms susceptible to AUGMENTIN should not require the addition of another antibiotic.

Bacteriological studies, to determine the causative organisms and their susceptibility to AUGMENTIN, should be performed together with any indicated surgical procedures.

Therapy may be instituted prior to obtaining the results from bacteriological and susceptibility studies to determine the causative organisms and their susceptibility to AUGMENTIN when there is reason to believe the infection may involve any of the β-lactamase producing organisms listed above. Once the results are known, therapy should be adjusted, if appropriate.

Contraindications: A history of allergic reactions to any penicillin is a contraindication.

Warnings: SERIOUS AND OCCASIONALLY FATAL HYPERSENSITIVITY (ANAPHYLACTOID) REACTIONS HAVE BEEN REPORTED IN PATIENTS ON PENICILLIN THERAPY. ALTHOUGH ANAPHYLAXIS IS MORE FREQUENT FOLLOWING PARENTERAL THERAPY, IT HAS OCCURRED IN PATIENTS ON ORAL PENICILLINS. THESE REACTIONS ARE MORE LIKELY TO OCCUR IN INDIVIDUALS WITH A HISTORY OF PENICILLIN HYPERSENSITIVITY AND/OR A HISTORY OF SENSITIVITY TO MULTIPLE ALLERGENS. THERE HAVE BEEN REPORTS OF INDIVIDUALS WITH A HISTORY OF PENICILLIN HYPERSENSITIVITY WHO HAVE EXPERIENCED SEVERE REACTIONS WHEN TREATED WITH CEPHALOSPORINS. BEFORE INITIATING THERAPY WITH ANY PENICILLIN, CAREFUL INQUIRY SHOULD BE MADE CONCERNING PREVIOUS HYPERSENSITIVITY REACTIONS TO PENICILLINS, CEPHALOSPORINS, OR OTHER ALLERGENS. IF AN ALLERGIC REACTION OCCURS, AUGMENTIN SHOULD BE DISCONTINUED AND THE APPROPRIATE THERAPY INSTITUTED. SERIOUS ANAPHYLACTOID REACTIONS REQUIRE IMMEDIATE EMERGENCY TREATMENT WITH EPINEPHRINE. OXYGEN INTRAVENOUS STEROIDS, AND AIRWAY MANAGEMENT, INCLUDING INTUBATION, SHOULD ALSO BE ADMINISTERED AS INDICATED.

Precautions:

General: While AUGMENTIN possesses the characteristic low toxicity of the penicillin group of antibiotics, period assessment of organ system functions, including renal, hepatic and hematopoietic function is advisable during prolonged therapy.

A high percentage of patients with mononucleosis who receive ampicillin develop a skin rash. Thus, ampicillin class antibiotics should not be administered to patients with mononucleosis.

The possibility of superinfections with mycotic or bacterial pathogens should be kept in mind during therapy. If superinfections occur (usually involving *Pseudomonas* or *Candida*), the drug should be discontinued and/or appropriate therapy instituted.

Drug Interactions: Probenecid decreases the renal tubular secretion of amoxicillin. Concurrent use with AUGMENTIN may result in increased and prolonged blood levels of amoxicillin.

The concurrent administration of allopurinol and ampicillin increases substantially the incidence of rashes in patients receiving both drugs as compared to patients receiving ampicillin alone. It is not known whether this potentiation of ampicillin rashes is due to allopurinol or the hyperuricemia present in these patients. There are no data with AUGMENTIN and allopurinol administered concurrently.

AUGMENTIN should not be co-administered with ANTABUSE® (disulfiram).

Drug/Laboratory Test Interactions: Oral administraion of AUGMENTIN will result in high urine concentrations of amoxicillin. High urine concentrations of ampicillin may result in false positive reactions when testing for the presence of glucose in urine using Clinitest™, Benedict's Solution or Fehling's Solution. Since this effect may also occur with amoxicillin and therefore AUGMENTIN, it is recommended that glucose tests based on enzymatic glucose oxidase reactions (such. as Clinistix™ or Testape™) be used.

Following administration of ampicillin to pregnant women a transient decrease in plasma concentration of total conjugated estriol, estriol-glucuronide, conjugated estrone and estradiol has been noted. This effect may also occur with amoxicillin and therefore AUGMENTIN.

Carcinogenesis, Mutagenesis, Impairment of Fertility: Long-term studies in animals have not been performed to evaluate carcinogenic or mutagenic potential.

Pregnancy (Category B): Reproduction studies have been performed in mice and rats at doses up to ten (10) times the human dose and have revealed no evidence of impaired fertility or harm to the fetus due to AUGMENTIN. There are, however, no adequate and well-controlled studies in pregnant women. Because animal reproduction studies are not always predictive of human response, this drug should be used during pregnancy only if clearly needed.

Labor and Delivery: Oral ampicillin class antibiotics are generally poorly absorbed during labor. Studies in guinea pigs have been shown that intravenous administration of ampicillin decreased the uterine tone, frequency of contractions, height of contractions and duration of contractions. However, it is not known whether the use of AUGMENTIN in humans during labor or delivery has immediate or delayed adverse effects on the fetus, prolongs the duration of labor or increases the likelihood that forceps delivery or other obstetrical intervention or resuscitation of the newborn will be necessary.

Nursing Mothers: Ampicillin class antibiotics are excreted in the milk; therefore, caution should be exercised when AUGMENTIN is administered to a nursing woman.

Adverse Reactions: AUGMENTIN is generally well tolerated. The majority of side effects observed in clinical trials were of a mild and transient nature and less than 3% of patients discontinued therapy because of drug related side effects. The most frequently reported adverse effects were diarrhea/loose stools (9%), nausea (3%), skin rashes and urticaria (3%), vomiting (1%), and vaginitis (1%). The overall incidence of side effects, and in particular diarrhea, increased with the higher recommended dose. Other less frequently reported reactions include: abdominal discomfort, flatulence and headache.

The following adverse reactions have been reported for ampicillin class antibiotics:

Gastrointestinal: Diarrhea, nausea, vomiting, gastritis, stomatitis, glossitis, black "hairy" tongue, enterocolitis and pseudomembraneous colitis.

Hypersensitivity reactions: Skin rashes, urticaria, erythema multiforme and an occasional case of exfoliative dermatitis have been reported. These reactions may be controlled with antihistamines and, if necessary, systemic corticosteroids. Whenever such reactions occur, the drug should be discontinued, unless the opinion of the physician dictates otherwise. Serious and occasional fatal hypersensitivity (anaphylactic) reactions can occur with oral penicillin (See Warnings).

Liver: A moderate rise in SGOT has been noted in patients treated with ampicillin class antibiotics as well as with AUGMENTIN, but the significance of these findings is unknown.

Hemic and Lymphatic Systems: Anemia, thrombocytopenia, thrombocytopenic purpura, eosinophilia, leukopenia and agranulocytosis have been reported during therapy with penicillins. These reactions are usually reversible on discontinuation of therapy and are believed to be hypersensitivity phenomena. A slight thrombocytosis was noted in less than 1% of the patients treated with AUGMENTIN.

Overdosage: Amoxicillin may be removed from circulation by hemodialysis.

The molecular weight, degree of protein binding and pharmacokinetic profile of clavulanic acid together with information from a single patient with renal insufficiency all suggest that this compound may also be removed by hemodialysis.

Dosage and Administration:

Dosage:

Adults: The usual adult dose is one AUGMENTIN '250' tablet every eight hours. For more severe infections and infections of the respiratory tract, the dose should be one AUGMENTIN '500' tablet every eight hours.

Since both the AUGMENTIN '250' and '500' tablets contain the same amount of clavulanic acid (125 mg, as the potassium salt), two AUGMENTIN '250' tablets are not equivalent to one AUGMENTIN '500' tablet. Therefore, two AUGMENTIN '250' tablets should not be substituted for one AUGMENTIN '500' tablet for treatment of more severe infections.

Children: The usual dose is 20 mg/kd/day, based on amoxicillin component, in divided doses every eight hours. For otitis media, sinusitis and lower respiratory infections, the dose should be 40 mg/kg/day, based on the amoxicillin component, in divided doses every eight hours. Severe infections should be treated with the higher recommended dose.

Children weighing 40 kg and more should be dosed according to the adult recommendations.

Directions For Mixing Oral Suspension: Prepare a suspension at time of dispensing as follows: Tap bottle until all the powder flows freely. Add approximately ⅓ of the total amount of water for reconstitution (see table below) and shake vigorously to suspend powder. Add remainder of the water and again shake vigorously.

Recommended AUGMENTIN Susceptibility Ranges[1,2]

ORGANISMS	RESISTANT	INTERMEDIATE	SUSCEPTIBLE	MIC[3] CORRELATES mcg/ml R	S
Gram Negative Enteric Bacteria	≤ 13 mm	14–17 mm	≥ 18 mm	> 32/16	< 8/4
Staphylococcus[4] and	≤ 19 mm	—	≥ 20 mm		< 8/4
Hemophilus spp					< 2/1

Continued on next page

Beecham Laboratories—Cont.

AUGMENTIN '125' Suspension
Amount of Water

Bottle Size	Required for Reconstitution
75 ml	70 ml
150 ml	140 ml

Each teaspoonful (5 ml) will contain 125 mg amoxicillin and 31.25 mg of clavulanic acid as the potassium salt.

AUGMENTIN '250' Suspension
Amount of Water

Bottle Size	Required for Reconstitution
75 ml	68 ml
150 ml	135 ml

Each teaspoonful (5 ml) will contain 250 mg amoxicillin and 62.5 mg of clavulanic acid as the potassium salt.

Note: SHAKE ORAL SUSPENSION WELL BEFORE USING.

Reconstituted suspension must be stored under refrigeration and discarded after 10 days.

Administration: The absorption of AUGMENTIN is unaffected by food. Therefore, AUGMENTIN may be administered without regard to meals.

How Supplied:
AUGMENTIN '250' TABLETS: Each tablet contains 250 mg amoxicillin as the trihydrate and 125 mg clavulanic acid as the potassium salt.
NDC 0029-6075-27 ....bottles of 30
NDC 0029-6075-30 ....bottles of 100
AUGMENTIN '500' TABLETS: Each tablet contains 500 mg amoxicillin as the trihydrate and 125 mg clavulanic acid as the potassium salt.
NDC 0029-6080-27 ....bottles of 30
NDC 0029-6080-30 ....bottles of 100
AUGMENTIN '125' FOR ORAL SUSPENSION:
Each 5 ml of reconstituted suspension contains 125 mg amoxicillin and 31.25 mg clavulanic acid as the potassium salt.
NDC 0029-6085-39 ....75 ml bottle
NDC 0029-6085-22 ....150 ml bottle
AUGMENTIN '250' FOR ORAL SUSPENSION:
Each 5 ml of reconstituted suspension contains 250 mg amoxicillin and 62.5 mg clavulanic acid as the potassium salt.
NDC 0029-6090-39 ....75 ml bottle
NDC 0029-6090-22 ....150 ml bottle
MAY, 1984
9417090

Shown in Product Identification Section, page 405

FASTIN® Capsules
[fǎs'tǐn]
(phentermine hydrochloride)

Description: Each Fastin (phentermine hydrochloride) capsule contains phentermine hydrochloride, 30 mg (equivalent to 24 mg phentermine).
Phentermine Hydrochloride is a white crystalline powder, very soluble in water and alcohol. Chemically, the product is phenyl-tertiary-butyl-amine hydrochloride.

Actions: FASTIN is a sympathomimetic amine with pharmacologic activity similar to the prototype drugs of this class used in obesity, the amphetamines. Actions include central nervous system stimulation and elevation of blood pressure. Tachyphylaxis and tolerance have been demonstrated with all drugs of this class in which these phenomena have been looked for.
Drugs of this class used in obesity are commonly known as "anorectics" or "anorexigenics." It has not been established that the action of such drugs in treating obesity is primarily one of appetite suppression. Other central nervous system actions, or metabolic effects may be involved, for example.
Adult obese subjects instructed in dietary management and treated with "anorectic" drugs, lose more weight on the average than those treated with placebo and diet, as determined in relatively short-term clinical trials.
The magnitude of increased weight loss of drug-treated patients over placebo-treated patients is only a fraction of a pound a week. The rate of weight loss is greatest in the first weeks of therapy for both drug and placebo subjects and tends to decrease in succeeding weeks. The possible origins of the increased weight loss due to the various drug effects are not established. The amount of weight loss associated with the use of an "anorectic" drug varies from trial to trial, and the increased weight loss appears to be related in part to variables other than the drugs prescribed, such as the physician-investigator, the population treated, and the diet prescribed. Studies do not permit conclusions as to the relative importance of the drug and nondrug factors on weight loss.
The natural history of obesity is measured in years, whereas the studies cited are restricted to a few weeks duration; thus, the total impact of drug-induced weight loss over that of diet alone must be considered clinically limited.

Indication: FASTIN is indicated in the management of exogenous obesity as a short term (a few weeks) adjunct in a regimen of weight reduction based on caloric restriction. The limited usefulness of agents of this class (see ACTIONS) should be measured against possible risk factors inherent in their use such as those described below.

Contraindications: Advanced arteriosclerosis, symptomatic cardiovascular disease, moderate to severe hypertension, hyperthyroidism, known hypersensitivity, or idiosyncrasy to the sympathomimetic amines, glaucoma.
Agitated states.
Patients with a history of drug abuse.
During or within 14 days following the administration of monoamine oxidase inhibitors (hypertensive crises may result).

Warnings: Tolerance to the anorectic effect usually develops within a few weeks. When this occurs, the recommended dose should not be exceeded in an attempt to increase the effect; rather, the drug should be discontinued.
FASTIN may impair the ability of the patient to engage in potentially hazardous activities such as operating machinery or driving a motor vehicle; the patient should therefore be cautioned accordingly.

Drug Dependence: FASTIN is related chemically and pharmacologically to the amphetamines. Amphetamines and related stimulant drugs have been extensively abused, and the possibility of abuse of FASTIN should be kept in mind when evaluating the desirability of including a drug as part of a weight reduction program. Abuse of amphetamines and related drugs may be associated with intense psychological dependence and severe social dysfunction. There are reports of patients who have increased the dosage to many times that recommended. Abrupt cessation following prolonged high dosage administration results in extreme fatigue and mental depression; changes are also noted on the sleep EEG. Manifestations of chronic intoxication with anorectic drugs include severe dermatoses, marked insomnia, irritability, hyperactivity, and personality changes. The most severe manifestation of chronic intoxications is psychosis, often clinically indistinguishable from schizophrenia.

Usage in Pregnancy: Safe use in pregnancy has not been established. Use of FASTIN by women who are or who may become pregnant, and those in the first trimester of pregnancy, requires that the potential benefit be weighed against the possible hazard to mother and infant.

Usage in Children: FASTIN is not recommended for use in children under 12 years of age.

Usage with Alcohol: Concomitant use of alcohol with FASTIN may result in an adverse drug interaction.

Precautions: Caution is to be exercised in prescribing FASTIN for patients with even mild hypertension.
Insulin requirements in diabetes mellitus may be altered in association with the use of FASTIN and the concomitant dietary regimen.
FASTIN may decrease the hypotensive effect of guanethidine.
The least amount feasible should be prescribed or dispensed at one time in order to minimize the possibility of overdosage.

Adverse Reactions:
Cardiovascular: Palpitation, tachycardia, elevation of blood pressure.
Central Nervous System: Overstimulation, restlessness, dizziness, insomnia, euphoria, dysphoria, tremor, headache, rarely psychotic episodes at recommended doses.
Gastrointestinal: Dryness of the mouth, unpleasant taste, diarrhea, constipation, other gastrointestinal disturbances.
Allergic: Urticaria.
Endocrine: Impotence, changes in libido.

Dosage and Administration:
Exogenous Obesity: One capsule at approximately 2 hours after breakfast for appetite control. Late evening medication should be avoided because of the possibility of resulting insomnia.
Administration of one capsule (30 mg.) daily has been found to be adequate in depression of the appetite for twelve to fourteen hours.
FASTIN is not recommended for use in children under 12 years of age.

Overdosage: Manifestations of acute overdosage with phentermine include restlessness, tremor, hyperreflexia, rapid respiration, confusion, assaultiveness, hallucinations, panic states. Fatigue and depression usually follow the central stimulation. Cardiovascular effects include arrhythmias, hypertension or hypotension, and circulatory collapse. Gastrointestinal symptoms include nausea, vomiting, diarrhea, and abdominal cramps. Fatal poisoning usually terminates in convulsions and coma.
Management of acute phentermine intoxication is largely symptomatic and includes lavage and sedation with a barbiturate. Experience with hemodialysis or peritoneal dialysis is inadequate to permit recommendations in this regard. Acidification of the urine increases phentermine excretion. Intravenous phentolamine (REGITINE) has been suggested for possible acute, severe hypertension, if this complicates phentermine overdosage.

Caution: Federal law prohibits dispensing without prescription.

How Supplied: Blue and clear capsules with blue and white beads containing 30 mg. phentermine hydrochloride (equivalent to 24 mg. Phentermine).
NDC 0029-2205-30 ....bottles of 100
NDC 0029-2205-29 ....bottles of 450
NDC 0029-2205-31 ....pack 5X30
Shown in Product Identification Section, page 000
Rev. Aug., 1982

NUCOFED®
[nū'cō-fěd]
SYRUP and CAPSULES

Description: Nucofed Syrup and Capsules is an antitussive-decongestant containing in each 5 ml (teaspoonful) and each capsule: Codeine Phosphate, 20 mg (Warning: May Be Habit Forming); Pseudoephedrine Hydrochloride, 60 mg. Nucofed Syrup contains no alcohol and contains 2.25 gm of sucrose per 5 ml (teaspoonful).

Clinical Pharmacology:
Nucofed Syrup and Capsules
The clinical pharmacology of this formulated product is thought to be due to the action of its ingredients, Codeine Phosphate and Pseudoephedrine Hydrochloride.
Codeine Phosphate. Codeine causes suppression of the cough reflex by a direct effect on the cough center in the medulla and appears to exert a drying effect on respiratory tract mucosa and to increase viscosity of bronchial secretions.
Codeine is well absorbed from the gastrointestinal tract. Following oral administration, peak antitussive effects usually can be expected to occur within 1-2 hours and may persist for a period of four hours. Codeine is metabolized in the liver. The drug undergoes O-demethylation, N-demethylation, and partial conjugation with glucuronic acid, and is excreted mainly in the urine as norcodeine and morphine in the free and conjugated forms.

Codeine appears in breast milk of nursing mothers and has been reported to cross the placental barrier.

Pseudoephedrine Hydrochloride. Pseudoephedrine is a physiologically active stereoisomer of ephedrine which acts directly on *alpha*, and, to a lesser degree, *beta*- adrenergic receptors. The *alpha*-adrenergic effects are believed to result from the reduced production of cyclic adenosine-3',5' monophosphate (cyclic 3',5'-AMP) by inhibition of the enzyme adenyl cyclase, where *beta*-adrenergic effects appear to be caused by the stimulation of adenyl cyclase activity.

Pseudoephedrine acts directly on *alpha*-adrenergic receptors in the respiratory tract mucosa producing vasoconstriction resulting in shrinkage of swollen nasal mucous membranes, reduction of tissue hyperemia, edema, and nasal congestion, and an increase in nasal airway patency. Drainage of sinus secretions is increased and obstructed eustachian ostia may be opened. Relaxation of bronchial smooth muscle by stimulation of $beta_2$ adrenergic receptors may also occur. Following oral administration significant broncho-dilation has not been demonstrated consistently.

Nasal decongestion usually occurs within 30 minutes and persists for 4–6 hours after oral administration of 60 mg of Pseudoephedrine Hydrochloride.

Although specific information is not available, Pseudoephedrine is presumed to cross the placenta and to enter cerebrospinal fluid. It is incompletely metabolized in the liver by N-demethylation to an inactive metabolite. Both are excreted in the urine with 55%–75% of a dose being unchanged.

Indications and Usage: NUCOFED is indicated for symptomatic relief when both coughing and congestion are associated with upper respiratory infections and related conditions such as common cold, bronchitis, influenza, and sinusitis.

Contraindications: Hypersensitivity to product's active ingredients.

Warnings: Persons with persistent cough such as occurs with smoking, asthma, emphysema, or where cough is accompanied by excessive secretions should not take this product except under the advice and supervision of a physician.

May cause or aggravate constipation.

Do not give this product to children taking other drugs except under the advice and supervision of a physician.

Persons with a chronic pulmonary disease or shortness of breath, high blood pressure, heart disease, diabetes or thyroid disease should not take this product except under the advice and supervision of a physician.

Do not exceed recommended dosage because at higher doses nervousness, dizziness, or sleeplessness may occur.

If symptoms do not improve within 7 days or are accompanied by high fever, consult a physician before continuing use.

Precautions:
General
Inasmuch as the active ingredients of Nucofed Syrup and Capsules consist of Codeine Phosphate and Pseudoephedrine Hydrochloride, this medication should be used with caution in the presence of the following:
- Cardiovascular disease (of any etiology)
- Diabetes mellitus
- Hypertension (of any severity)
- Abnormal thyroid function
- Prostatic hypertrophy
- Addison's disease
- Chronic ulcerative colitis
- History of drug abuse or dependence
- Chronic respiratory disease or impairment
- Functional impairment of the liver or kidney

Patients taking Nucofed Syrup and Capsules should be cautioned when driving or doing jobs requiring alertness and to get up slowly from a lying or sitting position, or to lie down if nausea occurs.

Possible Drug Interactions
Because of the potential for drug interactions, persons currently taking any of the following medications should take Nucofed Syrup and Capsules on the advice and under the supervision of a physician.

- Beta adrenergic blockers—concurrent use may increase the pressor effect of pseudoephedrine.
- Digitalis glycosides—concurrent use with pseudoephedrine may increase the possibility of cardiac arrhythmias.
- Antihypertensive agents including Veratrum alkaloids—hypotensive effects may be decreased by the concurrent use of pseudoephedrine.
- Monoamine oxidase (MAO) inhibitors— these agents may potentiate the pressor effect of Pseudoephedrine and may result in a hypertensive crisis; pseudoephedrine should not be administered during or within 14 days of MAO inhibitors.
- Sympathomimetics, other — sympathomimetics used concurrently may increase the effects either of these agents or of pseudoephedrine, thereby increasing the potential for side effects.
- Tricyclic antidepressants—the concurrent use of tricyclic antidepressants may antagonize the effects of pseudoephedrine and may increase the effects either of the antidepressants themselves or of the codeine component.
- CNS depressants
- Alcohol
- General anesthetics
- Anticholinergics—concurrent use may result in paralytic ileus.

Drug/Laboratory Test Interactions
- Codeine may cause an elevation in serum amylase levels due to the spasm producing potential of narcotic analgesics on the sphincter of Oddi.

Pregnancy: Category C
Animal reproduction studies of the components of Nucofed Syrup and Capsules (Codeine, Pseudoephedrine) have not been conducted. Thus, it is not known whether these agents can cause fetal harm when administered to pregnant women or whether they affect reproductive capacity. Accordingly, Nucofed Syrup and Capsules should be given to pregnant women only where clearly needed.

Nursing Mothers
Codeine and Pseudoephedrine are excreted in breast milk; therefore, caution should be exercised when this medication is prescribed for a nursing mother.

Pediatric Use
Do not give Nucofed Syrup and Capsules to children under two years of age except on the advice and under the supervision of a physician.

Adverse Reactions: Based on the composition of Nucofed Syrup and Capsules the following side effects may occur: nervousness, restlessness, trouble in sleeping, drowsiness, difficult or painful urination, dizziness or lightheadedness, headache, nausea and vomiting, constipation, trembling, troubled breathing, increase in sweating, unusual paleness, weakness, changes in heart rate.

Drug Abuse and Dependence: NUCOFED is placed in Schedule III of the Controlled Substances Act.

Overdosage: Nucofed Syrup and Capsules contain Codeine Phosphate and Pseudoephedrine Hydrochloride. Overdosage as a result of this product should be treated based upon the symptomatology of the patient as it relates to the individual ingredient. Treatment of acute overdosage would probably be based upon treating the patient for codeine toxicity which may be manifested as:

- Gradual drowsiness, dizziness, heaviness of the head, weariness, diminution of sensibility, loss of pain and other modalities of sensation.
- Nausea and vomiting.
- A transient excitement stage, characterized by extreme restlessness, delirium, and rarely epileptiform convulsions, is sometimes seen in children and rarely in adult women.
- Bilateral miosis, progressing to pinpoint pupils, which do not react to light or accommodation. The pupils may dilate during terminal asphyxia.
- Itching of the skin and nose, sometimes with skin rashes and urticaria.
- Coma, with muscular relaxation and depressed or absent superficial and deep reflexes. A Babinski toe sign may appear.
- Marked slowing of the respiratory rate with inadequate pulmonary ventilation and consequent cyanosis. Breathing becomes stertorous and irregular (Cheyne-Stokes or Biot).
- The pulse is slow and the blood pressure gradually falls to shock levels. Urine formation ceases or is reduced to a very low rate.

The lethal dose of codeine for an adult is about 0.5–1.0 gm. Treatment is as recommended for narcotics.

Dosage and Administration:
Recommended Dosage: Capsule
Adults: 1 capsule every 6 hours, not to exceed 4 capsules in 24 hours.
Recommended Dosage: Syrup
Adults: 1 teaspoonful every 6 hours, not to exceed 4 teaspoonfuls in 24 hours.
Children:
  6 to under 12 years: ½ teaspoonful every 6 hours, not to exceed 2 teaspoonfuls in 24 hours.
  2 to under 6 years: ¼ teaspoonful every 6 hours, not to exceed 1 teaspoonful in 24 hours.
Do not give this product to children under 2 years, except under the advice and supervision of a physician.

How Supplied:
Nucofed Syrup, Green, Mint Flavored
  NDC 0029-3135-34   Pints
Nucofed Capsules, Green Top, Clear Bottom
  NDC 0029-3138-39   Bottles of 60

Caution: Federal law prohibits dispensing without prescription.

Revised July, 1981
Shown in Product Identification Section, page 000

NUCOFED® EXPECTORANT
[nū'cō-fĕd]
SYRUP

Description: Nucofed Expectorant is an antitussive-decongestant-expectorant syrup for oral administration containing in each 5 ml (teaspoonful): Codeine Phosphate, 20 mg (Warning: May Be Habit Forming); Pseudoephedrine HCl, 60 mg; Guaifenesin, 200 mg; alcohol, 12.5%.

Clinical Pharmacology:
Nucofed Expectorant
The clinical pharmacology of this formulated product is thought to be due to the action of its ingredients, Codeine Phosphate, Pseudoephedrine Hydrochloride and Guaifenesin.

Codeine Phosphate. Codeine causes suppression of the cough reflex by a direct effect on the cough center in the medulla and appears to exert a drying effect on respiratory tract mucosa and to increase viscosity of bronchial secretions.

Codeine is well absorbed from the gastrointestinal tract. Following oral administration, peak antitussive effects can be expected to occur within one to two hours and may persist for a period of four hours. Codeine is metabolized in the liver. The drug undergoes O-demethylation, N-demethylation, and partial conjugation with glucuronic acid, and is excreted mainly in the urine as norcodeine and morphine in the free and conjugated forms.

Codeine appears in breast milk of nursing mothers and has been reported to cross the placental barrier.

Pseudoephedrine Hydrochloride. Pseudoephedrine is a physiologically active stereoisomer of ephedrine which acts directly on *alpha*, and to a lesser degree, *beta*-adrenergic receptors. The *alpha*-adrenergic effects are believed to result from the reduced production of cyclic adenosine-3',5' monophosphate (cyclic 3',5'-AMP) by inhibition of the enzyme adenyl cyclase, whereas *beta*-adrenergic effects appear to be caused by the stimulation of adenyl cyclase activity.

Pseudoephedrine acts directly on *alpha*-adrenergic receptors in the respiratory tract mucosa producing vasoconstriction resulting in shrinkage of swollen nasal mucous membranes, reduction of tissue hyperemia, edema, and nasal congestion, and an increase in nasal airway patency. Drainage of sinus secretions is increased and obstructed

Continued on next page

Beecham Laboratories—Cont.

eustachian ostia may be opened. Relaxation of bronchial smooth muscle by stimulation of $beta_2$ adrenergic receptors may also occur. Following oral administration significant broncho-dilation has not been demonstrated consistently.

Nasal decongestion usually occurs within 30 minutes and persists for 4–6 hours after oral administration of 60 mg of pseudoephedrine hydrochloride.

Although specific information is not available, pseudoephedrine is presumed to cross the placenta and to enter cerebrospinal fluid. It is incompletely metabolized in the liver by N-demethylation to an inactive metabolite. Both are excreted in the urine with 55%–75% of a dose being unchanged.

Guaifenesin. Guaifenesin, by increasing respiratory tract fluid, reduces the viscosity of tenacious secretions and acts as an expectorant.

Guaifenesin is excreted in the urine mainly as glucuronates and sulfonates.

Indications and Usage: NUCOFED EXPECTORANT is indicated for symptomatic relief when both coughing and congestion are associated with upper respiratory infections and related conditions such as common colds, bronchitis, influenza, and sinusitis.

Contraindications: Hypersensitivity to product's active ingredients.

Warnings: Persons with persistent cough such as occurs with smoking, asthma, emphysema, or where cough is accompanied by excessive secretions should not take this product except under the advice and supervision of a physician.

Do not give this product to children taking other drugs except under the advice and supervision of a physician.

Persons with a chronic pulmonary disease or shortness of breath, high blood pressure, heart disease, diabetes or thyroid disease should not take this product except under the advice and supervision of a physician.

Do not exceed recommended dosage because at higher doses nervousness, dizziness, or sleeplessness may occur.

If symptoms do not improve within 7 days or are accompanied by high fever, consult a physician before continuing use.

Precautions:

General. Inasmuch as the active ingredient of Nucofed Expectorant consist of Codeine Phosphate, Pseudoephedrine Hydrochloride and Guaifenesin, this medication should be used with caution in the presence of the following:
- Cardiovascular disease (of any etiology)
- Diabetes mellitus
- Hypertension (of any severity)
- Abnormal thyroid function
- Prostatic hypertrophy
- Addison's disease
- Chronic ulcerative colitis
- History of drug abuse or dependence
- Chronic respiratory disease or impairment
- Functional impairment of the liver or kidney

Patients taking Nucofed Expectorant should be cautioned when driving or doing jobs requiring alertness and to get up slowly from a lying or sitting position, or to lie down if nausea occurs.

Possible Drug Interactions. Because of the potential for drug interactions, persons currently taking any of the following medications should take Nucofed Expectorant only on the advice and under the supervision of a physician.
- Beta adrenergic blockers—concurrent use may increase the pressor effect of pseudoephedrine.
- Digitalis glycosides—concurrent use with pseudoephedrine may increase the possibility of cardiac arrhythmias.
- Antihypertensive agents including Veratrum alkaloids—hypotensive effects may be decreased by the concurrent use of pseudoephedrine.
- Monoamine oxidase (MAO) inhibitors—these agents may potentiate the pressor effect of pseudoephedrine and may result in a hypertensive crisis; pseudoephedrine should not be administered during or within 14 days of MAO inhibitors.
- Sympathomimetics, other — sympathomimetics used concurrently may increase the effects either of these agents or of pseudoephedrine, thereby increasing the potential for side effects.
- Tricyclic antidepressants—the concurrent use of tricyclic antidepressants may antagonize the effects of pseudoephedrine and may increase the effects either of the antidepressants themselves or of the codeine component.
- CNS depressants
- Alcohol
- General anesthetics
- Anticholinergics—concurrent use may result in paralytic ileus.

Drug/Laboratory Test Interactions
- Codeine may cause an elevation in serum amylase levels due to the spasm producing potential of narcotic analgesics on the sphincter of Oddi.
- Guaifenesin in known to interfere with the colorimetric determination of 5-hydroxy- indoleacetic acid (5-HIAA) and vanilmandelic acid (VMA).

Pregnancy: Category C

Animal reproduction studies of the components of Nucofed Expectorants (codeine, pseudoephedrine and guaifenesin) have not been conducted. Thus, it is not known whether these agents can cause fetal harm when administered to pregnant women or whether they affect reproductive capacity. Accordingly, Nucofed Expectorant should be given to pregnant women only where clearly needed.

Nursing Mothers

Codeine and Pseudoephedrine, two of the ingredients in Nucofed Expectorant, are excreted in breast milk; therefore, caution should be exercised when this medication is prescribed for a nursing mother.

Pediatric Use

Do not give Nucofed Expectorant to Children under two years of age except on the advice and under the supervision of a physician.

Adverse Reactions: Based on the composition of Nucofed Expectorant the following side effects may occur: nervousness, restlessness, trouble in sleeping, drowsiness, difficult or painful urination, dizziness or lightheadedness, headache, nausea or vomiting, constipation, trembling, troubled breathing, increase in sweating, unusual paleness, weakness, changes in heart rate.

Drug Abuse and Dependence: Nucofed Expectorant has been placed in Schedule III of the Controlled Substances Act.

Overdosage: Nucofed Expectorant contains Codeine Phosphate, Pseudoephedrine Hydrochloride and Guaifenesin. Overdosage as a result of this product should be treated based upon the symptomatology of the patient as it relates to the individual ingredient. Treatment of acute overdosage would probably be based upon treating the patient for codeine toxicity which may be manifested as:
- Gradual drowsiness, dizziness, heaviness of the head, weariness, diminution of sensibility, loss of pain and other modalities of sensation.
- Nausea and vomiting.
- A transient excitement stage, characterized by extreme restlessness, delirium, and rarely epileptiform convulsions, is sometimes seen in children and rarely in adult women.
- Bilateral miosis, progressing to pinpoint pupils, which do not react to light or accommodation. The pupils may dilate during terminal asphyxia.
- Itching of the skin and nose, sometimes with skin rashes and urticaria.
- Coma, with muscular relaxation and depressed or absent superficial and deep reflexes. A Babinski toe sign may appear.
- Marked slowing of the respiratory rate with inadequate pulmonary ventilation and consequent cyanosis. Breathing becomes stertorous and irregular (Cheyne-Stokes or Biot).
- The pulse is slow and the blood pressure gradually falls to shock levels. Urine formation ceases or is reduced to a very low rate.

The lethal dose of codeine for an adult is about 0.5–1.0 gram. Treatment is as recommended for narcotics.

Dosage and Administration:

Recommended Dosage:

Adults: 1 teaspoonful every 6 hours, not to exceed 4 teaspoonfuls in 24 hours.

Children:

6 to under 12 years: $\frac{1}{2}$ teaspoonful every 6 hours, not to exceed 2 teaspoonfuls in 24 hours.

2 to under 6 years: $\frac{1}{4}$ teaspoonful every 6 hours, not to exceed 1 teaspoonful in 24 hours.

Do not give this product to children under 2 years, except under the advice and supervision of a physician.

How Supplied:

Red, Wintergreen Flavored Syrup
NDC 0029-3142-34 Pints

Caution: Federal law prohibits dispensing without prescription.

NUCOFED®
[*nū'cō-fĕd*]
PEDIATRIC EXPECTORANT
Syrup

Description: Nucofed Pediatric Expectorant is an antitussive-decongestant-expectorant syrup for oral administration containing in each 5 ml (teaspoonful): Codeine Phosphate, 10 mg (Warning: May Be Habit Forming); Pseudoephedrine HCl, 30 mg; Guaifenesin, 100 mg; alcohol, 6%

Clinical Pharmacology:

Nucofed Pediatric Expectorant

The clinical pharmacology of this formulated product is thought to be due to the action of its ingredients, Codeine Phosphate, Pseudoephedrine Hydrochloride and Guaifenesin.

Codeine Phosphate. Codeine causes suppression of the cough reflex by a direct effect on the cough center in the medulla and appears to exert a drying effect on respiratory tract mucosa and to increase viscosity of bronchial secretions.

Codeine is well absorbed from the gastrointestinal tract. Following oral administration, peak antitussive effect usually can be expected to occur within one to two hours and may persist for a period of four hours. Codeine is metabolized in the liver. The drug undergoes 0-demethylation, N-demethylation, and partial conjugation with glucuronic acid, and is excreted mainly in the urine as norcodeine and morphine in the free and conjugated forms.

Codeine appears in breast milk of nursing mothers and has been reported to cross the placental barrier.

Psuedoephedrine Hydrochloride. Pseudoephedrine is a physiologically active stereoisomer of ephedrine which acts directly on *alpha*, and to a lesser degree, *beta*-adrenergic receptors. The *alpha*-adrenergic effects are believed to result from the reduced production of cyclic adenosine-3',5' monophosphate (cyclic 3',5'-AMP) by inhibition of the enzyme adenyl cyclase, whereas *beta*-adrenergic effects appear to be caused by the stimulation of adenyl cyclase activity.

Pseudoephedrine acts directly on *alpha*-adrenergic receptors in the respiratory tract mucosa producing vasoconstriction resulting in shrinkage of swollen nasal mucous membranes, reduction of tissue hyperemia, edema, and nasal congestion, and an incresase in nasal airway patency. Drainage of sinus secretions is increased and obstructed eustachian ostia may be opened. Relaxation of bronchial smooth muscle by stimulation $beta_2$ adrenergic receptors may also occur. Following oral administration significant broncho-dilation has not been demonstrated consistently.

Nasal decongestion usually occurs within 30 minutes and persists for 4–6 hours after oral administration of 30 mg of pseudoephedrine hydrochloride.

Although specific information is not available, pseudoephedrine is presumed to cross the placenta and to enter cerebrospinal fluid. It is incompletely metabolized in the liver by N-demethylation to an inactive metabolite. Both are excreted in the urine with 55%–75% of a dose being unchanged.

Guaifenesin. Guaifenesin, by increasing respiratory tract fluid, reduces the viscosity of tenacious secretions and acts as an expectorant.

Guaifenesin is excreted in the urine mainly as glucuronates and sulfonates.

Indications and Usage: NUCOFED PEDIATRIC EXPECTORANT is indicated for symptomatic relief when both coughing and congestion are associated with upper respiratory infections and related conditions such as common cold, bronchitis, influenza, and sinusitis.

Contraindications: Hypersensitivity to product's active ingredients.

Warnings: Persons with persistent cough such as occurs with smoking, asthma, emphysema, or where cough is accompanied by excessive secretions should not take this product except under the advice and supervision of a physician.

Do not give this product to children taking other drugs except under the advice and supervision of a physician.

Persons with a chronic pulmonary disease or shortness of breath, high blood pressure, heart disease, diabetes or thyroid disease should not take this product except under the advice and supervision of a physician.

Do not exceed recommended dosage because at higher doses nervousness, dizziness, or sleeplessness may occur.

If symptoms do not improve within 7 days or are accompanied by high fever, consult a physician before continuing use.

Precautions:
General. Inasmuch as the active ingredients of Nucofed Pediatric Expectorant consist of Codeine Phosphate, Pseudoephedrine Hydrochloride and Guaifenesin, this medication should be used with caution in the presence of the following:
- Cardiovascular disease (of any etiology)
- Diabetes mellitus
- Hypertension (of any severity)
- Abnormal thyroid function
- Prostatic hypertrophy
- Addison's disease
- Chronic ulcerative colitis
- History of drug abuse or dependence
- Chronic respiratory disease or impairment
- Functional impairment of the liver or kidney

Patients taking Nucofed Pediatric Expectorant should be cautioned when driving or doing jobs requiring alertness and to get up slowly from a lying or sitting position, or to lie down if nausea occurs.

Possible Drug Interactions. Because of the potential for drug interactions, persons currently taking any of the following medications should take Nucofed Pediatric Expectorant only on the advice and under the supervision of a physician.
- Beta adrenergic blockers—concurrent use may increase the pressor effect of pseudoephedrine.
- Digitalis glycosides—concurrent use with pseudoephedrine may increase the possibility of cardiac arrhythmias.
- Antihypertensive agents including Veratrum alkaloids—hypotensive effects may be decreased by the concurrent use of pseudoephedrine.
- Monoamine oxidase (MAO) inhibitors—these agents may potentiate the pressor effect of pseudoephedrine and may result in a hypertensive crisis; pseudoephedrine should not be administered during or within 14 days of MAO inhibitors.
- Sympathomimetics, other—sympathomimetics used concurrently may increase the effects either of these agents or of pseudoephedrine, thereby increasing the potential for side effects.
- Tricyclic antidepressants—the concurrent use of tricyclic antidepressants may antagonize the effects of pseudoephedrine and may increase the effects either of the antidepressants themselves or of the codeine component.
- CNS depressants
- Alcohol
- General anesthetics
- Anticholinergics—concurrent use may result in paralytic ileus.

TICARCILLIN SERUM LEVELS
mcg/ml

Dosage	Route	¼ hr.	½ hr.	1 hr.	2 hr.	3 hr.	4 hr.	6 hr.
Adults:								
500 mg	IM	—	7.7	8.6	6.0	4.0		2.9
1 Gm	IM	—	31.0	18.7	15.7	9.7		3.4
2 Gm	IM	—	63.6	39.7	32.3	18.9	—	3.4
3 Gm	IV	190.0	140.0	107.0	52.2	31.3	13.8	4.2
5 Gm	IV	327.0	280.0	175.0	106.0	63.0	28.5	9.6
3 Gm + 1 Gm Probenecid	IV Oral	223.0	166.0	123.0	78.0	54.0	35.4	17.1

		½ hr.	1 hr.	1½ hr.	2 hr.	4 hr.	8 hr.	
Neonates:								
50 mg/kg	IM	64.0	70.7	63.7	60.1	33.2	11.6	

Drug/Laboratory Test Interactions
- Codeine may cause an elevation in serum amylase levels due to the spasm producing potential of narcotic analgesics on the sphincter of Oddi.
- Guaifenesin is known to interfere with the colorimetric determination of 5-hydroxyindoleacetic acid (5-HIAA) and vanilmandelic acid (VMA).

Pregnancy: Category C
Animal reproduction studies of the components of Nucofed Pediatric Expectorant (codeine, pseudoephedrine and guaifensin) have not been conducted. Thus, it is not known whether these agents can cause fetal harm when administered to pregnant women or whether they affect reproductive capacity. Accordingly, Nucofed Pediatric Expectorant should be given to pregnant women only where clearly needed.

Nursing Mothers
Codeine and Pseudoephedrine, two of the ingredients in Nucofed Pediatric Expectorant, are excreted in breast milk; therefore, caution should be exercised when this medication is prescribed for a nursing mother.

Pediatric Use
Do not give Nucofed Pediatric Expectorant to Children under two years of age except on the advice and under the supervision of a physician.

Adverse Reactions: Based on the composition of Nucofed Pediatric Expectorant the following side effects may occur: nervousness, restlessness, trouble in sleeping, drowsiness, difficult or painful urination, dizziness or lightheadedness, headache, nausea or vomiting, constipation, trembling, troubled breathing, increase in sweating, unusual paleness, weakness, changes in heart rate.

Drug Abuse and Dependence: Nucofed Pediatric Expectorant has been placed in Schedule V of the Controlled Substances Act.

Overdosage: Nucofed Pediatric Expectorant contains Codeine Phosphate, Pseudoephedrine Hydrochloride and Guaifenesin. Overdosage as a result of this product should be treated based upon the symptomatology of the patient as it relates to the individual ingredient. Treatment of acute overdosage would probably be based upon treating the patient for codeine toxicity which may be manifested as:
- Gradual drowsiness, dizziness, heaviness of the head, weariness, diminution of sensibility, loss of pain and other modalities of sensation.
- Nausea and vomiting.
- A transient excitement stage, characterized by extreme restlessness, delirium, and rarely epileptiform convulsions, is sometimes seen in children and rarely in adult women.
- Bilateral miosis, progressing to pinpoint pupils, which do not react to light or accommodation. The pupils may dilate during terminal asphyxia.
- Itching of the skin and nose, sometimes with skin rashes and urticaria.
- Coma, with muscular relaxation and depressed or absent superficial and deep reflexes. A Babinski toe sign may appear.
- Marked slowing of the respiratory rate with inadequate pulmonary ventilation and consequent cyanosis. Breathing becomes stertorous and irregular (Cheyne-Stokes or Biot).
- The pulse is slow and the blood pressure gradually falls to shock levels. Urine formation ceases or is reduced to a very low rate.

The lethal dose of codeine for an adult is approximately 0.5–1.0 gm. Reliable information regarding the lethal dose in children is not available. Treatment is as recommended for narcotics.

Dosage and Administration:
Recommended Dosage:

Adults and Children 12 years of age and over: 2 teaspoonfuls every 6 hours, not to exceed 8 teaspoonfuls in 24 hours.

Children:

6 to under 12 years: 1 teaspoonful every 6 hours, not to exceed 4 teaspoonfuls in 24 hours.

2 to under 6 years: ½ teaspoonful every 6 hours, not to exceed 2 teaspoonfuls in 24 hours.

Do not give this product to children under 2 years, except under the advice and supervision of a physician.

How Supplied:
Red, Strawberry Flavored Syrup
NDC 0029-3130-39   Pints

Caution: Federal law prohibits dispensing without prescription.

TICAR® ℞
[tī′ kar]
(sterile ticarcillin disodium)
for Intramuscular or Intravenous Use

Description: TICAR (Ticarcillin Disodium) is a semisynthetic injectable penicillin derived from the penicillin nucleus, 6-amino-penicillanic acid. Chemically, it is 6-[(Carboxy-3-thienylacetyl) amino] -3,3-dimethyl-7-oxo-4-thia-1-azabicyclo [3.2.0] heptane-2-carboxylic acid disodium salt.

It is supplied as a white to pale yellow powder or lyophilized cake for reconstitution. The reconstituted solution is clear, colorless or pale yellow, having a pH of 6.0-8.0. Ticarcillin is very soluble in water, its solubility is greater than 600 mg/ml.

Actions:
PHARMACOLOGY
Ticarcillin is not absorbed orally, therefore, it must be given intravenously or intramuscularly. Following intramuscular administration, peak serum concentrations occur within ½–1 hour. Somewhat higher and more prolonged serum levels can be achieved with the concurrent administration of probenecid.

The minimum inhibitory concentrations (MIC) for many strains of *Pseudomonas* are relatively high by usual standards; serum levels of 60 mcg/ml or greater are required. However, the low degree of toxicity of Ticarcillin permits the use of doses large enough to achieve inhibitory levels for these strains in serum or tissues. Other susceptible organisms usually require serum levels in the 10–25 mcg/ml range.

[See table above]

As with other penicillins, Ticarcillin is eliminated by glomerular filtration and tubular secretion. It is not highly bound to serum protein (approxi-

Continued on next page

Beecham Laboratories—Cont.

mately 45%) and is excreted unchanged in high concentrations in the urine. After the administration of a 1–2 Gm I.M. dose, a urine concentration of 2000–4000 mcg/ml may be obtained in patients with normal renal function. The serum half-life of Ticarcillin in normal individuals is approximately 70 minutes.

An inverse relationship exists between serum half-life and creatinine clearance, but the dosage of TICAR need only be adjusted in cases of severe renal impairment (see DOSAGE AND ADMINISTRATION). The administered Ticarcillin may be removed from patients undergoing dialysis; the actual amount removed depends on the duration and type of dialysis.

Ticarcillin can be detected in tissues and interstitial fluid following parenteral administration. Penetration into the cerebrospinal fluid, bile and pleural fluid has been demonstrated.

MICROBIOLOGY

Ticarcillin is bactericidal and demonstrates substantial *in vitro* activity against both Gram-positive and Gram-negative organisms. Many strains of the following organisms were found to be susceptible to Ticarcillin *in vitro*:

Pseudomonas aeruginosa (and other species)
Escherichia coli
Proteus mirabilis
Proteus morganii
Proteus rettgeri
Proteus vulgaris
Enterobacter species
Haemophilus influenzae
Neisseria species
Salmonella species
Staphylococcus aureus (non-penicillinase producing)
Staphylococcus epidermidis
Beta-hemolytic streptococci (Group A)
Streptococcus faecalis (Enterococcus)
Streptococcus pneumoniae

Anaerobic bacteria, including:
Bacteroides species including *B. fragilis*
Fusobacterium species
Veillonella species
Clostridium species
Eubacterium species
Peptococcus species
Peptostreptococcus species

In vitro synergism between Ticarillin and gentamicin sulfate, tobramycin sulfate or amikacin sulfate against certain strains of *Pseudomonas aeruginosa* has been demonstrated.

Some strains of such microorganisms as *Mima-Herellea (Acinetobacter)*, *Citrobacter* and *Serratia* have shown susceptibility.

Ticarcillin is not stable in the presence of penicillinase.

Some strains of *Pseudomonas* have developed resistance fairly rapidly.

DISC SUSCEPTIBILITY TESTS

Susceptibility Test: Ticarcillin discs or powders should be used for testing susceptibility to ticarcillin. However, organisms, reportedly suspectible to carbenicillin are susceptible to ticarcillin.

Diffusion Techniques: For the disc diffusion method of suspectiblity testing a 75 mcg TICAR DISC should be used. The method for this test is the one outlined in NCCLS publication M2-A2* with the following interpretative criteria:
[See table below].

Dilution Techniques: Dilution techniques for determining the MIC (minimum inhibitory concentration) are published by NCCLS for the broth and agar dilution procedures. The MIC data should be interpreted in light of the concentrations present in serum, tissue, and body fluids. Organisms with MIC ≤ 64 are considered susceptible when they are in tissue but organisms with MIC ≤ 128 would be susceptible in urine where the TICAR concentrations are much greater. At present, only dilution methods can be recommended for testing antibiotic susceptibility of obligate anaerobes.

Susceptibility testing methods require the use of control organisms. The 75 mcg tricarcillin disc should give zone diameters between 21 and 27 mm for *P. aeruginosa* ATCC 27853 and 24 and 30 mm for *E. Coli* ATCC 25922. Reference strains are available for dilution testing of ticarcillin, 95% of the MIC's are expected to be within ± 1 dilution of the following:

S. aureus ATCC 29213, 4.0 mcg/ml; *S. faecalis* ATCC 29212, 32 mcg/ml; *E. coli* ATCC 25922, 2–4 mcg/ml; *P. aeruginosa* ATCC 27853, 16 mcg/ml.

* Performance standards for Antimicrobiotic Disc Susceptibility Tests, National Committee of Clinical Laboratory Standards, Vol. 2, pp 49–69, 1982.

Indications: TICAR (Ticarcillin Disodium) is indicated for the treatment of the following infections:

Bacterial septicemia (†)
Skin and soft-tissue infections (†)
Acute and chronic respiratory tract infections (†)(‡)

(†) caused by susceptible strains of *Pseudomonas aeruginosa*, *Proteus* species (both indole-positive and indole-negative) and *Escherichia coli*.

(‡) (Though clinical improvement has been shown, bacteriological cures cannot be expected in patients with chronic respiratory disease or cystic fibrosis.)

Genitourinary tract infections (complicated and uncomplicated) due to susceptible strains of *Pseudomonas aeruginosa*, *Proteus* species (both indole-positive and indole-negative), *Escherichia coli*, *Enterobacter* and *Streptococcus faecalis* (enterococcus).

Ticarcillin is also indicated in the treatment of the following infections due to susceptible anaerobic bacteria:

1. Bacterial septicemia.
2. Lower respiratory tract infections such as empyema, anaerobic pneumonitis and lung abscess.
3. Intra-abdominal infections such as peritonitis and intra-abdominal abscess (typically resulting from anaerobic organisms resident in the normal gastrointestinal tract).
4. Infections of the female pelvis and genital tract, such as endometritis, pelvic inflammatory disease, pelvic abscess and salpingitis.
5. Skin and soft-tissue infections.

Although Ticarcillin is primarily indicated in Gram-negative infections, its *in vitro* activity against Gram-positive organisms should be considered in treating infections caused by both Gram-negative and Gram-positive organisms (see MICROBIOLOGY).

Based on the *in vitro* synergism between Ticarcillin and gentamicin sulfate, tobramycin sulfate or amikacin sulfate against certain strains of *Pseudomonas aeruginosa*, combined therapy has been successful, using full therapeutic dosages. (For additional prescribing information, see the gentamicin sulfate, tobramycin sulfate and amikacin sulfate package inserts.)

NOTE: Culturing and susceptibility testing should be performed initially and during treatment to monitor the effectiveness of therapy and the susceptibility of the bacteria.

Contraindications: A history of allergic reaction to any of the penicillins is a contraindication.

Warnings: Serious and occasionally fatal hypersensitivity (anaphylactoid) reactions have been reported in patients receiving penicillin. These reactions are more likely to occur in persons with a history of sensitivity to multiple allergens.

There are reports of patients with a history of penicillin hypersensitivity reactions who experience severe hypersensitivity reactions when treated with a cephalosporin. Before therapy with a penicillin, careful inquiry should be made about previous hypersensitivity reactions to penicillins, cephalosporins, and other allergens. If a reaction occurs, the drug should be discontinued unless, in the opinion of the physician, the condition being treated is life-threatening and amenable only to Ticarcillin therapy. **Serious anaphylactoid reactions require immediate emergency treatment with epinephrine. Oxygen, intravenous steroids, airway management, including intubation, should also be administered as indicated.**

Some patients receiving high doses of Ticarcillin may develop hemorrhagic manifestations associated with abnormalities of coagulation tests, such as bleeding time and platelet aggregation. On withdrawal of the drug, the bleeding should cease and coagulation abnormalities revert to normal. Other causes of abnormal bleeding should also be considered. Patients with renal impairment, in whom excretion of Ticarcillin is delayed, should be observed for bleeding manifestations. Such patients should be dosed strictly according to recommendations (see DOSAGE AND ADMINISTRATION). If bleeding manifestations appear, Ticarcillin treatment should be discontinued and appropriate therapy instituted.

Precautions: Although TICAR (Ticarcillin Disodium) exhibits the characteristic low toxicity of the penicillins, as with any other potent agent, it is advisable to check periodically for organ system dysfunction (including renal, hepatic and hematopoietic) during prolonged treatment. If overgrowth of resistant organisms occurs, the appropriate therapy should be initiated.

Since the theoretical sodium content is 5.2 milliequivalents (120 mg) per gram of Ticarcillin, and the actual vial content can be as high as 6.5 mEq/Gm, electrolyte and cardiac status should be monitored carefully.

In a few patients receiving intravenous Ticarcillin, hypokalemia has been reported. Serum potassium should be measured periodically, and, if necessary, corrective therapy should be implemented.

As with any penicillin, the possibility of an allergic response, including anaphylaxis, exists, particularly in hypersensitive patients.

USAGE DURING PREGNANCY

Reproduction studies have been performed in mice and rats and have revealed no evidence of impaired fertility or harm to the fetus due to Ticarcillin. There are no well-controlled studies in pregnant women, but investigational experience does not include any positive evidence of adverse effects on the fetus. Although there is no clearly defined risk, such experience cannot exclude the possibility of infrequent or subtle damage to the fetus. Ticarcillin should be used in pregnant women only when clearly needed.

Adverse Reactions: The following adverse reactions may occur:

Hypersensitivity Reactions: Skin rashes, pruritus, urticaria, drug fever.

Gastrointestinal Disturbances: Nausea and vomiting.

Hemic and Lymphatic Systems: As with other penicillins, anemia, thrombocytopenia, leukopenia, neutropenia and eosinophilia.

Abnormalities of Blood, Hepatic and Renal Laboratory Studies: As with other semisynthetic penicillins, SGOT and SGPT elevations have been reported. To date, clinical manifestations of hepatic or renal disorders have not been observed which could be ascribed solely to Ticarcillin.

CNS: Patients, especially those with impaired renal function, may experience convulsions or neuromuscular excitability when very high doses of the drug are administered.

Other: Local reactions such as pain (rarely accompanied by induration) at the site of the injection have been reported.

Culture	Susceptible	Intermediate	Resistant
P. aeruginosa and *Enterobacteriaceae*	≥ 15 mm	12–14 mm	≤ 11 mm
The MIC Correlates are:	Resistant > 128 mcg/ml		
	Susceptible ≤ 64 mcg/ml		

TICAR

Dosage and Administration

Clinical experience indicates that in serious urinary tract and systemic infections, intravenous therapy in the higher doses should be used. Intramuscular injections should not exceed 2 grams per injection.

Adults:

Bacterial Septicemia Respiratory Tract Infections Skin and Soft-Tissue Infections Intra-Abdominal Infections Infections of the Female Pelvis and Genital Tract	200–300 mg/kg/day by I.V. infusion in divided doses every 3, 4 or 6 hours. [Usual recommended dosage: 3 grams every 3, 4 or 6 hours, depending on weight and the severity of the infection.]
Urinary Tract Infections Complicated:	150–200 mg/kg/day by I.V. infusion in divided doses every 4 or 6 hours. [Usual recommended dosage for average (70 kg) adults: 3 grams q.i.d.]
Uncomplicated:	1 gram I.M. or direct I.V. every 6 hours.

Infections complicated by renal insufficiency: (1)

Initial loading dose of 3 grams I.V. followed by I.V. doses, based on creatinine clearance and type of dialysis, as indicated below:

Creatinine clearance ml/min.:	
over 60	3 grams every 4 hours
30–60	2 grams every 4 hours
10–30	2 grams every 8 hours
less than 10	2 grams every 12 hours (or 1 gram I.M. every 6 hours)
less than 10 with hepatic dysfunction	2 grams every 24 hours (or 1 gram I.M. every 12 hours)
patients on peritoneal dialysis	3 grams every 12 hours
patients on hemodialysis	2 grams every 12 hours supplemented with 3 grams after each dialysis

To calculate creatinine clearance* from a serum creatinine value use the following formula:

$$C_{cr} = \frac{(140 - Age)(wt\ in\ kg)}{72 \times S_{cr}(mg/100\ ml)}$$

This is the calculated creatinine clearance for adult males; for females it is 15% less.

* Cockcroft, D.W., et al, "Prediction of Creatinine Clearance from Serum Creatinine" *Nephron* 16:31–41 (1976).

(1) The half-life of Ticarcillin in patients with renal failure is approximately 13 hours.

Children: Under 40 kg (88 lbs)

The daily dose for children should not exceed the adult dosage.

Bacterial Septicemia Respiratory Tract Infections Skin and Soft-Tissue Infections Intra-Abdominal Infections Infections of the Female Pelvis and Genital Tract	200–300 mg/kg/day by I.V. infusion in divided doses every 4 or 6 hours.
Urinary Tract Infections Complicated:	150–200 mg/kg/day by I.V. infusion in divided doses every 4 or 6 hours.
Uncomplicated:	50–100 mg/kg/day I.M. or direct I.V. in divided doses every 6 or 8 hours.

Infections complicated by renal insufficiency: Clinical data is insufficient to recommend an optimum dose.

Children weighing more than 40 kg (88 lbs) should receive adult dosages.

Neonates: In the neonate, for severe infections (sepsis) due to susceptible strains of *Pseudomonas, Proteus,* and *E. coli,* the following Ticarcillin dosages may be given I.M. or by 10–20 minutes I.V. infusion:

Infants under 2000 grams body weight:
Aged 0–7 days	75 mg/kg/12 hours (150 mg/kg/day)
Aged over 7 days	75 mg/kg/8 hours (225 mg/kg/day)

Infants over 2000 grams body weight:
Ages 0–7 days	75 mg/kg/8 hours (225 mg/kg/day)
Aged over 7 days	100 mg/kg/8 hours (300 mg/kg/day)

This dosage schedule is intended to produce peak serum concentrations of 125–150 mcg/ml one hour after a dose of Ticarcillin and trough concentrations of 25–50 mcg/ml immediately before the next dose.

NOTE: Gentamicin, tobramycin or amikacin may be used concurrently with Ticarcillin for initial therapy until results of culture and susceptibility studies are known.

Seriously ill patients should receive the higher doses. TICAR has proved to be useful in infections in which protective mechanisms are impaired, such as in acute leukemia and during therapy with immunosuppressive or oncolytic drugs.

Vein irritation and phlebitis can occur, particularly when undiluted solution is directly injected into the vein.
[See table above].

Directions For Use:

1 Gm, 3 Gm and 6 Gm Standard Vials:

Intramuscular Use: Each gram of Ticarcillin should be reconstituted with 2 ml of the desired intravenous solution listed below or 1% Lidocaine Hydrochloride solution (without epinephrine) **and used promptly.** Each 2.6 ml of the resulting solution will then contain 1 Gm of Ticarcillin.

[For full product information, refer to manufacturer's package insert for Lidocaine Hydrochloride.]

As with all intramuscular preparations, TICAR (Ticarcillin Disodium) should be injected well within the body of a relatively large muscle, using usual techniques and precautions.

Intravenous Use: Reconstitute each gram of Ticarcillin with 4 ml of the desired intravenous solution listed below; when dissolved, further dilute if desired. After the addition of 4 ml of diluent per gram of Ticarcillin each 1.0 ml of the resulting solution will have an approximate average concentration of 200 mg. Once dissolved, further dilute if desired.

Direct Intravenous Injection: In order to avoid vein irritation, administer solution as slowly as possible.

Intravenous Infusion: Administer by continuous or intermittent intravenous drip. Intermittent infusion should be administered over a 30 minute to 2 hour period in equally divided doses.

3 Gm Piggyback Bottles:

Direct Intravenous Injection:

The 3 gram bottle should be reconstituted with a minimum of 30 ml of the desired intravenous solution listed below.

Amount of Diluent	Concentration of Solution
100 ml	1 Gm/34 ml
60 ml	1 Gm/20 ml
30 ml	1 Gm/10 ml

In order to avoid vein irritation, the solution should be administered as slowly as possible. A dilution of approximately 1 Gm/20 ml or more will further reduce the incidence of vein irritation.

Intravenous Infusion: Stability studies in various intravenous solutions indicate that Ticarcillin Disodium will provide sufficient activity at room temperature within the stated time periods at concentrations between 10 mg/ml and 50 mg/ml:

STABILITY PERIOD

Intravenous Solution	Room Temperature (70–75°F)
* Sodium Chloride Injection	72 hours

Continued on next page

Beecham Laboratories—Cont.

* Dextrose Injection 5%   72 hours
* Lactated Ringer's Injection 48 hours

The above solutions remain stable for 14 days if stored under refrigeration (4°C); refrigerated solutions stored longer than 72 hours should *not* be used for multidose purposes.

(*) These solutions remain stable up to 100 mg/ml concentration. After reconstitution, they can be frozen (approx. 0°F) and stored for up to 30 days without loss of potency. The stabilities of the thawed solutions are identical to the unfrozen ones listed above.

Unused solutions should be discarded after the time periods mentioned above.

It is recommended that TICAR and gentamicin sulfate, tobramycin sulfate or amikacin sulfate *not* be mixed together in the same I.V. solution due to the gradual inactivation of gentamicin sulfate, tobramycin sulfate or amikacin sulfate under these circumstances. The therapeutic effect of TICAR and these aminoglycoside drugs remains unimpaired when administered separately.

How Supplied: TICAR (Sterile Ticarcillin Disodium). Each vial contains Ticarcillin Disodium equivalent to 1 Gm, 3 Gm, or 6 Gm Ticarcillin.

NDC 0029-6550-22 .... 1 Gm Vial
NDC 0029-6552-26 .... 3 Gm Vial
NDC 0029-6555-26 .... 6 Gm Vial
NDC 0029-6552-21 .... 3 Gm Piggyback Bottle
TICAR (Sterile Ticarcillin Disodium) Is also supplied as:
NDC 0029-6558-21 .... 20 Gm Bulk
                                          Pharmacy Package

Rev. September, 1983
7182/L

TIGAN® R
[tī'găn]
(trimethobenzamide HCl)

Description: Tigan is an antiemetic agent. Chemically, trimethobenzamide HCl is N-[p-[2-(dimethylamino)-ethoxy] benzyl]-3,4,5-trimethoxybenzamide hydrochloride. It has a molecular weight of 424.93.

Capsules; Blue, each containing 250 mg trimethobenzamide hydrochloride; blue and white, each containing 100 mg trimethobenzamide hydrochloride.

Suppositories: (200 mg): Each suppository contains 200 mg trimethobenzamide hydrochloride and 2% benzocaine in a base compounded with polysorbate 80, white beeswax and propylene glycol monostearate.

Suppositories, Pediatric (100 mg): Each suppository contains 100 mg trimethobenzamide hydrochloride and 2% benzocaine in a base compounded with polysorbate 80, white beeswax and propylene glycol monostearate.

Ampuls: Each 2-ml ampul contains 200 mg trimethobenzamide hydrochloride compounded with 0.2% parabens (methyl and propyl) as preservatives, 1 mg sodium citrate and 0.4 mg citric acid as buffers and pH adjusted to approximately 5.0 with sodium hydroxide.

Multiple Dose Vials: Each ml contains 100 mg trimethobenzamide hydrochloride compounded with 0.45% phenol as preservative, 0.5 mg sodium citrate and 0.2 mg citric acid as buffers and pH adjusted to approximately 5.0 with sodium hydroxide.

Thera-Ject™ (Disposable Syringes): Each 2 ml contains 200 mg trimethobenzamide hydrochloride compounded with 0.45% phenol as preservative, 1 mg sodium citrate and 0.4 mg citric acid as buffers, 0.2 mg disodium edetate as stabilizer and pH adjusted to approximately 5.0 with sodium hydroxide.

Actions: The mechanism of action of Tigan as determined in animals is obscure, but may be the chemoreceptor trigger zone (CTZ), an area in the medulla oblongata through which emetic impulses are conveyed to the vomiting center; direct impulses to the vomiting center apparently are not similarly inhibited. In dogs pretreated with trimethobenzamide HCl, the emetic response to apomorphine is inhibited, while little or no protection is afforded against emesis induced by intragastric copper sulfate.

Indications: Tigan is indicated for the control of nausea and vomiting.

Contraindications: The injectable form of Tigan in children, the suppositories in premature or newborn infants, and use in patients with known hypersensitivity to trimethobenzamide are contraindicated. Since the suppositories contain benzocaine they should not be used in patients known to be sensitive to this or similar local anesthetics.

Warnings:

> Caution should be exercised when administering Tigan to children for the treatment of vomiting. Antiemetics are not recommended for treatment of uncomplicated vomiting in children and their use should be limited to prolonged vomiting of known etiology. There are three principal reasons for caution:
> 1. There has been some suspicion that centrally acting antiemetics may contribute, in combination with viral illnesses (a possible cause of vomiting in children), to development of Reye's syndrome, a potentially fatal acute childhood encephalopathy with visceral fatty degeneration, especially involving the liver. Although there is no confirmation of this suspicion, caution is nevertheless recommended.
> 2. The extrapyramidal symptoms which can occur secondary to Tigan may be confused with the central nervous system signs of an undiagnosed primary disease responsible for the vomiting, e.g., Reye's syndrome or other encephalopathy.
> 3. It has been suspected that drugs with hepatotoxic potential, such as Tigan, may unfavorably alter the course of Reye's syndrome. Such drugs should therefore be avoided in children whose signs and symptoms (vomiting) could represent Reye's syndrome. It should also be noted that salicylates and acetaminophen are hepatotoxic at large doses. Although it is not known that at usual doses they would represent a hazard in patients with the underlying hepatic disorder of Reye's syndrome, these drugs, too, should be avoided in children whose signs and symptoms could represent Reye's syndrome, unless alternative methods of controlling fever are not successful.

Tigan may produce drowsiness. Patients should not operate motor vehicles or other dangerous machinery until their individual responses have been determined.

Reye's Syndrome has been associated with the use of TIGAN and other drugs, including antiemetics, although their contribution, if any, to the cause and course of the disease hasn't been established. This syndrome is characterized by an abrupt onset shortly following a nonspecific febrile illness, with persistent, severe vomiting, lethargy, irrational behavior, progressive encephalopathy leading to coma, convulsions and death.

Usage in Pregnancy: Trimethobenzamide hydrochloride was studied in reproduction experiments in rats and rabbits and no teratogenicity was suggested. The only effects observed were an increased percentage of embryonic resorptions or stillborn pups in rats administered 20 mg and 100 mg/kg and increased resorptions in rabbits receiving 100 mg/kg. In each study these adverse effects were attributed to one or two dams. The relevance to humans is not known. Since there is no adequate experience in pregnant or lactating women who have received this drug, safety in pregnancy or in nursing mothers has not been established.

Usage with Alcohol: Concomitant use of alcohol with Tigan may result in an adverse drug interaction.

Precautions: During the course of acute febrile illness, encephalitides, gastroenteritis, dehydration and electrolyte imbalance, especially in children and the elderly or debilitated, CNS reactions such as opisthotonos, convulsions, coma and extrapyramidal symptoms have been reported with and without use of Tigan or other antiemetic agents. In such disorders caution should be exercised in administering Tigan, particularly to patients who have recently received other CNS-acting agents (phenothiazines, barbiturates, belladonna derivatives). It is recommended that severe emesis should not be treated with an antiemetic drug alone; where possible the cause of vomiting should be established. Primary emphasis should be directed toward the restoration of body fluids and electrolyte balance, the relief of fever and relief of the causative disease process. Overhydration should be avoided since it may result in cerebral edema. The antiemetic effects of Tigan may render diagnosis more difficult in such conditions as appendicitis and obscure signs of toxicity due to overdosage of other drugs.

Adverse Reactions: There have been reports of hypersensitivity reactions and Parkinson-like symptoms. There have been instances of hypotension reported following parenteral administration to surgical patients. There have been reports of blood dyscrasias, blurring of vision, coma, convulsions, depression of mood, diarrhea, disorientation, dizziness, drowsiness, headache, jaundice, muscle cramps and opisthotonos. If these occur, the administration of the drug should be discontinued. Allergic-type skin reactions have been observed; therefore, the drug should be discontinued at the first sign of sensitization. While these symptoms will usually disappear spontaneously, symptomatic treatment may be indicated in some cases.

Dosage and Administration: (See WARNINGS and PRECAUTIONS.) Dosage should be adjusted according to the indication for therapy, severity of symptoms and the response of the patient.

Capsules, 250 mg and 100 mg
Usual Adult Dosage
  One 250-mg capsule t.i.d. or q.i.d.
Usual Children's Dosage
  30 to 90 lbs: One or two 100-mg capsules t.i.d. or q.i.d.

Suppositories, 200 mg (Not to be used in premature or newborn infants.)
Usual Adult Dosage
  One suppository (200 mg) t.i.d. or q.i.d.
Usual Children's Dosage
  Under 30 lbs: One-half suppository (100 mg) t.i.d. or q.i.d.
  30 to 90 lbs: One-half to one suppository (100 to 200 mg) t.i.d. or q.i.d.

SUPPOSITORIES, PEDIATRIC, 100 mg (Not to be used in Premature or newborn infants).
Usual Children's Dosage
  Under 30 lbs; One suppository
  (100 mg) t.i.d. or q.i.d.
  30 to 90 lbs; One to two suppositories
  (100 to 200 mg) t.i.d. or q.i.d.

Injectable, 100 mg/ml (Not recommended for use in children.)
Usual Adult Dosage: 2 ml (200 mg) t.i.d. or q.i.d. intramuscularly.

Intramuscular administration may cause pain, stinging, burning, redness and swelling at the site of injection. Such effects may be minimized by deep injection into the upper outer quadrant of the gluteal region, and by avoiding the escape of solution along the route.

Note: The injectable form is intended for intramuscular administration only; it is not recommended for intravenous use.

How Supplied:

Product	Package Sizes	NDC Numbers
Capsules		
100 mg.	100's	NDC-0029-4082-30
250 mg.	100's	NDC-0029-4083-30
	500's	NDC-0029-4083-32
Suppositories		
200 mg.	10's	NDC-0029-4084-38

	50's	NDC-0029-4084-39
Suppositories		
Pediatric		
100 mg.	10's	NDC-0029-4088-38
Injectable		
Ampuls		
2 ml,		
200 mg.	10's	NDC-0029-4085-22
Vials		
20 ml,		
100 mg./ml	Each	NDC-0029-4086-22
Thera-Ject®		
(Disposable Syringe)		
2 ml,		
100 mg./ml	25's	NDC-0029-4087-22

Shown in Product Identification Section, page 000

Berlex Laboratories, Inc.
300 FAIRFIELD ROAD
WAYNE, NJ 07470

DECONAMINE® Tablets ℞
[dē″con′uh-mēēn]
DECONAMINE® Elixir ℞
DECONAMINE® SR Capsules ℞
DECONAMINE® Syrup ℞

Description:
Tablets
Each scored, white tablet contains:
  chlorpheniramine maleate ....4 mg
  d-pseudoephedrine hydrochloride ....60 mg
Elixir
Each 5 ml (teaspoonful) blue liquid contains:
  chlorpheniramine maleate ....2 mg
  d-pseudoephedrine hydrochloride ....30 mg
  alcohol 15%
in a pleasant tasting aromatic vehicle.
SR Capsules
Each sustained release, blue and yellow capsule contains:
  chlorpheniramine maleate ....8 mg
  d-pseudoephedrine hydrochloride ....120 mg
The capsules are designed to provide prolonged release of medication.
Syrup—No alcohol, no dye
Each 5 ml (teaspoonful) clear, colorless liquid contains:
  chlorpheniramine maleate ....2 mg
  d-pseudoephedrine hydrochloride ....30 mg
in a grape-flavored, aromatic vehicle

Clinical Pharmacology: Chlorpheniramine maleate antagonizes the physiological action of histamine by acting as an H_1 receptor blocking agent.
Pseudoephedrine is an orally active sympathomimetic amine and exerts a decongestant action on the nasal mucosa. It does this by vasoconstriction, which results in reduction of tissue hyperemia, edema, nasal congestion and an increase in nasal airway patency. The vasoconstrictive action of pseudoephedrine is similar to that of ephedrine. In the usual dose it has minimal vasopressor effects.
Indications: For relief of nasal congestion associated with the common cold, hay fever and other allergies, sinusitis, eustachian tube blockage, and vasomotor and allergic rhinitis.
Contraindications: Patients with severe hypertension, severe coronary artery disease and patients on MAO inhibitor therapy. Deconamine® medication is also contraindicated in patients sensitive to antihistamines or sympathomimetic agents.
Warnings: Chlorpheniramine maleate should be used with extreme caution in patients with narrow angle glaucoma; stenosing peptic ulcer; pyloroduodenal obstruction; symptomatic prostatic hypertrophy; or bladder neck obstruction. Due to its mild atropine-like action, chlorpheniramine maleate should be used cautiously in patients with bronchial asthma.
Sympathomimetic amines should be used with caution in patients with hypertension, ischemic heart disease, diabetes mellitus, increased intraocular pressure, hyperthyroidism and prostatic hypertrophy. Sympathomimetics may produce central nervous system stimulation with convulsions or cardiovascular collapse with accompanying hypotension.
Precautions:
Information for patients:
Antihistamines may impair mental and physical abilities required for the performance of potentially hazardous tasks, such as driving a vehicle or operating machinery. Patients should also be warned about possible additive effects with alcohol and other central nervous system depressants (hypnotics, sedatives, tranquilizers).
Drug interactions:
Pseudoephedrine-containing drugs should not be given to patients treated with monoamine oxidase (MAO) inhibitors because of the possibility of precipitating a hypertensive crisis. MAO inhibitors also prolong and intensify the anticholinergic effects of antihistamines. Sympathomimetics may reduce the antihypertensive effect of methyldopa, reserpine, veratrum alkaloids and mecamylamine.
Alcohol and other sedative drugs will potentiate the sedative effects of chlorpheniramine.
Care should be taken in administering Deconamine® medication concomitantly with other sympathomimetic amines, since their combined effects on the cardiovascular system may be harmful to the patient.
Pregnancy:
Pregnancy Category C: Animal reproduction studies have not been conducted with Deconamine® medication. It is also not known whether Deconamine® medication can cause fetal harm when administered to a pregnant woman or can affect reproduction capacity. Deconamine® medication should be given to a pregnant woman only if clearly needed.
Nursing Mothers: Due to the possible passage of pseudoephedrine and chlorpheniramine into breast milk, and because of the higher than usual risk for infants from sympathomimetic amines and antihistamines, the benefit to the mother vs the potential risk should be considered, and a decision should be made whether to discontinue nursing or to discontinue the drug.
Pediatric Use: Deconamine® medication capsules or tablets should not be given to children under 12 years of age.
Adverse Reactions:
Chlorpheniramine maleate
Slight to moderate drowsiness may occur and is the most frequent side effect. Other possible side effects of antihistamines in general include:
General: urticaria, drug rash, anaphylactic shock, photosensitivity, excessive perspiration, chills, dryness of mouth, nose and throat.
Cardiovascular: hypotension, headache, palpitation, tachycardia, extrasystoles.
Hematological: hemolytic anemia, thrombocytopenia, agranulocytosis.
CNS: sedation, dizziness, disturbed coordination, fatigue, confusion, restlessness, excitation, nervousness, tremor, irritability, insomnia, euphoria, paresthesia, blurred vision, diplopia, vertigo, tinnitus, hysteria, neuritis, convulsion.
Gastrointestinal: epigastric distress, anorexia, nausea, vomiting, diarrhea, constipation.
Genitourinary: urinary frequency, difficult urination, urinary retention, early menses.
Respiratory: thickening of bronchial secretions, tightness of chest, wheezing and nasal stuffiness.
Pseudoephedrine hydrochloride
Pseudoephedrine may cause mild central nervous system stimulation especially in those patients who are hypersensitive to sympathomimetic drugs. Nervousness, excitability, restlessness, dizziness, weakness and insomnia may also occur. Headache and drowsiness have also been reported. Large doses may cause lightheadedness, nausea and/or vomiting. Sympathomimetic drugs have also been associated with certain untoward reactions including fear, anxiety, tenseness, restlessness, tremor, weakness, pallor, respiratory difficulty, dysuria, insomnia, hallucination, convulsion, CNS depression, arrhythmias and cardiovascular collapse with hypotension.

Overdosage: Acute overdosage may produce clinical signs of CNS stimulation and variable cardiovascular effects. Pressor amines should be used with great caution in the presence of pseudoephedrine. Patients with signs of stimulation should be treated conservatively.
Dosage and Administration:
Tablets
Adults and children over 12 years, 1 tablet three or four times daily.
Children under 12 years, Deconamine® Elixir or Syrup is recommended.
Elixir or Syrup
Adults and children over 12 years, 1 to 2 teaspoonfuls (5 to 10 ml) three or four times daily.
Children 6 to 12 years, ½ to 1 teaspoonful (2.5 to 5 ml) three or four times daily, not to exceed 4 teaspoonfuls in 24 hours.
Children 2 to 6 years, ½ teaspoonful (2.5 ml) three or four times daily, not to exceed 2 teaspoonfuls in 24 hours.
Children under two years, as directed by physician.
SR Capsules
Adults and children over 12 years, one capsule every 12 hours.
Children under 12 years, Deconamine® Elixir or Syrup is recommended.
How Supplied:
In bottles of:
Tablets
  100 ....NDC 50419-184-10
  500 ....NDC 50419-184-50
Elixir
  473 ml ....NDC 50419-182-16
SR Capsules
  100 ....NDC 50419-181-10
  500 ....NDC 50419-181-50
Syrup
  473 ml ....NDC 50419-185-16
Store at controlled room temperature.
Shown in Product Identification Section, page 406

ELIXICON® ℞
[ē″lix′i-con]
(theophylline)
Suspension

ELIXOPHYLLIN® ℞
[ē″lix′off′fil-in]
(theophylline)
Soft Gelatin Capsules

ELIXOPHYLLIN® SR ℞
(theophylline)
Soft Gelatin Capsules

ELIXOPHYLLIN® ℞
(theophylline)
Elixir

Description:
Elixicon® (theophylline) Suspension
Each 5 ml (teaspoonful) contains 100 mg anhydrous theophylline in an aqueous suspension. Contains no sugar or dye. Preserved with methylparaben and propylparaben.
Elixophyllin® (theophylline) Soft Gelatin Capsules
100 mg capsule—Each off-white, dye-free soft gelatin Elixophyllin® Capsule contains 100 mg anhydrous theophylline in a suspension of polyethylene glycol.
200 mg capsule—Each off-white, dye-free soft gelatin Elixophyllin® Capsule contains 200 mg anhy-

Continued on next page

Information on the Berlex products in the 1985 Annual is based on the labeling in effect on August 1, 1984. Further information on dosage and administration, side effects, precautions and contraindications for these and other Berlex products may be obtained from either the package insert or the Medical Affairs Department, Berlex Laboratories, Inc., 110 East Hanover Avenue, Cedar Knolls, New Jersey

Berlex—Cont.

drous theophylline in a suspension of polyethylene glycol.

Elixophyllin® (theophylline) SR Capsules
Elixophyllin® SR Capsules are designed to provide a prolonged therapeutic effect.
125 mg Capsule—Each white, opaque, dye-free capsule contains 125 mg anhydrous theophylline.
250 mg Capsule—Each clear, dye-free capsule contains 250 mg anhydrous theophylline.

Elixophyllin® (theophylline) Elixir
Each 15 ml (tablespoonful) of Elixophyllin® Elixir contains 80 mg anhydrous theophylline and 20% alcohol in a palatable aromatic base.
Theophylline (1H-purine-2,6-dione, 3,7-diydro-1,3-dimenthyl), a xanthine bronchodilator, is a white, odorless, crystalline powder having a bitter taste and is represented by the following structural formula:

Clinical Pharmacology: Theophylline directly relaxes the smooth muscle of the bronchial airways and pulmonary blood vessels, thus acting mainly as a bronchodilator and smooth muscle relaxant. The drug also produces other actions typical of xanthine derivatives: coronary vasodilation, cardiac stimulation, diuresis, cerebral stimulation and skeletal muscle stimulation. The actions of theophylline may be mediated through inhibition of phosphodiesterase and a resultant increase in intracellular cyclic AMP. In vivo studies indicate that xanthines improve the contractile properties of the diaphragm in normal human subjects.

In vitro theophylline has been shown to act synergistically with beta agonists that increase intracellular cyclic AMP through the stimulation of adenyl cyclase, but synergism has not been demonstrated in patient studies. More data are needed to determine if theophylline and beta agonists have clinically important additive effects in vivo.

Apparently, tolerance does not develop with chronic use of theophylline.

Pharmacokinetics: The half-life of theophylline is influenced by a number of known variables. It is prolonged in patients suffering from chronic alcoholism, impaired hepatic or renal function, congestive heart failure, and in patients receiving macrolide antibiotics or cimetidine. Older adults (over age 55) and patients with chronic obstructive pulmonary disease, with or without cor pulmonale, may also have much slower clearance rates. For such patients, the theophylline half-life may exceed 24 hours.

Newborns and neonates have extremely slow clearance rates compared with older infants (over 6 months) and children, and may also have a theophylline half-life of over 24 hours.

High fever for prolonged periods may also reduce the rate of theophylline elimination in adults as well as children.

THEOPHYLLINE ELIMINATION CHARACTERISTICS

	Theophylline Clearance Rates (mean±SD)	Half-life Average (mean±SD)
Children (over 6 months of age)	1.45 ± 0.58 ml/kg/min	3.7 ± 1.1 hr
Adult nonsmokers (uncomplicated asthma)	0.65 ± 0.19 ml/kg/min	8.7 ± 2.2 hr

The half-life of theophylline in smokers (1 to 2 packs/day) averages 4 to 5 hours, much shorter than the half-life in nonsmokers (which averages 7 to 9 hours). The increase in theophylline clearance caused by smoking is probably the result of induction of drug-metabolizing enzymes that do not readily normalize after cessation of smoking. It appears that between three months and two years may be necessary for the normalization of theophylline pharmacokinetics following cessation of smoking.

Indications: For relief and/or prevention of symptoms of asthma and reversible bronchospasm associated with chronic bronchitis and emphysema.

Contraindications: This product is contraindicated in individuals who have shown hypersensitivity to any of its components.

Warnings: Status asthmaticus should be considered a medical emergency and is defined as that degree of bronchospasm which is not rapidly responsive to usual doses of conventional bronchodilators. Optimal therapy for such patients frequently requires both *additional medication*, parenterally administered, and *close monitoring*, preferably in an intensive care setting.

Although increasing the theophylline dose may bring about relief, such treatment may be associated with toxicity. The likelihood of such toxicity developing increases significantly when the serum theophylline concentration exceeds 20 μg/ml. Therefore, determination of serum theophylline levels is recommended to assure maximum benefit without excessive risk.

Serum levels above 20 μg/ml are rarely found after appropriate administration of the recommended doses. However, in individuals in whom theophylline plasma clearance is reduced *for any reason*, even conventional doses may result in increased serum levels and potential toxicity. Reduced theophylline clearance has been documented in the following readily identifiable groups: 1) patients with impaired renal or liver function; 2) patients over 55 years of age, particularly males, and those with chronic lung disease; 3) patients with cardiac failure from any cause; 4) neonates and 5) those patients taking certain drugs (macrolide antibiotics or cimetidine). Decreased clearance of theophylline may be associated with either influenza immunization or active infection with influenza. Reduction of dosage and laboratory monitoring is especially appropriate in the above individuals.

Less serious signs of theophylline toxicity, eg, nausea and restlessness, may appear in up to 50% of patients. Unfortunately however, serious side effects (such as ventricular arrhythmias, convulsions or even death) may appear as the first sign of toxicity without any previous warning. *Serious toxicity is not reliably preceded by less severe side effects.*

Many patients who require theophylline may exhibit tachycardia due to their underlying disease process. Therefore, the cause/effect relationship of elevated serum theophylline concentrations may not be appreciated.

Theophylline products may cause an arrhythmia and/or worsen a preexisting arrhythmia. Any significant change in rate and/or rhythm warrants monitoring and further investigation.

Precautions:
General: Theophylline half-life is shorter in smokers than in nonsmokers. Therefore, smokers may require larger or more frequent doses. Theophylline should not be administered concurrently with other xanthine medications. Use with caution in patients with severe cardiac disease, severe hypoxemia, hypertension, hyperthyroidism, acute myocardial injury, cor pulmonale, congestive heart failure, liver disease, in the elderly (especially males) and in neonates. In particular, great caution should be used in giving theophylline to patients with congestive heart failure. Frequently, such patients have markedly prolonged theophylline serum levels, with theophylline persisting in serum for long periods following discontinuation of the drug.

Use theophylline cautiously in a patient with a history of peptic ulcer. Theophylline may occasionally act as a local irritant to the GI tract, although gastrointestinal symptoms are more commonly centrally mediated and are associated with serum drug concentrations exceeding 20 μg/ml.

Information for Patients: The physician should reinforce the importance of taking only the prescribed dose and only at the prescribed time interval between doses.

Drug Interactions: Toxic synergism with ephedrine has been documented and may occur with some other sympathomimetic bronchodilators. In addition, the following drug interactions have been demonstrated:

DRUG	EFFECT
Aminophylline with lithium carbonate	Increased excretion of lithium carbonate
Aminophylline with propranolol	Antagonism of propranolol effect
Theophylline with cimetidine	Increased theophylline blood levels
Theophylline with troleandomycin, erythromycin	Increased theophylline blood levels

Drug-Laboratory Test Interactions: When plasma levels of theophylline are measured by spectrophotometric methods, coffee, tea, cola beverages, chocolate and acetaminophen contribute to falsely high values.

Carcinogenesis, Mutagenesis and Impairment of Fertility: Long-term animal studies have not been performed to evaluate the carcinogenic potential, mutagenic potential or the effect on fertility of xanthine compounds.

Pregnancy: Category C—Animal reproduction studies have not been conducted with theophylline. It is not known whether theophylline can cause fetal harm when administered to a pregnant woman or whether it can affect reproductive capacity. Xanthines should be given to a pregnant woman only if clearly needed.

Nursing Mothers: It has been reported that theophylline distributes readily into breast milk and may cause adverse effects in the infant. Caution must be used if prescribing xanthines to a nursing mother, taking into account the risk-benefit of this therapy.

Pediatric Use: This drug is not recommended for infants under 6 months of age because of their marked variation in theophylline metabolism. The use of Elixophyllin® SR capsules is not recommended for children under 6 years of age.

Adverse Reactions: The most consistent adverse reactions are usually due to overdose and are:
1. **Gastrointestinal:** nausea, vomiting, epigastric pain, hematemesis, diarrhea.
2. **Central nervous system:** headaches, irritability, restlessness, insomnia, reflex hyperexcitability, muscle twitching, clonic and tonic generalized convulsions.
3. **Cardiovascular:** palpitations, tachycardia, extrasystoles, flushing, hypotension, circulatory failure, ventricular arrhythmias.
4. **Respiratory:** tachypnea.
5. **Renal:** albuminuria, increased excretion of renal tubular and red blood cells, potentiation of diuresis.
6. **Others:** hyperglycemia, inappropriate ADH secretion, rash

Overdosage:
Management:
If potential oral overdose is established and seizure has not occurred:
a. Induce vomiting.
b. Administer a cathartic (this is particularly important if a sustained-release preparation has been taken).
c. Administer activated charcoal.
If patient is having a seizure:
a. Establish an airway.
b. Administer oxygen.
c. Treat the seizure with intravenous diazepam, 0.1 to 0.3 mg/kg up to 10 mg.
d. Monitor vital signs, maintain blood pressure and provide adequate hydration.
Postseizure Coma:
a. Maintain airway and oxygenation.
b. If a result of oral medication, follow above recommendations to prevent absorption of the

Product Information

drug; however, intubation and lavage should be performed instead of inducing emesis. Any cathartic or charcoal should be introduced via a large bore gastric lavage tube.

c. Continue to provide full supportive care and adequate hydration while waiting for the drug to be metabolized. In general, the drug is rapidly metabolized and does not warrant consideration of dialysis. However, if serum levels exceed 50 µg/ml, charcoal hemoperfusion may be indicated.

Dosage and Administration: For most patients, *effective use* of theophylline, ie, use associated with optimal likelihood of benefit combined with minimal risk of toxicity, is considered to occur when serum levels are maintained between 10 and 20 µg/ml. Levels above 20 µg/ml may produce toxicity. In a small number of patients, toxicity may even be seen with serum levels between 15 and 20 µg/ml, particularly during initiation of therapy.

There is considerable variation among patients in the dosage required to achieve and maintain safe and therapeutic levels, primarily due to variable rates of elimination. Therefore, it is not only essential to individualize the dosage but also to titrate and monitor serum levels when possible. When serum concentration cannot be obtained, restriction of dosage to the amounts and intervals recommended in the guidelines listed below becomes essential. Dosage should be calculated on the basis of lean (ideal) body weight wherever mg/kg doses are presented. Theophylline does not distribute into fatty tissue.

Frequency of Dosing: When immediate-release products with rapid absorption (such as Elixophyllin® Soft Gelatin Capsules, Elixicon® Suspension and Elixophyllin® Elixir) are used, dosing to maintain serum levels generally requires administration every 6 hours. This is particularly true in children, but dosing intervals up to 8 hours may be satisfactory in adults, since they eliminate the drug at a slower rate. Some children and adults having rapid clearance rates (eg, half-lives of under 6 hours) require higher than average doses and may benefit from and be more effectively controlled during chronic therapy when given Elixophyllin® SR Capsules, since this provides longer dosing intervals and/or less fluctuation in serum concentration between dosing.

Elixophyllin® SR Capsules provide a prolonged therapeutic effect and should be used for chronic or long-term use, not for initial treatment in a patient with acute symptoms. It is recommended that the appropriate dosage be established using an immediate-release preparation (such as Elixophyllin® Elixir, Elixicon® Suspension or Elixophyllin® Soft Gelatin Capsules). Slow clinical titration is generally preferred to help assure medication acceptance and safety. If the total daily dose can be given by using a sustained-release product, the patient can usually be switched to Elixphyllin® SR Capsules. The total daily dose should be divided and administered at 12 hour intervals.

Elixicon® Suspension, Elixophyllin® Elixir, and Elixophyllin® Soft Gelatin Capsules®

	Oral Loading:	Followed by:	Maintenance:
1. Children 6 months to 9 years	6 mg/kg	4 mg/kg q4h × 3 doses	4 mg/kg q6h
2. Children 9-16 years and young adult smokers	6 mg/kg	3 mg/kg q4h × 3 doses	3 mg/kg q6h
3. Otherwise healthy nonsmoking adults	6 mg/kg	3 mg/kg q6h × 2 doses	3 mg/kg q8h
4. Older patients and patients with cor pulmonale	6 mg/kg	2 mg/kg q6h × 2 doses	2 mg/kg q8h
5. Patients with congestive heart failure	6 mg/kg	2 mg/kg q8h × 2 doses	1–2 mg/kg q12h

However, certain patients, such as the young, smokers and some nonsmoking adults, are likely to metabolize theophylline rapidly and require dosing at 8-hour intervals. Such patients can generally be identified as having trough serum concentrations lower than desired or repeatedly exhibit symptoms near the end of the dosing interval.

Dosage guidelines are only approximations. The wide range of theophylline clearance among individuals (particularly those with concomitant disease) makes indiscriminate usage hazardous. As a practical consideration, it is not always possible to determine serum levels. Under such conditions, the daily dosage in (otherwise healthy adults) should not be greater than 16 mg/kg/day of anhydrous theophylline taken in divided doses. This will result in relatively few patients exceeding a serum level of 20 µg/ml, the level at which toxicity may be manifested.

Dosage Guidelines:
I. Acute Symptoms of Asthma Requiring Rapid Theophyllinization:
   A. Patients not currently receiving theophylline products. Dosage recommendations are for anhydrous theophylline.
   [See table above].
   B. Patients currently receiving theophylline products:
   When possible, determine the time, amount, dosage form and route of administration of the patient's last dose.
   The loading dose for theophylline is based on the principle that each 0.5 mg/kg of theophylline administered as a loading dose will result in a 1.0 µg/ml increase in serum theophylline concentration. Ideally, the loading dose should be deferred if a serum theophylline concentration can be obtained rapidly.
   If this is not possible, the clinician must exercise judgment in selecting a dose based on the potential for benefit and risk. When there is sufficient respiratory distress to warrant a small risk, then 2.5 mg/kg of theophylline administered in rapidly absorbed form is likely to increase serum concentration by approximately 5 µg/ml. If the patient is not experiencing theophylline toxicity, this is unlikely to result in dangerous adverse effects.
   After modifying the loading dose for this group of patients, the maintenance dosage recommendations are the same as those described above.

II. Chronic Therapy
Theophylline administration is a treatment of first choice for the management of chronic asthma, (to prevent symptoms and maintain patent airways). Slow titration is generally preferred to assure safety and medication acceptance.
Initial Dose: 16 mg/kg/24 hr or 400 mg/24 hr (whichever is less) of anhydrous theophylline in divided doses at 6- or 8-hour intervals.
Increasing Dose: The above dosage may be increased in approximately 25% increments at 2- to 3-day intervals so long as the drug is tolerated, and until the maximum dose indicated in Section III (below) is reached.

III. Maximum Theophylline Dose When Serum Concentration is Not Measured:
WARNING: DO NOT ATTEMPT TO MAINTAIN ANY DOSE THAT IS NOT TOLERATED.

	Not to exceed the following:
Age < 9 years	24 mg/kg/day
Age 9–12 years	20 mg/kg/day
Age 12–16 years	18 mg/kg/day
Age > 16 years	13 mg/kg/day OR 900 mg (*WHICHEVER IS LESS*)

Note: Use ideal body weight for obese patients

IV. Measurement of Serum Theophylline Concentrations During Chronic Therapy:
If the above maximum doses are to be maintained or exceeded, serum theophylline measurement is recommended. The serum sample should be obtained at the time of peak absorption: 1 to 2 hours after administration for immediate-release products, and 4 hours after administration for most sustained-release formulations. It is important that the patient has not missed any doses during the previous 48 hours and that dosing intervals have been reasonably typical with no added doses being taken during that period. IF THESE INSTRUCTIONS HAVE NOT BEEN FOLLOWED, DOSAGE ADJUSTMENT BASED ON SERUM THEOPHYLLINE MEASUREMENTS MAY RESULT IN RECOMMENDATIONS THAT PRESENT RISK OF TOXICITY TO THE PATIENT.

V. Final Adjustment of Dosage: (See Table I) [See table left].

Continued on next page

Table I—Dosage adjustment after serum theophylline measurement[1]
Elixicon® Suspension, Elixophyllin® Elixir, Elixophyllin® Soft Gelatin Capsules and Elixophyllin® SR

If serum theophylline is:		Directions:
Within normal limits	10 to 20 µg/ml	Maintain dosage, if tolerated. Recheck serum theophylline concentration at 6- to 12-month intervals.*
Too high	20 to 25 µg/ml	Decrease doses by about 10%. Recheck serum theophylline concentration at 6- to 12-month intervals.*
	25 to 30 µg/ml	Skip next dose and decrease subsequent doses by about 25%. Recheck serum theophylline.
	Over 30 µg/ml	Skip next 2 doses and decrease subsequent doses by 50%. Recheck serum theophylline.
Too low	7.5 to 10 µg/ml	Increase dose by about 25%.** Recheck serum theophylline concentration at 6- to 12-month intervals.*
	5 to 7.5 µg/ml	Increase dose by about 25% to the nearest dose increment and recheck serum theophylline for guidance in further dosage adjustment. Another increase will probably be needed, but this provides a safety check.

* Finer adjustments in dosage may be needed for some patients
** The total daily dose may need to be administered at more frequent intervals if symptoms occur repeatedly at the end of a dosing interval.

Information on the Berlex products in the 1985 Annual is based on the labeling in effect on August 1, 1984. Further information on dosage and administration, side effects, precautions and contraindications for these and other Berlex products may be obtained from either the package insert or the Medical Affairs Department, Berlex Laboratories, Inc., 110 East Hanover Avenue, Cedar Knolls, New Jersey

Berlex—Cont.

[1] From the J Resp Dis, 1981; 2(7):16
Caution should be exercised in younger children who cannot complain of minor side effects. Older adults, and those with cor pulmonale, congestive heart failure and/or liver disease may have unusually low dosage requirements and thus may experience toxicity at the maximal dosage recommended above.

It is important that no patient be maintained on any dosage that is not tolerated. In instructing patients to increase dosage according to the above schedule, they should be instructed not to take a subsequent dose if apparent side effects occur and to resume therapy at a lower dose after adverse effects have disappeared.

How Supplied:
Elixicon® (theophylline) Suspension
Bottles of 237 ml ....NDC 50419-112-08
NSN 6505-01-104-0397
Avoid excessive heat. Store below 30 C (86 F). Do not freeze. Shake well before using.
Elixophyllin® (theophylline) Capsules
100 mg Capsules
Bottles of 100 ....NDC 50419-126-10
200 mg Capsules
Bottles of 100 ....NDC 50419-120-10
Bottles of 500 ....NDC 50419-120-50
Unit Dose Boxes
of 100 ....NDC 50419-120-11
Store at controlled room temperature. Avoid excessive heat.
Elixophyllin® (theophylline) SR Capsules
125 mg Capsules
Bottles of 100 ....NDC 50419-129-10
NSN 6505-01-049-6812
Bottles of 500 ....NDC 50419-129-50
Unit Dose Boxes
of 100 ....NDC 50419-129-11
250 mg Capsules
Bottles of 100 ....NDC 50419-123-10
NSN 6505-01-064-9555
Bottles of 500 ....NDC 50419-123-50
Unit Dose Boxes
of 100 ....NDC 50419-123-11
Store at controlled room temperature.
Elixophyllin® (theophylline) Elixir
Bottles of:
473 ml ....NDC 50419-121-16
946 ml ....NDC 50419-121-32
3785 ml ....NDC 50419-121-28
Store at controlled room temperature.
[Shown in Product Identification Section]
Mfd for
Berlex Laboratories, Inc.
Wayne, NJ 07470
Shown in Product Identification Section, page 406

ELIXOPHYLLIN®-GG ORAL LIQUID
[ē" lix-off' fil-in gēē-gēē"]
(theophylline - guaifenesin)

Description: Each 15 ml (tablespoonful) of Elixophyllin®-GG Liquid contains 100 mg anhydrous theophylline and 100 mg guaifenesin (glyceryl guaiacolate) in a cherry-berry flavored, non-alcoholic liquid. Elixophyllin®-GG Liquid does not contain sugar or dye.
(Please refer to Elixophyllin® [theophylline] Elixir for complete information on theophylline).
Clinical Pharmacology: Guaifenesin (glyceryl guaiacolate) exerts its expectorant action by reducing the viscosity of bronchial secretions, thereby increasing the efficiency of the cough reflex and of ciliary action in removing accumulated secretions from the trachea and bronchi. Unlike many other expectorants, guaifenesin rarely causes gastric irritation.
Indications: For relief and/or prevention of symptoms of asthma and reversible bronchospasm associated with chronic bronchitis and emphysema.
Precautions:
Drug Laboratory Test Interactions—Guaifenesin has been shown to produce a color interference with certain clinical laboratory determinations of 5-hydroxyindoleacetic acid (5-HIAA) and vanillylmandelic acid (VMA).
How Supplied: Elixophyllin®-GG Oral Liquid in bottles of:
237 ml ....NDC 50419-136-08
473 ml ....NDC 50419-136-16
Store at controlled room temperature.
Shown in Product Identification Section, page 406

KAY CIEL® Oral Solution 10%
[kā' sēēl"]
(potassium chloride)

KAY CIEL® Powder
(potassium chloride)

Description: Each 15 ml (tablespoonful) contains 1.5 g (20 mEq) potassium chloride in a palatable base. Alcohol 4%. Contains no sugar.
Each packet contains 1.5 g (20 mEq) potassium chloride. Contains no sugar.
Indications: Treatment and prevention of potassium deficiency occurring especially during thiazide diuretic or corticosteroid therapy, digitalis intoxication, low dietary intake of potassium, or as a result of excessive vomiting and diarrhea and for correction of associated hypochloremic alkalosis.
Contraindications: Impaired renal function, untreated Addison's Disease, dehydration, heat cramps and hyperkalemia.
Warnings: Do not use excessively.
Precautions: Administer with caution and adjust to the requirements of the individual patient. The patient should be checked frequently and periodic ECG recorded and/or plasma potassium levels determined. Use with caution in patients with cardiac disease. In hypokalemic states, attention should be directed toward correction of frequently associated hypochloremic alkalosis. **PATIENTS SHOULD BE CAUTIONED TO ADHERE TO DILUTION INSTRUCTIONS TO ASSURE AGAINST GASTROINTESTINAL INJURY.**
Adverse Reactions: Potassium intoxication indicated by listlessness, mental confusion, paresthesia of the extremities, weakness of the legs, flaccid paralysis, fall in blood pressure, cardiac depression, arrhythmias, arrest and heartblock. Vomiting, nausea, abdominal discomfort and diarrhea may occur.
Dosage and Administration:
Oral Solution
One tablespoonful (15 ml supplying 20 mEq) *diluted* in 4 ounces of cold water or fruit juice twice daily (preferably after a meal), or as directed by physician.
Powder:
Contents of 1 packet dissolved in 4 ounces of cold water or fruit juice twice daily (preferably after a meal), or as directed by physician.
Overdosage: In case of excessive use resulting in hyperkalemia or potassium intoxication, discontinue use of potassium chloride and/or take other steps to lower serum levels if indicated.
How Supplied:
Oral Solution: Bottles of:
118 ml.......................................NDC 50419-145-04
473 ml.......................................NDC 50419-145-16
3785 ml.....................................NDC 50419-145-28
Powder: Boxes of:
30 packets..........................NDC 50419-144-30
100 packets........................NDC 50419-144-11
500 packets........................NDC 50419-144-32
Store at controlled room temperature.

PYOCIDIN-OTIC®
[pī" ō-cī' dĭn ō' tĭk"]
(polymyxin B-hydrocortisone)
Sterile Otic Solution

Description: Each ml contains 10,000 USP units of polymyxin B sulfate and 5 mg hydrocortisone in a vehicle containing propylene glycol and water. Sodium hydroxide or hydrochloric acid may have been added to adjust pH.
Actions: Polymyxin B sulfate is effective against the gram-negative *Pseudomonas aeruginosa,* one of the most resistant microorganisms commonly causing otitis externa. The addition of hydrocortisone to the antibiotic affords an anti-inflammatory effect and relief against allergic manifestations and reduces the possibility of sensitivity and tissue reaction.
Indications: For the treatment of superficial bacterial infections of the external auditory canal caused by organisms susceptible to the action of the antibiotic.
Contraindications: This product is contraindicated in those individuals who have shown hypersensitivity to any of its components, and in herpes simplex, vaccinia and varicella.
Warnings: As with other antibiotic preparations, prolonged treatment may result in overgrowth of nonsusceptible organisms and fungi. If the infection is not improved after one week, cultures and susceptibility tests should be repeated to verify the identity of the organism and to determine whether therapy should be changed.
Patients who prefer to warm the medication before using should be cautioned against heating the solution above body temperature, in order to avoid loss of potency.
Precautions: If sensitization or irritation occurs, medication should be discontinued promptly.
Dosage and Administration: The external auditory canal should be thoroughly cleaned and dried with a sterile cotton applicator.
For adults, 4 drops of the solution should be instilled into the affected ear 3 or 4 times daily. For infants and children, 3 drops are suggested because of the smaller capacity of the ear canal.
The patient should lie with the affected ear upward and then the drops should be instilled. This position should be maintained for 5 minutes to facilitate penetration of the drops into the ear canal. Repeat, if necessary, for the opposite ear.
If preferred, a cotton wick may be inserted into the canal and then the cotton may be saturated with the solution. This wick should be kept moist by adding further solution every four hours. The wick should be replaced at least once every 24 hours.
How Supplied: 10 ml bottle with dropper.
NDC 50419-287-10.
Store at controlled room temperature.

QUINAGLUTE®
[kwĭn' uh-glōōt"]
(quinidine gluconate)
DURA-TABS®
(sustained-release tablets)

Description: Each Quinaglute® Dura-Tabs® tablet contains 324 mg quinidine gluconate (equivalent to 202 mg quinidine base) in a tablet matrix specially designed for the prolonged (8 to 12 hours) release of the drug in the gastrointestinal tract. Quinaglute® Dura-Tabs® tablets are to be administered orally.
Quinidine gluconate is the gluconate salt of quinidine (6-methoxy-α-(5-vinyl-2 quinuclidinyl)-4-quinoline-methanol), a dextrorotatory isomer of quinine. Quinidine gluconate is represented by the following structural formula:

Quinidine gluconate contains 62.3% of the anhydrous quinidine alkaloid, whereas quinidine sulfate contains 82.86%. In prescribing Quinaglute® Dura-Tabs® tablets, this factor should be considered.
Therapeutic category: Type I antiarrhythmic.
Clinical Pharmacology: The antiarrhythmic activity consists of the following basic actions:
1. In arrhythmias due to enhanced automaticity, quinidine decreases the rate of rise of slow diastolic (Phase 4) depolarization thereby depressing automaticity, particularly in ectopic foci.

2. In addition to the above, quinidine slows depolarization, repolarization and amplitude of the action potential, thus increasing its duration, leading to an increase in the refractoriness of atrial and ventricular tissue. Prolongation of the effective refractory period and an increase in conduction time may prevent the reentry phenomenon.
3. Quinidine exerts an indirect anticholinergic effect through blockade of vagal innervation. This anticholinergic effect may facilitate conduction in the atrioventricular junction.

Quinidine absorption from Quinaglute® Dura-Tabs® tablets proceeds at a slower rate than the immediate-release products. In a single-dose pharmacokinetic study conducted in normal volunteers, the time of peak quinidine serum concentration was 1.6 hours for quinidine sulfate tablets and 3.6 hours for Quinaglute® Dura-Tabs® tablets. The apparent elimination half-life of quinidine ranges from 4 to 10 hours in healthy persons with a usual mean value of 6 to 7 hours. The half-life may be prolonged in elderly persons.

From 60% to 80% of the dose is metabolized by the liver. Renal excretion of the intact drug comprises the remainder of the total clearance. Quinidine is approximately 75% bound to serum proteins.

In the past, plasma levels of 1.5 to 5 $\mu g/ml$ have been reported as therapeutic,[1] based on non-specific assay methodology which quantitates quinidine metabolites as well as intact quinidine. The therapeutic plasma level range using newer, more specific assays has not been definitively established; however, effective reduction of premature ventricular contractions has been reported with blood levels less than 1.0 $\mu g/ml$.[2] In general, plasma quinidine levels are lower using specific assays. Clinicians requesting serum quinidine determinations should therefore also ask that the method of analysis be specified.

Due to the wide individual variation in response to quinidine therapy, the usefulness of serum quinidine levels in the planning of optimal quinidine therapy has not been clearly established. A serum quinidine concentration within the reported therapeutic range may not necessarily be the optimal concentration for some patients. In the absence of toxicity, such patients may warrant an increase in dose to achieve the desired therapeutic effect. However, for those patients in which a high blood level has been achieved without significant therapeutic response, increasing the dose to potentially toxic levels is not warranted and consideration should be given to combination or alternate therapy. In all cases, the physician should carefully consider the patient response and evidence of toxicity along with blood levels in determining optimal quinidine therapy.

[1] Koch-Weser, Arch. Int. Med. 129:763-772, 1972.
[2] Carliner et al, Am. Heart Journ. 100:483-489, 1980.

Indications and Usage: Quinaglute® Dura-Tabs® tablets are indicated in the prevention and/or treatment of:
1. Ventricular arrhythmias
   Premature ventricular contractions
   Ventricular tachycardia (when not associated with complete heartblock)
2. Junctional (nodal) arrhythmias
   A-V junctional premature complexes
   Paroxysmal junctional tachycardia
3. Supraventricular (atrial) arrhythmias
   Premature atrial contractions
   Paroxysmal atrial tachycardia
   Atrial flutter
   Atrial fibrillation (chronic and paroxysmal)

Contraindications:
1. Idiosyncrasy or hypersensitivity to quinidine.
2. Complete A-V block.
3. Complete bundle branch block or other severe intraventricular conduction defects, especially those exhibiting a marked grade of QRS widening.
4. Digitalis intoxication manifested by A-V conduction disorders.
5. Myasthenia gravis.
6. Aberrant impulses and abnormal rhythms due to escape mechanisms.

Warnings:
1. In the treatment of atrial flutter, reversion to sinus rhythm may be preceded by a progressive reduction in the degree of A-V block to a 1:1 ratio resulting in an extremely rapid ventricular rate. This possible hazard may be reduced by digitalization prior to administration of quinidine.
2. Recent reports indicate that plasma concentrations of digoxin increase and may even double when quinidine is administered concurrently. Patients on concomitant therapy should be carefully monitored. Reduction of digoxin dosage may have to be considered.
3. Manifestations of quinidine cardiotoxicity such as excessive prolongation of the Q-T interval, widening of the QRS complex and ventricular tachyarrhythmias mandate immediate discontinuation of the drug and/or close clinical and electrocardiographic monitoring.
4. In susceptible individuals, such as those with marginally compensated cardiovascular disease, quinidine may produce clinically important depression of cardiac function such as hypotension, bradycardia, or heartblock. Quinidine therapy should be carefully monitored in such individuals.
5. Quinidine should be used with extreme caution in patients with incomplete A-V block since complete block and asystole may be produced. Quinidine may cause abnormalities of cardiac rhythm in digitalized patients and therefore should be used with caution in the presence of digitalis intoxication.
6. Quinidine should be used with caution in patients exhibiting renal, cardiac or hepatic insufficiency because of potential accumulation of quinidine in plasma leading to toxicity.
7. Patients taking quinidine occasionally have syncopal episodes which usually result from ventricular tachycardia or fibrillation. This syndrome has not been shown to be related to dose or plasma levels. Syncopal episodes frequently terminate spontaneously or in response to treatment, but sometimes are fatal.
8. A few cases of hepatotoxicity, including granulomatous hepatitis, due to quinidine hypersensitivity have been reported in patients taking quinidine. Unexplained fever and/or elevation of hepatic enzymes, particularly in the early stages of therapy, warrant consideration of possible hepatotoxicity. Monitoring liver function during the first 4–8 weeks should be considered. Cessation of quinidine in these cases usually results in the disappearance of toxicity.

Precautions: *General:* The precautions to be observed include all those applicable to quinidine. A preliminary test dose of a single tablet of quinidine sulfate may be administered to determine if the patient has an idiosyncrasy to quinidine. Hypersensitivity to quinidine, although rare, should constantly be considered, especially during the first weeks of therapy.

Hospitalization for close clinical observation, electrocardiographic monitoring, and possible determination of plasma quinidine levels is indicated when large doses are used, or with patients who present an increased risk.

Information for Patients: As with all solid oral dosage medications, Quinaglute® Dura-Tabs® tablets should be taken with an adequate amount of fluid, preferably in an upright position, to facilitate swallowing.

Drug Interactions:

Drug	Effect
Quinidine with anticholinergic drugs	Additive vagolytic effect
Quinidine with cholinergic drugs	Antagonism of cholinergic effects
Quinidine with carbonic anhydrase inhibitors, sodium bicarbonate, thiazide diuretics	Alkalinization of urine resulting in decreased excretion of quinidine
Quinidine with coumarin anticoagulants	Reduction of clotting factor concentrations
Quinidine with tubocurare, succinylcholine and decamethonium	Potentiation of neuromuscular blockade
Quinidine with phenothiazines and reserpine	Additive cardiac depressive effects
Quinidine with hepatic enzyme-inducing drugs (phenobarbital, phenytoin, rifampin)	Decreased plasma half-life of quinidine
Quinidine with digoxin	Increased plasma concentrations of digoxin (See WARNINGS)

Carcinogenesis, Mutagenesis and Impairment of Fertility: Long-term studies in animals have not been performed to evaluate the carcinogenic potential of quinidine. There is currently no evidence of quinidine-induced mutagenesis or impairment of fertility.

Pregnancy: Teratogenic Effects: Pregnancy Category C. Animal reproduction studies have not been conducted with quinidine. There are no adequate and well-controlled studies in pregnant women. Quinaglute® Dura-Tabs® tablets should be given to a pregnant woman only if clearly needed.

Nonteratogenic Effects: Like quinine, quinidine has been reported to have oxytocic properties. The significance of this property in the clinical setting has not been established.

Nursing Mothers: Caution should be exercised when Quinaglute® Dura-Tabs® tablets are administered to a nursing woman due to passage of the drug into breast milk.

Pediatric Use: There are no adequate and well-controlled studies establishing the safety and effectiveness of Quinaglute® Dura-Tabs® tablets in children.

Adverse Reactions: Symptoms of cinchonism, ringing in ears, headache, nausea, and/or disturbed vision may appear in sensitive patients after a single dose of the drug.

The most frequently encountered side effects to quinidine are gastrointestinal in nature. These gastrointestinal effects include nausea, vomiting, abdominal pain and diarrhea.

Less frequently encountered adverse reactions:
Cardiovascular: Widening of QRS complex, cardiac asystole, ventricular ectopic beats, idioventricular rhythms including ventricular tachycardia and fibrillation, paradoxical tachycardia, arterial embolism and hypotension.
Hematologic: Acute hemolytic anemia, hypoprothrombinemia, thrombocytopenia (purpura), agranulocytosis.
Central Nervous System: Headache, fever, vertigo, apprehension, excitement, confusion, delirium and syncope, disturbed hearing (tinnitus, decreased auditory acuity), disturbed vision (mydriasis, blurred vision, disturbed color perception, reduced vision field, photophobia, diplopia, night blindness, scotomata), optic neuritis.
Dermatologic: Rash, cutaneous flushing with intense pruritus, urticaria. Photosensitivity has also been reported.
Hypersensitivity Reactions: Angioedema, acute asthmatic episode, vascular collapse, respiratory arrest, hepatic toxicity including granulomatous hepatitis (See WARNINGS).

Although extremely rare, there have also been reports of lupus erythematosus in patients taking

Continued on next page

Information on the Berlex products in the 1985 Annual is based on the labeling in effect on August 1, 1984. Further information on dosage and administration, side effects, precautions and contraindications for these and other Berlex products may be obtained from either the package insert or the Medical Affairs Department, Berlex Laboratories, Inc., 110 East Hanover Avenue, Cedar Knolls, New Jersey

Berlex—Cont.

quinidine. A positive association with quinidine therapy has not been established.

Overdosage: If ingestion of quinidine is recent, gastric lavage, emesis and/or administration of activated charcoal may reduce absorption. Management of overdosage includes symptomatic treatment, ECG and blood pressure monitoring, cardiac pacing if indicated, and acidification of the urine. Artificial respiration and other supportive measures may be required.

IV infusion of $1/6$ molar sodium lactate reportedly reduces the cardiotoxic effects of quinidine. Since marked CNS depression may occur even in the presence of convulsions, CNS depressants should not be administered. Hypotension may be treated, if necessary, with metaraminol or norepinephrine after adequate fluid volume replacement. Hemodialysis has been reported to be effective in the treatment of quinidine overdosage in adults and children, but is rarely warranted.

Dosage and Administration: The dosage varies considerably depending upon the general condition and cardiovascular state of the patient. The quantity and frequency of administration of Quinaglute® Dura-Tabs® tablets that will achieve the desired clinical results must be determined for each patient.

The ideal dosage is the minimum amount of total dose and frequency of daily administration that will prevent premature contractions, paroxysmal tachycardias and maintain normal sinus rhythm.

Prevention of premature atrial, nodal or ventricular contractions:
1 to 2 tablets every 8 or 12 hours.

Maintenance of normal sinus rhythm following conversion of paroxysmal tachycardias:
2 tablets every 12 hours or 1 ½ to 2 tablets every 8 hours are usually required.

Although most patients may be maintained in normal rhythm on a dosage of 1 tablet every 8 or 12 hours; some patients may require larger doses or more frequent administration, ie, every 6 hours than the usually recommended schedule. Such increased dosage should be instituted only after careful clinical and laboratory evaluation of the patient including monitoring of plasma quinidine levels and, if possible, serial electrocardiograms. Quinaglute® Dura-Tabs® tablets are well tolerated with few gastrointestinal disturbances which, if they occur, may be minimized by administering the drug with food.

It is frequently desirable to determine if a patient can tolerate maintenance quinidine therapy prior to electrical conversion. Therefore, maintenance therapy may be initiated 2 to 3 days before electrical conversion is attempted. Quinaglute® Dura-Tabs® tablets are well suited for such a program and can be administered at a maintenance dose felt necessary for a given patient as indicated above.

Note: Dosage may be titrated by breaking the tablet in half. Do not crush or chew since sustained-release properties will be lost.

How Supplied:
White to off-white round tablet imprinted with:

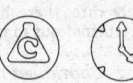

In bottles of:
100 Tablets .... NDC 50419-101-10
250 Tablets .... NDC 50419-101-25
500 Tablets .... NDC 50419-101-50
Unit Dose Boxes
  of 100 .... NDC 50419-101-11
Store at controlled room temperature.
Tablet designs are registered trademark of Berlex Laboratories, Inc.

Shown in Product Identification Section, page 406

SUS-PHRINE® ℞
[sŭs'frĭn"]
(epinephrine)
Aqueous Suspension for Subcutaneous Injection

Description: Each ml of Sus-Phrine® (brand of epinephrine) Suspension contains 5 mg epinephrine in a sterile aqueous vehicle containing ascorbic acid 10 mg and thioglycolic acid 6.6 mg (as sodium salts), phenol 5 mg and glycerin (USP) 325 mg. Sodium hydroxide is added to adjust the pH. Approximately 80% of the total epinephrine is in suspension.

Clinical Pharmacology: Sus-Phrine® Suspension (epinephrine) acts at both the alpha and beta receptor sites. Beta stimulation provides bronchodilator action by relaxing bronchial muscle. Alpha stimulation increases vital capacity by relieving congestion of the bronchial mucosa and by constricting pulmonary vessels.

Sus-Phrine® Suspension provides both rapid and sustained epinephrine activity. The rapid action is due to the epinephrine in solution, while the sustained activity is due to the crystalline epinephrine free base in suspension.

Indications: For the symptomatic treatment of bronchial asthma, and reversible bronchospasm associated with chronic bronchitis and emphysema.

Contraindications: Hypersensitivity to any of the components.

Narrow angle glaucoma, shock, cerebral arteriosclerosis and organic heart disease. Epinephrine is also contraindicated during general anesthesia with halogenated hydrocarbons or cyclopropane, and in local anesthesia of certain areas, e.g., fingers, toes, because of the danger of vasoconstriction producing sloughing of tissue, and in labor because the drug may delay the second stage.

Warnings: SUS-PHRINE SHOULD NOT BE EMPLOYED TO CORRECT DRUG INDUCED HYPOTENSION.

Administer with caution to elderly people; those with cardiovascular disease, diabetes, hypertension or hyperthyroidism; in psychoneurotic individuals and in pregnancy. Administer with extreme caution to patients with long-standing bronchial asthma and emphysema who have developed degenerative heart disease.

Cardiac arrhythmias may follow administration of epinephrine.

Anginal pain may be induced when coronary insufficiency is present.

Precautions: DO NOT USE IF PRODUCT IS DISCOLORED. Discoloration indicates the oxidation of epinephrine and possible loss of potency.

Use of Sus-Phrine® Suspension with digitalis, mercurial diuretics or other drugs that sensitize the heart to arrhythmias is not recommended.

Sus-Phrine® Suspension should not be administered concomitantly with other sympathomimetic agents, since their combined effects on the cardiovascular system may be deleterious to the patient. The effects of epinephrine may be potentiated by tricyclic antidepressants; sodium l-thyroxine, and certain antihistamines, e.g., diphenhydramine, tripelennamine or chlorpheniramine.

Adverse Reactions: In some individuals, restlessness, anxiety, headache, tremor, weakness, dizziness, pallor, respiratory difficulties, palpitation, nausea and vomiting may occur. These reactions may be exaggerated in hyperthyroidism. Occlusion of the central retinal artery and shock have also been reported.

Also, urticaria, wheal and hemorrhage at the site of injection may occur. Repeated injections at the same site may result in necrosis from vascular constriction.

Tolerance to epinephrine may occur with prolonged use.

Overdosage: Overdosage or inadvertent intravenous injection may cause cerebrovascular hemorrhage resulting from the sharp rise in blood pressure. Fatalities may also result from pulmonary edema because of peripheral constriction and cardiac stimulation produced. Rapidly acting vasodilators such as nitrites, or alpha blocking agents may counteract the marked pressor effects. Cardiac arrhythmias may be countered by administering rapidly acting antiarrhythmic or beta blocking agents.

Dosage and Administration:
NOTE: INJECT SUBCUTANEOUSLY.

It is suggested that Sus-Phrine® Suspension be administered with a tuberculin syringe and a 26 gauge, ½ inch needle.

A small initial test dose may be administered subcutaneously as a possible aid in determining patient sensitivity to epinephrine.

Site of injection should be varied to avoid necrosis at the site of injection.

Each time before withdrawing Sus-Phrine® Suspension into syringe, shake vial or ampul thoroughly to disperse particles and obtain a uniform suspension. Inject promptly subcutaneously to avoid settling of suspension in the syringe.

Adults:
Adult dosage range is 0.1 to 0.3 ml depending on patient response.

Subsequent doses should be administered only when necessary and not more frequently than every six hours.

Infants 1 month to 2 years and Children 2 to 12 years:
Pediatric dose is 0.005 ml/kg (2.2 lb) body weight injected subcutaneously.

FOR CHILDREN 30 kg OR LESS MAXIMUM SINGLE DOSE IS 0.15 ml.

Subsequent doses should be administered only when necessary and not more frequently than every six hours.

Clinical Studies: Controlled studies comparing the effectiveness of Sus-Phrine® Suspension and an aqueous solution of epinephrine 1:1000 were conducted in both pediatric and adult asthmatics. The studies demonstrated rapid bronchodilator acitivity following administration of either Sus-Phrine® Suspension or epinephrine 1:1000; however during the 6 hour study period, a greater improvement in FEV_1 and FEF_{25-75} was observed 4 to 6 hours subsequent to Sus-Phrine® Suspension administration. Improvement in WPEF was greater for Sus-Phrine® Suspension than epinephrine 1:1000 3 to 8 hours following administration (10 hour study duration).

How Supplied:
In boxes of
12 × 0.3 ml ampuls...................NDC 50419-137-12
25 × 0.3 ml ampuls...................NDC 50419-137-25
5.0 ml multiple dose vial ....NDC 50419-128-01
NSN 6505-01-022-2402
Store under refrigeration. Do not freeze. Do not expose to temperatures above 30° C (86°F).

Shown in Product Identification Section, page 406

EDUCATIONAL MATERIAL

Monographs—Cardiovascular

Ambulatory Electrocardiographic Monitoring: Its Role in the Management of Cardiac Disease. Fred J. Harris, MD, and Ezra A. Amsterdam, MD (professional education—free)

Approaches to the Management of Ventricular Arrhythmias. J. Thomas Bigger, MD (professional education—free)

Clinical Recognition, Significance and Management of Supraventricular Arrhythmias. Zakauddin Vera, MD (professional education—free)

Exercise Testing and Ambulatory Monitoring in the Diagnosis and Management of Cardiac Arrhythmias. Ezra A. Amsterdam, MD (professional education—free)

Long-Term Management of Cardiac Arrhythmias by Pharmacologic Therapy. Liaqat Zaman, MD and Robert J. Myerburg, MD (professional education—free)

Management of Arrhythmias After Acute Myocardial Infarction: Rationale for Therapy. Robert J. Capone, MD (professional education—free)

Use of Ventricular Stimulation and Intracardiac Recording. Mark E. Josephson, MD (professional education—free)

Medical Education Programs—Cardiovascular
Clinical Pharmacology and Differentiation of Conventional and Investigational Antiarrhythmic Agents. Dennis S. Miura, MD, Phd
Management of Cardiac Arrhythmias: Clinical Considerations and Therapeutic Objectives. Thomas B. Graboys, MD, and Philip J. Podrid, M.D.
Perspectives on Sudden Cardiac Death. Leonard N. Horowitz, MD, Scott R. Spielman, MD, and Allan M. Greenspan, MD
Stress and Sudden Cardiac Death. Robert S. Eliot, MD, and James C. Buell, MD
(All programs have CME credits. Lecturer is furnished with lecture guide, monograph and slides. All programs are available through your local Berlex Laboratories sales representative, or write to Berlex Laboratories, Inc.)
Patient Education Booklets—Cardiovascular
Information on Your Prescription. (Comes with samples of Quinaglute® Dura-Tabs® tablets. Available through your local Berlex Laboratories sales representative.)
Production Information—Cardiovascular
Quinaglute® Dura-Tabs® Tablets Product Information Monograph. (professional information—free)
Patient Education Booklets—Allergy/Respiratory
Living with Asthma. (Free. Available through your local Berlex Laboratories sales representative, or write to Berlex Laboratories, Inc.)
Product Samples
Professional samples are available through your local Berlex Laboratories sales representative, or by sending a completed prescription to Berlex Laboratories, Inc. 300 Fairfield Road, Wayne, New Jersey 07470

Beutlich, Inc.
7149 N. AUSTIN
NILES, IL 60648

CEO–TWO® SUPPOSITORIES
Composition: Each adult rectal suppository contains sodium bicarbonate and potassium bitartrate in a water soluble polyethylene glycol base.
Actions and Uses: The gentle pressure of the released CO_2 in the rectum stimulates peristalsis, and defecation usually results in 10 to 30 minutes. CEO-TWO® is successfully used as a bowel evacuant in spinal cord injury patients. It is gentle, effective, safe and predictable. Also used pre and post partum, pre and post operatively, or whenever the last 25cm of the lower bowel must be emptied.
Administration and Dosage: One or two suppositories can be used as needed. Moisten CEO-TWO with warm water before inserting. Patient should retain as long as possible. Dosage can be repeated in 4–6 hours if necessary.
Contraindications: As with other enemas or laxatives.
How Supplied: In packages of 10, white opaque suppositories. Keep in cool, dry place.
DO NOT REFRIGERATE

HURRICAINE® TOPICAL ANESTHETIC
LIQUID, GEL, and AEROSOL SPRAY
Composition: HURRICAINE® (20% Benzocaine)
Action and Indication: HURRICAINE® is a topical anesthetic for oral and mucosal application. To control pain as well as suppress the gag reflex and it tastes good.
Advantages: Safe, effective, 15-30 seconds, good tasting. The aerosol will not foam.
HURRICAINE® is probably the agent of choice in endoscopy since its onset is rapid, action is of short duration and virtually no systemic absorption occurs.
PATIENTS WITH A KNOWN HYPERSENSITIVITY TO BENZOCAINE SHOULD NOT USE HURRICAINE®
DO NOT USE IN EYES
NOT FOR INJECTION
KEEP OUT OF REACH OF CHILDREN
How Supplied:
AEROSOL SPRAY in 2 oz. can
LIQUID or GEL in 1 oz. bottles
LIQUID ¼cc Unit Dose
HURICAINE SPRAY KIT with 200 disposable extension tubes. These disposable extention tubes will minimize the risk of infection through cross contamination. Clean—quick and easy to attach.

MEVANIN-C CAPSULES
Composition: Each capsule contains: Ascorbic Acid 200 mg., Hesperidin Complex 30 mg., Calcium Lactate 300 mg., Cyanocobalamin 1 mcg., Ferrous Sulfate 65 mg., Folic Acid 0.1 mg., Vitamin A 3000 USP units, Vitamin D 300 USP units, Thiamine HCl 2 mg., Riboflavin 2 mg., Pyridoxine HCl 0.5 mg., Niacin 5 mg., plus trace amounts of copper, zinc, manganese, magnesium, potassium and iodine.
Administration and Dosage: One capsule daily.
How Supplied: In bottles of 90 and 450 red and white capsules.

PERIDIN-C®
Composition: Each tablet contains Hesperidin Methyl Chalcone 50 mg., Hesperidin Complex 150 mg., Ascorbic Acid 200 mg.
Dosage: 1 tablet daily.
How Supplied: In bottles of 100 and 500 orange tablets.

Biocraft Laboratories, Inc.
92 ROUTE 46
ELMWOOD PARK, NJ 07407

NDC 0332	PRODUCT	PROD. ID. NO.
	AMITRIPTYLINE HCL TABLETS ℞	
2120	10 mg.	22
2122	25 mg.	23
2124	50 mg.	24
2126	75 mg.	25
2128	100 mg.	26
	AMOXICILLIN CAPSULES ℞	
3107	250 mg.	01
3109	500 mg.	03
	AMOXICILLIN SUSPENSION ℞	
4150	125 mg./5 ml.	
4155	250 mg./5 ml.	
	AMPICILLIN CAPSULES ℞	
3111	250 mg.	05
3113	500 mg.	06
	AMPICILLIN SUSPENSION ℞	
4129	125 mg./5 ml.	
4131	250 mg./5 ml.	
	AMPICILLIN-PROBENECID SUSPENSION ℞	
4140	1 gm. Probenecid; 3.5 gm. Amp	
	CHLOROQUINE PHOSPHATE TABLETS ℞	
2160	250 mg.	38
	CLOXACILLIN CAPSULES ℞	
3119	250 mg.	28
3121	500 mg.	30
	CLOXACILLIN SOLUTION ℞	
4159	125 mg./5 ml.	
	DICLOXACILLIN CAPSULES ℞	
3123	250 mg.	02
3125	500 mg.	04
	IMIPRAMINE HCL TABLETS ℞	
2111	10 mg.	19
2113	25 mg.	20
2117	50 mg.	21
	NEOMYCIN SULFATE TABLETS ℞	
1177	500 mg.	18
	OXACILLIN CAPSULES ℞	
3115	250 mg.	12
3117	500 mg.	14
	OXACILLIN SOLUTION ℞	
4157	250 mg./5 ml.	
	PENICILLIN G POTASSIUM TABLETS ℞	
1117	200,000 Units	07
1121	250,000 Units	09
1123	400,000 Units	10
	PENICILLIN V POTASSIUM SOLUTION ℞	
4125	125 mg./5 ml.	
4127	250 mg./5 ml.	
	PENICILLIN V POTASSIUM TABLETS ℞	
1171	250 mg. ROUND	15
1172	250 mg. OVAL	16
1173	500 mg. ROUND	17
1174	500 mg. OVAL	49
	SULFAMETHOXAZOLE AND TRIMETHOPRIM TABLETS ℞	
2130	400 mg/80 mg (Single Strength)	32
2132	800 mg/160 mg (Double Strength)	33
	SULFAMETHOXAZOLE AND TRIMETHOPRIM PEDIATRIC SUSPENSION ℞	
6100	200 mg./40 mg. per 5 ml.	
	TRIMETHOPRIM TABLETS ℞	
2158	100 mg.	34

Bock Pharmacal Company
5435 HIGHLAND PARK DRIVE
ST. LOUIS, MO 63110

DOLPRN #3 TABLETS ℞ ⓒ
Analgesic

Each green layered tablet contains:
Acetaminophen .... 400 mg.
Aspirin .... 250 mg.
Magnesium Hydroxide .... 60 mg.
Dried Aluminum Hydroxide .... 60 mg.
Codeine Phosphate .... 30 mg.
How Supplied: Bottles of 40 and 250.

POLY-HISTINE EXPECTORANT ℞ ⓒ
WITH CODEINE

Each 5 ml. cherry flavored red syrup contains:
Codeine Phosphate .... 10.0 mg.
 (Warning: May be habit forming.)
Phenylpropanolamine HCl .... 12.5 mg.
Brompheniramine Maleate .... 2.0 mg.
Potassium Guaiacolsulfonate .... 100.0 mg.
How Supplied: Bottles of 16 oz. and 1 gallon.

POLY-HISTINE ℞
EXPECTORANT PLAIN

Each 5 ml. cherry flavored red syrup contains:
Phenylpropanolamine HCl .... 12.5 mg.
Brompheniramine Maleate .... 2.0 mg.
Potassium Guaiacolsulfonate .... 100.0 mg.
How Supplied: Bottles of 16 oz. and 1 gallon.

POLY-HISTINE–D CAPSULES ℞
Antihistamines + Decongestant

Each red-clear time release capsule imprinted BOCK contains:
Phenylpropanolamine HCl .... 50 mg.
Phenyltoloxamine Citrate .... 16 mg.
Pyrilamine Maleate .... 16 mg.
Pheniramine Maleate .... 16 mg.
How Supplied: Bottles of 100 and 1000.

POLY-HISTINE–D ELIXIR ℞
Antihistamines + Decongestant

Each 5 ml. wild cherry flavored red elixir contains:
Phenylpropanolamine HCl .... 12.5 mg.
Phenyltoloxamine Citrate .... 4.0 mg.
Pyrilamine Maleate .... 4.0 mg.
Pheniramine Maleate .... 4.0 mg.
How Supplied: Bottles of 16 oz. and 1 gallon.

POLY-HISTINE–D PEDIATRIC CAPSULES ℞
Antihistamine + Decongestant

Each clear time release capsule imprinted BOCK contains:

Continued on next page

Bock—Cont.

Phenylpropanolamine HCl ....25 mg.
Phenyltoloxamine Citrate .... 8 mg.
Pyrilamine Maleate .... 8 mg.
Pheniramine Maleate .... 8 mg.
How Supplied: Bottles of 100 and 1000

POLY-HISTINE-DX CAPSULES ℞
Antihistamine + Decongestant

Each purple-clear time release capsule imprinted BOCK contains:
Pseudoephedrine HCl ....120.0 mg.
Brompheniramine Maleate ....12.0 mg.
How Supplied: Bottles of 100 and 1000.

PRENATE 90 ℞
Vitamin-Mineral Supplement

Each white film coated tablet contains:
Iron (Ferrous Fumarate) .... 90 mg.
Iodine (Potassium Iodine) .... 0.15 mg.
Calcium (Calcium Carbonate) .... 250 mg.
Copper (Cupric Oxide) .... 2 mg.
Zinc (Zinc Oxide) .... 20 mg.
Folic Acid .... 1 mg.
Vitamin A (Acetate) .... 8000 I.U.
Vitamin D (Ergocalciferol) .... 400 I.U.
Vitamin E (Acetate) .... 30 I.U.
*Vitamin C (Ascorbic Acid) .... 200 mg.
Vitamin B_1 (Thiamine Mononitrate) .... 3 mg.
Vitamin B_2 (Riboflavin) .... 3.4 mg.
Vitamin B_6 (Pyridoxine HCl) .... 20 mg.
Vitamin B_{12} (Cyanocobalamin) .... 12 mcg.
Niacinamide .... 20 mg.
Docusate Sodium .... 50 mg.
How Supplied: Bottles of 100's and 1000's.

THEON SYRUP ℞

Each 5 ml. dye-free syrup contains:
Theophylline (Anhydrous) .... 50 mg.
Alcohol 1%
How Supplied: Bottles of 16 oz. and 1 gallon.

ZEPHREX TABLETS ℞

Each tablet contains:
Pseudoephedrine HCl ....60 mg.
Guaifenesin ....400 mg.
How Supplied: Bottles of 100 and 1000.

ZEPHREX-LA TABLETS ℞

Each tablet contains:
Pseudoephedrine HCl ....120 mg.
Guaifenesin ....600 mg.
How Supplied: Bottles of 100 and 1000.

Boehringer Ingelheim Ltd.
90 EAST RIDGE
POST OFFICE BOX 368
RIDGEFIELD, CT 06877

ALUPENT® ℞
[al'u-pent]
(metaproterenol sulfate)
Bronchodilator

Tablets 10 mg	BI-CODE 74
Tablets 20 mg	BI-CODE 72
Metered Dose Inhaler 15 ml	BI-CODE 70
Syrup 10mg/5ml	BI-CODE 73
Inhalant Solution 5%	BI-CODE 71
Inhalant Solution Unit Dose Vials 0.6%	BI-CODE 69

Description: Chemically, Alupent (metaproterenol sulfate) is 1-(3,5-dihydroxyphenyl) -2-isopropylamineothanol sulfate, a white, crystalline, racemic mixture of two optically active isomers. It differs from isoproterenol hydrochloride by having two hydroxyl groups attached at the meta positions on the benzene ring rather than one at the meta and one at the para position.

Clinical Pharmacology: Alupent (metaproterenol sulfate) is a potent beta-adrenergic stimulator. The Alupent Metered Dose Inhaler and Inhalant Solution have a rapid onset of action. It is postulated that beta-adrenergic stimulants produce many of their pharmacological effects by activation of adenyl cyclase, the enzyme which catalyzes the conversion of adenosine triphosphate to cyclic adenosine monophosphate.

Absorption, biotransformation and excretion studies following administration by inhalation have not been performed. Following oral administration in humans, an average of 40% of the drug is absorbed; it is not metabolized by catechol-O-methyltransferase or sulfatase enzymes in the gut, but is excreted primarily as glucuronic acid conjugates.

When administered orally or by inhalation, Alupent decreases reversible bronchospasm. Pulmonary function tests performed concomitantly usually show improvement following Alupent administration, e.g., an increase in the one-second forced expiratory volume (FEV_1), an increase in maximum expiratory flow rate, an increase in peak expiratory flow rate, an increase in forced vital capacity, and/or a decrease in airway resistance. The resultant decrease in airway obstruction may relieve the dyspnea associated with bronchospasm. In controlled single- and multiple-dose studies, the mean duration of effect of a single dose of 20 mg of Alupent Tablets or Alupent Syrup (15% or greater increase in FEV_1) was up to four hours. A controlled multiple-dose 60-day study comparing the effectiveness of Alupent Tablets with ephedrine tablets showed loss of efficacy with time for both Alupent Tablets and ephedrine. Therefore, the physician should take this phenomenon into account when evaluating the individual patients overall management. Further studies are in progress to adequately explain these results.

In controlled single-dose, studies with Alupent MDI, the duration of effect of 2 to 3 inhalations (20% or greater increase in mean FEV_1) has varied from 1 to 5 hours. In multiple-dosing studies (up to q.i.d.), the duration of effect for a similar dose of Alupent has ranged from about one to two-and-one-half hours. Present studies are inadequate to explain the divergence in duration of the FEV_1 effect between single- and multiple-dose studies.

In controlled single-dose studies with Alupent Inhalant Solution administered by an intermittent positive pressure breathing apparatus (IPPB) and by hand bulb nebulizers, significant improvement (15% or greater increase in FEV_1) occurred within 5 to 30 minutes and persisted for periods ranging from 2 to 6 hours. The longer duration of effect occurred in studies in which the drug was administered by IPPB, i.e., 6 hours versus 2 to 3 hours when administered by hand bulb nebulizer. The doses used were 0.3 ml by IPPB and 10 inhalations by hand bulb nebulizer.

In controlled repetitive-dosing studies by IPPB and by hand bulb nebulizer, the onset of effect occurred within 5 to 30 minutes and duration ranged from 4 to 6 hours. The doses used were 0.3 ml b.i.d. or t.i.d. when given by IPPB, and 10 inhalations q.i.d. (no more often than q4h) when given by hand bulb nebulizer. As in the single-dose studies, effectiveness was measured as a sustained increase in FEV_1 of 15% or greater. There was no apparent difference in duration between the two methods of delivery.

Clinical studies were conducted in which the effectiveness of Alupent Inhalant Solution was compared with that of isoproterenol hydrochloride over periods of two to three months. Both drugs continued to produce significant improvement in pulmonary function throughout this period of treatment.

Indications and Usage: Alupent (metaproterenol sulfate) is indicated as a bronchodilator for bronchial asthma, and for reversible bronchospasm which may occur in association with bronchitis and emphysema.

Contraindications: Use in patients with cardiac arrhythmias associated with tachycardia is contraindicated.

Although rare, immediate hypersensitivity reactions can occur. Therefore, Alupent (metaproterenol sulfate) is contraindicated in patients with a history of hypersensitivity to any of its components.

Warnings: Excessive use of adrenergic aerosols is potentially dangerous. Fatalities have been reported following excessive use of Alupent (metaproterenol sulfate) as with other sympathomimetic inhalation preparations, and the exact cause is unknown. Cardiac arrest was noted in several cases.

Paradoxical bronchoconstriction with repeated excessive administration has been reported with other sympathomimetic agents. Therefore, it is possible that this phenomenon could occur with Alupent.

Patients should be advised to contact their physician in the event that they do not respond to their usual dose of a sympathomimetic amine aerosol.

Precautions: Because Alupent (metaproterenol sulfate) is a sympathomimetic drug, it should be used with great caution in patients with hypertension, coronary artery disease, congestive heart failure, hyperthyroidism or diabetes, or when there is sensitivity to sympathomimetic amines.

Information for Patients: Extreme care must be exercised with respect to the administration of additional sympathomimetic agents. A sufficient interval of time should elapse prior to administration of another sympathomimetic agent.

Carcinogenesis: Long-term studies in mice and rats to evaluate the oral carcinogenic potential of metaproterenol sulfate have not been completed.

Pregnancy: *Teratogenic Effects: Pregnancy Category C.* Alupent has been shown to be teratogenic and embryocidal in rabbits when given orally in doses 620 times the human inhalation dose and 62 times the human oral dose; the teratogenic effects included skeletal abnormalities and hydrocephalus with bone separation. Oral reproduction studies in mice, rats and rabbits showed no teratogenic or embryocidal effect at 50 mg/kg, or 310 times the human inhalation dose and 31 times the human oral dose. There are no adequate and well-controlled studies in pregnant women. Alupent should be used during pregnancy only if the potential benefit justifies the potential risk to the fetus.

Nursing Mothers: It is not known whether this drug is excreted in human milk. Because many drugs are excreted in human milk, caution should be exercised when Alupent is administered to a nursing woman.

Pediatric Use: The safety and effectiveness of Alupent Metered Dose Inhaler and Inhalant Solution in children below the age of 12 have not been established. The safety and efficacy of Alupent Tablets in children below the age of 6 have not been established.

Adverse Reactions: Adverse reactions are similar to those noted with other sympathomimetic agents.

The most frequent adverse reactions to Alupent (metaproterenol sulfate) are nervousness, tachycardia, tremor and nausea. Less frequent adverse reactions are hypertension, palpitations, vomiting and bad taste.

Overdosage: The symptoms of overdosage are those of excessive beta adrenergic stimulation listed under **Adverse Reactions**. These reactions usually do not require treatment other than reduction of dosage and/or frequency of administration.

Dosage and Administration: If Alupent (metaproterenol sulfate) is administered before or after other sympathomimetic bronchodilators, caution should be exercised with respect to possible potentiation of adrenergic effects.

Tablets: *Adults* The usual dose is 20 mg three or four times a day. *Children* Aged six to nine years or weight under 60 lbs—10 mg three or four times a day. Over nine years or weight over 60 lbs—20 mg three or four times a day. Alupent Tablets are not recommended for use in children under six years of age.

Syrup: *Children* Aged six to nine years or weight under 60 lbs—one teaspoonful three or four times a day. Children over nine years or weight over 60 lbs—two teaspoonfuls three or four times a day.

Experience in children under the age of six is limited to seventy-eight children. Forty of these were treated with Alupent Syrup for at least one month, and daily doses of approximately 1.3 to 2.6 mg/kg were well tolerated. *Adults* Two teaspoonfuls three or four times a day.

Metered Dose Inhaler: The usual single dose is two to three inhalations. With repetitive dosing, inhalation should usually not be repeated more often than about every three or four hours. Total dosage per day should not exceed 12 inhalations. Alupent MDI is not recommended for use in children under 12 years of age.

Inhalant Solution: Usually, treatment need not be repeated more often than every four hours to relieve acute attacks of bronchospasm. As part of a total treatment program in chronic bronchospastic pulmonary diseases, Alupent Inhalant Solution may be administered three to four times a day. As with all medications, the physician should begin therapy with the lowest effective dose and then titrate the dosage according to the individual patient's requirements.

Alupent Inhalant Solution is not recommended for use in children under 12 years of age.

Inhalant Solution 5%: Alupent Inhalant Solution is administered by oral inhalation with the aid of a hand bulb nebulizer or an intermittent positive pressure breathing apparatus (IPPB). [See table above].

Inhalant Solution Unit Dose Vial 0.6%: Alupent Inhalant Solution Unit Dose Vial is administered by oral inhalation using an IPPB device. The usual adult dose is one vial per nebulization treatment. Each vial is equivalent to 0.3 ml Alupent Inhalant Solution 5% diluted to 2.5 ml with normal saline.

How Supplied: *Tablets:* Alupent (metaproterenol sulfate) is supplied in two dosage strengths as round, white, scored tablets in bottles of 100. Tablets of 10 mg coded B1/74. Tablets of 20 mg coded B1/72.

Syrup: Alupent is available as a cherry-flavored syrup. 10 mg per teaspoonful (5 ml), in 16 fl oz bottles.

Metered Dose Inhaler: Each Alupent Metered Dose Inhaler contains 225 mg of metaproterenol sulfate as a micronized powder in an inert propellant. This is sufficient medication for 300 inhalations. Each metered dose expressed from the inhaler delivers at the mouthpiece approximately 0.65 mg of metaproterenol sulfate. Alupent Metered Dose Inhaler with mouthpiece (15 ml). Alupent Metered Dose Inhaler refill (15 ml).

Inhalant Solution: Alupent Inhalant Solution is supplied as a 5% solution in bottles of 10 ml with accompanying calibrated dropper. Do not store above 77°F (25°C). Protect from light.

Alupent Inhalant Solution Unit Dose Vials are supplied as 0.6% clear, colorless or nearly colorless solution, each vial containing 2.5 ml, with 25 vials per box, 4 boxes per shipper.

Refrigerate unit dose vials at 36°–46°F (2°–8°C). Protect from light.

Do not use the solution if it is brown or has a precipitate.

AL-PI-11/84

CATAPRES® R
[*kah'tah-pres*]
brand of clonidine hydrochloride USP
Oral Antihypertensive

Tablets, 0.1 mg. ....BI-CODE 06
Tablets, 0.2 mg. ....BI-CODE 07
Tablets, 0.3 mg. ....BI-CODE 11

Description: Catapres, brand of clonidine hydrochloride, an antihypertensive agent, is an imidazoline derivative and exists as a mesomeric compound. Its chemical name is 2-(2,6-dichlorophenylamino)-2-imidazoline hydrochloride.

It is an odorless, bitter, white crystalline substance soluble in water and alcohol, with a molecular weight of 266.57. The 0.1 mg tablet is equivalent to 0.087 mg of the free base.

Actions: Catapres, brand of clonidine hydrochloride, is an antihypertensive agent whose mechanism of action appears to be central alpha-adrenergic stimulation as demonstrated in animal studies. This results in the inhibition of bulbar sympathetic cardioaccelerator and sympathetic vasoconstrictor centers, thereby causing a decrease in sympathetic outflow from the brain. Initially, Catapres, brand of clonidine hydrochloride, stimulates peripheral alpha-adrenergic receptors producing transient vasoconstriction.

Method of Administration	Usual Single Dose	Range	Dilution
Hand bulb nebulizer	10 inhalations	5–15 inhalations	No dilution
IPPB	0.3 ml	0.2–0.3 ml	Diluted in approx 2.5 ml of saline solution or other diluent

Catapres, brand of clonidine hydrochloride, acts relatively rapidly. The patient's blood pressure declines within 30 to 60 minutes after an oral dose, the maximum decrease occurring within 2 to 4 hours. The antihypertensive effect in humans lasts approximately 6 to 8 hours. The peak plasma level of Catapres, brand of clonidine hydrochloride, occurs in approximately 3 to 5 hours with a plasma half-life of 12 to 16 hours. Catapres, brand of clonidine hydrochloride, and its metabolites are excreted mainly in the urine. When labeled drug was administered, unchanged drug appearing in the urine accounted for about 32 percent of administered radioactivity.

Orthostatic effects are mild and infrequent since supine pressure is reduced to essentially the same extent as standing pressure. Catapres, brand of clonidine hydrochloride, does not alter normal hemodynamic responses to exercise. Acute studies with Catapres, brand of clonidine hydrochloride, in humans have demonstrated a moderate reduction (15 to 20%) of cardiac output in the supine position with no change in the peripheral resistance, while at a 45° tilt there is a smaller reduction in cardiac output and a decrease of peripheral resistance. Renal blood flow and the glomerular filtration rate remain essentially unchanged. During long-term therapy, cardiac output tends to return to control values, while peripheral resistance remains decreased. Slowing of the pulse rate has been observed in most patients given Catapres, brand of clonidine hydrochloride.

Other studies in humans have provided evidence of a reduction in plasma renin activity and in the excretion of aldosterone and catecholamines in patients treated with Catapres, brand of clonidine hydrochloride.

The exact relationship between these pharmacologic actions of Catapres, brand of clonidine hydrochloride, in humans, and its antihypertensive effect in individual patients, has not been fully elucidated at this time.

Catapres, brand of clonidine hydrochloride, has been administered together with hydralazine, guanethidine, methyldopa, reserpine, spironolactone, furosemide, chlorthalidone and thiazide diuretics without drug-to-drug interactions. The concomitant administration of a diuretic has been shown to enhance the antihypertensive efficacy of Catapres, brand of clonidine hydrochloride.

Indication: Catapres, brand of clonidine hydrochloride, is indicated in the treatment of hypertension. As an antihypertensive drug, Catapres, brand of clonidine hydrochloride, is mild to moderate in potency. It may be employed in a general treatment program with a diuretic and/or other antihypertensive agents as needed for proper patient response.

Warnings: Tolerance may develop in some patients, necessitating a reevaluation of therapy.

Use in Pregnancy: Reproduction studies have been performed with Catapres, brand of clonidine hydrochloride, in three animal species. The findings of these studies reflected no teratogenic effect but some embryotoxicity was evident at doses as low as 0.015 mg/kg (one-third the maximum recommended dose). In view of these findings, and since information on possible adverse effects in pregnant women is limited to uncontrolled clinical data, Catapres, brand of clonidine hydrochloride, is not recommended in women who are or may become pregnant unless the potential benefit outweighs the potential risk to mother and infant.

Use in Children: No clinical experience is available with the use of Catapres, brand of clonidine hydrochloride, in children. Studies are being performed to evaluate its use in the treatment of hypertension in children.

Precautions: When discontinuing Catapres, brand of clonidine hydrochloride, therapy the physician should reduce the dose gradually over 2 to 4 days to avoid a possible rapid rise in blood pressure and associated subjective symptoms such as nervousness, agitation, and headache. Patients on Catapres, brand of clonidine hydrochloride, therapy should be instructed not to discontinue therapy without consulting their physician. Rare instances of hypertensive encephalopathy and death have been recorded after abrupt cessation of Catapres, brand of clonidine hydrochloride, therapy. A causal relationship has not been established in these cases. It has been demonstrated that an excessive rise in blood pressure, should it occur, can be reversed by resumption of Catapres, brand of clonidine hydrochloride, therapy or by intravenous phentolamine.

Patients who engage in potentially hazardous activities, such as operating machinery or driving, should be advised of the sedative effect of Catapres, brand of clonidine hydrochloride. This drug may enhance the CNS-depressive effects of alcohol, barbiturates and other sedatives. Like any other antihypertensive agent, Catapres, brand of clonidine hydrochloride, should be used with caution in patients with severe coronary insufficiency, recent myocardial infarction, cerebrovascular disease or chronic renal failure.

As an integral part of their overall long-term care, patients treated with Catapres, brand of clonidine hydrochloride, should receive periodic eye examinations (see Toxicology).

Adverse Reactions: The most common reactions associated with Catapres, brand of clonidine hydrochloride, therapy are dry mouth (about 40%), drowsiness (about 35%), and sedation (about 8%). Constipation, dizziness, headache, and fatigue have been reported. Generally, these effects tend to diminish with continued therapy.

The following reactions have been associated with the drug, some of them rarely. In some instances an exact causal relationship has not been established.

Gastrointestinal: Anorexia, malaise, nausea, vomiting, parotid pain, mild transient abnormalities in liver function tests. There has been one report of possible drug-induced hepatitis without icterus and hyperbilirubinemia in a patient receiving Catapres, brand of clonidine hydrochloride, chlorthalidone and papaverine hydrochloride.

Metabolic: Weight gain, transient elevation of blood glucose or serum creatine phosphokinase, gynecomastia.

Cardiovascular: Congestive heart failure, Raynaud's phenomenon, and electrocardiographic abnormalities manifested as Wenckebach period or ventricular trigeminy.

Central Nervous System: Vivid dreams or nightmares, insomnia, other behavioral changes, nervousness, restlessness, anxiety, mental depression.

Dermatologic: Rash, angioneurotic edema, hives, urticaria, thinning of the hair, pruritus not associated with a rash.

Continued on next page

Boehringer Ingelheim—Cont.

Genitourinary: Impotence, urinary retention.
Other: Increased sensitivity to alcohol, dryness, itching or burning of the eyes, dryness of the nasal mucosa, pallor, or weakly positive Coombs' test.
Dosage and Administration: The dose of Catapres, brand of clonidine hydrochloride, must be adjusted according to the patient's individual blood pressure response. The following is a general guide to its administration.
Initial dose: One 0.1 mg tablet twice daily.
Maintenance dose: Further increments of 0.1 mg or 0.2 mg per day may be made until the desired response is achieved. The therapeutic doses most commonly employed have ranged from 0.2 mg to 0.8 mg per day given in divided doses. Studies have indicated that 2.4 mg is the maximum effective daily dose but doses as high as this have rarely been employed.
Overdosage: Profound hypotension, weakness, somnolence, diminished or absent reflexes and vomiting followed the accidental ingestion of Catapres, brand of clonidine hydrochloride, by several children from 19 months to 5 years of age. Gastric lavage and administration of an analeptic and vasopressor led to complete recovery within 24 hours. Tolazoline in intravenous doses of 10 mg at 30-minute intervals usually abolishes all effects of Catapres, brand of clonidine hydrochloride, overdosage.
Toxicology: In several studies Catapres, brand of clonidine hydrochloride, produced a dose-dependent increase in the incidence and severity of spontaneously occurring retinal degeneration in albino rats treated for six months or longer. Tissue distribution studies in dogs and monkeys revealed that Catapres, brand of clonidine hydrochloride, was concentrated in the choroid of the eye. In view of the retinal degeneration observed in rats, eye examinations were performed in 908 patients prior to the start of Catapres, brand of clonidine hydrochloride, therapy, who were then examined periodically thereafter. In 353 of these 908 patients, examinations were performed for periods of 24 months or longer. Except for some dryness of the eyes, no drug-related abnormal ophthalmologic findings were recorded and Catapres, brand of clonidine hydrochloride, did not alter retinal function as shown by specialized tests such as the electroretinogram and macular dazzle.
How Supplied: Catapres, brand of clonidine hydrochloride, is available as 0.1 mg (tan) and 0.2 mg (orange) oval, single-scored tablets in bottles of 100 and 1,000 and unit-dose packages of 100. Also available as 0.3 mg (peach) oval, single-scored tablets in bottles of 100.
Shown in Product Identification Section, page 406

COMBIPRES® ℞
[kom¹ be-pres]
Each tablet contains:
clonidine hydrochloride USP,
0.1 mg or 0.2 mg or 0.3 mg
and chlorthalidone USP, 15 mg
Oral Antihypertensive

Tablets 0.1	BI-CODE 08
Tablets 0.2	BI-CODE 09
Tablets 0.3	BI-CODE 10

WARNING

This fixed combination drug is not indicated for initial therapy of hypertension. Hypertension requires therapy titrated to the individual patient. If the fixed combination represents the dosage so determined, its use may be more convenient in patient management. The treatment of hypertension is not static, but must be reevaluated as conditions in each patient warrant.

Description: Combipres is a combination of clonidine hydrochloride and chlorthalidone. Clonidine hydrochloride, an antihypertensive agent, is an imidazoline derivative and exists as a mesomeric compound. The chemical name for clonidine hydrochloride is 2-(2,6-dichlorophenyl- amino)-2-imidazoline hydrochloride.
It is an odorless, bitter, white crystalline substance soluble in water and alcohol, with a molecular weight of 266.57. The 0.1 mg tablet is equivalent to 0.087 mg of the free base.
Chlorthalidone is 2-chloro-5-(1-hydroxy-3-oxo-1-isoindolinyl) benzenesulfonamide.
Chlorthalidone is an oral diuretic agent indicated for the treatment of edema and hypertension. The drug has a prolonged action. It differs from other sulfonamide diuretics in that a double ring system is incorporated in its chemical structure.
Actions: Combipres:
Combipres produces a more pronounced antihypertensive response than occurs after either clonidine hydrochloride or chlorthalidone alone in equivalent doses.
Clonidine hydrochloride:
Clonidine hydrochloride is an antihypertensive agent whose mechanism of action appears to be central alpha-adrenergic stimulation as demonstrated in animal studies. This results in the inhibition of bulbar sympathetic cardioaccelerator and sympathetic vasoconstrictor centers, thereby causing a decrease in sympathetic outflow from the brain. Initially, clonidine hydrochloride stimulates peripheral alpha-adrenergic receptors producing transient vasoconstriction.
Clonidine hydrochloride acts relatively rapidly. The patient's blood pressure declines within 30 to 60 minutes after an oral dose, the maximum decrease occurring within 2 to 4 hours. The antihypertensive effect in humans lasts approximately 6 to 8 hours. The peak plasma level of clonidine hydrochloride occurs in approximately 3 to 5 hours with a plasma half-life of 12 to 16 hours. Clonidine hydrochloride and its metabolites are excreted mainly in the urine. When labeled drug was administered, unchanged drug appearing in the urine accounted for about 32 percent of administered radioactivity.
Orthostatic effects are mild and infrequent since supine pressure is reduced to essentially the same extent as standing pressure. Clonidine hydrochloride does not alter normal hemodynamic responses to exercise. Acute studies with clonidine hydrochloride in humans have demonstrated a moderate reduction (15 to 20%) of cardiac output in the supine position with no change in the peripheral resistance, while at a 45° tilt there is a smaller reduction in cardiac output and a decrease of peripheral resistance. Renal blood flow and the glomerular filtration rate remain essentially unchanged. During long-term therapy, cardiac output tends to return to control values, while peripheral resistance remains decreased. Slowing of the pulse rate has been observed in most patients given clonidine hydrochloride.
Other studies in humans have provided evidence of a reduction in plasma renin activity and in the excretion of aldosterone and catecholamines in patients treated with clonidine hydrochloride.
The exact relationship between these pharmacologic actions of clonidine hydrochloride in humans and its antihypertensive effect in individual patients has not been fully elucidated at this time.
Clonidine hydrochloride has been administered together with hydralazine, guanethidine, methyldopa, reserpine, spironolactone, furosemide, chlorthalidone and thiazide diuretics without drug-to-drug interactions.
Chlorthalidone:
The diuretic action of chlorthalidone is thought to be due to inhibition of sodium and chloride reabsorption in the proximal tubule. It has been suggested that the initial antihypertensive action of the drug is due to a reduction of plasma volume.
Indication: Combipres is indicated in the treatment of hypertension (see box warning).
Contraindications: Combipres is contraindicated in patients with known hypersensitivity to chlorthalidone and in patients with severe renal or hepatic diseases.
Warnings: Tolerance may develop in some patients treated with Combipres. When this occurs therapy should be reevaluated.

Use in Pregnancy: No teratogenic changes have been observed following concomitant administration of chlorthalidone and clonidine hydrochloride to pregnant rats in doses up to 0.128 mg/kg of clonidine hydrochloride and 32 mg/kg of chlorthalidone. However, when animals were given clonidine hydrochloride alone in doses as low as 0.015 mg/kg (one-third the maximum recommended dose) some embryotoxicity was evident. In view of these findings and since information on possible adverse effects in pregnant women is limited to uncontrolled clinical data, Combipres is not recommended in women who are or may become pregnant unless the potential benefit outweighs the potential risk to mother and infant.
Use in Children: No clinical experience is available with the use of Combipres in children. Studies are being performed with clonidine hydrochloride to evaluate its use in the treatment of hypertension in children.
Precautions: Clonidine hydrochloride:
When discontinuing Combipres therapy, the physician should reduce the dose gradually over 2 to 4 days to avoid a possible rapid rise in blood pressure and associated subjective symptoms such as nervousness, agitation, and headache. Patients on Combipres therapy should be instructed not to discontinue therapy without consulting their physician. Rare instances of hypertensive encephalopathy and death have been recorded after abrupt cessation of clonidine hydrochloride therapy. A causal relationship has not been established in these cases. It has been demonstrated that an excessive rise in blood pressure, should it occur, can be reversed by resumption of Combipres therapy or by intravenous phentolamine.
Patients who engage in potentially hazardous activities, such as operating machinery or driving, should be advised of the sedative effect of the clonidine hydrochloride component. This drug may enhance the CNS-depressive effects of alcohol, barbiturates and other sedatives. Like any other antihypertensive agent, Combipres should be used with caution in patients with severe coronary insufficiency, recent myocardial infarction, cerebrovascular disease or chronic renal failure.
As an integral part of their overall long-term care, patients treated with Combipres should receive periodic eye examinations (see Toxicology).
Chlorthalidone:
Patients predisposed toward or affected by diabetes should be tested periodically while receiving Combipres, because of the hyperglycemic effect of chlorthalidone.
Because of the possibility of progression of renal failure, periodic determination of the BUN is indicated. If, in the physician's opinion, a rising BUN is significant, the drug should be stopped.
The chlorthalidone component of Combipres may lead to sodium and/or potassium depletion. Muscular weakness, muscle cramps, anorexia, nausea, vomiting, constipation, lethargy or mental confusion may occur. Severe dietary salt restriction is not recommended in patients receiving Combipres.
Periodic determinations of the serum potassium level will aid the physician in the detection of hypokalemia. Extra care should be given to detection of hypokalemia in patients receiving adrenal corticosteroids, ACTH or digitalis. Hypochloremic alkalosis often precedes other evidences of severe potassium deficiency. Frequently, therefore, more sensitive indicators than the potassium serum level are the serum bicarbonate and chloride concentrations. Also indicative of potassium depletion can be electrocardiographic alterations such as changes in conduction time, reduction in amplitude of the T wave, ST segment depression, prominent U wave. These abnormalities may appear with potassium depletion before the serum level of potassium decreases. To lessen the possibility of potassium deficiency, the diet, in addition to meat and vegetables, should include potassium-rich foods such as citrus fruits and bananas. If significant potassium depletion should occur during therapy, oral potassium supplements in the form of potassium chloride (3 to 4.5 g/day), fruit juice and bananas should be given.

Adverse Reactions: Combipres is generally well tolerated. The most common reactions associated with Combipres are dry mouth (about 40%), drowsiness (about 35%), and sedation (about 8%). Constipation, dizziness, headache, and fatigue have been reported. Generally, these effects tend to diminish with continued therapy.

In addition to the reactions listed above, certain adverse reactions associated with the component drugs of Combipres are shown below.

Clonidine hydrochloride:

Gastrointestinal: Anorexia, malaise, nausea, vomiting, parotid pain, mild transient abnormalities in liver function tests. One case of possible drug-induced hepatitis without icterus or hyperbilirubinemia has been reported in a patient receiving clonidine hydrochloride, chlorthalidone and papaverine hydrochloride.

Metabolic: Weight gain, transient elevation of blood glucose or serum creatine phosphokinase, gynecomastia.

Cardiovascular: Congestive heart failure, Raynaud's phenomenon, and electrocardiographic abnormalities manifested as Wenckebach period or ventricular trigeminy.

Central Nervous System: Vivid dreams or nightmares, insomnia, other behavioral changes, nervousness, restlessness, anxiety, mental depression.

Dermatologic: Rash, angioneurotic edema, hives, urticaria, thinning of the hair, pruritus not associated with a rash.

Genitourinary: Impotence, urinary retention.

Other: Increased sensitivity to alcohol, dryness, itching or burning of the eyes, dryness of the nasal mucosa, pallor, or weakly positive Coombs' test.

Chlorthalidone:

Symptoms such as nausea, gastric irritation, anorexia, constipation and cramping, weakness, dizziness, transient myopia and restlessness are occasionally observed. Headache and impotence or dysuria may occur rarely. Orthostatic hypotension has been reported and may be potentiated when chlorthalidone is combined with alcohol, barbiturates or narcotics. Skin rashes, urticaria and purpura have been reported in a few instances.

A decreased glucose tolerance evidenced by hyperglycemia and glycosuria may develop inconsistently. This condition, usually reversible on discontinuation of therapy, responds to control with antidiabetic treatment. Diabetics and those predisposed should be checked regularly.

As with other diuretic agents, hypokalemia may occur (see Precautions). Hyperuricemia may be observed on occasion and acute attacks of gout have been precipitated. In cases where prolonged and significant elevation of blood uric acid concentration is considered potentially deleterious, concomitant use of a uricosuric agent is effective in reversing hyperuricemia without loss of diuretic and/or antihypertensive activity.

Idiosyncratic drug reactions such as aplastic anemia, thrombocytopenia, leukopenia, agranulocytosis and necrotizing angiitis have occurred, but are rare.

The remote possibility of pancreatitis should be considered when epigastric pain or unexplained gastrointestinal symptoms develop after prolonged administration.

Other adverse reactions which have been reported with this general class of compounds include: jaundice, xanthopsia, paresthesia and photosensitization.

Dosage and Administration: *Dosage:* As determined by individual titration of clonidine hydrochloride and chlorthalidone (see box warning).

The following is a general guide to the administration of the individual components of Combipres:

Clonidine hydrochloride:

Initial dose: One 0.1 mg tablet twice daily.

Maintenance dose: Further increments of 0.1 mg or 0.2 mg per day may be made until the desired response is achieved. The therapeutic doses most commonly employed have ranged from 0.2 to 0.8 mg per day, given in divided doses. Studies have indicated that 2.4 mg is the maximum effective daily dose but doses as high as this have rarely been employed.

Chlorthalidone:

The usual initial dose is 50 mg daily, which may be given in divided doses.

If the individual doses of clonidine hydrochloride, and chlorthalidone determined by titration represent the dose contained in Combipres, for convenience the patient may then be given Combipres.

Overdosage: Clonidine hydrochloride:

Profound hypotension, weakness, somnolence, diminished or absent reflexes and vomiting followed the accidental ingestion of clonidine hydrochloride by several children from 19 months to 5 years of age. Gastric lavage and administration of an analeptic and vasopressor led to complete recovery within 24 hours. Tolazoline in intravenous doses of 10 mg at 30-minute intervals usually abolishes all effects of clonidine hydrochloride overdosage.

Chlorthalidone:

Symptoms of overdosage include nausea, weakness, dizziness, and disturbances of electrolyte balance. There is no specific antidote, but gastric lavage is recommended, followed by supportive treatment. Where necessary, this may include intravenous dextrose and saline with potassium, administered with caution.

Toxicology: In several studies, clonidine hydrochloride produced a dose-dependent increase in the incidence and severity of spontaneously occurring retinal degeneration in albino rats treated for 6 months or longer. Tissue distribution studies in dogs and monkeys revealed that clonidine hydrochloride was concentrated in the choroid of the eye. In view of the retinal degeneration observed in rats, eye examinations were performed in 908 patients prior to the start of clonidine hydrochloride therapy, who were then examined periodically thereafter. In 353 of these 908 patients, examinations were performed for periods of 24 months or longer. Except for some dryness of the eyes, no drug-related abnormal ophthalmologic findings were recorded and clonidine hydrochloride did not alter retinal function as shown by specialized tests such as the electroretinogram and macular dazzle.

How Supplied: Combipres® 0.1 (each tablet contains clonidine hydrochloride, 0.1 mg + chlorthalidone, 15 mg). It is available as pink, oval, single-scored compressed tablets in bottles of 100 and 1000.

Combipres® 0.2 (each tablet contains clonidine hydrochloride, 0.2 mg + chlorthalidone, 15 mg). It is available as blue, oval, single-scored compressed tablets in bottles of 100 and 1000.

Combipres® 0.3 (each tablet contains clonidine hydrochloride, 0.3 mg + chlorthalidone, 15 mg). It is available as white, oval, single-scored compressed tablets in bottles of 100.

Shown in Product Identification Section, page 406

DULCOLAX®
[dul'co-lax]
brand of bisacodyl USP
Tablets of 5 mg...BI-CODE 12
Suppositories of 10 mg..........................BI-CODE 52
Laxative

Description: Dulcolax is a contact laxative acting directly on the colonic mucosa to produce normal peristalsis throughout the large intestine. Its unique mode of action permits either oral or rectal administration, according to the requirements of the patient. Because of its gentleness and reliability of action without side effects, Dulcolax may be used whenever constipation is a problem. In preparation for surgery, proctoscopy, or radiologic examination, Dulcolax provides satisfactory cleansing of the bowel, obviating the need for an enema. Dulcolax is a colorless, tasteless compound that is practically insoluble in water and alkaline solution. It is designated chemically bis(p-acetoxyphenyl)-2-pyridylmethane.

Actions: Dulcolax differs markedly from other laxatives in its mode of action: it is virtually nontoxic, and its laxative effect occurs on contact with the colonic mucosa, where it stimulates sensory nerve endings to produce parasympathetic reflexes resulting in increased peristaltic contractions of the colon. Administered orally, Dulcolax is absorbed to a variable degree from the small bowel but such absorption is not related to the mode of action of the compound. Dulcolax administered rectally in the form of suppositories is negligibly absorbed. The contact action of the drug is restricted to the colon, and motility of the small intestine is not appreciably influenced. Local axon reflexes, as well as segmental reflexes, are initiated in the region of contact and contribute to the widespread peristaltic activity producing evacuation. For this reason, Dulcolax may often be employed satisfactorily in patients with ganglionic blockage or spinal cord damage (paraplegia, poliomyelitis, etc.).

Indications: *Acute Constipation:* Taken at bedtime, Dulcolax tablets are almost invariably effective the following morning. When taken before breakfast, they usually produce an effect within six hours. For a prompter response and to replace enemas, the suppositories, which are usually effective in 15 minutes to one hour, can be used.

Chronic Constipation and Bowel Retraining: Dulcolax is extremely effective in the management of chronic constipation, particularly in older patients. By gradually lengthening the interval between doses as colonic tone improves, the drug has been found to be effective in redeveloping proper bowel hygiene. There is no tendency to "rebound".

Preparation for Radiography: Dulcolax tablets are excellent in eliminating fecal and gas shadows from x-rays taken of the abdominal area. For barium enemas, no food should be given following the administration of the tablets, to prevent reaccumulation of material in the cecum, and a suppository should be given one to two hours prior to examination.

Preoperative Preparation: Dulcolax tablets have been shown to be an ideal laxative in emptying the G.I. tract prior to abdominal surgery or to other surgery under general anesthesia. They may be supplemented by suppositories to replace the usual enema preparation. Dulcolax will not replace the colonic irrigations usually given patients before intracolonic surgery, but is useful in the preliminary emptying of the colon prior to these procedures.

Postoperative Care: Suppositories can be used to replace enemas, or tablets given as an oral laxative, to restore normal bowel hygiene after surgery.

Antepartum Care: Either tablets or suppositories can be used for constipation in pregnancy without danger of stimulating the uterus.

Preparation for Delivery: Suppositories can be used to replace enemas in the first stage of labor provided that they are given at least two hours before the onset of the second stage.

Postpartum Care: The same indications apply as in postoperative care, with no contraindication in nursing mothers.

Preparation for Sigmoidoscopy or Proctoscopy: For unscheduled office examinations, adequate preparation is usually obtained with a single suppository. For sigmoidoscopy scheduled in advance, however, administration of tablets the night before in addition will result in adequate preparation almost invariably.

Colostomies: Tablets the night before or a suppository inserted into the colostomy opening in the morning will frequently make irrigations unnecessary, and in other cases will expedite the procedure.

Contraindication: There is no contraindication to the use of Dulcolax, other than an acute surgical abdomen.

Precaution: Dulcolax tablets contain FD&C Yellow No. 5 (tartrazine) which may cause allergic-type reactions (including bronchial asthma) in certain susceptible individuals. Although the overall incidence of FD&C Yellow No. 5 (tartrazine) sensitivity in the general population is low, it is frequently seen in patients who also have aspirin hypersensitivity.

Continued on next page

Boehringer Ingelheim—Cont.

Adverse Reactions: As with any laxative, abdominal cramps are occasionally noted, particularly in severely constipated individuals.

Dosage:
Tablets
Tablets must be swallowed whole, not chewed or crushed, and should not be taken within one hour of antacids or milk.
Adults: Two or three (usually two) tablets suffice when an ordinary laxative effect is desired. This usually results in one or two soft, formed stools. Up to six tablets may be safely given in preparation for special procedures when greater assurance of complete evacuation of the colon is desired. In producing such thorough emptying, these higher doses may result in several loose, unformed stools.
Children: One or two tablets, depending on age and severity of constipation, administered as above. Tablets should not be given to a child too young to swallow them whole.
Suppositories
Adults: One suppository at the time a bowel movement is required. Usually effective in 15 minutes to one hour.
Children: Half a suppository is generally effective for infants and children under two years of age. Above this age, a whole suppository is usually advisable.
Combined
In preparation for surgery, radiography and sigmoidoscopy, a combination of tablets the night before and a suppository in the morning is recommended (see Indications).
How Supplied: Dulcolax, brand of bisacodyl: Yellow, enteric-coated tablets of 5 mg in boxes of 24, bottles of 100, 1000 and unit strip packages of 100; suppositories of 10 mg in boxes of 2, 4, 8, 50 and 500.
Note: Dulcolax suppositories and tablets should be stored at temperatures not above 86°F (30°C).
Also Available: Dulcolax® Bowel Prep Kit. Each kit contains:
  1 Dulcolax suppository of 10 mg bisacodyl;
  4 Dulcolax tablets of 5 mg bisacodyl;
  Complete patient instructions.
Clinical Applications: Dulcolax can be used in virtually any patient in whom a laxative or enema is indicated. It has no effect on the blood picture, erythrocyte sedimentation rate, urinary findings, or hepatic or renal function. It may be safely given to infants and the aged, pregnant or nursing women, debilitated patients, and may be prescribed in the presence of such conditions as cardiovascular, renal, or hepatic diseases.

026-E (5/81)
Shown in Product Identification Section, page 406

PERSANTINE®
[per-san'tēn]
brand of dipyridamole USP
For Long-Term Therapy of
Chronic Angina Pectoris
Tablets of 25 mg..................BI-CODE 17
Tablets of 50 mg..................BI-CODE 18
Tablets of 75 mg..................BI-CODE 19

Description: Persantine, brand of dipyridamole, is classified as a coronary vasodilator. The drug is unrelated chemically to the nitrates or digitalis.
Chemistry: Persantine, brand of dipyridamole, is a homogeneous yellow crystalline powder, odorless but with a bitter taste. It is soluble in dilute acids, methanol, and chloroform. Its basic structure is a double ring of two condensed pyrimidine rings. It is designated chemically as 2,6-bis-(diethanolamino)-4,8-dipiperidino-pyrimido-(5,4-d) pyrimidine.
Actions: *Human:* Persantine, brand of dipyridamole, in therapeutic doses usually produces no significant alteration of systemic blood pressure or of blood flow in peripheral arteries; it increases coronary blood flow primarily by a selective dilation of the coronary arteries. The drug increases coronary sinus oxygen saturation without significantly altering myocardial oxygen consumption. A mild positive inotropic effect has been demonstrated in animals and man.
Animal: Experimental work in dogs subjected to artificial narrowing of one or both branches of the left coronary artery and chronically fed Persantine, brand of dipyridamole, has demonstrated an increase in intercoronary collateral circulation greater than that seen in placebo- or nitrate-treated animals exposed to identical conditions. A similar increase in collateral anastomoses over controls has been shown in healthy animals fed the drug.
In studies with heart preparations, the drug has been shown to protect against disturbances in function and fall in high-energy phosphate levels induced by hypoxia.
In animal (rat) studies using combination therapy with digitalis and dipyridamole, potentiation of digitalis toxicity occurred as measured by an augmentation of phosphorus exchange of the phosphorus-containing fractions of the myocardium. Experiments in cats, on the other hand, have shown that dipyridamole decreases the acute toxicity of digitoxin.
Studies with electron microscopy have demonstrated preservation of the anatomic structure of heart mitochondria (sarcosomes) in animals pretreated with the drug and exposed to hypoxia. Untreated animals showed dissolution of mitochondrial structure under similar conditions.

> **Indications:** Based on a review of this drug by the National Academy of Sciences—National Research Council and/or other information, FDA has classified the indication as follows:
> "Possibly" effective: For long-term therapy of chronic angina pectoris. Prolonged therapy may reduce the frequency of, or eliminate, anginal episodes, improve exercise tolerance, and reduce nitroglycerin requirements. The drug is not intended to abort the acute anginal attack.
> Final classification of the less-than-effective indications requires further investigation.

Contraindications: No specific contraindications are known.
Precautions: Since excessive doses can produce peripheral vasodilation, the drug should be used cautiously in patients with hypotension.
Adverse Reactions: Adverse reactions are minimal and transient at recommended dosages. Instances of headache, dizziness, nausea, flushing, weakness, or syncope, mild gastrointestinal distress and skin rash have been noted during therapy. Rare cases of what appeared to be an aggravation of angina pectoris have been reported, usually at the initiation of therapy.
On those uncommon occasions when adverse reactions have been persistent or intolerable to the patient, withdrawal of the medication has been followed promptly by cessation of the undesirable symptoms.
Dosage and Administration: The recommended dosage is 50 mg three times a day, taken at least one hour before meals. In some cases higher doses may be necessary but should be used with the knowledge that a significantly increased incidence of side effects is associated with increased dosage. Clinical response may not be evident before the second or third month of continuous therapy.
How Supplied:
Persantine (dipyridamole) is available as round, orange, sugar-coated tablets of 25 mg, coded 17. Bottles of 100 and 1000 and unit-dose packages of 100.
Persantine-50 (dipyridamole) is available as round, orange, sugar-coated tablets of 50 mg, coded 18. Bottles of 100 and 1000 and unit dose packages of 100.
Persantine-75 (dipyridamole) is available as round, orange, sugar-coated tablets of 75 mg, coded 19. Bottles of 100 and 500 and unit dose packages of 100.
Shown in Product Identification Section, page 406

PRELUDIN®
[pra-lu'din]
brand of phenmetrazine hydrochloride USP
Endurets® (prolonged-action
tablets, 75 mg..................BI-CODE 62

Description: Preludin, brand of phenmetrazine hydrochloride, belongs to the oxazine group of compounds and is designated chemically as 2-phenyl-3-methyltetrahydro-1,4-oxazine hydrochloride.
Phenmetrazine hydrochloride is a white, water-soluble, crystalline powder.
Actions: Preludin, brand of phenmetrazine hydrochloride, is a sympathomimetic amine with pharmacologic activity similar to the prototype drugs of this class used in obesity, the amphetamines. Actions include central nervous system stimulation and elevation of blood pressure. Tachyphylaxis and tolerance have been demonstrated with all drugs of this class in which these phenomena have been looked for.
Drugs of this class used in obesity are commonly known as "anorectics" or "anorexigenics". It has not been established, however, that the action of such drugs in treating obesity is primarily one of appetite suppression. Other central nervous system actions, or metabolic effects, may be involved, for example.
Adult obese subjects instructed in dietary management and treated with "anorectic" drugs, lose more weight on the average than those treated with placebo and diet, as determined in relatively short-term clinical trials.
The magnitude of increased weight loss of drug-treated patients over placebo-treated patients is only a fraction of a pound a week. The rate of weight loss is greatest in the first weeks of therapy for both drug and placebo subjects and tends to decrease in succeeding weeks. The possible origins of the increased weight loss due to the various drug effects are not established. The amount of weight loss associated with the use of an "anorectic" drug varies from trial to trial, and the increased weight loss appears to be related in part to variables other than the drug prescribed, such as the physician-investigator, the population treated, and the diet prescribed. Studies do not permit conclusions as to the relative importance of the drug and non-drug factors on weight loss.
The natural history of obesity is measured in years, whereas the studies cited are restricted to a few weeks' duration; thus, the total impact of drug-induced weight loss over that of diet alone must be considered clinically limited.
Preludin Endurets are formulated to release the active drug substance *in vivo* in a more gradual fashion than the standard formulation, as demonstrated by blood levels. The formulation has not been shown superior in effectiveness with respect to weight loss over the same dosage of the standard, noncontrolled-release formulations.
Indication: Preludin, brand of phenmetrazine hydrochloride, is indicated in the management of exogenous obesity as a short-term (a few weeks) adjunct in a regimen of weight reduction based on caloric restriction. The limited usefulness of agents of this class (see Actions) should be measured against possible risk factors inherent in their use such as those described below.
Contraindications: Advanced arteriosclerosis, symptomatic cardiovascular disease, moderate to severe hypertension, hyperthyroidism, known hypersensitivity or idiosyncrasy to sympathomimetic amines, glaucoma. Agitated states. Patients with a history of drug abuse. Concomitant use of CNS stimulants. During or within 14 days following the administration of monoamine oxidase inhibitors (hypertensive crises may result).
Warnings: Tolerance usually develops within a few weeks. When this occurs, the recommended dose should not be exceeded in an attempt to increase anorectic effect; rather, the drug should be discontinued.
Preludin, brand of phenmetrazine hydrochloride, may impair the ability of the patient to engage in potentially hazardous activities such as operating

machinery or driving a motor vehicle; the patient should therefore be cautioned accordingly.

Drug Dependence: Preludin, brand of phenmetrazine hydrochloride, is related chemically and pharmacologically to the amphetamines. Amphetamines and related stimulant drugs have been extensively abused, and the possibility of abuse of Preludin, brand of phenmetrazine hydrochloride, should be kept in mind when evaluating the desirability of including a drug as part of a weight reduction program. Abuse of amphetamines and related drugs may be associated with intense psychological dependence and severe social dysfunction. There are reports of patients who have increased the dosage to many times that recommended. Abrupt cessation following prolonged high dosage administration results in extreme fatigue and mental depression; changes are also noted on the sleep EEG. Manifestations of chronic intoxication with anorectic drugs include severe dermatoses, marked insomnia, irritability, hyperactivity, and personality changes. The most severe manifestation of chronic intoxication is psychosis, often clinically indistinguishable from schizophrenia.

Usage in Pregnancy: Safe use in pregnancy has not been established. Animal reproductive studies demonstrated no teratogenic effects. However, the conception rate was adversely affected, as well as survival and body weight of pups at weaning. There have been clinical reports of congenital malformation associated with the use of this compound but a causal relationship has not been proved. Until more information is available, Preludin, brand of phenmetrazine hydrochloride, should not be used by women who are or may become pregnant, particularly in the first trimester, unless in the opinion of the prescribing physician the potential benefits outweigh the possible risks.

Usage in Children: Preludin, brand of phenmetrazine hydrochloride, is not recommended for use in children under 12 years of age.

Precautions: Caution should be exercised in prescribing Preludin, brand of phenmetrazine hydrochloride, for patients with even mild hypertension. Insulin requirements in diabetes mellitus may be altered in association with the use of Preludin, brand of phenmetrazine hydrochloride, and the concomitant dietary regimen. Preludin, brand of phenmetrazine hydrochloride, may decrease the hypotensive effect of guanethidine. The least amount feasible should be prescribed or dispensed at one time in order to minimize the possibility of overdosage.

Preludin Endurets, 75 mg, contain FD&C Yellow No. 5 (tartrazine) which may cause allergic-type reactions (including bronchial asthma) in certain susceptible individuals. Although the overall incidence of FD&C Yellow No. 5 (tartrazine) sensitivity in the general population is low, it is frequently seen in patients who also have aspirin hypersensitivity.

Adverse Reactions: *Cardiovascular:* Palpitation, tachycardia, elevation of blood pressure.

Central Nervous System: Overstimulation, restlessness, dizziness, insomnia, euphoria, dysphoria, tremor, headache; rarely psychotic episodes at recommended doses.

Gastrointestinal: Dryness of the mouth, unpleasant taste, diarrhea, constipation, other gastrointestinal disturbances.

Allergic: Urticaria.

Endocrine: Impotence, changes in libido.

Dosage and Administration: Preludin, brand of phenmetrazine hydrochloride, is not recommended for use in children under 12 years of age. The maximum adult dosage is one 75 mg Endurets prolonged-action tablet taken daily. Since an Endurets tablet provides appetite suppression for approximately 12 hours, the time of administration should be determined by the period of the day over which the anorectic effect is desired.

Overdosage: Manifestations of acute overdosage with phenmetrazine hydrochloride include restlessness, tremor, hyperreflexia, rapid respiration, confusion, assaultiveness, hallucinations, panic states. Fatigue and depression usually follow the central stimulation. Cardiovascular effects include arrhythmias, hypertension, or hypotension and circulatory collapse. Gastrointestinal symptoms include nausea, vomiting, diarrhea and abdominal cramps. Poisoning may result in convulsions, coma, and death.

Management of acute phenmetrazine hydrochloride intoxication is largely symptomatic and includes lavage and sedation with a barbiturate. Experience with hemodialysis or peritoneal dialysis is inadequate to permit recommendation in this regard. As with the amphetamines, acidification of the urine should increase phenmetrazine hydrochloride excretion. Intravenous phentolamine has been suggested for possible acute, severe hypertension if this complicates phenmetrazine overdosage.

How Supplied: Preludin, brand of phenmetrazine hydrochloride, is available as pink, round Endurets prolonged-action tablets of 75 mg, for once-a-day administration. Bottles of 100 NDC 0597-0062-01.

Shown in Product Identification Section, page 406

PRELU-2®
[*pra¹lu (2)*]
brand of phendimetrazine tartrate
Timed Release Capsules   BI-CODE 64
105 mg

Description: Chemical name: phendimetrazine tartrate (+) 3, 4 dimethyl-2-phenylmorpholine tartrate. Phendimetrazine tartrate is a white, odorless powder with a bitter taste. It is soluble in water, methanol and ethanol. It has a molecular weight of 341.

The capsule is manufactured in a special base which is designed for prolonged release.

Clinical Pharmacology: Phendimetrazine tartrate is a sympathomimetic amine with pharmacologic activity similar to the prototype of drugs of this class used in obesity, the amphetamines. Actions include central nervous system stimulation and elevation of blood pressure. Tachyphylaxis and tolerance have been demonstrated with all drugs of this class in which these phenomena have been looked for.

Drugs of this class used in obesity are commonly known as 'anorectics' or 'anorexigenics.' It has not been established, however, that the action of such drugs in treating obesity is primarily one of appetite suppression. Other central nervous system actions, or metabolic effects, may be involved, for example.

Adult obese subjects instructed in dietary management and treated with 'anorectic' drugs lose more weight on the average than those treated with placebo and diet, as determined in relatively short-term clinical trials.

The magnitude of increased weight loss of drug-treated patients over placebo-treated patients is only a fraction of a pound a week. The rate of weight loss is greatest in the first weeks of therapy for both drug and placebo subjects and tends to decrease in succeeding weeks. The possible origins of the increased weight loss due to the various drug effects are not established. The amount of weight loss associated with the use of an 'anorectic' drug varies from trial to trial, and the increased weight loss appears to be related in part to variables other than the drug prescribed, such as the physician-investigator, the population treated, and the diet prescribed. Studies do not permit conclusions as to the relative importance of the drug and non-drug factors on weight loss.

The natural history of obesity is measured in years, whereas the studies cited are restricted to a few weeks duration; thus, the total impact of drug-induced weight loss over that of diet alone must be considered clinically limited.

The active drug 105 mg of phendimetrazine tartrate in each capsule of this special timed release dosage form approximates the action of three 35 mg non-timed doses taken at four hour intervals. The major route of elimination is via the kidneys where most of the drug and metabolites are excreted. Some of the drug is metabolized to phenmetrazine and also phendimetrazine-N-oxide.

The average half-life of elimination when studied under controlled conditions is about 3.7 hours for both the timed and non-timed forms. The absorption half-life of the drug from conventional non-timed 35 mg phendimetrazine tablets is appreciably more rapid than the absorption rate of the drug from the timed release formulation.

Indications and Usage: Phendimetrazine tartrate is indicated in the management of exogenous obesity as a short-term adjunct (a few weeks) in a regimen of weight reduction based on caloric restriction. The limited usefulness of agents of this class (see Clinical Pharmacology) should be measured against possible risk factors inherent in their use such as those described below.

Contraindications: Advanced arteriosclerosis, symptomatic cardiovascular disease, moderate to severe hypertension, hyperthyroidism, known hypersensitivity, or idiosyncrasy to the sympathomimetic amines, glaucoma.

Agitated states.

Patients with a history of drug abuse.

During or within 14 days following the administration of monoamine oxidase inhibitors (hypertensive crises may result).

Warnings: Tolerance to the anorectic effect usually develops within a few weeks. When this occurs, the recommended dose should not be exceeded in an attempt to increase the effect; rather, the drug should be discontinued.

Phendimetrazine tartrate may impair the ability of the patient to engage in potentially hazardous activities such as operating machinery or driving a motor vehicle; the patient should therefore be cautioned accordingly.

Drug Dependence: Phendimetrazine tartrate is related chemically and pharmacologically to the amphetamines. Amphetamines and related stimulant drugs have been extensively abused, and the possibility of abuse of phendimetrazine tartrate should be kept in mind when evaluating the desirability of including a drug as part of a weight reduction program. Abuse of amphetamines and related drugs may be associated with intense psychological dependence and severe social dysfunction. There are reports of patients who have increased the dosage to many times that recommended. Abrupt cessation following prolonged high dosage administration results in extreme fatigue and mental depression; changes are also noted on the sleep EEG. Manifestations of chronic intoxication with anorectic drugs include severe dermatoses, marked insomnia, irritability, hyperactivity, and personality changes. The most severe manifestation of chronic intoxications is psychosis, often clinically indistinguishable from schizophrenia.

Usage in Pregnancy: The safety of phendimetrazine tartrate in pregnancy and lactation has not been established. Therefore phendimetrazine tartrate should not be taken by women who are or may become pregnant.

Usage in Children: Phendimetrazine tartrate is not recommended for use in children under 12 years of age.

Precautions: Caution is to be exercised in prescribing phendimetrazine tartrate for patients with even mild hypertension.

Insulin requirements in diabetes mellitus may be altered in association with the use of phendimetrazine tartrate and the concomitant dietary regimen.

Phendimetrazine tartrate may decrease the hypotensive effect of guanethidine.

The least amount feasible should be prescribed or dispensed at one time in order to minimize the possibility of overdosage.

Adverse Reactions:

Cardiovascular: Palpitation, tachycardia, elevation of blood pressure.

Central Nervous System: Overstimulation, restlessness, dizziness, insomnia, euphoria, dysphoria, tremor, headache; rarely psychotic episodes at recommended doses.

Gastrointestinal: Dryness of the mouth, unpleasant taste, diarrhea, constipation, other gastrointestinal disturbances.

Continued on next page

Boehringer Ingelheim—Cont.

Allergic: Urticaria.
Endocrine: Impotence, changes in libido.

Overdosage: Manifestations of acute overdosage with phendimetrazine tartrate include restlessness, tremor, hyperreflexia, rapid respiration, confusion, assaultiveness, hallucinations, panic states.

Fatigue and depression usually follow the central stimulation.

Cardiovascular effects include arrhythmias, hypertension or hypotension and circulatory collapse. Gastrointestinal symptoms include nausea, vomiting, diarrhea, and abdominal cramps. Fatal poisoning usually terminates in convulsions and coma. Management of acute phendimetrazine tartrate intoxication is largely symptomatic and includes lavage and sedation with a barbiturate. Experience with hemodialysis or peritoneal dialysis is inadequate to permit recommendation in this regard. Acidification of the urine increases phendimetrazine tartrate excretion. Intravenous phentolamine (Regitine) has been suggested for possible acute, severe hypertension, if this complicates phendimetrazine tartrate overdosage.

Dosage and Administration: Since this product is a timed release dosage form, limit to one timed release capsule (105 mg phendimetrazine tartrate) in the morning.

Phendimetrazine tartrate is not recommended for use in children under 12 years of age.

How Supplied: 105 mg capsules (celery and green) in bottles of 100.

Federal law prohibits dispensing without a prescription.

Shown in Product Identification Section, page 406

RESPBID®
[resp′bid]
(theophylline)
Sustained release
Tablets of 250 mg and 500 mg
Oral Bronchodilator

Description: RESPBID® brand theophylline products are oral xanthine bronchodilators. Chemically, theophylline is 3,7-dihydro-1,3-dimethyl-1H-purine-2,6-dione.

RESPBID tablets contain 250 or 500 mg anhydrous theophylline, in a sustained-release formulation (see HOW SUPPLIED). Anhydrous theophylline is a white, odorless crystalline powder having a bitter taste.

Clinical Pharmacology: Theophylline directly relaxes the smooth muscle of the bronchial airways and pulmonary blood vessels, thus acting mainly as a bronchodilator and smooth muscle relaxant. The drug also has other actions typical of the xanthine derivatives: coronary vasodilation; diuresis; cardiac, cerebral, and skeletal muscle stimulation. The actions of theophylline may be mediated through inhibition of phosphodiesterase and a resultant increase in intracellular cyclic AMP which could mediate smooth muscle relaxation. At concentrations higher than those attained in vivo, theophylline also inhibits the release of histamine by mast cells.

In vitro, theophylline has been shown to act synergistically with beta agonists that increase intracellular cyclic AMP through the stimulation of adenyl cyclase, but synergism has not been demonstrated in patients. More data are needed to determine if theophylline and beta agonists have a clinically important additive effect in vivo.

Development of tolerance is not known to occur with chronic use of theophylline.

Pharmacokinetics: The half-life of theophylline is influenced by a number of known variables. It is prolonged in patients suffering from chronic alcoholism, impaired hepatic or renal function, congestive heart failure, and in patients receiving some macrolide antibiotics and cimetidine. Older adults (over age 55) and patients with chronic obstructive pulmonary disease, with or without cor pulmonale, may also have much slower clearance rates. infection with influenza (see Clinical Pharmacology—Pharmacokinetics).

Newborns and neonates have extremely slow clearance rates compared with older infants (over 6 months) and children, and may also have a theophylline half-life of over 24 hours. High fever for prolonged periods may also reduce the rate of theophylline elimination. Administration of influenza vaccine and infection with influenza virus have been associated with an impaired rate of theophylline elimination and consequent increases in serum theophylline levels, sometimes with toxic symptoms.

Theophylline Elimination Characteristics

	Theophylline Clearance Rates (mean ± S.D.)	Half-life Average (mean ± S.D.)
Children (over 6 months of age)	1.45 ± 0.58 ml/kg/min	3.7 ± 1.1 hrs.
Adult non-smokers with uncomplicated asthma	0.65 ± 0.19 ml/kg/min	8.7 ± 2.2 hrs.

The half-life of theophylline in smokers (one to two packs/day) averages four to five hours, much shorter than the half-life in nonsmokers which averages seven to nine hours. The increase in theophylline clearance caused by smoking is probably the result of induction of drug-metabolizing enzymes that do not readily normalize after cessation of smoking. It appears that between three months and two years may be necessary for normalization of the effect of smoking on theophylline pharmacokinetics.

In a single-dose study in eight fasted subjects, RESPBID tablets, 250 mg given at 7 mg/kg produced peak theophylline plasma levels of 9.1 ± 3.8 (SD) mcg/ml at 5.0 ± 1.5 hours following dose administration. The extent of theophylline absorption from RESPBID was complete in these subjects when compared with that from an immediate-release tablet. In a five-day, multiple-dose study involving 18 fasted subjects, RESPBID tablets, 250 mg given twice daily (11 mg/kg per day) produced mean minimum and maximum theophylline plasma levels of 7.3 ± 2.3 mcg/ml and 10.8 ± 3.1 mcg/ml, respectively.

Indications and Usage: For relief and/or prevention of symptoms of asthma and reversible bronchospasm associated with chronic bronchitis and emphysema.

Contraindications: RESPBID tablets are contraindicated in individuals who are hypersensitive to any of their components.

Warnings: Status asthmaticus should be considered a medical emergency and is defined as that degree of brochospasm which is not rapidly responsive to usual doses of conventional bronchodilators. Optimal therapy for such patients frequently requires both **additional medication,** parenterally administered, **and close monitoring,** preferably in an intensive care setting.

Although increasing the dose of theophylline may bring about relief, such treatment may be associated with toxicity. The likelihood of such toxicity developing increases significantly when the serum theophylline concentration exceeds 20 mcg/ml. Therefore, determination of serum theophylline levels is recommended to assure maximal benefit without excessive risk.

Serum levels above 20 mcg/ml are rarely found after appropriate administration of the recommended doses. However, in individuals in whom theophylline plasma clearance is reduced **for any reason,** even conventional doses may result in increased serum levels and potential toxicity. Reduced theophylline clearance has been documented in the following readily identifiable groups: 1) patients with impaired renal or liver function; 2) patients over 55 years of age, particularly males and those with chronic lung disease; 3) those with cardiac failure from any cause; 4) neonates; and 5) those patients taking certain drugs (some macrolide antibiotics and cimetidine). Decreased clearance of theophylline may be associated with either influenza immunization or active For such patients, the theophylline half-life may exceed 24 hours.

Reduction of dosage and laboratory monitoring are especially appropriate in the above individuals.

Less serious signs of theophylline toxicity, i.e., nausea and restlessness, may appear in up to 50% of patients. Unfortunately, however, serious side effects such as ventricular arrhythmias, convulsions or even death may appear as the first sign of toxicity without any previous warning. Stated differently, **serious toxicity is not reliably preceded by less severe side effects.**

Many patients who require theophylline may exhibit tachycardia due to their underlying disease process so that the cause/effect relationship to elevated serum theophylline concentrations may not be appreciated.

Theophylline products may cause dysrhythmia and/or worsen pre-existing arrhythmias, and any significant change in rate and/or rhythm warrants monitoring and further investigation.

The occurrence of arrhythmias and sudden death (with histological evidence of necrosis of the myocardium) has been recorded in laboratory animals (minipigs, rodents and dogs) when theophylline and beta agonists were administered concomitantly, although not when either was administered alone. The significance of these findings when applied to human usage is currently unknown.

Precautions: General Precautions: The half-life of theophylline is shorter in smokers than in non-smokers. Therefore smokers may require larger or more frequent doses. Morphine and curare should be used with caution in patients with airway obstruction as they may suppress respiration and stimulate histamine release. Alternative drugs should be used when possible. Theophylline should not be administered concurrently with other xanthine medications. Use with caution in patients with severe cardiac disease, severe hypoxemia, hypertension, hyperthyroidism, acute myocardial injury, cor pulmonale, congestive heart failure, liver disease, in the elderly (especially males) and in neonates. In particular, greater caution should be used in giving theophylline to patients with congestive heart failure. Frequently, such patients have markedly prolonged theophylline serum levels with theophylline persisting in serum for long periods following discontinuation of the drug. Use theophylline cautiously in patients with a history of peptic ulcer. Theophylline may occasionally act as a local irritant to the G.I. tract, although gastrointestinal symptoms are more commonly centrally mediated and associated with serum concentrations over 20 mcg/ml.

Information for Patients: If nausea, vomiting, restlessness, irregular heartbeat, or convulsions occur, contact a physician immediately.

Take only the amount of drug that has been prescribed. Do not take a larger dose, or take the drug more often, or for a longer time than recommended.

Do not take other medicines, especially those for pulmonary disorders, except on the advice of a physician.

Contact your physician if pulmonary symptoms occur repeatedly, especially at the end of a dosing interval.

Avoid drinking large amounts of caffeine-containing beverages, such as coffee, tea, cocoa, or cola, or eating large quantities of chocolate while taking this medicine, since these foods may increase the side effects of theophylline.

RESPBID tablets should not be chewed or crushed.

Laboratory Tests: Serum levels of theophylline should be monitored periodically to maintain optimum levels of 10 to 20 mcg/ml. The incidence of toxicity increases sharply above this range. For such measurements, serum should be obtained four to six hours after administration of RESPBID tablets. Patient compliance with the prescribed RESPBID regiment should have been good for the 48 hours preceding serum collection (i.e., no missed doses). ANY INCREASE IN DOSAGE BASED ON SERUM THEOPHYLLINE LEVEL WHEN THESE INSTRUCTIONS HAVE NOT BEEN FOLLOWED MAY INCREASE THE RISK OF TOXICITY. Because of the narrow range for therapeutic serum levels and great within-patient and between-patient variation in dosage necessary to produce and maintain such levels, measurement of serum theophylline is advised for individualization of dosage, both initially and during maintenance therapy. Certain patients may have slow elimination rates due to underlying conditions (see CLINICAL PHARMACOLOGY, WARNINGS and PRECAUTIONS, General Precautions); in such patients, conventional doses may produce high serum levels and associated signs of toxicity.

Drug Interactions: *Drug/Drug:* Toxic synergism with ephedrine has been documented and may occur with some other sympathomimetic bronchodilators. The administration of theophylline and sympathomimetic drugs concurrently is of particular concern in patients with cardiac arrhythmias. The following table lists drugs known to interact with theophylline and the effects of their concomitant use.

DRUG	EFFECT
Theophylline with lithium carbonate	Increased excretion of lithium carbonate
Theophylline with propranolol	Antagonism of propranolol effect
Theophylline with cimetidine	Increased theophylline blood levels
Theophylline with troleandomycin or erythromycin	Increased theophylline blood levels

Drug/Food: RESPBID tablets have not been adequately studied to determine whether their bioavailability is altered when they are given with food.

Available data suggest that drug administration at the time of food ingestion may influence the absorption characteristics of some or all theophylline controlled-release products resulting in serum values different from those found after administration in the fasting state.

A drug-food effect, if any, would likely have its greatest clinical significance when high theophylline serum levels are being maintained and/or when large single doses (greater than 13 mg/kg or 900 mg) of a controlled-release theophylline product are given. The influence of the type and amount of food on performance of controlled-release theophylline products is under study at this time.

Drug/Laboratory Test Interactions: When plasma levels of theophylline are measured by spectrophotometric methods, note that coffee, tea, cola beverages, chocolate, and acetaminophen can produce falsely high values.

Carcinogenesis, Mutagenesis, Impairment of Fertility: Long-term animal studies have not been performed to evaluate the carcinogenic potential, mutagenic potential, or the effect on fertility of xanthine compounds.

Pregnancy: Category C—Animal reproduction studies have not been conducted with theophylline. It is also not known whether theophylline can cause fetal harm when administered to a pregnant woman or can affect reproduction capacity. Xanthines should be given to a pregnant woman only if clearly needed.

Nursing Mothers: It has been reported that theophylline distributes readily into breast milk, and may cause adverse effects in the infant. Caution must be used if prescribing xanthines to a mother who is nursing, taking into account the risk-benefit of this therapy.

Pediatric Use: RESPBID tablets are not recommended for administration to children less than six years of age.

Adverse Reactions: The most consistent adverse reactions are usually due to overdose and are:
1. **Gastrointestinal:** nausea, vomiting, epigastric pain, hematemesis, diarrhea.
2. **Central nervous system:** headaches, irritability, restlessness, insomnia, reflex hyperexcitability, muscle twitching, clonic and tonic generalized convulsions.
3. **Cardiovascular:** palpitation, tachycardia, extrasystoles, flushing, hypotension, circulatory failure, ventricular arrhythmias.
4. **Respiratory:** tachypnea.
5. **Renal:** albuminuria, increased excretion of renal tubular and red blood cells, potentiation of diuresis.
6. **Others:** hyperglycemia and inappropriate ADH syndrome.

Drug Abuse and Dependence: Drug abuse and dependence have not been reported with theophylline.

Overdosage: Management: If potential overdose is established and seizure has not occurred:
1. Induce vomiting.
2. Administer a cathartic (this is particularly important if sustained-release preparations have been taken).
3. Administer activated charcoal.

If patient is having a seizure:
1. Establish an airway.
2. Administer oxygen.
3. Treat the seizure with intravenous diazepam, 0.1 to 0.3 mg/kg up to a maximum dose of 10 mg.
4. Monitor vital signs, maintain blood pressure and provide adequate hydration.

Post-seizure coma:
1. Maintain airway and oxygenation.
2. Follow above recommendations to prevent absorption of drug, but intubation and lavage will have to be performed instead of inducing emesis, and the cathartic and charcoal will need to be introduced via a large-bore gastric lavage tube.
3. Continue to provide full supportive care and adequate hydration while waiting for drug to be metabolized. In general, the drug is metabolized sufficiently rapidly so that dialysis is not required.

General: Serum theophylline should be monitored until the level is less than 20 mcg/ml. Electrolyte balance and hydration should be maintained by intravenous fluids.

If hypotension is not corrected by intravenous fluids, vasopressor drugs may be administered cautiously. (Caution: Sympathomimetic drugs may precipitate cardiac arrhythmia.)

Theophylline is dialyzable. However, in patients with very high serum theophylline levels and severe intoxication, charcoal hemoperfusion may be employed. This procedure is very effective in removing theophylline from the blood, and is to be preferred over peritoneal dialysis or hemodialysis.

Dosage and Administration: For most patients, effective use of theophylline, i.e., associated with optimal likelihood of benefit combined with minimal risk of toxicity, is considered to occur when serum levels are maintained between 10 and 20 mcg/ml. Levels above 20 mcg/ml may produce toxicity, and in a small number of patients, toxicity may even be seen with serum levels between 15 and 20 mcg/ml, particularly during initiation of therapy.

There is considerable variation from patient to patient in the dosage required to achieve and maintain therapeutic and safe levels, primarily because of variable rates of elimination. Therefore, it is essential not only that dosage be individualized, but also that titration and monitoring of serum levels be utilized where available. When serum concentration cannot be obtained, restriction of dosage to the amounts and intervals recommended in the guidelines listed below becomes essential.

Dosage should be calculated on the basis of lean (ideal) body weight where mg/kg doses are presented. Theophylline does not distribute into fatty tissue.

Dosage guidelines are approximations only and the wide range of theophylline clearance between individuals (particularly those with concomitant disease) makes indiscriminate usage hazardous. As a practical consideration, it is not always possible to obtain serum level determinations. Under such conditions, restriction of the daily dose (in otherwise healthy adults) to not greater than 13 mg/kg per day (of anhydrous theophylline) or 900 mg, whichever is less, in divided doses will result in relatively few patients exceeding serum levels of 20 mcg/ml and the resultant risk of toxicity.

RESPBID tablets have not been adequately studied for their bioavailability when administered with food (see PRECAUTIONS, Drug/Food Interactions).

RESPBID tablets should not be chewed or crushed.

Dosing Guidelines: Acute Symptoms—RESPBID tablets are not intended for patients experiencing an acute episode of bronchospasm (associated with asthma, chronic bronchitis, or emphysema). Such patients require **rapid** relief of symptoms and should be treated with an immediate-release theophylline preparation, an intravenous theophylline preparation or other bronchodilators, and not with controlled release products.

Chronic Symptoms—Theophylline administration is a treatment of first choice for the management of chronic asthma (to prevent symptoms and maintain patent airways) and is recommended for chronic bronchitis and emphysema. The appropriate dosage of theophylline can be established using an immediate-release preparation. Slow clinical titration is preferred to help assure acceptance and safety of the medication. When appropriate theophylline serum levels have been attained and clinical improvement has been maintained, the patient can usually be switched to RESPBID tablets by dividing the total daily dose of immediate-release theophylline by two and administering the appropriate RESPBID tablet every 12 hours (see conversion chart below). However, certain patients, such as the young, smokers, or some non-smoking adults, are likely to metabolize theophylline rapidly and require the total daily dose administered as three equal doses at eight-hour intervals. Such patients can generally be identified as having trough serum levels lower than desired or repeatedly exhibiting symptoms near the end of a dosing interval.

If the established daily dose is:	The q 12 hr regimen is: No. tablets:	strength:
500 mg	1	RESPBID 250 mg
1000 mg	1	RESPBID 500 mg

Alternatively, therapy of chronic bronchospasm can be initiated with RESPBID if the above dosage strengths permit titration and adjustment of dosage. It is recommended that for children under 25 kg, proper dosage be established with a liquid preparation to permit titration in small increments.

Recommended Doses for Chronic Bronchospasm: Initial Dose—As an initial dose, 16 mg/kg per 24 hours in divided doses at 8- or 12-hour intervals as appropriate.

Increasing Dose—The above daily dosage may be increased in approximately 25% increments at two- to three-day intervals so long as the drug is tolerated, until satisfactory clinical response is observed or the maximum dose indicated in the following section is reached.

Maximum Dose Where the Serum Concentration Is Not Measured:
WARNING: DO NOT ATTEMPT TO MAINTAIN ANY DOSE THAT IS NOT TOLERATED.

Do not exceed the following:
Age <9 years 24 mg/kg/day
Age 9–12 years 20 mg/kg/day
Age 12–16 years 18 mg/kg/day
Age >16 years 13 mg/kg/day or 900 mg, whichever is less

Measurement of Serum Theophylline: For measurement of serum theophylline levels during chronic therapy, see PRECAUTIONS—Laboratory Tests.

Dosage Adjustment after Serum Theophylline Measurement:
[See table on next page].
IT IS IMPORTANT THAT NO PATIENT BE MAINTAINED ON ANY DOSAGE THAT IS NOT TOLERATED. In instructing patients to increase dosage, they should be instructed not to take a subsequent dose if side effects occur and to resume therapy at a lower dose once adverse effects have disappeared.

Continued on next page

Boehringer Ingelheim—Cont.

Caution should be exercised for younger children who may not complain of minor side effects. Older adults, those with cor pulmonale, congestive heart failure, and/or liver disease may have unusually low dosage requirements and thus may experience toxicity at the maximal dosage recommended above.

HOW SUPPLIED: RESPBID® (theophylline) is supplied as 250 mg white, round, scored sustained release tablets imprinted with "BI 48" (NDC 0597-0048-01) and 500 mg white, capsule-shaped, scored sustained release tablets imprinted with "BI 49" (NDC 0597-0049-01) in bottles of 100. Store below 30°C (86°F).

Caution: Federal law prohibits dispensing without prescription.

RE-PI-11/84

SERENTIL®
[seh-ren'til]
brand of mesoridazine besylate

Tablets, 10 mg	BI-CODE 20
Tablets, 25 mg	BI-CODE 21
Tablets, 50 mg	BI-CODE 22
Tablets, 100 mg	BI-CODE 23
Concentrate of 25 mg/ml	BI-CODE 25
Ampuls of 1 ml (25 mg)	BI-CODE 27

Description: Serentil, brand of mesoridazine, the besylate salt of a metabolite of thioridazine, is a phenothiazine tranquilizer which is effective in the treatment of schizophrenia, organic brain disorders, alcoholism and psychoneuroses.

Serentil, brand of mesoridazine, is 10-[2(1-methyl-2-piperidyl) ethyl]-2- (methyl-sulfinyl)-phenothiazine [as the besylate].

Actions: Based upon animal studies Serentil, brand of mesoridazine, as with other phenothiazines, acts indirectly on reticular formation, whereby neuronal activity into reticular formation is reduced without affecting its intrinsic ability to activate the cerebral cortex. In addition, the phenothiazines exhibit at least part of their activities through depression of hypothalamic centers. Neurochemically, the phenothiazines are thought to exert their effects by a central adrenergic blocking action.

Indications: In clinical studies Serentil, brand of mesoridazine, has been found useful in the following disease states:

Schizophrenia: Serentil is effective in the treatment of schizophrenia. It substantially reduces the severity of emotional withdrawal, conceptual disorganization, anxiety, tension, hallucinatory behavior, suspiciousness and blunted affect in schizophrenic patients. As with other phenothiazines, patients refractory to previous medication may respond to Serentil, brand of mesoridazine.

Behavioral Problems in Mental Deficiency and Chronic Brain Syndrome: The effect of Serentil, brand of mesoridazine, was found to be excellent or good in the management of hyperactivity and uncooperativeness associated with mental deficiency and chronic brain syndrome.

Alcoholism—Acute and Chronic: Serentil, brand of mesoridazine, ameliorates anxiety, tension, depression, nausea and vomiting in both acute and chronic alcoholics without producing hepatic dysfunction or hindering the functional recovery of the impaired liver.

Psychoneurotic Manifestations: Serentil, brand of mesoridazine, reduces the symptoms of anxiety and tension, prevalent symptoms often associated with neurotic components of many disorders, and benefits personality disorders in general.

Contraindications: As with other phenothiazines, Serentil, brand of mesoridazine, is contraindicated in severe central nervous system depression or comatose states from any cause. Serentil, brand of mesoridazine, is contraindicated in individuals who have previously shown hypersensitivity to the drug.

Warnings: Where patients are participating in activities requiring complete mental alertness, (e.g., driving) it is advisable to administer the phenothiazines cautiously and to increase the dosage gradually.

Usage in Pregnancy: The safety of this drug in pregnancy has not been established; hence, it should be given only when the anticipated benefits to be derived from treatment exceed the possible risks to mother and fetus.

Usage in Children: The use of Serentil, brand of mesoridazine, in children under 12 years of age is not recommended, because safe conditions for its use have not been established.

Attention should be paid to the fact that phenothiazines are capable of potentiating central nervous system depressants (e.g., anesthetics, opiates, alcohol, etc.) as well as atropine and phosphorus insecticides.

Precautions: While ocular changes have not to date been related to Serentil, brand of mesoridazine, one should be aware that such changes have been seen with other drugs of this class.

Because of possible hypotensive effects, reserve parenteral administration for bedfast patients or for acute ambulatory cases, and keep patient lying down for at least one-half hour after injection.

Leukopenia and/or agranulocytosis have been attributed to phenothiazine therapy. A single case of transient granulocytopenia has been associated with Serentil, brand of mesoridazine. Since convulsive seizures have been reported, patients receiving anticonvulsant medication should be maintained on that regimen while receiving Serentil, brand of mesoridazine.

Neuroleptic drugs elevate prolactin levels; the elevation persists during chronic administration. Tissue culture experiments indicate that approximately one-third of human breast cancers are prolactin dependent in vitro, a factor of potential importance if the prescription of these drugs is contemplated in a patient with a previously detected breast cancer. Although disturbances such as galactorrhea, amenorrhea, gynecomastia, and impotence have been reported, the clinical significance of elevated serum prolactin levels is unknown for most patients. An increase in mammary neoplasms has been found in rodents after chronic administration of neuroleptic drugs. Neither clinical studies nor epidemiologic studies conducted to date, however, have shown an association between chronic administration of these drugs and mammary tumorigenesis; the available evidence is considered too limited to be conclusive at this time.

Serentil tablets contain FD&C Yellow No. 5 (tartrazine) which may cause allergic-type reactions (including bronchial asthma) in certain susceptible individuals. Although the overall incidence of FD&C Yellow No. 5 (tartrazine) sensitivity in the general population is low, it is frequently seen in patients who also have aspirin hypersensitivity.

Adverse Reactions: Drowsiness and hypotension were the most prevalent side effects encountered. Side effects tended to reach their maximum level of severity early with the exception of a few (rigidity and motoric effects) which occurred later in therapy.

With the exceptions of tremor and rigidity, adverse reactions were generally found among those patients who received relatively high doses early in treatment. Clinical data showed no tendency for the investigators to terminate treatment because of side effects.

Serentil, brand of mesoridazine, has demonstrated a remarkably low incidence of adverse reactions when compared with other phenothiazine compounds.

Central Nervous System: Drowsiness, Parkinson's syndrome, dizziness, weakness, tremor, restlessness, ataxia, dystonia, rigidity, slurring, akathisia, motoric reactions (opisthotonos) have been reported.

Autonomic Nervous System: Dry mouth, nausea and vomiting, fainting, stuffy nose, photophobia, constipation and blurred vision have occurred in some instances.

Genitourinary System: Inhibition of ejaculation, impotence, enuresis, incontinence have been reported.

Skin: Itching, rash, hypertrophic papillae of the tongue and angioneurotic edema have been reported.

Cardiovascular System: Hypotension and tachycardia have been reported. EKG changes have occurred in some instances (see Phenothiazine Derivatives: Cardiovascular Effects).

Phenothiazine Derivatives: It should be noted that efficacy, indications and untoward effects have varied with the different phenothiazines. The physician should be aware that the following have occurred with one or more phenothiazines and should be considered whenever one of these drugs is used:

Autonomic Reactions: Miosis, obstipation, anorexia, paralytic ileus.

Cutaneous Reactions: Erythema, exfoliative dermatitis, contact dermatitis.

Blood Dyscrasias: Agranulocytosis, leukopenia, eosinophilia, thrombocytopenia, anemia, aplastic anemia, pancytopenia.

Allergic Reactions: Fever, laryngeal edema, angioneurotic edema, asthma.

Hepatotoxicity: Jaundice, biliary stasis.

Cardiovascular Effects: Changes in the terminal portion of the electrocardiogram, including prolongation of the Q-T interval, lowering and inversion of the T wave and appearance of a wave tentatively identified as a bifid T or a U wave have been observed in some patients receiving the phenothiazine tranquilizers, including Serentil, brand of mesoridazine. To date, these appear to be due to altered repolarization and not related to myocardial damage. They appear to be reversible. While there is no evidence at present that these changes are in any way precursors of any significant disturbance of cardiac rhythm, it should be noted that sudden and unexpected deaths apparently due to cardiac arrest have occurred in patients previously showing characteristic electrocardiographic changes while taking the drug. The use of periodic electrocardiograms has been proposed but would appear to be of questionable value as a predictive device.

Hypotension, rarely resulting in cardiac arrest, has been noted.

Extrapyramidal Symptoms: Akathisia, agitation, motor restlessness, dystonic reactions, trismus, torticollis, opisthotonos, oculogyric crises, tremor, muscular rigidity, akinesia.

If serum theophylline is:		Directions:
Within normal limits	10 to 20 mcg/ml	Maintain dosage if tolerated. Recheck serum theophylline concentration at 6- to 12-month intervals.*
Too high	20 to 25 mcg/ml	Decrease doses by about 10%. Recheck serum theophylline concentration at 6- to 12-month intervals.*
Too high	25 to 30 mcg/ml	Skip next dose and decrease subsequent doses by about 25%.
Dangerous	Over 30 mcg/ml	Skip next two doses and decrease subsequent doses by 50%. Recheck serum theophylline.
Too low	7.5 to 10 mcg/ml	Increase dose by about 25%.** Recheck serum theophylline concentration at 6- to 12-month intervals.*
Too low	5 to 7.5 mcg/ml	Increase dose by about 25% to the nearest dose increment and recheck serum theophylline for guidance in further dosage adjustment (another increase will probably be needed, but this provides a safety check).

*Finer adjustments in dosage may be needed for some patients.
**If symptoms occur repeatedly at the end of a dosing interval, change the dosing regimen to q 8 hrs, not exceeding the recommended daily dose.

Persistent Tardive Dyskinesia: As with all antipsychotic agents, tardive dyskinesia may appear in some patients on long-term therapy or may occur after drug therapy has been discontinued. This risk seems to be greater in elderly patients on high-dose therapy, especially females. The symptoms are persistent and in some patients appear to be irreversible. The syndrome is characterized by rhythmical involuntary movements of the tongue, face, mouth or jaw (e.g., protrusion of tongue, puffing of cheeks, puckering of mouth, chewing movements). Sometimes these may be accompanied by involuntary movements of extremities.

There is no known effective treatment for tardive dyskinesia; antiparkinsonism agents usually do not alleviate the symptoms of this syndrome. It is suggested that all antipsychotic agents be discontinued if these symptoms appear.

Should it be necessary to reinstitute treatment, or increase the dosage of the agent, or switch to a different antipsychotic agent, the syndrome may be masked.

It has been reported that fine vermicular movements of the tongue may be an early sign of the syndrome and if the medication is stopped at that time, the syndrome may not develop.

Endocrine Disturbances: Menstrual irregularities, altered libido, gynecomastia, lactation, weight gain, edema. False positive pregnancy tests have been reported.

Urinary Disturbances: Retention, incontinence.

Others: Hyperpyrexia. Behavioral effects suggestive of a paradoxical reaction have been reported. These include excitement, bizarre dreams, aggravation of psychoses and toxic confusional states. More recently, a peculiar skin-eye syndrome has been recognized as a side effect following long-term treatment with phenothiazines. This reaction is marked by progressive pigmentation of areas of the skin or conjunctiva and/or accompanied by discoloration of the exposed sclera and cornea. Opacities of the anterior lens and cornea described as irregular or stellate in shape have also been reported. Systemic lupus erythematosus-like syndrome.

Dosage and Administration: The dosage of Serentil, brand of mesoridazine, as in most medications, should be adjusted to the needs of the individual. The lowest effective dosage should always be used. When maximum response is achieved, dosage may be reduced gradually to a maintenance level.

Schizophrenia: For most patients, regardless of severity, a starting dose of 50 mg t.i.d. is recommended. The usual optimum total daily dose range is 100-400 mg per day.

Behavioral Problems in Mental Deficiency and Chronic Brain Syndrome: For most patients a starting dose of 25 mg t.i.d. is recommended. The usual optimum total daily dose range is 75-300 mg per day.

Alcoholism: For most patients the usual starting dose is 25 mg b.i.d. The usual optimum total daily dose range is 50-200 mg per day.

Psychoneurotic Manifestations: For most patients the usual starting dose is 10 mg t.i.d. The usual optimum total daily dose range is 30-150 mg per day.

Injectable Form: In those situations in which an intramuscular form of medication is indicated, Serentil, brand of mesoridazine, injectable is available. For most patients a starting dose of 25 mg is recommended. The dose may be repeated in 30 to 60 minutes, if necessary. The usual optimum total daily dose range is 25-200 mg per day.

How Supplied:

Tablets: 10 mg, 25 mg, 50 mg, and 100 mg mesoridazine (as the besylate). Bottles of 100.

Ampuls: 1 ml [25 mg mesoridazine (as the besylate)]. Inactive ingredients: disodium edetate, USP, 0.5 mg; sodium chloride, USP, 7.2 mg; carbon dioxide gas (bone dry) q.s., water for injection, USP, q.s. to 1 ml. Boxes of 20 and 100.

Concentrate: Contains 25 mg mesoridazine (as the besylate) per ml; alcohol, USP, 0.61% by volume. Immediate containers: Amber glass bottles of 4 fl oz (118 ml) packaged in cartons of 12 bottles with an accompanying dropper graduated to de-

Serentil

Route	Mouse	Rat	Rabbit	Dog
Oral	560 ± 62.5	644 ± 48	MLD = 800	MLD = 800
I.M.	—	509M 584 F	405	—
I.V.	26 ± 0.08	—	—	—

liver 10 mg, 25 mg and 50 mg of mesoridazine (as the besylate).

Storage: Below 77°F. Protect from light. Dispense in amber glass bottles only.

The concentrate may be diluted with distilled water, acidified tap water, orange juice or grape juice.

Each dose should be so diluted just prior to administration. Preparation and storage of bulk dilutions is not recommended.

Additional information available to physicians.

Pharmacology: Pharmacological studies in laboratory animals have established that Serentil, brand of mesoridazine, has a spectrum of pharmacodynamic actions typical of a major tranquilizer. In common with other tranquilizers it inhibits spontaneous motor activity in mice, prolongs thiopental and hexobarbital sleeping time in mice and produces spindles and block of arousal reaction in the EEG of rabbits. It is effective in blocking spinal reflexes in the cat and antagonizes d-amphetamine excitation and toxicity in grouped mice. It shows a moderate adrenergic blocking activity in vitro and in vivo and antagonizes 5-hydroxytryptamine in vivo. Intravenously administered, it lowers the blood pressure of anesthetized dogs. It has a weak antiacetylcholine effect in vitro.

The most outstanding activity of Serentil, brand of mesoridazine, is seen in tests developed to investigate antiemotive activity of drugs. Such tests are those in which the rat reacts to acute or chronic stress by increased defecation (emotogenic defecation) or tests in which "emotional mydriasis" is elicited in the mouse by an electric shock. In both of these tests Serentil, brand of mesoridazine, is effective in reducing emotive reactions. Its ED_{50} in inhibiting emotogenic defecation in the rat is 0.053 mg/kg (subcutaneous administration). Serentil, brand of mesoridazine, has a potent antiemetic action. The intravenous ED_{50} against apomorphine-induced emesis in the dog is 0.64 mg/kg.

Serentil, brand of mesoridazine, in common with other phenothiazines, demonstrates antiarrhythmic activity in anesthetized dogs. Metabolic studies in the dog and rabbit with tritium labeled mesoridazine demonstrate that the compound is well absorbed from the gastrointestinal tract. The biological half-life of Serentil, brand of mesoridazine, in these studies appears to be somewhere between 24 to 48 hours. Although significant urinary excretion was observed following the administration of Serentil, brand of mesoridazine, these studies also suggest that biliary excretion is an important excretion route for mesoridazine and/or its metabolites.

Toxicity Studies

Acute LD_{50} (mg/kg):
[See table above].

Chronic toxicity studies were conducted in rats and dogs. Rats were administered Serentil, brand of mesoridazine, orally seven days per week for a period of seventeen months in doses up to 160 mg/kg per day. Dogs were administered Serentil, brand of mesoridazine, orally seven days per week for a period of thirteen months. The daily dosage of the drug was increased during the period of this test such that the "top-dose" group received a daily dose of 120 mg/kg of mesoridazine for the last month of the study. Untoward effects which occurred upon chronic administration of high dose-levels included:

Rats: Reduction of food intake, slowed weight gain, morphological changes in pituitary-supported endocrine organs, and melanin-like pigment deposition in renal tissues.

Dogs: Emesis, muscle tremors, decreased food intake and death associated with aspiration of oral-gastric contents into the respiratory system. Increased intrauterine resorptions were seen with Serentil, brand of mesoridazine, in rats at 70 mg/kg and in rabbits at 125 mg/kg but not at 60 and 100 mg/kg, respectively. No drug related teratology was suggested by these reproductive studies.

Local irritation from the intramuscular injection of Serentil, brand of mesoridazine, was of the same order of magnitude as with other phenothiazines.

Shown in Product Identification Section, page 406

THALITONE® ℞
[thal'ih-tōn]
brand of chlorthalidone USP
Tablets of 25 mg

Description: Thalitone, brand of chlorthalidone, is a monosulfamyl diuretic which differs chemically from thiazide diuretics in that a double-ring system is incorporated in its structure.

Actions: Chlorthalidone is an oral diuretic with prolonged action (48–72 hours) and low toxicity. The diuretic effect of the drug occurs within two hours of an oral dose and continues for up to 72 hours. It produces copious diuresis with greatly increased excretion of sodium and chloride. At maximal therapeutic dosage, chlorthalidone is approximately equal in its diuretic effect to comparable maximal therapeutic doses of benzothiadiazine diuretics. The site of action appears to be the cortical diluting segment of the ascending limb of Henle's loop of the nephron.

Indications: Diuretics such as Thalitone are indicated in the management of hypertension either as the sole therapeutic agent or to enhance the effect of other antihypertensive drugs in the more severe forms of hypertension. Thalitone is indicated as adjunctive therapy in edema associated with congestive heart failure, hepatic cirrhosis, and corticosteroid and estrogen therapy.

Thalitone has also been found useful in edema due to various forms of renal dysfunction such as nephrotic syndrome, acute glomerulonephritis, and chronic renal failure.

Usage in Pregnancy: The routine use of diuretics in an otherwise healthy woman is inappropriate and exposes mother and fetus to unnecessary hazard. Diuretics do not prevent development of toxemia of pregnancy, and there is no satisfactory evidence that they are useful in the treatment of developed toxemia. Edema during pregnancy may arise from pathological causes or from the physiologic and mechanical consequences of pregnancy. Chlorthalidone is indicated in pregnancy when edema is due to pathologic causes, just as it is in the absence of pregnancy, (however, see Warnings below). Dependent edema in pregnancy, resulting from restriction of venous return by the expanded uterus, is properly treated through elevation of the lower extremities and use of support hose; use of diuretics to lower intravascular volume in this case is illogical and unnecessary. There is hypervolemia during normal pregnancy which is harmful to neither the fetus nor the mother (in the absence of cardiovascular disease), but which is associated with edema, including generalized edema, in the majority of pregnant women. If this edema produces discomfort, increased recumbency will often provide relief. In rare instances, this edema may cause extreme discomfort which is not relieved by

Continued on next page

Boehringer Ingelheim—Cont.

rest. In these cases, a short course of diuretics may provide relief and may be appropriate.

Contraindications: Anuria. Hypersensitivity to chlorthalidone or other sulfonamide-derived drugs.

Warnings: Should be used with caution in severe renal disease. In patients with renal disease, chlorthalidone or related drugs may precipitate azotemia. Cumulative effects of the drug may develop in patients with impaired renal function.

Chlorthalidone should be used with caution in patients with impaired hepatic function or progressive liver disease, since minor alterations of fluid and electrolyte balance may precipitate hepatic coma.

Chlorthalidone may add to or potentiate the action of other antihypertensive drugs. Potentiation occurs with ganglionic or peripheral adrenergic blocking drugs.

Sensitivity reactions may occur in patients with a history of allergy or bronchial asthma.

The possibility of exacerbation or activation of systemic lupus erythematosus has been reported with thiazide diuretics, which are structurally related to chlorthalidone. However, systemic lupus erythematosus has not been reported following chlorthalidone administration.

Usage in Pregnancy: Reproduction studies in various animal species at multiples of the human dose showed no significant level of teratogenicity; no fetal or congenital abnormalities were observed. Animal data should not be extrapolated for clinical application.

Thiazides cross the placental barrier and appear in cord blood. The use of chlorthalidone and related drugs in pregnant women requires that the anticipated benefits of the drug be weighed against possible hazards to the fetus. These hazards include fetal or neonatal jaundice, thrombocytopenia, and possibly other adverse reactions which have occurred in the adult.

Nursing Mothers: Thiazides cross the placental barrier and appear in breast milk. If use of the drug is deemed essential, the patient should stop nursing.

Precautions: Periodic determination of serum electrolytes to detect possible electrolyte imbalance should be performed at appropriate intervals. All patients receiving chlorthalidone should be observed for clinical signs of fluid or electrolyte imbalance; namely, hyponatremia, hypochloremic alkalosis, and hypokalemia. Serum and urine electrolyte determinations are particularly important when the patient is vomiting excessively or receiving parenteral fluids. Medication such as digitalis may also influence serum electrolytes. Warning signs, irrespective of cause, are dryness of mouth, thirst, weakness, lethargy, drowsiness, restlessness, muscle pains or cramps, muscular fatigue, hypotension, oliguria, tachycardia, and gastrointestinal disturbances such as nausea and vomiting. Hypokalemia may develop with chlorthalidone as with any other potent diuretic, especially with brisk diuresis, when severe cirrhosis is present, or during concomitant use of corticosteroids or ACTH.

Interference with adequate oral electrolyte intake will also contribute to hypokalemia. Digitalis therapy may exaggerate metabolic effects of hypokalemia, especially with reference to myocardial activity.

Any chloride deficit is generally mild and usually does not require specific treatment except under extraordinary circumstances (as in liver disease or renal disease). Dilutional hyponatremia may occur in edematous patients in hot weather; appropriate therapy is water restriction, rather than administration of salt except in rare instances when the hyponatremia is life threatening. In actual salt depletion, appropriate replacement is the therapy of choice. Hyperuricemia may occur or frank gout may be precipitated in certain patients receiving chlorthalidone.

Insulin requirements in diabetic patients may be increased, decreased or unchanged. Latent diabetes mellitus may become manifest during chlorthalidone administration.

Chlorthalidone and related drugs may increase the responsiveness to tubocurarine. The antihypertensive effects of the drug may be enhanced in the postsympathectomy patient.

Chlorthalidone and related drugs may decrease arterial responsiveness to norepinephrine. This diminution is not sufficient to preclude effectiveness of the pressor agent for the therapeutic use. If progressive renal impairment becomes evident, as indicated by a rising non-protein nitrogen or blood urea nitrogen, a careful reappraisal of therapy is necessary with consideration given to withholding or discontinuing diuretic therapy.

Chlorthalidone and related drugs may decrease serum PBI levels without signs of thyroid disturbance.

Adverse Reactions: Gastrointestinal System Reactions: anorexia, gastric irritation, nausea, vomiting, cramping, diarrhea, constipation, jaundice (intrahepatic cholestatic jaundice), pancreatitis.

Central Nervous System Reactions: dizziness, vertigo, paresthesias, headache, xanthopsia.

Hematologic Reactions: leukopenia, agranulocytosis, thrombocytopenia, aplastic anemia.

Dermatologic-Hypersensitivity Reactions: purpura, photosensitivity, rash,urticaria, necrotizing angiitis (vasculitis) (cutaneous vasculitis), Lyell's syndrome (toxic epidermal necrolysis).

Cardiovascular Reactions: Orthostatic hypotension may occur and may be aggravated by alcohol, barbiturates or narcotics.

Other Adverse Reactions: hyperglycemia, glycosuria, hyperuricemia, muscle spasm, weakness, restlessness, impotence.

Whenever adverse reactions are moderate or severe, chlorthalidone dosage should be reduced or therapy withdrawn.

Dosage and Administration: Therapy should be initiated with the lowest possible dose. This dose should be titrated according to individual patient response to gain maximal therapeutic benefit while maintaining the minimal dosage possible. A single dose given in the morning with food is recommended; divided doses are unnecessary.

Hypertension. Initiation: Therapy, in most patients, should be initiated with a single daily dose of 25 mg. If the response is insufficient after a suitable trial, the dosage may be increased to a single daily dose of 50 mg. If additional control is required, the dosage of Thalitone may be increased to 100 mg once daily or a second antihypertensive drug (step-2 therapy) may be added. Dosage above 100 mg daily usually does not increase effectiveness. Increases in serum uric acid and decreases in serum potassium are dose-related over the 25–100 mg/day range.

Maintenance: Maintenance doses may be lower than initial doses and should be adjusted according to individual patient response. Effectiveness is well sustained during continued use.

Edema. Initiation: Adults, initially 50 to 100 mg daily, or 100 mg on alternate days. Some patients may require 150 to 200 mg at these intervals, or up to 200 mg daily. Dosages above this level, however, do not usually produce a greater response.

Maintenance: Maintenance doses may often be lower than initial doses and should be adjusted according to the individual patient. Effectiveness is well sustained during continued use.

Overdosage: Symptoms of overdosage include nausea, weakness, dizziness and disturbances of electrolyte balance. There is no specific antidote, but gastric lavage is recommended, followed by supportive treatment. Where necessary, this may include intravenous dextrose-saline with potassium, administered with caution.

How Supplied: White, kidney-shaped compressed tablets coded Bl/76 containing 25 mg of chlorthalidone in bottles of 100, NDC number 0597-0076-01.

Animal Pharmacology: Biochemical studies in animals have suggested reasons for the prolonged effect of chlorthalidone. Absorption from the gastro-intestinal tract is slow due to its low solubility. After passage to the liver, some of the drug enters the general circulation, while some is excreted in the bile, to be reabsorbed later. In the general circulation, it is distributed widely to the tissues, but is taken up in highest concentrations by the kidneys, where amounts have been found 72 hours after ingestion, long after it has disappeared from other tissues. The drug is excreted unchanged in the urine.

Store Below 30°C (86°F). 2/83

Shown in Product Identification Section, page 406

TORECAN® ℞
[tor'eh-can]
brand of thiethylperazine USP
Tablets, 10 mg ....BI-CODE 28
Suppositories, 10 mg ....BI-CODE 29
Injection, 10 mg/2 ml ampul ....BI-CODE 30
For IM use only.

Description: Torecan, brand of thiethylperazine, is a phenothiazine. Thiethylperazine is characterized by a substituted thioethyl group at position 2 in the phenothiazine nucleus, and a piperazine moiety in the side chain. The chemical designation is: 2-ethyl-mercapto-10-[3'-(1''-methyl-piperazinyl-4'')-propyl-1''] phenothiazine.

Actions: The pharmacodynamic action of Torecan, brand of thiethylperazine, in humans is unknown. However, a direct action of Torecan, brand of thiethylperazine, on both the CTZ and the vomiting center may be concluded from induced vomiting experiments in animals.

Indications: Torecan is indicated for the relief of nausea and vomiting.

Contraindications: Severe central nervous system (CNS) depression and comatose states. In patients who have demonstrated a hypersensitivity reaction (e.g., blood dyscrasias, jaundice) to phenothiazines.

Because severe hypotension has been reported after the intravenous administration of phenothiazines, this route of administration is contraindicated.

Usage in Pregnancy: Torecan, brand of thiethylperazine, is contraindicated in pregnancy.

Warnings: Phenothiazines are capable of potentiating CNS depressants (e.g., anesthetics, opiates, alcohol, etc.) as well as atropine and phosphorous insecticides.

Since Torecan, brand of thiethylperazine, may impair mental and/or physical ability required in the performance of potentially hazardous tasks such as driving a car or operating machinery, it is recommended that patients be warned accordingly.

Postoperative Nausea and Vomiting: With the use of this drug to control postoperative nausea and vomiting occurring in patients undergoing elective surgical procedures, restlessness and postoperative CNS depression during anesthesia recovery may occur. Possible postoperative complications of a severe degree of any of the known reactions of this class of drug must be considered.

Postural hypotension may occur after an initial injection, rarely with the tablet or suppository. The administration of epinephrine should be avoided in the treatment of drug-induced hypotension in view of the fact that phenothiazines may induce a reversed epinephrine effect on occasion. Should a vasoconstrictive agent be required, the most suitable are levarterenol and phenylephrine. The use of this drug has not been studied following intracardiac and intracranial surgery.

Usage in Pediatrics: The safety and efficacy of Torecan, brand of thiethylperazine, in children under 12 years of age has not been established.

Nursing Mothers: Information is not available concerning the secretion of Torecan, brand of thiethylperazine, in the milk of nursing mothers. As a general rule, nursing should not be undertaken while a patient is on a drug, since many drugs are secreted in human milk.

Precautions: Abnormal movements such as extrapyramidal symptoms (EPS) (e.g., dystonia, torticollis, dysphasia, oculogyric crises, akathisia) have occurred. Convulsions have also been reported. The varied symptom complex is more likely to occur in young adults and children. Extrapyramidal effects must be treated by reduction of dosage or cessation of medication.

Torecan tablets contain FD&C Yellow No. 5 (tartrazine) which may cause allergic-type reactions (including bronchial asthma) in certain susceptible individuals. Although the overall incidence of FD&C Yellow No. 5 (tartrazine) sensitivity in the general population is low, it is frequently seen in patients who also have aspirin hypersensitivity.

Postoperative Nausea and Vomiting: When used in the treatment of the nausea and/or vomiting associated with anesthesia and surgery, it is recommended that Torecan, brand of thiethylperazine, should be administered by deep intramuscular injection at or shortly before the termination of anesthesia.

Adverse Reactions: *Central Nervous System:-* Serious: Convulsions have been reported, Extrapyramidal symptoms (EPS) may occur, such as dystonia, torticollis, oculogyric crises, akathisia, and gait disturbances. Others: Occasional cases of dizziness, headache, fever and restlessness have been reported.

Drowsiness may occur on occasion, following an initial injection. Generally this effect tends to subside with continued therapy or is usually alleviated by a reduction in dosage.

Autonomic Nervous System: Dryness of the mouth and nose, blurred vision, tinnitus. An occasional case of sialorrhea together with altered gustatory sensation has been observed.

Endocrine System: Peripheral edema of the arms, hands and face.

Hepatotoxicity: An occasional case of cholestatic jaundice has been observed.

Others: An occasional case of cerebral vascular spasm and trigeminal neuralgia has been reported.

Phenothiazine Derivatives: The physician should be aware that the following have occurred with one or more phenothiazines and should be considered whenever one of these drugs is used:

Blood Dyscrasias: Serious: Agranulocytosis, leukopenia, thrombocytopenia, aplastic anemia, pancytopenia, Others: Eosinophilia, leukocytosis.

Autonomic Reactions: Miosis, obstipation, anorexia, paralytic ileus.

Cutaneous Reactions: Serious: Erythema, exfoliative dermatitis, contact dermatitis.

Hepatotoxicity: Serious: Jaundice, biliary stasis.

Cardiovascular Effects: Serious: Hypotension, rarely leading to cardiac arrest; electrocardiographic (ECG) changes.

Extrapyramidal Symptoms: Serious: Akathisia, agitation, motor restlessness, dystonic reactions, trismus, torticollis, opisthotonos, oculogyric crises, tremor, muscular rigidity, akinesia—some of which have persisted for several months or years especially in patients of advanced age with brain damage.

Endocrine Disturbances: Menstrual irregularities, altered libido, gynecomastia, weight gain. False positive pregnancy tests have been reported.

Urinary Disturbances: Retention, incontinence.

Allergic Reactions: Serious: Fever, laryngeal edema, angioneurotic edema, asthma.

Others: Hyperpyrexia. Behavioral effects suggestive of a paradoxical reaction have been reported. These include excitement, bizarre dreams, aggravation of psychoses and toxic confusional states. While there is no evidence at present that ECG changes observed in patients receiving phenothiazines are in any way precursors of any significant disturbance of cardiac rhythm, it should be noted that sudden and unexpected deaths apparently due to cardiac arrest have been reported in a few instances in hospitalized psychotic patients previously showing characteristic ECG changes. A peculiar skin-eye syndrome has also been recognized as a side effect following long-term treatment with certain phenothiazines. This reaction is marked by progressive pigmentation of areas of the skin or conjunctiva and/or accompanied by discoloration of the exposed sclera and cornea. Opacities of the anterior lens and cornea described as irregular or stellate in shape have also been reported.

Drug Interactions: Phenothiazines are capable of potentiating CNS depressants (e.g., anesthetics, opiates, alcohol, etc.) as well as atropine and phosphorous insecticides.

Phenothiazines may induce a reversed epinephrine effect on occasion.

Dosage and Administration:
Adult: Usual daily dose range is 10 mg to 30 mg.
Oral: One tablet, one to three times daily.
Intramuscular: 2 ml IM, one to three times daily. (See Precautions.)
Suppository: Insert one suppository, one to three times daily.
Children: Appropriate dosage of Torecan, brand of thiethylperazine, has not been determined in children.

How Supplied:
Tablets: Each tablet contains 10 mg thiethylperazine maleate, USP, bottles of 100.
Ampuls: Each 2 ml ampul contains in aqueous solution 10 mg thiethylperazine malate, USP; sodium metabisulfite, 0.5 mg; ascorbic acid, USP, 2.0 mg; sorbitol, NF, 40.0 mg; carbon dioxide gas q.s.; water for injection, USP, q.s. Boxes of 20 and 100.
Storage: Below 86° F; light-resistant container.
Administer only if clear and colorless.
Suppositories: Each containing 10 mg thiethylperazine maleate, USP and inactive ingredient —cocoa butter, NF; packages of 12.
Storage: Below 77° F; tight container (sealed foil).
TOR-Z17 (7/82)
Shown in Product Identification Section, page 406

Boots Pharmaceuticals, Inc.
6540 LINE AVENUE
SHREVEPORT, LA 71106 U.S.A.

PRODUCT INFORMATION WAS PREPARED IN AUGUST, 1984. FOR FURTHER INFORMATION ON THESE AND OTHER BOOTS PRODUCTS CONTACT YOUR BOOTS REPRESENTATIVE OR WRITE BOOTS PHARMACEUTICALS, INC., P. O. BOX 6750, SHREVEPORT, LA 71106.

REFORMULATED F-E-P CREME®
[f-e-p krēm]

Description: F-E-P Creme is a topical preparation containing Hydrocortisone acetate 1.0% and Pramoxine hydrochloride 1.0% in a hydrophilic cream base containing stearic acid, cetyl alcohol, aquaphor, isopropylpalmitate, polyoxyl-40-stearate, propylene glycol, potassium sorbate 0.1%, sorbic acid 0.1%, triethanolamine lauryl sulfate and water.

Topical corticosteroids are anti-inflammatory and anti-pruritic agents. The chemical structural formulas for active ingredients are presented below.

Hydrocortisone acetate
(Pregn-4-ene-3,20-dione,21-(acetyloxy)-11,17-dihydroxy-,(11β)-.

Pramoxine Hydrochloride
(4(3-(p-butyoxyphenoxyl))-propyl-morpholine hydrochloride.)

Clinical Pharmacology: Topical corticosteroids share anti-inflammatory, antipruritic and vasoconstrictive actions.

The mechanism of anti-inflammatory activity of the topical corticosteroids is unclear. Various laboratory methods, including vasoconstrictor assays, are used to compare and predict potencies and/or clinical efficacies of the topical corticosteroids. There is some evidence to suggest that a recognizable correlation exists between vasoconstrictor potency and therapeutic efficacy in humans.

Pramoxine hydrochloride is a topical anesthetic agent which provides temporary relief from itching and pain. It acts by stabilizing the neuronal membrane of nerve endings with which it comes into contact.

Pharmacokinetics: The extent of percutaneous absorption of topical corticosteroids is determined by many factors including the vehicle, the integrity of the epidermal barrier, and the use of occlusive dressings.

Topical corticosteroids can be absorbed from normal intact skin. Inflammation and/or other disease processes in the skin increase percutaneous absorption. Occlusive dressings substantially increase the percutaneous absorption of topical corticosteroids. Thus, occlusive dressings may be a valuable therapeutic adjunct for treatment of resistant dermatoses. (See **Dosage and Administration**).

Once absorbed through the skin, topical corticosteroids are handled through pharmacokinetic pathways similar to systemically administered corticosteroids. Corticosteroids are bound to plasma proteins in varying degrees. Corticosteroids are metabolized primarily in the liver and are then excreted by the kidneys. Some of the topical corticosteroids and their metabolites are also excreted into the bile.

Indications and Usage: Topical corticosteroids are indicated for the relief of the inflammatory and pruritic manifestations of corticosteroid-responsive dermatoses.

Contraindications: Topical corticosteroids are contraindicated in those patients with a history of hypersensitivity to any of the components of the preparation.

Precautions:
General: Systemic absorption of topical corticosteroids has produced reversible hypothalmic-pituitary-adrenal (HPA) axis suppression, manifestations of Cushing's syndrome, hyperglycemia, and glucosuria in some patients.

Conditions which augment systemic absorption include the applications of the more potent steroids, use over large surface areas, prolonged use, and the addition of occlusive dressings.

Therefore patients receiving a large dose of a potent topical steroid applied to a large surface area and under an occlusive dressing should be evaluated periodically for evidence of HPA axis suppression by using the urinary free cortisol and ACTH stimulation tests. If HPA axis suppression is noted, an attempt should be made to withdraw the drug, to reduce the frequency of application, or to substitute a less potent steroid.

Recovery of HPA axis function is generally prompt and complete upon discontinuation of the drug. Infrequently, signs and symptoms of steroid withdrawal may occur, requiring supplemental systemic corticosteroids.

Children may absorb proportionally large amounts of topical corticosteroids and thus be more susceptible to systemic toxicity. (See

Precautions—Pediatric Use).
If irritation develops, topical corticosteroids should be discontinued and appropriate therapy instituted.

In the presence of dermatological infections, the use of an appropriate antifungal or antibacterial agent should be instituted. If a favorable response does not occur promptly, the corticosteroid should

Continued on next page

Boots—Cont.

be discontinued until the infection has been adequately controlled.

Information for the Patient: Patients using topical corticosteroids should receive the following information and instructions:

1. This medication is to be used as directed by the physician. It is for external use only. Avoid contact with the eyes.
2. Patients should be advised not to use this medication for any disorder other than for which it was prescribed.
3. The treated skin area should not be bandaged or otherwise covered or wrapped as to be occlusive unless directed by the physician.
4. Patients should report any signs of adverse local reactions, especially under occlusive dressing.
5. Parents of pediatric patients should be advised not to use tightfitting diapers or plastic pants on a child being treated in the diaper area, as these garments may constitute occlusive dressings.

Laboratory Tests: The following tests may be helpful in evaluating the HPA axis suppression.
Urinary free cortisol test
ACTH stimulation test

Carcinogenesis, Mutagenesis, and Impairment of Fertility: Long-term animal studies have not been performed to evaluate the carcinogenic potential or the effect on fertility of topical corticosteroids. Studies to determine mutagenicity with prednisolone and hydrocortisone have revealed negative results.

Pregnancy Category C: Corticosteroids are generally teratogenic in laboratory animals when administered systemically at relatively low dosage levels. The more potent corticosteroids have been shown to be teratogenic after dermal application in laboratory animals. There are no adequate and well-controlled studies in pregnant women on teratogenic effects from topically applied corticosteroids. Therefore, topical corticosteroids should be used in pregnancy only if the potential benefit justifies the potential risk to the fetus. Drugs of this class should not be used extensively on pregnant patients, in large amounts, or for prolonged periods of time.

Nursing Mothers: It is not known whether topical administration of corticosteroids could result in sufficient systemic absorption to produce detectable amounts in breast milk. Systemically administered corticosteroids are secreted into breast milk in quantities NOT likely to have a deleterious effect on the infant. Nevertheless, caution should be exercised when topical corticosteroids are administered to a nursing woman.

Pediatric Use: Pediatric patients may demonstrate greater susceptibiliy to topical corticosteroid-induced HPA axis suppression and Cushing's syndrome than mature patients because of a larger skin surface area to body weight ratio. Hypothalmic-pituitary-adrenal (HPA) axis suppression, Cushing's syndrome, and intracranial hypertension have been reported in children receiving topical corticosteroids. Manifestations of adrenal suppression in children include linear growth retardation delayed weight gain, low plasma cortisol levels, and absence of response to ACTH stimulation. Manifestations of intracranial hypertension include bulging fontanelles, headaches, and bilateral papilledema.

Administration of topical corticosteroids to children should be limited to the least amount compatible with an effective therapeutic regimen. Chronic corticosteroid therapy may intefere with the growth and development of children.

Adverse Reactions: The following local adverse reactions are reported infrequently with topical corticosteroids, but may occur more frequently with the use of occlusive dressings. These reactions are listed in an approximate decreasing order of occurrence.

Burning
Itching
Irritation
Dryness
Folliculitis
Hypertrichosis
Acneiform eruptions
Hypopigmentation
Perioral dermatitis
Allergic contact dermatitis
Maceration of the skin
Secondary infection
Skin atrophy
Striae
Miliaria

Overdosage: Topically applied corticosteroids can be absorbed in sufficient amounts to produce systemic effects (See **Precautions**).

Dosage and Administration: Topical corticosteroids are generally applied to the affected area as a thin film 3–4 times daily depending on the severity of the condition.

Occlusive dressings may be used for the management of psoriasis or recalcitrant conditions.

If an infection develops, the use of occlusive dressings should be discontinued and appropriate antimicrobial therapy instituted.

How Supplied: ½ oz. (15 gm) tubes NDC 0524-2026-51

Caution: Federal law prohibits dispensng without prescription.

Manufactured by:
Ferndale Laboratories, Inc.
Ferndale, Michigan 48220

Distributed by:
Boots Pharmaceuticals, Inc.
Shreveport, Louisiana 71106 U.S.A.

LOPURIN®
[lō-pyoor-ĭn]
Allopurinol Tablets, USP

Description: LOPURIN® (Allopurinol U.S.P. in tablet form) is an orally administered xanthine oxidase inhibitor, with the chemical name 4-hydroxypyrazolo (3, 4-d) pyrimidine (HPP) (also described in U.S.P. XX as 1H-Pyrazolo (3, 4-d) pyrimidin-4-ol). The structural formula of allopurinol follows:

Clinical Pharmacology: Allopurinol acts on purine catabolism, without disrupting the biosynthesis of vital purines, thus reducing the production of uric acid by inhibiting the biochemical reactions immediately preceding its formation. Its action differs from that of uricosuric agents, which lower the serum uric acid level by increasing urinary excretion of uric acid. Allopurinol reduces both the serum and urinary uric acid levels by inhibiting the formation of uric acid. It thereby avoids the hazard of increased hyperuricosuria in patients with gouty nephropathy or with a predisposition to the formation of uric acid stones.

Allopurinol has produced a substantial reduction in serum and urinary uric acid levels in hitherto refractory patients even in the presence of renal damage marked enough to render uricosuric drugs virtually ineffective. Salicylates may be given conjointly for their antirheumatic effect without compromising the action of allopurinol. This is in contrast to the nullifying effect of salicylates on uricosuric drugs.

Allopurinol is a structural analogue of the natural purine base, hypoxanthine. It is a potent inhibitor of xanthine oxidase, the enzyme responsible for the conversion of hypoxanthine to xanthine and of xanthine to uric acid, the end product of purine metabolism in man. Allopurinol is metabolized to the corresponding xanthine analogue, oxipurinol (alloxanthine), which also is an inhibitor of xanthine oxidase.

Hyperuricemia may be primary, as in gout, or secondary to diseases such as acute and chronic leukemia, polycythemia vera, multiple myeloma, and psoriasis. It may occur with the use of diuretic agents, during renal dialysis, in the presence of renal damage, during starvation or reducing diets and in the treatment of neoplastic disease where rapid resolution of tissue masses may occur.

The major disease manifestations of gout—kidney stones, tophi in soft tissues, and deposits in joints and bones—result from the deposition of urates. If progressive deposition of urates is to be arrested or reversed, it is necessary to reduce the serum uric acid to a level below the saturation point to suppress urate precipitation. Reduction may be achieved by means of uricosuric agents. Uricosurics are less effective in the presence of renal disease, and some patients develop intolerance or sensitivity to these drugs. The use of allopurinol to block the formation of urate avoids the hazard of increased renal excretion of uric acid posed by uricosuric drugs.

The half-life of allopurinol in the body is determined both by renal excretion and by oxidation to 4, 6-dihydroxypyrazolo (3, 4-d) pyrimidine (oxipurinol). The latter is also an inhibitor of xanthine oxidase, but is somewhat weaker than allopurinol which is bound 15-fold more tightly to the enzyme than is the natural substrate, xanthine. The long half-life of oxipurinol in the plasma (18 to 30 hours), contributes significantly to the enzyme inhibition. Moreover, both allopurinol and oxipurinol tend to inactivate xanthine oxidase, thereby further controlling the level of its activity. Administration of allopurinol generally results in a fall in both serum and urinary uric acid within two to three days. The magnitude of this decrease can be manipulated almost at will since it is dose-dependent. A week or more of treatment with allopurinol may be required for the full effects of the drug to be manifest; likewise, uric acid may return to pretreatment levels slowly, usually after a period of 7 to 10 days following cessation of therapy. This reflects primarily the accumulation and slow clearance of oxipurinol. In some patients, particularly those with severe tophaceous gout and underexcretors, a dramatic fall in urinary uric acid excretion may not occur. It has been postulated that this may be due to the mobilization of urate from the tissue deposits as the serum uric acid level begins to fall.

The combined increase in hypoxanthine and xanthine excreted in the urine usually, but not always, is considerably less than the accompanying decline in urinary uric acid.

It has been shown that reutilization of both hypoxanthine and xanthine for nucleotide and nucleic acid synthesis is markedly enhanced when their oxidations are inhibited by allopurinol. This reutilization and the expected feedback inhibition which would result from an increase in available purine nucleotides serves to regulate purine biosynthesis, returning uric acid homeostasis to normal.

Primary deficiency of xanthine oxidase, which occurs in congenital xanthinuria as an inborn error of metabolism, has been shown to be compatible with normal health. While urinary levels of oxypurines attained with full doses of allopurinol may in exceptional cases equal those (250–600 mg per day) which in xanthinuric subjects have caused formation of urinary calculi, they usually fall in the range of 50–200 mg. Xanthine crystalluria has been reported in a few exceptional cases. Two of these had Lesch-Nyhan syndrome, which is characterized by excessive uric acid production combined with a deficiency in the enzyme, hypoxanthine-guanine phosphoribosyltransferase (HGPRTase). This enzyme is required for the conversion of hypoxanthine and guanine to their respective nucleotides. The third case occurred in a patient with lymphosarcoma, who produced an extremely large amount of uric acid because of rapid cell lysis during chemotherapy.

The serum concentration of oxypurines in patients receiving allopurinol is usually in the range of 0.3 mg to 0.4 mg percent compared to a normal level of approximately 0.15 mg percent. A maximum of 0.9 mg percent was observed when the serum urate was lowered to less than 2 mg percent by high doses of the drug. In one exceptional case a value of 2.7 mg percent was reached. These are far below the saturation level at which precipitation of xanthine or hypoxanthine would be expected to occur. The solubilities of uric acid and xanthine in the serum are similar (about 7 mg percent) while hypoxanthine is much more soluble. The finding that the renal clearance of oxypurines is at least 10 times greater than that of uric acid explains the relatively low serum oxypurine concentration at a time when the serum uric acid level has decreased markedly. At serum oxypurine levels of 0.3 mg to 0.9 mg percent, oxypurine: inulin clearance ratios were reported between 0.7 and 1.9. The glomerular filtration rate and urate clearance in patients receiving allopurinol do not differ significantly from those obtained prior to therapy. The rapid renal clearance of oxypurines suggests that allopurinol therapy should be of value in allowing a patient with gout to increase his total purine excretion.

Although the renal clearance of allopurinol is rapid, that of oxipurinol is slow and parallels that of uric acid but is higher by a factor of about three. The clearance of oxipurinol is increased by uricosuric drugs, and as a consequence, the addition of a uricosuric agent may reduce the degree of inhibition of xanthine oxidase by oxipurinol. However, such combined therapy may be useful in achieving minimum serum uric acid levels provided the total urinary uric acid load does not exceed the ability of the patients kidney to excrete it. In some patients, where renal function is severely impaired, normal serum urate levels may not be achievable.

The danger of uric acid calculi is diminished as the uric acid excretion is reduced. The amounts of xanthine and hypoxanthine excreted in the urine generally do not exceed the solubilities of these compounds in the urine, particularly if the urine is slightly alkaline. The amounts of allopurinol and oxipurinol excreted are likewise within the limits of their respective solubilities.

Allopurinol also inhibits the enzymatic oxidation of mercaptopurine, the sulfur-containing analogue of hypoxanthine, to 6-thiouric acid. This oxidation, which is catalyzed by xanthine oxidase, inactivates mercaptopurine. Hence, the inhibition of such oxidation by allopurinol may result in as much as 75 percent reduction in the therapeutic dose requirement of mercaptopurine when the two compounds are given together.

Indications and Use: This is not an innocuous drug and strict attention should be given to the indications for its use. Pending further investigation, its use in other hyperuricemic states is not indicated at this time.

Allopurinol is intended for:
1. treatment of gout, either primary, or secondary to the hyperuricemia associated with blood dyscrasias and their therapy;
2. treatment of primary or secondary uric acid nephropathy, with or without accompanying symptoms of gout;
3. treatment of patients with recurrent uric acid stone formation;
4. prophylactic treatment to prevent tissue urate deposition, renal calculi, or uric acid nephropathy in patients with leukemias, lymphomas and malignancies who are receiving cancer chemotherapy with its resultant elevating effect on serum uric acid levels.

Allopurinol, by promoting the resolution of tophi and urate crystals in the tissues, has relieved chronic joint pain, increased joint mobility and permitted urate sinuses to heal. The addition of allopurinol to a uricosuric regimen has reduced the size of tophi which have been refractory to uricosuric agents alone and increased joint mobility.

Allopurinol is particularly effective in preventing the occurrence and recurrence of uric acid stones and gravel. Allopurinol is useful in therapy and prophylaxis of acute urate nephropathy in patients with neoplastic disease who are particularly susceptible to hyperuricemia and uric acid stone formation, especially after radiation therapy or the use of antineoplastic drugs.

Contraindications: Pending further investigation this drug is contraindicated for use in children with the exception of those with hyperuricemia secondary to malignancy. The drug should not be employed in nursing mothers.

Patients who have developed a severe reaction to allopurinol should not be restarted on the drug.

Warnings: ALLOPURINOL SHOULD BE DISCONTINUED AT THE FIRST APPEARANCE OF SKIN RASH OR ANY SIGN OF ADVERSE REACTION. In some instances a skin rash may be followed by more severe hypersensitivity reactions such as exfoliative, urticarial and purpuric lesions as well as Stevens-Johnson syndrome (erythema multiforme) and very rarely a generalized vasculitis which may lead to irreversible hepatotoxicity and death.

A few cases of reversible clinical hepatotoxicity have been noted in patients taking allopurinol and in some patients asymptomatic rises in serum alkaline phosphatase or serum transaminase have been observed. Accordingly, periodic liver function tests should be performed during the early stages of therapy, particularly in patients with pre-existing liver disease.

Due to the occasional occurrence of drowsiness, patients should be alerted to the need for due precautions when engaging in activities where alertness is mandatory.

An increase in hepatic iron concentration has been reported in rats given allopurinol. However, laboratory experiments of several investigators show no effect of allopurinol on iron metabolism. Nevertheless, iron salts should not be given simultaneously with allopurinol. This drug should not be administered to immediate relatives of patients with idiopathic hemochromatosis.

In patients receiving mercaptopurine or azathioprine the concomitant administration of 300-600 mg of allopurinol per day will require a reduction in dose to approximately one-third to one-fourth of the usual dose of mercaptopurine or azathioprine. Subsequent adjustment of doses of mercaptopurine or azathioprine should be made on the basis of therapeutic response and any toxic effects.

USAGE IN PREGNANCY AND WOMEN OF CHILDBEARING AGE: Reproductive studies showed no adverse effect of allopurinol on animal litters.

However, since the effect of xanthine oxidase inhibition on the human fetus is still unknown, allopurinol should be used in pregnant women or women of childbearing age only if the potential benefits to the patient are weighed against the possible risk to the fetus.

Precautions: Some investigators have reported an increase in acute attacks of gout during the early stages of allopurinol administration, even when normal or subnormal serum uric acid levels have been attained. Accordingly, maintenance doses of colchicine (0.5 mg twice daily) generally should be given prophylactically when allopurinol is begun. In addition, it is recommended that the patient start with a low dose of allopurinol (100 mg daily) and increase at weekly intervals by 100 mg until a serum uric acid level of 6 mg per 100 ml or less is attained but without exceeding the maximal recommended dose. The use of therapeutic doses of colchicine or anti-inflammatory agents may be required to suppress attacks in some cases. The attacks usually become shorter and less severe after several months of therapy. A possible explanation for these flare-ups may be the mobilization of urates from tissue deposits followed by recrystallization, due to fluctuation in the serum uric acid level. Even with adequate therapy it may require several months to deplete the uric acid pool sufficiently to achieve control of the acute episodes.

The concomitant administration of a uricosuric agent with allopurinol may result in a decrease in urinary excretion of oxypurines as compared to their excretion with allopurinol alone. This may possibly be due to an increased excretion of oxipurinol and a lowering of the degree of inhibition of xanthine oxidase. Such combined therapy is not contraindicated, however, and for many patients, may provide optimum control. A report by Goldfinger, et al on a patient treated with sulfinpyrazone and salicylates in addition to allopurinol showed a marked decrease in the excretion of oxypurines which they suggested was due to interference with their clearance at the renal tubular level. However, subsequent studies have indicated no interference with oxypurine clearance by salicylates. Although clinical evidence to date has not demonstrated renal precipitation of oxypurines in patients either on allopurinol alone or in combination with uricosuric agents, the possibility should be kept in mind.

It has been reported that allopurinol prolongs the half-life of the anticoagulant, dicumarol. The clinical significance of this has not been established, but this interaction should be kept in mind when allopurinol is given to patients already on anticoagulant therapy, and the coagulation time should be reassessed.

A fluid intake sufficient to yield a daily urinary output of at least 2 liters and the maintenance of a neutral or, preferably, slightly alkaline urine are desirable to (1) avoid the theoretic possibility of formation of xanthine calculi under the influence of allopurinol therapy and (2) help prevent renal precipitation of urates in patients receiving concomitant uricosuric agents.

A few patients with pre-existing renal disease or poor urate clearance have shown a rise in BUN during allopurinol administration although a decrease in BUN has also been observed. Although the relationship of these observations to the drug has not been established, patients with impaired renal function require less drug and should be carefully observed during the early stages of allopurinol administration and the drug withdrawn if increased abnormalities in renal function appear. In patients with severely impaired renal function, or decreased urate clearance, the half-life of oxipurinol in the plasma is greatly prolonged. Therefore, a dose of 100 mg per day or 300 mg twice a week, or perhaps less, may be sufficient to maintain adequate xanthine oxidase inhibition to reduce serum urate levels. Such patients should be treated with the lowest effective dose, in order to minimize side effects.

Mild reticulocytosis has appeared in some patients, most of whom were receiving other therapeutic agents, so that significance of this observation is not known.

Periodic determination of liver and kidney function and complete blood counts should be performed especially during the first few months of therapy.

Adverse Reactions:
DERMATOLOGIC: Because in some instances skin rash has been followed by severe hypersensitivity reactions, it is recommended that therapy be discontinued at the first sign of rash or other adverse reaction (see WARNINGS).

Skin rash, usually maculopapular, is the adverse reaction most commonly reported.

Exfoliative, urticarial and purpuric lesions, Stevens-Johnson syndrome (erythema multiforme) and toxic epidermal necrolysis have also been reported.

A few cases of alopecia with and without accompanying dermatitis have been reported.

In some patients with a rash, restarting allopurinol therapy at lower doses has been accomplished without untoward incident.

Continued on next page

Boots—Cont.

GASTROINTESTINAL: Nausea, vomiting, diarrhea, and intermittent abdominal pain have been reported.
VASCULAR: There have been rare instances of a generalized hypersensitivity vasculitis or necrotizing angiitis which have led to irreversible hepatotoxicity and death.
HEMATOPOIETIC: Agranulocytosis, anemia, aplastic anemia, bone marrow depression, leukopenia, pancytopenia and thrombocytopenia have been reported in patients, most of whom received concomitant drugs with potential for causing these reactions. Allopurinol has been neither implicated nor excluded as a cause of these reactions.
NEUROLOGIC: There have been a few reports of peripheral neuritis occurring while patients were taking allopurinol. Drowsiness has also been reported in a few patients.
OPHTHALMIC: There have been a few reports of cataracts found in patients receiving allopurinol. It is not known if the cataracts predated the allopurinol therapy. "Toxic" cataracts were reported in one patient who also received an anti-inflammatory agent; again, the time of onset is unknown. In a group of patients followed by Gutman and Yu for up to five years on allopurinol therapy, no evidence of ophthalmologic effect attributable to allopurinol was reported.
DRUG IDIOSYNCRASY: Symptoms suggestive of drug idiosyncrasy have been reported in a few patients. This was characterized by fever, chills, leukopenia or leukocytosis, eosinophilia, arthralgias, skin rash, pruritus, nausea, and vomiting.
Overdosage: Massive overdosing, or acute poisoning, by allopurinol has not been reported.
Dosage and Administration: The dosage of allopurinol to accomplish full control of gout and to lower serum uric acid to normal or near-normal levels varies with the severity of the disease. The average is 200 to 300 mg per day for patients with mild gout and 400 to 600 mg per day for those with moderately severe tophaceous gout. The appropriate dosage may be administered in divided doses or as a single equivalent dose with the 300 mg tablet. Dosage requirements in excess of 300 mg should be supplemented in divided doses. It should also be noted that allopurinol is generally better tolerated if taken following meals. Similar considerations govern the regulation of dosage for maintenance purposes in secondary hyperuricemia. For the prevention of uric acid nephropathy during the vigorous therapy of neoplastic disease, treatment with 600 to 800 mg daily for two to three days is advisable together with a high fluid intake. The minimal effective dosage is 100 to 200 mg daily and the maximal recommended dosage is 800 mg daily. To reduce the possibility of flare-up of acute gouty attacks, it is recommended that the patient start with a low dose of allopurinol (100 mg daily) and increase at weekly intervals by 100 mg until a serum uric acid level of 6 mg per 100 ml or less is attained but without exceeding the maximal recommended dosage.
Normal serum urate levels are achieved in one to three weeks. The upper limit of normal is about 7 mg percent for men and postmenopausal women and 6 mg percent for premenopausal women. Too much reliance should not be placed on a single reading since, for technical reasons, estimation of uric acid may be difficult. By the selection of the appropriate dose, together with the use of uricosuric agents in certain patients, it is possible to reduce the serum uric acid level to normal and, if desired, to hold it as low as 2 to 3 mg percent indefinitely.
A fluid intake sufficient to yield a daily urinary output of at least 2 liters and the maintenance of a neutral or, preferably, slightly alkaline urine are desirable.
Since allopurinol and its metabolites are excreted only by the kidney, accumulation of the drug can occur in renal failure, and the dose of allopurinol should consequently be reduced. With a creatinine clearance of 20 to 10 ml/min, a daily dosage of 200 mg of allopurinol is suitable. When the creatinine clearance is less than 10 ml/min the daily dosage should not exceed 100 mg. With extreme renal impairment (creatinine clearance less than 3 ml/min) the interval between doses may also need to be lengthened.
The correct size and frequency of dosage for maintaining the serum uric acid just within the normal range is best determined by using the serum uric acid level as an index.
Children, 6 to 10 years of age, with secondary hyperuricemia associated with malignancies may be given 300 mg allopurinol daily while those under 6 years are generally given 150 mg daily. The response is evaluated after approximately 48 hours of therapy and a dosage adjustment is made if necessary.
In patients who are being treated with colchicine and/or anti-inflammatory agents, it is wise to continue this therapy while adjusting the dosage of allopurinol, until a normal serum uric acid and freedom from acute attacks have been maintained for several months.
In transferring a patient from a uricosuric agent to allopurinol, the dose of the uricosuric agent should be gradually reduced over a period of several weeks and the dose of allopurinol gradually increased to the required dose needed to maintain a normal serum uric acid level.
How Supplied: LOPURIN®:
100 mg (white) scored tablets, imprinted BOOTS/0051, unit dose, cartons of 100—NDC 0524-0051-61, bottles of 100—NDC 0524-0051-01, bottles of 1000—NDC 0524-0051-10.
300 mg (peach) scored tablets, imprinted BOOTS/0052, unit dose, cartons of 100—NDC 0524-0052-61 bottles of 30—NDC 0524-0052-30, bottles of 100—NDC 0524-0052-01, bottles of 500—NDC 0524-0052-05.
Animal Toxicology: In mice the LD50 is 160 mg/kg ip (with deaths delayed up to five days) and 700 mg/kg po (with deaths delayed up to three days). In rats the acute LD50 is 750 mg/kg ip >6000 mg/kg po.
In a 13 week feeding experiment in rats at a drug level of 72 mg/kg per day 2 of 10 rats died and at 225 mg/kg per day 4 of 10 died before the completion of the experiment. Both groups exhibited renal tubular damage due to the deposition of xanthine that was more extensive at the higher dose.
In chronic feeding experiments, rats showed no toxic effects at a level of 14 mg/kg per day after one year. At a level of 24 mg/kg per day for one year the rats showed very slight depression of weight gain and food intake, and 5 out of 10 of the animals showed minor changes in the kidney tubules of the type exhibited by the rats on the higher doses described above.
Dogs survived oral doses of 30 mg/kg per day for one year with nil to minor changes in the kidney and no other significant abnormalities. At 90 mg/kg per day for one year there was some accumulation of xanthine in the kidneys with resultant chronic irritation and slight tubular changes. Occasional hemosiderin-like deposits were seen in the reticuloendothelial system. A higher dose (270 mg/kg per day) resulted in large concretions in the renal pelves, with severe destructive changes in the kidney secondary to xanthine accumulation. The deposition of xanthine appears to be a function both of the metabolic turnover of purines (which is proportionately larger in the smaller animals) and the degree of inhibition of xanthine oxidase.
Reproductive studies in rats and rabbits indicated that allopurinol did not affect litter size, the mean weight of the progeny at birth or at three weeks postpartum, nor did it cause an increase in the number of animals born dead or with malformations.
Caution: Federal law prohibits dispensing without prescription.

Distributed by
Boots Pharmaceuticals, Inc.
SHREVEPORT, LOUISIANA 71106
Manufactured by
Boots Laboratories, Inc.
Palisades Park, N.J. 07650
Licensed for Use under U.S. Patent No. 3,624,205
Rev. November 1983

RUFEN®
[ōō′fĭn]
(ibuprofen)

Description: Rufen (ibuprofen) is $(\pm)$-2-(p-isobutylphenyl) propionic acid. It is a white powder with a melting point of 74–77°C and is very slightly soluble in water (<1 mg/ml) and readily soluble in organic solvents such as ethanol and acetone.
Its structural formula is:

$$(CH_3)_2CH-CH_2-C_6H_4-CH(CH_3)-COOH$$

Rufen is a nonsteroidal anti-inflammatory agent. It is available in 400 and 600 mg tablets for oral administration.
Clinical Pharmacology: Rufen (ibuprofen) is a nonsteroidal anti-inflammatory agent that possesses analgesic and antipyretic activities. Its mode of action, like that of other nonsteroidal anti-inflammatory agents, is not known; however, its therapeutic action is not due to pituitary-adrenal stimulation. Rufen does not alter the course of the underlying disease.
In patients treated with Rufen for rheumatoid arthritis and osteoarthritis, the anti-inflammatory action of Rufen has been shown by reduction in joint swelling, reduction in pain, reduction in duration of morning stiffness, reduction in disease activity as assessed by both the investigator and patient; and by improved functional capacity as demonstrated by an increase in grip strength, a delay in the time to onset of fatigue, and a decrease in time to walk 50 feet.
In clinical studies in patients with rheumatoid arthritis and osteoarthritis, Rufen has been shown to be comparable to aspirin in controlling the aforementioned signs and symptoms of disease activity and to be associated with a statistically significant reduction in the milder gastrointestinal side effects (see ADVERSE REACTIONS). Rufen may be well tolerated in some patients who have had gastrointestinal side effects with aspirin, but these patients when treated with Rufen should be carefully followed for signs and symptoms of gastrointestinal ulceration and bleeding.
Although it is not definitely known whether ibuprofen causes less peptic ulceration than aspirin, in one study involving 885 patients with rheumatoid arthritis treated for up to one year, there were no reports of gastric ulceration with ibuprofen whereas frank ulceration was reported in 13 patients in the aspirin group (statistically significant $p<.001$).
In clinical studies in patients with rheumatoid arthritis, Rufen has been shown to be comparable to indomethacin in controlling the aforementioned signs and symptoms of disease activity and to be associated with a statistically significant reduction of the milder gastrointestinal (see ADVERSE REACTIONS) and CNS side effects.
Rufen may be used in combination with gold salts and/or corticosteroids. When Rufen and placebo were compared in gold-treated rheumatoid arthritis patients, Rufen was consistently more effective in relieving symptoms than was placebo. However, it cannot be inferred that Rufen potentiates the effect of gold on the underlying disease. Whether or not Rufen can be used in conjunction with partially effective doses of corticosteroid for a "steroid-sparing" effect, and result in greater improvement, has not been adequately studied.
Controlled studies have demonstrated that Rufen is a more effective analgesic than propoxyphene for the relief of episiotomy pain, pain following

dental extraction procedures, and for the relief of the symptoms of primary dysmenorrhea.

In patients with primary dysmenorrhea Rufen has been shown to reduce elevated levels of prostaglandin activity in the menstrual fluid and to reduce resting and active intra-uterine pressure, as well as the frequency of uterine contractions. The probable mechanism of action is to inhibit prostaglandin synthesis rather than simply to provide analgesia.

Rufen is rapidly absorbed when administered orally. Peak serum ibuprofen levels are generally attained one to two hours after administration. With single doses ranging from 200 mg to 800 mg, a dose-response relationship exists between amount of drug administered and the integrated area under the serum drug concentration vs time curve. Above 800 mg, however, the area under the curve increases less than proportional to increases in dose. There is no evidence of drug accumulation or enzyme induction.

The administration of Rufen tablets either under fasting conditions or immediately before meals yields quite similar serum ibuprofen concentration-time profiles. When Rufen is administered immediately after a meal, there is a reduction in the rate of absorption but no appreciable decrease in the extent of absorption. The bioavailability of Rufen is minimally altered by the presence of food. Rufen is rapidly metabolized and eliminated in the urine. The excretion of Rufen is virtually complete 24 hours after the last dose. The serum half-life of Rufen is 1.8 to 2.0 hours.

Studies have shown that following ingestion of the drug 45% to 79% of the dose was recovered in the urine within 24 hours as metabolite A (25%), (+)-2-[p-(2hydroxymethylpropyl)phenyl] propionic acid and metabolite B(37%), (+)-2-[p-(2carboxypropyl)-phenyl] propionic acid, the percentages of free and conjugated ibuprofen were approximately 1% and 14%, respectively.

Indications and Usage: Rufen (ibuprofen) is indicated for relief of the signs and symptoms of rheumatoid arthritis and osteoarthritis. It is indicated in the treatment of acute flares and in the long-term management of these diseases.

Rufen is indicated for the relief of mild to moderate pain.

Rufen is also indicated for the treatment of primary dysmenorrhea.

Since there have been no controlled trials to demonstrate whether or not there is any beneficial effect or harmful interaction with the use of Rufen in conjunction with aspirin, the combination cannot be recommended (see **Drug Interactions**).

Controlled clinical trials to establish the safety and effectiveness of Rufen in children have not been conducted.

Contraindications: Rufen (ibuprofen) should not be used in patients who have previously exhibited hypersensitivity to it, or in individuals with the syndrome of nasal polyps, angioedema and bronchospastic reactivity to aspirin or other nonsteroidal anti-inflammatory agents (see WARNINGS).

Warnings: Anaphylactoid reactions have occurred in patients with known aspirin hypersensitivity (see CONTRAINDICATIONS).

Peptic ulceration and gastrointestinal bleeding, sometimes severe, have been reported in patients receiving Rufen (ibuprofen). Peptic ulceration, perforation, or severe gastrointestinal bleeding can have a fatal outcome, and although a few such reports have been received with ibuprofen, a cause and effect relationship has not been established. Rufen should be given under close supervision to patients with a history of upper gastrointestinal tract disease, and only after consulting the ADVERSE REACTIONS section.

In patients with active peptic ulcer and active rheumatoid arthritis, attempts should be made to treat the arthritis with nonulcerogenic drugs, such as gold. If Rufen must be given, the patient should be under close supervision for signs of ulcer perforation or gastrointestinal bleeding.

As with other nonsteroidal anti-inflammatory agents, chronic studies in rats and monkeys have shown histologic evidence of mild renal toxicity as demonstrated by papillary edema and papillary necrosis, in some animals. Renal papillary necrosis has been rarely reported in humans in association with Rufen treatment.

Precautions: Blurred and/or diminished vision, scotomata, and/or changes in color vision have been reported. If a patient develops such complaints while receiving Rufen (ibuprofen), the drug should be discontinued and the patient should have an ophthalmologic examination which includes central visual fields and color vision testing. Fluid retention and edema have been reported in association with Rufen; therefore, the drug should be used with caution in patients with a history of cardiac decompensation or hypertension.

As with other nonsteroidal anti-inflammatory drugs, borderline elevations of one or more liver tests may occur in up to 15% of patients. These abnormalities may progress, may remain essentially unchanged, or may be transient with continued therapy. The SGPT (ALT) test is probably the most sensitive indicator of liver dysfunction. Meaningful (3 times the upper limit of normal) elevations of SGPT or SGOT (AST) occurred in controlled clinical trials in less than 1% of patients. A patient with symptoms and/or signs suggesting liver dysfunction, or in whom an abnormal liver test has occurred, should be evaluated for evidence of the development of more severe hepatic reaction while on therapy with Rufen. Severe hepatic reactions, including jaundice and cases of fatal hepatitis, have been reported with ibuprofen as with other nonsteroidal anti-inflammatory drugs. Although such reactions are rare, if abnormal liver tests persist or worsen, if clinical signs and symptoms consistent with liver disease develop, or if systemic manifestations occur (e.g. eosinophilia, rash, etc.), Rufen should be discontinued.

Since Rufen is eliminated primarily by the kidneys, patients with significantly impaired renal function should be closely monitored and a reduction in dosage should be anticipated to avoid drug accumulation. Prospective studies on the safety of Rufen in patients with chronic renal failure have not been conducted.

Rufen, like other nonsteroidal anti-inflammatory agents, can inhibit platelet aggregation but the effect is quantitatively less and of shorter duration than that seen with aspirin. Ibuprofen has been shown to prolong bleeding time (but within the normal range) in normal subjects. Because this prolonged bleeding effect may be exaggerated in patients with underlying hemostatic defects, Rufen should be used with caution in persons with intrinsic coagulation defects and those on anticoagulant therapy.

Patients on Rufen should report to their physicians signs or symptoms of gastrointestinal ulceration or bleeding, blurred vision or other eye symptoms, skin rash, weight gain, or edema.

In order to avoid exacerbation of disease or adrenal insufficiency, patients who have been on prolonged corticosteroid therapy should have their therapy tapered slowly rather than discontinued abruptly when Rufen is added to the treatment program.

The antipyretic and anti-inflammatory activity of ibuprofen may reduce fever and inflammation, thus diminishing their utility as diagnostic signs in detecting complications of presumed noninfectious, noninflammatory painful conditions.

Drug-Interactions: *Coumarin-type anticoagulants.* Several short-term controlled studies failed to show that Rufen significantly affected prothrombin times or a variety of other clotting factors when administered to individuals on coumarin-type anticoagulants. However, because bleeding has been reported when Rufen and other nonsteroidal anti-inflammatory agents have been administered to patients on coumarin-type anticoagulants, the physician should be cautious when administering Rufen to patients on anticoagulants.

Aspirin. Animal studies show that aspirin given with nonsteroidal anti-inflammatory agents, including Rufen, yields a net decrease in anti-inflammatory activity with lowered blood levels of the non-aspirin drug. Single dose bioavailability studies in normal volunteers have failed to show an effect of aspirin on ibuprofen blood levels. Correlative clinical studies have not been done.

Pregnancy: Reproductive studies conducted in rats and rabbits at doses somewhat less than the maximal clinical dose did not demonstrate evidence of developmental abnormalities. These data are inadequate to provide reasonable assurance that the drug will not have an adverse effect on the fetus. Rufen (ibuprofen) has been shown to inhibit prostaglandin synthesis and release. The same effect has been demonstrated by other nonsteroidal and anti-inflammatory drugs and has been associated with an increased incidence of dystocia and delayed parturition in pregnant animals when such drugs were administered late in pregnancy. Administration of Rufen is not recommended during pregnancy.

Nursing Mothers: In limited studies, an assay capable of detecting 1 mcg/ml did not demonstrate ibuprofen in the milk of lactating mothers. However, because of the limited nature of the studies and the possible adverse effects of prostaglandin inhibiting drugs on neonates, Rufen is not recommended for use in nursing mothers.

Adverse Reactions: The most frequent type of adverse reaction occurring with Rufen (ibuprofen) is gastrointestinal. In controlled clinical trials the percentage of patients reporting one or more gastrointestinal complaints ranged from 4% to 16%. In controlled studies when ibuprofen was compared to aspirin and indomethacin in equally effective doses, the overall incidence of gastrointestinal complaints was about half that seen in either the aspirin-, or indomethacin-treated patients.

Reactions observed during controlled clinical trials which occurred in more than 1 in 100 patients were:

Incidence greater than 1%

Gastrointestinal: nausea*, epigastric pain*, heartburn*, diarrhea, abdominal distress, nausea and vomiting, indigestion, constipation, abdominal cramps or pain, fullness of the GI tract (bloating and flatulence).

Central Nervous System: dizziness*, headache, nervousness.

Dermatologic: rash* (including maculopapular type), pruritus.

Special Senses: tinnitus.

Metabolic: decreased appetite, edema, fluid retention. Fluid retention generally responds promptly to drug discontinuation (see PRECAUTIONS).

*Reactions occurring in 3% to 9% of patients treated with Rufen. (Those reactions occurring in less than 3% of the patients are unmarked.)

Incidence less than 1%

The following adverse reactions, occurring less frequently than 1 in 100, have been reported in controlled clinical trials and from marketing experience. The probability of a causal relationship exists between Rufen and these adverse reactions:

Gastrointestinal: gastric or duodenal ulcer with bleeding and/or perforation, gastrointestinal hemorrhage, melena, gastritis, hepatitis, jaundice, abnormal liver function tests.

Dermatologic: vesiculobullous eruptions, urticaria, erythema multiforme, Stevens-Johnson syndrome and alopecia.

Central Nervous System: depression, insomnia, confusion, emotional lability, somnolence, aseptic meningitis with fever and coma.

Special Senses: hearing loss, amblyopia (blurred and/or diminished vision), scotomata and/or changes in color vision). [see PRECAUTIONS].

Hematologic: neutropenia, agranulocytosis, aplastic anemia, hemolytic anemia (sometimes Coombs' positive), thrombocytopenia with or without purpura eosinophilia, decreases in hemoglobin and hematocrit.

Cardiovascular: congestive heart failure in patients with marginal cardiac function, elevated blood pressure and palpitations.

Continued on next page

Boots—Cont.

Allergic: syndrome of abdominal pain, fever, chills, nausea and vomiting, anaphylaxis, bronchospasms (see CONTRAINDICATIONS).
Renal: acute renal failure in patients with preexisting significantly impaired renal function, decreased creatinine clearance, polyuria, azotemia, cystitis, hematuria.
Miscellaneous: dry eyes and mouth, gingival ulcers, rhinitis.

Causal relationship unknown

Other reactions have been reported but occurred under circumstances where a causal relationship could not be established. However, in these rarely reported events, the possibility cannot be excluded. Therefore these observations are being listed to serve as alerting information to the physician.
Gastrointestinal: pancreatitis.
Central Nervous System: paresthesias, hallucinations, dream abnormalities, pseudotumor cerebri.
Dermatologic: toxic epidermal necrolysis, photoallergic skin reactions.
Special Senses: conjunctivitis, diplopia, optic neuritis.
Hematologic: bleeding episodes (e.g., epistaxis, menorrhagia).
Allergic: serum sickness, lupus erythematosus syndrome, Henoch-Schonlein vasculitis.
Endocrine: gynecomastia, hypoglycemic reaction.
Cardiovascular: arrhythmias (sinus tachycardia, sinus bradycardia).
Renal: renal papillary necrosis.
Overdosage: Approximately 1½ hours after the reported ingestion of from 7 to 10 ibuprofen tablets (400 mg), a 19-month old child weighing 12 kg was seen in the hospital emergency room, apneic and cyanotic, responding only to painful stimuli. This type of stimulus, however, was sufficient to induce respiration. Oxygen and parenteral fluids were given; a greenish-yellow fluid was aspirated from the stomach with no evidence to indicate the presence of ibuprofen. Two hours after ingestion the child's condition seemed stable; she still responded only to painful stimuli and continued to have periods of apnea lasting from 5 to 10 seconds. She was admitted to intensive care and sodium bicarbonate was administered as well as infusions of dextrose and normal saline. By four hours post-ingestion she could be aroused easily, sit by herself and respond to spoken commands. Blood level of ibuprofen was 102.9 mcg/ml approximately 8½ hours after accidental ingestion. At 12 hours she appeared to be completely recovered. In two other reported cases where children (each weighing approximately 10 kg) had taken six tablets for an estimated acute intake of approximately 120 mg/kg, there were no signs of acute intoxication or late sequelae. Blood level in one child 90 minutes after ingestion was 700 mcg/ml about 10 times the peak levels seen in absorption-excretion studies.

A 19-year old male who had taken 8,000 mg of ibuprofen over a period of a few hours complained of dizziness, and nystagmus was noted. After hospitalization, parenteral hydration and three days bed rest, he recovered with no reported sequelae.
In cases of acute overdosage, the stomach should be emptied by vomiting or lavage, though little drug will likely be recovered if more than an hour has elapsed since ingestion. Because the drug is acidic and is excreted in the urine, it is theoretically beneficial to administer alkali and induce diuresis.

Dosage and Administration: Rheumatoid arthritis and osteoarthritis, including flareups of chronic disease.

Suggested Dosage: 400 mg or 600 mg t.i.d. or q.i.d. The dose of Rufen (ibuprofen) should be tailored to each patient, and may be lowered or raised from the suggested doses depending on the severity of symptoms either at time of initiating drug therapy or as the patient responds or fails to respond.

In general, patients with rheumatoid arthritis seem to require higher doses of Rufen than do patients with osteoarthritis.
The smallest dose of Rufen that yields acceptable control should be employed.
A therapeutic response to Rufen therapy is sometimes seen in a few days to a week but most often is observed by two weeks. After a satisfactory response has been achieved, the patient's dose should be reviewed and adjusted as required.
Dysmenorrhea: For the treatment of dysmenorrhea, beginning with the earliest onset of such pain, Rufen should be given in a dose of 400 mg every 4 hours as necessary.
Mild to moderate pain: 400 mg every 4 to 6 hours as necessary for the relief of pain.
In controlled analgesic clinical trials, doses of Rufen greater than 400 mg were no more effective than the 400 mg dose.
Do not exceed 2,400 mg total daily dose. If gastrointestinal complaints occur, administer Rufen with meals or milk.
How Supplied: Rufen Tablets 400 mg; round magenta sugar-coated tablets printed RUFEN 400.
Bottles of 100   NDC 0524-0039-01
Bottles of 500   NDC 0524-0039-05

Manufactured for
Boots Pharmaceuticals, Inc.
Shreveport, Louisiana 71106, U.S.A.
By
The Boots Company P.L.C.
Nottingham, England

Rufen Tablets 600 mg: oblong white film-coated tablets printed RUFEN 6.
Bottles of 100   NDC 0524-0062-01
Bottles of 500   NDC 0524-0062-05

Manufactured and Distributed by:
Boots Pharmaceuticals, Inc.
Shreveport, Louisiana 71106 U.S.A.
Caution: Federal law prohibits dispensing without prescription. U.S. Patent No. 3,385,886.
Rev. 9/83

RU-TUSS® EXPECTORANT
[rōō′tŭs]

Description: Each fluid ounce of Ru-Tuss Expectorant contains:
Codeine Phosphate .... 59.1 mg
(WARNING: MAY BE HABIT FORMING)
Phenylephrine Hydrochloride .... 30 mg
Chlorpheniramine Maleate .... 12 mg
Ammonium Chloride .... 200 mg
Alcohol 5%
Ru-Tuss Expectorant is an oral antitussive, antihistaminic, nasal decongestant and expectorant preparation.
Actions: CODEINE PHOSPHATE is a well-known, centrally acting antitussive which calms the cough control center and relieves coughing.
CHLORPHENIRAMINE MALEATE is an antihistamine that antagonizes the effect of histamine.
PHENYLEPHRINE HYDROCHLORIDE is a nasal decongestant.
AMMONIUM CHLORIDE is an expectorant that increases mucus flow to help loosen phlegm (sputum).
Indications and Usage: Ru-Tuss Expectorant is indicated for the temporary relief of cough, and for the temporary relief of nasal congestion, due to the common cold.
Drug Interaction Precautions: Do not take this product if you are presently taking a prescription antihypertensive or antidepressant drug containing a monoamine oxidase inhibitor, except under the advice and supervision of a doctor.
Warnings: RU-TUSS Expectorant contains Codeine Phosphate which may cause or aggravate constipation, and may be habit forming.
Do not give RU-TUSS Expectorant to children taking other drugs, or to children under 6 years of age, except under the advice and supervision of a doctor.
Do not take RU-TUSS Expectorant for persistant or chronic cough such as occurs with smoking, asthma, emphysema, or where cough is accompanied by excessive secretions, except under the advice and supervision of a doctor.
A persistent cough may be a sign of a serious condition. If cough persists for more than one week, tends to reoccur or is accompanied by a high fever, rash or persistent headache, consult a doctor.
If your symptoms do not improve within 7 days or are accompanied by high fever, consult a doctor before continuing.
RU-TUSS Expectorant may cause marked drowsiness. Do not drive motor vehicles, operate heavy machinery, or consume alcoholic beverages while taking this product.
Do not take this product if you have asthma, glaucoma, high blood pressure, heart disease, diabetes, thyroid disease, or difficulty in urination due to the enlargement of the prostate gland, except under the advice and supervision of a doctor.
This product may cause excitability, especially in children.
Precautions: This package is not child resistant. Keep this and all medication out of the reach of children.
In case of accidental overdose, seek professional assistance or contact a poison control center immediately.
Dosage and Administration: Adults, 1 or 2 teaspoonfuls, orally, every 4 to 6 hours, not to exceed 10 teaspoonfuls in any 24-hour period.
Children 6 to 12 years of age, ½ teaspoonful-1 teaspoonful every 4 to 6 hours, not to exceed 6 teaspoonfuls in any 24-hour period.
Children under 6 years of age, consult a doctor before using.
How Supplied: Pint bottles (16 fl. oz.). NDC 0524-2010-16

Manufactured and Distributed by
Boots Pharmaceuticals, Inc.
Shreveport, Louisiana 71106 U.S.A.
Rev. 4/83

RU-TUSS® WITH HYDROCODONE
[rōō′tŭs]

Description: Each fluid ounce of Ru-Tuss with Hydrocodone contains:
Hydrocodone Bitartrate .... 10 mg
(Warning: May Be Habit Forming)
Phenylephrine Hydrochloride .... 30 mg
Phenylpropanolamine Hydrochloride .... 20 mg
Pheniramine Maleate .... 20 mg
Pyrilamine Maleate .... 20 mg
Alcohol 5%
Ru-Tuss with Hydrocodone is an oral antitussive, antihistaminic and nasal decongestant preparation.
Indications and Usage: Ru-Tuss with Hydrocodone is indicated for the temporary relief of symptoms associated with hay fever, allergies, nasal congestion and cough due to the common cold.
Contraindications: Hypersensitivity to antihistamines. Concomitant use of an antihypertensive or antidepressant drugs containing a monoamine oxidase inhibitor is contraindicated.
Ru-Tuss with Hydrocodone is contraindicated in patients with glaucoma, bronchial asthma and in women who are pregnant.
Warnings: Patients should be warned of the potential that Ru-Tuss with Hydrocodone may be habit forming.
Ru-Tuss with Hydrocodone may cause drowsiness. Patients should be warned of the possible additive effect caused by taking antihistamines with alcohol, hypnotics, sedatives and tranquilizers.
Precautions: Patients taking Ru-Tuss with Hydrocodone should avoid driving a motor vehicle or operating dangerous machinery (See Warnings).
Caution should be taken with patients having hypertension and cardiovascular disease.
Adverse Reactions: Ru-Tuss with Hydrocodone may cause drowsiness, lassitude, giddiness, dryness of mucous membranes, tightness of the chest, thickening of bronchial secretions, urinary frequency and dysuria, palpitation, tachycardia, hypotension/hypertension, faintness, dizziness, tinnitus, headache, incoordination, visual disturbances, mydriasis, xerostomia, blurred vision, anorexia, nausea, vomiting, diarrhea, constipation,

epigastric distress, hyperirritability, nervousness and insomnia.
Overdoses may cause restlessness, excitation, delirium, tremors, euphoria, stupor, tachycardia and even convulsions.

Dosage and Administration:
Adults: 2 teaspoonfuls, orally, every 4 to 6 hours.
Children 6 to 12 years of age: 1 teaspoonful every 4 to 6 hours.
Children 2 to 6 years of age: 1/2 to 1 teaspoonful ever 4 to 6 hours, according to age. Doses for children should not be repeated more than 4 times in any 24-hour period.

How Supplied:
Pint bottles (16 fl. oz) NDC 0524-1007-16
Federal law prohibits dispensing without prescription.

Manufactured and Distributed by
Boots Pharmaceuticals, Inc.
Shreveport, Louisiana 71106 U.S.A.
Rev. 10/80

RU-TUSS® PLAIN
[rōō′tŭs]

Description: Each fluid ounce of Ru-Tuss Plain contains:
Phenylephrine Hydrochloride .... 30 mg
Chlorpheniramine Maleate .... 12 mg
Alcohol 5%
Ru-Tuss Plain is an oral antihistaminic and nasal decongestant preparation.

Indications and Usage: Ru-Tuss Plain is indicated for the temporary relief of congestion, runny nose, sneezing, itching of nose or throat and itchy or watery eyes due to hay fever or the common cold.

Drug Interaction Precautions: Do not take this product if you are presently taking a prescription antihypertensive or antidepressant drug containing a monoamine oxidase inhibitor, except under the advice and supervision of a doctor.

Warnings: Do not exceed recommended dosage because at higher doses, nervousness, dizziness, or sleeplessness may occur.
If symptoms do not improve within 7 days or are accompanied by a high fever, consult a doctor before continuing use.
Do not take this product if you have high blood pressure, heart disease, diabetes, thyroid disease, asthma, glaucoma, or difficulty in urination due to enlargement of the prostate gland, except under the advice and supervision of a doctor.
May cause drowsiness. Avoid alcoholic beverages, driving a motor vehicle or operating heavy machinery while taking this product.
May cause excitability, especially in children.
Do not give to children under 6 years of age, except under the advice and supervision of a doctor.

Precautions: This package is not child resistant. Keep this and all medications out of reach of children.
In case of accidental overdose, seek professional assistance or contact a poison control center immediately.

Dosage and Administration: Adults, 2 teaspoonfuls, orally, every 4 to 6 hours, not to exceed 6 doses every 24 hours.
Children 6 to 12 years of age, 1 teaspoonful every 4 to 6 hours, not to exceed 6 doses every 24 hours. Children under 6 years of age, consult a doctor before using.

How Supplied: Pint bottles (16 fl. oz.) NDC 0524-1009-16

Manufactured and Distributed by
Boots Pharmaceuticals, Inc.
Shreveport, Louisiana 71106 U.S.A.
Rev. 6/83

RU-TUSS® TABLETS
[rōō′tŭs]

Description: Each prolonged action tablet contains:
Phenylephrine Hydrochloride .... 25 mg
Phenylpropanolamine Hydrochloride .... 50 mg
Chlorpheniramine Maleate .... 8 mg
Hyoscyamine Sulfate .... 0.19 mg
Atropine Sulfate .... 0.04 mg
Scopolamine Hydrobromide .... 0.01 mg
Ru-Tuss Tablets act continuously for 10 to 12 hours.
Ru-Tuss Tablets are an oral antihistaminic, nasal decongestant and anti-secretory preparation.

Indications and Usage: Ru-Tuss Tablets provide relief of the symptoms resulting from irritation of sinus, nasal and upper respiratory tract tissues. Phenylephrine and phenylpropanolamine combine to exert a vasoconstrictive and decongestive action while chlorpheniramine maleate decreases the symptoms of watering eyes, post nasal drip and sneezing which may be associated with an allergic-like response. The belladonna alkaloids, hyoscyamine, atropine and scopolamine further augment the anti-secretory activity of Ru-Tuss Tablets.

Contraindications: Hypersensitivity to antihistamines or sympathomimetics. Ru-Tuss Tablets are contraindicated in children under 12 years of age and in patients with glaucoma, bronchial asthma and women who are pregnant. Concomitant use of MAO inhibitors is contraindicated.

Warnings: Ru-Tuss Tablets may cause drowsiness. Patients should be warned of the possible additive effects caused by taking antihistamines with alcohol, hypnotics, sedatives or tranquilizers.

Precautions: Ru-Tuss Tablets contain belladonna alkaloids, and must be administered with care to those patients with urinary bladder neck obstruction. Caution should be exercised when Ru-Tuss Tablets are given to patients with hypertension, cardiac or peripheral vascular disease or hyperthyroidism. Patients should avoid driving a motor vehicle or operating dangerous machinery (See Warnings:).

Overdosage: Since the action of sustained release products may continue for as long as 12 hours, treatment of overdoses directed at reversing the effects of the drug and supporting the patient should be maintained for at least that length of time. Saline cathartics are useful for hastening evacuation of unreleased medication. In children and infants, antihistamine overdosage may produce convulsions and death.

Adverse Reactions: Hypersensitivity reactions such as rash, urticaria, leukopenia, agranulocytosis, and thrombocytopenia may occur. Other adverse reactions to Ru-Tuss Tablets may be drowsiness, lassitude, giddiness, dryness of the mucous membranes, tightness of the chest, thickening of bronchial secretions, urinary frequency and dysuria, palpitation, tachycardia, hypotension/hypertension, faintness, dizziness, tinnitus, headache, incoordination, visual disturbances, mydriasis, xerostomia, blurred vision, anorexia, nausea, vomiting, diarrhea, constipation, epigastric distress, hyperirritability, nervousness, dizziness and insomnia. Large overdoses may cause tachypnea, delirium, fever, stupor, coma and respiratory failure.

Dosage and Administration: Adults and children over 12 years of age, one tablet morning and evening. Not recommended for children under 12 years of age. Tablets are to be swallowed whole.

How Supplied:
Bottles of 100 Tablets   NDC 0524-0058-01
Bottles of 500 Tablets   NDC 0524-0058-05
Federal law prohibits dispensing without prescription.

Distributed by
Boots Pharmaceuticals, Inc.
Shreveport, Louisiana 71106
Manufactured by
Vitarine Company, Inc.
Springfield Gardens, New York, 11413
September 1981
Shown in Product Identification Section, page 407

RU-TUSS® II CAPSULES
[rōō′tus]

Description: Each sustained release capsule contains 12 mg of Chlorpheniramine Maleate, USP and 75 mg of Phenylpropanolamine Hydrochloride, USP in a base to provide prolonged activity.

CHLORPHENIRAMINE MALEATE
Category: Antihistaminic
Structural Formula:

Molecular Formula: $C_{16}H_{19}ClN_2 \cdot C_4H_4O_4$
Molecular Weight: 390.87
Chemical Name: 2 [p-chloro-a[2-(dimethylamino) ethyl]benzyl] pyridine maleate (1:1).

PHENYLPROPANOLAMINE HYDROCHLORIDE
Category: Adrenergic (vasoconstrictor).
Structural Formula:

Molecular Formula: $C_9H_{13}NO \cdot HCl$
Molecular Weight: 187.67
Chemical name: Benzenemethanol, a-(1-aminoethyl)-,hydrochloride (R*,S*), ($\pm$).

Clinical Pharmacology: Chlorpheniramine Maleate is an antihistamine with anticholinergic (drying) and sedative side effects. Antihistamines appear to compete with histamine for H_1 cell receptor sites on effector cells.
Chlorpheniramine Maleate does not prevent the release of histamine in response to injury, drugs, or antigens. Antihistamines effectively block most smooth muscle responses to histamine and act as an antagonism of the constrictor action of histamine on respiratory smooth muscle. Antihistamines counteract edema formation and whealing in response to injury, antigens, or histamine-liberating drugs. Antihistamines are readily absorbed from the gastrointestinal tract. The main site of metabolic transformation is the liver, but the lung and kidney can also metabolize the drug.
Phenylpropanolamine HCl acts similarly to ephedrine. It is effective orally for the symptomatic control of allergic manifestations, such as perennial hay fever and bronchial asthma. Its action is more prolonged than that of ephedrine, and it is not so apt to produce anxiety complex as is ephedrine.

Indications: For the treatment of the symptoms of seasonal and perennial allergic rhinitis and vasomotor rhinitis, including nasal obstruction (congestion).

Contraindications: Hypersensitivity to any of the components, concurrent MAO inhibitor therapy, severe hypertension, bronchial asthma, coronary artery disease, stenosing peptic ulcer, pyloroduodenal or bladder neck obstruction. Do not use in children under 12 years.
Do not use this drug in patients with narrow-angle glaucoma, obstructive or paralytic ileus, intestinal atony of the elderly or debilitated patient, unstable cardiovascular status in acute hemorrhage, severe ulcerative colitis, toxic megacolon complicating ulcerative colitis, myasthenia gravis.

Use in Nursing Mothers: Because of the higher risk of antihistamines for infants generally and for newborns and prematures in particular, antihistamine therapy is contraindicated in nursing mothers.

Use in Lower Respiratory Disease: Antihistamines should not be used to treat lower respiratory tract symptoms, including asthma. Antihistamines are also contraindicated in the following conditions: hypersensitivity to Chlorpheniramine Maleate and other antihistamines of similar chemical structure, monoamine oxidase inhibitor therapy. (See Drug Interactions Section.)

Use in The Elderly (Approximately 60 Years Or Older): Antihistamines are more likely to cause

Continued on next page

Boots—Cont.

dizziness, sedation, and hypotension in elderly patients.

Warnings: Caution patients about activities requiring alertness (e.g., operating vehicles or machinery). Patients should also be warned about the possible additive effects of alcohol and other CNS depressants.

Usage in Pregnancy: Safe use in pregnancy has not been established. This drug should be used in pregnancy, nursing mothers or by women who might bear children only when the potential benefits have been weighed against the possible hazards to the mother and child. However, this drug has had extensive clinical use in pregnant patients without known deleterious effect. Rat reproduction studies with low drug doses have shown no teratogenic effect. As with all anticholinergics, an inhibitory effect on lactation may occur.

Precautions: Chlorpheniramine Maleate has an atropine-like action and therefore should be used with caution in patients with a history of bronchial asthma, increased intraocular pressure, hyperthyroidism, cardiovascular disease, and/or hypertension.

In patients with functional or organic gastrointestinal hypermotility or malabsorption syndrome, this product is not the preferred therapy.

This drug should be used with caution when the following medical conditions exist: hiatal hernia with reflux esophagitis, intestinal atony of the elderly or debilitated, intestinal obstruction, myasthenia gravis, renal function impairment, and ulcerative colitis (severe).

Drug Interactions: Alcohol or CNS depressants, especially anesthetics, barbiturates, and narcotics. MAO inhibitors prolong and intensify the anticholinergic (drying) effects of antihistamines.

Adverse Reactions: Chlorpheniramine Maleate has a cocaine-like effect on sympathetic nervous transmission and thus prolongs the response to nervous stimulation, potentiates the response to norepinephrine, and inhibits the response to tyramine.

Slight to moderate drowsiness occurs relatively infrequently with Chlorpheniramine Maleate. Other possible side effects common to antihistamines in general include: perspiration, chills, dryness of mouth, nose and throat, urticaria, drug rash, anaphylactic shock, photosensitivity.

Cardiovascular System: Hypotension, hypertension, headache, palpitations, tachycardia, extrasystoles.

Hematologic System: Hemolytic anemia, thrombocytopenia, agranulocytosis, leukopenia.

Nervous Syatem: Sedation, dizziness, disturbed coordination, fatigue, confusion, restlessness, excitation, nervousness, tremor, irritability, insomnia, euphoria, paresthesias, blurred vision, diplopia, vertigo, tinnitus, acute labyrinthitis hysteria, neuritis, convulsions.

Gastrointestinal System: Epigastric distress, anorexia, nausea, vomiting, diarrhea, constipation.

Genitourinary System: Urinary frequency, difficult urination, urinary retention, early menses.

Respiratory System: Thickening of bronchial secretions, tightness of chest and wheezing, nasal stuffiness.

Dosage and Administration: Dosage should be individualized according to the needs and response of the patient. Adults: one capsule every 8 to 12 hours, not to exceed 3 capsules daily. Not for use in children under 12 years of age.

Overdosage: In the event of overdosage, emergency treatment should be started immediately.

Manifestations: May vary from central nervous system depression (sedation, apnea, cardiovascular collapse) to stimulation (insomnia, hallucinations, tremors or convulsions). Other signs and symptoms may be tinnitus, blurred vision, dizziness, ataxia and hypotension. Stimulation is particularly likely in children, as are atropine-like signs and symptoms (dry mouth, fixed dilated pupils, flushing, hyperthermia and gastrointestinal symptoms).

Treatment: The patient should be induced to vomit, even if emesis has occurred spontaneously. Vomiting by the administration of ipecac syrup is a preferred method. However, vomiting should not be induced in patients with impaired consciousness. The action of ipecac is facilitated by physical activity and by administering eight to twelve fluid ounces of water. If emesis does not occur within fifteen minutes, the dose of ipecac should be repeated. Precautions against aspiration must be taken, especially in infants and children. Following emesis, any drug remaining in the stomach may be absorbed by activated charcoal administered as a slurry with water. If vomiting is unsuccessful, or contraindicated, gastric lavage should be performed. Isotonic and one-half isotonic saline are the lavage solutions of choice. Saline cathartics, such as milk of magnesia, draw water into the bowel by osmosis and, therefore, may be valuable for their action in rapid dilution of bowel content. After emergency treatment, the patient should continue to be medically monitored. Treatment of the signs and symptoms of overdosage is symptomatic and supportive.

Special Note on "Sustained Release" Capsules: Since much of the "Sustained Release" capsule medication is coated for gradual release, therapy directed at reversing the effects of the ingested drugs and at supporting the patient should be continued for as long as overdosage symptoms remain. Saline cathartics are useful for hastening evacuation of pellets that have not already released medication.

Stimulants (analeptic agents) should **not** be used. Vasopressors may be used to treat hypotension. Short-acting barbiturates, diazepam or paraldehyde may be administered to control seizures. Hyperpyrexia, especially in children, may require treatment with tepid water sponge baths or a hypothermic blanket. Apnea is treated with ventilatory support.

If photophobia occurs, the patient should be kept in a darkened room.

How Supplied: Green and clear capsules with green and white beads.

Bottles of 100 capsules. NDC 0524-0031-01

Store at controlled room temperature 15–30°C (59–86°F).

Caution: Federal law prohibits dispensing without prescription.

Distributed By
Boots Pharmaceuticals, Inc.
Shreveport, LA 71106
Manufactured By
Cord Laboratories, Inc.
Broomfield, CO 80020

9/83

Shown in Product Identification Section, page 407

TWIN-K® ℞

Description: Each 15 ml (one tablespoonful) supplies 20 mEq of potassium ions as a combination of potassium gluconate and potassium citrate in a sorbitol and saccharin solution.

Indications and Usage: For use as oral potassium therapy in the prevention or treatment of hypokalemia which may occur secondary to diuretic or corticosteroid administration. It may be used in the treatment of cardiac arrhythmias due to digitalis intoxication.

Contraindications: Severe renal impairment with oliguria or azotemia, untreated Addison's disease, adynamia episodica hereditaria, acute dehydration, heat cramps and hyperkalemia from any cause. This product should not be used in patients receiving aldosterone antagonists or triamterene.

Warnings: TWIN-K (potassium gluconate and potassium citrate) is a palatable oral potassium replacement. It appears that little if any potassium gluconate-citrate is transported to the jejunum or ileum where enteric coated potassium chloride lesions have been noted. Excessive, undiluted doses of TWIN-K may cause a saline laxative effect.

Precautions: Potassium is a major intracellular cation which plays a significant role in body physiology. The serum level of potassium is normally 3.8–5.0 mEq/liter. While the serum or plasma level is a poor indicator of total body stores, a plasma or serum level below 3.5 mEq/liter is considered to be indicative of hypokalemia.

The most common cause of hypokalemia is excessive loss of potassium in the urine. However, hypokalemia can also occur with vomiting, gastric drainage and diarrhea.

Usually a potassium deficiency can be corrected by oral administration of potassium supplements. With normal kidney function, it is difficult to produce potassium intoxication by oral administration. However, potassium supplements must be administered with caution since, usually, the exact amount of the deficiency is not accurately known. Checks on the patient's clinical status and serum potassium levels should be made. High serum potassium levels may cause death by cardiac depression, arrhythmias or arrest.

In patients with hypokalemia who also have alkalosis and a chloride deficiency (hypokalemic-hypochloremic alkalosis), there will be a requirement for chloride ions. TWIN-K is not recommended for use in these patients.

Adverse Reactions: Symptoms of potassium intoxication include paresthesias of the extremities, flaccid paralysis, listlessness, mental confusion, weakness and heaviness of the legs, fall in blood pressure, cardiac arrhythmias and heart block. Hyperkalemia may exhibit the following electrocardiographic abnormalities: disappearance of the P wave, widening and slurring of the QRS complex, changes of the ST segment and tall peaked T waves.

TWIN-K taken on an empty stomach in undiluted doses larger than 30 ml (two tablespoons) can produce gastric irritation with nausea, vomiting, diarrhea, and abdominal discomfort.

Overdosage: The administration of oral potassium supplements to persons with normal kidney function rarely causes serious hyperkalemia. However, if the renal excretory function is impaired, potentially fatal hyperkalemia can result. It is important to note that hyperkalemia is usually asymptomatic and may be manifested only by an increased serum potassium concentration and characteristic E.K.G. changes.

Treatment measures include:
1. Elimination of potassium containing drugs or foods.
2. Elimination of potassium-sparing diuretics.
3. Intravenous administration of 300 to 500 ml/hr of a 10% dextrose solution containing 10–20 units of crystalline insulin per 1,000 milliliters.
4. Correction of acidosis, if present, with intravenous sodium bicarbonate.
5. Use of exchange resins, hemodialysis, or peritoneal dialysis.

In treating hyperkalemia, it should be noted that patients stabilized on digitalis can develop digitalis toxicity when the serum potassium concentration is lowered too rapidly.

Dosage and Administration: The usual adult dosage is one tablespoonful (15 ml) in 8 fluid ounces of water or fruit juice, two to four times a day. This will supply 40 to 80 mEq of potassium ions. The usual maintenance dose of potassium is 20 mEq per day while replacement doses range from 30 mEq to 100 mEq per day. Because of the potential for gastrointestinal irritation, undiluted large single doses (more than a tablespoonful or 15 ml) of TWIN-K are to be avoided.

To minimize gastrointestinal irritation, it is recommended that TWIN-K be taken with meals or diluted with water or fruit juice. A tablespoonful (15 ml) in 8 ounces of water is approximately isotonic. More than a single tablespoonful should not be taken without prior dilution.

Deviations from this schedule may be indicated, since no average total daily dose can be defined, but must be governed by close observation for clinical effects.

TWIN-K-Cl®

Description: Each 15 ml (one tablespoonful) supplies 15 mEq of potassium ions and 4 mEq of chloride ions as a combination of potassium gluconate, potassium citrate, and ammonium chloride, in a sorbitol and saccharin solution.

Indications and Usage: For use as oral potassium therapy in the prevention or treatment of hypokalemia which may occur secondary to diuretic or corticosteroid administration. It may be used in the treatment of cardiac arrhythmias due to digitalis intoxication.

Potassium and chloride are usually the salts of choice in the treatment of hypokalemia since chloride and potassium deficiencies are likely to be associated with each other.

In patients with hypokalemia who also have alkalosis and a chloride deficiency (hypokalemic-hypochloremic alkalosis), there will be a requirement for chloride ions. TWIN-K-CI is recommended for use in these patients.

Contraindications: Severe renal impairment with oliguria or azotemia, untreated Addison's disease, adynamia episodica hereditaria, acute dehydration, heat cramps and hyperkalemia from any cause. This product should not be used in patients receiving aldosterone antagonists or triamterene.

Warnings: TWIN-K-Cl is a palatable oral potassium replacement. Excessive, undiluted doses of TWIN-K-Cl may cause a saline laxative effect.

Precautions: Potassium is a major intracellular cation which plays a significant role in body physiology. The serum level of potassium is normally 3.8–5.0 mEq/liter. While the serum or plasma level is a poor indicator of total body stores, a plasma or serum level below 3.5 mEq/liter is considered to be indicative of hypokalemia.

The most common cause of hypokalemia is excessive loss of potassium in the urine. However, hypokalemia can also occur with vomiting, gastric drainage and diarrhea.

Usually a potassium deficiency can be corrected by oral administration of potassium supplements. With normal kidney function, it is difficult to produce potassium intoxication by oral administration. However, potassium supplements must be administered with caution since, usually, the exact amount of the deficiency is not accurately known. Checks on the patient's clinical status and serum potassium levels should be made. High serum potassium levels may cause death by cardiac depression, arrhythmias or arrest.

Adverse Reactions: Symptoms of potassium intoxication include paresthesias of the extremities, flaccid paralysis, listlessness, mental confusion, weakness and heaviness of the legs, fall in blood pressure, cardiac arrhythmias and heart block. Hyperkalemia may exhibit the following electrocardiographic abnormalities: disappearance of the P wave, widening and slurring of the QRS complex, changes of the ST segment and tall peaked T waves.

TWIN-K-Cl taken on an empty stomach in undiluted doses larger than 30 ml can produce gastric irritation with nausea, vomiting, diarrhea, and abdominal discomfort.

Overdosage: The administration of oral potassium supplements to persons with normal kidney function rarely causes serious hyperkalemia. However, if the renal excretory function is impaired potentially fatal hyperkalemia can result. It is important to note that hyperkalemia is usually asymptomatic and may be manifested only by an increased serum potassium concentration and characteristic E.K.G. changes.

Treatment measures include:
1. Elimination of potassium containing drugs or foods.
2. Elimination of potassium-sparing diuretics.
3. Intravenous administration of 300 to 500 ml/hr of a 10% dextrose solution containing 10–20 units of crystalline insulin per 1,000 milliliters.
4. Correction of acidosis, if present, with intravenous sodium bicarbonate.
5. Use of exchange resins, hemodialysis, or peritoneal dialysis.

In treating hyperkalemia, it should be noted that patients stabilized on digitalis can develop digitalis toxicity when the serum potassium concentration is lowered too rapidly.

Dosage and Administration: The usual adult dosage is one tablespoonful (15 ml) in 8 fluid ounces of water or fruit juice, two to four times a day. This will supply 30 to 60 mEq of potassium ions and 8 to 16 mEq of chloride ions. The usual maintenance dose of potassium is 20 mEq per day while replacement doses range from 30 mEq to 100 mEq per day. Because of the potential for gastrointestinal irritation, undiluted large single doses (more than a tablespoonful or 15 ml) of TWIN-K-Cl are to be avoided.

To minimize gastrointestinal irritation, it is recommended that TWIN-K-Cl be taken with meals or diluted with water or fruit juice. A tablespoonful (15 ml) in 8 ounces of water is approximately isotonic. More than a single tablespoonful should not be taken without prior dilution.

Deviations from this schedule may be indicated, since no average total daily dose can be defined, but must be governed by close observation for clinical effects.

How Supplied: Bottles of 1 pint (16 fl. oz.)
NDC 0524-0022-16

Caution: Federal law prohibits dispensing without prescription.

Manufactured and Distributed by
Boots Pharmaceuticals, Inc.
Shreveport, Louisiana 71106 U.S.A.

Rev. 11/83   0022-01

ZORPRIN®
(Aspirin)
(Zero-Order Release)

Description: Each capsule-shaped tablet of Zorprin contains 800 mg of aspirin, formulated in a special matrix to control the release of aspirin after ingestion. The controlled availability of aspirin provided by Zorprin approximates zero-order release; the in vitro release of aspirin from the tablet matrix is linear and independent of the concentration of the drug.

The structural formula of aspirin is

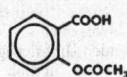

Clinical Pharmacology: Aspirin, as contained in Zorprin, is a salicylate that has demonstrated anti-inflammatory and analgesic activity. Its mode of action as an anti-inflammatory and analgesic agent may be due to the inhibition of synthesis of prostaglandins, although its exact mode of action is not known.

Zorprin dissolution is pH dependent. In vitro studies have shown very little aspirin to be released in acidic solutions; whereas, Zorprin releases the majority of its aspirin (90%) in a zero-order mode at a neutral to alkaline pH. It is this pH dependence of Zorprin that reduces direct contact between Zorprin and the gastric mucosa, resulting in a reduction of its gastrointestinal side-effect potential.

Bioavailability data for Zorprin have confirmed that plasma levels of salicylic acid and acetylsalicylic acid can be measured 24 hours after a single oral dose. This substantiates a twice daily dose regimen. Multiple dose bioavailability studies showed similar steady-state salicylate levels for Zorprin as for conventional release aspirin using the same total daily dose. Long-term monitoring of salicylate levels showed no signs of accumulation once steady-state levels were reached (4–6 days). Studies of in vivo prostaglandin levels (PGE2) have shown Zorprin plasma levels of salicylic acid and acetylsalicylic acid to reduce PGE2 levels 14 hours after a single oral 800 mg dose while an equivalent dose of aspirin produced a reduction of PGE2 levels only through six hours. Zorprin's effect on other prostaglandins than PGE2 has not been determined.

Salicylates are excreted mainly by the kidney, and from studies in humans it appears that salicylate is excreted in the urine as free salicylic acid (10%); salicyluric acid (75%); salicylic phenolic (10%); acyl glucuronides (5%) and gentisic acid (<1%).

Indications and Usage: Zorprin is indicated for the treatment of rheumatoid arthritis and osteoarthritis. The safety and efficacy of Zorprin have not been established in those rheumatoid arthritic patients who are designated by the American Rheumatism Association as Functional Class IV (incapacitated, largely or wholly bedridden, or confined to wheelchair, little or no self-care).

In patients treated with Zorprin for rheumatoid arthritis and osteoarthritis, the anti-inflammatory action of Zorprin has been shown by reduction in pain, morning stiffness and disease activity as assessed by both the investigators and patients.

In clinical studies in patients with rheumatoid arthritis and osteoarthritis, Zorprin has been shown to be comparable to conventional release aspirin in controlling the aforementioned signs and symptoms of disease activity and to be associated with a statistically significant reduction in the milder gastrointestinal side effects (see ADVERSE REACTIONS). Zorprin may be well tolerated in some patients who have had gastrointestinal side effects with conventional release aspirin, but these patients when treated with Zorprin should be carefully followed for signs and symptoms of gastrointestinal bleeding and ulceration. Since there have been no controlled trials to demonstrate whether or not there is any beneficial effect or harmful interaction with the use of Zorprin in conjunction with other nonsteroidal anti-inflammatory agents (NSAI), the combination cannot be recommended (see **Drug Interactions**).
Because of its relatively long onset of action, Zorprin is not recommended for antipyresis or for short-term analgesia.

Contraindications: Zorprin should not be used in patients known to be hypersensitive to salicylates or in individuals with the syndrome of nasal polyps, angioedema, bronchospastic reactivity to aspirin, renal or hepatic insufficiency, hypoprothrombinemia, or other bleeding disorders. Zorprin is not recommended for children under 12 years of age; it is contraindicated in all children with fever accompanied by dehydration.

Warnings: Zorprin should be used with caution when anticoagulants are prescribed concurrently, since aspirin may depress platelet aggregation and increase bleeding time. Large doses of salicylates may have hypoglycemic action and enhance the effect of the oral hypoglycemics; concomitant use therefore is not recommended. However, if such use is necessary, dosage of the hypoglycemic agent must be reduced. The hypoglycemic action of the salicylates may also necessitate adjustment of the insulin requirements of diabetics.

While salicylates in large doses have a uricosuric effect, smaller amounts may reduce urate excretion and increase serum uric acid.

USE IN PREGNANCY: Aspirin can harm the fetus when administered to pregnant women. Aspirin interferes with maternal and infant hemostasis and may lengthen the duration of pregnancy and parturition. Aspirin has produced teratogenic effects and increases the incidence of stillbirths and neonatal deaths in animals.

If this drug is used during pregnancy, or if the patient becomes pregnant while taking this drug, the patient should be apprised of the potential hazard to the fetus.

Continued on next page

How Supplied: Bottles of 1 pint (16 fl. oz.)
NDC 0524-0021-16

Caution: Federal law prohibits dispensing without prescription.

Manufactured and Distributed by
Boots Pharmaceuticals, Inc.
Shreveport, Louisiana 71106 U.S.A.

Rev. 11/83   0021-01

Boots—Cont.

Aspirin should not be taken during the last 3 months of pregnancy.

Precautions: Appropriate precautions should be taken in prescribing Zorprin (aspirin) for patients who are known to be sensitive to aspirin or salicylates. Particular care should be used when prescribing this medication for patients with erosive gastritis, peptic ulcer, mild diabetes or gout. As with all salicylate drugs, caution should be exercised in prescribing Zorprin (aspirin) for those patients with bleeding tendencies or those on anticoagulants.

In order to avoid exacerbation of disease or adrenal insufficiency, patients who have been on prolonged corticosteroid therapy should have their therapy tapered slowly rather than discontinued abruptly when Zorprin is made a part of the treatment program.

Patients receiving large doses of aspirin and/or prolonged therapy may develop mild salicylate intoxication (salicylism) that may be reversed by dosage reduction.

Salicylates can produce changes in thyroid function tests.

Salicylates should be used with caution in patients with severe hepatic damage, preexisting hypoprothrombinemia, Vitamin K deficiency and in those undergoing surgery.

Since aspirin release from Zorprin is pH dependent, it may change in those conditions where the gastric pH has been increased as a result of antacids, gastric secretion inhibitors or surgical procedures.

Drug Interactions: (See **Warnings**) Aspirin may interfere with some anticoagulant and antidiabetic drugs. Drugs which lower serum uric acid by increasing uric acid excretion (uricosurics) may be antagonized by the concomitant use of aspirin, particularly in doses less than 2.0 grams/day. Nonsteroidal anti-inflammatory drugs may be competitively displaced from their albumin binding sites by aspirin. This effect may negate the clinical efficacy of both drugs. Also, the gastrointestinal inflammatory potential of nonsteroidal anti-inflammatory drugs may be potentiated by aspirin. The combination of alcohol and aspirin may increase the risk of gastrointestinal bleeding. Aspirin may enhance the activity of methotrexate and increase its toxicity.

Sodium excretion produced by spironolactone may be decreased in the presence of salicylates. Concomitant administration of other anti-inflammatory drugs may increase the risk of gastrointestinal ulceration. Urinary alkalinizers decrease aspirin's effectiveness by increasing the rate of salicylate renal excretion. Phenobarbital decreases aspirin's effectiveness by enzyme induction.

Pregnancy Category D. See **Warnings** Section.

Nursing Mothers: Salicylates have been detected in the breast milk of nursing mothers. Because of the potential for serious adverse reactions in nursing infants from aspirin, a decision should be made whether to discontinue nursing or discontinue the drug, taking into account the benefit of the drug to the mother.

Adverse Reactions:

Hematologic: Aspirin interferes with hemostasis. Patients with a history of blood coagulation defects or receiving anticoagulant drugs or with severe anemia should avoid Zorprin. Aspirin used chronically may cause a persistent iron deficiency anemia.

Gastrointestinal: Aspirin may potentiate peptic ulcer, and cause stomach distress or heartburn. Aspirin can cause an increase in occult bleeding and in some patients massive gastrointestinal bleeding. However, the greatest release of active drug from Zorprin is designed to occur in the small intestine over a period of time. This has resulted in fewer symptomatic gastrointestinal side effects.

Allergic: Allergic and anaphylactic reactions have been noted when hypersensitive individuals have taken aspirin. Fatal anaphylactic shock, while not common, has been reported.

Respiratory: Aspirin intolerance, manifested by exacerbation of bronchospasm and rhinitis, may occur in patients with a history of nasal polyps, asthma, or rhinitis. The mechanism of this intolerance is unknown but may be the result of aspirin-induced shunting of prostaglandin synthesis to the lipoxygenase pathway and the liberation of leukotrienes, e.g., slow-reacting substance of anaphylaxis.

Dermatologic: Hives, rashes, and angioedema may occur, especially in patients suffering from chronic urticaria.

Central Nervous System: Taken in overdoses, aspirin provides stimulation which may be manifested by tinnitus. Following initial stimulation, depression of the central nervous system may be noted.

Renal: Aspirin rarely may aggravate chronic kidney disease.

Hepatic: High doses of aspirin have been reported to produce reversible hepatic dysfunction.

Overdosage: Overdosage, if it occurs would produce the usual symptoms of salicylism: tinnitus, vertigo, headache, confusion, drowsiness, sweating, hyperventilation, vomiting or diarrhea. Plasma salicylate levels in adults may range from 50 to 80 mg/dl in the mildly intoxicated patient to 110 to 160* mg/dl in the severely intoxicated patient. An arterial blood pH of 7.1 may indicate serious poisoning. The clearance of salicylates in children is much slower than adults and this should receive due consideration when aspirin overdosages occur in infants; salicylate half-lives of 30 hours have been reported in infants 4–8 months old. Treatment for mild intoxication should include emptying the stomach with an emetic, or gastric lavage with 5% sodium bicarbonate. Individuals suffering from severe intoxication should, in addition, have forced diuresis by intravenous infusions of sodium bicarbonate and dextrose or sodium lactate. In extreme cases, hemodialysis or peritoneal dialysis may be required. (*A plasma salicylate level of 160 mg/dl in an adult is usually considered lethal.)

Dosage and Administration:

In order to achieve a zero-order release, the tablets of Zorprin should be swallowed intact.
Breaking the tablets or disrupting the structure will alter the release profile of the drug.
It is recommended that Zorprin be taken with sufficient quantities of fluids (8 oz. or more).

Adult Dosage: For mild to moderate pain associated with rheumatoid arthritis and osteoarthritis, the recommended initial dose of Zorprin is 1600 mg (2-800 mg tablets) twice a day. Because of Zorprin's prolonged release of aspirin into the bloodstream, the tablets may be taken as a b.i.d. dose. Further adjustment of the dosage should be determined by the physician, based upon the patient's response and needs. Since it will take 4–6 days to reach steady-state levels of salicylic acid with Zorprin, it is recommended that dosages be given for at least one week before further adjustment. In general, patients with rheumatoid arthritis seem to require higher doses of Zorprin than do patients with osteoarthritis.

Zorprin is not recommended for children below the age of 12.

How Supplied: Zorprin Tablets 800 mg; plain, white capsule-shaped tablets.
Bottles of 100 Tablets—NDC 0524-0057-01

Caution: Federal law prohibits dispensing without prescription.

U.S. Patent No. 4,308,251

Manufactured and Distributed by:
Boots Pharmaceuticals, Inc.
Shreveport, Louisiana 71106 USA

Rev. 11/83   0057-04

Products are cross-indexed by generic and chemical names in the YELLOW SECTION

Boyle & Company
13260 MOORE STREET
CERRITOS, CA 90701

CITRA® FORTE SYRUP   ℞
CITRA® FORTE CAPSULES   ℞

Composition: Ea. 5cc   Ea. Cap.
Hydrocodone
 Bitartrate...5 mg.   5 mg.
 (Warning: May be habit forming)
Ascorbic Acid......................................30 mg.   50 mg.
Pheniramine
 Maleate...2.5 mg.   6.25 mg.
Potassium Citrate ....150 mg.
Pyrilamine Maleate.........................3.33 mg.   8.33 mg.
Chlorpheniramine Maleate ....1 mg.
Phenylephrine HCl ....10 mg.
Salicylamide......................................227 mg.
Caffeine Alkaloid................................30 mg.
Syrup in a palatable, alcohol 2% flavored base.

Action and Uses: *CITRA FORTE SYRUP:* Antitussive, Expectorant, Antihistaminic, Analgesic provides effective cough suppressant action, a sodium free expectorant, two antihistamines to help control allergic reactions. *CITRA FORTE CAPSULES:* Antitussive, Antihistaminic, decongestant, analgesic. Also provides cough relief and in addition three antihistamines (each in ⅓ their usual dosage) for fewer side effects and broader control of the patients allergic reaction to the cough/cold process. Decongestant action shrinks mucous membranes.

Administration and Dosage: *CITRA FORTE SYRUP: Usual Adult Dose.*—One or two teaspoonfuls every 3 or 4 hours. *Children* (6-12)—one-half adult dosage. *Children under 6 years*—according to standard method of calculation. *CITRA FORTE CAPSULES: Usual Adult Dose.*—One or two capsules every 3 or 4 hours.

Precautions: Patients should be advised to avoid using machinery or driving until response to antihistamines is established. Use with caution in patients with idiosyncrasies to formula ingredients. CITRA FORTE CAPSULES should be used with caution in patients with hypertension, cardiac disease, diabetes or hyperthyroidism.

How Supplied: CITRA FORTE SYRUP in pints and gallons; CITRA FORTE CAPSULES in bottles of 50 capsules.

GLYTINIC®
(For Iron Deficiency Anemia)
Tablets

Composition:
Each tablet contains:
Ferrous Gluconate ....3.4 gr.
 (Iron Content . . . 25 mg.)
Aminoacetic Acid N.F. (Glycine) ....325 mg.
Cobalamin Conc. N.F. (Vitamin B12) (Resin Adsorbed) 2.5 mcg.; Thiamine Mononitrate 1.9 mg.; Riboflavin 1.9 mg.; Pyridoxine Hydrochloride 0.56 mg.; Niacinamide 11.25 mg.; d-Pantothenyl alcohol 1.63 mg.; Liver Desiccated 1.25 gr.

Action and Uses: Ferrous Gluconate, inherently tolerable combined with amino acid, glycine, assures good toleration, assimilation, and utilization. Glycine supplies needed amino nitrogen for rapid, positive hemoglobin and hematocrit response. Patient acceptance is excellent. The liquid is surprisingly free from after-taste making it useful for all ages. Children and elderly patients will like the easy to swallow sugar coated tablet and the distinct freedom from gastric irritation. Glytinic is particularly useful for patients refractory or intolerant to iron preparations.

Administration and Dosage: Tablets, with or between meals: *Adults*—2 b.i.d.; *Children 6 to 12*—1 b.i.d.

How Supplied: Tablets —100's.

TRIVA® COMBINATION   ℞
TRIVA® DOUCHE POWDER
TRIVA® JEL   ℞

Composition: TRIVA COMBINATION combines therapeutic vaginal douche and jel in a convenient and complete treatment consisting of: TRIVA POWDER containing oxyquinoline sulfate 2%; alkyl aryl sulfonate 35%; disodium edetate 0.33%; sodium sulfate 53%; dispersant (lactose) 9.67% and TRIVA JEL containing per 5 Grams oxyquinoline benzoate 7.5 mg.; alkyl aryl sulfonate 62.5 mg.; disodium edetate 2.5 mg.; aminacrine HCl 10 mg.; copper sulfate .063 mg.; sodium sulfate 6.9 mg.; in an aqueous jel base of tragacanth, Irish moss, modified lanolin, glycerin, sodium bicarbonate preserved with methyl-propyl- and butyl-parahydroxy-benzoate.

Action and Uses: TRIVA COMBINATION effectively treats Monilial and Trichomonal as well as Non-specific Vulvovaginitis. Chronic, stubborn cases as well as Monilia and Trichomonas occurring together can be successfully treated. Organisms are eradicated along with symptoms. Vaginal flora and pH return to normal spontaneously. Fungicidal, trichomonacidal, bactericidal, detergent and chelating agents are provided for a safe, simple, patient-administered 16 day treatment without need for restraints on patient's activities. Flushing and detergent action of the douche combines with the continuous action of the jel to quickly destroy the infection and stop the symptoms.

Effectiveness of TRIVA COMBINATION has been demonstrated by clinical tests. Both diagnosis and cure were established by the use of special Papanicolaou smear and Sabouraud culture.

Administration and Dosage: TRIVA COMBINATION, ℞, sig: douche (1 packet in 1 qt water) at night followed immediately by one applicatorfull of JEL, continued for 15 nights followed on 16th morning by douche only. An additional course of treatment may be used if needed. Directions for complete mechanical use of product appear on each package.

TRIVA DOUCHE POWDER (individual packet dissolved in 1 qt water) alone is effective in most cases of Monilial, Trichomonal and Non-specific Vulvovaginitis. It provides rapid relief from symptoms. Particularly useful in pre- and post-operative and post-partum care. May be used adjunctively with oral treatment for Trichomonas.

TRIVA DOUCHE POWDER, sig, douche (1 packet in 1 qt water) morning and night for 12 days.

TRIVA JEL ℞, sig. one or two applicatorsful daily.

IMPORTANT: During menstruation, continue treatment as instructed.

Precautions: Occasionally, irritation occurs at the onset of treatment. In such cases it is recommended that the douche only be prescribed in one-half or less than usual strength for a day or two, then combined therapeutic treatment resumed as directed.

TRIVA COMBINATION, POWDER and JEL are spermicidal.

Side Effects: None.

Contraindications: None.

How Supplied: TRIVA COMBINATION contains 24 individual 3 Gm. packets douche powder, 1 tube 85 Gm. Jel with applicator.

TRIVA DOUCHE POWDER—Available individually, 24 individual 3 Gm. packets.

TRIVA JEL—Available individually, 1 tube 85 Gm. with applicator.

IDENTIFICATION PROBLEM?
Consult PDR's
Product Identification Section
where you'll find over 1200
products pictured actual size
and in full color.

Braintree Laboratories, Inc.
285 WASHINGTON STREET
BRAINTREE, MA 02184

GoLYTELY™ ℞
Polyethylene Glycol Electrolyte Lavage Solution

Description: A white powder for reconstitution containing 236 g polyethylene glycol 3350, 22.74 g sodium sulfate, 6.74 g sodium bicarbonate, 5.86 g sodium chloride, and 2.97 g potassium chloride. When dissolved in water to a volume of 4 liters, GoLYTELY is an isosmotic solution having a mildly salty taste. For oral administration.

Clinical Pharmacology: Orally administered GoLYTELY induces a diarrhea that rapidly cleanses the bowel, usually within four hours. Polyethylene glycol 3350 acts as an osmotic agent, and the electrolyte concentration results in virtually no net absorption or secretion of ions. Large volumes may be administered without significant changes in water or electrolyte balance.

Indication and Usage: GoLYTELY is indicated for bowel cleansing prior to colonoscopy and barium enema x-ray examination.

Contraindications: GoLYTELY is contraindicated in patients with gastrointestinal obstruction, gastric retention, bowel perforation, toxic colitis or megacolon.

Warnings: No additional ingredients, flavoring, etc, should be added to the solution before administration.

Precautions: Patients with impaired gag reflex or in an unconscious or semiconscious state, or who are otherwise prone to regurgitation or aspiration, should be observed during the administration of GoLYTELY, especially if it is given via nasogastric tube. If gastrointestinal obstruction or perforation is suspected, appropriate studies should be performed to rule out these contraindications before administering GoLYTELY.

Pregnancy Category C. Animal reproduction studies have not been conducted with GoLYTELY. It is also not known whether GoLYTELY can cause fetal harm when administered to a pregnant woman or can affect reproductive capacity. GoLYTELY should be given to a pregnant woman only if clearly needed.

Safety and effectiveness in children have not been established.

Long-term studies have not been done on animals to determine carcinogenic potential or effects on reproduction.

Adverse Reactions: GoLYTELY administration is associated with a low incidence of side effects—primarily nausea, abdominal fullness and bloating, and occasional cramps and vomiting. These side effects are transient and usually subside rapidly.

Dosage and Administration: The recommended dosage for adults is 4 liters of GoLYTELY solution prior to gastrointestinal examination. GoLYTELY is usually taken orally but may be given via nasogastric tube to patients who are unwilling or unable to drink the preparation. The rate of administration is 8 oz (240 mL) every ten minutes, until the 4 liters is consumed. It is preferred that each portion be ingested rapidly, not taken in small amounts. The first bowel movement should occur approximately one hour after the start of GoLYTELY administration.

Various regimens have been used. Ideally, the patient should fast approximately three to four hours prior to ingesting GoLYTELY, but in no case should solid foods be given for at least two hours before the solution is administered. One method is to schedule patients for examination at midmorning, allowing the patient three hours for drinking and a one-hour waiting period to complete bowel evacuation. Another method is to administer GoLYTELY on the evening before the examination, particularly if the patient is to have a barium enema. No foods except clear liquids are permitted after GoLYTELY administration and prior to examination.

How Supplied: In powdered form, for oral administration as a solution following reconstitution. Each disposable 4800 mL jug contains, in powdered form: polyethylene glycol 3350 236 g, sodium sulfate 22.74 g, sodium bicarbonate 6.74 g, sodium chloride 5.86 g, potassium chloride 2.97 g. When made up to 4 L volume with water, the solution contains PEG 3350 17.6 mmol/L, sodium 125 mmol/L, sulfate 40 mmol/L, chloride 35 mmol/L, bicarbonate 20 mmol/L, and potassium 10 mmol/L.

Caution: Federal law prohibits dispensing without prescription.

Storage: Store in sealed container at 59° to 86°F. When reconstituted, keep solution refrigerated. Use within 48 hours. Discard unused portion. (NDC 52268-0100-01).

Made by Lyne Laboratories,
Stoughton, MA 02072, for
BRAINTREE LABORATORIES, INC.
P.O. Box 361, Braintree, MA 02184
©1984 Rev. 10-29-84

Bristol Laboratories
(Division of Bristol-Myers Co.)
SYRACUSE, NY 13221-4755

AMIKIN® ℞
[ah-mi'kin]
(amikacin sulfate)

This is the full text of the latest Official Package Circular dated August 1979 [3015 DIMO-07].

WARNINGS

Patients treated with aminoglycosides should be under close clinical observation because of the potential ototoxicity and nephrotoxicity associated with their use.

Ototoxicity, both auditory and vestibular, can occur in patients treated at higher doses or for periods longer than those recommended. The risk of amikacin-induced ototoxicity is greater in patients with renal damage. High frequency deafness usually occurs first and can be detected only by audiometric testing. Vertigo may occur and may be evidence of vestibular injury.

The ototoxicity potential of amikacin in infants is not known. Until more safety reports become available, amikacin should be used in infants only in those specific circumstances when susceptibility testing indicates that other aminoglycosides cannot be used or are otherwise contraindicated, and when the infant can be observed closely for evidence of toxicity.

Aminoglycosides are potentially nephrotoxic. Renal and eighth-nerve function should be closely monitored in patients with known or suspected renal impairment and also in those whose renal function is initially normal but who develop signs of renal dysfunction during therapy. Such impairment may be characterized by decreased creatinine clearance, the presence of cells or casts, oliguria, proteinuria, decreased urine specific gravity, or evidence of increasing nitrogen retention (increasing BUN or creatinine).

Evidence of impairment in renal, vestibular, or auditory function requires discontinuation of the drug or dosage adjustment.

Serum concentrations should be monitored when feasible, and prolonged peak concentrations above 35 mcg./ml. should be avoided. Urine should be examined for increased excretion of protein, the presence of cells and casts, and decreased specific gravity.

Concurrent and/or sequential use of topically or systemically neurotoxic or nephrotoxic antibiotics, particularly kanamycin, gentamicin, tobramycin, neomycin, streptomycin, cephaloridine, paromomycin, viomycin, polymyxin B, colistin, and vancomycin should be avoided.

Continued on next page

Bristol—Cont.

AMIKIN should not be given concurrently with potent diuretics (ethacrynic acid, furosemide, meralluride sodium, sodium mercaptomerin, or mannitol). Some diuretics themselves cause ototoxicity, and intravenously administered diuretics enhance aminoglycoside toxicity by altering antibiotic concentrations in serum and tissue.

Description: Amikacin sulfate is a semi-synthetic aminoglycoside antibiotic derived from kanamycin. It is $C_{22}H_{43}N_5O_{13} \cdot 2H_2SO_4$. D-Streptamine, O-3-amino-3-deoxy-α-D-glucopyranosyl-(1→6) - O - [6-amino-6-deoxy-α-D-glucopyranosyl-(1→4)]-N[1]-(4-amino-2-hydroxyl-1-oxobutyl)-2 deoxy-, (S)-,sulfate (1:2) (salt).

The dosage form is supplied as a sterile, colorless to light straw colored solution. The 100 mg. per 2 ml. vial contains, in addition to amikacin sulfate, 0.13% sodium bisulfite and 0.5% sodium citrate with pH adjusted to 4.5 with sulfuric acid. The 500 mg. per 2 ml. vial and the 1 gram per 4 ml. vial contain 0.66% sodium bisulfite and 2.5% sodium citrate with pH adjusted to 4.5 with sulfuric acid.

Action:
Clinical-Pharmacology
Intramuscular Administration
AMIKIN is rapidly absorbed after intramuscular administration. In normal adult volunteers, average peak serum concentrations of about 12, 16, and 21 mcg/ml are obtained 1 hour after intramuscular administration of 250-mg (3.7 mg/Kg), 375-mg (5 mg/Kg), 500-mg (7.5 mg/Kg), single doses respectively. At 10 hours, serum levels are about 0.3 mcg/ml, 1.2 mcg/ml, and 2.1 mcg/ml, respectively. Tolerance studies in normal volunteers revealed that amikacin was well tolerated locally following repeated intramuscular dosing and, when given at maximally recommended doses, no ototoxicity or nephrotoxicity was reported. There was no evidence of drug accumulation with repeated dosing for 10 days when administered according to recommended doses.

With normal renal function about 91.9% of an intramuscular dose is excreted unchanged in the urine in the first 8 hours, and 98.2% within 24 hours. Mean urine concentrations for 6 hours are 563 mcg/ml following a 250-mg dose, 697 mcg/ml following a 375-mg dose, and 832 mcg/ml following a 500-mg dose.

Preliminary intramuscular studies in newborns of different weights (less than 1.5 Kg, 1.5 to 2.0 Kg, over 2.0 Kg) at a dose of 7.5 mg/Kg revealed that, like other aminoglycosides, serum half-life values were correlated inversely with post-natal age and renal clearances of amikacin. The volume of distribution indicates that amikacin, like other aminoglycosides, remains primarily in the extracellular fluid space of neonates. Repeated dosing every 12 hours in all the above groups did not demonstrate accumulation after 5 days.

Intravenous Administration
Single doses of 500 mg (7.5 mg/Kg) administered to normal adults as an infusion over a period of 30 minutes produced a mean peak serum concentration of 38 mcg/ml at the end of the infusion, and levels of 24 mcg/ml, 18 mcg/ml, and 0.75 mcg/ml at 30 minutes, 1 hour, and 10 hours post-infusion, respectively. Eighty-four percent of the administered dose was excreted in the urine in 9 hours and about 94% within 24 hours.

Repeat infusions of 7.5 mg/Kg every 12 hours in normal adults were well tolerated and caused no drug accumulation.

General
Pharmacokinetic studies in normal adult subjects reveal the mean serum half-life to be slightly over 2 hours with a mean total apparent volume of distribution of 24 liters (28% of the body weight). By the ultrafiltration technique, reports on serum protein binding range from 0 to 11%. The mean serum clearance rate is about 100 ml/min and the renal clearance rate is 94 ml/min in subjects with normal renal function.

Amikacin is excreted primarily by way of glomerular filtration. Patients with impaired renal function or diminished glomerular filtration pressure excrete the drug much more slowly (effectively prolonging the serum half-life). Therefore, renal function should be monitored carefully and dosage adjusted accordingly (see suggested dosage schedule under "Dosage and Administration").

Amikacin has been found in the cerebrospinal fluid, pleural fluid, and peritoneal cavity following parenteral administration.

Spinal fluid levels in normal infants are approximately 10 to 20% of the serum concentrations and may reach 50% when the meninges are inflamed. AMIKIN has been demonstrated to cross the placental barrier and yield significant concentrations in amniotic fluid. The peak fetal serum concentration is about 16% of the peak maternal serum concentration and maternal and fetal serum half-life values are about 2 and 3.7 hours, respectively.

Microbiology
Gram-negative—Amikacin is active in vitro against **Pseudomonas** species, **Escherichia coli**, **Proteus** species (indole-positive and indole-negative), **Providencia** species, **Klebsiella-Enterobacter-Serratia** species, **Acinetobacter** (formerly **Mima-Herellea**) species and **Citrobacter freundii**.

When strains of the above organisms are found to be resistant to other aminoglycosides, including gentamicin, tobramycin, and kanamycin, many are susceptible to amikacin in vitro.

Gram-positive—Amikacin is active in vitro against penicillinase and non-penicillinase-producing **Staphylococcus** species including methicillin-resistant strains. However, it has been shown to have a low order of activity against other Gram-positive organisms; viz, **Streptococcus pyogenes**, enterococci, and **Streptococcus pneumoniae** (formerly **Diplococcus pneumoniae**).

Amikacin resists degradation by most aminoglycoside inactivating enzymes known to affect gentamicin, tobramycin, and kanamycin.

Disc Susceptibility Tests
Quantitative methods that require measurement of zone diameters give the most precise estimates of antibiotic susceptibility. One such procedure* has been recommended for use with discs to test susceptibility to amikacin. Interpretation involves correlation of the diameters obtained in the disc test with MIC values for amikacin. When the causative organism is tested by the Kirby-Bauer methods of disc susceptibility, a 30-mcg amikacin disc should give a zone of 17 mm or greater to indicate susceptibility. Zone sizes of 14 mm or less indicate resistance. Zone sizes of 15 to 16 mm indicate intermediate susceptibility. With this procedure, a report from the laboratory of "susceptible" indicates that the infecting organism is likely to respond to therapy. A report of "resistant" indicates that the infecting organism is not likely to respond to therapy. A report of "intermediate susceptibility" suggests that the organism would be susceptible if the infection is confined to tissues and fluids (e.g., urine), in which high antibiotic levels are attained.

Indications and Usage:
AMIKIN is indicated in the short-term treatment of serious infections due to susceptible strains of Gram-negative bacteria, including **Pseudomonas** species, **Escherichia coli**, species of indole-positive and indole-negative **Proteus**, **Providencia** species, **Klebsiella-Enterobacter-Serratia** species, and **Acinetobacter** (**Mima-Herellea**) species.

Clinical studies have shown AMIKIN to be effective in bacteremia and septicemia (including neonatal sepsis); in serious infections of the respiratory tract, bones and joints, central nervous system (including meningitis) and skin and soft tissue; intra-abdominal infections (including peritonitis); and in burns and post-operative infections (including post-vascular surgery). Clinical studies have shown AMIKIN also to be effective in serious complicated and recurrent urinary tract infections due to these organisms. Aminoglycosides, including AMIKIN injectable, are not indicated in uncomplicated initial episodes of urinary tract infections unless the causative organisms are not susceptible to antibiotics having less potential toxicity.

Bacteriologic studies should be performed to identify causative organisms and their susceptibilities to amikacin. AMIKIN may be considered as initial therapy in suspected Gram-negative infections and therapy may be instituted before obtaining the results of susceptibility testing. Clinical trials demonstrated that AMIKIN was effective in infections caused by gentamicin and/or tobramycin resistant strains of Gram-negative organisms, particularly **Proteus rettgeri**, **Providencia stuartii**, **Serratia marcescens**, and **Pseudomonas aeruginosa**. The decision to continue therapy with the drug should be based on results of the susceptibility tests, the severity of the infection, the response of the patient, and the important additional considerations contained in the "Warning" box above.

AMIKIN has also been shown to be effective in staphylococcal infections and may be considered as initial therapy under certain conditions in the treatment of known or suspected staphylococcal disease such as, severe infections where the causative organism may be either a Gram-negative bacterium or a staphylococcus, infections due to susceptible strains of staphylococci in patients allergic to other antibiotics, and in mixed staphylococcal/Gram-negative infections.

Amikacin may be indicated in the treatment of neonatal sepsis when susceptibility testing indicates that other aminoglycosides cannot be used. In certain severe infections such as neonatal sepsis, concomitant therapy with a penicillin-type drug may be indicated because of the possibility of infections due to Gram-positive organisms such as streptococci or pneumococci.

Contraindications: A history of hypersensitivity to amikacin is a contraindication for its use.

Warning: See "Warning" box above.

Precautions: AMIKIN is potentially nephrotoxic, ototoxic, and neurotoxic. The concurrent or serial use of other ototoxic or nephrotoxic agents should be avoided either systemically or topically because of the potential for additive effects. Such agents include antibacterial drugs such as kanamycin, gentamicin, tobramycin, neomycin, streptomycin, cephaloridine, paromomycin, viomycin, polymyxin B, colistin, and vancomycin as well as certain diuretic agents such as ethacrynic acid or furosemide.

Ototoxicity
See "Warning" box.

Nephrotoxicity
Since AMIKIN is present in high concentrations in the renal excretory system, patients should be well hydrated to minimize chemical irritation of the renal tubules. Kidney function should be assessed by the usual methods prior to starting therapy and daily during the course of treatment.

If signs of renal irritation appear (casts, white or red cells or albumin), hydration should be increased. A reduction in dosage (see "Dosage and Administration") may be desirable if other evidence of renal dysfunction occurs such as decreased creatinine clearance, decreased urine specific gravity, increased BUN, creatinine, or oliguria. If azotemia increases or if a progressive decrease in urinary output occurs, treatment should be stopped.

Note: When patients are well hydrated and kidney function is normal the risk of nephrotoxic reactions with amikacin is low if the dosage recommendations (see "Dosage and Administration") are not exceeded.

Product Information

Neurotoxicity

Neuromuscular blockade and muscular paralysis have been demonstrated in the cat with high doses of amikacin (188 mg/Kg). The possibility of neuromuscular blockade and respiratory paralysis should be considered when amikacin is administered concomitantly with anesthetic or neuromuscular blocking drugs. If blockade occurs, calcium salts may reverse this phenomenon.

Other

Cross-allergenicity among aminoglycosides has been demonstrated. As with other antibiotics the use of amikacin may result in overgrowth of non-susceptible organisms. If this occurs, appropriate therapy should be instituted.

Pregnancy

Reproduction studies have been performed in rats and mice and have revealed no evidence of impaired fertility or harm to the fetus due to amikacin. There are no well-controlled studies in pregnant women but investigational experience does not include any positive evidence of adverse effects on the fetus. Although there is no clearly defined risk, such experience cannot exclude the possibility of infrequent or subtle damage to the fetus. AMIKIN should be used in pregnant women only when clearly needed.

It is not known whether this drug is excreted in human milk. As a general rule, nursing should not be undertaken while a patient is on a drug since many drugs are excreted in human milk.

Adverse Reactions:

Ototoxicity

See "Warning" box.

Nephrotoxocity

Albuminuria, presence of red and white cells, casts, azotemia, and oliguria have been reported.

Other

In addition to those described above, other adverse reactions which have been reported on rare occasions are skin rash, drug fever, headache, paresthesia, tremor, nausea and vomiting, eosinophilia, arthralgia, anemia, hypotension.

Overdosage

In the event of overdosage or toxic reaction, peritoneal dialysis or hemodialysis will aid in the removal of amikacin from the blood.

Dosage and Administration: The patient's pretreatment body weight should be obtained for calculation of correct dosage. AMIKIN may be given intramuscularly or intravenously.

Intramuscular Administration for Patients with Normal Renal Function

The recommended dosage for adults, children, and older infants (see Box "Warning") with normal renal function is 15 mg/Kg/day divided into 2 or 3 equal doses administered at equally-divided intervals, i.e., 7.5 mg/Kg q.12h. or 5 mg/Kg q.8h. Treatment of patients in the heavier weight classes shall not exceed 1.5 Gm/day.

When amikacin is indicated in newborns (see Box "Warning"), it is recommended that a loading dose of 10 mg/Kg be administered initially to be followed with 7.5 mg/Kg every 12 hours.

The usual duration of treatment is 7 to 10 days. The total daily dose by all routes of administration should not exceed 15 mg/Kg/day. In the unusual circumstances where treatment beyond 10 days is considered, the use of AMIKIN should be reevaluated and, if continued, renal and auditory functions should be monitored daily.

At the recommended dosage level, uncomplicated infections due to amikacin-sensitive organisms should respond in 24 to 48 hours. If definite clinical response does not occur within 3 to 5 days, therapy should be stopped and the antibiotic sensitivity pattern of the invading organism should be rechecked. Failure of the infection to respond may be due to resistance of the organism or to the presence of septic foci requiring surgical drainage.

When AMIKIN is indicated in uncomplicated urinary tract infections, a dose of 250 mg twice daily may be used.

Intramuscular Administration for Patients with Impaired Renal Function

Whenever possible, serum amikacin concentrations should be monitored by appropriate assay procedures. Doses may be adjusted in patients with impaired renal function either by administering normal doses at prolonged intervals or by administering reduced doses at a fixed interval.

Both methods are based on the patient's creatinine clearance or serum creatinine values since these have been found to correlate with aminoglycoside half-lives in patients with diminished renal function. These dosage schedules must be used in conjunction with careful clinical and laboratory observations of the patient and should be modified as necessary. Neither method should be used when dialysis is being performed.

Normal Dosage at Prolonged Intervals

If the creatinine clearance rate is not available and the patient's condition is stable, a dosage interval in hours for the normal dose can be calculated by multiplying the patient's serum creatinine by nine, e.g., if the serum creatinine concentration is 2 mg/100 ml the recommended single dose (7.5 mg/Kg) should be administered every 18 hours.

Reduced Dosage at Fixed Time Intervals

When renal function is impaired and it is desirable to administer AMIKIN at a fixed time interval, dosage must be reduced. In these patients serum AMIKIN concentrations should be measured to assure accurate administration of AMIKIN and to avoid concentrations above 35 mcg/ml. If serum assay determinations are not available and the patient's condition is stable, serum creatinine and creatinine clearance values are the most readily available indicators of the degree of renal impairment to use as a guide for dosage.

First, initiate therapy by administering a normal dose, 7.5 mg/Kg, as a loading dose. This loading dose is the same as the normally recommended dose which would be calculated for a patient with a normal renal function as described above.

To determine the size of maintenance doses administered every 12 hours, the loading dose should be reduced in proportion to the reduction in the patient's creatinine clearance rate:

$$\frac{\text{Maintenance Dose}}{\text{Every 12 Hours}} = \frac{\text{observed CC in ml/min}}{\text{normal CC in ml/min}} \times \frac{\text{calculated loading}}{\text{dose in mg}}$$

(CC—creatinine clearance rate)

An alternate rough guide for determining reduced dosage at twelve-hour intervals (for patients whose steady state serum creatinine values are known) is to divide the normally recommended dose by the patient's serum creatinine.

The above dosage schedules are not intended to be rigid recommendations but are provided as guides to dosage when the measurement of amikacin serum levels is not feasible.

Intravenous Administration

The individual dose, the total daily dose, and the total cumulative dose of AMIKIN are identical to the dose recommended for intramuscular administration. The solution for intravenous use is prepared by adding the contents of a 500-mg vial to 100 or 200 ml of sterile diluent such as normal saline or 5% Dextrose in Water or any other compatible solution.

The solution is administered to adults over a 30- to 60-minute period. The total daily dose should not exceed 15 mg/Kg/day and may be divided into either 2 or 3 equally-divided doses at equally-divided intervals.

In pediatric patients the amount of fluid used will depend on the amount ordered for the patient. It should be a sufficient amount to infuse the amikacin over a 30- to 60-minute period. Infants should receive a 1- to 2-hour infusion.

Amikacin should not be physically premixed with other drugs but should be administered separately according to the recommended dose and route.

Stability in IV Fluids

Amikin is stable for 24 hours at room temperature, at concentrations of 0.25 and 5.0 mg/ml in the following solutions:

5% Dextrose Injection, U.S.P.
5% Dextrose and 0.2% Sodium Chloride Injection, U.S.P.
5% Dextrose and 0.45% Sodium Chloride Injection, U.S.P.
0.9% Sodium Chloride Injection, U.S.P.
Lactated Ringer's Injection, U.S.P.
Normosol®M in 5% Dextrose Injection, U.S.P. (or Plasma-Lyte 56 Injection in 5% Dextrose in Water)
Normosol®R in 5% Dextrose Injection, U.S.P. (or Plasma-Lyte 148 Injection in 5% Dextrose in Water)

Supply: AMIKIN is supplied as a colorless solution which requires no refrigeration. It is stable at room temperature for at least two years. At times the solution may become a very pale yellow; this does not indicate a decrease in potency.

AMIKIN (amikacin sulfate injection)
NDC 0015-3015-20—100 mg per 2 ml
NDC 0015-3020-20—500 mg per 2 ml
NDC 0015-3020-21—Disposable Syringe (500 mg per 2 ml)
NDC 0015-3023-20—1.0 gm per 4 ml

For information on package sizes available, refer to the current price schedule.
[See table above].

*Bauer, A. W., Kirby, W. M. M., Sherris, J. C., and Turck, M.: Antibiotic Testing by a Standardized Single Disc Method, Am. J. Clin. Pathol., 45:493, 1966; Standardized Disc Susceptibility Test, FEDERAL REGISTER, 37:20527-29, 1972.

DOSAGE GUIDELINES
ADULTS AND CHILDREN WITH NORMAL RENAL FUNCTION

Patient Weight		Dosage	
lbs	kg	7.5 mg/kg q. 12h	5 mg/kg q. 8h
99	45	337.5 mg	225 mg
110	50	375 mg	250 mg
121	55	412.5 mg	275 mg
132	60	450 mg	300 mg
143	65	487.5 mg	325 mg
154	70	525 mg	350 mg
165	75	562.6 mg	375 mg
176	80	600 mg	400 mg
187	85	637.5 mg	425 mg
198	90	675 mg	450 mg
209	95	712.5 mg	475 mg
220	100	750 mg	500 mg

Available as: 500 mg/2 ml vial, 1 gm/4 ml vial, 500 mg/2 ml Disposable Syringe

---

BETAPEN®-VK
(penicillin V potassium)
Tablets (Film Coated) and Oral Solution

This is the full text of the latest Official Package Circular dated August 1980 [7506 DIR-07].

Continued on next page

Bristol—Cont.

Description: Betapen-VK is the potassium salt of penicillin V. The oral solutions contain in each 5 ml. (teaspoonful) 125 mg. or 250 mg. of penicillin V activity respectively.

Clinical Pharmacology: Penicillin V exerts a bactericidal action against penicillin-susceptible microorganisms during the stage of active multiplication. It acts through the inhibition of biosynthesis of cell wall mucopeptide. It is not active against the penicillinase-producing bacteria, which include many strains of staphylococci. The drug exerts high in vitro activity against staphylococci (except penicillinase-producing strains), streptococci (Groups A, C, G, H, L, and M) and pneumococci. Other organisms susceptible in vitro to penicillin V are **Corynebacterium diphtheriae, Bacillus anthracis,** Clostridia, **Actinomyces bovis, Streptobacillus moniliformis, Listeria monocytogenes,** Leptospira and **Neisseria gonorrhoeae. Treponema pallidum** is extremely susceptible.

Penicillin V has the distinct advantage over penicillin G in resistance to inactivation by gastric acid. It may be given with meals; however, blood levels are slightly higher when the drug is given on an empty stomach. Average blood levels are two to five times higher than the levels following the same dose of oral penicillin G and also show much less individual variation.

Once absorbed, penicillin V is about 80% bound to serum protein. Tissue levels are highest in the kidney, with lesser amounts in the liver, skin, and intestines. Small amounts are found in all other body tissues and the cerebrospinal fluid. The drug is excreted as rapidly as it is absorbed in individuals with normal renal function; however, recovery of the drug from the urine indicates that only about 25% of the dose is absorbed. In neonates, young infants, and individuals with impaired renal function, excretion is considerably delayed.

Indications and Usage: Betapen-VK is indicated in the treatment of mild to moderately severe infections due to penicillin G-susceptible microorganisms. Therapy should be guided by bacteriological studies (including susceptibility tests) and by clinical response.

Note: Severe pneumonia, empyema, bacteremia, pericarditis, meningitis, and arthritis should not be treated with oral penicillins during the acute stage.

Indicated surgical procedures should be performed.

The following infections will usually respond to adequate doses of penicillin V: Streptococcal Infections (without bacteremia), mild to moderate infections of the upper respiratory tract, scarlet fever, and mild erysipelas.

Note: Streptococci in Groups A, C, G, H, L, and M are very susceptible to penicillin. Other groups, including Group D (enterococcus) are resistant.

Pneumococcal Infections—Mild to moderately severe infections of the respiratory tract.

Staphylococcal Infections — penicillin G-susceptible. Mild infections of the skin and soft tissue.

Note: Reports indicate an increasing number of strains of staphylococci resistant to penicillin G, emphasizing the need for culture and susceptibility studies in treating suspected staphylococcal infections.

Fusospirochetosis (Vincent's gingivitis and pharyngitis)—Mild to moderately severe infections of the oropharynx usually respond to therapy with oral penicillin.

Note: Necessary dental care should be accomplished in infections involving gum tissue.

Medical conditions in which oral penicillin therapy is indicated as prophylaxis: For the prevention of recurrence following rheumatic fever and/or chorea. Prophylaxis with oral penicillin on a continuing basis has proven effective in preventing recurrence of these conditions.

Although no controlled clinical efficacy studies have been conducted penicillin V has been suggested by the American Heart Association and the American Dental Association for use as part of a parenteral-oral regimen and as an alternative oral regimen for prophylaxis against bacterial endocarditis in patients with congenital heart disease or rheumatic or other acquired valvular heart disease when they undergo dental procedures and surgical procedures of the respiratory tract.[1] Since it may happen that **alpha**-hemolytic streptococci, relatively resistant to penicillin, may be found when patients are receiving continuous oral penicillin for secondary prevention of rheumatic fever, prophylactic agents other than penicillin may be chosen for these patients and prescribed in addition to their continuous rheumatic fever prophylactic regimen. Oral penicillin should not be used as adjunctive prophylaxis for genitourinary instrumentation or surgery, lower intestinal tract surgery, sigmoidoscopy, and childbirth.

Note: When selecting antibiotics for the prevention of bacterial endocarditis the physician or dentist should read the full joint statement of the American Heart Association and the American Dental Association.[1]

Contraindications: A previous hypersensitivity reaction to any penicillin is a contraindication.

Warning: Serious and occasionally fatal hypersensitivity (anaphylactoid) reactions have been reported in patients on penicillin therapy. Although anaphylaxis is more frequent following parenteral therapy, it has occurred in patients on oral penicillins. These reactions are more apt to occur in individuals with a history of sensitivity to multiple allergens.

There have been well documented reports of individuals with a history of penicillin hypersensitivity reactions who experienced severe hypersensitivity reactions when treated with cephalosporins. Before therapy with a penicillin, careful inquiry should be made concerning previous hypersensitivity reactions to penicillins, cephalosporins, and other allergens. If an allergic reaction occurs, the drug should be discontinued and the patient treated with the usual agents, e.g., antihistamines, pressor amines, corticosteroids.

Precautions: Penicillins should be used with caution in individuals with a history of significant allergies and/or asthma.

The oral route of administration should not be relied upon in patients with severe illness, or with nausea, vomiting, gastric dilatation, cardiospasm or intestinal hypermotility.

Occasional patients will not absorb therapeutic amounts of orally administered penicillins.

In streptococcal infections, therapy must be sufficient to eliminate the organism (10 days minimum); otherwise the sequelae of streptococcal disease may occur. Cultures should be taken following completion of treatment to determine whether streptococci have been eradicated.

Prolonged use of antibiotics may promote the overgrowth of nonsusceptible organisms, including fungi. Should superinfection occur, appropriate measures should be taken.

Adverse Reactions: Although the incidence of reactions to oral penicillins has been reported with much less frequency than following parenteral therapy, it should be remembered that all degrees of hypersensitivity, including fatal anaphylaxis, have been reported with oral penicillin.

The most common reactions to oral penicillin are nausea, vomiting, epigastric distress, diarrhea, and black hairy tongue. The hypersensitivity reactions reported are skin eruptions (maculopapular to exfoliative dermatitis), urticaria and other serum sickness reactions, laryngeal edema and anaphylaxis. Fever and eosinophilia may frequently be the only reaction observed. Hemolytic anemia, leukopenia, thrombocytopenia, neuropathy, and nephropathy are infrequent reactions and usually associated with high doses of parenteral penicillin.

Administration and Dosage: The dosage of Betapen-VK should be determined according to the susceptibility of the causative organism and the severity of infection, and adjusted to the clinical response of the patient.

The usual dosage recommendations for adults and children 12 years and over are as follows:

Streptococcal Infections—mild to moderately severe—of the upper respiratory tract and including scarlet fever and erysipelas: 125 to 250 mg. (200,000 to 400,000 units) every 6 to 8 hours for 10 days.

Pneumococcal Infections—mild to moderately severe—of the respiratory tract, including otitis media: 250 mg. (400,000 units) every 6 hours until the patient has been afebrile for at least 2 days.

Staphylococcal Infections—mild infections of skin and soft tissue (culture and sensitivity tests should be performed): 250 mg. (400,000 units) every 6 to 8 hours.

Fusospirochetosis (Vincent's Infection) of the oropharynx—mild to moderately severe infections: 250 mg. (400,000 units) every 6 to 8 hours.

For the prevention of recurrence following rheumatic fever and/or chorea: 125 mg. (200,000 units) twice daily on a continuing basis.

For prophylaxis against bacterial endocarditis[1] in patients with congenital heart disease or rheumatic or other acquired valvular heart disease when undergoing dental procedures or surgical procedures of the upper respiratory tract, 1 of 2 regimens may be selected:

(1) For the oral regimen, give 2 grams of penicillin V (1 gram for children under 60 lbs) ½ to 1 hour before the procedure, and then, 500 mg (250 mg for children under 60 lbs) every 6 hours for 8 doses; or

(2) For the combined parenteral-oral regimen, give 1 million units of aqueous crystalline penicillin G (30,000 units/kg in children) intramuscularly mixed with 600,000 units procaine penicillin G (600,000 units for children) ½ to 1 hour before the procedure, and then, oral penicillin V, 500 mg for adults or 250 mg for children less than 60 lbs, every 6 hours for 8 doses. Doses for children should not exceed recommendations for adults for a single dose or for a 24-hour period.

Directions for Dispensing Oral Solutions: Prepare this formulation at the time of dispensing. For ease in preparation, add water to the bottle in two portions and shake well after each addition. Add the total amount of water as directed on the labeling of the package being dispensed. The reconstituted solutions are stable for 14 days under refrigeration.

How Supplied: BETAPEN-VK (penicillin V potassium) for Oral Solution. Each 5 ml. of reconstituted solution contains penicillin V potassium equivalent to 125 or 250 mg. penicillin V.

NDC 0015-7506—125 mg
NDC 0015-7507—250 mg

BETAPEN-VK (penicillin V potassium) Tablets (Film Coated). Each tablet contains penicillin V potassium equivalent to 250 or 500 mg. penicillin V.

NDC 0015-7508-250 mg.
NDC 0015-7509-500 mg.

For information on package sizes available, refer to the current price schedule.

Reference:
1. American Heart Association. 1977. Prevention of bacterial endocarditis. Circulation. 56:139A-143A.

Shown in Product Identification Section, page 407

BRISTOJECT®

The following products are available in pre-filled, disposable Bristoject® syringes:

NDC-0015	PRODUCT
	AMINOPHYLLIN
9314-87	250 mg in 10 ml 22 ga × 1½″
	ATROPINE SULFATE ℞
9410-87	0.5 mg in 5 ml, 22 ga × 1½″
9411-87	1 mg in 10 ml, 22 ga × 1½″
	CALCIUM CHLORIDE ℞
9422-78	1 gram in 10 ml (10%), 22 ga × 1½″
9422-75	1 gram in 10 ml (10%), 18 ga × 3½″

for possible revisions

Product Information

DEXAMETHASONE
9080-87 20 mg in 5 ml 22 ga × 1½"

DEXTROSE ℞
9424-87 50% (25 grams in 50 ml), 18 ga × 1½"

DIPHENHYDRAMINE HCl
9085-87 50 mg in 5 ml, 22 ga × 1½"

DOPAMINE HCl
9092-87 200 mg in 5 ml Inject-all® (40 mg/ml)
9093-87 400 mg in 10 ml Inject-all® (40 mg/ml)

EPHEDRINE
9090-87 50 mg in 10 ml 22 ga × 1½"

EPINEPHRINE ℞
9423-77 1 mg in 10 ml (1:10,000), 22 ga × 1½"
9423-87 1 mg in 10 ml (1:10,000), 18 ga × 3½"

LIDOCAINE HCl
9149-87 50 mg in 5 ml (1%), 22 ga × 1½"
9151-87 100 mg in 5 ml (2%), 22 ga × 1½"
9161-87 100 mg in 10 ml (1%), 22 ga × 1½"
9179-87 1 gram in 25 ml (4%), Inject-all®
9140-90 2 grams in 50 ml (4%), Inject-all®
9142-87 1 gram in 5 ml (20%) Inject-all®
9143-87 2 grams in 10 ml (20%) Inject-all®

MAGNESIUM SULFATE ℞
9266-87 50% (5 grams in 10 ml), 20 ga × 2½"

METARAMINOL BITARTRATE ℞
9440-90 100 mg in 10 ml (1%), Inject-all®

SODIUM BICARBONATE ℞
9121-87 44.6 mEq in 50 ml (7.5%), 18 ga × 1½"
9124-87 50 mEq in 50 ml (8.4%), 18 ga × 1½"
9125-87 (Ped) 10 mEq in 10 ml (8.4%), 22 ga × 1½"
9115-87 (Infant) 5 mEq in 10 ml (4.2%) 22 ga × 1½"

CEFADYL® ℞
[cef-a-dill]
(sterile cephapirin sodium)

This is the full text of the latest Official Package Circular dated October 1983 [7628DIR-25].

Description: Cefadyl (sterile cephapirin sodium) is a cephalosporin antibiotic intended for intramuscular or intravenous administration only. Each 500 mg contains 1.18 milli-equivalents of sodium.

Cefadyl is the sodium salt of 7-α-(4-pyridylthio)-acetamido-cephalosporanic acid and has the following structural formula.

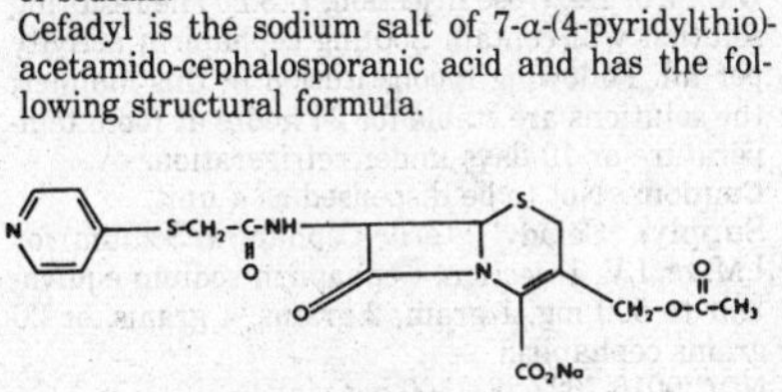

Clinical Pharmacology:
Human Pharmacology

TABLE I

Duration of Blood Levels of Cephapirin in Normal Volunteers
(Figures are mcg/ml)

	Time After Injection in Hours		
	½	4	6
Cefadyl 500 mg. I.M. (single dose)	9.0	0.7	0.2
Cefadyl 1 gram I.M. (single dose)	16.4	1.0	0.3

Cefadyl and its metabolites were excreted primarily by the kidneys. Antibiotic activity in the urine was equivalent to 35% of a 500-mg dose 6 hours after I.M. injection, and to 65% of a 500-mg dose 12 hours after injection. Following an I.M. dose of 500 mg, peak urine levels averaged 900 mcg/ml within the first 6 hours.

TABLE II

Duration of Blood Levels of Cephapirin in Normal Volunteers
(Figures are mcg/ml)

	Time After Injection in Minutes		
	5	30	180
Cefadyl 500 mg rapid I.V.	35	6.7	0.27
Cefadyl 1 gram rapid I.V.	67	14.0	0.61
Cefadyl 2 gram rapid I.V.	129	31.7	1.11

Seventy percent of the administered dose was recovered in the urine within 6 hours.
Repetitive intravenous administration of 1-gram doses over 6-hour periods produced serum levels between 4.5 and 5.5 mcg/ml.
At therapeutic drug levels, normal human serum binds Cefadyl to the extent of 44 to 50%. The average serum half-life of Cefadyl in patients with normal renal function is approximately 36 minutes. The major metabolite of cephapirin is desacetyl cephapirin which has been shown to contribute to antibacterial activity.
Controlled studies in normal adult volunteers revealed that Cefadyl was well tolerated intramuscularly. In controlled studies of volunteers and of patients receiving I.V. Cefadyl, the incidence of venous irritation was low.

Microbiology
In vitro tests demonstrate that the action of cephalosporins results from inhibition of cell-wall synthesis. Cefadyl is active against the following organisms **in vitro**:
  Beta-hemolytic streptococci and other streptococci.
  (Many strains of enterococci, e.g. **S. faecalis**, are relatively resistant.)
  Staphylococcus aureus (penicillinase and non-penicillinase-producing).
  Staphylococcus epidermidis (methicillin-susceptible strains).
  Streptococcus pneumoniae
    (formerly Diplococcus pneumoniae)
  Proteus mirabilis
  Haemophilus influenzae
  Escherichia coli
  Klebsiella species
Most strains of Enterobacter and indole-positive Proteus (**P. vulgaris, P. morganii, P. rettgeri**) are resistant to Cefadyl. Methicillin-resistant staphylococci, Serratia, Pseudomonas, Mima, and Herellea species are almost uniformly resistant to Cefadyl.

Disc Susceptibility Tests. — Quantitative methods that require measurement of zone diameters give the most precise estimates of antibiotic susceptibility. One such procedure* has been recommended for use with discs for testing susceptibility to cephalosporin class antibiotics. Interpretations correlate diameters of the disc test with MIC values for Cefadyl. With this procedure, a report from the laboratory of "susceptible" indicates that the infecting organism is likely to respond to therapy. A report of "resistant" indicates that the infecting organism is not likely to respond to therapy. A report of "intermediate susceptibility" suggests that the organism would be susceptible if high dosage is used, or if the infection is confined to tissues and fluid (e.g., urine), in which high antibiotic levels are attained.

Indications: Cefadyl is indicated in the treatment of infections caused by susceptible strains of the designated microorganisms in the diseases listed below. Culture and susceptibility studies should be performed. Therapy may be instituted before results of susceptibility studies are obtained.
Respiratory tract infections caused by **S. pneumoniae** (formerly **D. pneumoniae**); **Staphylococcus aureus** (penicillinase and nonpenicillinase-producing), **Klebsiella** species, **H. influenzae** and Group A beta-hemolytic streptococci.
Skin and skin structure infections caused by **Staphylococcus aureus** (penicillinase and non-penicillinase-producing), **Staphylococcus epidermidis** (methicillin-susceptible strains), **E. coli**, **P. mirabilis**, Klebsiella species, and Group A beta-hemolytic streptococci.
Urinary tract infections caused by **Staphylococcus aureus** (penicillinase and nonpenicillinase-producing), **E. coli**, **P. mirabilis**, and Klebsiella species.
Septicemia caused by **Staphylococcus aureus** (penicillinase and nonpenicillinase-producing), **S. viridans**, **E. coli**, Klebsiella species and Group A beta-hemolytic streptococci.
Endocarditis caused by **Streptococcus viridans** and **Staphylococcus aureus** (penicillinase and nonpenicillinase-producing).
Osteomyelitis caused by **Staphylococcus aureus** (penicillinase and nonpenicillinase-producing), Klebsiella species, **P. mirabilis**, and Group A beta-hemolytic streptococci.
Perioperative Prophylaxis—The prophylactic administration of Cefadyl preoperatively and postoperatively may reduce the incidence of certain postoperative infections in patients undergoing surgical procedures which are classified as contaminated or potentially contaminated, e.g., vaginal hysterectomy.
The perioperative use of Cefadyl may also be effective in surgical patients in whom infection at the operative site would present a serious risk, e.g., during open-heart surgery and prosthetic arthroplasty.
The prophylactic administration of Cefadyl should be discontinued within a 24 hour period after the surgical procedure. In surgery where the occurrence of infection may be particularly devastating, e.g., open-heart surgery and prosthetic arthroplasty, the prophylactic administration of Cefadyl may be continued for 3 to 5 days following completion of surgery. If there are signs of infection, specimens for culture should be obtained for the identification of the causative organism so that appropriate therapy may be instituted (See Dosage and Administration.)
Note: If the susceptibility tests show that the causative organism is resistant to Cefadyl, other appropriate therapy should be instituted.
Contraindications: Cefadyl is contraindicated in persons who have shown hypersensitivity to cephalosporin antibiotics.
Warnings: IN PENICILLIN-ALLERGIC PATIENTS, CEPHALOSPORINS SHOULD BE USED WITH GREAT CAUTION. THERE IS CLINICAL AND LABORATORY EVIDENCE OF PARTIAL CROSS-ALLERGENICITY OF THE PENICILLINS AND THE CEPHALOSPORINS, AND THERE ARE INSTANCES OF PATIENTS WHO HAVE HAD REACTIONS TO BOTH DRUGS (INCLUDING FATAL ANAPHYLAXIS AFTER PARENTERAL USE).
Any patient who has demonstrated some form of allergy, particularly to drugs, should receive antibiotics cautiously and then only when absolutely necessary. No exceptions should be made with regard to Cefadyl.
SERIOUS ANAPHYLACTOID REACTIONS REQUIRE IMMEDIATE EMERGENCY TREATMENT WITH EPINEPHRINE, OXYGEN, INTRAVENOUS STEROIDS, AND AIRWAY MANAGEMENT, INCLUDING INTUBATION, SHOULD ALSO BE ADMINISTERED AS INDICATED.

Continued on next page

Bristol—Cont.

Precautions: Usage in Pregnancy—Pregnancy Category B. Reproduction studies have been performed in rats and mice and have revealed no evidence of impaired fertility or harm to the fetus due to Cefadyl. There are however no well controlled studies in pregnant women. Because animal studies are not always predictive of human response, this drug should be used during pregnancy only if clearly indicated.

Nursing Mothers—Cefadyl may be present in human milk in small amounts. Caution should be exercised when Cefadyl is administered to a nursing woman.

The renal status of the patients should be determined prior to and during Cefadyl therapy, since in patients with impaired renal function, a reduced dose may be appropriate (see Dosage, Adults). When Cefadyl was given to patients with marked reduction in renal function and to renal transplant patients, no adverse effects were reported.

Prolonged use of Cefadyl may result in the overgrowth of nonsusceptible organisms. Careful observation of the patient is essential. If superinfection occurs during therapy, appropriate measures should be taken.

With high urine concentrations of cephapirin, false-positive glucose reactions may occur if Clinitest, Benedict's Solution, or Fehling's Solution are used. Therefore, it is recommended that glucose tests based on enzymatic glucose oxidase reactions (such as Clinistix or Tes-Tape) be used.

Increased nephrotoxicity has been reported following concomitant administration of cephalosporins and aminoglycoside antibiotics.

Adverse Reactions:
Hypersensitivity—Cephalosporins were reported to produce the following reactions: maculopapular rash, urticaria, reactions resembling serum sickness, and anaphylaxis. Eosinophilia and drug fever have been observed to be associated with other allergic reactions. These reactions are most likely to occur in patients with a history of allergy, particularly to penicillin.

Blood—During large scale clinical trials, rare instances of neutropenia, leukopenia, and anemia were reported. Some individuals, particularly those with azotemia, have developed positive direct Coombs' test during therapy with other cephalosporins.

Liver—Elevations in SGPT or SGOT, alkaline phosphatase, and bilirubin have been reported.

Kidney—Rises in BUN have been observed; their frequency increases in patients over 50 years old.

Dosage and Administration:
Adults—The usual dose is 500 mg to 1 gram every 4 to 6 hours intramuscularly or intravenously. The lower dose of 500 mg is adequate for certain infections, such as skin and skin structure and most urinary tract infections. However, the higher dose is recommended for more serious infections.

Very serious or life-threatening infections may require doses up to 12 grams daily. The intravenous route is preferable when high doses are indicated.

Depending upon the causative organism and the severity of infection, patients with reduced renal function (moderately severe oliguria or serum creatinine above 5.0 mg/100 ml) may be treated adequately with a lower dose 7.5 to 15 mg/Kg of cephapirin every 12 hours. Patients with severely reduced renal function and who are to be dialyzed should receive the same dose just prior to dialysis and every 12 hours thereafter.

Perioperative Prophylactic Use—To prevent postoperative infection in contaminated or potentially contaminated surgery. Recommended doses are:
a. 1 to 2 grams IM or IV administered ½ hour to 1 hour prior to the start of surgery.
b. 1 to 2 grams during surgery (administration modified depending on the duration of the operative procedure).
c. 1 to 2 grams IV or IM every 6 hours for 24 hours postoperatively.

It is important (1) the preoperative dose be given just prior to the start of surgery (½ to 1 hour) so that adequate antibiotic levels are present in the serum and tissues at the time of initial surgical incision, and (2) Cefadyl be administered, if necessary, at appropriate intervals during surgery to provide sufficient levels of the antibiotic at the anticipated moments of greatest exposure to infective organisms.

In surgery where the occurrence of infection may be particularly devastating, e.g., open-heart surgery and prosthetic arthroplasty, the prophylactic administration of Cefadyl may be continued for 3 to 5 days following completion of surgery.

Children—The dosage is in accordance with age, weight, and severity of infection. The recommended total daily dose is 40 to 80 mg/Kg (20 to 40 mg/lb) administered in four equally divided doses. The drug has not been extensively studied in infants, therefore, in the treatment of children under the age of three months the relative benefit/risk should be considered.

Therapy in beta-hemolytic streptococcal infections should continue for at least 10 days.

Where indicated surgical procedures should be performed in conjunction with antibiotic therapy. Cefadyl may be administered by the intramuscular or the intravenous routes.

Intramuscular Injection
The 500-mg and 1-gram vials should be reconstituted with 1 or 2 ml of Sterile Water for Injection, U.S.P., or Bacteriostatic Water for Injection, U.S.P., respectively. Each 1.2 ml contains 500 mg of cephapirin. All injections should be deep in the muscle mass.

Intravenous Injection
The intravenous route may be preferable for patients with bacteremia, septicemia, or other severe or life-threatening infections who may be poor risks because of lowered resistance resulting from such debilitating conditions as malnutrition, trauma, surgery, diabetes, heart failure, or malignancy, particularly if shock is present or impending. If patient has impaired renal function, a reduced dose may be indicated (see Dosage, Adults). In conditions such as septicemia, 6 to 8 grams per day may be given intravenously for several days at the beginning of therapy; then, depending on the clinical response and laboratory findings, the dosage may gradually be reduced.

When the infection has been refractory to previous forms of treatment and multiple sites have been involved, daily doses up to 12 grams have been used.

Intermittent Intravenous Injection
The contents of the 500-mg, 1-gram or 2-gram vial should be diluted with 10 ml or more of the specified diluent and administered slowly over a 3- to 5-minute period or may be given with intravenous infusions.

Intermittent Intravenous Infusion with Y-Tube
Intermittent intravenous infusion with a Y-type administration set can also be accomplished while bulk intravenous solutions are being infused. However, during infusion of the solution containing Cefadyl it is desirable to discontinue the other solution. When this technique is employed, careful attention should be paid to the volume of the solution containing Cefadyl so that the calculated dose will be infused. When a Y-tube hookup is used, the contents of the 4-gram vial of cephapirin should be diluted by addition of 40 ml of Bacteriostatic Water for Injection, U.S.P., Dextrose Injection, U.S.P., or Sodium Chloride Injection, U.S.P.

STABILITY
Utility Time For Cefadyl In Various Diluents At Concentrations Ranging From 20 to 400 mg/ml

Diluent	Approximate Concentration (mg/ml)	Utility Time 25°C	4°C
Water for Injection	50 to 400	12 hours	10 days
Bacteriostatic Water for Injection with Benzyl Alcohol or Parabens	250 to 400	48 hours	10 days
Normal Saline	20 to 100	24 hours	10 days
5% Dextrose in Water	20 to 100	24 hours	10 days

All of the above solutions can be frozen immediately after reconstitution and stored at −15°C for 60 days before use. After thawing at room temperature (25°C), all of the solutions are stable for at least 12 hours at room temperature or 10 days under refrigeration (4°C).

The pH of the resultant solution ranges from 6.5 to 8.5. During these storage conditions, no precipitation occurs. A change in solution color during this storage time does not affect the potency.

Compatibility with the Infusion Solution
Cefadyl is stable and compatible for 24 hours at room temperature at concentrations between 2 mg/ml and 30 mg/ml in the following solutions.
Sodium Chloride Injection, U.S.P.
5% W/V Dextrose in Water, U.S.P.
Sodium Lactate Injection, U.S.P.
5% Dextrose in Normal Saline, U.S.P.
10% Invert Sugar in Normal Saline
10% Invert Sugar in Water
5% Dextrose + 0.2% Sodium Chloride Injection, U.S.P.
Lactated Ringer's Injection, U.S.P.
Lactated Ringer's with 5% Dextrose
5% Dextrose + 0.45% Sodium Chloride Injection, U.S.P.
Ringer's Injection, U.S.P.
10% Dextrose Injection, U.S.P.
Sterile Water for Injection, U.S.P.
20% Dextrose Injection, U.S.P.
5% Sodium Chloride in Water
5% Dextrose in Ringer's Injection
Normosol® R
Normosol® R in 5% Dextrose Injection
Ionosol® D-CM
Ionosol® G in 10% Dextrose Injection

In addition, Cefadyl, at a concentration of 4 mg/ml, is stable and compatible for 10 days under refrigeration (4°C) or 14 days in the frozen state (15°C) followed by 24 hours at room temperature (25°C) in all of the intravenous solutions listed above.

"Piggyback" I.V. Package:
This glass vial contains the labeled quantity of Cefadyl and is intended for intravenous administration. The diluent and volume are specified on the label.

Hospital Bulk Package:
This glass vial contains 20 grams Cefadyl and is designed for use in the pharmacy in preparing I.V. additives. Add 67 ml of Sodium Chloride Injection, U.S.P., or Dextrose Injection, U.S.P. The resulting solution will contain 250 mg cephapirin activity per ml. Following reconstitution in this manner, the solutions are stable for 24 hours at room temperature or 10 days under refrigeration.
Caution: Not to be dispensed as a unit.
Supply: Cefadyl (Sterile Cephapirin Sodium) for I.M. or I.V. Injection. Cephapirin sodium equivalent to 500 mg, 1 gram, 2 grams, 4 grams, or 20 grams cephapirin.
NDC 0015-7627-28—500-mg vial
NDC 0015-7628-28—1-gram vial
NDC 0015-7629-30—2-gram vial
NDC 0015-7628-22—1-gram "piggyback" vial
NDC 0015-7629-28—2-gram "piggyback" vial
NDC 0015-7630-20—4-gram "piggyback" vial
NDC 0015-7613-20—20-gram Hospital Bulk Package
For information on package sizes available, refer to the current price schedule.

*Bauer, A. W., Kirby, W. M. M., Sherris, J. C. and Turck, M.: Antibiotic Testing by a Standardized Single Disc Method, Am. J. Clin. Pathol., 45:493, 1966; Standardized Disc Susceptibility Test, FEDERAL REGISTER 37:20527–29, 1972.

DYNAPEN®
[dĭn'ō-pĕn]
(dicloxacillin sodium)

DICLOXACILLIN SODIUM CAPSULES
125 mg, 250 mg and 500 mg

DICLOXACILLIN SODIUM FOR ORAL SUSPENSION
62.5 mg per 5 ml

This is the full text of the latest official Package Circular dated October 1983 [7856DIR-11].

Description: Dynapen (dicloxacillin sodium) is an antibacterial agent of the isoxazolyl penicillin series. It is a penicillinase-resistant, acid resistant semisynthetic penicillin suitable for oral administration. Dynapen is available as an oral suspension and capsules.

DICLOXACILLIN SODIUM

$C_{19}H_{16}Cl_2N_3NaO_5S \cdot H_2O$ 510.32 [CAS-13412 64-1] 4-Thia-1-azabicyclo [3.2.0]heptane-2-carboxylic acid,6-[[[3-(2,6-dichlorophenyl)-5-methyl-4-isoxazolyl]carbonyl]-amino]-3,3-dimethyl-7-oxo-, monosodium salt, monohydrate, [2S-(2α, 5α, 6β)]

Clinical Pharmacology:
Microbiology. Penicillinase-resistant penicillins exert a bactericidal action against penicillin-susceptible microorganisms during the state of active multiplication. All penicillins inhibit the biosynthesis of the bacterial cell wall.

The drugs in this class are highly resistant to inactivation by staphylococcal penicillinase and are active against penicillinase producing and non-penicillinase producing strains of **Staphylococcus aureus**. The penicillinase-resistant penicillins are active **in vitro** against a variety of other bacteria.

Susceptibility Plate Testing. Quantitative methods of susceptibility testing that require measurement of zone diameters or minimal inhibitory concentrations (M.I.C.'s) give the most precise estimates of antibiotic susceptibility. One such procedure has been recommended for use with discs to test susceptibility to this class of drugs.

Interpretations correlate diameters on the disc test with MIC values. A penicillinase-resistant class disc may be used to determine microbial susceptibility to cloxacillin, dicloxacillin, methicillin, nafcillin, and oxacillin. With this procedure, employing a 5 microgram methicillin sodium disc, a report from the laboratory of "susceptible" (zone of at least 14 mm) indicates that the infecting organism is likely to respond to therapy. A report of "resistant" (zone of less than 10 mm) indicates that the infecting organism is not likely to respond to therapy. A report of "intermediate susceptibility" (zone of 10–13 mm) suggests that the organism might be susceptible if high doses of the antibiotic are used, or if the infection is confined to tissues and fluids (e.g., urine), in which high antibiotic levels are attained.

In general, all staphylococci should be tested against the penicillin G disc and against the methicillin disc. Routine methods of antibiotic susceptibility testing may fail to detect strains of organisms resistant to the penicillinase-resistant penicillins. For this reason, the use of large inocula and 48-hour incubation periods may be necessary to obtain accurate susceptibility studies with these antibiotics. Bacterial strains which are resistant to one of the penicillinase-resistant penicillins should be considered resistant to all of the drugs in the class.

Pharmacokinetics. Dynapen (dicloxacillin sodium) is resistant to destruction by acid. Absorption of Dynapen after oral administration is rapid but incomplete. Studies with an oral dose of 125 mg gave average serum levels at 60 minutes of 4.74 mcg/ml. At four hours, average levels were 0.62 mcg/ml. In one study, single oral doses of Dynapen 500 mg produced peak serum concentrations of 10–17 mcg/ml at 1–1.5 hours.

Once absorbed, Dynapen (dicloxacillin sodium) binds to serum protein, mainly albumin. The degree of protein binding reported varies with the method of study and the investigator, but generally has been found to be 97.9 ± 0.6%. Oral absorption of dicloxacillin is delayed when the drug is administered after meals.

Dynapen, with normal doses, has insignificant concentrations in the cerebrospinal and ascitic fluids. It is found in therapeutic concentrations in the pleural, bile and amniotic fluids. Dynapen is rapidly excreted as unchanged drug in the urine by glomerular filtration and active tubular secretion. The elimination half-life for Dynapen is about 0.7 hours.

Indications and Usage: The penicillinase-resistant penicillins are indicated in the treatment of infections caused by penicillinase-producing staphylococci which have demonstrated susceptibility to the drugs. Cultures and susceptibility tests should be performed initially to determine the causative organism and their sensitivity to the drug (See **CLINICAL PHARMACOLOGY**—Susceptibility Plate Testing).

The penicillinase-resistant penicillins may be used to initiate therapy in suspected cases of resistant staphylococcal infections prior to the availability of laboratory test results. The penicillinase-resistant penicillins should not be used infections caused by organisms susceptible to penicillin G. If the susceptibility tests indicate that the infection is due to an organism other than a resistant staphylococcus, therapy should not be continued with a penicillinase-resistant penicillin.

Contraindications: A history of a hypersensitivity (anaphylactic) reaction to any penicillin is a contraindication.

Warnings: Serious and occasionally fatal hypersensitivity (anaphylactic shock with collapse) reactions have occurred in patients receiving penicillin. The incidence of anaphylactic shock in all penicillin-treated patients is between 0.015 and 0.04 percent. Anaphylactic shock resulting in death has occurred in approximately 0.002 percent of the patients treated. Although anaphylaxis is more frequent following a parenteral administration, it has occurred in patients receiving oral penicillins.

When penicillin therapy is indicated, it should be initiated only after a comprehensive patient drug and allergy history has been obtained. If an allergic reaction occurs, the drug should be discontinued and the patient should receive supportive treatment, e.g., artificial maintenance of ventilation, pressor amines, antihistamines, and corticosteroids. Individuals with a history of penicillin hypersensitivity may also experience allergic reactions when treated with a cephalosporin.

Precautions:
General. Penicillinase-resistant penicillins should generally not be administered to patients with a history of sensitivity to any penicillin.

Penicillin should be used with caution in individuals with histories of significant allergies and/or asthma. Whenever allergic reactions occur, penicillin should be withdrawn unless, in the opinion of the physician, the condition being treated is life-threatening and amenable only to penicillin therapy.

The oral route of administration should not be relied upon in patients with severe illness, or with nausea, vomiting, gastric dilation, cardiospasm, or intestinal hypermotility. Occasionally patients will not absorb therapeutic amounts of orally administered penicillin.

The use of antibiotics may result in overgrowth of nonsusceptible organisms. If new infections due to bacteria or fungi occur, the drug should be discontinued and appropriate measures taken.

Information for the Patient. Patients receiving penicillins should be given the following information and instructions by the physician:

1. Patients should be told that penicillin is an antibacterial agent which will work with the body's natural defenses to control certain types of infections. They should be told that the drug should not be taken if they have had an allergic reaction to any form of penicillin previously, and to inform the physician of any allergies or previous allergic reactions to any drugs they may have had (see **WARNINGS**).
2. Patients who have previously experienced an anaphylactic reaction to penicillin should be instructed to wear a medical identification tag or bracelet.
3. Because most antibacterial drugs taken by mouth are best absorbed on an empty stomach, patients should be directed, unless circumstances warrant otherwise, to take penicillin one hour before meals or two hours after eating (See **CLINICAL PHARMACOLOGY**—Pharmacokinetics).
4. Patients should be told to take the entire course of therapy prescribed, even if fever and other symptoms have stopped (See **PRECAUTIONS**—General).
5. If any of the following reactions occur, stop taking your prescription and notify the physician: shortness of breath, wheezing, skin rash, mouth irritation, black tongue, sore throat, nausea, vomiting, diarrhea, fever, swollen joints, or any unusual bleeding or bruising (See **ADVERSE REACTIONS**).
6. Do not take any additional medications without physician approval, including non-prescription drugs such as antacids, laxatives or vitamins.
7. Discard any liquid forms of penicillin after 7 days if stored at room temperature or after 14 days if refrigerated.

Laboratory Tests. Bacteriologic studies to determine the causative organisms and their susceptibility to the penicillinase-resistant penicillins should be performed (See **CLINICAL PHARMACOLOGY**—Microbiology). In the treatment of suspected staphylococcal infections, therapy should be changed to another active agent if culture tests fail to demonstrate the presence of staphylococci.

Periodic assessment of organ system function including renal, hepatic, and hematopoietic should be made during prolonged therapy with the penicillinase-resistant penicillins.

Blood cultures, white blood cell, and differential cell counts should be obtained prior to initiation of therapy and at least weekly during therapy with penicillinase-resistant penicillins.

Periodic urinalysis, blood urea nitrogen, and creatinine determinations should be performed during therapy with the penicillinase-resistant penicillins and dosage alterations should be considered if these values become elevated. If any impairment of renal function is suspected or known to exist, a reduction in the total dosage should be considered and blood levels monitored to avoid possible neurotoxic reactions (See **DOSAGE AND ADMINISTRATION**).

SGOT and SGPT values should be obtained periodically during therapy to monitor for possible liver function abnormalities.

Drug Interactions. Tetracycline, a bacteriostatic antibiotic, may antagonize the bactericidal effect of penicillin and concurrent use of these drugs should be avoided.

Carcinogenesis, Mutagenesis, Impairment of Fertility. No long-term animal studies have been conducted with these drugs.

Studies on reproduction (Nafcillin) in rats and rabbits reveal no fetal or maternal abnormalities before conception and continuously through weaning (one generation).

Pregnancy Category B. Reproduction studies performed in the mouse, rat, and rabbit have revealed no evidence of impaired fertility or harm to the fetus due to the penicillinase-resistant penicillins. Human experience with the penicillins during pregnancy has not shown any positive evidence of adverse effects on the fetus. There are, however, no adequate or well-controlled studies in pregnant women showing conclusively that harmful effects of these drugs on the fetus can be excluded. Because animal reproduction studies are

Continued on next page

Bristol—Cont.

not always predictive of human response, this drug should be used during pregnancy only if clearly needed.

Nursing Mothers. Penicillins are excreted in breast milk. Caution should be exercised when penicillins are administered to a nursing woman.

Pediatric Use. Because of incompletely developed renal function in newborns, penicillinase-resistant penicillins (especially methicillin) may not be completely excreted, with abnormally high blood levels resulting. Frequent blood levels are advisable in this group with dosage adjustments when necessary. All newborns treated with penicillins should be monitored closely for clinical and laboratory evidence of toxic or adverse effects (See **DOSAGE AND ADMINISTRATION**).

Adverse Reactions:

Body as a Whole: The reported incidence of allergic reactions to penicillin ranges from 0.7 to 10 percent (See **WARNINGS**). Sensitization is usually the result of treatment but some individuals have had immediate reactions to penicillin when first treated. In such cases, it is thought that the patients may have had prior exposure to the drug via trace amounts present in milk and vaccines. Two types of allergic reactions to penicillin are noted clinically, immediate and delayed.

Immediate reactions usually occur within 20 minutes of administration and range in severity from urticaria and pruritus to angioneurotic edema, laryngospasm, bronchospasm, hypotension, vascular collapse, and death. Such immediate anaphylactic reactions are very rare (See **WARNINGS**) and usually occur after parenteral therapy but have occurred in patients receiving oral therapy. Another type of immediate reaction, an accelerated reaction, may occur between 20 minutes and 48 hours after administration and may include urticaria, pruritus, and fever. Although laryngeal edema, laryngospasm, and hypotension occasionally occur, fatality is uncommon.

Delayed allergic reactions to penicillin therapy usually occur after 48 hours and sometimes as late as 2 to 4 weeks after initiation of therapy. Manifestations of this type of reaction include serum sickness-like symptoms (i.e., fever, malaise, urticaria, myalgia, arthralgia, abdominal pain) and various skin rashes. Nausea, vomiting, diarrhea, stomatitis, black or hairy tongue, and other symptoms of gastrointestinal irritation may occur, especially during oral penicillin therapy.

Nervous System Reactions: Neurotoxic reactions similar to those observed with penicillin G may occur with large intravenous doses of the penicillinase-resistant penicillins especially with patients with renal insufficiency.

Urogenital Reactions: Renal tubular damage and interstitial nephritis have been associated with the administration of methicillin sodium and infrequently with the administration of nafcillin and oxacillin. Manifestations of this reaction may include rash, fever, eosinophilia, hematuria, proteinuria, and renal insufficiency. Methicillin-induced nephropathy does not appear to be dose-related and is generally reversible upon prompt discontinuation of therapy.

Metabolic Reactions: Agranulocytosis, neutropenia, and bone marrow depression have been associated with the use of methicillin sodium, nafcillin, oxacillin, and cloxacillin. Hepatotoxicity, characterized by fever, nausea, and vomiting associated with abnormal liver function tests, mainly elevated SGOT levels, has been associated with the use of oxacillin and cloxacillin.

Dosage and Administration: The penicillinase-resistant penicillins are available for oral administration and for intramuscular and intravenous injection. The sodium salts of methicillin, oxacillin, and nafcillin may be administered parenterally and the sodium salts of cloxacillin, dicloxacillin, oxacillin, and nafcillin are available for oral use.

Bacteriologic studies to determine the causative organisms and their sensitivity to the penicillinase-resistant penicillins should always be performed. Duration of therapy varies with the type and severity of infection as well as the overall condition of the patient, therefore it should be determined by the clinical and bacteriological response of the patient. In severe staphylococcal infections, therapy with penicillinase-resistant penicillins should be continued for at least 14 days. Therapy should be continued for at least 48 hours after the patient has become afebrile, asymptomatic, and cultures are negative. The treatment of endocarditis and osteomyelitis may require a longer term of therapy.

Concurrent administration of the penicillinase-resistant penicillins and probenecid increases and prolongs serum penicillin levels. Probenecid decreases the apparent volume of distribution and slows the rate of excretion by competitively inhibiting renal tubular secretion of penicillin. Penicillin-probenecid therapy is generally limited to those infections where very high serum levels of penicillin are necessary.

Oral preparations of the penicillinase-resistant penicillins should not be used as initial therapy in serious, life-threatening infections (see **PRECAUTIONS**—General). Oral therapy with the penicillinase-resistant penicillins may be used to follow-up the previous use of a parenteral agent as soon as the clinical condition warrants. For intramuscular gluteal injections, care should be taken to avoid sciatic nerve injury. With intravenous administration, particularly in elderly patients, care should be taken because of the possibility of thrombophlebitis. [See table below].

Directions For Dispensing Oral Suspension: Prepare these formulations at the time of dispensing. For ease in preparation, add water to the bottle in two portions and shake well after each addition. Add the total amount of water as directed on the labeling of the package being dispensed. The reconstituted formulation is stable for 14 days under refrigeration.

How Supplied:
Dynapen (dicloxacillin sodium) for Oral Suspension, 62.5 mg per 5 ml.
NDC 0015-7856
Dynapen (dicloxacillin sodium) Capsules. Each capsule contains dicloxacillin sodium equivalent to 125, 250, or 500 mg dicloxacillin.
NDC 0015-7892—125 mg
NDC 0015-7893—250 mg
NDC 0015-7658—500 mg
For information on package sizes available, refer to the current price schedule.

7856DIR-10   October 1983
Shown in Product Identification Section, page 407

KANTREX® CAPSULES ℞
[kan' treks]
(kanamycin sulfate)
Not for Systemic Use

This is the full text of the latest Official Package Circular dated January 1978 [3506 DIRO-08].

Description: Kanamycin sulfate is a water soluble aminoglycoside antibiotic derived from Streptomyces kanamyceticus. It is supplied in oral formulation for topical effect within the gastrointestinal tract, because it is absorbed only very slightly when administered orally, and is excreted unchanged in the feces.

Actions: Kanamycin is poorly absorbed from the normal gastrointestinal tract. The small absorbed fraction is rapidly excreted with normal kidney function. The unabsorbed portion of the drug is eliminated unchanged in the feces.

Most intestinal bacteria are eliminated rapidly following oral administration of kanamycin, with bacterial suppression persisting for 48 to 72 hours.

Indications:
Suppression of Intestinal Bacteria—Kanamycin is indicated when supression of the normal bacterial flora of the bowel is desirable for short-term adjunctive therapy.

Hepatic Coma—Prolonged administration has been shown to be effective adjunctive therapy in **Hepatic Coma** by reduction of the ammonia-forming bacteria in the intestinal tract. The subsequent reduction in blood ammonia has resulted in neurologic improvement.

Contraindications: This drug is contraindicated in the presence of intestinal obstruction and in individuals with a history of hypersensitivity to the drug.

Warnings: Although negligible amounts of kanamycin are absorbed through intact intestinal mucosa (approximately 1 percent), the possibility of increased absorption from ulcerated or denuded areas should be considered. If renal insufficiency develops during treatment, the dosage should be reduced or the antibiotic discontinued. Urine and blood examinations and audiometric tests should be given prior to and during extended therapy in individuals with hepatic and/or renal disease.

Usage in Pregnancy: Safety for use in pregnancy has not been established.

Precautions: Caution should be taken in concurrent use of other ototoxic and/or nephrotoxic antimicrobial drugs while kanamycin is administered orally. These include streptomycin, neomycin, polymyxin B, colistin, viomycin, gentamicin, and cephaloridine.

The concurrent use of potent diuretics (e.g. ethacrynic acid, furosemide, and mannitol, particularly when the diuretics are given intravenously) should be avoided. They may cause cumulative adverse effects of the kanamycin on the kidney and auditory nerve.

Prolonged use of oral kanamycin may result in overgrowth of nonsusceptible organisms, particularly fungi. If this occurs, appropriate therapy should be instituted.

Adverse Reactions: The most common adverse reactions to oral kanamycin are nausea, vomiting, and diarrhea. The "Malabsorption Syndrome" characterized by increased fecal fat, decreased serum carotene, and fall in xylose absorption has been reported with prolonged therapy. Nephrotoxicity and ototoxicity have been reported following prolonged and high dosage therapy in hepatic coma.

Dosage and Administration For Oral Use Only:

Suppression of Intestinal Bacteria:
1. As an adjunct in therapy of Hepatic Coma for extended therapy: 8 to 12 Gm. per day in divided doses.
2. As an adjunct to mechanical cleansing of the large bowel in short term therapy: 1.0 Gm. (2 capsules) every hour for 4 hours followed by 1.0 Gm. (2 capsules) every 6 hours for 36 to 72 hours.

Duration of therapy within this range depends on the condition of the patient, the type and amount

---

RECOMMENDED DOSAGES FOR DYNAPEN (dicloxacillin sodium)
IN MILD TO MODERATE AND SEVERE INFECTIONS

DRUG	ADULTS		CHILDREN	
	Mild to Moderate	Severe	Mild to Moderate	Severe
Dicloxacillin	125 mg every 6 hours	250 mg every 6 hours	12.5 mg/kg/day[a] in equally divided doses every 6 hours	25 mg/kg/day[a] in equally divided doses every 6 hours

(a) Patients weighing less than 40 Kg (88 lbs)

of concurrent mechanical cleansing (catharsis and enemas), and the customary medical routine.
Supply: KANTREX (kanamycin sulfate) Capsules. Kanamycin sulfate equivalent to 500 mg kanamycin per capsule.
NDC 0015-3506—500mg
For information on package sizes available, refer to the current price schedule.
Shown in Product Identification Section, page 407

KANTREX® INJECTION ℞
[*kan'treks*]
(kanamycin sulfate injection)
500 mg. per 2 ml.; 1.0 Gm. per 3 ml.

KANTREX® PEDIATRIC INJECTION ℞
(kanamycin sulfate injection)
75 mg. per 2 ml.

This is the full text of the latest Official Package Circular dated November 1978 [3502DIM-09].

WARNING

Patients treated with aminoglycosides by any route should be under close clinical observation because of the potential toxicity associated with their use. As with other aminoglycosides, the major toxic effects of kanamycin sulfate are its action on the auditory and vestibular branches of the eighth nerve and the renal tubules. Loss of high frequency perception usually occurs before clinical hearing loss and can be detected by audiometric testing. There may not be clinical symptoms to warn of developing cochlear damage. Vertigo may occur and may be evidence of vestibular injury. Renal impairment may be characterized by decreased creatinine clearance, the presence of cells or casts, oliguria, proteinuria, decreased urine specific gravity, or evidence of increasing nitrogen retention (increasing BUN, NPN or serum creatinine).

In patients with impaired kidney function, the risks of severe ototoxic and nephrotoxic reactions are sharply increased. In such cases, either the total daily dosage should be reduced, or the interval between doses lengthened, or both. Assessment of renal function and audiograms should be obtained before treatment if possible and monitored frequently during the course of therapy (see "Precautions"). If there is evidence of progressive renal dysfunction (increasing NPN, BUN, serum creatinine or oliguria) during therapy, audiometric tests are advised and discontinuation of the drug should be considered.

Elderly patients, patients with preexisting tinnitus or vertigo or known subclinical deafness, those having received prior ototoxic drugs, and patients receiving a total dose of more than 15 g of kanamycin sulfate should be carefully observed for signs of eighth nerve damage. Loss of hearing may occur in such patients even with normal renal function.

Neuromuscular blockade with respiratory paralysis may occur when kanamycin sulfate is administered intraperitoneally concomitantly with anesthesia and muscle-relaxing drugs. Although there have been isolated reports of respiratory depression following intraperitoneal instillation of kanamycin, there is no conclusive proof that this side effect can be produced with recommended doses of the drug.

The concurrent and or sequential systemic or topical use of kanamycin and other potentially ototoxic, nephrotoxic, and/or neurotoxic drugs, particularly streptomycin, polymyxin B, colistin, neomycin, gentamicin, cephaloridine, paromomycin, tobramycin, amikacin, vancomycin and viomycin should be avoided because the toxicity may be additive.

Kanamycin sulfate should not be given concurrently with potent diuretics (ethacrynic acid, furosemide, meralluride sodium, sodium mercaptomerin, or mannitol). Some diuretics themselves cause ototoxicity, and intravenously administered diuretics may enhance aminoglycoside toxicity by altering antibiotic concentrations in serum and tissue.

Description: Kanamycin sulfate is an aminoglycoside antibiotic produced by **Streptomyces kanamyceticus**. It is $C_{18}H_{36}N_4O_{11} \cdot 2H_2SO_4$. D-Streptomine, 0-3- amino-3-deoxy-α-D-glucopyranosyl— $(1 \rightarrow 6)$-0-[6-amino-6-deoxy-α-D-glucopyranosyl-$(1 \rightarrow 4)$]-2-deoxy, sulfate 1:2 (salt). It consists of two amino sugars glycosidically linked to deoxystreptamine.

Kanamycin sulfate injection, sterile solution for parenteral administration, contains respectively: kanamycin sulfate 75 mg, 500 mg, and 1 g; sodium bisulfite, an antioxidant, 0.099%, 0.66%, and 0.45%, and sodium citrate, 0.33%, 2.2%, and 2.2% with pH of each dosage form adjusted to 4.5 with sulfuric acid.

Action:
Clinical Pharmacology
The drug is rapidly absorbed after intramuscular injection and peak serum levels are generally reached within approximately one hour. Doses of 7.5 mg/Kg give mean peak levels of 22 mcg/ml. At 8 hours following a 7.5 mg/Kg dose, mean serum levels are 3.2 mcg/ml. Intravenous administration of kanamycin over a period of one hour resulted in serum concentrations similar to those obtained by intramuscular administration.

Kanamycin diffuses rapidly into most body fluids including synovial and peritoneal fluids and bile. Significant levels of the drug appear in cord blood and amniotic fluid following intramuscular administration to pregnant patients. Spinal fluid concentrations in normal infants are approximately 10 to 20 percent of serum levels and may reach 50 percent when the meninges are inflamed. Studies in normal adult patients have shown only trace levels of kanamycin in spinal fluid. No data are available on adults with meningitis.

The drug is excreted almost entirely by glomerular filtration and is not reabsorbed by the renal tubules. Hence, high concentrations are attained in the nephron, and the urine may contain levels 10 to 20 times higher than those in serum. Renal excretion is extremely rapid. In patients with normal renal function, approximately one-half of the administered dose is cleared within 4 hours and excretion is complete within 24 to 48 hours. Patients with impaired renal function or with diminished glomerular filtration pressure excrete kanamycin more slowly. Such patients may build up excessively high blood levels which greatly increase the risk of ototoxic reactions.

Microbiology
Kanamycin sulfate is a bactericidal antibiotic which acts by inhibiting the synthesis of protein in susceptible microorganisms. Kanamycin sulfate is active **in vitro** against many strains of **Staphylococcus aureus** (including penicillinase and non-penicillinase-producing strains). **Staphylococcus epidermidis, N. gonorrhoeae, H. influenzae, E. coli, Enterobacter aerogenes, Shigella, Salmonella, K. pneumoniae, Serratia marcescens, Acinetobacter**, and many strains of both indole-positive and indole-negative **Proteus** that are frequently resistant to other antibiotics. Bacterial resistance to kanamycin develops slowly in most susceptible organisms. In vitro studies have demonstrated that an aminoglycoside combined with an antibiotic which interferes with cell wall synthesis (i.e., penicillins or cephalosporins) acts synergistically against some strains of Gram-negative organisms and enterococci (**Streptococcus faecalis**).

Susceptibility testing: The infecting organism should be cultured and its susceptibility demonstrated as a guide to therapy. If the Kirby-Bauer method of disc susceptibility is used, a 30-mcg kanamycin disc should give a zone of inhibition of 17 mm or more when tested against a kanamycin-susceptible bacterial strain. A zone of 16 mm or less indicates that the infecting organism is likely to be resistant. In certain conditions, it may be desirable to do additional susceptibility testing by the tube or Agar dilution method. Kanamycin reference standard is available for this purpose.

Indications and Usage: Kanamycin is indicated in the treatment of serious infections caused by susceptible strains of microorganisms. Bacteriological studies to identify the causative organisms and to determine their susceptibility to kanamycin should be performed. Therapy may be instituted prior to obtaining the results of susceptibility testing.

Kanamycin may be considered as initial therapy in the treatment of infections where one or more of the following are the known or suspected pathogens: E. coli, Proteus species (both indole-positive and indole-negative), Enterobacter aerogenes, Klebsiella pneumoniae, Serratia marcescens, Acinetobacter. The decision to continue therapy with the drug should be based on results of the susceptibility tests, the response of the infection to therapy, and the important additional concepts contained in the "Warning" box above.

In serious infections when the causative organisms are unknown, Kantrex may be administered as initial therapy in conjunction with a penicillin- or cephalosporin-type drug before obtaining results of susceptibility testing. If anaerobic organisms are suspected, consideration should be given to using other suitable antimicrobial therapy in conjunction with kanamycin.

Although kanamycin is not the drug of choice for staphylococcal infections, it may be indicated under certain conditions for the treatment of known or suspected staphylococcal disease. These situations include the initial therapy of severe infections where the organism is thought to be either a Gram-negative bacterium or a staphylococcus, infections due to susceptible strains of staphylococci in patients allergic to other antibiotics, and mixed staphylococcal/Gram-negative infections.

Contraindications: A history of hypersensitivity or toxic reaction to one aminoglycoside may also contraindicate the use of any other aminoglycoside, because of the known cross-sensitivity and cumulative effects of drugs in this category. THIS DRUG IS NOT INDICATED IN LONG-TERM THERAPY (e.g. Tuberculosis) BECAUSE OF THE TOXIC HAZARD ASSOCIATED WITH EXTENDED ADMINISTRATION.

Warning: See "Warning" box above.
Precautions:
Ototoxicity: In patients with renal dysfunction an audiogram should be obtained before treatment and repeated frequently during therapy. Therapy should be stopped if tinnitus or subjective hearing loss develops, or if follow-up audiograms show loss of high frequency perception.

It should be emphasized that since renal function may alter appreciably during therapy, the serum creatinine should be checked daily or more frequently. Changes in the concentration would, of course, necessitate changes in the dosage frequency.

Nephrotoxicity: Because of the high concentration of kanamycin sulfate in the urinary excretory system, patients should be well-hydrated to prevent chemical irritation of the renal tubules. Kidney function should be assessed by the usual methods, e.g., urinalysis, BUN, serum creatinine, prior to starting therapy and periodically during the course of treatment. If signs of renal irritation appear, such as casts, white or red cells, and albumin, hydration should be increased and a reduction in dosage may be desirable (see "Dosage and

Continued on next page

Bristol—Cont.

Administration"). These signs usually disappear when treatment is completed. However, if azotemia or a progressive decrease in urine output occurs, treatment should be stopped.

The possibility of neuromuscular blockade with respiratory paralysis should be considered if aminoglycosides are administered by any route in patients receiving anesthetics, in patients receiving neuromuscular-blocking agents such as tubocurarine, succinylcholine, decamethonium or in patients receiving massive transfusions of citrate-anticoagulated blood. In all cases, patients should be observed carefully for signs of respiratory depression. If blockade occurs, calcium salts or neostigmine may reverse this phenomenon.

NOTE: The risk of toxic reactions is low in well-hydrated patients with normal kidney function, who receive a total dose of 15 g of kanamycin or less.

Because of the possibility of additive effects of other potentially ototoxic, neurotoxic, and/or nephrotoxic drugs, the concurrent or sequential administration of these drugs with kanamycin sulfate should be avoided (see "Warning" box).

Increased nephrotoxicity has been reported following concomitant parenteral administration of aminoglycoside antibiotics and cephalothin.

Since kanamycin sulfate and methicillin inactivate each other in vitro, they should not be physically mixed together in the same solution intended for parenteral administration. However, this inactivation has not been demonstrated in patients who receive both drugs by different routes of administration. (See "Dosage and Administration.")

Elderly patients may have reduced renal function which may not be evident in the results of routine screening tests, such as BUN or serum creatinine. A creatinine clearance determination may be more helpful. Monitoring of renal function during treatment is particularly important in such patients.

Aminoglycosides should be used with caution in patients with myasthenia gravis since these drugs may aggravate muscle weakness because of their curare-like effect on the neuromuscular function. Kanamycin sulfate should not be given concurrently with potent diuretics (see "Warning" box).

Neurotoxic and nephrotoxic antibiotics may be absorbed from body surfaces after local irrigation or application. The potential toxic effect of aminoglycosides administered in this fashion should be considered (see "Warning" box).

Cross-allergenicity among aminoglycosides has been demonstrated.

As with other antibiotics, kanamycin sulfate administration may result in overgrowth of nonsusceptible organisms, including fungi. If superinfection occurs, appropriate therapy should be instituted.

Pregnancy:
Reproduction studies have been performed in rats and rabbits and have revealed no evidence of impaired fertility or teratogenic effects. Dosages of 200 mg/Kg/day in pregnant rats and pregnant guinea pigs led to hearing impairment in the offspring. There are no well-controlled studies in pregnant women but clinical experience does not include any positive evidence of adverse effects on the fetus. Although there is no clearly defined risk, such experience cannot exclude the possibility of infrequent or subtle damage to the fetus. Kantrex should be used in pregnant women only when clearly needed.

Adverse Reactions:
Nephrotoxicity—Albuminuria, presence of red and white cells, and granular casts; azotemia and oliguria have been reported.

Ototoxicity—Tinnitus, vertigo, and partial reversible to irreversible hearing loss have been reported, usually associated with higher than recommended dosage. Rapid development of hearing loss has been reported in patients with poor kidney function treated concurrently with kanamycin and one of the rapid-acting diuretic agents given intravenously. These have included ethacrynic acid, furosemide, and mannitol.

Other—Some local irritation or pain may follow intramuscular injection. Other adverse reactions of the drug reported on rare occasions are skin rash, drug fever, headache, and paresthesia.

Overdosage: In the event of overdosage or toxic reaction, hemodialysis or peritoneal dialysis will aid in the removal of kanamycin from the blood. In the newborn infant, exchange transfusions may also be considered.

Dosage and Administration:
Intramuscular Route: Inject deeply into the upper outer quadrant of the gluteal muscle. The recommended dose for adults or children is 15 mg/Kg/day in two equally divided dosages administered at equally divided intervals, i.e. 7.5 mg/Kg q12h. If continuously high blood levels are desired, the daily dose of 15 mg/Kg may be given in equally divided doses every 6 or 8 hours. Treatment of patients in the heavier weight classes, i.e. > 100 Kg, should not exceed 1.5 g/day.

In patients with impaired renal function, it is desirable to follow therapy by appropriate serum assays. If this is not feasible, a suggested method is to reduce the frequency of administration in patients with renal dysfunction. The interval between doses may be calculated with the following formula:

Serum creatinine (mg/100 ml) × 9 = Dosage Interval (in hours): e.g., if the serum creatinine is 2 mg, the recommended dose (7.5 mg/Kg) should be administered every 18 hours. Changes in creatinine concentration during therapy would, of course, necessitate changes in the dosage frequency.

The usual duration of treatment is 7 to 10 days. The total daily dose by all routes of administration should not exceed 1.5 g/day.

At the recommended dosage level, uncomplicated infections due to kanamycin-susceptible organisms should respond to therapy in 24 to 48 hours. If definite clinical response does not occur within 3 to 5 days, therapy should be stopped and the antibiotic susceptibility pattern of the invading organism should be rechecked. Failure of the infection to respond may be due to resistance of the organism or to the presence of septic foci requiring surgical drainage.

Intravenous Administration: The dose should not exceed 15 mg/Kg per day and must be administered slowly. The solution for intravenous use is prepared by adding the contents of a 500-mg vial to 100 to 200 ml of sterile diluent such as Normal Saline or 5% Dextrose in Water, or the contents of a 1 g vial to 200 to 400 ml of sterile diluent. The appropriate dose is administered over a 30- to 60-minute period. The total daily dose should be divided into two or three equally divided doses.

In pediatric patients the amount of diluent used should be sufficient to infuse the kanamycin sulfate over a 30- to 60-minute period.

Kanamycin sulfate injection should not be physically mixed with other antibacterial agents but each should be administered separately in accordance with its recommended route of administration and dosage schedule.

Intraperitoneal Use: (following exploration for established peritonitis or after peritoneal contamination due to fecal spill during surgery.)

Adults: 500 mg diluted in 20 ml sterile distilled water may be instilled through a polyethylene catheter sutured into the wound at closure. If possible, instillation should be postponed until the patient has fully recovered from the effects of anesthesia and muscle-relaxing drugs (see "Warning" box).

Aerosol Treatment: 250 mg two to four times a day. Withdraw 250 mg (1 ml) from 500-mg vial and dilute it with 3 ml Physiological Saline and nebulize.

Other Routes of Administration: Kantrex Injection in concentrations of 0.25 percent (2.5 mg/ml) has been used as an irrigating solution in abscess cavities, pleural space, peritoneal and ventricular cavities. Possible absorption of Kantrex by such routes must be taken into account and dosage adjustments should be arranged so that a maximum total dose of 1.5 g/day by all routes of administration is not exceeded.

PEDIATRIC DOSAGE GUIDE FOR KANTREX PEDIATRIC INJECTION,
75 mg/2 ml—
AMOUNT PER 24 HOURS
TO BE GIVEN IN DIVIDED DOSES

Weight in Pounds	Weight in Kilograms	Daily Dosage in Milligrams	Daily Dosage in Milliliters
2.2	1.00	15.0	0.4
2.8	1.25	18.8	0.5
3.3	1.50	22.5	0.6
3.9	1.75	26.2	0.7
4.4	2.00	30.0	0.8
5.0	2.25	33.8	0.9
5.5	2.50	37.5	1.0
6.0	2.75	41.2	1.1
6.6	3.00	45.0	1.2
7.7	3.50	52.5	1.4
8.8	4.00	60.0	1.6
9.9	4.50	67.5	1.8
11.0	5.00	75.0	2.0

Stability: Occasionally, some vials may darken during the shelf-life of the product, but this does not indicate a loss of potency.

How Supplied: KANTREX INJECTION (kanamycin sulfate injection)
NDC 0015-3502-20—500 mg per 2 ml
NDC 0015-3502-24—Disposable Syringe (500 mg per 2 ml)
NDC 0015-3503-20—1 g per 3 ml
KANTREX PEDIATRIC INJECTION (kanamycin sulfate injection)
NDC 0015-3512-20—75 mg per 2 ml
(activity assayed as kanamycin base)

NAFCIL™
[năf′sĭl]   ℞
(nafcillin sodium for injection)
For Intramuscular or Intravenous Injection

This is the full text of the latest Official Package Circular dated June 1984 [7224DIR-10].

Description: Nafcil (nafcillin sodium) is a semi-synthetic antibiotic substance derived from 6-amino-penicillanic acid. It is the sodium salt in a parenteral dosage form.

NAFCILLIN SODIUM

$C_{21}H_{21}N_2NaO_5S \cdot H_2O$ 454.47 [CAS 7177-50-6]
4-Thia-1-azabicyclo [3.2.0] heptane-2-carboxylic acid, 6[[(2-ethoxy-1-naphthalenyl) carbonyl] amino]-3,3-dimethyl-7-oxo-monosodium salt, monohydrate, $[2S(2\alpha, 5\alpha, 6\beta)]$.

Clinical Pharmacology
Microbiology: Penicillinase-resistant penicillins exert a bactericidal action against penicillin-susceptible microorganisms during the state of active multiplication. All penicillins inhibit the biosynthesis of the bacterial cell wall.

The drugs in this class are highly resistant to inactivation by staphylococcal penicillinase and are active against penicillinase producing and non-penicillinase producing strains of **Staphylococcus aureus.**

The penicillinase-resistant penicillins are active in *in vitro* against a variety of other bacteria.

Susceptibility Plate Testing: Quantitative methods of susceptibility testing that require measurement of zone diameters or minimal inhibitory concentrations (M.I.Cs) give the most precise estimates of antibiotic susceptibility. One such procedure has been recommended for use with discs to test susceptibility to this class of drugs. Interpretations correlate diameters on the disc test with MIC values. A penicillinase-resistant class disc may be used to determine microbial susceptibility to cloxacillin, dicloxacillin, methicillin, nafcillin, and oxacillin. With this procedure, employing a 5 microgram methicillin sodium disc, a report from the laboratory of "susceptible" (zone of at least 14 mm) indicates that the infecting organism is likely to respond to therapy. A report of "resistant" (zone of less than 10 mm) indicates that the infecting organism is not likely to respond to therapy. A report of "intermediate susceptibility" (zone of 10 to 13 mm) suggests that the organism might be susceptible if high doses of the antibiotic are used, or if the infection is confined to tissues and fluids (e.g., urine), in which high antibiotic levels are attained.

In general, all staphylococci should be tested against the penicillin G disc and against the methicillin disc. Routine methods of antibiotic susceptibility testing may fail to detect strains of organisms resistant to the penicillinase-resistant penicillins. For this reason, the use of large inocula and 48-hour incubation periods may be necessary to obtain accurate susceptibility studies with these antibiotics. Bacterial strains which are resistant to one of the penicillinase-resistant penicillins should be considered resistant to all of the drugs in the class.

Pharmacokinetics: Intramuscular injections of Nafcil (nafcillin sodium) 1 gram produced peak serum levels in 0.5 to 1 hour of 7.61 mcg/ml. The degree of protein binding reported has been 89.9 +/-1.5%. With normal doses Nafcil is found in therapeutic concentrations in the pleural, bile and amniotic fluids. Insignificant concentrations are found in the cerebrospinal fluid and aqueous humor. Blood concentrations may be tripled by the concurrent use of probenecid. Clinical studies with nafcillin sodium in infants under three days of age and prematures have revealed higher blood levels and slower rates of urinary excretion than in older children and adults. A high concentration of nafcillin sodium is excreted via the bile. About 30% of an intramuscular dose is excreted in the urine.

Indications and Usage: The penicillinase-resistant penicillins are indicated in the treatment of infections caused by penicillinase-producing staphylococci which have demonstrated susceptibility to the drugs. Cultures and susceptibility tests should be performed initially to determine the causative organism and their sensitivity to the drug (See **Clinical Pharmacology** — Susceptibility Plate Testing).

The penicillinase-resistant penicillins may be used to initiate therapy in suspected cases of resistant staphylococcal infections prior to the availability of laboratory test results. The penicillinase-resistant penicillins should not be used in infections caused by organisms susceptible to penicillin G. If the susceptibility tests indicate that the infection is due to an organism other than a resistant staphylococcus, therapy should not be continued with a penicillinase-resistant penicillin.

Contraindications: A history of a hypersensitivity (anaphylactic) reaction to any penicillin is a contraindication.

Warnings: Serious and occasionally fatal hypersensitivity (anaphylactic shock with collapse) reactions have occurred in patients receiving penicillin. The incidence of anaphylactic shock in all penicillin-treated patients is between 0.015 and 0.04 percent. Anaphylactic shock resulting in death has occurred in approximately 0.002 percent of the patients treated. Although anaphylaxis is more frequent following a parenteral administration, it has occurred in patients receiving oral penicillins.

When penicillin therapy is indicated, it should be initiated only after a comprehensive patient drug and allergy history has been obtained. If an allergic reaction occurs, the drug should be discontinued and the patient should receive supportive treatment, e.g., artificial maintenance of ventilations, pressor amines, antihistamines, and corticosteroids. Individuals with a history of penicillin hypersensitivity may also experience allergic reactions when treated with a cephalosporin.

Precautions

GENERAL: Penicillinase-resistant penicillins should generally not be administered to patients with a history of sensitivity to any penicillin.

Penicillin should be used with caution in individuals with histories of significant allergies and/or asthma. Whenever allergic reactions occur, penicillin should be withdrawn unless, in the opinion of the physician, the condition being treated is life-threatening and amenable only to penicillin therapy.

The oral route of administration should not be relied upon in patients with severe illness, or with nausea, vomiting, gastric dilation, cardiospasm, or intestinal hypermotility. Occasionally patients will not absorb therapeutic amounts of orally administered penicillin.

The use of antibiotics may result in overgrowth of nonsusceptible organisms. If new infections due to bacteria or fungi occur, the drug should be discontinued and appropriate measures taken.

Laboratory Tests: Bacteriologic studies to determine the causative organisms and their susceptibility to the penicillinase-resistant pencillins should be performed (See **Clinical Pharmacology** —Microbiology). In the treatment of suspected staphylococcal infections, therapy should be changed to another active agent if culture tests fail to demonstrate the presence of staphylococci.

Periodic assessment or organ system function including renal, hepatic, and hematopoietic should be made during prolonged therapy with the penicillinase-resistant penicillins.

Blood cultures, white blood cell, and differential cell counts should be obtained prior to initiation of therapy and at least weekly during therapy with penicillinase-resistant penicillins.

Periodic urinalysis, blood urea nitrogen, and creatinine determinations should be performed during therapy with the penicillinase-resistant penicillins and dosage alterations should be considered if these values become elevated. If any impairment of renal function is suspected or known to exist, a reduction in the total dosage should be considered and blood levels monitored to avoid possible neurotoxic reactions (See **Dosage and Administration**).

SGOT and SGPT values should be obtained periodically during therapy to monitor for possible liver function abnormalities.

Drug Interactions: Tetracycline, a bacteriostatic antibiotic, may antagonize the bactericidal effect of penicillin and concurrent use of these drugs should be avoided.

Carcinogenesis, Mutagensis, Impairment of Fertility: No long-term animal studies have been conducted with these drugs.

Studies on reproduction (nafcillin) in rats and rabbits reveal no fetal or maternal abnormalities before conception and continuously through weaning (one generation).

Pregnancy Category B: Reproduction studies performed in the mouse,rat, and rabbit have revealed no evidence of impaired fertility or harm to the fetus due to the penicillinase-resistant penicillins. Human experience with the penicillins during pregnancy has not shown any positive evidence of adverse effects on the fetus. There are, however, no adequate or well-controlled studies in pregnant women showing conclusively that harmful effects of these drugs on the fetus can be excluded. Because animal reproduction studies are not always predictive of human response, this drug should be used during pregnancy only if clearly needed.

Nursing Mothers: Penicillins are excreted in breast milk. Caution should be exercised when penicillins are administered to a nursing woman.

Pediatric Use: Because of incompletely developed renal function in newborns, penicillinase-resistant penicillins (especially methicillin) may not be completely excreted, with abnormally high blood levels resulting. Frequent blood levels are advisable in this group with dosage adjustments when necessary. All newborns treated with penicillins should be monitored closely for clinical and laboratory evidence of toxic or adverse effects (See **Dosage and Administration**).

Adverse Reactions

Body as a Whole: The reported incidence of allergic reactions to penicillins ranges from 0.7 to 10 percent (See **Warnings**). Sensitization is usually the result of treatment but some individuals have had immediate reactions to penicillin when first treated. In such cases, it is thought that the patients may have had prior exposure to the drug via trace amounts present in milk and vaccines.

Two types of allergic reactions to penicillin are noted clinically, immediate and delayed.

Immediate reactions usually occur within 20 minutes of administration and range in severity from urticaria and pruritus to angioneurotic edema, laryngospasm, bronchospasm, hypotension, vascular collapse, and death. Such immediate anaphylactic reactions are very rare (See **Warnings**) and usually occur after parenteral therapy but have occurred in patients receiving oral therapy. Another type of immediate reaction, an accelerated reaction, may occur between 20 minutes and 48 hours after administration and may include urticaria, pruritus, and fever. Although laryngeal edema, larynogospasm, and hypotension occasionally occur, fatality is uncommon.

Delayed allergic reactions to penicillin therapy usually occur after 48 hours and sometimes as late as 2 to 4 weeks after initiation of therapy. Manifestations of this type of reaction include serum sickness-like symptoms (i.e., fever, malaise, urticaria, myalgia, arthralgia, abdominal pain) and various skin rashes. Nausea, vomiting, diarrhea, stomatitis, black or hairy tongue and other symptoms of gastrointestinal irritation may occur, specially during oral penicillin therapy.

Nervous System Reactions: Neurotoxic reactions similar to those observed with penicillin G may occur with large intravenous doses of the penicillinase-resistant penicillins especially with patients with renal insufficiency.

Urogenital Reactions: Renal tubular damage and interstitial nephritis have been associated with the administration of methicillin sodium and infrequently with the administration of nafcillin and oxacillin. Manifestations of this reaction may include rash, fever, eosinophilia, hematuria, proteinuria, and renal insufficiency. Methicillin-induced nephropathy does not appear to be dose-related and is generally reversible upon prompt discontinuation of therapy.

Metabolic Reactions: Agranulocytosis, neutropenia, and bone marrow depression have been associated with the use of methicillin sodium, nafcillin, oxacillin, and cloxacillin. Hepatotoxicity, characterized by fever, nausea, and vomiting associated with abnormal liver function tests, mainly elevated SGOT levels, has been associated with the use of oxacillin and cloxacillin.

Dosage and Administration: The penicillinase-resistant penicillins are available for oral administration and for intramuscular and intravenous injection. The sodium salts of methicillin, oxacillin, and nafcillin may be administered parenterally and the sodium salts of cloxacillin, dicloxacillin, oxacillin, and nafcillin are available for oral use.

Bacteriologic studies to determine the causative organisms and their sensitivity to the penicillinase-resistant penicillins should always be performed. Duration of therapy varies with the type and severity of infection as well as the overall condition of the patient, therefore it should be determined by the clinical and bacteriological response of the patient. In severe staphylococcal infections, therapy with penicillinase-resistant penicillins should be continued for at least 14 days. Therapy should be continued for at least 48 hours after the patient has become afebrile, asymptomatic, and cultures are negative. The treatment of endocarditis and osteomyelitis may require a longer term of therapy.

Concurrent administration of the penicillinase-resistant penicillins and probenecid increases and prolongs serum penicillin levels. Probenecid decreases the apparent volume of distribution and

Continued on next page

Bristol—Cont.

slows the rate of excretion by competitively inhibiting renal tubular secretion of penicillin. Penicillin-probenecid therapy is generally limited to those infections where very high serum levels of penicillin are necessary.

Oral preparations of the penicillinase-resistant penicillins should not be used as initial therapy in serious, life threatening infections (See **Precautions — General**). Oral therapy with the penicillinase-resistant penicillins may be used to follow-up the previous use of a parenteral agent as soon as the clinical condition warrants. For intramuscular gluteal infections, care should be taken to avoid sciatic nerve injury. With intravenous administration, particularly in elderly patients, care should be taken because of the possibility of thrombophlebitis.

[See table below].

Directions For Use

For Intramuscular Use: Reconstitute with Sterile Water for Injection, USP 0.9% Sodium Chloride Injection, USP or Bacteriostatic Water for Injection, USP (with benzyl alcohol or parabens); add 1.8 ml to the 500 mg vial for 2 ml resulting solution; 3.4 ml to the 1 g vial for 4 ml resulting solution; 6.6 ml to the 2 g vial for 8 ml resulting solution. All reconstituted vials have a concentration of 250 mg per ml.

The clear solution should be administered by deep intragluteal injection immediately after reconstitution.

Reconstituted Stability: Reconstitute with the required amount of Sterile Water for Injection, USP, 0.9% Sodium Chloride Injection, USP or Bacteriostatic Water for Injection, USP (with benzyl alcohol or parabens). The resulting solutions are stable for 3 days at room temperature or 7 days under refrigeration and 90 days frozen.

For Direct Intravenous Use: The required amount of drug should be diluted in 15 to 30 ml of Sterile Water for Injection, USP or Sodium Chloride Injection, USP and injected over a 5- to 10-minute period. This may be accomplished through the tubing of an intravenous infusion if desirable.

For Administration by Intravenous Drip: Reconstitute as directed above (For intramuscular Use) prior to diluting with Intravenous Solution.

[See table above].

Only those solutions listed above should be used for the intravenous infusion of Nafcil (nafcillin sodium). The concentration of the antibiotic should fall within the range specified. The drug concentration and the rate and volume of the infusion should be adjusted so that the total dose of nafcillin is administered before the drug loses its stability in the solution in use.

There is no clinical experience available on the use of this agent in neonates or infants for this route of administration.

This route of administration should be used for relatively short-term therapy (24 to 48 hours) because of the occasional occurrence of thrombophlebitis particularly in elderly patients.

If another agent is used in conjunction with nafcillin therapy, **it should not be physically mixed with** nafcillin but should be administered separately.

"Piggyback" I.V. Package: This glass vial contains the labeled quantity of Nafcil and is intended for intravenous administration. The diluent and volume are specified on the label of each package.

STABILITY PERIODS FOR NAFCIL (nafcillin sodium)

Concentration Mg/Ml	Sterile H$_2$O for Injection	Isotonic Sodium Chloride	M/6 Molar Sodium Lactate Solution	5% Dextrose In H$_2$O	5% Dextrose In 0.45% NaCl	10% Invert Sugar	Lactated Ringers Solution
ROOM TEMPERATURE (25°C)							
10-200	24 Hrs	24 Hrs					
30			24 Hrs				
2-30				24 Hrs	24 Hrs		
10-30						24 Hrs	24 Hrs
REFRIGERATION (4°C)							
10-200	7 Days	7 Days					
10-30			7 Days	7 Days	7 Days	7 Days	7 Days
FROZEN (−15°C)							
250	90 Days	90 Days					
10-250			90 Days	90 Days	90 Days	90 Days	90 Days

When the "piggyback" vial is reconstituted with either Sterile Water for Injection, USP or 0.9% Sodium Chloride Injection, USP and the resulting solutions are in a concentration of 10 to 200 mg/ml, the solutions are stable for 24 hours at room temperature or 7 days under refrigeration and 90 days frozen.

Hospital Bulk Package: This glass vial contains 10 grams Nafcil and is designed for use in the pharmacy in preparing I.V. additives. Add 93 ml Sterile Water for Injection, USP or 0.9% Sodium Chloride Injection, USP. The resulting solution will contain 100 mg nafcillin activity per ml. Solutions in a concentration of 10 mg to 200 mg per ml are stable for 24 hours at room temperature or 7 days under refrigeration. Solutions in a concentration of 250 mg per ml are stable for 3 days at room temperature or 7 days under refrigeration and 90 days frozen.

Caution: NOT TO BE DISPENSED AS A UNIT.

Supply: Nafcil (nafcillin sodium) for Injection. Nafcillin sodium equivalent to 500 mg. 1 gram, 2 grams, or 10 grams nafcillin per vial.

NDC 0015-7224-20 — 500 mg vial
NDC 0015-7225-20 — 1 gram vial
NDC 0015-7226-20 — 2 gram vial
NDC 0015-7225-28 — 1 gram "piggyback" vial
NDC 0015-7226-28 — 2 gram "piggyback" vial
NDC 0015-7101-28 — 10 gram Hospital Bulk Package

For information on package sizes available, refer to the current price schedule.

NALDECON® B
[nal'dĕ-côn]
Tablets, Syrup, Pediatric Drops and Pediatric Syrup
For Oral Use Only

This is the full text of the latest Official Package Circular dated January 1983 [5600DIM-15].

Description:
Naldecon is a preparation containing:
[See table on top next page].

Clinical Pharmacology:

Phenylpropanolamine Hydrochloride
The drug may directly stimulate adrenergic receptors but probably indirectly stimulates both alpha (α) and beta (β) adrenergic receptors by releasing norepinephrine from its storage sites. Phenylpropanolamine increases heart rate, force of contraction and cardiac output, and excitability. It acts on α receptors in the mucosa of the respiratory tract, producing vasoconstriction which results in shrinkage of swollen mucous membranes, reduction of tissue, hyperemia, edema and nasal congestion, and an increase in nasal airway patency. Phenylpropanolamine causes CNS stimulation and reportedly has an anorexigenic effect.

Phenylephrine Hydrochloride
Phenylephrine acts predominantly by a direct action on alpha (α) adrenergic receptors. In therapeutic doses, the drug has no significant stimulant effect on the beta (β) adrenergic receptors of the heart. Following oral administration, constriction of blood vessels in the nasal mucosa may relieve nasal congestion. In therapeutic doses the drug causes little, if any, central nervous system stimulation.

Phenyltoloxamine Citrate
Phenyltoloxamine is an H$_1$ blocking agent which interferes with the action of histamine primarily in capillaries surrounding mucous tissues and sensory nerves of nasal and adjacent areas. It has the ability to interfere with certain actions of acetylcholine-inhibiting secretions in the nose, mouth and pharynx. It commonly causes CNS depression.

Chlorpheniramine Maleate
Chlorpheniramine competitively antagonizes most of the smooth muscle stimulating actions of histamine on the H$_1$ receptors of the GI tract, uterus, large blood vessels and bronchial muscle. It also antagonizes the action of histamine that results in increased capillary permeability and the formation of edema.

Indications and Usage: For the relief of nasal congestion and eustachian tube congestion associated with the common cold, sinusitis and acute upper respiratory infections. Also indicated symptomatic relief of perennial and seasonal allergic rhinitis, vasomotor rhinitis.

Decongestants in combination with antihistamines have been used to relieve eustachian tube congestion associated with acute eustachian salpingitis, aerotitis and serous otitis media.

Contraindications: Patients with severe hypertension, severe coronary artery disease, patients on MAO inhibitor therapy; patients with narrow angle glaucoma, urinary retention, peptic

RECOMMENDED DOSAGES FOR NAFCIL (nafcillin sodium)

Drug	Adults	Infants and Children < 40 kg (88 lbs)	Other Recommendations
Nafcillin	500 mg IM every 4 to 6 hrs. IV every 4 hrs.	25 mg/kg IM twice daily	Neonates 10 mg/kg IM twice daily
	1 gram IM or IV every 4 hrs. (severe infections)		

ulcer and during an asthmatic attack. Also contraindicated in patients with hypersensitivity or idiosyncrasy to sympathomimetic amines or antihistamines.

Warnings: Sympathomimetic amines should be used judiciously and sparingly in patients with hypertension, diabetes mellitus, ischemic heart disease, increased intraocular pressure, hyperthyroidism or prostatic hypertrophy. See, however, CONTRAINDICATIONS. Sympathomimetics may produce central nervous system stimulation with convulsions or cardiovascular collapse with accompanying hypotension.

Antihistamines may impair mental and physical abilities required for the performance of potentially hazardous tasks, such as driving a vehicle or operating machinery, and may impair mental alertness in children. Chlorpheniramine and phenyltoloxamine have an atropine-like action and should be used with caution in patients with increased intraocular pressure, cardiovascular disease, hypertension or in patients with a history of bronchial asthma. See, however, CONTRAINDICATIONS.

Do not exceed recommended dosage.

Precautions: Patients with diabetes, hypertension, cardiovascular disease and hyperreactivity to ephedrine. The antihistaminics may cause drowsiness and ambulatory patients who operate machinery or motor vehicles should be cautioned accordingly.

Drug Interactions: MAO inhibitors and beta adrenergic blockers increase the effect of sympathomimetics. Sympathomimetics may reduce the antihypertensive effects of methyldopa, mecamylamine, reserpine and veratrum alkaloids. Concomitant use of antihistamines with alcohol, tricyclic antidepressants, barbiturates and other CNS depressants may have an additive effect.

Pregnancy Category C: Animal reproduction studies have not been conducted with Naldecon. It is also not known whether Naldecon can cause fetal harm when administered to a pregnant woman or can effect reproductive capacity. Naldecon should be given to a pregnant woman only if clearly needed.

Nursing Mothers: Caution should be exercised when this drug is given to nursing mothers due to the higher than usual risk of the sympathomimetic amines in infants.

Adverse Reactions: Hyperreactive individuals may display ephedrine-like reactions such as tachycardia, palpitations, headache, dizziness or nausea. Patients sensitive to antihistamines may experience mild sedation. Sympathomimetics have been associated with certain untoward reactions including restlessness, tremor, weakness, pallor, respiratory difficulty, dysuria, insomnia, hallucinations, convulsions, CNS depression, arrhythmias and cardiovascular collapse with hypotension. Possible side effects of antihistamines are drowsiness, restlessness, dizziness, weakness, dry mouth, anorexia, nausea, vomiting, headache, nervousness, blurring of vision, polyuria, heartburn, dysuria and, very rarely, dermatitis.

Dosage and Administration: This chart represents single dosages for the products listed below. Usual dosage schedule for Naldecon Pediatric Drops, Naldecon Pediatric Syrup and Naldecon

Naldecon	For immediate action	For delayed action	Total contents
Each sustained-action tablet contains:			
Phenylpropanolamine hydrochloride	20.0 mg	20.0 mg	40.0 mg
Phenylephrine hydrochloride	5.0 mg	5.0 mg	10.0 mg
Phenyltoloxamine citrate	7.5 mg	7.5 mg	15.0 mg
Chlorpheniramine maleate	2.5 mg	2.5 mg	5.0 mg
Each teaspoonful (5 ml) of syrup contains:			
Phenylpropanolamine hydrochloride			20.0 mg
Phenylephrine hydrochloride			5.0 mg
Phenyltoloxamine citrate			7.5 mg
Chlorpheniramine maleate			2.5 mg

	Pediatric Syrup each 5-ml contains:	Pediatric Drops each 1-ml dropper contains:
Each pediatric formulation contains the following ingredients:		
Phenylpropanolamine hydrochloride	5.0 mg	5.0 mg
Phenylephrine hydrochloride	1.25 mg	1.25 mg
Phenyltoloxamine citrate	2.0 mg	2.0 mg
Chlorpheniramine maleate	0.5 mg	0.5 mg

Syrup is every 3 to 4 hours, not to exceed four doses in a 24-hour period. For sustained-action Naldecon Tablets, doses should be administered on arising, in midafternoon, and at bedtime. [See table below].

How Supplied:
NDC 0015-5600—Naldecon Tablets
NDC 0015-5601—Naldecon Syrup
NDC 0015-5615—Naldecon Pediatric Drops
NDC 0015-5616—Naldecon Pediatric Syrup
For information on package sizes available, refer to the current price schedule.
Shown in Product Identification Section, page 407

NALDECON–CX® SUSPENSION
[nal'dĕ-côn]
Decongestant/Expectorant/Antitussive

Description: Each teaspoonful (5 ml) of Naldecon-CX Suspension contains:
Phenylpropanolamine HCl .... 18 mg
Guaifenesin .... 200 mg
Codeine Phosphate
(Warning: May be Habit Forming) ...... 10 mg

Indications: Provide prompt relief from cough and nasal congestion due to the common cold, bronchitis, nasopharyngitis, and influenza. Codeine temporarily quiets non-productive coughing by its antitussive action while guaifenesin's expectorant action helps loosen phlegm and bronchial secretions. Phenylpropanolamine reduces swelling of nasal passages and shrinks swollen membranes. This combination production is antihistamine and alcohol free.

Contraindications: Hypersensitivity to guaifenesin, codeine or sympathomimetic amines.

Warnings: Nervousness, dizziness or sleeplessness may occur if recommended dosage is exceeded. Do not give this product to a child with high blood pressure, heart disease, diabetes or thyroid disease except under the advice and supervision of a physician. Do not give this product to a child presently taking a prescription drug containing a monamine oxidase inhibitor except under the advice and supervision of a physician. Do not administer this product for persistent or chronic cough associated with asthma or emphysema or when cough is accompanied by excessive secretions, except under the care and advice of a physician. A persistent cough may be a sign of a serious condition. If cough persists for more than 1 week, tends to recur, or is accompanied by high fever, rash or persistent headaches, consult a physician.

Dosage and Administration: Children 2 to 6 years—½ teaspoon 4 times daily. 6 to 12 years—1 teaspoon 4 times daily. Over 12 years—2 teaspoons 4 times daily.

How Supplied: Naldecon-CX Suspension—4 oz. and pint bottles.

(1) 5/81

NALDECON–DX® OTC
[nal'dĕ-côn Dx]
PEDIATRIC SYRUP

Description: Each teaspoonful (5 ml.) of Naldecon-DX Syrup contains:
dextromethorphan hydrobromide .... 7.5 mg
phenylpropanolamine hydrochloride ..... 9 mg
guaifenesin .... 100 mg
alcohol 5%

Indications: Provide prompt relief from cough and nasal congestion due to the common cold, bronchitis, nasopharyngitis and recurrent bronchial coughing. Dextromethorphan temporarily quiets non-productive coughing by its antitussive action while guaifenesin's expectorant action helps loosen phlegm and bronchial secretions. Phenylpropanolamine reduces swelling of nasal passages; shrinks swollen membranes. This combination product is antihistamine-free.

Contraindications: Hypersensitivity to guaifenesin, dextromethorphan or sympathomimetic amines.

Warnings: Nervousness, dizziness or sleeplessness may occur if recommended dosage is exceeded. Do not give this product to a child with high blood pressure, heart disease, diabetes or thyroid disease except under the advice and supervision of a physician. Do not give this product to a child presently taking a prescription drug containing a monamine oxidase inhibitor except under the advice and supervision of a physician. Do not administer this product for persistent or chronic cough such as occurs with asthma or emphysema or when cough is accompanied by excessive secretions except under the care and advice of a physician. A persistent cough may be a sign of a serious condition. If cough persists for more than 1 week, tends to recur, or is accompanied by high fever, rash or persistent headaches, consult a physician.

Dosage and Administration: Children 2 to 6 years—1 teaspoonful 4 times daily. Over 6 years—2 teaspoons 4 times daily.

Single Dosage for ...	Naldecon Pediatric Drops	Naldecon Pediatric Syrup	Naldecon Syrup	Naldecon Tablets
3 to 6 months (12–17 lbs)	¼ ml (0.25 ml)			
6 to 12 months (17–24 lbs)	½ ml (0.5 ml)	½ teaspoonful		
1 to 6 years (24–50 lbs)	1 ml (1.0 ml)	1 teaspoonful		
6 to 12 years (over 50 lbs)		2 teaspoonfuls	½ teaspoonful	½ tablet
over 12 years			1 teaspoonful	1 tablet

Continued on next page

Bristol—Cont.

How Supplied: Naldecon-DX Syrup in 4 oz. and pint bottles.

(1) 8/80

NALDECON-EX OTC
[nal'dĕ-côn Ex]
PEDIATRIC DROPS

Description: Each 1 ml. dropper of Naldecon-EX contains:
phenylpropanolamine hydrochloride ....9 mg
guaifenesin ....30 mg
alcohol 0.6%

Indications: Combined decongestant/expectorant designed specifically to promptly reduce the swelling of nasal membranes and to help loosen phlegm and bronchial secretions through productive coughing. This dual action is of particular value in infants with common cold, acute bronchitis, bronchiolitis, tracheobronchitis, nasopharyngitis and croup. This combination product is antihistamine-free.

Contraindications: Hypersensitivity to guaifenesin or sympathomimetic amines.

Warnings: Nervousness, dizziness or sleeplessness may occur if recommended dosage is exceeded. Do not give this product to a child with high blood pressure, heart disease, diabetes or thyroid disease except under the advice and supervision of a physician. Do not give this product to a child presently taking a prescription drug containing a monoamine oxidase inhibitor except under the advice and supervision of a physician. Do not administer this product for persistent or chronic cough such as occurs with asthma or emphysema or when cough is accompanied by excessive secretions except under the care and advice of a physician. A persistent cough may be a sign of a serious condition. If cough persists for more than 1 week, tends to recur, or is accompanied by high fever, rash or persistent headaches, consult a physician.

Dosage and Administration: Dose should be adjusted to age or weight and be given 4 times a day (see calibrations on dropper). Administer by mouth only.

1-3 Months: (8-12 lbs.)	¼ ml
4-6 Months: (13-17 lbs.)	½ ml
7-9 Months: (18-20 lbs.)	¾ ml
10 Months or over (21 lbs. or more)	1 ml

Bottle label dosage reads as follows: children under 2 years of age: use only as directed by a physician.

How Supplied: Naldecon-EX Pediatric Drops in 30 ml. bottles with calibrated dropper.

(1) 8/80

POLYCILLIN® ℞
[pol″e-cil'lin]
(ampicillin)
CAPSULES
250 mg. and 500 mg.
For Oral Suspension
125 mg. per 5 ml., 250 mg. per 5 ml., 500 mg. per 5 ml.
Pediatric Drops
100 mg. per ml.

POLYCILLIN-N® ℞
(sterile ampicillin sodium)
For Intramuscular or Intravenous Injection

This is the full text of the latest Combined Official Package Circulars dated October 1977 [7988DIRO-16 Polycillin] and May 1979 [7401DIRO-24 Polycillin-N].

(S 9/78)

Description: Polycillin (ampicillin) is a synthetic penicillin with a broad spectrum of bactericidal activity against both penicillin-susceptible Gram-positive organisms and many common Gram-negative pathogens.

Polycillin-N (sterile ampicillin sodium) contains 2.9 milliequivalents of sodium per 1 gram of drug.

Actions:
Pharmacology

Polycillin is stable in the presence of gastric acid and is well-absorbed from the gastrointestinal tract. It diffuses readily into most body tissues and fluids. However, penetration into the cerebrospinal fluid and brain occurs only when the meninges are inflamed. Ampicillin is excreted largely unchanged in the urine and its excretion can be delayed by concurrent administration of probenecid. The active form appears in the bile in higher concentrations than those found in serum. Ampicillin is the least serum-bound of all the penicillins, averaging about 20% compared to approximately 60 to 90% for other penicillins. Polycillin is well-tolerated by most patients and has been given in doses of 2 grams daily for many weeks without adverse reactions.

Microbiology
The following bacteria have been shown in **in vitro** studies to be susceptible to Polycillin:
GRAM-POSITIVE ORGANISMS: Hemolytic and nonhemolytic streptococci, **D. pneumoniae**, non-penicillinase-producing staphylococci, Clostridia spp., **B. anthracis, Listeria monocytogenes,** and most strains of enterococci.
GRAM-NEGATIVE ORGANISMS: H. influenzae, N. gonorrhoeae, N. meningitidis, Proteus mirabilis, and many strains of Salmonella, Shigella, and **E. coli.**
Polycillin does not resist destruction by penicillinase. Polycillin Susceptibility Test Discs, 10 mcg. should be used to estimate the **in vitro** susceptibility of bacteria to Polycillin.

Indications: Polycillin is indicated for the treatment of infections due to susceptible Gram-positive organisms including streptococci, pneumococci, penicillin G-susceptible staphylococci, and enterococci, and susceptible strains of Gram-negative bacteria including **H. influenzae, E. coli, Proteus mirabilis, N. gonorrhoeae, N. meningitidis,** Shigella, **S. typhosa** and other Salmonella.

Bacteriology studies to determine the causative organisms and their susceptibility to ampicillin should be performed. Therapy may be instituted prior to obtaining results of susceptibility testing. It is advisable to reserve the parenteral form of this drug for moderately severe and severe infections and for patients who are unable to take the oral forms. A change to oral Polycillin (ampicillin) may be made as soon as appropriate.

Indicated surgical procedures should be performed.

Contraindications: A history of a previous hypersensitivity reaction to any of the penicillins is a contraindication.

Warning: Serious and occasionally fatal hypersensitivity (anaphylactoid) reactions have been reported in patients on penicillin therapy. Although anaphylaxis is more frequent following parenteral therapy, it has occurred in patients on oral penicillins. These reactions are more apt to occur in individuals with a history of sensitivity to multiple allergens.

There have been well-documented reports of individuals with a history of penicillin hypersensitivity reactions who have experienced severe hypersensitivity reactions when treated with a cephalosporin. Before therapy with a penicillin, careful inquiry should be made concerning previous hypersensitivity reactions to penicillins, cephalosporins, and other allergens.

Serious anaphylactoid reactions require immediate emergency treatment with epinephrine. Oxygen, intravenous steroids, and airway management, including intubation, should also be administered as indicated.

USAGE IN PREGNANCY: Safety for use in pregnancy has not been established.

Precautions: The possibility of superinfections with mycotic organisms or bacterial pathogens should be kept in mind during therapy. In such cases, discontinue the drug and substitute appropriate treatment.

As with any potent drug, periodic assessment of organ system function, including renal, hepatic, and hematopoietic, should be made during prolonged therapy.

With high urine concentrations of ampicillin, false-positive glucose reactions may occur if Clinitest, Benedict's Solution, or Fehling's Solution are used. Therefore, it is recommended that glucose tests based on enzymatic glucose oxidase reactions (such as Clinistix or Tes-Tape) be used.

Adverse Reactions: As with other penicillins, it may be expected that untoward reactions will be essentially limited to sensitivity phenomena. They are more likely to occur in individuals who have previously demonstrated hypersensitivity to penicillins and in those with a history of allergy, asthma, hay fever, or urticaria.

The following adverse reactions have been reported as associated with the use of ampicillin.
Gastrointestinal—Glossitis, stomatitis, black "hairy" tongue, nausea, vomiting, enterocolitis, pseudomembranous colitis, and diarrhea. (These reactions are usually associated with oral dosage forms.)

Hypersensitivity reactions—Skin rashes and urticaria have been reported frequently. A few cases of exfoliative dermatitis and erythema multiforme have been reported. Anaphylaxis is the most serious reaction experienced and has usually been associated with the parenteral dosage form.

Note: Urticaria, other skin rashes, and serum sickness-like reactions may be controlled with antihistamines and, if necessary, systemic corticosteroids. Whenever such reactions occur, ampicillin should be discontinued, unless, in the opinion of the physician, the condition being treated is life threatening and amenable only to ampicillin therapy. Serious anaphylactic reactions require the immediate use of epinephrine, oxygen, and intravenous steroids.

Liver—A moderate rise in serum glutamic oxaloacetic transaminase (SGOT) has been noted, particularly in infants, but the significance of this finding is unknown. Mild transitory SGOT elevations have been observed in individuals receiving larger (two to four times) than usual and oft-repeated intramuscular injections. Evidence indicates that glutamic oxaloacetic transaminase (GOT) is released at the site of intramuscular injection of ampicillin sodium and that the presence of increased amounts of this enzyme in the blood does not necessarily indicate liver involvement.

Hemic and Lymphatic Systems—Anemia, thrombocytopenia, thrombocytopenic purpura, eosinophilia, leukopenia, and agranulocytosis have been reported during therapy with the penicillins. These reactions are usually reversible on discontinuation of therapy and are believed to be hypersensitivity phenomena.

Other—Since infectious mononucleosis is viral in origin, ampicillin should not be used in the treatment. A high percentage of patients with mononucleosis who received ampicillin developed a skin rash.

Dosage:
Infections of the respiratory tract and soft tissues:
Oral: Patients weighing 20 Kg. (44 lbs.) or more: 250 mg. every 6 hours.
Patients weighing less than 20 Kg. (44 lbs.): 50 mg./Kg./day in equally divided doses at 6-to 8-hour intervals.
Parenteral: Patients weighing 40 Kg. (88 lbs.) or more: 250 to 500 mg. every 6 hours.
Patients weighing less than 40 Kg. (88 lbs.): 25 to 50 mg./Kg./day in equally divided doses at 6-to 8-hour intervals.
Infections of the gastrointestinal and genitourinary tracts:
Oral: Patients weighing 20 Kg. (44 lbs.) or more: 500 mg. every 6 hours.
Patients weighing less than 20 Kg. (44 lbs.): 100 mg./Kg./day in equally divided doses at 6-to 8-hour intervals.
Infections of the gastrointestinal and genitourinary tracts (including those caused by Neisseria gonorrhoeae in females).

Parenteral: Patients weighing 40 Kg. (88 lbs.) or more: 500 mg. every 6 hours.
Patients weighing less than 40 Kg. (88 lbs.): 50 mg./Kg./day in equally divided doses at 6-to 8-hour intervals.
In the treatment of chronic urinary tract and intestinal infections, frequent bacteriological and clinical appraisal is necessary. Smaller doses than those recommended above should not be used. Higher doses should be used for stubborn or severe infections. In stubborn infections, therapy may be required for several weeks. It may be necessary to continue clinical and/or bacteriological follow-up for several months after cessation of therapy.
Urethritis in males or females due to N. gonorrhoeae:
Oral: 3.5 Grams, with 1.0 Gram probenecid, administered simultaneously.
Urethritis in males due to N. gonorrhoeae:
Parenteral: Adult: Two doses of 500 mg. each at an interval of 8 to 12 hours. Treatment may be repeated if necessary or extended if required.
In the treatment of complications of gonorrheal urethritis, such as prostatitis and epididymitis, prolonged and intensive therapy is recommended. Cases of gonorrhea with a suspected primary lesion of syphilis should have darkfield examinations before receiving treatment. In all other cases where concomitant syphilis is suspected, monthly serological tests should be made for a minimum of four months.
The parenteral doses for the preceding infections may be given by either the intramuscular or intravenous route. A change to oral Polycillin (ampicillin) may be made when appropriate.
Bacterial Meningitis
Parenteral ONLY: Adults and Children: 150 to 200 mg./Kg./day in equally divided doses every 3 to 4 hours. (Treatment may be initiated with intravenous drip therapy and continued with intramuscular injections.) The doses for other infections may be given by either the intravenous or intramuscular route.
Septicemia
Parenteral ONLY: Adults and Children: 150 to 200 mg./Kg./day. Start with intravenous administration for at least three days and continue with the intramuscular route every 3 to 4 hours. Treatment of all infections should be continued for a minimum of 48 to 72 hours beyond the time that the patient becomes asymptomatic or evidence of bacterial eradication has been obtained. A minimum of 10-days treatment is recommended for any infection caused by Group A beta-hemolytic streptococci to help prevent the occurrence of acute rheumatic fever or acute glomerulonephritis.
The following Dosage chart may be useful as a guide to therapy with the Pediatric Drops.
[See table above].
Note: For ease in administration, the dropper assembly is calibrated at the 62.5-mg. level (½ dropperful), at the 94-mg. level (¾ dropperful), and at the 125-mg. level (1 dropperful). Children over 10 Kg. (22 pounds) would generally be dosed with Polycillin for Oral Suspension.
Directions for Dispensing Oral Suspension and Pediatric Drops: Prepare these formulations at the time of dispensing. For ease in preparation, add water to the bottle in two portions and shake well after each addition. Add the total amount of water as directed on the labeling of the package being dispensed. The reconstituted formulation is stable for 14 days under refrigeration.

Pediatric Drops—Dosage Chart

Polycillin Weight		Infection	
Kg.	Lb.	Respiratory	GU/GI
Up to 5	Up to 11	62.5 mg. q. 6h. (½ dropperful q. 6h.)	125 mg. q. 6h. (1 dropperful q. 6h.)
5 to 7.5	11 to 16.5	94 mg. q. 6h. (¾ dropperful q. 6h.)	188 mg. q. 6h. (1½ dropperfuls q. 6h.)
7.6 to 10	16.6 to 22	125 mg. q. 6h. (1 dropperful q. 6h.)	250 mg. q. 6h. (2 dropperfuls q. 6h.)

Parenteral—Directions For Use: Use only freshly prepared solutions. Intramuscular and intravenous injections should be administered within one hour after preparation, since the potency may decrease significantly after this period.
For Intramuscular Use: Dissolve contents of a vial with the amount of Sterile Water for Injection, U.S.P. or Bacteriostatic Water for Injection, U.S.P., listed in the table below.
[See table below].
While Polycillin-N, 1.0 g. and 2.0 g., are primarily for intravenous use, they may be administered intramuscularly when the 250-mg. or 500-mg. vials are unavailable. In such instances, dissolve in 3.5 or 6.8 ml. Sterile Water for Injection, U.S.P. or Bacteriostatic Water for Injection, U.S.P., respectively. The resulting solution will provide a concentration of 250 mg. per ml.
Polycillin-N, 125 mg., is intended primarily for pediatric use. It also serves as a convenient dosage form when small parenteral doses of the antibiotic are required.
For Direct Intravenous Use: Add 5 ml. Sterile Water for Injection, U.S.P. or Bacteriostatic Water for Injection, U.S.P. to the 125-, 250-, and 500-mg. vials and administer slowly over a 3- to 5- minute period. Polycillin-N, 1.0 Gm. or 2.0 Gm., may also be given by direct intravenous administration. Dissolve in 7.4 or 14.8 ml. Sterile Water for Injection, U.S.P., or Bacteriostatic Water for Injection, U.S.P. respectively, and administer slowly over at least 10 to 15 minutes. CAUTION: More rapid administration may result in convulsive seizures.
For Administration by Intravenous Drip: Reconstitute as directed above (For Direct Intravenous Use) prior to diluting with Intravenous Solution. Stability studies on ampicillin sodium at several concentrations in various intravenous solutions indicate the drug will lose less than 10% activity at the temperatures noted for the time periods stated:
[See table on next page].
Only those solutions listed above should be used for the intravenous infusion of Polycillin-N. The concentrations should fall within the range specified. The drug concentration and the rate and volume of the infusion should be adjusted so that the total dose of ampicillin is administered before the drug loses its stability in the solution in use.
"Piggyback" I.V. Package: These glass vials contain the labeled quantity of POLYCILLIN-N and are intended for intravenous administration. The diluent and volume are specified on the label of each package.
Hospital Bulk Package: This glass vial contains 10 grams ampicillin and is designed for use in the pharmacy in preparing I.V. additives. Add 94 ml Sterile Water for Injection, U.S.P. The resulting solution will contain 100 milligrams ampicillin activity per ml, and is stable up to one hour at room temperature. Diluting further within one hour to 5 mg to 10 mg per ml, the resulting solution will remain stable for 8 hours at room temperature or 72 hours under refrigeration.
Caution: NOT TO BE DISPENSED AS A UNIT.
Supply: Polycillin (ampicillin) for Oral Suspension. Each 5 ml. of reconstituted suspension contains ampicillin trihydrate equivalent to 125, 250, or 500 mg. ampicillin.
NDC 0015-7988—125 mg., 80 ml., 100 ml., 150 ml. and 200 ml. bottles.
NDC 0015-7998—250 mg., 80 ml., 100 ml., 150 ml. and 200 ml. bottle
NDC 0015-7884—500 mg., 100 ml. bottle
Polycillin (ampicillin) Capsules. Ampicillin trihydrate equivalent to 250 or 500 mg. ampicillin per capsule.
NDC 0015-7992—250 mg.
NDC 0015-7993—500 mg.
Shown in Product Identification Section, page 407
Polycillin (ampicillin) for oral suspension. Each ml. of reconstituted pediatric drops contains ampicillin trihydrate equivalent to 100 mg. ampicillin.
NDC 0015-7884—100 mg., 20 ml. bottles.
Polycillin-N (sterile ampicillin sodium) for I.M. or I.V. Injection. Ampicillin sodium equivalent to 125, 250, 500 mg., 1 g or 2 g ampicillin per vial.
NDC 0015-7401-20—125-mg. vial.
NDC 0015-7402-20—250-mg. vial.
NDC 0015-7403-20—500-mg. vial.
NDC 0015-7404-20—1.0-Gm. vial.
NDC 0015-7405-20—2.0 Gm. vial.
NDC 0015-7403-31—500 mg. "piggyback" vial.
NDC 0015-7404-36—1.0 gram "piggyback" vial.
NDC 0015-7405-28—2.0 gram "piggyback" vial.
NDC 0015-7100-28—10 gram Hospital Bulk Package
For information on package sizes available, refer to the current price sheets.

POLYCILLIN-PRB® ℞
[pol"e-cil'lin]
(ampicillin-probenecid)
For Oral Suspension
Ampicillin Trihydrate equivalent to 3.5 Grams ampicillin with 1.0 Gram probenecid

This is the full text of the latest Official Package Circular dated October 1977 [7607 DIRO-06].
Description: Polycillin-PRB (ampicillin-probenecid) is a semisynthetic penicillin in combination with probenecid.
Actions:
Pharmacology
Ampicillin is stable in the presence of gastric acid and is well-absorbed from the gastrointestinal tract. It diffuses readily into most body tissues and fluids. However, penetration into the cerebrospinal fluid and brain occurs only when the meninges are inflamed. Ampicillin is excreted largely unchanged in the urine and its excretion can be delayed by concurrent administration of probenecid. The active form appears in the bile in higher concentrations than those found in serum. Ampicillin is the least serum-bound of all the penicillins, averaging about 20% compared to approximately 60 to 90% for other penicillins. Probenecid inhibits the renal tubular secretion of penicillins causing an increased serum level of the antibiotic.
Microbiology
Neisseria gonorrhoeae has been shown in **in vitro** studies to be susceptible to ampicillin.
Indications: Ampicillin-probenecid is indicated for the treatment of uncomplicated infections (ure-

Polycillin-N—Reconstitution Volumes

NDC 0015	Label Claim	Recommended Amount of Diluent	Withdrawable Volume	Concentration (in mg/ml)
7401-20	125 mg.	1.2 ml.	1.0 ml.	125 mg.
7402-20	250 mg.	1.0 ml.	1.0 ml.	250 mg.
7403-20	500 mg.	1.8 ml.	2.0 ml.	250 mg.
7404-20	1.0 gram	3.5 ml.	4.0 ml.	250 mg.
7405-20	2.0 gram	6.8 ml.	8.0 ml.	250 mg.

Continued on next page

Bristol—Cont.

thral, endocervical, or rectal) due to *N. gonorrhoeae* in males and females.
Susceptibility studies should be performed with recurrent infections or when resistant strains are encountered. Therapy may be instituted prior to obtaining results of susceptibility testing.

Contraindications:
Ampicillin
A history of previous hypersensitivity reactions to any of the penicillins is a contraindication.
Probenecid
Polycillin-PRB should not be given to individuals with a known hypersensitivity to probenecid. It is not recommended for patients with known blood dyscrasias, uric acid kidney stones or during an acute attack of gout.

Warnings: Serious and occasionally fatal hypersensitivity reactions have been reported in patients on penicillin therapy. Although anaphylaxis is more frequent following parenteral therapy, it has occurred in patients on oral penicillins. These reactions are more apt to occur in individuals with a history of sensitivity to multiple allergens.

There have been well-documented reports of individuals with a history of penicillin hypersensitivity reactions who have experienced severe hypersensitivity reactions when treated with a cephalosporin. Before therapy with a penicillin, careful inquiry should be made concerning previous hypersensitivity reactions to penicillins, cephalosporins, and other allergens. If an allergic reaction occurs, the patient should be treated with the usual agents, e.g., pressor amines, antihistamines, and corticosteroids. Serious anaphylactoid reactions require emergency treatment with epinephrine. Oxygen, intravenous steroids, and airway management, including intubation, should also be administered as indicated.

USAGE IN PREGNANCY: Safety for use in pregnancy has not been established.

Precautions: Cases of gonococcal infection with a suspected lesion of syphilis should have darkfield examinations ruling out syphilis before receiving ampicillin. Patients who do not have suspected lesions of syphilis and are treated with ampicillin should have a follow-up serologic test for syphilis each month for four months to detect syphilis that may have been masked by treatment for gonorrhea. Patients with gonorrhea who also have syphilis should be given additional appropriate parenteral penicillin treatment.

Adverse Reactions: As with other penicillins, it may be expected that untoward reactions to ampicillin will be essentially limited to sensitivity phenomena. They are more likely to occur in individuals who have previously demonstrated hypersensitivity to penicillins and in those with a history of allergy, asthma, hay fever, or urticaria.

The following adverse reactions have been reported as associated with the use of ampicillin:
Gastrointestinal—Glossitis, stomatitis, black "hairy" tongue, nausea, vomiting, enterocolitis, pseudomembranous colitis, and diarrhea. (These reactions are usually associated with oral dosage forms.)
Hypersensitivity reactions—Skin rashes and urticaria have been reported frequently. A few cases of exfoliative dermatitis and erythema multiforme have been reported. Anaphylaxis is the most serious reaction experienced and has usually been associated with the parenteral form.
Serious acute hypersensitivity reactions may require the use of epinephrine, oxygen, and airway management, which may include endotracheal intubation, intravenous steroids, and repletion of plasma volume.
Liver—A moderate rise in serum glutamic oxaloacetic transaminase (SGOT) has been noted, but the significance of this finding is unknown.
Hemic and Lymphatic Systems—Anemia, thrombocytopenia, thrombocytopenic purpura, eosinophilia, leukopenia, and agranulocytosis have been reported during therapy with the penicillins. These reactions are usually reversible on discontinuation of therapy and are believed to be hypersensitivity phenomena.

Dosage: Acute N. gonorrhoeae infections in adult males and females.
3.5 Grams ampicillin, with 1.0 Gram probenecid, administered simultaneously. One bottle contains enough of each drug for the required single dose. It is desirable that follow-up cultures be obtained from the original site(s) of infection 7 to 14 days after therapy.
In women, it is also desirable to obtain culture test-of-cure from both the endocervical and anal canal.
Directions For Dispensing Oral Suspension: Prepare this formulation at the time of dispensing. For ease in preparation, add water to the bottle in two portions and shake well after each addition. Add the total amount of water as directed on the labeling of the package being dispensed. The reconstituted formulation is stable for 24 hours at room temperature.
Supply: POLYCILLIN-PRB (Ampicillin-Probenecid) for Oral Suspension. Ampicillin Trihydrate equivalent to 3.5 Grams ampicillin with 1.0 Gram probenecid, single-dose bottle.
NDC 0015-7607

POLYMOX® ℞
[pol"e-mox]
(amoxicillin)
CAPSULES
250 mg. and 500 mg.
FOR ORAL SUSPENSION
125 mg. per 5 ml., 250 mg. per 5 ml.
PEDIATRIC DROPS
50 mg. per ml.

This is the full text of the latest Official Package Circular dated May 1976 [7276DIRO-07].

Polycillin-N IV Stability
Room Temperature (25°C.)

Diluent	Concentrations	Stability Periods
Sterile Water for Injection	up to 30 mg./ml.	8 hours
Isotonic Sodium Chloride	up to 30 mg./ml.	8 hours
M/6 Sodium Lactate Solution	up to 30 mg./ml.	8 hours
5% Dextrose in Water	10 to 20 mg./ml.	2 hours
5% Dextrose in Water	up to 2 mg./ml.	4 hours
5% Dextrose in 0.45% NaCl	up to 2 mg./ml.	4 hours
10% Invert Sugar in Water	up to 2 mg./ml.	4 hours
Lactated Ringer's Solution	up to 30 mg./ml.	8 hours

Refrigerated (4°C.)

Sterile Water for Injection	30 mg./ml.	48 hours
Sterile Water for Injection	up to 20 mg./ml.	72 hours
Isotonic Sodium Chloride	30 mg./ml.	48 hours
Isotonic Sodium Chloride	up to 20 mg./ml.	72 hours
Lactated Ringer's Solution	up to 30 mg./ml.	24 hours
M/6 Sodium Lactate	up to 30 mg./ml.	8 hours
5% Dextrose in Water	up to 20 mg./ml.	4 hours
5% Dextrose in 0.45% NaCl	up to 10 mg./ml.	4 hours
10% Invert Sugar	up to 20 mg./ml.	3 hours

Description: Polymox® (amoxicillin) is a semi-synthetic penicillin, an analogue of ampicillin, with a broad spectrum of bactericidal activity against Gram-positive organisms and many Gram-negative pathogens.

Actions:
Pharmacology
Polymox® is stable in the presence of gastric acid and is well absorbed from the gastrointestinal tract and may be given with no regard to food. It diffuses readily into most body tissues and fluids, with the exception of brain and spinal fluid, except when meninges are inflamed. The half-life of amoxicillin is 61.3 minutes. Most of the amoxicillin is excreted unchanged in the urine; its excretion can be delayed by concurrent administration of probenecid. Amoxicillin is not highly protein-bound. In blood serum, amoxicillin is approximately 20% protein-bound as compared to 60% for penicillin-G.
Orally administered doses of 250 mg. and 500 mg. amoxicillin capsules result in average peak blood levels one to two hours after administration in the range of 3.5 mcg./ml. to 5.0 mcg./ml. and 5.5 mcg./ml. to 7.5 mcg./ml. respectively.
Orally administered doses of amoxicillin suspension 125 mg./5 ml., and 250 mg./5 ml., result in average peak blood levels one to two hours after administration in the range of 1.5 mcg./ml. to 3.0 mcg./ml. and 3.5 mcg./ml. to 5.0 mcg./ml. respectively.
Detectable serum levels are observed up to 8 hours after an orally administered dose of amoxicillin. Approximately 60 percent of an orally administered dose of amoxicillin is excreted in the urine within six to eight hours.

Microbiology
Polymox® (amoxicillin) is similar to ampicillin in its bactericidal action against susceptible organisms during the stage of active multiplication. It acts through the inhibition of biosynthesis of cell wall mucopeptides. **In vitro** studies have demonstrated the susceptibility of most strains of the following Gram-positive bacteria: alpha- and beta-hemolytic streptococci, **Diplococcus pneumoniae**, nonpenicillinase-producing staphylococci, and **Streptococcus faecalis**. It is active in vitro against many strains of **Haemophilus influenzae, Neisseria gonorrhoeae, Escherichia coli** and **Proteus mirabilis.** Because it does not resist destruction by penicillinase, it is **not** effective against penicillinase-producing bacteria, particularly resistant staphylococci. All strains of Pseudomonas and most strains of Klebsiella and Enterobacter are resistant.

Disc Susceptibility Tests
Quantitative methods that require measurement of zone diameters give the most precise estimates of antibiotic susceptibility. One such procedure* has been recommended for use with discs for testing susceptibility to ampicillin-class antibiotics. Interpretations correlate diameters on the disc test with MIC values for amoxicillin. With this procedure, a report from the laboratory of "susceptible" indicates that the infecting organism is likely to respond to therapy. A report of "resistant" indicates that the infecting organism is not likely to respond to therapy. A report of "intermediate susceptibility" suggests that the organism would be susceptible if high dosage is used, or if the infection is confined to tissues and fluids (e.g., urine), in which high antibiotic levels are attained.

Indications: Polymox® (amoxicillin) is indicated in the treatment of infections due to susceptible strains of the following:
GRAM-NEGATIVE ORGANISMS—**H. influenzae, E. coli, P. mirabilis** and **N. gonorrhoeae.**
GRAM-POSITIVE ORGANISMS—Streptococci (including **Streptococcus faecalis**), **D. pneumoniae**, and nonpenicillinase-producing staphylococci.
Therapy may be instituted prior to obtaining results from bacteriological and susceptibility studies to determine the causative organisms and their susceptibility to amoxicillin.
Indicated surgical procedures should be performed.

Contraindications: A history of a previous hypersensitivity reaction to any of the penicillins is a contraindication.

Warning: Serious and occasionally fatal hypersensitivity (anaphylactoid) reactions have been reported in patients on penicillin therapy. Although anaphylaxis is more frequent following parenteral therapy, it has occurred in patients on oral penicillins. These reactions are more apt to occur in individuals with a history of sensitivity to multiple allergens.

There have been well-documented reports of individuals with a history of penicillin hypersensitivity reactions who have experienced severe hypersensitivity reactions when treated with a cephalosporin. Before therapy with a penicillin, careful inquiry should be made concerning previous hypersensitivity reactions to penicillins, cephalosporins, and other allergens.

SERIOUS ANAPHYLACTOID REACTIONS REQUIRE IMMEDIATE EMERGENCY TREATMENT WITH EPINEPHRINE. OXYGEN, INTRAVENOUS STEROIDS, AND AIRWAY MANAGEMENT, INCLUDING INTUBATION, SHOULD ALSO BE ADMINISTERED AS INDICATED.

Usage In Pregnancy: Safety for use in pregnancy has not been established.

Precautions: The possibility of superinfections with mycotic organisms or bacterial pathogens should be kept in mind during therapy. In such cases, discontinue the drug and substitute appropriate treatment.

As with any potent drug, periodic assessment of organ system function, including renal, hepatic, and hematopoietic, should be made during prolonged therapy.

Adverse Reactions: As with other penicillins, it may be expected that untoward reactions will be essentially limited to sensitivity phenomena. They are more likely to occur in individuals who have previously demonstrated hypersensitivity to penicillins and in those with a history of allergy, asthma, hay fever, or urticaria.

The following adverse reactions have been reported as associated with the use of penicillin:

Gastrointestinal—Glossitis, stomatitis, black "hairy" tongue, nausea, vomiting, and diarrhea. (These reactions are usually associated with oral dosage forms.)

Hypersensitivity Reactions—Skin rashes and urticaria have been reported frequently. A few cases of exfoliative dermatitis and erythema multiforme have been reported. Anaphylaxis is the most serious reaction experienced and has usually been associated with the parenteral dosage form.

Note: Urticaria, other skin rashes, and serum sickness-like reactions may be controlled with antihistamines and, if necessary, systemic corticosteroids. Whenever such reactions occur, penicillin should be discontinued unless, in the opinion of the physician, the condition being treated is life threatening and amenable only to penicillin therapy. Serious anaphylactic reactions require the immediate use of epinephrine, oxygen, and intravenous steroids.

Liver—A moderate rise in serum glutamic oxaloacetic transaminase (SGOT) has been noted, particularly in infants, but the significance of this finding is unknown.

Hemic and Lymphatic Systems—Anemia, thrombocytopenia, thrombocytopenic purpura, eosinophilia, leukopenia, and agranulocytosis have been reported during therapy with the penicillins. These reactions are usually reversible on discontinuation of therapy and are believed to be hypersensitivity phenomena.

Dosage and Administration: Infections of the ear, nose, and throat due to streptococci, pneumococci, nonpenicillinase-producing staphylococci and **H. influenzae:**

Infections of the genitourinary tract due to **E. coli, Proteus mirabilis,** and **Streptococcus faecalis;**

Infections of the skin and soft-tissues due to streptococci, susceptible staphylococci, and **E. coli:**
Usual Dosage: Adults: 250 mg. every 8 hours.

Children: 20 mg./Kg./day in divided doses every 8 hours.

Children weighing 20 Kg. or more should be dosed according to the adult recommendations. In severe infections or those caused by less susceptible organisms: 500 mg. every 8 hours for adults, and 40 mg./Kg./day in divided doses every 8 hours for children may be needed.

Infections of the lower respiratory tract, due to streptococci, pneumococci, nonpenicillinase-producing staphylococci, and **H. influenzae:**

Usual Dosage: Adults: 500 mg. every 8 hours.
Children: 40 mg./Kg./day in divided doses every 8 hours.

Children weighing 20 Kg. or more should be dosed according to the adult recommendations. Larger doses may be required for stubborn or severe infections.

The children's dosage is intended for individuals whose weight will not cause a dosage to be calculated greater than that recommended for adults.

Gonorrhea, acute uncomplicated ano-genital and urethral infections due to **N. gonorrhoeae:** (males and females) 3 grams as a single oral dose.

Cases of gonorrhea with a suspected lesion of syphilis should have dark-field examinations before receiving amoxicillin, and monthly serological tests for a minimum of four months.

It should be recognized that in the treatment of chronic urinary tract infections, frequent bacteriological and clinical appraisals are necessary. Smaller doses than those recommended above should not be used. Even higher doses may be needed at times. In stubborn infections, therapy may be required for several weeks. It may be necessary to continue clinical and/or bacteriological follow-up for several months after cessation of therapy. Except for gonorrhea, treatment should be continued for a minimum of 48 to 72 hours beyond the time that the patient becomes asymptomatic or evidence of bacterial eradication has been obtained. It is recommended that there be at least 10 days treatment for any infection caused by hemolytic streptococci to prevent the occurrence of acute rheumatic fever or glomerulonephritis.

Dosage and Administration of Pediatric Drops: Usual dosage for all indications except infections of the lower respiratory tract:

Under 6 Kg. (13 lbs.): 0.5 ml. every 8 hours.
6-8 Kg. (13 to 18 lbs.): 1 ml. every 8 hours.

Infections of the lower respiratory tract:
Under 6 Kg. (13 lbs.): 1 ml. every 8 hours.
6-8 Kg. (13 to 18 lbs.): 2 ml. every 8 hours.

Children weighing more than 8 Kg. (18 lbs.) should receive the appropriate dose of the Oral Suspension 125 mg. or 250 mg./5 ml.

After reconstitution, the required amount of suspension should be placed directly on the child's tongue for swallowing. Alternate means of administration are to add the required amount of suspension to formula, milk, fruit juice, water, ginger ale, or cold drinks. These preparations should then be taken immediately. To be certain the child is receiving full dosage, such preparations should be consumed in entirety.

Directions For Dispensing Oral Suspension and Pediatric Drops:
Prepare these formulations at the time of dispensing. For ease in preparation, add water to the bottle in two portions and shake well after each addition. Add the total amount of water as directed on the labeling of the package being dispensed.

The reconstituted formulation is stable for 14 days at either room temperature or refrigeration.

How Supplied:
Polymox (amoxicillin) Capsules. Each capsule contains amoxicillin trihydrate equivalent to 250 or 500 mg. amoxicillin.
NDC 0015-7278—250 mg., bottles of 100 and 500.
NDC 0015-7279—500 mg., bottles of 50 and 100.
Shown in Product Identification Section, page 407
Polymox (amoxicillin) for Oral Suspension. Each 5 ml. of reconstituted suspension contains amoxicillin trihydrate equivalent to 125 or 250 mg. amoxicillin.
NDC 0015-7276—125 mg., 80 ml., 100 ml. and 150 ml. bottles.
NDC 0015-7277—250 mg., 80 ml., 100 ml. and 150 ml. bottles.
Polymox (amoxicillin) for Oral Suspension. Each ml. of reconstituted pediatric drops contains amoxicillin trihydrate equivalent to 50 mg. amoxicillin.
NDC 0015-7277—50 mg.
For information on package sizes available, refer to the current price sheets.

*Bauer, A.W., Kirby, W.M.M., Sherris, J.C., and Turck, M.: Antibiotic Testing by a Standardized Single Disc Method, Am. J. Clin. Pathol., 45:493, 1966; Standardized Disc Susceptibility Test, FEDERAL REGISTER 37:20527-29, 1972.

PRECEF®
[pree-sef]
ceforanide for injection

This is the full text of the latest Official Package Circular dated July 1984 [7351DIR-06].

Description: Precef (ceforanide) is a semisynthetic broad spectrum cephalosporin antibiotic for parenteral administration. It is provided as a sterile sodium-free mixture of 7-[0-(aminomethyl)-phenylacetamido)-]3-[((1-(carboxymethyl)-1H-tetrazol-5-yl)thio)methyl)-3-cephem-4-carboxylic acid and lysine. When reconstituted the lysine salt is formed. Solutions of Precef range in color from light yellow to amber depending on the concentration and diluent used. The pH of the solution ranges from 5.5-8.5. The structural formula is as shown below:

Clinical Pharmacology: Mean peak plasma concentrations of 40 and 76 mcg/ml occurred at 1 hr. after intramuscular administration of doses of 0.5 and 1.0 g. respectively, of Precef to normal subjects. These concentrations declined to 3.9 and 6.7 mcg/ml at 12 hours. Following 30-minute intravenous infusions of 1.0 and 2.0 g doses of Precef, respectively, the mean plasma concentrations were 125 and 240 mcg/ml, declining to 5.9 and 9.0 mcg/ml in 12 hours.

The terminal plasma half-life was 2.9 hours after intravenous and intramuscular administration. Plasma protein binding was 80% at plasma concentrations achieved after 0.5-2.0 g doses. There was no evidence of drug accumulation and plasma pharmacokinetics did not change after twice daily administration of 0.5-2.0 g for 9.5 days.

Precef was not metabolized prior to elimination and was primarily excreted by the kidneys. After intramuscular administration of 0.5 and 1.0 g doses, mean peak urinary concentrations of 1250 and 2900 mcg/ml occurred within 2 hours. Urine levels were 110 and 265 mcg/ml, respectively, at 9-12 hours. Intravenous doses of 1.0 and 2.0 g of Precef produced mean urinary concentrations of 2550 and 5130 mcg/ml, respectively, within 2 hours after administration. Urine levels were 190 and 440 mcg/ml, respectively, at 9-12 hours. Excretion kinetics and clearance rates did not change following twice daily administration of these doses for 9.5 days. Urinary excretion accounted for 78-95% of the 0.5-2.0 g intramuscular and/or intravenous dose in 12 hours.

Probenecid has no effect on serum concentrations of Precef.

Precef reaches therapeutic levels in the gall bladder, myocardium, bone, skeletal muscle, and vaginal tissue. Therapeutic levels are also achieved in pericardial fluid, synovial fluid and bile.

Microbiology: The bactericidal activity of Precef results from inhibition of cell wall synthesis. Celoranide has a high degree of stability in the presence of some *beta*-lactamases. Celoranide is

Continued on next page

Bristol—Cont.

usually active against the following microorganisms in vitro.

Aerobes:

Gram-negative: **Escherichia coli; Klebsiella** species; **Proteus mirabilis; Providencia** species (including Providencia rettgeri, formerly **Proteus rettgeri); Citrobacter** species; **Haemophilus influenzae; Haemophilus parainfluenzae; Enterobacter** species; **Salmonella typhi; Neisseria gonorrhoeae.**

Gram-positive: Staphylococci, including penicillinase-producing strains. **Note:** Methicillin-resistant staphylococci as well as some strains of **Staphylococcus epidermidis** are resistant. **Streptococcus pneumoniae** (Formerly **Diplococcus pneumoniae**) Group A and Group B streptococci. **Streptococcus viridans.** Note: Most strains of enterococci, e.g. **Streptococcus faecalis,** are resistant.

Anaerobes:

Fusobacterium species, **Clostridium** species, Note: Most strains of **Clostridium difficile** are resistant. **Peptococcus** species, **Peptostreptococcus species.** While most strains of **B. fragilis** are resistant, ceforanide demonstrates in vitro activity against some bacteroides species. **Note; Pseudomonas, Acinetobacter calcoaceticus** (formerly **Mima** and **Herellea**) species and most **Serratia** strains are resistant to ceforanide.

Disc susceptibility tests: Quantitative methods that require measurement of zone diameters give the most precise estimate of antibiotic susceptibility. One such procedure† has been recommended for use with discs to test susceptibility to ceforanide.

Reports from the laboratory giving results of the standard single-disc susceptibility test with a 30-mcg cefamandole disc should be interpreted according to the following criteria:

Susceptible organisms produce zones of 18 mm or greater, indicating that the test organism is likely to respond to therapy.

Organisms that produce zones of 15 to 17 mm are expected to be susceptible if high dosage is used or if the infection is confined to tissues and fluids (e.g. urine) in which high antibiotic levels are attained. Resistant organisms produce zones of 14 mm or less, indicating that other therapy should be selected.

For gram-positive isolates, the test may be performed with either the cephalosporin-class disc (30 mcg cephalothin) or the cefamandole disc (30 mcg cefamandole), and a zone of 18 mm is indicative of a ceforanidie-susceptible organisms. Gram-negative organisms should be tested with the cefamandole disc (using the above criteria) since ceforanide has been shown by in vitro tests to have activity against certain strains of **Enterobacteriaeceae** found resistant when tested with the cephalosporin-class disc. Gram-negative organisms having zones of less than 18 mm around the cephalothin disc are not necessarily moderately susceptible or resistant to ceforanide.

In other susceptibility testing procedures, e.g. ICS agar dilution‡ or the equivalent, a bacterial isolate may be considered susceptible if the MIC value for ceforanide is not more than 16 mcg/ml. Organisms are considered resistant to ceforanide if the MIC is greater than 32 mcg/ml. Organisms having an MIC value of 32 mcg/ml or less than 32 mcg/ml, but greater than 16 mcg/ml, are expected to be susceptible if high dosage is used or if the infection is confined to tissues and fluids (e.g. urine) in which high antibiotic levels are attained.

Indications and Usage: Precef is indicated for the treatment of serious infections caused by susceptible strains of the designated microorganisms in the diseases listed below:

1. Bone and Joint Infections—caused by **Staphylococcus aureus** (penicillinase and non-penicillinase producing strains).
2. Endocarditis—caused by **Staphylococcus aureus** (penicillinase and non-penicillinase producing strains).
3. Lower Respiratory Tract Infections—caused by **Staphylococcus aureus** (penicillinase and non-penicillinase producing strains), **Streptococcus pneumoniae** (formerly **D. pneumoniae), Klebsiella pneumoniae,** and **Haemophilus influenzae.**
4. Bacterial Septicemia—caused by **Staphylococcus aureus** (penicillinase and non-penicillinase producing strains), **Streptococcus pneumoniae,** and **Escherichia coli.**
5. Skin and Skin Structure Infections—caused by **Staphylococcus aureus** (penicillinase and non-penicillinase producing strains), **Staphylococcus epidermidis,** Group A and Group B streptococci, **Escherichia coli, Proteus mirabilis,** and **Klebsiella pneumoniae.**
6. Urinary Tract Infections—caused by **Escherichia coli, Proteus mirabilis,** and **Klebsiella pneumoniae.**

NOTE: Injectible Penicillin G Benzathine is considered to be the drug of choice in the treatment and prevention of streptococcal infections including prophylaxis of rheumatic fever.

Specimens for bacteriologic cultures should be obtained in order to isolate and identify causative organisms and to determine their susceptibilities to ceforanide. Therapy may be instituted before results of susceptibility studies are known; however, once these results become available, the antibiotic treatment should be adjusted accordingly.

Prophylactic Use: PERIOPERATIVE PROPHYLAXIS: The preoperative prophylactic administration of Precef may prevent the growth of susceptible organisms and thereby may reduce the incidence of certain postoperative infections in patients undergoing surgical procedures which are classified as contaminated or potentially contaminated, e.g., vaginal hysterectomy. Effective prophylactic use of an antibiotic in surgery depends upon the time of administration. Precef should usually be administered sixty minutes before the operation to allow sufficient time to achieve an effective antibiotic concentration in the wound tissues during the procedure: Prophylactic administration is usually not required after the surgical procedure ends and should be discontinued within a 24 hour period. In the majority of surgical procedures, continuing prophylactic administration of any antibiotic does not reduce the incidence of subsequent infections but will increase the possibility of adverse reactions and the development of bacterial resistance.

The perioperative use of Precef may also be effective in surgical patients in whom infections at the operative site would present a serious risk, e.g. during prosthetic anthroplasty and open-heart surgery. Although ceforanide has been shown to be as effective as cephalothin in the prevention of infections following coronary artery bypass surgery, no placebo controlled trials have been conducted to evaluate any cephalosporin antibiotic in the prevention of infection following either coronary artery bypass surgery or prosthetic heart valve replacement. In these procedures where the occurrence of infection may be particularly devastating, the prophylactic administration of Precef may be continued for 2 days, administered every 12 hours following completion of surgery. If there are signs of infection, specimens for culture should be obtained for the identification of the causative organism so that the appropriate therapy may be instituted. (See Dosage and Administration).

Contraindication: Precef is contraindicated in patients with known hypersensitivity to ceforanide and the cephalosporin group of antibiotics.

Warnings: BEFORE THERAPY WITH PRECEF IS INSTITUTED, CAREFUL INQUIRY SHOULD BE MADE TO DETERMINE WHETHER THE PATIENT HAS HAD PREVIOUS HYPERSENSITIVITY REACTIONS TO CEPHALOSPORINS, PENICILLINS, OR OTHER DRUGS. THIS PRODUCT SHOULD BE GIVEN CAUTIOUSLY TO PENICILLIN-SENSITIVE PATIENTS. ANTIBIOTICS SHOULD BE ADMINISTERED WITH CAUTION TO ANY PATIENT WHO HAS DEMONSTRATED SOME FORM OF ALLERGY, PARTICULARLY TO DRUGS IF AN ALLERGIC REACTION TO PRECEF OCCURS, DISCONTINUE THE DRUG. SERIOUS ACUTE HYPERSENSITIVITY REACTIONS MAY REQUIRE EPINEPHRINE ADMINISTRATION AND OTHER EMERGENCY MEASURES.

Pseudomembranous colitis has been reported with the use of cephalosporins (and other broad spectrum antibiotics); therefore, it is important to consider its diagnosis in patients in whom diarrhea develops in association with cephalosporin use.

Treatment with broad spectrum antibiotics alters the normal flora of the colon and may permit overgrowth of clostridia. Studies indicate a toxin produced by **Clostridium difficile** is one primary cause of antibiotic-associated colitis. Cholestyramine and colestipol HCl resins have been shown to bind the toxin in vitro.

Mild cases of colitis may respond to drug discontinuance alone.

Moderate to severe cases should be managed with fluid, electrolyte, and protein supplementation as indicated.

When the colitis is not relieved by drug discontinuance or when it is severe, oral vancomycin is effective in treatment of the antibiotic-associated pseudomembranous colitis produced by **C. difficile.** Other causes of colitis should also be considered.

Precautions: Although Precef rarely produces alterations in kidney function, evaluation of renal status during therapy is recommended, especially in seriously ill patients receiving the maximum dosage. The total daily dose of Precef should be reduced in patients with transient or persistent renal insufficiency (see Dosage) because high and prolonged serum antibiotic concentrations can occur in such individuals from usual dosage.

Cephalosporins should be given with caution to patients receiving concurrent treatment with potent diuretics as these regimens are suspected of adversely affecting renal function. Nephrotoxicity has been reported following concomitant administration of cephalosporins and aminoglycoside antibiotics.

Precef should be prescribed with caution in individuals with a history of gastrointestinal disease, particularly colitis.

As with other antibiotics, prolonged use of Precef may result in over-growth of non-susceptible organisms. Repeated evaluation of the patient's condition is essential. If superinfection occurs during therapy, appropriate measures should be taken.

Usage in Pregnancy—Pregnancy Category B—In a study in which rats were treated prior to mating and through pregnancy and lactation at dose levels (1600 mg/kg/day) 50 times the usual Precef dose (30 mg/kg/day), there was no evidence of impaired male or female fertility or reproductive performance. Results of teratogenicity tests in mice and rats employing doses as high as 25 times the human dose were also negative. In a peripostnatal study, female rats treated subcutaneously with Precef at 50 times the usual human dose had a higher number of resorption sites than controls and there was a decrease in viability of the offspring. These phenomena may well have been secondary to the effects on the maternal animals of the high volume of solution injected (8 ml/kg/day), rather than representing a direct effect on the conceptus; neither was evident at lower dosage levels (e.g., 25 times human dose). There are, however, no adequate and well controlled studies in pregnant women. Because animal reproduction studies are not always predictive of human response, Precef should be used during pregnancy only if clearly needed.

Labor and Delivery—There are no data concerning the administration of Precef to women during labor or prior to delivery.

Nursing Mothers—It is not known whether Precef is excreted in human milk. Because many drugs are, caution should be exercised when Precef is administered to a nursing woman.

Pediatric Use—Safety and effectiveness of Precef in children below the age of one year have not been established. Therefore, if Precef is administered to infants, the physician should determine if the potential benefits of the product's use outweigh the possible risks of administration. Precef has been effectively used in children between the age of 1–17 years.

Adverse Reactions:

Allergic Reactions: Rash (one in 45 patients), pruritus (one in 200 patients) and eosinophilia (in about one in 12 patients) have been reported. Reactions are more likely to occur in patients with a history of hypersensitivity, particularly to penicillins.

Hematopoietic: As occurs during therapy with other cephalosporin antibiotics, therapy with Precef has been associated with transient thrombocytosis (in about one in 5 patients). Some individuals (one in 40 patients) have developed positive direct Coombs Tests during treatment with ceforanide without clinical or laboratory evidence of hemolysis.

Gastrointestinal: Nausea (one in 270 patients), vomiting (one in 2,000 patients) and diarrhea (one in 140 patients) have been reported.

Symptoms of pseudomembranous colitis may appear during or after cephalosporin treatment.

Laboratory Changes: Transient elevation in SGOT (one in 16 patients), SGPT (one in 9 patients), and alkaline phosphatase levels (one in 27 patients) have been reported.

As with other cephalosporins, transient elevations in serum creatinine and BUN levels have been observed (in one in 9 and one in 50 patients, respectively). As may occur with intramuscular injections, the administration of Precef by this route has been associated with an elevation of CPK (in about one in 3 patients).

Local Effects: Local effects were reported in less than one percent of patients and included pain (one in 155 patients) and phlebitis (one in 140 patients).

Other reactions which have been reported in less than one percent of patients are local swelling, lethargy, confusion, headache, and hypotension.

Dosage and Administration:

Dosage: Adults—The usual dose range for Precef is 0.5 to 1.0 g twice daily depending on the severity of the infection. Precef is administered every 12 hours by either the intramuscular or intravenous route. The route of administration should be dictated by the condition of the patient and anticipated ease of administration.

Children—Administration of 20–40 mg/kg/day in equally divided doses every 12 hours has been effective for most infections susceptible to Precef.

Perioperative Prophylactic Use—To prevent postoperative infection in contaminated or potentially contaminated surgery a 0.5 to 1 g IM or IV dose administered 1 hour prior to the start of surgery is recommended.

It is important that the preoperative dose be given 1 hour prior to the start of surgery so that adequate antibiotic levels are present in the serum and tissues at the time of initial surgical incision. In surgery where the occurrence of infection may be particularly devastating, e.g. prosthetic anthroplasty and open-heart surgery, the prophylactic administration of Precef may be continued for 2 days following completion of surgery.

Impaired Renal Function—Dosage should be determined by the degree of renal impairment, the severity of infection, the susceptibility of the causative organism, and therapeutic monitoring. If the creatinine clearance rate (CL_{cr}) is 60 ml/min/1.73 m² or greater, the normal 12-hour dosing interval is maintained. When Cl_{cr} is 20–59 ml/min 1.73 m² a 24-hour dosing interval is recommended, and when Cl_{cr} is 5–19 ml/min/1.73 m² a 48-hour dosing interval is recommended. If Cl_{cr} is less than 5 ml/min/1.73 m², a 48–72 hour dosing interval may be used with monitoring of plasma ceforanide concentrations.

If only serum creatinine is available, creatinine clearance may be calculated from the following formula when renal function and serum creatinine levels are at steady state.

Males $Cl_{cr} = \frac{(140 - \text{age}) \times \text{Wt (kg)}}{72 \times \text{serum creatinine (mg/100 ml)}}$

Females: 0.85 of the above value

Note: As with antibiotic therapy in general, administration of Precef should be continued for a minimum of 48 to 72 hours after the patient becomes asymptomatic or after evidence of bacterial eradication has been obtained. A minimum of 10 days of treatment is recommended in infections caused by group A beta-hemolytic streptococci in order to guard against the risk of rheumatic fever or glomerulonephritis.

Administration: Precef may be administered by either the intramuscular or the intravenous routes. Controlled clinical studies performed in normal adult volunteers and patients demonstrated that ceforanide was very well tolerated intramuscularly. In normal volunteers and patients receiving intravenous therapy, a low incidence of venous irritation was attributed to ceforanide.

Intramuscular Injection: The 500 mg and 1 gram vials should be reconstituted with 1.7 ml and 3.2 ml, respectively, of Bacteriostatic Water for Injection, 0.9% Sodium Chloride Injection, Sterile Water for Injection, or Bacteriostatic Sodium Chloride Injection. Each 1.0 ml contains 250 mg of ceforanide. All injections should be administered deep into the muscle mass.

Intravenous Administration: The intravenous route may be preferable for patients with bacterial septicemia, or other severe or life-threatening infections. These patients may be poor risks because of lowered resistance resulting from such debilitating conditions as malnutrition, trauma, surgery, diabetes, heart failure, or malignancy, particularly if shock is present or impending.

Intravenous Infusion: The contents of the 500 mg vial should be diluted in 5 ml or more of the specified diluent; the 1 gram vial should be diluted in 10 ml or more of the specified diluent, and both may be administered slowly by direct I.V. administration over a 3 to 5 minute period or may be given with intravenous infusion over a 30-minute period.

Intermittent intravenous infusion with Y-Tube: Intermittent intravenous infusion with a Y-type administration set can also be accomplished while bulk intravenous solutions are being infused. However, during infusion of the solution containing ceforanide, it is desirable to discontinue the other solution. When this technique is employed, careful attention should be paid to the volume of the solution containing ceforanide so that the calculated dose will be infused. When a Y-tube hookup is used, the contents of the 0.5 gram and 1 gram vial or StrapKap Piggyback of ceforanide should be diluted by the addition of the appropriate volume of diluent solution.

Stability and Compatibility

Intramuscular Solutions: The 500 mg and 1 gram vials when reconstituted with 1.7 ml and 3.2 ml, respectively, of (1) Bacteriostatic Water for Injection, (2) 0.9% Sodium Chloride Injection, (3) Sterile Water for Injection, or (4) Bacteriostatic Sodium Chloride Injection, are stable for 48 hours at room temperature (25°C), 14 days at refrigerator temperature (4°C), and 90 days in the frozen state (−15°C). After thawing, the solution is stable for 48 hours at room temperature.

Intravenous Solutions: Precef is stable and compatible for 24 hours at room temperature at concentrations between **0.5 mg/ml** and **200 mg/ml** in the following infusion solutions:

Sterile Water for Injection; 0.9% Sodium Chloride Injection; 5% Dextrose in Water; 5% Dextrose and 0.45% Sodium Chloride Injection; 5% Dextrose and 0.2% Sodium Chloride Injection; Lactated Ringer's Injection; 5% Dextrose in Lactated Ringer's Injection; 10% Dextrose in Water.

StrapKap® Piggyback I.V. Package: The StrapKap piggyback I.V. dosage form is available in 500 mg and 1 gram StrapKap piggyback glass containers. This package is intended for intravenous administration. Reconstitute with 10 ml or more of the appropriate diluent as secified on the container labels. Following reconstitution, the solutions are stable for 24 hours at room temperature. Upon reconstitution, the initial Precef Injection appears somewhat cloudy but will de-aerate upon brief standing to provide a clear solution. Parenteral drug products should be inspected visually for particulate matter and discoloration prior to administration, whenever solution and container permit.

How Supplied: Precef (ceforanide for injection) for I.M. or I.V. use. Ceforanide as the sodium-free lysine salt equivalent to 500 mg or 1 gram ceforanide.

NDC 0015-7351-20—500 mg vial
NDC 0015-7352-20—1 gram vial
NDC 0015-7351-28—500 mg StrapKap piggyback container
NDC 0015-7352-28—1 gram StrapKap piggyback container

For information on package sizes available, refer to the current price schedule.

† Bauer, et al., Am J Clin Path 1966; 45:493 and Federal Register 1972 Sep 30; 37:20525-20529.

‡ Determine by the ICS agar-dilution method (Ericsson H M, and Sherris J C: Acta Pathol Microbiol Scand 1971 (B), Supplement No. 217) or any other method that has been shown to give equivalent results.

PROSTAPHLIN®   B
(oxacillin sodium)
Capsules, Oral Solution, I.M. or I.V.

This is the full text of the latest Combined Official Package Circular dated June 1984 [7977DIRO-10] *and* [7979DIRO-26]   (17) 11/84

Description: Prostaphlin (oxacillin sodium) is an antibacterial agent of the isoxazolyl penicillin series. It is a penicillinase-resistant, acid-resistant, semi-synthetic penicillin. Each 1 gram of Prostaphlin for injection contains approximately 2.8 mEq of sodium and is buffered with 40 mg of dibasic sodium phosphate.

$C_{19}H_{18}N_3NaO_5S \cdot H_2O$ 441.43   [CAS 7240-38-2]
4-Thia-1-azabicyclo[3.2.0]heptane-2-carboxylic acid, 3,3
dimethyl-6-[[(5-methyl-3-phenyl-4-isoxazolyl)carbonyl] amino]
7 oxo-, monosodium salt, monohydrate, $[2S(2\alpha,5\alpha,6\beta)]$.

Clinical Pharmacology:

Microbiology

Penicillinase-resistant penicillins exert a bactericidal action against penicillin-susceptible microorganisms during the state of active multiplication. All penicillins inhibit the biosynthesis of the bacterial cell wall.

The drugs in this class are highly resistant to inactivation by staphylococcal penicillinase and are active against penicillinase producing and nonpenicillinase producing strains of *Staphylococcus aureus*.

The penicillinase-resistant penicillins are active *in vitro* against a variety of other bacteria.

Susceptibility Plate Testing

Quantitative methods of susceptibility testing that require measurement of zone diameters or minimal inhibitory concentrations (M.I.C.s) give the most precise estimates of antibiotic susceptibility. One such procedure has been recommended for use with discs to test susceptibility to this class of drugs. Interpretations correlate diameters on the disc test with MIC values. A penicillinase-resistant class disc may be used to determine microbial susceptibility to cloxacillin, dicloxacillin, methicillin, nafcillin, and oxacillin. With this procedure, employing a 5 microgram methicillin sodium disc, a report from the laboratory of "susceptible" (zone of at least 14 mm) indicates that the infecting organism is likely to respond to therapy. A report of "resistant" (zone of less than 10 mm) indicates that the infecting organism is not likely to respond to therapy. A report of "intermediate susceptibility" (zone of 10–13 mm) suggests that the organism might be susceptible if high doses of the antibiotic are used, or if the infection is confined to tissues and fluids (e.g., urine), in which high antibiotic levels are attained.

In general, all staphylococci should be tested against the penicillin G disc and against the methicillin disc. Routine methods of antibiotic suscepti-

Continued on next page

Bristol—Cont.

bility testing may fail to detect strains of organisms resistant to the penicillinase-resistant penicillins. For this reason, the use of large inocula and 48-hour incubation periods may be necessary to obtain accurate susceptibility studies with these antibiotics. Bacterial strains which are resistant to one of the penicillinase-resistant penicillins should be considered resistant to all of the drugs in the class.

Pharmacokinetics: Prostaphlin, with normal doses, has insignificant concentrations in the cerebrospinal and ascitic fluids. It is found in therapeutic concentrations in the pleural, bile and amniotic fluids. Prostaphlin is rapidly excreted as unchanged drug in the urine by glomerular filtration and active tubular secretion.

Prostaphlin (oxacillin sodium) binds to serum protein, mainly albumin. The degree of protein binding reported varies with the method of study and the investigator, but generally has been found to be $94.2 \pm 2.1\%$.

Prostaphlin (oxacillin sodium) is resistant to destruction by acid. Absorption of Prostaphlin after oral administration is rapid but incomplete. A single 250-mg oral dose gives a 1-hour peak serum level of 1.65 mcg/ml. A 500-mg dose peaks at about 2.6 mcg/ml. Peak serum levels with the oral solution occur somewhat earlier, about one-half hour after dosing. A single dose of 250-mg oral solution gives a peak serum level of 1.9 mcg/ml; of 500-mg, 4.8 mcg/ml. Oral absorption is delayed when the drug is administered after meals.

Intramuscular injections give peak serum levels 30 minutes after injection. A 250 mg dose gives a level of 5.3 mcg/ml while a 500 mg dose peaks at 10.9 mcg/ml. Intravenous injection gives a peak about 5 minutes after the injection is completed. Slow I.V. dosing with 500 mg gives a 5 minute peak of 43 mcg/ml with a half-life of 20 to 30 minutes.

Indications and Usage: The penicillinase-resistant penicillins are indicated in the treatment of infections caused by penicillinase-producing staphylococci which have demonstrated susceptibility to the drugs. Culture and susceptibility tests should be performed initially to determine the causative organisms and their sensitivity to the drug (See CLINICAL PHARMACOLOGY—Susceptibility Plate Testing).

The penicillinase-resistant penicillins may be used to initiate therapy in suspected cases of resistant staphylococcal infections prior to the availability of laboratory test results. The penicillinase-resistant penicillins should not be used in infections caused by organisms susceptible to penicillin G. If the susceptibility tests indicate that the infection is due to an organism other than a resistant staphylococcus, therapy should not be continued with a penicillinase-resistant penicillin.

Contraindications: A history of hypersensitivity (anaphylactic) reaction to any penicillin is a contraindication.

Warnings: Serious and occasionally fatal hypersensitivity (anaphylactic shock with collapse) reactions have occurred in patients receiving penicillin. The incidence of anaphylactic shock in all penicillin-treated patients is between 0.015 and 0.04 percent. Anaphylactic shock resulting in death has occurred in approximately 0.002 percent of the patients treated. Although anaphylaxis is more frequent following a parenteral administration, it has occurred in patients receiving oral penicillins.

When penicillin therapy is indicated, it should be initiated only after a comprehensive patient drug and allergy history has been obtained. If an allergic reaction occurs, the drug should be discontinued and the patient should receive supportive treatment, e.g., artificial maintenance of ventilation, pressor amines, antihistamines, and corticosteroids. Individuals with a history of penicillin hypersensitivity may also experience allergic reactions when treated with a cephalosporin.

Precautions:
General
Penicillinase-resistant penicillins should generally not be administered to patients with a history of sensitivity to any penicillin.

Penicillin should be used with caution in individuals with histories of significant allergies and/or asthma. Whenever allergic reactions occur, penicillin should be withdrawn unless, in the opinion of the physician, the condition being treated is life-threatening and amenable only to penicillin therapy.

The oral route of administration should not be relied upon in patients with severe illness, or with nausea, vomiting, gastric dilation, cardiospasm, or intestinal hypermotility. Occasionally patients will not absorb therapeutic amounts of orally administered penicillin.

The use of antibiotics may result in overgrowth of nonsusceptible organisms. If new infections due to bacteria or fungi occur, the drug should be discontinued and appropriate measures taken.

Laboratory Tests
Bacteriologic studies to determine the causative organisms and their susceptibility to the penicillinase-resistant penicillins should be performed (See **Clinical Pharmacoogy—Microbiology**). In the treatment of suspected staphylococcal infections, therapy should be changed to another active agent if culture tests fail to demonstrate the presence of staphylococci.

Periodic assessment of organ system function including renal, hepatic, and hematopoietic should be made during prolonged therapy with the penicillinase-resistant penicillins.

Blood cultures, white blood cell, and differential cell counts should be obtained prior to initiation of therapy and at least weekly during therapy with penicillinase-resistant penicillins.

Periodic urinalysis, blood urea nitrogen; and creatinine determinations should be performed during therapy with the penicillinase-resistant penicillins and dosage alterations should be considered if these values become elevated. If any impairment of renal function is suspected or known to exist, a reduction in the total dosage should be considered and blood levels monitored to avoid possible neurotoxic reactions (See **Dosage and Administration**).

SGOT and SGPT values should be obtained periodically during therapy to monitor for possible liver function abnormalities.

Drug Interactions
Tetracycline, a bacteriostatic antibiotic, may antagonize the bactericidal effect of penicillin and concurrent use of these drugs should be avoided.

Carcinogenesis, Mutagenesis, Impairment of Fertility
No long-term animal studies have been conducted with these drugs. Studies on reproduction (nafcillin) in rats and rabbits reveal no fetal or maternal abnormalities before conception and continuously through weaning (one generation).

Pregnancy Category B
Reproduction studies performed in the mouse, rat, and rabbit have revealed no evidence of impaired fertility or harm to the fetus due to the penicillinase-resistant penicillins. Human experience with the penicillins during pregnancy has not shown any positive evidence of adverse effects on the fetus. There are, however, no adequate or well-controlled studies in pregnant women showing conclusively that harmful effects of these drugs on the fetus can be excluded. Because animal reproduction studies are not always predictive of human response, this drug should be used during pregnancy only if clearly needed.

Nursing Mothers
Penicillins are excreted in breast milk. Caution should be exercised when penicillins are administered to a nursing woman.

Pediatric Use
Because of incompletely developed renal function in newborns, penicillinase-resistant penicillins (especially methicillin) may not be completely excreted, with abnormally high blood levels resulting. Frequent blood levels are advisable in this group with dosage adjustments when necessary.

All newborns treated with penicillins should be monitored closely for clinical and laboratory evidence of toxic or adverse effects (See **Dosage and Administration**).

Adverse Reactions:
Body as a Whole:
The reported incidence of allergic reactions to penicillins ranges from 0.7 to 10 percent (See WARNINGS). Sensitization is usually the result of treatment but some individuals have had immediate reactions to penicillin when first treated. In such cases, it is thought that the patients may have had prior exposure to the drug via trace amounts present in milk and vaccines.

Two types of allergic reactions to penicillin are noted clinically, immediate and delayed.

Immediate reactions usually occur within 20 minutes of administration and range in severity from urticaria and pruritus to angioneurotic edema, laryngospasm, bronchospasm, hypotension, vascular collapse, and death. Such immediate anaphylactic reactions are very rare (See WARNINGS) and usually occur after parenteral therapy but have occurred in patients receiving oral therapy. Another type of immediate reaction, an accelerated reaction, may occur between 20 minutes and 48 hours after administration and may include urticaria, pruritus, and fever. Although laryngeal edema, laryngospasm, and hypotension occasionally occur, fatality is uncommon.

Delayed allergic reactions to penicillin therapy usually occur after 48 hours and sometimes as late as 2 to 4 weeks after initiation of therapy. Manifestations of this type of reaction include serum sickness-like symptoms (i.e., fever, malaise, urticaria, myalgia, arthralgia, abdominal pain) and various skin rashes. Nausea, vomiting, diarrhea, stomatitis, black or hairy tongue, and other symptoms of gastrointestinal irritation may occur, especially during oral penicillin therapy.

Nervous System Reactions:
Neurotoxic reactions similar to those observed with Penicillin G may occur with large intravenous doses of the penicillinase-resistant penicillins especially with patients with renal insufficiency.

Urogenital Reactions:
Renal tubular damage and interstitial nephritis have been associated with the administration of methicillin sodium and infrequently with the administration of nafcillin and oxacillin. Manifestations of this reaction may include rash, fever, eosinophilia, hematuria, proteinuria, and renal insufficiency. Methicillin-induced nephropathy does not appear to be dose-related and is generally reversible upon prompt discontinuation of therapy.

Gastrointestinal Reactions
Pseudomembranous colitis has been reported with the use of Prostaphlin (and other broad spectrum antibiotics); therefore, it is important to consider its diagnosis in patients who develop diarrhea in association with antibiotic use.

Treatment with broad spectrum antibiotics alters normal flora of the colon and may permit overgrowth of clostridia. Studies indicate a toxin produced by *Clostridium difficile* is one primary cause of antibiotic-associated colitis. Cholestyramine and colestipol resins have been shown to bind the toxin *in vitro*.

Mild cases of colitis may respond to drug discontinuance alone.

Moderate to severe cases should be managed with fluid, electrolyte and protein supplementation as indicated.

When the colitis is not relieved by drug discontinuance or when it is severe, oral vancomycin is the treatment of choice for antibiotic-associated pseudomembranous colitis produced by *C. difficile*. Other causes of colitis should also be considered.

Metabolic Reactions:
Agranulocytosis, neutropenia, and bone marrow depression have been associated with the use of methicillin sodium, nafcillin, oxacillin, and cloxacillin. Hepatotoxicity, characterized by fever, nausea, and vomiting associated with abnormal liver function tests, mainly elevated SGOT levels, has been associated with the use of oxacillin and cloxacillin.

Dosage and Administration: The penicillinase-resistant penicillins are available for oral administration and for intramuscular and intravenous injection. The sodium salts of methicillin, oxacillin, and nafcillin may be administered parenterally and the sodium salts of cloxacillin, dicloxacillin, oxacillin, and nafcillin are available for oral use.

Bacteriologic studies to determine the causative organisms and their sensitivity to the penicillinase-resistant penicillins should always be performed. Duration of therapy varies with the type and severity of infection as well as the overall condition of the patient, therefore it should be determined by the clinical and bacteriological response of the patient. In severe staphylococcal infections, therapy with penicillinase-resistant penicillins should be continued for at least 14 days. Therapy should be continued for at least 48 hours after the patient had become afebrile, asymptomatic, and cultures are negative. The treatment of endocarditis and osteomyelitis may require a longer term of therapy.

Concurrent administration of the penicillinase-resistant penicillins and probenecid increases and prolongs serum penicillin levels. Probenecid decreases the apparent volume of distribution and slows the rate of excretion by competitively inhibiting renal tubular secretion of penicillin. Penicillin-probenecid therapy is generally limited to those infections where very high serum levels of penicillin are necessary.

Oral preparations of the penicillinase-resistant penicillins should not be used as initial therapy in serious, life-threatening infections (See **Precautions—General**). Oral therapy with the penicillinase-resistant penicillins may be used to follow-up the previous use of a parenteral agent as soon as the clinical condition warrants. For intramuscular gluteal injections, care should be taken to avoid sciatic nerve injury. With intravenous administration, particularly in elderly patients, care should be taken because of the possibility of thrombophlebitis.
[See table above].

Directions For Dispensing Oral Solution: Prepare these formulations at the time of dispensing. For ease in preparation, add water to the bottle in two portions and shake well after each addition. Add the total amount of water as directed on the labeling of the package being dispensed. The reconstituted formulation is stable for 3 days at room temperature or 14 days under refrigeration. [See table below].

Directions For Use:
For Intramuscular Use: Use Sterile Water for Injection, USP. Add 1.4 ml to the 250 mg vial, 2.7 ml to the 500 mg vial, 5.7 ml to the 1 gram vial, 11.5 ml to the 2 gram vial, and 23 ml to the 4 gram vial. Shake well until a clear solution is obtained. After reconstitution, vials will contain 250 mg of active drug per 1.5 ml of solution. The reconstituted solution is stable for 3 days at 70°F or for one week under refrigeration (40°F).

For Direct Intravenous Use: Use Sterile Water for Injection, USP or Sodium Chloride Injection, USP. Add 5 ml to the 250 mg and 500 mg vials; 10 ml to the 1 gram vial; 20 ml to the 2 gram vial; and 40 ml to the 4 gram vial. Withdraw the entire contents and administer slowly over a period of approximately 10 minutes.

RECOMMENDED ORAL DOSAGES FOR PROSTAPHLIN (oxacillin sodium) IN MILD TO MODERATE AND SEVERE INFECTIONS

DRUG	ADULTS Mild to Moderate	ADULTS Severe	CHILDREN Mild to Moderate	CHILDREN Severe
Oxacillin	500 mg every 4–6 hours	1 gram every 4–6 hours (followup of parenteral therapy)	50 mg/kg/day[a] in equally divided doses every 6 hours	100 mg/kg/day[a] in equally divided doses every 4–6 hours (followup of parenteral therapy)

[a] Patients weighing less than 40 Kg (88 lbs)

(For Direct Intravenous Use) prior to diluting with Intravenous Solution.
[See table on next page].
Stability studies on Prostaphlin at concentrations of 0.5 mg/ml and 2 mg/ml in various intravenous solutions listed below indicate the drug will lose less than 10% activity at room temperature (70°F) during a 6 hour period.
I.V. Solution:
5% Dextrose in Normal Saline
10% D-Fructose in Water
10% D-Fructose in Normal Saline
Lactated Potassic Saline Injection
10% Invert Sugar in Normal Saline
10% Invert Sugar Plus 0.3% Potassium Chloride in Water
Travert 10% Electrolyte #1
Travert 10% Electrolyte #2
Travert 10% Electrolyte #3
Only those solutions listed above should be used for the intravenous infusion of Prostaphlin. The concentration of the antibiotic should fall within the range specified. The drug concentration and the rate and volume of the infusion should be adjusted so that the total dose of oxacillin is administered before the drug loses its stability in the solution in use.
If another agent is used in conjunction with oxacillin therapy, **it should not be physically mixed** with oxacillin but should be administered separately.
"Piggyback" I.V. Package: This glass vial contains the labeled quantity of Prostaphlin and is intended for intravenous administration. The diluent and volume are specified on the label of each package.
Discard solution after 24 hours at room temperature.
Hospital Bulk Package: This glass vial contains 10 grams Prostaphlin and is designed for use in the pharmacy in preparing I.V. additives. Add 93 ml Sterile Water for Injection, USP or Sodium Chloride Injection, USP. The resulting solution will contain 100 mg oxacillin sodium per ml.
Following reconstitution in this manner, the resulting solutions are stable for 4 days at room temperature or 7 days under refrigeration.
CAUTION: NOT TO BE DISPENSED AS A UNIT.
Supply: Prostaphlin (oxacillin sodium) for Injection. Oxacillin sodium equivalent to 250, 500 mg, 1, 2, 4 or 10 grams oxacillin per vial.
NDC 0015-7978-20—250 mg vial
NDC 0015-7979-20—500 mg vial
NDC 0015-7981-20—1 gram vial
NDC 0015-7970-20—2 gram vial
NDC 0015-7300-20—4 gram vial
NDC 0015-7981-28—1 gram "Piggyback" vial
NDC 0015-7970-28–2 gram "Piggyback" vial
NDC 0015-7300-28–4 gram "Piggyback" vial
NDC 0015-7103-28–10 gram Hospital Bulk Package
Also available: PROSTAPHLIN (oxacillin sodium) Capsules. Oxacillin sodium equivalent to 250 or 500 mg oxacillin per capsule.
NDC 0015-7977—250 mg
NDC 0015-7982—500 mg
PROSTAPHLIN (oxacillin sodium) for Oral Solution. Each 5 ml of reconstituted solution contains oxacillin sodium equivalent to 250 mg oxacillin.
NDC 0015-7985—250 mg
For information on package sizes available, refer to the current price schedule.
Shown in Product Identification Section, page 407

SALURON® ℞
[săl-ū-rŏn]
(hydroflumethiazide)

This is the full text of the latest Official Package Circular dated December 1976 [5410DIRO-10].
Description: Saluron (hydroflumethiazide) is a potent oral diuretic-antihypertensive agent of low toxicity developed by Bristol Laboratories.
Action: The mechanism of action results in an interference with the renal tubular mechanism of electrolyte reabsorption. At maximal therapeutic dosage all thiazides are approximately equal in their diuretic potency. The mechanism whereby thiazides function in the control of hypertension is unknown.
Indications: Saluron is indicated as adjunctive therapy in edema associated with congestive heart failure, hepatic cirrhosis, and corticosteroid and estrogen therapy.
Saluron has also been found useful in edema due to various forms of renal dysfunction such as nephrotic syndrome, acute glomerulonephritis, and chronic renal failure.
Saluron is indicated in the management of hypertension either as the sole therapeutic agent or to enhance the effectiveness of other antihypertensive drugs in the more severe forms of hypertension.
Usage in Pregnancy: The routine use of diuretics in an otherwise healthy woman is inappropriate and exposes mother and fetus to unnecessary hazard. Diuretics do not prevent development of toxemia of pregnancy, and there is no satisfactory evidence that they are useful in the treatment of developed toxemia.
Edema during pregnancy may arise from pathological causes or from the physiologic and mechanical consequences of pregnancy. Thiazides are indicated in pregnancy when edema is due to pathologic causes, just as they are in the absence of pregnancy (however, see Warnings, below). Dependent edema in pregnancy, resulting from restriction of venous return by the expanded uterus, is properly treated through elevation of the lower extremities and use of support hose; use of diuretics to lower intravascular volume in this case is illogical and unnecessary. There is hypervolemia during normal pregnancy which is harmful to neither the fetus nor the mother (in the absence of cardiovascular disease), but which is associated with edema, including generalized edema, in the majority of pregnant women. If this edema produces discomfort, increased recumbency will often provide re-

RECOMMENDED PARENTERAL DOSAGES FOR PROSTAPHLIN (oxacillin sodium)

Drug	Adults	Infants and Children 40 kg (88 lbs)	Other Recommendations
Oxacillin	250–500 mg IM or IV every 4–6 hours (mild to moderate infections)	50 mg/kg/day IM or IV in equally divided doses every 6 hours (mild to moderate infections)	
	1 gram IM or IV every 4–6 hours (severe infections)	100 mg/kg/day IM or IV in equally divided doses every 4–6 hours (severe infections)	Premature and Neonates 25 mg/kg/day IM or IV

Continued on next page

Bristol—Cont.

lief. In rare instances, this edema may cause extreme discomfort which is not relieved by rest. In these cases, a short course of diuretics may provide relief and may be appropriate.

Contraindications: Patients with anuria or hypersensitivity to this or other sulfonamide derived drugs.

Warnings: Saluron should be used with caution in severe renal disease. In patients with renal disease, thiazides may precipitate azotemia. Cumulative effects of the drug may develop in patients with impaired renal function.

Thiazides should be used with caution in patients with impaired hepatic function or progressive liver disease, since minor alterations of fluid and electrolyte balance may precipitate hepatic coma.

Thiazides may be additive or potentiative of the action of other antihypertensive drugs. Potentiation occurs with ganglionic or peripheral adrenergic blocking drugs.

Sensitivity reactions may occur in patients with a history of allergy or bronchial asthma.

The possibility of exacerbation or activation of systemic lupus erythematosus has been reported.

Usage in Pregnancy: Thiazides cross the placental barrier and appear in cord blood. The use of thiazides in pregnant women requires that the anticipated benefit be weighed against possible hazards to the fetus. These hazards include fetal or neonatal jaundice, thrombocytopenia, and possibly other adverse reactions which have occurred in the adult.

Nursing Mothers: Thiazides appear in breast milk. If use of the drug is deemed essential, the patient should stop nursing.

Precautions: Periodic determination of serum electrolytes to detect possible electrolyte imbalance should be performed at appropriate intervals. All patients receiving thiazide therapy should be observed for clinical signs of fluid or electrolyte imbalance; namely, hyponatremia, hypochloremic alkalosis, and hypokalemia. Serum and urine electrolyte determinations are particularly important when the patient is vomiting excessively or receiving parenteral fluids. Medication such as digitalis may also influence serum electrolytes. Warning signs, irrespective of cause, are: Dryness of mouth, thirst, weakness, lethargy, drowsiness, restlessness, muscle pains or cramps, muscular fatigue, hypotension, oliguria, tachycardia, and gastrointestinal disturbances such as nausea and vomiting.

Hypokalemia may develop with thiazides as with any other potent diuretic, especially with brisk diuresis, when severe cirrhosis is present, or during concomitant use of corticosteroids or ACTH. Interference with adequate oral electrolyte intake will also contribute to hypokalemia. Digitalis therapy may exaggerate metabolic effects of hypokalemia especially with reference to myocardial activity.

Any chloride deficit is generally mild and usually does not require specific treatment except under extraordinary circumstances (as in liver disease or renal disease). Dilutional hyponatremia may occur in edematous patients in hot weather; appropriate therapy is water restriction, rather than administration of salt except in rare instances when the hyponatremia is life-threatening. In actual salt depletion, appropriate replacement is the therapy of choice.

Hyperuricemia may occur or frank gout may be precipitated in certain patients receiving thiazide therapy.

Insulin requirements in diabetic patients may be increased, decreased, or unchanged. Latent diabetes mellitus may become manifested during thiazide administration.

Thiazide drugs may increase the responsiveness to tubocurarine.

The antihypertensive effects of the drug may be enhanced in the postsympathectomy patient.

Thiazides may decrease arterial responsiveness to norepinephrine. This diminution is not sufficient to preclude effectiveness of the pressor agent for therapeutic use.

If progressive renal impairment becomes evident, as indicated by a rising nonprotein nitrogen or blood urea nitrogen, a careful reappraisal of therapy is necessary with consideration given to withholding or discontinuing diuretic therapy.

Thiazides may decrease serum PBI levels without signs of thyroid disturbance.

Adverse Reactions:
A. Gastrointestinal system reactions: Anorexia, gastric irritation, nausea, vomiting, cramping, diarrhea, constipation, jaundice (intrahepatic cholestatic jaundice), pancreatitis.
B. Central nervous system reactions: Dizziness, vertigo, parasthesias, headache, xanthopsia.
C. Hematologic reactions: Leukopenia, agranulocytosis, thrombocytopenia, aplastic anemia.
D. Dermatologic-hypersensitivity reactions: Purpura, photo-sensitivity, rash, urticaria, necrotizing angiitis (vasculitis) (cutaneous vasculitis).
E. Cardiovascular reaction: Orthostatic hypotension may occur and may be aggravated by alcohol, barbiturates, or narcotics.
F. Other: Hyperglycemia, glycosuria, hyperuricemia, muscle spasm, weakness, restlessness.

Whenever adverse reactions are moderate or severe, thiazide dosage should be reduced or therapy withdrawn.

Dosage and Administration: The average adult diuretic dose is 25 to 200 mg. per day. The average adult antihypertensive dose is 50 to 100 mg. per day.

Therapy should be individualized according to patient response. This therapy should be titrated to gain maximal therapeutic response as well as the minimal dose possible to maintain that therapeutic response.

How Supplied: NDC 0015-5410—Saluron Tablets, scored, 50 mg., bottles of 100.

For information on package sizes available refer to the current price schedule.

Shown in Product Identification Section, page 407

SALUTENSIN® ℞
SALUTENSIN–Demi®
[săl-ū-tĕn'sĭn]
(hydroflumethiazide, reserpine Antihypertensive Formulation)

This is the full text of the latest Official Package Circular dated July 1984 [5436 DIR-09].

> **WARNING**
> This fixed combination drug is not indicated for initial therapy of hypertension. Hypertension requires therapy titrated to the individual patient. If the fixed combination represents the dosage so determined, its use may be more convenient in patient management. The treatment of hypertension is not static, but must be reevaluated as conditions in each patient warrant.

Description: Salutensin combines two antihypertensive agents: Saluron® (hydroflumethiazide) and reserpine. The chemical name for hydroflumethiazide is 3, 4-dihydro-7-sulfamyl-6-trifluoromethyl-2H-1, 2, 4-benzothiadiazine-1, 1-dioxide. Reserpine (3,4,5-trimethoxybenzoyl methyl reserpate) is a crystalline alkaloid derived from Rauwolfia serpentina.

Each Salutensin tablet contains:
  Saluron (hydroflumethiazide).......... 50 mg
  Reserpine............................. 0.125 mg
Each Salutensin-Demi tablet contains:
  Saluron (hydroflumethiazide).......... 25 mg
  Reserpine............................. 0.125 mg

Actions: Hydroflumethiazide is an oral diuretic-antihypertensive agent. It exerts its effect by inhibiting renal tubular reabsorption, inducing increased excretion of sodium and chloride and water with variable concomitant loss of potassium and bicarbonate as well. When used alone as an antihypertensive agent, hydroflumethiazide usually induces a gradual but sustained decrease in abnormally elevated blood pressure—both systolic and diastolic. Hypertensive patients who have been maintained on chlorothiazide or hydrochlorothiazide may also be maintained on hydroflumethiazide.

The component, reserpine, probably produces its antihypertensive effects through depletion of tissue stores of catecholamines (epinephrine and norepinephrine) from peripheral sites. By contrast, its sedative and tranquilizing properties are thought to be related by depletion of 5-hydroxytryptamine from the brain.

Reserpine is characterized by slow onset of action and sustained effect. Both its cardiovascular and central nervous system effects may persist following withdrawal of the drug.

Careful observation for changes in blood pressure must be made when Salutensin is used with other antihypertensive drugs. The dosage of other agents must be reduced by at least 50 percent as soon as Salutensin is added to the regimen to prevent excessive drop in blood pressure. As the blood pressure falls under the potentiating effect of Salutensin, a further reduction in dosage or even discontinuation of other antihypertensive drugs may be necessary.

STABILITY PERIODS
PROSTAPHLIN
M/6 Molar

Concentration Mg/Ml	Sterile H₂O for Injection	Isotonic Sodium Chloride	Sodium Lactate Solution	5% Dextrose in H₂O	5% Dextrose in 0.45% NaCl	10% Invert Sugar	Lactated Ringers Solution
ROOM TEMPERATURE (25°C)							
10–100	4 Days	4 Days					
10–30			24 Hrs		24 Hrs		
0.5–2				6 Hrs		6 Hrs	6 Hrs
REFRIGERATION (4°C)							
10–100	7 Days	7 Days					
10–30			4 Days	4 Days	4 Days	4 Days	4 Days
FROZEN (−15°C)							
50–100	30 Days						
250/1.5 ml	30 Days						
100		30 Days					
10–100			30 Days	30 Days	30 Days	30 Days	30 Days

Hypertension therapy requires therapy titrated to the individual patient. If a fixed combination represents the dosage so determined its use may be more convenient in patient management.

Indications: Hypertension (see box warning).

Contraindications: Salutensin is contraindicated in patients who have previously demonstrated hypersensitivity to its components. Patients with anuria or oliguria should not be given this medication. The presence of an active peptic ulcer, ulcerative colitis, or severe depression contraindicates the use of reserpine. It is also contraindicated in patients receiving electroconvulsive therapy.

Warnings: Azotemia may be precipitated or increased by hydroflumethiazide. Special caution is necessary in patients with impaired renal function to avoid cumulative or toxic effects.

Since in hepatic cirrhosis, minor alterations of fluid and electrolyte balance may precipitate coma, hydroflumethiazide should be given with caution.

The possibility of sensitivity reactions should be considered in patients with a history of allergy or bronchial asthma.

Hydroflumethiazide potentiates the action of other antihypertensive drugs. Therefore, the dosage of these agents, especially the ganglion blockers, must be reduced by at least 50 percent as soon as hydroflumethiazide is added to the regimen.

The possibility of exacerbation or activation of systemic lupus erythematosus has been reported for sulfonamide derivatives (including thiazides) and reserpine.

The occurrence of mental depression due to reserpine in doses of 0.25 mg daily or less is unusual. In any event, Salutensin should be discontinued at the first sign of depression.

Usage in Pregnancy and the Child-Bearing Age

Since thiazides and reserpine appear in breast milk, Salutensin is contraindicated in nursing mothers. If use of the drug is deemed essential, the patient should stop nursing. Reserpine has been demonstrated to cross the placental barrier in guinea pigs with depression of adrenal catecholamine stores in the newborn. There is some evidence that side effects such as nasal congestion, lethargy, depressed Moro reflex, and bradycardia may appear in infants born of reserpine-treated mothers. Thiazides cross the placental barrier and appear in cord blood. When Salutensin is used in women of child-bearing age, the potential benefits of the drug should be weighed against the possible hazards to the fetus. These hazards include fetal or neonatal jaundice, thrombocytopenia, and possibly other adverse reactions which have occurred in the adult.

Precautions:

Hydroflumethiazide

Careful check should be kept for signs of fluid and electrolyte imbalance. Serum and urine electrolyte determinations are particularly important when the patient is vomiting excessively or receiving parenteral fluids. Warning signs, irrespective of cause, are: dryness of mouth, thirst, weakness, lethargy, drowsiness, restlessness, muscle pains or cramps, muscular fatigue, hypotension, oliguria, tachycardia, and gastrointestinal disturbances.

Potassium excretion is usually minimal. However, hypokalemia may develop with hydroflumethiazide as with any other potent diuretic, especially with brisk diuresis, when severe cirrhosis is present, or during concomitant use of steroids or ACTH. Interference with adequate electrolyte intake will contribute to hypokalemia. Digitalis therapy may exaggerate metabolic effects of hypokalemia especially with reference to myocardial activity. If dietary salt is unduly restricted, especially during hot weather, in severely edematous patients with congestive failure or renal disease, a low salt syndrome may complicate therapy with thiazides.

Hypokalemia may be avoided or treated by use of potassium chloride or giving foods with a high potassium content. Any chloride deficit may similarly be corrected by use of ammonium chloride (excepting patients with hepatic disease) and largely prevented by a near normal salt intake.

Thiazide drugs may increase the responsiveness to tubocurarine. The antihypertensive effect of the drug may be enhanced in the post-sympathectomy patient. Hydroflumethiazide decreases arterial responsiveness to norepinephrine, as do other thiazides, necessitating due care in surgical patients. It is recommended that thiazides be discontinued 48 hours before elective surgery. Orthostatic hypotension may occur and may be potentiated by alcohol, barbiturates, or narcotics.

Pathological changes in the parathyroid glands with hypercalcemia and hypophosphatemia have been observed in a few patients on prolonged thiazide therapy. The common complications of hyperparathyroidism such as renal lithiasis, bone resorption, and peptic ulceration have not been seen. The effect of discontinuation of thiazide therapy on serum calcium and phosphorus levels may be helpful in assessing the need for parathyroid surgery in such patients. Parathyroidectomy has been followed by subjective clinical improvement in most patients, but is without effect on the hypertension. Following surgery, thiazide therapy may be resumed.

Caution is necessary in patients with hyperuricemia or a history of gout, since gout may be precipitated. Insulin requirements in diabetic patients may be increased, decreased, or unchanged. In latent diabetics, hydroflumethiazide, in common with other benzothiadiazines, may cause hyperglycemia and glycosuria.

Reserpine

Since reserpine may increase gastric secretion and motility, it should be used cautiously in patients with a history of peptic ulcer, ulcerative colitis, or other gastrointestinal disorder. This compound may precipitate biliary colic in patients with gallstones, or bronchial asthma in susceptible persons. Reserpine may cause hypotension including orthostatic hypotension. In hypertensive patients on reserpine therapy significant hypotension and bradycardia may develop during surgical anesthesia. Therefore, the drug should be discontinued two weeks before giving anesthesia. For emergency surgical procedures, it may be necessary to give vagal blocking agents parenterally to prevent or reverse hypotension and/or bradycardia.

Anxiety or depression, as well as psychosis, may develop during reserpine therapy. If depression is present when therapy is begun, it may be aggravated. Mental depression is unusual with reserpine doses of 0.25 mg daily or less. In any case, Salutensin should be discontinued at the first sign of depression. Extreme caution should be used in treating patients with a history of mental depression, and the possibility of suicide should be kept in mind.

As with most antihypertensive therapy, caution should be exercised when treating hypertensive patients with renal insufficiency, since they adjust poorly to lowered blood pressure levels. Use reserpine cautiously with digitalis and quinidine; cardiac arrhythmias have occurred with reserpine preparations. Thiazides may decrease serum P.B.I. levels without signs of thyroid disturbance.

Animal Tumorigenicity

Rodent studies have shown that reserpine is an animal tumorigen, causing an increased incidence of mammary fibroadenomas in female mice, malignant tumors of the seminal vesicles in male mice, and malignant adrenal medullary tumors in male rats. These findings arose in 2 year studies in which the drug was administered in the feed at concentrations of 5 and 10 ppm—about 100 to 300 times the usual human dose. The breast neoplasms are thought to be related to reserpine's prolactin-elevating effect. Several other prolactin-elevating drugs have also been associated with an increased incidence of mammary neoplasia in rodents.

The extent to which these findings indicate a risk to humans is uncertain. Tissue culture experiments show that about one-third of human breast tumors are prolactin-dependent in vitro, a factor of considerable importance if the use of the drug is contemplated in a patient with previously detected breast cancer. The possibility of an increased risk of breast cancer in reserpine users has been studied extensively; however, no firm conclusion has emerged. Although a few epidemiologic studies have suggested a slightly increased risk (less than two-fold in all studies except one) in women who have used reserpine, other studies of generally similar design have not confirmed this. Epidemiologic studies conducted using other drugs (neuroleptic agents) that, like reserpine, increase prolactin levels and therefore would be considered rodent mammary carcinogens, have not shown an association between chronic administration of the drug and human mammary tumorigenesis. While long-term clinical observation has not suggested such an association, the available evidence is considered too limited to be conclusive at this time. An association of reserpine intake with pheochromocytoma or tumors of the seminal vesicles has not been explored.

Adverse Reactions:

Hydroflumethiazide

A. Gastrointestinal System Reactions: Anorexia, gastric irritation, nausea, vomiting, cramping, diarrhea, constipation, jaundice (intrahepatic cholestatic jaundice), pancreatitis, hyperglycemia, and glycosuria.

B. Central Nervous System Reactions: dizziness, vertigo, parasthesias, headache, and xanthopsia.

C. Hematologic Reactions: leukopenia, thrombocytopenia, agranulocytosis, and aplastic anemia.

D. Dermatologic-Hypersensitivity Reactions: purpura, photosensitivity, rash, urticaria, and necrotizing angiitis (vasculitis) (cutaneous vasculitis).

E. Cardiovascular Reaction: orthostatic hypotension may occur and may be aggravated by alcohol, barbiturates or narcotics.

F. Miscellaneous: muscle spasm, weakness, and restlessness.

Whenever adverse reactions are moderate or severe, thiazide dosage should be reduced or therapy withdrawn.

Reserpine

Side effects due to reserpine often disappear with continued use and most can be controlled by reducing the dosage. Rarely, it may be necessary to discontinue therapy. The reactions most often reported include: excessive sedation, nightmares, nasal congestion, conjunctival injection, enhanced susceptibility to colds, muscular aches, headache, dizziness, dyspnea, anorexia, nausea, increased intestinal motility, diarrhea, weight gain, dryness of the mouth, blurred vision, flushing of the skin and pruritus. Skin rash, dysuria, syncope, non-puerperal lactation, impotence or decreased libido, increased salivation, vomiting, bradycardia, mental depression, nervousness, paradoxical anxiety, epistaxis, purpura due to thrombocytopenia, angina pectoris and other direct cardiac effects (e.g., premature ventricular contractions, fluid retention, congestive failure), and central nervous system sensitization manifested by dull sensorium, deafness, glaucoma, uveitis, and optic atrophy also have been noted. In some patients reserpine has produced a syndrome similar to Parkinson's disease, though this effect usually is reversible with decreased dosage or discontinuation of therapy. Salutensin should be given with caution to hypertensive patients who also have coronary artery disease to avoid a precipitous drop in blood pressure.

Dosage: As determined by individual titration (see box warning).

The usual adult dose of Salutensin is one tablet once or twice daily. If a smaller amount of thiazide diuretic is desired, Salutensin-Demi, one tablet once or twice daily, can be given. Most patients will respond to this dosage level. In refractory cases, the physician may carefully increase the dose to three or four tablets per day in divided doses providing the proper precautions are observed—careful attention to serum uric acid, fasting blood sugar, BUN or NPN, and serum electrolyte levels. (See sections on Precautions and Warnings above.) When the desired blood pressure reduction

Continued on next page

Bristol—Cont.

has been achieved, the dose should be reduced to the minimum effective dose for the individual patient.

Careful observation for changes in blood pressure must be made when Salutensin is used with other antihypertensive drugs. The dosage of other agents must be reduced by at least 50 percent as soon as Salutensin is added to the regimen to prevent excessive drop in blood pressure. As the blood pressure falls under the potentiating effect of Salutensin, a further reduction in dosage or even discontinuation of other antihypertensive drugs may be necessary.

Supply:
Salutensin Tablets—NDC 0015-5436
Salutensin-Demi Tablets—NDC 0015-5455
For information on package sizes available, refer to the current price schedule.

Shown in Product Identification Section, page 407

STADOL® ℞
[stā'dŏl]
(butorphanol tartrate)

This is the full text of the latest Official Package Circular dated October 1979 [5644DIM-04].

Description: Stadol (butorphanol tartrate), sterile, parenteral, narcotic agonist-antagonist, analgesic, is a member of the phenanthrene series. The chemical name is levo-N- cyclobutylmethyl-6, 10aβ-dihydroxy-1,2,3,9,10, 10a-hexahydro- (4H) 10, 4a-iminoethanophenanthrene tartrate. It is a white crystalline substance soluble in aqueous solution. The dose is expressed as the salt. One milligram of tartrate salt is equivalent to 0.68 milligram of base. In addition to Stadol (butorphanol tartrate), each ml contains 3.3 mg citric acid, 6.4 mg sodium citrate and 6.4 mg sodium chloride. The structural formula is

The molecular weight is 477.56 and the molecular formula is $C_{21}H_{29}NO_2 \cdot C_4H_6O_6$

Clinical Pharmacology: Stadol is a potent analgesic. The duration of analgesia is generally 3 to 4 hours and is approximately equivalent to that of morphine. The onset time for analgesia is within 10 minutes following intramuscular injection and very rapidly following intravenous administration. Peak analgesic activity is obtained at 30 to 60 minutes following intramuscular injection and more rapidly following intravenous administration.

Narcotic Antagonist Activity
Stadol has narcotic antagonist activity which is approximately equivalent to that of nalorphine, 30 times that of pentazocine and 1/40 that of naloxone (Narcan®) as measured by the antagonism of morphine analgesia in the rat tail flick test.

Mechanism of Analgesic Action
The exact mechanism of action of Stadol is unknown. It is felt that the class of narcotic antagonist analgesics exert their analgesic effect via a central nervous system mechanism. Currently, it is believed the site of action of centrally acting analgesics is subcortical, possibly in the limbic system.

Effect on Respiration
At the analgesic dose of 2 mg, Stadol depresses respiration to a degree equal to 10 mg morphine. The magnitude of respiratory depression with Stadol is not appreciably increased at doses of 4 mg. In contrast to the magnitude of respiratory depression, the duration of respiratory depression with Stadol is dose-related. Any respiratory depression produced by Stadol is reversible by naloxone which is a specific antagonist.

Cardiovascular Effects
The hemodynamic changes after the intravenous administration of Stadol are similar to the reported hemodynamic changes after pentazocine. The changes include increased pulmonary artery pressure, pulmonary wedge pressure, left ventricular end-diastolic pressure, systemic arterial pressure, and pulmonary vascular resistance. Although smaller than those following pentazocine, these changes are nevertheless in a direction which increases the work of the heart, especially in the pulmonary circuit.

Indications and Usage: Stadol is recommended for the relief of moderate to severe pain. Stadol can also be used for preoperative or preanesthetic medication, as a supplement to balanced anesthesia, and for the relief of prepartum pain.

Contraindications: Stadol should not be administered to patients who have been shown to be hypersensitive to it.

Warnings:
Patients Physically Dependent on Narcotics
Because of its antagonist properties, Stadol is not recommended for patients physically dependent on narcotics. Detoxification in such patients is required prior to use.

Due to the difficulty in assessing addiction in patients who have recently received substantial amounts of narcotic medication, caution should be used in the administration of Stadol. Detoxification of such patients prior to usage should be carefully considered.

Drug Dependence
Special care should be exercised in administering Stadol to emotionally unstable patients and to those with a history of drug misuse. When long-term therapy is contemplated, such patients should be closely supervised. Even though Stadol has a low physical dependence liability, care should be taken that individuals who may be prone to drug abuse are closely supervised. It is important to avoid increases in dose and frequency of injections by the patient and to prevent the use of the drug in anticipation of pain rather than for the relief of pain.

Head Injury and Increased Intracranial Pressure
Although there is no clinical experience in patients with head injury, it can be assumed that Stadol, like other potent analgesics, elevates cerebrospinal fluid pressure. Therefore the use of Stadol in cases of head injury can produce effects (e.g., miosis) which may obscure the clinical course of patients with head injuries. In such patients Stadol must be used with extreme caution and only if its use is deemed essential.

Cardiovascular Effects
Because Stadol increases the work of the heart, especially the pulmonary circuit, (see Clinical Pharmacology), the use of this drug in acute myocardial infarction or in cardiac patients with ventricular dysfunction or coronary insufficiency should be limited to those who are hypersensitive to morphine sulfate or meperidine.

Precautions:
Certain Respiratory Conditions
Because Stadol causes some respiratory depression, it should be administered only with caution and low dosage to patients with respiratory depression (e.g., from other medication, uremia, or severe infection), severely limited respiratory reserve, bronchial asthma, obstructive respiratory conditions, or cyanosis.

Impaired Renal or Hepatic Function
Although laboratory tests have not indicated that Stadol causes or increases renal or hepatic impairment, the drug should be administered with caution to patients with such impairment. Extensive liver disease may predispose to greater side effects and greater activity from the usual clinical dose, possibly the result of decreased metabolism of the drug by the liver.

Biliary Surgery
Clinical studies have not been done to establish the safety of Stadol administration to patients about to undergo surgery of the biliary tract.

Usage as a Pre-Operative or Pre-Anesthetic Medication
Slight increases in systolic blood pressure may occur, therefore caution should be employed when Stadol is used in the hypertensive patient.

Usage in Balanced Anesthesia
The use of pancuronium in combination with Stadol may cause an increase in conjunctival changes.

Usage in Pregnancy
The safety of Stadol for use in pregnancy prior to the labor period has not been established; therefore, this drug should be used in pregnant patients only when in the judgment of the physician its use is deemed essential to the welfare of the patient. Reproduction studies have been performed in rats, mice, and rabbits and have revealed no evidence of impaired fertility or harm to the fetus due to Stadol at about 2.5 to 5 times the human dose.

Usage in Labor and Delivery
Safety to the mother and fetus following the administration of Stadol during labor has been established. Patients receiving Stadol during labor have experienced no adverse effects other than those observed with commonly used analgesics. Stadol should be used with caution in women delivering premature infants.

Usage in Nursing Mothers
The use of Stadol in lactating mothers who are nursing their infants is not recommended, since it is not known whether this drug is excreted in milk. Stadol has been used safely for labor pain in mothers who subsequently nursed their infants.

Usage in Children
Safety and efficacy in children below age 18 years have not been established at present.

Adverse Reactions: The most frequent adverse reactions in 1250 patients treated with Stadol are: sedation (503, 40%), nausea (82, 6%), clammy/sweating (76, 6%).

Less frequent reactions are: headache (35, 3%), vertigo (33, 3%), floating feeling (33, 3%), dizziness (23, 2%), lethargy (19, 2%), confusion (15, 1%), lightheadedness (12, 1%).

Other adverse reactions which may occur (reported incidence of less than 1%) are:

CNS: nervousness, unusual dreams, agitation, euphoria, hallucinations
Autonomic: flushing and warmth, dry mouth, sensitivity to cold
Cardiovascular: palpitation, increase or decrease of blood pressure
Gastrointestinal: vomiting
Respiratory: slowing of respiration, shallow breathing
Dermatological: rash or hives
Eye: diplopia or blurred vision

Overdosage:
Manifestations
Although there have been no experiences of overdosage with Stadol during clinical trials, this may occur due to accidental or intentional misuse as well as therapeutic use. Based on the pharmacology of Stadol, overdosage could produce some degree of respiratory depression and variable cardiovascular and central nervous system effects.

Treatment
The immediate treatment of suspected Stadol overdosage is intravenous naloxone. The respiratory and cardiac status of the patient should be evaluated constantly and appropriate supportive measures instituted, such as oxygen, intravenous fluids, vasopressors, and assisted or controlled respiration.

Dosage and Administration:
Adults:
Intramuscular—The usual recommended single dose is 2 mg. This may be repeated every three to four hours, as necessary. The effective dosage range, depending on the severity of pain, is 1 to 4 mg repeated every three to four hours. At this time, there is insufficient clinical data to recommend single doses beyond 4 mg.

Intravenous—The usual recommended single dose for intravenous administration is 1 mg repeated every three to four hours as necessary. The effective dosage range, depending on the severity of pain, is 0.5 to 2 mg repeated every three to four hours.

Concomitant Use with Tranquilizers
According to accepted procedure, the dose of Stadol should be reduced when administered concomitantly with phenothiazines and other tranquilizers which may potentiate the action of Stadol.

Children:
Since there is no clinical experience in children under 18 years, Stadol is not recommended in this age group.

Storage Conditions
Store at room temperature.

Supply: Stadol (butorphanol tartrate) Injection for I.M. or I.V. use, is available as follows:
NDC 0015-5644-20—2 mg per ml, 2-ml vial
NDC 0015-5645-20—1 mg per ml, 1-ml vial
NDC 0015-5646-20—2 mg per ml, 1-ml vial
NDC 0015-5646-23—2 mg per ml, 1-ml Disposable Syringe
NDC 0015-5648-20—2 mg per ml, 10-ml multi-dose vial

For information on package sizes available, refer to the current price schedule.

STAPHCILLIN® ℞
[stăf' sĭl-ĭn]
(methicillin sodium for Injection)
Buffered
For I.M. Or I.V. Use

This is the full text of the latest Official Package Circular dated June 1984 [7961DIR-18].

Description: Staphcillin (methicillin sodium) is a semisynthetic antibiotic substance derived from 6-amino penicillanic acid. It is the sodium salt in a parenteral dosage form. Each gram of Staphcillin is equivalent to 900 mg methicillin activity and is buffered with 50 mg sodium citrate.

METHICILLIN SODIUM

$C_{17}H_{19}N_2NaO_6S \cdot H_2O$ 420.41 [CAS 7246-14 2]
4-Thia-1 azabicyclo[3.2.0]heptane-2 carboxylic acid, 6-[(2,6-dimethoxybenzoyl)amino]- 3, 3-dimethyl-7-oxo, mono-sodium salt, monohydrate, [2S-(2α,5α,6β)]-.

Clinical Pharmacology:
Microbiology: Penicillinase-resistant penicillins exert a bactericidal action against penicillin-susceptible microorganisms during the state of active multiplication. All penicillins inhibit the biosynthesis of the bacterial cell wall.

The drugs in this class are highly resistant to inactivation by staphylococcal penicillinase and are active against penicillinase producing and non-penicillinase producing strains of **Staphylococcus aureus.**

The penicillinase-resistant penicillins are active *in vitro* against a variety of other bacteria.

Susceptibility Plate Testing: Quantitative methods of susceptibility testing that require measurement of zone diameters or minimal inhibitory concentrations (MIC's) give the most precise estimates of antibiotic susceptibilty. One such procedure has been recommended for use with discs to test susceptibility to this class of drugs. Interpretations correlate diameters on the disc test with MIC values. A penicillinase-resistant class disc may be used to determine microbial susceptibility to cloxacillin, dicloxacillin, methicillin, nafcillin, and oxacillin. With this procedure, employing a 5 microgram methicillin sodium disc, a report from the laboratory of "susceptible" (zone of at least 14 mm) indicates that the infecting organism is likely to respond to therapy. A report of "resistant" (zone of less than 10 mm) indicates that the infecting organism is not likely to respond to therapy. A report of "intermediate susceptibility" (zone of 10 to 13 mm) suggests that the organism might be susceptible if high doses of the antibiotic are used, or if the infection is confined to tissues and fluids (e.g., urine), in which high antibiotic levels are attained. In general, all staphylococci should be tested against the penicillin G disc and against the methicillin disc. Routine methods of antibiotic susceptibility testing may fail to detect strains of organisms resistant to the penicillinase-resistant penicillins. For this reason, the use of large inocula and 48-hour incubation periods may be necessary to obtain accurate susceptibility studies with these antibiotics. Bacterial strains which are resistant to one of the penicillinase-resistant penicillins should be considered resistant to all of the drugs in the class.

Pharmacokinetics: Staphcillin (methicillin sodium) is not acid-resistant and must be administered by intramuscular or intravenous injection. A 1-Gram intramuscular dose gives a peak blood level of approximately 12 mcg/ml which drops off to about 1 mcg/ml within a 4-hour period. Methicillin is rapidly excreted unchanged in the urine in individuals with normal kidney function. Impairment in kidney function results in elevated blood levels which may require adjustment of dosage and treatment intervals. Protein binding of methicillin is approximately 40%. The drug penetrates body tissues well, and diffuses readily into pleural, pericardial, and synovial fluids. As with all penicillins, absorption into spinal fluids is poor under normal conditions. However, higher concentrations may be attained in the presence of meningeal inflammation.

Indications and Usage: The penicillanse-resistant penicillins are indicated in the treatment of infections caused by penicillinase-producing staphylococci which have demonstrated susceptibility to the drugs. Culture and susceptibility tests should be performed initially to determine the causative organism and their sensitivity to the drug (See **Clinical Pharmacology**—Susceptibility Plate Testing).

The penicillinase-resistant penicillins may be used to initiate therapy in suspected cases of resistant staphylococcal infections prior to the availability of laboratory test results. The penicillinase-resistant penicillins should not be used in infections caused by organisms susceptible to penicillin G. If the susceptibility tests indicate that the infection is due to an organism other than a resistant staphylococcus, therapy should not be continued with a penicillinase-resistant penicillin.

Contraindications: A history of a hypersensitivity (anaphylactic) reaction to any penicillin is a contraindication.

Warnings: Serious and occasionally fatal hypersensitivity (anaphylactic shock with collapse) reactions have occurred in patients receiving penicillin. The incidence of anaphylactic shock in all penicillin-treated patients is between 0.015 and 0.04 percent. Anaphylactic shock resulting in death has occurred in approximately 0.002 percent of the patients treated. Although anaphylaxis is more frequent following a parenteral administration, it has occurred in patients receiving oral penicillins.

When penicillin therapy is indicated, it should be initiated only after a comprehensive patient drug and allergy history has been obtained. If an allergic reaction occurs, the drug should be discontinued and the patient should receive supportive treatment, e.g., artificial maintenance of ventilation, pressor amines, antihistamines, and corticosteroids. Individuals with a history of penicillin hypersensitivity may also experience allergic reactions when treated with cephalosporin.

Precautions
General: Penicillinase-resistant penicillins should generally not be administered to patients with a history of sensitivity to any penicillin.

Penicillin should be used with caution in individuals with histories of significant allergies and/or asthma. Whenever allergic reactions occur, penicillin should be withdrawn unless, in the opinion of the physician, the condition being treated is life-threatening and amenable only to penicillin therapy.

The oral route of administration should not be relied upon in patients with severe illness, or with nausea, vomiting, gastric dilation, cardiospasm, or intestinal hypermotility. Occasionally patients will not absorb therapeutic amounts of orally administered penicillin.

The use of antibiotics may result in overgrowth of nonsusceptible organisms. If new infections due to bacteria or fungi occur, the drug should be discontinued and appropriate measures taken.

Laboratory Tests: Bacteriologic studies to determine the causative organisms and their susceptibility to the penicillinase-resistant penicillins should be performed (See **Clinical Pharmacology**—Microbiology). In the treatment of suspected staphylococcal infections, therapy should be changed to another active agent if culture tests fail to demonstrate the presence of staphylococci. Periodic assessment of organ system function including renal, hepatic, and hematopoietic should be made during prolonged therapy with the penicillinase-resistant penicillins.

Blood cultures, white blood cell, and differential cell counts should be obtained prior to initiation of therapy and at least weekly during therapy with penicillinase-resistant penicillins.

Periodic urinalysis, blood urea nitrogen, and creatinine determinations should be performed during therapy with the penicillinase resistant penicillins and dosage alterations should be considered if these values become elevated. If any impairment of renal function is suspected or known to exist, a reduction in the total dosage should be considered and blood levels monitored to avoid possible neurotoxic reactions (See **DOSAGE AND ADMINISTRATION**).

SGOT and SGPT values should be obtained periodically during therapy to monitor for possible liver function abnormalities.

Drug Interactions: Tetracycline, a bacteriostatic antibiotic, may antagonize the bactericidal effect of penicillin and concurrent use of these drugs should be avoided.

Carcinogenesis, Mutagenesis, Impairment of Fertility: No long-term animal studies have been conducted with these drugs.

Studies on reproduction (nafcillin) in rats and rabbits reveal no fetal or maternal abnormalities before conception and continuously through weaning (one generation).

Pregnancy Category B: Reproduction studies performed in the mouse, rat, and rabbit have revealed no evidence of impaired fertility or harm to the fetus due to the penicillinase-resistant penicillins. Human experience with the penicillins during pregnancy has not shown any positive evidence of adverse effects on the fetus. There are, however, no adequate or well-controlled studies in pregnant women showing conclusively that harmful effects of these drugs on the fetus can be excluded. Because animal reproduction studies are not always predictive of human response, this drug should be used during pregnancy only if clearly needed.

Nursing Mothers: Penicillins are excreted in breast milk. Caution should be exercised when penicillins are administered to a nursing woman.

Pediatric Use: Because of incompletely developed renal function in newborns, penicillinase-resistant penicillins (especially methicillin) may not be completely excreted, with abnormally high blood levels resulting. Frequent blood levels are advisable in this group with dosage adjustments when necessary. All newborns treated with penicillins should be monitored closely for clinical and laboratory evidence of toxic or adverse effects (See **DOSAGE AND ADMINISTRATION**).

Adverse Reactions
Body as a Whole: The reported incidence of allergic reactions to penicillins ranges from 0.7 to 10 percent (See **WARNINGS**). Sensitization is usually the result of treatment but some individuals have had immediate reactions to penicillin when first treated. In such cases, it is thought that the patients may have had prior exposure to the drug via trace amounts present in milk and vaccines.

Two types of allergic reactions to penicillin are noted clinically, immediate and delayed.

Continued on next page

Bristol—Cont.

Immediate reactions usually occur within 20 minutes of administration and range in severity from urticaria and pruritus to angioneurotic edema, laryngospasm, bronchospasm, hypotension, vascular collapse, and death. Such immediate anaphylactic reactions are very rare (See **WARNINGS**) and usually occur after parenteral therapy but have occurred in patients receiving oral therapy. Another type of immediate reaction, an accelerated reaction, may ocur between 20 minutes and 48 hours after administration and may include urticaria, pruritus, and fever. Although laryngeal edema, laryngospasm, and hypotension occasionally occur, fatality is uncommon.

Delayed allergic reactions to penicillin therapy usually occur after 48 hours and sometimes as late as 2 to 4 weeks after initiation of therapy. Manifestations of this type of reaction include serum sickness-like symptoms (i.e., fever, malaise, urticaria, myalgia, arthralgia, abdominal pain) and various skin rashes. Nausea, vomiting, diarrhea, stomatitis, black or hairy tongue, and other symptoms of gastrointestinal irritation may occur, especially during oral penicillin therapy.

Nervous System Reactions: Neurotoxic reactions similar to those observed with penicillin G may occur with large intravenous doses of the penicillinase-resistant penicillins especially in patients with renal insufficiency.

Urogenital Reactions: Renal tubular damage and interstitial nephritis have been associated with the administration of methicillin sodium and infrequently with the administration of nafcillin and oxacillin. Manifestations of this reaction may include rash, fever, eosinophilia, hematuria, proteinuria, and renal insufficiency. Methicillin-induced nephropathy does not appear to be dose-related and is generally reversible upon prompt discontinuation of therapy.

Metabolic Reactions: Agranulocytosis, neutropenia, and bone marrow depression have been associated with the use of methicillin sodium, nafcillin, oxacillin, and cloxacillin. Hepatotoxicity, characterized by fever, nausea, and vomiting associated with abnormal liver function tests, mainly elevated SGOT levels, has been associated with the use of oxacillin and cloxacillin.

Dosage and Administration: The penicillinase-resistant penicillins are available for oral administration and for intramuscular and intravenous injection. The sodium salts of methicillin, oxacillin, and nafcillin may be administered parenterally and the sodium salts of cloxacillin, dicloxacillin, oxacillin, and nafcillin are available for oral use.

Bacteriologic studies to determine the causative organisms and their sensitivity to the penicillinase-resistant penicillins should always be performed. Duration of therapy varies with the type and severity of infection as well as the overall condition of the patient, therefore it should be determined by the clinical and bacteriological response of the patient. In severe staphylococcal infections, therapy with penicillinase-resistant penicillins should be continued for at least 14 days. Therapy should be continued for at least 48 hours after the patient has become afebrile, asymptomatic, and cultures are negative. The treatment of endocarditis and osteomyelitis may require a longer term of therapy.

Concurrent administration of the penicillinase-resistant penicillins and probenecid increases and prolongs serum penicillin levels. Probenecid decreases the apparent volume of distribution and slows the rate of excretion by competitively inhibiting renal tubular secretion of penicillin. Penicillin-probenecid therapy is generally limited to those infections where very high serum levels of penicillin are necessary.

Oral preparations of the penicillinase-resistant penicillins should not be used as initial therapy in serious, life-threatening infections (See **PRECAUTIONS**—General). Oral therapy with the penicillinase-resistant penicillins may be used to follow-up the previous use of a parenteral agent as soon as the clinical condition warrants. For intramuscular gluteal injections, care should be taken to avoid sciatic nerve injury. With intravenous administration, particularly in elderly patients, care should be taken because of the possibility of thrombophlebitis.

[See table below].

Directions For Use

For Intramuscular Use: Use Sterile Water for Injection, USP or Sodium Chloride Injection, USP. Add 1.5 ml to the 1 gram vial, 5.7 ml to the 4 gram vial, and 8.6 ml to the 6 gram vial and withdraw the entire contents. Each 1 ml will contain approximately 500 mg of Staphcillin. The solutions are stable for 24 hours at room temperature or 4 days under refrigeration.

For Direct Intravenous Use: Further dilute each 1 ml of solution, reconstituted as above, with 25 ml of Sodium Chloride Injection, USP and inject at the rate of 10 ml per minute.

For Administration by Intravenous Drip: Reconstitute as directed above (For Intramuscular Use) prior to diluting with Intravenous Solution.

[See table above].

Stability studies on Staphcillin at concentrations of 2 mg/ml, 10 mg/ml and 20 mg/ml in various intravenous solutions listed below indicate the drug will lose less than 10% activity at room temperature (70°F) during an 8-hour period.

I.V. Solution:
5% Dextrose in Normal Saline
10% D-Fructose in Water
10% D-Fructose in Normal Saline
Lactated Potassic Saline Injection
5% Plasma Hydrolysate in Water
*10% Invert Sugar in Normal Saline
10% Invert Sugar Plus 0.3% Potassium Chloride in Water
Travert 10% Electrolyte #1
Travert 10% Electrolyte #2
Travert 10% Electrolyte #3

Only those solutions listed above should be used for the intravenous infusion of Staphcillin. The concentration of the antibiotic should fall within the range specified. The drug concentration and the rate and volume of the infusion should be adjusted so that the total dose of methicillin is administered before the drug loses its stability in the solution in use.

If another agent is used in conjunction with methicillin therapy. **It should not be physically mixed** with methicillin but should be administered separately.

*At a concentration of 2 mg/ml, Staphcillin is stable for only 4 hours in this solution. Concentrations between 10 mg/ml and 30 mg/ml are stable for 8 hours.

"Piggyback" I.V. Package: This glass vial contains the labeled quantity of Staphcillin and is intended for intravenous administration. The diluent and volume are specified on the label of each package.

Discard solution after 24 hours at room temperature.

Hospital Bulk Package: This glass vial contains 10 grams Staphcillin and is designed for use in the pharmacy in preparing I.V. additives. Add 94 ml Sterile Water for Injection, USP or Sodium Chloride Injection, USP. The resulting solution will contain 100 mg methicillin sodium per ml, which is equivalent to 90 mg per ml methicillin activity. Following reconstitution in this manner, the resulting solutions are stable for 24 hours at room temperature or 7 days under refrigeration.

CAUTION: NOT TO BE DISPENSED AS A UNIT.

Supply: STAPHCILLIN (methicillin sodium for injection) buffered.
NDC 0015-7961-20—1 gram vial
NDC 0015-7964-20—4 gram vial
NDC 0015-7965-20—6 gram vial
NDC 0015-7961-28—1 gram "piggyback" vial
NDC 0015-7964-28—4 gram "piggyback" vial
NDC 0015-7102-28—10 gram Hospital Bulk Package

For information on package sizes available, refer to the current price schedule.

STABILITY PERIODS STAPHCILLIN

Concentration Mg/Ml	Sterile H₂O for Injection	Isotonic Sodium Chloride	M/6 Molar Sodium Lactate Solution	5% Dextrose in H₂O	5% Dextrose in 0.45% NaCl	10% Invert Sugar	Lactated Ringers Solution
ROOM TEMPERATURE (25°C)								
10–200	24 Hrs	24 Hrs					
2–20			8 Hrs	8 Hrs		8 Hrs	8 Hrs
10–30					24 hrs		
REFRIGERATION (4°C)								
10–200	7 Days	7 Days					
10–30			7 Days	7 Days	7 Days	7 Days	7 Days
FROZEN (−15°C)								
19–500	30 Days						
20–100		30 Days	30 Days	30 Days	30 Days	30 Days	30 Days

RECOMMENDED DOSAGES FOR STAPHCILLIN (methicillin sodium)

Drug	Adults	Infants and Children < 40 kg (88 lbs)
Methicillin Sodium	1 gram IM every 4 or 6 hours IV every 6 hours	25 mg/kg IM every 6 hours IV not recommended

TEGOPEN® ℞

[těg'ō-pěn]
Cloxacillin Sodium
CLOXACILLIN SODIUM CAPSULES
250 mg and 500 mg
CLOXACILLIN SODIUM FOR
ORAL SOLUTION
125 mg/5 ml

This is the full text of the latest Official Package Circular dated June 1984 [7935DIR-11].

Description: Tegopen (cloxacillin sodium) is an antibacterial agent of the isoxazolyl penicillin series. It is a penicillinase-resistant, acid resistant semisynthetic penicillin suitable for oral administration. Tegopen is available as an oral solution and capsules.

CLOXACILLIN SODIUM

$C_{19}H_{17}ClN_3NaO_5S \cdot H_2O$ 475.88 [CAS 7081 44 9]4-Thia-1-azabicyclo[3.2.0]heptane-2-carboxylic acid, 6 [[[3 (2-chlorophenyl)-5-methyl-4-isoxazolyl] carbonyl] amino] 3,3-dimethyl-7-oxo-, monosodium salt, monohydrate, [2 $S(2\alpha5\alpha, 6\beta)$]-.

Clinical Pharmacology:
Microbiology: Penicillinase-resistant penicillins exert a bactericidal action against penicillin-susceptible microorganisms during the state of active multiplication. All penicillins inhibit the biosynthesis of the bacterial cell wall.

The drugs in this class are highly resistant to inactivation by staphylococcal penicillinase and are active against penicillinase producing and non-penicillinase producing strains of **Staphylococcus aureus**. The penicillinase-resistant penicillins are active in vitro against a variety of other bacteria.

Susceptibility Plate Testing: Quantitative methods of susceptibility testing that require measurement of zone diameters or minimal inhibitory concentrations (MIC's) give the most precise estimates of antibiotic susceptibility. One such procedure has been recommended for use with discs to test susceptibility to this class of drugs.

Interpretations correlate diameters on the disc test with MIC values. A penicillinase-resistant class disc may be used to determine microbial susceptibility to cloxacillin, dicloxacillin, methicillin, nafcillin, and oxacillin. With this procedure, employing a 5 microgram methicillin sodium disc, a report from the laboratory of "susceptible" (zone of at least 14 mm) indicates that the infecting organism is likely to respond to therapy. A report of "resistant" (zone of less than 10 mm) indicates that the infecting organism is not likely to respond to therapy. A report of "intermediate susceptibility" (zone of 10 to 13 mm) suggests that the organism might be susceptible if high doses of the antibiotic are used, or if the infection is confined to tissues and fluids (e.g., urine), in which high antibiotic levels are attained.

In general, all staphylococci should be tested against the penicillin G disc and against the methicillin disc. Routine methods of antibiotic susceptibility testing may fail to detect strains of organisms resistant to the penicillinase-resistant penicillins. For this reason, the use of large inocula and 48-hour incubation periods may be necessary to obtain accurate susceptibility studies with these antibiotics. Bacterial strains which are resistant to one of the penicillinase-resistant penicillins should be considered resistant to all of the drugs in the class.

Pharmacokinetics: Tegopen (cloxacillin sodium) is resistant to destruction by acid. Absorption of Tegopen after oral administration is rapid but incomplete. Studies with an oral dose of 1 gram gave average serum levels at 60 minutes of 14.4 mcg/ml. At four hours, average levels were 2 mcg/ml. In one study, single oral doses of Tegopen 500 mg produced peak serum concentrations of 7.5 to 14.4 mcg/ml at 1 to 1.5 hours.

Once absorbed, Tegopen (cloxacillin sodium) binds to serum protein, mainly albumin. The degree of protein binding reported varies with the method of study and the investigator, but generally has been found to be $95.2 \pm 0.5\%$. Oral absorption of cloxacillin is delayed when the drug is administered after meals.

Tegopen, with normal doses, has insignificant concentrations in the cerebrospinal and ascitic fluids. It is found in the therapeutic concentrations in the pleural, bile and amniotic fluids. Tegopen is rapidly excreted as unchanged drug in the urine by glomerular filtration and active tubular secretion.

Indications and Usage: The penicillinase-resistant penicillins are indicated in the treatment of infections caused by penicillinase-producing staphylococci which have demonstrated susceptibility to the drugs. Cultures and susceptibility tests should be performed initially to determine the causative organisms and their sensitivity to the drug (See **Clinical Pharmacology—Susceptibility Plate Testing**).

The penicillinase-resistant penicillins may be used to initiate therapy in suspected cases of resistant staphylococcal infections prior to the availability of laboratory test results. The penicillinase-resistant penicillins should not be used in infections caused by organisms susceptible to penicillin G. If the susceptibility tests indicate that the infection is due to an organism other than a resistant staphylococcus, therapy should not be continued with a penicillinase-resistant penicillin.

Contraindications: A history of a hypersensitivity (anaphylactic) reaction to any penicillin is a contraindication.

Warnings: Serious and occasionally fatal hypersensitivity (anaphylactic shock with collapse) reactions have occurred in patients receiving penicillin. The incidence of anaphylactic shock in all penicillin-treated patients is between 0.015 and 0.04 percent. Anaphylactic shock resulting in death has occured in approximately 0.002 percent of the patients treated. Although anaphylaxis is more frequent following a parenteral administration, it has occurred in patients receiving oral penicillins.

When penicillin therapy is indicated, it should be initiated only after a comprehensive patient drug and allergy history has been obtained. If an allergic reaction occurs, the drug should be discontinued and the patient should receive supportive treatment, e.g., artificial maintenance of ventilation, pressor amines, antihistamines, and corticosteroids. Individuals with a history of penicillin hypersensitivity may also experience allergic reactions when treated with a cephalosporin.

Precautions:
General: Penicillinase-resistant penicillins should generally not be administered to patients with a history of sensitivity to any penicillin.

Penicillin should be used with caution in individuals with histories of significant allergies and/or asthma. Whenever allergic reactions occur, penicillin should be withdrawn unless, in the opinion of the physician, the condition being treated is life-threatening and amenable only to penicillin therapy.

The oral route of administration should not be relied upon in patients with severe illness, or with nausea, vomiting, gastric dilation, cardiospasm, or intestinal hypermotility. Occasionally patients will not absorb therapeutic amounts of orally administered penicillin.

The use of antibiotics may result in overgrowth of nonsusceptible organisms. If new infections due to bacteria or fungi occur, the drug should be discontinued and appropriate measures taken.

Information for the Patient: Patients receiving penicillins should be given the following information and instructions by the physician:

1. Patients should be told that penicillin is an antibacterial agent which will work with the body's natural defenses to control certain types of infections. They should be told that the drug should not be taken if they have had an allergic reaction to any form of penicillin previously, and to inform the physician of any allergies or previous allergic reactions to any drugs they may have had (see **Warnings**).

2. Patients who have previously experienced an anaphylactic reaction to penicillin should be instructed to wear a medical identification tag or bracelet.

3. Because most antibacterial drugs taken by mouth are best absorbed on an empty stomach, patients should be directed, unless circumstances warrant otherwise, to take penicillin one hour before meals or two hours after eating (See **Clinical Pharmacology—Pharmacokinetics**).

4. Patients should be told to take the entire course of therapy prescribed, even if fever and other symptoms have stopped (See **Precautions—General**).

5. If any of the following reactions occur, stop taking your prescription and notify the physician: shortness of breath, wheezing, skin rash, mouth irritation, black tongue, sore throat, nausea, vomiting, diarrhea, fever, swollen joints, or any unusual bleeding or bruising (See **Adverse Reactions**).

6. Do not take any additional medications without physician approval, including non-prescription drugs such as antacids, laxatives or vitamins.

7. Discard any liquid forms of penicillin after 7 days if stored at room temperature or after 14 days if refrigerated.

Laboratory Tests: Bacteriologic studies to determine the causative organisms and their susceptibility to the penicillinase-resistant penicillins should be performed (See **Clinical Pharmacology—Microbiology**). In the treatment of suspected staphylococcal infections, therapy should be changed to another active agent if culture tests fail to demonstrate the presence of staphylococci.

Periodic assessment of organ system function including renal, hepatic, and hematopoietic should be made during prolonged therapy with the penicillinase-resistant penicillins.

Blood cultures, white blood cell, and differential cell counts should be obtained prior to initiation of therapy and at least weekly during therapy with penicillinase-resistant penicillins.

Periodic urinalysis, blood urea nitrogen, and creatinine determinations should be performed during therapy with the penicillinase-resistant penicillins and dosage alterations should be considered if these values become elevated. If any impairment of renal function is suspected or known to exist, a reduction in the total dosage should be considered and blood levels monitored to avoid possible neurotoxic reactions (See **Dosage and Administration**).

SGOT and SGPT values should be obtained periodically during therapy to monitor for possible liver function abnormalities.

Drug Interactions: Tetracycline, a bacteriostatic antibiotic, may antagonize the bactericidal effect of penicillin and concurrent use of these drugs should be avoided.

Carcinogenesis, Mutagenesis, Impairment of Fertility: No long-term animal studies have been conducted with these drugs.

Studies on reproduction (Nafcillin) in rats and rabbits reveal no fetal or maternal abnormalities before conception and continuously through weaning (one generation).

Pregnancy Category B: Reproduction studies performed in the mouse, rat, and rabbit have revealed no evidence of impaired fertility or harm to the fetus due to the penicillinase-resistant penicillins. Human experience with the penicillins during pregnancy has not shown any positive evidence of adverse effects on the fetus. There are, however, no adequate or well-controlled studies in pregnant women showing conclusively that harmful effects of these drugs on the fetus can be excluded. Because animal reproduction studies are not always predictive of human response, this

Continued on next page

Bristol—Cont.

drug should be used during pregnancy only if clearly needed.

Nursing Mothers: Penicillins are excreted in breast milk. Caution should be exercised when penicillins are administered to a nursing woman.

Pediatric Use: Because of incompletely developed renal function in newborns penicillinase-resistant penicillins (especially methicillin) may not be completely excreted, with abnormally high blood levels resulting. Frequent blood levels are advisable in this group with dosage adjustments when necessary. All newborns treated with penicillins should be monitored closely for clinical and laboratory evidence of toxic or adverse efects (See **Dosage and Administration**).

Adverse Reactions:

Body as a Whole: The reported incidence of allergic reactions to penicillin ranges from 0.7 to 10 percent (See **Warnings**). Sensitization is usually the result of treatment but some individuals have had immediate reactions to penicillin when first treated. In such cases, it is thought that the patients may have had prior exposure to the drug via trace amounts present in milk and vaccines.

Two types of allergic reactions to penicillin are noted clinically, immediate and delayed.

Immediate reactions usually occur within 20 minutes of administration and range in severity from urticaria and pruritus to angioneurotic edema, laryngospasm, bronchospasm, hypotension, vascular collapse, and death. Such immediate anaphylactic reactions are very rare (See **Warnings**) and usually occur after parenteral therapy but have occurred in patients receiving oral therapy. Another type of immediate reaction, an accelerated reaction, may occur between 20 minutes and 48 hours after administration and may include urticaria, pruritus, and fever. Although laryngeal edema, laryngospasm, and hypotension occasionally occur, fatality is uncommon.

Delayed allergic reactions to penicillin therapy usually occur after 48 hours and sometimes as late as 2 to 4 weeks after initiation of therapy. Manifestations of this type of reaction include serum sickness-like symptoms (i.e., fever, malaise, urticaria, myalgia, arthralgia, abdominal pain) and various skin rashes. Nausea, vomiting, diarrhea, stomatitis, black or hairy tongue, and other symptoms of gastrointestinal irritation may occur, especially during oral penicillin therapy.

Nervous System Reactions: Neurotoxic reactions similar to those observed with penicillin G may occur with large intravenous doses of the penicillinase-resistant penicillins especially in patients with renal insufficiency.

Urogenital Reactions: Renal tubular damage and interstitial nephritis have been associated with the administration of methicillin sodium and infrequently with the administration of nafcillin and oxacillin. Manifestations of this reaction may include rash, fever, eosinophilia, hematuria, proteinuria, and renal insufficiency. Methicillin-induced nephropathy does not appear to be dose-related and is generally reversible upon prompt discontinuation of therapy.

Metabolic Reactions: Agranulocytosis, neutropenia, and bone marrow depression have been associated with the use of methicillin sodium, nafcillin, oxacillin, and cloxacillin. Hepatotoxicity, characterized by fever, nausea, and vomiting associated with abnormal liver function tests, mainly elevated SGOT levels, has been associated with the use of oxacillin and cloxacillin.

Dosage and Administration: The penicillinase-resistant penicillins are available for oral administration and for intramuscular and intravenous injection. The sodium salts of methicillin, oxacillin, and nafcillin may be administered parenterally and the sodium salts of cloxacillin, dicloxacillin, oxacillin, and nafcillin are available for oral use.

Bacteriologic studies to determine the causative organisms and their sensitivity to the penicillinase resistant penicillins should always be performed. Duration of therapy varies with the type and severity of infection as well as the overall condition of the patient, therefore it should be determined by the clinical and bacteriological response of the patient. In severe staphylococcal infections, therapy with penicillinase-resistant penicillins should be continued for at least 14 days. Therapy should be continued for at least 48 hours after the patient has become afebrile, asymptomatic, and cultures are negative. The treatment of endocarditis and osteomyelitis may require a longer term of therapy.

Concurrent administration of the penicillinase-resistant penicillins and probenecid increases and prolongs serum penicillin levels. Probenecid decreases the apparent volume of distribution and slows the rate of excretion by competitively inhibiting renal tubular secretion of penicillin. Penicillin-probenecid therapy is generally limited to those infections where very high serum levels of penicillin are necessary.

Oral preparations of the penicillinase-resistant penicillins should not be used as initial therapy in serious, life-threatening infections (see **Precautions—General**). Oral therapy with the penicillinase-resistant penicillins may be used to follow-up the previous use of a parenteral agent as soon as the clinical condition warrants. For intramuscular gluteal injections, care should be taken to avoid sciatic nerve injury. With intravenous administration, particularly in elderly patients, care should be taken because of the possibility of thrombophlebitis.

[See table below].

Directions For Dispensing Oral Solution: Prepare solution at the time of dispensing. For ease in preparation, add the water in two portions, shaking well after each addition. Add the total amount of water as directed on the labeling of the package being dispensed. Refrigerated, the solution is stable for 14 days.

How Supplied: Tegopen (cloxacillin sodium) for Oral Solution, 125 mg per 5 ml.
NDC 0015-7941—125 mg per 5 ml
Tegopen (cloxacillin sodium) Capsules. Each capsule contains cloxacillin sodium equivalent to 250 or 500 mg cloxacillin.
NDC 0015-7935—250 mg
NDC 0015-7496—500 mg

For information on package sizes available, refer to the current price schedule.

Shown in Product Identification Section, page 407

ULTRACEF®
[ul-trah-sef]
cefadroxil
CAPSULES, TABLETS AND ORAL SUSPENSION

This is the full text of the latest Office Package Circular dated November, 1981 [7271DIR-09].

Description: ULTRACEF (cefadroxil) is a semi-synthetic cephalosporin antibiotic intended for oral administration. It is a white to yellowish-white crystalline powder. It is soluble in water and it is acid-stable. It is chemically designated as 7-[[D-2-amino-2-(4-hydroxyphenyl) acetyl]amino]-3-methyl-8-oxo-5-thia-1-azabicyclo [4.2.0]oct-2-ene-2-carboxylic acid monohydrate. It has the following structural formula.

Clinical Pharmacology: ULTRACEF (cefadroxil) is rapidly absorbed after oral administration. Following single doses of 500 and 1000 mg, average peak serum concentrations were approximately 16 and 28 mcg/ml, respectively. Measurable levels were present 12 hours after administration. Over 90 percent of the drug is excreted unchanged in the urine within 24 hours. Peak urine concentrations are approximately 1800 mcg/ml during the period following a single 500-mg oral dose. Increases in dosage generally produce a proportionate increase in ULTRACEF urinary concentration. The urine antibiotic concentration, following a 1-gram dose, was maintained well above the MIC of susceptible urinary pathogens for 20 to 22 hours.

Microbiology: In vitro tests demonstrate that the cephalosporins are bactericidal because of their inhibition of cell-wall synthesis. ULTRACEF is active against the following organisms **in vitro**:
  Beta-hemolytic streptococci
  Staphylococci, including coagulase-positive, coagulase-negative, and penicillinase-producing strains
  Streptococcus (Diplococcus) pneumoniae
  Escherichia coli
  Proteus mirabilis
  Klebsiella species

Note: Most strains of Enterococci (**Streptococcus faecalis** and **S. faecium**) are resistant to ULTRACEF. It is not active against most strains of **Enterobacter** species. **P. Morganii**, and **P. vulgaris**. It has no activity against **Pseudomonas** species and **Acinetobacter calcoaceticus** (formerly **Mima** and **Herellea** species).

Disc Susceptibility Tests—Quantitative methods that require measurement of zone diameters give the most precise estimates of antibiotic susceptibility. One recommended procedure (CFR Section 460.1) uses a cephalosporin-class disc for testing susceptibility; interpretations correlate zone diameters of this disc test with MIC values for ULTRACEF. With this procedure, a report from the laboratory of "resistant" indicates that the infecting organism is not likely to respond to therapy. A report of "intermediate susceptibility" suggests that the organism would be susceptible if the infection is confined to the urinary tract, as ULTRACEF produces high antibiotic levels in the urine.

Indications: ULTRACEF (cefadroxil) is indicated for the treatment of the following infections when caused by susceptible strains of the designated microorganisms:

Urinary tract infections caused by **E. coli, P. mirabilis,** and **Klebsiella** species.
Skin and skin structure infections caused by staphylococci and/or streptococci.

RECOMMENDED DOSAGES FOR TEGOPEN (cloxacillin sodium) IN MILD TO MODERATE AND SEVERE INFECTIONS

DRUG	ADULTS		CHILDREN	
	Mild to Moderate	Severe	Mild to Moderate	Severe
Cloxacillin	250 mg every 6 hours	500 mg or higher every 6 hours	50 mg/kg/day[a] in equally divided doses every 6 hours	100 mg/kg/day[a] or higher in equally divided doses every 6 hours

[a] Patients weighing less than 20 Kg (44 lbs)

Pharyngitis and tonsillitis caused by Group A beta-hemolytic streptococci. (Penicillin is the usual drug of choice in the treatment and prevention of streptococcal infections, including the prophylaxis of rheumatic fever. ULTRACEF is generally effective in the eradication of streptococci from the nasopharynx; however substantial data establishing the efficacy of ULTRACEF in the subsequent prevention of rheumatic fever are not available at present.)

Note: Culture and susceptibility tests should be initiated prior to and during therapy. Renal function studies should be performed when indicated.

Contraindications: ULTRACEF (cefadroxil) is contraindicated in patients with known allergy to the cephalosporin group of antibiotics.

Warning:
IN PENICILLIN-ALLERGIC PATIENTS, CEPHALOSPORIN ANTIBIOTICS SHOULD BE USED WITH GREAT CAUTION. THERE IS CLINICAL AND LABORATORY EVIDENCE OF PARTIAL CROSS-ALLERGENICITY OF THE PENICILLINS AND THE CEPHALOSPORINS, AND THERE ARE INSTANCES OF PATIENTS WHO HAVE HAD REACTIONS TO BOTH DRUGS (INCLUDING FATAL ANAPHYLAXIS AFTER PARENTERAL USE).

Any patient who had demonstrated a history of some form of allergy, particularly to drugs, should receive antibiotics cautiously and then only when absolutely necessary. No exception should be made with regard to ULTRACEF (cefadroxil).

Pseudomembranous colitis has been reported with the use of cephalosporins (and other broad spectrum antibiotics); therefore, it is important to consider its diagnosis in patients who develop diarrhea in association with antibiotic use.

Treatment with broad spectrum antibiotics alters normal flora of the colon and may permit overgrowth of clostridia. Studies indicate a toxin produced by **Clostridium difficile** is one primary cause of antibiotic-associated colitis. Cholestyramine and colestipol resins have been shown to bind the toxin in vitro.

Mild cases of colitis may respond to drug discontinuance alone.

Moderate to severe cases should be managed with fluid, electrolyte and protein supplementation as indicated.

When the colitis is not relieved by drug discontinuance or when it is severe, oral vancomycin is the treatment of choice for antibiotic-associated pseudomembranous colitis produced by **C. difficile**. Other causes of colitis should also be considered.

Precautions: Patients should be followed carefully so that any side effects or unusual manifestations of drug idiosyncrasy may be detected. If a hypersensitivity reaction occurs, the drug should be discontinued and the patient treated with the usual agents (e.g., epinephrine or other pressor amines, antihistamines, or corticosteroids).

ULTRACEF (cefadroxil) should be used with caution in the presence of markedly impaired renal function (creatinine clearance rate of less than 50 ml/min/1.73M^2). (See DOSAGE AND ADMINISTRATION.) In patients with known or suspected renal impairment, careful clinical observation and appropriate laboratory studies should be made prior to and during therapy.

Prolonged use of ULTRACEF may result in the overgrowth of nonsusceptible organisms. Careful observation of the patient is essential. If superinfection occurs during therapy, appropriate measures should be taken.

Positive direct Coombs' tests have been reported during treatment with the cephalosporin antibiotics. In hematologic studies or in transfusion cross-matching procedures when antiglobulin tests are performed on the minor side or in Coombs' testing of newborns whose mothers have received cephalosporin antibiotics before parturition, it should be recognized that a positive Coombs' test may be due to the drug.

ULTRACEF should be prescribed with caution in individuals with a history of gastrointestinal disease, particularly colitis.

Usage in Pregnancy: Pregnancy Category B: Reproduction studies have been performed in mice and rats at doses up to 11 times the human dose and have revealed no evidence of impaired fertility or harm to the fetus due to cefadroxil. There are, however, no adequate and well controlled studies in pregnant women. Because animal reproduction studies are not always predictive of human response, this drug should be used during pregnancy only if clearly needed.

Nursing Mothers: Caution should be exercised when cefadroxil is administered to a nursing mother.

Adverse Reactions:

Gastrointestinal — Symptoms of pseudomembranous colitis can appear during antibiotic treatment. Nausea and vomiting have been reported rarely. Administration with food decreases nausea and does not decrease absorption. Diarrhea and dysuria have also occurred.

Hypersensitivity — Allergies (in the form of rash, urticaria, and angioedema) have been observed. These reactions usually subsided upon discontinuation of the drug.

Other reactions have included genital pruritus, genital moniliasis, vaginitis, and moderate transient neutropenia.

Dosage and Administration: ULTRACEF (cefadroxil) is acid stable and may be administered orally without regard to meals. Administration with food may be helpful in diminishing potential gastrointestinal complaints occasionally associated with oral cephalosporin therapy.

Adults

Urinary Tract Infections — for uncomplicated lower urinary tract infections (i.e. cystitis) the usual dosage is 1 or 2 grams per day in single (q.d.) or divided doses (b.i.d.).

For all other urinary tract infections the usual dosage is 2 grams per day in divided doses (b.i.d.).

Skin and Skin Structure Infections — For skin and skin structure infections the usual dosage is 1 gram per day in single (q.d.) or divided doses (b.i.d.).

Pharyngitis and Tonsillitis — Treatment of Group A beta-hemolytic streptococcal pharyngitis and tonsillitis — 1 gram per day in divided doses (b.i.d.) for 10 days.

Children — The recommended daily dosage for children is 30 mg/kg/day in divided doses every 12 hours as indicated:

Ultracef Oral Suspension

Child's Weight			
lbs	Kg	125 mg/5 ml	250 mg/5 ml
10	4.5	½ tsp. b.i.d.	
20	9.1	1 tsp. b.i.d.	½ tsp. b.i.d.
30	13.6	1 ½ tsp. b.i.d.	¾ tsp. b.i.d.
40	18.2	2 tsp. b.i.d.	1 tsp. b.i.d.
50	22.7	2 ½ tsp. b.i.d.	1 ¼ tsp. b.i.d.

In the treatment of beta-hemolytic, streptococcal infections, a therapeutic dosage of Ultracef should be administered for at least ten days.

In patients with renal impairment, the dosage of cefadroxil should be adjusted according to creatinine clearance rates to prevent drug accumulation. The following schedule is suggested. In adults, the initial dose is 1000 mg of ULTRACEF (cefadroxil) and the maintenance dose (based on the creatinine clearance rate [ml/min/1.73M^2]) is 500 mg at the time intervals listed below.

Creatinine Clearances	Dosage Interval
0-10 ml/min	36 hours
10-25 ml/min	24 hours
25-50 ml/min	12 hours

Patients with creatinine clearance rates over 50 ml/min may be treated as if they were patients having normal renal function.

How Supplied: ULTRACEF (cefadroxil) tablets. Each tablet contains cefadroxil monohydrate equivalent to 1 gram cefadroxil.

NDC 0015-7286—1 gram—Bottles of 24's ULTRACEF (cefadroxil) capsules. Each capsule contains cefadroxil monohydrate equivalent to 500 mg cefadroxil.

NDC 0015-7271—500 mg—Bottles of 50's and 100's ULTRACEF (cefadroxil) for oral suspension. Each 5 ml of reconstituted suspension contains cefadroxil monohydrate equivalent to 125 mg or 250 mg cefadroxil.

NDC 0015-7283—125 mg—available in 50 and 100 ml

NDC 0015-7284—250 mg—available in 50 and 100ml

Directions for mixing are included on the label. Shake well before using. Keep container tightly closed.

Store reconstituted suspension in refrigerator, discard unused portion after 14 days.

For information on package sizes available, refer to the current price schedule.

Shown in Product Identification Section, page 407

VERSAPEN®-K CAPSULES
[ver'sa-pen]
(hetacillin potassium)
VERSAPEN® ℞
(hetacillin)
Oral Suspension, Pediatric Drops

This is the full text of the latest Official Package Circular dated April 1979 [7805DIR-15].

Description: Versapen (hetacillin) is a semisynthetic antibiotic derived from the penicillin nucleus, 6-aminopenicillanic acid. **The antibiotic activity of hetacillin is provided by its rapid conversion to ampicillin.**

Actions:
Pharmacology

Oral preparations of hetacillin are acid stable and, therefore, well absorbed. Food retards absorption. In the conversion of hetacillin to ampicillin at a pH of 7.1, the hetacillin half-life is 20 minutes. Oral formulations of hetacillin and hetacillin potassium equivalent to 225 mg. and 450 mg. of ampicillin activity provide peak blood levels in the range of 1.7 to 2.1 mcg./ml. and 2.5 to 2.7 mcg./ml., respectively.

Ampicillin diffuses readily into most body tissues and fluids. However, penetration into the cerebrospinal fluid and brain occurs only when the meninges are inflamed. Ampicillin is excreted largely unchanged in the urine and its excretion can be delayed by concurrent administration of probenecid. The active form appears in the bile in higher concentrations than those found in the serum. Ampicillin is the least serum-bound of all the penicillins, averaging about 20% compared to approximately 60 to 90% for other penicillins.

Microbiology

No antibacterial activity has been demonstrated for the hetacillin moiety itself. Hetacillin, upon conversion to the active drug, ampicillin, is similar to benzyl penicillin in its bactericidal action against susceptible organisms during the stage of active multiplication.

The following bacteria have been shown in **in vitro** studies to be susceptible to ampicillin.

Gram-Positive Organisms—Hemolytic and non-hemolytic streptococci, **D. pneumoniae,** non-penicillinase-producing staphylococci, Clostridia spp., **B. anthracis, Listeria monocytogenes,** and most strains of enterococci.

Gram-Negative Organisms—H. influenzae, N. gonorrhoeae, N. meningitidis, Proteus mirabilis, and many strains of Salmonella, Shigella, and E. coli.

The drug does not resist destruction by penicillinase and hence is not effective against penicillin G-resistant staphylococci. Ampicillin Susceptibility Test Discs, 10 micrograms, should be used to estimate the **in vitro** susceptibility of bacteria to hetacillin.

Indications: Versapen is indicated in the treatment of susceptible strains of the following organisms in the diseases listed. Bacteriology studies to determine the causative organisms and their sus-

Continued on next page

Bristol—Cont.

ceptibility should be performed. Therapy may be instituted prior to obtaining results of susceptibility testing.

Group A beta-hemolytic streptococcus: Tonsillitis, pharyngitis, otitis media, skin and soft tissue infections. (Injectable benzathine penicillin is considered to be the drug of choice in treatment and prevention of streptococcal pharyngitis and in long-term prophylaxis of rheumatic fever. Versapen is effective in the eradication of streptococci from the nasopharynx; however, data establishing the efficacy of orally administered Versapen in the subsequent prevention of rheumatic fever are not available at present.)

Diplococcus pneumoniae: Broncho- and lobar pneumonia, otitis media.

Non-penicillinase-producing Staphylococcus aureus: Skin and soft tissue infections, otitis media.

Haemophilus influenzae: Bronchitis, bronchopneumonia, otitis media.

Escherichia coli: Cystitis, pyelonephritis, prostatitis/urethritis, skin and soft tissue infections.

Proteus mirabilis: Cystitis, pyelonephritis, skin and soft tissue infections.

Enterococcus (Streptococcus faecalis): Cystitis, pyelonephritis, prostatitis/urethritis.

Shigella species: Shigellosis.

Indicated surgical procedures should be performed.

Contraindications: A history of a previous hypersensitivity reaction to any of the penicillins is a contraindication.

Warnings: Serious and occasionally fatal hypersensitivity (anaphylactic) reactions have been reported in patients on penicillin therapy. Although anaphylaxis is more frequent following parenteral therapy, it has occurred in patients on oral penicillins. These reactions are more apt to occur in individuals with a history of sensitivity to multiple allergens.

There have been reports of individuals with a history of penicillin hypersensitivity reactions who experienced severe hypersensitivity reactions when treated with cephalosporins. Before therapy with a penicillin, careful inquiry should be made concerning previous hypersensitivity reactions to penicillins, cephalosporins, and other allergens.

Serious anaphylactoid reactions require immediate emergency treatment with epinephrine. Oxygen, intravenous steroids, and airway management, including intubation, should also be administered as indicated.

Usage in Pregnancy: Safety for use in pregnancy has not been established.

Precautions: The possibility of superinfection with mycotic or bacterial pathogens should be kept in mind during therapy. In such cases, discontinue the drug and substitute appropriate treatment.

As with any potent drug, periodic assessment of renal, hepatic, and hematopoietic function should be made during prolonged therapy.

This oral preparation should not be relied upon in patients with severe illness or with nausea, vomiting, gastric dilatation, cardiospasm, or intestinal hypermotility.

Adverse Reactions: As with other penicillins, it may be expected that untoward reactions will be essentially limited to sensitivity phenomena. They are more likely to occur in individuals who have previously demonstrated hypersensitivity to penicillins and in those with a history of allergy, asthma, hay fever, or urticaria.

The following adverse reactions have been reported:

Gastrointestinal: Glossitis, stomatitis, black "hairy" tongue, nausea, vomiting, enterocolitis, pseudomembranous colitis, and diarrhea. (These reactions are usually associated with oral dosage forms.)

Hypersensitivity reactions: Skin rashes and urticaria have been reported frequently. A few cases of exfoliative dermatitis and erythema multiforme have been reported. Anaphylaxis is the most serious reaction experienced and has usually been associated with the parenteral dosage form.

Note: Urticaria, other skin rashes, and serum sickness-like reactions may be controlled with antihistamines and, if necessary, systemic corticosteroids. Whenever such reactions occur, the drug should be discontinued, unless, in the opinion of the physician, the condition being treated is life threatening and amenable only to this therapy.

Liver: A moderate rise in serum glutamic oxaloacetic transaminase (SGOT) has been noted, particularly in infants, but the significance of this finding is unknown.

Hemic and Lymphatic Systems: Anemia, thrombocytopenia, thrombocytopenic purpura, eosinophilia, leukopenia, and agranulocytosis have been reported during therapy with the penicillins. These reactions are usually reversible on discontinuation of therapy and are believed to be hypersensitivity phenomena.

Other: Since infectious mononucleosis is viral in origin, hetacillin should not be used in the treatment. A high percentage of patients with mononucleosis who received ampicillin developed a skin rash.

Dosage: Infections of the upper and lower respiratory tracts; those of the skin and soft tissue; and infections of the gastrointestinal and genitourinary tracts due to susceptible organisms:

Patients weighing 88 lbs. (40 Kg.) or more: 225 to 450 mg. q.i.d., depending on the severity of the infection.

Patients weighing less than 88 lbs. (40 Kg.): 22.5 to 45 mg./Kg./day or 10 to 20 mg./lb./day, depending on the severity of the infection.

Urinary and gastrointestinal tract infections may require prolonged and intensive therapy at doses higher than those recommended above. It may be necessary to maintain therapy for several weeks and to continue bacteriologic and/or clinical follow-up for several months after cessation of therapy.

The oral drug should be administered in a fasting state to insure maximum absorption.

For very severe infections in adults or children, treatment should be initiated with parenteral ampicillin.

INFECTIONS DUE TO GROUP A BETA-HEMOLYTIC STREPTOCOCCI SHOULD BE TREATED FOR A MINIMUM OF TEN DAYS.

Directions for Dispensing Oral Suspension and Pediatric Drops

Prepare these formulations at the time of dispensing. For ease in preparation, add water to the bottle in two portions and shake well after each addition. Add the total amount of water as directed on the labeling of the package being dispensed. The reconstituted formulation is stable 14 days under refrigeration.

Supply: VERSAPEN-K (hetacillin potassium) Capsules. Hetacillin potassium equivalent to 225 or 450 mg. ampicillin per capsule.

NDC 0015-7805—225 mg.
NDC 0015-7806—450 mg.

Shown in Product Identification Section, page 407
VERSAPEN (hetacillin) for Oral Suspension. Each 5 ml. of reconstituted oral suspension contains hetacillin equivalent to 112.5 or 225 mg. ampicillin.

NDC 0015-7808—112.5 mg., 100 ml. bottle
NDC 0015-7809—225 mg., 100 ml. bottle
VERSAPEN (hetacillin) Pediatric Drops. Each ml. of reconstituted pediatric drops contains hetacillin equivalent to 112.5 mg. ampicillin.

NDC 0015-7807—112.5 mg.

For information on package sizes available, refer to the current price schedule.

Products are cross-indexed by generic and chemical names in the **YELLOW SECTION**

Bristol-Myers Oncology Division
(Bristol-Myers Company)
P.O. BOX 4755
THOMPSON ROAD
SYRACUSE, NY 13221

BiCNU®   ℞
[bĭk′ nū]
(carmustine [BCNU])

This is the full text of the latest Official Package Circular dated November 1981 [3012 DIM-07].

> **WARNING**
> BiCNU should be administered preferably by individuals experienced in antineoplastic therapy. Since delayed bone marrow toxicity is the major toxicity, complete blood counts should be monitored frequently for at least 6 weeks after a dose. Repeat doses of BiCNU should not be given more frequently than every 6 weeks. The bone marrow toxicity of BiCNU is cumulative, and therefore dosage adjustment must be considered on the basis of nadir blood counts from prior dose (see dosage adjustment table under **Dosage**).
> It is recommended that liver function, pulmonary function, and renal function tests also be monitored.

Description: BiCNU (1,3-bis (2-chloroethyl)-1-nitrosourea) is one of the nitrosoureas. It is a white lyophilized powder with a molecular weight of 214.06. It is highly soluble in alcohol and poorly soluble in water. It is also highly soluble in lipids.

Action: BiCNU alkylates DNA and RNA and has also been shown to inhibit several enzymes by carbamoylation of amino acids in proteins.

Intravenously administered BiCNU is rapidly degraded, with no intact drug detectable after 15 minutes. However, in studies with C^{-14} labeled drug, prolonged levels of the isotope were observed in the plasma and tissue, probably representing radioactive fragments of the parent compound. It is thought that the antineoplastic and toxic activities of BiCNU may be due to metabolites. Approximately 60 to 70% of a total dose is excreted in the urine in 96 hours and about 10% as respiratory CO_2. The fate of the remainder is undetermined. Because of the high lipid solubility and the relative lack of ionization at a physiological pH, BiCNU crosses the blood brain barrier quite effectively. Levels of radioactivity in the CSF are 50% or greater than those measured concurrently in plasma.

Indications: BiCNU is indicated as palliative therapy as a single agent or in established combination therapy with other approved chemotherapeutic agents in the following:

1. **Brain tumors**—glioblastoma, brainstem glioma, medulloblastoma, astrocytoma, ependymoma, and metastatic brain tumors.
2. **Multiple myeloma**—in combination with prednisone.
3. **Hodgkin's Disease**—as secondary therapy in combination with other approved drugs in patients who relapse while being treated with primary therapy, or who fail to respond to primary therapy.
4. **Non-Hodgkin's lymphomas**—as secondary therapy in combination with other approved drugs for patients who relapse while being treated with primary therapy, or who fail to respond to primary therapy.

Contraindications: BiCNU should not be given to individuals who have demonstrated a previous hypersensitivity to it.

BiCNU should not be given to individuals with decreased circulating platelets, leukocytes, or erythrocytes either from previous chemotherapy or other causes.

Warnings: Safe use in pregnancy has not been established. BiCNU is embryotoxic and teratogenic in rats and embryotoxic in rabbits at dose levels equivalent to the human dose. BiCNU also affects fertility in male rats at doses somewhat higher than the human dose.

BiCNU is carcinogenic in rats and mice, producing a marked increase in tumor incidence in doses approximating those employed clinically.

Nitrosourea therapy does have carcinogenic potential. The occurrence of acute leukemia and bone marrow dysplasias have been reported in patients following nitrosourea therapy.

Precautions: BiCNU should be administered preferably by individuals experienced in antineoplastic therapy. Since delayed bone marrow toxicity is the major toxicity, complete blood counts should be monitored frequently for at least 6 weeks after a dose. Repeat doses of BiCNU should not be given more frequently than every 6 weeks. The bone marrow toxicity of BiCNU is cumulative, and therefore dosage adjustment must be considered on the basis of nadir blood counts from prior dose (see Dosage Adjustment Table under DOSAGE).

It is recommended that liver function tests also be monitored.

Safe Use in Pregnancy has not been established. Therefore, the benefit to risk of toxicity must be carefully weighed.

See "Warnings" section for information on carcinogenesis.

Adverse Reactions:

Hematopoietic—The most frequent and most serious toxicity of BiCNU is delayed myelosuppression. It usually occurs 4 to 6 weeks after drug administration and is dose-related. Platelet nadirs occur at 4 to 5 weeks; leukocyte nadirs occur at 5 to 6 weeks post therapy. Thrombocytopenia is generally more severe than leukopenia. However both may be dose limiting toxicities. Anemia also occurs, but is generally less severe.

Gastrointestinal—Nausea and vomiting after IV administration of BiCNU are noted frequently. This toxicity appears within 2 hours of dosing, usually lasting 4 to 6 hours, and is dose-related. Prior administration of antiemetics is effective in diminishing and sometimes preventing this side effect.

Hepatic—When high doses of BiCNU have been employed, a reversible type of hepatic toxicity, manifested by increased transaminase, alkaline phosphatase and bilirubin levels, has been reported in a small percentage of patients.

Pulmonary—Pulmonary toxicity characterized by pulmonary infiltrate and/or fibrosis have been reported in some patients receiving prolonged therapy with BiCNU.

Renal—Renal abnormalities consisting of decrease in kidney size, progressive azotemia and renal failure have been reported in patients who received large cumulative doses after prolonged therapy with BiCNU and related nitrosoureas. Kidney damage has also been reported occasionally in patients receiving lower total doses.

Local—Burning at the site of injection is common but true thrombosis is rare.

Other—Rapid IV infusion of BiCNU may produce intensive flushing of the skin and suffusion of the conjunctiva within 2 hours, lasting about 4 hours. Accidental contact of reconstituted BiCNU with the skin has caused burning and hyperpigmentation of the affected areas.

Dosage: The recommended dose of BiCNU as single agent in previously untreated patients is 200 mg/m^2 intravenously every 6 weeks. This may be given as a single dose or divided into daily injections such as 100 mg/m^2 on 2 successive days. When BiCNU is used in combination with other myelosuppressive drugs or in patients in whom bone marrow reserve is depleted, the doses should be adjusted accordingly.

A repeat course of BiCNU should not be given until circulating blood elements have returned to acceptable levels (platelets above 100,000/mm^3; leukocytes above 4,000/mm^3), and this is usually in 6 weeks. Blood counts should be monitored frequently and repeat courses should not be given before 6 weeks because of delayed toxicity.

Doses subsequent to the initial dose should be adjusted according to the hematologic response of the patient to the preceding dose. The following schedule is suggested as a guide to dosage adjustment:

Nadir After Prior Dose		Percentage of Prior Dose to be Given
Leukocytes	Platelets	
> 4000	> 100,000	100%
3000-3999	75,000-99,999	100%
2000-2999	25,000-74,999	70%
< 2000	< 25,000	50%

Preparation of Intravenous Solutions: Dissolve BiCNU with 3 ml of the supplied sterile diluent and then aseptically add 27 ml of Sterile Water for Injection, U.S.P., to the alcohol solution. Each ml of the resulting solution will contain 3.3 mg of BiCNU in 10% ethanol having a pH of 5.6 to 6.0. Accidental contact of reconstituted BiCNU with the skin has caused transient hyperpigmentation of the affected areas.

Reconstitution as recommended results in a clear, colorless solution which may be further diluted with Sodium Chloride for Injection, U.S.P., or 5% Dextrose for Injection, U.S.P.

The reconstituted solution should be used intravenously only and should be administered by IV drip over a 1 to 2 hour period. Injection of BiCNU over shorter periods of time may produce intense pain and burning at the site of injection.

Important Note: The lyophilized dosage formulation contains no preservatives and is not intended as a multiple dose vial.

Stability: Unopened vials of the dry powder must be stored in a refrigerator (2°C to 8°C). The recommended storage of unopened vials prevents significant decomposition for at least 2 years.

After reconstitution as recommended, decomposition of BiCNU at room temperature is linear with time. After 3 hours, approximately 6% of the solution has decomposed and after 6 hours, approximately 8%.

Refrigeration (4°C) of the reconstituted BiCNU significantly increases the stability of the solution. After 24 hours, when protected from light, there is only 4% decomposition. Further dilution of the reconstituted solution with 500 ml. of Sodium Chloride for Injection, U.S.P., or 5% Dextrose for Injection, U.S.P., results in a solution which is stable for 48 hours when protected from light and refrigerated.

Important Note: BiCNU has a low melting point (approximately 30.5°C–32.0°C). Exposure of the drug to this temperature or above will cause the drug to liquify and appear as an oil film in the bottom of the vials. This is a sign of decomposition and vials should be discarded.

Supply: BiCNU (Carmustine [BCNU]). Each package contains a vial containing 100 mg. carmustine and a vial containing 3 ml. sterile diluent. NDC 0015-3012

For information on package sizes available, refer to the current price schedule.

BLENOXANE® ℞
[blĕ-nŏk'săn]
(sterile bleomycin sulfate)

This is the full text of the latest Official Package Circular dated October 1983 [3010 DIR-14].

WARNING

It is recommended that Blenoxane be administered under the supervision of a qualified physician experienced in the use of cancer chemotherapeutic agents.

Appropriate management of therapy and complications is possible only when adequate diagnostic and treatment facilities are readily available.

Pulmonary fibrosis is the most severe toxicity associated with Blenoxane. The most frequent presentation is pneumonitis occasionally progressing to pulmonary fibrosis. Its occurrence is higher in elderly patients and in those receiving greater than 400 units total dose, but pulmonary toxicity has been observed in young patients and those treated with low doses.

A severe idiosyncratic reaction consisting of hypotension, mental confusion, fever, chills, and wheezing has been reported in approximately 1% of lymphoma patients treated with Blenoxane.

Description: Blenoxane (sterile bleomycin sulfate) is a mixture of cytotoxic glycopeptide antibiotics isolated from a strain of *Streptomyces verticillus*. It is freely soluble in water.

Note: A unit of bleomycin is equal to the formerly used milligram activity. The term milligram activity is a misnomer and was changed to units to be more precise.

Action: Although the exact mechanism of action of Blenoxane is unknown, available evidence would seem to indicate that the main mode of action is the inhibition of DNA synthesis with some evidence of lesser inhibition of RNA and protein synthesis.

In mice, high concentrations of Blenoxane are found in the skin, lungs, kidneys, peritoneum, and lymphatics. Tumor cells of the skin and lungs have been found to have high concentrations of Blenoxane in contrast to the low concentrations found in hematopoietic tissue. The low concentrations of Blenoxane found in bone marrow may be related to high levels of Blenoxane degradative enzymes found in that tissue.

In patients with a creatinine clearance of > 35 ml. per minute, the serum or plasma terminal elimination half-life of bleomycin is approximately 115 minutes. In patients with a creatinine clearance of < 35 ml. per minute, the plasma or serum terminal elimination half-life increases exponentially as the creatinine clearance decreases. In humans, 60 to 70% of an administered dose is recovered in the urine as active bleomycin.

Indications: Blenoxane should be considered a palliative treatment. It has been shown to be useful in the management of the following neoplasms either as a single agent or in proven combinations with other approved chemotherapeutic agents:

Squamous Cell Carcinoma—Head and neck including mouth, tongue, tonsil, nasopharynx, oropharynx, sinus, palate, lip, buccal mucosa, gingiva, epiglottis, skin, larynx, penis, cervix, and vulva. The response to Blenoxane is poorer in patients with head and neck cancer previously irradiated.

Lymphomas—Hodgkin's, reticulum cell sarcoma, lymphosarcoma.

Testicular Carcinoma—Embryonal cell, choriocarcinoma, and teratocarcinoma.

Contraindications: Blenoxane is contraindicated in patients who have demonstrated a hypersensitive or an idiosyncratic reaction to it.

Warnings: Patients receiving Blenoxane must be observed carefully and frequently during and after therapy. It should be used with extreme caution in patients with significant impairment of renal function or compromised pulmonary function.

Pulmonary toxicities occur in 10% of treated patients. In approximately 1%, the nonspecific pneumonitis induced by Blenoxane progresses to pulmonary fibrosis, and death. Although this is age and dose related, the toxicity is unpredictable. Frequent roentgenograms are recommended.

Idiosyncratic reactions similar to anaphylaxis have been reported in 1% of lymphoma patients treated with Blenoxane. Since these usually occur after the first or second dose, careful monitoring is essential after these doses.

Renal or hepatic toxicity, beginning as a deterioration in renal or liver function tests, have been reported, infrequently. These toxicities may occur, however, at any time after initiation of therapy.

Usage in Pregnancy: Safe use of Blenoxane in pregnant women has not been established.

Adverse Reactions:

Pulmonary—This is potentially the most serious side effect, occurring in approximately 10% of

Continued on next page

Bristol-Myers Oncology—Cont.

treated patients. The most frequent presentation is pneumonitis occasionally progressing to pulmonary fibrosis. Approximately 1% of patients treated have died of pulmonary fibrosis. Pulmonary toxicity is both dose and age-related, being more common in patients over 70 years of age and in those receiving over 400 units total dose. This toxicity, however, is unpredictable and has been seen occasionally in young patients receiving low doses.

Because of lack of specificity of the clinical syndrome, the identification of patients with pulmonary toxicity due to Blenoxane has been extremely difficult. The earliest symptom associated with Blenoxane pulmonary toxicity is dyspnea. The earliest sign is fine rales.

Radiographically, Blenoxane-induced pneumonitis produces nonspecific patchy opacities, usually of the lower lung fields. The most common changes in pulmonary function tests are a decrease in total lung volume and a decrease in vital capacity. However, these changes are not predictive of the development of pulmonary fibrosis.

The microscopic tissue changes due to Blenoxane toxicity include bronchiolar squamous metaplasia, reactive macrophages, atypical alveolar epithelial cells, fibrinous edema, and interstitial fibrosis. The acute stage may involve capillary changes and subsequent fibrinous exudation into alveoli producing a change similar to hyaline membrane formation and progressing to a diffuse interstitial fibrosis resembling the Hamman-Rich syndrome. These microscopic findings are nonspecific, e.g., similar changes are seen in radiation pneumonitis, pneumocystic pneumonitis.

To monitor the onset of pulmonary toxicity, roentgenograms of the chest should be taken every 1 to 2 weeks. If pulmonary changes are noted, treatment should be discontinued until it can be determined if they are drug related. Recent studies have suggested that sequential measurement of the pulmonary diffusion capacity for carbon monoxide (DL_{co}) during treatment with Blenoxane may be an indicator of subclinical pulmonary toxicity. It is recommended that the DL_{co} be monitored monthly if it is to be employed to detect pulmonary toxicities, and thus the drug should be discontinued when the DL_{co} falls below 30 to 35% of the pretreatment value.

Because of bleomycin's sensitization of lung tissue, patients who have received bleomycin are at greater risk of developing pulmonary toxicity when oxygen is administered at surgery. While long exposure to very high oxygen concentrations is a known cause of lung damage, after bleomycin administration, lung damage can occur at lower concentrations than usually would be considered safe. Suggestive preventive measures are:

(1) Maintain Fl O_2 at concentrations approximating that of room air (25%) during surgery and the post operative period.
(2) Monitor carefully fluid replacement, focusing more on colloid administration rather than crystalloid.

Idiosyncratic Reactions—In approximately 1% of the lymphoma patients treated with Blenoxane an idiosyncratic reaction, similar to anaphylaxis clinically, has been reported. The reaction may be immediate or delayed for several hours, and usually occurs after the first or second dose. It consists of hypotension, mental confusion, fever, chills, and wheezing. Treatment is symptomatic including volume expansion, pressor agents, antihistamines, and corticosteroids.

Integument and Mucus Membranes—These are the most frequent side effects, being reported in approximately 50% of treated patients. These consist of erythema, rash, striae, vesiculation, hyperpigmentation, and tenderness of the skin. Hyperkeratosis, nail changes, alopecia, pruritus, and stomatitis have also been reported. It was necessary to discontinue Blenoxane therapy in 2% of treated patients because of these toxicities.

Skin toxicity is a relatively late manifestation usually developing in the 2nd and 3rd week of treatment after 150 to 200 units of Blenoxane has been administered and appears to be related to the cumulative dose.

Other—Fever, chills, and vomiting were frequently reported side effects. Anorexia and weight loss are common and may persist long after termination of this medication. Pain at tumor site, phlebitis, and other local reactions were reported infrequently.

There are isolated reports of Raynaud's phenomenon occurring in patients with testicular carcinomas treated with a combination of Blenoxane and Velban®. It is currently unknown if the cause for the Raynaud's phenomenon in these cases is the disease, Blenoxane, Velban, or a combination of any or all of these.

Dosage: Because of the possibility of an anaphylactoid reaction, lymphoma patients should be treated with 2 units or less for the first 2 doses. If no acute reaction occurs, then the regular dosage schedule may be followed.

The following dose schedule is recommended:
Squamous cell carcinoma, lymphosarcoma, reticulum cell sarcoma, testicular carcinoma—0.25 to 0.50 units/Kg. (10 to 20 units/M^2) given intravenously, intramuscularly, or subcutaneously weekly or twice weekly.

Hodgkin's Disease—0.25 to 0.50 units/Kg. (10 to 20 units/M^2) given intravenously, intramuscularly, or subcutaneously weekly or twice weekly. After a 50% response, a maintenance dose of 1 unit daily or 5 units weekly intravenously or intramuscularly should be given.

Pulmonary toxicity of Blenoxane appears to be dose-related with a striking increase when the total dose is over 400 units. Total doses over 400 units should be given with great caution.

Note: When Blenoxane is used in combination with other antineoplastic agents, pulmonary toxicities may occur at lower doses.

Improvement of Hodgkin's Disease and testicular tumors is prompt and noted within two weeks. If no improvement is seen by this time, improvement is unlikely. Squamous cell cancers respond more slowly, sometimes requiring as long as three weeks before any improvement is noted.

Administration: Blenoxane may be given by the intramuscular, intravenous, or subcutaneous routes.

Intramuscular or Subcutaneous—Dissolve the contents of a Blenoxane vial in 1 to 5 ml. of Sterile Water for Injection, U.S.P., Sodium Chloride for Injection, U.S.P., 5% Dextrose Injection, U.S.P., or Bacteriostatic Water for Injection, U.S.P.

Intravenous—Dissolve the contents of the vial in 5 ml. or more of a solution suitable for injection, e.g., physiologic saline or glucose, and administer slowly over a period of ten minutes.

Stability: The sterile powder is stable under refrigeration (2°-8°C) and should not be used after the expiration date is reached.

Blenoxane is stable for 24 hours at room temperature in Sodium Chloride or 5% Dextrose Solution.

Blenoxane is stable for 24 hours in 5% Dextrose containing heparin 100 units per ml. or 1000 units per ml.

Supply: Each vial contains 15 units of Blenoxane as sterile bleomycin sulfate.
NDC 0015-3010-20
For information on package sizes available, refer to the current price sheet.

CeeNU®
[cē'nū]
(lomustine [CCNU])

This is the full text of the latest Official Package Circular dated February 1983 [3030 DIM-10].

WARNING
CeeNU should be administered by individuals experienced in the use of antineoplastic therapy.
Since the major toxicity is delayed bone marrow suppression, blood counts should be monitored weekly for at least 6 weeks after a dose. (See "Adverse Reactions.") At the recommended dosage, courses of CeeNU should not be given more frequently than 6 weeks.
Caution should be used in administering CeeNU to patients with decreased circulating platelets, leukocytes, or erythrocytes. (See "Dosage and Administration.")
Liver function should be monitored periodically. (See "Adverse Reactions.")

Description: CeeNU 1-(2-chloroethyl)-3-cyclohexyl-1-nitrosoureal is one of a group of nitrosoureas. It is a yellow powder with the empirical formula of $C_9H_{16}ClN_3O_2$ and a molecular weight of 233.71. CeeNU is soluble in 10% ethanol (0.05 mg. per ml.) and in absolute alcohol (70 mg. per ml.). CeeNU is relatively insoluble in water (<0.05 mg. per ml.). It is relatively unionized at a physiological pH.

Action: It is generally agreed that CeeNU acts as an alkylating agent but, as with other nitrosoureas, it may also inhibit several key enzymatic processes.

CeeNU may be given orally. Following oral administration of radioactive CeeNU at doses ranging from 30 mg/M^2 to 100 mg/M^2, about half of the radioactivity given was excreted within 24 hours. The serum half-life of the drug and/or metabolites ranges from 16 hours to 2 days. Tissue levels are comparable to plasma levels at 15 minutes after intravenous administration.

Because of the high lipid solubility and the relative lack of ionization at a physiological pH, CeeNU crosses the blood brain barrier quite effectively. Levels of radioactivity in the CSF are 50% or greater than those measured concurrently in plasma.

Indications: CeeNU is indicated as palliative therapy to be employed in addition to other modalities, or in established combination therapy with other approved chemotherapeutic agents in the following:

Brain tumors—both primary and metastatic, in patients who have already received appropriate surgical and/or radiotherapeutic procedures;
Hodgkin's Disease—as a secondary therapy.

Contraindications: CeeNU should not be given to individuals who have demonstrated a previous hypersensitivity to it.

Warnings: Safe use in pregnancy has not been established. CeeNU is embryotoxic and teratogenic in rats and embryotoxic in rabbits at dose levels equivalent to the human dose. CeeNU also affects fertility in male rats at doses somewhat higher than the human dose.

CeeNU is carcinogenic in rats and mice, producing a marked increase in tumor incidence in doses approximating those employed clinically.

Nitrosourea therapy does have carcinogenic potential. The occurrence of acute leukemia and bone marrow dysplasias have been reported in patients following nitrosourea therapy.

Pulmonary Toxicity—Three cases of pulmonary infiltrates and/or fibrosis have been reported with CeeNU, to date. Onset of toxicity has occurred after an interval of six months or longer from the start of therapy with cumulative doses ranging from 600 to 1040 mg.

Related nitrosoureas are also associated with pulmonary toxicity.

Precautions: CeeNU should be administered by individuals experienced in the use of antineoplastic therapy.

Since the major toxicity is delayed bone marrow suppression blood counts should be monitored weekly for at least 6 weeks after a dose. (See "Adverse Reactions".)

At the recommended dosage, courses of CeeNU should not be given more frequently than every 6 weeks.

Caution should be used in administering CeeNU to patients with decreased circulating platelets, leukocytes, or erythrocytes. (See "Dosage and Administration".)

Liver function should be monitored periodically. (See "Adverse Reactions".)

See "Warnings" section for information on carcinogenesis.

Adverse Reactions: Nausea and vomiting may occur 3 to 6 hours after an oral dose and usually last less than 24 hours. The frequency and duration may be reduced by the use of antiemetics prior to dosing and by the administration of CeeNU to fasting patients.

Thrombocytopenia occurs at about 4 weeks after a dose of CeeNU and persists for 1 to 2 weeks.

Leukopenia occurs at about 6 weeks after a dose of CeeNU and persists for 1 to 2 weeks. Approximately 65% of patients develop white blood counts below 5000 wbc/mm^3 and 36% develop white blood counts below 3000 wbc/mm^3.

CeeNU may produce cumulative myelosuppression, manifested by more depressed indices or longer duration of suppression after repeated doses.

Other toxicities: Stomatitis, alopecia, anemia, and hepatic toxicity, manifested by transient reversible elevation of liver function tests, have been reported infrequently.

Neurological reactions such as disorientation, lethargy, ataxia, and dysarthria have been noted in some patients receiving CeeNU. However, the relationship to medication in these patients is unclear.

Renal abnormalities consisting of decrease in kidney size, progressive azotemia and renal failure have been reported in patients who received large cumulative doses after prolonged therapy with CeeNU and related nitrosoureas. Kidney damage has also been reported occasionally in patients receiving lower total doses.

Dosage and Administration: The recommended dose of CeeNU in adults and children is 130 mg/M^2 as a single dose by mouth every 6 weeks.

In individuals with compromised bone marrow function, the dose should be reduced to 100 mg/M^2 every 6 weeks.

A repeat course of CeeNU should not be given until circulating blood elements have returned to acceptable levels (platelets above 100,000/mm^3; leukocytes above 4,000/mm^3). Blood counts should be monitored weekly and repeat courses should not be given before 6 weeks because the hematologic toxicity is delayed and cumulative.

Doses subsequent to the initial dose should be adjusted according to the hematologic response of the patient to the preceding dose. The following schedule is suggested as a guide to dosage adjustment:

Nadir After Leukocytes	Prior Dose Platelets	Percentage of Prior Dose to be Given
> 4000	> 100,000	100%
3000-3999	75,000-99,999	100%
2000-2999	25,000-74,999	70%
< 2000	> 25,000	50%

When CeeNU is used in combination with myelosuppressive drugs, the doses should be adjusted accordingly.

Stability: CeeNU capsules are stable for at least 2 years when stored at room temperature in well closed containers. Avoid excessive heat (over 40°C).

Supply: The dose pack of CeeNU (Lomustine [CCNU]) Capsules contains;

NDC 0015-3032-13—2—100 mg capsules (Green/Green)

NDC 0015-3031-13—2—40 mg capsules (Purple/Green)

NDC 0015-3030-13—2—10 mg capsules (Purple/Purple)

Directions to the Pharmacist

The capsules are to provide enough medication for a single dose. The total dose prescribed by the physician can be obtained (to within 10 mg) by determining the appropriate combination of the enclosed capsule strengths.

The appropriate number of capsules of each size should be placed in a single vial to which the patient information label (gummed label provided) explaining the differences in the appearance of the capsules is affixed.

Example: A patient dose of 240 mg can be obtained by combining two 100 mg capsules and one 40 mg capsule. The remaining capsules (if any) should be discarded.

A patient information sticker, to be placed on dispensing container, is enclosed.

Also Available: Individual bottles of 20 capsules each.

NDC 0015-3032-20—20—100 mg. capsules (Green/Green)

NDC 0015-3031-20—20—40 mg. capsules (Purple/Green)

NDC 0015-3030-20—20—10 mg. capsules (Purple/Purple)

Shown in Product Identification Section, page 407

CYTOXAN®
[sī-taks'an]
(Cyclophosphamide)

Description: CYTOXAN (cyclophosphamide) is supplied as a sterile powder for parenteral use containing 45 mg sodium chloride per 100 mg cyclophosphamide (anhydrous), a sterile lyophilizate for parenteral use containing 75 mg mannitol per 100 mg cyclophosphamide (anhydrous), a tablet for oral use containing 25 mg cyclophosphamide (anhydrous), and a tablet for oral use containing 50 mg cyclophosphamide (anhydrous). Cyclophosphamide is a synthetic antineoplastic drug chemically related to the nitrogen mustards. Cyclophosphamide is a white crystalline powder with the molecular formula of $C_7H_{15}Cl_2N_2O_2P \cdot H_2O$ and a molecular weight of 279.1. The chemical name for cyclophosphamide is 2-bis[(2-chloroethyl)amino]-tetrahydro-2H-1, 3, 2-oxazaphosphorine 2-oxide monohydrate. Cyclophosphamide is soluble in water, saline, or ethanol and has the following structural formula:

Actions: Although it is classified generally as an alkylating agent, cyclophosphamide itself is not an alkylating agent or irritant. It interferes with the growth of susceptible neoplasms and, to some extent, certain normal tissues. Its mechanism of action is not known.

Cyclophosphamide is absorbed from the gastrointestinal tract and parenteral sites. It is metabolized (the details of metabolism are not fully known) and the drug and its metabolites are distributed throughout the body, including the brain. Intravenously administered, cyclophosphamide is reported to have a serum half-life of about four hours; however the drug and/or its metabolites may be detected in plasma up to seventy-two hours.

Cyclophosphamide and its metabolites are excreted by the kidneys, but the extent to which they are excreted by other routes is not known. Of three alkylating metabolites found in urine, only one (nor-nitrogen mustard) has been identified definitely.

Indications: Cyclophosphamide, though effective alone in susceptible malignancies, is more frequently used concurrently or sequentially with other antineoplastic drugs. The following malignancies are often susceptible to cyclophosphamide treatment:

1. Malignant lymphomas (Stages III and IV of the Ann Arbor staging system); Hodgkin's disease; lymphocytic lymphoma (nodular or diffuse); mixed-cell type lymphoma; histiocytic lymphoma; Burkitt's lymphoma.
2. Multiple myeloma.
3. Leukemias: chronic lymphocytic leukemia; chronic granulocytic leukemia (it is ineffective in acute blastic crisis); acute myelogenous and monocytic leukemia; acute lymphoblastic (stem-cell) leukemia in children (cyclophosphamide given during remission is effective in prolonging its duration).
4. Mycosis fungoides (advanced disease).
5. Neuroblastoma (disseminated disease).
6. Adenocarcinoma of the ovary.
7. Retinoblastoma.
8. Carcinoma of the breast.

Warnings:

Cardiac Toxicity: Although a few instances of cardiac dysfunction have been reported following use of recommended doses of cyclophosphamide, no causal relationship has been established. Cardiotoxicity has been observed in some patients receiving high doses of cyclophosphamide ranging from 120 to 270 mg/kg administered over a period of a few days, usually as a portion of an intensive antineoplastic multidrug regimen or in conjunction with transplantation procedures. In a few instances with high doses of cyclophosphamide, severe, and sometimes fatal, congestive heart failure has occurred within a few days after the first cyclophosphamide dose. Histopathologic examination has primarily shown hemorrhagic myocarditis.

No residual cardiac abnormalities as evidenced by electrocardiogram or echocardiogram appear to be present in patients surviving episodes of apparent cardiac toxicity associated with high doses of cyclophosphamide.

Cyclophosphamide has been reported to potentiate doxorubicin-induced cardiotoxicity.

Adrenalectomy: Since cyclophosphamide has been reported to be more toxic in adrenalectomized dogs, adjustment of the doses of both replacement steroids and cyclophosphamide may be necessary for the adrenalectomized patient.

Other:

Barbiturates: The rate of metabolism and the leukopenic activity of cyclophosphamide reportedly are increased by chronic administration of high doses of phenobarbital.

Combined Drug Actions: The physician should be alert for possible combined drug actions, desirable or undesirable, involving cyclophosphamide even though cyclophosphamide has been used successfully concurrently with other drugs, including other cytotoxic drugs.

Wound Healing: Cyclophosphamide may interfere with normal wound healing.

Usage in Pregnancy: Cyclophosphamide can be teratogenic or cause fetal resorption in experimental animals. It should not be used in pregnancy, particularly in early pregnancy, unless in the judgment of the physician the potential benefits outweigh the possible risks. Cyclophosphamide is excreted in breast milk and breast-feeding should be terminated prior to institution of cyclophosphamide therapy.

Patients, male or female, capable of conception ordinarily should be advised of the mutagenic potential of cyclophosphamide. Adequate methods of contraception appear desirable for such patients receiving cyclophosphamide.

Precautions: Cyclophosphamide should be given cautiously to patients wih any of the following conditions.

1. Leukopenia
2. Thrombocytopenia
3. Tumor cell infiltration of bone marrow
4. Previous X-ray therapy
5. Previous therapy with other cytotoxic agents
6. Impaired hepatic function
7. Impaired renal function

Because cyclophosphamide may exert a suppressive action on immune mechanisms, the interruption or modification of dosage should be considered for patients who develop bacterial, fungal or viral infections. This is especially true for patients receiving concomitant steroid therapy and perhaps those with a recent history of steroid therapy, since infections in some of these patients have been fatal. Varicella zoster infections appear to be particularly dangerous under these circumstances.

Adverse Reactions:

Secondary Neoplasia. Secondary malignancies have developed in some patients treated with cy-

Continued on next page

Bristol-Myers Oncology—Cont.

cyclophosphamide alone or in association with other antineoplastic drugs and/or modalities. These malignancies most frequently have been urinary bladder, myeloproliferative, and lymphoproliferative malignancies. Secondary malignancies most frequently have developed in the cyclophosphamide-treated patients with primary myeloproliferative and lymphoproliferative malignancies and primary nonmalignant diseases in which immune processes are believed to be involved pathologically. In some cases, the secondary malignancy was detected up to several years after cyclophosphamide treatment was discontinued. The secondary urinary bladder malignancies generally have occurred in patients who previously developed hemorrhagic cystitis (see Genitourinary under Adverse Reactions). Although no cause-effect relationship has been established between cyclophosphamide and the development of malignancy in humans, the possibility of secondary malignancy, based on available data, should be considered in any benefit-to-risk assessment for the use of the drug.

Hematopoietic. Leukopenia is an expected effect and ordinarily is used as a guide to therapy. Thrombocytopenia or anemia may occur in a few patients. These effects are almost always reversible when therapy is interrupted.

Gastrointestinal. Anorexia, nausea, or vomiting are common and related to dose as well as individual susceptibility. There are isolated reports of hemorrhagic colitis, oral mucosal ulceration and jaundice occurring during therapy.

Genitourinary. Sterile hemorrhagic cystitis can result from the administration of cyclophosphamide. **This can be severe, even fatal, and is probably due to metabolites in the urine.** Nonhemorrhagic cystitis and/or fibrosis of the bladder also have been reported to result from cyclophosphamide administration. Atypical epithelial cells may be found in the urinary sediment. **Ample fluid intake and frequent voiding help to prevent the development of cystitis,** but when it occurs it is ordinarily necessary to interrupt cyclophosphamide therapy. Hematuria usually resolves spontaneously within a few days after cyclophosphamide therapy is discontinued, but may persist for several months. In severe cases replacement of blood loss may be required. The application of electrocautery to telangiectatic areas of the bladder and diversion of urine flow have been successful methods used in treatment of protracted cases. Cryosurgery has also been used. (See also Secondary Neoplasia under Adverse Reactions.) Nephrotoxicity, including hemorrhage and clot formation in the renal pelvis, has been reported.

Gonadal suppression, resulting in amenorrhea or azoospermia, has been reported in a number of patients treated with cyclophosphamide and appears to be related to dosage and duration of therapy. This side effect, possibly irreversible, should be anticipated in patients treated with cyclophosphamide. It is not known to what extent cyclophosphamide may affect prepubertal gonads. Fibrosis of the ovary following cyclophosphamide therapy has been reported also.

Integument. It is ordinarily advisable to inform patients in advance of possible alopecia, a frequent complication of cyclophosphamide therapy. Regrowth of hair can be expected although occasionally the new hair may be of a different color or texture. The skin and fingernails may become darker during therapy. Non-specific dermatitis has been reported to occur with cyclophosphamide.

Pulmonary: Interstitial pulmonary fibrosis has been reported in patients receiving high doses of cyclophosphamide over a prolonged period.

Dosage and Administration: Chemotherapy with cyclophosphamide, as with other drugs used in cancer chemotherapy, is potentially hazardous and fatal complications can occur. It is recommended that it be administered only by physicians aware of the associated risks. Therapy may be aimed at either induction or maintenance of remission.

Induction Therapy: The usual initial intravenous loading dose for patients with no hematologic deficiency is 40–50 mg/kg. This total initial intravenous loading dose usually is given in divided doses over a period of two to five days.

Patients with any previous treatment that may have compromised the functional capacity of the bone marrow, such as X ray or cytotoxic drugs, and patients with tumor infiltration of the bone marrow may require reduction of the initial loading dose by $\frac{1}{3}$ to $\frac{1}{2}$.

A marked leukopenia is usually associated with the above doses, but recovery usually begins after 7–10 days. The white blood cell count should be monitored closely during induction therapy.

If initial therapy is given orally, a dose of 1–5 mg/kg/day can be administered depending on tolerance by the patient.

Maintenance Therapy: It is frequently necessary to maintain chemotherapy in order to suppress or retard neoplastic growth. A variety of schedules has been used:
(1) 1–5 mg/kg p.o. daily
(2) 10–15 mg/kg i.v. every 7–10 days
(3) 3–5 mg/kg i.v. twice weekly

Unless the disease is unusually sensitive to cyclophosphamide, it is advisable to give the largest maintenance dose that can be reasonably tolerated by the patient. The total leukocyte count is a good objective guide for regulating the maintenance dose. Ordinarily a leukopenia of 3000–4000 cells/cu. mm. can be maintained without undue risk of serious infection or other complications.

Preparation and Handling of Solutions: Parenteral drug products should be inspected visually for particulate matter and discoloration prior to administration, whenever solution and container permit.

CYTOXAN for Injection and Lyophilized CYTOXAN for Injection should be prepared for parenteral use by adding Bacteriostatic Water for Injection, U.S.P. (paraben preserved only) or Sterile Water for Injection, U.S.P. to the vial and shaking to dissolve. Use the quantity of diluent shown below to reconstitute the product.

Dosage Strength	Quantity of Diluent
100 mg	5 ml
200 mg	10 ml
500 mg	25 ml
1.0 g	50 ml
2.0 g	100 ml

Solutions of CYTOXAN for Injection and Lyophilized CYTOXAN for Injection may be injected intravenously, intramuscularly, intraperitoneally, or intrapleurally or they may be infused intravenously in the following:
Dextrose Injection, U.S.P. (5% dextrose)
Dextrose and Sodium Chloride Injection, U.S.P. (5% dextrose and 0.9% sodium chloride)
5% Dextrose and Ringer's Injection
Lactated Ringer's Injection, U.S.P.
Sodium Chloride Injection, U.S.P. (0.45% sodium chloride)
Sodium Lactate Injection, U.S.P. ($\frac{1}{6}$ molar sodium lactate)

Reconstituted CYTOXAN for Injection and Lyophilized CYTOXAN for Injection are chemically and physically stable for 24 hours at room temperature or for six days in the refrigerator; they do not contain any antibacterial agent and thus care must be taken to assure the sterility of prepared solutions.

CYTOXAN for Injection and Lyophilized CYTOXAN prepared by adding Bacteriostatic Water for Injection U.S.P. (paraben preserved only) should be used within 24 hours if stored at room temperature or within 6 days if stored under refrigeration.

If CYTOXAN for Injection or Lyophilized CYTOXAN for Injection is not prepared by adding Bacteriostatic Water for Injection U.S.P. (paraben preserved only), it is recommended that the solution be used promptly (preferably within six hours). The osmolarities of solutions of CYTOXAN for Injection, Lyophilized CYTOXAN for Injection, and normal saline are compared in the following table:

	mOsm/L
Lyophilized CYTOXAN for Injection	172
CYTOXAN for Injection	380
Normal saline	287

Lyophilized CYTOXAN for Injection is slightly hypotonic with respect to normal saline.

Extemporaneous liquid preparations of CYTOXAN for oral administration may be prepared by dissolving CYTOXAN for Injection or Lyophilized CYTOXAN for Injection in Aromatic Elixir, N.F. Such preparations should be stored under refrigeration and used within 14 days.

Overdosage: No specific antidote for CYTOXAN products is known. Management of overdosage would include general supportive measures to sustain the patient through any period of toxicity that might occur.

How Supplied: CYTOXAN for Injection contains 45 mg of sodium chloride per 100 mg of cyclophosphamide (anhydrous).

CYTOXAN® for Injection (cyclophosphamide with sodium chloride).
 NDC 0087-0500-41 100 mg vials, carton of 12, case of 1 carton
 NDC 0087-0501-41 200 mg vials, carton of 12, case of 1 carton
 NDC 0087-0502-41 500 mg vials, carton of 12, case of 1 carton
 NDC 0087-0505-41 1.0 g vials, carton of 6
 NDC 0087-0506-41 2.0 g vials, carton of 6

Lyophilized CYTOXAN for Injection contains 75 mg of mannitol per 100 mg of cyclophosphamide (anhydrous) and is supplied in vials for single dose use.

Lyophilized CYTOXAN® (cyclophosphamide) for Injection.
 NDC 0087-0547-41 500 mg vials, carton of 12, case of 1 carton

CYTOXAN Tablets, 25 mg, and CYTOXAN Tablets, 50 mg, are white tablets with blue flecks containing 25 mg and 50 mg cyclophosphamide (anhydrous), respectively.

CYTOXAN® (cyclophosphamide) tablets.
 NDC 0087-0503-01 50 mg, bottles of 100
 NDC 0087-0503-02 50 mg, bottles of 1000
 NDC 0087-0503-03 50 mg, Unit Dose cartons of 100
 NDC 0087-0504-01 25 mg, bottles of 100

Storage at or below 77°F (25°C) is recommended; this product will withstand brief exposure to temperatures up to 86°F (30°C) but should be protected from temperatures above 86°F (30°C).

Shown in Product Identification Section, page 407

LYSODREN® ℞
[li'sō-drĕn"]
(mitotane)

This is the full text of the latest Official Package Circular dated August 1978 [3080DIM-01].

Treatment should be instituted in the hospital until a stable dosage regimen is achieved. Lysodren should be temporarily discontinued immediately following shock or severe trauma since adrenal suppression is its prime action. Exogenous steroids should also be administered in such circumstances, since the depressed adrenal may not immediately start to secrete steroids.

LYSODREN (mitotane) is an oral chemotherapeutic agent.

Description: LYSODREN (mitotane) is best known by its trivial name, o,p'-DDD, and is chemically, 1.1 dichloro-2 (o-chlorophenyl)-2- (p-chlorophenyl) ethane.

LYSODREN is a white granular solid composed of clear colorless crystals.

LYSODREN is tasteless and has a slight pleasant aromatic odor.

Action: LYSODREN (mitotane) can best be described as an adrenal cytotoxic agent, although it can cause adrenal inhibition, apparently without cellular destruction. Its biochemical mechanism of action is unknown. Data are available to suggest that the drug modifies the peripheral metabolism of steroids as well as directly suppressing the adrenal cortex. The administration of LYSODREN alters the extra-adrenal metabolism of cortisol in man, leading to a reduction in measurable 17-hydroxy corticosteroids, even though plasma levels of corticosteroids do not fall. The drug apparently causes increased formation of 6-β-hydroxy cortisol.

Indications: LYSODREN is indicated only in the treatment of inoperable adrenal cortical carcinoma of both functional and non-functional types.

Contraindications: The only contraindication for LYSODREN is known hypersensitivity to the drug.

Warnings: Lysodren should be temporarily discontinued immediately following shock or severe trauma, since adrenal suppression is its prime action. Exogenous steroids should also be administered in such circumstances, since the depressed adrenal may not immediately start to secrete steroids.

LYSODREN should be administered with care to patients with liver disease other than metastatic lesions from the adrenal cortex, since the metabolism of LYSODREN may be interfered with and the drug may accumulate.

All possible tumor tissue should be surgically removed from large metastatic masses before LYSODREN administration is instituted. This is necessary to minimize the possibility of infarction and hemorrhage in the tumor due to a rapid positive effect of the drug.

Long-term continuous administration of high doses of LYSODREN may lead to brain damage and impairment of function. Behavioral and neurological assessments should be made at regular intervals when continuous LYSODREN treatment exceeds two years.

Uses in Pregnancy and Lactation: The safety of LYSODREN in pregnancy or lactation has not been established. Treatment of women who are, or who may become pregnant, should be undertaken only after consideration of the benefits versus the possibility of harm to mother and child.

Precautions: Adrenal insufficiency may develop in patients treated with LYSODREN, and adrenal steroid replacement should be considered for these patients.

Since sedation, lethargy, vertigo, and other CNS side effects can occur, ambulatory patients should be cautioned about driving, operating machinery, and other hazardous pursuits requiring mental and physical alertness.

Adverse Reactions: A very high percentage of patients treated with LYSODREN have shown at least one type of side effect. The main types of adverse reactions consist of the following:
1. Gastrointestinal disturbances, which consisted of anorexia, nausea or vomiting, and in some cases diarrhea, occurred in about 80% of the patients.
2. Central nervous system side effects occurred in 40% of the patients. These consisted primarily of depression as manifested by lethargy and somnolence (25%), and dizziness or vertigo (15%).
3. Skin toxicity was observed in about 15% of the cases. In some instances, however, this side effect subsided while the patients were maintained on drug.

Infrequently occurring side effects involve the eye (visual blurring, diplopia, lens opacity, toxic retinopathy); the genitourinary system (hematuria, hemorrhagic cystitis, and albuminuria); cardiovascular system (hypertension, orthostatic hypotension, and flushing); and some miscellaneous complaints including generalized aching, hyperpyrexia, and lowered PBI.

Dosage and Administration: The recommended treatment schedule is to start the patient at 9-10 grams of LYSODREN per day in divided doses, either q.i.d. or t.i.d. If severe side effects appear, the dose should be reduced until the maximum tolerated dose is achieved. If the patient can tolerate higher doses and improved clinical response appears possible, the dose should be increased until adverse reactions interfere. Experience has shown that the maximum tolerated dose (MTD) will vary from 2-16 grams per day, but has usually been 8-10 grams per day. The highest doses used in the studies to date were 18-19 grams per day.

Treatment should be instituted in the hospital until a stable dosage regimen is achieved.

Treatment should be continued as long as clinical benefits are observed. Maintenance of clinical status or slowing of growth of metastatic lesions can be considered clinical benefits if they can clearly be shown to have occurred.

If no clinical benefits are observed after three months at the maximum tolerated dose, the case may be considered a clinical failure. However, 10% of the patients who showed a measurable response required more than three months at the MTD. Early diagnosis and prompt institution of treatment improve the probability of a positive clinical response.

How Supplied: LYSODREN is available as a 500 mg. scored tablet in bottles of 100. NDC 15-3080-60—500 mg. tablets

Animal Studies: Dogs were used for much of the experimental work with LYSODREN (1). Doses as low as 4 mg/kg/day may produce some effects upon the canine adrenals. However, most of the data suggest that toxicity occurs between 80-200 mg/kg/day, primarily as a result of LYSODREN'S effect upon the adrenals. At doses of 100 mg/kg/day and higher of LYSODREN, deaths occurred in some of the dogs after two to four weeks of administration.

The primary action of LYSODREN is upon the adrenal cortex. The toxicity observed in animals appears to result from suppression of the activity of the adrenal cortex. The production of adrenal steroids has been shown to be reduced in most of the studies.

A toxicity study was conducted in rats at doses as high as 300 mg/kg/day for 28 days. There were no deaths nor was there any evidence of organ changes in these animals. In this study even the adrenal cortex showed no evidence of change, indicating that the rodent appears to be highly resistant to LYSODREN.

In both dogs and rats, there was a dose-related rise in alkaline phosphatase. In dogs, there were signs of histological changes in the liver at the high doses (50-100 mg/kg/day).

A dose of 300 mg/kg/day administered to guinea pigs resulted in death in one of three animals and reduction in cortisol levels. Death was probably due to adrenal insufficiency (2).

Metabolic Studies of LYSODREN in Man: One study (3) with adrenal carcinoma patients indicated that about 40% of oral LYSODREN was absorbed, and approximately 10% was recovered in the urine as a water-soluble metabolite. A small amount was excreted in the bile and the balance was apparently stored in the tissues. When administered parenterally, approximately 25% of the dose was found in the urine as a water-soluble metabolite.

Blood levels were determined during and following administration of LYSODREN. Both unchanged drug and metabolite were measured. The levels in patients receiving doses from 5-15 grams per day varied from 7-90 micrograms/ml of unchanged LYSODREN and 29-54 micrograms/ml of the metabolite. These studies indicated no relationship between blood levels and therapeutic and/or toxic effects.

Following discontinuation of the drug, LYSODREN blood levels fell, but persisted for several weeks. In most patients blood levels became undetectable after six to nine weeks. In one patient who had received a total of 1900 grams of LYSODREN, high blood levels were found ten weeks after stopping the drug. Autopsy data have provided evidence that LYSODREN is found in most tissues of the body. Fat tissues were the primary site of storage. In one patient a very large number of tissues were examined and the drug was found in essentially every tissue. LYSODREN appears to be converted, in part, to a water-soluble metabolite. This material has not been characterized, but is only found in the urine and blood of patients receiving LYSODREN. Examination of bile was made and found to contain no unchanged LYSODREN. There was metabolite in the bile, and this would indicate that biliary excretion is a significant route of removal of this metabolite from the body.

Clinical Studies: Hutter and Kayhoe (4) reported on the clinical features and the results of LYSODREN treatment of 138 patients with adrenal cortical carcinoma, and compared their findings with 48 treated patients previously reported in the literature. Subsequent to their report, 115 patients given drug were studied. There is no evidence of a cure as a consequence of the administration of LYSODREN. A number of patients have been treated intermittently, treatment being restarted when severe symptoms reappeared. Patients often do not respond after the third or fourth such course. Experience accumulated to date suggests that continuous treatment with the maximum possible dosage of LYSODREN would be the best approach.

A substantial percentage of the patients treated showed signs of adrenal insufficiency. It therefore appears necessary to watch for and institute steroid replacement in those patients. It has been shown that the metabolism of exogenous steroids is modified and consequently somewhat higher doses than just replacement therapy may be required.

There was significant reduction in tumor mass following LYSODREN administration in about 50%, and a significant reduction in elevated steroid excretion in about 80% of the evaluable patients studied to date (4). Clinical effectiveness can be shown by reduction in tumor mass, reduction in pain, weakness or anorexia, and reduction of steroid symptoms.

Bibliography:
1. a) Nelson, A A, Woodward, G: *Archives of Pathology*, 48:387, 1949.
   b) Nichols, D J: Studies on an Adrenal Cortical Inhibitor, in *The Adrenal Cortex*, Scranton, Pa., Harper and Row, 1961, p 83.
2. Kupfer, D, *et al: Life Sciences*, 3:959, 1964.
3. Moy, R H: *J Lab Clin Med*, 58:296, 1961.
4. Hutter, A M, Kahoe, D E: *Am J Med*, 41:572, 581, 1966.

Shown in Product Identification Section, page 407

MEGACE® tablets   ℞
[měg'ace]
(megestrol acetate)
U.S. Patent No. 3,356,573

This is the full text of the latest Official Package Circular dated July 1984 (P-1450-03)

THE USE OF PROGESTATIONAL AGENTS DURING THE FIRST FOUR MONTHS OF PREGNANCY IS NOT RECOMMENDED

Progestational agents have been used beginning with the first trimester of pregnancy in an attempt to prevent habitual abortion or treat threatened abortion. There is no adequate evidence that such use is effective and there is evidence of potential harm to the fetus when such drugs are given during the first four months of pregnancy.

Furthermore, in the vast majority of women, the cause of abortion is a defective ovum, which progestational agents could not be expected to influence. In addition, the use of progestational agents, with their uterine-relaxant properties, in patients with fertilized defective ova may cause a delay in spontaneous abortion. Therefore, the use of such drugs during the first four months of pregnancy is not recommended.

Several reports suggest an association between intrauterine exposure to female sex hormones and congenital anomalies, including congenital heart defects and limb reduction defects.[1-5] One study[4] estimated a 4.7-fold

Continued on next page

Bristol-Myers Oncology—Cont.

increased risk of limb reduction defects in infants exposed *in utero* to sex hormones (oral contraceptives, hormone withdrawal tests for pregnancy, or attempted treatment for threatened abortion).

Some of these exposures were very short and involved only a few days of treatment. The data suggest that the risk of limb reduction defects in exposed fetuses is somewhat less than 1 to 1,000.

If the patient is exposed to Megace during the first four months of pregnancy or if she becomes pregnant while taking this drug, she should be apprised of the potential risks to the fetus.

Description: Megestrol acetate is a white, crystalline solid chemically described as 17α-acetoxy-6-methylpregna-4, 6-diene-3, 20-dione. Its molecular weight is 384.5. The empirical formula is $C_{24}H_{32}O_4$ and the chemical structure is:

MEGESTROL ACETATE*
*U.S. Patent No. 3,356,573

Actions: While the precise mechanism by which Megace (megestrol acetate) produces its antineoplastic effects against endometrial carcinoma is unknown at the present time, an antiluteinizing effect mediated via the pituitary has been postulated. There is also evidence to suggest a local effect as a result of the marked changes brought about by the direct instillation of progestational agents into the endometrial cavity. Likewise, the antineoplastic action of Megace (megestrol acetate) on carcinoma of the breast is unclear.

Indications: Megace (megestrol acetate) is indicated for the palliative treatment of advanced carcinoma of the breast or endometrium (i.e., recurrent, inoperable, or metastatic disease). It should not be used in lieu of currently accepted procedures such as surgery, radiation, or chemotherapy.

Contraindications: As a diagnostic test for pregnancy.

Warnings

Administration for up to 7 years of megestrol acetate to female dogs is associated with an increased incidence of both benign and malignant tumors of the breast. Comparable studies in rats and ongoing studies in monkeys are not associated with an increased incidence of tumors. The relationship of the dog tumors to humans is unknown but should be considered in assessing the benefit-to-risk ratio when prescribing Megace and in surveillance of patients on therapy.

The use of Megace (megestrol acetate) in other types of neoplastic disease is not recommended.

Precautions: There are no specific precautions identified for the use of Megace (megestrol acetate) when used as recommended. Close, customary surveillance is indicated for any patient being treated for recurrent or metastatic cancer. Use with caution in patients with a history of thrombophlebitis.

Adverse Reactions: No untoward effects have been ascribed to Megace (megestrol acetate) therapy. Reports have been received of patients developing carpal tunnel syndrome, deep vein thrombophlebitis and alopecia while taking megestrol acetate.

Overdosage: No serious side effects have resulted from studies involving Megace (megestrol acetate) administered in dosages as high as 800 mg/day.

Dosage and Administration:
Breast cancer: 160 mg/day (40 q.i.d.)
Endometrial carcinoma: 40—320 mg/day in divided doses.
At least two months of continuous treatment is considered an adequate period for determining the efficacy of Megace (megestrol acetate).

How Supplied: Megace® is available as light blue, scored tablets containing 20 mg or 40 mg megestrol acetate.
NDC 0087-0595-01, Bottles of 100 20 mg tablet
NDC 0087-0596-41, Bottles of 100 40 mg tablet
NDC 0087-0596-45, Bottles of 500 40 mg tablet
6505-01-070-1493 (Bottles of 100) (Defense)

References:
1. Gal I, Kirman B and Stern J: "Hormonal Pregnancy Tests and Congenital Malformation," Nature 216:83, 1967.
2. Levy EP, Cohen A and Fraser FC: "Hormone Treatment During Pregnancy and Congenital Heart Defects," Lancet 1:611, 1973.
3. Nora J and Nora A: "Birth Defects and Oral Contraceptives," Lancet 1:941, 1973.
4. Janerich DT, Piper JM and Glebatis DM: "Oral Contraceptives and Congenital Limb-Reduction Defects," N Eng J Med, 291:697, 1974.
5. Heinonen OP, Slone D, Monson RR, Hook EB and Shapiro S: "Cardiovascular Birth Defects and Antenatal Exposure to Female Sex Hormones," N Eng J Med, 296:67, 1977.

Shown in Product Identification Section, page 407

MEXATE®
[měk'sāt]
(methotrexate sodium)
FOR INJECTION

This is the full text of the latest Official Package Circular dated July 1984 [3050 DIM-08].

WARNINGS

MEXATE (METHOTREXATE SODIUM) SHOULD BE ADMINISTERED UNDER THE SUPERVISION OF A QUALIFIED PHYSICIAN EXPERIENCED IN THE USE OF CANCER CHEMOTHERAPEUTIC AGENTS.

BECAUSE OF THE POSSIBILITY OF FATAL OR SEVERE TOXIC REACTIONS THE PATIENT SHOULD BE FULLY INFORMED BY THE PHYSICIAN OF THE RISKS INVOLVED AND SHOULD BE UNDER HIS CONSTANT SUPERVISION.

DEATHS HAVE BEEN REPORTED WITH THE USE OF METHOTREXATE IN THE TREATMENT OF PSORIASIS. IN THE TREATMENT OF PSORIASIS METHOTREXATE SHOULD BE RESTRICTED TO SEVERE, RECALCITRANT, DISABLING PSORIASIS WHICH IS NOT ADEQUATELY RESPONSIVE TO OTHER FORMS OF THERAPY, BUT ONLY WHEN THE DIAGNOSIS HAS BEEN ESTABLISHED AS BY BIOPSY AND/OR AFTER DERMATOLOGIC CONSULTATION.

1. Bone marrow suppression, notably thrombocytopenia and leukopenia, which may contribute to bleeding and overwhelming infections in an already compromised patient, is the most common and severe of the toxic effects of Mexate (see "WARNINGS" and "ADVERSE REACTIONS").

2. Methotrexate may be hepatotoxic, particularly at high dosage or with prolonged therapy. Liver atrophy, necrosis, cirrhosis, fatty changes, and periportal fibrosis have been reported. Since changes may occur without previous signs of gastrointestinal or hematologic toxicity, it is imperative that hepatic function be determined prior to initiation of treatment and monitored regularly throughout therapy. Special caution is indicated in the presence of preexisting liver damage or impaired hepatic function. Concomitant use of other drugs with hepatotoxic potential (including alcohol) should be avoided.

3. Methotrexate has caused fetal death and/or congenital anomalies, therefore, it is not recommended in women of childbearing potential unless there is appropriate medical evidence that the benefits can be expected to outweigh the considered risks. Pregnant psoriatic patients should not receive methotrexate.

4. Impaired renal function is usually a contraindication.

5. Diarrhea and ulcerative stomatitis are frequent toxic effects and require interruption of therapy; otherwise hemorrhagic enteritis and death from intestinal perforation may occur.

METHOTREXATE HAS BEEN ADMINISTERED IN VERY HIGH DOSAGE FOLLOWED BY LEUCOVORIN RESCUE IN EXPERIMENTAL TREATMENT OF CERTAIN NEOPLASTIC DISEASES. THIS PROCEDURE IS INVESTIGATIONAL AND HAZARDOUS.

Description: Mexate (methotrexate sodium) is an antimetabolite used in the treatment of certain neoplastic diseases. It is the sodium salt of 4-amino-10-methylfolic acid. The structural formula is:

Mexate for Injection is available in 20, 50, 100, and 250 mg single dose vials of lyophilized sterile powder, containing no preservatives, to be administered parenterally.

Each 20 mg vial contains methotrexate, 20 mg, prepared as the sodium salt; sodium hydroxide to adjust pH to about 8.5.

Each 50 mg vial contains methotrexate, 50 mg, prepared as the sodium salt; sodium hydroxide to adjust pH to about 8.5.

Each 100 mg vial contains methotrexate, 100 mg, prepared as the sodium salt; sodium hydroxide to adjust pH to about 8.5.

Each 250 mg vial contains methotrexate, 250 mg, prepared as the sodium salt; sodium hydroxide to adjust the pH to about 8.5.

Clinical Pharmacology: Methotrexate competitively inhibits dihydrofolate reductase, the enzyme responsible for converting folic acid to reduced folate cofactors. Reduced folates are necessary for the metabolic transfer of one-carbon units in a variety of biochemical reactions. Those reactions which are of special importance in cellular proliferation are the biosynthesis of thymidylic acid, the nucleotide specific to DNA, and the biosynthesis of inosinic acid, the precursor of purines necessary for both DNA and RNA synthesis. In human synthesis, methotrexate appears to inhibit DNA synthesis to a greater extent than RNA synthesis, suggesting that inhibition of thymidylate synthesis is the most important mechanism of methotrexate cytotoxicity. Hence the drug is highly cell cycle dependent, acting primarily during DNA synthesis (S-phase). Actively proliferating tissues such as malignant cells, bone marrow cells, and cells of the dermal epithelium, buccal and intestinal mucosa, are in general more sensitive to this effect of methotrexate.

After parenteral injection, peak serum levels are seen in about 30 to 60 minutes. Approximately one-half the absorbed methotrexate is reversibly bound to serum protein but exchanges with body fluids easily and diffuses into the body tissue cells. The terminal half-life is of the order of 24 hours. Approximately 41% of an intravenously administered dose is excreted unchanged in the urine within 6 hours after administration, 90% within 24 hours, and 95% within 30 hours. One to 2% is excreted in the stool as the parent compound and metabolites. The methotrexate metabolites account for less than 10% of the total dose administered when methotrexate is given intravenously. Repeated daily doses result in more sustained serum levels and some retention of methotrexate over each 24-hour period which may result in accumulation of the drug within the tissues. The liver cells appear to retain certain amounts of the drug for prolonged periods even after a single therapeutic dose. Methotrexate is retained in the presence of impaired renal function and may increase rapidly in the serum and in the tissue cells under such conditions.

Distribution of methotrexate into interstitial fluid spaces, such as cerebrospinal fluid, pleural and peritoneal cavities, occurs slowly and with characteristics that resemble a passive transport system. If these "third spaces" are pathologically increased as in ascites and pleural effusion, they may act as reservoirs and prolong the presence of methotrexate in the plasma compartment. Methotrexate does not penetrate the blood cerebrospinal fluid barrier in therapeutic amounts when given parenterally. High concentrations of the drug when needed may be attained by direct intrathecal administration.

Indications and Usage:
Antineoplastic Chemotherapy:
Trophoblastic Tumors:
Mexate is indicated for the treatment of gestational choriocarcinoma, and hydatidiform mole.
Leukemia:
Mexate is indicated for the treatment of acute lymphocytic leukemia and in the treatment and prophylaxis of meningeal leukemia. Greatest effect has been observed in the treatment of acute lymphoblastic (stem-cell) leukemias in children. In combination with other anticancer drugs or suitable agents Mexate may be used for induction of remission, but it is most commonly used, as described in the literature, in the maintenance of induced remission.
Lymphomas:
Mexate is effective in the treatment of the advanced stages (III and IV) of non-Hodgkin's lymphoma, particularly in children and in advanced cases of mycosis fungoides.
Psoriasis Chemotherapy (See "BOX WARNINGS"):
Because of high risk attending its use, Mexate is only indicated in the symptomatic control of severe, recalcitrant, disabling psoriasis which is not adequately responsive to other forms of therapy, but only when the diagnosis has been established, as by biopsy and/or after dermatologic consultation.
Contraindications: Patients with known hypersensitivity to methotrexate; pregnant psoriatic patient; psoriatic patients with severe renal or hepatic disorders; and psoriatic patients with preexisting blood dyscrasias, such as bone marrow hypoplasia, leukopenia, thrombocytopenia or anemia, should not receive Mexate.
Warnings: See "BOX WARNINGS".
Precautions:
General:
Mexate has a high potential for serious toxicity which is usually dose-related. The physician should be familiar with the various characteristics of the drug and its established clinical usage. Patients undergoing therapy should be subject to appropriate supervision so that signs or symptoms of possible adverse reactions may be detected and evaluated with minimal delay. Pretreatment and periodic hematologic studies are essential to the use of Mexate in chemotherapy because of its common effect of hematopoietic suppression. This may occur abruptly and on apparent safe dosage, and any profound drop in blood-cell count indicates immediate stopping of the drug. In patients with malignant disease who have preexisting bone marrow aplasia, leukopenia, thrombocytopenia or anemia, other than that caused by bone marrow involvement with tumor, the drug should be used with caution, if at all.

Mexate is excreted principally by the kidneys. Its use in the presence of impaired renal function may result in accumulation of toxic amounts or even additional renal damage. The patient's renal status should be determined prior to and during methotrexate therapy and proper caution exercised should significant renal impairment be disclosed. Drug dosage should be reduced or discontinued until renal function is improved or restored. Mexate should be used with extreme caution in the presence of infection, peptic ulcer, ulcerative colitis, debility and in extreme youth or old age.

If profound leukopenia occurs during therapy, bacterial infection may occur or become a threat. Cessation of the drug and appropriate antibiotic therapy is usually indicated. In severe bone marrow depression, blood or platelet transfusions may be necessary.

Since it is reported that methotrexate may have an immunosuppressive action, this factor must be taken into consideration in evaluating the use of the drug where immune responses in a patient may be important or essential.

In all instances where the use of Mexate is considered for chemotherapy, the physician must evaluate the need and usefulness of the drug against the risk for adverse reactions. Most such adverse reactions are reversible if detected early. If severe reactions occur, the drug should be reduced in dosage or discontinued and appropriate corrective measures should be taken according to the clinical judgment of the physician. Reinstitution of Mexate therapy should be carried out with caution, with adequate consideration of further need for the drug and alertness as to possible recurrence of toxicity.

Laboratory Tests:
In general, the following laboratory tests are recommended as part of essential clinical evaluation and appropriate monitoring of patients chosen for or receiving methotrexate therapy; complete hemogram, urinalysis, renal function tests, and liver function tests. A chest x-ray is also recommended to determine the presence of pleural effusion. The tests should be performed prior to therapy, at appropriate periods during therapy and after termination of therapy.

Drug Interactions:
Methotrexate is bound in part to serum albumin after absorption and toxicity may be increased because of displacement by certain drugs such as salicylates, sulfonamides, phenytoin, phenylbutazone, and some antibacterials such as tetracycline, chloramphenicol. These drugs, especially salicylates, phenylbutazone, and sulfonamides, whether antibacterial, hypoglycemic or diuretic, should not be given concurrently until the significance of these findings is established.

Weak acids like salicylates and probenecid may compete with methotrexate for renal tubular secretion. As a result, concomitant administration with these agents may prolong the serum half-life of methotrexate.

Carcinogenesis, Mutagenesis, Impairment of Fertility:
Like most other anticancer agents, Mexate might have a carcinogenic potential (see "BOX WARNINGS")

Pregnancy:
Pregnancy "Category D"—Methotrexate has caused fetal death and/or congenital anomalies and is therefore not recommended in women of childbearing potential unless there is appropriate medical evidence that the benefits to the mother can be expected to outweigh the considered risks to the fetus. Pregnant psoriatic patients should not receive Mexate (see "BOX WARNINGS").

Nursing Mothers:
Because of the potential for serious adverse reactions in nursing infants from Mexate, a decision should be made whether to discontinue nursing or to discontinue the drug, taking into account the importance of the drug to the mother.

Adverse Reactions: The most common adverse reactions include ulcerative stomatitis, leukopenia, nausea and abdominal distress. Others reported are malaise, undue fatigue, chills and fever, dizziness and decreased resistance to infection. In general, the incidence and severity of side effects are considered to be dose-related. Adverse reactions as reported for the various systems are as follows:

Blood: bone marrow depression, leukopenia, thrombocytopenia, anemia, hypogammaglobulinemia, hemorrhage from various sites, septicemia.

Alimentary System: gingivitis, pharyngitis, stomatitis, anorexia, vomiting, diarrhea, hematemesis, melena, gastrointestinal ulceration and bleeding, enteritis, hepatic toxicity resulting in acute liver atrophy, necrosis, fatty metamorphosis, periportal fibrosis, or hepatic cirrhosis.

Urogenital System: renal failure, azotemia, cystitis, hematuria; defective oogenesis or spermatogenesis, transient oligospermia, menstrual dysfunction; infertility, abortion, fetal defect, severe nephropathy.

Skin: erythematous rashes, pruritus, urticaria, photosensitivity, depigmentation, alopecia, ecchymosis, telangiectasia, acne, furunculosis. Lesions of psoriasis may be aggravated by concomitant exposure to ultraviolet radiation.

Central Nervous System: headaches, drowsiness, blurred vision. Aphasia, hemiparesis, paresis and convulsions have also occurred following administration of methotrexate.

There have been reports of leucoencephalopathy following intravenous administration of methotrexate to patients who have had craniospinal irradiation.

After the intrathecal use of methotrexate, the central nervous system toxicity which may occur can be classified as follows:

(1) chemical arachnoiditis manifested by such symptoms as headache, back pain, vomiting, nuchal rigidity, fever, and cerebrospinal fluid pleocytosis mimicking bacterial meningitis.

(2) motor dysfunction of the brain or the spinal cord. Paraplegia, quadraplegia, cerebellar dysfunction, cranial nerve palsies and seizures may occur a few weeks after starting treatment.

(3) leucoencephalopathy manifested by confusion, dysarthria, irritability, somnolence, ataxia, dementia, and occasionally major convulsions and coma. The risk for this toxicity seems to be proportional to the amount of methotrexate given.

Other reactions related to or attributed to the use of methotrexate, such as interstitial pneumonitis; metabolic changes precipitating diabetes; osteoporotic effects, abnormal tissue cell changes, and even sudden death, have been reported.

Overdosage: Leucovorin Calcium Injection, USP (citrovorum factor) is a potent agent for neutralizing the immediate toxic effects of Mexate on the hematopoietic system. Where large doses or overdoses are given, Leucovorin Calcium Injection, USP may be administered by intravenous infusion in doses up to 75 mg within 12 hours, followed by 12 mg intramuscularly every six hours for four doses. Where average doses of Mexate appear to have an adverse effect, 2 to 4 ml (6 to 12 mg) of Leucovorin Calcium Injection, USP may be given intramuscularly every six hours for four doses. In general, where overdosage is suspected, the dose of Leucovorin Calcium Injection, USP should be equal to or higher than the offending dose of Mexate and should best be administered within the first hour. Use of Leucovorin Calcium Injection, USP after an hour delay is much less effective.

Dosage and Administration:
Antineoplastic Chemotherapy
Mexate for injection may be given by intramuscular, intravenous, intraarterial or intrathecal route. Initial treatment is usually undertaken with the patient under hospital care.

Choriocarcinoma and similar trophoblastic diseases: Mexate is administered intramuscularly in doses of 15 to 30 mg daily for a five-day course. Such courses are usually repeated three to five times as required, with rest periods of one or more weeks interposed between courses, to allow any manifesting toxic symptoms to subside. The effectiveness of therapy is ordinarily evaluated by serum 24-hour quantitative analysis of beta-chorionic gonadotropin hormone (β-HCG) which should

Continued on next page

Bristol-Myers Oncology—Cont.

return to normal, usually after the 3rd or 4th course. The complete resolution of measurable lesions usually occurs within 4 to 6 weeks. One to two courses of Mexate after normalization of β-HCG is usually recommended. Before each course of the drug, careful clinical assessment is essential. Cyclic combination therapy of Mexate with other antitumor drugs has been reported as being useful.

Since hydatidiform mole may precede choriocarcinoma, prophylactic chemotherapy with Mexate has been recommended. Mexate is administered in these disease states in doses similar to those recommended for choriocarcinoma.

Leukemia: Acute lymphatic (lymphoblastic) leukemia in children and young adolescents is the most responsive to present-day chemotherapy. In young adults and older patients, clinical remission is more difficult to obtain and early relapse is more common. In chronic lymphatic leukemia, the prognosis for adequate response is less encouraging. Mexate alone or in combination with other agents appears to be the drug of choice for securing maintenance of drug-induced remissions. When remission is achieved and supportive care has been produced general clinical improvement, maintenance therapy may be initiated, as follows: Mexate is administered two times weekly intramuscularly in doses of 30 mg/M^2. It has also been given in doses of 2.5 mg/kg intravenously every 14 days. If and when relapse does occur, reinduction of remission can usually be obtained by repeating the initial induction regimen. A variety of dosage schedules exist for both induction and maintenance of remission with various combinations of alkylating agents plant products and antimetabolites. The physician should be familiar with the new advances in antileukemic therapy.

Meningeal leukemia: Patients with leukemia are subject to leukemic invasion of the central nervous system. This may manifest characteristic signs or symptoms or may remain silent and be diagnosed only by examination of the cerebrospinal fluid (CSF) which contains leukemic cells in such cases. Therefore, the CSF should be examined in all pediatric acute lymphoblastic leukemia patients. Since penetration of Mexate from the blood to the cerebrospinal fluid is minimal, the drug is administered intrathecally for adequate therapy. It is now common practice because of the noted increased frequency of meningeal leukemia to administer Mexate intrathecally as prophylaxis in all cases of lymphocytic leukemia.

For intrathecal injection, the sodium salt of Mexate is administered in solution as a 12 mg/M^2 dose. The solution is made in a strength of up to 2.5 mg/ml with an appropriate, sterile, preservative-free medium such as 0.9% Sodium Chloride Injection, USP.

For the treatment of meningeal leukemia, Mexate is given at intervals of two to five days. Mexate is administered until the leukemia cell count of the cerebrospinal fluid disappears. At this point one additional dose is advisable. For prophylaxis against meningeal leukemia, the dosage is the same as for treatment except for the intervals of administration. On this subject, it is advisable for the physician to consult the medical literature. Large doses may cause convulsions. Untoward side effects may occur with any given intrathecal injection and are commonly neurological in character. Mexate given by intrathecal route appears in significant concentrations in the systemic circulation and may cause systemic Mexate toxicity. Therefore concurrent systemic antileukemic therapy should be appropriately adjusted. Focal leukemic involvement of the central nervous system may not respond to intrathecal chemotherapy and is best treated with radiotherapy.

Lymphomas: In stage III and IV non-Hodgkins lymphomas, Mexate is commonly given concomitantly with other antitumor agents. Treatment usually consists of several courses of the drug interposed with seven to ten day rest periods. Mexate may be used in combination therapy in doses of 0.625 to 2.5 mg/Kg per day.

In mycosis fungoides therapy with Mexate appears to produce clinical remissions in about one-half of the cases treated. Dosage is usually daily by mouth for weeks or months. Drug dose levels and their subsequent adjustment are guided by patient response and hematologic monitoring. Mexate has also been given intramuscularly in doses of 50 mg once weekly or 25 mg two times weekly.

Psoriasis Chemotherapy:
The patient should be fully informed of the risks involved and should be under the constant supervision of a physician.

Assessment of renal function, liver function, and blood elements should be made by history, physical examination, and laboratory tests (such as CBC, urinalysis, serum creatinine, liver function studies, and liver biopsy if indicated) before beginning Mexate, periodically during Mexate therapy, and before reinstituting Mexate therapy after a rest period. Appropriate steps should be taken to avoid conception during and for at least 8 weeks following Mexate therapy.

There are 3 commonly used general types of dosage schedules:
1. weekly oral or parenteral intermittent large doses
2. divided dose intermittent oral schedule over a 36-hour period
3. daily oral with a rest period

All schedules should be continually tailored to the individual patient. Dose schedules cited below pertain to an average 70 Kg adult.
Recommended starting dose schedule:
Weekly single IM or IV dose schedule:
10 to 25 mg per week until adequate response is achieved. With this dosage schedule, 50 mg per week should ordinarily not be exceeded.

Special Note: Available data suggest that schedule 3 (daily oral dose with a rest period) may carry an increased risk of serious liver pathology. Dosages may be gradually adjusted to achieve optimal clinical response, but not to exceed the maximum stated in the schedule.

Once optimal clinical response has been achieved, the dosage schedule should be reduced to the lowest possible amount of drug and to the longest possible rest period. The use of Mexate may permit the return to conventional topical therapy, which should be encouraged.

Caution:
Pharmacist: Because of its potential to cause severe toxicity, Mexate therapy requires close supervision of the patient by the physician.
Parenteral drug products should be inspected visually for particulate matter and discoloration prior to administration, whenever solution and container permit.

Directions for Use: Intramuscular or intravenous administration: reconstitute with 2 to 10 ml of Sterile Water for Injection, USP, 0.9% Sodium Chloride Injection, USP, or Bacteriostatic Water for Injection, USP with Parabens or Benzyl Alcohol.

Intrathecal administration: reconstitute immediately prior to use with an appropriate sterile, preservative-free medium such as 0.9% Sodium Chloride Injection, USP. The concentration for intrathecal injection should be 1 mg to 2.5 mg ml.

As with other potentially toxic compounds, caution should be exercised in handling the powder and preparing the solution of methotrexate. Skin reactions associated with accidental exposure to Mexate may occur. The use of gloves is recommended. If Mexate powder or solution contact skin or mucosa, immediately wash the skin or mucosa thoroughly with soap and water.

Stability
Mexate for Injection is stable for four weeks at room temperature (25°C) at concentrations of 2 to 125 mg/ml in Sterile Water for Injection, USP, 0.9% Sodium Chloride Injection, USP or Bacteriostatic Water for Injection, USP with Parabens or Benzyl Alcohol. These solutions are stable for three months under refrigeration (4°C) or frozen (−15°C). For intrathecal use, reconstitute immediately prior to use.

How Supplied: Mexate (methotrexate sodium) for Injection.
NDC 0015-3050-20—20 mg vial
NDC 0015-3051-20—50 mg vial
NDC 0015-3052-20—100 mg vial
NDC 0015-3053-20—250 mg vial

MUTAMYCIN® ℞
[mū″-tĕ-mī′-sĭn]
(mitomycin for injection)

This is the full text of the latest Official Package Circular dated October 1983 [3001DIM-17].

WARNING

Mutamycin should be administered under the supervision of a qualified physician experienced in the use of cancer chemotherapeutic agents. Appropriate management of therapy and complications is possible only when adequate diagnostic and treatment facilities are readily available.

Bone marrow suppression, notably thrombocytopenia and leukopenia, which may contribute to overwhelming infections in an already compromised patient, is the most common and severe of the toxic effects of Mutamycin (see "Warnings" and "Adverse Reactions" sections).

Description: Mutamycin (also known as mitomycin and/or mitomycin-C) is an antibiotic isolated from the broth of **Streptomyces caespitosus** which has been shown to have antitumor activity. The compound is heat stable, has a high melting point, and is freely soluble in organic solvents.

Action: Mutamycin selectively inhibits the synthesis of deoxyribonucleic acid (DNA). The guanine and cytosine content correlates with the degree of Mutamycin-induced cross-linking. At high concentrations of the drug, cellular RNA and protein synthesis are also suppressed.

In humans, Mutamycin is rapidly cleared from the serum after intravenous administration. Time required to reduce the serum concentration by 50% after a 30 mg. bolus injection is 17 minutes. After injection of 30 mg., 20 mg., or 10 mg. I.V., the maximal serum concentrations were 2.4 mcg./ml., 1.7 mcg./ml., and 0.52 mcg./ml., respectively. Clearance is effected primarily by metabolism in the liver, but metabolism occurs in other tissues as well. The rate of clearance is inversely proportional to the maximal serum concentration because, it is thought, of saturation of the degradative pathways.

Approximately 10% of a dose of Mutamycin is excreted unchanged in the urine. Since metabolic pathways are saturated at relatively low doses, the percent of a dose excreted in urine increases with increasing dose. In children, excretion of intravenously administered Mutamycin is similar.

Animal Toxicology—Mutamycin has been found to be carcinogenic in rats and mice. At doses approximating the recommended clinical dose in man, it produces a greater than 100 percent increase in tumor incidence in male Sprague-Dawley rats, and a greater than 50 percent increase in tumor incidence in female Swiss mice.

Indications: Mutamycin is not recommended as single-agent, primary therapy. It has been shown to be useful in the therapy of disseminated adenocarcinoma of the stomach or pancreas in proven combinations with other approved chemotherapeutic agents and as palliative treatment when other modalities have failed. Mutamycin is not recommended to replace appropriate surgery and/or radiotherapy.

Contraindications: Mutamycin is contraindicated in patients who have demonstrated a hypersensitive or idiosyncratic reaction to it in the past. Mutamycin is contraindicated in patients with thrombocytopenia, coagulation disorder, or an increase in bleeding tendency due to other causes.

Warnings: Patients being treated with Mutamycin must be observed carefully and frequently during and after therapy.

The use of Mutamycin results in a high incidence of bone marrow suppression, particularly thrombocytopenia and leukopenia. Therefore, the following studies should be obtained repeatedly during therapy and for at least 8 weeks following therapy: platelet count, white blood cell count, differential, and hemoglobin. The occurrence of a platelet count below 150,000/MM^3 or a WBC below 4,000/MM^3 or a progressive decline in either is an indication for interruption of therapy.

Patients should be advised of the potential toxicity of this drug, particularly bone marrow suppression. Deaths have been reported due to septicemia as a result of leukopenia due to the drug.

Patients receiving Mutamycin should be observed for evidence of renal toxicity. Mutamycin should not be given to patients with a serum creatinine greater than 1.7 mg. percent.

Usage in Pregnancy—Safe use of Mutamycin in pregnant women has not been established. Teratological changes have been noted in animal studies. The effect of Mutamycin on fertility is unknown.

Adverse Reactions: Bone Marrow Toxicity— This was the most common and most serious toxicity, occurring in 605 of 937 patients (64.4%). Thrombocytopenia and/or leukopenia may occur anytime within 8 weeks after onset of therapy with an average time of 4 weeks. Recovery after cessation of therapy was within 10 weeks. About 25% of the leukopenic or thrombocytopenic episodes did not recover. Mutamycin produces cumulative myelosuppression.

Integument and Mucus Membrane Toxicity— This has occurred in approximately 4% of patients treated with Mutamycin. Delayed erythema and/or ulceration have occured either at or distant from the injection site weeks to months after Mutamycin. However, no obvious evidence of extravasation was observed at the time of administration. Skin grafting has been required in some cases. Cellulitis at the injection site has been reported and is occasionally severe. Stomatitis and alopecia also occurred frequently.

Renal Toxicity—2% of 1,281 patients demonstrated a statistically significant rise in creatinine. There appeared to be no correlation between total dose administered or duration of therapy and the degree of renal impairment.

Pulmonary Toxicity—This has occurred infrequently but can be severe. Dyspnea with a nonproductive cough and radiographic evidence of pulmonary infiltrates may be indicative of Mutamycin-induced pulmonary toxicity. If other etiologies are eliminated, Mutamycin therapy should be discontinued. Steroids have been employed as treatment of this toxicity, but the therapeutic value has not been determined.

Microangiopathic Hemolytic Anemia—A syndrome consisting of microangiopathic hemolytic anemia, thrombocytopenia, renal failure and hypertension have been reported in patients receiving Mutamycin. Most of these patients received long-term therapy (6 to 12 months) with Mutamycin in combination with fluorouracil; however, some patients received Mutamycin in combination with other drugs or were treated for less than 6 months.

Acute Side Effects Due to Mutamycin were fever, anorexia, nausea, and vomiting. They occurred in about 14% of 1,281 patients.

Other Undesirable Side Effects that have been reported during Mutamycin therapy have been headache, blurring of vision, confusion, drowsiness, syncope, fatigue, edema, thrombophlebitis, hematemesis, diarrhea, and pain. These did not appear to be dose related and were not unequivocally drug related. They may have been due to the primary or metastatic disease processes.

Dosage and Administration: Mutamycin should be given intravenously only, using care to avoid extravasation of the compound. If extravasation occurs, cellulitis, ulceration, and slough may result.

Each vial contains either mitomycin 5 mg. and mannitol 10 mg. or mitomycin 20 mg. and mannitol 40 mg. To administer, add Sterile Water for Injection, 10 ml. or 40 ml. respectively. Shake to dissolve. If product does not dissolve immediately, allow to stand at room temperature until solution is obtained.

After full hematological recovery (see guide to dosage adjustment) from any previous chemotherapy, the following dosage schedule may be used at 6 to 8 week intervals.

20 mg./M.^{2} intravenously as a single dose via a functioning intravenous catheter.

Because of cumulative myelosuppression, patients should be fully reevaluated after each course of Mutamycin, and the dose reduced if the patient has experienced any toxicities. Doses greater than 20 mg./M.^{2} have not been shown to be more effective, and are more toxic than lower doses.

The following schedule is suggested as a guide to dosage adjustment:

Nadir After Prior Dose		Percentage of Prior Dose to be Given
Leukocytes	Platelets	
>4000	>100,000	100%
3000–3999	75,000–99,999	100%
2000–2999	25,000–74,999	70%
<2000	<25,000	50%

No repeat dosage should be given until leukocyte count has returned to 3000 and platelet count to 75,000.

When Mutamycin is used in combination with other myelosuppressive agents, the doses should be adjusted accordingly. If the disease continues to progress after two courses of Mutamycin, the drug should be stopped since chances of response are minimal.

Stability:
1. **Unreconstituted** Mutamycin is stable at room temperature. Avoid excessive heat (over 40°C).
2. **Reconstituted** with Sterile Water for Injection to a concentration of 0.5 mg. per ml., Mutamycin is stable for 14 days refrigerated or 7 days at room temperature.
3. **Diluted** in various IV fluids at room temperature, to a concentration of 20 to 40 micrograms per ml:

IV Fluid	Stability
5% Dextrose Injection	3 hours
0.9% Sodium Chloride Injection	12 hours
Sodium Lactate Injection	24 hours

4. **The combination** of Mutamycin (5 mg. to 15 mg.) and heparin (1,000 units to 10,000 units) in 30 ml. of 0.9% Sodium Chloride Injection is stable for 48 hours at room temperature.

Supply:
Mutamycin (mitomycin) for Injection.
NDC 0015-3001-20—Each vial contains 5 mg. mitomycin.
NDC 0015-3002-20—Each vial contains 20 mg. mitomycin.

PLATINOL® ℞
[plā' tĭ-nŏl″]
(cisplatin for injection)

This is the full text of the latest Official Package Circular dated June 1983 [3070DIM-19].

WARNING
Platinol (cisplatin) should be administered under the supervision of a qualified physician experienced in the use of cancer chemotherapeutic agents. Appropriate management of therapy and complications is possible only when adequate diagnostic and treatment facilities are readily available.
Cumulative renal toxicity associated with Platinol is severe. Other major dose-related toxicities are myelosuppression and nausea and vomiting.
Ototoxicity, which may be more pronounced in children, and is manifested by tinnitus, and/or loss of high frequency hearing and occasionally deafness, is significant.
Anaphylactic-like reactions to Platinol have been reported. Facial edema, bronchoconstriction, tachycardia, and hypotension may occur within minutes of Platinol administration. Epinephrine, corticosteroids, and antihistamines have been effectively employed to alleviate symptoms (see "Warnings" and "Adverse Reactions" sections).

Description: Platinol (cisplatin) (cis-diamminedichloroplatinum) is a heavy metal complex containing a central atom of platinum surrounded by two chloride atoms and two ammonia molecules in the cis position. It is a white lyophilized powder with the molecular formula Pt $Cl_2H_6N_2$, and a molecular weight of 300.1. It is soluble in water or saline at 1 mg/ml and in dimethylformamide at 24 mg/ml. It has a melting point of 207°C.

Action: Platinol has biochemical properties similar to that of bifunctional alkylating agents producing interstrand and intrastrand crosslinks in DNA. It is apparently cell-cycle non-specific. Following a single I.V. dose, Platinol concentrates in liver, kidneys, and large and small intestines in animals and humans. Platinol apparently has poor penetration into the CNS.

Plasma levels of radioactivity decay in a biphasic manner after an I.V. bolus dose of radioactive Platinol to patients. The initial plasma half-life is 25 to 49 minutes, and the post-distribution plasma half-life is 58 to 73 hours. During the post-distribution phase, greater than 90% of the radioactivity in the blood is protein bound. Platinol is excreted primarily in the urine. However, urinary excretion is incomplete with only 27 to 43% of the radioactivity being excreted within the first 5 days post-dose in human beings. There are insufficient data to determine whether biliary or intestinal excretion occurs.

Indications: Platinol is indicated as palliative therapy to be employed as follows:

Metastatic Testicular Tumors—in established combination therapy with other approved chemotherapeutic agents in patients with metastatic testicular tumors who have already received appropriate surgical and/or radiotherapeutic procedures. An established combination therapy consists of Platinol, Blenoxane (Bleomycin Sulfate) and Velban (Vinblastine Sulfate).

Metastatic Ovarian Tumors—in established combination therapy with other approved chemotherapeutic agents in patients with metastatic ovarian tumors who have already received appropriate surgical and/or radiotherapeutic procedures. An established combination consists of Platinol and Adriamycin (Doxorubicin Hydrochloride). Platinol, as a single agent, is indicated as secondary therapy in patients with metastatic ovarian tumors refractory to standard chemotherapy who have not previously received Platinol therapy.

Advanced Bladder Cancer—Platinol is indicated as a single agent for patients with transitional cell bladder cancer which is no longer amenable to local treatments such as surgery and/or radiotherapy.

Contraindications: Platinol is contraindicated in patients with preexisting renal impairment. Platinol should not be employed in myelosuppressed patients, or patients with hearing impairment.

Platinol is contraindicated in patients with a history of allergic reactions to Platinol or other platinum-containing compounds.

Warnings: Platinol produces cumulative nephrotoxicity which is potentiated by aminoglycoside antibiotics. The serum creatinine, BUN, creatinine clearance and magnesium, potassium and calcium levels should be measured prior to initiating therapy, and prior to each subsequent course. At the recommended dosage, Platinol should not be given more frequently than once every 3 to 4 weeks (see "Adverse Reactions").

Anaphylactic-like reactions to Platinol have been

Continued on next page

Memorandum

Bristol-Myers Oncology—Cont.

reported. These reactions have occurred within minutes of administration to patients with prior exposure to Platinol, and have been alleviated by administration of epinephrine, corticosteroids and antihistamines.

Since ototoxicity of Platinol is cumulative, audiometric testing should be performed prior to initiating therapy and prior to each subsequent dose of drug (see "Adverse Reactions").

Safe use in human pregnancy has not been established. Platinol is mutagenic in bacteria and produces chromosome aberrations in animal cells in tissue culture. In mice Platinol is teratogenic and embryotoxic.

Platinol has not been studied for its carcinogenic potential but compounds with similar mechanisms of action and mutagenicity have been reported to be carcinogenic.

Precautions: Peripheral blood counts should be monitored weekly. Liver function should be monitored periodically. Neurologic examination should also be performed regularly (see "Adverse Reactions").

Adverse Reactions:
Nephrotoxicity
Dose-related and cumulative renal insufficiency is the major dose-limiting toxicity of Platinol. Renal toxicity has been noted in 28 to 36% of patients treated with a single dose of 50 mg/M^2. It is first noted during the second week after a dose and is manifested by elevations in BUN and creatinine, serum uric acid and/or a decrease in creatinine clearance. **Renal toxicity becomes more prolonged and severe with repeated courses of the drug. Renal function must return to normal before another dose of Platinol can be given.**

Impairment of renal function has been associated with renal tubular damage. The administration of Platinol using a 6- to 8-hour infusion with intravenous hydration, and mannitol has been used to reduce nephrotoxicity. However, renal toxicity still can occur after utilization of these procedures.

Ototoxicity
Ototoxicity has been observed in up to 31% of patients treated with a single dose of Platinol 50 mg/M^2, and is manifested by tinnitus and/or hearing loss in the high frequency range (4,000 to 8,000 Hz). Decreased ability to hear normal conversational tones may occur occasionally. Ototoxic effects may be more severe in children receiving Platinol. Hearing loss can be unilateral or bilateral and tends to become more frequent and severe with repeated doses. It is unclear whether Platinol-induced ototoxicity is reversible. Careful monitoring of audiometry should be performed prior to initiation of therapy and prior to subsequent doses of Platinol.

Hematologic
Myelosuppression occurs in 25 to 30% of patients treated with Platinol. The nadirs in circulating platelets and leukocytes occur between days 18 to 23 (range 7.5 to 45) with most patients recovering by day 39 (range 13 to 62). Leukopenia and thrombocytopenia are more pronounced at higher doses (>50 mg/M^2). Anemia (decrease of >2 g hemoglobin/100 ml) occurs at approximately the same frequency and with the same timing as leukopenia and thrombocytopenia.

Gastrointestinal
Marked nausea and vomiting occur in almost all patients treated with Platinol, and are occasionally so severe that the drug must be discontinued. Nausea and vomiting usually begin within one to four hours after treatment and last up to 24 hours. Various degrees of nausea and anorexia may persist for up to one week after treatment.

Other Toxicities:
Serum Electrolyte Disturbances
Hypomagnesemia, hypocalcemia, hypokalemia and hypophosphatemia have been reported to occur in patients treated with Platinol and are probably related to renal tubular damage. Tetany has occasionally been reported in those patients with hypocalcemia and hypomagnesemia. Generally, normal serum electrolyte levels are restored by

administering supplemental electrolytes and discontinuing Platinol.

Hyperuricemia

Hyperuricemia has been reported to occur at approximately the same frequency as the increases in BUN and serum creatinine. It is more pronounced after doses greater than 50 mg/M^2, and peak levels of uric acid generally occur between 3 to 5 days after the dose. Allopurinol therapy for hyperuricemia effectively reduces uric acid levels.

Neurotoxicity

Neurotoxicity, usually characterized by peripheral neuropathies, has occurred in some patients. Optic neuritis, papilledema and cerebral blindness have been reported rarely. Improvement and/or total recovery usually occurs after discontinuing Platinol. Steroids with or without mannitol have been used; however, the efficacy is not established. Loss of taste and seizures have also been reported. Neuropathies resulting from Platinol treatment may occur after prolonged therapy (4 to 7 months); however, neurologic symptoms have been reported to occur after a single dose.

Platinol therapy should be discontinued when the symptoms are first observed. Preliminary evidence suggests peripheral neuropathy may be irreversible in some patients.

Anaphylactic-like Reactions

Anaphylactic-like reactions have been occasionally reported in patients previously exposed to Platinol. The reactions consist of facial edema, wheezing, tachycardia and hypotension within a few minutes of drug administration. Reactions may be controlled by intravenous epinephrine, corticosteroids or antihistamines. Patients receiving Platinol should be observed carefully for possible anaphylactic-like reactions and supportive equipment and medication should be available to treat such a complication.

Other toxicities reported to occur infrequently are cardiac abnormalities, anorexia and elevated SGOT.

Dosage and Administration:

Note: Needles or intravenous sets containing aluminum parts that may come in contact with Platinol should not be used for preparation or administration. Aluminum reacts with Platinol, causing precipitate formation and a loss of potency.

Metastatic Testicular Tumors—An effective combination for the treatment of patients with metastatic testicular carcinomas includes Platinol, Blenoxane (Bleomycin Sulfate) and Velban (Vinblastine Sulfate). Remission induction therapy consists of Platinol, Blenoxane (Bleomycin Sulfate) and Velban (Vinblastine Sulfate) in the following doses:

    PLATINOL—20 mg/M^2 I.V. daily for 5 days (days 1–5) every three weeks for three courses.
    BLENOXANE® (Bleomycin Sulfate)—30 units I.V. weekly (Day 2 of each week) for 12 consecutive doses.
    VELBAN® (Vinblastine Sulfate)—0.15 to 0.2 mg/Kg I.V. twice weekly (Days 1 and 2) every three weeks for four courses (a total of eight doses).

Maintenance therapy for patients who respond to the above regimen consists of Velban (Vinblastine Sulfate) 0.3 mg/Kg I.V. every 4 weeks for a total of 2 years.

For directions for the administration of Blenoxane (Bleomycin Sulfate) and Velban (Vinblastine Sulfate), refer to their respective package insert.

Metastatic Ovarian Tumors—An effective combination for the treatment of patients with metastatic ovarian tumors includes Platinol and Adriamycin (Doxorubicin Hydrochloride) in the following doses:

    PLATINOL—50 mg/M^2 I.V. once every 3 weeks (Day 1).
    ADRIAMYCIN™ (Doxorubicin Hydrochloride)—50 mg/M^2 I.V. once every 3 weeks (Day 1).

For directions for the administration of Adriamycin (Doxorubicin Hydrochloride), refer to the Adriamycin (Doxorubicin Hydrochloride) package insert.

In combination therapy, Platinol and Adriamycin (Doxorubicin Hydrochloride) are administered sequentially.

As a single agent, Platinol should be administered at a dose of 100 mg/M^2 I.V. once every 4 weeks.

Advanced Bladder Cancer—Platinol should be administered as a single agent at a dose of 50-70 mg/m^2 I.V. once every 3 to 4 weeks depending on the extent of prior exposure to radiation therapy and/or prior chemotherapy. For heavily pretreated patients an initial dose of 50 mg/m^2 repeated every 4 weeks is recommended.

Pretreatment hydration with 1 to 2 liters of fluid infused for 8 to 12 hours prior to a Platinol dose is recommended. The drug is then diluted in 2 liters of 5% Dextrose in ½ or ⅓N Saline containing 37.5 g of mannitol, and infused over a 6- to 8-hour period. Adequate hydration and urinary output must be maintained during the following 24 hours. A repeat course of Platinol should not be given until the serum creatinine is below 1.5 mg/100 ml, and/or the BUN is below 25 mg/100 ml. A repeat course should not be given until circulating blood elements are at an acceptable level (platelets $\geq 100,000/mm^3$, WBC $\geq 4,000/mm^3$). Subsequent doses of Platinol should not be given until an audiometric analysis indicates that auditory acuity is within normal limits.

As with other potentially toxic compounds, caution should be exercised in handling the powder and preparing the solution of cisplatin. Skin reactions associated with accidental exposure to cisplatin may occur. The use of gloves is recommended. If cisplatin powder or solution contact skin or mucosae, immediately wash the skin or mucosae thoroughly with soap and water.

Preparation of Intravenous Solutions: The 10 mg and 50 mg vials should be reconstituted with 10 ml or 50 ml of Sterile Water for Injection, U.S.P., respectively. Each ml of the resulting solution will contain 1 mg of Platinol.

Reconstitution as recommended results in a clear, colorless solution.

The reconstituted solution should be used intravenously only and should be administered by I.V. infusion over a 6- to 8-hour period. (See Dosage and Administration.)

Stability: Unopened vials of the dry powder are stable for 2 years at room temperature (27°C).

The reconstituted solution is stable for 20 hours at room temperature (27°C).

Important Note: Once reconstituted, the solution should be kept at room temperature (27°C). If the reconstituted solution is refrigerated a precipitate will form.

Supply: PLATINOL (cisplatin) for Injection
    NDC 0015-3070-20—Each amber vial contains 10 mg of cisplatin.
    NDC 0015-3072-20—Each amber vial contains 50 mg of cisplatin.

VEPESID® ℞
[vĕ′pĭ-sĭd]
(etoposide [VP-16-213])
INJECTION

This is the full text of the latest Official Package Circular dated November 1983 [3095 DIM-05].

WARNINGS

VePesid (etoposide) should be administered under the supervision of a qualified physician experienced in the use of cancer chemotherapeutic agents. Severe myelosuppression with resulting infection or bleeding may occur.

Description: VePesid (etoposide) (VP-16-213) is a semisynthetic derivative of podophyllotoxin used in the treatment of certain neoplastic diseases. It is 4′-Demethylepipodophyllotoxin 9-[4,6-0-(R)-ethylidene-β-D-glucopyranoside]. It is very soluble in methanol and chloroform, slightly soluble in ethanol and sparingly soluble in water and ether. It is made more miscible with water by means of organic solvents. It has a molecular weight of 588.58 and a molecular formula of $C_{29}H_{32}O_{13}$. VePesid is administered by intravenous infusion. VePesid Injection is available in 100 mg (5 ml) sterile multiple dose vials. The pH of the clear yellow solution is 3 to 4.

Each ml contains 20 mg etoposide, 2 mg citric acid, 30 mg benzyl alcohol, 80 mg polysorbate 80/Tween 80, 650 mg polyethylene glycol 300, and 30.5 percent (v/v) alcohol.

The structural formula is:

Clinical Pharmacology: VePesid has been shown to cause metaphase arrest in chick fibroblasts. Its main effect, however, appears to be at the G_2 portion of the cell cycle in mammalian cells. Two different dose-dependent responses are seen. At high concentrations (10 μg/ml or more), lysis of cells entering mitosis is observed. At low concentrations (0.3 to 10μg/ml), cells are inhibited from entering prophase. It does not interfere with microtubular assembly. The predominant macromolecular effect of VePesid appears to be DNA synthesis inhibition.

Pharmacokinetics: In adult patients, VePesid is cleared from the plasma in a biphasic manner. The terminal half-life ($T^{1}\!/_{2}\beta$) is 7 hours with a range of 3 to 12 hours. The steady state volume of distribution is approximately 28% of body weight. Approximately 94% of the drug is bound to human serum proteins at etoposide concentrations of 10 μg/ml. The distribution of etoposide and metabolites into the CSF is low and variable. During the 72 hours after intravenous infusion of radioactive etoposide, 44 to 60% of the radioactivity was recovered in the urine with 67% of the total amount as unchanged drug and the remainder as metabolites. Recovery in the feces ranges from less than 2 to 16% over 3 days.

In a limited number of children, VePesid administered in a dose of 200–250 mg/m^2 produced peak serum concentrations between 17 and 88 μg/ml and showed a terminal half-life ($T^{1}\!/_{2}\beta$) of 5.7±1.3 hours. Mean plasma clearance was 21.5 ml/min/m^2 and CSF concentrations 24 hours post-infusion ranged from less than 10 ng/ml to 45 μg/ml.

Indication and Usage: VePesid has been shown to be useful in the management of the following neoplasms:

Refractory Testicular Tumors—in combination therapy with other approved chemotherapeutic agents in patients with refractory testicular tumors who have already received appropriate surgical, chemotherapeutic and radiotherapeutic therapy.

Contraindications: VePesid is contraindicated in patients who have demonstrated a previous hypersensitivity to it.

Warnings: Patients being treated with VePesid must be observed for myelosuppression carefully and frequently both during and after therapy. Dose limiting bone marrow suppression is the most significant toxicity associated with VePesid therapy. Therefore, the following studies should be obtained at the start of therapy and prior to each subsequent dose of VePesid: platelet count, hemoglobin, white blood cell count and differential. The occurrence of a platelet count below 50,000/mm^3 or an absolute neutrophil count below 500/mm^3 is an indication to withhold further therapy until the blood counts have sufficiently recovered.

Continued on next page

Bristol-Myers Oncology—Cont.

Physicians should be aware of the possible occurrence of an anaphylactic reaction manifested by chills, fever, tachycardia, bronchospasm, dyspnea and hypotension. Treatment is symptomatic. The infusion should be terminated immediately, followed by the administration of pressor agents, corticosteroids, antihistamines, or volume expanders at the discretion of the physician.

VePesid should be given only by slow intravenous infusion (usually over a 30 to 60 minute period) since hypotension has been reported as a possible side effect of rapid intravenous injection.

Pregnancy: Pregnancy "Category D". VePesid can cause fetal harm when administered to a pregnant woman. VePesid has been shown to be teratogenic in mice and rats. There are no adequate and well-controlled studies in pregnant women. If this drug is used during pregnancy, or if the patient becomes pregnant while receiving this drug, the patient should be apprised of the potential hazard to the fetus. Women of childbearing potential should be advised to avoid becoming pregnant.

VePesid is teratogenic and embryocidal in rats and mice at doses of 1 to 3% of the recommended clinical dose based on body surface area.

VePesid was subjected to a teratology study in SPF rats at doses of 0.13, 0.4, 1.2 and 3.6 mg/kg/day administered intravenously on Days 6 to 15 of gestation. VePesid caused a dose-related maternal toxicity, embryotoxicity, and teratogenicity at dose levels of 0.4 mg/kg/day and higher. Embryonic resorptions were 90 and 100% at the 2 highest dosages. At 0.4 and 1.2 mg/kg, fetal weights were decreased and fetal abnormalities occurred including major skeletal abnormalities, exencephaly, encephalocele and anophthalmia. Even at the lowest dose tested, 0.13 mg/kg, a significant increase in retarded ossification was observed.

A study by Sieber, et. al. in Swiss-Albino mice given a single intraperitoneal injection of VePesid at dosages of 1, 1.5 and 2 mg/kg on Days 6, 7 or 8 of gestation disclosed dose-related embryotoxicity, cranial abnormalities and major skeletal malformations.

Precautions:
General: In all instances where the use of VePesid is considered for chemotherapy, the physician must evaluate the need and usefulness of the drug against the risk of adverse reactions. Most such adverse reactions are reversible if detected early. If severe reactions occur, the drug should be reduced in dosage or discontinued and appropriate corrective measures should be taken according to the clinical judgment of the physician. Reinstitution of VePesid therapy should be carried out with caution, and with adequate consideration of the further need for the drug and alertness as to possible recurrence of toxicity.

Laboratory Tests: Periodic complete blood counts should be done during the course of VePesid treatment. They should be performed prior to therapy and at appropriate periods during therapy. At least one determination should be done prior to each dose of VePesid.

Carcinogenesis, Mutagenesis, Impairment of Fertility: Carcinogenicity tests with VePesid have not been conducted in laboratory animals. Given its mechanism of action, it should be considered a possible carcinogen in humans.

VePesid induced aberrations in chromosome number and structure in embryonic murine cells.

Treatment of swiss albino mice with 1.5 mg/kg IP of VePesid on day 7 of gestation increased the incidence of intrauterine death and fetal malformations as well as significantly decreasing the average fetal body weights. Maternal weight gain was not affected.

Treatment of pregnant SPF rats with 1.2 mg/kd/day IV for 10 days of VePesid led to a prenatal mortality of 92%, and 50% of the implanting fetuses were abnormal.

Pregnancy: Pregnancy "Category D". See "WARNINGS" section.

Nursing Mothers: It is not known whether this drug is excreted in human milk. Because many drugs are excreted in human milk and because of the potential for serious adverse reactions in nursing infants from VePesid, a decision should be made whether to discontinue nursing or to discontinue the drug, taking into account the importance of the drug to the mother.

Pediatric Use: Safety and effectiveness in children have not been established.

Adverse Reactions: The following data on adverse reactions is based on intravenous administration of VePesid as a single agent on several different dose schedules for treatment of a wide variety of malignancies. The incidences of adverse reactions are derived from two different data bases—Bristol-sponsored studies comprised of a population of 148 patients and studies reported in the published literature comprised of a population of 1,393 patients.

In the paragraphs below, the incidence of adverse reactions is reported for each of the two data bases.

Hematological Toxicity: Myelotoxicity is most often dose limiting, with granulocyte nadirs occurring 7 to 14 days and platelet nadirs occurring 9 to 16 days after drug administration. Bone marrow recovery is usually complete by day 20, and no cumulative toxicity has been reported. Leukopenia was observed in 91% of patients in Bristol-sponsored studies and 60% of patients in the published literature. Severe leukopenia (less than 1,000 WBC/mm^3) was observed in 17% of patients in Bristol-sponsored studies and 7% of patients in the published literature. Thrombocytopenia was reported in 41% of patients in the Bristol-sponsored studies and 28% of patients in the published literature. Severe thrombocytopenia (less than 50,000 platelets/mm^3) was reported in 20% of patients in Bristol-sponsored studies and 4% of patients in the published literature.

Gastrointestinal Toxicity: Nausea and vomiting are the major gastrointestinal toxicities. The incidence was 32% in patients in Bristol-sponsored studies and 31% in patients in the published literature. Nausea and vomiting can usually be controlled with standard antiemetic therapy. Anorexia was reported in 10% and 13%, respectively, of patients in Bristol-sponsored studies and patients in the published literature. Diarrhea was reported in 1% of patients in Bristol-sponsored studies and 13% of patients in the published literature. Stomatitis was reported in 1% of patients in Bristol-sponsored studies but was not reported in the literature. Liver toxicity was not reported in Bristol-sponsored studies, but a 3% incidence was reported in the literature.

Alopecia: Reversible alopecia, sometimes progressing to total baldness, was observed in 8% of patients in Bristol-sponsored studies and 20% of patients in the published literature.

Hypotension: Temporary hypotension following rapid intravenous administration has been reported in 1% of patients in Bristol-sponsored studies and 2% of patients in the published literature. It has not been associated with cardiac toxicity or electrocardiographic changes. No delayed hypotension has been noted. To prevent this rare occurrence, it is recommended that VePesid be administered by slow intravenous infusion over a 30 to 60 minute period. If hypotension occurs, it usually responds to stopping the infusion and administering fluids or other supportive therapy as appropriate. When restarting the infusion, a slower administration rate should be used.

Allergic Reactions: Anaphylactic-like reactions characterized by chills, fever, tachycardia, bronchospasm, dyspnea and hypotension have been reported to occur in 0.7% of patients in Bristol-sponsored studies and 2% of patients in the published literature. These reactions have usually responded promptly to the cessation of the infusion and administration of pressor agents, corticosteroids, antihistamines or volume expanders as appropriate. One fatal acute reaction associated with bronchospasm has been reported.

Neurotoxicity: Peripheral neuropathy was reported in 0.7% of patients. Central nervous system toxicity (somnolence and fatigue) was reported in 3% of patients in Bristol-sponsored studies and none was reported in the published literature.

Other Toxicities: The following adverse reactions have been rarely reported: aftertaste, hypertension, rash and a single report of radiation recall dermatitis.

Overdosage: No proven antidotes have been established for VePesid overdosage.

Dosage and Administration: The usual dose for VePesid is 50 to 100 mg/M^2/day, days 1 to 5 or 100 mg/M^2/day, days 1, 3 and 5 every 3 to 4 weeks in combination with other drugs approved for use in the disease to be treated. Dosage should be modified to take into account the myelosuppressive effects of other drugs in the combination or the effects of prior x-ray therapy or chemotherapy which may have compromised bone marrow reserve.

Administration Precautions: As with other potentially toxic compounds, caution should be exercised in handling and preparing the solution of VePesid. Skin reactions associated with accidental exposure to VePesid may occur. The use of gloves is recommended. If VePesid solution contacts the skin or mucosa, immediately wash the skin or mucosa thoroughly with soap and water.

Preparation for Intravenous Administration: VePesid Injection may be diluted with either 5% Dextrose Injection, USP or 0.9% Sodium Chloride Injection, USP to give a final concentration of 0.2 or 0.4 mg/ml. Hypertension following rapid intravenous administration has been reported, hence, it is recommended that the VePesid solution be administered over a 30 to 60 minute period. **VePesid SHOULD NOT BE GIVEN BY RAPID INTRAVENOUS PUSH.**

Parenteral drug products should be inspected visually for particulate matter and discoloration (see DESCRIPTION section) prior to administration whenever solution and container permit.

Stability: Unopened vials of VePesid Injection are stable for 24 months at room temperature (25°C). VePesid vials when diluted as recommended to a concentration of 0.2 or 0.4 mg/ml are stable for 96 and 48 hours, respectively, at room temperature (25°C) under normal room fluorescent light in both glass and plastic containers.

How Supplied:
VePesid (etoposide) Injection
NDC 0015-3095-19—100 mg/5 ml Multiple Dose Vial,

For information on package sizes available, refer to the current price schedule.

Bristol-Myers Products
(Div. of Bristol-Myers Co.)
345 PARK AVENUE
NEW YORK, NY 10154

ARTHRITIS STRENGTH BUFFERIN®
[bŭf′fĕr-ĭn]
Analgesic

Composition: Aspirin 7½ gr. (486 mg.) in a formulation buffered with Di-Alminate,® Bristol-Myers' brand of Aluminum Glycinate and Magnesium Carbonate.

Action and Uses: For the temporary relief from the minor aches and pains, stiffness, swelling and inflammation of arthritis and rheumatism. ARTHRITIS STRENGTH BUFFERIN also reduces pain and fever of colds and "flu" and provides fast, effective pain relief for: simple headache, lower back muscular aches from fatigue, sinusitis, neuralgia, neuritis, tooth extraction, muscle strain, athletic soreness, painful distress associated with normal menstrual periods.

Contraindications: Hypersensitivity to salicylates.

Caution: If pain persists for more than 10 days or redness is present or in arthritic or rheumatic conditions affecting children under 12, consult physician immediately. Do not take without consulting physician if under medical care.

Warning: KEEP THIS AND ALL MEDICINES OUT OF CHILDREN'S REACH, IN CASE OF AC-

Product Information

	COMTREX Tablets	COMTREX Liquid	COMTREX Capsules
Acetaminophen	325 mg.	650 mg.	325 mg.
Phenylpropanolamine HCl:	12 ½ mg.	25 mg.	12 ½ mg.
Chlorpheniramine Maleate:	1 mg.	2 mg.	1 mg.
Dextromethorphan HBr	10 mg.	20 mg.	10 mg.
Alcohol:	—	20% by Volume	—

CIDENTAL OVERDOSE, CONSULT A PHYSICIAN IMMEDIATELY. As with any drug, if you are pregnant or nursing a baby, seek the advice of a health professional before using this product.
Administration and Dosage: Two tablets with water. Repeat after four hours if necessary. Do not exceed 8 tablets in any 24 hour period. If dizziness, impaired hearing or ringing in ear occurs, discontinue use. Not recommended for children.
Overdose: (Symptoms and treatment) Typical of aspirin.
How Supplied: Tablets in bottles of 40 and 100. Samples available upon request.
Product Identification: Plain white elongated tablet.

BUFFERIN® Analgesic
[bŭf'fĕr-ĭn]

Composition: Each tablet and capsule contains Aspirin 5 gr. (324 mg.). Tablets are buffered with Di-Alminate®, Bristol-Myers's brand of Aluminum Glycinate, and Magnesium Carbonate. Capsules are buffered with Calcium Carbonate, Magnesium Oxide, Magnesium Carbonate.
Action and Uses: For relief of simple headache; and for temporary relief of: toothache, minor arthritic pain, the painful discomforts and fever of colds and "flu", menstrual cramps, and muscular aches from fatigue.
Contraindications: Hypersensitivity to salicylates.
Caution: If pain persists for more than 10 days or redness is present or, in arthritic or rheumatic conditions affecting children under 12, consult physician immediately. Do not take without consulting physician if under medical care. Consult a dentist for toothache promptly.
Warning: KEEP THIS AND ALL MEDICINES OUT OF CHILDREN'S REACH. IN CASE OF ACCIDENTAL OVERDOSE, CONSULT A PHYSICIAN IMMEDIATELY. As with any drug, if you are pregnant or nursing a baby, seek the advice of a health professional before using this product.
Administration and Dosage: 2 tablets every four hours as needed. Do not exceed 12 tablets in 24 hours, unless directed by a physician. For children 6-12, one-half dose. Under 6, consult physician.
Overdose: (Symptoms and treatment) Typical of aspirin.
How Supplied: Tablets in bottles of 12, 36, 60, 100, 165, 225, and 375. For hospital and clinical use: bottle—1,000; boxed 200x2 tablet foil packets. Capsules in bottles of 30, 50 and 75. Samples available on request.
Product Identification Mark: Tablet is white with letter "B" on one surface. Capsule is white with BUFFERIN on four sides of outer half of capsule.

EXTRA–STRENGTH BUFFERIN®
[bŭf'fĕr-ĭn]
Analgesic

Composition: Each tablet and capsule contains aspirin 500 mg. Tablets are buffered with Di-Alminate®, Bristol-Myers' brand of Aluminum Glycinate and Magnesium Carbonate. Capsules are buffered with Calcium Carbonate, Magnesium Oxide and Magnesium Carbonate.
Action and Uses: Extra-Strength BUFFERIN is formulated to provide the maximum quantity of aspirin recommended without a prescription. For relief of headaches, menstrual cramps, muscular aches, painful discomforts and fever of colds or flu, and temporary relief from toothache and the minor aches, pain and inflammation of arthritis and rheumatism.
Contraindications: Hypersensitivity to salicylates.
Caution: If pain persists for more than 10 days, or redness is present, or in arthritic or rheumatic conditions affecting children under 12, consult a physician immediately. Do not take without consulting a physician if under medical care. Consult a dentist for toothache promptly.

Warning: KEEP THIS AND ALL MEDICINES OUT OF CHILDREN'S REACH. IN CASE OF ACCIDENTAL OVERDOSE, CONSULT A PHYSICIAN IMMEDIATELY. As with any drug, if you are pregnant or nursing a baby, seek the advice of a health professional before using this product.
Administration and Dosage: Tablets—Capsules 2 every 4 hours as needed. Do not exceed 8 in 24 hours, or give to children 12 or under, unless directed by a physician.
Overdose: (Symptoms and treatment) Typical of aspirin.
How Supplied: Tablets in bottles of 30, 60 and 100. Capsules in bottles of 24's, 50's and 75's. All sizes packaged in child resistant closures except 60's (for tablets); 50's (for capsules) which are sizes not recommended for households with young children.
Product Identification Mark: White, elongated tablets with "ESB" imprinted on one side. White and blue capsules with "EXTRA-STRENGTH BUFFERIN" imprinted on 3 sides.

COMTREX®
[cŏm'trĕx]
Multi-Symptom Cold Reliever

Composition: Each tablet, fluid ounce (30 ml.), and capsule contains:
[See table above].
Action and Uses: COMTREX contains a combination of ingredients including a non-aspirin analgesic, a decongestant, an antihistamine and a non-narcotic antitussive. COMTREX is of value in relieving the following cold symptoms when they occur together: nasal and sinus congestion, post nasal drip, coughing due to minor throat and bronchial irritation, fever, minor sore throat pain (systemically), headache, body aches and pain.
Contraindications: Hypersensitivity to acetaminophen or antihistamines.
Caution: Do not take without consulting a physician if under medical care. Do not drive a car or operate machinery while taking this cold remedy as it may cause drowsiness.
Warning: Keep this and all medicine out of children's reach. In case of accidental overdose, consult a physician immediately. Persistent cough may indicate the presence of a serious condition. Persons with a high fever or persistent cough, or with high blood pressure, diabetes, heart or thyroid disease, asthma, glaucoma or difficulty in urination due to enlargement of the prostate gland should not use this preparation unless directed by a physician. Do not use for more than 10 days unless directed by a physician. As with any drug, if you are pregnant or nursing a baby, seek the advice of a health professional before using this product.
Administration and Dosage:
Tablets—Adults: 2 tablets every 4 hours as needed not to exceed 12 tablets in 24 hours. Children 6-12 years: ½ the adult dose. Under 6, consult a physician.
Liquid—Adults: 1 fluid ounce (30 ml.) every 4 hours as needed, not to exceed 6 fluid ounces (180 ml.) in 24 hours. Children 6-12 years: ½ the adult dose. Under 6, consult a physician.
Capsules—Adults 2 capsules every 4 hours as needed not to exceed 12 capsules in 24 hours. Children 6–12 years: ½ the adult dose. Under 6, consult a physician.
Overdose: In case of overdose, contact regional poison control center immediately.
How Supplied: Tablets in bottles of 12's, 24's, 50's, 100's. Capsules in bottles of 16's and 36's. Liquid in 6 oz. and 10 oz. plastic bottles. Samples available on request.

Product Identification Mark: Yellow tablet with letter "C" on one surface. Orange and Yellow capsules with "Bristol-Myers" and "Comtrex" on one side. Liquid is orange in color.

CONGESPIRIN® Aspirin Free
[cŏn"gĕs'pĭr-ĭn]
Chewable Cold Tablets for Children

Composition: Each tablet contains 81 mg. (1¼ grains) acetaminophen, 1¼ mg phenylephrine hydrochloride.
Action and Uses: A non-aspirin analgesic/nasal decongestant to temporarily reduce fever and relieve aches, pains and nasal congestion associated with colds and flu.
Warnings: KEEP THIS AND ALL MEDICATIONS OUT OF CHILDREN'S REACH. IN CASE OF ACCIDENTAL OVERDOSE, CONTACT A PHYSICIAN IMMEDIATELY.
Caution: If child is under medical care, do not administer without consulting physician. Do not exceed recommended dosage. Consult your physician if symptoms persist or if high blood pressure, heart disease, diabetes or thyroid disease is present. Do not administer for more than 10 days unless directed by physician.
Dosage and Administration: Under 2, consult your physician.
2–3 years ....2 tablets
4–5 years ....3 tablets
6–8 years ....4 tablets
9–10 years ....5 tablets
10–2 years ....6 tablets
12 years ....8 tablets
Repeat dose in four hours if necessary. Do not give more than four doses per day unless prescribed by your physician.
Overdose: In case of overdose contact a regional poison control center immediately.
Product Identification: Scored orange tablet with "C" on one side.
How Supplied: Tablets, in bottles of 24.

CONGESPIRIN®
[cŏn"gĕs'pĭr-ĭn]
Chewable Cold Tablets for Children

Composition: Each tablet contains aspirin 81 mg. (1¼ grains) phenylephrine hydrochloride (1¼ mg.).
Action and Uses: For the temporary relief of fever, aches and pains of the common cold or "flu". Plus an effective nasal decongestant to help relieve stuffiness, runny nose and sneezing from colds.
Dosage and Administration:
Under Age 2 consult your physician.
2–3 YRS. ....2 TABLETS
4–5 YRS. ....3 TABLETS
6–8 YRS. ....4 TABLETS
9–10 YRS. ....5 TABLETS
11 YRS. ....6 TABLETS
12 YRS. ....8 TABLETS
Repeat dose in four hours if necessary. Do not give more than four doses per day unless prescribed by your physician.
Caution: If child is under medical care, do not administer without consulting physician.
Warning: KEEP THIS AND ALL MEDICINES OUT OF CHILDREN'S REACH. IN CASE OF ACCIDENTAL OVERDOSAGE, CONTACT A PHYSICIAN IMMEDIATELY. Do not exceed recommended dosage. Consult your physician if symptoms persist or if high fever, high blood pressure, heart disease, diabetes or thyroid disease is pre-

Continued on next page

Bristol-Myers Products—Cont.

sent. Do not administer for more than 10 days unless directed by your physician.
Overdose: In case of overdose contact a regional poison control center immediately.
How Supplied: Tablets in bottles of 36.
Product Identification Mark: Two layer (orange/white) circular tablet with letter "C" imprinted on the orange side.

CONGESPIRIN® for Children
[cŏn″gĕs′pir-in]
COUGH SYRUP

Composition: Each 5 ml teaspoon contains Dextromethorphan hydrobromide—5 mg.
Actions and Uses: Contains a non-narcotic antitussive comparable in potency to codeine, in an orange flavored syrup. Reduces coughs due to colds and to minor throat irritations.
Warning: Do not administer without consulting a physician if child is under medical care. Persistent cough may indicate the presence of a serious condition. Children with a cough persisting for more than 10 days, with high fever, or with fever lasting more than 3 days should not be given this preparation unless directed by a physician. Do not administer to children under two years of age, except as directed by physician. KEEP THIS AND ALL MEDICINES OUT OF THE REACH OF CHILDREN.
Administration and Dosage: Children 2–6, one teaspoon every 4 hours as needed. Do not exceed 6 teaspoons in 24 hours. Children 6–12, two teaspoons every 4 hours as needed. Do not exceed 12 teaspoons in 24 hours.
Overdose: In case of overdose contact a regional poison control center immediately.
How Supplied: Available in 3 oz plastic bottles
Product Identification: Clear Orange Liquid

CONGESPRIN®
[con″ges′pir-in]
Liquid Cold Medicine

Composition: Each 5 ml. teaspoon contains Acetaminophen 130 mg., Phenylpropanolamine Hydrochloride 6 1/4 mg., Alcohol 10% by volume.
Action and Uses: A non-aspirin analgesic/nasal decongestant to temporarily reduce fever and relieve aches, pains and nasal congestion associated with cold and flu.
Dosage and Administration:
Children 3–5, 1 teaspoon every 3–4 hours.
Children 6–12, 2 teaspoons every 3–4 hours.
Children under 3 years use only as directed by your physician.
Do not give more than 4 doses a day unless directed by your physician.
Caution: If child is under medical care, do not administer without consulting physician.
Warning: KEEP THIS AND ALL MEDICINES OUT OF CHILDREN'S REACH. IN CASE OF ACCIDENTAL OVERDOSAGE, CONTACT A PHYSICIAN IMMEDIATELY. Do not exceed recommended dosage. Consult your physician if symptoms persist or if high fever, high blood pressure, heart disease, diabetes or thyroid disease is present. Do not administer for more than 10 days unless directed by your physician.
Overdose: In case of overdose contact regional poison control center immediately.
How Supplied: In 3 oz. plastic, unbreakable bottles.
Product Identification: Clear red liquid.

EXTRA-STRENGTH DATRIL®
[dā′tril]
Analgesic

Composition: Each tablet and capsule contain acetaminophen, 500 mg.
Actions and Uses: Extra-Strength DATRIL contains non-aspirin acetominophen which is less likely to irritate the stomach than plain aspirin. Extra-Strength DATRIL is intended for the temporary relief of minor aches, pains, headaches and fever. For most persons with peptic ulcer Extra-Strength DATRIL may be used when taken as directed for recommended conditions.
Contraindictions: There have been rare reports of skin rash or glossitis attributed to acetaminophen. Discontinue use if a sensitivity reaction occurs. However, acetaminophen is usually well tolerated by aspirin-sensitive patients.
Caution: Severe or recurrent pain or high or continued fever may be indicative of serious illness. Under these conditions consult a physician. Do not take without consulting a physician if under medical care.
Warning: Do not give to children 12 and under or use for more than 10 days unless directed by a physician. Keep this and all medicines out of reach of children. In case of accidental overdose contact a physician immediately. As with any drug, if you are pregnant or nursing a baby, seek the advice of a health professional before using this product.
Dosage: Adults: Two tablets. May be repeated in 4 hours if needed. Do not exceed 8 tablets in any 24 hour period.
Overdose: In case of overdose contact a regional poison control center immediately.
How Supplied: Tablets in bottles of 24's, 50's and 72's. Capsules in bottles of 24's and 50's. Samples available on request.
Product Identification Mark: White tablet with DATRIL on one surface. Green and white capsule with Bristol-Myers on green half and DATRIL 500 mg on white half.

EXCEDRIN® Extra-Strength Analgesic
[ĕx″cĕd′rin]

Composition: Each tablet and capsule contains Acetaminophen 250 mg.; Aspirin 250 mg.; and Caffeine 65 mg.
Action and Uses: Extra-Strength Excedrin is intended for the relief of pain from: headache, sinusitis, colds or 'flu', muscular aches and menstrual discomfort. Also recommended for temporary relief of toothaches and minor arthritic pains.
Contraindications: Hypersensitivity to salicylates or acetaminophen.
Caution: If sinus or arthritis pain persists (for a week), or if skin redness is present, or in arthritic conditions affecting children under 12, consult physician immediately. Consult dentist for toothache promptly. Do not take without consulting physician if under medical care. Store at room temperature.
Warning: Do not exceed 8 tablets/capsules in 24 hours or use for more than 10 days unless directed, or give to children under 12. Keep this and all medicines out of children's reach. In case of accidental overdose, contact a physician immediately. As with any drug, if you are pregnant or nursing a baby, seek the advice of a health professional before using this product.
Administration and Dosage: Tablets—Individuals 12 and over, take 2 tablets every 4 hours as needed. Capsules—Individuals 12 and over, take 2 capsules every 4 hours as needed.
How Supplied: Bottles of 12, 36, 60, 100, 165, 225, and 375 tablets. Capsules in bottles of 24's, 40's and 60's. A metal tin of 12 tablets. All sizes packaged in child resistant closures except 100's (for tablets); 60's (for capsules) which are sizes not recommended for households with young children.
Overdose: In case of overdose contact a regional poison control center immediately.
Product Identification Mark: White, circular tablet with letter "E" imprinted on both sides. Red capsules with "EXCEDRIN" printed on 2 sides.

EXCEDRIN P.M.®
[ĕx″cĕd′rin]
Analgesic Sleeping Aid

Composition: Each tablet and capsule contain Acetaminophen 500 mg. and Diphenhydramine citrate 38 mg.
Action and Uses: For the temporary relief of occasional headaches and minor aches and pains with accompanying sleeplessness. Also for fever with accompanying sleeplessness.
Contraindications: Hypersensitivity to acetaminophen or antihistamines.
Caution: Do not drive a car or operate machinery while taking this medication. Do not take without consulting physician if under medical care. Store at room temperature.
Warning: Do not exceed 2 tablets in 24 hours, or give to children under 12 or use for more than 10 days unless directed by physician. KEEP THIS AND ALL MEDICINES OUT OF CHILDREN'S REACH. IN CASE OF ACCIDENTAL OVERDOSE, CONTACT A PHYSICIAN IMMEDIATELY. Consult your physician if symptoms persist or new ones occur or if fever persists more than 3 days (72 hours) or recurs or if sleeplessness persists continuously for more than two weeks. Insomnia may be a symptom of serious underlying medical illness. Take this product with caution if alcohol is being consumed. DO NOT TAKE THIS PRODUCT IF YOU HAVE ASTHMA, GLAUCOMA OR ENLARGEMENT OF THE PROSTATE GLAND EXCEPT UNDER THE ADVICE AND SUPERVISION OF A PHYSICIAN. As with any drug, if you are pregnant or nursing a baby, seek the advice of a health professional before using this product.
Administration and Dosage: Adults take two tablets at bedtime or as directed by a physician. Do not exceed recommended dosage.
Overdose: In case of overdose contact a regional poison control center immediately.
How Supplied: Bottles of 10, 30, 50, and 80 tablets. All sizes packaged in child resistant closures except 50's, which is a size not recommended for households with young children.
Product Identification Mark: Blue/green circular tablet with letters "PM" imprinted on one side.

4-WAY® Cold Tablets

Composition: Each tablet contains aspirin 324 mg., phenylpropanolamine HCl 12 1/2 mg., and chlorpheniramine maleate 2 mg.
Action and Uses: For temporary relief of minor aches and pains, fever, nasal congestion and runny nose as may occur in the common cold.
Dosage and Administration:
Adults—2 tablets every 4 hours, if needed. Do not exceed 6 tablets in 24 hours. Children 6–12 years—1 tablet every 4 hours. Do not exceed 4 tablets in 24 hours. Under age 6, consult a physician.
Caution: This preparation may cause drowsiness. Do not drive or operate machinery while taking this medication.
Warning: Keep this and all medicines out of children's reach. In case of accidental overdose, consult a physician immediately. Do not exceed recommended dosage or use for more than 10 days unless directed by a physician. Individuals with high blood pressure, diabetes, heart or thyroid disease, asthma, glaucoma or difficulty in urination due to enlargement of the prostate gland should not use this preparation unless directed by a physician. Do not take without consulting a physician if under medical care. As with any drug, if you are pregnant or nursing a baby, seek the advice of a health professional before using this product.
Overdose: In case of overdose contact a regional poison control center immediately.
How Supplied: Carded 15's and bottles of 36's and 60's.
Product Identification Mark: Pink and White tablet with number "4" on one surface.

4-WAY® Nasal Spray

Composition: Phenylephrine hydrochloride 0.5%, naphazoline hydrochloride 0.05%, pyrilamine maleate 0.2%, in a buffered isotonic aqueous solution with thimerosal 0.005% added as a preservative. Also available in a mentholated formula.

Action and Uses: For temporary relief of nasal congestion due to the common cold, sinusitis, hay fever or other upper respiratory allergies.
Dosage and Administration: With head in a normal upright position, put atomizer tip into nostril. Squeeze atomizer with firm, quick pressure while inhaling. Adults-spray twice into each nostril. Children 6-12-spray once. Under 6-consult physician. Repeat in three hours, if needed.
Warning: Overdosage in young children may cause marked sedation. Do not exceed recommended dosage because symptoms may occur such as burning, stinging, sneezing or increase of nasal discharge. Follow directions carefully. Do not use this product for more than 3 days. If symptoms persist, consult physician. The use of this dispenser by more than one person may spread infection. Keep out of children's reach.
Store at room temperature.
How Supplied: Atomizers of ½ fluid ounce and 1 fluid ounce.

4-WAY® Long Acting Nasal Spray

Composition: Oxymetazoline Hydrochloride 0.05% in a buffered isotonic aqueous solution. Thimerosal, 0.005% added as a preservative.
Action and Uses: Provides temporary relief of nasal congestion due to the common cold, sinusitis, hayfever or other upper respiratory allergies.
Dosage and Administration: With head in a normal upright position, put atomizer tip into nostril. Squeeze atomizer with firm, quick pressure while inhaling. Adults: Spray 2 or 3 times in each nostril twice daily. For children under 12, consult physician.
Warning: For adult use only. Do not give this product to children under 12 years except under the advice and supervision of a physician. Do not exceed recommended dosage because symptoms may occur such as burning, stinging, sneezing, or an increase of nasal discharge. Do not use this product for more than 3 days. If symptoms persist, consult a physician. The use of this dispenser by more than one person may spread infection.
KEEP OUT OF CHILDREN'S REACH.
How Supplied: Atomizers of ½ fluid ounce.

NO DOZ® TABLETS
[nō'dōz]

Composition: Each tablet contains 100 mg. Caffeine.
Action and Uses: Helps restore mental alertness.
Dosage and Administration:
For Adults: 2 tablets initially, thereafter, 1 tablet every three hours should be sufficient.
Caution: Do not take without consulting physician if under medical care. No stimulant should be substituted for normal sleep in activities requiring physical alertness.
Warning: KEEP THIS AND ALL MEDICINES OUT OF THE REACH OF CHILDREN. As with any drug, if you are pregnant or nursing a baby, seek the advice of a health professional before using this product.
Overdose: Typical of caffeine.
How Supplied: Carded 15's and 36's and bottles of 60's.
Product Identification Mark: A white tablet with No Doz on one side.

NUPRIN™
(ibuprofen)
Analgesic

Composition: Each tablet contains ibuprofen USP, 200 mg.
Action and Uses: For the temporary relief of minor aches and pains associated with the common cold, headache, toothache, muscular aches, backache, for the minor pain of arthritis, for the pain of menstrual cramps and for reduction of fever.
Contraindications: ASPIRIN SENSITIVE PATIENTS should not take this product if they have had a severe allergic reaction to aspirin, e.g. —asthma, swelling, shock or hives, because even though this product contains no aspirin or salicylates, cross-reactions may occur in patients allergic to aspirin.
Warnings: The following warnings are stated on the Nuprin label: Do not take for pain for more than 10 days or for fever for more than 3 days unless directed by a doctor. If pain or fever persists or gets worse, if new symptoms occur, or if the painful area is red or swollen, consult a doctor. These could be signs of serious illness. If you are under a doctor's care for any serious condition, consult a doctor before taking this product. As with aspirin and acetaminophen, if you have any condition which requires you to take prescription drugs or if you have had any problems or serious side effects from taking any non-prescription pain reliever, do not take NUPRIN without first discussing it with your doctor. If you experience any symptoms which are unusual or seem unrelated to the condition for which you took ibuprofen, consult a doctor before taking any more of it. Although ibuprofen is indicated for the same conditions as aspirin and acetaminophen, it should not be taken with them except under a doctor's direction. Before using any drug, including NUPRIN, you should seek the advice of a health professional if you are pregnant or nursing a baby. IT IS ESPECIALLY IMPORTANT NOT TO USE IBUPROFEN DURING THE LAST 3 MONTHS OF PREGNANCY UNLESS SPECIFICALLY DIRECTED TO DO SO BY A DOCTOR BECAUSE IT MAY CAUSE PROBLEMS IN THE UNBORN CHILD OR COMPLICATIONS DURING DELIVERY. Keep this and all drugs out of the reach of children. In case of accidental overdose, seek professional assistance or contact a poison control center immediately.
Caution: Store at room temperature. Avoid excessive heat 40°C (104°F).
Administration and Dosage:
Directions. Adults: Take 1 tablet every 4 to 6 hours while symptoms persist. If pain or fever does not respond to 1 tablet, 2 tablets may be used but do not exceed 6 tablets in 24 hours, unless directed by a doctor. The smallest effective dose should be used. Take with food or milk if occasional and mild heartburn, upset stomach, or stomach pain occurs with use. Consult a doctor if these symptoms are more than mild or if they persist. Children: Do not give this product to children under 12 except under the advice and supervision of a doctor.
Overdosage: In case of overdose please contact a regional poison control center immediately.
How Supplied: Tablets in bottles of: Trial size 8, 24's, 50's and 100's.
Product Identification: Golden yellow round tablet with NUPRIN 200 printed on one side.
Nuprin is a trademark of The Upjohn Company
Manufactured by The Upjohn Company
Distributed by Bristol-Myers Company

The Brown Pharmaceutical Company, Inc.
2500 WEST SIXTH STREET
P.O. BOX 57925
LOS ANGELES, CA 90057

ANDROID-5® ℞
(Methyltestosterone Buccal Tablets U.S.P., 5 mg.)
ANDROID-10® ℞
(Methyltestosterone Tablets U.S.P., 10 mg.)
ANDROID-25® ℞
(Methyltestosterone Tablets U.S.P., 25 mg.)

Description: Methyltestosterone is an androgenic steroid which occurs as white or creamy white crystals or crystalline powder. The androgens are steroids that develop and maintain primary and secondary male sex characteristics.
Structural Formula and Chemical Name:
(See next column)
Clinical Pharmacology: Endogenous androgens are responsible for the normal growth and development of the male sex organs and for maintenance of secondary sex characteristics. These

METHYLTESTOSTERONE

$C_{20}H_{30}O_2$ m.w. 302.46 (CAS-58-18-4)
17β-Hydroxy-17-methylandrost-4-en-3-one

effects include the growth and maturation of prostate, seminal vesicles, penis, and scrotum; the development of male hair distribution, such as beard, pubic, chest and axillary hair; laryngeal enlargement, vocal cord thickening, alterations in body musculature, and fat distribution. Drugs in this class also cause retention of nitrogen, sodium, potassium, phosphorus, and decreased urinary excretion of calcium. Androgens have been reported to increase protein anabolism and decrease protein catabolism. Nitrogen balance is improved only when there is sufficient intake of calories and protein.

Androgens are responsible for the growth spurt of adolescence and eventual termination of linear growth which is brought about by fusion of the epiphyseal growth centers. In children, exogenous androgens accelerate linear growth rates, but may cause a disproportionate advancement in bone maturation. Use over long periods may result in fusion of the epiphyseal growth centers and termination of growth process. Androgens have been reported to stimulate the production of red blood cells by enhancing the production of erythropoietic stimulating factor. During exogenous testosterone release is inhibited through feedback inhibition of pituitary luteinizing hormone (LH). At large doses of exogenous androgens, spermatogenesis may also be suppressed through feedback inhibition of pituitary follicle stimulating hormone (FSH).

There is a lack of substantial evidence that androgens are effective in fractures, surgery, convalescence, and functional uterine bleeding.
Pharmacokinetics
Testosterone given orally is metabolized by the gut and 44 percent is cleared by the liver in the first pass. Oral doses as high as 400 mg per day are needed to achieve clinically effective blood levels for full replacement therapy. The synthetic androgens (methyltestosterone) are less extensively metabolized by the liver and have longer half-lives. They are more suitable than testosterone for oral administration.

Testosterone in plasma is 98 percent bound to a specific testosterone-estradiol binding globulin, and about 2 percent is free. Generally, the amount of this sex-hormone binding globulin in the plasma will determine the distribution of testosterone between free and bound forms, and the free testosterone concentration will determine its half-life. About 90 percent of a dose of testosterone is excreted in the urine as glucuronic and sulfuric acid conjugates of testosterone and its metabolites; about 6 percent of a dose is excreted in the feces, mostly in the unconjugated form. Inactivation of testosterone occurs primarily in the liver. Testosterone is metabolized to various 17-keto steroids through two different pathways. There are considerable variations of the half-life of testosterone as reported in the literature, ranging from 10 to 100 minutes.

In many tissues the activity of testosterone appears to depend on reduction to dihydrotestosterone, which binds to cytosol receptor proteins. The steroid-receptor complex is transported to the nucleus where it initiated transcription events and cellular changes related to androgen action.
Indications and Usage:
1. Males
Androgens are indicated for replacement therapy in conditions associated with a deficiency or absence of endogenous testosterone:

Continued on next page

Brown—Cont.

a. Primary hypogonadism (congenital or acquired)-testicular failure due to cryptorchidism, bilateral torsion, orchitis, vanishing testis syndrome; or orchidectomy.
b. Hypogonadotropic hypogonadism (congenital or acquired)—idiopathic gonadotropin or LHRH deficiency, or pituitary-hypothalamic injury from tumors, trauma, or radiation.

If the above conditions occur prior to puberty, androgen replacement therapy will be needed during the adolescent years for development of secondary sexual characteristics. Prolonged androgen treatment will be required to maintain sexual characteristics in these and other males who develop testosterone deficiency after puberty.

c. Androgens may be used to stimulate puberty in carefully selected males with clearly delayed puberty. These patients usually have a familial pattern of delayed puberty that is not secondary to a pathological disorder; puberty is expected to occur spontaneously at a relatively late date. Brief treatment with conservative doses may occasionally be justified in these patients if they do not respond to psychological support. The potential adverse effect on bone maturation should be discussed with the patient and parents prior to androgen administration. An X-ray of the hand and wrist to determine bone age should be obtained every 6 months to assess the effect of treatment on the epiphyseal centers (see WARNINGS).

2. Females
Androgens may be used secondarily in women with advancing inoperable metastatic (skeletal) mammary cancer who are 1 to 5 years postmenopausal. Primary goals of therapy in these women include ablatio of the ovaries. Other methods of counteracting estrogen activity are adronalectomy, hypophysectomy, and/or antiestrogen therapy. This treatment has also been used in premenopausal women with breast cancer who benefited from oophorectomy and are considered to have a hormone-responsive tumor. Judgment concerning adrogen therapy should be made by an oncologist with expertise in this field.

Androgens (including Methyltestosterone) have been used for the management of postpartum breast pain and engorgement.

Contraindications: Androgens are contraindicated in men with carcinomas of the breast or with known or suspected carcinomas of the prostate, and in women who are or may become pregnant. When administered to pregnant women, androgens cause virilization of the external genitalia of the female fetus. This virilization includes clitoromegaly, abnormal vaginal development, and fusion of genital folds to form a scrotal-like structure. The degree of masculinization is related to the amount of drug given and the age of the fetus, and is most likely to occur in the female fetus when the drugs are given in the first trimester. If the patient becomes pregnant while taking these drugs, she should be apprised of the potential hazard to the fetus.

Warnings: In patients with breast cancer, androgen therapy may cause hypercalcemia by stimulating osteolysis. In this case, the drug should be discontinued.

Prolonged use of high doses of androgens have been associated with the development of peliosis hepatis and hepatic neoplasms including hepatocellular carcinoma. See PRECAUTIONS—Carcinogenesis). Peliosis hepatis can be life-threatening or fatal complication.

Cholestatic hepatitis and jaundice occur with 17-alpha-alkylandrogens at a relatively low dose. If cholestatic hepatitis with jaundice appears or if liver function tests become abnormal, the androgen should be discontinued and the etiology should be determined. Drug-induced jaundice is reversible when the medication is discontinued.

Geriatric patients treated with androgens may be at an increased risk for the development of prostatic hypertropy and prostatic carcinoma.

Edema with or without congestive heart failure may be a serious complication in patients with preexisting cardiac, renal, or hepatic disease. In addition to discontinuation of the drug, diuretic therapy may be required.

Gynecomastia frequently developes and occasionally persists in patients being treated for hypogonadism.

Androgen therapy should be used cautiously in healthy males with delayed puberty. The effect on bone maturation should be monitored by assessing bone age of the wrist and hand every 6 months. In children, androgen treatment may accelerate bone maturation without producing compensatory gain in linear growth. This adverse effect may result in compromised adult stature. The younger the child the greater the risk of compromising final mature height.

Precautions:
General
Women should be observed for signs of virilization (deepening of the voice, hirsutism, acne, clitoromegaly and menstrual irregularities). Discontinuation of drug therapy at the time of evidence of mild virilism is necessary to prevent irreversible virilization. Such virilization is usual following androgen use at high doses. A decision may be made by the patient and the physician that some virilization will be tolerated during treatment for breast carcinoma.

Information for the Patient
The physician should instruct patients to report any of the following side effects of androgens:
Adult or Adolescent Males: Too frequent or persistent erections of the penis.
Women: Hoarseness, acne, changes in menstrual periods, or more hair on the face.
All Patients: Any nausea, vomiting, changes in skin color or ankle swelling. Any male adolescent patient receiving androgens for delayed puberty should have bone development checked every six months.

Laboratory Tests
1. Women with disseminated breast carcinoma should have frequent determination of urine and serum calcium levels during the course of androgen therapy. (See WARNINGS).
2. Because of the hepatotoxicity associated with the use of 17-alpha-alkylated androgens, liver function tests should be obtained periodically.
3. Periodic (every 6 months) x-ray examinations of bone age should be made during treatment of prepubertal males to determine the rate of bone maturation and the effects of androgen therapy on the epiphyseal centers.
4. Hemoglobin and hematocrit should be checked periodically for polycythemia in patients who are receiving high doses of androgens.

Drug Interactions
1. Anticoagulants. C-17 substituted derivatives of testosterone, such as methandrostenolone, have been reported to decrease the anticoagulant requirements of patients receiving oral anticoagulants. Patients receiving anticoagulant therapy require close monitoring, especially when androgens are started or stopped.
2. Oxyphenbutazone. Concurrent administration of oxyphenbutazone and androgens may result in elevated serum levels of oxyphenbutazone.
3. Insulin. In diabetic patients the metabolic effects of androgens may decrease blood glucose and insulin requirements.

Drub/Laboratory Test Interferences
Androgens may decrease levels of thyroxine-binding globulin, resulting in decreased total T_4 serum levels and increased resin uptake of T_3 and T_4. Free thyroid hormone levels remain unchanged, however, and there is no clinical evidence of thyroid dysfunction.

Carcinogenesis
Animal Data. Testosterone has been tested by subcutaneous injection and implantation in mice and rats. The implant induced cervical-uterine tumors in mice, which metastasized in some cases. There is suggestive evidence that injection of testosterone into some strains of female mice increases their susceptibility to hepatoma. Testosterone is also known to increase the number of tumors and decrease the degree of differenton of chemically induced carcinomas of the liver in rats.

Human Data. There are rare reports of hepatocellular carcinoma in patients receiving long-term therapy with androgens in high doses. Withdrawal of the drugs did not lead to regression of the tumors in all cases.

Geriatric patients treated with androgens may be at an increased risk for the development of prostatic hypertrophy and prostatic carcinoma.

Nursing Mothers
It is not known whether androgens are excreted in human milk. Because many drugs are excreted in human milk and because of the potential for serious adverse reactions in nursing infants from androgens, a decision should be made whether to discontinue nursing or to discontinue the drug, taking into account the importance of the drug to the mother.

Pediatric Use
Androgen therapy should be used very cautiously in children and only by specialists who are aware of the adverse effects on bone maturation. Skeletal maturation must be monitored every six months by an x-ray of hand and wrist.

Adverse Reactions:
Endocrine and Urogenital
Female. The most common side effects of androgen therapy are amenorrhea and other menstrual irregularities, inhibition of gonadotropin secretion, and virilization, including deepening of the voice and clitoral enlargement. The latter usually is not reversible after androgens are discontinued. When administered to a pregnant woman androgens cause virilization of external genitalia of the female fetus.

Male. Gynecomastia, and excessive frequency and duration of penile erections. Oligospermia may occur at high doses.

Skin and appendates: Hirsutism, male pattern of baldness, and acne.

Fluid and Electrolyte Disturbances: Retention of sodium, chloride, water, potassium, calcium, and inorganic phosphates.

Gastrointestinal: Nausea, cholestatic jaundice, alterations in liver function tests, rarely hepatocellular neoplasms and peliosis hepatis.

Hematologic: Suppression of clotting factors, II, V, VII, and X, bleeding in patients on concomitant anticoagulant therapy, and polycythemia.

Nervous System: Increased or decrease libido, headache, anxiety, depression, and generalized paresthesia.

Metabolic: Increased serum cholesterol.

Overdosage: There have been no reports of acute overdosage with the androgens.

Dosage and Administration: The suggested dosage for androgens varies depending on the age, sex, and diagnosis of the individual patient. Dosage is adjusted according to the patient's response and the appearance of adverse reactions. See Table 1 for guidelines for replacement therapy in androgen-deficient males. Various dosage regimens have been used to induce pubertal changes in hypogonadal males: some experts have advocated lower dosages initially, gradually increasing the dose as puberty progresses, with or without a decrease to maintenance levels. Other experts emphasize that higher dosages are needed to induce pubertal changes and lower dosages can be used for maintenance after puberty. The chronological and skeletal ages must be taken into consideration, both in determining the initial dose and in adjusting the dose.

Dosages used in delayed puberty generally are in the lower ranges of those given in Table 1, and for a limited duration, for example 4 to 6 months.

Women with metastatic breast carcinoma must be followed closely because androgen therapy occasionally appears to accelerate the disease. Thus, many experts prefer to use the shorter acting androgen preparations rather than those with prolonged activity for treating breast carcinoma, particularly during the early stages of androgen therapy.

Guideline dosages of androgens for use in the palliative treatment of women with metastatic breast carcinoma are given in Table 2.

TABLE 1
Guidelines for Androgen Replacement Therapy in the Male

Drug	Route	Dose	Frequency
Methyltestosterone	Oral	10-50 mg	Daily
	Buccal	5-25 mg	Daily

TABLE 2
Guidelines for Androgen Therapy in Breast Carcinoma in Females

Drug	Route	Dose	Frequency
Methyltestosterone	Oral	50-200 mg	Daily
	Buccal	25-100 mg	Daily

Suggested dosages of androgens for use in the prevention of postpartum breast pain and engorement are: methyltestosterone, buccal tablets 40 mg daily, or oral tablets 80 mg daily for 3 to 5 days after delivery.
[See table above].

How Supplied:
Android 5 mg Buccal Tablets are oblong white unscored tablets, imprinted BP 956, and are supplied in bottles of 60 and 250 tablets.

Android 10 mg Oral Tablets are square green unscored tablets, imprinted BP 958. and are supplied in bottles of 60 and 250 tablets.

Android 25 mg Oral Tablets are square yellow unscored tablets, imprinted BP 996, and are supplied in bottles of 60.

Literature Available: Samples.
Shown in Product Identification Section, page 407

ANDROID-F®
(Fluoxymesterone Tablets U.S.P., 10mg.)

Description: Fluoxymesterone is an adrogenic steroid which occurs as white or creamy white crystals or crystalline powder. The androgens are steroids that develop and maintain primary and secondary male sex characteristics.

Structural Formula and Chemical Name:

FLUOXYMESTERONE

$C_{20}H_{29}FO_3$ m.w. 336.45 (CAS-76-43-7)
9-Fluoro-11β, 17β-dihydroxy-17-methylandrost-4-en-3-one

See preceding **Android** product information for **Clinical Pharmacology, Indications and Usage, Contraindications, Warnings, Precautions, Adverse Reactions,** and **Overdosage.**

Dosage and Administration: The suggested dosage for androgens varies depending on the age, sex, and diagnosis of the individual patient. Dosage is adjusted according to the patient's response and the appearance of adverse reactions. See Table 1 for guidelines for replacement therapy in androgen-deficient males. Various dosage regimens have been used to induce pubertal changes in hypogonadal males: some experts have advocated lower dosages intially, gradually increasing the dose as puberty progresses, with or without a decrease to maintenance levels. Other experts emphasize that higher dosages are needed to induce pubertal changes and lower dosages can be used for maintenance after puberty. The chronological and skeletal ages must be taken into consideration, both in determining the initial dose and in adjusting the dose.

Dosages used in delayed puberty generally are in the lower ranges of those given in Table I, and for a limited duration, for example 4 to 6 months.
Women with metastatic breast carcinoma must be followed closely because androgen therapy occasionally appears to accelerate the disease. Thus, many experts prefer to use the shorter acting androgen preparations rather than those with prolonged activity for treating breast carcinoma, particularly during the early stage of androgen therapy.

Guideline dosages of androgens for use in the palliative treatment of women with metastatic breast carcinoma are given Table 2.

Suggested dosages of androgens for use in the prevention of postpartum breast pain and engorement are: Fluoxymesterone, 2.5 mg oral tablets starting shortly after delivery; thereafter, 5 to 10 mg daily, preferably in divided doses for 4 to 5 days.
[See table below].

How Supplied: Android F (Fluoxymesterone 10 mg.) is supplied as a round white scored oral tablet, imprinted BP 998, and is supplied in bottles of 60.

Literature Available: Samples.
Shown in Product Identification Section, page 407

LIPO-NICIN®/100 mg. Tablets
LIPO-NICIN®/250 mg. Tablets
LIPO-NICIN®/300 mg. Timed Caps

Composition:
LIPO-NICIN®/100 mg.
Each blue tablet contains:
Nicotinic Acid .... 100 mg.
Niacinamide .... 75 mg.
Ascorbic Acid .... 150 mg.
Thiamine HCl (B-1) .... 25 mg.
Riboflavin (B-2) .... 2 mg.
Pyridoxine HCl (B-6) .... 10 mg.
LIPO-NICIN /250 mg.
Each yellow tablet contains:
Nicotinic Acid .... 250 mg.
Niacinamide .... 75 mg.
Ascorbic Acid .... 150 mg.
Thiamine HCl (B-1) .... 25 mg.
Riboflavin (B-2) .... 2 mg.
Pyridoxine HCl (B-6) .... 10 mg.
LIPO-NICIN®/300 mg. Timed Caps
Each red capsule contains:
Nicotinic Acid .... 300 mg.
Vitamin C (Ascorbic Acid) .... 150 mg.
Vitamin B_1 (Thiamine HCl) .... 25 mg.
Vitamin B_2 (Riboflavin) .... 2 mg.
Pyridoxine HCl (B_6) .... 10 mg.
In a special base so prepared that the active ingredients are released over a period of 6 to 8 hours.

Action and Uses: For use as a vasodilator in the symptoms of cold feet, leg cramps, dizziness, memory loss or tinnitus when associated with impaired peripheral circulation. Also provides concomitant administration of the listed vitamins.
The warm tingling flush which may follow each dose is one of the therapeutic effects that often produce psychologic benefits to the patient.

Side Effects: Flushing with heat and itching, in some cases followed by sweating, nausea and abdominal cramps. This reaction is usually transient. Nausea caused by high acidity can be relieved by nonabsorbable antacid.

Caution: Federal law prohibits dispensing without prescription.

Administration and Dosage:
LIPO-NICIN /100 mg.—1 to 5 tablets daily.
LIPO-NICIN /250 mg.—1 to 3 tablets daily.
LIPO-NICIN® /300 mg Timed— 1 to 2 capsules daily.

Available: Bottles of 100.
Literature Available: Samples.

Burroughs Wellcome Co.
3030 CORNWALLIS ROAD
RESEARCH TRIANGLE PARK,
NC 27709

LITERATURE AVAILABLE: Folders, packaging inserts, file cards, films, slides, lecture guides and monographs.

ACTIFED® TABLETS and SYRUP
[ăk'tĭ-fĕd"]
(See PDR For Nonprescription Drugs)

ACTIFED® With CODEINE
[ăk'tĭ-fĕd" with kō'dēn]
Cough Syrup

Description: Each 5 ml (1 teaspoonful) contains: codeine phosphate 10 mg (Warning—may be habit-forming), Actidil® (triprolidine hydrochloride) 1.25 mg, Sudafed® (pseudoephedrine hydrochloride) 30 mg and alcohol 4.3%. Sodium benzoate 0.1% and methylparaben 0.1% are added as preservatives. This medication is intended for oral administration.

Actifed with Codeine Cough Syrup has antitussive, antihistaminic and nasal decongestant effects. The components of Actifed with Codeine Cough Syrup have the following chemical names and structural formulae:

Codeine Phosphate, U.S.P.:
7, 8-didehydro-4, 5α- epoxy-3-methoxy-17-methyl-morphinan-6α-ol phosphate (1:1) (salt) hemihydrate

Triprolidine Hydrochloride Monohydrate:
(E)-2-[3-(1-pyrrolidinyl) -1-(p-tolyl)propenyl]pyridine monohydrochloride monohydrate

Pseudoephedrine Hydrochloride:
[S- (R *,R *)]-α-[1- (methylamino)ethyl]benzenemethanol hydrochloride

Clinical Pharmacology:
Codeine: Codeine probably exerts its antitussive activity by depressing the medullary (brain) cough center, thereby raising its threshold for incoming cough impulses.

TABLE I
Guidelines for Androgen Replacement Therapy in the Male

Drug	Route	Dose	Frequency
Fluoxymesterone	Oral	5-20 mg	Daily

TABLE 2
Guidelines for Androgen Therapy in Breast Carcinoma in Females

Drug	Route	Dose	Frequency
Fluoxymesterone	Oral	10-40 mg	Daily

Continued on next page

Burroughs Wellcome—Cont.

Codeine is readily absorbed from the gastrointestinal tract, with a therapeutic dose reaching peak antitussive effectiveness in about 2 hours and persisting for 4 to 6 hours. Codeine is rapidly distributed from blood to body tissues and taken up preferentially by parenchymatous organs such as liver, spleen and kidney. It passes the blood brain barrier and is found in fetal tissue and breast milk. The drug is not bound by plasma proteins nor is it accumulated in body tissues. Codeine is metabolized in the liver to morphine and norcodeine, each representing about 10 percent of the administered codeine dose. About 90 percent of the dose is excreted within 24 hours, primarily through the kidneys. Urinary excretion products are free and glucuronide-conjugated codeine (about 70%), free and conjugated norcodeine (about 10%), free and conjugated morphine (about 10%), normorphine (under 4%) and hydrocodone (< 1%). The remainder of the dose appears in the feces.

Triprolidine: Antihistamines such as triprolidine hydrochloride act as antagonists of the H_1 histamine receptor. Consequently, they prevent histamine from eliciting typical immediate hypersensitivity responses in the nose, eyes, lungs and skin. Animal distribution studies have shown localization of triprolidine in lung, spleen and kidney tissue. Liver microsome studies have revealed the presence of several metabolites with an oxidized product of the toluene methyl group predominating.

Pseudoephedrine: Pseudoephedrine acts as an indirect sympathomimetic agent by stimulating sympathetic (adrenergic) nerve endings to release norepinephrine. Norepinephrine in turn stimulates alpha and beta receptors throughout the body. The action of pseudoephedrine hydrochloride is apparently more specific for the blood vessels of the upper respiratory tract and less specific for the blood vessels of the systemic circulation. The vasoconstriction elicited at these sites results in the shrinkage of swollen tissues in the sinuses and nasal passages.

Pseudoephedrine is rapidly and almost completely absorbed from the gastrointestinal tract. Considerable variation in half-life has been observed (from about 4½ to 10 hours), which is attributed to individual differences in absorption and excretion. Excretion rates are also altered by urine pH, increasing with acidification and decreasing with alkalinization. As a result, mean half-life falls to about 4 hours at pH 5 and increases to 12 to 13 hours at pH 8.

After administration of a 60 mg tablet, 87 to 96% of the pseudoephedrine is cleared from the body within 24 hours. The drug is distributed to body tissues and fluids, including fetal tissue, breast milk and the central nervous system (CNS). About 55 to 75% of an administered dose is excreted unchanged in the urine; the remainder is apparently metabolized in the liver to inactive compounds by N-demethylation, parahydroxylation and oxidative deamination.

The pharmacokinetic properties of codeine, triprolidine and pseudoephedrine from 10 ml of Actifed with Codeine Cough Syrup were investigated compared to a reference preparation of equal component doses in 18 healthy adults. The results of this study showed that Actifed with Codeine Cough Syrup and the reference preparation were bioequivalent.

Pharmacokinetic parameters for Actifed with Codeine Cough Syrup are as follows: [See table below].

Indications and Usage: Actifed with Codeine Cough Syrup is indicated for temporary relief of coughs and upper respiratory symptoms, including nasal congestion, associated with allergy or the common cold.

Contraindications: Actifed with Codeine Cough Syrup is contraindicated under the following conditions:

Use in Newborn or Premature Infants: This drug should *not* be used in newborn or premature infants.

Use in Lower Respiratory Disease: Antihistamines should *not* be used to treat lower respiratory tract symptoms, including asthma.

Hypersensitivity to: 1) codeine phosphate or other narcotics; 2) triprolidine hydrochloride or other antihistamines of similar chemical structure; 3) sympathomimetic amines, including pseudoephedrine.

Sympathomimetic amines are contraindicated in patients with severe hypertension, severe coronary artery disease and in patients on monoamine oxidase (MAO) inhibitor therapy (see Drug Interaction Section).

Warnings: Actifed with Codeine Cough Syrup should be used with considerable caution in patients with increased intraocular pressure (narrow angle glaucoma), stenosing peptic ulcer, pyloroduodenal obstruction, symptomatic prostatic hypertrophy, bladder neck obstruction, hypertension, diabetes mellitus, ischemic heart disease, and hyperthyroidism.

In the presence of head injury or other intracranial lesions, the respiratory depressant effects of codeine and other narcotics may be markedly enhanced, as well as their capacity for elevating cerebrospinal fluid pressure.

Narcotics also produce other CNS depressant effects, such as drowsiness, that may further obscure the clinical course of patients with head injuries. Codeine or other narcotics may obscure signs on which to judge the diagnosis or clinical course of patients with acute abdominal conditions.

Precautions:

General: Actifed with Codeine Cough Syrup should be prescribed with caution for certain special-risk patients, such as the eldery or debilitated, and for those with severe impairment of renal or hepatic function, gallbladder disease or gallstones, respiratory impairment, cardiac arrhythmias, history of bronchial asthma, prostatic hypertrophy or urethral stricture, and in patients known to be taking other antitussive, antihistamine or decongestant medications. Patients' self-medication habits should be investigated to determine their use of such medications. Actifed with Codeine Cough Syrup is intended for short-term use only.

Information for Patients:

1. Patients should be warned about engaging in activities requiring mental alertness such as driving a car, operating dangerous machinery or hazardous appliances.
2. Patients with a history of glaucoma, peptic ulcer, urinary retention or pregnancy should be cautioned before starting Actifed.
3. Patients should be told not to take alcohol, sleeping pills, sedatives or tranquilizers while taking Actifed.
4. Antihistamines as in Actifed, may cause dizziness, drowsiness, dry mouth, blurred vision, weakness, nausea, headache or nervousness in some patients.
5. Patients should be told to store this medicine in a tightly closed container in a dry, cool place away from heat or direct sunlight and out of the reach of children.
6. **Nursing Mothers** refer to following section titled "Nursing Mothers."

Actifed with Codeine Cough Syrup should not be used by persons intolerant to sympathomimetics used for the relief of nasal congestion. Such drugs include ephedrine, epinephrine, phenylpropanolamine, and phenylphrine. Symptoms of intolerance include drowsiness, dizziness, weakness, difficulty in breathing, tenseness, muscle tremors or palpitations.

Codeine may be habit-forming when used over long periods or in high doses. Patients should take the drug only for as long, in the amounts, and as frequently as prescribed.

Drug Interactions: Actifed with Codeine Cough Syrup may **enhance** the effects of:

1. monoamine oxidase (MAO) inhibitors;
2. other narcotic analgesics, alcohol, general anesthetics, tranquilizers, sedative-hypnotics, surgical skeletal muscle relaxants, or other CNS depressants, by causing increased CNS depression.

Actifed with Codeine Cough Syrup may **diminish:** the antihypertensive effects of guanethidine, bethanidine, methyldopa, and reserpine.

Drug/Laboratory Test Interactions:

Codeine: Narcotic administration may increase serum amylase levels.

Carcinogenesis, Mutagenesis, Impairment of Fertility: No adequate studies have been conducted in animals to determine whether the components of Actifed with Codeine Cough Syrup have a potential for carcinogenesis, mutagenesis or impairment of fertility.

Pregnancy: *Teratogenic Effects:* Pregnancy Category C. Animal reproduction studies have not been conducted with Actifed with Codeine Cough Syrup. It is also not known whether Actifed with Codeine Cough Syrup can cause fetal harm when administered to a pregnant woman or can affect reproduction capacity. Actifed with Codeine Cough Syrup should be given to a pregnant woman only if clearly needed.

Teratology studies have been conducted with three of the ingredients of Actifed with Codeine Cough Syrup. Pseudoephedrine studies were conducted in rats at doses up to 150 times the human dose; triprolidine was studied in rats and rabbits at doses up to 125 times the human dose and codeine studies were conducted in rats and rabbits at doses up to 150 times the human dose. No evidence of teratogenic harm to the fetus was revealed in any of these studies. However, overt signs of toxicity were observed in the dams which received pseudoephedrine. This was reflected in reduced average weight and length and rate of skeletal ossification in their fetuses.

Nursing Mothers: The components of Actifed with Codeine Cough Syrup are excreted in breast milk in small amounts, but the significance of their effects on nursing infants is not known. Because of the potential for serious adverse reactions in nursing infants from maternal ingestion of Actifed with Codeine Cough Syrup, a decision should be made whether to discontinue nursing or to discontinue the drug, taking into account the importance of the drug to the mother.

Pediatric Use: As in adults, the combination of an antihistamine, sympathomimetic amine and codeine can elicit mild stimulation or mild sedation in children. In infants and children particularly, the ingredients in this drug product **in overdosage** may produce hallucinations, convulsions and death. Symptoms of toxicity in children may include fixed dilated pupils, flushed face, dry mouth, fever, excitation, hallucinations, ataxia, incoordination, athetosis, tonic clonic convulsions and postictal depression, (see CONTRAINDICATIONS and OVERDOSAGE sections).

Use in Elderly (approximately 60 years or older): The ingredients in Actifed with Codeine Cough Syrup are more likely to cause adverse reactions in elderly patients.

Parameter	Codeine*	Triprolidine†	Pseudoephedrine‡
Elimination Half Life (hr)	2.7 ± 0.4§	4.0 ± 2.2	5.5 ± 0.9
Time to Maximum Concentration (hr)	1.2 ± 0.5	1.8 ± 0.7	2.6 ± 1.0
Maximum Plasma Concentration (ng/ml)	44.8 ± 11.7	4.9 ± 1.8	189 ± 44
Area Under Plasma Curve from $t = 0$ to $t = \infty$ (ng/ml·hr) (ng/ml·hr)	226 ± 41	42.5 ± 34.0	1938 ± 440

* 20 mg Codeine Phosphate hemihydrate (equivalent to 14.7 mg free base)
† 2.5 mg Triprolidine HCl monohydrate (equivalent to 2.1 mg free base)
‡ 60 mg Pseudoephedrine HCl (equivalent to 49.1 mg free base)
§ Means ± S.D.

Adverse Reactions: (The most frequent adverse reactions are underlined.)
General: Dryness of mouth, dryness of nose, dryness of throat, urticaria, drug rash, anaphylactic shock, photosensitivity, excessive perspiration and chills.
Cardiovascular System: Hypotension, headache, palpitations, tachycardia, extrasystoles.
Hematologic System: Hemolytic anemia, thrombocytopenia, agranulocytosis.
Nervous System: Sedation, sleepiness, dizziness, disturbed coordination, fatigue, confusion, restlessness, excitation, anxiety, nervousness, tremor, irritability, insomnia, euphoria, paresthesias, blurred vision, diplopia, vertigo, tinnitus, acute labyrinthitis, hysteria, neuritis, convulsions, CNS depression, hallucination.
G.I. System: Epigastric distress, anorexia, nausea, vomiting, diarrhea, constipation.
G.U. System: Urinary frequency, difficult urination, urinary retention, early menses.
Respiratory System: Thickening of bronchial secretions, tightness of chest and wheezing, nasal stuffiness, respiratory depression.
Drug Abuse and Dependence: Like other medications containing a narcotic, Actifed with Codeine Cough Syrup is controlled by the Drug Enforcement Administration and is classified under Schedule V.
Actifed with Codeine Cough Syrup can produce drug dependence of the morphine type, and therefore it has a potential for being abused. Psychic dependence, physical dependence and tolerance may develop on repeated administration.
The dependence liability of codeine has been found to be too small to permit a full definition of its characteristics. Studies indicate that addiction to codeine is extremely uncommon and requires very high parenteral doses.
When dependence on codeine occurs at therapeutic doses, it appears to require from one to two months to develop, and withdrawal symptoms are mild. Most patients on long-term oral codeine therapy show no signs of physical dependence upon abrupt withdrawal.
Overdosage: Since Actifed with Codeine Cough Syrup is comprised of three pharmacologically different compounds, it is difficult to predict the exact manifestation of symptoms in a given individual. Reaction to an overdosage of Actifed with Codeine Cough Syrup may vary from CNS depression to stimulation. A detailed description of symptoms which are likely to appear after ingestion of an excess of the individual components follows.
Overdosage with codeine can cause transient euphoria, drowsiness, dizziness, weariness, diminution of sensibility, loss of sensation, vomiting, transient excitement in children and occasionally in adult women, miosis progressing to nonreactive pinpoint pupils, itching sometimes with skin rashes and urticaria, and clammy skin with mottled cyanosis. In more severe cases, muscular relaxation with depressed or absent superficial and deep reflexes and a positive Babinski sign may appear. Marked slowing of the respiratory rate with inadequate pulmonary ventilation and consequent cyanosis may occur. Terminal signs include shock, pulmonary edema, hypostatic or aspiration pneumonia and respiratory arrest, with death occurring within 6–12 hours following ingestion.
Overdoses of antihistamines may cause hallucinations, convulsions, or possibly death, especially in infants and children. Antihistamines are more likely to cause dizziness, sedation, and hypotension in elderly patients.
Overdoses with triprolidine may produce reactions varying from depression to stimulation of the Central Nervous System (CNS); the latter is particularly likely in children. Atropine-like signs and symptoms (dry mouth, fixed dilated pupils, flushing, tachycardia, hallucinations, convulsions, urinary retention, cardiac arrthymias and coma) may occur.
Overdosage with pseudoephedrine can cause excessive CNS stimulation resulting in excitement, nervousness, anxiety, tremor, restlessness and insomnia. Other effects include tachycardia, hypertension, pallor, mydriasis, hyperglycemia and urinary retention. Severe overdosage may cause tachypnea or hyperpnea, hallucinations, convulsions, or delirium, but in some individuals there may be CNS depression with somnolence, stupor or respiratory depression. Arrhythmias (including ventricular fibrillation) may lead to hypotension and circulatory collapse. Severe hypokalemia can occur probably due to compartmental shift rather than depletion of potassium. No organ damage or significant metabolic derangement is associated with pseudoephedrine overdosage.
The toxic plasma concentration of codeine is not known with certainty. Experimental production of mild to moderate CNS depression in healthy, non-tolerant subjects occurs at plasma concentrations of 0.5–1.9 µg/ml when codeine is given by intravenous infusion. The single lethal dose of codeine in adults is estimated to be from 0.5 to 1.0 gram. It is also estimated that 5 mg/kg could be fatal in children.
The LD$_{50}$ (single, oral dose) of triprolidine is 163 to 308 mg/kg in the mouse (depending upon strain) and 840 mg/kg in the rat.
Insufficient data are available to estimate the toxic and lethal doses of triprolidine in humans. No reports of acute poisoning with triprolidine have appeared.
The LD$_{50}$ (single, oral dose) of pseudoephedrine is 726 mg/kg in the mouse, 2206 mg/kg in the rat and 1177 mg/kg in the rabbit. The toxic and lethal concentrations in human biologic fluids are not known. Excretion rates increase with urine acidification and decrease with alkalinization. Few reports of toxicity due to pseudoephedrine have been published and no case of fatal overdosage is known.
Therapy, if instituted within 4 hours of overdosage, is aimed at reducing further absorption of the drug. In the conscious patient, vomiting should be induced even though it may have occurred spontaneously. If vomiting cannot be induced, gastric lavage is indicated. Adequate precautions must be taken to protect against aspiration, especially in infants and children. Charcoal slurry or other suitable agents should be instilled into the stomach after vomiting or lavage. Saline cathartics or milk of magnesia may be of additional benefit.
In the unconscious patient, the airway should always be secured with a cuffed endotracheal tube before attempting to evacuate the gastric contents. Intensive supportive and nursing care is indicated, as for any comatose patients.
If breathing is significantly impaired, maintenance of adequate airway and mechanical support of respiration is the most effective means of providing adequate oxygenation.
Hypotension is an early sign of inpending cardiovascular collapse and should be treated vigorously. Do not use CNS stimulants. Convulsions should be controlled by careful administration of diazepam or short-acting barbiturate, repeated as necessary. Physostigmine may be also considered for use in controlling medicated convulsions.
Ice packs and cooling sponge baths, not alcohol, can aid in reducing the fever commonly seen in children.
For codeine, continuous stimulation that arouses, but does not exhaust, the patient is useful in preventing coma. Continuous or intermittent oxygen therapy is usually indicated, while Naloxone is useful as a codeine antidote. Close nursing care is essential.
Saline cathartics, such as Milk of Magnesia, help to dilute the concentration of the drugs in the bowel by drawing water into the gut, thereby hastening drug elimination.
Adrenergic receptor blocking agents are antidotes to pseudoephedrine. In practice, the most useful is the beta-blocker propranolol, which is indicated when there are signs of cardiac toxicity.
There are no specific antidotes to triprolidine. Histamine should not be given.
Pseudoephedrine and codeine are theoretically dialyzable, but the procedures have not been clinically established.
In severe cases of overdosage, it is essential to monitor both the heart (by electrocardiograph) and plasma electrolytes and to give intravenous potassium as indicated by these continuous controls. Vasopressors may be used to treat hypotension, and excessive CNS stimulation may be counteracted with parenteral diazepam. Stimulants should not be used.

Dosage and Administration: DOSAGE SHOULD BE INDIVIDUALIZED ACCORDING TO THE NEEDS AND RESPONSE OF THE PATIENT.
Usual Dose:

	Teaspoonfuls (5 ml)	
Adults and children 12 years and older	2	every 4–6 hours not to exceed 4 doses in a 24-hour period
Children 6 to under 12 years	1	
Children 2 to under 6 years	½	

How Supplied: Bottles of one pint (NDC-0081-0025-96), and one gallon (NDC-0081-0025-57). Store at 15°–30°C (59°–86°F) and protect from light.

AEROSPORIN® ℞
[air'ō-spor"ĭn]
brand Polymyxin B Sulfate
Sterile Powder
Polymyxin B Sulfate for Parenteral and/or Ophthalmic Administration

---
WARNING
CAUTION: WHEN THIS DRUG IS GIVEN INTRAMUSCULARLY AND/OR INTRATHECALLY, IT SHOULD BE GIVEN ONLY TO HOSPITALIZED PATIENTS, SO AS TO PROVIDE CONSTANT SUPERVISION BY A PHYSICIAN.
RENAL FUNCTION SHOULD BE CAREFULLY DETERMINED AND PATIENTS WITH RENAL DAMAGE AND NITROGEN RETENTION SHOULD HAVE REDUCED DOSAGE. PATIENTS WITH NEPHROTOXICITY DUE TO POLYMYXIN B SULFATE USUALLY SHOW ALBUMINURIA, CELLULAR CASTS, AND AZOTEMIA. DIMINISHING URINE OUTPUT AND A RISING BUN ARE INDICATIONS FOR DISCONTINUING THERAPY WITH THIS DRUG.
NEUROTOXIC REACTIONS MAY BE MANIFESTED BY IRRITABILITY, WEAKNESS, DROWSINESS, ATAXIA, PERIORAL PARESTHESIA, NUMBNESS OF THE EXTREMITIES, AND BLURRING OF VISION. THESE ARE USUALLY ASSOCIATED WITH HIGH SERUM LEVELS FOUND IN PATIENTS WITH IMPAIRED RENAL FUNCTION AND/OR NEPHROTOXICITY. THE CONCURRENT USE OF OTHER NEPHROTOXIC AND NEUROTOXIC DRUGS, PARTICULARLY KANAMYCIN, STREPTOMYCIN, CEPHALORIDINE, PAROMOMYCIN, TOBRAMYCIN, POLYMYXIN E (COLISTIN), NEOMYCIN, GENTAMICIN, AND VIOMYCIN, SHOULD BE AVOIDED.
THE NEUROTOXICITY OF POLYMYXIN B SULFATE CAN RESULT IN RESPIRATORY PARALYSIS FROM NEUROMUSCULAR BLOCKADE, ESPECIALLY WHEN THE DRUG IS GIVEN SOON AFTER ANESTHESIA AND/OR MUSCLE RELAXANTS.
USAGE IN PREGNANCY: THE SAFETY OF THIS DRUG IN HUMAN PREGNANCY HAS NOT BEEN ESTABLISHED.

Description: Polymyxin B sulfate is one of a group of basic polypeptide antibiotics derived from *B polymyxa* (*B aerosporous*).
Aerosporin brand Sterile Polymyxin B Sulfate is in powder form suitable for preparation of sterile solutions for intramuscular, intravenous drip, intrathecal, or ophthalmic use.
In the medical literature, dosages have frequently been given in terms of equivalent weight of pure polymyxin B base. Each milligram of pure polymyxin B base is equivalent to 10,000 units of poly-

Continued on next page

Burroughs Wellcome—Cont.

myxin B and each microgram of pure polymyxin B base is equivalent to 10 units of polymyxin B.
Aqueous solutions of Aerosporin brand Polymyxin B Sulfate may be stored up to 12 months without significant loss of potency if kept under refrigeration. In the interest of safety, solutions for parenteral use should be stored under refrigeration and any unused portion should be discarded after 72 hours. Polymyxin B sulfate should not be stored in alkaline solutions since they are less stable.
Actions: Aerosporin brand Polymyxin B Sulfate has a bactericidal action against almost all gram-negative bacilli except the *Proteus* group. Polymyxins increase the permeability of bacterial cell wall membranes. All gram-positive bacteria, fungi, and the gram-negative cocci, *N gonorrhoeae* and *N meningitidis*, are resistant.
Susceptibility plate testing: If the Kirby-Bauer method of disc susceptibility testing is used, a 300-unit polymyxin B disc should give a zone of over 11 mm when tested against a polymyxin B-susceptible bacterial strain.
Polymyxin B sulfate is not absorbed from the normal alimentary tract. Since the drug loses 50 percent of its activity in the presence of serum, active blood levels are low. Repeated injections may give a cumulative effect. Levels tend to be higher in infants and children. The drug is excreted slowly by the kidneys. Tissue diffusion is poor and the drug does not pass the blood brain barrier into the cerebrospinal fluid. In therapeutic dosage, polymyxin B sulfate causes some nephrotoxicity with tubule damage to a slight degree.
Indications: Acute Infections Caused by Susceptible Strains of *Pseudomonas aeruginosa*. Polymyxin B sulfate is a drug of choice in the treatment of infections of the urinary tract, meninges, and bloodstream caused by susceptible strains of *Ps aeruginosa*. It may also be used topically and subconjunctivally in the treatment of infections of the eye caused by susceptible strains of *Ps aeruginosa*.
It may be indicated in serious infections caused by susceptible strains of the following organisms, when less potentially toxic drugs are ineffective or contraindicated:
H. influenzae, specifically meningeal infections.
Escherichia coli, specifically urinary tract infections.
Aerobacter aerogenes, specifically bacteremia.
Klebsiella pneumoniae, specifically bacteremia.
Note. In Meningeal Infections, Polymyxin B Sulfate Should Be Administered Only by the Intrathecal Route.
Contraindications: This drug is contraindicated in persons with a prior history of hypersensitivity reactions to the polymyxins.
Precautions: See "Warning" box.
Baseline renal function should be done prior to therapy, with frequent monitoring of renal function and blood levels of the drug during parenteral therapy.
Avoid concurrent use of a curariform muscle relaxant and other neurotoxic drugs (ether, tubocurarine, succinylcholine, gallamine, decamethonium and sodium citrate) which may precipitate respiratory depression. If signs of respiratory paralysis appear, respiration should be assisted as required, and the drug discontinued.
As with other antibiotics, use of this drug may result in overgrowth of nonsusceptible organisms, including fungi. If superinfection occurs, appropriate therapy should be instituted.
Adverse Reactions: See "Warning" box.
Nephrotoxic reactions: Albuminuria, cylinduria, azotemia, and rising blood levels without any increase in dosage.
Neurotoxic reactions: Facial flushing, dizziness progressing to ataxia, drowsiness, peripheral paresthesias (circumoral and stocking-glove), apnea due to concurrent use of curariform muscle relaxants and other neurotoxic drugs or inadvertent overdosage, and signs of meningeal irritation with intrathecal administration, e.g., fever, headache,

stiff neck and increased cell count and protein cerebrospinal fluid.
Other reactions occasionally reported: Drug fever, urticarial rash, pain (severe) at intramuscular injection sites, and thrombophlebitis at intravenous injection sites.
Dosage and Administration:
PARENTERAL:
Intravenous. Dissolve 500,000 units polymyxin B sulfate in 300-500 cc of 5 percent dextrose in water for continuous intravenous drip.
Adults and children. 15,000-25,000 units/kg body weight/day in individuals with normal kidney function. This amount should be reduced from 15,000 units/kg downward for individuals with kidney impairment. Infusions may be given every 12 hours; however, the total daily dose must not exceed 25,000 units/kg/day.
Infants. Infants with normal kidney function may receive up to 40,000 units/kg/day without adverse effects.
Intramuscular. Not recommended routinely because of severe pain at injection sites, particularly in infants and children. Dissolve 500,000 units polymyxin B sulfate in 2 cc sterile distilled water (Water for Injection, U.S.P.) or sterile physiologic saline (Sodium Chloride Injection, U.S.P.) or 1 percent procaine hydrochloride solution.
Adults and children. 25,000-30,000 units/kg/ day. This should be reduced in the presence of renal impairment. The dosage may be divided and given at either 4- or 6-hour intervals.
Infants. Infants with normal kidney function may receive up to 40,000 units/kg/day without adverse effects.
Note. Doses as high as 45,000 units/kg/day have been used in limited clinical studies in treating prematures and newborn infants for sepsis caused by *Ps aeruginosa*.
Intrathecal. A treatment of choice for *Ps aeruginosa* meningitis. Dissolve 500,000 units polymyxin B sulfate in 10 cc of sterile physiologic saline (Sodium Chloride Injection, U.S.P.) for 50,000 units per ml dosage unit.
Adults and children over 2 years of age. Dosage is 50,000 units once daily intrathecally for 3-4 days, then 50,000 units once every other day for at least 2 weeks after cultures of the cerebrospinal fluid are negative and sugar content has returned to normal.
Children under 2 years of age. 20,000 units once daily, intrathecally for 3-4 days or 25,000 units once every other day. Continue with a dose of 25,000 units once every other day for at least 2 weeks after cultures of the cerebrospinal fluid are negative and sugar content has returned to normal.
IN THE INTEREST OF SAFETY, SOLUTIONS FOR PARENTERAL USE SHOULD BE STORED UNDER REFRIGERATION, AND ANY UNUSED PORTIONS SHOULD BE DISCARDED AFTER 72 HOURS.

TOPICAL:
Ophthalmic. Dissolve 500,000 units polymyxin B sulfate in 20-50 cc sterile distilled water (Water for Injection, U.S.P.) or sterile physiologic saline (Sodium Chloride Injection U.S.P.) for a 10,000-25,000 units per cc concentration.
For the treatment of *Ps aeruginosa* infections of the eye, a concentration of 0.1 percent to 0.25 percent (10,000 units to 25,000 units per cc) is administered 1-3 drops every hour, increasing the intervals as response indicates.
Subconjunctival injection of up to 10,000 units/- day may be used for the treatment of *Ps aeruginosa* infections of the cornea and conjunctiva.
Note. Avoid total systemic and ophthalmic instillation over 25,000 units/kg/day.
AVAILABLE DOSAGE FORM
500,000 units.
Rubber-stoppered vial with flip off cap.
Vial—VA NSN 6505-00-913-3124

ALKERAN®
[al-kur'an]
(Melphalan)
2 mg Scored Tablets

> **WARNING:** Melphalan is leukemogenic in humans.
> Melphalan produces chromosomal aberrations *in vitro* and *in vivo* and therefore should be considered potentially mutagenic in humans.
> Melphalan produces amenorrhea.

Description: Alkeran (melphalan), also known as L-phenylalanine mustard, phenylalanine mustard, L-PAM, or L-sarcolysin, is a phenylalanine derivative of nitrogen mustard. Alkeran is a bifunctional alkylating agent which is active against selective human neoplastic diseases. It is known chemically as 4-[bis(2-chloroethyl)amino]-*L*-phenylalanine and has the following structural formula:

$$(ClCH_2CH_2)_2N\text{-}\text{-}CH_2\text{-}\underset{H}{\overset{NH_2}{C}}\text{-}COOH$$

Melphalan is the active L-isomer of the compound and was first synthesized in 1953 by Bergel and Stock; the D-isomer, known as medphalan, is less active against certain animal tumors, and the dose needed to produce effects on chromosomes is larger than that required with the L-isomer. The racemic (DL-) form is known as merphalan or sarcolysin. Melphalan is insoluble in water and has a pKa_1 of ~ 2.1.
Alkeran (melphalan) is available in 2 mg scored tablets for oral administration.
Clinical Pharmacology: Alberts et al[1] found that plasma melphalan levels are highly variable after oral dosing, both with respect to the time of the first appearance of melphalan in plasma (range 0 to 336 minutes) and to the peak plasma concentration (range 0.166 to 3.741 µg/ml) achieved.[2] These results may be due to incomplete intestinal absorption, a variable "first pass" hepatic metabolism, or to rapid hydrolysis. Five patients were studied after both oral and intravenous dosing with 0.6 mg/kg as a single bolus dose by each route. The areas under the plasma concentration-time curves after oral administration averaged $61 \pm 26\%$ ($\pm$ standard deviation; range 25 to 89%) of those following intravenous administration. In 18 patients given a single oral dose of 0.6 mg/kg of melphalan, the terminal plasma half-disappearance time of parent drug was 89.5 ± 50 minutes. The 24-hour urinary excretion of parent drug in these patients was $10 \pm 4.5\%$, suggesting that renal clearance is not a major route of elimination of parent drug.
Tattersall et al,[3] using universally labeled ^{14}C-melphalan, found substantially less radioactivity in the urine of patients given the drug by mouth (30% of administered dose in nine days) than in the urine of those given it intravenously (35 to 65% in seven days). Following either oral or intravenous administration, the pattern of label recovery was similar, with the majority being recovered in the first 24 hours. Following oral administration, peak radioactivity occurred in plasma at two hours and then disappeared with a half-life of approximately 160 hours. In one patient where parent drug (rather than just radiolabel) was determined, the melphalan half-disappearance time was 67 minutes.[3]
Indications and Usage: Alkeran (melphalan) is indicated for the palliative treatment of multiple myeloma and for the palliation of non-resectable epithelial carcinoma of the ovary.
Contraindications: Melphalan should not be used in patients whose disease has demonstrated a prior resistance to this agent. Patients who have demonstrated hypersensitivity to melphalan should not be given the drug.

Warnings: As with other nitrogen mustard drugs, excessive damage will produce marked bone marrow depression. Frequent blood counts are essential to determine optimal dosage and to avoid toxicity. The drug should be discontinued or the dosage reduced upon evidence of depression of the bone marrow.

There are many reports of patients with multiple myeloma who have developed acute, non-lymphatic leukemia following therapy with alkylating agents (including melphalan). Evaluation of published reports strongly suggests that melphalan is leukemogenic in patients with multiple myeloma. The potential benefits from the drug and potential risk of carcinogenesis must be evaluated on an individual basis.

Pregnancy: "Pregnancy Category D." Melphalan may cause fetal harm when administered to a pregnant woman. Animal reproduction studies have not been conducted with melphalan. There are no adequate and well-controlled studies in pregnant women. If this drug is used during pregnancy, or if the patient becomes pregnant while taking this drug, the patient should be apprised of the potential hazard to the fetus. Women of childbearing potential should be advised to avoid becoming pregnant.

Precautions:
General: Melphalan should be used with extreme caution in patients whose bone marrow reserve may have been compromised by prior irradiation or chemotherapy, or whose marrow function is recovering from previous cytotoxic therapy. If the leukocyte count falls below 3,000/µl, or the platelet count below 100,000 µl, the drug should be discontinued until the peripheral blood cell counts have recovered.

A recommendation as to whether or not dosage reduction should be made routinely in patients with impaired creatinine clearance cannot be made because:
(a) There is considerable inherent patient-to-patient variability in the systemic availability of melphalan in patients with normal renal function.
(b) There is only a small amount of the administered dose that appears as parent drug in the urine of patients with normal renal function.

Patients with azotemia should be closely observed, however, in order to make dosage reductions, if required, at the earliest possible time.

Information for Patients: Patients should be informed that the major toxicities of melphalan are related to myelosuppression, hypersensitivity, gastrointestinal toxicity, pulmonary toxicity, infertility, and non-lymphocytic leukemia. Patients should never be allowed to take the drug without close medical supervision and should be advised to consult their physician if they experience skin rash, vasculitis, bleeding, fever, persistent cough, nausea, vomiting, amenorrhea, weight loss, or unusual lumps/masses. Women of childbearing potential should be advised to avoid becoming pregnant.

Laboratory Tests: Weekly examination of the blood should be made to determine hemoglobin levels, total and differential leukocyte counts, and platelet enumeration. Patients may develop symptoms of anemia if the hemoglobin falls below 9–10 gm/dl, and are at risk of severe infection if the absolute neutrophil count is below 1,000/mm^3, and may bleed if the platelet count falls below 50,000/mm^3.

Drug Interactions: There are no known drug/drug interactions with melphalan.

Carcinogenesis, Mutagenesis, Impairment of Fertility: In an animal study to evaluate carcinogenesis, rats were given melphalan i.p. 3 times weekly for six months in doses ten to twenty times greater than the recommended dose in man. Fifty percent (50%) of the animals developed peritoneal sarcomas. Males and females developed lung tumors in excess of controls.[4] In a 39-week test melphalan produced a dose-related increase in lung tumors in mice.[5]

There are several reports of acute non-lymphocytic leukemia arising in patients with multiple myeloma and ovarian carcinoma following melphalan treatment.[6,7,8] In many instances, these patients also received other chemotherapeutic agents or some form of radiation therapy. The quantitation of the risk of melphalan-induction of leukemia or carcinoma in humans is not possible. Evaluation of published reports of leukemia developing in patients who have received melphalan (and other alkylating agents) suggests that the risk of leukemogenesis increases with both chronicity of treatment and large cumulative doses. However, it has proved impossible to find a cumulative dose below which there is no risk of the induction of secondary malignancy. The potential benefits from melphalan therapy must be weighed on an individual basis against the possible risk of the induction of a second malignancy.

Melphalan has been shown to cause chromatid or chromosome damage in man.[9] Melphalan causes suppression of ovarian function in pre-menopausal women, resulting in amenorrhea in a significant number of patients.[10,11]

Pregnancy: *Teratogenic Effects:* Pregnancy Category D: See WARNINGS section.

Nursing Mothers: It is not known whether this drug is excreted in human milk. Because many drugs are excreted in human milk and because of the potential for serious adverse reactions in nursing infants from melphalan, a decision should be made whether to discontinue nursing or to discontinue the drug, taking into account the importance of the drug to the mother.

Pediatric Use: The safety and effectiveness in children have not been established.

Adverse Reactions:
Hematologic Effects: The most common side effect is bone marrow suppression.[12] Although bone marrow suppression frequently occurs, it is usually reversible if melphalan is withdrawn early enough. However, irreversible bone marrow failure has been reported.[13,14]

Gastrointestinal: Gastrointestinal disturbances such as nausea and vomiting, diarrhea and oral ulceration occur infrequently.

Miscellaneous: Other reported adverse reactions include: pulmonary fibrosis[15,16] and interstitial pneumonitis, skin hypersensitivity, vasculitis, alopecia, hemolytic anemia, and allergic reaction.

Overdosage: Immediate effects are likely to be vomiting, ulceration of the mouth, diarrhea and hemorrhage of the gastrointestinal tract. The main toxic effect is on the bone marrow, and there is no known antidote. The blood picture should be closely followed for three to six weeks. General supportive measures, together with appropriate blood transfusions and antibiotics, should be instituted if necessary. This drug is not removed from plasma to any significant degree by hemodialysis.[17]

The oral LD$_{50}$ dose in mice is 21 mg/kg.

Dosage and Administration:
Multiple Myeloma: The usual oral dose is 6 mg (3 tablets) daily. The entire daily dose may be given at one time. It is adjusted, as required, on the basis of blood counts done at approximately weekly intervals. After two to three weeks of treatment, the drug should be discontinued for up to four weeks during which time the blood count should be followed carefully. When the white blood cell and platelet counts are rising, a maintenance dose of 2 mg daily may be instituted. Because of the patient-to-patient variation in melphalan plasma levels following oral administration of the drug, several investigators have recommended that melphalan dosage be cautiously escalated until some myelosuppression is observed, in order to assure that potentially therapeutic levels of the drug have been reached.[1,3]

Other dosage regimens have been used by various investigators. Osserman and Takatsuki have used an initial course of 10 mg/day for seven to ten days.[18,19] They report that maximal suppression of the leukocyte and platelet counts occurs within three to five weeks and recovery within four to eight weeks. Continuous maintenance therapy with 2 mg/day is instituted when the white blood cell count is greater than 4,000 and the platelet count is greater than 100,000. Dosage is adjusted to between 1 and 3 mg/day depending upon the hematological response. It is desirable to try to maintain a significant degree of bone marrow depression so as to keep the leukocyte count in the range of 3,000 to 3,500 cells/µl.

Hoogstraten et al have started treatment with 0.15 mg/kg/day for seven days.[20] This is followed by a rest period of at least 14 days, but it may be as long as five to six weeks. Maintenance therapy is started when the white blood cell and platelet counts are rising. The maintenance dose is 0.05 mg/kg per day or less and is adjusted according to the blood count.

Available evidence suggests that about one third to one half of the patients with multiple myeloma show a favorable response to oral administration of the drug.

One study by Alexanian et al has shown that the use of melphalan in combination with prednisone significantly improves the percentage of patients with multiple myeloma who achieve palliation.[21] One regimen has been to administer courses of melphalan at 0.25 mg/kg/day for four consecutive days (or, 0.20 mg/kg/day for five consecutive days) for a total dose of 1 mg/kg per course. These four- to five-day courses are then repeated every four to six weeks if the granulocyte count and the platelet count have returned to normal levels.

It is to be emphasized that response may be very gradual over many months; it is important that repeated courses or continuous therapy be given since improvement may continue slowly over many months, and the maximum benefit may be missed if treatment is abandoned too soon.

In patients with moderate to severe renal impairment, currently available pharmacokinetic data does not justify an absolute recommendation on dosage reduction to those patients, but it may be prudent to use a reduced dose initially.[22,23]

Epithelial Ovarian Cancer: One commonly employed regimen for the treatment of ovarian carcinoma has been to administer melphalan at a dose of 0.2 mg/kg daily for five days as a single course. Courses are repeated every four to five weeks depending upon hematologic tolerance.[24,25]

How Supplied: White, scored tablets containing 2 mg melphalan, imprinted with "ALKERAN" and "A2A"; in bottle of 50 (NDC-0081-0045-35). Store at 15°–25°C (59°–77°F) in a dry place and protect from light.

References:
1. Alberts DS et al: Oral Melphalan Kinetics. *Clin Pharmacol Ther*, 26(6):737–745, 1979.
2. Alberts DS et al: Unpublished Data on File with Burroughs Wellcome Co., 1981.
3. Tattersall MHN et al: Pharmacokinetics of Melphalan Following Oral or Intravenous Administration in Patients with Malignant Disease. *Europ J Cancer*, 11:507–513, 1977.
4. Weisburger JH et al: The Carcinogenic Properties of Some of the Principal Drugs used in Clinical Cancer Chemotherapy. *Recent Results Cancer Res*, 52:1–17, 1975.
5. Shimkin MB et al: Bioassay of 29 Alkylating Chemicals by the Pulmonary-Tumor Response in Strain A Mice. *J Natl Cancer Inst*, 36:915–935, 1966.
6. Meytes D, Seligsohn U and Ramot B: Multiple Myeloma with Terminal Erythroleukemia. *Acta Haemat*, 55:358–362, 1976.
7. Reimer RR et al: Acute Leukemia after Alkylating-Agent Therapy of Ovarian Cancer. *N Engl J Med*, 297(4):177–181, 1977.
8. Einhorn N et al: Acute Leukemia After Chemotherapy (Melphalan). *Cancer*, 41:444–447, 1978.
9. Sharpe HB: Observations on the Effect of Therapy with Nitrogen Mustard or a Derivative on Chromosomes of Human Peripheral Blood Lymphocytes. *Cell Tissue Kinet*, 4:501–504, 1971.
10. Rose DP and David TE: Ovarian Function in Patients Receiving Adjuvant Chemotherapy for Breast Cancer. *Lancet*, 1:1174–1176, 1977.
11. Ahmann DL et al: Repeated Adjuvant Chemotherapy with Phenylalanine Mustard or 5-

Continued on next page

Burroughs Wellcome—Cont.

Fluorouracil, Cyclophosphamide and Prednisone With or Without Radiation, After Mastectomy for Breast Cancer. *Lancet, 1:* 893–896, 1978.
12. Speed DE *et al:* Melphalan in the Treatment of Myelomatosis. *Br Med J, 1:* 1664–1669, 1964.
13. Smith JP and Rutledge F: Chemotherapy in the Treatment of Cancer of the Ovary. *Am J Obstet Gynecol, 107:* 691–703, 1970.
14. Bergsagel DE *et al:* The Treatment of Plasma Cell Myeloma. *Adv Cancer Research, 10:* 311–359, 1967.
15. Taetle R, Dickman PS and Feldman PS. Pulmonary Histopathologic Changes Associated with Melphalan Therapy. *Cancer, 42:* 1239–1245, 1978.
16. Westerfield BT *et al:* Reversible Melphalan-Induced Lung Damage. *Am J Med, 68:* 767–771, 1980.
17. Pallante SL *et al:* Quantitation by Gas Chromatography-Chemical Ionization-Mass Spectrometry of Phenylalanine Mustard in Plasma of Patients. *Cancer Res, 40:* 2268–2272, 1980.
18. Osserman EF: Therapy of Plasma Cell Myeloma with Melphalan. *Proc Am Assoc Cancer Res, 4:* 50, 1963.
19. Osserman EF and Takatsuki K: Plasma Cell Myeloma: Gamma Globulin Synthesis and Structure. *Medicine, 42:* 357–384, 1963.
20. Hoogstraten B *et al:* Melphalan in Multiple Myeloma. *Blood, 30(1):* 74–83, 1967.
21. Alexanian R *et al:* Treatment for Multiple Myeloma. *JAMA, 208(9):* 1680–1685, 1969.
22. Alberts DS *et al:* Comparative Pharmokinetics of Chlorambucil and Melphalan in Man. *Recent Results Cancer Res, 74:* 124–131, 1980.
23. Alberts DS *et al:* Effect of Renal Dysfunction in Dogs on the Disposition and Marrow Toxicity of Melphalan. *Brit J Cancer, 43:* 330–334, 1981.
24. Smith JP and Rutledge FN: Chemotherapy in Advanced Ovarian Cancer. *Natl Cancer Inst Monogr, 42:* 141–143, 1975.
25. Young RC *et al:* Advanced Ovarian Adenocarcinoma. *N Engl J Med, 299(23):* 1261–1266, 1978.

Shown in Product Identification Section, page 407

ANECTINE®
[ă-nĕk'tēn]
(Succinylcholine Chloride)
Injection, USP

ANECTINE®
(Succinylcholine Chloride)
Sterile Powder Flo-Pack®

This drug should be used only by individuals familiar with its actions, characteristics and hazards.

Description: Anectine (succinylcholine chloride) is an ultra short-acting depolarizing-type, skeletal muscle relaxant for intravenous administration. Succinylcholine chloride is a white, odorless, slightly bitter powder and very soluble in water. The drug is unstable in alkaline solutions but relatively stable in acid solutions, depending upon the concentration of the solution and the storage temperature. Solutions of succinylcholine chloride should be stored under refrigeration to preserve potency. Anectine Injection is a sterile solution for intravenous injection, containing 20 mg succinylcholine chloride in each ml and made isotonic with sodium chloride. The pH is adjusted to 3.5 with hydrochloric acid. Methylparaben (0.1%) is added as a preservative. Anectine® Flo-Pack is a sterile powder, containing either 500 mg or 1000 mg of succinylcholine chloride in each vial. The chemical name for succinylcholine chloride is 2,2'-[(1,4-dioxo-1,4-butanediyl)bis(oxy)]bis[N,N,N-trimethylethanaminium] dichloride.

Clinical Pharmacology: Succinylcholine is a depolarizing skeletal muscle relaxant. As does acetylcholine, it combines with the cholinergic receptors of the motor end plate to produce depolarization. This depolarization may be observed as fasciculations. Subsequent neuromuscular transmission is inhibited so long as adequate concentration of succinylcholine remains at the receptor site. Onset of flaccid paralysis is rapid (less than one minute after intravenous administration), and with single administration lasts approximately 4–6 minutes.

Succinylcholine is rapidly hydrolyzed by plasma pseudocholinesterase to succinylmonocholine (which possesses nondepolarizing muscle relaxant properties) and then more slowly to succinic acid and choline. About 10% of the drug is excreted unchanged in the urine. The paralysis following administration of succinylcholine is selective, initially involving consecutively the levator muscles of the face, muscles of the glottis and finally the intercostals and the diaphragm and all other skeletal muscles.

Succinylcholine has no direct action on the uterus or other smooth muscle structures. Because it is highly ionized and has low fat solubility, it does not readily cross the placenta.

Tachyphylaxis occurs with repeated administration.

When succinylcholine is given over a prolonged period of time, the characteristic depolarizing neuromuscular block (Phase 1 block) may change to a block with characteristics superficially resembling a non-depolarizing block (Phase II block). This may be associated with prolonged respiratory depression or apnea in patients who manifest the transition to Phase II block. When this diagnosis is confirmed by peripheral nerve stimulation, it may be reversed with anticholinesterase drugs such as neostigmine (See Precautions).

While succinylcholine has no direct effect on the myocardium, changes in rhythm may result from vagal stimulation, such as may result from surgical procedures (particularly in children) or from potassium-mediated alterations in electrical conductivity. These effects are enhanced by cyclopropane and halogenated anesthetics.

Succinylcholine causes a slight, transient increase in intraocular pressure immediately after its injection and during the fasciculation phase, and slight increases may persist after onset of complete paralysis. This suggests that the drug should not be used in the presence of open eye injuries.

Succinylcholine has no effect on consciousness, pain threshold or cerebration. It should be used only with adequate anesthesia.

Indications and Usage: Succinylcholine chloride is indicated as an adjunct to general anesthesia, to facilitate endotracheal intubation, and to provide skeletal muscle relaxation during surgery or mechanical ventilation.

Contraindications: Succinylcholine is contraindicated for persons with genetically determined disorders of plasma pseudocholinesterase, personal or familial history of malignant hyperthermia, myopathies associated with elevated creatine phosphokinase (CPK) values, known hypersensitivity to the drug, acute narrow angle glaucoma, and penetrating eye injuries.

Warnings: Succinylcholine should be used only by those skilled in the management of artificial respiration and only when facilities are instantly available for endotracheal intubation and for providing adequate ventilation of the patient, including the administration of oxygen under positive pressure and the elimination of carbon dioxide. The clinician must be prepared to assist or control respiration.

Succinylcholine should not be mixed with short-acting barbiturates in the same syringe or administered simultaneously during intravenous infusion through the same needle. Solutions of succinylcholine have an acid pH, whereas those of barbiturates are alkaline. Depending upon the resultant pH of a mixture of solutions of these drugs, either free barbituric acid may be precipitated or succinylcholine hydrolyzed.

Succinylcholine administration has been associated with acute onset of fulminant hypermetabolism of skeletal muscle known as malignant hyperthermic crisis. This frequently presents as intractable spasm of the jaw muscles which may progress to generalized rigidity, increased oxygen demand, tachycardia, tachypnea and profound hyperpyrexia. Successful outcome depends on recognition of early signs, such as jaw muscle spasm, lack of laryngeal relaxation or generalized rigidity to initial administration of succinylcholine for endotracheal intubation, or failure of tachycardia to respond to deepening anesthesia. Skin mottling, rising temperature and coagulopathies occur late in the course of the hypermetabolic process. Recognition of the syndrome is a signal for discontinuance of anesthesia, attention to increased oxygen consumption, correction of metabolic acidosis, support of circulation, assurance of adequate urinary output and institution of measures to control rising temperature. Dantrolene sodium, intravenously, is recommended as an adjunct to supportive measures in the management of this problem. Consult literature references or the dantrolene prescribing information for additional information about the management of malignant hyperthermic crisis. Routine, continuous monitoring of temperature is recommended as an aid to early recognition of malignant hyperthermia.

Precautions:
General: Low levels or abnormal variants of pseudocholinesterase may be associated with prolonged respiratory depression or apnea following the use of succinylcholine. Low levels of pseudocholinesterase may occur in patients with the following conditions: burns, severe liver disease or cirrhosis, cancer, severe anemia, pregnancy, malnutrition, severe dehydration, collagen diseases, myxedema, and abnormal body temperature. Also, exposure to neurotoxic insecticides, antimalarial or anti-cancer drugs, monoamine oxidase inhibitors, contraceptive pills, pancuronium, chlorpromazine, ecothiopate iodide, or neostigmine may result in low levels of pseudocholinesterase. Succinylcholine should be administered with extreme care to such patients. If low pseudocholinesterase activity is suspected, a small test dose of from 5 to 10 mg of succinylcholine may be administered, or relaxation may be produced by the cautious administration of a 0.1% solution of the drug by intravenous drip. Apnea or prolonged muscle paralysis should be treated with controlled respiration. Succinylcholine should be administered with great caution to patients recovering from severe trauma, those suffering from electrolyte imbalance, those receiving quinidine, and those who have been digitalized recently or who may have digitalis toxicity, because in these circumstances it may induce serious cardiac arrhythmias or cardiac arrest. Great caution should be observed also in patients with pre-existing hyperkalemia, those who are paraplegic, or have suffered extensive or severe burns, extensive denervation of skeletal muscle due to disease or injury of the central nervous system, or have degenerative or dystrophic neuromuscular disease, because such patients tend to become severely hyperkalemic when given succinylcholine.

When succinylcholine is given over a prolonged period of time, the characteristic depolarization block of the myoneural junction (Phase I block) may change to a block with characteristics superficially resembling a non-depolarizing block (Phase II block). Prolonged respiratory depression or apnea may be observed in patients manifesting this transition to Phase II block. The transition from Phase I to Phase II block has been reported in 7 of 7 patients studied under halothane anesthesia after an accumulated dose of 2 to 4 mg/kg succinylcholine (administered in repeated, divided doses). The onset of Phase II block coincided with the onset of tachyphylaxis and prolongation of spontaneous recovery. In another study, using balanced anesthesia (N_2O/O_2/narcotic-thiopental) and succinylcholine infusion, the transition was less abrupt, with great individual variability in the dose of succinylcholine required to produce Phase II block. Of 32 patients studied, 24 developed

ANTEPAR

TABLE I

Dosage Form	Contains	Equivalency in Terms of Piperazine Hexahydrate
Syrup	Piperazine Citrate Anhydrous 550 mg per 5 cc (1 teaspoonful)	500 mg per teaspoonful
Scored Tablet	Piperazine Citrate Anhydrous 550 mg per tablet	500 mg per tablet

Phase II block. Tachyphylaxis was not associated with the transition to Phase II block, and 50% of the patients who developed Phase II block experienced prolonged recovery.

When Phase II block is suspected in cases of prolonged neuromuscular blockage, positive diagnosis should be made by peripheral nerve stimulation, prior to administration of any anticholinesterase drug. Reversal of Phase II block is a medical decision which must be made upon the basis of the individual clinical pharmacology and the experience and judgment of the physician. The presence of Phase II block is indicated by fade of responses to successive stimuli (preferably "train of four"). The use of anticholinesterase drugs to reverse Phase II block should be accompanied by appropriate doses of atropine to prevent disturbances of cardiac rhythm. After adequate reversal of Phase II block with an anticholinesterase agent, the patient should be continually observed for at least 1 hour for signs of return of muscle relaxation. Reversal should not be attempted unless: (1) a peripheral nerve stimulator is used to determine the presence of Phase II block (since anti-cholinesterase agents will potentiate succinylcholine-induced Phase I block), and (2) spontaneous recovery of muscle twitch has been observed for at least 20 minutes and has reached a plateau with further recovery proceeding slowly; this delay is to ensure complete hydrolysis of succinylcholine by pseudocholinesterase prior to administration of the anticholinesterase agent. Should the type of block be misdiagnosed, depolarization of the type initially induced by succinylcholine, that is depolarizing block, will be prolonged by an anticholinesterase agent.

Succinylcholine should be used with caution, if at all, during ocular surgery and in patients with glaucoma. The drug should be employed with caution in patients with fractures or muscle spasm because the initial muscle fasciculations may cause additional trauma.

Neuromuscular blockade may be prolonged in patients with hypokalemia or hypocalcemia.

Drug Interactions: Drugs which may enhance the neuromuscular blocking action of succinylcholine include: phenelzine, promazine, oxytocin, aprotinin, certain nonpenicillin antibiotics, quinidine, β-adrenergic blockers, procainamide, lidocaine, trimethaphan, lithium carbonate, magnesium salts, quinine, chloroquin, propanidid, diethylether, and isoflurane.

If other relaxants are to be used during the same procedure, the possibility of a synergistic or antagonistic effect should be considered.

Pregnancy: *Teratogenic Effects:* Pregnancy Category C.

Animal reproduction studies have not been conducted with succinylcholine chloride. It is also not known whether succinylcholine can cause fetal harm when administered to a pregnant woman or can affect reproduction capacity. Succinylcholine should be given to a pregnant woman only if clearly needed.

Nonteratogenic Effects: Pseudocholinesterase levels are decreased by approximately 24% during pregnancy and for several days postpartum. Therefore, a higher proportion of patients may be expected to show sensitivity (prolonged apnea) to succinylcholine when pregnant than when nonpregnant.

Labor and Delivery: Succinylcholine is commonly used to provide muscle relaxation during delivery by caesarean section. While small amounts of succinylcholine are known to cross the placental barrier, under normal conditions the quantity of drug that enters fetal circulation after a single dose of 1 mg/kg to the mother will not endanger the fetus. However, since the amount of drug that crosses the placental barrier is dependent on the concentration gradient between the maternal and fetal circulations, residual neuromuscular blockade (apnea and flaccidity) may occur in the neonate after repeated high doses to, or in the presence of, atypical pseudocholinesterase in the mother.

Adverse Reactions: Adverse reactions consist primarily of an extension of the drug's pharmacological actions. It causes profound muscle relaxation resulting in respiratory depression to the point of apnea; this effect may be prolonged. Hypersensitivity to the drug may exist in rare instances. The following additional adverse reactions have been reported: cardiac arrest, malignant hyperthermia, arrhythmias, bradycardia, tachycardia, hypertension, hypotension, hyperkalemia, prolonged respiratory depression or apnea, increased intraocular pressure, muscle fasciculation, postoperative muscle pain, myoglobinemia, excessive salivation, and rash.

Dosage and Administration: The dosage of succinylcholine is essentially individualized and its administration should always be determined by the clinician after careful assessment of the patient. To avoid distress to the patient, succinylcholine should not be administered before unconsciousness has been induced. Succinylcholine should not be mixed with short-acting barbiturates in the same syringe or administered simultaneously during intravenous infusion through the same needle.

For Short Surgical Procedures: The average dose for relaxation of short duration is 0.6 mg/kg (~2.0 ml) Anectine (succinylcholine chloride) Injection given intravenously. The optimum dose will vary among individuals and may be from 0.3 to 1.1 mg/kg for adults (1.0 to 4.0 ml). Following administration of doses in this range, relaxation develops in about 1 minute; maximum muscular paralysis may persist for about 2 minutes, after which recovery takes place within 4 to 6 minutes. However, very large doses may result in more prolonged apnea. An initial test dose of 0.1 mg/kg (~0.5 ml) may be used to determine the sensitivity of the patient and the individual recovery time.

For Long Surgical Procedures: The dosage of succinylcholine administered by infusion depends upon the duration of the surgical procedure and the need for muscle relaxation. The average rate for an adult ranges between 2.5 and 4.3 mg per minute.

Solutions containing from 0.1% to 0.2% (1 to 2 mg per ml) succinylcholine have commonly been used for continuous intravenous drip. Solutions of 0.1% or 0.2% may conveniently be prepared by adding 1 g succinylcholine (the contents of one Anectine Sterile Powder Flo-Pack unit containing 1 g succinylcholine chloride) respectively to 1,000 or 500 ml of sterile solution, such as sterile 5% dextrose solution or sterile isotonic saline solution. The more dilute solution (0.1% or 1 mg per ml) is probably preferable from the standpoint of ease of control of the rate of administration of the drug and, hence, of relaxation. This intravenous drip solution containing 1 mg per ml may be administered at a rate of 0.5 mg (0.5 ml) to 10 mg (10 ml) per minute to obtain the required amount of relaxation. The amount required per minute will depend upon the individual response as well as the degree of relaxation required. The 0.2% solution may be especially useful in those cases where it is desired to avoid overburdening the circulation with a large volume of fluid. It is recommended that neuromuscular function be carefully monitored with a peripheral nerve stimulator when using succinylcholine by infusion in order to avoid overdose, detect development of Phase II block, follow its rate of recovery, and assess the effects of reversing agents.

Solutions of succinylcholine must be used within 24 hours after preparation. Discard unused solutions.

Intermittent intravenous injections of succinylcholine may also be used to provide muscle relaxation for long procedures. An intravenous injection of 0.3 to 1.1 mg/kg may be given initially, followed, at appropriate intervals, by further injections of 0.04 to 0.07 mg/kg to maintain the degree of relaxation required.

The intravenous dose of succinylcholine is 2 mg/kg for infants and small children. For older children and adolescents the dose is 1 mg/kg.

Intramuscular Use: If necessary, succinylcholine may be given intramuscularly to infants, older children or adults when a suitable vein is inaccessible. A dose of up to 3 to 4 mg/kg may be given, but not more than 150 mg total dose should be administered by this route. The onset of effect of succinylcholine given intramuscularly is usually observed in about 2 to 3 minutes.

How Supplied: For immediate injection of single doses for short procedures:

Anectine® Injection, 20 mg succinylcholine chloride in each ml.

Multiple-dose vials of 10 ml.

Box of 12 vials, NDC-0081-0071-95.

DoD & VA NSN 6505-00-133-4309

Store in refrigerator at 2°-8°C (36°-46°F). The multi-dose vials are stable for up to 14 days at room temperature without significant loss of potency.

For preparation of intravenous drip solutions only:

Anectine® Flo-Pack®, 500 mg sterile succinylcholine chloride powder.

Box of 12 vials, NDC-0081-0085-15.

Anectine® Flo-Pack®, 1000 mg sterile succinylcholine chloride powder.

Box of 12 vials, NDC-0081-0086-15.

DoD & VA NSN 6505-01-028-2260

Anectine Flo-Pack does not require refrigeration. Solutions of succinylcholine must be used within 24 hours after preparation. Discard unused solutions.

ANTEPAR® ℞
[ăn'tuh-par]
(Piperazine Citrate)
Syrup/Tablets

Description: [See table above].
Piperazine hexahydrate is a white, crystalline substance.

Actions: Clinical investigations in man have demonstrated its activity against the human pinworm, *Enterobius vermicularis,* and against the "common roundworm," *Ascaris lumbricoides.*

Piperazine produces a paralysis of ascaris muscle with resultant expulsion of the worm through intestinal peristalsis.

Systemic absorption of piperazine is variable and the drug is excreted essentially unchanged.

Indications: For the treatment of ascariasis ("common roundworm" infection) and enterobiasis (pinworm infection).

Contraindications: This product is contraindicated in patients with impaired renal or hepatic function, convulsive disorders, or a history of hypersensitivity reactions from piperazine and its salt.

Warnings: Because of potential neurotoxicity of this drug, especially in children, prolonged or repeated treatment in excess of that recommended should be avoided.

Usage in Pregnancy: Safety of this drug for use during pregnancy has not been established.

Continued on next page

Burroughs Wellcome—Cont.

Precautions: If CNS, significant gastrointestinal, or hypersensitivity reactions occur, the drug should be discontinued.

In patients with severe malnutrition, or anemia, appropriate caution should be exercised.

Adverse Reactions: The following reactions have been reported, usually due to excessive dosage:

Gastrointestinal—nausea, vomiting, abdominal cramps, and diarrhea.

Central Nervous System—headache, vertigo, ataxia, tremors, choreiform movement, muscular weakness, hyporeflexia, paresthesia, blurring of vision, paralytic strabismus, convulsion, EEG abnormalities, sense of detachment, and memory defect.

Hypersensitivity—urticaria, erythema multiforme, purpura, fever, and arthralgia.

Dosage and Administration:

For ascariasis ("common roundworm" infection):

Adults—a single daily dose of 3.5 g (hexahydrate equivalent) for 2 consecutive days.

Children—a single daily dose of 75 mg (hexahydrate equivalent)/kg of body weight/day for 2 consecutive days, with maximum daily dose of 3.5 g. In severe infections, the treatment course may be repeated after a one week interval. In circumstances where it is desired to apply mass therapy of ascariasis as a public health measure and where repeated therapy is not practicable, one single dose of 70 mg per pound of body weight, up to a maximum dose of 3 g may be used, as described by Swartzwelder and Goodwin.* This procedure is successful in removing ascarids in the great majority of cases. However, the maximum cure rate is usually obtained with the multiple-dose regimen.

For enterobiasis (pinworm infection):

Adults and children—a single daily dose of 65 mg (hexahydrate equivalent)/kg of body weight/day, with a maximum daily dose of 2.5 g, for 7 consecutive days. In severe infections, the treatment course may be repeated after a one week interval. Use of laxatives or enema and dietary restriction are not necessary.

To prevent reinfection practice of personal and environmental hygiene should be recommended.

How Supplied:

ANTEPAR® (Piperazine Citrate) SYRUP 550 mg per 5 cc (equivalent to 500 mg piperazine hexahydrate). Bottle of 1 pint.

ANTEPAR® (Piperazine Citrate) TABLETS 550 mg scored (equivalent to 500 mg piperazine hexahydrate). Bottle of 100. Imprinted Y4A for identification.

Antepar Syrup
Pint DoD NSN 6505-00-598-8561

*References:

Swartzwelder C, Miller JH, Sappenfield RW: Treatment of ascariasis in children with a single dose of piperazine citrate. Pediatrics 16(1):115, 1955

Goodwin LG, Standen OD: Treatment of roundworm with piperazine citrate (Antepar). Brit MJ 2:1332, 1954

Shown in Product Identification Section, page 407

A.P.C. with Codeine Tablets   ℞ ©
[ā' pē' sē' with kō'dēn]
TABLOID® BRAND

Description: Tabloid A.P.C. with Codeine is supplied in tablet form for oral administration. Each tablet contains aspirin (acetylsalicylic acid) 227 mg, phenacetin 162 mg, and caffeine 32 mg, plus codeine phosphate in one of the following strengths: No. 3–30 mg, and No. 4–60 mg. (Warning—may be habit-forming.)

Tabloid A.P.C. with Codeine has analgesic, antipyretic and anti-inflammatory effects.

Clinical Pharmacology:

Aspirin: The analgesic, anti-inflammatory and antipyretic effects of aspirin are believed to result from inhibition of the synthesis of certain prostaglandins. Aspirin interferes with clotting mechanisms primarily by diminishing platelet aggregation; at high doses prothrombin synthesis can be inhibited.

Aspirin in solution is rapidly absorbed from the stomach and from the upper small intestine. About 50 percent of an oral dose is absorbed in 30 minutes and peak plasma concentrations are reached in about 40 minutes. Higher than normal stomach pH or the presence of food slightly delays absorption.

Once absorbed, aspirin is mainly hydrolyzed to salicylic acid and distributed to all body tissues and fluids, including fetal tissue, breast milk and the central nervous system (CNS). Highest concentrations are found in plasma, liver, renal cortex, heart and lung.

From 50 to 80 percent of the salicylic acid and its metabolites in the plasma are loosely bound to plasma proteins. The plasma half-life of total salicylate is about 30 hours, with a 650 mg dose. Higher doses of aspirin cause increases in plasma salicylate half-life. Metabolism occurs primarily in the hepatocytes. The major metabolites are salicyluric acid (75%), the phenolic and acyl glucuronides of salicylate (15%), and gentisic and gentisuric acid (<1%).

Almost all of a therapeutic dose of aspirin is excreted through the kidneys, either as salicylic acid or the above-mentioned metabolic products. Renal clearance of salicylates is greatly augmented by an alkaline urine, as is produced by concurrent administration of sodium bicarbonate or potassium citrate.

Toxic salicylate blood levels are usually above 30 mg/100 ml. The single lethal dose of aspirin in normal adults is approximately 25–30 g, but patients have recovered from much larger doses with appropriate treatment.

Phenacetin: The mechanism through which phenacetin relieves pain is uncertain.

Phenacetin is rapidly absorbed from the gastrointestinal tract and reaches peak plasma concentrations in one-half to two hours. The physiologic half-life of phenacetin varies from about one-half to one and one-half hours: the drug is almost completely cleared from the body five hours after ingestion. About 30 to 40 percent of phenacetin is bound to plasma protein. Phenacetin and its pharmacologically active metabolite, acetaminophen, are distributed throughout the body tissues and fluids, including fetal tissue, breast milk and the CNS. Their concentration in body fluids, including milk, is relatively uniform, but the extent to which phenacetin and acetaminophen are taken up by various body tissues has not been established. About 75 to 80 percent of phenacetin is rapidly deethylated in the liver to acetaminophen, which reaches peak plasma concentration in one to two hours and has a half-life of one to three hours. The therapeutic plasma concentration of acetaminophen is reported to be 0.5–2.0 mg/100 ml and the lethal concentration is 150 mg/100 ml. About 80 percent of the derived acetaminophen is excreted in urine after conjugation, primarily as the glucuronide; 3 percent is excreted unchanged. Other metabolites are formed by deacetylation and hydroxylation.

Phenacetin is metabolized by deacetylation (to para-phenetidin) and hydroxylation to a number of breakdown products; traces of phenacetin are eliminated unchanged. Toxic effects (sedation, dizziness) have been seen with single doses of 2 g. The minimum lethal dose has been estimated to be 5–20 g, but adults have recovered completely from acute overdoses of 50–60 g.

Caffeine: In ordinary doses, caffeine stimulates the CNS to elevate mood, decrease fatigue, promote alertness and improve motor skills. Caffeine also reduces susceptibility to fatigue by increasing the strength of skeletal muscle contractions. At higher doses or in the presence of medullary depressants, caffeine has been shown to stimulate respiration.

Caffeine exerts central and peripheral effects on heart rate that tend to offset each other except at high doses, when its direct positive chronotropic action predominates and an increased heart rate results. Caffeine also causes a moderate increase in myocardial contractility. While the balance between its central and peripheral effects on blood vessels generally favors vasodilation, caffeine causes vasoconstriction in the cerebral circulation. This effect is thought to explain its efficacy in relieving headache. In addition, caffeine has mild diuretic and smooth-muscle relaxant properties. Like most xanthines, caffeine is rapidly absorbed and distributed in all body tissues and fluids, including the CNS, fetal tissues and breast milk. About 90 percent of an administered dose is metabolized in the liver to approximately equal amounts of 1-methyl-xanthine and 1-methyluric acid; the remainder is excreted unchanged in the urine.

Caffeine achieves its peak effect in about 2 hours; the plasma half-life is about 1.5 hours. The dose level at which toxicity occurs is about 1 g. The single lethal dose is estimated to be over 10 g.

Codeine: Codeine probably exerts its analgesic effect through actions on opiate receptors in the CNS.

Codeine is readily absorbed from the gastrointestinal tract, and a therapeutic dose reaches peak analgesic effectiveness in about 2 hours and persists for 4 to 6 hours. Oral codeine (60 mg) given to healthy males has been shown to achieve peak blood levels of 0.016 mg/100 ml at approximately one hour post-dose. The codeine plasma half-life for a 60 mg oral dose is about 2.9 hours. Blood levels causing CNS depression begin at 0.05–0.19 mg/100 ml. The single lethal dose of codeine in adults is estimated to be approximately 0.5–1.0 g. Codeine is rapidly distributed from blood to body tissues and taken up preferentially by parenchymatous organs such as liver, spleen and kidney. It passes the blood-brain barrier and is found in fetal tissue and breast milk.

The drug is not bound by plasma protein nor is it accumulated in body tissues. Codeine is metabolized in the liver to morphine and norcodeine, each representing about 10 percent of the administered dose of codeine. About 90 percent of the dose is excreted within 24 hours, primarily through the kidneys. Urinary excretion products are free and glucuronide-conjugated codeine (about 70%), free and conjugated norcodeine (about 10%), free and conjugated morphine (about 10%), normorphine (under 4%) and hydrocodone (<1%). The remainder of the dose appears in the feces.

Indications and Usage: Tabloid A.P.C. with Codeine is indicated for the relief of mild, moderate, and moderate to severe pain.

Contraindications: Tabloid A.P.C. with Codeine is contraindicated under the following conditions:

(1) hypersensitivity or intolerance to aspirin, phenacetin, caffeine or codeine.
(2) severe bleeding, disorders of coagulation or primary hemostasis, including hemophilia, hypoprothrombinemia, von Willebrand's disease, the thrombocytopenias, thrombasthenia and other ill-defined hereditary platelet dysfunctions, as well as such associated conditions as severe vitamin K deficiency and severe liver damage.
(3) anticoagulant therapy, and
(4) peptic ulcer, or other serious gastrointestinal lesions.

Warnings: Therapeutic doses of aspirin can cause anaphylactic shock and other severe allergic reactions. A history of allergy is often lacking. Significant bleeding can result from aspirin therapy in patients with peptic ulcer or other gastrointestinal lesions, and in patients with bleeding disorders. Aspirin administered pre-operatively may prolong the bleeding time.

Nephrotoxicity (renal papillary necrosis), frequently accompanied by urinary tract infection, has been reported in a small percentage of individuals consuming analgesic mixtures regularly in large amounts for long periods. Carcinoma of the renal pelvis and urinary bladder has been associated with chronic abuse of analgesic mixtures.

In the presence of head injury or other intracranial lesions, the respiratory depressant effects of codeine and other narcotics may be markedly enhanced, as well as their capacity for elevating cerebrospinal fluid pressure. Narcotics also produce other CNS depressant effects, such as drowsiness, that may further obscure the clinical course of patients with head injuries.

Codeine or other narcotics may obscure signs on which to judge the diagnosis or clinical course of patients with acute abdominal conditions.

Precautions:

General: Tabloid A.P.C. with Codeine should be prescribed with caution for certain special-risk patients such as the elderly or debilitated, and for those with severe impairment of renal or hepatic function, gallbladder disease or gallstones, respiratory impairment, cardiac arrhythmias, inflammatory disorders of the gastrointestinal tract, hypothyroidism. Addison's disease, prostatic hypertrophy or urethral stricture, coagulation disorders, head injuries, acute abdominal conditions and patients known to be taking other analgesic-antipyretic medications. Patients' self-medication habits should be investigated to determine their use of such medications. Tabloid A.P.C. with Codeine should not be prescribed for long-term therapy unless specifically indicated.

Precautions should be taken when administering salicylates to persons with known allergies. Hypersensitivity to aspirin is particularly likely in patients with nasal polyps, and relatively common in those with asthma.

In persons with glucose-6-phosphate dehydrogenase deficiency, phenacetin can cause acute hemolytic anemia.

In persons with renal insufficiency, a typically mild but progressive hemolytic anemia can occur with long-term use of phenacetin. Patients with renal insufficiency appear to be especially susceptible to renal inflammatory lesions characteristic of so-called analgesic nephropathy associated with chronic abuse of analgesic medications.

Patients with severe heart disease should not receive high doses of caffeine, since it can cause tachycardia or extrasystoles and thus precipitate cardiac failure.

Palpitations that may be caused by caffeine are usually of significance only in patients with severe heart disease. Caffeine may cause gastrointestinal irritation and, in susceptible persons, overstimulation, "jitters" or insomnia.

Information for Patients: Tabloid A.P.C. with Codeine may impair the mental and/or physical abilities required for performance of potentially dangerous tasks such as driving a car or operating machinery. Such tasks should be avoided while taking Tabloid A.P.C. with Codeine.

Alcohol and other CNS depressants may produce an additive CNS depression when taken with Tabloid A.P.C. with Codeine, and should be avoided. Patients with severe heart disease should be advised to reduce their total intake of caffeine.

Codeine may be habit-forming when used over long periods or in high doses. Chronic use of Tabloid A.P.C. with Codeine at high doses for long periods of time may result in kidney or liver damage. Patients should take this drug only for as long as prescribed, in the amounts prescribed, and no more frequently than prescribed.

Laboratory Tests: Hypersensitivity to aspirin cannot be detected by skin testing or radioimmunoassay procedures.

The primary screening tests for detecting a bleeding tendency are platelet count, bleeding time, activated partial thromboplastin time and prothrombin time.

In patients with severe hepatic or renal disease, effects of therapy should be monitored with serial liver and/or renal function tests.

Drug Interactions: Tabloid A.P.C. with Codeine may *enhance* the effects of:
(1) monoamine oxidase (MAO) inhibitors,
(2) oral anticoagulants, causing bleeding by inhibiting prothrombin formation in the liver and displacing anticoagulants from plasma protein binding sites,
(3) oral antidiabetic agents and insulin, causing hypoglycemia by contributing an additive effect, and by displacing the oral antidiabetic agents from secondary binding sites,
(4) 6-mercaptopurine and methotrexate, causing bone marrow toxicity and blood dyscrasias by displacing these drugs from secondary binding sites,
(5) penicillins and sulfonamides, increasing their blood levels by displacing these drugs from protein binding sites,
(6) non-steroidal anti-inflammatory agents, increasing the risk of peptic ulceration and bleeding by contributing additive effects,
(7) other narcotic analgesics, alcohol, general anesthetics, tranquilizers such as chlor- diazepoxide, sedative-hypnotics, or other CNS depressants, causing increased CNS depression,
(8) corticosteroids, potentiating steroid anti-inflammatory effects by displacing steroids from protein binding sites. Aspirin intoxication may occur with corticosteroid withdrawal because steroids promote renal clearance of salicylates.

Tabloid A.P.C. with Codeine may *diminish* the effects of:
(1) uricosuric agents such as probenecid and sulfinpyrazone, reducing their effectiveness in the treatment of gout. Aspirin competes with these agents for protein binding sites.

Aspirin and its metabolites may be caused to accumulate in the body, perhaps to toxic levels, by para-amino-salicylic acid, furosemide, and vitamin C. Phenobarbital decreases the effects of phenacetin by accelerating its excretion. Sorbitol and polysorbate accelerate the absorption of phenacetin. High doses of caffeine can cause a potentially lethal hypertensive reaction in the presence of MAO inhibitors. Caffeine and stimulants such as amphetamines may combine to cause excessive excitation or "nervousness".

Drug/Laboratory Test Interactions:

Aspirin: Aspirin may interfere with the following laboratory determinations in blood: serum amylase, fasting blood glucose, carbon dioxide, cholesterol, protein, protein bound iodine, uric acid, prothrombin time, bleeding time, and spectrophotometric detection of barbiturates. Aspirin may interfere with the following laboratory determinations in urine: glucose, 5-hydroxyindoleacetic acid, Gerhardt ketone, vanillylmandelic acid (VMA), protein, uric acid, and diacetic acid.

Phenacetin: Phenacetin may interfere with laboratory determinations of 5-hydroxyindoleacetic acid and glucose in urine.

Caffeine: Caffeine may interfere with laboratory determinations of bilirubin, fasting blood glucose, and uric acid in blood, and catecholamines and 5-hydroxyindoleacetic acid in urine.

Codeine: Codeine may increase serum amylase levels.

Carcinogenesis, Mutagenesis, Impairment of Fertility: No adequate long-term studies have been conducted in animals to determine whether codeine has a potential for carcinogenesis, mutagenesis, or impairment of fertility.

Adequate long-term studies have been conducted in mice and rats with aspirin, phenacetin and caffeine given alone or in combination. No evidence of carcinogenesis was seen in these studies. No adequate animal studies have been conducted with aspirin, phenacetin or caffeine to determine whether they have a potential for mutagenesis or impairment of fertility.

Pregnancy: *Teratogenic Effects:* Pregnancy Category C. Animal reproduction studies have not been conducted with Tabloid A.P.C. with Codeine. It is also not known whether Tabloid A.P.C. with Codeine can cause fetal harm when administered to a pregnant woman or can affect reproduction capacity. Tabloid A.P.C. with Codeine should be given to a pregnant woman only if clearly needed. Reproductive studies in rats and mice have shown aspirin to be teratogenic and embryocidal at four to six times the human therapeutic dose. Studies in pregnant women, however, have not shown that aspirin increases the risk of abnormalities when administered during the first trimester of pregnancy. In controlled studies involving 41,337 pregnant women and their offspring, there was no evidence that aspirin taken during pregnancy caused stillbirth, neonatal death or reduced birthweight. In controlled studies of 50,282 pregnant women and their offspring, aspirin administration in moderate and heavy doses during the first four lunar months of pregnancy showed no teratogenic effect. Reproduction studies have been performed in rats and mice at doses up to 10 times the human dose and have revealed no evidence of impaired fertility or harm to the fetus due to caffeine.

Reproduction studies have been performed in rabbits and rats at doses up to 150 times the human dose and have revealed no evidence of impaired fertility or harm to the fetus due to codeine.

Nonteratogenic Effects: Therapeutic doses of aspirin in pregnant women close to term may cause bleeding in mother, fetus, or neonate. During the last six months of pregnancy, regular use of aspirin in high doses may prolong pregnancy and delivery.

The risk of methemoglobinemia or hemolytic anemia occurring in the fetus may be increased by: (1) regular ingestion of high doses of phenacetin during pregnancy, (2) renal insufficiency in the mother and/or fetus, (3) glucose-6-phosphate dehydrogenase deficiency, or (4) a genetically acquired abnormality in phenacetin metabolism.

Labor and Delivery: Ingestion of aspirin prior to delivery may prolong delivery or lead to bleeding in the mother or neonate. Ingestion of phenacetin may cause methemoglobinemia or hemolytic anemia. Use of codeine during labor may lead to respiratory depression in the neonate.

Nursing Mothers: All components of Tabloid A.P.C. with Codeine are excreted in breast milk in small amounts, but the significance of their effects on nursing infants is not known. Because of the potential for serious adverse reactions in nursing infants from Tabloid A.P.C. with Codeine, a decision should be made whether to discontinue nursing or to discontinue the drug, taking into account the importance of the drug to the mother.

Adverse Reactions:

Codeine: The most frequently observed adverse reactions to codeine include light-headedness, dizziness, drowsiness, nausea, vomiting, constipation and depression of respiration. Less common reactions to codeine include euphoria, dysphoria, pruritus and skin rashes.

Aspirin: Mild intoxication (salicylism) can occur in response to chronic use of large doses. Manifestations include nausea, vomiting, hearing impairment, tinnitus, diminished vision, headache, dizziness, drowsiness, metal confusion, hyperpnea, hyperventilation, tachycardia, sweating and thirst.

Therapeutic doses of aspirin can induce mild or severe allergic reactions manifested by skin rashes, urticaria, angioedema, rhinorrhea, asthma, abdominal pain, nausea, vomiting, or anaphylactic shock. A history of allergy is often lacking, and allergic reactions may occur in patients who have previously taken aspirin without any ill effects. Allergic reactions to aspirin are most likely to occur in patients with a history of allergic disease, especially in patients with nasal polyps or asthma.

Some patients are unable to take aspirin or other salicylates without developing nausea or vomiting. Occasional patients respond to aspirin (usually in large doses) with dyspepsia or heartburn, which may be accompanied by occult bleeding. Excessive bruising or bleeding is sometimes seen in patients with mild disorders of primary hemostasis who regularly use low doses of aspirin.

Prolonged use of aspirin can cause painless erosion of gastric mucosa, occult bleeding and, infrequently, iron-deficiency anemia. High doses of aspirin can exacerbate symptoms of peptic ulcer and, occasionally cause extensive bleeding.

Excessive bleeding can follow injury or surgery in patients with or without known bleeding disorders who have taken therapeutic doses of aspirin within the preceding 10 days.

Hepatotoxicity has been reported in association with prolonged use of large doses of aspirin in patients with lupus erythematosus, rheumatoid arthritis, or rheumatic disease.

Continued on next page

Burroughs Wellcome—Cont.

Bone-marrow depression, manifested by weakness, fatigue, or abnormal bruising or bleeding, has occasionally been reported.

In patients with glucose-6-phosphate dehydrogenase deficiency, aspirin can cause a mild degree of hemolytic anemia.

In hyperuricemic persons, low doses of aspirin may reduce the effectiveness of uricosuric therapy or precipitate an attack of gout.

Phenacetin: In therapeutic doses, side effects of phenacetin are generally limited to occasional sedation, skin rashes or, uncommonly, drug fever. Adverse reactions to phenacetin are usually the result of acute overdosage or chronic abuse of analgesic mixtures containing phenacetin. Toxic doses can cause dizziness, drowsiness or stimulation, methemoglobinemia and sulfhemoglobinemia (cyanosis, fatigue), and, rarely, hepatic necrosis (gastrointestinal symptoms possibly followed by general obtundation) or nephropathy (cloudy urine due to cells, casts, organism, sloughed tissue, edema of lower legs).

Caffeine: Usual doses of caffeine may cause gastric disturbances in some persons. Side effects are usually due to hyperresponsiveness or overdosage, actue or chronic. Toxic doses can cause nervousness, excitement, insomnia, muscle tenderness or tremors, tinnitus, scintillating scotomas, headache on withdrawal of the drug, diuresis, tachycardia and extrasystoles.

Drug Abuse and Dependence: Like other medications containing a narcotic analgesic, Tabloid A.P.C. with Codeine is controlled by the Drug Enforcement Administration and is classified under Schedule III.

Tabloid A.P.C. with Codeine can produce drug dependence of the morphine type; therefore, it has the potential for being abused. Psychic dependence, physical dependence and tolerance may develop on repeated administration.

The dependence liability of codeine has been found to be too small to permit a full definition of its characteristics. Studies indicate that addiction to codeine is extremely uncommon and requires very high parenteral doses.

When dependence on codeine occurs at therapeutic doses, it appears to require from one to two months to develop, and withdrawal symptoms are mild. Most patients on long-term oral codeine therapy show no signs of physical dependence upon abrupt withdrawal.

Overdosage: Severe intoxication, caused by overdose of Tabloid A.P.C. with Codeine may produce: skin eruptions, dyspnea, vertigo, double vision, delusions, hallucinations, garbled speech, excitability, restlessness, delirium, constricted pupils, a positive Babinski sign, respiratory depression (slow and shallow breathing, Cheyne-Stokes respiration), cyanosis, clammy skin, muscle flaccidity, circulatory collapse, stupor and coma. In children, difficulty in hearing, tinnitus, dim vision, headache, dizziness, drowsiness, confusion, rapid breathing, sweating, thirst, nausea, vomiting, hyperpyrexia, dehydration and convulsions are prominent signs. The most severe manifestations from A.P.C. result from cardiovascular and respiratory insufficiency secondary to aspirin-induced acid-base and electrolyte disturbances, complicated by hyperthermia and dehydration. The most severe manifestations from codeine are associated with respiratory depression.

Respiratory alkalosis is characteristic of the early phase of intoxication with aspirin while hyperventilation is occurring, and is quickly followed by metabolic acidosis in most people with severe intoxication. This occurs more readily in children. Hypoglycemia may occur in children who have taken large overdoses. Other laboratory findings associated with aspirin intoxication include ketonuria, hyponatremia, hypokalemia, and occasionally proteinuria. A slight rise in lactic dehydrogenase and hydroxybutyric dehydrogenase may occur.

Hemolytic anemia due to phenacetin is possible and should be monitored by periodic laboratory tests.

Methemoglobin and sulfhemoglobin formation are seldom clinically significant in adults but may contribute to general toxicity. When prominent, they appear as a grayish cyanosis seen most clearly in the lips and nailbeds. Definitive diagnosis is made by spectroscopic analysis of a water-diluted (1:100) blood specimen, which shows an abnormal band at 630 m for methemoglobin and at 618 m for sulfhemoglobin.

Concentrations of aspirin in plasma above 30 mg/100 ml are associated with toxicity. (See Clinical Pharmacology section for information on factors influencing aspirin blood levels.) The single lethal dose of aspirin in adults is probably about 25–30 g, but is not known with certainty.

Toxic and lethal concentrations of phenacetin in human fluids are not known with certainty. Patient response per phenacetin dose may be greater than usual in infants, in patients with renal insufficiency or hepatic insufficiency and in those with a glucose-6-phosphate dehydrogenase deficiency or a decreased ability to convert phenacetin to acetaminophen. Toxic effects (e.g. sedation) have been seen with single doses of 2 g. The minimum lethal dose has been estimated to be 5–20 g, but adults have recovered from acute overdoses of 50–60 g.

Toxic and lethal concentrations of caffeine in human fluids are not known with certainty. Patient response per dose is increased in the presence of renal or hepatic insufficiency. Toxic manifestations may appear with a caffeine dose of 1 g. The single lethal dose in man is generally estimated to be over 10 g, but the lowest reported lethal dose was 3.2 g or 57 mg/kg.

The toxic plasma concentration of codeine is not known with certainty. Experimental production of mild to moderate CNS depression in healthy, non-tolerant subjects occurred at plasma concentrations of 0.05–0.19 mg/100 ml when codeine was given by intravenous infusion. The single lethal dose of codeine in adults is estimated to be from 0.5–1.0 g. It is also estimated that 5 mg/kg could be fatal in children.

Hemodialysis and peritoneal dialysis can be performed to reduce the body aspirin content. Phenacetin is dialyzable, but dialysis of the drug and its major metabolite, acetaminophen, has not yet been established as an effective means of altering the consequences of acute phenacetin overdosage. Caffeine and codeine are theoretically dialyzable but the procedure has not been clinically established for either.

Treatment of overdosage consists primarily of support of vital functions, management of codeine-induced respiratory depression, increasing salicylate elimination, and correcting the acid-base imbalance due primarily to salicylism.

In a comatose patient, primary attention should be given to establishment of adequate respiratory exchange through provision of a patent airway and the institution of assisted or controlled ventilation. The narcotic antagonist naloxone is a specific antidote for respiratory depression which may result from overdosage or unusual sensitivity to narcotics. Therefore, an appropriate dose of an antagonist should be administered, preferably by the intravenous route, simultaneously with efforts at respiratory resuscitation. Since the duration of action of Tabloid A.P.C. with Codeine may exceed that of the antagonist, the patient should be kept under continued surveillance and repeated doses of the antagonist should be administered as needed to maintain adequate respiration.

A narcotic antagonist should not be administered in absence of clinically significant respiratory or cardiovascular depression.

Gastric emptying (Syrup of Ipecac) and/or lavage is recommended as soon as possible after ingestion, even if the patient has vomited spontaneously. (Apomorphine should not be used as an emetic for Tabloid A.P.C. with Codeine, since it may potentiate hypotension and respiratory depression.) Administration of activated charcoal as a slurry is beneficial after lavage and/or emesis, if less than three hours have passed since ingestion. Charcoal adsorption should *not* be employed prior to emesis or lavage.

Severity of aspirin intoxication is determined by measuring the blood salicylate level. Acid-base status should be closely followed with serial blood gas and serum pH measurements. Fluid and electrolyte balance should also be regularly monitored.

A serum salicylate level of 30 mg/100 ml or higher indicates a need for enhanced salicylate excretion that can be achieved through body-fluid supplementation and urine alkalinization if renal function is normal. In mild intoxication, urine flow can be increased by forcing oral fluids and giving potassium citrate capsules. (DO NOT GIVE BICARBONATE BY MOUTH SINCE IT INCREASES THE RATE OF SALICYLATE ABSORPTION.)

In severe cases, hyperthermia and hypovolemia as well as respiratory depression are the major immediate threats to life. Children should be sponged with tepid water. Replacement fluid should be administered intravenously in adequate amount and augmented with sufficient bicarbonate to correct acidosis, with monitoring of plasma electrolytes and pH, to promote alkaline diuresis of salicylate if renal function is normal. Complete control may also require infusion of glucose to control hypoglycemia.

Potassium deficiency may also be corrected through the infusion, once adequate urinary output is assured. Plasma or plasma expanders may be needed if fluid replacement is insufficient to maintain normal blood pressure or adequate urinary output.

In patients with renal insufficiency or in cases of life-threatening intoxication, dialysis is usually required. Peritoneal dialysis or exchange transfusion is indicated in infants and young children, and hemodialysis in older patients.

Oxygen, intravenous fluids, vasopressors and other supportive measures should be employed as needed.

Dosage and Administration: Dosage is adjusted according to the severity of pain and the response of the patient. It may occasionally be necessary to exceed the usual dosage recommended below when pain is severe or the patient has become tolerant to the analgesic effect of codeine. Tabloid A.P.C. with Codeine is given orally. The usual adult dose for Tabloid A.P.C. with Codeine No. 3 is one or two tablets every four hours as required. The usual adult dose for Tabloid A.P.C. with Codeine No. 4 is one tablet every four hours as required.

Tabloid A.P.C. with Codeine should be taken with food or a full glass of milk or water to lessen gastric irritation.

How Supplied:
Tabloid A.P.C. with Codeine No. 3: (white tablet embossed with "TABLOID BRAND" and "3")
   Bottle of 100   NDC 0081-0356-55
   Bottle of 1000   NDC 0081-0356-75
Tabloid A.P.C. with Codeine No. 4: (white tablet embossed with "TABLOID BRAND" and "4")
   Bottle of 100   NDC 0081-0369-55
   Bottle of 1000   NDC 0081-0369-75
Store at 15°–30°C (59°–86°F) in a dry place and protect from light.

Shown in Product Identification Section, page 407

CARDILATE® TABLETS ℞
[kar′dĭ-lāt]
(Erythrityl Tetranitrate)

Description: Cardilate (erythrityl tetranitrate) is an antianginal drug that belongs to the organic nitrate class of pharmaceutical agents. Erythrityl tetranitrate is soluble in alcohol, ether and glycerol, but insoluble in water. It has the empirical formula $C_4H_6N_4O_{12}$, molecular weight of 302.12 and melting point of 61°C.

Erythrityl tetranitrate is known chemically as (R*S*)-1,2,3,4-butanetetrol tetranitrate and has the following structural formula:
(See next column)

In the pure state, erythrityl tetranitrate will explode upon percussion, but properly diluted with lactose, as in Cardilate tablets, it is nonexplosive. Since it is a low melting solid, erythrityl tetranitrate does not evaporate from the Cardilate tablets.

Cardilate Oral/Sublingual Tablets contain either 5 or 10 mg erythrityl tetranitrate dispersed in lactose, with disintegration characteristics that permit sublingual or oral (swallowed) administration. Cardilate Chewable Tablets contain 10 mg erythrityl tetranitrate and lactose, with wintergreen flavoring to enhance patient acceptance.

Clinical Pharmacology: Cardilate exerts its effects by relaxation of vascular smooth muscle.[1] The action is maximal on the post-capillary vessels, including the large veins. Venodilatation results in peripheral blood pooling, which decreases venous return to the heart, central venous pressure and pulmonary capillary wedge pressure (preload reduction).[2] Pulmonary arteriolar dilatation causes a reduction in pulmonary vascular resistance.[2] A decrease in systemic arterial pressure (afterload reduction) can also occur, but is usually less pronounced. Augmentation of cardiac output generally occurs in those patients with increased filling pressures and high resting systemic vascular resistance.[2]

Mechanism of Action: The inadequate myocardial oxygenation that precipitates angina can be corrected by: (1) increasing the supply of oxygen to ischemic myocardium through direct dilatation of the large coronary conductance vessels or (2) decreasing the myocardial oxygen demand secondary to a reduction of cardiac work (preload and afterload reduction).[3] The beneficial effect of Cardilate probably involves both mechanisms.

Pharmacokinetics and Metabolism: Cardilate is readily absorbed from the sublingual, buccal and gastrointestinal mucosae. The peak effect from a swallowed dose is diminished but of longer duration when compared to the sublingual route.[4] The biotransformation of Cardilate is thought to occur by reductive hydrolysis catalyzed by the hepatic enzyme glutathione-organic nitrate reductase.[3] Differences in response among various nitrates may relate to both intrinsic potency at cardiovascular sites, as well as factors related to pharmacokinetics and biotransformation.[5]

Time to onset of effect is approximately 5 minutes for the sublingual and chewable routes and 15 to 30 minutes for swallowed tablets, with peak effect in 15 minutes and 60 minutes, respectively. Duration of action will vary, but vasodilatory effects have been demonstrated for up to 3 hours after sublingual and chewable administration[4,6] and for 6 hours after the oral (swallowed) route.[4]

Indications and Usage: Cardilate (Erythrityl Tetranitrate) is intended for the prophylaxis and long-term treatment of patients with frequent or recurrent anginal pain and reduced exercise tolerance associated with angina pectoris, rather than for the treatment of the acute attack of angina pectoris, since its onset is somewhat slower than that of nitroglycerin.

Contraindications: Cardilate should not be administered to individuals with a known hypersensitivity or idiosyncratic reaction to organic nitrates.

Warnings: The use of nitrates in acute myocardial infarction or congestive heart failure should be undertaken only under close clinical observation and/or in conjunction with hemodynamic monitoring.

Precautions:
General: Cardilate should be used with caution in patients with severe liver or renal disease. Development of tolerance and cross-tolerance to the effects of erythrityl tetranitrate and other organic nitrates may occur. However, recent studies in patients with chronic heart failure[1] indicate that nitrates produce sustained beneficial hemodynamic effects.

Carcinogenesis, Mutagenesis, Impairment of Fertility: No long-term studies in animals have been performed.

Pregnancy: *Teratogenic Effects.* Pregnancy Category C. Animal reproduction studies have not been conducted with Cardilate. It is also not known whether Cardilate can cause fetal harm when administered to a pregnant woman or can affect reproduction capacity. Cardilate should be given to a pregnant woman only if clearly needed.

Nursing Mothers: It is not known whether this drug is excreted in human milk. Because many drugs are excreted in human milk, caution should be exercised when Cardilate is administered to a nursing woman.

Pediatric Use: Safety and effectiveness in children have not been established.

Adverse Reactions: The most frequent adverse reaction in patients treated with Cardilate is headache. Lowering the dose and the use of analgesics will help control headaches, which usually diminish or disappear as therapy is continued. Other adverse reactions occurring are the following: cutaneous vasodilatation with flushing, and transient episodes of dizziness and weakness, plus other signs of cerebral ischemia associated with postural hypotension. Occasional individuals exhibit marked sensitivity to the hypotensive effects of organic nitrates, and severe responses (e.g., nausea, vomiting, weakness, restlessness, pallor, perspiration and collapse) can occur even with the usual therapeutic dose. Alcohol may enhance this effect. Drug rash and/or exfoliative dermatitis may occasionally occur.

Overdosage: Accidental overdosage of Cardilate may result in severe hypotension and reflex tachycardia, which can be treated by laying the patient down and elevating the legs. If further treatment is required, the administration of intravenous fluids or other means of treating hypotension should be considered.

Dosage and Administration:
Oral/Sublingual Tablets: The Cardilate Oral/Sublingual Tablet can be placed under the tongue or swallowed. Sublingual therapy may be initiated with a dose of 5 to 10 mg prior to each anticipated physical or emotional stress, and at bedtime for patients subject to nocturnal attacks of angina. The dose may be increased as needed.

If the patient is to swallow the tablet, therapy may be initiated with 10 mg before each meal, as well as mid-morning and mid-afternoon if needed, and at bedtime for patients subject to nocturnal attacks. The dose may be increased or decreased as needed. Dosage titration up to 100 mg daily has been well tolerated, but temporary headache is more apt to occur with increasing doses. When headache occurs, the dose should be reduced for a few days. If headache is troublesome during adjustment of dosage, it may be effectively relieved with an analgesic.

Chewable Tablets: Cardilate Chewable Tablets offer the advantages of the sublingual tablet in a wintergreen-flavored tablet. Dosage, time of onset and maximum effect are the same as for the sublingual tablet, if the tablet is thoroughly chewed and kept in the mouth for as long as possible.

How Supplied:
CARDILATE (Erythrityl Tetranitrate) ORAL/SUBLINGUAL TABLETS (scored).

5 mg: Bottles of 100 (NDC-0081-0166-55), Imprint "CARDILATE P2B" (round, white).

10 mg: Bottles of 100 (NDC-0081-0168-55) and 1000 (NDC-0081-0168-75). Imprint "CARDILATE X7A" (square, white).

CARDILATE (Erythrityl Tetranitrate) CHEWABLE TABLETS (scored),

10 mg: Bottles of 100 (NDC-0081-0161-55). Imprint "CARDILATE X7A" (round, white).

All tablets should be stored at 15°-25°C (59°- 77°F) in a dry place and dispensed in glass.

References:
1. Chatterjee K, Parmley WW: Vasodilator Therapy for Chronic Heart Failure. *Ann Rev Pharmacol Toxicol,* 20:475-512, 1980.
2. Goldberg S, Mann T, Grossman W: Nitrate Therapy of Heart Failure in Valvular Heart Disease. *Am J Med,* 66:161-66, 1978.
3. Needleman P, Johnson EM: Vasodilators and the Treatment of Angina. In: AG Gilman, LS Goodman, A Gilman, eds. The Pharmacological Basis of Therapeutics, 6th Edition, New York: Macmillan Publishing Co., Inc. 819–33, 1980.
4. Hannemann RE, Erb RJ, Stoltman WP, Bronson EC, Williams EJ, Long RA, Hull JH, Starbuck RR: Digital Plethysmograph for Assessing Erythrityl Tetranitrate Bioavailability. *Clin Pharmacol Ther,* 29:35–9, 1981.
5. Wastila WB, Namm DH, Maxwell RA: Comparison of the Vascular Effects of Several Organic Nitrates in Anesthetized Rats and Dogs after Intravenous and Intraportal Administration. Vascular Neuroeffector Mechanisms. 2nd Int. Symp., Odense. Basel: Karger Publishing Co. 216–25, 1975.
6. Haffty GB, Nakamura Y, Spodick DH, Long RA, Hull JH: Bioavailability of Organic Nitrates: a Comparison of Methods for Evaluating Plethysmographic Responses. *J Clin Pharmacol.* 22:117–124, 1982.

Shown in Product Identification Section, page 407

CORTISPORIN® CREAM ℞
[*kor′ ti-spor″ in krēm*]
(Polymyxin B-Neomycin-Gramicidin-Hydrocortisone)

Description: Each gram contains: Aerosporin® brand Polymyxin B Sulfate 10,000 units; neomycin sulfate 5 mg (equivalent to 3.5 mg neomycin base); gramicidin 0.25 mg; hydrocortisone acetate 5 mg (0.5%); preservative—methylparaben 0.25%.

The base contains the inactive ingredients liquid petrolatum, white petrolatum, propylene glycol, polyoxyethylene polyoxypropylene compound, emulsifying wax and purified water.

The base is a smooth vanishing cream with a pH of approximately 5.0. The acid pH helps restore normal cutaneous acidity. The cream is cosmetically acceptable and may be easily removed with water. Owing to its excellent spreading and penetrating properties, the cream facilitates treatment of hairy and intertriginous areas. It may also be of value in selective cases where the lesions are moist. The antibiotics diffuse readily from the base into fluids of the skin or tissues.

Action: The cream is useful wherever the antiinflammatory and antipruritic action of hydrocortisone is indicated in conjunction with the bactericidal action of polymyxin B, neomycin, and gramicidin. For anti-inflammatory action, the acetate salt of the naturally-occurring adrenal corticosteroid hydrocortisone is used.

Wide range antibacterial action, approaching the ideal, is provided by the overlapping spectra of polymyxin B, neomycin, and gramicidin. The range of action of this combination includes virtually all pathogenic bacteria found topically, and the three antibacterials are bactericidal, rather than bacteriostatic. The index of allergenicity of this combination has been shown over the years to be low and the rarity of topical irritation has been well demonstrated.

Polymyxin B is one of a group of closely related substances produced by various strains of *Bacillus polymyxa.* Its activity is sharply restricted to gram-negative bacteria, including many strains of *Pseudomonas aeruginosa.*

Neomycin, isolated from *Streptomyces fradiae,* has antibacterial activity *in vitro* against a wide range of gram-negative and gram-positive organisms, with effectiveness against many strains of *Proteus.* Gramicidin has particular action *in vitro* against certain gram-positive bacteria.

Indications: Based on a review of this drug by the National Academy of Sciences—National Research Council and/or other infor-

Continued on next page

Burroughs Wellcome—Cont.

mation, FDA has classified the indications as follows:

"Possibly" effective: General: The cream is indicated in the treatment of topical bacterial infections caused by organisms sensitive to the antibiotic ingredients, and when the anti-inflammatory and/or anti-allergic action of the hydrocortisone is indicated as in burns, wounds, and skin grafts; otitis externa; also following surgical procedures. Dermatologic: Atopic, contact, stasis and infectious eczematoid dermatitis; neurodermatitis; eczema; anogenital pruritus. It may also be useful as an adjunct in certain pyodermas, such as impetigo, during specific systemic antibiotic therapy for these infections.

Final classification of the less-than-effective indications requires further investigation.

Contraindications: Not for use in the eyes or in the external ear canal if the eardrum is perforated. This drug is contraindicated in tuberculous, fungal or viral lesions of the skin (herpes simplex, vaccinia and varicella). This product is contraindicated in those individuals who have shown hypersensitivity to any of its components.

Warning: Because of the potential hazard of nephrotoxicity and ototoxicity due to neomycin, care should be exercised when using this product in treating extensive burns, trophic ulceration and other extensive conditions where absorption of neomycin is possible. In burns where more than 20 percent of the body surface is affected, especially if the patient has impaired renal function or is receiving other aminoglycoside antibiotics concurrently, not more than one application a day is recommended.

When using neomycin-containing products to control secondary infection in the chronic dermatoses, such as chronic otitis externa or stasis dermatitis, it should be borne in mind that the skin in these conditions is more liable than is normal skin to become sensitized to many substances, including neomycin. The manifestation of sensitization to neomycin is usually a low grade reddening with swelling, dry scaling and itching; it may be manifest simply as a failure to heal. During long-term use of neomycin-containing products, periodic examination for such signs is advisable and the patient should be told to discontinue the product if they are observed. These symptoms regress quickly on withdrawing the medication. Neomycin-containing applications should be avoided for that patient thereafter.

Precautions: As with other antibacterial preparations, prolonged use may result in overgrowth of nonsusceptible organisms, including fungi. Appropriate measures should be taken if this occurs. Use of steroids on infected areas should be supervised with care as anti-inflammatory steroids may encourage spread of infection. If this occurs steroid therapy should be stopped and appropriate antibacterial drugs used. Generalized dermatological conditions may require systemic corticosteroid therapy. As the safety of topical steroid preparations during pregnancy has not been fully established, they should not be used unnecessarily, on extended areas, in large amounts, or for prolonged periods of time, in pregnancy.

Adverse Reactions: When steroid preparations are used for long periods of time in intertriginous areas or over extensive body areas, with or without occlusive non-permeable dressings, striae may occur; also there exists the possibility of systemic side effects when steroid preparations are used over larger areas or for a long period of time. Neomycin is a not uncommon cutaneous sensitizer. Articles in the current literature indicate an increase in the prevalence of persons allergic to neomycin. Ototoxicity and nephrotoxicity have been reported (see Warning section).

Dosage and Administration: A small quantity of the cream should be applied 2 to 4 times daily, as required. The cream should, if conditions permit, be gently rubbed into the affected areas. In chronic conditions, withdrawal of treatment is carried out by decreasing the frequency of application, until the cream finally is applied as infrequently as once a week.

How Supplied: Tube of 7.5 g.

CORTISPORIN® OINTMENT ℞
[kor' ti-spor" in]
(Polymyxin B-Bacitracin-Neomycin-Hydrocortisone)

Description: Each gram contains:
Aerosporin® brand Polymyxin B Sulfate 5,000 units; bacitracin zinc 400 units; neomycin sulfate 5 mg (equivalent to 3.5 mg neomycin base); hydrocortisone 10 mg (1%); special white petrolatum qs.

Action: The ointment is useful wherever the anti-inflammatory and antipruritic action of hydrocortisone is indicated in conjunction with the bactericidal action of polymyxin B, neomycin, and bacitracin. For anti-inflammatory action, the naturally occurring adrenal corticosteriod hydrocortisone was selected.

The combination of Aerosporin brand Polymyxin B Sulfate with neomycin and bacitracin was selected because it most nearly meets the criteria for an ideal topical antibacterial preparation. The spectrum of action encompasses most pathogenic bacteria found topically, and the three antibiotics are bactericidal rather than bacteriostatic. When used topically, polymyxin B, neomycin and bacitracin are rarely irritating, and absorption from skin or mucous membrane is insignificant. The index of allergenicity of this combination has been shown over the years to be low. And finally, since these antibiotics are seldom used systemically, the patient is spared sensitization to those antibiotics which might later be required systemically.

Polymyxin B is one of a group of closely related substances produced by various strains of *Bacillus polymyxa*. Its activity is sharply restricted to gram-negative bacteria, including many strains of *Pseudomonas aeruginosa*.

Neomycin, isolated from *Streptomyces fradiae*, has antibacterial activity *in vitro* against a wide range of gram-negative and gram-positive organisms, with effectiveness against many strains of *Proteus*. Bacitracin, an antibiotic substance derived from cultures of *Bacillus subtilis* (Tracy), exerts antibacterial action *in vitro* against a variety of gram-positive and a few gram-negative organisms.

Indications: For the treatment of corticosteroid-responsive dermatoses with secondary infection. It has not been demonstrated that this steroid-antibiotic combination provides better benefit than the steroid component alone after 7 days of treatment (see WARNINGS section).

Contraindications: This product is contraindicated in those individuals who have shown hypersensitivity to any of its components. Do not use in the external ear canal if the eardrum is perforated.

Warning: Because of the concern of nephrotoxicity and ototoxicity associated with neomycin, this combination product should not be used over a wide area or for extended periods of time.

When using neomycin-containing products to control secondary infection in the chronic dermatoses, such as chronic otitis externa or stasis dermatitis, it should be borne in mind that the skin in these conditions is more liable than is normal skin to become sensitized to many substances, including neomycin. The manifestation of sensitization to neomycin is usually a low grade reddening with swelling, dry scaling and itching; it may be manifest simply as a failure to heal. During long-term use of neomycin-containing products, periodic examination for such signs is advisable and the patient should be told to discontinue the product if they are observed. These symptoms regress quickly on withdrawing the medication. Neomycin-containing applications should be avoided for that patient thereafter.

Precautions: As with any antibiotic preparation, prolonged use may result in the overgrowth of nonsusceptible organisms, including fungi. Appropriate measures should be taken if this occurs. Use of steroids on infected areas should be supervised with care as anti-inflammatory steroids may encourage spread of infection. If this occurs steroid therapy should be stopped and appropriate antibacterial drugs used. Generalized dermatological conditions may require systemic corticosteroid therapy. As the safety of topical steroid preparations during pregnancy has not been fully established, they should not be used unnecessarily, on extended areas, in large amounts, or for prolonged periods of time, in pregnancy.

Adverse Reactions: When steroid preparations are used for long periods of time in intertriginous areas or over extensive body areas, with or without occlusive nonpermeable dressings, striae may occur; also there exists the possibility of systemic side effects when steroid preparations are used over larger areas or for a long period of time. Neomycin is a not uncommon cutaneous sensitizer. Articles in the current literature indicate an increase in the prevalence of persons allergic to neomycin. Ototoxicity and nephrotoxicity have been reported (see Warning section).

Dosage and Administration: A thin film is applied 2 to 4 times daily. In chronic conditions, withdrawal of treatment is carried out by decreasing the frequency of application, until the ointment is applied as infrequently as once a week.

How Supplied: Tube of ½ oz with applicator tip.

CORTISPORIN® OPHTHALMIC ℞
[kor' ti-spor' in]
OINTMENT Sterile
(Polymyxin B Sulfate-Bacitracin Zinc-Neomycin Sulfate-Hydrocortisone)

Description: Cortisporin® Ophthalmic Ointment (polymyxin B sulfate-bacitracin zinc-neomycin sulfate-hydrocortisone) is a sterile antimicrobial and anti-inflammatory ointment for ophthalmic use. Each gram contains Aerosporin® (polymyxin B sulfate) 10,000 units, bacitracin zinc 400 units, neomycin sulfate equivalent to 3.5 mg neomycin base, hydrocortisone 10 mg (1%) and special white petrolatum, qs.

Polymyxin B sulfate is the sulfate salt of polymyxin B_1 and B_2 which are produced by the growth of *Bacillus polymyxa* (Prazmowski) Migula (Fam. Bacillaceae). It has a potency of not less than 6,000 Polymyxin B units per mg, calculated on an anhydrous basis.

Bacitracin zinc is the zinc salt of bacitracin, a mixture of related cyclic polypeptides (mainly bacitracin A) produced by the growth of an organism of the *licheniformis* group of *Bacillus subtilis* (Fam. Bacillaceae). It has a potency of not less than 40 bacitracin units per mg.

Neomycin sulfate is the sulfate salt of neomycin B and C, which are produced by the growth of *Streptomyces fradiae* Waksman (Fam. Streptomycetaceae). It has a potency equivalent of not less than 600 µg of neomycin standard per mg, calculated on an anhydrous basis.

Hydrocortisone, 11β, 17, 21-trihydroxypregn-4-ene-3, 20-dione, is an anti-inflammatory hormone.

Clinical Pharmacology: Corticoids suppress the inflammatory response to a variety of agents and they may delay healing. Since corticoids may inhibit the body's defense mechanism against infection, a concomitant antimicrobial drug may be used when this inhibition is considered to be clinically significant in a particular case.

The anti-infective components in the combination are included to provide action against specific organisms susceptible to them. Polymyxin B sulfate, bacitracin zinc and neomycin sulfate together are considered active against the following microorganisms: *Staphylococcus aureus*, streptococci, including *Streptococcus pneumoniae*, *Escherichia coli*, *Haemophilus influenzae*, *Klebsiella-Enterobacter* species, *Neisseria* species and *Pseudomonas aeruginosa*.

When used topically, polymyxin B, bacitracin and neomycin are rarely irritating, and absorption from the intact skin or mucous membrane is insignificant. The incidence of skin sensitization to this combination has been shown to be low on normal skin.[1,2] Since these antibiotics are seldom used systemically, the patient is spared sensitization to those antibiotics which might later be required systemically.

When a decision to administer both a corticoid and antimicrobials is made, the administration of such drugs in combination has the advantage of greater patient compliance and convenience, with the added assurance that the appropriate dosage of both drugs is administered, plus assured compatibility of ingredients when both types of drug are in the same formulation and, particularly, that the intended volume of each drug is delivered simultaneously, thereby avoiding dilution of either medication by sucessive applications.

The relative potency of corticosteroids depends on the molecular structure, concentration, and release from the vehicle.

Indications and Usage: For steroid-responsive inflammatory ocular conditions for which a corticosteroid is indicated and where bacterial infection or a risk of bacterial ocular infection exists. Ocular steroids are indicated in inflammatory conditions of the palpebral and bulbar conjunctiva, cornea and anterior segment of the globe where the inherent risk of steroid use in certain infective conjunctivitides is accepted to obtain a diminution in edema and inflammation. They are also indicated in chronic anterior uveitis and corneal injury from chemical, radiation, or thermal burns, or penetration of foreign bodies.

The use of a combination drug with an anti-infective component is indicated where the risk of infection is high or where there is an expectation that potentially dangerous numbers of bacteria will be present in the eye.

The particular anti-infective drugs in this product are active against the following common bacterial eye pathogens: *Staphylococcus aureus*, streptococci, including *Streptococcus pneumoniae, Escherichia coli, Haemophilus influenzae, Klebsiella-Enterobacter* species, *Neisseria* species and *Pseudomonas aeruginosa.*

The product does not provide adequate coverage against *Serratia marcescens.*

Contraindications: Epithelial herpes simplex keratitis (dendritic keratitis), vaccinia, varicella, and many other viral diseases of the cornea and conjunctiva. Mycobacterial infection of the eye. Fungal diseases of ocular structures. Hypersensitivity to a component of the medication. (Hypersensitivity to the antibiotic component occurs at a higher rate than for other components.)

The use of these combinations is contraindicated after uncomplicated removal of a corneal foreign body.

Warnings: Prolonged use may result in glaucoma, with damage to the optic nerve, defects in visual acuity and fields of vision, and posterior subcapsular cataract formation. Prolonged use may suppress the host response and thus increase the hazard of secondary ocular infections. In those diseases causing thinning of the cornea or sclera, perforations have been known to occur with the use of topical steroids. In acute purulent conditions of the eye, steroids may mask infection or enhance existing infection. If these products are used for 10 days or longer, intraocular pressure should be routinely monitored even though it may be difficult in children and uncooperative patients. Employment of steroid medication in the treatment of herpes simplex requires great caution.

Neomycin sulfate may cause cutaneous sensitization. A precise incidence of hypersensitivity reactions (primarily skin rash) due to topical neomycin is not known.

The manifestations of sensitization to neomycin are usually itching, reddening and edema of the conjunctiva and eyelid. It may be manifest simply as a failure to heal. During long-term use of neomycin-containing products, periodic examination for such signs is advisable, and the patient should be told to discontinue the product if they are observed. These symptoms subside quickly on withdrawing the medication. Neomycin-containing applications should be avoided for the patient thereafter.

Precautions:
General: The initial prescription and renewal of the medication order beyond 8 grams should be made by a physician only after examination of the patient with the aid of magnification, such as slit lamp biomicroscopy and, where appropriate, fluorescein staining.

The possibility of persistent fungal infections of the cornea should be considered after prolonged steroid dosing.

Allergic cross-reactions may occur which could prevent the use of any or all of the following antibiotics for the treatment of future infections: kanamycin, paromomycin, streptomycin, and possibly gentamicin.

Carcinogenesis, Mutagenesis, Impairment of Fertility: Long-term studies in animals (rats, rabbits, mice) showed no evidence of carcinogenicity attributable to oral administration of corticosteroids.

Pregnancy: *Teratogenic Effects:* Pregnancy Category C. Corticosteriods have been shown to be teratogenic in rabbits when applied topically at concentrations of 0.5% on days 6-18 of gestation and in mice when applied topically at a concentration of 15% on days 10-13 of gestation. There are no adequate and well-controlled studies in pregnant women. Corticosteroids should be used during pregnancy only if the potential benefit justifies the potential risk to the fetus.

Nursing Mothers: Hydrocortisone appears in human milk following oral administration of the drug. Since systemic absorption of hydrocortisone may occur when applied topically, caution should be exercised when Cortisporin Ophthalmic Ointment is used by a nursing woman.

Adverse Reactions: Adverse reactions have occurred with steriod/anti-infective combination drugs which can be attributed to the steriod component, the anti-infective component, or the combination. Reactions occurring most often from the presence of the anti-infective ingredient are localized hypersensitivity, including itching, swelling and conjunctival erythema. Local irritation on instillation has also been reported. Exact incidence figures are not available since no denominator of treated patients is available.

The reactions due to the steriod component in decreasing order of frequency are: elevation of introcular pressure (IOP) with possible development of glaucoma, and infrequent optic nerve damage; posterior subcapsular cataract formation; and delayed wound healing.

Secondary Infection: The development of secondary infection has occurred after use of combinations containing steriods and antimicrobials. Fungal infections of the cornea are particularly prone to develop coincidentally with long-term applications of steriod. The possibility of fungal invasion must be considered in any persistent corneal ulceration where steriod treatment has been used. Secondary bacterial ocular infection following suppression of host responses also occurs.

Dosage and Administration: Apply the ointment in the affected eye every 3 or 4 hours, depending on the severity of the condition.

Not more than 8 grams should be prescribed initially and the prescription should not be refilled without further evaluation as outlined in PRECAUTIONS above.

How Supplied: Tube of 1/8 oz with ophthalmic tip (NDC-0081-0197-86).

Store at 15°–30°C (59°–86°F).

DoD NSN 6505-01-102-4303
References:
1. Leyden JJ and Kligman AM. Contact Dermatitis to Neomycin Sulfate *JAMA* 242 (12):1276-1278, 1979.
2. Prystowsky SD, Allen AM, Smith RW, Nonomura JH, Odom RB and Akers WA. Allergic Contact Hypersensitivity to Nickel, Neomycin, Ethylenediamine, and Benzocaine. *Arch Dermatol* 115:959-962, 1979.

CORTISPORIN®
[kor' ti-spor" in]
OPHTHALMIC SUSPENSION Sterile
(Polymyxin B Sulfate-Neomycin Sulfate-Hydrocortisone)

Description: Cortisporin® Ophthalmic Suspension (polymyxin B sulfate-neomycin sulfate-hydrocortisone) is a sterile antimicrobial and anti-inflammatory suspension for ophthalmic use. Each ml contains: Aerosporin® (polymyxin B sulfate) 10,000 units, neomycin sulfate equivalent to 3.5 mg neomycin base and hydrocortisone, 10 mg (1%). The vehicle contains thimerosal 0.001% (added as a preservative) and the inactive ingredients cetyl alcohol, glyceryl monostearate, mineral oil, polyoxyl 40 stearate, propylene gylcol and water for injection.

Polymyxin B Sulfate is the sulfate salt of polymyxin B_1 and B_2 which are produced by the growth of *Bacillus polymyxa* (Prazmowski) Migula (Fam. Bacillaceae). It has a potency of not less than 6,000 Polymyxin B units per mg, calculated on an anhydrous basis.

Clinical Pharmacology: Corticoids suppress the inflammatory response to a variety of agents and they may delay healing. Since corticoids may inhibit the body's defense mechanism against infections, a concomitant antimicrobial drug may be used when this inhibition is considered to be clinically significant in a particular case.

The anti-infective components in the combination are included to provide action against specific organisms susceptible to them. Polymyxin B sulfate and neomycin sulfate together are considered active against the following microorganisms: *Staphylococcus aureus, Escherichia coli, Haemophilus influenzae, Klebsiella-Enterobacter* species, *Neisseria* species and *Pseudomonas aeruginosa.*

When used topically, polymyxin B and neomycin are rarely irritating, and absorption from the intact skin or mucous membrane is insignificant. The incidence of skin sensitization to this combination has been shown to be low on normal skin.[1,2] Since these antibiotics are seldom used systemically, the patient is spared sensitization to those antibiotics which might later be required systemically.

When a decision to administer both a corticoid and antimicrobials is made, the administration of such drugs in combination has the advantage of greater patient compliance and convenience, with the added assurance that the intended dosage of both drugs is administered, plus assured compatibility of ingredients when both types of drug are in the same formulation and, particularly, that the intended volume of each drug is delivered and simultaneously, thereby avoiding dilution of either medication by successive installations.

The relative potency of corticosteroids depends on the molecular structure, concentration, and release from the vehicle.

Indications and Usage: For steroid-responsive inflammatory ocular conditions for which a corticosteroid is indicated and where bacterial infection or a risk of bacterial ocular infection exists. Ocular steroids are indicated in inflammatory conditions of the palpebral and bulbar conjunctiva, cornea and anterior segment of the globe where the inherent risk of steroid use in certain infective conjunctivitides is accepted to obtain a diminution in edema and inflammation. They are also indicated in chronic anterior uveitis and corneal injury from chemical, radiation, or thermal burns, or penetration of foreign bodies.

The use of a combination drug with an anti-infective component is indicated where the risk of infection is high or where there is an expectation that potentially dangerous numbers of bacteria will be present in the eye.

The particular anti-infective drugs in this product are active against the following common bacterial eye pathogens: *Staphylococcus aureus, Escherichia coli, Haemophilus influenzae, Klebsiella-Enterobacter* species, *Neisseria* species, and *Pseudomonas aeruginosa.*

Continued on next page

Burroughs Wellcome—Cont.

The product does not provide adequate coverage against: *Serratia marcescens* and Streptococci, including *Streptococcus pneumoniae*.

Contraindications: Epithelial herpes simplex keratitis (dendritic keratitis), vaccinia, varicella, and many other viral diseases of the cornea and conjunctiva. Mycobacterial infection of the eye. Fungal diseases of ocular structures. Hypersensitivity to a component of the medication. (Hypersensitivity to the antibiotic component occurs at a higher rate than for other components.)

The use of these combinations is always contraindicated after uncomplicated removal of a corneal foreign body.

Warnings: Prolonged use may result in glaucoma, with damage to the optic nerve, defects in visual acuity and fields of vision, and posterior subcapsular cataract formation. Prolonged use may suppress the host response and thus increase the hazard of secondary ocular infections. In those diseases causing thinning of the cornea or sclera, perforations have been known to occur with the use of topical steroids. In acute purulent conditions of the eye, steroids may mask infection or enhance existing infection. If these products are used for 10 days or longer, intraocular pressure should be routinely monitored even though it may be difficult in children and uncooperative patients. Employment of steroid medication in the treatment of herpes simplex requires great caution.

Neomycin sulfate may cause cutaneous sensitization. A precise incidence of hypersensitivity reactions (primarily skin rash) due to topical neomycin is not known.

The manifestations of sensitization to neomycin are usually itching, reddening and edema of the conjunctiva and eyelid. It may be manifest simply as a failure to heal. During long-term use of neomycin-containing products, periodic examination for such signs is advisable, and the patient should be told to discontinue the product if they are observed. These symptoms subside quickly on withdrawing the medication. Neomycin-containing applications should be avoided for the patient thereafter.

Precautions: General: The initial prescription and renewal of the medication order beyond 20 milliliters should be made by a physician only after examination of the patient with the aid of magnification, such as slit lamp biomicroscopy and, where appropriate, fluorescein staining.

The possibility of persistent fungal infections of the cornea should be considered after prolonged steroid dosing.

Allergic cross-reactions may occur which could prevent the use of any or all of the following antibiotics for the treatment of future infections: kanamycin, paromomycin, streptomycin, and possibly gentamicin.

Carcinogenesis, Mutagenesis, Impairment of Fertility: Long-term studies in animals (rats, rabbits, mice) showed no evidence of carcinogenicity attributable to oral administration of corticosteroids.

Pregnancy: *Teratogenic Effects:* Pregnancy Category C. Corticosteroids have been shown to be teratogenic in rabbits when applied topically at concentrations of 0.5% on days 6–18 of gestation and in mice when applied topically at a concentration of 15% on days 10–13 of gestation. There are no adequate and well-controlled studies in pregnant women. Corticosteroids should be used during pregnancy only if the potential benefit justifies the potential risk to the fetus.

Nursing Mothers: Hydrocortisone appears in human milk following oral administration of the drug. Since systemic absorption of hydrocortisone may occur when applied topically, caution should be exercised when Cortisporin Ophthalmic Suspension is used by a nursing woman.

Adverse Reactions: Adverse reactions have occurred with steroid/anti-infective combination drugs which can be attributed to the steroid component, the anti-infective component, or the combination. Reactions occurring most often from the presence of the anti-infective ingredient are localized hypersensitivity, including itching, swelling and conjunctival erythema. Local irritation on instillation has also been reported. Exact incidence figures are not available since no denominator of treated patients is available.

The reactions due to the steroid component in decreasing order of frequency are: elevation of intraocular pressure (IOP) with possible development of glaucoma, and infrequent optic nerve damage; posterior subcapsular cataract formation; and delayed wound healing.

Secondary Infection: The development of secondary infection has occurred after use of combinations containing steroids and antimicrobials. Fungal infections of the cornea are particularly prone to develop coincidentally with long-term applications of steroid. The possibility of fungal invasion must be considered in any persistent corneal ulceration where steroid treatment has been used.

Secondary bacterial ocular infection following suppression of host responses also occurs.

Dosage and Administration: One or two drops in the affected eye every 3 or 4 hours, depending on the severity of the condition. The suspension may be used more frequently if necessary.

No more than 20 milliliters should be prescribed initially and the prescription should not be refilled without further evaluation as outlined in PRECAUTIONS above.

SHAKE WELL BEFORE USING.

How Supplied: Bottle of 5 ml with Sterile Dropper (NDC-0081-0193-84).

Store at 15°–25°C (59°–77°F).

DOD NSN 6505-00-764-9042

References:
1. Leyden JJ and Kligman AM, Contact Dermatitis to Neomycin Sulfate. *JAMA 242 (12)*: 1276–1278, 1979.
2. Prystowsky SD, Allen AM, Smith RW, Nonomura JH, Odom RB and Akers WA, Allergic Contact Hypersensitivity to Nickel, Neomycin, Ethylenediamine, and Benzocaine, *Arch Dermatol 115*:959–962, 1979.

CORTISPORIN® OTIC SOLUTION   ℞
[*kor' tĭ-spor" ĭn ō-tĭk*]
Sterile
(Polymyxin B-Neomycin-Hydrocortisone)

Description: Each ml contains:
Aerosporin® brand Polymyxin B
  Sulfate ....10,000 Units
Neomycin sulfate ....5 mg
  (equivalent to 3.5 mg neomycin base)
Hydrocortisone ....10 mg (1%)
The vehicle contains the inactive ingredients cupric sulfate, glycerin, hydrochloric acid, propylene glycol, water for injection and potassium metabisulfite (preservative) 0.1%.

Action: Hydrocortisone, the naturally occurring adrenal corticosteroid, affords antiallergic, antipruritic and anti-inflammatory activity.

Polymyxin B is one of a group of closely related substances produced by various strains of *Bacillus polymyxa*. Its activity is sharply restricted to gram-negative bacteria, including many strains of *Pseudomonas aeruginosa*.

Neomycin, isolated from *Streptomyces fradiae*, has antibacterial activity *in vitro* against a wide range of gram-negative and gram-positive organisms, with effectiveness against many strains of *Proteus*.

Indications: For the treatment of superficial bacterial infections of the external auditory canal caused by organisms susceptible to the action of the antibiotics.

Contraindications: This product is contraindicated in those individuals who have shown hypersensitivity to any of its components, and in herpes simplex, vaccinia and varicella.

Warnings: As with other antibiotic preparations, prolonged treatment may result in overgrowth of nonsusceptible organisms and fungi.

If the infection is not improved after one week, cultures and susceptibility tests should be repeated to verify the identity of the organism and to determine whether therapy should be changed.

When using neomycin-containing products to control secondary infection in the chronic dermatoses, such as chronic otitis externa, it should be borne in mind that the skin in these conditions is more liable than is normal skin to become sensitized to many substances, including neomycin. The manifestation of sensitization to neomycin is usually a low grade reddening with swelling, dry scaling and itching; it may be manifest simply as a failure to heal. During long-term use of neomycin-containing products, periodic examination for such signs is advisable and the patient should be told to discontinue the product if they are observed. These symptoms regress quickly on withdrawing the medication. Neomycin-containing applications should be avoided for that patient thereafter.

Precautions: If sensitization or irritation occurs, medication should be discontinued promptly. This drug should be used with care when the integrity of the tympanic membrane is in question because of the possibility of ototoxicity caused by neomycin.

Patients who prefer to warm the medication before using should be cautioned against heating the solution above body temperature, in order to avoid loss of potency.

Treatment should not be continued for longer than ten days.

Allergic cross-reactions may occur which could prevent the use of any or all of the following antibiotics for the treatment of future infections: kanamycin, paromomycin, streptomycin, and possibly gentamicin.

Adverse Reactions: Neomycin is a not uncommon cutaneous sensitizer. There are articles in the current literature that indicate an increase in the prevalence of persons sensitive to neomycin.

Stinging and burning have been reported when this drug has gained access to the middle ear.

Dosage and Administration: The external auditory canal should be thoroughly cleansed and dried with a sterile cotton applicator.

For adults, 4 drops of the solution should be instilled into the affected ear 3 or 4 times daily. For infants and children, 3 drops are suggested because of the smaller capacity of the ear canal.

The patient should lie with the affected ear upward and then the drops should be instilled. This position should be maintained for 5 minutes to facilitate penetration of the drops into the ear canal. Repeat, if necessary, for the opposite ear.

If preferred, a cotton wick may be inserted into the canal and then the cotton may be saturated with the solution. This wick should be kept moist by adding further solution every four hours. The wick should be replaced at least once every 24 hours. The patient should be instructed to avoid contaminating the dropper with material from the ear, fingers, or other source. This caution is necessary if the sterility of the drops is to be preserved.

How Supplied: Bottle of 10 ml with sterilized dropper.

10 ml—DoD & VA   NSN 6505-01-014-1378

CORTISPORIN® OTIC SUSPENSION   ℞
[*kor' tĭ-spor" ĭn ō-tĭk*]
Sterile
(Polymyxin B-Neomycin-Hydrocortisone)

Description: Each ml contains: Aerosporin® brand Polymyxin B Sulfate 10,000 units; neomycin sulfate 5 mg (equivalent to 3.5 mg neomycin base); hydrocortisone 10 mg (1%).

The vehicle contains the inactive ingredients cetyl alcohol, propylene glycol, polysorbate 80, water for injection and thimerosal (preservative) 0.01%.

Action: Hydrocortisone, the naturally occurring adrenal corticosteroid, affords antiallergic, antipruritic and anti-inflammatory activity.

Polymyxin B is one of a group of closely related substances produced by various strains of *Bacillus polymyxa*. Its activity is sharply restricted to gram-negative bacteria, including many strains of *Pseudomonas aeruginosa*.

Neomycin, isolated from *Streptomyces fradiae*, has antibacterial activity *in vitro* against a wide range of gram-negative and gram-positive organisms, with effectiveness against many strains of *Proteus*.

combination has been shown to be low on normal skin.[1,2] Since these antibiotics are seldom used systemically, the patient is spared sensitization to those antibiotics which might later be required systemically.

When a decision to administer both a corticoid and antimicrobials is made, the administration of such drugs in combination has the advantage of greater patient compliance and convenience, with the added assurance that the appropriate dosage of both drugs is administered, plus assured compatibility of ingredients when both types of drug are in the same formulation and, particularly, that the intended volume of each drug is delivered simultaneously, thereby avoiding dilution of either medication by sucessive applications.

The relative potency of corticosteroids depends on the molecular structure, concentration, and release from the vehicle.

Indications and Usage: For steroid-responsive inflammatory ocular conditions for which a corticosteroid is indicated and where bacterial infection or a risk of bacterial ocular infection exists. Ocular steroids are indicated in inflammatory conditions of the palpebral and bulbar conjunctiva, cornea and anterior segment of the globe where the inherent risk of steroid use in certain infective conjunctivitides is accepted to obtain a diminution in edema and inflammation. They are also indicated in chronic anterior uveitis and corneal injury from chemical, radiation, or thermal burns, or penetration of foreign bodies.

The use of a combination drug with an anti-infective component is indicated where the risk of infection is high or where there is an expectation that potentially dangerous numbers of bacteria will be present in the eye.

The particular anti-infective drugs in this product are active against the following common bacterial eye pathogens: *Staphylococcus aureus*, streptococci, including *Streptococcus pneumoniae*, *Escherichia coli*, *Haemophilus influenzae*, *Klebsiella-Enterobacter* species, *Neisseria* species and *Pseudomonas aeruginosa*.

The product does not provide adequate coverage against *Serratia marcescens*.

Contraindications: Epithelial herpes simplex keratitis (dendritic keratitis), vaccinia, varicella, and many other viral diseases of the cornea and conjunctiva. Mycobacterial infection of the eye. Fungal diseases of ocular structures. Hypersensitivity to a component of the medication. (Hypersensitivity to the antibiotic component occurs at a higher rate than for other components.)

The use of these combinations is contraindicated after uncomplicated removal of a corneal foreign body.

Warnings: Prolonged use may result in glaucoma, with damage to the optic nerve, defects in visual acuity and fields of vision, and posterior subcapsular cataract formation. Prolonged use may suppress the host response and thus increase the hazard of secondary ocular infections. In those diseases causing thinning of the cornea or sclera, perforations have been known to occur with the use of topical steroids. In acute purulent conditions of the eye, steroids may mask infection or enhance existing infection. If these products are used for 10 days or longer, intraocular pressure should be routinely monitored even though it may be difficult in children and uncooperative patients. Employment of steroid medication in the treatment of herpes simplex requires great caution.

Neomycin sulfate may cause cutaneous sensitization. A precise incidence of hypersensitivity reactions (primarily skin rash) due to topical neomycin is not known.

The manifestations of sensitization to neomycin are usually itching, reddening and edema of the conjunctiva and eyelid. It may be manifest simply as a failure to heal. During long-term use of neomycin-containing products, periodic examination for such signs is advisable, and the patient should be told to discontinue the product if they are observed. These symptoms subside quickly on withdrawing the medication. Neomycin-containing applications should be avoided for the patient thereafter.

Precautions:
General: The initial prescription and renewal of the medication order beyond 8 grams should be made by a physician only after examination of the patient with the aid of magnification, such as slit lamp biomicroscopy and, where appropriate, fluorescein staining.

The possibility of persistent fungal infections of the cornea should be considered after prolonged steroid dosing.

Allergic cross-reactions may occur which could prevent the use of any or all of the following antibiotics for the treatment of future infections: kanamycin, paromomycin, streptomycin, and possibly gentamicin.

Carcinogenesis, Mutagenesis, Impairment of Fertility: Long-term studies in animals (rats, rabbits, mice) showed no evidence of carcinogenicity attributable to oral administration of corticosteroids.

Pregnancy: *Teratogenic Effects:* Pregnancy Category C. Corticosteriods have been shown to be teratogenic in rabbits when applied topically at concentrations of 0.5% on days 6-18 of gestation and in mice when applied topically at a concentration of 15% on days 10-13 of gestation. There are no adequate and well-controlled studies in pregnant women. Corticosteroids should be used during pregnancy only if the potential benefit justifies the potential risk to the fetus.

Nursing Mothers: Hydrocortisone appears in human milk following oral administration of the drug. Since systemic absorption of hydrocortisone may occur when applied topically, caution should be exercised when Cortisporin Ophthalmic Ointment is used by a nursing woman.

Adverse Reactions: Adverse reactions have occurred with steriod/anti-infective combination drugs which can be attributed to the steriod component, the anti-infective component, or the combination. Reactions occurring most often from the presence of the anti-infective ingredient are localized hypersensitivity, including itching, swelling and conjunctival erythema. Local irritation on instillation has also been reported. Exact incidence figures are not available since no denominator of treated patients is available.

The reactions due to the steriod component in decreasing order of frequency are: elevation of introcular pressure (IOP) with possible development of glaucoma, and infrequent optic nerve damage; posterior subcapsular cataract formation; and delayed wound healing.

Secondary Infection: The development of secondary infection has occurred after use of combinations containing steriods and antimicrobials. Fungal infections of the cornea are particularly prone to develop coincidentally with long-term applications of steriod. The possibility of fungal invasion must be considered in any persistent corneal ulceration where steriod treatment has been used. Secondary bacterial ocular infection following suppression of host responses also occurs.

Dosage and Administration: Apply the ointment in the affected eye every 3 or 4 hours, depending on the severity of the condition.

Not more than 8 grams should be prescribed initially and the prescription should not be refilled without further evaluation as outlined in PRECAUTIONS above.

How Supplied: Tube of 1/8 oz with ophthalmic tip (NDC-0081-0197-86).

Store at 15°-30°C (59°-86°F).

DoD NSN 6505-01-102-4303

References:
1. Leyden JJ and Kligman AM. Contact Dermatitis to Neomycin Sulfate *JAMA* 242 (12):1276-1278, 1979.
2. Prystowsky SD, Allen AM, Smith RW, Nonomura JH, Odom RB and Akers WA. Allergic Contact Hypersensitivity to Nickel, Neomycin, Ethylenediamine, and Benzocaine. *Arch Dermatol* 115:959-962, 1979.

CORTISPORIN®
[kor′ ti-spor″ in]
OPHTHALMIC SUSPENSION Sterile
(Polymyxin B Sulfate-Neomycin Sulfate-Hydrocortisone)

Description: Cortisporin® Ophthalmic Suspension (polymyxin B sulfate-neomycin sulfate-hydrocortisone) is a sterile antimicrobial and anti-inflammatory suspension for ophthalmic use. Each ml contains: Aerosporin® (polymyxin B sulfate) 10,000 units, neomycin sulfate equivalent to 3.5 mg neomycin base and hydrocortisone, 10 mg (1%). The vehicle contains thimerosal 0.001% (added as a preservative) and the inactive ingredients cetyl alcohol, glyceryl monostearate, mineral oil, polyoxyl 40 stearate, propylene gylcol and water for injection.

Polymyxin B Sulfate is the sulfate salt of polymyxin B_1 and B_2 which are produced by the growth of *Bacillus polymyxa* (Prazmowski) Migula (Fam. Bacillaceae). It has a potency of not less than 6,000 Polymyxin B units per mg, calculated on an anhydrous basis.

Clinical Pharmacology: Corticoids suppress the inflammatory response to a variety of agents and they may delay healing. Since corticoids may inhibit the body's defense mechanism against infections, a concomitant antimicrobial drug may be used when this inhibition is considered to be clinically significant in a particular case.

The anti-infective components in the combination are included to provide action against specific organisms susceptible to them. Polymyxin B sulfate and neomycin sulfate together are considered active against the following microorganisms: *Staphylococcus aureus*, *Escherichia coli*, *Haemophilus influenzae*, *Klebsiella-Enterobacter* species, *Neisseria* species and *Pseudomonas aeruginosa*.

When used topically, polymyxin B and neomycin are rarely irritating, and absorption from the intact skin or mucous membrane is insignificant. The incidence of skin sensitization to this combination has been shown to be low on normal skin.[1,2] Since these antibiotics are seldom used systemically, the patient is spared sensitization to those antibiotics which might later be required systemically.

When a decision to administer both a corticoid and antimicrobials is made, the administration of such drugs in combination has the advantage of greater patient compliance and convenience, with the added assurance that the intended dosage of both drugs is administered, plus assured compatibility of ingredients when both types of drug are in the same formulation and, particularly, that the intended volume of each drug is delivered and simultaneously, thereby avoiding dilution of either medication by successive installations.

The relative potency of corticosteroids depends on the molecular structure, concentration, and release from the vehicle.

Indications and Usage: For steroid-responsive inflammatory ocular conditions for which a corticosteroid is indicated and where bacterial infection or a risk of bacterial ocular infection exists. Ocular steroids are indicated in inflammatory conditions of the palpebral and bulbar conjunctiva, cornea and anterior segment of the globe where the inherent risk of steroid use in certain infective conjunctivitides is accepted to obtain a diminution in edema and inflammation. They are also indicated in chronic anterior uveitis and corneal injury from chemical, radiation, or thermal burns, or penetration of foreign bodies.

The use of a combination drug with an anti-infective component is indicated where the risk of infection is high or where there is an expectation that potentially dangerous numbers of bacteria will be present in the eye.

The particular anti-infective drugs in this product are active against the following common bacterial eye pathogens: *Staphyloccus aureus*, *Escherichia coli*, *Haemophilus influenzae*, *Klebsiella-Enterobacter* species, *Neisseria* species, and *Pseudomonas aeruginosa*.

Continued on next page

Burroughs Wellcome—Cont.

The product does not provide adequate coverage against: *Serratia marcescens* and Streptococci, including *Streptococcus pneumoniae*.

Contraindications: Epithelial herpes simplex keratitis (dendritic keratitis), vaccinia, varicella, and many other viral diseases of the cornea and conjunctiva. Mycobacterial infection of the eye. Fungal diseases of ocular structures. Hypersensitivity to a component of the medication. (Hypersensitivity to the antibiotic component occurs at a higher rate than for other components.)

The use of these combinations is always contraindicated after uncomplicated removal of a corneal foreign body.

Warnings: Prolonged use may result in glaucoma, with damage to the optic nerve, defects in visual acuity and fields of vision, and posterior subcapsular cataract formation. Prolonged use may suppress the host response and thus increase the hazard of secondary ocular infections. In those diseases causing thinning of the cornea or sclera, perforations have been known to occur with the use of topical steroids. In acute purulent conditions of the eye, steroids may mask infection or enhance existing infection. If these products are used for 10 days or longer, intraocular pressure should be routinely monitored even though it may be difficult in children and uncooperative patients. Employment of steroid medication in the treatment of herpes simplex requires great caution.

Neomycin sulfate may cause cutaneous sensitization. A precise incidence of hypersensitivity reactions (primarily skin rash) due to topical neomycin is not known.

The manifestations of sensitization to neomycin are usually itching, reddening and edema of the conjunctiva and eyelid. It may be manifest simply as a failure to heal. During long-term use of neomycin-containing products, periodic examination for such signs is advisable, and the patient should be told to discontinue the product if they are observed. These symptoms subside quickly on withdrawing the medication. Neomycin-containing applications should be avoided for the patient thereafter.

Precautions: General: The initial prescription and renewal of the medication order beyond 20 milliliters should be made by a physician only after examination of the patient with the aid of magnification, such as slit lamp biomicroscopy and, where appropriate, fluorescein staining.

The possibility of persistent fungal infections of the cornea should be considered after prolonged steroid dosing.

Allergic cross-reactions may occur which could prevent the use of any or all of the following antibiotics for the treatment of future infections: kanamycin, paromomycin, streptomycin, and possibly gentamicin.

Carcinogenesis, Mutagenesis, Impairment of Fertility: Long-term studies in animals (rats, rabbits, mice) showed no evidence of carcinogenicity attributable to oral administration of corticosteroids.

Pregnancy: *Teratogenic Effects:* Pregnancy Category C. Corticosteroids have been shown to be teratogenic in rabbits when applied topically at concentrations of 0.5% on days 6–18 of gestation and in mice when applied topically at a concentration of 15% on days 10–13 of gestation. There are no adequate and well-controlled studies in pregnant women. Corticosteroids should be used during pregnancy only if the potential benefit justifies the potential risk to the fetus.

Nursing Mothers: Hydrocortisone appears in human milk following oral administration of the drug. Since systemic absorption of hydrocortisone may occur when applied topically, caution should be exercised when Cortisporin Ophthalmic Suspension is used by a nursing woman.

Adverse Reactions: Adverse reactions have occurred with steroid/anti-infective combination drugs which can be attributed to the steroid component, the anti-infective component, or the combination. Reactions occurring most often from the presence of the anti-infective ingredient are localized hypersensitivity, including itching, swelling and conjunctival erythema. Local irritation on instillation has also been reported. Exact incidence figures are not available since no denominator of treated patients is available.

The reactions due to the steroid component in decreasing order of frequency are: elevation of intraocular pressure (IOP) with possible development of glaucoma, and infrequent optic nerve damage; posterior subcapsular cataract formation; and delayed wound healing.

Secondary Infection: The development of secondary infection has occurred after use of combinations containing steroids and antimicrobials. Fungal infections of the cornea are particularly prone to develop coincidentally with long-term applications of steroid. The possibility of fungal invasion must be considered in any persistent corneal ulceration where steroid treatment has been used. Secondary bacterial ocular infection following suppression of host responses also occurs.

Dosage and Administration: One or two drops in the affected eye every 3 or 4 hours, depending on the severity of the condition. The suspension may be used more frequently if necessary.

No more than 20 milliliters should be prescribed initially and the prescription should not be refilled without further evaluation as outlined in PRECAUTIONS above.

SHAKE WELL BEFORE USING.

How Supplied: Bottle of 5 ml with Sterile Dropper (NDC-0081-0193-84).

Store at 15°–25°C (59°–77°F).

DOD NSN 6505-00-764-9042

References:
1. Leyden JJ and Kligman AM, Contact Dermatitis to Neomycin Sulfate. *JAMA 242 (12):* 1276–1278, 1979.
2. Prystowsky SD, Allen AM, Smith RW, Nonomura JH, Odom RB and Akers WA, Allergic Contact Hypersensitivity to Nickel, Neomycin, Ethylenediamine, and Benzocaine, *Arch Dermatol 115:*959–962, 1979.

CORTISPORIN® OTIC SOLUTION ℞
[kor′ tĭ-spor″ ĭn ō-tĭk]
Sterile
(Polymyxin B-Neomycin-Hydrocortisone)

Description: Each ml contains:
Aerosporin® brand Polymyxin B
Sulfate ....10,000 Units
Neomycin sulfate ....5 mg
 (equivalent to 3.5 mg neomycin base)
Hydrocortisone ....10 mg (1%)
The vehicle contains the inactive ingredients cupric sulfate, glycerin, hydrochloric acid, propylene glycol, water for injection and potassium metabisulfite (preservative) 0.1%.

Action: Hydrocortisone, the naturally occurring adrenal corticosteroid, affords antiallergic, antipruritic and anti-inflammatory activity.

Polymyxin B is one of a group of closely related substances produced by various strains of *Bacillus polymyxa*. Its activity is sharply restricted to gram-negative bacteria, including many strains of *Pseudomonas aeruginosa*.

Neomycin, isolated from *Streptomyces fradiae,* has antibacterial activity *in vitro* against a wide range of gram-negative and gram-positive organisms, with effectiveness against many strains of *Proteus*.

Indications: For the treatment of superficial bacterial infections of the external auditory canal caused by organisms susceptible to the action of the antibiotics.

Contraindications: This product is contraindicated in those individuals who have shown hypersensitivity to any of its components, and in herpes simplex, vaccinia and varicella.

Warnings: As with other antibiotic preparations, prolonged treatment may result in overgrowth of nonsusceptible organisms and fungi.

If the infection is not improved after one week, cultures and susceptibility tests should be repeated to verify the identity of the organism and to determine whether therapy should be changed.

When using neomycin-containing products to control secondary infection in the chronic dermatoses, such as chronic otitis externa, it should be borne in mind that the skin in these conditions is more liable than is normal skin to become sensitized to many substances, including neomycin. The manifestation of sensitization to neomycin is usually a low grade reddening with swelling, dry scaling and itching; it may be manifest simply as a failure to heal. During long-term use of neomycin-containing products, periodic examination for such signs is advisable and the patient should be told to discontinue the product if they are observed. These symptoms regress quickly on withdrawing the medication. Neomycin-containing applications should be avoided for that patient thereafter.

Precautions: If sensitization or irritation occurs, medication should be discontinued promptly. This drug should be used with care when the integrity of the tympanic membrane is in question because of the possibility of ototoxicity caused by neomycin.

Patients who prefer to warm the medication before using should be cautioned against heating the solution above body temperature, in order to avoid loss of potency.

Treatment should not be continued for longer than ten days.

Allergic cross-reactions may occur which could prevent the use of any or all of the following antibiotics for the treatment of future infections: kanamycin, paromomycin, streptomycin, and possibly gentamicin.

Adverse Reactions: Neomycin is a not uncommon cutaneous sensitizer. There are articles in the current literature that indicate an increase in the prevalence of persons sensitive to neomycin.

Stinging and burning have been reported when this drug has gained access to the middle ear.

Dosage and Administration: The external auditory canal should be thoroughly cleansed and dried with a sterile cotton applicator.

For adults, 4 drops of the solution should be instilled into the affected ear 3 or 4 times daily. For infants and children, 3 drops are suggested because of the smaller capacity of the ear canal.

The patient should lie with the affected ear upward and then the drops should be instilled. This position should be maintained for 5 minutes to facilitate penetration of the drops into the ear canal. Repeat, if necessary, for the opposite ear.

If preferred, a cotton wick may be inserted into the canal and then the cotton may be saturated with the solution. This wick should be kept moist by adding further solution every four hours. The wick should be replaced at least once every 24 hours. The patient should be instructed to avoid contaminating the dropper with material from the ear, fingers, or other source. This caution is necessary if the sterility of the drops is to be preserved.

How Supplied: Bottle of 10 ml with sterilized dropper.

10 ml—DoD & VA   NSN 6505-01-014-1378

CORTISPORIN® OTIC SUSPENSION ℞
[kor′ tĭ-spor″ ĭn ō-tĭk]
Sterile
(Polymyxin B-Neomycin-Hydrocortisone)

Description: Each ml contains: Aerosporin® brand Polymyxin B Sulfate 10,000 units; neomycin sulfate 5 mg (equivalent to 3.5 mg neomycin base); hydrocortisone 10 mg (1%).

The vehicle contains the inactive ingredients cetyl alcohol, propylene glycol, polysorbate 80, water for injection and thimerosal (preservative) 0.01%.

Action: Hydrocortisone, the naturally occurring adrenal corticosteroid, affords antiallergic, antipruritic and anti-inflammatory activity.

Polymyxin B is one of a group of closely related substances produced by various strains of *Bacillus polymyxa*. Its activity is sharply restricted to gram-negative bacteria, including many strains of *Pseudomonas aeruginosa*.

Neomycin, isolated from *Streptomyces fradiae,* has antibacterial activity *in vitro* against a wide range of gram-negative and gram-positive organisms, with effectiveness against many strains of *Proteus*.

Indications: For the treatment of superficial bacterial infections of the external auditory canal caused by organisms susceptible to the action of the antibiotics, and for the treatment of infections of mastoidectomy and fenestration cavities caused by organisms susceptible to the antibiotics.

Contraindications: This product is contraindicated in those individuals who have shown hypersensitivity to any of its components, and in herpes simplex, vaccinia and varicella.

Warnings: As with other antibiotic preparations, prolonged treatment may result in overgrowth of nonsusceptible organisms and fungi.

If the infection is not improved after one week, cultures and susceptibility tests should be repeated to verify the identity of the organism and to determine whether therapy should be changed. When using neomycin-containing products to control secondary infection in the chronic dermatoses, such as chronic otitis externa, it should be borne in mind that the skin in these conditions is more liable than is normal skin to become sensitized to many substances, including neomycin. The manifestation of sensitization by neomycin is usually a low grade reddening with swelling, dry scaling and itching; it may be manifest simply as a failure to heal. During long-term use of neomycin-containing products, periodic examination for such signs is advisable and the patient should be told to discontinue the product if they are observed. These symptoms regress quickly on withdrawing the medication. Neomycin-containing applications should be avoided for that patient thereafter.

Precautions: If sensitization or irritation occurs, medication should be discontinued promptly.

This drug should be used with care in cases of perforated eardrum and in longstanding cases of chronic otitis media because of the possibility of ototoxicity caused by neomycin.

Patients who prefer to warm the medication before using should be cautioned against heating the solution above body temperature, in order to avoid loss of potency.

Treatment should not be continued for longer than ten days.

Allergic cross-reactions may occur which could prevent the use of any or all of the following antibiotics for the treatment of future infections: kanamycin, paromomycin, streptomycin, and possibly gentamicin.

Adverse Reactions: Neomycin is a not uncommon cutaneous sensitizer. There are articles in the current literature that indicate an increase in the prevalence of persons sensitive to neomycin.

Dosage and Administration: The external auditory canal should be thoroughly cleansed and dried with a sterile cotton applicator.

For adults, 4 drops of the suspension should be instilled into the affected ear 3 or 4 times daily. For infants and children, 3 drops are suggested because of the smaller capacity of the ear canal. The patient should lie with the affected ear upward and then the drops should be instilled. This position should be maintained for 5 minutes to facilitate penetration of the drops into the ear canal. Repeat, if necessary, for the opposite ear.

If preferred, a cotton wick may be inserted into the canal and then the cotton may be saturated with the suspension. This wick should be kept moist by adding further suspension every four hours. The wick should be replaced at least once every 24 hours.

The patient should be instructed to avoid contaminating the dropper with material from the ear, fingers, or other source. This caution is necessary if the sterility of the drops is to be preserved.

SHAKE WELL BEFORE USING.

How Supplied: Bottle of 10 ml with sterilized dropper.

10 ml DoD & VA   NSN 6505-01-043-0230

DARAPRIM®   R
[dair'ah-prim"]
(Pyrimethamine)

Description: Daraprim (Pyrimethamine) is chemically known as 2, 4-diamino-5-p-chlorophenyl-6-ethylpyrimidine. It is a tasteless and odorless substance.

Actions and Benefits: Daraprim is a folic acid antagonist and the rationale for its therapeutic action is based on the differential requirement between host and parasite for nucleic acid precursors involved in growth. This activity is highly selective against plasmodia and *Toxoplasma gondii*.

Pyrimethamine possesses blood schizonticidal and some tissue schizonticidal activity against malaria parasites of man. However, its blood schizonticidal activity may be slower than that of 4-aminoquinoline compounds. It does not destroy gametocytes, but arrests sporogony in the mosquito.

The action of Daraprim against *Toxoplasma gondii* is greatly enhanced when used in conjunction with sulfonamides. This was demonstrated by Eyles and Coleman in the treatment of experimental toxoplasmosis in the mouse. Jacobs *et at* demonstrated that combination of the two drugs effectively prevented the development of severe uveitis in most rabbits following the inoculation of the anterior chamber of the eye with toxoplasma.

Indications: Daraprim (Pyrimethamine) is indicated for the chemoprophylaxis of malaria due to susceptible strains of plasmodia. Fast-acting schizonticides (chloroquine, amodiaquin, quinacrine or quinine) are indicated and preferable for the treatment of acute attacks. However, conjoint use of Daraprim will initiate *transmission control* and *suppressive cure*.

Daraprim is also indicated for the treatment of toxoplasmosis. For this purpose the drug should be used conjointly with a sulfonamide since synergism exists with this combination.

Warnings: The dosage of pyrimethamine required for the treatment of toxoplasmosis is 10 to 20 times the recommended antimalarial dosage and approaches the toxic level. If signs of folic or folinic acid deficiency develop (see Adverse Reactions) reduce the dosage or discontinue the drug according to the response of the patient. Folinic acid (leucovorin) may be administered in a dosage of 3 to 9 mg intramuscularly daily for 3 days, or as required to produce a return of depressed platelet or white blood cell counts to safe levels.

Patients should be warned to keep Daraprim out of the reach of children since accidental ingestion has led to fatality.

Use in Pregnancy: Pyrimethamine, like other folic acid antagonists, may, in large doses, produce teratogenic effects in laboratory animals. The large doses required to treat toxoplasmosis should be used only after a definitive diagnosis of acute toxoplasmosis has been made, and the possibility of teratogenic effects from the drug has been carefully weighed against the possible risks of permanent damage to the fetus from the infection. Concurrent administration of folinic acid is recommended when pyrimethamine is used for treatment of toxoplasmosis during pregnancy.

Precautions: The recommended dosage for malaria suppression should not be exceeded. In patients receiving high dosage, as for the treatment of toxoplasmosis, semi-weekly blood counts, including platelet counts, should be made. In patients with convulsive disorders a small "starting" dose (for toxoplasmosis) is recommended to avoid the potential nervous system toxicity of pyrimethamine.

Adverse Reactions: With large doses, anorexia and vomiting may occur. Vomiting may be minimized by giving the medication with meals; it usually disappears promptly upon reduction of dosage. Also, large doses as used in toxoplasmosis may produce megaloblastic anemia, leukopenia, thrombocytopenia, pancytopenia and atrophic glossitis. Acute intoxication may follow the ingestion of an excessive amount of pyrimethamine; this may involve central nervous system stimulation including convulsions. In such cases a parenteral barbiturate may be indicated followed by folinic acid (leucovorin).

Dosage and Administration:

For Chemoprophylaxis of Malaria: Adults and children over 10 years—25 mg (1 tablet) once weekly.

Children 4 through 10 years—12.5 mg (½ tablet) once weekly.

Infants and children under 4 years—6.25 mg (¼ tablet) once weekly.

Regimens planned to include *suppressive cure* should be extended through any characteristic periods of early recrudescence and late relapse for at least 10 weeks in each case.

For Treatment of Acute Attacks: Daraprim is recommended in areas where only susceptible plasmodia exist. The drug is not recommended alone in the treatment of acute attacks of malaria in non-immune persons. Fast-acting schizonticides (chloroquine, amodiaquin, quinacrine or quinine) are indicated for treatment of acute attacks. However, conjoint Daraprim dosage of 25 mg daily for two days will initiate *transmission control* and *suppressive cure*. Should circumstances arise wherein Daraprim must be used alone in semi-immune persons, the adult dosage for an acute attack is 50 mg daily for 2 days; children 4 through 10 years old may be given 25 mg daily for 2 days. In any event, clinical cure should be followed by the once-weekly regimen described above.

For Toxoplasmosis: The dosage of Daraprim (Pyrimethamine) in the treatment of toxoplasmosis must be carefully adjusted so as to provide maximum therapeutic effect and a minimum of side effects. At the high dosage required, there is a marked variation in the tolerance to the drug. Young patients may tolerate higher doses than older individuals.

The adult *starting* dose is 50 to 75 mg of the drug daily, together with 1 to 4 g daily of a sulfonamide drug of the sulfapyrimidine type, e.g., sulfadiazine, triple-sulfa. This dosage is ordinarily continued for 1 to 3 weeks, depending on the response of the patient and his tolerance of the therapy. The dosage may then be reduced to about one-half that previously given for each drug and continued for an additional 4 or 5 weeks.

The pediatric dosage of Daraprim is 1 mg/kg per day divided into 2 equal daily doses; after 2 to 4 days this dose may be reduced to one-half and continued for approximately one month. The usual pediatric sulfonamide dosage is used in conjunction with Daraprim.

Supplied: Tablets, scored, 25 mg, bottles of 100. Tablets bear identification, A3A.

100—DoD   NSN 6505-00-926-4765

Shown in Product Identification Section, page 407

EMPIRIN®
[ĭm'per-ĭn" or ĭmp'prĭn]
ASPIRIN TABLETS
ASPIRIN—325 mg (5 grs)

(See PDR for Nonprescription Drugs)

EMPIRIN® with Codeine Tablets   R
[ĭm'per-ĭn with kō'dēn]

Description: Empirin with Codeine is supplied in tablet form for oral administration. Each tablet contains aspirin (acetylsalicylic acid) 325 mg plus codeine phosphate in one of the following strengths: No. 2–15 mg, No. 3–30 mg, and No. 4–60 mg. (Warning—may be habit-forming).

Empirin with Codeine has analgesic, antipyretic and anti-inflammatory effects.

Clinical Pharmacology:

Aspirin: The analgesic, anti-inflammatory and antipyretic effects of aspirin are believed to result from inhibition of the synthesis of certain prostaglandins. Aspirin interferes with clotting mechanisms primarily by diminishing platelet aggregation; at high doses prothrombin synthesis can be inhibited.

Aspirin in solution is rapidly absorbed from the stomach and from the upper small intestine. About 50 percent of an oral dose is absorbed in 30 minutes and peak plasma concentrations are reached in about 40 minutes. Higher than normal stomach pH or the presence of food slightly delays absorption.

Continued on next page

Burroughs Wellcome—Cont.

Once absorbed, aspirin is mainly hydrolyzed to salicylic acid and distributed to all body tissues and fluids, including fetal tissue, breast milk and the central nervous system (CNS). Highest concentrations are found in plasma, liver, renal cortex, heart and lung.

From 50 to 80 percent of the salicylic acid and its metabolites in plasma are loosely bound to proteins. The plasma half-life of total salicylate is about 3.0 hours, with a 650 mg dose. Higher doses of aspirin cause increases in plasma salicylate half-life. Metabolism occurs primarily in the hepatocytes. The major metabolites are salicyluric acid (75%), the phenolic and acyl glucuronides of salicylate (15%), and gentisic and gentisuric acid (<1%).

Almost all of a therapeutic dose of aspirin is excreted through the kidneys, either as salicylic acid or the above mentioned metabolic products. Renal clearance of salicylates is greatly augmented by an alkaline urine, as is produced by concurrent administration of sodium bicarbonate or potassium citrate.

Toxic salicylate blood levels are usually above 30 mg/100 ml. The single lethal dose of aspirin in normal adults is approximately 25–30 g, but patients have recovered from much larger doses with appropriate treatment.

Codeine: Codeine probably exerts its analgesic effect through actions on opiate receptors in the CNS.

Codeine is readily absorbed from the gastrointestinal tract, and a therapeutic dose reaches peak analgesic effectiveness in about 2 hours and persists for 4 to 6 hours. Oral codeine (60 mg) given to healthy males has been shown to achieve peak blood levels of 0.016 mg/100 ml at approximately one hour post-dose. The codeine plasma half-life for a 60 mg oral dose is about 2.9 hours. Blood levels causing CNS depression begin at 0.05–0.19 mg/100 ml. The single lethal dose of codeine in adults is estimated to be approximately 0.5–1.0 g. Codeine is rapidly distributed from blood to body tissues and taken up preferentially by parenchymatous organs such as liver, spleen and kidney. It passes the blood-brain barrier and is found in fetal tissue and breast milk.

The drug is not bound by plasma proteins nor is it accumulated in body tissues. Codeine is metabolized in liver to morphine and norcodeine, each representing about 10 percent of the administered dose of codeine. About 90 percent of the dose is excreted within 24 hours, primarily through the kidneys. Urinary excretion products are free and glucuronide-conjugated codeine (about 70%), free and conjugated norcodeine (about 10%), free and conjugated morphine (about 10%), normorphine (under 4%) and hydrocodone (<1%). The remainder of the dose appears in the feces.

Indications and Usage: Empirin® with Codeine is indicated for the relief of mild, moderate, and moderate to severe pain.

Contraindications: Emprin with Codeine is contraindicated under the following conditions:
(1) hypersensitivity or intolerance to aspirin or codeine,
(2) severe bleeding, disorders of coagulation or primary hemostasis, including hemophilia, hypoprothrombinemia, von Willebrand's disease, the thrombocytopenias, thrombasthenia and other ill-defined hereditary platelet dysfunctions, and well as such associated conditions as severe vitamin K deficiency and severe liver damage,
(3) anticoagulant therapy, and
(4) peptic ulcer, or other serious gastrointestinal lesions.

Warnings: Therapeutic doses of aspirin can cause analphylactic shock and other severe allergic reactions. A history of allergy is often lacking. Significant bleeding can result from aspirin therapy in patients with peptic ulcer or other gastrointestinal lesions, and in patients with bleeding disorders. Aspirin administered preoperatively may prolong the bleeding time.

In the presence of head injury or other intracranial lesions, the respiratory depressant effects of codeine and other narcotics may be markedly enhanced, as well as their capacity for elevating cerebrospinal fluid pressure. Narcotics also produce other CNS depressant effects, such as drowsiness, that may further obscure the clinical course of patients with head injuries.

Codeine or other narcotics may obscure signs on which to judge the diagnosis or clinical course of patients with acute abdominal conditions.

Precautions:

General: Empirin® with Codeine should be prescribed with caution for certain special-risk patients such as the elderly or debilitated, and those with severe impairment of renal or hepatic function, gallbladder disease or gallstones, respiratory impairment, cardiac arrhythmias, inflammatory disorders of the gastrointestinal tract, hypothyroidism, Addison's disease, prostatic hypertrophy or urethral stricture, coagulation disorders, head injuries, or acute abdominal conditions. Empirin® with Codeine should not be prescribed for long-term therapy unless specifically indicated.

Precautions should be taken when administering salicylates to persons with known allergies. Hypersensitivity to aspirin is particularly likely in patients with nasal polyps, and relatively common in those with asthma.

Information for Patients: Empirin with Codeine may impair the mental and/or physical abilities required for the performance of potentially hazardous tasks such as driving a car or operating machinery. Such tasks should be avoided while taking Empirin with Codeine.

Alcohol and other CNS depressants may produce an additive CNS depression when taken with Empirin with Codeine, and should be avoided.

Codeine may be habit-forming when used over long periods or in high doses. Patients should take the drug only for as long as it is prescribed, in the amounts prescribed, and no more frequently than prescribed.

Laboratory Tests: Hypersensitivity to aspirin cannot be detected by skin testing or radioimmunoassay procedures.

The primary screening tests for detecting a bleeding tendency are platelet count, bleeding time, activated partial thromboplastin time and prothrombin time.

In patients with severe hepatic or renal disease, effects of therapy should be monitored with serial liver and/or renal function tests.

Drug Interactions: Empirin® with Codeine may *enhance* the effects of:
(1) monoamine oxidase (MAO) inhibitors,
(2) oral anticoagulants, causing bleeding by inhibiting prothrombin formation in the liver and displacing anticoagulants from plasma protein binding sites,
(3) oral antidiabetic agents and insulin, causing hypoglycemia by contributing an additive effect, and by displacing the oral antidiabetic agents from secondary binding sites,
(4) 6-mercaptopurine and methotrexate, causing bone marrow toxicity and blood dyscrasias by displacing these drugs from secondary binding sites,
(5) penicillins and sulfonamides, increasing their blood levels by displacing these drugs from protein binding sites,
(6) non-steroidal anti-inflammatory agents, increasing the risk of peptic ulceration and bleeding by contributing additive effects.
(7) other narcotic analgesics, alcohol, general anesthetics, tranquilizers such as chlordiazepoxide, sedative-hypnotics, or other CNS depressants, causing increased CNS depression,
(8) corticosteroids, potentiating steroid anti-inflammatory effects by displacing steroids from protein binding sites. Aspirin intoxication may occur with corticosteroid withdrawal because steroids promote renal clearance of salicylates.

Empirin® with Codeine may *diminish* the effects of:
(1) uricosuric agents such as probenecid and sulfinpyrazone, reducing their effectiveness in the treatment of gout. Aspirin competes with these agents for protein binding sites.

Aspirin and its metabolites may be caused to accumulate in the body, perhaps to toxic levels, by para-aminosalicylic acid, furosemide, and vitamin C.

Drug/Laboratory Test Interactions:

Aspirin: Aspirin may interfere with the following laboratory determinations in blood: serum amylase, fasting blood glucose, carbon dioxide, cholesterol, protein, protein bound iodine, uric acid, prothrombin time, bleeding time, and spectrophotometric detection of barbiturates. Aspirin may interfere with the following laboratory determinations in urine: glucose, 5-hydroxyindoleacetic acid, Gerhardt ketone, vanillylmandelic acid (VMA), protein, uric acid, and diacetic acid.

Codeine: Codeine may increase serum amylase levels.

Carcinogenesis, Mutagenesis, Impairment of Fertility: No adequate long-term studies have been conducted in animals to determine whether codeine has a potential for carcinogenesis, mutagenesis, or impairment of fertility.

Adequate long-term studies have been conducted in mice and rats with aspirin, alone or in combination with other drugs, in which no evidence of carcinogenesis was seen. No adequate studies have been conducted in animals to determine whether aspirin has a potential for mutagenesis or impairment of fertility.

Pregnancy: *Teratogenic Effects:* Pregnancy Category C. Animal reproduction studies have not been conducted with Empirin® with Codeine. It is also not known whether Empirin with Codeine can cause fetal harm when administered to a pregnant woman or can affect reproduction capacity. Empirin with Codeine should be given to a pregnant woman only if clearly needed.

Reproductive studies in rats and mice have shown aspirin to be teratogenic and embryocidal at four to six times the human therapeutic dose. Studies in pregnant women, however, have not shown that aspirin increases the risk of abnormalities when administered during the first trimester of pregnancy. In controlled studies involving 41,337 pregnant women and their offspring, there was no evidence that aspirin taken during pregnancy caused stillbirth, neonatal death or reduced birthweight. In controlled studies of 50,282 pregnant women and their offspring, aspirin administration in moderate and heavy doses during the first four lunar months of pregnancy showed no teratogenic effect. Reproduction studies have been performed in rabbits and rats at doses up to 150 times the human dose and have revealed no evidence of impaired fertility or harm to the fetus due to codeine.

Nonteratogenic Effects: Therapeutic doses of aspirin in pregnant women close to term may cause bleeding in mother, fetus, or neonate. During the last six months of pregnancy, regular use of aspirin in high doses may prolong pregnancy and delivery.

Labor and Delivery: Ingestion of aspirin prior to delivery may prolong delivery or lead to bleeding in the mother or neonate. Use of codeine during labor may lead to respiratory depression in the neonate.

Nursing Mothers: Aspirin and codeine are excreted in breast milk in small amounts, but the significance of their effects on nursing infants is not known. Because of the potential for serious adverse reactions in nursing infants from Empirin® with Codeine, a decision should be made whether to discontinue nursing or to discontinue the drug, taking into account the importance of the drug to the mother.

Adverse Reactions:

Codeine: The most frequently observed adverse reactions to codeine include light-headedness, dizziness, drowsiness, nausea, vomiting, constipation and depression of respiration. Less common reactions to codeine include euphoria, dysphoria, pruritis and skin rashes.

Aspirin: Mild aspirin intoxication (salicylism) can occur in response to chronic use of large doses. Manifestations include nausea, vomiting, hearing impairment, tinnitus, diminished vision, headache, dizziness, drowsiness, mental confusion, hyperpnea, hyperventilation, tachycardia, sweating and thirst.

Therapeutic doses of aspirin can induce mild or severe allergic reactions manifested by skin rashes, urticaria, angioedema, rhinorrhea, asthma, abdominal pain, nausea, vomiting, or anaphylactic shock. A history of allergy is often lacking, and allergic reactions may occur even in patients who have previously taken aspirin without any ill effects. Allergic reactions to aspirin are most likely to occur in patients with a history of allergic disease, especially in patients with nasal polyps or asthma.

Some patients are unable to take aspirin or other salicylates without developing nausea or vomiting. Occasional patients respond to aspirin (usually in large doses) with dyspepsia or heartburn, which may be accompanied by occult bleeding. Excessive bruising or bleeding is sometimes seen in patients with mild disorders of primary hemostasis who regularly use low doses of aspirin.

Prolonged use of aspirin can cause painless erosion of gastric mucosa, occult bleeding and, infrequently, iron-deficiency anemia. High doses of aspirin can exacerbate symptoms of peptic ulcer and, occasionally, cause extensive bleeding.

Excessive bleeding can follow injury or surgery in patients with or without known bleeding disorders who have taken therapeutic doses of aspirin within the preceding 10 days.

Hepatotoxicity has been reported in association with prolonged use of large doses of aspirin in patients with lupus erythematosus, rheumatoid arthritis and rheumatic disease.

Bone marrow depression, manifested by weakness, fatigue, or abnormal bruising or bleeding, has occasionally been reported.

In patients with glucose-6-phosphate dehydrogenase deficiency, aspirin can cause a mild degree of hemolytic anemia.

In hyperuricemic persons, low doses of aspirin may reduce the effectiveness of uricosuric therapy or precipitate an attack of gout.

Drug Abuse and Dependence:
Like other medications containing a narcotic analgesic, Empirin® with Codeine is controlled by the Drug Enforcement Administration and is classified under Schedule III.

Empirin with Codeine can produce drug dependence of the morphine type; therefore, it has a potential for being abused. Psychic dependence, physical dependence and tolerance may develop on repeated administration.

The dependence liability of codeine has been found to be too small to permit a full definition of its characteristics. Studies indicate that addiction to codeine is extremely uncommon and requires very high parenteral doses.

When dependence on codeine occurs at therapeutic doses, it appears to require from one to two months to develop, and withdrawal symptoms are mild. Most patients on long-term oral codeine therapy show no signs of physical dependence upon abrupt withdrawal.

Overdosage: Severe intoxication, caused by overdose of Empirin® with Codeine may produce: skin eruptions, dyspnea, vertigo, double vision, delusions, hallucinations, garbled speech, excitability, restlessness, delirium, constricted pupils, a positive Babinski sign, respiratory depression (slow and shallow breathing; Cheyne-Stokes respiration), cyanosis, clammy skin, muscle flaccidity, circulatory collapse, stupor and coma. In children, difficulty in hearing, tinnitus, dim vision, headache, dizziness, drowsiness, confusion, rapid breathing, sweating, thirst, nausea, vomiting, hyperpyrexia, dehydration and convulsions are prominent signs. The most severe manifestations from aspirin result from cardiovascular and respiratory insufficiency secondary to acid-base and electrolyte disturbances, complicated by hyperthermia and dehydration. The most severe manifestations from codeine are associated with respiratory depression.

Respiratory alkalosis is characteristic of the early phase of intoxication with aspirin while hyperventilation is occurring, but is quickly followed by metabolic acidosis in most people with severe intoxication. This occurs more readily in children. Hypoglycemia may occur in children who have taken large overdoses. Other laboratory findings associated with aspirin intoxication include ketonuria, hyponatremia, hypokalemia, and occasionally proteinuria. A slight rise in lactic dehydrogenase and hydroxybutyric dehydrogenase may occur.

Concentrations of aspirin in plasma above 30 mg/100 ml are associated with toxicity. (See Clinical Pharmacology Section for information on factors influencing aspirin blood levels.) The single lethal dose of aspirin in adults is probably about 25–30 g, but is not known with certainty.

The toxic plasma concentration of codeine is not known with certainty. Experimental production of mild to moderate CNS depression in healthy, non-tolerant subjects occurred at plasma concentrations of 0.05–0.19 mg/100 ml when codeine was given by intravenous infusion. The single lethal dose of codeine in adults is estimated to be from 0.5–1.0 g. It is also estimated that 5 mg/kg could be fatal in children. Hemodialysis and peritoneal dialysis can be performed to reduce the body aspirin content. Codeine is theoretically dialyzable but the procedure has not been clinically established.

Treatment of overdosage consists primarily of support of vital functions, management of codeine-induced respiratory depression, increasing salicylate elimination, and correcting the acid-base imbalance due primarily to salicylism.

In a comatose patient, primary attention should be given to establishment of adequate respiratory exchange through provisions of a patent airway and the institution of assisted or controlled ventilation. The narcotic antagonist naloxone is a specific antidote for respiratory depression which may result from overdose or unusual sensitivity to narcotics. Therefore, an appropriate dose of an antagonist should be administered, preferably by the intravenous route, simultaneously with efforts at respiratory resuscitation. Since the duration of action of Empirin® with Codeine may exceed that of the antagonist, the patient should be kept under continued surveillance and repeated doses of the antagonist should be administered as needed to maintain adequate respiration.

A narcotic antagonist should not be administered in the absence of clinically significant respiratory or cardiovascular depression.

Gastric emptying (Syrup of Ipecac) and/or lavage is recommended as soon as possible after ingestion, even if the patient has vomited spontaneously. (Apomorphine should not be used as an emetic for Empirin® with Codeine, since it may potentiate hypotension and respiratory depression.) Administration of activated charcoal as a slurry is beneficial after lavage and/or emesis, if less than three hours have passed since ingestion. Charcoal adsorption should *not* be employed prior to emesis or lavage.

Severity of aspirin intoxication is determined by measuring the blood salicylate level. Acid-base status should be closely followed with serial blood gas and serum pH measurements. Fluid and electrolyte balance should also be regularly monitored.

A serum salicylate level of 30 mg/100 ml or higher indicates a need for enhanced salicylate excretion that can be achieved through body-fluid supplementation and urine alkalinization if renal function is normal. In mild intoxication, urine flow can be increased by forcing oral fluids and giving potassium citrate capsules. (DO NOT GIVE BICARBONATE BY MOUTH SINCE IT INCREASES THE RATE OF SALICYLATE ABSORPTION.)

In severe cases, hyperthermia and hypovolemia, as well as respiratory depression are the major immediate threats to life. Children should be sponged with tepid water. Replacement fluid should be administered intravenously and augmented with sufficient bicarbonate to correct acidosis, with monitoring of plasma electrolytes and pH, to promote alkaline diuresis of salicylate if renal function is normal. Complete control may also require infusion of glucose to control hypoglycemia.

Potassium deficiency may also be corrected through the infusion, once adequate urinary output is assured. Plasma or plasma expanders may be needed if fluid replacement is insufficient to maintain normal blood pressure or adequate urinary output.

In patients with renal insufficiency or in cases of life-threatening intoxication, dialysis is usually required. Peritoneal dialysis or exchange transfusion is indicated in infants and young children, and hemodialysis in older patients.

Oxygen, intravenous fluids, vasopressors and other supportive measures should be employed as needed.

Dosage and Administration: Dosage is adjusted according to the severity of pain and the response of the patient. It may occasionally be necessary to exceed the usual dosage recommended below when pain is severe or the patient has become tolerant to the analgesic effect of codeine. Empirin® with Codeine is given orally. The usual adult dose for Empirin with Codeine No. 2 and No. 3 is one or two tablets every four hours as required. The usual adult dose for Empirin with Codeine No. 4 is one tablet every four hours as required.

Empirin® with Codeine should be taken with food or a full glass of milk or water to lessen gastric irritation.

How Supplied:
Empirin with Codeine 15 mg No. 2: (white tablet imprinted with "EMPIRIN" and "2")
    Bottle of 100   NDC 0081-0215-55
    Bottle of 1000   NDC 0081-0215-75
Empirin with Codeine 30 mg No. 3: (white tablet imprinted with "EMPIRIN" and "3")
    Bottle of 100   NDC 0081-0220-55
    VA NSN 6505-00-959-4431
    Bottle of 500   NDC 0081-0220-70
    Bottle of 1000   NDC 0081-0220-75
    DoD NSN 6505-00-149-0116
Dispenserpak®
of 25   NDC 0081-0220-25
    DoD NSN 6505-06-118-2347
Empirin with Codeine 60 mg No. 4: (white tablet imprinted with "EMPIRIN" and "4")
    Bottle of 100   NDC 0081-0225-55
    Bottle of 500   NDC 0081-0225-70
    Bottle of 1000   NDC 0081-0225-75
Dispenserpak®
of 25   NDC 0081-0225-25

Store at 15°–30°C (59°–86°F) in a dry place and protect from light.

Shown in Product Identification Section, page 408

EMPRACET® with Codeine Phosphate ℞ @
[*im'prah-set"*]
30 mg, No. 3; 60 mg, No. 4

Description: Each Empracet with Codeine Phosphate tablet contains codeine phosphate* 30 mg in No. 3 and 60 mg in No. 4 (**WARNING:** May be habit-forming) and acetaminophen 300 mg.

Acetaminophen occurs as a white, odorless crystalline powder, possessing a slightly bitter taste. Codeine is an alkaloid, obtained from opium or prepared from morphine by methylation. Codeine occurs as colorless or white crystals, effloresces slowly in dry air and is affected by light.

Actions: Acetaminophen is a nonopiate, non-salicylate analgesic and antipyretic. Codeine is an opiate analgesic and antitussive. Codeine retains at least one-half of its analgesic activity when administered orally.

Indications: No. 3—for relief of mild to moderate pain; No. 4—for the relief of moderate to moderately severe pain.

Contraindications: Hypersensitivity to acetaminophen or codeine.

Continued on next page

Burroughs Wellcome—Cont.

Warnings:
Drug Dependence: Codeine can produce drug dependence of the morphine type, and therefore has the potential for being abused. Psychic dependence, physical dependence and tolerance may develop upon repeated administration of this drug and it should be prescribed and administered with the same degree of caution appropriate to the use of other oral narcotic medications. This acetaminophen and codeine dosage form is subject to the Federal Controlled Substances Act (Schedule III).
Precautions:
General:
Head injury and increased intracranial pressure: The respiratory depressant effects of narcotics and their potential to elevate cerebrospinal fluid pressure may be markedly exaggerated in the presence of head injury, other intracranial lesions or a pre-existing increase in intracranial pressure. Furthermore, narcotics produce adverse reactions which may obscure the clinical course of patients with head injuries.
Acute abdominal conditions: The administration of products containing codeine or other narcotics may obscure the diagnosis or clinical course in patients with acute abdominal conditions.
Special risk patients: Acetaminophen with codeine should be given with caution to certain patients, such as the elderly or debilitated, and those with severe impairment of hepatic or renal function, hypothyroidism, Addison's disease, and prostatic hypertrophy or urethral stricture.
Information for Patients: Codeine may impair the mental and/or physical abilities required for the performance of potentially hazardous tasks such as driving a car or operating machinery. The patient taking this drug should be cautioned accordingly.
Drug Interactions: Patients receiving other narcotic analgesics, antipsychotics, antianxiety, or other CNS depressants (including alcohol) concomitantly with acetaminophen and codeine may exhibit additive CNS depression due to the codeine component. When such therapy is contemplated, the dose of one or both agents should be reduced. The use of MAO inhibitors or tricyclic antidepressants with codeine preparations may increase the effect of either the antidepressant or codeine.
The concurrent use of anticholinergics with codeine may produce paralytic ileus.
Usage in Pregnancy: Safe use in pregnancy has not been established relative to possible adverse effects on fetal development. Therefore, acetaminophen and codeine should not be used in pregnant women unless, in the judgment of the physician, the potential benefits outweigh the possible hazards.
Nursing Mothers: It is not known whether the components of this drug are excreted in human milk. Because many drugs are excreted in human milk, caution should be exercised when acetaminophen and codeine is administered to a nursing woman.
Adverse Reactions: The most frequently observed adverse reactions include light-headedness, dizziness, sedation, shortness of breath, nausea and vomiting. These effects seem to be more prominent in ambulatory than in non-ambulatory patients, and some of these adverse reactions may be alleviated if the patient lies down.
Other adverse reactions include euphoria, dysphoria, constipation and pruritus. At higher doses, codeine has most of the disadvantages of morphine, including respiratory depression.
Overdosage:
Acetaminophen:
Signs and Symptoms: Acetaminophen in massive overdosage may cause hepatic toxicity in some patients. In all cases of suspected overdose, immediately call your regional poison center or the Rocky Mountain Poison Center's toll-free number (800-525-6115) for assistance in diagnosis and for directions in the use of N-acetylcysteine as an antidote, a use currently restricted to investigational status.
In adults, hepatic toxicity has rarely been reported with acute overdoses of less than 10 grams and fatalities with less than 15 grams. Importantly, young children seem to be more resistant than adults to the hepatotoxic effect of an acetaminophen overdose. Despite this, the measures outlined below should be initiated in any adult or child suspected of having ingested an acetaminophen overdose.
Early symptoms following a potentially hepatotoxic overdose may include: nausea, vomiting, diaphoresis and general malaise. Clinical and laboratory evidence of hepatic toxicity may not be apparent until 48 to 72 hours post-ingestion.
Treatment: The stomach should be emptied promptly by lavage or by induction of emesis with syrup of ipecac. Patients' estimates of the quantity of a drug ingested are notoriously unreliable. Therefore, if an acetaminophen overdose is suspected, a serum acetaminophen assay should be obtained as early as possible, but no sooner than four hours following ingestion. Liver function studies should be obtained initially and repeated at 24-hour intervals.
The antidote, N-acetylcysteine, should be administered as early as possible, and within 16 hours of the overdose ingestion for optimal results. Following recovery, there are no residual, structural or functional hepatic abnormalities.
Codeine:
Signs and Symptoms: Serious overdose with codeine is characterized by respiratory depression (a decrease in respiratory rate and/or tidal volume. Cheyne-Stokes respiration, cyanosis), extreme somnolence progressing to stupor or coma, skeletal muscle flaccidity, cold and clammy skin, and sometimes bradycardia and hypotension. In severe overdosage, apnea, circulatory collapse, cardiac arrest, and death may occur.
Treatment: Primary attention should be given to the reestablishment of adequate respiratory exchange through provision of a patent airway and the institution of assisted or controlled ventilation. The narcotic antagonist naloxone is a specific antidote against respiratory depression which may result from overdosage or unusual sensitivity to narcotics, including codeine. Therefore, an appropriate dose of naloxone (see package insert) should be administered, preferably by the intravenous route, and simultaneously with efforts at respiratory resuscitation. Since the duration of action of codeine may exceed that of the antagonist, the patient should be kept under continued surveillance and repeated doses of the antagonist should be administered as needed to maintain adequate respiration.
An antagonist should not be administered in the absence of clinically significant respiratory or cardiovascular depression. Oxygen, intravenous fluids, vasopressors and other supportive measures should be employed as indicated.
Gastric emptying may be useful in removing unabsorbed drug.
Dosage and Administration: Dosage should be adjusted according to severity of pain and response of the patient. However, it should be kept in mind that tolerance to codeine can develop with continued use and that the incidence of untoward effects is dose related. This product is inappropriate even in high doses for severe or intractable pain. Adult doses of codeine higher than 60 mg fail to give commensurate relief of pain, but merely prolong analgesia and are associated with an appreciably increased incidence of undesirable side effects. Equivalently high doses in children would have similar effects.
The usual adult dose of Empracet with Codeine phosphate 30 mg, No. 3 is one or two tablets every four hours, as required.
The usual adult dose of Empracet with Codeine phosphate 60 mg, No. 4 is one tablet every four hours, as required.
How Supplied: Empracet® with Codeine phosphate 30 mg. No. 3 is available in tablets (peach) coded with "Empracet 3" and "K9B." Bottles of 100, (NDC-0081-0315-55) 500 (NDC-0081-0315-70) and Dispenserpak® of 25 (NDC-0081-0315-25). Empracet® with Codeine Phosphate 60 mg, No. 4, is available in tablets (peach), coded with "EMPRACET 4" and "L9B." Bottles of 100 (NDC-0081-0327-55) and 500 (NDC-0081-0327-70).
Shown in Product Identification Section, page 408

FEDRAZIL® TABLETS
[fĕd'rah-zĭl"]
(See PDR for Nonprescription Drugs).

IMURAN® R
[ĭm'ū-ran"]
(Azathioprine)
50 mg Scored Tablets
20 ml vial (as the sodium salt) for I.V. injection, equivalent to 100 mg Azathioprine sterile lyophilized material.

> **Warning:** Chronic immunosuppression with this purine antimetabolite increases *risk of neoplasia* in humans. Physicians using this drug should be very familiar with this risk as well as with the mutagenic potential to both men and women and with possible hematologic toxicities. See below under WARNINGS.

Description: Azathioprine is chemically 6-[(1-methyl-4-nitro-imidazol-5-yl)thio] purine. It is an imidazolyl derivative of 6-mercaptopurine (Purinethol®) and many of its biological effects are similar to those of the parent compound.
Azathioprine is insoluble in water, but may be dissolved with addition of one molar equivalent of alkali. The sodium salt of azathioprine is sufficiently soluble to make a 10 mg/ml water solution which is stable for 24 hours at 59° to 86°F (15° to 30°C). Azathioprine is stable in solution at neutral or acid pH but hydrolysis to mercaptopurine occurs in excess sodium hydroxide (0.1N), especially on warming. Conversion to mercaptopurine also occurs in the presence of sulfhydryl compounds such as cysteine, glutathione and hydrogen sulfide.
Clinical Pharmacology and Actions
Metabolism[1]: Azathioprine is well absorbed following oral administration. Maximum serum radioactivity occurs at one to two hours after oral ^{35}S-azathioprine and decays with a half-life of five hours. This is not an estimate of the half-life of azathioprine itself but is the decay rate for all ^{35}S-containing metabolites of the drug. Because of extensive metabolism, only a fraction of the radioactivity is present as azathioprine. Usual doses produce blood levels of azathioprine, and of mercaptopurine derived from it, which are low (<1 mcg/ml). Blood levels are of little predictive value for therapy since the magnitude and duration of clinical effects correlate with thiopurine nucleotide levels in tissues rather than with plasma drug levels. Azathioprine and mercaptopurine are moderately bound to serum proteins (30%) and are partially dialyzable.
Azathioprine is cleaved *in vivo* to mercaptopurine. Both compounds are rapidly eliminated from blood and are oxidized or methylated in erythrocytes and liver, no azathioprine or mercaptopurine is detectable in urine after eight hours. Conversion to inactive 6-thiouric acid by xanthine oxidase is an important degradative pathway, and the inhibition of this pathway in patients receiving allopurinol (Zyloprim®) is the basis for the azathioprine dosage reduction required in these patients (see DOSAGE AND ADMINISTRATION). Proportions of metabolites are different in individual patients, and this presumably accounts for variable magnitude and duration of drug effects. Renal clearance is probably not important in predicting biological effectiveness or toxicities, although dose reduction is practiced in patients with poor renal function.
Homograft Survival[1,2]: Summary information from transplant centers and registries indicates relatively universal use of Imuran® with or without other immunosuppressive agents.[3,4,5] Although the use of azathioprine for inhibition of

renal homograft rejection is well established, the mechanism(s) for this action are somewhat obscure. The drug suppresses hypersensitivities of the cell-mediated type and causes variable alterations in antibody production. Suppression of T-cell effects, including ablation of T-cell suppression, is dependent on the temporal relationship to antigenic stimulus or engraftment. This agent has little effect on established graft rejections or secondary responses.

Alterations in specific immune responses or immunologic functions in transplant recipients are difficult to relate specifically to immunosuppression by azathioprine. These patients have subnormal responses to vaccines, low numbers of T-cells, and abnormal phagocytosis by peripheral blood cells, but their mitogenic responses, serum immunoglobulins and secondary antibody responses are usually normal. Transplant recipients on azathioprine also receive corticosteroids and may be given antilymphocyte globulin; there are no known hazards or toxicities due to interactions of these agents.

Immunoinflammatory Response: Azathioprine suppresses disease manifestations as well as underlying pathology in animal models of auto-immune disease. For example, the severity of adjuvant arthritis is reduced by azathioprine.

The mechanisms whereby azathioprine affects auto-immune diseases are not known. Azathioprine is immunosuppressive, delayed hypersensitivity and cellular cytotoxicity tests being suppressed to a greater degree than are antibody responses. In the rat model of adjuvant arthritis, azathioprine has been shown to inhibit the lymph node hyperplasia which precedes the onset of the signs of the disease. Both the immunosuppressive and therapeutic effects in animal models are dose-related. Azathioprine is considered a slow acting drug and effects may persist after the drug has been discontinued.

Indications and Usage: Imuran® is indicated as an adjunct for the prevention of rejection in renal homotransplantation. It is also indicated for the management of severe, active rheumatoid arthritis unresponsive to rest, aspirin or other nonsteroidal anti-inflammatory drugs, or to agents in the class of which gold is an example.

Renal Homotransplantation: Imuran is indicated as an adjunct for the prevention of rejection in renal homotransplantation. Experience with over 16,000 transplants shows a five-year patient survival of 35% to 55%, but this is dependent on donor, match for HLA antigens, anti-donor or anti B-cell alloantigen antibody and other variables. The effect of Imuran on these variables has not been tested in controlled trials.

Rheumatoid Arthritis[6,7]**:** Imuran is indicated only in adult patients meeting criteria for classic or definite rheumatoid arthritis as specified by the American Rheumatism Association[8]. Imuran should be restricted to patients with severe, active and erosive disease not responsive to conventional management including rest, aspirin or other nonsteroidal drugs or to agents in the class of which gold is an example. Rest, physiotherapy and salicylates should be continued while Imuran is given, but it may be possible to reduce the dose of corticosteroids in patients on Imuran. The combined use of Imuran with gold, antimalarials or penicillamine has not been studied for either added benefit or unexpected adverse effects. The use of Imuran with these agents cannot be recommended.

Contraindications: Imuran should not be given to patients who have shown hypersensitivity to the drug.

Imuran should not be used for treating rheumatoid arthritis in pregnant women.

Patients with rheumatoid arthritis previously treated with alkylating agents (cyclophosphamide, chlorambucil, melphalan or others) may have a prohibitive risk of neoplasia if treated with Imuran.

Warnings: Severe *leukopenia and/or thrombocytopenia* may occur in patients on Imuran. Macrocytic anemia and severe bone marrow depression may also occur. Hematologic toxicities are dose related and may be more severe in renal transplant patients whose homograft is undergoing rejection. It is suggested that patients on Imuran have complete blood counts, including platelet counts, weekly during the first month, twice monthly for the second and third months of treatment, then monthly or more frequently if dosage alterations or other therapy changes are necessary. Delayed hematologic suppression may occur. Prompt reduction in dosage or temporary withdrawal of the drug may be necessary if there is a rapid fall in, or persistently low leukocyte count or other evidence of bone marrow depression. Leukopenia does not correlate with therapeutic effect, therefore the dose should not be increased intentionally to lower the white blood cell count.

Serious infections are a constant hazard for patients on chronic immunosuppression, especially for homograft recipients. Fungal, viral, bacterial and protozoal infections may be fatal and should be treated vigorously. Reduction of azathioprine dosage and/or use of other drugs should be considered.

Imuran® is mutagenic in animals and humans, carcinogenic in animals, and may increase the patient's *risk of neoplasia*. Renal transplant patients are known to have an increased risk of malignancy, predominantly skin cancer and reticulum cell or lymphomatous tumors.[9] Information is available on the spontaneous neoplasia risk in Rheumatoid Arthritis[11], and on neoplasia following immunosuppressive therapy of other autoimmune diseases[12]. It has not been possible to define the precise risk of neoplasia due to Imuran[10], but the risk is lower for patients with rheumatoid arthritis than for transplant recipients. However, acute myelogenous leukemia as well as solid tumors have been reported in patients with rheumatoid arthritis who have received azathioprine. Data on neoplasia in patients receiving Imuran can be found under Adverse Reactions.

Pregnancy Warning[13]**:** Imuran should not be given during pregnancy without careful weighing of risk versus benefit. Whenever possible, use of Imuran in pregnant patients should be avoided. Imuran has been shown to be mutagenic in both male and female animals. Chromosomal abnormalities have also been documented in patients, however, the abnormalities in humans were reversed upon discontinuance of the drug.[14]

Imuran is teratogenic in rodents. Transplacental transmission of azathioprine and its metabolites has been reported in man.[15] Limited immunologic and other abnormalities have occurred in some infants born of renal homograft recipients on Imuran. Benefit versus risk must be weighed carefully before use of Imuran in patients of reproductive potential. This drug should not be used for treating rheumatoid arthritis in pregnant women.

Precautions: Patient information: Patients being started on Imuran should be informed of the necessity of periodic blood counts while they are receiving the drug and should be encouraged to report any unusual bleeding or bruising to their physician. They should be advised of the danger of infection while receiving Imuran and encouraged to report signs and symptoms of infection to their physician. Careful dosage instructions should be given to the patient, especially when Imuran is being administered in the presence of impaired renal function or concomitantly with allopurinol (see DOSAGE AND ADMINISTRATION). Patients should be advised of the potential risks of the use of Imuran during pregnancy and during the nursing period. The increased risk of neoplasia following Imuran therapy should be explained to the patient.

Adverse Reactions: The principal and potentially serious toxic effects of Imuran® are hematologic and gastrointestinal. The risks of secondary infection and neoplasia are also important. The frequency and severity of adverse reactions depend on the dose and duration of Imuran as well as on the patient's underlying disease or concomitant therapies. The incidence of hematologic toxicities and neoplasia encountered in groups of renal homograft recipients is significantly higher than that in studies employing Imuran for rheumatoid arthritis. The relative incidences in clinical studies are summarized below:

Toxicity	Renal Homograft	Rheumatoid Arthritis
Leukopenia		
Any Degree	<50%	28 %
<2500/mm^3	16%	5.3%
Neoplasia		
Lymphoma	0.5%	
Others	2.8%	*

*18 reported cases; denominator unknown.

Hematologic: Leukopenia and/or thrombocytopenia are dose dependent and may occur late in the course of Imuran therapy. Dose reduction or temporary withdrawal allows reversal of these toxicities. Infection may occur as a secondary manifestation of bone marrow suppression or leukopenia, but the incidence of infection in renal homotransplantation is 30 to 60 times that in rheumatoid arthritis. Macrocytic anemia and/or bleeding have been reported in two patients on Imuran.

Gastrointestinal: Nausea and vomiting may occur within the first few months of Imuran therapy, and occurred in approximately 12% of 676 rheumatoid arthritis patients. The frequency of gastric disturbance can be reduced by administration of the drug in divided doses and/or after meals. Vomiting with abdominal pain may occur rarely with a hypersensitivity pancreatitis. Hepatotoxicity with elevated serum alkaline phosphatase and bilirubin is known to occur with thiopurines including Imuran and 6-mercaptopurine (Purinethol®). This toxic hepatitis with biliary stasis is known to occur in homograft recipients and has been generally reversible after interruption of Imuran. Hepatotoxicity has been uncommon in rheumatoid arthritis patients on Imuran (less than 1%).

Others: Additional side effects of low frequency have been reported. These include skin rashes (approximately 2%), alopecia, fever, arthralgias, diarrhea, steatorrhea and negative nitrogen balance (all less than 1%).

Dosage and Administration: Renal Homotransplantation: The dose of Imuran® required to prevent rejection and minimize toxicity will vary with individual patients; this necessitates careful management. Initial dose is usually 3 to 5 mg/kg daily, beginning at the time of transplant. Imuran is usually given as a single daily dose on the day of, and in a minority of cases one to three days before, transplantation. Imuran is often initiated with the intravenous administration of the sodium salt, with subsequent use of tablets (at the same dose level) after the post-operative period. Intravenous administration of the sodium salt is indicated only in patients unable to tolerate oral medications. Dose reduction to maintenance levels of 1 to 3 mg/kg daily is usually possible. The dose of Imuran should not be increased to toxic levels because of threatened rejection. Discontinuation may be necessary for severe hematologic or other toxicity, even if rejection of the homograft may be a consequence of drug withdrawal.

Rheumatoid Arthritis: Imuran is usually given on a daily basis. The initial dose should be approximately 1.0 mg/kg (50 to 100 mg) given as a single dose or on a twice daily schedule. The dose may be increased, beginning at six to eight weeks and thereafter by steps at four-week intervals, if there are no serious toxicities and if initial response is unsatisfactory. Dose increments should be 0.5 mg/kg daily, up to a maximum dose of 2.5 mg/kg/day. Therapeutic response occurs after several weeks of treatment, usually six to eight; an adequate trial should be a minimum of 12 weeks. Patients not improved after twelve weeks can be considered refractory. Imuran may be continued long-term in patients with clinical response, but patients should be monitored carefully, and gradual dosage reduction should be attempted to reduce risk of toxicities. Maintenance therapy should be at the lowest effective dose, and the dose given can be lowered incrementally with changes of 0.5 mg/kg or approximately 25 mg daily every

Continued on next page

Burroughs Wellcome—Cont.

four weeks while other therapy is kept constant. The optimum duration of maintenance Imuran has not been determined. Imuran can be discontinued abruptly, but delayed effects are possible.

Use in Renal Dysfunction: Relatively oliguric patients, especially those with tubular necrosis in the immediate post-cadaveric transplant period, may have delayed clearance of Imuran or its metabolites, may be particularly sensitive to this drug and may require lower doses.

Use with Allopurinol (Zyloprim®): The principal pathway for detoxification of Imuran is inhibited by allopurinol (Zyloprim). Patients receiving Imuran and Zyloprim concomitantly should have a dose reduction of Imuran, to approximately $\frac{1}{3}$ to $\frac{1}{4}$ the usual dose.

Parenteral Administration: Add 10 ml of sterile Water for Injection, and swirl until a clear solution results. This solution is for intravenous use only; it has a pH of approximately 9.6, and it should be used within twenty-four hours. Further dilution into sterile saline or dextrose is usually made for infusion; the final volume depends on time for the infusion, usually 30-60 minutes but as short as 5 minutes and as long as 8 hours for the daily dose.

How Supplied: 50 mg oval-shaped, yellow, scored tablets imprinted with "IMURAN" and "50" on each tablet; bottle of 100. **DoD & VA NSN 6505-00-119-9317**

20 ml vial containing the equivalent of 100 mg azathioprine (as the sodium salt). The sterile, lyophilized sodium salt is yellow, and should be dissolved in sterile Water for Injection (see Parenteral Administration under DOSAGE AND ADMINISTRATION).

References:
1. Elion, G.B. and G.H. Hitchings, "Azathioprine" in *Handbook of Experimental Pharmacology*, Vol. 38, ed. by Sartorelli and Johns, Springer Verlag, New York, 1975.
2. McIntosh, J., P. Hansen et al., "Defective Immune and Phagocytic Functions in Uremia and Renal Transplantation," *Int. Arch. Allergy Appl. Immunol.*, 51:544–559, 1976.
3. Advisory Committee, Renal Transplant Registry, "The 12th Report of the Human Renal Transplant Registry," *JAMA*, 233:787–796, 1975.
4. McGeown, M., "Immunosuppression for Kidney Transplantation," *Lancet*, ii:310–312, 1973.
5. Simmons, R.L., E.J. Thompson et al., "115 Patients with First Cadaver Kidney Transplants Followed Two to Seven and a Half Years," *Am. J. Med.*, 62:234–242, 1977.
6. Fye, K. and N. Talal, "Cytotoxic Drugs in the Treatment of Rheumatoid Arthritis," *Ration. Drug Ther.*, 9(4): 1–5, 1975.
7. Davis, J.D., H.B. Muss, and R.A. Turner, "Cytotoxic Agents in the Treatment of Rheumatoid Arthritis," *South. Med. J.*, 71(1): 58–64, 1978.
8. McEwen, C., "The Diagnosis and Differential Diagnosis of Rheumatoid Arthritis," *Arthritis and Allied Conditions*, Philadelphia, Lea and Febiger, pp. 403–418, 1972.
9. Hoover, R. and J.F. Fraumeni, "Risk of Cancer in Renal Transplant Recipients," *Lancet*, 2:55–57, 1973.
10. Sieber, S.M. and R.H. Adamson, "Toxicity of Antineoplastic Agents in Man," *Adv. Cancer Res.*, 22:57–155, 1975.
11. Lewis, R.B., C.W. Castor, R.E. Knisley, and G.C. Bole, "Frequency of Neoplasia in Systemic Lupus Erythematosus and Rheumatoid Arthritis," *Arthritis Rheum.*, 19(6): 1256–1260, 1976.
12. Louie, S. and R.S. Schwartz, "Immunodeficiency and the Pathogenesis of Lymphoma and Leukemia," *Semin. Hematol.*, 15(2): 117–138, 1978.
13. Tagatz, G.E. and R.L. Simmons, "Pregnancy After Renal Transplantation," *Ann. Intern. Med.*, 82:113–114, 1975 (Editorial).
14. Hunter, T., M.B. Urowitz, D.A. Gordon, H.A. Smythe and M.A. Ogryzlo, Azathioprine in Rheumatoid Arthritis. A Long-Term Follow-Up Study, *Arthritis Rheum.*, 18(1): 15–20, 1975.
15. Saarikoski, S. and M. Sepalla, Immunosuppressive During Pregnancy: Transmission of Azathioprine and its Metabolites from the Mother to the Fetus, *Am. J. Obstet, Gynecol.*, 115(8): 1100–1106, 1973.

Shown in Product Identification Section, page 408

KEMADRIN®
[kĕm'ah-drĭn]
(Procyclidine Hydrochloride)

Description: Kemadrin (Procyclidine Hydrochloride) is a synthetic antispasmodic compound of relatively low toxicity. It has been shown to be useful for the symptomatic treatment of parkinsonism (paralysis agitans) and extrapyramidal dysfunction caused by tranquilizer therapy. Procyclidine hydrochloride was developed at The Wellcome Research Laboratories as the most promising of a series of antiparkinsonism compounds produced by chemical modification of antihistamines. Chemically it is 1-cyclohexyl-1-phenyl-3-pyrrolidinopropan-1-ol hydrochloride, a white crystalline substance, soluble in water and almost tasteless. It is stable at normal temperatures and has the following structural formula:

Pharmacologic Action: Pharmacologic tests have shown that procyclidine hydrochloride has an atropine-like action and exerts an antispasmodic effect on smooth muscle. It is a potent mydriatic and inhibits salivation. It has no sympathetic ganglion blocking activity in doses as high as 4 mg/kg, as measured by the lack of inhibition of the response of the nictitating membrane to preganglionic electrical stimulation.

The intravenous LD_{50} in mice was about 60 mg/kg. Subcutaneously, doses of 300 mg/kg were not toxic. In dogs the intraperitoneal administration of procyclidine hydrochloride in doses of 5 mg/kg caused maximal dilation of the pupil and inhibition of salivation, but had no toxic action. When the dose was increased to 20 mg/kg the same symptoms occurred, and in addition there were tremors and ataxia lasting 4 to 5 hours. In one animal convulsions occurred which were controlled by pentobarbital. In all animals behavior returned to normal within 24 hours.

Chronic toxicity tests in rats showed that the compound caused only a very slight retardation in growth, and no change in the erythrocyte count or the histological appearance of the lungs, liver, spleen and kidney when as much as 10 mg/kg body weight was given subcutaneously daily for 9 weeks.

Indications: Kemadrin (Procyclidine Hydrochloride) is indicated for the treatment of parkinsonism including the postencephalitic, arteriosclerotic and idiopathic types. Partial control of the parkinsonism symptoms is the usual therapeutic accomplishment. Procyclidine hydrochloride is usually more efficacious in the relief of rigidity than tremor; but tremor, fatigue, weakness and sluggishness are frequently beneficially influenced. It can be substituted for all previous medications in mild and moderate cases. For the control of more severe cases other drugs may be added to procyclidine therapy as indications warrant. Clinical reports indicate that procyclidine often successfully relieves the symptoms of extrapyramidal dysfunction (dystonia, dyskinesia, akathisia and parkinsonism) which accompany the therapy of mental disorders with phenothiazine and rauwolfia compounds. In addition to minimizing the symptoms induced by tranquilizing drugs, the drug effectively controls sialorrhea resulting from neuroleptic medication. At the same time freedom from the side effects induced by tranquilizer drugs, as provided by the administration of procyclidine, permits a more sustained treatment of the patient's mental disorder.

Clinical results in the treatment of parkinsonism indicate that most patients experience subjective improvement characterized by a feeling of well-being and increased alertness, together with diminished salivation and a marked improvement in muscular coordination as demonstrated by objective tests of manual dexterity and by increased ability to carry out ordinary self-care activities. While the drug exerts a mild atropine-like action and therefore causes mydriasis, this may be kept minimal by careful adjustment of the daily dosage.

Contraindications: Procyclidine hydrochloride should not be used in angle-closure glaucoma although simple type glaucomas do not appear to be adversely affected.

Warnings:
Use in Children
Safety and efficacy have not been established in the pediatric age group; therefore, the use of procyclidine hydrochloride in this age group requires that the potential benefits be weighed against the possible hazards to the child.
Pregnancy Warning
The safe use of this drug in pregnancy has not been established; therefore, the use of procyclidine hydrochloride in pregnancy, lactation or in women of childbearing age requires that the potential benefits be weighed against the possible hazards to the mother and child.

Precautions: Conditions in which inhibition of the parasympathetic nervous system is undesirable such as tachycardia and urinary retention (such as may occur with marked prostatic hypertrophy) require special care in the administration of the drug. Hypotensive patients who receive the drug should be observed closely. Occasionally, particularly in older patients, mental confusion and disorientation may occur with the development of agitation, hallucinations and psychotic-like symptoms.

Patients with mental disorders occasionally experience a precipitation of a psychotic episode when the dosage of antiparkinsonism drugs is increased to treat the extrapyramidal side effects of phenothiazine and rauwolfia derivatives.

Adverse Reactions: Anticholinergic effects can be produced by therapeutic doses although these can frequently be minimized or eliminated by careful dosage. They include: dryness of the mouth, mydriasis, blurring of vision, giddiness, light headedness and gastrointestinal disturbances such as nausea, vomiting, epigastric distress and constipation. Occasionally an allergic reaction such as a skin rash may be encountered. Feelings of muscular weakness may occur. Acute suppurative parotitis as a complication of dry mouth has been reported.

Dosage and Administration:
For Parkinsonism
The dosage of the drug for the treatment of parkinsonism depends upon the age of the patient, the etiology of the disease, and individual responsiveness. Therefore, the dosage must remain flexible to permit adjustment to the individual tolerance and requirements of each patient. In general, younger and postencephalitic patients require and tolerate a somewhat higher dosage than older patients and those with arteriosclerosis.

For Patients Who Have Received No Other Therapy
The usual dose of procyclidine hydrochloride for initial treatment is 2.5 mg administered three times daily after meals. If well tolerated, this dose may be gradually increased to 5 mg three times a day and occasionally 5 mg given before retiring. In some cases smaller doses may be employed with good therapeutic results.

Occasionally a patient is encountered who cannot tolerate a bedtime dose of the drug. In such cases it may be desirable to adjust dosage so that the bedtime dose is omitted and the total daily requirement is administered in three equal daytime doses. It is best administered during or after meals to minimize the development of side reactions.

To Transfer Patients to Kemadrin brand Procyclidine Hydrochloride from Other Therapy
Patients who have been receiving other drugs may be transferred to procyclidine hydrochloride. This is accomplished gradually by substituting 2.5 mg three times a day for all or part of the original drug. The dose of procyclidine is then increased as required while that of the other drug is correspondingly omitted or decreased until complete replacement is achieved. The total daily dosage may then be adjusted to the level which produces maximum benefit.

For Drug-Induced Extrapyramidal Symptoms
For treatment of symptoms of extrapyramidal dysfunction induced by tranquilizer drugs during the therapy of mental disorders, the dosage of procyclidine hydrochloride will depend on the severity of side effects associated with tranquilizer administration. In general the larger the dosage of the tranquilizer the more severe will be the associated symptoms, including rigidity and tremors. Accordingly, the drug dosage should be adjusted to suit the needs of the individual patient and to provide maximum relief of the induced symptoms. A convenient method to establish the daily dosage of procyclidine is to begin with the administration of 2.5 mg three times daily. This may be increased by 2.5 mg daily increments until the patient obtains relief of symptoms. In most cases excellent results will be obtained with 10 to 20 mg daily.

How Supplied: Scored tablets of 5 mg, bottles of 100. Tablets bear imprint KEMADRIN, S3A.
Shown in Product Identification Section, page 408

LANOXICAPS® R
[lă-nŏx'ĭ-kăps"]
(Digoxin Solution in Capsules)
50 µg (0.05 mg) I.D. Imprint A2C (red)
100 µg (0.1 mg) I.D. Imprint B2C (yellow)
200 µg (0.2 mg) I.D. Imprint C2C (green)

Description: Digoxin is one of the cardiac (or digitalis) glycosides, a closely related group of drugs having in common specific effects on the myocardium. These drugs are found in a number of plants. Digoxin is extracted from the leaves of *Digitalis lanata*. The term "digitalis" is used to designate the whole group. The glycosides are composed of two portions: a sugar and a cardenolide (hence "glycosides").

Digoxin has the molecular formula $C_{41}H_{64}O_{14}$, a molecular weight of 780.95 and melting and decomposition points above 235°C. The drug is practically insoluble in water and in ether; slightly soluble in diluted (50%) alcohol and in chloroform; and freely soluble in pyridine. Digoxin powder is composed of odorless white crystals.

Digoxin has the chemical name: 3β-[(O-2,6-dideoxy- β -D-ribo-hexopyranosyl-(1→4)-O-2,6-dideoxy- β -D-ribo-hexopyranosyl-(1→4)- 2,6-dideoxy-β-D-ribo-hexopyranosyl) oxy]-12β, 14-dihydroxy-5β-card-20(22)-enolide, and the structure shown: (See next column)

Lanoxicaps is a stable solution of digoxin enclosed within a soft gelatin capsule for oral use. Each capsule contains the labeled amount of digoxin USP dissolved in a solvent comprised of polyethylene glycol 400 USP, 8 percent ethyl alcohol, propylene glycol USP and purified water USP.

Clinical Pharmacology:
Mechanism of Action: The influence of digitalis glycosides on the myocardium is dose-related, and involves both a direct action on cardiac muscle and the specialized conduction system, and indirect actions on the cardiovascular system mediated by the autonomic nervous system. The indirect actions mediated by the autonomic nervous system involve a vagomimetic action, which is responsible for the effects of digitalis on the sino-atrial (SA) and atrioventricular (AV) nodes; and also a baroreceptor sensitization which results in increased carotid sinus nerve activity and enhanced sympathetic withdrawal for any given increment in mean arterial pressure. The pharmacologic consequences of these direct and indirect effects are: 1) an increase in the force and velocity of myocardial systolic contraction (positive inotropic action); 2) a slowing of heart rate (negative chronotropic effect); and 3) decreased conduction velocity through the AV node. In higher doses, digitalis increases sympathetic outflow from the central nervous system (CNS) to both cardiac and peripheral sympathetic nerves. This increase in sympathetic activity may be an important factor in digitalis cardiac toxicity. Most of the extracardiac manifestations of digitalis toxicity are also mediated by the CNS.

Pharmacokinetics:
Absorption—Gastrointestinal absorption of digoxin is a passive process. Absorption of digoxin from Lanoxicaps capsules has been demonstrated to be 90 to 100% complete compared to an identical intravenous dose of digoxin. Conventional digoxin tablets are absorbed 60 to 80%. The enhanced absorption from Lanoxicaps compared to digoxin tablets and elixir is associated with reduced between-patient and within-patient variability in steady-state serum concentrations. The peak serum concentrations are higher than those observed after tablets. When digoxin tablets or capsules are taken after meals, the rate of absorption is slowed, but the total amount of digoxin absorbed is usually unchanged. When taken with meals high in bran fiber, however, the amount absorbed from an oral dose may be reduced. Comparisons of the systemic availability and equivalent doses for digoxin preparations are shown in the following table:
[See table above].

LANOXICAPS PRODUCT	BIOAVAILABILITY		EQUIVALENT DOSES (IN MG)*	
Lanoxin® Tablet	60–80%	0.125	0.25	0.5
Lanoxin Elixir	70–85%	0.125	0.25	0.5
Lanoxin Injection/IM	70–85%	0.125	0.25	0.5
Lanoxin Injection/IV	100%	0.1	0.2	0.4
Lanoxicaps Capsules	90–100%	0.1	0.2	0.4

*1 mg = 1000 µg

In some patients, orally administered digoxin is converted to cardioinactive reduction products (e.g., dihydrodigoxin) by colonic bacteria in the gut. Data suggest that one in ten patients treated with digoxin tablets will degrade 40% or more of the ingested dose. This phenomenon is minimized with Lanoxicaps because they are rapidly absorbed in the upper gastrointestinal tract.

Distribution—Following drug administration, a 6 to 8 hour distribution phase is observed. This is followed by a much more gradual serum concentration decline, which is dependent on digoxin elimination from the body. The peak height and slope of the early portion (absorption/distribution phases) of the serum concentration-time curve are dependent upon the route of administration and the absorption characteristics of the formulation. Clinical evidence indicates that the early high serum concentrations (particularly high for digoxin capsules) do not reflect the concentration of digoxin at its site of action, but that with chronic use, the steady-state post-distribution serum levels are in equilibrium with tissue levels and correlate with pharmacologic effects. In individual patients, these post-distribution serum concentrations are linearly related to maintenance dosage and may be useful in evaluating therapeutic and toxic effects (see Serum Digoxin Concentrations in DOSAGE AND ADMINISTRATION section).

Digoxin is concentrated in tissues and therefore has a large apparent volume of distribution. Digoxin crosses both the blood-brain barrier and the placenta. At delivery, serum digoxin concentration in the newborn is similar to the serum level in the mother. Approximately 20 to 25% of plasma digoxin is bound to protein. Serum digoxin concentrations are not significantly altered by large changes in fat tissue weight, so that its distribution space correlates best with lean (ideal) body weight, not total body weight.

Pharmacologic Response—The approximate times to onset of effect and to peak effect of all the Lanoxin and Lanoxicaps preparations are given in the following table:
[See table below].

Excretion—Elimination of digoxin follows first-order kinetics (that is, the quantity of digoxin eliminated at any time is proportional to the total body content). Following intravenous administration to normal subjects, 50 to 70% of a digoxin dose is excreted unchanged in the urine. Renal excretion of digoxin is proportional to glomerular filtration rate and is largely independent of urine flow. In subjects with normal renal function, digoxin has a half-life of 1.5 to 2.0 days. The half-life in anuric patients is prolonged to 4 to 6 days. Digoxin is not effectively removed from the body by dialysis, exchange transfusion or during cardiopulmonary bypass because most of the drug is in tissue rather than circulating in the blood.

Indications and Usage:
Heart Failure: The increased cardiac output resulting from the inotropic action of digoxin ameliorates the disturbances characteristic of heart failure (venous congestion, edema, dyspnea, orthopnea and cardiac asthma).

Digoxin is more effective in "low output" (pump) failure than in "high output" heart failure secondary to arteriovenous fistula, anemia, infection or hyperthyroidism.

LANOXICAPS PRODUCT	TIME TO ONSET OF EFFECT*	TIME TO PEAK EFFECT*
Lanoxin® Tablet	0.5–2 hours	2–6 hours
Lanoxin Elixir	0.5–2 hours	2–6 hours
Lanoxin Injection/IM	0.5–2 hours	2–6 hours
Lanoxin Injection/IV	5–30 minutes†	1–4 hours
Lanoxicaps Capsules	0.5–2 hours	2–6 hours

*Documented for ventricular response rate in atrial fibrillation, inotropic effect and electrocardiographic changes.
†Depending upon rate of infusion.

Continued on next page

Burroughs Wellcome—Cont.

Digoxin is usually continued after failure is controlled, unless some known precipitating factor is corrected. Studies have shown, however, that even though hemodynamic effects can be demonstrated in almost all patients, corresponding improvement in the signs and symptoms of heart failure is not necessarily apparent. Therefore, in patients in whom digoxin may be difficult to regulate, or in whom the risk of toxicity may be great (e.g., patients with unstable renal function or whose potassium levels tend to fluctuate) a cautious withdrawal of digoxin may be considered. If digoxin is discontinued, the patient should be regularly monitored by clinical evidence of recurrent heart failure.

Atrial Fibrillation: Digoxin reduces ventricular rate and thereby improves hemodynamics. Palpitation, precordial distress or weakness are relieved and concomitant congestive failure ameliorated. Digoxin should be continued in doses necessary to maintain the desired ventricular rate.

Atrial Flutter: Digoxin slows the heart and regular sinus rhythm may appear. Frequently the flutter is converted to atrial fibrillation with a controlled ventricular response. Digoxin treatment should be maintained if atrial fibrillation persists. (Electrical cardioversion is often the treatment of choice for atrial flutter. See discussion of cardioversion in PRECAUTIONS section.)

Paroxysmal Atrial Tachycardia (PAT): Digoxin may convert PAT to sinus rhythm by slowing conduction through the AV node. If heart failure has ensued or paroxysms recur frequently, digoxin should be continued. In infants, digoxin is usually continued for 3 to 6 months after a single episode of PAT to prevent recurrence.

Contraindications: Digitalis glycosides are contraindicated in ventricular fibrillation.

In a given patient, an untoward effect requiring permanent discontinuation of other digitalis preparations usually constitutes a contraindication to digoxin. Hypersensitivity to digoxin itself is a contraindication to its use. Allergy to digoxin, though rare, does occur. It may not extend to all such preparations, and another digitalis glycoside may be tried with caution.

Warnings: Digitalis alone or with other drugs has been used in the treatment of obesity. This use of digoxin or other digitalis glycosides is unwarranted. Moreover, since they may cause potentially fatal arrhythmias or other adverse effects, the use of these drugs solely for the treatment of obesity is dangerous.

It is recommended that digoxin in soft capsules be administered in divided daily doses to minimize any potential adverse reactions, since peak serum digoxin concentrations resulting from the capsules are approximately twice those after bioequivalent tablet doses (400 μg of Lanoxicaps are bioequivalent to 500 μg of tablets). Studies are underway to determine if there are any increased risks associated with the higher peaks that occur with single daily dosing of soft gelatin capsules.

Anorexia, nausea, vomiting and arrhythmias may accompany heart failure or may be indications of digitalis intoxication. Clinical evaluation of the cause of these symptoms should be attempted before further digitalis administration. In such circumstances determination of the serum digoxin concentration may be an aid in deciding whether or not digitalis toxicity is likely to be present. If the possibility of digi- talis intoxication cannot be excluded, cardiac glycosides should be temporarily withheld, if permitted by the clinical situation.

Patients with renal insufficiency require smaller than usual maintenance doses of digoxin (see DOSAGE AND ADMINISTRATION section).

Heart failure accompanying acute glomerulonephritis requires extreme care in digitalization. Relatively low loading and maintenance doses and concomitant use of antihypertensive drugs may be necessary and careful monitoring is essential. Digoxin should be discontinued as soon as possible.

Patients with severe carditis, such as carditis associated with rheumatic fever or viral myocarditis, are especially sensitive to digoxin-induced disturbances of rhythm.

Newborn infants display considerable variability in their tolerance to digoxin. Premature and immature infants are particularly sensitive, and dosage must not only be reduced but must be individualized according to their degree of maturity.

Note: Digitalis glycosides are an important cause of accidental poisoning in children.

Precautions:

General: Digoxin toxicity develops more frequently and lasts longer in patients with renal impairment because of the decreased excretion of digoxin. Therefore, it should be anticipated that dosage requirements will be decreased in patients with moderate to severe renal disease (see DOSAGE AND ADMINISTRATION section). Because of the prolonged half-life, a longer period of time is required to achieve an initial or new steady-state concentration in patients with renal impairment than in patients with normal renal function.

In patients with hypokalemia, toxicity may occur despite serum digoxin concentrations within the "normal range", because potassium depletion sensitizes the myocardium to digoxin. Therefore, it is desirable to maintain normal serum potassium levels in patients being treated with digoxin. Hypokalemia may result from diuretic, amphotericin B or corti- costeroid therapy, and from dialysis or mechanical suction of gastrointestinal secretions. It may also accompany malnutrition, diarrhea, prolonged vomiting, old age and long-standing heart failure. In general, rapid changes in serum potassium or other electrolytes should be avoided, and intravenous treatment with potassium should be reserved for special circumstances as described below (see TREATMENT OF ARRHYTHMIAS PRODUCED BY OVERDOSAGE section).

Calcium, particularly when administered rapidly by the intravenous route, may produce serious arrhythmias in digitalized patients. Hypercalcemia from any cause predisposes the patient to digitalis toxicity. On the other hand, hypocalcemia can nullify the effects of digoxin in man; thus, digoxin may be ineffective until serum calcium is restored to normal. These interactions are related to the fact that calcium affects contractility and excitability of the heart in a manner similar to digoxin.

Hypomagnesemia may predispose to digitalis toxicity. If low magnesium levels are detected in a patient on digoxin, replacement therapy should be instituted.

Quinidine and verapamil cause a rise in serum digoxin concentration, with the implication that digitalis intoxication may result. This rise appears to be proportional to the dose. The effect is mediated by a reduction in the digoxin clearance and, in the case of quinidine, decreased volume of distribution as well. Due to considerable variability of these interactions, digoxin dosage should be carefully individualized when patients receive coadministration medications.

Certain antibiotics may increase digoxin absorption in patients who convert digoxin to inactive metabolites in the gut (see Pharmacokinetics portion of the CLINICAL PHARMACOLOGY section). Recent studies have shown that specific colonic bacteria in the lower gastrointestinal tract convert digoxin to cardioinactive reduction products, thereby reducing its bioavailability. Although inactivation of these bacteria by antibiotics is rapid, the serum digoxin concentration will rise at a rate consistent with the elimination half-life of digoxin. The magnitude of rise in serum digoxin concentration relates to the extent of bacterial inactivation, and may be as much as two-fold in some cases. This interaction is significantly reduced if digoxin is given as Lanoxicaps.

Patients with acute myocardial infarction or severe pulmonary disease may be unusually sensitive to digoxin-induced disturbances of rhythm.

Atrial arrhythmias associated with hypermetabolic states (e.g. hyperthyroidism) are particularly resistant to digoxin treatment. Large doses of digoxin are not recommended as the only treatment of these arrhythmias and care must be taken to avoid toxicity if large doses of digoxin are required. In hypothyroidism, the digoxin requirements are reduced. Digoxin responses in patients with compensated thyroid disease are normal.

Reduction of digoxin dosage may be desirable prior to electrical cardioversion to avoid induction of ventricular arrhythmias, but the physician must consider the consequences of rapid increase in ventricular response to atrial fibrillation if digoxin is withheld 1 to 2 days prior to cardioversion. If there is a suspicion that digitalis toxicity exists, elective cardioversion should be delayed. If it is not prudent to delay cardioversion, the energy level selected should be minimal at first and carefully increased in an attempt to avoid precipitating ventricular arrhythmias.

Incomplete AV block, especially in patients with Stokes-Adams attacks, may progress to advanced or complete heart block if digoxin is given.

In some patients with sinus node disease (i.e. Sick Sinus Syndrome), digoxin may worsen sinus bradycardia or sino-atrial block.

In patients with Wolff-Parkinson-White Syndrome and atrial fibrillation, digoxin can enhance transmission of impulses through the accessory pathway. This effect may result in extremely rapid ventricular rates and even ventricular fibrillation.

Digoxin may worsen the outflow obstruction in patients with idiopathic hypertrophic subaortic stenosis (IHSS). Unless cardiac failure is severe, it is doubtful whether digoxin should be employed.

Patients with chronic constrictive pericarditis may fail to respond to digoxin. In addition, slowing of the heart rate by digoxin in some patients may further decrease cardiac output.

Patients with heart failure from amyloid heart disease or constrictive cardiomyopathies respond poorly to treatment with digoxin.

Digoxin is not indicated for the treatment of sinus tachycardia unless it is associated with heart failure.

Digoxin may produce false positive ST-T changes in the electrocardiogram during exercise testing.

Intramuscular injection of digoxin is extremely painful and offers no advantages unless other routes of administration are contraindicated.

Laboratory Tests: Patients receiving digoxin should have their serum electrolytes and renal function (BUN and/or serum creatinine) assessed periodically; the frequency of assessments will depend on the clinical setting. For discussion of serum digoxin concentrations, see DOSAGE AND ADMINISTRATION section.

Drug Interactions: Potassium-depleting *corticosteroids* and *diuretics* may be major contributing factors to digitalis toxicity. *Calcium,* particularly if administered rapidly by the intravenous route, may produce serious arrhythmias in digitalized patients. *Quinidine* and *verapamil* cause a rise in serum digoxin concentration, with the implication that digitalis intoxication may result. Certain *antibiotics* increase digoxin absorption in patients who inactivate digoxin by bacterial metabolism in the lower intestine, so that digitalis intoxication may result. *Propantheline* and *diphenoxylate,* by decreasing gut motility, may increase digoxin absorption. *Antacids, kaolin-pectin, sulfasalazine, neomycin, cholestyramine* and certain *anticancer drugs* may interfere with intestinal digoxin absorption, resulting in unexpectedly low serum concentrations. *Thyroid* administration to a digitalized, hypothyroid patient may increase the dose requirement of digoxin. Concomitant use of digoxin and *sympathomimetics* increases the risk of cardiac arrhythmias, because both enhance ectopic pacemaker activity. *Succinylcholine* may cause a sudden extrusion of potassium from muscle cells, and may thereby cause arrhythmias in digitalized patients. Although β adrenergic blockers or calcium channel blockers and digoxin may be useful in combination to control atrial fibrillation, their additive effects on AV node conduction can result in complete heart block.

Carcinogenesis, Mutagenesis, Impairment of Fertility: There have been no long-term studies performed in animals to evaluate carcinogenic potential.

Pregnancy: *Teratogenic Effects:* Pregnancy Category C. Animal reproduction studies have not been conducted with digoxin. It is also not known whether digoxin can cause fetal harm when administered to a pregnant woman or can affect reproduction capacity. Digoxin should be given to a pregnant woman only if clearly needed.

Nursing Mothers: Studies have shown that digoxin concentrations in the mother's serum and milk are similar. However, the estimated daily dose to a nursing infant will be far below the usual infant maintenance dose. Therefore, this amount should have no pharmacologic effect upon the infant. Nevertheless, caution should be exercised when digoxin is administered to a nursing woman.

Adverse Reactions: The frequency and severity of adverse reactions to digoxin depend on the dose and route of administration, as well as on the patient's underlying disease or concomitant therapies (see PRECAUTIONS section). The overall incidence of adverse reactions has been reported as 5 to 20%, with 15 to 20% of them being considered serious (one to four percent of patients receiving digoxin). Evidence suggests that the incidence of toxicity has decreased since the introduction of the serum digoxin assay and improved standardization of digoxin tablets. Cardiac toxicity accounts for about one-half, gastrointestinal disturbances for about one-fourth, and CNS and other toxicity for about one-fourth of these adverse reactions.

Adults:

Cardiac—Unifocal or multiform ventricular premature contractions, especially in bigeminal or trigeminal patterns, are the most common arrhythmias associated with digoxin toxicity in adults with heart disease. Ventricular tachycardia may result from digitalis toxicity. Atrioventricular (AV) dissociation, accelerated junctional (nodal) rhythm and atrial tachycardia with block are also common arrhythmias caused by digoxin overdosage.

Excessive slowing of the pulse is a clinical sign of digoxin overdosage. AV block (Wenckebach) of increasing degree may proceed to complete heart block.

Note: The electrocardiogram is fundamental in determining the presence and nature of these cardiac disturbances. Digoxin may also induce other changes in the ECG (e.g. PR prolongation, ST depression), which represent digoxin effect and may or may not be associated with digitalis toxicity.

Gastrointestinal—Anorexia, nausea, vomiting and, less commonly, diarrhea are common early symptoms of overdosage. However, uncontrolled heart failure may also produce such symptoms.

CNS—Visual disturbances (blurred or yellow vision), headache, weakness, apathy and psychosis can occur.

Other—Gynecomastia is occasionally observed.

Infants and Children: Toxicity differs from the adult in a number of respects. Anorexia, nausea, vomiting, diarrhea and CNS disturbances may be present but are rare as initial symptoms in infants. Cardiac arrhythmias are more reliable signs of toxicity. Digoxin in children may produce any arrhythmia. The most commonly encountered are conduction disturbances or supraventricular tachyarrhythmias, such as atrial tachycardia with or without block, and junctional (nodal) tachycardia. Ventricular arrhythmias are less common. Sinus bradycardia may also be a sign of impending digoxin intoxication, especially in infants, even in the absence of first degree heart block. Any arrhythmia or alteration in cardiac conduction that develops in a child taking digoxin should initially be assumed to be a consequence of digoxin intoxication.

Treatment of Arrhythmias Produced By Overdosage:

Adults: Digoxin should be discontinued until all signs of toxicity are gone. Discontinuation may be all that is necessary if toxic manifestations are not severe and appear only near the expected time for maximum effect of the drug.

Potassium salts are commonly used, particularly if hypokalemia is present. Potassium chloride in divided oral doses totaling 3 to 6 grams of the salt (40 to 80 mEq K +) for adults may be given provided renal function is adequate (see below for potassium recommendations in Infants and Children).

When correction of the arrhythmia is urgent and the serum potassium concentration is low or normal, potassium should be administered intravenously in 5% dextrose injection. For adults, a total of 40 to 80 mEq (diluted to a concentration of 40 mEq per 500 ml) may be given at a rate not exceeding 20 mEq per hour, or slower if limited by pain due to local irritation. Additional amounts may be given if the arrhythmia is uncontrolled and potassium well-tolerated. ECG monitoring should be performed to watch for any evidence of potassium toxicity (e.g. peaking of T waves) and to observe the effect on the arrhythmia. The infusion may be stopped when the desired effect is achieved.

Note: Potassium should not be used and may be dangerous in heart block due to digoxin, unless primarily related to supraventricular tachycardia. Other agents that have been used for the treatment of digoxin intoxication include lidocaine, procainamide, propranolol and phenytoin, although use of the latter must be considered experimental. In advanced heart block, temporary ventricular pacing may be beneficial. Rapid reversal of potentially life-threatening digitalis intoxication unresponsive to other therapy has been reported* following intravenous administration of digoxin-specific (ovine) antibody fragments (Fab); this therapy should also be considered investigational at this time. (New Engl J Med. 1982; *307*: 1357–1362.)

Infants and Children: See Adult section for general recommendations for the treatment of arrhythmias produced by overdosage and for cautions regarding the use of potassium.

If a potassium preparation is used to treat toxicity, it may be given orally in divided doses totaling 1 to 1.5 mEq K + per kilogram (kg) body weight (1 gram of potassium chloride contains 13.4 mEq K +).

When correction of the arrhythmia with potassium is urgent, approximately 0.5 mEq/kg of potassium per hour may be given intravenously, with careful ECG monitoring. The intravenous solution of potassium should be dilute enough to avoid local irritation; however, especially in infants, care must be taken to avoid intravenous fluid overload.

Dosage and Administration: Recommended dosages are average values that may require considerable modification because of individual sensitivity or associated conditions. Diminished renal function is the most important factor requiring modification of recommended doses.

Due to the more complete absorption of digoxin from soft capsules, recommended oral doses are only 80 percent of those for Tablets, Elixir and I.M. Injection.

Because the significance of the higher peak serum concentrations associated with once daily capsules is not established, divided daily dosing is presently recommended for:

1. Infants and children under 10 years of age;
2. Patients requiring a daily dose of 300 µg (0.3 mg) or greater;
3. Patients with a previous history of digi- talis toxicity;
4. Patients considered likely to become toxic;
5. Patients in whom compliance is not a problem.

Where compliance is considered a problem, single daily dosing may be appropriate.

In deciding the dose of digoxin, several factors must be considered:

1. The disease being treated Atrial arrhythmias may require larger doses than heart failure.
2. The body weight of the patient. Doses should be calculated based upon lean or ideal body weight.
3. The patient's renal function, preferably evaluated on the basis of creatinine clearance.
4. Age is an important factor in infants and children.
5. Concomitant disease states, drugs or other factors likely to alter the expected clinical response to digoxin (see PRECAUTIONS and Drug Interactions sections).

Digitalization may be accomplished by either of two general approaches that vary in dosage and frequency of administration, but reach the same endpoint in terms of total amount of digoxin accumulated in the body.

1. Rapid digitalization may be achieved by administering a loading dose based upon projected body digoxin stores, then calculating the maintenance dose as a percentage of the loading dose.
2. More gradual digitalization may be obtained by beginning an appropriate maintenance dose, thus allowing digoxin body stores to accumulate slowly. Steady-state serum digoxin concentrations will be achieved in approximately 5 half-lives of the drug for the individual patient. Depending upon the patient's renal function, this will take between one and three weeks.

Adults:

Adults—Rapid Digitalization with a Loading Dose: Peak body digoxin stores of 8 to 12 µg/kg should provide therapeutic effect with minimum risk of toxicity in most patients with heart failure and normal sinus rhythm. Larger stores (10 to 15 µg/kg) are ofter required for adequate control of ventricular rate in patients with atrial flutter or fibrillation. Because of altered digoxin distribution and elimination, projected peak body stores for patients with renal insufficiency should be conservative (i.e. 6 to 10 µg/kg) [see PRECAUTIONS section].

The loading dose should be based on the projected peak body stores and administered in several portions, with roughly half the total given as the first dose. Additional fractions of this planned total dose may be given at 6 to 8 hour intervals, **with careful assessment of clinical response before each additional dose.**

If the patient's clinical response necessitates a change from the calculated dose of digoxin, then calculation of the maintenance dose should be based upon the amount actually given.

In previously undigitalized patients, a single initial Lanoxicaps dose of 400 to 600 µg (0.4 to 0.6 mg) usually produces a detectable effect in 0.5 to 2 hours that becomes maximal in 2 to 6 hours. Additional doses of 100 to 300 µg (0.1 to 0.3 mg) may be given cautiously at 6 to 8 hour intervals until clinical evidence of an adequate effect is noted. The usual amount of Lanoxicaps that a 70 kg patient required to achieve 8 to 15 µg/kg peak body stores is 600 to 1000 µg (0.6 to 1.0 mg).

Although peak body stores are mathematically related to loading doses and are utilized to calculate maintenance doses, they do not correlate with measured serum concentrations. This discrepancy is caused by digoxin distribution within the body during the first 6 to 8 hours following a dose. Serum concentrations drawn during this time are usually not interpretable.

The maintenance dose should be based upon the percentage of the peak body stores lost each day through elimination. The following formula has had wide clinical use:

$$\text{Maintenance Dose} = \text{Peak Body Stores (i.e. Loading Dose)} \times \frac{\% \text{ Daily Loss}}{100}$$

Where: % Daily Loss = 14 + Ccr/5

Ccr is creatinine clearance, corrected to 70 kg body weight or 1.73 m² body surface area. **For adults,** if only serum creatinine concentrations (Scr) are available, a Ccr (corrected to 70 kg body weight) may be estimated in men as (140 − Age)/Scr. For women, this result should be multiplied by 0.85.

Note: This equation cannot be used for estimating creatinine clearance in infants or children.

A common practice involves the use of Lanoxin® Injection to achieve rapid digitalization, with conversion to Lanoxicaps or Lanoxin Tablets for

Continued on next page

Burroughs Wellcome—Cont.

maintenance therapy. If patients are switched from IV to oral digoxin formulations, allowances must be made for differences in bioavailability when calculating maintenance dosages (see table, CLINICAL PHARMACOLOGY section).

Adults—Gradual Digitalization with a Maintenance Dose: The following table provides average Lanoxicaps daily maintenance dose requirements for patients with heart failure based upon lean body weight and renal function:
[See table below].

Example—based on the above table, a patient in heart failure with an estimated lean body weight of 70 kg and a Ccr of 60 ml/min, should be given 200 µg (0.2 mg) of Lanoxicaps per day, usually taken as a 100 µg (0.1 mg) capsule after the morning and evening meals. Steady-state serum concentrations should not be anticipated before 11 days.

Infants and Children: Digitalization must be individualized. Divided daily dosing is recommended for infants and young children. In these patients, where dosage adjustment is frequent and outside the fixed dosages available, Lanoxicaps may not be the formulation of choice. Children over 10 years of age require adult dosages in proportion to their body weight.

In the newborn period, renal clearance of digoxin is diminished and suitable dosage adjustments must be observed. This is especially pronounced in the premature infant. Beyond the immediate newborn period, children generally require proportionally larger doses than adults on the basis of body weight or body surface area.

Lanoxin® Injection Pediatric can be used to achieve rapid digitalization, with conversion to an oral Lanoxin formulation for maintenance therapy. If patients are switched from IV to oral digoxin tablets or elixir, allowances must be made for differences in bioavailability when calculating maintenance dosages (see bioavailability table in CLINICAL PHARMACOLOGY section and dosing table above).

Intramuscular injection of digoxin is extremely painful and offers no advantages unless other routes of administration are contraindicated.

Digitalizing and daily maintenance doses for each age group are given below and should provide therapeutic effect with minimum risk of toxicity in most patients with heart failure and normal sinus rhythm. Larger doses are often required for adequate control of ventricular rate in patients with atrial flutter or fibrillation.

The loading dose should be administered in several portions, with roughly half the total given as the first dose. Additional fractions of this planned total dose may be given at 6 to 8 hour intervals, with careful assessment of clinical response before each additional dose. If the patient's clinical response necessitates a change from the calculated dose of digoxin, then calculation of the maintenance dose should be based upon the amount actually given.
[See table above].

More gradual digitalization can also be accomplished by beginning an appropriate maintenance dose. The range of percentages provided above can be used in calculating this dose for patients with normal renal function. In children with renal disease, digoxin dosing must be carefully titrated based upon desired clinical response.

Long-term use of digoxin is indicated in many children who have been digitalized for acute heart failure, unless the cause is transient. Children with severe congenital heart disease, even after surgery, may require digoxin for prolonged periods.

It cannot be overemphasized that both the adult and pediatric dosage guidelines provided are based upon average patient response and substantial individual variation can be expected. Accordingly, ultimate dosage selection must be based upon clinical assessment of the patient.

Serum Digoxin Concentrations: Measurement of serum digoxin concentrations can be helpful to the clinician in determining the state of digitalization and in assigning certain probabilities to the likelihood of digoxin intoxication. Studies in adults considered adequately digitalized (without evidence of toxicity) show that about two-thirds of such patients have serum digoxin levels ranging from 0.8 to 2.0 ng/ml. Patients with atrial fibrillation or atrial flutter require and appear to tolerate higher levels than do patients with other indications. On the other hand, in adult patients with clinical evidence of digoxin toxicity, about two-thirds will have serum digoxin levels greater than 2.0 ng/ml. Thus, whereas levels less than 0.8 ng/ml are infrequently associated with toxicity, levels greater than 2.0 ng/ml are often associated with toxicity. Values in between are not very helpful in deciding whether a certain sign or symptom is more likely caused by digoxin toxicity or by something else. There are rare patients who are unable to tolerate digoxin even at serum concentrations below 0.8 ng/ml. Some researchers suggest that infants and young children tolerate slightly higher serum concentrations than do adults.

To allow adequate time for equilibration of digoxin between serum and tissue, **sampling of serum concentrations for clinical use should be at least 6 to 8 hours after the last dose**, regardless of the route of administration or formulation used. On a twice daily dosing schedule, there will be only minor differences in serum digoxin concentrations whether sampling is done at 8 or 12 hours after a dose. After a single daily dose, the concentration will be 10 to 25% lower when sampled at 24 versus 8 hours, depending upon the patient's renal function. Ideally, sampling for assessment of steady-state concentrations should be done just before the next dose.

If a discrepancy exists between the reported serum concentration and the observed clinical response, the clinician should consider the following possibilities:
1. Analytical problems in the assay procedure.
2. Inappropriate serum sampling time.
3. Administration of a digitalis glycoside other than digoxin.
4. Conditions (described in WARNINGS and PRECAUTIONS sections) causing an alteration in the sensitivity of the patient to digoxin.
5. The patient falls outside the norm in his response to or handling of digoxin. This decision should only be reached after exclusion of the other possibilities and generally should be confirmed by additional correlations of clinical observations with serum digoxin concentrations.

The serum concentration data should always be interpreted in the overall clinical context and an isolated serum concentration value should not be used alone as a basis for increasing or decreasing digoxin dosage.

Adjustment of Maintenance Dose in Previously Digitalized Patients: Lanoxicaps maintenance doses in individual patients on steady-state digoxin can be adjusted upward or downward in proportion to the ratio of the desired versus the measured serum concentration. For example, a patient at steady-state on 100 µg (0.1 mg) of Lanoxicaps per day with a measured serum concentration of 0.7 ng/ml, should have the dose increased to 200 µg (0.2 mg) per day to achieve a steady-state serum concentration of 1.4 ng/ml, **assuming the serum digoxin concentration measurement is correct, renal function remains stable during this time and the needed adjustment is not the result of a problem with compliance.**

Dosage Adjustment When Changing Preparations: The absolute bioavailability of the capsule formulation is greater than that of the standard tablets and very near that of the intravenous dosage form. As a result the doses recommended for Lanoxicaps capsules are the same as those for Lanoxin® Injection (see CLINICAL PHARMACOLOGY section). Adjustments in dosage will seldom be necessary when converting a patient from intravenous to Lanoxicaps formulation. The differences in bioavailability between injectable Lanoxin or Lanoxicaps, and Lanoxin Elixir Pediatric or Lanoxin Tablets must be considered when changing patients from one dosage form to another.

Lanoxin Injection and Lanoxicaps doses of 100 µg (0.1 mg) and 200 µg (0.2 mg) are approximately equivalent to 125 µg (0.125 mg) and 250 µg (0.25 mg) doses of Lanoxin Tablets and Elixir Pediatric (see table in CLINICAL PHARMACOLOGY section). Intramuscular injection of digoxin is extremely painful and offers no advantages unless other routes of administration are contraindicated.

How Supplied:
LANOXICAPS (DIGOXIN SOLUTION IN CAPSULES), 50 µg (0.05 mg): bottles of 100, Imprint A2C (red), NDC-0081-0270-55
LANOXICAPS (DIGOXIN SOLUTION IN CAPSULES), 100 µg (0.1 mg)* bottles of 100, and Unit Dose Pack of 100, NDC 0081-0272-77. Imprint B2C (yellow). NDC 0081-0272-55

Usual Digitalizing and Maintenance Dosages for Lanoxicaps in Children with Normal Renal Function Based on Lean Body Weight

Age	Digitalizing* Dose (µg/kg)	Daily † Maintenance Dose (µg/kg)
2–5 Years	25–35	25–35% of the oral or IV loading dose ‡
5–10 Years	15–30	
Over 10 years	8–12	

*IV digitalizing doses are the same as Lanoxicaps digitalizing doses.
†Divided daily dosing is recommended for children under 10 years of age.
‡Projected or actual digitalizing dose providing desired clinical response.

Usual Lanoxicaps Daily Maintenance Dose Requirements (µg) for Estimated Peak Body Stores of 10 µg/kg

		Lean Body Weight (kg/lbs)					
		50/110	60/132	70/154	80/176	90/198	100/220
	0	50	100	100	100	150	150	22
	10	100	100	100	150	150	150	19
	20	100	100	150	150	150	200	16
Corrected	30	100	150	150	150	200	200	14	Number of
Ccr	40	100	150	150	200	200	250	13	Days
(ml/min	50	150	150	200	200	250	250	12	Before
per 70 kg)	60	150	150	200	200	250	300	11	Steady-State
	70	150	200	200	250	250	300	10	Achieved
	80	150	200	200	250	300	300	9
	90	150	200	250	250	300	350	8
	100	200	200	300	300	300	350	7

for possible revisions **Product Information** 797

LANOXICAPS (DIGOXIN SOLUTION IN CAPSULES), 200 μg (0.2 mg)* bottles of 100, and Unit Dose Pack of 100, NDC 0081-0274-77. Imprint C2C (green). NDC-0081-0274-55
Store at 15°–30°C (59°–86°F) in a dry place and protect from light.
Also Available:
LANOXIN® (DIGOXIN) TABLETS, Scored 125 μg (0.125 mg): Bottles of 100 and 1000: Unit Dose Pack of 1000; Unit of Use Bottles of 30. Imprinted with LANOXIN and Y3B (yellow).
LANOXIN (DIGOXIN) TABLETS, Scored 250 μg (0.25 mg): Bottles of 100, 1000 and 5000; Unit Dose Pack of 100; Unit of Use bottles of 30 and 100. Imprinted with LANOXIN and X3A (white).
LANOXIN (DIGOXIN) TABLETS Scored 500 μg (0.5 mg): Bottles of 100. Imprinted with LANOXIN and T9A (Green)
LANOXIN (DIGOXIN) ELIXIR PEDIATRIC, 50 μg (0.05 mg) per ml; bottle of 60 ml with calibrated dropper.
LANOXIN (DIGOXIN) INJECTION, 500 μg (0.5 mg) in 2 ml (250 μg [0.25 mg] per ml); boxes of 12 and 100 ampuls.
LANOXIN (DIGOXIN) INJECTION PEDIATRIC, 100 μg (0.1 mg) in 1 ml; box of 50 ampuls.
*U.S. Patent No. 4088750
Shown in Product Identification Section, page 408

LANOXIN® ℞
[lă-nŏx'ĭn"]
(Digoxin)
Tablets/Injections/Elixir Pediatric

Description: Digoxin is one of the cardiac (or digitalis) glycosides, a closely related group of drugs having in common specific effects on the myocardium. These drugs are found in a number of plants. Digoxin is extracted from the leaves of *Digitalis lanata*. The term "digitalis" is used to designate the whole group. The glycosides are composed of two portions: a sugar and a cardenolide (hence "glycosides").
Digoxin has the molecular formula $C_{41}H_{64}O_{14}$, a molecular weight of 780.95 and melting and decomposition points above 235°C. The drug is practically insoluble in water and in ether, slightly soluble in diluted (50%) alcohol and in chloroform; and freely soluble in pyridine. Digoxin powder is composed of odorless white crystals.
Digoxin has the chemical name: 3β-[(O-2,6-dideoxy-β-D-ribo-hexopyranosyl-(1→4)-O-2,6-dideoxy-β-D-ribo-hexopyranosyl-(1→4)-2,6-dideoxy-β-D-ribo-hexopyranosyl) oxy]-12β, 14-dihydroxy-5β-card-20(22)-enolide.
Lanoxin Tablets with 125μg (0.125 mg), 250 μg (0.25 mg) or 500 μg (0.5 mg) digoxin USP are intended for oral use. Each tablet contains the labeled amount of digoxin USP dispersed in lactose and other inert ingredients.
Lanoxin (Digoxin) Injection and Injection Pediatric are sterile solutions of digoxin for intravenous or intramuscular injection. The vehicle contains 40% propylene glycol and 10% alcohol. The injection is buffered to a pH of 6.8 to 7.2 with 0.3 percent sodium phosphate and 0.08 percent anhydrous citric acid. Each 2 ml ampul of Lanoxin Injection contains 500 μg (0.5 mg) digoxin [250 μg (0.25 mg) per ml]. Each 1 ml ampul of Lanoxin Injection Pediatric contains 100 μg (0.1 mg) digoxin. Dilution is not required.
Lanoxin Elixir Pediatric is a stable solution of digoxin specially formulated for oral use in infants and children. Each ml contains 50 μg (0.05 mg)

PRODUCT	ABSOLUTE BIOAVAILABILITY	EQUIVALENT DOSES (IN MG*)		
Lanoxin Tablet	60–80%	0.125	0.25	0.5
Lanoxin Elixir	70–85%	0.125	0.25	0.5
Lanoxin Injection/IM	70–85%	0.125	0.25	0.5
Lanoxin Injection/IV	100%	0.1	0.2	0.4
Lanoxicaps Capsules	90–100%	0.1	0.2	0.4

*1 mg = 1000 μg

digoxin USP. The lime-flavored elixir contains 10% alcohol and 0.1% methylparaben added as a preservative. Each package is supplied with a specially calibrated dropper to facilitate the administration of accurate dosage even in premature infants. Starting at 0.2 ml, this 1 ml dropper is marked in divisions of 0.1 ml, each corresponding to 5 μg (0.005 mg) digoxin.

Clinical Pharmacology:
Mechanism of Action:
The influence of digitalis glycosides on the myocardium is dose-related, and involves both a direct action on cardiac muscle and the specialized conduction system, and indirect actions on the cardiovascular system mediated by the autonomic nervous system. The indirect actions mediated by the autonomic nervous system involve a vagomimetic action, which is responsible for the effects of digitalis on the sino-atrial (SA) and atrioventricular (AV) nodes; and also a baroreceptor sensitization which results in increased carotid sinus nerve activity and enhanced sympathetic withdrawal for any given increment in mean arterial pressure. The pharmacologic consequences of these direct and indirect effects are: 1) an increase in the force and velocity of myocardial systolic contraction (positive inotropic action); 2) a slowing of heart rate (negative chronotropic effect); and 3) decreased conduction velocity through the AV node. In higher doses, digitalis increases sympathetic outflow from the central nervous system (CNS) to both cardiac and peripheral sympathetic nerves. This increase in sympathetic activity may be an important factor in digitalis cardiac toxicity. Most of the extracardiac manifestations of digitalis toxicity are also mediated by the CNS.

Pharmacokinetics:
Note: The following data are from studies performed in adults, unless otherwise stated.
Absorption—Gastrointestinal absorption of digoxin is a passive process. Absorption of digoxin from the Lanoxin® tablet formulation has been demonstrated to be 60 to 80% complete and absorption of digoxin from the Lanoxin® Elixir Pediatric formulation, 70 to 85% complete compared to an identical intravenous dose of digoxin (absolute bioavailability). When digoxin elixir or tablets are taken after meals, the rate of absorption is slowed, but the total amount of digoxin absorbed is usually unchanged. When taken with meals high in bran fiber, however, the amount absorbed from an oral dose may be reduced. Comparison of the systemic availability and equivalent doses for digoxin preparations are shown in the following table:
[See table above].
In some subjects, orally administered digoxin is converted to cardioinactive reduction products (e.g., dihydrodigoxin) by colonic bacteria in the gut. Data suggest that one in ten patients treated with digoxin tablets will degrade 40% or more of the ingested dose.

Distribution—Following drug administration, a 6 to 8 hour distribution phase is observed. This is followed by a much more gradual serum concentration decline, which is dependent on digoxin elimination from the body. The peak height and slope of the early portion (absorption/distribution phases) of the serum concentration-time curve are dependent upon the route of administration and the absorption characteristics of the formulation. Clinical evidence indicates that the early high serum concentrations do not reflect the concentration of digoxin at its site of action, but that with chronic use, the steady-state post-distribution serum levels are in equilibrium with tissue levels and correlate with pharmacologic effects. In individual patients, these post-distribution serum concentrations are linearly related to maintenance dosage and may be useful in evaluating therapeutic and toxic effects (see Serum Digoxin Concentrations in DOSAGE AND ADMINISTRATION section).
Digoxin is concentrated in tissues and therefore has a large apparent volume of distribution. Digoxin crosses both the blood-brain barrier and the placenta. At delivery, serum digoxin concentration in the newborn is similar to the serum level in the mother. Approximately 20 to 25% of plasma digoxin is bound to protein. Serum digoxin concentrations are not significantly altered by large changes in fat tissue weight, so that its distribution space correlates best with lean (ideal) body weight, not total body weight.
Pharmacologic Response—The approximate times to onset of effect and to peak effect of all the Lanoxin® preparations are given in the following table:
[See table below].
Excretion—Elimination of digoxin follows first-order kinetics (that is, the quantity of digoxin eliminated at any time is proportional to the total body content). Following intravenous administration to normal subjects, 50 to 70% of a digoxin dose is excreted unchanged in the urine. Renal excretion of digoxin is proportional to glomerular filtration rate and is largely independent of urine flow. In subjects with normal renal function, digoxin has a half-life of 1.5 to 2.0 days. The half-life in anuric patients is prolonged to 4 to 6 days. Digoxin is not effectively removed from the body by dialysis, exchange transfusion or during cardiopulmonary bypass because most of the drug is in tissue rather than circulating in the blood.

Indications and Usage:
Heart Failure:
The increased cardiac output resulting from the inotropic action of digoxin ameliorates the disturbances characteristic of heart failure (venous congestion, edema, dyspnea, orthopnea and cardiac asthma).
Digoxin is more effective in "low output" (pump) failure than in "high output" heart failure secondary to arteriovenous fistula, anemia, infection or hyperthyroidism.
Digoxin is usually continued after failure is controlled, unless some known precipitating factor is corrected. Studies have shown, that even though hemodynamic effects can be demonstrated in almost all patients, corresponding improvement in the signs and symptoms of heart failure is not necessarily apparent. Therefore, in patients in whom digoxin may be difficult to regulate, or in whom the risk of toxicity may be great (e.g., patients with unstable renal function or whose potassium levels tend to fluctutate) a cautious withdrawal of di-

PRODUCT	TIME TO ONSET OF EFFECT*	TIME TO PEAK EFFECT*
Lanoxin Tablet	0.5–2 hours	2–6 hours
Lanoxin Elixir	0.5–2 hours	2–6 hours
Lanoxin Injection/IM	0.5–2 hours	2–6 hours
Lanoxin Injection/IV	5–30 minutes†	1–4 hours
Lanoxicaps Capsules	0.5–2 hours	2–6 hours

*Documented for ventricular response rate in atrial fibrillation, inotropic effect and electrocardiographic changes.
†Depending upon rate of infusion.

Continued on next page

Burroughs Wellcome—Cont.

goxin may be considered. If digoxin is discontinued, the patient should be regularly monitored for clinical evidence or recurrent heart failure.

Atrial Fibrillation:
Digoxin reduces ventricular rate and thereby improves hemodynamics. Palpitation, precordial distress or weakness are relieved and concomitant congestive failure ameliorated. Digoxin should be continued in doses necessary to maintain the desired ventricular rate.

Atrial Flutter:
Digoxin slows the heart and regular sinus rhythm may appear. Frequently the flutter is converted to atrial fibrillation with a controlled ventricular response. Digoxin treatment should be maintained if atrial fibrillation persists. (Electrical cardioversion is often the treatment of choice for atrial flutter. See discussion of cardioversion in PRECAUTIONS section.)

Paroxysmal Atrial Tachycardia (PAT):
Digoxin may convert PAT to sinus rhythm by slowing conduction through the AV node. If heart failure has ensued or paroxysms recur frequently, digoxin should be continued. In infants, digoxin is usually continued for 3 to 6 months after a single episode of PAT to prevent recurrence.

Contraindications:
Digitalis glycosides are contraindicated in ventricular fibrillation.

In a given patient, an untoward effect requiring discontinuation of other digitalis preparations usually constitutes a contraindication to digoxin. Hypersensitivity to digoxin itself is a contraindication to its use. Allergy to digoxin, though rare, does occur. It may not extend to all such preparations, and another digitalis glycoside may be tried with caution.

Warnings:
Digitalis alone or with other drugs has been used in the treatment of obesity. This use of digoxin or other digitalis glycosides is unwarranted. Moreover, since they may cause potentially fatal arrhythmias or other adverse effects, the use of these drugs solely for the treatment of obesity is dangerous.

Anorexia, nausea, vomiting and arrhythmias may accompany heart failure or may be indications of digitalis intoxication. Clinical evaluation of the cause of these symptoms should be attempted before further digitalis administration. In such circumstances determination of the serum digoxin concentration may be an aid in deciding whether or not digitalis toxicity is likely to be present. If the possibility of digitalis intoxication cannot be excluded, cardiac glycosides should be temporarily withheld, if permitted by the clinical situation. Patients with renal insufficiency require smaller than usual maintenance doses of digoxin (see DOSAGE AND ADMINISTRATION section).

Heart failure accompanying acute glomerulonephritis requires extreme care in digitalization. Relatively low loading and maintenance doses and concomitant use of antihypertensive drugs may be necessary and careful monitoring is essential. Digoxin should be discontinued as soon as possible. Patients with severe carditis, such as carditis associated with rheumatic fever or viral myocarditis, are especially sensitive to digoxin-induced disturbances of rhythm.

Newborn infants display considerable variability in their tolerance to digoxin. Premature and immature infants are particularly sensitive, and dosage must not only be reduced but must be individualized according to their degree of maturity.

Note: Digitalis glycosides are an important cause of accidental poisoning in children.

Precautions:
General:
Digoxin toxicity develops more frequently and lasts longer in patients with renal impairment because of the decreased excretion of digoxin. Therefore, it should be anticipated that dosage requirements will be decreased in patients with moderate to severe renal disease (see DOSAGE AND ADMINISTRATION section). Because of the prolonged half-life, a longer period of time is required to achieve an initial or new steady-state concentration in patients with renal impairment than in patients with normal renal function.

In patients with hypokalemia, toxicity may occur despite serum digoxin concentrations within the "normal range", because potassium depletion sensitizes the myocardium to digoxin. Therefore, it is desirable to maintain normal serum potassium levels in patients being treated with digoxin. Hypokalemia may result from diuretic, amphotericin B or corticosteroid therapy, and from dialysis or mechanical suction of gastrointestinal secretions. It may also accompany malnutrition, diarrhea, prolonged vomiting, old age and long-standing heart failure. In general, rapid changes in serum potassium or other electrolytes should be avoided, and intravenous treatment with potassium should be reserved for special circumstances as described below (see TREATMENT OF ARRHYTHMIAS PRODUCED BY OVERDOSAGE section).

Calcium, particularly when administered rapidly by the intravenous route, may produce serious arrhythmias in digitalized patients. Hypercalcemia from any cause predisposes the patient to digitalis toxicity. On the other hand, hypocalcemia can nullify the effects of digoxin in man; thus, digoxin may be ineffective until serum calcium is restored to normal. These interactions are related to the fact that calcium affects contractility and excitability of the heart in a manner similar to digoxin.

Hypomagnesemia may predispose to digitalis toxicity. If low magnesium levels are detected in a patient on digoxin, replacement therapy should be instituted.

Quinidine and verapamil cause a rise in serum digoxin concentration, with the implication that digitalis intoxication may result. This rise appears to be proportional to the dose. The effect is mediated by a reduction in the digoxin clearance and, in the case of quinidine, decreased volume of distribution as well. Due to the considerable variability of these interactions, digoxin dosage should be carefully individualized when patients receive coadministered medications.

Certain antibiotics may increase digoxin absorption in patients who convert digoxin to inactive metabolites in the gut (see Pharmacokinetics portion of the CLINICAL PHARMACOLOGY section). Recent studies have shown that specific colonic bacteria in the lower gastrointestinal tract convert digoxin to cardioinactive reduction products, thereby reducing its bioavailability. Although inactivation of these bacteria by antibiotics is rapid, the serum digoxin concentration will rise at a rate consistent with the elimination half-life of digoxin. The magnitude of rise in serum digoxin concentration relates to the extent of bacterial inactivation, and may be as much as two-fold in some cases. This interaction is significantly reduced if digoxin is given as Lanoxicaps.

Patients with acute myocardial infarction or severe pulmonary disease may be unusually sensitive to digoxin-induced disturbances of rhythm.

Atrial arrhythmias associated with hypermetabolic states (e.g. hyperthyroidism) are particularly resistant to digoxin treatment. Large doses of digoxin are not recommended as the only treatment of these arrhythmias and care must be taken to avoid toxicity if large doses of digoxin are required. In hypothyroidism, the digoxin requirements are reduced. Digoxin responses in patients with compensated thyroid disease are normal.

Reduction of digoxin dosage may be desirable prior to electrical cardioversion to avoid induction of ventricular arrhythmias, but the physician must consider the consequences of rapid increase in ventricular response to atrial fibrillation if digoxin is withheld 1 to 2 days prior to cardioversion. If there is a suspicion that digitalis toxicity exists, elective cardioversion should be delayed. If it is not prudent to delay cardioversion, the energy level selected should be minimal at first and carefully increased in an attempt to avoid precipitating ventricular arrhythmias.

Incomplete AV block, especially in patients with Stokes-Adams attacks, may progress to advanced or complete heart block if digoxin is given.

In some patients with sinus node disease (i.e. Sick Sinus Syndrome), digoxin may worsen sinus bradycardia or sino-atrial block.

In patients with Wolff-Parkinson-White Syndrome and atrial fibrillation, digoxin can enhance transmission of impulses through the accessory pathway. This effect may result in extremely rapid ventricular rates and even ventricular fibrillation. Digoxin may worsen the outflow obstruction in patients with idiopathic hypertrophic subaortic stenosis (IHSS). Unless cardiac failure is severe, it is doubtful whether digoxin should be employed. Patients with chronic constrictive pericarditis may fail to respond to digoxin. In addition, slowing of the heart rate by digoxin in some patients may further decrease cardiac output.

Patients with heart failure from amyloid heart disease or constrictive cardiomyopathies respond poorly to treatment with digoxin.

Digoxin is not indicated for the treatment of sinus tachycardia unless it is associated with heart failure.

Digoxin may produce false positive ST-T changes in the electrocardiogram during exercise testing. Intramuscular injection of digoxin is extremely painful and offers no advantages unless other routes of administration are contraindicated.

Laboratory Tests:
Patients receiving digoxin should have their serum electrolytes and renal function (BUN and/or serum creatinine) assessed periodically; the frequency of assessments will depend on the clinical setting. For discussion of serum digoxin concentrations, see DOSAGE AND ADMINISTRATION section.

Drug Interactions:
Potassium-depleting *corticosteroids* and *diuretics* may be major contributing factors to digitalis toxicity. *Calcium*, particularly if administered rapidly by the intravenous route, may produce serious arrhythmias in digitalized patients. *Quinidine* and *verapamil* cause a rise in serum digoxin concentration, with the implication that digitalis may result. Certain *antibiotics* increase digoxin absorption in patients who inactivate digoxin by bacterial metabolism in the lower intestine, so that digitalis intoxication may result. *Propantheline* and *diphenoxylate*, by decreasing gut motility, may increase digoxin absorption. *Antacids*, *kaolin-pectin*, *sulfasalazine*, *neomycin*, *cholestyramine* and certain *anticancer drugs* may interfere with intestinal digoxin absorption, resulting in unexpectedly low serum concentrations. *Thyroid* administration to a digitalized, hypothyroid patient may increase the dose requirement of digoxin. Concomitant use of digoxin and *sympathomimetics* increases the risk of cardiac arrhythmias because both enhance ectopic pacemaker activity. *Succinylcholine* may cause a sudden extrusion of potassium from muscle cells, and may therefore cause arrhythmias in digitalized patients. Although β adrenergic blockers or calcium channel blockers and digoxin may be useful in combination to control atrial fibrillation, their additive effects on AV node conduction can result in complete heart block.

Carcinogenesis, Mutagenesis, Impairment of Fertility:
There have been no long-term studies in animals to evaluate carcinogenic potential.

Pregnancy: *Teratogenic Effects:*
Pregnancy Category C. Animal reproduction studies have not been conducted with digoxin. It is also not known whether digoxin can cause fetal harm when administered to a pregnant woman or can affect reproduction capacity. Digoxin should be given to a pregnant woman only if clearly needed.

Nursing Mothers:
Studies have shown that digoxin concentrations in the mother's serum and milk are similar. However, the estimated daily dose to a nursing infant will be far below the usual infant maintenance dose. Therefore, this amount should have no pharmacologic effect upon the infant. Nevertheless, caution should be exercised when digoxin is administered to a nursing woman.

Adverse Reactions:
The frequency and severity of adverse reactions to digoxin depend on the dose

and route of administration, as well as on the patient's underlying disease or concomitant therapies (see PRECAUTIONS section). The overall incidence of adverse reactions has been reported as 5 to 20%, with 15 to 20% of them being considered serious (one to four percent of patients receiving digoxin). Evidence suggests that the incidence of toxicity has decreased since the introduction of the serum digoxin assay and improved standardization of digoxin tablets. Cardiac toxicity accounts for about one-half, gastrointestinal disturbances for about one-fourth, and CNS and other toxicity for about one-fourth of these adverse reactions.

Adults:
Cardiac—Unifocal or multiform ventricular premature contractions, especially in begeminal or trigeminal patterns, are the most common arrhythmias associated with digoxin toxicity in adults with heart disease. Ventricular tachycardia may result from digitalis toxicity. Atrioventricular (AV) dissociation, accelerated junctional (nodal) rhythm and atrial tachycardia with block are also common arrhythmias caused by digoxin overdosage.

Excessive slowing of the pulse is a clinical sign of digoxin overdosage. AV block (Wenckebach) of increasing degree may proceed to complete heart block.

Note: The electrocardiogram is fundamental in determining the presence and nature of these cardiac disturbances. Digoxin may also induce other changes in the ECG (e.g. PR prolongation, ST depression), which represent digoxin effect and may or may not be associated with digitalis toxicity.

Gastrointestinal—Anorexia, nausea, vomiting and less commonly diarrhea are common early symptoms of overdosage. However, uncontrolled heart failure may also produce such symptoms.

CNS—Visual disturbances (blurred or yellow vision), headache, weakness, apathy and psychosis can occur.

Other—Gynecomastia is occasionally observed.

Infants and Children:
Toxicity differs from the adult in a number of respects. Anorexia, nausea, vomiting, diarrhea and CNS disturbances may be present but are rare as initial symptoms in infants. Cardiac arrhythmias are more reliable signs of toxicity. Digoxin in children may produce any arrhythmia.

Cardiac—Conduction disturbances or supraventricular tachyarrhythmias, such as atrioventricular (AV) block (Wenckebach), atrial tachycardia with or without block and junctional (nodal) tachycardia are the most common arrhythmias associated with digoxin toxicity in children. Ventricular arrhythmias, such as unifocal or multiform ventricular premature contractions, especially in bigeminal or trigeminal patterns, are less common. Ventricular tachycardia may result from digitalis toxicity. Sinus bradycardia may also be a sign of impending digoxin intoxication, especially in infants, even in the absence of first degree heart block. Any arrhythmias or alteration in cardiac conduction that develops in a child taking digoxin should initially be assumed to be a consequence of digoxin intoxication.

Note: The electrocardiogram is fundamental in determining the presence and nature of these cardiac disturbances. Digoxin may also induce other changes in the ECG (e.g. PR prolongation ST depression), which represent digoxin effect and may or may not be associated with digitalis toxicity.

Gastrointestinal—Anorexia, nausea, vomiting and diarrhea may be early symptoms of overdosage. However, uncontrolled heart failure may also produce such symptoms.

CNS—Visual disturbances (blurred or yellow vision), headache, weakness, apathy and psychosis can occur. These may be difficult to recognize in infants and children.

Other—Gynecomastia is occasionally observed.

Treatment of Arrhythmias Produced by Overdosage:

Adults:
Digoxin should be discontinued until all signs of toxicity are gone. Discontinuation may be all that is necessary if toxic manifestations are not severe and appear only near the expected time for maximum effect of the drug.

Potassium salts are commonly used, particularly if hypokalemia is present. Potassium chloride in divided oral doses totaling 3 to 6 grams of the salt (40 to 80 mEq K+) for adults may be given provided renal function is adequate (see below for potassium recommendations in Infants and Children).

When correction of the arrhythmia is urgent and the serum potassium concentration is low or normal, potassium should be administered intravenously in 5% dextrose injection. For adults, a total of 40 to 80 mEq (diluted to a concentration of 40 mEq per 500 ml) may be given at a rate not exceeding 20 mEq per hour, or slower if limited by pain due to local irritation. Additional amounts may be given if the arrhythmia is uncontrolled and potassium well-tolerated. ECG monitoring should be performed to watch for any evidence of potassium toxicity (e.g. peaking of T waves) and to observe the effect on the arrhythmia. The infusion may be stopped when the desired effect is achieved.

Note: Potassium should not be used and may be dangerous in heart block due to digoxin, unless primarily related to supraventricular tachycardia.

Other agents that have been used for the treatment of digoxin intoxication include lidocaine, procainamide, propranolol and phenytoin, although use of the latter must be considered experimental. In advanced heart block, temporary ventricular pacing may be beneficial. Rapid reversal of potentially life-threatening digitalis intoxication unresponsive to other therapy has been reported* following intravenous administration of digoxin-specific (ovine) antibody fragments (Fab); this therapy should also be considered investigational at this time. (*New Engl J Med, 1982; 307; 1357-1362.

Infants and Children:
See Adult section for general recommendations for the treatment of arrhythmias produced by overdosage and for cautions regarding the use of potassium.

If a potassium preparation is used to treat toxicity, it may be given orally in divided doses totaling 1 to 1.5 mEq K+ per kilogram (kg) body weight (1 gram of potassium chloride contains 13.4 mEq K+).

When correction of the arrhythmia with potassium is urgent, approximately 0.5 mEq/kg of potassium per hour may be given intravenously, with careful ECG monitoring. The intravenous solution of potassium should be dilute enough to avoid local irritation; however, especially in infants, care must be taken to avoid intravenous fluid overload.

Dosage and Administration: Recommended dosages are average values that may require considerable modification because of individual sensitivity or associated conditions. Diminished renal function is the most important factor requiring modification of recommended doses.

Parenteral administration of digoxin should be used only when the need for rapid digitalization is urgent or when the drug cannot be taken orally. Intramuscular injection can lead to severe pain at the injection site, thus intravenous administration is preferred. If the drug must be administered by the intramuscular route, it should be injected deep into the muscle followed by massage. No more than 500 μg (2 ml) of Lanoxin Injection or 200 μg (2 ml) of Lanoxin Injection Pediatric should be injected into a single site.

Lanoxin® Injection and Injection Pediatric can be administered undiluted or diluted with a 4-fold or greater volume of sterile water for injection, 0.9% sodium chloride injection or 5% dextrose injection. The use of less than a 4-fold volume of diluent could lead to precipitation of the digoxin. Immediate use of the diluted product is recommended.

If tuberculin syringes are used to measure very small doses, one must be aware of the problem of inadvertent overadministration of digoxin. The syringe should *not* be flushed with the parenteral solution after its contents are expelled into an indwelling vascular catheter.

Slow infusion of Lanoxin® Injection or Injection Pediatric is preferable to bolus administration. Rapid infusion of digitalis glycosides has been shown to cause systemic and coronary arteriolar constriction, which may be clinically undesirable. Caution is thus advised and Lanoxin Injection or Injection Pediatric should probably be administered over a period of 5 minutes or longer. Mixing of Lanoxin Injections with other drugs in the same container or simultaneous administration in the same intravenous line is not recommended.

In deciding the dose of digoxin, several factors must be considered:
1. The disease being treated. Atrial arrhythmias may require larger doses than heart failure.
2. The body weight of the patient. Doses should be calculated based upon lean or ideal body weight.
3. The patient's renal function, preferably evaluated on the basis of creatinine clearance.
4. Age is an important factor in infants and children.
5. Concomitant disease states, drugs or other factors likely to alter the expected clinical response to digoxin (see PRECAUTIONS and Drug Interactions sections).

Digitalization may be accomplished by either of two general approaches that vary in dosage and frequency of administration, but reach the same endpoint in terms of total amount of digoxin accumulated in the body.
1. Rapid digitalization may be achieved by administering a loading dose based upon projected peak body digoxin stores, then calculating the maintenance dose as a percentage of the loading dose.
2. More gradual digitalization may be obtained by beginning an appropriate maintenance dose, thus allowing digoxin body stores to accumulate slowly. Steady-state serum digoxin concentration will be achieved in approximately 5 half-lives of the drug for the individual patient. Depending upon the patient's renal function, this will take between one and three weeks.

Adults:
Adults—Rapid Digitalization with a Loading Dose. Peak body digoxin stores of 8 to 12 μg/kg should provide therapeutic effect with minimum risk of toxicity in most patients with heart failure and normal sinus rhythm. Larger stores (10 to 15 μg/kg) are often required for adequate control of ventricular rate in patients with atrial flutter or fibrillation. Because of altered digoxin distribution and elimination, projected peak body stores for patients with renal insufficiency should be conservative (i.e. 6 to 10 μg/kg) [see PRECAUTIONS section].

The loading dose should be based on the projected peak body stores and administered in several portions, with roughly half the total given as the first dose. Additional fractions of this planned total dose may be given at 4 to 8 hour intervals IV or 6 to 8 hour intervals orally, with **careful assessment of clinical response before each additional dose.**

If the patient's clinical response necessitates a change from the calculated dose of digoxin, then calculation of the maintenance dose should be based upon the amount actually given.

In previously undigitalized patients, a single initial intravenous Lanoxin® Injection dose of 400 to 600 μg (0.4 to 0.6 mg) usually produces a detectable effect in 5 to 30 minutes that becomes maximal in 1 to 4 hours. Additional doses of 100 to 300 μg (0.1 to 0.3 mg) may be given cautiously at 4 to 8 hour intervals until clinical evidence of an adequate effect is noted. The usual amount of Lanoxin Injection that a 70 kg patient requires to achieve 8 to 15

Continued on next page

Burroughs Wellcome—Cont.

μg/kg peak body stores is 600 to 1000 μg (0.6 to 1.0 mg).

A single initial Lanoxin® Tablet or Elixir Pediatric dose of 500 to 750 μg (0.5 to 0.75 mg) usually produces a detectable effect in 0.5 to 2 hours that becomes maximal in 2 to 6 hours. Additional doses of 125 to 375 μg (0.125 to 0.375 mg) may be given cautiously at 6 to 8 hour intervals until clinical evidence of an adequate effect is noted. The usual amount of Lanoxin Tablets or Elixir that a 70 kg patient requires to achieve 8 to 15 μg peak body stores is 750 to 1250 μg (0.75 to 1.25 mg).

Although peak body stores are mathematically related to loading doses and are utilized to calculate maintenance doses, they do not correlate with measured serum concentrations. This discrepancy is caused by digoxin distribution within the body during the first 6 to 8 hours following a dose. Serum concentrations drawn during this time are usually not interpretable.

The maintenance dose should be based upon the percentage of the peak body stores lost each day through elimination. The following formula has had wide clinical use:

[See table below].

Ccr is creatinine clearance, corrected to 70 kg body weight or 1.73 m^2 body surface area. *For adults*, if only serum creatinine concentrations (Scr) are available, a Ccr (corrected to 70 kg body weight) may be estimated in men as (140 – Age)/Scr. For women, this result should be multiplied by 0.85.

Note: This equation cannot be used for estimating creatinine clearance in infants or children.

A common practice involves the use of Lanoxin® Injection to achieve rapid digitalization, with conversion to Lanoxin Tablets or Lanoxicaps for maintenance therapy. If patients are switched from IV to oral digoxin formulations, allowances must be made for differences in bioavailability when calculating maintenance dosages (see table, CLINICAL PHARMACOLOGY section).

Adults—Gradual Digitalization with a Maintenance Dose: The following table provides average Lanoxin Tablet daily maintenance dose requirements for patients with heart failure based upon lean body weight and renal function:

[See table above].

Infants and Children:

Digitalization must be individualized. Divided daily dosing is recommended for infants and young children. Children over 10 years of age require adult dosages in proportion to their body weight. In the newborn period, renal clearance of digoxin is diminished and suitable dosage adjustments must be observed. This is especially pronounced in the premature infant. Beyond the immediate newborn period, children generally require proportionally larger doses than adults on the basis of body weight or body surface area.

Infants and Children— Rapid Digitalization with a Loading Dose: Lanoxin Injection Pediatric can be used to achieve rapid digitalization, with conversion to an oral Lanoxin formulation for maintenance therapy. If patients are switched from IV to oral digoxin tablets or elixir, allowances must be made for differences in bioavailability when calculating maintenance dosages (see bioavailability table in CLINICAL PHARMACOLOGY section and dosing tables below).

Intramuscular injection of digoxin is extremely painful and offers no advantages unless other routes of administration are contraindicated.

Digitalizing and daily maintenance doses for each age group are given below and should provide therapeutic effect with minimum risk of toxicity in most patients with heart failure and normal sinus rhythm. Larger doses are often required for adequate control of ventricular rate in patients with atrial flutter or fibrillation.

The loading dose should be administered in several portions, with roughly half the total given as the first dose. Additional fractions of this planned total dose may be given at 6 to 8 hour intervals with Lanoxin Tablets or Elixir or at 4 to 8 hour intervals with Lanoxin Injection or Injection Pediatric **with careful assessment of clinical response before each additional dose.** If the patient's clinical response necessitates a change from the calculated dose of digoxin, then calculation of the maintenance dose should be based upon the amount actually given.

[See table on next page].

Infants and Children—Gradual Digitalization With A Maintenance Dose: More gradual digitalization can also be accomplished by beginning an appropriate maintenance dose. The range of percentages provided above can be used in calculating this dose for patients with normal renal function. In children with renal disease, digoxin dosing must be carefully titrated based upon clinical response.

Long-term use of digoxin is indicated in many children who have been digitalized for acute heart failure, unless the cause is transient. Children with severe congenital heart disease, even after surgery, may require digoxin for prolonged periods.

It cannot be overemphasized that both the adult and pediatric dosage guidelines provided are based upon average patient response and substantial individual variation can be expected. Accordingly, ultimate dosage selection must be based upon clinical assessment of the patient.

Serum Digoxin Concentrations:

Measurement of serum digoxin concentrations can be helpful to the clinician in determining the state of digitalization and in assigning certain probabilities to the likelihood of digoxin intoxication. Studies in adults considered adequately digitalized (without evidence of toxicity) show that about two-thirds of such patients have serum digoxin levels ranging from 0.8 to 2.0 ng/ml. Patients with atrial fibrillation or atrial flutter require and appear to tolerate higher levels than do patients with other indications. On the other hand, in adult patients with clinical evidence of digoxin toxicity, about two-thirds will have serum digoxin levels greater than 2.0 ng/ml. Thus, whereas levels less than 0.8 ng/ml are infrequently associated with toxicity, levels greater than 2.0 ng/ml are often associated with toxicity. Values in between are not very helpful in deciding whether a certain sign or symptom is more likely caused by digoxin toxicity or by something else. There are rare patients who are unable to tolerate digoxin even at serum concentrations below 0.8 ng/ml. Some researchers suggest that infants and young children tolerate slightly higher serum concentrations than do adults.

To allow adequate time for equilibration of digoxin between serum and tissue, **sampling of serum concentrations for clinical use should be at least 6 to 8 hours after the last dose**, regardless of the route of administration or formulation used. On a twice daily dosing schedule, there will be only minor differences in serum digoxin concentrations whether sampling is done at 8 or 12 hours after a dose. After a single daily dose, the concentration will be 10 to 25% lower when sampled at 24 versus 8 hours, depending upon the patient's renal function. Ideally, sampling for assessment of steady-state concentrations should be done just before the next dose.

If a discrepancy exists between the reported serum concentration and the observed clinical response, the clinician should consider the following possibilities:

1. Analytical problems in the assay procedure.
2. Inappropriate serum sampling time.
3. Administration of a digitalis glycoside other than digoxin.
4. Conditions (described in WARNINGS and PRECAUTIONS sections) causing an alteration in the sensitivity of the patient to digoxin.
5. The patient falls outside the norm in his response to or handling of digoxin. This decision should only be reached after exclusion of the other possibilities and generally should be confirmed by additional correlations of clinical observations with serum digoxin concentrations.

The serum concentration data should always be interpreted in the overall clinical context and an isolated serum concentration value should not be used alone as a basis for increasing or decreasing digoxin dosage.

Adjustment of Maintenance Dose in Previously Digitalized Patients:

Maintenance doses in individual patients on steady-state digoxin can be adjusted upward or downward in proportion to the ratio of the desired versus the measured serum concentration. For example, a patient at steady-state on 125 μg (0.125 mg) of Lanoxin Tablets per day with a measured serum concentration of 0.7 ng/ml, should have the dose increased to 250 μg (0.25 mg) per day to achieve a steady-state serum concentration of 1.4 ng/ml, **assuming the serum digoxin concentration measurement is correct, renal function remains stable during this time and the needed adjustment is not the result of a problem with compliance.**

Dosage Adjustment When Changing Preparations:

The differences in bioavailability between injectable Lanoxin or Lanoxicaps and Lanoxin Elixir

---

Usual Lanoxin Daily Maintenance Dose Requirements (μg)
For Estimated Peak Body Stores of 10 μg/kg

		\multicolumn{6}{c}{Lean Body Weight (kg/lbs)}		
		50/110	60/132	70/154	80/176	90/198	100/200		
	0	63*†	125	125	125	188††	188	22	
	10	125	125	125	188	188	188	19	
	20	125	125	188	188	188	250	16	
Corrected	30	125	188	188	188	250	250	14	Number of
Ccr	40	125	188	188	250	250	250	13	Days
(ml/min	50	188	188	250	250	250	250	12	Before
per 70 kg)	60	188	188	250	250	250	375	11	Steady-State
	70	188	250	250	250	250	375	10	Achieved
	80	188	250	250	250	375	375	9	
	90	188	250	250	250	375	500	8	
	100	250	250	250	375	375	500	7	

* 63 μg = 0.063 mg
† ½ of 125 μg tablet or 125 μg every other day
†† 1½ of 125 μg tablet.

Example—based on the above table, a patient in heart failure with an estimated lean body weight of 70 kg and a Ccr of 60 ml/min, should be given a 250 μg (0.25 mg) Lanoxin® Tablet each day, usually taken after the morning meal. Steady-state serum concentrations should not be anticipated before 11 days.

Lanoxin   Maintenance Dose = Peak Body Stores (i.e. Loading Dose) × $\dfrac{\%\ \text{Daily Loss}}{100}$

Where: % Daily Loss = 14 + Ccr/5

Pediatric or Lanoxin Tablets must be considered when changing patients from one dosage form to another.

Lanoxin Injection and Lanoxicaps doses of 100 µg (0.1 mg) and 200 µg (0.2 mg) are approximately equivalent to 125 µg (0.125 mg) and 250 µg (0.25 mg) doses of Lanoxin Tablets and Elixir Pediatric (see table in CLINICAL PHARMACOLOGY section). Intramuscular injection of digoxin is extremely painful and offers no advantages unless other routes of administration are contraindicated.

How Supplied:
LANOXIN® (DIGOXIN) TABLETS, Scored 125 µg (0.125 mg): Bottles of 100 (NDC-0081-0242-55) and 1000 (NDC-0081-0242-75); Unit dose pack of 1000 (200 x 5's) (NDC-0081-0242-72); Unit of Use bottles of 30 (NDC-0081-0242-30) **VA NSN** 6505-01-049-6807. Imprinted with LANOXIN and Y3B (yellow). Store at 15°–30°C (59°–86°F) in a dry place and protect from light.

LANOXIN (DIGOXIN) TABLETS, Scored 250 µg (0.25 mg): Bottles of 100 (NDC-0081-0249-55) **DoD NSN** 6505-00-116-7750, 500 (NDC-0081-0249-70), 1000 (NDC-0081-0249-75) **VA NSN** 6505-00-611-7898 and 5000 (NDC-0081-0249-80); Unit dose pack of 100 (10 x 10) (NDC-0081-0249-77) **DoD NSN** 6505-00-117-5689; Unit of Use bottles of 30 (NDC-0081-0249-30) **VA NSN** 6505-01-035-2104 and 100 (NDC-0081-0249-17). Imprinted with LANOXIN and X3A (white). Store at 15°–30°C (59°–86°F) in a dry place.

LANOXIN (DIGOXIN) TABLETS, Scored 500 µg (0.5 mg): Bottles of 100 (NDC-0081-0253-55). Imprinted with LANOXIN and T9A (green). Store at 15°–30°C (59°–86°F) in a dry place and protect from light.

LANOXIN (DIGOXIN) INJECTION, 500 µg (0.5 mg) in 2 ml [250 µg (0.25 mg) per ml]; boxes of 12 (NDC-0081-0260-15) **DoD NSN** 6505-00-531-7761 and 100 ampuls (NDC-0081-0260-55). Store at 15°–30°C (59°–86°F) and protect from light.

LANOXIN (DIGOXIN) INJECTION PEDIATRIC, 100 µg (0.1 mg) in 1 ml; box of 50 ampuls (NDC-0081-0262-35). Store at 15°–30°C (59°– 86°F) and protect from light.

LANOXIN (DIGOXIN) ELIXIR PEDIATRIC, 50 µg (0.05 mg) per ml; bottle of 60 ml with calibrated dropper (NDC-0081-0264-27) **DoD NSN** 6505-00-890-1726. Store at 15°–25°C (59°–77°F) and protect from light.

Tablets Shown in Product Identification Section, page 408

LEUKERAN® ℞
(Chlorambucil)
2 mg Sugar-coated Tablets

> **WARNING:** Leukeran (chlorambucil) can severely suppress bone marrow function. Chlorambucil is a carcinogen in humans. Chlorambucil is probably mutagenic and teratogenic in humans. Chlorambucil produces human infertility. See "WARNINGS" and "PRECAUTIONS" sections.

Description: Leukeran (chlorambucil) was first synthesized by Everett et al.[1] It is a bifunctional alkylating agent of the nitrogen mustard type that has been found active against selected human neoplastic diseases. Chlorambucil is known chemically as 4-[bis(2-chloroethyl)amino]benzenebutanoic acid and has the following structural formula:

(ClCH₂CH₂)₂N—⟨phenyl⟩—CH₂CH₂CH₂COOH

Chlorambucil hydrolyzes in water and has a pKa of 5.8.

Leukeran (chlorambucil) is available in 2 mg sugar-coated tablets for oral administration.

Clinical Pharmacology: Chlorambucil is rapidly and completely absorbed from the gastrointestinal tract. After single oral doses of 0.6–1.2 mg/kg, peak plasma chlorambucil levels are reached within one hour and the terminal half-life of the parent drug is estimated at 1.5 hours. Chlorambucil undergoes rapid metabolism to phenylacetic acid mustard, the major metabolite, and the combined chlorambucil and phenylacetic acid mustard urinary excretion is extremely low—less than 1% in 24 hours. The peak plasma levels of chlorambucil and phenylacetic acid mustard are similar, approximately 1 µg/ml; however, the metabolite's half-life is 1.6 times greater than the parent drug.[2,3]

Chlorambucil and its metabolites are extensively bound to plasma and tissue proteins. In vitro, chlorambucil is 99% bound to plasma proteins, specifically albumin.[4] Cerebrospinal fluid levels of chlorambucil have not been determined. Evidence of human teratogenicity suggests that the drug crosses the placenta.[5,6]

Chlorambucil is extensively metabolized in the liver primarily to phenylacetic acid mustard which has antineoplastic activity.[2,3] Chlorambucil and its major metabolite spontaneously degrade in vivo forming monohydroxy and dihydroxy derivatives.[2] After a single dose of radiolabeled chlorambucil (¹⁴C) approximately 15% to 60% of the radioactivity appears in the urine after 24 hours. Again, less than 1% of the urinary radioactivity is in the form of chlorambucil or phenylacetic acid mustard.[2] In summary, the pharmacokinetic data suggest that oral chlorambucil undergoes rapid gastrointestinal absorption and plasma clearance and that it is almost completely metabolized, having extremely low urinary excretion.

Indications and Usage: Leukeran (chlorambucil) is indicated in the treatment of chronic lymphatic (lymphocytic) leukemia, malignant lymphomas including lymphosarcoma, giant follicular lymphoma and Hodgkin's disease. It is not curative in any of these disorders but may produce clinically useful palliation.

Contraindications: Chlorambucil should not be used in patients whose disease has demonstrated a prior resistance to the agent. Patients who have demonstrated hypersensitivity to chlorambucil should not be given the drug.[7] There may be cross-hypersensitivity (skin rash) between chlorambucil and other alkylating agents.[8]

Warnings: Because of its carcinogenic properties, chlorambucil should not be given to patients with conditions other than chronic lymphatic leukemia or malignant lymphomas. Convulsions,[9] infertility,[10] leukemia[11,12] and secondary malignancies[13] have been observed when chlorambucil was employed in the therapy of malignant and non-malignant diseases.

There are many reports of acute leukemia arising with both malignant[15] and non-malignant[16] diseases following chlorambucil treatment. In many instances, these patients also received other chemotherapeutic agents or some form of radiation therapy. The quantitation of the risk of chlorambucil-induction of leukemia or carcinoma in humans is not possible.

Evaluation of published reports of leukemia developing in patients who have received chlorambucil (and other alkylating agents) suggests that the risk of leukemogenesis increases with both chronicity of treatment and large cumulative doses. However, it has proved impossible to define a cumulative dose below which there is no risk of the induction of secondary malignancy. The potential benefits from chlorambucil therapy must be weighed on an individual basis against the possible risk of the induction of a secondary malignancy. Chlorambucil has been shown to cause chromatid or chromosome damage in man.[17,18] Both reversible and permanent sterility have been observed in both sexes receiving chlorambucil.

A high incidence of sterility has been documented when chlorambucil is administered to prepubertal and pubertal males.[19] Prolonged or permanent azoospermia has also been observed in adult males.[20] While most reports of gonadal dysfunction secondary to chlorambucil have related to males, the induction of amenorrhea in females with alkylating agents is well documented and chlorambucil is capable of producing amenorrhea. Autopsy studies of the ovaries from women with malignant lymphoma treated with combination chemotherapy including chlorambucil have shown varying degrees of fibrosis, vasculitis, and depletion of primordial follicles.[21,22]

Pregnancy: *"Pregnancy Category D":* Chlorambucil can cause fetal harm when administered to a pregnant woman. Unilateral renal agenesis has been observed in two offspring whose mothers received chlorambucil during the first trimester.[5,6] Urogenital malformations including absence of a kidney were found in fetuses of rats given chlorambucil.[14] There are no adequate and well-controlled studies in pregnant women. If this drug is used during pregnancy, or if the patient becomes pregnant while taking this drug, the patient should be apprised of the potential hazard to

Continued on next page

Usual Digitalizing and Maintenance Dosages for **Lanoxin® Tablets or Lanoxin® Elixir Pediatric** in Children with **Normal Renal Function Based on Lean Body Weight**

Age	Digitalizing* Dose (µg/kg)	Daily† Oral Maintenance Dose (µg/kg)
Premature	20–30	20–30% of *oral* loading dose††
Full-Term	25–35	
1–24 Months	35–60	
2–5 Years	30–40	25–35% of *oral* loading dose††
5–10 Years	20–35	
Over 10 years	10–15	

Usual Digitalizing and Maintenance Dosages for **Lanoxin® Injection or Lanoxin® Injection Pediatric** in Children with **Normal Renal Function Based on Lean Body Weight**

Age	Digitalizing* Dose (µg/kg)	Daily† IV Maintenance Dose (µg/kg)
Premature	15–25	20–30% of the IV loading dose††
Full-Term	20–30	
1–24 Months	30–50	
2–5 Years	25–35	25–35% of the IV loading dose††
5–10 Years	15–30	
Over 10 Years	8–12	

* IV digitalizing doses are 80% of oral digitalizing doses.
† Divided daily dosing is recommended for children under 10 years of age.
†† Projected or actual digitalizing dose providing clinical response.

Burroughs Wellcome—Cont.

the fetus. Women of childbearing potential should be advised to avoid becoming pregnant.

Precautions:

General: Many patients develop a slowly progressive lymphopenia during treatment. The lymphocyte count usually rapidly returns to normal levels upon completion of drug therapy. Most patients have some neutropenia after the third week of treatment and this may continue for up to ten days after the last dose. Subsequently, the neutrophil count usually rapidly returns to normal. Severe neutropenia appears to be related to dosage and usually occurs only in patients who have received a total dosage of 6.5 mg/kg or more in one course of therapy with continuous dosing. About one-quarter of all patients receiving the continuous-dose schedule, and one-third of those receiving this dosage in eight weeks or less may be expected to develop severe neutropenia.[23]

While it is not necessary to discontinue chlorambucil at the first evidence of a fall in neutrophil count, it must be remembered that the fall may continue for ten days after the last dose and that as the total dose approaches 6.5 mg/kg there is a risk of causing irreversible bone marrow damage. The dose of chlorambucil should be decreased if leukocyte or platelet counts fall below normal values and should be discontinued for more severe depression.

Chlorambucil should **not** be given at full dosages before four weeks after a full course of radiation therapy or chemotherapy because of the vulnerability of the bone marrow to damage under these conditions. If the pretherapy leukocyte or platelet counts are depressed from bone marrow disease process prior to institution of therapy, the treatment should be instituted at a reduced dosage.

Persistently low neutrophil and platelet counts or peripheral lymphocytosis suggest bone marrow infiltration. If confirmed by bone marrow examination, the daily dosage of chlorambucil should not exceed 0.1 mg/kg. Chlorambucil appears to be relatively free from gastrointestinal side effects or other evidence of toxicity apart from the bone marrow depressant action. In humans, single oral doses of 20 mg or more may produce nausea and vomiting.

Information for Patients: Patients should be informed that the major toxicities of chlorambucil are related to hypersensitivity, drug fever, myelosuppression, hepatotoxicity, infertility, seizures, gastrointestinal toxicity, and secondary malignancies. Patients should never be allowed to take the drug without medical supervision and should consult their physician if they experience skin rash, bleeding, fever, jaundice, persistent cough, seizures, nausea, vomiting, amenorrhea, or unusual lumps/masses. Women of childbearing potential should be advised to avoid becoming pregnant.

Laboratory Tests: Patients must be followed carefully to avoid life-endangering damage to the bone marrow during treatment. Weekly examination of the blood should be made to determine hemoglobin levels, total and differential leukocyte counts, and quantitative platelet counts. Also, during the first 3 to 6 weeks of therapy, it is recommended that white blood cell counts be made 3 or 4 days after each of the weekly complete blood counts. Galton et al[23] have suggested that in following patients it is helpful to plot the blood counts on a chart at the same time that body weight, temperature, spleen size, etc., are recorded. It is considered dangerous to allow a patient to go more than two weeks without hematological and clinical examination during treatment.

Drug Interactions: There are no known drug/drug interactions with chlorambucil.

Carcinogenesis, Mutagenesis, Impairment of Fertility: See WARNINGS section for information on carcinogenesis, mutagenesis and impairment of fertility.

Pregnancy: *Teratogenic Effects:* Pregnancy Category D: See WARNINGS section.

Nursing Mothers: It is not known whether this drug is excreted in human milk. Because many drugs are excreted in human milk and because of the potential for serious adverse reactions in nursing infants from chlorambucil, a decision should be made whether to discontinue nursing or to discontinue the drug, taking into account the importance of the drug to the mother.

Pediatric Use: The safety and effectiveness in children have not been established.

Adverse Reactions:

Hematologic Effects: The most common side effect is bone marrow suppression.[24] Although bone marrow suppression frequently occurs, it is usually reversible if the chlorambucil is withdrawn early enough. However, irreversible bone marrow failure has been reported.[25,26]

Gastrointestinal: Gastrointestinal disturbances such as nausea and vomiting, diarrhea and oral ulceration occur infrequently.

Miscellaneous: Other reported adverse reactions include: pulmonary fibrosis, hepatotoxicity and jaundice, drug fever, skin hypersensitivity, peripheral neuropathy, interstitial pneumonia, sterile cystitis, infertility, leukemia and secondary malignancies (see WARNINGS). Seizures have occurred in children with nephrotic syndrome and dose-related focal fits have been reported in adults.[9,27]

Overdosage: Reversible pancytopenia was the main finding of inadvertent overdoses of chlorambucil.[28,29] Neurological toxicity ranging from agitated behavior and ataxia to multiple grand mal seizures has also occurred.[28,30] As there is no known antidote, the blood picture should be closely monitored and general supportive measures should be instituted, together with appropriate blood transfusions if necessary. Chlorambucil is not dialyzable.

Oral LD$_{50}$ single doses in mice are 123 mg/kg. In rats, a single intraperitoneal dose of 12.5 mg/kg of chlorambucil produces typical nitrogen-mustard effects; these include atrophy of the intestinal mucous membrane and lymphoid tissues, severe lymphopenia becoming maximal in four days, anemia and thrombocytopenia. After this dose, the animals begin to recover within three days and appear normal in about a week although the bone marrow may not become completely normal for about three weeks. An intraperitoneal dose of 18.5 mg/kg kills about 50% of the rats with development of convulsions. As much as 50 mg/kg has been given orally to rats as a single dose, with recovery. Such a dose causes bradycardia, excessive salivation, hematuria, convulsions, and respiratory dysfunction.

Dosage and Administration: The usual oral dosage is 0.1 to 0.2 mg/kg body weight daily for three to six weeks as required. This usually amounts to 4 to 10 mg a day for the average patient. The entire daily dose may be given at one time. These dosages are for initiation of therapy or for short courses of treatment. The dosage must be carefully adjusted according to the response of the patient and must be reduced as soon as there is an abrupt fall in the white blood cell count. Patients with Hodgkin's disease usually require 0.2 mg/kg daily whereas patients with other lymphomas or chronic lymphocytic leukemia usually require only 0.1 mg/kg daily. When lymphocytic infiltration of the bone marrow is present, or when the bone marrow is hypoplastic, the daily dose should not exceed 0.1 mg/kg (about 6 mg for the average patient).

Alternate schedules for the treatment of chronic lymphocytic leukemia employing intermittent, biweekly or once monthly pulse doses of chlorambucil have been reported.[31,32] Intermittent schedules of chlorambucil begin with an initial single dose of 0.4 mg/kg. Doses are generally increased by 0.1 mg/kg until control of lymphocytosis or toxicity is observed. Subsequent doses are modified to produce mild hematologic toxicity. It is felt that the response rate of chronic lymphocytic leukemia to the bi-weekly or once monthly schedule of chlorambucil administration is similar to or better to that previously reported with daily administration and that hematologic toxicity was less than or equal to that encountered in studies using daily chlorambucil.

Radiation and cytotoxic drugs render the bone marrow more vulnerable to damage and chlorambucil should be used with particular caution within four weeks of a full course of radiation therapy or chemotherapy. However, small doses of palliative radiation over isolated foci remote from the bone marrow will not usually depress the neutrophil and platelet count. In these cases chlorambucil may be given in the customary dosage.

It is presently felt that short courses of treatment are safer than continuous maintenance therapy although both methods have been effective. It must be recognized that continuous therapy may give the appearance of "maintenance" in patients who are actually in remission and have no immediate need for further drug. If maintenance dosage is used, it should not exceed 0.1 mg/kg daily and may well be as low as 0.03 mg/kg daily. A typical maintenance dose is 2 mg to 4 mg daily, or less, depending on the status of the blood counts. It may, therefore, be desirable to withdraw the drug after maximal control has been achieved since intermittent therapy reinstituted at time of relapse may be as effective as continuous treatment.

How Supplied: White sugar-coated tablet containing 2 mg chlorambucil; bottle of 50 (NDC-0081-0635-35).

Store at 15°–30°C (59°–86°F) in a dry place.

References:

1. Everett JL, Roberts JR, and Ross WCJ: Aryl-2-halogen-oalkylamines. Part XII. Some Carboxylic Derivatives of NN-Di-2-chloroethylaniline. *J Chem Soc, 3:*2386, 1953.
2. Alberts DS *et al:* Pharmokinetics and Metabolism of Chlorambucil in Man: A Preliminary Report. *Cancer Treat Rev, 6* (Suppl.):9, 1979.
3. McLean A *et al:* Pharmokinetics and Metabolism of Chlormabucil in Patients with Malignant Disease. *Cancer Treat Rev, 6* (Suppl.):33, 1979.
4. Ehrsson H *et al:* Degradation of Chlorambucil in Aqueous Solution - Influence of Human Albumin Binding. *J Pharm Pharmacol, 33:*313, 1981.
5. Shotton D and Monie IW: Possible Teratogenic Effect of Chlorambucil on a Human Fetus. *JAMA, 186:*74, 1963.
6. Steege JF and Caldwell DS: Renal Agenesis after First Trimester Exposure to Chlorambucil. *South Med J, 73:*1414, 1980.
7. Knisley RE *et al:* Unusual Reaction to Chlorambucil in a Patient with Chronic Lymphocytic Leukemia. *Arch Dermatol, 104:*77, 1971.
8. Weiss RB and Bruno S: Hypersensitivity Reactions to Cancer Chemotherapeutic Agents. *Ann Intern Med, 94:*66, 1981.
9. Williams SA *et al:* Seizures: A Significant Side Effect of Chlorambucil Therapy in Children. *J Pediatr, 93:*516, 1978.
10. Freckman HA *et al:* Chlorambucil-Prednisolone Therapy for Disseminated Breast Carcinoma. *JAMA 189:*23, 1964.
11. Aymard JP *et al:* Acute Leukemia after Prolonged Chlorambucil Treatment for Non-Malignant Disease: A Report of a New Case and Literature Survey. *Acta Haematol* (Basel), *63:*283, 1980.
12. Berk PD *et al:* Increased Incidence of Acute Leukemia in Polycythermia Vera Associated with Chlorambucil Therapy. *N Engl J Med, 304:*441, 1981.
13. Lerner HJ: Acute Myelogenous Leukemia in Patients Receiving Chlorambucil as Long-Term Adjuvant Chemotherapy for Stage II Breast Cancer. *Cancer Treat Rep, 62:*1135, 1978.
14. Monie IW: Chlorambucil-Induced Abnormalities of the Urogenital System of Rat Fetuses. *Anat Rec, 139:*145–153, 1961.
15. Zarrabi MH *et al:* Chronic Lymphocytic Leukemia Terminating in Acute Leukemia. *Arch Intern Med, 137:*1059, 1977.
16. Cameron S: Chlorambucil and Leukemia. *N Eng J Med, 296:*1065, 1977.
17. Lawler SD and Lele KP: Chromosomal Damage Induced by Chlorambucil in Chronic Lym-

phocytic Leukemia. *Scand J Hematol, 9:*603, 1972.
18. Stevenson AC and Patel C: Effects of Chlorambucil on Human Chromosomes. *Mutat Res, 18:*333, 1973.
19. Guesry P, Lenoir G, and Broyer M: Gonadal Effects of Chlorambucil Given to Prepubertal and Pubertal Boys for Nephrotic Syndrome. *J Pediatr, 92:*299, 1978.
20. Richter, P et al: Effect of Chlorambucil on Spermatogenesis in the Human with Malignant Lymphoma. *Cancer, 25:*1026, 1970.
21. Morgenfeld MC et al: Ovarian Lesions Due to Cytostatic Agents During the Treatment of Hodgkin's Disease. *Surg Gynecol Obstet, 134:*826, 1972.
22. Sobrinho LG et al: Amenorrhea in Patients with Hodgkin's Disease Treated with Antineoplastic Agents. *Am J Obstet Gynecol, 109:*135, 1971.
23. Galton DAG, Israels LG, Nabarro JDN, and Till M: Clinical Trials of p-(Di-2-chloroethylamino)-phenylbutyric Acid (CB 1348) in Malignant Lymphoma. *Brit Med J, 2:*1172, 1955.
24. Moore GE et al: Effects of Chlorambucil (NSC-3088) in 374 Patients with Advanced Cancer. *Cancer Chemother Rep, (Part 1) 52:*661 (1968).
25. Galton DAG et al: The Use of Chlorambucil and Steroids in the Treatment of Chronic Lymphocytic Leukemia. *Br J Haematol, 7:*73, 1961.
26. Rudd P et al: Irreversible Bone Marrow Failure with Chlorambucil. *J Rheumatol, 2:*421, 1975.
27. Naysmith A and Robson RH: Focal Fits During Chlorambucil Therapy. *Postgrad Med J, 55:*806, 1979.
28. Green AA and Naiman JL: Chlorambucil Poisoning. *Am J. Dis Child, 116:*190, 1968.
29. Enck RE and Bennett JM: Inadvertant Chlorambucil Overdose in Adults. *NY State J Med, 77:*1480, 1977.
30. Wolfson S and Olney MB: Accidental Ingestion of a Toxic Dose of Chlorambucil: Report of a Case in a Child. *JAMA, 165:*239, 1957.
31. Knospe WH et al: Bi-Weekly Chlorambucil Treatment of Chronic Lymphocytic Leukemia. *Cancer, 33:*555, 1974.
32. Sawitsky A et al: Comparison of Daily Versus Intermittent Chlorambucil and Prednisone Therapy in the Treatment of Patients with Chronic Lymphocytic Leukemia. *Blood, 50:*1049-1059, 1977.

Shown in Product Identification Section, page 408

MANTADIL® CREAM
[măn' tah-dĭl"]

Description: Mantadil® Cream contains the antihistamine chlorcyclizine hydrochloride 2% and the corticosteroid hydrocortisone acetate 0.5%, preserved with methylparaben 0.25% in a vanishing cream base. The inactive ingredients are liquid and white petrolatum, emulsifying wax and purified water.
Mantadil Cream is an ANTIPRURITIC-ANTI-INFLAMMATORY-ANESTHETIC for topical administration.
Chlorcyclizine hydrochloride is known chemically as 1-[(4-Chlorophenyl) phenylmethyl]-4-methylpiperazine monohydrochloride.
Hydrocortisone acetate is the acetate ester of cortisol, known chemically as 17-hydroxycorticosterone 21-acetate.
The pH of this product is approximately 4.5.
Clinical Pharmacology: Chlorcylizine hydrochloride is an H_1 histamine-receptor antagonist that will occupy receptor sites in effector cells to the exclusion of histamine. It blocks most of the effects of histamine mediated by H_1 receptors, including contraction of smooth muscle and increased capillary permeability. Absorption of chlorcyclizine hydrochloride into the skin is rapid following topical application, whereas systemic absorption from the skin is minimal. Chlorcyclizine hydrochloride prevents local edema and provides local anesthetic and antipruritic action in the skin.
Hydrocortisone acetate administered topically suppresses most inflammatory and allergic responses in the skin. Following topical application, it is absorbed rapidly into the skin, where it reduces local heat, redness, swelling, and tenderness. A small part of the dose applied to broken skin is absorbed systemically and metabolized by the liver.
Indications and Usage: Mantadil Cream is indicated for the treatment of pruritic skin eruptions and other dermatoses including: eczema (allergic, nuchal and nummular); dermatitis (atopic, lichenoid and seborrheic); contact dermatitis including poison ivy, poison oak and poison sumac; localized neurodermatitis; insect bites; sunburn; intertrigo; and anogenital pruritus.
Contraindications: This preparation is contraindicated in patients who are hypersensitive to any of its components; in tuberculosis of the skin, vaccinia, varicella, and herpes simplex. As with other topical products containing hydrocortisone, the cream should not be used in bacterial infections of the skin unless antibacterial therapy is concomitant.
Not for ophthalmic use.
Warnings: Oral chlorcyclizine is teratogenic in animals. Long-term reproduction studies of topical chlorcyclizine have not been conducted in humans.
Precautions:
General: If signs of irritation develop with use of this cream, treatment should be discontinued and appropriate therapy instituted.
Any of the side effects reported following systemic use of corticosteroids, including adrenal suppression, may also occur following their topical use, especially in infants and children. Systemic absorption of topically applied steroids will be increased if extensive body surface areas are treated or if the occlusive technique is used. Under these circumstances, suitable precautions should be taken when long-term use is anticipated, particularly in infants and children.
Carcinogenesis, Mutagenesis, Impairment of Fertility:
Oral chlorcyclizine is teratogenic in animals. Long-term reproduction studies of topical chlorcyclizine have not been conducted. It is poorly absorbed percutaneously.
Pregnancy: **Teratogenic Effects:**
Pregnancy Category C. Animal reproduction studies have not been conducted with Mantadil Cream. It is also not known whether Mantadil Cream can cause fetal harm when administered to a pregnant woman or can affect reproduction capacity. Mantadil Cream should be given to a pregnant woman only if clearly needed.
Nursing Mothers: Hydrocortisone acetate appears in human milk following oral administration of the drug.
Caution should be exercised when hydrocortisone acetate is administered to a nursing woman.
It is not known whether chlorcyclizine hydrochloride is excreted in human milk. Because many drugs are excreted in human milk, caution should be exercised when chlorcyclizine hydrochloride is administered to a nursing woman.
Adverse Reactions: Allergic contact dermatitis may occur with topical application of chlorcyclizine hydrochloride. Systemic side effects have been reported after topical application of antihistamines to large areas of skin.
The following local adverse reactions have been reported with topical corticosteroids, especially under occlusive dressings: irritation, folliculitis, hypertrichosis, acneiform eruptions, hypopigmentation, allergic contact dermatitis, secondary infection, skin atrophy, striae and miliaria.
Overdosage: With continued application of topical corticosteroid on large areas of damaged skin and under occlusion, there is a remote possibility that sufficient absorption could occur to produce Cushing's syndrome. This is more likely in children.
Systemic toxicity following application of chlorcyclizine has never been reported.
The oral LD_{50} of chlorcyclizine hydrochloride in the mouse is 300 mg/kg.
The intraperitoneal LD_{50} of hydrocortisone acetate in the mouse is 2300 mg/kg.
Dosage and Administration: Apply to the skin two to five times daily. If the condition of the skin will permit, the cream should be well rubbed in.
How Supplied: Mantadil Cream (Chlorcyclizine hydrochloride 2% and hydrocortisone acetate 0.5%) is available in 15 gram tubes (NDC-0081-0650-94).
Store at 15°-30°C (59°-86°F).

MAREZINE®
[mair' uh-zēn"]
(Cyclizine Lactate)
Injection
50 mg in 1 ml

Description: Chemically, cyclizine is N-benzhydryl-N' methylpiperazine, and has a molecular weight of 266.4.
It is a white crystalline solid having a bitter taste, and is soluble in water and isotonic saline.
Marezine (Cyclizine Lactate) Injection is a sterile solution for INTRAMUSCULAR INJECTION ONLY.
Action: Marezine (Cyclizine Lactate) has antiemetic, anticholinergic and antihistaminic properties. It also reduces the sensitivity of the labyrinthine apparatus. The exact mechanism of action is unknown. In dogs the drug prevents emesis from intravenous threshold doses of apomorphine, but it is much less effective in blocking emesis from orally administered copper sulfate. These data suggest that the action is mediated through the chemoreceptive trigger zone.
Indications: For the treatment of nausea and vomiting of motion sickness when the oral route cannot be used.
Contraindications: Marezine is contraindicated in individuals who have shown a previous hypersensitivity to the drug.
Warnings: Patients may become drowsy while taking Marezine and should be cautioned against engaging in activities requiring mental alertness, e.g., driving a car or operating heavy machinery or appliances.
Use in Children: Clinical studies establishing safety and efficacy in children have not been done; therefore, usage in this age group and nursing mothers cannot be recommended.
Use with CNS Depressants: May have additive effects with alcohol and other CNS depressants (hypnotics, sedatives, tranquilizers, antianxiety agents, etc.).
Precautions: Because of its anticholinergic action, Marezine should be used with caution and appropriate monitoring in patients with glaucoma, obstructive disease of the gastrointestinal or genitourinary tract, and in elderly males with possible prostatic hypertrophy. Incipient glaucoma may be precipitated by anticholinergic drugs such as Marezine. The drug may have a hypotensive action. This may be confusing or dangerous in postoperative patients and should influence the decision on using the drug postoperatively.
Adverse Reactions: Urticaria, drug rash, dryness of mouth, nose and throat, drowsiness, restlessness, excitation, nervousness, insomnia, euphoria, anorexia, nausea, vomiting, diarrhea, constipation, hypotension, blurred vision, diplopia, vertigo, tinnitus, palpitation, tachycardia, urinary frequency, difficult urination, urinary retention, auditory and visual hallucinations have been reported, particularly when dosage recommendations are exceeded. Cholestatic jaundice has occurred in association with the use of Marezine.
Dosage and Administration: Marezine (Cyclizine Lactate) Injection is administered INTRAMUSCULARLY. The usual dose is 1 ml (50 mg) every 4 to 6 hours as necessary.
Overdosage:
Symptoms of Overdosage: Moderate overdosage may cause hyperexcitability alternating with

Continued on next page

Burroughs Wellcome—Cont.

drowsiness. Massive overdosage may cause convulsions; hallucinations; respiratory paralysis.
Treatment: Appropriate supportive and symptomatic treatment. Consider dialysis.
Caution: Do not use morphine or other respiratory depressants.
[See table below].
How Supplied:
MAREZINE® (CYCLIZINE LACTATE) INJECTION
50 mg in 1 ml
Boxes of 100 ampuls
The injection should be stored in a cold place. It may develop a slight yellow tint if stored at room temperature for several months; however, it retains full potency.
Also Available:
MAREZINE® (CYCLIZINE HYDROCHLORIDE)
50 mg Scored TABLETS
Boxes of 12
Bottle of 100
Shown in Product Identification Section, page 408

MYLERAN® ℞
[mī'lah-ran"]
(Busulfan)
2 mg Scored Tablets

Warnings: Myleran® (busulfan) is a potent drug. It should not be used unless a diagnosis of chronic myelogenous leukemia has been adequately established and the responsible physician is knowledgeable in assessing response to chemotherapy.
Myleran (busulfan) can induce severe bone marrow hypoplasia. Reduce or discontinue the dosage immediately at the first sign of any unusual depression of bone marrow function as reflected by an abnormal decrease in any of the formed elements of the blood. A bone marrow examination should be performed if the bone marrow status is uncertain.
SEE "WARNINGS" SECTION FOR INFORMATION REGARDING BUSULFAN-INDUCED LEUKEMOGENESIS IN HUMANS.

Description: Myleran (busulfan) (1,4-butanediol dimethanesulfonate) is a bifunctional alkylating agent. It is the most clinically useful member of a series of sulfonic acid esters of dihydric, straight chain aliphatic alcohols synthesized by Haddow and Timmis at the Chester Beatty Research Institute. It is the tetramethylene member (n = 4) of the series $CH_3SO_2O(-CH_2-)_n OSO_2CH_3$. It is not a structural analog of the nitrogen mustards.
The activity of busulfan in chronic myelogenous leukemia was first reported by D.A.G. Galton in 1953.[1]
Clinical Pharmacology: No analytical method has been found which permits the quantitation of unmetabolized busulfan or its metabolites in biological tissues or plasma. All studies of the pharmacokinetics of busulfan in humans have employed radiolabeled drug using either sulfur-35 (labeling the "carrier" portion of the molecule) or carbon-14 or tritium in the alkane portion of the 4-carbon chain (labels in the "alkylating" portion of the molecule).
Studies with ^{35}S-busulfan.[3] Following the intravenous administration of a single therapeutic dose of ^{35}S-busulfan, there was rapid disappearance of radioactivity from the blood; 90 to 95% of the ^{35}S-label disappeared within three to five minutes after injection. Thereafter, a constant, low level of radioactivity (1 to 3% of the injected dose) was maintained during the subsequent forty-eight hour period of observation. Following the oral administration of ^{35}S-busulfan, there was a lag period of one-half to two hours prior to the detection of radioactivity in the blood. However, at four hours the (low) level of circulating radioactivity was comparable to that obtained following intravenous administration.
After either oral or intravenous administration of ^{35}S-busulfan to humans, 45 to 60% of the radioactivity was recovered in the urine in the forty-eight hours after administration; the majority of the total urinary excretion occurred in the first twenty-four hours. In man, over 95% of the urinary sulfur-35 occurs as ^{35}S-methanesulfonic acid. The fact that urinary recovery of sulfur-35 was equivalent, irrespective of whether the drug was given intravenously or orally, suggests virtually complete absorption by the oral route.
Studies with ^{14}C-busulfan.[3] Oral and intravenous administration of 1,4-^{14}C-busulfan showed the same rapid initial disappearance of plasma radioactivity with a subsequent low-level plateau as observed following the administration of ^{35}S-labeled drug. Cumulative radioactivity in the urine after forty-eight hours was 25 to 30% of the administered dose (contrasting with 45 to 60% for ^{35}S-busulfan) and suggests a slower excretion of the alkylating portion of the molecule and its metabolites than for the sulfonoxymethyl moieties. Regardless of the route of administration, 1,4-^{14}C-busulfan yielded a complex mixture of at least 12 radiolabeled metabolites in urine; the main metabolite being 3-hydroxytetrahydrothiophene-1, 1-dioxide.
Studies with ^{3}H-busulfan.[4] Human pharmacokinetic studies have been conducted employing busulfan labeled with tritium on the tetramethylene chain. These experiments confirmed a rapid initial clearance of the radioactivity from plasma, irrespective of whether the drug was given orally or intravenously, and showed a gradual accumulation of radioactivity in the plasma after repeated doses. Urinary excretion of less than 50% of the total dose given suggested a slow elimination of the metabolic products from the body.
There is no experience with the use of dialysis in an attempt to modify the clinical toxicity of busulfan. One technical difficulty would derive from the extremely poor water solubility of busulfan. Additionally, all studies of the metabolism of busulfan employing radiolabeled materials indicate rapid chemical reactivity of the parent compound with prolonged retention of some of the metabolites (particularly the metabolites arising from the "alkylating" portion of the molecule). The effectiveness of dialysis at removing significant quantities of unreacted drug would be expected to be minimal in such a situation.
No information is available regarding the penetration of busulfan into brain or cerebrospinal fluid.
Biochemical Pharmacology: In aqueous media, busulfan undergoes a wide range of nucleophilic substitution reactions. While this chemical reactivity is relatively non-specific, alkylation of the DNA is felt to be an important biological mechanism for its cytotoxic effect.[3] Coliphage T7 exposed to busulfan was found to have the DNA crosslinked by intrastrand crosslinkages, but no interstrand linkages were found.
The metabolic fate of busulfan has been studied in rats and humans using ^{14}C- and ^{35}S-labeled materials.[3,6,7] In man,[3] as in the rat,[7] almost all of the radioactivity in ^{35}S-labeled busulfan is excreted in the urine in the form of ^{35}S-methanesulfonic acid. No unchanged drug was found in human urine,[3] although a small amount has been reported in rat urine.[7] Roberts and Warwick demonstrated that the formation of methanesulfonic acid in vivo in the rat is not due to a simple hydrolysis of busulfan to 1,4-butanediol, since only about 4% of 2,3-^{14}C-busulfan was excreted as carbon dioxide whereas 2,3-^{14}C-1,4-butanediol was converted almost exclusively to carbon dioxide.[6] The predominant reaction of busulfan in the rat is the alkylation of sulfhydryl groups (particularly cysteine and cysteine-containing compounds) to produce a cyclic sulfonium compound which is the precursor of the major urinary metabolite of the 4-carbon portion of the molecule, 3-hydroxytetrahydrothiophene-1, 1-dioxide.[6] This has been termed a "sulfur-stripping" action of busulfan and it may modify the function of certain sulfur-containing amino acids, polypeptides, and proteins; whether this action makes an important contribution to the cytotoxicity of busulfan is unknown.
The biochemical basis for acquired resistance to busulfan is largely a matter of speculation. Although altered transport of busulfan into the cell is one possibility, increased intracellular inactivation of the drug before it reaches the DNA is also possible. Experiments with other alkylating agents have shown that resistance to this class of compounds may reflect an acquired ability of the resistant cell to repair alkylation damage more effectively.[5]
Indications and Usage: Myleran® (busulfan) is indicated for the palliative treatment of chronic myelogenous (myeloid, myelocytic, granulocytic) leukemia. Although not curative, busulfan reduces the total granulocyte mass, relieves symptoms of the disease, and improves the clinical state of the patient. Approximately 90% of adults with previously untreated chronic myelogenous leukemia will obtain hematologic remission with regression or stabilization of organomegaly following the use of busulfan. It has been shown to be superior to splenic irradiation with respect to survival times and maintenance of hemoglobin levels, and to be equivalent to irradiation at controlling splenomegaly.[8]
It is not clear whether busulfan unequivocally prolongs the survival of responding patients beyond the 31 months experienced by an untreated group of historical controls.[9] Median survival figures of 31–42 months have been reported for several groups of patients treated with busulfan, but concurrent control groups of comparable, untreated patients are not available.[8,10,11,12] The median survival figures reported from different studies will be influenced by the percentage of "poor risk" patients initially entered into the particular study. Patients who are alive two years following the diagnosis of chronic myelogenous leukemia, and who have been treated during that period with busulfan, are estimated to have a mean annual mortality rate during the second to fifth year which is approximately two-thirds that of patients who received either no treatment, conventional x-ray or ^{32}P-irradiation, or chemotherapy with minimally active drugs.[13]

Compatibility Table
Marezine (Cyclizine Lactate) Injection

A clear solution with:	Is not compatible with:
Can be mixed with)	(requires separate injection)
... sulfate	Oxytetracycline hydrochloride
... idine hydrochloride (Demerol)	Chlortetracycline hydrochloride
... ine sulfate	Penicillin
... cline hydrochloride	Any solution with pH of 6.8
... mycin sulfate	or higher (this includes
... ine hydrochloride*	Pentothal sodium and other
... phosphate and sulfate	soluble barbiturates)
... drone HCl (Nisentil)	
... mine hydrobromide*	
... on (Hydrochlorides of	
... alkaloids)*	
... morphone (Dilaudid)*	

*Administer within 4–10 minutes

Busulfan is clearly less effective in patients with chronic myelogenous leukemia who lack the Philadelphia (Ph[1]) chromosome.[14] Also, the so-called "juvenile" type of chronic myelogenous leukemia, typically occurring in young children and associated with the absence of a Philadelphia chromosome, responds poorly to busulfan.[15] The drug is of no benefit in patients whose chronic myelogenous leukemia has entered a "blastic" phase.

Contraindications: Myleran® (busulfan) should not be used unless a diagnosis of chronic myelogenous leukemia has been adequately established and the responsible physician is knowledgeable in assessing response to chemotherapy.

Myleran should not be used in patients whose chronic myelogenous leukemia has demonstrated prior resistance to this drug.

Myleran is of no value in chronic lymphocytic leukemia, acute leukemia, or in the "blastic crisis" of chronic myelogenous leukemia.

Warnings: The most frequent, serious side effect of treatment with busulfan is the induction of bone marrow failure (which may or may not be anatomically hypoplastic) resulting in severe pancytopenia. The pancytopenia caused by busulfan may be more prolonged than that induced with other alkylating agents. It is generally felt that the usual cause of busulfan-induced pancytopenia is the failure to stop administration of the drug soon enough; individual idiosyncrasy to the drug does not seem to be an important factor. *Myleran should be used with extreme caution and exceptional vigilance in patients whose bone marrow reserve may have been compromised by prior irradiation or chemotherapy, or whose marrow function is recovering from previous cytotoxic therapy.* Although recovery from busulfan-induced pancytopenia may take from one month to two years, this complication is potentially reversible and the patient should be vigorously supported through any period of severe pancytopenia.[16]

A rare, important complication of busulfan therapy is the development of bronchopulmonary dysplasia with pulmonary fibrosis.[17] Symptoms have been reported to occur within eight months to ten years after initiation of therapy—the average duration of therapy being four years. The histologic findings associated with "busulfan lung" mimic those seen following pulmonary irradiation. Clinically, patients have reported the insidious onset of cough, dyspnea, and low-grade fever. Pulmonary function studies have revealed diminished diffusion capacity and decreased pulmonary compliance. It is important to exclude more common conditions (such as opportunistic infections or leukemic infiltration of the lungs) with appropriate diagnostic techniques. If measures such as sputum cultures, virologic studies, and exfoliative cytology fail to establish an etiology for the pulmonary infiltrates, lung biopsy may be necessary to establish the diagnosis. Treatment of established busulfan-induced pulmonary fibrosis is unsatisfactory; in most cases the patients have died within six months after the diagnosis was established. There is no specific therapy for this complication other than the immediate discontinuation of busulfan. The administration of corticosteroids has been suggested, but the results have not been impressive or uniformly successful.

Busulfan may cause cellular dysplasia in many organs in addition to the lung. Cytologic abnormalities characterized by giant, hyperchromatic nuclei have been reported in lymph nodes, pancreas, thyroid, adrenal glands, liver, and bone marrow. This cytologic dysplasia may be severe enough to cause difficulty in interpretation of exfoliative cytologic examinations from the lung, bladder, breast, and the uterine cervix.

In addition to the widespread epithelial dysplasia that has been observed during busulfan therapy, chromosome aberrations have been reported in cells from patients receiving busulfan.

Busulfan is mutagenic in mice and, possibly, in man.

A number of malignant tumors have been reported in patients on busulfan therapy and this drug may be a human carcinogen. Four cases of acute leukemia occurred among 243 patients treated with busulfan as adjuvant chemotherapy following surgical resection of bronchogenic carcinoma. All four cases were from a subgroup of 19 of these 243 patients who developed pancytopenia while taking busulfan five to eight years before leukemia became clinically apparent. These findings suggest that busulfan is leukemogenic, although its mode of action is uncertain.[18]

Busulfan may cause fetal harm when administered to a pregnant woman. Although there have been a number of cases reported where apparently normal children have been born after busulfan treatment during pregnancy,[19] one case has been cited where a malformed baby was delivered by a mother treated with busulfan. During the pregnancy that resulted in the malformed infant, the mother received x-ray therapy early in the first trimester, mercaptopurine until the third month, then busulfan until delivery.[20] In pregnant rats, busulfan produces sterility in both male and female offspring due to the absence of germinal cells in testes and ovaries.[21] Germinal cell aplasia or sterility in offspring of mothers receiving busulfan during pregnancy has not been reported in humans. If this drug is used during pregnancy or if the patient becomes pregnant while taking this drug, the patient should be apprised of the potential hazard to the fetus.

Ovarian suppression and amenorrhea with menopausal symptoms commonly occur during busulfan therapy in premenopausal patients. Busulfan interferes with spermatogenesis in experimental animals, and there have been clinical reports of sterility, azoospermia and testicular atrophy in male patients.

Precautions: General: The most consistent, dose-related toxicity is bone marrow suppression. This may be manifest by anemia, leukopenia, thrombocytopenia, or any combination of these. It is imperative that patients be instructed to report promptly the development of fever, sore throat, signs of local infection, bleeding from any site, or symptoms suggestive of anemia. Any one of these findings may indicate busulfan toxicity; however, they may also indicate transformation of the disease to an acute "blastic" form. Since busulfan may have a delayed effect, it is important to withdraw the medication temporarily at the first sign of an abnormally large or exceptionally rapid fall in any of the formed elements of the blood. *Patients should never be allowed to take the drug without close medical supervision.*

Laboratory Tests: It is recommended that evaluation of the hemoglobin or hematocrit, total white blood cell count and differential count, and quantitative platelet count be obtained weekly while the patient is on busulfan therapy. In cases where the cause of fluctuation in the formed elements of the peripheral blood is obscure, bone marrow examination may be useful for evaluation of marrow status. A decision to increase, decrease, continue, or discontinue a given dose of busulfan must be based not only on the absolute hematologic values, but also on the rapidity with which changes are occurring. The dosage of busulfan may need to be reduced if this agent is combined with other drugs whose primary toxicity is myelosuppression. Occasional patients may be unusually sensitive to busulfan administered at standard dosage and suffer neutropenia or thrombocytopenia after a relatively short exposure to the drug. Busulfan should not be used where facilities for complete blood counts, including quantitative platelet counts, are not available at weekly (or more frequent) intervals.

Carcinogenesis, Mutagenesis, Impairment of Fertility: See "WARNINGS" section.

Pregnancy: ***Teratogenic effects:*** Pregnancy Category D. See "WARNINGS" section.

Non-Teratogenic effects: There have been reports in the literature of small infants being born after the mothers received busulfan during pregnancy, in particular, during the third trimester.[22] One case was reported where an infant had mild anemia and neutropenia at birth after busulfan was administered to the mother from the eighth week of pregnancy to term.[19]

Nursing Mothers: It is not known whether this drug is excreted in human milk. Because of the potential for tumorigenicity shown for Myleran (busulfan) in animal and human studies, a decision should be made whether to discontinue nursing or to discontinue the drug, taking into account the importance of the drug to the mother.

Adverse Reactions:

Hematological Effects: The most frequent, serious, toxic effect of busulfan is myelosuppression resulting in leukopenia, thrombocytopenia, and anemia. Myelosuppression is most frequently the result of a failure to discontinue dosage in the face of an undetected decrease in leukocyte or platelet counts.[16]

Pulmonary: Interstitial pulmonary fibrosis has been reported rarely, but it is a clinically significant adverse effect when observed and calls for immediate discontinuation of further administration of the drug. The role of corticosteroids in arresting or reversing the fibrosis has been reported to be beneficial in some cases and without effect in others.[17]

Cardiac: One case of endocardial fibrosis has been reported in a 79-year-old woman who received a total dose of 7,200 mg of busulfan over a period of nine years for the management of chronic myelogenous leukemia.[23] At autopsy, she was found to have endocardial fibrosis of the left ventricle in addition to interstitial pulmonary fibrosis.

Ocular: Busulfan is capable of inducing cataracts in rats and there have been several reports indicating that this is a rare complication in humans. In the few cases reported in humans, cataracts have occurred only after prolonged administration of busulfan.[24]

Dermatologic: Hyperpigmentation is the most common adverse skin reaction and occurs in 5–10% of patients, particularly those with a dark complexion.

Metabolic: In a few cases, a clinical syndrome closely resembling adrenal insufficiency and characterized by weakness, severe fatigue, anorexia, weight loss, nausea and vomiting, and melanoderma has developed after prolonged busulfan therapy. The symptoms have sometimes been reversible when busulfan was withdrawn. Adrenal responsiveness to exogenously administered ACTH has usually been normal. However, pituitary function testing with metyrapone revealed a blunted urinary 17-hydroxycorticosteroid excretion in two patients.[25] Following the discontinuation of busulfan (which was associated with clinical improvement), rechallenge with metyrapone revealed normal pituitary-adrenal function.

Hyperuricemia and/or hyperuricosuria are not uncommon in patients with chronic myelogenous leukemia. Additional rapid destruction of granulocytes may accompany the initiation of chemotherapy and increase the urate pool. Adverse effects can be minimized by increased hydration, urine alkalinization, and the prophylactic administration of a xanthine oxidase inhibitor such as Zyloprim® (allopurinol).

Miscellaneous: Other reported adverse reactions include: urticaria, erythema multiforme, erythema nodosum, alopecia, porphyria cutanea tarda, excessive dryness and fragility of the skin with anhidrosis, dryness of the oral mucous membranes and cheilosis, gynecomastia, cholestatic jaundice, and myasthenia gravis. Most of these are single case reports, and in many a clear cause and effect relationship with busulfan has not been demonstrated.

Overdosage: There is no known antidote to busulfan. The principal toxic effect is on the bone marrow. Survival after a single 140 mg dose has been reported in an 18 kg, 4 year old child,[26] but hematologic toxicity is likely to be more profound with chronic overdosage. The hematologic status should be closely monitored and vigorous supportive measures instituted if necessary.

Dosage and Administration: Busulfan is administered orally. The usual adult dose for *remis-*

Continued on next page

Burroughs Wellcome—Cont.

sion induction is four to eight mg total dose, daily. Dosing on a weight basis (mg/kg) is the same for both children and adults, approximately 60 μg per kg of body weight or 1.8 mg per square meter of body surface, daily. Since the rate of fall of the leukocyte count is dose related, daily doses exceeding four mg per day should be reserved for patients with the most compelling symptoms; the greater the total daily dose, the greater is the possibility of inducing bone marrow aplasia.

A decrease in the leukocyte count is not usually seen during the first ten to fifteen days of treatment; the leukocyte count may actually increase during this period and it should not be interpreted as resistance to the drug, nor should the dose be increased.[27] Since the leukocyte count may continue to fall for more than one month after discontinuing the drug, it is important that busulfan be discontinued *prior* to the total leukocyte count falling into the normal range. When the total leukocyte count has declined to approximately 15,000/μl the drug should be withheld.

With a constant dose of busulfan, the total leukocyte count declines exponentially; a weekly plot of the leukocyte count on semilogarithmic graph paper aids in predicting the time when therapy should be discontinued.[28] With the recommended dose of busulfan, a normal leukocyte count is usually achieved in twelve to twenty weeks.

During remission, the patient is examined at monthly intervals and treatment resumed with the induction dosage when the total leukocyte count reaches approximately 50,000/μl. When remission is shorter than three months, maintenance therapy of 1 to 3 mg daily may be advisable in order to keep the hematological status under control and prevent rapid relapse.

How Supplied: White, scored tablets containing 2 mg busulfan, imprinted with "WELLCOME" and "K2A" on each tablet; in bottle of 25.

References:
1. Haddow, A., and Timmis, G.M.: Myleran in Chronic Myeloid Leukaemia; Chemical Constitution and Biological Action. Lancet *1*: 207–208, 1953.
2. Galton, D.A.G.: Myleran in Chronic Myeloid Leukaemia, Lancet *1*: 208–213, 1953.
3. Nadkarni, M.V., Trams, E.G., and Smith, P.K.: Preliminary Studies on the Distribution and Fate of TEM, TEPA, and Myleran in the Human. Cancer Res. *19*: 713–718, 1959.
4. Vodopick, H., Hamilton, H.E., Jackson, H.L., Peng, C.T., and Sheets, R.F.: Metabolic Fate of Tritiated Busulfan in Man. J. Lab. & Clin. Med. *73*: 266–276, 1969.
5. Fox, B.W.: Mechanism of Action of Methanesulfonates. In, *Antineoplastic and Immunosuppressive Agents,* Part II. (Edited by A.C. Sartorelli and D.G. Johns) Berlin, Springer-Verlag, 35–46, 1975.
6. Roberts, J.J., and Warwick, G.P.: The Mode of Action of Alkylating Agents—III. The Formation of 3-hydroxytetrahydrothiophene-1:1-dioxide from 1:4-dimethanesulphonyloxybutane (Myleran), S-β-L-alanyltetrahydrothiophenium mesylate, tetrahydrothiophene and tetrahydrothiophene-1:1-dioxide in the Rat, Rabbit and Mouse. Biochem. Pharmacol. *6*: 217–227, 1961.
7. Peng, C.T.: Distribution and Metabolic Fate of S-35 Labeled Myleran (Busulfan) in Normal and Tumor Bearing Rats. J. Pharmac. Exp. Therap. *120*: 229–238, 1957.
8. Medical Research Council's Working Party for Therapeutic Trials in Leukemia: Chronic Granulocytic Leukaemia: Comparison of Radiotherapy and Busulphan Therapy, Brit. Med. J. *1*: 201–208, 1968.
9. Minot, G.R., Buckman, T.E., and Isaacs, R.: Chronic Myelogenous Leukemia: Age Incidence, Duration, and Benefit Derived From Irradiation, JAMA *82*: 1489–1494, 1924.
10. Haut, A., Abbott, W.S., Wintrobe, M.M., and Cartwright, G.E.: Busulfan in the Treatment of Chronic Myelocytic Leukemia. The Effect of Long Term Intermittent Therapy. Blood *17*: 1–19, 1961.
11. Monfardini, S., Gee, T., Fried J. and Clarkson, B.: Survival in Chronic Myelogenous Leukemia: Influence of Treatment and Extent of Disease at Diagnosis. Cancer *31*: 492–501, 1973.
12. Conrad, F.G.: Survival in Chronic Granulocytic Leukemia. Arch. Intern. Med. *131*: 684–685, 1973.
13. Sokal, J.E.: Evaluation of Survival Data for Chronic Myelocytic Leukemia. Am. J. Hematol. *1*: 493–500, 1976.
14. Ezdinli, E.Z., Sokal, J.E., Crosswhite, L., and Sandberg, A.A.: Philadelphia-Chromosome-Positive and -Negative Chronic Myelocytic Leukemia. Ann. Intern. Med. *72*: 175–182, 1970.
15. Smith, K.L., and Johnson, W.: Classification of Chronic Myelocytic Leukemia in Children. Cancer *34*: 670–679, 1974.
16. Stuart, J.J., Crocker, D.L., and Roberts, H.R.: Treatment of Busulfan-Induced Pancytopenia. Arch. Intern. Med. *136*: 1181–1183, 1976.
17. Sostman, H.D., Matthay, R.A., and Putman, C.E.: Cytotoxic Drug-Induced Lung Disease. Am. J. Med. *62*: 608–615, 1977.
18. Stott, H., Fox, W., Girling, D.J., Stephens, R.J., and Galton, D.A.G.: Acute Leukemia After Busulphan. Brit. Med. J. *2*: 1513–1517, 1977.
19. Dugdale, M. and Fort, A.T.: Busulfan Treatment of Leukemia During Pregnancy. Case Report and Review of the Literature. JAMA *199*: 131–133, 1967.
20. Diamond, I., Anderson, M.M. and McCreadie, S.R.: Transplacental Transmission of Busulfan (Myleran®) in a Mother with Leukemia. Pediatrics *25*: 85–90, 1960.
21. Bollag, W.: Cytostatica in der Schwangershaft, Schweiz. Med. Wochenschr. *84*: 393–395, 1954.
22. Boros, S.J. and Reynolds, J.W.: Intrauterine Growth Retardation Following Third-Trimester-Exposure to Busulfan. Am. J. Obstet. Gynecol. *129*: 111–112, 1977.
23. Weinberger, A., Pinkhas, J., Sandbank, U., Shaklai, M., and Vries, A. de: Endocardial Fibrosis Following Busulfan Treatment. JAMA *231*: 495, 1975.
24. Ravindranathan, M.P., Paul, V.J., and Kuriakose, E.T.: Cataract after Busulphan Treatment. Brit. Med. J. *1*: 218–219, 1972.
25. Vivacqua, R.J., Haurani, F.I., and Erslev, A.J.: "Selective", Pituitary Insufficiency Secondary to Busulfan. Ann. Intern. Med. *67*: 380–387, 1967.
26. Oliveira, H.P. de, Cruz, E., Fonseca, A. de S., and Medeiros, M.: Accidental Ingestion of a Toxic Dose of Myleran by a Child. Acta Haemat. (Basel) *29*: 249–255, 1963.
27. Stryckmans, P.A.: Current Concepts in Chronic Myelogenous Leukemia. Semin. Hematol. *11*: 101–139, 1974.
28. Galton, D.A.G.: Chemotherapy of Chronic Myelocytic Leukaemia. Semin. Hematol. *6*: 323–343, 1969.

Shown in Product Identification Section, page 408

NEOSPORIN® AEROSOL
[nē″ō-spor′ĭn]
(Polymyxin B-Bacitracin-Neomycin Powder)
For Topical Use Only (Not Sterile)

Description: Each aerosol spray packing of 90 g contains: Aerosporin® brand Polymyxin B Sulfate 100,000 units; bacitracin zinc 8,000 units; neomycin sulfate 100 mg (equivalent to 70 mg neomycin base).
Inert propellant: dichlorodifluoromethane and trichloromonofluoromethane.
Approximate spraying time of the container is 100 seconds.
Neosporin® Aerosol (Polymyxin B-Bacitracin-Neomycin Powder) is useful for the treatment of certain bacterial infections of the skin. Infections of the deeper tissues will not be controlled by topical medication, but require more vigorous measures such as surgery, or systemic therapy. The propellant evaporates quickly, leaving only a fine white layer of soluble antibiotic powder. This triple antibiotic powder is adherent even to dry skin, since the extremely small antibiotic particles lodge in crevices and irregularities in the skin. Another advantage of this mode of application is that the concentration of antibiotics at the treated area can be varied simply by spraying the same area repeatedly. In addition, the cool, nonirritating spray is especially suited to treating tender, sensitive lesions with the least patient discomfort. Substantial time and effort are saved through such aerosol treatment as compared to applying other forms of topical medication.

Action: The combination of Aerosporin brand Polymyxin B Sulfate with neomycin and bacitracin was selected because it most nearly meets the criteria for an ideal topical antibacterial preparation. The spectrum of action encompasses most pathogenic bacteria found topically, and the three antibiotics are bactericidal rather than bacteriostatic. When used topically, polymyxin B, neomycin and bacitracin are rarely irritating, and absorption from skin or mucous membrane is insignificant. The index of allergenicity of this combination has been shown over the years to be low. And finally, since these antibiotics are seldom used systemically, the patient is spared sensitization to those antibiotics which might later be required systemically.

Polymyxin B is one of a group of closely related substances produced by various strains of *Bacillus polymyxa*. Its activity is sharply restricted to gram-negative bacteria, including many strains of *Pseudomonas aeruginosa*.

Neomycin, isolated from *Streptomyces fradiae*, has antibacterial activity *in vitro* against a wide range of gram-negative and gram-positive organisms, with effectiveness against many strains of *Proteus*. Bacitracin, an antibiotic substance derived from cultures of *Bacillus subtilis* (Tracy), exerts antibacterial action *in vitro* against a variety of gram-positive and a few gram-negative organisms.

Indications: Based on a review of this drug by the National Academy of Sciences-National Research Council and/or other information, FDA has classified the indications as follows:

"Possibly" effective: For topical administration for the treatment of the listed localized infections or for suppressive therapy in such conditions:

Biopsy sites	Abrasions
Vascular ulcers	Cuts
Decubitus ulcers	Lacerations
Burns	Infected eczemas
Dermabrasion	Infected dermatoses
	Skin grafts and donor sites

Final classification of the less-than-effective indications requires further investigation.

Contraindications: This product is contraindicated in those individuals who have shown hypersensitivity to any of its components.

Warning: Because of the potential hazard of nephrotoxicity and ototoxicity due to neomycin, care should be exercised when using this product in treating extensive burns, trophic ulceration and other extensive conditions where absorption of neomycin is possible. In burns where more than 20 percent of the body surface is affected, especially if the patient has impaired renal function or is receiving other aminoglycoside antibiotics concurrently, not more than one application a day is recommended.

When using neomycin-containing products to control secondary infection in the chronic dermatoses, such as chronic otitis externa or stasis dermatitis, it should be borne in mind that the skin in these conditions is more liable than is normal skin to become sensitized to many substances, including neomycin. The manifestation of sensitization to neomycin is usually a low grade reddening with swelling, dry scaling and itching; it may be manifest simply as failure to heal. During long-term use of neomycin-containing products, periodic examination for such signs is advisable and the patient should be told to discontinue the product if they are observed. These symptoms regress quickly on withdrawing the medication. Neomycin-containing applications should be avoided for that patient thereafter.

Precautions: As with other antibiotic preparations, prolonged use may result in overgrowth of nonsusceptible organisms including fungi. Appropriate measures should be taken if this occurs. Do not spray in the eyes. Contents are under pressure, but are not flammable. Do not puncture or incinerate container.

Adverse Reactions: Neomycin is a not uncommon cutaneous sensitizer. Articles in the current literature indicate an increase in the prevalence of persons allergic to neomycin. Ototoxicity and nephrotoxicity have been reported (see Warning section).

Dosage and Administration: SHAKE WELL before each spraying. Remove cap, twist off tamper-proof seal and press button to spray affected area. Container will operate in either upright or inverted position. Use one-second intermittent sprays from a distance of about 8 inches. Prolonged spraying is unnecessary and wastes medication.

How Supplied: Aerosol spray can of 90 g.

NEOSPORIN®-G CREAM ℞
[nē″ō-spor′in]
(Polymyxin B-Neomycin-Gramicidin)

Description: Each gram contains:
Aerosporin® (Polymyxin B Sulfate) 10,000 units; neomycin sulfate 5 mg (equivalent to 3.5 mg neomycin base); gramicidin 0.25 mg.
Inactive ingredients: liquid petrolatum, white petrolatum, purified water, propylene glycol, polyoxyethylene polyoxypropylene compound, emulsifying wax, and 0.25% methylparaben as preservative.

The base is a smooth vanishing cream with a pH of approximately 5.0. The acid pH helps restore normal cutaneous acidity. The cream is cosmetically acceptable and may be easily removed with water. Owing to its excellent spreading and penetrating properties, the cream facilitates treatment of hairy and intertriginous areas. It may also be of value in selective cases where the lesions are moist. The antibiotics diffuse readily from the base into fluids of the skin or tissues.

Action: Wide range antibacterial action, approaching the ideal, is provided by the overlapping spectra of polymyxin B, neomycin, and gramicidin. The range of action of this combination includes virtually all pathogenic bacteria found topically, and the three antibacterials are bactericidal, rather than bacteriostatic. The index of allergenicity of this combination has been shown over the years to be low and the rarity of topical irritation has been well demonstrated.

Polymyxin B is one of a group of closely related substances produced by various strains of *Bacillus polymyxa*. Its activity is sharply restricted to gram-negative bacteria, including many strains of *Pseudomonas aeruginosa*.

Neomycin, isolated from *Streptomyces fradiae*, has antibacterial activity *in vitro* against a wide range of gram-negative and gram-positive organisms, with effectiveness against many strains of *Proteus*. Gramicidin has particular action *in vitro* against certain gram-positive bacteria.

Indications: Based on a review of this drug by the National Academy of Sciences—National Research Council and/or other information, FDA has classified the indications as follows:

"Possibly" effective: For topical administration for the treatment of the listed localized infections or for suppressive therapy in such conditions: primary pyodermas (impetigo, ecthyma, sycosis vulgaris, paronychia); secondary infected dermatoses (eczema, herpes and seborrheic dermatitis); traumatic lesions (inflamed or suppurating as a result of bacterial infection).

Final classification of the less-than-effective indications requires further investigation.

Contraindications: Not for use in the eyes or in the external ear canal if the eardrum is perforated. This product is contraindicated in those individuals who have shown hypersensitivity to any of its components.

Warning: Because of the potential hazard of nephrotoxicity and ototoxicity due to neomycin, care should be exercised when using this product in treating extensive burns, trophic ulceration and other extensive conditions where absorption of neomycin is possible. In burns where more than 20 percent of the body surface is affected, especially if the patient has impaired renal function or is receiving other aminoglycoside antibiotics concurrently, not more than one application a day is recommended.

When using neomycin-containing products to control secondary infection in the chronic dermatoses, such as chronic otitis externa or stasis dermatitis, it should be borne in mind that the skin in these conditions is more liable than is normal skin to become sensitized to many substances, including neomycin. The manifestation of sensitization to neomycin is usually a low grade reddening with swelling, dry scaling and itching; it may be manifest simply as a failure to heal. During long-term use of neomycin-containing products, periodic examination for such signs is advisable and the patient should be told to discontinue the product if they are observed. These symptoms regress quickly on withdrawing the medication. Neomycin-containing applications should be avoided for that patient thereafter.

Precautions: As with other antibacterial preparations, prolonged use may result in overgrowth of nonsusceptible organisms, including fungi. Appropriate measures should be taken if this occurs.

Adverse Reactions: Neomycin is a not uncommon cutaneous sensitizer. Articles in the current literature indicate an increase in the prevalence of persons allergic to neomycin. Ototoxicity and nephrotoxicity have been reported (see Warning section).

Dosage and Administration: A small quantity of the cream should be applied 2 to 5 times daily, as required. The cream should, if conditions permit, be gently rubbed into the affected areas.

How Supplied: Tube of 15 g.
15 g—DoD & VA   NSN 6505-00-926-2159

NEOSPORIN® G.U. IRRIGANT ℞
[ne″o-spor′in]
**STERILE
(Neomycin Sulfate-Polymyxin B Sulfate Solution For Irrigation)
NOT FOR INJECTION**

Description: Neosporin G.U. Irrigant is a concentrated sterile antibiotic solution to be diluted for urinary bladder irrigation. Each ml contains neomycin sulfate equivalent to 40 mg neomycin base, 200,000 units polymyxin B sulfate and water for injection. The 20-ml multiple-dose vial contains, in addition to the above, 1 mg methylparaben (0.1%) added as a preservative.

Neomycin sulfate, an antibiotic of the aminoglycoside group, is the sulfate salt of neomycin B and C produced by *Streptomyces fradiae*. It has a potency equivalent to not less than 600 μg of neomycin per mg. The structural formulae are:
(See preceding column)

Polymyxin B sulfate, a polypeptide antibiotic, is the sulfate salt of polymyxin B_1 and B_2 produced by the growth of *Bacillus polymyxa*. It has a potency of not less than 6,000 polymyxin B units per mg. The structural formulae are:

Polymyxin B Sulfate

Polymyxin B_1 (R = CH_3)
Polymyxin B_2 (R = H)

Clinical Pharmacology: After prophylactic irrigation of the intact urinary bladder, neomycin and polymyxin are absorbed in clinically insignificant quantities. A neomycin serum level of 0.1 μg/ml was observed in three of 33 patients receiving the rinse solution. This level is well below that which has been associated with neomycin-induced toxicity.

When used topically, polymyxin B sulfate and neomycin are rarely irritating.

Microbiology: The prepared Neosporin G.U. Irrigant Sterile solution is bactericidal. The aminoglycosides act in inhibiting normal protein synthesis in susceptible microorganisms. Polymyxins increase the permeability of bacterial cell wall membranes. The solution is active *in vitro* against

Escherichia coli
Staphylococcus aureus
Haemophilus influenzae
Klebsiella and *Enterobacter* species
Neisseria species, and
Pseudomonas aeruginosa

It is not active *in vitro* against *Serratia marcescens* and streptococci.
Bacterial resistance may develop following the use of the antibiotics in the catheter-rinse solution.

Indications and Usage: Neosporin G.U. Irrigant is indicated for short-term use (up to 10 days) as a continuous irrigant or rinse in the urinary bladder of abacteriuric patients to help prevent bacteriuria and gram-negative rod septicemia associated with the use of indwelling catheters.

Since organisms gain entrance to the bladder by way of, and around the catheter, significant bacteriuria is induced by bacterial multiplication in the bladder urine, in the mucoid film often present between catheter and urethra, and in other sites. Urinary tract infection may result from the repeated presence in the urine of large numbers of pathogenic bacteria. The use of closed systems with indwelling catheters has been shown to reduce the risk of infection. A three-way closed catheter system with constant neomycin-polymyxin B bladder rinse is indicated to prevent the development of infection while using indwelling catheters. If uropathogens are isolated, they should be identified and tested for susceptibility so that appropriate antimicrobial therapy for systemic use can be initiated.

Contraindications: Hypersensitivity to neomycin, the polymyxins, or any ingredient in the solution is a contraindication to its use. A history of hypersensitivity or serious toxic reaction to an aminoglycoside may also contraindicate the use of any other aminoglycoside because of the known cross-sensitivity of patients to drugs of this class.

Warnings: PROPHYLACTIC BLADDER CARE WITH NEOSPORIN G.U. IRRIGANT STERILE SHOULD NOT BE GIVEN WHERE THERE IS A POSSIBILITY OF SYSTEMIC ABSORPTION.

Continued on next page

Burroughs Wellcome—Cont.

NEOSPORIN G.U. IRRIGANT STERILE SHOULD NOT BE USED FOR IRRIGATION OTHER THAN FOR THE URINARY BLADDER. Systemic absorption after topical application of neomycin to open wounds, burns, and granulating surfaces is significant and serum concentrations comparable to and often higher than those attained following oral and parenteral therapy have been reported. Absorption of neomycin from the denuded bladder surface has been reported.

However, the likelihood of toxicity following topical irrigation of the intact urinary bladder with Neosporin G.U. Irrigant Sterile is low since no appreciable amounts of these antibiotics enter the systemic circulation by this route if irrigation does not exceed ten days.

Neosporin G.U. Irrigant is intended for continuous prophylactic irrigation of the lumen of the intact urinary bladder of patients with indwelling catheters. Patients should be under constant supervision by a physician. Irrigation should be avoided in patients with defects in the bladder mucosa or bladder wall, such as vesical rupture, or in association with operative procedures on the bladder wall, because of the risk of toxicity due to systemic absorption following diffusion into absorptive tissues and spaces. When absorbed, neomycin and polymyxin B are nephrotoxic antibiotics, and the nephrotoxic potentials are additive. In addition, both antibiotics, when absorbed, are neurotoxins: neomycin can destroy fibers of the acoustic nerve causing permanent bilateral deafness; neomycin and polymyxin B are additive in their neuromuscular blocking effects, not only in terms of potency and duration but also in terms of characteristics of the blocks produced.

Aminoglycosides, when absorbed, can cause fetal harm when administered to a pregnant woman. Aminoglycoside antibiotics cross the placenta and there have been reports of total, irreversible, bilateral, congenital deafness in children whose mothers received streptomycin during pregnancy. Although serious side effects have not been reported in the treatment of pregnant women with other aminoglycosides, the potential for harm exists. If Neosporin G.U. Irrigant Sterile is used during pregnancy, the patient should be apprised of the potential hazard to the fetus (See PRECAUTIONS).

Precautions:
General: Ototoxicity, nephrotoxicity, and neuromuscular blockade may occur if Neosporin G.U. Irrigant ingredients are systemically absorbed (See WARNINGS). Absorption of neomycin from the denuded bladder surface has been reported. Patients with impaired renal function, infants, dehydrated patients, elderly patients, and patients receiving high doses of prolonged treatment are especially at risk for the development of toxicity. Irrigation of the bladder with Neosporin G.U. Irrigant may result in overgrowth of nonsusceptible organisms, including fungi. Appropriate measures should be taken if this occurs. The safety and effectiveness of the preparation for use in the care of patients with recent lower urinary tract surgery have not been established. Urine specimens should be collected during prophylactic bladder care for urinalysis, culture, and susceptibility testing. Positive cultures suggest the presence of organisms which are resistant to the bladder rinse antibiotics.

Pregnancy: Teratogenic Effects: Pregnancy Category D. (See WARNINGS section).

Adverse Reactions: Neomycin occasionally causes skin sensitization when applied topically; however, topical application to mucus membranes rarely results in local or systemic hypersensitivity reactions.

Irritation of the urinary bladder mucosa has been reported.

Signs of ototoxicity and nephrotoxicity have been reported following parenteral use of these drugs and following the oral and topical use of neomycin (See WARNINGS).

Dosage and Administration: This preparation is specifically designed for use with "three-way" catheters or with other catheter systems permitting continuous irrigation of the urinary bladder. The usual irrigation dose is one 1-ml ampul a day for up to ten days.

Using strict aseptic techniques, the contents of one 1-ml ampul of Neosporin G.U. Irrigant Sterile (Neomycin Sulfate-Polymyxin B Sulfate Solution for Irrigation) should be added to a 1,000-ml container of isotonic saline solution. This container should then be connected to the inflow lumen of the "three-way" catheter which has been inserted with full aseptic precautions; use of a sterile lubricant is recommended during insertion of the catheter. The outflow lumen should be connected, via a sterile disposable plastic tube, to a disposable plastic collection bag. Stringent procedures, such as taping the inflow and outflow junction at the catheter, should be observed when necessary to insure the junctional integrity of the system.

For most patients, the inflow rate of the 1,000-ml saline solution of neomycin and polymyxin B should be adjusted to a slow drip to deliver about 1,000 ml every twenty-four hours. If the patient's urine output exceeds 2 liters per day, it is recommended that the inflow rate should be adjusted to deliver 2,000 ml of the solution in a twenty-four hour period.

It is important that the rinse of the bladder be continuous; the inflow or rinse solution should not be interrupted for more than a few minutes.
Preparation of the irrigation solution should be performed with strict aseptic techniques. The prepared solution should be stored at 4°C, and should be used within 48 hours following preparation to reduce the risk of contamination with resistant microorganisms.

How Supplied: 1-ml ampuls, boxes of 12 (NDC-0081-0748-15) and 100 ampuls (NDC-0081-0748-55); 20-ml multi-dose vial (NDC-0081-0748-93).
Store at 2° to 8°C (36° to 46°F).

NEOSPORIN®
[nē″ō-spor′ĭn]
OINTMENT
(Polymyxin B-Bacitracin-Neomycin)

Description: Each gram contains:
Aerosporin® (Polymyxin B Sulfate) 5,000 units; bacitracin zinc 400 units; neomycin sulfate 5 mg (equivalent to 3.5 mg neomycin base); special white petrolatum qs.

Action: The overlapping spectra of the antibiotics provide effective antibacterial action against most commonly occurring bacteria known to be topical invaders. The range of antibacterial activity encompasses many bacteria which are, or have become, resistant to other antibiotics or chemicals—notably *Pseudomonas* and *Staphylococcus*. In susceptible organisms, resistance rarely develops, even on repeated or prolonged use.

Indications: *Therapeutically*, (as an adjunct to systemic therapy when indicated), for topical infections, primary or secondary, due to susceptible organisms, as in: infected burns, skin grafts, surgical incisions, otitis externa; primary pyodermas (impetigo, ecthyma, sycosis vulgaris, paronychia); secondarily infected dermatoses (eczema, herpes, and seborrheic dermatitis); traumatic lesions, inflamed or suppurating as a result of bacterial infection.

Prophylactically, the ointment may be used to prevent bacterial contamination in burns, skin grafts, incisions, and other clean lesions. For abrasions, minor cuts and wounds accidentally incurred, its use may prevent the development of infection and permit wound healing.

Contraindications: Not for use in the eyes or external ear canal if the eardrum is perforated. This product is contraindicated in those individuals who have shown hypersensitivity to any of its components.

Warning: Because of the potential hazard of nephrotoxicity and ototoxicity due to neomycin, care should be exercised when using this product in treating extensive burns, trophic ulceration and other extensive conditions where absorption of neomycin is possible. In burns where more than 20 percent of the body surface is affected, especially if the patient has impaired renal function or is receiving other aminoglycoside antibiotics concurrently, not more than one application a day is recommended.

When using neomycin-containing products to control secondary infection in the chronic dermatoses, such as chronic otitis externa or stasis dermatitis, it should be borne in mind that the skin in these conditions is more liable than is normal skin to become sensitized to many substances, including neomycin. The manifestation of sensitization to neomycin is usually a low grade reddening with swelling, dry scaling and itching; it may be manifest simply as a failure to heal. During long term use of neomycin-containing products, periodic examination for such signs is advisable and the patient should be told to discontinue the product if they are observed. These symptoms regress quickly on withdrawing the medication. Neomycin-containing applications should be avoided for that patient thereafter.

Precautions: As with other antibacterial products, prolonged use may result in overgrowth of nonsusceptible organisms, including fungi. Appropriate measures should be taken if this occurs.

Adverse Reactions: Neomycin is a not uncommon cutaneous sensitizer. Articles in the current literature indicate an increase in the prevalence of persons allergic to neomycin. Ototoxicity and nephrotoxicity have been reported (see Warning section).

Dosage and Administration: Apply a small quantity to the affected area 2 to 5 times daily, depending on the severity of the condition. May be left exposed or covered with a dressing, as indicated.

How Supplied: Tubes of 1 oz and ½ oz and foil packet of 1/32 oz (approx.) in box of 144 for topical use only.
1oz DoD NSN 6505-00-254-8361

NEOSPORIN® ℞
[nē″ō-spor′ĭn]
OPHTHALMIC OINTMENT Sterile
(Polymyxin B Sulfate-Bacitracin Zinc-Neomycin Sulfate)

Description: Neosporin Ophthalmic Ointment (polymyxin B sulfate-bacitracin zinc-neomycin sulfate) is a sterile antimicrobial ointment for ophthalmic use. Each gram contains: Aerosporin® (polymyxin B sulfate) 10,000 units, bacitracin zinc 400 units, neomycin sulfate equivalent to 3.5 mg neomycin base and special white petrolatum, qs. Polymyxin B sulfate is the sulfate salt of polymyxin B_1 and B_2 which are produced by the growth of *Bacillus polymyxa* (Prazmowski) Migula (Fam. Bacillaceae). It has a potency of not less than 6,000 polymyxin B units per mg, calculated on an anhydrous basis. The structural formulae are:

Polymyxin B Sulfate

$$RCH_2CH(CH_2)_4CO-Dab-Thr-Dab-Dab\begin{array}{c}\gamma-NH_2\\|\\Dab-D-Phe-Leu\\|\\\gamma-NH_2\ \gamma-NH_2\ \ -Thr-Dab-Dab\\|\\\gamma-NH_2\ \gamma-NH_2\end{array}\cdot xH_2SO_4$$

Polymyxin B_1 (R = CH_3)
Polymyxin B_2 (R = H)

Bacitracin zinc is the zinc salt of bacitracin, a mixture of related cyclic polypeptides (mainly bacitracin A) produced by the growth of an organism of the *licheniformis* group of *Bacillus subtilis* (Fam. Bacillacea). It has a potency of not less than 40 bacitracin units per mg. The precise formula is not known.

Neomycin sulfate is the sulfate salt of neomycin B and C, which are produced by the growth of *Streptomyces fradiae* Waksman (Fam. Streptomycetaceae). It has a potency equivalent of not less than 600 µg of neomycin standard per mg, calculated on an anhydrous basis. The structural formulae are:

Neomycin Sulfate

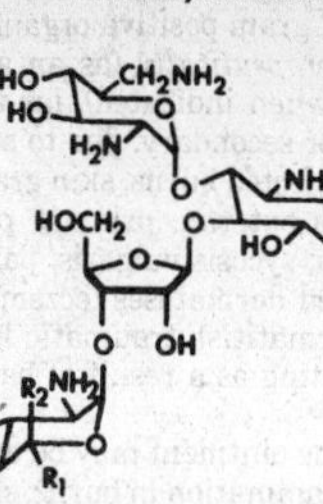

Neomycin B (R₁= H, R₂= CH₂NH₂)
Neomycin C (R₁= CH₂NH₂, R₂= H)

Clinical Pharmacology: A wide range of antibacterial action is provided by the overlapping spectra of polymyxin B sulfate, bacitracin and neomycin. The spectrum of action encompasses most bacterial pathogens capable of causing external infections of the eye and its adnexa.

Polymyxin B is a bactericidal for a variety of gram negative organisms. It increases the permeability of the bacterial cell membrane by interacting with the phospholipid components of the membrane.

Bacitracin is bactericidal for a variety of gram-positive and gram-negative organisms. It interferes with bacterial cell wall synthesis by inhibition of the regeneration of phospholipid receptors involved in peptidoglycan synthesis.

Neomycin is bactericidal for many gram-positive and gram-negative organisms. It is an aminoglycoside antibiotic which inhibits protein synthesis by binding with ribosomal RNA and causing misreading of the bacterial genetic code.

When used topically, polymyxin B, bacitracin and neomycin are rarely irritating, and absorption from the intact skin or mucous membrane is insignificant. The incidence of skin sensitization to this combination has been shown to be low on normal skin.[1,2] Since these antibiotics are seldom used systemically, the patient is spared sensitization to those antibiotics which might later be required systemically.

Microbiology: Polymyxin B sulfate, bacitracin zinc and neomycin sulfate together are considered active against the following microorganisms: *Staphylococcus aureus*, streptococci, including *Streptococcus pneumoniae*, *Escherichia coli*, *Haemophilus influenzae*, *Klebsiella-Enterobacter* species, *Neisseria* species and *Pseudomonas aeruginosa*. The product dose not provide adequate coverage against *Serratia marcescens*.

Indications and Usage: Neosporin Ophthalmic Ointment is indicated in the short-term treatment of superficial external ocular infections caused by organisms susceptible to one or more of the antibiotics contained therein.

Contraindications: This product is contraindicated in those persons who have shown hypersensitivity to any of its components.

Warnings: The manifestations of sensitization to neomycin are usually itching, reddening and edema of the conjunctiva and eyelid. It may be manifest simply as a failure to heal. During long-term use of neomycin-containing products, periodic examination for such signs are advisable, and the patient should be told to discontinue the product if they are observed. These symptoms subside quickly on withdrawing the medication. Neomycin-containing applications should be avoided for the patient thereafter.

Precautions:
General: As with other antibiotic preparations, prolonged use may result in overgrowth of nonsusceptible organisms including fungi. Appropriate measures should be taken if this occurs.

Allergic cross-reactions may occur which could prevent the use of any or all of the following antibiotics for the treatment of future infections: kanamycin, paromomycin, streptomycin, and possibly gentamicin.

Information for Patients: If redness, irritation, swelling or pain persists or increases, discontinue use and contact your physician.

Avoid contaminating the applicator tip with material from the eye, fingers or other source. This caution is necessary if the sterility of the ointment is to be preserved.

Adverse Reactions: Neomycin Sulfate may cause cutaneous and conjunctival sensitization. A precise incidence of hypersensity reactions (primarily skin rash) due to topical neomycin is not known.

Dosage and Administration: Apply the ointment every 3 or 4 hours for 7 to 10 days, depending on the severity of the infection.

How Supplied: Tube of ⅛ oz with ophthalmic tip. (NDC 0081-0732-86)
Store at 15°-30°C (59°-86°F).
⅛ oz. × 12—DoD   NSN 6505-01-143-4644

References:
1. Leyden JJ, and Kligman AM. Contact Dermatitis to Neomycin Sulfate, *JAMA 242* (12): 1276-1278, 1979.
2. Prystowsky SD, Allen AM, Smith RW, Nonomura JH, Odom RB, and Akers WA. Allergic Hypersensitivity to Nickle, Neomycin, Ethylenediamine, and Benzocaine. *Arch Dermatol 115:* 959-962, 1979.

NEOSPORIN® OPHTHALMIC SOLUTION Sterile   ℞
[nē′ō-spor′ĭn]
(Polymyxin B Sulfate-Neomycin Sulfate-Gramicidin)

Description: Neosporin Ophthalmic Solution (polymyxin B sulfate-neomycin sulfate-gramicidin) is a sterile antimicrobial solution for ophthalmic use. Each ml contains: Aerosporin® (polymyxin B sulfate) 10,000 units, neomycin sulfate equivalent to 1.75 mg neomycin base and gramicidin 0.025 mg. The vehicle contains alcohol 0.5%, thimerosal 0.001% (added as a preservative) and the inactive ingredients propylene glycol, polyoxyethylene polyoxypropylene compound, sodium chloride and water for injection.

Polymyxin B sulfate is the sulfate salt of polymyxin B₁ and B₂ which are produced by the growth of *Bacillus polymyxa* (Prazmowski) Migula (Fam. Bacillaceae). It has a potency of not less than 6,000 polymyxin B units per mg, calculated on an anhydrous basis. The structural formulae are:

Polymyxin B Sulfate

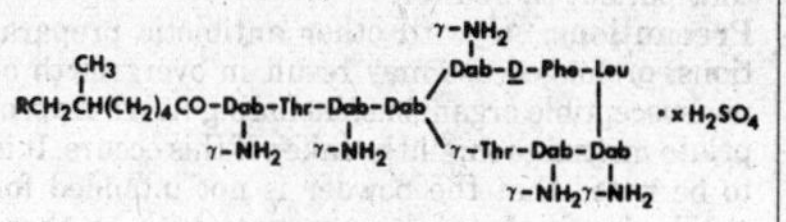

Polymyxin B₁(R = CH₃)
Polymyxin B₂(R = H)

Neomycin sulfate is the sulfate salt of neomycin B and C, which are produced by the growth of *Streptomyces fradiae* Waksman (Fam. Streptomycetaceae). It has a potency equivalent of not less than 600 μg of neomycin standard per mg, calculated on an anhydrous basis. The structural formulae are:

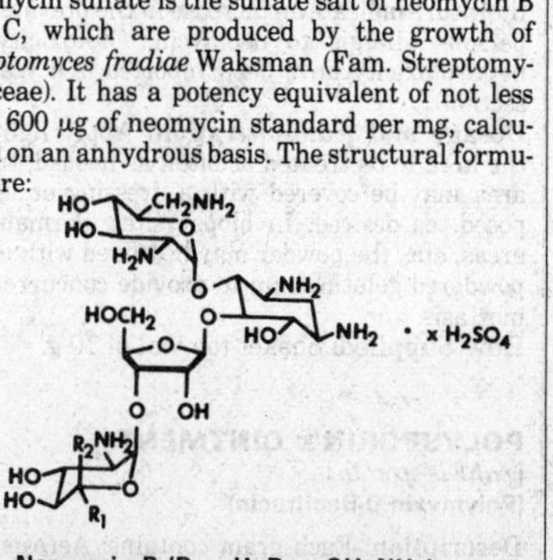

Neomycin B (R₁=H, R₂=CH₂NH₂)
Neomycin C (R₁=CH₂NH₂, R₂=H)

Gramicidin (also called Gramicidin D) is a mixture of three pairs of antibacterial substances (Gramicidin A, B and C) produced by the growth of *Bacillus brevis* Dubos (Fam. Bacillaeae). It has a potency of not less than 900 μg of standard gramicidin per mg. The structural formulae are:

Gramicidin D

O
‖
HC-X-Gly-Ala-D-Leu-Ala-D-Val-Val-D-Val-Trp-D-Leu-Y-D-Leu-Trp-D-Leu-Trp-NHCH₂CH₂OH

	X	Y
Valine - gramicidin A	Val	Trp
Isoleucine - gramicidin A	Ileu	Trp
Valine - gramicidin D	Val	Phe
Isoleucine - gramicidin B	Ileu	Phe
Valine - gramicidin C	Val	Tyr
Isoleucine - gramicidin C	Ileu	Tyr

Clinical Pharmacology: A wide range of antibacterial action is provided by the overlapping spectra of polymyxin B sulfate, neomycin and gramicidin. The spectrum of action encompasses most bacterial pathogens capable of causing external infections of the eye and its adnexa.

Polymyxin B is a bactericidal for a variety of gram-negative organisms. It increases the permeability of the bacterial cell membrane by interacting with the phospholipid components of the membrane.

Neomycin is bactericidal for many gram-positive and gram-negative organisms. It is an aminoglycoside antibiotic which inhibits protein synthesis by binding with ribosomal RNA and causing misreading of the bacterial genetic code.

Gramicidin is bactericidal for a variety of gram-positive organisms. It increases the permeability of the bacterial cell membrane to inorganic cations by forming a network of channels through the normal lipid bilayer of the membrane.

When used typically, polymyxin B, neomycin and gramicidin are rarely irritating, and absorption from the intact skin or mucous membrane is insignificant. The incidence of skin sensitization to this combination has been shown to be low on normal skin.[1,2] Since these antibiotics are seldom used systemically, the patient is spared sensitization to those antibiotics which might later be required systemically.

Microbiology: Polymyxin B sulfate, neomycin sulfate and gramicidin together are considered active against the following microorganisms: *Staphylococcus aureus*, streptococci, including *Streptococcus pneumoniae*, *Escherichia coli*, *Haemophilus influenzae*, *Klebsiella-Enterobacter* species, *Neisseria* species and *Pseudomonas aeruginosa*. The product does not provide adequate coverage against *Serratia marcescens*.

Indications and Usage: Neosporin Ophthalmic Solution is indicated in the short-term treatment of superficial external ocular infections caused by organisms susceptible to one or more of the antibiotics contained therein.

Contraindications: This product is contraindicated in those individuals who have shown hypersensitivity to any of its components.

Warnings: The manifestations of sensitization to neomycin are usually itching, reddening and edema of the conjunctiva and eyelid. It may be manifest simply as a failure to heal. During long-term use of neomycin-containing products, periodic examination for such signs is advisable, and the patient should be told to discontinue the product if they are observed. These symptoms subside quickly on withdrawing the medication. Neomycin-containing applications should be avoided for the patient thereafter.

Precautions:
General: As with other antibiotic preparations, prolonged use may result in overgrowth of nonsusceptible organisms including fungi. Appropriate measures should be taken if this occurs.

Allergic cross-reactions may occur which could prevent the use of any or all of the following antibi-

Continued on next page

Burroughs Wellcome—Cont.

otics for the treatment of future infections: kanamycin, paromomycin, streptomycin, and possibly gentamicin.
Information for Patients: If redness, irritation, swelling or pain persists or increases, discontinue use and contact your physician.
Avoid contaminating the dropper with material from the eye, fingers, or other sources. This caution is necessary if the sterility of the drops is to be preserved.
Adverse Reactions: Neomycin Sulfate may cause cutaneous and conjunctival sensitization. A precise incidence of hypersensitivity reactions (primarily skin rash) due to topical neomycin is not known.
Dosage and Administration: The suggested dosage is one or two drops in the affected eye two to four times daily, or more frequently as required, for 7 to 10 days. In acute infections, initiate therapy with one or two drops every 15 to 30 minutes, reducing the frequency of instillation gradually as the infection is controlled.
How Supplied: Drop Dose® of 10 ml (plastic dispenser bottle). (NDC-0081-0728-69)
Store at 15°-30°C (59°-86°F) and protect from light.
10 ml-DoD & VA   NSN 6505-01-143-4643
References:
1. Leyden JJ, and Kligman AM. Contact Dermatitis to Neomycin Sulfate. JAMA 242(12): 1276-1278, 1979.
2. Prystowsky SD, Allen AM, Smith RW, Nonomura JH, Odom RB and Akers WA, Allergic Contact Hypersensitivity to Nickel, Neomycin, Ethylenediamine, and Benzocaine. Arch Dermatol 115:959-962, 1979.

NEOSPORIN® POWDER ℞
[ne"ō-spor'in pow'dŭr]
(Polymyxin B-Bacitracin-Neomycin)
For Topical Use Only (Not Sterile)

Description: Each gram contains:
Aerosporin® brand Polymyxin B Sulfate 5,000 units; bacitracin zinc 400 units; neomycin sulfate 5 mg (equivalent to 3.5 mg neomycin base); in a special lactose base.
Action: The powder is a combination of polymyxin B sulfate, bacitracin and neomycin sulfate for topical use in mixed infections of the skin and mucous membrane, due to susceptible organisms. It is especially useful where the drying effect of a powder is desirable, as in the treatment of suppurating or serous discharging lesions, infected ulcers, moist or oozing lesions, and intertriginous areas. It may also be used as an insufflation in certain external body cavities.
The combination of Aerosporin brand Polymyxin B Sulfate with neomycin and bacitracin was selected because it most nearly meets the criteria for an ideal topical antibacterial preparation. The spectrum of action encompasses virtually all pathogenic bacteria found topically; and the three antibiotics are bactericidal rather than bacteriostatic. When used topically, polymyxin B sulfate, neomycin and bacitracin are rarely irritating, and absorption from skin or mucous membrane is insignificant. The index of allergenicity of this combination has been shown over the years to be very low. And finally, since these antibiotics are seldom used systemically, the patient is spared sensitization to those antibiotics which might later be required systemically.
Polymyxin B is one of a group of closely related substances produced by various strains of *Bacillus polymyxa*. Its activity is sharply restricted to gram-negative bacteria, including many strains of *Pseudomonas aeruginosa*.
Neomycin, isolated from *Streptomyces fradiae*, has antibacterial activity *in vitro* against a wide range of gram-negative and gram-positive organisms, with effectiveness against many strains of *Proteus*.
Bacitracin, an antibiotic substance derived from cultures of *Bacillus subtilis*(Tracy), exerts antibacterial action *in vitro* against a variety of gram-positive and a few gram-negative organisms.

Indications: Based on a review of this drug by the National Academy of Sciences—National Research Council and/or other information, FDA has classified the indications as follows:
"Possibly" effective: For topical administration for the treatment of the listed localized infections or for suppressive therapy in such conditions:
Prophylactic:
Postoperative and traumatic surface wounds
Biopsy sites
Skin grafts and donor sites
Dermabrasion
Therapeutic (when infected by susceptible organisms):
Vascular ulcers
Decubitus ulcers
Pyodermas
Infected eczemas
Infected dermatoses
Final classification of the less-than-effective indications requires further investigation.

Contraindications: This product is contraindicated in those individuals who have shown hypersensitivity to any of its components.
Warning: Because of the potential hazard of nephrotoxicity and ototoxicity due to neomycin, care should be exercised when using this product in treating extensive burns, trophic ulceration and other extensive conditions where absorption of neomycin is possible. In burns where more than 20 percent of the body surface is affected, especially if the patient has impaired renal function or is receiving other aminoglycoside antibiotics concurrently, not more than one application a day is recommended.
When using neomycin-containing products to control secondary infection in the chronic dermatoses, such as chronic otitis externa or stasis dermatitis, it should be borne in mind that the skin in these conditions is more liable than is normal skin to become sensitized to many substances, including neomycin. The manifestation of sensitization to neomycin is usually a low grade reddening with swelling, dry scaling and itching; it may be manifest simply as a failure to heal. During long term use of neomycin-containing products, periodic examination for such signs is advisable and the patient should be told to discontinue the product if they are observed. These symptoms regress quickly on withdrawing the medication. Neomycin-containing applications should be avoided for that patient thereafter.
Precautions: As with other antibiotic preparations, prolonged use may result in overgrowth of nonsusceptible organisms, including fungi. Appropriate measures should be taken if this occurs. It is to be noted that the powder is not intended for sterile use in surgical procedures such as those involving abdominal or thoracic body cavities.
Adverse Reactions: Neomycin is a not uncommon cutaneous sensitizer. Articles in the current literature indicate an increase in the prevalence of persons allergic to neomycin. Ototoxicity and nephrotoxicity have been reported (see Warning section).
Dosage and Administration: Apply lightly to the area to be treated as often as needed; treated area may be covered with a dressing or left exposed, as desired. In biopsy sites, dermabraded areas, etc., the powder may be mixed with a little powdered gelatin foam to provide concurrent hemostasis.
How Supplied: Shaker-top vial of 10 g.

POLYSPORIN® OINTMENT
[pah" lē-spor'in]
(Polymyxin B-Bacitracin)

Description: Each gram contains: Aerosporin® (Polymyxin B Sulfate) 10,000 units; bacitracin zinc 500 units in a special white petrolatum qs.

Action: Combined antibiotic action against gram-negative and gram-positive organisms.
Indications: *Therapeutically*, (as an adjunct to systemic therapy when indicated), for topical infections, primary or secondary, due to susceptible organisms, as in: infected burns, skin grafts, surgical incisions, otitis externa; primary pyodermas (impetigo, ecthyma, sycosis vulgaris, paronychia); secondarily infected dermatoses (eczema, herpes, and seborrheic dermatitis); traumatic lesions, inflamed or suppurating as a result of bacterial infection.
Prophylactically, the ointment may be used to prevent bacterial contamination in burns, skin grafts, incisions, and other clean lesions. For abrasions, minor cuts and wounds accidentally incurred, its use may prevent the development of infection and permit wound healing.
Contraindication: This product is contraindicated in those individuals who have shown hypersensitivity to any of its components.
Precaution: As with other antibiotic products, prolonged use may result in overgrowth of nonsusceptible organisms including fungi. Appropriate measures should be taken if this occurs.
Dosage and Administration: Apply 2 to 5 times daily, depending on the severity of the infection.
How Supplied: Tubes of ½ oz, 1 oz and 1/32 oz (approx.) foil packet in box of 144.
1 oz-VA   NSN 6505-00-579-9110

POLYSPORIN® OPHTHALMIC
OINTMENT ℞
(Polymyxin B-Bacitracin)
Sterile

Description: Each gram contains:
Aerosporin® (Polymyxin B Sulfate) 10,000 units, bacitracin zinc 500 units, special white petrolatum qs.
Actions: Polymyxin B attacks gram-negative bacilli, including virtually all strains of *Pseudomonas aeruginosa* and *H influenzae* species.
Bacitracin is active against most gram-positive bacilli and cocci, including hemolytic streptococci.
Indications: For the treatment of superficial ocular infections involving the conjunctiva and/or cornea caused by organisms susceptible to polymyxin B sulfate and bacitracin zinc.
Contraindications: This product is contraindicated in those individuals who have shown hypersensitivity to any of its components.
Warnings: Ophthalmic ointments may retard corneal healing.
Precautions: As with other antibiotic preparations, prolonged use may result in overgrowth of nonsusceptible organisms, including fungi. Appropriate measures should be taken if this occurs.
Dosage and Administration: Apply the ointment every 3 or 4 hours, depending on the severity of the infection.
How Supplied: Tube of ⅛ oz with ophthalmic tip.

PROLOPRIM® ℞
[prō'lah-prim"]
(Trimethoprim)
100 mg and 200 mg Scored Tablets

Description: Proloprim® (trimethoprim)* is a synthetic antibacterial, available in scored white tablets, each containing 100 mg trimethoprim and scored yellow tablets, each containing 200 mg trimethoprim. Trimethoprim is 2, 4-diamino-5-(3,4,5,-trimethoxybenzyl) pyrimidine. It is a white to light yellow, odorless, bitter compound with a molecular weight of 290.3.
Clinical Pharmacology: Trimethoprim is rapidly absorbed following oral administration. Mean peak serum levels of approximately 1.0 mcg/ml occur 1 to 4 hours after oral administration of a single 100 mg dose. A single 200 mg dose will result in serum levels approximately twice as high. The half-life of trimethoprim is 8 to 10 hours.
Trimethoprim exists in the blood as free, protein-bound and metabolized forms. Approximately 44% of trimethoprim is protein-bound in the

blood. The free form is considered to be the therapeutically active form. Excretion of trimethoprim is chiefly by the kidneys through glomerular filtration and tubular secretion. Urine concentrations of trimethoprim are considerably higher than are the concentrations in the blood.

Trimethoprim urine levels, after a single oral dose of 100 mg, ranged from 30 to 160 mcg/ml during the 0 to 4 hour period and declined to approximately 18 to 91 mcg/ml during the 8 to 24 hour period. After oral administration, 50% to 60% of trimethoprim is excreted in the urine within 24 hours, approximately 80% of this being unmetabolized trimethoprim.

Microbiology: Proloprim blocks the production of tetrahydrofolic acid from dihydrofolic acid by binding to and reversibly inhibiting the enzyme dihydrofolate reductase. This binding is very much stronger for the bacterial enzyme than for the corresponding mammalian enzyme. Thus, Proloprim selectively interferes with bacterial biosynthesis of nucleic acids and proteins.

In vitro serial dilution tests have shown that the spectrum of antibacterial activity of Proloprim includes the common urinary tract pathogens with the exception of *Pseudomonas aeruginosa*.

REPRESENTATIVE MINIMUM INHIBITORY CONCENTRATIONS FOR TRIMETHOPRIM-SUSCEPTIBLE ORGANISMS

Bacteria	Trimethoprim MIC—mcg/ml (Range)
Escherichia coli	0.05–1.5
Proteus mirabilis	0.5 –1.5
Klebsiella pneumoniae	0.5 –5.0
Enterobacter species	0.5 –5.0
Staphylococcus species, coagulase-negative	0.15–5.0

The recommended quantitative disc susceptibility method[1,2] may be used for estimating the susceptibility of bacteria to Proloprim.

Reports from the laboratory giving results of the standardized test using the 5 mcg trimethoprim disc should be interpreted according to the following criteria:

Organisms producing zones of 16 mm or greater are classified as susceptible whereas those producing zones of 11 to 15 mm are classified as having intermediate susceptibility. A report from the laboratory of "Susceptible" to trimethoprim or "Intermediate" susceptibility to trimethoprim indicates that the infection is likely to respond when, as in uncomplicated urinary tract infections, effective therapy is dependent upon the urine concentration of trimethoprim.

Organisms producing zones of 10 mm or less are reported as resistant, indicating that other therapy should be selected.

Dilution methods for determining susceptibility are also used, and results are reported as the minimum drug concentration inhibiting microbial growth (MIC)[3].

If the MIC is 8 mcg per ml or less, the microorganism is considered "susceptible". If the MIC is 16 mcg per ml or greater the microorganism is considered "resistant".

Normal vaginal and fecal flora are the source of most pathogens causing urinary tract infections. It is therefore relevant to consider the suppressive effect of trimethoprim in these sites.

Concentrations of trimethoprim in vaginal secretions are consistently greater than those found simultaneously in the serum, being typically 1.6 times the concentration of simultaneously obtained serum samples. Sufficient trimethoprim is excreted in the feces to markedly reduce or eliminate trimethoprim susceptible organisms from the fecal flora.

The dominant fecal organisms (non-*Enterobacteriaceae*), *Bacteroides* spp. and *Lactobacillus* spp., are not susceptible to trimethoprim levels obtained with the recommended dosage.

Indications and Usage: For the treatment of initial episodes of uncomplicated urinary tract infections due to susceptible strains of the following organisms: *Escherichia coli, Proteus mirabilis, Klebsiella pneumoniae* and *Enterobacter* species and coagulase-negative *Staphylococcus* species, including *S. saprophyticus.*

Cultures and susceptibility tests should be performed to determine the susceptibility of the bacteria to trimethoprim. Therapy may be initiated prior to obtaining the results of these tests.

Contraindications: Proloprim is contraindicated in individuals hypersensitive to trimethoprim and in those with documented megaloblastic anemia due to folate deficiency.

Warnings: Experience with trimethoprim alone is limited, but it has been reported rarely to interfere with hematopoiesis, especially when administered in large doses and/or for prolonged periods. The presence of clinical signs such as sore throat, fever, pallor or purpura may be early indications of serious blood disorders. Complete blood counts should be obtained if any of these signs are noted in a patient receiving trimethoprim and the drug discontinued if a significant reduction in the count of any formed blood element is found.

Precautions:

General: Trimethoprim should be given with caution to patients with possible folate deficiency. Folates may be administered concomitantly without interfering with the antibacterial action of trimethoprim. Trimethoprim should also be given with caution to patients with impaired renal or hepatic function.

Pregnancy: *Teratogenic Effects: Pregnancy Category C.* Trimethoprim has been shown to be teratogenic in the rat when given in doses 40 times the human dose. In some rabbit studies, an overall increase in fetal loss (dead and resorbed and malformed conceptuses) was associated with doses 6 times the human therapeutic dose. While there are no large well-controlled studies on the use of trimethoprim in pregnant women, Brumfitt and Pursell[4] reported the outcome of 186 pregnancies during which the mother received either placebo or trimethoprim in combination with sulfamethoxazole. The incidence of congenital abnormalities was 4.5% (3 of 66) in those who received placebo and 3.3% (4 of 120) in those receiving trimethoprim plus sulfamethoxazole. There were no abnormalities in the 10 children whose mothers received the drug during the first trimester. In a separate survey, Brumfitt and Pursell also found no congenital abnormalities in 35 children whose mothers had received trimethoprim plus sulfamethoxazole at the time of conception or shortly thereafter.

Because trimethoprim may interfere with folic acid metabolism, Proloprim should be used during pregnancy only if the potential benefit justifies the potential risk to the fetus.

Nursing Mothers: Trimethoprim is excreted in human milk. Because trimethoprim may interfere with folic acid metabolism, caution should be exercised when Proloprim is administered to a nursing mother.

Pediatric Use: The safety of trimethoprim in infants under 2 months has not been demonstrated. The effectiveness of trimethoprim has not been established in children under 12 years of age.

Adverse Reactions: The adverse effects encountered most often with trimethoprim are rash and pruritus. Other adverse effects reported involved the gastrointestinal and hematopoietic systems.

Dermatologic Reactions: Rash, pruritus and exfoliative dermatitis. At the recommended dosage regimens of 100 mg b.i.d. or 200 mg q.d., the incidence of rash is 2.9% to 6.7%. In clinical studies which employed high doses of Proloprim, an elevated incidence of rash was noted. These rashes were maculopapular, morbilliform, pruritic and generally mild to moderate, appearing 7 to 14 days after the initiation of therapy.

Gastrointestinal Reactions: Epigastric distress, nausea, vomiting, and glossitis.

Hematologic Reactions: Thrombocytopenia, leukopenia, neutropenia, megaloblastic anemia, and methemoglobinemia.

Miscellaneous Reactions: Fever, elevation of serum transaminases and bilirubin, and increases in BUN and serum creatinine levels.

Overdosage:

Acute: Signs of acute overdosage with trimethoprim may appear following ingestion of 1 gram or more of the drug and include nausea, vomiting, dizziness, headaches, mental depression, confusion and bone marrow depression (SEE CHRONIC OVERDOSAGE). Treatment consists of gastric lavage and general supportive measures. Acidification of the urine will increase renal elimination of trimethoprim. Peritoneal dialysis is not effective and hemodialysis only moderately effective in eliminating the drug.

Chronic: Use of trimethoprim at high doses and/or for extended periods of time may cause bone marrow depression manifested as thrombocytopenia, leukopenia and/or megaloblastic anemia. If signs of bone marrow depression occur, trimethoprim should be discontinued and the patient should be given leucovorin, 3 to 6 mg intramuscularly daily for three days, or as required to restore normal hematopoiesis.

Dosage and Administration: The usual oral adult dosage is 100 mg of Proloprim every 12 hours or 200 mg of Proloprim every 24 hours, each for 10 days.

The use of trimethoprim in patients with a creatinine clearance of less than 15 ml/min is not recommended. For patients with a creatinine clearance of 15 to 30 ml/min, the dose should be 50 mg every 12 hours. The effectiveness of trimethoprim has not been established in children under 12 years of age.

How Supplied: 100 mg (white) scored tablets, imprinted with "PROLOPRIM 09A"— bottle of 100 (NDC-0081-0820-55) and unit dose pack of 100 (NDC-0081-0820-56). Store at 15°– 30°C (59°–86°F) in a dry place. 200 mg (yellow) scored tablets, imprinted with "PROLOPRIM 200"—bottle of 100 (NDC-0081-0825-55). Store at 15°–30°C (59°–86°F) in a dry place and protect from light.

References:

1. Bauer AW, Kirby WMM, Sherris JC, Turck M: Antibiotic Susceptibility Testing by Standardized Single Disk Method. Am J Clin Path 45: 493–496, 1966.
2. Approved Standard ASM-2 Performance Standards for Antimicrobial Disc Susceptibility Test: National Committee for Clinical Laboratory Standards, 771 East Lancaster Avenue, Villanova, Pennsylvania 19085.
3. Ericsson HM and Sherris JC: Antibiotic Sensitivity Testing. Report of an International Collaborative Study. Acta Pathologica et Microbiologica Scandinavica, Section B, Suppl. 217, 1971, pp. 1–90.
4. Brumfitt W and Pursell R: Trimethoprim/Sulfamethoxazole in the Treatment of Bacteriuria in Women. J Inf Dis Suppl 128: S657–S663, 1973.

*Mfd. under Pat. #3,956,327.

Shown in Product Identification Section, page 408

PURINETHOL®
[pur'in-thawl']
(Mercaptopurine)
50 mg Scored Tablets

Caution: Purinethol® (mercaptopurine) is a potent drug. It should not be used unless a diagnosis of acute leukemia or chronic myelogenous leukemia has been adequately established and the responsible physician is knowledgeable in assessing response to chemotherapy.

Description: Purinethol® (mercaptopurine) (6-mercaptopurine) was synthesized and developed by Hitchings, Elion, and associates at the Wellcome Research Laboratories.[1] It is one of a large series of purine analogues which interfere with nucleic acid biosynthesis. Mercaptopurine is an analogue of the purine bases adenine and hypoxanthine.

Biochemical Pharmacology: Mercaptopurine competes with hypoxanthine and guanine for the

Continued on next page

Burroughs Wellcome—Cont.

enzyme hypoxanthine-guanine phosphoribosyltransferase (HGPRTase) and is itself converted to thioinosinic acid (TIMP). This intracellular nucleotide inhibits several reactions involving inosinic acid (IMP), including the conversion of IMP to xanthylic acid (XMP) and the conversion of IMP to adenylic acid (AMP) via adenylosuccinate (SAMP). In addition, 6-methylthioinosinate (MTIMP) is formed by the methylation of TIMP. Both TIMP and MTIMP have been reported to inhibit glutamine-5-phosphoribosylpyrophosphate amidotransferase, the first enzyme unique to the de novo pathway for purine ribonucleotide synthesis.[2] Experiments indicate that radiolabeled mercaptopurine may be recovered from the DNA in the form of deoxythioguanosine.[3] Some mercaptopurine is converted to nucleotide derivatives of 6-thioguanine (6-TG) by the sequential actions of inosinate (IMP) dehydrogenase and xanthylate (XMP) aminase, converting TIMP to thioguanylic acid (TGMP).

Animal tumors that are resistant to mercaptopurine have lost the ability to convert mercaptopurine to TIMP. However, it is clear that resistance to mercaptopurine may be acquired by other means as well, particularly in human leukemias. It is not known exactly which of any one or more of the biochemical effects of mercaptopurine and its metabolites are directly or predominantly responsible for cell death.[4]

The catabolism of mercaptopurine and its metabolites is complex. In man, after oral administration of ^{35}S-6-mercaptopurine, urine contains intact mercaptopurine, thiouric acid (formed by direct oxidation by xanthine oxidase, probably via 6-mercapto-8-hydroxypurine) and a number of 6-methylated thiopurines. The methylthiopurines yield appreciable amounts of inorganic sulfate.[2] The importance of the metabolism by xanthine oxidase relates to the fact that Zyloprim® (allopurinol) inhibits this enzyme and retards the catabolism of mercaptopurine and its active metabolites. A significant reduction in mercaptopurine dosage is mandatory if a potent xanthine oxidase inhibitor and Purinethol (mercaptopurine) are used simultaneously in a patient (see "WARNINGS").

Clinical Pharmacology: Clinical studies have shown that the absorption of an oral dose of mercaptopurine in man is incomplete and variable, averaging approximately 50% of the administered dose.[5] The factors influencing absorption are unknown. Intravenous administration of an investigational preparation of mercaptopurine revealed a plasma half-disappearance time of 21 minutes in children and 47 minutes in adults. The volume of distribution usually exceeded that of the total body water.[5]

Following the oral administration of ^{35}S-6-mercaptopurine in one subject, a total of 46% of the dose could be accounted for in the urine (as parent drug and metabolites) in the first 24 hours. Metabolites of mercaptopurine were found in urine within the first 2 hours after administration. Radioactivity (in the form of sulfate) could be found in the urine for weeks afterwards.[2]

There is negligible entry of mercaptopurine into cerebrospinal fluid.

Plasma protein binding averages 19% over the concentration range 10 to 50 micrograms per milliliter (a concentration only achieved by intravenous administration of mercaptopurine at doses exceeding 5 to 10 mg/kg).[5]

Monitoring plasma levels of mercaptopurine during therapy is of questionable value.[2] It is technically difficult to determine plasma concentrations which are seldom greater than 1 to 2 micrograms per milliliter after a therapeutic oral dose. More significantly, mercaptopurine enters rapidly into the anabolic and catabolic pathways for purines and the active intracellular metabolites have appreciably longer half-lives than the parent drug. The biochemical effects of a single dose of mercaptopurine are evident long after the parent drug has disappeared from plasma. Because of this rapid metabolism of mercaptopurine to active intracellular derivatives, hemodialysis would not be expected to appreciably reduce toxicity of the drug. There is no known pharmacologic antagonist to the biochemical actions of mercaptopurine in vivo.

Indications and Usage: Purinethol (mercaptopurine) is indicated for remission induction, remission consolidation, and maintenance therapy of the acute leukemias. The response to this agent depends upon the particular sub-classification of the acute leukemia (lymphatic, myelogenous, undifferentiated, etc.) and the age of the patient (child or adult). Purinethol (mercaptopurine) is also indicated for the palliative treatment of chronic myelogenous (granulocytic) leukemia.

a) **Acute Lymphatic (Lymphocytic, Lymphoblastic) Leukemia:** Acute lymphatic leukemia occurring in children responds, in general, more favorably to mercaptopurine than the same disorder occuring in adults. Given as a single agent for remission induction, mercaptopurine induces complete remission in approximately 25% of children and 10% of adults. These results can be improved upon considerably by using multiple, carefully selected agents in combination. Reliance upon mercaptopurine alone is seldom justified. The duration of complete remission induced in children with acute lymphatic leukemia is so brief without the use of maintenance therapy that some form of drug therapy is considered essential following remission induction. Mercaptopurine, as a single agent, is capable of significantly prolonging complete remission duration in children; however, combination therapy with multiple agents has produced results superior to that achieved with mercaptopurine alone. The effectiveness of mercaptopurine in maintenance programs in adult acute lymphatic leukemia has not been established.

b) **Acute Myelogenous (and Acute Myelomonocytic) Leukemia:** As a single agent, mercaptopurine will induce complete remission in approximately 10% of children and adults with acute myelogenous leukemia or its sub-classifications. These results are inferior to those achieved with combination chemotherapy employing optimum treatment schedules.

c) **Chronic Myelogenous (Granulocytic) Leukemia:** Mercaptopurine is one of several agents with demonstrated efficacy in the treatment of chronic myelogenous leukemia. Approximately 30 to 50% of patients with chronic myelogenous leukemia obtain an objective response to mercaptopurine. This is less than the 90% objective responses with busulfan, and, of these two agents, Myleran® (busulfan) is usually regarded as the preferred drug for initial therapy.

d) **Central Nervous System Leukemia:** Mercaptopurine is not effective for prophylaxis or treatment of central nervous system leukemia.

e) **Other Neoplasms:** Purinethol (mercaptopurine) is not effective in chronic lymphatic leukemia, the lymphomas (including Hodgkin's Disease), or solid tumors.

Contraindications: Purinethol (mercaptopurine) should not be used unless a diagnosis of acute leukemia or chronic myelogenous leukemia has been adequately established and the responsible physician is knowledgeable in assessing response to chemotherapy.

Mercaptopurine should not be used in patients whose disease has demonstrated prior resistance to this drug. In animals and man there is usually complete cross-resistance between Purinethol (mercaptopurine) and Tabloid® brand thioguanine.

Warnings:
a) **Bone Marrow Toxicity:** The most consistent, dose-related toxicity is bone marrow suppression. This may be manifest by anemia, leukopenia, thrombocytopenia, or any combination of these. Any of these findings may also indicate progression of the underlying disease. It is imperative that patients be instructed to report promptly the development of fever, sore throat, signs of local infection, bleeding from any site, or symptoms suggestive of anemia. Since mercaptopurine may have a delayed effect, it is important to withdraw the medication temporarily at the first sign of an abnormally large fall in any of the formed elements of the blood.

b) **Hepatotoxicity:**[5] Purinethol (mercaptopurine) is hepatotoxic in animals and man; deaths have been reported from hepatic necrosis. Hepatic injury can occur with any dosage, but seems to occur with greatest frequency when doses of 2.5 mg/kg/day are exceeded. The histologic pattern of mercaptopurine hepatotoxicity includes features of both intrahepatic cholestasis and parenchymal cell necrosis, either of which may predominate. It is not clear how much of the hepatic damage is due to direct toxicity from the drug and how much may be due to a hypersensitivity reaction. In some patients jaundice has cleared following withdrawal of mercaptopurine and reappeared with its reintroduction.

Published reports have cited widely varying incidences of overt hepatotoxicity; several reports have indicated that as many as 10 to 40% of patients with acute leukemia develop jaundice while receiving treatment with mercaptopurine. Usually, clinically detectable jaundice appears early in the course of treatment (one to two months). However, jaundice has been reported as early as one week and as late as eight years after the start of treatment with mercaptopurine.

Monitoring of serum transaminase levels, alkaline phosphatase, and bilirubin levels may allow early detection of hepatotoxicity. It is advisable to monitor these liver function tests at weekly intervals when first beginning therapy and at monthly intervals thereafter. Liver function tests may be advisable more frequently in patients who are receiving mercaptopurine with other hepatotoxic drugs or with known pre-existing liver disease.

The concomitant administration of mercaptopurine with other hepatotoxic agents requires especially careful clinical and biochemical monitoring of hepatic function. Combination therapy involving mercaptopurine with other drugs not felt to be hepatotoxic should nevertheless be approached with caution. The combination of mercaptopurine with doxorubicin (Adriamycin®) was reported to be hepatotoxic in 19 of 20 patients undergoing remission-induction therapy for leukemia resistant to previous therapy.

The hepatotoxicity has been associated in some cases with anorexia, diarrhea, jaundice, and ascites. Hepatic encephalopathy has occurred.

The onset of clinical jaundice, hepatomegaly, or anorexia with tenderness in the right hypochondrium are immediate indications for withholding mercaptopurine until the exact etiology can be identified. Likewise, any evidence of deterioration in liver function studies, toxic hepatitis, or biliary stasis should prompt discontinuation of the drug and lead to a search for an etiology of the hepatotoxicity.

c) **Interaction with Zyloprim® (Allopurinol): When allopurinol and mercaptopurine are administered concomitantly, it is imperative that the dose of mercaptopurine be reduced to one-third to one-quarter of the usual dose. Failure to observe this dosage reduction will result in a delayed catabolism of mercaptopurine and the strong likelihood of inducing severe toxicity.**

d) **Immunosuppression:** Mercaptopurine recipients may manifest decreased cellular hypersensitivities and impaired allograft rejection. Induction of immunity to infectious agents or vaccines will be subnormal in these patients; the degree of immunosuppression will depend on antigen dose and temporal relationship to drug. This drug effect is similar to that of Imuran® (azathioprine) and should be carefully considered with regard to intercurrent infections and risk of subsequent neoplasia.

e) **Mutagenesis and Carcinogenesis:** Purinethol (mercaptopurine) causes chromosomal aberrations in animals and man and induces dominant-lethal mutations in male mice. Carcinogenic potential exists in man, but the extent of the risk is unknown.

f) **Teratogenesis:** Mercaptopurine has embryopathic effects in rats. Women receiving mercaptopurine in the first trimester of pregnancy have an increased incidence of abortion; the risk of malformation in offspring surviving first trimester exposure is not accurately known. In a series of twenty-eight women receiving mercaptopurine after the first trimester of pregnancy, three mothers died undelivered, one delivered a stillborn child, and one aborted; there were no cases of macroscopically abnormal fetuses. Since such experience cannot exclude the possibility of fetal damage, mercaptopurine should be used during pregnancy only if the benefit clearly justifies the possible risk to the fetus, and particular caution should be given to the use of mercaptopurine in the first trimester of pregnancy.

g) **Effects on Fertility:** The effect of mercaptopurine on human fertility is unknown for either males or females.

Precautions: The safe and effective use of Purinethol demands a thorough knowledge of the natural history of the condition being treated. For example, remission induction of adult acute leukemia virtually always necessitates the production of moderate to severe bone marrow hypoplasia. The degree of myelosuppression acceptable in this disease would not be desirable in the management of chronic granulocytic leukemia. After selection of an initial dosage schedule, therapy will frequently need to be modified depending upon the patient's response and manifestations of toxicity. The most frequent, serious, toxic effect of mercaptopurine is myelosuppression resulting in leukopenia, thrombocytopenia, and anemia. These toxic effects are often unavoidable during the induction phase of adult acute leukemia if remission induction is to be successful. Whether or not these manifestations demand modification or cessation of dosage depends both upon the response of the underlying disease and a careful consideration of supportive facilities (granulocyte and platelet transfusions) which may be available. Life-threatening infections and bleeding have been observed as a consequence of mercaptopurine induced granulocytopenia and thrombocytopenia. Severe hematologic toxicity may require supportive therapy with platelet transfusions for bleeding, and antibiotics and granulocyte transfusions if sepsis is documented.

If it is not the intent to intentionally induce bone marrow hypoplasia, it is important to discontinue the drug temporarily at the first evidence of an abnormally large fall in white blood cell count, platelet count, or hemoglobin concentration. In many patients with severe depression of the formed elements of the blood due to mercaptopurine, the bone marrow appears hypoplastic on aspiration or biopsy, whereas in other cases it may appear normocellular. The qualitative changes in the erythroid elements toward the megaloblastic series, characteristically seen with the folic acid antagonists and some other antimetabolites, are not seen with this drug.

It is recommended that evaluation of the hemoglobin or hematocrit, total white blood cell count and differential count, and quantitative platelet count be obtained weekly while the patient is on mercaptopurine therapy. In cases where the cause of fluctuations in the formed elements in the peripheral blood is obscure, bone marrow examination may be useful for the evaluation of marrow status. The decision to increase, decrease, continue, or discontinue a given dosage of mercaptopurine must be based not only on the absolute hematologic values, but also upon the rapidity with which changes are occurring. In many instances, particularly during the induction phase of acute leukemia, complete blood counts will need to be done more frequently than once weekly in order to evaluate the effect of the therapy. The dosage of mercaptopurine may need to be reduced when this agent is combined with other drugs whose primary toxicity is myelosuppression.

It is probably advisable to start with smaller dosages in patients with impaired renal function, since the latter might result in slower elimination of the drug and a greater cumulative effect.

See "WARNINGS" section for information on immunosuppression, mutagenesis and carcinogenesis, teratogenesis, and effects on fertility.

Adverse Reactions: Intestinal ulceration has been reported.[8] Nausea, vomiting and anorexia are uncommon during initial administration, but they may occur during toxicity. Mild diarrhea and sprue-like symptoms have been noted occasionally, but it is difficult at present to attribute these to the medication. Oral lesions are rarely seen, and when they occur they resemble thrush rather than antifolic ulcerations.

Hyperuricemia frequently occurs in patients receiving mercaptopurine as a consequence of rapid cell lysis accompanying the antineoplastic effect. Adverse effects can be minimized by increased hydration, urine alkalinization, and the prophylactic administration of a xanthine oxidase inhibitor such as Zyloprim® (allopurinol). The dosage of mercaptopurine should be reduced to one-third to one-quarter of the usual dose if Zyloprim® (allopurinol) is given concurrently.

Drug fever has been very rarely reported with mercaptopurine. Before attributing fever to mercaptopurine, every attempt should be made to exclude more common causes of pyrexia, such as sepsis, in patients with acute leukemia.

Overdosage: There is no known pharmacologic antagonist of mercaptopurine. The drug should be discontinued immediately if unintended toxicity occurs during treatment. If a patient is seen immediately following an accidental overdosage of the drug, induced emesis may be useful. Hemodialysis is thought to be of marginal use due to the rapid intracellular incorporation of mercaptopurine into active metabolites with long persistence.

Dosage and Administration:

a) **Induction and Consolidation Therapy:** Purinethol (mercaptopurine) is administered orally. The dosage which will be tolerated or will be effective varies from patient-to-patient, and therefore careful titration is necessary to obtain the optimum therapeutic effect without incurring excessive, unintended toxicity. The usual initial dosage for children and adults is 2.5 mg/kg of body weight per day (100 to 200 mg in the average adult and 50 mg in an average 5 year old child). Children with acute leukemia have tolerated this dose without difficulty in most cases; it may be continued daily for several weeks or more in some patients. If, after four weeks at this dosage, there is no clinical improvement and no definite evidence of leukocyte or platelet depression, the dosage may be increased up to 5 mg/kg daily.

A dosage of 2.5 mg/kg per day may result in a rapid fall in leukocyte count within 1 to 2 weeks in some adults with acute leukemia and high total leukocyte counts, as well as in certain adults with chronic myelocytic leukemia. The total daily dosage may be given at one time. It is calculated to the nearest multiple of 25 mg. The dosage of mercaptopurine should be reduced to one-third to one-quarter of the usual dose if Zyloprim® (allopurinol) is given concurrently. Since the drug may have a delayed action, it should be discontinued at the first sign of an abnormally large or rapid fall in the leukocyte or platelet count. If subsequently the leukocyte count or platelet count remains constant for two or three days, or rises, treatment may be resumed.

b) **Maintenance Therapy:** If a complete hematologic remission is obtained with mercaptopurine, either alone or in combination with other agents, maintenance therapy should be considered. This is indicated in children with acute lymphatic leukemia. The use of mercaptopurine in maintenance schedules for adults with acute leukemia has not been established to be effective. If remission is achieved, maintenance doses will vary from patient-to-patient. A usual daily maintenance dose of mercaptopurine is 1.5 to 2.5 mg/kg/day as a single dose. It is to be emphasized that in children with acute lymphatic leukemia in remission, superior results have been obtained when mercaptopurine has been combined with other agents (most frequently with methotrexate) for remission maintenance. Mercaptopurine should rarely be relied upon as a single agent for the maintenance of remissions induced in acute leukemia.

How Supplied: Cream-colored, scored tablets containing 50 mg mercaptopurine, imprinted with "WELLCOME" and "04A" on each tablet; bottles of 25 and 250.

References:

1. New York Academy of Sciences: 6-mercaptopurine. ANN NY ACAD SCI 60: 359-507 (1954).
2. Elion GB: Biochemistry and pharmacology of purine analogues. FED PROC 26: 898-904 (1967).
3. Scannell JP, Hitchings GH: Thioguanine in deoxyribonucleic acid from tumors of 6-mercaptopurine-treated mice. PROC SOC EXP BIOL MED 122: 627-629 (1966).
4. Paterson ARP, Tidd DM: 6-thiopurines. pp. 384-403. In: Sartorelli AC, Johns DG, ed. Antineoplastic and Immunosuppressive Agents, Part II, Berlin, Springer-Verlag, 1975.
5. Loo TL, Luce JK, Sullivan MP, Frei E: Clinical pharmacologic observations on 6-mercaptopurine and 6-methylthiopurine ribonucleoside. CLIN PHARMACOL THER 9: 180-194 (1968).
6. Schein PS, Winokur SH: Immunosuppressive and cytotoxic chemotherapy: long-term complications. ANN INTERN MED 82: 84-95 (1975).
7. Stern MH, Minow MD, Casey MD: Hepatotoxicity in patients treated with adriamycin and 6-mercaptopurine for refractory leukemia. AM J CLIN PATHOL 63: 758-759 (1975).
8. Clark PA, Hsia YE, Huntsman RG: Toxic complications of treatment with 6-mercaptopurine. BR MED J 1: 393-395 (1960).

Shown in Product Identification Section, page 408

SEPTRA®
[sĕp' trah]
I.V. INFUSION
(Trimethoprim-Sulfamethoxazole)

Description: Septra I.V. Infusion, a sterile solution for intravenous infusion only, is a synthetic antibacterial combination product. Each 5 ml contains 80 mg trimethoprim* (16 mg/ml) and 400 mg sulfamethoxazole (80 mg/ml) compounded with 40% propylene glycol, 10% ethyl alcohol and 0.3% diethanolamine; 1% benzyl alcohol and 0.1% sodium metabisulfite as preservatives, water for injection, and pH adjusted to approximately 10 with sodium hydroxide.

Trimethoprim is 2,4-diamino-5-(3,4,5-trimethoxybenzyl)pyrimidine. It is a white to light yellow, odorless, bitter compound with a molecular weight of 290.3.

Sulfamethoxazole is N^1-(5-methyl-3-isoxazolyl) sulfanilamide. It is an almost white in color, odorless, tasteless compound with a molecular weight of 253.28.

Clinical Pharmacology: Following a one-hour intravenous infusion of a single dose of 160 mg trimethoprim plus 800 mg sulfamethoxazole to 11 patients whose weight ranged from 105 lbs. to 165 lbs. (mean, 143 lbs.), the mean peak plasma concentrations of trimethoprim and sulfamethoxazole were 3.4 ± 0.3 µg/ml and 46.3 ± 2.7 µg/ml, respectively. Following repeated intravenous administration of the same dose at eight-hour intervals, the mean plasma concentrations just prior to and immediately after each infusion at steady state

Continued on next page

Burroughs Wellcome—Cont.

were 5.6 ± 0.6 µg/ml and 8.8 ± 0.9 µg/ml for trimethoprim and 70.6 ± 7.3 µg/ml and 105.6 ± 10.9 µg/ml for sulfamethoxazole. The mean plasma half-life was 11.3 ± 0.7 hours for trimethoprim and 12.8 ± 1.8 hours for sulfamethoxazole. All of these 11 patients had normal renal function and their age ranged from 17 to 78 years (median, 60 years)[1].

Pharmacokinetic studies in children and adults suggest an age dependent half-life of trimethoprim as indicated in the following table.[2]

Age (yrs.)	No. of Patients	Mean TMP Half-life (hours)
<1	2	7.67
1–10	9	5.49
10–20	5	8.19
20–63	6	12.82

Sulfamethoxazole exists in the blood as free, conjugated and protein-bound forms; trimethoprim is present as free and protein-bound and metabolized forms. The free forms are considered to be the therapeutically active forms. Approximately 44 percent of trimethoprim and 70 percent of sulfamethoxazole are protein-bound in blood. The presence of 10 mg percent sulfamethoxazole in plasma decreases the protein binding of trimethoprim to an insignificant degree; trimethoprim does not influence the protein binding of sulfamethoxazole.

Excretion of Septra is chiefly by the kidneys through both glomerular filtration and tubular secretion. Urine concentrations of both sulfamethoxazole and trimethoprim are considerably higher than are the concentrations in the blood. When administered together as in Septra, neither sulfamethoxazole nor trimethoprim affects the urinary excretion pattern of the other.

Microbiology: Sulfamethoxazole inhibits bacterial synthesis of dihydrofolic acid by competing with *para*-aminobenzoic acid. Trimethoprim blocks the production of tetrahydrofolic acid from dihydrofolic acid by binding to and reversibly inhibiting the required enzyme, dihydrofolate reductase. Thus, Septra blocks two consecutive steps in the biosynthesis of nucleic acids and proteins essential to many bacteria.

In vitro studies have shown that bacterial resistance develops more slowly with Septra than with trimethoprim or sulfamethoxazole alone.

In vitro serial dilution tests have shown that the spectrum of antibacterial activity of Septra includes common bacterial pathogens with the exception of *Pseudomonas aeruginosa.* The following organisms are usually susceptible: *Escherichia coli, Klebsiella-Enterobacter, Proteus mirabilis,* indole-positive *Proteus* species, *Haemophilus influenzae (including ampicillin-resistant strains), Streptococcus, pneumoniae, Shigella flexneri* and *Shigella sonnei.* It should be noted, however, that there are little clinical data on the use of Septra I.V. infusion in serious systemic infections due to *Haemophilus influenzae* and *Streptococcus pneumoniae.*

[See table below].

The recommended quantitative disc susceptibility method may be used for estimating the susceptibility of bacteria to Septra.[3,4] With this procedure, a report from the laboratory of "Susceptible to trimethoprim-sulfamethoxazole" indicates that the infection is likely to respond to therapy with Septra. If the infection is confined to the urine, a report of "Intermediate susceptibility to trimethoprim-sulfamethoxazole" also indicates that the infection is likely to respond. A report of "Resistant to trimethoprim-sulfamethoxazole" indicates that the infection is unlikely to respond to therapy with Septra.

Indications and Usage:
PNEUMOCYSTIS CARINII PNEUMONITIS: Septra I.V. Infusion is indicated in the treatment of *Pneumocystis carinii* pneumonitis in children and adults.

SHIGELLOSIS: Septra I.V. Infusion is indicated in the treatment of enteritis caused by susceptible strains of *Shigella flexneri* and *Shigella sonnei* in children and adults.

URINARY TRACT INFECTIONS: Septra I.V. Infusion is indicated in the treatment of severe or complicated urinary tract infections due to susceptible strains of *Escherichia coli, Klebsiella-Enterobacter* and *Proteus* sp. when oral administration of Septra is not feasible and when the organism is not suceptible to single agent antibacterials effective in the urinary tract.

Cultures and susceptibility tests should be performed to determine the susceptibility of the bacteria to Septra. Therapy may be initiated prior to obtaining the results of these tests.

Contraindications: Hypersensitivity to trimethoprim or sulfonamides. Patients with documented megaloblastic anemia due to folate deficiency. Pregnancy at term and during the nursing period, because sulfonamides pass the placenta and are excreted in the milk and may cause kernicterus.

Infants less than two months of age.

Warnings: SEPTRA I.V. INFUSION SHOULD NOT BE USED IN THE TREATMENT OF STREPTOCOCCAL PHARYNGITIS. Clinical studies have documented that patients with Group A, β-hemolytic streptococcal tonsillopharyngitis have a greater incidence of bacteriologic failure when treated with Septra than do those patients treated with penicillin as evidenced by failure to eradicate this organism from the tonsillopharyngeal area. Deaths associated with the administration of sulfonamides have been reported from hypersensitivity reactions, agranulocytosis, aplastic anemia and other blood dyscrasias. Experience with trimethoprim alone is much more limited, but it has been reported to interfere with hematopoiesis in occasional patients. In elderly patients concurrently receiving certain diuretics, primarily thiazides, as increased incidence of thrombopenia with purpura has been reported.

The presence of clinical signs such as sore throat, fever, pallor, purpura or jaundice may be early indications of serious blood disorders.

Precautions:
General: Septra should be given with caution to patients with impaired renal or hepatic function, to those with possible folate deficiency and to those with severe allergy or bronchial asthma. In glucose-6-phosphate dehydrogenase-deficient individuals, hemolysis may occur. This reaction is frequently dose-related. Adequate fluid intake must be maintained in order to prevent crystalluria and stone formation.

Local irritation and inflammation due to extravascular infiltration of the infusion has been observed with Septra I.V. Infusion. If this occurs the infusion should be discontinued and restarted at another site.

Laboratory Tests: Appropriate culture and susceptibility studies should be performed before and throughout treatment. Complete blood counts should be done frequently in patients receiving Septra; if a significant reduction in the count of any formed blood element is noted, Septra should be discontinued. Urinalyses with careful microscopic examination and renal function tests should be performed during therapy, particularly for those patients with impaired renal function.

Drug Interactions: It has been reported that Septra may prolong the prothrombin time in patients who are receivng the anticoagulant warfarin. This interaction should be kept in mind when Septra is given to patients already on anticoagulant therapy, and the coagulation time should be reassessed.

Carcinogenesis, Mutagenesis, Impairment of Fertility:

Carcinogenesis: Long-term studies in animals to evaluate carcinogenic potential have not been conducted with Septra I.V. Infusion.

Mutagenesis: Bacterial mutagenic studies have not been performed with sulfamethoxazole and trimethoprim in combination. Trimethoprim was demonstrated to be non-mutagenic in the Ames assay. No chromosomal damage was observed in human leukocytes cultured *in vitro* with sulfamethoxazole and trimethoprim alone or in combination; the concentrations used exceeded blood levels of these compounds following therapy with Septra. Observations of leukocytes obtained from patients treated with Septra revealed no chromosomal abnormalities.

Impairment of Fertility: Septra I.V. Infusion has not been studied in animals for evidence of impairment of fertility. However, studies in rats at oral dosages as high as 70 mg/kg trimethoprim plus 350 mg/kg sulfamethoxazole daily showed no adverse effects on fertility or general reproductive performance.

Pregnancy: Teratogenic Effects: Pregnancy Category C. In rats, oral doses of 533 mg/kg sulfamethoxazole or 200 mg/kg trimethoprim produced teratological effects manifested mainly as cleft palates.

The highest dose which did not cause cleft palates in rats was 512 mg/kg sulfamethoxazole or 192 mg/kg trimethoprim when administered separately. In two studies in rats, no teratology was observed when 512 mg/kg of sulfamethoxazole was used in combination with 128 mg/kg of trimethoprim. In one study, however, cleft palates were observed in one litter out of 9 when 355 mg/kg of sulfamethoxazole was used in combination with 88 mg/kg of trimethoprim.

In some rabbit studies, an overall increase in fetal loss (dead and resorbed and malformed concep-

---

REPRESENTATIVE MINIMUM INHIBITORY CONCENTRATION VALUES FOR SEPTRA SUSCEPTIBLE ORGANISMS
(MIC-mcg/ml)

Bacteria	TMP Alone	SMX Alone	TMP/SMX (1:19) TMP	SMX
Escherichia coli	0.05–1.5	1.0–245	0.05–0.5	0.95–9.5
Proteus species (indole positive)	0.5–5.0	7.35–300	0.05–1.5	0.95–28.5
Proteus mirabilis	0.5–1.5	7.35–30	0.05–0.15	0.95–2.85
Klebsiella-Enterobacter	0.15–5.0	2.45–245	0.05–1.5	0.95–28.5
Haemophilus influenzae	0.15–1.5	2.85–95	0.015–0.15	0.285–2.85
Streptococcus pneumoniae	0.15–1.5	7.35–24.5	0.05–1.5	0.95–2.85
Shigella flexneri†	<0.01–0.04	<0.16–>320	<0.002–0.03	0.04–0.625
Shigella sonnei†	0.02–0.08	0.625–>320	0.004–0.06	0.08–1.25

TMP = Trimethoprim   SMX = Sulfamethoxazole

†Rudoy, R.C., Nelson, J.D., Haltalin, K.C. Antimicrobial Agents and Chemotherapy 5:439-43, 1974.

tuses) was associated with doses of trimethoprim 6 times the human therapeutic dose.

While there are no large, well-controlled studies on the use of trimethoprim plus sulfamethoxazole in pregnant women. Brumfitt and Pursell[5] reported the outcome of 186 pregnancies during which the mother received either placebo or oral trimethoprim in combination with sulfamethoxazole. The incidence of congenital abnormalities was 4.5% (3 of 66) in those who received placebo and 3.3% (4 of 120) in those receiving trimethoprim plus sulfamethoxazole. There were no abnormalities in the 10 children whose mothers received the drug during the first trimester. In a separate survey, Brumfitt and Pursell also found no congenital abnormalities in 35 children whose mothers had received oral trimethoprim plus sulfamethoxazole at the time of conception or shortly thereafter.

Because trimethoprim plus sulfamethoxazole may interfere with folic acid metabolism, Septra I.V. Infusion should be used during pregnancy only if the potential benefit justifies the potential risk to the fetus.

Nonteratogenic Effects: See "CONTRAINDICATIONS" section.

Nursing Mothers: See "CONTRAINDICATIONS" section.

Adverse Reactions: The most frequent adverse reactions reported for Septra I.V. Infusion are nausea and vomiting, thrombocytopenia, and rash. These occurred in less than one in twenty patients. Local reaction, pain and slight irritation on I.V. administration are infrequent. Thrombophlebitis has rarely been observed. For completeness, all major reactions to sulfonamides and to trimethoprim are included below, even though they may not have been reported with Septra I.V. Infusion.

Allergic Reactions: Generalized skin eruptions, pruritus, urticaria, erythema multiforme, Stevens-Johnson syndrome, epidermal necrolysis, serum sickness, exfoliative dermatitis, anaphylactoid reactions, periorbital edema, conjunctival and scleral injection, photosensitization, arthralgia and allergic myocarditis.

Blood Dyscrasias: Megaloblastic anemia, hemolytic anemia, purpura, thrombopenia, leukopenia, agranulocytosis, aplastic anemia, hypoprothrombinemia and methemoglobinemia.

Gastrointestinal Reactions: Glossitis, stomatitis, nausea, emesis, abdominal pains, hepatitis, diarrhea, pseudomembranous colitis and pancreatitis.

C.N.S. Reactions: Headache, peripheral neuritis, mental depression, ataxia, convulsions, hallucinations, tinnitus, vertigo, insomnia, apathy, fatigue, muscle weakness and nervousness.

Miscellaneous Reactions: Drug fever, chills, and toxic nephrosis with oliguria and anuria. Periarteritis nodosa and L. E. phenomenon have occurred. The sulfonamides bear certain chemical similarities to some goitrogens, diuretics (acetazolamide and the thiazides) and oral hypoglycemic agents. Cross-sensitivity may exist with these agents. Diuresis and hypoglycemia have occurred rarely in patients receiving sulfonamides.

Overdosage: Since there has been no extensive experience in humans with single doses of Septra I.V. Infusion in excess of 25 ml (400 mg trimethoprim and 2000 mg sulfamethoxazole), the maximum tolerated dose in humans is unknown.

Use of Septra I.V. Infusion at high doses and/or for extended periods of time may cause bone marrow depression manifested as thrombopenia, leukopenia, and/or megaloblastic anemia. If signs of bone marrow depression occur, the patient should be given leucovorin 3 to 6 mg intramuscularly daily for three days, or as required to restore normal hematopoiesis.

Peritoneal dialysis is not effective and hemodialysis only moderately effective in eliminating trimethoprim and sulfamethoxazole.

The LD_{50} of Septra I.V. Infusion in mice is 700 mg/kg or 7.3 ml/kg; in rats and rabbits the LD_{50} is > 500 mg/kg or > 5.2 ml/kg. The vehicle produced the same LD_{50} in each of these species as the active drug.

The signs and symptoms noted in mice, rats and rabbits with Septra I.V. Infusion or its vehicle at the high I.V. doses used in acute toxicity studies included ataxia, decreased motor activity, loss of righting reflex, tremors or convulsions, and/or respiratory depression.

Dosage and Administration: [CONTRAINDICATED IN INFANTS LESS THAN TWO MONTHS OF AGE.] CAUTION—SEPTRA I.V. INFUSION MUST BE DILUTED IN 5% DEXTROSE IN WATER SOLUTION PRIOR TO ADMINISTRATION. DO NOT MIX SEPTRA I.V. INFUSION WITH OTHER DRUGS OR SOLUTIONS. RAPID OR BOLUS INJECTION MUST BE AVOIDED.

Children and Adults:
PNEUMOCYSTIS CARINII PNEUMONITIS:
Total daily dose is 15 to 20 mg/kg (based on the trimethoprim component) given in three to four equally divided doses every 6 or 8 hours for up to 14 days. One investigator noted that a total daily dose of 10 to 15 mg/kg was sufficient in 10 adult patients with normal renal function.[6]

SEVERE URINARY TRACT INFECTIONS AND SHIGELLOSIS: Total daily dose is 8 to 10 mg/kg (based on the trimethoprim component) given in two to four equally divided doses every 6, 8 or 12 hours for up to 14 days for severe urinary tract infections and 5 days for shigellosis.

For Patients with Impaired Renal Function: When renal function is impaired, a reduced dosage should be employed using the following table:

Creatinine Clearance (ml/min)	Recommended Dosage Regimen
Above 30	Use Standard Regimen
15–30	½ the Usual Regimen
Below 15	Use Not Recommended

Method of Preparation: Septra I.V. Infusion must be diluted. EACH 5 ml SHOULD BE ADDED TO 125 ml OF 5% DEXTROSE IN WATER. After diluting with 5% dextrose in water the solution should not be refrigerated and should be used within 6 hours. If upon visual inspection there is cloudiness or evidence of crystallization after mixing, the solution should be discarded and a fresh solution prepared.

The following infusion sets have been tested and found satisfactory: unit-dose glass containers (McGaw Laboratories, Cutter Laboratories, Inc., and Abbott Laboratories); unit-dose plastic containers (Viaflex™ from Travenol Laboratories and Accumed™ from McGaw Laboratories). No other systems have been tested and therefore no others can be recommended.

NOTE: In those instances where fluid restriction is desirable, each 5 ml may be added to 75 ml of 5% dextrose in water. Under these circumstances the solution should be mixed just prior to use and should be administered within two (2) hours. If upon visual inspection there is cloudiness or evidence of crystallization after mixing, the solution should be discarded and a fresh solution prepared.

Administration: The solution should be given by intravenous infusion over a period of 60 to 90 minutes. Rapid infusion or bolus injections must be avoided. Septra I.V. Infusion should not be given intramuscularly.

How Supplied: 5 ml ampuls, containing 80 mg trimethoprim (16 mg/ml) and 400 mg sulfamethoxazole (80 mg/ml) for infusion with 5% dextrose in water. Boxes of 10 (NDC-0081-0856-10)

10 ml vials, containing 160 mg trimethoprim (16 mg/ml) and 800 mg sulfamethoxazole (80 mg/ml) for infusion with 5% dextrose in water. Box of 10 (NDC-0081-0856-95)

20 ml multiple dose vial, containing 320 mg trimethoprim (16 mg/ml) and 1600 mg sulfamethoxazole (80 mg/ml) for infusion with 5% dextrose in water. Box of 1 (NDC-0081-0856-93)

STORE AT ROOM TEMPERATURE 15°–30°C (59°–86°F). DO NOT REFRIGERATE.

Also available in tablets containing 80 mg trimethoprim and 400 mg sulfamethoxazole (bottles of 100 and 500 tablets; unit dose pack of 100); oral suspension containing 40 mg trimethoprim and 200 mg sulfamethoxazole in each 5 ml (bottle of 473 ml; Unit of Use: bottle of 100 ml with child-resistant cap) and double strength, oval-shaped,

pink, scored tablets containing 160 mg trimethoprim and 800 mg sulfamethoxazole (bottles of 100 and 250, unit dose pack of 100, and Compliance™ Pak of 20).

References:
1. Grose WE, Bodey GP, Loo TL: Clinical Pharmacology of Intravenously Administered Trimethoprim-Sulfamethoxazole. Antimicrob Agents Chemother 15: 447, 1979.
2. Siber GR, Gorham C, Durbin W, Lesko L, Levin MJ: Pharmacology of Intravenous Trimethoprim-Sulfamethoxazole in Children and Adults. Current Chemotherapy and Infectious Diseases, American Society for Microbiology, Washington, D.C., 1980, Vol. 1, pp. 691–692.
3. Bauer AW, Kirby WMM, Sherris JC, Turck M: Antibiotic Susceptibility Testing by Standardized Single Disk Method. Am J Clin Path 45: 493, 1966.
4. Approved Standard ASM-2 Performance Standards for Antimicrobial Disc Susceptibility Test: National Committee for Clinical Laboratory Standards, 771 East Lancaster Avenue, Villanova, Pennsylvania 19085.
5. Brumfitt W and Pursell R: Trimethoprim/Sulfamethoxazole in the Treatment of Bacteriuria in Women. J Inf Dis Suppl 128: S657, 1973.
6. Winston DJ, Lau WK, Gale RP, Young LS: Trimethoprim-Sulfamethoxazole for the Treatment of Pneumocystis carinii pneumonia. Ann Int Med 92: 762–769, 1980.

*Mfd. under Pat. 3,956,327

SEPTRA® TABLETS and SUSPENSION ℞
[sĕp'trah]
SEPTRA® DS TABLETS Double Strength
(Trimethoprim-Sulfamethoxazole)

Description: Septra is a synthetic antibacterial combination product, available in scored pink tablets, each containing 80 mg trimethoprim* and 400 mg sulfamethoxazole and in double strength, pink, scored tablets, each containing 160 mg trimethoprim and 800 mg sulfamethoxazole.

*Mfd. under Pat. 3,956,327

Also available as a pink, cherry flavored oral suspension, each teaspoonful (5 ml) containing the equivalent of 40 mg trimethoprim and 200 mg sulfamethoxazole compounded with 0.26% alcohol.

Trimethoprim is 2,4-diamino-5-(3,4,5-trimethoxybenzl) pyrimidine. It is a white to light yellow, odorless, bitter compound with a molecular weight of 290.3.

Sulfamethoxazole is N^1-(5-methyl-3-isoxazolyl) sulfanilamide. It is an almost white in color, odorless, tasteless compound with a molecular weight of 253.28.

Clinical Pharmacology:

Septra is rapidly absorbed following oral administration. The blood levels of trimethoprim and sulfamethoxazole are similar to those achieved when each component is given alone. Peak blood levels for the individual components occur one to four hours after oral administration. The half-lives of sulfamethoxazole and trimethoprim, 10 and 8 to 10 hours respectively, are relatively the same regardless of whether these compounds are administered as individual components or as Septra. Detectable amounts of trimethoprim and sulfamethoxazole are present in the blood 24 hours after drug administration. Free sulfamethoxazole and trimethoprim blood levels are proportionately dose-dependent. On repeated administration, the steady-state ratio of trimethoprim to sulfamethoxazole levels in the blood is about 1:20.

Sulfamethoxazole exists in the blood as free, conjugated and protein-bound forms; trimethoprim is present as free, protein-bound and metabolized forms. The free forms are considered to be the therapeutically active forms. Approximately 44 percent of trimethoprim and 70 percent of sulfamethoxazole are protein-bound in the blood. The presence of 10 mg percent sulfamethoxazole in plasma decreases the protein

Continued on next page

Burroughs Wellcome—Cont.

binding of trimethoprim to an insignificant degree; trimethoprim does not influence the protein binding of sulfamethoxazole.

Excretion of Septra is chiefly by the kidneys through both glomerular filtration and tubular secretion. Urine concentrations of both sulfamethoxazole and trimethoprim are considerably higher than are the concentrations in the blood. When administered together as in Septra, neither sulfamethoxazole nor trimethoprim affects the urinary excretion pattern of the other.

Microbiology: Sulfamethoxazole inhibits bacterial synthesis of dihydrofolic acid by competing with *para*-aminobenzoic acid. Trimethoprim blocks the production of tetrahydrofolic acid from dihydrofolic acid by binding to and reversibly inhibiting the required enzyme, dihydrofolate reductase. Thus, Septra blocks two consecutive steps in the biosynthesis of nucleic acids and proteins essential to many bacteria.

In vitro studies have shown that bacterial resistance develops more slowly with Septra than with trimethoprim or sulfamethoxazole alone.

In vitro serial dilution tests have shown that the spectrum of antibacterial activity of Septra includes the common urinary tract pathogens with the exception of *Pseudomonas aeruginosa*. The following organisms are usually susceptible: *Escherichia coli, Klebsiella-Enterobacter, Proteus mirabilis* and indole-positive *Proteus* species.

In addition, the usual spectrum of antimicrobial activity of Septra includes the following bacterial pathogens isolated from middle ear exudate and bronchial secretions: *Haemophilus influenzae*, including ampicillin resistant strains, and *Streptococcus pneumoniae*.

Shigella flexneri and *Shigella sonnei* are also usually susceptible.

[See table below].

The recommended quantitative disc susceptibility method (Federal Register *37:*20527-29, 1972; Bauer AW, Kirby WMM, Sherris JC, Turck M: Antibiotic susceptibility testing by a standardized single disk method, Am J Clin Path *45:*493, 1966) may be used for estimating the susceptibility of bacteria to Septra. With this procedure, a report from the laboratory of "Susceptible to trimethoprim-sulfamethoxazole" indicates that the infection is likely to respond to therapy with Septra. If the infection is confined to the urine, a report of "Intermediate susceptibility to trimethoprim-sulfamethoxazole" also indicates that the infection is likely to respond. A report of "Resistant to trimethoprim-sulfamethoxazole" indicates that the infection is unlikely to respond to therapy with Septra.

Indications and Usage:

URINARY TRACT INFECTIONS: For the treatment of urinary tract infections due to susceptible strains of the following organisms: *Escherichia coli, Klebsiella-Enterobacter, Proteus mirabilis, Proteus vulgaris, Proteus morganii.* It is recommended that initial episodes of uncomplicated urinary tract infections be treated with a single effective antibacterial agent rather than the combination.

Note: Currently, the increasing frequency of resistant organisms is a limitation of the usefulness of all antibacterial agents, especially in the treatment of these urinary tract infections.

ACUTE OTITIS MEDIA: For the treatment of acute otitis media in children due to susceptible strains of *Haemophilus influenzae* or *Streptococcus pneumoniae* when in the judgment of the physician Septra offers some advantage over the use of other antimicrobial agents. To date, there are limited data on the safety of repeated use of Septra in children under two years of age. Septra is not indicated for prophylactic or prolonged administration in otitis media at any age.

ACUTE EXACERBATIONS OF CHRONIC BRONCHITIS IN ADULTS: For the treatment of acute exacerbations of chronic bronchitis due to susceptible strains of *Haemophilus influenzae* or *Streptococcus pneumoniae*, when in the judgment of the physician, Septra offers some advantage over the use of a single antimicrobial agent.

SHIGELLOSIS: For the treatment of enteritis caused by susceptible strains of *Shigella flexneri* and *Shigella sonnei* when antibacterial therapy is indicated.

PNEUMOCYSTIS CARINII PNEUMONITIS: Septra is also indicated in the treatment of documented *Pneumocystis carinii* pneumonitis.

Contraindications:
Hypersensitivity to trimethoprim or sulfonamides. Patients with documented megaloblastic anemia due to folate deficiency. Pregnancy at term and during the nursing period, because sulfonamides pass the placenta and are excreted in the milk and may cause kernicterus. Infants less than two months of age.

Warnings:
SEPTRA SHOULD NOT BE USED IN THE TREATMENT OF STREPTOCOCCAL PHARYNGITIS. Clinical studies have documented that patients with Group A β-hemolytic streptococcal tonsillopharyngitis have a greater incidence of bacteriologic failure when treated with Septra than do those patients treated with penicillin as evidenced by failure to eradicate this organism from the tonsillopharyngeal area. Deaths associated with the administration of sulfonamides have been reported from hypersensitivity reactions, agranulocytosis, aplastic anemia and other blood dyscrasias. Experience with trimethoprim alone is much more limited, but it has been reported to interfere with hematopoiesis in occasional patients. In elderly patients concurrently receiving certain diuretics, primarily thiazides, an increased incidence of thrombopenia with purpura has been reported.

The presence of clinical signs such as sore throat, fever, pallor, purpura or jaundice may be early indications of serious blood disorders. Complete blood counts should be done frequently in patients receiving Septra. If a significant reduction in the count of any formed blood element is noted, Septra should be discontinued.

Precautions:
General: Septra should be given with caution to patients with impaired renal or hepatic function, to those with possible folate deficiency and to those with severe allergy or bronchial asthma. In glucose-6-phosphate dehydrogenase-deficient individuals, hemolysis may occur. This reaction is frequently dose-related. Adequate fluid intake must be maintained in order to prevent crystalluria and stone formation. Urinalyses with careful microscopic examination and renal function tests should be performed during therapy, particularly for those patients with impaired renal function.

It has been reported that Septra may prolong the prothrombin time of patients who are receiving the anticoagulant warfarin. This interaction should be kept in mind when Septra is given to patients already on anticoagulant therapy, and the coagulation time should be reassessed.

Pregnancy: Teratogenic Effects: Pregnancy Category C. In rats, doses of 533 mg/kg sulfamethoxazole or 200 mg/kg trimethoprim produced teratological effects manifested mainly as cleft palates. The highest dose which did not cause cleft palates in rats was 512 mg/kg sulfamethoxazole or 192 mg/kg trimethoprim when administered separately. In two studies in rats, no teratology was observed when 512 mg/kg of sulfamethoxazole was used in combination with 128 mg/kg of trimethoprim. In one study, however, cleft palates were observed in one litter out of 9 when 355 mg/kg of sulfamethoxazole was used in combination with 88 mg/kg of trimethoprim.

In some rabbit studies, an overall increase in fetal loss (dead and resorbed and malformed conceptuses) was associated with doses of trimethoprim 6 times the human therapeutic dose.

While there are no large well-controlled studies on the use of trimethoprim plus sulfamethoxazole in pregnant women, Brumfitt and Pursell (Trimethoprim/Sulfamethoxazole in the Treatment of Bacteriuria in Women. J Inf Dis Suppl 128:S657-S663, 1973.) reported the outcome of 186 pregnancies during which the mother received either placebo or trimethoprim in combination with sulfamethoxazole. The incidence of congenital abnormalities was 4.5% (3 of 66) in those who received placebo and 3.3% (4 of 120) in those receiving trimethoprim plus sulfamethoxazole. There were no abnormalities in the 10 children whose mothers received the drug during the first trimester. In a separate survey, Brumfitt and Pursell also found no congenital abnormalities in 35 children whose mothers had received trimethoprim plus sulfamethoxazole at the time of conception or shortly thereafter.

Because trimethoprim plus sulfamethoxazole may interfere with folic acid metabolism, Septra should be used during pregnancy only if the potential benefit justifies the potential risk to the fetus.

Nonteratogenic Effects: See "CONTRAINDICATIONS" section.

Nursing Mothers: See "CONTRAINDICATIONS" section.

Adverse Reactions:
For completeness, all major reactions to sulfonamides and to trimethoprim are included below even though they may not have been with Septra.

Blood Dyscrasias: Agranulocytosis, aplastic anemia, megaloblastic anemia, thrombopenia, leukopenia, hemolytic anemia, purpura, hypoprothrombinemia and methemoglobinemia.

REPRESENTATIVE MINIMUM INHIBITORY CONCENTRATION VALUES FOR SEPTRA SUSCEPTIBLE ORGANISMS
(MIC-mcg/ml)

Bacteria	TMP Alone	SMX Alone	TMP/SMX (1:19) TMP	TMP/SMX (1:19) SMX
Escherichia coli	0.05–1.5	1.0 –245	0.05 –0.5	0.95 – 9.5
Proteus species (indole positive)	0.5 –5.0	7.35 –300	0.05 –1.5	0.95 –28.5
Proteus mirabilis	0.5 –1.5	7.35 – 30	0.05 –0.15	0.95 – 2.85
Klebsiella-Enterobacter	0.15–5.0	2.45 –245	0.05 –1.5	0.95 –28.5
Haemophilus influenzae	0.15–1.5	2.85 – 95	0.015 –0.15	0.285 – 2.85
Streptococcus pneumoniae	0.15–1.5	7.35 – 24.5	0.05 –0.15	0.95 – 2.85
Shigella flexneri†	<0.01–0.04	<0.16 –>320	<0.002 –0.03	0.04 –0.625
Shigella sonnei†	0.02–0.08	0.625 –>320	0.004 –0.06	0.08 –1.25

TMP = Trimethoprim   SMX = Sulfamethoxazole
†Rudoy, R.C., Nelson, J.D., Haltalin, K.C. *Antimicrobial Agents and Chemotherapy* 5:439–43, 1974.

Allergic Reactions: Erythema multiforme, Stevens-Johnson syndrome, generalized skin eruptions, epidermal necrolysis, urticaria, serum sickness, pruritus, exfoliative dermatitis, anaphylactoid reactions, periorbital edema, conjutival and scleral injection, photosensitization, arthralgia and allergic myocarditis.

Gastrointestinal Reactions: Glossitis, stomatitis, nausea, emesis, abdominal pains, hepatitis, diarrhea, pseudomembranous colitis and pancreatitis.

C.N.S. Reactions: Headache, peripheral neuritis, mental depression, convulsions, ataxia, hallucinations, tinnitus, vertigo, insomnia, apathy, fatigue, muscle weakness and nervousness.

Miscellaneous Reactions: Drug fever, chills, and toxic nephrosis with oliguria and anuria. Periarteritis nodosa and L.E. phenomenon have occurred.

The sulfonamides bear certain chemical similarities to some goitrogens, diuretics (acetazolamide and the thiazides) and oral hypoglycemic agents. Goiter production, diuresis and hypoglycemia have occurred rarely in patients receiving sulfonamides. Cross-sensitivity may exist with these agents. Rats appear to be especially susceptible to the goitrogenic effects of sulfonamides, and long-term administration has produced thyroid malignancies in the species.

Dosage and Administration: Not recommended for use in infants less than two months of age.

URINARY TRACT INFECTIONS AND SHIGELLOSIS IN ADULTS AND CHILDREN, ACUTE OTITIS MEDIA IN CHILDREN.

Adults: The usual adult dosage for the treatment of urinary tract infections is one Septra DS Tablet or two Septra Tablets or four teaspoonfuls (20 ml) Septra Suspension every 12 hours for 10 to 14 days. An identical daily dosage is used for 5 days in the treatment of shigellosis.

Children: The recommended dose for children with urinary tract infections or acute otitis media is 8 mg/kg trimethoprim and 40 mg/kg sulfamethoxazole per 24 hours, given in two divided doses every 12 hours for 10 days. In children weighing 88 lbs (40 kg) or more, the dosage is one Septra DS Tablet or two Septra Tablets every 12 hours for 10 days. An identical daily dosage is used for 5 days in the treatment of shigellosis. The following table is a guideline for the attainment of this dosage using Septra Tablets or Suspension.

Children: Two months of age or older

Weight		Dose—every 12 hours	
lb	kg	Teaspoonfuls	Tablets
22	10	1 (5 ml)	
44	20	2 (10 ml)	1
66	30	3 (15 ml)	1 ½
88	40	4 (20 ml)	2 (or 1 DS Tablet)

For patients with renal impairment:

Creatinine Clearance (ml/min)	Recommended Dosage Regimen
Above 30	Usual Standard Regimen
15–30	Half of the usual dosage regimen
Below 15	Use Not Recommended

Acute Exacerbations of Chronic Bronchitis in Adults: The usual adult dosage in the treatment of acute exacerbations of chronic bronchitis is one Septra DS tablet or two Septra tablets or four teaspoonfuls (20 ml) of Septra Suspension every 12 hours for 14 days.

PNEUMOCYSTIS CARINII **PNEUMONITIS:**
The recommended dosage for patients with documented *Pneumocystis carinii* pneumonitis is 20 mg/kg trimethoprim and 100 mg/kg sulfamethoxazole per 24 hours given in equally divided doses every 6 hours for 14 days. The following table is a guideline for the attainment of this dosage in children.

Weight		Dose—every 6 hours	
lb	kg	Teaspoonfuls	Tablets
18	8	1 (5 ml)	½
35	16	2 (10 ml)	1
53	24	3 (15 ml)	1 ½
70	32	4 (20 ml)	2 (or 1 DS Tablet)

How Supplied: TABLETS, containing 80 mg trimethoprim and 400 mg sulfamethoxazole—bottles of 100 and 500, tablets; unit dose pack of 100. Regular strength tablets bear identification, SEPTRA Y2B.
ORAL SUSPENSION, containing the equivalent of 40 mg trimethoprim and 200 mg sulfamethoxazole in each teaspoonful (5 ml), cherry flavored—bottles of 100 ml and 473 ml.
Also available in double strength, oval-shaped, pink, scored tablets containing 160 mg trimethoprim and 800 mg sulfamethoxazole—Compliance™ Pak of 20, bottles of 100 and 250 and unit dose pack of 100. Double strength tablets bear identification, SEPTRA DS O2C.

Tablets Shown in Product Identification Section, page 408

SUDAFED® COUGH SYRUP
[sū'dah-fēd"]
Decongestant/Cough Suppressant/Expectorant

(See PDR for Nonprescription Drugs)

SUDAFED® SYRUP/TABLETS
[sū'dah-fēd"]
(See PDR for Nonprescription Drugs)

SUDAFED® PLUS SYRUP/TABLETS
(See PDR for Nonprescription Drugs)

TABLOID® brand THIOGUANINE ℞
[tab'loid]
40 mg Scored Tablets

CAUTION: Tabloid brand thioguanine is a potent drug. It should not be used unless a diagnosis of acute nonlymphocytic leukemia has been adequately established and the responsible physician is knowledgeable in assessing response to chemotherapy.

Description: Tabloid brand thioguanine was synthesized and developed by Hitchings, Elion, and associates at the Wellcome Research Laboratories. It is one of a large series of purine analogues which interfere with nucleic acid biosynthesis, and has been found active against selective human neoplastic diseases.[1]

Thioguanine, known chemically as 2-amino-1,7-dihydro-6H-purine-6-thione, is an analogue of the nucleic acid constituent guanine, and is closely related structurally and functionally to Purinethol® (mercaptopurine). Its structural formula is:

Tabloid brand thioguanine is available in 40 mg scored tablets for oral administration.

Clinical Pharmacology: Clinical studies have shown that the absorption of an oral dose of thioguanine in man is incomplete and variable, averaging approximately 30% of the administered dose (range: 14–46%).[2,3] Following oral administration of ^{35}S-6-thioguanine, total plasma radioactivity reached a maximum at eight hours and declined slowly thereafter. Parent drug represented only a very small fraction of the total plasma radioactivity at any time, being virtually undetectable throughout the period of measurements. The oral administration of radiolabeled thioguanine revealed only trace quantities of parent drug in the urine. However, a methylated metabolite, 2-amino-6-methylthiopurine (MTG), appeared very early, rose to a maximum six to eight hours after drug administration, and was still being excreted after 12 to 22 hours. Radiolabeled sulfate appeared somewhat later than MTG but was the principal metabolite after eight hours. Thiouric acid and some unidentified products were found in the urine in small amounts.[3] Intravenous administration of ^{35}S-6-thioguanine disclosed a median plasma half-disappearance time of 80 minutes (range: 25–240 minutes) when the compound was given in single doses of 65 to 300 mg/m². Although initial plasma levels of thioguanine did correlate with the dose level, there was no correlation between the plasma half-disappearance time and the dose.[2]

Thioguanine is incorporated into the DNA and the RNA of human bone marrow cells. Studies with intravenous ^{35}S-6-thioguanine have shown that the amount of thioguanine incorporated into nucleic acids is more than 100 times higher after five daily doses than after a single dose. With the 5-dose schedule, from one-half to virtually all of the guanine in the residual DNA was replaced by thioguanine.[2] Tissue distribution studies of ^{35}S-6-thioguanine in mice showed only traces of radioactivity in brain after oral administration. No measurements have been made of thioguanine concentrations in human cerebrospinal fluid, but observations on tissue distribution in animals, together with the lack of CNS penetration by the closely related compound, mercaptopurine, suggest that thioguanine does not reach therapeutic concentrations in the CSF.

Monitoring of plasma levels of thioguanine during therapy is of questionable value.[3] There is technical difficulty in determining plasma concentrations, which are seldom greater than 1 to 2 micrograms per ml after a therapeutic oral dose. More significantly, thioguanine enters rapidly into the anabolic and catabolic pathways for purines, and the active intracellular metabolites have appreciably longer half-lives than the parent drug. The biochemical effects of a single dose of thioguanine are evident long after the parent drug has disappeared from plasma. Because of this rapid metabolism of thioguanine to active intracellular derivatives, hemodialysis would not be expected to appreciably reduce toxicity of the drug.

Thioguanine competes with hypoxanthine and guanine for the enzyme hypoxanthine-guanine phosphoribosyltransferase (HGPRTase) and is itself converted to 6-thioguanylic acid (TGMP). This nucleotide reaches high intracellular concentrations at therapeutic doses. TGMP interferes at several points with the synthesis of guanine nucleotides. It inhibits *de novo* purine biosynthesis by pseudo-feedback inhibition of glutamine-5-phosphoribosylpyrophosphate amidotransferase—the first enzyme unique to the *de novo* pathway for purine ribonucleotide synthesis. TGMP also inhibits the conversion of inosinic acid (IMP) to xanthylic acid (XMP) by competition for the enzyme, IMP dehydrogenase. At one time TGMP was felt to be a significant inhibitor of ATP:GMP phosphotransferase (guanylate kinase),[4] but recent results have shown this not to be so.[5]

Thioguanylic acid is further converted to the di- and tri-phosphates, thioguanosine diphosphate (TGDP) and thioguanosine triphosphate (TGTP) (as well as their 2′-deoxyribosyl analogues) by the same enzymes which metabolize guanine nucleotides.[6] Thioguanine nucleotides are incorporated into both the RNA and the DNA by phosphodiester linkages[2] and it has been argued that incorporation of such fraudulent bases contributes to the cytotoxicity of thioguanine.

Thus, thioguanine has multiple metabolic effects and at present it is not possible to designate one major site of action. Its tumor inhibitory properties may be due to one or more of its effects on (a) feedback inhibition of *de novo* purine synthesis; (b) inhibition of purine nucleotide interconversions;

Continued on next page

Burroughs Wellcome—Cont.

or (c) incorporation into the DNA and the RNA. The net consequence of its actions is a sequential blockade of the synthesis and utilization of the purine nucleotides.[4,6,7]

The catabolism of thioguanine and its metabolites is complex and shows significant differences between man and the mouse.[2,3] In both humans and mice, after oral administration of ^{35}S-6-thioguanine, urine contains virtually no detectable intact thioguanine. While deamination and subsequent oxidation to thiouric acid occurs only to a small extent in man, it is the main pathway in mice. The product of deamination by guanase, 6-thioxanthine, is inactive, having negligible antitumor activity. This pathway of thioguanine inactivation is not dependent on the action of xanthine oxidase and an inhibitor of that enzyme (such as allopurinol), will not block the detoxification of thioguanine even though the inactive 6-thioxanthine is normally further oxidized by xanthine oxidase to thiouric acid before it is eliminated. In man, methylation of thioguanine is much more extensive than in the mouse. The product of methylation, 2-amino-6-methylthiopurine, is also substantially less active and less toxic than thioguanine and its formation is likewise unaffected by the presence of allopurinol. Appreciable amounts of inorganic sulfate are also found in both murine and human urine, presumably arising from further metabolism of the methylated derivatives.

In some animal tumors, resistance to the effect of thioguanine correlates with the loss of HGPRTase activity and the resulting inability to convert thioguanine to thioguanylic acid. However, other resistance mechanisms, such as increased catabolism of TGMP by a nonspecific phosphatase, may be operative. Although not invariable, it is usual to find cross-resistance between thioguanine and its close analogue, Purinethol® (mercaptopurine).

Indications and Usage:

a) Acute Nonlymphocytic Leukemias: Tabloid brand thioguanine is indicated for remission induction, remission consolidation, and maintenance therapy of acute nonlymphocytic leukemias.[8,9] The response to this agent depends upon the age of the patient (younger patients faring better than older), and whether or not thioguanine is used in previously treated or previously untreated patients. Reliance upon thioguanine alone is seldom justified for initial remission induction of acute nonlymphocytic leukemias because combination chemotherapy including thioguanine results in more frequent remission induction and longer duration of remission than thioguanine alone.

b) Other Neoplasms: Tabloid brand thioguanine is not effective in chronic lymphocytic leukemia, Hodgkin's lymphoma, multiple myeloma, or solid tumors. Although thioguanine is one of several agents with activity in the treatment of the chronic phase of chronic myelogenous leukemia, more objective repsonses are observed with Myleran® (busulfan), and therefore busulfan is usually regarded as the preferred drug.

Contraindications: Thioguanine should not be used in patients whose disease has demonstrated prior resistance to this drug. In animals and man, there is usually complete cross-resistance between Purinethol® (mercaptopurine) and Tabloid® brand thioguanine.

Warnings: SINCE DRUGS USED IN CANCER CHEMOTHERAPY ARE POTENTIALLY HAZARDOUS, IT IS RECOMMENDED THAT ONLY PHYSICIANS EXPERIENCED WITH THE RISKS OF THIOGUANINE AND KNOWLEDGEABLE IN THE NATURAL HISTORY OF ACUTE NONLYMPHOCYTIC LEUKEMIAS ADMINISTER THIS DRUG.

The most consistent, dose-related toxicity is bone marrow suppression. This may be manifest by anemia, leukopenia, thrombocytopenia, or any combination of these. Any one of these findings may also reflect progression of the underlying disease. Since thioguanine may have a delayed effect, it is important to withdraw the medication temporarily at the first sign of an abnormally large fall in any of the formed elements of the blood.

It is recommended that evaluation of the hemoglobin concentration or hematocrit; total white blood cell count and differential count; and quantitative platelet count be obtained frequently while the patient is on thioguanine therapy. In cases where the cause of fluctuations in the formed elements in the peripheral blood is obscure, bone marrow examination may be useful for the evaluation of marrow status. The decision to increase, decrease, continue or discontinue a given dosage of thioguanine must be based not only on the absolute hematologic values, but also upon the rapidity with which changes are occurring. In many instances, particularly during the induction phase of acute leukemia, complete blood counts will need to be done more frequently in order to evaluate the effect of the therapy. The dosage of thioguanine may need to be reduced when this agent is combined with other drugs whose primary toxicity is myelosuppression.

Myelosuppression is often unavoidable during the induction phase of adult acute nonlymphocytic leukemias if remission induction is to be successful. Whether or not this demands modification or cessation of dosage depends both upon the response of the underlying disease and a careful consideration of supportive facilities (granulocyte and platelet transfusions) which may be available. Life-threatening infections and bleeding have been observed as consequences of thioguanine-induced granulocytopenia and thrombocytopenia. The effect of thioguanine on the immunocompetence of patients is unknown.

Pregnancy: *"Pregnancy Category D":* Drugs such as thioguanine are potential mutagens and teratogens. Thioguanine may cause fetal harm when administered to a pregnant woman. Thioguanine has been shown to be teratogenic in rats when given in doses five (5) times the human dose. When given to the rat on the 4th and 5th days of gestation, 13% of surviving placentas did not contain fetuses, and 19% of offspring were malformed or stunted. The malformations noted included generalized edema, cranial defects and general skeletal hypoplasia, hydrocephalus, ventral hernia, situs inversus, and incomplete development of the limbs.[10] There are no adequate and well-controlled studies in pregnant women. If this drug is used during pregnancy, or if the patient becomes pregnant while taking the drug, the patient should be apprised of the potential hazard to the fetus. Women of childbearing potential should be advised to avoid becoming pregnant.

Precautions:

General: Although the primary toxicity of thioguanine is myelosuppression, other toxicities have occasionally been observed, particularly when thioguanine is used in combination with other cancer chemotherapeutic agents.

A few cases of jaundice have been reported in patients with leukemia receiving thioguanine. Among these were two adult male patients and four children with acute myelogenous leukemia and an adult male with acute lymphocytic leukemia who developed veno-occlusive hepatic disease while receiving chemotherapy for their leukemia.[11,12] Six patients had received cytarabine prior to treatment with thioguanine, and some were receiving other chemotherapy in addition to thioguanine when they became symptomatic. While veno-occlusive hepatic disease has not been reported in patients treated with thioguanine alone, it is recommended that thioguanine be withheld if there is evidence of toxic hepatitis or biliary stasis, and that appropriate clinical and laboratory investigations be initiated to establish the etiology of the hepatic dysfunction. Deterioration in liver function studies during thioguanine therapy should prompt discontinuation of treatment and a search for an explanation of the hepatotoxicity.

Information For Patients: It is imperative that patients be instructed to report promptly the development of fever, sore throat, signs of local infection, bleeding from any site, or symptoms suggestive of anemia. Women of childbearing potential should be advised to avoid becoming pregnant.

Laboratory Tests: It is advisable to monitor liver function tests (serum transaminases, alkaline phosphatase, bilirubin) at weekly intervals when first beginning therapy and at monthly intervals thereafter. It may be advisable to perform liver function tests more frequently in patients with known pre-existing liver disease or in patients who are receiving thioguanine and other hepatotoxic drugs. Patients should be instructed to discontinue thioguanine immediately if clinical jaundice is detected. (See WARNINGS section).

Drug Interactions: There is usually complete cross-resistance between Purinethol® (mercaptopurine) and Tabloid® brand thioguanine.

Carcinogenesis, Mutagenesis, Impairment of Fertility: In view of its action on cellular DNA, thioguanine is potentially mutagenic and carcinogenic, and consideration should be given to the theoretical risk of carcinogenesis when thioguanine is administered. (See WARNINGS section)

Pregnancy: *Teratogenic Effects:* Pregnancy Category D. See WARNINGS section.

Nursing Mothers: It is not known whether this drug is excreted in human milk. Because of the potential for tumorigenicity shown for thioguanine, a decision should be made whether to discontinue nursing or to discontinue the drug, taking into account the importance of the drug to the mother.

Adverse Reactions: The most frequent adverse reaction to thioguanine is myelosuppression. The induction of complete remission of acute myelogenous leukemia usually requires combination chemotherapy in dosages which produce marrow hypoplasia.[13] Since consolidation and maintenance of remission are also effected by multiple drug regimens whose component agents cause myelosuppression, pancytopenia is observed in nearly all patients. Dosages and schedules must be adjusted to prevent life-threatening cytopenias whenever these adverse reactions are observed. Hyperuricemia frequently occurs in patients receiving thioguanine as a consequence of rapid cell lysis accompanying the antineoplastic effect. Adverse effects can be minimized by increased hydration, urine alkalinization, and the prophylactic administration of a xanthine oxidase inhibitor such as Zyloprim® (allopurinol). Unlike Purinethol® (mercaptopurine) and Imuran® (azathioprine), thioguanine may be continued in the usual dosage when allopurinol is used conjointly to inhibit uric acid formation.

Less frequent adverse reactions include nausea, vomiting, anorexia and stomatitis. Liver enzyme and other liver function studies are occasionally abnormal. If jaundice, hepatomegaly or anorexia with tenderness in the right hypochondrium occurs, thioguanine should be withheld until the exact etiology can be determined. There have been reports of veno-occlusive liver disease occuring in patients who received combination chemotherapy including thioguanine.[11,12] Intestinal necrosis and perforation have been reported also in patients who received multiple drug chemotherapy including thioguanine.

Overdosage: Signs and symptoms of overdosage may be immediate, such as nausea, vomiting, malaise, hypertension and diaphoresis; or delayed, such as myelosuppression and azotemia.[14] It is not known whether thioguanine is dialyzable. Hemodialysis is thought to be of marginal use due to the rapid intracellular incorporation of thioguanine into active metabolites with long persistence. The oral LD$_{50}$ of thioguanine was determined to be 823 mg/kg ± 50.73 mg/kg and 740 mg/kg ± 45.24 mg/kg for male and female rats respectively.[15] Symptoms of overdosage may occur after a single dose of as little as 2.0 to 3.0 mg/kg thioguanine. As much as 35 mg/kg has been given in a single oral dose with reversible myelosuppression observed. There is no known pharmacologic antagonist of thioguanine. The drug should be discontinued immediately if unintended toxicity occurs during treatment. Severe hematologic toxicity may require supportive therapy with platelet transfusions for bleeding, and granulocyte transfusions and antibiotics if sepsis is documented. If a patient is seen immediately following an accidental overdosage of the drug, it may be useful to induce emesis.

Dosage and Administration: Tabloid brand thioguanine is administered orally. The dosage which will be tolerated and effective varies according to the stage and type of neoplastic process being treated. Because the usual therapies for adult and childhood acute nonlymphocytic leukemias involve the use of thioguanine with other agents in combination, physicians responsible for administering these therapies should be experienced in the use of cancer chemotherapy and in the chosen protocol.

Ninety-six (59%) of one hundred sixty-three children with previously untreated acute nonlymphocytic leukemia obtained complete remission with a multiple drug protocol including thioguanine, prednisone, cytarabine, cyclophosphamide, and vincristine. Remission was maintained with daily thioguanine, four-day pulses of cytarabine and cyclophosphamide, and a single dose of vincristine every 28 days. The median duration of remission was 11.5 months.[8]

Fifty-three percent of previously untreated adults with acute nonlymphocytic leukemias attained remission following use of the combination of thioguanine and cytarabine according to a protocol developed at The Memorial Sloan-Kettering Cancer Center. A median duration of remission of 8.8 months was achieved with the multiple drug maintenance regimen which included thioguanine.[9]

On those occasions when single agent chemotherapy with thioguanine may be appropriate, the usual initial dosage for children and adults is approximately 2 mg/kg of body weight per day. If, after four weeks on this dosage, there is no clinical improvement and no leukocyte or platelet depression, the dosage may be cautiously increased to 3 mg/kg per day. The total daily dose may be given at one time.

The dosage of thioguanine used does not depend on whether or not the patient is receiving Zyloprim® (allopurinol); **this is in contradistinction to the dosage reduction which is mandatory when Purinethol® (mercaptopurine) or IMURAN® (azathioprine) is used simultaneously with allopurinol.**

How Supplied: Greenish-yellow, scored tablets containing 40 mg thioguanine, imprinted with "WELLCOME" and "U3B" on each tablet; in bottle of 25 (NDC-0081-0880-25). Store at 15°-25°C (59°-77°F) in a dry place.

References:
1. Hitchings GH, and Elion GB: The Chemistry and Biochemistry of Purine Analogs. *Ann NY Acad Sci* 60:195-199, 1954.
2. LePage GA, and Whitecar JP, Jr.: Pharmacology of 6-Thioguanine in Man. *Cancer Res* 31:1627-1631, 1971.
3. Elion GB: Biochemistry and Pharmacology of Purine Analogues. *Fed Proc* 26:898-904, 1967.
4. Miech RP, Parks RE, Jr. and Sartorelli AC: An Hypothesis on the Mechanism of Action of 6-thioguanine. *Biochem Pharmacol* 16:2222-2227, 1967.
5. Miller RL, Adamczyk DL, and Spector T: Reassessment of the Inter-Actions of Guanylate Kinase and 6-thioguanine 5'-phosphate. *Proc Am Assoc Cancer Res* 18:6, 1977. Abstract.
6. Paterson ARP, and Tidd DN: 6-thiopurines. In: *Antineoplastic and Immunosuppressive Agents*, Part II. (Edited by AC Sartorelli and DG Johns.) Berlin, Springer-Verlag, 384-403, 1975.
7. Nelson JA, Carpenter JW, Rose LN, and Adamson DJ: Mechanisms of Action of 6-thioguanine, 6-mercaptopurine, and 8-azaguanine. *Cancer Res* 35:2872-2878, 1975.
8. Chard RL, Finkelstein JZ, Sonley MJ, *et al*.: Increased Survival in Childhood Acute Nonlymphocytic Leukemia after Treatment with Prednisone, Cytosine Arabinoside, 6-thioguanine, Cyclophosphamide, and Oncovin (PATCO) Combination Chemotherapy. *Med Ped Oncol* 4:263-273, 1978.
9. Mertelsmann R, Drapkin RL, Gee TS, *et al*.: Treatment of Acute Nonlymphocytic Leukemia in Adults. *Cancer* 48:2136-2142, 1981.
10. Theiresch JB: Effect of 2-6 Diamino-purine (2-6 DP): 6 Chlorpurine (CIP) and Thioguanine (ThG) on Rat Litter *in utero*. *Proc Soc Exp Biol Med* 94:40-43, 1957.
11. Griner PF, Elbadawi A, and Packman CH: Veno-Occlusive Disease of the Liver After Chemotherapy of Acute Leukemia. *Ann Inter Med* 85:578-582, 1976.
12. Gill RA, Onstad GR, Cardamone, JM, *et al*.: Hepatic Veno-Occlusive Disease Caused by 6-thioguanine. *Ann Intern Med* 96:58-60, 1982.
13. Clarkson B, Dowling MD, Gee TS, *et al*.: Treatment of Acute Leukemia in Adults. *Cancer* 36:775-795, 1975.
14. Presant CA, Denes AE, Klein L, *et al*.: Phase I and Preliminary Phase II Observations of High-dose Intermittent 6-thioguanine. *Cancer Treat Rep* 64(10-11):1109-1113, 1980.
15. Unplublished data on file with Burroughs Wellcome Co.

Shown in Product Identification Section, page 408

VASOXYL® ℞
[văz″ŏx′ŭl]
(Methoxamine Hydrochloride)
INJECTION
20 mg in 1 ml

Description: Vasoxyl (Methoxamine Hydrochloride) Injection is a sterile solution for intramuscular or intravenous injection, made isotonic with sodium chloride. Each ml contains 20 mg methoxamine hydrochloride. Citric acid anhydrous 0.3% and sodium citrate 0.3% are added as buffers and potassium metabisulfite 0.1% is added as an antioxidant.

Methoxamine is a sympathomimetic amine. Chemically, methoxamine is α-(1-aminoethyl)-2,5-dimethoxybenzenemethanol hydrochloride. It is available as the hydrochloride in sterile aqueous solution for parenteral use.

The structural formula is as follows:

Actions: Vasoxyl (Methoxamine Hydrochloride) Injection is a vasopressor agent which produces a prompt and prolonged rise in blood pressure following parenteral administration. It is especially useful for maintaining blood pressure during operations under spinal anesthesia; it may also safely be used during general anesthesia.

The outstanding characteristic is potent, prolonged pressor action following parenteral administration. Unlike most pressor amines, there is no increase in cardiac rate but rather on occasions a decrease in rate develops as the blood pressure increases. This bradycardia is apparently caused by a carotid sinus reflex mediated over the vagus nerve. It is abolished by atropine.

The pressor action appears to be due primarily to peripheral vasoconstriction. Dripps has pointed out that evidence for direct action on blood vessels is provided by the observation of intense constriction along the course of a vein into which methoxamine has been injected. Taube and Fassett have shown that methoxamine increases central venous pressure. Methoxamine hydrochloride has the distinct advantage of being free of central stimulating action. This has been demonstrated by de Beer in laboratory studies as well as by Fassett in electroencephalogram tracings of patients receiving the drug. Pressor action without central stimulation may be especially desirable in patients undergoing surgery under spinal anesthesia.

Of special significance is the conclusion of Stutzman, Pettinga and Fruggiero that "Methoxamine does not increase the irritability of the cyclopropane-sensitized heart. It is a safe pressor agent for use during cyclopropane anesthesia." It has already been noted that it tends to slow the ventricular rate; large doses may produce bradycardia, but do not cause ventricular tachycardia, fibrillation, or an increased sinoauricular rate.

Finally, tachyphylaxis does not appear to be a factor clinically; Dripps states that he has never observed true tachyphylaxis to methoxamine.

Indications: For supporting, restoring or maintaining blood pressure during anesthesia (including cyclopropane anesthesia).

For terminating some episodes of paroxysmal supraventricular tachycardia.

Contraindications: Methoxamine is contraindicated as a combination with local anesthetics to prolong their action at local sites.

Precautions: The use of Vasoxyl (Methoxamine Hydrochloride) Injection is not a substitute for the replacement of blood, plasma, fluids and electrolytes which should promptly be restored when loss has occurred.

Caution should be observed when used closely following the parenteral injection of ergot alkaloids, to prevent an excessive rise in blood pressure. Caution should be exercised to avoid overdosage so that undesirably high blood pressure or excessive bradycardia will not occur. (Bradycardia may be abolished with atropine.) While 20 mg Vasoxyl (Methoxamine Hydrochloride) Injection intramuscularly has been used by some anesthesiologists, with favorable results, most studies indicate that 10 to 15 mg intramuscularly is adequate to give a satisfactory pressor response. A second dose should not be given until the previous one has had time to act (about 15 minutes). The intravenous route should be reserved for emergencies where a strong immediate pressor response is imperative, in which case not more than 5 mg may be given slowly.

Vasoxyl (Methoxamine Hydrochloride) Injection, like other vasopressor agents, should be used with care in patients with hyperthyroidism or severe hypertension. It is to be noted, however, that patients with hypertension may suffer greater or more serious fall in blood pressure than those with normal blood pressure when under spinal anesthesia, hence a pressor drug may be especially valuable properly used under these circumstances.

The possibility exists that the increase in peripheral resistance produced by methoxamine may produce or exacerbate heart failure associated with a diseased myocardium, due to the production of an increased workload.

Adverse Reactions: Methoxamine may on occasion produce sustained excessive blood pressure elevations with severe headache, pilomotor response, a desire to void and projectile vomiting, particularly with high dosage.

Dosage: (Methoxamine Hydrochloride) Injection is administered by either intramuscular or intravenous administration.

The usual intravenous dose of methoxamine for emergencies is 3 to 5 mg, injected slowly. Intravenous injection may be supplemented by intramuscular injections to provide a more prolonged effect. The usual intramuscular dose is 10 to 15 mg. This may be given shortly before or at the time of administering spinal anesthesia to prevent a fall in blood pressure. The tendency for the blood pressure to fall is greater with higher levels of spinal anesthesia, hence the dosage may be adjusted accordingly; 10 mg may be adequate at lower spinal levels while 15 to 20 mg may be required at high levels of spinal anesthesia. Repeated doses may be given if necessary but time should be allowed for the previous dose to act (see Precautions).

For purposes of correcting a fall in blood pressure an intramuscular injection of 10 to 15 mg methoxamine hydrochloride may be given depending upon the degree of fall. In cases where the systolic pressure falls to 60 mm or less, or whenever an emergency exists, an intravenous injection of 3 to 5 mg Vasoxyl (Methoxamine Hydrochloride) Injection is indicated. This may be accompanied by 10 to 15 mg intramuscularly to provide more prolonged effect.

Continued on next page

Burroughs Wellcome—Cont.

For preoperative and postoperative use in cases of only moderate hypotension 5 to 10 mg intramuscularly may be adequate. In paroxysmal supraventricular tachycardia the average dose is 10 mg intravenously injected slowly.

How Supplied: Vasoxyl (Methoxamine Hydrochloride) Injection 20 mg in 1 ml: 1 ml ampuls; boxes of 12.

VIROPTIC® OPHTHALMIC R
[vī-rŏp'tĭk"]
SOLUTION, 1%
(trifluridine) Sterile

Description: Viroptic® is the brand name for trifluridine (also known as trifluorothymidine, F_3TdR, F_3T), an antiviral drug for topical treatment of epithelial keratitis caused by Herpes simplex virus. The chemical name of trifluridine is 2'-deoxy-5-(trifluoromethyl)uridine.

Viroptic sterile ophthalmic solution contains 1% trifluridine in an aqueous solution with acetic acid and sodium acetate (buffers), sodium chloride, and thimerosal 0.001% (added as a preservative).

Clinical Pharmacology: Trifluridine is a fluorinated pyrimidine nucleoside with *in vitro* and *in vivo* activity against Herpes simplex virus, types 1 and 2 and vacciniavirus. Some strains of Adenovirus are also inhibited *in vitro*.

Trifluridine interferes with DNA synthesis in cultured mammalian cells. However, its antiviral mechanism of action is not completely known.

In vitro perfusion studies on excised rabbit corneas have shown that trifluridine penetrates the intact cornea as evidenced by recovery of parental drug and its major metabolite, 5-carboxy-2'-deoxyuridine, on the endothelial side of the cornea. Absence of the corneal epithelium enhances the penetration of trifluridine approximately two-fold.

Intraocular penetration of trifluridine occurs after topical instillation of Viroptic into human eyes. Decreased corneal integrity or stromal or uveal inflammation may enhance the penetration of trifluridine into the aqueous humor. Unlike the results of ocular penetration of trifluridine *in vitro*, 5-carboxy-2'-deoxyuridine was not found in detectable concentrations within the aqueous humor of the human eye.

Systemic absorption of trifluridine following therapeutic dosing with Viroptic appears to be negligible. No detectable concentrations of trifluridine or 5-carboxy-2'-deoxyuridine were found in the sera of adult healthy normal subjects who had Viroptic instilled into their eyes seven times daily for 14 consecutive days.

Indications and Usage: Viroptic (Trifluridine) Ophthalmic Solution, 1% is indicated for the treatment of primary keratoconjunctivitis and recurrent epithelial keratitis due to Herpes simplex virus, types 1 and 2. Viroptic is also effective in the treatment of epithelial keratitis that has not responded clinically to the topical administration of idoxuridine or when ocular toxicity or hypersensitivity to idoxuridine has occurred. In a smaller number of patients found to be resistant to topical vidarabine, Viroptic was also effective.

The clinical efficacy of Viroptic in the treatment of stromal keratitis and uveitis due to Herpes simplex virus or ophthalmic infections caused by vacciniavirus and Adenovirus has not been established by well-controlled clinical trials. Viroptic has not been shown to be effective in the prophylaxis of Herpes simplex virus keratoconjunctivitis and epithelial keratitis by well-controlled clinical trials. Viroptic is not effective against bacterial, fungal or chlamydial infections of the cornea or nonviral trophic lesions.

During controlled multicenter clinical trials, 92 of 97 (95%) patients (78 of 81 with dendritic and 14 of 16 with geographic ulcers) responded to Viroptic therapy as evidenced by complete corneal re-epithelialization within the 14 day therapy period. In these controlled studies, 56 of 75 (75%) patients (49 of 58 with dendritic and 7 of 17 with geographic ulcers) responded to idoxuridine therapy. The mean time to corneal re-epithelialization of dendritic ulcers (6 days) and geographic ulcers (7 days) was similar for both therapies. In other clinical studies, Viroptic was evaluated in the treatment of Herpes simplex virus keratitis in patients who were unresponsive or intolerant to the topical administration of idoxuridine or vidarabine. Viroptic was effective in 138 of 150 (92%) patients (109 of 114 with dendritic and 29 of 36 with geographic ulcers) as evidenced by corneal re-epithelialization. The mean time to corneal re-epithelialization was 6 days for patients with dendritic ulcers and 12 days for patients with geographic ulcers.

Contraindications: Viroptic (Trifluridine) Ophthalmic Solution, 1%, is contraindicated for patients who develop hypersensitivity reactions or chemical intolerance to trifluridine.

Warnings:
The recommended dosage and frequency of administration should not be exceeded (see Dosage and Administration).

Precautions:
General: Viroptic (Trifluridine) Ophthalmic Solution, 1% should be prescribed only for patients who have a clinical diagnosis of herpetic keratitis.

Viroptic may cause mild local irritation of the conjunctiva and cornea when instilled but these effects are usually transient.

Although documented *in vitro* viral resistance to trifluridine has not been reported following multiple exposure to Viroptic, the possibility exists of viral resistance development.

Drug Interactions: The following drugs have been administered topically to the eye and concurrently with Viroptic in a limited number of patients without apparent evidence of adverse interaction: antibiotics—chloramphenicol, erythromycin, polymyxin B sulfate, bacitracin, gentamicin sulfate, tetracycline HCl, sodium sulfacetamide, neomycin sulfate; steroids—dexamethasone, dexamethasone sodium phosphate, prednisolone acetate, prednisolone sodium phosphate, hydrocortisone, fluorometholone; and other ophthalmic drugs—atropine sulfate, scopolamine hydrobromide, naphazoline hydrochloride, cyclopentolate hydrochloride, homatropine hydrobromide, pilocarpine, 1-epinephrine hydrochloride, sodium chloride.

Carcinogenesis, Mutagenesis, Impairment of Fertility: *Mutagenic Potential.* Trifluridine has been shown to exert mutagenic, DNA damaging and cell transforming activities in various standard *in vitro* test systems, and clastogenic activity in *Vicia faba* cells.

Although the significance of these test results is not clear or fully understood, there exists the possibility that mutagenic agents may cause genetic damage in humans.

Oncogenic Potential. The oncogenic potential of trifluridine is unknown at this time. The oncogenic potential of trifluridine in rodents is being evaluated.

Pregnancy: The drug should not be prescribed for pregnant women unless the potential benefits outweigh the potential risks.

Teratogenic Potential: Kury and Crosby[1] found that trifluridine was teratogenic when injected directly into the yolk sac of developing chick embryos. Itoi *et al*[2] found that topical application of 1% trifluridine ophthalmic solution to the eyes of rabbits on days 6–18 of pregnancy produced no teratogenic effects. Trifluridine was not teratogenic when given subcutaneously to rats at doses up to 5.0 mg/kg/day although drug induced fetal toxicity (delayed ossification of portions of the skeletal system) was observed at the 2.5 mg/kg/day dose level. Trifluridine was not teratogenic when given subcutaneously to rabbits at doses up to 5.0 mg/kg/day. Drug induced fetal toxicity (delayed ossification of portions of the skeletal system) was observed at the 2.5 mg/kg/day dose level. A 1.0 mg/kg/day dose was considered to be a no effect level in both rats and rabbits. Based upon these findings in animals, it is unlikely that Viroptic would cause embryonic or fetal damage if given in the recommended ophthalmic dosage to pregnant women. A safe dose, however, has not been established for the human embryo or fetus.

Nursing Mothers: It is unlikely that trifluridine is excreted in human milk after ophthalmic instillation of Viroptic because of the relatively small dosage (<5.0 mg/day), its dilution in body fluids and its extremely short half-life (approximately 12 minutes). The drug should not be prescribed for nursing mothers unless the potential benefits outweigh the potential risks.

Adverse Reactions: The most frequent adverse reactions reported during controlled clinical trials were mild, transient burning or stinging upon instillation (4.6%) and palpebral edema (2.8%). Other adverse reactions in decreasing order of reported frequency were superficial punctate keratopathy, epithelial keratopathy, hypersensitivity reaction, stromal edema, irritation, keratitis sicca, hyperemia, and increased intraocular pressure.

Overdosage: Overdosage by ocular instillation is unlikely because any excess solution should be quickly expelled from the conjunctival sac.

Acute overdosage by accidental oral ingestion of Viroptic has not occurred. However, should such ingestion occur, the 75 mg dosage of trifluridine in a 7.5 ml bottle of Viroptic is not likely to produce adverse effects. Single intravenous doses of 15–30 mg/kg/day in children and adults with neoplastic disease produce reversible bone marrow depression as the only potentially serious toxic effect and only after 3–5 courses of therapy.[3] The acute oral LD_{50} in the mouse and rat was 4379 mg/kg or higher.

Dosage and Administration: Instill one drop of Viroptic Ophthalmic Solution, 1% onto the cornea of the affected eye every two hours while awake for a maximum daily dosage of nine drops until the corneal ulcer has completely re-epithelialized. Following re-epithelialization, treatment for an additional seven days of one drop every four hours while awake for a minimum daily dosage of five drops is recommended.

If there are no signs of improvement after seven days of therapy or complete re-epithelialization has not occurred after 14 days of therapy, other forms of therapy should be considered. Continuous administration of Viroptic for periods exceeding 21 days should be avoided because of potential ocular toxicity.

How Supplied: Viroptic Opthalmic Solution, 1% is supplied as a sterile ophthalmic solution in a plastic Drop-Dose® dispenser bottle of 7.5 ml. (NDC-0081-0968-02)

Store under refrigeration 2° to 8°C (36° to 46°F)

Animal Pharmacology and Animal Toxicology: Corneal wound healing studies in rabbits showed that Viroptic did not significantly retard closure of epithelial wounds. However, mild toxic changes such as intracellular edema of the basal cell layer, mild thinning of the overlying epithelium and reduced strength of stromal wounds were observed.

Whereas instillation of Viroptic into rabbit eyes during a subchronic toxicity study produced some degree of corneal epithelial thinning, a 12-month chronic toxicity study in rabbits in which Viroptic was instilled into eyes in intermittent, multiple, full-therapy courses showed no drug related changes in the cornea.

DoD NSN 6505-01-142-8314

References:
1. Kury, G. and R.J. Crosby—The teratogenic effect of 5-trifluoromethyl-2'-deoxyuridine in chicken embryos. *Toxicol. Appl. Pharmacol.* 1/(1):72–80, 1967.
2. Itoi, M., J.W. Gefter, N. Kaneko, Y. Ishii, R.M. Ramer and A.R. Gasset—Teratogenicities of ophthalmic drugs. I. Antiviral ophthalmic drugs. *Arch. Ophthalmol.* 93(1):46–51, 1975.
3. Ansfield, F.J. and G. Ramirez—Phase I and II Studies of 2'-deoxy-5-(trifluoromethyl)-uridine (NSC-75520). *Cancer Chemother. Rep.* (Pt. 1) 55(2):205–208, 1971.

WELLCOVORIN® INJECTION ℞
[wĕl″ kō-vor′ ĭn]
(Leucovorin Calcium)

Description: Wellcovorin® (leucovorin calcium) Injection, a sterile aqueous solution for intramuscular or intravenous administration, contains 5 mg leucovorin per ml, as the calcium salt of N-[p-[[(2-amino-5-formyl-1,4,5,6,7,8-hexahydro-4-oxo-6-pteridinyl) methyl]amino]benzoyl]-L-glutamic acid. This is the equivalent to 5.40 mg of anhydrous leucovorin calcium. The vehicle contains methylparaben 0.08% and propylparaben 0.02% added as preservatives; hydrochloric acid or sodium hydroxide q.s. to adjust the pH to approximately 7.8 and water for injection, q.s.

Leucovorin is a water soluble vitamin in the folate group; it is useful as an anitdote to drugs which act as folic acid antagonists. The structural formula of leucovorin calcium (which normally exists as a hydrate, 8% to 15% water) is:

Clinical Pharmacology: Leucovorin is a mixture of the diastereoisomers of the 5-formyl derivative of tetrahydrofolic acid. The biologically active component of the mixture is the (-)-L-isomer, known as *Citrovorum factor*, or (-)-folinic acid. Leucovorin does *not* require reduction by the enzyme dihydrofolate reductase in order to participate in reactions utilizing folates as a source of "one-carbon" moieties. Following parenteral administration, leucovorin rapidly enters the general body pool of reduced folates[1]. The increase in plasma and serum folate activity (determined microbiologically with *Lactobacillus casei*) seen after parenteral administration of leucovorin is predominantly due to 5-methyl-tetrahydrofolate.[1,2,3,4,5]

Twenty normal men were given a single, intramuscular (gluteus maximus) 15 mg dose (7.5 mg/m²) of leucovorin calcium and serum folate concentrations were assayed with *L casei*[6]. Mean values observed (± one standard error) were:[4]
a) Time to peak serum folate concentration: 0.71 ± .09 hrs.,
b) Peak serum folate concentration achieved: 241 ± 17 ng/ml,
c) Serum folate half-disappearance time: 3.7 hours.

Intragluteally administered leucovorin yielded areas under the serum folate concentration-time curves (AUC's) that were 8 percent less than an equal amount of leucovorin administered in the deltoid muscle, and 12% less than with an intravenous injection.

Indications and Usage: Wellcovorin (leucovorin calcium) Injection is indicated to diminish the toxicity and counteract the effect of inadvertently administered overdosages of folic acid antagonists. (See Warnings)

Contraindications: Leucovorin is improper therapy for pernicious anemia and other megaloblastic anemias secondary to the lack of vitamin B_{12}. A hematologic remission may occur while neurologic manifestations remain progressive.

Warnings: In the treatment of accidental overdosage of folic acid antagonists, leucovorin should be administered as promptly as possible. As the time interval between antifolate administration (e.g. methotrexate) and leucovorin rescue increases, leucovorin's effectiveness in counteracting hematologic toxicity diminishes.

Precautions:
General: Following chemotherapy with folic acid antagonists, parenteral administration of leucovorin is preferable to oral dosing if there is a possibility that the patient may vomit and not absorb the leucovorin. In the presence of pernicious anemia a hematologic remission may occur while neurologic manifestations remain progressive.

Pregnancy: Teratogenic Effects: Pregnancy Category C. Animal reproduction studies have not been conducted with Wellcovorin. It is also not known whether Wellcovorin can cause fetal harm when administered to a pregnant woman or can affect reproduction capacity. Wellcovorin should be given to a pregnant woman only if clearly needed.

Nursing Mothers: It is not known whether this drug is excreted in human milk. Because many drugs are excreted in human milk, caution should be exercised when Wellcovorin is administered to a nursing mother.

Adverse Reactions: Allergic sensitization has been reported following both oral and parenteral administration of folic acid.

Overdosage: Excessive amounts of leucovorin may nullify the chemotherapeutic effect of folic acid antagonists.

Dosage and Administration: Wellcovorin Injection is intended for intramuscular or intravenous injection. Leucovorin is a specific antidote for the hematopoietic toxicity of methotrexate and other strong inhibitors of the enzyme dihydrofolate reductase. Leucovorin rescue of high-dose methotrexate therapy is usally begun within 24 hours of administration. A conventional leucovorin rescue dosage schedule is 10 mg/m² I.M. or I.V. followed by 10 mg/m² orally every six hours for seventy-two hours. If, however, at 24 hours following methotrexate administration the serum creatinine is 50% or greater than the pretreatment serum creatinine, the leucovorin dose should be immediately increased to 100 mg/m² every three hours until the serum methotrexate level is below 5×10^{-8}.[7,8]

The recommended dose of leucovorin to counteract hematologic toxicity from folic acid antagonists with less affinity for mammalian dihydrofolate reductase than methotrexate (i.e. trimethoprim, pyrimethamine) is a substantially less and 5 to 15 mg of leucovorin per day has been recommended by some investigators.[9,10,11]

How Supplied: Wellcovorin® Injection is available in ampuls containing 5 mg leucovorin per ml, as a calcium salt.
1 ml amber ampuls, Box of 12 (NDC-0081-0633-15).
5 ml amber ampuls, Box of 10 (NDC-0081-0633-10).
Store at 15°-30°C (59°-86°F).
Also available in 5 mg tablets, bottles of 100, and in 25 mg tablets, bottles of 25.

References:
1. Nixon PF and Bertino JR: Effective Absorption and Utilization of Oral Formyltetrahydrofolate in Man. N Engl J Med 286(4): 175–179, Jan. 27, 1972.
2. Baker H, Frank O, Feingold S et al: The Fate of Orally and Parenterally Administered Folates. Am J Clin Nutr 17:88–95, 1965.
3. Mehta BM, Gisolfi AL, Hutchison DJ, Nirenberg A, Kellick MG and Rosen G: Serum Distribution of Citrovorum Factor and 5-methyltetrahydrofolate Following Oral and I.M. Administration of Calcium Leucovorin in Normal Adults. Cancer Treat Rep 62(3): 345–350, Mar. 1978.
4. Data on file, Medical Division, Burroughs Wellcome Co., Research Triangle Park, N.C. 27709, USA.
5. Whitehead VM, Pratt R, Viallet A and Cooper BA: Intestinal Conversion of Folinic Acid to 5-methyltetrahydrofolate in Man. Br J Haematol 22 63–72, 1972.
6. Herbert V: Aseptic Addition of *Lactobacillus casei* Assay of Folate Activity in Human Serum. J Clin Path 19: 12–16, 1966.
7. Bleyer WA: The Clinical Pharmacology of Methotrexate. Cancer, 41(1): 36–51, 1978.
8. Frei E, Blum RH, Pitman SW, et al: High Dose Methotrexate with Leucovorin Rescue: Rationale and Spectrum of Antitumor Activity. Am J Med, 68: 370–376, 1980.
9. Golde DW, Bersch N, Quan SG: Trimethoprim and Sulphamethoxazole Inhibition of Haematopoiesis *in vitro*. Br J Haematol, 40(3): 363–367, 1978.
10. Steinberg SE, Campbell CL, Rabinovitch PS, et al: The Effect of Trimethoprim/Sulfamethoxazole on Friend Erythroleukemia Cells. Blood, 55(3): 501–504, 1980.
11. Mahmoud AAF and Warren KS: Algorithms in the Diagnosis and Management of Exotic Disease. XX. Toxoplasmosis. J Infect Dis, 135(3): 493–496, 1977.

WELLCOVORIN® TABLETS ℞
[wĕl″ kō-vor′ ĭn]
(Leucovorin Calcium)

Description: Wellcovorin (leucovorin calcium) Tablets contain either 5 mg or 25 mg leucovorin as the calcium salt of N-[p-[[(2-amino-5-formyl-1,4,5,6,7,8-hexahydro-4-oxo-6-pteridinyl) - methyl] amino]benzoyl]-L-glutamic acid. This is equivalent to 5.40 mg or 27.01 mg of anhydrous leucovorin calcium.

Leucovorin is a water soluble vitamin in the folate group; it is useful as an antidote to drugs which act as folic acid antagonists. These tablets are intended for oral administration only. The structural formula of leucovorin clacium (which normally exists as a hydrate, 8% to 15% water) is:

Clinical Pharmacology: Leucovorin is a mixture of the diastereoisomers of the 5-formyl derivative of tetrahydrofolic acid. The biologically active component of the mixture is the (-)-L-isomer, known as *Citrovorum factor*, or (-)-folinic acid. Leucovorin does *not* require reduction by the enzyme dihydrofolate reductase in order to participate in reactions utilizing folates as a source of "one-carbon" moieties. Following oral administration, leucovorin is rapidly absorbed and enters the general body pool of reduced folates.[1] The increase in plasma and serum folate activity (determined microbiologically with *Lactobacillus casei*) seen after oral administration of leucovorin is predominantly due to 5-methyltetrhydrofolate.[1,2,3,4,5]

Twenty normal men were given a single, oral 15 mg dose (7.5 mg/m²) of leucovorin calcium and serum folate concentrations were assayed with *L casei*.[6] Mean values observed (± one standard error) were:[4]
a) Time to peak serum folate concentration: 1.72 ± 0.08 hrs.,
b) Peak serum folate concentration achieved: 268 ± 18 ng/ml,
c) Serum folate half-disappearance time: 3.5 hours.

Oral tablets yielded areas under the serum folate concentration-time curves (AUC's) that were 12% greater than equal amounts of leucovorin given intramuscularly and equal to the same amounts given intravenously.

Indications and Usage: Wellcovorin (leucovorin calcium) is indicated for the prophylaxis and treatment of undesired hematopoietic effects of folic acid antagonists (see WARNINGS).

Contraindications: Leucovorin is improper therapy for pernicious anemia and other megaloblastic anemias secondary to the lack of vitamin B_{12}. A hematologic remission may occur while neurologic manifestations remain progressive.

Warnings In the treatment of accidental overdosage of folic acid antagonists, leucovorin should be administered as promptly as possible. As the time interval between antifolate administration (e.g. methotrexate) and leucovorin rescue increases, leucovorin's effectiveness in counteracting hematologic toxicity diminishes.

Precautions:
General: Following chemotherapy with folic acid antagonists, parenteral administration of leucovorin is preferable to oral dosing if there is a possibility that the patient may vomit and not absorb the leucovorin. In the presence of pernicious anemia a hematologic remission may occur while neurologic

Continued on next page

Burroughs Wellcome—Cont.

manifestations remain progressive. Leucovorin has no effect on other toxicities of methotrexate, such as the nephrotoxicity resulting from drug precipitation in the kidney.
Drug Interactions: Folic acid in large amounts may counteract the antiepileptic effect of phenobarbital, phenytoin and primidone, and increase the frequency of seizures in susceptible children.
Pregnancy: *Teratogenic Effects:* Pregnancy Category C. Animal reproduction studies have not been conducted with Wellcovorin. It is also not known whether Wellcovorin can cause fetal harm when administered to a pregnant woman or can affect reproduction capacity. Wellcovorin should be given to a pregnant woman only if clearly needed.
Nursing Mothers: It is not known whether this drug is excreted in human milk. Because many drugs are excreted in human milk, caution should be exercised when Wellcovorin is administered to a nursing mother.
Pediatric Use: See "Drug Interactions".
Adverse Reactions: Allergic sensitization has been reported following both oral and parenteral administration of folic acid.
Overdosage: Excessive amounts of luecovorin may nullify the chemotherapeutic effect of folic acid antagonists.
Dosage and Administration: Leucovorin is a specific antidote for the hematopoietic toxicity of methotrexate and other strong inhibitors of the enzyme dihydrofolate reductase. Leucovorin rescue must begin within 24 hours of antifolate administration. A conventional leucovorin rescue dosage schedule is 10 mg/m^2 orally or parenterally followed by 10 mg/m^2 orally every six hours for seventy-two hours. If, however, at 24 hours following methotrexate administration the serum creatinine is 50% or greater than the premethotrexate serum creatinine, the leucovorin dose should be immediately increased to 100 mg/m^2 every three hours until the serum methotrexate level is below 5×10^{-8}M.[7,8]
The recommended dose of leucovorin to counteract hematologic toxicity from folic acid antagonists with less affinity for mammalian dihydrofolate reductase than methotrexate (i.e. trimethoprim, pyrimethamine) is substantially less and 5 to 15 mg of leucovorin per day has been recommended by some investigators.[9,10,11]
How Supplied: 5 mg (off-white) tablets containing 5 mg leucovorin as the calcium salt imprinted with "WELLCOVORIN" and "R3C"; bottle of 100 (NDC-0081-0631-55).

25 mg (peach) scored tablets containing 25 mg leucovorin as the calcium salt imprinted with "WELLCOVORIN" and "T3C"; bottle of 25 (NDC-0081-0632-25).

Store at 15°–30°C (59°–86°F) in a dry place and protect from light and moisture.
Also available: Wellcovorin Injection in 1 ml and 5 ml ampuls each containing 5 mg per ml.

References:
1. Nixon PF and Bertino JR; Effective Absorption and Utilization of Oral Formyltetrahydrofolate in Man. *N Engl J Med* 286(4):175–179, Jan. 27, 1972.
2. Ratanasthien K, Blair JA, Leeming RJ, Cooke WT and Melikian V: Folates in Human Serum. *J Clin Pathol* 27:875–879, 1974.
3. Mehta BM, Gisolfi AL, Hutchison DJ, Nirenberg A, Kellick MG and Rosen G: Serum Distribution of Citrovorum Factor and 5-methyltetrahydrofolate Following Oral and I.M. Administration of Calcium Leucovorin in Normal Adults. *Cancer Treat Rep* 62(3):345–350. Mar. 1978.
4. Data on file, Medical Division, Burroughs Wellcome Co., Research Triangle Park, N.C. 27709, USA.
5. Whitehead VM, Pratt R, Viallet A and Cooper BA: Intestinal Conversion of Folinic Acid to 5-methyltetrahydrofolate in Man. *Br J Haematol* 22:63–72, 1972.
6. Herbert V: Aseptic Addition for *Lactobacillus casei* Assay of Folate Activity in Human Serum. *J Clin Path* 19:12–16, 1966.
7. Bleyer WA: The Clinical Pharmacology of Methotrexate. *Cancer:*41(1):36–51, 1978.
8. Frei E, Blum RH, Pitman SW, *et al:* High Dose Methotrexate with Leucovorin Rescue: Rationale and Spectrum of Antitumor Activity. *Am J Med.* 68:370–376, 1980.
9. Golde DW, Bersch N, Quan SG: Trimethoprim and Sulphamethoxazole Inhibition of Haematopoiesis *in Vitro. Br J Haematol,* 40(3):363–367, 1978.
10. Steinberg SE, Campbell CL, Rabinovitch PS, *et al:* The Effect of Trimethoprim/Sulfamethoxazole on Friend Erythroleukemia Cells. *Blood,* 55(3):501–504, 1980.
11. Mahmoud AAF and Warren KS: Algorithms in the Diagnosis and Management of Exotic Disease. XX. Toxoplasmosis. *J Infect Dis.* 135(3):493–496, 1977.

Shown in Product Identification Section, page 408

ZOVIRAX® (Acyclovir) ℞
[zō″ vī′ răx]
Ointment 5%

Description: Zovirax is the brand name for acyclovir, an antiviral drug against herpes viruses. Zovirax Ointment 5% is a formulation for topical administration. Each gram of Zovirax Ointment 5% contains 50 mg of acyclovir in a polyethylene glycol (PEG) base.
The chemical name of acyclovir is 9-[(2-hydroxyethoxy)methyl]guanine.
Acyclovir is a white, crystalline powder with a molecular weight of 225 Daltons, and a maximum solubility in water of 1.3 mg/ml.
Clinical Pharmacology: Acyclovir is a synthetic acyclic purine nucleoside analogue with *in vitro* inhibitory activity against Herpes simplex types 1 and 2 (HSV-1 and HSV-2), varicella-zoster, Epstein-Barr and cytomegalovirus. In cell cultures, the inhibitory activity of acyclovir for Herpes simplex virus is highly selective. Cellular thymidine kinase does not effectively utilize acyclovir as a substrate. Herpes simplex virus-coded thymidine kinase, however, converts acyclovir into acyclovir monophosphate, a nucleotide. The monophosphate is further converted into diphosphate by cellular guanylate kinase and into triphosphate by a number of cellular enzymes.[1] Acyclovir triphosphate interferes with Herpes simplex virus DNA polymerase and inhibits viral DNA replication. Acyclovir triphosphate also inhibits cellular α-DNA polymerase but to a lesser degree. *In vitro,* acyclovir triphosphate can be incorporated into growing chains of DNA by viral DNA polymerase and to a much smaller extent by cellular α-DNA polymerase.[2] When incorporation occurs, the DNA chain is terminated.[3] Acyclovir is preferentially taken up and selectively converted to the active triphosphate form by herpesvirus-infected cells. Thus, acyclovir is much less toxic *in vitro* for normal uninfected cells because: 1) less is taken up; 2) less is converted to the active form; 3) cellular α-DNA polymerase is less sensitive to the effects of the active form.
The relationship between *in vitro* susceptibility of Herpes simplex virus to antiviral drugs and clinical response has not been established. The techniques and cell culture types used for determining *in vitro* susceptibility may influence the results obtained. Using a quantitative assay to determine the acyclovir concentration producing 50% inhibition of viral cytopathic effect (ID$_{50}$), 28 HSV-1 clinical isolates had a mean ID$_{50}$ of 0.17 μg/ml and 32 HSV-2 clinical isolates had a mean ID$_{50}$ of 0.46 μg/ml.* Results from other studies using different assays have yielded mean ID$_{50}$ values for clinical HSV-1 isolates of 0.018, 0.03 and 0.043 μg/ml and for clinical HSV-2 isolates of 0.027, 0.36 and 0.03 μg/ml, respectively.[4,5,6]
Two clinical pharmacology studies were performed with Zovirax Ointment 5% in adult immunocompromised patients, at risk of developing mucocutaneous Herpes simplex virus infections or with localized varicella-zoster infections. These studies were designed to evaluate the dermal tolerance, systemic toxicity and percutaneous absorption of acyclovir. In one of these studies, which included 16 inpatients, the complete ointment or its vehicle were randomly administered in a dose of 1 cm strips (25 mg acyclovir) four times a day for seven days to an intact skin surface area of 4.5 square inches. No local intolerance, systemic toxicity or contact dermatitis were observed. In addition, no drug was detected in blood and urine by radioimmunoassay (sensitivity, 0.01 μg/ml).
The other study included eleven patients with localized varicella-zoster. In this uncontrolled study, acyclovir was detected in the blood of 9 patients and in the urine of all patients tested. Acyclovir levels in plasma ranged from <0.01 to 0.28 μg/ml in eight patients with normal renal function, and from <0.01 to 0.78 μg/ml in one patient with impaired renal function. Acyclovir excreted in the urine ranged from <0.02 to 9.4 percent of the daily dose. Therefore, systemic absorption of acyclovir after topical application is minimal.
Indications And Usage: Zovirax (Acyclovir) Ointment 5% is indicated in the management of initial herpes genitalis and in limited nonlife-threatening mucocutaneous Herpes simplex virus infections in immunocompromised patients. In clinical trials of initial herpes genitalis, Zovirax Ointment 5% has shown a decrease in healing time and in some cases a decrease in duration of viral shedding and duration of pain. In studies in immunocompromised patients with mainly herpes labialis, there was a decrease in duration of viral shedding and a slight decrease in duration of pain. By contrast, in studies of recurrent herpes genitalis and of herpes labialis in nonimmunocompromised patients, there was no evidence of clinical benefit; there was some decrease in duration of viral shedding.
Diagnosis: Whereas cutaneous lesions associated with Herpes simplex infections are often characteristic, the finding of multinucleated giant cells in smears prepared from lesion exudate or scrapings may assist in the diagnosis.[7] Positive cultures for Herpes simplex virus offer a reliable means for confirmation of the diagnosis. In genital herpes, appropriate examinations should be performed to rule out other sexually transmitted diseases.
Contraindications: Zovirax Ointment 5% is contraindicated for patients who develop hypersensitivity or chemical intolerance to the components of the formulation.
Warnings: Zovirax Ointment 5% is intended for cutaneous use only and should not be used in the eye.
Precautions:
General: The recommended dosage, frequency of applications, and length of treatment should not be exceeded (see DOSAGE AND ADMINISTRATION). There exist no data which demonstrate that the use of Zovirax Ointment 5% will either prevent transmission of infection to other persons or prevent recurrent infections when applied in the absence of signs and symptoms. Zovirax Ointment 5% should not be used for the prevention of recurrent HSV infections. Although clinically significant viral resistance associated with the use of Zovirax Ointment 5% has not been observed, this possibility exists.
Drug Interactions: Clinical experience has identified no interactions resulting from topical or systemic administration of other drugs concomitantly with Zovirax Ointment 5%.
Carcinogenesis, Mutagenesis, Impairment of Fertility: Acyclovir was tested in lifetime bioassays in rats and mice at single daily doses of 50, 150 and 450 mg/kg/day given by gavage. These studies showed no statistically significant difference in the incidence of benign and malignant tumors produced in drug-treated as compared to control animals, nor did acyclovir induce the occurrence of tumors earlier in drug-treated animals as compared to controls. In 2 *in vitro* cell transformation assays, used to provide preliminary assessment of potential oncogenicity in advance of these more definitive lifetime bioassays in rodents, conflicting results were obtained. Acyclovir was positive at the highest dose used in one system and the result-

ing morphologically transformed cells formed tumors when inoculated into immunosuppressed, syngeneic, weanling mice. Acyclovir was negative in another transformation system.

No chromosome damage was observed at maximum tolerated parenteral doses of 100 mg/kg acyclovir in rats or Chinese hamsters; higher doses of 500 and 1000 mg/kg were clastogenic in Chinese hamsters. In addition, no activity was found in a dominant lethal study in mice. In 9 of 11 microbial and mammalian cell assays, no evidence of mutagenicity was observed. In 2 mammalian cell assays (human lymphocytes and L5178Y mouse lymphoma cells *in vitro*), positive response for mutagenicity and chromosomal damage occurred, but only at concentrations at least 1000 times the plasma levels achieved in man following topical application.

Acyclovir does not impair fertility or reproduction in mice at oral doses up to 450 mg/kg/day or in rats at subcutaneous doses up to 25 mg/kg/day. In rabbits given a high dose of acyclovir (50 mg/kg/day, s.c.), there was a statistically significant decrease in implantation efficiency.

Pregnancy: *Teratogenic Effects. Pregnancy Category C.* Acyclovir has been known to cause a statistically significant decrease in implantation efficiency in rabbits, when given at subcutaneous doses providing mean plasma levels of drug 2.2 times those expected from use in patients with normal renal function.

Reproduction studies were negative for impairment of fertility or harm to the fetus in mice given oral doses, and in rats given subcutaneous doses providing mean plasma levels of drug 84 times and 4 times (respectively) greater than those expected from use in patients with normal renal function. Acyclovir was not teratogenic after subcutaneous administration of up to 50 mg/kg/day during the period of organogenesis in rats and rabbits; doses up to 450 mg/kg given daily by gavage to mice were not teratogenic. There are, however, no adequate and well-controlled studies in pregnant women. Acyclovir should be used during pregnancy only if the potential benefit justifies the potential risk to the fetus.

Nursing Mothers: It is not known whether this drug is excreted in human milk. Because many drugs are excreted in human milk, caution should be exercised when Zovirax is administered to a nursing woman.

Adverse Reactions: Because ulcerated genital lesions are characteristically tender and sensitive to any contact or manipulation, patients may experience discomfort upon application of ointment. In the controlled clinical trials, mild pain (including transient burning and stinging) was reported by 103 (28.3%) of 364 patients treated with acyclovir and by 115 (31.1%) of 370 patients treated with placebo; treatment was discontinued in 2 of these patients. Other local reactions among acyclovir-treated patients included pruritis in 15 (4.1%), rash in 1 (0.3%) and vulvitis in 1 (0.3%). Among the placebo-treated patients, pruritus was reported by 17 (4.6%) and rash by 1 (0.3%).

In all studies, there was no significant difference between the drug and placebo group in the rate or type of reported adverse reactions nor were there any differences in abnormal clinical laboratory findings.

Overdosage: Overdosage by topical application of Zovirax Ointment 5% is unlikely because of limited transcutaneous absorption (see Clinical Pharmacology).

Dosage And Administration: Apply sufficient quantity to adequately cover all lesions every 3 hours 6 times per day for 7 days. The dose size per application will vary depending upon the total lesion area but should approximate a one-half inch ribbon of ointment per 4 square inches of surface area. A finger cot or rubber glove should be used when applying Zovirax to prevent autoinoculation of other body sites and transmission of infection to other persons. **Therapy should be initiated as early as possible following onset of signs and symptoms.**

How Supplied: Zovirax Ointment 5% is supplied in 15 g tubes (NDC 0081-0993-94). Each gram contains 50 mg acyclovir in a polyethylene glycol base. Store at 15°–25°C (59°–77°F) in a dry place.

Animal Pharmacology And Animal Toxicology: Topical treatment of guinea pigs with 10% acyclovir in polyethylene glycol ointment for three weeks did not result in cutaneous irritation or systemic toxicity. Also, a wide variety of animal tests by parenteral routes demonstrated that acyclovir has a low order of toxicity. Acyclovir did not cause dermal sensitization in guinea pigs.

References
1. Miller WH and Miller RL. J Biol Chem 255(15):7204–7207, 1980.
2. Furman PA et al. J Virol 32(1):72–77, 1979.
3. Derse D et al. J Biol Chem 256(22): 11447–11451, 1981.
4. Collins P and Bauer DJ. J Antimicrob Chemother 5:431–436, 1979.
5. Crumpacker CS et al. Antimicrob Agents Chemother 15:642–645, 1979.
6. De Clercq E et al. J Infect Dis 141:563–574, 1980.
7. Naib ZM et al. Cancer Res 33:1452–1463, 1973.
*Data on file at Burroughs Wellcome Co.

U.S. Patent No. 4199574

ZOVIRAX® Sterile Powder ℞
[zō″ vī′răx]
(Acyclovir Sodium)
FOR INTRAVENOUS INFUSION ONLY

Description: Zovirax is the brand name for acyclovir, an antiviral drug active against herpesviruses. Zovirax Sterile Powder is a formulation for intravenous administration. Each vial of Zovirax Sterile Powder contains 549 mg of sterile lyophilized acyclovir sodium equivalent to 500 mg of acyclovir.

The chemical name of acyclovir sodium is 9-[(2-hydroxyethoxy)methyl]guanine sodium; it has the following structural formula:

Acyclovir sodium is a white, crystalline powder with a molecular weight of 247 daltons, and a solubility in water exceeding 100 mg/ml. Recommended reconstitution with 10 ml diluent per vial yields 50 mg/ml acyclovir (pH approximately 11). Further dilution in any appropriate intravenous solution must be performed before infusion (see Method of Preparation). At physiologic pH, acyclovir exists as the un-ionized form with a molecular weight of 225 daltons and a maximum solubility of 2.5 mg/ml at 37°C.

Clinical Pharmacology: Acyclovir is a synthetic acyclic purine nucleoside analogue with *in vitro* and *in vivo* inhibitory activity against Herpes simplex, varicella-zoster, Epstein-Barr and cytomegalovirus. In cell cultures, the inhibitory activity of acyclovir for Herpes simplex virus is highly selective. Cellular thymidine kinase does not effectively utilize acyclovir as a substrate. Herpes simplex virus-coded thymidine kinase, however, converts acyclovir into acyclovir monophosphate, a nucleotide analogue. The monophosphate is further converted into diphosphate by cellular guanylate kinase and into triphosphate by a number of cellular enzymes.[1] Acyclovir triphosphate interferes with Herpes simplex virus DNA polymerase and inhibits viral DNA replication. Acyclovir triphosphate also inhibits cellular α-DNA polymerase but to a lesser degree. *In vitro*, acyclovir triphosphate can be incorporated into growing chains of DNA by viral DNA polymerase and to a much smaller extent by cellular α-DNA polymerase.[2] When incorporation occurs, the DNA chain is terminated.[3] Acyclovir is preferentially taken up and selectively converted to the active triphosphate form by herpesvirus-infected cells. Thus, acyclovir is much less toxic *in vitro* for normal uninfected cells because: 1) less is taken up; 2) less is converted to the active form; 3) cellular α-DNA polymerase is less sensitive to the effects of the active form.

The relationship between *in vitro* susceptibility of Herpes simplex virus to antiviral drugs and clinical response has not been established. The techniques and cell types used for determining *in vitro* susceptibility may influence the results obtained. With a quantitative assay to determine the acyclovir concentration producing 50% inhibition of viral cytopathic effect (ID_{50}), 28 HSV-1 clinical isolates had a mean ID_{50} of 0.17 µg/ml and 32 HSV-2 clinical isolates had a mean ID_{50} of 0.46 µg/ml. Results from other studies using different assays have yielded mean ID_{50} values for clinical HSV-1 isolates of 0.018, 0.03 and 0.043 µg/ml and for clinical HSV-2 isolates of 0.027, 0.36 and 0.03 µg/ml, respectively.[4,5,6]

Pharmacokinetics: The pharmacokinetics of acyclovir has been evaluated in 95 patients (9 studies). Results were obtained in adult patients with normal renal function during Phase I/II studies after single doses ranging from 0.5 to 15 mg/kg and after multiple doses ranging from 2.5 to 15 mg/kg every 8 hours. Pharmacokinetics was also determined in pediatric patients with normal renal function ranging in age from 1 to 17 years at doses of 250 mg/M^2 or 500 mg/M^2 every 8 hours. In these studies, dose-independent pharmacokinetics is observed in the range of 0.5 to 15 mg/kg. Proportionality between dose and plasma levels is seen after single doses or at steady state after multiple dosing.[7] When Zovirax was administered to adults at 5 mg/kg (approximately 250 mg/M^2) by 1-hr infusions every 8 hours, mean steady-state peak and trough concentrations of 9.8 µg/ml (5.5 to 13.8 µg/ml) and 0.7 µg/ml (0.2 to 1.0 µg/ml), respectively, were achieved. Similar concentrations are achieved in children over 1 year of age when doses of 250 mg/M^2 are given every 8 hours. Concentrations achieved in the cerebrospinal fluid are approximately 50% of plasma values. Plasma protein binding is relatively low (9% to 33%) and drug interactions involving binding site displacement are not anticipated.[7]

Renal excretion of unchanged drug by glomerular filtration and tubular secretion is the major route of acyclovir elimination accounting for 62 to 91% of the dose as determined by ^{14}C-labelled drug. The only major urinary metabolite detected is 9-carboxymethoxymethylguanine. This may account for up to 14.1% of the dose in patients with normal renal function. An insignificant amount of drug is recovered in feces and expired CO_2 and there is no evidence to suggest tissue retention.[7] However, postmortem examinations have shown that acyclovir is widely distributed in tissues and body fluids including brain, kidney, lung, liver, muscle, spleen, uterus, vaginal mucosa, vaginal secretions, cerebrospinal fluid and herpetic vesicular fluid.

In a Phase I study in 3 adult volunteers, 1 g of probenecid was administered orally prior to a single 1-hour 5 mg/kg intravenous infusion of acyclovir. The acyclovir half-life and area under the plasma concentration-time curve increased by 18 and 40%, respectively, compared to a control infusion of acyclovir without probenecid. The mean urinary excretion of acyclovir decreased from 79% to 69% of the dose indicating that probenecid can influence the renal excretion of acyclovir.[8]

Continued on next page

Burroughs Wellcome—Cont.

The half-life and total body clearance of acyclovir is dependent on renal function as shown below.[7]

Creatinine Clearance (ml/min/1.73M²)	Half-Life (hr)	Total Body Clearance (ml/min/1.73M²)
>80	2.5	327
50–80	3.0	248
15–50	3.5	190
0 (Anuric)	19.5	29

Zoviraz was administered at a dose of 2.5 mg/kg to 6 adult patients with severe renal failure. The peak and trough plasma levels during the 47 hours preceding hemodialysis were 8.5 µg/ml and 0.7 µg/ml, respectively.

Consult DOSAGE AND ADMINISTRATION section for recommended adjustments in dosing based upon creatinine clearance.

The half-life and total body clearance of acyclovir in pediatric patients over 1 year of age is similar to those in adults with normal renal function (see DOSAGE AND ADMINISTRATION).

Indications and Usage: Zovirax Sterile Powder is indicated for the treatment of initial and recurrent mucosal and cutaneous Herpes simplex (HSV-1 and HSV-2) infections in immunocompromised adults and children. It is also indicated for severe initial clinical episodes of herpes genitalis in patients who are not immunocompromised.

These indications are based on the results of several double-blind, placebo-controlled studies which evaluated the drug's effect on virus excretion, complete healing of lesions, and relief of pain.

Herpes Simplex Infections in Immunocompromised Patients

A multicenter trial of Zovirax Sterile Powder at a dose of 250 mg/M² every 8 hours (750 mg/M²/day) for 7 days was conducted in 97 immunocompromised patients with oro-facial, esophageal, genital and other localized infections (50 treated with Zovirax and 47 with placebo). Zoviraz significantly decreased virus excretion, reduced pain, and promoted scabbing and rapid healing of lesions.[9,10,11]

Initial Episodes of Herpes Genitalis

A controlled trial was conducted in 28 patients with severe initial episodes of herpes genitalis with a Zovirax dosage of 5 mg/kg every 8 hours for 5 days (12 patients treated with Zovirax and 16 with placebo). Significant treatment effects were seen in elimination of virus from lesions and in reduction of healing times.[12]

In a similar study, 15 patients with initial episodes of genital herpes were treated with Zovirax 5 mg/kg every 8 hours for 5 days and 15 with placebo. Zovirax decreased the duration of viral excretion, new lesion formation, duration of vesicles and promoted more rapid healing of all lesions.[13]

Diagnosis

The use of appropriate laboratory diagnostic procedures will help to establish the etiologic diagnosis. Positive cultures for Herpes simplex virus offer a reliable means for confirmation of the diagnosis. In initial episodes of genital herpes, appropriate examinations should be performed to rule out other sexually transmitted diseases. Whereas cutaneous lesions associated with Herpes simplex infections are often characteristic, the finding of multinucleated giant cells in smears prepared from lesion exudate or scrapings may assist in the diagnosis.[14]

Contraindications: Zovirax Sterile Powder is contraindicated for patients who develop hypersensitivity to the drug.

Warnings: Zovirax Sterile Powder is intended for intravenous infusion only, and should not be administered topically, intramuscularly, orally, subcutaneously, or in the eye. Intravenous infusions must be given over a period of at least 1 (one) hour to prevent renal tubular damage (see PRECAUTIONS and DOSAGE AND ADMINISTRATION).

Precautions:

General: The recommended dosage, frequency and length of treatment should not be exceeded (see DOSAGE AND ADMINISTRATION).

Although the aqueous solubility of acyclovir sodium (for infusion) is > 100 mg/ml, precipitation of acyclovir crystals in renal tubules can occur if the maximum solubility of free acyclovir (2.5 mg/ml at 37°C in water) is exceeded or if the drug is administered by bolus injection. This complication causes a rise in serum creatinine and blood urea nitrogen (BUN), and a decrease in renal creatinine clearance. Ensuing renal tubular damage can produce acute renal failure.

Abnormal renal function (decreased creatinine clearance) can occur as a result of acyclovir administration and depends on the state of the patient's hydration, other treatments, and the rate of drug administration. Bolus administration of the drug leads to a 10% incidence of renal dysfunction, while in controlled studies, infusion of 5 mg/kg (250 mg/M²) over an hour was associated with a lower frequency—4.6%. Concomitant use of other nephrotoxic drugs, pre-existing renal disease, and dehydration make further renal impairment with acyclovir more likely. In most instances, alterations of renal function were transient and resolved spontaneously or with improvement of water and electrolyte balance, drug dosage adjustment or discontinuation of drug administration. However, in some instances, these changes may progress to acute renal failure.

Administration of Zovirax by intravenous infusion must be accompanied by adequate hydration. Since maximum urine concentration occurs within the first 2 hours following infusion, particular attention should be given to establishing sufficient urine flow during that period in order to prevent precipitation in renal tubules.

When dosage adjustments are required they should be based on estimated creatinine clearance (See DOSAGE AND ADMINISTRATION).

Approximately 1% of patients receiving intravenous acyclovir have manifested encephalopathic changes characterized by either lethargy, obtundation, tremors, confusion, hallucinations, agitation, seizures or coma. Zovirax should be used with caution in those patients who have underlying neurologic abnormalities and those with serious renal, hepatic, or electrolyte abnormalities or significant hypoxia. It should also be used with caution in patients who have manifested prior neurologic reactions to cytotoxic drugs or those receiving concomitant intrathecal methotrexate or interferon.

Exposure of HSV isolates to acyclovir *in vitro* can lead to the emergence of less sensitive viruses. These viruses usually are deficient in thymidine kinase (required for acyclovir activation) and are less pathogenic in animals. Similar isolates have been observed in 6 severely immunocompromised patients during the course of controlled and uncontrolled studies of intravenously administered Zovirax. These occurred in patients with congenital severe combined immunodeficiencies or following bone marrow transplantation. The presence of these viruses was not associated with a worsening of clinical illness and, in some instances, the virus disappeared spontaneously. The possibility of the appearance of less sensitive viruses must be borne in mind when treating such patients. The relationship between the *in vitro* sensitivity of herpesviruses to acyclovir and clinical response to therapy has yet to be established.

Drug Interactions: Co-administration of probenecid with acyclovir has been shown to increase the mean half-life and the area under the concentration-time curve. Urinary excretion and renal clearance were correspondingly reduced. Clinical experience has identified no other significant interactions resulting from administration of other drugs concomitantly with Zovirax Sterile Powder.

Carcinogenesis, Mutagenesis, Impairment of Fertility: Acyclovir was tested in lifetime bioassays in rats and mice at single daily doses of 50, 150 and 450 mg/kg given by gavage. There was no statistically significant difference in the incidence of tumors between treated and control animals, nor did acyclovir appear to shorten the latency of tumors. In 2 *in vitro* cell transformation assays, used to provide preliminary assessment of potential oncogenicity in advance of these more definitive lifetime bioassays in rodents, conflicting results were obtained. Acyclovir was positive at the highest dose used in one system and the resulting morphologically transformed cells formed tumors when inoculated into immunosuppressed, syngeneic, weanling mice. Acyclovir was negative in another transformation system.

No chromosome damage was observed at maximum tolerated parenteral doses of 100 mg/kg acyclovir in rats or Chinese hamsters; higher doses of 500 and 1000 mg/kg were clastogenic in Chinese hamsters. In addition, no activity was found in a dominant lethal study in mice. In 9 of 11 microbial and mammalian cell assays, no evidence of mutagenicity was observed. In 2 mammalian cell assays (human lymphocytes and L5178Y mouse lymphoma cells *in vitro*), positive responses for mutagenicity and chromosomal damage occurred, but only at concentrations at least 25 times the acyclovir plasma levels achieved in man.

Acyclovir does not impair fertility or reproduction in mice at oral doses up to 450 mg/kg/day. In female rabbits treated subcutaneously with acyclovir subsequent to mating, there was a statistically significant decrease in implantation efficiency but no concomitant decrease in litter size at a dose of 50 mg/kg/day.

Pregnancy: Teratogenic Effects. Pregnancy Category C. Acyclovir was not teratogenic in the mouse (450 mg/kg/day, p.o.), rabbit (50 mg/kg/day, s.c.) or rat (50 mg/kg/day, s.c.). Although maximum tolerated doses were tested in the teratology studies, the plasma levels obtained did not exaggerate maximum plasma levels that might occur with clinical use of intravenous acyclovir.

There have been no adequate and well-controlled studies in pregnant women. Acyclovir should be used during pregnancy only if the potential benefit justifies the potential risk to the fetus.

Nursing Mothers: It is not known whether this drug is excreted in human milk. Because many drugs are excreted in human milk, caution should be exercised when Zovirax is administered to a nursing woman.

Adverse Reactions: The most frequent adverse reactions reported during controlled clinical trials of Zovirax in 64 patients were inflammation or phlebitis at the injection site following infiltration of the I.V. fluid in 9 (14.0%), transient elevations of serum creatinine in 3 (4.7%), and rash or hives in 3 (4.7%). Less frequent adverse reactions were diaphoresis, hematuria, hypotension, headache and nausea, each of which occurred in 1 patient (1.6%). Of the 63 patients receiving placebo, 3 (4.8%) experienced inflammation/phlebitis and 3 (4.8%) experienced rash or itching. Hematuria and nausea were experienced by placebo recipients at the same frequency.

Among 51 immunocompromised patients, one, a bone marrow transplant recipient with pneumonitis, developed seizures, cerebral edema, coma and expired with changes consistent with cerebral anoxia on postmortem biopsy; another immunocompromised patient exhibited coarse tremor and clonus.

Additional adverse reactions were reported in uncontrolled trials. The most frequent adverse reaction was elevated serum creatinine. This occurred in 9.8 percent of patients, usually following rapid (less than 10 minutes) intravenous infusion. Less frequent adverse experiences were thrombocytosis and jitters, each in 0.4% of patients.

Approximately 1% of patients receiving intravenous acyclovir have manifested encephalopathic changes characterized by either lethargy, obtundation, tremors, confusion, hallucinations, agitation, seizures or coma (see PRECAUTIONS).

Overdosage: Overdosage has been reported following administration of bolus injections, or inappropriately high doses, and in patients whose fluid and electrolyte balance was not properly monitored. This has resulted in elevations in BUN, serum creatinine and subsequent renal failure.

Precipitation of acyclovir in renal tubules may occur when the solubility (2.5 mg/ml) in the intratubular fluid is exceeded (see PRECAUTIONS). A six hour hemodialysis results in a 60% decrease in plasma acyclovir concentration. Data concerning peritoneal dialysis are incomplete but indicate that this method may be significantly less efficient in removing acyclovir from the blood. In the event of acute renal failure and anuria, the patient may benefit from hemodialysis until rena function is restored (see DOSAGE AND ADMINISTRATION).

Dosage and Administration: CAUTION—RAPID OR BOLUS INTRAVENOUS AND INTRAMUSCULAR OR SUBCUTANEOUS INJECTION MUST BE AVOIDED.

Dosage: *MUCOSAL AND CUTANEOUS HERPES SIMPLEX (HSV-1 and HSV-2) INFECTIONS IN IMMUNOCOMPROMISED PATIENTS*—5 mg/kg infused at a constant rate over 1 hour, every 8 hours (15 mg/kg/day) for 7 days in adult patients with normal renal function. In children under 12 years of age, more accurate dosing can be attained by infusing 250 mg/M^2 at a constant rate over 1 hour, every 8 hours (750 mg/M^2/day) for 7 days. *SEVERE INITIAL CLINICAL EPISODES OF HERPES GENITALIS*—The same dose given above——administered for 5 days.

Therapy should be initiated as early as possible following onset of signs and symptoms.

PATIENTS WITH ACUTE OR CHRONIC RENAL IMPAIRMENT: Refer to DOSAGE AND ADMINISTRATION section for recommended doses, and adjust the dosing interval as indicated in the table below.

Creatinine Clearance (ml/min/1.73M^2)	Dose (mg/kg)	Dosing Interval (hours)
>50	5	8
25–50	5	12
10–25	5	24
0–10	2.5	24

Hemodialysis: For patients who require dialysis, the mean plasma half-life of acyclovir during hemodialysis is approximately 5 hours. This results in a 60% decrease in plasma concentrations following a 6 hour dialysis period. Therefore, the patient's dosing schedule should be adjusted so that a dose is administered after each dialysis.

Method of Preparation: Each 10 ml vial contains acyclovir sodium equivalent to 500 mg of acyclovir. The contents of the vial should be dissolved in 10 ml of sterile water for injection or bacteriostatic water for injection containing benzyl alcohol. yielding a final concentration of 50 mg/ml of acyclovir (pH approximately 11). Shake the vial well to assure complete dissolution before measuring and transferring each individual dose. DO NOT USE BACTERIOSTATIC WATER FOR INJECTION CONTAINING PARABENS. It is incompatible with Zovirax Sterile Powder and may cause precipitation.

Administration: The calculated dose should then be removed and added to any appropriate intravenous solution at a volume selected for administration during each 1 hour infusion. Infusion concentrations of approximately 7 mg/ml or lower are recommended. In clinical studies, the average 70 kg adult received approximately 60 ml of fluid per dose. Higher concentrations (e.g., 10 mg/ml) may produce phlebitis or inflammation at the injection site upon inadvertent extravasation. Standard, commercially available electrolyte and glucose solutions are suitable for intravenous administration; biologic or colloidal fluids (e.g., blood products, protein solutions, etc.) are not recommended. Once in solution in the vial at a concentration of 50 mg/ml, the drug should be used within 12 hours. Once diluted for administration, each dose should be used within 24 hours. Refrigeration of reconstituted solutions may result in formation of a precipitate which will redissolve at room temperature.

How Supplied: ZOVIRAX Sterile Powder is supplied in 10 ml sterile vials, each containing acyclovir sodium equivalent to 500 mg of acyclovir, cartons of 5 (NDC 0081-0995-46) and 25 (NDC 0081-0995-95). Store at 15°–30°C (59°–86°F).

Also available: ZOVIRAX Ointment, 5% in 15 g tubes. Each gram contains 50 mg acyclovir in a polyethylene glycol base.

U.S. Patent No. 4199574

References
1. W.H. Miller and R.L. Miller, J. Biol. Chem. 225(15): 7204–7207, 1980.
2. P.A. Furman, et al., J. Virol. 32(1): 72–77, 1979.
3. D. Derse, et al., J. Biol. Chem. 256(22): 11447–11451, 1981.
4. P. Collins and D.J. Bauer. J. Antimicrob. Chemother. 15:431–436, 1979.
5. C.S. Crumpacker, et al., Antimicrob. Agents Chemother. 15:642–645, 1979.
6. E. De Clercq. et al., J. Infect. Dis. 141:563–574, 1980.
7. M.R. Blum, et al., Am. J. Med. 73(1A): 186–192, Jul. 20, 1982.
8. O.L. Laskin, et al., Antimicrob. Agents Chemother. 21(5): 804–807, May 1982.
9. C.D. Mitchell, et al., Lancet 1(8235): 1389–1392, Jun. 27, 1981.
10. J.C. Wade, et al., Ann. Intern. Med. 96(3): 265–269, Mar. 1982.
11. J.D. Meyers, et al., Am. J. Med. 73(1A): 229–235, Jul. 20, 1982.
12. Data on file, Burroughs Wellcome Co.
13. A. Mindel, et al., Lancet 1(8274): 697–700, Mar. 27, 1982.
14. Z.M. Naib, et al., Cancer Res. 33:1452–1463, 1973.

ZYLOPRIM ®
[zī'lō-prĭm"]
(Allopurinol)
100 mg Scored Tablets and 300 mg Scored Tablets

Description: Allopurinol is a xanthine oxidase inhibitor with the chemical name 4-hydroxypyrazolo (3,4-d) pyrimidine (HPP).

Clinical Pharmacology: Zyloprim (Allopurinol) acts on purine catabolism, without disrupting the biosynthesis of vital purines, thus reducing the production of uric acid by inhibiting the biochemical reactions immediately preceding its formation. Its action differs from that of uricosuric agents, which lower the serum uric acid level by increasing urinary excretion of uric acid. Zyloprim reduces both the serum and urinary uric acid levels by inhibiting the formation of uric acid. It thereby avoids the hazard of increased hyperuricosuria in patients with gouty nephropathy or with a predisposition to the formation of uric acid stones.

Zyloprim has produced a substantial reduction in serum and urinary uric acid levels in hitherto refractory patients even in the presence of renal damage marked enough to render uricosuric drugs virtually ineffective. Salicylates may be given conjointly for their antirheumatic effect without compromising the action of allopurinol. This is in contrast to the nullifying effect of salicylates on uricosuric drugs.

Zyloprim is a structural analogue of the natural purine base, hypoxanthine. It is a potent inhibitor of xanthine oxidase, the enzyme responsible for the conversion of hypoxanthine to xanthine and of xanthine to uric acid, the end product of purine metabolism in man. Zyloprim is metabolized to the corresponding xanthine analogue, oxipurinol (alloxanthine), which also is an inhibitor of xanthine oxidase.

Hyperuricemia may be primary, as in gout, or secondary to diseases such as acute and chronic leukemia, polycythemia vera, multiple myeloma, and psoriasis. It may occur with the use of diuretic agents, during renal dialysis, in the presence of renal damage, during starvation or reducing diets and in the treatment of neoplastic disease where rapid resolution of tissue masses may occur.

The major disease manifestations in gout—kidney stones, tophi in soft tissues, and deposits in joints and bones—result from the deposition of urates. If progressive deposition of urates is to be arrested or reversed, it is necessary to reduce the serum uric acid to a level below the saturation point to suppress urate precipitation. Reduction may be achieved by means of uricosuric agents. Uricosurics are less effective in the presence of renal disease, and some patients develop intolerance or sensitivity to these drugs. The use of allopurinol to block the formation of urate avoids the hazard of increased renal excretion of uric acid posed by uricosuric drugs.

The half-life of Zyloprim in the body is determined both by renal excretion and by oxidation to 4,6-dihydroxypyrazolo (3,4-d) pyrimidine (oxipurinol). The latter is also an inhibitor of xanthine oxidase, but is somewhat weaker than allopurinol which is bound 15-fold more tightly to the enzyme than is the natural substrate, xanthine. The long half-life of oxipurinol in the plasma (18 to 30 hours), contributes significantly to the enzyme inhibition. Moreover, both allopurinol and oxipurinol tend to inactivate xanthine oxidase, thereby further controlling the level of its activity. Administration of Zyloprim generally results in a fall in both serum and urinary uric acid within two to three days. The magnitude of this decrease can be manipulated almost at will since it is dose-dependent. A week or more of treatment with allopurinol may be required for the full effects of the drug to be manifest; likewise, uric acid may return to pretreatment levels slowly, usually after a period of seven to 10 days following cessation of therapy. This reflects primarily the accumulation and slow clearance of oxipurinol. In some patients, particularly those with severe tophaceous gout and underexcretors, a dramatic fall in urinary uric acid excretion may not occur. It has been postulated that this may be due to the mobilization of urate from the tissue deposits as the serum uric acid level begins to fall.

The combined increase in hypoxanthine and xanthine excreted in the urine usually, but not always, is considerably less than the accompanying decline in urinary uric acid.

It has been shown that reutilization of both hypoxanthine and xanthine for nucleotide and nucleic acid synthesis is markedly enhanced when their oxidations are inhibited by allopurinol. This reutilization and the normal feedback inhibition which would result from an increase in available purine nucleotides serve to regulate purine biosynthesis and, in essence, the defect of the overproducer of uric acid is thereby compensated.

Innate deficiency of xanthine oxidase, which occurs in congenital xanthinuria as an inborn error of metabolism, has been shown to be compatible with normal health. While urinary levels of oxypurines attained with full doses of allopurinol may in exceptional cases equal those (250–600 mg per day) which in xanthinuric subjects have caused formation of urinary calculi, they usually fall in the range of 50–200 mg. Xanthine crystalluria has been reported in a few exceptional cases. Two of these had Lesch-Nyhan syndrome, which is characterized by excessive uric acid production combined with a deficiency in the enzyme, hypoxanthine-guanine phosphoribosyltransferase (HG-PRTase). This enzyme is required for the conversion of hypoxanthine and guanine to their respective nucleotides. The third case was a patient with lymphosarcoma, who produced an extremely large amount of uric acid because of rapid cell lysis during chemotherapy.

The serum concentration of oxypurines in patients receiving allopurinol is usually in the range of 0.3 mg to 0.4 mg percent compared to a normal level of approximately 0.15 mg percent. A maximum of 0.9 mg percent was observed when the serum urate was lowered to less than 2 mg percent by high doses of the drug. In one exceptional case a value of 2.7 mg percent was reached. These are far below

Continued on next page

Burroughs Wellcome—Cont.

the saturation level at which precipitation of xanthine or hypoxanthine would be expected to occur. The solubilities of uric acid and xanthine in the serum are similar (about 7 mg percent) while hypoxanthine is much more soluble. The finding that the renal clearance of oxypurines is at least 10 times greater than that of uric acid explains the relatively low serum oxypurine concentration at a time when the serum uric acid level has decreased markedly. At serum oxypurine levels of 0.3 mg to 0.9 mg percent, oxypurine: inulin clearance ratios were between 0.7 and 1.9. The glomerular filtration rate and urate clearance in patients receiving allopurinol do not differ significantly from those obtained prior to therapy. The rapid renal clearance of oxypurines suggests that allopurinol therapy should be of value in allowing a patient with gout to increase his total purine excretion.

Although the renal clearance of allopurinol is rapid, that of oxipurinol is slow and parallels that of uric acid but is higher by a factor of about three. The clearance of oxipurinol is increased by uricosuric drugs, and as a consequence, the addition of a uricosuric agent may reduce the degree of inhibition of xanthine oxidase by oxipurinol. However, such combined therapy may be useful in achieving minimum serum uric acid levels provided the total urinary uric acid load does not exceed the competence of the patient's renal function. In some patients, where renal function is severely impaired, normal serum urate levels may not be achievable. The danger of uric acid calculi is diminished as the uric acid excretion is reduced. The amounts of xanthine and hypoxanthine excreted in the urine generally do not exceed the solubilities of these compounds in the urine, particularly if the urine is slightly alkaline. The amounts of allopurinol and oxipurinol excreted are likewise within the limits of their respective solubilities.

Zyloprim also inhibits the enzymatic oxidation of mercaptopurine, the sulfur-containing analogue of hypoxanthine, to 6-thiouric acid. This oxidation, which is catalyzed by xanthine oxidase, inactivates mercaptopurine. Hence, the inhibition of such oxidation by allopurinol may result in as much as 75 percent reduction in the therapeutic dose requirement of mercaptopurine when the two compounds are given together.

Indications and Use: This is not an innocuous drug and strict attention should be given to the indications for its use. Pending further investigation, its use in other hyperuricemic states is not indicated at this time.

Zyloprim® (allopurinol) is intended for:
1. treatment of gout, either primary, or secondary to the hyperuricemia associated with blood dyscrasias and their therapy;
2. treatment of primary or secondary uric acid nephropathy, with or without accompanying symptoms of gout;
3. treatment of patients with recurrent uric acid stone formation;
4. prophylactic treatment to prevent tissue urate deposition, renal calculi, or uric acid nephropathy in patients with leukemias, lymphomas and malignancies who are receiving cancer chemotherapy with its resultant elevating effect on serum uric acid levels.

Allopurinol, by promoting the resolution of tophi and urate crystals in the tissues, has relieved chronic joint pain, increased joint mobility and permitted urate sinuses to heal. The addition of allopurinol to a uricosuric regimen has reduced the size of tophi which have been refractory to uricosuric agents alone and increased joint mobility.

Zyloprim is particularly effective in preventing the occurrence and recurrence of uric acid stones and gravel. Zyloprim is useful in therapy and prophylaxis of acute urate nephropathy in patients with neoplastic disease who are particularly susceptible to hyperuricemia and uric acid stone formation, especially after radiation therapy or the use of antineoplastic drugs.

Contraindications: Pending further investigation this drug is contraindicated for use in children with the exception of those with hyperuricemia secondary to malignancy. The drug should not be employed in nursing mothers.

Patients who have developed a severe reaction to Zyloprim should not be restarted on the drug.

Warnings: ZYLOPRIM SHOULD BE DISCONTINUED AT THE FIRST APPEARANCE OF SKIN RASH OR ANY SIGN OF ADVERSE REACTION. In some instances a skin rash may be followed by more severe hypersensitivity reactions such as exfoliative, urticarial and purpuric lesions as well as Stevens-Johnson syndrome (erythema multiforme) and very rarely a generalized vasculitis which may lead to irreversible hepatotoxicity and death.

A few cases of reversible clinical hepatotoxicity have been noted in patients taking Zyloprim and in some patients asymptomatic rises in serum alkaline phosphatase or serum transaminase have been observed. Accordingly, periodic liver function tests should be performed during the early stages of therapy, particularly in patients with pre-existing liver disease.

Due to the occasional occurrence of drowsiness, patients should be alerted to the need for due precautions when engaging in activities where alertness is mandatory.

Occasional cases of hypersensitivity have been reported in patients with renal compromise receiving thiazides and Zyloprim concurrently. For this reason, in this clinical setting, such combination should be administered with caution.

In patients receiving Purinethol® (mercaptopurine) or Imuran® (azathioprine), the concomitant administration of 300–600 mg of Zyloprim per day will require a reduction in dose to approximately one-third to one-fourth of the usual dose of mercaptopurine or azathioprine. Subsequent adjustment of doses of Purinethol or Imuran should be made on the basis of therapeutic response and any toxic effects.

Usage in Pregnancy and Women of Childbearing Age: Reproductive studies showed no adverse effect of Zyloprim on animal litters. However, since the effect of xanthine oxidase inhibition on the human fetus is still unknown, Zyloprim should be used in pregnant women or women of childbearing age only if the potential benefits to the patient are weighed against the possible risk to the fetus.

Precautions: Some investigators have reported an increase in acute attacks of gout during the early stages of allopurinol administration, even when normal or subnormal serum uric acid levels have been attained. Accordingly, maintenance doses of colchicine (0.5 mg twice daily) generally should be given prophylactically when allopurinol is begun. In addition, it is recommended that the patient start with a low dose of allopurinol (100 mg daily) and increase at weekly intervals by 100 mg until a serum uric acid level of 6 mg per 100 ml or less is attained but without exceeding the maximal recommended dose. The use of therapeutic doses of colchicine or anti-inflammatory agents may be required to suppress attacks in some cases. The attacks usually become shorter and less severe after several months of therapy. A possible explanation for these flare-ups may be the mobilization of urates from tissue deposits followed by recrystallization, due to fluctuation in the serum uric acid level. Even with adequate therapy it may require several months to deplete the uric acid pool sufficiently to achieve control of the acute episodes.

The concomitant administration of a uricosuric agent with Zyloprim may result in a decrease in urinary excretion of oxypurines as compared to their excretion with allopurinol alone. This may possibly be due to an increased excretion of oxipurinol and a lowering of the degree of inhibition of xanthine oxidase. Such combined therapy is not contraindicated, however, and for many patients, may provide optimum control. A report by Goldfinger, et al on a patient treated with sulfinpyrazone and salicylates in addition to allopurinol showed a marked decrease in the excretion of oxypurines which they suggested was due to interference with their clearance at the renal tubular level. However, subsequent studies in our laboratories have indicated no interference with oxypurine clearance by salicylates. Although clinical evidence to date has not demonstrated renal precipitation of oxypurines in patients either on Zyloprim alone or in combination with uricosuric agents, the possiblity should be kept in mind.

It has been reported that allopurinol prolongs the half-life of the anticoagulant, dicumarol. The clinical significance of this has not been established, but this interaction should be kept in mind when allopurinol is given to patients already on anticoagulant therapy, and the coagulation time should be reassessed.

A fluid intake sufficient to yield a daily urinary output of at least 2 liters and the maintenance of a neutral or, preferably, slightly alkaline urine are desirable to (1) avoid the theoretic possibility of formation of xanthine calculi under the influence of Zyloprim therapy and (2) help prevent renal precipitation of urates in patients receiving concomitant uricosuric agents.

A few patients with preexisting renal disease or poor urate clearance have shown a rise in BUN during Zyloprim administration although a decrease in BUN has also been observed. Although the relationship of these observations to the drug has not been established, patients with impaired renal function require less drug and should be carefully observed during the early stages of Zyloprim administration and the drug withdrawn if increased abnormalities in renal function appear.

In patients with severely impaired renal function, or decreased urate clearance, the half-life of oxipurinol in the plasma is greatly prolonged. Therefore, a dose of 100 mg per day or 300 mg twice a week, or perhaps less, may be sufficient to maintain adequate xanthine oxidase inhibition to reduce serum urate levels. Such patients should be treated with the lowest effective dose, in order to minimize side effects.

Mild reticulocytosis has appeared in some patients, most of whom were receiving other therapeutic agents, so that the significance of this observation is not known.

Periodic determination of liver and kidney function and complete blood counts should be performed especially during the first few months of therapy.

Adverse Reactions:

Dermatologic: Because in some instances skin rash has been followed by severe hypersensitivity reactions, it is recommended that therapy be discontinued at the first sign of rash or other adverse reaction (see WARNINGS).

Skin rash, usually maculopapular, is the adverse reaction most commonly reported. The incidence of skin rash may be increased in the presence of renal disorders.

Exfoliative, urticarial and purpuric lesions, Stevens-Johnson syndrome (erythema multiforme) and toxic epidermal necrolysis have also been reported.

A few cases of alopecia with and without accompanying dermatitis have been reported.

In some patients with a rash, restarting Zyloprim therapy at lower doses has been accomplished without untoward incident.

Gastrointestinal: Nausea, vomiting, diarrhea, and intermittent abdominal pain have been reported.

Hepatic: Rare cases of granulomatous hepatitis and hepatic necrosis have been reported.

Vascular: There have been rare instances of a generalized hypersensitivity vasculitis or necrotizing angiitis which have led to irreversible hepatotoxicity and death.

Hematopoietic: Agranulocytosis, anemia, aplastic anemia, bone marrow depression, leukopenia, pancytopenia and thrombocytopenia have been reported in patients, most of whom received concomitant drugs with potential for causing these reactions. Zyloprim has been neither implicated nor excluded as a cause of these reactions.

Renal: Rare cases of renal failure have been reported in hypertensive patients who received thiazides and Zyloprim concurrently. Some patients had evidence of hypersensitivity to allopurinol.

Neurologic: There have been a few reports of peripheral neuritis occurring while patients were taking Zyloprim.

Drowsiness has also been reported in a few patients.

Ophthalmic: There have been a few reports of cataracts found in patients receiving Zyloprim. It is not known if the cataracts predated the Zyloprim therapy. "Toxic" cataracts were reported in one patient who also received an anti-inflammatory agent; again, the time of onset is unknown. In a group of patients followed by Gutman and Yu for up to five years on Zyloprim therapy, no evidence of ophthalmologic effect attributable to Zyloprim was reported.

Drug Idiosyncrasy: Symptoms suggestive of drug idiosyncrasy have been reported in a few patients. This was characterized by fever, chills, leukopenia or leukocytosis, eosinophilia, arthralgias, skin rash, pruritus, nausea and vomiting.

Overdosage: Massive overdosing, or acute poisoning, by Zyloprim has not been reported.

Dosage and Administration: The dosage of Zyloprim brand Allopurinol to accomplish full control of gout and to lower serum uric acid to normal or near-normal levels varies with the severity of the disease. The average is 200 to 300 mg per day for patients with mild gout and 400 to 600 mg per day for those with moderately severe tophaceous gout. The appropriate dosage may be administered in divided doses or as a single equivalent dose with the 300 mg tablet. Dosage requirements in excess of 300 mg should be supplemented in divided doses. It should also be noted that allopurinol is generally better tolerated if taken following meals. Similar considerations govern the regulation of dosage for maintenance purposes in secondary hyperuricemia. For the prevention of uric acid nephropathy during the vigorous therapy of neoplastic disease, treatment with 600 to 800 mg daily for two or three days is advisable together with a high fluid intake. The minimal effective dosage is 100 to 200 mg daily and the maximal recommended dosage is 800 mg daily. To reduce the possiblity of flare-up of acute gouty attacks, it is recommended that the patient start with a low dose of allopurinol (100 mg daily) and increase at weekly intervals by 100 mg until a serum uric acid level of 6 mg per 100 ml or less is attained but without exceeding the maximal recommended dosage. Normal serum urate levels are achieved in one to three weeks. The upper limit of normal is about 7 mg percent for men and postmenopausal women and 6 mg percent for premenopausal women. Too much reliance should not be placed on a single reading since, for technical reasons, estimation of uric acid may be difficult. By the selection of the appropriate dose, together with the use of uricosuric agents in certain patients, it is possible to reduce the serum uric acid level to normal and, if desired, to hold it as low as 2 to 3 mg percent indefinitely.

A fluid intake sufficient to yield a daily urinary output of at least 2 liters and the maintenance of a neutral or, preferably, slightly alkaline urine are desirable.

Since allopurinol and its metabolites are excreted only by the kidney, accumulation of the drug can occur in renal failure, and the dose of allopurinol should consequently be reduced. With a creatinine clearance of 20 to 10 ml/min, a daily dosage of 200 mg of Zyloprim is suitable. When the creatinine clearance is less than 10 ml/min the daily dosage should not exceed 100 mg. With extreme renal impairment (creatinine clearance less than 3 ml/min) the interval between doses may also need to be lengthened.

The correct size and frequency of dosage for maintaining the serum uric acid just within the normal range is best determined by using the serum uric acid level as an index.

Children, 6 to 10 years of age, with secondary hyperuricemia associated with malignancies may be given 300 mg allopurinol daily while those under 6 years are generally given 150 mg daily. The response is evaluated after approximately 48 hours of therapy and a dosage adjustment is made if necessary.

In patients who are being treated with colchicine and/or anti-inflammatory agents, it is wise to continue this therapy while adjusting the dosage of Zyloprim, until a normal serum uric acid and freedom from acute attacks have been maintained for several months.

In transferring a patient from a uricosuric agent to Zyloprim, the dose of the uricosuric agent should be gradually reduced over a period of several weeks and the dose of allopurinol gradually increased to the required dose needed to maintain a normal serum uric acid level.

How Supplied: 100 mg (white) scored tablets, bottles of 100 and 1000; unit dose pack of 1000. Tablets bear identification, ZYLOPRIM U4A. 300 mg (peach) scored tablets, bottles of 30, 100, 500 and unit dose pack of 1000. Tablets bear identification, ZYLOPRIM C9B.

100 mg × 100—DoD & VA
                  NSN 6505-00-998-4381
300 mg × 30—VA
                  NSN 6505-01-006-5974
300 mg × 100—DoD & VA
                  NSN 6505-01-004-3952
300 mg × 100 (UDP)
                  NSN 6505-01-044-9395

Animal Toxicology: In mice the LD_{50} is 160 mg/kg ip (with deaths delayed up to five days) and 700 mg/kg po (with deaths delayed up to three days). In rats the acute LD_{50} is 750 mg/kg ip > 6000 mg/kg po.

In a 13 week feeding experiment in rats at a drug level of 72 mg/kg per day 2 of 10 rats died and at 225 mg/kg per day 4 of 10 died before the completion of the experiment. Both groups exhibited renal tubular damage due to the deposition of xanthine that was more extensive at the higher dose.

In chronic feeding experiments, rats showed no toxic effects at a level of 14 mg/kg per day after one year. At a level of 24 mg/kg per day for one year the rats showed very slight depression of weight gain and food intake, and 5 out of 10 of the animals showed minor changes in the kidney tubules of the type exhibited by the rats on the higher doses described above.

Dogs survived oral doses of 30 mg/kg per day for one year with nil to minor changes in the kidney and no other significant abnormalities. At 90 mg/kg per day for one year there was some accumulation of xanthine in the kidneys with resultant chronic irritation and slight tubular changes. Occasional hemosiderin-like deposits were seen in the reticuloendothelial system. A higher dose (270 mg/kg per day) resulted in large concretions in the renal pelves, with severe destructive changes in the kidney secondary to xanthine accumulation. The deposition of xanthine appears to be a function both of the metabolic turnover of purines (which is proportionately larger in the smaller animals) and the degree of inhibition of xanthine oxidase.

Reproductive studies in rats and rabbits indicated that Zyloprim did not affect litter size, the mean weight of the progeny at birth or at three weeks postpartum, nor did it cause an increase in the number of animals born dead or with malformations.

U.S. Patent No. 3,624,205 (Use Patent)

Shown in Product Identification Section, page 408

EDUCATIONAL MATERIAL

The following is a selected list of materials loaned free or available without charge to medical personnel, pharmacists, or patients. To order or obtain information regarding availability of continuing medical education credit, contact your area Burroughs Wellcome Co. Representative or write:

Burroughs Wellcome Co., Educational Services, 3030 Cornwallis Road, Research Triangle Park, NC 27709.

CONTINUING MEDICAL EDUCATION MATERIAL AVAILABLE FROM BURROUGHS WELLCOME CO.

AAFP Annual Series
AAFP Monograph Series
Monographs in Urology Series
Pediatric Emergency Casebook Series
Wellcome Programs in Pharmacy
Review Series
    Essential Otolaryngology, Second Edition
    Essential Otolaryngology, Third Edition
    Cardiology Specialty Board Review
    Handbook of Ophthalmological Emergencies
    Cardiovascular Disease Book
Film/Monograph Programs
    Sex and the Heart Patient
    Sports Injuries of the Knee
    Sports Injuries of the Ankle
    Pitfalls in Digoxin Therapy
    Gout Learning System
    Gout: A Clinical Comprehensive
    Gout: A Management Update
    Update on the Management of Otitis Media
    Update on the Management of Acute Exacerbations of Chronic Bronchitis
    Update on the Management of Recurrent Renal Stones
    Update on the Diagnosis and Management of Genital Herpes
    Herpes Simplex Infections in the Immunocompromised Patient
    Atracurium: Update on a New Intermediate-Acting Nondepolarizing Muscle Relaxant
Selected Monographs
    The Wellcome Atlas of Sexually Transmitted Diseases
    AIDS: Diagnosis and Management
    Diffuse External Otitis
    Treatment of Urinary Tract Infection and Its Prevention
    Treatment of Acute, Uncomplicated Urinary Tract Infections
    Treatment of Hyperuricemia Associated with Gout/Other Conditions
Collections of Symposia Presentations Covering the Following Medical Topics
    Therapeutic Workshop Modifying the Disease Process in Rheumatoid Arthritis
    Review of Infectious Diseases
    Proceedings of a Symposium on Acyclovir
    Proceedings of a Symposium on Atracurium
    Proceedings of a Symposium on Antimicrobial Chemotherapy
    Digoxin Therapy
Medical Notes on the Following Disease States
    The Common Cold
    External Otitis
    Selected Skin Diseases
    Heart Failure
    Angina Pectoris
    Hyperuricemia
    Parkinsonism and Pseudoparkinsonism
    Medical Terminology
Learning Units
    "Pathophysiology of Gout"
    "Virology—A Basic Science Learning Unit"
    "Virology and Herpetic Diseases"
    "Atracurium Learning Unit"—For Hospital Pharacists
Patient Instructions/Information
    "How to Eliminate Pinworms and Roundworms"
    "How to Administer Ear Drops" (English or Spanish)
    "Do You Have Arthritis?"
    "Treating Empetigo" (English or Spanish)
    Urinary Tract Infection
    "How to Administer Eye Drops & Ointment" (English or Spanish)

Continued on next page

Burroughs Wellcome—Cont.

Visual Acuity Chart—Child
"Ocular Herpes Simplex Infection"
Understanding Gout (English or Spanish)
"Herpes Alert"—Public Service Pamphlet (English or Spanish)
"Patient Instructions For Treating Genital Herpes" (English or Spanish)
"Straight Talk About Herpes" (English or Spanish)

C & M Pharmacal, Inc.
1519 E. EIGHT MILE ROAD
HAZEL PARK, MI 48030-2696

POD-BEN-25 (C&M) ℞
[päd-bĕn-25]
for the removal of warts (including condylomas)

Description: 25% Podophyllin (Podophyllum resin, Indian) in Tincture of Benzoin, USP
Note: Podophyllin is a powerful caustic. It is a resin whose principal constituents are various podophyllotoxins, peltatins and flavonoids. Indian podophyllin is more potent than U.S. due to its higher content of podophyllotoxins.
Action: Podophyllin's topical effectiveness is due to its cytotoxic, antimitotic action[1,2].
Indications: Pod-Ben-25 is to be used for the removal of warts (including condylomas).
Cautions: **Pod-Ben-25 is an extremely potent medicinal and is to be used (applied) only by the doctor.** Do not use if wart or surrounding tissue is inflamed or irritated. Care and caution should be used in selection of patients to be treated with Pod-Ben-25. Do not use for pregnant women, diabetics, or people with poor blood-circulation; nor on moles, birthmarks, or unusual warts with hair growing from them. It is recommended that patient be advised of effect and possible results of treatment. Keep away from the eyes; if any contacts eye flush with warm water thoroughly and treat as condition indicates.
A noteworthy summary of the position and problem of podophyllin therapy was given by Dr. A.A. Fisher in the opening paragraphs of his Sept. 1981 article in *Cutis:* "Podophyllum resin remains the treatment of choice for condylomata acuminata (venereal warts). As a rule, an intense inflammatory reaction occurs which may become quite painful for a few days. Usually the treatment is successful and there are no local or systemic sequelae. Occasionally, however, severe systemic and local reactions do occur.... Although many dermatologists have used topical podophyllum resin for many years without encountering systemic reactions in their patients, a review of the literature reveals several reports of severe systemic reactions. Among the various systemic effects that have been reported from the use of topically applied podophyllum resin are the following: paresthesia, polyneuritis, paralytic ileus, pyrexia leukopenia, thrombocytopenia, coma, and death."[3]
Method: Pod-Ben-25 is applied to cleansed lesion, using appropriate applicator and allowed to dry thoroughly. Only intact (no bleeding) lesions should be treated and contact with healthy tissue is to be avoided. Due to possible extra-sensitivity to the drug it is recommended that the lotion be first left in contact for a short time (30 to 40 minutes) to determine patient's reaction, if any. To avoid systemic absorption, time of contact should be minimum time necessary to produce the desired result (1 to 4 hours, depending on condition of lesion and of patient), the doctor developing his own experience and technique. Large areas or numerous warts should not be treated at once.
The dried lotion can be removed by alcohol or soap and water; removal should be complete.
How Supplied: 1 fl. oz. bottle NDC 0398-0087-01
Note: **Pod-Ben-25 is available from C&M ONLY by direct shipment to physician.**

References:
1. Bettley: The treatment of skin carcinoma with podophyllum derivatives; Brit. J. Dermat., *84*, 74 (1971)
2. Zackheim: Hazards of topical mitotic-blocking agents; Arch. Dermat., *113*, 234 (1977)
3. Fisher: Severe systemic and local reactions to topical podophyllum resin; Cutis, *28*, 233 (1981)*

* An extensive list of references to podophyllin in the literature is provided at the end of Dr. Fisher's article.

VERR–CANTH–C&M ℞
[vĕr-kănth]
for the removal of benign epithelial growths

Description: Cantharidin 0.7% in an adherent-film-forming base of ethylcellulose, cellosolve, collodion, castor oil, penederm (octylphenyl-polyethylene glycol), acetone.
Note: Cap tightly immediately after use. Keep away from heat and flame. If Verr-Canth thickens (loss of solvent by evaporation) add minimum amount of acetone needed to obtain original consistency, mixing well.
Action: The well-known vesicating and macerating effect of cantharidin is enhanced by the adherency of the film and by the penederm which facilitates its release from the film.
Indications: Verr-Canth is to be used topically for the removal of benign epithelial growths such as verruca vulgaris or molluscum contagiosum. For unusually resistant warts see Verrusol-C&M.
Cautions: **Verr-Canth is a potent vesicant and is to be used (applied) only by the doctor.** It is recommended that care be used in the selection of patients to be treated with Verr-Canth and method used, the doctor developing his own experience and technique. Care should be used in selection of site of application since residual pigmentation may occur (rarely). It is recommended that patients be advised of effect and possible results of treatment and that no more than one or two lesions be treated until patient tolerance is known. Do not use on mucosal tissue. Do not use if growth or surrounding tissue is inflamed or irritated. Do not use for diabetics, or people with poor blood-circulation, nor for moles, birthmarks, or unusual warts with hair growing from them, or if lesion is being treated with other agents. There are no studies of use in pregnant women.
If any Verr-Canth contacts eye or mucosal tissue or normal skin, flush immediately with water for 15 minutes, removing the film precipitated by the water.
Method: Using the thin-tipped applicator provided, apply Verr-Canth to the growth, one drop at a time, covering it completely; allow each drop to dry before applying the next. When completely dry, cover with a non-porous, slightly elastic tape, making sure that none of the medicinal is able to escape. (Prior to the application of the Verr-Canth some of the growth's surface may be removed, if deemed advisable, by paring or by gentle abrasion with a coarse cloth or emery board. Bleeding is to be avoided.) Tape should be left on as long as possible up to 24 hours for warts, up to 6 hours for molluscum. If any Verr-Canth film is still present it should be covered with a Band-aid or similar covering. When treating palpebral warts great care must be used in applying Verr-Canth making certain that film is thoroughly dry and warning patient not to touch the eyelid.
Removal of necrotic material should be done by the doctor. Growth is usually removed with the tape or it may be pared out. If necessary, repeat applications of Verr-Canth can be made when area is free of irritation or inflammation. After the removal of the growth, the use of a mild antibacterial until area heals is advisable.
How Supplied: 7.5 cc bottle with thin-tipped applicator attached to inside of cap. NDC 0398-0085-75.

VERREX–C&M ℞
[vĕr-rĕks]
for the removal of benign epithelial growths such as common warts

Description: Salicylic acid 30.0%, podophyllin 10.0%, penederm 0.5% (octylphenylpolyethylene glycol) in an adherent-film-forming vehicle of ethylcellulose, cellosolve, collodion, castor oil, acetone.
Caution: Federal law prohibits dispensing without prescription.
Action: The well-known keratolytic salicylic acid and roentgomimetic, antimetasticizing podophyllin are present at maximum levels; the surfactant penederm facilitates release from the film and penetration.
Indications: Verrex is to be used topically for the removal of benign epithelial growths such as common warts.
Cautions: Verrex is an extremely potent medicinal and it is recommended that care be used in the selection of patients to use Verrex, as well as location of warts to be treated. Do not use near eyes or on mucosal tissue (genital, anal). Do not use if wart or surrounding skin is inflamed or irritated. Large areas should not be treated at one time since discomfort may be excessive and systemic absorption may result. It is recommended that Verrex not be used for pregnant women, diabetics, or people with poor blood-circulation; nor on moles, birthmarks, or unusual warts with hair growing from them. Care should be used in selection of site of application since residual pigmentation may occur. It is recommended that the patient be advised of effect and possible results of treatment. Do not use if wart is being treated with other agents. Verrex is very flammable: keep away from fire or flame. Cap tightly immediately after use. Store at room temperature away from heat.
If any Verrex contacts eyes or mucosal tissue flush with water for 15 minutes, removing film precipitated by the water.
KEEP OUT OF REACH OF CHILDREN
Method: Wash affected area and soak in warm water for 5 minutes, then dry. Apply one or two drops of Verrex to growth allowing each drop to dry completely. Do not allow Verrex to contact normal skin. Cover with appropriate adhesive bandage which will cover but not adhere to the wart itself making sure that none of the Verrex film escapes. Use once daily for two days to a week, as required. After the removal of the growth the use of a mild anti-bacterial agent until area heals is advisable.
Note: When Verrex is applied by the doctor some of the growth's surface may be removed by rubbing gently with a coarse cloth or emery board after soaking with warm water and drying just prior to initial application. Bleeding is to be avoided.
How Supplied: 7.5 cc bottle with thin-tipped applicator attached to inside of cap. NDC 0398-0080-75.

VERRUSOL–C&M ℞
[vĕr′ yŭ-sol]
for the removal of benign epithelial growths such as common warts

Description: Salicylic acid 30.0%, podophyllin 5.0%, cantharidin 1.0%, penederm 0.5% (octylphenylpolyethylene glycol) in an adherent-film-forming vehicle of ethylcellulose, cellosolve, collodion, castor oil, acetone.
Note: If Verrusol thickens (loss of solvent by evaporation) add minimum amount of acetone needed to obtain original consistency, mixing well.
Action: Verrusol provides a convenient combination in a single vehicle of well-known wart-removing agents. Salicylic acid and cantharidin, both at maximum levels, serve as keratolytic and vesicating agents, respectively; podophyllin provides roentgomimetic and antimetasticizing effects and the surfactant penederm facilitates release from the film and penetration.
Indications: Verrusol is to be used by the doctor (see below) topically for the removal of warts.

Cautions: <u>Verrusol is an extremely potent medicinal and is to be used (applied) only by the doctor.</u> Do not use near eyes or on mucosal tissue (genital, anal). Do not use if wart or surrounding skin is inflamed or irritated. Large areas should not be treated at one time since discomfort may be excessive and systemic absorption may result. Care and caution should be used in selection of patients to be treated with Verrusol and method used, the doctor developing his own experience and technique. It is recommended that Verrusol not be used for pregnant women, diabetics, or people with poor blood-circulation; nor on moles, birthmarks, or unusual warts with hair growing from them. Care should be used in selection of site of application since residual pigmentation may occur. It is recommended that the patient be advised of effect and possible results of treatment, and that no more than one or two warts be treated until patient tolerance is known.

Verrusol is very flammable: keep away from fire or flame. Cap tightly immediately after use. Store at room temperature away from heat. If any Verrusol contacts eyes or mucosal tissue flush with warm water for 15 minutes, removing film precipitated by the water. Do not use if wart is being treated with other agents. Annular warts, if they develop (rare), can be treated with Verrusol (or Verr-Canth).

Method: Using the thin-tipped applicator provided, apply Verrusol to the wart one drop at a time until it is covered: allow each drop to dry before adding the next. When completely dry, cover with a non-porous, slightly elastic tape making sure none of the dried Verrusol is able to escape. Blister forms within 24 hours. It is often painful and inflamed. (Aspirin with codeine or other analgesics may be needed during this period.) Tape should be left on only as long as is necessary up to 24 hours (3 or 4 hours until patient tolerance is known). Growth is usually removed with the tape; or it is pared out after tape is removed. The use of a mild antibacterial agent until area heals is recommended.

<u>Verrusol has been in active use since 1962—with very gratifying results.</u>

How Supplied: 7.5 cc bottle with thin-tipped applicator attached to inside of cap. NDC 0398-0081-75.

Campbell Laboratories Inc.
300 EAST 51st STREET
P.O. BOX 812, F.D.R. STATION
NEW YORK, NY 10022

HERPECIN-L® Cold Sore Lip Balm   OTC
[*her" puh-sin-el"*]

Composition: A soothing, emollient, cosmetically pleasant lip balm incorporating pyridoxine HCl; allantoin; the sunscreen, octyl p-(dimethylamino)-benzoate (Padimate O); and titanium dioxide in a balanced, acidic lipid system. (All ingredients appear on the package. Does not contain any "caines", antibiotics, phenol or camphor.) (NDC 38083-777-31)

Actions and Uses: HERPECIN-L® relieves dryness and chapping by providing a lipid barrier to help restore normal moisture balance to labial tissues. The sunscreen is effective in 2900-3200 AU range while titanium dioxide helps to block, scatter and reflect the sun's rays.

Administration: (1) *Recurrent "cold sores, sun and fever blisters"*: Simply put, users report the sooner and more often applied, the better the results. Frequent sufferers report that with *prophylactic* use (B.I.D./P.R.N.), their attacks are fewer and less severe. Most recurrent herpes labialis patients are aware of the *prodromal* symptoms: tingling, itching, burning. At this stage, or if the lesion has already developed, HERPECIN-L should be applied liberally as often as convenient—at least *every hour* (qq. hor.). The prodrome will often persist and remind the patient to continue to reapply HERPECIN-L. (2) *Outdoor sun/winter protection:* Apply during and after exposure (and after swimming) and again at bedtime (h.s.). (3) *Dry, chapped lips:* Apply as needed.

Note: HERPECIN-L is for peri-oral use only; not for "canker sores" (aphthous stomatitis). Primary attacks, usually in children and young adults, are normally intra-oral and accompanied by foul breath, pain and fever. Lasting up to six weeks, they are resistant to most treatments. Adjunctive therapy for pain, fever and secondary infection may be indicated. "Mouth breathing" is often causative of excessive chapping.

Adverse Reactions: A few, rare instances of topical sensitivity to pyridoxine HCl (Vitamin B_6) have been reported. Discontinue use if allergic reaction develops.

Contraindications: HERPECIN-L does not contain any steroids. (Corticosteroids are normally contraindicated in *herpes* infections.)

How Supplied: 2.8 gm. swivel tubes. O.T.C.
Samples Available: Yes. (Request on letterhead.)

The Carlton Corporation
(See Glenwood, Inc.)

Carnrick Laboratories, Inc.
65 HORSE HILL ROAD
CEDAR KNOLLS, NJ 07927

AMEN®   ℞
[*ā' men'*]
(medroxyprogesterone acetate tablet U.S.P. 10 mg)

Caution: Federal Law Prohibits Dispensing Without Prescription

Warning:
THE USE OF PROGESTATIONAL AGENTS DURING THE FIRST FOUR MONTHS OF PREGNANCY IS NOT RECOMMENDED.

Progestational agents have been used beginning with the first trimester of pregnancy in an attempt to prevent habitual abortion or treat threatened abortion. There is no adequate evidence that such use is effective and there is evidence of potential harm to the fetus when such drugs are given during the first four months of pregnancy. Furthermore, in the vast majority of women, the cause of abortion is a defective ovum, which progestational agents could not be expected to influence. In addition, the use of progestational agents, with their uterine-relaxant properties, in patients with fertilized defective ova may cause a delay in spontaneous abortion. Therefore, the use of such drugs during the first four months of pregnancy is not recommended.

Several reports suggest an association between intrauterine exposure to female sex hormones and congenital anomalies, including congenital heart defects and limb reduction defects (Refs. 1-5). One study (Ref. 4) estimated a 4.7-fold increased risk of limb reduction defects in infants exposed in utero to sex hormones (oral contraceptives, hormone withdrawal test for pregnancy, or attempted treatment for threatened abortion). Some of these exposures were very short and involved only a few days of treatment. The data suggest that the risk of limb reduction defects in exposed fetuses is somewhat less than 1 in 1,000.

If the patient is exposed to Amen® during the first four months of pregnancy or if she becomes pregnant while taking this drug, she should be apprised of the potential risks to the fetus.

Description: Amen® (medroxyprogesterone acetate U.S.P.) is a derivative of progesterone. It is a white to off-white, odorless crystalline powder, stable in air, melting between 200° and 210°C. It is freely soluble in chloroform, soluble in acetone and in dioxane, sparingly soluble in alcohol and in methanol, slightly soluble in ether, and insoluble in water.

The chemical name for medroxyprogesterone acetate is Pregn-4-ene-3,20-dione,17-(acetyloxy)-6-methyl-, (6α)-. The structural formula is:

[Structural formula of medroxyprogesterone acetate]

Actions: Amen® (medroxyprogesterone acetate), administered orally in the recommended dose to women with adequate endogenous estrogen, transforms proliferative endometrium into secretory endometrium. Androgenic and anabolic effects have been noted, but the drug is apparently devoid of significant estrogenic activity.

Indications: Amen® (medroxyprogesterone acetate) is indicated in secondary amenorrhea and abnormal uterine bleeding due to hormonal imbalance in the absence of organic pathology, such as submucous fibroids or uterine cancer.

Contraindications: 1. Thrombophlebitis, thromboembolic disorders, cerebral apoplexy or patients with a past history of these conditions. **2.** Liver dysfunction or disease. **3.** Known or suspected malignancy of breast or genital organs. **4.** Undiagnosed vaginal bleeding. **5.** Missed abortion. **6.** As a diagnostic test for pregnancy. **7.** Known sensitivity to medroxyprogesterone acetate.

Warnings: 1. The physician should be alert to the earliest manifestations of thrombotic disorders (thrombophlebitis, cerebrovascular disorders, pulmonary embolism, and retinal thrombosis). Should any of these occur or be suspected, the drug should be discontinued immediately.
2. Beagle dogs treated with medroxyprogesterone acetate developed mammary nodules, some of which were malignant. Although nodules occasionally appeared in control animals, they were intermittent in nature, whereas the nodules in the drug treated animals were larger, more numerous, persistent, and there were some breast malignancies with metastases, their significance with respect to humans has not been established.
3. Discontinue medication pending examination if there is sudden partial or complete loss of vision, or if there is sudden onset of proptosis, diplopia or migraine. If examination reveals papilledema, or retinal vascular lesions, medication should be withdrawn.

Detectable amounts of progestin have been identified in the milk of mothers receiving the drug. The effect of this on the nursing infant has not been determined. Masculinization of the female fetus has occurred when progestins have been used in pregnant women.
4. Retrospective studies of morbidity and mortality in Great Britain and studies of morbidity in the United States have shown a statistically significant association between thrombophlebitis, pulmonary embolism, and cerebral thrombosis and embolism and the use of oral contraceptives. There have been three principal studies in Great Britain[6-8] leading to this conclusion and one[9] in this country. The estimate of the relative risk of thromboembolism in the study by Vessey and Doll[8] was about sevenfold, while Sartwell and Associates[9] in the United States found a relative risk of 4.4, meaning that the users are several times as likely to undergo thromboembolic disease without evident cause as non-users. The American study also indicated that the risk did not persist after discontinuation of administration, and that it was not enhanced by long continued administration. The American study was not designed to evaluate a difference between products.

Continued on next page

Carnrick—Cont.

Precautions: 1. The pretreatment physical examination should include special reference to breast and pelvic organs, as well as Papanicolaou smear.
2. Because this drug may cause some degree of fluid retention, conditions which might be influenced by this factor, such as epilepsy, migraine, asthma, cardiac or renal dysfunction require careful observation.
3. In cases of breakthrough bleeding, as in all cases of irregular bleeding per vaginum, nonfunctional causes should be borne in mind. In cases of undiagnosed vaginal bleeding adequate diagnostic measures are indicated.
4. Patients who have a history of psychic depression should be carefully observed and the drug discontinued if the depression recurs to a serious degree.
5. Any possible influence of prolonged progestin therapy on pituitary, ovarian, adrenal, hepatic or uterine functions awaits further study.
6. A decrease in glucose tolerance has been observed in a small percentage of patients on estrogen-progestin combination drugs. The mechanism of this decrease is obscure. For this reason, diabetic patients should be carefully observed while receiving progestin therapy.
7. The age of the patient constitutes no absolute limiting factor although treatment with progestins may mask the onset of the climacteric.
8. The pathologist should be advised of progestin therapy when relevant specimens are submitted.
9. Because of the occasional occurence of thrombotic disorders, (thrombophlebitis, pulmonary embolism, retinal thrombosis, and cerebrovascular disorders) in patients taking estrogen-progestin combinations and since the mechanism is obscure, the physician should be alert to the earliest manifestation of these disorders.
10. Information for the patient. See text of Patient Information which is printed at the end of this insert.

Adverse Reactions: The following adverse reactions have been associated with the use of medroxyprogesterone acetate.
Breast: In a few instances, breast tenderness or galactorrhea have occurred.
Pregnancy: A few cases of clitoral hypertrophy have been reported in new born females, whose mothers received medroxyprogesterone acetate during pregnancy. Prolonged postpartum bleeding, postabortal bleeding and missed abortion have been reported. (See WARNING box for possible adverse effects on the fetus).
Psychic: An occasional patient has experienced nervousness, insomnia, somnolence, fatigue or dizziness.
Thromboembolic phenomena: Thromboembolic phenomena including thrombophlebitis and pulmonary embolism have been reported.
Skin and mucous membranes: Sensitivity reactions ranging from pruritus, urticaria, angioneurotic edema to generalized rash and anaphylaxis have occasionally been reported. Acne, alopecia, or hirsutism have been reported in a few cases.
Gastrointestinal: Rarely, nausea has been reported. Jaundice, including neonatal jaundice, has been noted in a few instances.
Miscellaneous: Rare cases of headache and hyperpyrexia have been reported. The following adverse reactions have been observed in women taking progestins including medroxyprogesterone acetate: breakthrough bleeding; spotting; change in menstrual flow; amenorrhea; edema; change in weight (increase or decrease); changes in cervical erosion and cervical secretions; cholestatic jaundice; rash (allergic) with and without pruritus; melasma or chloasma; mental depression.
A statistically significant association has been demonstrated between use of estrogen-progestin combination drugs and the following serious adverse reactions; thrombophlebitis, pulmonary embolism and cerebral thrombosis and embolism.

For this reason patients on progestin therapy should be carefully observed.
Although available evidence is suggestive of an association, such a relationship has been neither confirmed nor refuted for the following serious adverse reactions: neuro-ocular lesions, e.g., retinal thrombosis and optic neuritis.
The following adverse reactions have been observed in patients receiving estrogen-progestin combination drugs; rise in blood pressure in susceptible individuals; premenstrual-like syndrome; changes in libido; changes in appetite; cystitis-like syndrome; headache; nervousness; dizziness; fatigue; backache; hirsutism; loss of scalp hair; erythema multiforme; erythema nodosum; hemorraghic eruption; itching.
In view of these observations, patients on progestin therapy should be carefully observed.
Female fetal masculinization has been observed in patients receiving progestins. The following laboratory results may be altered by the use of estrogen-progestin combination drugs: Increased sulfobromophthalein and other hepatic function tests; Coagulation tests: increase in prothrombin factors VII, VIII, IX and X; Metyrapone test; Pregnanediol determination.

Dosage and Administration: Secondary Amenorrhea—Amen® (medroxyprogesterone acetate) may be given in dosages of 5 to 10 mg daily for from 5 to 10 days. A dose for inducing an optimum secretory transformation of an endometrium that has been adequately primed with either endogenous or exogenous estrogen is 10 mg of Amen® daily for 10 days. In cases of secondary amenorrhea, therapy may be started at any time. Progestin withdrawal bleeding usually occurs within three to seven days after discontinuing therapy with Amen®.

Abnormal Uterine Bleeding Due to Hormonal Imbalance in the Absence of Organic Pathology—Beginning on the calculated 16th or 21st day of the menstrual cycle, 5 to 10 mg of Amen® may be given daily for from 5 to 10 days. To produce an optimum secretory transformation of an endometrium that has been adequately primed with either endogenous or exogenous estrogen, 10 mg of Amen® daily for 10 days beginning on the 16th day of the cycle is suggested. Progestin withdrawal bleeding usually occurs within three to seven days after discontinuing therapy with Amen®. Patients with a past history of recurrent episodes of abnormal uterine bleeding may benefit from planned menstrual cycling with Amen®.

References: 1. Gal, I., B. Kirman, and J. Stern, "Hormonal Pregnancy Tests and Congenital Malformation," Nature, 216:83, 1967.
2. Levy, E. P., A. Cohen, and F. C. Fraser, "Hormone Treatment During Pregnancy and Congenital Heart Defects," Lancet, 1:611, 1973.
3. Nora, J. and A. Nora, "Birth Defects and Oral Contraceptives," Lancet, 1:941, 1973.
4. Janerich, D. T., J. M. Piper, and D. M. Glebatis, "Oral Contraceptives and Congenital Limb-Reduction Defects," New England Journal of Medicine, 291:697, 1974.
5. Heinonen, O. P., D. Slone, R. R. Monson, E. B. Hook, and S. Shapiro, "Cardiovascular Birth Defects and Antenatal Exposure to Female Sex Hormones," New England Journal of Medicine, 296:67, 1977.
6. Royal College of General Practitioners; Oral Contraception and Thromboembolic Disease. J. Coll. Gen. Prac., 13:267–279, 1967.
7. Inman, W. H. W. and Vessey, M. P.: Investigation of Deaths From Pulmonary Coronary and Cerebral Thrombosis and Embolism in Women in Child-Bearing Age, Brit. Med. J., 2:193–199, 1968.
8. Vessey, M. P. and Doll, R.: Investigation in Relation Between Use of Oral Contraceptives and Thromboembolic Disease. A Further Report, Brit. Med. J., 2:651–657, 1969.
9. Sartwell, P. E., Masi, A. T., Arthes, G. R., Greene, R. R., and Smith, H. E.: Thromboembolism and Oral Contraceptives: An Epidemiological Case-Control Study, Am. J. Epidem., 90: 365–380, (Nov.) 1969.

Patient Information for Amen®—Warning for Women

There is an increased risk of birth defects in children whose mothers take this drug during the first four months of pregnancy.
Amen® is similar to the progesterone hormones naturally produced by the body. Progesterone and progesterone-like drugs are used to treat menstrual disorders, to test if the body is producing certain hormones, and to treat some forms of cancer in women.
They have been used as a test for pregnancy but such use is no longer considered safe because of possible damage to a developing baby. Also, more rapid methods for testing for pregnancy are now available. These drugs have also been used to prevent miscarriage in the first few months of pregnancy. No adequate evidence is available to show that they are effective for this purpose and there is evidence of an increased risk of birth defects, such as heart or limb defects, if these drugs are taken during the first four months of pregnancy. Furthermore, most cases of early miscarriage are due to causes which could not be helped by these drugs. The exact risk of taking this drug early in pregnancy and having a baby with a birth defect is not known. However, one study found that babies born to women who had taken sex hormones (such as progesterone-like drugs) during the first three months of pregnancy were 4 to 5 times more likely to have abnormalities of the arms or legs than if their mothers had not taken such drugs. Some of these women had taken these drugs for only a few days. The chance that an infant whose mother had taken this drug will have this type of defect is about 1 in 1,000.
If you take Amen® and later find you were pregnant when you took it, be sure to discuss this with your doctor as soon as possible.

How Supplied: Two-layered peach and white scored tablet with "C" on one side and "AMEN" on the other. Amen® tablets containing 10 mg. of medroxyprogesterone acetate U.S.P. are available in bottles of 50 (NDC 0086-0049-05) 100 (NDC 0086-0049-10) and 1000 (NDC 0086-0049-90).
The most recent revision of this labeling is April 1984.
Manufactured for Carnrick Laboratories, Inc.
Shown in Product Identification Section, page 408

BONTRIL® PDM
[bŏn'tril]
(brand of phendimetrazine tartrate 35 mg. tablets)

Dosage and Administration: Usual Adult Dosage: Dosage should be individualized to obtain an adequate response with the lowest effective dose. In some cases 17½ mg. per dose may be adequate. 1 tablet (35 mg.) b.i.d. or t.i.d. one hour before meals. Dosage should not exceed 2 tablets t.i.d.
How Supplied: Three layered green, white and yellow tablets with 8648 on the scored side and the letter "C" on the other. Bottles of 100, NDC 0086-0048-10. Bottles of 1,000, NDC 0086-0048-90.
Caution: Federal law prohibits dispensing without prescription.
See product insert for complete information.
Manufactured for Carnrick Laboratories, Inc.
Shown in Product Identification Section, page 408

BONTRIL® SLOW-RELEASE
[bŏn'tril]
(brand of phendimetrazine tartrate slow–release capsules 105 mg)

Description: Phendimetrazine tartrate, as the dextro isomer, has the chemical name of (+)-3,4-Dimethyl-2-phenylmorpholine Tartrate.
The structural formula is as follows:

M.W. 341

Phendimetrazine tartrate is a white, odorless powder with a bitter taste. It is soluble in water, methanol and ethanol.

Actions: Phendimetrazine tartrate is a sympathomimetic amine with pharmacological activity similar to the prototype drugs of this class used in obesity, the amphetamines. Actions include central nervous system stimulation and elevation of blood pressure. Tachyphylaxis and tolerance have been demonstrated with all drugs of this class in which these phenomena have been looked for.

Drugs of this class used in obesity are commonly known as "anorectics" or "anorexigenics". It has not been established, however, that the action of such drugs in treating obesity is primarily one of appetite suppression. Other central nervous system actions or metabolic effects may be involved. Adult obese subjects instructed in dietary management and treated with anorectic drugs lose more weight on the average than those treated with placebo and diet, as determined in relatively short term clinical trials.

The magnitude of increased weight loss of drug-treated patients over placebo-treated patients is only a fraction of a pound a week. The rate of weight loss is greatest in the first weeks of therapy for both drug and placebo subjects and tends to decrease in succeeding weeks. The possible origin of the increased weight loss due to the various drug effects is not established. The amount of weight loss associated with the use of an anorectic drug varies from trial to trial, and the increased weight loss appears to be related in part to variables other than the drug prescribed, such as the physician investigator, the population treated, and the diet prescribed. Studies do not permit conclusions as to the relative importance of the drug and non-drug factors on weight loss.

The natural history of obesity is measured in years, whereas the studies cited are restricted to a few weeks duration; thus, the total impact of drug-induced weight loss over that of diet alone must be considered clinically limited.

The active dose 105 mg of phendimetrazine tartrate in each capsule of this special slow-release dosage form approximates the action of three 35 mg non-time release doses taken at 4 hours intervals.

The major route of elimination is via the kidneys where most of the drug and metabolites are excreted. Some of the drug is metabolized to phenmetrazine and also phendimetrazine-N-oxide.

The average half-life of elimination when studied under controlled conditions is about 1.9 hours for the non-time and 9.8 hours for the slow-release dosage form. The absorption half-life of the drug from conventional non-time 35 mg phendimetrazine tablets is approximately the same. These data indicate that the slow-release product has a similar onset of action to the conventional non-time-release product and, in addition, has a prolonged therapeutic effect.

Indications: Phendimetrazine tartrate is indicated in the management of exogenous obesity as a short term adjunct (a few weeks) in a regimen of weight reduction based on caloric restriction. The limited usefulness of agents of this class (see ACTIONS) should be measured against possible risk factors inherent in their use such as those described below.

Contraindications: Advanced arteriosclerosis, symptomatic cardiovascular disease, moderate and severe hypertension, hyperthyroidism, known hypersensitivity, or idiosyncrasy to the sympathomimetic amines. Agitated states. Patients with a history of drug abuse. Use in Patients taking other CNS stimulants including monoamine oxidase inhibitors.

Warnings: Tolerance to the anorectic effect usually develops within a few weeks. When this occurs, the recommended dose should not be exceeded in an attempt to increase the effect; rather, the drug should be discontinued.

Use of phendimetrazine within 14 days following the administration of monoamine oxidase inhibitors may result in a hypertensive crisis.

Abrupt cessation of administration following prolonged high dosage results in extreme fatigue and depression. Because of the effect on the central nervous system phendimetrazine tartrate may impair the ability of the patient to engage in potentially hazardous activities such as operating machinery or driving a motor vehicle; the patient should therefore be cautioned accordingly.

Precautions: Caution is to be exercised in prescribing phendimetrazine for patients with even mild hypertension.

Insulin requirements in diabetes mellitus may be altered in association with the use of phendimetrazine and the concomitant dietary regimen.

Phendimetrazine may decrease the hypotensive effect of guanethidine.

The least amount feasible should be prescribed or dispensed at one time in order to minimize the possibility of overdosage.

Usage in Pregnancy: Safe use in pregnancy has not been established. Until more information is available, phendimetrazine tartrate should not be taken by women who are or may become pregnant unless, in the opinion of the physician, the potential benefits outweigh the possible hazards.

Usage in Children: Phendimetrazine tartrate is not recommended for use in children under 12 years of age.

Adverse Reactions: Cardiovascular: Palpitation, tachycardia, elevation of blood pressure.

Central Nervous System: Overstimulation, restlessness, dizziness, insomnia, tremor, headache, rarely psychotic episodes at recommended doses, agitation, flushing, sweating, blurring of vision.

Gastrointestinal: Dryness of the mouth, diarrhea, constipation, nausea, stomach pain.

Genitourinary: Changes in libido, urinary frequency, dysuria.

Drug Abuse and Dependence:

Controlled Substance: Phendimetrazine is a Schedule III controlled substance.

Dependence: Phendimetrazine Tartrate is related chemically and pharmacologically to the amphetamines. Amphetamines and related stimulant drugs have been extensively abused, and the possibility of abuse of phendimetrazine should be kept in mind when evaluating the desirability of including a drug as part of a weight reduction program. Abuse of amphetamines and related drugs may be associated with intense psychological dependence and severe social dysfunction. There are reports of patients who have increased the dosage to many times that recommended. Abrupt cessation following prolonged high dosage administration results in extreme fatigue and mental depression; changes are also noted on the sleep EEG. Manifestations of chronic intoxication with anorectic drugs include severe dermatoses, marked insomnia, irritability, hyperactivity and personality changes. The most severe manifestation of chronic intoxications is psychosis, often clinically indistinguishable from schizophrenia.

Overdosage: Manifestations of acute overdosage may include restlessness, tremor, hyperreflexia, rapid respiration, confusion, assaultiveness, hallucinations, panic states.

Fatigue and depression usually follow the central stimulation.

Cardiovascular effects include arrhythmias, hypertension, or hypotension and circulatory collapse. Gastrointestinal symptoms include nausea, vomiting, diarrhea, and abdominal cramps. Poisoning may result in convulsions, coma, and death. Management of acute intoxication is largely symptomatic and includes lavage and sedation with a barbiturate. Experience with hemodialysis or peritoneal dialysis is inadequate to permit recommendation in this regard.

Acidification of the urine increases phendimetrazine tartrate excretion.

Intravenous phentolamine (Regitine) has been suggested for possible acute, severe hypertension, if this complicates overdosage.

Dosage and Administration: One Slow-Release Capsule (105 mg) in the morning, taken 30-60 minutes before the morning meal.

Phendimetrazine Tartrate is not recommended for use in children under twelve years of age.

How Supplied: Phendimetrazine Slow-Release Capsules, 105 mg is supplied in bottles of 100 opaque green and clear yellow capsules, imprinted with the letter "C" and 8647. NDC # 0086-0047-10.

Store at controlled room temperature, 15°-30°C(59°-86°F).

The most recent revision of this labeling is Oct. 1984.

Caution: Federal law prohibits dispensing without prescription.

Manufactured For: Carnrick Laboratories, Inc.

Shown in Product Identification Section, page 408

CAPITAL® with CODEINE
(acetaminophen with codeine)
Tablets ℞ Suspension ℞

Caution: Federal law prohibits dispensing without prescription.

Description:

Each CAPITAL® with CODEINE tablet contains:
Codeine Phosphate*   30 mg
*WARNING: May be habit forming
Acetaminophen   325 mg

CAPITAL® with CODEINE suspension contains (in each 5ml):
Codeine Phosphate*   12 mg
*WARNING: May be habit forming
Acetaminophen   120 mg

Acetaminophen occurs as a white, odorless crystalline powder, possessing a slightly bitter taste. Codeine is an alkaloid, obtained from opium or prepared from morphine by methylation. Codeine occurs as colorless or white crystals, efforesces slowly in dry air and is affected by light.

Actions: Acetaminophen is a nonopiate, nonsalicylate analgesic and antipyretic. Codeine is an opiate analgesic and antitussive. Codeine retains at least one-half of its analgesic activity when administered orally.

Indications: CAPITAL® with CODEINE tablets are indicated for the relief of mild to moderately severe pain. CAPITAL® with CODEINE suspension is indicated for the relief of mild to moderate pain.

Contraindications: Hypersensitivity to acetaminophen or codeine.

Warnings:

Drug Dependence: Codeine can produce drug dependence of the morphine type, and therefore, has the potential for being abused. Psychic dependence, physical dependence and tolerance may develop upon repeated administration of this drug and it should be prescribed and administered with the same degree of caution appropriate to the use of other oral narcotic medications.

CAPITAL® with CODEINE tablets is subject to the Federal Controlled Substances Act (Schedule III). CAPITAL® with CODEINE suspension is subject to the Federal Controlled Substances Act (Schedule V).

Precautions:

1. **General:**

   Head Injury and increased intracranial pressure: The respiratory depressant effects of narcotics and their capacity to elevate cerebrospinal fluid pressure may be markedly exaggerated in the presence of head injury, other intracranial lesions or a pre-existing increase in intracranial pressure. Furthermore, narcotics produce adverse reactions which may obscure the clinical course of patients with head injuries.

   Acute abdominal conditions: The administration of products containing codeine or other narcotics may obscure the diagnosis or clinical course in patients with acute abdominal conditions.

   Special risk patients: Acetaminophen with codeine should be given with caution to certain patients such as elderly or debilitated, and those with severe impairment of hepatic or renal funcion, hypothyroidism, Addison's disease, and prostatic hypertrophy or urethral stricture.

Continued on next page

Carnrick—Cont.

2. **Information for Patients:**
Codeine may impair the mental and/or physical abilities required for the performance of potentially hazardous tasks such as driving a car or operating machinery. The patient taking this drug should be cautioned accordingly.

3. **Drug Interactions:**
Patients receiving other narcotic analgesics, antipsychotics, antianxiety, or other CNS depressants (including alcohol) concomitantly with acetaminophen and codeine may exhibit additive CNS depression due to the codeine component. When such therapy is contemplated, the dose of one or both agents should be reduced. The use of MAO inhibitors or tricyclic antidepressants with codeine preparations may increase the effect of either the antidepressant or codeine.

The concurrent use of anticholinergics with codeine may produce paralytic ileus.

4. **Usage in Pregancy:**
Safe use in pregnancy has not been established relative to possible adverse effects on fetal development. Therefore, acetaminophen and codeine should not be used in pregnant women unless, in the judgment of the physician, the potential benefits outweigh the possible hazards.

5. **Nursing Mothers:**
Problems in humans have not been documented; however, risk-benefit must be considered since acetaminophen (in very low concentrations) and codeine are excreted in breast milk.

6. **Pediatric Use:**
Safety and effectiveness of the suspension in children below the age of 3 have not been established. Tablets should not be administered to children under 12.

Adverse Reactions: The most frequently observed adverse reactions include light-headedness, dizziness, sedation, shortness of breath, nausea, and vomiting. These effects seem to be more prominent in ambulatory than in non-ambulatory patients, and some of these adverse reactions may be alleviated if the patient lies down.

Other adverse reactions include euphoria, dysphoria, constipation and pruritus. At higher doses codeine has most of the disadvantages of morphine including respiratory depression.

Overdosage:
Acetaminophen:
Signs and Symptoms: Acetaminophen in massive overdosage may cause hepatic toxicity in some patients. In all cases of suspected overdose, immediately call your regional poison center or the Rocky Mountain Poison Center's toll-free number (800 525-6115) for assistance in diagnosis and for directions in the use of N-acetylcysteine as an antidote, a use currently restricted to investigational status. In adults, hepatic toxicity has rarely been reported with acute overdoses of less than 10 grams and fatalities with less than 15 grams. Importantly, young children seem to be more resistant than adults to the hepatotoxic effect of an acetaminophen overdose. Despite this, the measures outlined below should be initiated in any adult or child suspected of having ingested an acetaminophen overdose.

Early symptoms following a potentially hepatotoxic overdose may include: nausea, vomiting, diaphoresis and general malaise. Clinical and laboratory evidence of hepatic toxicity may not be apparent until 48 to 72 hours post-ingestion.

Treatment: The stomach should be emptied promptly by lavage or by induction of emesis with syrup of ipecac. Patients' estimates of the quantity of a drug ingested are notoriously unreliable. Therefore, if an acetaminophen overdose is suspected, a serum acetaminophen assay should be obtained as early as possible, but no sooner than four hours following ingestion. Liver function studies should be obtained initially and repeated at 24-hour intervals.

The antidote, N-acetylcysteine, should be administered as early as possible, and within 16 hours of the overdose ingestion for optimal results. Following recovery, there are no residual, structural or functional hepatic abnormalities.

Codeine:
Signs and Symptoms: Serious overdose with codeine is characterized by respiratory depression (a decrease in respiratory rate and/or tidal volume, Cheyne-Stokes respiration, cyanosis), extreme somnolence progressing to stupor or coma, skeletal muscle flaccidity, cold and clammy skin, and sometimes bradycardia and hypotension. In severe overdosage, apnea, circulatory collapse, cardiac arrest and death may occur.

Treatment: Primary attention should be given to the reestablishment of adequate respiratory exchange through provision of a patent airway and the institution of assisted or controlled ventilation. The narcotic antagonist naloxone is a specific antidote against respiratory depression which may result from overdosage or unusual sensitivity to narcotics, including codeine. Therefore, an appropriate dose of naloxone (see package insert) should be administered, preferably by the intravenous route, and simultaneously with efforts at respiratory resuscitation. Since the duration of acion of codeine may exceed that of the antagonist, the patient should be kept under continued surveillance and repeated doses of the antagonist should be administered as needed to maintain adequate respiration.

An antagonist should not be administered in the absence of clinically significant respiratory or cardiovascular depression. Oxygen, intravenous fluids, vasopressors and other supportive measures should be employed as indicated.

Gastric emptying may be useful in removing unabsorbed drug.

Dosage and Administration: Dosage should be adjusted according to severity of pain and response of the patient. However, it should be kept in mind that tolerance to codeine can develop with continued use and that the incidence of untoward effects is dose related. This product is inappropriate even in high doses for severe or intractable pain. Adult doses of codeine higher than 60 mg. fail to give commensurate relief of pain but merely prolong analgesia and are associated with an appreciably increased incidence of undesirable side effects. Equivalently high doses in children would have similar effects.

CAPITAL® with CODEINE tablets are given orally. Adults: One tablet for mild to moderate pain. Two tablets for moderate to moderately severe pain. Doses can be repeated up to every 4 hours as required.

CAPITAL® with CODEINE suspension is given orally. The usual doses are: Children (3 to 6 years): One teaspoonful (5 ml) 3 or 4 times daily. (7 to 12 years): Two teaspoonfuls (10 ml) 3 or 4 times daily. Adults: One tablespoonful (15 ml) every 4 hours as needed.

SHAKE WELL BEFORE USING

How Supplied: CAPITAL® with CODEINE tablets: Pale blue scored tablet imprinted with 8644 and a sunburst on the scored side and the letter "C" on the other. Bottle of 100 tablets, NDC 0086-0044-10. Store at Controlled Room Temperature 15°-30°C (59°-86°F) in a dry place.

CAPTIAL® with CODEINE suspension: a pink, pleasantly flavored suspension—16 oz. bottles, NDC 0086-0046-16. Store at Controlled Room Temperature 15°-30°C (59°-86°F)

The most recent revision of this labeling is September 1983.

Manufactured for: Carnrick Laboratories, Inc.
Shown in Product Identification Section, page 408

MIDRIN®
[mid′rin]

Caution: Federal law prohibits dispensing without prescription.

Description: Each red capsule with pink band contains Isometheptene Mucate 65 mg., Dichloralphenazone 100 mg., and Acetaminophen 325 mg. Isometheptene Mucate is a white crystalline powder having a characteristic aromatic odor and bitter taste. It is an unsaturated aliphatic amine with sympathomimetic properties.

Dichloralphenazone is a white, microcrystalline powder, with slight odor and tastes saline at first, becoming acrid. It is a mild sedative.

Acetaminophen, a non-salicylate, occurs as a white, odorless, crystalline powder possessing a slightly bitter taste.

Actions: Isometheptene Mucate, a sympathomimetic amine, acts by constricting dilated cranial and cerebral arterioles, thus reducing the stimuli that lead to vascular headaches. Dichloralphenazone, a mild sedative, reduces the patient's emotional reaction to the pain of both vascular and tension headaches. Acetaminophen raises the threshold to painful stimuli, thus exerting an analgesic effect against all types of headaches.

Indications: For relief of tension and vascular headaches.*

* Based on a review of this drug (isometheptene mucate) by the National Academy of Sciences-National Research Council and/or other information, FDA has classified the other indication as "Possibly" effective in the treatment of migraine headache.

Final classification of the less-than-effective indication requires further investigation.

Contraindications: Midrin is contraindicated in glaucoma and/or severe cases of renal disease, hypertension, organic heart disease, hepatic disease and in those patients who are on monoamine-oxidase (MAO) inhibitor therapy.

Precautions: Caution should be observed in hypertension, peripheral vascular disease and after recent cardiovascular attacks.

Adverse Reactions: Transient dizziness and skin rash may appear in hypersensitive patients. This can usually be eliminated by reducing the dose.

Dosage and Administration: FOR RELIEF OF MIGRAINE HEADACHE: The usual adult dosage is two capsules at once, followed by one capsule every hour until relieved, up to 5 capsules within a twelve hour period.

FOR RELIEF OF TENSION HEADACHE: The usual adult dosage is one or two capsules every four hours up to 8 capsules a day.

How Supplied: Red capsules imprinted with pink band, the letter "C" and 86120. Bottles of 50 capsules, NDC 0086-0120-05. Bottles of 100 capsules, NDC 0086-0120-10. Store at controlled room temperature 15–30°C (59–86°F) in a dry place.

The most recent revision of this labeling is Dec. 1983.

Manufactured for Carnrick Laboratories, Inc.
Shown in Product Identification Section, page 408

NOLAHIST®
[nō′lă-hist]
(phenindamine tartrate)

Description: Each tablet contains:
Phenindamine Tartrate .... 25 mg
Indications: For temporary relief of running nose, sneezing, itching of the nose or throat and itchy and watery eyes as may occur in allergic rhinitis (such as hay fever).

Dosage: Adult oral dosage is one tablet every 4 to 6 hours not to exceed six tablets in 24 hours. Children 6 to under 12 years oral dosage is one-half tablet every 4 to 6 hours not to exceed 3 tablets in 24 hours. For children under 6 years, there is no recommended dosage except under the advice and supervision of a physician.

Warnings: May cause drowsiness. May cause excitability espcially in children. Do not take this product if you have asthma, glaucoma or difficulty in urination due to enlargement of the prostate gland except under the advice and supervision of a physician. Do not give this product to children under 6 years except under the advise and supervision of a physician. As with any drug, if you are pregnant or nursing a baby, seek the advice of a health professional before using this product. Keep this and all medication out of the reach of children. In case of accidental overdose, seek professional assistance or contact a Poison Control Center immediately.

Cautions: May cause nervousness and insomnia in some individuals. Avoid driving a motor vehicle or operating heavy machinery. Avoid alcoholic beverages while taking this product.

How Supplied: White, capsule-shaped, scored tablet inscribed with 8652 on one side and the letter C on the other side in bottles of 100. Each tablet contains phenindamine tartrate 25 mg. (NDC 0086-0052-10)

Store at 15°–30°C (59°–86°F) and keep tightly closed away from light.

Manufactured for Carnrick Laboratories, Inc.

Shown in Product Identification Section, page 408

NOLAMINE® ℞
[nō' lă-mēn']

Description:
Each timed release tablet contains:
Phenindamine tartrate .... 24 mg
Chlorpheniramine maleate .... 4 mg
Phenylpropanolamine hydrochloride .... 50 mg
Formulated to provide 8 to 12 hours of continuous relief.

Caution: Federal law prohibits dispensing without prescription.

Indications: As a nasal decongestant associated with the common cold, sinusitis, hay fever and other allergies.

Contraindications: Hypersensitivity to any of the components. Contraindicated in concurrent MAO inhibitor therapy.

Side Effects: Nervousness, insomnia, tremors, dizziness and drowsiness may occur occasionally.

Precautions: Antihistamines may cause drowsiness and should be used with caution in patients who operate motor vehicles or dangerous machinery. Use with caution in patients with hypertension, cardiovascular disease, diabetes or hyperthyroidism. Ths product should be used with caution in patients with prostatic hypertrophy or glaucoma.

Dosage: Usual adult dose: Orally, one tablet every 8 hours. In mild cases, one tablet every 10 to 12 hours.

How Supplied: Pink, timed release tablets coded C 86204 in bottles of 100 (NDC 0086-0204-10) and 250 (NDC 0086-0204-25). Store at room temperature.

Manufactured for Carnrick Laboratories, Inc.

Shown in Product Identification Section, page 408

PHRENILIN® ℞
[fren' ĭ-lin]
and
PHRENILIN® FORTE ℞

Caution: Federal Law Prohibits Dispensing Without Prescription

Description: PHRENILIN®: Each PHRENILIN® tablet, an analgesic-sedative combination for oral administration contains: butalbital, USP 50 mg., (Warning—May be habit forming); acetaminophen, USP 325 mg.

PHRENILIN® FORTE: Each PHRENILIN® FORTE capsule, an analgesic-sedative combination for oral administration, contains: butalbital, USP 50 mg., (Warning—May be habit forming); acetaminophen, USP 650 mg.

Butalbital
Butalbital, 5-allyl-5-isobutyl-barbituric acid, a white odorless crystalline powder, is a short to intermediate acting barbiturate.

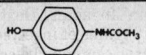

Acetaminophen
Acetaminophen, N-acetyl-p-amino-phenol, occurs as a white, odorless, crystalline powder, possessing a slightly bitter taste. Acetaminophen is a non-salicylate, non-narcotic analgesic, and antipyretic.

Clinical Pharmacology: Pharmacologically, Butalbital-Acetaminophen combines the analgesic properties of acetaminophen with the anxiolytic and muscle relaxant properties of butalbital.

Butalbital is a short to intermediate acting barbiturate which produces mild sedation. Barbiturates are capable of producing all levels of CNS mood alteration from excitation to mild sedation, to hypnosis, and deep coma. Overdosage can produce death.

Barbiturates depress the sensory cortex, decrease motor activity, alter cerebellar function, and produce drowsiness, sedation, and hypnosis. Barbiturates are respiratory depressants. The degree of respiratory depression is dependent on dose.

Barbiturates do not impair normal hepatic function, but have been shown to induce liver microsomal enzymes, thus increasing and/or altering the metabolism of barbiturates and other drugs.

Acetaminophen is a non-narcotic analgesic and antipyretic. Acetaminophen produces analgesia by elevation of the pain threshold and antipyresis through action on the hypothalamic heat-regulating center.

Pharmacokinetics: The onset and duration of action, which is related to the rate at which the barbiturates are redistributed throughout the body, varies among persons and in the same person from time to time. Butalbital has a duration of action from 3 to 6 hours.

Barbiturates are weak acids that are absorbed and rapidly distributed to all tissues and fluids with high concentrations in the brain, liver, and kidneys. The more lipid soluble the barbiturate, the more rapidly it penetrates all tissues of the body. Barbiturates are bound to plasma and tissue proteins to a varying degree with the degree of binding increasing directly as a function of lipid solubility. Barbiturates are metabolized primarily by the hepatic microsomal enzyme system and the metabolic products are excreted in the urine, and less commonly, in the feces. The inactive metabolites of the barbiturates are excreted as conjugates of glucoronic acid.

Acetaminophen is rapidly and almost completely absorbed from the gastrointestinal tract, producing maximum serum concentrations within 30 minutes to one hour. The plasma half-life varies from one to four hours. Acetaminophen is relatively uniformly distributed throughout most body fluids and is approximately 25% protein bound. Approximately 90 to 95% of a dose is metabolized in the liver, primarily by conjugation with glucuronic acid, sulfuric acid, and cysteine. An intermediate metabolite is hepatotoxic. Excretion is renal; primarily as conjugates. About 3% of a dose may be excreted unchanged.

Indications and Usage: PHRENILIN® and PHRENILIN® FORTE are indicated for the relief of the symptom complex of tension (or muscle contraction) headache.

Contraindications: Hypersensitivity to any of the components. Patients with porphyria.

Warnings: Acetaminophen in massive overdosage may cause hepatotoxicity in some patients. (See OVERDOSAGE.)

Habit Forming: Barbiturates may be habit forming. Tolerance, psychological and physical dependence may occur with continued use. (See DRUG ABUSE AND DEPENDENCE.) Abrupt cessation after prolonged use in the dependent person may result in withdrawal symptoms, including delirium, convulsions, and possibly death. Barbiturates should be withdrawn gradually from any patient known to be taking excessive dosage over long periods of time.

Acute or Chronic Pain: Caution should be exercised when barbiturates are administered to patients with acute or chronic pain, because paradox-ical excitement could be induced or important symptoms could be masked.

Use in Pregnancy: (See PRECAUTIONS section.)

Synergistic Effects: The concomitant use of alcohol or other CNS depressants may produce additive CNS depressant effects.

Precautions:
General: Barbiturates may be habit forming. Tolerance and psychological and physical dependence may occur with continuing use. (See DRUG ABUSE AND DEPENDENCE.) Barbiturates should be administered with caution, if at all, to patients who are mentally depressed, have suicidal tendencies, or a history of drug abuse.

Elderly or debilitated patients may react to barbiturates with marked excitement, depression, and confusion. In some persons, barbiturates repeatedly produce excitement rather than depression.

In patients with hepatic damage, barbiturates should be administered with caution and initially in reduced doses. Barbiturates should not be administered to patients showing the premonitory signs of hepatic coma.

Use with caution in patients with severe renal function impairment.

Do not exceed recommended dosage. Excessive or prolonged use should be avoided.

Information for Patients: Practitioners should give the following information and instructions to patients receiving barbiturates.

1. The use of barbiturates carries with it an associated risk of psychological and/or physical dependence. The patient should be warned against increasing the dose of the drug without consulting a physician.
2. Barbiturates may impair mental and/or physical abilities required for the performance of potentially hazardous tasks (e.g., driving, operating machinery, etc.).
3. Alcohol should not be consumed while taking barbiturates. Concurrent use of the barbiturates with other CNS depressants (e.g., alcohol, narcotics, tranquilizers, and antihistamines) may result in additional CNS depressant effects.

Drug Interactions: The concomitant use of other central nervous system depressants, including other sedatives or hypnotics, antihistamines, tranquilizers, or alcohol, may produce additive depressant effects. When such combined therapy is necessary, the dose of one or more agents may need to be reduced.

The presence of barbiturates decreases the effects of oral anticoagulants, griseofulvin, doxycycline, corticosteroids, and possibly phenytoin. Monoamine oxidase inhibitors (MAOI) prolong the effects of barbiturates.

Use in Pregnancy: Animal reproduction studies have not been conducted with PHRENILIN® or PHRENILIN® FORTE. It is also not known whether PHRENILIN® or PHRENILIN® FORTE can cause fetal harm when administered to a pregnant woman or can affect reproduction capacity.

BUTALBITAL:

First trimester: The teratogenic potential of butalbital has not been studied in either animals or humans. Although teratogenic effects with this combination medication have not been reported clinically, risk-benefit must be considered since other barbiturates have been shown to increase the risk of fetal abnormalities in humans. If this drug is used during pregnancy, or if the patient becomes pregnant while taking this drug, the patient should be apprised of the potential hazard to the fetus.

Third trimester: Use of barbiturates throughout the last trimester of pregnancy may cause physical dependence with resulting withdrawal symptoms (convulsions and hyperirritability) in the neonate. These withdrawal symptoms may occur up to 14 days after birth. (See DRUG ABUSE AND DEPENDENCE.) Also, one study in humans has shown that prenatal exposure to barbiturates may be associated with an increased incidence of brain

Continued on next page

Carnrick—Cont.

tumors. In addition, use of barbiturates during pregnancy may be associated with neonatal hemorrhage due to reduction in levels of vitamin K-dependent clotting factors in the neonate.

Labor and delivery: Use of barbiturates just prior to or during delivery may cause respiratory depression in the neonate, especially the premature neonate, because of immature hepatic function.

ACETAMINOPHEN:
Problems in humans have not been documented; however, controlled studies have not been done. Risk-benefit must be considered since acetaminophen crosses the placenta.

Nursing Mothers:
BUTALBITAL
Barbiturates are excreted in breast milk; use by nursing mothers may cause CNS depression, bradycardia, or respiratory depression in the infant.

ACETAMINOPHEN
Problems in humans have not been documented; however, risk-benefit must be considered. Although peak concentrations of 10 to 15 mcg per ml have been measured in breast milk 1 to 2 hours following maternal ingestion of a single 650-mg dose, neither acetaminophen nor its metabolites were detected in the urine of the nursing infants. The half-life in breast milk is 1.35 to 3.5 hours. Caution should be exercised when PHRENILIN® or PHRENILIN® FORTE is administered to a nursing woman.

Pediatric Use: Safety and effectiveness in children below the age of 12 have not been established.

Adverse Reactions: Drowsiness, dizziness, nausea, vomiting, constipation and skin rash may occur.

Drug Abuse and Dependence: Barbiturates may be habit forming. Tolerance, psychological dependence, and physical dependence may occur especially following prolonged use of high doses of barbiturates.

The average daily dose for the barbiturate addict is usually about 1.5 grams. As tolerance to barbiturates develops, the amount needed to maintain the same level of intoxication increases; tolerance to a fatal dosage, however, does not increase more than two-fold. As this occurs, the margin between an intoxicating dosage and fatal dosage becomes smaller.

Symptoms of acute intoxication with barbiturates include unsteady gait, slurred speech, and sustained nystagmus. Mental signs of chronic intoxication include confusion, poor judgment, irritability, insomnia, and somatic complaints.

Symptoms of barbiturate dependence are similar to those of chronic alcoholism. If an individual appears to be intoxicated with alcohol to a degree that is radically disproportionate to the amount of alcohol in his or her blood the use of barbiturates should be suspected. The lethal dose of a barbiturate is far less if alcohol is also ingested.

The symptoms of barbiturate withdrawal can be severe and may cause death. Major withdrawal symptoms (convulsions and delirium) may occur within 16 hours and last up to 5 days after abrupt cessation of these drugs. Intensity of withdrawal symptoms gradually declines over a period of approximately 15 days. Individuals susceptible to barbiturate abuse and dependence include alcoholics and opiate abusers, as well as other sedative-hypnotic and amphetamine abusers.

Treatment of barbiturate dependence consists of cautious and gradual withdrawal of the drug. Barbiturate-dependent patients can be withdrawn by using a number of different withdrawal regimens. One method involves initiating treatment at the patient's regular dosage level and decreasing the daily dosage by 10 percent if tolerated by the patient.

Overdosage:
BARBITURATES:
Signs and Symptoms: The toxic dose of barbiturates varies considerably. In general, an oral dose of 1 gram of most barbiturates produces serious poisoning in an adult. Death commonly occurs after 2 to 10 grams of ingested barbiturate. Barbiturate intoxication may be confused with alcoholism, bromide intoxication, and with various neurological disorders.

Acute overdosage with barbiturates is manifested by CNS and respiratory depression which may progress to Cheyne-Stokes respiration, areflexia, constriction of the pupils to a slight degree (though in severe poisoning they may show paralytic dilation), oliguria, tachycardia, hypotension, lowered body temperature, and coma. Typical shock syndrome (apnea, circulatory collapse, respiratory arrest, and death) may occur.

In extreme overdose, all electrical activity in the brain may cease, in which case a "flat" EEG normally equated with clinical death cannot be accepted. This effect is fully reversible unless hypoxic damage occurs. Consideration should be given to the possibility of barbiturate intoxication even in situations that appear to involve trauma.

Complications such as pneumonia, pulmonary edema, cardiac arrhythmias, congestive heart failure, and renal failure may occur. Uremia may increase CNS sensitivity to barbiturates if renal function is impaired. Differential diagnosis should include hypoglycemia, head trauma, cerebrovascular accidents, convulsive states, and diabetic coma.

Treatment: Treatment of barbiturate overdosage is mainly supportive and consists of the following: 1. Maintenance of an adequate airway, with assisted respiration and oxygen administration as necessary. 2. Monitoring of vital signs and fluid balance. 3. If the patient is conscious and has not lost the gag reflex, emesis may be induced with ipecac. Care should be taken to prevent pulmonary aspiration of vomitus. After completion of vomiting, 30 grams activated charcoal in a glass of water may be administered. 4. If emesis is contraindicated, gastric lavage may be performed with a cuffed endotracheal tube in place with the patient in the face down position. Activated charcoal may be left in the emptied stomach and a saline cathartic administered. 5. Fluid therapy and other standard treatment for shock, if needed. 6. If renal function is normal, forced diuresis may aid in the elimination of the barbiturate. Alkalinization of the urine increases renal excretion of some barbiturates. 7. Although not recommended as a routine procedure, hemodialysis may be used in severe barbiturate intoxications or if the patient is anuric or in shock. 8. Patient should be rolled from side to side every 30 minutes. 9. Antibiotics should be given if pneumonia is suspected. 10. Appropriate nursing care to prevent hypostatic pneumonia, decubiti, aspiration, and other complications of patients with altered states of consciousness.

ACETAMINOPHEN:
Signs and Symptoms: Acetaminophen in massive overdosage may cause hepatic toxicity in some patients. In all cases of suspected overdose, immediately call your regional poison center or the Rocky Mountain Poison Center's toll-free number (800-525-6115) for assistance in diagnosis and for directions in the use of N-acetylcysteine as an antidote, a use currently restricted to investigational status.

In adults, hepatic toxicity has rarely been reported with acute overdoses of less than 10 grams and fatalities with less than 15 grams. Importantly, young children seem to be more resistant than adults to the hepatotoxic effect of an acetaminophen overdose. Despite this, the measures outlined below should be initiated in any adult or child suspected of having ingested an acetaminophen overdose.

Early symptoms following a potentially hepatotoxic overdose may include: nausea, vomiting, diaphoresis, and general malaise. Clinical and laboratory evidence of hepatic toxicity may not be apparent until 48 to 72 hours post-ingestion.

Treatment: The stomach should be emptied promptly by lavage or by induction of emesis with syrup of ipecac. Patients' estimates of the quantity of a drug ingested are notoriously unreliable. Therefore, if an acetaminophen overdose is suspected, a serum acetaminophen assay should be obtained as early as possible, but no sooner than four hours following ingestion. Liver function studies should be obtained initially and repeated at 24-hour intervals.

The antidote, N-acetylcysteine, should be administered as early as possible, and within 16 hours of the overdose ingestion for optimal results. Following recovery, there are no residual, structural or functional hepatic abnormalities.

Dosage and Administration:
PHRENILIN®: One or two tablets every four hours. Total daily dosage should not exceed six tablets.
PHRENILIN® FORTE: One capsule every 4-6 hours. Total daily dosage should not exceed three capsules.

How Supplied:
PHRENILIN®: Pale violet scored tablets with the letter 'C' on one side and 8650 on the other, in bottles of 100 (NDC 0086-0050-10).
PHRENILIN® FORTE: Amethyst, opaque capsules imprinted with the letter 'C' and 8656, in bottles of 100 (NDC 0086-0056-10).
The most recent revision of this labeling is 11/82.
Manufactured for Carnrick Laboratories, Inc.
Shown in Product Identification Section, page 408

PHRENILIN® with CODEINE No. 3
[fren′ĭ-lin]

Caution: Federal Law Prohibits Dispensing Without Prescription.

Description: Each capsule contains: butalbital, USP 50 mg. (Warning—May be habit forming), acetaminophen, USP 325 mg; and codeine phosphate, USP 30 mg, (Warning—May be habit forming).

Dosage and Administration: Adult oral dosage —One capsule, repeated if necessary every 4-6 hours. Total daily dosage should not exceed four capsules.

How Supplied: Amethyst and white, opaque capsules imprinted with the letter "C" and 8655. Supplied in bottles of 100 capsules NDC 0086-0055-10. Store at controlled room temperature, 15°–30°C (59°–86°F).
See package insert for prescribing information.
Manufactured for Carnrick Laboratories, Inc.
Shown in Product Identification Section, page 409

PROPAGEST® and PROPAGEST®
SYRUP
(Phenylpropanolamine HCl)

Description:
PROPAGEST™—Each tablet contains:
Phenylpropanolamine HCl .... 25 mg.
PROPAGEST™ SYRUP —Each 5 ml. (one teaspoonful) contains:
Phenylpropanolamine HCl .... 12.5 mg.

Indications: For the temporary relief of nasal congestion associated with the common cold, sinusitis, hay fever or other upper respiratory allergies.

Dosage:
PROPAGEST™
Adult oral dosage is one tablet every 4 hours not to exceed 6 tablets in 24 hours. Children 6 to under 12 years oral dosage is one-half tablet every 4 hours not to exceed 3 tablets in 24 hours. Children 2 to under 6 years, use PROPAGEST™ SYRUP.
PROPAGEST™ SYRUP
Indicated dosage may be given every 4 hours.
Do not exceed 6 doses in 24 hours.
Adult oral dosage ....2 teaspoonfuls
Children 6 to under 12 years
oral dosage ....1 teaspoonful
Children 2 to under 6 years
oral dosage ....½ teaspoonful
For children under 2 years, there is no recommended dosage except under the advice and supervision of a physician.

Warnings: Do not exceed recommended dosage because at higher doses nervousness, dizziness, sleeplessness, rapid pulse or high blood pressure may occur.
If symptoms do not improve within 7 days or are accompanied by high fever, consult a physician

before continuing use. Do not take this product if you have high blood pressure, heart disease, diabetes or thyroid disease except under the advice and supervision of a physician. As with any drug, if you are pregnant or nursing a baby, seek the advice of a health professional before using this product.

DRUG INTERACTION PRECAUTION: Do not take this product if you are presently taking a prescription antihypertensive or antidepressant drug containing a monoamine oxidase inhibitor except under the advice and supervision of a physician. Consult your physician if you are taking other medication.

Our labeling states:
KEEP THIS AND ALL MEDICATION OUT OF THE REACH OF CHILDREN.
In case of accidental overdose, seek professional assistance or contact a Poison Control Center immediately.
Keep tightly closed away from light and store at room temperature.

How Supplied: PROPAGEST™—White, oval scored tablets containing 25 mg. phenylpropanolamine HCl in bottles of 100. (NDC 0086-0051-10) PROPAGEST™ SYRUP —Orange-flavored, colorless, syrup containing 12.5 mg. phenylpropanolamine HCl per 5 ml. in bottles of 16 fluid ounces (NDC 0086-0053-16) and in bottles of 4 fluid ounces (NDC 0086-0053-04).
Manufactured for Carnrick Laboratories, Inc.
Shown in Product Identification Section, page 408

SINULIN®

Description: Each tablet contains: phenylpropanolamine HCl 37.5 mg., chlorpheniramine maleate 2 mg., acetaminophen 325 mg., salicylamide 250 mg., homatropine methylbromide 0.75 mg.
Indications: For relief of sinus congestion and headache.
Warning: Not to be used by persons with high blood pressure, diabetes, heart or thyroid disease, glaucoma or excessive pressure within the eye. Elderly persons and children under 12 use only as directed by a physician. As with any drug, if you are pregnant or nursing a baby, seek the advice of a health professional before using this product.
Precaution: If drowsiness occurs, do not drive a car or operate machinery. Discontinue use if rapid pulse, dizziness or blurring of vision occurs. If dryness of mouth occurs reduce dosage. Not for frequent or prolonged use. If eye pain occurs, discontinue and see your physician immediately as this can indicate glaucoma.
Overdosage: In case of accidental overdose, seek professional assistance or contact a poison control center immediately.
Dosage: Adults: 1 tablet every 4 hours. Not more than 4 tablets daily. If symptoms persist for more than 10 days consult physician.
How Supplied: Peach color, scored tablets inscribed with 8625 on one side and C logo on the other. Bottles of 20 (NDC 0086-0250-02), 7 boxes of 24 blisters (NDC 0086-0250-24) and Bottles of 100 (NDC 0086-0250-10).
Manufactured for Carnrick Laboratories, Inc.
Shown in Product Identification Section, page 408

SKELAXIN® ℞
brand of metaxalone

Caution: Federal law prohibits dispensing without prescription.
Description: Each pale rose, scored tablet contains: metaxalone, 400 mg.
Skelaxin (metaxalone) has the following chemical structure and name:
5-[(3,4-dimethylphenoxy)methyl]-2 oxazolidinone

Actions: The mechanism of action of metaxalone in humans has not been established, but may be due to general central nervous system depression. It has no direct action on the contractile mechanism of striated muscle, the motor end plate or the nerve fiber.
Indications: Skelaxin (metaxalone) is indicated as an adjunct to rest, physical therapy, and other measures for the relief of discomforts associated with acute, painful musculoskeletal conditions. The mode of action of this drug has not been clearly identified, but may be related to its sedative properties. Metaxalone does not directly relax tense skeletal muscles in man.
Contraindications: Metaxalone is contraindicated in individuals who have shown hypersensitivity to the drug. Metaxalone should not be administered to patients with a known tendency to drug-induced, hemolytic, or other anemias. It is contraindicated in patients with significantly impaired renal or hepatic function.
Precautions: Elevation in cephalin flocculation tests without concurrent changes in other liver function parameters have been noted. Hence, it is recommended that metaxalone be administered with great care to patients with pre-existing liver damage and that serial liver function studies be performed as required.
False-positive Benedict's tests, due to an unknown reducing substance, have been noted. A glucose-specific test will differentiate findings.
Pregnancy: Reproduction studies have been performed in rats and have revealed no evidence of impaired fertility or harm to the fetus due to metaxalone. Reactions reports from marketing experience have not revealed evidence of fetal injury, but such experience cannot exclude the possibility of infrequent or subtle damage to the human fetus. As with all drugs, metaxalone should be used in women who are or may become pregnant only when clearly needed.
Nursing Mothers: It is not known whether this drug is secreted in human milk. As a general rule, nursing should not be undertaken while a patient is on a drug since many drugs are excreted in human milk.
Pediatric Use: Safety and effectiveness in children 12 years of age and below have not been established.
Adverse Reactions: The most frequent reactions to metaxalone include nausea, vomiting, gastrointestinal upset, drowsiness, dizziness, headache, and nervousness or "irritability." Other adverse reactions are: hypersensitivity reaction, characterized by a light rash with or without pruritus; leukopenia; hemolytic anemia; jaundice.
Dosage: The recommended dose for adults and children over 12 years of age is two tablets (800 mg) three to four times a day.
Management of Overdosage: Gastric lavage and supportive therapy as indicated. (When determining the LD$_{50}$ in rats and mice, progressive sedation, hypnosis and finally respiratory failure were noted as the dosage increased. In dogs, no LD$_{50}$ could be determined as the higher doses produced an emetic action in 15 to 30 minutes). No documented case of major toxicity has been reported.
How Supplied: Skelaxin (metaxalone) is available as a 400 mg. pale rose tablet, inscribed with 8662 on the scored side and "C" on the other. Available in bottles of 100 (NDC 0086-0062-10). Store at Controlled Room Temperature, between 15°C and 30°C (59°F and 86°F).
Manufactured for
CARNRICK LABORATORIES, INC.
Shown in Product Identification Section, page 409

Products are cross-indexed by generic and chemical names in the
YELLOW SECTION

Center Laboratories
Division of EM Industries, Inc.
35 CHANNEL DRIVE
PORT WASHINGTON, NY 11050

EPIPEN®/EPIPEN® Jr. ℞
Epinephrine Auto–Injectors

Description: EpiPen provides epinephrine for intramuscular auto-injection in a sterile solution prepared from epinephrine with the aid of hydrochloric acid in pyrogen-free water. The EpiPen Auto-Injector is designed to deliver a dose of 0.3 mg epinephrine.
The EpiPen Jr. Auto-Injector will deliver a dose of 0.15 mg epinephrine.
Clinical Pharmacology: Epinephrine is a sympathomimetic drug, acting on both alpha and beta receptors. It is the drug of choice for the emergency treatment of severe allergic reactions such as the sting of Hymenoptera insects: bees, wasps, hornets, and yellow jackets. The strong vasoconstrictor action of epinephrine acts quickly to counter vasodilation and resulting increased capillary permeability. By its effect on smooth muscle, epinephrine relaxes the bronchioles, thereby relieving wheezing and dyspnea. Its action also relieves angioedema or hives.
Indications and Usage: Epinephrine is indicated in the emergency treatment of anaphylactic reactions to insect stings. The EpiPen Auto-Injector is intended for immediate self-administration by individuals with a history of hypersensitivity to insect stings. It is designed as emergency supportive therapy only and is not a replacement or substitute for subsequent medical or hospital care, nor is it intended to supplant insect venom hyposensitization.
Contraindications: Epinephrine is contraindicated in individuals with organic brain damage.
Warnings: Epinephrine is sensitive to light and heat. Store EpiPen in a cool dark place. Before using, check EpiPen to make sure solution in Auto-Injector is not brown in color. If it is discolored or contains a precipitate, do not use. Every effort should be made to avoid possible inadvertent intravascular administration through appropriate selection of an injection site such as the thigh or deltoid. Do not inject into buttock.
Large doses or accidental intravenous injection of epinephrine may result in cerebral hemorrhage due to sharp rise in blood pressure. Rapidly acting vasodilators can counteract the marked pressor effects of epinephrine.
Epinephrine should be administered with extreme caution to patients who have developed degenerative heart disease. Use of epinephrine with drugs that sensitize the heart to arrhythmias is not recommended. Anginal pain may be induced by epinephrine in patients with coronary insufficiency.
Precautions: The effects of epinephrine may be potentiated by tricyclic antidepressants; certain antihistamines, e.g., diphenhydramine, tripelennamine, d-chlorpheniramine; and sodium l-thyroxine.
Administer with caution to hyperthyroid individuals, psychoneurotic individuals, individuals with cardiovascular disease, hypertension, or diabetes, elderly individuals and pregnant women.
Adverse Reactions: Transient and minor side effects of epinephrine include palpitation, respiratory difficulty, pallor, dizziness, weakness, tremor, headache, throbbing, restlessness, tenseness, anxiety and fear.
Ventricular arrhythmias may follow administration of epinephrine.
Dosage and Administration: Dosage in any specific patient should be based on body weight in addition to the patient's risk of anaphylaxis and ability to tolerate epinephrine. Usual epinephrine adult dosage for allergic emergencies is 0.3 mg. Usual pediatric dose is 0.01/kg body weight.
A physician who prescribes EpiPen should take appropriate steps to insure that his patient under-

Continued on next page

Center—Cont.

stands the indications and use of this device thoroughly. The physician should review with the patient, in detail, the package insert and operation of the EpiPen Auto-Injector. Inject the required dose of the EpiPen/EpiPen Jr. Auto-Injector intramuscularly into the anteriolateral aspect of the thigh or the deltoid region of the arm. See detailed Directions for Use.

How Supplied: Package containing one or two (twin pack) EpiPen/EpiPen Jr. Auto-Injectors. Also available in packages of six units. Training Device for patient instruction purposes also available.

Caution: Federal (U.S.A.) law prohibits dispensing without a prescription.

Central Pharmaceuticals, Inc.
SEYMOUR, IN 47274

CODICLEAR DH SYRUP
[kō'di-klēr'']

Description: A clear, colorless, sweet-tasting syrup which is alcohol-free, sugar-free and dye-free.
Each teaspoonful (5 ml.) contains:
Hydrocodone bitartrate ....5 mg.
(Warning - May be habit forming)
Potassium guaiacolsulfonate ....300 mg.

Clinical Pharmacology: Hydrocodone bitartrate is a potent antitussive which causes suppression of the cough reflex by direct action on the cough center. Hydrocodone is approximately three times as potent as codeine on a weight basis and has a higher addiction potential also. Potassium guaiacolsulfonate has been used empirically for many decades as an expectorant.

Indications: For the temporary relief of dry, nonproductive cough due to colds, pertussis or influenza.

Contraindications: Hypersensitivity to any of the ingredients.

Warnings: Hydrocodone can produce drug dependence and therefore has the potential for being abused. Codiclear DH should be prescribed and administered with the degree of caution appropriate for this type product.

Precautions:
General: The hydrocodone in this product may exhibit additive effects with other CNS depressants, including alcohol. Respiratory depression can be a real hazard so caution should be used, especially in patients with chronic obstructive pulmonary disease.

Information for Patients: The hydrocodone may cause drowsiness and ambulatory patients who operate machinery or motor vehicles should be cautioned accordingly.

Drug Interactions: Concomitant use of hydrocodone with alcohol and/or other CNS depressants may have an additive effect.

Usage in Pregnancy: Pregnancy Category C. Hydrocodone has been shown to be teratogenic in hamsters when given in doses 700 times the human dose. There are no adequate and well-controlled studies in pregnant women. CODICLEAR DH Syrup should be used during pregnancy only if the potential benefit justifies the potential risk to the fetus.

Adverse Reactions: Adverse reactions include drowsiness, lassitude, nausea, giddiness, constipation, respiratory depression and addiction.

Drug Abuse and Dependence: This product is a Schedule III Controlled Substance. Because of the hydrocodone content, some abuse might be expected. Psychic dependence, physical dependence and tolerance may develop upon repeated administration. It should be prescribed and administered with the degree of caution appropriate for this type product.

Overdosage: Symptoms of overdosage include respiratory depression, extreme somnolence progressing to stupor or coma, skeletal muscle flaccidity, cold and clammy skin and other symptoms common with narcotic overdosage.

Primary treatment consists of insuring adequate respiration through provision of a patent airway and the institution of assisted or controlled ventilation. Naloxone hydrochloride should be administered in small intravenous doses (consult specific product labeling before use). In addition, oxygen, intravenous fluids, vasopressors and other supportive measures should be employed as indicated. Gastric emptying may be useful in removing unabsorbed drug. Activated charcoal may also be of benefit.

Dosage and Administration: Adults and older children–1 to 1½ teaspoonfuls; children, 6 to 12 years of age–½ to 1 teaspoonful; children, 3 to 6 years of age–¼ to ½ teaspoonful. These doses may be given four times daily as needed. Not recommended for children under 3 years of age.

How Supplied:
Bottles of 4 fl. oz.–NDC 0131-5034-64
Bottles of 1 pint–NDC 0131-5034-70

CODIMAL® DH
[kō'di-mahl'']
CODIMAL® DM
CODIMAL® PH
CODIMAL® EXPECTORANT

Description: Each teaspoonful (5 ml) of CODIMAL DH contains: Hydrocodone Bitartrate 1.66 mg. (Warning—May be habit forming); Phenylephrine Hydrochloride 5.0 mg.; Pyrilamine Maleate 8.33 mg.

Each teaspoonful (5 ml) of CODIMAL DM contains: Dextromethorphan hydrobromide 10 mg.; Phenylephrine hydrochloride 5 mg.; Pyrilamine maleate 8.33 mg.; Alcohol 4%. Sugar-free.

Each teaspoonful (5 ml) of CODIMAL PH contains: Codeine Phosphate 10 mg. (Warning—May be habit forming); Phenylephrine Hydrochloride 5 mg.; Pyrilamine Maleate 8.33 mg.

Each teaspoonful (5 ml) of CODIMAL EXPECTORANT contains: Phenylpropanolamine Hydrochloride 25 mg.; Guaifenesin 100 mg.

Indications and Usage: For temporary relief of cough due to the common cold or other upper respiratory infection or irritation.

Contraindications: In persons with a known hypersensitivity to any of the ingredients.

Precautions: Should be administered with extreme caution to patients with hypertension, heart disease, diabetes, thyroid disease or vascular disease, or those receiving MAO inhibitors. Codeine and its derivative, Hydrocodone Bitartrate, are narcotic agents and the usual precautions in their use should be observed, particularly in infants and elderly patients.

Side Effects: Occasional drowsiness, blurred vision, palpitation, flushing, nervousness or gastrointestinal upsets.

Warnings: Patients should be instructed not to drive or operate machinery while taking the medication; and not to administer it to patients with a high fever or persistent cough unless so directed by a physician.

Administration and Dosage: Codimal DH, Codimal DM and Codimal PH: Adults and older children—1 to 2 teaspoonfuls; children 6 to 12—1 teaspoonful; children 2 to 6—½ teaspoonful. These doses may be taken every 4 hours. Children 6 months to 2 years—¼ teaspoonful every 6 hours.

Codimal Expectorant: Adults and older children—1 teaspoonful; children, 6 to 12 years—½ teaspoonful; children, 2 to 6—¼ teaspoonful. This dose may be taken every four hours.

How Supplied: Bottles of 4 ounces, pints and gallons. Codimal Expectorant not available in gallons.

CODIMAL®-L.A. CAPSULES
[kō'di-mahl'']

Description: Each Timed Release Capsule contains:
Chlorpheniramine maleate ....8 mg.
Pseudoephedrine
   hydrochloride ....120 mg.
in a specially prepared base to provide prolonged action.

How Supplied:
Bottle of 100 Capsules NDC 0131-4213-37
Bottle of 1000 Capsules NDC 0131-4213-43
Shown in Product Identification Section, page 409

CO-GESIC®
[kō'je''zik]

Description: Each tablet contains:
Hydrocodone Bitartrate ....5 mg.
   (WARNING—May be habit forming)
Acetaminophen ....500 mg.

Acetaminophen is a nonopiate, non-salicylate analgesic and antipyretic which occurs as a white, odorless crystalline powder possessing a slightly bitter taste. Hydrocodone bitartrate is an opioid analgesic and antitussive and occurs as fine, white crystals or as a crystalline powder. It is affected by light.

Clinical Pharmacology: Hydrocodone is a semisynthetic narcotic analgesic and antitussive with multiple actions qualitatively similar to those of codeine. Most of these involve the central nervous system and smooth muscle. The precise mechanism of action of hydrocodone and other opiates is not known, although it is believed to relate to the existence of opiate receptors in the central nervous system. In addition to analgesia, narcotics may produce drowsiness, changes in mood and mental clouding.

Radioimmunoassay techniques have recently been developed for the analysis of hydrocodone in human plasma. After a 10 mg oral dose of hydrocodone bitartrate, a mean peak serum drug level of 23.6 ng/ml and an elimination half-life of 3.8 hours were found.

The analgesic action of acetaminophen involves peripheral and central influences, but the specific mechanism is as yet undetermined. Antipyretic activity is mediated through hypothalmic heat regulating centers. Acetaminophen inhibits prostaglandin synthetase. Therapeutic doses of acetaminophen have negligible effects on the cardiovascular or respiratory systems; however, toxic doses may cause circulatory failure and rapid, shallow breathing. Acetaminophen is rapidly and almost completely absorbed from the gastrointestinal tract, producing maximum serum concentrations within 30 minutes to one hour. The plasma half-life in adults and children ranges from 0.90 hours to 3.25 hours with an average of approximately 2 hours. The drug distributes uniformly in most body fluids and is approximately 25% protein bound. Acetaminophen is conjugated in the liver, with less than 3% of the dose excreted unchanged in 24 hours. The primary metabolic pathway is conjugation to sulfate and glucuronide by-products. A minor oxidative pathway forms cysteine and mercapturic acid. These compounds are subsequently excreted by the kidneys into the urine.

Indications and Usage: For the relief of moderate to moderately severe pain.

Contraindications: Hypersensitivity to acetaminophen or hydrocodone.

Warnings: Respiratory Depression: At high doses or in sensitive patients, hydrocodone may produce dose-related respiratory depression by acting directly on brain stem respiratory centers. Hydrocodone also effects centers that control respiratory rhythm, and may produce irregular and periodic breathing.

Head Injury and Increased Intracranial Pressure: The respiratory depressant effects of narcotics and their capacity to elevate cerebrospinal fluid pressure may be markedly exaggerated in the presence of head injury, other intracranial lesions or a preexisting increase in intracranial pressure. Furthermore, narcotics produce adverse reactions which may obscure the clinical course of patients with head injuries.

Acute Abdominal Conditions: The administration of narcotics may obscure the diagnosis or clinical course of patients with acute abdominal conditions.

Precautions: Special Risk Patients: As with any narcotic analgesic agent, CO-GESIC Tablets should be used with caution in elderly or debilitated patients and those with severe impairment of hepatic or renal function, hypothyroidism, Addison's disease, prostatic hypertrophy or urethral stricture. The usual precautions should be observed and the possibility of respiratory depression should be kept in mind.

Information for Patients: CO-GESIC Tablets, like all narcotics, may impair the mental and/or physical abilities required for the performance of potentially hazardous tasks such as driving a car or operating machinery; patients should be cautioned accordingly.

Cough Reflex: Hydrocodone suppresses the cough reflex; as with all narcotics, caution should be exercised when CO-GESIC Tablets are used postoperatively and in patients with pulmonary disease.

Drug Interactions: Patients receiving other narcotic analgesics, antipsychotics, antianxiety agents, or other CNS depressants (including alcohol) concomitantly with CO-GESIC Tablets may exhibit an additive CNS depression. When combined therapy is contemplated, the dose of one or both agents should be reduced.

The use of MAO inhibitors or tricyclic antidepressants with hydrocodone preparations may increase the effect of either the antidepressant or hydrocodone.

The concurrent use of anticholinergics with hydrocodone may produce paralytic ileus.

Usage in Pregnancy: Pregnancy Category C. Hydrocodone has been shown to be teratogenic in hamsters when given doses 700 times the human dose. There are no adequate and well-controlled studies in pregnant women. CO-GESIC Tablets should be used during pregnancy only if the potential benefit justifies the potential risk to the fetus.

Nonteratogenic Effects: Babies born to mothers who have been taking opioids regularly prior to delivery will be physically dependent. The withdrawal signs include irritability and excessive crying, tremors, hyperactive reflexes, increased respiratory rate, increased stools, sneezing, yawning, vomiting, and fever. The intensity of the syndrome does not always correlate with the duration of maternal opioid use or dose. There is no consensus on the best method of managing withdrawal. Chlorpromazine 0.7 to 1.0 mg/kg q6h, and paregoric 2 to 4 drops/kg q4h, have been used to treat withdrawal symptoms in infants. The duration of therapy is 4 to 28 days, with the dosage decreased as tolerated.

Labor and Delivery: As with all narcotics, administration of CO-GESIC Tablets to the mother shortly before delivery may result in some degree of respiratory depression in the newborn, especially if higher doses are used.

Nursing Mothers: It is not known whether this drug is excreted in human milk. Because many drugs are excreted in human milk and because of the potential for serious adverse reactions in nursing infants from CO-GESIC Tablets, a decision should be made whether to discontinue nursing or to discontinue the drug, taking into account the importance of the drug to the mother.

Pediatric Use: Safety and effectiveness in children have not been established.

Adverse Reactions: Central Nervous System: Sedation, drowsiness, mental clouding, lethargy, impairment of mental and physical performance, anxiety, fear, dysphoria, dizziness, psychic dependence, mood changes.

Gastronintestinal System: Nausea and vomiting may occur; they are more frequent in ambulatory than in recumbent patients. The antiemetic phenothiazines are useful in suppressing these effects; however, some phenothiazine derivatives seem to be antianalgesic and to increase the amount of narcotic required to produce pain relief, while other phenothiazines reduce the amount of narcotic required to produce a given level of analgesia. Prolonged administration of CO-GESIC Tablets may produce constipation.

Genitourinary System: Ureteral spasm, spasm of vesical sphincters and urinary retention have been reported.

Respiratory Depression: CO-GESIC Tablets may produce dose-related respiratory depression by acting directly on brain stem respiratory centers. Hydrocodone also affects centers that control respiratory rhythm, and may produce irregular and periodic breathing. If significant respiratory depression occurs, it may be antagonized by the use of naloxone hydrochloride. Apply other supportive measures when indicated.

Drug Abuse and Dependence: CO-GESIC Tablets are subject to the Federal Controlled Substance Act (Schedule III). Psychic dependence, physical dependence, and tolerance may develop upon repeated administration of narcotics; therefore CO-GESIC Tablets should be prescribed and administered with caution. However, psychic dependence is unlikely to develop when CO-GESIC Tablets are used for a short time for the treatment of pain. Physical dependence, the condition in which continued administration of the drug is required to prevent the appearance of a withdrawal syndrome, assumes clinically significant proportions only after several weeks of continued narcotic use, although some mild degree of physical dependence may develop after a few days of narcotic therapy. Tolerance, in which increasingly large doses are required in order to produce the same degree of analgesia, is manifested initially by a shortened duration of analgesic effect, and subsequently by decreases in the intensity of analgesia. The rate of development of tolerance varies among patients.

Overdosage: Acetaminophen: Signs and Symptoms: Acetaminophen in massive overdosage may cause hepatic toxicity in some patients. In all cases of suspected overdose, immediately call your regional poison center or the Rocky Mountain Poison Center's toll-free number (800-525-5115) for assistance in diagnosis and for directions in the use of N-acetylcysteine as an antidote, a use currently restricted to investigational status.

In adults, hepatic toxicity has rarely been reported with acute overdoses of less than 10 grams and fatalities with less than 15 grams. Importantly, young children seem to be more resistant than adults to the hepatotoxic effect of an acetaminophen overdose. Despite this, the measures outlined below should be initiated in any adult or child suspected of having ingested an acetaminophen overdose.

Early symptoms following a potentially hepatotoxic overdose may include: nausea, vomiting, diaphoresis and general malaise. Clinical and laboratory evidence of hepatic toxicity may not be apparent until 48 to 72 hours post-ingestion.

Treatment: The stomach should be emptied promptly by lavage or by induction of emesis with syrup of ipecac. Patients' estimates of the quantity of a drug ingested are notoriously unreliable. Therefore, if an acetaminophen overdose is suspected, a serum acetaminophen assay should be obtained as early as possible, but no sooner than four hours following ingestion. Liver function studies should be obtained initially and repeated at 24-hour intervals.

The antidote, N-acetylcysteine, should be administered as early as possible, and within 16 hours of the overdose ingestion for optimal results. Following recovery, there are no residual, structural or functional hepatic abnormalities.

Hydrocodone: Signs and Symptoms: Serious overdose with hydrocodone is characterized by respiratory depression (a decrease in respiratory rate and/or tidal volume, Cheyne-Stokes respiration, cyanosis), extreme somnolence progressing to stupor or coma, skeletal muscle flaccidity, cold and clammy skin, and sometimes bradycardia and hypotension. In severe overdosage, apnea, circulatory collapse, cardiac arrest and death may occur.

Treatment: Primary attention should be given to the reestablishment of adequate respiratory exchange through provision of a patent airway and the institution of assisted or controlled ventilation. The narcotic antagonist naloxone is a specific antidote against respiratory depression which may result from overdosages or unusual sensitivity to narcotics, including hydrocodone. Therefore, an appropriate dose of naloxone (see package insert) should be administered, preferably by the intravenous route, and simultaneously with efforts at respiratory resuscitation. Since the duration of action of hydrocodone may exceed that of the antagonist, the patient should be kept under continued surveillance and repeated doses of the antagonist should be administered as needed to maintain adequate respiration.

An antagonist should not be administered in the absence of clinically significant respiratory or cardiovascular depression. Oxygen, intravenous fluids, vasopressors and other supportive measures should be employed as indicated.

Gastric emptying may be useful in removing unabsorbed drug.

Dosage and Administration: Dosage should be adjusted according to the severity of the pain and the response of the patient. However, it should be kept in mind that tolerance to hydrocodone can develop with continued use and that the incidence of untoward effects is dose related.

The usual adult dose is one tablet every six hours as needed for pain. If necessary, this dose may be repeated at four hour intervals. In cases of more severe pain, two tablets every six hours (up to 8 tablets in 24 hours) may be required.

How Supplied: Oval shaped white compressed tablet with 500 and 5 separated by bisect on one side and Central logo on the other.

Bottles of 100 tablets: NDC 0131-2104-37

Shown in Product Identification Section, page 409

DIA-GESIC™ ℞
[di″ah-jē′zik]

Description: Each tablet contains:
Hydrocodone bitartrate .... 5 mg.
  (WARNING—May be habit forming)
Aspirin .... 230 mg.
Acetaminophen .... 150 mg.
Caffeine .... 30 mg.

How Supplied: Flat, truncated oval, bisected white tablets inscribed with the Central logo on one side and the number 31 and the score on the other side.

Bottles of 100 tablets—NDC 0131-2810-37
Bottles of 1000 tablets—NDC 0131-2810-43

Shown in Product Identification Section, page 409

MONO–GESIC® ℞
[mon″o-je′zik]
(salsalate)
(salicylsalicylic acid)

Description: Each pink film coated tablet contains:
Salsalate (salicylsalicylic acid) .... 750 mg.
The ingredient in this product is of the following classes: non-steroidal anti-inflammatory agent, analgesic and antipyretic.

Clinical Pharmacology: Due to the poor solubility of salsalate in gastric fluid, most will pass through the stomach unhydrolyzed and unabsorbed. In the small intestine, it is partially hydrolyzed to two molecules of salicylic acid and rapidly absorbed both as the parent compound and as salicylic acid. A small proportion is excreted unchanged while the remainder is excreted as salicylic acid and its metabolites. Salsalate has a greater half-life of elimination than salicylic acid. The mode of action of salsalate and other non-steroidal anti-inflammatory drugs is unresolved. It does, however, appear to be involved with the inhibition of prostaglandin synthesis. Unlike aspirin, salsalate has not been associated with reactions causing asthmatic attacks in susceptible people. Also, it is not known to effect the platelet adhesiveness involved in the clotting mechanism. Salsalate also does not cause the gastrointestinal blood loss

Continued on next page

Central—Cont.

common to other nonsteroidal anti-inflammatory agents.

Indications and Usage: MONO-GESIC is indicated for the temporary relief of symptoms of rheumatoid arthritis, osteoarthritis and related rheumatic disorders.

Contraindications: Hypersensitivity to salsalate.

Precautions:

General: To avoid potentially toxic concentrations, the plasma salicylic acid levels should be monitored to maintain the therapeutically effective levels of 10 to 30 mg/100 ml. Changes in urinary pH can have significant effects on the plasma level of salsalate. Acidification can result in an increase in the plasma level resulting in toxicity while an increase in urinary pH will increase renal clearance and urinary excretion of salsalate, thus lowering plasma levels.

Information for Patients: Patients on long-term treatment should be warned not to take other salicylates. They should also be warned that if symptoms of overdosage, such as tinnitus, vertigo, headache, confusion, drowsiness, sweating, hyperventilation, vomiting or diarrhea appear, the drug should be stopped and physician notified.

Drug Interactions: Salicylates antagonize the uricosuric action of drugs used to treat gout. Salicylates will be additive to MONO-GESIC and could increase plasma concentrations to toxic levels. Drugs and foods that raise urine pH will increase renal clearance and urinary excretion of salicylic acid, thus lowering plasma levels; acidifying drugs or foods will decrease urinary excretion and increase plasma levels. Salicylates may competitively displace anticoagulant drugs from plasma protein binding sites and thereby predispose to systemic bleeding. Salicylates may enhance the hypoglycemic effect of oral antidiabetic drugs of the sulfonylurea class. Salicylate competes with a number of drugs for protein binding sites, notably penicillin, thiopental, thyroxine, triiodothyronine, phenytoin, sulfinpyrazone, naproxen, warfarin, methotrexate, and possibly corticosteroids.

Drug/Laboratory Test Interactions: Salicylate competes with thyroid hormone for binding to plasma proteins, which may be reflected in a depressed plasma T_4 value in some patients; thyroid function and basal metabolism are unaffected.

Carcinogenesis: No long-term animal studies have been performed with MONO-GESIC to evaluate its carcinogenic potential; however, several such studies using aspirin and other salicylates have failed to demonstrate any association of these agents with cancerous cell changes.

Use in Pregnancy: Pregnancy Category C: Salsalate and salicylic acid have been shown to be teratogenic and embryocidal in rats when given in doses four to five times the usual human dose. These effects were not observed at doses twice as great as the usual human dose. There are no adequate and well controlled studies in pregnant women. MONO-GESIC should be used during pregnancy only if the potential benefit justifies the potential risk to the fetus.

Labor and Delivery: There exists no adequate and well-controlled studies in pregnant women. Although adverse effects on mother or infant have not been reported with MONO-GESIC use during labor, caution is advised when anti-inflammatory dosage is involved. However, other salicylates have been associated with prolonged gestation and labor, maternal and neonatal bleeding sequelae, potentiation of narcotic and barbiturate effects (respiratory or cardiac arrest in the mother), delivery problems and stillbirth.

Nursing Mothers: It is not known whether salsalate per se is excreted in human milk; salicylic acid, the primary metabolite of MONO-GESIC, has been shown to appear in human milk in concentrations approximating the maternal blood level. Thus the infant of a mother on MONO-GESIC therapy might ingest in mother's milk 30 to 80% as much salicylate per kg body weight as the mother is taking. Accordingly, caution should be exercised when MONO-GESIC is administered to a nursing woman.

Pediatric Use: Not recommended for use in children.

Adverse Reactions: Adverse reactions are usually the result of overdosage and may include tinnitus and temporary hearing loss, vertigo, headache, confusion, drowsiness, sweating, hyperventilation, vomiting and diarrhea.

Drug Abuse and Dependence: Drug abuse and dependence have not been reported with MONO-GESIC.

Overdosage: No deaths after overdosage have been reported for MONO-GESIC. Death has followed ingestion of 10 to 30 g of other salicylates in adults, but much larger amounts have been ingested without fatal outcome.

Symptoms: The usual symptoms of salicylism, tinnitus, vertigo, headache, confusion, drowsiness, sweating, hyperventilation, vomiting and diarrhea will occur. More severe intoxication will lead to disruption of electrolyte balance and blood pH, and hyperthermia and dehydration.

Treatment: Further absorption of MONO-GESIC from the G.I. tract should be prevented by emesis (syrup of ipecac) and, if necessary, by gastric lavage.

Fluid and electrolyte imbalance should be corrected by the administration of appropriate I.V. therapy. Adequate renal function should be maintained. Hemodialysis or peritoneal dialysis may be required in extreme cases.

Dosage and Administration: Dosage should be adjusted according to the severity of the disease and the response of the patient. Response will be gradual and full benefits may not be evident for three to four days when plasma salsalate levels have achieved steady state.

The usual dosage is 3,000 mg. daily, given in divided doses, such as two tablets twice daily or one tablet four times daily.

How Supplied: An oval, pink film coated tablet embossed with Central logo on one side and 750/mg on the other side.

Bottles of 100 tablets - NDC 0131-2164-37

Shown in Product Identification Section, page 409

NEOLAX® TABLETS ℞
[ne'o-lax"]

Description: Each NEOLAX Tablet contains: Dehydrocholic Acid 240 mg. and Docusate sodium 50 mg.

Clinical Pharmacology: The actions of NEOLAX are the result of the combination of complementary activities of its ingredients. Dehydrocholic acid, the oxidation product of cholic acid, is a potent hydrocholeretic. It is a mild laxative that has shown very low toxicity in both experimental animals and in clinical use. The mechanism by which dehydrocholic acid increases the frequency of bowel movements is unknown. Docusate sodium affects the surface tension and increases the water content of the stool, making it softer and, therefore, easier to pass. This softening, combined with the laxative effect of dehydrocholic acid, alleviates both of these symptoms of constipation.

Indications and Usage: A mild laxative and fecal softener as an aid in the treatment of chronic functional constipation, particularly in the elderly.

Contraindications: Biliary tract obstruction, acute hepatitis, or sensitivity to any of its ingredients.

Precautions: Patients should be examined periodically to prevent fluid and electrolyte deficiencies due to excessive laxative effects or inadequate intake.

Administration and Dosage: One or two tablets three times daily with meals. This dosage should be reduced as the condition is relieved.

How Supplied:
Bottles of 100   NDC 0131-2187-37
Bottles of 1000   NDC 0131-2187-43
Unit Dose Pkg. of 100   NDC 0131-2187-86

NIFEREX® TABLETS/ELIXIR
[ni'fer"ex]
NIFEREX®-150 CAPSULES
NIFEREX® with VITAMIN C TABLETS
(polysaccharide-iron complex)

Description: NIFEREX is a highly water-soluble complex of iron and a low molecular weight polysaccharide. Each NIFEREX-150 Capsule contains 150 mg. elemental iron. Each NIFEREX Film Coated Tablet and each NIFEREX with Vitamin C Chewable Tablet contains 50 mg. elemental iron. In addition, each NIFEREX with Vitamin C tablet contains Ascorbic acid, U.S.P., 100 mg. and Sodium ascorbate, 168.75 mg. Each 5 ml. (teaspoonful) NIFEREX Elixir contains 100 mg. elemental iron, alcohol 10% (sugar free).

Action and Uses: NIFEREX is an easily assimilated source of iron for treatment of uncomplicated iron deficiency anemia. Because NIFEREX is a polysaccharide bound iron complex, it is relatively nontoxic and there are relatively few, if any, of the gastrointestinal side effects associated with iron therapy, thus permitting full therapeutic dosage (150 to 300 mg. elemental iron daily) in a single dose if desirable. There is no staining of teeth and no metallic aftertaste.

Indications and Usage: For treatment of uncomplicated iron deficiency anemia.

Contraindications: In patients with hemochromatosis and hemosiderosis, and in those with a known hypersensitivity to any of the ingredients.

Administration and Dosage: ADULTS: One or two NIFEREX-150 Capsules daily, or one or two NIFEREX or NIFEREX with Vitamin C Tablets twice daily, *or* one to two teaspoonfuls NIFEREX Elixir daily. CHILDREN 6 to 12 years of age: One or two NIFEREX *or* one NIFEREX with Vitamin C Tablet daily, or one teaspoonful NIFEREX Elixir daily; Children 2 to 6 years of age: ½ teaspoonful NIFEREX Elixir daily. Children under 2 years: ¼ teaspoonful daily.

How Supplied: NIFEREX-150 Capsules: Bottles of 100 and 1,000. NIFEREX Elixir: Bottles of 8 ounces. NIFEREX Tablets: Bottles of 100. NIFEREX with Vitamin C Chewable Tablets: Bottles of 50.

Shown in Product Identification Section, page 409

NIFEREX®-150 FORTE CAPSULES ℞
[ni'fer"ex for'ta]
NIFEREX® FORTE ELIXIR ℞

Description: Each capsule Niferex®-150 Forte contains:
Iron (Elemental) .... 150 mg.
   (as polysaccharide-iron complex)
Folic Acid .... 1 mg.
Vitamin B$_{12}$ .... 25 mcg.

Each teaspoon (5 ml) Niferex® Forte Elixir contains:
Iron (Elemental) .... 100 mg.
   (as polysaccharide-iron complex)
Folic Acid .... 1 mg.
Vitamin B$_{12}$ .... 25 mcg.
Alcohol 10%
Sugar-Free

How Supplied:
NIFEREX-150 FORTE CAPSULES
Bottle of 100   NDC 0131-4330-37
Bottle of 1000   NDC 0131-4330-43
NIFEREX FORTE ELIXIR
Bottle of 4 fl. oz.   NDC 0131-5065-64

Capsules Shown in Product Identification Section, page 409

NIFEREX®—PN TABLETS ℞
[ni'fer"ex]

Description: Each film-coated tablet contains:
Iron (Elemental) .... 60 mg.
   (as polysaccharide-iron complex)
Folic acid .... 1 mg.
Ascorbic acid .... 50 mg.
   (as sodium ascorbate)
Cyanocobalamin (Vitamin B$_{12}$) .... 3 mcg.
Vitamin A .... 4000 I.U.
Vitamin D$_2$ .... 400 I.U.
Thiamine mononitrate .... 3 mg.

Riboflavin ....3 mg.
Pyridoxine hydrochloride ....2 mg.
Niacinamide ....10 mg.
Calcium carbonate ....312 mg.
Zinc sulfate USP ....80 mg.
(as 50 mg. dried zinc sulfate)

Indications and Usage: For the prevention and/or treatment of dietary vitamin and mineral deficiencies associated with pregnancy and lactation.
Contraindications: Hypersensitivity to any of the ingredients.
Warnings: Folic acid alone is improper therapy in the treatment of pernicious anemia and other megaloblastic anemias where vitamin B_{12} is deficient.
Precautions: Folic acid, especially in doses above 0.1 mg. daily may obscure pernicious anemia, in that hematologic remission may occur while neurological manifestations remain progressive.
Adverse Reactions: Allergic sensitization has been reported following both oral and parenteral administration of folic acid.
Dosage and Administration: One tablet daily or as prescribed by a physician.
How Supplied:
Bottles of 100 tablets—NDC 0131-2209-37
Bottles of 1000 tablets—NDC 0131-2209-43
Shown in Product Identification Section, page 409

SYNOPHYLATE® Elixir ℞
[sin-ah'fil-āt'']
(theophylline sodium glycinate)
SYNOPHYLATE®-GG Tablets/Syrup ℞
(theophylline sodium glycinate and guaifenesin)

SYNOPHYLATE (theophylline sodium glycinate) Elixir contains per tbsp. (15 ml.): theophylline sodium glycinate, 330 mg. (equivalent to 150 mg. theophylline). Alcohol 20%.
SYNOPHYLATE-GG Syrup or Tablets contain per tbsp. (15 ml.) or per tablet: theophylline sodium glycinate, 300 mg. (equivalent to 137 mg. theophylline); guaifenesin 100 mg. (Alcohol 10% in the syrup).
How Supplied:
SYNOPHYLATE ELIXIR
Pint   NDC 0131-5089-70
Gallon   NDC 0131-5089-72
SYNOPHYLATE-GG TABLETS
100   NDC 0131-2253-37
SYNOPHYLATE-GG SYRUP
Pint   NDC 0131-5092-70
Gallon   NDC 0131-5092-72

THEOCLEAR® L.A.–260 CAPSULES ℞
[the'ō-klēr'']
THEOCLEAR® L.A.–130 CAPSULES ℞
THEOCLEAR®–80 Syrup ℞
(theophylline anhydrous)

Description: THEOCLEAR L.A.-260 and THEOCLEAR L.A.-130: Each capsule contains 260 mg. or 130 mg. of theophylline anhydrous in a sustained release bead formulation.
THEOCLEAR-80: Each 15 ml. (1 tablespoonful) contains 80 mg. Anhydrous Theophylline as the active ingredient. Other ingredients are saccharin sodium; tartaric acid; benzoic acid; citric acid; sorbitol; glycerin; propylene glycol; artificial flavor and purified water q.s. This formulation provides an alcohol-free, dye-free, and sugar-free vehicle containing no corn by-products.
How Supplied:
THEOCLEAR L.A.-260 CAPSULE
Bottle of 100   NDC 0131-4248-37
Bottle of 1000   NDC 0131-4248-43
THEOCLEAR L.A.-130 CAPSULE
Bottle of 100   NDC 0131-4247-37
THEOCLEAR-80 SYRUP
One Pint   NDC 0131-5098-70
One Gallon   NDC 0131-5098-72
Shown in Product Identification Section, page 409

Cetylite Industries, Inc.
P.O. BOX CN6
9051 RIVER ROAD
PENNSAUKEN, NJ 08110

CETACAINE® ℞
[set'a-cane'']
TOPICAL ANESTHETIC
A BRAND OF
Benzocaine 14.0%
Butyl Aminobenzoate............................. 2.0%
Tetracaine Hydrochloride 2.0%
Benzalkonium Chloride 0.5%
Cetyl Dimethyl Ethyl
  Ammonium Bromide 0.005%
In a bland water soluble base.
Action: Cetacaine produces anesthesia rapidly in approximately 30 seconds.
Indications: Cetacaine is a topical anesthetic indicated for the production of anesthesia of accessible mucous membrane.
Cetacaine Spray is indicated for use to control pain or gagging. Cetacaine in all forms is indicated for use to control pain.
Dosage and Administration: Cetacaine Spray should be applied for approximately one second or less for normal anesthesia. Only limited quantity of Cetacaine is required for anesthesia and a spray in excess of 2 seconds is contraindicated. Average expulsion rate of residue from spray, at normal temperatures, is 200 mg. per second.
Tissue need not be dried prior to application of Cetacaine.
Cetacaine should be applied directly to the site where pain control is required.
Cetacaine Liquid or Cetacaine Ointment may be applied with a cotton pledget or directly to tissue. Cotton pledget should not be held in position for extended periods of time, since local reactions to benzoate topical anesthetics are related to the length of time of application.
Adverse Reactions: Although systemic reactions to Cetacaine have not been reported, local reactions to benzoate topical anesthetics may be associated with the condition of the mucous membrane treated and the length of time of application. Dehydration of the epithelium or a slight escharotic effect may result from prolonged contact. Allergic reactions are known to occur in some patients with preparations containing benzocaine.
Usage in Pregnancy: Safe use of Cetacaine has not been established with respect to possible adverse effects upon fetal development. Therefore Cetacaine should not be used during early pregnancy, unless in the judgment of a physician the potential benefits outweigh the unknown hazards.
Routine precaution for the use of any topical anesthetic should be observed when Cetacaine is used.
Contraindications:
Cetacaine is not for injection.
Do not use in the eyes.
To avoid excessive systemic absorption, Cetacaine should not be applied to large areas of denuded or inflamed tissue.
Cetacaine should not be administered to patients who are hypersensitive to any of its ingredients.
Individual dosage of tetracaine hydrochloride in excess of 20 mg. is contraindicated. Cetacaine should not be used under dentures or cotton rolls, as retention of the active ingredients under a denture or cotton roll could possibly cause a slight escharotic effect.
Jetco Cannula: The Jetco cannula for Cetacaine Spray is specially designed for accessibility and application of Cetacaine, at the required site of pain control.
The Jetco cannula is supplied in various sizes and shapes.
The Jetco cannula is inserted firmly onto the protruding plastic tubing on each bottle of Cetacaine Spray.
The Jetco cannula may be removed and re-inserted as many times as required for cleansing or sterilization.

Packaging Available:
Aerosol Spray 56 gm., including propellant.
Liquid 56 gm. bottle.
Ointment, flavored, 37 gram jar.
Hospital Gel, 29 grams in polyethylene tube.
Caution: Federal law prohibits dispensing Cetacaine without prescription.
Keep out of reach of children.

CETYLCIDE® SOLUTION
[see'til-side'']
Composition:
Cetyl Dimethyl Ethyl
  Ammonium Bromide 6.5%
Benzalkonium Chloride U.S.P. 6.5%
Isopropyl Alcohol.. 13.0%
Inert Ingredients 74.0%
Formulation contains Sodium Nitrite
Indications and Uses: Cetylcide is for use in the chemical disinfection of dental and surgical instruments. Cetylcide, when diluted, is a potent germicidal solution combining high bactericidal and bacteriostatic action against most kinds of pathogenic bacteria.
Germicides containing a Quarternary Ammonium derivative should not be relied upon to destroy spore bearing organisms, mycobacterium tuberculosis or the etiologic agent of viral hepatitis. Thus, instruments suspected of such contamination should be sterilized by heat. Needles, hypodermic syringes, corroded instruments or those with deep narrow crevices, as well as hinged or defective plated instruments, should be sterilized by heat. To maintain disinfection they may then be immersed in Cetylcide Solution.
How Supplied: 10 cc ampules, 32 ounce bottles, and 16 ounce bottles.

Chemi-Tech Labs, Inc.
74-80 MARINE STREET
FARMINGDALE, NY 11735

HVS 1 + 2™   OTC

Description: Viscous, translucent lotion containing benzalkonium chloride *complex* in a special, synergistically formulated base, for use in the mouth and topically.
Indications and Usage: Treatment and relief of herpes simplex. Relieves pain and discomfort, reduces frequency of outbreaks, promotes fast healing.
Contraindications: Avoid contact with eyes. In case of accidental contact with eyes, flush immediately with cool water for ten minutes and seek immediate medical attention.
Warnings: In case of accidental ingestion, seek professional assistance or contact a poison control center immediately.
Dosage and Administration: Apply up to 6 times daily until completely healed or as directed by physician.
How Supplied: ½ fl. oz. container and finger cots.

Important Notice
Before prescribing or administering any product described in PHYSICIANS' DESK REFERENCE always consult the PDR Supplement for possible new or revised information

CIBA Pharmaceutical Company
Division of CIBA-GEIGY Corporation
SUMMIT, NJ 07901

To provide a convenient and accurate means of identifying CIBA solid dosage form products, a code number has been imprinted on all tablets and capsules. To help you quickly identify a CIBA Tablet or Capsule by its code number, a numerical listing of codes (with corresponding product names) and an alphabetical listing of products (with corresponding codes and list numbers) have been compiled below.

CIBA Code #	ALPHABETICAL LISTING	List Number
	Antrenyl® bromide (oxyphenonium bromide)	
15	TABLETS, 5 mg (white, scored)	
	100s	2410
	Anturane® (sulfinpyrazone USP)	
41	TABLETS (white, single-scored) each containing 100 mg sulfinpyrazone USP	
	100s	1910
168	CAPSULES (green) each containing 200 mg sulfinpyrazone USP	
	100s	1920
	Apresazide® (hydralazine HCl and hydrochlorothiazide)	
139	CAPSULES 25/25 (light blue and white opaque), each containing 25 mg hydralazine HCl and 25 mg hydrochlorothiazide	
	100s	3131
149	CAPSULES 50/50 (pink and white opaque), each containing 50 mg hydralazine HCl and 50 mg hydrochlorothiazide	
	100s	3132
159	CAPSULES 100/50 (pink flesh and white opaque), each containing 100 mg hydralazine HCl and 50 mg hydrochlorothiazide	
	100s	3133
	Apresoline® hydrochloride (hydralazine hydrochloride USP)	
37	TABLETS, 10 mg (pale yellow, dry-coated)	
	100s	2629
	1000s	2627
	Consumer Pack	
	100s	2603
39	TABLETS, 25 mg (deep blue, dry-coated)	
	100s	2611
	500s	2613
	1000s	2615
	Accu-Pak® 100s	2647
	Consumer Pack	
	100s	2606
73	TABLETS, 50 mg (light blue, dry-coated)	
	100s	2619
	500s	2621
	1000s	2623
	Accu-Pak® 100s	2648
	Consumer Pack	
	100s	2643
101	TABLETS, 100 mg (peach, dry-coated)	
	100s	2638
	Apresoline®-Esidrix® (hydralazine hydrochloride and hydrochlorothiazide)	
129	TABLETS (orange, dry-coated), each containing 25 mg hydralazine hydrochloride and 15 mg hydrochlorothiazide	
	100s	3120
	Cytadren® (aminoglutethamide)	
24	TABLETS-250 mg (white, round, scored into quarters)	
	100s	2120

	Esidrix® (hydrochlorothiazide USP)	
22	TABLETS, 25 mg (pink, scored)	
	100s	4310
	1000s	4313
	Accu-Pak®	
	100s	4312
	Consumer Pack	
	100s	4325
46	TABLETS, 50 mg (yellow, scored)	
	100s	4315
	1000s	4318
	Accu-Pak®	
	100s	4317
	Consumer Pack	
	30s	4328
	60s	4331
	100s	4330
192	TABLETS, 100 mg (blue, scored)	
	100s	4340
	Esimil®	
47	TABLETS (white, scored), each containing 10 mg guanethidine monosulfate and 25 mg hydrochlorothiazide	
	100s	4503
	Consumer Pack	
	100s	4512
	Ismelin® sulfate (guanethidine monosulfate)	
49	TABLETS, 10 mg (pale yellow, scored)	
	100s	5010
	1000s	5012
	Consumer Pack	
	100s	5003
103	TABLETS, 25 mg (white, scored)	
	100s	5020
	1000s	5022
	Consumer Pack	
	100s	5026
	Lithobid® (lithium carbonate)	
65	TABLETS, 300 mg (peach colored)	
	100s	0210
	1000s	0220
	Accu-Pak® 100s	0230
	Ludiomil® (maprotiline hydrochloride)	
110	TABLETS, 25 mg (oval, dark orange, coated)	
	100s	1710
	Accu-Pak®	
	100s	1714
26	TABLETS, 50 mg (round, dark orange, coated)	
	100s	1720
	Accu-Pak®	
	100s	1721
135	TABLETS, 75 mg (oval, white, coated)	
	100s	1730
	Accu-Pak®	
	100s	1732
	Metandren® (methyltestosterone USP)	
30	TABLETS, 10 mg (white, scored)	
	100s	1414
32	TABLETS, 25 mg (pale yellow, scored)	
	100s	1418
51	LINGUETS®, 5 mg (white)	
	100s	1432
64	LINGUETS®, 10 mg (yellow)	
	100s	1438
	Metopirone® (metyrapone USP)	
130	TABLETS, 250 mg (white, scored)	
	18s	5403
	Rimactane® (rifampin USP)	
154	CAPSULES, 300 mg (opaque scarlet and caramel)	
	30s	8903
	60s	8904
	100s	8901
	Rimactane®/INH Dual Pack (rifampin USP) (isoniazid USP)	
8912	Each Dual Pack contains two Rimactane 300-mg CAPSULES and one INH 300-mg TABLET	8912

	Ritalin® hydrochloride ℂ (methylphenidate hydrochloride USP)	
07	TABLETS, 5 mg (yellow)	
	100s	7410
	500s	7412
	1000s	7414
03	TABLETS, 10 mg (pale green, scored)	
	100s	7416
	500s	7418
	1000s	7420
	Accu-Pak® 100s	7415
34	TABLETS, 20 mg (pale yellow, scored)	
	100s	7422
	1000s	7426
	Ritalin-SR® ℂ (methylphenidate hydrochloride) sustained-release tablets	
16	TABLETS, 20 mg (round, white, scored)	
	100s	7442
71	**Ser-Ap-Es®** TABLETS (light salmon pink, dry-coated), each containing 0.1 mg reserpine, 25 mg hydralazine hydrochloride and 15 mg hydrochlorothiazide	
	100s	6610
	1000s	6612
	Accu-Pak® 100s	6605
	Consumer Pack	
	100s	6617
	Serpasil® (reserpine USP)	
35	TABLETS, 0.1 mg (white)	
	100s	7610
	1000s	7614
36	TABLETS, 0.25 mg (white, scored)	
	100s	7616
	500s	7618
	1000s	7620
	Consumer Pack	
	100s	7607
	Serpasil®-Apresoline® (reserpine and hydralazine hydrochloride)	
40	TABLETS #1 (yellow, dry-coated), each containing 0.1 mg reserpine and 25 mg hydralazine hydrochloride	
	100s	7721
104	TABLETS #2 (yellow, dry-coated), each containing 0.2 mg reserpine and 50 mg hydralazine hydrochloride	
	100s	7709
	Serpasil®-Esidrix® (reserpine and hydrochlorothiazide)	
13	TABLETS #1 (light orange), each containing 0.1 mg reserpine and 25 mg hydrochlorothiazide	
	100s	7010
	1000s	7012
97	TABLETS #2 (light orange), each containing 0.1 mg reserpine and 50 mg hydrochlorothiazide	
	100s	7020
	1000s	7022
	Slow-K® (potassium chloride)	
165	TABLETS (pale orange, sugar-coated), each containing 8 mEq (600 mg) potassium chloride	
	100s	2807
	1000s	2811
	Accu-Pak®	
	100s	2817
	Consumer Pack	
	100s	2815
	[See table on next page].	
	Transderm® Scōp	
4345	Package of 3 cartons (4 discs per carton)	5921

CIBA Code #	NUMERICAL LISTING	
	Ritalin® hydrochloride ℂ (methylphenidate hydrochloride USP)	
03	TABLETS, 10 mg (pale green, scored)	
07	TABLETS, 5 mg (yellow)	

Product Information

		Serpasil®-Esidrix®
		(reserpine and hydrochlorothiazide)
13		TABLETS #1 (light orange), each containing 0.1 mg reserpine and 25 mg hydrochlorothiazide
		Antrenyl® bromide
		(oxyphenonium bromide)
15		TABLETS, 5 mg (white, scored)
		Ritalin-SR® ©
		(methylphenidate hydrochloride) sustained-release tablets
16		TABLETS, 20 mg (round, white, scored)
		Esidrix®
		(hydrochlorothiazide USP)
22		TABLETS, 25 mg (pink, scored)
		Cytadren®
		(aminoglutethamide)
24		TABLETS, 250 mg (white, round, scored into quarters)
		Ludiomil®
		(maprotiline hydrochloride)
26		TABLETS, 50 mg (round, dark orange, coated)
		Metandren®
		(methyltestosterone USP)
30		TABLETS, 10 mg (white, scored)
		Metandren®
		(methyltestosterone USP)
32		TABLETS, 25 mg (pale yellow, scored)
		Ritalin® hydrochloride ©
		(methylphenidate hydrochloride USP)
34		TABLETS, 20 mg (pale yellow, scored)
		Serpasil®
		(reserpine USP)
35		TABLETS, 0.1 mg (white)
36		TABLETS, 0.25 mg (white, scored)
		Apresoline® hydrochloride
		(hydralazine hydrochloride USP)
37		TABLETS, 10 mg (pale yellow, dry-coated)
39		TABLETS, 25 mg (deep blue, dry-coated)
		Serpasil®-Apresoline®
		(reserpine and hydralazine hydrochloride)
40		TABLETS #1 (yellow, dry-coated), each containing 0.1 mg reserpine and 25 mg hydralazine hydrochloride
		Anturane®
		(sulfinpyrazone USP)
41		TABLETS (white, single-scored) each containing 100 mg sulfinpyrazone USP
		Esidrix®
		(hydrochlorothiazide USP)
46		TABLETS, 50 mg (yellow, scored)
		Esimil®
47		TABLETS (white, scored), each containing 10 mg guanethidine monosulfate and 25 mg hydrochlorothiazide
		Ismelin® sulfate
		(guanethidine monosulfate)
49		TABLETS, 10 mg (pale yellow, scored)
		Metandren®
		(methyltestosterone USP)
51		LINGUETS®, 5 mg (white)
		Metandren®
		(methyltestosterone USP)
64		LINGUETS®, 10 mg (yellow)
		Lithobid®
		(lithium carbonate)
65		TABLETS, 300 mg (peach colored)
		Ser-Ap-Es®
71		TABLETS (light salmon pink, dry-coated), each containing 0.1 mg reserpine, 25 mg hydralazine hydrochloride and 15 mg hydrochlorothiazide
		Apresoline® hydrochloride
		(hydralazine hydrochloride USP)
73		TABLETS, 50 mg (light blue, dry-coated)
		Serpasil®-Esidrix®
		(reserpine and hydrochlorothiazide)
97		TABLETS #2 (light orange), each containing 0.1 mg reserpine and 50 mg hydrochlorothiazide
		Apresoline® hydrochloride
		(hydralazine hydrochloride USP)
101		TABLETS, 100 mg (peach, dry-coated)

Transderm®-Nitro (Nitroglycerin)

Code	Transderm-Nitro System Rated Release in vivo	Total Nitroglycerin in System	System Size	List No.	Carton Size
2025	2.5 mg/24 hr	12.5 mg	5 cm^2	2901	30 Systems
2105	5 mg/24 hr	25 mg	10 cm^2	2903	30 Systems
	5 mg/24 hr	25 mg	10 cm^2	2905	7 Systems
2110	10 mg/24 hr	50 mg	20 cm^2	2902	30 Systems
2115	15 mg/24 hr	75 mg	30 cm^2	2904	30 Systems

		Ismelin® sulfate
		(guanethidine monosulfate)
103		TABLETS, 25 mg (white, scored)
		Serpasil®-Apresoline®
		(reserpine and hydralazine hydrochloride)
104		TABLETS #2 (yellow, dry-coated), each containing 0.2 mg reserpine and 50 mg hydralazine hydrochloride
		Ludiomil®
		(maprotiline hydrochloride)
110		TABLETS, 25 mg (oval, dark orange coated)
		Apresoline®-Esidrix®
		(hydralazine hydrochloride and hydrochlorothiazide)
129		TABLETS (orange, dry-coated), each containing 25 mg hydralazine hydrochloride and 15 mg hydrochlorothiazide
		Metopirone®
		(metyrapone USP)
130		TABLETS, 250 mg (white, scored)
		Ludiomil®
		(maprotiline hydrochloride)
135		TABLETS, 75 mg (oval, white, coated)
		Apresazide®
		(hydralazine HCl and hydrochlorothiazide)
139		CAPSULES 25/25 (light blue and white opaque), each containing 25 mg hydralazine hydrochloride and 25 mg hydrochlorothiazide
149		CAPSULES 50/50 (pink and white opaque), each containing 50 mg hydralazine hydrochloride and 50 mg hydrochlorothiazide
		Rimactane®
		(rifampin USP)
154		CAPSULES, 300 mg (opaque scarlet and caramel)
		Rimactane®/INH® Dual Pack
		(rifampin USP) (isoniazid USP)
8912		Each Dual Pack contains two Rimactane 300-mg CAPSULES and one INH 300-mg TABLET
		Apresazide®
		(hydralazine HCl and hydrochlorothiazide)
159		CAPSULES 100/50 (pink flesh and white opaque), each containing 100 mg hydralazine hydrochloride and 50 mg hydrochlorothiazide
		Slow-K®
		(potassium chloride)
165		TABLETS (buff colored, sugar-coated), each containing 8 mEq (600 mg) potassium chloride
		Anturane®
		(sulfinpyrazone USP)
168		CAPSULES (green) each containing 200 mg sulfinpyrazone USP
		Esidrix®
		(hydrochlorothiazide USP)
192		TABLETS, 100 mg (blue, scored)
		Transderm®-Nitro
		(nitroglycerin)
2025	2.5 mg		30 systems
2105	5 mg		30 systems
2110	10 mg		30 systems
2115	15 mg		30 systems
		Transderm® Scōp
4345		Package of 3 cartons (4 discs per carton)

ANTRENYL® bromide ℞
[ann′tre-nill]
(oxyphenonium bromide)

Indications: Peptic Ulcer, as adjunctive therapy.

Contraindications: Glaucoma; obstructive uropathy (for example, bladder neck obstruction due to prostatic hypertrophy); obstructive disease of the gastrointestinal tract (as in achalasia, paralytic ileus, pyloroduodenal stenosis, etc.); intestinal atony of the elderly or debilitated patient; unstable cardiovascular status in acute hemorrhage; severe ulcerative colitis; toxic megacolon complicating ulcerative colitis; myasthenia gravis; hypersensitivity.

Warnings: In the presence of a high environmental temperature, heat prostration can occur with drug use (fever and heat stroke due to decreased sweating).

Diarrhea may be an early symptom of incomplete intestinal obstruction, especially in patients with ileostomy or colostomy. In this instance, treatment with Antrenyl would be inappropriate and possibly harmful.

Anticholinergics may produce drowsiness or blurred vision. Therefore, patients should be warned not to engage in activities requiring mental alertness (such as operating a motor vehicle or other machinery) or perform hazardous work while taking Antrenyl.

Usage in Pregnancy
The safe use of this drug in pregnant women or during lactation has not been established. Therefore, the benefits must be weighed against the potential hazards.

Precautions: Give cautiously to patients with autonomic neuropathy; hepatic or renal disease; early evidence of ileus (as in peritonitis); ulcerative colitis (large doses may suppress intestinal motility to the point of producing a paralytic ileus and the use of anticholinergics may precipitate or aggravate the serious complication of toxic megacolon); hyperthyroidism; coronary heart disease; congestive heart failure; cardiac arrhythmias; hypertension; nonobstructing prostatic hypertrophy; hiatal hernia associated with reflux esophagitis, since anticholinergic drugs may aggravate this condition.

It should be noted that the use of anticholinergic drugs in the treatment of gastric ulcer may produce a delay in gastric emptying time and may complicate such therapy (antral stasis). Do not rely on the use of Antrenyl in the presence of biliary tract disease. Investigate any tachycardia before giving anticholinergic (atropine-like) drugs, since they may increase the heart rate.

With overdosage, a curare-like action may occur. Use cautiously in debilitated patients with chronic lung disease, because reduction in bronchial secretions can lead to inspissation and formation of bronchial plugs. All anticholinergic agents should be used with caution in patients over 40 years of age because of the increased incidence of glaucoma in this age group.

Adverse Reactions: Anticholinergics produce certain effects which may be physiologic or toxic, depending upon the individual patient's response. The physician must delineate these.

Continued on next page

The full prescribing information for each CIBA drug is contained herein and is that in effect as of October 1, 1984.

CIBA—Cont.

Adverse reactions may include xerostomia; urinary hesitancy and retention; blurred vision; tachycardia; palpitations; mydriasis; dilatation of the pupil; cycloplegia; increased ocular tension; loss of taste; headaches; nervousness; drowsiness; weakness; dizziness; insomnia; nausea; vomiting; impotence; suppression of lactation; constipation; bloated feeling; severe allergic reaction or drug idiosyncrasies, including anaphylaxis, urticaria, and other dermal manifestation; some degree of mental confusion and/or excitement, especially in elderly persons.

Decreased sweating is another adverse reaction that may occur. It should be noted that adrenergic innervation of the eccrine sweat glands on the palms and soles make complete control of sweating impossible. An end point of complete anhidrosis cannot occur because large doses of drug would be required, and this would produce severe side effects from parasympathetic paralysis.

Dosage and Administration: Average adult dosage is 10 mg (2 tablets) 4 times daily for several days. Dosage may then be reduced, depending on patient's response.

Not for use in children.

Overdosage: Treatment is the same as for atropine overdosage. Gastric lavage or, in the absence of coma, an emetic should be given, and activated charcoal slurry instilled into the stomach. If central nervous system excitation occurs, a short-acting barbiturate may be used. Avoid long-acting sedatives; the central depressive action of these agents may coincide with depression produced by oxyphenonium in later stages. Fever may be combated with ice bags, alcohol sponges, and other appropriate measures.

How Supplied: *Tablets,* 5 mg (white, scored); bottles of 100. C77-16 Rev. 3/77

Shown in Product Identification Section, page 409

ANTURANE®
[ann'too-rain]
(sulfinpyrazone USP)
Tablets Capsules

Indications: Anturane is indicated for the treatment of:
1. Chronic gouty arthritis
2. Intermittent gouty arthritis

Contraindications: Patients with an active peptic ulcer or symptoms of gastrointestinal inflammation or ulceration should not receive the drug.

The drug is contraindicated in patients with a history or the presence of:
1. Hypersensitivity to phenylbutazone or other pyrazoles
2. Blood dyscrasias

Warnings: Studies on the teratogenicity of pyrazole compounds in animals have yielded inconclusive results. Up to the present time, however, there have been no reported cases of human congenital malformation proved to be due to the use of the drug.

It is suggested that Anturane be used with caution in pregnant women, weighing the potential risks against the possible benefits.

Precautions: As with all pyrazole compounds, patients receiving Anturane should be kept under close medical supervision and periodic blood counts are recommended. It may be administered with care to patients with a history of healed peptic ulcer.

Recent reports have indicated that Anturane potentiates the action of certain sulfonamides, such as sulfadiazine and sulfisoxazole. In addition, other pyrazole compounds (phenylbutazone) have been observed to potentiate the hypoglycemic sulfonylurea agents, as well as insulin. In view of these observations, it is suggested that Anturane be used with caution in conjunction with sulfa drugs, the sulfonylurea hypoglycemic agents and insulin.

Because Anturane is a potent uricosuric agent, it may precipitate urolithiasis and renal colic, especially in the initial stages of therapy. For this reason, an adequate fluid intake and alkalinization of the urine are recommended. In cases with significant renal impairment, periodic assessment of renal function is indicated. Occasional cases of renal failure have been reported; but a cause-and-effect relationship has not always been clearly established.

Salicylates antagonize the uricosuric action of Anturane and for this reason their concomitant use is contraindicated in gouty arthritis.

Anturane may accentuate the action of coumarin-type anticoagulants and further depress prothrombin activity when these medications are employed simultaneously.

Note: Anturane has minimal anti-inflammatory effect and is not intended for the relief of an acute attack of gout.

In the initial stages of therapy, because of the marked ability of Anturane to mobilize urates, acute attacks of gouty arthritis may be precipitated.

Adverse Reactions: The most frequently reported adverse reactions with Anturane have been upper gastrointestinal disturbances. In these patients it is advisable to administer the drug with food, milk, or antacids. Despite this precaution, Anturane may aggravate or reactivate peptic ulcer.

Rash has been reported. In most instances, this reaction did not necessitate discontinuance of therapy. In general, Anturane has not been observed to affect electrolyte balance.

Blood dyscrasias (anemia, leukopenia, agranulocytosis, thrombocytopenia and aplastic anemia) have rarely been reported. There has also been a published report associating Anturane, administered concomitantly with other drugs including colchicine, with leukemia following long-term treatment of patients with gout. However, the circumstances involved in the two cases reported are such that a cause-and-effect relationship to Anturane has not been clearly established.

Overdosage:

Symptoms: Nausea, vomiting, diarrhea, epigastric pain, ataxia, labored respiration, convulsions, coma. Possible symptoms, seen after overdosage with other pyrazolone derivatives: anemia, jaundice, ulceration.

Treatment: No specific antidote. Induce emesis; gastric lavage; supportive treatment (intravenous glucose infusions, analeptics).

Dosage and Administration:

Initial: 200–400 mg daily in two divided doses, with meals or milk, gradually increasing when necessary to full maintenance dosage in one week.

Maintenance:

400 mg daily, given in two divided doses, as above. This dosage may be increased to 800 mg daily, if necessary, and may sometimes be reduced to as low as 200 mg daily after the blood urate level has been controlled. Treatment should be continued without interruption even in the presence of acute exacerbations, which can be concomitantly treated with phenylbutazone or colchicine. Patients previously controlled with other uricosuric therapy may be transferred to Anturane at full maintenance dosage.

How Supplied: White, single-scored tablets of 100 mg, bottles of 100 (NDC 0083-0041-30). Green capsules of 200 mg, bottles of 100 (NDC 0083-0168-30).

Dispense in tight container (USP).

C80-24 (1/81)

Shown in Product Identification Section, page 409

APRESAZIDE®
[a-press'ă-zyde]
(hydralazine HCl and hydrochlorothiazide)
25/25 Capsules
50/50 Capsules
100/50 Capsules

Warning

This fixed combination drug is not indicated for initial therapy of hypertension. Hypertension requires therapy titrated to the individual patient. If the fixed combination represents the dosage so determined, its use may be more convenient in patient management. The treatment of hypertension is not static, but must be reevaluated as conditions in each patient warrant.

Indications
Hypertension. (See box warning.)
Contraindications
Hydralazine
Hypersensitivity to hydralazine; coronary artery disease; and mitral valvular rheumatic heart disease.
Hydrochlorothiazide
Anuria; hypersensitivity to this or other sulfonamide-derived drugs.
Warnings
Hydralazine

Hydralazine may produce in a few patients a clinical picture simulating systemic lupus erythematosus. In such patients hydralazine should be discontinued unless the benefit-to-risk determination requires continued antihypertensive therapy with this drug. Symptoms and signs usually regress when the drug is discontinued but residua have been detected many years later. Long-term treatment with steroids may be necessary.

Complete blood counts, L.E. cell preparations, and antinuclear antibody titer determinations are indicated before and periodically during prolonged therapy with hydralazine even though the patient is asymptomatic. These studies are also indicated if the patient develops arthralgia, fever, chest pain, continued malaise or other unexplained signs or symptoms.

A positive antinuclear antibody titer and/or positive L.E. cell reaction requires that the physician carefully weigh the implications of the test results against the benefits to be derived from antihypertensive therapy with hydralazine.

Use MAO inhibitors with caution in patients receiving hydralazine.

When other potent parenteral antihypertensive drugs, such as diazoxide, are used in combination with hydralazine, patients should be continuously observed for several hours for any excessive fall in blood pressure. Profound hypotensive episodes may occur when diazoxide injection and hydralazine are used concomitantly.

Hydrochlorothiazide

Use with caution in severe renal disease. In patients with renal disease, thiazides may precipitate azotemia. Cumulative effects of the drug may develop in patients with impaired renal function. Thiazides should be used with caution in patients with impaired hepatic function or progressive liver disease, since minor alterations of fluid and electrolyte imbalance may precipitate hepatic coma.

Thiazides may add to or potentiate the action of other antihypertensive drugs. Potentiation occurs with ganglionic or peripheral adrenergic blocking drugs.

Sensitivity reactions are more likely to occur in patients with a history of allergy or bronchial asthma.

The possibility of exacerbation or activation of systemic lupus erythematosus has been reported.
Usage in Pregnancy
Hydralazine
Animal studies indicate that hydralazine is teratogenic in mice, possibly in rabbits, and not in rats. Teratogenic effects observed were cleft palate and malformations of facial and cranial bones. Although clinical experience does not include any positive evidence of adverse effects on the human fetus, hydralazine should not be used during pregnancy unless the expected benefit clearly justifies the potential risk to the fetus.
Hydrochlorothiazide
Thiazides cross the placental barrier and appear in cord blood. The use of thiazides in pregnant women requires that the anticipated benefit be weighed against possible hazards to the fetus. These hazards include fetal or neonatal jaundice,

thrombocytopenia, and possibly other adverse reactions which have occurred in the adult.
Nursing Mothers: Thiazides appear in breast milk. If the use of the drug is deemed essential, the patient should stop nursing.
Precautions
Hydralazine
Myocardial stimulation produced by hydralazine can cause anginal attacks and ECG changes of myocardial ischemia. The drug has been implicated in the production of myocardial infarction. It must, therefore, be used with caution in patients with suspected coronary artery disease.

The "hyperdynamic" circulation caused by hydralazine may accentuate specific cardiovascular inadequacies. An example is that hydralazine may increase pulmonary artery pressure in patients with mitral valvular disease. The drug may reduce the pressor responses to epinephrine. Postural hypotension may result from hydralazine but is less common than with ganglionic blocking agents. Use with caution in patients with cerebral vascular accidents.

In hypertensive patients with normal kidneys who are treated with hydralazine, there is evidence of increased renal blood flow and a maintenance of glomerular filtration rate. In some instances improved renal function has been noted where control values were below normal prior to hydralazine administration. However, as with any antihypertensive agent, hydralazine should be used with caution in patients with advanced renal damage.

Peripheral neuritis, evidenced by paresthesias, numbness, and tingling, has been observed. Published evidence suggests an antipyridoxine effect and the addition of pyridoxine to the regimen if symptoms develop.

Blood dyscrasias, consisting of reduction in hemoglobin and red cell count, leukopenia, agranulocytosis, and purpura, have been reported. If such abnormalities develop, discontinue therapy. Periodic blood counts are advised during prolonged therapy.

Hydrochlorothiazide
Periodic determination of serum electrolytes to detect possible electrolyte imbalance should be performed at appropriate intervals. All patients receiving thiazide therapy should be observed for clinical signs of fluid or electrolyte imbalance; namely, hyponatremia, hypochloremic alkalosis, and hypokalemia. Serum and urine electrolyte determinations are particularly important when the patient is vomiting excessively or receiving parenteral fluids. Medication such as digitalis may also influence serum electrolytes. Warning signs are dryness of mouth, thirst, weakness, lethargy, drowsiness, restlessness, muscle pains or cramps, muscular fatigue, hypotension, oliguria, tachycardia, and gastrointestinal disturbance such as nausea or vomiting.

Hypokalemia may develop, especially with brisk diuresis, when severe cirrhosis is present, or during concomitant use of steroids or ACTH.

Interference with adequate oral intake of electrolytes will also contribute to hypokalemia. Hypokalemia can sensitize or exaggerate the response of the heart to the toxic effects of digitalis (*eg*, increased ventricular irritability).

Any chloride deficit is generally mild and usually does not require specific treatment except under extraordinary circumstances (as in liver disease or renal disease). Dilutional hyponatremia may occur in edematous patients in hot weather; appropriate therapy is water restriction rather than administration of salt, except in rare instances when the hyponatremia is life-threatening. In actual salt depletion, appropriate replacement is the therapy of choice.

Hyperuricemia may occur or frank gout may be precipitated in certain patients receiving thiazide therapy.

Insulin requirements in diabetic patients may be increased, decreased, or unchanged. Latent diabetes may become manifest during thiazide administration.

Thiazide drugs may increase the responsiveness to tubocurarine.

The antihypertensive effects of the drug may be enhanced in the postsympathectomy patient.
Thiazides may decrease arterial responsiveness to norepinephrine. This diminution is not sufficient to preclude effectiveness of the pressor agent for therapeutic use.

If progressive renal impairment becomes evident, withholding or discontinuing diuretic therapy should be considered.

Thiazides may decrease serum PBI levels without signs of thyroid disturbance.

Calcium excretion is decreased by thiazides. Pathological changes in the parathyroid gland with hypercalcemia and hypophosphatemia have been observed in a few patients on prolonged thiazide therapy. The common complications of hyperparathyroidism such as renal lithiasis, bone resorption, and peptic ulceration have not been seen. Thiazides should be discontinued before carrying out tests for parathyroid function.

The Apresazide capsules (100/50) contain FD&C Yellow No. 5 (tartrazine) which may cause allergic-type reactions (including bronchial asthma) in certain susceptible individuals. Although the overall incidence of FD&C Yellow No. 5 (tartrazine) sensitivity in the general population is low, it is frequently seen in patients who also have aspirin hypersensitivity.

Adverse Reactions
Hydralazine
Adverse reactions with hydralazine are usually reversible when dosage is reduced. However, in some cases it may be necessary to discontinue the drug.

Common: Headache; palpitations; anorexia; nausea; vomiting; diarrhea; tachycardia; angina pectoris.

Less frequent: Nasal congestion; flushing; lacrimation; conjunctivitis; peripheral neuritis, evidenced by paresthesias, numbness, and tingling; edema; dizziness; tremors; muscle cramps; psychotic reactions characterized by depression, disorientation, or anxiety; hypersensitivity (including rash, urticaria, pruritus, fever, chills, arthralgia, eosinophilia, and, rarely, hepatitis); constipation; difficulty in micturition; dyspnea; paralytic ileus; lymphadenopathy; splenomegaly; blood dyscrasias, consisting of reduction in hemoglobin and red cell count, leukopenia, agranulocytosis and purpura; hypotension; paradoxical pressor response.

Hydrochlorothiazide
Gastrointestinal: Anorexia, gastric irritation, nausea, vomiting, cramping, diarrhea, constipation, jaundice (intrahepatic cholestatic), pancreatitis, sialadenitis.
Central Nervous System: Dizziness, vertigo, paresthesias, headache, xanthopsia.
Hematologic: Leukopenia, thrombocytopenia, agranulocytosis, aplastic anemia.
Cardiovascular: Orthostatic hypotension (may be potentiated by alcohol, barbiturates, or narcotics).
Hypersensitivity: Purpura, photosensitivity, rash, urticaria, necrotizing angiitis, Stevens-Johnson syndrome, and other hypersensitivity reactions.
Other: Hyperglycemia, glycosuria, hyperuricemia, muscle spasm, weakness, restlessness.
When adverse reactions are moderate or severe, thiazide dosage should be reduced or therapy withdrawn.

Dosage and Administration:
As determined by individual titration (see box warning).
Usual dosage is one Apresazide Capsule twice daily, the strength depending upon individual requirement following titration. For maintenance, adjust dosage to lowest effective level.
When necessary, other antihypertensives such as sympathetic inhibitors may be added gradually in reduced dosages; watch effects carefully.

How Supplied:
25/25 Capsules (light blue and white opaque), each containing 25 mg hydralazine hydrochloride and 25 mg hydrochlorothiazide; bottles of 100.
50/50 Capsules (pink and white opaque), each containing 50 mg hydralazine hydrochloride and 50 mg hydrochlorothiazide; bottles of 100.
100/50 Capsules (pink flesh and white opaque), each containing 100 mg hydralazine hydrochloride and 50 mg hydrochlorothiazide; bottles of 100.
Dispense in tight, light-resistant container (USP).
C80-11 (1/80)
Shown in Product Identification Section, page 409

APRESOLINE® hydrochloride ℞
[*a-press'oh-leen*]
(hydralazine hydrochloride USP)
Tablets
Listed in USP, a Medicare designated compendium.

Indications: Essential hypertension, alone or as an adjunct.
Contraindications: Hypersensitivity to hydralazine; coronary artery disease; and mitral valvular rheumatic heart disease.
Warnings: Hydralazine may produce in a few patients a clinical picture simulating systemic lupus erythematosus. In such patients hydralazine should be discontinued unless the benefit-to-risk determination requires continued antihypertensive therapy with this drug. Symptoms and signs usually regress when the drug is discontinued but residua have been detected many years later. Long-term treatment with steroids may be necessary.

Complete blood counts, L. E. cell preparations, and antinuclear antibody titer determinations are indicated before and periodically during prolonged therapy with hydralazine even though the patient is asymptomatic. These studies are also indicated if the patient develops arthralgia, fever, chest pain, continued malaise or other unexplained signs or symptoms.

A positive antinuclear antibody titer and/or positive L.E. cell reaction requires that the physician carefully weigh the implications of the test results against the benefits to be derived from antihypertensive therapy with hydralazine.

Use MAO inhibitors with caution in patients receiving hydralazine.

When other potent parenteral antihypertensive drugs, such as diazoxide, are used in combination with hydralazine, patients should be continuously observed for several hours for any excessive fall in blood pressure. Profound hypotensive episodes may occur when diazoxide injection and Apresoline (hydralazine hydrochloride) are used concomitantly.

Usage in Pregnancy: Animal studies indicate that hydralazine is teratogenic in mice, possibly in rabbits, and not in rats. Teratogenic effects observed were cleft palate and malformations of facial and cranial bones. Although clinical experience does not include any positive evidence of adverse effects on the human fetus, hydralazine should not be used during pregnancy unless the expected benefit clearly justifies the potential risk to the fetus.

Precautions: Myocardial stimulation produced by Apresoline can cause anginal attacks and ECG changes of myocardial ischemia. The drug has been implicated in the production of myocardial infarction. It must, therefore, be used with caution in patients with suspected coronary artery disease. The "hyperdynamic" circulation caused by Apresoline may accentuate specific cardiovascular inadequacies. An example is that Apresoline may increase pulmonary artery pressure in patients with mitral valvular disease. The drug may reduce the pressor responses to epinephrine. Postural hypotension may result from Apresoline, but is less common than with ganglionic blocking agents. Use with caution in patients with cerebral vascular accidents.

In hypertensive patients with normal kidneys who are treated with Apresoline, there is evidence of increased renal blood flow and a maintenance of

Continued on next page

The full prescribing information for each CIBA drug is contained herein and is that in effect as of October 1, 1984.

CIBA—Cont.

glomerular filtration rate. In some instances improved renal function has been noted where control values were below normal prior to Apresoline administration. However, as with any antihypertensive agent, Apresoline should be used with caution in patients with advanced renal damage.
Peripheral neuritis, evidenced by paresthesias, numbness, and tingling, has been observed. Published evidence suggests an antipyridoxine effect and the addition of pyridoxine to the regimen if symptoms develop.
Blood dyscrasias, consisting of reduction in hemoglobin and red cell count, leukopenia, agranulocytosis, and purpura, have been reported. If such abnormalities develop, discontinue therapy. Periodic blood counts are advised during prolonged therapy.
The Apresoline tablets (10 and 100 mg) contain FD&C Yellow No. 5 (tartrazine) which may cause allergic-type reactions (including bronchial asthma) in certain susceptible individuals. Although the overall incidence of FD&C Yellow No. 5 (tartrazine) sensitivity in the general population is low, it is frequently seen in patients who also have aspirin hypersensitivity.
Adverse Reactions: Adverse reactions with Apresoline are usually reversible when dosage is reduced. However, in some cases it may be necessary to discontinue the drug.
Common: Headache; palpitations; anorexia; nausea; vomiting; diarrhea; tachycardia; angina pectoris.
Less Frequent: Nasal congestion; flushing; lacrimation; conjunctivitis; peripheral neuritis, evidenced by paresthesias, numbness, and tingling; edema; dizziness; tremors; muscle cramps; psychotic reactions characterized by depression, disorientation, or anxiety; hypersensitivity (including rash, urticaria, pruritus, fever, chills, arthralgia, eosinophilia, and, rarely, hepatitis); constipation; difficulty in micturition; dyspnea; paralytic ileus; lymphadenopathy; splenomegaly; blood dyscrasias, consisting of reduction in hemoglobin and red cell count, leukopenia, agranulocytosis, and purpura; hypotension; paradoxical pressor response.
Dosage and Administration
Initiate therapy in gradually increasing dosages; adjust according to individual response. Start with 10 mg 4 times daily for the first 2 to 4 days, increase to 25 mg 4 times daily for balance of first week. For second and subsequent weeks, increase dosage to 50 mg 4 times daily. For maintenance, adjust dosage to lowest effective levels.
The incidence of toxic reactions, particularly the L. E. cell syndrome, is high in the group of patients receiving large doses of Apresoline.
In a few resistant patients, up to 300 mg Apresoline daily may be required for a significant antihypertensive effect. In such cases, a lower dosage of Apresoline combined with a thiazide, reserpine, or both may be considered. However, when combining therapy, individual titration is essential to insure the lowest possible therapeutic dose of each drug.
Overdosage
Signs and Symptoms
Hypotension, tachycardia, headache and generalized skin flushing are to be expected. Myocardial ischemia and cardiac arrhythmia can develop; profound shock can occur in severe overdosage.
Treatment
Evacuate gastric contents, taking adequate precautions against aspiration and for protection of the airway; instill activated charcoal slurry, if general conditions permit. These manipulations may have to be omitted or carried out after cardiovascular status has been stabilized, since they might precipitate cardiac arrhythmias or increase the depth of shock.
Support of the cardiovascular system is of primary importance. Shock should be treated with volume expanders without resorting to use of vasopressors, if possible. If a vasopressor is required, use one that is least likely to precipitate or aggravate cardiac arrhythmia. Digitalization may be necessary. Renal function must be monitored and supported as required.
No experience has been reported with extracorporeal or peritoneal dialysis.
How Supplied: *Tablets,* 10 mg (pale yellow, dry-coated); bottles of 100 and 1000. *Tablets,* 25 mg (deep blue, dry-coated) and 50 mg (light blue, dry-coated); bottles of 100, 500, 1000 and Accu-Pak® blister units of 100. *Tablets,* 100 mg (peach, dry-coated); bottles of 100.
Dispense in tight, light-resistant container (USP).
C80-15 (1/80)
Shown in Product Identification Section, page 409

APRESOLINE® hydrochloride ℞
[a-press'oh-leen]
(hydralazine hydrochloride USP)
Parenteral
Listed in USP, a Medicare designated compendium.
Indications
Severe essential hypertension when the drug cannot be given orally or when there is an urgent need to lower blood pressure.
Contraindications: Hypersensitivity to hydralazine; coronary artery disease; and mitral valvular rheumatic heart disease.
Warnings: Hydralazine may produce in a few patients a clinical picture simulating systemic lupus erythematosus. In such patients hydralazine should be discontinued unless the benefit-to-risk determination requires continued antihypertensive therapy with this drug. Symptoms and signs usually regress when the drug is discontinued but residua have been detected many years later. Long-term treatment with steroids may be necessary.
Complete blood counts, L. E. cell preparations, and antinuclear antibody titer determinations are indicated before and periodically during prolonged therapy with hydralazine even though the patient is asymptomatic. These studies are also indicated if the patient develops arthralgia, fever, chest pain, continued malaise, or other unexplained signs or symptoms.
A positive antinuclear antibody titer and/or positive L.E. cell reaction requires that the physician carefully weigh the implications of the test results against the benefits to be derived from antihypertensive therapy with hydralazine.
Use MAO inhibitors with caution in patients receiving hydralazine.
When other potent parenteral antihypertensive drugs, such as diazoxide, are used in combination with hydralazine, patients should be continuously observed for several hours for any excessive fall in blood pressure. Profound hypotensive episodes may occur when diazoxide injection and Apresoline (hydralazine hydrochloride) are used concomitantly.
Usage in Pregnancy
Animal studies indicate that hydralazine is teratogenic in mice, possibly in rabbits, and not in rats. Teratogenic effects observed were cleft palate and malformations of facial and cranial bones. Although clinical experience does not include any positive evidence of adverse effects on the human fetus, hydralazine should not be used during pregnancy unless the expected benefit clearly justifies the potential risk to the fetus.
Precautions: Myocardial stimulation produced by Apresoline can cause anginal attacks and ECG changes of myocardial ischemia. The drug has been implicated in the production of myocardial infarction. It must, therefore, be used with caution in patients with suspected coronary artery disease. The "hyperdynamic" circulation caused by Apresoline may accentuate specific cardiovascular inadequacies. An example is that Apresoline may increase pulmonary artery pressure in patients with mitral valvular disease. The drug may reduce the pressor responses to epinephrine. Postural hypotension may result from Apresoline, but is less common than with ganglionic blocking agents. Use with caution in patients with cerebral vascular accidents.
In hypertensive patients with normal kidneys who are treated with Apresoline, there is evidence of increased renal blood flow and a maintenance of glomerular filtration rate. In some instances improved renal function has been noted where control values were below normal prior to Apresoline administration. However, as with any antihypertensive agent, Apresoline should be used with caution in patients with advanced renal damage.
Peripheral neuritis, evidenced by paresthesias, numbness, and tingling, has been observed. Published evidence suggests an antipyridoxine effect and the addition of pyridoxine to the regimen if symptoms develop.
Blood dyscrasias, consisting of reduction in hemoglobin and red cell count, leukopenia, agranulocytosis, and purpura, have been reported. If such abnormalities develop, discontinue therapy. Periodic blood counts are advised during prolonged therapy.
Adverse Reactions: Adverse reactions with Apresoline are usually reversible when dosage is reduced. However, in some cases it may be necessary to discontinue the drug.
Common: Headache; palpitations; anorexia; nausea; vomiting; diarrhea; tachycardia; angina pectoris.
Less Frequent: Nasal congestion; flushing; lacrimation; conjunctivitis; peripheral neuritis, evidenced by paresthesias, numbness, and tingling; edema; dizziness; tremors; muscle cramps; psychotic reactions characterized by depression, disorientation, or anxiety; hypersensitivity (including rash, urticaria, pruritus, fever, chills, arthralgia, eosinophilia, and, rarely, hepatitis); constipation; difficulty in micturition; dyspnea; paralytic ileus; lymphadenopathy; splenomegaly; blood dyscrasias, consisting of reduction in hemoglobin and red cell count, leukopenia, agranulocytosis, and purpura; hypotension; paradoxical pressor response.
Dosage and Administration: When there is urgent need, therapy in the hospitalized patient may be initiated intravenously or intramuscularly. Use parenteral Apresoline only when the drug cannot be given orally. Usual dose is 20 to 40 mg, repeated as necessary. Certain patients (especially those with marked renal damage) may require a lower dose. Check blood pressure frequently. It may begin to fall within a few minutes after injection, with an average maximal decrease occurring in 10 to 80 minutes. In cases where there is a previously existing increased intracranial pressure, lowering the blood pressure may increase cerebral ischemia. Most patients can be transferred to oral Apresoline within 24 to 48 hours.
Overdosage
Signs and Symptoms
Hypotension, tachycardia, headache and generalized skin flushing are to be expected. Myocardial ischemia and cardiac arrhythmia can develop; profound shock can occur in severe overdosage.
Treatment
Support of the cardiovascular system is of primary importance. Shock should be treated with volume expanders without resorting to use of vasopressors, if possible. If a vasopressor is required, use one that is least likely to precipitate or aggravate cardiac arrhythmia. Digitalization may be necessary. Renal function must be monitored and supported as required.
No experience has been reported with extracorporeal or peritoneal dialysis.
How Supplied: *Ampuls,* 1 ml, each ml containing 20 mg hydralazine hydrochloride, 0.1 ml propylene glycol with 0.065% methyl-p-hydroxybenzoate and 0.035% propyl-p-hy- droxybenzoate as preservatives in water; cartons of 5. C80-42 (5/80)

APRESOLINE®-ESIDRIX® ℞
[a-press'oh-leen ess'a-dricks]
(hydralazine hydrochloride and hydrochlorothiazide)

Warning
This fixed combination drug is not indicated for initial therapy of hypertension. Hyperten-

sion requires therapy titrated to the individual patient. If the fixed combination represents the dosage so determined, its use may be more convenient in patient management. The treatment of hypertension is not static, but must be reevaluated as conditions in each patient warrant.

Indications
Hypertension. (See box warning.)

Contraindications
Hydralazine
Hypersensitivity to hydralazine; coronary artery disease; and mitral valvular rheumatic heart disease.

Hydrochlorothiazide
Anuria; hypersensitivity to this or other sulfonamide-derived drugs.

Warnings
Hydralazine
Hydralazine may produce in a few patients a clinical picture simulating systemic lupus erythematosus. In such patients hydralazine should be discontinued unless the benefit-to-risk determination requires continued antihypertensive therapy with this drug. Symptoms and signs usually regress when the drug is discontinued but residua have been detected many years later. Long-term treatment with steroids may be necessary.

Complete blood counts, L. E. cell preparations, and antinuclear antibody titer determinations are indicated before and periodically during prolonged therapy with hydralazine even though the patient is asymptomatic. These studies are also indicated if the patient develops arthralgia, fever, chest pain, continued malaise or other unexplained signs or symptoms.

A positive antinuclear antibody titer and/or positive L. E. cell reaction requires that the physician carefully weigh the implications of the test results against the benefits to be derived from antihypertensive therapy with hydralazine.

Use MAO inhibitors with caution in patients receiving hydralazine.

When other potent parenteral antihypertensive drugs, such as diazoxide, are used in combination with hydralazine, patients should be continuously observed for several hours for any excessive fall in blood pressure. Profound hypotensive episodes may occur when diazoxide injection and Apresoline (hydralazine hydrochloride) are used concomitantly.

Hydrochlorothiazide
Use with caution in severe renal disease. In patients with renal disease, thiazides may precipitate azotemia. Cumulative effects of the drug may develop in patients with impaired renal function. Thiazides should be used with caution in patients with impaired hepatic function or progressive liver disease, since minor alterations of fluid and electrolyte imbalance may precipitate hepatic coma.

Thiazides may add to or potentiate the action of other antihypertensive drugs. Potentiation occurs with ganglionic or peripheral adrenergic blocking drugs.

Sensitivity reactions are more likely to occur in patients with a history of allergy or bronchial asthma.

The possibility of exacerbation or activation of systemic lupus erythematosus has been reported.

Usage in Pregnancy
Hydralazine
Animal studies indicate that hydralazine is teratogenic in mice, possibly in rabbits, and not in rats. Teratogenic effects observed were cleft palate and malformations of facial and cranial bones. Although clinical experience does not include any positive evidence of adverse effects on the human fetus, hydralazine should not be used during pregnancy unless the expected benefit clearly justifies the potential risk to the fetus.

Hydrochlorothiazide
Thiazides cross the placental barrier and appear in cord blood. The use of thiazides in pregnant women requires that the anticipated benefit be weighed against possible hazards to the fetus. These hazards include fetal or neonatal jaundice, thrombocytopenia, and possibly other adverse reactions which have occurred in the adult.

Nursing Mothers: Thiazides appear in breast milk. If the use of the drug is deemed essential, the patient should stop nursing.

Precautions
Hydralazine
Myocardial stimulation produced by hydralazine can cause anginal attacks and ECG changes of myocardial ischemia. The drug has been implicated in the production of myocardial infarction. It must, therefore, be used with caution in patients with suspected coronary artery disease.

The "hyperdynamic" circulation caused by hydralazine may accentuate specific cardiovascular inadequacies. An example is that hydralazine may increase pulmonary artery pressure in patients with mitral valvular disease. The drug may reduce the pressor responses to epinephrine. Postural hypotension may result from hydralazine but is less common than with ganglionic blocking agents. Use with caution in patients with cerebral vascular accidents.

In hypertensive patients with normal kidneys who are treated with hydralazine, there is evidence of increased renal blood flow and a maintenance of glomerular filtration rate. In some instances improved renal function has been noted where control values were below normal prior to hydralazine administration. However, as with any antihypertensive agent, hydralazine should be used with caution in patients with advanced renal damage. Peripheral neuritis, evidenced by paresthesias, numbness, and tingling, has been observed. Published evidence suggests an antipyridoxine effect and the addition of pyridoxine to the regimen if symptoms develop.

Blood dyscrasias, consisting of reduction in hemoglobin and red cell count, leukopenia, agranulocytosis, and purpura, have been reported. If such abnormalities develop, discontinue therapy. Periodic blood counts are advised during prolonged therapy.

Hydrochlorothiazide
Periodic determination of serum electrolytes to detect possible electrolyte imbalance should be performed at appropriate intervals. All patients receiving thiazide therapy should be observed for clinical signs of fluid or electrolyte imbalance; namely, hyponatremia, hypochloremic alkalosis, and hypokalemia. Serum and urine electrolyte determinations are particularly important when the patient is vomiting excessively or receiving parenteral fluids. Medication such as digitalis may also influence serum electrolytes. Warning signs are dryness of mouth, thirst, weakness, lethargy, drowsiness, restlessness, muscle pains or cramps, muscular fatigue, hypotension, oliguria, tachycardia, and gastrointestinal disturbance such as nausea or vomiting.

Hypokalemia may develop, especially with brisk diuresis, when severe cirrhosis is present, or during concomitant use of steroids or ACTH.

Interference with adequate oral intake of electrolytes will also contribute to hypokalemia. Hypokalemia can sensitize or exaggerate the response of the heart to the toxic effects of digitalis (*eg*, increased ventricular irritability).

Any chloride deficit is generally mild and usually does not require specific treatment except under extraordinary circumstances (as in liver disease or renal disease). Dilutional hyponatremia may occur in edematous patients in hot weather; appropriate therapy is water restriction rather than administration of salt, except in rare instances when the hyponatremia is life-threatening. In actual salt depletion, appropriate replacement is the therapy of choice.

Hyperuricemia may occur or frank gout may be precipitated in certain patients receiving thiazide therapy.

Insulin requirements in diabetic patients may be increased, decreased, or unchanged. Latent diabetes may become manifest during thiazide administration.

Thiazide drugs may increase the responsiveness to tubocurarine.

The antihypertensive effects of the drug may be enhanced in the postsympathectomy patient. Thiazides may decrease arterial responsiveness to norepinephrine. This diminution is not sufficient to preclude effectiveness of the pressor agent for therapeutic use.

If progressive renal impairment becomes evident, withholding or discontinuing diuretic therapy should be considered.

Thiazides may decrease serum PBI levels without signs of thyroid disturbance.

Calcium excretion is decreased by thiazides. Pathological changes in the parathyroid gland with hypercalcemia and hypophosphatemia have been observed in a few patients on prolonged thiazide therapy. The common complications of hyperparathyroidism such as renal lithiasis, bone resorption, and peptic ulceration have not been seen. Thiazides should be discontinued before carrying out tests for parathyroid function.

Adverse Reactions
Hydralazine
Adverse reactions with hydralazine are usually reversible when dosage is reduced. However, in some cases it may be necessary to discontinue the drug.

Common: Headache; palpitations; anorexia; nausea; vomiting; diarrhea; tachycardia; angina pectoris.

Less frequent: Nasal congestion; flushing; lacrimation; conjunctivitis; peripheral neuritis, evidenced by paresthesias, numbness, and tingling; edema; dizziness; tremors; muscle cramps; psychotic reactions characterized by depression, disorientation, or anxiety; hypersensitivity (including rash, urticaria, pruritus, fever, chills, arthralgia, eosinophilia, and, rarely, hepatitis); constipation; difficulty in micturition; dyspnea; paralytic ileus; lymphadenopathy; splenomegaly; blood dyscrasias, consisting of reduction in hemoglobin and red cell count, leukopenia, agranulocytosis and purpura; hypotension; paradoxical pressor response.

Hydrochlorothiazide
Gastrointestinal: Anorexia, gastric irritation, nausea, vomiting, cramping, diarrhea, constipation, jaundice (intrahepatic cholestatic), pancreatitis, sialadenitis.
Central Nervous System: Dizziness, vertigo, paresthesia, headache, xanthopsia.
Hematologic: Leukopenia, thrombocytopenia, agranulocytosis, aplastic anemia.
Cardiovascular: Orthostatic hypotension (may be potentiated by alcohol, barbiturates, or narcotics).
Hypersensitivity: Purpura, photosensitivity, rash, urticaria, necrotizing angiitis, Stevens-Johnson syndrome, and other hypersensitivity reactions.
Other: Hyperglycemia, glycosuria, hyperuricemia, muscle spasm, weakness, restlessness.

When adverse reactions are moderate or severe, thiazide dosage should be reduced or therapy withdrawn.

Dosage and Administration: As determined by individual titration (see box warning).

Usual dosage is 1 tablet t.i.d. (maximal dosage is 2 tablets t.i.d.). For maintenance, adjust dosage to lowest effective level.

When necessary, other antihypertensives may be added gradually in reduced dosages. When the drug is given in conjunction with ganglionic blocking agents, dosage must be reduced by at least 50% and effects should be watched carefully.

Overdosage
Hydralazine
Signs and Symptoms
Hypotension, tachycardia, headache and generalized skin flushing are to be expected. Myocardial ischemia and cardiac arrhythmia can develop; profound shock can occur in severe overdosage.

Continued on next page

The full prescribing information for each CIBA drug is contained herein and is that in effect as of October 1, 1984.

CIBA—Cont.

Treatment
Evacuate gastric contents, taking adequate precautions against aspiration and for protection of the airway; instill activated charcoal slurry, if general conditions permit. These manipulations may have to be omitted or carried out after cardiovascular status has been stabilized, since they might precipitate cardiac arrhythmias or increase the depth of shock.

Support of the cardiovascular system is of primary importance. Shock should be treated with volume expanders without resorting to use of vasopressors, if possible. If a vasopressor is required, use one that is least likely to precipitate or aggravate cardiac arrhythmia. Digitalization may be necessary. Renal function must be monitored and supported as required.

No experience has been reported with extracorporeal or peritoneal dialysis.

Hydrochlorothiazide
Signs and Symptoms
Diuresis is to be expected; lethargy of varying degree may appear and may progress to coma within a few hours, with minimal depression of respiration and cardiovascular function and without significant serum electrolyte changes or dehydration. The mechanism of CNS depression with thiazide overdosage is unknown.

GI irritation and hypermotility may occur; temporary elevation of BUN has been reported and serum electrolyte changes could occur, especially in patients with impairment of renal function.

Treatment
Evacuate gastric contents but take care to prevent aspiration, especially in the stuporous or comatose patient. GI effects are usually of short duration, but may require symptomatic treatment.

Monitor serum electrolyte levels and renal function; institute supportive measures as required individually to maintain hydration, electrolyte balance, respiration and cardiovascular-renal function.

How Supplied: *Tablets* (orange, dry-coated), each containing 25 mg hydralazine hydrochloride and 15 mg hydrochlorothiazide; bottles of 100.

C78-52 (1/79)

Shown in Product Identification Section, page 409

CORAMINE® ℞
[córe-a-meen]
(nikethamide)
Solution
Ampuls

Description: Coramine, nikethamide, is a central nervous system (CNS) stimulant, available as an aqueous solution (25% w/w) for oral administration and in 1.5-ml ampuls for parenteral administration. Nikethamide is N,N-diethyl-3-pyridinecarboxamide.

Nikethamide is a clear, colorless to pale yellow, somewhat viscous liquid that crystallizes in the cold and melts again as the temperature rises. It has a faint, characteristic, aromatic odor and a peculiar, bitter taste. Its solutions are clear and nearly colorless and have a faint amine-like odor. Nikethamide is miscible with water, with alcohol, and with ether. Its molecular weight is 178.24.

Clinical Pharmacology: The mechanism of action of Coramine is unknown. Coramine stimulates the CNS at all levels of the cerebrospinal axis; it also acts as a respiratory and circulatory stimulant.

Coramine is generally given by the intravenous or intramuscular route, but it is absorbed from all routes of administration. Nikethamide is converted to nicotinamide and then excreted as n-methylnicotinamide.

Pharmacokinetic data in humans are not available.

Indications and Usage: Coramine is indicated for the treatment of CNS depression, respiratory depression, and circulatory failure, particularly when these are due to the effects of CNS depressant drugs.

Combined with electroshock therapy, Coramine helps restore respiration more quickly and may reduce the number of treatments required in cases of psychotic excitement.

Contraindications: Coramine is contraindicated in patients with hypersensitivity to nikethamide or related compounds.

Warnings: Coramine should not be injected intra-arterially, as arterial spasm and thrombosis may result.

Precautions:
Carcinogenesis, Mutagenesis, Impairment of Fertility
Long-term carcinogenicity studies in animals have not been conducted with Coramine.

Pregnancy Category C
Animal reproduction studies have not been conducted with Coramine. It is also not known whether Coramine can cause fetal harm when administered to a pregnant woman or can affect reproduction capacity. Coramine should be given to a pregnant woman only if clearly needed.

Labor and Delivery
The effect of Coramine on labor and delivery or on the newborn is unknown.

Nursing Mothers
It is not known whether this drug is excreted in human milk. Because many drugs are excreted in human milk, caution should be exercised when Coramine is administered to a nursing woman.

Pediatric Use
Safety and effectiveness in children have not been established.

Adverse Reactions: The difference between the clinically effective dose and that producing side effects varies but is often small. The following side effects that have been reported may, in fact, be the result of overdosage.

The most common side effect is an unpleasant feeling or burning or itching, especially at the back of the nose. Occasionally, flushing or a subjective feeling of warmth, sneezing, coughing, sweating, nausea, vomiting, generalized restlessness, fearfulness, changing depth and frequency of respiration, tachycardia, elevated blood pressure, tics (especially facial), and convulsions have also been reported.

Overdosage:
Acute Toxicity
The highest known doses survived are 6,250 mg orally (17-year-old woman) and 375 mg intramuscularly (3-year-old girl).

Intravenous LD_{50} in rats: 152 mg/kg.

Signs and Symptoms
Coughing, sneezing, hyperpnea, and muscle tremors can occur. Heart rate and blood pressure may increase, although probably not markedly. With severe overdosage, as may occur with injection, generalized muscle spasm and convulsive seizures can occur.

Treatment
Treatment is usually not required, except in severe overdosage. In such cases, a short-acting barbiturate is effective in controlling the generalized muscle spasm and convulsions that may be present.

Since the oral solution is rapidly absorbed, attempts to induce emesis or to perform gastric lavage are of little value and, in the presence of paroxysmal coughing or sneezing, could result in complications from aspiration.

Dosage and Administration: Although Coramine is readily absorbed after oral, subcutaneous, or intramuscular administration, it is most effective by the intravenous route.

Parenteral
Anesthetic Overdosage. To Shorten Narcosis: 4 ml intravenously or intramuscularly.

To Increase Amplitude of Respiration: 2-5 ml intravenously.

To Overcome Respiratory Depression: 5-10 ml intravenously, repeated as necessary.

To Combat Respiratory Paralysis: 15 ml intravenously as the minimal initial dose, repeated as required. Other methods of resuscitation, including artificial respiration, should also be employed as indicated. If cardiac arrest is also present, 0.5-1.0 ml administered intracardially may be of some benefit.

Narcotic, Hypnotic, and Carbon Monoxide Poisoning. The initial dose is 5-10 ml intravenously, followed by 5 ml every 5 minutes for the first hour, depending on the response. Thereafter, 5-ml booster doses may be given every hour if needed or, in more serious cases, as often as every half hour. Artificial respiration, gastric lavage, oxygen, and other means of stimulation should also be employed.

Cardiac Decompensation and Coronary Occlusion. In emergencies 5-10 ml intravenously or intramuscularly may be given.

Shock. The primary treatment of shock requires oxygen and adequate solutions, including blood or plasma, for volume replacement. Given in doses of 10-15 ml intravenously or intramuscularly initially and repeated as indicated by the response, Coramine may be of value in compensating peripheral circulation until blood or plasma is available.

Acute Alcoholism. The initial dose is 5-20 ml intravenously to overcome CNS depression, repeated as necessary.

Electroshock Therapy. The recommended dose is 5 ml of Coramine diluted with an equal volume of sterile, distilled water in a 10-ml syringe and injected rapidly into an antecubital vein. The electrical stimulus is applied when the patient's face flushes and the respiratory rate increases noticeably, usually within 1 minute after injection.

Oral
For maintenance therapy, 3-5 ml of the oral solution may be given every 4-6 hours, when indicated.

How Supplied
Available as 25% (by weight) aqueous solution.
Ampuls 1.5 ml
Cartons of 20 ....NDC 0082-3212-20
Oral Solution
Bottles of 3 fluid ounces (approx. 90 ml) ......NDC 0083-3234-61
Dispense in tight, light-resistant container (USP).

C82-22 (8/82)

CYTADREN® ℞
[sight'a-dren]
(aminoglutethimide)

Description: Cytadren is available as 250-mg tablets of aminoglutethimide for oral administration. It acts as an inhibitor of adrenal cortical steroid synthesis. The chemical name is α-(p-aminophenyl)-α-ethylglutarimide.

Empirical formula: $C_{13}H_{16}N_2O_2$. Molecular weight: 232.28. Melting point: 149°-150°C. It is very slightly soluble in water but is readily soluble in most organic solvents.

Clinical Pharmacology: Cytadren inhibits the enzymatic conversion of cholesterol to Δ^5-pregnenolone, thereby reducing the synthesis of adrenal glucocorticoids, mineralocorticoids and other steroids. Evidence suggests that aminoglutethimide acts by binding to the hemoprotein, cytochrome P_{450}, and that it may also affect other steps in the synthesis and metabolism of steroids.

In human volunteers the major portion of aminoglutethimide is excreted unchanged in the urine within 24 hours. The N-acetyl derivative of aminoglutethimide also has been found in the urine of subjects receiving the parent drug. The half-life of the drug in man is not known.

Aminoglutethimide was marketed previously as an anticonvulsant but was withdrawn from marketing for that indication in 1966 because of the effects on the adrenal gland.

Indications and Usage: Cytadren is indicated for the suppression of adrenal function in selected patients with Cushing's syndrome. Plasma cortisol levels (morning) in patients with adrenal carcinoma and ectopic ACTH-producing tumors were reduced on the average to about one-half the pretreatment levels, and in patients with adrenal hyperplasia to about two-thirds of the pretreatment levels during one to three months on Cytadren. Data available from the few patients with adrenal adenoma who were treated suggest similar reductions in plasma cortisol levels. Measurements of plasma cortisol showed reductions to at least 50% of baseline or to normal levels in one-third or more of patients studied, depending on diagnostic groups and time of measurement.

Because aminoglutethimide does not affect the underlying disease process, it has been used primarily during clinical investigations either as an interim measure until more definitive therapy such as surgery can be undertaken, or in cases where such therapy is not appropriate. Only small numbers of patients have been treated for longer than 3 months. A decreased effect or escape from a favorable effect seems to occur more frequently in pituitary dependent Cushing's syndrome, probably because of increasing ACTH levels in response to decreasing glucocorticoid levels.

Cytadren should be used only in those patients who are demonstrated to respond to it.

Contraindications: Cytadren is contraindicated in those patients with serious forms and/or more severe manifestations of hypersensitivity to glutethimide or aminoglutethimide.

Warnings: Cytadren may cause adrenal cortical hypofunction, especially under conditions of stress such as surgery, trauma, or acute illness. Patients should be carefully monitored and given hydrocortisone and mineralocorticoid supplements as indicated. Dexamethasone should not be used. (See Drug Interactions.)

Cytadren also may suppress aldosterone production by the adrenal cortex and may cause orthostatic or persistent hypotension. The blood pressure should be followed in all patients at appropriate intervals. Patients should be advised of the possible occurrence of weakness and dizziness as symptoms of hypotension, and of measures to be taken should they occur.

Cytadren can cause fetal harm when administered to a pregnant woman. In about 5000 patients in the earlier experience with the drug, two cases of pseudohermaphroditism were reported in female infants whose mothers took Cytadren and concomitant anticonvulsants. Normal pregnancies have also occurred during the administration of Cytadren. When administered to rats at doses $\frac{1}{2}$ and $1\frac{1}{4}$ times the maximum human dose Cytadren caused a decrease in fetal implantation, increase in fetal deaths and a variety of teratogenic effects. The compound also caused pseudohermaphroditism in rats treated with approximately three times the highest recommended human dose. If this drug must be used during pregnancy, or if the patient becomes pregnant while taking the drug, the patient should be apprised of the potential hazard to the fetus.

Precautions:
1. *General:* This drug should be administered only by physicians familiar with its use and hazards. Therapy should be initiated in a hospital. See Dosage and Administration.
2. *Information for Patients:* Patients should be warned that drowsiness may occur and that in its presence they should not drive, operate potentially dangerous machinery, or engage in other activities with possibly harmful effects.

    Patients should also be warned of the possibility of hypotension and its symptoms (see Warnings).
3. *Laboratory Tests:* Hypothyroidism may occur in association with aminoglutethimide; hence, appropriate clinical observations should be made and laboratory studies of thyroid function performed as indicated. Supplementary thyroid hormone may be required.

    Hematologic abnormalities in patients receiving Cytadren have been reported (see Adverse Reactions). Therefore, baseline hematologic studies should be followed by periodic hematologic checks.

    Since elevations in SGOT, alkaline phosphatase, and bilirubin have been reported, appropriate clinical observations and regular laboratory studies should be performed before and during therapy.

    Serum electrolytes should be determined periodically.
4. *Drug Interactions:* Cytadren accelerates the metabolism of dexamethasone; therefore, if glucocorticoid replacement is needed, hydrocortisone should be prescribed.
5. *Carcinogenesis, Mutagenesis, Impairment of Fertility:* No mutagenesis studies or animal carcinogenicity studies have been performed. Cytadren affects fertility in female rats. (See Warnings.) Whether it does so in humans has not been determined.
6. *Pregnancy:* Pregnancy category D. See Warnings section.
7. *Pediatric Use:* Safety and effectiveness have not been established by adequate and well-controlled studies in children. See Clinical Studies section for additional information.

Adverse Reactions: Untoward effects have been reported in about two out of three patients treated with Cytadren as the only adrenal cortical suppressant for four or more weeks in Cushing's syndrome. The most frequent and reversible side effects such as drowsiness (approximately one in three), morbilliform skin rash (one in six), nausea and anorexia (each approximately one in eight) often disappear spontaneously within one or two weeks of continued therapy.

Other effects observed are:
Hematologic abnormalities: In four of 27 patients with adrenal carcinoma who were treated with Cytadren for at least four weeks, there were single occurrences of neutropenia, leukopenia (patient received o,p'DDD concomitantly), pancytopenia (5-fluorouracil also administered), and agranulocytosis. The latter two were considered by the investigators not to be related to the administration of Cytadren. One patient with adrenal hyperplasia showed decreased hemoglobin and hematocrit during the course of treatment with Cytadren. In 1214 non-Cushingoid patients, transient leukopenia, the only hematological effect, was reported once. Coombs-negative hemolytic anemia was reported in one patient. In approximately 300 patients with nonadrenal malignancy, 10 to 12 cases showed some degree of anemia and two developed pancytopenia while taking Cytadren.

Endocrine effects: Adrenal insufficiency occurred during four or more weeks of Cytadren therapy in one of thirty patients with Cushing's syndrome. This may involve the glucocorticoids as well as the mineralocorticoids. Hypothyroidism, occasionally associated with thyroid enlargement, may be detected early or confirmed by measuring the plasma levels of the thyroid hormones. Masculinization and hirsutism have occasionally occurred in females as has precocious sex development in males.

CNS effects: Headache and dizziness, possibly caused by lowered vascular resistance or orthostasis have occurred in about one in twenty patients.

Cardiovascular effects: Hypotension, occasionally orthostatic, occurred in one of thirty patients receiving Cytadren, and tachycardia in one of forty.

Gastrointestinal and liver: Vomiting occurred in one of thirty cases. Isolated instances of abnormal liver function tests have been reported. Suspected hepatotoxicity occurred in less than one in a thousand.

Skin: In addition to a rash (one in six cases and often reversible on continued therapy), pruritus was reported in one of twenty cases. These may be allergic or hypersensitivity reactions. Urticaria has occurred rarely.

Miscellaneous: Fever, possibly related to therapy, has been reported in several patients on Cytadren therapy for less than four weeks in duration and with the administration of other drugs. Myalgia occurred in one of 30 patients.

Overdosage: Intentional overdosage with aminoglutethimide has caused ataxia, sedation, and deep coma with hyperventilation and hypotension. No reports of death have been found following doses estimated to have been as high as 7 grams. Gastric lavage and unspecified supportive treatment have been employed. Full consciousness following deep coma was regained forty hours or less after ingestion of three or four grams without lavage. No evidence of hematologic, renal, or hepatic effects were subsequently found. Dialysis may be considered in severe intoxication.

Extreme weakness has been reported with divided doses of 3 grams/day in patients.

A parenteral glucocorticoid, preferably hydrocortisone, and/or a mineralocorticoid, such as fludrocortisone, may be indicated in the event of extreme prostration due to adrenocortical hypofunction.

Dosage and Administration:
Adults: Treatment should be instituted in a hospital until a stable dosage regimen is achieved. Therapy should be initiated with 250 mg orally q.i.d., preferably at 6-hour intervals. Adrenal cortical response should be followed by careful monitoring of plasma cortisol until the desired level of suppression is achieved. If cortisol suppression is inadequate, the dosage may be increased in increments of 250 mg daily at intervals of one to two weeks to a total daily dose of 2 grams. Dose reduction or temporary discontinuation may be required in the event of adverse responses, including extreme drowsiness, severe skin rash, or excessively low cortisol levels. If a skin rash persists for longer than five to eight days, or becomes severe, the drug should be discontinued. It may be possible to reinstate therapy at a lower dosage following the disappearance of a mild or moderate rash.

Mineralocorticoid replacement therapy (e.g., fludrocortisone) may be necessary. If glucocorticoid replacement therapy is needed, 20–30 mg of hydrocortisone orally in the morning will replace endogenous secretion.

How Supplied: Tablets 250 mg (white, round and scored into quarters) bottles of 100 (NDC 0083-0024-30).

Clinical Studies: Clinical investigations included 9 patients in the age range $2\frac{1}{2}$ to 16 years; 4 of these were aged 10 or less. However, of the 9, seven received other therapies (drugs or irradiation) either concomitantly or within a short period prior to Cytadren. Diagnoses included 5 with adrenal carcinoma, 3 with adrenal hyperplasia, and one with ectopic ACTH-producing tumor. Treatment duration in this group ranged from 3 days to $6\frac{1}{2}$ months. Dosages ranged from 0.375 gm daily to 1.5 gm daily. In general, smaller doses were used for younger patients; for example, a $2\frac{1}{2}$-year-old received 0.5–0.75 gm/day, a $3\frac{8}{12}$-year-old received 0.5 gm/day, and all of the others over 10 years of age were given 0.75–1.5 gm daily. Results are difficult to evaluate because of the concomitant therapy, duration of therapy, or inadequate laboratory documentation. Most did show decreases of plasma or urinary steroids at some time during treatment, but these may have been due to other therapeutic modalities or their combinations.

Dispense in tight, light-resistant container (USP).

C80-36 (11/80)

Shown in Product Identification Section, page 409

DESFERAL® mesylate   R
[des'fer-all]
(deferoxamine mesylate USP)

Description: Desferal is available as the mesylate salt of deferoxamine. Its solubility in water is greater than 25%; 500 mg will dissolve in 2 ml distilled water.

Chemically, it is N-[5-[3-[(5-Aminopentyl) hydroxycarbamoyl] propionamido] pentyl] -3 - [[5-(N-hydroxyacetamido) pentyl] carbamoyl] propionohydroxamic acid monomethanesulfonate (salt).

Actions: Desferal is a compound with a specific ability to chelate iron, forming a stable complex which prevents the iron from entering into further chemical reactions. This chelate is readily soluble in water and passes easily through the kidney, giving the urine a characteristic reddish color. Some is also excreted in the feces via the bile. Theoretically, 100 parts by weight of Desferal are capable of binding approximately 8.5 parts by weight

Continued on next page

The full prescribing information for each CIBA drug is contained herein and is that in effect as of October 1, 1984.

CIBA—Cont.

of ferric iron. In studies thus far in man and animals, Desferal does not cause any demonstrable increase in the excretion of electrolytes and trace metals.

Indications: To facilitate the removal of iron in the treatment of acute iron intoxication and in chronic iron overload due to transfusion-dependent anemias.

ACUTE IRON INTOXICATION

Desferal is an adjunct to, and not a substitute for, standard measures generally used in treating acute iron intoxication which may include the following:

1. Induction of emesis with syrup of ipecac.
2. Gastric lavage.
3. Suction and maintenance of clear airway.
4. Control of shock with intravenous fluids, blood, oxygen, and vasopressors.
5. Correction of acidosis.

CHRONIC IRON OVERLOAD

Desferal can promote iron excretion in patients who have secondary iron overload from multiple transfusions (such as occur in some chronic anemias including thalassemia). One controlled study has found that long-term therapy with Desferal slows accumulation of hepatic iron and retards or eliminates progression of hepatic fibrosis. Iron mobilization by Desferal is relatively poor in patients under the age of three with relatively small degrees of iron overload. The drug should ordinarily be withheld in such patients unless a demonstration of significant iron mobilization (eg, one mg of iron per day or more) can be demonstrated.

Desferal is not indicated for the treatment of primary hemochromatosis, since phlebotomy is the method of choice for removing excess iron in this indication.

Contraindications: Desferal is contraindicated in patients with severe renal disease or anuria, since the drug and the chelate which it forms with iron are excreted primarily by the kidney.

Warnings: Rarely, cataracts have been observed in patients who received the drug over prolonged periods in the treatment of chronic iron storage diseases. Slit-lamp examinations performed in patients treated with Desferal for acute iron intoxication have not revealed cataracts. Slit-lamp examinations are recommended periodically in patients treated for chronic iron overload.

Usage in Pregnancy

Skeletal anomalies were noted in the fetuses of two animal species at doses just above those recommended for humans. Therefore, Desferal should not be administered to women of childbearing potential, particularly during early pregnancy, except when in the judgment of the physician the potential benefits outweigh the possible hazards.

Precautions: Flushing of the skin, urticaria, hypotension, and even shock have occurred in a few patients when Desferal has been administered by rapid intravenous injection. To avoid these reactions, DESFERAL SHOULD BE GIVEN INTRAMUSCULARLY, OR BY SLOW SUBCUTANEOUS OR INTRAVENOUS INFUSION.

Adverse Reactions: Occasionally, pain and induration at the site of injection have been reported. Side effects reported in patients treated for acute iron intoxication include generalized erythema, urticaria, and hypotension, which occurred with rapid intravenous injection. Adverse effects reported in patients receiving long-term therapy for chronic iron storage diseases include allergic-type reactions (cutaneous wheal formation, generalized itching, rash, anaphylactic reaction), blurring of vision, dysuria, abdominal discomfort, diarrhea, leg cramps, tachycardia, and fever. Adverse effects reported in patients receiving subcutaneous therapy include localized pain, pruritus, erythema, skin irritation and swelling. These reactions might also occur in an occasional patient treated for acute iron intoxication.

Dosage and Administration: Since little of the drug is absorbed when administered orally, it is necessary to administer Desferal parenterally to chelate the iron that has been absorbed.

ACUTE IRON INTOXICATION

Intramuscular Administration

Intramuscular administration is preferred and should be used for ALL PATIENTS NOT IN SHOCK.

Dose: One gm should be administered initially. This may be followed by 0.5 gm every four hours for two doses. Depending upon the clinical response, subsequent doses of 0.5 gm may be administered every four to twelve hours. The total amount administered should not exceed 6 gm in twenty-four hours.

Preparation of Solution for Intramuscular Administration: Dissolve the Desferal by adding 2 ml sterile water for injection to each vial. Make sure that the drug is completely dissolved and then withdraw the drug and administer intramuscularly.

Intravenous Administration

This route should be used ONLY FOR PATIENTS IN A STATE OF CARDIOVASCULAR COLLAPSE and then ONLY BY SLOW INFUSION. THE RATE OF INFUSION SHOULD NOT EXCEED 15 mg/kg/hour.

Dose: An initial dose of 1 gm should be administered at a rate NOT TO EXCEED 15 mg/kg/hour. This may be followed by 0.5 gm every four hours for two doses. Depending upon the clinical response, subsequent doses of 0.5 gm may be administered every four to twelve hours. The total amount administered should not exceed 6 gm in twenty-four hours.

As soon as the clinical condition of the patient permits, intravenous administration should be discontinued and the drug administered intramuscularly.

Preparation of Solution for Intravenous Administration: Dissolve the Desferal by adding 2 ml sterile water for injection to each vial. Make sure that the drug is completely dissolved and then withdraw the drug and add to physiologic saline, glucose in water, or Ringer's lactate solution and administer at a rate NOT TO EXCEED 15 mg/kg/hour.

CHRONIC IRON OVERLOAD

The more effective of the following two routes of administration must be individualized for each patient.

Intramuscular Administration: 0.5 to 1.0 gm daily administered intramuscularly. In addition, 2.0 gm should be administered intravenously with each unit of blood transfused. However, Desferal should be administered separately from blood. The rate of intravenous infusion must not exceed 15 mg/kg/hour.

Subcutaneous Administration: 1.0 gm to 2.0 gm (20-40 mg/kg/day) administered daily over 8 to 24 hours utilizing a small portable pump capable of providing continuous mini-infusion. The duration of infusion must be individualized. In some patients iron excretion will be as great after a short infusion of 8 to 12 hours as it is if the same dose is given over a 24-hour period.

Preparation of Solution for Subcutaneous Administration: Dissolve the Desferal by adding 2.0 ml sterile water to each vial. Make sure that the drug is completely dissolved and then withdraw the drug in syringe to be used for administration.

Note: Desferal reconstituted with sterile water may be stored under sterile conditions and protected from light at room temperature for not longer than one week.

How Supplied: Vials, each containing 500 mg lyophilized deferoxamine mesylate sterile, for INTRAMUSCULAR, SUBCUTANEOUS, OR INTRAVENOUS administration; cartons of 4.

C80-22 (1/80)

ESIDRIX® ℞
[ess'a-dricks]
(hydrochlorothiazide USP)

Listed in USP, a Medicare designated compendium.

Indications:

Hypertension: In the management of hypertension either as the sole therapeutic agent or to enhance the effect of other antihypertensive drugs in the more severe forms of hypertension.

Edema: As adjunctive therapy in edema associated with congestive heart failure, hepatic cirrhosis, and corticosteroid and estrogen therapy.

Esidrix has also been found useful in edema due to various forms of renal dysfunction, such as the nephrotic syndrome, acute glomerulonephritis, and chronic renal failure.

Usage in Pregnancy: The routine use of diuretics in an otherwise healthy woman is inappropriate and exposes mother and fetus to unnecessary hazard. Diuretics do not prevent development of toxemia of pregnancy, and there is no satisfactory evidence that they are useful in the treatment of developed toxemia.

Edema during pregnancy may arise from pathological causes or from the physiologic and mechanical consequences of pregnancy. Thiazides are indicated in pregnancy when edema is due to pathologic causes, just as they are in the absence of pregnancy (however, see WARNINGS). Dependent edema in pregnancy, resulting from restriction of venous return by the expanded uterus, is properly treated through elevation of the lower extremities and use of support hose; use of diuretics to lower intravascular volume in this case is illogical and unnecessary. There is hypervolemia during normal pregnancy which is not harmful to either the fetus or the mother (in the absence of cardiovascular disease) but which is associated with edema, including generalized edema, in the majority of pregnant women. If this edema produces discomfort, increased recumbency will often provide relief. In rare instances, this edema may cause extreme discomfort which is not relieved by rest. In these cases, a short course of diuretics may provide relief and may be appropriate.

Contraindications: Anuria; hypersensitivity to this or other sulfonamide-derived drugs.

Warnings: Use with caution in severe renal disease. In patients with renal disease, thiazides may precipitate azotemia. Cumulative effects of the drug may develop in patients with impaired renal function.

Thiazides should be used with caution in patients with impaired hepatic function or progressive liver disease, since minor alterations of fluid and electrolyte imbalance may precipitate hepatic coma.

Thiazides may add to or potentiate the action of other antihypertensive drugs. Potentiation occurs with ganglionic or peripheral adrenergic blocking drugs.

Sensitivity reactions are more likely to occur in patients with a history of allergy or bronchial asthma.

The possibility of exacerbation or activation of systemic lupus erythematosus has been reported.

Usage in Pregnancy

Thiazides cross the placental barrier and appear in cord blood. The use of thiazides in pregnant women requires that the anticipated benefit be weighed against possible hazards to the fetus. These hazards include fetal or neonatal jaundice, thrombocytopenia, and possibly other adverse reactions which have occurred in the adult.

Nursing Mothers: Thiazides appear in breast milk. If the use of the drug is deemed essential, the patient should stop nursing.

Precautions: Periodic determination of serum electrolytes to detect possible electrolyte imbalance should be performed at appropriate intervals. All patients receiving thiazide therapy should be observed for clinical signs of fluid or electrolyte imbalance: namely, hyponatremia, hypochloremic alkalosis, and hypokalemia. Serum and urine electrolyte determinations are particularly important when the patient is vomiting excessively or receiving parenteral fluids. Medication such as digitalis may also influence serum electrolytes. Warning signs are dryness of mouth, thirst, weakness, lethargy, drowsiness, restlessness, muscle pains or cramps, muscular fatigue, hypotension, oliguria, tachycardia, and gastrointestinal disturbance such as nausea or vomiting.

Hypokalemia may develop, especially with brisk diuresis, when severe cirrhosis is present, or during concomitant use of steroids or ACTH.

Interference with adequate oral intake of electrolytes will also contribute to hypokalemia. Hypokalemia can sensitize or exaggerate the response of the heart to the toxic effects of digitalis (eg, increased ventricular irritability).

Any chloride deficit is generally mild and usually does not require specific treatment except under extraordinary circumstances (as in liver disease or renal disease). Dilutional hyponatremia may occur in edematous patients in hot weather; appropriate therapy is water restriction, rather than administration of salt except in rare instances when the hyponatremia is life-threatening. In actual salt depletion, appropriate replacement is the therapy of choice.

Hyperuricemia may occur or frank gout may be precipitated in certain patients receiving thiazide therapy.

Insulin requirements in diabetic patients may be increased, decreased, or unchanged. Latent diabetes may become manifest during thiazide administration.

Thiazide drugs may increase the responsiveness to tubocurarine.

The antihypertensive effects of the drug may be enhanced in the postsympathectomy patient. Thiazides may decrease arterial responsiveness to norepinephrine. This diminution is not sufficient to preclude effectiveness of the pressor agent for therapeutic use.

If progressive renal impairment becomes evident, withholding or discontinuing diuretic therapy should be considered.

Thiazides may decrease serum PBI levels without signs of thyroid disturbance.

Calcium excretion is decreased by thiazides. Pathological changes in the parathyroid gland with hypercalcemia and hypophosphatemia have been observed in a few patients on prolonged thiazide therapy. The common complications of hyperparathyroidism such as renal lithiasis, bone resorption, and peptic ulceration have not been seen. Thiazides should be discontinued before carrying out tests for parathyroid function.

Adverse Reactions:
Gastrointestinal: Anorexia, gastric irritation, nausea, vomiting, cramping, diarrhea, constipation, jaundice (intrahepatic cholestatic), pancreatitis, sialadenitis
Central Nervous System: Dizziness, vertigo, paresthesias, headache, xanthopsia
Hematologic: Leukopenia, agranulocytosis, thrombocytopenia, aplastic anemia
Cardiovascular: Orthostatic hypotension (may be potentiated by alcohol, barbiturates, or narcotics)
Hypersensitivity: Purpura, photosensitivity, rash, urticaria, necrotizing angiitis, Stevens-Johnson syndrome, and other hypersensitivity reactions
Other: Hyperglycemia, glycosuria, hyperuricemia, muscle spasm, weakness, restlessness

Whenever adverse reactions are moderate or severe, thiazide dosage should be reduced or therapy withdrawn.

Dosage and Administration: Therapy should be individualized according to patient response. Dosage should be titrated to gain maximal therapeutic response as well as the minimal dose possible to maintain that therapeutic response.

Adults
Hypertension
To Initiate Therapy: Usual dose is 75 mg daily. May be given as a single dose every morning.
Maintenance: After a week dosage may be adjusted downward to as little as 25 mg a day, or upward to as much as 100 mg daily.
Combined Therapy: When necessary, other antihypertensive agents may be added cautiously. Since this drug potentiates the antihypertensive effect of other agents, such additions should be gradual. Dosages of ganglionic blockers in particular should be halved initially.

Edema
To Initiate Diuresis: 25 to 200 mg daily for several days, or until dry weight is attained.
Maintenance: 25 to 100 mg daily or intermittently depending on patient's response. A few refractory patients may require up to 200 mg daily.

Infants and Children
The usual pediatric dosage is administered twice daily.
The total daily dosage for infants up to 2 years of age: 12.5 to 37.5 mg; for children 2 to 12 years of age: 37.5 to 100 mg. Dosage should be based on body weight at the rate of 1 mg per pound, but infants below 6 months of age may require 1.5 mg per pound.

Overdosage
Signs and Symptoms
Diuresis is to be expected; lethargy of varying degree may appear and may progress to coma within a few hours, with minimal depression of respiration and cardiovascular function and without significant serum electrolyte changes or dehydration. The mechanism of CNS depression with thiazide overdosage is unknown.
GI irritation and hypermotility may occur; temporary elevation of BUN has been reported and serum electrolyte changes could occur, especially in patients with impairment of renal function.

Treatment
Evacuate gastric contents but take care to prevent aspiration, especially in the stuporous or comatose patient. GI effects are usually of short duration, but may require symptomatic treatment.
Monitor serum electrolyte levels and renal function; institute supportive measures as required individually to maintain hydration, electrolyte balance, respiration and cardiovascular-renal function.

How Supplied: *Tablets,* 100 mg (blue, scored): bottles of 100. *Tablets,* 50 mg (yellow, scored); bottles of 30, 60, 100, 1000, 5000 and Accu-Pak® blister units of 100.
Tablets, 25 mg (pink, scored); bottles of 100, 1000 and 5000.   C78-1 (Rev. 1/78)
Shown in Product Identification Section, page 409

ESIMIL®   ℞
[*ess'a-mill*]
guanethidine monosulfate 10 mg
hydrochlorothiazide 25 mg

Warning
This fixed combination drug is not indicated for initial therapy of hypertension. Hypertension requires therapy titrated to the individual patient. If the fixed combination represents the dosage so determined, its use may be more convenient in patient management. The treatment of hypertension is not static, but must be reevaluated as conditions in each patient warrant.

Indications
Hypertension. (See box warning.)
Contraindications
Guanethidine
Known or suspected pheochromocytoma; hypersensitivity; frank congestive heart failure not due to hypertension; use of MAO inhibitors.
Hydrochlorothiazide
Anuria; hypersensitivity to this or other sulfonamide-derived drugs.
Warnings: Guanethidine and hydrochlorothiazide are potent drugs and their use can lead to disturbing and serious clinical problems. Physicians should be familiar with both drugs and their combination before prescribing, and patients should be warned not to deviate from instructions.
Guanethidine

Orthostatic hypotension can occur frequently and patients should be properly instructed about this potential hazard. Fainting spells may occur unless the patient is forewarned to sit or lie down with the onset of dizziness or weakness. Postural hypotension is most

marked in the morning and is accentuated by hot weather, alcohol, or exercise. Dizziness or weakness may be particularly bothersome during the initial period of dosage adjustment and with postural changes, such as arising in the morning. The potential occurrence of these symptoms may require alteration of previous daily activity. The patient should be cautioned to avoid sudden or prolonged standing or exercise while taking the drug.

Concurrent use of guanethidine and rauwolfia derivatives may cause excessive postural hypotension, bradycardia, and mental depression.

If possible, withdraw therapy two weeks prior to surgery to reduce the possibility of vascular collapse and cardiac arrest during anesthesia. If emergency surgery is indicated, preanesthetic and anesthetic agents should be administered cautiously in reduced dosage. Oxygen, atropine, vasopressors, and adequate solutions for volume replacement should be ready for immediate use to counteract vascular collapse in the surgical patient. Vasopressors should be used only with extreme caution, since guanethidine augments the responsiveness to exogenously administered norepinephrine and vasopressors with respect to blood pressure and their propensity for the production of cardiac arrhythmias.

Dosage requirements may be reduced in the presence of fever.

Exercise special care when treating patients with a history of bronchial asthma; asthmatics are more apt to be hypersensitive to catecholamine depletion and their condition may be aggravated.
Hydrochlorothiazide
Use with caution in severe renal disease. In patients with renal disease, thiazides may precipitate azotemia. Cumulative effects of the drug may develop in patients with impaired renal function. Thiazides should be used with caution in patients with impaired hepatic function or progressive liver disease, since minor alterations of fluid and electrolyte imbalance may precipitate hepatic coma.

Thiazides may add to or potentiate the action of other antihypertensive drugs. Potentiation occurs with ganglionic or peripheral adrenergic blocking drugs.

Sensitivity reactions are more likely to occur in patients with a history of allergy or bronchial asthma.

The possibility of exacerbation or activation of systemic lupus erythematosus has been reported.
Usage in Pregnancy
Guanethidine
The safety of guanethidine for use in pregnancy has not been established; therefore, this drug should be used in pregnant patients only when, in the judgment of the physician, its use is deemed essential to the welfare of the patient.
Hydrochlorothiazide
Thiazides cross the placental barrier and appear in cord blood. The use of thiazides in pregnant women requires that the anticipated benefit be weighed against possible hazards to the fetus. These hazards include fetal or neonatal jaundice, thrombocytopenia, and possibly other adverse reactions which have occurred in the adult.
Nursing Mothers: Thiazides appear in breast milk. If the use of the drug is deemed essential, the patient should stop nursing.
Precautions
Guanethidine
The effects of guanethidine are cumulative over long periods; initial doses should be small and increased gradually in small increments.
Use very cautiously in hypertensive patients with: renal disease and nitrogen retention or rising BUN levels, since decreased blood pressure may

Continued on next page

The full prescribing information for each CIBA drug is contained herein and is that in effect as of October 1, 1984.

CIBA—Cont.

further compromise renal function; coronary disease with insufficiency or recent myocardial infarction; cerebral vascular disease, especially with encephalopathy.

Do not give to patients with severe cardiac failure except with extreme caution since guanethidine may interfere with the compensatory role of the adrenergic system in producing circulatory adjustment in patients with congestive heart failure.

In patients with incipient cardiac decompensation, watch for weight gain or edema, which may be averted by the concomitant administration of a thiazide.

Remember that both digitalis and guanethidine slow the heart rate.

Use cautiously in patients with a history of peptic ulcer or other chronic disorders which may be aggravated by a relative increase in parasympathetic tone.

Amphetamine-like compounds, stimulants (eg, ephedrine, methylphenidate), tricyclic antidepressants (eg, amitriptyline, imipramine, desipramine) and other psychopharmacologic agents (eg, phenothiazines and related compounds), and oral contraceptives may reduce the hypotensive effect of guanethidine.

MAO inhibitors should be discontinued for at least one week before starting therapy with guanethidine.

Hydrochlorothiazide

Periodic determination of serum electrolytes to detect possible electrolyte imbalance should be performed at appropriate intervals. All patients receiving thiazide therapy should be observed for clinical signs of fluid or electrolyte imbalance; namely, hyponatremia, hypochloremic alkalosis, and hypokalemia. Serum and urine electrolyte determinations are particularly important when the patient is vomiting excessively or receiving parenteral fluids. Medication such as digitalis may also influence serum electrolytes. Warning signs are dryness of mouth, thirst, weakness, lethargy, drowsiness, restlessness, muscle pains or cramps, muscular fatigue, hypotension, oliguria, tachycardia, and gastrointestinal disturbance such as nausea or vomiting.

Hypokalemia may develop, especially with brisk diuresis, when severe cirrhosis is present, or during concomitant use of steroids or ACTH.

Interference with adequate oral intake of electrolytes will also contribute to hypokalemia. Hypokalemia can sensitize or exaggerate the response of the heart to the toxic effects of digitalis (eg, increased ventricular irritability).

Any chloride deficit is generally mild and usually does not require specific treatment except under extraordinary circumstances (as in liver disease or renal disease). Dilutional hyponatremia may occur in edematous patients in hot weather; appropriate therapy is water restriction rather than administration of salt, except in rare instances when the hyponatremia is life-threatening. In actual salt depletion, appropriate replacement is the therapy of choice.

Hyperuricemia may occur or frank gout may be precipitated in certain patients receiving thiazide therapy.

Insulin requirements in diabetic patients may be increased, decreased, or unchanged. Latent diabetes may become manifest during thiazide administration.

Thiazide drugs may increase the responsiveness to tubocurarine.

The antihypertensive effects of the drug may be enhanced in the postsympathectomy patient.

Thiazides may decrease arterial responsiveness to norepinephrine. This diminution is not sufficient to preclude effectiveness of the pressor agent for therapeutic use.

If progressive renal impairment becomes evident, withholding or discontinuing diuretic therapy should be considered.

Thiazides may decrease serum PBI levels without signs of thyroid disturbance.

Calcium excretion is decreased by thiazides. Pathological changes in the parathyroid gland with hypercalcemia and hypophosphatemia have been observed in a few patients on prolonged thiazide therapy. The common complications of hyperparathyroidism such as renal lithiasis, bone resorption, and peptic ulceration have not been seen. Thiazides should be discontinued before carrying out tests for parathyroid function.

Adverse Reactions

Guanethidine

Frequent reactions due to sympathetic blockade: dizziness, weakness, lassitude, and syncope resulting from either postural or exertional hypotension.

Frequent reactions due to unopposed parasympathetic activity: bradycardia, increase in bowel movements, and diarrhea. Diarrhea may be severe at times and necessitate discontinuance of the medication.

Other common reactions: inhibition of ejaculation, a tendency toward fluid retention and edema with occasional development of congestive heart failure.

Other less common reactions: dyspnea, fatigue, nausea, vomiting, nocturia, urinary incontinence, dermatitis, scalp hair loss, dry mouth, rise in BUN, ptosis of the lids, blurring of vision, parotid tenderness, myalgia, muscle tremor, mental depression, chest pains (angina), chest paresthesias, nasal congestion, weight gain, and asthma in susceptible individuals. Although a causal relationship has not been established, a few instances of blood dyscrasias (anemia, thrombocytopenia, and leukopenia) and of priapism have been reported.

Hydrochlorothiazide

Gastrointestinal: Anorexia, gastric irritation, nausea, vomiting, cramping, diarrhea, constipation, jaundice (intrahepatic cholestatic), pancreatitis, sialadenitis

Central Nervous System: Dizziness, vertigo, paresthesias, headache, xanthopsia

Hematologic: Leukopenia, thrombocytopenia, agranulocytosis, aplastic anemia

Cardiovascular: Orthostatic hypotension (may be potentiated by alcohol, barbiturates, or narcotics)

Hypersensitivity: Purpura, photosensitivity, rash, urticaria, necrotizing angiitis, Stevens-Johnson syndrome, and other hypersensitivity reactions

Other: Hyperglycemia, glycosuria, hyperuricemia, muscle spasm, weakness, restlessness

Whenever adverse reactions are moderate or severe, thiazide dosage should be reduced or therapy withdrawn.

Dosage and Administration: As determined by individual titration (see box warning).

The usual dosage of Esimil is 2 tablets daily. As with any antihypertensive, dosage should be individually titrated for the patient. Depending upon the degree of hypertension, the patient should be started on the lowest possible dose (usually 1 tablet daily) and then gradually increased at weekly intervals until the desired response is obtained. Blood pressure should be recorded with the patient in the supine position and again after 10 minutes of standing. Dosage should be increased only if the standing blood pressure has not been reduced to desired levels. Dosage adjustment should be made at not less than weekly intervals; maximal dosage should not exceed 4 tablets daily. If additional effect is desirable, supplement individually with guanethidine tablets.

Do not give MAO inhibitors with Esimil. Stop ganglionic blockers before instituting therapy with Esimil. Wait at least one week after one drug is discontinued before starting Esimil.

When Esimil is to be substituted for other antihypertensive agents, the change should be made gradually. In general, dosage of the agent to be discontinued should be discontinued by one-half, and Esimil should be started at 1 tablet daily. Follow this schedule for at least one week; then, dosage of the previous therapy may be halved again and dosage of Esimil increased to 2 tablets daily. At the next week interval, the previously used drugs can generally be discontinued. Titrate dosage of Esimil at weekly intervals as mentioned above.

Patients receiving more than 75 mg guanethidine alone may do well on a smaller dose if also given hydrochlorothiazide. Because of the ratio of the combination, they are probably not candidates for Esimil.

Overdosage

Guanethidine

Signs and Symptoms

Postural hypotension [with dizziness, blurring of vision, etc., possibly progressing to syncope when standing] and bradycardia are most likely to occur; diarrhea, possibly severe, also may occur. Unconsciousness is unlikely if adequate blood pressure and cerebral perfusion can be maintained by appropriate positioning [supine] and by other treatment as required.

Treatment

In previously normotensive patients, treatment has consisted essentially of restoring blood pressure and heart rate to normal by keeping patient in supine position. Normal homeostatic control usually returns gradually over a 72-hour period in these patients.

In previously hypertensive patients, particularly those with impaired cardiac reserve or other cardiovascular-renal disease, intensive treatment may be required to support vital functions and/or to control cardiac irregularities that might be present. Supine position must be maintained; if vasopressors are required, it must be remembered that guanethidine may increase responsiveness as to blood pressure rise and occurrence of cardiac arrhythmias.

Diarrhea, if severe or persistent, should be treated symptomatically to reduce intestinal hypermotility, with due attention to maintenance of hydration and electrolyte balance.

Hydrochlorothiazide

Signs and Symptoms

Diuresis is to be expected; lethargy of varying degree may appear and may progress to coma within a few hours, with minimal depression of respiration and cardiovascular function and without significant serum electrolyte changes or dehydration. The mechanism of CNS depression with thiazide overdosage is unknown.

GI irritation and hypermotility may occur; temporary elevation of BUN has been reported and serum electrolyte changes could occur, especially in patients with impairment of renal function.

Treatment

Evacuate gastric contents but take care to prevent aspiration, especially in the stuporous or comatose patient. GI effects are usually of short duration, but may require symptomatic treatment.

Monitor serum electrolyte levels and renal function; institute supportive measures as required individually to maintain hydration, electrolyte balance, respiration and cardiovascular-renal function.

How Supplied:

Tablets—round, white, scored (imprinted CIBA 47)
10 mg guanethidine monosulfate
25 mg hydrochlorothiazide
Bottles of 100 ....NDC 0083-0047-30
Consumer Pack—One Unit
   12 bottles—
   100 tablets each ....NDC 0083-0047-65
Dispense in tight container (USP)   C82-15 (7/82)
Shown in Product Identification Section, page 409

INH (isoniazid USP)   ℞
[*eye-enn-aitch*]
Tablets

Warning

Severe and sometimes fatal hepatitis associated with isoniazid therapy may occur and may develop even after many months of treatment. The risk of developing hepatitis is age related. Approximate case rates by age are: 0 per 1,000 for persons under 20 years of age, 3 per 1,000 for persons in the 20-34 year age group, 12 per 1,000 for persons in the 35-49 year age group, 23 per 1,000 for persons in the 50-64 year age group, and 8 per 1,000 for persons over 65 years of age. The risk of hepatitis is increased with daily consumption of alcohol. Precise data to assess a fatality rate for isoniazid-related hepatitis is not available; however, in a U.S. Public Health Service Surveillance Study of 13,838 persons taking isoniazid, there were 8 deaths among 174 cases of hepatitis.

Therefore, patients given isoniazid should be carefully monitored and interviewed at monthly intervals. Serum transaminase concentration becomes elevated in about 10–20 percent of patients, usually during the first few months of therapy but it can occur at any time. Usually enzyme levels return to normal despite continuance of drug but in some cases progressive liver dysfunction occurs. Patients should be instructed to report immediately any of the prodromal symptoms of hepatitis, such as fatigue, weakness, malaise, anorexia, nausea, or vomiting. If these symptoms appear or if signs suggestive of hepatic damage are detected, isoniazid should be discontinued promptly, since continued use of the drug in these cases has been reported to cause a more severe form of liver damage.

Patients with tuberculosis should be given appropriate treatment with alternative drugs. If isoniazid must be reinstituted, it should be reinstituted only after symptoms and laboratory abnormalities have cleared. The drug should be restarted in very small and gradually increasing doses and should be withdrawn immediately if there is any indication of recurrent liver involvement.

Preventive treatment should be deferred in persons with acute hepatic diseases.

Indications: For all forms of tuberculosis in which organisms are susceptible.

For preventive therapy for the following groups, in order of priority:

1. Household members and other close associates of persons with recently diagnosed tuberculous disease.
2. Positive tuberculin skin test reactors with findings on the chest roentgenogram consistent with nonprogressive tuberculous disease, in whom there are neither positive bacteriologic findings nor a history of adequate chemotherapy.
3. Newly infected persons.
4. Positive tuberculin skin test reactors in the following special clinical situations: prolonged therapy with adrenocorticosteroids; immunosuppressive therapy; some hematologic and reticuloendothelial diseases, such as leukemia or Hodgkin's disease; diabetes mellitus; silicosis; after gastrectomy.
5. Other positive tuberculin reactors under 35 years of age.

The risk of hepatitis must be weighed against the risk of tuberculosis in positive tuberculin reactors over the age of 35. However, the use of isoniazid is recommended for those with the additional risk factors listed above (1–4) and on an individual basis in situations where there is likelihood of serious consequences to contacts who may become infected.

Contraindications: Isoniazid is contraindicated in patients who develop severe hypersensitivity reactions, including drug-induced hepatitis. Previous isoniazid-associated hepatic injury: severe adverse reactions to isoniazid, such as drug fever, chills, and arthritis; acute liver disease of any etiology.

Warnings: See the boxed warning.

Ophthalmologic examinations (including ophthalmoscopy) should be done *before* INH is started and periodically thereafter, even without occurrence of visual symptoms.

Carcinogenesis

Isoniazid has been reported to induce pulmonary tumors in a number of strains of mice.

Usage in Pregnancy and Lactation

It has been reported that in both rats and rabbits, isoniazid may exert an embryocidal effect when administered orally during pregnancy, although no isoniazid-related congenital anomalies have been found in reproduction studies in mammalian species (mice, rats, and rabbits). Isoniazid should be prescribed during pregnancy only when therapeutically necessary. The benefit of preventive therapy should be weighed against a possible risk to the fetus. Preventive treatment generally should be started after delivery because of the increased risk of tuberculosis for new mothers.

Since isoniazid is known to cross the placental barrier and to pass into maternal breast milk, neonates and breast-fed infants of isoniazid treated mothers should be carefully observed for any evidence of adverse effects.

Precautions: Use of isoniazid should be carefully monitored in the following:

1. Patients who are receiving phenytoin concurrently. Isoniazid may decrease the excretion of phenytoin or may enhance its effects. To avoid phenytoin intoxication, appropriate adjustment of the anticonvulsant should be made.
2. Daily users of alcohol. Daily ingestion of alcohol may be associated with a higher incidence of isoniazid hepatitis.
3. Patients with current chronic liver disease or severe renal dysfunction.

Adverse Reactions: The most frequent reactions are those affecting the nervous system and the liver.

Nervous system reactions: Peripheral neuropathy is the most common toxic effect. It is dose-related, occurs most often in the malnourished and in those predisposed to neuritis (*eg,* alcoholics and diabetics), and is usually preceded by paresthesias of the feet and hands. The incidence is higher in "slow inactivators".

Other neurotoxic effects, which are uncommon with conventional doses, are convulsions, toxic encephalopathy, optic neuritis and atrophy, memory impairment, and toxic psychosis.

Gastrointestinal reactions: Nausea, vomiting, epigastric distress.

Hepatic reactions: Elevated serum transaminases (SGOT; SGPT), bilirubinemia, bilirubinuria, jaundice and occasionally severe and sometimes fatal hepatitis. The common prodromal symptoms are anorexia, nausea, vomiting, fatigue, malaise, and weakness. Mild and transient elevation of serum transaminase levels, occurs in 10 to 20 percent of persons taking isoniazid. The abnormality usually occurs in the first 4 to 6 months of treatment but can occur at any time during therapy. In most instances, enzyme levels return to normal with no necessity to discontinue medication. In occasional instances, progressive liver damage occurs, with accompanying symptoms. In these cases, the drug should be discontinued immediately. The frequency of progressive liver damage increases with age. It is rare in persons under 20, but occurs in up to 2.3 percent of those over 50 years of age.

Hematologic reactions: Agranulocytosis; hemolytic, sideroblastic, or aplastic anemia; thrombocytopenia; and eosinophilia.

Hypersensitivity reactions: Fever, skin eruptions (morbilliform, maculopapular, purpuric, or exfoliative), lymphadenopathy and vasculitis.

Metabolic and endocrine reactions: Pyridoxine deficiency, pellagra, hyperglycemia, metabolic acidosis, and gynecomastia

Miscellaneous reactions: Rheumatic syndrome and systemic lupus erythematosus-like syndrome.

Overdosage:

Signs and Symptoms

Isoniazid overdosage produces signs and symptoms within 30 minutes to 3 hours after ingestion. Nausea, vomiting, dizziness, slurring of speech, blurring of vision, and visual hallucinations (including bright colors and strange designs), are among the early manifestations. With marked overdosage, respiratory distress and CNS depression, progressing rapidly from stupor to profound coma, are to be expected, along with severe, intractable seizures. Severe metabolic acidosis, acetonuria, and hyperglycemia are typical laboratory findings.

Treatment

Untreated or inadequately treated cases of gross isoniazid overdosage can terminate fatally, but good response has been reported in most patients brought under adequate treatment within the first few hours after drug ingestion.

Secure the airway and establish adequate respiratory exchange. Gastric lavage within the first 2 to 3 hours is advised, but should not be attempted until convulsions are under control. To control convulsions administer I.V. short-acting barbiturates and I.V. pyridoxine (usually 1 mg/1mg isoniazid ingested).

Obtain blood samples for immediate determination of gases, electrolytes, BUN, glucose, etc.; type and crossmatch blood in preparation for possible hemodialysis.

Rapid control of metabolic acidosis is fundamental to management. Give I.V. sodium bicarbonate at once and repeat as needed, adjusting subsequent dosage on the basis of laboratory findings (*ie,* serum sodium, pH, etc.).

Forced osmotic diuresis must be started early and should be continued for some hours after clinical improvement to hasten renal clearance of drug and help prevent relapse; monitor fluid intake and output.

Hemodialysis is advised for severe cases; if this is not available, peritoneal dialysis can be used along with forced diuresis.

Along with measures based on initial and repeated determination of blood gases and other laboratory tests as needed, utilize meticulous respiratory and other intensive care to protect against hypoxia, hypotension, aspiration pneumonitis, etc.

Dosage and Administration (See also indications):

NOTE—For preventive therapy of tuberculous infection it is recommended that physicians be familiar with the joint recommendations of the American Thoracic Society, American Lung Association, and the Center for Disease Control, as published in the American Review of Respiratory Diseases Vol. 110, No. 3, September 1974, or CDC's Morbidity and Mortality Weekly Report, Vol. 24, No. 8, February 22, 1975.

For treatment of active tuberculosis: Isoniazid is used in conjunction with other effective antituberculous agents.

If the bacilli become resistant, therapy must be changed to agents to which the bacilli are susceptible.

Usual oral dosage

Adults: 5 mg/kg up to 300 mg daily in a single dose.

Infants and children: 10–20 mg/kg depending on severity of infection, (up to 300–500 mg daily) in a single dose.

For preventive therapy

Adults: 300 mg/day in a single dose.

Infants and children: 10 mg/kg (up to 300 mg daily) in a single dose.

Continuous administration of isoniazid for a sufficient period is an essential part of the regimen because relapse rates are higher if chemotherapy is stopped prematurely. In the treatment of tuberculosis, resistant organisms may multiply and the emergence of resistant organisms during the treatment may necessitate a change in the regimen. Concomitant administration of pyridoxine (B_6) is recommended in the malnourished and in those predisposed to neuropathy (*eg,* alcoholics and diabetics).

How Supplied: *Tablets,* 300 mg (white, scored); available as Rimactane® (rifampin USP)/INH Dual Pack containing 30 INH Tablets and 60 Rimactane 300-mg Capsules.

C78-15 (Rev. 3/78)

ISMELIN® sulfate ℞
[*iz'mel-lin*]
(guanethidine monosulfate)

Listed in USP, a Medicare designated compendium.

Continued on next page

The full prescribing information for each CIBA drug is contained herein and is that in effect as of October 1, 1984.

CIBA—Cont.

Indications: *Moderate and severe hypertension* either alone or as an adjunct.
Renal hypertension, including that secondary to pyelonephritis, renal amyloidosis, and renal artery stenosis.

Contraindications: Known or suspected pheochromocytoma; hypersensitivity; frank congestive heart failure not due to hypertension; use of MAO inhibitors.

Warnings: Ismelin is a potent drug and can lead to disturbing and serious clinical problems. Before prescribing, physicians should familiarize themselves with the details of its use and warn patients not to deviate from instructions.

> Orthostatic hypotension can occur frequently and patients should be properly instructed about this potential hazard. Fainting spells may occur unless the patient is forewarned to sit or lie down with the onset of dizziness or weakness. Postural hypotension is most marked in the morning and is accentuated by hot weather, alcohol, or exercise. Dizziness or weakness may be particularly bothersome during the initial period of dosage adjustment and with postural changes, such as arising in the morning. The potential occurrence of these symptoms may require alteration of previous daily activity. The patient should be cautioned to avoid sudden or prolonged standing or exercise while taking the drug.

Concurrent use of Ismelin and rauwolfia derivatives may cause excessive postural hypotension, bradycardia, and mental depression.

If possible, withdraw therapy two weeks prior to surgery to reduce the possibility of vascular collapse and cardiac arrest during anesthesia. If emergency surgery is indicated, preanesthetic and anesthetic agents should be administered cautiously in reduced dosage. Oxygen, atropine, vasopressors, and adequate solutions for volume replacement should be ready for immediate use to counteract vascular collapse in the surgical patient. Vasopressors should be used only with extreme caution, since Ismelin augments the responsiveness to exogenously administered norepinephrine and vasopressors with respect to blood pressure and their propensity for the production of cardiac arrhythmias.

Dosage requirements may be reduced in the presence of fever.

Exercise special care when treating patients with a history of bronchial asthma; asthmatics are more apt to be hypersensitive to catecholamine depletion and their condition may be aggravated.

Usage in Pregnancy
The safety of Ismelin for use in pregnancy has not been established; therefore this drug should be used in pregnant patients only when, in the judgment of the physician, its use is deemed essential to the welfare of the patient.

Precautions: The effects of guanethidine are cumulative over long periods; initial doses should be small and increased gradually in small increments.

Use very cautiously in hypertensive patients with: renal disease and nitrogen retention or rising BUN levels, since decreased blood pressure may further compromise renal function; coronary disease with insufficiency or recent myocardial infarction; cerebral vascular disease, especially with encephalopathy.

Do not give to patients with severe cardiac failure except with extreme caution since Ismelin may interfere with the compensatory role of the adrenergic system in producing circulatory adjustment in patients with congestive heart failure.

In patients with incipient cardiac decompensation, watch for weight gain or edema, which may be averted by the concomitant administration of a thiazide.

Remember that both digitalis and Ismelin slow the heart rate.

Use cautiously in patients with a history of peptic ulcer or other chronic disorders which may be aggravated by a relative increase in parasympathetic tone.

Amphetamine-like compounds, stimulants (*eg,* ephedrine, methylphenidate), tricyclic antidepressants (*eg,* amitriptyline, imipramine, desipramine) and other psychopharmacologic agents (*eg,* phenothiazines and related compounds), and oral contraceptives may reduce the hypotensive effect of guanethidine.

MAO inhibitors should be discontinued for at least one week before starting therapy with Ismelin.

Adverse Reactions:
Frequent reactions due to sympathetic blockade: dizziness, weakness, lassitude, and syncope resulting from either postural or exertional hypotension.

Frequent reactions due to unopposed parasympathetic activity: bradycardia, increase in bowel movements, and diarrhea. Diarrhea may be severe at times and necessitate discontinuance of the medication.

Other common reactions: inhibition of ejaculation, a tendency toward fluid retention and edema with occasional development of congestive heart failure.

Other less common reactions: dyspnea, fatigue, nausea, vomiting, nocturia, urinary incontinence, dermatitis, scalp hair loss, dry mouth, rise in BUN, ptosis of the lids, blurring of vision, parotid tenderness, myalgia, muscle tremor, mental depression, chest pains (angina), chest paresthesias, nasal congestion, weight gain, and asthma in susceptible individuals. Although a causal relationship has not been established, a few instances of blood dyscrasias (anemia, thrombocytopenia, and leukopenia) and of priapism have been reported.

Dosage and Administration: Better control may be obtained, especially in the initial phases of treatment, if the patient can have his blood pressure recorded regularly at home.

Ambulatory Patients. Begin treatment with small doses (10 mg). Increase gradually, depending upon the patient's response. Ismelin has a long duration of action; therefore, dosage increases should not be made more often than every 5 to 7 days, unless the patient is hospitalized.

Take blood pressure in the supine position, after standing for ten minutes, and immediately after exercise if feasible. Increase dosage only if there has been *no* decrease in standing blood pressure from the previous levels. The average daily dose is 25 to 50 mg; only 1 dose a day is usually required.

Dosage Chart for Ambulatory Patients

Visits at Intervals of 5 to 7 Days	Daily Dose
Visit No. 1 (Start with 10-mg tablets)	10 mg
Visit No. 2	20 mg
Visit No. 3 (Patient can be changed to 25-mg tablets whenever convenient)	30 mg (three 10-mg tablets) or 37.5 mg (one and one-half 25-mg tablets)
Visit No. 4	50 mg

Visit No. 5 (and subsequent). Dosage may be increased by 12.5 mg or 25 mg if necessary.
Reduce dosage in any of the following 3 situations:
1. *Normal supine pressure*
2. *Excessive orthostatic fall in pressure*
3. *Severe diarrhea*

Hospitalized Patients. Initial oral dose is 25 to 50 mg, increased by 25 or 50 mg daily or every other day as indicated. This higher dosage is possible because hospitalized patients can be watched carefully. Unless absolutely impossible, take the standing blood pressure regularly. Patients should not be discharged from the hospital until the effect of the drug on the standing blood pressure is known.
Patients should be told about the possibility of orthostatic hypotension and warned not to get out of bed without help during the period of dosage adjustment.

Combination Therapy. Ismelin may be added gradually to thiazides and/or hydralazine. Thiazide diuretics enhance the effectiveness of Ismelin and may reduce the incidence of edema. When thiazide diuretics are added to the regimen in patients on Ismelin, it is usually necessary to reduce the dosage of Ismelin. After control is established, reduce dosage of all drugs to the lowest effective level.

When replacing MAO inhibitors, at least one week should elapse before commencing treatment with Ismelin.

In many cases ganglionic blockers will have been stopped before Ismelin is started. It may be advisable, however, to withdraw the blocker gradually to prevent a spiking blood pressure response during the transfer period.

Overdosage
Signs and Symptoms
Postural hypotension [with dizziness, blurring of vision, etc., possibly progressing to syncope when standing] and bradycardia are most likely to occur; diarrhea, possibly severe, also may occur. Unconsciousness is unlikely if adequate blood pressure and cerebral perfusion can be maintained by appropriate positioning [supine] and by other treatment as required.

Treatment
In previously normotensive patients, treatment has consisted essentially of restoring blood pressure and heart rate to normal by keeping patient in supine position. Normal homeostatic control usually returns gradually over a 72-hour period in these patients.

In previously hypertensive patients, particularly those with impaired cardiac reserve or other cardiovascular-renal disease, intensive treatment may be required to support vital functions and/or to control cardiac irregularities that might be present. Supine position must be maintained; if vasopressors are required, it must be remembered that Ismelin may increase responsiveness as to blood pressure rise and occurrence of cardiac arrhythmias.

Diarrhea, if severe or persistent, should be treated symptomatically to reduce intestinal hypermotility, with due attention to maintenance of hydration and electrolyte balance.

How Supplied:
Tablets 10 mg — pale yellow, scored (imprinted 49 CIBA)
Bottles of 100 ....NDC 0083-0049-30
Bottles of 1000 ....NDC 0083-0049-40
Consumer Pack—One Unit
 (12 bottles - 100 tablets
 each) ....NDC 0083-0049-65
Accu-Pak® Unit Dose (blister pack)
 Box of 100 (strips of 10) ....NDC 0083-0049-32
Tablets 25 mg — white, scored (imprinted 103 CIBA)
Bottles of 100 ....NDC 0083-0103-30
Bottles of 1000 ....NDC 0083-0103-40
Consumer Pack—One Unit
 (12 bottles-100 tablets
 each) ....NDC 0083-0103-65
Accu-Pak® Unit Dose (blister pack)
 Box of 100 (strips of 10) ....NDC 0083-0103-32
Dispense in tight container (USP)

C81-20 (6/81)
Shown in Product Identification Section, page 409

LITHOBID® ℞
[lith'oh-bidd]
(lithium carbonate)
slow-release tablets (not USP)

CIBALITH-S™ Syrup ℞
[see'ba-lith-ess]
(lithium citrate)

> **WARNING**
> Lithium toxicity is closely related to serum lithium levels, and can occur at doses close to therapeutic levels. Facilities for prompt and accurate serum lithium determinations should be available before initiating therapy.

Description:

Lithobid: Each film-coated slow-release tablet contains 300 mg of lithium carbonate, 40 mg of sodium chloride, equivalent to 15.7 mg of sodium. This slowly dissolving film-coated tablet is designed to give postadministration serum lithium peaks lower than obtained with conventional oral lithium dosage forms.

Cibalith-S: Each 5 ml of this lithium citrate syrup contains 8 mEq of lithium ion (Li+), equivalent to the amount of lithium in 300 mg of lithium carbonate.

Lithium carbonate is a white, light alkaline powder with molecular formula Li_2CO_3 and molecular weight 73.89. Lithium is an element of the alkali-metal group with atomic number 3, atomic weight 6.94 and an emission line at 671 nm on the flame photometer.

Lithium citrate is prepared in solution from lithium hydroxide and citric acid in a ratio approximating di-lithium citrate.

Indications: Lithium is indicated in the treatment of manic episodes of manic-depressive illness. Maintenance therapy prevents or diminishes the intensity of subsequent episodes in those manic-depressive patients with a history of mania.

Typical symptoms of mania include pressure of speech, motor hyperactivity, reduced need for sleep, flight of ideas, grandiosity, elation, poor judgment, aggressiveness, and possibly hostility. When given to a patient experiencing a manic episode, lithium may produce a normalization of symptomatology within 1 to 3 weeks.

Warnings: Lithium should generally not be given to patients with significant renal or cardiovascular disease, severe debilitation or dehydration, or sodium depletion, and to patients receiving diuretics, since the risk of lithium toxicity is very high in such patients. If the psychiatric indication is life-threatening, and if such a patient fails to respond to other measures, lithium treatment may be undertaken with extreme caution, including daily serum lithium determinations and adjustment to the usually low doses ordinarily tolerated by these individuals. In such instances, hospitalization is a necessity.

Lithium toxicity is closely related to serum lithium levels, and can occur at doses close to therapeutic levels (see DOSAGE AND ADMINISTRATION).

Lithium therapy has been reported in some cases to be associated with morphologic changes in the kidneys. The relationship between such changes and renal function has not been established.

Outpatients and their families should be warned that the patient must discontinue lithium therapy and contact his physician if such clinical signs of lithium toxicity as diarrhea, vomiting, tremor, mild ataxia, drowsiness, or muscular weakness occur.

Lithium may prolong the effects of neuromuscular blocking agents. Therefore, neuromuscular blocking agents should be given with caution to patients receiving lithium.

Lithium may impair mental and/or physical abilities. Caution patients about activities requiring alertness (*e.g.*, operating vehicles or machinery).

Combined use of haloperidol and lithium: An encephalopathic syndrome (characterized by weakness, lethargy, fever, tremulousness and confusion, extrapyramidal symptoms, leucocytosis, elevated serum enzymes, BUN and FBS) followed by irreversible brain damage has occurred in a few patients treated with lithium plus haloperidol. A causal relationship between these events and the concomitant administration of lithium and haloperidol has not been established; however, patients receiving such combined therapy should be monitored closely for early evidence of neurological toxicity and treatment discontinued promptly if such signs appear. The possibility of similar adverse interactions with other antipsychotic medications exists.

Usage in Pregnancy

Adverse effects on nidation in rats, embryo viability in mice, and metabolism *in vitro* of rat testis and human spermatozoa have been attributed to lithium, as have teratogenicity in submammalian species and cleft palates in mice. Studies in rats, rabbits and monkeys have shown no evidence of lithium-induced teratology.

There are lithium birth registries in the United States and elsewhere; however there are at the present time insufficient data to determine the effects of lithium on human fetuses. Therefore, at this point, lithium should not be used in pregnancy, especially the first trimester, unless in the opinion of the physician, the potential benefits outweigh the possible hazards.

Usage in Nursing Mothers

Lithium is excreted in human milk. Nursing should not be undertaken during lithium therapy except in rare and unusual circumstances where, in the view of the physician, the potential benefits to the mother outweigh possible hazards to the child.

Usage in Children

Since information regarding the safety and effectiveness of lithium in children under 12 years of age is not available, its use in such patients is not recommended at this time.

Precautions: The ability to tolerate lithium is greater during the acute manic phase and decreases when manic symptoms subside (see DOSAGE AND ADMINISTRATION).

The distribution space of lithium approximates that of total body water. Lithium is primarily excreted in urine with insignificant excretion in feces. Renal excretion of lithium is proportional to its plasma concentration. The half-elimination time of lithium is approximately 24 hours. Lithium decreases sodium reabsorption by the renal tubules which could lead to sodium depletion. Therefore, it is essential for the patient to maintain a normal diet, including salt, and an adequate fluid intake (2500–3000 ml) at least during the initial stabilization period. Decreased tolerance to lithium has been reported to ensue from protracted sweating or diarrhea and, if such occur, supplemental fluid and salt should be administered.

In addition to sweating and diarrhea, concomitant infection with elevated temperatures may also necessitate a temporary reduction or cessation of medication.

Previously existing underlying disorders do not necessarily constitute a contraindication to lithium treatment; where hypothyroidism exists, careful monitoring of thyroid function during lithium stabilization and maintenance allows for correction of changing thyroid parameters, if any, where hypothroidism occurs during lithium stabilization and maintenance, supplemental thyroid treatment may be used.

Indomethacin (50 mg t.i.d.) has been reported to increase steady-state plasma lithium levels from 30 to 59 percent. There is also some evidence that other nonsteroidal, anti-inflammatory agents may have a similar effect. When such combinations are used, increased plasma lithium level monitoring is recommended.

Adverse Reactions: Adverse reactions are seldom encountered at serum lithium levels below 1.5 mEq/l, except in the occasional patient sensitive to lithium. Mild-to-moderate toxic reactions may occur at levels from 1.5–2.5 mEq/l, and moderate-to-severe reactions may be seen at levels from 2.0–2.5 mEq/l, depending upon individual response to the drug.

Fine hand tremor, polyuria and mild thirst may occur during initial therapy for the acute manic phase, and may persist throughout treatment. Transient and mild nausea and general discomfort may also appear during the first few days of lithium administration.

These side effects are an inconvenience rather than a disabling condition, and usually subside with continued treatment or a temporary reduction or cessation of dosage. If persistent, a cessation of dosage is indicated.

Diarrhea, vomiting, drowsiness, muscular weakness and lack of coordination may be early signs of lithium intoxication, and can occur at lithium levels below 2.0 mEq/l. At higher levels, giddiness, ataxia, blurred vision, tinnitus and a large output of dilute urine may be seen. Serum lithium levels above 3.0 mEq/l may produce a complex clinical picture involving multiple organs and organ systems. Serum lithium levels should not be permitted to exceed 2.0 mEq/l during the acute treatment phase.

The following toxic reactions have been reported and appear to be related to serum lithium levels, including levels within the therapeutic range.

Neuromuscular: tremor, muscle hyperirritability (fasciculations, twitching, clonic movements of whole limbs), ataxia, choreoathetotic movements, hyperactive deep tendon reflexes.

Central Nervous System: blackout spells, epileptiform seizures, slurred speech, dizziness, vertigo, incontinence of urine or feces, somnolence, psychomotor retardation, restlessness, confusion, stupor, coma.

Cardiovascular: cardiac arrhythmia, hypotension, peripheral circulatory collapse.

Gastrointestinal: anorexia, nausea, vomiting, diarrhea.

Genitourinary: albuminuria, oliguria, polyuria, glycosuria.

Dermatologic: drying and thinning of hair, anesthesia of skin, chronic folliculitis, xerosis cutis, alopecia, exacerbation of psoriasis.

Autonomic Nervous System: blurred vision, dry mouth.

Miscellaneous: fatigue, lethargy, tendency to sleep, dehydration, weight loss, transient scotomata.

Thyroid Abnormalities: euthyroid goiter and/or hypothyroidism (including myxedema) accompanied by lower T_3 and T_4. I_{131} iodine uptake may be elevated (See Precautions). Paradoxically, rare cases of hyperthyroidism have been reported.

EEG Changes: diffuse slowing, widening of frequency spectrum, potentiation and disorganization of background rhythm.

EKG Changes: reversible flattening, isoelectricity or inversion of T-waves.

Miscellaneous reactions unrelated to dosage are: transient electroencephalographic and electrocardiographic changes, leucocytosis, headache, diffuse nontoxic goiter with or without hypothyroidism, transient hyperglycemia, generalized pruritus with or without rash, cutaneous ulcers, albuminuria, worsening of organic brain syndromes, excessive weight gain, edematous swelling of ankles or wrists, and thirst or polyuria, sometimes resembling diabetes insipidus and metallic taste. A single report has been received of the development of painful discoloration of fingers and toes and coldness of the extremities within one day of the starting of treatment of lithium. The mechanism through which these symptoms (resembling Raynaud's Syndrome) developed is not known. Recovery followed discontinuance.

Dosage and Administration:

Acute Mania: Optimal patient response can usually be established and maintained with the following dosages:

Lithobid ....900 mg b.i.d. or 600 mg t.i.d.
(1800 mg per day)

Cibalith-S ....10 ml (2 teaspoons)
(16 mEq of lithium) t.i.d.

Such doses will normally produce an effective serum lithium level ranging between 1.0 and 1.5 mEq/l. Dosage must be individualized according to serum levels and clinical response. Regular monitoring of the patient's clinical state and of serum lithium levels is necessary. Serum levels should be determined twice per week during the acute phase, and until the serum level and clinical condition of the patient have been stabilized.

Long-Term Control: The desirable serum lithium levels are 0.6 to 1.2 mEq/l. Dosage will vary from one individual to another, but usually the following dosages will maintain this level:

Continued on next page

The full prescribing information for each CIBA drug is contained herein and is that in effect as of **October 1, 1984.**

CIBA—Cont.

Lithobid ....900 mg to 1200 mg per day given in two or three divided doses.
Cibalith-S ....5 ml (1 teaspoon) (8 mEq of lithium) t.i.d. or q.i.d.

Serum lithium levels in uncomplicated cases receiving maintenance therapy during remission should be monitored at least every two months. Patients abnormally sensitive to lithium may exhibit toxic signs at serum levels of 1.0 to 1.5 mEq/l. Elderly patients often respond to reduced dosage, and may exhibit signs of toxicity at serum levels ordinarily tolerated by other patients.

N.B.: Blood samples for serum lithium determinations should be drawn immediately prior to the next dose when lithium concentrations are relatively stable (i.e., 8–12 hours after previous dose). Total reliance must not be placed on serum levels alone. Accurate patient evaluation requires both clinical and laboratory analysis.

Overdosage: The toxic levels for lithium are close to the therapeutic levels. It is therefore important that patients and their families be cautioned to watch for early toxic symptoms and to discontinue the drug and inform the physician should they occur. Toxic symptoms are listed in detail under ADVERSE REACTIONS.

Treatment: No specific antidote for lithium poisoning is known. Early symptoms of lithium toxicity can usually be treated by reduction or cessation of dosage of the drug and resumption of the treatment at a lower dose after 24 to 48 hours. In severe cases of lithium poisoning, the first and foremost goal of treatment consists of elimination of this ion from the patient.

Treatment is essentially the same as that used in barbiturate poisoning: 1) gastric lavage 2) correction of fluid and electrolyte imbalance and 3) regulation of kidney functioning. Urea, mannitol, and aminophylline all produce significant increases in lithium excretion. Hemodialysis is an effective and rapid means of removing the ion from the severely toxic patient. Infection prophylaxis, regular chest x-rays, and preservation of adequate respiration are essential.

How Supplied:
Lithobid, lithium carbonate 300 mg, peach-colored, slow-release tablets are supplied in bottles of 100's & 1000's and in unit-dose boxes of 100's.
Shown in Product Identification Section, page 409
Cibalith-S, lithium citrate syrup, 8 mEq of lithium ion per 5 ml (1 teaspoon) is supplied as a sugar-free, raspberry-flavored syrup in bottles of 480 ml.

C81-70 (1/82)
Dist. by: CIBA Pharmaceutical Company
Div. of CIBA-GEIGY Corporation
Summit, NJ 07901

LUDIOMIL® ℞
[*loó-dee-oh-mill*]
(maprotiline hydrochloride)
Tablets

Description: Ludiomil®, maprotiline hydrochloride, is an antidepressant for oral administration which belongs to a new chemical series, dibenzo-bicyclo-octadienes. Its molecular weight is 315.5, and its empirical formula is $C_{20}H_{24}Cl N$. Ludiomil is a white, odorless, stable, crystalline powder which is slightly soluble in water. It melts at 236–246°C.

Clinical Pharmacology: The mechanism of action of Ludiomil is not precisely known. It does not act primarily by stimulation of the central nervous system and is not a monoamine oxidase inhibitor. The postulated mechanism of Ludiomil is that it acts primarily by potentiation of central adrenergic synapses by blocking reuptake of norepinephrine at nerve endings. This pharmacologic action is thought to be responsible for the drug's antidepressant and anxiolytic effects.

The mean time to peak is 12 hours.[1] The half-life of elimination averages 51 hours.[1,2]

Steady-state levels measured prior to the morning dose on a one-dosage regimen are summarized as follows:[2]

Regimen	Average Minimum Concentration ng/ml	95% Confidence Limits ng/ml
50 mg x 3 daily	238	181–295

Indications and Usage: Ludiomil is indicated for the treatment of depressive illness in patients with depressive neurosis (dysthymic disorder) and manic-depressive illness, depressed type (major depressive disorder). Ludiomil is also effective for the relief of anxiety associated with depression.

Contraindications: Ludiomil is contraindicated in patients hypersensitive to Ludiomil and in patients with known or suspected seizure disorders. It should not be given concomitantly with monoamine oxidase (MAO) inhibitors. A minimum of 14 days should be allowed to elapse after discontinuation of MAO inhibitors before treatment with Ludiomil is initiated. Effects should be monitored with gradual increase in dosage until optimum response is achieved. The drug is not recommended for use during the acute phase of myocardial infarction.

Warnings: Extreme caution should be used when this drug is given to:
—patients with a history of myocardial infarction;
—patients with a history or presence of cardiovascular disease because of the possibility of conduction defects, arrhythmias, myocardial infarction, strokes and tachycardia.

Precautions:
General: The possibility of suicide in seriously depressed patients is inherent in their illness and may persist until significant remission occurs. Therefore, patients must be carefully supervised during all phases of treatment with Ludiomil, and prescriptions should be written for the smallest number of tablets consistent with good patient management.

Seizures have been reported in patients treated with Ludiomil with the incidence of direct reports at less than 1/10 of 1%. Most of the seizures occurred in patients without a known history of seizures. However, in some of these patients other confounding factors were present including concomitant medications known to lower the seizure threshold, rapid escalation of Ludiomil dosage and dosage which exceeded the recommended therapeutic range. While it must be noted that a cause-and-effect relationship has not been established, the risk of seizures may be reduced by initiating therapy at low dosage. Because of the long half-life of Ludiomil (average 51 hours) initial dosage should be maintained for two weeks before being raised gradually in small increments (see **Dosage and Administration**).

Hypomanic or manic episodes have been known to occur in some patients taking tricyclic antidepressant drugs, particularly in patients with cyclic disorders. Such occurrences have also been noted, rarely, with Ludiomil.

Prior to elective surgery, Ludiomil should be discontinued for as long as clinically feasible, since little is known about the interaction between Ludiomil and general anesthetics.

Ludiomil should be administered with caution in patients with increased intraocular pressure, history of urinary retention, or history of narrow-angle glaucoma because of the drug's anticholinergic properties.

Information for Patients: Warn patients to exercise caution about potentially hazardous tasks, or operating automobiles or machinery since the drug may impair mental and/or physical abilities. Ludiomil may enhance the response to alcohol, barbiturates, and other CNS depressants, requiring appropriate caution of administration.

Laboratory Tests: Although not observed with Ludiomil, the drug should be discontinued if there is evidence of pathologic neutrophil depression. Leukocyte and differential counts should be performed in patients who develop fever and sore throat during therapy.

Drug Interactions: Close supervision and careful adjustment of dosage are required when administering Ludiomil concomitantly with anticholinergic or sympathomimetic drugs because of the possibility of additive atropine-like effects.

Concurrent administration of Ludiomil with electroshock therapy should be avoided because of the lack of experience in this area.

Caution should be exercised when administering Ludiomil to hyperthyroid patients or those on thyroid medication because of the possibility of enhanced potential for cardiovascular toxicity of Ludiomil.

Ludiomil should be used with caution in patients receiving guanethidine or similar agents since it may block the pharmacologic effects of these drugs.
(See "Information for Patients")

Carcinogenesis, Mutagenesis, Impairment of Fertility: Carcinogenicity and chronic toxicity studies have been conducted in laboratory rats and dogs. No drug- or dose-related occurrence of carcinogenesis was evident in rats receiving daily oral doses up to 60 mg/kg of Ludiomil for eighteen months or in dogs receiving daily oral doses up to 30 mg/kg of Ludiomil for one year. In addition, no evidence of mutagenic activity was found in offspring of female mice mated with males treated with up to 60 times the maximum daily human dose.

Pregnancy Category B: Reproduction studies have been performed in female laboratory rabbits, mice, and rats at doses up to 1.3, 7, and 9 times the maximum daily human dose respectively and have revealed no evidence of impaired fertility or harm to the fetus due to Ludiomil. There are, however, no adequate and well-controlled studies in pregnant women. Because animal reproduction studies are not always predictive of human response, this drug should be used during pregnancy only if clearly needed.

Labor and Delivery: Although the effect of Ludiomil on labor and delivery is unknown, caution should be exercised as with any drug with CNS depressant action.

Nursing Mothers: Ludiomil is excreted in breast milk. At steady state, the concentrations in milk correspond closely to the concentrations in whole blood. Caution should be exercised when Ludiomil is administered to a nursing woman.

Pediatric Use: Safety and effectiveness in children below the age of 18 have not been established.

Adverse Reactions: The following adverse reactions have been noted with Ludiomil and are generally similar to those observed with tricyclic antidepressants.

Cardiovascular: Rare occurrences of hypotension, hypertension, tachycardia, palpitation, arrhythmia, heart block, and syncope have been reported with Ludiomil.

Psychiatric: Nervousness (6%), anxiety (3%), insomnia (2%), and agitation (2%); rarely, confusional states (especially in the elderly), hallucinations, disorientation, delusions, restlessness, nightmares, hypomania, mania, exacerbation of psychosis, decrease in memory, and feelings of unreality.

Neurological: Drowsiness (16%), dizziness (8%), tremor (3%), and, rarely, numbness, tingling, motor hyperactivity, akathisia, seizures, EEG alterations, tinnitus, extrapyramidal symptoms, ataxia, and dysarthria.

Anticholinergic: Dry mouth (22%), constipation (6%), and blurred vision (4%); rarely, accommodation disturbances, mydriasis, urinary retention, and delayed micturition.

Allergic: Rare instances of skin rash, petechiae, itching, photosensitization, edema, and drug fever.

Gastrointestinal: Nausea (2%) and, rarely, vomiting, epigastric distress, diarrhea, bitter taste, abdominal cramps and dysphagia.

Endocrine: Rare instances of increased or decreased libido, impotence, and elevation or depression of blood sugar levels.

Other: Weakness and fatigue (4%) and headache (4%); rarely, altered liver function, jaundice, weight loss or gain, excessive perspiration, flushing, urinary frequency, increased salivation, and nasal congestion.

Note: Although the following adverse reactions have not been reported with Ludiomil, its pharmacologic similarity to tricyclic antidepressants requires that each reaction be considered when administering Ludiomil.

—Bone marrow depression, including agranulocytosis, eosinophilia, purpura, and thrombocytopenia, myocardial infarction, stroke, peripheral neuropathy, sublingual adenitis, black tongue, stomatitis, paralytic ileus, gynecomastia in the male, breast enlargement and galactorrhea in the female, and testicular swelling.

Overdosage:
Animal Oral LD$_{50}$: The oral LD$_{50}$ of Ludiomil is 600-750 mg/kg in mice, 760-900 mg/kg in rats, > 1000 mg/kg in rabbits, > 300 mg/kg in cats, and > 30 mg/kg in dogs.

Signs and Symptoms: Data dealing with overdosage in humans are limited with only a few cases on record. Symptoms are drowsiness, tachycardia, ataxia, vomiting, cyanosis, hypotension, shock, restlessness, agitation, hyperpyrexia, muscle rigidity, athetoid movements, mydriasis, cardiac arrhythmias, impaired cardiac condition. In severe cases, loss of consciousness and generalized convulsions may occur. Since congestive heart failure has been seen with overdosages of tricyclic antidepressants, it should be considered with Ludiomil overdosage.

Treatment: There is no specific antidote. Induced emesis and gastric lavage are recommended. It may be helpful to leave the tube in the stomach with irrigation and continual aspiration of stomach contents possibly promoting more rapid elimination of the drug from the body. The room should be darkened, allowing only minimal external stimulation to reduce the tendency to convulsions.

1. The intravenous administration of 1 to 3 mg of physostigmine has been reported to reverse the signs and symptoms of overdosage with tricyclic antidepressants. Repeat doses at intervals of 30 to 60 minutes may be necessary.
2. Hyperirritability and convulsions may be treated with carefully titrated parenteral barbiturates. Barbiturates should not be employed, however, if drugs that inhibit monoamine oxidase have also been taken by the patient in overdosage or in recent therapy. Similarly, barbiturates may induce respiratory depression, particularly in children. It is therefore advisable to have equipment available for artificial ventilation and resuscitation when barbiturates are employed. Paraldehyde may be used effectively in some children to counteract muscular hypertonus and convulsions with less likelihood of causing respiratory depression.
3. Shock (circulatory collapse) should be treated with supportive measures such as intravenous fluids, oxygen, and corticosteroids.
4. Hyperpyrexia should be controlled by whatever means available, including ice packs if necessary.
5. Signs of congestive heart failure may be satisfactorily treated by rapid digitalization.
6. Dialysis is of little value because of the low plasma concentration of this drug.

Dosage and Administration: A single daily dose is an alternative to divided daily doses. Therapeutic effects are sometimes seen within 3 to 7 days, although as long as 2 to 3 weeks are usually necessary.

Initial Adult Dosage: An initial dosage of 75 mg daily is suggested for outpatients with mild-to-moderate depression. However, in some patients, particularly the elderly, an initial dosage of 25 mg daily may be used. Because of the long half-life of Ludiomil, the initial dosage should be maintained for two weeks. The dosage may then be increased gradually in 25-mg increments as required and tolerated. In most outpatients a maximum dose of 150 mg daily will result in therapeutic efficacy. It is recommended that this dose not be exceeded except in the most severely depressed patients. In such patients, dosage may be gradually increased to a maximum of 225 mg.

More severely depressed, hospitalized patients should be given an initial daily dose of 100 mg to 150 mg which may be gradually increased as required and tolerated. Most hospitalized patients with moderate-to-severe depression respond to a daily dosage of 150 mg although dosages as high as 225 mg may be required in some cases. Daily dosage of 225 mg should not be exceeded.

Elderly Patients: In general, lower dosages are recommended for patients over 60 years of age. Dosages of 50 mg to 75 mg daily are usually satisfactory as maintenance therapy for elderly patients who do not tolerate higher amounts.

Maintenance: Dosage during prolonged maintenance therapy should be kept at the lowest effective level. Dosage may be reduced to levels of 75 mg to 150 mg daily during such periods, with subsequent adjustment depending on therapeutic response.

How Supplied:
Tablets 25 mg—oval, dark orange, coated (imprinted CIBA 110)
Bottle of 100—NDC 0083-0110-30
Accu-Pak® Unit Dose (blister pack)
Box of 100 (strips of 10)—NDC 0083-0110-32
Tablets 50 mg—round, dark orange, coated (imprinted CIBA 26)
Bottle of 100—NDC 0083-0026-30
Accu-Pak® Unit Dose (blister pack)
Box of 100 (strips of 10)—NDC 0083-0026-32
Tablets 75 mg—oval, white, coated (imprinted CIBA 135)
Bottles of 100—NDC 0083-0135-30
Accu-Pak® Unit Dose (blister pack)
Box of 100 (strips of 10)—NDC 0083-0135-32
Dispense in tight container (USP).

1. Alkalay D, et al. Bioavailability and kinetics of maprotiline. *Clin Pharmacol Ther* 1980; **27** (5): 697–703.
2. Riess W, et al. The pharmacokinetic properties of maprotiline (Ludiomil®) in man. *J Int Med Res* 1975; **3** (2): 16–41.

C83-22 (Rev. 7/83)
Shown in Product Identification Section, page 409

METANDREN® R
[*meh-tan'dren*]
(methyltestosterone USP)
Linguets® and Tablets
Listed in USP, a Medicare designated compendium.

Indications
In the Male
1. Eunuchoidism and eunuchism.
2. Climacteric symptoms when these are secondary to androgen deficiency.
3. Impotence due to androgen deficiency.
4. Postpuberal cryptorchidism with evidence of hypogonadism.

In the Female
1. Prevention of postpartum breast pain and engorgement. There is no satisfactory evidence that this drug prevents or suppresses lactation.
2. Palliation of androgen-responsive, advancing, inoperable mammary cancer, in women who are more than 1 year, but less than 5 years postmenopausal or who have been proven to have a hormone-dependent tumor as shown by previous beneficial response to castration.

Contraindications: Carcinoma of the male breast; known or suspected carcinoma of the prostate; cardiac, hepatic, or renal decompensation; hypercalcemia; impaired liver function; prepuberal males; patients easily stimulated; pregnancy; and breast feeding.

Warnings: Hypercalcemia may occur in immobilized patients and in breast cancer patients. In patients with cancer hypercalcemia may indicate progression of bony metastasis, in which case the drug should be discontinued.

Watch female patients closely for signs of virilization. Some effects such as voice changes may not be reversible even when the drug is stopped.

Discontinue the drug if cholestatic hepatitis with jaundice appears or liver function tests become abnormal.

Precautions: Patients with cardiac, renal, or hepatic derangement may retain sodium and water with resulting edema formation.

Males, especially the elderly, may become overly stimulated.

Priapism or excessive sexual stimulation may develop.

Oligospermia and reduced ejaculatory volume may occur after prolonged administration or excessive dosage.

Hypersensitivity and gynecomastia may occur.

Alterations in liver function tests (eg, increased BSP retention and SGOT levels) and rarely jaundice have been reported and appear to be directly related to the dose of the drug.

When any of these effects appear, the androgen should be stopped; if restarted, a lower dosage should be utilized.

Use cautiously in young boys to avoid possible premature epiphyseal closure or precocious sexual development.

The PBI may decrease during androgen therapy without clinical significance.

The Metandren Linguets® (10 mg) and tablets (25 mg) contain FD&C Yellow No. 5 (tartrazine) which may cause allergic-type reactions (including bronchial asthma) in certain susceptible individuals. Although the overall incidence of FD&C Yellow No. 5 (tartrazine) sensitivity in the general population is low, it is frequently seen in patients who also have aspirin hypersensitivity.

Adverse Reactions: Hypersensitivity, including skin manifestations and anaphylactoid reactions; acne; decreased ejaculatory volume; oligospermia; gynecomastia; edema; priapism; hypercalcemia, especially in immobile patients and those with metastatic breast carcinoma; virilization in females; cholestatic jaundice. There have been rare reports of hepatocellular neoplasms and peliosis hepatis in association with long-term androgenic-anabolic steroid therapy.

Dosage and Administration: Dosage must be strictly individualized. Daily requirements are best administered in divided doses. The following chart is suggested as an average daily dosage guide. Duration of therapy will depend upon the response of the condition being treated and the appearance of adverse reactions.

NOTE: Linguets have approximately twice the potency of the orally ingested hormone.

INDICATIONS	AVERAGE DAILY DOSAGE	
	Linguets	*Tablets*
In the Male		
Eunuchoidism and eunuchoidism	5 to 20 mg	10 to 40 mg
Male climacteric and male impotence	5 to 20 mg	10 to 40 mg
Cryptorchidism—postpuberal	15 mg	30 mg
In the Female		
Postpartum breast pain and engorgement (3 to 5 days)	40 mg	80 mg
Breast cancer	100 mg	200 mg

Administration of Linguets
Linguets should not be swallowed since the hormone is meant to be absorbed through the mucous membranes. Place Linguet in the upper or lower buccal pouch between the gum and cheek. Avoid eating, drinking, chewing, or smoking while the Linguet is in place. Proper oral hygienic measures are particularly important after the use of Linguets.

How Supplied: *Linguets,* 5 mg (white); bottles of 100. *Linguets,* 10 mg (yellow); bottles of 100. *Tablets,* 10 mg (white, scored) and 25 mg (pale yellow, scored); bottles of 100.

LINGUETS® (tablets for mucosal absorption CIBA)

Dispense in tight, light-resistant container (USP).

C80-18 (1/80)
Shown in Product Identification Section, page 409

Continued on next page

The full prescribing information for each CIBA drug is contained herein and is that in effect as of October 1, 1984.

CIBA—Cont.

METOPIRONE® ℞
[met-oh-pie′rone]
(metyrapone USP)
Tablets
Diagnostic Test of Pituitary
Adrenocorticotropic Function

Description: Metopirone, metyrapone USP, is an inhibitor of endogenous adrenal corticosteroid synthesis, available as 250-mg tablets for oral administration. Its chemical name is 2-methyl-1,2-di-3-pyridyl-1-propanone, and its structural formula is:

Metyrapone USP is a white to light amber, fine, crystalline powder, having a characteristic odor. It is sparingly soluble in water, and soluble in methanol and in chloroform. It forms water-soluble salts with acids. Its molecular weight is 226.28.

Clinical Pharmacology: The pharmacological effect of Metopirone is to reduce cortisol and corticosterone production by inhibiting the 11-β-hydroxylation reaction in the adrenal cortex. Removal of the strong inhibitory feedback mechanism exerted by cortisol results in an increase in adrenocorticotropic hormone (ACTH) production by the pituitary. With continued blockade of the enzymatic steps leading to production of cortisol and corticosterone, there is a marked increase in adrenocortical secretion of their immediate precursors, 11-deoxycortisol and desoxycorticosterone, which are weak suppressors of ACTH release, and a corresponding elevation of these steroids in the plasma and of their metabolites in the urine. These metabolites are readily determined by measuring urinary 17-hydroxycorticosteroids (17-OHCS) or 17-ketogenic steroids (17-KGS). Because of these actions, Metopirone is used as a diagnostic test, with urinary 17-OHCS measured as an index of pituitary ACTH responsiveness. Metopirone may also suppress biosynthesis of aldosterone, resulting in a mild natriuresis.

The response to Metopirone does not occur immediately. Following oral administration, peak steroid excretion occurs during the subsequent 24-hour period. Metopirone is absorbed rapidly and well when administered orally as prescribed. Plasma concentrations during the period of treatment are 0.5–1 µg/ml. The major biotransformation is reduction of the ketone to an alcohol and conjugation of metyrapone and reduced metyrapone to the corresponding glucuronides. The apparent half-life of elimination averages 1–2.5 hours. Within 2 days after initiation of treatment, about 40% of the administered dose is excreted in the urine, mostly in the form of glucuronides.

Indications and Usage: A diagnostic drug for testing hypothalamic-pituitary ACTH function.

Contraindications: Adrenal cortical insufficiency, hypersensitivity to Metopirone.

Warnings: Metopirone may induce acute adrenal insufficiency in patients with reduced adrenal secretory capacity.

Precautions:
General
Ability of adrenals to respond to exogenous ACTH should be demonstrated before Metopirone is employed as a test. In the presence of hypo- or hyperthyroidism, response to the Metopirone test may be subnormal.

Laboratory Tests
See INTERPRETATION.

Drug Interactions
All corticosteroid therapy must be discontinued prior to and during testing with Metopirone. The metabolism of Metopirone is accelerated by phenytoin; therefore, results of the test may be inaccurate in patients taking phenytoin within two weeks before. A subnormal response may occur in patients on estrogen therapy.

Carcinogenesis, Mutagenesis, Impairment of Fertility
Long-term carcinogenicity and reproduction studies in animals have not been conducted.

Pregnancy Category C
A subnormal response to Metopirone may occur in pregnant women. Animal reproduction studies have not been conducted with Metopirone. The Metopirone test was administered to 20 pregnant women in their second and third trimester of pregnancy and evidence was found that the fetal pituitary responded to the enzymatic block. It is not known if Metopirone can affect reproduction capacity. Metopirone should be given to a pregnant woman only if clearly needed.

Nursing Mothers
It is not known whether this drug is excreted in human milk. Because many drugs are excreted in human milk, a decision should be made whether a woman undergoing the Metopirone test should discontinue nursing for the duration of the test.

Pediatric Use
See DOSAGE AND ADMINISTRATION.

Adverse Reactions:
Gastrointestinal System: Nausea, abdominal discomfort
Central Nervous System: Headache, dizziness, sedation
Dermatologic System: Allergic rash

Overdosage:
Acute Toxicity
One case has been recorded in which a 6-year-old girl died after two doses of Metopirone, 2 g. Oral LD$_{50}$ in animals (mg/kg): rats, 521; maximum tolerated intravenous dose in one dog, 300.

Signs and Symptoms
The clinical picture of poisoning with Metopirone is characterized by gastrointestinal symptoms and by signs of acute adrenocortical insufficiency.
Cardiovascular System: Cardiac arrhythmias, hypotension, dehydration.
Nervous System and Muscles: Anxiety, confusion, weakness, impairment of consciousness.
Gastrointestinal System: Nausea, vomiting, epigastric pain, diarrhea.
Laboratory Findings: Hyponatremia, hypochloremia, hyperkalemia.

Combined Poisoning
In patients under treatment with insulin or oral antidiabetics, the signs and symptoms of acute poisoning with Metopirone may be aggravated or modified.

Treatment
There is no specific antidote. Besides general measures to eliminate the drug and reduce its absorption, a large dose of hydrocortisone should be administered at once, together with saline and glucose infusions.
Surveillance: For a few days blood pressure and fluid and electrolyte balance should be monitored.

Dosage and Administration:
Day 1: Control period—Collect 24-hour urine for measurement of 17-OHCS or 17-KGS.
Day 2: ACTH test to determine the ability of adrenals to respond—Standard ACTH test such as infusion of 50 units ACTH over 8 hours and measurement of 24-hour urinary steroids. If results indicate adequate response, the Metopirone test may proceed.
Day 3–4: Rest period.
Day 5: Administration of Metopirone:
Recommended with milk or snack.
Adults: 750 mg orally, every 4 hours for 6 doses. A single dose is approximately equivalent to 15 mg/kg.
Children: 15 mg/kg orally every 4 hours for 6 doses. A minimal single dose of 250 mg is recommended.
Day 6: After administration of Metopirone—Determination of 24-hour urinary steroids for effect.

Interpretation:
ACTH Test
The normal 24-hour urinary excretion of 17-OHCS ranges from 3 to 12 mg. Following continuous intravenous infusion of 50 units ACTH over a period of 8 hours, 17-OHCS excretion increases to 15 to 45 mg per 24 hours.

Metopirone
Normal response: In patients with a normally functioning pituitary, administration of Metopirone is followed by a two-to four-fold increase of 17-OHCS excretion or doubling of 17-KGS excretion.
Subnormal response: Subnormal response in patients without adrenal insufficiency is indicative of some degree of impairment of pituitary function, either panhypopituitarism or partial hypopituitarism (limited pituitary reserve).
1. *Panhypopituitarism* is readily diagnosed by the classical clinical and chemical evidences of hypogonadism, hypothyroidism, and hypoadrenocorticism. These patients usually have subnormal basal urinary steroid levels. Depending upon the duration of the disease and degree of adrenal atrophy, they may fail to respond to exogenous ACTH in the normal manner. Administration of Metopirone is not essential in the diagnosis, but if given, it will not induce an appreciable increase in urinary steroids.
2. *Partial hypopituitarism* or limited pituitary reserve is the more difficult diagnosis as these patients do not present the classical signs and symptoms of hypopituitarism. Measurements of target organ functions often are normal under basal conditions. The response to exogenous ACTH is usually normal, producing the expected rise of urinary steroids (17-OHCS or 17-KGS). The response, however, to Metopirone is *subnormal;* that is, no significant increase in 17-OHCS or 17-KGS excretion occurs.
This failure to respond to metyrapone may be interpreted as evidence of impaired pituitary-adrenal reserve. In view of the normal response to exogenous ACTH, the failure to respond to metyrapone is inferred to be related to a defect in the CNS-pituitary mechanisms which normally regulate ACTH secretions. Presumably the ACTH secreting mechanisms of these individuals are already working at their maximal rates to meet everyday conditions and possess limited "reserve" capacities to secrete additional ACTH either in response to stress or to decreased cortisol levels occurring as a result of metyrapone administration.
Subnormal response in patients with Cushing's syndrome is suggestive of either autonomous adrenal tumors that suppress the ACTH-releasing capacity of the pituitary or nonendocrine ACTH-secreting tumors.

Excessive response: An excessive excretion of 17-OHCS or 17-KGS after administration of Metopirone is suggestive of Cushing's syndrome associated with adrenal hyperplasia. These patients have an elevated excretion of urinary corticosteroids under basal conditions and will often, but not invariably, show a "supernormal" response to ACTH and also to Metopirone, excreting more than 35 mg per 24 hours of either 17-OHCS or 17-KGS.

How Supplied:
Tablets 250 mg—round, white, scored (imprinted CIBA 130)
Bottles of 18 ....NDC 0083-0130-11
Dispense in tight, light-resistant container (USP).
C82-40 (Rev. 5/83)
Shown in Product Identification Section, page 409

NUPERCAINAL®
[new-purr-cayne′ull]
Anesthetic Ointment
Pain-Relief Cream

Caution:
Nupercainal products are not for prolonged or extensive use and should never be applied in or near the eyes.
Consult labels before using.
Keep this and all medications out of reach of children.
NUPERCAINAL SHOULD NOT BE SWALLOWED. SWALLOWING OR USE OF A LARGE QUANTITY IS HAZARDOUS, PARTICULARLY TO CHILDREN. CONSULT A

PHYSICIAN OR POISON CONTROL CENTER IMMEDIATELY.

Indications: Nupercainal Ointment and Cream are fast-acting, long-lasting pain relievers that you can use for a number of painful skin conditions. **Nupercainal Anesthetic Ointment** is for hemorrhoids and for general use. **Nupercainal Pain-Relief Cream** is for general use only. The **Cream** is half as strong as the **Ointment**.

How to use Nupercainal Anesthetic Ointment (for general use). This soothing Ointment helps lubricate dry, inflamed skin and gives fast, temporary relief of pain and itching. It is recommended for sunburn, nonpoisonous insect bites, minor burns, cuts, and scratches. **DO NOT USE THIS PRODUCT IN OR NEAR YOUR EYES.**
Apply to affected areas gently. If necessary, cover with a light dressing for protection. Do not use more than 1 ounce of Ointment in a 24-hour period for an adult, do not use more than one-quarter of an ounce in a 24-hour period for a child. If irritation develops, discontinue use and consult your doctor.

How to use Nupercainal Anesthetic Ointment for fast, temporary relief of pain and itching due to hemorrhoids (also known as piles).
Remove cap from tube and set it aside. Attach the white plastic applicator to the tube. Squeeze the tube until you see the Ointment begin to come through the little holes in the applicator. Using your finger, lubricate the applicator with the Ointment. Now insert the entire applicator gently into the rectum. Give the tube a good squeeze to get enough Ointment into the rectum for comfort and lubrication. Remove applicator from rectum and wipe it clean. Apply additional Ointment to anal tissues to help relieve pain, burning, and itching. For best results use Ointment morning and night and after each bowel movement. After each use detach applicator, and wash it off with soap and water. Put cap back on tube before storing. In case of rectal bleeding, discontinue use and consult your doctor.

Pain-Relief Cream for general use. This Cream is particularly effective for fast, temporary relief of pain and itching associated with sunburn, cuts, scratches, minor burns and nonpoisonous insect bites. **DO NOT USE THIS PRODUCT IN OR NEAR YOUR EYES.** Apply liberally to affected area and rub in gently. This Cream is water-washable, be sure to reapply after bathing, swimming or sweating. If irritation develops, discontinue use and consult your doctor.

Nupercainal Anesthetic Ointment contains 1% (one percent) dibucaine USP in a lubricant base. Available in tubes of 1 and 2 ounces.

Nupercainal Pain-Relief Cream contains 0.5% (one-half of one percent) dibucaine USP in a water-soluble base. Available in 1 1/2 ounce tubes.

Dibucaine USP is officially classified as a "topical anesthetic" and is one of the strongest and longest lasting of all pain relievers. It is not a narcotic.

C81-17 (5/81)

NUPERCAINAL®
[new-purr-cayne′ ull]
Suppositories

Caution:
Nupercainal Suppositories are not for prolonged or extensive use. Contact with the eyes should be avoided.
Consult labels before using.
Keep this and all medications out of reach of children.
NUPERCAINAL SUPPOSITORIES SHOULD NOT BE SWALLOWED. SWALLOWING CAN BE HAZARDOUS, PARTICULARLY TO CHILDREN. IN THE EVENT OF ACCIDENTAL SWALLOWING CONSULT A PHYSICIAN OR POISON CONTROL CENTER IMMEDIATELY.

Indications: Nupercainal Suppositories are for the temporary relief from itching, burning, and discomfort due to hemorrhoids or other anorectal disorders.

How to use Nupercainal Suppositories for hemorrhoids (also known as piles) or other anorectal disorders.
Tear off one suppository along the perforated line. Remove foil wrapper. Insert the suppository, rounded end first, well into the anus until you can feel it moving into your rectum. For best results, use one suppository after each bowel movement and as needed, but not to exceed 6 in a 24-hour period. Each suppository is sealed in its own foil packet to reduce danger of leakage when carried in pocket or purse. **To prevent melting, do not store above 86°F (30°C).**

Nupercainal Suppositories contain 2.4 gram cocoa butter, .25 gram zinc oxide, .1 gram bismuth subgallate, and acetone sodium bisulfite as preservative.

Dist. by:
CIBA Pharmaceutical Company
Division of CIBA-GEIGY Corporation
Summit, New Jersey 07901

C82-56 (12/82)

NUPERCAINE® hydrochloride   ℞
[new-purr-cayne′]
(dibucaine hydrochloride USP)
1:200 (0.5%)

Listed in USP, a Medicare designated compendium.
Specially Prepared for Isobaric Spinal Anesthesia According to the Method of Keyes and McLellan*

*Keyes, E. L., and McLellan, A. M.: *Amer J Surg* 9:1 (July) 1930. Not to be confused with the method of Howard Jones wherein the technique is somewhat different and the dibucaine hydrochloride solution is much weaker (1:1500) or with the Heavy Solution Nupercaine® hydrochloride (dibucaine hydrochloride).

Principle: A small volume of this concentrated solution of dibucaine hydrochloride is mixed with cerebrospinal fluid and injected in a final concentration of 1:1000.

Solution: Nupercaine hydrochloride 1:200 is an isobaric, isotonic, phosphate-buffered solution.

Specific Gravity
1.0062 (15.5°C) 1.0060 (20.0°C) 1.0059 (37.0°C)

Equipment
Syringe: Luer-Lok all-glass syringe, capacity 10 ml.
Needles: One needle of convenient size to transfer solution from the ampul into the syringe.
One spinal needle with an accurately fitted stylet. It is suggested that a needle no larger than No. 22 be used. Larger sizes, permitting loss of spinal fluid, contribute to postinjection headache.
The bevel of the needle is important. It should be short with an angle of no less than 45° to decrease the possibility that part of the dibucaine hydrochloride solution might escape into the extradural space during the injection.
Because dibucaine hydrochloride is precipitated by minute amounts of alkali, syringes and needles should be rinsed with acidified distilled water to remove traces of alkaline salts and small foreign particles.
Ampuls: As part of the meticulous technique for administration of any spinal anesthetic agent, ampuls should be prepared as follows: Autoclave sterilization, considered by several authorities to be the best method. Dibucaine hydrochloride 1:200 solution (method of Keyes and McLellan) is stable as to pH, color and chemical assay when subjected to 3 repeated sterilizations at 121°C for 30 minutes.

Preparation of the Patient: Food and liquid, unless otherwise contraindicated, may be given freely up to the night before surgery. Enemas may be given.
It is recommended that a mild hypnotic be given the night before the operation. One-half to one hour before the patient is brought into the operating room, $\frac{1}{4}$ grain (15 mg) of morphine sulfate [with 1/200 gr (0.33 mg) of scopolamine hydrobromide as recommended by Keyes and McLellan] is administered. If necessary, $\frac{1}{6}$ gr (10 mg) of morphine is given shortly before spinal puncture.

Position of the Patient: The sitting position facilitates injection. If necessary, the lateral position may be employed; care must be taken so that the vertebral column is straight and without lateral curvature.

Insertion of the Spinal Needle: The patient sits bending well forward, and the puncture is made at the L_3-L_4 interspace. (If he is in the lateral position he should be fully flexed.) The D_{12}-L_1 interspace can be the site of injection for upper abdominal operations and L_1-L_2 for gynecologic surgery. When the spinal needle is in the correct position, the stylet is removed and about 2 ml cerebrospinal fluid is allowed to escape. The stylet is replaced. If the tapped fluid is bloody after 2 ml have flowed or if there is radiating pain, there has been incorrect placement of the needle. It should be withdrawn and inserted at another interspace.
Once the needle is correctly inserted, it is very important to avoid displacing it from the subdural space.

Suggested Dosages

Surgical Area	Dose (mg)	Volume (ml)
Perineum and lower limbs	2.5 to 5	0.5 to 1
Lower abdomen	5 to 7.5	1 to 1.5
Upper abdomen	10	2

The size of the individual, the degree of anesthesia desired and particularly the experience of the physician may modify these recommended dosages.

Note: The maximum dose should never be more than 10 mg (2 ml).

Injection: The desired amount of Nupercaine hydrochloride (dibucaine hydrochloride) 1:200 is drawn up into the syringe by the "transfer" needle. With the stylet removed from the positioned spinal needle, the syringe is attached. If the patient is in the upright position, cerebrospinal fluid pressure usually will force the fluid out into the syringe to mix with the dibucaine hydrochloride 1:200 solution. If fluid does not flow easily, gentle aspiration may be used. The appropriate volume of cerebrospinal fluid (4 times the volume of the dibucaine hydrochloride 1:200 solution) is withdrawn and allowed to mix with the dibucaine hydrochloride.
[See table 1 above].
About one-third of the mixture is then injected, after which spinal fluid is again aspirated. Following this, one-half of the remaining contents of the syringe is injected. Another aspiration is then followed by injection of the remainder of the mixture.

Continued on next page

Table 1
Dilution of Dibucaine Hydrochloride 1:200 by Cerebrospinal Fluid

Ml Dibucaine Hydrochloride 1:200	Ml Cerebrospinal Fluid	Final Concentration Dibucaine Hydrochloride	Mg Dibucaine Hydrochloride Per Dose
0.5	2	1:1000	2.5
1	4	1:1000	5
1.5	6	1:1000	7.5
2	8	1:1000	10

The full prescribing information for each CIBA drug is contained herein and is that in effect as of October 1, 1984.

CIBA—Cont.

The whole injection should be carried out very slowly.

Regulation of Anesthesia: When injection is complete, the needle is removed, the skin swabbed with antiseptic, sterile gauze fixed, and the patient is placed in Trendelenburg position.

Immediately after dibucaine hydrochloride is injected subdurally, it is advisable to inject ¾ to 1½ gr (50 to 100 mg) ephedrine intramuscularly. This usually prevents a fall in blood pressure in case the anesthetic solution ascends higher than desired.

For operations on the abdominal viscera a 20° Trendelenburg position is used; with surgery on the lower abdomen, perineum and lower limbs, the tilt may be decreased to 10° to 15°.

The level of anesthesia should be determined after 1 or 2 minutes so that the tilt of the table can be adjusted for the desired level of anesthesia.

With correct technique and dosage, anesthesia with Nupercaine hydrochloride (dibucaine hydrochloride) should be sufficiently developed after 10 to 15 minutes. Failure of this to occur suggests either:

(1) Separation of dibucaine hydrochloride because of alkalinity of the syringe or needle.
(2) Extradural injection of the anesthetic solution.

Anesthesia lasts, on the average, up to six hours. This is followed by a period of slowly returning sensibility during which the patient is free from postoperative discomfort.

General Contraindications

Absolute
1. Disease of the cerebrospinal system, such as meningitis, cranial hemorrhage, tumors, poliomyelitis.
2. Moribund patients.
3. Blood stream infection.
4. Pernicious anemia with cord symptoms.
5. Arthritis, spondylitis, and other diseases of the spinal column rendering spinal puncture impossible. The presence of tuberculosis or metastatic lesions in the column is also a contraindication.
6. Pyogenic infection of the skin at or adjacent to the site of puncture.

Relative
1. **Hysteria or excessive nervous tension.** This difficulty may frequently be overcome by the preoperative administration of morphine sulfate ⅙ to ¼ gr (10 to 15 mg), scopolamine 1/150 to 1/100 gr (0.43 to 0.65 mg), or a sedative.
2. **Chronic backache.** The patient may blame any exacerbation of symptoms, either immediate or late, on the spinal anesthesia.
3. **Preoperative headache of long duration or history of migraine.** Exacerbation of symptoms may follow spinal injection.
4. **Hypersensitivity to drugs.** This drug may be used frequently in patients who have shown a sensitivity to procaine. However, in all patients in whom drug sensitivity is suspected, a skin test should be performed by injecting intradermally a small amount (0.1 ml) of dibucaine hydrochloride and at the same time injecting intradermally a small amount (0.1 ml) of physiologic salt solution as a control. Reaction may be local (redness), or systemic (dyspnea, agitation). Use of the drug is absolutely contraindicated in the presence of local reaction if there is a history of drug idiosyncrasy.
5. **Possibility of severe hemorrhage during operation.** Judgment in this case must include consideration of the amount of possible hemorrhage, the height of anesthesia to be induced, and the facilities available to control shock.
6. **Shock.** All forms of anesthesia are poorly borne by patients in shock. Systolic blood pressure should be raised to at least 105 mm Hg before operation is contemplated.
7. **Hypotension.** In cases not due to Addison's disease or associated with severe shock, this has become of relatively little importance because of the effectiveness of ephedrine in restoring pressure to normal (see *Complications:* Hypotension).
8. **Hemorrhagic spinal fluid.** Where clear spinal fluid cannot be obtained, the needle should be withdrawn and puncture made at another interspace. This is important in order to avoid the possibility of intravenous injection of the drug.
9. **Cardiac decompensation, massive pleural effusions, and markedly increased intra-abdominal pressure** as in massive ascites and tumors.

Warnings
1. An extremely potent anesthetic agent and therefore is to be used in much smaller concentrations than other local anesthetics.
2. As is true for any spinal anesthetic agent, the anesthetist should remain in constant attendance. Ephedrine and oxygen should be held in readiness in order to effectively combat a sudden fall in blood pressure should such occur. Likewise, a quick-acting barbiturate should be readily available so that any evidence of toxicity, as manifested by excitement, may be treated promptly.
3. Persons with known drug sensitivity should be pretested before using any of the local anesthetic agents.

Cautions: Authorities agree that spinal anesthesia should not be induced unless the anesthetist is: (1) equipped to provide a rigidly aseptic technique; (2) prepared to remain in constant attendance; (3) equipped to deal with complications or side effects that may arise; (4) familiar with the contraindications to spinal anesthesia.

Complications and Side Effects
1. **Respiratory.** Cessation of respiration may occur from spread of the anesthetic into the cervical region. This is absolutely prevented by following the technique described. It may also occur because of medullary anoxia which follows the circulatory collapse incident to severe hypotension.
   Treatment: Intubation to assure an adequate airway; artificial respiration; oxygen; respiratory stimulant repeated as necessary.
2. **Hypotension.** The fall of blood pressure produced by spinal anesthesia is due to a number of factors, most important of which are: (1) sudden vasodilatation incident to paralysis of sympathetic vasomotor fibers and (2) loss of muscle tone with decrease in venous pressure, venous return, and cardiac output. The degree of fall therefore depends upon the number of segments involved, being greatest in high spinal anesthesia and practically nonexistent when the effect is confined to the perineal area alone.
   There have been several reports indicating that Nupercaine hydrochloride (dibucaine hydrochloride) has less effect upon blood pressure than does a comparable degree of anesthesia produced by procaine.
   Treatment: The prophylactic use of 25 mg ephedrine given intramuscularly before the anesthetic is injected is advised by many authorities. It may be omitted in low spinals. An additional dose of 25 mg should be given *intravenously* if a fall below 100 mm Hg occurs. This dose may be repeated; total should not exceed 100 mg.
   Fluids, plasma, or whole blood should be administered intravenously when severe fall of blood pressure occurs. In *obstetrical patients,* raising the legs to the vertical position is the most effective initial procedure to increase blood pressure.
3. **Postanesthetic Headache.** Since this is usually due to leakage of spinal fluid, incidence will decrease as technique improves.
   Prophylaxis: A needle of small caliber (not over 20 or 22 gauge) should be used. Some authorities recommend special needles, one of 20 gauge to penetrate the skin and fascia and an inner needle of 24 gauge to pierce the dura. It has also been recommended that the needle be introduced with the bevel held laterally so as to cut fewer fibers of the dura. The needle should remain in place for several seconds after injection to allow time for equalization of pressure.
   Treatment: Tight abdominal binder. Hydration of the patient with either oral or intravenous fluids. One ml surgical pituitrin or 100 mg ephedrine. Rapid relief has been reported after intraspinal or caudal injection of 30 ml sterile saline.
4. **Nausea and Vomiting.** These may occur from psychic causes, drop in blood pressure, or intra-abdominal manipulation.
   Treatment: When caused by hypotension, inhalations of 100 percent oxygen in conjunction with a vasopressor may be found effective. Light cyclopropane or an intravenous barbiturate will control that which is due to intra-abdominal manipulation.
5. **Palsies.** Transient nerve palsies, usually involving the abducens, have occasionally been reported. This very uncommon complication generally occurs during the second week and clears up by the third or fourth week. Temporary or permanent transverse myelitis may follow the use of spinal anesthetic agents (see *Warnings*).
6. **Meningitis.** An aseptic technique should practically preclude the occurrence of this complication. Aseptic meningitis or meningismus, usually of rapid and benign course, has occurred after spinal anesthesia as it has also in cases where no spinal puncture has been carried out. Lundy has called attention to the fact that meningitides following spinal anesthesia may occur without relation to the method but due to pathologically proved metastases from distant foci. However, even the remote possibility of this complication reinforces the necessity for an absolutely sterile technique.
7. **Drug Idiosyncrasy.** The use of this drug is exceptionally free of this hazard. Patients giving a history of hypersensitivity to drugs, however, should be skin tested (see *Contraindications*).
   Treatment: The occurrence of motor excitement requires the anticonvulsant action of an intravenous barbiturate.

How Supplied: *Ampuls,* for spinal anesthesia, 2 ml, 1:200 (method of Keyes and McLellan), each ampul containing 10 mg dibucaine hydrochloride, 10 mg sodium chloride, 4 mg sodium phosphate monobasic, 0.9 mg sodium phosphate dibasic, and water q.s.; cartons of 10.

C80-50 (7/80)

NUPERCAINE® hydrochloride ℞
[*new-purr-cayn'*]
(dibucaine hydrochloride USP)
1:1500

Listed in USP, a Medicare designated compendium.
Specially Prepared for Hypobaric Spinal Anesthesia According to the Method of Howard Jones*

*Not to be confused with the method of Keyes and McLellan wherein the technique is completely different and the dibucaine hydrochloride solution is much more concentrated.

Principle: A relatively large volume of this solution of dibucaine hydrochloride with a specific gravity *less* than that of the cerebrospinal fluid (hypobaric) is injected without previous removal of fluid.

Solution: Nupercaine hydrochloride 1:1500 in saline. Specific Gravity: 1.0038 (15.5°C), 1.0036 (37°C).

Equipment
Syringe: Luer-Lok syringe with a capacity of 20 ml, accurately gauged, made of neutral glass.
Needles: Rustless needles, 20 gauge and 3½ inches in length; short bevels.

Large needles inflict unnecessary trauma; their use is apt to be followed by postinjection backache and headache, presumably due to trauma and leakage of spinal fluid. With a needle as slender as 22 gauge or more, longer than $3\frac{1}{2}$ inches, bending is apt to occur when the needle is held by the hub and attempt made to puncture the skin; on the other hand, needles less than $3\frac{1}{2}$ inches long may be too short for obese patients. The bevel of the needle is of importance; if it is less than 45 degrees, the chance of having a portion of the lumen outside the dura is increased, although the tip lies in the subdural space; the result being that a part or all of the anesthetic solution escapes extradurally when the attempt is made to inject it. The spinal puncture needle should be furnished with an accurately fitting stylet. The needle should be carefully examined and tested by bending before sterilization.

Syringes and needles are sterilized, preferably in an autoclave, then rinsed in slightly acidulated distilled water or 95% alcohol (2 to 3 drops of dilute hydrochloric acid to the liter), and covered with a sterile towel. This procedure is of importance, both for removing any small foreign particles and also to neutralize any alkalinity.

Ampuls: As part of the meticulous technique for administration of any spinal anesthetic agent, ampuls should be prepared as follows: Autoclave sterilization, considered by several authorities to be the best method. Dibucaine hydrochloride 1:1500 solution (method of Howard Jones) is stable as to pH, color and chemical assay when subjected to 3 repeated sterilizations at 121°C for 30 minutes.

Preoperative Procedure: The patient's confidence should be gained. Food and liquids, unless contraindicated, may be given freely up to the night preceding surgery; enemas may be given.

A mild hypnotic is indicated in order to provide sleep the night preceding the operation; $\frac{1}{4}$ gr morphine sulfate is administered $\frac{1}{2}$ to 1 hour before the patient is brought to the operating room. If necessary, $\frac{1}{6}$ gr morphine may be given shortly before puncture.

Administration: The patient is placed in the right lateral position, after his back has been painted with tincture of iodine over an area extending a palm's breadth below the scapular angle to the gluteal cleft, washed with 70% alcohol and draped with sterile cloth or towels.

It is important to have the patient in a lateral position when making the subdural injection, because the solution with the specific gravity lighter than the one of the spinal fluid (usually 1.005 to 1.007) will ascend rapidly in the canal, with possible involvement of the medullary centers, if the sitting position is adopted.

The lumbar puncture is made between the 2nd and 3rd vertebrae or between the 3rd and 4th, according to the level of the operation. The needle, inserted in the proper interspace, is pushed 1 mm further after the first appearance of cerebrospinal fluid, and a few drops are allowed to escape. The syringe is then attached, care being taken not to displace the needle. The injection is made very slowly and should be discontinued for 3 to 4 seconds when an increasing resistance is encountered. The needle is, under these circumstances, maintained strictly in the position adopted to minimize leakage. No efforts should be made to decrease the resistance by moving the needle, but pauses are made after the injection of each succeeding 2 ml of the solution.

While barbotage is practiced in the administration of the buffered (1:200) solution of Nupercaine hydrochloride (dibucaine hydrochloride), it should *never* be employed with the hypobaric (1:1500) concentration.

Upon the completion of the injection, that is, the selected volume of the solution (see dosage), the needle is allowed to remain in place for 1 or 2 minutes to permit increased subdural pressure to return to normal.

Position Following Injection: The needle withdrawn, the patient is immediately turned flat in the prone position for 5 to 10 minutes to enable the light solution to impregnate the posterior roots. If there is a pronounced degree of dorsal curvature, the table may be tilted, fastened down with the head-piece flexed to bring the head below the level of the dorsal region.

The patient is then turned on his back in a slight Trendelenburg position (head 2 inches below feet), which is maintained throughout the operation.

Dosage: For anesthesia of the lower extremities as high as the pelvis, 4 mg (6 ml solution, 1:1500) are usually sufficient. 7.5 to 10 mg (11 to 15 ml) will be required for most abdominal operations.

Usually, dosage above 15 ml is not necessary. The volume of solution to pass the level of D_5 is roughly calculated by subtracting from the number of inches given by the measurement of the distance from the spine C_7 to the interiliac line (4 for males and 6 for females). For caudal block, 6 ml is usually sufficient; 10 ml for the level D_{10}, 12 ml for D_7-D_8. For operations of longer duration on the stomach or duodenum, up to 20 ml may be required (16 ml for a 5-foot woman, 17 ml for a 5-foot man with 1 ml added for every 3 inches over 5 feet—to a maximum of 20 ml). For anesthesia in the lower part of the abdomen, divide 100 by the number of the uppermost thoracic nerve segment which is to be anesthetized. The result is the amount (in ml) of Nupercaine hydrochloride (dibucaine hydrochloride) solution to be used.

Approximate Dosage

Dosage for:	Concentration	Amount
Upper Abdominal	1:1500	15 to 18 ml
Lower Abdominal	1:1500	10 to 15 ml
Simple Caudal Block	1:1500	6 ml

Obstetrical Contraindications To Spinal Anesthesia: (1) Pelvic disproportion, (2) placenta praevia, (3) abruptio placenta, (4) unengaged head, and (5) necessity for intrauterine manipulations such as podalic version.

General Contraindications

Absolute
1. Disease of the cerebrospinal system, such as meningitis, cranial hemorrhage, tumors, poliomyelitis.
2. Moribund patients.
3. Blood stream infection.
4. Pernicious anemia with cord symptoms.
5. Arthritis, spondylitis, and other diseases of the spinal column rendering spinal puncture impossible. The presence of tuberculosis or metastatic lesions in the column is also a contraindication.
6. Pyogenic infection of the skin at or adjacent to the site of puncture.

Relative
1. **Hysteria or excessive nervous tension.** This difficulty may frequently be overcome by the preoperative administration of morphine sulfate $\frac{1}{6}$ to $\frac{1}{4}$ gr (10 to 15 mg), scopolamine 1/150 to 1/100 gr (0.43 to 0.65 mg), or a sedative.
2. **Chronic backache.** The patient may blame any exacerbation of symptoms, either immediate or late, on the spinal anesthesia.
3. **Preoperative headache of long duration or history of migraine.** Exacerbation of symptoms may follow spinal injection.
4. **Hypersensitivity to drugs.** This drug may be used frequently in patients who have shown a sensitivity to procaine. However, in all patients in whom drug sensitivity is suspected, a skin test should be performed by injecting intradermally a small amount (0.1 ml) of dibucaine hydrochloride and at the same time injecting intradermally a small amount (0.1 ml) of physiological salt solution as a control. Reaction may be local (redness), or systemic (dyspnea, agitation). Use of the drug is absolutely contraindicated in the presence of local reaction if there is a history of drug idiosyncrasy.
5. **Possibility of severe hemorrhage during operation.** Judgment in this case must include consideration of the amount of possible hemorrhage, the height of anesthesia to be induced, and the facilities available to control shock.
6. **Shock.** All forms of anesthesia are poorly borne by patients in shock. Systolic blood pressure should be raised to at least 105 mm Hg before operation is contemplated.
7. **Hypotension.** In cases not due to Addison's disease or associated with severe shock, this has become of relatively little importance because of the effectiveness of ephedrine in restoring pressure to normal (see *Complications:* Hypotension).
8. **Hemorrhagic spinal fluid.** Where clear spinal fluid cannot be obtained, the needle should be withdrawn and puncture made at another interspace. This is important in order to avoid the possibility of intravenous injection of the drug.
9. **Cardiac decompensation, massive pleural effusions, and markedly increased intra-abdominal pressure** as in massive ascites and tumors.

Warnings
1. An extremely potent anesthetic agent and therefore is to be used in much smaller concentrations than other local anesthetics.
2. As is true for any spinal anesthetic agent, the anesthetist should remain in constant attendance. Ephedrine and oxygen should be held in readiness in order to effectively combat a sudden fall in blood pressure should such occur. Likewise, a quick-acting barbiturate should be readily available so that any evidence of toxicity, as manifested by excitement, may be treated promptly.
3. Persons with known drug sensitivity should be pretested before using any of the local anesthetic agents.

Cautions: Authorities agree that spinal anesthesia should not be induced unless the anesthetist is: (1) equipped to provide a rigidly aseptic technique; (2) prepared to remain in constant attendance; (3) equipped to deal with complications or side effects that may arise; (4) familiar with the contraindications to spinal anesthesia.

Complications and Side Effects
1. **Respiratory.** Cessation of respiration may occur from spread of the anesthetic into the cervical region. This is absolutely prevented by following the technique described. It may also occur because of medullary anoxia which follows the circulatory collapse incident to severe hypotension.
   Treatment: Intubation to assure an adequate airway; artificial respiration; oxygen; respiratory stimulant repeated as necessary.
2. **Hypotension.** The fall of blood pressure produced by spinal anesthesia is due to a number of factors, most important of which are: (1) sudden vasodilatation incident to paralysis of sympathetic vasomotor fibers and (2) loss of muscle tone with decrease in venous pressure, venous return, and cardiac output. The degree of fall therefore depends upon the number of segments involved, being greatest in high spinal anesthesia and practically nonexistent when the effect is confined to the perineal area alone.
   There have been several reports indicating that Nupercaine hydrochloride (dibucaine hydrochloride) has less effect upon blood pressure than does a comparable degree of anesthesia produced by procaine.
   Treatment: The prophylactic use of 25 mg ephedrine given intramuscularly before the anesthetic is injected is advised by many authorities. It may be omitted in low spinals. An additional dose of 25 mg should be given *intravenously* if a fall below 100 mm Hg occurs. This dose may be repeated; total should not exceed 100 mg.
   Fluids, plasma, or whole blood should be administered intravenously when severe fall of blood pressure occurs. In *obstetrical patients,*

Continued on next page

The full prescribing information for each CIBA drug is contained herein and is that in effect as of October 1, 1984.

CIBA—Cont.

raising the legs to the vertical position is the most effective initial procedure to increase blood pressure.

3. **Postanesthetic Headache.** Since this is usually due to leakage of spinal fluid, incidence will decrease as technique improves.
   Prophylaxis: A needle of small caliber (not over 20 or 22 gauge) should be used. Some authorities recommend special needles, one of 20 gauge to penetrate the skin and fascia and an inner needle of 24 gauge to pierce the dura. It has also been recommended that the needle be introduced with the bevel held laterally so as to cut fewer fibers of the dura. The needle should remain in place for several seconds after injection to allow time for equalization of pressure.
   Treatment: Tight abdominal binder. Hydration of the patient with either oral or intravenous fluids. One ml surgical pituitrin or 100 mg ephedrine. Rapid relief has been reported after intraspinal or caudal injection of 30 ml sterile saline.
4. **Nausea and Vomiting.** These may occur from psychic causes, drop in blood pressure, or intra-abdominal manipulation.
   Treatment: When caused by hypotension, inhalations of 100 percent oxygen in conjunction with a vasopressor may be found effective. Light cyclopropane or an intravenous barbiturate will control that which is due to intra-abdominal manipulation.
5. **Palsies.** Transient nerve palsies, usually involving the abducens, have occasionally been reported. This very uncommon complication generally occurs during the second week and clears up by the third or fourth week. Temporary or permanent transverse myelitis may follow the use of spinal anesthetic agents (see *Warnings*).
6. **Meningitis.** An aseptic technique should practically preclude the occurrence of this complication. Aseptic meningitis or meningismus, usually of rapid and benign course, has occurred after spinal anesthesia as it has also in cases where no spinal puncture has been carried out. Lundy has called attention to the fact that meningitides following spinal anesthesia may occur without relation to the method but due to pathologically proved metastases from distant foci. However, even the remote possibility of this complication reinforces the necessity for an absolutely sterile technique.
7. **Drug Idiosyncrasy.** The use of this drug is exceptionally free of this hazard. Patients giving a history of hypersensitivity to drugs, however, should be skin tested (see *Contraindications*).
   Treatment: The occurrence of motor excitement requires the anticonvulsant action of an intravenous barbiturate.

How Supplied: *Ampuls*, for spinal anesthesia, 20 ml, 1:1500 (method of Howard Jones), each ml containing 0.667 mg dibucaine hydrochloride, 5 mg sodium chloride, and water q.s.; cartons of 12.

C80-54 (7/80)

HEAVY SOLUTION NUPERCAINE® hydrochloride
[*new-purr-cayne'*]
(dibucaine hydrochloride)
with Dextrose 5%
For Spinal Anesthesia

Indications: Heavy Solution Nupercaine hydrochloride is indicated for the production of low spinal anesthesia.

Contraindications: Shock, hypovolemia due to hemorrhage, and severe anemia; septicemia; pernicious anemia with evidence of spinal cord involvement; infection of the skin or subcutaneous tissue at or near the puncture site; tuberculosis or metastatic lesions in the lumbar spine; history of hypersensitivity to dibucaine or related com-

pounds; in obstetrics: abruptio placenta, placenta praevia with significant bleeding, and early stages of labor (see Dosage and Administration); diseases, syndromes, or situations causing increased intra-abdominal pressure, such as ascites, tumors, or advanced pregnancy (unless in preparation for vaginal delivery).

Warnings: Nupercaine hydrochloride is a highly potent agent and therefore is to be used in lower concentration and lower total dosage than certain other local anesthetic drugs.

Pooling of a concentrated solution of Nupercaine hydrochloride or any other anesthetic agent in the conus may cause irreversible nerve damage. Therefore, the patient must not be kept in the sitting position for more than one minute following injection of the drug.

Do not inject Nupercaine during uterine contractions since spinal fluid currents may carry the drug further cephalad than desired.

The possibility of severe bleeding during planned surgery and the facilities available to manage the resulting complications must be considered in the selection of anesthesia.

To avoid intravascular injection, do not administer spinal anesthesia in the presence of blood noted in attempting lumbar puncture. If the fluid does not clear after entering the dural space, repeat lumbar puncture is recommended; use of another interspace should be considered.

Low spinal anesthesia of the type provided by Heavy Nupercaine is not recommended for delivery involving abdominal operation, nor does it provide the uterine relaxation necessary for obstetrical manipulations such as internal podalic version.

Precautions: Spinal anesthesia should not be undertaken unless the anesthesiologist is familiar with techniques of and contraindications to spinal anesthesia, equipped to provide a rigidly aseptic technique, prepared to remain in constant attendance, monitoring patient's condition continuously, and equipped to deal with any complications that may arise.

Impairment of respiration may result from spread of the anesthetic above the desired level; this can be minimized by following the administration techniques described. It can also occur because of medullary hypoxia associated with circulatory collapse incident to severe hypotension, requiring intensive supportive treatment.

Hypotension during spinal anesthesia may be related to a number of factors, most important of which are sudden vasodilation incident to paralysis of sympathetic vasomotor fibers and loss of muscle tone with decrease in venous pressure, venous return, and cardiac output. The degree of hypotension relates to the number of vasoconstrictor fibers blocked, being greater in a higher level of spinal anesthesia.

If the operative conditions permit, it may be possible to restore blood pressure to an acceptable level without drugs by repositioning the patient and administering intravenous fluids. In obstetrics, lateral displacement of the uterus to the left may raise the blood pressure by improving venous return to the heart. If a vasopressor is necessary, one having both central and peripheral actions (*eg*, ephedrine) should be administered as needed. Plasma expanders or whole blood may also be required; adequate respiratory exchange must be maintained.

The use of spinal anesthesia in patients with cardiac disease depends upon the practitioner's evaluation of the type and severity of the physiological disturbance weighed against the possible pharmacological changes resulting from the anesthesia, and upon his ability to manage any possible complications.

In the presence of neurological disease (*eg*, meningitis, spinal block, hemorrhage, poliomyelitis, migraine, headache of long duration) or conditions involving the back (*eg*, arthritis, spondylitis, chronic backache), the decision to use spinal anesthesia will depend upon the practitioner's evaluation of the disease process and its possible implications. In these circumstances, the patient may ascribe signs and symptoms of previously existing

disease or exacerbations of chronic backache to the spinal anesthetic.

Selection of another form of anesthesia should be considered if the patient is uncooperative, hysterical, or excessively nervous or apprehensive. Use of spinal anesthesia in such cases will depend upon the practitioner's ability to evaluate and to manage the individual situation.

Adverse Reactions
Postanesthetic Headache. This can be minimized by use of small caliber needles (24 to 26 gauge) specially designed to prevent spinal fluid leakage and by keeping patient flat on back, without a pillow, for appropriate period after delivery or operation.

Nausea and Vomiting. These may result from psychic causes, fall in blood pressure, intra-abdominal manipulation, or concomitant medication.

Palsies. Nerve palsies, involving extra-ocular muscles, legs, vesical and anal sphincters, have occasionally been reported. These usually are transient and clear completely, but in rare instances a permanent residual has been reported.

Meningitis, Myelitis. Careful selection of patients, use of strictest aseptic techniques, and scrupulous care to avoid injury to meninges and cord during anesthetic drug injection should prevent infectious and traumatic complications almost entirely. Instances of aseptic meningitis or myelitis have occurred, occasionally with permanent residual and fatal termination. Aseptic meningitis or myelitis also have been reported in rare instances following diagnostic lumbar puncture without spinal anesthesia, following various operations for which spinal anesthesia was not used and spinal tap was done, and following pregnancy and delivery without use of spinal anesthesia or spinal tap. Meningismus also has been reported, evidently without infection, and usually clears promptly.

Dosage and Administration: Heavy Solution Nupercaine hydrochloride has a specific gravity greater than that of spinal fluid. When introduced into the spinal subarachnoid space, it will gravitate toward the lowest point; with the patient in sitting position, it settles toward the conus.

If injection is made with patient recumbent and the Trendelenburg position is immediately assumed, flow of anesthetic will be cephalad. Extent of upward spread will depend upon rate, force and volume of fluid injected, and length of time the Trendelenburg position is maintained. **Level of anesthesia and extent of involvement must be precisely regulated by careful attention to the various techniques described herein.**

Syringe should be filled with required amount of solution prior to lumbar puncture in order to reduce possibility of dislodgment of needle. Injection is made as rapidly as gentle pressure will permit, with needle held firmly to prevent dislodgment. The latter detail is of utmost importance, because failure to obtain anesthesia after an apparently satisfactory lumbar puncture may be due to dislodgment of needle during injection of solution. Needle should be kept in place for a few seconds after injection to permit equalization of pressure. **Directions for amount of solution, rapidity of injection, and positioning of patient following injection must be followed precisely to obtain desired level of anesthesia and to minimize complications.**

Inasmuch as Nupercaine hydrochloride is readily precipitated by even the slightest amount of alkali, needles and syringes must be thoroughly rinsed in distilled water prior to autoclaving. As part of the meticulous technique for administration of any spinal anesthetic agent, ampuls should be autoclaved to assure sterility of exterior surface. Heavy Solution Nupercaine hydrochloride can be resterilized once at 121° C for 30 minutes; repeated autoclaving produces progressive lowering of pH and darkening of color, probably from caramelization of the dextrose contained. Any ampul showing discoloration after resterilization must be discarded.

Heavy Solution Nupercaine hydrochloride should be used only in accordance with the following techniques:

Obstetric Analgesia Not Involving Abdominal Operation

Dose: 1 ml Heavy Solution Nupercaine hydrochloride is the amount most frequently used. However, greater duration of anesthesia will result from the use of 2 ml.

Time of Injection: Low spinal anesthesia is not intended to relieve the pains of early labor; these can be controlled adequately by other methods. There is general agreement that the injection should not be made until the cervix is well effaced, the head fixed in the pelvis, and the labor progressing satisfactorily. Parmley and Adriani advise injection after the cervix is 5 to 6 cm dilated and 60 to 80 percent effaced.

Injection must not be made during uterine contractions, since currents in the spinal fluid may carry solution cephalad.

Position of Patient at Injection: Sitting with legs over side of bed or delivery table, supported by an attendant. Downward pressure on the head to increase flexion should be avoided.

Injection: Draw Heavy Solution Nupercaine into syringe before lumbar puncture. After introduction of needle into subarachnoid space, make injection to count of 1-and-2-and-3 (approximately 2 to 3 seconds). Keep patient sitting for exactly 30 seconds, then place her flat, with head supported by two pillows, or in Fowler's position of 5 degrees. Under no circumstances is patient allowed to remain in sitting position for more than one minute after injection of the hyperbaric solution, since pooling in the conus can produce irreversible nerve damage.

Saddle Block Anesthesia in Rectal and Urologic Surgery Not Involving Abdominal Surgery

Position of Patient at Injection: *Sitting.* Under no circumstances should the patient be allowed to remain in the sitting position for longer than one minute after injection of the hyperbaric solution since pooling of the anesthetic in the conus may produce irreversible nerve damage.

Dose: For anesthesia of the perineum, rectum, lower scrotum, and penis, inject 1 ml Heavy Solution Nupercaine hydrochloride and allow the patient to sit upright for only 60 seconds.

For anesthesia of fundus of the uterus, dome of the bladder, and other pelvic structures, in addition to the areas previously mentioned, inject 2 ml Heavy Solution Nupercaine hydrochloride and allow patient to sit upright for 0 to 5 seconds.

Position Following Injection: Place patient down immediately at expiration of the required number of seconds, with head supported by two pillows and table placed in Fowler's position at an angle of 5 degrees. After allowing at least 10 minutes for fixation of the anesthetic level, determining by sensory testing (as by pin-prick) that the level has ceased to rise, place patient in desired position for operation.

How Supplied: *Ampuls,* 2 ml, each ampul containing 5 mg Nupercaine hydrochloride (0.25%) and 100 mg dextrose in water.
Cartons of 10 .... NDC 0083-5662-10
C82-18 (5/82)

PERCORTEN® acetate ℞
[*per-core' ten*]
(desoxycorticosterone acetate pellets USP)
Pellets

Description: Percorten acetate, desoxycorticosterone acetate USP, is a mineralocorticoid hormone available as pellets for subcutaneous implantation in the infrascapular region.

Each pellet consists only of sterile, uniformly compressed, crystalline desoxycorticosterone acetate and weighs approximately 125 mg (the accurate weight of each pellet is stated on the label).

Desoxycorticosterone acetate is 21-hydroxy-4-pregnene-3,20-dione acetate, and its structural formula is:

Desoxycorticosterone acetate USP is an odorless, white or creamy white, crystalline powder. It is practically insoluble in water; slightly soluble in vegetable oils; and sparingly soluble in alcohol, in acetone, and in dioxane. It melts between 155°C and 161°C. Its molecular weight is 372.50.

Clinical Pharmacology: Percorten acetate is an adrenocortical hormone. In recommended doses, it acts as a mineralocorticoid and is devoid of glucocorticoid activity. It has more prolonged activity than the unesterified desoxycorticosterone because of the addition of the acetate radical.

The principal action of the mineralocorticoids is on the distal tubules of the kidney where the reabsorption of sodium ions from tubular fluid into the plasma is enhanced and urinary excretion of both potassium and hydrogen ion is increased. After several days of administration, intact or adrenalectomized subjects may "escape" from the sodium-retaining action of the drug and come into sodium balance. However, potassium continues to be excreted despite developing hypokalemia.

Desoxycorticosterone is unique among the corticosteroids in that it is ineffective when given orally. The sterile crystalline desoxycorticosterone acetate pellets, when implanted in the subcutaneous tissue, provide a repository for slow release of active drug over a period of 8–12 months. There is extensive, competitive, reversible plasma protein binding among the corticosteroids, with highest affinity for globulin. Metabolism is primarily oxidative, with metabolites excreted in the urine.

Indications and Usage: Percorten acetate is indicated as partial replacement therapy for primary and secondary adrenocortical insufficiency in Addison's disease and for the treatment of salt-losing adrenogenital syndrome.

Contraindications: Percorten acetate is contraindicated in patients with hypersensitivity to desoxycorticosterone acetate, hypertension, congestive heart failure, or cardiac disease.

Warnings: Use of mineralocorticoids should be accompanied by adequate glucocorticoid therapy in adrenal insufficiency or the salt-losing form of the adrenogenital syndrome.

Precautions:
General
Patients receiving Percorten acetate should be watched for evidence of intercurrent infection. Should infection occur, appropriate anti-infective therapy should be initiated.

Since Percorten acetate is a potent adrenocortical preparation, which may produce side effects, patients should be closely watched. Patients with Addison's disease are more sensitive to the action of the hormone and may exhibit side effects to an exaggerated degree. Treatment should be stopped in the event of a significant increase in weight or blood pressure, or the development of edema or cardiac enlargement.

Sodium retention and the loss of potassium are accelerated by a high intake of sodium. Hence, it may be necessary to restrict the intake of sodium and increase that of potassium. Especially if edema occurs, dietary sodium restriction may be required.

Information For Patients
Patients should be clearly informed about the nature of their condition, the action of the hormone, and the possibility of unwanted side effects. A medical identification card should be carried during long-term therapy.

Laboratory Tests
Serum electrolyte determinations and blood pressure and weight measurements should be performed frequently; potassium supplementation may be necessary.

Only if absolutely necessary should a glucose tolerance test (particularly intravenous) be performed, as patients with Addison's disease tend to react with severe hypoglycemia within 3 hours, whether or not they are receiving desoxycorticosterone therapy.

Drug/Drug Interactions
Excessive potassium loss may result from the concomitant use of potassium-depleting diuretics such as thiazides. By induction of hepatic enzymes, concomitant use of drugs such as phenobarbital, phenytoin, or rifampin may increase the metabolism of corticosteroids. Adverse effects from cardiac glycosides may be enhanced by corticosteroids.

Drug/Laboratory Test Interactions
See **Laboratory Tests.**

Carcinogenesis, Mutagenesis, Impairment of Fertility
Long-term carcinogenicity studies in animals have not been performed with Percorten acetate.

Pregnancy Category C
Animal reproduction studies have not been conducted with Percorten acetate. It is also not known whether Percorten acetate can cause fetal harm when administered to a pregnant woman or can affect reproduction capacity. Percorten acetate should be given to a pregnant woman only if clearly needed. If it is necessary to give steroids to a pregnant woman, the newborn infant should be watched closely for signs of hypoadrenalism, and appropriate therapy instituted if such signs are present.

Nursing Mothers
Corticosteroids are excreted in breast milk. Caution should be exercised when Percorten acetate is administered to a nursing woman.

Pediatric Use
Safety and effectiveness in children have not been established.

Adverse Reactions:
Cardiovascular: Generalized edema; hypertension and cardiac enlargement, especially if hypertension was present before the onset of adrenal insufficiency; cardiac arrhythmias.
Neurologic: Frontal or occipital headaches; extreme weakness of extremities with ascending paralysis secondary to low serum potassium.
Musculoskeletal: Arthralgia and tendon contractures.
Other: Hypersensitive reactions; rarely, irritation at the site of pellet implantation.

Overdosage:
Acute Toxicity
No cases of acute overdosage with Percorten acetate have been reported.
Oral LD_{50} in rats is > 1000 mg/kg.

Possible Signs and Symptoms
Since Percorten acetate is available only for infrascapular implantation, acute poisoning is most unlikely to occur. In the improbable event of such poisoning, however, the patient might develop clinical manifestations that represent extensions of its therapeutic effect, such as disturbances in fluid and electrolyte balance, hypokalemia, edema, hypertension, and cardiac insufficiency.

Treatment
There is no specific antidote.
In cases of acute poisoning, symptomatic treatment, together with measures to correct fluid and electrolyte imbalance, would be indicated.
In case of hypokalemia, digitalis should be used only with caution.

Dosage and Administration: Mineralocorticoid therapy may not be necessary if the patient's condition can be controlled with adequate salt intake and glucocorticoid therapy.

If mineralocorticoid therapy is necessary, dosage must be chosen according to the severity of the disease and the response of the patient, and it should be accompanied by adequate amounts of glucocorticoid hormone.

Percorten acetate pellets should be implanted only after the optimal daily maintenance dose of desoxycorticosterone acetate in oil has been carefully determined. Implantation of a number of pellets not exactly calculated on the basis of the optimal

Continued on next page

The full prescribing information for each CIBA drug is contained herein and is that in effect as of October 1, 1984.

CIBA—Cont.

daily maintenance dose by injection may lead to irreparable damage.

For determination of the ultimate optimal maintenance dose, several weeks are required. It is advisable, however, in order to eliminate the possibility of overdosage, that the patient be maintained on desoxycorticosterone acetate in oil for at least 2–3 months prior to pellet implantation.

Calculation of Pellet Requirement
One pellet is implanted for each 0.5 mg of the daily injected maintenance dose of desoxycorticosterone acetate in oil. For example, a patient with Addison's disease whose optimal daily maintenance requirement is 5 mg of desoxycorticosterone acetate in oil should receive a maximum of ten pellets.

Technique of Pellet Implantation
Pellets should be implanted only in a fully equipped operating room. Aseptic precautions and careful hemostasis are primary requirements for successful implantation.

The infrascapular region is the most suitable site for the implantation. Strict asepsis is observed. The operative field is prepared with iodine and alcohol, and the site of incision is anesthetized. A 2- to 4-cm transverse incision is made a few centimeters below the inferior angle of the scapula. A number of small pockets, determined by the number of pellets to be implanted, are prepared in the subcutaneous tissue by blunt dissection, radiating from the incision.

The pellets, which have been removed from the vial under sterile conditions and kept close at hand on a sterile towel, are placed in the pockets with forceps. The use of a nasal dilator, introduced into the opening of the pocket, permits placement of the pellet sufficiently far away from the incision. If the pellet is not placed a least 2 cm away from the incision, the chances are greatly increased that it may be extruded later. No pellet should be extruded spontaneously if implanted aseptically and sufficiently far away from the incision and if careful hemostasis is observed. It is a matter of technique and experience whether each single pellet pocket should be closed with an individual suture or whether the skin incision only should be closed with subcuticular sutures of fine black silk. As many as 15 pellets may be inserted through a single incision by this technique.

Observation After Implantation
The pellets are effective for an average period of 8–12 months. In case of infection, disease, or other stress, supplementary injections of desoxycorticosterone acetate in oil may be necessary until the patient has returned to the condition established when the pellets were implanted.

In a few instances, it has been necessary to remove pellets even though the maintenance dose was adequately determined prior to implantation. The occurrence of edema, excessive weight gain, and rise in blood pressure are signs of overdosage.

Reimplantation of Pellets
The effect of the implanted pellets fades after approximately 8–12 months. A gradual decrease in blood pressure and weight, increased fatigue, and loss of appetite are usually the first indications of this decrease in hormonal supply, and the patient must be carefully watched. It may be necessary to resume daily injections of desoxycorticosterone acetate in oil with slowly increasing doses. Over a period of 4–6 weeks, the maintenance requirement of desoxycorticosterone acetate in oil can be reestablished; from this dosage the number of new pellets to be implanted can be calculated. Under no circumstances should pellets be arbitrarily implanted on the basis of the initial assay, as the condition of the patient may have undergone a change in hormone requirement during the year.

How Supplied:
Pellets—White, oval—each consisting of approximately 125 mg of desoxycorticosterone acetate.
Cartons of 1 ....NDC 0083-2232-01
C83-33 (Rev. 7/83)

PERCORTEN® pivalate ℞
[*purr-core'ten*]
(desoxycorticosterone pivalate)

Not USP, differs in pH range (5.0-8.5)
INTRAMUSCULAR REPOSITORY

Indications: As partial replacement therapy for primary and secondary adrenocortical insufficiency in Addison's disease and for treatment of salt-losing adrenogenital syndrome.

Contraindications: Hypersensitivity to Percorten pivalate suspension or any of its ingredients. Patients with hypertension or cardiac disease.

Warnings: Since Percorten pivalate is potent and long-acting, do not administer more frequently than once per month.

Usage in Pregnancy
The safe use of this drug in pregnant women or during lactation has not been established. Therefore, the benefits must be weighed against the potential hazards.

Precautions: Patients with Addison's disease are more sensitive to the action of the hormone and may exhibit side effects in an exaggerated degree. Since Percorten pivalate is a potent adrenocortical preparation which may produce side effects, patients should be closely watched. Treatment should be stopped in the event of a significant increase in weight or blood pressure, or the development of edema or cardiac enlargement.

Sodium retention and the loss of potassium are accelerated by a high intake of sodium. Hence, it may be necessary to restrict intake of sodium and increase that of potassium.

Only if absolutely necessary should a glucose tolerance test (particularly intravenous) be performed, as addisonian patients with or without desoxycorticosterone therapy have the tendency to react with severe hypoglycemia within 3 hours.

Adverse Reactions: Like other adrenocortical hormones, Percorten pivalate may cause severe side effects if dosage is too high or prolonged. It may cause increased blood volume, edema, elevation of blood pressure, and enlargement of the heart shadow. In patients with essential hypertension or a tendency toward its development, a marked rise in blood pressure may follow administration of this drug.

Headache, arthralgia, weakness, ascending paralysis, low potassium syndrome, and hypersensitivity may occur.

On rare occasions, irritation at the site of injection has been reported.

Dosage and Administration: In treating Addison's disease, Percorten pivalate should be used only in conjunction with other supplemental measures (*eg,* other hormonal agents, electrolytes, control of infection).

At initiation of treatment, the daily requirement for maintenance therapy should be determined with desoxycorticosterone acetate in oil. For each mg of desoxycorticosterone acetate in oil, 1 ml (25 mg) Percorten pivalate suspension is to be injected intramuscularly through a 20-gauge needle into the upper outer quadrant of one or both buttocks. The average dose is 25 to 100 mg every 4 weeks.

How Supplied: *Multiple-Dose Vials,* 4 ml, each ml containing 25 mg desoxycorticosterone pivalate, 10.5 mg methylcellulose, 3 mg sodium carboxymethylcellulose, 1 mg polysorbate 80, and 8 mg sodium chloride with 0.002% thimerosal added as preservative in aqueous suspension.
Cartons of 1 ....NDC 0083-2222-01
For intramuscular use only.
Shake well before using.

C81-12 (2/81)

PRISCOLINE® hydrochloride ℞
[*priss'coe-leen*]
(tolazoline hydrochloride USP)
Parenteral/Intra-Arterial

Listed in USP, a Medicare designated compendium.

Indications
Based on a review of this drug by the National Academy of Sciences-National Research Council and/or other information, FDA has classified the indications as follows:

"Possibly" effective: Spastic peripheral vascular disorders associated with acrocyanosis, acroparesthesia, arteriosclerosis obliterans, Buerger's disease, causalgia, diabetic arteriosclerosis, gangrene, endarteritis, frostbite (sequelae), post-thrombotic conditions (thrombophlebitis), Raynaud's disease, and scleroderma.

Final classification of the less-than-effective indications requires further investigation.

Contraindications: Priscoline is contraindicated following a cerebrovascular accident; known or suspected coronary artery disease; hypersensitivity to tolazoline.

Warnings: Priscoline stimulates gastric secretion and may activate peptic ulcers. Use cautiously in patients with gastritis or known or suspected peptic ulcer.

In patients with mitral stenosis, parenterally administered Priscoline may produce either a fall or a rise in pulmonary artery pressure and total pulmonary resistance, hence must be used with caution in known or suspected mitral stenosis.

Usage in Pregnancy
The safe use of this drug in pregnant women or during lactation has not been established. Therefore, the benefits must be weighed against the potential hazards.

Precautions: Because of the risks involved, intraarterial administration should be used only by those thoroughly familiar with the procedure and, preferably, only in the hospital or a clinic facility (see Dosage and Administration).

Adverse Reactions: Although side effects are generally mild and may decrease progressively during continued therapy, cardiac ar- rhythmias, anginal pain, and marked hypertension have been reported. Exacerbations of peptic ulcer have also occurred.

Other side effects include nausea, vomiting, diarrhea, epigastric discomfort, tachycardia, flushing, slight rise or fall in blood pressure, increased pilomotor activity with tingling or chilliness, rash and edema.

Thrombocytopenia, leukopenia, psychiatric reactions characterized by confusion or hallucinations, hepatitis, oliguria and hematuria have been reported rarely.

Intra-arterial administration, in addition to the above, may also produce a feeling of warmth or a "burning sensation" in the injected extremity, transient weakness, transient postural vertigo, palpitations, formication, and apprehension. Rarely, a paradoxical response (further decrease in an already impaired blood supply) may occur in a seriously damaged limb with incipient or established gangrene. This usually disappears with continued treatment and may usually be prevented by prior administration of histamine.

Dosage and Administration: Dosage should be individualized according to the condition being treated and the response of the patient.

Subcutaneous, Intramuscular, or *Intravenous:* 10 to 50 mg 4 times daily. Start with low doses, increasing with patient under close observation until optimal dosage (as determined by appearance of flushing) is established. Keeping patient warm will often increase effectiveness of drug.

Intra-arterial: This approach should not be used except in carefully selected cases and only after it has been determined that maximal benefit has been achieved with other forms of parenteral administration.

Caution: Because of the risks involved, and because of the special technique and strict aseptic precautions required with intra-arter- ial injection, this approach should be used only by those thoroughly familiar with the procedure and, preferably, only in the hospital or a clinic facility.

Initially, 25 mg (1 ml) is given slowly as a test dose to determine the response. Subsequently, the average single dose may be 50 to 75 mg (2 to 3 ml) per injection, depending on the observed response.

One or 2 injections daily are usually required initially to achieve maximum response. For maintenance, 2 or 3 injections weekly may be enough to sustain improved circulation, but more may be needed.

Overdosage

Signs and Symptoms: Increased pilomotor activity, peripheral vasodilatation and skin flushing, and, in rare instances, hypotension to shock levels.

Treatment: In treating hypotension, placement of the patient in the head-low position and the administration of intravenous fluids is most important. If a vasopressor is necessary, one having both central and peripheral action (*eg,* ephedrine) may be administered as needed. Do not use epinephrine or norepinephrine, since large doses of Priscoline may cause "epinephrine reversal" (further reduction in blood pressure followed by an exaggerated rebound).

How Supplied: *Multiple-dose Vials,* 10 ml, each ml containing 25 mg tolazoline hydrochloride, 0.65% sodium citrate, 0.65% tartaric acid, and 0.5% chlorobutanol as preservative in water; cartons of 1.   C82-5 (3/82)

PRIVINE®
[*pri-veen´*]
0.05% Nasal Solution
0.05% Nasal Spray

Caution: Do not use Privine if you have glaucoma. Privine is an effective nasal decongestant **when you use it in the recommended dosage.** If you use too much, too long, or too often, Privine may be harmful to your nasal mucous membranes and cause burning, stinging, sneezing or an increased runny nose.

Do not use Privine by mouth.

Keep this and all medications out of the reach of children. Do not use Privine with children under 6 years of age, except with the advice and supervision of a doctor.

OVERDOSAGE IN YOUNG CHILDREN MAY CAUSE MARKED SEDATION AND IF SEVERE, EMERGENCY TREATMENT MAY BE NECESSARY.

IF NASAL STUFFINESS PERSISTS AFTER 3 DAYS OF TREATMENT, DISCONTINUE USE AND CONSULT A DOCTOR.

Privine is a nasal decongestant that comes in two forms: Nasal Solution (in a bottle with a dropper) and Nasal Spray (in a plastic squeeze bottle). Both are for prompt, and prolonged relief of nasal congestion due to common colds, sinusitis, hay fever, etc.

How to use Nasal Solution: Squeeze rubber bulb to fill dropper with proper amount of medication. For best results, tilt head as far back as possible and put two drops of solution into your right nostril. Then lean head forward, inhaling and turning your head to the left. Refill dropper by squeezing bulb. Now tilt head as far back as possible and put two drops of solution into your left nostril. Then lean head forward, inhaling, and turning your head to the right.

Use only 2 drops in each nostril. Do not repeat this dosage more than every 3 hours.

The Privine dropper bottle is designed to make administration of the proper dosage easy and to prevent accidental overdosage. Privine will not cause sleeplessness, so you may use it before going to bed.

Important: After use, be sure to rinse the dropper with very hot water. This helps prevent contamination of the bottle with bacteria from nasal secretions. Use of the dispenser by more than one person may spread infection.

Note: Privine Nasal Solution may be used on contact with glass, plastic, stainless steel and specially treated metals used in atomizers. Do not let the solution come in contact with reactive metals, especially aluminum. If solution becomes discolored, it should be discarded.

How to use Nasal Spray: For best results do **not** shake the plastic squeeze bottle.

Remove cap. With head held upright, spray twice into each nostril. Squeeze the bottle sharply and firmly while sniffing through the nose.

For best results use every 4 to 6 hours. Do not use more often than every 3 hours.

Avoid overdosage. Follow directions for use carefully.

Privine Nasal Solution contains 0.05% naphazoline hydrochloride USP with benzalkonium chloride as a preservative. Available in bottles of .66 fl. oz. (20 ml) with dropper, and bottles of 16 fl. oz. (473 ml). Privine Nasal Spray contains 0.05% naphazoline hydrochloride USP with benzalkonium chloride as a preservative. Available in plastic squeeze bottles of ½ fl. oz. (15 ml).

C80-5 (1/80)

REGITINE® ℞
[*rej´a-teen*]
(phentolamine mesylate USP)

Listed in USP a Medicare designated compendia.

Indications
Parenteral Regitine

Prevention or control of hypertensive episodes that may occur in a patient with pheochromocytoma as a result of stress or manipulation during preoperative preparation and surgical excision.

Prevention and treatment of dermal necrosis and sloughing following intravenous administration or extravasation of norepinephrine.

Diagnosis of pheochromocytoma—Regitine blocking test.

Contraindications: Myocardial infarction, history of myocardial infarction, coronary insufficiency, angina or other evidence suggestive of coronary artery disease. Hypersensitivity to phentolamine or related compounds.

Warnings: Myocardial infarction, cerebrovascular spasm, and cerebrovascular occlusion have been reported to occur following the administration of phentolamine, usually in association with marked hypotensive episodes with shock-like states which occasionally follow parenteral administration.

For screening tests in patients with hypertension, the generally available urinary assay of catecholamines or other biochemical assays have largely supplanted the Regitine and other pharmacological tests for reasons of accuracy and safety. None of the chemical or pharmacological tests is infallible in the diagnosis of pheochromocytoma. The Regitine test is not the procedure of choice and should be reserved for cases in which additional confirmatory evidence is necessary, and the relative risks involved in conducting the test have been considered.

Usage in Pregnancy: The safe use of this drug in pregnant women or during lactation has not been established. Therefore, the benefits must be weighed against the potential hazards.

Precautions: Tachycardia and cardiac arrhythmias may occur with the use of Regitine or other alpha adrenergic blocking agents. When possible, defer administration of cardiac glycosides until cardiac rhythm returns to normal.

Adverse Reactions: Acute and prolonged hypotensive episodes, tachycardia, and cardiac arrhythmias have been reported, most frequently after parenteral administration. In addition, weakness, dizziness, flushing, orthostatic hypotension, nasal stuffiness, nausea, vomiting, and diarrhea may occur.

Dosage and Administration

1. Prevention or control of hypertensive episodes in the patient with pheochromocytoma.

For use in preoperative reduction of elevated blood pressure, inject 5 mg of Regitine mesylate (1 mg for children) intravenously or intramuscularly 1 or 2 hours before surgery (and repeat if necessary). During surgery administer Regitine mesylate (5 mg for adults, 1 mg for children) intravenously as indicated to help prevent or control paroxysms of hypertension, tachycardia, respiratory depression, convulsions, or other effects of epinephrine intoxication. (Postoperatively, norepinephrine may be given to control the hypotension which commonly follows complete removal of a pheochromocytoma.)

2. Prevention and treatment of dermal necrosis and sloughing following intravenous administration or extravasation of norepinephrine.

For prevention, add 10 mg Regitine mesylate to each liter of solution containing norepinephrine. The pressor effect of norepinephrine is not affected.

For treatment, inject Regitine mesylate (5 to 10 mg in 10 ml saline) into the area of extravasation within 12 hours.

3. Diagnosis of pheochromocytoma—Regitine blocking test.

a. Intravenous

Preparation.

Review the *Contraindications, Warnings,* and *Precautions.* Withhold sedatives, analgesics, and all other medication not deemed essential (such as digitalis and insulin) for at least 24 hours (preferably 48 to 72 hours) prior to the test. Withhold antihypertensive drugs until blood pressure returns to the untreated, hypertensive level. Do not perform test on a patient who is normotensive.

Procedure.

1. Keep patient at rest in the supine position throughout the test, preferably in a quiet, darkened room. Delay Regitine injection until blood pressure is stabilized, as evidenced by blood pressure readings taken every 10 minutes for at least one-half hour.
2. Dissolve 5 mg Regitine mesylate in 1 ml Sterile Water for Injection. Dose for adults is 5 mg; for children, 1 mg.
3. Insert the syringe needle into vein, delay injection until pressor response to venipuncture has subsided.
4. Inject Regitine rapidly. Record blood pressure immediately after injection, at 30-second intervals for the first 3 minutes, and at 60-second intervals for the next 7 minutes.

Interpreting the Test

Positive response, suggestive of pheochromocytoma, is indicated by a drop in blood pressure of more than 35 mm Hg systolic and 25 mm Hg diastolic pressure. A typical positive response may be a drop of 60 mm Hg systolic and 25 mm Hg diastolic. Maximal depressor pressure effect usually is evident within 2 minutes after injection. Return to pre-injection pressure commonly occurs within 15 to 30 minutes, but may return more rapidly. If blood pressure falls to a dangerous level, treat patient as outlined under "Overdosage."

A positive response should always be confirmed by other diagnostic procedures, preferably the measurement of urinary catecholamines or their metabolites.

Negative response is indicated when the blood pressure is unchanged, elevated, or is reduced less than 35 mm Hg systolic and 25 mm Hg diastolic after injection of Regitine. A negative response to this test does not exclude the diagnosis of pheochromocytoma, especially in patients with paroxysmal hypertension in whom the incidence of false negative responses is high.

b. Intramuscular

If the intramuscular test for pheochromocytoma is preferred, preparation is the same as for the intravenous test. Then dissolve 5 mg Regitine mesylate in 1 ml Sterile Water for Injection. Dose for adults is 5 mg intramuscularly; for children, 3 mg. Record blood pressure every 5 minutes for 30 to 45 minutes following intramuscular injection. Positive response is indicated by a drop in blood pressure of 35 mm Hg systolic and 25 mm Hg diastolic or greater within 20 minutes following injection.

Continued on next page

The full prescribing information for each CIBA drug is contained herein and is that in effect as of October 1, 1984.

CIBA—Cont.

c. Reliability
The test is most reliable in detecting pheochromocytoma in patients with sustained hypertension, and least reliable in those with paroxysmal hypertension. False positive tests may occur in patients with hypertension without pheochromocytoma.

Overdosage: In the event of a drop in blood pressure to dangerous level or other evidence of shock-like conditions, treat vigorously and promptly. Include intravenous infusion of norepinephrine, titrated to maintain blood pressure to normotensive level, and all available supportive measures. Do not use epinephrine since it may cause a paradoxical fall in blood pressure.

How Supplied
Vials, each containing 5 mg phentolamine mesylate USP and 25 mg mannitol in lyophilized form.
Cartons of 2 ....NDC 0083-6830-02
Cartons of 6 ....NDC 0083-6830-06
The reconstituted solution should be used upon preparation and should not be stored.

C84-8 (Rev. 3/84)

RIMACTANE®
[re-mack' tayne]
(rifampin USP)

Indications
Pulmonary Tuberculosis
In the initial treatment and in the retreatment of pulmonary tuberculosis, Rimactane must be used in conjunction with at least one other antituberculous drug.
Frequently used regimens have been the following:
  isoniazid and Rimactane
  ethambutol and Rimactane
  isoniazid, ethambutol, and Rimactane

Neisseria Meningitidis Carriers
Rimactane is indicated for the treatment of asymptomatic carriers of *N. meningitidis* to eliminate meningococci from the nasopharynx.
Rimactane is not indicated for the treatment of meningococcal infection.
To avoid the indiscriminate use of Rimactane, diagnostic laboratory procedures, including serotyping and susceptibility testing, should be performed to establish the carrier state and the correct treatment. In order to preserve the usefulness of Rimactane in the treatment of asymptomatic meningococcal carriers, it is recommended that the drug be reserved for situations in which the risk of meningococcal meningitis is high.
Both in the treatment of tuberculosis and in the treatment of meningococcal carriers, small numbers of resistant cells, present within large populations of susceptible cells, can rapidly become the predominating type. Since rapid emergence of resistance can occur, culture and susceptibility tests should be performed in the event of persistent positive cultures.

Contraindications: A history of previous hypersensitivity reaction to any of the rifamycins.

Warnings: Rifampin has been shown to produce liver dysfunction. There have been fatalities associated with jaundice in patients with liver disease or receiving rifampin concomitantly with other hepatotoxic agents. Since an increased risk may exist for individuals with liver disease, benefits must be weighed carefully against the risk of further liver damage. Periodic liver function monitoring is mandatory.
The possibility of rapid emergence of resistant meningococci restricts the use of Rimactane to short-term treatment of the asymptomatic carrier state. Rimactane is not to be used for the treatment of meningococcal disease.
Several studies of tumorigenicity potential have been done in rodents. In one strain of mice known to be particularly susceptible to the spontaneous development of hepatomas, rifampin given at a level 2–10 times the maximum dosage used clinically, resulted in a significant increase in the occurrence of hepatomas in female mice of this strain after one year of administration. There was no evidence of tumorigenicity in the males of this strain, in males or females of another mouse strain, or rats.

Usage in Pregnancy: Although rifampin has been reported to cross the placental barrier and appear in cord blood, the effect of Rimactane, alone or in combination with other antituberculous drugs, on the human fetus is not known. An increase in congenital malformations, primarily spina bifida and cleft palate, has been reported in the offspring of rodents given oral doses of 150-250 mg/kg/day of rifampin during pregnancy.
The possible teratogenic potential in women capable of bearing children should be carefully weighed against the benefits of therapy.

Precautions: Rimactane is not recommended for intermittent therapy; the patient should be cautioned against intentional or accidental interruption of the daily dosage regimen since rare renal hypersensitivity reactions have been reported when therapy was resumed in such cases.
Rifampin has been observed to increase the requirements for anticoagulant drugs of the coumarin type. The cause of this phenomenon is unknown. In patients receiving anticoagulants and rifampin concurrently, it is recommended that the prothrombin time be performed daily or as frequently as necessary to establish and maintain the required dose of anticoagulant.
Urine, feces, saliva, sputum, sweat, and tears may be colored red-orange by rifampin and its metabolites. Soft contact lenses may be permanently stained. Individuals to be treated should be made aware of these possibilities.
It has been reported that the reliability of oral contraceptives may be affected in some patients being treated for tuberculosis with rifampin in combination with at least one other antituberculous drug. In such cases, alternative contraceptive measures may need to be considered.
Rifampin has been reported to diminish the effects of concurrently administered methadone, oral hypoglycemics, corticosteroids, dapsone, and digitalis preparations; appropriate dosage adjustments may be necessary if indicated by the patient's clinical condition.
When rifampin is taken in combination with PAS, decreased rifampin serum levels may result. Therefore, the drugs should be given at least 4 hours apart.
Therapeutic levels of rifampin have been shown to inhibit standard assays for serum folate and vitamin B_{12}. Alternative methods must be considered when determining folate and vitamin B_{12} concentrations in the presence of rifampin.
Since rifampin has been reported to cross the placental barrier and appear in cord blood, neonates of rifampin-treated mothers should be carefully observed for any evidence of adverse effects. Rifampin is excreted in breast milk.

Adverse Reactions: Gastrointestinal disturbances such as heartburn, epigastric distress, anorexia, nausea, vomiting, gas, cramps, and diarrhea have been noted in some patients. Rarely, pseudomembranous enterocolitis has been reported. Headache, drowsiness, fatigue, ataxia, dizziness, inability to concentrate, mental confusion, visual disturbances, muscular weakness, fever, pains in extremities, generalized numbness, and menstrual disturbances have also been noted.
Hypersensitivity reactions have been reported. Encountered occasionally have been pruritus, urticaria, rash, pemphigoid reaction, eosinophilia, sore mouth, sore tongue, and exudative conjunctivitis. Rarely, hepatitis or a shock-like syndrome with hepatic involvement and abnormal liver function tests have been reported. Transient abnormalities in liver function tests (eg, elevations in serum bilirubin, BSP, alkaline phosphatase, serum transaminases) have also been observed. The BSP test should be performed prior to the morning dose of rifampin to avoid false-positive results.
Thrombocytopenia, transient leukopenia, hemolytic anemia, and decreased hemoglobin have been observed. Thrombocytopenia has occurred when rifampin and ethambutol were administered concomitantly according to an intermittent dose schedule twice weekly and in high doses.
Elevations in BUN and serum uric acid have occurred. Rarely, hemolysis, hemoglobinuria, hematuria, renal insufficiency or acute renal failure have been reported and are generally considered to be hypersensitivity reactions. These have usually occurred during intermittent therapy or when treatment was resumed following intentional or accidental interruption of a daily dosage regimen and were reversible when rifampin was discontinued and appropriate therapy instituted.
Although rifampin has been reported to have an immunosuppressive effect in some animal experiments, available human data indicate that this has no clinical significance.

Dosage and Administration: It is recommended that Rimactane be administered once daily, either one hour before or two hours after a meal.
Data are not available for determination of dosage for children under 5.

Pulmonary Tuberculosis
Adults: 600 mg (two 300-mg Capsules) in a single daily administration.
Children: 10 to 20 mg/kg, not to exceed 600 mg/day.
In the treatment of pulmonary tuberculosis, Rimactane must be used in conjunction with at least one other antituberculous agent. In general, therapy should be continued until bacterial conversion and maximal improvement have occurred.

Meningococcal Carriers
It is recommended that Rimactane be administered once daily for four consecutive days in the following doses:
Adults: 600 mg (two 300-mg Capsules) in a single daily administration.
Children: 10 to 20 mg/kg, not to exceed 600 mg/day.

Susceptibility Testing
Pulmonary Tuberculosis: Rifampin susceptibility powders are available for both direct and indirect methods of determining the susceptibility of strains of mycobacteria. The MIC's of susceptible clinical isolates when determined in 7H10 or other non-egg-containing media have ranged from 0.1 to 2 mcg/ml.
Meningococcal Carriers: Susceptibility discs containing 5 mcg rifampin are available for susceptibility testing of *N. meningitidis*.
Quantitative methods that require measurement of zone diameters give the most precise estimates of antibiotic susceptibility. One such procedure[1] has been recommended for use with discs for testing susceptibility to rifampin. Interpretations correlate zone diameters from the disc test with MIC (minimal inhibitory concentration) values for rifampin. A range of MIC's from 0.1 to 1 mcg/ml has been found *in vitro* for susceptible strains of *N. meningitidis*. With this procedure, a report from the laboratory of "resistant" indicates that the organism is not likely to be eradicated from the nasopharynx of asymptomatic carriers.

How Supplied: *Capsules,* 300 mg (opaque scarlet and caramel); bottles of 30, 60, and 100. Also available, Rimactane®/INH (isoniazid USP) Dual Pack containing 60 Rimactane Capsules and 30 INH 300-mg Tablets.

Reference:
1. Bauer, A. W., Kirby, W. M. M., Sherris, J. C., and Turck, M. Antibiotic susceptibility testing by a standardized single disk method. Am. J. Clin. Path. 45:493-496, 1966.

C83-8 (Rev. 7/83)
Shown in Product Identification Section, page 409

RITALIN® hydrochloride
[rit' ah-lin]
(methylphenidate hydrochloride USP)
tablets

RITALIN-SR®
(methylphenidate hydrochloride)
sustained-release tablets

Description: Ritalin is a white, odorless, fine crystalline powder, solutions of which are acid to litmus. It is freely soluble in water.

Clinical Pharmacology: Ritalin is a mild central nervous system stimulant.

The mode of action in man is not completely understood, but Ritalin presumably activates the brain stem arousal system and cortex to produce its stimulant effect.

There is neither specific evidence which clearly establishes the mechanism whereby Ritalin produces its mental and behavioral effects in children, nor conclusive evidence regarding how these effects relate to the condition of the central nervous system.

Ritalin in the SR tablets is more slowly but as extensively absorbed as in the regular tablets. Relative bioavailability of the SR tablet compared to the Ritalin tablet, measured by the urinary excretion of Ritalin major metabolite (α-phenyl-2-piperidine acetic acid) was 105% (49–168%) in children and 101% (85–152%) in adults. The time to peak rate in children was 4.7 hours (1.3–8.2 hours) for the SR tablets and 1.9 hours (0.3–4.4 hours) for the tablets. An average of 67% of SR tablet dose was excreted in children as compared to 86% in adults.

Indications
Attention Deficit Disorders, Narcolepsy (previously known as Minimal Brain Dysfunction in Children). Other terms being used to describe the behavioral syndrome below include: Hyperkinetic Child Syndrome, Minimal Brain Damage, Minimal Cerebral Dysfunction, Minor Cerebral Dysfunction.

Ritalin is indicated as an integral part of a total treatment program which typically includes other remedial measures (psychological, educational, social) for a stabilizing effect in children with a behavioral syndrome characterized by the following group of developmentally inappropriate symptoms: moderate-to-severe distractibility, short attention span, hyperactivity, emotional lability, and impulsivity. The diagnosis of this syndrome should not be made with finality when these symptoms are only of comparatively recent origin. Nonlocalizing (soft) neurological signs, learning disability, and abnormal EEG may or may not be present, and a diagnosis of central nervous system dysfunction may or may not be warranted.

Special Diagnostic Considerations
Specific etiology of this syndrome is unknown, and there is no single diagnostic test. Adequate diagnosis requires the use not only of medical but of special psychological, educational, and social resources.

Characteristics commonly reported include: chronic history of short attention span, distractibility, emotional lability, impulsivity, and moderate-to-severe hyperactivity; minor neurological signs and abnormal EEG. Learning may or may not be impaired. The diagnosis must be based upon a complete history and evaluation of the child and not solely on the presence of one or more of these characteristics.

Drug treatment is not indicated for all children with this syndrome. Stimulants are not intended for use in the child who exhibits symptoms secondary to environmental factors and/or primary psychiatric disorders, including psychosis. Appropriate educational placement is essential and psychosocial intervention is generally necessary. When remedial measures alone are insufficient, the decision to prescribe stimulant medication will depend upon the physician's assessment of the chronicity and severity of the child's symptoms.
Contraindications: Marked anxiety, tension, and agitation are contraindications to Ritalin, since the drug may aggravate these symptoms. Ritalin is contraindicated also in patients known to be hypersensitive to the drug, in patients with glaucoma, and in patients with motor tics or with a family history or diagnosis of Tourette's syndrome.
Warnings: Ritalin should not be used in children under six years, since safety and efficacy in this age group have not been established.

Sufficient data on safety and efficacy of long-term use of Ritalin in children are not yet available. Although a causal relationship has not been established, suppression of growth (*ie,* weight gain, and/or height) has been reported with the long-term use of stimulants in children. Therefore, patients requiring long-term therapy should be carefully monitored.

Ritalin should not be used for severe depression of either exogenous or endogenous origin. Clinical experience suggests that in psychotic children, administration of Ritalin may exacerbate symptoms of behavior disturbance and thought disorder.

Ritalin should not be used for the prevention or treatment of normal fatigue states.

There is some clinical evidence that Ritalin may lower the convulsive threshold in patients with prior history of seizures, with prior EEG abnormalities in absence of seizures, and, very rarely, in absence of history of seizures and no prior EEG evidence of seizures. Safe concomitant use of anticonvulsants and Ritalin has not been established. In the presence of seizures, the drug should be discontinued.

Use cautiously in patients with hypertension. Blood pressure should be monitored at appropriate intervals in all patients taking Ritalin, especially those with hypertension.

Symptoms of visual disturbances have been encountered in rare cases. Difficulties with accommodation and blurring of vision have been reported.

Drug Interactions
Ritalin may decrease the hypotensive effect of guanethidine. Use cautiously with pressor agents and MAO inhibitors.

Human pharmacologic studies have shown that Ritalin may inhibit the metabolism of coumarin anticoagulants, anticonvulsants (phenobarbital, diphenylhydantoin, primidone), phenylbutazone, and tricyclic antidepressants (imipramine, desipramine). Downward dosage adjustments of these drugs may be required when given concomitantly with Ritalin.

Usage in Pregnancy
Adequate animal reproduction studies to establish safe use of Ritalin during pregnancy have not been conducted. Therefore, until more information is available, Ritalin should not be prescribed for women of childbearing age unless, in the opinion of the physician, the potential benefits outweigh the possible risks.

Drug Dependence
Ritalin should be given cautiously to emotionally unstable patients, such as those with a history of drug dependence or alcoholism, because such patients may increase dosage on their own initiative.

Chronically abusive use can lead to marked tolerance and psychic dependence with varying degrees of abnormal behavior. Frank psychotic episodes can occur, especially with parenteral abuse. Careful supervision is required during drug withdrawal, since severe depression as well as the effects of chronic overactivity can be unmasked. Long-term follow-up may be required because of the patient's basic personality disturbances.

Precautions: Patients with an element of agitation may react adversely; discontinue therapy if necessary.

Periodic CBC, differential, and platelet counts are advised during prolonged therapy.

Drug treatment is not indicated in all cases of this behavioral syndrome and should be considered only in light of the complete history and evaluation of the child. The decision to prescribe Ritalin should depend on the physician's assessment of the chronicity and severity of the child's symptoms and their appropriateness for his/her age. Prescription should not depend solely on the presence of one or more of the behavioral characteristics. When these symptoms are associated with acute stress reactions, treatment with Ritalin is usually not indicated.

Long-term effects of Ritalin in children have not been well established.

Adverse Reactions: Nervousness and insomnia are the most common adverse reactions but are usually controlled by reducing dosage and omitting the drug in the afternoon or evening. Other reactions include hypersensitivity (including skin rash, urticaria, fever, arthralgia, exfoliative dermatitis, erythema multiforme with histopathological findings of necrotizing vasculitis, and thrombocytopenic purpura); anorexia; nausea; dizziness; palpitations; headache; dyskinesia; drowsiness; blood pressure and pulse changes, both up and down; tachycardia; angina; cardiac arrhythmia; abdominal pain; weight loss during prolonged therapy. There have been rare reports of Tourette's syndrome. Toxic psychosis has been reported. Although a definite causal relationship has not been established, the following have been reported in patients taking this drug: leukopenia and/or anemia; a few instances of scalp hair loss. In children, loss of appetite, abdominal pain, weight loss during prolonged therapy, insomnia, and tachycardia may occur more frequently; however, any of the other adverse reactions listed above may also occur.
Dosage and Administration: Dosage should be individualized according to the needs and responses of the patient.
Adults
Tablets: Administer in divided doses 2 or 3 times daily, preferably 30 to 45 minutes before meals. Average dosage is 20 to 30 mg daily. Some patients may require 40 to 60 mg daily. In others, 10 to 15 mg daily will be adequate. Patients who are unable to sleep if medication is taken late in the day should take the last dose before 6 p.m.
SR Tablets: Ritalin SR Tablets have a duration of action of approximately 8 hours. Therefore, Ritalin SR tablets may be used in place of Ritalin tablets when the 8 hour dosage of Ritalin SR corresponds to the titrated 8 hour dosage of Ritalin.
Children (6 years and over)
Ritalin should be initiated in small doses, with gradual weekly increments. Daily dosage above 60 mg is not recommended.

If improvement is not observed after appropriate dosage adjustments over a one-month period, the drug should be discontinued.

Tablets: Start with 5 mg twice daily (before breakfast and lunch) with gradual increments of 5 to 10 mg weekly.

SR Tablets: Ritalin SR tablets have a duration of action of approximately 8 hours. Therefore, Ritalin SR tablets may be used in place of Ritalin tablets when the 8 hour dosage of Ritalin SR corresponds to the titrated 8 hour dosage of Ritalin.

If paradoxical aggravation of symptoms or other adverse effects occur, reduce dosage, or, if necessary, discontinue the drug.

Ritalin should be periodically discontinued to assess the child's condition. Improvement may be sustained when the drug is either temporarily or permanently discontinued.

Drug treatment should not and need not be indefinite and usually may be discontinued after puberty.
Overdosage: Signs and symptoms of acute overdosage, resulting principally from overstimulation of the central nervous system and from excessive sympathomimetic effects, may include the following: vomiting, agitation, tremors, hyperreflexia, muscle twitching, convulsions (may be followed by coma), euphoria, confusion, hallucinations, delirium, sweating, flushing, headache, hyperpyrexia, tachycardia, palpitations, cardiac arrhythmias, hypertension, mydriasis, and dryness of mucous membranes.

Treatment consists of appropriate supportive measures. The patient must be protected against self-injury and against external stimuli that would aggravate overstimulation already present.

Continued on next page

The full prescribing information for each CIBA drug is contained herein and is that in effect as of October 1, 1984.

CIBA—Cont.

If signs and symptoms are not too severe and the patient is conscious, gastric contents may be evacuated by induction of emesis or gastric lavage. In the presence of severe intoxication, use a carefully titrated dosage of a *short-acting* barbiturate *before* performing gastric lavage.

Intensive care must be provided to maintain adequate circulation and respiratory exchange; external cooling procedures may be required for hyperpyrexia.

Efficacy of peritoneal dialysis or extracorporeal hemodialysis for Ritalin overdosage has not been established.

How Supplied:
Tablets 20 mg—round, pale yellow, scored (imprinted CIBA 34)

Bottles of 100	NDC 0083-0034-30
Bottles of 1000	NDC 0083-0034-40

Tablets 10 mg —round, pale green, scored (imprinted CIBA 3)

Bottles of 100	NDC 0083-0003-30
Bottles of 500	NDC 0083-0003-35
Bottles of 1000	NDC 0083-0003-40

Accu-Pak® Unit Dose (blister pack)
Box of 100 (strips of 10) NDC 0083-0003-32

Tablets 5 mg—round, yellow (imprinted CIBA 7)

Bottles of 100	NDC 0083-0007-30
Bottles of 500	NDC 0083-0007-35
Bottles of 1000	NDC 0083-0007-40

SR Tablets 20 mg—round, white, coated (imprinted CIBA 16)

Bottles of 100	NDC 0083-0016-30

Note: SR Tablets are color-additive free.
Do not store above 86°F (30°C). Protect from moisture.

Dispense in tight, light-resistant container (USP).
C84-29 (Rev. 6/84)
Shown in Product Identification Section, page 409

SER-AP-ES® ℞
[*su-rapp'ess*]
reserpine 0.1 mg
hydralazine hydrochloride 25 mg
hydrochlorothiazide 15 mg
Combination Tablets

> **Warning**
> This fixed combination drug is not indicated for initial therapy of hypertension. Hypertension requires therapy titrated to the individual patient. If the fixed combination represents the dosage so determined, its use may be more convenient in patient management. The treatment of hypertension is not static, but must be reevaluated as conditions in each patient warrant.

Indications
Hypertension. (See box warning.)
Contraindications
Reserpine
Known hypersensitivity, mental depression (especially with suicidal tendencies), active peptic ulcer, ulcerative colitis, and patients receiving electroconvulsive therapy.
Hydralazine
Hypersensitivity to hydralazine; coronary artery disease; and mitral valvular rheumatic heart disease.
Hydrochlorothiazide
Anuria; hypersensitivity to this or other sulfonamide-derived drugs.
Warnings
Reserpine
Extreme caution should be exercised in treating patients with a history of mental depression. Discontinue the drug at first sign of despondency, early morning insomnia, loss of appetite, impotence, or self-deprecation. Drug-induced depression may persist for several months after drug withdrawal and may be severe enough to result in suicide.

MAO inhibitors should be avoided or used with extreme caution.
Hydralazine
Hydralazine may produce in a few patients a clinical picture simulating systemic lupus erythematosus. In such patients hydralazine should be discontinued unless the benefit-to-risk determination requires continued antihypertensive therapy with this drug. Symptoms and signs usually regress when the drug is discontinued but residua have been detected many years later. Long-term treatment with steroids may be necessary.

Complete blood counts, L. E. cell preparations, and antinuclear antibody titer determinations are indicated before and periodically during prolonged therapy with hydralazine, even though the patient is asymptomatic. These studies are also indicated if the patient develops arthralgia, fever, chest pain, continued malaise or other unexplained signs or symptoms.

A positive antinuclear antibody titer and/or positive L. E. cell reaction requires that the physician carefully weigh the implications of the test results against the benefits to be derived from antihypertensive therapy with hydralazine.

Use MAO inhibitors with caution in patients receiving hydralazine.

When other potent parenteral antihypertensive drugs, such as diazoxide, are used in combination with hydralazine, patients should be continuously observed for several hours for any excessive fall in blood presssure. Profound hypotensive episodes may occur when diazoxide injection and hydralazine are used concomitantly.
Hydrochlorothiazide
Use with caution in severe renal disease. In patients with renal disease, thiazides may precipitate azotemia. Cumulative effects of the drug may develop in patients with impaired renal function.
Thiazides should be used with caution in patients with impaired hepatic function or progressive liver disease, since minor alterations of fluid and electrolyte imbalance may precipitate hepatic coma.

Thiazides may add to or potentiate the action of other antihypertensive drugs. Potentiation occurs with ganglionic or peripheral adrenergic blocking drugs.

Sensitivity reactions are more likely to occur in patients with a history of allergy or bronchial asthma.

The possibility of exacerbation or activation of systemic lupus erythematosus has been reported.
Usage in Pregnancy
Reserpine
The safety of reserpine for use during pregnancy or lactation has not been established; therefore, the drug should be used in pregnant patients or in women of childbearing potential only when, in the judgment of the physician, it is essential to the welfare of the patient. Increased respiratory tract secretions, nasal congestion, cyanosis, and anorexia may occur in neonates and breast-fed infants of reserpine-treated mothers since reserpine crosses the placental barrier and appears in maternal breast milk.
Hydralazine
Animal studies indicate that hydralazine is teratogenic in mice, possibly in rabbits, and not in rats. Teratogenic effects observed were cleft palate and malformations of facial and cranial bones. Although clinical experience does not include any positive evidence of adverse effects on the human fetus, hydralazine should not be used during pregnancy unless the expected benefit clearly justifies the potential risk to the fetus.
Hydrochlorothiazide
Thiazides cross the placental barrier and appear in cord blood. The use of thiazides in pregnant women requires that the anticipated benefit be weighed against possible hazards to the fetus. These hazards include fetal or neonatal jaundice, thrombocytopenia, and possibly other adverse reactions which have occurred in the adult.
Nursing Mothers: Thiazides appear in breast milk. If the use of the drug is deemed essential, the patient should stop nursing.

Precautions
Reserpine
Since reserpine increases gastrointestinal motility and secretion, it should be used cautiously in patients with a history of peptic ulcer, ulcerative colitis, or gallstones (biliary colic may be precipitated).

Caution should be exercised when treating hypertensive patients with renal insufficiency since they adjust poorly to lowered blood pressure levels.

Use reserpine cautiously with digitalis and quinidine, since cardiac arrhythmias have occurred with rauwolfia preparations.

Preoperative withdrawal of reserpine does not assure that circulatory instability will not occur. It is important that the anesthesiologist be aware of the patient's drug intake and consider this in the overall management, since hypotension has occurred in patients receiving rauwolfia preparations. Anticholinergic and/or adrenergic drugs (*eg,* metaraminol, norepinephrine) have been employed to treat adverse vagocirculatory effects.

Animal tumorigenicity: rodent studies have shown that reserpine is an animal tumorigen, causing an increased incidence of mammary fibroadenomas in female mice, malignant tumors of the seminal vesicles in male mice, and malignant adrenal medullary tumors in male rats. These findings arose in 2 year studies in which the drug was administered in the feed at concentrations of 5 and 10 ppm—about 100 to 300 times the usual human dose. The breast neoplasms are thought to be related to reserpine's prolactin-elevating effect. Several other prolactin-elevating drugs have also been associated with an increased incidence of mammary neoplasia in rodents.

The extent to which these findings indicate a risk to humans is uncertain. Tissue culture experiments show that about one-third of human breast tumors are prolactin-dependent in vitro, a factor of considerable importance if the use of the drug is contemplated in a patient with previously detected breast cancer. The possibility of an increased risk of breast cancer in reserpine users has been studied extensively, however, no firm conclusion has emerged. Although a few epidemiologic studies have suggested a slightly increased risk (less than twofold in all studies except one) in women who have used reserpine, other studies of generally similar design have not confirmed this. Epidemiologic studies conducted using other drugs (neuroleptic agents) that, like reserpine, increase prolactin levels and therefore would be considered rodent mammary carcinogens, have not shown an association between chronic administration of the drug and human mammary tumorigenesis. While long-term clinical observation has not suggested such an association, the available evidence is considered too limited to be conclusive at this time. An association of reserpine intake with pheochromocytoma or tumors of the seminal vesicles has not been explored.
Hydralazine
Myocardial stimulation produced by hydralazine can cause anginal attacks and ECG changes of myocardial ischemia. The drug has been implicated in the production of myocardial infarction. It must, therefore, be used with caution in patients with suspected coronary artery disease.

The "hyperdynamic" circulation caused by hydralazine may accentuate specific cardiovascular inadequacies. An example is that hydralazine may increase pulmonary artery pressure in patients with mitral valvular disease. The drug may reduce the pressor responses to epinephrine. Postural hypotension may result from hydralazine but is less common than with ganglionic blocking agents. Use with caution in patients with cerebral vascular accidents.

In hypertensive patients with normal kidneys who are treated with hydralazine, there is evidence of increased renal blood flow and a maintenance of glomerular filtration rate. In some instances improved renal function has been noted where control values were below normal prior to hydralazine administration. However, as with any antihypertensive agent, hydralazine should be used with caution in patients with advanced renal damage. Peripheral neuritis, evidenced by paresthesias, numbness, and tingling, has been observed. Published evidence suggests an antipyridoxine effect and the addition of pyridoxine to the regimen if symptoms develop.

Blood dyscrasias, consisting of reduction in hemoglobin and red cell count, leukopenia, agranulocytosis, and purpura, have been reported. If such abnormalities develop, discontinue therapy. Periodic blood counts are advised during prolonged therapy.

Hydrochlorothiazide

Periodic determination of serum electrolytes to detect possible electrolyte imbalance should be performed at appropriate intervals. All patients receiving thiazide therapy should be observed for clinical signs of fluid or electrolyte imbalance; namely, hyponatremia, hypochloremic alkalosis, and hypokalemia. Serum and urine electrolyte determinations are particularly important when the patient is vomiting excessively or receiving parenteral fluids. Medication such as digitalis may also influence serum electrolytes. Warning signs are dryness of mouth, thirst, weakness, lethargy, drowsiness, restlessness, muscle pains or cramps, muscular fatigue, hypotension, oliguria, tachycardia, and gastrointestinal disturbance such as nausea or vomiting.

Hypokalemia may develop, especially with brisk diuresis, when severe cirrhosis is present, or during concomitant use of steroids or ACTH.

Interference with adequate oral intake of electrolytes will also contribute to hypokalemia. Hypokalemia can sensitize or exaggerate the response of the heart to the toxic effects of digitalis (eg, increased ventricular irritability).

Any chloride deficit is generally mild and usually does not require specific treatment except under extraordinary circumstances (as in liver disease or renal disease). Dilutional hyponatremia may occur in edematous patients in hot weather; appropriate therapy is water restriction rather than administration of salt, except in rare instances when the hyponatremia is life-threatening. In actual salt depletion, appropriate replacement is the therapy of choice.

Hyperuricemia may occur or frank gout may be precipitated in certain patients receiving thiazide therapy.

Insulin requirements in diabetic patients may be increased, decreased, or unchanged. Latent diabetes may become manifest during thiazide administration.

Thiazide drugs may increase the responsiveness to tubocurarine.

The antihypertensive effects of the drug may be enhanced in the postsympathectomy patient. Thiazides may decrease arterial responsiveness to norepinephrine. This diminution is not sufficient to preclude effectiveness of the pressor agent for therapeutic use.

If progressive renal impairment becomes evident, withholding or discontinuing diuretic therapy should be considered.

Thiazides may decrease serum PBI levels without signs of thyroid disturbance.

Calcium excretion is decreased by thiazides. Pathological changes in the parathyroid gland with hypercalcemia and hypophosphatemia have been observed in a few patients on prolonged thiazide therapy. The common complications of hyperparathyroidism such as renal lithiasis, bone resorption, and peptic ulceration have not been seen. Thiazides should be discontinued before carrying out tests for parathyroid function.

Adverse Reactions
Reserpine

Rauwolfia preparations have caused gastrointestinal reactions including hypersecretion, nausea, vomiting, anorexia, and diarrhea; cardiovascular reactions including angina-like symptoms, arrhythmias (particularly when used concurrently with digitalis or quinidine), and bradycardia; central nervous system reactions including drowsiness, depression, nervousness, paradoxical anxiety, nightmares, rare parkinsonian syndrome and other extrapyramidal tract symptoms, and CNS sensitization manifested by dull sensorium, deafness, glaucoma, uveitis, and optic atrophy. Nasal congestion is a frequent occurrence. Pruritus, rash, dryness of mouth, dizziness, headache, dyspnea, syncope, epistaxis, purpura and other hematologic reactions, impotence or decreased libido, dysuria, muscular aches, conjunctival injection, weight gain, breast engorgement, pseudolactation, and gynecomastia have been reported. These reactions are usually reversible and disappear after the drug is discontinued.

Water retention with edema in patients with hypertensive vascular disease may occur rarely, but the condition generally clears with cessation of therapy or with the administration of a diuretic agent.

Hydralazine

Adverse reactions with hydralazine are usually reversible when dosage is reduced. However, in some cases it may be necessary to discontinue the drug.

Common: Headache; palpitations; anorexia; nausea; vomiting; diarrhea; tachycardia; angina pectoris.

Less Frequent: Nasal congestion; flushing; lacrimation; conjunctivitis; peripheral neuritis, evidenced by paresthesias, numbness, and tingling; edema; dizziness; tremors; muscle cramps; psychotic reactions characterized by depression, disorientation, or anxiety; hypersensitivity (including rash, urticaria, pruritus, fever, chills, arthralgia, eosinophilia, and, rarely, hepatitis); constipation; difficulty in micturition; dyspnea; paralytic ileus; lymphadenopathy; splenomegaly; blood dyscrasias, consisting of reduction in hemoglobin and red cell count, leukopenia, agranulocytosis, and purpura; hypotension; paradoxical pressor response.

Hydrochlorothiazide

Gastrointestinal: Anorexia, gastric irritation, nausea, vomiting, cramping, diarrhea, constipation, jaundice (intrahepatic cholestatic), pancreatitis, sialadenitis

Central Nervous System: Dizziness, vertigo, paresthesias, headache, xanthopsia

Hematologic: Leukopenia, thrombocytopenia, agranulocytosis, aplastic anemia

Cardiovascular: Orthostatic hypotension (may be potentiated by alcohol, barbiturates, or narcotics)

Hypersensitivity: Purpura, photosensitivity, rash, urticaria, necrotizing angiitis, Stevens-Johnson syndrome, and other hypersensitivity reactions

Other: Hyperglycemia, glycosuria, hyperuricemia, muscle spasm, weakness, restlessness

Whenever adverse reactions are moderate or severe, thiazide dosage should be reduced or therapy withdrawn.

Dosage and Administration: As determined by individual titration (see box warning). Usual dosage is 1 to 2 tablets t.i.d.

Since the antihypertensive effects of reserpine are not immediately apparent, maximal reduction in blood pressure from a given dosage may not occur for 2 weeks. For maintenance, adjust dosage to lowest patient requirement.

When necessary, more potent antihypertensives may be added gradually in dosages reduced by at least 50 percent. Watch effects carefully.

Overdosage
Reserpine
Signs and Symptoms

Impairment of consciousness may occur and may range from drowsiness to coma, depending upon the severity of overdosage. Flushing of the skin, conjunctival injection, and pupillary constriction are to be expected. Hypotension, hypothermia, central respiratory depression, and bradycardia may develop in cases of severe overdosage. Diarrhea may also occur.

Treatment

Evacuate stomach contents, taking adequate precautions against aspiration and for the protection of the airway; instill activated charcoal slurry. Treat the effect of reserpine overdosage symptomatically. If hypotension is severe enough to require treatment with a vasopressor, use one having a direct action upon vascular smooth muscle (eg phenylephrine, levarterenol, metaraminol). Since reserpine is long-acting, observe the patient carefully for at least 72 hours, administering treatment as required.

Hydralazine
Signs and Symptoms

Hypotension, tachycardia, headache and generalized skin flushing are to be expected. Myocardial ischemia and cardiac arrhythmia can develop; profound shock can occur in severe overdosage.

Treatment

Evacuate gastric contents, taking adequate precautions against aspiration and for protection of the airway; instill activated charcoal slurry, if general conditions permit. These manipulations may have to be omitted or carried out after cardiovascular status has been stabilized, since they might precipitate cardiac arrhythmias or increase the depth of shock.

Support of the cardiovascular system is of primary importance. Shock should be treated with volume expanders without resorting to use of vasopressors, if possible. If a vasopressor is required, use one that is least likely to precipitate or aggravate cardiac arrhythmia. Digitalization may be necessary. Renal function must be monitored and supported as required.

No experience has been reported with extracorporeal or peritoneal dialysis.

Hydrochlorothiazide
Signs and Symptoms

Diuresis is to be expected; lethargy of varying degree may appear and may progress to coma within a few hours, with minimal depression of respiration and cardiovascular function and without significant serum electrolyte changes or dehydration. The mechanism of CNS depression with thiazide overdosage is unknown.

GI irritation and hypermotility may occur; temporary elevation of BUN has been reported and serum electrolyte changes could occur, especially in patients with impairment of renal function.

Treatment

Evacuate gastric contents but take care to prevent aspiration, especially in the stuporous or comatose patient. GI effects are usually of short duration, but may require symptomatic treatment.

Monitor serum electrolyte levels and renal function; institute supportive measures as required individually to maintain hydration, electrolyte balance, respiration and cardiovascular-renal function.

How Supplied: *Tablets* (light salmon pink, dry-coated), each containing 0.1 mg reserpine, 25 mg hydralazine hydrochloride, and 15 mg hydrochlorothiazide; bottles of 100, 1000 and Accu-Pak® blister units of 100.

C83-28 (Rev. 9/83)

Shown in Product Identification Section, page 409

SERPASIL® ℞
[sir′pah-sill]
(reserpine USP) Tablets

Listed in USP, a Medicare designated compendium.

Indications

Mild essential hypertension; also useful as adjunctive therapy with other antihypertensive agents in the more severe forms of hypertension; relief of symptoms in agitated psychotic states (eg, schizophrenia), primarily in those individuals unable to tolerate phenothiazine derivatives or those who also require antihypertensive medication.

Contraindications: Known hypersensitivity, mental depression (especially with suicidal tendencies), active peptic ulcer, ulcerative colitis, and patients receiving electroconvulsive therapy.

Warnings: Extreme caution should be exercised in treating patients with a history of mental depression. Discontinue the drug at first sign of despondency, early morning insomnia, loss of appe-

Continued on next page

The full prescribing information for each CIBA drug is contained herein and is that in effect as of October 1, 1984.

CIBA—Cont.

tite, impotence, or self-deprecation. Drug-induced depression may persist for several months after drug withdrawal and may be severe enough to result in suicide.

MAO inhibitors should be avoided or used with extreme caution.

Usage in Pregnancy

The safety of reserpine for use during pregnancy or lactation has not been established; therefore, the drug should be used in pregnant patients or in women of childbearing potential only when, in the judgment of the physician, it is essential to the welfare of the patient. Increased respiratory tract secretions, nasal congestion, cyanosis, and anorexia may occur in neonates and breast-fed infants of reserpine-treated mothers since reserpine crosses the placental barrier and also appears in maternal breast milk.

Precautions: Since Serpasil increases gastrointestinal motility and secretion, it should be used cautiously in patients with a history of peptic ulcer, ulcerative colitis, or gallstones (biliary colic may be precipitated).

Caution should be exercised when treating hypertensive patients with renal insufficiency since they adjust poorly to lowered blood pressure levels.

Use Serpasil cautiously with digitalis and quinidine since cardiac arrhythmias have occurred with rauwolfia preparations.

Preoperative withdrawal of reserpine does not assure that circulatory instability will not occur. It is important that the anesthesiologist be aware of the patient's drug intake and consider this in the overall management, since hypotension has occurred in patients receiving rauwolfia preparations. Anticholinergic and/or adrenergic drugs (eg, metaraminol, norepinephrine) have been employed to treat adverse vagocirculatory effects.

Animal tumorigenicity: rodent studies have shown that reserpine is an animal tumorigen, causing an increased incidence of mammary fibroadenomas in female mice, malignant tumors of the seminal vesicles in male mice, and malignant adrenal medullary tumors in male rats. These findings arose in 2 year studies in which the drug was administered in the feed at concentrations of 5 and 10 ppm—about 100 to 300 times the usual human dose. The breast neoplasms are thought to be related to reserpine's prolactin-elevating effect. Several other prolactin-elevating drugs have also been associated with an increased incidence of mammary neoplasia in rodents.

The extent to which these findings indicate a risk to humans is uncertain. Tissue culture experiments show that about one-third of human breast tumors are prolactin-dependent in vitro, a factor of considerable importance if the use of the drug is contemplated in a patient with previously detected breast cancer. The possibility of an increased risk of breast cancer in reserpine users has been studied extensively, however, no firm conclusion has emerged. Although a few epidemiologic studies have suggested a slightly increased risk (less than twofold in all studies except one) in women who have used reserpine, other studies of generally similar design have not confirmed this. Epidemiologic studies conducted using other drugs (neuroleptic agents) that, like reserpine, increase prolactin levels and therefore would be considered rodent mammary carcinogens, have not shown an association between chronic administration of the drug and human mammary tumorigenesis. While long-term clinical observation has not suggested such an association, the available evidence is considered too limited to be conclusive at this time. An association of reserpine intake with pheochromocytoma or tumors of the seminal vesicles has not been explored.

Adverse Reactions: Rauwolfia preparations have caused gastrointestinal reactions including hypersecretion, nausea, vomiting, anorexia, and diarrhea; cardiovascular reactions including angina-like symptoms, arrhythmias (particularly when used concurrently with digitalis or quinidine), bradycardia; central nervous system reactions including drowsiness, depression, nervousness, paradoxical anxiety, nightmares, rare parkinsonian syndrome and other extrapyramidal tract symptoms, and CNS sensitization manifested by dull sensorium, deafness, glaucoma, uveitis, and optic atrophy. Nasal congestion is a frequent occurrence. Pruritus, rash, dryness of mouth, dizziness, headache, dyspnea, syncope, epistaxis, purpura and other hematologic reactions, impotence or decreased libido, dysuria, muscular aches, conjunctival injection, weight gain, breast engorgement, pseudolactation, and gynecomastia have been reported. These reactions are usually reversible and usually disappear after the drug is discontinued.

Water retention with edema in patients with hypertensive vascular disease may occur rarely, but the condition generally clears with cessation of therapy or with the administration of a diuretic agent.

Dosage and Administration

For Hypertension: In the average patient not receiving other antihypertensive agents, the usual initial dose is 0.5 mg daily for 1 or 2 weeks. For maintenance, reduce to 0.1 mg to 0.25 mg daily. Higher doses should be used cautiously, because serious mental depression and other side effects may be increased considerably.

For Psychiatric Disorders: The usual initial dose is 0.5 mg, with a range of 0.1 mg to 1.0 mg. Adjust dosage upward or downward according to the patient's response.

Concomitant use of Serpasil with ganglionic blocking agents, guanethidine, veratrum, hydralazine, methyldopa, chlorthalidone, or thiazides necessitates careful titration of dosage with each agent.

Overdosage

Signs and Symptoms

Impairment of consciousness may occur and may range from drowsiness to coma, depending upon the severity of overdosage. Flushing of the skin, conjunctival injection, and pupillary constriction are to be expected. Hypotension, hypothermia, central respiratory depression, and bradycardia may develop in cases of severe overdosage. Diarrhea may also occur.

Treatment

Evacuate stomach contents, taking adequate precautions against aspiration and for the protection of the airway; instill activated charcoal slurry.

Treat the effects of reserpine overdosage symptomatically. If hypotension is severe enough to require treatment with a vasopressor, use one having a direct action upon vascular smooth muscle (eg, phenylephrine, levarterenol, metaraminol). Since reserpine is long-acting, observe the patient carefully for at least 72 hours, administering treatment as required.

How Supplied

Tablets 0.1 mg — white (imprinted 35 CIBA)
Bottles of 100 ....NDC 0083-0035-30
Bottles of 1000 ....NDC 0083-0035-40
Tablets 0.25 mg — white, scored (imprinted 36 CIBA)
Bottles of 100 ....NDC 0083-0036-30
Bottles of 500 ....NDC 0083-0036-35
Bottles of 1000 ....NDC 0083-0036-40
Consumer Pack — One Unit
(12 bottles — 100 tablets
 each) ....NDC 0083-0036-65
Dispense in tight, light-resistant container (USP).
C83-24 (Rev. 9/83)
Shown in Product Identification Section, page 409

SERPASIL® ℞
[sir′pah-sill]
(reserpine USP)
Parenteral Solution

Listed in USP, a Medicare designated compendium.

Indications: Hypertensive emergencies, such as acute hypertensive encephalopathy, in which it is desired to reduce blood pressure rapidly; psychiatric conditions only to initiate treatment in those patients unable to accept oral medication or to control symptoms of extreme agitation.

Contraindications: Known hypersensitivity, mental depression (especially with suicidal tendencies), active peptic ulcer, ulcerative colitis, and patients receiving electroconvulsive therapy.

Warnings: Extreme caution should be exercised in treating patients with a history of mental depression. Discontinue the drug at first sign of despondency, early morning insomnia, loss of appetite, impotence, or self-deprecation. Drug-induced depression may persist for several months after drug withdrawal and may be severe enough to result in suicide.

MAO inhibitors should be avoided or used with extreme caution.

Usage in Pregnancy

The safety of reserpine for use during pregnancy or lactation has not been established; therefore, the drug should be used in pregnant patients or in women of childbearing potential only when, in the judgment of the physician, it is essential to the welfare of the patient. Increased respiratory tract secretions, nasal congestion, cyanosis, and anorexia may occur in neonates and breast-fed infants of reserpine-treated mothers since reserpine crosses the placental barrier and also appears in maternal breast milk.

Precautions: Since Serpasil increases gastrointestinal motility and secretion, it should be used cautiously in patients with a history of peptic ulcer, ulcerative colitis, or gallstones (biliary colic may be precipitated).

Caution should be exercised when treating hypertensive patients with renal insufficiency since they adjust poorly to lowered blood pressure levels.

Use Serpasil cautiously with digitalis and quinidine since cardiac arrhythmias have occurred with rauwolfia preparations.

Preoperative withdrawal of reserpine does not assure that circulatory instability will not occur. It is important that the anesthesiologist be aware of the patient's drug intake and consider this in the overall management, since hypotension has occurred in patients receiving rauwolfia preparations. Anticholinergic and/or adrenergic drugs (eg, metaraminol, norepinephrine) have been employed to treat adverse vagocirculatory effects.

Animal tumorigenicity: rodent studies have shown that reserpine is an animal tumorigen, causing an increased incidence of mammary fibroadenomas in female mice, malignant tumors of the seminal vesicles in male mice, and malignant adrenal medullary tumors in male rats. These findings arose in 2 year studies in which the drug was administered in the feed at concentrations of 5 and 10 ppm—about 100 to 300 times the usual human dose. The breast neoplasms are thought to be related to reserpine's prolactin-elevating effect. Several other prolactin-elevating drugs have also been associated with an increased incidence of mammary neoplasia in rodents.

The extent to which these findings indicate a risk to humans is uncertain. Tissue culture experiments show that about one-third of human breast tumors are prolactin-dependent in vitro, a factor of considerable importance if the use of the drug is contemplated in a patient with previously detected breast cancer. The possibility of an increased risk of breast cancer in reserpine users has been studied extensively, however, no firm conclusion has emerged. Although a few epidemiologic studies have suggested a slightly increased risk (less than twofold in all studies except one) in women who have used reserpine, other studies of generally similar design have not confirmed this. Epidemiologic studies conducted using other drugs (neuroleptic agents) that, like reserpine, increase prolactin levels and therefore would be considered rodent mammary carcinogens, have not shown an association between chronic administration of the drug and human mammary tumorigenesis. While long-term clinical observation has not suggested such an association, the available evidence is considered too limited to be conclusive at this time. An association of reserpine intake with pheochromocytoma or tumors of the seminal vesicles has not been explored.

Adverse Reactions: Rauwolfia preparations have caused gastrointestinal reactions including hypersecretion, nausea, vomiting, anorexia, and diarrhea; cardiovascular reactions including angina-like symptoms, arrhythmias (particularly when used concurrently with digitalis or quinidine), bradycardia; central nervous system reactions including drowsiness, depression, nervousness, paradoxical anxiety, nightmares, rare parkinsonian syndrome and other extrapyramidal tract symptoms, and CNS sensitization manifested by dull sensorium, deafness, glaucoma, uveitis, and optic atrophy. Nasal congestion is a frequent occurrence. Pruritus, rash, dryness of mouth, dizziness, headache, dyspnea, syncope, epistaxis, purpura and other hematologic reactions, impotence or decreased libido, dysuria, muscular aches, conjunctival injection, weight gain, breast engorgement, pseudolactation, and gynecomastia have been reported. These reactions are usually reversible and usually disappear after the drug is discontinued.

Water retention with edema in patients with hypertensive vascular disease may occur rarely, but the condition generally clears with cessation of therapy or with the administration of a diuretic agent.

Dosage and Administration: Serpasil may be administered intramuscularly in the short-term treatment of hypertensive crises. Because of the varying responsiveness, a titration procedure should be used. An initial dose of 0.5 to 1 mg intramuscularly is followed at intervals of 3 hours, if necessary, by doses of 2 and 4 mg until the blood pressure falls to the desired level. If the 4-mg dose is ineffective, other antihypertensive agents should be used. An initial dose larger than 0.5 mg may induce severe hypotension, particularly in patients with cerebral hemorrhage.

Serpasil may be administered intramuscularly in psychiatric emergencies to initiate treatment in those patients unable to accept oral medication or to control extreme agitation. The usual dose is from 2.5 mg to 5.0 mg, following a small initial dose to test patient responsiveness.

Concomitant use of Serpasil with ganglionic blocking agents, guanethidine, veratrum, hydralazine, methyldopa, chlorthalidone, or thiazides necessitates careful titration of dosage with each agent.

Overdosage
Signs and Symptoms
Impairment of consciousness may occur and may range from drowsiness to coma, depending upon the severity of overdosage. Flushing of the skin, conjunctival injection, and pupillary constriction are to be expected. Hypotension, hypothermia, central respiratory depression, and bradycardia may develop in cases of severe overdosage. Diarrhea may also occur.

Treatment
Hypotension is likely to require major therapeutic attention. If a vasopressor is necessary, use one having a direct action upon vascular smooth muscle (eg, phenylephrine, levarterenol, metaraminol).

If bradycardia becomes marked, especially with cardiac arrhythmia, consider use of vagal blocking agents along with other appropriate measures. Treat other effects of reserpine overdosage symptomatically. Since reserpine is long-acting, observe the patient carefully for at least 72 hours, administering treatment as required.

How Supplied
Parenteral Solution: Each ml contains 2.5 mg reserpine, 0.1 ml dimethylacetamide, 10 mg adipic acid, 0.1 mg versene, 0.01 ml benzyl alcohol, 0.05 ml polyethylene glycol, 0.5 mg ascorbic acid, and 0.1 mg sodium sulfite in water. *Ampuls,* 2 ml; cartons of 5.

C83-25 (Rev. 9/83)

SERPASIL®-APRESOLINE® ℞
[*sir'pah-sill a-press'oh-leen*]
hydrochloride
(reserpine and hydralazine hydrochloride)
Combination Tablets

Warning
This fixed combination drug is not indicated for initial therapy of hypertension. Hypertension requires therapy titrated to the individual patient. If the fixed combination represents the dosage so determined, its use may be more convenient in patient management. The treatment of hypertension is not static, but must be reevaluated as conditions in each patient warrant.

Indications
Hypertension. (See box warning.)
Contraindications
Reserpine
Known hypersensitivity, mental depression (especially with suicidal tendencies), active peptic ulcer, ulcerative colitis, and patients receiving electroconvulsive therapy.
Hydralazine
Hypersensitivity to hydralazine; coronary artery disease; and mitral valvular rheumatic heart disease.
Warnings
Reserpine
Extreme caution should be exercised in treating patients with a history of mental depression. Discontinue the drug at first sign of despondency, early morning insomnia, loss of appetite, impotence, or self-deprecation. Drug-induced depression may persist for several months after drug withdrawal and may be severe enough to result in suicide.
MAO inhibitors should be avoided or used with extreme caution.
Hydralazine
Hydralazine may produce in a few patients a clinical picture simulating systemic lupus erythematosus. In such patients hydralazine should be discontinued unless the benefit-to- risk determination requires continued antihypertensive therapy with this drug. Symptoms and signs usually regress when the drug is discontinued but residua have been detected many years later. Long-term treatment with steroids may be necessary.
Complete blood counts, L. E. cell preparations, and antinuclear antibody titer determinations are indicated before and periodically during prolonged therapy with hydralazine, even though the patient is asymptomatic. These studies are also indicated if the patient develops arthralgia, fever, chest pain, continued malaise, or other unexplained signs or symptoms.
A positive antinuclear antibody titer and/or positive L. E. cell reaction requires that the physician carefully weigh the implications of the test results against the benefits to be derived from antihypertensive therapy with hydralazine.
Use MAO inhibitors with caution in patients receiving hydralazine.
When other potent parenteral antihypertensive drugs, such as diazoxide, are used in combination with hydralazine, patients should be continuously observed for several hours for any excessive fall in blood pressure. Profound hypotensive episodes may occur when diazoxide injection and Apresoline (hydralazine hydrochloride) are used concomitantly.
Usage in Pregnancy
Reserpine
The safety of reserpine for use during pregnancy or lactation has not been established; therefore, the drug should be used in pregnant patients or in women of childbearing potential only when, in the judgment of the physician, it is essential to the welfare of the patient. Increased respiratory tract secretions, nasal congestion, cyanosis, and anorexia may occur in neonates and breast-fed infants of reserpine-treated mothers since reserpine crosses the placental barrier and appears in maternal breast milk.
Hydralazine
Animal studies indicate that hydralazine is teratogenic in mice, possibly in rabbits, and not in rats. Teratogenic effects observed were cleft palate and malformations of facial and cranial bones. Although clinical experience does not include any positive evidence of adverse effects on the human fetus, hydralazine should not be used during pregnancy unless the expected benefit clearly justifies the potential risk to the fetus.
Precautions
Reserpine
Since reserpine increases gastrointestinal motility and secretion, it should be used cautiously in patients with a history of peptic ulcer, ulcerative colitis, or gallstones (biliary colic may be precipitated).
Caution should be exercised when treating hypertensive patients with renal insufficiency, since they adjust poorly to lowered blood pressure levels.
Use reserpine cautiously with digitalis and quinidine since cardiac arrhythmias have occurred with rauwolfia preparations.
Preoperative withdrawal of reserpine does not assure that circulatory instability will not occur. It is important that the anesthesiologist be aware of the patient's drug intake and consider this in the overall management, since hypotension has occurred in patients receiving rauwolfia preparations. Anticholinergic and/or adrenergic drugs (eg, metaraminol, norepinephrine) have been employed to treat adverse vagocirculatory effects.
Animal tumorigenicity: rodent studies have shown that reserpine is an animal tumorigen, causing an increased incidence of mammary fibroadenomas in female mice, malignant tumors of the seminal vesicles in male mice, and malignant adrenal medullary tumors in male rats. These findings arose in 2 year studies in which the drug was administered in the feed at concentrations of 5 and 10 ppm—about 100 to 300 times the usual human dose. The breast neoplasms are thought to be related to reserpine's prolactin-elevating effect. Several other prolactin-elevating drugs have also been associated with an increased incidence of mammary neoplasia in rodents.
The extent to which these findings indicate a risk to humans is uncertain. Tissue culture experiments show that about one-third of human breast tumors are prolactin-dependent in vitro, a factor of considerable importance if the use of the drug is contemplated in a patient with previously detected breast cancer. The possibility of an increased risk of breast cancer in reserpine users has been studied extensively, however, no firm conclusion has emerged. Although a few epidemiologic studies have suggested a slighty increased risk (less than twofold in all studies except one) in women who have used reserpine, other studies of generally similar design have not confirmed this. Epidemiologic studies conducted using other drugs (neuroleptic agents) that, like reserpine, increse prolactin levels and therefore would be considered rodent mammary carcinogens, have not shown an association between chronic administration of the drug and human mammary tumorigenesis. While long-term clinical observation has not suggested such an association, the available evidence is considered too limited to be conclusive at this time. An association of reserpine intake with pheochromocytoma or tumors of the seminal vesicles has not been explored.
Hydralazine
Myocardial stimulation produced by hydralazine can cause anginal attacks and ECG changes of myocardial ischemia. The drug has been implicated in the production of myocardial infarction. It

Continued on next page

The full prescribing information for each CIBA drug is contained herein and is that in effect as of October 1, 1984.

CIBA—Cont.

must, therefore, be used with caution in patients with suspected coronary artery disease.

The "hyperdynamic" circulation caused by hydralazine may accentuate specific cardiovascular inadequacies. An example is that hydralazine may increase pulmonary artery pressure in patients with mitral valvular disease. The drug may reduce the pressor responses to epinephrine. Postural hypotension may result from hydralazine but is less common than with ganglionic blocking agents. Use with caution in patients with cerebral vascular accidents.

In hypertensive patients with normal kidneys who are treated with hydralazine, there is evidence of increased renal blood flow and a maintenance of glomerular filtration rate. In some instances improved renal function has been noted where control values were below normal prior to hydralazine administration. However, as with any antihypertensive agent, hydralazine should be used with caution in patients with advanced renal damage.

Peripheral neuritis, evidenced by paresthesias, numbness, and tingling, has been observed. Published evidence suggests an antipyridoxine effect and the addition of pyridoxine to the regimen if symptoms develop.

Blood dyscrasias, consisting of reduction in hemoglobin and red cell count, leukopenia, agranulocytosis, and purpura, have been reported. If such abnormalities develop, discontinue therapy. Periodic blood counts are advised during prolonged therapy.

The Serpasil-Apresoline tablets (#1 and #2) contain FD&C Yellow No. 5 (tartrazine) which may cause allergic-type reactions (including bronchial asthma) in certain susceptible individuals. Although the overall incidence of FD&C Yellow No. 5 (tartrazine) sensitivity in the general population is low, it is frequently seen in patients who also have aspirin hypersensitivity.

Adverse Reactions
Reserpine
Rauwolfia preparations have caused gastrointestinal reactions including hypersecretion, nausea, vomiting, anorexia, and diarrhea; cardiovascular reactions including angina-like symptoms, arrhythmias (particularly when used concurrently with digitalis or quinidine), and bradycardia; central nervous system reactions including drowsiness, depression, nervousness, paradoxical anxiety, nightmares, rare parkinsonian syndrome and other extrapyramidal tract symptoms, and CNS sensitization manifested by dull sensorium, deafness, glaucoma, uveitis, and optic atrophy. Nasal congestion is a frequent occurrence. Pruritus, rash, dryness of mouth, dizziness, headache, dyspnea, syncope, epistaxis, purpura and other hematologic reactions, impotence or decreased libido, dysuria, muscular aches, conjunctival injection, weight gain, breast engorgement, pseudolactation, and gynecomastia have been reported. These reactions are usually reversible and disappear after the drug is discontinued.

Water retention with edema in patients with hypertensive vascular disease may occur rarely, but the condition generally clears with cessation of therapy or with the administration of a diuretic agent.

Hydralazine
Adverse reactions with hydralazine are usually reversible when dosage is reduced. However, in some cases it may be necessary to discontinue the drug.

Common: Headache; palpitations; anorexia; nausea; vomiting; diarrhea; tachycardia; angina pectoris.

Less Frequent: Nasal congestion; flushing; lacrimation; conjunctivitis; peripheral neuritis, evidenced by paresthesias, numbness, and tingling; edema; dizziness; tremors; muscle cramps; psychotic reactions characterized by depression, disorientation, or anxiety; hypersensitivity (including rash, urticaria, pruritus, fever, chills, arthralgia, eosinophilia, and, rarely, hepatitis); constipation; difficulty in micturition; dyspnea; paralytic ileus; lymphadenopathy; splenomegaly; blood dyscrasias, consisting of reduction in hemoglobin and red cell count, leukopenia, agranulocytosis, and purpura; hypotension; paradoxical pressor response.

Dosage and Administration: As determined by individual titration (see box warning).

Step 1:
a. Start with reserpine alone. Average dosage: 0.5 mg daily.
b. Continue for at least one week. If results prove satisfactory—as they will in many cases—no other medication is required. For maintenance, reduce dosage to 0.25 mg or less daily.

Step 2:
a. Should more than the therapeutic action of reserpine be indicated, therapy with Tablet #2 (reserpine 0.2 mg/hydralazine hydrochloride 50 mg) should be initiated—one tablet 4 times a day.
b. When reduction of dosage is indicated, Tablet #1 (reserpine 0.1 mg/hydralazine hydrochloride 25 mg) should be used—one tablet 4 times a day.

Side effects associated with hydralazine (headache, tachycardia, palpitation) are seldom encountered when the patient has been "primed" with reserpine before combination therapy is begun. Should side effects appear, however, reduction of dosage to one Tablet #1 two to four times a day for a few days will usually alleviate them.

In cases where further individualization of dosage is necessary, the adjustment may be made by increasing or decreasing the dosage of reserpine and/or hydralazine.

For maintenance, daily dosage of hydralazine should probably not exceed 200 mg, nor should the dosage of reserpine exceed 1 mg.

For Patients on Hydralazine.
Patients already on this drug may be given a combination tablet as required. With the addition of reserpine, it is usually possible to reduce the dose of hydralazine.

Overdosage
Reserpine
Signs and Symptoms
Impairment of consciousness may occur and may range from drowsiness to coma, depending upon the severity of overdosage. Flushing of the skin, conjunctival injection, and pupillary constriction are to be expected. Hypotension, hypothermia, central respiratory depression, and bradycardia may develop in cases of severe overdosage. Diarrhea may also occur.

Treatment
Evacuate stomach contents, taking adequate precautions against aspiration and for the protection of the airway; instill activated charcoal slurry. Treat the effects of reserpine overdosage symptomatically. If hypotension is severe enough to require treatment with a vasopressor, use one having a direct action upon vascular smooth muscle (eg, phenylephrine, levarterenol, metaraminol). Since reserpine is long-acting, observe the patient carefully for at least 72 hours, administering treatment as required.

Hydralazine
Signs and Symptoms
Hypotension, tachycardia, headache and generalized skin flushing are to be expected. Myocardial ischemia and cardiac arrhythmia can develop; profound shock can occur in severe overdosage.

Treatment
Evacuate gastric contents, taking adequate precautions against aspiration and for protection of the airway; instill activated charcoal slurry, if general conditions permit. These manipulations may have to be omitted or carried out after cardiovascular status has been stabilized, since they might precipitate cardiac arrhythmias or increase the depth of shock.

Support of the cardiovascular system is of primary importance. Shock should be treated with volume expanders without resorting to use of vasopressors, if possible. If a vasopressor is required, use one that is least likely to precipitate or aggravate cardiac arrhythmia. Digitalization may be necessary. Renal function must be monitored and supported as required.

No experience has been reported with extracorporeal or peritoneal dialysis.

How Supplied
Tablets #2 (yellow, dry-coated), each containing 0.2 mg reserpine and 50 mg hydralazine hydrochloride; bottles of 100.
Tablets #1 (yellow, dry-coated), each containing 0.1 mg reserpine and 25 mg hydralazine hydrochloride; bottles of 100.
Dispense in tight, light-resistant container (USP).

C83-26 (Rev. 9/83)
Shown in Product Identification Section, page 409

SERPASIL®-ESIDRIX®   ℞
[sir'pah-sill ess'ah-dricks]
(reserpine and hydrochlorothiazide)
Combination Tablets

> **Warning**
> This fixed combination drug is not indicated for initial therapy of hypertension. Hypertension requires therapy titrated to the individual patient. If the fixed combination represents the dosage so determined, its use may be more convenient in patient management. The treatment of hypertension is not static, but must be reevaluated as conditions in each patient warrant.

Indications
Hypertension. (See box warning.)

Contraindications
Reserpine
Known hypersensitivity, mental depression (especially with suicidal tendencies), active peptic ulcer, ulcerative colitis, and patients receiving electroconvulsive therapy.

Hydrochlorothiazide
Anuria; hypersensitivity to this or other sulfonamide-derived drugs.

Warnings
Reserpine
Extreme caution should be exercised in treating patients with a history of mental depression. Discontinue the drug at first sign of despondency, early morning insomnia, loss of appetite, impotence, or self-deprecation. Drug-induced depression may persist for several months after drug withdrawal and may be severe enough to result in suicide.

MAO inhibitors should be avoided or used with extreme caution.

Hydrochlorothiazide
Use with caution in severe renal disease. In patients with renal disease, thiazides may precipitate azotemia. Cumulative effects of the drug may develop in patients with impaired renal function. Thiazides should be used with caution in patients with impaired hepatic function or progressive liver disease, since minor alterations of fluid and electrolyte imbalance may precipitate hepatic coma.

Thiazides may add to or potentiate the action of other antihypertensive drugs. Potentiation occurs with ganglionic or peripheral adrenergic blocking drugs.

Sensitivity reactions are more likely to occur in patients with a history of allergy or bronchial asthma.

The possibility of exacerbation or activation of systemic lupus erythematosus has been reported.

Usage in Pregnancy
Reserpine
The safety of reserpine for use during pregnancy or lactation has not been established; therefore, the drug should be used in pregnant patients or in women of childbearing potential only when, in the judgment of the physician, it is essential to the welfare of the patient. Increased respiratory tract secretions, nasal congestion, cyanosis, and anorexia may occur in neonates and breast-fed infants of reserpine-treated mothers, since reserpine crosses the placental barrier and appears in maternal breast milk.

Hydrochlorothiazide

Thiazides cross the placental barrier and appear in cord blood. The use of thiazides in pregnant women requires that the anticipated benefit be weighed against possible hazards to the fetus. These hazards include fetal or neonatal jaundice, thrombocytopenia, and possibly other adverse reactions which have occurred in the adult.

Nursing Mothers: Thiazides appear in breast milk. If the use of the drug is deemed essential, the patient should stop nursing.

Precautions
Reserpine

Since reserpine increases gastrointestinal motility and secretion, it should be used cautiously in patients with a history of peptic ulcer, ulcerative colitis, or gallstones (biliary colic may be precipitated).

Caution should be exercised when treating hypertensive patients with renal insufficiency since they adjust poorly to lowered blood pressure levels.

Use reserpine cautiously with digitalis and quinidine since cardiac arrhythmias have occurred with rauwolfia preparations.

Preoperative withdrawal of reserpine does not assure that circulatory instability will not occur. It is important that the anesthesiologist be aware of the patient's drug intake and consider this in the overall management, since hypotension has occurred in patients receiving rauwolfia preparations. Anticholinergic and/or adrenergic drugs (*eg*, metaraminol, norepinephrine) have been employed to treat adverse vagocirculatory effects.

Animal tumorigenicity: rodent studies have shown that reserpine is an animal tumorigen, causing an increased incidence of mammary fibroadenomas in female mice, malignant tumors of the seminal vesicles in male mice, and malignant adrenal medullary tumors in male rats. These findings arose in 2 year studies in which the drug was administered in the feed at concentrations of 5 and 10 ppm—about 100 to 300 times the usual human dose. The breast neoplasms are thought to be related to reserpine's prolactin-elevating effect. Several other prolactin-elevating drugs have also been associated with an increased incidence of mammary neoplasia in rodents.

The extent to which these findings indicate a risk to humans is uncertain. Tissue culture experiments show that about one-third of human breast tumors are prolactin-dependent in vitro, a factor of considerable importance if the use of the drug is contemplated in a patient with previously detected breast cancer. The possibility of an increased risk of breast cancer in reserpine users has been studied extensively, however, no firm conclusion has emerged. Although a few epidemiologic studies have suggested a slightly increased risk (less than twofold in all studies except one) in women who have used reserpine, other studies of generally similar design have not confirmed this. Epidemiologic studies conducted using other drugs (neuroleptic agents) that, like reserpine, increase prolactin levels and therefore would be considered rodent mammary carcinogens, have not shown an association between chronic administration of the drug and human mammary tumorigenesis. While long-term clinical observation has not suggested such an association, the available evidence is considered too limited to be conclusive at this time. An association of reserpine intake with pheochromocytoma or tumors of the seminal vesicles has not been explored.

Hydrochlorothiazide

Periodic determination of serum electrolytes to detect possible electrolyte imbalance should be performed at appropriate intervals. All patients receiving thiazide therapy should be observed for clinical signs of fluid or electrolyte imbalance; namely, hyponatremia, hypochloremic alkalosis, and hypokalemia. Serum and urine electrolyte determinations are particularly important when the patient is vomiting excessively or receiving parenteral fluids. Medication such as digitalis may also influence serum electrolytes. Warning signs are dryness of mouth, thirst, weakness, lethargy, drowsiness, restlessness, muscle pains or cramps, muscular fatigue, hypotension, oliguria, tachycardia, and gastrointestinal disturbance such as nausea or vomiting.

Hypokalemia may develop, especially with brisk diuresis, when severe cirrhosis is present, or during concomitant use of steroids or ACTH. Interference with adequate oral intake of electrolytes will also contribute to hypokalemia. Hypokalemia can sensitize or exaggerate the response of the heart to the toxic effects of digitalis (*eg*, increased ventricular irritability).

Any chloride deficit is generally mild and usually does not require specific treatment except under extraordinary circumstances (as in liver disease or renal disease). Dilutional hyponatremia may occur in edematous patients in hot weather; appropriate therapy is water restriction rather than administration of salt, except in rare instances when the hyponatremia is life-threatening. In actual salt depletion, appropriate replacement is the therapy of choice.

Hyperuricemia may occur or frank gout may be precipitated in certain patients receiving thiazide therapy.

Insulin requirements in diabetic patients may be increased, decreased, or unchanged. Latent diabetes may become manifest during thiazide administration.

Thiazide drugs may increase the responsiveness to tubocurarine.

The antihypertensive effects of the drug may be enhanced in the postsympathectomy patient. Thiazides may decrease arterial responsiveness to norepinephrine. This diminution is not sufficient to preclude effectiveness of the pressor agent for therapeutic use.

If progressive renal impairment becomes evident, withholding or discontinuing diuretic therapy should be considered.

Thiazides may decrease serum PBI levels without signs of thyroid disturbance.

Calcium excretion is decreased by thiazides. Pathological changes in the parathyroid gland with hypercalcemia and hypophosphatemia have been observed in a few patients on prolonged thiazide therapy. The common complications of hyperparathyroidism such as renal lithiasis, bone resorption, and peptic ulceration have not been seen. Thiazides should be discontinued before carrying out tests for parathyroid function.

The Serpasil-Esidrix tablets (#1 and #2) contain FD&C Yellow No. 5 (tartrazine) which may cause allergic-type reactions (including bronchial asthma) in certain susceptible individuals. Although the overall incidence of FD&C Yellow No. 5 (tartrazine) sensitivity in the general population is low, it is frequently seen in patients who also have aspirin hypersensitivity.

Adverse Reactions
Reserpine

Rauwolfia preparations have caused gastrointestinal reactions including hypersecretion, nausea, vomiting, anorexia, and diarrhea; cardiovascular reactions including angina-like symptoms, arrhythmias (particularly when used concurrently with digitalis or quinidine), and bradycardia; central nervous system reactions including drowsiness, depression, nervousness, paradoxical anxiety, nightmares, rare parkinsonian syndrome and other extrapyramidal tract symptoms, and CNS sensitization manifested by dull sensorium, deafness, glaucoma, uveitis, and optic atrophy. Nasal congestion is a frequent occurrence. Pruritus, rash, dryness of mouth, dizziness, headache, dyspnea, syncope, epistaxis, purpura and other hematologic reactions, impotence or decreased libido, dysuria, muscular aches, conjunctival injection, weight gain, breast engorgement, pseudolactation, and gynecomastia have been reported. These reactions are usually reversible and disappear after the drug is discontinued.

Water retention with edema in patients with hypertensive vascular disease may occur rarely, but the condition generally clears with cessation of therapy or with the administration of a diuretic agent.

Hydrochlorothiazide

Gastrointestinal: Anorexia, gastric irritation, nausea, vomiting, cramping, diarrhea, constipation, jaundice (intrahepatic cholestatic), pancreatitis, sialadenitis

Central Nervous System: Dizziness, vertigo, paresthesias, headache, xanthopsia

Hematologic: Leukopenia, thrombocytopenia, agranulocytosis, aplastic anemia

Cardiovascular: Orthostatic hypotension (may be potentiated by alcohol, barbiturates, or narcotics)

Hypersensitivity: Purpura, photosensitivity, rash, urticaria, necrotizing angiitis, Stevens-Johnson syndrome, and other hypersensitivity reactions

Other: Hyperglycemia, glycosuria, hyperuricemia, muscle spasm, weakness, restlessness

Whenever adverse reactions are moderate or severe, thiazide dosage should be reduced or therapy withdrawn.

Dosage and Administration: As determined by individual titration (see box warning).

Usual dosage is 2 Tablets #2 daily in single or divided doses. For patients requiring less hydrochlorothiazide, substitute Tablets #1.

Since antihypertensive effects of reserpine are not immediately apparent, maximal reduction in blood pressure from a given dosage may not occur for 2 weeks. For maintenance, reduce dosage to lowest effective level; as little as 1 tablet daily may suffice.

When necessary, more potent antihypertensive agents may be added gradually in reduced dosages. Watch effects carefully.

Overdosage
Reserpine
Signs and Symptoms

Impairment of consciousness may occur and may range from drowsiness to coma, depending upon the severity of overdosage. Flushing of the skin, conjunctival injection, and pupillary constriction are to be expected. Hypotension, hypothermia, central respiratory depression, and bradycardia may develop in cases of severe overdosage. Diarrhea may also occur.

Treatment

Evacuate stomach contents, taking adequate precautions against aspiration and for the protection of the airway; instill activated charcoal slurry.

Treat the effects of reserpine overdosage symptomatically. If hypotension is severe enough to require treatment with a vasopressor, use one having a direct action upon vascular smooth muscle (*eg*, phenylephrine, levarterenol, metaraminol). Since reserpine is long-acting, observe the patient carefully for at least 72 hours, administering treatment as required.

Hydrochlorothiazide
Signs and Symptoms

Diuresis is to be expected; lethargy of varying degree may appear and may progress to coma within a few hours, with minimal depression of respiration and cardiovascular function and without significant serum electrolyte changes or dehydration. The mechanism of CNS depression with thiazide overdosage is unknown.

GI irritation and hypermotility may occur; temporary elevation of BUN has been reported and serum electrolyte changes could occur, especially in patients with impairment of renal function.

Treatment

Evacuate gastric contents but take care to prevent aspiration, especially in the stuporous or comatose patient. GI effects are usually of short duration, but may require symptomatic treatment.

Monitor serum electrolyte levels and renal function; institute supportive measures as required individually to maintain hydration, electrolyte balance, respiration and cardiovascular-renal function.

Continued on next page

The full prescribing information for each CIBA drug is contained herein and is that in effect as of October 1, 1984.

CIBA—Cont.

How Supplied: *Tablets #1* (light orange), each containing 0.1 mg reserpine and 25 mg hydrochlorothiazide; bottles of 100 and 1000.
Tablets #2 (light orange), each containing 0.1 mg reserpine and 50 mg hydrochlorothiazide; bottles of 100 and 1000.
Dispense in tight, light-resistant container (USP).
C83-27 (Rev. 9/83)
Shown in Product Identification Section, page 409

SLOW-K® ℞
[sloe-kay]
(potassium chloride)
slow-release tablets

Description: Slow-K is a sugar-coated (not enteric-coated) tablet containing 600 mg potassium chloride (equivalent to 8 mEq) in a wax matrix. This formulation is intended to provide a controlled release of potassium from the matrix to minimize the likelihood of producing high localized concentrations of potassium within the gastrointestinal tract.

Actions: Potassium ion is the principal intracellular cation of most body tissues. Potassium ions participate in a number of essential physiological processes, including the maintenance of intracellular tonicity, the transmission of nerve impulses, the contraction of cardiac, skeletal, and smooth muscle and the maintenance of normal renal function.

Potassium depletion may occur whenever the rate of potassium loss through renal excretion and/or loss from the gastrointestinal tract exceeds the rate of potassium intake. Such depletion usually develops slowly as a consequence of prolonged therapy with oral diuretics, primary or secondary hyperaldosteronism, diabetic ketoacidosis, severe diarrhea, or inadequate replacement of potassium in patients on prolonged parenteral nutrition. Potassium depletion due to these causes is usually accompanied by a concomitant deficiency of chloride and is manifested by hypokalemia and metabolic alkalosis. Potassium depletion may produce weakness, fatigue, disturbances of cardiac rhythm (primarily ectopic beats), prominent U-waves in the electrocardiogram, and in advanced cases flaccid paralysis and/or impaired ability to concentrate urine.

Potassium depletion associated with metabolic alkalosis is managed by correcting the fundamental causes of the deficiency whenever possible and administering supplemental potassium chloride, in the form of high potassium food or potassium chloride solution or tablets.

In rare circumstances (eg, patients with renal tubular acidosis) potassium depletion may be associated with metabolic acidosis and hyperchloremia. In such patients potassium replacement should be accomplished with potassium salts other than the chloride, such as potassium bicarbonate, potassium citrate, or potassium acetate.

Indications: BECAUSE OF REPORTS OF INTESTINAL AND GASTRIC ULCERATION AND BLEEDING WITH SLOW-RELEASE POTASSIUM CHLORIDE PREPARATIONS, THESE DRUGS SHOULD BE RESERVED FOR THOSE PATIENTS WHO CANNOT TOLERATE OR REFUSE TO TAKE LIQUID OR EFFERVESCENT POTASSIUM PREPARATIONS OR FOR PATIENTS IN WHOM THERE IS A PROBLEM OF COMPLIANCE WITH THESE PREPARATIONS.

1. For therapeutic use in patients with hypokalemia with or without metabolic alkalosis; in digitalis intoxication and in patients with hypokalemic familial periodic paralysis.
2. For prevention of potassium depletion when the dietary intake of potassium is inadequate in the following conditions: Patients receiving digitalis and diuretics for congestive heart failure; hepatic cirrhosis with ascites; states of aldosterone excess with normal renal function; potassium-losing nephropathy, and certain diarrheal states.
3. The use of potassium salts in patients receiving diuretics for uncomplicated essential hypertension is often unnecessary when such patients have a normal dietary pattern. Serum potassium should be checked periodically, however, and, if hypokalemia occurs, dietary supplementation with potassium-containing foods may be adequate to control milder cases. In more severe cases supplementation with potassium salts may be indicated.

Contraindications: Potassium supplements are contraindicated in patients with hyperkalemia since a further increase in serum potassium concentration in such patients can produce cardiac arrest. Hyperkalemia may complicate any of the following conditions: chronic renal failure, systemic acidosis such as diabetic acidosis, acute dehydration, extensive tissue breakdown as in severe burns, adrenal insufficiency, or the administration of a potassium-sparing diuretic (eg, spironolactone, triamterene).

Wax-matrix potassium chloride preparations have produced esophageal ulceration in certain cardiac patients with esophageal compression due to an enlarged left atrium.

All solid dosage forms of potassium supplements are contraindicated in any patient in whom there is cause for arrest or delay in tablet passage through the gastrointestinal tract. In these instances, potassium supplementation should be with a liquid preparation.

Warnings:
Hyperkalemia
In patients with impaired mechanisms for excreting potassium, the administration of potassium salts can produce hyperkalemia and cardiac arrest. This occurs most commonly in patients given potassium by the intravenous route but may also occur in patients given potassium orally. Potentially fatal hyperkalemia can develop rapidly and be asymptomatic.

The use of potassium salts in patients with chronic renal disease, or any other condition which impairs potassium excretion, requires particularly careful monitoring of the serum potassium concentration and appropriate dosage adjustment.

Interaction with Potassium-Sparing Diuretics
Hypokalemia should not be treated by the concomitant administration of potassium salts and a potassium-sparing diuretic (eg, spironolactone or triamterene), since the simultaneous administration of these agents can produce severe hyperkalemia.

Gastrointestinal lesions
Potassium chloride tablets have produced stenotic and/or ulcerative lesions of the small bowel and deaths. These lesions are caused by a high localized concentration of potassium ion in the region of a rapidly dissolving tablet, which injures the bowel wall and thereby produces obstruction, hemorrhage, or perforation. Slow-K is a wax-matrix tablet formulated to provide a controlled rate of release of potassium chloride and thus to minimize the possibility of a high local concentration of potassium ion near the bowel wall. While the reported frequency of small-bowel lesions is much less with wax-matrix tablets (less than one per 100,000 patient-years) than with enteric-coated potassium chloride tablets (40-50 per 100,000 patient-years) cases associated with wax-matrix tablets have been reported both in foreign countries and in the United States. In addition, perhaps because the wax-matrix preparations are not enteric-coated and release potassium in the stomach, there have been reports of upper gastrointestinal bleeding associated with these products. The total number of gastrointestinal lesions remains approximately one per 100,000 patient-years. Slow-K should be discontinued immediately and the possibility of bowel obstruction or perforation considered if severe vomiting, abdominal pain, distention, or gastrointestinal bleeding occurs.

Metabolic acidosis
Hypokalemia in patients with metabolic *acidosis* should be treated with an alkalinizing potassium salt such as potassium bicarbonate, potassium citrate, or potassium acetate.

Precautions: The diagnosis of potassium depletion is ordinarily made by demonstrating hypokalemia in a patient with a clinical history suggesting some cause for potassium depletion. In interpreting the serum potassium level, the physician should bear in mind that acute alkalosis *per se* can produce hypokalemia in the absence of a deficit in total body potassium, while acute acidosis *per se* can increase the serum potassium concentration into the normal range even in the presence of a reduced total body potassium. The treatment of potassium depletion, particularly in the presence of cardiac disease, renal disease, or acidosis, requires careful attention to acid-base balance and appropriate monitoring of serum electrolytes, the electrocardiogram, and the clinical status of the patient.

Adverse Reactions: The most common adverse reactions to oral potassium salts are nausea, vomiting, abdominal discomfort, and diarrhea. These symptoms are due to irritation of the gastrointestinal tract and are best managed by diluting the preparation further, taking the dose with meals, or reducing the dose.

One of the most severe adverse effects is hyperkalemia (see Contraindications, Warnings and Overdosage). There also have been reports of upper and lower gastrointestinal conditions including obstruction, bleeding, ulceration and perforation (see Contraindications and Warnings); other factors known to be associated with such conditions were present in many of these patients.

Skin rash has been reported rarely.

Overdosage: The administration of oral potassium salts to persons with normal excretory mechanisms for potassium rarely causes serious hyperkalemia. However, if excretory mechanisms are impaired or if potassium is administered too rapidly intravenously, potentially fatal hyperkalemia can result (see Contraindications and Warnings). It is important to recognize that hyperkalemia is usually asymptomatic and may be manifested only by an increased serum potassium concentration and characteristic electrocardiographic changes (peaking of T-waves, loss of P-wave, depression of S-T segment, and prolongation of the QT interval). Late manifestations include muscle paralysis and cardiovascular collapse from cardiac arrest.

Treatment measures for hyperkalemia include the following: (1) elimination of foods and medications containing potassium and of potassium-sparing diuretics; (2) intravenous administration of 300 to 500 ml/hr of 10% dextrose solution containing 10-20 units of insulin per 1,000 ml; (3) correction of acidosis, if present, with intravenous sodium bicarbonate; (4) use of exchange resins, hemodialysis, or peritoneal dialysis.

In treating hyperkalemia, it should be recalled that in patients who have been stabilized on digitalis, too rapid a lowering of the serum potassium concentration can produce digitalis toxicity.

Dosage and Administration: The usual dietary intake of potassium by the average adult is 40 to 80 mEq per day. Potassium depletion sufficient to cause hypokalemia usually requires the loss of 200 or more mEq of potassium from the total body store. Dosage must be adjusted to the individual needs of each patient but is typically in the range of 20 mEq per day for the prevention of hypokalemia to 40-100 mEq per day or more for the treatment of potassium depletion.

Note: Slow-K slow-release tablets must be swallowed whole and never crushed or chewed.

How Supplied:
Tablets 600 mg potassium chloride (equiv. to 8 mEq)—round, buff colored, sugar-coated (imprinted CIBA 165)
    Bottles of 100 ....NDC 0083-0165-30
    Bottles of 1000 ....NDC 0083-0165-40
    Consumer Pack—One Unit
      (12 Bottles—100 tablets each) ....NDC 0083-0165-65
    Accu-Pak® Unit Dose (Blister pack)
      Box of 100 (strips of 10) ...NDC 0083-0165-32
Protect from moisture. Protect from light. Do not store above 86°F (30°C).

Dispense in tight, light-resistant container (USP).
C82-58 (Rev. 1/83)
Shown in Product Identification Section, page 409

TRANSDERM®-NITRO ℞
[*trans' derm nye' trow*]
(nitroglycerin)
Transdermal Therapeutic System

Description: Transderm-Nitro (nitroglycerin) transdermal therapeutic system is a flat unit designed to provide controlled release of nitroglycerin through a semipermeable membrane continuously for 24 hours following application to intact skin. Nitroglycerin (glyceryl trinitrate) is a prompt-acting vasodilator for the relief and prevention of anginal attacks. Systems are rated to release *in vivo* 2.5, 5, 10 and 15 mg nitroglycerin over 24 hours and are in sizes of 5, 10, 20 and 30 cm^2 respectively.

One-fifth of the total nitroglycerin in the system is delivered transdermally to the patient over 24 hours; the remainder serves as the reservoir to release the drug and remains in the system. The rated release of drug is dependent upon the area of the system; 0.5 mg nitroglycerin is delivered *in vivo* for every cm^2 of system size.

The Transderm-Nitro system comprises four layers as shown below. Proceeding from the visible surface towards the surface attached to the skin, these layers are: 1) a tan-colored backing layer (aluminized plastic) that is impermeable to nitroglycerin; 2) a drug reservoir containing nitroglycerin adsorbed on lactose, colloidal silicon dioxide, and silicone medical fluid; 3) an ethylene/vinyl acetate copolymer membrane that is permeable to nitroglycerin; and 4) a layer of hypoallergenic silicone adhesive. Prior to use, a protective peel strip is removed from the adhesive surface.

Cross section of the system:

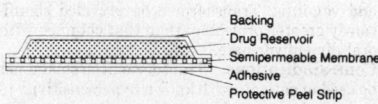
Backing
Drug Reservoir
Semipermeable Membrane
Adhesive
Protective Peel Strip

Actions: When the Transderm-Nitro system is applied to the skin, nitroglycerin is absorbed continuously through the skin into the systemic circulation. This results in active drug reaching the target organs (heart, extremities) before being inactivated by the liver. Nitroglycerin is a smooth muscle relaxant with vascular effects manifested predominantly by venous dilatation and pooling. The major beneficial effect of nitroglycerin in angina pectoris is a reduction in myocardial oxygen consumption secondary to vascular smooth muscle relaxation and consequent reduced cardiac preload and afterload. In recent years there has been an increasing recognition of a direct vasodilator effect of nitroglycerin on the coronary vessels.

In healthy volunteers transdermal absorption of nitroglycerin from a nitroglycerin system occurred in a continuous and well-controlled manner for a minimum of 24 hours. Steady-state plasma levels are attained within 2 hours after application, and continue for the duration of wearing the system. Precise definition of "therapeutic plasma level" is not known at this time. Plasma levels of nitroglycerin fall to approximately one-half the steady-state values 1 hour after system removal and are undetectable after 2 hours.

The amount of nitroglycerin released (2.5 mg, 5 mg, 10 mg, or 15 mg per 24 hours) represents the mean release rate of nitroglycerin from the system as determined from healthy volunteers, and hence, the amount potentially available for absorption through the skin. Absorption will vary among individuals.

Indications and Usage
This drug product has been conditionally approved by the FDA for the prevention and treatment of angina pectoris due to coronary artery disease. The conditional approval reflects a determination that the drug may be marketed while further investigation of its effectiveness is undertaken. A final evaluation of the effectiveness of the product will be announced by the FDA.

Transderm-Nitro System Rated Release *in vivo*	Total Nitroglycerin in System	System Size	Carton Size
2.5 mg/24 hr	12.5 mg	5 cm^2	30 systems (NDC 0083-2025-26)
5 mg/24 hr	25 mg	10 cm^2	30 Systems (NDC 0083-2105-26)
5 mg/24 hr	25 mg	10 cm^2	7 Systems (NDC 0083-2105-07)
10 mg/24 hr	50 mg	20 cm^2	30 Systems (NDC 0083-2110-26)
15 mg/24 hr	75 mg	30 cm^2	30 Systems (NDC 0083-2115-26)

Contraindications: Intolerance of organic nitrate drugs, marked anemia, increased intraocular pressure or increased intracranial pressure.

Warnings: In patients with acute myocardial infarction or congestive heart failure, Transderm-Nitro system should be used under careful clinical and/or hemodynamic monitoring.

In terminating treatment of anginal patients, both the dosage and frequency of application must be gradually reduced over a period of 4 to 6 weeks to prevent sudden withdrawal reactions, which are characteristic of all vasodilators in the nitroglycerin class.

Transdermal nitroglycerin systems should be removed before attempting defibrillation or cardioversion because of the potential for altered electrical conductivity which may enhance the possibility of arcing, a phenomenon associated with the use of defibrillators.

Precautions: Symptoms of hypotension, such as faintness, weakness or dizziness, particularly orthostatic hypotension may be due to overdosage. When these symptoms occur, the dosage should be reduced or use of the product discontinued.

Transderm-Nitro system is not intended for immediate relief of anginal attacks. For this purpose occasional use of the sublingual preparations may be necessary.

Adverse Reactions: Transient headaches are the most common side effect, especially when higher doses of the drug are used. These headaches should be treated with mild analgesics while Transderm-Nitro therapy is continued. When such headaches are unresponsive to treatment, the nitroglycerin dosage should be reduced or use of the product discontinued.

Adverse reactions reported less frequently include hypotension, increased heart rate, faintness, flushing, dizziness, nausea, vomiting, and dermatitis. These symptoms are attributable to the known pharmacologic effects of nitroglycerin, but may be symptoms of overdosage. When they persist the dose should be reduced or use of the product discontinued.

Dosage and Administration: Therapy should be initiated with application of one Transderm-Nitro 5 system to the desired area of skin. Many patients prefer the chest; if hair is likely to interfere with system adhesion or removal, it can be clipped prior to placement of the system. Each system is designed to remain in place for 24 hours, and each successive application should be to a different skin area. Transderm-Nitro system should not be applied to the distal parts of the extremities. The usual dosage is one Transderm-Nitro 5 system every 24 hours. Some patients, however, may require the Transderm-Nitro 10 system. If a single Transderm-Nitro 5 system fails to provide adequate clinical response, the patient should be instructed to remove it and apply either two Transderm-Nitro 5 systems or one Transderm-Nitro 10 system. More systems may be added as indicated by continued careful monitoring of clinical response. The Transderm-Nitro 2.5 system is useful principally for decreasing the dosage gradually, though it may provide adequate therapy for some patients when used alone.

The optimal dosage should be selected based upon the clinical response, side effects, and the effects of therapy upon blood pressure. The greatest attainable decrease in resting blood pressure that is not associated with clinical symptoms of hypotension especially during orthostasis indicates the optimal dosage. To decrease adverse reactions, the size and/or number of systems should be tailored to the individual patient's needs.

Do not store above 86°F (30°C).

Patient Instructions For Applications: A patient leaflet is supplied with the systems.

How Supplied:
[See table above].

Dist. by   CIBA Pharmaceutical Company
Division of CIBA-GEIGY
Corporation
Summit, New Jersey 07901
C84-7 (Rev. 2/84)

PATIENT INSTRUCTION SHEET
How to use

Transderm®-Nitro
nitroglycerin
Transdermal Therapeutic System

The usual starting dose is one Transderm-Nitro 5 system. The dose may vary, however, depending on your individual response to the system. For instance, your doctor may decide to increase or decrease the size of the system, or prescribe a combination of systems, to suit your particular needs.

Where to place Transderm-Nitro

Select any area of skin on the body, **EXCEPT** the extremities below the knee or elbow. The chest is the preferred site, but the back is an excellent alternative because it is usually free of hair, skin folds, and excessive muscular movement. The area should be clean, dry, and hairless. If hair is likely to interfere with system adhesion or removal, clip the hair prior to applying the system. Do not shave. Take care to avoid areas with cuts or irritations. Do **NOT** apply the system immediately after showering or bathing. It is best to wait until you are certain the skin is completely dry.

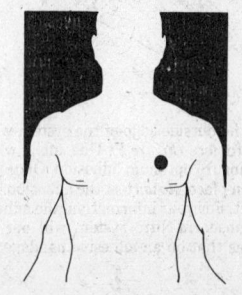

Continued on next page

The full prescribing information for each CIBA drug is contained herein and is that in effect as of October 1, 1984.

CIBA—Cont.

How to apply Transderm-Nitro

1. Open the package containing the system by tearing at the indicated indentations: then remove the system from the package *(Figure A)*.

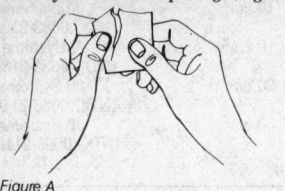

Figure A

2. Carefully pick up the system lengthwise with the tab up *(Figure B)*.

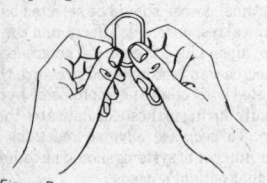

Figure B

3. Bend tab forward with thumb. With both thumbs, begin to remove the **clear plastic** backing from the system at the tab *(Figure C)*. Do not touch the inside of the exposed system, because the adhesive covers the entire surface.

clear plastic backing

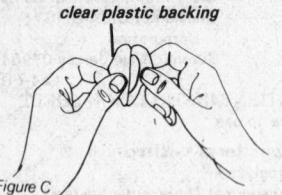

Figure C

4. Continue to remove the **clear plastic** backing *slowly* along the length of the system, allowing the system to rest on the outside of your fingers *(Figure D)*.

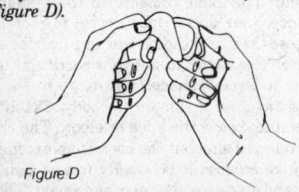

Figure D

5. Place the exposed, adhesive side of the system on the chosen skin site. It is extremely important to *press firmly* in place with the palm of your hand, and maintain the pressure for 10–15 seconds *(Figure E)*.

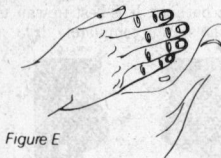

Figure E

6. Circle the outside edge of the system with one or two fingers *(Figure F)*. This, along with step 5, will insure optimum adhesion. Once the system is in place, *do not* test the adhesion by pulling on it. For your information, the adhesive in the Transderm-Nitro system will not feel as sticky as that on an adhesive bandage.

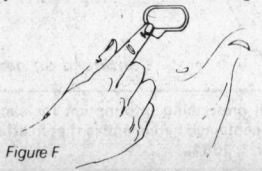

Figure F

7. Remove and discard the system after 24 hours. Dispose of the system by conventional means, such as in a trash container. Place a new system on a different skin site, following steps 1–6.

Please note:
Contact with water, as in bathing, swimming, or showering will not affect the system. In the unlikely event that a system falls off, discard it and put a new one on a different skin site.

Precautions: The most common side effect that is encountered is transient headaches. These often decrease as therapy is continued, but may require treatment with a mild analgesic. Although uncommon, faintness, flushing, and dizziness may occur, especially when suddenly rising from the recumbent (lying horizontal) position. If these latter symptoms do occur, the system should be removed from the skin and your physician should be notified. For changes in dosage and frequency of application, consult your physician.
Keep these systems and all drugs out of the reach of children.

DO NOT STORE ABOVE 86°F (30°C).
Dist. by:
CIBA Pharmaceutical Company
Division of CIBA-GEIGY Corporation
Summit, New Jersey 07901
C83-40 (Rev. 12/83)
Shown in Product Identification Section, page 410

TRANSDERM® SCŌP   ℞
[*trans-derm scōpe*]
scopolamine
(formerly Transderm-V)

Transdermal Therapeutic System

Programmed delivery *in vivo* **of 0.5 mg of scopolamine over 3 days**

This product is now marketed by CIBA Consumer Pharmaceutical Company, Division of CIBA-GEIGY Corporation.

Description: The Transderm Scōp system is a circular flat disc designed for continuous release of scopolamine following application to an area of intact skin on the head, behind the ear. Clinical evaluation has demonstrated that the system provides effective antiemetic and antinauseant actions when tested against motion-sickness stimuli in adults.
The Transderm Scōp system is a film 0.2 mm thick and 2.5cm^2, with four layers. Proceeding from the visible surface towards the surface attached to the skin, these layers are: (1) a backing layer of tan-colored, aluminized, polyester film; (2) a drug reservoir of scopolamine, mineral oil, and polyisobutylene; (3) a microporous polypropylene membrane that controls the rate of delivery of scopolamine from the system to the skin surface; and (4) an adhesive formulation of mineral oil, polyisobutylene, and scopolamine. A protective peel strip of siliconized polyester, which covers the adhesive layer, is removed before the system is used. The inactive components, mineral oil (12.4 mg) and polyisobutylene (11.4 mg), are not released from the system.

Cross section of the system:

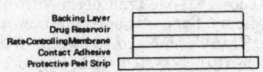

Release-Rate Concept: The Transderm Scōp system contains 1.5 mg of scopolamine. The system is programmed to deliver 0.5 mg of scopolamine at an approximately constant rate to the systemic circulation over the 3-day lifetime of the system. An initial priming dose of scopolamine, released from the adhesive layer of the system, saturates the skin binding sites and rapidly brings the plasma concentration of scopolamine to the required steady-state level. A continuous controlled release of scopolamine, which flows from the drug reservoir through the rate-controlling membrane, maintains the plasma level constant.

Clinical Pharmacology: The sole active agent of Transderm Scōp is scopolamine, a belladonna alkaloid with well-known pharmacological properties. The drug has a long history of oral and parenteral use for central anticholinergic activity, including prophylaxis of motion sickness. The mechanism of action of scopolamine in the central nervous system (CNS) is not definitely known but may include anticholinergic effects. The ability of scopolamine to prevent motion-induced nausea is believed to be associated with inhibition of vestibular input to the CNS, which results in inhibition of the vomiting reflex. In addition, scopolamine may have a direct action on the vomiting center within the reticular formation of the brain stem. Applied to the postauricular skin, Transderm Scōp provides for a gradual release of scopolamine from an adhesive matrix of mineral oil and polyisobutylene.

Indications and Usage: Transderm Scōp is indicated for prevention of nausea and vomiting associated with motion sickness in adults. The disc should be applied only to skin in the postauricular area.

Clinical Results: Transderm Scōp provides antiemetic protection within several hours following application of the disc behind the ear. In 195 adult subjects of different racial origins who participated in clinical efficacy studies at sea or in a controlled motion environment, there was a 75% reduction in the incidence of motion-induced nausea and vomiting. Transderm Scōp provided significantly greater protection than that obtained with oral dimenhydrinate.

Contraindications: Transderm Scōp should not be used in patients with known hypersensitivity to scopolamine or any of the components of the adhesive matrix making up the therapeutic system, or in patients with glaucoma.

Warnings: Transderm Scōp should not be used in children and should be used with special caution in the elderly. See **PRECAUTIONS**.
Since drowsiness, disorientation, and confusion may occur with the use of scopolamine, patients should be warned of the possibility and cautioned against engaging in activities that require mental alertness, such as driving a motor vehicle or operating dangerous machinery.
Potentially alarming idiosyncratic reactions may occur with ordinary therapeutic doses of scopolamine.

Precautions:
General
Scopolamine should be used with caution in patients with pyloric obstruction, or urinary bladder neck obstruction. Caution should be exercised when administering an antiemetic or antimuscarinic drug to patients suspected of having intestinal obstruction.
Transderm Scōp should be used with special caution in the elderly or in individuals with impaired metabolic, liver, or kidney functions, because of the increased likelihood of CNS effects.

Information for Patients
Since scopolamine can cause temporary dilation of the pupils and blurred vision if it comes in contact with the eyes, patients should be strongly advised to wash their hands thoroughly with soap and water immediately after handling the disc.
Patients should be warned against driving a motor vehicle or operating dangerous machinery. A patient brochure is available.

Drug Interactions
Scopolamine should be used with care in patients taking drugs, including alcohol, capable of causing CNS effects. Special attention should be given to drugs having anticholinergic properties, e.g., belladonna alkaloids, antihistamines (including meclizine), and antidepressants.

Product Information

Carcinogenesis, Mutagenesis, Impairment of Fertility
No long-term studies in animals have been performed to evaluate carcinogenic potential.
Fertility studies were performed in female rats and revealed no evidence of impaired fertility or harm to the fetus due to scopolamine hydrobromide administered by daily subcutaneous injection. In the highest-dose group (plasma level approximately 500 times the level achieved in humans using a transdermal system), reduced maternal body weights were observed.

Pregnancy Category C
Teratogenic studies were performed in pregnant rats and rabbits with scopolamine hydrobromide administered by daily intravenous injection. No adverse effects were recorded in the rats. In the rabbits, the highest dose (plasma level approximately 100 times the level achieved in humans using a transdermal system) of drug administered had a marginal embryotoxic effect.
Transderm Scōp should be used during pregnancy only if the anticipated benefit justifies the potential risk to the fetus.

Nursing Mothers
It is not known whether scopolamine is excreted in human milk. Because many drugs are excreted in human milk, caution should be exercised when Transderm Scōp is administered to a nursing woman.

Pediatric Use
Children are particularly susceptible to the side effects of belladonna alkaloids. Transderm Scōp should not be used in children because it is not known whether this system will release an amount of scopolamine that could produce serious adverse effects in children.

Adverse Reactions:
The most frequent adverse reaction to Transderm Scōp is dryness of the mouth. This occurs in about two thirds of the people. A less frequent adverse reaction is drowsiness, which occurs in less than one sixth of the people. Transient impairment of eye accommodation, including blurred vision and dilation of the pupils, is also observed.
The following adverse reactions have also been reported on infrequent occasions during the use of Transderm Scōp: disorientation; memory disturbances; dizziness; restlessness; hallucinations; confusion; difficulty urinating; rashes and erythema; acute narrow-angle glaucoma; and dry, itchy, or red eyes. In a few cases, dizziness has been reported when use of the drug was discontinued after 3 or more days of therapy; however, a causal relationship to the drug has not been established.

Overdosage:
Overdosage with scopolamine may cause disorientation, memory disturbances, dizziness, restlessness, hallucinations, or confusion. Should these symptoms occur, the Transderm Scōp disc should be immediately removed. Appropriate parasympathomimetic therapy should be initiated if these symptoms are severe.

Dosage and Administration:
Initiation of Therapy: One Transderm Scōp disc (programmed to deliver 0.5 mg of scopolamine over 3 days) should be applied to the hairless area behind one ear at least 4 hours before the antiemetic effect is required. Only one disc should be worn at any time.
Handling: After the disc is applied on dry skin behind the ear, the hands should be washed thoroughly with soap and water and dried. Upon removal of the disc, it should be discarded, and the hands and application site washed thoroughly with soap and water and dried, to prevent any traces of scopolamine from coming into direct contact with the eyes. (A patient brochure is available.)
Continuation of Therapy: Should the disc become displaced, it should be discarded, and a fresh one placed on the hairless area behind the other ear. If therapy is required for longer than 3 days, the first disc should be discarded, and a fresh one placed on the hairless area behind the other ear.

How Supplied:
The Transderm Scōp system is a tan-colored disc, 2.5 cm², on a clear, oversized, hexagonal peel strip, which is removed prior to use. Each Transderm Scōp system contains 1.5 mg of scopolamine and is programmed to deliver *in vivo* 0.5 mg of scopolamine over 3 days.
Transderm Scōp is available in packages of four discs. Each disc is foil wrapped. Patient instructions are included.
1 Package (4 discs) ....NDC 0083-4345-04
The system should be stored at room temperature.
C83-12 (Rev. 5/83)

Information for the Patient About—
TRANSDERM® SCŌP
Generic Name: scopolamine,
pronounced skoe-POL-a-meen
(formerly Transderm-V)
Transdermal Therapeutic System

The Transderm Scōp system helps to prevent the nausea and vomiting of motion sickness for up to 3 days. It is an adhesive disc that you place behind your ear several hours before you travel. Wear only one disc at any time.
Be sure to wash your hands thoroughly with soap and water immediately after handling the disc, so that any drug that might get on your hands will not come into contact with your eyes.
Avoid drinking alcohol while using Transderm Scōp. Also, be careful about driving or operating any machinery while using the system because the drug might make you drowsy.
TRANSERM SCOP SHOULD NOT BE USED IN CHILDREN AND SHOULD BE USED WITH SPECIAL CAUTION IN THE ELDERLY.

How the Transderm Scop System Works
A group of nerve fibers deep inside the ear helps people keep their balance. For some people, the motion of ships, airplanes, trains, automobiles, and buses increases the activity of these nerve fibers. This increased activity causes the *dizziness, nausea, and vomiting* of motion sickness. People may have only some, or all of these symptoms. Transderm Scōp contains the drug scopolamine, which helps reduce the activity of the nerve fibers in the inner ear. When a Transderm Scōp disc is placed on the skin behind one of the ears, scopolamine passes through the skin and into the bloodstream. One disc may be kept in place for 3 days if needed.

Precautions:
Before using Transderm Scop be sure to tell your doctor if you—
- Are pregnant or nursing (or planning to become pregnant)
- Have glaucoma (increased pressure in the eyeball)
- Have (or have had) any metabolic, liver, or kidney disease
- Have any obstructions of the stomach or intestine
- Have trouble urinating or any bladder obstruction
- Have any skin allergy or have had a skin reaction such as a rash or redness to any drug, especially scopolamine, or chemical or food substance.

Any of these conditions could make Transderm Scōp unsuitable for you. Also tell your doctor if you are taking any other medicines.
Transderm Scōp should not be used in children. The safety of its use in children has not been determined. Children and the elderly may be particularly sensitive to the effects of scopolamine.

Side Effects:
The most common side effect experienced by people using Transderm Scōp is dryness of the mouth. This occurs in about two thirds of the people. A less frequent side effect is drowsiness, which occurs in less than one sixth of the people. Temporary blurring of vision and dilation (widening) of the pupils may occur, especially if the drug is on your hands and comes in contact with the eyes. On infrequent occasions, disorientation, memory disturbances, dizziness, restlessness, hallucinations, confusion, difficulty urinating, skin rashes or redness, and dry, itchy, or red eyes have been reported. If these effects do occur, remove the disc and call your doctor. Since drowsiness, disorientation, and confusion may occur with the use of scopolamine, be careful driving or operating any dangerous machinery, especially when you first start using the drug system.

How to Use Transderm Scop
Transderm Scōp may be kept at room temperature until you are ready to use it.
1. Plan to apply one Transderm Scōp disc at least 4 hours before you need it. **Wear only one disc at any time.**
2. Select a hairless area of skin behind one ear, taking care to avoid any cuts or irritations. Wipe the area with a clean, dry tissue.
3. Peel the package open and remove the disc (Figure 1).

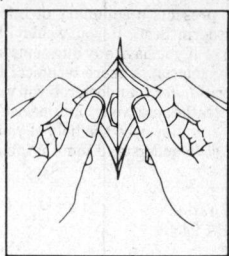

(Figure 1)

4. Remove the clear plastic six-sided backing from the round system. Try not to touch the adhesive surface on the disc with your hands (Figure 2).

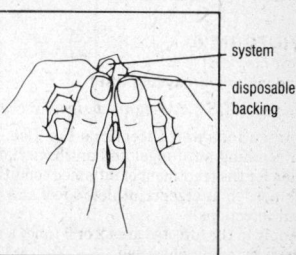

(Figure 2)

5. Firmly apply the adhesive surface (metallic side) to the dry area of skin behind the ear so that the tan-colored side is showing (Figure 3). Make good contact, especially around the edge. Once you have placed the disc behind your ear, do not move it for as long as you want to use it (up to 3 days).

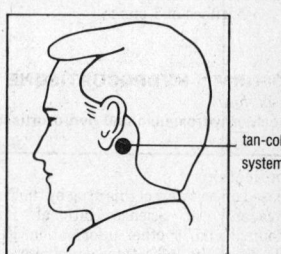

(Figure 3)

6. *Important:* After the disc is in place, be sure to wash your hands thoroughly with soap and water to remove any scopolamine. If this drug were to contact your eyes, it could cause temporary blurring of vision and dilation (widening) of the pupils (the dark circles in the center of your eyes). This is not serious, and your pupils should return to normal.
7. Remove the disc after 3 days and throw it away. (You may remove it sooner if you are no longer concerned about motion sickness). After removing the disc, be sure to wash your hands and the area behind your ear thoroughly with soap and water.

Continued on next page

The full prescribing information for each CIBA drug is contained herein and is that in effect as of October 1, 1984.

CIBA—Cont.

8. If you wish to control nausea for longer than 3 days, *remove* the first disc after 3 days, and place a new one *behind the other ear*, repeating instructions 2 to 7.
9. Keep the disc dry, if possible, to prevent it from falling off. Limited contact with water, however, as in bathing or swimming, will not affect the system. In the unlikely event that the disc falls off, throw it away and put a new one behind the other ear.

This leaflet presents a summary of information about Transderm Scōp. If you would like more information or if you have any questions, ask your doctor or pharmacist. A more technical leaflet is available, written for your doctor. If you would like to read the leaflet, ask your pharmacist to show you a copy. You may need the help of your doctor or pharmacist to understand some of the information.

Mfd. by:
ALZA Corporation
Palo Alto, CA 94304
Dist. by:
CIBA Consumer Pharmaceutical Co.
Division of CIBA-GEIGY Corp.
Summit, NJ 07901

C83-13 (Rev. 5/83)
Shown in Product Identification Section, page 409

VIOFORM®
[*vye-oh-form*]
(iodochlorhydroxyquin USP)

Listed in USP, a Medicare designated compendium.

Indications and Directions For Use:
A soothing antifungal and antibacterial preparation for the treatment of inflamed conditions of the skin, such as eczema, athlete's foot and other fungal infections.
Apply to the affected area 2 or 3 times a day or use as directed by physician.
Caution: May prove irritating to sensitized skin in rare cases. If this should occur, discontinue treatment and consult physician. May stain.
KEEP OUT OF REACH OF CHILDREN.
How Supplied:
Ointment, 3% iodochlorhydroxyquin in a petrolatum base; tubes of 1 ounce.
Cream, 3% iodochlorhydroxyquin in a water-washable base; tubes of 1 ounce.

(7/80)

VIOFORM®-HYDROCORTISONE   ℞
[*vye-oh-form*]
(iodochlorhydroxyquin and hydrocortisone)

Indications
Based on a review of this drug by the National Academy of Sciences-National Research Council and/or other information, FDA has classified the indications as follows:
"Possibly" effective: Contact or atopic dermatitis; impetiginized eczema; nummular eczema; infantile eczema; endogenous chronic infectious dermatitis; stasis dermatitis; pyoderma; nuchal eczema and chronic eczematoid otitis externa; acne urticata; localized or disseminated neurodermatitis; lichen simplex chronicus; anogenital pruritus (vulvae, scroti, ani); folliculitis; bacterial dermatoses; mycotic dermatoses such as tinea (capitis, cruris, corporis, pedis); moniliasis; intertrigo.
Final classification of the less-than-effective indications requires further investigation.

Contraindications: Hypersensitivity to Vioform-Hydrocortisone, or any of its ingredients or related compounds; lesions of the eye; tuberculosis of the skin; most viral skin lesions (including herpes simplex, vaccinia, and varicella).
Warnings: *This product is not for ophthalmic use.*
In the presence of systemic infections, appropriate systemic antibiotics should be used.

Usage in Pregnancy: Although topical steroids have not been reported to have an adverse effect on pregnancy, the safety of their use in pregnant women has not been absolutely established. In laboratory animals, increases in incidence of fetal abnormalities have been associated with exposure of gestating females to topical corticosteroids, in some cases at rather low dosage levels. Therefore, drugs of this class should not be used extensively on pregnant patients in large amounts or for prolonged periods of time.
Precautions: May prove irritating to sensitized skin in rare cases. If irritation occurs, discontinue therapy. Staining of skin and fabrics may occur. Additionally, there are rare reports of discoloration of hair and nails.
Signs and symptoms of systemic toxicity, electrolyte imbalance, or adrenal suppression have not been reported with Vioform-Hydrocortisone. Nevertheless, the possibility of suppression of the pituitary-adrenal axis during therapy should be kept in mind, especially when the drug is used under occlusive dressings, for a prolonged period, or for treating extensive cutaneous areas since significant absorption of corticosteroid may occur under these conditions, particularly in children and infants.
Vioform may be absorbed through the skin and interfere with thyroid function tests. If such tests are contemplated, wait at least one month between discontinuation of therapy and performance of these tests. The ferric chloride test for phenylketonuria (PKU) can yield a false-positive result if Vioform is present in the diaper or urine.
Prolonged use may result in overgrowth of nonsusceptible organisms requiring appropriate therapy.
Adverse Reactions: There have been a few reports of rash and hypersensitivity.
The following local adverse reactions have been reported with topical corticosteroids, especially under occlusive dressings: burning; itching; irritation; dryness; folliculitis; hypertrichosis; acneiform eruptions; hypopigmentation; perioral dermatitis; allergic contact dermatitis; maceration of the skin; secondary infection; skin atrophy; striae; miliaria. Discontinue therapy if any untoward reaction occurs.
Dosage and Administration: Apply a thin layer to the affected parts 3 or 4 times daily.
The *Cream,* because of its slight drying effect, is primarily useful for moist, weeping lesions; the *Lotion* is particularly suitable for application behind the ears and in intertriginous areas of the body; the *Ointment* is best used for dry lesions accompanied by thickening and scaling of the skin.
The *Mild Cream* and *Mild Ointment* should be used when treating lesions involving extensive body areas or less severe dermatoses.
How Supplied: *Cream,* 3% iodochlorhydroxyquin and 1% hydrocortisone in a water-washable base containing stearyl alcohol, cetyl alcohol, stearic acid, petrolatum, sodium lauryl sulfate, and glycerin in water; tubes of 5 and 20 Gm.
Ointment, 3% iodochlorhydroxyquin and 1% hydrocortisone in a petrolatum base; tubes of 20 Gm.
Lotion, 3% iodochlorhydroxyquin and 1% hydrocortisone in a water-washable base containing stearic acid, cetyl alcohol, lanolin, propylene glycol, sorbitan trioleate, polysorbate 60, triethanolamine, methylparaben, propylparaben, and perfume Flora in water; plastic squeeze bottles of 15 ml.
Mild Cream, 3% iodochlorhydroxyquin and 0.5% hydrocortisone in a water-washable base containing stearyl alcohol, cetyl alcohol, stearic acid, petrolatum, sodium lauryl sulfate, and glycerin in water; tubes of ½ and 1 ounce.
Mild Ointment, 3% iodochlorhydroxyquin and 0.5% hydrocortisone in a petrolatum base; tubes of 1 ounce.

C79-1 (5/79)

Clinical Nutrition Division
Sandoz Nutrition Corporation
5320 WEST TWENTY THIRD STREET
P.O. BOX 370
MINNEAPOLIS, MN 55440

CITROTEIN®
[*sit'ro-tēn*]
Powder
Protein · Vitamin · Mineral Food

Fortifies the clear liquid diet to help prevent nutrition related complications.
Usage: A good-tasting fruit flavored supplement for oral feeding to fortify clear liquid and other modified diets. Specifically prescribed as: Fortification for Special Diets—clear liquid, lactose free, bland, sodium restricted, low fat, cholesterol free, low purine, gluten free, low residue. Supplementary Nourishment—in rapid growth periods, pre- and postoperative states, convalescence, chronic illness, geriatrics, pediatrics, anorexia, pregnancy and postpartum.
Features: High quality protein—egg albumin; three eight fl oz servings provide 70% or more of the RDA for protein and essential vitamins and minerals; easily digested and well tolerated; a caloric distribution of 25% protein, 73% carbohydrate and 2% fat; appropriate for clear liquid diet supplementation; lactose free; three refreshing fruit flavors; recipe variations available upon request.
Ingredients (Orange): Sucrose, pasteurized egg white solids, maltodextrin, calcium glycerophosphate, citric acid, natural and artificial flavor, mono and diglycerides, partially hydrogenated soybean oil, FD&C Yellow No. 5 and No. 6, vitamins and minerals.
Administration and Dosage: 3 servings (3-1.57 oz packets) provide 70% or more of the RDA for protein, vitamins and minerals, providing 510 Calories, 31.5 g highest biological value egg protein, 93.3 g carbohydrate and 1.2 g fat. Fortification of Clear Liquid Diets—5 servings (5-1.57 oz packets) provide 100% or more of the U.S. RDA and NRC RDA for protein, vitamins and minerals, providing 850 Calories, 52.5 g protein, 156 g carbohydrate and 2.0 g fat.
How Supplied: In 14.16 oz cans and 1.57 oz individual serving packets in ORANGE, GRAPE and PUNCH Flavors.

COMPLEAT® MODIFIED FORMULA
[*kom'plēt*]
Low Sodium Meat Base Blenderized Tube Feeding

Usage: Tube feeding with the benefits of normal foods providing optimal nutritional support for head and neck surgery, stroke and comatose patients, who require a modified diet low in sodium, fat, cholesterol, lactose free and isotonic.
Features: Nutritionally complete, balanced diet of natural foods containing normal proportions of meat, vegetables and fruit, uniform in consistency for gravity or pump feeding. Is low in sodium, fat and cholesterol, lactose and gluten free and isotonic. Clinical trials confirm excellent tolerance and utilization for patients with a broad range of clinical conditions (see COMPLEAT-B®) requiring total nutrition or supplementation by tube feeding and who may also require a low sodium, low fat or lactose free intake.
• Caloric Distribution:
  16% Calories from protein
  54% Calories from carbohydrate
  30% Calories from fat
• Fiber—9.3 g (1500 ml)
Ingredients: Deionized water, hydrolyzed cereal solids, beef puree, pea puree, green bean puree, corn oil, peach puree, calcium caseinate, orange juice, mono and diglycerides, carrageenan, vitamins and minerals.
Administration and Dosage: Six cans (1500 ml) meet or exceed the RDA for protein and essential vitamins and minerals including trace minerals, providing 1600 Calories, 64 g high quality protein (meat and milk), 212 g carbohydrate and 55 g fat. At standard dilution the caloric concentration

is 1.07 Cal/ml; osmolality is 300 mOsm/Kg. Feed slowly at room temperature through nasogastric, gastrostomy or jejunostomy tubes. Do not administer parenterally. Provide additional water to meet fluid requirements, especially for patients with limited renal concentrating capacity, fever, dehydration or who are comatose. Postoperative feedings should not be initiated until small bowel function is re-established. If intake of food has been limited prior to initiation of tube feeding, initial feedings should be of reduced volume. For children under 10, reduce amount fed downward to match Recommended Dietary Allowances for the age group involved. Use only under medical supervision.

How Supplied: 250 ml cans.

COMPLEAT-B®
[kom'plēt-bē]
Meat Base Blenderized Tube Feeding Formula

Usage: Tube feeding with the benefits of normal foods providing optimal nutritional support for head and neck surgery, stroke and comatose patients.

Features: Nutritionally complete, balanced diet of natural foods with normal proportions of meat, vegetables, milk and fruit in a blenderized feeding, uniform in consistency for gravity or pump feeding. Indicated for patients with normal GI tracts requiring tube feeding.
- Caloric Distribution:
  16% Calories from protein
  48% Calories from carbohydrate
  36% Calories from fat
- Fiber—9.3 g (1500 ml)

Clinical trials confirm excellent tolerance and utilization for patients with a broad range of clinical conditions requiring total nutrition or supplementation by tube feeding.

Ingredients: Deionized water, beef puree, hydrolyzed cereal solids, green bean puree, pea puree, nonfat milk, corn oil, maltodextrin, peach puree, orange juice, mono and diglycerides, carrageenan, vitamins and minerals.

Administration and Dosage: Six bottles or cans (1500 ml) meet or exceed the RDA for protein, vitamins and minerals including trace minerals, providing 1600 Calories, 64 g high quality protein (meat and milk), 192 g carbohydrate and 64 g fat. At standard dilution the caloric concentration is 1.07 Cal/ml; osmolality is 405 mOsm/Kg. Feed slowly at room temperature through nasogastric gastrostomy or jejunostomy tubes.

Do not administer parenterally. Provide additional water to meet fluid requirements, especially for patients with limited renal concentrating capacity, fever, dehydration or who are comatose. Postoperative feedings should not be initiated until small bowel function is re-established. If intake of food has been limited prior to initiation of tube feeding, initial feedings should be of reduced volume and concentration. For children under 10, reduce amount fed downward to match Recommended Dietary Allowances for the age group involved.

Use only under medical supervision.

How Supplied: 250 ml cans and bottles for use with Ready To Use Disposable Doyle Tube Feeding Sets™.

ISOTEIN HN®
[i'so-tēn]
Nutritional Complete High Protein Isotonic Formula

Usage: Optimum nutrition for rapid recovery of catabolic cancer and burn patients.

Features: A high protein, isotonic, good tasting formula, nutritionally concentrated in a small volume. Formulated for patients with catabolic conditions including severe cancer and burns, which necessitate a high protein, isotonic feeding. Easy to administer for tube feeding and well accepted for oral feeding. ISOTEIN HN is lactose, purine and gluten free, contains low levels of residue, cholesterol and sodium, and is moderate in fat content.

- High Quality Protein—delactosed lactalbumin
- Nitrogen: Calorie Ratio—1:112
- Nitrogen: Non-protein Calorie Ratio—1:86
- 1.2 Cal/ml
- Caloric Distribution:
  23% Calories from protein
  52% Calories from carbohydrate
  25% Calories from fat

Ingredients: Maltodextrin, delactosed lactalbumin, partially hydrogenated soy oil with BHA, fructose, medium chain triglycerides, artificial flavor, sodium caseinate, mono and diglycerides, vitamins and minerals.

Administration and Dosage: Six servings (6-2.9 oz packets) meet or exceed 100% of the RDA for protein, vitamins and minerals including trace minerals, providing 2100 Calories, 120 g protein (18.8 g nitrogen), 276 g carbohydrate and 60 g fat (25% as medium chain triglycerides). Oral Feeding—have patient drink slowly within 4 hours. Tube Feeding—administer at a slow rate within 4 hours. May be fed through nasogastric, gastrostomy or jejunostomy tubes. Provide additional water to meet fluid requirements, especially for patients with limited renal concentrating capacity, fever, dehydration or who are comatose. Postoperative feedings should not be initiated until small bowel function is re-established. For children under 10, reduce amount fed downward to match Recommended Dietary Allowances for the age group involved. Use only under medical supervision.

How Supplied: In 2.9 oz individual serving packets in good tasting VANILLA Flavor.

MERITENE® Liquid
[mer'i-tēn]
Protein-Vitamin-Mineral Food

Provides high quality protein and essential nutrients for repletion of debilitated geriatric, convalescent and oral surgery patients.

Usage: Concentrate high quality protein·vitamin·mineral food prescribed for patients whose nutritional requirements are high or whose appetite or tolerance for sufficient ordinary food results in inadequate intake. Specifically prescribed as: Supplementary Nourishment—in debilitation and stress conditions—pre- and postoperative, convalescence, chronic illnesses, anemias, geriatrics, anorexia, underweight, pregnancy, postpartum and rapid growth periods; or for Fortification of Modified Diets—liquid, bland, high protein, low sodium, high calorie and gluten free.

NOTE: Complimentary Professional Diet Service and recipe variations available upon request.

Features: High quality protein—milk and caseinate; 14.4 grams of protein (32% of U.S. RDA) per serving; a variety of excellent tasting flavors; convenient, ready-to-serve liquid; easily digested; well tolerated; a caloric distribution of 24% protein, 46% carbohydrate and 30% fat; 5 servings (1200 ml) provide 100% or more of the U.S. RDA and NRC RDA for protein and essential vitamins and minerals.

Ingredients (Vanilla): Concentrated sweet skim milk, corn syrup solids, corn oil, sodium caseinate, sucrose, artificial flavor, cellulose flour, mono and diglycerides, salt, cellulose gum, carrageenan, vitamins and minerals.

Administration and Dosage: Supplemental Feeding—2 or 3 servings (250 ml/serving) per day between meals and at bedtime provide 40-60% of the RDA for protein and essential vitamins and minerals.

Do not administer parenterally. For children under 10, reduce amount fed downward to match Recommended Dietary Allowances for the age group involved. Use only under medical supervision.

How Supplied: In 250 ml, ready-to-serve, pull-tab cans in VANILLA, CHOCOLATE, EGG NOG and VANILLA SUPREME Flavors.

MERITENE® Powder
[mer'i-tēn]
Protein-Vitamin-Mineral Food

Provides high quality protein and essential nutrients for repletion of debilitated geriatric, convalescent and oral surgery patients.

Usage: Concentrated high quality protein·vitamin·mineral food prescribed for patients whose nutritional requirements are high or whose appetite or tolerance for sufficient ordinary food results in inadequate intake. Specifically prescribed as: Supplementary Nourishment—in debilitation and stress conditions—pre- and postoperative, convalescence, chronic illnesses, anemias, geriatrics, anorexia, underweight, pregnancy, postpartum and rapid growth periods; or for Fortification of Modified Diets—liquid, bland, high protein, low sodium, high calorie and gluten free.

NOTE: Complimentary Professional Diet Service and recipe variations available upon request.

Features: High quality protein—milk and caseinate; 18 grams of protein (40% of U.S. RDA) per serving; a variety of excellent tasting flavors; easily digested and well tolerated; a caloric distribution of 26% protein, 45% carbohydrate, 29% fat; four servings (1040 ml) provide 100% or more of the U.S. RDA and NRC RDA for protein and essential vitamins and minerals.

Ingredients (Vanilla): Specially processed nonfat dry milk, sucrose, calcium caseinate, corn syrup solids, fructose, sodium chloride, natural and artificial flavor, lecithin, vitamins and minerals.

Administration and Dosage: Supplemental Feeding—2-3 servings (1.14 oz powder in 8 fl oz whole milk/serving) per day between meals and at bedtime provide 50-75% of the RDA for protein and essential vitamins and minerals. Do not administer parenterally. For children under 10, reduce amount fed downward to match Recommended Dietary Allowances for the age group involved. Use only under medical supervision.

How Supplied: In 1 lb cans, 4½ lb cans and 25 lb drums in PLAIN, VANILLA, CHOCOLATE, EGG NOG and MILK CHOCOLATE Flavors.

NUTRISOURCE® Modular System

Usage: NUTRISOURCE provides the freedom and flexibility to tailor nutritional support for the critically ill patient with precise nutritional requirements.

Features: The NUTRISOURCE Modular System is a clinically proven, well-tolerated complete enteral system of individual nutrient components for tube feeding formulas, including a source of nitrogen as either whole protein, amino acids or amino acids-high branched chain; a ready to use, concentrated source of carbohydrate; a ready to use, concentrated source of fat as either medium chain triglycerides or long chain triglycerides; a vitamin module providing 100% of the NRC-RDA for essential vitamins; and standard as well as electrolyte-restricted mineral modules providing 100% of the NRC-RDA for essential minerals and recommended safe and adequate intakes of trace minerals which complement the protein and amino acid components.

The availability of separate modular components allows the formulation of specific enteral formulas for critically ill patients with precise nutritional requirements and altered nutrient metabolism as well as the flexibility to alter the nutrient prescription in response to changes in the patient's clinical condition or laboratory values.

Administration and Dosage: NUTRISOURCE Modular System components are intended for use as a complete enteral system and should not be used individually as the sole source of nutrition. Protein, fat, carbohydrate, vitamins and minerals should be provided from the appropriate NUTRISOURCE Modular System components to meet individual nutritional requirements. NUTRISOURCE formulas are intended for tube feeding only; components are not flavored for oral feed-

Continued on next page

Clinical Nutrition—Cont.

ing. Use only under medical supervision. Do not administer parenterally. Provide additional water to met fluid requirements especially for patients with limited renal concentrating capacity, fever, dehydration or who are comatose. Post-operative feedings should not be initiated until small bowel function is re-established. Formulation of feedings with extremely high or low levels of individual nutrient components or excessively high osmolalities necessitates careful patient monitoring to adjust the nutritional formula, fluid and electrolyte intake and/or flow rate based on tolerance and utilization.

Ingredients: NUTRISOURCE® Protein: Delactosed lactalbumin, egg white solids, mono and diglycerides, polysorbate 80.
How Supplied: 19.8 g packets.
Ingredients: NUTRISOURCE® Amino Acids: L-leucine, L-glutamic acid, L-lysine acetate, L-phenylalanine, L-isoleucine, L-valine, L-alanine, glycine, L-arginine, L-aspartic acid, L-threonine, L-proline, L-methionine, L-histidine, L-serine, L-tryptophan, L-cysteine, L-tyrosine.
How Supplied: 15.4 g packets.
Ingredients: NUTRISOURCE® Amino Acids-High Branched Chain: L-leucine, L-isoleucine, L-valine, L-lysine acetate, L-glutamic acid, L-arginine, L-alanine, L-threonine, L-phenylalanine, L-histidine, L-aspartic acid, L-methionine, glycine, L-serine, L-proline, L-tryptophan, L-cysteine, L-tyrosine.
How Supplied: 15.4 g packets.
Ingredients: NUTRISOURCE® Lipid-Long Chain Triglycerides: Deionized water, soybean oil, polyglycerol esters of fatty acids.
How Supplied: 250 ml cans.
Ingredients: NUTRISOURCE® Lipid-Medium Chain Triglycerides: Deionized water, medium chain triglycerides, polyglycerol esters of fatty acids, hydroxylated lecithin, mono and diglycerides.
How Supplied: 250 ml cans.
Ingredients: NUTRISOURCE® Carbohydrate: Deionized corn syrup solids, deionized water.
How Supplied: 10 g packets.
Ingredients: NUTRISOURCE® Vitamins: Maltodextrin, choline bitartrate, ascorbic acid, niacinamide, alpha tocopheryl acetate, D-calcium pantothenate, vitamin A palmitate, pyridoxine hydrochloride, thiamin hydrochloride, riboflavin, folic acid, D-biotin, phytonadione, vitamin D, cyanocobalamin.
How Supplied: 10 g packets.
Ingredients: NUTRISOURCE® Minerals for Protein Formulas: Magnesium gluconate, maltodextrin, calcium glycerophosphate, potassium citrate, sodium chloride, potassium phosphate, potassium chloride, high selenium yeast, high chromium yeast, ferrous sulfate, zinc sulfate, manganese gluconate, copper gluconate, sodium molybdate, potassium iodide.
How Supplied: 24 g packets.
Ingredients: NUTRISOURCE® Minerals for Protein Formulas-Electrolyte Restricted: Maltodextrin, magnesium gluconate, calcium glycerophosphate, monoammonium phosphate, high selenium yeast, high chromium yeast, ferrous sulfate, zinc sulfate, manganese gluconate, copper gluconate, sodium molybdate, potassium iodide.
How Supplied: 24 g packets.
Ingredients: NUTRISOURCE® Minerals for Amino Acid Formulas: Magnesium gluconate, calcium glycerophosphate, potassium citrate, maltodextrin, sodium chloride, sodium citrate, potassium phosphate, potassium chloride, high selenium yeast, high chromium yeast, ferrous sulfate, zinc sulfate, manganese gluconate, copper gluconate, sodium molybdate, potassium iodide.
How Supplied: 24 g packets.
Ingredients: NUTRISOURCE® Minerals for Amino Acids Formulas-Electrolyte Restricted: Maltodextrin, magnesium gluconate, calcium glycerophosphate, monoammonium phosphate, high selenium yeast, high chromium yeast, ferrous sulfate, zinc sulfate, manganese gluconate, copper gluconate, sodium molybdate, potassium iodide.
How Supplied: 24 g packets.

BCAA STRESSTEIN™
[stres′tēn]
Nutritionally Complete Branched Chain Enriched Modified Amino Acid Formula

Usage: Minimizes the catabolic response by meeting the unique fuel requirements of patients with polytrauma, sepsis and severe postsurgical stress.
Features: Clinically proven enteral modified amino acid formula enriched with 44% branched chain amino acids with a Isoleucine: Leucine: Valine ratio of 1:2:1 and a Nitrogen:Non-protein Calorie Ratio of 1:97. Provides a balance of amino acids, carbohydrate and fat developed to meet the unique fuel requirements of patients with polytrauma, sepsis and severe postsurgical stress. STRESSTEIN is a nutritionally complete, well tolerated and easy to administer tube feeding formula.
- 1.2 Cal/ml
- Caloric Distribution:
  23% Calories from protein
  57% Calories from carbohydrate
  20% Calories from fat

Ingredients: Maltodextrin, medium chain triglycerides, L-leucine, soybean oil, L-isoleucine, L-valine, L-glutamic acid, L-arginine, L-lysine acetate, L-alanine, L-threonine, L-phenylalanine, L-aspartic acid, L-histidine, L-methionine, glycine, polyglycerol esters of fatty acids, L-serine, L-proline, sodium chloride, L-tryptophan, L-cysteine, sodium citrate, L-tyrosine, vitamins and minerals.

Amino Acid Content:
(grams per 100 g protein as amino acids)
Essential Amino Acids

L-Isoleucine	11.0
L-Leucine	22.0
L-Lysine	6.5
L-Methionine	3.0
L-Phenylalanine	4.0
L-Threonine	5.0
L-Tryptophan	1.5
L-Valine	11.0

Non Essential Amino Acids

L-Alanine	5.5
L-Arginine	7.0
L-Aspartic Acid	3.5
L-Cysteine	1.0
L-Glutamic Acid	7.8
Glycine	3.0
L-Histidine	3.5
L-Proline	2.0
L-Serine	2.0
L-Tyrosine	0.7

Administration and Dosage: Six servings (6-3.4 oz. packets) provide 2400 Calories, 140 g protein (as amino acids) containing 19 g nitrogen, 340 g carbohydrate, 56 g fat (61.9% as medium chain triglycerides) and 100% of the U.S. RDA and NRC-RDA for essential vitamins and minerals. Specifically designed for tube feeding—administer at a slow rate, use within 4 hours. May be fed through nasogastric, gastrostomy or jejunostomy tubes.
Do not administer parenterally. Provide additional water to meet fluid requirements especially for patients with limited renal concentrating capacity, fever, dehydration or who are comatose. Post-operative feeding should not be initiated until small bowel function is re-established. Individuals who demonstrate osmotic or volume sensitivity may require reduced rates of diluted formula during the first 24-48 hours. Use only for patients with severe metabolic stress (sepsis, polytrauma and severe postsurgical stress). Use only under medical supervision.
How Supplied: In 3.4 oz individual serving packets.

Colgate-Hoyt Laboratories
(Formerly Hoyt Laboratories)
Division of Colgate-Palmolive Co.
575 UNIVERSITY AVENUE
NORWOOD, MA 02062 U.S.A.

LURIDE® Drops ℞
brand of Sodium Fluoride

Description: Each drop contains 0.125 ($^1/_8$) mg fluoride ion (F^-) from 0.275 mg sodium fluoride (NaF) for use as a dental caries preventive in children. Sugar-free. Saccharin-free.
Clinical Pharmacology: Sodium fluoride acts systemically (before tooth eruption) and topically (post-eruption) by increasing tooth resistance to acid dissolution, by promoting remineralization, and by inhibiting the cariogenic microbial process.
Indications and Usage: It has been established that ingestion of fluoridated drinking water (1 ppm F) during the period of tooth development results in a significant decrease in the incidence of dental caries.[1] LURIDE Drops was developed to provide systemic fluoride for use as a supplement in infants and children from birth to age 3 and older, living in areas where the drinking water fluoride level does not exceed 0.7 ppm.
Contraindications: Do not use in areas where the drinking water exceeds 0.7 ppm F.
Warnings: See "Contraindications" above. As in the case of all medications, keep out of reach of children.
Precautions: See "Overdosage" section below. Incompatibility of fluoride with dairy foods has been reported due to formation of calcium fluoride which is poorly absorbed.
Adverse Reactions: Allergic rash and other idiosyncrasies have been rarely reported.
Overdosage: Prolonged daily ingestion of excessive fluoride will result in varying degrees of dental fluorosis. (The total amount of sodium fluoride in a bottle of 30 ml LURIDE Drops (67.5 mg F)* conforms with the recommendations of the American Dental Association for the maximum to be dispensed at one time for safety purposes.)
Dosage[2] and Administration: Invert bottle vertically for proper drop delivery.

F-Content of Drinking Water	Daily Dosage Birth to Age 2	Age 2–3	Age 3–12
<0.3 ppm	2 drops	4 drops	8 drops
0.3–0.7 ppm	One-half above dosage.		
>0.7 ppm	Fluoride supplements contraindicated.		

LURIDE Drops may be administered orally undiluted or mixed with fluids.
How Supplied: Squeeze-bottles of 30 ml. (peach flavor—NDC#0126-0003-31)
Caution: Federal (U.S.A.) law prohibits dispensing without prescription.
References:
1. *Accepted Dental Therapeutics*, Ed. 39, American Dental Association, Chicago, 1982, p.347–350.
2. Ibid., p.321; American Academy of Pediatrics, Pediatrics 63:150–152, 1979.

*Revised Drop Size 4/84.

LURIDE® Lozi-Tabs® Tablets ℞
brand of Sodium Fluoride
Full-strength 1.0 mg F
Luride-SF (no artificial flavor or color) 1.0 mg F
Half-strength 0.5 mg F
Quarter-strength 0.25 mg F

Description: LURIDE® brand of sodium fluoride Lozi-Tabs® brand of lozenge/chewable tablets for use as a dental caries preventive in children. Sugar-free. Saccharin-free.
Each LURIDE 1.0 mg F tablet (full-strength) contains 1.0 mg fluoride (F) from 2.2 mg sodium fluoride.
Each LURIDE -SF 1.0 mg F tablet (SF for Special Formula: no artificial color or flavor) contains 1.0 mg F from 2.2 mg NaF.
Each LURIDE 0.5 mg F tablet (half-strength) contains 0.5 mg F from 1.1 mg NaF.

Each Luride 0.25 mg F tablet (quarter-strength) contains 0.25 mg F from 0.55 mg NaF.

Clinical Pharmacology: Sodium fluoride acts systemically (before tooth eruption) and topically (post-eruption) by increasing tooth resistance to acid dissolution, by promoting remineralization, and by inhibiting the cariogenic microbial process.

Indications and Usage: It is well established that ingestion of fluoridated drinking water (1 ppm F) during the period of tooth development results in a significant decrease in the incidence of dental caries.[1] LURIDE tablets were developed to provide fluoride for children living in areas where the water fluoride level is 0.7 ppm or less.

Contraindications: LURIDE and LURIDE-SF 1.0 mg F tablets are contraindicated when the F-content of drinking water is 0.3 ppm or more and should not be administered to children under age 3. LURIDE 0.5 mg F and .25 mg F tablets are contraindicated when the F-content of drinking water exceeds 0.7 ppm.

Warnings: Do not use LURIDE or LURIDE-SF 1.0 mg F tablets for children under age 3, nor in areas where the F-content of the drinking water is 0.3 ppm or more. Do not use LURIDE 0.5 mg F or LURIDE 0.25 mg F in areas where the F-content of the drinking water is more than 0.7 ppm. As in the case of all medications, keep out of reach of children.

Precautions: See "Overdosage" section below. Incompatibility of fluoride with dairy foods has been reported due to formation of calcium fluoride which is poorly absorbed.

Adverse Reactions: Allergic rash and other idiosyncrasies have been rarely reported.

Overdosage: Prolonged daily ingestion of excessive fluoride will result in varying degrees of dental fluorosis. (The total amount of sodium fluoride in a bottle of 120 LURIDE tablets (all strengths) conforms with the recommendations of the American Dental Association for the maximum to be dispensed at one time for safety purposes.)

Dosage[2] and Administration:

F-Content of Drinking Water	Daily Dosage (F ion) Birth to Age 2	Age 2–3	Age 3–12
<0.3 ppm	0.25 mg	0.5 mg	1.0 mg.
0.3–0.7 ppm	One-half above dosages.		
>0.7 ppm	Fluoride supplements contraindicated.		

One tablet daily, to be dissolved in the mouth or chewed before swallowing, preferably at bedtime after brushing teeth.

How Supplied:
[See table above].
(1) cherry, orange, lemon, lime
(2) Special Formula: no artificial flavor or coloring
* FOR DISPENSING ONLY

Caution: Federal (U.S.A.) law prohibits dispensing without prescription.

References:
1. *Accepted Dental Therapeutics*, Ed. 39, American Dental Association, Chicago, 1982, p. 347–350.
2. Ibid., p. 321; American Academy of Pediatrics, Pediatrics 63:150–152, 1979

Shown in Product Identification Section, page 410

ORABASE® Plain
"THE ORAL BANDAGE"™
Oral Protective Paste

(See PDR For Nonprescription Drugs)

ORABASE® with Benzocaine
"THE ORAL BANDAGE"™
Analgesic Oral Protective Paste

(See PDR For Nonprescription Drugs)

ORABASE® HCA   ℞
Oral Paste

Description: ORABASE HCA is an adrenocorticoid topical dental paste for application to the oral mucosa. Each gram contains hydrocortisone acetate 5mg (0.5%) in a paste vehicle containing pectin, gelatin, sodium carboxymethylcellulose dispersed in a plasticized hydrocarbon gel composed of 5% polyethylene in mineral oil, flavored with imitation vanilla.

Hydrocortisone is also known as cortisol, $11\beta, 17\alpha$, 21-trihydroxy-Δ^4-pregnene-3, 20-dione.

Clinical Pharmacology: Hydrocortisone acetate is a natural corticosteroid and possesses properties of an anti-inflammatory, antipruritic, and antiallergic nature. The paste acts as an adhesive vehicle for applying the active medication to oral tissues. The protective action of the adhesive vehicle may serve to reduce the pain associated with oral irritation.

Indications and Usage: Indicated for adjunctive treatment and for temporary relief of symptoms associated with oral inflammatory lesions and ulcerative lesions resulting from trauma.

Contraindications: Fungal, viral, or bacterial infections of the oral mucosa. Hypersensitivity to any component. This preparation is not for ophthalmic use.

Warnings: Patients with tuberculosis, peptic ulcer, or diabetes mellitus should not be routinely treated with this steroid preparation.
If significant regeneration or repair of oral tissues does not occur within 7 days of treatment, additional investigation of the oral lesion is advised.
Keep Out of Reach of Children

Precautions: It should be borne in mind that the normal defensive responses of the oral tissues are depressed in patients receiving topical corticosteroid therapy. Virulent strains of oral microorganisms may multiply without producing the usual warning symptoms of oral infections.
Pregnancy Category C. Animal reproduction studies have not been conducted with ORABASE HCA. It is also not known whether ORABASE HCA can cause fetal harm when administered to a pregnant woman or can affect reproduction capacity. ORABASE HCA should be given to a pregnant woman only if clearly needed.
Nursing mothers: It is not known whether this drug is excreted in human milk. Because many drugs are excreted in human milk, caution should be exercised when ORABASE HCA is administered in a nursing woman.

Adverse Reactions: Prolonged administration may elicit the adverse reactions known to occur with systemic hydrocortisone preparations; for example, adrenal suppression, alteration of glucose metabolism, protein catabolism, peptic ulcer activations, and others. These are usually reversible and disappear when the drug is discontinued.

Dosage and Administration: Dab, do not rub, on the lesion until the paste adheres. (Rubbing this preparation on lesions may result in a granular, gritty sensation.) After application, a smooth, slippery film develops.
Usual adult dose: Topical, to the oral mucous membrane, 2 or 3 times a day following meals and at bedtime.
Usual pediatric dose: Dosage has not been established.

How Supplied: Net weight 5-Gm. tubes (NDC #0126-0101-45). Available for office use in 0.75-Gm. chair-side packets in boxes of 100 (NDC #0126-0101-01).

Caution: Federal (U.S.A.) law prohibits dispensing without prescription.

PEROXYL®
brand of Hydrogen Peroxide
MOUTHRINSE

(See PDR For Nonprescription Drugs)

PHOS–FLUR® Oral Rinse/Supplement   ℞
brand of Acidulated Phosphate Fluoride

Description: Each teaspoonful (5 ml) contains 1.0 mg fluoride ion (F^-) from 2.2 mg sodium fluoride (NaF), in a 0.1 Molar phosphate solution at pH 4, for use as a dental caries preventive in children. Cherry, orange, lime–sugar and saccharin free. Cinnamon–contains saccharin but is sugar free.

Clinical Pharmacology: Sodium fluoride acts systemically (before tooth eruption) and topically (post-eruption) by increasing tooth resistance to acid dissolution, by promoting remineralization, and by inhibiting the cariogenic microbial process. Acidulation provides greater topical fluoride uptake by dental enamel than neutral solutions.[1] Phosphate protects enamel from demineralization by the acidulated formulation (common ion effect).[1]

Indications and Usage: It has been well established that ingestion of fluoridated drinking water (1 ppm F) during the period of tooth development results in a significant decrease in the incidence of dental caries.[2] PHOS-FLUR was developed to provide topical and systemic fluoride for use as a rinse/supplement (rinse-and-swallow) in children age 3 and older living in areas where the water fluoride level does not exceed 0.7 ppm. Where the drinking water contains more than 0.7 ppm F, PHOS-FLUR provides benefits as a topical fluoride dental rinse only (rinse-and-expectorate) for children age 6 and older.[3] Pioneering clinical studies on PHOS-FLUR were published by Frankl et al.[4] and Aasenden et al,[5] in 1972.

Contraindications: DO NOT SWALLOW in areas where the F-content of drinking water exceeds 0.7 ppm, nor in children under age 3.

Warnings: Do not use as a rinse in children under age 6. Do not use as a supplement in children under age 3, nor in areas where the drinking water exceeds 0.7 ppm F. As in the case of all medications, keep out of reach of children.

Precautions: See "Overdosage" section below. Incompatibility of systemic fluoride with dairy foods has been reported due to formation of calcium fluoride which is poorly absorbed.

Adverse Reactions: Allergic reactions and other idiosyncrasies have been rarely reported.

LURIDE

Strength (F ion)	Tablets per Bottle	Flavor	NDC Number 0126-
1.0mg F (full strength)	120	cherry	0006-21
		assorted[1]	0143-21
		SF[2]	0007-21
	1000*	cherry	0006-10
		assorted[1]	0143-10
	5000*	cherry	0006-51
0.5mg F (half-strength)	120	grape	0014-21
	1200*	grape	0014-81
0.25mg F (quarter-strength)	120	vanilla	0186-21

Continued on next page

Colgate-Hoyt—Cont.

Overdosage: Prolonged daily ingestion of excessive fluoride will result in varying degrees of dental fluorosis. (The total amount of sodium fluoride in a bottle of 500ml PHOS-FLUR Rinse/Supplement conforms to the recommendations of the American Dental Association for the maximum to be dispensed at one time for safety purposes).

Dosage and Administration:
As A Daily Dental Rinse—Children age 6 and over, preferably at bedtime after thoroughly brushing the teeth, rinse one teaspoonful (5 ml) or two teaspoonfuls (10 ml) vigorously around and between teeth for one minute, then expectorate.

As A Daily Supplement—Children age 3 and over, in areas where the drinking water contains less than 0.3 ppm F, rinse one teaspoonful (5 ml) as above and swallow. When drinking water contains 0.3 to 0.7 ppm F, inclusive, reduce dosage to ½ teaspoonful.

How Supplied:

Bottles of	Flavors	NDC# 0126
5 ml	cherry	0129-01
	cinnamon	0126-01
250 ml	cherry	0129-99
500 ml	cherry	0129-46
	cinnamon	0126-46
	lime	0017-46
	orange	0128-46
1 gallon	cherry	0129-28

Caution: Federal (U.S.A.) law prohibits dispensing without prescription.
References:
[1] F. Brudevold et al. Arch. Oral Biol. 8:167–177, 1963. [2] Accepted Dental Therapeutics, American Dental Association, Chicago, 1982, p.346. [3] Ibid., p. 351. [4] S.N. Frankl, S. Fleisch, and R. P. Diodati. J.A.D.A. 85:882–886, 1972. [5] R. Aasenden, P.F. DePaola, and F. Brudevold. Arch. Oral Biol. 17:1705–1714, 1972.

POINT-TWO® Dental Rinse ℞
brand of Sodium Fluoride

Description: 0.2% sodium fluoride (NaF) in a mint-flavored, neutral aqueous solution containing 6% alcohol. For weekly use as a caries preventive in children.
Clinical Pharmacology: Topical application of sodium fluoride increases tooth resistance to acid dissolution, promotes remineralization, and inhibits the cariogenic microbial process.
Indications and Usage: It has been established that weekly rinsing with a neutral 0.2% sodium fluoride solution protects against dental caries in children.[1] POINT-TWO Rinse was developed to provide a ready-to-use, flavored preparation for convenient administration and favorable compliance.
Contraindications: None. (May be used whether drinking water is fluoridated or not, since topical fluoride cannot produce fluorosis).
Warnings: DO NOT SWALLOW. Do not use in children under age 6, since younger children frequently cannot perform the rinse process without significant swallowing. As in the case of all medications, keep out of reach of children.
Precautions: Not for systemic use. (Each 5 ml contains 5 mg fluoride ion).
Adverse Reactions: In patients with mucositis, gingival tissues may be hypersensitive to flavor or alcohol present in formulation.
Overdosage: In the event a dose is accidentally swallowed, nausea and/or vomiting may result (treat with milk or antacids).
Dosage and Administration: For caries,[2] children age 6 to 12, one teaspoonful (5 ml); over age 12, 2 teaspoonfuls (10 ml). Once a week, preferably at bedtime after thoroughly brushing the teeth, rinse vigorously around and between the teeth for one minute, then expectorate. DO NOT SWALLOW. For maximum benefit, do not eat, drink, or rinse mouth for at least 30 minutes afterwards.
How Supplied:
Bottles of 8 fl. oz. with child-resistant closure. (Mint—NDC #0126-0178-99)
Gallon (with pump dispenser) (Mint—NDC #0126-0178-28)
Caution. Federal (U.S.A.) law prohibits dispensing without prescription.
References: [1] Accepted Dental Therapeutics, Ed. 39, American Dental Association, Chicago, 1982, p.353. [2] Ibid.

PREVIDENT™ Brush-On Gel ℞
brand of Neutral Sodium Fluoride

Description: Prescription-strength self-topical neutral fluoride containing 1.1% sodium fluoride for use as a dental caries preventive in children and adults. This product is not a dentifrice.
Clinical Pharmacology: Prescription-strength, high frequency topical applications of sodium fluoride to the teeth enhance tooth resistance to acid dissolution. Release of enamel deposited fluoride inhibits the cariogenic microbial process and stimulates remineralization of early carious lesions.
Indications and Usage: It is well established that 1.1% sodium fluoride is safe and extraordinarily effective as a caries preventive when applied frequently with mouthpiece applicators[1-4]. PreviDent Brush-On Gel in a squeeze-tube is a particularly convenient dosage form which permits the application of a thin ribbon of gel onto a toothbrush as well as a mouthpiece tray.
Contraindications: None (May be used in areas where drinking water is fluoridated or not, because topical fluoride cannot produce fluorosis).
Warnings: As with all medications, keep out of reach of children. Use in children under age 6 requires special supervision to prevent repeated swallowing of gel which could cause dental fluorosis.
Overdose: Accidental ingestion of a usual treatment dose (1-2 mgF) is not harmful.
Dosage and Administration: Adults and children 6 years of age and older. Apply daily a thin ribbon of gel to the teeth with a toothbrush or mouthtrays, for at least one minute preferably at bedtime, after brushing with toothpaste. After use, expectorate gel and rinse mouth thoroughly.
How Supplied: 2 ounce (60Gm) plastic tube
Fresh mint flavor—NDC #0126-0088-02
Cool lime flavor—NDC #0126-0089-02
Caution: Federal (U.S.A.) law prohibits dispensing without prescription.
References:
1. Accepted Dental Therapeutics, Ed. 39, ADA, Chicago, p. 353–356, 1982.
2. Englander HR, Keyes PH and Gestwicki M: JADA 75:638–644, 1967.
3. Englander HR et al: JADA 78:783–787, 1969.
4. Englander HR et al: JADA 82:354–358, 1971.

THERA-FLUR® Topical Gel-Drops ℞
brand of Acidulated Phosphate Fluoride
THERA-FLUR®-N Topical Gel-Drops ℞
brand of Neutral Sodium Fluoride

Description: THERA-FLUR (acidulated) gel-drops contains 0.5% fluoride ion (F^-) from 1.1% sodium fluoride (NaF) in a lime-flavored aqueous solution containing 0.1 Molar phosphate at pH 4.5. THERA-FLUR-N (neutral) also contains 0.5% (F^-) from 1.1% NaF, but with no acid phosphate, nor artificial flavor or color, at neutral pH. For daily self-topical use as a dental caries preventive.
Clinical Pharmacology: High-potency, high-frequency topical applications of sodium fluoride to the teeth increase tooth resistance to acid dissolution. Acidulation of topical fluoride increases deposition and penetration of the fluoride ion into tooth enamel. Phosphate acts as a common ion to inhibit demineralization of enamel by acidulated fluoride. Release of enamel-deposited fluoride inhibits the cariogenic microbial process and stimulates remineralization. Neutral fluoride provides less fluoride uptake by enamel, but diminished clinical efficacy has not been detected after high-potency, high-frequency treatment.
Indications and Usage: It is well established that 1.1% sodium fluoride is a safe and effective caries preventive when applied frequently with mouthpiece applicators.[1] Pioneering clinical studies with THERA-FLUR and THERA-FLUR-N Gel-Drops in schoolchildren were conducted by Englander et al.[2,3,4]
Both neutral and acidulated phosphate fluoride gels have been effective in controlling rampant dental decay which frequently follows xerostomia-producing radiotherapy of tumors in the head and neck region.[5,6]
Contraindications: None (May be used in areas where drinking water is fluoridated or not, because topical fluoride cannot produce fluorosis).
Warnings: As with all medications, keep out of reach of children.
Precautions: Laboratory tests indicate that use of acidulated fluoride may cause dulling of porcelain and ceramic restorations. Therefore, THERA-FLUR-N (neutral) is recommended for this type of patient.
Adverse Reactions: In patients with mucositis, gingival tissues may be hypersensitive to the acidity of THERA-FLUR, but will tolerate THERA-FLUR-N (neutral).
Overdosage: Accidental ingestion of a usual treatment dose (2–4 mg F) is not harmful.
Dosage and Administration: Age 3 and older. For daily use with applicators supplied by the dentist.[2] Apply 4 to 8 drops as required to cover inner surface of each applicator. Spread gel-drops with tip of bottle. Place applicators over upper and lower teeth at the same time. Bite down lightly for 6 minutes. Remove applicators and rinse mouth. Clean applicators with cold water.
How Supplied: 24 ml and 60 ml plastic squeeze bottles.

	NDC# 0126
THERA-FLUR (new lime flavor)	24ml 0048-54
	60ml 0048-02
THERA-FLUR-N (no artificial flavor or color)	24ml 0196-54
	60ml 0196-02

Caution: Federal (U.S.A.) law prohibits dispensing without prescription.
References:
[1] Accepted Dental Therapeutics, Ed.39, American Dental Association, Chicago, 1982, p.353–356. [2] H. R. Englander, P. H. Keyes, and M. Gestwicki. J.A.D.A. 75:638–644, 1967. [3] H. R. Englander et al. J.A.D.A. 78:783–787, 1969. [4] H. R. Englander et al. J.A.D.A. 82:354–358, 1971. [5] E. Johansen and T. O. Olsen in "Continuing Evaluation of the Use of Fluorides" (AAAS Selected Symposium 11), Westview Press, Boulder, CO, 1979, p.66. [6] S. Dreizen et al. J. Dent. Res. 56:99–104, 1977.

Consolidated Chemical, Inc.
**3224 SOUTH KINGSHIGHWAY BLVD.
ST. LOUIS, MO 63139**

FORMULA MAGIC®
Antibacterial Nursing Lubricant

Composition: ACTIVE INGREDIENT: Benzethonium Chloride INACTIVE INGREDIENTS: Talc, Mineral Oil, Magnesium Carbonate, Fragrance, DMDM Hydantoin
NDC 46706-202
Action: Talc based body powder and nursing lubricant. Aids in preventing excoriation and friction chafing. Aids in controlling odor.
Precautions: Non-irritating to skin. Practically non-toxic. Slight eye irritant. In case of eye contact flush with water.
Dosage and Administration: Apply liberally to patient's body. Provides a protective barrier against chafing.
How Supplied: 4 oz., 12 oz.

PERINEAL/OSTOMY SPRAY CLEANER™

Composition: Water, Cocamidopropylamine Oxide, Witch Hazel, Coco Betaine, DMDM Hydantoin, Fragrance, D&C Red #33, FD&C Blue #1.

Action: A gentle, effective spray cleaner for cleaning, refreshing, and deodorizing the perineal area, stoma sites, and stoma appliances.

Precautions: Non-irritating to skin. Practically non-toxic. May cause slight eye discomfort. In case of eye contact flush with water.

Dosage and Administration: Spray directly on entire perineal area, or peristomal skin or in stoma appliance for quick odor control and thorough cleaning. See label for full instructions.

How Supplied: 8 oz., 1 gallon.

SATIN®
Antibacterial Skin Cleanser

Composition: ACTIVE INGREDIENT: Chloroxylenol
INACTIVE INGREDIENTS: Water, Sodium Laureth Sulfate, Cocamidoproply Betaine, PEG-8, Cocamide DEA, Glycol Stearate, Lanolin Oil, Fragrance, Citric Acid, Tetrasodium EDTA, D&C Yellow #10.
NDC 46706-101

Action: Skin cleanser and shampoo for daily use. Reduces bacteria on the skin. Aids in reducing odor.

Precautions: Non-irritating to skin. Practically non-toxic. Moderate eye irritant. In case of eye contact flush with water.

Dosage and Administration: Apply directly to skin or hair or to dampened washcloth. Wash in normal manner. Rinse thoroughly.

How Supplied: 8 oz., 16 oz., 1 gallon.

SKIN MAGIC™
Antibacterial Body Rub and Skin Lotion

Composition: ACTIVE INGREDIENTS: Chloroxylenol INACTIVE INGREDIENTS: Water, Stearic Acid, Mineral Oil, Propylene Glycol, Isostearyl Alcohol, Glycol Stearate, Stearamide DEA, Triethanolamine, Cetyl Alcohol, Myristyl Propionate, Lanolin Oil, Fragrance, Propylparaben, DMDM Hydantoin, Methylparaben, Carbomer 934. NDC 46706-201.

Action: Emollient body rub and skin lotion. Soothes and moisturizes dry irritated skin. Aids in reducing odor.

Precautions: Non-irritating to skin. Practically non-toxic. Slight eye irritant. In case of eye contact flush with water.

Dosage and Administration: Apply liberally and massage into skin.

How Supplied: 4 oz., 8 oz., 1 gallon.

Cook-Waite Laboratories, Inc.
90 PARK AVENUE
NEW YORK, NEW YORK 10016

CARBOCAINE® ℞
hydrochloride 3% Injection
(mepivacaine hydrochloride injection, USP)

CARBOCAINE® ℞
hydrochloride 2%
with NEO–COBEFRIN®
1:20,000 Injection
(mepivacaine hydrochloride and levonordefrin injection, USP)

THESE SOLUTIONS ARE INTENDED FOR DENTAL USE ONLY.

Description: Mepivacaine hydrochloride is 1-methyl-2', 6'-pipecoloxylidide monohydrochloride. It is a white, crystalline, odorless powder soluble in water, but very resistant to both acid and alkaline hydrolysis.

Levonordefrin is $(-)$-α-(1-Aminoethyl)-3, 4-dihydroxybenzyl alcohol.

It is a white or buff-colored crystalline solid, freely soluble in aqueous solutions of mineral acids, but practically insoluble in water.

DENTAL CARTRIDGES MAY NOT BE AUTOCLAVED.

COMPOSITION	CARTRIDGE	
Each ml contains:	2%	3%
mepivacaine hydrochloride	20.0 mg	30.0 mg
levonordefrin	0.05 mg	—
sodium chloride	4.0 mg	3.0 mg
acetone sodium bisulfite not more than	2.0 mg	—
water for injection qs ad	1.0 ml	1.0 ml

The pH of the 2% cartridge solution is adjusted between 3.3 and 5.5 with NaOH or HCl.
The pH of the 3% cartridge solution is adjusted between 4.5 and 6.8 with NaOH or HCl.

Clinical Pharmacology: Carbocaine stabilizes the neuronal membrane and prevents the initiation and transmission of nerve impulses, thereby effecting local anesthesia.

CARBOCAINE is rapidly metabolized, with only a small percentage of the anesthetic (5 to 10 per cent) being excreted unchanged in the urine. CARBOCAINE, because of its amide structure, is not detoxified by the circulating plasma esterases. The liver is the principal site of metabolism, with over 50 per cent of the administered dose being excreted into the bile as metabolites. Most of the metabolized mepivacaine is probably resorbed in the intestine and then excreted into the urine since only a small percentage is found in the feces. The principal route of excretion is via the kidney. Most of the anesthetic and its metabolites are eliminated within 30 hours. It has been shown that hydroxylation and N-demethylation, which are detoxification reactions, play important roles in the metabolism of the anesthetic. Three metabolites of mepivacaine have been identified from adult humans: two phenols, which are excreted almost exclusively as their glucuronide conjugates, and the N-demethylated compound (2',6'-pipecoloxylidide).

The onset of action is rapid (30 to 120 seconds in the upper jaw; 1 to 4 minutes in the lower jaw) and CARBOCAINE Hydrochloride 3% without vasoconstrictor will ordinarily provide operating anesthesia of 20 minutes in the upper jaw and 40 minutes in the lower jaw.

CARBOCAINE hydrochloride 2% with Neo-Cobefrin 1:20,000 (brand of mepivacaine hydrochloride and levonordefrin injection) provides anesthesia of longer duration for more prolonged procedures, 1 hour to 2.5 hours in the upper jaw and 2.5 hours to 5.5 hours in the lower jaw.

CARBOCAINE does not ordinarily produce irritation or tissue damage.

Neo-Cobefrin (brand of levonordefrin) is a sympathomimetic amine used as a vasoconstrictor in local anesthetic solutions. It has pharmacologic activity similar to that of epinephrine but it is more stable than epinephrine. In equal concentrations, Neo-Cobefrin is less potent than epinephrine in raising blood pressure, and as a vasoconstrictor.

Indications: Carbocaine is indicated for the production of local anesthesia for dental procedures by infiltration injection or nerve block.

Contraindications: Mepivacaine is contraindicated in patients with a known hypersensitivity to amide type local anesthetics.

Warnings: RESUSCITATIVE EQUIPMENT AND DRUGS SHOULD BE IMMEDIATELY AVAILABLE. (See Adverse Reactions).

Reactions resulting in fatality have occurred on rare occasions with the use of local anesthetics, even in the absence of a history of hypersensitivity.

The solution which contains a vasoconstrictor should be used with extreme caution for patients whose medical history and physical evaluation suggest the existence of hypertension, arteriosclerotic heart disease, cerebral vascular insufficiency, heart block, thyrotoxicosis and diabetes, etc. The solution which contains a vasoconstrictor, should also be used with extreme caution in patients receiving drugs known to produce blood pressure alterations (i.e., MAO inhibitors, tricyclic anti-depressants, phenothiazines, etc.) as either sustained hypotension or hypertension may occur.

Usage in Children. Great care must be exercised in adhering to safe concentrations and dosages for pedodontic administration (see Dosage and Administration).

Usage in Pregnancy. Safe use of mepivacaine has not been established with respect to adverse effects on fetal development. Careful consideration should be given to this fact before administration during pregnancy.

Local anesthetic procedures should be used with caution when there is inflammation and/or sepsis in the region of the proposed injection.

Precautions: The safety and effectiveness of mepivacaine depend upon proper dosage, correct technique, adequate precautions, and readiness for emergencies.

The lowest dose that results in effective anesthesia should be used to avoid high plasma levels and possible adverse effects. Injection of repeated doses of mepivacaine may cause significant increase in blood levels with each repeated dose due to slow accumulation of the drug or its metabolites, or due to slower metabolic degradation than normal.

Tolerance varies with the status of the patient. Debilitated, elderly patients, acutely ill patients, and children should be given reduced doses commensurate with their weight and physical status. Mepivacaine should be used with caution in patients with a history of severe disturbances of cardiac rhythm or heart block.

INJECTIONS SHOULD ALWAYS BE MADE SLOWLY WITH ASPIRATION TO AVOID INTRAVASCULAR INJECTION AND THEREFORE SYSTEMIC REACTION TO BOTH LOCAL ANESTHETIC AND VASOCONSTRICTOR.

If sedatives are employed to reduce patient apprehension, use reduced doses, since local anesthetic agents, like sedatives, are central nervous system depressants which in combination may have an additive effect. Young children should be given minimal doses of each agent.

Changes in sensorium such as excitation, disorientation, drowsiness, may be early indications of a high blood level of the drug and may occur following inadvertent intravascular administration or rapid absorption of mepivacaine.

Solutions containing a vasoconstrictor should be used cautiously in the presence of diseases which may adversely affect the patient's cardiovascular system. Serious cardiac arrhythmias may occur if preparations containing a vasoconstrictor are employed in patients during or following the administration of chloroform, halothane, cyclopropane, trichloroethylene, or other related agents.

Mepivacaine SHOULD BE USED WITH CAUTION IN PATIENTS WITH KNOWN DRUG ALLERGIES AND SENSITIVITIES. A thorough history of the patient's prior experience with mepivacaine or other local anesthetics as well as concomitant or recent drug use should be taken (see Contraindications). Patients allergic to methylparaben or para-aminobenzoic acid derivatives (procaine, tetracaine, benzocaine, etc.) have not shown cross-sensitivity to agents of the amide type such as mepivacaine. Since mepivacaine is metabolized in the liver and excreted by the kidneys, it should be used cautiously in patients with liver and renal disease.

Adverse Reactions: Systemic adverse reactions involving the central nervous system and the cardiovascular system usually result from high plasma levels due to excessive dosage, rapid absorption, or inadvertent intravascular injection. A small number of reactions may result from hypersensitivity, idiosyncrasy or diminished tolerance to normal dosage on the part of the patient. Reactions involving the *central nervous system* are characterized by excitation and/or depression. Nervousness, dizziness, blurred vision, or tremors

Continued on next page

Cook-Waite—Cont.

may occur followed by drowsiness, convulsions, unconsciousness, and possibly respiratory arrest. Since excitement may be transient or absent, the first manifestations may be drowsiness merging into unconsciousness and respiratory arrest.

Reactions involving the *cardiovascular system* include depression of the myocardium, hypotension, bradycardia, and even cardiac arrest.

Allergic reactions are rare and may occur as a result of sensitivity to the local anesthetic and are characterized by cutaneous lesions of delayed onset or urticaria, edema and other manifestations of allergy. The detection of sensitivity by skin testing is of limited value. As with other local anesthetics, anaphylactoid reactions to CARBOCAINE have occurred rarely. The reaction may be abrupt and severe and is not usually dose related.

Treatment of a patient with toxic manifestations consists of assuring and maintaining a patent airway and supporting ventilation (respiration) as required. This usually will be sufficient in the management of most reactions. Should a convulsion persist despite ventilatory therapy, small increments of anticonvulsive agents may be given intravenously, such as benzodiazepine (e.g., diazepam) or ultra-short acting barbiturates (e.g., thiopental or thiamylal) or short-acting barbiturate (e.g., pentobarbital or secobarbital). Cardiovascular depression may require circulatory assistance with intravenous fluids and/or vasopressor (e.g., ephedrine) as dictated by the clinical situation. Allergic reactions should be managed by conventional means.

Dosage and Administration: As with all local anesthetics, the dose varies and depends upon the area to be anesthetized, the vascularity of the tissues, individual tolerance and the technique of anesthesia. The lowest dose needed to provide effective anesthesia should be administered. For specific techniques and procedures refer to standard dental manuals and textbooks.

For infiltration and block injections in the upper or lower jaw, the average dose of 1 cartridge will usually suffice.

Each cartridge contains 1.8 ml. (36 mg. of 2% or 54 mg. of 3%).

Five cartridges (180 mg. of the 2% solution or 270 mg. of the 3% solution) are usually adequate to effect anesthesia of the entire oral cavity. Whenever a larger dose seems to be necessary for an extensive procedure, the maximum dose should be calculated according to that patient's weight. A dose of up to 3 mg. per pound of body weight may be administered. At any single dental sitting the total dose for all injected sites should not exceed 400 mg. in adults.

The maximum pediatric dose should be *carefully calculated* and should not exceed 5 cartridges (180 mg. of the 2% solution and 270 mg. of the 3% solution). The maximum pediatric dose should be calculated as:

Maximum Dose for Children =
Child's Weight (lbs.)
─────────────── × Maximum Recommended Dose
150   for Adults (400 mg.)

When using CARBOCAINE for infiltration or regional block anesthesia, injection should always be made slowly and with frequent aspiration.

Any unused portion of a cartridge should be discarded.

Disinfection of Cartridges: As in the case of any cartridge, the diaphragm should be disinfected before needle puncture. The diaphragm should be thoroughly swabbed with either pure 91% isopropyl alcohol or 70% ethyl alcohol, USP just prior to use. Many commercially available alcohol solutions contain ingredients which are injurious to container components, and therefore, should not be used. Cartridges should not be immersed in any solution.

How Supplied: Both formulas are available in 1.8 ml. cartridges, containers of 50, to fit the Carpule® Aspirator.

The 2% solution should be stored at controlled room temperature, between 15° and 30° C (59° and 86° F).

Marketed by:
COOK-WAITE LABORATORIES, INC.
Mfg. by Sterling Drug Inc.
New York, N.Y. 10016
Carbocaine and Neo-Cobefrin
are the registered trademarks
of Sterling Drug Inc.
Revised March 1982 CO 160/0382

For full prescribing information on the medical use of Carbocaine, see Winthrop-Breon Laboratories product listing in this publication.

Cooper Dermatology Laboratories, Inc.
3145 PORTER DRIVE
PALO ALTO, CA 94304

AVEENO® BATH
REGULAR FORMULA AND OILATED FOR DRY SKIN

AVEENO® BATHS contain Colloidal Oatmeal, a natural oat derivative developed specially for soothing and cleansing itchy, sore, sensitive skin. AVEENO® BATHS contain no soaps or synthetic detergents that may be harmful to the skin. They cleanses naturally because of their unique adsorptive properties.

Infants and children with sensitive skin will also benefit from soothing, calming AVEENO® Colloidal Oatmeal baths.

Ingredients: Aveeno Bath Regular: 100% colloidal oatmeal; Aveeno Bath Oilated: 43% colloidal oatmeal, liquid petrolatum, and a specially selected emollient.

Aveeno®bar
Regular for normal to oily skin

Aveeno®bar Regular is made especially for sensitive skin that is irritated by ordinary soaps.

More than 50% of this mild skin cleanser is colloidal oatmeal, noted for its soothing and protective qualities.

Aveeno®bar Regular is completely soapfree. It leaves no harsh alkaline film to irritate delicate skin... it leaves it feeling soft and comfortable.

Ingredients: Aveeno® Colloidal Oatmeal, 50%; specially selected lanolin derivative; in a sudsing soapfree base containing a mild surfactant.

Aveeno®bar
MEDICATED FOR ACNE
(FORMERLY ACNAVEEN®)

Aveeno®bar Medicated is a special soapfree cleansing bar for acne. It contains colloidal oatmeal, 2% sulfur, and 2% salicylic acid, to help cleanse and soothe irritated skin.

Ingredients: Aveeno® Colloidal Oatmeal, 50%; sulfur, 2%; salicylic acid, 2%; in a sudsing soapfree base containing a mild surfactant.

Aveeno®bar
OILATED FOR DRY SKIN
(FORMERLY EMULAVE®)

Aveeno®bar Oilated is a unique, soapfree cleanser for dry, sensitive skin that is irritated by ordinary soaps. Aveeno®bar Oilated contains over 29% skin-softening emollients to help replace natural skin oils and 30% colloidal oatmeal, recommended for its soothing and protective qualities.

Ingredients: A combination of vegetable oils, specially selected lanolin derivative and glycerine 29%, Aveeno® Colloidal Oatmeal, 30%; in a sudsing soap-free base containing a mild surfactant.

PENTRAX®
Tar Shampoo with Fractar®

Description: Pentrax Tar Shampoo contains 8.75% Fractar® (which is equal to 4.3% crude coal tar), a standardized tax extract, a blend of highly concentrated detergents, and conditioning agents. Spectrophotometric standardization, based on hydrocarbon analysis assures uniform tar content from batch to batch. Pentrax Tar Shampoo does not contain hexachlorophene, parabens or other preservatives.

Action and Indications: Coal tar helps correct abnormalities of keratinization by decreasing epidermal proliferation and dermal infiltration. Pentrax Tar Shampoo is indicated for the adjunctive, topical management of dandruff, seborrheic dermatitis, psoriasis and subacute and chronic eczematous dermatoses of the scalp.

Advantages: Pentrax Tar Shampoo contains all the desirable crude coal tar fractions without undesirable pitch. It has excellent lathering qualities and leaves hair clean and manageable.

Contraindications: Pentrax Tar Shampoo is contraindicated in patients with a history of hypersensitivity to tar and other components of the formulation.

Precautions: Not for ophthalmic use. Minor dermatologic side effects have been reported from the use of topical tar preparations. These include irritation, folliculitis from long-term use, allergic contact dermatitis and phototoxicity. May stain dyed or colored hair. Keep of the reach of children.

Directions: Apply Pentrax® Tar Shampoo to wet hair; massage, adding water liberally to produce lather. Rinse. Reapply. Second lather may be allowed to remain up to 10 minutes. Rinse. Shampoo twice weekly.

Packaging:
4 fluid ounce plastic bottles.
NDC 0041-3916-04
8 fluid ounce plastic bottles.
NDC 0041-3916-08

TEXACORT® Scalp Lotion   ℞

Caution: Federal law prohibits dispensing without prescription.

Texacort Scalp Lotion contains hydrocortisone in a concentration of 1% (10 mg per gram). Hydrocortisone (cortisol) has the chemical formula of pregn-4-ene-3,20-dione, 11,17,21-trihydroxy, (11β)-. The vehicle contains: 33% alcohol, propylene glycol, polysorbate 20, benzalkonium chloride, and purified water. Texacort Scalp Lotion is lipid-free and paraben-free.

Actions: Topical steroids are primarily effective because of their antiinflammatory, antipruritic and vasoconstrictive actions.

Indications: For relief of the inflammatory manifestations of corticosteroid responsive dermatoses.

Contraindications: Topical steroids are contraindicated in those patients with a history of hypersensitivity to any components of the preparation.

Precautions: If irritation develops, Texacort Scalp Lotion should be discontinued and appropriate therapy instituted.

In the presence of an infection the use of an appropriate antifungal or antibacterial agent should be instituted. If a favorable response does not occur promptly, the corticosteroid should be discontinued until the infection has been adequately controlled.

If extensive areas are treated or if the occlusive technique is used there will be increased systemic absorption of the corticosteroid and suitable precautions should be taken, particularly in children and infants.

Although topical steroids have not been reported to have an adverse effect on human pregnancy, the safety of their use in pregnant women has not been absolutely established. In laboratory animals, increases in incidence of fetal abnormalities have been associated with exposure of gestating females to topical corticosteroids, in some cases at rather low dosage levels. Therefore, drugs of this class should not be used extensively on pregnant patients, in large amounts, or for prolonged periods of time.

Texacort Scalp Lotion is not for ophthalmic use.

Adverse Reactions: The following local adverse reactions have been reported with topical corticosteroids, especially under occlusive dressings: burning, itching, irritation, dryness, folliculitis, hypertrichosis, acneform eruptions, hypopigmentation, perioral dermatitis, allergic contact dermatitis, maceration of the skin, secondary infection, skin atrophy, striae and miliaria.

Dosage and Administration: Apply to affected areas 2 or 4 times daily. When a favorable response is obtained, gradually reduce dosage and eventually discontinue.

How Supplied: Texacort Scalp Lotion is supplied in 1 fl oz bottles with dropper (N 0064-3912-01).

Store between 59°–86° F [15°–30° C].

CooperVision Pharmaceuticals Inc.
SAN GERMAN, PUERTO RICO 00753

OPHTHALMIC PRODUCTS

For information on CooperVision Pharmaceuticals Inc. prescription and OTC ophthalmic products, consult the Physicians' Desk Reference For Ophthalmology. For literature, service items or sample material, contact your CooperVision Pharmaceuticals Inc. representative. See a complete listing of products in the Manufacturers' Index section of this book.

Cutter Biological
Div. Miles Laboratories, Inc.
2200 POWELL STREET
EMERYVILLE, CA 94662

GAMASTAN® ℞
[găm'as-tan"]
(Immune Serum Globulin—Human U.S.P.)
2 ml., 10 ml. vials

IMMUNE GLOBULIN ℞
INTRAVENOUS, 5%
(In 10% Maltose)
GAMIMUNE®
[gam'i-mūne"]

Description: Immune Globulin Intravenous, 5% in 10% Maltose (IGIV,5%-Maltose)-Gamimune® is a sterile $5 \pm 1\%$ solution of human protein stabilized with $10 \pm 2\%$ maltose; it contains no preservatives. The immunoglobulin is selectively reduced under controlled conditions using dithiothreitol and alkylated with iodoacetamide to render it suitable for intravenous administration.[1-3] Each 10 mL contains approximately 500 mg of protein, not less than 90% of which is immunoglobulin. Thus, there are approximately 450 mg of immunoglobulin in each 10 mL of IGIV,5%-Maltose. The pH is 5.25 ± 0.25. The calculated osmolality is 327 milliosmoles per kilogram of solvent (water) and the calculated osmolarity is 292 milliosmoles per liter of solution. The product is prepared by cold alcohol fractionation from large pools of human venous plasma. Each individual unit of plasma has been tested and found non-reactive for hepatitis B surface antigen (HBsAg) using a test with third-generation sensitivity.

Clinical Pharmacology: Gamimune® supplies IgG antibodies for prevention or attenuation of infectious diseases.[4-12] The half-life of Gamimune® is approximately three weeks[13] but individual patient variation in half-life has been observed.[14] Thus, this variable as well as the amount of immunoglobulin administered per dose is important in determining the frequency of administration of the drug for each patient.

Maltose is added to the solution in a 10% concentration for stabilization of the protein.[15] A comparative clinical study of IGIV with and without maltose showed the incidence of adverse effects was significantly less with the maltose-containing preparation.[16]

The intravenous administration of solutions of maltose has been studied by several investigators.[17-21] Healthy subjects tolerated the infusions well and no adverse effects were observed at a rate of 0.25 g maltose/kg per hour.[18] In safety studies conducted by Cutter Laboratories, infusions of 10% maltose administered at 0.27 to 0.62 g maltose/kg per hour[21] to normal subjects produced either mild side effects (e.g., headache) or no adverse reaction.[22] Following intravenous infusions of maltose, maltose was detected in the peripheral blood, there was a dose dependent excretion of maltose and glucose in the urine and a mild diuretic effect.[22] These alterations were tolerated without significant adverse effects.[22]

Since one milliliter of IGIV,5%-Maltose contains 0.1 g of maltose, the recommended dose of 0.1 g to 0.2 g IGIV,5%-Maltose per kilogram body weight (see Dosage and Administration) would result in the patient receiving a total of 0.2 g to 0.4 g maltose per kilogram body weight given over 2 to 4 hours. These amounts are within those levels tolerated in the Cutter safety studies cited above.

Indications and Usage: Immune Globulin Intravenous,5% in 10% Maltose (IGIV,5%-Maltose)-Gamimune® is indicated for the maintenance treatment of patients who are unable to produce sufficient amounts of IgG antibodies. Usage of Gamimune may be preferred to that of intramuscular immunoglobulin preparations especially in patients who require an immediate increase in intravascular immunoglobulin levels, in patients with a small muscle mass, and in patients with bleeding tendencies in whom intramuscular injections are contraindicated. It may be used in disease states such as congenital agammaglobulinemia (e.g., x-linked agammaglobulinemia), common variable hypogammaglobulinemia, x-linked immunodeficiency with hyper IgM, and combined immunodeficiency.[4,9-11,14,16,22-24]

Contraindications: IGIV,5%-Maltose is contraindicated in individuals who are known to have had an anaphylactic or severe systemic response to Immune Serum Globulin (Human). Individuals with selective IgA deficiencies who have known anti-IgA antibody should not receive IGIV,5%-Maltose since these patients may experience severe anaphylactic reactions to even small amounts of immune globulin preparations.[25]

Warnings: IGIV,5%-Maltose should be administered only intravenously as the intramuscular route has not yet been evaluated.

IGIV,5%-Maltose can, on occasion, cause a precipitous fall in blood pressure and the clinical picture of anaphylaxis even when the patient is not known to be sensitive to immune globulin preparations. These reactions appear to be related to the rate of infusion. Accordingly, the infusion rate given under Dosage and Administration should be closely followed, at least until the physician has had sufficient experience with a given patient. The patient's vital signs should be monitored continuously and careful observation made for any symptoms throughout the entire infusion. Epinephrine should be available for treatment of any acute anaphylactoid reaction.

Precautions:
General: Any vial that has been entered should be used promptly. Partially used vials should be discarded. Do not use if turbid.
Drug Interactions: If dilution is required Immune Globulin Intravenous,5% in 10% Maltose (IGIV,5%-Maltose)-Gamimune® may be diluted with 5% dextrose. No other drug interactions or compatibilities have been evaluated. It is recommended that the infusion of Gamimune be given via separate line, by itself, without mixing with other intravenous fluids or medications the patient might be receiving.

Pregnancy Category C:
Animal reproduction studies have not been conducted with Gamimune. It is also not known whether Gamimune can cause fetal harm when administered to a pregnant woman or can affect reproduction capacity. Gamimune should be given to a pregnant woman only if clearly needed.

Adverse Reactions: In a small safety study of IGIV,5%-Maltose, pH 5.25 in ten patients with primary immunodeficiency diseases, who received a total of 28 infusions at a dose of 400 mg per kg body weight, there were no adverse reactions reported during any of the infusions. Post-infusion, three patients reported adverse effects "possibly" or "definitely" related to the IGIV infusion; two patients experienced post-infusion headache, and one had a flu-like syndrome consisting of joint pain, red ees, and fatigue following the infusion.[22] During additional investigational studies, eleven other patients with hematologic disorders received a total of 91 infusions of IGIV,5%-Maltose, pH 5.25. Most of these infusions were at doses of 400 mg/kg body weight for 5 consecutive days; however, some patients received 800 mg/kg body weight as a single infusion intermittently. In this group, 6 out of 11 patients (55%) reported generally mild reactions in 11 out of 91 infusions (12%). The most common symptom noted was headache (occasionally during infusion but more commonly post-infusion); other less frequent side effects were low grade fever, nausea, emesis and chest tightness.[22]

Other types of adverse reactions have not been reported to date with IGIV,5%-Maltose, pH 5.25. It may be, however, that adverse effects will be similar to those seen with IGIV,5%-Maltose, pH 6.8, to which it is identical except for a slight difference in pH and the absence of glycine.

Potential reactions, therefore, may also include anxiety, flushing, chills, wheezing, abdominal cramps, back pain, myalgia, arthralgia, malaise and dizziness; rash has been reported only rarely. These reactions tend to be related to the rate of infusion; their management is described under Dosage and Administration. The over-all reaction rate for IGIV,5%-Maltose, pH 5.25 of approximately 11% is similar to that previously reported with infusions of IGIV,5%-Maltose, pH 6.8.[16,22,23,26-37]

True anaphylactic reactions to IGIV,5%-Maltose may occur in recipients with documented prior histories of severe allergic reactions to intramuscular immune seum globulin, but some patients may tolerate cautiously administered IGIV without adverse effects.[22,38] Very rarely an anaphylactoid reaction may occur in patients with no prior history of severe allergic reactions to either intramuscular or intravenous immune serum globulin.[22]

Dosage and Administration: The usual dose of Immune Globulin Intravenous,5% in 10% Maltose (IGIV,5%-Maltose)-Gamimune® for prophylaxis in immunodeficiency syndromes is 100 mg/kg of body weight (i.e., 2 mL/kg body weight) administered once a month by intravenous infusion. If the clinical response is inadequate or the level of IgG achieved (in the circulation) is felt to be insufficient, the dosage may be increased to 200 mg/kg body weight (i.e., 4 mL/kg body weight) or the infusion may be repeated more frequently than once a month.

Recent investigations confirm that Gamimune is well tolerated and less likely to produce side effects when infused at the indicated rate.[16] It is recommended that Gamimune be infused, by itself, at a rate of 0.01 to 0.02 mL/kg body weight per minute for 30 minutes. If the patient does not experience any discomfort, the rate may be gradually increased to between 0.02 and 0.04 mL/kg body weight per minute. If side effects occur, the rate should be reduced or the infusion interrupted until the symptoms subside. The infusion may

Continued on next page

Cutter—Cont.

then be resumed at a rate which is tolerated by the patient.

Parenteral drug products should be inspected visually for particulate matter and discoloration prior to administration whenever solution and container permit.

How Supplied: Gamimune® is supplied in 10, 50 and 100 ml single dose vials.

Storage: Store at 2 to 8°C (35 to 46°F). Do not freeze. Solution that has been frozen should not be used. Do not use after expiration date.

Caution: U.S. Federal law prohibits dispensing without a prescription.

Limited Warranty: A number of factors beyond our control could reduce the efficacy of this product or event result in an ill effect following its use. These include improper storage and handling of the product after it leaves our hands, diagnosis, dosage, method of administration, and biological differences in individual patients. Because of these factors, it is important that this product be stored properly and the directions be followed carefully during use.

The foregoing statement is made in lieu of any other warranty, expressed or implied, including any warranty of merchantibility or fitness. Representatives of the Company are not authorized to vary the terms of this warranty or the contents of any printed labeling for this product except by printed notice from the Company's Berkeley office. The prescriber and user of this product must accept the terms hereof.

References:
1. Pappenhagen AR, Lundblad JL, Schroeder DD, inventors; Cutter Laboratories, Inc., assignee. Pharmaceutical compositions comprising intravenously injectable modified serum globulin, its productions and use. U.S. patent 3,903,262 1975 September 2.
2. Schroeder DD, Tankersley DL, Lundblad JL: A new preparation of modified immune serum globulin (human) suitable for intravenous administration. I. Standardization of the reduction and alkylation reaction. *Vox Sang* 40:373-82, 1981.
3. Schroeder DD, Tankersley DL, Lundblad JL: A new generation of modified immune serum globulin (human) suitable for intravenous administration. II. Functional characterization. *Vox Sang* 40:383-94, 1981.
4. Ochs HD, Davis SD, Wedgwood RJ: Intravenous gamma globulin (IVGG) therapy in immunodeficiency syndromes. *Clin Res* 22:124A, 1974.
5. Davis SD: Efficacy of modified human immune serum globulin in the treatment of experimental murine infections with seven immunotypes of *Pseudomonas aeruginosa*. *J Infect Dis* 131(6):717-21, 1975.
6. Scheiermann N, Duwert EK: Untersuchung menschlicher Gammaglobulinpraparate. I. (Mitteilung): Virales Antikoerperprofil. *Med Klin* 74(21):820-4, 1979.
7. Scheiermann N, Duwert EK: Untersuchung menschlicher Gammaglobulinpraparte. II. Reinheitsgrad und Zusammensetzung. *Med Klin* 74(21):825-9, 1979.
8. Collins MS, Zuffi C, Fox EN: Group B streptococcal bactericidal properties of modified human immune globulin. Abstract. Annual Meeting of the American Society for Microbiology, Los Angeles, May 4-9, 1979.
9. Nolte MT, Pirofsky B, Gerritz GA, et al: Intravenous immunogloulin therapy for antibody deficiency. *Clin Exp Immunol* 36:237-43, 1979.
10. Pirofsky B, Campbell SM, Montanaro A: Individual patient variations in the kinetics of intravenous immune globulin administration. *J Clin Immunol* 2(2:Suppl):7S-14S, 1982.
11. Ochs HD, Fischer SH, Wedgwood RJ: Modified immune globulin: Its use in the prophylactic treatment of patients with immune deficiency. *J Clin Immunol* 2(2:Suppl):22S-30S, 1982.
12. Ammann AJ, Ashman RF, Buckley RH, et al: Use of intravenous gammaglobulin in antibody immunodeficiency: results of a multicenter controlled trial. *Clin Immunol Immunopath* 22:60-7, 1982.
13. Wells JV, Stites DP, Wybran J, et al: New preparation of therapeutic intravenous gamma-globulin: normal survival in acquired hypogammaglobulinemia. *Clin Res* 20:521, 1972.
14. Buckley RH: Immunoglobulin replacement therapy: indications and contraindications for use and variable IgG levels achieved. In: Alving BM (ed): Immunoglobulins: characteristics and uses of intravenous preparations. Washington, D.C., U.S. Government Printing Office [1980], pp 3-8.
15. Lundblad JL, Warner WL, Fernandes PM, inventors; Cutter Laboratories, Inc., assignee. Stabilized immune serum globulin. U.S. patent 4,186,192 1980 January 29.
16. Ochs HD, Buckley RH, Pirofsky B, et al: Safety and patient acceptability of intravenous immune globulin in 10% maltose. *Lancet* 2(8205):1158-9, 1980.
17. Berg G, Matzkies F: Wirkung von Maltose nach intravenoser Dauerinfusion auf den Stoffwechsel. *Z Ernahrungswiss* 15:255-62, 1976.
18. Forster H, Hoos I, Boecker S: Versuche mit Probanden zur parenteralen Verwertung von Maltose. *Z Ernahrungswiss* 15(3):284-93, 1976.
19. Finke C, Reinauer H: Utilization of maltose and oligosaccharides after intravenous infusion in man. *Nutr Metab* 21(Supp 1):115-7, 1977.
20. Young EA, Drummond A, Cioletti L, et al: Metabolism of continuously infused intravenous maltose. *Clin Res* 25(3):543A, 1977.
21. Soroff HS, Hansen LM, Sasvary D, et al: Clinical pharmacology and metabolism of maltose in normal human volunteers. *Clin Res* 26(3):286A, 1978.
22. Unpublished data in the files of Cutter Biological.
23. Pirofsky B, Anderson CJ, Bardana EJ Jr.: Therapeutic and detrimental effects of intravenous immunoglobulin therapy. In: Alving BM (ed): Immunoglobins: characteristics and uses of intravenous preparations. Washington, D.C., U.S. Government Printing Office [1980], pp 15-22.
24. Ochs HD: Intravenous immunoglobulin therapy of patients with primary immunodeficiency syndromes: efficacy and safety of a new modified immune globulin preparation. In: Alving BM (ed): Immunoglobulins: characteristics and uses of intravenous preparations. Washington, DC, U.S. Government Printing Office, [1980], pp 9-14.
25. Molleson, PL: Blood Transfusion in Clinical Medicine, 6th Edition, Oxford, The Oxford Press, [1979], pp 626-7.
26. Montanaro A, Pirofsky B: Prolonged interval high-dose intravenous immunoglobulin in patients with primary immunodeficiency states. *Am J Med* 76(3A):67-72, 1984.
27. Sorensen RU, Tomford JW, Gyves MT, et al: Use of intravenous immunoglobulin in pregnant women with common variable hypogammaglobulinemia. *Am J Med* 76(3A):73-7, 1984.
28. Gordon DS, Hearn EB, Spira TJ, et al: Phase I study of intravenous gammaglobulin in multiple myeloma. *Am J Med* 76(3A):111-16, 1984
29. Winston DJ, Ho WG, Lin C-H, et al: Intravenous immune globulin for modification of cytomegalovirus infections associated with bone marrow transplantations. Preliminary results of a controlled trial. *Am J Med* 76(3A):128-33, 1984.
30. Warrier AI, Lusher JM: Intravenous gammaglobulin treatment of chronic idiopathic thrombocytopenic purpura in children. *Am J Med* 76(3A):193-8, 1984.
31. Besa EC: Use of immunoglobulin in chronic lymphocytic leukemia: *Am J Med* 76(3A):209-18, 1984.
32. Preiksaitis JK, Rosno S, Rasmussen L, et al: Cytomegalovirus infection in heart transplant recipients: preliminary results of a controlled trial of intravenous gamma globulin. *J Clin Immun* 2(2):365-415, 1982.
33. Winston DJ, Ho WG, Rasmussen LE, et al: Use of intravenous immune globulin in patients receiving bone marrow transplants. *J Clin Immun* 2(2):42S-47S, 1982.
34. Carroll RR, Noyes WD, Kitchens CS: High-dose intravenous immunoglobulin therapy in patients with immune thrombocytopenic purpura. *JAMA* 249:1748-50, 1983.
35. Dau PC: Immunoglobulin intravenous replacement after plasma exchange. *J Clin Aphereis* 1:104-8, 1983.
36. Kekomaki R, Elfenbeing G, Gardner R, et al: Improved response of patients refractory to random-donor platelet transfusions by intravenous gamma globulin. *Am J Med* 76(3A):199-203, 1984.
37. Shirani KZ, Vaughan GM, McManus AT, et al: Replacement therapy with modified immunoglobulin G in burn patients: preliminary kinetic studies. *Am J Med* 76(3A):175-80, 1984.
38. Peerless AG, Stiehm ER: Intravenous gammaglobulin for reaction to intramuscular preparation. *Lancet* 2(8347):461, 1983.

U.S. License No. 8
Canadian License No. 24

HYPERAB® ℞
[hī'per-ab"]
(Rabies Immune Globulin—Human)
2 ml. (300 IU) pediatric vial
10 ml. (1500 IU) adult vial

HYPERHEP® ℞
[hī'per-hep"]
(Hepatitis B Immune Globulin—Human)
1 ml., 5 ml. vials

HYPER-TET® ℞
[hī'per-tet"]
(Tetanus Immune Globulin—Human U.S.P.)
250 units vial or prefilled disposable syringe

HYPERTUSSIS® ℞
[hī'per-tus"is]
(Pertussis Immune Globulin—Human, U.S.P.)
1.25 ml. vial

HypRho®–D Mini-Dose ℞
[hī"prō-d']
Rh₀(D) Immune Globulin (Human), USP

Description: Rh₀(D) Immune Globulin (Human)—HypRho®-D Mini-Dose—is a sterile solution of immune globulin containing antibodies to Rh₀(D) which is for intramuscular injection only. It is prepared from human venous plasma collected from carefully screened donors. It contains 16.5 ± 1.5% protein stabilized with 0.3 M glycine and preserved with 1:10,000 thimerosal (a mercury derivative). The pH is adjusted with sodium carbonate.

One dose of HypRho-D Mini-Dose contains not less than one-sixth the quantity of Rh₀(D) antibody contained in one standard dose of Rh₀(D) Immune Globulin (Human), and it will suppress the immunizing potential of 2.5 ml of Rh₀(D) positive or D^u positive packed red blood cells or the equivalent of whole blood (5 ml). HypRho-D Mini-Dose has been titered against and the quantity of Rh₀(D) antibody found to be not less than one-sixth of that contained in 1 ml of the U.S. Food and Drug Administration Reference Rh₀(D) Immune Globulin (Human).

Each individual unit of plasma used in the manufacturing of this product has been found nonreactive for hepatitis B surface antigen (HBsAg) using a U.S. Federally approved test with third-generation sensitivity.

Clinical Pharmacology: Rh sensitization may occur in nonsensitized $Rh_o(d)$ negative. D^u negative women following transplacental hemorrhage resulting from spontaneous or induced abortions.[1-2] The risk of sensitization is higher in women undergoing induced abortions than in those aborting spontaneously.[1-3]

HypRho-D Mini-Dose is used to prevent the formation of anti-$Rh_o(D)$ antibody in $Rh_o(D)$ negative, D^u negative women who are exposed to the $Rh_o(D)$ antigen at the time of spontaneous or induced abortion (up to 12 weeks gestation).[3-5] HypRho-D Mini-Dose suppresses the stimulation of active immunity by $Rh_o(D)$ positive or D^u positive fetal erythrocytes that may enter the maternal circulation at the time of termination of the pregnancy. The amount of anti-$Rh_o(D)$ in HypRho-D Mini-Dose has been shown to effectively prevent maternal isosensitization to the $Rh_o(D)$ or D^u antigens following spontaneous or induced abortion occurring up to the 12th week of gestation.[6-8] After the 12th week of gestation, a standard dose of $Rh_o(D)$ Immune Globulin (Human)—HypRho®-D is indicated.

Indications and Usage: HypRho-D Mini-Dose is recommended to prevent the isoimmunization of $Rh_o(D)$ negative, D^u negative women at the time of spontaneous or induced abortion of up to 12 weeks gestation provided the following criteria are met:
1. The mother must be $Rh_o(D)$ negative and D^u negative and must not already be sensitized to the $Rh_o(D)$ antigen.
2. The father is not known to be $Rh_o(D)$ negative and D^u negative.
3. Gestation is not more than 12 weeks at termination.

Note: $Rh_o(D)$ Immune Globulin (Human) prophylaxis is not indicated if the fetus or father can be determined to be Rh negative. If the Rh status of the fetus is unknown, the fetus must be assumed to be $Rh_o(D)$ positive or D^u positive, and HypRho-D Mini-Dose should be administered to the mother. FOR ABORTIONS OR MISCARRIAGES OCCURRING AFTER 12-WEEKS GESTATION, A STANDARD DOSE OF $RH_o(D)$ IMMUNE GLOBULIN (HUMAN) IS INDICATED.

HypRho-D Mini-Dose should be administered within three hours or as soon as possible after spontaneous passage or surgical removal of the products of conception. However, if HypRho-D Mini-Dose is not given within this time period, consideration should still be given to its administration since clinical studies in male volunteers have demonstrated the effectiveness of $Rh_o(D)$ Immune Globulin (Human) in preventing isoimmunization as long as 72 hours after infusion of $Rh_o(D)$ positive red cells.[9]

Contraindications: HypRho-D Mini-Dose is contraindicated for use in:
1. An $Rh_o(D)$ positive or D^u positive individual.
2. An $Rh_o(D)$ negative and D^u negative individual previously sensitized to the $Rh_o(D)$ or D^u antigen.

Warnings: HypRho-D Mini-Dose should be given with caution to patients with a history of prior systemic allergic reactions following the administration of human immune globulin preparations.

Precautions: INJECT ONLY INTRAMUSCULARLY. NEVER ADMINISTER HYPRHO-D MINI-DOSE INTRAVENOUSLY. DO NOT SKIN TEST. ADMINISTER ONLY TO WOMEN POST-ABORTION OR POST-MISCARRIAGE OF UP TO 12 WEEKS GESTATION.

Adverse Reactions: Reactions to $Rh_o(D)$ Immune Globulin (Human) are infrequent in $Rh_o(D)$ negative, D^u negative individuals and consist primarily of slight soreness at the site of injection and slight temperature elevation. While sensitization to repeated injections of human globulin is extremely rare, it has occurred.

No instances of transmission of hepatitis have been reported from the use of human immune globulin prepared by the fractionation methods employed by Cutter Biological.

Dosage and Administration: One syringe of HypRho-D Mini-Dose provides sufficient antibody to prevent Rh sensitization to 2.5 ml $Rh_o(D)$ positive or D^u positive packed red cells or the equivalent (5 ml) of whole blood. This dose is sufficient to provide protection against maternal Rh sensitization for women undergoing spontaneous or induced abortion of up to 12 weeks gestation.

HypRho-D Mini-Dose should be administered within three hours or as soon as possible following spontaneous or induced abortion. If prompt administration is not possible, HypRho-D Mini-Dose should be given within 72 hours following termination of the pregnancy.

How Supplied: Each HypRho-D Mini-Dose package contains:
Ten single dose prefilled syringes of HypRho-D Mini-Dose, a package insert giving directions for use, and patient identification cards. Product Code 621-05.

Storage: Store at 2–8°C (35–46°F). Do not freeze. Do not use after expiration date.

Caution: U.S. Federal law prohibits dispensing without prescription.

Limited Warranty: A number of factors beyond our control could reduce the efficacy of this product or even result in an ill effect following its use. These include storage and handling of the product after it leaves our hands, diagnosis, dosage, method of administration, and biological differences in individual patients. Because of these factors, it is important that this product be stored properly and that the directions be followed carefully during use.

The foregoing statement is made in lieu of any other warranty, express or implied, including any warranty of merchantability or fitness. Representatives of the company are not authorized to vary the terms of this warranty or the contents of any printed labeling for this product except by printed notice from the Company's Berkeley office. The prescriber and user of this product must accept the terms hereof.

References:
1. Queenan JT, Shah S. Kubarych SF, et al: Role of induced abortion in rhesus immunisation. *Lancet* 1(7704):815-7, 1971.
2. Goldman JA, Eckerling B: Prevention of Rh immunization after abortion with anti-$Rh_o(D)$-immunoglobulin. *Obstet Gynecol* 40(3):366-70, 1972.
3. The selective use of $Rh_o(D)$ immune globulin (RhIG). *ACOG Tech Bull* 61, 1981.
4. Prevention of Rh sensitization. *WHO Tech Rep Ser* 468, 1971.
5. Recommendation of the Public Health Service Advisory Committee on Immunization Practices: Rh immune globulin. *Morbid Mortal Wkly Rep* 21(15):126–7, 1972.
6. Stewart FH, Burnhill MS, Bozorgi N: Reduced dose of Rh immunoglobulin following first trimester pregnancy termination. *Obstet Gynecol* 51(3):318–22, 1978.
7. McMaster conference on prevention of Rh immunization. 28–30 September, 1977. *Vox Sang* 36(1):50–64, 1979.
8. Simonovits I: Efficiency of anti-D IgG prevention after induced abortion, *Vox Sang* 26(4):361–7, 1974.
9. Freda VJ, Gorman JG, Pollack W: Prevention of Rh-hemolytic disease with Rh-immune globulin. *Am J Obstet Gynecol* 128(4):456–60, 1977.

HypRho®-D R
[hī″prō-d′]
$Rh_o(D)$ Immune
Globulin (Human)

Description: $Rh_o(D)$ Immune Globulin (Human)—HypRho®-D is a sterile solution of immune globulin containing antibodies to $Rh_o(D)$ prepared from human venous plasma collected from carefully screened donors. It contains 16.5 ± 1.5% protein stabilized with 0.3 M glycine and preserved with 1:10,000 thimerosal (a mercury derivative). The pH is adjusted with sodium carbonate. HypRho-D has been titered against and the potency found equal to or greater than that of the U.S. Food and Drug Administration Reference $Rh_o(D)$ Immune Globulin (Human). One vial or syringe has been shown to effectively suppress the immunizing potential of 15 ml of $Rh_o(D)$ positive or D^u positive packed red blood cells.

This product has been prepared from large pools of human venous plasma. Each individual unit of plasma has been found nonreactive for hepatitis B surface antigen (HBsAg) using a U.S. Federally approved test of at least third-generation sensitivity.

Clinical Pharmacology: HypRho-D is used to prevent isoimmunization in the $Rh_o(D)$ negative, D^u negative individual exposed to $Rh_o(D)$ positive or D^u positive blood as the result of a fetomaternal hemorrhage occuring during a delivery of a $Rh_o(D)$ positive or D^u positive infant, abortion (either spontaneous or induced), or following amniocentesis. Similarly, immunization resulting in the production of anti-$Rh_o(D)$ following transfusion of Rh positive red cells to a $Rh_o(D)$ negative recipient may be prevented by administering $Rh_o(D)$ immune globulin.

Rh hemolytic disease of the newborn is the result of the active immunization of a $Rh_o(D)$ negative, D^u negative mother by $Rh_o(D)$ positive or D^u positive red cells entering the maternal circulation during a previous delivery, abortion or amniocentesis or as a result of red cell transfusion. HypRho-D acts by suppressing the specific immune response of $Rh_o(D)$ negative individuals to $Rh_o(D)$ positive red blood cells.

The administration of $Rh_o(D)$ Immune Globulin within 72 hours of a full-term delivery of an infant to a $Rh_o(D)$ negative, D^u negative mother at risk reduced the incidence of Rh isoimmunization from 12–13% reduces 1–2%. The 1–2% treatment failures are probably due to isoimmunization occurring during the latter part of pregnancy or following delivery. Bowman, et al, have reported that the incidence of isoimmunization can be further reduced from approximately 1.6% to less than 0.1% by administering $Rh_o(D)$ Immune Globulin in two doses, one antenatal at 28 weeks gestation and another following delivery.

Indications and Usage:
Pregnancy and Other Obstetric Conditions
HypRho-D is recommended for the prevention of Rh hemolytic disease of the newborn by its administration to the $Rh_o(D)$ negative, D^u negative mother within 72 hours after birth of a $Rh_o(D)$ positive or D^u positive infant, providing the following criteria are met:
1. The mother must be $Rh_o(D)$ negative, D^u negative and must not already be sensitized to the $Rh_o(D)$ factor.
2. Her child must be $Rh_o(D)$ positive or D^u positive, and should have a negative direct Coombs test. A positive direct Coombs test may be caused by antibodies other than $Rh_o(D)$ and while this does not contraindicate therapy with HypRho-D, it should be investigated. A positive direct Coombs test due to anti-$Rh_o(D)$ is a contraindication to the use of HypRho-D.

Even though Rh hemolytic disease of the newborn is less frequent when there is ABO incompatibility between the $Rh_o(D)$ negative mother and the $Rh_o(D)$ positive fetus, protection against $Rh_o(D)$ sensitization may be incomplete, and treatment of the mother with HypRho-D is indicated in such cases.

If $Rh_o(D)$ Immune Globulin (Human)—HypRho®-D is administered antepartum, it is essential that the mother receive another dose of HypRho-D after delivery of a $Rh_o(D)$ positive or D^u positive infant.

HypRho-D should be administered within 72 hours to all nonimmunized $Rh_o(D)$ negative, D^u negative women who have undergone spontaneous or induced abortion, following ruptured tubal pregnancy or following amniocentesis unless the blood type of the fetus or the father is known to be $Rh_o(D)$ negative, R^u negative. If the fetal blood type is unknown, one must assume that it is $Rh_o(D)$

Continued on next page

Cutter—Cont.

positive, and HypRho-D should be administered to the mother.

Transfusion

HypRho-D may be used to prevent isoimmunization in $Rh_o(D)$ negative, D^u negative individuals who have been transfused with $Rh_o(D)$ positive or D^u positive red blood cells or blood components containing red blood cells.

Contraindications: HypRho-D is contraindicated for use in:
1. A $Rh_o(D)$ positive or D^u positive individual.
2. A $Rh_o(D)$ negative or D^u negative individual previously sensitized to the $Rh_o(D)$ or D^u antigen.

Warnings:
1. Solutions which have been frozen should not be used.
2. Partially used vials or syringes must be discarded.
3. Babies born of women given Rh immune globulin antepartum may have a weakly positive direct Coomb's test at birth.

Precautions: NEVER ADMINISTER HypRho-D INTRAVENOUSLY. NEVER ADMINISTER TO THE NEONATE.

The presence of fetal cells in a maternal blood sample, or passive antibody given to the mother antepartum can affect the interpretation of laboratory tests to identify and monitor the patient for HypRho-D. If in doubt as to the patient's Rh type or immune status, HypRho-D should be administered.

Adverse Reactions: Reactions to $Rh_o(D)$ Immune Globulin (Human) are infrequent in $Rh_o(D)$ negative, D^u negative individuals and consist primarily of slight soreness at the site of injection and slight temperature elevation. While sensitization to repeated injections of human immune globulin is extremely rare, it has occurred. Elevated bilirubin levels have been reported in some individuals receiving multiple doses of $Rh_o(D)$ Immune Globulin (Human) following mismatched tranfusions. This is believed to be due to a relatively rapid rate of foreign red cell destruction.

No instances of transmission of hepatitis have been reported from the use of human immune globulin prepared by the fractionation methods employed at Cutter Laboratories, Inc.

Dosage and Administration:

Pregnancy and Other Obstetric Conditions
1. For postpartum prophylaxis, administer one vial or syringe of HypRho-D intramuscularly, preferably within 72 hours of delivery. Although a lesser degree of protection is afforded if Rh antibody is administered beyond the 72-hour period, HypRho-D may still be given. However, full-term deliveries can vary in their dosage requirements depending on the magnitude of the fetomaternal hemorrhage. One vial or syringe of HypRho-D provides sufficient antibody to prevent Rh sensitization if the **packed red blood cell** volume that has entered the circulation is 15 ml or less. In instances where a large (greater than 30 ml of whole blood or 15 ml **packed red blood cells**) fetomaternal hemorrhage is suspected, a fetal red cell count by an approved laboratory technique (e.g. Modified Kleihauer-Betke acid elution stain technique) should be performed to determine the dosage of immune globulin required. The **packed red blood cell** volume of the calculated fetomaternal hemorrhage is divided by 15 ml to obtain the number of vials or syringes of HypRho-D for administration.
2. For antenatal prophylaxis, one vial or syringe of $Rh_o(D)$ Immune Globulin (Human)—HypRho®D is administered intramuscularly at approximately 28 weeks. This must be followed by another full dose (one vial or one syringe), preferably within 72 hours following delivery, if the infant is Rh positive.
3. Following miscarriage, abortion, or ectopic pregnancy, it is recommended that one vial or syringe of HypRho-D be given. If more than 15 ml of packed red cells is suspected, due to fetomaternal hemorrhage, the same dose modification in #1 above applies.

Transfusion

In the case of a transfusion of $Rh_o(D)$ positive or D^u positive red cells to a $Rh_o(D)$ negative, D^u negative recipient, the volume of Rh positive whole blood administered is multiplied by the hematocrit of the donor unit giving the volume of **packed red blood cells** transfused. The volume of **packed red blood cells** is divided by 15 ml which provides the number of vials or syringes of HypRho-D to be administered.

If the dose calculated results in a fraction, the next whole number of vials or syringes should be administered (e.g., if 1.4, give 2 vials or 2 syringes). HypRho-D should be administered within 72 hours after the red cell transfusion, but preferably as soon as possible.

Injection Procedure

DO NOT INJECT INTRAVENOUSLY. DO NOT INJECT NEONATE.

A. Single Vial or Syringe Dose
INJECT ENTIRE CONTENTS OF THE VIAL OR SYRINGE INTO THE INDIVIDUAL INTRAMUSCULARLY.

B. Multiple Vial or Syringe Dose
1. Calculate the number of vials or syringes of HypRho-D to be given (See Dosage section).
2. The total volume of HypRho-D can be given in divided doses at different sites at one time or the total dose may be divided and injected at intervals, provided the total dosage is given within 72 hours of the fetomaternal hemorrhage or transfusion. USING STERILE TECHNIQUE, INJECT THE ENTIRE CONTENTS OF THE CALCULATED NUMBER OF VIALS OR SYRINGES INTRAMUSCULARLY INTO THE PATIENT.

Storage: Store at 2–8°C (35–46°F). Do not freeze. Do not use after expiration date. Do not store after entry.

How Supplied: HypRho-D is available in vials and in syringes as follows:

Product Code	Contents
621-10	Ten single dose vials of HypRho-D. Package insert giving directions for use and patient identification cards.
621-15	One single dose vial of HypRho-D. Package insert giving directions for use, patient identification cards, and injection form.
621-22	Ten single dose syringes of HypRho-D. Package insert giving directions for use and patient identification cards.
621-05	Ten single dose prefilled syringes of HypRho-D Mini-Dose. Package insert giving directions for use, and patient identification cards.

Caution: U.S. Federal law prohibits dispensing without a prescription.

14-7621-102
(Rev May 1982)

KOĀTE®-HT ℞
[kō'ate]
Antihemophilic Factor (Human)
(Factor VIII, AHF, AHG)

A heat-treated, stable, purified dried concentrate of human Antihemophilic Factor.

250 AHF units, approx., with 10 ml. Sterile Water for Injection, U.S.P., sterile filter needle, and transfer needle.
500 AHF units, approx., with 20 ml. Sterile Water for Injection, U.S.P., sterile filter needle, and transfer needle.
1000 AHF units, approx., with 40 ml Sterile Water for Injection, U.S.P., sterile filter needle, and transfer needle.
1500 AHF units, approx., with 40 ml Sterile Water for Injection, U.S.P., sterile filter needle, and transfer needle.

KONYNE® ℞
[kō'nine]
(Factor IX Complex—Human—Factors II, VII, IX and X)

500 unit vial, approx., with 20 ml. Sterile Water for Injection, U.S.P., sterile filter needle, and transfer needle.
1000 unit vial, approx., with 40 ml. Sterile Water for Injection, U.S.P., sterile filter needle, and transfer needle.

PLAGUE VACCINE, U.S.P. ℞
20 ml. vials

Dalin Pharmaceuticals, Inc.
74-80 MARINE STREET
FARMINGDALE, NY 11735

CELLUZYME™
[sel'u-zime]
Chewable Digestive Enzyme Tablets with Simethicone

Description: Green, spearmint-flavored, chewable, palatable tablets. Each tablet contains Cellulase 9 mg., Amylase 30 mg., Protease 6 mg., Lipase 20 mg., Simethicone 25 mg.

Action and Uses: To relieve the discomfort of: Intestinal Gas • Vegetable Bezoars • Functional Gastrointestinal Disorders • Pancreatic Insufficiency • Dyspepsia • Flatulence • Bloating.

Contraindications: A known sensitivity to any ingredient.

Dosage: Chew or swallow 1 or 2 tablets with meals and at bedtime.

How Supplied: 100 tablets. Hospital Unit Dose Available.

Remarks: DOES NOT CONTAIN PANCREATIN.

DALIDYNE™
[dal'e-dine]
Lotion
Effective Treatment and Prompt Relief

Composition: Methylbenzethonium Chloride, Benzocaine, Tannic Acid, Camphor, Chlorothymol, Menthol, Benzyl Alcohol in a Specially Prepared Aromatized Base. Alcohol 61%.

Action and Uses: A cooling, soothing, quick-drying lotion possessing anesthetic, astringent, germicidal, fungicidal and healing properties used in the treatment of: Aphthous Stomatitis • Herpes Simplex • Herpes Genitalis • Trench Mouth • Thrush • Gingivitis • Denture Irritations • Teething Pain • Throat Irritations (as mouth wash or gargle).

Administration and Dosage: Topical Application: Dry area and apply several times a day with cotton applicator. As Gargle or Mouth Wash: ½ teaspoonful in ½ glass of warm water several times a day.

How Supplied: 1 fl. oz.

SORBUTUSS®
[sor'bew-tus]
Sugar Free for the Diabetic Cough Patient
Alcohol Free for the Alcoholic Patient

Composition: Each teaspoonful (5 cc.) contains d-methorphan hydrobromide 10 mg., glycerol guaiacolate 100 mg., potassium citrate 85 mg., citric acid 35 mg., in a palatable, mint-flavored, glycerin-sorbitol vehicle.

Action and Uses: Effective sugar-free and alcohol-free antitussive and expectorant with mucolytic properties for relief of coughs and coughs due to colds.

No • Sugar • Decongestants
   • Alcohol • Sodium
   • Antihistamines

Recommended for all patients including diabetic, cardiac, hypertensive, geriatric and alcoholic. Soothing for coughs due to smoking.

Product Information

Administration and Dosage: Adults—2 teaspoonfuls every 3 to 4 hours. Children—in proportion.

How Supplied: Bottles of 4 fl. oz., pints and gallons.

Remarks: SUGAR-FREE and SODIUM-FREE, NON-NARCOTIC and NON-ALCOHOLIC.

Danbury Pharmacal, Inc.
131 WEST STREET
P.O. BOX 296
DANBURY, CT 06810

PRODUCT IDENTIFICATION CODE

Danbury Prescription Capsules and Tablets are identified with a symbol DAN and the NDC Product Number.

Controlled Substance Products are identified with the Danbury NDC Number 591-followed by a letter identifying the product.

To quickly identify a product, a compilation of most of Danbury's products is listed below in alphabetical order with corresponding product codes.

NDC# 0591-	PRODUCT	IMPRINT
5543	Allopurinol Tablets, 100 mg.	U: DAN L: 5543
5544	Allopurinol Tablets, 300 mg.	U: DAN L: 5544
5370	Bethanechol Chloride Tablets, 5 mg.	U: DAN L: 5370
5369	Bethanechol Chloride Tablets, 10 mg.	U: DAN L: 5369
5402	Bethanechol Chloride Tablets, 25 mg.	U: DAN L: 5402
5515	Bethanechol Chloride Tablets, 50 mg.	U: DAN L: 5515
5519	Butalbital and Acetaminophen Tablets, 50 mg/325 mg.	591F
5541	Carisoprodol Compound Tablets	U: DAN L: 5541
5513	Carisoprodol Tablets, 350 mg.	U: DAN L: 5513
5548	Chloroquine Phosphate Tablets, 250 mg.	U: DAN L: 5548
5549	Chloroquine Phosphate Tablets, 500 mg.	U: DAN L: 5549
5444	Chlorothiazide Tablets, 250 mg.	U: DAN L: 5444
5579	Chlorpropamide Tablets, 100 mg.	U: DAN L: 5579
5455	Chlorpropamide Tablets, 250 mg.	U: DAN L: 5455
5507	Chlorthalidone Tablets, 25 mg.	U: DAN L: 5507
5518	Chlorthalidone Tablets, 50 mg.	U: DAN L: 5518
5495	Chlorzoxazone Tablets, 250 mg.	U: DAN L: 5495
5509	Chlorzoxazone with APAP Tablets, 250 mg.	U: DAN L: 5509
0944	Colchicine Tablets, 0.6 mg.	U: DAN L: 944
5325	Col-Probenecid Tablets, 0.5 mg./500 mg.	U: DAN L: 5325
5484	Cyproheptadine HCl. Tablets, 4 mg.	U: DAN L: 5484
5309	Dicyclomine HCl. Capsules, 10 mg.	DAN/ 5309
5383	Dicyclomine HCl. Tablets, 20 mg.	U: DAN L: 5383
5002	Diphenhydramine HCl. Capsules, 25 mg.	DAN/ 5002
5003	Diphenhydramine HCl. Capsules, 50 mg.	DAN/ 5003
5510	Dipyridamole Tablets, 25 mg.	DAN/ 5510
5376	Disulfiram Tablets, 250 mg.	U: DAN L: 5376
5368	Disulfiram Tablets, 500 mg.	U: DAN L: 5368
5535	Doxycycline Hyclate Capsules (Equivalent to 50 mg. Doxycycline)	DAN/ 5535
5440	Doxycycline Hyclate Capsules (Equivalent to 100 mg. Doxycycline)	DAN/ 5440
5553	Doxycycline Hyclate Tablets (Equivalent to 100 mg. Doxycycline)	U: DAN L: 5553
5504	Ergoloid Mesylates Oral Tablets 1.0 mg.	U: DAN L: 5504
5502	Ergoloid Mesylates Sublingual Tablets, 0.5 mg.	U: DAN L: 5502
5501	Ergoloid Mesylates Sublingual Tablets, 1.0 mg.	U: DAN L: 5501
5479	Erythromycin Estolate Capsules, 250 mg.	DAN/ 5479
5216	Folic Acid Tablets, 1.0 mg.	U: DAN L: 5216
5493	Glycopyrrolate Tablets, 1 mg.	U: DAN L: 5493
5494	Glycopyrrolate Tablets, 2 mg.	U: DAN L: 5494
5050	Hydralazine HCl. Tablets, 25 mg.	U: DAN L: 5050
5055	Hydralazine HCl. Tablets, 50 mg.	U: DAN L: 5055
5428	Hydrochlorothiazide, Hydralazine HCl., Reserpine Tablets, 15 mg., 25 mg. 0.1 mg.	L: 5428
5406	Hydrochlorothiazide/Reserpine Tablets, 25 mg./0.125 mg.	U: DAN L: 5406
5407	Hydrochlorothiazide/Reserpine Tablets 50 mg./0.125 mg.	U: DAN L: 5407
5345	Hydrochlorothiazide Tablets, 50 mg.	U: DAN L: 5345
5183	Hydrocortisone Tablets, 20 mg.	U: DAN L: 5183
5522	Hydroxyzine Hydrochloride Tablets, 10 mg.	U: DAN L: 5522
5523	Hydroxyzine Hydrochloride Tablets, 25 mg.	U: DAN L: 5523
5565	Hydroxyzine Hydrochloride Tablets, 50 mg.	U: DAN L: 5565
5532	Hydroxyzine Pamoate Capsules (Equivalent to 50 mg. Hydroxyzine HCl.)	DAN/ 5532
5537	Hydroxyzine Pamoate Capsules (Equivalent to 100 mg. Hydroxyzine HCl.)	DAN/ 5537
0528	Isoniazid Tablets, 50 mg.	U: DAN L: 528
0525	Isoniazid Tablets, 100 mg.	U: DAN L: 525
0526	Isoniazid Tablets, 300 mg.	U: DAN L: 526
5374	Isosorbide Dinitrate Oral Tablets, 5 mg.	U: DAN L: 5374
5373	Isosorbide Dinitrate Oral Tablets, 10 mg.	U: DAN L: 5373
5387	Isosorbide Dinitrate Sublingual Tablets, 2.5 mg.	U: DAN L: 5387
5385	Isosorbide Dinitrate Sublingual Tablets, 5 mg.	U: DAN L: 5385
5400	Isoxsuprine HCl. Tablets, 10 mg.	U: 10 L: DAN/ 5400
5401	Isoxsuprine HCl. Tablets, 20 mg.	U: 20 L: DAN/ 5401
5381	Methocarbamol Tablets, 500 mg.	U: DAN L: 5381
5382	Methocarbamol Tablets, 750 mg.	U: DAN L: 5382
5540	Metronidazole Tablets, 250 mg.	U: DAN L: 5540
5552	Metronidazole Tablets, 500 mg.	U: DAN L: 5552
5342	Nylidrin HCl. Tablets, 6 mg.	U: DAN L: 5342
5390	Nylidrin HCl. Tablets, 12 mg.	U: DAN L: 5390
0938	Papaverine HCl. Tablets, 100 mg.	U: DAN L: 938
5196	Papaverine HCl. T.D. Capsules, 150 mg.	DAN/ 5196
5521	Phenylbutazone Tablets, 100 mg.	U: DAN L: 5521
5059	Prednisolone Tablets, 5 mg.	U: DAN L: 5059
5052	Prednisone Tablets, 5 mg.	U: DAN L: 5052
5442	Prednisone Tablets, 10 mg.	U: DAN L: 5442
5443	Prednisone Tablets, 20 mg.	U: DAN L: 5443
5490	Prednisone Tablets, 50 mg.	U: DAN L: 5490
5321	Primidone Tablets, 250 mg.	U: DAN L: 5321
5347	Probenecid Tablets, 500 mg.	U: DAN L: 5347
5026	Procainamide HCl. Capsules, 250 mg.	DAN/ 5026
5350	Procainamide HCl. Capsules, 375 mg.	DAN/ 5350
5333	Procainamide HCl. Capsules, 500 mg.	DAN/ 5333
5257	Propantheline Bromide Tablets, 15 mg.	DAN/ 5257
5204	Pseudoephedrine HCl. Tablets, 60 mg.	U: DAN L: 5204
5516	Quindan Tablets (Quinine Sulfate Tablets, 260 mg.)	U: DAN L: 5516
5538	Quinidine Gluconate Sustained Action Tablets, 324 mg.	L: 5538
5453	Quinidine Sulfate Tablets, 100 mg.	U: DAN L: 5453
5438	Quinidine Sulfate Tablets, 200 mg.	U: DAN L: 5438
5454	Quinidine Sulfate Tablets, 300 mg.	U: DAN L: 5454
5496	Spironolactone/Hydrochlorothiazide Tablets	U: DAN L: 5496
5546	Sulfamethoxazole 400 mg. with Trimethoprim 80 mg. Tablets	U: DAN L: 5546
5547	Sulfamethoxazole 800 mg. with Trimethoprim 160 mg. Tablets (Double Strength)	U: DAN L: 5547
5503	Sulfasalazine Tablets, 500 mg.	DAN/ 5503
5514	Sulfinpyrazone Tablets, 100 mg.	U: DAN L: 5514
5162	Tetracycline HCl. Capsules, 250 mg.	DAN/ 5162
5520	Tetracycline HCl. Capsules, 500 mg.	DAN/ 5520
5481	Theofedral Tablets	U: DAN L: 5481
5566	Thioridazine HCl. Tablets, 10 mg.	U: DAN L: 5566
5572	Thioridazine HCl. Tablets, 15 mg.	U: DAN L: 5572
5542	Thioridazine HCl. Tablets, 25 mg.	U: DAN L: 5542
5568	Thioridazine HCl. Tablets, 50 mg.	U: DAN L: 5568
5569	Thioridazine HCl 100 mg.	U: DAN L: 5569
5508	Tolbutamide Tablets, 500 mg.	U: DAN L: 5508
5388	Triamcinolone Tablets, 4 mg.	U: DAN L: 5388
5335	Trihexyphenidyl HCl. Tablets, 2 mg.	U: DAN L: 5335
5337	Trihexyphenidyl HCl. Tablets, 5 mg.	U: DAN L: 5337
5058	Tripelennamine HCl. Tablets, 50 mg.	U: DAN L: 5058
5434	Tripodrine Tablets	U: DAN L: 5434

Continued on next page

Danbury—Cont.

CONTROLLED SUBSTANCE PRODUCTS

NDC#	SCHEDULE#	PRODUCT	IMPRINT
5238	C-IV	Meprobamate Tablets, 400 mg.	591-A
5239	C-IV	Meprobamate Tablets, 200 mg.	591-B
5069	C-IV	Phenobarbital Tablets, 1/4 gr.	591-C
5180	C-IV	Phenobarbital Tablets, 1/2 gr.	591-D
5073	C-IV	Phenobarbital Tablets, 1/8 gr.	591-E
5366	C-III	Glutethimide Tablets, 500 mg.	591-J
5346	C-IV	Phenobarbital Tablets, 1½ gr.	591-O
5476	C-IV	Phenobarbital Tablets, 30 mg.	591-T
5478	C-IV	Phenobarbital Tablets, 60 mg.	591-V

Delmont Laboratories, Inc.
P.O. BOX AA
SWARTHMORE, PA 19081

STAPHAGE LYSATE (SPL)™
[staf'faj lī'sāt]
BACTERIAL ANTIGEN MADE FROM STAPHYLOCOCCUS

Description: STAPHAGE LYSATE (SPL)™ is a whole culture vaccine, in solution, of two strains of lysed *Staphylococcus aureus*, Serologic Types I & III, specially selected for their broad antigenic spectrum.
How Supplied: 1-ml ampules, boxes of 10 (NDC 48532-0299-2), for subcutaneous, aerosol, topical, and oral use; 10-ml multiple-dose vials (NDC 48532-0299-1) for aerosol, topical, and oral use. For complete prescribing information and literature, please write, or call (215) 543-3365 or 543-2747.

Dermik Laboratories, Inc.
500 VIRGINIA DRIVE
FT. WASHINGTON, PA 19034

ANTHRA–DERM® Ointment
[anthra-derm]
(anthralin) 1%, ½%, ¼%, 1/10%
FOR TOPICAL USE ONLY

Description: Each gram of Anthra-Derm® (anthralin) Ointment 1/10%, ¼%, ½% and 1.0% contains 1 mg, 2.5 mg, 5 mg and 10 mg, respectively of anthralin in a base consisting of mineral oil and white petrolatum. Anthralin is an antipsoriatic agent with cytostatic, irritant and weak antimicrobial properties.
Clinical Pharmacology: Although the exact mechanism of anthralin's activity is unknown, there is experimental evidence that anthralin binds DNA, inhibiting synthesis of nucleic protein, and thus reduces mitotic activity.
Absorption in man has not been determined. However, based on a study in piglets it would appear to be quite low.
Indications and Usage: For the topical treatment of psoriasis.
Contraindications: Anthra-Derm® (anthralin) Ointment is contraindicated in patients with acute psoriasis or where inflammation is present, and in those patients with a history of hypersensitivity to any of the ingredients.
Warnings: Although no renal, hepatic or hematologic abnormalities have been reported as a result of topical application of Anthra-Derm® (anthralin) Ointment, caution is advised in patients with renal disease. Patients with renal disease and those having extensive and prolonged applications should have periodic urine tests for albuminuria. Discontinue use if sensitivity reactions occur.
Precautions: General: When redness is observed on adjacent normal skin, reduce frequency of application. For external use only. Do not apply to face, genitalia or intertriginous areas. Wash area thoroughly and carefully after using. Keep out of the reach of children. Anthralin is a tumor-promoting agent in 2-stage carcinogenesis on mouse skin. However, there have not been any reports of such effects in humans at the usual dosages.
Pregnancy: Pregnancy Category C. Animal reproduction studies have not been conducted with anthralin. It is also not known whether anthralin can cause fetal harm when administered to a pregnant woman or can affect reproduction capacity. Anthra-Derm® Ointment should be given to a pregnant woman only if clearly needed.
Nursing mothers: It is not known whether this drug is excreted in human milk. Because many drugs are excreted in milk and because of the potential for tumorigenicity shown for anthralin in animal studies, a decision should be made whether to discontinue nursing or to discontinue the drug, taking into account the importance of the drug to the mother.
Pediatric use: Safety and effectiveness in children have not been established.
Adverse Reactions: Irritation of normal skin is the most frequently reported adverse reaction. Anthra-Derm® may, temporarily, stain skin and hair.
Dosage and Administration: The usual dosage regimen begins with the lowest concentration (1/10%) and is gradually increased until the desired effect is obtained. Apply in a thin layer to affected areas once or twice daily, or as directed by a physician.
How Supplied: Anthra-Derm® (anthralin) Ointment 1/10%, ¼%, ½% and 1.0% is available in 1.5 oz (42.5 g) tubes.

5 BENZAGEL® MICROGEL™
[ben-za-jel]
(5% benzoyl peroxide) and
10 BENZAGEL® FORMULA
(10% benzoyl peroxide)
Acne Gels

Description: Each gram of 5 Benzagel® and 10 Benzagel® contains 50 mg and 100 mg respectively, of benzoyl peroxide in a gel vehicle of purified water, carbomer 940, sodium hydroxide, dioctyl sodium sulfosuccinate, alkyl polyglycol ether, fragrance and alcohol 14%.
Benzoyl peroxide is an antibacterial and keratolytic agent.
Clinical Pharmacology: Benzoyl peroxide is an antibacterial agent which has been shown to be effective against *Propionibacterium* acnes. This action is believed to be responsible for its usefulness in acne. One study in the rhesus monkey demonstrated a percutaneous absorption of about 1.8 μg per cm^2 of benzoyl peroxide or 45% of the applied dose in a 24-hour period. The absorbed benzoyl peroxide was completely converted in the skin to benzoic acid.
Indication and Usage: 5 & 10 Benzagel® may be used alone topically for mild to moderate acne and as an adjunct in acne treatment regimens which might include retinoic acid products, systemic antibiotics, and/or sulfur and salicylic acid containing preparations. The active ingredient, benzoyl peroxide, exerts a desquamative and antibacterial action. It provides mild peeling and keratolytic activity.
Contraindications: Benzagel® should not be used by patients having known sensitivity to benzoyl peroxide or any of its components.
Warnings: If itching, redness, burning, swelling or undue dryness occurs, discontinue use.
Precautions: For external use only. Not for ophthalmic use. Keep away from eyes and mucosae. Very fair individuals should begin with a single application at bedtime allowing overnight medication. May bleach colored fabrics. Keep this and all medications out of the reach of children.
Carcinogenesis, Mutagenesis and Impairment of Fertility—Long-term studies in animals have not been performed to evaluate carcinogenic potential.
Pregnancy Category C—Animal reproduction studies have not been conducted with benzoyl peroxide. It is also not known whether benzoyl peroxide can cause fetal harm when administered to a pregnant woman or can affect reproduction capacity. Benzoyl peroxide should be given to a pregnant woman only if clearly needed.
Nursing Mothers—It is not known whether this drug is excreted in human milk. Because many drugs are excreted in human milk, caution should be exercised when benzoyl peroxide is administered to a nursing woman.
Pediatric Use: Safety and effectiveness in children under the age of 12 have not been established.
Adverse Reactions: Irritation and contact dermatitis are the most frequent side reactions to benzoyl peroxide.
Dosage and Administration: Wash and dry affected areas prior to application. Apply sparingly one or more times daily.
How Supplied: 5 & 10 Benzagel® are available in 1.5 oz (42.5 g) and 3 oz (85 g) plastic tubes; 5 Benzagel® contains 50 mg benzoyl peroxide per gram and 10 Benzagel® contains 100 mg benzoyl peroxide per gram.
Caution: Federal law prohibits dispensing without prescription.

DURRAX™ Tablets
[Door-ax]
(hydroxyzine HCl)

Description: Durrax™, hydroxyzine hydrochloride, has the chemical name of Ethanol, 2-[2-[4-[(4-chlorophenyl) phenylmethyl]-1-piperazinyl]-ethoxy]-,dihydrochloride.
Hydroxyzine hydrochloride occurs as a white, odorless powder which is very soluble in water.
Clinical Pharmacology: Hydroxyzine hydrochloride is unrelated chemically to phenothiazine, reserpine, meprobamate or the benzodiazepines. Hydroxyzine is not a cortical depressant, but its action may be due to a suppression of activity in certain key regions of the subcortical area of the central nervous system.
Primary skeletal muscle relaxation has been demonstrated experimentally. Bronchodilator activity, and antihistaminic and analgesic effects have been demonstrated experimentally and confirmed clinically. An antiemetic effect, both by the apomorphine test and the veriloid test, has been demonstrated.
Pharmacological and clinical studies indicate that hydroxyzine, in therapeutic dosage, does not increase gastric secretion or acidity and in most cases has mild antisecretory activity.
Hydroxyzine hydrochloride is rapidly absorbed in the gastrointestinal tract and its effects are usually noted within 15 to 30 minutes after oral administration.
Indications: For symptomatic relief of anxiety and tension associated with psychoneurosis and as an adjunct in organic disease states in which anxiety is manifested.
Useful in the management of pruritus due to allergic conditions such as chronic urticaria and atopic and contact dermatoses and in histamine-mediated pruritus.
As a sedative when used as a premedication and following general anesthesia. Hydroxyzine may potentiate meperidine and barbiturates, so their use in pre-anesthetic adjunctive therapy should be modified on an individual basis. Atropine and other belladonna alkaloids are not affected by the drug. Hydroxyzine is not known to interfere with the action of digitalis in any way and it may be used concurrently with this agent.
The effectiveness of hydroxyzine as an anti-anxiety agent for long term use, that is more than 4 months, has not been assessed by systematic clinical studies. The physician should reassess periodically the usefulness of the drug for the individual patient.

Contraindications: Hydroxyzine, when administered to the pregnant mouse, rat, and rabbit induced fetal abnormalities in the rat and mouse at doses substantially above the human therapeutic range. Clinical data in human beings are inadequate to establish safety in early pregnancy. Until such data are available, hydroxyzine is contraindicated in early pregnancy.

Hydroxyzine hydrochloride is contraindicated for patients who have shown a previous hypersensitivity to it.

Precautions: The potentiating action of hydroxyzine must be considered when the drug is used in conjunction with central nervous system depressants. Therefore, when central nervous system depressants are administered concomitantly with hydroxyzine their dosage should be reduced.

Since drowsiness may occur with use of this drug, patients should be warned of this possibility and cautioned against driving a car or operating dangerous machinery while taking hydroxyzine. Patients should also be advised against the simultaneous use of other CNS depressant drugs, and cautioned that the effect of alcohol may be increased.

Nursing Mothers: It is not known whether this drug is excreted in human milk. Since many drugs are so excreted, hydroxyzine should not be given to nursing mothers.

Adverse Reactions: Side effects reported with the administration of hydroxyzine are usually mild and transitory in nature.

Anticholinergic: Dry mouth.

Central Nervous System: Drowsiness is usually transitory and may disappear in a few days of continued therapy or upon reduction of the dose. Involuntary motor activity including rare instances of tremor and convulsions have been reported, usually with doses considerably higher than those recommended. Clinically significant respiratory depression has not been reported at recommended doses.

Overdosage: The most common manifestation of hydroxyzine overdosage is hypersedation. As in the management of overdosage with any drug, it should be borne in mind that multiple agents may have been taken.

If vomiting has not occurred spontaneously, it should be induced. Immediate gastric lavage is also recommended. General supportive care, including frequent monitoring of the vital signs and close observation of the patient, is indicated. Hypotension, though unlikely, may be controlled with intravenous fluids and norepinephrine or metaraminol. Do not use epinephrine as hydroxyzine counteracts its pressor action. Caffeine and Sodium Benzoate Injection, U.S.P. may be used to counteract central nervous system depressant effects.

There is no specific antidote. It is doubtful that hemodialysis would be of any value in the treatment of overdosage with hydroxyzine. However, if other agents such as barbiturates have been ingested concomitantly, hemodialysis may be indicated. There is no practical method to quantitate hydroxyzine in body fluids or tissue after its ingestion or administration.

Dosage and Administration: For symptomatic relief of anxiety and tension associated with psychoneurosis and as an adjunct in organic disease states in which anxiety is manifested: Adults, 50–100 mg q.i.d.; children under 6 years, 50 mg daily in divided doses; children over 6 years, 50–100 mg daily in divided doses.

For use in the management of pruritus due to allergic conditions such as chronic urticaria and atopic and contact dermatoses and in histamine-mediated pruritus: Adults, 25 mg t.i.d. or q.i.d.; children under 6 years, 50 mg daily in divided doses; children over 6 years, 50–100 mg daily in divided doses.

As a sedative when used as a premedication and following general anesthesia: 50–100 mg for adults, and 0.6 mg/kg of body weight in children. When treatment is initiated by the intramuscular route of administration, subsequent doses may be administered orally.

As with all potent medication, the dosage should be adjusted according to the patient's response to therapy.

Caution: Federal law prohibits dispensing without prescription.

Store below 86°F (30°C) and dispense in tight, light-resistant container as defined in the U.S.P.

How Supplied: 10 mg—light lavender colored, coated tablets in bottles of 100 (NDC 0066-0044-68); 25 mg—dark lavender colored, coated tablets in bottles of 100 (NDC 0066-0045-68).

Manufactured by PAR PHARMACEUTICAL, INC.
Upper Saddle River, NJ 07458
FOR
DERMIK LABORATORIES, INC.
Fort Washington, PA 19034

FLORONE® ℞
[flŏr-ōhn]
(brand of diflorasone diacetate cream and diflorasone diacetate ointment 0.05%)

Description: Each gram of FLORONE Cream and FLORONE Ointment contains 0.5 mg diflorasone diacetate in a cream or ointment base.

Chemically, diflorasone diacetate is: 6α, 9α-difluoro-11β,17,21-trihydroxy-16β-methylpregna-1,4-diene-3,20-dione 17,21 diacetate.

FLORONE Cream contains diflorasone diacetate in an emulsified and hydrophilic cream base consisting of propylene glycol, stearic acid, polysorbate 60, sorbitan monostearate and monooleate, sorbic acid, citric acid and water. The corticosteroid is formulated as a solution in the vehicle using 15 percent propylene glycol to optimize drug delivery.

FLORONE Ointment contains diflorasone diacetate in an emollient, occlusive base consisting of polyoxypropylene 15-stearyl ether, stearic acid, lanolin alcohol and white petrolatum.

Clinical Pharmacology: Topical corticosteroids share anti-inflammatory, antipruritic and vasoconstrictive actions.

The mechanism of anti-inflammatory activity of the topical corticosteroids is unclear. Various laboratory methods, including vasoconstrictor assays, are used to compare and predict potencies and/or clinical efficacies of the topical corticosteroids. There is some evidence to suggest that a recognizable correlation exists between vasoconstrictor potency and therapeutic efficacy in man.

Pharmacokinetics: The extent of percutaneous absorption of topical corticosteroids is determined by many factors including the vehicle, the integrity of the epidermal barrier and the use of occlusive dressings.

Topical corticosteroids can be absorbed from normal intact skin. Inflammation and/or other disease processes in the skin increase percutaneous absorption. Occlusive dressings substantially increase the percutaneous absorption of topical corticosteroids. Thus, occlusive dressings may be a valuable therapeutic adjunct for treatment of resistant dermatoses. (See DOSAGE AND ADMINISTRATION).

Once absorbed through the skin, topical corticosteroids are handled through pharmacokinetic pathways similar to systemically administered corticosteroids. Corticosteroids are bound to plasma proteins in varying degrees. They are metabolized primarily in the liver and are then excreted by the kidneys. Some of the topical corticosteroids and their metabolites are also excreted into the bile.

Indications and Usage: Topical corticosteroids are indicated for relief of the inflammatory and pruritic manifestations of corticosteroid responsive dermatoses.

Contraindications: Topical steroids are contraindicated in those patients with a history of hypersensitivity to any of the components of the preparation.

Precautions:
General:
Systemic absorption of topical corticosteroids has produced reversible hypothalamic-pituitary-adrenal (HPA) axis suppression, manifestations of Cushing's syndrome, hyperglycemia, and glucosuria in some patients.

Conditions which augment systemic absorption include the application of the more potent steroids, use over large surface areas, prolonged use, and the addition of occlusive dressings.

Therefore, patients receiving a large dose of a potent topical steroid applied to a large surface area or under an occlusive dressing should be evaluated periodically for evidence of HPA axis suppression by using the urinary free cortisol and ACTH stimulation tests. If HPA axis suppression is noted, an attempt should be made to withdraw the drug, to reduce the frequency of application, or to substitute a less potent steroid.

Recovery of HPA axis function is generally prompt and complete upon discontinuation of the drug. Infrequently, signs and symptoms of steroid withdrawal may occur, requiring supplemental systemic corticosteroids.

Children may absorb proportionally larger amounts of topical corticosteroids and thus be more susceptible to systemic toxicity. (See PRECAUTIONS—Pediatric Use)

If irritation develops, topical corticosteroids should be discontinued and appropriate therapy instituted.

In the presence of dermatological infections, the use of an appropriate antifungal or antibacterial agent should be instituted. If a favorable response does not occur promptly, the corticosteroid should be discontinued until the infection has been adequately controlled.

Information for the Patient: Patients using topical corticosteroids should receive the following information and instructions:

1. This medication is to be used as directed by the physician. It is for external use only. Avoid contact with the eyes.
2. Patients should be advised not to use this medication for any disorder other than for which it was prescribed.
3. The treated skin area should not be bandaged or otherwise covered or wrapped as to be occlusive unless directed by the physician.
4. Patients should report any signs of local adverse reactions especially under occlusive dressing.
5. Parents of pediatric patients should be advised not to use tight-fitting diapers or plastic pants on a child being treated in the diaper area, as these garments may constitute occlusive dressings.

Laboratory Tests: The following tests may be helpful in evaluating the HPA axis suppression:
Urinary free cortisol test
ACTH stimulation test

Carcinogenesis, Mutagenesis, and Impairment of Fertility: Long-term animal studies have not been performed to evaluate the carcinogenic potential or the effect on fertility of topical corticosteroids. Studies to determine mutagenicity with prednisolone and hydrocortisone have revealed negative results.

Pregnancy Category C: Corticosteroids are generally teratogenic in laboratory animals when administered systemically at relatively low dosage levels. The more potent corticosteroids have been shown to be teratogenic after dermal application in laboratory animals. There are no adequate and well-controlled studies in pregnant women on teratogenic effects from topically applied corticosteroids. Therefore, topical corticosteroids should be used during pregnancy only if the potential benefit justifies the potential risk to the fetus. Drugs of this class should not be used extensively on pregnant patients, in large amounts, or for prolonged periods of time.

Nursing Mothers: It is not known whether topical administration of corticosteroids could result in sufficient systemic absorption to produce detectable quantities in breast milk. Systemically administered corticosteroids are secreted into breast milk in quantities **not** likely to have a deleterious effect on the infant. Nevertheless, caution should

Continued on next page

Dermik—Cont.

be exercised when topical corticosteroids are administered to a nursing woman.
Pediatric Use *Pediatric patients may demonstrate greater susceptibility to topical corticosteroid-induced HPA axis suppression and Cushing's syndrome than mature patients because of a larger skin surface area to body weight ratio.*
Hypothalamic-pituitary-adrenal (HPA) axis suppression, Cushing's syndrome, and intracranial hypertension have been reported in children receiving topical corticosteroids. Manifestations of adrenal suppression in children include linear growth retardation, delayed weight gain, low plasma cortisol levels, and absence of response to ACTH stimulation. Manifestations of intracranial hypertension include bulging fontanelles, headaches, and bilateral papilledema.
Administration of topical corticosteroids to children should be limited to the least amount compatible with an effective therapeutic regimen. Chronic corticosteroid therapy may interfere with the growth and development of children.
Adverse Reactions: The following local adverse reactions have been reported with topical corticosteroids, but may occur more frequently with the use of occlusive dressings. These reactions are listed in an approximate decreasing order of occurrence:
1. Burning
2. Itching
3. Irritation
4. Dryness
5. Folliculitis
6. Hypertrichosis
7. Acneiform eruptions
8. Hypopigmentation
9. Perioral dermatitis
10. Allergic contact dermatitis
11. Maceration of the skin
12. Secondary infection
13. Skin atrophy
14. Striae
15. Miliaria

Overdosage: Topically applied corticosteroids can be absorbed in sufficient amounts to produce systemic effects (See PRECAUTIONS).
Dosage and Administration: Topical corticosteroids are generally applied to the affected area as a thin film from one to four times daily depending on the severity of the condition.
Occlusive dressings may be used for the management of psoriasis or recalcitrant conditions.
If an infection develops, the use of occlusive dressings should be discontinued and appropriate antimicrobial therapy instituted.
How Supplied:
FLORONE Cream is available as follows:
  15 gram tube NDC 0066-0074-17
  30 gram tube NDC 0066-0074-31
  60 gram tube NDC 0066-0074-60
FLORONE Ointment is available as follows:
  15 gram tube NDC 0066-0075-17
  30 gram tube NDC 0066-0075-31
  60 gram tube NDC 0066-0075-60

HYTONE® Cream, Lotion and Ointment   ℞
[*hi-tōne*]
(hydrocortisone)

Description: *Cream*—Each gram of 1% and 2½% Cream contains 10 mg or 25 mg, respectively, of hydrocortisone in a water-washable base of purified water, propylene glycol, glyceryl monostearate SE, cholesterol and related sterols, isopropyl myristate, polysorbate 60, cetyl alcohol, sorbitan monostearate, polyoxyl 40 stearate and sorbic acid.
Lotion—Each ml of 1% and 2½% Lotion contains 10 mg or 25 mg, respectively, of hydrocortisone in a vehicle consisting of carbomer 940, propylene glycol, polysorbate 40, propylene glycol stearate, cholesterol and related sterols, isopropyl myristate, sorbitan palmitate, cetyl alcohol, triethanolamine, sorbic acid, simethicone and purified water.
Ointment—Each gram of 1% and 2½% contains 10 mg or 25 mg, respectively, of hydrocortisone in a topical emollient base of mineral oil, white petrolatum and sorbitan sesquioleate.
Chemically, hydrocortisone is 11, 17, 21-trihydroxypregn-4-ene 3, 20-dione.
The topical corticosteroids including hydrocortisone, constitute a class of primarily synthetic steroids used as anti-inflammatory and antipruritic agents.

Clinical Pharmacology: Topical corticosteroids share anti-inflammatory, antipruritic and vasoconstrictive actions. The mechanism of anti-inflammatory activity of the topical corticosteroids is unclear. Various laboratory methods, including vasoconstrictor assays, are used to compare and predict potencies and/or clinical efficacies of the topical corticosteroids. There is some evidence to suggest that a recognizable correlation exists between vasoconstrictor potency and therapeutic efficacy in man.

Pharmacokinetics
The extent of percutaneous absorption of topical corticosteroids is determined by many factors including the vehicle, the integrity of the epidermal barrier, and the use of occlusive dressings.
Topical corticosteroids can be absorbed from normal intact skin. Inflammation and/or other disease processes in the skin increase percutaneous absorption. Occlusive dressings substantially increase the percutaneous absorption of topical corticosteroids. Thus, occlusive dressings may be a valuable therapeutic adjunct for treatment of resistant dermatoses.
(See *DOSAGE AND ADMINISTRATION*.)
Once absorbed through the skin, topical corticosteroids are handled through pharmacokinetic pathways similar to systemically administered corticosteroids. Corticosteroids are bound to plasma proteins in varying degrees. Corticosteroids are metabolized primarily in the liver and are then excreted by the kidneys. Some of the topical corticosteroids and their metabolites are also excreted into the bile.

Indications and Usage: Topical corticosteroids are indicated for the relief of the inflammatory and pruritic manifestations of corticosteroid-responsive dermatoses.
Contraindications: Topical corticosteroids are contraindicated in those patients with a history of hypersensitivity to any of the components of the preparation.
Precautions:
General — Systemic absorption of topical corticosteroids has produced reversible hypothalamic-pituitary-adrenal (HPA) axis suppression, manifestations of Cushing's syndrome, hyperglycemia, and glucosuria in some patients.
Conditions which augment systemic absorption include the application of the more potent steroids, use over large surface areas, prolonged use, and the addition of occlusive dressings.
Therefore, patients receiving a large dose of a potent topical steroid applied to a large surface area or under an occlusive dressing should be evaluated periodically for evidence of HPA axis suppression by using the urinary free cortisol and ACTH stimulation tests. If HPA axis suppression is noted, an attempt should be made to withdraw the drug, to reduce the frequency of application, or to substitute a less potent steroid.
Recovery of HPA axis function is generally prompt and complete upon discontinuation of the drug. Infrequently, signs and symptoms of steroid withdrawal may occur, requiring supplemental systemic corticosteroids.
Children may absorb proportionally larger amounts of topical corticosteroids and thus be more susceptible to systemic toxicity (See PRECAUTIONS—Pediatric Use).
If irritation develops, topical corticosteroids should be discontinued and appropriate therapy instituted.
In the presence of dermatological infections, the use of an appropriate antifungal or antibacterial agent should be instituted. If a favorable response does not occur promptly, the corticosteroid should be discontinued until the infection has been adequately controlled.
Information for the Patient — Patients using topical corticosteroids should receive the following information and instructions:
1. This medication is to be used as directed by the physician. It is for external use only. Avoid contact with the eyes.
2. Patients should be advised not to use this medication for any disorder other than for which it was prescribed.
3. The treated skin area should not be bandaged or otherwise covered or wrapped as to be occlusive unless directed by the physician.
4. Patients should report any signs of local adverse reactions, especially under occlusive dressing.
5. Parents of pediatric patients should be advised not to use tight-fitting diapers or plastic pants on a child being treated in the diaper area, as these garments may constitute occlusive dressings.

Laboratory Tests — The following tests may be helpful in evaluating the HPA axis suppression:
  Urinary free cortisol test
  ACTH stimulation test
Carcinogenesis, Mutagenesis, and Impairment of Fertility — Long-term animal studies have not been performed to evaluate the carcinogenic potential or the effect on fertility of topical corticosteroids.
Studies to determine mutagenicity with prednisolone and hydrocortisone have revealed negative results.
Pregnancy Category C — Corticosteroids are generally teratogenic in laboratory animals when administered systemically at relatively low dosage levels. The more potent corticosteroids have been shown to be teratogenic after dermal application in laboratory animals. There are no adequate and well-controlled studies in pregnant women on teratogenic effects from topically applied corticosteroids. Therefore, topical corticosteroids should be used during pregnancy only if the potential benefit justifies the potential risk to the fetus. Drugs of this class should not be used extensively on pregnant patients, in large amounts, or for prolonged periods of time.
Nursing Mothers — It is not known whether topical administration of corticosteroids could result in sufficient systemic absorption to produce detectable quantities in breast milk. Systemically administered corticosteroids are secreted into breast milk in quantities *not* likely to have a deleterious effect on the infant. Nevertheless, caution should be exercised when topical corticosteroids are administered to a nursing woman.
Pediatric Use —Pediatric patients may demonstrate greater susceptibility to topical corticosteroid-induced HPA axis suppression and Cushing's syndrome than mature patients because of a larger skin surface area to body weight ratio.
Hypothalamic-pituitary-adrenal (HPA) axis suppression, Cushing's syndrome, and intracranial hypertension have been reported in children receiving topical corticosteroids. Manifestations of adrenal suppression in children include linear growth retardation, delayed weight gain, low plasma cortisol levels, and absence of response to ACTH stimulation. Manifestations of intracranial hypertension include bulging fontanelles, headaches, and bilateral papilledema.
Administration of topical corticosteroids to children should be limited to the least amount compatible with an effective therapeutic regimen. Chronic corticosteroid therapy may interfere with the growth and development of children.
Adverse Reactions: The following local adverse reactions are reported infrequently with topical corticosteroids, but may occur more frequently with the use of occlusive dressings. These reactions are listed in an approximate decreasing order of occurrence:

Burning	Perioral dermatitis
Itching	Allergic contact dermatitis
Irritation	Maceration of the skin
Dryness	Secondary infection
Folliculitis	Skin atrophy

Hypertrichosis, Striae, Acneiform eruptions, Miliaria, Hypopigmentation

Overdosage: Topically applied corticosteroids can be absorbed in sufficient amounts to produce systemic effects (See PRECAUTIONS).

Dosage and Administration: Topical corticosteroids are generally applied to the affected area as a thin film from two to four times daily depending on the severity of the condition. Occlusive dressings may be used for the management of psoriasis or recalcitrant conditions.

If an infection develops, the use of occlusive dressings should be discontinued and appropriate antimicrobial therapy instituted.

How Supplied: Cream—2½% - tube 1 oz NDC 0066-0095-01; 1% - tube 1 oz NDC 0066-0083-01 and jar 4 oz NDC 0066-0083-04; ½% - tube 1 oz (OTC) NDC 0066-0082-01.

Lotion—2½% - bottle 2 fl oz NDC 0066-0098-02; 1% - bottle 4 fl oz NDC 0066-0090-04.

Ointment—2 ½% - tube 1 oz NDC 0066-0085-01; 1% - tube 1 oz NDC 0066-0087-01 and jar 4 oz NDC 0066-0087-04.

SULFACET-R® Acne Lotion ℞
[sul-fa-set]
(sodium sulfacetamide 10% and sulfur 5%)

Description: Each gram of Sulfacet-R® Acne Lotion (sodium sulfacetamide 10% and sulfur 5%) as dispensed, contains 100 mg of sodium sulfacetamide and 50 mg of sulfur in a flesh-tinted lotion of purified water, alkylaryl sulfonic acid salts, hydroxyethylcellulose, propylene glycol, xanthan gum, lauric myristic diethanolamide, polyoxyethylene laurate, butylparaben, methylparaben, silicone emulsion, talc, zinc oxide, titanium dioxide, attapulgite, iron oxides, pH buffers and 2-bromo-2-nitropropane-1, 3 diol.

Sodium sulfacetamide is a sulfonamide with antibacterial activity while sulfur acts as a keratolytic agent. Chemically sodium sulfacetamide is N'-[(4-aminophenyl)sulfonyl]-acetamide, monosodium salt, monohydrate.

Clinical Pharmacology: The most widely accepted mechanism of action of sulfonamides is the Woods-Fildes theory which is based on the fact that sulfonamides act as competitive antagonists to para-aminobenzoic acid (PABA), an essential component for bacterial growth. While absorption through intact skin has not been determined, sodium sulfacetamide is readily absorbed from the gastrointestinal tract when taken orally and excreted in the urine, largely unchanged. The biological half-life has variously been reported as 7 to 12.8 hours.

The exact mode of action of sulfur in the treatment of acne is unknown, but it has been reported that it inhibits the growth of p. acnes and the formation of free fatty acids.

Indications: Sulfacet-R® is indicated in the topical control of acne vulgaris, acne rosacea and seborrheic dermatitis.

Contraindications: Sulfacet-R® Acne Lotion is contraindicated for use by patients having known hypersensitivity to sulfonamides, sulfur, or any other component of this preparation. Sulfacet-R® Acne Lotion is not to be used by patients with kidney disease.

Warnings: Although rare, sensitivity to sodium sulfacetamide may occur. Therefore, caution and careful supervision should be observed when prescribing this drug for patients who may be prone to hypersensitivity to topical sulfonamides. Systemic toxic reactions such as agranulocytosis, acute hemolytic anemia, purpura hemorrhagica, drug fever, jaundice, and contact dermatitis indicate hypersensitivity to sulfonamides. Particular caution should be employed if areas of denuded or abraded skin are involved.

Precautions: General—if irritation develops, use of the product should be discontinued and appropriate therapy instituted. For external use only. Keep away from eyes. Patients should be carefully observed for possible local irritation or sensitization during long-term therapy. The object of this therapy is to achieve desquamation without irritation, but sodium sulfacetamide and sulfur can cause reddening and scaling of epidermis. These side effects are not unusual in the treatment of acne vulgaris, but patients should be cautioned about the possibility. Keep out of the reach of children.

Carcinogenesis, Mutagenesis and Impairment of Fertility—Long-term studies in animals have not been performed to evaluate carcinogenic potential.

Pregnancy—Pregnancy Category C. Animal reproduction studies have not been conducted with Sulfacet-R® Acne Lotion. It is also not known whether Sulfacet-R® Acne Lotion can cause fetal harm when administered to a pregnant woman or can affect reproduction capacity. Sulfacet-R® Acne Lotion should be given to a pregnant woman only if clearly needed.

Nursing Mothers—It is not known whether sodium sulfacetamide is excreted in the human milk following topical use of Sulfacet-R® Acne Lotion. However, small amounts of orally administered sulfonamides have been reported to be eliminated in human milk. In view of this and because many drugs are excreted in human milk, caution should be exercised when Sulfacet-R® Acne Lotion is administered to a nursing woman.

Pediatric Use—Safety and effectiveness in children under the age of 12 have not been established.

Adverse Reactions: Although rare, sodium sulfacetamide may cause local irritation.

Dosage and Administration: Shake well before using. Apply a thin film to affected areas with light massaging to blend in each application 1 to 3 times daily. Each package contains a Dermik Color Blender™ which enables the patient to alter the basic shade of the lotion so that it matches the skin color exactly.

(Important to the Pharmacist—At the time of dispensing, add contents of vial* to the bottle. Shake well and/or stir with a glass rod to insure uniform dispersion. Place expiration date of four (4) months on bottle label.)

*Sulfa-Pak™ vial contains 2.4 grams of sodium sulfacetamide.

How Supplied: 1 oz (28.35 g) bottles

VANOXIDE-HC® Acne Lotion ℞
[van-ox-īd]
(Clear)

Description: Each gram of Vanoxide-HC® Lotion contains, as dispensed, 50 mg benzoyl peroxide, and 5 mg hydrocortisone. It is incorporated in a water-washable lotion of purified water, calcium phosphate, propylene glycol, caprylic/capric triglyceride, propylene glycol monostearate, laneth-10 acetate, decyl oleate, polysorbate 20, cetyl alcohol, mineral oil, lanolin alcohol, sodium phosphate, sodium biphosphate, stearyl heptanoate, hydroxyethylcellulose, tetrasodium EDTA, cyclohexanediamine tetraacetic acid, propylparaben, methylparaben, vegetable oil, monoglyceride citrate, simethicone, BHT, sodium hydroxide, BHA, propyl gallate, FD&C colors.

Clinical Pharmacology: Benzoyl peroxide is an antibacterial agent which has been shown to be effective against *Propionibacterium acnes*. This action is believed to be largely responsible for its usefulness. In addition, benzoyl peroxide exerts a desquamative and keratolytic action. One study in the rhesus monkey demonstrated a percutaneous absorption of about 1.8 μg per cm^2 of benzoyl peroxide or 45% of the applied dose in a 24-hour period. The absorbed benzoyl peroxide was completely converted in the skin to benzoic acid.

Topical steroids are primarily effective because of their anti-inflammatory, antipruritic and vasoconstrictive actions.

Indications and Usage: Treatment of acne vulgaris and oily skin.

Contraindications: Vanoxide-HC® Lotion is contraindicated in individuals having known sensitivity to benzoyl peroxide, hydrocortisone or any of the components of the product. Topical steroids are contraindicated in viral diseases of the skin, such as varicella or vaccinia.

Warnings: If itching, redness, swelling or undue dryness occurs, discontinue use.

Precautions: For external use only. Keep away from the eyes and mucosae. Very fair individuals should begin with a single application at bedtime allowing overnight medication. May bleach colored fabrics.

Carcinogenesis, Mutagenesis, Impairment of Fertility—Long-term studies in animals have not been performed to evaluate carcinogenic potential.

Pregnancy, Category C—Animal reproduction studies have not been conducted with Vanoxide-HC® Lotion. It is not known whether Vanoxide-HC® Lotion can cause fetal harm when administered to a pregnant woman or can affect reproduction capacity. Vanoxide-HC® Lotion should be given to a pregnant woman only if clearly needed.

Nursing Mothers—It is not known whether this drug is excreted in human milk. Because many drugs are excreted in human milk, caution should be exercised when Vanoxide-HC® Lotion is administered to a nursing woman.

Pediatric Use—Safety and effectiveness in children under the age of 12 have not been established.

Adverse Reactions: Irritation and contact dermatitis are the most frequent side reactions to benzoyl peroxide. Although 0.5% hydrocortisone is considered safe, the following adverse reactions have been reported with topical corticosteroids, especially under occlusive dressings: burning, itching, irritation, dryness, folliculitis, hypertrichosis, acneform eruptions, hypopigmentation, perioral dermatitis, allergic contact dermatitis, maceration of the skin, secondary infection, skin atrophy, striae, miliaria.

Dosage and Administration: Shake well before using. Apply a thin film 1 to 3 times daily with gentle massaging to blend with skin, or as directed by physician.

How Supplied: Bottles, 25 grams net weight as dispensed. Package contains a bottle of lotion base and a Benzie-Pak™ vial containing a mixture of benzoyl peroxide, 35%, and calcium phosphate, 65%. Net weight of vial is 3.8 grams.

To the Pharmacist—At the time of dispensing, add contents of Benzie-Pak™ to the lotion in the bottle. Shake well and/or stir with glass rod to ensure uniform dispersion. Place expiration date of three (3) months on bottle label.

VLEMASQUE®
[vle-mask]
(6% sulfurated lime topical solution)

Description: Contains sulfurated lime topical solution 6%, S.D. alcohol 7% in a drying clay mask.

Indication: For the treatment of acne.

Directions: Daily, apply generous layer over entire face and neck, or as directed by physician. Avoid eyes, nostrils and lips. Leave on for 20-25 minutes. Remove with lukewarm water, using a gentle circular motion. Pat dry.

Warnings: Keep away from eyes. In case of contact, flush eyes thoroughly. For external use only. If any irritation appears, stop treatment immediately and consult physician.

How Supplied: 4 oz. jars

VYTONE® CREAM ℞
[vī-tone]
(hydrocortisone-iodoquinol)

Description: Each gram of Vytone® Cream ½% and 1% contains 5 mg or 10 mg of hydrocortisone, respectively, and 10 mg of iodoquinol in a greaseless base of purified water, propylene glycol, glyceryl monostearate SE, cholesterol and related sterols, isopropyl myristate, polysorbate 60, cetyl alcohol, sorbitan monostearate, polyoxyl 40 stearate, sorbic acid, and polysorbate 20.

Chemically, hydrocortisone is 11, 17, 21-trihydroxypregn-4-ene-3, 20-dione and iodoquinol, 5,7-diiodo-8-quinolinol.

Continued on next page

Dermik—Cont.

Hydrocortisone is an anti-inflammatory and antipruritic agent, while iodoquinol is an antifungal and antibacterial agent.

Clinical Pharmacology: Hydrocortisone has anti-inflammatory, antipruritic and vasoconstrictor properties. The mechanism of anti-inflammatory activity is unclear. There is some evidence to suggest that a recognizable correlation exists between vasoconstrictor potency and therapeutic efficacy in man.

Iodoquinol has both antifungal and antibacterial properties.

Pharmacokinetics

The extent of percutaneous absorption of topical corticosteroids is determined by many factors including vehicle, the integrity of the epidermal barrier, and the use of occlusive dressings.

Hydrocortisone can be absorbed from normal intact skin. Inflammation and/or other inflammatory disease processes in the skin increase percutaneous absorption. Occlusive dressings substantially increase the percutaneous absorption of topical corticosteroids.

Once absorbed through the skin, hydrocortisone is metabolized in the liver and most body tissues to hydrogenated and degraded forms such as tetrahydrocortisone and tetrahydrocortisol. These are excreted in the urine, mainly conjugated as glucuronides, together with a very small proportion of unchanged hydrocortisone.

There are no data available regarding the percutaneous absorption of iodoquinol; however, following oral administration, 3–5% of the dose was recovered in the urine as a glucuronide.

Indications and Usage: Based on a review of a related drug by the National Research Council and subsequent FDA classification for that drug, the indications are as follows: "Possibly" Effective: Contact or atopic dermatitis; impetiginized eczema; nummular eczema; infantile eczema; endogenous chronic infectious dermatitis; stasis dermatitis; pyoderma; nuchal eczema and chronic eczematoid otitis externa; acne urticata; localized or disseminated neurodermatitis; lichen simplex chronicus; anogenital pruritus (vulvae, scroti, ani); folliculitis, bacterial dermatoses; mycotic dermatoses such as tinea (capitis, cruris, corporis, pedis); moniliasis, intertrigo. Final classification of the less-than-effective indications requires further investigation.

Contraindications: Vytone® Cream is contraindicated in those patients with a history of hypersensitivity to hydrocortisone, iodoquinol or any other components of the preparation.

Warnings and Precautions: For external use only. Keep away from eyes. If irritation develops, the use of Vytone® Cream should be discontinued and appropriate therapy instituted. Staining of the skin and fabrics may occur. If extensive areas are treated or if the occlusive technique is used, the possibility of increased systemic absorption of the corticosteroid, and suitable precautions should be taken. Children may absorb proportionally larger amounts of topical corticosteroids and thus be more susceptible to systemic toxicity. Parents of pediatric patients should be advised not to use tight-fitting diapers or plastic pants on a child being treated in the diaper area, as these garments may constitute occlusive dressings. Iodoquinol may be absorbed through the skin and interfere with thyroid function tests. If such tests are contemplated, wait at least one month after discontinuance of therapy to perform these tests. The ferric chloride test for phenylketonuria (PKU) can yield a false positive result if iodoquinol is present in the diaper or urine.

Prolonged use may result in overgrowth of non-susceptible organisms requiring appropriate therapy. Keep out of reach of children.

Carcinogenesis, Mutagenesis and Impairment of Fertility: Long-term animal studies have not been performed to evaluate the carcinogenic potential or the effect on fertility of hydrocortisone or iodoquinol.

In vitro studies to determine mutagenicity with hydrocortisone have revealed negative results. Mutagenicity studies have not been conducted with iodoquinol.

Pregnancy Category C: Animal reproductive studies have not been conducted with Vytone® Cream. It is not known whether Vytone® Cream can cause fetal harm when administered to a pregnant woman or can affect reproductive capacity. Vytone® Cream should be given to a pregnant woman only if clearly needed.

Nursing Mothers: It is not known whether this drug is excreted in human milk. Because many drugs are excreted in human milk, caution should be exercised when Vytone® Cream is administered to a nursing woman.

Pediatric Use: Safety and effectiveness in children under the age of 12 have not been established.

Adverse Reactions: The following local adverse reactions are reported infrequently with topical corticosteroids. These reactions are listed in an approximate decreasing order of occurrence.

Burning	Perioral dermatitis
Itching	Allergic contact dermatitis
Irritation	Maceration of the skin
Dryness	Secondary infection
Folliculitis	Skin atrophy
Hypertrichosis	Striae
Acneiform eruptions	Miliaria

Hypopigmentation

Dosage and Administration: Apply to affected area 3 to 4 times daily in accordance with physician's directions.

How Supplied:
½%-Tube 1 oz NDC 0066-0049-01,
1%-Tube 1 oz NDC 0066-0051-01

ZETAR® EMULSION (Coal Tar) ℞
[zē-tar]

Description: Zetar® Emulsion, coal tar, is a liquid for topical application, following dilution in aqueous media. Each ml contains 300 mg whole coal tar in polysorbates. It is a topical anti-eczematic. The complete chemical composition of coal tar has not been ascertained; components are grouped into six categories: aromatic hydrocarbons, acidic phenolic compounds, cyclic nitrogen compounds, organic sulfur compounds, nonacidic phenolics and nonbasic nitrogen compounds.

Clinical Pharmacology: There is no confirmed scientific evidence as to the clinical pharmacologic effects of coal tar. Its actions in humans have been reported in the literature as antiseptic, antipruritic, antiparasitic, antifungal, antibacterial, keratoplastic and antiacanthotic. Vasoconstrictive activity of coal tar has also been reported.

Indications and Usage: Zetar® Emulsion is indicated for the relief of symptoms associated with generalized, persistent dermatoses such as psoriasis, eczema, atopic dermatitis and seborrheic dermatitis.

Contraindications: Not to be used on open or infected lesions.

Warnings: Application of coal tar may elicit a pustular eruption or a cyst (epidermal) like reaction.

Patients who have previously exhibited sensitivity to tars must be under careful and continuous supervision by the physician.

Precautions: For external (topical) use only. Keep away from the eyes. When used in the bath, add lukewarm water (not hot water). For 72 hours following treatment with coal tar, patients should avoid exposure to either direct sunlight or sunlamps (ultra-violet A and/or B) unless directed by physician, as this drug may photoactivate the skin. Prior to exposure to sunlight, completely remove all tar from skin. Sensitization or dermatitis may occur after prolonged use. If irritation develops or increases, discontinue use and consult physician. Keep out of the reach of children.

While no known drug interactions have been reported pertaining to the clinical use of this drug in patients, the concomitant use of drugs with phototoxic and/or photoactivating potential is not recommended (i.e. tetracyclines, psoralens, topical retinoic acid).

Carcinogenesis—Coal tar applied to the skin of mice resulted in an increase in epidermal carcinomas. Painting rabbit ears with coal tar appears to increase self-limiting keratoacanthomas. To date, existing reports do not suggest an increased incidence of skin cancer in psoriatics treated with coal tar.

Pregnancy Category C—Animal reproduction studies have not been conducted with Zetar® Emulsion (coal tar). It is also not known whether Zetar® Emulsion can cause fetal harm when administered to a pregnant woman or can affect reproduction capacity. Zetar® Emulsion should be given to a pregnant woman only if clearly needed.

Nursing Mothers—It is not known whether this drug is excreted in human milk. Because of the tumorigenicity shown for coal tar in animal studies, a decision should be made whether to discontinue nursing or to discontinue the drug, taking into account the importance of the drug to the mother.

Adverse Reactions: Application of coal tar may result in superficial folliculitis. Patients hypersensitive to coal tar may exhibit a pustular or keratocystic response.

Dosage and Administration: Add 3 to 5 teaspoonfuls of Zetar® Emulsion to a bath of lukewarm water. This is mixed throughout the bath. The patient immerses in the bath for 15 to 20 minutes. The interval recommended between dosing is from once-a-day to once every third day, and usual duration of treatment is 30 to 45 days.

If the physician decides to administer supplemental ultraviolet irradiation (Goeckerman treatment) to the patient (ultraviolet B; A or A/B), this may be accomplished between 2 and 72 hours. A determination of minimal erythemal dosage (MED) should be made for each patient; initial irradiation should be suberythemal, not to exceed MED.

Compounding: Zetar® Emulsion (coal tar) may be utilized in compounding prescriptions in aqueous based vehicles requiring coal tar. Each ml of Zetar® Emulsion contains 300 mg whole coal tar.

How Supplied: Zetar® Emulsion (coal tar) is available in 6 fl oz (177 ml) plastic bottles. The strength of the preparation is 300 mg coal tar/ml. **SHAKE WELL** before each use. No special handling or storage conditions are required.

ZETAR® SHAMPOO
[zē-tar]

Description: WHOLE Coal Tar (as Zetar®) 1.0% in a golden foam shampoo which produces soft, fluffy abundant lather.

Actions and Indications: Antiseptic, antibacterial, antiseborrheic. Loosens and softens scales and crusts. Indicated in psoriasis, seborrhea, dandruff, cradle-cap and other oily, itchy conditions of the body and scalp.

Contraindications: Acute inflammation, open or infected lesions.

Precautions: If undue skin irritation develops or increases, discontinue use and consult physician. In rare instances, temporary discoloration of blond, bleached, or tinted hair may occur. Avoid contact with eyes.

Dosage and Administration: Massage into moistened scalp. Rinse. Repeat; leave on 5 minutes. Rinse thoroughly.

How Supplied: 6 oz. Plastic Bottles.

Products are cross-indexed by
generic and chemical names
in the
YELLOW SECTION

Dista Products Company
Division of Eli Lilly and Company
307 EAST McCARTY STREET
INDIANAPOLIS, IN 46285

LEGEND
Hyporets®—*Disposable Syringes, Dista*
Identi-Code®—*Formula Identification Code, Dista*
Identi-Dose®—*Unit Dose Medication, Dista*
Pulvules®—*Filled Gelatin Capsules, Dista*
℞Pak—*Prescription Package, Dista*
Traypak™—*Multivial Carton, Dista*

IDENTI-CODE® Index

Illustrations of examples of products bearing Identi-Code® appear in the Product Identification Section.

Identi-Code® Product Name

C03-C22 (Coated Tablets)

C03 Ilotycin®
Composition (Each Enteric-Coated Tablet): Erythromycin, USP, 250 mg

C19 Mi-Cebrin®
Composition (Each Coated Tablet): Thiamine (vitamin B_1), 10 mg; riboflavin (vitamin B_2), 5 mg; pyridoxine (vitamin B_6), 1.7 mg; pantothenic acid, 10 mg; niacinamide, 30 mg; vitamin B_{12} (activity equivalent), 3 mcg; ascorbic acid (vitamin C), 100 mg; dl-alpha tocopheryl acetate (vitamin E), 5.5 IU (5.5 mg); vitamin A, 10,000 IU (3 mg); vitamin D, 400 IU (10 mcg); contains also (approximately): iron (as ferrous sulfate), 15 mg; copper (as the sulfate), 1 mg; iodine (as potassium iodide), 0.15 mg; manganese (as the glycerophosphate), 1 mg; magnesium (as the hydroxide), 5 mg; zinc (as the chloride), 1.5 mg

C20 Mi-Cebrin T®
Composition (Each Coated Tablet): Thiamine mononitrate (vitamin B_1), 15 mg; riboflavin (vitamin B_2), 10 mg; pyridoxine hydrochloride (vitamin B_6), 2 mg; pantothenic acid (as calcium pantothenate), 10 mg; niacinamide, 100 mg; vitamin B_{12} (activity equivalent), 7.5 mcg; ascorbic acid (vitamin C), 150 mg; dl-alpha tocopheryl acetate (vitamin E), 5.5 IU (5.5 mg); vitamin A, 10,000 IU (3 mg); vitamin D, 400 IU (10 mcg); contains also (approximately): iron (as ferrous sulfate), 15 mg; copper (as the sulfate), 1 mg; iodine (as potassium iodide), 0.15 mg; manganese (as the glycerophosphate), 1 mg; magnesium (as the hydroxide), 5 mg; zinc (as the chloride), 1.5 mg

C22 Becotin®-T
Composition (Each Coated Tablet): Thiamine mononitrate (vitamin B_1), 15 mg; riboflavin (vitamin B_2), 10 mg; pyridoxine hydrochloride (vitamin B_6), 5 mg; niacinamide, 100 mg; pantothenic acid (as calcium pantothenate), 20 mg; vitamin B_{12} (activity equivalent), 4 mcg; ascorbic acid (vitamin C) (as sodium ascorbate), 300 mg

---

F62-H77 (Pulvules®)

F62 Becotin®
Composition (Each Pulvule®): Thiamine hydrochloride (vitamin B_1), 10 mg; riboflavin (vitamin B_2), 10 mg; pyridoxine (vitamin B_6), 4.1 mg; niacinamide, 50 mg; pantothenic acid, 25 mg; vitamin B_{12} (activity equivalent), 1 mcg

F77 Becotin® with Vitamin C
Composition (Each Pulvule®): Thiamine hydrochloride (vitamin B_1), 10 mg; riboflavin (vitamin B_2), 10 mg; pyridoxine (vitamin B_6), 4.1 mg; niacinamide, 50 mg; pantothenic acid, 25 mg; vitamin B_{12} (activity equivalent), 1 mcg; ascorbic acid (vitamin C), 150 mg

3055 Cinobac®
Composition (Each Pulvule®): Cinoxacin, USP, 250 mg

3056 Cinobac®
Composition (Each Pulvule®): Cinoxacin, USP, 500 mg

3122 Co-Pyronil®2, Pediatric
Composition (Each Pulvule®): chlorpheniramine maleate, 2 mg; pseudoephedrine hydrochloride, 30 mg

3123 Co-Pyronil® 2
Composition (Each Pulvule®): chlorpheniramine maleate, 4 mg; pseudoephedrine hydrochloride, 60 mg

---

H07 Ilosone®
Composition (Each Pulvule®): Erythromycin Estolate, USP, 125 mg (equiv. to erythromycin)

H09 Ilosone®
Composition (Each Pulvule®): Erythromycin Estolate, USP, 250 mg (equiv. to erythromycin)

H69 Keflex®
Composition (Each Pulvule®): Cephalexin, USP, 250 mg

H71 Keflex®
Composition (Each Pulvule®): Cephalexin, USP, 500 mg

©H74 Valmid®
Composition (Each Pulvule®): Ethinamate, USP, 500 mg

H76 Nalfon® 200
Composition (Each Pulvule®): Fenoprofen Calcium, USP, 200 mg (equiv. to fenoprofen)

H77 Nalfon®
Composition (Each Pulvule®): Fenoprofen Calcium, USP, 300 mg (equiv. to fenoprofen)

U05-U60 (Compressed Tablets)

U05 Ilosone® Chewable
Composition (Each Compressed Tablet): Erythromycin Estolate, USP, 125 mg (equiv. to erythromycin)

U25 Ilosone® Chewable
Composition (Each Compressed Tablet): Erythromycin Estolate, USP, 250 mg (equiv. to erythromycin)

U26 Ilosone®
Composition (Each Compressed Tablet): Erythromycin Estolate, USP, 500 mg (equiv. to erythromycin)

U59 Nalfon®
Composition (Each Compressed Tablet): Fenoprofen Calcium, USP, 600 mg (equiv. to fenoprofen)

U60 Keflex®
Composition (Each Compressed Tablet): Cephalexin, 1 g

W03-W68 (Miscellaneous)

W03 Ilosone®, for Oral Suspension
Composition (When Mixed as Directed): Each 5 ml contain erythromycin estolate equivalent to 125 mg erythromycin (USP).

W14 Cordran® Tape
Composition: Flurandrenolide, USP, 4 mcg/sq cm

W15 Ilosone® Liquid, Oral Suspension
Composition: Each 5 ml contain erythromycin estolate equivalent to 125 mg erythromycin (USP).

W17 Ilosone® Liquid, Oral Suspension
Composition: Each 5 ml contain erythromycin estolate equivalent to 250 mg erythromycin (USP).

W18 Ilosone® Ready-Mixed Drops
Composition: Each ml contains erythromycin estolate equivalent to 100 mg erythromycin (USP).

W21 Keflex®, for Oral Suspension
Composition (When Mixed as Directed): Each 5 ml contain 125 mg cephalexin (USP).

W22 Keflex®, for Pediatric Drops
Composition (When Mixed as Directed): Each ml contains 100 mg cephalexin (USP).

W68 Keflex®, for Oral Suspension
Composition (When Mixed as Directed): Each 5 ml contain 250 mg cephalexin (USP).

UNIT-DOSE PACKAGING

Identi-Dose® (unit dose medication, Dista)
Closed-circuit control of medication from pharmacy to nurse to patient and return. Simplifies counting and dispensing whether in single-unit or prescription-size quantities. Fits into any dispensing system for ready identification and legibility, better inventory control, protection from contamination, easier handling and recording under Medicare, prevention of drug loss through pilferage or spilling, better control of Federal Controlled Substances, and less chance of medication errors.
The following products are available through normal channels of supply:

Identi-Dose®
Pulvules® No.
325 Becotin® with Vitamin C
375 Ilosone®, 250 mg
402 Keflex®, 250 mg
403 Keflex®, 500 mg

Tablets No.
1790 Mi-Cebrin®
1807 Mi-Cebrin T®
1810 Becotin®-T
1896 Keflex®, 1 g

Miscellaneous No.
M-201 Keflex®, for Oral Suspension, 125 mg/5 ml
M-202 Keflex®, for Oral Suspension, 250 mg/5 ml

BECOTIN®   OTC
[bĕk′ō-tĭn]
(vitamin B complex)

Description: Each Pulvule® contains—
Thiamine Hydrochloride
(Vitamin B_1)..................................10 mg
Riboflavin
(Vitamin B_2)..................................10 mg
Pyridoxine (Vitamin B_6)..............4.1 mg
Niacinamide......................................50 mg
Pantothenic Acid.............................25 mg
Vitamin B_{12} (Activity Equivalent).............1 mcg

Indications: Prophylaxis or treatment of vitamin B complex deficiencies. Acute B complex deficiencies may be precipitated by concurrent diseases or by surgical procedures, particularly of the gastrointestinal tract. The following symptoms of vitamin B complex deficiencies have been described: loss of appetite, nausea, burning tongue, vomiting, headache, general uneasiness or indis-

Continued on next page

Dista—Cont.

position, nervousness, apprehensive mental depression, hypersensitivity to noise, mental confusion, fatigue, burning sensation of the skin, sore mouth and tongue, and burning and itching of the eyes.

Dosage: *Prophylaxis*—1 Pulvule a day. *Treatment*—2 or 3 Pulvules a day, or as directed by the physician.

How Supplied: *Pulvules No. 300, Becotin® (vitamin B complex, Dista), F62**(No. 0, Dark-Blue), in bottles of 100 (NDC 0777-0662-02). [030183]

*Identi-Code® symbol.

BECOTIN®-T   OTC
[běk'ō-tĭn tē]
(vitamin B complex with vitamin C, therapeutic)

Description: Becotin-T is an easy-to-swallow, cinnamon-brown tablet which provides therapeutic quantities of vitamin B complex and vitamin C. Each tablet contains—
Thiamine Mononitrate (Vitamin B₁)............15 mg
Riboflavin (Vitamin B₂) ....10 mg
Pyridoxine Hydrochloride
  (Vitamin B₆)... 5 mg
Niacinamide ....100 mg
Pantothenic Acid
  (as Calcium Pantothenate)........................20 mg
Vitamin B₁₂ (Activity Equivalent)................4 mcg
Ascorbic Acid (Vitamin C)
  (as Sodium Ascorbate)..............................300 mg

Becotin-T is especially useful as an adjunct to specific therapy in medical or surgical aftercare. By restoring normal tissue levels of these easily depleted water-soluble vitamins, Becotin-T reduces morbidity—helps shorten convalescence.

Indications: For the prevention or treatment of concurrent vitamin B complex and vitamin C deficiencies.

Dosage: 1 or 2 tablets a day, or as directed by the physician.

How Supplied: *Tablets No. 1810, Becotin®-T (vitamin B complex with vitamin C, therapeutic, Dista), C22,** Coated, Cinnamon Brown, in bottles of 100 (NDC 0777-0322-02) and 1000 (NDC 0777-0322-04) and in 10 strips of 10 individually labeled blisters each containing 1 tablet (ID100) (NDC 0777-0322-33). [030183]

*Identi-Code® symbol.

BECOTIN® WITH VITAMIN C   OTC
[běk'ō-tĭn with vī'ta-mĭn sē]
(vitamin B complex with vitamin C)

Description: Each Pulvule® contains—
Thiamine Hydrochloride
  (Vitamin B₁)..10 mg
Riboflavin
  (Vitamin B₂)...10 mg
Pyridoxine
  (Vitamin B₆)..4.1 mg
Niacinamide ....50 mg
Pantothenic Acid ....25 mg
Vitamin B₁₂ (Activity Equivalent)................1 mcg
Ascorbic Acid
  (Vitamin C) ....150 mg

Indications: For the prevention or treatment of concurrent vitamin B complex and vitamin C deficiencies. See also under Becotin®.

Dosage: *Prophylaxis*—1 Pulvule a day. *Treatment*—2 or 3 Pulvules a day, or as directed by the physician.

How Supplied: *Pulvules No. 325, Becotin® with Vitamin C (vitamin B complex with vitamin C, Dista), F77** (No. 0, Green Body, Dark-Blue Cap), in bottles of 100 (NDC 0777-0677-02), 500 (NDC 0777-0677-03), and 1000 (NDC 0777-0677-04) and in 10 strips of 10 individually labeled blisters each containing 1 Pulvule (ID100) (NDC 0777-0677-33). [030183]

*Identi-Code® symbol.

CINOBAC®   ℞
[sĭn'ō-băk]
(cinoxacin)
Capsules, USP

Description: Cinobac® (cinoxacin, Dista) is a synthetic antimicrobial agent for oral administration. It is 1-ethyl-1,4-dihydro-4-oxo-[1,3] dioxolo[4,5-g]cinnoline-3-carboxylic acid and occurs as white or very light-yellow needle-shaped crystals. Cinobac is available as 250 and 500-mg Pulvules®. Examples of other antibacterial drugs in this class are nalidixic acid and oxolinic acid.

Clinical Pharmacology: Cinoxacin is rapidly absorbed after oral administration. A 500-mg dose produced a peak serum concentration of 15 mcg/ml, which declined to approximately 1 to 2 mcg/ml six hours after administration, as determined by fluorometric assay. A 500-mg dose produced an average urine concentration of approximately 300 mcg/ml during the first four hours and approximately 100 mcg/ml during the second four-hour period. These urine concentrations are many times greater than the minimum inhibitory concentration (MIC) of cinoxacin for most gram-negative organisms commonly found in urinary tract infections.

Ninety-seven percent of a 500-mg oral dose of radiolabeled cinoxacin was recovered in the urine within 24 hours, 60 percent of which was present as unaltered cinoxacin and the remainder as inactive metabolic products.

The presence of food did not affect the total absorption of cinoxacin. Peak serum concentrations were reduced, but the 24-hour urinary recovery of antibacterial activity was unaltered. The mean serum half-life is 1.5 hours.

Microbiology—Cinoxacin has in vitro activity against a wide variety of aerobic gram-negative bacilli, particularly strains of *Enterobacteriaceae*. In vitro tests demonstrate that cinoxacin is bactericidal. The mode of action has been shown to be inhibition of bacterial DNA replication. It is active within the range of urinary pH.

Cinoxacin is active against most strains of the following organisms: *Escherichia coli, Klebsiella* species, *Enterobacter* species (including *E. aerogenes, E. cloacae*, and *E. hafniae*), *Proteus mirabilis*, and *P. vulgaris*.

Cinoxacin is not active against *Pseudomonas*, enterococci, or staphylococci. Cross-resistance with drugs in this class (nalidixic acid and oxolinic acid) has been demonstrated. Bacterial resistance to cinoxacin has been reported in less than 4 percent of patients treated with recommended doses; however, bacterial resistance to cinoxacin has not been shown to be transferable via R-factor.

Susceptibility Tests—Quantitative methods give the most precise estimates of susceptibility to antibacterial drugs. For purposes of judging susceptibility of bacterial isolates to cinoxacin, minimum inhibitory concentration and disc test breakpoints were established on the basis of (1) human drug bioavailability studies and (2) test results obtained with normally susceptible strains compared with results from resistant strains. The breakpoints have been verified by comparison with results of the clinical trials with cinoxacin.

One quantitative method, a standardized disc test, has been recommended.* Reports from the laboratory giving results of the standardized test using the 100-mcg cinoxacin disc should be interpreted according to the following criteria:

Organisms producing zones of 19 mm or greater are classified as susceptible, whereas those producing zones of 15 to 18 mm are classified as having intermediate susceptibility. Organisms in either of these categories are likely to respond to therapy if the infection is confined to the urinary tract.

Organisms producing zones of 14 mm or less are reported as resistant, indicating that other therapy should be selected.

Certain strains of *Enterobacteriaceae* exhibit heterogeneity of resistance to cinoxacin. These strains produce isolated colonies within the inhibition zone. When such strains are encountered, the clear inhibition zone should be measured *within* the isolated colonies.

Dilution methods for determining susceptibility are also used, and results are reported as the minimum drug concentration inhibiting microbial growth (MIC).

If the MIC is 16 mcg/ml or less, the microorganism is considered "susceptible"; if greater than 16 mcg/ml and less than 64 mcg/ml, it is "intermediate"; and it is "resistant" if the MIC is 64 mcg/ml or greater.

---
* Approved Standard ASM-2 Performance Standards for Antimicrobial Disc Susceptibility Tests; National Committee for Clinical Laboratory Standards, 771 East Lancaster Avenue, Villanova, Pennsylvania 19085.

Indications and Usage: Cinobac® (cinoxacin, Dista) is indicated for the treatment of initial and recurrent urinary tract infections in adults caused by the following susceptible microorganisms: *E. coli, P. mirabilis, P. vulgaris, Klebsiella pneumoniae* and *Klebsiella* species, and *Enterobacter* species.

In vitro susceptibility testing should be performed prior to administration of the drug and, when clinically indicated, during treatment.

Contraindication: Cinobac® (cinoxacin, Dista) is contraindicated in patients with a history of hypersensitivity to cinoxacin.

Warnings: The use of cinoxacin in prepubertal children and during pregnancy is not recommended. The oral administration of a single 250-mg/kg dose of cinoxacin caused lameness in immature dogs. Histologic examination of the weight-bearing joints of these dogs revealed permanent lesions of the cartilage. Related drugs (e.g., nalidixic acid, oxolinic acid) also produce erosions of the cartilage in weight-bearing joints and other signs of arthropathy in immature animals of various species.

Precautions: *General*—Since Cinobac® (cinoxacin, Dista) is eliminated primarily by the kidney, the usual dosage should be lower in patients with reduced renal function (*see* Dosage and Administration). Administration of Cinobac is not recommended for anuric patients.

Cinobac should be used with caution in patients with a history of hepatic disease.

Pregnancy—Pregnancy Category B—Reproduction studies have been performed in rats and rabbits at doses up to ten times the daily human dose and have revealed no evidence of impaired fertility or harm to the fetus due to cinoxacin. There are, however, no adequate and well-controlled studies in pregnant women. **Since cinoxacin, like other drugs in its class, causes arthropathy in immature animals, its use during pregnancy is not recommended** (*see* **Warnings**).

Nursing Mothers—It is not known whether cinoxacin is excreted in human milk. Because other drugs in this class are excreted in human milk and because of the potential for serious adverse reactions from cinoxacin in nursing infants, a decision should be made to discontinue nursing or to discontinue the drug, taking into account the importance of the drug to the mother.

Pediatric Use—Cinoxacin is not recommended for use in prepubertal children (*see* Warnings).

Adverse Reactions: In clinical studies in 1118 patients, the following adverse effects were considered related to cinoxacin therapy:

Gastrointestinal—Nausea was reported most commonly and occurred in less than 3 in 100 patients. Other side effects, occurring less frequently (1 in 100), were anorexia, vomiting, abdominal cramps, and diarrhea.

Central Nervous System—The most frequent side effects were headache and dizziness, reported by 1 in 100 patients. Other adverse reactions possibly related to Cinobac® (cinoxacin, Dista) include insomnia, tingling sensation, perineal burning, photophobia, and tinnitus, and these were reported by less than 1 in 100 patients.

Hypersensitivity—Rash, urticaria, pruritus, and edema were reported by less than 3 in 100 patients.

Laboratory values that were reported to be abnormal were, in order of frequency, BUN (1 in 100) and SGOT, SGPT, serum creatinine, and alkaline phosphatase (each less than 1 in 100). Although not observed in the 1118 patients treated with cinoxacin, the following side effects have been reported for other drugs in the same pharmacologically active and chemically related class: restlessness, nervousness, over- brightness of lights, change in color perception, difficulty in focusing, decrease in visual acuity, double vision, abdominal pain, weakness, constipation, angioedema, erythema and bullae, feelings of disorientation or agitation or acute anxiety, palpitation, soreness of the gums, drowsiness, joint stiffness, swelling of the extremities, metallic taste, toxic psychosis or convulsions (rare), reduction in hematocrit/ hemoglobin, and eosinophilia.

All adverse reactions observed with drugs in this class were reversible.

Dosage and Administration: The usual adult dosage for the treatment of urinary tract infections is 1 g daily, administered orally in two or four divided doses (500 mg b.i.d. or 250 mg q.i.d.) for seven to 14 days. Although susceptible organisms may be eradicated within a few days after therapy has begun, the full treatment course is recommended.

Impaired Renal Function—When renal function is impaired, a reduced dosage must be employed. After an initial dose of 500 mg, a maintenance dosage schedule should be used (*see* table).

MAINTENANCE DOSAGE GUIDE
FOR PATIENTS WITH RENAL
IMPAIRMENT

Creatinine Clearance (ml/min/1.73 m²)	Renal Function	Dosage
>80	Normal	500 mg b.i.d.
80–50	Mild Impairment	250 mg t.i.d.
50–20	Moderate Impairment	250 mg b.i.d.
<20	Marked Impairment	250 mg q.d.

Administration of Cinobac® (cinoxacin, Dista) to anuric patients is not recommended.

When only serum creatinine is available, the following formula (based on sex, weight, and age of the patient) may be used to convert this value into creatinine clearance. The serum creatinine should represent a steady state of renal function.

Males: Weight (kg) x (140 − age)
　　　　　 72 x serum creatinine
Females: 0.9 x male value

How Supplied: Pulvules:
250 mg, orange and green (No. 3055)—40 (NDC 0777-3055-40).
500 mg, orange and green (No. 3056)—50 (NDC 0777-3056-50).

Animal Pharmacology: Crystalluria, sometimes associated with secondary urinary tract pathology, occurs in laboratory animals treated orally with cinoxacin. In the rhesus monkey, crystalluria (without urinary tract pathology) has been noted at doses as low as 50 mg/kg/day (lowest dose tested). Cinoxacin-related crystalluria has not been observed in humans receiving twice the recommended daily dosage.

Cinoxacin and related drugs have been shown to cause arthropathy in immature animals of most species tested (*see* Warnings).

Some drugs of this class have been shown to have oculotoxic potential. Cinoxacin administered to cats at high dosages (200 mg/kg/day) resulted in retinal degeneration and other ocular changes. The dog appeared to be somewhat resistant to these effects, but high dosages (500 mg/kg/day) resulted in mild retinal atrophy. No cinoxacin-related ocular changes were noted in the rabbit, rat, or monkey or in human studies. (In one of the studies in the monkey, cinoxacin was administered for one year at ten times the recommended clinical dose.) [060783]

Shown in Product Identification Section, page 410

CO-PYRONIL® 2 DOSAGE TABLE

Directions[a]	Pulvules Adults	Liquid Adults	Liquid Children 6 to Under 12 Yr[c]	Pediatric Pulvules Children 6 to Under 12 Yr[c]
	1 Pulvule q.6 h.[b]	2 tsp q. 6 h.	1 tsp q. 6 h.	1 Pulvule q. 6 h.

[a]Or as directed by a physician. Do not exceed four doses in a 24-hour period.
[b]Not recommended at this dosage for children under 12 years of age.
[c]For children under age six, consult a physician.

CO-PYRONIL® 2　　　　OTC
[*kō-pī′rō-nĭl too*]
(chlorpheniramine maleate and pseudoephedrine hydrochloride)
Co-Pyronil 2 is an Antihistaminic and Nasal Decongestant

Description: Each Pulvule® of Co-Pyronil® 2 contains—
　Chlorpheniramine maleate ....4 mg
　Pseudoephedrine hydrochloride ....60 mg
Each Pulvule of Co-Pyronil 2, Pediatric, contains—
　Chlorpheniramine maleate ....2 mg
　Pseudoephedrine hydrochloride ....30 mg
Each 5 ml (approximately 1 teaspoonful) of Co-Pyronil 2, liquid, contains—
　Chlorpheniramine maleate ....2 mg
　Pseudoephedrine hydrochloride ....30 mg

Indications: Alleviates, decreases, or provides temporary relief of running nose, sneezing, itching of the nose or throat, and itchy and watery eyes as may occur in allergic rhinitis (such as hay fever). For temporary relief of nasal congestion due to hay fever or other upper respiratory allergies.

Warnings: May cause drowsiness. May cause excitability, especially in children. Do not take this product if you have asthma, glaucoma, high blood pressure, heart disease, diabetes, thyroid disease, or difficulty in urination due to enlargement of the prostate gland, and do not give to children under six years, except under the advice and supervision of a physician. Do not exceed recommended dosage because at higher doses nervousness, dizziness, or sleeplessness may occur. If symptoms do not improve within seven days or are accompanied by high fever, consult a physician before continuing use. Keep this and all drugs out of reach of children. In case of accidental overdose, seek professional assistance or contact a Poison Control Center immediately. As with any drug, if you are pregnant or nursing a baby, seek the advice of a health professional before using this product.

Caution: Avoid driving a motor vehicle or operating heavy machinery. Avoid alcoholic beverages while taking this product.

Drug Interaction Precaution: Do not take this product if you are presently taking a prescription antihypertensive or antidepressant drug containing a monoamine oxidase inhibitor except under the advice and supervision of a physician.
[See table above].

How Supplied: *Pulvules No. 3123, Co-Pyronil® 2 (chlorpheniramine maleate and pseudoephedrine hydrochloride, Dista)*(No. 3, Yellow Opaque Body, Green Opaque Cap), in bottles of 100 (NDC 0777-3123-02) and 1000 (NDC 0777-3123-04).
Pulvules No. 3122, Co-Pyronil 2, Pediatric (No. 4, Dark Red), in bottles of 100 (NDC 0777-3122-02).
Liquid No. 5122, Co-Pyronil 2, in 16-fl-oz bottles (NDC 0777-5122-05). *Avoid freezing.*

[080184]

CORDRAN® and　　　　R
CORDRAN® SP
[*kôr′drăn and kôr′drăn ĕs pē*]
(flurandrenolide) USP

Description: Cordran® (Flurandrenolide, USP, Dista) is a potent corticosteroid intended for topical use. It occurs as white to off-white, fluffy, crystalline powder and is odorless. Cordran is practically insoluble in water and in ether. One g dissolves in 72 ml of alcohol and in 10 ml of chloroform. The molecular weight of Cordran is 436.52. The chemical name of Cordran is 6α-fluoro-16α-hydroxyhydrocortisone-16, 17-acetonide; its empirical formula is $C_{24}H_{33}FO_6$.

Each g of Cream Cordran® SP (Flurandrenolide Cream, USP, Dista) contains 0.5 mg (0.05 percent) or 0.25 mg (0.025 percent) flurandrenolide in an emulsified base composed of cetyl alcohol, citric acid, mineral oil, polyoxyl 40 stearate, propylene glycol, sodium citrate, stearic acid, and purified water.

Each g of Ointment Cordran® (Flurandrenolide Ointment, USP, Dista) contains 0.5 mg (0.05 percent) or 0.25 mg (0.025 percent) flurandrenolide in a base composed of white wax, cetyl alcohol, sorbitan sesquioleate, and white petrolatum.

Each ml of Lotion Cordran® (Flurandrenolide Lotion, USP, Dista) contains 0.5 mg (0.05 percent) flurandrenolide in an oil-in-water emulsion base composed of glycerin, cetyl alcohol, stearic acid, glyceryl monostearate, mineral oil, polyoxyl 40 stearate, menthol, benzyl alcohol, and purified water.

Clinical Pharmacology: Cordran® (flurandrenolide, Dista) is primarily effective because of its anti-inflammatory, antipruritic, and vasoconstrictive actions.

The mechanism of the anti-inflammatory effect of topical corticosteroids is not completely understood. Various laboratory methods, including vasoconstrictor assays, are used to compare and predict potencies and/or clinical efficacies of the topical corticosteroids. There is some evidence to suggest that a recognizable correlation exists between vasoconstrictor potency and therapeutic efficacy in man. Corticosteroids with anti-inflammatory activity may stabilize cellular and lysosomal membranes. There is also the suggestion that the effect on the membranes of lysosomes prevents the release of proteolytic enzymes and, thus, plays a part in reducing inflammation.

Evaporation of water from the lotion vehicle produces a cooling effect which is often desirable in the treatment of acutely inflamed or weeping lesions.

Pharmacokinetics—The extent of percutaneous absorption of topical corticosteroids is determined by many factors, including the vehicle, the integrity of the epidermal barrier, and the use of occlusive dressings.

Topical corticosteroids can be absorbed from normal intact skin. Inflammation and/or other disease processes in the skin increase percutaneous absorption. Occlusive dressings substantially increase the percutaneous absorption of topical corticosteroids. Thus, occlusive dressings may be a valuable therapeutic adjunct for treatment of resistant dermatoses. *See* Dosage and Administration.

Continued on next page

Dista—Cont.

Once absorbed through the skin, topical corticosteroids are handled through pharmacokinetic pathways similar to those of systemically administered corticosteroids. Corticosteroids are bound to plasma proteins in varying degrees. Corticosteroids are metabolized primarily in the liver and then excreted in the kidneys. Some of the topical corticosteroids and their metabolites are also excreted into the bile.

Indications and Usage: Cordran® (flurandrenolide, Dista) is indicated for the relief of the inflammatory and pruritic manifestations of corticosteroid-responsive dermatoses.

Contraindications: Topical corticosteroids are contraindicated in patients with a history of hypersensitivity to any of the components of these preparations.

Precautions: *General Precautions*—Systemic absorption of topical corticosteroids has produced reversible hypothalamic-pituitary-adrenal (HPA) axis suppression, manifestations of Cushing's syndrome, hyperglycemia, and glucosuria in some patients.

Conditions which augment systemic absorption include application of the more potent steroids, use over large surface areas, prolonged use, and the addition of occlusive dressings.

Therefore, patients receiving a large dose of a potent topical steroid applied to a large surface area or under an occlusive dressing should be evaluated periodically for evidence of HPA axis suppression by using urinary-free cortisol and ACTH stimulation tests. If HPA axis suppression is noted, an attempt should be made to withdraw the drug, to reduce the frequency of application, or to substitute a less potent steroid.

Recovery of HPA axis function is generally prompt and complete upon discontinuation of the drug. Infrequently, signs and symptoms of steroid withdrawal may occur, so that supplemental systemic corticosteroids are required.

Children may absorb proportionately larger amounts of topical corticosteroids and thus be more susceptible to systemic toxicity See Precautions—Usage in Children.

If irritation develops, topical corticosteroids should be discontinued and appropriate therapy instituted.

In the presence of dermatologic infections, the use of an appropriate antifungal or antibacterial agent should be instituted. If a favorable response does not occur promptly, Cordran should be discontinued until the infection has been adequately controlled.

Information for the Patient—Patients using topical corticosteroids should receive the following information and instructions.

1. This medication is to be used as directed by the physician. It is for external use only. Avoid contact with the eyes.
2. Patients should be advised not to use this medication for any disorder other than that for which it was prescribed.
3. The treated skin area should not be bandaged or otherwise covered or wrapped in order to be occlusive unless the patient is directed to do so by the physician.
4. Patients should report any signs of local adverse reactions, especially under occlusive dressing.
5. Parents of pediatric patients should be advised not to use tight-fitting diapers or plastic pants on a child being treated in the diaper area, because these garments may constitute occlusive dressings.

Laboratory Tests—The following tests may be helpful in evaluating the HPA axis suppression:
   Urinary-free cortisol test
   ACTH stimulation test

Carcinogenesis, Mutagenesis, and Impairment of Fertility—Long-term animal studies have not been performed to evaluate the carcinogenic potential or the effect on fertility of topical corticosteroids.

Studies to determine mutagenicity with prednisolone and hydrocortisone have revealed negative results.

Usage in Pregnancy—Pregnancy Category C—Corticosteroids are generally teratogenic in laboratory animals when administered systemically at relatively low dosage levels. The more potent corticosteroids have been shown to be teratogenic after dermal application in laboratory animals. There are no adequate and well-controlled studies in pregnant women on teratogenic effects from topically applied corticosteroids. Therefore, topical corticosteroids should be used during pregnancy only if the potential benefit justifies the potential risk to the fetus. Drugs of this class should not be used extensively on pregnant patients or in large amounts or for prolonged periods of time.

Nursing Mothers—It is not known whether topical administration of corticosteroids could result in sufficient systemic absorption to produce detectable quantities in breast milk. Systemically administered corticosteroids are secreted into breast milk in quantities *not* likely to have a deleterious effect on the infant. Nevertheless, caution should be exercised when topical corticosteroids are administered to a nursing woman.

Usage in Children—Pediatric patients may demonstrate greater susceptibility to topical corticosteroid-induced HPA axis suppression and Cushing's syndrome than do mature patients because of a larger skin surface area to body weight ratio.

Hypothalamic-pituitary-adrenal (HPA) axis suppression, Cushing's syndrome, and intracranial hypertension have been reported in children receiving topical corticosteroids. Manifestations of adrenal suppression in children include linear growth retardation, delayed weight gain, low plasma cortisol levels, and absence of response to ACTH stimulation. Manifestations of intracranial hypertension include bulging fontanelles, headaches, and bilateral papilledema.

Administration of topical corticosteroids to children should be limited to the least amount compatible with an effective therapeutic regimen. Chronic corticosteroid therapy may interfere with the growth and development of children.

Adverse Reactions: The following local adverse reactions are reported infrequently with topical corticosteroids but may occur more frequently with the use of occlusive dressings. These reactions are listed in an approximate decreasing order of occurrence:
Burning
Itching
Irritation
Dryness
Folliculitis
Hypertrichosis
Acneiform eruptions
Hypopigmentation
Perioral dermatitis
Allergic contact dermatitis
Maceration of the skin
Secondary infection
Skin atrophy
Striae
Miliaria

Overdosage: Topically applied corticosteroids can be absorbed in sufficient amounts to produce systemic effects (*See* Precautions).

Dosage and Administration: For moist lesions, a small quantity of the cream or lotion should be rubbed gently into the affected areas two or three times a day. For dry, scaly lesions, the ointment is applied as a thin film to affected areas two or three times daily.

Occlusive dressings may be used for the management of psoriasis or recalcitrant conditions.

If an infection develops, the use of occlusive dressings should be discontinued and appropriate antimicrobial therapy instituted.

Topical corticosteroids are generally applied to the affected area as a thin film one to four times daily, depending on the severity of the condition.

Use with Occlusive Dressings

The technique of occlusive dressings (for management of psoriasis and other persistent dermatoses) is as follows:

1. Remove as much as possible of the superficial scaling before applying Cream Cordran® SP (flurandrenolide, Dista) or Ointment or Lotion Cordran. Soaking in a bath will help soften the scales and permit easier removal by brushing, picking, or rubbing.
2. Rub Cream Cordran SP or Ointment or Lotion Cordran thoroughly into the affected areas.
3. Cover with an occlusive plastic film, such as polyethylene, Saran Wrap™, or Handi-Wrap®. (When Cream Cordran SP or Lotion Cordran is used, added moisture may be provided by placing a slightly dampened cloth or gauze over the lesion before the plastic film is applied.)
4. Seal the edges to adjacent normal skin with tape or hold in place by a gauze wrapping.
5. For convenience, the patient may remove the dressing during the day. The dressing should then be reapplied each night.
6. For daytime therapy, the condition may be treated by rubbing Cream Cordran SP or Ointment or Lotion Cordran sparingly into the affected areas.
7. In more resistant cases, leaving the dressing in place for three to four days at a time may result in a better response.
8. Thin polyethylene gloves are suitable for treatment of the hands and fingers; plastic garment bags may be utilized for treating lesions on the trunk or buttocks. A tight shower cap is useful in treating lesions on the scalp.

Occlusive Dressings Have the Following Advantages—1. Percutaneous penetration of the corticosteroid is enhanced.

2. Medication is concentrated on the areas of skin where it is most needed.

3. This method of administration frequently is more effective in very resistant dermatoses than is the conventional application of Cordran® (flurandrenolide, Dista).

Precautions to Be Observed in Therapy with Occlusive Dressings—Treatment should be continued for at least a few days after clearing of the lesions. If it is stopped too soon, a relapse may occur. Reinstitution of treatment frequently will cause remission.

Because of the increased hazard of secondary infection from resistant strains of staphylococci among hospitalized patients, it is suggested that the use of occlusive plastic films for corticosteroid therapy in such cases be restricted.

Generally, occlusive dressings should not be used on weeping, or exudative, lesions.

When large areas of the body are covered, thermal homeostasis may be impaired. If elevation of body temperature occurs, use of the occlusive dressing should be discontinued.

Rarely, a patient may develop miliaria, folliculitis, or a sensitivity to either the particular dressing material or a combination of Cordran® (flurandrenolide, Dista) and the occlusive dressing. If miliaria or folliculitis occurs, use of the occlusive dressing should be discontinued. Treatment by inunction with a corticosteroid such as Cordran may be continued. If the sensitivity is caused by the particular material of the dressing, substitution of a different material may be tried.

Warnings—Some plastic films are readily flammable. Patients should be cautioned against the use of any such material.

When plastic films are used on infants and children, the persons caring for the patients must be reminded of the danger of suffocation if the plastic material accidentally covers the face.

How Supplied:
(℞) *Cordran® (Flurandrenolide, USP), 0.05%, Lotion No. M-128*, in 15-ml (NDC 0777-2352-47) and 60-ml (NDC 0777-2352-97) plastic squeeze bottles. *Avoid freezing.*
(℞) *Cordran® (Flurandrenolide, USP), 0.025%, Ointment No. 79*, in 30-g (NDC 0777-1824-67) and 60-g (NDC 0777-1824-97) tubes and in 225-g (NDC 0777-1824-88) jars.

for possible revisions — **Product Information** — 897

(℞) *Cordran® (Flurandrenolide, USP), 0.05%, Ointment No. 85,* in 15-g (NDC 0777-1826-47), 30-g (NDC 0777-1826-67), and 60-g (NDC 0777-1826-97) tubes and in 225-g (NDC 0777-1826-88) jars.
(℞) *Cordran® (Flurandrenolide, USP), 0.025%, Cream No. 9,* in 30-g (NDC 0777-6034-67) and 60-g (NDC 0777-6034-97) tubes and in 225-g (NDC 0777-6034-88) jars.
(℞) *Cordran® SP (Flurandrenolide, USP), 0.05%, Cream No. 11,* in 15-g (NDC 0777-6035-47), 30-g (NDC 0777-6035-67), and 60-g (NDC 0777-6035-97) tubes and in 225-g (NDC 0777-6035-88) jars.
Cream No. 11, 0.05%—15 g—6505-00-890-1554(A); 60 g—6505-00-728-2623A; 225 g—6505-00-728-2624
Lotion No. M-128, 0.05%—15 ml—6505-00-926-9110
Ointment No. 85, 0.05%—15 g—6505-00-728-2626
[050283]

CORDRAN®-N ℞
[kôr′drăn ĕn]
(flurandrenolide with neomycin sulfate)

Description: Cordran® (Flurandrenolide, USP, Dista) is a potent corticosteroid intended for topical use. The chemical formula of Cordran is 6α-fluoro-16α-hydroxyhydrocortisone 16,17-acetonide.
Each g of Cordran-N cream contains 0.5 mg (0.05 percent) flurandrenolide and 5 mg neomycin sulfate (equivalent to 3.5 mg neomycin base) in a base composed of stearic acid, cetyl alcohol, mineral oil, polyoxyl 40 stearate, ethylparaben, glycerin, and purified water.
Each g of Cordran-N ointment contains 0.5 mg (0.05 percent) flurandrenolide and 5 mg neomycin sulfate (equivalent to 3.5 mg neomycin base) in a base composed of white wax, cetyl alcohol, sorbitan sesquioleate, and white petrolatum.
Actions: Cordran® (flurandrenolide, Dista) is primarily effective because of its anti-inflammatory, antipruritic, and vasoconstrictive actions.
The addition of neomycin broadens the usefulness of Cordran so that dermatoses complicated by actual skin infections may be treated more effectively and with safety.
For the treatment of corticosteroid-responsive dermatoses with secondary infection. It has not been demonstrated that ths steroid antiboitic combination provides greater benefit than the steroid component alone after seven days of treatment (*see* Warning section).
Contraindications: Topical corticosteroids are contraindicated in patients with a history of hypersensitivity to any of the components of these preparations.
Warning: Because of the concern of nephrotoxicity and ototoxicity associated with neomycin, this combination product should not be used over a wide area or for extended periods of time.
Precautions: If irritation develops, the product should be discontinued and appropriate therapy instituted.
Patients with superficial fungus or yeast infections should be treated with additional appropriate methods and observed frequently.
Prolonged use of neomycin preparations may result in the overgrowth of nonsusceptible organisms. If this occurs, appropriate measures should be taken.
There are articles in the current medical literature that indicate an increase in the prevalence of persons who are sensitive to neomycin.
If extensive areas are treated or if the occlusive technique is used, there will be increased systemic absorption of the corticosteroid, and suitable precautions should be taken, particularly in children and infants.
Although topical corticosteroids have not been reported to have an adverse effect on human pregnancy, the safety of their use on pregnant women has not been absolutely established. In laboratory animals, increases in incidence of fetal abnormalities have been associated with exposure of gestating females to topical corticosteroids, in some cases at rather low dosage levels. Therefore, drugs of this class should not be used extensively, in large amounts, or for prolonged periods of time on pregnant patients.
These products are not for ophthalmic use.
Adverse Reactions: The following local adverse reactions have been reported with topical corticosteroid formulations:
  Acneform eruptions
  Allergic contact dermatitis
  Burning
  Dryness
  Folliculitis
  Hypertrichosis
  Hypopigmentation
  Irritation
  Itching
  Perioral dermatitis
The following may occur more frequently with occlusive dressings:
  Maceration of the skin
  Miliaria
  Secondary infection
  Skin atrophy
  Striae
Topical neomycin has been reported to cause allergic contact dermatitis, ototoxicity, and nephrotoxicity.
Dosage and Administration: For moist lesions, a small quantity of the cream should be rubbed gently into the affected areas two or three times a day. For dry, scaly lesions, the ointment is applied as a thin film to affected areas two or three times daily.
Use with Occlusive Dressings—See under Cordran and Cordran SP.
How Supplied: (℞) *Cordran®-N (flurandrenolide with neomycin sulfate, Dista), Cream No. 12,* in 15 (NDC 0777-1884-47), 30 (NDC 0777-1884-67), and 60-g (NDC 0777-1884-97) tubes.
(℞) *Cordran®-N (flurandrenolide with neomycin sulfate, Dista), Ointment No. 86,* in 15 (NDC 0777-1827-47), 30 (NDC 0777-1827-67), and 60-g (NDC 0777-1827-97) tubes.
[042384]

CORDRAN® TAPE ℞
[kôr′drăn tăp]
(flurandrenolide tape)
USP

Description: Cordran Tape is a transparent, inconspicuous, plastic surgical tape, impervious to moisture. It contains Cordran® (flurandrenolide, Dista), a potent corticosteroid for topical use. *See also under* Cordran® and Cordran SP.
Each square centimeter contains 4 mcg of flurandrenolide uniformly distributed in the adhesive layer. The tape is made of a thin, matte-finish polyethylene film which is slightly elastic and highly flexible.
The adhesive is a synthetic copolymer of acrylate ester and acrylic acid which is free from substances of plant origin. The pressure-sensitive adhesive surface is covered with a protective paper liner to permit handling and trimming before application.
Clinical Pharmacology: Cordran® (flurandrenolide, Dista) is primarily effective because of its anti-inflammatory, antipruritic, and vasoconstrictive actions.
See also under Cordran and Cordran SP.
The tape serves as both a vehicle and an occlusive dressing. Retention of insensible perspiration by the tape results in hydration of the stratum corneum and improved diffusion of the medication. The skin is protected from scratching, rubbing, desiccation, and chemical irritation. The tape acts as a mechanical splint to fissured skin. Since it prevents removal of the medication by washing or the rubbing action of clothing, the tape formulation provides a sustained action.
Pharmacokinetics—See under Cordran and Cordran SP.
Indications and Usage: For relief of the inflammatory and pruritic manifestations of corticosteroid-responsive dermatoses, particularly dry, scaling localized lesions.
Contraindications: Topical corticosteroids are contraindicated in patients with a history of hypersensitivity to any of the components of this preparation.
Use of Cordran® Tape (flurandrenolide tape, Dista) is not recommended for lesions exuding serum or in intertriginous areas.
Precautions, Adverse Reactions, and **Overdosage:** *See under* Cordran and Cordran SP.
Dosage and Administration: Occlusive dressings may be used for the management of psoriasis or recalcitrant conditions.
If an infection develops, the use of occlusive dressings should be discontinued and appropriate antimicrobial therapy instituted.
Replacement of the tape every 12 hours produces the lowest incidence of adverse reactions, but it may be left in place for 24 hours if it is well tolerated and adheres satisfactorily. When necessary, the tape may be used at night only and removed during the day.
If ends of the tape loosen prematurely, they may be trimmed off and replaced with fresh tape.
The directions given below are included on a separate package insert for the patient to follow unless otherwise instructed by the physician.

Application of Cordran Tape

IMPORTANT: Skin should be clean and dry before tape is applied. Tape should always be cut, never torn.

DIRECTIONS FOR USE:
1. Prepare skin as directed by your physician or as follows: Gently clean the area to be covered to remove scales, crusts, dried exudates, and any previously used ointments or creams. A germicidal soap or cleanser should be used to prevent the development of odor under the tape. Shave or clip the hair in the treatment area to allow good contact with the skin and comfortable removal. If shower or tub baths are to be taken, they should be completed before the tape is applied. The skin should be dry before application of the tape.
2. Remove tape from package and cut a piece slightly larger than area to be covered. Round off corners.
3. Pull white paper from transparent tape. Be careful that tape does not stick to itself.
4. Apply tape, keeping skin smooth; press tape into place.
REPLACEMENT OF TAPE:
Unless instructed otherwise by your physician, replace tape after 12 hours. Cleanse skin and allow it to dry for one hour before applying new tape.
IF IRRITATION OR INFECTION DEVELOPS, REMOVE TAPE AND CONSULT PHYSICIAN.

How Supplied: (℞) *Cordran® Tape (Flurandrenolide Tape, USP), M-170, W14,*[*] 4 mcg flurandrenolide/sq cm, in Small Rolls 24 inches long and 3 inches wide (60 cm x 7.5 cm) (NDC 0777-2314-24) and in Large Rolls 80 inches long and 3 inches wide (200 cm x 7.5 cm) (NDC 0777-2314-28), in single packages.
Directions for the patient are included in each package. [062182]
Cordran Tape is manufactured by Minnesota Mining and Mfg. Co., St. Paul, Minnesota 55101, for Dista Products Company.
M-170—Cordran Tape, 80 in × 3 in—6505-00-168-6813

*Identi-Code® symbol.

ILOSONE® ℞
[ī-lō-sōn]
(erythromycin estolate)
USP

WARNING
Hepatic dysfunction with or without jaundice has occurred, chiefly in adults, in association

Continued on next page

Dista—Cont.

with erythromycin estolate administration. It may be accompanied by malaise, nausea, vomiting, abdominal colic, and fever. In some instances, severe abdominal pain may simulate an abdominal surgical emergency.

If the above findings occur, discontinue Ilosone® (erythromycin estolate, Dista) promptly.

Ilosone is contraindicated for patients with a known history of sensitivity to this drug and for those with preexisting liver disease.

Description: Erythromycin is produced by a strain of *Streptomyces erythraeus* and belongs to the macrolide group of antibiotics. It is basic and readily forms salts with acids. The base, the stearate salt, and the esters are poorly soluble in water and are suitable for oral administration.

Ilosone® (erythromycin estolate, Dista) is the lauryl sulfate salt of the propionyl ester of erythromycin.

Actions: Erythromycin inhibits protein synthesis without affecting nucleic acid synthesis. Some strains of *Haemophilus influenzae* and staphylococci have demonstrated resistance to erythromycin. Some strains of *H. influenzae* that are resistant in vitro to erythromycin alone are susceptible to erythromycin and sulfonamides used concomitantly.

Culture and susceptibility testing should be done. If the Bauer-Kirby method of disc susceptibility testing is used, a 15-mcg erythromycin disc should give a zone diameter of at least 18 mm when tested against an erythromycin-susceptible organism.

Orally administered erythromycin estolate is readily and reliably absorbed. Because of acid stability, serum levels are comparable whether the estolate is taken in the fasting state or after food. After a single 250-mg dose, blood concentrations average 0.29, 1.2, and 1.2 mcg/ml respectively at two, four, and six hours. Following a 500-mg dose, blood concentrations average 3, 1.9, and 0.7 mcg/ml respectively at two, six, and 12 hours.

After oral administration, serum antibiotic levels consist of erythromycin base and propionyl erythromycin ester. The propionyl ester continuously hydrolyzes to the base form of erythromycin to maintain an equilibrium ratio of approximately 20 percent base and 80 percent ester in the serum.

After absorption, erythromycin diffuses readily into most body fluids. In the absence of meningeal inflammation, low concentrations are normally achieved in the spinal fluid, but passage of the drug across the blood-brain barrier increases in meningitis. In the presence of normal hepatic function, erythromycin is concentrated in the liver and excreted in the bile; the effect of hepatic dysfunction on excretion of erythromycin by the liver into the bile is not known. After oral administration, less than 5 percent of the administered dose can be recovered as the active form in the urine. Erythromycin crosses the placental barrier, but fetal plasma levels are low.

Indications: *Streptococcus pyogenes* (Group A Beta-Hemolytic)—Upper and lower respiratory tract, skin, and soft-tissue infections of mild to moderate severity.

Injectable penicillin G benzathine is considered by the American Heart Association to be the drug of choice in the treatment and prevention of streptococcal pharyngitis and in long-term prophylaxis of rheumatic fever.

When oral medication is preferred for treating the above-mentioned conditions, penicillin G or V or erythromycin is the alternate drug of choice.

The importance of the patient's strict adherence to the prescribed dosage regimen must be stressed when oral medication is given. A therapeutic dose should be administered for at least ten days.

Alpha-Hemolytic Streptococci (Viridans Group) —Although no controlled clinical efficacy trials have been conducted, oral erythromycin has been suggested by the American Heart Association and American Dental Association for use in a regimen for prophylaxis against bacterial endocarditis in patients hypersensitive to penicillin who have congenital heart disease or rheumatic or other acquired valvular heart disease when they undergo dental procedures and surgical procedures of the upper respiratory tract.[1] Erythromycin is not suitable for such prophylaxis prior to genitourinary or gastrointestinal tract surgery.

Note: When selecting antibiotics for the prevention of bacterial endocarditis, the physician or dentist should read the full joint statement of the American Heart Association and the American Dental Association.[1]

Staphylococcus aureus—Acute infections of skin and soft tissue which are mild to moderately severe. Resistance may develop during treatment.

S. (Diplococcus) pneumoniae—Infections of the upper respiratory tract (e.g., otitis media, pharyngitis) and lower respiratory tract (e.g., pneumonia) of mild to moderate severity.

Mycoplasma pneumoniae (Eaton Agent, PPLO) —In the treatment of respiratory tract infections due to this organism.

H. influenzae—May be used concomitantly with adequate doses of sulfonamides in treating upper respiratory tract infections of mild to moderate severity. Not all strains of this organism are susceptible at the erythromycin concentrations ordinarily achieved (see appropriate sulfonamide labeling for prescribing information).

Treponema pallidum—Erythromycin is an alternate choice of treatment for primary syphilis in penicillin-allergic patients. In primary syphilis, spinal-fluid examinations should be done before treatment and as part of follow-up after therapy.

Corynebacterium diphtheriae—As an adjunct to antitoxin, to prevent establishment of carriers, and to eradicate the organism in carriers.

C. minutissimum—In the treatment of erythrasma.

Entamoeba histolytica—In the treatment of intestinal amebiasis only. Extraenteric amebiasis requires treatment with other agents.

Listeria monocytogenes—Infections due to this organism.

Bordetella pertussis—Erythromycin is effective in eliminating the organism from the nasopharynx of infected individuals, rendering them noninfectious. Some clinical studies suggest that erythromycin may be helpful in the prophylaxis of pertussis in exposed susceptible individuals.

Legionnaires' Disease—Although no controlled clinical efficacy studies have been conducted, in vitro and limited preliminary clinical data suggest that erythromycin may be effective in treating Legionnaires' disease.

Chlamydia trachomatis—Erythromycins are indicated for treatment of the following infections caused by *C. trachomatis:* conjunctivitis of the newborn, pneumonia of infancy, urogenital infections during pregnancy (*see* Warnings). When tetracyclines are contraindicated or not tolerated, erythromycin is indicated for the treatment of adults with uncomplicated urethral, endocervical, or rectal infections due to *C. trachomatis.*[2]

Contraindication: Erythromycin is contraindicated in patients with known hypersensitivity to this antibiotic.

Warnings: (*See* Warning box above.) The administration of erythromycin estolate has been associated with the infrequent occurrence of cholestatic hepatitis. Laboratory findings have been characterized by abnormal hepatic function test values, peripheral eosinophilia, and leukocytosis. Symptoms may include malaise, nausea, vomiting, abdominal cramps, and fever. Jaundice may or may not be present. In some instances, severe abdominal pain may simulate the pain of biliary colic, pancreatitis, perforated ulcer, or an acute abdominal surgical problem. In other instances, clinical symptoms and results of liver function tests have resembled findings in extrahepatic obstructive jaundice.

Initial symptoms have developed in some cases after a few days of treatment but generally have followed one or two weeks of continuous therapy. Symptoms reappear promptly, usually within 48 hours after the drug is readministered to sensitive patients. The syndrome seems to result from a form of sensitization, occurs chiefly in adults, and has been reversible when medication is discontinued.

Usage in Pregnancy—Safety of this drug for use during pregnancy has not been established.

Therefore, the physician should consider carefully the benefits and risks of use of this drug during pregnancy.

Precautions: Since erythromycin is excreted principally by the liver, caution should be exercised in administering the antibiotic to patients with impaired hepatic function.

The use of erythromycin in patients who are receiving high doses of theophylline may be associated with an increase in serum theophylline levels and potential theophylline toxicity. In case of theophylline toxicity and/or elevated serum theophylline levels, the dose of theophylline should be reduced while the patient is receiving concomitant erythromycin therapy.

Surgical procedures should be performed when indicated.

Adverse Reactions: The most frequent side effects of erythromycin preparations are gastrointestinal (e.g., abdominal cramping and discomfort) and are dose related. Nausea, vomiting, and diarrhea occur infrequently with usual oral doses.

During prolonged or repeated therapy, there is a possibility of overgrowth of nonsusceptible bacteria or fungi. If such infections arise, the drug should be discontinued and appropriate therapy instituted.

Mild allergic reactions, such as urticaria and other skin rashes, have occurred. Serious allergic reactions, including anaphylaxis, have been reported. There have been isolated reports of reversible hearing loss occurring chiefly in patients with renal insufficiency and in patients receiving high doses of erythromycin.

Dosage and Administration: *Adults*—The usual dosage is 250 mg every six hours. This may be increased up to 4 g or more/day according to the severity of the infection.

Children—Age, weight, and severity of the infection are important factors in determining the proper dosage. The usual regimen is 30 to 50 mg/kg/day in divided doses. For more severe infections, this dosage may be doubled.

If administration is desired on a twice-a-day schedule in either adults or children, one-half of the total daily dose may be given every 12 hours.

Twice-a-day dosing is not recommended when doses larger than 1 g daily are administered.

Streptococcal Infections—For the treatment of streptococcal pharyngitis and tonsillitis, the usual dosage range is 20 to 50 mg/kg/day in divided doses.

Body Weight	Total Daily Dose
10 kg or less (less than 25 lb)	250 mg
11–18 kg (25–40 lb)	375 mg
18–25 kg (40–55 lb)	500 mg
25–36 kg (55–80 lb)	750 mg
36 kg or more (more than 80 lb)	1000 mg (adult dose)

In the treatment of group A beta-hemolytic streptococcal infections, a therapeutic dosage of erythromycin should be administered for at least ten days. In continuous prophylaxis of streptococcal infections in persons with a history of rheumatic heart disease, the dosage is 250 mg twice a day. For prophylaxis against bacterial endocarditis[1] in patients with congenital heart disease or rheumatic or other acquired valvular heart disease when undergoing dental procedures or surgical procedures of the upper respiratory tract, the dosage schedule for adults is 1 g (20 mg/kg for children) orally one and one-half to two hours before the procedure and then 500 mg (10 mg/kg for children) orally every six hours for eight doses.

Primary Syphilis—A regimen of 20 g of erythromycin estolate in divided doses over a period of ten days has been shown to be effective in the treatment of primary syphilis.

Dysenteric Amebiasis—Dosage for adults is 250 mg four times daily for ten to 14 days; for children, 30 to 50 mg/kg/day in divided doses for ten to 14 days.

Pertussis—Although optimum dosage and duration have not been established, the dosage of erythromycin utilized in reported clinical studies was 40 to 50 mg/kg/day, given in divided doses for five to 14 days.

Legionnaires' Disease—Although optimum doses have not been established, doses utilized in reported clinical data were those recommended above (1 to 4 g erythromycin estolate daily in divided doses).

Conjunctivitis of the Newborn Caused by C. trachomatis—Oral erythromycin suspension, 50mg/kg/day in four divided doses for at least two weeks.[2]

Pneumonia of Infancy Caused by C. trachomatis—Although the optimum duration of therapy has not been established, the recommended therapy is oral erythromycin suspension, 50 mg/kg/day in four divided doses for at least three weeks.[2]

Urogenital Infections During Pregnancy Due to C. trachomatis—Although the optimum dose and duration of therapy have not been established, the suggested treatment is erythromycin, 500 mg orally four times a day for at least seven days. For women who cannot tolerate this regimen, a decreased dose of 250 mg orally four times a day should be used for at least 14 days.[2]

For adults with uncomplicated urethral, endocervical, or rectal infections caused by *C. trachomatis* in whom tetracyclines are contraindicated or not tolerated: 500 mg orally four times a day for at least seven days.[2]

References: 1. American Heart Association: Prevention of Bacterial Endocarditis, Circulation, 56:139A, 1977.
2. Sexually Transmitted Diseases Treatment Guidelines 1982. Centers for Disease Control, Morbidity and Mortality Weekly Report, U.S. Department of Health and Human Services, Atlanta, 31:355, 1982.

How Supplied: (℞) *Pulvules® Ilosone® (Erythromycin Estolate Capsules, USP)*: No. 374, H07,* 125 mg (equivalent to erythromycin) (No. 2, Ivory Opaque Body, Red Opaque Cap), in bottles of 24 (NDC 0777-0807-24) and 100 (NDC 0777-0807-02); No. 375, H09,* 250 mg (equivalent to erythromycin) (No. 0, Ivory Opaque Body, Red Opaque Cap), in bottles of 24 (NDC 0777-0809-24) and 100 (NDC 0777-0809-02) and in 10 strips of 10 individually labeled blisters each containing 1 Pulvule (ID100) (NDC 0777-0809-33).

Shown in Product Identification Section, page 410
(℞) *Tablets Ilosone® (Erythromycin Estolate Tablets, USP)*, No. 1863, U26,* 500 mg (equivalent to erythromycin), Specially Coated, Light-Pink (capsule-shaped, scored), in bottles of 50 (NDC 0777-2126-50).

(℞) *Tablets Ilosone® Chewable (Erythromycin Estolate Tablets, USP)*, No. 1834, U05,* 125 mg (equivalent to erythromycin), Light-Pink, in bottles of 50 (NDC 0777-2105-50); No. 1865, U25,* 250 mg (equivalent to erythromycin), Light-Pink, in bottles of 50 (NDC 0777-2125-50).

(℞) *Ilosone® Liquid (Erythromycin Estolate Oral Suspension, USP)*, M-148, W15,* in 100-ml (NDC 0777-2315-48) and 16-fl-oz (NDC 0777-2315-05) bottles.

Each 5 ml contain erythromycin estolate equivalent to 125 mg erythromycin in an orange-flavored vehicle. *Shake well before using. Refrigerate to maintain optimum taste.*

(℞) *Ilosone® Liquid (Erythromycin Estolate Oral Suspension, USP)*, M-153, W17,* in 100-ml (NDC 0777-2317-48) and 16-fl-oz (NDC 0777-2317-05) bottles.

Each 5 ml contain erythromycin estolate equivalent to 250 mg erythromycin in a cherry-flavored vehicle. *Shake well before using. Refrigerate to maintain optimum taste.*

(℞) *Ilosone® (Erythromycin Estolate for Oral Suspension, USP)*, M-104, W03,* in 60 (NDC 0777-2303-97) and 150-ml-size (NDC 0777-2303-68) packages.

Each 60-ml-size package consists of a bottle containing erythromycin estolate equivalent to 1.5 g erythromycin. At the time of dispensing, 48 ml of water are added to provide 60 ml of an oral suspension.

Each 150-ml-size package consists of a bottle containing erythromycin estolate equivalent to 3.75 g erythromycin. At the time of dispensing, 120 ml of water are added to provide 150 ml of an oral suspension.

When mixed as directed, each 5 ml (approximately 1 teaspoonful) will contain erythromycin estolate equivalent to 125 mg erythromycin. After being mixed, the suspension may be kept at room temperature for 14 days without significant loss of potency. *Shake well before using. Keep tightly closed.*

(℞) *Ilosone® Ready-Mixed Drops (Erythromycin Estolate Oral Suspension, USP)*, M-159, W18,* in 10-ml bottles (NDC 0777-2318-37).

Each package consists of a bottle containing erythromycin estolate equivalent to 1 g erythromycin in a pleasantly flavored vehicle and a special dropper calibrated at approximately 25 mg and 50 mg.

Each ml contains erythromycin estolate equivalent to 100 mg erythromycin. *Shake well before using. Refrigerate to maintain optimum taste.*

[060684]

*Identi-Code® symbol.

ILOTYCIN® ℞

[*ī-lō-tī'sĭn*]
(erythromycin)
Ophthalmic Ointment, USP

Description: Ilotycin® (erythromycin, Dista) is a wide-range antibiotic discovered in the research laboratories of Eli Lilly and Company and produced from a strain of *Streptomyces erythraeus*. The special sterile ophthalmic ointment base, containing mineral oil and white petrolatum, flows freely over the conjunctiva.

Indications: For the treatment of superficial ocular infections involving the conjunctiva and/or cornea caused by organisms susceptible to Ilotycin® (erythromycin, Dista).

For prophylaxis of ophthalmia neonatorum due to *Neisseria gonorrhoeae* or *Chlamydia trachomatis*. The Centers for Disease Control (U.S.P.H.S.) and the Committee on Drugs, the Committee on Fetus and Newborn, and the Committee on Infectious Diseases of the American Academy of Pediatrics recommend 1 percent silver nitrate solution in single-dose ampoules or single-use tubes of an ophthalmic ointment containing 0.5 percent erythromycin or 1 percent tetracycline as "effective and acceptable regimens for prophylaxis of gonococcal ophthalmia neonatorum."[1] (For infants born to mothers with clinically apparent gonorrhea, intravenous or intramuscular injections of aqueous crystalline penicillin G should be given: a single dose of 50,000 units for term infants or 20,000 units for infants of low birth weight. Topical prophylaxis alone is inadequate for these infants.[1]) Ophthalmic Ointment Ilotycin also has been effective for prevention of neonatal conjunctivitis due to *C. trachomatis*,[2] a condition that may develop one to several weeks after delivery in infants of mothers whose birth canals harbor the organism.

Contraindication: This drug is contraindicated in patients with a history of hypersensitivity to erythromycin.

Precautions: The use of antimicrobial agents may be associated with the overgrowth of antibiotic-resistant organisms; in such a case, antibiotic administration should be stopped and appropriate measures taken.

Adverse Reactions: As with any other medicament intended for topical use, there is always the possibility that sensitivity reactions will occur in certain individuals. If such reactions develop, the medication should be discontinued.

Dosage and Administration: In the treatment of external ocular infections, Ophthalmic Ointment Ilotycin® (erythromycin, Dista) should be applied directly to the infected structure one or more times daily, depending on the severity of the infection.

For prophylaxis of neonatal gonococcal or chlamydial conjunctivitis, a ribbon of ointment approximately 0.5 to 1 cm in length should be instilled into each conjunctival sac. The ointment should not be flushed from the eye following instillation. A new tube should be used for each infant. Infants born by cesarean section as well as those delivered by the vaginal route should receive prophylaxis.

References: 1. American Academy of Pediatrics: Prophylaxis and Treatment of Neonatal Gonococcal Infections, Pediatrics, 65:1047, 1980. 2. Hammerschlag, M. R., et al.: Erythromycin Ointment for Ocular Prophylaxis of Neonatal Chlamydial Infection, J.A.M.A., 244:2291, 1980.

How Supplied: (℞) *Sterile Ophthalmic Ointment No. 52, Ilotycin® (Erythromycin Ophthalmic Ointment, USP)*, 5 mg/g, in 1/8-oz tamperproof tubes (NDC 0777-1863-17) and 1-g plastic containers (ID24) (NDC 0777-1863-52). *Store at controlled room temperature, 15° to 30°C (59° to 86°F).*

[101283]

ILOTYCIN® ℞

[*ī-lō-tī'sĭn*]
(erythromycin)
Tablets, USP
(Enteric-Coated)

Description: Erythromycin is produced by a strain of *Streptomyces erythraeus* and belongs to the macrolide group of antibiotics. It is basic and readily forms salts with acids. The base, the stearate salt, and the esters are poorly soluble in water and are suitable for oral administration.

Tablets Ilotycin® (erythromycin, Dista) are specially coated to protect the contents from the inactivating effect of gastric acid and to permit efficient absorption of the antibiotic in the small intestine.

Each enteric-coated tablet contains 250 mg erythromycin.

Actions: Erythromycin inhibits protein synthesis without affecting nucleic acid synthesis. Some strains of *Haemophilus influenzae* and staphylococci have demonstrated resistance to erythromycin. Some strains of *H. influenzae* that are resistant in vitro to erythromycin alone are susceptible to erythromycin and sulfonamides used concomitantly. Culture and susceptibility testing should be done. If the Bauer-Kirby method of disc susceptibility testing is used, a 15-mcg erythromycin disc should give a zone diameter of at least 18 mm when tested against an erythromycin-susceptible organism.

Tablets Ilotycin® (erythromycin, Dista) are well absorbed and may be given without regard to meals.

After absorption, erythromycin diffuses readily into most body fluids. In the absence of meningeal inflammation, low concentrations are normally achieved in the spinal fluid, but passage of the drug across the blood-brain barrier increases in meningitis. In the presence of normal hepatic function, erythromycin is concentrated in the liver and excreted in the bile; the effect of hepatic dysfunction on excretion of erythromycin by the liver into the bile is not known. After oral administration, less than 5 percent of the administered dose can be recovered as the active form in the urine. Erythromycin crosses the placental barrier, but fetal plasma levels are low.

Indications: *Streptococcus pyogenes* (Group A Beta-Hemolytic)—Upper and lower respiratory tract, skin, and soft-tissue infections of mild to moderate severity.

Injectable penicillin G benzathine is considered by the American Heart Association to be the drug of choice in the treatment and prevention of streptococcal pharyngitis and in long-term prophylaxis of rheumatic fever.

When oral medication is preferred for treating the above-mentioned conditions, penicillin G or V or erythromycin is the alternate drug of choice.

Continued on next page

Dista—Cont.

The importance of the patient's strict adherence to the prescribed dosage regimen must be stressed when oral medication is given. A therapeutic dose should be administered for at least ten days.

Alpha-Hemolytic Streptococci (Viridans Group)—Although no controlled clinical efficacy trials have been conducted, oral erythromycin has been suggested by the American Heart Association and American Dental Association for use in a regimen for prophylaxis against bacterial endocarditis in patients hypersensitive to penicillin who have congenital heart disease or rheumatic or other acquired valvular heart disease when they undergo dental procedures and surgical procedures of the upper respiratory tract.[1] Erythromycin is not suitable for such prophylaxis prior to genitourinary or gastrointestinal tract surgery.

Note: When selecting antibiotics for the prevention of bacterial endocarditis, the physician or dentist should read the full joint statement of the American Heart Association and the American Dental Association.[1]

Staphylococcus aureus—Acute infections of skin and soft tissue which are mild to moderately severe. Resistance may develop during treatment.

S. (Diplococcus) pneumoniae—Infections of the upper respiratory tract (e.g., otitis media, pharyngitis) and lower respiratory tract (e.g., pneumonia) of mild to moderate severity.

Mycoplasma pneumoniae (Eaton Agent, PPLO)—In the treatment of respiratory tract infections due to this organism.

H. influenzae—May be used concomitantly with adequate doses of sulfonamides in treating upper respiratory tract infections of mild to moderate severity. Not all strains of this organism are susceptible at the erythromycin concentrations ordinarily achieved (see appropriate sulfonamide labeling for prescribing information).

Treponema pallidum—Erythromycin is an alternate choice of treatment for primary syphilis in penicillin-allergic patients. In primary syphilis, spinal-fluid examinations should be done before treatment and as part of follow-up after therapy.

Corynebacterium diphtheriae—As an adjunct to antitoxin, to prevent establishment of carriers, and to eradicate the organism in carriers.

C. minutissimum—In the treatment of erythrasma.

Entamoeba histolytica—In the treatment of intestinal amebiasis only. Extraenteric amebiasis requires treatment with other agents.

Listeria monocytogenes—Infections due to this organism.

Neisseria gonorrhoeae—In female patients with a history of sensitivity to penicillin, a parenteral erythromycin (such as the gluceptate) may be administered in conjunction with an oral erythromycin as alternate therapy in acute pelvic inflammatory disease caused by *N. gonorrhoeae*. In the treatment of gonorrhea, patients suspected of having concomitant syphilis should have microscopic examinations (by immunofluorescence or darkfield) before receiving erythromycin and monthly serologic tests for a minimum of four months.

Bordetella pertussis—Erythromycin is effective in eliminating the organism from the nasopharynx of infected individuals and in rendering them noninfectious. Some clinical studies suggest that erythromycin may be helpful in the prophylaxis of pertussis in exposed susceptible individuals.

Legionnaires' Disease—Although no controlled clinical efficacy studies have been conducted, in vitro and limited preliminary clinical data suggest that erythromycin may be effective in treating Legionnaires' disease.

Chlamydia trachomatis—Erythromycins are indicated for treatment of the following infections caused by *C. trachomatis:* conjunctivitis of the newborn, pneumonia of infancy, urogenital infections during pregnancy (*see* Warning). When tetracyclines are contraindicated or not tolerated, erythromycin is indicated for the treatment of adults with uncomplicated urethral, endocervical, or rectal infections due to *C. trachomatis.*[2]

Contraindication: Erythromycin is contraindicated in patients with known hypersensitivity to this antibiotic.

Warning: *Usage in Pregnancy*—Safety of this drug for use during pregnancy has not been established. Therefore, the physician should consider carefully the benefits and risks of the use of this drug during pregnancy.

Precautions: Since erythromycin is excreted principally by the liver, caution should be exercised in administering the antibiotic to patients with impaired hepatic function. There have been reports of hepatic dysfunction, with or without jaundice, occurring in patients taking oral erythromycin products.

The use of erythromycin in patients who are receiving high doses of theophylline may be associated with an increase in serum theophylline levels and potential theophylline toxicity. In case of theophylline toxicity and/or elevated serum theophylline levels, the dose of theophylline should be reduced while the patient is receiving concomitant erythromycin therapy.

Surgical procedures should be performed when indicated.

Adverse Reactions: The most frequent side effects of erythromycin preparations are gastrointestinal (e.g., abdominal cramping and discomfort) and are dose related. Nausea, vomiting, and diarrhea occur infrequently with usual oral doses.

During prolonged or repeated therapy, there is a possibility of overgrowth of nonsusceptible bacteria or fungi. If such infections arise, the drug should be discontinued and appropriate therapy instituted.

Mild allergic reactions, such as urticaria and other skin rashes, have occurred. Serious allergic reactions, including anaphylaxis, have been reported. There have been isolated reports of reversible hearing loss occurring chiefly in patients with renal insufficiency and in patients receiving high doses of erythromycin.

Dosage and Administration: Tablets Ilotycin® (erythromycin, Dista) are well absorbed whether given immediately after meals or between meals on an empty stomach.

Adults—The usual dose is 250 mg every six hours. This may be increased up to 4 g or more/day according to the severity of the infection.

Children—Age, weight, and severity of the infection are important factors in determining the proper dosage. The usual regimen is 30 to 50 mg/kg/day in divided doses. For more severe infections, this dosage may be doubled.

If administration is desired on a twice-a-day schedule in either adults or children, one-half of the total daily dose may be given every 12 hours.

Streptococcal Infections—In the treatment of group A beta-hemolytic streptococcal infections, a therapeutic dosage of erythromycin should be administered for at least ten days. In continuous prophylaxis of streptococcal infections in persons with a history of rheumatic heart disease, the dosage is 250 mg twice a day.

For prophylaxis against bacterial endocarditis[1] in patients with congenital heart disease or rheumatic or other acquired valvular heart disease when undergoing dental procedures or surgical procedures of the upper respiratory tract, the dosage schedule for adults is 1 g (20 mg/kg for children) orally one and one-half to two hours before the procedure and then 500 mg (10 mg/kg for children) orally every six hours for eight doses.

Primary Syphilis—30 to 40 g given in divided doses over a period of ten to 15 days.

Acute Pelvic Inflammatory Disease Caused by N. gonorrhoeae—Ilotycin® Gluceptate (Sterile Erythromycin Gluceptate, USP, Dista), 500 mg intravenously every six hours for at least three days, followed by Ilotycin, 250 mg every six hours for seven days.

Dysenteric Amebiasis—250 mg four times daily for ten to 14 days for adults; 30 to 50 mg/kg/day in divided doses for ten to 14 days for children.

Pertussis—Although optimum dosage and duration of treatment have not been established, the dosage of erythromycin utilized in reported clinical studies was 40 to 50 mg/kg/day, given in divided doses for five to 14 days.

Legionnaires' Disease—Although optimum doses have not been established, doses utilized in reported clinical data were those recommended above (1 to 4 g erythromycin base daily in divided doses).

Conjunctivitis of the Newborn Caused by C. trachomatis—Oral erythromycin suspension, 50 mg/kg/day in four divided doses for at least two weeks.[2]

Pneumonia of Infancy Caused by C. trachomatis—Although the optimum duration of therapy has not been established, the recommended therapy is oral erythromycin suspension, 50 mg/kg/day in four divided doses for at least three weeks.[2]

Urogenital Infections during Pregnancy Due to C. trachomatis—Although the optimum dose and duration of therapy have not been established, the suggested treatment is erythromycin, 500 mg orally four times a day for at least seven days. For women who cannot tolerate this regimen, a decreased dose of 250 mg orally four times a day should be used for at least 14 days.[2]

For adults with uncomplicated urethral, endocervical, or rectal infections caused by *C. trachomatis* in whom tetracyclines are contraindicated or not tolerated: 500 mg orally four times a day for at least seven days.[2]

References: 1. American Heart Association: Prevention of Bacterial Endocarditis, Circulation, 56: 139A, 1977.
2. Sexually Transmitted Diseases Treatment Guidelines 1982. Centers for Disease Control, Morbidity and Mortality Weekly Report, U.S. Department of Health and Human Services, Atlanta, 31 (Supplement):355, 1982.

How Supplied: (℞) *Tablets No. 23, Ilotycin® (Erythromycin Tablets, USP) (Enteric-Coated), C03,** 250 mg, Orange, in bottles of 24 (NDC 0777-0303-24), 100 (NDC 0777-0303-02), and 500 (NDC 0777-0303-03).

[072183]

*Identi-Code® symbol.

ILOTYCIN® GLUCEPTATE ℞
[ĭ-lō-tĭ'sĭn gloo-sĕp'tāt]
(erythromycin gluceptate)
Sterile, USP
IntraVenous

Description: Erythromycin is produced by a strain of *Streptomyces erythraeus* and belongs to the macrolide group of antibiotics. It is basic and readily forms salts with acids.

Actions: Erythromycin inhibits protein synthesis without affecting nucleic acid synthesis. Some strains of *Haemophilus influenzae* and staphylococci have demonstrated resistance to erythromycin. Culture and susceptibility testing should be done. If the Bauer-Kirby method of disc susceptibility testing is used, a 15-mcg erythromycin disc should give a zone diameter of at least 18 mm when tested against an erythromycin-susceptible organism.

Intravenous injection of 200 mg of erythromycin produces peak serum levels of 3 to 4 mcg/ml at one hour and 0.5 mcg/ml at six hours.

Erythromycin diffuses readily into the body fluids. Only low concentrations are normally achieved in the spinal fluid, but passage of the drug across the blood-brain barrier increases in meningitis. In the presence of normal hepatic function, erythromycin is concentrated in the liver and excreted in the bile; the effect of hepatic dysfunction on excretion of erythromycin by the liver into the bile is not known. From 12 to 15 percent of intravenously administered erythromycin is excreted in active form in the urine.

Erythromycin crosses the placental barrier, but fetal plasma levels are low.

Indications: *Streptococcus pyogenes* (Group A Beta-Hemolytic)—Upper and lower respiratory tract, skin, and soft-tissue infections of mild to moderate severity.

Injectable penicillin G benzathine is considered by the American Heart Association to be the drug of choice in the treatment and prevention of streptococcal pharyngitis and in long-term prophylaxis of rheumatic fever.

Staphylococcus aureus—Acute infections of skin and soft tissue which are mild to moderately severe. Resistance may develop during treatment.

S. (Diplococcus) pneumoniae—Infections of the upper respiratory tract (e.g., otitis media, pharyngitis) and lower respiratory tract (e.g., pneumonia) of mild to moderate severity.

Mycoplasma pneumoniae (Eaton Agent, PPLO) —In the treatment of respiratory tract infections due to this organism.

H. influenzae—May be used concomitantly with adequate doses of sulfonamides in treating upper respiratory tract infections of mild to moderate severity. Not all strains of this organism are susceptible at the erythromycin concentrations ordinarily achieved (see appropriate sulfonamide labeling for prescribing information).

Corynebacterium diphtheriae—As an adjunct to antitoxin.

Listeria monocytogenes—Infections due to this organism.

Neisseria gonorrhoeae—In female patients with a history of sensitivity to penicillin, a parenteral erythromycin (such as the gluceptate) may be administered in conjunction with an oral erythromycin as alternate therapy in acute pelvic inflammatory disease caused by *N. gonorrhoeae*. In the treatment of gonorrhea, patients suspected of having concomitant syphilis should have microscopic examinations (by immunofluorescence or darkfield) before receiving erythromycin and monthly serologic tests for a minimum of four months.

Legionnaires' Disease—Although no controlled clinical efficacy studies have been conducted, in vitro and limited preliminary clinical data suggest that erythromycin may be effective in treating Legionnaires' disease.

Contraindication: Intravenous erythromycin is contraindicated in patients with known hypersensitivity to this antibiotic.

Warning: *Usage in Pregnancy*—Safety of this drug for use during pregnancy has not been established.

Precautions: Side effects following the use of intravenous erythromycin are rare. Occasional venous irritation has been encountered, but if the injection is given slowly, in dilute solution, preferably by continuous intravenous infusion over 20 to 60 minutes, pain and vessel trauma are minimized.

Since erythromycin is excreted principally by the liver, caution should be exercised in administering the antibiotic to patients with impaired hepatic function.

Recent data from studies of erythromycin reveal that its use in patients who are receiving high doses of theophylline may be associated with an increase in serum theophylline levels and potential theophylline toxicity. In case of theophylline toxicity and/or elevated serum theophylline levels, the dose of theophylline should be reduced while the patient is receiving concomitant erythromycin therapy.

Surgical procedures should be performed when indicated.

Adverse Reactions: Allergic reactions, ranging from urticaria and mild skin eruptions to anaphylaxis, have occurred with intravenously administered erythromycin.

During prolonged or repeated therapy, there is a possibility of overgrowth of nonsusceptible bacteria or fungi. If such infections arise, the drug should be discontinued and appropriate therapy instituted.

Variations in liver function have been observed following daily doses at high levels or after prolonged therapy. Hepatic function tests should be performed when such therapy is given.

Reversible hearing loss associated with the intravenous infusion of 4 g or more/day of erythromycin has been reported rarely.

Dosage and Administration: Prepare the initial solution of Ilotycin® Gluceptate (erythromycin gluceptate, Dista) by (1) adding at least 10 ml of Sterile Water for Injection to the 250 or 500-mg vial or at least 20 ml of Sterile Water for Injection to the 1-g vial of Ilotycin Gluceptate and (2) shaking the vial until all of the drug is dissolved.

It is important that the product be diluted only with Sterile Water for Injection without preservatives.

After reconstitution, the sterile solutions should be stored in a refrigerator and used within seven days.

When all of the drug is dissolved, the solution may then be added to 0.9% Sodium Chloride Injection or to 5% Dextrose in Water to give 1 g/liter for slow, continuous infusion. IV fluid admixtures with a pH below 5.5 tend to lose potency rapidly. Therefore, such solutions should be administered completely within four hours after dilution.

If the period of administration is prolonged, the pH of the infusion fluid should be buffered to neutrality with a sterile agent such as Neut® (Sodium Bicarbonate 4% Additive Solution, Abbott) or Buff™ (Phosphate-Carbonate Buffer, Travenol). For administration of the antibiotic in 500 or 1000 ml of 5% Dextrose in Water, add one ampoule fullstrength Buff or 5 ml of Neut; for administration of the antibiotic in the same volumes of 0.9% Sodium Chloride Injection, add one ampoule half-strength Buff or 5 ml of Neut. These solutions should be completely administered within 24 hours after dilution.

If the medication is to be given in 100 to 250 ml of fluid by a volume control set such as Metriset® (McGaw), Volu-Trole® "B" (Cutter), Soluset® (Abbott), or Buretrol® (Baxter-Travenol), the IV fluid should be buffered in its primary container before being added to the volumetric administration set.

If the medication is to be given by intermittent injection, one-fourth of the total daily dose can be given in 20 to 60 minutes by slow intravenous injection of 250 to 500 mg in 100 to 250 ml of 0.9% Sodium Chloride Injection or 5% Dextrose in Water. Injection should be sufficiently slow to avoid pain along the vein.

The recommended IV dosage for severe infections in adults and children is 15 to 20 mg/kg of body weight/day. Higher doses (up to 4 g/day) may be given in very severe infections. Continuous infusion is preferable, but administration in divided doses at intervals of no more than every six hours is also effective.

For treatment of acute pelvic inflammatory disease caused by *N. gonorrhoeae*, administer 500 mg Ilotycin Gluceptate intravenously every six hours for at least three days, followed by 250 mg Ilotycin® (Erythromycin Tablets, USP, Dista) every six hours for seven days.

Patients receiving intravenous erythromycin should be changed to the oral dosage form as soon as possible.

For Treatment of Legionnaires' Disease—Although optimum doses have not been established, doses utilized in reported clinical data were those recommended above (1 to 4 g daily in divided doses).

How Supplied: (℞) *Vials Ilotycin® Gluceptate (Sterile Erythromycin Gluceptate, USP), IV*, rubberstoppered (Dry Powder): *No. 524*, 250 mg (equivalent to erythromycin), 30-ml size (NDC 0777-1404-01); *No. 538*, 500 mg (equivalent to erythromycin), 30-ml size (NDC 0777-1409-01); and *No. 646*, 1 g (equivalent to erythromycin), 30-ml size (NDC 0777-1441-01), in singles (10 per carton).

[020582]

KEFLEX® ℞
[kĕf'lĕks]
(cephalexin)
USP

Description: Keflex® (cephalexin, Dista) is a semisynthetic cephalosporin antibiotic intended for oral administration. It is 7-(D-α-amino-α-phenylacetamido) - 3 - methyl - 3 - cephem - 4 - carboxylic acid, monohydrate.

The nucleus of cephalexin is related to that of other cephalosporin antibiotics. The compound is a zwitterion; i.e., the molecule contains both a basic and an acidic group. The isoelectric point of cephalexin in water is approximately 4.5 to 5.

The crystalline form of cephalexin which is available is a monohydrate. It is a white crystalline solid having a bitter taste. Solubility in water is low at room temperature; 1 or 2 mg/ml may be dissolved readily, but higher concentrations are obtained with increasing difficulty.

The cephalosporins differ from penicillins in the structure of the bicyclic ring system. Cephalexin has a D-phenylglycyl group as substituent at the 7-amino position and an unsubstituted methyl group at the 3-position.

Clinical Pharmacology: *Human Pharmacology* —Keflex® (cephalexin, Dista) is acid stable and may be given without regard to meals. It is rapidly absorbed after oral administration. Following doses of 250 mg, 500 mg, and 1 g, average peak serum levels of approximately 9, 18, and 32 mcg/ml respectively were obtained at one hour. Measurable levels were present six hours after administration. Cephalexin is excreted in the urine by glomerular filtration and tubular secretion. Studies showed that over 90 percent of the drug was excreted unchanged in the urine within eight hours. During this period, peak urine concentrations following the 250-mg, 500-mg, and 1-g doses were approximately 1000, 2200, and 5000 mcg/ml respectively.

Microbiology—In vitro tests demonstrate that the cephalosporins are bactericidal because of their inhibition of cell-wall synthesis. Keflex is active against the following organisms in vitro:

Beta-hemolytic streptococci
Staphylococci, including coagulase-positive, coagulase-negative, and penicillinase-producing strains
Streptococcus (Diplococcus) pneumoniae
Escherichia coli
Proteus mirabilis
Klebsiella sp.
Haemophilus influenzae
Neisseria catarrhalis

Note—Most strains of enterococci *(S. faecalis)* and a few strains of staphylococci are resistant to Keflex. It is not active against most strains of *Enterobacter* sp., *P. morganii*, and *P. vulgaris*. It has no activity against *Pseudomonas* or *Herellea* species. When tested by in vitro methods, staphylococci exhibit cross-resistance between Keflex and methicillin-type antibiotics.

Disc Susceptibility Tests—Quantitative methods that require measurement of zone diameters give the most precise estimates of antibiotic susceptibility. One such procedure (*Am. J. Clin. Pathol.*, 45:493, 1966; *Federal Register*, 39:19182–19184, 1974) has been recommended for use with discs for testing susceptibility to cephalothin. Interpretations correlate zone diameters of the disc test with MIC values for Keflex. With this procedure, a report from the laboratory of "resistant" indicates that the infecting organism is not likely to respond to therapy. A report of "intermediate susceptibility" suggests that the organism would be susceptible if the infection is confined to the urine, in which high antibiotic levels can be obtained, or if high dosage is used in other types of infection.

Indications and Usage: Keflex® (cephalexin, Dista) is indicated for the treatment of the following infections when caused by susceptible strains of the designated microorganisms:

Respiratory tract infections caused by *S. pneumoniae* and group A beta-hemolytic streptococci (Penicillin is the usual drug of choice in the treatment and prevention of streptococcal infections, including the prophylaxis of rheumatic fever. Keflex is generally effective in the eradication of streptococci from the nasopharynx; however, substantial data establishing the efficacy of Keflex in the subsequent prevention of rheumatic fever are not available at present.)

Otitis media due to *S. pneumoniae*, *H. influenzae*, staphylococci, streptococci, and *N. catarrhalis*

Continued on next page

Dista—Cont.

Skin and skin-structure infections caused by staphylococci and/or streptococci

Bone infections caused by staphylococci and/or *P. mirabilis*

Genitourinary tract infections, including acute prostatitis, caused by *E. coli, P. mirabilis*, and *Klebsiella* sp.

Note—Culture and susceptibility tests should be initiated prior to and during therapy. Renal function studies should be performed when indicated.

Contraindication: Keflex® (cephalexin, Dista) is contraindicated in patients with known allergy to the cephalosporin group of antibiotics.

Warnings: BEFORE CEPHALEXIN THERAPY IS INSTITUTED, CAREFUL INQUIRY SHOULD BE MADE CONCERNING PREVIOUS HYPERSENSITIVITY REACTIONS TO CEPHALOSPORINS AND PENICILLIN. CEPHALOSPORIN C DERIVATIVES SHOULD BE GIVEN CAUTIOUSLY TO PENICILLIN-SENSITIVE PATIENTS.

SERIOUS ACUTE HYPERSENSITIVITY REACTIONS MAY REQUIRE EPINEPHRINE AND OTHER EMERGENCY MEASURES.

There is some clinical and laboratory evidence of partial cross-allergenicity of the penicillins and the cephalosporins. Patients have been reported to have had severe reactions (including anaphylaxis) to both drugs.

Any patient who has demonstrated some form of allergy, particularly to drugs, should receive antibiotics cautiously. No exception should be made with regard to Keflex® (cephalexin, Dista).

Pseudomembranous colitis has been reported with virtually all broad-spectrum antibiotics (including macrolides, semisynthetic penicillins, and cephalosporins); therefore, it is important to consider its diagnosis in patients who develop diarrhea in association with the use of antibiotics. Such colitis may range in severity from mild to life-threatening.

Treatment with broad-spectrum antibiotics alters the normal flora of the colon and may permit overgrowth of clostridia. Studies indicate that a toxin produced by *Clostridium difficile* is one primary cause of antibiotic-associated colitis.

Mild cases of pseudomembranous colitis usually respond to drug discontinuance alone. In moderate to severe cases, management should include sigmoidoscopy, appropriate bacteriologic studies, and fluid, electrolyte, and protein supplementation. When the colitis does not improve after the drug has been discontinued, or when it is severe, oral vancomycin is the drug of choice for antibiotic-associated pseudomembranous colitis produced by *C. difficile*. Other causes of colitis should be ruled out.

Usage in Pregnancy—Safety of this product for use during pregnancy has not been established.

Precautions: *General Precautions*—Patients should be followed carefully so that any side effects or unusual manifestations of drug idiosyncrasy may be detected. If an allergic reaction to Keflex® (cephalexin, Dista) occurs, the drug should be discontinued and the patient treated with the usual agents (e.g., epinephrine or other pressor amines, antihistamines, or corticosteroids).

Prolonged use of Keflex may result in the overgrowth of nonsusceptible organisms. Careful observation of the patient is essential. If superinfection occurs during therapy, appropriate measures should be taken.

Positive direct Coombs' tests have been reported during treatment with the cephalosporin antibiotics. In hematologic studies or in transfusion crossmatching procedures when antiglobulin tests are performed on the minor side or in Coombs' testing of newborns whose mothers have received cephalosporin antibiotics before parturition, it should be recognized that a positive Coombs' test may be due to the drug.

Keflex should be administered with caution in the presence of markedly impaired renal function. Under such conditions, careful clinical observation and laboratory studies should be made because safe dosage may be lower than that usually recommended.

Indicated surgical procedures should be performed in conjunction with antibiotic therapy.

As a result of administration of Keflex, a false-positive reaction for glucose in the urine may occur. This has been observed with Benedict's and Fehling's solutions and also with Clinitest® tablets but not with Tes-Tape® (Glucose Enzymatic Test Strip, USP, Lilly).

Broad-spectrum antibiotics should be prescribed with caution in individuals with a history of gastrointestinal disease, particularly colitis.

Usage in Pregnancy—Pregnancy Category B—The daily oral administration of cephalexin to rats in doses of 250 or 500 mg/kg prior to and during pregnancy, or to rats and mice during the period of organogenesis only, had no adverse effect on fertility, fetal viability, fetal weight, or litter size. Note that the safety of cephalexin during pregnancy in humans has not been established.

Cephalexin showed no enhanced toxicity in weanling and newborn rats as compared with adult animals. Nevertheless, because the studies in humans cannot rule out the possibility of harm, Keflex should be used during pregnancy only if clearly needed.

Nursing Mothers—The excretion of cephalexin in the milk increased up to four hours after a 500-mg dose; the drug reached a maximum level of 4 mcg/ml, then decreased gradually, and had disappeared eight hours after administration. Caution should be exercised when Keflex is administered to a nursing woman.

Adverse Reactions: *Gastrointestinal*—Symptoms of pseudomembranous colitis may appear either during or after antibiotic treatment. Nausea and vomiting have been reported rarely. The most frequent side effect has been diarrhea. It was very rarely severe enough to warrant cessation of therapy. Dyspepsia and abdominal pain have also occurred.

Hypersensitivity—Allergies (in the form of rash, urticaria, and angioedema) have been observed. These reactions usually subsided upon discontinuation of the drug. Anaphylaxis has also been reported.

Other reactions have included genital and anal pruritus, genital moniliasis, vaginitis and vaginal discharge, dizziness, fatigue, and headache. Eosinophilia, neutropenia, and slight elevations in SGOT and SGPT have been reported.

Dosage and Administration: Keflex® (cephalexin, Dista) is administered orally.

Adults—The adult dosage ranges from 1 to 4 g daily in divided doses. The usual adult dose is 250 mg every six hours. For the following infections, a dosage of 500 mg may be administered every 12 hours: streptococcal pharyngitis, skin and skin-structure infections, and uncomplicated cystitis in patients over 15 years of age. Cystitis therapy should be continued for seven to 14 days. For more severe infections or those caused by less susceptible organisms, larger doses may be needed. If daily doses of Keflex greater than 4 g are required, parenteral cephalosporins, in appropriate doses, should be considered.

Children—The usual recommended daily dosage for children is 25 to 50 mg/kg in divided doses. For streptococcal pharyngtitis in patients over one year of age and for skin and skin-structure infections, the total daily dose may be divided and administered every 12 hours.

[See table below].

In severe infections, the dosage may be doubled. In the therapy of otitis media, clinical studies have shown that a dosage of 75 to 100 mg/kg/day in four divided doses is required.

In the treatment of beta-hemolytic streptococcal infections, a therapeutic dosage of Keflex should be administered for at least ten days.

How Supplied: (℞) For Oral Suspension, Keflex® (Cephalexin for Oral Suspension, USP), M-201, W21,* in 60 (NDC 0777-2321-97), 100 (NDC 0777-2321-48), and 200-ml-size (NDC 0777-2321-89) packages and in unit-dose bottles of 100 (ID100) (NDC 0777-2321-33).

Each 60-ml-size package contains 1.5 g cephalexin in a dry, pleasantly flavored mixture. At the time of dispensing, add 36 ml of water in *two* portions to the dry mixture in the bottle. Shake well after each addition.

Each 100-ml-size package contains 2.5 g cephalexin in a dry, pleasantly flavored mixture. At the time of dispensing, add 60 ml of water in *two* portions to the dry mixture in the bottle. Shake well after each addition.

Each 200-ml-size package contains 5 g cephalexin in a dry, pleasantly flavored mixture. At the time of dispensing, add 120 ml of water in *two* portions to the dry mixture in the bottle. Shake well after each addition.

When mixed as directed, each 5 ml (approximately 1 teaspoonful) will contain 125 mg cephalexin. After mixing, store in a refrigerator. The mixture may be kept for 14 days without significant loss of potency. *Shake well before using. Keep tightly closed.*

(℞) For Oral Suspension, Keflex® (Cephalexin for Oral Suspension, USP), M-202, W68,* in 100 (NDC 0777-2368-48) and 200-ml-size (NDC 0777-2368-89) packages and in unit-dose bottles of 100 (ID100) (NDC 0777-2368-33).

Each 100-ml-size package contains 5 g cephalexin in a dry, pleasantly flavored mixture. At the time of dispensing, add 60 ml of water in *two* portions to the dry mixture in the bottle. Shake well after each addition.

Each 200-ml-size package contains 10 g cephalexin in a dry, pleasantly flavored mixture. At the time of dispensing, add 124 ml of water in *two* portions to the dry mixture in the bottle. Shake well after each addition.

When mixed as directed, each 5 ml (approximately 1 teaspoonful) will contain 250 mg cephalexin. After mixing, store in a refrigerator. The mixture may be kept for 14 days without significant loss of potency. *Shake well before using. Keep tightly closed.*

(℞) For Pediatric Drops, Keflex® (Cephalexin for Oral Suspension, USP), M-204, W22,* in 10-ml-size packages (NDC 0777-2322-37).

This package contains 1 g cephalexin in a dry, pleasantly flavored mixture and a special dropper calibrated at approximately 25 and 50 mg.

At the time of dispensing, add 5.5 ml of water to the dry mixture in the bottle. Close with original bottle cap and shake promptly until all of the powder is in suspension. Remove detachable portion of bottle label but leave white tab affixed.

When mixed as directed, each ml will contain 100 mg cephalexin. After being mixed, the suspension may be kept in a refrigerator for 14 days without significant loss of potency. *Shake well before using. Keep tightly closed.*

(℞) Pulvules® Keflex® (Cephalexin Capsules, USP): No. 402, H69,* 250 mg (No. 0, White Opaque Body, Dark-Green Opaque Cap), and No. 403, H71,* 500 mg (No. 0, Light-Green Opaque Body, Dark-Green Opaque Cap), in bottles of 20 (NDC 0777-0869-20 and 0871-20) and 100 (NDC 0777-0869-02 and 0871-02) and in 10 strips of 10 individ-

Keflex Suspension

Child's Weight	125 mg/5 ml	250 mg/5 ml
10 kg (22 lb)	½ to 1 tsp q.i.d.	¼ to ½ tsp q.i.d.
20 kg (44 lb)	1 to 2 tsp q.i.d.	½ to 1 tsp q.i.d.
40 kg (88 lb)	2 to 4 tsp q.i.d.	1 to 2 tsp q.i.d.

or

Child's Weight	125 mg/5 ml	250 mg/5 ml
10 kg (22 lb)	1 to 2 tsp b.i.d.	½ to 1 tsp. b.i.d.
20 kg (44 lb)	2 to 4 tsp b.i.d.	1 to 2 tsp b.i.d.
40 kg (88 lb)	4 to 8 tsp b.i.d.	2 to 4 tsp b.i.d.

ually labeled blisters each containing 1 Pulvule (ID100) (NDC 0777-0869-33 and 0871-33).

(℞) *Tablets No. 1896, Keflex® (Cephalexin Tablets, USP), U60,* *1 g, Green (capsule-shaped), in bottles of 24 (NDC 0777-2160-24) and in 10 strips of 10 individually labeled blisters each containing 1 tablet (ID100) (NDC 0777-2160-33). [092083]
Shown in Product Identification Section, page 410
Pulvules No. 402, 250 mg—100's—6505-00-165-6545(A); ID100's—6505-00-197-9200(A)
Pulvules No. 403, 500 mg—100's—6505-00-183-8543A; ID100's—6505-00-171-1213(A)
M-201—For Oral Suspension—100-ml size—6505-00-009-1833

* Identi-Code® symbol.

MI-CEBRIN® OTC
[*mī-sē' brĭn*]
(vitamins-minerals)

Description: Each tablet contains—
Thiamine (Vitamin B₁)................................10 mg
Riboflavin (Vitamin B₂).................................5 mg
Pyridoxine (Vitamin B₆)...............................1.7 mg
Pantothenic Acid...10 mg
Niacinamide..30 mg
Vitamin B₁₂ (Activity Equivalent)..............3 mcg
Ascorbic Acid
 (Vitamin C)..100 mg
dl-Alpha Tocopheryl
 Acetate (Vitamin E).......................5.5 IU (5.5 mg)
Vitamin A...................................10,000 IU (3 mg)
Vitamin D......................................400 IU (10 mcg)
Contains also—   approximately
Iron (as Ferrous
 Sulfate)..15 mg
Copper (as the Sulfate)....................................1 mg
Iodine (as Potassium
 Iodide)..0.15 mg
Manganese (as the
 Glycerophosphate)..1 mg
Magnesium (as the Hydroxide)........................5 mg
Zinc (as the Chloride)..................................1.5 mg

Mi-Cebrin offers a comprehensive vitamin-mineral formula in a yellow tablet of convenient size. The use of synthetic vitamins A and D eliminates any unpleasant fish-liver-oil odor or taste.
Indications: For the prevention or treatment of multiple vitamin and mineral deficiencies and in states of subnutrition. Both vitamins and minerals are essential components of vital physiologic mechanisms, including many enzyme systems. Although trace elements are known constituents of foodstuffs, their exact role in nutrition has not been defined. Studies have shown that foodstuffs may be lacking in these elements when grown in soil notably deprived of its normal constituents.
Dosage: 1 tablet a day, or as directed by the physician.
How Supplied: *Tablets No. 1790, Mi-Cebrin® (vitamins-minerals, Dista), C19,* *Coated, Yellow, in bottles of 60 (NDC 0777-0319-60), 100 (NDC 0777-0319-02), and 1000 (NDC 0777-0319-04) and in 10 strips of 10 individually labeled blisters each containing 1 tablet (ID100) (NDC 0777-0319-33).
[030183]

*Identi-Code® symbol.

MI-CEBRIN T® OTC
[*mī-sē' brĭn tē*]
(vitamin-minerals therapeutic)

Description: Each tablet contains—
Thiamine Mononitrate
 (Vitamin B₁)..15 mg
Riboflavin (Vitamin B₂)................................10 mg
Pyridoxine Hydrochloride
 (Vitamin B₆)..2 mg
Pantothenic Acid (as Calcium
 Pantothenate)..10 mg
Niacinamide...100 mg
Vitamin B₁₂ (Activity
 Equivalent)...7.5 mcg
Ascorbic Acid (Vitamin C)..........................150 mg

dl-Alpha Tocopheryl
 Acetate (Vitamin E).......................5.5 IU (5.5 mg)
Vitamin A...................................10,000 IU (3 mg)
Vitamin D......................................400 IU (10 mcg)
Contains also—   approximately
Iron (as Ferrous Sulfate)...............................15 mg
Copper (as the Sulfate)....................................1 mg
Iodine (as Potassium Iodide).......................0.15 mg
Manganese (as the
 Glycerophosphate)..1 mg
Magnesium (as the Hydroxide)........................5 mg
Zinc (as the Chloride)..................................1.5 mg

Mi-Cebrin T is an extended-range therapeutic vitamin-mineral tablet formulated to aid patient recovery. Each tablet contains ten vitamins and six minerals and is specially coated to protect the full potency of the ingredients.
Indications: For the therapeutic management of surgical patients and patients with burns or injuries, febrile diseases, or poor dietary intake.
Precaution: Rarely, vitamins A and D in large doses daily for several months or longer cause toxicity.
Dosage: 1 tablet a day, or as directed by the physician.
How Supplied: *Tablets No. 1807, Mi-Cebrin T® (vitamin-minerals therapeutic, Dista), C20,* *Coated, Orange, in bottles of 30 (NDC 0777-0320-30), 100 (NDC 0777-0320-02), and 1000 (NDC 0777-0320-04) and in 10 strips of 10 individually labeled blisters each containing 1 tablet (ID100) (NDC 0777-0320-33).
[030183]

*Identi-Code® symbol.

NALFON® ℞
[*năl' fŏn*]
NALFON® 200
(fenoprofen calcium)
USP

Description: Nalfon® (fenoprofen calcium, Dista) is a nonsteroidal, anti-inflammatory, antiarthritic drug. Pulvules® and Tablets Nalfon contain fenoprofen calcium as the dihydrate in an amount equivalent to 200 mg or 300 mg (Pulvules) or 600 mg (Tablets) of fenoprofen. Chemically, Nalfon is an arylacetic acid derivative.
Nalfon is a white crystalline powder, soluble in alcohol (95%) to the extent of approximately 15 mg/ml at 25°C, slightly soluble in water, and insoluble in benzene.
The pK_a of Nalfon is 4.5 at 25°C.
Clinical Pharmacology: Nalfon® (fenoprofen calcium, Dista) is a nonsteroidal, anti-inflammatory, antiarthritic drug that also possesses analgesic and antipyretic activities. Its exact mode of action is unknown, but it is thought that prostaglandin synthetase inhibition is involved. Nalfon has been shown to inhibit prostaglandin synthetase isolated from bovine seminal vesicles. Reproduction studies in rats have shown Nalfon to be associated with prolonged labor and difficult parturition when given during late pregnancy. Evidence suggests that this may be due to decreased uterine contractility resulting from the inhibition of prostaglandin synthesis. Its action is not mediated through the adrenal gland.
Fenoprofen shows anti-inflammatory effects in rodents by inhibiting the development of redness and edema in acute inflammatory conditions and by reducing soft-tissue swelling and bone damage associated with chronic inflammation. It exhibits analgesic activity in rodents by inhibiting the writhing response caused by the introduction of an irritant into the peritoneal cavities of mice and by elevating pain thresholds to pressure in edematous hindpaws of rats. In rats made febrile by the subcutaneous administration of brewer's yeast, fenoprofen produces antipyretic action. These effects are characteristic of nonsteroidal, anti-inflammatory, antipyretic, analgesic drugs.
The results in humans confirmed the anti-inflammatory and analgesic actions found in animals. The emergence and degree of erythemic response were measured in adult male volunteers exposed to ultraviolet irradiation. The effects of Nalfon, aspirin, and indomethacin were compared separately with those of a placebo. All three drugs demonstrated antierythemic activity.

In patients with rheumatoid arthritis, the anti-inflammatory action of Nalfon has been evidenced by relief of pain; by increase in grip strength; by reductions in joint swelling, duration of morning stiffness, and disease activity (as assessed by both the investigator and the patient); and by increased mobility (a decrease in the number of joints having limited motion).
The use of Nalfon® (fenoprofen calcium, Dista) in combination with gold salts or corticosteroids has been studied in patients with rheumatoid arthritis. The studies, however, were inadequate in demonstrating whether further improvement is obtained by adding Nalfon to maintenance therapy with gold salts or steroids. Whether or not Nalfon, used in conjunction with partially effective doses of a corticosteroid, has a "steroid-sparing" effect is unknown.
In patients with osteoarthritis, the anti-inflammatory and analgesic effects of Nalfon have been demonstrated by reduction in tenderness on pressure; relief of pain with motion and at rest; reductions in night pain, stiffness, swelling, and overall disease activity (as assessed by both the patient and the investigator); and increased range of motion in involved joints.
In patients with rheumatoid arthritis and osteoarthritis, clinical studies have shown Nalfon to be comparable to aspirin in controlling the aforementioned measures of disease activity, but mild gastrointestinal adverse reactions (nausea, dyspepsia) and tinnitus occurred less frequently than in aspirin-treated patients. It is not known whether Nalfon causes less peptic ulceration than does aspirin.
In patients with pain, the analgesic action of Nalfon has produced a reduction in pain intensity, an increase in pain relief, improvement in total analgesia scores, and a sustained analgesic effect.
Under fasting conditions, Nalfon is rapidly absorbed, and peak plasma levels of 50 mcg/ml are achieved within two hours after oral administration of 600-mg doses. Good dose proportionality was observed between 200-mg and 600-mg doses in fasting male volunteers. The plasma half-life is approximately three hours. About 90% of a single oral dose is eliminated within 24 hours as fenoprofen glucuronide and 4'-hydroxyfenoprofen glucuronide, the major urinary metabolites of fenoprofen. Fenoprofen is highly bound (99%) to albumin.
The concomitant administration of antacid (containing both aluminum and magnesium hydroxide) does not interfere with absorption of Nalfon. There is less suppression of collagen-induced platelet aggregation with single doses of Nalfon than there is with aspirin.
Indications and Usage: Nalfon® (fenoprofen calcium, Dista) is indicated for relief of the signs and symptoms of rheumatoid arthritis and osteoarthritis. It is recommended for the treatment of acute flares and exacerbations and for the long-term management of these diseases.
Nalfon is also indicated for the relief of mild to moderate pain.
Controlled trials are currently in progress to establish the safety and efficacy of Nalfon in children.
Contraindications: Nalfon® (fenoprofen calcium, Dista) is contraindicated in patients who have shown hypersensitivity to it.
The drug should not be administered to patients with a history of significantly impaired renal function.
Nalfon should not be given to patients in whom aspirin and other nonsteroidal anti-inflammatory drugs induce the symptoms of asthma, rhinitis, or urticaria, because cross-sensitivity to these drugs occurs in a high proportion of such patients.
Warnings: Nalfon® (fenoprofen calcium, Dista) should be given under close supervision to patients

Continued on next page

Dista—Cont.

with a history of upper gastrointestinal tract disease and only after the Adverse Reactions section has been consulted. Gastrointestinal bleeding, sometimes severe (with fatalities having been reported), may occur in patients receiving Nalfon as with other nonsteroidal anti-inflammatory drugs. If Nalfon must be given to patients with an active peptic ulcer, the patient should be on a vigorous anti-ulcer treatment regimen and under close supervision for signs of ulcer perforation or severe gastrointestinal bleeding.

Since Nalfon has been marketed, there have been reports of genitourinary tract problems in patients taking it. The most frequently reported problems have been episodes of dysuria, cystitis, hematuria, interstitial nephritis, and the nephrotic syndrome. This syndrome may be preceded by the appearance of fever, rash, arthralgia, oliguria, and azotemia and may progress to anuria. There may also be substantial proteinuria, and, on renal biopsy, electron microscopy has shown foot process fusion and T-lymphocyte infiltration in the renal interstitium. Early recognition of the syndrome and withdrawal of the drug have been followed by rapid recovery. Administration of steroids and the use of dialysis have also been included in the treatment. Because a syndrome with some of these characteristics has also been reported with other nonsteroidal anti-inflammatory drugs, it is recommended that patients who have had these reactions with other such drugs not be treated with Nalfon. In patients with possibly compromised renal function, periodic renal function examinations should be done.

Precautions: In chronic studies in rats, high doses of Nalfon®(fenoprofen calcium, Dista) caused elevation of serum transaminase and hepatocellular hypertrophy. In clinical trials, some patients developed elevation of serum transaminase, LDH, and alkaline phosphatase that persisted for some months and usually, but not always, declined despite continuation of the drug. The significance of this is unknown. It is recommended, therefore, that Nalfon be discontinued if any significant liver abnormalities occur.

As with other nonsteroidal anti-inflammatory drugs, borderline elevations of one or more liver tests may occur in up to 15 percent of patients. These abnormalities may progress, may remain essentially unchanged, or may be transient with continued therapy. The SGPT (ALT) test is probably the most sensitive indicator of liver dysfunction. Meaningful (three times the upper limit of normal) elevations of SGPT or SGOT (AST) occurred in controlled clinical trials in less than 1 percent of patients. A patient with symptoms and/or signs suggesting liver dysfunction, or in whom an abnormal liver test has occurred, should be evaluated for evidence of the development of more severe hepatic reaction while on therapy with Nalfon. Severe hepatic reactions, including jaundice and cases of fatal hepatitis, have been reported with Nalfon as with other nonsteroidal anti-inflammatory drugs. Although such reactions are rare, if abnormal liver tests persist or worsen, if clinical signs and symptoms consistent with liver disease develop, or if systemic manifestations occur (e.g., eosinophilia, rash, etc.), Nalfon should be discontinued.

Safe use of Nalfon during pregnancy and lactation has not been established; therefore, administration to pregnant patients and nursing mothers is not recommended. Reproduction studies have been performed in rats and rabbits. When fenoprofen was given to rats during pregnancy and continued to the time of labor, parturition was prolonged. Similar results have been found with other nonsteroidal anti-inflammatory drugs that inhibit prostaglandin synthetase.

In patients receiving Nalfon and a steroid concomitantly, any reduction in steroid dosage should be gradual in order to avoid the possible complications of sudden steroid withdrawal.

Patients with initial low hemoglobin values who are receiving long-term therapy with Nalfon should have a hemoglobin determination at reasonable intervals.

Peripheral edema has been observed in some patients taking Nalfon; therefore, Nalfon should be used with caution in patients with compromised cardiac function or hypertension. The possibility of renal involvement should be considered.

Studies to date have not shown changes in the eyes attributable to the administration of Nalfon. However, adverse ocular effects have been observed with other anti-inflammatory drugs. Eye examinations, therefore, should be performed if visual disturbances occur in patients taking Nalfon.

Caution should be exercised by patients whose activities require alertness if they experience central-nervous-system side effects from Nalfon.

Since the safety of Nalfon has not been established in patients with impaired hearing, these patients should have periodic tests of auditory function during chronic therapy with Nalfon.

Nalfon decreases platelet aggregation and may prolong bleeding time. Patients who may be adversely affected by prolongation of the bleeding time should be carefully observed when Nalfon is administered.

Drug Interactions: The coadministration of aspirin decreases the biologic half-life of fenoprofen because of an increase in metabolic clearance that results in a greater amount of hydroxylated fenoprofen in the urine. Although the mechanism of interaction between fenoprofen and aspirin is not totally known, enzyme induction and displacement of fenoprofen from plasma albumin binding sites are possibilities. Because Nalfon® (fenoprofen calcium, Dista) has not been shown to produce any additional effect beyond that obtained with aspirin alone and because aspirin increases the rate of excretion of Nalfon, the concomitant use of Nalfon and salicylates is not recommended.

Chronic administration of phenobarbital, a known enzyme inducer, may be associated with a decrease in the plasma half-life of fenoprofen. When phenobarbital is added or withdrawn, dosage adjustment of Nalfon may be required.

In vitro studies have shown that fenoprofen, because of its affinity for albumin, may displace from their binding sites other drugs which are also albumin bound, and this may lead to drug interaction. Theoretically, fenoprofen could likewise be displaced. Patients receiving hydantoin, sulfonamides, or sulfonylureas should be observed for increased activity of these drugs and, therefore, signs of toxicity to these drugs. In patients receiving coumarin-type anticoagulants, the addition of Nalfon to therapy could prolong the prothrombin time. Patients receiving both drugs should be under careful observation.

Adverse Reactions: During clinical studies for rheumatoid arthritis or osteoarthritis, complaints were compiled from a checklist of potential adverse reactions, from which the following data emerged. These encompass observations in 3391 patients, including 188 observed for at least 52 weeks. During short-term studies for analgesia, the incidence of adverse reactions was markedly lower than that seen in longer-term studies.

INCIDENCE GREATER THAN 1%
Probable Causal Relationship

Digestive System—During clinical trials with Nalfon® (fenoprofen calcium, Dista), the most common adverse reactions were gastrointestinal in nature and occurred in about 14% of patients. In descending order of frequency, these reactions included dyspepsia,* constipation,* nausea,* vomiting,* abdominal pain, anorexia, occult blood in the stool, diarrhea, flatulence, and dry mouth. The drug was discontinued because of adverse gastrointestinal reactions in less than 2% of patients.

Nervous System—The most frequent adverse neurologic reactions were headache and somnolence, which occurred in about 15% of patients. Dizziness,* tremor, confusion, and insomnia were noted less frequently.

Nalfon was discontinued in less than 0.5% of patients because of these side effects.

Skin and Appendages—Pruritus,* rash, increased sweating, and urticaria.

Nalfon was discontinued in about 1% of patients because of an adverse effect related to the skin.

Special Senses—Tinnitus, blurred vision, and decreased hearing.

Nalfon was discontinued in less than 0.5% of patients because of adverse effects related to the special senses.

Cardiovascular—Palpitations* and tachycardia. Nalfon was discontinued in about 0.5% of patients because of adverse cardiovascular reactions.

Miscellaneous—Nervousness,* asthenia,* dyspnea, fatigue, and malaise.

* Reactions in 3% to 9% of patients treated with Nalfon. (Those reactions occurring in less than 3% of the patients are unmarked.)

INCIDENCE LESS THAN 1%
Probable Causal Relationship

The following adverse reactions, occurring in less than 1% of patients, were reported in controlled clinical trials and through voluntary reports since Nalfon® (fenoprofen calcium, Dista) was initially marketed. The probability of a causal relationship exists between Nalfon and these adverse reactions:

Digestive System—Gastritis, peptic ulcer with/without perforation, and/or gastrointestinal hemorrhage. Increases in alkaline phosphatase, LDH, and SGOT, jaundice, and cholestatic hepatitis were observed (*see* Precautions).

Genitourinary Tract—Dysuria, cystitis, hematuria, oliguria, azotemia, anuria, interstitial nephritis, nephrosis, and papillary necrosis (*see* Warnings).

Hematologic—Purpura, bruising, hemorrhage, thrombocytopenia, hemolytic anemia, agranulocytosis, and pancytopenia.

Miscellaneous—Peripheral edema and anaphylaxis.

INCIDENCE LESS THAN 1%
Causal Relationship Unknown

Other reactions have been reported but occurred in circumstances in which a causal relationship could not be established. However, with these rarely reported reactions, the possibility of such a relationship cannot be excluded. Therefore, these observations are listed to alert the physician.

Skin and Appendages—Stevens-Johnson syndrome, angioneurotic edema, exfoliative dermatitis, and alopecia.

Digestive System—Aphthous ulcerations of the buccal mucosa, metallic taste, and pancreatitis.

Cardiovascular—Atrial fibrillation, pulmonary edema, electrocardiographic changes, and supraventricular tachycardia.

Nervous System—Depression, disorientation, seizures, and trigeminal neuralgia.

Special Senses—Burning tongue, diplopia, and optic neuritis.

Hematologic—Aplastic anemia.

Miscellaneous—Personality change, lymphadenopathy, mastodynia, and fever.

Overdosage: No specific information is available on the treatment of overdosage with Nalfon® (fenoprofen calcium, Dista). If it should occur, standard procedures to evacuate gastric contents and to support vital functions should be employed. Since Nalfon is acidic and is excreted in the urine, it may be beneficial to administer alkali and charcoal and induce diuresis. Furosemide did not lower blood levels.

Dosage and Administration: *Analgesia*— For the treatment of mild to moderate pain, the recommended dosage is 200 mg every four to six hours, as needed.

Rheumatoid Arthritis and Osteoarthritis—The suggested dosage is 300 to 600 mg three or four times a day. The dose should be tailored to the needs of the patient and may be increased or decreased depending on the severity of the symptoms. Dosage adjustments may be made after initiation of drug therapy or during exacerbations of the disease. Total daily dosage should not exceed 3200 mg.

If gastrointestinal complaints occur, Nalfon® (fenoprofen calcium, Dista) may be administered with meals or with milk. Although the total amount absorbed is not affected, peak blood levels are delayed and diminished.

Patients with rheumatoid arthritis generally seem to require larger doses of Nalfon than do those with osteoarthritis. The smallest dose that yields acceptable control should be employed.

Although improvement may be seen in a few days in many patients, an additional two to three weeks may be required to gauge the full benefits of therapy.

How Supplied: (℞) *Pulvules Nalfon®* 200 *(Fenoprofen Calcium Capsules, USP):* No. 415, H76, * 200 mg (equivalent to fenoprofen) (No. 1, White Opaque Body, Ocher Opaque Cap), in an ℞Pak of 100 (NDC 0777-0876-02). All ℞Paks have safety closures.

(℞) *Pulvules Nalfon,* No. 416, H77, * 300 mg (equivalent to fenoprofen) (No. 0, Yellow Opaque Body, Ocher Opaque Cap), in an ℞Pak of 100 (NDC 0777-0877-02) and in bottles of 500 (NDC 0777-0877-03).

(℞) *Tablets Nalfon®* (*Fenoprofen Calcium Tablets, USP),* No. 1900, U59, * 600 mg (equivalent to fenoprofen), Yellow (paracapsule-shaped, scored), in an ℞Pak of 100 (NDC 0777-2159-02) and in bottles of 500 (NDC 0777-2159-03). All ℞Paks have safety closures.

[061984]

Shown in Product Identification Section, page 410

---

* Identi-Code® symbol.

NEBCIN® ℞
[nĕb'sĭn]
(tobramycin sulfate)
Injection, USP

WARNINGS

Patients treated with Nebcin® (Tobramycin Sulfate Injection, USP, Dista) and other aminoglycosides should be under close clinical observation, because these drugs have an inherent potential for causing ototoxicity and nephrotoxicity.

Neurotoxicity, manifested as both auditory and vestibular ototoxicity, can occur. The auditory changes are irreversible, are usually bilateral, and may be partial or total. Eighth-nerve impairment and nephrotoxicity may develop, primarily in patients having preexisting renal damage and in those with normal renal function to whom aminoglycosides are administered for longer periods or in higher doses than those recommended. Other manifestations of neurotoxicity may include numbness, skin tingling, muscle twitching, and convulsions. The risk of aminoglycoside-induced hearing loss increases with the degree of exposure to either high peak or high trough serum concentrations. Patients who develop cochlear damage may not have symptoms during therapy to warn them of eighth-nerve toxicity, and partial or total irreversible bilateral deafness may continue to develop after the drug has been discontinued. Rarely, nephrotoxicity may not become manifest until the first few days after cessation of therapy. Aminoglycoside-induced nephrotoxicity usually is reversible.

Renal and eighth-nerve function should be closely monitored in patients with known or suspected renal impairment and also in those whose renal function is initially normal but who develop signs of renal dysfunction during therapy. Peak and trough serum concentrations of aminoglycosides should be monitored periodically during therapy to assure adequate levels and to avoid potentially toxic levels. Prolonged serum concentrations above 12 mcg/ml should be avoided. Rising trough levels (above 2 mcg/ml) may indicate tissue accumulation. Such accumulation, excessive peak concentrations, advanced age, and cumulative dose may contribute to ototoxicity and nephrotoxicity (*see* Precautions). Urine should be examined for decreased specific gravity and increased excretion of protein, cells, and casts. Blood urea nitrogen, serum creatinine, and creatinine clearance should be measured periodically. When feasible, it is recommended that serial audiograms be obtained in patients old enough to be tested, particularly high-risk patients. Evidence of impairment of renal, vestibular, or auditory function requires discontinuation of the drug or dosage adjustment.

Nebcin should be used with caution in premature and neonatal infants because of their renal immaturity and the resulting prolongation of serum half-life of the drug.

Concurrent and sequential use of other neurotoxic and/or nephrotoxic antibiotics, particularly other aminoglycosides (e.g., amikacin, streptomycin, neomycin, kanamycin, gentamicin, and paromomycin), cephaloridine, viomycin, polymyxin B, colistin, cisplatin, and vancomycin, should be avoided. Other factors that may increase patient risk are advanced age and dehydration.

Aminoglycosides should not be given concurrently with potent diuretics, such as ethacrynic acid and furosemide. Some diuretics themselves cause ototoxicity, and intravenously administered diuretics enhance aminoglycoside toxicity by altering antibiotic concentrations in serum and tissue.

Aminoglycosides can cause fetal harm when administered to a pregnant woman (*see* Precautions).

Description: Tobramycin sulfate, a water-soluble antibiotic of the aminoglycoside group, is derived from the actinomycete *Streptomyces tenebrarius.* Nebcin® (tobramycin sulfate, Dista), Injection, is a clear and colorless sterile aqueous solution for parenteral administration.

Each ml also contains 5 mg phenol as a preservative, 3.2 mg sodium bisulfite, 0.1 mg edetate disodium, and water for injection, q.s. Sulfuric acid and/or sodium hydroxide may have been added to adjust the pH. Tobramycin is 4-0-[2,6-diamino-2, 3, 6-trideoxy-α-D-glucopyranosyl]-6- 0- [3-amino -3-deoxy-α-D-glucopyranosyl] -2- deoxystreptamine.

Clinical Pharmacology: Tobramycin is rapidly absorbed following intramuscular administration. Peak serum concentrations of tobramycin occur between 30 and 90 minutes after intramuscular administration. Following an intramuscular dose of 1 mg/kg of body weight, maximum serum concentrations reach about 4 mcg/ml, and measurable levels persist for as long as eight hours. Therapeutic serum levels are generally considered to range from 4 to 6 mcg/ml. When Nebcin® (tobramycin sulfate, Dista) is administered by intravenous infusion over a one-hour period, the serum concentrations are similar to those obtained by intramuscular administration. Nebcin is poorly absorbed from the gastrointestinal tract.

In patients with normal renal function, except neonates, Nebcin administered every eight hours does not accumulate in the serum. However, in those with reduced renal function and in neonates, the serum concentration of the antibiotic is usually higher and can be measured for longer periods of time than in normal adults. Dosage for such patients must, therefore, be adjusted accordingly (*see* Dosage and Administration).

Following parenteral administration, little, if any, metabolic transformation occurs, and tobramycin is eliminated almost exclusively by glomerular filtration. Renal clearance is similar to that of endogenous creatinine. Ultrafiltration studies demonstrate that practically no serum protein binding occurs. In patients with normal renal function, up to 84 percent of the dose is recoverable from the urine in eight hours and up to 93 percent in 24 hours.

Peak urine concentrations ranging from 75 to 100 mcg/ml have been observed following the intramuscular injection of a single dose of 1 mg/kg. After several days of treatment, the amount of tobramycin excreted in the urine approaches the daily dose administered. When renal function is impaired, excretion of Nebcin is slowed, and accumulation of the drug may cause toxic blood levels. The serum half-life in normal individuals is two hours. An inverse relationship exists between serum half-life and creatinine clearance, and the dosage schedule should be adjusted according to the degree of renal impairment (*see* Dosage and Administration). In patients undergoing dialysis, 25 to 70 percent of the administered dose may be removed, depending on the duration and type of dialysis.

Tobramycin can be detected in tissues and body fluids after parenteral administration. Concentrations in bile and stools ordinarily have been low, which suggests minimum biliary excretion. Tobramycin has appeared in low concentration in the cerebrospinal fluid following parenteral administration, and concentrations are dependent on dose, rate of penetration, and degree of meningeal inflammation. It has also been found in sputum, peritoneal fluid, synovial fluid, and abscess fluids, and it crosses the placental membranes. Concentrations in the renal cortex are several times higher than the usual serum levels.

Probenecid does not affect the renal tubular transport of tobramycin.

Microbiology—In vitro tests demonstrate that tobramycin is bactericidal and that it acts by inhibiting the synthesis of protein in bacterial cells. Tobramycin is usually active against most strains of the following organisms in vitro and in clinical infections:

Pseudomonas aeruginosa
Proteus species (indole-positive and indole-negative), including *Proteus mirabilis, P. morganii, P. rettgeri,* and *P. vulgaris*
Escherichia coli
Klebsiella-Enterobacter-Serratia group
Citrobacter species
Providencia species
Staphylococci, including *Staphylococcus aureus* (coagulase-positive and coagulase-negative)

Aminoglycosides have a low order of activity against most gram-positive organisms, including *Streptococcus pyogenes, S. pneumoniae,* and enterococci.

Although most strains of group D streptococci demonstrate in vitro resistance, some strains in this group are susceptible. In vitro studies have shown that an aminoglycoside combined with an antibiotic which interferes with cell-wall synthesis affects some group D streptococcal strains synergistically. The combination of penicillin G and tobramycin results in a synergistic bactericidal effect in vitro against certain strains of *S. faecalis.* However, this combination is not synergistic against other closely related organisms, e.g., *S. faecium.* Speciation of group D streptococci alone cannot be used to predict susceptibility. Susceptibility testing and tests for antibiotic synergism are emphasized.

Cross-resistance between aminoglycosides occurs and depends largely on inactivation by bacterial enzymes.

Susceptibility Tests—If the FDA Standardized Disc Test method (formerly the Bauer-Kirby-Sherris-Turck method) of disc susceptibility testing is used, a disc containing 10 mcg tobramycin should give a zone of at least 15 mm when tested against a tobramycin-susceptible bacterial strain, a zone of 13 to 14 mm against strains of intermediate susceptibility, and a zone of 12 mm or less against resistant organisms. The minimum inhibitory concentration correlates are ≤ 4 mcg/ml for susceptibility and ≥ 8 mcg/ml for resistance.

Indications and Usage: Nebcin® (tobramycin sulfate, Dista) is indicated for the treatment of serious bacterial infections caused by susceptible strains of the designated microorganisms in the diseases listed below:

Septicemia in the neonate, child, and adult caused by *P. aeruginosa, E. coli,* and *Klebsiella* species

Continued on next page

Dista—Cont.

Lower respiratory tract infections caused by *P. aeruginosa*, *Klebsiella* species, *Enterobacter* species, *Serratia* species, *E. coli*, and *S. aureus* (penicillinase and non-penicillinase-producing strains)

Serious central-nervous-system infections (meningitis) caused by susceptible organisms

Intra-abdominal infections, including peritonitis, caused by *E. coli*, *Klebsiella* species, and *Enterobacter* species.

Skin, bone, and skin-structure infections caused by *P. aeruginosa*, *Proteus* species, *E. coli*, *Klebsiella* species, *Enterobacter* species, and *S. aureus*

Complicated and recurrent urinary tract infections caused by *P. aeruginosa*, *Proteus* species (indole-positive and indole-negative), *E. coli*, *Klebsiella* species, *Enterobacter* species, *Serratia* species, *S. aureus*, *Providencia* species, and *Citrobacter* species

Aminoglycosides, including Nebcin, are not indicated in uncomplicated initial episodes of urinary tract infections unless the causative organisms are not susceptible to antibiotics having less potential toxicity. Nebcin may be considered in serious staphylococcal infections when penicillin or other potentially less toxic drugs are contraindicated and when bacterial susceptibility testing and clinical judgment indicate its use.

Bacterial cultures should be obtained prior to and during treatment to isolate and identify etiologic organisms and to test their susceptibility to tobramycin. If susceptibility tests show that the causative organisms are resistant to tobramycin, other appropriate therapy should be instituted. In patients in whom a serious life-threatening gram-negative infection is suspected, including those in whom concurrent therapy with a penicillin or cephalosporin and an aminoglycoside may be indicated, treatment with Nebcin may be initiated before the results of susceptibility studies are obtained. The decision to continue therapy with Nebcin® (tobramycin sulfate, Dista) should be based on the results of susceptibility studies, the severity of the infection, and the important additional concepts discussed in the WARNINGS box above.

Contraindications: A hypersensitivity to any aminoglycoside is a contraindication to the use of tobramycin. A history of hypersensitivity or serious toxic reactions to aminoglycosides may also contraindicate the use of any other aminoglycoside because of the known cross-sensitivity of patients to drugs in this class.

Warnings: See WARNINGS box above.

Precautions: Serum and urine specimens for examination should be collected during therapy, as recommended in the WARNINGS box. Serum calcium, magnesium, and sodium should be monitored.

Peak and trough serum levels should be measured periodically during therapy. Prolonged concentrations above 12 mcg/ml should be avoided. Rising trough levels (above 2 mcg/ml) may indicate tissue accumulation. Such accumulation, advanced age, and cumulative dosage may contribute to ototoxicity and nephrotoxicity. It is particularly important to monitor serum levels closely in patients with known renal impairment.

A useful guideline would be to perform serum level assays after two or three doses, so that the dosage could be adjusted if necessary, and also at three to four-day intervals during therapy. In the event of changing renal function, more frequent serum levels should be obtained and the dosage or dosage interval adjusted according to the guidelines provided in the Dosage and Administration section.

In order to measure the peak level, a serum sample should be drawn about 30 minutes following intravenous infusion or one hour after an intramuscular injection. Trough levels are measured by obtaining serum samples at eight hours or just prior to the next dose of Nebcin®(tobramycin sulfate, Dista). These suggested time intervals are intended only as guidelines and may vary according to institutional practices. It is important, however, that there be consistency within the individual patient program unless computerized pharmacokinetic dosing programs are available in the institution. These serum-level assays may be especially useful for monitoring the treatment of severely ill patients with changing renal function or of those infected with less sensitive organisms or those receiving maximum dosage.

Neuromuscular blockade and respiratory paralysis have been reported in cats receiving very high doses of tobramycin (40 mg/kg). The possibility that prolonged or secondary apnea may occur should be considered if tobramycin is administered to anesthetized patients who are also receiving neuromuscular blocking agents, such as succinylcholine, tubocurarine, or decamethonium, or to patients receiving massive transfusions of citrated blood. If neuromuscular blockade occurs, it may be reversed by the administration of calcium salts.

Cross-allergenicity among aminoglycosides has been demonstrated.

In patients with extensive burns, altered pharmacokinetics may result in reduced serum concentrations of aminoglycosides. In such patients treated with Nebcin, measurement of serum concentration is especially recommended as a basis for determination of appropriate dosage.

Elderly patients may have reduced renal function that may not be evident in the results of routine screening tests, such an BUN or serum creatinine. A creatinine clearance determination may be more useful. Monitoring of renal function during treatment with aminoglycosides is particularly important in such patients.

An increased incidence of nephrotoxicity has been reported following concomitant administration of aminoglycoside antibiotics and cephalosporins.

Aminoglycosides should be used with caution in patients with muscular disorders, such as myasthenia gravis or parkinsonism, since these drugs may aggravate muscle weakness because of their potential curare-like effect on neuromuscular function.

Aminoglycosides may be absorbed in significant quantities from body surfaces after local irrigation or application and may cause neurotoxicity and nephrotoxicity.

See WARNINGS box regarding concurrent use of potent diuretics and concurrent and sequential use of other neurotoxic or nephrotoxic drugs.

The inactivation of tobramycin and other aminoglycosides by beta-lactam-type antibiotics (penicillins or cephalosporins) has been demonstrated in vitro and in patients with severe renal impairment. Such inactivation has not been found in patients with normal renal function who have been given the drugs by separate routes of administration.

Therapy with tobramycin may result in overgrowth of nonsusceptible organisms. If overgrowth of nonsusceptible organisms occurs, appropriate therapy should be initiated.

Pregnancy Category D—Aminoglycosides can cause fetal harm when administered to a pregnant woman. Aminoglycoside antibiotics cross the placenta, and there have been several reports of total irreversible bilateral congenital deafness in children whose mothers received streptomycin during pregnancy. Serious side effects to mother, fetus, or newborn have not been reported in the treatment of pregnant women with other aminoglycosides. If tobramycin is used during pregnancy or if the patient becomes pregnant while taking tobramycin, she should be apprised of the potential hazard to the fetus.

Usage in Children—See Indications and Usage and Dosage and Administration.

Adverse Reactions: *Neurotoxicity*—Adverse effects on both the vestibular and auditory branches of the eighth nerve have been noted, especially in patients receiving high doses or prolonged therapy, in those given previous courses of therapy with an ototoxin, and in cases of dehydration. Symptoms include dizziness, vertigo, tinnitus, roaring in the ears, and hearing loss. Hearing loss is usually irreversible and is manifested initially by diminution of high-tone acuity. Tobramycin and gentamicin sulfates closely parallel each other in regard to ototoxic potential.

Nephrotoxicity—Renal function changes, as shown by rising BUN, NPN, and serum creatinine and by oliguria, cylindruria, and increased proteinuria, have been reported, especially in patients with a history of renal impairment who are treated for longer periods or with higher doses than those recommended. Adverse renal effects can occur in patients with initially normal renal function.

Clinical studies and studies in experimental animals have been conducted to compare the nephrotoxic potential of tobramycin and gentamicin. In some of the clinical studies and in the animal studies, tobramycin caused nephrotoxicity significantly less frequently than gentamicin. In some other clinical studies, no significant difference in the incidence of nephrotoxicity between tobramycin and gentamicin was found.

Other reported adverse reactions possibly related to Nebcin® (tobramycin sulfate, Dista) include anemia, granulocytopenia, and thrombocytopenia; and fever, rash, itching, urticaria, nausea, vomiting, headache, lethargy, pain at the injection site, mental confusion, and disorientation. Laboratory abnormalities possibly related to Nebcin include increased serum transaminases (SGOT, SGPT); increased serum LDH and bilirubin; decreased serum calcium, magnesium, sodium, and potassium; and leukopenia, leukocytosis, and eosinophilia.

Overdosage: In the event of overdosage or toxic reaction, hemodialysis or peritoneal dialysis will reduce serum levels. Hemodialysis is preferable because it is more efficient in reducing serum levels.

Dosage and Administration: Nebcin® (tobramycin sulfate, Dista) may be given intramuscularly or intravenously. Recommended dosages are the same for both routes. The patient's pretreatment body weight should be obtained for calculation of correct dosage. It is desirable to measure both peak and trough serum concentrations (see WARNINGS box and Precautions).

Administration for Patients with Normal Renal Function—Adults with Serious Infections: 3 mg/kg/day in three equal doses every eight hours (see Table 1).

Adults with Life-Threatening Infections: Up to 5 mg/kg/day may be administered in three or four equal doses (see Table 1). The dosage should be reduced to 3 mg/kg/day as soon as clinically indicated. To prevent increased toxicity due to excessive blood levels, dosage should not exceed 5 mg/kg/day unless serum levels are monitored. [See table on next page].

Children: 6 to 7.5 mg/kg/day in three or four equally divided doses (2 to 2.5 mg/kg every eight hours or 1.5 to 1.89 mg/kg every six hours).

Premature or Full-Term Neonates One Week of Age or Less: Up to 4 mg/kg/day may be administered in two equal doses every 12 hours.

It is desirable to limit treatment to a short term. The usual duration of treatment is seven to ten days. A longer course of therapy may be necessary in difficult and complicated infections. In such cases, monitoring of renal, auditory, and vestibular functions is advised, because neurotoxicity is more likely to occur when treatment is extended longer than ten days.

Administration for Patients with Impaired Renal Function—Whenever possible, serum tobramycin concentrations should be monitored during therapy.

Following a loading dose of 1 mg/kg, subsequent dosage in these patients must be adjusted, either with reduced doses administered at eight-hour intervals or with normal doses given at prolonged intervals. Both of these methods are suggested as guides to be used when serum levels of tobramycin cannot be measured directly. They are based on either the creatinine clearance or the serum creatinine of the patient, because these values correlate with the half-life of tobramycin. The dosage schedules derived from either method should be used in conjunction with careful clinical and laboratory observations of the patient and should be modified as necessary. Neither method should be used when dialysis is being performed.

<u>Reduced dosage at eight-hour intervals</u>: When the creatinine clearance rate is 70 ml or less per minute or when the serum creatinine value is known, the amount of the reduced dose can be determined by multiplying the normal dose from Table 1 by the percent of normal dose from the accompanying nomogram.

REDUCED DOSAGE NOMOGRAM*

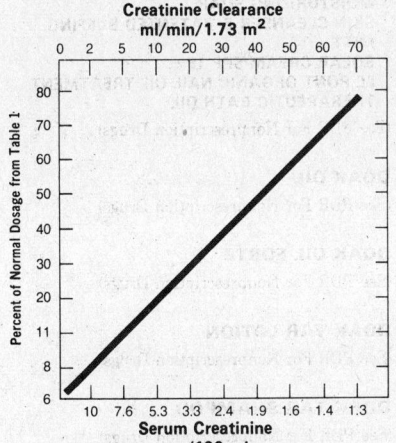

*Scales have been adjusted to facilitate dosage calculations.

An alternate rough guide for determining reduced dosage at eight-hour intervals (for patients whose steady-state serum creatinine values are known) is to divide the normally recommended dose by the patient's serum creatinine.

<u>Normal dosage at prolonged intervals</u>: If the creatinine clearance rate is not available and the patient's condition is stable, a dosage frequency *in hours* for the dosage given in Table 1 can be determined by multiplying the patient's serum creatinine by six.

Dosage in Obese Patients—The appropriate dose may be calculated by using the patient's estimated lean body weight plus 40 percent of the excess as the basic weight on which to figure mg/kg.

Intramuscular Administration—Nebcin may be administered by withdrawing the appropriate dose directly from a vial or by using a prefilled Hyporet® (disposable syringe, Dista).

Intravenous Administration—For intravenous administration, the usual volume of diluent (0.9% Sodium Chloride Injection or 5% Dextrose Injection) is 50 to 100 ml for adult doses. For children, the volume of diluent should be proportionately less than for adults. The diluted solution usually should be infused over a period of 20 to 60 minutes. Infusion periods of less than 20 minutes are not recommended, because peak serum levels may exceed 12 mcg/ml (see WARNINGS box).

Nebcin® (tobramycin sulfate, Dista) should not be physically premixed with other drugs but should be administered separately according to the recommended dose and route.

How Supplied: (℞) *Vials (Multiple Dose) Nebcin® (Tobramycin Sulfate Injection, USP): No. 781,* 80 mg (equivalent to tobramycin) per 2 ml, 2 ml, rubber-stoppered, in singles (10 per carton) (NDC 0777-1499-01) and in Traypak™ (multivial carton, Dista) of 25 (NDC 0777-1499-25); *No. 7090,* 1.2 g (equivalent to tobramycin) per 30 ml (Pharmacy Bulk Package), rubber-stoppered, in Traypak of 6 (NDC 0777-7090-16).

(℞) *Vials (Multiple Dose) No. 782, Nebcin® (Tobramycin Sulfate Injection, USP), Pediatric,* 20 mg (equivalent to tobramycin) per 2 ml, 2 ml, rubber-stoppered, in singles (10 per carton) (NDC 0777-0501-01).

(℞) *Hyporets® (disposable syringes, Dista) Nebcin® (Tobramycin Sulfate Injection, USP): No. 55,* 60 mg (equivalent to tobramycin) per 1.5 ml, 1.5 ml, in packages of 24 (NDC 0777-0509-24), and *No.*

TABLE 1. DOSAGE SCHEDULE GUIDE FOR NEBCIN® (TOBRAMYCIN SULFATE) IN ADULTS WITH NORMAL RENAL FUNCTION
(Dosage at Eight-Hour Intervals)

For Patient Weighing		Usual Dose for Serious Infections 1 mg/kg q. 8 h. (Total, 3 mg/kg/day)		Maximum Dose for Life-Threatening Infections (Reduce as soon as possible) 1.66 mg/kg q. 8 h. (Total, 5 mg/kg/day)	
kg	lb	mg/dose	ml/dose* q. 8 h.	mg/dose	ml/dose* q. 8 h.
120	264	120 mg	3 ml	200 mg	5 ml
115	253	115 mg	2.9 ml	191 mg	4.75 ml
110	242	110 mg	2.75 ml	183 mg	4.5 ml
105	231	105 mg	2.6 ml	175 mg	4.4 ml
100	220	100 mg	2.5 ml	166 mg	4.2 ml
95	209	95 mg	2.4 ml	158 mg	4 ml
90	198	90 mg	2.25 ml	150 mg	3.75 ml
85	187	85 mg	2.1 ml	141 mg	3.5 ml
80	176	80 mg	2 ml	133 mg	3.3 ml
75	165	75 mg	1.9 ml	125 mg	3.1 ml
70	154	70 mg	1.75 ml	116 mg	2.9 ml
65	143	65 mg	1.6 ml	108 mg	2.7 ml
60	132	60 mg	1.5 ml	100 mg	2.5 ml
55	121	55 mg	1.4 ml	91 mg	2.25 ml
50	110	50 mg	1.25 ml	83 mg	2.1 ml
45	99	45 mg	1.1 ml	75 mg	1.9 ml
40	88	40 mg	1 ml	66 mg	1.6 ml

*Applicable to all product forms except Nebcin, Pediatric, Injection (see How Supplied).

42, 80 mg (equivalent to tobramycin) per 2 ml, 2 ml, in packages of 24 (NDC 0777-0503-24). Each Hyporet is scored with a 10-mg (0.25-ml) fractional dose scale. [061184]

NEBCIN® ℞
[nĕb′sĭn]
(tobramycin sulfate)
Sterile

This vial is intended for use by the hospital pharmacist in the extemporaneous preparation of IV solutions.

Warnings: See under Nebcin, Injection, USP.

Description: Tobramycin sulfate, a water-soluble antibiotic of the aminoglycoside group, is derived from the actinomycete *Streptomyces tenebrarius.* Nebcin® (tobramycin sulfate, Dista), Sterile, is supplied as a sterile dry powder and is intended for solution in Sterile Water for Injection, USP. Sulfuric acid and/or sodium hydroxide may have been added during manufacture to adjust the pH. Each vial contains 1200 mg of tobramycin activity. After dilution, the solution will contain 40 mg of tobramycin per ml. The product contains no preservative. See also under Nebcin, Injection, USP.

Clinical Pharmacology, Indications and Usage, Contraindications, Warnings, Precautions, Adverse Reactions, and **Overdosage:** See under Nebcin, Injection, USP.

Dosage and Administration: The patient's pretreatment body weight should be obtained for calculation of correct dosage. It is desirable to measure both peak and trough serum concentrations (*see* WARNINGS box and Precautions *under* Nebcin, Injection, USP).

Administration for Patients with Normal Renal Function—Adults with Serious Infections: 3 mg/kg/day in three equal doses every eight hours (*see* Table 1 under Nebcin, Injection, USP).

Adults with Life-Threatening Infections: Up to 5 mg/kg/day may be administered in three or four equal doses (*see* Table 1). The dosage should be reduced to 3 mg/kg/day as soon as clinically indicated. To prevent increased toxicity due to excessive blood levels, dosage should not exceed 5 mg/kg/day unless serum levels are monitored.

Children: 6 to 7.5 mg/kg/day in three or four equally divided doses (2 to 2.5 mg/kg every eight hours or 1.5 to 1.89 mg/kg every six hours).

Premature or Full-Term Neonates One Week of Age or Less: Up to 4 mg/kg/day may be administered in two equal doses every 12 hours.

It is desirable to limit treatment to a short term. The usual duration of treatment is seven to ten days. A longer course of therapy may be necessary in difficult and complicated infections. In such cases, monitoring of renal, auditory, and vestibular functions is advised, because neurotoxicity is more likely to occur when treatment is extended longer than ten days.

Administration for Patients with Impaired Renal Function—Whenever possible, serum tobramycin concentrations should be monitored during therapy.

Following a loading dose of 1 mg/kg, subsequent dosage in these patients must be adjusted, either with reduced doses administered at eight-hour intervals or with normal doses given at prolonged intervals. Both of these methods are suggested as guides to be used when serum levels of tobramycin cannot be measured directly. They are based on either the creatinine clearance or the serum creatinine of the patient, because these values correlate with the half-life of tobramycin. The dosage schedules derived from either method should be used in conjunction with careful clinical and laboratory observations of the patient and should be modified as necessary. Neither method should be used when dialysis is being performed.

<u>Reduced dosage at eight-hour intervals</u>: When the creatinine clearance rate is 70 ml or less per minute or when the serum creatinine value is known, the amount of the reduced dose can be determined by multiplying the normal dose from Table 1 by the percent of normal dose from the nomogram *under* Nebcin, Injection, USP.

An alternate rough guide for determining reduced dosage at eight-hour intervals (for patients whose steady-state serum creatinine values are known) is to divide the normally recommended dose by the patient's serum creatinine.

<u>Normal dosage at prolonged intervals</u>: If the creatinine clearance rate is not available and the patient's condition is stable, a dosage frequency *in hours* for the dosage given in Table 1 can be determined by multiplying the patient's serum creatinine by six.

Dosage in Obese Patients—The appropriate dose may be calculated by using the patient's estimated

Continued on next page

Dista—Cont.

lean body weight plus 40 percent of the excess as the basic weight on which to figure mg/kg.

Intravenous Administration—For intravenous administration, the usual volume of diluent (0.9% Sodium Chloride Injection or 5% Dextrose Injection) is 50 to 100 ml for adult doses. For children, the volume of diluent should be proportionately less than for adults. The diluted solution usually should be infused over a period of 20 to 60 minutes. Infusion periods of less than 20 minutes are not recommended, because peak serum levels may exceed 12 mcg/ml (*see* WARNINGS box).

Nebcin® (tobramycin sulfate, Dista) should not be physically premixed with other drugs but should be administered separately according to the recommended dose and route.

Preparation and Storage of Solution: Nebcin, Sterile, is supplied as a dry powder. The contents of the vial (No. 7040) should be diluted with 30 ml of Sterile Water for Injection, USP, to provide a solution containing 40 mg of tobramycin per ml. Prior to reconstitution, the vial should be stored at controlled room temperature, 59° to 86°F (15° to 30°C). After reconstitution, the solution should be kept in a refrigerator and used within 96 hours. If kept at room temperature, the solution must be used within 24 hours.

How Supplied: (℞) Vials No. 7040, Nebcin® (tobramycin sulfate, Dista), Sterile, 1.2 g (equivalent to tobramycin), 40-ml size, rubber-stoppered (Dry Powder), in a Traypak™ (multivial carton, Dista) of 6 (NDC 0777-7040-16).

[050682]

VALMID®
[văl′mĭd]
(ethinamate)
Capsules, USP

Description: Valmid® (ethinamate, Dista) is 1-ethinyl-cyclohexyl-carbamate. It is a nonirritating, colorless, faintly bitter, stable crystalline powder with a melting point of 96°-98° C. Valmid is relatively insoluble in water but quite soluble in many alcohols and oils.

Valmid is a hypnotic agent for oral administration. Its site and mechanism of action are unknown.

Clinical Pharmacology: Valmid® (ethinamate, Dista) is rapidly absorbed after oral administration. Following a single oral dose of 1 g, peak plasma levels are reached in approximately 36 minutes and decline to negligible values over the next eight hours. Approximately 36 percent of the administered dose appears in the urine within 24 hours. The effect of multiple doses and prolonged administration on pharmacodynamics and pharmacokinetics is not known.

Indications and Usage: Valmid® (ethinamate, Dista) is a short-acting hypnotic. It has not been sufficiently well studied with currently available sleep laboratory techniques to delimit its value in specific types of insomnia. Valmid is best used for limited periods. Should insomnia persist, drug-free intervals of one week or more should elapse before re-treatment is considered. Attempts should be made to find alternative nondrug therapy for chronic insomnia. The prolonged administration of Valmid is not recommended, since it has not been shown to be effective for a period of more than seven days.

Contraindication: Valmid® (ethinamate, Dista) is contraindicated in patients with known hypersensitivity to the drug.

Warnings: Patients receiving Valmid® (ethinamate, Dista) should be cautioned about possible additive effects when it is taken in combination with alcohol or other CNS depressants. Patients should be cautioned against becoming involved in hazardous occupations requiring complete mental alertness, such as operating machines or driving a motor vehicle, shortly after ingestion of the drug.

Precautions: *Drug Interactions*—If Valmid is to be administered in combination with other drugs known to have a hypnotic or CNS-depressant effect, consideration should be given to the potential additive effects.

Carcinogenesis—Long-term studies in animals have *not* been performed to evaluate carcinogenic potential.

Usage in Pregnancy—Pregnancy Category C—Animal reproduction studies have not been conducted with Valmid. It is also not known whether the drug can cause fetal harm when administered to a pregnant woman or can affect reproduction capacity. Valmid should be given to a pregnant woman only if clearly needed.

Nursing Mothers—It is not known whether this drug is excreted in human milk. Because many drugs are excreted in human milk, caution should be exercised when Valmid is administered to a nursing woman.

Usage in Children—Safety and effectiveness in children below the age of 15 years have not been established.

Adverse Reactions: Rare cases of thrombocytopenic purpura and drug idiosyncrasy with fever have been reported. Paradoxical excitement in children, mild gastrointestinal symptoms, and skin rashes have occurred after the use of Valmid® (ethinamate, Dista).

Drug Abuse and Dependence: *Controlled Substance*—Valmid® (ethinamate, Dista) is a Schedule IV drug.

Dependence—Drug dependence characterized by both a psychologic and a physical dependence has occurred when Valmid has been taken at higher than recommended doses for prolonged intervals. It is, therefore, desirable to exercise caution in administering Valmid to individuals who are addiction-prone and to those whose history suggests that they may increase dosage on their own initiative. It is advisable to limit repeated prescriptions without adequate medical supervision.

In the event that an individual has established dependence on Valmid, withdrawal must be accomplished with extreme care. Abrupt withdrawal may cause a typical abstinence syndrome accompanied by convulsions. Withdrawal may be accomplished by hospitalizing the patient and reducing the addictive daily dose at a rate of 500 to 1000 mg every two or three days. Psychiatric follow-up is indicated.

Overdosage: In suicidal overdosage, CNS and respiratory depression should be treated in the same manner as barbiturate intoxication. Valmid® (ethinamate, Dista) is dialyzable.

Dosage and Administration: For insomnia, 1 or 2 Pulvules (500 mg or 1 g) of Valmid® (ethinamate, Dista) should be taken 20 minutes before retiring.

Special Patient Population—Since the risk of oversedation, dizziness, confusion, and/or ataxia substantially increases with the administration of large doses of sedatives and hypnotics in the elderly and debilitated, it is recommended that a single 500-mg Pulvule be the dose given to such individuals. Should this dose prove to be ineffective, clinical judgment must weigh the risk of increasing the dosage against the potential hazards mentioned above.

How Supplied: (©) *Pulvules No. 399, Valmid® (Ethinamate Capsules, USP), H74,* *500 mg (No. 0, Light-Blue Opaque Body, Blue Opaque Cap), in bottles of 100 (NDC 0777-0874-02). [051982]

Shown in Product Identification Section, page 410.

*Identi-Code® symbol.

Products are
listed alphabetically
in the
PINK SECTION.

Doak Pharmacal Co., Inc.
128 MAGNOLIA AVENUE
WESTBURY, NY 11590

FORMULA 405 SKIN CARE PRODUCTS
BODY SMOOTHING LOTION
ENRICHED CREAM
EYE CREAM
LIGHT TEXTURED MOISTURIZER
MOISTURIZING LOTION
MOISTURIZING SOAP
SKIN CLEANSER & PATENTED BUFFING MITT
SOLAR CREAM SPF 15+
LE PONT ORGANIC NAIL OIL TREATMENT
THERAPEUTIC BATH OIL

(See PDR For Nonprescription Drugs)

DOAK OIL
(See PDR For Nonprescription Drugs)

DOAK OIL FORTE
(See PDR For Nonprescription Drugs)

DOAK TAR LOTION
(See PDR For Nonprescription Drugs)

DOAK TAR SHAMPOO
(See PDR For Nonprescription Drugs)

LAVATAR TAR BATH
(See PDR For Nonprescription Drugs)

TARPASTE
(See PDR For Nonprescription Drugs)

TERSASEPTIC HYGIENIC SKIN CLEANSER
(See PDR For Nonprescription Drugs)

Dorsey Laboratories
Division of Sandoz, Inc.
LINCOLN, NE 68501

ACID MANTLE® CREME AND LOTION
[ă′sĭd-mănt′l]

Description: A greaseless, water-miscible preparation containing buffered aluminum acetate.
Indications: Provides relief from mild skin irritation due to exposure to soaps, detergents, chemicals, alkalis. Aids in the treatment of diaper rash, acne, eczema and dry, rough, scaly skin from varied causes.
Application: Apply several times daily, especially after wet work.
Caution: Limited compatibility and stability with Vitamin A, neomycin and water-soluble antibiotics. For external use only. Not for ophthalmic use.
How Supplied: Creme: 1 oz tubes; 4 oz and 1 lb jars. Lotion: 4 oz bottles.

CAMA® ARTHRITIS PAIN RELIEVER
[kă′măh]

Description: Each CAMA Arthritis Pain Reliever Tablet contains: aspirin, USP, 500 mg (7.7 grains); magnesium oxide, USP, 150 mg; aluminum hydroxide dried gel, USP, 150 mg.
Indications: For temporary relief of minor arthritis pain and for the management of arthritic conditions under the supervision of a physician.
Contraindications: Hypersensitivity to salicylates.
Warnings: The antipyretic effect of salicylates may mask the diagnostic importance of persistent fever.

Precautions: The occasional occurrence of mild salicylism may require adjustment of dosage. Use with caution in pregnant or nursing mothers.

Drug Interaction Precaution: Use with caution in patients taking anticoagulants, uricosuric agents, antidiabetic agents, anticonvulsants or methotrexate.

Adverse Reactions: Overdosage of salicylates will cause tinnitus, hearing loss, nausea, vomiting and gastrointestinal upsets and bleeding.

Dosage and Administration: Adults: 2 tablets with a full glass of water every 6 hours. Physicians may increase the dosage as required to provide satisfactory relief of symptoms.

How Supplied: CAMA Arthritis Pain Reliever Tablets (white with salmon inlay), imprinted "CAMA 500" on one side, "DORSEY" on the other, in bottles of 100 and 250.

DORCOL® CHILDREN'S COUGH SYRUP
[door'call]

Description: Each teaspoonful (5 ml) of DORCOL Children's Cough Syrup contains: pseudoephedrine hydrochloride 15 mg, guaifenesin 50 mg and dextromethorphan hydrobromide 5 mg. Inactive ingredients: alcohol (5%), benzoic acid, edetate disodium, FD&C Blue No. 1, FD&C Red No. 40, flavors, purified water, saccharin sodium, sodium hydroxide, sucrose, tartaric acid.

Indications: Provides prompt relief of cough and nasal congestion due to the common cold. The expectorant component helps loosen bronchial secretions. The decongestant, expectorant and antitussive are provided in an antihistamine-free formula.

Contraindications: Hypersensitivity to any of the ingredients. The use of sympathomimetic agents such as pseudoephedrine hydrochloride is contraindicated in patients with severe hypertension, severe coronary artery disease or in those taking monoamine oxidase inhibitors.

Precautions: Exercise prescribing caution in patients with persistent or chronic cough such as occurs with chronic bronchitis or bronchial asthma. Use with caution in patients with hypertension, hyperthyroidism, cardiovascular disease, diabetes mellitus, elevated intraocular pressure or prostatic hypertrophy.

Adverse Reactions: Occasional blurred vision, cardiac palpitations, flushing, gastrointestinal upsets, nervousness, dizziness, or sleeplessness may occur.

Dosage and Administration: Children 6–12 years—2 teaspoonfuls every 4 hours. Children 2–6 years—1 teaspoonful every 4 hours. The suggested dosage for pediatric patients 3 months to under 12 months of age is 3 drops per kilogram of body weight administered every 4 hours. The suggested dosage for patients 12 months to under 24 months of age is 7 drops (0.2 ml) per kilogram of body weight administered every 4 hours. A maximum of 4 doses per 24 hours is recommended

How Supplied: DORCOL Children's Cough Syrup (grape colored) in 4 fl oz and 8 fl oz plastic bottles with tamper-evident band around child-resistant cap.

DORCOL™ CHILDREN'S DECONGESTANT LIQUID
[door'call]

Description: Each teaspoonful (5 ml) of DORCOL Children's Decongestant Liquid contains pseudoephedrine hydrochloride 15 mg. Inactive ingredients: benzoic acid, D&C Yellow No. 10, edetate disodium, FD&C Yellow No. 6, flavors, purified water, sodium hydroxide, sorbitol solution, sucrose.

Indications: Provides temporary relief of nasal congestion due to the common cold, hay fever or other upper respiratory allergies, or associated with sinusitis. Promotes nasal and sinus drainage.

Contraindications: Hypersensitivity to any of the components. The use of sympathomimetic agents such as pseudoephedrine hydrochloride is contraindicated in patients with severe hypertension, severe coronary artery disease or in those taking monoamine oxidase inhibitors.

Precautions: Exercise prescribing caution in patients with hypertension, cardiovascular disease, diabetes mellitus, hyperthyroidism, elevated intraocular pressure or prostatic hypertrophy.

Adverse Reactions: Mild CNS stimulation, nervousness, dizziness, excitability, weakness, insomnia or restlessness may occur. Large doses may cause lightheadedness, nausea and/or vomiting.

Dosage and Administration:
By age:
  Children 2 to under 6 years: 1 teaspoonful
  Children 6 years: 2 teaspoonfuls
By weight:
  Children 25 to 45 pounds: 1 teaspoonful
  Children 46 to 85 pounds: 2 teaspoonfuls

The suggested dosage for pediatric patients 3 months to under 12 months of age is 3 drops per kilogram of body weight. The suggested dosage for patients 12 months to under 24 months of age is 7 drops (0.2 ml) per kilogram of body weight.
Give dose every 4 hours. A maximum of 4 doses per 24 hours is recommended.

How Supplied: DORCOL Children's Decongestant Liquid (pale orange) in 4 fl oz bottles with tamper-evident band around child-resistant cap.

DORCOL™ CHILDREN'S FEVER & PAIN REDUCER
[door'call]

Description: Each teaspoonful (5 ml) of DORCOL Children's Fever & Pain Reducer contains: acetaminophen 160 mg. Inactive ingredients: alcohol (10%), benzoic acid, edetate disodium, FD&C Red No. 40, flavors, glycerin, polyethylene glycol, povidone, purified water, saccharin sodium, sodium chloride, sorbitol solution, sucrose,

Indications: Provides analgesic/antipyretic action for infants and children with conditions requiring relief of pain or reduction of fever.

Contraindications: Hypersensitivity to any of the ingredients. Repeated administration of acetaminophen is contraindicated in patients with anemia or cardiac, pulmonary, renal or hepatic disease.

Precautions: Acetaminophen is relatively nontoxic in therapeutic doses. However, it should be used with caution in patients with preexisting anemia, since cyanosis may not be apparent despite very high levels of methemoglobin.

Adverse Reactions: Acetaminophen has rarely been found to produce any side effects. Sensitivity reactions have been reported.

Dosage and Administration:
By Age:
  Children 2 to under 4 years: 1 teaspoonful
  Children 4 to under 6 years: 1½ teaspoonfuls
  Children 6 years: 2 teaspoonfuls
By Weight:
  Children 25 to 35 pounds: 1 teaspoonful
  Children 36 to 45 pounds: 1½ teaspoonfuls
  Children 46 to 60 pounds: 2 teaspoonfuls

The suggested dosage for pediatric patients 3 months to under 12 months of age is 3 drops per kilogram of body weight. The suggested dosage for patients 12 months to under 24 months of age is 7 drops (0.2 ml) per kilogram of body weight.
Give dose every 4 hours while symptoms persist. A maximum of 5 doses per 24 hours is recommended.

How Supplied: DORCOL Children's Fever & Pain Reducer (red) in 4 fl oz bottles with tamper-evident band around child-resistant cap.

Dosage	Amount of Calcium Supplied Daily	Percentage of U.S. Recommended Daily Allowance (U.S. RDA) Children 1 to under 4 (800 mg)	Children 4 to 6 (1000 mg)
1 teaspoonful 3 times daily	345 mg	45%	35%
2 teaspoonfuls 3 times daily	690 mg	90%	70%

(Part of need is supplied by diet.)

DORCOL™ CHILDREN'S LIQUID CALCIUM SUPPLEMENT
[door'call]

Description: Each teaspoonful (5 ml) of DORCOL Children's Liquid Calcium Supplement contains: glubionate calcium 1.8 gm (calcium content 115 mg). Also contains: benzoic acid, citric acid, flavors, purified water, saccharin sodium, sorbitol solution, sucrose.

Indications: As a dietary supplement for the prevention of calcium deficiency which may be associated with childhood growth periods and inadequate dietary intake.

Contraindications: Hypersensitivity to any of the ingredients. Calcium salts are contraindicated in patients with hypercalcemia or renal calculi.

Adverse Reactions: DORCOL Children's Liquid Calcium Supplement is exceptionally well tolerated. Gastrointestinal disturbances are rare. Symptoms of hypercalcemia include anorexia, nausea, vomiting, constipation, abdominal pain, dryness of the mouth, thirst and polyuria.

Dosage and Administration: As a dietary supplement for prevention of calcium deficiency: [See table above].

How Supplied: DORCOL Children's Liquid Calcium Supplement (straw yellow) in 4 fl oz bottles with tamper-evident band around child-resistant cap.

DORCOL™ CHILDREN'S LIQUID COLD FORMULA
[door'call]

Description: Each teaspoonful (5 ml) of DORCOL Children's Liquid Cold Formula contains pseudoephedrine hydrochloride 15 mg and chlorpheniramine maleate 1 mg. Inactive ingredients: benzoic acid, D&C Yellow No. 10, FD&C Blue No. 1, FD&C Red No. 40, flavors, purified water, sorbitol solution, sucrose.

Indications: Provides temporary relief of nasal congestion due to the common cold, hay fever or other upper respirtory allergies, or associated with sinusitis. For relief of sneezing and rhinorrhea as may occur in allergic rhinitis. Promotes nasal and sinus drainage.

Contraindications: Hypersensitivity to any of the ingredients. The use of sympathomimetic agents such as pseudoephedrine hydrochloride is contraindicated in patients with severe hypertension, severe coronary artery disease or in those taking monoamine oxidase inhibitors.

Precautions: Exercise prescribing caution in patients with hypertension, cardiovascular disease, diabetes mellitus, hyperthyroidism, elevated intraocular pressure, prostatic hypertrophy, stenosing peptic ulcer, pyloroduodenal obstruction, bladder neck obstruction, angle-closure glaucoma, or bronchial asthma.

Adverse Reactions: Drowsiness, blurred vision, palpitations, flushing, gastrointestinal upsets, nervousness, dizziness, or sleeplessness may occur. May cause excitability especially in children.

Dosage and Administration:
By age:
  Children 6 to 12 years: 2 teaspoonfuls
By weight:
  Children 45 to 85 pounds: 2 teaspoonfuls

The suggested dosage for pediatric patients 3 months to under 12 months of age is 2 drops per kilogram of body weight. The suggested dosage for patients 12 months to under 24 months of age is 5 drops (0.2 ml) per kilogram of body weight. The

Continued on next page

Dorsey Labs.—Cont.

suggested dosage for patients 2 years to under 6 years is 1 teaspoonful.
Give dose every 4 to 6 hours. A maximum of 4 doses per 24 hours is recommended.
How Supplied: DORCOL Children's Liquid Cold Formula (light brown) in 4 fl oz bottles with tamper-evident band around child-resistant cap.

TOTAL ECLIPSE® Sunscreen (SPF 15)
[ē clips']
**Moisturizing Lotion and
Cooling Alcohol Lotion**

Description: A nongreasy, noncomedogenic moisturizing lotion containing padimate O (octyl dimethyl PABA), octyl salicylate and oxybenzone (benzophenone-3). A nongreasy, noncomedogenic cooling alcohol lotion containing oxybenzone (benzophenone-3), padimate O (octyl dimethyl PABA) and glyceryl PABA.
Indications: Prevention of sunburn and long term harmful effects of the sun. Overexposure to the sun may lead to premature aging of the skin and skin cancer. The liberal and regular use over the years of this product may help reduce the chance of these harmful effects.
Actions: Absorbs ultraviolet radiation from the UV-A band and from the burning UV-B band. Total ECLIPSE prevents tanning and sunburn. Affords the most protection against sunburn for highly sun-sensitive skin. Provides fifteen times the skin's natural protection from sunburn.
Warnings: For external use only. Do not use if sensitive to benzocaine, sulfonamides, aniline dyes, PABA or related compounds. Avoid contact with eyes or eyelids. Discontinue use if signs of irritation or rash appear. Keep out of the reach of children. May stain some fabrics.
Dosage and Administration: Apply liberally before sun exposure. ECLIPSE Sunscreens resist washoff from swimming and perspiration. Reapplication is recommended after 40 minutes in the water or after excessive sweating.
How Supplied: Moisturizing Lotion: 4 oz and 6 oz plastic bottles; Cooling Alcohol Lotion: 4 oz plastic bottles.

KANULASE® TABLETS
[căn' ū-lāce]

Description: Each KANULASE Tablet contains: Dorase® (cellulase) standardized to 9 mg; Pancreatin (equivalent to the following enzyme activities: Lipase 1000 USP units, Amylase 1000 USP units, Protease 12,000 USP units); Glutamic acid hydrochloride 200 mg; Ox bile extract 100 mg; Pepsin 150 mg.
Indications: For relief of discomforts of intestinal gas such as belching, bloating and flatulence.
Caution: KANULASE contains glutamic acid hydrochloride which is not usually given to patients with peptic ulcer. Use with caution in pregnant and nursing mothers.
Warning: Keep this and all medicines out of the reach of children.
Dosage and Administration: Adults—1 or 2 tablets, swallowed whole, with meals. If looseness of stools occurs, decrease the dosage.
How Supplied: KANULASE Tablets (pink) in bottles of 50.

METAPREL® R
[me' ta-prel]
**(metaproterenol sulfate)
Inhalant Solution
Metered Dose Inhaler
Syrup
Tablets**

Description: Chemically, METAPREL (metaproterenol sulfate) is 1-(3,5-dihydroxyphenyl)-2-isopropylaminoethanol sulfate, a white crystalline, racemic mixture of two optically active isomers. It differs from isoproterenol hydrochloride by having two hydroxyl groups attached at the meta positions on the benzene ring rather than one at the meta and one at the para position.
Clinical Pharmacology: METAPREL (metaproterenol sulfate) is a potent beta-adrenergic stimulator with the aerosol and inhalant solution having a rapid onset of action. It is postulated that beta-adrenergic stimulants produce many of their pharmacological effects by activation of adenyl cyclase, the enzyme which catalyzes the conversion of adenosine triphosphate to cyclic adenosine monophosphate.
Absorption, biotransformation and excretion studies following administration by inhalation have not been performed. Following oral administration in humans, an average of 40% of the drug is absorbed; it is not metabolized by catechol-O-methyltransferase or sulfatase enzymes in the gut, but is excreted primarily as glucuronic acid conjugates.
Indications and Usage: METAPREL (metaproterenol sulfate) is indicated as a bronchodilator for bronchial asthma, and for reversible bronchospasm which may occur in association with bronchitis and emphysema.
When administered orally or by inhalation, METAPREL (metaproterenol sulfate) decreases reversible bronchospasm. Pulmonary function tests performed concomitantly usually show improvement following METAPREL (metaproterenol sulfate) administration, e.g., an increase in the one-second forced expiratory volume (FEV_1), an increase in maximum expiratory flow rate, an increase in peak expiratory flow rate, an increase in forced vital capacity, and/or a decrease in airway resistance. The resultant decrease in airway obstruction may relieve the dyspnea associated with bronchospasm.
Controlled single- and multiple-dose studies have been performed with pulmonary function monitoring. The mean duration of effect of a single dose of 20 mg of METAPREL (metaproterenol sulfate) Tablets or Syrup, (i.e., the period of time during which there is a 15% or greater increase in FEV_1) was up to 4 hours. Four controlled multiple-dose 60-day studies, comparing the effectiveness of METAPREL Tablets with ephedrine tablets, have been performed. Because of difficulties in study design, only one study was available which could be analyzed in depth. This study showed a loss of efficacy with time for both METAPREL Tablets and ephedrine. Therefore, the physician should take this phenomenon into account in evaluating the individual patient's overall management. Further studies are in progress to adequately explain these results.
The duration of effect of a single dose of 2 to 3 inhalations of METAPREL (metaproterenol sulfate) (i.e., the period of time during which there is a 15% or greater increase in mean FEV_1) has varied from 1 to 5 hours. In repetitive-dosing studies (up to q.i.d.) the duration of effect for a similar dose of METAPREL (metaproterenol sulfate) has ranged from about 1 to 2½ hours. Present studies are inadequate to explain the divergence in duration of the FEV_1 effect between single- and repetitive-dosing studies, respectively.
Following controlled single-dose studies with METAPREL Inhalant Solution by an intermittent positive pressure breathing apparatus (IPPB) and by hand bulb nebulizers, significant improvement (15% or greater increase in FEV_1) occurred within 5 to 30 minutes and persisted for periods varying from 2 to 6 hours. In these studies the longer duration of effect occurred in the studies in which the drug was administered by IPPB, i.e., 6 hours versus 2 to 3 hours when administered by hand bulb nebulizer. In these studies the doses used were 0.3 ml by IPPB and 10 inhalations by hand bulb nebulizer.
In controlled repetitive-dosing studies by IPPB and by hand bulb nebulizer, the onset of effect occurred within 5 to 30 minutes and duration ranged from 4 to 6 hours. In these studies the doses used were 0.3 ml b.i.d. or t.i.d. when given by IPPB, and 10 inhalations q.i.d. (no more often than q4h) when given by hand bulb nebulizer. As in the single-dose studies, effectiveness was measured as a sustained increase in FEV_1 of 15% or greater. In these repetitive-dosing studies there was no apparent difference in duration between the two methods of delivery.
Clinical studies were conducted in which the effectiveness of METAPREL (metaproterenol sulfate) Inhalant Solution was evaluated by comparison with that of isoproterenol hydrochloride over periods of two to three months. Both drugs continued to produce significant improvement in pulmonary function throughout this period of treatment.
Contraindications: Use in patients with cardiac arrhythmias associated with tachycardia is contraindicated.
Warnings: Excessive use of adrenergic aerosols is potentially dangerous. Fatalities have been reported following excessive use of METAPREL (metaproterenol sulfate) as with other sympathomimetic inhalation preparations, and the exact cause is unknown. Cardiac arrest was noted in several cases.
Paradoxical bronchoconstriction with repeated excessive administration has been reported with other sympathomimetic agents. Therefore, it is possible that this phenomenon could occur with METAPREL (metaproterenol sulfate).
Patients should be advised to contact their physician in the event that they do not respond to their usual dose of a sympathomimetic amine aerosol.
Precautions: Because METAPREL (metaproterenol sulfate) is a sympathomimetic drug, it should be used with great caution in patients with hypertension, coronary artery disease, congestive heart failure, hyperthyroidism or diabetes, or when there is sensitivity to sympathomimetic amines.
Information For Patients: Extreme care must be exercised with respect to the administration of additional sympathomimetic agents. A sufficient interval of time should elapse prior to administration of another sympathomimetic agent.
Carcinogenesis: Long-term studies in mice and rats to evaluate the oral carcinogenic potential of metaproterenol sulfate have not been completed.
Pregnancy: *Teratogenic Effects: Pregnancy Category C.* METAPREL (metaproterenol sulfate) has been shown to be teratogenic and embryocidal in rabbits when given orally in doses 620 times the human inhalation dose and 62 times the human oral dose; the teratogenic effects included skeletal abnormalities and hydrocephalus with bone separation. Oral reproduction studies in mice, rats and rabbits showed no teratogenic or embryocidal effect at 50 mg/kg, or 310 times the human inhalation dose and 31 times the human oral dose. There are no adequate and well-controlled studies in pregnant women. METAPREL (metaproterenol sulfate) should be used during pregnancy only if the potential benefit justifies the potential risk to the fetus.
Nursing Mothers: It is not known whether this drug is excreted in human milk. Because many drugs are excreted in human milk, caution should be exercised when METAPREL (metaproterenol sulfate) is administered to a nursing woman.
Pediatric Use: Safety and effectiveness of METAPREL Metered Dose Inhaler and Inhalant Solution in children below the age of 12 have not been established. The safety and efficacy of METAPREL Tablets in children below the age of 6 have not been established.
Adverse Reactions: Adverse reactions are similar to those noted with other sympathomimetic agents.
The most frequent adverse reactions to METAPREL (metaproterenol sulfate) are nervousness, tachycardia, tremor and nausea. Less frequent adverse reactions are hypertension, palpitations, vomiting and bad taste.
Overdosage: The symptoms of overdosage are those of excessive beta adrenergic stimulation listed under Adverse Reactions. These reactions usually do not require treatment other than reduction of dosage and/or frequency of administration.
Dosage and Administration:
Tablets: Adults: The usual dose is 20 mg 3 or 4 times a day. Children: Aged 6 to 9 years or weight under 60 lbs—10 mg 3 or 4 times a day. Over 9

years or weight over 60 lbs—20 mg 3 or 4 times a day.

Syrup: Children: Aged 6 to 9 years or weight under 60 lbs—1 teaspoonful 3 or 4 times a day. Children over 9 years or weight over 60 lbs—2 teaspoonfuls 3 or 4 times a day. Experience in children under the age of 6 is limited to 78 children. Of this number, 40 were treated with METAPREL Syrup for at least one month. In this group, daily doses of approximately 1.3 to 2.6 mg/kg were well tolerated. Adults: 2 teaspoonfuls 3 or 4 times a day.

Metered Dose Inhaler: The usual single dose is 2 to 3 inhalations. With repetitive dosing, inhalation should usually not be repeated more often than about every 3 to 4 hours. Total dosage per day should not exceed 12 inhalations.

METAPREL (metaproterenol sulfate) Metered Dose Inhaler is not recommended for children under 12 years of age because there is not sufficient data on administration of this dosage form in this age group.

Inhalant Solution: METAPREL (metaproterenol sulfate) Inhalant Solution is administered by oral inhalation with the aid of a hand bulb nebulizer or an intermittent positive pressure breathing apparatus (IPPB).

Usually, treatment need not be repeated more often than every 4 hours to relieve acute attacks of bronchospasm. As part of a total treatment program in chronic bronchospastic pulmonary disease. METAPREL (metaproterenol sulfate) Inhalant Solution may be administered 3 to 4 times a day.

As with all medications, the physician should begin therapy with the lowest effective dose and then titrate the dosage according to the individual patient's requirements.

[See table above].

METAPREL (metaproterenol sulfate) Inhalant Solution is not recommended for use in children under 12 years of age.

How Supplied: Inhalant Solution: METAPREL (metaproterenol sulfate) Inhalant Solution is supplied as a 5% solution in bottles of 10 ml with accompanying calibrated dropper. Store at room temperature; avoid excessive heat. Protect from light.

Metered Dose Inhaler: Each METAPREL (metaproterenol sulfate) Metered Dose Inhaler contains 225 mg of metaproterenol sulfate as a micronized powder in an inert propellant. This is sufficient medication for 300 inhalations. Each metered dose expressed from the inhaler delivers at the mouthpiece approximately 0.65 mg of metaproterenol sulfate. METAPREL Metered Dose Inhaler with mouthpiece (15 ml). METAPREL Metered Dose Inhaler refill (15 ml).

Syrup: METAPREL (metaproterenol sulfate) is available as a cherry-flavored syrup, 10 mg per teaspoonful (5 ml), in pint bottles.

Tablets: METAPREL (metaproterenol sulfate) Tablets, 10 mg, white, scored, round, imprinted "Dorsey" on one side and "10" on the other. METAPREL (metaproterenol sulfate) Tablets, 20 mg, white, scored, round, imprinted "Dorsey" on one side and "20" on the other. Both strengths are available in bottles of 100.

TRIAMINIC® ALLERGY TABLETS
[trī″ah-mĭn′ĭc]

(See PDR For Nonprescription Drugs)

TRIAMINIC® CHEWABLES
[trī″ah-mĭn′ĭc]

(See PDR For Nonprescription Drugs)

TRIAMINIC® COLD SYRUP
[trī″ah-mĭn′ĭc]

Description: Each teaspoonful (5 ml) of TRIAMINIC Cold Syrup contains: phenylpropanolamine hydrochloride 12.5 mg and chlorpheniramine maleate 2 mg in a nonalcoholic vehicle.

Indications: For the temporary relief of nasal congestion, sneezing, and itchy watery eyes that

Method of Administration	Usual Single Dose	Range	Dilution
Hand bulb nebulizer	10 inhalations	5–15 inhalations	No dilution
IPPB	0.3 ml	0.2–0.3 ml	Diluted in approximately 2.5 ml of saline solution or other diluent

may occur in hay fever or other upper respiratory allergies, the common cold and sinusitis.

Contraindications: TRIAMINIC Cold Syrup is contraindicated in the presence of hypersensitivity to any of the ingredients. The use of pressor amines such as phenylpropanolamine hydrochloride is contraindicated in those patients taking monoamine oxidase inhibitors for antihypertensive or antidepressant indications.

Precautions: Caution should be observed in operating a motor vehicle or performing potentially hazardous tasks requiring mental alertness. Alcoholic beverages and other CNS depressants may potentiate the sedative effects of antihistamines. Caution should be observed in the presence of hypertension, hyperthyroidism, cardiovascular disease or diabetes mellitus. Because of the anticholinergic action of antihistamines, they should be administered with caution to patients with bronchial asthma, narrow angle glaucoma, stenosing peptic ulcer, pyloroduodenal obstruction, prostatic hypertrophy or other bladder neck obstruction. Use with caution in pregnant and nursing mothers.

Adverse Reactions: Drowsiness, blurred vision, palpitations, flushing, gastrointestinal upsets, nervousness, dizziness, or sleeplessness may occur. May cause excitability especially in children.

Dosage and Administration: Adults—2 teaspoonfuls every 4 hours. Children 6–12 years—1 teaspoonful every 4 hours. Children 2–6 years—½ teaspoonful every 4 hours. The suggested dosage for pediatric patients 3 months to under 12 months of age is 1 drop per kilogram of body weight administered every 4 hours. The suggested dosage for patients 12 months to under 24 months of age is 3 drops per kilogram of body weight administered every 4 hours.

How Supplied: TRIAMINIC Cold Syrup (orange), in 4 fl oz and 8 fl oz plastic bottles with tamper-evident band around child-resistant cap.

TRIAMINIC® COLD TABLETS
[trī″ah-mĭn′ĭc]

Description: Each TRIAMINIC Cold Tablet contains: phenylpropanolamine hydrochloride 12.5 mg and chlorpheniramine maleate 2 mg.

Indications: For the temporary relief of nasal congestion, sneezing and itchy watery eyes that may occur in hay fever or other upper respiratory allergies, the common cold and sinusitis.

Contraindications: TRIAMINIC Cold Tablets are contraindicated in the presence of hypersensitivity to any of the ingredients. The use of pressor amines such as phenylpropanolamine hydrochloride is contraindicated in those patients taking monoamine oxidase inhibitors for antihypertensive or antidepressant indications.

Precautions: Caution should be observed in operating a motor vehicle or performing potentially hazardous tasks requiring mental alertness. Alcoholic beverages and other CNS depressants may potentiate the sedative effects of antihistamines. Caution should be observed in the presence of hypertension, hyperthyroidism, cardiovascular disease or diabetes mellitus. Because of anticholinergic action of antihistamines, they should be administered with caution to patients with bronchial asthma, narrow angle glaucoma, stenosing peptic ulcer, pyloroduodenal obstruction, prostatic hypertrophy or other bladder neck obstruction. Use with caution in pregnant and nursing mothers.

Adverse Reactions: Drowsiness, blurred vision, palpitations, flushing, gastrointestinal upsets, nervousness, dizziness, or sleeplessness may occur. May cause excitability expecially in children.

Dosage and Administration: Adults — 2 tablets every 4 hours. Children 6-12 years — 1 tablet every 4 hours.

How Supplied: TRIAMINIC Cold Tablets (orange), imprinted "DORSEY" on one side, "TRIAMINIC" on the other, in blister packs of 24 and 48.

TRIAMINIC® EXPECTORANT
[trī″ah-mĭn′ĭc]

Description: Each teaspoonful (5 ml) of TRIAMINIC Expectorant contains: phenylpropanolamine hydrochloride 12.5 mg, guaifenesin 100 mg, alcohol 5%.

Indications: Provides prompt relief of cough and nasal congestion due to the common cold. The expectorant component helps loosen bronchial secretions. The decongestant and expectorant are provided in an antihistamine-free formula.

Contraindications: TRIAMINIC Expectorant is contraindicated in the presence of hypersensitivity to any of the ingredients. The use of pressor amines such as phenylpropanolamine hydrochloride is contraindicated in those patients taking monoamine oxidase inhibitors.

Precautions: Exercise prescribing caution in patients with persistent or chronic cough such as occurs with smoking, chronic bronchitis, bronchial asthma, or emphysema. Use with caution in patients with hypertension, hyperthyroidism, cardiovascular disease or diabetes mellitus. Use with caution in pregnant and nursing mothers.

Adverse Reactions: Occasional blurred vision, cardiac palpitations, flushing, gastrointestinal upsets, nervousness, dizziness, or sleeplessness may occur.

Dosage and Administration: Adults—2 teaspoonfuls every 4 hours. Children 6–12 years—1 teaspoonful every 4 hours. Children 2–6 years—½ teaspoonful every 4 hours. The suggested dosage for pediatric patients 3 months to under 12 months of age is 2 drops per kilogram of body weight administered every 4 hours. The suggested dosage for patients 12 months to under 24 months of age is 3 drops per kilogram of body weight administered every 4 hours.

How Supplied: TRIAMINIC Expectorant (yellow) in 4 fl oz and 8 fl oz plastic bottles with tamper-evident band around child-resistant cap.

TRIAMINIC® EXPECTORANT WITH CODEINE
[trī″ah-mĭn′ĭc]

Description: Each teaspoonful (5 ml) of TRIAMINIC Expectorant with Codeine contains: codeine phosphate 10 mg (Warning: May be habit forming), phenylpropanolamine hydrochloride 12.5 mg, guaifenesin 100 mg, alcohol 5%.

Indications: For use in providing temporary relief of coughs and nasal congestion due to the common cold, when the antitussive properties of codeine are desired. The expectorant component helps loosen bronchial secretions. The ingredients are provided in an antihistamine-free formula.

Contraindications: TRIAMINIC Expectorant with Codeine is contraindicated in the presence of hypersensitivity to any of the ingredients. The use of pressor amines such as phenylpropanolamine hydrochloride is contraindicated in those patients taking monoamine oxidase inhibitors for antihy-

Continued on next page

Dorsey Labs.—Cont.

pertensive or antidepressant indications. Continuous dosage over an extended period is generally contraindicated since codeine phosphate may cause addiction.

Precautions: Exercise prescribing caution in patients with persistent or chronic cough such as occurs with chronic bronchitis, bronchial asthma, or emphysema. Use with caution in patients with hypertension, hyperthyroidism, cardiovascular disease, diabetes mellitus, chronic pulmonary disease or shortness of breath. Exercise caution in prescribing this product to children taking other drugs. Use with caution in pregnant and nursing mothers.

Adverse Reactions: Occasional blurred vision, cardiac palpitations, flushing, gastrointestinal upsets, nervousness, dizziness, sleeplessness and drowsiness. May cause or aggravate constipation.

Dosage and Administration: Adults—2 teaspoonfuls every 4 hours. Children 6 to 12 years—1 teaspoonful every 4 hours. Children 2 to 6 years—½ teaspoonful every 4 hours. The suggested dosage in pediatric patients 3 months to 2 years of age is 2 drops per kilogram of body weight administered every 4 hours.

How Supplied: TRIAMINIC Expectorant with Codeine (green) in 4 fl oz and pint bottles. TRIAMINIC Expectorant with Codeine is a Schedule V controlled substance.

TRIAMINIC JUVELETS®
[trī″ah min′ic joov′ah-lets′]
(Timed Release)

TRIAMINIC® TR TABLETS
(Timed Release)

Description: TRIAMINIC JUVELETS (Timed Release): Each tablet contains phenylpropanolamine hydrochloride 25 mg, pheniramine maleate 12.5 mg, pyrilamine maleate 12.5 mg.
TRIAMINIC TR TABLETS (Timed Release): Each tablet contains phenylpropanolamine hydrochloride 50 mg, pheniramine maleate 25 mg, pyrilamine maleate 25 mg.
These products combine the nasal decongestant properties of phenylpropanolamine hydrochloride with the antihistaminic activities of pheniramine maleate and pyrilamine maleate.
Phenylpropanolamine hydrochloride, a sympathomimetic drug, is structurally related to ephedrine and amphetamine. Pheniramine maleate is an antihistamine of the alkylamine class while pyrilamine maleate belongs to the ethylenediamine class.

Clinical Pharmacology: Phenylpropanolamine presumably acts on α-adrenergic receptors in the mucosa of the respiratory tract producing vasoconstriction which results in shrinkage of swollen mucous membranes, reduction of tissue hyperemia, edema and nasal congestion, and an increase in nasal airway patency. Its pharmacologic properties are analogous to those of ephedrine. Antihistamines competitively act as H_1 receptor antagonists of histamine. They exhibit anticholinergic (drying) and sedative side effects. There are several classes of antihistamines which vary with respect to potency, dosage and the relative incidence of side effects. Antihistamines inhibit the effects of histamine on capillary permeability and on vascular, bronchial and many other types of smooth muscle. This accounts for the predominant use of antihistamines in hypersensitivity states.

Indications and Usage: For relief from such symptoms as nasal congestion, and postnasal drip associated with colds, allergies, sinusitis and rhinitis. Also for the relief of symptoms associated with allergic rhinitis such as sneezing, rhinorrhea, pruritus and lacrimation.

Contraindications: These formulas are contraindicated in patients exhibiting hypersensitivity to any of the components. Antihistamines are contraindicated in patients receiving monoamine oxidase inhibitors since these agents prolong and intensify the anticholinergic effects of antihistamines (see Drug Interactions). Antihistamines should not be used to treat lower respiratory tract symptoms. Sympathomimetic preparations are contraindicated in patients with severe hypertension, severe coronary artery disease and in patients receiving monoamine oxidase inhibitor therapy due to potentiation of the pressor effects of phenylpropanolamine.

Nursing Mothers: Because of the higher risk of antihistamines for newborns and prematures in particular, antihistamine therapy is contraindicated in nursing mothers.

Warnings: Sympathomimetics should be used with caution in patients with hypertension, hyperthyroidism, diabetes mellitus and cardiovascular disease. Antihistamines should be used with caution in patients with narrow angle glaucoma, stenosing peptic ulcer, pyloroduodenal obstruction, symptomatic prostatic hypertrophy and bladder neck obstruction.
Antihistamines have additive effects with alcohol and other CNS depressants (hypnotics, sedatives, tranquilizers, etc.). Patients should be warned about engaging in activities requiring mental alertness such as driving a car or operating machinery.

Use In The Elderly (approximately 60 years or older): Antihistamines are more likely to cause dizziness, sedation and hypertension in elderly patients. Overdosages of sympathomimetics in this age group may cause hallucinations, convulsions, CNS depression and death in elderly patients.

Precautions:
General: Use with caution in patients with hypertension, hyperthyroidism, diabetes mellitus, cardiovascular disease, bronchial asthma, increased intraocular pressure (see WARNINGS).

Information For Patients: Patients should be informed of the potential for sedation or drowsiness and warned about driving or operating machinery. The concomitant consumption of alcoholic beverages or other sedative drugs should be avoided.

Drug Interactions:
(1) Monoamine oxidase inhibitors: MAO inhibitors prolong and intensify the anticholinergic effects of antihistamines and potentiate the pressor effects of sympathomimetics.
(2) Alcohol and CNS depressants: These agents potentiate the sedative effects of antihistamines.
(3) Certain antihypertensives: Sympathomimetics may reduce the antihypertensive effects of methyldopa, mecamylamine, reserpine and veratrum alkaloids.

Carcinogenesis, Mutagenesis, Impairment Of Fertility: No data are available on the long-term potential for carcinogenicity, mutagenicity or impairment of fertility in animals or humans.

Pregnancy: *Pregnancy Category C*—Animal reproduction studies have not been conducted. Safe use in pregnancy has not been established relative to possible adverse effects on fetal development. Therefore, TRIAMINIC should not be used in pregnant patients unless, in the judgment of the physician, the potential benefits outweigh possible hazards.

Nursing Mothers: See CONTRAINDICATIONS.

Pediatric Use: TRIAMINIC JUVELETS are intended for administration to children 6 to 12 years of age (see DOSAGE AND ADMINISTRATION). It is important to note the variability of response infants and small children exhibit to antihistamines and sympathomimetics. As in adults, the combination of an antihistamine and sympathomimetic can elicit either mild stimulation or mild sedation in children. In the young child, mild stimulation is the response most frequently seen. In infants and children, overdosage of antihistamines may cause hallucinations, convulsions or death.

Adverse Reactions: The most frequent adverse reactions are underlined.
(1) *General:* Urticaria, drug rash, anaphylactic shock, photosensitivity, excessive perspiration, chills, dryness of mouth, nose and throat.
(2) *Cardiovascular System:* Hypotension, headache, palpitations, tachycardia, extrasystoles.
(3) *Hematologic System:* Hemolytic anemia, thrombocytopenia, agranulocytosis.
(4) *Nervous System:* <u>Sedation, sleepiness, dizziness, disturbed coordination</u>, fatigue, confusion, <u>restlessness, excitation, nervousness</u>, tremor, irritability, <u>insomia</u>, euphoria, paresthesias, blurred vision, diplopia, vertigo, tinnitus, acute labyrinthitis, hysteria, neuritis, convulsion, CNS depression, hallucinations.
(5) *GI System:* <u>Epigastric distress</u>, anorexia, nausea, vomiting, diarrhea, constipation.
(6) *GU System:* Urinary frequency, difficult urination, urinary retention, early menses.
(7) *Respiratory System:* Thickening of bronchial secretions, tightness of chest and wheezing, nasal stuffiness.

Overdosage: Overdosage reactions may vary from central nervous system depression to stimulation. Stimulation is particularly likely in children. Atropine-like signs and symptoms: dry mouth; fixed, dilated pupils; flushing; and gastrointestinal symptoms may also occur.
If vomiting has not occurred spontaneously, the conscious patient should be induced to vomit. This is best done by having the patient drink a glass of water or milk after which they should be made to gag. Precautions against aspiration must be taken, especially in infants and children.
If vomiting is unsuccessful gastric lavage is indicated within three hours after ingestion and even later if large amounts of milk or cream were given beforehand. Isotonic and ½ isotonic saline is the lavage solution of choice.
Saline cathartics, such as milk of magnesia, by osmosis draw water into the bowel and therefore, are valuable for their action in rapid dilution of bowel content.
Stimulants should *not* be used. Vasopressors may be used to treat hypotension.

Dosage and Administration: TRIAMINIC JUVELETS (Timed Release): Children 6 to 12 years—1 tablet, swallowed whole, in the morning, midafternoon and before retiring. Adults—2 tablets on same dosage schedule.
TRIAMINIC TR Tablets (Timed Release): Adults and children over 12 years—1 tablet swallowed whole, in the morning, midafternoon and before retiring.

How Supplied: TRIAMINIC JUVELETS (Timed Release) (pink, round, film-coated, imprinted "Dorsey" on one side) in bottles of 50.
TRIAMINIC TR Tablets (Timed Release) (yellow, round, film-coated, imprinted "Dorsey" on one side) in bottles of 100 and 250.

TRIAMINIC® ORAL INFANT DROPS
[trī″ah-min′ic]

Description: TRIAMINIC Oral Infant Drops: Each ml contains phenylpropanolamine hydrochloride 20 mg, pheniramine maleate 10 mg, pyrilamine maleate 10 mg.
This product combines the nasal decongestant properties of phenylpropanolamine hydrochloride with the antihistaminic activities of pheniramine maleate and pyrilamine maleate.
Phenylpropanolamine hydrochloride, a sympathomimetic drug, is structurally related to ephedrine and amphetamine. Pheniramine maleate is an antihistamine of the alkylamine class while pyrilamine maleate belongs to the ethylenediamine class.

Clinical Pharmacology: Phenylpropanolamine presumably acts on α-adrenergic receptors in the mucosa of the respiratory tract producing vasoconstriction which results in shrinkage of swollen mucous membranes, reduction of tissue hyperemia, edema and nasal congestion, and an increase in nasal airway patency. Its pharmacologic properties are analogous to those of ephedrine. Antihistamines competitively act as H_1 receptor antagonists of histamine. They exhibit anticholinergic (drying) and sedative side effects. There are several classes of antihistamines which vary with respect to potency, dosage and the relative incidence of side effects. Antihistamines inhibit the effects of histamine on capillary permeability and on vascular, bronchial and many other types of smooth muscle. This accounts for the predominant use of antihistamines in hypersensitivity states.

Indications and Usage: For relief from such symptoms as nasal congestion, and postnasal drip associated with colds, allergies, sinusitis and rhinitis. Also for the relief of symptoms associated with allergic rhinitis such as sneezing, rhinorrhea, pruritus and lacrimation.

Contraindications: TRIAMINIC Oral Infant Drops are contraindicated in patients exhibiting hypersensitivity to any of the components. Antihistamines are contraindicated in patients receiving monoamine oxidase inhibitors since these agents prolong and intensify the anticholinergic effects of antihistamines (see Drug Interactions). Antihistamines should not be used to treat lower respiratory tract symptoms. Sympathomimetic preparations are contraindicated in patients with severe hypertension, severe coronary artery disease and in patients receiving monoamine oxidase inhibitor therapy due to potentiation of the pressor effects of phenylpropanolamine.

Warnings: Sympathomimetics should be used with caution in patients with hypertension, hyperthyroidism, diabetes mellitus and cardiovascular disease. Antihistamines should be used with caution in patients with narrow angle glaucoma, stenosing peptic ulcer, pyloroduodenal obstruction, symptomatic prostatic hypertrophy and bladder neck obstruction.

Antihistamines have additive effects with other CNS depressants (hypnotics, sedatives, tranquilizers, alcohol, etc.). Warn mothers that drowsiness may occur. When prescribing antihistamine preparations, patients should be cautioned against mechanical activity requiring alertness.

Precautions:

General: Use with caution in patients with hypertension, hyperthyroidism, diabetes mellitus, cardiovascular disease, bronchial asthma, increased intraocular pressure (see WARNINGS).

Information For Patients: Mothers should be informed of the potential for sedation or drowsiness.

Drug Interactions:

(1) Monoamine oxidase inhibitors: MAO inhibitors prolong and intensify the anticholinergic effects of antihistamines and potentiate the pressor effects of sympathomimetics.

(2) Alcohol and CNS depressants: These agents potentiate the sedative effects of antihistamines.

(3) Certain antihypertensives: Sympathomimetics may reduce the antihypertensive effects of methyldopa, mecamylamine, reserpine and veratrum alkaloids.

Carcinogenesis, Mutagenesis, Impairment Of Fertility: No data are available on the long-term potential for carcinogenicity, mutagenicity or impairment of fertility in animals or humans.

Pediatric Use: TRIAMINIC Oral Infant Drops have been formulated to provide safe and effective symptomatic relief for infants and small children. Precise dosage (on a body weight basis) is facilitated through the use of the plastic squeeze bottle with attached dropper tip (see DOSAGE AND ADMINISTRATION). It is important to note the variability of response infants and small children exhibit to antihistamines and sympathomimetics. As in adults, the combination of an antihistamine and sympathomimetic can elicit either mild stimulation or mild sedation in children. In the young child, mild stimulation is the response most frequently seen. In infants and children, overdosage of antihistamines may cause hallucinations, convulsions or death.

Adverse Reactions: The most frequent adverse reactions are underlined.

(1) *General:* Urticaria, drug rash, anaphylactic shock, photosensitivity, excessive perspiration, chills, dryness of mouth, nose, and throat.

(2) *Cardiovascular System:* Hypotension, headache, palpitations, tachycardia, extrasystoles.

(3) *Hematologic System:* Hemolytic anemia, thrombocytopenia, agranulocytosis.

(4) *Nervous System:* Sedation, sleepiness, dizziness, disturbed coordination, fatigue, confusion, restlessness, excitation, nervousness, tremor, irritability, insomnia, euphoria, paresthesias, blurred vision, diplopia, vertigo, tinnitus, acute labyrinthitis, hysteria, neuritis, convulsions, CNS depression, hallucinations.

(5) *GI System:* Epigastric distress, anorexia, nausea, vomiting, diarrhea, constipation.

(6) *GU System:* Urinary frequency, difficult urination, urinary retention.

(7) *Respiratory System:* Thickening of bronchial secretions, tightness of chest and wheezing, nasal stuffiness.

Overdosage: TRIAMINIC product overdosage reactions may vary from central nervous system depression to stimulation. Stimulation is particularly likely in children. Atropine-like signs and symptoms: dry mouth; fixed, dilated pupils; flushing; and gastrointestinal symptoms may also occur.

If vomiting has not occurred spontaneously the conscious patient should be induced to vomit. This is best done by having the patient drink a glass of water or milk after which they should be made to gag. Precautions against aspiration must be taken, especially in infants and children.

If vomiting is unsuccessful gastric lavage is indicated within three hours after ingestion and even later if large amounts of milk or cream were given beforehand. Isotonic and ½ isotonic saline is the lavage solution of choice.

Saline cathartics such as milk of magnesia, by osmosis draw water into the bowel and therefore, are valuable for their action in rapid dilution of bowel content.

Stimulants should *not* be used. Vasopressors may be used to treat hypotension.

Dosage and Administration: TRIAMINIC Oral Infant Drops: 1 drop per 2 pounds of body weight administered orally 4 times daily. The prescribed number of drops may be put directly into child's mouth or on a spoon for administration.

How Supplied: TRIAMINIC Oral Infant Drops in 15 ml plastic squeeze bottles which deliver approximately 24 drops per ml. Store TRIAMINIC Oral Infant Drops at room temperature.

TRIAMINIC–DM® COUGH FORMULA
[trī″ah-mĭn′ĭc]

Description: Each teaspoonful (5 ml) of TRIAMINIC-DM Cough Formula contains: phenylpropanolamine hydrochloride 12.5 mg and dextromethorphan hydrobromide 10 mg in a nonalcoholic vehicle.

Indications: Provides prompt, temporary relief of cough and nasal congestion due to the common cold. The decongestant and antitussive are provided in an antihistamine-free formula.

Contraindications: TRIAMINIC-DM Cough Formula is contraindicated in the presence of hypersensitivity to any of the ingredients. The use of pressor amines such as phenylpropanolamine hydrochloride is contraindicated in those patients taking monoamine oxidase inhibitors.

Precautions: Exercise prescribing caution in patients with persistent or chronic cough such as occurs with smoking, chronic bronchitis, bronchial asthma, or emphysema. Use with caution in patients with hypertension, hyperthyroidism, cardiovascular disease or diabetes mellitus. Use with caution in pregnant and nursing mothers.

Adverse Reactions: Occasional blurred vision, cardiac palpitations, flushing, gastrointestinal upsets, nervousness, dizziness, or sleeplessness may occur.

Dosage and Administration: Adults—2 teaspoonfuls every 4 hours. Children 6–12 years—1 teaspoonful every 4 hours. Children 2–6 years—½ teaspoonful every 4 hours. The suggested dosage for pediatric patients 3 months to under 12 months of age is 1 drop per kilogram of body weight administered every 4 hours. The suggested dosage for patients 12 months to under 24 months of age is 3 drops per kilogram of body weight administered every 4 hours.

How Supplied: TRIAMINIC-DM Cough Formula (dark red) in 4 fl oz and 8 fl oz plastic bottles with tamper-evident band around child-resistant cap.

TRIAMINIC-12® TABLETS
[trī″ah-mĭn′ĭc]

Description: Each TRIAMINIC-12 Tablet contains: phenylpropanolamine hydrochloride 75 mg and chlorpheniramine maleate 12 mg. TRIAMINIC-12 Tablets contain the nasal decongestant phenylpropanolamine and the antihistamine chlorpheniramine, in a formulation providing 12 hours of symptomatic relief.

Indications: For the temporary relief of nasal congestion due to the common cold, hay fever or other upper respiratory allergies and associated with sinusitis. Helps decongest sinus openings, sinus passages; promotes nasal and/or sinus drainage; temporarily restores freer breathing through the nose.

For temporary relief of running nose, sneezing, itching of the nose or throat and itchy and watery eyes as may occur in allergic rhinitis (such as hay fever).

Dosage: Adults and children over 12 years of age—1 tablet swallowed whole every 12 hours. NOTE: The nonactive portion of the tablet that supplies the active ingredients may occasionally appear in the stool as a soft mass.

Warnings: This product is not recommended for use in children under 12 years of age. Use with caution in patients with high blood pressure, heart disease, diabetes, thyroid disease, asthma, glaucoma or difficulty in urination due to enlargement of the prostate gland. Do not exceed the recommended dosage because at higher doses nervousness, dizziness, or sleeplessness may occur. This preparation may cause drowsiness; this preparation may cause excitability, especially in children.

Caution: Patients should be advised to avoid driving a motor vehicle or operating heavy machinery. Patients should also be advised to avoid alcoholic beverages while taking this product. Use with caution in pregnant and nursing mothers.

Drug Interaction Precaution: Use with caution in patients presently taking a prescription antihypertensive or antidepressant drug containing a monoamine oxidase inhibitor.

How Supplied: TRIAMINIC-12 Tablets (orange), imprinted "DORSEY" on one side, "TRIAMINIC 12" on the other, in blister packs of 10 and 20.

TRIAMINICIN® TABLETS
[trī″ah-mĭn′ĭ-sĭn]

(See PDR For Nonprescription Drugs)

TRIAMINICOL® MULTI-SYMPTOM COLD SYRUP
[trī″ah-mĭn′ĭ-call]

Description: Each teaspoonful (5 ml) of TRIAMINICOL Multi-Symptom Cold Syrup contains: phenylpropanolamine hydrochloride 12.5 mg, chlorpheniramine maleate 2 mg, and dextromethorphan hydrobromide 10 mg, in a palatable nonalcoholic vehicle.

Indications: For the temporary relief of nasal congestion, sneezing and itchy watery eyes that may occur in hay fever or other upper respiratory allergies, the common cold and sinusitis. For the temporary relief of cough due to minor throat and bronchial irritation as may occur with the common cold or with inhaled irritants.

Contraindications: TRIAMINICOL Multi-Symptom Cold Syrup is contraindicated in the presence of hypersensitivity to any of the ingredients. The use of pressor amines such as phenylpropanolamine hydrochloride is contraindicated in those patients taking monoamine oxidase inhibitors.

Precautions: Caution should be observed in operating a motor vehicle or performing poten-

Continued on next page

Dorsey Labs.—Cont.

tially hazardous tasks requiring mental alertness. Alcoholic beverages and other CNS depressants may potentiate the sedative effects of antihistamines. Exercise prescribing caution in patients with persistent or chronic cough such as occurs with smoking, chronic bronchitis, bronchial asthma or emphysema. Caution should be observed in the presence of hypertension, hyperthyroidism, cardiovascular disease or diabetes mellitus. Because of anticholinergic action of antihistamines, they should be administered with caution to patients with bronchial asthma, narrow angle glaucoma, stenosing peptic ulcer, pyloroduodenal obstruction, prostatic hypertrophy or other bladder neck obstruction. Use with caution in pregnant and nursing mothers.

Adverse Reactions: Blurred vision, palpitations, flushing, gastrointestinal upsets, nervousness, dizziness, or sleeplessness may occur. May cause excitability especially in children. May cause marked drowsiness.

Dosage and Administration: Adults—2 teaspoonfuls every 4 hours. Children 6–12 years—1 teaspoonful every 4 hours. Children 2–6 years—½ teaspoonful every 4 to 6 hours. The suggested dosage for pediatric patients 3 months to under 12 months of age is 1 drop per kilogram of body weight administered every 4 hours. The suggested dosage for patients 12 months to under 24 months of age is 3 drops per kilogram of body weight administered every 4 hours.

How Supplied: TRIAMINICOL Multi-Symptom Cold Syrup (red), in 4 fl oz and 8 fl oz plastic bottles with tamper-evident band around child-resistant cap.

TRIAMINICOL® MULTI-SYMPTOM COLD TABLETS
[trī″ah-mǐn′ĭ-call]

Description: Each TRIAMINICOL Multi-Symptom Cold Tablet contains: phenylpropanolamine hydrochloride 12.5 mg, chlorpheniramine maleate 2 mg, and dextromethorphan hydrobromide 10 mg.

Indications: For the temporary relief of nasal congestion, sneezing and itchy watery eyes that may occur in hay fever or other upper respiratory allergies, the common cold and sinusitis. For the temporary relief of cough due to minor throat and bronchial irritation as may occur with the common cold or with inhaled irritants.

Contraindications: TRIAMINICOL Multi-Symptom Cold Tablets are contraindicated in the presence of hypersensitivity to any of the ingredients. The use of pressor amines such as phenylpropanolamine hydrochloride is contraindicated in those patients taking monoamine oxidase inhibitors for antihypertensive or antidepressant indications.

Precautions: Caution should be observed in operating a motor vehicle or performing potentially hazardous tasks requiring mental alertness. Alcoholic beverages and other CNS depressants may potentiate the sedative effects of antihistamines. Exercise prescribing caution in patients with chronic bronchitis, bronchial asthma or emphysema. Caution should be observed in the presence of hypertension, hyperthyroidism, cardiovascular disease or diabetes mellitus. Because of anticholinergic action of antihistamines, they should be administered with caution to patients with bronchial asthma, narrow angle glaucoma, stenosing peptic ulcer, pyloroduodenal obstruction, prostatic hypertrophy or other bladder neck obstruction. Use with caution in pregnant and nursing mothers.

Adverse Reactions: Blurred vision, palpitations, flushing, gastrointestinal upsets, nervousness, dizziness, or sleeplessness may occur. May cause excitability especially in children. May cause marked drowsiness.

Dosage and Administration: Adults—2 tablets every 4 hours. Children 6–12 years—1 tablet every 4 hours.

How Supplied: TRIAMINICOL Multi-Symptom Cold Tablets (cherry pink), imprinted "DORSEY" on one side, "TRIAMINICOL" on the other, in blister packs of 24 and 48.

TUSSAGESIC®
TABLETS AND SUSPENSION
[tuss″ah-gee′zĭk]

(See PDR For Nonprescription Drugs)

URSINUS® INLAY-TABS®
[yer-sī′nus]

(See PDR For Nonprescription Drugs)

Drug Industries Co., Inc.
3237 HILTON ROAD
FERNDALE, MI 48220

Products Available

Al-Vite
BC-Vite
Bilax
C-Caps 500
Calfer-Vite
Day-Vite
Di-Sosul
Di-Sosul Forte
E-Plus
Hemo-Vite
Hemo-Vite Liquid
Sinovan Timed
Trilax
Vanodonnal Timed
Vicef

AL-VITE ℞
[ol′vīt]
(high potency vitamin formula with intrinsic factor + Vitamin D$_3$)

Composition: Each capsule shaped tablet contains: Vitamin A Palmitate, 10,000 USP Units, Vitamin D$_3$ (activ. 7-Dehydrocholestrol), 400 USP Units, Vitamin E (from D-Alpha Tocopheryl Acetate Concentrate), 25 int. Units, Vitamin C (Ascorbic Acid), 200 mg., Vitamin B$_1$ (Thiamine Mononitrate), 20 mg., Vitamin B$_2$ (Riboflavin), 10 mg., Vitamin B$_6$ (Pyridoxine Hydrochloride), 6 mg., Calcium Pantothenate, 20 mg., Niacinamide, 100 mg., Vitamin B$_{12}$ with Intrinsic Factor Concentrate, ½ N.F. Unit (oral).

Action and Uses: Provides Vitamins A, D, C and B Complex factors in therapeutic amounts. For use in multiple vitamin deficiencies.

Administration and Dosage: One or two tablets daily or as directed by the physician.

Side Effects: None known when taken as directed.

Caution: This preparation is not a reliable substitute for parenterally administered cyanocobalamin (vitamin B$_{12}$) in the management of pernicious anemia. Periodic examinations and laboratory studies of pernicious anemia patients are essential.

Contraindications: Idiosyncrasy to any component.

How Supplied: Bottles of 100 and 500 light orange capsule shaped tablets.

BILAX CAPSULES™ ℞
[bī′laks]

Composition: Each Bilax Capsule contains:
Dehydrocholic Acid .... 50 mg.
Dioctyl Sodium Sulfosuccinate .... 100 mg.

Action and Uses: The actions of Bilax are the result of the combination of complementary activities of its ingredients. Dioctyl Sodium Sulfosuccinate effects the surface tension and increases the water content of the stool, making it softer and therefore, easier to pass. The softening, combined with the laxative effect of Dehydrocholic Acid, alleviates symptoms of constipation.

Indications: A mild laxative and fecal softener designed as an aid in the treatment of functional constipation, particularly in the elderly.

Contraindications: Biliary tract obstruction, acute hepatitis, or sensitivity to any of its ingredients.

Precautions: Patients should be examined periodically to prevent fluid and electrolyte deficiencies due to excessive laxative effects or inadequate intake.

Administration and Dosage: One or two capsules three times daily with meals. This dosage should be reduced as the condition is relieved.

How Supplied: Bottles of 100.
Bottles of 500.

NDC 261-0157-01

HEMO-VITE ℞
[hē′mō-vīt]
(hematinic with vitamins and intrinsic factor)

Composition: Each tablet contains: Ferrous Fumarate, 240.0 mg., Copper Sulfate, 1.0 mg., Vitamin C (ascorbic acid) 150.0 mg., Vitamin B$_1$ (Thiamine Hydrochloride) 5.0 mg., Vitamin B$_2$ (Riboflavin), 5.0 mg., Vitamin B$_6$ (Pyridoxine Hydrochloride), 1.0 mg., Calcium Pantothenate, 10.0 mg., Niacinamide, 50.0 mg., Folic Acid, .2 mg., Vitamin B$_{12}$ (Crystalline with Intrinsic Factor Concentrate), ½ N.F. Unit (oral).

Action and Uses: For the treatment and prevention of iron deficiency anemias. Contains the well tolerated effective fumarate salt of iron.

Administration and Dosage: One or two tablets daily after meals or as directed by the physician.

Precautions: If any symptoms of intolerance appear, the medication should be discontinued. Prolonged administration requires closer medical supervision. Folic acid may obscure the symptoms of pernicious anemia while neurological destruction is progressive. Patients with pernicious anemia should be treated with parenteral B$_{12}$
HEMO-VITE should not be used in cases of serious folic acid deficiency where therapeutic amounts of folic acid are needed.

Side Effects: None known when used as directed.

Contraindications: Idiosyncrasy to any component.

How Supplied: Bottles of 100 and 500 black capsule shaped tablets.
Also available in Hemo-Vite Liquid—pint bottles.

HEMO–VITE LIQUID ℞
[hē′mō′vīt]

Composition: Each 5 ml., (one teaspoonful) contains:
Vitamin B-12, crystalline .... 8.34 mcg.
Vitamin B-6 (Pyridoxine Hydrochloride) 2.0 mg.
Ferric Pyrophosphate, soluble .... 100.00 mg.
Folic Acid .... 0.25 mg.
Niacinamide .... 13.3 mg.
In a base of Sorbitol Solution

Important: Dispense only in amber bottle. This product is light sensitive.

Store in a cool place but avoid freezing.

Indications: For the prevention of Vitamin B-12, Vitamin B-6 and iron deficiencies.

Contraindications: Hemovite should not be used in patients with pernicious anemia. In the recommended dosage Hemovite supplies 1.5 mg. of folic acid daily. The use of folic acid in patients who have or may develop pernicious anemia involves a serious hazard of permitting progressive degeneration of the spinal cord while treating the anemia characteristic of the disease. Furthermore the absorption of the Vitamin B-12 in Hemovite is not enhanced in patients with pernicious anemia. Parenterally administered cyanocobalamine (Vitamin B-12) is the therapy of choice in pernicious anemia and should be employed in patients receiving folic acid unless pernicious anemia has been ruled out.

Dosage and Administration: In both adults and older children, one teaspoonful (5 ml.) three times daily or one tablespoonful (15 ml.) once a day if preferred. Children up to 2 years of age may be given one teaspoonful (5 ml.) twice daily.
NOTE: In some infants large doses of Hemovite may produce the diarrhea often associated with concentrated sugars.
Important: If particularly rapid B-12 response is desired, an injection of 100 mcg. B-12 intramuscularly can be given initially. Oral Hemovite on a daily basis will then maintain the levels quickly achieved with B-12 Injection.
Caution: FEDERAL LAW PROHIBITS DISPENSING WITHOUT A PRESCRIPTION.
Warning: Like other iron preparations, this preparation should be stored out of the reach of children to guard against accidental iron poisoning.
How Supplied: Pint bottles.
NDC-0261-0076-01

SINOVAN TIMED™ ℞
[si′nō′van]

Composition: Each black and clear timed capsule contains 8 mg. Chlorpheniramine Maleate, 20 mg. of Phenylephrine Hydrochloride, and 2.5 mg. of Methscopolamine Nitrate in a special base that provides a prolonged therapeutic effect of from about 10 to 12 hours.
Action and Uses: Provides temporary relief of the distressing symptoms accompanying the common cold, hay fever, and similar allergic conditions.
Contraindications: Pyloric obstruction, prostatic hypertrophy, intolerance to anticholinergic or antisecretory drugs, glaucoma, hepatitis, asthma, and toxemia of pregnancy.
Administration and Dosage: One capsule in the morning and at bedtime.
How Supplied: In bottles of 100 and 1000.

TRILAX™ ℞
[trī′laks]
(laxative, fecal softener, choleretic)

Composition: Each blue and white capsule contains:
Dioctyl Sodium Sulfosuccinate .... 200 mg.
Yellow Phenolphthalein .... 30 mg.
Dehydrocholic Acid .... 20 mg.
Action and Uses: Provides softening of the feces, homogenization, and laxative action without the discomfort of bowel distention, pain, cramping, or interference of vitamin absorption. For use in geriatric, obstetric, cardiac and surgical patients, and in those with hepatic or biliary disease or other conditions causing biliary stasis without complete mechanical obstruction of the common duct where increase in volume of fluid bile is desired.
Contraindications: TRILAX is contraindicated in patients with biliary tract obstruction and severe acute hepatitis.
Administration and Dosage: One or two capsules at bedtime for 2 or 3 days. Dosage may then be adjusted to meet individual needs.
How Supplied: Bottles of 100.
Bottles of 500.
NDC 261-0103-01

Products are cross-indexed
by product classifications
in the
BLUE SECTION

Du Pont Pharmaceuticals
E.I. duPont de Nemours & Co. (Inc.)
WILMINGTON, DE 19898

Du Pont Pharmaceuticals Caribe Inc.
Subsidiary of E.I. duPont de Nemours & Co. (Inc.)
P.O. BOX 12
MANATI, PUERTO RICO 00701

Du Pont Pharmaceuticals, Inc.
Subsidiary of E.I. duPont de Nemours & Co. (Inc.)
P.O. BOX 363
MANATI, PUERTO RICO 00701

Products indicated by a dagger are products of Du Pont Pharmaceuticals Caribe, Inc.

PRODUCT IDENTIFICATION
The DuPont logo and product name and strength (where applicable) is imprinted on all DuPont tablets and capsules as listed below.

PRODUCT

COUMADIN® (crystalline warfarin sodium) Tablets
  2 mg
  2½ mg
  5 mg
  7½ mg
  10 mg
ENDECON® (decongestant, analgesic, antipyretic) Tablets
HYCODAN® (hydrocodone bitartrate/homatropine methylbromide combination) Tablets ⓒ
HYCOMINE® COMPOUND (hydrocodone bitartrate/chlorpheniramine maleate/phenylephrine hydrochloride/APAP/caffeine) Tablets ⓒ
MOBAN® (molindone hydrochloride) Tablets
  5 mg
  10 mg
  25 mg
  50 mg
  100 mg
†**PERCOCET®** (oxycodone/APAP combination) Tablets ⓒ
†**PERCODAN®** (oxycodone/aspirin combination) Tablets ⓒ
†**PERCODAN®-DEMI** (oxycodone/aspirin combination) Tablets ⓒ
REMSED® (promethazine hydrochloride) Tablets
  50 mg
SYMMETREL® (amantadine hydrochloride) Capsules
  100 mg
VALPIN® 50 (anisotropine methylbromide) Tablets
  50 mg
VALPIN® 50-PB (anisotropine methylbromide with phenobarbital) Tablets

COUMADIN® ℞
[ku′ma-din]
(crystalline warfarin sodium, U.S.P.)*

Description: COUMADIN (crystalline warfarin sodium), a prothrombinopenic anticoagulant, is chemically crystalline sodium warfarin isopropanol clathrate. The crystallization of warfarin sodium virtually eliminates trace impurities present in amorphous warfarin sodium, thus achieving a crystalline product of the highest purity. Warfarin* is the coined generic name for 3-(α-Acetonylbenzyl)-4-hydroxycoumarin. On a dose-for-dose basis, COUMADIN (crystalline warfarin sodium) is therapeutically equivalent to amorphous warfarin sodium.
Actions: COUMADIN and other coumarin anticoagulants act by depressing synthesis in the liver of several factors which are known to be active in the coagulation mechanisms in a variety of diseases characterized by thromboembolic phenomena. The resultant **in vivo** effect is a sequential depression of Factors VII, IX, X and II. The degree of depression is dependent upon the dosage administered. Anticoagulants have no direct effect on an established thrombus, nor do they reverse ischemic tissue damage. However, once a thrombosis has occurred, anticoagulant treatment aims to prevent further extension of the formed clot and prevents secondary thromboembolic complications which may result in serious and possible fatal sequelae.
After oral administration, absorption is essentially complete, and maximal plasma concentrations are reached in 1 to 9 hours. Approximately 97% is bound to albumin within the plasma. COUMADIN usually induces hypoprothrombinemia in 36 to 72 hours, and its duration of action may persist for 4 to 5 days, thus producing a smooth, long lasting response curve. Little is known of the metabolic pathways involved in the biotransformation of oral anticoagulants in man. However, their metabolites appear to be eliminated principally in the urine.
Indications: COUMADIN is indicated for the prophylaxis and treatment of venous thrombosis and its extension, the treatment of atrial fibrillation with embolization, the prophylaxis and treatment of pulmonary embolism, and as an adjunct in the treatment of coronary occulsion.
Contraindications: Anticoagulation is contraindicated in any localized or general physical condition or personal circumstance in which the hazard of hemorrhage might be greater than its potential clinical benefits, such as:
Pregnancy—COUMADIN is contraindicated in pregnancy because the drug passes through the placental barrier and may cause fatal hemorrhage to the fetus in utero. Furthermore, there have been reports of birth malformations in children born to mothers who have been treated with warfarin during pregnancy. Women of childbearing potential who are candidates for anticoagulant therapy should be carefully evaluated and the indications critically reviewed with the patient. If the patient becomes pregnant while taking this drug, she should be apprised of the potential risks to the fetus, and the possibility of termination of the pregnancy should be discussed in light of those risks.
Hemorrhagic tendencies or blood dyscrasias.
Recent or contemplated surgery of: (1) central nervous system; 2) eye; (3) traumatic surgery resulting in large open surfaces.
Bleeding tendencies associated with active ulceration or overt bleeding of: (1) gastrointestinal, genitourinary or respiratory tracts; (2) cerebrovascular hemorrhage; (3) aneurysms—cerebral, dissecting aorta; (4) pericarditis and pericardial effusions; (5) subacute bacterial endocarditis.
Threatened abortion, eclampsia and preeclampsia.
Inadequate laboratory facilities or unsuper- vised senility, alcoholism, psychosis; or lack of patient cooperation.
Spinal puncture and other diagnostic or therapeutic procedures with potential for uncontrollable bleeding.
Miscellaneous: major regional, lumbar block anesthesia and malignant hypertension.
Warnings: Warfarin sodium is a potent drug with a half-life of 2½ days; therefore its effects may become more pronounced as daily maintenance doses overlap. It cannot be emphasized too strongly that treatment of each patient is a highly individualized matter. Dosage should be controlled by periodic determinations of prothrombin time or other suitable coagulation tests. Determinations of

Continued on next page

DuPont—Cont.

whole blood clotting and bleeding times are not effective measures for control of therapy. Heparin prolongs the one-stage prothrombin time. Therefore, to obtain a valid prothrombin time when heparin and COUMADIN (crystalline warfarin sodium) are given together, a period of at least 5 hours should elapse after the last intravenous dose and 24 hours after the last subcutaneous dose of heparin, before blood is drawn.

Caution should be observed when warfarin sodium is administered in any situation or physical condition where added risk of hemorrhage is present. Administration of anticoagulants in the following conditions will be based upon clinical judgment in which the risks of anticoagulant therapy are weighed against the risk of thrombosis or embolization in untreated cases. The following may be associated with these increased risks:

Lactation—coumarins may pass into the milk of mothers and cause a prothrombinopenic state in the nursing infant.
Severe to moderate hepatic or renal insufficiency.
Infectious diseases or disturbances of intestinal flora—sprue, antibiotic therapy.
Trauma which may result in internal bleeding.
Surgery or trauma resulting in large exposed raw surfaces.
Indwelling catheters.
Severe to moderate hypertension.
Miscellaneous: polycythemia vera, vasculitis, severe diabetes, severe allergic and anaphylactic disorders.

Patients with congestive heart failure may become more sensitive to COUMADIN, thereby requiring more frequent laboratory monitoring, and reduced doses of COUMADIN.

Concurrent use of anticoagulants with streptokinase or urokinase is not recommended and may be hazardous. (Please note recommendations accompanying these preparations.)

Abrupt cessation of anticoagulant therapy is not generally recommended; taper dose gradually over three to four weeks.

Precautions: Periodic determination of prothrombin time or other suitable coagulation test is essential.

Numerous factors, alone or in combination, including travel, changes in diet, environment, physical state and medication may influence response of the patient to anticoagulants. It is generally good practice to monitor the patient's response with additional prothrombin time determinations in the period immediately after discharge from the hospital, and whenever other medications are initiated, discontinued or taken haphazardly. The following factors are listed for your reference; however, other factors may also affect the prothrombin response.

The following factors, alone or in combination, may be responsible for increased prothrombin time response:

ENDOGENOUS FACTORS: Carcinoma; collagen disease; congestive heart failure; diarrhea; elevated temperature; hepatic disorders—infectious hepatitis, hyperthyroidism; jaundice; poor nutritional state; vitamin K deficiency—steatorrhea.

EXOGENOUS FACTORS: Alcohol†; allopurinol; aminosalicylic acid; anabolic steroids; antibiotics; bromelains; chloral hydrate†; chlorpropamide; chymotrypsin; cimetidine; cinchophen; clofibrate; COUMADIN overdosage; dextran; dextrothyroxine; diazoxide; dietary deficiencies; diuretics†; disulfiram; drugs affecting blood elements; ethacrynic acid; fenoprofen; glucagon; hepatotoxic drugs; ibuprofen; indomethacin; inhalation anesthetics; mefenamic acid; methyldopa; methylphenidate; metronidazole; monoamine oxidase inhibitors; nalidixic acid: naproxen; oxolinic acid; oxyphenbutazone; pyrazolones; phenylbutazone; phenyramidol; phenytoin; prolonged hot weather; prolonged narcotics; quinidine; quinine; salicylates; sulfinpyrazone; sulfonamides, long acting; sulindac; thyroid drugs; tolbutamide; triclofos sodium; trimethoprim/sulfamethoxazole; unreliable prothrombin time determinations.
†Increased and decreased prothrombin time responses have been reported.

The following factors, alone or in combination, may be responsible for decreased prothrombin time response:

ENDOGENOUS FACTORS: Edema; hereditary resistance to coumarin therapy; hyperlipemia; hypothyroidism.

EXOGENOUS FACTORS: Adrenocortical steroids; alcohol†; antacids; antihistamines; barbiturates; carbamazepine; chloral hydrate†; chlordiazepoxide; cholestyramine; COUMADIN underdosage; diet high in vitamin K; diuretics†; ethchorvynol; glutethimide; griseofulvin; haloperidol; meprobamate; oral contraceptives; paraldehyde; primidone; rifampin; unreliable prothrombin time determinations; vitamin C.
† Increased and decreased prothrombin time responses have been reported.

A patient may be exposed to a combination of the above factors, some of which may increase and some decrease his sensitivity to COUMADIN (crystalline warfarin sodium). Because the net effect on his prothrombin time response may be unpredictable under these circumstances, more frequent laboratory monitoring is advisable.

Drugs not yet shown to interact or not to interact with coumarins are best regarded with suspicion, and when their administration is started or stopped, the prothrombin time should be determined more often than usual.

Coumarins also affect the action of other drugs. Hypoglycemic agents (chlorpropamide and tolbutamide) and anticonvulsants (phenytoin and phenobarbital) may accumulate in the body as a result of interference with either their metabolism or excretion.

Adverse Reactions: Potential side effects of COUMADIN (crystalline warfarin sodium) include:

1. Minor or major hemorrhage from any tissue or organ—which is an extension of the physiologic activity of prothrombinopenia. The signs and symptoms will vary according to the location and degree or extent of the bleeding. Therefore the possibility of hemorrhage should be considered in evaluating the condition of any anticoagulated patient with complaints which do not indicate an obvious diagnosis. Bleeding during anticoagulant therapy does not always correlate with prothrombin activity. (See TREATMENT FOR OVERDOSAGE.)
Bleeding which occurs when the prothrombin time is within the therapeutic range warrants diagnostic investigation since it may unmask a previously unsuspected lesion, e.g., tumor, ulcer etc.

2. Side effects other than hemorrhage are infrequent and consist of alopecia, urticaria, dermatitis, fever, nausea, diarrhea, abdominal cramping, a syndrome called "purple toes," hypersensitivity reactions and a reaction consisting of hemorrhagic infarction and necrosis of the skin.

3. Priapism has been associated with anticoagulant administration, however, a causal relationship has not been established.

Dosage and Laboratory Control: The aim of anticoagulant therapy is to impede the coagulation or clotting mechanism to such an extent that thrombosis will not occur, but at the same time avoiding such extensive impairment as might produce spontaneous bleeding. Effective therapeutic levels with minimal complications can best be achieved in cooperative and well-instructed patients, who keep the doctor informed of their status between visits. COUMADIN patient aids are available to physicians on request.

The administration and dosage of COUMADIN must be individualized for each patient according to the particular patient's sensitivity to the drug as indicated by the prothrombin time. The prothrombin time reflects the depression of vitamin K dependent Factors VII, X and II. These factors, in addition to Factor IX, are affected by coumarin anticoagulants. There are several modifications of the Quick one-stage prothrombin time and the physician should become familiar with the specific method used in his laboratory.

Administration of COUMADIN should be gauged according to prothrombin time determinations by a suitable method. The blood prothrombin time should usually be determined daily after the administration of the initial dose until prothrombin time results stabilize in the therapeutic range. Intervals between subsequent prothrombin time determinations should be based upon the physician's judgment of the patient's reliability and response to warfarin in order to maintain the individual within the therapeutic range. Acceptable intervals for prothrombin time determinations have usually fallen within the range of one to four weeks. Satisfactory levels for maintenance of therapeutic anticoagulation are $1\frac{1}{2}$ to $2\frac{1}{2}$ times the normal prothrombin time (e.g. 18 to 30 seconds, with a control of 12 seconds).

Induction—Induction may be initiated with 10 to 15 mg daily and thereafter (usually 2 or 3 days) adjusted according to prothrombin time response. The basis for this no-loading dose regimen is that the depression of Factors II, IX, and X is not accelerated by the administration of a loading dose. Avoidance of a large priming dose may minimize the possibility of excessive increases in prothrombin time.

Alternatively, 40 to 60 mg for average adult or 20 to 30 mg for elderly and/or debilitated patients for one dose only administered orally, intravenously, or intramuscularly.

Maintenance—Most patients are satisfactorily maintained at a dose of 2 to 10 mg daily. Flexibility of dosage is provided by breaking scored tablets in half. The individual dose and interval should be gauged by the patient's prothrombin response.

Duration of therapy—The duration of therapy in each patient should be individualized. In general, anticoagulant therapy should be continued until the danger of thrombosis and embolism has passed.

Treatment during dentistry and surgery—The management of patients who undergo dental and surgical procedures requires close liaison between attending physicians, surgeons and dentists. Interruption of anticoagulant therapy may precipitate thromboembolism, and conversely, if anticoagulants are maintained at full doses, some patients may hemorrhage excessively. If it is elected to administer anticoagulants prior to, during, or immediately following dental or surgical procedures, it is recommended that the dosage of COUMADIN (crystalline warfarin sodium) be adjusted to maintain the prothrombin time at approximately $1\frac{1}{2}$ to $2\frac{1}{2}$ times the control level. The operative site should be sufficiently limited to permit the effective use of local procedures for hemostasis including absorbable hemostatic agents, sutures, and pressure dressings if necessary. Under these conditions dental and surgical procedures may be performed without undue risk of hemorrhage.

COUMADIN with Heparin—Since a delay intervenes between the administration of the initial dose and the therapeutic prolongation of prothrombin time, it may be advisable in emergency situations to administer sodium heparin initially along with COUMADIN. The initial dose of heparin and injectable COUMADIN may be administered together in the same syringe.

It should be noted that heparin may affect the prothrombin time, and therefore, when patients are receiving both heparin and COUMADIN, the blood sample for prothrombin time determination should be drawn just prior to the next heparin dosage, at least 5 hours after the last intravenous injection or 24 hours after the last subcutaneous injection.

Treatment For Overdosage: Excessive prothrombinopenia, with or without bleeding, is readily controlled by discontinuing COUMADIN (crystalline warfarin sodium), and if necessary, the oral or parenteral administration of vitamin K_1. The appearance of microscopic hematuria, excessive menstrual bleeding, melena, petechiae or oozing from nicks made while shaving are early manifestations of hypoprothrombinemia beyond a safe and satisfactory level.

for possible revisions — Product Information

In excessive prothrombinopenia with mild or no bleeding, omission of one or more doses of COUMADIN may suffice; and if necessary, small doses of vitamin K_1 orally, 2.5 to 10 mg will usually correct the problem.

If minor bleeding persists, or progresses to frank bleeding, vitamin K_1 in doses of 5 to 25 mg may be given parenterally. (Please note recommendations accompanying vitamin K preparations prior to use.)

Fresh whole blood transfusions should be considered in cases of severe bleeding or prothrombinopenic states unresponsive to vitamin K_1.

Resumption of COUMADIN administration reverses the effect of vitamin K_1, and a therapeutic hypoprothrombinemia level can again be obtained.

Supplied: Tablets: COUMADIN (crystalline warfarin sodium, USP). For oral use, single scored, imprinted numerically in bottles with potencies and colors as follows:

[See table above].

Also available in Military Depot:
2 mg.   NSN 6505-00-982-4230
5 mg.   NSN 6505-00-982-4229

In VA Depot:
2 mg.   NSN 6505-00-982-4230A
5 mg.   NSN 6505-00-982-4229B

Also available in Hospital Unit-Dose blister package of 100:
2 mg   NDC 0056-0170-75
2½ mg   NDC 0056-0171-75
5 mg   NDC 0056-0172-75
7½   NDC 0056-0173-75
10 mg   NDC 0056-0174-75

Also available in Military Depot:
5 mg   NSN 6505-00-149-0317

In VA Depot:
5 mg   NSN 6505-00-149-0317A

Injection: Available as single injection units of amorphous warfarin sodium lyophilized for intravenous or intramuscular use in a box of 6 units (NDC 0056-0330-06) for use immediately after reconstitution.

50 mg: Unit consists of 1 vial, 50 mg; sodium chloride, 10 mg; thimerosal, 0.2 mg. pH is adjusted with sodium hydroxide, accompanied by a 2 ml ampul Sterile Water for Injection.

Sterile Water for Injection contains no antimicrobial or other substance, and it is not suitable for intravascular injection without first having been made approximately isotonic by the addition of a suitable solute. Use only for reconstitution of the lyophilized product.

---

* Present as crystalline sodium warfarin isopropanol clathrate.

Injection manufactured by Lypho-Med, Inc., Chicago, Illinois 60651 for Du Pont Pharmaceuticals. COUMADIN® is a registered trademark of E.I. duPont de Nemours & Co. (Inc.)
6136-3
Shown in Product Identification Section, page 410

HYCODAN®
[hī-kō-dan]
Tablets and Syrup

Description: Each HYCODAN® Tablet or teaspoonful (5 ml) contains:

	COUMADIN		
	100's		1000's
2 mg lavender	NDC 0056-0170-70		NDC 0056-0170-90
2½ mg orange	NDC 0056-0171-70		NDC 0056-0171-90
5 mg peach	NDC 0056-0172-70		NDC 0056-0172-90
7½ mg yellow	NDC 0056-0173-70		
10 mg white	NDC 0056-0174-70		

Hydrocodone bitartrate .... 5 mg
  WARNING: May be habit forming
Homatropine methylbromide .... 1.5 mg
Hydrocodone is 7,8-dihydrocodeinone, a derivative of codeine.

Actions: Hydrocodone is a centrally acting narcotic antitussive providing cough relief for up to 6 hours.

Indications: Based on a review of this drug by the National Academy of Sciences-National Research Council and/or other information, FDA has classified HYCODAN® Tablets and Syrup as follows:
"Probably" effective: for the symptomatic relief of cough.
Final classification of this "probably" effective indication requires further investigation.

Contraindications: HYCODAN® should not be used in patients with glaucoma or hypersensitivity to hydrocodone or homatropine methylbromide.

Warnings: HYCODAN® should be pre-scribed and administered with the same degree of caution appropriate for the use of other oral narcotic-containing medications since it can produce drug dependence and, therefore, has the potential for abuse. Patients should be warned not to drive a car or operate machinery if they become drowsy or show impaired mental and/or physical abilities while taking HYCODAN®. Patients receiving narcotic analgesics, phenothiazines, other tranquilizers, sedative-hypnotics or other central nervous system depressants (including alcohol) concomitantly with HYCODAN® may exhibit an additive central nervous system depression. When such combined therapy is contemplated, the dose of one or both agents should be reduced.

Precautions: Before prescribing medication to suppress or modify cough, it is important to ascertain that the underlying cause of cough is identified, that modification of cough does not increase the risk of clinical or physiologic complications, and that appropriate therapy for the primary disease is provided.

Adverse Reactions: Adverse reactions when they occur include sedation, nausea, vomiting and constipation.

Dosage and Administration: HYCODAN® should be taken after meals and at bedtime, with food, not less than 4 hours apart. Treatment should be started with the suggested initial dose and subsequent doses adjusted if required.
[See table below].

Drug Interactions: The central nervous system depressant effects of HYCODAN® may be additive with that of other central nervous system depressants. See WARNINGS.

Management of Overdosage:
Signs and Symptoms: Serious overdose with HYCODAN® may be characterized by respiratory depression, extreme somnolence progressing to stupor or coma, skeletal muscle flaccidity, cold and clammy skin, and sometimes bradycardia and hypotension. In severe overdosage, apnea, circulatory collapse, cardiac arrest and death may occur. The ingestion of very large amounts of HYCODAN® may, in addition, result in acute homatropine intoxication.

Treatment: Primary attention should be given to the reestablishment of adequate respiratory exchange through provision of a patent airway and the institution of assisted or controlled ventilation. The narcotic antagonist naloxone hydrochloride (NARCAN®) is a specific antidote against respiratory depression which may result from overdosage or unusual sensitivity to narcotics including hydrocodone. Therefore, an appropriate dose of naloxone hydrochloride should be administered, (usual initial adult dose: 0.4 mg) preferably by the intravenous route and simultaneously with efforts at respiratory resuscitation. Since the duration of action of hydrocodone may exceed that of the antagonist, the patient should be kept under continued surveillance and repeated doses of the antagonist should be administered as needed to maintain adequate respiration. Oxygen, intravenous fluids, vasopressors and other supportive measures should be employed as indicated, including treatment for anticholinergic drug intoxication. Gastric emptying may be useful in removing unabsorbed drug. Activated charcoal may be of benefit.

How Supplied:
As white, scored tablets available in
  Bottles of 100   NDC 0056-0042-70
  Bottles of 500   NDC 0056-0042-85
As a red-colored, wild cherry flavored syrup available in
  Bottles of one pint   NDC 0056-0234-16
  Bottles of one gallon NDC 0056-0234-82
Oral prescription where permitted by State law.
HYCODAN® is a registered trademark of E.I. du Pont de Nemours & Co. (Inc.) NARCAN® is a registered U.S. trademark of Du Pont Pharmaceuticals, Inc.
6014-12
Shown in Product Identification Section, page 410

HYCOMINE®
[hī-ko-mēn]
Pediatric Syrup

HYCOMINE®
Syrup

Description: Hycomine® contains hydrocodone (dihydrocodeinone) bitartrate, a semi-synthetic centrally-acting narcotic antitussive and phenylpropanolamine hydrochloride, a sympathomimetic amine decongestant for oral administration.

	Hycomine® Pediatric Syrup	Hycomine® Syrup
Each teaspoonful (5 ml) contains:		
Hydrocodone bitartrate	2.5 mg	5 mg
Warning: May be habit forming		
Phenylpropanolamine hydrochloride	12.5 mg	25 mg.

Clinical Pharmacology: Clinical trials have proven hydrocodone bitartrate to be an effective antitussive agent which is pharmacologically 2 to 8 times as potent as codeine. At equi-effective doses, its sedative action is greater than codeine. The precise mechanism of action of hydrocodone and other opiates is not known, however, hydrocodone is believed to act by directly depressing the

Continued on next page

HYCODAN® DOSAGE AND ADMINISTRATION
Usual Dosage

	TABLETS		SYRUP teaspoonful (5 ml)	
	Initial dose	Maximum single dose	Initial dose	Maximum single dose
Adults	1	3	1 tsp.	3 tsps.
Children				
over 12 years	1	2	1 tsp.	2 tsps.
2 to 12 years	½	1	½ tsp.	1 tsp.
under 2 years	¼	½	¼ tsp.	½ tsp.

DuPont—Cont.

cough center. In excessive doses, hydrocodone, like other opium derivatives, will depress respiration. The effects of hydrocodone in therapeutic doses on the cardiovascular system is insignificant. The constipation effects of hydrocodone are much weaker than that of morphine and no stronger than that of codeine. Hydrocodone can produce miosis, euphoria, physical and psychological dependence. At therapeutic antitussive doses, it does exert analgesic effects. Following a 10 mg oral dose of hydrocodone administered to five adult male subjects, the mean peak concentration was 23.6 ± 5.2 ng/ml. Maximum serum levels were achieved at 1.3 ± 0.3 hours and the half-life was determined to be 3.8 ± 0.3 hours. Hydrocodone exhibits a complex pattern of metabolism including O-demethylation, N-demethylation and 6-keto reduction to the corresponding 6-α- and 6-β-hydroxymetabolites.

Phenylpropanolamine effects its vasoconstrictor activity by releasing noradrenaline from sympathetic nerve endings, and from direct stimulation of α-adrenoreceptors in blood vessels.

Indications and Usage: Hycomine® is indicated for the symptomatic relief of cough and nasal congestion.

Contraindications: Hycomine® is contraindicated in patients hypersensitive to hydrocodone or phenylpropanolamine, and in patients on concurrent MAO inhibitor therapy. Patients known to be hypersensitive to other opioids or sympathomimetic amines may exhibit cross sensitivity to Hycomine®. Phenylpropanolamine is contraindicated in patients with heart disease, hypertension, diabetes or hyperthyroidism. Hydrocodone is contraindicated in the presence of an intracranial lesion associated with increased intracranial pressure; and whenever ventilatory function is depressed.

Warnings: May be habit forming. Hydrocodone can produce drug dependence of the morphine type and, therefore, has the potential for being abused. Psychic dependence, physical dependence and tolerance may develop upon repeated administration of Hycomine® and it should be prescribed and administered with the same degree of caution appropriate to the use of other narcotic drugs (See DRUG ABUSE AND DEPENDENCE).

Respiratory Depression: Hycomine® produces dose-related respiratory depression by directly acting on brain stem respiratory centers. If respiratory depression occurs, it may be antagonized by the use of Narcan® (naloxone hydrochloride) and other supportive measures when indicated.

Head Injury and Increased Intracranial Pressure: The respiratory depression properties of narcotics and their capacity to elevate cerebrospinal fluid pressure may be markedly exaggerated in the presence of head injury, other intracranial lesions or a preexisting increase in intracranial pressure. Furthermore, narcotics produce adverse reactions which may obscure the clinical course of patients with head injuries.

Acute Abdominal Conditions: The administration of Hycomine® or other narcotics may obscure the diagnosis or clinical course of patients with acute abdominal conditions.

Phenylpropanolamine: Hypertensive crises can occur with concurrent use of phenylpropanolamine and monoamine oxidase (MAO) inhibitors, indomethacin or with beta-blockers and methyldopa.

If a hypertensive crisis occurs, these drugs should be discontinued immediately and therapy to lower blood pressure should be instituted immediately. Fever should be managed by means of external cooling.

Precautions: Before prescribing medication to suppress or modify cough, it is important to ascertain that the underlying cause of cough is identified, that modification of cough does not increase the risk of clinical or physiologic complications, and that appropriate therapy for the primary disease is provided.

Usage in Ambulatory Patients: Hydrocodone, like all narcotics, may impair the mental and/or physical abilities required for the performance of potentially hazardous tasks such as driving a car or operating machinery; phenylpropanolamine may produce a rapid pulse, dizziness or palpitations; patients should be cautioned accordingly.

Drug Interactions: Patients receiving other narcotic analgesics, general anesthetics, phenothiazines, other tranquilizers, sedative-hypnotics or other CNS depressants (including alcohol) concomitantly with hydrocodone may exhibit an additive CNS depression. When such combined therapy is contemplated, the dose of one or both agents should be reduced. The use of phenylpropanolamine with other sympathomimetic amines and MAO inhibitors may produce an additive elevation of blood pressure (See WARNINGS).

Carcinogenesis, Mutagenesis, Impairment of Fertility: Carcinogenicity, mutagenicity and reproduction studies have not been conducted with Hycomine®.

Usage in Pregnancy: Pregnancy Category C: Animal reproduction studies have not been conducted with Hycomine®. It is also not known whether Hycomine® can cause fetal harm when administered to a pregnant woman or can affect reproductive capacity. Hycomine® should be given to a pregnant woman only if clearly needed.

Nonteratogenic Effects: Babies born to mothers who have been taking opioids regularly prior to delivery will be physically dependent. The withdrawal signs include irritability and excessive crying, tremors, hyperactive reflexes, increased respiratory rate, increased stools, sneezing, yawning, vomiting and fever. The intensity of the syndrome does not always correlate with the duration of maternal opioid use or dose. There is no consensus on the best method of managing withdrawal. Chlorpromazine 0.7–1.0 mg/kg q 6 h, phenobarbital 2 mg/kg q 6 h, and paregoric 2–4 drops/kg q 4 h, have been used to treat withdrawal symptoms in infants. The duration of therapy is 4 to 28 days, with the dosages decreased as tolerated.

Nursing Mothers: It is not known whether this drug is excreted in human milk. Because many drugs are excreted in human milk and because of the potential for serious adverse reactions in nursing infants from Hycomine®, a decision should be made whether to discontinue nursing or discontinue the drug, taking into account the importance of the drug to the mother.

Usage in Patients Below the Age of 6 Years: Safety and effectiveness in this group have not been established.

Adverse Reactions:

Respiratory System: Hydrocodone produces dose-related respiratory depression by acting directly on brain stem respiratory centers.

Cardiovascular System: Hypertension, postural hypotension, tachycardia and palpitations.

Genitourinary System: Ureteral spasm, spasm of vesical sphincters and urinary retention have been reported with opiates.

Central Nervous System: Sedation, drowsiness, mental clouding, lethargy, impairment of mental and physical performance, anxiety, fear, dysphoria, dizziness, psychic dependence, mood changes and blurred vision.

Gastrointestinal System: Nausea and vomiting occur more frequently in ambulatory than in recumbent patients.

Drug Abuse and Dependence: Special care should be exercised in prescribing hydrocodone for emotionally unstable patients and for those with a history of drug misuse. Such patients should be closely supervised when long-term therapy is contemplated.

Hycomine® is a Schedule III narcotic. Psychic dependence, physical dependence, and tolerance may develop upon repeated administration of narcotics; therefore, Hycomine® should always be prescribed and administered with caution. Physical dependence is the condition in which continued administration of the drug is required to prevent the appearance of a withdrawal syndrome.

Patients physically dependent on opioids will develop an abstinence syndrome upon abrupt discontinuation of the opioid or following the administration of a narcotic antagonist. The character and severity of the withdrawal symptoms are related to the degree of physical dependence. Manifestations of opioid withdrawal are similar to but milder than that of morphine and include lacrimation, rhinorrhea, yawning, sweating, restlessness, dilated pupils, anorexia, gooseflesh, irritability and tremor. In more severe forms, nausea vomiting, intestinal spasm and diarrhea, increased heart rate and blood pressure, chills, and pains in bones and muscles of the back and extremities may occur. Peak effects will usually be apparent at 48 to 72 hours.

Treatment of withdrawal is usually managed by providing sufficient quantities of an opioid to suppress severe withdrawal symptoms and then gradually reducing the dose of opioid over a period of several days.

Overdosage:

Signs and Symptoms: Serious overdosage with Hycomine® is characterized by respiratory depression (a decrease in respiratory rate and/or tidal volume, Cheyne-Stokes respiration, cyanosis), extreme somnolence progressing to stupor to coma, skeletal muscle flaccidity, cold and clammy skin, and sometims bradycardia and hypotension. In severe overdosage apnea, circulatory collapse, cardiac arrest, and death may occur.

The signs and symptoms of overdosage of the individual components of Hycomine® may be modified in varying degrees by the presence of other active ingredients. Overdosage with phenylpropanolamine alone may result in tremor, restlessness, increased motor activity, agitation and hallucinations.

Treatment: Primary attention should be given to the reestablishment of adequate respiratory exchange through provision of a patent airway and the institution of assisted or controlled ventilation. The narcotic antagonist naloxone hydrochloride (Narcan®) is a specific antidote against respiratory depression which may result from overdosage or unusual sensitivity to narcotics including hydrocodone. Therefore, an appropriate dose of naloxone hydrochloride should be administered (Usual initial dose: 0.4 mg; usual initial child dose: 0.01 mg/kg body weight. For further information see Narcan® full prescribing information.) preferably by the intravenous route, simultaneously with efforts at respiratory resuscitation. Since the duration of action of hydrocodone may exceed that of the antagonist, the patient should be kept under continued surveillance and repeated doses of the antagonist should be administered as needed to maintain adequate respiration. Oxygen, intravenous fluids, vasopressors and other supportive measures should be employed as indicated.

Gastric emptying may be useful in removing unabsorbed drug. Activated charcoal may be of benefit.

Dosage and Administration:

Usual Dosage:

	Hycomine® Pediatric Syrup	Hycomine® Syrup
Adults	—	1 tsp. (5 ml)
Children		
6 to 12 years	1 tsp. (5 ml)	

After meals and at bedtime, not less than 4 hours apart (not to exceed 6 teaspoonfuls in a 24 hour period).

How Supplied: Hycomine® Syrup is available as an orange-colored, fruit-flavored syrup in bottles as follows:
One Pint: NDC 0056-0246-16
One Gallon: NDC 0056-0246-82

Hycomine® Pediatric Syrup is available as a green-colored, fruit-flavored syrup in bottles as follows:
One Pint: NDC 0056-0247-16

Store at controlled room temprature (59°–86°F, 15°–30°C).

Hycomine® is a Registered Trademark of E. I. du Pont de Nemours & Co. (Inc.)

Narcan® is a Registered Trademark of Du Pont Pharmaceuticals, Inc.

HYCOMINE® COMPOUND
[hī-ko-mēn kom'pound]

Description: HYCOMINE Compound tablets contain hydrocodone (dihydrocodeinone) bitartrate, a semi-synthetic centrally-acting narcotic antitussive; chlorpheniramine maleate, an antihistamine; phenylephrine hydrochloride, a sympathomimetic amine decongestant; acetaminophen, an analgesic/antipyretic; and caffeine, a centrally-acting stimulant; for oral administration.

Each HYCOMINE Compound tablet contains:
Hydrocodone bitartrate .... 5 mg
WARNING: May be habit forming
Chlorpheniramine maleate .... 2 mg
Phenylephrine hydrochloride ...... 10 mg
Acetaminophen ....250 mg
Caffeine .... 30 mg

Clinical Pharmacology: Clinical trials have proven hydrocodone bitartrate to be an effective antitussive agent which is pharmacologically 2 to 8 times as potent as codeine. At equi-antitussive doses, its sedative action is greater than codeine. The precise mechanism of action of hydrocodone and other opiates is not known, however, hydrocodone is believed to act by directly depressing the cough center. In excessive doses hydrocodone, like other opium derivatives, will depress respiration. The effects of hydrocodone in therapeutic doses on the cardiovascular system is insignificant. The constipation effects of hydrocodone are much weaker than that of morphine and no stronger than that of codeine. Hydrocodone can produce miosis, euphoria, physical and psychological dependence. At therapeutic antitussive doses, it does exert analgesic effects. Following a 10 mg oral dose of hydrocodone administered to five adult male human subjects, the mean peak concentration was 23.6 ± 5.2 ng/ml. Maximum serum levels were achieved at 1.3 ± 0.3 hours and the half-life was determined to be $3.8 \pm$ hours. Hydrocodone exhibits a complex pattern of metabolism including O-demethylation, N-demethylation and 6-keto reduction to the corresponding 6-α- and 6-β-hydroxymetabolites.

Chlorpheniramine maleate is a competitive H_1-receptor histamine blocking drug, thereby counteracting the effects of histamine release associated with allergic manifestations of upper respiratory tract inflammatory disorders. H_1-blocking drugs inhibit the actions of histamine on smooth muscle, capillary permeability, and can both stimulate and depress the central nervous system. Phenylephrine hydrochloride effects its vasoconstrictor activity by releasing noradrenaline from sympathetic nerve endings, and from direct stimulation of α-adreno-receptors in blood vessels. Acetaminophen is an antipyretic and peripherally acting analgesic. Caffeine is a central nervous system stimulant.

Indications and Usage: HYCOMINE Compound is indicated for the symptomatic relief of cough, nasal congestion, and discomfort associated with upper respiratory tract infections.

Contraindications: HYCOMINE Compound is contraindicated in patients hypersensitive to any component of the drug, and concurrent MAO inhibitor therapy. Patients known to be hypersensitive to other opioids, antihistamines, or sympathomimetic amines may exhibit cross sensitivity with HYCOMINE Compound. Phenylephrine is contraindicated in patients with heart disease, hypertension, diabetes or hyperthyroidism. Hydrocodone is contraindicated in the presence of an intracranial lesion associated with increased intracranial pressure; and whenever ventilatory function is depressed.

Warnings: May be habit forming. Hydrocodone can produce drug dependence of the morphine type and therefore has the potential for being abused. Psychic dependence, physical dependence and tolerance may develop upon repeated administration of HYCOMINE Compound and it should be prescribed and administered with the same degree of caution appropriate to the use of other narcotic drugs. (See DRUG ABUSE AND DEPENDENCE.)

Respiratory Depression: HYCOMINE Compound produces dose-related respiratory depression by directly acting on brain stem respiratory centers. If respiratory depression occurs, it may be antagonized by the use of NARCAN® (naloxone hydrochloride) and other supportive measures when indicated.

Head Injury and Increased Intracranial Pressure: The respiratory depressant properties of narcotics and their capacity to elevate cerebrospinal fluid pressure may be markedly exaggerated in the presence of head injury, other intracranial lesions or a pre-existing increase in intracranial pressure. Furthermore, narcotics produce adverse reactions which may obscure the clinical course of patients with head injuries.

Acute abdominal conditions: The administration of HYCOMINE Compound or other narcotics may obscure the diagnosis or clinical course of patients with acute abdominal conditions.

Phenylephrine: Hypersensitive crises can occur with concurrent use of phenylephrine and monoamine oxidase (MAO) inhibitors, indomethacin or with beta-blockers and methyldopa.

If a hypertensive crisis occurs these drugs should be discontinued immediately and therapy to lower blood pressure should be instituted immediately. Fever should be managed by means of external cooling.

Chlorpheniramine: Antihistamines may produce drowsiness or excitation, particularly in children and elderly patients.

Precautions: Before prescribing medication to suppress or modify cough, it is important to ascertain that the underlying cause of cough is identified, that modification of cough does not increase the risk of clinical or physiologic complications, and that appropriate therapy for the primary disease is provided.

Usage in Ambulatory Patients: Hydrocodone, like all narcotics, and antihistamines such as chlorpheniramine maleate, may impair the mental and/or physical abilities required for the performance of potentially hazardous tasks such as driving a car or operating machinery; phenylephrine may produce a rapid pulse, dizziness or palpitations; patients should be cautioned accordingly.

Drug Interactions: Patients receiving other narcotic analgesics, general anesthetics, phenothiazines, other tranquilizers, sedative-hypnotics or other CNS depressants (including alcohol) concomitantly with hydrocodone may exhibit an additive CNS depression. When such combined therapy is contemplated, the dose of one or both agents should be reduced. The use of phenylephrine with other sympathomimetic amines and MAO inhibitors may produce an additive elevation of blood pressure. MAO inhibitors may prolong the anticholinergic effects of antihistamines. (See WARNINGS).

Carcinogenesis, mutagenesis, impairment of fertility: Carcinogenicity, mutagenicity, and reproduction studies have not been conducted with HYCOMINE Compound.

Usage in Pregnancy: Pregnancy Category C. Animal reproduction studies have not been conducted with HYCOMINE Compound. It is also not known whether HYCOMINE Compound can cause fetal harm when administered to a pregnant woman or can affect reproductive capacity. HYCOMINE Compound should be given to a pregnant woman only if clearly needed.

Nonteratogenic effects: Babies born to mothers who have been taking opioids regularly prior to delivery will be physically dependent. The withdrawal signs include irritability and excessive crying, tremors, hyperactive reflexes, increased respiratory rate, increased stools, sneezing, yawning, vomiting and fever. The intensity of the syndrome does not always correlate with the duration of maternal opioid use or dose. Chlorpromazine 0.7–1.0 mg/kg q 6 h, phenobarbital 2 mg/kg q 6 h, and paregoric 2–4 drops/kg q 4 h, have been used to treat withdrawal symptoms in infants. The duration of therapy is 4 to 28 days, with the dosages decreased as tolerated.

Nursing mothers: It is not known whether this drug is excreted in human milk. Because many drugs are excreted in human milk and because of the potential for serious adverse reactions in nursing infants from HYCOMINE Compound, a decision should be made whether to discontinue nursing or discontinue the drug, taking into account the importance of the drug to the mother.

Pediatric use: Safety and effectiveness in children below the age of 2 years have not been established.

Adverse Reactions:
Respiratory System: Hydrocodone produces dose-related respiratory depression by acting directly on brain stem respiratory centers.
Cardiovascular System: Hypertension, postural hypotension, tachycardia and palpitations.
Genitourinary System: Ureteral spasm, spasm of vesical sphincters and urinary retention have been reported with opiates.
Central Nervous System: Sedation, drowsiness, mental clouding, lethargy, impairment of mental and physical performance, anxiety, fear, dysphoria, dizziness, psychic dependence, mood changes, and blurred vision.
Gastrointestinal System: Nausea and vomiting occur more frequently in ambulatory than in recumbent patients.

Drug Abuse and Dependence: Special care should be exercised in prescribing hydrocodone for emotionally unstable patients and for those with a history of drug misuse. Such patients should be closely supervised when long-term therapy is contemplated.

HYCOMINE Compound is a Schedule III narcotic. Psychic dependence, physical dependence, and tolerance may develop upon repeated administration of narcotics; therefore, HYCOMINE Compound should always be prescribed and administered with caution. Physical dependence is the condition in which continued administration of the drug is required to prevent the appearance of a withdrawal syndrome.

Patients physically dependent on opioids will develop an abstinence syndrome upon abrupt discontinuation of the opioid or following the administration of a narcotic antagonist. The character and severity of the withdrawal symptoms are related to the degree of physical dependence. Manifestations of opioid withdrawal are similar to but milder than that of morphine and include lacrimation, rhinorrhea, yawning, sweating, restlessness, dilated pupils, anorexia, gooseflesh, irritability and tremor. In more severe forms, nausea, vomiting, intestinal spasms and diarrhea, increased heart rate and blood pressure, chills, and pains in bones and muscles of the back and extremities may occur. Peak effects will usually be apparent at 48 to 72 hours.

Treatment of withdrawal is usually managed by providing sufficient quantities of an opioid to suppress **severe** withdrawal symptoms and then gradually reducing the dose of opioid over a period of several days.

Overdosage: The signs and symptoms of overdosage of the individual components of HYCOMINE Compound may be modified in varying degrees by the presence of other active ingredients.

Signs and Symptoms: Serious overdosage with hydrocodone is characterized by respiratory depression (a decrease in respiratory rate and/or tidal volume. Cheyne-Stokes respiration, cyanosis), extreme somnolence progressing to stupor or coma, skeletal muscle flaccidity, cold and clammy skin, and sometimes bradycardia and hypotension. In severe overdosage apnea, circulatory collapse, cardiac arrest, and death may occur. The ingestion of large amounts of acetaminophen may produce hepatic toxicity.

The signs and symptoms of overdosage of the individual components of HYCOMINE Compound may be modified in varying degrees by the presence of other active ingredients. Overdosage with phenylephrine alone may result in tremor, restlessness, increased motor activity, agitation and hallucinations.

Continued on next page

DuPont—Cont.

Treatment: Primary attention should be given to the reestablishment of adequate respiratory exchange through provision of a patent airway and the institution of assisted or controlled ventilation. The narcotic antagonist naloxone hydrochloride (NARCAN®) is a specific antidote against respiratory depression which may result from overdosage or unusual sensitivity to narcotics including hydrocodone. Therefore, an appropriate dose of naloxone hydrochloride should be administered (usual initial adult dose: 0.4 mg; usual initial child dose is 0.01 mg/kg body weight. For further information see NARCAN® full prescribing information) preferably by the intravenous route, simultaneously with efforts at respiratory resuscitation. Since the duration of action of hydrocodone may exceed that of the antagonist, the patient should be kept under continued surveillance and repeated doses of the antagonist should be administered as needed to maintain adequate respiration. Oxygen, intravenous fluids, vasopressors and other supportive measures should be employed as indicated.

Gastric emptying may be useful in removing unabsorbed drug. Activated charcoal may be of benefit. Treatment of acute acetaminophen overdosage is purely symptomatic.

Dosage and Administration: Usual dosage, not less than 4 hours apart:
Adults: 1 tablet 4 times a day
Children: 6 to 12 years: ½ tablet 4 times a day
Children: 2 to 6 years: ½ tablet twice daily

How Supplied: HYCOMINE® Compound is available as a coral pink, scored tablet in bottles as follows:

Bottles of 100   NDC 0056-0048-70
Bottles of 500   NDC 0056-0048-85

Store at controlled room temperature (59°–86° F, 15°–30° C)

HYCOMINE® is a Registered Trademark of E. I. du Pont de Nemours & Co. (Inc.)
NARCAN® is a Registered U.S. Trademark of Du Pont Pharmaceuticals, Inc.
6015-8

HYCOTUSS®
[*hī-kō-tus*]
Expectorant

Description: HYCOTUSS Expectorant Syrup contains hydrocodone (dihydrocodeinone) bitartrate, a semi-synthetic centrally-acting narcotic, antitussive and guaifenesin, an expectorant for oral administration.

Each teaspoonful (5 ml) contains:
Hydrocodone bitartrate .... 5 mg
  Warning: May be habit forming
Guaifenesin .... 100 mg
Alcohol U.S.P. 10% v/v ....

Clinical Pharmacology: Clinical trials have proven hydrocodone bitartrate to be an effective antitussive agent which is pharmacologically 2 to 8 times as potent as codeine. At equi-effective doses, its sedative action is greater than codeine. The precise mechanism of action of hydrocodone and other opiates is not known, however, hydrocodone is believed to act by directly depressing the cough center. In excessive doses hydrocodone, like other opium derivatives, can depress respiration. The effects of hydrocodone in therapeutic doses on the cardiovascular system is insignificant. The constipation effects of hydrocodone are much weaker than that of morphine and no stronger than that of codeine. Hydrocodone can produce miosis, euphoria, physical and psychological dependence. At therapeutic antitussive doses, it does exert analgesic effects. Following a 10 mg oral dose of hydrocodone administered to five male human subjects, the mean peak concentration was 23.6 ± 5.2 ng/ml. Maximum serum levels were achieved at 1.3 ± 0.3 hours and half-life was determined to be 3.8 ± 0.3 hours. Hydrocodone exhibits a complex pattern of metabolism including O-demethylation, N-demethylation and 6-keto reduction to the corresponding 6-α- and 6-β-hydroxymetabolites.

The exact mechanism of action is not established but guaifenesin is believed to act by stimulating receptors in the gastric mucosa that initiates a reflex secretion of respiratory tract fluid, thereby increasing the volume and decreasing the viscosity of bronchial secretions. Studies with guaifenesin indicate that it is rapidly absorbed from the gastrointestinal tract and has a half-life of one hour.

Indications and Usage: HYCOTUSS Expectorant is indicated for the symptomatic relief of irritating non-productive cough associated with upper and lower respiratory tract congestion.

Contraindications: HYCOTUSS Expectorant is contraindicated in patients hypersensitive to hydrocodone or guaifenesin. Patients known to be hypersensitive to other opioids may exhibit cross sensitivity to HYCOTUSS Expectorant. Hydrocodone is contraindicated in the presence of an intracranial lesion associated with increased intracranial pressure; and whenever ventilatory function is depressed.

Warnings: May be habit forming. Hydrocodone can produce drug dependence of the morphine type and therefore has the potential for being abused. Psychic dependence, physical dependence and tolerance may develop upon repeated administration of HYCOTUSS Expectorant and it should be prescribed and administered with the same degree of caution appropriate to the use of other narcotic drugs (See DRUG ABUSE AND DEPENDENCE).

Respiratory Depression: HYCOTUSS Expectorant produces dose-related respiratory depression by directly acting on the brain stem respiratory centers. If respiratory depression occurs, it may be antagonized by the use of NARCAN® (naloxone hydrochloride) and other supportive measures when indicated.

Head Injury and Increased Intracranial Pressure: The respiratory depressant properties of narcotics and their capacity to elevate cerebrospinal fluid pressure may be markedly exaggerated in the presence of head injury, other intracranial lesions or a pre-existing increase in intracranial pressure. Furthermore, narcotics produce adverse reactions which may obscure the clinical course of patients with head injuries.

Acute Abdominal Conditions: The administration of HYCOTUSS Expectorant or other opioids may obscure the diagnosis or clinical course of patients with acute abdominal conditions.

Precautions: Before prescribing medication to suppress or modify cough, it is important to ascertain that the underlying cause of cough is identified, that modification of cough does not increase the risk of clinical or physiologic complications, and that appropriate therapy for the primary disease is provided.

Usage in Ambulatory Patients: Hydrocodone, like all narcotics, may impair the mental and/ or physical abilities required for the performance of potentially hazardous tasks such as driving a car or operating machinery, and patients should be warned accordingly.

Drug Interactions: Patients receiving other narcotic analgesics, general anesthetics, phenothiazines, other tranquilizers, sedative hypnotics or other CNS depressants (including alcohol) concomitantly with hydrocodone may exhibit an additive CNS depression. When such combined therapy is contemplated, the dose of one or both agents should be reduced. (See WARNINGS).

Laboratory Interactions: The metabolite of guaifenesin has been found to produce an apparent increase in urinary 5-hydroxyindolea- cetic acid, and guaifenesin therefore may interfere with the interpretation of this test for the diagnosis of carcinoid syndrome. Guaifenesin administration should be discontinued 24 hours prior to the collection of urine specimens for the determination of 5-hydroxyindoleacetic acid.

Carcinogenesis, mutagenesis, impairment of fertility: Carcinogenicity, mutagenicity and reproduction studies have not been conducted with HYCOTUSS Expectorant.

Usage in Pregnancy: Pregnancy Category C. Animal reproduction studies have not been conducted with HYCOTUSS Expectorant. It is also not known whether HYCOTUSS Expectorant can cause fetal harm when administered to a pregnant woman or can affect reproductive capacity. HYCOTUSS Expectorant should be given to a pregnant woman only if clearly needed.

Nonteratogenic effects: Babies born to mothers who have been taking opioids regularly prior to delivery will be physically dependent. The withdrawal signs include irritability and excessive crying, tremors, hyperactive reflexes, increased respiratory rate, increased stools, sneezing, yawning, vomiting and fever. The intensity of the syndrome does not always correlate with the duration of maternal opioid use or dose. There is no consensus on the best method of managing withdrawal. Chlorpromazine 0.7–1.0 mg/kg q 6 h, phenobarbital 2 mg/kg q 6 h, and paregoric 2–4 drops/kg q 4 h, have been used to treat withdrawal symptoms in infants. The duration of therapy is 4 to 28 days, with the dosages decreased as tolerated.

Nursing mothers: It is not known whether this drug is excreted in human milk. Because many drugs are excreted in human milk and because of the potential for serious adverse reactions in nursing infants from HYCOTUSS Expectorant, a decision should be made whether to discontinue nursing or discontinue the drug, taking into account the importance of the drug to the mother.

Adverse Reactions:

Respiratory System: Hydrocodone produces dose-related respiratory depression by acting directly on brain stem respiratory centers.

Cardiovascular System: Hypertension, postural hypotension and palpitations.

Genitourinary System: Ureteral spasm, spasm of vesical sphincters and urinary retention have been reported with opiates.

Central Nervous System: Sedation, drowsiness, mental clouding, lethargy, impairment of mental and physical performance, anxiety, fear, dysphoria, dizziness, psychic dependence, mood changes and blurred vision.

Gastrointestinal System: Nausea and vomiting occur more frequently in ambulatory than in recumbent patients.

Drug Abuse and Dependence: Special care should be exercised in prescribing hydrocodone for emotionally unstable patients and for those with a history of drug misuse. Such patients should be closely supervised when long-term therapy is contemplated.

HYCOTUSS Expectorant is a Schedule III narcotic. Psychic dependence, physical dependence and tolerance may develop upon repeated administration of narcotics; therefore, HYCOTUSS Expectorant should always be prescribed and administered with caution. Physical dependence is the condition in which continued administration of the drug is required to prevent the appearance of a withdrawal syndrome.

Patients physically dependent on opioids will develop an abstinence syndrome upon abrupt discontinuation of the opioid or following the administration of a narcotic antagonist. The character and severity of the withdrawal symptoms are related to the degree of physical dependence. Manifestations of opioid withdrawal are similar to but milder than that of morphine and include lacrimation, rhinorrhea, yawning, sweating, restlessness, dilated pupils, anorexia, gooseflesh, irritability and tremor. In more severe forms, nausea, vomiting, intestinal spasm and diarrhea, increased heart rate and blood pressure, chills, and pains in bones and muscles of the back and extremities may occur. Peak effects will usually be apparent at 48 to 72 hours.

Treatment of withdrawal is usually managed by providing sufficient quantities of an opioid to suppress **severe** withdrawal symptoms and then gradually reducing the dose of opioid over a period of several days.

Overdosage:

Signs and Symptoms: Serious overdosage with HYCOTUSS Expectorant is characterized by respiratory depression (a decrease in respiratory rate and/or tidal volume, Cheyne-Stokes respiration, cyanosis), extreme somnolence progressing to stupor or coma, skeletal muscle flaccidity, cold and clammy skin, and sometimes bradycardia and hypotension. In severe overdosage apnea, circulatory collapse, cardiac arrest, and death may occur.

Treatment: Primary attention should be given to the reestablishment of adequate respiratory exchange through provision of a patent airway and the institution of assisted or controlled ventilation. The narcotic antagonist naloxone hydrochloride (NARCAN®) is a specific antidote against respiratory depression which may result from overdosage or unusual sensitivity to narcotics including hydrocodone. Therefore, an appropriate dose of naloxone hydrochloride should be administered (usual initial adult dose: 0.4 mg. For further information see NARCAN® full prescribing information) preferably by the intravenous route, simultaneously with efforts at respiratory resuscitation. Since the duration of action of hydrocodone may exceed that of the antagonist, the patient should be kept under continued surveillance and repeated doses of the antagonist should be administered as needed to maintain adequate respiration. Oxygen, intravenous fluids, vasopressors and other supportive measures should be employed as indicated.

Gastric emptying may be useful in removing unabsorbed drug. Activated charcoal may be of benefit.

Dosage and Administration:
Usual Adult Dose: One teaspoonful (5 ml) after meals and at bedtime, not less than 4 hours apart (not to exceed 6 teaspoonsful in a 24 hour period). Treatment should be initiated with one teaspoonful and subsequent doses, up to a maximum single dose of 3 teaspoonsful, adjusted if required.

Usual Children's Dose:
Over 12 years: Initial dose 1 teaspoonful; maximum single dose, 2 teaspoonsful.
2 to 12 years: Initial dose ½ teaspoonful; maximum single dose, 1 teaspoonful.
Under 2 years: Dosage should be calculated as Hydrocodone, 0.3 mg/kg/24 hours, divided into four equal doses.

How Supplied: HYCOTUSS Expectorant is available as an orange-colored, butterscotch flavored syrup in bottles as follows:
One pint: NDC 0056-0235-16
Store at controlled room temperature (59°–86° F, 15°–30° C).
HYCOTUSS® is a Registered Trademark of E.I. du Pont de Nemours & Co. (Inc.)
NARCAN® is a Registered Trademark of Du Pont Pharmaceuticals, Inc.
6131-2

MOBAN®
[mō′ ban]
(molindone hydrochloride)
Tablets and Concentrate

Description: MOBAN (molindone hydrochloride) is a dihydroindolone compound which is not structurally related to the phenothiazines, the butyrophenones or the thioxanthenes.
MOBAN is 3-ethyl-6, 7-dihydro-2-methyl-5-(morpholinomethyl) indol-4(5H)-one hydrochloride. It is a white crystalline powder, freely soluble in water and alcohol and has a molecular weight of 312.67.

Actions: MOBAN (molindone hydrochloride) has a pharmacological profile in laboratory animals which predominantly resembles that of major tranquilizers causing reduction of spontaneous locomotion and aggressiveness, suppression of a conditioned response and antagonism of the bizarre stereotyped behavior and hyperactivity induced by amphetamines. In addition, MOBAN antagonizes the depression caused by the tranquilizing agent tetrabenazine.

In human clinical studies tranquilization is achieved in the absence of muscle relaxing or incoordinating effects. Based on EEG studies, MOBAN exerts its effect on the ascending reticular activating system.

Human metabolic studies show MOBAN (molindone hydrochloride) to be rapidly absorbed and metabolized when given orally. Unmetabolized drug reached a peak blood level at 1.5 hours. Pharmacological effect from a single oral dose persists for 24–36 hours. There are 36 recognized metabolites with less than 2–3% unmetabolized MOBAN being excreted in urine and feces.

Indications: MOBAN is indicated for the management of the manifestations of psychotic disorders. The antipsychotic efficacy of MOBAN was established in clinical studies which enrolled newly hospitalized and chronically hospitalized, acutely ill, schizophrenic patients as subjects.

Contraindications: MOBAN (molindone hydrochloride) is contraindicated in severe central nervous system depression (alcohol, barbiturates, narcotics, etc.) or comatose states, and in patients with known hypersensitivity to the drug.

Warnings:
Usage in Pregnancy: Studies in pregnant patients have not been carried out. Reproduction studies have been performed in the following animals:

Pregnant Rats oral dose—	20	mg/kg/day —10 days
no adverse effect		
	40	mg/kg/day —10 days
no adverse effect		
Pregnant Mice oral dose—	20	mg/kg/day —10 days
slight increase resorptions		
	40	mg/kg/day —10 days
slight increase resorptions		
Pregnant Rabbits oral dose—	5	mg/kg/day —12 days
no adverse effect		
	10	mg/kg/day —12 days
no adverse effect		
	20	mg/kg/day —12 days
no adverse effect		

Animal reproductive studies have not demonstrated a teratogenic potential. The anticipated benefits must be weighed against the unknown risks to the fetus if used in pregnant patients.

Nursing Mothers: Data are not available on the content of MOBAN (molindone hydrochloride) in the milk of nursing mothers.

Usage in Children: Use of MOBAN (molindone hydrochloride) in children below the age of twelve years is not recommended because safe and effective conditions for its usage have not been established.

Moban has not been shown effective in the management of behavorial complications in patients with mental retardation.

Precautions: Some patients receiving MOBAN (molindone hydrochloride) may note drowsiness initially and they should be advised against activities requiring mental alertness until their response to the drug has been established.

Increased activity has been noted in patients receiving MOBAN. Caution should be exercised where increased activity may be harmful.

MOBAN does not lower the seizure threshold in experimental animals to the degree noted with more sedating antipsychotic drugs. However, in humans convulsive seizures have been reported in a few instances.

The physician should be aware that this tablet preparation contains calcium sulfate as an excipient and that calcium ions may interfere with the absorption of preparations containing phenytoin sodium and tetracyclines.

MOBAN has an antiemetic effect in animals. A similar effect may occur in humans and may obscure signs of intestinal obstruction or brain tumor.

Neuroleptic drugs elevate prolactin levels; the elevation persists during chronic administration. Tissue culture experiments indicate that approximately one-third of human breast cancers are prolactin dependent in vitro, a factor of potential importance if the prescription of these drugs is contemplated in a patient with a previously detected breast cancer. Although disturbances such as galactorrhea, amenorrhea, gynecomastia, and impotence have been reported, the clinical significance of elevated serum prolactin levels is unknown for most patients. An increase in mammary neoplasms has been found in rodents after chronic administration of neuroleptic drugs. Neither clinical studies nor epidemiologic studies conducted to date however, have shown an association between chronic administration of these drugs and mammary tumorigenesis; the available evidence is considered too limited to be conclusive at this time.

Adverse Reactions:
CNS Effects
The most frequently occurring effect is initial drowsiness that generally subsides with continued usage of the drug or lowering of the dose.
Noted less frequently were depression, hyperactivity and euphoria.

Neurological
Extrapyramidal Reactions
Extrapyramidal reactions noted below may occur in susceptible individuals and are usually reversible with appropriate management.

Akathisia
Motor restlessness may occur early.

Parkinson Syndrome
Akinesia, characterized by rigidity, immobility and reduction of voluntary movements and tremor, have been observed. Occurrence is less frequent than akathisia.

Dystonic Syndrome
Prolonged abnormal contractions of muscle groups occur infrequently. These symptoms may be managed by the addition of a synthetic antiparkinson agent (other than L-dopa), small doses of sedative drugs, and/or reduction in dosage.

Tardive Dyskinesia
Neuroleptic drugs are known to cause a syndrome of dyskinetic movements commonly referred to as tardive dyskinesia. The movements may appear during treatment or upon withdrawal of treatment and may be either reversible or irreversible (i.e., persistent) upon cessation of further neuroleptic administration. Reports of reversible tardive dyskinesia in association with MOBAN therapy have been received. Reports of the irreversible variety have not been received, but this cannot be used to predict that MOBAN cannot cause an irreversible dyskinetic syndrome.

The syndrome is known to have a variable latency for development and the duration of the latency cannot be determined reliably. It is thus wise to assume that any neuroleptic agent has the capacity to induce the syndrome and act accordingly until sufficient data has been collected to settle the issue definitively for a specific drug product. In the case of neuroleptics known to produce the irreversible syndrome, the following has been observed: Tardive dyskinesia associated with other agents has appeared in some patients on long-term therapy and has also appeared after drug therapy has been discontinued. The risk appears to be greater in elderly patients on high-dose therapy, especially females. The symptoms are persistent and in some patients appear to be irreversible. The syndrome is characterized by rhythmical involuntary movements of the tongue, face, mouth or jaw (e.g., protrusion of tongue, puffing of cheeks, puckering of mouth, chewing movements). There may be involuntary movements of extremities.

There is no known effective treatment of tardive dyskinesia; antiparkinsonism agents usually do not alleviate the symptoms of this syndrome. It is suggested that all antipsychotic agents be discontinued if these symptoms appear. Should it be necessary to reinstitute treatment, or increase the dosage of the agent, or switch to a different antipsychotic agent, the syndrome may be masked. It has been reported that fine vermicular movements of the tongue may be an early sign of the syndrome and if the medication is stopped at that time the syndrome may not develop.

Autonomic Nervous System
Occasionally blurring of vision, tachycardia, nausea, dry mouth and salivation have been reported.

Continued on next page

DuPont—Cont.

Urinary retention and constipation may occur particularly if anticholinergic drugs are used to treat extrapyramidal symptoms.

Hematological
There have been rare reports of leucopenia and leucocytosis. If such reactions occur, treatment with MOBAN may continue if clinical symptoms are absent. Alterations of blood glucose, liver function tests, B.U.N., and red blood cells have not been considered clinically significant.

Metabolic and Endocrine Effects
Alteration of thyroid function has not been significant. Amenorrhea has been reported infrequently. Resumption of menses in previously amenorrheic women has been reported. Initially heavy menses may occur. Galactorrhea and gynecomastia have been reported infrequently. Increase in libido has been noted in some patients. Although both weight gain and weight loss have been in the direction of normal or ideal weight, excessive weight gain has not occurred with MOBAN.

Cardiovascular
Rare, transient, non-specific T wave changes have been reported on E.K.G. Association with a clinical syndrome has not been established. Rarely has significant hypotension been reported.

Ophthalmological
Lens opacities and pigmentary retinopathy have not been reported where patients have received MOBAN® (molindone hydrochloride). In some patients, phenothiazine induced lenticular opacities have resolved following discontinuation of the phenothiazine while continuing therapy with MOBAN.

Skin
Early, non-specific skin rash, probably of allergic origin, has occasionally been reported. Skin pigmentation has not been seen with MOBAN usage alone.

MOBAN (molindone hydrochloride) has certain pharmacological similarities to other antipsychotic agents. Because adverse reactions are often extensions of the pharmacological activity of a drug, all of the known pharmacological effects associated with other antipsychotic drugs should be kept in mind when MOBAN is used. Upon abrupt withdrawal after prolonged high dosage an abstinence syndrome has not been noted.

Dosage and Administration: Initial and maintenance doses of MOBAN (molindone hydrochloride) should be individualized.

Initial Dosage Schedule: The usual starting dosage is 50–75 mg/day.
—Increase to 100 mg/day in 3 or 4 days.
—Based on severity of symptomatology, dosage may be titrated up or down depending on individual patient response.
—An increase to 225 mg/day may be required in patients with severe symptoma- tology.

Elderly and debilitated patients should be started on lower dosage.

Maintenance Dosage Schedule:
1. Mild—5 mg-15 mg three or four times a day.
2. Moderate—10 mg-25 mg three or four times a day.
3. Severe—225 mg/day may be required.

Drug Interactions: Potentiation of drugs administered concurrently with MOBAN (molindone hydrochloride) has not been reported. Additionally, animal studies have not shown increased toxicity when MOBAN is given concurrently with representative members of three classes of drugs (i.e., barbiturates, chloral hydrate and antiparkinson drugs).

Management of Overdosage: Symptomatic, supportive therapy should be the rule.
Gastric lavage is indicated for the reduction of absorption of MOBAN (molindone hydrochloride) which is freely soluble in water.
Since the adsorption of MOBAN (molindone hydrochloride) by activated charcoal has not been determined, the use of this antidote must be considered of theoretical value.

Emesis in a comatose patient is contraindicated. Additionally, while the emetic effect of apomorphine is blocked by MOBAN® in animals, this blocking effect has not been determined in humans.

A significant increase in the rate of removal of unmetabolized MOBAN from the body by forced diuresis, peritoneal or renal dialysis would not be expected. (Only 2% of a single ingested dose of MOBAN is excreted unmetabolized in the urine.) However, poor response of the patient may justify use of these procedures.

While the use of laxatives or enemas might be based on general principles, the amount of unmetabolized MOBAN in feces is less than 1%. Extrapyramidal symptoms have responded to the use of diphenhydramine (Benadryl*), Amantadine HCl (Symmetrel®) and the synthetic anticholinergic antiparkinson agents, (i.e., Artane*, Cogentin*, Akineton*).

How Supplied: As tablets in bottles of 100 with potencies and colors as follows:

5 mg orange	NDC 0056-0072-70
10 mg lavender	NDC 0056-0073-70
25 mg light green	NDC 0056-0074-70
50 mg blue	NDC 0056-0076-70
100 mg tan	NDC 0056-0077-70

As a concentrate containing 20 mg molindone hydrochloride per ml in 4 oz. (120 ml) bottles, NDC 0056-0460-04.

---

*Benadryl—Trademark, Parke-Davis and Co.
*Artane—Trademark, Lederle Laboratories
*Cogentin—Trademark, Merck Sharp & Dohme
*Akineton—Trademark, Knoll Pharmaceutical Co.
*Symmetrel—Trademark of E.I. du Pont de Nemours & Co. (Inc.)
6145-3
MOBAN® is a registered U.S. trademark of E.I. duPont de Nemours & Co. (Inc.)
Shown in Product Identification Section, page 410

NARCAN® INJECTION R
[nar'kan]
NARCAN® NEONATAL INJECTION R
(naloxone hydrochloride)
Narcotic Antagonist

Description: NARCAN (naloxone hydrochloride), a narcotic antagonist, is a synthetic congener of oxymorphone. In structure it differs from oxymorphone in that the methyl group on the nitrogen atom is replaced by an allyl group.

Naloxone hydrochloride occurs as a white to slightly off-white powder, and is soluble in water, in dilute acids, and in strong alkali; slightly soluble in alcohol; practically insoluble in ether and in chloroform.

NARCAN injection is available as a sterile solution for intravenous, intramuscular and subcutaneous administration in two concentrations, 0.02 mg and 0.4 mg of naloxone hydrochloride per ml. Each ml of either strength contains 8.6 mg of sodium chloride; and 2.0 mg of methylparaben and propylparaben as preservatives in a ratio of 9 to 1. pH is adjusted to 3.5 ± 0.5 with hydrochloric acid.

Clinical Pharmacology: NARCAN (naloxone hydrochloride) prevents or reverses the effects of opioids including respiratory depression, sedation and hypotension. Also, it can reverse the psychotomimetic and dysphoric effects of agonist-antagonist such as pentazocine.

NARCAN (naloxone hydrochloride) is an essentially pure narcotic antagonist, i.e., it does not possess the "agonistic" or morphine-like properties characteristic of other narcotic antagonists; NARCAN does not produce respiratory depression, psychotomimetic effects or pupillary constriction. In the absence of narcotics or agonistic effects of other narcotic antagonists it exhibits essentially no pharmacologic activity.

NARCAN has not been shown to produce tolerance nor to cause physical or psychological dependence.

In the presence of physical dependence on narcotics NARCAN will produce withdrawal symptoms.

Mechanisms of Action: While the mechanism of action of NARCAN is not fully understood, the preponderance of evidence suggests that NARCAN antagonizes the opioid effects by competing for the same receptor sites.

When NARCAN is administered intravenously the onset of action is generally apparent within two minutes; the onset of action is only slightly less rapid when it is administered subcutaneously or intramuscularly. The duration of action is dependent upon the dose and route of administration of NARCAN. Intramuscular administration produces a more prolonged effect than intravenous administration. The requirement for repeat doses of NARCAN, however, will also be dependent upon the amount, type and route of administration of the narcotic being antagonized.

Following parenteral administration NARCAN is rapidly distributed in the body. It is metabolized in the liver, primarily by glucuronide conjugation and excreted in urine. In one study the serum half-life in adults ranged from 30 to 81 minutes (mean 64 ± 12 minutes). In a neonatal study the mean plasma half-life was observed to be 3.1 ± 0.5 hours.

Indications and Usage: NARCAN is indicated for the complete or partial reversal of narcotic depression, including respiratory depression, induced by opioids including natural and synthetic narcotics, propoxyphene, methadone and the narcotic-antagonist analgesics: nalbuphine, pentazocine and butorphanol. NARCAN is also indicated for the diagnosis of suspected acute opioid overdosage.

Contraindications: NARCAN is contraindicated in patients known to be hypersensitive to it.

Warnings: NARCAN should be administered cautiously to persons including newborns of mothers who are known or suspected to be physically dependent on opioids. In such cases an abrupt and complete reversal of narcotic effects may precipitate an acute abstinence syndrome.

The patient who has satisfactorily responded to NARCAN should be kept under continued surveillance and repeated doses of NARCAN should be administered, as necessary, since the duration of action of some narcotics may exceed that of NARCAN.

NARCAN is not effective against respiratory depression due to non-opioid drugs.

Precautions: In addition to NARCAN, other resuscitative measures such as maintenance of a free airway, artificial ventilation, cardiac massage, and vasopressor agents should be available and employed when necessary to counteract acute narcotic poisoning.

Several instances of hypotension, hypertension, ventricular tachycardia and fibrillation, and pulmonary edema have been reported. These have occurred in postoperative patients most of whom had pre-existing cardiovascular disorders or received other drugs which may have similar adverse cardiovascular effects. Although a direct cause and effect relationship has not been established, NARCAN should be used with caution in patients with pre-existing cardiac disease or patients who have received potentially cardiotoxic drugs.

Carcinogenesis, Mutagenesis, Impairment of Fertility: Carcinogenicity and mutagenicity studies have not been performed with NARCAN. Reproductive studies in mice and rats demonstrated no impairment of fertility.

Use in Pregnancy: Pregnancy Catagory B: Reproduction studies performed in mice and rats at doses up to 1,000 times the human dose, revealed no evidence of impaired fertility or harm to the fetus due to NARCAN. There are, however, no adequate and well controlled studies in pregnant women. Because animal reproduction studies are not always predictive of human response, NARCAN should be used during pregnancy only if clearly needed.

Nursing Mothers: It is not known whether NARCAN is excreted in human milk. Because many drugs are excreted in human milk, caution should be exercised when NARCAN is administered to a nursing woman.

Adverse Reactions: Abrupt reversal of narcotic depression may result in nausea, vomiting, sweating, tachycardia, increased blood pressure, and tremulousness. In postoperative patients, larger than necessary dosage of NARCAN may result in significant reversal of analgesia, and in excitement. Hypotension, hypertension, ventricular tachycardia and fibrillation, and pulmonary edema have been associated with the use of NARCAN postoperatively (see PRECAUTIONS & USAGE IN ADULTS-POSTOPERATIVE NARCOTIC DEPRESSION). Seizures have been reported to occur infrequently after the administration of naloxone; however, a causal relationship has not been established.

Overdosage: There is no clinical experience with NARCAN overdosage in humans.
In the mouse and rat the intravenous LD_{50} is 150 $\pm$ 5 mg/kg and 109 $\pm$ 4 mg/kg respectively. In acute subcutaneous toxicity studies in newborn rats the LD_{50} (95% CL) is 260 (228-296) mg/kg. Subcutaneous injection of 100 mg/kg/day in rats for 3 weeks produced only transient salivation and partial ptosis following injection: no toxic effects were seen at 10 mg/kg/day for 3 weeks.

Dosage and Administration: NARCAN (naloxone hydrochloride) may be administered intravenously, intramuscularly, or subcutaneously. The most rapid onset of action is achieved by intravenous administration and it is recommended in emergency situations.

Since the duration of action of some narcotics may exceed that of NARCAN the patient should be kept under continued surveillance and repeated doses of NARCAN should be administered, as necessary.

Intravenous Infusion: NARCAN may be diluted for intravenous infusion in normal saline or 5% dextrose solutions. The addition of 2 mg of NARCAN in 500 ml of either solution provides a concentration of 0.004 mg/ml. Mixtures should be used within 24 hours. After 24 hours, the remaining unused solution must be discarded. The rate of administration should be titrated in accordance with the patient's response.

Parenteral drug products should be inspected visually for particulate matter and discoloration prior to administration whenever solution and container permit. NARCAN should not be mixed with preparations containing bisulfite, metabisulfite, long-chain or high molecular weight anions, or any solution having an alkaline pH. No drug or chemical agent should be added to NARCAN unless its effect on the chemical and physical stability of the solution has first been established.

Usage in Adults:
Narcotic Overdose—Known or Suspected: An initial dose of 0.4 mg to 2 mg of NARCAN may be administered intravenously. If the desired degree of counteraction and improvement in respiratory functions is not obtained, it may be repeated at 2 to 3 minute intervals. If no response is observed after 10 mg of NARCAN have been administered, the diagnosis of narcotic induced or partial narcotic induced toxicity should be questioned. Intramuscular or subcutaneous administration may be necessary if the intravenous route is not available.

Postoperative Narcotic Depression: For the partial reversal of narcotic depression following the use of narcotics during surgery, smaller doses of NARCAN are usually sufficient. The dose of NARCAN should be titrated according to the patient's response. For the initial reversal of respiratory depression, NARCAN should be injected in increments of 0.1 to 0.2 mg intravenously at two to three minute intervals to the desired degree of reversal i.e. adequate ventilation and alertness without significant pain or discomfort. Larger than necessary dosage of NARCAN may result in significant reversal of analgesia and increase in blood pressure. Similarly, too rapid reversal may induce nausea, vomiting, sweating or circulatory stress.

Repeat doses of NARCAN may be required within one to two hour intervals depending upon the amount, type (i.e., short or long acting) and time interval since last administration of narcotic. Supplemental intramuscular doses have been shown to produce a longer lasting effect.

Usage in Children:
Narcotic Overdose—Known or Suspected: The usual initial dose in children is 0.01 mg/kg body weight given I.V. If this dose does not result in the desired degree of clinical improvement, a subsequent dose of 0.1 mg/kg body weight may be administered. If an I.V. route of administration is not available, NARCAN may be administered I.M. or S.C. in divided doses. If necessary, NARCAN can be diluted with sterile water for injection.

Postoperative Narcotic Depression: Follow the recommendations and cautions under Adult Postoperative Depression. For the initial reversal of respiratory depression NARCAN should be injected in increments of 0.005 mg to 0.01 mg intravenously at two to three minute intervals to the desired degree of reversal.

Usage in Neonates:
Narcotic-Induced Depression: The usual initial dose is 0.01 mg/kg body weight administered I.V., I.M., or S.C. This dose may be repeated in accordance with adult administration guidelines for postoperative narcotic depression.

HOW SUPPLIED: 0.4 mg/ml of NARCAN® (naloxone hydrochloride) for intravenous, intramuscular and subcutaneous administration. Available as follows:
1 ml ampuls in
  boxes of 10   NDC 0590-0365-10
Also available in Military Depot and VA Depot:
  box of 10   NSN 6505-00-079-7867
1 ml disposable prefilled syringes.
  boxes of 10   NDC 0590-0365-15
10 ml vials   NDC 0590-0365-05
0.02 mg/ml of NARCAN® (naloxone hydrochloride) NEONATAL INJECTION for intravenous, intramuscular and subcutaneous administration.
Available as:
2 ml ampuls in
  boxes of 10   NDC 0590-0367-10
NARCAN® is a Registered U.S. Trademark of DuPont Pharmaceuticals, Inc.
6108-5
Shown in Product Identification Section, page 410

NUBAIN®   ℞
[nū′ bān]
(nalbuphine hydrochloride)

Description: NUBAIN (nalbuphine hydrochloride) is a synthetic narcotic agonist-antagonist analgesic of the phenanthrene series. It is chemically related to both the widely used narcotic antagonist, naloxone, and the potent narcotic analgesic, oxymorphone.

Nalbuphine hydrochloride is (-)-17-(cyclobutylmethyl)-4, 5α-epoxy-morphinan-3,6α, 14-triol, hydrochloride.

Nubain® is available in two concentrations, 10 mg and 20 mg of nalbuphine hydrochloride per ml. Both strengths contain .94% sodium citrate, 1.26% citric acid anhydrous, 0.1% sodium metabisulfite, and 0.2% of a 9:1 mixture of methylparaben and propylparaben as preservatives: pH is adjusted, if necessary, with hydrochloric acid. Sodium chloride may be added to adjust isotonicity in the 10 mg ml concentration.

Actions: NUBAIN is a potent analgesic. Its analgesic potency is essentially equivalent to that of morphine on a milligram basis.

Its onset of action occurs within 2 to 3 minutes after intravenous administration, and in less than 15 minutes following subcutaneous or intramuscular injection. The plasma half-life of nalbuphine is 5 hours and in clinical studies the duration of analgesic activity has been reported to range from 3 to 6 hours.

The narcotic antagonist activity of NUBAIN is one-fourth as potent as nalorphine and 10 times that of pentazocine.

Indications: For the relief of moderate to severe pain. NUBAIN can also be used for preoperative analgesia, as a supplement to surgical anesthesia, and for obstetrical analgesia during labor.

Contraindications: NUBAIN should not be administered to patients who are hypersensitive to it.

Warnings:
Drug Dependence NUBAIN has been shown to have a low abuse potential which is approximate to that of pentazocine. When compared with drugs which are not mixed agonist-antagonists, it has been reported that nalbuphine's potential for abuse would be less than that of codeine and propoxyphene. Psychological and physical dependence and tolerance may follow the abuse or misuse of nalbuphine. Therefore, caution should be observed in prescribing it for emotionally unstable patients, or for individuals with a history of narcotic abuse. Such patients should be closely supervised when long-term therapy is contemplated. Care should be taken to avoid increases in dosage or frequency of administration which in susceptible individuals might result in physical dependence.

Abrupt discontinuation of NUBAIN following prolonged use has been followed by symptoms of narcotic withdrawal, i.e., abdominal cramps, nausea and vomiting, rhinorrhea, lacrimation, restlessness, anxiety, elevated temperature and piloerection.

Use in Ambulatory Patients NUBAIN may impair the mental or physical abilities required for the performance of potentially dangerous tasks such as driving a car or operating machinery. Therefore, NUBAIN should be administered with caution to ambulatory patients who should be warned to avoid such hazards.

Use in Emergency Procedures Maintain patient under observation until recovered from NUBAIN effects that would affect driving or other potentially dangerous tasks.

Use in Children Clinical experience to support administration to patients under 18 years is not available at present.

Use in Pregnancy (other than labor) Safe use of NUBAIN in pregnancy has not been established. Although animal reproductive studies have not revealed teratogenic or embryotoxic effects, nalbuphine should only be administered to pregnant women when, in the judgment of the physician, the potential benefits outweigh the possible hazards.

Use During Labor and Delivery NUBAIN can produce respiratory depression in the neonate. It should be used with caution in women delivering premature infants.

Head Injury and Increased Intracranial Pressure The possible respiratory depressant effects and the potential of potent analgesics to elevate cerebrospinal fluid pressure (resulting from vasodilation following CO_2 retention) may be markedly exaggerated in the presence of head injury, intracranial lesions or a pre-existing increase in intracranial pressure. Furthermore, potent analgesics can produce effects which may obscure the clinical course of patients with head injuries. Therefore, NUBAIN should be used in these circumstances only when essential, and then should be administered with extreme caution.

Interaction With Other Central Nervous System Depressants Although NUBAIN possesses narcotic antagonist activity, there is evidence that in nondependent patients it will not antagonize a narcotic analgesic administered just before, concurrently, or just after an injection of NUBAIN. Therefore, patients receiving a narcotic analgesic, general anesthetics, phenothiazines, or other tranquilizers, sedatives, hypnotics, or other CNS depressants (including alcohol) concomitantly with NUBAIN may exhibit an additive effect. When such combined therapy is contemplated, the dose of one or both agents should be reduced.

Precautions:
Impaired Respiration At the usual adult dose of 10 mg/70 kg, NUBAIN causes some respiratory depression approximately equal to that produced by equal doses of morphine. However, in contrast to morphine, respiratory depression is not appre-

Continued on next page

DuPont—Cont.

ciably increased with higher doses of NUBAIN. Respiratory depression induced by NUBAIN can be reversed by NARCAN® (naloxone hydrochloride) when indicated. NUBAIN should be administered with caution at low doses to patients with impaired respiration (e.g., from other medication, uremia, bronchial asthma, severe infection, cyanosis or respiratory obstructions).

Impaired Renal or Hepatic Function Because NUBAIN is metabolized in the liver and excreted by the kidneys, patients with renal or liver dysfunction may over-react to custom- ary doses. Therefore, in these individuals, NUBAIN should be used with caution and administered in reduced amounts.

Myocardial Infarction As with all potent analgesics, NUBAIN should be used with caution in patients with myocardial infarction who have nausea or vomiting.

Biliary Tract Surgery As with all narcotic analgesics, NUBAIN should be used with caution in patients about to undergo surgery of the biliary tract since it may cause spasm of the sphincter of Oddi.

Adverse Reactions: The most frequent adverse reaction in 1066 patients treated with NUBAIN is sedation 381(36%).
Less frequent reactions are: sweaty/clammy 99(9%), nausea/vomiting 68(6%), dizziness/ vertigo 58(5%), dry mouth 44(4%), and headache 27(3%).
Other adverse reactions which may occur (reported incidence of 1% or less) are:
CNS Effects nervousness, depression, restlessness, crying, euphoria, floating, hostility, unusual dreams, confusion, faintness, hallucinations, dysphoria, feeling of heaviness, numbness, tingling, unreality. The incidence of psychotomimetic effects, such as unreality, depersonalization, delusions, dysphoria and hallucinations has been shown to be less than that which occurs with pentazocine.
Cardiovascular Hypertension, hypotension, bradycardia, tachycardia.
Gastrointestinal Cramps, dyspepsia, bitter taste.
Respiration Depression, dyspnea, asthma.
Dermatological Itching, burning, urticaria.
Miscellaneous Speech difficulty, urinary urgency, blurred vision, flushing and warmth.

Dosage and Administration: The usual recommended adult dose is 10 mg for a 70 kg individual, administered subcutaneously, intramuscularly or intravenously; this dose may be repeated every 3 to 6 hours as necessary. Dosage should be adjusted according to the severity of the pain, physical status of the patient, and other medications which the patient may be receiving. (See Interaction with Other Central Nervous System Depressants under WARNINGS). In non-tolerant individuals, the recommended single maximum dose is 20 mg, with a maximum total daily dose of 160 mg.

Patients Dependent on Narcotics Patients who have been taking narcotics chronically may experience withdrawal symptoms upon the administration of NUBAIN. If unduly troublesome, narcotic withdrawal symptoms can be controlled by the slow intravenous administration of small increments of morphine, until relief occurs. If the previous analgesic was morphine, meperidine, codeine, or other narcotic with similar duration of activity, one-fourth of the anticipated dose of NUBAIN can be administered initially and the patient observed for signs of withdrawal, i.e., abdominal cramps, nausea and vomiting, lacrimation, rhinorrhea, anxiety, restlessness, elevation of temperature or piloerection. If untoward symptoms do not occur, progressively larger doses may be tried at appropriate intervals until the desired level of analgesia is obtained with NUBAIN.

Management of Overdosage The immediate intravenous administration of NARCAN® (naloxone hydrochloride) is a specific antidote. Oxygen, intravenous fluids, vasopressors and other supportive measures should be used as indicated.

The administration of single doses of 72 mg of NUBAIN subcutaneously to eight normal subjects has been reported to have resulted primarily in symptoms of sleepiness and mild dysphoria.

How Supplied: NUBAIN® (nalbuphine hydrochloride) injection for intramuscular, subcutaneous, or intravenous use is available in:
NDC 0590-0385-10
   10 mg/ml, 1 ml ampuls (box of 10)
NDC 0590-0386-01
   10 mg/ml, 10 ml ampuls (box of 1)
NDC 0590-0396-10
   20 mg/ml, 1 ml ampuls (box of 10)
NDC 0590-0396-15
   20 mg/ml, 1 ml disposable pre-filled syringes (box of 10)
NDC 0590-0339-01
   20 mg/ml, 10 ml vials (box of 1)
Also available in Military Depot:
10 mg/ml, 1 ml box of 10
   NSN 6505-01-115-9852
10 mg/ml, 10 ml box of 1
   NSN 6505-01-117-9690
NARCAN® is a Registered U.S. Trademark of DuPont Pharmaceuticals, Inc.
6109-4
Shown in Product Identification Section, page 410

NUMORPHAN®
[nū-mor'fan]
(oxymorphone hydrochloride) injection

Description: NUMORPHAN (oxymorphone hydrochloride), a semisynthetic narcotic substitute for morphine, is a potent analgesic.
NUMORPHAN is 4,5α-Epoxy-3, 14-dihydroxy-17-methylmorphinan-6-one hydrochloride.
Oxymorphone hydrochloride occurs as a white or slightly off-white, odorless powder, sparingly soluble in alcohol and ether, but freely soluble in water.
NUMORPHAN injection is available in two concentrations, 1.0 mg and 1.5 mg of oxymorphone hydrochloride per ml. Both strengths contain sodium chloride 0.8%; with methylparaben 0.18%, propylparaben 0.02% and sodium dithionite 0.1%, as preservatives. pH is adjusted with sodium hydroxide.

Actions: NUMORPHAN (oxymorphone hydrochloride) is a potent narcotic analgesic. Administered parenterally, one mg of NUMORPHAN is approximately equivalent in analgesic activity to 10 mg of morphine sulfate.
The onset of action is rapid; initial effects are usually perceived within 5 to 10 minutes. Its duration of action is approximately 3 to 6 hours.
NUMORPHAN produces mild sedation and causes little depression of the cough reflex. These properties make it particularly useful in postoperative patients.

Indications: NUMORPHAN (oxymorphone hydrochloride) is indicated for the relief of moderate to severe pain. This drug is also indicated parenterally for preoperative medication, for support of anesthesia, for obstetrical analgesia, and for relief of anxiety in patients with dyspnea associated with acute left ventricular failure and pulmonary edema.

Contraindications: Safe use of NUMORPHAN (oxymorphone hydrochloride) in children under 12 years of age has not been established. This drug should not be used in patients known to be hypersensitive to morphine analogs.

Warnings: *May be habit forming.* As with other narcotic drugs, tolerance and addiction may develop. The addicting potential of the drug appears to be about the same as for morphine. Like other narcotic-containing medications, NUMORPHAN is subject to the Federal Controlled Substances Act.
Interaction with other central nervous system depressants: Patients receiving other narcotic analgesics, general anesthetics, phenothiazines, other tranquilizers, sedatives, hypnotics or other CNS depressants (including alcohol) concomitantly with NUMORPHAN may exhibit an additive CNS depression. When such combined therapy is contemplated, the dose of one or both agents should be reduced.

Safe use in pregnancy has not been established (relative to possible adverse effects on fetal development). As with other analgesics, the use of NUMORPHAN (oxymorphone hydrochloride) in pregnancy, in nursing mothers, or in women of childbearing potential requires that the possible benefits of the drug be weighed against the possible hazards to the mother and the fetus.

Precautions: The same care and caution should be taken when administering NUMORPHAN (oxymorphone hydrochloride) as when other potent narcotic analgesics are used. It should be borne in mind that some respiratory depression may occur as with all potent narcotics especially when other analgesic and/or anesthetic drugs with depressant action have been given shortly before administration of NUMORPHAN.
The respiratory depressant effects of narcotics and their capacity to elevate cerebrospinal fluid pressure may be markedly exaggerated in the presence of head injury, other intracranial lesions or a preexisting increase in intracranial pressure. Furthermore narcotics produce adverse reactions which may obscure the clinical course of patients with head injuries.
As with other analgesics, caution must also be exercised in elderly and debilitated patients and in patients who are known to be sensitive to central nervous system depressants, such as those with cardiovascular, pulmonary, or hepatic disease, in hypothyroidism (myxedema), acute alcoholism, delirium tremens, convulsive disorders, bronchial asthma and kyphoscoliosis. Debilitated and elderly patients and those with severe liver diseases should receive smaller doses of NUMORPHAN.

Adverse Reactions: As with all potent narcotic analgesics, possible side effects include drowsiness, nausea, vomiting, miosis, itching, dysphoria, light-headedness, and headache. Respiratory depression may occur with oxymorphone as with other narcotics.

Dosage and Administration: Usual Adult Dosage of NUMORPHAN (oxymorphone hydrochloride) Injection: Subcutaneous or intramuscular administration: initially 1 mg to 1.5 mg, repeated every 4 to 6 hours as needed. Intravenous: 0.5 mg initially. In nondebilitated patients the dose can be cautiously increased until satisfactory pain relief is obtained. For analgesia during labor 0.5 mg to 1 mg intramuscularly is recommended.

Management of Overdosage: *Signs and Symptoms:* Serious overdosage with NUMORPHAN is characterized by respiratory depression (a decrease in respiratory rate and/or tidal volume, Cheyne-Stokes respiration, cyanosis), extreme somnolence progressing to stupor or coma, skeletal muscle flaccidity, cold and clammy skin, and sometimes bradycardia and hypotension. In severe overdosage, apnea, circulatory collapse, cardiac arrest and death may occur.
Treatment: Primary attention should be given to the reestablishment of adequate respiratory exchange through provision of a patent airway and the institution of assisted or controlled ventilation. The narcotic antagonist naloxone hydrochloride (NARCAN®) is a specific antidote against respiratory depression which may result from overdosage or unusual sensitivity to narcotics including oxymorphone. Therefore, an appropriate dose of naloxone hydrochloride should be administered (usual initial adult dose: 0.4 mg) preferably by the intravenous route and simultaneously with efforts at respiratory resuscitation. Since the duration of action of oxymorphone may exceed that of the antagonist, the patient should be kept under continued surveillance and repeated doses of the antagonist should be administered as needed to maintain adequate respiration.
Oxygen, intravenous fluids, vasopressors and other supportive measures should be employed as indicated.

How Supplied:
For Injection: DEA Order Form Required
1 mg/ml   1 ml ampuls (box of 10)
   NDC 0590-0370-10
1.5 mg/ml   1 ml ampuls (box of 10)

NDC 0590-0373-10
10 ml multiple dose vial (box of 1)
NDC 0590-0374-01
NARCAN® is a Registered Trademark of DuPont Pharmaceuticals, Inc.
6110-2

†PERCOCET®
[perk'o-set]

Description:
Each tablet of PERCOCET® contains:
Oxycodone hydrochloride ....5 mg
WARNING: May be habit forming
Acetaminophen (APAP) ....325 mg
The oxycodone component is 14-hydroxydihydrocodeinone, a white, odorless crystalline powder which is derived from the opium alkaloid, thebaine.

Actions: The principal analgesic ingredient, oxycodone, is a semisynthetic narcotic with multiple actions qualitatively similar to those of morphine; the most prominent of these involve the central nervous system and organs composed of smooth muscle. The principal actions of therapeutic value of the oxycodone in PERCOCET® are analgesia and sedation.
Oxycodone is similar to codeine and methadone in that it retains at least one half of its analgesic activity when administered orally.
PERCOCET® also contains the non-narcotic antipyretic-analgesic acetaminophen.

Indications: For the relief of moderate to moderately severe pain.

Contraindications: Hypersensitivity to oxycodone or acetaminophen.

Warnings:
Drug Dependence: Oxycodone can produce drug dependence of the morphine type and, therefore, has the potential for being abused. Psychic dependence, physical dependence and tolerance may develop upon repeated administration of PERCOCET®, and it should be prescribed and administered with the same degree of caution appropriate to the use of other oral narcotic-containing medications. Like other narcotic-containing medications, PERCOCET® is subject to the Federal Controlled Substances Act.

Usage in ambulatory patients: Oxycodone may impair the mental and/or physical abilities required for the performance of potentially hazardous tasks such as driving a car or operating machinery. The patient using PERCOCET® should be cautioned accordingly.

Interaction with other central nervous system depressants: Patients receiving other narcotic analgesics, general anesthetics, phenothiazines, other tranquilizers, sedative-hypnotics or other CNS depressants (including alcohol) concomitantly with PERCOCET® may exhibit an additive CNS depression. When such combined therapy is contemplated, the dose of one or both agents should be reduced.

Usage in pregnancy: Safe use in pregnancy has not been established relative to possible adverse effects on fetal development. Therefore, PERCOCET® should not be used in pregnant women unless, in the judgment of the physician, the potential benefits outweigh the possible hazards.

Usage in children: PERCOCET® should not be administered to children.

Precautions:
Head injury and increased intracranial pressure: The respiratory depressant effects of narcotics and their capacity to elevate cerebrospinal fluid pressure may be markedly exaggerated in the presence of head injury, other intracranial lesions or a pre-existing increase in intracranial pressure. Furthermore, narcotics produce adverse reactions which may obscure the clinical course of patients with head injuries.

Acute abdominal conditions: The administration of PERCOCET® or other narcotics may obscure the diagnosis or clinical course in patients with acute abdominal conditions.

Special risk patients: PERCOCET® should be given with caution to certain patients such as the elderly or debilitated, and those with severe impairment of hepatic or renal function, hypothyroidism, Addison's disease, and prostatic hypertrophy or urethral stricture.

Adverse Reactions: The most frequently observed adverse reactions include light headedness, dizziness, sedation, nausea and vomiting. These effects seem to be more prominent in ambulatory than in nonambulatory patients, and some of these adverse reactions may be alleviated if the patient lies down.
Other adverse reactions include euphoria, dysphoria, constipation, skin rash and pruritus.

Dosage and Administration: Dosage should be adjusted according to the severity of the pain and the response of the patient. It may occasionally be necessary to exceed the usual dosage recommended below in cases of more severe pain or in those patients who have become tolerant to the analgesic effect of narcotics. PERCOCET® is given orally. The usual adult dose is one tablet every 6 hours as needed for pain.

Drug Interactions: The CNS depressant effects of PERCOCET® may be additive with that of other CNS depressants. See WARNINGS.

Management of Overdosage:
Signs and Symptoms: Serious overdose with PERCOCET® is characterized by respiratory depression (a decrease in respiratory rate and/or tidal volume, Cheyne-Stokes respiration, cyanosis), extreme somnolence progressing to stupor or coma, skeletal muscle flaccidity, cold and clammy skin, and sometimes bradycardia and hypotension. In severe overdosage, apnea, circulatory collapse, cardiac arrest and death may occur. The ingestion of very large amounts of PERCOCET® may, in addition, result in acute hepatic toxicity.

Treatment: Primary attention should be given to the reestablishment of adequate respiratory exchange through provision of a patent airway and the institution of assisted or controlled ventilation. The narcotic antagonist naloxone hydrochloride (NARCAN®) is a specific antidote against respiratory depression which may result from overdosage or unusual sensitivity to narcotics including oxycodone. Therefore, an appropriate dose of naloxone hydrochloride should be administered (usual adult dose: 0.4 mg) preferably by the intraveous route, simultaneously with efforts at respiratory resuscitation. Since the duration of action of oxycodone may exceed that of the antagonist, the patient should be kept under continued surveillance and repeated doses of the antagonist should be administered as needed to maintain adequate respiration.
Oxygen, intravenous fluids, vasopressors and other supportive measures should be employed as indicated.
Gastric emptying may be useful in removing unabsorbed drug.
Acetaminophen in massive overdosage may cause hepatotoxicity in some patients. Clinical and laboratory evidence of hepatotoxicity may be delayed for up to one week. Close clinical monitoring and serial hepatic enzyme determinations are therefore recommended.
Treatment of acute acetaminophen overdosage is purely symptomatic.

How Supplied:
As white, scored tablets available in:
  Bottles of 100   NDC 0060-0127-70
  Bottles of 500   NDC 0060-0127-85
  Hospital blister pack of 25 NDC 0060-0127-25
  (available in units of 250 and 1,000)
Also available in Military Depot:
Bottle of 100 NSN 6505-01-082-5509
Blister Pack (250) NSN 6505-01-071-8405
DEA Order Form Required
PERCOCET® is a registered Trademark of DuPont Pharmaceuticals Caribe, Inc. NARCAN® is a Registered U.S. Trademark of DuPont Pharmaceuticals, Inc.
6090-4

†Product of DuPont Pharmaceuticals Caribe, Inc.
Shown in Product Identification Section, page 410

†PERCODAN®
[perk'o-dan]
†PERCODAN®-DEMI
Tablets

Description:
Each tablet of PERCODAN® contains:
Oxycodone hydrochloride ....4.50 mg
  WARNING: May be habit forming
Oxycodone terephthalate ....0.38 mg
  WARNING: May be habit forming
Aspirin ....325 mg
Each tablet of PERCODAN®-Demi contains:
Oxycodone hydrochloride ....2.25 mg
  WARNING: May be habit forming
Oxycodone terephthalate ....0.19 mg
  WARNING: May be habit forming
Aspirin ....325 mg
The oxycodone component is 14-hydroxydihydrocodeinone, a white odorless crystalline powder which is derived from the opium alkaloid, thebaine.

Actions: The principal ingredient, oxycodone, is a semisynthetic narcotic analgesic with multiple actions qualitatively similar to those of morphine; the most prominent of these involve the central nervous system and organs composed of smooth muscle. The principal actions of therapeutic value of the oxycodone in PERCODAN® and PERCODAN®-Demi are analgesia and sedation.
Oxycodone is similar to codeine and methadone in that it retains at least one half of its analgesic activity when administered orally.
PERCODAN® and PERCODAN®-Demi also contain the non-narcotic antipyretic-analgesic, aspirin.

Indications: For the relief of moderate to moderately severe pain.

Contraindications: Hypersensitivity to oxycodone or aspirin.

Warnings:
Drug Dependence: Oxycodone can produce drug dependence of the morphine type and, therefore, has the potential for being abused. Psychic dependence, physical dependence and tolerance may develop upon repeated administration of PERCODAN® and PERCODAN®-Demi, and it should be prescribed and administered with the same degree of caution appropriate to the use of other oral narcotic-containing medications. Like other narcotic-containing medications, PERCODAN® and PERCODAN®-Demi are subject to the Federal Controlled Substances Act.

Usage in ambulatory patients: Oxycodone may impair the mental and/or physical abilities required for the performance of potentially hazardous tasks such as driving a car or operating machinery. The patient using PERCODAN® and PERCODAN®-Demi should be cautioned accordingly.

Interaction with other central nervous system depressants: Patients receiving other narcotic analgesics, general anesthetics, phenothiazines, other tranquilizers, sedative-hypnotics or other CNS depressants (including alcohol) concomitantly with PERCODAN® and PERCODAN®-Demi may exhibit an additive CNS depression. When such combined therapy is contemplated, the dose of one or both agents should be reduced.

Usage in pregnancy: Safe use in pregnancy has not been established relative to possible adverse effects on fetal development. Therefore, PERCODAN® and PERCODAN®-Demi should not be used in pregnant women unless, in the judgment of the physician, the potential benefits outweigh the possible hazards.

Usage in children: PERCODAN® should not be administered to children. PERCODAN®-Demi, containing half the amount of oxycodone, can be considered. (See Dosage and Administration for PERCODAN®-Demi).
Salicylates should be used with caution in the presence of peptic ulcer or coagulation abnormalities.

Continued on next page

DuPont—Cont.

Precautions:
Head injury and increased intracranial pressure: The respiratory depressant effects of narcotics and their capacity to elevate cerebrospinal fluid pressure may be markedly exaggerated in the presence of head injury, other intracranial lesions or a pre-existing increase in intracranial pressure. Furthermore, narcotics produce adverse reactions which may obscure the clinical course of patients with head injuries.
Acute abdominal conditions: The administration of PERCODAN® and PERCODAN®-Demi or other narcotics may obscure the diagnosis or clinical course in patients with acute abdominal conditions.
Special risk patients: PERCODAN® and PERCODAN®-Demi should be given with caution to certain patients such as the elderly or debilitated, and those with severe impairment of hepatic or renal function, hypothyroidism, Addison's disease, and prostatic hypertrophy or urethral stricture.
Adverse Reactions: The most frequently observed adverse reactions include light headedness, dizziness, sedation, nausea and vomiting. These effects seem to be more prominent in ambulatory than in nonambulatory patients, and some of these adverse reactions may be alleviated if the patient lies down.
Other adverse reactions include euphoria, dysphoria, constipation and pruritus.
Dosage and Administration: Dosage should be adjusted according to the severity of the pain and the response of the patient. It may occasionally be necessary to exceed the usual dosage recommended below in cases of more severe pain or in those patients who have become tolerant to the analgesic effect of narcotics. PERCODAN® and PERCODAN®-Demi are given orally.
PERCODAN®: The usual adult dose is one tablet every 6 hours as needed for pain.
PERCODAN®-Demi: Adults—One or two tablets every six hours. Children 12 years and older—One-half tablet every six hours. Children 6 to 12 years—One-quarter tablet every six hours. PERCODAN®-Demi is not indicated for children under 6 years of age.
Drug Interactions: The CNS depressant effects of PERCODAN® and PERCODAN®-Demi may be additive with that of other CNS depressants. See WARNINGS.
Aspirin may enhance the effect of anticoagulants and inhibit the uricosuric effects of uricosuric agents.
Management of Overdosage:
Signs and Symptoms: Serious overdose with PERCODAN® or PERCODAN®-Demi is characterized by respiratory depression (a decrease in respiratory rate and/or tidal volume, Cheyne-Stokes respiration, cyanosis), extreme somnolence progressing to stupor or coma, skeletal muscle flaccidity, cold and clammy skin, and sometimes bradycardia and hypotension. In severe overdosage, apnea, circulatory collapse, cardiac arrest and death may occur. The ingestion of very large amounts of PERCODAN® or PERCODAN®-Demi may, in addition, result in acute salicylate intoxication.
Treatment: Primary attention should be given to the reestablishment of adequate respiratory exchange through provision of a patent airway and the institution of assisted or controlled ventilation. The narcotic antagonist naloxone hydrochloride (NARCAN®) is a specific antidote against respiratory depression which may result from overdosage or unusual sensitivity to narcotics, including oxycodone. Therefore, an appropriate dose of naloxone hydrochloride should be administered (usual adult dose: 0.4 mg) preferably by the intravenous route, simultaneously with efforts at respiratory resuscitation. Since the duration of action of oxycodone may exceed that of the antagonist, the patient should be kept under continued surveillance and repeated doses of the antagonist should be administered as needed to maintain adequate respiration.
Oxygen, intravenous fluids, vasopressors and other supportive measures should be employed as indicated.
Gastric emptying may be useful in removing unabsorbed drug.
How Supplied:
Percodan®—As yellow, scored tablets, available in:

Bottles of 100	NDC 0060-0135-70
Bottles of 500	NDC 0060-0135-85
Bottles of 1000	NDC 0060-0135-90
Hospital blister pack of 25	NDC 0060-0135-65
(available in units of 250 and 1000)	

Also available in Military Depot:
Btl's of 100 NSN 6505-01-030-9493
Blister Pack (250) NSN 6505-01-030-9492
Percodan®-Demi—As pink, scored tablets available in:

Bottles of 100	NDC 0060-0136-70
Bottles of 500	NDC 0060-0136-85

DEA Order Form Required
Shown in Product Identification Section, page 410
PERCODAN is a registered U.S. trademark of DuPont Pharmaceuticals Caribe, Inc.
†Products of DuPont Pharmaceuticals Caribe, Inc. 6117-3/6118-3
NARCAN is a Registered U.S. Trademark of DuPont Pharmaceuticals, Inc.

REMSED® TABLETS   R
[rem'sed]
(promethazine hydrochloride)

Description: REMSED (promethazine hydrochloride) is a phenothiazine derivative.
Actions: REMSED, a phenothiazine, possesses antihistaminic, sedative, anti-motion, antiemetic and anticholinergic effects. The duration of action is generally from 4 to 6 hours. As an antihistamine it acts by competitive antagonism, but does not block the release of histamine. It antagonizes in varying degrees most, but not all, of the pharmacological effects of histamine.
Indications: REMSED (promethazine hydrochloride) is indicated for the production of light sleep from which the patient can be easily aroused. In addition, REMSED can provide:
 a) sedation in both children and adults.
 b) relief of apprehension
 c) preoperative, postoperative, and obstetric sedation.
REMSED can also be of clinical use as follows:
 a) adjunctive therapy with meperidine or other analgesics for control of postoperative pain.
 b) for prevention and control of nausea and vomiting associated with anesthesia and surgery.
 c) as an antiemetic in postoperative patients.
 d) for active and prophylactic treatment of motion sickness.
Contraindications: REMSED is contraindicated in comatose patients. It is also contraindicated in patients receiving monoamine oxidase inhibitors and in patients who have received large amounts of central nervous system depressants (alcohol, barbiturates, narcotics, etc.). Additionally, the drug is contraindicated in patients who have demonstrated an idiosyncrasy or hypersensitivity to REMSED or to other phenothiazines.
REMSED is contraindicated in patients with bone marrow depression, narrow-angle glaucoma, bladder neck obstruction, prostatic hypertrophy, pyloroduodenal obstruction and stenosing peptic ulcer. The drug should not be used in patients during asthmatic attacks or to treat lower respiratory tract symptoms.
REMSED is contraindicated in newborn or premature infants. It should not be used in acutely ill or dehydrated children because there is an increased susceptibility to dystonias.
Warnings: REMSED may impair the mental and/or physical abilities required for the performance of potentially hazardous tasks such as driving a vehicle or operating machinery. Similarly, it may impair mental alertness in children. The concomitant use of alcohol or other central nervous system depressants may have an additive effect. Patients should be warned accordingly.
Usage in Pregnancy: The safe use of REMSED has not been established with respect to the possible adverse effects upon fetal development. Therefore, it should not be used in women of childbearing potential, particularly during early pregnancy, or in lactating women unless in the judgment of the physician the potential benefits outweigh the possible risks. There are reports of jaundice and prolonged extrapyramidal symptoms in infants whose mothers received phenothiazines during pregnancy. Therefore, the use of this drug during early pregnancy, or in lactating women, should be undertaken only after weighing possible risks against potential benefit. REMSED may interfere with the accuracy of diagnostic tests for pregnancy.

Caution should be exercised when administering REMSED to children for the treatment of vomiting. Antiemetics are not recommended for treatment of uncomplicated vomiting in children and their use should be limited to prolonged vomiting of known etiology. There are three principal reasons for caution:
1. There has been some suspicion that centrally acting antiemetics may contribute, in combination with viral illnesses (a possible cause of vomiting in children), to development of Reye's syndrome, a potentially fatal acute childhood encephalopathy with visceral fatty degeneration, especially involving the liver. Although there is no confirmation of this suspicion, caution is nevertheless recommended.
2. The extrapyramidal symptoms which can occur secondary to REMSED may be confused with the central nervous system signs of an undiagnosed primary disease responsible for the vomiting, e.g., Reye's syndrome or other encephalopathy.
3. It has been suspected that drugs with hepatotoxic potential, such as REMSED, may unfavorably alter the course of Reye's syndrome. Such drugs should therefore be avoided in children whose signs and symptoms (vomiting) could represent Reye's syndrome.
It should also be noted that salicylates and acetaminophen are hepatotoxic at large doses. Although it is not known that at usual doses they would represent a hazard in patients with the underlying hepatic disorder of Reye's syndrome, these drugs, too, should be avoided in children whose signs and symptoms could represent Reye's syndrome, unless alternative methods of controlling fever are not successful.

Precautions: REMSED (promethazine hydrochloride) may significantly affect the actions of other drugs. It may increase, prolong or intensify the sedative action of central nervous system depressants such as anesthetics, barbiturates or alcohol. The dose of a narcotic or barbiturate may be reduced to $\frac{1}{4}$ or $\frac{1}{2}$ the usual amount when REMSED is administered concomitantly. Excessive amounts of REMSED, relative to a narcotic, may lead to restlessness and motor hyperactivity in the patient with pain.
REMSED can block and even reverse some of the actions of epinephrine.
The drug should also be used cautiously in persons with acute or chronic respiratory impairment, particularly children, because of possible suppression of the cough reflex.
REMSED should be used cautiously in persons with cardiovascular disease, impairment of liver function or a history of ulcer disease.
Because of its antiemetic effect, REMSED may mask signs of overdosage of toxic drugs or may obscure conditions such as brain tumor or intestinal obstruction.
Neuroleptic drugs elevate prolactin levels; the elevation persists during chronic administration. Tissue culture experiments indicate that approxi-

mately one-third of human breast cancers are prolactin dependent in vitro, a factor of potential importance if the prescription of these drugs is contemplated in a patient with a previously detected breast cancer. Although disturbances such as galactorrhea, amenorrhea, gynecomastia, and impotence have been reported, the clinical significance of elevated serum prolactin levels is unknown for most patients. An increase in mammary neoplasms has been found in rodents after chronic administration of neuroleptic drugs. Neither clinical studies nor epidemiologic studies conducted to date, however, have shown an association between chronic administration of these drugs and mammary tumorigenesis; the available evidence is considered too limited to be conclusive at this time.

Adverse Reactions:
Note: Not all of the following adverse reactions have been reported with this specific drug; however, pharmacological similarities among phenothiazine derivatives require that each be considered when REMSED is administered. There have been occasional reports of sudden death in patients receiving phenothiazine derivatives chronically.

CNS Effects: Drowsiness is the most prominent CNS effect of this drug. Extrapyramidal reactions occur, particularly with high dosages. Hyperreflexia has been reported in the newborn when a phenothiazine was used during pregnancy. Other reported reactions include blurred vision, diplopia, dizziness, euphoria, fatigue, grand mal seizures, incoordination, insomnia, lassitude, nervousness, tinnitus and tremors.

Cardiovascular Effects: Postural hypotension is the most common cardiovascular effect of REMSED. Reflex tachycardia may be seen. Bradycardia, faintness, dizziness and cardiac arrest have been reported. EKG changes, including blunting of T waves and prolongation of the Q-T interval, may be seen.

Gastrointestinal: Anorexia, constipation, dry mouth, epigastric distress, nausea and vomiting may occur.

Genitourinary: Urinary frequency and dysuria may occur.

Allergic Reactions: These include anaphylactoid reactions, angioedema, asthma, dermatitis, laryngeal edema and urticaria.

The following adverse reactions have been reported with all phenothiazines but are less common with REMSED: agranulocytosis, leukopenia, jaundice and extrapyramidal reactions.

Dosage and Administration: The usual adult daytime dose is 12.5 mg to 25 mg, 3 to 4 times daily. The usual adult bedtime dose is 50 mg. The dose for preoperative, postoperative and obstetrical sedation is 25 mg to 50 mg; 50 mg will provide sedation and relief of apprehension in early stages of labor.

Pediatric and geriatric doses may be adjusted according to age and weight.

When used prophylactically for motion sickness, the usual adult dose is 12.5 mg to 25 mg, 3 or 4 times daily. An initial dose of 25 mg should be taken ½ to 1 hour before anticipated travel.

Overdosage: Signs of overdosage include excitation, ataxia, incoordination, athetosis, convulsion and coma. Common signs in children are fixed, dilated pupils, fever and a flushed face. The treatment is symptomatic and supportive.

Drug Interactions: Phenothiazine medications include a large number of related molecular structures with many pharmacologic actions, including antihistaminic, antinauseant, antihypertensive, sedative and tranquilizing properties. As a result, they may interact with other medications, potentiating those drugs having similar pharmacologic effects, and antagonizing others having the opposite actions. Whenever REMSED is used concomitantly with other medications, the patient should be observed carefully for drug interactions.

How Supplied: REMSED is available as: Tablets—50 mg (light blue, scored) in bottles of 100 NDC 0056-0051-70.

REMSED® is a U.S. Trademark of E.I. duPont de Nemours & Co. (Inc.)

6048-5

SYMMETREL® ℞
[sim'e-trel"]
(amantadine hydrochloride)

Description SYMMETREL is designated generically as amantadine hydrochloride and chemically as 1-adamantanamine hydrochloride.

Amantadine hydrochloride is a stable white or nearly white crystalline powder, freely soluble in water and soluble in alcohol and in chloroform.

Amantadine hydrochloride has pharmacological actions as both an anti-Parkinson and an antiviral drug.

SYMMETREL is available in capsules and syrup.

Clinical Pharmacology: SYMMETREL is readily absorbed, is not metabolized, and is excreted unchanged in the urine.

After oral administration of a single dose of 100 mg. maximum blood levels are reached, based on the mean time of the peak urinary excretion rate, in approximately 4 hours; the peak excretion rate is approximately 5 mg/hr; the mean half-life of the excretion rate approximates 15 hours.

The mechanism of action of SYMMETREL in the treatment of Parkinson's disease and drug-induced extrapyramidal reactions is not known. It has been shown to cause an increase in dopamine release in the animal brain. The drug does not possess anticholinergic activity in animal tests at doses similar to those used clinically. The antiviral activity of SYMMETREL against influenza A virus is not completely understood. The mode of action of SYMMETREL appears to be the prevention of the release of infectious viral nucleic acid into the host cell. SYMMETREL does not appear to interfere with the immunogenicity of inactivated influenza A virus vaccine.

Indications and Usage: Parkinson's Disease/Syndrome and Drug-Induced Extrapyramidal Reactions: SYMMETREL is indicated in the treatment of idiopathic Parkinson's disease (Paralysis Agitans), postencephalitic parkinsonism, drug-induced extrapyramidal reactions, and symptomatic parkinsonism which may follow injury to the nervous system by carbon monoxide intoxication. It is indicated in those elderly patients believed to develop parkinsonism in association with cerebral arteriosclerosis. In the treatment of Parkinson's disease, SYMMETREL is less effective than levodopa, (1)-3-(3, 4-dihydroxyphenyl)-L-ala- nine, and its efficacy in comparison with the anticholinergic antiparkinson drugs has not yet been established. Although anticholinergic type side effects have been noted with SYMMETREL when used in patients with drug-induced extrapyramidal reactions, there is a lower incidence of these side effects than that observed with anticholinergic antiparkinson drugs.

Influenza A Virus Respiratory Tract Illness: SYMMETREL (amantadine hydrochloride) is indicated in the prevention and treatment of respiratory tract illness caused by influenza A virus strains. SYMMETREL should be considered especially for high risk patients, close household or hospital ward contacts of index cases and patients with severe influenza A virus illness. In the prophylaxis of influenza due to A virus strains, early immunization as periodically recommended by the Public Health Service Advisory Committee on Immunization Practices is the method of choice. When early immunization is not feasible, or when the vaccine is contraindicated or not available. SYMMETREL can be used for chemoprophylaxis against influenza A virus illness. Because SYMMETREL does not appear to suppress antibody response, it can be used chemoprophylactically in conjunction with inactivated influenza A virus vaccine until protective antibody responses develop. There is no clinical evidence that this drug has efficacy in the prophylaxis or treatment of viral respiratory tract illnesses other than those caused by influenza A virus strains.

Contraindications: SYMMETREL in contraindicated in patients with known hypersensitivity to the drug.

Warnings: Patients with a history of epilepsy or other "seizures" should be observed closely for possible increased seizure activity.

Patients with a history of congestive heart failure or peripheral edema should be followed closely as there are patients who developed congestive heart failure while receiving SYMMETREL.

Patients with Parkinson's disease improving on SYMMETREL should resume normal activities gradually and cautiously, consistent with other medical considerations, such as the presence of osteoporosis or phlebothrombosis.

Patients receiving SYMMETREL who note central nervous system effects or blurring of visions should be cautioned against driving or working in situations where alertness is important.

Precautions: SYMMETREL (amantadine hydrochloride) should not be discontinued abruptly since a few patients with Parkinson's disease experienced a parkinsonian crisis, i.e., a sudden marked clinical deterioration, when this medication was suddenly stopped. The dose of anticholinergic drugs or of SYMMETREL should be reduced if atropine-like effects appear when these drugs are used concurrently.

The dose of SYMMETREL may need careful adjustment in patients with renal impairment, congestive heart failure, peripheral edema, or orthostatic hypotension. Since SYMMETREL is not metabolized and is mainly excreted in the urine, it may accumulate when renal function is inadequate.

Care should be exercised when administering SYMMETREL to patients with liver disease, a history of recurrent eczematoid rash, or to patients with psychosis or severe psychoneurosis not controlled by chemotherapeutic agents. Careful observation is required when SYMMETREL is administered concurrently with central nervous system stimulants.

No long-term studies in animals have been performed to evaluate the carcinogenic potential of SYMMETREL.

The mutagenic potential of the drug has not yet been determined in experimental systems.

Pregnancy Category C: SYMMETREL (amantadine hydrochloride) has been shown to be embryotoxic and teratogenic in rats at 50 mg/kg/day, about 12 times the recommended human dose, but not at 37 mg/kg/day. Embryotoxic and teratogenic drug effects were not seen in rabbits which received up to 25 times the recommended human dose. There are no adequate and well-controlled studies in pregnant women.

SYMMETREL should be used during pregnancy only if the potential benefit justifies the potential risk to the embryo or the fetus.

Nursing Mothers: SYMMETREL is excreted in human milk. Caution should be exercised when SYMMETREL is administered to a nursing woman.

Pediatric Use: The safety and efficacy of SYMMETREL in newborn infants, and infants below the age of 1 year have not been established.

Adverse Reactions: The most frequently occurring serious adverse reactions are depression, congestive heart failure, orthostatic hypotensive episodes, psychosis, and urinary retention. Rarely convulsions, leukopenia, and neutropenia have been reported.

Other adverse reactions of a less serious nature which have been observed are the following: hallucinations, confusion, anxiety and irritability, anorexia, nausea, and constipation; ataxia and dizziness (lightheadedness); livedo reticularis and peripheral edema. Adverse reactions observed less frequently are the following: vomiting; dry mouth; headache; dyspnea; fatigue, insomnia, and a sense of weakness. Infrequently, skin rash, slurred speech, and visual disturbances have been observed. Rarely eczematoid dermatitis and oculogyric episodes have been reported.

Overdosage: There is no specific antidote. However, slowly administered intravenous physostigmine in 1 and 2 mg doses in an adult[1] at 1 to 2 hour intervals and 0.5 mg doses in a child[2] at 5 to 10 minute intervals up to a maximum of 2 mg/hour have been reported to be effective in the control of

Continued on next page

DuPont—Cont.

central nervous system toxicity caused by amantadine hydrochloride. For acute overdosing, general supportive measures should be employed along with immediate gastric lavage or induction of emesis. Fluids should be forced, and if necessary, given intravenously. The pH of the urine has been reported to influence the excretion rate of SYMMETREL. Since the excretion rate of SYMMETREL increases rapidly when the urine is acidic, the administration of urine acidifying drugs may increase the elimination of the drug from the body. The blood pressure, pulse, respiration and temperature should be monitored. The patient should be observed for hyperactivity and convulsions; if required, sedation, and anticonvulsant therapy should be administered. The patient should be observed for the possible development of arrhythmias and hypotension, if required, appropriate antiarrhythmic and antihypotensive therapy should be given. The blood electrolytes, urine pH and urinary output should be monitored. If there is no record of recent voiding, catheterization should be done. The possibility of multiple drug ingestion by the patient should be considered.

[1] D.F. Casey, N. Engl. J. Med. 298:516, 1978.
[2] C.D. Berkowitz, J. Pediatr. 95:144, 1979.

Dosage and Administration:
Dosage for Parkinsonism:
Adult: The usual dose of SYMMETREL (amantadine hydrochloride) is 100 mg twice a day when used alone. SYMMETREL has an onset of action usually within 48 hours.
The initial dose of SYMMETREL is 100 mg daily for patients with serious associated medical illnesses or who are receiving high doses of other antiparkinson drugs. After one to several weeks at 100 mg once daily, the dose may be increased to 100 mg twice daily, if necessary.
Occasionally, patients whose responses are not optimal with SYMMETREL at 200 mg daily may benefit from an increase up to 400 mg daily in divided doses. However, such patients should be supervised closely by their physicians.
Patients initially deriving benefit from SYMMETREL not uncommonly experience a fall-off of effectiveness after a few months. Benefit may be regained by increasing the dose to 300 mg daily. Alternatively, temporary discontinuation of SYMMETREL for several weeks, followed by reinitiation of the drug, may result in regaining benefit in some patients. A decision to use other antiparkinson drugs may be necessary.
Dosage for Concomitant Therapy
Some patients who do not respond to anticholinergic antiparkinson drugs may respond to SYMMETREL. When SYMMETREL or anticholinergic antiparkinson drugs are each used with marginal benefit, concomitant use may produce additional benefit.
When SYMMETREL and levodopa are initiated concurrently, the patient can exhibit rapid therapeutic benefits. SYMMETREL should be held constant at 100 mg daily or twice daily while the daily dose of levodopa is gradually increased to optimal benefit.
When SYMMETREL is added to optimal well-tolerated doses of levodopa, additional benefit may result, including smoothing out the fluctuations in improvement which sometimes occur in patients on levodopa alone. Patients who require a reduction in their usual dose of levodopa because of development of side effects may possibly regain lost benefit with the addition of SYMMETREL.

Dosage for Drug-induced Extrapyramidal Reactions:
Adult: The usual dose of SYMMETREL (amantadine hydrochloride) is 100 mg twice a day. Occasionally, patients whose responses are not optimal with SYMMETREL at 200 mg daily may benefit from an increase up to 300 mg daily in divided doses.

Dosage for Prophylaxis and Treatment of Influenza A Virus Respiratory Tract Illness:
Adult: The adult daily dosage of SYMMETREL (amantadine hydrochloride) is 200 mg; two 100 mg capsules (or four teaspoonfuls of syrup) as a single daily dose, or the daily dosage may be split into one capsule of 100 mg (or two teaspoonfuls of syrup) twice a day. If central nervous system effects develop on once-a-day dosage, a split dosage schedule may reduce such complaints.
Children: 1 yr.–9 yrs. of age: The total daily dose should be calculated on the basis of 2 to 4 mg/lb/day (4.4 to 8.8 mg/kg/day), but not to exceed 150 mg per day.
9 yrs.–12 yrs. of age: The total daily dose is 200 mg given as one capsule of 100 mg (or two teaspoonfuls of syrup) twice a day.
Prophylactic dosing should be started in anticipation of contact or as soon as possible after contact with individuals with influenza A virus respiratory illness. SYMMETREL should be continued daily for at least 10 days following a known exposure. If SYMMETREL is used chemoprophylactically in conjunction with inactivated influenza A virus vaccine until protective antibody responses develop, then it should be administered for 2 to 3 weeks after the vaccine has been given. When inactivated influenza A virus vaccine is unavailable or contraindicated, SYMMETREL should be administered for up to 90 days in case of possible repeated and unknown exposures. Treatment of influenza A virus illness should be started as soon as possible after onset of symptoms and should be continued for 24 to 48 hours after the disappearance of symptoms.

How Supplied: SYMMETREL (amantadine hydrochloride) is available as capsules (each red, soft gelatin capsule contains 100 mg amantadine hydrochloride) in

Bottles of 100   NDC 0056-0105-70
Bottles of 500   NDC 0056-0105-85
Hospital Unit-Dose blister package of 100
       NDC 0056-0105-75
As a syrup (each 5 ml [1 teaspoonful] contains 50 mg amantadine hydrochloride) in 16 oz. (480 ml) bottles NDC 0056-0205-16.
Also available in Military Depot:
Btl's of 100 NSN 6505-00-148-4624
In VA Depot:
Btls. of 100 NSN 6505-00-148-4624A
SYMMETREL is a Registered U.S. Trademark of E.I. duPont de Nemours & Co. (Inc.)
Capsules manufactured by
R.P. Scherer-North America,
St. Petersburg, Florida 33733
For DuPont Pharmaceuticals
6043-14

Shown in Product Identification Section, page 410

TESSALON® ℞
[*tes'a-lon''*]
(benzonatate USP)

Description: TESSALON®, a nonnarcotic antitussive agent, is 2, 5, 8, 11, 14, 17, 20, 23, 26-nonaoxaoctacosan-28-yl p-(butylamino) benzoate.
Actions: TESSALON® acts peripherally by anesthetizing the stretch receptors located in the respiratory passages, lungs, and pleura by dampening their activity and thereby reducing the cough reflex at its source. It begins to act within 15 to 20 minutes and its effect lasts for 3 to 8 hours. TESSALON® has no inhibitory effect on the respiratory center in recommended dosage.
Indications: Symptomatic relief of cough.
Contraindications: Hypersensitivity to benzonatate or related compounds.
Warnings: Usage in Pregnancy: The safe use of this drug in pregnant women or during lactation has not been established. Therefore, the benefits must be weighed against the potential hazards.
Precautions: Release of TESSALON® from the perle in the mouth can produce a temporary local anesthesia of the oral mucosa. Therefore, the perles should be swallowed without chewing.
Adverse Reactions: Sedation, headache, mild dizziness, pruritus and skin eruptions, nasal congestion, constipation, nausea, gastrointestinal upset, sensation of burning in the eyes, a vague "chilly" sensation, numbness in the chest, and hypersensitivity have been reported.
Dosage and Administration: *Adults and Children over 10:* Usual dose is one 100 mg perle t.i.d. as required. If necessary, up to 6 perles daily may be given.
Overdosage: No clinically significant cases have been reported, to our knowledge. The drug is chemically related to tetracaine and other topical anesthetics and shares various aspects of their pharmacology and toxicology. Drugs of this type are generally well absorbed after ingestion.
Signs and Symptoms
If perles are chewed or dissolved in the mouth, oropharyngeal anesthesia will develop rapidly. CNS stimulation may cause restlessness and tremors which may proceed to clonic convulsions followed by profound CNS depression.
Treatment
Evacuate gastric contents and administer copious amounts of activated charcoal slurry. Even in the conscious patient, cough and gag reflexes may be so depressed as to necessitate special attention to protection against aspiration of gastric contents and orally administered materials.
Convulsions should be treated with a *short-acting* barbiturate given intravenously and carefully titrated for the smallest effective dosage.
Intensive support of respiration and cardiovascular-renal function is an essential feature of the treatment of severe intoxication from overdosage.
Do not use CNS stimulants.
How Supplied: Perles, 100 mg (yellow); bottles of 100 NDC 0056-0010-70.
Also available in Military Depot:
Btls. of 100 NSN 6505-00-660-1798
6075-9
TESSALON is manufactured by R.P. Scherer-North America, St. Petersburg, Florida 33702 for DuPont Pharmaceuticals.

Shown in Product Identification Section, page 411

VALPIN® 50 ℞
[*val'pin*]
anisotropine methylbromide 50 mg

Description: VALPIN® 50 is anisotropine methylbromide, a quaternary ammonium salt which differs chemically from atropine and most other anticholinergics in the substitution of an aliphatic for an aromatic side chain in the acid moiety of the ester.
Chemically, VALPIN® 50 is 2-propyl pentanoyl tropinium methylbromide. Its stability both to acid and alkaline hydrolysis minimizes inactivation.
Actions: VALPIN® 50 inhibits gastric acid secretion and reduces gastrointestinal motility.
Indications: For use as adjunctive therapy in the treatment of peptic ulcer.
AS WITH ALL ANTICHOLINERGICS, IT SHOULD BE NOTED THAT AT THE PRESENT TIME THERE IS LACK OF CONCURRENCE AS TO THEIR VALUE IN THE TREATMENT OF GASTRIC ULCER. IT HAS NOT BEEN SHOWN CONCLUSIVELY WHETHER ANTICHOLINERGIC DRUGS AID IN THE HEALING OF A PEPTIC ULCER, DECREASE THE RATE OF RECURRENCES OR PREVENT COMPLICATION.
Contraindications: Glaucoma; obstructive uropathy (for example, bladder neck obstruction due to prostatic hypertrophy); obstructive disease of the gastrointestinal tract (as in achalasia, pyloroduodenal stenosis, etc.); paralytic ileus, intestinal atony of the elderly or debilitated patient; unstable cardiovascular status in acute hemorrhage; severe ulcerative colitis; toxic megacolon complicating ulcerative colitis; myasthenia gravis.
Warnings:
Use in Pregnancy Since the safety of these preparations in pregnancy, lactation or in women of child-bearing age has not been established, use of the drugs in such patients requires that the potential benefits of the drug be weighed against possible hazards to the mother and child.

In the presence of a high environmental temperature, heat prostration can occur with drug use (fever and heat stroke due to decreased sweating). Diarrhea may be an early symptom of incomplete intestinal obstruction, especially in patients with ileostomy or colostomy. In this instance treatment with this drug would be inappropriate and possibly harmful.

VALPIN® 50 may produce drowsiness or blurred vision. In this event, the patient should be warned not to engage in activities requiring mental alertness such as operating a motor vehicle or other machinery or perform hazardous work while taking this drug.

Precautions:
Use with caution in patients with:
—Autonomic neuropathy.
—Hepatic or renal disease.
—Ulcerative colitis—large doses may suppress intestinal motility to the point of producing a paralytic ileus and the use of this drug may precipitate or aggravate the serious complication of toxic megacolon.
—Hyperthyroidism, coronary heart disease, congestive heart failure, cardiac ar- rhythmias, hypertension and non-obstructing prostatic hypertrophy.
—Hiatal hernia associated with reflux esophagitis since anticholinergic drugs may aggravate this condition.

It should be noted that the use of anticholinergic drugs in the treatment of gastric ulcer may produce a delay in gastric emptying time and may complicate such therapy (antral stasis).

Do not rely on the use of the drug in the presence of complication of biliary tract disease.

Investigate any tachycardia before giving anticholinergic (atropine-like) drugs since they may increase the heart rate.

With overdosage, a curare-like action may occur.

Adverse Reactions: Anticholinergic drugs produce certain effects which may be physiologic or toxic depending upon the individual patient's response. The physician must delineate these.

Adverse reactions may include xerostomia; urinary hesitancy and retention; blurred vision and tachycardia; palpitations; mydriasis; cycloplegia; increased ocular tension; loss of taste; headaches; nervousness; drowsiness; weakness; dizziness; insomnia; nausea; vomiting; impotence; suppression of lactation; constipation; bloated feeling; severe allergic reaction or drug idiosyncrasies including anaphylaxis; urticaria and other dermal manifestations; some degree of mental confusion and/or excitement especially in elderly persons. Decreased sweating is another adverse reaction that may occur.

Dosage and Administration: To be effective dosage must be titrated to individual patient needs. Usual adult dosage—VALPIN® 50 mg tablet; one tablet 3 times daily.

Management of Overdosage: While overdosage intoxication with anisotropine methylbromide has not been reported, theoretically it could occur since anisotropine methylbromide is an anticholinergic drug. When anticholinergic drugs are taken in sufficient overdose to produce severe symptoms, prompt treatment should be instituted. If the drug has been taken orally, gastric lavage and other measures to limit intestinal absorption should be initiated without delay. Physostigmine administered parenterally may be necessary for treatment of the serious manifestations of intoxication. Additionally, symptomatic therapy, including oxygen, sedatives, and control of hyperthermia may be necessary.

How Supplied: VALPIN® 50: 50 mg anisotropine methylbromide in each scored, beige tablet. Bottles of 100 tablets NDC 0056-0161-70

Animal Pharmacology and Toxicology: VALPIN® 50 (anisotropine methylbromide) is a relatively non-toxic drug. In dogs, mice, rats and guinea pigs both acute toxic and chronic toxic dose-levels are at many times in excess of the clinically useful range.

Both **in vitro** and oral **in vivo** data in mice and rats indicate that VALPIN® 50 (anisotropine methylbromide) is at least 2 or 3 times as potent as homatropine methylbromide in antispasmodic action while it is less than two-thirds as active in mydriatic effect. It has less than one-fiftieth of the mydriatic activity of atropine sulfate. In inhibition of salivary flow, VALPIN® 50 (anisotropine methylbromide) is one-fifth as active as homatropine methylbromide and only one-hundredth as active as atropine sulfate. This pharmacologic profile is consistent with relative specificity of action on the gastrointestinal smooth muscle and the lesser tendency to produce side effects.

VALPIN® is a registered U.S. trademark of E.I. duPont de Nemours & Co. (Inc.)
6083-7

Dura Pharmaceuticals, Inc.
P.O. BOX 28331
SAN DIEGO, CA 92128

DURA-TAP/PD™ CAPSULES ℞

Description: Each timed release capsule contains:
Brompheniramine Maleate ....6 mg.
Phenylephrine Hydrochloride ....10 mg.
Phenylpropanolamine Hydrochloride ....10 mg.
in specially prepared base to provide prolonged action.

How Supplied: Dura-Tap/PD™ capsules are supplied in bottles of 100. NDC 51479-004-01. Dispense in tight, light resistant container. Store between 59°–86°F.

DURA-VENT™ CAPSULES ℞

Description: Each continuous release blue and clear capsule imprinted "Dura-Vent™" contains:
Phenylpropanolamine Hydrochloride ....75 mg
Guaifenesin ....400 mg
in a special base to provide a prolonged therapeutic effect.

How Supplied: Dura-Vent™ capsules are supplied in bottles of 100. NDC 51479-001-01. Dispense in tight, light resistant container. Store between 59°–86°F.

DURA-VENT™/A CAPSULES ℞

Description: Each continuous release clear capsule imprinted "Dura-Vent™/A" contains:
Phenylpropanolamine Hydrochloride ....75 mg.
Chlorpheniramine Maleate ....10 mg.
in a specially prepared base to provide prolonged action.

How Supplied: Dura-Vent™/A capsules are supplied in bottles of 100. NDC 51479-002-01. Dispense in tight, light resistant container. Store between 59°–86°F.

DURA-VENT™/DA CAPSULES ℞

Description: Each brown and clear capsule contains:
Chlorpheniramine Maleate ....8 mg.
Phenylephrine Hydrochloride ....20 mg.
Methscopolamine Nitrate ....2.5 mg.
in a specially prepared base to provide prolonged action.

How Supplied: Dura-Vent™/DA capsules are supplied in bottles of 100. NDC 51479-003-01. Dispense in tight light resistant container. Store between 59°–86°F.

Products are cross-indexed by generic and chemical names in the **YELLOW SECTION**

Eaton Laboratories
See NORWICH EATON PHARMACEUTICALS, INC.

Ecological Formulas
Division of Cardiovascular Research, Inc.
1061 SHARY CIRCLE
CONCORD, CA 94518

CAPRYSTATIN™
(Caprylic Acid)

Description: Each Caprystatin tablet consists of enterically-coated caprylic acid (octanoic acid) adsorbed to a non-resinous ion exchange moiety. Caprystatin is designed for slow release of caprylic acid throughout the small and large intestine.

Clinical Pharmacology: Caprylic acid exhibits fungicidal and fungistatic properties *in vitro* and *in vivo*. Proposed mechanisms of action include caprylic acid rapidly permeating Candida cell membranes and binding irreversibly to certain respiratory enzymes, completely inhibiting them at 0.01 mM concentration.

Indications: Caprystatin is indicated as primary or adjunctive therapy for enteric Candida overgrowth syndromes, including irritable bowel syndrome associated with this organism. Caprystatin may be used as an adjunctive therapy for disseminated Candidiasis.

Contraindications: Caprystatin is contraindicated in the presence of hypersensitivity to any component of the preparation.

Adverse Reactions: Mild gastrointestinal distress has been reported after Caprystatin use but the incidence is low. As with other fungicidal anti-Candida therapies, the possibility of a Herxheimer-like reaction to lysed yeast cells should be considered.

Dosage and Administration: The tablet must be swallowed intact to protect the enteric coating. Caprystatin is preferably administered at least one hour before or two hours after meals. If gastrointestinal discomfort is noted, Caprystatin may be taken with meals.

Adult Dose: First week: one tablet, two times daily. Second week: two tablets, twice daily. Third week: three tablets twice daily. Maintenance: minimal effective dose determined from titration schedule.

How Supplied: Bottles of 90 and 500 tablets.
Literature Available: Upon request.
Also available: Orithrush preparations for the treatment of oral thrush and yeast vaginitis.

Elder Pharmaceuticals Inc.
222 N. Vincent Ave.
Covina, CA 91722

BENOQUIN® ℞
[*berĺ ō-kwin*]
(Monobenzone USP 20% Cream)

Federal (U.S.A.) law prohibits dispensing without prescription.

Contains: Each gram of Benoquin Cream contains 200 mg. of monobenzone, USP, in a water-washable base consisting of purified water, cetyl alcohol, propylene glycol, sodium lauryl sulfate and beeswax.

Action: Potent Depigmenting Agent.

Indications: For final depigmentation in extensive vitiligo.

BENOQUIN is not recommended for freckling, hyperpigmentation due to photosensitization following use of certain perfumes (berlock dermatitis), melasma (chloasma) of pregnancy, and hyperpigmentation following inflammation of the skin. BENOQUIN is of no value in the treatment of cafe-au-lait spots, pigmented nevi, malignant mela-

Continued on next page

Elder—Cont.

noma, or pigment resulting from pigments other than melanin, including, bile, silver, and artificial pigments.
Warning: BENOQUIN is a potent depigmenting agent, not a mild cosmetic bleach. Do not use except for final depigmentation in extensive vitiligo.
Adverse Reactions: Discontinue use if irritation, burning sensation, or dermatitis occurs.
Dosage and Administration: Apply and rub into the pigmented areas to be treated, two or three times daily.
Note: Depigmentation is usually observed after one to four months of therapy. If satisfactory results have not been obtained within four months, treatment should be discontinued.
How Supplied: BENOQUIN Cream, 20% in 1¼ oz. tubes (NDC 0163-0380-34).
BENOQUIN Cream should be stored at room temperature (15-30°C) (59-86°F)

ELAQUA® XX CREAM
[el'äk-wah]
Description: Elaqua XX contains urea 20%, water, mineral oil, white petrolatum, micro-crystalline cellulose, polyethylene glycol 400, cetyl alcohol, cetearyl alcohol and ceteareth 20, imidazolidinyl urea, p-hydroxybenzoic acid esters.
Indications: Moisturizing Cream.
How Supplied: Cream—1½ oz. plastic squeeze tube (NDC 0163-0367-39) and 8 oz. plastic jar (NDC 0163-0367-38).
Elaqua XX should be stored at room temperature (15–30°C) (59–86°F).

ELDECORT® CREAM 1%, 2.5%   ℞
[él-duh-cort"]
(hydrocortisone USP topical cream)
Description: Eldecort contains hydrocortisone in a water-washable cream base of water, stearic acid, PEG-25 propylene glycol stearate, PEG-40 stearate, propylene glycol, glyceryl stearate, mineral oil, squalane, allantoin, citric acid, and potassium sorbate.
The content of hydrocortisone in milligrams per gram of cream for each product is as follows:

% Hydrocortisone	mg. Hydrocortisone/gm. Cream
1	10
2½	25

How Supplied:

Concentration	Size/Tubes	NDC Number
1%	1 ounce	0163-0386-31
2½%	1 ounce	0163-0351-31

Eldecort should be stored at room temperature (59–86° F).

ELDER PSORALITE®
[sor'a-līte"]
The Elder Psoralite is an ultraviolet phototherapy medical device available in both full-body and smaller units to meet the physician's requirements. For complete model and specifications information, contact manufacturer.

ELDOPAQUE Forte® 4% Cream   ℞
[él-do-pāk" for' tā]
(Hydroquinone 4% USP)
Skin Bleaching Cream With SunBlock
CAUTION: FEDERAL LAW (U.S.A.) PROHIBITS DISPENSING WITHOUT A PRESCRIPTION.
FOR EXTERNAL USE ONLY
Description: Each gram of Eldopaque Forte 4% Cream contains 40 mg of hydroquinone in a tinted sunblocking base of water, stearic acid, talc, PEG-40 stearate, PEG-25 propylene glycol stearate, propylene glycol, glyceryl stearate, iron oxides, mineral oil, squalane, disodium EDTA, sodium metabisulfite, and potassium sorbate.
Clinical Pharmacology: Topical application of hydroquinone produces a reversible depigmentation of the skin by inhibition of the enzymatic oxidation of tyrosine to 3, 4-dihydroxyphenylalanine (dopa) and suppression of other melanocyte metabolic processes. Exposure to sunlight or ultraviolet light will cause repigmentation which may be prevented by the sunblocking agents contained in Eldopaque Forte.
Indications and Usage: Eldopaque Forte 4% Cream is indicated for the gradual bleaching of hyperpigmented skin conditions such as chloasma, melasma, freckles, senile lentigines, and other unwanted areas of melanin hyperpigmentation.
Contraindications: Prior history of sensitivity or allergic reaction to this product or any of its ingredients. The safety of topical hydroquinone use during pregnancy or in children (12 years and under) has not been established.
Warnings:
A. CAUTION: Hydroquinone is a skin bleaching agent which may produce unwanted cosmetic effects if not used as directed. The physician should be familiar with the contents of this insert before prescribing or dispensing this medication.
B. Test for skin sensitivity before using Eldopaque 4% Cream by applying a small amount to an unbroken patch of skin and check in 24 hours. Minor redness is not a contraindication, but where there is itching or vesicle formation or excessive inflammatory response, further treatment is not advised. Close patient supervision is recommended.
Contact with the eyes should be avoided. If no bleaching or lightening effect is noted after 2 months of treatment use, Eldopaque Forte 4% Cream should be discontinued. Eldopaque Forte 4% Cream is formulated for use as a skin bleaching agent and should not be used for the prevention of sunburn.
C. Sunscreen use is an essential aspect of hydroquinone therapy because even minimal sunlight exposure sustains melanocytic activity. The sunscreens in Eldopaque Forte 4% Cream provide the necessary sun protection during skin bleaching therapy. After clearing and during maintenance therapy, sun exposure should be avoided on bleached skin by application of a sunscreen or sunblock agent, or protective clothing to prevent repigmentation.
D. Keep this and all medications out of the reach of children. In case of accidental ingestion, call a physician or a poison control center immediately.
Precautions: SEE WARNINGS.
A. Pregnancy Category C. Animal reproduction studies have not been conducted with topical hydroquinone. It is also not known whether hydroquinone can cause fetal harm when used topically on a pregnant woman or affect reproductive capacity. It is not known to what degree, if any, topical hydroquinone is absorbed systemically. Topical hydroquinone should be used in women only when clearly indicated.
B. Nursing mothers. It is not known whether topical hydroquinone is absorbed or excreted in human milk. Caution is advised when topical hydroquinone is used by a nursing mother.
C. Pediatric usage. Safety and effectiveness in children below the age of 12 years have not been established.
Adverse Reactions: No systemic adverse reactions have been reported. Occasional hypersensitivity (localized contact dermatitis) may occur in which case the medication should be discontinued and the physician notified immediately.
Overdosage: There have been no systemic reactions from the use of topical hydroquinone or the sunblockers in Eldopaque Forte 4% Cream. However, treatment should be limited to relatively small areas of the body at one time since some patients experience a transient skin reddening and a mild burning sensation which does not preclude treatment.
Drug Dosage and Administration: A thin application of Eldopaque Forte 4% Cream should be applied to the affected area twice daily or as directed by a physician. Do not rub in. There is no recommendation for children under 12 years of age except under the advice and supervision of a physician.
How Supplied: Eldopaque Forte 4% Cream is available as follows:

Size	NDC Number
0.5 ounce tube	0163-0395-35
1.0 ounce tube	0163-0395-31

Available without prescription for maintenance therapy: Eldopaque® (2% Hydroquinone) in ½ ounce (NDC 0163-0518-35) and 1 ounce (NDC 0163-0518-31) tubes.
Eldopaque Forte 4% Cream should be stored at room temperature (15-30°C) (59-86°F).

ELDOQUIN Forte® 4% Cream   ℞
[el'-dō-kwin" for' tā]
(Hydroquinone 4% USP)
Skin Bleaching Cream
CAUTION: FEDERAL LAW (U.S.A.) PROHIBITS DISPENSING WITHOUT A PRESCRIPTION.
FOR EXTERNAL USE ONLY
Description: Each gram of Eldoquin Forte 4% Cream contains 40 mg of hydroquinone in a vanishing cream base of water, stearic acid, propylene glycol, polyethylene glycol-40 stearate, propylene glycol-25 stearate, glyceryl stearate, mineral oil, squalane, propylparaben, and sodium metabisulfite.
Clinical Pharmacology: Topical application of hydroquinone produces a reversible depigmentation of the skin by inhibition of the enzymatic oxidation of tyrosine to 3, 4-dihydroxyphenylalanine (dopa) and suppression of the other melanocyte metabolic processes. Exposure to sunlight or ultraviolet light will cause repigmentation of the bleached areas.
Indications and Usage:
Eldoquin Forte 4% Cream is indicated for the gradual bleaching of hyperpigmented skin conditions such as chloasma, melasma, freckles, senile lentigines, and other unwanted areas of melanin hyperpigmentation. It is intended for night-time use only since it contains no sunblocking agents. For daytime usage, Solaquin Forte™ 4% Cream or Eldopaque® 4% Cream should be prescribed.
Contraindications: Prior history of sensitivity or allergic reaction to this product or any of its ingredients. The safety of topical hydroquinone use during pregnancy or in children (12 years and under) has not been established.
Warnings:
A. CAUTION: Hydroquinone is a skin bleaching agent which may produce unwanted cosmetic effects if not used as directed. The physician should be familiar with the contents of this insert before prescribing or dispensing this medication.
B. Test for skin sensitivity before using Eldoquin Forte 4% Cream by applying a small amount to an unbroken patch of skin and check in 24 hours. Minor redness is not a contraindication, but where there is itching or vesicle formation or excessive inflammatory response, further treatment is not advised. Close patient supervision is recommended.
Contact with the eyes should be avoided. If no bleaching or lightening effect is noted after 2 months of treatment, the medication should be discontinued.
C. There are no sunblocking or sunscreening agents in Eldoquin Forte 4% Cream and since minimal sunlight exposure may reverse the bleaching effect of this preparation, it should be used only at night or on areas of the body covered by protective clothing. During the daytime, sunblocking or broad spectrum sunscreen preparations or protective clothing should be used to prevent the bleached areas from repigmentation. For daytime bleaching of unwanted pigmented areas, the use of Solaquin Forte™ 4% Cream or Eldopaque Forte® 4% Cream should be considered.
D. Keep this and all medication out of the reach of children. In case of accidental ingestion, call a

physician or a poison control center immediately.
Precautions: SEE WARNINGS.
A. Pregnancy Category C. Animal reproduction studies have not been conducted with topical hydroquinone. It is also not known whether hydroquinone can cause fetal harm when used topically on a pregnant woman or affect reproductive capacity. It is not known to what degree, if any, topical hydroquinone is absorbed systemically. Topical hydroquinone should be used in women only when clearly indicated.
B. Nursing mothers. It is not known whether topical hydroquinone is absorbed or excreted in human milk. Caution is advised when topical hydroquinone is used by a nursing mother.
C. Pediatric usage. Safety and effectiveness in children below the age of 12 years have not been established.
Adverse Reactions: No systemic adverse reactions have been reported. Occasional hypersensitivity (localized contact dermatitis) may occur in which case the medication should be discontinued and the physician notified immediately.
Overdosage: There have been no systemic reactions from the use of topical hydroquinone in Eldoquin Forte 4% Cream. However, treatment should be limited to relatively small areas of the body at one time since some patients experience a transient skin reddening and a mild burning sensation which does not preclude treatment.
Drug Dosage and Administration: Eldoquin Forte 4% Cream should be applied to the affected area and rubbed in well twice daily or as directed by a physician. There is no recommended dosage for children under 12 years of age except under the advice and supervision of a physician.
How Supplied: ELDOQUIN FORTE 4% Cream is available as follows:

Size	NDC Number
0.5 ounce tube	0163-0394-35
1.0 ounce tube	0163-0394-31

Available without prescription for maintenance therapy: Eldoquin® (2% Hydroquinone) in ½ ounce (NDC 0163-0382-35) and 1 ounce tubes (NDC 0163-0382-31); Eldoquin Lotion (2% Hydroquinone) in ½ ounce bottles (NDC 0163-0423-35). Eldoquin Forte 4% Cream should be stored at room temperature (15–30°C) (59–86°F).

FOTOTAR® CREAM
[fōtō' tar]
(coal tar USP, 1.6%)
Therapeutic Coal Tar Cream
FOR EXTERNAL USE ONLY
CAUTION: FEDERAL (U.S.A.) LAW PROHIBITS DISPENSING WITHOUT A PRESCRIPTION.
Description: Each gram of Fototar Cream contains 20 mg. of Eldotar® Coal Tar extract (equivalent to 16 mg. of Coal Tar, USP) in an emollient moisturizing cream base containing purified water, white petrolatum, mineral oil, microcrystalline cellulose, PEG 8, stearyl alcohol, glyceryl stearate PEG 100 stearate blend, coceth 6, imidazolidinyl urea, methylparaben, and propylparaben.
Clinical Pharmacology: The mechanism of action of coal tar products is largely unknown. Coal tars have antiseptic qualities, because they contain many substituted phenols. Coal tars also act as mild irritants and have a keratoplastic and antipruritic action. Coal tars have a photosensitizing effect and have been used for years with sunlight or ultraviolet (UV) radiation (Goeckerman Therapy) for the treatment of psoriasis. Coal tars have been successfully used in the treatment of seborrhea, eczema, psoriasis, lichen simplex chronicus, and other chronic skin diseases with lichenification. Refinement of the crude coal tars has not lessened their therapeutic effectiveness and has increased patient acceptability.
Indications: Fototar is indicated in chronic skin disorders that are responsive to coal tars such as psoriasis, infantile and atopic eczema, seborrhea, lichen simplex chronicus, and other chronic skin disorders exhibiting lichenification. Fototar is useful in the Goeckerman program (tars plus UV radiation) in the treatment of psoriasis or other conditions responding to this combined therapy.
Contraindications:
A. Fototar is contraindicated in patients with a history of sensitivity to this product or with a history of sensitivity to coal tar products.
B. Fototar should not be used on patients who have a disease characterized by photosensitivity such as lupus erythematosus or allergy to sunlight.
Warnings:
A. Fototar should not be applied to inflamed or broken skin except on the advice of a physician.
B. Since Fototar is photosensitizing, care must be exercised in exposing the areas of application to excessive UV or sunlight for 24 hours. In the Goeckerman treatment of psoriasis or other skin conditions, care must be taken against overexposure of the areas of application during therapeutic UV radiation or subsequent to such treatment because serious burns may result. Sunscreening or sunblocking agents or protective clothing for at least 24 hours after treatment is recommended to protect the treated areas against additional UV exposure from sunlight.
C. Fototar contains a coal tar derivative. Coal tar preparations should not be used in patients with an exacerbation of psoriasis since this may precipitate total body exfoliation.
D. In psoriatic patients receiving Goeckerman therapy, care should be taken that Fototar application and/or subsequent sunlight exposure be avoided over normal skin since this may cause the appearance of new psoriatic lesions in areas of skin trauma (Koebner Phenomenon).
E. Contact with the eyes should be avoided.
F. Staining of clothing may occur which is normally removed by standard laundry methods. Use on the scalp may cause temporary staining of light colored hair.
Precautions:
A. Patients should be advised of the photosensitizing effect of Fototar.
B. Laboratory tests—none required.
C. Carcinogenesis. Skin cancer following the use of Fototar has not been seen. The use of crude coal tar combined with UV radiation in the production of skin cancer has been studied with conflicting results. Stern, et al, 1980, estimated an increased risk for such cancer in patients with high exposure to tar and ultraviolet radiation compared with those lacking high exposure. They recommended continued surveillance for tumors among psoriatic patients who receive long-term tar and/or UV radiation therapy. However, Pittelkow, et al, 1981, did a 25 year follow-up study on patients receiving combined crude coal tar and UV radiation for psoriasis at the Mayo Clinic and found the incidence of skin cancer not appreciably increased above the expected incidence for the general population, and concluded that this combined regimen (Goeckerman) could be used with minimal risk for skin cancer in the treatment of psoriasis.
D. Pregnancy Category C. Animal reproduction studies have not been conducted with Fototar. It is not known whether Fototar can cause fetal harm when administered to a pregnant woman or can affect reproductive capacity. Fototar should be given to a pregnant woman only if clearly indicated.
E. Nursing Mothers. The absorption of Fototar in nursing mothers has not been studied and caution should be exercised when Fototar is administered to a nursing woman.
F. Pediatric Use. Safety and effectiveness of Fototar in children have not been established.
Adverse Reactions:
A. SEE WARNINGS
B. Chemical folliculitis has been observed in areas of skin which have received long term coal tar applications. This phenomenon has not been observed with the use of Fototar, but its possibility should be borne in mind. This reaction normally clears if coal tar is discontinued or frequency of application reduced.

Overdosage:
A. SEE WARNINGS about use on normal skin.
B. If Fototar is accidentally ingested, call a physician or a poison control center for instructions.
Dosage and Administration: Fototar should be rubbed in the desired area well prior to UV radiation. After several minutes, the excess cream remaining on the skin can be patted with paper tissues to remove the excess.
How Supplied: Fototar (NDC 0163-0373-03) is supplied in 3.0 ounce plastic tubes.
Fototar Cream should be stored at room temperature (15–30°C) (59–86°F).

FOTOTAR® STIK 5%
[fōtō' tar stik]
(Coal Tar USP, 5%)
Therapeutic Coal Tar Stick
FOR EXTERNAL USE ONLY
CAUTION: FEDERAL (U.S.A.) LAW PROHIBITS DISPENSING WITHOUT A PRESCRIPTION.
Description: Each gram of Fototar Stik 5% contains 62.5 mg of Eldotar® (equivalent to 50 mg of Coal Tar, USP) in a hydrophilic wax base containing methyl gluceth-20 sesquistearate, C_{18-36} acid triglyceride, methyl sesquistearate, C_{18-36} acid glycol ester, steareth 2, and polysorbate 80.
Clinical Pharmacology: The mechanism of action of coal tar products is largely unknown. Coal tars have antiseptic qualities because they contain many substituted phenols. Coal tars also act as mild irritants and have a keratoplastic and antipruritic action. Coal tars have a photosensitizing effect and have been used for years with sunlight or ultraviolet (UV) radiation (Goeckerman Therapy) for the treatment of psoriasis. Coal tars have been successfully used in the treatment of seborrhea, eczema, psoriasis, lichen simplex chronicus, and other chronic skin diseases with lichenification. Refinement of the crude coal tars has not lessened their therapeutic effectiveness and has increased patient acceptability.
Indications: Fototar Stik 5% is indicated in chronic skin disorders that are responsive to coal tars such as psoriasis, infantile and atopic eczema, seborrhea, lichen simplex chronicus, and other chronic skin disorders exhibiting lichenification. Fototar Stik 5% is useful in the Goeckerman program (tars plus UV radiation) in the treatment of psoriasis or other conditions responding to this combined therapy.
Contraindications:
A. Fototar Stik 5% is contraindicated in patients with a history of sensitivity to this product or with a history of sensitivity to coal tar products.
B. Fototar Stik 5% should not be used on patients who have a disease characterized by photosensitivity such as lupus erythematosus or allergy to sunlight.
Warnings:
A. Fototar Stik 5% should not be applied to inflamed or broken skin except on the advice of a physician.
B. Since Fototar Stik 5% is photosensitizing, care must be exercised in exposing the areas of application to excessive UV or sunlight for 24 hours. In the Goeckerman treatment of psoriasis or other skin conditions, care must be taken against overexposure of the areas of application during therapeutic UV radiation or subsequent to such treatment because serious burns may result. Sunscreening or sunblocking agents or protective clothing for at least 24 hours after treatment is recommended to protect the treated areas against additional UV exposure from sunlight.
C. Fototar Stik 5% contains a coal tar derivative. Coal tar preparations should not be used in patients with an exacerbation of psoriasis since this may precipitate total body exfoliation.
D. In psoriatic patients receiving Goeckerman therapy, care should be taken that Fototar Stik 5% application and/or subsequent sunlight

Continued on next page

Elder—Cont.

exposure be avoided over normal skin since this may cause the appearance of new psoriatic lesions in areas of skin trauma (Koebner Phenomenon).
E. Contact with the eyes should be avoided.
F. Staining of clothing may occur which is normally removed by standard laundry methods. Use on the scalp may cause temporary staining of light colored hair.

Precautions:
A. Patients should be advised of the photosensitizing effect of Fototar Stik 5%.
B. Laboratory tests - none required.
C. Carcinogenesis. Skin cancer following the use of Fototar Stik 5% has not been seen. The use of crude coal tar combined with UV radiation in the production of skin cancer has been studied with conflicting results. Stern, et al, 1980, estimated an increased risk for such cancer in patients with high exposure to tar and ultraviolet radiation compared with those lacking high exposure. They recommended continued surveillance for tumors among psoriatic patients who receive long-term tar and/or UV radiation therapy. However, Pittelkow, et al, 1981, did a 25 year follow-up study on patients receiving combined crude coal tar and UV radiation for psoriasis at the Mayo Clinic and found the incidence of skin cancer not appreciably increased above the expected incidence for the general population, and concluded that this combined regimen (Goeckerman) could be used with minimal risk for skin cancer in the treatment of psoriasis.
D. Pregnancy Category C. Animal reproduction studies have not been conducted with Fototar Stik 5%. It is not known whether Fototar Stik 5% can cause fetal harm when administered to a pregnant woman or can affect reproductive capacity. Fototar Stik 5% should be given to a pregnant woman only if clearly indicated.
E. Nursing Mothers. The absorption of Fototar Stik 5% in nursing mothers has not been studied and caution should be exercised when Fototar Stik 5% is administered to a nursing woman.
F. Pediatric Use. Safety and effectiveness of Fototar Stik 5% in children have not been established.

Adverse Reactions:
A. SEE WARNINGS
B. Chemical folliculitis has been observed in areas of skin which have received long term coal tar applications. This phenomenon has not been observed with the use of Fototar Stik 5%, but its possibility should be borne in mind. This reaction normally clears if coal tar is discontinued or frequency of application reduced.

Overdosage:
A. SEE WARNINGS about use on normal skin.
B. If Fototar Stik 5% is accidentially ingested, call a physician or a poison control center for instructions.

Dosage and Administration
Fototar Stik 5% should be applied on the desired area well prior to UV radiation.
How Supplied: Fototar Stik 5% (NDC 0163-0522-35) is supplied in 0.5 ounce (15 gram) plastic stick applicator container.
Fototar Stik 5% should be stored at room temperature (15–30°C) (59–86°F).

OXSORALEN® CAPSULES ℞
[ox'-sore"a-len]
(Methoxsalen, USP, 10 mg)

CAUTION: FEDERAL LAW PROHIBITS DISPENSING WITHOUT PRESCRIPTION.
CAUTION: METHOXSALEN IS A POTENT DRUG. READ ENTIRE BROCHURE BEFORE PRESCRIBING OR DISPENSING THIS MEDICATION.

Methoxsalen with UV radiation should be used only by physicians who have special competence in the diagnosis and treatment of psoriasis and vitiligo and who have special training and experience in photochemotherapy. Psoralen and ultraviolet radiation therapy should be under constant supervision of such a physician. For the treatment of patients with psoriasis, photochemotherapy should be restricted to patients with severe, recalcitrant, disabling psoriasis which is not adequately responsive to other forms of therapy, and only when the diagnosis has been supported by biopsy. Because of the possibilities of ocular damage, aging of the skin, and skin cancer (including melanoma), the patient should be fully informed by the physician of the risks inherent in this therapy.

Description: Oxsoralen (Methoxsalen, 8-Methoxypsoralen) Capsules, 10 mg. Methoxsalen is a naturally occuring photoactive substance found in the seeds of the <u>Ammi majus</u> (Umbelliferae) plant. It belongs to a group of compounds known as psoralens, or furocoumarins. The chemical name of methoxsalen is 9-methoxy-7H-furo[3,2-g][1]-benzopyran-7-one.

Clinical Pharmacology: The combination treatment regimen of psoralen (P) and ultraviolet radiation of 320-400 nm wavelength commonly referred to as UVA is known by the acronym, PUVA. Skin reactivity to UVA (320-400 nm) radiation is markedly enhanced by the ingestion of methoxsalen. The drug reaches its maximum bioavailability 1½-3 hours after oral administration and may last for up to 8 hours (Pathak et al, 1974). Methoxsalen is reversibly bound to serum albumen and is also preferentially taken up by epidermal cells (Artuc et al, 1979). At a dose which is six times larger than that used in humans, it induces mixed function oxidases in the liver of mice (Mandula et al, 1978). In both mice and man, methoxsalen is rapidly metabolized. Approximately 95% of the drug is excreted as a series of metabolites in the urine within 24 hours (Pathak et al, 1977).

The exact mechanism of action of methoxsalen with the epidermal melanocytes and keratinocytes is not known. The best known biochemical reaction of methoxsalen is with DNA. Methoxsalen, upon photoactivation, conjugates and forms covalent bonds with DNA which leads to the formation of both monofunctional (addition to a single strand of DNA) and bifunctional adducts (crosslinking of psoralen to both strands of DNA)(Dall'Acqua et al, 1971; Cole, 1970; Musajo et al, 1974; Dall'Acqua et al, 1979). Reactions with proteins have also been described (Yoshikawa et al, 1979).

Methoxsalen acts as a photosensitizer. Administration of the drug and subsequent exposure to UVA can lead to cell injury. Orally administered methoxsalen reaches the skin via the blood and UVA penetrates well into the skin. If sufficient cell injury occurs in the skin, an inflammatory reaction occurs. The most obvious manifestation of this reaction is delayed erythema, which may not begin for several hours and peaks at 48-72 hours. The inflammation is followed, over several days to weeks, by repair which is manifested by increased melanization of the epidermis and thickening of the stratum corneum. The mechanisms of therapy are not known. In the treatment of vitiligo, it has been suggested that melanocytes in the hair follicle are stimulated to move up the follicle and to repopulate the epidermis (Ortonne et al, 1979). In the treatment of psoriasis, the mechanism is most often assumed to be DNA photodamage and resulting decrease in cell proliferation but other vascular, leukocyte, or cell regulatory mechanisms may also be playing some role. Psoriasis is a hyperproliferative disorder and other agents known to be therapeutic for psoriasis are known to inhibit DNA synthesis.

Indications and Usage:
A. Photochemotherapy (methoxsalen with long wave UVA radiation) is indicated for the symptomatic control of severe, recalcitrant, disabling psoriasis not adequately responsive to other forms of therapy and when the diagnosis has been supported by biopsy. Photochemotherapy is intended to be administered only in conjunction with a schedule of controlled doses of long wave ultraviolet radiation.
B. Photochemotherapy (methoxsalen with long wave ultraviolet radiation) is indicated for the repigmentation of idiopathic vitiligo.

Contraindications:
A. Patients exhibiting idiosyncratic reactions to psoralen compounds.
B. Patients possessing a specific history of light sensitive disease states should not initiate methoxsalen therapy. Diseases associated with photosensitivity include lupus erythematosus, porphyria cutanea tarda, erythropoietic protoporphyria, variegate porphyria, xeroderma pigmentosum, and albinism.
C. Patients exhibiting melanoma or possessing a history of melanoma.
D. Patients exhibiting invasive squamous cell carcinomas.
E. Patients with aphakia, because of the significantly increased risk of retinal damage due to the absence of lenses.

Warnings—General:
A. **Skin Burning:** Serious burns from either UVA or sunlight (even through window glass) can result if the recommended dosage of the drug and/or exposure schedules are not maintained.
B. **Carcinogenicity:**
1. ANIMAL STUDIES: Topical or intraperitoneal methoxsalen has been reported to be a potent photocarcinogen in albino mice and hairless mice. However, methoxsalen given by the oral route to albino mice or by any route in pigmented mice is considerably less phototoxic or carcinogenic (Hakim et al, 1960; Pathak et al, 1959).
2. HUMAN STUDIES: A prospective study of 1380 patients over 5 years revealed an approximately nine-fold increase in risks of squamous cell carcinoma among PUVA treated patients. (Stern et al, 1979 and Stern et al, 1980) This increase in risk appears greatest among patients who are fair skinned or had pre-PUVA exposure to 1) prolonged tar and UVB treatment, 2) ionizing radiation, or 3) arsenic.

In addition, an approximately two-fold increase in the risk of basal cell carcinoma was noted in this study. Roenigk et al, 1980 studied 690 patients for up to 4 years and found no increase in the risk of non-melanoma skin cancer. However, patients in this cohort had significantly less exposure to PUVA than in the Stern et al study. After 5 years, two of 1380 patients in the Stern et al PUVA study have developed malignant melanoma. In addition, more than 1/5 of patients in this cohort have developed macular pigmented lesions on the buttocks. While there is no evidence that an increased risk of melanoma exists in PUVA treated patients, these observations indicate the need for continued evaluation of melanoma risk in PUVA treated patients.

In a study in Indian patients treated for 4 years for vitiligo, 12 percent developed keratoses, but not cancer, in the depigmented, vitiliginous areas (Mosher, 1980). Clinically, the keratoses were keratotic papules, actinic keratosis-like macules, non-scaling dome-shaped papules, and lichenoid porokeratotic-like papules.

C. **Cataractogenicity:**
1. ANIMAL STUDIES: Exposure to large doses of UVA causes cataracts in animals, and this effect is enhanced by the administration of methoxsalen (Cloud et al, 1960; Cloud et al, 1961; Freeman et al, 1969).
2. HUMAN STUDIES: It has been found that the concentration of methoxsalen in the lens is proportional to the serum level. If the lens is exposed to UVA during the time methoxsalen is present in the lens, photochemical action may lead to irreversible binding of methoxsalen to proteins and the DNA components of the lens (Lerman et al, 1980). However, if the lens

is shielded from UVA, the methoxsalen will diffuse out of the lens in a 24 hour period. Patients should be told emphatically to wear UVA-absorbing, wrap-around sunglasses for the twenty-four (24) hour period following ingestion of methoxsalen, whether exposed to direct or indirect sunlight in the open or through a window glass.

Among patients using proper eye protection, there is no evidence for a significantly increased risk of cataracts in association with PUVA therapy. Thirty-five of 1380 patients have developed cataracts in the five years since their first PUVA treatment. This incidence is comparable to that expected in a population of this size and age distribution. No relationship between PUVA dose and cataract risk in this group has been noted.

D. **Actinic Degeneration:** Exposure to sunlight and/or ultraviolet radiation may result in "premature aging" of the skin.

E. **Basal Cell Carcinomas:** Patients exhibiting multiple basal cell carcinomas or having a history of basal cell carcinomas should be diligently observed and treated.

F. **Radiation Therapy:** Patients having a history of previous x-ray therapy or grenz ray therapy should be diligently observed for signs of carcinoma.

G. **Arsenic Therapy:** Patients having a history of previous arsenic therapy should be diligently observed for signs of carcinoma.

H. **Hepatic Diseases:** Patients with hepatic insufficiency should be treated with caution since hepatic biotransformation is necessary for drug urinary excretion.

I. **Cardiac Diseases:** Patients with cardiac diseases or others who may be unable to tolerate prolonged standing or exposure to heat stress should not be treated in a vertical UVA chamber.

J. **Total Dosage:** The total cumulative dose of UVA that can be given over long periods of time with safety has not as yet been established.

K. **Concomitant Therapy:** Special care should be exercised in treating patients who are receiving concomitant therapy (either topically or systemically) with known photosensitizing agents such as anthralin, coal tar or coal tar derivatives, griseofulvin, phenothiazines, nalidixic acid, halogenated salicylanilides (bacteriostatic soaps), sulfonamides, tetracyclines, thiazides and certain organic staining dyes such as methylene blue, toluidine blue, rose bengal, and methyl orange.

Precautions: This product contains FD&C Yellow No. 5 (tartrazine) as a color additive which may cause allergic-type reactions (including bronchial asthma) in certain susceptible individuals. Although the overall incidence of FD&C Yellow #5 (tartrazine) sensitivity is low it is frequently seen in patients who also have aspirin hypersensitivity.

A. **General-Applicable To Both Vitiligo and Psoriasis Treatment**
1. BEFORE METHOXSALEN INGESTION
Patients must not sunbathe during the 24 hours prior to methoxsalen ingestion and UV exposure. The presence of a sunburn may prevent an accurate evaluation of the patient's response to photochemotherapy.
2. AFTER METHOXSALEN INGESTION
a. UVA-absorbing wrap-around sunglasses should be worn during daylight for 24 hours after methoxsalen ingestion. The protective eyewear must be designed to prevent entry of stray radiation to the eyes, including that which may enter from the sides of the eyewear. The protective eyewear is used to prevent the irreversible binding of methoxsalen to the proteins and DNA components of the lens. Cataracts form when enough of the binding occurs. Visual discrimination should be permitted by the eyewear for patient well-being and comfort.
b. Patients must avoid sun exposure, even through window glass or cloud cover, for at least 8 hours after methoxsalen ingestion. If sun exposure cannot be avoided, the patient should wear protective devices such as a hat and gloves, and/or apply sunscreens which contain ingredients that filter out UVA radiation (e.g. sunscreens containing benzophenone and/or PABA esters which exhibit a sun protective factor equal to or greater than 15). These chemical sunscreens should be applied to all areas that might be exposed to the sun (including lips). Sunscreens should not be applied to areas affected by psoriasis until after the patient has been treated in the UVA chamber.
3. DURING PUVA THERAPY
a. Total UVA-absorbing/blocking goggles mechanically designed to give maximal ocular protection must be worn. Failure to do so may increase the risk of cataract formation. A reliable radiometer can be used to verify elimination of UVA transmission through the goggles.
b. Abdominal skin, breasts, genitalia, and other sensitive areas should be protected for approximately 1/3 of the initial exposure time until tanning occurs.
c. Unless affected by disease, male genitalia should be shielded.
4. AFTER COMBINED METHOXSALEN/UVA THERAPY
a. UVA-absorbing wrap-around sunglasses should be worn during the daylight for 24 hours after combined methoxsalen/UVA therapy.
b. Patients should not sunbathe for 48 hours after therapy. Erythema and/or burning due to photochemotherapy and sunburn due to sun exposure are additive.
5. VITILIGO THERAPY
a. The dosage of methoxsalen should not be increased above 0.6 mg/kg since overdosage may result in serious burning of the skin.
b. Eye and skin sun protection as described in the Precautions-General section should be observed.

B. **Information For Patients:** See Patient Package Insert.

C. **Laboratory Tests:**
1. Patients should have an ophthalmologic examination prior to start of therapy, and thence yearly.
2. Patients should have the following tests prior to the start of therapy and should be retested 6-12 months subsequently. Additional tests at more extended time periods should be conducted as clinically indicated.
   a. Complete Blood Count (Hemoglobin or Hematocrit; White Blood Count-if abnormal, a differential count).
   b. Anti-nuclear Antibodies.
   c. Liver Function Tests.
   d. Renal Function Tests (Creatinine or Blood Urea Nitrogen).

D. **Drug Interactions:** See Warnings Section.
E. **Carcinogenesis:** See Warnings Section.
F. **Pregnancy:**
Pregnancy Category C. Animal reproduction studies have not been conducted with methoxsalen. It is also not known whether methoxsalen can cause fetal harm when administered to a pregnant woman or can affect reproduction capacity. Methoxsalen should be given to a woman only if clearly needed.

G. **Nursing Mothers:**
It is not known whether this drug is excreted in human milk. Because many drugs are excreted in human milk, caution should be exercised when methoxsalen is administered to a nursing woman.

H. **Pediatric Use:**
Safety in children has not been established. Potential hazards of long-term therapy include the possibilities of carcinogenicity and cataractogenicity as described in the Warnings Section as well as the probability of actinic degeneration which is also described in the Warnings Section.

Adverse Reactions:
A. **Methoxsalen**
The most commonly reported side effect of methoxsalen alone is nausea, which occurs with approximately 10% of all patients. This effect may be minimized or avoided by instructing the patient to take methoxsalen with milk or food, or to divide the dose into two portions, taken approximately one-half hour apart. Other effects include nervousness, insomnia, and psychological depression.

B. **Combined Methoxsalen/UVA Therapy**
1. PRURITUS: This adverse reaction occurs with approximately 10% of all patients. In most cases, pruritus can be alleviated with frequent application of bland emollients or other topical agents; severe pruritus may require systemic treatment. If pruritus is unresponsive to these measures, shield pruritic areas from further UVA exposure until the condition resolves. If intractable pruritus is generalized, UVA treatment should be discontinued until the pruritus disappears.
2. ERYTHEMA: Mild, transient erythema at 24-48 hours after PUVA therapy is an expected reaction and indicates that a therapeutic interaction between methoxsalen and UVA occurred. Any area showing moderate erythema (greater than Grade 2—See Table 1 for grades of erythema) should be shielded during subsequent UVA exposures until the erythema has resolved. Erythema greater than Grade 2 which appears within 24 hours after UVA treatment may signal a potentially severe burn. Erythema may become progressively worse over the next 24 hours, since the peak erythemal reaction characteristically occurs 48 hours or later after methoxsalen ingestion. The patient should be protected from further UVA exposures and sunlight, and should be monitored closely.
3. IMPORTANT DIFFERENCES BETWEEN PUVA ERYTHEMA AND SUNBURN: PUVA-induced inflammation differs from sunburn or UVB phototherapy in several ways. The *in situ* depth of photochemistry is deeper within the tissue because UVA is transmitted further into the skin. The DNA lesions induced by PUVA are very different from UV-induced thymine dimers and may lead to a DNA crosslink. This DNA lesion may be more problematic to the cell because crosslinks are more lethal and psoralen-DNA photoproducts may be "new" or unfamiliar substrates for DNA repair enzymes. DNA synthesis is also suppressed longer after PUVA. The time course of delayed erythema is different with PUVA and may not involve the usual mediators seen in sunburn. PUVA-induced redness may be just beginning at 24 hours, when UVB erythema has already passed its peak. The erythema dose-response curve is also steeper for PUVA. Compared to equally erythemogenic doses of UVB, the histologic alterations induced by PUVA show more dermal vessel damage and longer duration of epidermal and dermal abnormalities.
4. OTHER ADVERSE REACTIONS: Those reported include edema, dizziness, headache, malaise, depression, hypopigmentation, vesiculation and bullae formation, non-specific rash, herpes simplex, miliaria, urticaria, folliculitis, gastrointestinal disturbances, cutaneous tenderness, leg cramps, hypotension, and extension of psoriasis.

Overdosage: In the event of methoxsalen overdosage, induce emesis and keep the patient in a darkened room for at least 24 hours. Emesis is beneficial only within the first 2 to 3 hours after ingestion of methoxsalen, since maximum blood levels are reached by this time.

Drug Dosage & Administration:
A. **Vitiligo Therapy**
1. DRUG DOSAGE: Two capsules (10 mg each) in one dose taken with milk or in food two to four hours before ultraviolet light exposure.
2. LIGHT EXPOSURE: The exposure time to sunlight should comply with the following guide:

	Basic Skin Color		
	Light	Medium	Dark
Initial Exposure	15 min	20 min	25 min
Second Exposure	20 min	25 min	30 min

Continued on next page

Elder—Cont.

Third Exposure	25 min	30 min	35 min
Fourth Exposure	30 min	35 min	40 min

Subsequent Exposure: Gradually increase exposure based on erythema and tenderness of the amelanotic skin.

Therapy should be on alternate days and never two consecutive days.

B. Psoriasis Therapy

1. DRUG DOSAGE-INITIAL THERAPY: The methoxsalen capsules should be taken two hours before UVA exposure with some food or milk according to the following table:

Patient's Weight (kg.)	(lbs.)	Dose (mg.)
< 30	< 65	10
30-50	65-100	20
51-65	101-145	30
66-80	146-175	40
81-90	176-200	50
91-115	201-250	60
> 115	> 250	70

Additional drug dosage directions are as follows:

a. Weight Change: In the event that the weight of a patient changes during treatment such that he/she falls into an adjacent weight range/dose category, no change in the dose of methoxsalen is usually required. If, in the physician's opinion, however, a weight change is sufficiently great to modify the drug dose, then an adjustment in the time of exposure to UVA should be made.

b. Dose/Week: The number of doses per week of methoxsalen capsules will be determined by the patient's schedule of UVA exposures. In no case should treatments be given more often than once every other day because the full extent of phototoxic reactions may not be evident until 48 hours after each exposure.

c. Dosage Increase: Dosage may be increased by 10 mg. after the fifteenth treatment under the conditions outlined in the section titled PUVA Treatment Protocol, part B)4)b).

UVA Radiation Source Specifications & Information:

A. Irradiance Uniformity

The following specifications should be met with the window of the detector held in a vertical plane:

1. Vertical variation: For readings taken at any point along the vertical center axis of the chamber (to within 15 cm from the top and bottom), the lowest reading should not be less than 70 percent of the highest reading.

2. Horizontal variation: Throughout any specific horizontal plane, the lowest reading must be at least 80 percent of the highest reading, excluding the peripheral 3 cm of the patient treatment space.

B. Patient Safety Features

The following safety features should be present: (1) Protection from electrical hazard: All units should be grounded and conform to applicable electrical codes. The patient or operator should not be able to touch any live electrical parts. There should be ground fault protection. (2) Protective shielding of lamps: The patient should not be able to come in contact with the bare lamps. In the event of lamp breakage, the patient should not be exposed to broken lamp components. (3) Hand rails and hand holds: Appropriate supports should be available to the patient. (4) Patient viewing window: A window which blocks UV should be provided for viewing the patient during treatment. (5) Door and latches: Patients should be able to open the door from the inside with only slight pressure to the door. (6) Non-skid floor: The floor should be of a non-skid nature. (7) Thermoregulation: Sufficient air flow should be provided for patient safety and comfort, limiting temperature within the UVA radiator cabinet to approximately less than 100°F. (8) Timer: The irradiator should be equipped with an automatic timer which terminates the exposure at the conclusion of a pre-set time interval. (9) Patient alarm device: An alarm device within the UVA irradiator chamber should be accessible to the patient for emergency activation. (10) Danger label: The unit should have a label prominently displayed which reads as follows:

Danger-Ultraviolet radiation-Follow your physicians instructions-Failure to use protective eyewear may result in eye injury.

C. UVA Exposure Dosimetry Measurements:

The maximum radiant exposure or irradiance (within ± 15 percent) of UVA (320-400 nm) delivered to the patient should be determined by using an appropriate radiometer calibrated to be read in Joules/cm^2 or mW/cm^2. In the absence of a standard measuring technique approved by the National Bureau of Standards, the system should use a detector corrected to a cosine spatial response. The use and recalibration frequency of such a radiometer for a specific UVA irradiator chamber should be specified by the manufacturer because the UVA dose (exposure) is determined by the design of the irradiator, the number of lamps, and the age of the lamps. If irradiance is measured, the radiometer reading in mW/cm^2 is used to calculate the exposure time in minutes to deliver the required UVA dose in Joules/cm^2 to a patient in the UVA irradiator cabinet. The equation is:

$$\text{Exposure Time in Minutes} = \frac{\text{Desired UVA Dose (J/cm}^2\text{)}}{0.06 \times \text{Irradiance (mW/cm}^2\text{)}}$$

Overexposure due to human error should be minimized by using an accurate automatic timing device, which is set by the operator and controlled by energizing and de-energizing the UVA irradiator lamp. The timing device calibration interval should be specified by the manufacturer. Safety systems should be included to minimize the possibility of delivering a UVA exposure which exceeds the prescribed dose, in the event that the timer of radiometer should malfunction.

D. UVA Spectral Output Distribution

The spectral distributions of the lamps should meet the following specifications:

Wavelength band (nanometers)	Output[1]
< 310	< 1
310 to 320	1 to 3
320 to 330	4 to 8
330 to 340	11 to 17
340 to 350	18 to 25
350 to 360	19 to 28
360 to 370	15 to 23
370 to 380	8 to 12
380 to 390	3 to 7
390 to 400	1 to 3

[1] As a percentage of total irradiance between 320 and 400 nanometers.

PUVA Treatment Protocol:

A. Initial Exposure:
The initial UVA exposure radiation level and corresponding time of exposure is determined by the patient's skin characteristics for sun burning and tanning as follows:

[See table below].

B. Clearing Phase:
Specific recommendations for patient treatment are as follows:

1. SKIN TYPES I, II, and III. Patients with skin types I, II, and III may be treated 2 or 3 times per week. UVA exposure may be held constant or increased by up to 1.0 Joule/cm^2 at each treatment, according to the patient's response. If erythema occurs, however, do not increase exposure time until erythema resolves. The severity and extent of the patient's erythema may be used to determine whether the next exposure should be shortened, omitted, or maintained at the previous dosage. See Adverse Reactions section for additional information.

2. SKIN TYPES IV, V, and VI. Patients with skin types IV, V, and VI may be treated 2 or 3 times per week. UVA exposure may be held constant or increased by up to 1.5 Joules/cm^2 at each treatment unless erythema occurs. If erythema occurs, follow instructions outlined above in the procedures for patients with skin types I, II, and III.

3. ERYTHRODERMIC PSORIASIS. Patients with erythrodermic psoriasis should be treated with special attention because pre-existing erythema may obscure observations of possible treatment-related phototoxic erythema. These patients may be treated 2 or 3 times per week, as a Type I patient.

4. MISCELLANEOUS SITUATIONS:

a. If there is no response after a total of 10 treatments, the exposure of UVA energy may be increased by an additional 0.5-1.0 Joules/cm^2 above the prior incremental increases for each treatment. (Example: a patient whose exposure dosage is being increased by 1.0 Joule/cm^2 may now have all subsequent doses increased by 1.5-2.0 Joules/cm^2.)

b. If there is no response, or only minimal response, after 15 treatments, the dosage of methoxsalen may be increased by 10 mg. (a one-time increase in dosage). This increased dosage may be continued for the remainder of the course of treatment but should not be exceeded.

c. If a patient misses a treatment, the UVA exposure time of the next treatment should not be increased. If more than one treatment is missed, reduce the exposure by 0.5 Joule/cm^2 for each treatment missed.

d. If the lower extremities are not responding as well as the rest of the body and do not show erythema, cover all other body areas and give 25 percent of the present exposure dose as an additional exposure to the lower extremities. This additional exposure to the lower extremities should be terminated if erythema develops on these areas.

e. Non-responsive psoriasis: If a patient's generalized psoriasis is not responding, or if the condition appears to be worsening during treatment, the possibility of a generalized phototoxic reaction should be considered. This may be confirmed by the improvement of the condition following temporary discontinuance of this therapy for two weeks. If no improvement occurs during the interruption of treatment, this patient may be considered a treatment failure.

C. Alternative Exposure Schedule:
As an alternative to increasing the UVA exposure at each treatment, the following schedule may be followed; this schedule may reduce the total number of Joules/cm^2 received by the patient over the entire course of therapy.

1. Incremental increases in UVA exposure for all patients may range from 0.5 to 1.5 Jou-

OXSORALEN

Skin Type	History	Recommended Joules/cm^2
I	Always burn, never tan (Patients with erythrodermic psoriasis are to be classed as Type I for determination of UVA dosage.)	0.5 J/cm^2
II	Always burn, but sometimes tan	1.0 J/cm^2
III	Sometimes burn, but always tan	1.5 J/cm^2
IV	Never burn, always tan	2.0 J/cm^2
	Physician Examination	
V*	Moderately pigmented	2.5 J/cm^2
VI*	Blacks	3.0 J/cm^2

[*Patients with natural pigmentation of these types should be classified into a lower skin type category if the sunburning history so indicates.]

les/cm^2, according to the patient's response to therapy.

2. Once Grade 2 clearing (see Table 2) has been reached and the patient is progressing adequately, UVA dosage is held constant. The dosage is maintained until Grade 4 clearing is reached.

3. If the rate of clearing significantly decreases, exposure dosage may be increased at each treatment (0.1-1.5 Joules/cm^2) until Grade 3 clearing and a satisfactory progress rate is attained. The UVA exposure will be held constant again until Grade 4 clearing is attained. These increases may be used also if the rate of clearing significantly decreases between Grade 3 and Grade 4 response. However, the possibility of a phototoxic reaction should be considered; see Nonresponsive Psoriasis, above.

4. In summary, this schedule raises slightly the increments (Joules/cm^2) of UVA dosage, but limits these increases to those periods when the patient is not responding adequately. Otherwise, the UVA exposure is held at the lowest effective dose.

D. Maintenance Phase:
The goal of maintenance treatment is to keep the patient symptom-free as possible with the least amount of UVA exposure.

1. SCHEDULE OF EXPOSURES: When patients have achieved 95 percent clearing, or Grade 4 response (Table 2), they may be placed on the following maintenance schedules (M_1-M_4), in sequence. It is recommended that each maintenance schedule be adhered to for at least 2 treatments (unless erythema or psoriatic flare occurs, in which case see (2a) and (2b) below).

Maintenance Schedules
M_1–once/week
M_2–once/2 weeks
M_3–once/3 weeks
M_4–p.r.n. (i.e. for flares)

2. LENGTH OF EXPOSURE: The UVA exposure for the first maintenance treatment of any schedule (except M_4 as noted below) is the same as that of the patient's last treatment under the previous schedule. For skin types I-IV, however, it is recommended that the maximum UVA dosage during maintenance treatments not exceed the following:

Skin Type	Joules/cm^2/treatment
I	12
II	14
III	18
IV	22

If the patient develops erythema or new lesions of psoriasis, proceed as follows:

a. Erythema: During maintenance therapy, the patient's tan and threshold dose for erythema may gradually decrease. If maintenance treatments produce significant erythema, the exposure to UVA should be decreased by 25 percent until further treatments no longer produce erythema.

b. Psoriasis: If the patient develops new areas of psoriasis during maintenance therapy (but still is classified as having a Grade 4 response), the exposure to UVA may be increased by 0.5-1.5 Joules/cm^2 at each treatment; this is appropriate for all types of patients. These increases are continued until the psoriasis is brought under control and the patient is again clear. The exposure being administered when this clearing is reached should be used for further maintenance treatment.

3. FLARES DURING MAINTENANCE: If the patient flares during maintenance treatment (i.e., develops psoriasis on more than 5 percent of the originally involved areas of the body) his maintenance treatment schedule may be changed to the preceding maintenance or clearing schedule. The patient may be kept on his schedule until again 95 percent clear. If the original maintenance treatment schedule is unable to control the psoriasis, the schedule may be changed to a more frequent regimen. If a flare occurs less than 6 weeks after the last treatment, 25 percent of the maximum exposure received during the clearing phase may be used and proceed with the clearing schedule previously followed for this patient. (At 95 percent clearing follow regular maintenance until the optimum maintenance schedule is determined for the patient.) If more than 6 weeks have elapsed since the last treatment was given, treat patients as if they were beginning therapy insofar as exposure dosages are concerned, since their threshold for erythema may have decreased.

Table 1.—Grades of Erythema

Grade	Erythema Level
0	No erythema
1	Minimally perceptible erythema— faint pink
2	Marked erythema but with no edema
3	Fiery erythema with edema
4	Fiery erythema with edema and blistering

[See table above].

How Supplied: Oxsoralen Capsules, each containing 10 mg. of methoxsalen packaged in amber glass bottles are available as follows:

Unit Count	NDC Number
30	NDC 0163-0600-30
100	NDC 0163-0600-01

Oxsoralen should be stored at room temperature (15–30°C) (59–86°F).

Shown in Product Identification Section, page 411

OXSORALEN® LOTION 1% ℞
[*ox'sore"a-len*]
(methoxsalen USP, 1%)

CAUTION: FEDERAL LAW PROHIBITS DISPENSING WITHOUT A PRESCRIPTION.
CAUTION: METHOXSALEN LOTION IS A POTENT DRUG. READ ENTIRE BROCHURE BEFORE PRESCRIBING OR USING THIS MEDICATION.
WARNING: METHOXSALEN LOTION IS A POTENT DRUG CAPABLE OF PRODUCING SEVERE BURNS IF IMPROPERLY USED. IT SHOULD BE APPLIED ONLY BY A PHYSICIAN UNDER CONTROLLED CONDITIONS FOR LIGHT EXPOSURE AND SUBSEQUENT LIGHT SHIELDING. THIS PREPARATION SHOULD NEVER BE DISPENSED TO A PATIENT.

Description: Each ml. of Oxsoralen Lotion contains 10 mg. methoxsalen in an inert vehicle containing alcohol (71% v/v), propylene glycol, acetone, and water.
Methoxsalen is a naturally occurring substance found in the seeds of the Ammi majus (Umbelliferae) plant; it belongs to a group of compounds known as psoralens or furocoumarins. The chemical name of methoxsalen is 9-methoxy-7H-furo(3, 2g) (1)-benzopyran-7-one. It has the following structure:

Clinical Pharmacology: The exact mechanism of action of methoxsalen with the epidermal melanocytes and keratinocytes is not known. Psoralens given orally are preferentially taken up by epidermal cells (Artuc et al, 1979). The best known biochemical reaction of methoxsalen is with DNA. Methoxsalen, upon photoactivation, conjugates and forms covalent bonds with DNA which leads to the formation of both monofunctional (addition to a single strand of DNA) and bifunctional adducts (crosslinking of psoralen to both strands of DNA) (Dall'Acqua et al, 1971). Reactions with proteins have also been described (Yoshikawa et al, 1979).

Methoxsalen acts as a photosensitizer. Topical application of this drug and subsequent exposure to UVA, whether artificial or sunlight, can cause cell injury. If sufficient cell injury occurs in the skin an inflammatory reaction will result. The most obvious manifestation of this reaction is delayed erythema which may not begin for several hours and may not peak for 2 to 3 days or longer. It is crucial to realize that the length of time the skin remains sensitized or when the maximum erythema will occur is quite variable from person to person. The erythematous reaction is followed over several days or weeks by repair which is manifested by increased melanization of the epidermis and thickening of the stratum corneum. The exact mechanics are unknown but it has been suggested melanocytes in the hair follicles are stimulated to move up the follicle and to repopulate the epidermis. (Ortonne, et al, 1979)

Indications and Usage: As a topical repigmenting agent in vitiligo in conjunction with controlled doses of ultraviolet A (320–400 nm) or sunlight.

Contraindications:
A. Patients exhibiting idiosyncratic reactions to psoralen compounds or a history of sensitivity reactions to them.
B. Patients exhibiting melanoma or with a history of melanoma.
C. Patients exhibiting invasive skin carcinoma generally.
D. Patients with photosensitivity diseases such as porphyria, acute lupus erythematosus, xeroderma pigmentosum, etc.
E. Children under 12 since clinical studies to determine the efficacy and safety of treatment in this age group have not been done.

Warnings:
A. Skin Burns
Serious skin burns from either UVA or sunlight (even through window glass) can result if recommended exposure schedule is exceeded and/or protective covering or sunscreens are not used. The blistering of the skin sometimes encountered after UV exposure generally heals without complication or scarring. (Farrington Daniels, Jr, M.D., personal communication). Suitable covering of the area of application or a topical sunblock should follow the therapeutic UVA exposure.

B. Carcinogenicity
1. Animal Studies. Topical methoxsalen has been reported to be a potent photocarcinogen in certain strains of mice. (Pathak et al 1959).
2. Human Studies. None of our clinical investigators reported skin cancers as a complication of topical treatment for vitiligo. However, it is recommended that caution be exercised when the patient is fair-skinned or has a history of prior coal tar UV treatment, or has had ionizing radiation or taken arsenical compounds. Such patients who subsequently have oral psoralen—UVA treatment (PUVA) are at increased risk for developing skin cancer.

OXSORALEN   Table 2.—Response to Therapy

Grade	Criteria	Percent Improvement (compared to original extent of disease)
–1	Psoriasis worse	0
0	No change	0
1	Minimal improvement—slightly less scale and/or erythema	5-20
2	Definite improvement—partial flattening of all plagues—less scaling and less erythema	20-50
3	Considerable improvement—nearly complete flattening of all plagues but borders of plagues still palpable	50-95
4	Clearing; complete flattening of plagues including borders; plagues may be outlined by pigmentation	95

Continued on next page

Elder—Cont.

C. Concomitant Therapy

Special care should be exercised in treating patients who are receiving concomitant therapy (either topically or systemically) with known photosensitizing agents such as anthralin, coal tar or coal tar derivatives, griseofulvin, phenothiazines, nalidixic acid, halogenated salicylanilides (bacteriostatic soaps), sulfonamides, tetracyclines, thiazides and certain organic staining dyes such as methylene blue, toluidine blue, rose bengal, and methyl orange.

Precautions:

A. This product should be applied only in small well defined lesions and preferably on lesions which can be protected by clothing or a sunscreen from subsequent exposure to radiant UVA. If this product is used to treat vitiligo of face or hands, be very emphatic when instructing patient to keep the treated areas protected from light by use of protective clothing or sunscreening agents. The area of application may be highly photosensitive for several days and may result in severe burn injury if exposed to additional UV or sunlight.
B. CARCINOGENESIS: See Warning Section
C. Pregnancy Category C. Animal reproduction studies have not been conducted with topical methoxsalen. It is also not known whether methoxsalen can cause fetal harm when used topically on a pregnant woman or affect reproductive capacity. It is not known to what degree, if any, topical methoxsalen is absorbed systemically. Topical methoxsalen should be used in women only when clearly indicated.
D. Nursing Mothers. It is not known whether topical methoxsalen is absorbed or excreted in human milk. Caution is advised when topical methoxsalen is used in a nursing mother.
E. Pediatric Usage. Safety and effectiveness in children below the age of 12 years have not been established.

Adverse Reactions: Systemic adverse reactions have not been reported. The most common adverse reaction is severe burns of the treated area from overexposure to UVA, including sunlight. TREATMENT MUST BE INDIVIDUALIZED. Minor blistering of the skin is not a contraindication to further treatment and generally heals without incident. Treatment would be the standard for burn therapy. Since 1953, many studies have demonstrated the safety and effectiveness of topical methoxsalen and UVA for the treatment of vitiligo when used as directed. (Lerner, A.B., et al, 1953) (Fitzpatrick, T.B., et al, 1966) (Fulton, James F. et al, 1969)

Overdosage: This does not apply to topical usage. In the unlikely event that the lotion is ingested, standard procedures for poisoning should be followed, including gastric lavage. Protection from UVA or daylight for hours or days would also be necessary and the patient kept in a darkened room.

Administration: The OXSORALEN® Lotion is applied to a well-defined area of vitiligo by the physician and the area is then exposed to a suitable source of UVA. Initial exposure time should be conservative and not exceed that which is predicted to be one-half the minimal erythema dose. Treatment intervals should be regulated by the erythema response and once a week is recommended or less often depending on the results. The hands and fingers of the person applying the medication should be protected by gloves or finger cots to avoid photosensitization and possible burns.

Pigmentation may begin after a few weeks but significant repigmentation may require up to 6 to 9 months of treatment. Periodic re-treatment may be necessary to retain all of the new pigment. Idiopathic vitiligo is reversible but not equally reversible in every patient. Treatment must be individualized. Repigmentation will vary in completeness, time of onset, and duration. Repigmentation occurs more rapidly in fleshy areas such as face, abdomen, and buttocks and less rapidly over less fleshy areas such as the dorsum of the hands or feet.

How Supplied: Oxsoralen Lotion containing 1% methoxsalen (8-methoxypsoralen) packaged in 1 ounce amber glass bottles (NDC 0163-0402-31). Oxsoralen Lotion 1% should be stored at room temperature (15–30°C) (59–86°F).

PSORANIDE® CREAM 0.025%   ℞
[sor'a-nīde"]
(fluocinolone acetonide)

Description: Each gram of Psoranide Cream contains 0.25 mg. of Fluocinolone Acetonide ((Pregna-1,4-diene-3,20-dione, 6,9-difluro-11,21-dihydroxy -16,17- ((1-methylethylidene)bis(oxy))-6a)) possessing an empirical formula of $C_{24}H_{30}F_2O_6$ and an empirical weight of 452.9.49 daltons in a water-washable cream base of water, propylene glycol, propylene glycol stearate, mineral oil lanolin alcohol, isopropyl palmitate, polysorbate 60, cetyl alcohol, sorbitan stearate, PEG-40 stearate, sorbic acid, methylparaben and propylparaben.

How Supplied: Psoranide Cream is available as follows:

Size	NDC Number
½ ounce tube	0163-0521-35
2 ounce tube	0163-0521-02

Psoranide should be stored at room temperature (15–30°C) (59–86°F).

RVP® OINTMENT
(Red Petrolatum-ELDER)

Composition: Red petrolatum, paraben and lanolin-free sunscreen. Now improved with 2.5% surfactants for easier application and easier removal with soap and water.

Action and Use: Topical sunscreen. Absorbs erythemal spectrum through 340 nanometers, but allows the tanning rays to pass. RVP gives sun protection and sun tanning when applied before sun exposure in the thinnest possible film. Resists water and perspiration; safe around the eyes and on the lips.

How Supplied: 2 ounce tube (NDC 0163-0384-02). RVP should be stored at room temperature (15–30°C) (59–86°F).

RVPaba® LIP STICK
5% ParaAminobenzoic Acid (PABA) + Red Petrolatum (RVP)

Actions and Uses: RVPaba LIP STICK is a topical sunscreen and protectant for lips and small areas of exposed dermis. ParaAminobenzoic Acid (Paba) in Red Petrolatum (RVP) absorbs burning UV in a wide spectrum. Protects against sunburn, windburn and chapping winter or summer. RVPaba LIP STICK contains no perfumes or colors.

Dosage and Administration: Apply to lips and other sensitive areas of the face and hands before exposure to the sun. Reapply as needed.

Caution: Individuals sensitive to Paba should not use RVPaba LIP STICK.

Supply: 1/7 oz. lipstick tubes (NDC 0163-0505-41).
Military—Cold Climate Stock #6508-00-116-1479.
Hot Climate Stock #6508-00-116-1473.
RVPaba should be stored at room temperature (15–30°C) (59–86°F).

RVPaque® OINTMENT
[r-v-pāk']
(Physical Sunscreen)

Composition: Red petrolatum, zinc oxide, and 2-ethoxyethyl p-methoxycinnamate in a greaseless, water-resistant base.

Actions and Uses: Unlike chemical sunscreens, RVPaque functions by reflecting instead of absorbing incident solar radiation. It therefore provides a significant barrier to a wide range of solar wavelengths including visible light. Tinted to blend with most skin tones.

Indications: RVPaque provides extra sun protection in any condition in which ultraviolet and visible light are contraindicated. It may be used adjunctively with depigmenting and skin bleaching agents.

To Use: Apply in a uniformly thin film which is visible to areas requiring exclusion of light. Reapply if removed by abrasion.

Contraindications: None reported; discontinue use if reaction develops.

How Supplied: ½ ounce (NDC 0163-0397-35) and 1¼ ounce tubes (NDC 0163-0397-34).
RVPaque should be stored at room temperature (15–30°C) (59–86°F).

SOLAQUIN FORTE® 4% Cream   ℞
[sōl'a-kwin" for'tā]
(HYDROQUINONE USP, 4%)
Skin Bleaching Cream with Sunscreens

CAUTION: FEDERAL (U.S.A.) LAW PROHIBITS DISPENSING WITHOUT PRESCRIPTION.
FOR EXTERNAL USE ONLY.

Description: Each gram of Solaquin Forte 4% Cream contains 40 mg hydroquinone, 50 mg ethyl dihydroxypropyl PABA, 30 mg dioxybenzone and 20 mg oxybenzone in a bland emollient cream of water, glyceryl stearate, octyldodecyl stearoyl stearate, glyceryl dilaurate, quaternium-26, coceth-6, stearyl alcohol, diethylaminoethyl stearate, dimethicone, polysorbate-80, lactic acid, ascorbic acid, hydroxyethylcellulose, quaternium-14, myristylkonium chloride, disodium EDTA, and sodium metabisulfite.

Clinical Pharmacology: Topical application of hydroquinone produces a reversible depigmentation of the skin by inhibition of the enzymatic oxidation of tyrosine to 3, 4-dihy- droxyphenylalanine (dopa) and suppression of other melanocyte metabolic processes. Exposure to sunlight or ultraviolet light will cause repigmentation which may be prevented by the broad spectrum sunscreen agents contained in Solaquin Forte.

Indications and Usage: Solaquin Forte 4% Cream is indicated for the gradual bleaching of hyperpigmented skin conditions such as chloasma, melasma, freckles, senile lentigines, and other unwanted areas of melanin hyperpigmentation.

Contraindications: Prior history of sensitivity or allergic reaction to this product or any of its ingredients. The safety of topical hydroquinone use during pregnancy or in children (12 years and under) has not been established.

Warnings:

A. CAUTION: Hydroquinone is a skin bleaching agent which may produce unwanted cosmetic effects if not used as directed. The physician should be familiar with the contents of this insert before prescribing or dispensing this medication.
B. Test for skin sensitivity before using Solaquin Forte 4% Cream by applying a small amount to an unbroken patch of skin and check in 24 hours. Minor redness is not a contraindication, but where there is itching or vesicle formation or excessive inflammatory response further treatment is not advised. Close patient supervision is recommended. Contact with the eyes should be avoided. If no bleaching or lightening effect is noted after 2 months of treatment use, Solaquin Forte 4% Cream should be discontinued. Solaquin Forte 4% Cream is formulated for use as a skin bleaching agent and should not be used for the prevention of sunburn.
C. Sunscreen use is an essential aspect of hydroquinone therapy because even minimal sunlight exposure sustains melanocytic activity. The sunscreens in Solaquin Forte 4% Cream provide the necessary sun protection during skin bleaching therapy. After clearing and during maintenance therapy, sun exposure should be avoided on bleached skin by application of a sunscreen or sunblock agent or protective clothing to prevent repigmentation.
D. Keep this and all medication out of the reach of children. In case of accidental ingestion, call a physician or a poison control center immediately.

Precautions: SEE WARNINGS.
A. Pregnancy Category C. Animal reproduction studies have not been conducted with topical hydroquinone. It is also not known whether hydroquinone can cause fetal harm when used topically on a pregnant woman or affect reproductive capacity. It is not known to what degree, if any, topical hydroquinone is absorbed systemically. Topical hydroquinone should be used in women only when clearly indicated.
B. Nursing mothers. It is not known whether topical hydroquinone is absorbed or excreted in human milk. Caution is advised when topical hydroquinone is used by a nursing mother.
C. Pediatric usage. Safety and effectiveness in children below the age of 12 years have not been established.

Adverse Reactions: No systemic adverse reactions have been reported. Occasional hypersensitivity (localized contact dermatitis) may occur in which case the medication should be discontinued and the physician notified immediately.

Overdosage: No systemic reactions from the topical use of Solaquin Forte 4% Cream have been noted. However, treatment should be limited to relatively small areas of the body at one time since some patients experience a transient skin reddening and a mild burning sensation which does not preclude treatment.

Drug Dosage and Administration: Solaquin Forte 4% Cream should be applied to the affected area and rubbed in well twice daily or as directed by a physician. There is no recommended dosage for children under 12 years of age except under the advice and supervision of a physician.

How Supplied: SOLAQUIN FORTE 4% Cream is available as follows:

Size	NDC Number
0.5 ounce tube	0163-0396-35
1.0 ounce tube	0163-0396-31

Available without prescription for maintenance therapy: Solaquin (2% Hydroquinone) in 1 ounce tubes (NDC 0163-0372-31).

Solaquin Forte 4% Cream should be stored at room temperature (15–30°C) (59–86°F).

SOLAQUIN FORTE® 4% GEL ℞
[sōl′a-kwin for′tā]
(Hydroquinone USP, 4%)
Skin Bleaching Gel with Sunscreens

CAUTION: FEDERAL (U.S.A.) LAW PROHIBITS DISPENSING WITHOUT A PRESCRIPTION.
FOR EXTERNAL USE ONLY

Description: Each gram of Solaquin Forte 4% Gel contains 40 mg of Hydroquinone, 50 mg Ethyl Dihydroxypropyl-p-aminobenzoate and 30 mg Dioxybenzone in a hydroalcoholic base of alcohol, purified water, propylene glycol, tetrahydroxypropyl ethylenediamine, carbomer 940, disodium EDTA and sodium metabisulfite.

Clinical Pharmacology: Topical application of hydroquinone produces a reversible depigmentation of the skin by inhibition of the enzymatic oxidation of tyrosine to 3,4-dihydroxyphenylalanine (dopa) and suppression of other melanocyte metabolic processes. Exposure to sunlight or ultraviolet light will cause repigmentation which may be prevented by the broad spectrum sunscreen agents contained in Solaquin Forte 4% Gel.

Indications and Usage: Solaquin Forte 4% Gel is indicated for the gradual bleaching of hyperpigmented skin conditions such as chloasma, melasma, freckles, senile lentigines and other unwanted areas of melanin hyperpigmentation.

Contraindications: Prior history of sensitivity or allergic reaction to this product or any of its ingredients. The safety of topical hydroquinone use during pregnancy or in children (12 years and under) has not been established.

Warnings:
A. CAUTION: Hydroquinone is a skin bleaching agent which may produce unwanted cosmetic effects if not used as directed. The physician should be familiar with the contents of this insert before prescribing or dispensing this medication.
B. Test for skin sensitivity before using Solaquin Forte 4% Gel by applying a small amount to an unbroken patch of skin and check in 24 hours. Minor redness is not a contraindication, but where there is itching or vesicle formation or excessive inflammatory response further treatment is not advised. Close patient supervision is recommended. Contact with the eyes should be avoided. If no bleaching or lightening effect is noted after 2 months of treatment use, Solaquin Forte 4% Gel should be discontinued. Solaquin Forte 4% Gel is formulated for use as a skin bleaching agent and should not be used for the prevention of sunburn.
C. Sunscreen use is an essential aspect of hydroquinone therapy because even minimal sunlight sustains melanocytic activity. The sunscreens in Solaquin Forte 4% Gel provide the necessary sun protection during skin bleaching therapy. After clearing and during maintenance therapy, sun exposure should be avoided on bleached skin by application of a sunscreen or sunblock agent or protective clothing to prevent repigmentation.
D. Keep this and all medication out of the reach of children. In case of accidental ingestion, call a physician or a poison control center immediately.

Precautions:
SEE WARNINGS
A. Pregnancy Category C. Animal reproduction studies have not been conducted with topical hydroquinone. It is also not known whether hydroquinone can cause fetal harm when used topically on a pregnant woman or affect reproductive capacity. It is not known to what degree, if any, topical hydroquinone is absorbed systemically. Topical hydroquinone should be used in pregnant women only when clearly indicated.
B. Nursing mothers. It is not known whether topical hydroquinone is absorbed or excreted in human milk. Caution is advised when topical hydroquinone is used by a nursing mother.
C. Pediatric usage. Safety and effectiveness in children below the age of 12 years have not been established.

Adverse Reactions: No systemic adverse reactions have been reported. Occasional hypersensitivity (localized contact dermatitis) may occur in which case the medication should be discontinued and the physician notified immediately.

Overdosage: There have been no systemic reactions from the use of topical hydroquinone in Solaquin Forte 4% Gel. However, treatment should be limited to relatively small areas of the body at one time since some patients experience a transient skin reddening and a mild burning sensation which does not preclude treatment.

Drug Dosage and Administration: Solaquin Forte 4% Gel should be applied to the affected area and rubbed in well twice daily or as directed by a physician. There is no recommended dosage for children under 12 years of age except under the advice and supervision of a physician.

How Supplied: SOLAQUIN FORTE 4% Gel is available as follows:

Size	NDC Number
0.5 ounce tube (15 grams)	0163-0523-35
1.0 ounce tube (30 grams)	0163-0523-31

Solaquin Forte 4% Gel should be stored at room temperature (15–30°C) (59–86°F).

TRISORALEN® TABLETS ℞
[trī′sore″a-len]
(Trioxsalen USP, 5 mg)

To facilitate repigmentation in vitiligo, increase tolerance to solar exposure and enhance pigmentation.

Caution: THIS IS A POTENT DRUG.
Caution: Federal (U.S.A.) law prohibits dispensing without prescription.
Description: Trisoralen Tablets 5 mg.
TRISORALEN is the first synthetic psoralen compound made available to the medical profession. It possesses greater activity than Methoxsalen, yet the LD 50 is six times that of Methoxsalen.

Contains color additives including FD&C Yellow No. 5 (Tartrazine).

Actions: Pigment formation with TRISORALEN.
The normal pigmentation of the skin is due to melanin which is produced in the cytoplasm of the melanocytes located in the basal layers of the epidermis at its junction with the dermis. Melanin is formed by the oxidation of tyrosine to DOPA (Dihydroxyphenylalanine) with tyrosinase as catalyst. This enzymatic reaction, however, must be activated by radiant energy in the form of ultraviolet light, preferably between 2900 and 3800 angstroms (black light).

The exact mechanism of the action of psoralens in the process of melanogenesis is not known. One group of investigators feel that the psoralens have a specific effect on the epidermis or, more specifically, on the melanocytes. Another group feels that the primary response to the psoralens is an inflammatory one and that the process of melanogenesis is secondary.

Indications: TRISORALEN taken approximately two hours before measured periods of exposure to ultraviolet facilitates:

1. Repigmentation of idiopathic vitiligo. Repigmentation, not equally reversible in every patient, will vary in completeness, time of onset, and duration. The rate of completeness of pigmentation with respect to locations of lesions, occurs more rapidly on fleshy regions, such as the face, abdomen, and buttocks, and less rapidly over bony areas such as the dorsum of the hands and feet. Repigmentation may begin after a few weeks; however, significant results may take as long as six to nine months, and repigmentation, at the optimum level, may, in some cases, require maintenance dosage to retain the new pigment. If follicular repigmentation is not apparent after three months of daily treatment, treatment should be discontinued as a failure.

2. Increasing tolerance to sunlight. In blond persons and those with fair complexions who suffer painful reactions when exposed to sunlight, TRISORALEN aids in increasing resistance to solar damage. Certain persons who are allergic to sunlight or exhibit sun sensitivity may be benefited by the protective action of TRISORALEN. In albinism, TRISORALEN will increase the tolerance of the skin to sunlight, although no pigment is formed. This protective action seems to be related to the thickening of the horny layer and retention of melanin which produces a thickened melanized stratum corneum and formation of a stratum lucidum.

3. Enhancing pigmentation. The use of TRISORALEN accelerates pigmentation only when the administration of the drug is followed by exposure of the skin to sunlight or ultraviolet irradiation. The increase in pigmentation is not immediate but occurs gradually within a few days of repeated exposure and may become equivalent in a degree to that achieved by a full summer of sun exposure. Since sufficient pigment will have been formed within two weeks of continuous therapy, the use of TRISORALEN should not be continued beyond this period. Pigmentation can be maintained by periodic exposure to sunlight.

Contraindications: In those diseases associated with photosensitivity, such as porphyria, acute lupus erythematosus, or leukoderma of infectious origin. To date, the safety of this drug in young persons (12 and under), has not been established and is, therefore contraindicated. No preparation with any photosensitizing capacity, internal or external should be used concomitantly with TRISORALEN therapy.

Warnings: TRISORALEN IS A POTENT DRUG.
Read entire brochure before prescribing or dispensing this medication. The dosage of this medication should not be increased.

The dosage of TRISORALEN and exposure time should not be increased. Overdosage and/or overexposure may result in serious burning and blis-

Continued on next page

Elder—Cont.

tering. When used to increase tolerance to sunlight or accelerate tanning, TRISORALEN total dosage should not exceed 28 tablets, taken in daily single doses of two tablets on a continuous or interrupted regimen. To prevent harmful effects, the physician should carefully instruct the patient to adhere to the prescribed dosage schedule and procedure.

Precautions: Accidental Overdosage:
If an overdose of TRISORALEN or ultraviolet light has been taken, emesis should be encouraged. The individual should be kept in a darkened room for eight hours or until cutaneous reactions subside. The treatment for severe reactions resulting from overdosage or over-exposure should follow accepted procedures for treatment of severe burns. There have not been any clinical reports or tests to verify that more severe reactions may result from the concomitant ingestion of furocoumarin-containing food while on TRISORALEN therapy; but the physician should warn the patient that taking limes, figs, parsley, parsnips, mustard, carrots and celery, might be dangerous.

This product contains FD&C Yellow No. 5 (Tartrazine) which may cause allergic-type reactions (including bronchial asthma) in certain susceptible individuals. Although the overall incidence of FD&C Yellow No. 5 (Tartrazine) sensitivity is low, it is frequently seen in patients who also have aspirin hypersensitivity.

Adverse Reactions and Side Effects: Severe burns can result from excessive sunlight or sun lamp ultraviolet exposure.

Occasionally, there may occur gastric discomfort; to minimize this gastric effect, the tablets may be taken with milk or after a meal. Some patients who are unable to tolerate 10 mg. will tolerate 5 mg. This dosage produces the same therapeutic effect but more slowly.

Dosage: (Adults and children over 12 years of age)
VITILIGO: Two tablets daily, taken two to four hours before measured periods of ultraviolet exposure or fluorescent black light. (See suggested sun exposure guide.)

To increase tolerance to sunlight and/or enhance pigmentation: Two tablets daily, taken two hours before measured periods of exposure to sun or ultraviolet irradiation. Not to be continued for longer than 14 days. The dosage should NOT be increased, as severe burning may occur. (See suggested sun exposure guide.)

SUGGESTED SUN EXPOSURE GUIDE
The exposure time to sunlight should be limited according to the following plan:

	Basic Skin Color	
	Light	Medium
Initial Exposure	15 min.	20 min.
Second Exposure	20 min.	25 min.
Third Exposure	25 min.	30 min.
Fourth Exposure	30 min.	35 min.
Subsequent Exposure:	Gradually increase exposure based on erythema and tenderness.	

Sunglasses should be worn during exposure and the lips protected with a light-screening lipstick.

SUN-LAMP EXPOSURE: Should be initiated according to directions of the sun-lamp manufacturer.

How Supplied: TRISORALEN Tablets 5 mg. in bottles of 28 (NDC 0163-0303-28) and 100 (NDC 0163-0303-01).
Military—TRIOXSALEN Tablets 5 mg. stock # 6505-00-560-7022.
Trisoralen should be stored at room temperature (15–30°C) (59–86°F).

Shown in Product Identification Section, page 411

VITADYE® LOTION
[vīta'dī]
(Cosmetic Cover for hypopigmented skin)

Composition: Dihydroxyacetone (5%), water, isopropyl alcohol, acetone, sodium metabisulfite, disodium edetate. FD&C yellow #5, FD&C red #40, FD&C blue #1.

Use: To cover light colored or white patches of skin. For external use only.

Administration: Use the applicator and apply Vitadye to affected skin areas as often as necessary. To obtain darker shades repeated applications may be necessary. Allow previous applications to dry before reapplying.

Concomitant Therapy: Vitadye transmits most UVA radiation so it can be used concurrently with psoralens in vitiligo therapy.

Precaution: If rash or irritation of the skin develops, discontinue use and contact a physician. Avoid contact with the eyes. Avoid flame. VITADYE will stain, avoid contact with clothing until dry.

Warning: Keep this and all drugs out of the reach of children. In case of accidental ingestion, seek professional assistance or contact a poison control center immediately. Avoid open flame.

How Supplied: Vitadye is available in ½ fluid ounce (NDC 0163-0413-35) and 2 fluid ounce (NDC 0163-0413-02) packages.
Vitadye should be stored at room temperature (15–30°C) (59–86°F).

Elkins-Sinn, Inc.
A subsidiary of A. H. Robins Company
2 ESTERBROOK LANE
CHERRY HILL, NJ 08034

Elkins-Sinn's DOSETTE® line offers a broad spectrum of injectable products in a variety of single-dose containers—DOSETTE vials, DOSETTE ampuls, and DOSETTE syringes. Easily adaptable to any hospital pharmacy set-up, the DOSETTE system combines easily identifiable, clearly printed product labeling with space-conserving packaging. Each DOSETTE single-dose container is characterized by product name and strength in large, bold-faced type, important usage and storage data, lot identification number, and expiration date.
Elkins-Sinn also produces a vast number of multiple dose vials. Listed below are some major ESI products. Additional syringe products are currently being marketed. For a complete catalog and price list, direct inquiries to Customer Service. For specific product information, direct inquiries to the Professional Services Department.

DOSETTE® SYRINGES
Dexamethasone Sodium Phosphate Injection, USP
 4 mg/1 ml
 10 mg/1ml
Gentamicin Sulfate Injection, USP
 60 mg/1.5 ml
 80 mg/2 ml
Hydroxyzine Hydrochloride Intramuscular Injection
 25 mg/1 ml
 50 mg/1 ml
 100 mg/2 ml

DOSETTE® VIALS
Aminophylline Injection, USP
 250 mg/10 ml
 500 mg/20 ml
Atropine Sulfate Injection, USP
 400 mcg/1ml (0.4 mg, 1/150 gr)
 1.0 mg/1 ml
 1.2 mg/1 ml
Codeine Phosphate Injection, USP
 30 mg/1 ml
 60 mg/1 ml
Cyanocobalamin Injection, USP (Vit. B-12)
 1 mg/1 ml (1000 mcg)
Dexamethasone Sodium Phosphate Injection, USP
 4 mg/1 ml
 10 mg/1 ml

Dexpanthenol Injection
 500 mg/2 ml
Dextrose Injection, USP
 50%-50 ml
Diphenhydramine Hydrochloride Injection, USP
 50 mg/1 ml
Dopamine Hydrochloride Injection
 200 mg/5 ml
 400 mg/5 ml
Doxycycline Hyclate for Injection, USP
 100 mg
 200 mg
Furosemide Injection, USP
 20 mg/2 ml
 40 mg/4 ml
 100 mg/10 ml
Gentamicin Sulfate Injection, USP
 20 mg/2 ml (Pediatric)
 80 mg/2 ml
Hep-Lock® PF (Preservative-Free Heparin Lock Flush Solution, USP)
 10 USP units/1ml
 100 USP units/1ml
Hep-Lock® (Heparin Lock Flush Solution, USP)
 10 USP units/ml-1ml and 2 ml
 100 USP units/ml-1ml and 2 ml
Heparin Sodium Injection, USP
 1000 USP units/ml-1 ml and 2 ml
 5000 USP units/1 ml
 10,000 USP units/1 ml
Hydromorphone Hydrochloride Injection, USP
 2 mg/1 ml
Hydroxyzine Hydrochloride Intramuscular Injection
 25 mg/1 ml
 50 mg/1ml
 75 mg/1.5 ml
 100 mg/2 ml
Lidocaine Hydrochloride Injection, USP
 1%-2 ml
 2%-2 ml
Lidocaine Hydrochloride Injection, USP (Preservative-free)
 1%-5 ml
 2%-5 ml
Lidocaine Hydrochloride Injection for Intravenous Use in Cardiac Arrhythmias
 50 mg/5 ml
 100 mg/5 ml
 1 gram/25 ml
 2 grams/50 ml
Meperidine Hydrochloride Injection, USP
 25 mg/1 ml
 50 mg/1 ml
 75 mg/1 ml
 100 mg/1 ml
Metronidazole Redi-Infusion™
 500 mg/100 ml (With IV set)
 500 mg/100 ml (w/o IV set)
Mineral Oil, Sterile Light
 10 ml
 30 ml
Morphine Sulfate Injection, USP
 5 mg/1 ml (1/12 gr)
 8 mg/1 ml (1/8 gr)
 10 mg/1 ml (1/6 gr)
 15 mg/1 ml (1/4 gr)
Pentobarbital Sodium Injection, USP
 100 mg/2 ml
Phenobarbital Sodium Injection, USP
 65 mg/1 ml
 130 mg/1 ml
Phenytoin Sodium Injection, USP
 100 mg/2 ml
 250 mg/5 ml
Sodium Chloride Injection, USP (Preservative-free)
 0.9%-2 ml
Scopolamine Hydrobromide Injection, USP
 400 mcg/1 ml (0.4 mg, 1/150 gr)
Sodium Nitroprusside (Sterile), USP
 50 mg
Thiamine Hydrochloride Injection, USP
 100 mg/1 ml
Vials, Sterile Empty
 2 ml

DOSETTE® AMPULS

Aminophylline Injection, USP
 250 mg/10 ml
 500 mg/20 ml
Atropine Sulfate Injection, USP
 400 mcg/ml (0.4 mg, 1/150 gr)
 400 mcg/0.5 ml (0.4 mg, 1/150 gr)
Calcium Chloride Injection, USP
 1 gram/10 ml (10%)
Calcium Gluconate Injection, USP
 1 gram/10 ml (10%)
Chlorpromazine Hydrochloride Injection, USP
 25 mg/1 ml
 50 mg/2 ml
Cyanocobalamin Injection, USP (Vit. B-12)
 1 mg/1 ml (1000 mcg)
Digoxin Injection, USP
 0.5 mg/2 ml
Dopamine Hydrochloride Injection
 200 mg/5 ml
 400 mg/5 ml
Duramorph®PF (Preservative-free morphine sulfate injection, USP)
 5 mg/10 ml
 10 mg/10 ml
Epinephrine Injection, USP
 1 mg/1 ml (1:1000)
Fentanyl Citrate Injection, USP
 100 mcg/2 ml
 250 mcg/5 ml
 500 mcg/10 ml
 1 mg/20 ml
Furosemide Injection, USP
 20 mg/2 ml
 40 mg/4 ml
 100 mg/10 ml
Isoproterenol Hydrochloride Injection, USP
 1 mg/5 ml (1:5000)
Magnesium Sulfate Injection, USP
 50% 1 gram/2 ml
Meperidine Hydrochloride Injection, USP
 25 mg/1 ml
 50 mg/1 ml
 75 mg/1 ml
 100 mg/1 ml
Methylene Blue Injection, USP
 1%-10 ml
Morphine Sulfate Injection, USP
 8 mg/1 ml (1/8 gr)
 10 mg/1 ml (1/6 gr)
 15 mg/1 ml (1/4 gr)
Paraldehyde Sterile, USP
 5 ml
Phenytoin Sodium Injection, USP (formerly Sodium Diphenylhydantoin)
 100 mg/2 ml
 250 mg/5 ml
Potassium Chloride Injection, USP
 20 mEq/10 ml
 40 mEq/20 ml
Prochlorperazine Edisylate Injection, USP
 10 mg/2 ml
Promethazine Hydrochloride Injection, USP
 25 mg/1 ml
 50 mg/1 ml
Sodium Chloride Injection, USP (Preservative-free)
 0.9%-5 ml
 0.9%-10 ml
Sotradecol® (Sodium Tetradecyl Sulfate)
 1%-2 ml
 3%-2 ml
Water for Injection, Sterile, USP (Preservative-free)
 5 ml
 10 ml

MULTIPLE DOSE VIAL

Aminocaproic Acid Injection, USP
 250 mg/ml-20 ml
Atropine Sulfate Injection, USP
 400 mcg/ml (0.4 mg, 1/150 gr)-20 ml
Chloramphenicol Sodium Succinate (Sterile), USP
 1 Gram
Chlorpromazine Hydrochloride Injection, USP
 25 mg/ml-10 ml
Cyanocobalamin Injection, USP (Vit. B-12)
 1 mg/ml (1000 mcg)-10 ml and 30 ml
Dexamethasone Sodium Phosphate Injection, USP
 4 mg/ml-5 ml and 25 ml
 10 mg/ml-10 ml
Gentamicin Sulfate Injection, USP
 40 mg/ml-20 ml
Hep-Lock® (Heparin Lock Flush Solution, USP)
 10 USP units/ml-10 ml and 30 ml
 100 USP units/ml-10 ml and 30 ml
Heparin Sodium Injection, USP
 1000 USP units/ml-10 ml and 30 ml
 5000 USP units/ml-10 ml
 10,000 USP units/ml-4 ml
Hydrocortisone Sodium Succinate For Injection, USP
 100 mg
 250 mg
 500 mg
 1000 mg (1 gram)
Hydroxyzine Hydrochloride Intramuscular Injection
 50 mg/ml-10 ml
Lidocaine Hydrochloride Injection, USP
 1%-30 ml and 50 ml
 2%-30 ml and 50 ml
Lidocaine Hydrochloride and Epinephrine 1:100,000 Injection, USP
 1%-30 ml
 2%-30 ml
Methylprednisolone Sodium Succinate for Injection, USP
 40 mg
 125 mg
 500 mg
 1000 mg (1 gram)
Neostigmine Methylsulfate Injection, USP
 1:1000 (1 mg/1 ml)-10 ml
Potassium Chloride Injection, USP
 2 mEq/ml-30 ml
Procaine Hydrochloride Injection, USP
 1%-30 ml
 2%-30 ml
Sodium Chloride Injection, Bacteriostatic, USP
 0.9%-30 ml
Vials, Sterile Empty
 5 ml
 10 ml
 30 ml
Water for Injection, Bacteriostatic, USP
 30 ml

DURAMORPH® PF
(morphine sulfate injection, USP)
Preservative-Free

Description: Preservative-free DURAMORPH® PF (Morphine Sulfate Injection, USP) is a sterile, pyrogen-free, isobaric solution free of antioxidants, preservatives or other potentially neurotoxic additives, and is intended for intravenous, epidural or intrathecal administration as a narcotic analgesic. Each milliliter contains morphine sulfate 0.5 mg or 1 mg (Warning: May Be Habit Forming) and sodium chloride 9 mg in Water for Injection. pH range is 2.5-6.0. Ampuls are sealed under nitrogen. Each Dosette® ampul is intended for SINGLE USE ONLY. Discard any unused portion. DO NOT AUTOCLAVE.

Clinical Pharmacology: Morphine exerts its primary effects on the central nervous system and organs containing smooth muscle. Pharmacologic effects include analgesia, drowsiness, alteration in mood (euphoria), reduction in body temperature (at low doses), dose-related depression of respiration, interference with adrenocortical response to stress (at high doses), reduction in peripheral resistance with little or no effect on cardiac index and miosis.

Morphine, as other opioids, acts as an agonist interacting with stereospecific and saturable binding sites/receptors in the brain, spinal cord and other tissues. These sites have been classified as μ receptors and are widely distributed throughout the central nervous system being present in highest concentration in the limbic system (frontal and temporal cortex, amygdala and hippocampus), thalamus, striatum, hypothalamus, midbrain and laminae I, II, IV and V of the dorsal horn in the spinal cord. It has been postulated that exogenously administered morphine exerts its analgesic effect, in part, by altering the central release of neurotransmitter from afferent nerves sensitive to noxious stimuli. Peripheral threshold or responsiveness to noxious stimuli is unaffected leaving monosynaptic reflexes such as the patellar or the Achilles tendon reflex intact.

Autonomic reflexes are not affected by epidural or intrathecal morphine, however morphine exerts spasmogenic effects on the gastrointestinal tract that result in decreased peristaltic activity.

Central nervous sysem effects of intravenously administered morphine sulfate are influenced by ability to cross the blood-brain barrier.

The delay in the onset of analgesia following epidural or intrathecal injection may be attributed to its relatively poor lipid solubility (i.e., an oil/water partition coefficient of 1.42), and its slow access to the receptor sites. The hydrophilic character of morphine may also explain its retention in the CNS and is slow release into the systemic circulation, resulting in a prolonged effect.

Nausea and vomiting may be prominent and are thought to be the result of central stimulation of the chemoreceptor trigger zone. Histamine release is common; allergic manifestations of urticaria and, rarely, anaphylaxis may occur. Bronchoconstriction may occur either as an idiosyncratic reaction or from large dosages.

Approximately one-third of intravenous morphine is bound to plasma proteins. Free morphine is rapidly redistributed in parenchymatous tissues. The major metabolic pathway is through conjugation with glucuronic acid in the liver. Elimination half-life is approximately 1.5 to 2 hours in healthy volunteers. For intravenously administered morphine, 90% is excreted in the urine within 24 hours and traces are detectable in urine up to 48 hours. About 7-10% of administered morphine eventually appears in the feces as conjugated morphine.

Peak serum levels following epidural or intrathecal administration of DURAMORPH® PF are reached within 30 minutes in most subjects and decline to very low levels during the next 2 to 4 hours. The onset of action occurs in 15 to 60 minutes following epidural administration or intrathecal administration; analgesia may last up to 24 hours. Due to this extended duration of action, sustained pain relief can be provided with lower daily doses (by these two routes) than are usually required with intravenous or intramuscular morphine administration.

Indications and Usage: Preservative-free DURAMORPH® PF is a systemic narcotic analgesic for administration by the intravenous, epidural or intrathecal routes. It is used for the management of pain not responsive to non-narcotic analgesics. Morphine sulfate, administered epidurally or intrathecally, provides pain relief for extended periods without attendant loss of motor, sensory or sympathetic funtion.

Contraindications: DURAMORPH® PF is contraindicated in those medical conditions which would preclude the administration of opioids by the intravenous route—allergy to morphine or other opiates, acute bronchial asthma, upper airway obstruction.

Administration of morphine by the epidural or intrathecal route is contraindicated in the presence of infection at the injection site, anticoagulant therapy, bleeding diathesis, parenterally administered corticosteroids within a two week period or other concomitant drug therapy or medical condition which would contraindicate the technique of epidural or intrathecal analgesia.

Warnings: DURAMORPH® PF administration should be limited to use by those familiar with the management of respiratory depression, and in the case of epidural or intrathecal administration, familiar with the techniques and patient manage-

Continued on next page

Elkins-Sinn—Cont.

ment problems associated with epidural or intrathecal drug administration. Because epidural administration has been associated with lessened potential for immediate or late adverse effects than intrathecal administration, the epidural route should be used whenever possible. Rapid intravenous administration may result in chest wall rigidity. FACILITIES WHERE DURAMORPH® PF IS ADMINISTERED MUST BE EQUIPPED WITH RESUSCITATIVE EQUIPMENT, OXYGEN, NALOXONE INJECTION, AND OTHER RESUSCITATIVE DRUGS. WHEN THE EPIDURAL OR INTRATHECAL ROUTE OF ADMINISTRATION IS EMPLOYED, PATIENTS MUST BE OBSERVED IN A FULLY EQUIPPED AND STAFFED ENVIRONMENT FOR AT LEAST 24 HOURS.
SEVERE RESPIRATORY DEPRESSION UP TO 24 HOURS FOLLOWING EPIDURAL OR INTRATHECAL ADMINISTRATION HAS BEEN REPORTED.
Morphine sulfate may be habit forming. (See Drug Abuse and Dependence section.)
Precautions:
GENERAL
Preservative-free DURAMORPH® PF (Morphine Sulfate Injection, USP) should be administered with extreme caution in aged or debilitated patients, in the presence of increased intracranial-/intraocular pressure and in patients with head injury. Pupilliary changes (miosis) may obscure the course of intracranial pathology. Care is urged in patients who have a decreased respiratory reserve (e.g., emphysema, severe obesity, kyphoscoliosis).
Seizures may result from high doses. Patients with known seizure disorders should be carefully observed for evidence of morphine-induced seizure activity.
It is recommended that administration of DURAMORPH® PF by the epidural or intrathecal routes be limited to the lumbar area. Intrathecal use has been associated with a higher incidence of respiratory depression than epidural use.
Smooth muscle hypertonicity may result in biliary colic, difficulty in urination and possible urinary retention requiring catheterization. Consideration should be given to risks inherent in urethral catheterization, e.g., sepsis, when epidural or intrathecal administration is considered, especially in the perioperative period.
Elimination half-life may be prolonged in patients with reduced metabolic rates and with hepatic or renal dysfunction. Hence, care should be exercised in administering morphine in these conditions, particularly with repeated dosing.
Patients with reduced circulating blood volume, impaired myocardial function or on sympatholytic drugs should be observed carefully for orthostatic hypotension, particularly in transport.
Patients with chronic obstructive pulmonary disease and patients with acute asthmatic attack may develop acute respiratory failure with administration of morphine. Use in these patients should be reserved for those whose conditions require endotracheal intubation and respiratory support or control of ventilation.
DRUG INTERACTIONS
Depressant effects of morphine are potentiated by either concomitant administration or in the presence of other CNS depressants such as alcohol, sedatives, antihistaminics or psychotropic drugs (e.g., MAO inhibitors, phenothiazines, butyrophenones and tricyclic antidepressants). Premedication or intra-anesthetic use of neuroleptics with morphine may increase the risk of respiratory depression.
CARCINOGENESIS, MUTAGENESIS, IMPAIRMENT OF FERTILITY
Studies of morphine sulfate in animals to evaluate the carcinogenic and mutagenic potential or the effect on fertility have not been conducted.

PREGNANCY
Teratogenic effects—Pregnancy Category C. Animal reproduction studies have been conducted with morphine sulfate. It is also not known whether morphine sulfate can cause fetal harm when administered to a pregnant woman or can affect reproduction capacity. Morphine sulfate should be given to a pregnant woman only if clearly needed.
Nonteratogenic effects. Infants born from mothers who have been taking morphine chronically may exhibit withdrawal symptoms.
LABOR AND DELIVERY
Intravenous morphine readily passes into the fetal circulation and may result in respiratory depression in the neonate. Naloxone and resuscitative equipment should be available for reversal of narcotic-induced respiratory depression in the neonate. In addition, intravenous morphine may reduce the strength, duration and frequency of uterine contraction resulting in prolonged labor.
Epidurally and intrathecally administered morphine readily passes into the fetal circulation and may result in respiratory depression of the neonate. Controlled clinical studies have shown that *epidural* administration has little or no effect on the relief of labor pain.
However, studies have suggested that in most cases 0.2 to 1 mg of morphine *intrathecally* provides adequate pain relief with little effect on the duration of first stage labor. The second stage labor, though, may be prolonged if the parturient is not encouraged to bear down. A continuous intravenous infusion of naloxone, 0.6 mg/hr, for 24 hours after intrathecal injection may be employed to reduce the incidence of potential side effects.
NURSING MOTHERS
Morphine is excreted in maternal milk. Effect on the nursing infant is not known.
PEDIATRIC USE
Safety and effectiveness in children have not been established.
Adverse Reactions: The most serious side effect is respiratory depression. Because of delay in maximum CNS effect with intravenously administered drug (30 min), rapid administration may result in overdosing. Bolus administration by the epidural or intrathecal route may result in early respiratory depression due to direct venous redistribution of morphine to the respiratory centers in the brain. Late (up to 24 hours) onset of acute respiratory depression has been reported with administration by the epidural or intrathecal route and is believed to be the result of rostral spread. Reports of respiratory depression following intrathecal administration have been more frequent, but the dosage used in most of these cases has been considerably higher than that recommended. This depression may be severe and could require intervention (see Warnings and Overdosage sections). Even without clinical evidence of ventilatory inadequacy, a diminished CO_2 ventilation response may be noted for up to 22 hours following epidural or intrathecal administration.
While low doses of intravenously administered morphine have little effect on cardiovascular stability, high doses are excitatory, resulting from sympathetic hyperactivity and increase in circulating catecholamines. Excitation of the central nervous system resulting in convulsions may accompany high doses of morphine given intravenously. Dysphoric reactions may occur and toxic psychoses have been reported.
Epidural or intrathecal administration is accompanied by a high incidence of pruritus which is dose related but not confined to site of administration. Nausea and vomiting are frequently seen in patients following morphine administration. Urinary retention which may persist for 10-20 hours following single epidural or intrathecal administration has been reported in approximately 90% of males. Incidence is somewhat lower in females. Patients may require catheterization (see Precautions). Pruritus, nausea/vomiting and urinary retention frequently can be alleviated by the intravenous administration of low doses of naloxone (0.2 mg).

Tolerance and dependence to chronically administered morphine, by whatever route, is known to occur (see Drug Abuse and Dependence section). Miscellaneous side effects include constipation, headache, anxiety, depression of cough reflex, interference with thermal regulation and oliguria. Evidence of histamine release such as urticaria, wheals and/or local tissue irritation may occur. In general, side effects are amenable to reversal by narcotic antagonists. NALOXONE INJECTION AND RESUSCITATIVE EQUIPMENT SHOULD BE IMMEDIATELY AVAILABLE FOR ADMINISTRATION IN CASE OF LIFE-THREATENING OR INTOLERABLE SIDE EFFECTS.
Drug Abuse and Dependence:
CONTROLLED SUBSTANCE
Morphine sulfate is a Schedule II substance under the Drug Enforcement Administration classification.
ABUSE
Morphine has recognized abuse and dependence potential.
DEPENDENCE
Cerebral and spinal receptors may develop tolerance/dependence independently, as a function of local dosage. Care must be taken to avert withdrawal in those patients who have been maintained on parenteral/oral narcotics when epidural or intrathecal administration is considered. Withdrawal may occur following chronic epidural or intrathecal administration, as well as the development of tolerance to morphine by these routes. (See nonteratogenic effects under Pregnancy.)
Overdosage: Overdosage is characterized by respiratory depression with or without concomitant CNS depression. Since respiratory arrest may result either through direct depression of the respiratory center or as the result of hypoxia, primary attention should be given to the establishment of adequate respiratory exchange through provision of a patent airway and institution of assisted or controlled ventilation. The narcotic antagonist, naloxone, is a specific antidote. Naloxone (usually 0.4 mg) should be administered intravenously, simultaneously with respiratory resuscitation. *As the duration of effect of naloxone is considerably shorter than that of epidural or intrathecal morphine, repeated administration may be necessary.* Patients should be closely observed for evidence of renarcotization. *Note: Respiratory depression may be delayed in onset up to 24 hours* following epidural or intrathecal administration. In painful conditions, reversal of narcotic effect may result in acute onset of pain and release of catecholamines. Careful administration of naloxone may permit reversal of side effects without affecting analgesia. Parenteral administration of narcotics in patients receiving epidural or intrathecal morphine may result in overdosage.
Dosage and Administration: Preservative-free DURAMORPH® PF (Morphine Sulfate Injection, USP) is intended for intravenous, epidural or intrathecal administration.
INTRAVENOUS ADMINISTRATION
Dosage: The initial dose of morphine should be 2 mg to 10 mg/70 kg of body weight. Patients under the age of 18; no information available.
EPIDURAL ADMINISTRATION
DURAMORPH® PF SHOULD BE ADMINISTERED EPIDURALLY ONLY BY PHYSICIANS EXPERIENCED IN THE TECHNIQUES OF EPIDURAL ADMINISTRATION AND WHO ARE THOROUGHLY FAMILIAR WITH THE LABELING. IT SHOULD BE ADMINISTERED ONLY IN SETTINGS WHERE ADEQUATE PATIENT MONITORING IS POSSIBLE. RESUSCITATIVE EQUIPMENT AND A SPECIFIC ANTAGONIST (NALOXONE INJECTION) SHOULD BE IMMEDIATELY AVAILABLE FOR THE MANAGEMENT OF RESPIRATORY DEPRESSION AS WELL AS COMPLICATIONS WHICH MIGHT RESULT FROM INADVERTENT INTRATHECAL OR INTRAVASCULAR INJECTION. [NOTE: INTRATHECAL DOSAGE IS USUALLY 1/10 THAT OF EPIDURAL DOSAGE.] **PATIENT MONITORING SHOULD BE CONTINUED FOR AT LEAST 24 HOURS AFTER EACH DOSE, SINCE**

DELAYED RESPIRATORY DEPRESSION MAY OCCUR.

Proper placement of a needle or catheter in the epidural space should be verified before DURAMORPH® PF is injected. Acceptable techniques for verifying proper placement include: a) aspiration to check for absence of blood or cerebrospinal fluid, or b) administration of 5 mL (3 mL in obstetric patients) of 1.5% UNPRESERVED Lidocaine and Epinephrine (1:200,000) Injection and then observe the patient for lack of tachycardia (this indicates that vascular injection has *not* been made) and lack of sudden onset of segmental anesthesia (this indicates that intrathecal injection has *not* been made.)

Epidural Adult Dosage: Initial injection of 5 mg in the lumbar region may provide satisfactory pain relief for up to 24 hours. If adequate pain relief is not achieved within one hour, careful administration of incremental doses of 1 to 2 mg at intervals sufficient to assess effectiveness may be given. No more than 10 mg/24 hr should be administered.

Thoracic administration has been shown to dramatically increase the incidence of early and late respiratory depression even at doses of 1 to 2 mg.

For continuous infusion an initial dose of 2 to 4 mg/24 hours is recommended. Further doses of 1 to 2 mg may be given if pain relief is not achieved initially.

Aged or debilitated patients—Administer with extreme caution (see Precautions section). Doses of less than 5 mg may provide satisfactory pain relief for up to 24 hours.

Epidural Pediatric Use: No information on use in pediatric patients is available.

INTRATHECAL ADMINISTRATION

NOTE: INTRATHECAL DOSAGE IS USUALLY 1/10 THAT OF EPIDURAL DOSAGE.

DURAMORPH® PF SHOULD BE ADMINISTERED INTRATHECALLY ONLY BY PHYSICIANS EXPERIENCED IN THE TECHNIQUES OF INTRATHECAL ADMINISTRATION AND WHO ARE THOROUGHLY FAMILIAR WITH THE LABELING. IT SHOULD BE ADMINISTERED ONLY IN SETTINGS WHERE ADEQUATE PATIENT MONITORING IS POSSIBLE. RESUSCITATIVE EQUIPMENT AND A SPECIFIC ANTAGONIST (NALOXONE INJECTION) SHOULD BE IMMEDIATELY AVAILABLE FOR THE MANAGEMENT OF RESPIRATORY DEPRESSION AS WELL AS COMPLICATIONS WHICH MIGHT RESULT FROM INADVERTENT INTRAVASCULAR INJECTION. PATIENT MONITORING SHOULD BE CONTINUED FOR AT LEAST 24 HOURS AFTER EACH DOSE, SINCE DELAYED RESPIRATORY DEPRESSION MAY OCCUR. RESPIRATORY DEPRESSION (BOTH EARLY AND LATE ONSET) HAS OCCURRED MORE FREQUENTLY FOLLOWING INTRATHECAL ADMINISTRATION.

Intrathecal Adult Dosage: A single injection of 0.2 to 1 mg may provide satisfactory pain relief for up to 24 hours. (CAUTION: THIS IS ONLY 0.4 TO 2 ML OF THE 5 MG/10 ML AMPUL OR 0.2 TO 1 ML OF THE 10 MG/10 ML AMPUL OF DURAMORPH® PF.) DO NOT INJECT INTRATHECALLY MORE THAN 2 ML OF THE 5 MG/10 ML AMPUL OR 1 ML OF THE 10 MG/10 ML AMPUL. USE IN THE LUMBAR AREA ONLY IS RECOMMENDED. Repeated intrathecal injections of DURAMORPH® PF are not recommended. A constant intravenous infusion of naloxone, 0.6 mg/hr, for 24 hours after intrathecal injection may be used to reduce the incidence of potential side effects.

Aged or debilitated patients—Administer with extreme caution (see Precautions section). A lower dosage is usually satisfactory.

Repeat Dosage: If pain recurs, alternative routes of administration should be considered, since experience with repeated doses of morphine by the intrathecal route is limited.

Intrathecal Pediatric Use: No information on use in pediatric patients is available.

Parenteral drug products should be inspected for particulate matter and discoloration prior to administration, whenever solution and container permit.

How Supplied: Amber Dosette® ampuls for intravenous, epidural and intrathecal administration.

5 mg/10 mL (0.5 mg/mL) packaged in 10s (NDC 0641-1113-33)

10 mg/10 mL (1 mg/1 mL) packaged in 10s (NDC 0641-1115-33)

Storage: Protect from light. Store in carton at controlled room temperature, 15°C to 30°C (59°F to 86°F) until ready to use. DURAMORPH® PF contains no perservative. DISCARD ANY UNUSED PORTION. DO NOT AUTOCLAVE.

Caution: Federal law prohibits dispensing without prescription.

SOTRADECOL® ℞
[sō'trah"de'kol"]
(Sodium Tetradecyl Sulfate)
For Intravenous Use Only

Description: Sotradecol (sodium tetradecyl sulfate) Injection is a sterile solution containing in each ml sodium tetradecyl sulfate 10 mg (1%) or 30 mg (3%) in Water for Injection with 0.02 ml benzyl alcohol and buffered with dibasic sodium phosphate. pH is adjusted to 7–8.1 with monobasic sodium phosphate or sodium hydroxide.

Actions: The product is a mild sclerosing agent which acts by irritation of the vein intimal endothelium.

Indications: Indicated in the treatment of small uncomplicated varicose veins of the lower extremities.

The benefit-to-risk ratio should be considered in selected patients who are great surgical risks due to conditions such as old age.

Contraindications: Contraindicated in acute superficial thrombophlebitis; underlying arterial disease; varicosities caused by abdominal and pelvic tumors, uncontrolled diabetes mellitus, thyrotoxicosis, tuberculosis, neoplasms, asthma, sepsis, blood dyscrasias, acute respiratory or skin diseases; and any condition which causes the patient to be bedridden. Do not use if precipitated.

Warnings: Sotradecol (sodium tetradecyl sulfate) should be used in pregnant women only when clearly needed. See Precautions.

Precautions: For varicosities, sclerotherapy should not be undertaken if tests such as the Trendelenberg and Perthes, and angiography show significant valvular or deep venous incompetence. The physician should bear in mind the fact that injection necrosis may result from direct injection of sclerosing agents.

The drug should be administered by physicians who are familiar with an acceptable injection technique. Because of the danger of extension of thrombosis into the deep venous system, thorough pre-injection evaluation for valvular competency should be carried out, and slow injections with a small amount (not over 2 ml) of the preparation should be injected into the varicosity. In particular, deep venous patency must be determined by angiography and/or the Perthes test before sclerotherapy is undertaken.

No well controlled studies have been performed on patients taking anti-ovulatory agents. The physician must use judgment and evaluate any patient taking anti-ovulatory drugs prior to initiating treatment with Sotradecol (sodium tetradecyl sulfate). See Adverse Reactions.

Pregnancy category C. Adequate reproduction studies have not been performed in animals to determine whether this drug affects fertility in males or females, has teratogenic potential, or has other adverse effects on the fetus. There are no well-controlled studies in pregnant women, but investigational and marketing experience does not include any positive evidence of adverse effects on the fetus. Although there is no clearly defined risk, such experience cannot exclude the possibility of infrequent or subtle damage to the human fetus.

Adverse Reactions: Post-operative complication of sloughing may occur. A permanent discoloration, usually small and hardly noticeable may occur at the site of injection, and may be objectionable from a cosmetic viewpoint. Allergic reactions have been reported. Therefore, as a precaution against anaphylactic shock, it is recommended that an injection of 0.5 ml of the product into a varicosity be followed by observance of the patient for several hours before a larger injection is administered. The possibility of an anaphylactic reaction should always be kept in mind, and the physician should be prepared to treat it appropriately. In extreme emergencies, 0.25 ml of a 1:1000 solution of epinephrine (0.25 mg) intravenously should be used and side reactions controlled with antihistamines.

One death has been reported in a patient who received Sotradecol (sodium tetradecyl sulfate) and who had been receiving an anti-ovulatory agent. Another death (fatal pulmonary embolism) has been reported in a 36-year-old female treated with sodium tetradecyl acetate and who was not taking oral contraceptives.

Dosage and Administration: For intravenous use only. Do not use if precipitated. The strength of solution required depends on the size and degree of varicosity. In general, the 3% solution will be found most useful, with the 1% solution preferred for small varicosities. The dosage should be kept small, using 0.5 to 2 ml for each injection, and the maximum single treatment should not exceed 10 ml.

Literature describing various current techniques of administration is available upon request from the Professional Services Department.

How Supplied:
1% — 2 ml Dosette® Ampuls, 5's — #1514-34 (NDC 0641-1514-34)
3% — 2 ml Dosette® Ampuls, 5's — #1516-34 (NDC 0641-1516-34)

Everett Laboratories, Inc.
76 FRANKLIN STREET
EAST ORANGE, NEW JERSEY 07017

ANAFED Capsules and Syrup ℞
Antihistamine-Decongestant

Each timed release capsule contains: Chlorpheniramine Maleate 8 mg., Pseudoephedrine HCl. 120 mg.

Each tsp. contains: Chlorpheniramine Maleate 2 mg., Pseudoephedrine HCl. 30 mg.

Supplied: Bottles of 100 yellow/clear capsules; Pints, pineapple flavor.

BEROVITE PLUS TABLETS ℞
Multivitamin/Mineral
Prophylactic or Therapeutic
Nutritional Supplement

Supplied: Bottles of 100.

FLORVITE Chewable Tablets 0.5 mg & 1 mg ℞
Children's Vitamins+ Fluoride

Supplied: Multiflavored chewable tablets in bottles of 100 and 1000.

FLORVITE Drops ℞
Children's Vitamins+ Fluoride

Supplied: Bottles of 50 ml.

FLORVITE + IRON Chewable Tablets 1 mg ℞
Children's Vitamins + Iron + Fluoride

Supplied: Grape flavored chewable tablets in bottles of 100.

FLORVITE + IRON Drops ℞
Children's Vitamins-Iron-Fluoride

Supplied: Bottles of 50 ml.

Continued on next page

Everett—Cont.

LIBIDINAL Soft Gel Capsules   OTC

Each capsule contains: Zinc Gluconate 150 mg., Vitamin E 400 I.U.
Supplied: Bottles of 60 sugar and salt free capsules.

PAVATYM Capsules   ℞

Each timed release capsule contains: Papaverine HCl. 150 mg.
Supplied: Bottles of 100 and 1000 capsules and Unit Dose packs of 100. Capsules imprinted EVERETT.

REPAN Tablets   ℞

Each tablet contains: Butalbital 50 mg. (Warning: May be habit forming.), Caffeine (Anhydrous) 40 mg., Acetaminophen 325 mg.
Supplied: Bottles of 100 tablets imprinted EVERETT and 162.

VITAFOL Tablets   ℞
Vitamins, Minerals, Iron, Folic Acid Supplement
Supplied: Bottles of 100 and 1000 pink film coated tablets.

Ferndale Laboratories, Inc.
780 W. EIGHT MILE ROAD
FERNDALE, MI 48220

AQUAPHYLLIN SYRUP   ℞
(Theophylline, anhydrous 80 mg/15 ml)
Dye-Free, Alcohol-free and saccharin-free.

Actions and Uses: Theophylline is most effective in relaxing smooth muscles of bronchi, particularly if there is bronchial constriction, as in asthma. AQUAPHYLLIN is indicated for relief of acute bronchial asthma and for reversible bronchospasm associated with chronic asthma, bronchitis and emphysema.
Dosage and Administration:
AQUAPHYLLIN SYRUP:
Severe Asthma Attack: Adults—75 ml (5 tablespoonfuls). Children—One ml per kg. body weight, Do not repeat within six hours.
Maintenance 24-Hour Therapy: Adults for first six doses—45 ml (3 tablespoonfuls) upon every 6–8 hours, then 30 ml (2 tablespoonfuls) doses every 6–8 hours.
Children 3 to 5 mg. of theophylline per kg. body weight every 6–8 hours. It is recommended that dosage increases be based on serum theophylline determinations, particularly when exceeding the usual dosage range.
Adverse Effects: Nausea, vomiting, epigastric or substernal pain, palpitation, headache, dizziness may occur.
How Supplied:
Liquid: Pints, gallons and unit dose vials.

KRONOFED–A–JR KRONOCAPS*   ℞
Dye-Free, Sustained Release

Each capsule contains:
Pseudoephedrine HCl .... 60 mg.
Chlorpheniramine Maleate .... 4 mg.
How Supplied: Bottles of 100 and 500 capsules.
*Detailed information is available upon request.

KRONOFED–A KRONOCAPS*   ℞
Dye-Free, Sustained Release

Each capsule contains:
Pseudoephedrine HCl .... 120 mg.
Chlorpheniramine maleate .... 8 mg.
How Supplied: Bottles of 100 and 500 capsules.
*Detailed information is available upon request.

KRONOHIST KRONOCAPS*   ℞
Timed Disintegration Capsules.

Each Capsule contains:
Chlorpheniramine Maleate .... 4 mg.
Pyrilamine Maleate .... 25 mg.
Phenylpropanolamine HCl .... 50 mg.
How Supplied: Bottles of 100 and 1000 capsules.
*Detailed information is available upon request.

LIQUI–DOSS*

Contains: Dioctyl Sodium Sulfosuccinate and mineral oil in a self-emulsifying, pleasantly flavored base.
How Supplied: Pints and unit dose vials.
*Detailed information is available upon request.

PRAMOSONE CREAM, LOTION AND OINTMENT   ℞

Description: Pramosone Cream: Contains Hydrocortisone acetate 0.5%, 1% or 2.5% and Pramoxine HCl 1% in a hydrophilic base containing stearic acid, cetyl alcohol, aquaphor, isopropyl palmitate, polyoxyl 40 stearate, propylene glycol, potassium sorbate 0.1%, sorbic acid 0.1%, triethanolamine lauryl sulfate and water.
Pramosone Lotion: Contains Hydrocortisone acetate 0.5%, 1% or 2.5% and Pramoxine HCl 1% in a base containing forlan-L, cetyl alcohol, stearic acid, di-isopropyl adipate, polyoxyl 40 stearate, silicon, triethanolamine, glycerine, polyvinylpyrolidone, potassium sorbate 0.1%, sorbic acid 0.1% and water.
Pramosone Ointment: Contains Hydrocortisone acetate 1% and Pramoxine HCl 1% in an emollient ointment base containing Sorbitan sesquioleate, Water, Aquaphor and White petrolatum.
Actions: Hydrocortisone acetate is a corticosteroid. Topically, it is primarily effective because of its anti-inflammatory, anti-pruritic and vaso-constrictive actions. Pramoxine hydrochloride is a topical anesthetic which provides temporary relief from itching and pain.
Indications and Usage: Topical corticosteroids are indicated for the relief of the inflammatory and pruritic manifestations of corticosteroid-responsive dermatoses.
Contraindications: Topical steroids are contraindicated in viral diseases of the skin, such as varicella and vaccinia. Topical steroids are contraindicated in those patients with a history of hypersensitivity to any of the components of the preparation. Topical steroids should not be used when circulation is markedly impaired.
Precautions: If irritation develops, the product should be discontinued and appropriate therapy instituted. In the presence of an infection, the use of appropriate antifungal or antibacterial agents should be instituted. If a favorable response does not occur promptly, the corticosteroid should be discontinued until the infection has been adequately controlled. If extensive areas are treated or if the occlusive technique is used, the possibility exists of increased systemic absorption of the corticosteroid and suitable precautions should be taken.
The product is not for opthalmic use.
Warnings: USAGE IN PREGNANCY: Although topical steroids have not been reported to have an adverse effect on the fetus, the safety of their use in pregnant females has not absolutely been established. Therefore, they should not be used extensively on pregnant patients, or in large amounts, or for prolonged periods of time.
Caution: Federal law prohibits despensing without prescription.
Adverse Reactions: The following local adverse reactions have been reported with topical corticosteroids, especially under occlusive dressings. Burning, Itching, Irritation, Dryness, Folliculitis, Hypertrichosis, Acneiform eruptions, Hypopigmentation, Perioral dermatitis, Allergic Contact Dermatitis, Maceration of the skin, Secondary infection, Skin atrophy, Striae, and Miliaria.
Dosage and Administration: Apply to affected area 3 or 4 times daily.

How Supplied: CREAM: ½% or 1% in 1 oz. tubes, 4 oz. jars and lb. jars. LOTION: ½% or 1% in 1¼ fl. oz., 4 fl. oz., and 8 fl. oz., and HIGH POTENCY: 2½% in 2 fl. oz. plastic dispenser bottles.
OINTMENT: 1 oz. tubes, 4 oz. jars and lb jars.

PRAX CREAM AND LOTION*
(Pramoxine HCl 1% in a hydrophilic lotion base)

Available: CREAM: 1 oz. tubes, 4 oz. jars and lb. jars. LOTION: 15 mL. and 120 mL. dispenser bottles.
*Additional information available upon request.

The Fielding Company
2384 CENTERLINE INDUSTRIAL DRIVE
ST. LOUIS, MO 63146

IROSPAN® Tablets/Capsules

Each tablet or capsule contains:
Ferrous Sulfate (exsic.)   200 mg.
Ascorbic Acid (Vit. C)   150 mg.
Description: Irospan is a unique presentation of sustained release ferrous sulfate and ascorbic acid. Irospan is of particular value during pregnancy and lactation providing excellent tolerance and absorption.
Dosage: One tablet or capsule daily or as prescribed by the physician.
How Supplied: Irospan Tablets—bottles of 100. Irospan Capsules—bottles of 60.

METRIC® 21   ℞
(metronidazole)

Description: An antiprotozoal and antibacterial agent for use in the treatment of trichomoniasis in both the female and male patient.
Dosage: Metric 21 (250 mg) one tablet three times a day for seven days. The seven day course of treatment appears to provide a higher cure rate than the one day treatment regimen.
How Supplied: Metric 21 (250 mg) in bottles of 100.
NDC 0421-8282-01

NESTABS® FA TABLETS   ℞
Prenatal Tablets

Description: East tablet contains: U.S. RDA

Vitamin A	8000 Units	100%
Vitamin D	400 Units	100%
Vitamin E	30 Units	100%
Vitamin C	120 mg.	200%
Folic Acid	1 mg.	125%
Thiamine	3 mg.	176%
Riboflavin	3 mg.	125%
Niacinamide	20 mg.	100%
Pyridoxine	3 mg.	120%
Vitamin B12	8 mcg.	100%
Calcium Carbonate	500 mg.	15%
Iodine	150 mcg.	100%
Ferrous Fumarate	110 mg.	200%
Zinc	15 mg.	100%

A comprehensive vitamin-mineral supplement expressly formulated for use during pregnancy and lactation.
Dosage: One tablet daily, or as prescribed by the physician.
Precaution: Folic acid may obscure pernicious anemia in that hematologic remission can occur while neurological manifestations remain progressive.
How Supplied: Bottles of 100 tablets.
NDC 0421-1594-01

Products are cross-indexed by generic and chemical names in the **YELLOW SECTION**

Fisons Corporation
Pharmaceutical Division
TWO PRESTON COURT
BEDFORD, MA 01730

In addition to the products described in this section, Fisons also distributes the following products. On these and all Fisons products, information may be obtained by addressing Fisons Corporation, 2 Preston Court, Bedford, MA 01730.

BACID® CAPSULES OTC
lactobacillus acidophilus

ERGOMAR® SUBLINGUAL TABLETS ℞
ergotamine tartrate
2.0 mg sublingual tablet

KONDREMUL® OTC
KONDREMUL® with CASCARA
KONDREMUL® with PHENOLPHTHALEIN
mineral oil microemulsion

NEO-CULTOL® OTC
refined mineral oil, jelly, chocolate flavored

PERSISTIN® OTC
salicylsalicylic acid - 7 ½ gr
aspirin - 2 ½ gr

PROFERDEX™ ℞
iron dextran injection, USP
complex of ferric hydroxide and dextran in a 0.9% sodium chloride solution.

VAPO-ISO® ℞
isoproterenol HCl
solution 0.5% (1:200)

VAPONEFRIN® SOLUTION OTC
(racepinephrine)

VITRON-C® OTC
ferrous fumarate - 200 mg
ascorbic acid - 125 mg

VITRON-C PLUS® OTC
ferrous fumarate - 400 mg
ascorbic acid - 250 mg

INTAL® Nebulizer Solution ℞
[ĭn'tăl]
(cromolyn sodium, USP)
For Inhalation Use Only—Not for Injection

Description: Each ampule of Intal (cromolyn sodium, USP) Nebulizer Solution contains 20 mg cromolyn sodium in 2 ml of purified water for inhalation. Chemically, cromolyn sodium is the disodium salt of 1,3-bis (2-carboxychromon-5-yloxy)-2-hydroxypropane. Intal Nebulizer Solution is clear, colorless, sterile and has a pH of 4.0-7.0. The molecular structure is:

Pharmacological Category: Mast cell stabilizer/antiallergic.
Therapeutic Category: Antiasthmatic.

Clinical Pharmacology: *In vitro* and *in vivo* animal studies have shown that cromolyn sodium inhibits the degranulation of sensitized mast cells which occurs after exposure to specific antigens. Cromolyn sodium inhibits the release of histamine and SRS-A (the slow-reacting substance of anaphylaxis). Bronchial asthma induced by the inhalation of specific antigens can be inhibited to varying degrees by pretreatment with cromolyn sodium. Another activity demonstrated *in vitro* is the capacity of cromolyn sodium to inhibit the degranulation of non-sensitized rat mast cells by phospholipase A and the subsequent release of chemical mediators. An additional *in vitro* study showed that cromolyn sodium did not inhibit the enzymatic activity of released phospholipase A on its specific substrate.
Cromolyn sodium has no intrinsic bronchodilator, antihistaminic or anti-inflammatory activity. Because of its prophylactic mechanism of action, Intal Nebulizer Solution has no role in the treatment of an acute attack of asthma.
Cromolyn sodium is poorly absorbed from the gastrointestinal tract. After inhalation of Intal capsules, about 8 percent of the total dose administered is deposited in the lung, absorbed, and rapidly excreted unchanged in the bile and urine. The remainder of the dose is either exhaled or deposited in the oropharynx, swallowed and excreted via the alimentary tract.

Indications and Usage: Intal Nebulizer Solution is indicated in the management of patients with bronchial asthma in whom the frequency, intensity and predictability of episodes indicate the use of a continuing program of symptomatic medication. Such patients must have a significant bronchodilator-reversible component to their airway obstruction as demonstrated by a generally accepted pulmonary function test of airway mechanics.
If improvement occurs, it will ordinarily occur within the first 4 weeks of administration as manifested by a decrease in the severity of clinical symptoms of asthma, or in the need for concomitant therapy, or both.
A decision to continue the administration of Intal Nebulizer Solution on a long term basis is justified if introduction of the drug into the patient's regime:
   produces a significant reduction in the severity of the symptoms of asthma, or
   permits a significant reduction in or elimination of steroids, or
   permits better management of patients who have intolerable side effects to sympathomimetic agents or methylxanthines.

Contraindications: Intal Nebulizer Solution is contraindicated in those patients who have shown hypersensitivity to cromolyn sodium.

Warnings: Intal (cromolyn sodium, USP) Nebulizer Solution has no role in the treatment of an acute attack of asthma, especially status asthmaticus.
The prophylactic effect of cromolyn sodium is usually evident after several weeks of treatment, although some patients show an almost immediate response.

Precautions: General: In view of the biliary and renal routes of excretion for cromolyn sodium, consideration should be given to decreasing the dosage or discontinuing the administration of the drug in patients with impaired renal or hepatic function.
If eosinophilic pneumonia (pulmonary infiltrates with eosinophilia) occurs during the course of Intal Nebulizer Solution therapy, the drug should be discontinued.
Occasionally patients may experience cough and/or bronchospasm following cromolyn sodium inhalation. At times, patients with cromolyn sodium induced bronchospasm may not be able to continue its administration despite prior bronchodilator administration. Rarely very severe bronchospasm has been encountered.
Symptoms of asthma may recur if Intal® Nebulizer Solution is reduced below the recommended dosage, or discontinued.

Carcinogenesis, Mutagenesis, and Impairment of Fertility: Long term studies in mice (12 months intraperitoneal treatment followed by 6 months observation), hamsters (12 months intraperitoneal treatment followed by 12 months observation), and rats (18 months subcutaneous treatment) showed no neoplastic effect of cromolyn sodium.
No evidence of chromosomal damage or cytotoxicity was obtained in various mutagenesis studies.
No evidence of impaired fertility was shown in laboratory animal reproduction studies.

Pregnancy: Pregnancy Category B. Reproduction studies with cromolyn sodium administered parenterally to pregnant mice, rats and rabbits in doses up to 338 times the human clinical doses produced no evidence of fetal malformations. Adverse fetal effects (increased resorptions and decreased fetal weight) were noted only at the very high parenteral doses that produced maternal toxicity. There are, however, no adequate and well-controlled studies in pregnant women. Because animal reproduction studies are not always predictive of human response, this drug should be used in pregnancy only if clearly needed.

Drug Interaction During Pregnancy: Cromolyn sodium and isoproterenol were studied following subcutaneous injections in pregnant mice. Cromolyn sodium alone in doses of 60 to 540 mg/kg (38 to 338 times the human dose) did not cause significant increases in resorptions or major malformations. Isoproterenol alone at a dose of 2.7 mg/kg (90 times the human dose) increased both resorptions and malformations. The addition of cromolyn sodium (338 times the human dose) to isoproterenol (90 times the human dose) appears to have increased the incidence of both resorptions and malformations.

Nursing Mothers: It is not known whether this drug is excreted in human milk. Because many drugs are excreted in human milk, caution should be exercised when INTAL Nebulizer Solution is administered to a nursing woman.

Pediatric Use: Safety and effectiveness in children below the age of 2 years have not been established.

Adverse Reactions: The adverse reactions which have been observed in clinical trials with Intal Nebulizer Solution are noted as follows: Cough, Nasal Congestion, Nausea, Sneezing, Wheezing.
Other reactions have been reported in clinical trials; however, a causal relationship could not be established: Drowsiness, Nasal itching, Nose bleed, Nose burning, Serum sickness, Stomach ache.
In addition, adverse reactions have been reported with Intal (cromolyn sodium) 20 mg Capsules. The most frequently reported adverse reactions attributed to Intal capsules (on the basis of reoccurrence following readministration) involve the respiratory tract and include: Bronchospasm, Cough, Laryngeal edema (rare), Nasal congestion, Pharyngeal irritation, Wheezing.
Other adverse reactions which have also been attributed to Intal capsules (on the basis of reoccurrence following readministration) are: Angioedema, Dizziness, Dysuria and urinary frequency, Joint swelling and pain, Lacrimation, Nausea and headache, Rash, Swollen parotid gland, Urticaria.
In addition, the following adverse reactions have been reported as rare events and it is unclear whether these are attributable to Intal capsules: Anaphylaxis, Anemia, Exfoliative dermatitis, Hemoptysis, Hoarseness, Myalgia, Nephrosis, Periarteritic vasculitis, Pericarditis, Peripheral neuritis, Photodermatitis, Polymyositis, Pulmonary infiltrates with eosinophilia, Vertigo.

Overdosage: No action other than medical observation should be necessary.

Dosage and Administration: The usual starting dosage for adults and children 2 years of age and over is the contents of one ampule administered by nebulization four times a day. One ampule contains 20 mg cromolyn sodium. Intal Nebulizer Solution should be administered from a power-operated nebulizer having an adequate flow rate, equipped with a suitable face mask. Hand operated nebulizers are not suitable for the administration of Intal Nebulizer Solution. Patients should be advised that the effect of Intal Nebulizer Solution therapy is dependent upon its administration at regular intervals, as directed. Intal Nebulizer Solution should be introduced into the patient's therapeutic regimen when the acute episode has been controlled, the airway cleared and the patient is able to inhale adequately.
Once a patient is stabilized on Intal® Nebulizer Solution, if there is no need for steroids, the frequency of administration may be titrated downward to the least frequent level consistent with the desired effect. The usual decrease is from four to three Intal Nebulizer Solution ampules per day. It is important that the dosage be reduced slowly, maintaining close supervision of the patient, to avoid exacerbation of asthma. It should be emphasized that in patients who have been titrated to

Continued on next page

Fisons—Cont.

less than four ampules per day, an increase in dosage may be needed if the patient's clinical condition worsens.

Corticosteroid treatment and its relation to Intal Nebulizer Solution use: An attempt to decrease corticosteroid administration and particularly to institute an alternate day regimen should be made in asthmatic patients receiving corticosteroids. Concomitant corticosteroids, as well as bronchodilators, should be continued following the introduction of Intal Nebulizer Solution. If the patient improves, an attempt to decrease corticosteroids should be made. Even if the steroid-dependent patient fails to improve following Intal Nebulizer Solution administration, gradual tapering of steroid dosage may nonetheless be attempted. It is important that the dose be reduced slowly, maintaining close supervision of the patient to avoid an exacerbation of asthma. It should be borne in mind that prolonged corticosteroid therapy frequently causes a reduction in the activity and size of the adrenal cortex. Relative adrenocortical insufficiency upon discontinuation of therapy may be avoided by gradual reduction of dosage.

However, a potentially critical degree of insufficiency may persist asymptomatically for some time even after gradual discontinuation of adrenocortical steroids. Therefore, if a patient is subjected to significant stress, such as a severe asthmatic attack, surgery, trauma or severe illness while being treated or within one year (occasionally up to two years) after corticosteroid treatment has been terminated, consideration should be given to reinstituting corticosteroid therapy. When the inhalation of Intal Nebulizer Solution is impaired, as may occur in severe exacerbation of asthma, a temporary increase in the amount of corticosteroids and/or other medications may be required.

It is particularly important that great care be exercised if for any reason Intal Nebulizer Solution is withdrawn in cases where its use has permitted a reduction in the maintenance dose of steroids. In such cases, continued close supervision of the patient is essential since there may be sudden reappearance of severe manifestations of asthma which will require immediate therapy and possible reintroduction of corticosteroids.

How Supplied: Intal Nebulizer Solution is supplied in a double ended glass ampule containing 20 mg cromolyn sodium in 2 ml purified water.

NDC 0585-0673-02   60 ampules × 2 ml
NDC 0585-0673-03   120 ampules × 2 ml

Intal Nebulizer Solution should be stored below 30°C (86°F) and protected from direct light.

Please see package insert for complete information.   Rev. 6/83

Also available as:

INTAL®   ℞
(cromolyn sodium)
20 mg Capsules
For Inhalation Only
For Use With The SPINHALER®
TURBO-INHALER

Description: Chemically, cromolyn sodium is the disodium salt of 1,3-bis (2-carboxychromon-5-yloxy)-2-hydroxypropane.

It is soluble in water. Each capsule contains 20 mg cromolyn sodium in micronized form together with 20 mg of lactose powder added to improve the flow properties of the material. The contents of the capsule are intended for inhalation only, with the SPINHALER® turbo-inhaler.

Please see package insert for complete instructions.

ISOCLOR® Timesule®   ℞
[ĭs′ō-klŏr]
Capsules

Description: Each sustained-action Timesule capsule contains 8 mg chlorpheniramine maleate and 120 mg pseudoephedrine HCl in a special form providing a prolonged therapeutic effect.

Indications: For temporary relief of upper respiratory and nasal congestion associated with the common cold, hay fever and allergies, sinusitis, and vasomotor and allergic rhinitis.

Contraindications: Severe hypertension or severe cardiac disease. Sensitivity to antihistamines or sympathomimetic agents.

Precautions: Use with caution in patients with hyperthyroidism. Patients susceptible to the soporific effects of chlorpheniramine should be warned against driving or operating machinery which requires complete mental alertness.

Dosage: *Adults*—1 Timesule capsule every 12 hrs.

Supplied: Bottles of 100 and 500.

Isoclor® and Timesule® are registered trademarks of American Hospital Supply Corporation

Distributed by FISONS CORPORATION
Bedford, MA 01750

NASALCROM®   ℞
[năz′ŭl-krōm″]
(cromolyn sodium, USP)
NASAL SOLUTION

Description: Each milliliter of NASALCROM® (cromolyn sodium, USP) Nasal Solution contains 40 mg cromolyn sodium in purified water with benzalkonium chloride 0.01% and EDTA (disodium edetate) 0.01% added to stabilize and to provide antimicrobial protection for the solution. NASALCROM possesses a natural pH of 4.5–6.5 and negligible titratable acidity. Chemically, cromolyn sodium is the disodium salt of 1,3-bis (2-carboxychromon-5-yloxy)-2-hydroxypropane.

The molecular structure is:

Pharmacologic Category: Mast cell stabilizer/antiallergic.

Therapeutic Category: Antiallergic.

After priming the delivery system for NASALCROM, each actuation of the unit delivers a metered spray containing 5.2 mg of cromolyn sodium. The contents of one nasal spray bottle delivers at least 100 sprays.

Clinical Pharmacology: *In vitro* and *in vivo* animal studies have shown that cromolyn sodium inhibits the degranulation of sensitized mast cells which occurs after exposure to specific antigens. Cromolyn sodium inhibits the release of histamine and SRS-A (the slow-reacting substance of anaphylaxis). Rhinitis induced by the inhalation of specific antigens can be inhibited to varying degrees by pretreatment with NASALCROM.

Another activity demonstrated *in vitro* is the capacity of cromolyn sodium to inhibit the degranulation of non-sensitized rat mast cells by phospholipase A and the subsequent release of chemical mediators. An additional *in vitro* study showed that cromolyn sodium did not inhibit the enzymatic activity of released phospholipase A on its specific substrate.

Cromolyn sodium has no intrinsic bronchodilator, antihistaminic or anti-inflammatory activity.

Cromolyn sodium is poorly absorbed from the gastrointestinal tract. After instillation of NASALCROM, less than 7% of the total dose administered is absorbed and is rapidly excreted unchanged in the bile and urine. The remainder of the dose is expelled from the nose, or swallowed and excreted via the alimentary tract.

Indications: NASALCROM is indicated for the prevention and treatment of the symptoms of allergic rhinitis.

Contraindications: NASALCROM is contraindicated in those patients who have shown hypersensitivity to any of the ingredients.

Precautions: General: Some patients may experience transient nasal stinging and/or sneezing immediately following instillation of NASALCROM. Except in rare occurrences, these experiences have not caused discontinuation of therapy.

In view of the biliary and renal routes of excretion for cromolyn sodium, consideration should be given to decreasing the dosage or discontinuing the administration of the drug in patients with impaired renal or hepatic function.

Carcinogenesis, Mutagenesis, and Impairment of Fertility: Long term studies in mice (12 months intraperitoneal treatment followed by 6 months observation), hamsters (12 months intraperitoneal treatment followed by 12 months observation), and rats (18 months subcutaneous treatment) showed no neoplastic effect of cromolyn sodium.

No evidence of chromosomal damage or cytotoxicity was obtained in various mutagenesis studies. No evidence of impaired fertility was shown in laboratory animal reproduction studies.

Pregnancy: Pregnancy Category B. Reproduction studies with cromolyn sodium administered parenterally to pregnant mice, rats, and rabbits in doses up to 338 times the human clinical doses produced no evidence of fetal malformations. Adverse fetal effects (increased resorptions and decreased fetal weight) were noted only at the very high parenteral doses that produced maternal toxicity. There are, however, no adequate and well-controlled studies in pregnant women. Because animal reproduction studies are not always predictive of human response, this drug should be used during pregnancy only if clearly needed.

Drug Interaction During Pregnancy: Cromolyn sodium and isoproterenol were studied following subcutaneous injections in pregnant mice. Cromolyn sodium alone in doses of 60 to 540 mg/kg (38 to 338 times the human dose) did not cause significant increases in resorptions or major malformations. Isoproterenol alone at a dose of 2.7 mg/kg (90 times the human dose) increased both resorptions and malformations. The addition of cromolyn sodium (338 times the human dose) to isoproterenol (90 times the human dose) appears to have increased the incidence of both resorptions and malformations.

Nursing Mothers: It is not known whether this drug is excreted in human milk. Because many drugs are excreted in human milk, caution should be exercised when NASALCROM is administered to a nursing woman.

Pediatric Use: Safety and effectiveness in children below the age of 6 years have not been established.

Adverse Reactions: The most frequent adverse reactions occurring in the 430 patients included in the clinical trials with NASALCROM were sneezing (1 in 10 patients), nasal stinging (1 in 20), nasal burning (1 in 25), and nasal irritation (1 in 40). Headaches and bad taste were reported in about 1 in 50 patients. Epistaxis, postnasal drip, and rash were reported in less than one percent of the patients. One patient in the clinical trials developed anaphylaxis.

Adverse reactions which have occurred in the use of other cromolyn sodium formulations for inhalation include angioedema, joint pain and swelling, urticaria, cough, and wheezing. Other reactions reported rarely are serum sickness, periarteritic vasculitis, polymyositis, pericarditis, photodermatitis, exfoliative dermatitis, peripheral neuritis, and nephrosis.

Dosage and Administration: The dose for adults and children 6 years and older is one spray in each nostril 3–4 times daily at regular intervals. If needed, this dose may be increased to one spray to each nostril 6 times daily. The patient should be instructed to clear the nasal passages before administering the spray and should inhale through the nose during administration.

In the management of seasonal (pollenotic) rhinitis, and for prevention of rhinitis caused by exposure to other types of specific inhalant allergens, treatment with NASALCROM will be more effective if started prior to expected contact with the offending allergen. Treatment should be continued throughout the period of exposure, i.e., until the pollen season is over or until exposure to the offending allergen is terminated.

In the management of perennial allergic rhinitis, the effects of treatment with NASALCROM may become apparent only after two to four weeks of treatment. The concomitant use of antihistamine and/or nasal decongestant may be necessary during the initial phase of treatment, but the need for this type of medication should diminish and may be eliminated when the full benefit of NASALCROM is achieved.

How Supplied: Each 13 ml NASALCROM (cromolyn sodium, USP) Nasal Solution spray bottle contains 520 mg (40 mg/ml) of cromolyn sodium and is to be used with the Nasalmatic™ metered spray device. The Nasalmatic device consists of a pump unit, plastic case and a patient leaflet of instructions. The cleaning of this device is not recommended. The pump device should be replaced at six month intervals. NASALCROM should be stored at controlled room temperature (15°-30°C).

NDC 0585-0671-02 Complete pack (13 ml bottle, metered spray device)
NDC 0585-0671-01 Refill (13 ml bottle)

Caution: Federal law prohibits dispensing without prescription.

Rev.5/83
FC7102A

SOMOPHYLLIN®-CRT CAPSULES ℞
[sŏm″áh-fĭ-lĭn]
(theophylline anhydrous controlled release capsules)

Description: Each capsule contains anhydrous theophylline, USP, in a formulation to provide a prolonged therapeutic effect. Somophyllin-Controlled Release Theophylline capsules contain not less than 90.0 percent and not more than 110.0 percent of the labelled amount of anhydrous theophylline ($C_7H_8N_4O_2$). Theophylline, a xanthine compound, is a white, odorless crystalline powder having a bitter taste.

Somophyllin-CRT capsules are supplied in 100 mg, 200 mg, 250 mg and 300 mg strengths.

Clinical Pharmacology: Theophylline directly relaxes the smooth muscle of the bronchial airways and pulmonary blood vessels, thus acting mainly as a bronchodilator, pulmonary vasodilator and smooth muscle relaxant. The drug also possesses other actions typical of the xanthine derivatives: coronary vasodilation; diuresis; cardiac, cerebral and skeletal muscle stimulation. The actions of theophylline may be mediated through inhibition of phosphodiesterase and a resultant increase in intracellular cyclic AMP which could mediate smooth muscle relaxation. At concentrations higher than those attained *in vivo*, theophylline also inhibits the release of histamine by mast cells.

In vitro, theophylline has been shown to act synergistically with beta agonists (isoproterenol) that increase intracellular cyclic AMP through the stimulation of adenyl cyclase, but synergism has not been demonstrated in patient studies. More data are needed to determine if theophylline and beta agonists have a clinically important additive effect *in vivo*. Apparently, no development of tolerance occurs with chronic use of theophylline.

The half-life of theophylline is shortened with cigarette smoking. It is prolonged in alcoholism, reduced hepatic or renal function, congestive heart failure, and in patients receiving antibiotics such as TAO (troleandomycin), erythromycin and clindamycin. High fever for prolonged periods may reduce the rate of theophylline elimination.

Theophylline Elimination Characteristics:

	Theophylline Clearance Rates (mean ± SD)	Half-life Average (mean ± SD)
Children (over 6 months of age)	1.45 ± 0.58 ml/kg/min	3.7 ± 1.1 hrs
Adult nonsmokers with uncomplicated asthma	0.65 ± 0.19 ml/kg/min	8.7 ± 2.2 hrs

Newborn infants have extremely slow theophylline clearance rates. The theophylline half-life in newborn infants may exceed 24 hours. Not until 3-6 months of age do these rates approach those seen in older children.

Older adults with chronic obstructive pulmonary disease, any patients with cor pulmonale or other causes of heart failure, and patients with liver pathology may have much slower clearance rates with a half-life that may exceed 24 hours.

The half-life of theophylline in smokers (1 to 2 packs/day) averaged 4-5 hours among various studies, much shorter than the half-life in nonsmokers which averaged about 7-9 hours. The increase in theophylline clearance caused by smoking is probably the result of induction of drug-metabolizing enzymes that do not readily normalize after cessation of smoking. It appears that between 3 months and 2 years may be necessary for normalization of the effect of smoking on theophylline pharmacokinetics.

Indications: For relief and/or prevention of symptoms of reversible bronchospasm associated with asthma, chronic bronchitis, and emphysema.

Contraindications: This product is contraindicated in individuals who have shown hypersensitivity to its components.

Warnings: *Status asthmaticus is a medical emergency. Intravenous or rapidly absorbed oral liquid formulations of theophylline are preferred over slower releasing controlled release forms in this condition. Optimal therapy frequently requires additional medication including corticosteroids when the patient is not rapidly responsive to bronchodilators.*

Excessive theophylline doses may be associated with toxicity. The determination of serum theophylline levels is recommended to assure maximal benefit without excessive risk. Incidence of toxicity increases at serum theophylline levels greater than 20 mcg/ml. Morphine, curare, and stilbamidine should be used with caution in patients with airflow obstruction because they stimulate histamine release and they can induce asthmatic attacks. These drugs may also suppress respiration leading to respiratory failure. Alternative drugs should be chosen whenever possible.

There is an excellent correlation between high blood levels of theophylline resulting from conventional doses and associated clinical manifestations of toxicity in (1) patients with lowered body plasma clearances (due to transient cardiac decompensation), (2) patients with liver dysfunction or chronic obstructive lung disease, (3) patients who are older than 55 years of age, particularly males.

Less serious signs of theophylline toxicity such as nausea, and restlessness may appear in up to 50 percent of patients. However, serious side effects such as ventricular arrhythmias and convulsions may appear without warning as the first signs of toxicity.

Many patients who have higher theophylline serum levels exhibit tachycardia.

Theophylline products may aggravate pre-existing arrhythmias.

Usage in Pregnancy: Safe use in pregnancy has not been established relative to possible adverse effects on fetal development, but neither have adverse effects on fetal development been established. This is true for most anti-asthmatic medications. Use of theophylline in pregnant women should be balanced against the risk of uncontrolled asthma.

Precautions: Mean half-life in smokers is shorter than nonsmokers, therefore, smokers may require larger doses of theophylline. Theophylline should not be administered concurrently with other xanthine medications. Use with caution in patients with severe cardiac disease, severe hypoxemia, hypertension, hyperthyroidism, acute myocardial injury, cor pulmonale, congestive heart failure, liver disease, in the elderly (especially males) and in neonates. In particular, great caution should be used in giving theophylline to patients with congestive heart failure. Frequently, such patients have markedly prolonged theophylline serum levels with theophylline persisting in serum for long periods following discontinuation of the drug.

Use theophylline cautiously in patients with history of peptic ulcer. Theophylline may occasionally act as a local irritant to G.I. tract although gastrointestinal symptoms are more commonly centrally mediated and associated with serum drug concentrations over 20 mcg/ml.

Adverse Reactions: The most consistent adverse reactions are usually due to overdose and are:
1. Gastrointestinal: nausea, vomiting, epigastric pain, hematemesis, diarrhea.
2. Central nervous system: headaches, irritability, restlessness, insomnia, reflex hyperexcitability, muscle twitching, clonic and tonic generalized convulsions.
3. Cardiovascular: palpitation, tachycardia, extra systoles, flushing, hypotension, circulatory failure, life threatening ventricular arrhythmias.
4. Respiratory: tachypnea.
5. Renal: albuminuria, increased excretion of renal tubular and red blood cells, potentiates diuresis.
6. Others: hyperglycemia and inappropriate ADH syndrome.

Drug Interactions: Toxic synergism with ephedrine has been documented and may occur with some other sympathomimetic bronchodilators.

Drug	Effect
Aminophylline with lithium carbonate	Increased excretion of lithium carbonate
Aminophylline with propranolol	Antagonism of propranolol effect
Theophylline with clindamycin, troleandomycin, erythromycin, lincomycin, cimetidine	Increased theophylline plasma levels

Overdose:
Management:
A. If potential oral overdose is established and seizure has not occurred:
  1. Induce vomiting.
  2. Administer a cathartic (THIS IS PARTICULARLY IMPORTANT IF CONTROLLED RELEASE PREPARATIONS SUCH AS SOMOPHYLLIN®-CRT CAPSULES HAVE BEEN TAKEN).
  3. Administer activated charcoal.
B. If patient is having a seizure:
  1. Establish an airway.
  2. Administer oxygen.
  3. Treat the seizure with intravenous diazepam, 0.1 to 0.3 mg/kg up to 10 mg.
  4. Monitor vital signs, maintain blood pressure, and provide adequate hydration.
C. Post-seizure coma:
  1. Maintain an airway and oxygenation.
  2. If a result of oral medication, follow above recommendations to prevent absorption of drug, but intubation and lavage will have to be performed instead of inducing emesis, and the cathartic and charcoal will need to be introduced via a large bore gastric lavage tube.
  3. Continue to provide full supportive care and adequate hydration while waiting for drug to be metabolized. In general, the drug is metabolized sufficiently rapidly so as not to warrant consideration of dialysis.
D. Animal studies suggest that phenobarbital may decrease theophylline toxicity. There is as yet, however, insufficient data to recommend pretreatment of an overdosage with phenobarbital.

Dosage and Administration: Therapeutic serum levels associated with optimal likelihood for benefit and minimal risk of toxicity are considered to be between 10 mcg/ml and 20 mcg/ml. Levels above 20 mcg/ml may produce toxic effects. There is great variation from patient to patient in dosage needed in order to achieve a therapeutic blood level because of variable rates of elimination. Because of this wide interpatient variation and the

Continued on next page

Fisons—Cont.

relatively narrow therapeutic blood level range, dosage must be individualized. Monitoring of theophylline serum levels is highly recommended. Dosage should be calculated on the basis of lean (ideal) body weight where mg/kg doses are stated. Theophylline does not distribute into fatty tissue.
NOTE: Somophyllin®-CRT capsules are designed to release theophylline slowly but completely. It is recommended that the daily dosage requirement first be established by monitoring serum theophylline levels while the patient has been receiving an immediately available oral liquid such as Somophyllin® Oral Liquid for several days. Thereafter, conversion to Somophyllin®-CRT capsules can be accomplished by administering one half of the total daily theophylline requirement every 12 hours. Rapid theophyllinization should not be attempted using controlled release formulations.
For maximum maintenance dose without measurement of serum concentration or without prior stabilization on an immediately bioavailable form, do not exceed the following:

Age <9 yrs	24 mg/kg/day
Age 9–12 yrs	20 mg/kg/day
Age 12–16 yrs	18 mg/kg/day
Age >16 yrs	13 mg/kg/day or 900 mg/day

(WHICHEVER IS LESS)
Use ideal body weight for obese patients.
If higher doses than those contrained in the above dose schedule are necessary, it is essential that serum theophylline levels be monitored as a clinical guide.
Warning: Do not attempt to maintain any dose that is not tolerated.
Measurement of serum theophylline concentration during chronic therapy: If the above maximum doses are to be maintained or exceeded, serum theophylline measurement is recommended. This should be obtained at the approximate time of peak absorption (4–6 hours) during chronic therapy. It is important that the patient will have missed *no* doses during the previous 72 hours and that dosing intervals will have been reasonably typical with no added doses during that period of time. *Dosage Adjustment Based on Serum Theophylline Measurements When These Instructions Have Not Been Followed May Result in Recommendations That Present Risk of Toxicity to the Patient.*
Comments: It is recommended that serum theophylline concentrations be monitored in order to obtain optimal therapeutic theophylline dosage. However, it is not always possible or practical to obtain a serum theophylline level. Therefore, patients should be closely monitored for signs of toxicity. The present data suggest that the above dosage recommendations will achieve therapeutic serum concentrations with minimal risk of toxicity for most patients. However, some risk of toxic serum concentrations is still present.
Adverse reactions to theophylline often occur when serum theophylline levels exceed 20 mcg/ml.
Caution should be exercised for younger children who cannot complain of minor side effects. Older adults, those with cor pulmonale, congestive heart failure, and/or liver disease, may have unusually low dosage requirements and thus may experience toxicity at maximal dosages.
It is important that no patient be maintained on any dosage that is not tolerated. In instructing patients to increase dosage, they should be instructed not to take a subsequent dose if apparent side effects occur and to resume therapy at a lower dose once adverse effects have disappeared.
How Supplied: Somophyllin-CRT capsules, 100 mg, 200 mg, 250 mg, and 300 mg, in white and clear, imprinted gelatin capsules.

Unit dose boxes of 100
100 mg capsules: NDC 0585-6218-72–imprinted S-CRT 100
200 mg capsules: NDC 0585-6219-03–imprinted S-CRT 200
250 mg capsules: NDC 0585-7218-77–imprinted S-CRT 250
300 mg capsules: NDC 0585-7219-12–imprinted S-CRT 300

Bottles of 100
100 mg capsules: NDC 0585-6218-70–imprinted S-CRT 100
200 mg capsules: NDC 0585-6219-01–imprinted S-CRT 200
250 mg capsules: NDC 0585-7218-75–imprinted S-CRT 250
300 mg capsules: NDC 0585-7219-10–imprinted S-CRT 300

Manufactured for:
FISONS CORPORATION
BEDFORD, MA 01730 U.S.A.
By: DM Graham Laboratories, Inc.
Hobart, NY 13788 U.S.A.

Revised 11/82
FC1888D

Additional Somophyllin® Products are:
SOMOPHYLLIN® Oral Liquid ℞
SOMOPHYLLIN®-DF Oral Liquid ℞
(aminophylline oral solution)
SOMOPHYLLIN® Rectal Solution ℞
(aminophylline enema, USP)
SOMOPHYLLIN®-T Capsules ℞
(theophylline anhydrous capsules)
Please see package inserts for full prescribing information.

EDUCATIONAL MATERIAL

Booklets:
"Asthma Answer Book"—written in lay terminology outlining asthma, medications, triggers, etc. (Free)
"Allergy Fact Book"—written in lay terminology outlining allergic rhinitis and other allergies. Answer book about Nasalcrom®. (Free)
Monographs—for Nasalcrom®. (Free)

Pictures—Charts:
Intal® Sticker Calendar—intended for children on Intal®, to keep daily record of doses with stickers. Colorful and fun. (Free)
Instructional Wall Charts—for Intal® via Spinhaler® and Intal® Nebulizer Solution. (Free)

Samples:
Intal®, Spinhaler® Demo Kit, Intal® Nebulizer Solution, Nasalcrom® Sample Pack, Somophyllin®-CRT (100mg, 200mg, 250mg, 300mg), Somophyllin®-Oral Liquid and -DF (dye free) Oral Liquid, Isoclor® Timesule® Capsules, and Liquid. Available in limited quantities.

C. B. Fleet Co., Inc.
4615 MURRAY PL.
LYNCHBURG, VA. 24502-2235

FLEET® BABYLAX®

Active Ingredient: Glycerin (USP)
Indications: For temporary relief of constipation in young children. Children under 1 year old, consult physician.
Actions: The exact mode of action of glycerin administered rectally as a laxative is not known. It has been suggested that glycerin causes dehydration of exposed tissues to produce an irritant effect which results in a laxative response.
Warning: For rectal use only. Glycerin administered rectally may produce rectal discomfort in some individuals. Frequent or prolonged use of laxatives may result in dependence. Do not use when nausea, vomiting or abdominal pain is present. If use results in unusual pain or side effects, consult a physician. Keep this and all drugs out of the reach of children. If a sudden change in bowel habits persists over two weeks, consult a physician before using a laxative. This product should not be used longer than one week except under a physician's advice.
Dosage and Administration: Children under 1 year old: consult physician. Children 1–6 years of age: 1 rectal applicator containing 4 ml. of glycerin as needed or as directed by physician. Hold unit upright. Remove protective shield and discard. With steady pressure, gently insert stem with tip pointing toward navel. Squeeze unit until nearly all liquid is expelled. Remove tip from rectum. Note: A small amount of liquid will remain in unit. Usually produces a bowel movement within 30 minutes. Store and use at room temperature.
How Supplied: Six 4 ml. rectal applicators per package.
Is This Product O.T.C.: Yes.
Literature Available: Yes.

FLEET® BISACODYL ENEMA
(bisacodyl U.S.P.)

Composition: Each 30 ml (delivered dose) contains 10 mg. of bisacodyl, U.S.P. suspended in an aqueous medium. The FLEET® Bisacodyl Enema unit, with a 2-inch prelubricated Comfortip®, contains 1¼ fl. oz. of enema suspension in a ready-to-use plastic squeeze bottle. Designed for quick, convenient administration by nurse or patient according to instructions. Disposable after single use.
Action and Uses: FLEET® Bisacodyl Enema is a contact laxative acting directly on the colonic mucosa to produce peristalsis. FLEET® Bisacodyl Enema actually produces peristalsis and evacuation of the large intestine by stimulating sensory nerve endings in the colonic mucosa to produce parasympathetic reflexes. FLEET® Bisacodyl Enema is very effective usually producing an evacuation within 15 minutes to 1 hour. FLEET® Bisacodyl Enema may be used whenever a laxative or enema is indicated. It is useful as a laxative for relief of constipation, in bowel cleansing before X-ray and endoscopic examination.
Warning: Frequent or prolonged use of any laxative may result in dependence. Do not use when nausea, vomiting or abdominal pain is present. If use results in unusual pain or other side effects, contact a physician. Keep this and all medication out of the reach of children. In case of accidental overdose or ingestion, contact the nearest poison control center.
Precautions: Do not administer to children under two years of age.
Dosage and Administration: Adults—one unit or as directed by a physician. This dosage is not recommended for children under two years of age. Administration: Preferred position—Lying on left side with left knee slightly bent and the right leg drawn up, or knee-chest position. Rubber diaphragm at base of tube prevents accidental leakage and assures controlled flow of the enema solution. May be used at room temperature.
How Supplied: FLEET® Bisacodyl Enema is supplied in 1¼ fl. oz. ready-to-use squeeze bottle.
Is this Product OTC: Yes.
Literature Available: Professional literature mailed on request.

FLEET® ENEMA

Composition: Each 118 ml (delivered dose) contains 19 g. sodium biphosphate and 7 g. sodium phosphate. The FLEET Enema unit, with a 2-inch, prelubricated Comfortip™, contains 4½ fl. oz. of enema solution in a hand-size plastic squeeze bottle. Designed for quick, convenient administration by nurse or patient according to instructions. Disposable after single use.
Action and Uses: FLEET Enema is useful as a laxative in the relief of constipation, and as a bowel evacuant for a variety of diagnostic, surgical, and therapeutic indications. FLEET Enema provides thorough yet safe cleansing action and induces complete emptying of the left colon usually within 2 to 5 minutes without pain or spasm. FLEET Enema may be used for the relief of constipation; as a routine enema; preparation for rectal examination; during pregnancy and pre- and postnatally; preoperative cleansing and general post-

operative care; to help relieve fecal or barium impaction.
Contraindications: Do not use when nausea, vomiting, or abdominal pain is present.
Warnings: Frequent or prolonged use of enemas may result in dependence. Do not use in patients with megacolon, as hypernatremic dehydration may occur. Use with caution in patients with impaired renal function as hyperphosphatemia and hypocalcemia may occur. As with any drug, if you are pregnant or nursing a baby, seek the advice of a health professional before using this product.
Precautions: Do not administer to children under two years of age unless directed by a physician.
Administration and Dosage: Preferred position: Lying on left side with left knee slightly bent and the right leg drawn up, or knee-chest position. Dosage: Adults, 4 fl. oz.; Children two years or older, 2 fl. oz., or as directed by physician. Rubber diaphragm at base of tube prevents accidental leakage and assures controlled flow of the enema solution. May be used at room temperature. Each 118 ml. (delivered dose) contains 4.4 g. sodium.
How Supplied: FLEET Enema is supplied in 4½ fl. oz. ready-to-use squeeze bottle. Pediatric size, 2¼ fl. oz.
Is This Product O.T.C.: Yes.
Literature Available: Professional literature mailed on request.

FLEET® MINERAL OIL ENEMA

Composition: The FLEET Mineral Oil Enema unit, with a 2-inch, prelubricated Comfortip™, contains 4½ fl.oz. (133 ml.) mineral oil USP in a hand-size plastic squeeze bottle.
Action and Uses: Serves to soften and lubricate hard stools, easing their passage without irritating the mucosa. Results approximate a normal bowel movement in that only the rectum, sigmoid, and part or all of the descending colon are evacuated. Indicated for relief of fecal impaction; valuable in relief of constipation when straining must be avoided (in hypertension, coronary occlusion, proctologic procedures, postoperative care); for removal of barium sulfate residues from the colon after barium administration for GI series or outlining the left atrium; to obtain the laxative benefits of mineral oil while avoiding possible untoward effects of oral administration such as (1) interference with intestinal absorption of fat-soluble vitamins A, D, E and K and other nutrients (2) danger of systemic absorption (3) possible risk of lipid pneumonia due to aspiration.
Contraindications: Do not use when nausea, vomiting, or abdominal pain is present.
Warnings: Frequent or prolonged use of enemas may result in dependence. Take only when needed or when prescribed by a physician. As with any drug, if you are pregnant or nursing a baby, seek the advice of a health professional before using this product.
Precautions: Do not administer to children under two years of age unless directed by a physician.
Administration and Dosage: For rectal administration only. Ready-to-use unit permits easy, rapid administration by physician, nurse, or patient; disposable after single use. *Adults,* 4 fl.oz. *Children two years or older,* one quarter to one half the adult dose, or as directed by physician.
How Supplied: FLEET Mineral Oil Enema is supplied in 4½ fl.oz. ready-to-use squeeze bottle.
Is This Product O.T.C.: Yes.
Literature Available: Professional literature available on request.

FLEET® PHOSPHO®-SODA
Buffered Laxative

Composition: Each 100 ml. of regular or flavored PHOSPHO-SODA contains 48 g. sodium biphosphate and 18 g. sodium phosphate in a stable, buffered aqueous solution.
Action and Uses: Versatile in action as a gentle laxative or purgative, according to dosage. Usually works within one hour when taken before meals, or overnight when taken at bedtime. Virtually free from likelihood of GI discomfort and irritation, PHOSPHO-SODA is pleasant to take, safe for all age groups. Useful before diagnostic examinations or bowel surgery.
Contraindications: Do not use when nausea, vomiting, or abdominal pain is present.
Warnings: Frequent or prolonged use of this preparation may result in dependence on laxatives. Do not use in patients with megacolon, as hypernatremic dehydration may occur. Use with caution in patients with impaired renal function as hyperphosphatemia and hypocalcemia may occur. As with any drug, if you are pregnant or nursing a baby, seek the advice of a health professional before using this product.
Administration and Dosage: Mix required dose with one-half glass cold clear liquid and follow with a full glass of water, preferably on arising or at least 30 minutes before a meal, or at bedtime for overnight action.
As a laxative: 4 teaspoonfuls, diluted as directed.
As a purgative: 8 teaspoonfuls, diluted as directed.
Children: One half the adult dose for children 10 years old or older; one quarter the adult dose for children between 5 and 10 years of age.
Each recommended dose (4 teaspoonfuls) contains 96.4 meq. sodium.
How Supplied: Regular or Flavored, in bottles of 3 and 8 fl. oz.; 1½ fl. oz. size for hospitals.
Is This Product O.T.C.: Yes.
Literature Available: Professional literature on request.

FLEET® PREP KITS
Bowel Evacuant

Description: FLEET® Prep Kit No. 1 contains:
1. FLEET® Phospho®-Soda—1½ fl. oz. Ingredients: Each teaspoonful (5 ml) contains: Active Ingredients: Sodium Biphosphate 2.4 Gm. and Sodium Phosphate 0.9 Gm.
2. FLEET® Bisacodyl—4 laxative tablets. Ingredients: Each enteric-coated tablet contains Bisacodyl, USP, 5 mg.
3. FLEET® Bisacodyl—1 laxative suppository. Ingredients: Bisacodyl, USP, 10 mg.
4. 1 Patient Instruction Sheet.

FLEET® Prep Kit No. 2 contains:
1. FLEET® Phospho®-Soda—1½ fl. oz.
2. FLEET® Bisacodyl—4 tablets.
3. FLEET® Bagenema—1. Ingredients: Liquid castile soap ⅔ fl. oz.
4. 1 Patient Instruction Sheet.

FLEET® Prep Kit No. 3 contains:
1. FLEET® Phospho®-Soda—1½ fl. oz.
2. FLEET® Bisacodyl—4 tablets.
3. FLEET® Bisacodyl Enema—1 laxative enema. Ingredients: 1–30 ml. dose containing 10 mg. of Bisacodyl.
4. 1 Patient Instruction Sheet.

FLEET® Prep Kit No. 4 contains:
1. FLEET® Flavored Castor Oil Emulsion-1½ fl. oz.
Ingredients: Each tablespoonful (15 ml.) contains: Active Ingredients: Castor Oil U.S.P. 10 ml.
2. FLEET® Bisacodyl—4 tablets.
3. FLEET® Bisacodyl—1 suppository.
4. 1 Patient Instruction Sheet.

FLEET® Prep Kit No. 5 contains:
1. FLEET® Flavored Castor Oil Emulsion-1½ fl. oz.
2. FLEET® Bisacodyl—4 tablets.
3. FLEET® Bagenema—1.
4. 1 Patient Instruction Sheet.

FLEET® Prep Kit No. 6 contains:
1. FLEET® Flavored Castor Oil Emulsion-1½ fl. oz.
2. FLEET® Bisacodyl—4 tablets.
3. FLEET® Bisacodyl Enema—30 ml.
4. 1 Patient Instruction Sheet.
Actions: Bowel Evacuant.
Indications: Preparation of the colon for radiology (prior to barium enemas or I.V.P.'s), surgery, and many proctologic and colonoscopic procedures.
Warnings: Each recommended dose ((1½ fl. oz.) (45ml)) of Phospho®-Soda contains 216.9 milliequivalents (mEq) of Sodium. Persons on a low salt diet should consult a health professional before use.
Do not use in patients with megacolon, as hypernatremic dehydration may occur. Use with caution in patients with impaired renal function as hyperphosphatemia and hypocalcemia may occur. Castor Oil affects the small intestine, and regular use may cause excessive loss of water and body salts which can have debilitating effects.
General Warnings: Do not use when nausea, vomiting, or abdominal pain is present. Frequent or prolonged use may result in a dependence on laxatives.
These Kits should not be used by patients under 6 years of age, except on advice of physician.
As with any drug, if you are pregnant or nursing a baby, seek the advice of a health professional before using this product.
Dosage and Administration: See Patient Instruction Sheet for 12, 24, and 48 hour preparation schedule in each kit.
How Supplied: See "Description" for contents of each kit.
Shipping Unit: 48 FLEET® Prep Kits per carton.
For full prescribing information on specific products, see individual listings (FLEET® Phospho®-Soda, FLEET® Bisacodyl Enema and FLEET® Flavored Castor Oil Emulsion).
Is this Product O.T.C: Yes.
Literature Available: Yes.

FLEET® FLAVORED CASTOR OIL EMULSION

Ingredients: Each tablespoonful (15 ml.) contains:
Active Ingredients: Castor oil U.S.P. 10 ml.
Inactive Ingredients: Water, flavoring, emulsifying agents, propylene glycol, sodium benzoate, citric acid and sodium saccharin.
Indications: For the treatment of constipation and preparation of the colon for x-ray and endoscopic examination. (See FLEET® Prep Kit listings.)
Actions: Works directly on the small intestine to promote bowel movement.
Dosage and Administration: Adults: Purgative: 6 tablespoonfuls (90 ml.) Laxative: 3 tablespoonfuls (45 ml.) Children 2 to 12 years: 1 tablespoonful (15 ml.) Children up to 2 years: 1 teaspoonful (5 ml.) For best results, take on an empty stomach. Follow with one full glass of cool water. May be chilled to enhance taste.
General Warnings: Do not use when nausea, vomiting or abdominal pain is present. Frequent or prolonged use may result in a dependence on laxatives. Not to be used on a daily basis, except under the direction of a physician. If you have noticed a sudden change in bowel habits that persists over a period of two weeks, consult a physician before using a laxative. If the recommended use of this product for one week has had no effect, discontinue use and consult a physician. Castor oil affects the small intestine and regular use may cause excessive loss of water and body salts, which can have a debilitating effect. Keep this and all drugs out of the reach of children. In case of accidental overdose, consult a physician immediately. As with any drug, if you are pregnant or nursing a baby, seek the advice of a health professional before using this product.
How Supplied: Bottles of 1½ and 3 fl. oz.
Is This Product O.T.C.: Yes.
Literature Available: Yes.

FLEET® RELIEF   OTC
Anesthetic Hemorrhoidal Ointment

Active Ingredient: Pramoxine Hydrochloride 1%.
Actions: Pramoxine hydrochloride is a topical anesthetic proven to be safe and effective in hospital tests. Delivered in a water soluble base that is greaseless, stainless, and odorless, it begins to

Continued on next page

Fleet—Cont.

work immediately to relieve hemorrhoidal discomforts.
Warning: If bleeding is present, consult physician. Certain persons can develop allergic reactions to ingredients in this product. During treatment, if condition worsens or persists more than seven days, consult physician. If introduction of this product into the rectum causes additional pain, stop use and consult physician promptly. As with any drug, if you are pregnant or nursing a baby, seek the advice of a health professional before using this product.
Dosage and Administration: Disposable Prefilled Applicator—Remove protective cap and gently insert prelubricated stem into the rectum. Squeeze gently until applicator is empty. Remove and discard unit. Use one unit as needed each morning and night and after bowel movements. Do not exceed five applications in 24 hours. Tube—Apply Fleet Relief Ointment generously to the affected area up to five times daily. If accompanying applicator is used, attach to tube and lubricate with small amount of ointment. Insert gently into rectum and squeeze tube. Cleanse applicator after each use.
How Supplied: Six 4 ml. rectal applicators per package or single one ounce tube with applicator.
Is This Product OTC: Yes.

SUMMER'S EVE®
MEDICATED DOUCHE

Active Ingredient: Povidone-iodine provided as a .23 percent solution when packet and sanitized fluid are mixed.
Indications: For symptomatic relief of minor vaginal irritation and itching due to Candida albicans, Trichomonas vaginalis, and Gardnerella vaginalis.
Actions: Povidone-iodine is an effective broad spectrum anti-microbial agent used in treatment of both gram negative and gram positive bacteria, fungi, yeast, and protozoa.
Warnings: Douching does not prevent pregnancy. Do not use during pregnancy or if nursing a baby except with the approval of a physician. If douching results in pain, soreness, itching, excessive dryness, or irritation, stop douching. If symptoms persist after seven days, consult a physician. Keep out of reach of children. Women with iodine sensitivity should not use this product.
Dosage and Administration: Dosage is contained in a single-unit concentrate packet to be added to 4.5 fluid ounces of sanitized solution supplied in a disposable unit. Remove the sanitary overwrap. Unscrew nozzle cap. Carefully open medicated packet and pour contents into bottle. Screw nozzle cap back on to bottle. Swirl gently to assure complete mixing. Pull up the flexible nozzle until it clicks and locks, and Summer's Eve® Medicated Douche is ready to use. After use, the unit is discarded.
Use once daily for seven days even if symptoms disappear.
How Supplied: 4.5 fluid ounce single pack with one 0.14 fluid ounce medicated packet or twin pack containing two 4.5 fluid ounce units and two 0.14 fluid ounce packets.
Is This Product O.T.C.: Yes.

Products are
listed alphabetically
in the
PINK SECTION.

Fleming & Company
1600 FENPARK DR.
FENTON, MO 6

AEROLATE SR & JR & III Capsules ℞
(theophylline, anhydrous T.D.)
AEROLATE LIQUID
(theophylline, anhydrous)

Composition: Contains theophylline 4 grs. (260 mg) as SR, 2 grs (130 mg) as JR, 1 gr. as III (65 mg), in red/clear capsules. Liquid has 160 mg theophyllin/15cc in a non-sugar, non-alcoholic, non-saccharin tangerine flavored base.
Action and Uses: Timed action pellets by-pass stomach to prevent gastric upset. Bronchodilation is achieved through bowel absorption only. Liquid is for the acute attack primarily.
Administration and Dosage: One capsule every 12 hours. Every 8 hours in severe attacks. Liquid—adults—40 ml (2.5 tablespoonfuls) for acute attack. Children—0.25 ml/lb. Maintainance therapy—adults—for the first 6 doses, 25 ml (1.5 tablespoonfuls) before breakfast, at 3 p.m., at bedtime. Then 15 ml doses at above times. Children—0.15ml/lb. at these times, then 0.1ml/lb per dose.
Side Effects: Nausea, vomiting, epigastric or substernal pain, palpitation, headache, dizziness may occur.
How Supplied: Capsules in bottles of 100 and 1000.
Liquid in pints and gallons.

CONGESS SR & JR Capsules ℞
Expectorant/Decongestant T.D.

Composition: Contains guaifenesin 250 mgs/pseudoephedrine 120 mgs as SR; guaifenesin 125 mgs/pseudoephedrine 60 mgs as JR in blue/pink capsules.
Action and Uses: To loosen mucus plugs in upper respiratory tract and congestion in acute pulmonary disorders, and in coughing. Nasal decongestion and alleviation of bronchospasm is also achieved up to 12 hrs. that accompany most coughs, especially during the nocturnal period.
Indications: Nasal congestion, sinusitis, acute aerotitis media, bronchial asthma, serous otitis media, and symptoms of the common cold.
Dosage: Adults and children over 12 yrs. one SR capsule every 12 hrs. Under 12 yrs. one JR capsule as prescribed by physician.
Precaution and Side Effects: Use with care in severe hypertension, heart disease, hyperthyroidism, diabetes. Low grade sensitivity to drugs may be experienced.
Contraindications: Glaucoma, prostatic hypertrophy, patients receiving MAO inhibitors.
How Supplied: Plastic bottles of 100 and 1000 capsules.

EXTENDRYL ℞
T.D. Capsules SR & JR, Syrup and Tablets

Each timed action SR capsule contains phenylepherine HCl 20 mg; methscopolamine nitrate 2.5 mg; chlorpheniramine maleate 8 mg. The JR potency is exactly half-strength. Green/red color for both. Each 5 cc of root beer flavored syrup and tablet contains: phenylephrine HCl 10 mg; methscopolamine nitrate 1.25 mg; chlorpheniramine maleate 2 mg.
Action and Uses: Antihistaminic-decongestant for relief of respiratory congestion; allergic rhinitis; allergic skin reactions of urticaria and angioedema.
Administration and Dosage: Capsules—one every 12 hrs of the SR for adults; one JR every 12 hrs for children 6–12 yrs. Syrup-two teaspoonfuls every 4 hrs for adults; children 1 teaspoonful every 4 hrs. Tablets—adults two and children one every 4 hrs. Do not exceed 4 doses in 24 hrs.
Children under 6 yrs. as recommended by a physician.

Precautions: Withdraw therapy if drowsiness occurs. Patients are cautioned against driving or operating mechanical devices.
Contraindications: Glaucoma, cardiac disease, hyperthyroidism and hypertension.
How Supplied: Capsules and tablets in bottles of 100 and 1000. Syrup in pints and gallons.

MARBLEN
Suspensions and Tablet
(See PDR For Nonprescription Drugs)

NEPHROCAPS   OTC
Dialysis Vitamin Supplement

Description: Each black oval gelatin 'liquid' capsule provides:
Thiamin 1.5 mg; Riboflavin 1.7 mg; Niacin 20 mg; Pantothenic acid 5 mg; Biotin 150 mcg; Cyanocobalamin 6 mcg; Pyridoxin 10 mg; Ascorbic acid 100 mg and Folic acid 0.95 mg.
Indications: the wasting syndrome in chronic renal failure; uremia; impaired metabolic functions of the kidney.
Dosage: One capsule daily. On dialysis days, one Nephrocap must be taken after treatment.
Supplied: Plastic bottles of 100 only.

NEPHROX SUSPENSION
(aluminum hydroxide)
Antacid Suspension
(See PDR For Nonprescription Drugs)

NICOTINEX Elixir
nicotinic acid
(See PDR For Nonprescription Drugs)

OCEAN MIST
(buffered saline)
(See PDR For Nonprescription Drugs)

PIMA Syrup ℞
potassium iodide)

Composition: Contains KI 5 grs./tsp., in a black raspberry flavored base.
Action and Uses: An expectorant in the symptomatic treatment of chronic pulmonary diseases where tenacious mucus complicates the problem, including bronchial asthma, bronchitis and pulmonary emphysema.
Administration and Dosage: Children—one half to one tsp. and adults one or two tsp. every 4-6 hours.
Side Effects: May include gastrointestinal upset, metallic taste, minor skin eruptions, nausea, vomiting and epigastric pain. Therapy should be withdrawn.
Precautions: In patients sensitive to iodides, in hyperthyroidism, and in rare cases iodine-induced goiter may occur.
How Supplied: Plastic pints and gallons.

PURGE
(flavored castor oil)
(See PDR For Nonprescription Drugs)

RUM-K ℞
(potassium chloride 15% conc.)

Description: Each 10 ml. contains 1.5 Gm. potassium chloride (20 mEq) in a butter/rum synthetic flavored base that is alcohol and sugar free.
Indications: Hypokalemic-hypochloremic alkalosis; digitalis toxicity; hypokalemia prevention secondary to corticosteroid or diuretic administration.
Contraindications: Impaired renal function, untreated Addison's Disease, acute dehydration, heat cramps, hyperkalemia.
Precautions: Do not use in patients with low urinary output or renal decompensation. Potassium replacements vary and should be individualized. Patients should be checked frequently, ECG and plasma K+ levels should be made. High serum

concentrations of K+ cause death thru cardiac depression, arrhythmias or arrest. Use with caution in cardiac disease.

Adverse Reactions: Vomiting, nausea, abdominal discomfort, diarrhea may occur. Symptoms and signs of potassium overdose include paresthesias of extremities, flaccid paralysis, listlessness, fall in blood pressure, weakness and heaviness of the legs, cardiac arrhythmias and heart block. Hyperkalemia may cause ECG changes as disappearance of the P wave, widening and slurring of QRS complex, changes of the S-T segment, tall peaked T waves.

Dosage and Administration: Adults—two teaspoonful (10ml) in 4–6 oz water 2 to 4 times daily after meals to supply 40–80 mEq of elemental potassium and chloride. Larger doses may be required and administered under close supervision due to possible potassium intoxication or saline laxative effect.

How Supplied: 2 oz; 4 oz; pints and gallons.

S-P-T
(Pork thyroid "liquid" capsules USP)

Composition: S-P-T is prepared by special process from cleaned, fresh pork thyroid glands, deprived of connective tissue, defatted and suspended in soy bean oil and encapsulated in gelatin for greater oral absorption. The active hormones (T4 and T3) are available in their natural state in a ratio of approximately 2.5:1, as in humans, to insure therapeutic availability. Capsules are standardized by USP method for iodine content and also biologically to insure 100% metabolic potency.

Action: To increase metabolic rate of body tissues. S-P-T is replacement therapy for diminished or absent thyroid function. Effect develops slowly and is fully reached in 10—14 days per grain increase in most instances.

Indications: As replacement therapy in hypothyroidism, cretinism, myxedema, and after surgery following complete thyroidectomy.

Contraindications: In thyrotoxicosis, angina pectoris, myocardial infarction and hypertension unless complicated by hypothyroidism, and uncorrected adrenal insufficiency.

Precaution and Side Effects: Overdosage may cause tachycardia, angina pectoris, diarrhea, nervousness, sweating, headache and increased pulse action. In most cases, reduction of dosage overcomes side effects.

Dosage and Administration: Patients should be titrated starting at lower levels and increasing by 1 gr every 2 weeks until mild thyromimetic effects are noted. Then lower the dose to the level at which the patient felt best, as patients vary widely as to thyroid need.

> **Warnings:** Drugs with thyroid hormone activity, alone or together with other therapeutic agents, have been used for the treatment of obesity. In euthyroid patients, doses within the range of daily hormonal requirements are ineffective for weight reduction. Larger doses may produce serious or even life-threatening manifestations of toxicity, particularly when given in association with sympathomimetic amines such as those used for their anorectic effects.

How Supplied: As 1 gr (green); 2 gr (brown); 3 gr (red); 5 gr (black) gelatin sealed capsules in bottles of 100 and 1000.

Products are cross-indexed by product classifications in the **BLUE SECTION**

Flint
Division of Travenol Laboratories, Inc.
ONE BAXTER PKWY.
DEERFIELD, IL 60015

CHOLOXIN®
[kō" lŏcks' ĭn]
(Dextrothyroxine Sodium Tablets, USP) Flint

Description: CHOLOXIN (dextrothyroxine sodium) is the sodium salt of the dextrorotatory isomer of thyroxine. It is chemically described as D-3,5,3',5'-tetraiodothyronine sodium salt.

Clinical Pharmacology: The predominant effect of CHOLOXIN (dextrothyroxine sodium) is the reduction of serum cholesterol levels in hyperlipidemic patients. Beta lipoprotein and triglyceride fractions may also be reduced from previously elevated levels.
Available evidence indicates that CHOLOXIN (dextrothyroxine sodium) stimulates the liver to increase catabolism and excretion of cholesterol and its degradation products via the biliary route into the feces. Cholesterol synthesis is not inhibited and abnormal metabolic end-products do not accumulate in the blood.

Indication and Usage: For treatment of hyperlipidemia in patients with no known heart disease. **This is not an innocuous drug. Strict attention should be paid to the indications and contraindications.**
CHOLOXIN (dextrothyroxine sodium) is an antilipidemic agent used as an adjunct to diet and other measures for the reduction of elevated serum cholesterol (low density lipoproteins) in euthyroid patients with no known evidence of organic heart disease.
It has not been clearly established whether the drug-induced lowering of serum cholesterol or lipid levels has a detrimental, beneficial, or no effect on the morbidity or mortality due to atherosclerosis or coronary heart disease. Several years will be required before current investigations will yield an answer to this question.

Contraindications: The administration of CHOLOXIN (dextrothyroxine sodium) to euthyroid patients with one or more of the following conditions is contraindicated:
1. Known organic heart disease, including angina pectoris; history of myocardial infarction; cardiac arrhythmia or tachycardia, either active or in patients with demonstrated propensity for arrhythmias; rheumatic heart disease; history of congestive heart failure; and decompensated or borderline compensated cardiac status.
2. Hypertensive states (other than mild, labile systolic hypertension).
3. Advanced liver or kidney disease.
4. Pregnancy.
5. Nursing mothers.
6. History of iodism.

Warnings:

> Drugs with thyroid hormone activity, alone or together with other therapeutic agents, have been used for the treatment of obesity. In euthyroid patients, doses within the range of daily hormonal requirements are ineffective for weight reduction. Larger doses may produce serious or even life threatening manifestations of toxicity, particularly when given in association with sympathomimetic amines such as those used for their anorectic effects.

CHOLOXIN (dextrothyroxine sodium) may potentiate the effects of anticoagulants on prothrombin time. Reductions of anticoagulant dosage by as much as 30% have been required in some patients. Consequently, the dosage of anticoagulants should be reduced by one-third upon initiation of CHOLOXIN (dextrothyroxine sodium) therapy and the dosage subsequently readjusted on the basis of prothrombin time. The prothrombin time of patients receiving anticoagulant therapy concomitantly with CHOLOXIN (dextrothyroxine sodium) therapy should be observed as frequently as necessary, at least weekly during the first few weeks of treatment.
In the surgical patient, it is wise to consider withdrawal of the drug two weeks prior to surgery if the use of anticoagulants during surgery is contemplated.
Special consideration must be given to the dosage of other thyroid medications used concomitantly with CHOLOXIN (dextrothyroxine sodium). As with all thyroactive drugs, hypothyroid patients are more sensitive than euthyroid patients to a given dose of dextrothyroxine sodium.
The injection of epinephrine into patients with coronary artery disease may precipitate an episode of coronary insufficiency. This condition may be enhanced in patients receiving thyroid analogues. These phenomena should be kept in mind when catecholamine injections are required in dextrothyroxine sodium-treated patients with coronary artery disease.
Since the possibility of precipitating cardiac arrhythmias during surgery may be greater in patients treated with thyroid hormones, it may be wise to discontinue CHOLOXIN (dextrothyroxine sodium) in euthyroid patients at least two weeks prior to an elective operation. During emergency surgery in euthyroid patients, the patients should be carefully observed.
There are reports that dextrothyroxine sodium in diabetic patients is capable of increasing blood sugar levels with a resultant increase in requirements of insulin or oral hypoglycemic agents. Special attention should be paid to parameters necessary for good control of the diabetic state in dextrothyroxine sodium-treated subjects and to dosage requirements of insulin or other antidiabetic drugs. If dextrothyroxine sodium is later withdrawn from patients who had required a dosage increase of insulin or oral hypoglycemic agents during its administration, the dosage of antidiabetic drugs should be reduced and adjusted to maintain good control of the diabetic state.
When impaired liver and/or kidney function are present, the advantages of CHOLOXIN (dextrothyroxine sodium) therapy must be weighed against the possibility of deleterious results.

Precautions: It is expected that patients on CHOLOXIN (dextrothyroxine sodium) therapy will show increased serum thyroxine levels. These increased serum thyroxine values are evidence of absorption and transport of the drug, and should NOT be interpreted as evidence of hypermetabolism; therefore, they may not be used to determine the effective dose of dextrothyroxine sodium. Thyroxine values in the range of 10 to 25 mcg% in dextrothyroxine sodium-treated patients are common.
If signs or symptoms of iodism develop during dextrothyroxine sodium therapy, the drug should be discontinued.
A few children with familial hypercholesterolemia have been treated with CHOLOXIN (dextrothyroxine sodium) for periods of one year or longer with no adverse effects on growth. However, it is recommended that the drug be continued in patients in this age group only if a significant serum cholesterol-lowering effect is observed.
The 2 mg and 6 mg tablets of CHOLOXIN (dextrothyroxine sodium) contain FD&C Yellow No. 5 (tartrazine) which may cause allergic-type reactions (including bronchial asthma) in certain susceptible individuals. Although the overall incidence of FD&C Yellow No. 5 (tartrazine) sensitivity in the general population is low, it is frequently seen in patients who also have aspirin hypersensitivity.

Usage in Women of Childbearing Age: Women of childbearing age with familial hypercholesterolemia or hyperlipemia should not be deprived of the use of this drug; it can be given to those patients exercising strict birth control procedures. Since pregnancy may occur despite the use of birth control procedures, administration of CHOLOXIN (dextrothyroxine sodium) to women of this age

Continued on next page

Flint—Cont.

group should be undertaken only after weighing the possible risk to the fetus against the possible benefits to the mother. Teratogenic studies in two animal species have resulted in no abnormalities in the offspring.

Adverse Reactions: The side effects attributed to CHOLOXIN (dextrothyroxine sodium) therapy are, for the most part, due to increased metabolism, and may be minimized by following the recommended dosage schedule. Adverse effects are least commonly seen in euthyroid patients with no signs or symptoms of organic heart disease.

In the absence of known organic heart disease, some cardiac changes may be precipitated during dextrothyroxine sodium therapy. Angina pectoris, extrasystoles, ectopic beats, supraventricular tachycardia, ECG evidence of ischemic myocardial changes and increase in heart size have all been observed. Myocardial infarctions, both fatal and nonfatal, have occurred, but these are not unexpected in untreated patients in the age groups studied. It is not known whether any of these infarcts were drug related.

Changes in clinical status that may be related to the metabolic action of the drug include the development of insomnia, nervousness, palpitations, tremors, loss of weight, lid lag, sweating, flushing, hyperthermia, hair loss, diuresis, and menstrual irregularities. Gastrointestinal complaints during therapy have included dyspepsia, nausea and vomiting, constipation, diarrhea, and decrease in appetite.

Other side effects reported to be associated with dextrothyroxine sodium therapy include the development of headache, changes in libido (increase or decrease), hoarseness, tinnitus, dizziness, peripheral edema, malaise, tiredness, visual disturbances, psychic changes, paresthesia, muscle pain, and various bizarre subjective complaints. Skin rashes, including a few which appeared to be due to iodism, and itching have been attributed to dextrothyroxine sodium by some investigators. Gallstones have been discovered in occasional dextrothyroxine sodium-treated patients and cholestatic jaundice has occurred in one patient, although its relationship to dextrothyroxine sodium therapy was not established.

In several instances, the previously existing conditions of the patient appeared to continue or progress during the administration of dextrothyroxine sodium. A worsening of peripheral vascular disease, sensorium, exophthalmos and retinopathy have been reported.

Dextrothyroxine sodium potentiates the effects of anticoagulants on prothrombin time, thus indicating a decrease in the dosage requirements of the anticoagulants. On the other hand, dosage requirements of antidiabetic drugs have been reported to be increased during dextrothyroxine sodium therapy (see WARNINGS section).

Dosage and Administration: For **adult** euthyroid hypercholesterolemic patients, the recommended maintenance dose of CHOLOXIN (dextrothyroxine sodium) is 4 to 8 mg per day. The initial dose should be 1 to 2 mg daily, to be increased in 1 to 2 mg increments at intervals of not less than one month to a maximal level of 4 to 8 mg daily.

For **pediatric** hypercholesterolemic patients, the recommended maintenance dose of CHOLOXIN (dextrothyroxine sodium) is approximately 0.1 mg (100 mcg) per kilogram. The initial dosage should be approximately 0.05 mg (50 mcg) per kilogram daily, increased at not more than 0.05 mg (50 mcg) per kilogram increments at monthly intervals. The recommended maximal dose is 4 mg daily.

If signs or symptoms of cardiac disease develop during the treatment period, the drug should be withdrawn.

How Supplied: CHOLOXIN (dextrothyroxine sodium) Tablets are supplied as scored, color-coded tablets in 4 concentrations: 1 mg-orange... 2 mg-yellow... 4 mg-white... 6 mg-green.

Literature Available: Upon request.

Shown in Product Identification Section, page 411

FLINT SSD™
(1% Silver Sulfadiazine Cream)

Description: Flint SSD™ (1% Silver Sulfadiazine Cream) is a topical antibacterial preparation which has as its active antimicrobial ingredient silver sulfadiazine. The active moiety is contained within an opaque, white, water-miscible cream base.

Each 1000 grams of Flint SSD™ Cream contains 10 grams of silver sulfadiazine. The cream base contains White Petrolatum, USP; Stearyl Alcohol, NF; Isopropyl Myristate, NF; Sorbitan Monooleate, NF; Polyoxyl 40 Stearate, NF; Propylene Glycol, USP; and Purified Water, USP; with 0.3% Methylparaben, NF, as a preservative.

Silver sulfadiazine has an empirical formula of $C_{10}H_9AgN_4O_2S$, molecular weight of 357.14, and structural formula as shown:

Clinical Pharmacology: Flint SSD™ Cream has demonstrated *in vitro* antimicrobial activity against actual clinical burn wound isolates. Representative organisms included numerous strains of gram-negative and gram-positive bacteria and yeasts. *In vitro* test results evaluating the antimicrobial effectiveness of silver sulfadiazine are summarized in Table 1. All microorganisms analyzed for susceptibility are isolates from burn patients obtained nationwide.

[See table below].

Flint SSD™ (1% Silver Sulfadiazine Cream) exerts its principal antimicrobial effect at the level of the cell membrane and cell wall. The mechanism and site of action differ from sodium sulfadiazine and silver nitrate. *In vitro* analysis has demonstrated that the bactericidal activity exerted by Flint SSD™ (1% Silver Sulfadiazine Cream) is superior to sulfadiazine alone.

Flint SSD™ Cream may be especially applicable to the treatment of pediatric burn patients, because it is not a carbonic anhydrase inhibitor. There have been no reports of acidosis attributable to treatment with Flint SSD™ Cream.

Indications and Usage: Flint SSD™ Cream is a topical antibacterial preparation which is indicated as an adjunct to currently accepted principles of burn wound care, for the prevention and treatment of burn wound sepsis in patients with partial and full thickness burns.

Contraindications: Since sulfonamide derivatives are known to increase the possibility of kernicterus[1], Flint SSD™ Cream should not be used in pregnant women approaching or at term, premature infants, or neonates less than two months of age.

Warnings: Flint SSD™ Cream should be administered with caution to patients with a history of hypersensitivity to silver sulfadiazine. It is not known whether prior sensitivity to other sulfonamides will precipitate an allergic response to Flint SSD™ Cream.

Should manifestation of allergic response to Flint SSD™ Cream be observed, continuation of therapy must be weighed against the potential hazards of the particular allergic reaction.

While Flint SSD™ Cream is exerting a bacteriostatic effect on the burn wound, fungal proliferation in and below the eschar may occur. However, the incidence of clinically reported fungal superinfection is low.

Flint SSD™ Cream should be used with caution in patients with a history of glucose-6-phosphate dehydrogenase deficiency, as hemolysis may occur.

When treatment with Flint SSD™ Cream involves prolonged administration and /or large burn surfaces, considerable amounts of silver sulfadiazine are absorbed. Serum sulfa concentrations may approach adult therapeutic levels (8-12 mg%).

In extensively burned patients, serum sulfa concentrations and renal function should be closely monitored, and urine should be analyzed for presence of sulfa crystals.

Precautions: Following administration of Flint SSD™ (1% Silver Sulfadiazine Cream), absorption of sulfadiazine has been reported. In addition, small amounts of silver are absorbed over the course of repeated application of Flint SSD™ Cream. Impairment of hepatic and renal functions which results in diminished excretion of

TABLE 1
NUMBER OF SENSITIVE BURN ISOLATED STRAINS/
TOTAL BURN ISOLATED STRAINS TESTED
CONCENTRATION OF SILVER SULFADIAZINE

Genus & Species	62.5 mcg/ml	125 mcg/ml
Pseudomonas aeruginosa	46/54	50/54
Pseudomonas cepacia	2/3	2/3
Pseudomonas species	2/3	2/3
Enterobacter cloacae	6/14	6/14
Enterobacter aerogenes	4/6	4/6
Enterobacter agglomerans	1/1	1/1
Klebsiella pneumoniae	4/4	4/4
Klebsiella species	1/3	1/3
Escherichia coli	11/15	11/15
Serratia liquifaciens	3/3	3/3
Serratia marcescens	6/6	6/6
Serratia rubidea	2/2	2/2
Serratia species	0/1	1/1
Proteus mirabilis	8/8	8/8
Proteus morganii	8/9	8/9
Proteus rettgeri	1/1	1/1
Proteus vulgaris	3/4	4/4
Providencia species	3/3	3/3
Citrobacter diversus	0/2	0/2
Shigella species	1/2	1/2
Acinetobacter anitratum	2/2	2/2
Aeromonas hydrophilia	3/3	3/3
Arizona hinshawii	1/1	1/1
Alcaligenes faecalis	2/2	2/2
Staphylococcus aureus	7/7	7/7
Streptococcus Group D (including *Enterococcus*)	17/18	18/18
Bacillus species	0/1	1/1
Candida albicans	1/3	3/3
Candida species	0/1	1/1

drug constituents may lead to accumulation of silver and sulfadiazine moieties. In the presence of hepatic and/or renal dysfunction, the therapeutic benefits of continued silver sulfadiazine administration must be assessed in light of the possibility of accumulation of by-products.

When utilizing topical enzymatic preparations for debridement of partial and full thickness burn wounds, concomitant or alternating topical antimicrobial therapy must be employed.

Pregnancy Category C. Animal reproduction studies have not been conducted with Flint SSD™ Cream. It is also not known whether Flint SSD™ Cream can cause fetal harm when administered to a pregnant woman or can affect reproduction capacity. Flint SSD™ Cream should be given to a pregnant woman only if clearly needed. To date, there are no reports in the medical literature which associate Flint SSD™ Cream therapy with adverse effects on the fetus or reproductive capacity.

Flint SSD™ Cream should be administered to pregnant women only when the physician decides that the potentially life-saving benefits of silver sulfadiazine therapy in the larger burn (extent greater than 20% body surface area) outweigh possible hazard to the fetus.

There is no evidence that topical application of Flint SSD™ Cream results in excretion of any of its constituents in human milk. However, since all sulfonamide derivatives are known to increase the possibility of kernicterus, caution should be exercised when Flint SSD™ Cream is administered to nursing women.

Adverse Reactions: Several cases of transient leukopenia have been reported in patients receiving silver sulfadiazine therapy. Leukopenia associated with silver sulfadiazine administration is primarily characterized by decreased neutrophil count. Maximal white blood cell depression occurs within two to four days of initiation of therapy. Rebound to normal leukocyte levels follows onset within two to three days. Recovery is not influenced by continuation of silver sulfadiazine therapy. This reaction has been reported to occur in approximately one in twenty patients.[6,7]

A low incidence of other adverse reactions has been reported. These include burning sensation, rashes and pruritus, and rarely, interstitial nephritis.

It is often difficult to differentiate topical reactions which are precipitated by Flint SSD™ (1% Silver Sulfadiazine Cream) from those resulting from routine burn wound effects, or caused by hypersensitivity to other therapeutic agents being administered concurrently to the patient.

During the treatment of burns over large body surfaces (greater than 20% body surface area), significant amounts of silver sulfadiazine are systemically absorbed. Therefore, it is possible that any adverse reactions associated with sulfonamides may occur.

Dosage and Administration: In the patients with a major burn, evaluation of airway and fluid replacement needs should precede treatment of the burn wound. After appropriate resuscitative measures are instituted, the burn wound is evaluated for extent and depth, and an appropriate treatment regimen is instituted.

Flinit SSD™ Cream should be applied to a thickness of at least 1/16 inch, to selected burned surfaces once or twice daily.

It is recommended that a protocol for management of the burn wound using accepted principles and techniques of debridement be followed. Flint SSD™ Cream should be applied with sterile gloves.

Flint SSD™ Cream will provide antimicrobial protection when used with either open treatment or occlusive dressing regimens. When treating patients utilizing the open method, care must be taken to promptly reapply Flint SSD™ Cream whenever it is removed by patient movement.

Daily hydrotherapy facilitates debridement of loosened eschar and removal of accumulated debris. Flint SSD™ Cream should be reapplied immediately after hydrotherapy.

Treatment of burns with topical antimicrobial agents has been reported to allow spontaneous healing of deep partial thickness burn wounds, by preventing bacterial proliferation which could otherwise cause conversion to full thickness loss. However, delayed separation of eschar associated with the use of topical antimicrobial agents such as Flint SSD™ Cream may require definitive surgical treatment of the eschar.

should be applied continually until either spontaneous healing or grafting of the burn wound is achieved.

In order to avoid the possibility of infection, Flint SSD™ Cream should not be withdrawn from the therapeutic regimen until definitive wound closure is accomplished, unless there is a significant adverse reaction to the drug.

How Supplied: Flint SSD™ (1% Silver Sulfadiazine Cream) is supplied in plastic jars containing 50 and 400 grams.

Store between 15°–30° C (59°–86° F).

References:
1. **AMA Drug Evaluations,** Fourth Edition: Chapter 77, Sulfonamides and related compounds. 1980, p 1305.
2. Delaveau P, Freidrich-Noue P: Cutaneous absorption and urinary elimination of silver sulfadiazine compounds used in the treatment of burns. **Therapy** 32:563-572, 1977.
3. Dimick AR: Experience with the use of proteolytic enzyme (Travase®) in burn patients. **J Trauma** 17:948-955, 1977.
4. Fox CL Jr: Silver Sulfadiazine - A new topical therapy for Pseudomonas in burns. Therapy of Pseudomonas infection in burns. **Arch Surg** 96:184-188, 1968.
5. Fox CL, Modak SM: Mechanism of silver sulfadiazine action of burn wound infections. **Antimicrobial Agents for Chemotherapy** 5:582-588, 1974.
6. Harrison HN: Pharmacology of sulfadiazine silver - its attachment to burned human and rat skin and studies of gastrointestinal absorption and extension. **Arch Surg** 114:281-285, 1979.
7. Jarret F, Ellerbe S, Demling R: Acute leukopenia during topical burn therapy with silver sulfadiazine. **Amer J Surg** 135:818-819, 1978.
8. Kiker RG, Carvajal HF, Mlcak RP, Larson DL: A controlled study of the effects of silver sulfadiazine on white blood cell counts in burned children. **J Trauma** 17:835-836, 1977.
9. Krizek TJ: Emergency nonsurgical escharotomy in the burned extremity. **Ortho Rev,** July 1975, p 53-55.
10. Pennisi VR, Abril F, Cappozzi A: The combined efficacy of Travase and silver sulphadiazine in the acute burn. **Burns** 2:169-172, 1976.
11. Rodeheaver G: Proteolytic enzymes as adjuncts to antimicrobial prophylaxis of contaminated wounds. **Amer J Surg** 129:537-544, 1975.

Literature Available: Upon request.

Shown in Product Identification Section, page 411

SYNTHROID®   ℞

[sin'throid]
(Levothyroxine Sodium, USP) Flint
Synthroid Tablets—for oral administration
Synthroid Injection—for parenteral administration after reconstitution

Description: SYNTHROID (levothyroxine sodium) Tablets and SYNTHROID Injection contain synthetic crystalline levothyroxine sodium (L-thyroxine). L-thyroxine is the principal hormone secreted by the normal thyroid gland.

Pharmacologic Category: SYNTHROID (levothyroxine sodium) Tablets, taken orally, provide hormone that is absorbed readily from the gastrointestinal tract. SYNTHROID Injection is effective by any parenteral route. Following absorption, the synthetic L-thyroxine provided by SYNTHROID (levothyroxine sodium) products cannot be distinguished from L-thyroxine that is secreted endogenously. Each is bound to the same serum proteins forming a reservoir of circulating L-thyroxine.

Both SYNTHROID (levothyroxine sodium) products will provide L- thyroxine (T_4) as a substrate for physiologic deiodination to L-triiodothyronine (T_3). Therefore, patients taking properly adjusted doses of both SYNTHROID (levothyroxine sodium) products will demonstrate normal blood levels of L- triiodothyronine even when the thyroid gland has been removed surgically or destroyed by radioiodine. Administration of levothyroxine sodium alone will result in complete physiologic thyroid replacement.

Indications and Usage: SYNTHROID (levothyroxine sodium) products serve as specific replacement therapy for reduced or absent thyroid function of any etiology. SYNTHROID (levothyroxine sodium) Injection can be used intravenously whenever a rapid onset of effect is critical, and either intravenously or intramuscularly in hypothyroid patients whenever the oral route is precluded for long periods of time.

Contraindications: There are no absolute contraindications to SYNTHROID (levothyroxine sodium) therapy. Relative contraindications include acute myocardial infarction, uncorrected adrenal insufficiency and thyrotoxicosis (see WARNINGS).

Warnings:

> Drugs with thyroid hormone activity, alone or together with other therapeutic agents, have been used for the treatment of obesity. In euthyroid patients, doses within the range of daily hormonal requirements are ineffective for weight reduction. Larger doses may produce serious or even life threatening manifestations of toxicity, particularly when given in association with sympathomimetic amines such as those used for their anorectic effects.

Patients with cardiovascular diseases warrant particularly close attention during the restoration of normal thyroid function by any thyroid drug. In such cases, low initial dosage increased slowly by small increments is indicated. Occasionally, the cardiovascular capacity of the patient is so compromised that the metabolic demands of the normal thyroid state cannot be met. Clinical judgment will then dictate a less-than-complete restoration of thyroid status.

Endocrine disorders such as diabetes mellitus, adrenal insufficiency (Addison's disease), hypopituitarism and diabetes insipidus are characterized by signs and symptoms which may be diminished in severity or obscured by hypothyroidism. SYNTHROID (levothyroxine sodium) therapy for such patients may aggravate the intensity of previously obscured symptoms and require appropriate adjustment of therapeutic measures directed at these concomitant disorders.

Thyroid replacement may potentiate the effects of anticoagulants. Patients on anticoagulant therapy should have frequent prothrombin determinations when instituting thyroid replacement to gauge the need to reduce anticoagulant dosage.

Precautions: Overdosage with any thyroid drug may produce the signs and symptoms of thyrotoxicosis, but resistance to such factitious thyrotoxicosis is the general rule. With SYNTHROID (levothyroxine sodium) Tablets, the relatively slow onset of action minimizes the risk of overdose but close observation in the weeks following institution of a dosage regimen is advised. Treatment of thyroid hyperactivity induced by oral medication is confined to interruption of therapy for a week, followed by reinstitution of daily therapy at an appropriately reduced dosage.

Close observation of the patient following the administration of SYNTHROID (levothyroxine sodium) Injection is advised, and appropriate adjustment of repeated dosage is recommended.

The 100 mcg (0.1 mg) and 300 mcg (0.3 mg) tablets of SYNTHROID (levothyroxine sodium) contain FD&C Yellow No. 5 (tartrazine) which may cause allergic-type reactions (including bronchial asthma) in certain susceptible individuals. Al-

Continued on next page

Flint—Cont.

though the overall incidence of FD&C Yellow No. 5 (tartrazine) sensitivity in the general population is low, it is frequently seen in patients who also have aspirin hypersensitivity.

Adverse Reactions: Adverse reactions are due to overdose and are those of induced hyperthyroidism.

Dosage and Administration: For most adults, a final dosage of 100 mcg. (0.1 mg.) to 200 mcg. (0.2 mg.) of SYNTHROID (levothyroxine sodium) **Tablets** daily will provide adequate thyroid replacement, and only occasionally will patients require larger doses. Failure to respond adequately to a daily oral intake of 400 mcg. (0.4 mg.) or more is rare and should prompt reconsideration of the diagnosis of hypothyroidism, special investigation of the patient in terms of malabsorption of L-thyroxine from the gastrointestinal tract or evaluation of patient compliance to therapy.

The concomitant appearance of other diseases, especially cardiovascular diseases, usually dictates a replacement regimen with initial doses smaller than 100 mcg. (0.1 mg.) per day.

In otherwise healthy adults with relatively recent onset of hypothyroidism, full replacement doses of 150 mcg. (0.15 mg.) or 200 mcg. (0.2 mg.) have been instituted immediately without untoward effect and with good therapeutic response. General experience, however, favors a more cautious approach in view of the possible presence of subclinical disorders of the cardiovascular system or other endocrinopathies.

The age and general physical condition of the patient and the severity and duration of hypothyroid symptoms determine the starting dosage and the rate of incremental dosage increase leading to a final maintenance dosage. In the elderly patient with long standing disease, evidence of myxedematous infiltration and symptomatic, functional or electrocardiographic evidence of cardiovascular dysfunction, the starting dose may be as little as 25 mcg. (0.025 mg.) per day. Further incremental increases of 25 mcg. (0.025 mg.) per day may be instituted at three to four week intervals depending on patient response. Conversely, otherwise healthy adults may be started at higher daily doses and raised to a full replacement dose in two to three weeks. Clearly it is the physician's judgment of the severity of the disease and close observation of patient response which determine the rate and extent of dosage increase.

Appropriate laboratory tests are beneficial in monitoring thyroid replacement therapy. Although measurements of normal blood levels of thyroxine in patients on oral replacement regimens frequently coincide with clinical impressions of normal thyroid status, higher than normal levels occur occasionally and should not be considered evidence of overdosage per se. In all cases, clinical impressions of the well-being of the patient take precedence over laboratory determinations of appropriate individual dosage.

In infants and children, there is a great urgency to achieve full thyroid replacement because of the critical importance of thyroid hormone in sustaining growth and maturation. Despite the smaller body size, the dosage needed to sustain a full rate of growth, development and general thriving is higher in the child than in the adult.

The recommended daily replacement dosage of levothyroxine sodium in childhood is: 0-1 years: 9 mcg/kg; 1-5 years: 6 mcg/kg; 6-10 years: 4 mcg/kg; 11-20 years: 3 mcg/kg. Dose is administered once daily only. Optimal maintenance levels should be adjusted individually to obtain normal serum T_3, T_4, free T_4 index and Thyroid Stimulating Hormone (TSH) values after several weeks of therapy for hypothyroidism. The patient's clinical status is most important and some patients may be clinically euthyroid with individual laboratory values that are not within normal range (i.e. elevated total T_4 with normal T_3). An exception may be seen in congenital hypothyroidism where elevated serum TSH values may persist for the first 2-3 years of life despite normalization of free T_4 measurements. In such cases, it generally is recommended that maintenance of normal serum free T_4 values alone should be considered therapeutically sufficient.

In myxedema coma or stupor, without concomitant severe heart disease, 200 to 500 mcg. of SYNTHROID (levothyroxine sodium) **Injection** may be administered intravenously as a solution containing 100 mcg./ml. DO NOT ADD TO OTHER INTRAVENOUS FLUIDS. Although the patient may show evidence of increased responsivity within six to eight hours, full therapeutic effect may not be evident until the following day. An additional 100 to 300 mcg. or more may be given on the second day if evidence of significant and progressive improvement has not occurred. Like the oral dosage form, SYNTHROID (levothyroxine sodium) **Injection** produces a predictable increase in the reservoir level of hormone with a seven day half-life. This usually precludes the need for multiple injections but continued daily administration of lesser amounts parenterally should be maintained until the patient is fully capable of accepting a daily oral dose. A daily maintenance dose of 50 to 100 mcg parenterally should suffice to maintain the euthyroid state, once established.

In the presence of concomitant heart disease, the sudden administration of such large doses of L-thyroxine intravenously is clearly not without its cardiovascular risks. Under such circumstances, intravenous therapy should not be undertaken without weighing the alternative risks of the myxedema coma and the cardiovascular disease. Clinical judgment in this situation may dictate smaller intravenous doses of SYNTHROID (levothyroxine sodium) **Injection**.

SYNTHROID (levothyroxine sodium) **Injection** by intravenous or intramuscular routes can be substituted for the oral dosage form when ingestion of SYNTHROID (levothyroxine sodium) **Tablets** is precluded for long periods of time. The initial parenteral dosage should be approximately one half of the previously established oral dosage of levothyroxine sodium tablets. Close observation of the patient, with individual adjustment of the dosage as needed, is recommended.

How Supplied: SYNTHROID (levothyroxine sodium) **Tablets** are supplied as scored, color-coded potency-marked tablets in 8 strengths: 25 mcg. (0.025 mg.)—orange ... 50 mcg. (0.05 mg.)—white ... 75 mcg. (0.075 mg.)—violet ... 100 mcg. (0.1 mg.)—yellow ... 125 mcg. (0.125 mg)—brown ... 150 mcg. (0.15 mg.)—blue ... 200 mcg. (0.2 mg.)—pink ... 300 mcg. (0.3 mg.)—green.

SYNTHROID (levothyroxine sodium) **Injection** is lyophilized in the final container with 10 mg Mannitol, USP and 0.7 mg tribasic sodium phosphate anhydrous. pH may be adjusted with sodium hydroxide. It is supplied in color-coded 10 ml vials in 3 strengths: 100 mcg — blue... 200 mcg—gray... 500 mcg—yellow.

Directions for Reconstitution: Reconstitute the lyophilized levothyroxine sodium by aseptically adding 5 ml. of 0.9% Sodium Chloride Injection, USP or Bacteriostatic Sodium Chloride Injection, USP with Benzyl Alcohol, only. Shake vial to insure complete mixing. **Use immediately** after reconstitution. Do not add to other intravenous fluids. Discard any unused portion.

Literature Available: Upon request.

Shown in Product Identification Section, page 411

TRAVASE® OINTMENT R
[trăv'āz]
(Sutilains Ointment, USP)

Description: TRAVASE Ointment (Sutilains Ointment, USP) is a sterile preparation of proteolytic enzymes, elaborated by **Bacillus subtilis**, in a hydrophobic ointment base consisting of 95% white petrolatum and 5% polyethylene. One gram of ointment contains approximately 82,000 casein units* of proteolytic activity.

*A casein unit is the amount of enzyme required to produce the same optical density at 275 mμ as that of a solution of 1.5 mcg. tyrosine/ml. after the enzyme has been incubated with 35 mg. of casein at 37° C. for one minute.

Action: TRAVASE Ointment selectively digests necrotic soft tissues by proteolytic action. It dissolves and facilitates the removal of necrotic tissues and purulent exudates that otherwise impair formation of granulation tissue and delay wound healing.

At body temperatures these proteolytic enzymes have optimal activity in the pH range from 6.0 to 6.8.

Indications: For wound debridement—TRAVASE Ointment is indicated as an adjunct to established methods of wound care for biochemical debridement of the following lesions:
  Second and third degree burns,
  Decubitus ulcers,
  Incisional, traumatic, and pyogenic wounds,
  Ulcers secondary to peripheral vascular disease.

Contraindications: Application of TRAVASE Ointment is contraindicated in the following conditions:
  Wounds communicating with major body cavities,
  Wounds containing exposed major nerves or nervous tissue,
  Fungating neoplastic ulcers,
  Wounds in women of child-bearing potential—because of lack of laboratory evidence of effects of TRAVASE Ointment upon the developing fetus.

Warning: Do not permit TRAVASE Ointment to come into contact with the eyes. In treatment of burns or lesions about the head or neck, should the ointment inadvertently come into contact with the eyes, the eyes should be immediately rinsed with copious amounts of water, preferably sterile.

Precautions: A moist environment is essential to optimal activity of the enzyme. Enzyme activity may also be impaired by certain agents. **In vitro**, several detergents and antiseptics (benzalkonium chloride, hexachlorophene, iodine, and nitrofurazone) may render the substrate indifferent to the action of the enzyme. Compounds such as thimerosal, containing metallic ions, interfere directly with enzyme activity to a slight degree, whereas neomycin, sulfamylon, streptomycin, and penicillin do not affect enzyme activity. In cases where adjunctive topical therapy has been used and no dissolution of slough occurs after treatment with TRAVASE Ointment for 24 to 48 hours, further application, because of interference by the adjunctive agents, is unlikely to be rewarding.

In cases where there is existent or threatening invasive infection, appropriate systemic antibiotic therapy should be instituted concurrently.

Although there have been no reports of systemic allergic reaction to TRAVASE Ointment in humans, studies have shown that there may be an antibody response in humans to absorbed enzyme material.

Adverse Reactions: Adverse reactions consist of mild, transient pain, paresthesias, bleeding and transient dermatitis. Pain usually can be controlled by administration of mild analgesics. Side effects severe enough to warrant discontinuation of therapy occasionally have occurred.

If bleeding or dermatitis occurs as a result of the application of TRAVASE Ointment, therapy should be discontinued. No systemic toxicity has been observed as a result of the topical application of TRAVASE Ointment.

Dosage and Administration:
STRICT ADHERENCE TO THE FOLLOWING IS REQUIRED FOR EFFECTIVE RESULTS OF TREATMENT
1. Thoroughly cleanse and irrigate wound area with sodium chloride or water solutions. Wound MUST be cleansed of antiseptics or heavy-metal antibacterials which may denature enzyme or alter substrate characteristics (e.g., hexachlorophene, silver nitrate, benzalkonium chloride, nitrofurazone).
2. Thoroughly moisten wound area either through tubbing, showering, or wet soaks (e.g., sodium chloride or water solutions).
3. Apply TRAVASE Ointment in a thin layer assuring intimate contact with necrotic tis-

sue and complete wound coverage extending to ¼ to ½ inch beyond the area to be debrided.
4. Apply loose moist dressings.
5. Repeat entire procedure 3 to 4 times per day for best results.

How Supplied: TRAVASE Ointment (Sutilains Ointment, USP) is supplied sterile in one-half ounce (14.2 g) tubes. Each gram contains 82,000 casein units of proteolytic activity in a hydrophobic ointment base.
The ointment must be refrigerated at 2° to 8° C (35° to 46° F).

Shown in Product Identification Section, page 411

EDUCATIONAL MATERIAL

Booklet-Pamphlet
"Thyroid Today" various authors, publication issued 4 times per year. Publication provides information written by physicians for physicians concerning thyroid disease diagnosis and treatment. Free to Physicians and Pharmacists.
Samples
Provide physicians with professional supply of Synthroid® (Levothyroxine Sodium, USP) when written prescription is included. (Allow 8 wks. delivery.) Strengths include 0.025 mg., 0.05 mg., 0.1 mg., 0.15 mg., 0.2 mg., 0.3 mg., in unit size of 100 tablets per bottle. Only 2 samples per order.

Fluoritab Corporation
P.O. BOX 381
FLINT, MICHIGAN 48501

FLUORITAB® ℞
[*floor'a tab*]
sodium fluoride (Active Ingredient)

Composition:
Sodium fluoride .... 2.2 mg.
Inert organic filler .... 75.8 mg.
Each tablet contains 1 mg. of fluorine (as fluoride ion)

Action and Uses: FLUORITAB dietary fluoride products are straight fluoride and contain no other active ingredients. They are to provide optimum fluoride where water supplies are deficient in fluorine. Dietary fluoride is beneficial in providing teeth that are more resistant to decay. Fluorine combines with calcium to form the apatite molecule of teeth and bone to form fluorapatite crystals.
Administration and Dosage: FLUORITAB dietary fluoride can be given in baby formulas, or in any liquid. They can be swallowed quickly, or permitted to remain in the mouth to dissolve, which may provide surface benefit to tooth enamel. Fluoride must be taken on a continued basis throughout the period of tooth formation to be fully effective.
Dosage should provide the child with ½ mg. per day from birth to 3 years of age and 1 mg. per day from 3 years of age up.
Water supplies with 0.2 parts per million or less require supplementing with ½ mg. and 1 mg. dosage per day for children under and over 3, respectively. Water supplies with 0.2 to 0.6 parts per million require ¼ mg. and ½ mg. dosage per day for children under 3 and over 3 respectively.
Side Effects: Excess fluoride is to be avoided, as it may cause dental fluorosis (mottling of the teeth).
Precautions: Where water with 0.7 P.P.M. of fluoride is used, dietary fluoride ought not be used.
Contraindications: None.
Overdosage: (*Symptoms and Treatment*): The total contents of our safety limited packages can be taken without any effect.
How Supplied: FLUORITAB TABLETS are supplied in bottles of 100, scored, easily divided 1.2 grain tablets, 1 mg. fluorine per tablet. FLUORITAB LIQUID is supplied in 19 cc. (480 drop) (.25 mg. fluorine per drop) polyethelene squeeze type dropper bottles.
Product Identification Mark(s): FLUORITAB products have the "FLUORITAB" name on all packages.
Remarks: FLUORITAB dietary fluoride was the first dietary fluoride product given A.D.A. acceptance (July, 1958). We adhere rigidly to their recommendation of restricting our package size to their safety admonition: *Never* to sell packages containing more than 264 mg. of sodium fluoride.
Literature Available: Reprints, educational folders and prescription instructions will be sent free, on request.

Forest Laboratories, Inc.
919 THIRD AVENUE
NEW YORK, NEW YORK 10022

ISOCHRON® TABLETS ℞
[*ī'sō-kron"*]
(Isosorbide Dinitrate in Controlled Release)

Description: Isosorbide Dinitrate has the following structural formula:

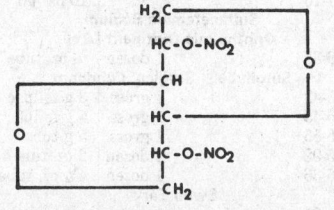

(1,4:3,6-dianhydro-d-glucitol-dinitrate)

It is a white, crystalline, odorless compound, stable in air and in solution with a melting point of 70°C and optical rotation of +134° (c=1.0, alcohol, 20°C).
Actions: The basic action of Isosorbide Dinitrate is that of all nitrates, the relaxation of smooth muscle. How this relates to its clinical usefulness in the treatment of angina pectoris (pain of coronary artery disease) is not clear, since the exact cause of this pain is also obscure.
The objective of therapy is a decrease in the frequency and severity of attacks of angina pectoris and a decrease in the need to use nitroglycerin. This is the only practical way to judge the effects of therapy, especially since there is a wide variation in symptomatic response to treatment. Isosorbide Dinitrate is widely accepted as a safe and useful therapeutic agent in the treatment of angina pectoris.

Indications: Based on a review of this drug by the National Academy of Sciences-National Research Council and/or other information, FDA has classified the indications as follows:
"Possibly" effective: When taken by the oral route, Isosorbide Dinitrate is indicated for the relief of angina pectoris (pain of coronary artery disease).
It is not intended to abort the acute anginal episode, but is widely regarded as useful in prophylactic treatment of angina pectoris.
Final classification of the less-than effective indications requires further investigation.

Contraindication: Idiosyncrasy to this drug.
Warnings: Data supporting the use of nitrites during the early days of the acute phase of myocardial infarction (the period during which clinical and laboratory findings are unstable) are insufficient to establish safety.
Precautions: Tolerance to this drug, and cross-tolerance to other nitrites and nitrates may occur. In patients with functional or organic gastrointestinal hypermotility or malabsorption syndrome it is suggested that 2.5 mg. or 5 mg. sublingual or chewable tablets be the preferred therapy.
Adverse Reactions:
1. Cutaneous vasodilation with flushing.
2. Headache is common and may be severe and persistent.
3. Transient episodes of dizziness and weakness, as well as other signs of cerebral ischemia associated with postural hypotension, may occasionally develop.
4. This drug can act as a physiological antagonist to norepinephrine, acetylcholine, histamine, and many other agents.
5. An occasional individual exhibits marked sensitivity to the hypotensive effects of nitrite, and severe responses (nausea, vomiting, weakness, restlessness, pallor, perspiration and collapse) can occur even with the usual therapeutic dose. Alcohol may enhance this effect.
6. Drug rash and/or exfoliative dermatitis may occasionally occur.

Dosage and Administration: These sustained action medications are administered one tablet orally every 6 to 12 hours according to need. They are indicated for sustained prophylaxis against angina pectoris attacks including nocturnal angina. Although the latter condition is relatively infrequent, it is nonetheless angina, i.e., pain of coronary artery disease. Although experiencing a reduction in the number of anginal attacks while under therapy, patients may still have an attack under stressful conditions. In such cases, therapy should be supplemented with sublingual nitroglycerin. Isosorbide Dinitrate in Controlled Release Tablets SHOULD NOT BE CHEWED.
How Supplied: Isochron™ Tablets (Isosorbide Dinitrate in Controlled Release) 40 mg. are available in green capsule shaped scored tablets in bottles of 60, 100, 500 and 1000.
White, capsule-shaped scored 20 mg. Isochron® Tablets in Controlled Release are available in bottles of 100, 500, and 1000.
Storage: Preserve in well closed containers and prevent exposure to excessive heat.
Caution: Federal law prohibits dispensing without prescription.

E. Fougera & Company
Division of Altana Inc.
60 BAYLIS ROAD
MELVILLE, NY 11747

NDC 0168	PRODUCT		
	Analgesic Balm		
0036-31			1 oz. tube
0036-16			1 lb. jar
	Analgesic Balm (Greaseless)		
0219-31			1 oz. tube
0219-16			1 lb. jar
	Atropine Sulfate Ophthalmic Ointment, U.S.P. 1% (*Rx*)		
0065-38		1 dozen	⅛ oz. tube
	Bacitracin Ointment U.S.P. 500 units per g		
0011-09		1 gross	1/32 oz. foilpac
0011-35			½ oz. tube
0011-31			1 oz. tube
0011-04			4 oz. tube
0011-16			1 lb. jar
	Bacitracin Ophthalmic Ointment U.S.P. (*Rx*)		
0026-38		1 dozen	⅛ oz. tube
	Bacitracin-Neomycin-Polymyxin Ointment		
0012-09		1 gross	1/32 oz. foilpac
0012-35			½ oz. tube
0012-31			1 oz. tube
	Bacitracin-Neomycin-Polymyxin Ophthalmic Ointment (*Rx*)		
0027-38		1 dozen	⅛ oz. tube

Continued on next page

Fougera—Cont.

Bacitracin-Polymyxin Ointment
0021-35   ½ oz. tube
0021-31   1 oz. tube

Betamethasone Valerate Cream, U.S.P. 0.1% (Rx)
0040-15   15 g tube
0040-46   45 g tube

Betamethasone Valerate Ointment U.S.P. 0.1% (Rx)
0033-15   15 g tube
0033-46   45 g tube

Betamethasone Valerate Lotion U.S.P. 0.1% (Rx)
0041-60   60 ml bottle

Boric Acid Ointment
0042-31   1 oz. tube
0042-02   2 oz. tube

Boric Acid Ophthalmic Ointment 5%
0066-38   1 dozen   ⅛ oz. tube

Cold Cream U.S.P.
0045-31   1 oz. tube
0045-16   1 lb. jar

Dibucaine Ointment, U.S.P. 1%
0046-31   1 oz. tube

Efodine® Ointment (Povidone-Iodine)
0090-09   1 gross   1/32 oz. foilpac
0090-31   1 oz. tube
0090-16   1 lb. jar

Erythromycin Ophthalmic Ointment U.S.P. (Rx)
0070-38   1 dozen   ⅛ oz. tube

Fluocinolone Acetonide Cream, U.S.P. 0.01% (Rx)
0058-15   15 g tube
0058-60   60 g tube

Fluocinolone Acetonide Topical Solution, U.S.P. 0.01% (Rx)
0059-60   60 ml bottle

Fluocinolone Acetonide Cream, U.S.P. 0.025% (Rx)
0060-15   15 g tube
0060-60   60 g tube

Fluocinolone Acetonide Ointment, U.S.P. 0.025% (Rx)
0064-15   15 g tube
0064-50   60 g tube

Hydrocortisone Cream, U.S.P. 0.5%
0014-31   1 oz. tube

Hydrocortisone Ointment, U.S.P. 0.5%
0016-31   1 oz. tube

Hydrocortisone Cream, U.S.P. 1% (Rx)
0015-29   20 g tube
0015-31   1 oz. tube
0015-04   4 oz. jar
0015-16   1 lb. jar

Hydrocortisone Ointment, U.S.P. 1% (Rx)
0020-31   1 oz. tube
0020-16   1 lb. jar

Hydrophilic Ointment
0047-16   1 lb. jar

Ichthammol Ointment U.S.P. 10%
0048-31   1 oz. tube

Ichthammol Ointment 20%
0049-31   1 oz. tube

Iodochlorhydroxyquin 3% with Hydrocortisone 0.5% Cream (Rx)
0010-31   1 oz. tube

Iodochlorhydroxyquin 3% with Hydrocortisone 1% Cream (Rx)
0022-29   20 g tube

Lanolin Anhydrous U.S.P.
0052-16   1 lb. jar

Lanolin U.S.P.
0051-31   1 oz. tube
0051-16   1 lb. jar

Lidocaine Ointment, U.S.P. 5% (Rx)
0204-37   1¼ oz. tube

Nitroglycerin Ointment 2% (Rx)
0038-30   30 g tube
0038-60   60 g tube

Nystatin Cream U.S.P. (Rx)
0054-15   100,000 U/g   15 g tube
0054-30   30 g tube

Nystatin Ointment U.S.P. (Rx)
0007-15   100,000 U/g   15 g tube

Nystatin Vaginal Tablets U.S.P. (Rx) 100,000 Units
0031-15   box of 15
0031-30   box of 30

Nystatin-Neomycin-Gramicidin-Triamcinolone Cream (Rx)
0024-15   15 g tube
0024-30   30 g tube
0024-60   60 g tube
0024-04   120 g jar

Nystatin-Neomycin-Gramicidin-Triamcinolone Ointment (Rx)
0025-15   15 g tube
0025-30   30 g tube
0025-60   60 g tube

Petrolatum (White) U.S.P.
0053-45   1 gross   5 g foilpac
0053-21   1 oz. tube
0053-31   Hospital Pak   1 gross   1 oz. tube
0053-16   1 lb. jar

Petrolatum (White) Ophthalmic Ointment
0053-38   1 dozen   ⅛ oz. tube

Polysorb® Hydrate Cream
0217-02   2 oz. tube
0217-16   16 oz. jar

Sulfacetamide Sodium Ophthalmic Ointment (Rx)
0079-38   1 dozen   ⅛ oz. tube

Surgilube® Surgical Lubricant
0205-43   1 gross   3 g foilpac
0205-45   1 gross   5 g foilpac
0205-55   1 gross   5 g tube
0205-02   1 dozen   2 oz. tube
0205-36   1 dozen   4¼ oz. tube

Swim Ear®
7931-91   1 dozen   1 oz. bottle

Triamcinolone Acetonide Cream, U.S.P. 0.025% (Rx)
0003-15   15 g tube
0003-80   80 g tube
0003-16   1 lb. jar

Triamcinolone Acetonide Ointment, U.S.P. 0.025% (Rx)
0005-15   15 g tube
0005-80   80 g tube

Triamcinolone Acetonide Cream, U.S.P. 0.1% (Rx)
0004-15   15 g tube
0004-80   80 g tube
0004-16   1 lb. jar

Triamcinolone Acetonide Ointment, U.S.P. 0.1% (Rx)
0006-15   15 g tube
0006-80   80 g tube

Triamcinolone Acetonide Cream, U.S.P. 0.5% (Rx)
0002-15   15 g tube

Triple Sulfa Vaginal Cream (Rx)
0018-33   (Sulfathiazole 3.42%, Sulfacetamide 2.86%, Sulfabenzamide 3.7% and Urea 0.64%)   2¾ oz. tube w/applicator
0018-34   Disposable Applicators for single-dose use   1 dozen

Vitamin A + Vitamin D Ointment
0035-45   1 gross   5 g foilpac
0035-01   2 oz. tube
0035-02   Hospital Pak   6 dozen   2 oz. tube
0035-04   4 oz. tube
0035-16   1 lb. jar

Whitfield's Ointment
0061-31   (Benzoic & Salicylic Acid Ointment U.S.P.)   1 oz. tube

Yellow Mercuric Oxide Ophthalmic Ointment 1%
0075-38   1 dozen   ⅛ oz. tube

Yellow Mercuric Oxide Ophthalmic Ointment 2%
0076-38   1 dozen   ⅛ oz. tube

Zinc Oxide Ointment U.S.P.
0062-31   1 oz. tube
0062-02   2 oz. tube
0062-16   1 lb. jar

GEIGY Pharmaceuticals
Division of CIBA-GEIGY Corporation
ARDSLEY, NY 10502

GY-CODE® INDEX

GEIGY Pharmaceuticals has established a Drug Identity Code System entitled GY-CODE. This system affords a convenient and accurate means of uniquely identifying each Geigy solid dosage form on which the GY-CODE number and the name "Geigy" appear. The GY-CODE number also appears as part of the National Drug Code number.

GY-CODE NUMBER	PROD. DESCRIPTION	NATIONAL DRUG CODE
11 Tofranil® Tablets	imipramine hydrochloride USP	25 mg.
	Coral-colored (black Geigy imprint) coated tablets	
	100's	0028-0011-01
	1000's	0028-0011-10
	100's Unit Dose Pkg.	0028-0011-61
	Gy-Pak® 100's	
	One unit (12 × 100)	0028-0011-65
	Six units (72 × 100)	0028-0011-65
14 Butazolidin® Tablets	phenylbutazone USP	100 mg.
	Red, film-coated tablets	
	100's	0028-0014-01
	1000's	0028-0014-10
	100's Unit Dose Pkg.	0028-0014-61
20 Tofranil-PM® Capsules	imipramine pamoate 75 mg.	
	Coral-colored capsules	
	30's	0028-0020-26
	100's	0028-0020-01
	1000's	0028-0020-10
	100's Unit Dose Pkg.	0028-0020-61
21 Tofranil® Tablets	imipramine hydrochloride USP	10 mg.
	Triangular, coral-colored, coated tablets	
	100's	0028-0021-01
	1000's	0028-0021-10
22 Tofranil-PM® Capsules	imipramine pamoate	150 mg.
	Coral-colored capsules	
	30's	0028-0022-26
	100's	0028-0022-01
	100's Unit Dose Pkg.	0028-0022-61
23 Lioresal® Tablets	baclofen	10 mg.
	White, oval, scored tablets	
	100's	0028-0023-01
	100's Unit Dose Pkg.	0028-0023-61
33 Lioresal® Tablets	baclofen	20 mg.
	White, capsule shaped, scored tablets	
	100's	0028-0033-01
	100's Unit Dose Pkg.	0028-0033-61
40 Tofranil-PM® Capsules	imipramine pamoate	100 mg.
	Dark yellow/coral-colored capsules	
	30's	0028-0040-26
	100's	0028-0040-01
42 Constant-T™ Tablets	theophylline (anhydrous)	200 mg.
	Light pink, oval, scored tablets	
	100's	0028-0042-01
	100's Unit Dose Pkg.	0028-0042-61
	Gy-Pak® 60's	
	One Unit (12 × 60)	0028-0042-73
	Six Units (72 × 60)	0028-0042-73
43 PBZ® Tablets	tripelennamine hydrochloride USP	50 mg.
	Light blue, scored tablets	
	100's	0028-0043-01
	1000's	0028-0043-10
44 Butazolidin® Capsules	phenylbutazone USP	100 mg.
	Orange/white capsules	
	100's	0028-0044-01
	1000's	0028-0044-10

for possible revisions — Product Information

```
                100's Unit Dose Pkg.        0028-0044-61
            Gy-Pak® 100's
                One Unit (12 × 100)         0028-0044-65
                Six Units (72 × 100)        0028-0044-65
45 Tofranil-PM® Capsules
            imipramine pamoate              125 mg.
            Light yellow/coral-colored capsules
                30's                        0028-0045-26
                100's                       0028-0045-01
47 Tegretol® Chewable Tablets
            carbamazepine USP
            Round, red-speckled, pink, single-scored
            tablets
                100's                       0028-0047-01
                100's Unit Dose Pkg.        0028-0047-61
48 PBZ-SR® Tablets
            tripelennamine hydrochloride
                                            100 mg.
            Lavender-colored tablets
                100's                       0028-0048-01
51 Lopressor® Tablets
            metoprolol tartrate             50 mg.
            Light red, capsule-shaped, scored tablets
                100's                       0028-0051-01
                1000's                      0028-0051-10
                100's Unit Dose Pkg.        0028-0051-61
            Gy-Pak® 60's
                One Unit (12 × 60)          0028-0051-73
                Six Units (72 × 60)         0028-0051-73
            Gy-Pak® 100's
                One Unit (12 × 100)         0028-0051-65
                Six Units (72 × 100)        0028-0051-65
57 Constant-T™ Tablets
            theophylline (anhydrous)        300 mg.
            Light blue, oval, scored tablets
                100's                       0028-0057-01
                100's Unit Dose Pkg.        0028-0057-61
            Gy-Pak® 60's
                One Unit (12 × 60)          0028-0057-73
                Six Units (72 × 60)         0028-0057-73
67 Tegretol® Tablets
            carbamazepine USP               200 mg.
            White, single-scored tablets
                100's                       0028-0067-01
                1000's                      0028-0067-10
                100's Unit Dose Pkg.        0028-0067-61
            Gy-Pak® 100's
                One Unit (12 × 100)         0028-0067-65
                Six Units (72 × 100)        0028-0067-65
71 Lopressor® Tablets
            metoprolol tartrate             100 mg.
            Light blue, capsule-shaped, scored tablets
                100's                       0028-0071-01
                1000's                      0028-0071-10
                100's Unit Dose Pkg.        0028-0071-61
            Gy-Pak® 60's
                One Unit (12 × 60)          0028-0071-73
                Six Units (72 × 60)         0028-0071-73
            Gy-Pak® 100's
                One Unit (12 × 100)         0028-0071-65
                Six Units (72 × 100)        0028-0071-65
72 Brethine® Tablets
            terbutaline sulfate USP         2.5 mg.
            Oval, white, scored tablets
                100's                       0028-0072-01
                1000's                      0028-0072-10
                100's Unit Dose Pkg.        0028-0072-61
            Gy-Pak® 90's
                One Unit (12 × 90)          0028-0072-90
                Six Units (72 × 90)         0028-0072-90
            Gy-Pak® 100's
                One Unit (12 × 100)         0028-0072-65
                Six Units (72 × 100)        0028-0072-65
74 Tofranil® Tablets
            imipramine hydrochloride USP
                                            50 mg.
            Coral-colored (white Geigy im-
            print) coated tablets
                100's                       0028-0074-01
                1000's                      0028-0074-10
                100's Unit Dose Pkg.        0028-0074-61
            Gy-Pak® 100's
                One unit (12 × 100)         0028-0074-65
                Six units (72 × 100)        0028-0074-65
85 Tandearil® Tablets
            oxyphenbutazone USP             100 mg.
            Tan, coated tablets
                100's                       0028-0085-01
                1000's                      0028-0085-10
                100's Unit Dose Pkg.        0028-0085-61
95 PBZ® Tablets
            tripelennamine hydrochloride
                                            25 mg.
            Green, sugar-coated tablets
                100's                       0028-0095-01
105 Brethine® Tablets
            terbutaline sulfate USP         5 mg.
            Round, scored, white tablets
                100's                       0028-0105-01
                1000's                      0028-0105-10
                100's Unit Dose Pkg.        0028-0105-61
            Gy-Pak® 90's
                One Unit (12 × 90)          0028-0105-90
                Six Units (72 × 90)         0028-0105-90
            Gy-Pak® 100's
                One unit (12 × 100)         0028-0105-65
                Six units (72 × 100)        0028-0105-65
6114 Otrivin® Nasal Drops (0.1%)
            xylometazoline hydrochloride USP
                20 ml.                      0028-6114-58
6116 Otrivin® Pediatric (0.05%)
            xylometazoline hydrochloride USP
                20 ml.                      0028-6116-58
6118 Otrivin® Spray (0.1%)
            xylometazoline hydrochloride USP
                15 ml.                      0028-6118-57
6925 PBZ® Elixir
            Per 5-ml. teaspoon:
                tripelennamine citrate
                USP                         37.5 mg.
                (equivalent to 25 mg.
                tripelennamine hydrochloride)
                473 ml.                     0028-6925-16
6946 PBZ® Antihistamine Cream
            tripelennamine hydrochloride
            Cream 2% (water-washable base)
                1 oz.                       0028-6946-76
```

BRETHINE® ℞
[breth-een']
terbutaline sulfate USP
Tablets of 5 mg   GY-CODE 105
Tablets of 2.5 mg   GY-CODE 72

Description: Brethine, a synthetic sympathomimetic amine, may be chemically described as α-[(tert-Butylamino) methyl] -3,5- dihydroxybenzyl alcohol sulfate.

Brethine, terbutaline sulfate, is a water soluble, colorless, crystalline solid. Tablets containing terbutaline sulfate should be stored at controlled room temperature.

Each scored, white tablet contains 5 mg (equivalent to 4.1 mg of free base) or 2.5 mg (equivalent to 2.05 mg of free base) of terbutaline sulfate.

Actions: Brethine is a β-adrenergic receptor agonist which has been shown by *in vitro* and *in vivo* pharmacological studies in animals to exert a preferential effect on β_2-adrenergic receptors such as those located in bronchial smooth muscle. Controlled clinical studies in patients who were administered the drug orally have revealed proportionally greater changes in pulmonary function parameters than in heart rate or blood pressure. While this *suggests* a relative preference for the β_2 receptor in man, the usual cardiovascular effects commonly associated with sympathomimetic agents were also observed with Brethine.

Brethine has been shown in controlled clinical studies to relieve bronchospasm in chronic obstructive pulmonary disease.

This action is manifested by a clinically significant increase in pulmonary function as demonstrated by an increase of 15% or more in FEV_1 and in $FEF_{25-75\%}$. Following administration of Brethine tablets, a measurable change in flow rate is usually observed in 30 minutes, and a clinically significant improvement in pulmonary function occurs at 60–120 minutes. The maximum effect usually occurs within 120-180 minutes. Brethine also produces a clinically significant decrease in airway and pulmonary resistance which persists for at least four hours or longer. Significant bronchodilator action, as measured by various pulmonary function determinations (airway resistance, $FEF_{25-75\%}$, or PEFR), has been demonstrated in some studies for periods up to eight hours.

Clinical studies were conducted in which the effectiveness of Brethine was evaluated in comparison with ephedrine over periods up to three months. Both drugs continued to produce significant improvement in pulmonary function throughout this period of treatment.

Indications: Brethine is indicated as a bronchodilator for bronchial asthma and for reversible bronchospasm which may occur in association with bronchitis and emphysema.

Contraindications: Brethine is contraindicated when there is known hypersensitivity to sympathomimetic amines.

Warnings: *Usage in Pregnancy:* Animal reproductive studies have been negative with respect to adverse effects on fetal development. The safe use of Brethine has not, however, been established in human pregnancy. As with any medication, the use of the drug in pregnancy, lactation, or women of childbearing potential requires that the expected therapeutic benefit of the drug be weighed against its possible hazards to the mother or child.

Usage in Pediatrics: Brethine tablets are not presently recommended for children below the age of 12 years due to insufficient clinical data in this pediatric group.

Precautions: Brethine should be used with caution in patients with diabetes, hypertension, hyperthyroidism, and a history of seizures.

As with other sympathomimetic bronchodilator agents, Brethine should be administered cautiously to cardiac patients, especially those with associated arrhythmias.

The concomitant use of Brethine with other sympathomimetic agents is not recommended, since their combined effect on the cardiovascular system may be deleterious to the patient. However, this does not preclude the use of an aerosol bronchodilator of the adrenergic stimulant type for the relief of an acute bronchospasm in patients receiving chronic oral Brethine therapy.

Adverse Reactions: Commonly observed side effects include nervousness and tremor. Other reported reactions include headache, increased heart rate, palpitations, drowsiness, nausea, vomiting, sweating, and muscle cramps. These reactions are generally transient in nature and usually do not require treatment. The frequency of these side effects appears to diminish with continued therapy. In general, all the side effects observed are characteristic of those commonly seen with sympathomimetic amines.

Dosage and Administration: The usual oral dose of Brethine for adults is 5 mg administered at approximately six-hour intervals, three times daily, during the hours the patient is usually awake. If side effects are particularly disturbing, the dose may be reduced to 2.5 mg three times daily, and still provide a clinically significant improvement in pulmonary function. A dose of 2.5 mg, three times daily, also is recommended for children in the 12- to 15-year group. Brethine is not recommended at present for use in children below the age of 12 years. In adults, a total dose of 15 mg should not be exceeded in a 24-hour period. In children, a total dose of 7.5 mg should not be exceeded in a 24-hour period.

Overdosage: Overdosage experience is limited. Excessive beta-adrenergic receptor stimulation may augment the signs or symptoms listed under **Adverse Reactions** and they may be accompanied by other adrenergic effects. Treat the alert patient who has taken excessive oral medication by emptying the stomach by means of induced emesis, followed by gastric lavage. In the unconscious patient, secure the airway with a cuffed endotracheal tube before beginning lavage (do not induce emesis). Instillation of activated charcoal slurry

Continued on next page

The full prescribing information for each GEIGY drug is contained herein and is that in effect as of October 1, 1984.

Geigy—Cont.

may help reduce absorption of terbutaline sulfate. Maintain adequate respiratory exchange. Provide cardiac and respiratory support as needed. Continue observation until symptom-free.

How Supplied: Round, scored, white tablets of 5 mg are supplied in bottles of 100 and 1,000 and Unit Dose Packages of 100; and oval, scored, white tablets of 2.5 mg are supplied in bottles of 100 and 1,000 and Unit Dose Packages of 100.

C80-57 (12/80)

Shown in Product Identification Section, page 411

BRETHINE® ℞
[*breth-een'*]
terbutaline sulfate USP   GY-CODE 7507
Ampuls
A sterile aqueous solution
for subcutaneous injection.

Description: Brethine, α-[(*tert*-Butylamino)methyl]-3,5-dihydroxybenzyl alcohol sulfate is a synthetic sympathomimetic amine.

Brethine is a water soluble colorless crystalline solid. Solutions are sensitive to excessive heat and light, and ampuls should therefore be stored at controlled room temperature with protection from light by storage in their original carton until dispensed. Solutions should not be used if discolored. Each milliliter of sterile isotonic solution contains 1.0 mg of terbutaline sulfate (equivalent to 0.82 mg of free base), 8.9 mg of sodium chloride, and hydrochloric acid to adjust the pH to 3.0–5.0.

Actions: Brethine is a β-adrenergic receptor agonist which has been shown by *in vitro* and *in vivo* pharmacological studies in animals to exert a preferential effect on β_2-adrenergic receptors such as those located in bronchial smooth muscle. However, controlled clinical studies in patients who were administered the drug subcutaneously have not revealed a preferential β_2 adrenergic effect.

Brethine has been shown in controlled clinical studies to relieve acute bronchospasm in acute and chronic obstructive pulmonary disease, resulting in a clinically significant increase in pulmonary flow rates, e.g., an increase of 15% or greater in FEV_1. Following administration of 0.25 mg of subcutaneous Brethine, a measurable change in flow rate is usually observed within five minutes, and a clinically significant increase in FEV_1 occurs by 15 minutes following the injection. The maximum effect usually occurs within 30–60 minutes and clinically significant bronchodilator activity has been observed to persist for 90 minutes to four hours. The duration of clinically significant improvement is comparable to that found with equimilligram doses of epinephrine.

Indications: Brethine is indicated as a bronchodilator for bronchial asthma and for reversible bronchospasm which may occur in association with bronchitis and emphysema.

Contraindications: Brethine is contraindicated when there is known hypersensitivity to sympathomimetic amines.

Precautions: Brethine should be used with caution in patients with diabetes, hypertension, hyperthyroidism, and a history of seizures.

As with other sympathomimetic bronchodilator agents, Brethine should be administered cautiously to cardiac patients, especially those with associated arrhythmias.

The concomitant use of Brethine with other sympathomimetic agents is not recommended, since their combined effect on the cardiovascular system may be deleterious to the patient.

Preparation of Other Dosage Forms: Use of the subcutaneous injection for preparation of other dosage forms, i.e., I.V. infusion, is inappropriate. Sterility and accurate dosing cannot be assured if the ampuls are not used in accordance with **Dosage and Administration.**

Carcinogenesis, Mutagenesis, Impairment of Fertility: An 18-month oral (feeding) carcinogenicity study of terbutaline (5, 50, and 200 mg/kg, corresponding to 500x, 5000x, and 20,000x the clinical subcutaneous dose) in NMRI strain mice revealed no drug-related tumorigenicity. Mutagenicity and fertility studies were not performed.

Pregnancy Category B: Reproduction studies have been performed in mice and rats at doses up to 1,000 times the human dose and have revealed no evidence of impaired fertility or harm to the fetus due to terbutaline. There are, however, no adequate and well-controlled studies in pregnant women. Because animal reproduction studies are not always predictive of human response, this drug should be used during pregnancy only if clearly needed.

Usage in Labor and Delivery: Serious adverse reactions have been reported following administration of terbutaline sulfate to women in labor. These reports have included transient hypokalemia, pulmonary edema and hypoglycemia in the mother and hypoglycemia in the neonatal children of women treated with terbutaline parenterally.

Pediatric Use: Studies are in progress to define the safe and effective dose of Brethine in children. Therefore, until such studies are completed and evaluated, Brethine is not recommended for use in pediatrics.

Adverse Reactions: Commonly observed side effects include increases in heart rate, nervousness, tremor, palpitations and dizziness. These occur more frequently at doses in excess of 0.25 mg. Other reported reactions include headache, nausea, vomiting, anxiety, and muscle cramps. These reactions are transient in nature and usually do not require treatment. In general, all side effects are characteristic of those commonly seen with sympathomimetic amines such as epinephrine.

Dosage and Administration: The usual subcutaneous dose of Brethine is 0.25 mg injected into the lateral deltoid area. If significant clinical improvement does not occur by 15–30 minutes, a second dose of 0.25 mg may be administered. A total dose of 0.5 mg should not be exceeded within a four-hour period. If a patient fails to respond to a second 0.25-mg dose of Brethine within 15–30 minutes, other therapeutic measures should be considered.

Overdosage: Overdosage experience is limited. Excessive beta-adrenergic receptor stimulation may augment the signs or symptoms listed under **Adverse Reactions** and they may be accompanied by other adrenergic effects. In the case of subcutaneous injectable terbutaline overdosage, the patient should be treated symptomatically under guidelines for sympathomimetic overdosage.

How Supplied:
Ampuls 1-mg/ml (2-ml size ampul, expiration-dated)

Box of 10 .... NDC 0028-7507-23
Box of 100 .... NDC 0028-7507-01

Protect from light by storing ampuls in original carton until dispensed.

Keep at controlled room temperature (59°–86°F) 15°–30°C. Do not use if solution is discolored.

C83-5 (Rev. 6/83)

BUTAZOLIDIN® ℞
[*bew-ta-zahl'eh-dinn*]
phenylbutazone USP   GY-CODE 14
Tablets
Capsules
Nonhormonal Antiarthritic
Anti-Inflammatory Agent

Important Note: Butazolidin cannot be considered a simple analgesic and should never be administered casually. Each patient should be carefully evaluated before treatment is started and should remain constantly under the close supervision of the physician. The following cautions should be observed:

1. Therapy should not be initiated until a careful detailed history and complete physical and laboratory examination, including a complete hemogram and urinalysis, etc., of the patient have been made. These examinations should be made at regular, frequent intervals throughout the duration of this drug therapy.
2. Patients should be carefully selected, avoiding those in whom it is contraindicated as well as those who will respond to ordinary therapeutic measures, or those who cannot be observed at frequent intervals.
3. Patients taking this drug should be warned not to exceed the recommended dosage, since this may lead to toxic effects, and should discontinue the drug and report to the physician immediately any sign of:
   a. Fever, sore throat, lesions in the mouth (symptoms of blood dyscrasia).
   b. Dyspepsia, epigastric pain, symptoms of anemia, unusual bleeding, unusual bruising, black or tarry stools or other evidence of intestinal ulceration.
   c. Skin rashes.
   d. Significant weight gain or edema.
4. A trial period of one week of therapy is considered adequate to determine the therapeutic effect of the drug. In the absence of a favorable response, therapy should be discontinued.
   a. In the elderly (sixty years and over) the drug should be restricted to short-term treatment periods only—if possible, *one week* maximum.
5. **Before prescribing Butazolidin for an individual patient, read thoroughly the information contained under each heading which follows:**

Description: Butazolidin should not be considered as a simple analgesic that can be prescribed for indiscriminate use. Butazolidin is closely related chemically and pharmacologically, including toxic effects, to the well-known pyrazolines (pyrazole compounds) amidopyrine and antipyrine.

Butazolidin is 4-Butyl-1,2-diphenyl-3,5-pyrazolidinedione, with a molecular weight of 308.38. It is very slightly soluble in water; freely soluble in acetone and in ether; soluble in alcohol.

Clinical Pharmacology: Butazolidin is a nonsalicylate, nonsteroidal, anti-inflammatory drug. It has anti-inflammatory, antipyretic, analgesic and mild uricosuric properties that produce symptomatic relief but do not alter the disease process. The exact mechanism of the anti-inflammatory effects of Butazolidin has not been elucidated, but clinical pharmacology studies have shown that Butazolidin inhibits certain factors believed to be involved in the inflammatory process. These processes are (1) prostaglandin synthesis; (2) leucocyte migration; (3) release and/or activity of lysosomal enzymes.

Phenylbutazone is rapidly absorbed after oral administration of Butazolidin. Tests conducted in 18 healthy adult male volunteers indicated that a peak plasma concentration of 43.3 ($\pm$3.1) mg/l was attained within 2.5 ($\pm$1.4) hours after the ingestion of three 100-mg tablets. In these same volunteers, the apparent elimination half-life was 84 ($\pm$23) hours. About 98% of the drug is bound to human serum albumin.

Twenty-one days after oral administration of ^{14}C-labelled drug, 61% was recovered from the urine and 27% from the feces. However, only about 1% of total urinary radioactivity represents unchanged drug. The sum of nonconjugated urinary metabolites (oxyphenbutazone, γ-hydroxyphenylbutazone, p,γ-dihydroxyphenylbutazone), and phenylbutazone itself amounted to only about 10%. About 40% of the total urinary radioactivity was excreted as the C(4)-glucuronide of phenylbutazone and an additional 12% was identified as the C(4)-glucuronide of γ-hydroxyphenylbutazone.

The major metabolite of phenylbutazone in human plasma is oxyphenbutazone; steady-state plasma levels about 50% of those of phenylbutazone. Less than 2% of the dose of phenylbutazone appears in the urine as oxyphenbutazone.

Indications: The indications for Butazolidin are:

Acute Gouty Arthritis
Active Rheumatoid Arthritis
Active Ankylosing Spondylitis
Short-term treatment of acute attacks of degenerative joint disease of the hips and knees not responsive to other treatment.
Painful Shoulder (peritendinitis, capsulitis, bursitis, and acute arthritis of that joint)

Product Information

Contraindications:

1. *Age:* Butazolidin is contraindicated in children 14 years of age or younger since controlled clinical trials in patients of this age group have not been conducted.
2. *Other Medical Conditions:* Butazolidin is contraindicated in patients with incipient cardiac failure, blood dyscrasias, pancreatitis, parotitis, stomatitis, polymyalgia rheumatica, temporal arteritis, senility, drug allergy, and in the presence of severe renal, cardiac and hepatic disease, and in patients with a history of peptic ulcer disease, or symptoms of gastrointestinal inflammation or active ulceration because serious adverse reactions or aggravation of existing medical problems can occur.
3. *Concomitant Medications:* Butazolidin should not be used in combination with other drugs which accentuate or share a potential for similar toxicity.

It is also inadvisable to administer Butazolidin in combination with other potent drugs because of the possibility of increased toxic reactions from Butazolidin and other agents. (see also *Drug/Drug Interactions.*)

Butazolidin is contraindicated in patients with a history or suggestion of prior toxicity, sensitivity, or idiosyncrasy to phenylbutazone or oxyphenbutazone.

Warnings: Based on reports of clinical experience with phenylbutazone and related compounds, the following warnings should be considered by the physician prior to prescribing the drug:

1. *Gastrointestinal:* Upper G.I. diagnostic tests should be performed in patients with persistent or severe dyspepsia. Peptic ulceration, reactivation of latent peptic ulcer, perforation and gastrointestinal bleeding, sometimes severe, have been reported.

   As with other nonsteroidal anti-inflammatory drugs, borderline elevations of values measured by one or more liver tests may occur in up to 15% of patients. These abnormalities may progress, may remain essentially unchanged, or may be transient with continued therapy. The SGPT (ALT) test is probably the most sensitive indicator of liver dysfunction. Meaningful elevations (three times the upper limit of normal) of SGPT or SGOT (AST) have occurred in controlled clinical trials in less than 1% of patients. A patient with symptoms and/or signs suggesting liver dysfunction, or in whom an abnormal liver test has occurred, should be evaluated for evidence of the development of more severe hepatic reactions while on therapy with Butazolidin. Severe hepatic reactions, including jaundice and cases of fatal hepatitis, have been reported with Butazolidin as with other nonsteroidal anti-inflammatory drugs. Although such reactions are rare, if abnormal liver tests persist or worsen, if clinical signs and symptoms consistent with liver disease develop, or if systemic manifestations (e.g., eosinophilia, rash, etc.) occur, therapy with Butazolidin be discontinued.

2. *Hematologic: Frequent and regular hematologic evaluations should be performed on patients receiving the drug for periods over one week.* Any significant change in the total white count, relative decrease in granulocytes, appearance of immature forms or fall in hematocrit should be a signal for immediate cessation of therapy and a complete hematologic investigation. Serious, sometimes fatal blood dyscrasias, including aplastic anemia have been reported to occur. Hematologic toxicity may occur suddenly or many days or weeks after cessation of treatment as manifest by the appearance of anemia, leukopenia, thrombocytopenia or clinically significant hemorrhagic diathesis. There have been published reports associating phenylbutazone with leukemia. However, the circumstances involved in these reports are such that a cause-and-effect relationship to the drug has not been clearly established.

3. *Pregnancy:* Reproductive studies in animals, although inconclusive, exhibited evidence of possible embryotoxicity. It is, therefore, recommended that this drug should be used with caution during pregnancy. The benefits should be weighed against the potential risk to the fetus.

4. *Nursing Mothers:* Caution is also advised in prescribing Butazolidin in nursing mothers since the drug may appear in cord blood and breast milk.

5. Patients reporting visual disturbances while receiving the drug should discontinue treatment and have an ophthalmologic examination because ophthalmologic adverse reactions have been reported (see **Adverse Reactions:** *Special Senses*)

6. In the aging (forty years and over), there appears to be an increase in the possibility of adverse reactions. Butazolidin should be used with commensurately greater care in the elderly and should be avoided altogether in the senile patient.

7. Like other drugs with prostaglandin synthetase inhibition activity, Butazolidin may precipitate acute episodes of asthmatic attacks in patients with asthma.

8. Butazolidin increases sodium retention. Evidence of fluid retention in patients in whom there is danger of cardiac decompensation is an indication to discontinue the drug.

Precautions: Because of potential serious adverse reactions to Butazolidin, the following precautions should be observed in the use of the drug:

—A careful diagnostic physical examination and history should be performed on all patients at regular intervals while the patient is receiving the drug.

—Butazolidin is not recommended for chronic use in the elderly.

—Hematologic evaluation should be performed at frequent and regular intervals and additional laboratory examinations performed as indicated.

—Patients should be instructed to report immediately the occurrence of high fever, severe sore throat, stomatitis, salivary gland enlargement, tarry stools, unusual bleeding or bruising, sudden weight gain, or edema.

—The drug reduces iodine uptake by the thyroid and may interfere with laboratory tests of thyroid function (see **Adverse Reactions:** *Endocrine-Metabolic*).

—The patient should be cautioned regarding participation in activities requiring alertness and coordination and that the concomitant ingestion of alcohol with Butazolidin may further impair psychomotor skills.

Drug/Drug Interactions: Butazolidin competitively displaces other drugs, e.g., other anti-inflammatory agents, oral anticoagulants, oral antidiabetics, sulfonamides, sodium valproate, and phenytoin, from serum-binding sites. The activity, duration of effect, and toxicity of the displaced drugs may thus be increased. Butazolidin accentuates the prothrombin depression produced by coumarin-type anticoagulants. When administered alone, Butazolidin does not affect prothrombin activity.

Butazolidin may induce the hepatic microsomal metabolism of dicoumarol, amidopyrine, digitoxin, hexobarbital, and cortisone. Conversely, it may inhibit the metabolism of phenytoin.

Concomitant administration of phenylbutazone and phenytoin may result in increased serum levels of phenytoin which could lead to increased phenytoin toxicity.

Inducers of hepatic microsomal enzymes, e.g., barbiturates, promethazine, chlorpheniramine, rifampin, and corticosteroids (prednisone), may decrease the half-life of Butazolidin.

The effects of methotrexate, insulin, antidiabetic and sulfonamide drugs may be potentiated by Butazolidin. Butazolidin increases the serum concentration of lithium by increasing tubular reabsorption, and it reduces the renal clearance of sulfonylureas.

Methylphenidate is reported to prolong the half-life of Butazolidin and to increase the serum level of oxyphenbutazone.

Cholestyramine reduces the enteral absorption of Butazolidin. See CONTRAINDICATIONS.

Adverse Reactions: Based upon reports of clinical experience with phenylbutazone and related compounds, the following adverse reactions have been reported.

The adverse reactions listed in the following table have been arranged into three groups: (1) incidence greater than 1%, (2) incidence less than 1% and (3) causal relationship unknown. The incidence for group (1) was obtained from sixty-eight (68) clinical trials reported in the literature (5369 patients). The incidence for group (2) was based on reports in clinical trials, in the literature, and on voluntary reports since marketing. The reactions in group (3) have been reported but occurred under circumstances where a causal relationship could not be established. In some patients the reported reactions may have been unrelated to the administration of Butazolidin. However, in these reported events, the possibility cannot be excluded. Therefore these observations are being listed to serve as alerting information to physicians. Before prescribing this drug for an individual patient, the physician should be familiar with the following:

(1) Incidence greater than 1%	(2) Incidence less than 1%
GASTROINTESTINAL (See **Warnings**)	
nausea	vomiting
dyspepsia/including indigestion and heartburn	abdominal distention with flatulence constipation
abdominal discomfort/distress *(See Note)*	diarrhea esophagitis gastritis salivary gland enlargement stomatitis, sometimes with ulceration ulceration and perforation of the intestinal tract including acute and reactivated peptic ulcer with perforation, hemorrhage and hematemesis anemia due to gastrointestinal bleeding which may be occult hepatitis, both fatal and nonfatal, sometimes associated with evidence of cholestasis
HEMATOLOGICAL (See **Warnings**)	
None	anemia leukopenia thrombocytopenia with associated purpura, petechiae, and hemorrhage pancytopenia aplastic anemia bone marrow depression agranulocytosis and agranulocytic anginal syndrome hemolytic anemia
HYPERSENSITIVITY	
None	urticaria anaphylactic shock arthralgia, drug fever hypersensitivity angiitis (polyarteritis) and vasculitis

Continued on next page

The full prescribing information for each GEIGY drug is contained herein and is that in effect as of October 1, 1984.

Geigy—Cont.

rash	Lyell's syndrome serum sickness Stevens-Johnson syndrome activation of systemic lupus erythematosus aggravation of temporal arteritis in patients with polymyalgia rheumatica **DERMATOLOGIC** pruritus erythema nodosum erythema multiforme nonthrombocytopenic purpura
CARDIOVASCULAR, FLUID AND ELECTROLYTE	
edema/water retention (See Note)	sodium and chloride retention fluid retention and plasma dilution cardiac decompensation (congestive heart failure) with edema and dyspnea metabolic acidosis respiratory alkalosis hypertension pericarditis interstitial myocarditis with muscle necrosis and perivascular granulomata
RENAL	
None	hematuria proteinuria ureteral obstruction with uric acid crystals anuria glomerulonephritis acute tubular necrosis cortical necrosis renal stones nephrotic syndrome impaired renal function and renal failure associated with azotemia acute allergic and chronic interstitial nephritis
CENTRAL NERVOUS SYSTEM	
None	headache drowsiness agitation confusional states and lethargy tremors numbness weakness
ENDOCRINE-METABOLIC (See **Precautions**)	
None	hyperglycemia
SPECIAL SENSES (See **Warnings**)	
Ocular: None	
Otic: None	hearing loss tinnitus

(3) **Causal relationship unknown—incidence less than 1%:** *Hematological* (see **Warnings**)—Leukemia (There have been reports associating phenylbutazone with leukemia. However, the circumstances involved in these reports are such that a cause-and-effect relationship to the drug has not been clearly established.) *Endocrine—Metabolic* (see **Precautions**)—Thyroid hyperplasia; goiters associated with hyperthyroidism and hypothyroidism; pancreatitis. *Special Senses* (see **Warnings**)—Blurred vision; optic neuritis; toxic amblyopia; scotomata; retinal detachment; retinal hemorrhage; oculomotor palsy.

Overdosage: *Signs and Symptoms:* Include any of the following: nausea, vomiting, epigastric pain, excessive perspiration, euphoria, psychosis, headaches, giddiness, vertigo, hyperventilation, insomnia, tinnitus, difficulty in hearing, edema (sodium retention), hypertension, cyanosis, respiratory depression, agitation, hallucinations, stupor, convulsions, coma, hematuria, and oliguria. Hepatomegaly, jaundice, and ulceration of the buccal or gastrointestinal mucosa have been reported as late manifestations of massive overdosage.

Reported laboratory abnormalities following overdosage include: respiratory or metabolic acidosis, impaired hepatic or renal function, and abnormalities of formed blood elements.

Treatment: In the alert patient, empty the stomach promptly by induced emesis followed by lavage. In the obtunded patient, secure the airway with a cuffed endotracheal tube before beginning lavage (do not induce emesis). Maintain adequate respiratory exchange, do not use respiratory stimulants. Treat shock with appropriate supportive measures. Control seizures with intravenous diazepam or short-acting barbiturates. Dialysis may be helpful if renal function is impaired.

Dosage and Administration: Butazolidin should be used at the smallest effective dosage to afford rapid relief of severe symptoms. It is contraindicated in children under 14 years of age and in senile patients.

If a favorable symptomatic response to treatment is not obtained after one week, the drug should be discontinued. When a favorable therapeutic response has been obtained, the dosage should be reduced and then discontinued as soon as possible. In elderly patients (sixty years and over) every effort must be made to discontinue therapy on, or as soon as possible after, the seventh day, because of the exceedingly high risk of severe fatal toxic reactions in this age group.

To minimize gastric upset, the drug should be taken with milk or with meals.

In selecting the appropriate dosage in any specific case, consideration should be given to the patient's age, weight, general health, and any other factors that may influence his response to the drug.

Rheumatoid Arthritis, Ankylosing Spondylitis, Acute Attacks of Degenerative Joint Disease, and Painful Shoulder: Initial Dosage: The initial daily dose in adult patients is 300 to 600 mg as 3 to 4 divided doses. Maximum therapeutic response is usually obtained at a total daily dose of 400 mg. A trial period of one week of therapy is considered adequate to determine the therapeutic effect of the drug. In the absence of a favorable response, therapy should be discontinued.

Maintenance Dosage: When improvement is obtained, dosage should be promptly decreased to the minimum effective level necessary to maintain relief, not exceeding 400 mg daily because of the possibility of cumulative toxicity. A satisfactory clinical response may be obtained with daily doses as low as 100 to 200 mg daily.

Acute Gouty Arthritis: Satisfactory results are obtained after an initial dose of 400 mg followed by 100 mg every 4 hours. The articular inflammation usually subsides within 4 days and treatment should not be continued longer than one week.

How Supplied:
Tablets 100 mg—round, red, film-coated (imprinted GEIGY 14)
Bottles of 100 ....NDC 0028-0014-01
Bottles of 1000 ....NDC 0028-0014-10
Unit Dose (blister pack)
Box of 100 (strips of 10) ....NDC 0028-0014-61
Capsules 100 mg—orange and white (imprinted GEIGY 44)
Bottles of 100 ....NDC 0028-0044-01
Bottles of 1000 ....NDC 0028-0044-10
Gy-Pak® — One Unit
(12 bottles — 100
 capsules each) ....NDC 0028-0044-65
Unit Dose (blister pack)
Box of 100 (strips of 10) ....NDC 0028-0044-61
Dispense in tight, light-resistant container (USP).
NOTE: Reactions occurring in 3% to 9% of patients treated with phenylbutazone (those reactions occurring in less than 3% of the patients are unmarked).
C83-18 (Rev. 12/83)
Shown in Product Identification Section, page 411

CONSTANT-T® ℞
[*kahn-stant' tee'*]
theophylline (anhydrous)
Sustained-Action Tablets
Tablets
200 mg
300 mg

Description: Constant-T Sustained-Action Tablets contain anhydrous theophylline. Constant-T is available in two strengths: 200-mg and 300-mg oval, scored tablets. Theophylline, a xanthine compound, is a white, odorless crystalline powder, having a bitter taste.

Actions: The pharmacologic actions of Constant-T are as a bronchodilator, pulmonary vasodilator and smooth muscle relaxant, since the drug directly relaxes the smooth muscle of the bronchial airways and pulmonary blood vessels. Theophylline also possesses other actions typical of the xanthine derivatives: coronary vasodilator, diuretic, cardiac stimulant, cerebral stimulant and skeletal muscle stimulant. The actions of theophylline may be mediated through inhibition of phosphodiesterase and a resultant increase in intracellular cyclic AMP which could mediate smooth muscle relaxation. No development of tolerance appears to occur with chronic use of theophylline.

The half-life is shortened with cigarette smoking and prolonged in alcoholism, reduced hepatic or renal function, congestive heart failure, and in patients receiving certain antibiotics (see **Drug Interactions**). High fever for prolonged periods may decrease theophylline elimination. Children over six months of age have rapid clearances with average half-lives of approximately 3–5 hours. Newborn infants have extremely slow clearances and half-lives exceeding 24 hours. Older adults with chronic obstructive pulmonary disease, any patients with cor pulmonale or other causes of heart failure, and patients with liver pathology may have much lower clearances with half-lives that exceed 24 hours. The half-life of theophylline in smokers (1–2 packs per day) averages 4–5 hours; the half-life in nonsmokers averages 7–9 hours.

In single-dose studies, adjusting the data to dosing equivalent to 8 mg/kg body weight, Constant-T produced mean peak theophylline blood levels of 9.1 ± 0.7 µg/ml at 5.0 ± 1.2 hours with the 200-mg dosage form, and 9.8 ± 0.9 µg/ml at 4.6 ± 0.9 hours with the 300-mg dosage form. In a multidose, steady-state, 5-day study, Constant-T achieved constant intrasubject theophylline levels with an average peak-trough difference of only 3.4 µg/ml. This is indicative of smooth and stable maintenance therapeutic theophylline levels throughout a 12-hour dosing interval.

Indications: Symptomatic relief and/or prevention of asthma and reversible bronchospasm associated with chronic bronchitis and emphysema.

Contraindications: Constant-T is contraindicated in individuals who have shown hypersensitivity to any of its components or to xanthine derivatives.

Warnings: Excessive theophylline doses may be associated with toxicity; serum theophylline levels should be monitored to assure maximum benefit with minimum risk. Incidence of toxicity increases at serum levels greater than 20 µg/ml. High blood levels of theophylline resulting from conventional doses are correlated with clinical manifestations of toxicity in: patients with lowered body plasma clearances; patients with liver dysfunction or chronic obstructive lung disease, and patients who are older than 55 years of age, particularly males. There are often no early signs of less serious theophylline toxicity such as nausea and restlessness, which may appear in up to 50% of patients prior to onset of convulsions. Ventricular arrhythmias or seizures may be the first signs of toxicity. Many patients who have higher theophylline serum levels exhibit a tachycardia. Theophylline products may worsen preexisting arrhythmias.

Usage in Pregnancy: Safe use in pregnancy has not been established relative to possible adverse effects on fetal development, but neither have adverse effects on fetal development been established. This is, unfortunately, true for most antiasthmatic medications. Therefore, use of theophylline in pregnant women should be balanced against the risk of uncontrolled asthma.

Precautions: CONSTANT-T TABLETS SHOULD NOT BE CHEWED OR CRUSHED. Theophyllines should not be administered concurrently with other xanthine medications. It should be used with caution in patients with severe cardiac disease, severe hypoxemia, hypertension, hyperthyroidism, acute myocardial injury, cor pulmonale, congestive heart failure, liver disease and in the elderly, particularly males, and in neonates. Great caution should be used in giving theophylline to patients in congestive heart failure since these patients show markedly prolonged theophylline blood level curves. Use theophylline cautiously in patients with history of peptic ulcer. Theophylline may occasionally act as a local irritant to GI tract although gastrointestinal symptoms are more commonly central and associated with high serum concentrations above 20 μg/ml.

Adverse Reactions: The most consistent adverse reactions are usually due to overdose and are:

Gastrointestinal: Nausea, vomiting, epigastric pain, hematemesis, diarrhea.

Central Nervous System: Headaches, irritability, restlessness, insomnia, reflex hyperexcitability, muscle twitching, clonic and tonic generalized convulsions.

Cardiovascular: Palpitation, tachycardia, extrasystoles, flushing, hypotension, circulatory failure, life-threatening ventricular arrhythmias.

Respiratory: Tachypnea.

Renal: Albuminuria, increased excretion of renal tubular cells and red blood cells; potentiation of diuresis.

Others: Hyperglycemia and inappropriate ADH syndrome.

Drug Interactions:

Drug	Effect
Theophylline with Furosemide	Increased Diuresis
Theophylline with Hexamethonium	Decreased Chronotropic Effect
Theophylline with Reserpine	Tachycardia
Theophylline with Cyclamycin (TAO), Erythromycin, or Lincomycin	Increased Theophylline Blood Levels

Overdosage

Management:

A. If potential oral overdose is established and seizure has not occurred:
 1) Induce vomiting.
 2) Administer a cathartic (this is particularly important if sustained-release preparations have been taken).
 3) Administer activated charcoal.

B. If patient is having a seizure:
 1) Establish an airway.
 2) Administer O₂.
 3) Treat the seizure with intravenous diazepam, 0.1 to 0.3 mg/kg up to 10 mg.
 4) Monitor vital signs, maintain blood pressure and provide adequate hydration.

C. Postseizure coma:
 1) Maintain airway and oxygenation.
 2) If a result of oral medication, follow above recommendations to prevent absorption of the drug, but intubation and lavage will have to be performed instead of inducing emesis, and the cathartic and charcoal will need to be introduced via a large-bore gastric lavage tube.
 3) Continue to provide full supportive care and adequate hydration while waiting for drug to be metabolized. In general, the drug is metabolized sufficiently rapidly so as to not warrant consideration of dialysis.

Dosage and Administration: Therapeutic serum levels associated with optimal likelihood for benefit and minimal risk of toxicity are considered to be between 10 and 20 μg/ml. There is a great variation from patient to patient in dosage needed in order to achieve a therapeutic blood level due to variable rates of elimination. Because of this wide variation from patient to patient, and the relatively narrow therapeutic range, dosage must be individualized.

THE AVERAGE INITIAL CHILDREN'S (15 to 20 kg) DOSE IS ONE-HALF OF A CONSTANT-T 200-mg TABLET q12h.

THE AVERAGE INITIAL CHILDREN'S (20 to 25 kg) DOSE IS ONE-HALF (150 mg) OF A CONSTANT-T 300-mg TABLET q12h.

THE AVERAGE INITIAL ADULT AND CHILDREN'S (OVER 25 kg) DOSE IS ONE CONSTANT-T 200-mg TABLET q12h.

If the desired response is not achieved with the above AVERAGE INITIAL DOSAGE recommendations, and there are no adverse reactions, the dose may be increased, after 3 days, to the following MAXIMUM DOSE WITHOUT MEASUREMENT OF SERUM CONCENTRATION.

MAXIMUM DOSE WITHOUT MEASUREMENT OF SERUM CONCENTRATION

	Dose Per Interval
Children (15–20 kg)	150 mg q12h
Children (20–25 kg)	200 mg q12h
Children (25–35 kg)	250 mg q12h
Adults and Children (over 35 kg)	300 mg q12h

If increased dose is not tolerated because of headaches or stomach upset (nausea, vomiting, diarrhea, etc.), decrease dose to AVERAGE INITIAL DOSE. If tolerated, the dose may be increased, after 3 days, to the following MINIMUM DOSE REQUIRING MEASUREMENT OF SERUM CONCENTRATION.

MINIMUM DOSE REQUIRING MEASUREMENT OF SERUM CONCENTRATION

	Dose Per Interval
Children (15–20 kg)	200 mg q12h
Children (20–30 kg)	250 mg q12h
Children (30–35 kg)	300 mg q12h
Children (35–40 kg)	350 mg q12h
Adults and Children (over 40 kg)	400 mg q12h

CHECK SERUM CONCENTRATION BETWEEN 3 AND 8 HOURS AFTER A DOSE WHEN NONE HAVE BEEN MISSED OR ADDED FOR AT LEAST 3 DAYS.

If serum theophylline concentration is between 10 and 20 μg/ml, maintain dose, if tolerated. RECHECK SERUM THEOPHYLLINE CONCENTRATION AT 6- TO 12-MONTH INTERVALS.*

* Finer adjustments in dosage may be needed for some patients.

Take the following action if the serum theophylline concentration is too high.

20 to 25 μg/ml—Decrease dose by 50 mg q12h.

25 to 30 μg/ml—Skip next dose and decrease subsequent doses by 25% to the nearest 50 mg q12h.

Over 30 μg/ml—Skip next 2 doses and decrease subsequent doses by 50% to nearest 50 mg q12h. RECHECK SERUM THEOPHYLLINE CONCENTRATION.

Take the following action if the serum theophylline concentration is too low.

7.5 to 10 μg/ml—Increase dose by 25% to the nearest 50 mg.†

5 to 7.5 μg/ml—Increase dose by 25% to the nearest 50 mg and RECHECK SERUM THEOPHYLLINE FOR GUIDANCE IN FURTHER DOSAGE ADJUSTMENT.

† Dividing the daily dosage into 3 doses administered at 8-hour intervals may be indicated if symptoms occur repeatedly at the end of a dosing interval.

DOSAGE ADJUSTMENT, BASED ON SERUM THEOPHYLLINE CONCENTRATION MEASUREMENTS WHEN THESE INSTRUCTIONS HAVE NOT BEEN FOLLOWED, MAY RESULT IN RECOMMENDATIONS THAT PRESENT RISK OF TOXICITY TO THE PATIENT.

How Supplied:

Sustained-Action Tablets 200 mg—
 light pink, oval, scored (imprinted Geigy 42)
 Bottles of 100 ....NDC 0028-0042-01
 Bottles of 1000 ....NDC 0028-0042-10
Gy-Pak®—One Unit
 12 bottles—
  60 tablets each ....NDC 0028-0042-73
Unit Dose (blister pack)
 Box of 100 (strips of 10) ....NDC 0028-0042-61

Sustained-Action Tablets 300 mg—
 light blue, oval, scored (imprinted Geigy 57)
 Bottles of 100 ....NDC 0028-0057-01
 Bottles of 1000 ....NDC 0028-0057-10
Gy-Pak®—One Unit
 12 bottles—
  60 tablets each ....NDC 0028-0057-73
Unit Dose (blister pack)
 Box of 100
  (strips of 10) ....NDC 0028-0057-61

Storage Conditions:
Do not store above 86°F. Protect from moisture.
Dispense in tight, light-resistant container (USP).

C84-6 (Rev. 4/84)

Dist. by:
GEIGY Pharmaceuticals
Div. of CIBA-GEIGY Corp.
Ardsley, New York 10502

Shown in Product Identification Section, page 411

LIORESAL® 10 mg ℞
[*lye-oar'eh-sal*]
baclofen
Muscle Relaxant, Antispastic 20 mg ℞

Description: Lioresal is 4-amino-3-(*p*-chlorophenyl) butyric acid, a white to off-white crystalline substance.

It is slightly soluble in water and poorly soluble in organic solvents. Molecular weight: 213.67.

Actions: The precise mechanism of action of Lioresal is not fully known. Lioresal is capable of inhibiting both monosynaptic and polysynaptic reflexes at the spinal level, possibly by hyperpolarization of afferent terminals, although actions at supraspinal sites may also occur and contribute to its clinical effect. Although Lioresal is an analog of the putative inhibitory neurotransmitter gamma-aminobutyric acid (GABA), there is no conclusive evidence that actions on GABA systems are involved in the production of its clinical effects. In studies with animals, Lioresal has been shown to have general CNS depressant properties as indicated by the production of sedation with tolerance, somnolence, ataxia, and respiratory and cardiovascular depression. Lioresal is rapidly and extensively absorbed and eliminated. Absorption may be dose-dependent, being reduced with increasing doses. Lioresal is excreted primarily by the kidney in unchanged form and there is relatively large intersubject variation in absorption and/or elimination.

Indications: Lioresal is useful for the alleviation of signs and symptoms of spasticity resulting from multiple sclerosis, particularly for the relief of flexor spasms and concomitant pain, clonus, and muscular rigidity.

Patients should have reversible spasticity so that Lioresal treatment will aid in restoring residual function.

Lioresal may also be of some value in patients with spinal cord injuries and other spinal cord diseases. Lioresal is not indicated in the treatment of skeletal muscle spasm resulting from rheumatic disorders.

The efficacy of Lioresal in stroke, cerebral palsy, and Parkinson's disease has not been established

Continued on next page

The full prescribing information for each GEIGY drug is contained herein and is that in effect as of October 1, 1984.

Geigy—Cont.

and, therefore, it is not recommended for these conditions.

Contraindications: Hypersensitivity to baclofen.

Warnings:
a. *Abrupt Drug Withdrawal:* Hallucinations and seizures have occurred on abrupt withdrawal of Lioresal. Therefore, except for serious adverse reactions, the dose should be reduced slowly when the drug is discontinued.
b. *Impaired Renal Function:* Because Lioresal is primarily excreted unchanged through the kidneys, it should be given with caution, and it may be necessary to reduce the dosage.
c. *Stroke:* Lioresal has not significantly benefited patients with stroke. These patients have also shown poor tolerability to the drug.
d. *Pregnancy:* Lioresal has been shown to increase the incidence of omphaloceles (ventral hernias) in fetuses of rats given approximately 13 times the maximum dose recommended for human use, at a dose which caused significant reductions in food intake and weight gain in dams. This abnormality was not seen in mice or rabbits. There was also an increased incidence of incomplete sternebral ossification in fetuses of rats given approximately 13 times the maximum recommended human dose, and an increased incidence of unossified phalangeal nuclei of forelimbs and hindlimbs in fetuses of rabbits given approximately 7 times the maximum recommended human dose. In mice, no teratogenic effects were observed, although reductions in mean fetal weight with consequent delays in skeletal ossification were present when dams were given 17 or 34 times the human daily dose. There are no studies in pregnant women. Lioresal should be used during pregnancy only if the benefit clearly justifies the potential risk to the fetus.

Precautions: Safe use of Lioresal in children under age 12 has not been established, and it is, therefore, not recommended for use in children.

Because of the possibility of sedation, patients should be cautioned regarding the operation of automobiles or other dangerous machinery, and activities made hazardous by decreased alertness. Patients should also be cautioned that the central nervous system effects of Lioresal may be additive to those of alcohol and other CNS depressants.

Lioresal should be used with caution where spasticity is utilized to sustain upright posture and balance in locomotion or whenever spasticity is utilized to obtain increased function.

In patients with epilepsy, the clinical state and electroencephalogram should be monitored at regular intervals, since deterioration in seizure control and EEG have been reported occasionally in patients taking Lioresal.

It is not known whether this drug is excreted in human milk. As a general rule, nursing should not be undertaken while a patient is on a drug since many drugs are excreted in human milk.

A dose-related increase in incidence of ovarian cysts and a less marked increase in enlarged and/or hemorrhagic adrenal glands was observed in female rats treated chronically with Lioresal.

Ovarian cysts have been found by palpation in about 4% of the multiple sclerosis patients that were treated with Lioresal for up to one year. In most cases these cysts disappeared spontaneously while patients continued to receive the drug. Ovarian cysts are estimated to occur spontaneously in approximately 1% to 5% of the normal female population.

The clinical relevance of these findings is not known.

Adverse Reactions: The most common is transient drowsiness (10–63%). In one controlled study of 175 patients, transient drowsiness was observed in 63% of those receiving Lioresal compared to 36% of those in the placebo group. Other common adverse reactions are dizziness (5–15%), weakness (5–15%) and fatigue (2–4%). Others reported:

Neuropsychiatric: Confusion (1–11%), headache (4–8%), insomnia (2–7%); and, rarely, euphoria, excitement, depression, hallucinations, paresthesia, muscle pain, tinnitus, slurred speech, coordination disorder, tremor, rigidity, dystonia, ataxia, blurred vision, nystagmus, strabismus, miosis, mydriasis, diplopia, dysarthria, epileptic seizure.

Cardiovascular: Hypotension (0–9%). Rare instances of dyspnea, palpitation, chest pain, syncope.

Gastrointestinal: Nausea (4–12%), constipation (2–6%); and, rarely, dry mouth, anorexia, taste disorder, abdominal pain, vomiting, diarrhea, and positive test for occult blood in stool.

Genitourinary: Urinary frequency (2–6%); and, rarely, enuresis, urinary retention, dysuria, impotence, inability to ejaculate, nocturia, hematuria.

Other: Instances of rash, pruritus, ankle edema, excessive perspiration, weight gain, nasal congestion.

Some of the CNS and genitourinary symptoms may be related to the underlying disease rather than to drug therapy.

The following laboratory tests have been found to be abnormal in a few patients receiving Lioresal: increased SGOT, elevated alkaline phosphatase, and elevation of blood sugar.

Overdosage: *Signs and Symptoms:* Vomiting, muscular hypotonia, drowsiness, accommodation disorders, coma, respiratory depression, and seizures.

Treatment: In the alert patient, empty the stomach promptly by induced emesis followed by lavage. In the obtunded patient, secure the airway with a cuffed endotracheal tube before beginning lavage (do not induce emesis). Maintain adequate respiratory exchange, do not use respiratory stimulants.

Dosage and Administration: The determination of optimal dosage requires individual titration. Start therapy at a low dosage and increase gradually until optimum effect is achieved (usually between 40–80 mg daily).

The following dosage titration schedule is suggested:

5 mg t.i.d. for 3 days
10 mg t.i.d. for 3 days
15 mg t.i.d. for 3 days
20 mg t.i.d. for 3 days

Thereafter additional increases may be necessary but the total daily dose should not exceed a maximum of 80 mg daily (20 mg q.i.d.).

The lowest dose compatible with an optimal response is recommended. If benefits are not evident after a reasonable trial period, patients should be slowly withdrawn from the drug (see **Warnings** *Abrupt Drug Withdrawal*).

How Supplied:
Tablets 10 mg—white, oval, single scored (imprinted 23 Geigy)
  Bottles of 100 ....NDC 0028-0023-01
  Unit Dose (blister pack)
  Box of 100 (strips of 10) ....NDC 0028-0023-61
Tablets 20 mg—white, capsule shaped, scored (imprinted 33 Geigy)
  Bottles of 100 ....NDC 0028-0033-01
  Unit Dose (blister pack)
  Box of 100 (strips of 10)   NDC 0028-0033-61
Dispense in tight container (USP).
C84-10 (Rev. 1/84)
Shown in Product Identification Section, page 411

LOPRESSOR®   ℞
metoprolol tartrate
Tablets of 50 mg   GY-CODE 51
Tablets of 100 mg   GY-CODE 71
Ampuls 5 ml
An antihypertensive beta-blocking agent

Description: Lopressor, metoprolol tartrate, is a selective beta$_1$-adrenoreceptor blocking agent, available as 50- and 100-mg tablets for oral administration and in 5-ml ampuls for intravenous administration. Each ampul contains a sterile solution of metoprolol tartrate, 5 mg, and sodium chloride USP, 45 mg. Metoprolol tartrate is 1-isopropylamino-3-[*p*-(2-methoxyethyl) phenoxyl-2-propanol 2:1 *dextro*-tartrate.

Metoprolol tartrate is a white, practically odorless, crystalline powder with a molecular weight of 684.82. It is readily soluble in chloroform, in methylene chloride, and in water; soluble in ethanol; and sparingly soluble in acetone.

Clinical Pharmacology: Lopressor is a beta-adrenergic receptor blocking agent. *In vitro* and *in vivo* animal studies have shown that it has a preferential effect on beta$_1$ adrenoreceptors, chiefly located in cardiac muscle. This preferential effect is not absolute, however, and at higher doses, Lopressor also inhibits beta$_2$ adrenoreceptors, chiefly located in the bronchial and vascular musculature.

Clinical pharmacology studies have confirmed the beta-blocking activity of metoprolol in man, as shown by (1) reduction in heart rate and cardiac output at rest and upon exercise, (2) reduction of systolic blood pressure upon exercise, (3) inhibition of isoproterenol-induced tachycardia, and (4) reduction of reflex orthostatic tachycardia.

Relative beta$_1$ selectivity has been confirmed by the following: (1) In normal subjects, Lopressor is unable to reverse the beta$_2$-mediated vasodilating effects of epinephrine. This contrasts with the effect of nonselective (beta$_1$ plus beta$_2$) beta blockers, which completely reverse the vasodilating effects of epinephrine. (2) In asthmatic patients, Lopressor reduces FEV$_1$ and FVC significantly less than a nonselective beta blocker, propranolol, at equivalent beta$_1$-receptor blocking doses.

Lopressor has no intrinsic sympathomimetic activity, and membrane-stabilizing activity is detectable only at doses much greater than required for beta blockade. Lopressor crosses the blood-brain barrier and has been reported in the CSF in a concentration 78% of the simultaneous plasma concentration. Animal and human experiments indicate that Lopressor slows the sinus rate and decreases AV nodal conduction.

In controlled clinical studies, Lopressor has been shown to be an effective antihypertensive agent when used alone or as concomitant therapy with thiazide-type diuretics, at dosages of 100–450 mg daily. In controlled, comparative, clinical studies, Lopressor has been shown to be as effective an antihypertensive agent as propranolol, methyldopa, and thiazide-type diuretics, and to be equally effective in supine and standing positions.

The mechanism of the antihypertensive effects of beta-blocking agents has not been elucidated. However, several possible mechanisms have been proposed: (1) competitive antagonism of catecholamines at peripheral (especially cardiac) adrenergic neuron sites, leading to decreased cardiac output; (2) a central effect leading to reduced sympathetic outflow to the periphery; and (3) suppression of renin activity.

In a large (1,395 patients randomized), double-blind, placebo-controlled clinical study, Lopressor was shown to reduce 3-month mortality by 36% in patients with suspected or definite myocardial infarction.

Patients were randomized and treated as soon as possible after their arrival in the hospital, once their clinical condition had stabilized and their hemodynamic status had been carefully evaluated. Subjects were ineligible if they had hypotension, bradycardia, peripheral signs of shock, and/or more than minimal basal rales as signs of congestive heart failure. Initial treatment consisted of intravenous followed by oral administration of Lopressor or placebo, given in a coronary care or comparable unit. Oral maintenance therapy with Lopressor or placebo was then continued for 3 months. After this double-blind period, all patients were given Lopressor and followed up to 1 year. The median delay from the onset of symptoms to the initiation of therapy was 8 hours in both the Lopressor and placebo treatment groups. Among patients treated with Lopressor, there were comparable reductions in 3-month mortality for those treated early ($\leq$ 8 hours) and those in whom treatment was started later. Significant reductions in the incidence of ventricular fibrillation and in chest pain following initial intravenous therapy were also observed with Lopressor and were independent of the interval between onset of symptoms and initiation of therapy.

The precise mechanism of action of Lopressor in patients with suspected or definite myocardial infarction is not known.

In this study, patients treated with metoprolol received the drug both very early (intravenously) and during a subsequent 3-month period, while placebo patients received no beta-blocker treatment for this period. The study thus was able to show a benefit from the overall metoprolol regimen but cannot separate the benefit of very early intravenous treatment from the benefit of later beta-blocker therapy. Nonetheless, because the overall regimen showed a clear beneficial effect on survival without evidence of an early adverse effect on survival, one acceptable dosage regimen is the precise regimen used in the trial. Because the specific benefit of very early treatment remains to be defined however, it is also reasonable to administer the drug orally to patients at a later time as is recommended for certain other beta blockers.

Pharmacokinetics

In man, absorption of Lopressor is rapid and complete. Plasma levels following oral administration, however, approximate 50% of levels following intravenous administration, indicating about 50% first-pass metabolism.

Plasma levels achieved are highly variable after oral administration. Only a small fraction of the drug (about 12%) is bound to human serum albumin. Elimination is mainly by biotransformation in the liver, and the plasma half-life ranges from approximately 3 to 7 hours. Less than 5% of an oral dose of Lopressor is recovered unchanged in the urine; the rest is excreted by the kidneys as metabolites that appear to have no clinical significance. The systemic availability and half-life of Lopressor in patients with renal failure do not differ to a clinically significant degree from those in normal subjects. Consequently, no reduction in dosage is usually needed in patients with chronic renal failure.

Significant beta-blocking effect (as measured by reduction of exercise heart rate) occurs within 1 hour after oral administration, and its duration is dose-related. For example, a 50% reduction of the maximum registered effect after single oral doses of 20, 50, and 100 mg occurred at 3.3, 5.0, and 6.4 hours, respectively, in normal subjects. After repeated oral dosages of 100 mg twice daily, a significant reduction in exercise systolic blood pressure was evident at 12 hours.

Following intravenous administration of Lopressor, the half-life of the distribution phase is approximately 12 minutes; the urinary recovery of unchanged drug is approximately 10%. When the drug was infused over a 10-minute period, in normal volunteers, maximum beta blockade was achieved at approximately 20 minutes. Doses of 5 mg and 15 mg yielded a maximal reduction in exercise-induced heart rate of approximately 10% and 15%, respectively. The effect on exercise heart rate decreased linearly with time at the same rate for both doses, and disappeared at approximately 5 hours and 8 hours for the 5-mg and 15-mg doses, respectively.

Equivalent maximal beta-blocking effect is achieved with oral and intravenous doses in the ratio of approximately 2.5:1.

There is a linear relationship between the log of plasma levels and reduction of exercise heart rate. However, antihypertensive activity does not appear to be related to plasma levels. Because of variable plasma levels attained with a given dose and lack of a consistent relationship of antihypertensive activity to dose, selection of proper dosage requires individual titration.

In several studies of patients with acute myocardial infarction, intravenous followed by oral administration of Lopressor caused a reduction in heart rate, systolic blood pressure, and cardiac output. Stroke volume, diastolic blood pressure, and pulmonary artery end diastolic pressure remained unchanged.

Indications and Usage:

Hypertension

Lopressor tablets are indicated for the treatment of hypertension. They may be used alone or in combination with other antihypertensive agents.

Myocardial Infarction

Lopressor ampuls and tablets are indicated in the treatment of hemodynamically stable patients with definite or suspected acute myocardial infarction to reduce cardiovascular mortality. Treatment with intravenous Lopressor can be initiated as soon as the patient's clinical condition allows (see **Dosage and Administration, Contraindications,** and **Warnings**). Alternatively, treatment can begin within 3 to 10 days of the acute event (see **Dosage and Administration**).

Contraindications:

Hypertension

Lopressor is contraindicated in sinus bradycardia, heart block greater than first degree, cardiogenic shock, and overt cardiac failure (see **Warnings**).

Myocardial Infarction

Lopressor is contraindicated in patients with a heart rate < 45 beats/min; significant heart block greater than first degree (P-R interval ≥ 0.24 sec); systolic blood pressure < 100 mmHg; or moderate-to-severe cardiac failure (see **Warnings**).

Warnings:

Hypertension

Cardiac Failure: Sympathetic stimulation is a vital component supporting circulatory function in congestive heart failure, and beta blockade carries the potential hazard of further depressing myocardial contractility and precipitating more severe failure. In hypertensive patients who have congestive heart failure controlled by digitalis and diuretics, Lopressor should be administered cautiously. Both digitalis and Lopressor slow AV conduction.

In Patients Without a History of Cardiac Failure: Continued depression of the myocardium with beta-blocking agents over a period of time can, in some cases, lead to cardiac failure. At the first sign or symptom of impending cardiac failure, patients should be fully digitalized and/or given a diuretic. The response should be observed closely. If cardiac failure continues, despite adequate digitalization and diuretic therapy, Lopressor should be withdrawn.

Ischemic Heart Disease: Following abrupt cessation of therapy with certain beta-blocking agents, exacerbations of angina pectoris and, in some cases, myocardial infarction have been reported. Even in the absence of overt angina pectoris, when discontinuing therapy, Lopressor should not be withdrawn abruptly, and patients should be cautioned against interruption of therapy without the physician's advice (see **Precautions, Information for Patients**).

Bronchospastic Diseases: PATIENTS WITH BRONCHOSPASTIC DISEASES SHOULD, IN GENERAL, NOT RECEIVE BETA BLOCKERS. Because of its relative beta$_1$ selectivity, however, Lopressor may be used with caution in patients with bronchospastic disease who do not respond to, or cannot tolerate, other antihypertensive treatment. Since beta$_1$ selectivity is not absolute, a beta$_2$-stimulating agent should be administered concomitantly, and the lowest possible dose of Lopressor should be used. In these circumstances it would be prudent initially to administer Lopressor in smaller doses three times daily, instead of larger doses two times daily, to avoid the higher plasma levels associated with the longer dosing interval. (See Dosage and Administration.)

Major Surgery: The necessity or desirability of withdrawing beta-blocking therapy prior to major surgery is controversial; the impaired ability of the heart to respond to reflex adrenergic stimuli may augment the risks of general anesthesia and surgical procedures.

Lopressor, like other beta blockers, is a competitive inhibitor of beta-receptor agonists, and its effects can be reversed by administration of such agents, e.g., dobutamine or isoproterenol. However, such patients may be subject to protracted severe hypotension. Difficulty in restarting and maintaining the heart beat has also been reported with beta blockers.

Diabetes and Hypoglycemia: Lopressor should be used with caution in diabetic patients if a beta-blocking agent is required. Beta blockers may mask tachycardia occurring with hypoglycemia, but other manifestations such as dizziness and sweating may not be significantly affected.

Thyrotoxicosis: Beta-adrenergic blockade may mask certain clinical signs (e.g., tachycardia) of hyperthyroidism. Patients suspected of developing thyrotoxicosis should be managed carefully to avoid abrupt withdrawal of beta blockade, which might precipitate a thyroid storm.

Myocardial Infarction

Cardiac Failure: Sympathetic stimulation is a vital component supporting circulatory function, and beta blockade carries the potential hazard of depressing myocardial contractility and precipitating or exacerbating minimal cardiac failure. During treatment with Lopressor, the hemodynamic status of the patient should be carefully monitored. If heart failure occurs or persists despite appropriate treatment, Lopressor should be discontinued.

Bradycardia: Lopressor produces a decrease in sinus heart rate in most patients; this decrease is greatest among patients with high initial heart rates and least among patients with low initial heart rates. Acute myocardial infarction (particularly inferior infarction) may in itself produce a significant lowering of the sinus rate. If the sinus rate decreases to < 40 beats/min, particularly if associated with evidence of lowered cardiac output, atropine (0.25–0.5 mg) should be administered intravenously. If treatment with atropine is not successful, Lopressor should be discontinued, and cautious administration of isoproterenol or installation of a cardiac pacemaker should be considered.

AV Block: Lopressor slows AV conduction and may produce significant first- (P-R interval ≥ 0.26 sec), second-, or third-degree heart block. Acute myocardial infarction also produces heart block. If heart block occurs, Lopressor should be discontinued and atropine (0.25–0.5 mg) should be administered intravenously. If treatment with atropine is not successful, cautious administration of isoproterenol or installation of a cardiac pacemaker should be considered.

Hypotension: If hypotension (systolic blood pressure ≤ 90 mmHg) occurs, Lopressor should be discontinued, and the hemodynamic status of the patient and the extent of myocardial damage carefully assessed. Invasive monitoring of central venous, pulmonary capillary wedge, and arterial pressures may be required. Appropriate therapy with fluids, positive inotropic agents, balloon counterpulsation, or other treatment modalities should be instituted. If hypotension is associated with sinus bradycardia or AV block, treatment should be directed at reversing these (see above).

Bronchospastic Diseases: PATIENTS WITH BRONCHOSPASTIC DISEASES SHOULD, IN GENERAL, NOT RECEIVE BETA BLOCKERS. Because of its relative beta$_1$ selectivity, Lopressor may be used with extreme caution in patients with bronchospastic disease. Because it is unknown to what extent beta$_2$-stimulating agents may exacerbate myocardial ischemia and the extent of infarction, these agents should *not* be used prophylactically. If bronchospasm not related to congestive heart failure occurs, Lopressor should be discontinued. A theophylline derivative or a beta$_2$ agonist may be administered cautiously, depending on the clinical condition of the patient. Both theophyl-

Continued on next page

The full prescribing information for each GEIGY drug is contained herein and is that in effect as of October 1, 1984.

Geigy—Cont.

line derivatives and beta$_2$ agonists may produce serious cardiac arrhythmias.

Precautions:
General
Lopressor should be used with caution in patients with impaired hepatic function.

Information for Patients
Patients should be advised to take Lopressor regularly and continuously, as directed, with or immediately following meals. If a dose should be missed, the patient should take only the next scheduled dose (without doubling it). Patients should not discontinue Lopressor without consulting the physician.

Patients should know how they react to this medicine before they operate automobiles and machinery or engage in other tasks requiring alertness. Patients should contact the physician if any difficulty in breathing occurs, and before surgery of any type, the patient should inform the physician or dentist that he or she is taking Lopressor.

Laboratory Tests
Clinical laboratory findings may include elevated levels of serum transaminase, alkaline phosphatase, and lactate dehydrogenase.

Drug Interactions
Catecholamine-depleting drugs (e.g., reserpine) may have an additive effect when given with beta-blocking agents. Patients treated with Lopressor plus a catecholamine depletor should therefore be closely observed for evidence of hypotension or marked bradycardia, which may produce vertigo, syncope, or postural hypotension.

Carcinogenesis, Mutagenesis, Impairment of Fertility
Long-term studies in animals have been conducted to evaluate toxic effects and carcinogenic potential. In a 1-year study in dogs, there was no evidence of drug-induced toxicity at or below oral dosages of 105 mg/kg per day. In 2-year studies in rats at three oral dosage levels of up to 800 mg/kg per day, there was no increase in the development of spontaneously occurring benign or malignant neoplasms of any type. The only histologic changes that appeared to be drug-related were an increased incidence of generally mild focal accumulation of foamy macrophages in pulmonary alveoli and a slight increase in biliary hyperplasia. Neither finding represents symptoms of a known disease entity in man. In a 21-month study in mice at three oral dosage levels of up to 750 mg/kg per day, benign lung tumors (small adenomas) occurred more frequently in female mice receiving the highest dose than in untreated control animals. There was no increase in malignant or total (benign plus malignant) lung tumors, nor in the overall incidence of tumors or malignant tumors. This 21-month study was repeated, and no statistically or biologically significant differences were observed between treated and control mice of either sex for any type of tumor.

Pregnancy Category B
Reproduction studies have been performed in rats at doses up to 55.5 times the maximum daily human dose of 450 mg and have revealed no evidence of impaired fertility or teratogenicity due to Lopressor. Increased postimplantation loss and decreased neonatal survival did occur in the rats (threshold between 50 and 500 mg/kg), and distribution studies in mice confirm exposure of the fetus when Lopressor is administered to the pregnant animal. There are no adequate and well-controlled studies in pregnant women. Because animal reproduction studies are not always predictive of human response, this drug should be used during pregnancy only if clearly needed.

Nursing Mothers
Lopressor is excreted in breast milk in very small quantity. An infant consuming 1 liter of breast milk daily would receive a dose of less than 1 mg of the drug. Caution should be exercised when Lopressor is administered to a nursing woman.

Pediatric Use
Safety and effectiveness in children have not been established.

Adverse Reactions:
Hypertension
Most adverse effects have been mild and transient.

Central Nervous System: Tiredness and dizziness have occurred in about 10 of 100 patients. Depression has been reported in about 5 of 100 patients. Mental confusion and short-term memory loss have been reported. Headache, nightmares, and insomnia have also been reported, but a drug relationship is not clear.

Cardiovascular: Shortness of breath and bradycardia have occurred in approximately 3 of 100 patients. Cold extremities; arterial insufficiency, usually of the Raynaud type; palpitations; and congestive heart failure have been reported. (See **Contraindications, Warnings,** and **Precautions.**)

Respiratory: Wheezing (bronchospasm) has been reported in fewer than 1 of 100 patients (see **Warnings**).

Gastrointestinal: Diarrhea has occurred in about 5 of 100 patients. Nausea, gastric pain, constipation, flatulence, and heartburn have been reported in 1 of 100, or fewer, patients.

Hypersensitive Reactions: Pruritus has occurred in fewer than 1 of 100 patients. Rash has been reported.

Miscellaneous: Peyronie's disease has been reported in fewer than 1 of 100,000 patients. Alopecia has been reported.

The oculomucocutaneous syndrome associated with the beta blocker practolol has not been reported with Lopressor.

Myocardial Infarction
Central Nervous System: Tiredness has been reported in about 1 of 100 patients. Vertigo, sleep disturbances, hallucinations, headache, dizziness, visual disturbances, confusion, and reduced libido have also been reported, but a drug relationship is not clear.

Cardiovascular: In the randomized comparison of Lopressor and placebo described in the **Clinical Pharmacology** section, the following adverse reactions were reported:

	Lopressor	Placebo
Hypotension (systolic BP < 90 mmHg)	27.4%	23.2%
Bradycardia (heart rate < 40 beats/min)	15.9%	6.7%
Second- or third-degree heart block	4.7%	4.7%
First-degree heart block (P-R ≥ 0.26 sec)	5.3%	1.9%
Heart failure	27.5%	29.6%

Respiratory: Dyspnea of pulmonary origin has been reported in fewer than 1 of 100 patients.

Gastrointestinal: Nausea and abdominal pain have been reported in fewer than 1 of 100 patients.

Dermatologic: Rash and worsened psoriasis have been reported, but a drug relationship is not clear.

Miscellaneous: Unstable diabetes and claudication have been reported, but a drug relationship is not clear.

Potential Adverse Reactions
A variety of adverse reactions not listed above have been reported with other beta-adrenergic blocking agents and should be considered potential adverse reactions to Lopressor.

Central Nervous System: Reversible mental depression progressing to catatonia; an acute reversible syndrome characterized by disorientation for time and place, short-term memory loss, emotional lability, slightly clouded sensorium, and decreased performance on neuropsychometrics.

Cardiovascular: Intensification of AV block (See **Contraindications**).

Hematologic: Agranulocytosis, nonthrombocytopenic purpura, thrombocytopenic purpura.

Hypersensitive Reactions: Fever combined with aching and sore throat, laryngospasm, and respiratory distress.

Overdosage:
Acute Toxicity
Several cases of overdosage have been reported, some leading to death.

Oral LD$_{50}$'s (mg/kg): mice, 1158–2460; rats, 3090–4670.

Signs and Symptoms
Potential signs and symptoms associated with overdosage with Lopressor are bradycardia, hypotension, bronchospasm, and cardiac failure.

Treatment
There is no specific antidote.
In general, patients with acute or recent myocardial infarction may be more hemodynamically unstable than other patients and should be treated accordingly (see **Warnings, Myocardial Infarction**).
On the basis of the pharmacologic actions of Lopressor, the following general measures should be employed:

Elimination of the Drug: Gastric lavage should be performed.

Bradycardia: Atropine should be administered. If there is no response to vagal blockade, isoproterenol should be administered cautiously.

Hypotension: A vasopressor should be administered, e.g., levarterenol or dopamine.

Bronchospasm: A beta$_2$-stimulating agent and/or a theophylline derivative should be administered.

Cardiac Failure: A digitalis glycoside and diuretic should be administered. In shock resulting from inadequate cardiac contractility, administration of dobutamine, isoproterenol, or glucagon may be considered.

Dosage and Administration:
Hypertension
The dosage of Lopressor should be individualized. Lopressor should be taken with or immediately following meals.

The usual initial dosage is 100 mg daily in single or divided doses, whether used alone or added to a diuretic. The dosage may be increased at weekly (or longer) intervals until optimum blood pressure reduction is achieved. In general, the maximum effect of any given dosage level will be apparent after 1 week of therapy. The effective dosage range is 100 to 450 mg per day. Dosages above 450 mg per day have not been studied. While once-daily dosing is effective and can maintain a reduction in blood pressure throughout the day, lower doses (especially 100 mg) may not maintain a full effect at the end of the 24-hour period, and larger or more frequent daily doses may be required. This can be evaluated by measuring blood pressure near the end of the dosing interval to determine whether satisfactory control is being maintained throughout the day. Beta$_1$ selectivity diminishes as the dose of Lopressor is increased.

Myocardial Infarction
Early Treatment: During the early phase of definite or suspected acute myocardial infarction, treatment with Lopressor can be initiated as soon as possible after the patient's arrival in the hospital. Such treatment should be initiated in a coronary care or similar unit immediately after the patient's hemodynamic condition has stabilized. Treatment in this early phase should begin with the intravenous administration of three bolus injections of 5 mg of Lopressor each; the injections should be given at approximately 2-minute intervals. During the intravenous administration of Lopressor, blood pressure, heart rate, and electrocardiogram should be carefully monitored.

In patients who tolerate the full intravenous dose (15 mg), Lopressor tablets, 50 mg every 6 hours, should be initiated 15 minutes after the last intravenous dose and continued for 48 hours. Thereafter, patients should receive a maintenance dosage of 100 mg twice daily (see *Late Treatment* below). Patients who appear not to tolerate the full intravenous dose should be started on either 25 mg or 50 mg every 6 hours (depending on the degree of intolerance) 15 minutes after the last intravenous dose or as soon as their clinical condition allows. In patients with severe intolerance, treatment with Lopressor should be discontinued (see **Warnings**).

Late Treatment: Patients with contraindications to treatment during the early phase of suspected or definite myocardial infarction, patients who appear not to tolerate the full early treatment, and patients in whom the physician wishes to delay therapy for any other reason should be started on Lopressor tablets, 100 mg twice daily, as soon as their clinical condition allows. Therapy should be continued for at least 3 months. Although the efficacy of Lopressor beyond 3 months has not been conclusively established, data from studies with other beta blockers suggest that treatment should be continued for 1–3 years.

Note: **Parenteral drug products should be inspected visually for particulate matter and discoloration prior to administration, whenever solution and container permit.**

How Supplied:
Tablets 50 mg—capsule-shaped, light red, scored (imprinted GEIGY 51)
Bottles of 100 ....NDC 0028-0051-01
Bottles of 1000 ....NDC 0028-0051-10
Gy-Pak®—One Unit
  12 bottles—60 tablets each...NDC 0028-0051-73
  12 bottles—100 tablets each.................................
                                           NDC 0028-0051-65
Unit Dose (blister pack)
  Box of 100 (strips of 10) ....NDC 0028-0051-61
Tablets 100 mg—capsule-shaped, light blue, scored (imprinted GEIGY 71)
Bottles of 100 ....NDC 0028-0071-01
Bottles of 1000 ....NDC 0028-0071-10
Gy-Pak®—One Unit
  12 bottles—60 tablets each...NDC 0028-0071-73
  12 bottles—100 tablets each.................................
                                           NDC 0028-0071-65
Unit Dose (blister pack)
  Box (strips of 10) ....NDC 0028-0071-61
Store at controlled room temperature and protect from moisture.
Dispense in tight, light-resistant container (USP).
Ampuls 5 ml—each containing 5 mg of metoprolol tartrate
  Box of 12 ampuls....................NDC 0028-4201-12
Protect from light.
                                           C84-15 (Rev. 4/84)

OTRIVIN®
[oh′ trah-vinn]
xylometazoline hydrochloride USP
Nasal Spray and Nasal Drops 0.1%
Pediatric Nasal Drops 0.05%

One application provides rapid and long-lasting relief of nasal congestion for up to 10 hours.
Quickly clears stuffy noses due to common cold, sinusitis, hay fever.
Nasal congestion can make life miserable—you can't breathe, smell, taste or sleep comfortably. That is why Otrivin is so helpful. It clears away that stuffy feeling, usually within 5 to 10 minutes, and your head feels clear for hours.
Otrivin has been prescribed by doctors for many years. Here is how you use it:
Nasal Spray 0.1%—Spray 2 to 3 times into each nostril every 8–10 hours. With head upright, squeeze sharply and firmly while inhaling (sniffing) through the nose.
Nasal Drops 0.1%—for adults and children 12 years and older. Put 2 or 3 drops into each nostril every 8 to 10 hours. Tilt head as far back as possible. Immediately bend head forward toward knees, hold for a few seconds, then return to upright position.
Do not give Nasal Spray 0.1% or Nasal Drops 0.1% to children under 12 years except under the advice and supervision of a physician.
Pediatric Nasal Drops 0.05%—for children 2 to 12 years of age. Put 2 to 3 drops into each nostril every 8 to 10 hours. Tilt head as far back as possible. Immediately bend head forward toward knees, hold a few seconds, then return to upright position.
Do not give this product to children under 2 years except under the advice and supervision of a physician.
Otrivin Nasal Spray/Nasal Drops are available in unbreakable plastic spray package of ½ fl oz (15 ml) and in plastic dropper bottle of .66 fl oz (20ml).
Otrivin Pediatric Nasal Drops
Available in plastic dropper bottle of .66 fl oz (20ml).
Warnings: Do not exceed recommended dosage, because symptoms such as burning, stinging, sneezing, or increase of nasal discharge may occur. Do not use this product for more than 3 days. If symptoms persist, consult a physician. The use of this dispenser by more than one person may cause infection.
Keep this and all medicines out of the reach of children. In case of accidental ingestion, seek professional assistance or contact a Poison Control Center immediately.
                                           C80-47 (8/80)

PBZ-SR® GY-CODE 48   ℞
tripelennamine HCl
sustained-release tablets
Tablets of 100 mg

Description: PBZ-SR Tablets are available as the hydrochloride salt of tripelennamine, 2-[benzyl[2-(dimethylamino)ethyl]-amino]pyridine, in a wax matrix. This formulation is intended to provide a gradual and prolonged release of tripelennamine from the matrix. Tripelennamine hydrochloride is an antihistamine occurring as a white, crystalline powder that slowly darkens on exposure to light and is freely soluble in water and alcohol.
Actions: Antihistamines are competitive antagonists of histamine, which also produce central nervous system effects (both stimulant and depressant) and peripheral anticholinergic, atropine-like effects (e.g., drying).
Indications: Perennial and seasonal allergic rhinitis; vasomotor rhinitis; allergic conjunctivitis due to inhalant allergens and foods; mild, uncomplicated allergic skin manifestations of urticaria and angioedema; amelioration of allergic reactions to blood or plasma; dermographism; anaphylactic reactions as adjunctive therapy to epinephrine and other standard measures after the acute manifestations have been controlled.
Contraindications: PBZ-SR should not be used in premature infants, neonates, or nursing mothers; patients receiving MAO inhibitors; patients with narrow-angle glaucoma, stenosing peptic ulcer, symptomatic prostatic hypertrophy, bladder neck obstruction, pyloroduodenal obstruction, lower respiratory tract symptoms (including asthma), or hypersensitivity to tripelennamine or related compounds.
Warnings: Antihistamines often produce drowsiness and may reduce mental alertness in children and adults. Patients should be warned about engaging in activities requiring mental alertness (*e.g.*, driving a car, operating machinery or hazardous appliances). In elderly patients, approximately 60 years or older, antihistamines are more likely to cause dizziness, sedation and hypotension.
Patients should be warned that the central nervous system effects of PBZ-SR may be additive with those of alcohol and other CNS depressants (e.g., hypnotics, sedatives, tranquilizers, antianxiety agents).
Antihistamines may produce excitation, particularly in children.
Usage in Pregnancy
Although no tripelennamine-related teratogenic potential or other adverse effects on the fetus have been observed in limited animal reproduction studies, the safe use of this drug in pregnancy or during lactation has not been established. Therefore, the drug should not be used during pregnancy or lactation unless, in the judgment of the physician, the expected benefits outweigh the potential hazards.
Usage in Children
In infants and children particularly, antihistamines in overdosage may produce hallucinations, convulsions and/or death.
Precautions: PBZ-SR, like other antihistamines, has atropine-like, anticholinergic activity and should be used with caution in patients with increased intraocular pressure, hyperthyroidism, cardiovascular disease, hypertension, or history of bronchial asthma.
Adverse Reactions: The most frequent adverse reactions to antihistamines are sedation or drowsiness; sleepiness; dryness of the mouth, nose, and throat; thickening of bronchial secretions; dizziness; disturbed coordination; epigastric distress.

Other adverse reactions which may occur are: fatigue; chills; confusion; restlessness; excitation; hysteria; nervousness; irritability; insomnia; euphoria; anorexia; nausea; vomiting; diarrhea; constipation; hypotension; tightness in the chest; wheezing; blurred vision; diplopia; vertigo; tinnitus; convulsions; headache; palpitations; tachycardia; extrasystoles; nasal stuffiness; urinary frequency; difficult urination; urinary retention; leukopenia; hemolytic anemia; thrombocytopenia; agranulocytosis; aplastic anemia; allergic or hypersensitivity reactions, including drug rash, urticaria, anaphylactic shock, and photosensitivity.
Although the following may have been reported to occur in association with some antihistamines, they have not been known to result from the use of PBZ-SR: excessive perspiration, tremor, paresthesias, acute labyrinthitis, neuritis and early menses.
Dosage and Administration: Dosage should be individualized according to the needs and response of the patient.
Adults: One 100-mg PBZ-SR Tablet in the morning and one in the evening is generally adequate. In difficult cases, one 100-mg PBZ-SR Tablet every 8 hours may be required.
Children: PBZ-SR Tablets are not intended for use in children.
Overdosage:
Signs and Symptoms
The greatest danger from acute overdosage with antihistamines is their central nervous system effects which produce depression and/or stimulation.
In children, stimulation predominates initially in a syndrome which may include excitement, hallucinations, ataxia, incoordination, athetosis, and convulsions followed by postictal depression. Dry mouth, fixed dilated pupils, flushing of the face, and fever are common and resemble the syndrome of atropine poisoning.
In adults, CNS depression (i.e., drowsiness, coma) is more common. CNS stimulation is rare; fever and flushing are uncommon.
In both children and adults, there can be a terminal deepening of coma and cardiovascular collapse; death can occur, especially in infants and children.
Treatment
There is no specific therapy for acute overdosage with antihistamines. General symptomatic and supportive measures should be instituted promptly and maintained for as long as necessary. In the conscious patient, vomiting should be induced even though it may have occurred spontaneously. If vomiting cannot be induced, gastric lavage is indicated. Adequate precautions must be taken to protect against aspiration, especially in infants and children. Charcoal slurry or other suitable agent should be instilled into the stomach after vomiting or lavage. Saline cathartics or milk of magnesia may be of additional benefit.
In the unconscious patient, the airway should be secured with a cuffed endotracheal tube before attempting to evacuate the gastric contents. Intensive supportive and nursing care is indicated, as for any comatose patient.
If breathing is significantly impaired, maintenance of an adequate airway and mechanical support of respiration is the safest and most effective means of providing for adequate oxygenation of tissues to prevent hypoxia (especially brain hypoxia during convulsions).
Hypotension is an early sign of impending cardiovascular collapse and should be treated vigorously. Although general supportive measures are important, specific treatment with intravenous infusion of a vasopressor (e.g., levarterenol bitartrate) titrated to maintain adequate blood pressure is also necessary.

Continued on next page

The full prescribing information for each GEIGY drug is contained herein and is that in effect as of October 1, 1984.

Geigy—Cont.

Do *not* use CNS stimulants.
Convulsions should be controlled by careful titration of a short-acting barbiturate, repeated as necessary.
Ice packs and cooling sponge baths can aid in reducing the fever commonly seen in children.
How Supplied: *PBZ-SR Tablets,* 100 mg (lavender), each containing 100 mg tripelennamine hydrochloride; bottles of 100.
Dispense in tight container (USP).

C78-44 (12/78)

Shown in Product Identification Section, page 411

PBZ® ℞
tripelennamine
Tablets   GY-CODE 95
Elixir   GY-CODE 6925

Listed in USP, a Medicare designated compendium.

Description: PBZ Tablets are available as the hydrochloride salt and PBZ Elixir as the citrate salt of 2-[benzyl[2-(dimethylamino) ethyl]-amino]-pyridine. Tripelennamine hydrochloride is an antihistamine occurring as a white, crystalline powder that slowly darkens on exposure to light and is freely soluble in water and alcohol.
Actions: Antihistamines are competitive antagonists of histamine, which also produce central nervous system effects (both stimulant and depressant) and peripheral anticholinergic, atropine-like effects (e.g., drying).
Indications: Perennial and seasonal allergic rhinitis; vasomotor rhinitis; allergic conjunctivitis due to inhalant allergens and foods; mild, uncomplicated allergic skin manifestations of urticaria and angioedema; amelioration of allergic reactions to blood or plasma; dermographism; anaphylactic reactions as adjunctive therapy to epinephrine and other standard measures after the acute manifestations have been controlled.
Contraindications: PBZ should not be used in premature infants, neonates, or nursing mothers; patients receiving MAO inhibitors; patients with narrow-angle glaucoma, stenosing peptic ulcer, symptomatic prostatic hypertrophy, bladder neck obstruction, pyloroduodenal obstruction, lower respiratory tract symptoms (including asthma), or hypersensitivity to tripelennamine or related compounds.
Warnings: Antihistamines often produce drowsiness and may reduce mental alertness in children and adults. Patients should be warned about engaging in activities requiring mental alertness (e.g., driving a car, operating machinery or hazardous appliances). In elderly patients, approximately 60 years or older, antihistamines are more likely to cause dizziness, sedation and hypotension.
Patients should be warned that the central nervous system effects of PBZ may be additive with those of alcohol and other CNS depressants (e.g., hypnotics, sedatives, tranquilizers, antianxiety agents).
Antihistamines may produce excitation, particularly in children.
Usage in Pregnancy
Although no tripelennamine-related teratogenic potential or other adverse effects on the fetus have been observed in limited animal reproduction studies, the safe use of this drug in pregnancy or during lactation has not been established. Therefore, the drug should not be used during pregnancy or lactation unless, in the judgment of the physician, the expected benefits outweigh the potential hazards.
Usage in Children
In infants and children particularly, antihistamines in overdosage may produce hallucinations, convulsions and/or death.
Precautions: PBZ, like other antihistamines, has atropine-like, anticholinergic activity and should be used with caution in patients with increased intraocular pressure, hyperthyroidism, cardiovascular disease, hypertension, or history of bronchial asthma.

Adverse Reactions: The most frequent adverse reactions to antihistamines are sedation or drowsiness; sleepiness; dryness of the mouth, nose, and throat; thickening of bronchial secretions; dizziness; disturbed coordination; epigastric distress. Other adverse reactions which may occur are: fatigue; chills; confusion; restlessness; excitation; hysteria; nervousness; irritability; insomnia; euphoria; anorexia; nausea; vomiting; diarrhea; constipation; hypotension; tightness in the chest; wheezing; blurred vision; diplopia; vertigo; tinnitus; convulsions; headache; palpitations; tachycardia; extrasystoles; nasal stuffiness; urinary frequency; difficult urination; urinary retention; leukopenia; hemolytic anemia; thrombocytopenia; agranulocytosis; aplastic anemia; allergic or hypersensitivity reactions, including drug rash, urticaria, anaphylactic shock, and photosensitivity.
Although the following may have been reported to occur in association with some antihistamines, they have not been known to result from the use of PBZ: excessive perspiration, tremor, paresthesias, acute labyrinthitis, neuritis and early menses.
Dosage and Administration: Dosage should be individualized.
Usual Adult Dose: 25 to 50 mg every four to six hours. As little as 25 mg may control symptoms, but as much as 600 mg daily may be given in divided doses, if necessary.
Children and Infants: 5 mg/kg/24 hours or 150 mg/m^2/24 hours divided into four to six doses. Do not exceed maximum total dose of 300 mg/24 hours.
Note: Recommended dosages are based on the hydrochloride salt; each ml of Elixir (tripelennamine citrate) is equivalent to 5 mg tripelennamine hydrochloride.
Overdosage
Signs and Symptoms
The greatest danger from acute overdosage with antihistamines is their central nervous system effects which produce depression and/or stimulation.
In children, stimulation predominates initially in a syndrome which may include excitement, hallucinations, ataxia, incoordination, athetosis, and convulsions followed by postictal depression. Dry mouth, fixed dilated pupils, flushing of the face, and fever are common and resemble the syndrome of atropine poisoning. In adults, CNS depression (i.e., drowsiness, coma) is more common. CNS stimulation is rare; fever and flushing are uncommon.
In both children and adults, there can be a terminal deepening of coma and cardiovascular collapse; death can occur, especially in infants and children.
Treatment
There is no specific therapy for acute overdosage with antihistamines. General symptomatic and supportive measures should be instituted promptly and maintained for as long as necessary.
In the conscious patient, vomiting should be induced even though it may have occurred spontaneously. If vomiting cannot be induced, gastric lavage is indicated. Adequate precautions must be taken to protect against aspiration, especially in infants and children. Charcoal slurry or other suitable agent should be instilled into the stomach after vomiting or lavage. Saline cathartics or milk of magnesia may be of additional benefit.
In the unconscious patient, the airway should be secured with a cuffed endotracheal tube before attempting to evacuate the gastric contents. Intensive supportive and nursing care is indicated, as for any comatose patient.
If breathing is significantly impaired, maintenance of an adequate airway and mechanical support of respiration is the safest and most effective means of providing for adequate oxygenation of tissues to prevent hypoxia (especially brain hypoxia during convulsions).
Hypotension is an early sign of impending cardiovascular collapse and should be treated vigorously. Although general supportive measures are important, specific treatment with intravenous infusion of a vasopressor (e.g., levarterenol bitartrate) titrated to maintain adequate blood pressure may be necessary.

Do *not* use CNS stimulants.
Convulsions should be controlled by careful titration of a short-acting barbiturate, repeated as necessary.
Ice packs and cooling sponge baths can aid in reducing the fever commonly seen in children.
How Supplied:
Tablets 25 mg—round, white, scored (imprinted Geigy 111)
Bottles of 100 .... NDC 0028-0111-01
Tablets 50 mg—round, light blue, scored (imprinted Geigy 43)
Bottles of 100 .... NDC 0028-0043-01
Bottles of 1000 .... NDC 0028-0043-10
Elixir—green, cinnamon-flavored—37.5 mg tripelennamine citrate USP (equivalent to 25 mg tripelennamine hydrochloride) per 5 ml
Bottles of 473 ml .... NDC 0028-6925-16
Dispense in tight, light-resistant container.

C84-14 (Rev. 2/84)

Shown in Product Identification Section, page 411

PBZ® hydrochloride
tripelennamine hydrochloride
Cream   GY-CODE 6946
Antihistamine

Indications: For the temporary relief of itching due to minor skin disorders, ivy and oak poisoning, hives, sunburn, insect bites (non-poisonous), and stings.
Directions: Apply gently to the affected area 3 or 4 times daily or according to physician's directions.
Caution: If the condition persists or irritation develops, discontinue use and consult physician. Do not use in eyes.
KEEP OUT OF REACH OF CHILDREN.
How Supplied:
Cream, 2% tripelennamine hydrochloride in a water-washable base; tubes of 1 ounce.

(1/80)

TANDEARIL® ℞
[*tan-deer' ill*]
oxyphenbutazone USP
A Potent Anti-Inflammatory Agent
Tablets of 100 mg   GY-CODE 85

Important Note: Tandearil cannot be considered a simple analgesic and should never be administered casually. Each patient should be carefully evaluated before treatment is started and should remain constantly under the close supervision of the physician. The following cautions should be observed:

1. Therapy should not be initiated until a careful detailed history and complete physical and laboratory examination, including a complete hemogram and urinalysis, etc., of the patient have been made. These examinations should be made at regular, frequent intervals throughout the duration of this drug therapy.
2. Patients should be carefully selected, avoiding those in whom it is contraindicated as well as those who will respond to ordinary therapeutic measures, or those who cannot be observed at frequent intervals.
3. Patients taking this drug should be warned not to exceed the recommended dosage, since this may lead to toxic effects, and should discontinue the drug and report to the physician immediately any sign of:
    a. Fever, sore throat, lesions in the mouth (symptoms of blood dyscrasia).
    b. Dyspepsia, epigastric pain, symptoms of anemia, unusual bleeding, unusual bruising, black or tarry stools or other evidence of intestinal ulceration.
    c. Skin rashes.
    d. Significant weight gain or edema.
4. A trial period of one week of therapy is considered adequate to determine the therapeutic effect of the drug. In the absence of a favorable response, therapy should be discontinued.
    a. In the elderly (sixty years and over) the drug should be restricted to short-term

treatment periods only—if possible, *one week* maximum.
5. **Before prescribing Tandearil for an individual patient, read thoroughly the information contained under each heading which follows:**

Description: Tandearil should not be considered as a simple analgesic that can be prescribed for indiscriminate use. Tandearil is closely related chemically and pharmacologically, including toxic effects, to the well-known pyrazolines (pyrazole compounds) amidopyrine and antipyrine.

Chemically, Tandearil is 4-Butyl-1-(p-hydroxyphenyl) 2-phenyl-3,5-pyrazolidinedione monohydrate, the parahydroxy analog of Butazolidin®, brand of phenylbutazone USP.

It has anti-inflammatory and antipyretic action as well as analgesic and mild uricosuric properties resulting in symptomatic relief only. **The disease process itself is unaltered by this drug.**

Clinical Pharmacology: In man, oxyphenbutazone is completely absorbed after oral administration of Tandearil. After ingestion of three 100-mg tablets, peak plasma concentration of oxyphenbutazone has been measured at 34.9 ($\pm$ 5.3) mg/l within six hours. After therapeutic doses, about 98 percent of the drug is bound to human serum albumin. Elimination is mainly by biotransformation in the liver, and the plasma half-life has been measured as 72 ($\pm$ 15 hours). Urinary excretion consists mostly of metabolites.

Indications: The indications for Tandearil are:
Acute Gouty Arthritis
Active Rheumatoid Arthritis
Active Ankylosing Spondylitis
Short-term treatment of acute attacks of degenerative joint disease of the hips and knees not responsive to other treatment.
Painful Shoulder (peritendinitis, capsulitis, bursitis, and acute arthritis of that joint)

Contraindications:
1. *Age:* Tandearil is contraindicated in children 14 years of age or younger since controlled clinical trials in patients of this age group have not been conducted.
2. *Other Medical Conditions:* Tandearil is contraindicated in patients with incipient cardiac failure, blood dyscrasias, pancreatitis, parotitis, stomatitis, polymyalgia rheumatica, temporal arteritis, senility, drug allergy, and in the presence of severe renal, cardiac and hepatic disease, and in patients with a history of peptic ulcer disease, or symptoms of gastrointestinal inflammation or active ulceration because serious adverse reactions or aggravation of existing medical problems can occur.
3. *Concomitant Medications:* Tandearil should not be used in combination with other drugs which accentuate or share a potential for similar toxicity.
It is also inadvisable to administer Tandearil in combination with other potent drugs because of the possibility of increased toxic reactions from Tandearil and other agents. (See also *Drug/Drug Interactions.*)
Tandearil is contraindicated in patients with a history or suggestion of prior toxicity, sensitivity, or idiosyncrasy to phenylbutazone or oxyphenbutazone.

Warnings: Based on reports of clinical experience with oxyphenbutazone and related compounds, the following warnings should be considered by the physician prior to prescribing the drug:
1. *Gastrointestinal:* Upper G.I. diagnostic tests should be performed in patients with persistent or severe dyspepsia. Peptic ulceration, reactivation of latent peptic ulcer, perforation and gastrointestinal bleeding, sometimes severe, have been reported.
As with other nonsteroidal anti-inflammatory drugs, borderline elevations of values measured by one or more liver tests may occur in up to 15% of patients. These abnormalities may progress, may remain essentially unchanged, or may be transient with continued therapy. The SGPT (ALT) test is probably the most sensitive indicator of liver dysfunction. Meaningful elevations (three times the upper limit of normal) of SGPT or SGOT (AST) have occurred in controlled clinical trials in less than 1% of patients. A patient with symptoms and/or signs suggesting liver dysfunction, or in whom an abnormal liver test has occurred, should be evaluated for evidence of the development of more severe hepatic reactions while on therapy with Tandearil. Severe hepatic reactions, including jaundice and cases of fatal hepatitis, have been reported with Tandearil as with other nonsteroidal anti-inflammatory drugs. Although such reactions are rare, if abnormal liver tests persist or worsen, if clinical signs and symptoms consistent with liver disease develop, or if systemic manifestations (e.g., eosinophilia, rash, etc.) occur, therapy with Tandearil should be discontinued.

2. *Hematologic:* Frequent and regular hematologic evaluations should be performed on patients receiving the drug for periods over one week. Any significant change in the total white count, relative decrease in granulocytes, appearance of immature forms, or fall in hematocrit should be a signal for immediate cessation of therapy and a complete hematologic investigation. Serious, sometimes fatal blood dyscrasias, including aplastic anemia have been reported to occur. Hematologic toxicity may occur suddenly or many days or weeks after cessation of treatment as manifest by the appearance of anemia, leukopenia, thrombocytopenia or clinically significant hemorrhagic diathesis. There have been published reports associating oxyphenbutazone with leukemia. However, the circumstances involved in these reports are such that a cause-and-effect relationship to the drug has not been clearly established.

3. *Pregnancy:* Reproductive studies in animals, although inconclusive, exhibited evidence of possible embryotoxicity. It is, therefore, recommended that this drug should be used with caution during pregnancy. The benefits should be weighed against the potential risk to the fetus.

4. *Nursing Mothers:* Caution is also advised in prescribing Tandearil in nursing mothers since the drug may appear in cord blood and breast milk.

5. Patients reporting visual disturbances while receiving the drug should discontinue treatment and have an ophthalmologic examination because ophthalmologic adverse reactions have been reported (see **Adverse Reactions:** *Special Senses*).

6. In the aging (forty years and over), there appears to be an increase in the possibility of adverse reactions. Tandearil should be used with commensurately greater care in the elderly and should be avoided altogether in the senile patient.

7. Like other drugs with prostaglandin synthetase inhibition activity, Tandearil may precipitate acute episodes of asthmatic attacks in patients with asthma.

8. Tandearil increases sodium retention. Evidence of fluid retention in patients in whom there is danger of cardiac decompensation is an indication to discontinue the drug.

Precautions: Because of potential serious adverse reactions to Tandearil, the following precautions should be observed in the use of the drug:
—A careful diagnostic physical examination and history should be performed on all patients at regular intervals while the patient is receiving the drug.
—Tandearil is not recommended for chronic use in the elderly.
—Hematologic evaluation should be performed at frequent and regular intervals and additional laboratory examinations performed as indicated.
—Patients should be instructed to report immediately the occurrence of high fever, severe sore throat, stomatitis, salivary gland enlargement, tarry stools, unusual bleeding or bruising, sudden weight gain, or edema.
—The drug reduces iodine uptake by the thyroid and may interfere with laboratory tests of thyroid function (see **Adverse Reactions:** *Endocrine-Metabolic*).
—The patient should be cautioned regarding participation in activities requiring alertness and coordination, and that the concomitant ingestion of alcohol with Tandearil may further impair psychomotor skills.

Drug/Drug Interactions: Tandearil competitively displaces other drugs, e.g., other anti-inflammatory agents, oral anticoagulants, oral antidiabetics, sulfonamides, sodium valproate, and phenytoin, from serum-binding sites. The activity, duration of effect, and toxicity of the displaced drugs may be thus increased.

Tandearil accentuates the prothrombin depression produced by the coumarin-type anti-coagulants. When administered alone, Tandearil does not affect prothrombin activity.

Tandearil may induce the hepatic microsomal metabolism of dicoumarol, amidopyrine, digitoxin, hexobarbital, and cortisone. Conversely, it may inhibit the metabolism of phenytoin.

Concomitant administration of oxyphenbutazone and phenytoin may result in increased serum levels of phenytoin which could lead to increased phenytoin toxicity.

Inducers of hepatic microsomal enzymes, e.g., barbiturates, promethazine, chlorpheniramine, rifampin, and corticosteroids (prednisone), may decrease the half-life of Tandearil.

The effects of methotrexate, insulin, antidiabetic and sulfonamide drugs may be potentiated by Tandearil. Tandearil increases the serum concentration of lithium by increasing tubular reabsorption, and it reduces the renal clearance of sulfonylureas.

Methylphenidate is reported to increase the serum level of Tandearil.

Cholestyramine reduces the enteral absorption of Tandearil. See CONTRAINDICATIONS.

Adverse Reactions: Based upon reports of clinical experience with oxyphenbutazone and related compounds, the following adverse reactions have been reported.

The adverse reactions listed in the following table have been arranged into three groups: (1) incidence greater than 1%, (2) incidence less than 1% and (3) causal relationship unknown. The incidence for group (1) was obtained from fifty-seven (57) clinical trials reported in the literature (3713 patients). The incidence for group (2) was based on reports in clinical trials, in the literature, and on voluntary reports since marketing. The reactions in group (3) have been reported but occurred under circumstances where a causal relationship could not be established. In some patients the reported reactions may have been unrelated to the administration of Tandearil. However, in these reported events, the possibility cannot be excluded. Therefore these observations are being listed to serve as alerting information to physicians. Before prescribing this drug for an individual patient, the physician should be familiar with the following:

(1) Incidence greater than 1%	(2) Incidence less than 1%
GASTROINTESTINAL (See **Warnings**)	
gastrointestinal upset	nausea dyspepsia/including indigestion and heartburn abdominal and epigastric distress vomiting abdominal distention with flatulence

Continued on next page

The full prescribing information for each GEIGY drug is contained herein and is that in effect as of October 1, 1984.

Geigy—Cont.

	constipation
	diarrhea
	esophagitis
	gastritis
	salivary gland enlargement
	stomatitis, sometimes with ulceration
	ulceration and perforation of the intestinal tract including acute and reactivated peptic ulcer with perforation, hemorrhage and hematemesis
	anemia due to gastrointestinal bleeding which may be occult
	hepatitis, both fatal and nonfatal, sometimes associated with evidence of cholestasis
HEMATOLOGICAL (See **Warnings**)	
None	anemia
	leukopenia
	thrombocytopenia with associated purpura, petechiae, and hemorrhage
	pancytopenia
	aplastic anemia
	bone marrow depression
	agranulocytosis and agranulocytic anginal syndrome
	hemolytic anemia
HYPERSENSITIVITY	
None	urticaria
	anaphylactic shock
	arthralgia, drug fever
	hypersensitivity angiitis (polyarteritis) and vasculitis
	Lyell's syndrome
	serum sickness
	Stevens-Johnson syndrome
	activation of systemic lupus erythematosus
	aggravation of temporal arteritis in patients with polymyalgia rheumatica
DERMATOLOGIC	
None	pruritus
	drug rashes
	erythema nodosum
	erythema multiforme
	nonthrombocytopenic purpura
CARDIOVASCULAR, FLUID AND ELECTROLYTE	
None	sodium and chloride retention
	fluid retention and plasma dilution
	cardiac decompensation (congestive heart failure) with edema and dyspnea
	metabolic acidosis
	respiratory alkalosis
	hypertension
	pericarditis
	interstitial myocarditis with muscle necrosis and perivascular granulomata
RENAL	
None	hematuria
	proteinuria
	ureteral obstruction with uric acid crystals
	anuria
	glomerulonephritis
	acute tubular necrosis
	cortical necrosis
	renal stones
	nephrotic syndrome
	impaired renal function and renal failure associated with azotemia
	acute allergic and chronic interstitial nephritis
CENTRAL NERVOUS SYSTEM	
None	headache
	drowsiness
	agitation
	confusional states and lethargy
	tremors
	numbness
	weakness
ENDOCRINE-METABOLIC (See **Precautions**)	
None	None
SPECIAL SENSES (See **Warnings**)	
Ocular: None	None
Otic: None	hearing loss
	tinnitus

(3) **Causal relationship unknown—Incidence less than 1%:** *Hematological* (see **Warnings**)— Leukemia (There have been reports associating oxyphenbutazone with leukemia. However, the circumstances involved in these reports are such that a cause-and-effect relationship to the drug has not been clearly established) *Endocrine—Metabolic* (see **Precautions**)— Thyroid hyperplasia; goiters associated with hyperthyroidism and hypothyroidism; pancreatitis; hyperglycemia. *Special Senses* (see **Warnings**)— Blurred vision; optic neuritis; toxic amblyopia; scotomata; retinal detachment; retinal hemorrhage; oculomotor palsy.

Overdosage: *Signs and Symptoms:* Include any of the following: nausea, vomiting, epigastric pain, excessive perspiration, euphoria, psychosis, headaches, giddiness, vertigo, hyperventilation, insomnia, tinnitus, difficulty in hearing, edema (sodium retention), hypertension, cyanosis, respiratory depression, agitation, hallucinations, stupor, convulsions, coma, hematuria, and oliguria. Hepatomegaly, jaundice, and ulceration of the buccal or gastrointestinal mucosa have been reported as late manifestations of massive overdosage.

Reported laboratory abnormalities following overdosage include: respiratory or metabolic acidosis, impaired hepatic or renal function, and abnormalities of formed blood elements.

Treatment: In the alert patient, empty the stomach promptly by induced emesis followed by lavage. In the obtunded patient, secure the airway with a cuffed endotracheal tube before beginning lavage (do not induce emesis). Maintain adequate respiratory exchange, do not use respiratory stimulants. Treat shock with appropriate supportive measures. Control seizures with intravenous diazepam or short-acting barbiturates. Dialysis may be helpful if renal function is impaired.

Dosage and Administration: Tandearil should be used at the smallest effective dosage to afford rapid relief of severe symptoms. It is contraindicated in children under 14 years of age and in senile patients.

If a favorable symptomatic response to treatment is not obtained after one week, the drug should be discontinued. When a favorable therapeutic response has been obtained, the dosage should be reduced and then discontinued as soon as possible.

In elderly patients (sixty years and over) every effort must be made to discontinue therapy on, or as soon as possible after, the seventh day, because of the exceedingly high risk of severe fatal toxic reactions in this age group.

To minimize gastric upset, the drug should be taken with milk or with meals.

In selecting the appropriate dosage in any specific case, consideration should be given to the patient's age, weight, general health, and any other factors that may influence his response to the drug.

Rheumatoid Arthritis, Ankylosing Spondylitis, Acute Attacks of Degenerative Joint Disease, and Painful Shoulder: Initial Dosage: The initial daily dose in adult patients is 300 to 600 mg as 3 to 4 divided doses. Maximum therapeutic response is usually obtained at a total daily dose of 400 mg. A trial period of one week of therapy is considered adequate to determine the therapeutic effect of the drug. In the absence of a favorable response, therapy should be discontinued.

Maintenance Dosage: When improvement is obtained, dosage should be promptly decreased to the minimum effective level necessary to maintain relief, not exceeding 400 mg daily because of the possibility of cumulative toxicity. A satisfactory clinical response may be obtained with daily doses as low as 100 to 200 mg daily.

Acute Gouty Arthritis: Satisfactory results are obtained after an initial dose of 400 mg followed by 100 mg every 4 hours. The articular inflammation usually subsides within 4 days and treatment should not be continued longer than one week.

How Supplied:
Tablets 100 mg—round, biconvex, light brown to beige, film coated (imprinted Geigy 85)
Bottle of 100 ....NDC 0028-0085-01
Bottle of 1000 ....NDC 0028-0085-10
Unit Dose—(blister-pack)
Box of 100 (strips of 10)............NDC 0028-0085-61
Dispense in tight container (USP).

C84-17 (Rev. 4/84)
Shown in Product Identification Section, page 411

TEGRETOL® ℞
[teg′ rit-tall]
carbamazepine USP
Chewable Tablets of 100 mg—red-speckled,
pink   GY-CODE 47
Tablets of 200 mg—white   GY-CODE 67

> **WARNING**
> SERIOUS AND SOMETIMES FATAL ABNORMALITIES OF BLOOD CELLS (APLASTIC ANEMIA, AGRANULOCYTOSIS, THROMBOCYTOPENIA, AND LEUKOPENIA) HAVE BEEN REPORTED FOLLOWING TREATMENT WITH TEGRETOL, CARBAMAZEPINE. EARLY DETECTION OF HEMATOLOGIC CHANGE IS IMPORTANT SINCE, IN SOME PATIENTS, APLASTIC ANEMIA IS REVERSIBLE.
> COMPLETE PRETREATMENT BLOOD COUNTS, INCLUDING PLATELET AND POSSIBLY RETICULOCYTE AND SERUM IRON, SHOULD BE OBTAINED. ANY SIGNIFICANT ABNORMALITIES SHOULD RULE OUT USE OF THE DRUG. THESE SAME TESTS SHOULD BE REPEATED AT FREQUENT INTERVALS, POSSIBLY WEEKLY DURING THE FIRST THREE MONTHS OF THERAPY AND MONTHLY THEREAFTER FOR AT LEAST TWO TO THREE YEARS. THE DRUG SHOULD BE STOPPED IF ANY EVIDENCE OF BONE MARROW DEPRESSION DEVELOPS.
> PATIENTS SHOULD BE MADE AWARE OF THE EARLY TOXIC SIGNS AND SYMPTOMS OF A POTENTIAL HEMATOLOGIC PROBLEM, SUCH AS FEVER, SORE THROAT, ULCERS IN THE MOUTH, EASY BRUISING, PETECHIAL OR PURPURIC HEMORRHAGE, AND SHOULD BE ADVISED TO DISCONTINUE THE DRUG AND TO REPORT TO THE PHYSICIAN IMMEDI-

ATELY IF ANY SUCH SIGNS OR SYMPTOMS APPEAR.

This drug is not a simple analgesic and should not be used for the relief of trivial aches or pains. Treatment of epilepsy should be restricted to those classifications listed under "INDICATIONS AND USAGE."

Before prescribing Tegretol, the physician should be thoroughly familiar with the details of this prescribing information, particularly regarding use with other drugs, especially those which accentuate toxicity potential.

Description: Tegretol, carbamazepine USP, is an anticonvulsant and specific analgesic for trigeminal neuralgia, available as chewable tablets of 100 mg and tablets of 200 mg for oral administration. Its chemical name is 5H-dibenz[b,f]azepine-5-carboxamide.

Carbamazepine USP is a white to off-white powder, practically insoluble in water and soluble in alcohol and in acetone.

Clinical Pharmacology: In controlled clinical trials, Tegretol has been shown to be effective in the treatment of psychomotor and grand mal seizures, as well as trigeminal neuralgia.

It has demonstrated anticonvulsant properties in rats and mice with electrically and chemically induced seizures. It appears to act by reducing polysynaptic response and blocking the posttetanic potentiation. Tegretol greatly reduces or abolishes pain induced by stimulation of the infraorbital nerve in cats and rats. It depresses thalamic potential and bulbar and polysynaptic reflexes, including the linguomandibular reflex in cats. Tegretol is chemically unrelated to other anticonvulsants or other drugs used to control the pain of trigeminal neuralgia. The mechanism of action remains unknown.

Tegretol tablets are adequately absorbed after oral administration at a slower rate than a solution, thus avoiding undesirably high peak concentrations. Tegretol in blood is 76% bound to plasma proteins. Plasma levels of Tegretol are variable and may range from 0.5-25 µg/ml, with no apparent relationship to the daily intake of the drug. Usual adult therapeutic levels are between 4 and 12 µg/ml. Following oral administration, serum levels peak at 4 to 5 hours. The CSF/serum ratio is 0.22, similar to the 22% unbound Tegretol in serum. Because Tegretol may induce its own metabolism, the half-life is also variable. Initial half-life values range from 25-65 hours, with 12-17 hours on repeated doses. Tegretol is metabolized in the liver. After oral administration of ^{14}C-carbamazepine, 72% of the administered radioactivity was found in the urine and 28% in the feces. This urinary radioactivity was composed largely of hydroxylated and conjugated metabolites, with only 3% of unchanged Tegretol. Transplacental passage of Tegretol is rapid (30 to 60 minutes), and the drug is accumulated in fetal tissues, with higher levels found in liver and kidney than in brain and lungs.

Indications and Usage:

Epilepsy: Tegretol is indicated for the following conditions in patients who have not responded satisfactorily to treatment with other agents such as phenytoin, phenobarbital, or primidone:
1. Partial seizures with complex symptomatology (psychomotor, temporal lobe). Patients with these seizures appear to show greater improvement than those with other types.
2. Generalized tonic-clonic seizures (grand mal).
3. Mixed seizure patterns which include the above, or other partial or generalized seizures. Absence seizures (petit mal) do not appear to be controlled by Tegretol.

Because of the necessity for frequent laboratory evaluation for potentially serious side effects, Tegretol is not recommended as the drug of first choice in seizure disorders. It should be reserved for patients whose seizures are difficult to control or patients experiencing marked side effects (e.g., excessive sedation).

Trigeminal Neuralgia: Tegretol is indicated in the treatment of the pain associated with true trigeminal neuralgia.

Beneficial results have also been reported in glossopharyngeal neuralgia.

Contraindications: Tegretol should not be used in patients with a history of previous bone marrow depression, hypersensitivity to the drug, or known sensitivity to any of the tricyclic compounds, such as amitriptyline, desipramine, imipramine, protriptyline, nortriptyline, etc. Likewise, on theoretical grounds its use with monoamine oxidase inhibitors is not recommended. Before administration of Tegretol, MAO inhibitors should be discontinued for a minimum of fourteen days, or longer if the clinical situation permits.

Warnings: The drug should be discontinued if evidence of significant bone marrow depression occurs, as follows:

1) Erythrocytes   less than 4,000,000/cu mm
   Hematocrit   less than 32%
   Hemoglobin   less than 11 gm/100 ml
2) Leukocytes   less than 4000/cu mm
3) Platelets   less than 100,000/cu mm
4) Reticulocytes less than 0.3% (20,000/cu mm)
5) Serum iron greater than 150 µg/100 ml

Patients with a history of adverse hematologic reaction to any drug may be particularly at risk. Tegretol has shown mild anticholinergic activity; therefore, patients with increased intraocular pressure should be closely observed during therapy.

Because of the relationship of the drug to other tricyclic compounds, the possibility of activation of a latent psychosis and, in elderly patients, of confusion or agitation should be borne in mind.

Precautions:

General: Before initiating therapy, a detailed history and physical examination should be made. Therapy should be prescribed only after critical benefit-to-risk appraisal in patients with a history of cardiac, hepatic or renal damage, adverse hematologic reaction to other drugs, or interrupted courses of therapy with Tegretol.

Information for Patients: Since dizziness and drowsiness may occur, patients should be cautioned about the hazards of operating machinery or automobiles or engaging in other potentially dangerous tasks.

Laboratory Tests: Complete pretreatment blood counts, including platelets and possibly reticulocytes and serum iron, should be obtained. Any significant abnormalities should rule out use of the drug. These same tests should be repeated at frequent intervals, possibly weekly, during the first three months of therapy and monthly thereafter for at least two to three years.

Baseline and periodic evaluations of liver function, particularly in patients with a history of liver disease, must be performed during treatment with this drug since liver damage may occur. The drug should be discontinued immediately in cases of aggravated liver dysfunction or active liver disease.

Baseline and periodic eye examinations, including slit-lamp, funduscopy and tonometry, are recommended since many phenothiazines and related drugs have been shown to cause eye changes.

Baseline and periodic complete urinalysis and BUN determinations are recommended for patients treated with this agent because of observed renal dysfunction.

Monitoring of blood levels (see **CLINICAL PHARMACOLOGY**) has increased the efficacy and safety of anticonvulsants. This monitoring may be particularly useful in cases of dramatic increase in seizure frequency and for verification of compliance. In addition, measurement of drug serum levels may aid in determining the cause of toxicity when more than one medication is being used.

Thyroid function tests have been reported to show decreased values with Tegretol administered alone.

Drug Interactions: The simultaneous administration of phenobarbital, phenytoin, or primidone, or a combination of two, produces a marked lowering of serum levels of Tegretol. The half-lives of phenytoin, warfarin, doxycycline were significantly shortened when administered concurrently with Tegretol. The doses of these drugs may therefore have to be increased when Tegretol is added to the therapeutic regime.

Concomitant administration of Tegretol and erythromycin has been reported to result in elevated plasma levels of carbamazepine resulting in toxicity in some cases.

Alterations of thyroid function have been reported in combination therapy with other anticonvulsant medications.

Breakthrough bleeding has been reported among patients receiving concomitant oral contraceptives and their reliability may be adversely affected.

Carcinogenicity, Mutagenesis, Impairment of Fertility: Carbamazepine, when administered to Sprague-Dawley rats for two years in the diet at doses of 25, 75, and 250 mg/kg/day, resulted in a dose-related increase in the incidence of hepatocellular tumors in females and of benign interstitial cell adenomas in the testes of males.

Carbamazepine must, therefore, be considered to be carcinogenic in Sprague-Dawley rats. Bacterial and mammalian mutagenicity studies using carbamazepine produced negative results. The significance of these findings relative to the use of carbamazepine in humans is, at present, unknown.

Pregnancy Category C: Tegretol has been shown to have adverse effect in reproduction studies in rats when given orally in dosages 10–25 times the maximum human daily dosage of 1200 mg. In rat teratology studies, 2 of 135 offspring showed kinked ribs at 250 mg/kg and 4 of 119 offspring at 650 mg/kg showed other anomalies (cleft palate, 1; talipes, 1; anophthalmos, 2). In reproduction studies in rats, nursing offspring demonstrated a lack of weight gain and an unkempt appearance at a maternal dosage level of 200 mg/kg.

There are no adequate and well-controlled studies in pregnant women. Tegretol should be used during pregnancy only if the potential benefit justifies the potential risk to the fetus. It is important to note that anticonvulsant drugs should not be discontinued in patients in whom the drug is administered to prevent major seizures because of the strong possibility of precipitating status epilepticus with attendant hypoxia and threat to life. In individual cases where the severity and frequency of the seizure disorder are such that removal of medication does not pose a serious threat to the patient, discontinuation of the drug may be considered prior to and during pregnancy, although it cannot be said with any confidence that even minor seizures do not pose some hazard to the developing embryo or fetus.

Labor and Delivery: The effect of Tegretol on human labor and delivery is unknown.

Nursing Mothers: During lactation, concentration of Tegretol in milk is approximately 60% of the maternal plasma concentration.

Because of the potential for serious adverse reactions in nursing infants from carbamazepine, a decision should be made whether to discontinue nursing or to discontinue the drug, taking into account the importance of the drug to the mother.

Pediatric Use: Safety and effectiveness in children below the age of 6 years have not been established.

Adverse Reactions: If adverse reactions are of such severity that the drug must be discontinued, the physician must be aware that abrupt discontinuation of any anticonvulsant drug in a responsive epileptic patient may lead to seizures or even status epilepticus with its life-threatening hazards.

Continued on next page

The full prescribing information for each GEIGY drug is contained herein and is that in effect as of October 1, 1984.

Geigy—Cont.

The most severe adverse reactions have been observed in the hemopoietic system (see boxed WARNING), the skin and the cardiovascular system.

The most frequently observed adverse reactions, particularly during the initial phases of therapy, are dizziness, drowsiness, unsteadiness, nausea, and vomiting. To minimize the possibility of such reactions, therapy should be initiated at the low dosage recommended.

The following additional adverse reactions have been reported:

Hemopoietic System: Aplastic anemia, agranulocytosis, thrombocytopenia, leukopenia, leukocytosis, eosinophilia.

Skin: Pruritic and erythematous rashes, urticaria, Stevens-Johnson syndrome, photosensitivity reactions, alterations in skin pigmentation, exfoliative dermatitis, erythema multiforme and nodosum, purpura, aggravation of disseminated lupus erythematosus, alopecia, and diaphoresis. In certain cases, discontinuation of therapy may be necessary.

Cardiovascular System: Congestive heart failure, edema, aggravation of hypertension, hypotension, syncope and collapse, aggravation of coronary artery disease, arrhythmias and A-V block, primary thrombophlebitis, recurrence of thrombophlebitis, and adenopathy or lymphadenopathy. Some of these cardiovascular complications have resulted in fatalities. Myocardial infarction has been associated with other tricyclic compounds.

Liver: Abnormalities in liver function tests, cholestatic and hepatocellular jaundice, hepatitis.

Respiratory System: Pulmonary hypersensitivity characterized by fever, dyspnea, pneumonitis or pneumonia.

Genitourinary System: Urinary frequency, acute urinary retention, oliguria with elevated blood pressure, azotemia, renal failure, and impotence. Albuminuria, glycosuria, elevated BUN and microscopic deposits in the urine have also been reported.

Testicular atrophy occurred in rats receiving Tegretol orally from 4 to 52 weeks at dosage levels of 50 to 400 mg/kg/day. Additionally, rats receiving Tegretol in the diet for two years at dosage levels of 25, 75, and 250 mg/kg/day had a dose-related incidence of testicular atrophy and aspermatogenesis. In dogs, it produced a brownish discoloration, presumably a metabolite, in the urinary bladder at dosage levels of 50 mg/kg and higher. Relevance of these findings to humans is unknown.

Nervous System: Dizziness, drowsiness, disturbances of coordination, confusion, headache, fatigue, blurred vision, visual hallucinations, transient diplopia, oculomotor disturbances, nystagmus, speech disturbances, abnormal involuntary movements, peripheral neuritis and paresthesias, depression with agitation, talkativeness, tinnitus, and hyperacusis.

There have been reports of associated paralysis and other symptoms of cerebral arterial insufficiency, but the exact relationship of these reactions to the drug has not been established.

Digestive System: Nausea, vomiting, gastric distress and abdominal pain, diarrhea, constipation, anorexia, and dryness of the mouth and pharynx, including glossitis and stomatitis.

Eyes: Scattered, punctate, cortical lens opacities, as well as conjunctivitis have been reported. Although a direct causal relationship has not been established, many phenothiazines and related drugs have been shown to cause eye changes.

Musculoskeletal System: Aching joints and muscles and leg cramps.

Metabolism: Fever and chills. Inappropriate antidiuretic hormone syndrome has been reported.

Drug Abuse and Dependence: No evidence of abuse potential has been associated with Tegretol, nor is there evidence of psychological or physical dependence in humans.

Overdosage:
Acute Toxicity
Lowest known lethal dose: adults, > 60 g (39-year-old man). Highest known doses survived: adults, 30 g (31-year-old woman); children, 10 g (6-year-old boy); small children, 5 g (3-year-old girl).
Oral LD_{50} in animals (mg/kg); mice, 1100-3750; rats, 3850-4025; rabbits, 1500-2680; guinea pigs, 920.

Signs and Symptoms
The first signs and symptoms appear after 1-3 hours. Neuromuscular disturbances are the most prominent. Cardiovascular disorders are generally milder, and severe cardiac complications occur only when very high doses (> 60 g) have been ingested.

Respiration: Irregular breathing, respiratory depression.

Cardiovascular System: Tachycardia, hypotension or hypertension, shock, conduction disorders.

Nervous System and Muscles: Impairment of consciousness ranging in severity to deep coma. Convulsions, especially in small children. Motor restlessness, muscular twitching, tremor, athetoid movements, opisthotonos, ataxia, drowsiness, dizziness, mydriasis, nystagmus, adiadochokinesia, ballism, psychomotor disturbances, dysmetria. Initial hyperreflexia, followed by hyporeflexia.

Gastrointestinal Tract: Nausea, vomiting.

Kidneys and Bladder: Anuria or oliguria, urinary retention.

Laboratory Findings: Isolated instances of overdosage have included leukocytosis, reduced leukocyte count, glycosuria and acetonuria. EEG may show dysrhythmias.

Combined Poisoning: When alcohol, tricyclic antidepressants, barbiturates or hydantoins are taken at the same time, the signs and symptoms of acute poisoning with Tegretol may be aggravated or modified.

Treatment
The prognosis in cases of severe poisoning is critically dependent upon prompt elimination of the drug, which may be achieved by inducing vomiting, irrigating the stomach, and by taking appropriate steps to diminish absorption. If these measures cannot be implemented without risk on the spot, the patient should be transferred at once to a hospital, while ensuring that vital functions are safeguarded. There is no specific antidote.

Elimination of the Drug: Induction of vomiting. Gastric lavage. Even when more than 4 hours have elapsed following ingestion of the drug, the stomach should be repeatedly irrigated, especially if the patient has also consumed alcohol.

Measures to Reduce Absorption: Activated charcoal, laxatives.

Measures to Accelerate Elimination: Forced diuresis.

Dialysis is indicated only in severe poisoning associated with renal failure. Replacement transfusion is indicated in severe poisoning in small children.

Respiratory Depression: Keep the airways free; resort, if necessary, to endotracheal intubation, artificial respiration, and administration of oxygen.

Hypotension, Shock: Keep the patient's legs raised and administer a plasma expander. If blood pressure fails to rise despite measures taken to increase plasma volume, use of vasoactive substances should be considered.

Convulsions: Diazepam or barbiturates.

Warning: Diazepam or barbiturates may aggravate respiratory depression (especially in children), hypotension, and coma. However, barbiturates should not be used if drugs that inhibit monoamine oxidase have also been taken by the patient either in overdosage or in recent therapy (within one week).

Surveillance: Respiration, cardiac function (ECG monitoring), blood pressure, body temperature, pupillary reflexes, and kidney and bladder function should be monitored for several days.

Treatment of Blood Count Abnormalities: If evidence of bone marrow depression develops, the following recommendations are suggested: 1) stop the drug, (2) perform daily CBC, platelet and reticulocyte counts, (3) do a bone marrow aspiration and trephine biopsy immediately and repeat with sufficient frequency to monitor recovery.

Special periodic studies might be helpful as follows: (1) white cell and platelet antibodies, (2) ^{59}Fe—ferrokinetic studies, (3) peripheral blood cell typing, (4) cytogenetic studies on marrow and peripheral blood, (5) bone marrow culture studies for colony-forming units, (6) hemoglobin electrophoresis for A_2 and F hemoglobin, and (7) serum folic acid and B_{12} levels.

A fully developed aplastic anemia will require appropriate, intensive monitoring and therapy, for which specialized consultation should be sought.

Dosage and Administration: Monitoring of blood levels has increased the efficacy and safety of anticonvulsants (see **PRECAUTIONS** Laboratory Tests). Dosage should be adjusted to the needs of the individual patient. A low initial daily dosage with a gradual increase is advised. As soon as adequate control is achieved, the dosage may be reduced very gradually to the minimum effective level. Tablets should be taken with meals.

Epilepsy (see INDICATIONS AND USAGE)

Adults and children over 12 years of age—Initial: 200 mg b.i.d. on the first day. Increase gradually by adding up to 200 mg per day using a t.i.d. or q.i.d. regimen until the best response is obtained. Dosage should generally not exceed 1000 mg daily in children 12 to 15 years of age, and 1200 mg daily in patients above 15 years of age. Doses up to 1600 mg daily have been used in adults in rare instances. *Maintenance:* Adjust dosage to the minimum effective level, usually 800-1200 mg daily.

Children 6-12 years of age—Initial: 100 mg b.i.d. on the first day. Increase gradually by adding 100 mg per day using a t.i.d. or q.i.d. regimen until the best response is obtained. Dosage should generally not exceed 1000 mg.

Maintenance: Adjust dosage to the minimum effective level, usually 400–800 mg daily.

Combination Therapy: Tegretol may be used alone or with other anticonvulsants. When added to existing anticonvulsant therapy, the drug should be added gradually while the other anticonvulsants are maintained or gradually decreased, except phenytoin, which may have to be increased. (see **PRECAUTIONS** Drug Interactions).

Trigeminal Neuralgia (see INDICATIONS AND USAGE)

Initial: 100 mg b.i.d. on the first day for a total daily dose of 200 mg. This daily dose may be increased by up to 200 mg a day using increments of 100 mg every 12 hours only as needed to achieve freedom from pain. Do not exceed 1200 mg daily.

Maintenance: Control of pain can be maintained in most patients with 400 mg to 800 mg daily. However, some patients may be maintained on as little as 200 mg daily, while others may require as much as 1200 mg daily. At least once every 3 months throughout the treatment period, attempts should be made to reduce the dose to the minimum effective level or even to discontinue the drug.

How Supplied:
Chewable Tablets 100 mg—round, red-speckled, pink, single-scored (imprinted Geigy 47)
Bottles of 100 .... NDC 0028-0047-01
Unit Dose (blister pack)
Box of 100
(strips of 10) .... NDC 0028-0047-61
Tablets 200 mg—round, white, single-scored (imprinted Geigy 67)
Bottles of 100 .... NDC 0028-0067-01
Bottles of 1000 .... NDC 0028-0067-10
Gy-Pak®—One Unit
12 bottles—100 tablets each ....
.... NDC 0028-0067-65
Unit Dose (blister pack)
Box of 100
(strips of 10) .... NDC 0028-0067-61
Protect from moisture.
Dispense in tight container (USP).

C82-48 (1/83)

Shown in Product Identification Section, page 411

TOFRANIL®
[toe-fray'nill]
imipramine hydrochloride USP
Tablets of 10 mg — GY-CODE 21
Tablets of 25 mg — GY-CODE 11
Tablets of 50 mg — GY-CODE 74
For oral administration
Ampuls, 2 cc
For intramuscular administration

Each 2 cc ampul contains: imipramine hydrochloride USP, 25 mg; ascorbic acid, 2 mg; sodium bisulfite, 1 mg; sodium sulfite, anhydrous, 1 mg

Description: Tofranil, the original tricyclic antidepressant, is a member of the dibenzazepine group of compounds. It is designated 5-[3-(Dimethylamino)propyl]-10, 11-dihydro-5H-dibenz[b,f] azepine Monohydrochloride. Its molecular weight is 316.9 and its empirical formula is $C_{19}H_{25}N_2Cl$. Tofranil is a white, crystalline substance that turns yellowish or reddish on long exposure to light. It is easily soluble in water, fairly soluble in acetone or alcohol, but almost insoluble in ether. It melts at 170–174° C.

Clinical Pharmacology: The mechanism of action of Tofranil is not definitely known. However, it does not act primarily by stimulation of the central nervous system. The clinical effect is hypothesized as being due to potentiation of adrenergic synapses by blocking uptake of norepinephrine at nerve endings. The mode of action of the drug in controlling childhood enuresis is thought to be apart from its antidepressant effect.

Indications: *Depression:* For the relief of symptoms of depression. Endogenous depression is more likely to be alleviated than other depressive states. One to three weeks of treatment may be needed before optimal therapeutic effects are evident.

Childhood Enuresis: May be useful as temporary adjunctive therapy in reducing enuresis in children aged 6 years and older, after possible organic causes have been excluded by appropriate tests. In patients having daytime symptoms of frequency and urgency, examination should include voiding cystourethrography and cystoscopy, as necessary. The effectiveness of treatment may decrease with continued drug administration.

Contraindications: The concomitant use of monoamine oxidase inhibiting compounds is contraindicated. Hyperpyretic crises or severe convulsive seizures may occur in patients receiving such combinations. The potentiation of adverse effects can be serious, or even fatal. When it is desired to substitute Tofranil in patients receiving a monoamine oxidase inhibitor, as long an interval should elapse as the clinical situation will allow, with a minimum of 14 days. Initial dosage should be low and increases should be gradual and cautiously prescribed.

The drug is contraindicated during the acute recovery period after a myocardial infarction. Patients with a known hypersensitivity to this compound should not be given the drug. The possibility of cross-sensitivity to other dibenzazepine compounds should be kept in mind.

Warnings:
Children: A dose of 2.5 mg/kg/day of imipramine hydrochloride should not be exceeded in childhood. ECG changes of unknown significance have been reported in pediatric patients with doses twice this amount.

Extreme caution should be used when this drug is given to:
- patients with cardiovascular disease because of the possibility of conduction defects, arrhythmias, congestive heart failure, myocardial infarction, strokes and tachycardia. These patients require cardiac surveillance at all dosage levels of the drug;
- patients with increased intraocular pressure, history of urinary retention, or history of narrow-angle glaucoma because of the drug's anticholinergic properties;
- hyperthyroid patients or those on thyroid medication because of the possibility of cardiovascular toxicity;
- patients with a history of seizure disorder because this drug has been shown to lower the seizure threshold;
- patients receiving guanethidine, clonidine, or similar agents, since imipramine hydrochloride may block the pharmacologic effects of these drugs;
- patients receiving methylphenidate hydrochloride. Since methylphenidate hydrochloride may inhibit the metabolism of imipramine hydrochloride, downward dosage adjustment of imipramine hydrochloride may be required when given concomitantly with methylphenidate hydrochloride.

Tofranil may enhance the CNS depressant effects of alcohol. Therefore, it should be borne in mind that the dangers inherent in a suicide attempt or accidental overdosage with the drug may be increased for the patient who uses excessive amounts of alcohol. (See **Precautions**.)

Since imipramine hydrochloride may impair the mental and/or physical abilities required for the performance of potentially hazardous tasks, such as operating an automobile or machinery, the patient should be cautioned accordingly.

Precautions: An ECG recording should be taken prior to the initiation of larger-than-usual doses of imipramine hydrochloride and at appropriate intervals thereafter until steady state is achieved. (Patients with any evidence of cardiovascular disease require cardiac surveillance at all dosage levels of the drug. See **Warnings**.) Elderly patients and patients with cardiac disease or a prior history of cardiac disease are at special risk of developing the cardiac abnormalities associated with the use of imipramine hydrochloride.

It should be kept in mind that the possibility of suicide in seriously depressed patients is inherent in the illness and may persist until significant remission occurs. Such patients should be carefully supervised during the early phase of treatment with imipramine hydrochloride, and may require hospitalization. Prescriptions should be written for the smallest amount feasible.

Hypomanic or manic episodes may occur, particularly in patients with cyclic disorders. Such reactions may necessitate discontinuation of the drug. If needed, imipramine hydrochloride may be resumed in lower dosage when these episodes are relieved. Administration of a tranquilizer may be useful in controlling such episodes.

An activation of the psychosis may occasionally be observed in schizophrenic patients and may require reduction of dosage and the addition of a phenothiazine.

Concurrent administration of imipramine hydrochloride with electroshock therapy may increase the hazards; such treatment should be limited to those patients for whom it is essential, since there is limited clinical experience.

Usage During Pregnancy and Lactation:
Animal reproduction studies have yielded inconclusive results. (See also **Animal Pharmacology & Toxicology**.)

There have been no well-controlled studies conducted with pregnant women to determine the effect of imipramine hydrochloride on the fetus. However, there have been clinical reports of congenital malformations associated with the use of the drug. Although a causal relationship between these effects and the drug could not be established, the possibility of fetal risk from the maternal ingestion of imipramine hydrochloride cannot be excluded. Therefore, imipramine hydrochloride should be used in women who are or might become pregnant only if the clinical condition clearly justifies potential risk to the fetus.

Limited data suggest that imipramine hydrochloride is likely to be excreted in human breast milk. As a general rule, a woman taking a drug should not nurse since the possibility exists that the drug may be excreted in breast milk and be harmful to the child.

Usage in Children: The effectiveness of the drug in children for conditions other than nocturnal enuresis has not been established.

The safety and effectiveness of the drug as temporary adjunctive therapy for nocturnal enuresis in children less than 6 years of age has not been established.

The safety of the drug for long-term, chronic use as adjunctive therapy for nocturnal enuresis in children 6 years of age or older has not been established; consideration should be given to instituting a drug-free period following an adequate therapeutic trial with a favorable response.

A dose of 2.5 mg/kg/day should not be exceeded in childhood. ECG changes of unknown significance have been reported in pediatric patients with doses twice this amount.

Patients should be warned that imipramine hydrochloride may enhance the CNS depressant effects of alcohol. (See **Warnings**.)

Imipramine hydrochloride should be used with caution in patients with significantly impaired renal or hepatic function.

Patients who develop a fever and a sore throat during therapy with imipramine hydrochloride should have leukocyte and differential blood counts performed. Imipramine hydrochloride should be discontinued if there is evidence of pathological neutrophil depression.

Prior to elective surgery, imipramine hydrochloride should be discontinued for as long as the clinical situation will allow.

In occasional susceptible patients or in those receiving anticholinergic drugs (including antiparkinsonism agents) in addition, the atropine-like effects may become more pronounced (e.g., paralytic ileus). Close supervision and careful adjustment of dosage is required when imipramine hydrochloride is administered concomitantly with anticholinergic drugs.

Avoid the use of preparations, such as decongestants and local anesthetics, which contain any sympathomimetic amine (e.g., epinephrine, norepinephrine), since it has been reported that tricyclic antidepressants can potentiate the effects of catecholamines.

Caution should be exercised when imipramine hydrochloride is used with agents that lower blood pressure.

Imipramine hydrochloride may potentiate the effects of CNS depressant drugs.

Patients taking imipramine hydrochloride should avoid excessive exposure to sunlight since there have been reports of photosensitization.

Both elevation and lowering of blood sugar levels have been reported with imipramine hydrochloride use.

The Tofranil tablets (10, 25, 50 mg) contain FD&C Yellow No. 5 (tartrazine) which may cause allergic-type reactions (including bronchial asthma) in certain susceptible individuals. Although the overall incidence of FD&C Yellow No. 5 (tartrazine) sensitivity in the general population is low, it is frequently seen in patients who also have aspirin hypersensitivity.

Adverse Reactions: Note: Although the listing which follows includes a few adverse reactions which have not been reported with this specific drug, the pharmacological similarities among the tricyclic antidepressant drugs require that each of the reactions be considered when imipramine is administered.

Cardiovascular: Orthostatic hypotension, hypertension, tachycardia, palpitation, myocardial infarction, arrhythmias, heart block, ECG changes, precipitation of congestive heart failure, stroke.

Psychiatric: Confusional states (especially in the elderly) with hallucinations, disorientation, delusions; anxiety, restlessness, agitation; insomnia and nightmares; hypomania; exacerbation of psychosis.

Continued on next page

The full prescribing information for each GEIGY drug is contained herein and is that in effect as of October 1, 1984.

Geigy—Cont.

Neurological: Numbness, tingling, paresthesias of extremities; incoordination, ataxia, tremors; peripheral neuropathy; extrapyramidal symptoms; seizures, alterations in EEG patterns; tinnitus.
Anticholinergic: Dry mouth, and, rarely, associated sublingual adenitis; blurred vision, disturbances of accommodation, mydriasis; constipation, paralytic ileus; urinary retention, delayed micturition, dilation of the urinary tract.
Allergic: Skin rash, petechiae, urticaria, itching, photosensitization; edema (general or of face and tongue); drug fever; cross-sensitivity with desipramine.
Hematologic: Bone marrow depression including agranulocytosis; eosinophilia; purpura; thrombocytopenia.
Gastrointestinal: Nausea and vomiting, anorexia, epigastric distress, diarrhea; peculiar taste, stomatitis, abdominal cramps, black tongue.
Endocrine: Gynecomastia in the male; breast enlargement and galactorrhea in the female; increased or decreased libido, impotence; testicular swelling; elevation or depression of blood sugar levels; inappropriate antidiuretic hormone (ADH) secretion syndrome.
Other: Jaundice (simulating obstructive); altered liver function; weight gain or loss; perspiration; flushing; urinary frequency; drowsiness; dizziness, weakness and fatigue; headache, parotid swelling; alopecia; proneness to falling.
Withdrawal Symptoms: Though not indicative of addiction, abrupt cessation of treatment after prolonged therapy may produce nausea, headache and malaise.
Note: In enuretic children treated with Tofranil the most common adverse reactions have been nervousness, sleep disorders, tiredness, and mild gastrointestinal disturbances. These usually disappear during continued drug administration or when dosage is decreased. Other reactions which have been reported include constipation, convulsions, anxiety, emotional instability, syncope, and collapse. All of the adverse effects reported with adult use should be considered.

Dosage and Administration:
Depression: Lower dosages are recommended for elderly patients and adolescents. Lower dosages are also recommended for outpatients as compared to hospitalized patients who will be under close supervision. Dosage should be initiated at a low level and increased gradually, noting carefully the clinical response and any evidence of intolerance. Following remission, maintenance medication may be required for a longer period of time, at the lowest dose that will maintain remission.
Parenteral administration should be used only for starting therapy in patients unable or unwilling to use oral medication. The oral form should supplant the injectable as soon as possible.
Oral:—Usual Adult Dose: Hospitalized patients— Initially, 100 mg/day in divided doses gradually increased to 200 mg/day as required. If no response after two weeks, increase to 250-300 mg/day.
*Outpatients—*Initially, 75 mg/day increased to 150 mg/day. Dosages over 200 mg/day are not recommended. Maintenance, 50-150 mg/day.
*Adolescent and geriatric patients—*Initially, 30–40 mg/day; it is generally not necessary to exceed 100 mg/day.
Parenteral: Initially, up to 100 mg/day intramuscularly in divided doses.
Childhood Enuresis: Initially, an oral dose of 25 mg/day should be tried in children aged 6 and older. Medication should be given one hour before bedtime. If a satisfactory response does not occur within one week, increase the dose to 50 mg nightly in children under 12 years; children over 12 may receive up to 75 mg nightly. A daily dose greater than 75 mg does not enhance efficacy and tends to increase side effects. Evidence suggests that in early night bedwetters, the drug is more effective given earlier and in divided amounts, i.e., 25 mg in midafternoon, repeated at bedtime. Consideration should be given to instituting a drug-free period following an adequate therapeutic trial with a favorable response. Dosage should be tapered off gradually rather than abruptly discontinued; this may reduce the tendency to relapse. Children who relapse when the drug is discontinued do not always respond to a subsequent course of treatment.
A dose of 2.5 mg/kg/day should not be exceeded. ECG changes of unknown significance have been reported in pediatric patients with doses twice this amount.
The safety and effectiveness of Tofranil as temporary adjunctive therapy for nocturnal enuresis in children less than 6 years of age has not been established.

Overdosage: Children have been reported to be more sensitive than adults to an acute overdosage of imipramine hydrochloride. An acute overdose of any amount in infants or young children, especially, must be considered serious and potentially fatal.
Signs and Symptoms: These may vary in severity depending upon factors such as the amount of drug absorbed, the age of the patient, and the interval between drug ingestion and the start of treatment. Blood and urine levels of imipramine may not reflect the severity of poisoning; they have chiefly a qualitative rather than quantitative value, and are unreliable indicators in the clinical management of the patient.
CNS abnormalities may include drowsiness, stupor, coma, ataxia, restlessness, agitation, hyperactive reflexes, muscle rigidity, athetoid and choreiform movements, and convulsions.
Cardiac abnormalities may include arrhythmia, tachycardia, ECG evidence of impaired conduction, and signs of congestive failure.
Respiratory depression, cyanosis, hypotension, shock, vomiting, hyperpyrexia, mydriasis, and diaphoresis may also be present.
Treatment: Because CNS involvement, respiratory depression and cardiac arrhythmia can occur suddenly, hospitalization and close observation are necessary, even when the amount ingested is thought to be small or the initial degree of intoxication appears slight or moderate. All patients with ECG abnormalities should have continuous cardiac monitoring for at least 72 hours and be closely observed until well after cardiac status has returned to normal; relapses may occur after apparent recovery.
The *slow* intravenous administration of physostigmine salicylate has been reported to reverse most of the cardiovascular and CNS effects of overdosage with tricyclic antidepressants. In adults, 1 to 3 mg has been reported to be effective. In children, start with 0.5 mg and repeat at 5-minute intervals to determine the minimum effective dose; do not exceed 2 mg. Because of the short duration of action of physostigmine, repeat the effective dose at 30- to 60-minute intervals, as necessary. Avoid rapid injection to reduce the possibility of physostigmine-induced convulsions.
In the alert patient, empty the stomach promptly by induced emesis followed by lavage. In the obtunded patient, secure the airway with a cuffed endotracheal tube before beginning lavage (do not induce emesis). Continue lavage for 24 hours or longer, depending on the apparent severity of intoxication. Use normal or half-normal saline to avoid water intoxication, especially in children. Instillation of activated charcoal slurry may help reduce absorption of imipramine.
Minimize external stimulation to reduce the tendency to convulsions. If anticonvulsants are necessary, diazepam, short-acting barbiturates, paraldehyde or methocarbamol may be useful. Do not use barbiturates if MAO inhibitors have been taken recently.
Maintain adequate respiratory exchange. Do not use respiratory stimulants.
Shock should be treated with supportive measures, such as intravenous fluids, oxygen and corticosteroids. Digitalis may increase conduction abnormalities and further irritate an already sensitized myocardium. If congestive heart failure necessitates rapid digitalization, particular care must be exercised.
Hyperpyrexia should be controlled by whatever external means are available, including ice packs and cooling sponge baths, if necessary.
Hemodialysis, peritoneal dialysis, exchange transfusions and forced diuresis have been generally reported as ineffective because of the rapid fixation of imipramine in tissues. Blood and urine levels of imipramine may not correlate with the degree of intoxication, and are unreliable indicators in the clinical management of the patient.

How Supplied
Tablets 10 mg — triangular, coral, coated (imprinted Geigy 21)
  Bottles of 100 ....NDC 0028-0021-01
  Bottles of 1000 ....NDC 0028-0021-10
Tablets 25 mg — round, coral, coated (imprinted Geigy 11)
  Bottles of 100 ....NDC 0028-0011-01
  Bottles of 1000 ....NDC 0028-0011-10
  Gy-Pak®—One Unit
    12 bottles - 100 tablets each
  ....NDC 0028-0011-65
  Unit Dose (blister pack)
    Box of 100 (strips of 10)
  ....NDC 0028-0011-61
Tablets 50 mg — round, coral, coated (imprinted Geigy 74)
  Bottles of 100 ....NDC 0028-0074-01
  Bottles of 1000 ....NDC 0028-0074-10
  Gy-Pak®—One Unit
    12 bottles - 100 tablets each
  ....NDC 0028-0074-65
  Unit Dose (blister pack)
    Box of 100 (strips of 10)
  ....NDC 0028-0074-61
Dispense in tight container (USP).
Ampuls 2 ml - For intramuscular administration only
  25 mg imipramine hydrochloride, 2 mg ascorbic acid, 1 mg sodium bisulfite, 1 mg sodium sulfite
  Boxes of 10 ....NDC 0028-0065-23
Note: Upon storage, minute crystals may form in some ampuls. This has no influence on the therapeutic efficacy of the preparation, and the crystals redissolve when the affected ampuls are immersed in hot tap water for one minute.

Animal Pharmacology & Toxicology:
A. *Acute:* Oral LD$_{50}$ ranges are as follows:
  Rat   355 to 682 mg/kg
  Dog   100 to 215 mg/kg
Depending on the dosage in both species, toxic signs proceeded progressively from depression, irregular respiration and ataxia to convulsions and death.
B. *Reproduction/Teratogenic:* The overall evaluation may be summed up in the following manner:
Oral: Independent studies in three species (rat, mouse and rabbit) revealed that when Tofranil is administered orally in doses up to approximately 2½ times the maximum human dose in the first 2 species and up to 25 times the maximum human dose in the third species, the drug is essentially free from teratogenic potential. In the three species studied, only one instance of fetal abnormality occurred (in the rabbit) and in that study there was likewise an abnormality in the control group. However, evidence does exist from the rat studies that some systemic and embryotoxic potential is demonstrable. This is manifested by reduced litter size, a slight increase in the stillborn rate and a reduction in the mean birth weight.
Parenteral: In contradistinction to the oral data, Tofranil does exhibit a slight but definite teratogenic potential when administered by the subcutaneous route. Drug effects on both the mother and fetus in the rabbit are manifested in higher resorption rates and decrease in mean fetal birth weights, while teratogenic findings occurred at a level of 5 times the maximum human dose. In the mouse, teratogenicity occurred at 1½ and 6½ times the maximum human dose, but no teratogenic effects were seen at levels 3 times the maximum human dose. Thus, in the mouse, the findings are equivocal.

Dispense in tight container (USP).
C84-3 (Rev. 1/84)
Shown in Product Identification Section, page 411

For full prescribing information on Enuresis, please refer to Tofranil® imipramine hydrochloride USP, on page 969

TOFRANIL–PM®
[*toe-fray' nil-pee-emm*] ℞
imipramine pamoate

Capsules of 75 mg	GY-CODE 20
Capsules of 100 mg	GY-CODE 40
Capsules of 125 mg	GY-CODE 45
Capsules of 150 mg	GY-CODE 22

For oral administration

Each 75-mg capsule contains imipramine pamoate equivalent to 75 mg of imipramine hydrochloride.
Each 100-mg capsule contains imipramine pamoate equivalent to 100 mg of imipramine hydrochloride.
Each 125-mg capsule contains imipramine pamoate equivalent to 125 mg of imipramine hydrochloride.
Each 150-mg capsule contains imipramine pamoate equivalent to 150 mg of imipramine hydrochloride.

Description: Tofranil-PM is the pamoate salt of imipramine. It is designated bis 5-[3-(Dimethylamino)propyl]-10, 11-dihydro-5H-dibenz[b,f] azepine compound (2:1) with 4,4-methylene-bis-[3-hydroxy-2-naphthoic acid] with the empirical formula $C_{61}H_{64}N_4O_6$.

Tofranil-PM is a fine, yellow, tasteless and odorless powder. It is soluble in ethyl alcohol, acetone, ethyl ether, chloroform and carbon tetrachloride. It is insoluble in water.

Clinical Pharmacology: The mechanism of action of imipramine is not definitely known. However, it does not act primarily by stimulation of the central nervous system. The clinical effect is hypothesized as being due to potentiation of adrenergic synapses by blocking uptake of norepinephrine at nerve endings.

Indications: For the relief of symptoms of depression. Endogenous depression is more likely to be alleviated than other depressive states. One to three weeks of treatment may be needed before optimal therapeutic effects are evident.

Contraindications: The concomitant use of monoamine oxidase inhibiting compounds is contraindicated. Hyperpyretic crises or severe convulsive seizures may occur in patients receiving such combinations. The potentiation of adverse effects can be serious, or even fatal. When it is desired to substitute Tofranil-PM in patients receiving a monoamine oxidase inhibitor, as long an interval should elapse as the clinical situation will allow, with a minimum of 14 days. Initial dosage should be low and increases should be gradual and cautiously prescribed.

The drug is contraindicated during the acute recovery period after a myocardial infarction. Patients with a known hypersensitivity to this compound should not be given the drug. The possibility of cross-sensitivity to other dibenzazepine compounds should be kept in mind.

Warnings: Extreme caution should be used when this drug is given to:

patients with cardiovascular disease because of the possibility of conduction defects, arrhythmias, congestive heart failure, myocardial infarction, strokes and tachycardia. These patients require cardiac surveillance at all dosage levels of the drug;

patients with increased intraocular pressure, history of urinary retention, or history of narrow-angle glaucoma because of the drug's anticholinergic properties;

hyperthyroid patients or those on thyroid medication because of the possibility of cardiovascular toxicity;

patients with a history of seizure disorder because this drug has been shown to lower the seizure threshold;

patients receiving guanethidine, clonidine, or similar agents, since imipramine pamoate may block the pharmacologic effects of these drugs;

patients receiving methylphenidate hydrochloride. Since methylphenidate hydrochloride may inhibit the metabolism of imipramine pamoate, downward dosage adjustment of imipramine pamoate may be required when given concomitantly with methylphenidate hydrochloride.

Since imipramine pamoate may impair the mental and/or physical abilities required for the performance of potentially hazardous tasks, such as operating an automobile or machinery, the patient should be cautioned accordingly.

Tofranil-PM may enhance the CNS depressant effects of alcohol. Therefore, it should be borne in mind that the dangers inherent in a suicide attempt or accidental overdosage with the drug may be increased for the patient who uses excessive amounts of alcohol. (See **Precautions**.)

Usage in Children: Tofranil-PM should not be used in children of any age because of the increased potential for acute overdosage due to the high unit potency (75 mg, 100 mg, 125 mg and 150 mg). Each capsule contains imipramine pamoate equivalent to 75 mg, 100 mg, 125 mg or 150 mg imipramine hydrochloride.

Precautions: An ECG recording should be taken prior to the initiation of larger-than-usual doses of imipramine pamoate and at appropriate intervals thereafter until steady state is achieved. (Patients with any evidence of cardiovascular disease require cardiac surveillance at all dosage levels of the drug. See **Warnings**.) Elderly patients and patients with cardiac disease or a prior history of cardiac disease are at special risk of developing the cardiac abnormalities associated with the use of imipramine pamoate. It should be kept in mind that the possibility of suicide in seriously depressed patients is inherent in the illness and may persist until significant remission occurs. Such patients should be carefully supervised during the early phase of treatment with imipramine pamoate and may require hospitalization. Prescriptions should be written for the smallest amount feasible. Hypomanic or manic episodes may occur, particularly in patients with cyclic disorders. Such reactions may necessitate discontinuation of the drug. If needed, imipramine pamoate may be resumed in lower dosage when these episodes are relieved. Administration of a tranquilizer may be useful in controlling such episodes.

An activation of the psychosis may occasionally be observed in schizophrenic patients and may require reduction of dosage and the addition of a phenothiazine.

Concurrent administration of imipramine pamoate with electroshock therapy may increase the hazards; such treatment should be limited to those patients for whom it is essential, since there is limited clinical experience.

Usage During Pregnancy and Lactation:
Animal reproduction studies have yielded inconclusive results. (See also **Animal Pharmacology & Toxicology**.)

There have been no well-controlled studies conducted with pregnant women to determine the effect of imipramine on the fetus. However, there have been clinical reports of congenital malformations associated with the use of the drug. Although a causal relationship between these effects and the drug could not be established, the possibility of fetal risk from the maternal ingestion of imipramine cannot be excluded. Therefore, imipramine should be used in women who are or might become pregnant only if the clinical condition clearly justifies potential risk to the fetus.

Limited data suggest that imipramine is likely to be excreted in human breast milk. As a general rule, a woman taking a drug should not nurse since the possibility exists that the drug may be excreted in breast milk and be harmful to the child.

Patients should be warned that imipramine pamoate may enhance the CNS depressant effects of alcohol. (See **Warnings**.)

Imipramine pamoate should be used with caution in patients with significantly impaired renal or hepatic function.

Patients who develop a fever and a sore throat during therapy with imipramine pamoate should have leukocyte and differential blood counts performed. Imipramine pamoate should be discontinued if there is evidence of pathological neutrophil depression.

Prior to elective surgery, imipramine pamoate should be discontinued for as long as the clinical situation will allow.

In occasional susceptible patients or in those receiving anticholinergic drugs (including antiparkinsonism agents) in addition, the atropine-like effects may become more pronounced (e.g., paralytic ileus). Close supervision and careful adjustment of dosage is required when imipramine pamoate is administered concomitantly with anticholinergic drugs.

Avoid the use of preparations, such as decongestants and local anesthetics, which contain any sympathomimetic amine (e.g., epinephrine, norepinephrine), since it has been reported that tricyclic antidepressants can potentiate the effects of catecholamines.

Caution should be exercised when imipramine pamoate is used with agents that lower blood pressure.

Imipramine pamoate may potentiate the effects of CNS depressant drugs.

Patients taking imipramine pamoate should avoid excessive exposure to sunlight since there have been reports of photosensitization.

Both elevation and lowering of blood sugar levels have been reported with imipramine pamoate use.

The Tofranil-PM capsules (100 and 125 mg) contain FD&C Yellow No. 5 (tartrazine) which may cause allergic-type reactions (including bronchial asthma) in certain susceptible individuals. Although the overall incidence of FD&C Yellow No. 5 (tartrazine) sensitivity in the general population is low, it is frequently seen in patients who also have aspirin hypersensitivity.

Adverse Reactions: Note: Although the listing which follows includes a few adverse reactions which have not been reported with this specific drug, the pharmacological similarities among the tricyclic antidepressant drugs require that each of the reactions be considered when imipramine is administered.

Cardiovascular: Orthostatic hypotension, hypertension, tachycardia, palpitation, myocardial infarction, arrhythmias, heart block, ECG changes, precipitation of congestive heart failure, stroke.

Psychiatric: Confusional states (especially in the elderly) with hallucinations, disorientation, delusions; anxiety, restlessness, agitation; insomnia and nightmares; hypomania; exacerbation of psychosis.

Neurological: Numbness, tingling, paresthesias of extremities; incoordination, ataxia, tremors; peripheral neuropathy; extrapyramidal symptoms; seizures, alterations in EEG patterns; tinnitus.

Continued on next page

The full prescribing information for each GEIGY drug is contained herein and is that in effect as of October 1, 1984.

Geigy—Cont.

Anticholinergic: Dry mouth, and, rarely, associated sublingual adenitis; blurred vision, disturbances of accommodation, mydriasis; constipation, paralytic ileus; urinary retention, delayed micturition, dilation of the urinary tract.
Allergic: Skin rash, petechiae, urticaria, itching, photosensitization; edema (general or of face and tongue); drug fever; cross-sensitivity with desipramine.
Hematologic: Bone marrow depression including agranulocytosis; eosinophilia; purpura; thrombocytopenia.
Gastrointestinal: Nausea and vomiting, anorexia, epigastric distress, diarrhea; peculiar taste, stomatitis, abdominal cramps, black tongue.
Endocrine: Gynecomastia in the male; breast enlargement and galactorrhea in the female; increased or decreased libido, impotence; testicular swelling; elevation or depression of blood sugar levels; inappropriate antidiuretic hormone (ADH) secretion syndrome.
Other: Jaundice (simulating obstructive); altered liver function; weight gain or loss; perspiration; flushing; urinary frequency; drowsiness, dizziness, weakness and fatigue; headache; parotid swelling; alopecia; proneness to falling.
Withdrawal Symptoms: Though not indicative of addiction, abrupt cessation of treatment after prolonged therapy may produce nausea, headache and malaise.
Dosage and Administration: The following recommended dosages for Tofranil-PM should be modified as necessary by the clinical response and any evidence of intolerance.
Initial Adult Dosage:
Outpatients—Therapy should be initiated at 75 mg/day. Dosage may be increased to 150 mg/day which is the dose level at which optimum response is usually obtained. If necessary, dosage may be increased to 200 mg/day.
Dosage higher than 75 mg/day may also be administered on a once-a-day basis after the optimum dosage and tolerance have been determined. The daily dosage may be given at bedtime. In some patients it may be necessary to employ a divided-dose schedule.
As with all tricyclics, the antidepressant effect of imipramine may not be evident for one to three weeks in some patients.
Hospitalized Patients—Therapy should be initiated at 100-150 mg/day and may be increased to 200 mg/day. If there is no response after two weeks, dosage should be increased to 250-300 mg/day.
Dosage higher than 150 mg/day may also be administered on a once-a-day basis after the optimum dosage and tolerance have been determined. The daily dosage may be given at bedtime. In some patients it may be necessary to employ a divided-dose schedule.
As with all tricyclics, the antidepressant effect of imipramine may not be evident for one to three weeks in some patients.
Adult Maintenance Dosage: Following remission, maintenance medication may be required for a longer period of time at the lowest dose that will maintain remission after which the dosage should gradually be decreased.
The usual maintenance dosage is 75-150 mg/day. The total daily dosage can be administered on a once-a-day basis, preferably at bedtime. In some patients it may be necessary to employ a divided-dose schedule.
In cases of relapse due to premature withdrawal of the drug, the effective dosage of imipramine should be reinstituted.
Adolescent and Geriatric Patients: Therapy in these age groups should be initiated with Tofranil®, brand of imipramine hydrochloride, tablets at a total daily dosage of 25-50 mg, since Tofranil-PM capsules are not available in these strengths. Dosage may be increased according to response and tolerance, but it is generally unnecessary to exceed 100 mg/day in these patients.
Tofranil-PM capsules may be used when total daily dosage is established at 75 mg or higher.
The total daily dosage can be administered on a once-a-day basis, preferably at bedtime. In some patients it may be necessary to employ a divided-dose schedule.
As with all tricyclics, the antidepressant effect of imipramine may not be evident for one to three weeks in some patients.
Adolescent and geriatric patients can usually be maintained at lower dosage. Following remission, maintenance medication may be required for a longer period of time at the lowest dose that will maintain remission after which the dosage should gradually be decreased.
The total daily maintenance dosage can be administered on a once-a-day basis, preferably at bedtime. In some patients it may be necessary to employ a divided-dose schedule.
In cases of relapse due to premature withdrawal of the drug, the effective dosage of imipramine should be reinstituted.
Overdosage: Children have been reported to be more sensitive than adults to an acute overdosage of imipramine pamoate. An acute overdose of any amount in infants or young children, especially, must be considered serious and potentially fatal.
Signs and Symptoms: These may vary in severity depending upon factors such as the amount of drug absorbed, the age of the patient, and the interval between drug ingestion and the start of treatment. Blood and urine levels of imipramine may not reflect the severity of poisoning; they have chiefly a qualitative rather than quantitative value, and are unreliable indicators in the clinical management of the patient.
CNS abnormalities may include drowsiness, stupor, coma, ataxia, restlessness, agitation, hyperactive reflexes, muscle rigidity, athetoid and choreiform movements, and convulsions.
Cardiac abnormalities may include arrhythmia, tachycardia, ECG evidence of impaired conduction, and signs of congestive failure.
Respiratory depression, cyanosis, hypotension, shock, vomiting, hyperpyrexia, mydriasis, and diaphoresis may also be present.
Treatment: Because CNS involvement, respiratory depression and cardiac arrhythmia can occur suddenly, hospitalization and close observation are necessary, even when the amount ingested is thought to be small or the initial degree of intoxication appears slight or moderate. All patients with ECG abnormalities should have continuous cardiac monitoring for at least 72 hours and be closely observed until well after cardiac status has returned to normal; relapses may occur after apparent recovery.
The *slow* intravenous administration of physostigmine salicylate has been reported to reverse most of the cardiovascular and CNS effects of overdosage with tricyclic antidepressants. In adults, 1 to 3 mg has been reported to be effective. In children, start with 0.5 mg and repeat at 5-minute intervals to determine the minimum effective dose; do not exceed 2 mg. Because of the short duration of action of physostigmine, repeat the effective dose at 30- to 60-minute intervals, as necessary. Avoid rapid injection to reduce the possibility of physostigmine-induced convulsions.
In the alert patient, empty the stomach promptly by induced emesis followed by lavage. In the obtunded patient, secure the airway with a cuffed endotracheal tube before beginning lavage (do not induce emesis). Continue lavage for 24 hours or longer, depending on the apparent severity of intoxication. Use normal or half-normal saline to avoid water intoxication, especially in children. Instillation of activated charcoal slurry may help reduce absorption of imipramine.
Minimize external stimulation to reduce the tendency to convulsions. If anticonvulsants are necessary, diazepam, short-acting barbiturates, paraldehyde or methocarbamol may be useful. Do not use barbiturates if MAO inhibitors have been taken recently.
Maintain adequate respiratory exchange. Do not use respiratory stimulants.
Shock should be treated with supportive measures, such as intravenous fluids, oxygen and corticosteroids. Digitalis may increase conduction abnormalities and further irritate an already sensitized myocardium. If congestive heart failure necessitates rapid digitalization, particular care must be exercised.
Hyperpyrexia should be controlled by whatever external means are available, including ice packs and cooling sponge baths, if necessary.
Hemodialysis, peritoneal dialysis, exchange transfusions and forced diuresis have been generally reported as ineffective because of the rapid fixation of imipramine in tissues. Blood and urine levels of imipramine may not correlate with the degree of intoxication, and are unreliable indicators in the clinical management of the patient.

How Supplied
Capsules 75 mg — coral (imprinted Geigy 20) equivalent to 75 mg imipramine hydrochloride
    Bottles of 30 ....NDC 0028-0020-26
    Bottles of 100 ....NDC 0028-0020-01
    Bottles of 1000 ....NDC 0028-0020-10
    Unit Dose (blister pack)
      Box of 100 (strips of 10)
    ....NDC 0028-0020-61
Capsules 100 mg — dark yellow/coral (imprinted Geigy 40) equivalent to 100 mg imipramine hydrochloride
    Bottles of 30 ....NDC 0028-0040-26
    Bottles of 100 ....NDC 0028-0040-01
Capsules 125 mg — light yellow/coral (imprinted Geigy 45) equivalent to 125 mg imipramine hydrochloride
    Bottles of 30 ....NDC 0028-0045-26
    Bottles of 100 ....NDC 0028-0045-01
Capsules 150 mg — coral (imprinted Geigy 22) equivalent to 150 mg imipramine hydrochloride
    Bottles of 30 ....NDC 0028-0022-26
    Bottles of 100 ....NDC 0028-0022-01
    Unit Dose (blister pack)
      Box of 100 (strips of 10)
    ....NDC 0028-0022-61

Animal Pharmacology & Toxicology
A. *Acute:* Oral LD_{50}:
Mouse	2185 mg/kg
Rat (F)	1142 mg/kg
(M)	1807 mg/kg
Rabbit	1016 mg/kg
Dog	693 mg/kg (Emesis ED_{50})

B. *Subacute:*
Two three-month studies in dogs gave evidence of an adverse drug effect on the testes, but only at the highest dose level employed, i.e., 90 mg/kg (10 times the maximum human dose). Depending on the histological section of the testes examined, the findings consisted of a range of degenerative changes up to and including complete atrophy of the seminiferous tubules, with spermatogenesis usually arrested.
Human studies show no definitive effect on sperm count, sperm motility, sperm morphology or volume of ejaculate.
Rat
One three-month study was done in rats at dosage levels comparable to those of the dog studies. No adverse drug effect on the testes was noted in this study, as confirmed by histological examination.
C. *Reproduction/Teratogenic:*
Oral: Imipramine pamoate was fed to male and female albino rats for 28 weeks through two breeding cycles at dose levels of 15 mg/kg/day and 40 mg/kg/day (equivalent to 2½ and 7 times the maximum human dose). No abnormalities which could be related to drug administration were noted in gross inspection. Autopsies performed on pups from the second breeding likewise revealed no pathological changes in organs or tissues; however, a decrease in mean litter size from both matings was noted in the drug-treated groups and significant growth suppression occurred in the nursing pups of both sexes in the high group as well as in the females of the low-level group. Finally, the lactation index (pups weaned divided by number left to nurse) was significantly lower in the second litter of the high-level group.
Dispense in tight container (USP).

C84-4 (Rev.1/84)
Shown in Product Identification Section, page 411

for possible revisions

Product Information

Geneva Generics
2599 W. MIDWAY BLVD.
BROOMFIELD, CO 80020

NDC 0781	PRODUCT
	APAP w/CODEINE TABLETS #3 ℞ ℂ
1752-01	½ gr., 100's
1752-13	Unit Dose 100's
	APAP w/CODEINE #4 ℞ ℂ
1654-01	1 gr., 100's
1654-13	Unit Dose 100's
	AMINOPHYLLINE TABLETS
1214-01	100 mg., 100's
1318-01	200 mg., 100's
	AMITRIPTYLINE HCl. TABLETS ℞
1486-01	10mg., 100's
1487-01	25mg., 100's
1487-13	Unit Dose 100's
1488-01	50mg., 100's
1489-01	75mg., 100's
1490-01	100mg., 100's
1491-01	150mg., 100's
7210-70	**ANTIBIOTIC EAR DROPS** ℞
	10 cc
	ASPIRIN (325mg.) ℞ ℂ
	w/CODEINE TABLETS
1660-01	30mg. (½ gr.), 100's
1875-01	60mg. (1 gr.), 100's
1225-01	**AZO-SULFISOXAZOLE TABLETS** ℞
	100's
7023-01	**BISACODYL SUPPOSITORIES** OTC
	10mg., 100's
1050-01	**CARISOPRODOL TABLETS** ℞
	100's
2235-01	**CHLORAL HYDRATE** ℞ ℂ
	CAPSULES
	500mg., 100's
	CHLORDIAZEPOXIDE ℞ ℂ
	CAPSULES
2080-01	5mg., 100's
2082-01	10mg., 100's
2082-13	Unit Dose 100's
2084-01	25 mg., 100's
	CHLOROTHIAZIDE TABLETS ℞
1944-01	250mg., 100's
1940-01	500mg., 100's
1970-01	**CHLOROTHIAZIDE (250mg.)** ℞
	w/RESERPINE TABLETS
	0.125mg., 100's
	CHLORPHENIRAMINE MALEATE ℞
	T.D. CAPSULES
2602-01	8mg., 100's
2699-01	12 mg., 100's
	CHLORPROMAZINE HCl. ℞
	TABLETS
1715-01	10mg., 100's
1715-13	Unit Dose 100's
1716-01	25mg., 100's
1716-13	Unit Dose 100's
1717-01	50mg., 100's
1717-13	Unit Dose 100's
1718-01	100mg., 100's
1718-13	Unit Dose 100's
1719-01	200mg., 100's
1719-13	Unit Dose 100's
4009-08	**CHLORPROMAZINE CONCEN-** ℞
	TRATE SYRUP
	100mg./cc., 8 oz.
	CHLORPROPAMIDE TABLETS ℞
1613-01	100 mg., 100's
1623-01	250 mg., 100's
1623-25	250's
1698-01	**CHLORAXAZONE (250mg.)** ℞
	w/APAP TABLETS
	300mg., 100's
	CONJUGATED ESTROGENS ℞
	TABLETS
1135-01	0.625mg., 100's
1835-01	1.25mg., 100's
1625-01	2.5mg., 100's
	CYCLANDELATE CAPSULES ℞
2668-01	200mg., 100's
2670-01	400mg., 100's

1125-01	**CYPROHEPTADINE HCl.** ℞
	TABLETS
	4mg., 100's
	DANTHRON TABLETS ℞
1574-01	75mg., 100's
1574-13	75mg., Unit Dose 100's
6606-04	**DEPROIST EXPECTORANT** ℞ ℂ
	w/CODEINE
	(Codeine Phosphate, Pseudoephe-
	drine, Guaifenesin, Alcohol)
	4 oz.
	DIPHENHYDRAMINE CAPSULES ℞
2458-01	25mg., 100's
2498-01	50mg., 100's
	DIPYRIDAMOLE TABLETS ℞
1890-01	25mg., 100's
1890-13	Unit Dose 100's
1678-01	50mg., 100's
1478-01	75mg., 100's
1600-01	**DISOBROM TABLETS**
	(Dexbrompheniramine Maleate,
	Pseudoephedrine) 100's
1060-01	**DISULFIRAM TABLETS** ℞
	250mg., 100's
	DOXYCYCLINE HYCLATE
2525-50	50mg., 50's, Capsules
2522-50	100mg., 50's, Capsules
1075-50	100mg., 50's, Tablets
	ERGOLOID MESYLATES
	TABLETS ℞
1990-01	0.5mg., 100's (Sublingual)
1255-01	1.0mg., 100's (Sublingual)
1155-01	1.0mg., 100's (Oral)
1608-01	**FLUOXYMESTERONE TABLETS** ℞
	10mg., 100's
	FUROSEMIDE TABLETS ℞
1818-01	20mg., 100's
1818-13	20mg., Unit Dose 100's
1966-01	40mg., 100's
1966-13	40mg., Unit Dose 100's
1446-01	80 mg., 100's
1827-01	**GLUTETHIMIDE TABLETS** ℞ ℂ
	500mg., 100's
	HYDRALAZINE HCl. TABLETS ℞
1732-01	10mg., 100's
1733-01	25mg., 100's
1734-01	50mg., 100's
	HYDRALAZINE w/HYDRO-
	CHLOROTHIAZIDE CAPSULES
2610-01	25mg., 100's
2612-01	50mg., 100's
	HYDROCHLOROTHIAZIDE
	TABLETS
1480-01	25mg., 100's
1481-01	50mg., 100's
1481-13	50 mg., Unit Dose 100's
1735-01	100mg., 100's
1010-01	**HYDROCHLOROTHIAZIDE 25 mg.** ℞
	w/RESERPINE TABLETS
	0.125mg., 100's
1011-01	**HYDROCHLOROTHIAZIDE 50 mg.** ℞
	w/RESERPINE TABLETS
	0.125mg., 100's
1772-01	**HYDROFLUMETHIAZIDE 25 mg.** ℞
	w/RESERPINE 0.125 mg. TABLETS
	100's
1774-01	**HYDROFLUMETHIAZIDE 50 mg.** ℞
	w/RESERPINE 0.125 mg. TABLETS
	100's
	HYDROXYZINE TABLETS ℞
1332-01	10mg., 100's
1334-01	25mg., 100's
1336-01	50mg., 100's
	IMIPRAMINE TABLETS ℞
1762-01	10mg., 100's
1764-01	25mg., 100's
1764-13	Unit Dose 100's
1766-01	50mg., 100's
	INDOMETHACIN CAPSULES ℞
2325-01	25 mg., 100's
2350-01	50 mg., 100's
	ISOSORBIDE DINITRATE ℞
	TABLETS
1635-01	5mg., 100's (Oral)
1565-01	5mg., 100's (Sublingual)
1556-01	10mg., 100's (Oral)
1695-01	20mg., 100's

2520-01	**ISOSORBIDE DINITRATE T.D.** ℞
	CAPSULES
	40mg., 100's
1417-01	**ISOSORBIDE DINITRATE T.D.** ℞
	TABLETS
	40mg., 100's
	ISOXSUPRINE TABLETS ℞
1840-01	10mg., 100's
1840-13	Unit Dose 100's
1842-01	20mg., 100's
1842-13	Unit Dose 100's
1262-01	**LONOX TABLETS** ℞ ℂ
	(Diphenoxylate HCl., Atropine
	Sulfate), 100's
	MECLIZINE HCl. TABLETS OTC
1345-01	12.5mg., 100's
1345-13	12.5mg., Unit Dose 100's
1410-01	**MEPROBAMATE TABLETS** ℞ ℂ
	400mg., 100's
	METHOCARBAMOL TABLETS ℞
1760-01	500mg., 100's
1750-01	750mg., 100's
	METHYLDOPA TABLETS ℞
1320-01	250 mg., 100's
1322-01	500 mg., 100's
	METRONIDAZOLE TABLETS ℞
1740-01	250 mg., 100's
1745-01	500 mg., 100's
6532-42	**MYGEL SUSPENSION** OTC
	(Aluminum Hydroxide, Magnesium
	Hydroxide, Simethicone), 12 oz
	NITROGLYCERIN S.R. ℞
	CAPSULES
2718-60	2.5mg., 60's
2786-01	6.5mg., 100's
2798-60	9mg., 60's
	NYLIDRIN TABLETS ℞
1406-01	6mg., 100's
1413-01	12mg., 100's
1370-01	**P.E.T.N. S.R. TABLETS** ℞
	80mg., 100's
2000-01	**PAPAVERINE T.D. CAPSULES** ℞
	150mg., 100's
2440-01	**PHENYLBUTAZONE CAPSULES** ℞
	100mg., 100's
1440-01	**PHENYLBUTAZONE TABLETS** ℞
	100mg., 100's
6003-52	**POLYVITE WITH FLUORIDE DROPS**
	(Vitamin A, Vitamin D, Vitamin E, Vi-
	tamin C, Thiamine, Riboflavin, Niacin,
	Vitamin B-6, Vitamin B-12, Fluoride),
	50ml.
	POTASSIUM CHLORIDE ℞
6040-16	10% Sugar Free, 16 oz.
6790-16	20% Sugar Free, 16 oz.
1540-01	**PREDNISOLONE TABLETS** ℞
	5mg., 100's
	PREDNISONE TABLETS ℞
1495-01	5mg., 100's
1500-01	10mg., 100's
1485-01	20mg., 100's
1450-01	50mg., 100's
1040-01	**PRIMIDONE TABLETS** ℞
	250mg. 100's
1021-01	**PROBENECID TABLETS** ℞
	0.5gm., 100's
1023-01	**PROBENECID & COLCHICINE** ℞
	TABLETS
	0.5gm., 100's
2315-01	**PROCAINAMIDE CAPSULES** ℞
	500mg., 100's
	PROCHLORPERAZINE TABLETS ℞
1120-01	5mg., 100's
1122-01	10mg., 100's
1124-01	25mg., 100's
2060-01	**PRO-ISO CAPSULES** ℞
	(Prochlorperazine as the Maleate,
	Isopropamide as the Iodide), 100's
6030-16	**PROMETHAZINE DM (Ped)** ℞
	EXPECTORANT
	16 oz.
6930-16	**PROMETHAZINE w/CODEINE** ℞ ℂ
	EXPECTORANT
	16 oz.

Continued on next page

Geneva—Cont.

Code	Product
6635-16	**PROMETHAZINE VC EXPECTORANT** ℞ 16 oz.
6950-16	**PROMETHAZINE VC w/CODEINE EXPECTORANT** ℞ ⓒ 16 oz.
1855-01	**PROPANTHELINE BROMIDE TABLETS** ℞ 15mg., 100's
2140-01	**PROPOXYPHENE HCl. CAPSULES** ℞ ⓒ 65mg., 100's
2367-01	**PROPOXYPHENE-AC** ℞ ⓒ 100's
1378-01	**PROPOXYPHENE HCl 65 w/APAP** ℞ ⓒ 650mg., 100's
1535-01	**PSEUDOEPHEDRINE TABLETS** OTC 60mg., 100's
1804-01	**QUINIDINE GLUCONATE S.R. TABLETS** ℞ 324mg., 100's
1900-01	**QUINIDINE SULFATE TABLETS** ℞ 3 gr., 100's
2995-01	**QUININE SULFATE CAPSULES** OTC 200mg., 100's
2997-01	**QUININE SULFATE CAPSULES** OTC 5 gr., 100's
1926-01	**QUIPHILE TABLETS** ℞ Quinine Sulfate 260 mg., 100's
2427-01	**RESAID T.D. CAPSULES** ℞ (Phenylpropanolamine HCl., Chlorpheniramine Maleate) 100's
2847-01	**RESCAPS-D T.D. CAPSULES** ℞ (Caramiphen Edisylate, Phenylpropanolamine HCl.), 100's
1598-01	**SPIRONOLACTONE TABLETS** ℞ 25mg., 100's
1150-01	**SPIRONOLACTONE (25mg.) w/HYDROCHLOROTHIAZIDE TABLETS** ℞ 25mg., 100's
1261-01	**SULFAMETHOXAZOLE TABLETS** ℞ 500mg., 100's
1063-01	**SULFAMETHOXAZOLE w/ TRIMETHOPRIM DS** ℞ 100's
1062-01	**SULFAMTHOXAZOLE w/ TRIMETHOPRIM SS** ℞ 100's
1045-01	**SULFASALAZINE TABLETS** ℞ 500mg., 100's
1015-01	**SULFISOXAZOLE TABLETS** ℞ 500mg., 100's
1988-01	**T.E.H. TABLETS** ℞ (Ephedrine Sulfate, Theophylline, Hydroxyzine HCl.), 100's
1325-01	**T.E.P. TABLETS** OTC (Theophylline Anhydrous, Ephedrine HCl., Phenobarbital), 100's
6710-16	**TAMINE ELIXIR** ℞ 16 oz.
1153-01	**TAMINE S.R. TABLETS** ℞ (Brompheniramine Maleate, Phenylephrine Hydrochloride, Phenylpropanolamine Hydrochloride), 100's
6600-16	**THEOPHYLLINE ELIXIR** ℞ 16 oz.
	THEOPHYLLINE S.R. TABLETS ℞
1003-01	100 mg., 100's
1004-01	200 mg., 100's
1005-01	300mg., 100's
	THIORIDAZINE TABLETS
1604-01	10mg., 100's
1604-10	10mg., 1000's
1614-01	15mg., 100's
1614-10	15mg., 1000's
1624-01	25mg., 100's
1624-10	25mg., 1000's
1634-01	50mg., 100's
1634-10	50mg., 1000's
1644-01	100 mg., 100's
1644-10	100 mg., 1000's
1704-01	**TOLBUTAMIDE TABLETS** ℞ 0.5gm., 100's
	TRIAMCINOLONE ACETONIDE CREAM ℞
7036-16	0.1%, 16 oz.
7030-16	0.025%, 16 oz.
1670-01	**TRIAMCINOLONE TABLETS** 4mg., 100's
1180-01	**TRICHLORMETHIAZIDE TABLETS** ℞ 4mg., 100's
1663-01	**TRIFED TABLETS** ℞ (Triprolidine HCl., Pseudoephedrine HCl.), 100's
6510-16	**TRIFED SYRUP** ℞ 16 oz.
	TRIFLUOPERAZINE TABLETS ℞
1030-01	1mg., 100's
1030-13	Unit Dose 100's
1032-01	2mg., 100's
1032-13	Unit Dose 100's
1034-01	5mg., 100's
1034-13	Unit Dose 100's
1036-01	10mg., 100's
1036-13	Unit Dose 100's
6005-52	**TRIPLEVITE WITH FLUORIDE DROPS** ℞ (Vitamin A, Vitamin D, Vitamin C, Fluoride), 1-50cc.
1340-01	**UROBLUE TABLETS** ℞ (Atropine Sulfate, Hyoscyamine, Methenamine, Methylene Blue, Phenyl Salicylate, Benzoic Acid), 100's

Products are cross-indexed by generic and chemical names in the **YELLOW SECTION**

Gerber Products Company
FREMONT, MI 49412

MBF* (Meat Base Formula) Liquid Hypoallergenic Infant Feeding Formula, Gerber

Ingredients: Water, beef hearts, cane sugar, sesame oil, modified tapioca starch, tricalcium phosphate, calcium citrate, potassium chloride, iodized salt, sodium ascorbate, magnesium chloride, ferrous sulfate, zinc sulfate, tocopheryl acetate, thiamin hydrochloride, calcium pantothenate, niacinamide, cupric sulfate, pyridoxine hydrochloride, vitamin A palmitate, riboflavin, phytonadione (vitamin K_1), folic acid, manganese sulfate, potassium iodide, biotin, vitamin D and vitamin B_{12}.
[See table below].

Action and Uses: A nutritionally adequate formula for infants and children intolerant to cow's and goat's milk whose symptoms may be diarrhea, colic, eczema, upper respiratory, etc. Useful in the management of milk sensitivity, lactase deficiency and milk induced steatorrhea.

Administration and Dosage: Provides 20 cal/fl.oz. when diluted 1:1; similar to other milk-based and soy-based infant formulas. Concentrated liquid added to previously boiled (not hot) water is to be divided among prescribed number of bottles, easily fed thru cross-cut nipples.
MBF's content of essential nutrients conforms to the infant formula standard established by the U.S. Food and Drug Administration in 1971 and the 1980 American Academy of Pediatrics infant formula recommendations.

Side Effects: None.
Precautions: None.
Contraindications: None.

How Supplied: Concentrated Liquid, 15 fl. oz. cans.

Literature Available: Yes.
*Trademark

	Undiluted Percentage Composition	Undiluted One 15 Fl. Oz. Can Contains	Diluted 1 to 1 5 Fl. Oz. Contain
Calories	40 per fl. oz.	600	100
Protein	5.1%	24g	4.0g
Fat	6.5%	30.6g	5.1g
Carbohydrates	12.0%	57.0g	9.5g
Water	75.5%	357g	133.4g
Linoleic Acid		1800mg	300mg
Vitamins:			
Vitamin A		1600IU	268IU
Vitamin D		240IU	40IU
Vitamin E		6.6IU	1.1IU
Vitamin K		24µg	4µg
Thiamin (Vitamin B_1)		540µg	90µg
Riboflavin (Vitamin B_2)		900µg	150µg
Vitamin B_6		780µg	130µg
Vitamin B_{12}		7.8µg	1.3µg
Niacin		3600µg	600µg
Folic Acid (Folacin)		24.0µg	4.0µg
Pantothenic Acid		1800µg	300µg
Biotin		9.0µg	1.5µg
Vitamin C (Ascorbic Acid)		54.0mg	9.0mg
Choline		90.0mg	15.0mg
Inositol		150.0mg	25.0mg
Minerals:			
Calcium		900mg	150mg
Phosphorus		600mg	100mg
Magnesium		36.0mg	2.0mg
Iron		12.0mg	6.0mg
Zinc		3.0mg	0.5mg
Manganese		30.0µg	5.0µg
Copper		360.0µg	60.0µg
Iodine		30.0µg	5.0µg
Sodium		246mg	41mg
Potassium		486mg	81mg
Chloride		438mg	73mg

Geneva Generics
2599 W. MIDWAY BLVD.
BROOMFIELD, CO 80020

NDC 0781	PRODUCT
	APAP w/CODEINE TABLETS #3 ℞ ©
1752-01	½ gr., 100's
1752-13	Unit Dose 100's
	APAP w/CODEINE #4 ℞ ©
1654-01	1 gr., 100's
1654-13	Unit Dose 100's
	AMINOPHYLLINE TABLETS ℞
1214-01	100 mg., 100's
1318-01	200 mg., 100's
	AMITRIPTYLINE HCl. TABLETS ℞
1486-01	10mg., 100's
1487-01	25mg., 100's
1487-13	Unit Dose 100's
1488-01	50mg., 100's
1489-01	75mg., 100's
1490-01	100mg., 100's
1491-01	150mg., 100's
7210-70	**ANTIBIOTIC EAR DROPS** ℞ 10 cc
	ASPIRIN (325mg.) w/CODEINE TABLETS ℞ ©
1660-01	30mg. (½ gr.), 100's
1875-01	60mg. (1 gr.), 100's
1225-01	**AZO-SULFISOXAZOLE TABLETS** ℞ 100's
7023-01	**BISACODYL SUPPOSITORIES** OTC 10mg., 100's
1050-01	**CARISOPRODOL TABLETS** ℞ 100's
2235-01	**CHLORAL HYDRATE CAPSULES** ℞ © 500mg., 100's
	CHLORDIAZEPOXIDE CAPSULES ℞ ©
2080-01	5mg., 100's
2082-01	10mg., 100's
2082-13	Unit Dose 100's
2084-01	25 mg., 100's
	CHLOROTHIAZIDE TABLETS ℞
1944-01	250mg., 100's
1940-01	500mg., 100's
1970-01	**CHLOROTHIAZIDE (250mg.) w/RESERPINE TABLETS** ℞ 0.125mg., 100's
	CHLORPHENIRAMINE MALEATE T.D. CAPSULES ℞
2602-01	8mg., 100's
2699-01	12 mg., 100's
	CHLORPROMAZINE HCl. TABLETS ℞
1715-01	10mg., 100's
1715-13	Unit Dose 100's
1716-01	25mg., 100's
1716-13	Unit Dose 100's
1717-01	50mg., 100's
1717-13	Unit Dose 100's
1718-01	100mg., 100's
1718-13	Unit Dose 100's
1719-01	200mg., 100's
1719-13	Unit Dose 100's
4009-08	**CHLORPROMAZINE CONCENTRATE SYRUP** ℞ 100mg./cc., 8 oz.
	CHLORPROPAMIDE TABLETS ℞
1613-01	100 mg., 100's
1623-01	250 mg., 100's
1623-25	250's
1698-01	**CHLORAXAZONE (250mg.) w/APAP TABLETS** ℞ 300mg., 100's
	CONJUGATED ESTROGENS TABLETS ℞
1135-01	0.625mg., 100's
1835-01	1.25mg., 100's
1625-01	2.5mg., 100's
	CYCLANDELATE CAPSULES ℞
2668-01	200mg., 100's
2670-01	400mg., 100's

1125-01	**CYPROHEPTADINE HCl. TABLETS** ℞ 4mg., 100's
	DANTHRON TABLETS ℞
1574-01	75mg., 100's
1574-13	75mg., Unit Dose 100's
6606-04	**DEPROIST EXPECTORANT w/CODEINE** ℞ © (Codeine Phosphate, Pseudoephedrine, Guaifenesin, Alcohol) 4 oz.
	DIPHENHYDRAMINE CAPSULES ℞
2458-01	25mg., 100's
2498-01	50mg., 100's
	DIPYRIDAMOLE TABLETS ℞
1890-01	25mg., 100's
1890-13	Unit Dose 100's
1678-01	50mg., 100's
1478-01	75mg., 100's
1600-01	**DISOBROM TABLETS** ℞ (Dexbrompheniramine Maleate, Pseudoephedrine) 100's
1060-01	**DISULFIRAM TABLETS** ℞ 250mg., 100's
	DOXYCYCLINE HYCLATE
2525-50	50mg., 50's, Capsules
2522-50	100mg., 50's, Capsules
1075-50	100mg., 50's, Tablets
	ERGOLOID MESYLATES TABLETS ℞
1990-01	0.5mg., 100's (Sublingual)
1255-01	1.0mg., 100's (Sublingual)
1155-01	1.0mg., 100's (Oral)
1608-01	**FLUOXYMESTERONE TABLETS** ℞ 10mg., 100's
	FUROSEMIDE TABLETS ℞
1818-01	20mg., 100's
1818-13	20mg., Unit Dose 100's
1966-01	40mg., 100's
1966-13	40mg., Unit Dose 100's
1446-01	80 mg., 100's
1827-01	**GLUTETHIMIDE TABLETS** ℞ © 500mg., 100's
	HYDRALAZINE HCl. TABLETS ℞
1732-01	10mg., 100's
1733-01	25mg., 100's
1734-01	50mg., 100's
	HYDRALAZINE w/HYDROCHLOROTHIAZIDE CAPSULES
2610-01	25mg., 100's
2612-01	50mg., 100's
	HYDROCHLOROTHIAZIDE TABLETS ℞
1480-01	25mg., 100's
1481-01	50mg., 100's
1481-13	50 mg., Unit Dose 100's
1735-01	100mg., 100's
1010-01	**HYDROCHLOROTHIAZIDE 25 mg. w/RESERPINE TABLETS** ℞ 0.125mg., 100's
1011-01	**HYDROCHLOROTHIAZIDE 50 mg. w/RESERPINE TABLETS** ℞ 0.125mg., 100's
1772-01	**HYDROFLUMETHIAZIDE 25 mg. w/RESERPINE 0.125 mg. TABLETS** ℞ 100's
1774-01	**HYDROFLUMETHIAZIDE 50 mg. w/RESERPINE 0.125 mg. TABLETS** ℞ 100's
	HYDROXYZINE TABLETS ℞
1332-01	10mg., 100's
1334-01	25mg., 100's
1336-01	50mg., 100's
	IMIPRAMINE TABLETS ℞
1762-01	10mg., 100's
1764-01	25mg., 100's
1764-13	Unit Dose 100's
1766-01	50mg., 100's
	INDOMETHACIN CAPSULES
2325-01	25 mg., 100's
2350-01	50 mg., 100's
	ISOSORBIDE DINITRATE TABLETS ℞
1635-01	5mg., 100's (Oral)
1565-01	5mg., 100's (Sublingual)
1556-01	10mg., 100's (Oral)
1695-01	20mg., 100's

2520-01	**ISOSORBIDE DINITRATE T.D. CAPSULES** ℞ 40mg., 100's
1417-01	**ISOSORBIDE DINITRATE T.D. TABLETS** ℞ 40mg., 100's
	ISOXSUPRINE TABLETS ℞
1840-01	10mg., 100's
1840-13	Unit Dose 100's
1842-01	20mg., 100's
1842-13	Unit Dose 100's
1262-01	**LONOX TABLETS** ℞ © (Diphenoxylate HCl., Atropine Sulfate), 100's
	MECLIZINE HCl. TABLETS OTC
1345-01	12.5mg., 100's
1345-13	12.5mg., Unit Dose 100's
1410-01	**MEPROBAMATE TABLETS** ℞ © 400mg., 100's
	METHOCARBAMOL TABLETS
1760-01	500mg., 100's
1750-01	750mg., 100's
	METHYLDOPA TABLETS ℞
1320-01	250 mg., 100's
1322-01	500 mg., 100's
	METRONIDAZOLE TABLETS ℞
1740-01	250 mg., 100's
1745-01	500 mg., 100's
6532-42	**MYGEL SUSPENSION** OTC (Aluminum Hydroxide, Magnesium Hydroxide, Simethicone), 12 oz
	NITROGLYCERIN S.R. CAPSULES ℞
2718-60	2.5mg., 60's
2786-01	6.5mg., 100's
2798-60	9mg., 60's
	NYLIDRIN TABLETS ℞
1406-01	6mg., 100's
1413-01	12mg., 100's
1370-01	**P.E.T.N. S.R. TABLETS** ℞ 80mg., 100's
2000-01	**PAPAVERINE T.D. CAPSULES** ℞ 150mg., 100's
2440-01	**PHENYLBUTAZONE CAPSULES** ℞ 100mg., 100's
1440-01	**PHENYLBUTAZONE TABLETS** ℞ 100mg., 100's
6003-52	**POLYVITE WITH FLUORIDE DROPS** (Vitamin A, Vitamin D, Vitamin E, Vitamin C, Thiamine, Riboflavin, Niacin, Vitamin B-6, Vitamin B-12, Fluoride), 50ml.
	POTASSIUM CHLORIDE ℞
6040-16	10% Sugar Free, 16 oz.
6790-16	20% Sugar Free, 16 oz.
1540-01	**PREDNISOLONE TABLETS** ℞ 5mg., 100's
	PREDNISONE TABLETS ℞
1495-01	5mg., 100's
1500-01	10mg., 100's
1485-01	20mg., 100's
1450-01	50mg., 100's
1040-01	**PRIMIDONE TABLETS** ℞ 250mg. 100's
1021-01	**PROBENECID TABLETS** ℞ 0.5gm., 100's
1023-01	**PROBENECID & COLCHICINE TABLETS** ℞ 0.5gm., 100's
2315-01	**PROCAINAMIDE CAPSULES** ℞ 500mg., 100's
	PROCHLORPERAZINE TABLETS ℞
1120-01	5mg., 100's
1122-01	10mg., 100's
1124-01	25mg., 100's
2060-01	**PRO-ISO CAPSULES** ℞ (Prochlorperazine as the Maleate, Isopropamide as the Iodide), 100's
6030-16	**PROMETHAZINE DM (Ped) EXPECTORANT** ℞ 16 oz.
6930-16	**PROMETHAZINE w/CODEINE EXPECTORANT** ℞ © 16 oz.

Continued on next page

Geneva—Cont.

Code	Product
6635-16	PROMETHAZINE VC EXPECTORANT ℞ 16 oz.
6950-16	PROMETHAZINE VC ℞ © w/CODEINE EXPECTORANT 16 oz.
1855-01	PROPANTHELINE BROMIDE ℞ TABLETS 15mg., 100's
2140-01	PROPOXYPHENE HCl. ℞ © CAPSULES 65mg., 100's
2367-01	PROPOXYPHENE-AC ℞ © 100's
1378-01	PROPOXYPHENE HCl 65 ℞ © w/APAP 650mg., 100's
1535-01	PSEUDOEPHEDRINE TABLETS OTC 60mg., 100's
1804-01	QUINIDINE GLUCONATE S.R. TAB- ℞ LETS 324mg., 100's
1900-01	QUINIDINE SULFATE TABLETS ℞ 3 gr., 100's
2995-01	QUININE SULFATE CAPSULES OTC 200mg., 100's
2997-01	QUININE SULFATE CAPSULES OTC 5 gr., 100's
1926-01	QUIPHILE TABLETS ℞ Quinine Sulfate 260 mg., 100's
2427-01	RESAID T.D. CAPSULES ℞ (Phenylpropanolamine HCl., Chlorpheniramine Maleate) 100's
2847-01	RESCAPS-D T.D. CAPSULES ℞ (Caramiphen Edisylate, Phenylpropanolamine HCl.), 100's
1598-01	SPIRONOLACTONE TABLETS ℞ 25mg., 100's
1150-01	SPIRONOLACTONE (25mg.) ℞ w/HYDRO- CHLOROTHIAZIDE TABLETS 25mg., 100's
1261-01	SULFAMETHOXAZOLE TABLETS ℞ 500mg., 100's
1063-01	SULFAMETHOXAZOLE w/ ℞ TRIMETHOPRIM DS 100's
1062-01	SULFAMTHOXAZOLE w/ ℞ TRIMETHOPRIM SS 100's
1045-01	SULFASALAZINE TABLETS ℞ 500mg., 100's
1015-01	SULFISOXAZOLE TABLETS ℞ 500mg., 100's
1988-01	T.E.H. TABLETS ℞ (Ephedrine Sulfate, Theophylline, Hydroxyzine HCl.), 100's
1325-01	T.E.P. TABLETS OTC (Theophylline Anhydrous, Ephedrine HCl., Phenobarbital), 100's
6710-16	TAMINE ELIXIR ℞ 16 oz.
1153-01	TAMINE S.R. TABLETS ℞ (Brompheniramine Maleate, Phenylephrine Hydrochloride, Phenylpropanolamine Hydrochloride), 100's
6600-16	THEOPHYLLINE ELIXIR ℞ 16 oz.
	THEOPHYLLINE S.R. TABLETS ℞
1003-01	100 mg., 100's
1004-01	200 mg., 100's
1005-01	300mg., 100's
	THIORIDAZINE TABLETS
1604-01	10mg., 100's
1604-10	10mg., 1000's
1614-01	15mg., 100's
1614-10	15mg., 1000's
1624-01	25mg., 100's
1624-10	25mg., 1000's
1634-01	50mg., 100's
1634-10	50mg., 1000's
1644-01	100 mg., 100's
1644-10	100 mg., 1000's
1704-01	TOLBUTAMIDE TABLETS ℞ 0.5gm., 100's
	TRIAMCINOLONE ACETONIDE ℞ CREAM
7036-16	0.1%, 16 oz.
7030-16	0.025%, 16 oz.
1670-01	TRIAMCINOLONE TABLETS ℞ 4mg., 100's
1180-01	TRICHLORMETHIAZIDE ℞ TABLETS 4mg., 100's
1663-01	TRIFED TABLETS ℞ (Triprolidine HCl., Pseudoephedrine HCl.), 100's
6510-16	TRIFED SYRUP ℞ 16 oz.
	TRIFLUOPERAZINE TABLETS ℞
1030-01	1mg., 100's
1030-13	Unit Dose 100's
1032-01	2mg., 100's
1032-13	Unit Dose 100's
1034-01	5mg., 100's
1034-13	Unit Dose 100's
1036-01	10mg., 100's
1036-13	Unit Dose 100's
6005-52	TRIPLEVITE WITH FLUORIDE ℞ DROPS (Vitamin A, Vitamin D, Vitamin C, Fluoride), 1-50cc.
1340-01	UROBLUE TABLETS ℞ (Atropine Sulfate, Hyoscyamine, Methenamine, Methylene Blue, Phenyl Salicylate, Benzoic Acid), 100's

Products are cross-indexed by generic and chemical names in the **YELLOW SECTION**

Gerber Products Company
FREMONT, MI 49412

MBF* (Meat Base Formula) Liquid Hypoallergenic Infant Feeding Formula, Gerber

Ingredients: Water, beef hearts, cane sugar, sesame oil, modified tapioca starch, tricalcium phosphate, calcium citrate, potassium chloride, iodized salt, sodium ascorbate, magnesium chloride, ferrous sulfate, zinc sulfate, tocopheryl acetate, thiamin hydrochloride, calcium pantothenate, niacinamide, cupric sulfate, pyridoxine hydrochloride, vitamin A palmitate, riboflavin, phytonadione (vitamin K_1), folic acid, manganese sulfate, potassium iodide, biotin, vitamin D and vitamin B_{12}.
[See table below].

Action and Uses: A nutritionally adequate formula for infants and children intolerant to cow's and goat's milk whose symptoms may be diarrhea, colic, eczema, upper respiratory, etc. Useful in the management of milk sensitivity, lactase deficiency and milk induced steatorrhea.

Administration and Dosage: Provides 20 cal/fl.oz. when diluted 1:1; similar to other milk-based and soy-based infant formulas. Concentrated liquid added to previously boiled (not hot) water is to be divided among prescribed number of bottles, easily fed thru cross-cut nipples.

MBF's content of essential nutrients conforms to the infant formula standard established by the U.S. Food and Drug Administration in 1971 and the 1980 American Academy of Pediatrics infant formula recommendations.

Side Effects: None.
Precautions: None.
Contraindications: None.

How Supplied: Concentrated Liquid, 15 fl. oz. cans.

Literature Available: Yes.
*Trademark

	Undiluted Percentage Composition	Undiluted One 15 Fl. Oz. Can Contains	Diluted 1 to 1 5 Fl. Oz. Contain
Calories	40 per fl. oz.	600	100
Protein	5.1%	24g	4.0g
Fat	6.5%	30.6g	5.1g
Carbohydrates	12.0%	57.0g	9.5g
Water	75.5%	357g	133.4g
Linoleic Acid		1800mg	300mg
Vitamins:			
Vitamin A		1600IU	268IU
Vitamin D		240IU	40IU
Vitamin E		6.6IU	1.1IU
Vitamin K		24µg	4µg
Thiamin (Vitamin B_1)		540µg	90µg
Riboflavin (Vitamin B_2)		900µg	150µg
Vitamin B_6		780µg	130µg
Vitamin B_{12}		7.8µg	1.3µg
Niacin		3600µg	600µg
Folic Acid (Folacin)		24.0µg	4.0µg
Pantothenic Acid		1800µg	300µg
Biotin		9.0µg	1.5µg
Vitamin C (Ascorbic Acid)		54.0mg	9.0mg
Choline		90.0mg	15.0mg
Inositol		150.0mg	25.0mg
Minerals:			
Calcium		900mg	150mg
Phosphorus		600mg	100mg
Magnesium		36.0mg	6.0mg
Iron		12.0mg	2.0mg
Zinc		3.0mg	0.5mg
Manganese		30.0µg	5.0µg
Copper		360.0µg	60.0µg
Iodine		30.0µg	5.0µg
Sodium		246mg	41mg
Potassium		486mg	81mg
Chloride		438mg	73mg

Geriatric Pharm. Corp.
149 COVERT AVENUE
P.O. BOX 1098
NEW HYDE PARK, NY 11040

B-C-BID CAPSULES
B Complex with Vitamin C
SUSTAINED RELEASE
BY MICRODIALYSIS DIFFUSION

Composition: Each capsule contains: Vitamin B-1 15 mg., Vitamin B-2 10 mg., Vitamin B-6 5 mg., Niacinamide 50 mg., Calcium Pantothenate 10 mg., Vitamin C 300 mg., and Vitamin B-12 (Cyanocobalamin) 5 mcg.
Medication is released at a smooth, continuous, predictable rate dependent only upon the presence of fluid in the G.I. tract, and not dependent on pH and other variables. *No regurgitation; no aftertaste.*
On b.i.d. dosage, this smooth, continuous release of B-C-BID's essential vitamins frees your patient from the "peak and valley" effect of ordinary capsules or tablets.
Dosage: For continuous 24 hour therapy, one capsule after breakfast and one after supper.

CEVI-BID Capsules (500 mg. Vitamin C)
SUSTAINED RELEASE
BY MICRO-DIALYSIS DIFFUSION

Composition: Each CEVI-BID capsule contains 500 mg. Vitamin C.
Action and Uses: For treatment of Vitamin C deficiency. CEVI-BID maintains optimal blood levels of Vitamin C around the clock on b.i.d. dosage, and avoids "peak and valley" effects of ordinary Vitamin C tablets. Medication is released at a smooth, continuous, predictable rate dependent only upon the presence of fluid in the G.I. tract and independent of pH or other variables.
Dosage: For continuous 24 hour therapy, one capsule after breakfast and one after supper.

CEVI-FER CAPSULES ℞
Hematinic with 300 mg Vitamin C
SUSTAINED RELEASE BY
MICRO-DIALYSIS DIFFUSION

Composition: CEVI-FER capsules contain *Ferrous Fumarate 60 mg. (Equivalent to 20 mg. elemental iron), *Ascorbic Acid 300 mg., Folic Acid 1 mg.
*Prepared in a special base for prolonged therapeutic effect.
Ferrous fumarate and ascorbic acid are released at a smooth, continuous, predictable rate dependent only upon the presence of fluid in the G.I. tract; not dependent on the variable digestive processes.
Action and Uses: Acute and/or severe iron deficiency anemia, also as a maintenance hematinic where daily supplementation is required.
Advantages: The special medication release pattern (sustained release by micro-dialysis diffusion) provides continuous release of ascorbic acid and ferrous fumarate over a 24 hour period on b.i.d. dosage. Thus gastric distress and constipation are largely avoided.
Clinical studies have proven that ascorbic acid tends to enhance iron absorption. The ferrous form of iron is better absorbed and utilized than the ferric form. Virtually eliminates black stools.
Precautions: Folic acid in doses above 0.1 mg. daily may obscure pernicious anemia, in that hematologic remission may occur while neurological manifestations remain progressive.
Adverse Reactions: Allergic sensitivity reactions may occur.
Dosage: One capsule a day. In severe anemias, one capsule after breakfast and supper for two weeks, then one capsule a day.

GER-O-FOAM™ Analgesic Anesthetic Foam

Composition: Aerosol foam containing methyl salicylate 30% and benzocaine 3% in a specially-processed oil emulsion.
Action and Uses: For topical application in alleviating minor pains of musculoskeletal conditions such as rheumatoid and osteoarthritis and low back pain. GER-O-FOAM permits increased range of motion by decreasing pain.
Administration and Dosage: Massage into affected area 2 or 3 times daily.
Precautions: If a rash or irritation occurs, discontinue. Avoid application in or near eyes, mucous membranes or open wounds.
How Supplied: 4 oz. Aerosol cans.

GUSTASE®
Gastrointestinal Enzyme Tablets

Composition: Each GUSTASE tablet contains GERILASE (standardized amylolytic enzyme) 30 mg., GERIPROTASE (standardized proteolytic enzyme) 6 mg., GERICELLULASE (standardized cellulolytic enzyme) 2 mg.
Action and Uses: GUSTASE is indicated in dyspepsia, colitis, flatulence, diverticulitis, abdominal distension, etc. GUSTASE is effective in a broad pH spectrum (3–10), and is not enteric coated.
Administration and Dosage: One tablet during or immediately after meals.

ISO–BID® CAPSULES 40 mg. ℞
SUSTAINED RELEASE BY
MICRO-DIALYSIS DIFFUSION

Composition: Each ISO-BID SUSTAINED-MEDICATION CAPSULE contains 40 mg. Isosorbide Dinitrate. Medication is released at a smooth, continuous, predictable rate dependent only upon the presence of fluid in the G.I. tract; not dependent on the variable digestive processes.
Mode of Action: The mechanism of action of ISO-BID, like all nitrates, is the relaxation of smooth muscle. The relationship between this and its clinical usefulness is obscure, since the exact cause of anginal pain is presently unknown. ISO-BID is intended to decrease the frequency and severity of anginal attacks, and thus effect a decrease in the need for nitroglycerin. These should be the criteria for the success of ISO-BID therapy, since there is a wide variation in symptomatic response to treatment. Isosorbide Dinitrate is widely accepted as a safe and useful therapeutic agent in the treatment of angina pectoris.

> **Indications:** Based on a review of this drug by the National Academy of Sciences—National Research Council and/or other information, FDA has classified the indications as follows:
> *Effective:* When taken orally ISO-BID SUSTAINED MEDICATION CAPSULES are indicated for the relief of angina pectoris (pain of coronary artery disease). ISO-BID SUSTAINED RELEASE CAPSULES are not intended to abort the acute anginal episode, but are widely regarded as useful in the prophylactic treatment of angina pectoris. Final classification of the less-than-effective indication requires further investigation.

Contraindication: Idiosyncrasy to this drug.
Warnings: Data supporting the use of nitrites during the early days of the acute phase of myocardial infarction (the period during which clinical and laboratory findings are unstable) are insufficient to establish safety.
Precautions: Use with caution in patients with glaucoma. Tolerance to this drug, and cross-tolerance to other nitrites and nitrates may occur.
Patients with gastric hypermotility for any reason, where the duration of passage through the gastrointestinal tract may be less than normal, should take sublingual nitroglycerin rather than sustained release medications.
Adverse Reactions: Cutaneous vasodilation with flushing. Headache may commonly occur, and may be both severe and persistent. Transient dizziness and weakness, in addition to other signs of cerebral ischemia associated with postural hypotension may occasionally be seen. ISO-BID can act as a physiological antagonist to norepinephrine, histamine, acetylcholine and many other medications. An occasional patient may show marked sensitivity to the hypotensive effects of nitrite; severe responses (nausea, vomiting, weakness, restlessness, pallor, excessive sweating and collapse) can occur, even with the usual therapeutic dosage. Alcohol may enhance this effect. A drug rash and/or exfoliative dermatitis is occasionally seen.
Dosage: One 40mg. ISO-BID CAPSULE every 12 hours on an empty stomach according to need, for continuous 24-hour therapy. This dosage schedule is particularly convenient in the management of nocturnal angina. Some patients may require higher dosage levels. In these patients, dosage should be titrated, and may require two ISO-BID - CAPSULES b.i.d.

EDUCATIONAL MATERIAL

Brochures and samples available on all Geriatric Phamaceutical Products.

Gilbert Laboratories
31 FAIRMOUNT AVENUE
CHESTER, NEW JERSEY 07930

ESGIC® ℞
[es'jik]
Tablets and Capsules

Description: Each ESGIC tablet or capsule for oral administration contains:
Butalbital*   50 mg.
   (isobutylallylbarbituric acid)
***Warning:** May be habit forming
Acetaminophen   325 mg.
Caffeine   40 mg.
Butalbital, 5-allyl-5-isobutyl-barbituric acid, a white, odorless crystalline powder having a slightly bitter taste, is an intermediate-acting barbiturate.
Acetaminophen, N-acetyl-p-aminophenol, occurs as a white, odorless crystalline powder, possessing a slightly bitter taste. Acetaminophen is a non-salicylate, non-narcotic analgesic, and antipyretic.
Caffeine, 1,3,7-trimethylxanthine, is a white crystalline, glistening substance soluble in water to the extent of 1:50.
Clinical Pharmacology: Pharmacologically, ESGIC combines the analgesic properties of acetaminophen-caffeine with the anxiolytic and muscle relaxant properties of butalbital (isobutylallylbarbituric acid). Acetaminophen may be used safely by most persons sensitive to aspirin.
Indications: ESGIC is indicated for the relief of the symptom complex of stress (or muscle contraction) headache.
Contraindications: Hypersensitivity to acetaminophen, caffeine, or barbiturates. Patients with porphyria.
Precautions:
1. **General:** Barbiturates should be administered with caution, if at all, to patients who are mentally depressed, have suicidal tendencies, or a history of drug abuse.
Elderly or debilitated patients may react to barbiturates with marked excitement, depression, and confusion. In some persons, barbiturates repeatedly produce excitement rather than depression.
2. **Information for the Patient:** Practitioners should give the following information and instructions to patients receiving barbiturates.
   1. The use of barbiturates carries with it an associated risk of psychological and/or physical dependence. The patient should be warned against increasing the dose of the drug without consulting a physician.

Continued on next page

Gilbert—Cont.

2. Barbiturates may impair mental and/or physical abilities required for the performance of potentially hazardous tasks (e.g., driving, operating machinery, etc.).
3. Alcohol should not be consumed while taking barbiturates. Concurrent use of the barbiturates with other CNS depressants (e.g., alcohol, narcotics, tranquilizers, and antihistamines) may result in additional CNS depressant effects.

3. **Drug Interactions:** Patients receiving narcotic analgesics, antipsychotics, antianxiety agents, or other CNS depressants (including alcohol) concomitantly with ESGIC may exhibit additive CNS depressant effects.

DRUGS	EFFECT
Butalbital with coumarin anticoagulants	Decreased effect of anticoagulant because of increased metabolism resulting from enzyme induction
Butalbital with tricyclic antidepressants	Decreased blood levels of the antidepressant

4. **Usage in Pregnancy:** Adequate studies have not been performed in animals to determine whether this drug affects fertility in males or females, has teratogenic potential or has other adverse effects on the fetus. There are no well-controlled studies in pregnant women. Although there is no clearly defined risk, one cannot exclude the possibility of infrequent or subtle damage to the human fetus. ESGIC should be used in pregnant women only when clearly needed.
5. **Nursing Mothers:** The effects of ESGIC on infants of nursing mothers are not known. Barbiturates are excreted in the breast milk of nursing mothers. The serum levels in infants are believed to be insignificant with therapeutic doses.
6. **Pediatric Use:** Safety and effectiveness in children below the age of 12 have not been established.

Adverse Reactions: The most frequent adverse reactions are drowsiness and dizziness. Less frequent adverse reactions are lightheadedness and nausea. Mental confusion or depression can occur due to intolerance or overdosage of butalbital.

Drug Abuse and Dependence: Prolonged use of barbiturates can produce drug dependence, characterized by psychic dependence and tolerance. The abuse liability of ESGIC is similar to that of other barbiturate-containing drug combinations. Caution should be exercised when prescribing medication for patients with a known propensity for taking excessive quantities of drugs, which is not uncommon in patients with chronic stress headache.

Overdosage: The toxic effects of acute overdosage of ESGIC are attributable mainly to its barbiturate component, and, to a lesser extent, acetaminophen. Because toxic effects of caffeine occur in very high dosages only, the possibility of significant caffeine toxicity from ESGIC overdosage is unlikely.

Barbiturate Poisoning:
Symptoms: Drowsiness, confusion, coma; respiratory depression; hypotension; shock.
Treatment:
1. Maintenance of an adequate airway, with assisted respiration and oxygen administration as necessary.
2. Monitoring of vital signs and fluid balance.
3. If the patient is conscious and has not lost the gag reflex, emesis may be induced with ipecac. Care should be taken to prevent pulmonary aspiration of vomitus. After completion of vomiting, 30 grams activated charcoal in a glass of water may be administered.
4. If emesis is contraindicated, gastric lavage may be performed with a cuffed endotracheal tube in place with the patient in the face down position. Activated charcoal may be left in the emptied stomach and a saline cathartic administered.
5. Fluid therapy and other standard treatment for shock, if needed.
6. If renal function is normal, forced diuresis may aid in the elimination of the barbiturate. Alkalinization of the urine increases renal excretion of some barbiturates.
7. Although not recommended as a routine procedure, hemodialysis may be used in severe barbiturate intoxications or if the patient is anuric or in shock.

Acetaminophen Poisoning:
Symptoms: Acetaminophen in massive overdosage may cause hepatic toxicity in some patients. In all cases of suspected overdose, immediately call your regional poison center or The Rocky Mountain Poison Center's toll-free number (800-525-6115) for assistance in diagnosis and for directions in the use of N-acetylcysteine as an antidote, a use currently restricted to investigational status.
In adults, hepatic toxicity has rarely been reported with acute overdoses of less than 10 grams and fatalities with less than 15 grams. Importantly, young children seem to be more resistant than adults to the hepatotoxic effect of an acetaminophen overdose.
Early symptoms following a potentially hepatotoxic overdose may include: nausea, vomiting, diaphoresis and general malaise. Clinical and laboratory evidence of hepatic toxicity may not be apparent until 48 to 72 hours post-ingestion.
Treatment: The stomach should be emptied promptly by lavage or by induction of emesis with syrup of ipecac. Patients' estimates of the quantity of a drug ingested are notoriously unreliable. Therefore, if an acetaminophen overdose is suspected, a serum acetaminophen assay should be obtained as early as possible, but no sooner than four hours following ingestion. Liver function studies should be obtained initially and repeated at 24-hour intervals.
The antidote, N-acetylcysteine, should be administered as early as possible, and within 16 hours of the overdose ingestion for optimal results. Following recovery, there are no residual, structural or functional hepatic abnormalities.

Dosage and Administration:
Oral: One or two tablets or capsules every four hours as needed. Do not exceed six tablets or capsules per day.

How Supplied:
ESGIC tablets: white, round, compressed tablet imprinted with Gilbert Laboratories logo on one side and NDC 535-11 on the opposite side. Supplied in bottles of 100 tablets. NDC #0535-0011-01.
ESGIC capsules: white, opaque capsules imprinted with Gilbert Laboratories logo and NDC 535-12 in black print. Supplied in bottles of 100 capsules. NDC #0535-0012-01.
Revised 07/84
Shown in Product Identification Section, page 411

EDUCATIONAL MATERIAL

Brochures:
Gilbert Headache Questionnaire
(Diagnostic aid for patient to fill out)
Patient Headache Information Brochure
(A handout for doctor to give patient)
ESGIC SAMPLES available on physician request

Products are
listed alphabetically
in the
PINK SECTION.

Glaxo Inc.
FIVE MOORE DRIVE
RESEARCH TRIANGLE PARK, NC
27709

B C G VACCINE, USP ℞
For Intradermal Use Only
Freeze-Dried

Description: BCG Vaccine, USP, is a standardized preparation of dried living culture of the bacillus Calmette-Guérin (BCG) strain of *Mycobacterium tuberculosis* var. *bovis* for use in immunization against tuberculosis using the intradermal route. It is prepared from a Glaxo culture of the Danish 1077 substrain of BCG. The organisms are harvested, suspended in a medium consisting of suitable concentrations of dextran, glucose, and Triton WR 1339 (90% tyloxapol in water), and then freeze-dried to give a product free from microorganisms other than BCG. This vaccine, when reconstituted as directed, contains not less than 8 million and not more than 26 million colony-forming units per ml.

Clinical Pharmacology: BCG Vaccine induces active immunity to tuberculosis. After proper intradermal injection of the immunizing dose, the initial skin lesion usually appears within 7 to 10 days. The normal lesion consists of a small red papule at the site of injection: it reaches its maximum diameter of approximately 8 mm after about 5 weeks. The top of the papule scales, ulcerates and dries, and the whole lesion gradually shrinks to a smooth or scaly pink or bluish scar approximately 3 months after vaccination and becomes a smooth or pitted white scar in approximately 6 months.
Vaccinated persons normally become tuberculin positive (Mantoux test) after a period of 8 weeks has elapsed, but sometimes up to 14 weeks are needed.
A postvaccinal tuberculin test should be conducted 2 to 3 months after vaccination. If the test is negative, the vaccination should be repeated.

Indications and Usage: BCG Vaccine is indicated for the prevention of tuberculosis. The Advisory Committee on Immunization Practices of the U.S. Public Health Service has made the following specific recommendations[1] for the use of BCG Vaccine.
1. BCG vaccination should be seriously considered for persons who have negative tuberculin skin tests and repeated exposure to persistently untreated or ineffectively treated sputum-positive cases of pulmonary tuberculosis.
2. BCG vaccination should be considered for well-defined communities or groups if an excessive rate of new infections can be demonstrated and the usual surveillance and treatment programs have failed or have been shown not to be applicable.

Contraindications: BCG Vaccine is contraindicated in tuberculin-positive individuals, subjects with fresh smallpox vaccinations, and burn patients. In addition, BCG Vaccine should not be given to individuals being given prolonged treatment with corticosteroids or other immunosuppressive therapy or to those with hypogammaglobulinemia or any other disorder in which the natural immunologic capacity of the host may be altered (eg, AIDS).

Warnings: BCG vaccination has been associated with adverse reactions, including severe or prolonged ulceration at the vaccination site, lymphadenitis, osteomyelitis, disseminated BCG infection, and death. Systemic treatment with anti-tubercular chemotherapy (such as isoniazid, rifampin or streptomycin) should be given where generalized infection with BCG is suspected. In cases of severe local reactions with abscess formation, aspiration should be carried out, perhaps with streptomycin replacement.

Precautions: General: There has been the occasional report of an anaphylactic reaction after BCG Vaccine but, in keeping with good medical practice, epinephrine should be available.

Geriatric Pharm. Corp.
149 COVERT AVENUE
P.O. BOX 1098
NEW HYDE PARK, NY 11040

B-C-BID CAPSULES
B Complex with Vitamin C
SUSTAINED RELEASE
BY MICRODIALYSIS DIFFUSION

Composition: Each capsule contains: Vitamin B-1 15 mg., Vitamin B-2 10 mg., Vitamin B-6 5 mg., Niacinamide 50 mg., Calcium Pantothenate 10 mg., Vitamin C 300 mg., and Vitamin B-12 (Cyanocobalamin) 5 mcg.

Medication is released at a smooth, continuous, predictable rate dependent only upon the presence of fluid in the G.I. tract, and not dependent on pH and other variables. *No regurgitation; no aftertaste.*

On b.i.d. dosage, this smooth, continuous release of B-C-BID's essential vitamins frees your patient from the "peak and valley" effect of ordinary capsules or tablets.

Dosage: For continuous 24 hour therapy, one capsule after breakfast and one after supper.

CEVI-BID Capsules (500 mg. Vitamin C)
SUSTAINED RELEASE
BY MICRO-DIALYSIS DIFFUSION

Composition: Each CEVI-BID capsule contains 500 mg. Vitamin C.

Action and Uses: For treatment of Vitamin C deficiency. CEVI-BID maintains optimal blood levels of Vitamin C around the clock on b.i.d. dosage, and avoids "peak and valley" effects of ordinary Vitamin C tablets. Medication is released at a smooth, continuous, predictable rate dependent only upon the presence of fluid in the G.I. tract and independent of pH or other variables.

Dosage: For continuous 24 hour therapy, one capsule after breakfast and one after supper.

CEVI–FER CAPSULES ℞
Hematinic with 300 mg Vitamin C
SUSTAINED RELEASE BY
MICRO-DIALYSIS DIFFUSION

Composition: CEVI-FER capsules contain *Ferrous Fumarate 60 mg. (Equivalent to 20 mg. elemental iron), *Ascorbic Acid 300 mg., Folic Acid 1 mg.
*Prepared in a special base for prolonged therapeutic effect.

Ferrous fumarate and ascorbic acid are released at a smooth, continuous, predictable rate dependent only upon the presence of fluid in the G.I. tract; not dependent on the variable digestive processes.

Action and Uses: Acute and/or severe iron deficiency anemia, also as a maintenance hematinic where daily supplementation is required.

Advantages: The special medication release pattern (sustained release by micro-dialysis diffusion) provides continuous release of ascorbic acid and ferrous fumarate over a 24 hour period on b.i.d. dosage. Thus gastric distress and constipation are largely avoided.

Clinical studies have proven that ascorbic acid tends to enhance iron absorption. The ferrous form of iron is better absorbed and utilized than the ferric form. Virtually eliminates black stools.

Precautions: Folic acid in doses above 0.1 mg. daily may obscure pernicious anemia, in that hematologic remission may occur while neurological manifestations remain progressive.

Adverse Reactions: Allergic sensitivity reactions may occur.

Dosage: One capsule a day. In severe anemias, one capsule after breakfast and supper for two weeks, then one capsule a day.

GER-O-FOAM™ Analgesic Anesthetic Foam

Composition: Aerosol foam containing methyl salicylate 30% and benzocaine 3% in a specially-processed oil emulsion.

Action and Uses: For topical application in alleviating minor pains of musculoskeletal conditions such as rheumatoid and osteoarthritis and low back pain. GER-O-FOAM permits increased range of motion by decreasing pain.

Administration and Dosage: Massage into affected area 2 or 3 times daily.

Precautions: If a rash or irritation occurs, discontinue. Avoid application in or near eyes, mucous membranes or open wounds.

How Supplied: 4 oz. Aerosol cans.

GUSTASE®
Gastrointestinal Enzyme Tablets

Composition: Each GUSTASE tablet contains GERILASE (standardized amylolytic enzyme) 30 mg., GERIPROTASE (standardized proteolytic enzyme) 6 mg., GERICELLULASE (standardized cellulolytic enzyme) 2 mg.

Action and Uses: GUSTASE is indicated in dyspepsia, colitis, flatulence, diverticulitis, abdominal distension, etc. GUSTASE is effective in a broad pH spectrum (3–10), and is not enteric coated.

Administration and Dosage: One tablet during or immediately after meals.

ISO–BID® CAPSULES 40 mg. ℞
SUSTAINED RELEASE BY
MICRO-DIALYSIS DIFFUSION

Composition: Each ISO-BID SUSTAINED-MEDICATION CAPSULE contains 40 mg. Isosorbide Dinitrate. Medication is released at a smooth, continuous, predictable rate dependent only upon the presence of fluid in the G.I. tract; not dependent on the variable digestive processes.

Mode of Action: The mechanism of action of ISO-BID, like all nitrates, is the relaxation of smooth muscle. The relationship between this and its clinical usefulness is obscure, since the exact cause of anginal pain is presently unknown. ISO-BID is intended to decrease the frequency and severity of anginal attacks, and thus effect a decrease in the need for nitroglycerin. These should be the criteria for the success of ISO-BID therapy, since there is a wide variation in symptomatic response to treatment. Isosorbide Dinitrate is widely accepted as a safe and useful therapeutic agent in the treatment of angina pectoris.

> **Indications:** Based on a review of this drug by the National Academy of Sciences—National Research Council and/or other information, FDA has classified the indications as follows:
> *Effective:* When taken orally ISO-BID SUSTAINED MEDICATION CAPSULES are indicated for the relief of angina pectoris (pain of coronary artery disease). ISO-BID SUSTAINED RELEASE CAPSULES are not intended to abort the acute anginal episode, but are widely regarded as useful in the prophylactic treatment of angina pectoris. Final classification of the less-than-effective indication requires further investigation.

Contraindication: Idiosyncrasy to this drug.

Warnings: Data supporting the use of nitrites during the early days of the acute phase of myocardial infarction (the period during which clinical and laboratory findings are unstable) are insufficient to establish safety.

Precautions: Use with caution in patients with glaucoma. Tolerance to this drug, and cross-tolerance to other nitrites and nitrates may occur.

Patients with gastric hypermotility for any reason, where the duration of passage through the gastrointestinal tract may be less than normal, should take sublingual nitroglycerin rather than sustained release medications.

Adverse Reactions: Cutaneous vasodilation with flushing. Headache may commonly occur, and may be both severe and persistent. Transient dizziness and weakness, in addition to other signs of cerebral ischemia associated with postural hypotension may occasionally be seen. ISO-BID can act as a physiological antagonist to norepinephrine, histamine, acetylcholine and many other medications. An occasional patient may show marked sensitivity to the hypotensive effects of nitrite; severe responses (nausea, vomiting, weakness, restlessness, pallor, excessive sweating and collapse) can occur, even with the usual therapeutic dosage. Alcohol may enhance this effect. A drug rash and/or exfoliative dermatitis is occasionally seen.

Dosage: One 40mg. ISO-BID CAPSULE every 12 hours on an empty stomach according to need, for continuous 24-hour therapy. This dosage schedule is particularly convenient in the management of nocturnal angina. Some patients may require higher dosage levels. In these patients, dosage should be titrated, and may require two ISO-BID - CAPSULES b.i.d.

EDUCATIONAL MATERIAL

Brochures and samples available on all Geriatric Phamaceutical Products.

Gilbert Laboratories
31 FAIRMOUNT AVENUE
CHESTER, NEW JERSEY 07930

ESGIC® ℞
[es′jik]
Tablets and Capsules

Description: Each ESGIC tablet or capsule for oral administration contains:
Butalbital*   50 mg.
 (isobutylallylbarbituric acid)
*Warning: May be habit forming
Acetaminophen   325 mg.
Caffeine   40 mg.

Butalbital, 5-allyl-5-isobutyl-barbituric acid, a white, odorless crystalline powder having a slightly bitter taste, is an intermediate-acting barbiturate.

Acetaminophen, N-acetyl-p-aminophenol, occurs as a white, odorless crystalline powder, possessing a slightly bitter taste. Acetaminophen is a non-salicylate, non-narcotic analgesic, and antipyretic.

Caffeine, 1,3,7-trimethylxanthine, is a white crystalline, glistening substance soluble in water to the extent of 1:50.

Clinical Pharmacology: Pharmacologically, ESGIC combines the analgesic properties of acetaminophen-caffeine with the anxiolytic and muscle relaxant properties of butalbital (isobutylallylbarbituric acid). Acetaminophen may be used safely by most persons sensitive to aspirin.

Indications: ESGIC is indicated for the relief of the symptom complex of stress (or muscle contraction) headache.

Contraindications: Hypersensitivity to acetaminophen, caffeine, or barbiturates. Patients with porphyria.

Precautions:
1. **General:** Barbiturates should be administered with caution, if at all, to patients who are mentally depressed, have suicidal tendencies, or a history of drug abuse.
   Elderly or debilitated patients may react to barbiturates with marked excitement, depression, and confusion. In some persons, barbiturates repeatedly produce excitement rather than depression.
2. **Information for the Patient:** Practitioners should give the following information and instructions to patients receiving barbiturates.
   1. The use of barbiturates carries with it an associated risk of psychological and/or physical dependence. The patient should be warned against increasing the dose of the drug without consulting a physician.

Continued on next page

Gilbert—Cont.

2. Barbiturates may impair mental and/or physical abilities required for the performance of potentially hazardous tasks (e.g., driving, operating machinery, etc.).
3. Alcohol should not be consumed while taking barbiturates. Concurrent use of the barbiturates with other CNS depressants (e.g., alcohol, narcotics, tranquilizers, and antihistamines) may result in additional CNS depressant effects.
3. **Drug Interactions:** Patients receiving narcotic analgesics, antipsychotics, antianxiety agents, or other CNS depressants (including alcohol) concomitantly with ESGIC may exhibit additive CNS depressant effects.

DRUGS	EFFECT
Butalbital with coumarin anticoagulants	Decreased effect of anticoagulant because of increased metabolism resulting from enzyme induction
Butalbital with tricyclic antidepressants	Decreased blood levels of the antidepressant

4. **Usage in Pregnancy:** Adequate studies have not been performed in animals to determine whether this drug affects fertility in males or females, has teratogenic potential or has other adverse effects on the fetus. There are no well-controlled studies in pregnant women. Although there is no clearly defined risk, one cannot exclude the possibility of infrequent or subtle damage to the human fetus. ESGIC should be used in pregnant women only when clearly needed.
5. **Nursing Mothers:** The effects of ESGIC on infants of nursing mothers are not known. Barbiturates are excreted in the breast milk of nursing mothers. The serum levels in infants are believed to be insignificant with therapeutic doses.
6. **Pediatric Use:** Safety and effectiveness in children below the age of 12 have not been established.

Adverse Reactions: The most frequent adverse reactions are drowsiness and dizziness. Less frequent adverse reactions are lightheadedness and nausea. Mental confusion or depression can occur due to intolerance or overdosage of butalbital.

Drug Abuse and Dependence: Prolonged use of barbiturates can produce drug dependence, characterized by psychic dependence and tolerance. The abuse liability of ESGIC is similar to that of other barbiturate-containing drug combinations. Caution should be exercised when prescribing medication for patients with a known propensity for taking excessive quantities of drugs, which is not uncommon in patients with chronic stress headache.

Overdosage: The toxic effects of acute overdosage of ESGIC are attributable mainly to its barbiturate component, and, to a lesser extent, acetaminophen. Because toxic effects of caffeine occur in very high dosages only, the possibility of significant caffeine toxicity from ESGIC overdosage is unlikely.

Barbiturate Poisoning:
Symptoms: Drowsiness, confusion, coma; respiratory depression; hypotension; shock.
Treatment:
1. Maintenance of an adequate airway, with assisted respiration and oxygen administration as necessary.
2. Monitoring of vital signs and fluid balance.
3. If the patient is conscious and has not lost the gag reflex, emesis may be induced with ipecac. Care should be taken to prevent pulmonary aspiration of vomitus. After completion of vomiting, 30 grams activated charcoal in a glass of water may be administered.
4. If emesis is contraindicated, gastric lavage may be performed with a cuffed endotracheal tube in place with the patient in the face down position. Activated charcoal may be left in the emptied stomach and a saline cathartic administered.
5. Fluid therapy and other standard treatment for shock, if needed.
6. If renal function is normal, forced diuresis may aid in the elimination of the barbiturate. Alkalinization of the urine increases renal excretion of some barbiturates.
7. Although not recommended as a routine procedure, hemodialysis may be used in severe barbiturate intoxications or if the patient is anuric or in shock.

Acetaminophen Poisoning:
Symptoms: Acetaminophen in massive overdosage may cause hepatic toxicity in some patients. In all cases of suspected overdose, immediately call your regional poison center or The Rocky Mountain Poison Center's toll-free number (800-525-6115) for assistance in diagnosis and for directions in the use of N-acetylcysteine as an antidote, a use currently restricted to investigational status.
In adults, hepatic toxicity has rarely been reported with acute overdoses of less than 10 grams and fatalities with less than 15 grams. Importantly, young children seem to be more resistant than adults to the hepatotoxic effect of an acetaminophen overdose.
Early symptoms following a potentially hepatotoxic overdose may include: nausea, vomiting, diaphoresis and general malaise. Clinical and laboratory evidence of hepatic toxicity may not be apparent until 48 to 72 hours post-ingestion.
Treatment: The stomach should be emptied promptly by lavage or by induction of emesis with syrup of ipecac. Patients' estimates of the quantity of a drug ingested are notoriously unreliable. Therefore, if an acetaminophen overdose is suspected, a serum acetaminophen assay should be obtained as early as possible, but no sooner than four hours following ingestion. Liver function studies should be obtained initially and repeated at 24-hour intervals.
The antidote, N-acetylcysteine, should be administered as early as possible, and within 16 hours of the overdose ingestion for optimal results. Following recovery, there are no residual, structural or functional hepatic abnormalities.

Dosage and Administration:
Oral: One or two tablets or capsules every four hours as needed. Do not exceed six tablets or capsules per day.
How Supplied:
ESGIC tablets: white, round, compressed tablet imprinted with Gilbert Laboratories logo on one side and NDC 535-11 on the opposite side. Supplied in bottles of 100 tablets. NDC #0535-0011-01.
ESGIC capsules: white, opaque capsules imprinted with Gilbert Laboratories logo and NDC 535-12 in black print. Supplied in bottles of 100 capsules. NDC #0535-0012-01.
Revised 07/84
Shown in Product Identification Section, page 411

EDUCATIONAL MATERIAL

Brochures:
Gilbert Headache Questionnaire
(Diagnostic aid for patient to fill out)
Patient Headache Information Brochure
(A handout for doctor to give patient)
ESGIC SAMPLES available on physician request

Products are
listed alphabetically
in the
PINK SECTION.

Glaxo Inc.
FIVE MOORE DRIVE
RESEARCH TRIANGLE PARK, NC
27709

B C G VACCINE, USP ℞
For Intradermal Use Only
Freeze–Dried

Description: BCG Vaccine, USP, is a standardized preparation of dried living culture of the bacillus Calmette-Guérin (BCG) strain of *Mycobacterium tuberculosis* var. *bovis* for use in immunization against tuberculosis using the intradermal route. It is prepared from a Glaxo culture of the Danish 1077 substrain of BCG. The organisms are harvested, suspended in a medium consisting of suitable concentrations of dextran, glucose, and Triton WR 1339 (90% tyloxapol in water), and then freeze-dried to give a product free from microorganisms other than BCG. This vaccine, when reconstituted as directed, contains not less than 8 million and not more than 26 million colony-forming units per ml.

Clinical Pharmacology: BCG Vaccine induces active immunity to tuberculosis. After proper intradermal injection of the immunizing dose, the initial skin lesion usually appears within 7 to 10 days. The normal lesion consists of a small red papule at the site of injection: it reaches its maximum diameter of approximately 8 mm after about 5 weeks. The top of the papule scales, ulcerates and dries, and the whole lesion gradually shrinks to a smooth or scaly pink or bluish scar approximately 3 months after vaccination and becomes a smooth or pitted white scar in approximately 6 months.
Vaccinated persons normally become tuberculin positive (Mantoux test) after a period of 8 weeks has elapsed, but sometimes up to 14 weeks are needed.
A postvaccinal tuberculin test should be conducted 2 to 3 months after vaccination. If the test is negative, the vaccination should be repeated.

Indications and Usage: BCG Vaccine is indicated for the prevention of tuberculosis. The Advisory Committee on Immunization Practices of the U.S. Public Health Service has made the following specific recommendations[1] for the use of BCG Vaccine.
1. BCG vaccination should be seriously considered for persons who have negative tuberculin skin tests and repeated exposure to persistently untreated or ineffectively treated sputum-positive cases of pulmonary tuberculosis.
2. BCG vaccination should be considered for well-defined communities or groups if an excessive rate of new infections can be demonstrated and the usual surveillance and treatment programs have failed or have been shown not to be applicable.

Contraindications: BCG Vaccine is contraindicated in tuberculin-positive individuals, subjects with fresh smallpox vaccinations, and burn patients. In addition, BCG Vaccine should not be given to individuals being given prolonged treatment with corticosteroids or other immunosuppressive therapy or to those with hypogammaglobulinemia or any other disorder in which the natural immunologic capacity of the host may be altered (eg, AIDS).

Warnings: BCG vaccination has been associated with adverse reactions, including severe or prolonged ulceration at the vaccination site, lymphadenitis, osteomyelitis, disseminated BCG infection, and death. Systemic treatment with anti-tubercular chemotherapy (such as isoniazid, rifampin or streptomycin) should be given where generalized infection with BCG is suspected. In cases of severe local reactions with abscess formation, aspiration should be carried out, perhaps with streptomycin replacement.

Precautions: General: There has been the occasional report of an anaphylactic reaction after BCG Vaccine but, in keeping with good medical practice, epinephrine should be available.

Although chronic diseases involving the skin are not contraindications, individuals with such conditions should be vaccinated in a healthy area of skin.

BCG vaccination is not normally undertaken without prior determination that the patient is nonreactive to a tuberculin skin test. The individual to be vaccinated should first be tuberculin-tested by a suitable method. A Mantoux test at 5 T.U. of Tuberculin P.P.D. (Purified Protein Derivative) is suitable. If this test is negative, the person may be vaccinated immediately. The test should be performed within the 6-week period preceding vaccination. The protection from tuberculosis afforded by BCG vaccination is only relative and is not permanent or entirely predictable. If the tuberculin test again becomes negative and the risk of infection continues, BCG vaccination may need to be repeated.

Interpretation of Tuberculin Test—After BCG vaccination, it is usually not possible to distinguish between a tuberculin reaction caused by virulent supra-infection and a reaction resulting from persistent postvaccination sensitivity. Therefore, caution is advised in attributing a positive skin test to BCG (except in the immediate postvaccination period), especially if the vaccinee has recently been exposed to infective tuberculosis.

Tuberculosis in Vaccinated Persons—Since full, lasting protection from BCG vaccination cannot be assured, tuberculosis should be included in the differential diagnosis of any tuberculosis-like illness in a BCG vaccinee.

Drug Interactions: BCG Vaccine will not be effective if given during treatment with isoniazid, rifampin, streptomycin or other drugs, which inhibit multiplication of BCG.

BCG Vaccine may be given at the same time as oral poliomyelitis vaccine. With other live vaccines it is preferable to allow an interval of three weeks between administration of BCG and the other vaccine, but the interval can be reduced to ten days if a longer period is not available.

In general, vaccines containing toxoids or killed organisms should be given at least seven days before BCG Vaccine, or ten days after. However, diphtheria/tetanus vaccine has been given at the same time as BCG Vaccine (but in different arms) with satisfactory results.[2]

Usage in Pregnancy: Pregnancy Category C: Animal reproduction studies have not been conducted with BCG Vaccine. It is also not known whether BCG Vaccine can cause fetal harm when administered to a pregnant woman or can affect reproduction capacity. BCG Vaccine should be given to a pregnant woman only if clearly needed.

Adverse Reactions: The Glaxo BCG strain used has proved to be associated with a very low incidence of untoward reactions.

However, BCG vaccination has been associated with adverse reactions, including severe or prolonged ulceration at the vaccination site, lymphadenitis, osteomyelitis, disseminated BCG infection, and death. The reported frequency of complications, mostly from other countries, has varied greatly, depending on the substrain of BCG used and on the extent of the surveillance effort. For example, the occurrence of ulceration and lymphadenitis has been reported to range from 1 to 10% depending on the vaccine, the dosage, and the age of vaccinees. Osteomyelitis has been noted in 1 per 1,000,000 vaccinees, although recent information indicates that the rate may be as high as 5 per 100,000 in newborns. Disseminated BCG infection and death are very rare; they range from 1 to 10 per 10,000,000 vaccinees and occur almost exclusively in children with impaired immune response.

Autoinoculation ulcers are seen occasionally. Abscesses in the skin at the site of inoculation may occur from secondary infection. Rarely, abscesses may develop in the regional lymph nodes draining the site of the BCG vaccination. Most local reactions are excessive hypersensitivity responses not related to BCG infections. These should be treated with a local corticosteroid and, perhaps, with a broad spectrum antibacterial agent. Granulomas, appearing approximately 4 to 6 weeks following the vaccination, have been reported at the site of the injection. They may result from application of irritating dressings to a normal BCG reaction or may occur occasionally as an idiosyncrasy. Such granulomas may persist for variable periods of time and may have a keloid scar after final healing. Rarely, persistent lupus reactions of the skin that required treatment have been reported. For these, isoniazid in a daily dose of 4 mg per kg of body weight taken for three months has been recommended. One case of histiocytoma at the vaccination site required excision[3]. Transient urticaria has been observed and there have been occasional reports of anaphylaxis, erythema nodosum and erythema multiforme following BCG vaccination. Very much larger doses of BCG by other routes have resulted in one anecdotal report of Guillain-Barre Syndrome and one of aplastic anemia.

Dosage and Administration: After the vaccine has been prepared, the immunizing dose of 0.1 ml is given by *intradermal* injection (subcutaneous injection must be avoided). A 0.05 ml dose may be given to infants under 28 days of age. The recommended vaccination site is the arm—over the insertion of the deltoid muscle.

The vaccine must not be contaminated with any antiseptic or detergent. If alcohol is used to swab the skin, it must be allowed to evaporate before the vaccine is injected.

Vaccinees should be advised to leave the vaccinated lesion open to the air and keep it dry and clean to facilitate healing.

A postvaccinal tuberculin test should be conducted 2 to 3 months after vaccination. If the test is negative, the vaccination should be repeated.

Preparation of vaccine: Using appropriate aseptic technique, add 1 ml of Sterile Water for Injection USP to each 1 ml size multiple dose ampule of vaccine. Allow to stand for approximately 1 minute. Avoid shaking, since this results in foaming. The process of withdrawing the solution from the ampule will yield a homogeneous suspension.

Parenteral drug products should be inspected visually for particulate matter and discoloration prior to administration, whenever solution and container permit.

Following reconstitution, the liquid vaccine should be used immediately and any material remaining should be discarded, and preferably incinerated or treated with a disinfectant such as strong hypochlorite solution.

How Supplied: BCG Vaccine, USP is supplied in individually boxed 1 ml multi-dose ampules (NDC 0173-0339-65).

Before use, the product should be stored at a uniform temperature between 2° and 8°C (36° and 46°F), preferably at the lower limit. This vaccine contains live bacteria and should be protected against exposure to light.

References:
1. U.S. Department of Health, Education, and Welfare: BCG Vaccines, Morbidity and Mortality Weekly Report, 28:21, 1979.
2. Brit. Med. J., 2:193, 1971.
3. Hartston W.: Uncommon Skin Reactions after BCG Vaccination, Tubercle, 40:265, 1959.

BECLOVENT® ORAL INHALER ℞
[bec′ lō-vent]
(beclomethasone dipropionate, USP)
For Oral Inhalation Only

Description: Beclomethasone dipropionate, USP, the active component of BECLOVENT® (beclomethasone dipropionate) Oral Inhaler, is an anti-inflammatory steroid having the chemical name 9-Chloro-11β, 17, 21-trihydroxy-16β-methylpregna-1, 4-diene-3, 20-dione 17, 21-dipropionate.

BECLOVENT® Oral Inhaler is a metered-dose aerosol unit containing a microcrystalline suspension of beclomethasone dipropionate-trichloromonofluoromethane clathrate in a mixture of propellants (trichloromonofluoromethane and dichlorodifluoromethane) with oleic acid. Each canister contains beclomethasone dipropionate – trichloromonofluoromethane clathrate having a molecular proportion of beclomethasone dipropionate to trichloromonofluoromethane between 3:1 and 3:2. Each actuation delivers from the mouthpiece a quantity of clathrate equivalent to 42 mcg of beclomethasone dipropionate. The contents of one canister provide at least 200 oral inhalations.

Clinical Pharmacology: Beclomethasone 17, 21-dipropionate is a diester of beclomethasone, a synthetic corticosteroid which is chemically related to prednisolone. Beclomethasone differs from prednisolone only in having a chlorine at the 9-alpha and a methyl group at the 16-beta position in place of hydrogen. Animal studies showed that beclomethasone dipropionate has potent anti-inflammatory activity. When administered systemically to mice, the anti-inflammatory activity was accompanied by other typical features of glucocorticoid action including thymic involution, liver glycogen deposition, and pituitary-adrenal suppression. However, after systemic administration to rats, the anti-inflammatory action was associated with little or no effect on other tests of glucocorticoid activity.

Beclomethasone dipropionate is sparingly soluble and is poorly mobilized from subcutaneous or intramuscular injection sites. However, systemic absorption occurs after all routes of administration. When given to animals in the form of an aerosolized suspension of the trichloromonofluoromethane clathrate, the drug is deposited in the mouth and nasal passages, the trachea and principal bronchi, and in the lung; a considerable portion of the drug is also swallowed. Absorption occurs rapidly from all respiratory and gastrointestinal tissues, as indicated by the rapid clearance of radioactively labeled drug from local tissues and appearance of tracer in the circulation. There is no evidence of tissue storage of beclomethasone dipropionate or its metabolites. Lung slices can metabolize beclomethasone dipropionate rapidly to beclomethasone 17-monopropionate and more slowly to free beclomethasone (which has very weak anti-inflammatory activity). However, irrespective of the route of administration (injection, oral, or aerosol), the principal route of excretion of the drug and its metabolites is the feces. Less than 10% of the drug and its metabolites is excreted in the urine. In humans, 12% to 15% of an orally administered dose of beclomethasone dipropionate was excreted in the urine as both conjugated and free metabolites of the drug.

The mechanisms responsible for the anti-inflammatory action of beclomethasone dipropionate are unknown. The precise mechanism of the aerosolized drug's action in the lung is also unknown.

Indications: BECLOVENT® (beclomethasone dipropionate) Oral Inhaler is indicated only for patients who require chronic treatment with corticosteroids for control of the symptoms of bronchial asthma. Such patients would include those already receiving systemic corticosteroids, and selected patients who are inadequately controlled on a non-steroid regimen and in whom steroid therapy has been withheld because of concern over potential adverse effects.

BECLOVENT® Oral Inhaler is NOT indicated:
1. For relief of asthma which can be controlled by bronchodilators and other non-steroid medications.
2. In patients who require systemic corticosteroid treatment infrequently.
3. In the treatment of non-asthmatic bronchitis.

Contraindications: BECLOVENT® Oral Inhaler is contraindicated in the primary treatment of status asthmaticus or other acute episodes of asthma where intensive measures are required.

Continued on next page

Glaxo—Cont.

Hypersensitivity to any of the ingredients of this preparation contraindicates its use.

Warnings:
Particular care is needed in patients who are transferred from systemically active corticosteroids to BECLOVENT® Oral Inhaler because deaths due to adrenal insufficiency have occurred in asthmatic patients during and after transfer from systemic corticosteroids to aerosol beclomethasone dipropionate. After withdrawal from systemic corticosteroids, a number of months are required for recovery of hypothalamic-pituitary-adrenal (HPA) function. During this period of HPA suppression, patients may exhibit signs and symptoms of adrenal insufficiency when exposed to trauma, surgery or infections, particularly gastroenteritis. Although BECLOVENT® Oral Inhaler may provide control of asthmatic symptoms during these episodes, it does NOT provide the systemic steroid which is necessary for coping with these emergencies.

During periods of stress or a severe asthmatic attack, patients who have been withdrawn from systemic corticosteroids should be instructed to resume systemic steroids (in large doses) immediately and to contact their physician for further instruction. These patients should also be instructed to carry a warning card indicating that they may need supplementary systemic steroids during periods of stress or a severe asthma attack. To assess the risk of adrenal insufficiency in emergency situations, routine tests of adrenal cortical function, including measurement of early morning resting cortisol levels, should be performed periodically in all patients. An early morning resting cortisol level may be accepted as normal only if it falls at or near the normal mean level.

Localized infections with *Candida albicans* or *Aspergillus niger* have occurred frequently in the mouth and pharynx and occasionally in the larynx. Positive cultures for oral *Candida* may be present in up to 75% of patients. Although the frequency of clinically apparent infection is considerably lower, these infections may require treatment with appropriate antifungal therapy or discontinuance of treatment with BECLOVENT® Oral Inhaler.
BECLOVENT® Oral Inhaler is not to be regarded as a bronchodilator and is not indicated for rapid relief of bronchospasm.
Patients should be instructed to contact their physician immediately when episodes of asthma which are not responsive to bronchodilators occur during the course of treatment with BECLOVENT® (beclomethasone dipropionate) Oral Inhaler. During such episodes, patients may require therapy with systemic corticosteroids.
There is no evidence that control of asthma can be achieved by the administration of BECLOVENT® Oral Inhaler in amounts greater than the recommended doses.
Transfer of patients from systemic steroid therapy to BECLOVENT® Oral Inhaler may unmask allergic conditions previously suppressed by the systemic steroid therapy, eg, rhinitis, conjunctivitis, and eczema.

Precautions: During withdrawal from oral steroids, some patients may experience symptoms of systemically active steroid withdrawal, e g , joint and/or muscular pain, lassitude and depression, despite maintenance or even improvement of respiratory function (See **Dosage and Administration** for details).
In responsive patients, beclomethasone dipropionate may permit control of asthmatic symptoms without suppression of HPA function. Since beclomethasone dipropionate is absorbed into the circulation and can be systemically active, the beneficial effects of BECLOVENT® Oral Inhaler in minimizing or preventing HPA dysfunction may be expected only when recommended dosages are not exceeded.
The long-term effects of beclomethasone dipropionate in human subjects are still unknown. In particular, the local effects of the agent on developmental or immunologic processes in the mouth, pharynx, trachea, and lung are unknown. There is also no information about the possible long-term systemic effects of the agent.
The potential effects of BECLOVENT® Oral Inhaler on acute, recurrent, or chronic pulmonary infections, including active or quiescent tuberculosis, are not known. Similarly, the potential effects of long-term administration of the drug on lung or other tissues are unknown.
Pulmonary infiltrates with eosinophilia may occur in patients on BECLOVENT® Oral Inhaler therapy. Although it is possible that in some patients this state may become manifest because of systemic steroid withdrawal when inhalational steroids are administered, a causative role for beclomethasone dipropionate and/or its vehicle cannot be ruled out.

Use in Pregnancy: Glucocorticoids are known teratogens in rodent species and beclomethasone dipropionate is no exception.
Teratology studies were done in rats, mice, and rabbits treated with subcutaneous beclomethasone dipropionate. Beclomethasone dipropionate was found to produce fetal resorption, cleft palate, agnathia, microstomia, absence of tongue, delayed ossification and partial agenesis of the thymus. Well-controlled trials relating to fetal risk in humans are not available. Glucocorticoids are secreted in human milk. It is not known whether beclomethasone dipropionate would be secreted in human milk but it is safe to assume that it is likely. The use of beclomethasone dipropionate in pregnancy, nursing mothers, or women of childbearing potential requires that the possible benefits of the drug be weighed against the potential hazards to the mother, embryo, or fetus. Infants born of mothers who have received substantial doses of corticosteroids during pregnancy should be carefully observed for hypoadrenalism.

Adverse Reactions: Deaths due to adrenal insufficiency have occurred in asthmatic patients during and after transfer from systemic corticosteroids to aerosol beclomethasone dipropionate (see **Warnings**).
Suppression of HPA function (reduction of early morning plasma cortisol levels) has been reported in adult patients who received 1600 mcg daily doses of BECLOVENT® (beclomethasone dipropionate) Oral Inhaler for one month. A patients on BECLOVENT® Oral Inhaler have complained of hoarseness or dry mouth. Bronchospasm and rash have been reported rarely.

Dosage and Administration: Adults: The usual dosage is two inhalations (84 mcg) given three or four times a day. In patients with severe asthma, it is advisable to start with 12 to 16 inhalations a day and adjust the dosage downward according to the response of the patient. The maximal daily intake should not exceed 20 inhalations, 840 mcg (0.84 mg), in adults.
Children 6 to 12 years of age: The usual dosage is one or two inhalations (42 to 84 mcg) given three or four times a day according to the response of the patient. The maximal daily intake should not exceed ten inhalations, 420 mcg (0.42 mg), in children 6 to 12 years of age. Insufficient clinical data exist with respect to the administration of BECLOVENT® Oral Inhaler in children below the age of 6.
Rinsing the mouth after inhalation is advised.
Patients receiving bronchodilators by inhalation should be advised to use the bronchodilator before BECLOVENT® Oral Inhaler in order to enhance penetration of beclomethasone dipropionate into the bronchial tree. After use of an aerosol bronchodilator, several minutes should elapse before use of the BECLOVENT® Oral Inhaler to reduce the potential toxicity from the inhaled fluorocarbon propellants in the two aerosols.

Different considerations must be given to the following groups of patients in order to obtain the full therapeutic benefit of BECLOVENT® Oral Inhaler.
Patients not receiving systemic steroids: The use of BECLOVENT® Oral Inhaler is straightforward in patients who are inadequately controlled with non-steroid medications but in whom systemic steroid therapy has been withheld because of concern over potential adverse reactions. In patients who respond to BECLOVENT® Oral Inhaler, an improvement in pulmonary function is usually apparent within one to four weeks after the start of BECLOVENT® Oral Inhaler.
Patients receiving systemic steroids: In those patients dependent on systemic steroids, transfer to BECLOVENT® Oral Inhaler and subsequent management may be more difficult because recovery from impaired adrenal function is usually slow. Such suppression has been known to last for up to 12 months. Clinical studies, however, have demonstrated that BECLOVENT® Oral Inhaler may be effective in the management of these asthmatic patients and may permit replacement or significant reduction in the dosage of systemic corticosteroids.
The patient's asthma should be reasonably stable before treatment with BECLOVENT® Oral Inhaler is started. Initially, the aerosol should be used concurrently with the patient's usual maintenance dose of systemic steroid. After approximately one week, gradual withdrawal of the systemic steroid is started by reducing the daily or alternate daily dose. The next reduction is made after an interval of one or two weeks, depending on the response of the patient. Generally, these decrements should not exceed 2.5 mg of prednisone or its equivalent. A slow rate of withdrawal cannot be overemphasized. During withdrawal, some patients may experience symptoms of systemically active steroid withdrawal, eg, joint and/or muscular pain, lassitude and depression, despite maintenance or even improvement of respiratory function. Such patients should be encouraged to continue with the Inhaler but should be watched carefully for objective signs of adrenal insufficiency, such as hypotension and weight loss. If evidence of adrenal insufficiency occurs, the systemic steroid dose should be boosted temporarily and thereafter further withdrawal should continue more slowly.
During periods of stress or a severe asthma attack, transfer patients will require supplementary treatment with systemic steroids. Exacerbations of asthma which occur during the course of treatment with BECLOVENT® (beclomethasone dipropionate) Oral Inhaler should be treated with a short course of systemic steroid which is gradually tapered as these symptoms subside. There is no evidence that control of asthma can be achieved by administration of BECLOVENT® Oral Inhaler in amounts greater than the recommended doses.

Directions for Use: Illustrated patient instructions for proper use accompany each package of BECLOVENT® Oral Inhaler.
CONTENTS UNDER PRESSURE. Do not puncture. Do not use or store near heat or open flame. Exposure to temperatures above 120°F may cause bursting. Never throw container into fire or incinerator. Keep out of reach of children.
How Supplied: BECLOVENT® Oral Inhaler 16.8 g canister with oral adapter and patient's instructions (NDC 0173-0312-88) and BECLOVENT Oral Inhaler Refill 16.8 g canister only with patient's instructions (NDC 0173-0312-98).

Shown in Product Identification Section, page 411

BECONASE® Nasal Inhaler
[bek'on-as"]
(beclomethasone dipropionate, USP)
For Nasal Inhalation Only

Description: Beclomethasone dipropionate, USP, the active component of BECONASE Nasal Inhaler, is an anti-inflammatory steroid having the chemical name, 9-Chloro-11β, 17, 21-trihydroxy-16β-methylpregna-1, 4-diene-3, 20-dione 17,21-dipropionate.

Beclomethasone dipropionate is a white to creamy-white, odorless powder with a molecular weight of 521.25. It is very slightly soluble in water; very soluble in chloroform; and freely soluble in acetone and in alcohol.

BECONASE Nasal Inhaler is a metered-dose aerosol unit containing a microcrystalline suspension of beclomethasone dipropionate-trichloromonofluoromethane clathrate in a mixture of propellants (trichloromonofluoromethane and dichlorodifluoromethane) with oleic acid. Each canister contains beclomethasone dipropionate-trichloromonofluoromethane clathrate having a molecular proportion of beclomethasone dipropionate to trichloromonofluoromethane between 3:1 and 3:2. Each actuation delivers from the nasal adapter a quantity of clathrate equivalent to 42 mcg of beclomethasone dipropionate, USP. The contents of one canister provide at least 200 metered doses.

Clinical Pharmacology: Beclomethasone 17,21-dipropionate is a diester of beclomethasone, a synthetic corticosteroid which is chemically related to dexamethasone. Beclomethasone differs from dexamethasone only in having a chlorine at the 9-alpha position in place of a fluorine. Animal studies showed that beclomethasone dipropionate has potent glucocorticoid and weak mineralocorticoid activity.

The mechanisms for the anti-inflammatory action of beclomethasone dipropionate are unknown. The precise mechanism of the aerosolized drug's action in the nose is also unknown. Biopsies of nasal mucosa obtained during clinical studies showed no histopathologic changes when beclomethasone dipropionate was administered intranasally.

The effects of beclomethasone dipropionate on hypothalamic-pituitary-adrenal (HPA) function have been evaluated in adult volunteers by other routes of administration. Studies are currently being undertaken with beclomethasone dipropionate by the intranasal route, which may demonstrate that there is more or that there is less absorption by this route of administration. There was no suppression of early morning plasma cortisol concentrations when beclomethasone dipropionate was administered in a dose of 1000 mcg/day for one month as an oral aerosol or for three days by intramuscular injection. However, partial suppression of plasma cortisol concentration was observed when beclomethasone dipropionate was administered in doses of 2000 mcg/day either by oral aerosol or intramuscularly. Immediate suppression of plasma cortisol concentrations was observed after single doses of 4000 mcg of beclomethasone dipropionate. Suppression of HPA function (reduction of early morning plasma cortisol levels) has been reported in adult patients who received 1600 mcg daily doses of oral beclomethasone dipropionate for one month. In clinical studies using beclomethasone dipropionate intranasally, there was no evidence of adrenal insufficiency.

Beclomethasone dipropionate is sparingly soluble. When given by nasal inhalation in the form of an aerosolized suspension, the drug is deposited primarily in the nasal passages. A portion of the drug is swallowed. Absorption occurs rapidly from all respiratory and gastrointestinal tissues. There is no evidence of tissue storage of beclomethasone dipropionate or its metabolites. *In vitro* studies have shown that tissue other than the liver (lung slices) can rapidly metabolize beclomethasone dipropionate to beclomethasone 17-monopropionate and more slowly to free beclomethasone (which has very weak anti-inflammatory activity). However, irrespective of the route of entry the principal route of excretion of the drug and its metabolites is the feces. In humans, 12% to 15% of an orally administered dose of beclomethasone dipropionate is excreted in the urine as both conjugated and free metabolites of the drug. The half-life of beclomethasone dipropionate in humans is approximately 15 hours. Studies have shown that the degree of binding to plasma proteins is 87%.

Indications and Usage: BECONASE Nasal Inhaler is indicated for the relief of the symptoms of seasonal or perennial rhinitis in those cases poorly responsive to conventional treatment.

Clinical studies have shown that improvement is usually apparent within a few days. However, symptomatic relief may not occur in some patients for as long as 2 weeks. Although systemic effects are minimal at recommended doses, BECONASE Nasal Inhaler should not be continued beyond 3 weeks in the absence of significant symptomatic improvement. BECONASE Nasal Inhaler should not be used in the presence of untreated localized infection involving the nasal mucosa.

Contraindications: Hypersensitivity to any of the ingredients of this preparation contraindicates its use.

Warnings: The replacement of a systemic corticosteroid with BECONASE Nasal Inhaler can be accompanied by signs of adrenal insufficiency.

When transferred to BECONASE Nasal Inhaler, careful attention must be given to patients previously treated for prolonged periods with systemic corticosteroids. This is particularly important in those patients who have associated asthma or other clinical conditions, where too rapid a decrease in systemic corticosteroids may cause a severe exacerbation of their symptoms.

Studies have shown that the combined administration of alternate-day prednisone systemic treatment and orally inhaled beclomethasone increase the likelihood of HPA suppression compared to a therapeutic dose of either one alone. Therefore, BECONASE Nasal Inhaler treatment should be used with caution in patients already on alternate day prednisone regimens for any disease.

Precautions: General: During withdrawal from oral steroids, some patients may experience symptoms of withdrawal, eg, joint and/or muscular pain, lassitude, and depression.

In clinical studies with beclomethasone dipropionate administered intranasally, the development of localized infections of the nose and pharynx with *Candida albicans* has occurred only rarely. When such an infection develops, it may require treatment with appropriate local therapy or discontinuation of treatment with BECONASE Nasal Inhaler.

Beclomethasone dipropionate is absorbed into the circulation. Use of excessive doses of BECONASE Nasal Inhaler may suppress HPA function.

BECONASE Nasal Inhaler should be used with caution, if at all, in patients with active or quiescent tuberculous infections of the respiratory tract, or in untreated fungal, bacterial, systemic viral infections or ocular herpes simplex.

Because of the inhibitory effect of corticosteroids on wound healing, patients who have experienced recent nasal septal ulcers, nasal surgery, or trauma should not use a nasal corticosteroid until healing has occurred.

Although systemic effects have been minimal with recommended doses, this potential increases with excessive doses. Therefore, larger than recommended doses should be avoided.

Information for Patients: Patients should use BECONASE Nasal Inhaler at regular intervals since its effectiveness depends on its regular use. The patient should take the medication as directed. It is not acutely effective and the prescribed dosage should not be increased. Instead nasal vasoconstrictors or oral antihistamines may be needed until the effects of BECONASE Nasal Inhaler are fully manifested. One to two weeks may pass before full relief is obtained. The patient should contact the doctor if symptoms do not improve, or if the condition worsens, or if sneezing or nasal irritation occurs. For the proper use of this unit and to attain maximum improvement, the patient should read and follow the accompanying Patient's Instructions carefully.

Carcinogenesis, Mutagenesis, Impairment of Fertility: Treatment of rats for a total of 95 weeks, 13 weeks by inhalation and 82 weeks by the oral route, resulted in no evidence of carcinogenic activity. Mutagenic studies have not been performed.

Impairment of fertility, as evidenced by inhibition of the estrous cycle in dogs, was observed following treatment by the oral route. No inhibition of the estrous cycle in dogs was seen following treatment with beclomethasone dipropionate by the inhalation route.

Pregnancy Category C: Like other corticoids, parenteral (subcutaneous) beclomethasone dipropionate has been shown to be teratogenic and embryocidal in the mouse and rabbit when given in doses approximately ten times the human dose. In these studies, beclomethasone was found to produce fetal resorption, cleft palate, agnathia, microstomia, absence of tongue, delayed ossification, and agenesis of the thymus. No teratogenic or embryocidal effects have been seen in the rat when beclomethasone dipropionate was administered by inhalation at 10 times the human dose or orally at 1000 times the human dose. There are no adequate and well-controlled studies in pregnant women. Beclomethasone dipropionate should be used during pregnancy only if the potential benefit justifies the potential risk to the fetus.

Nonteratogenic Effects: Hypoadrenalism may occur in infants born of mothers receiving corticosteroids during pregnancy. Such infants should be carefully observed.

Nursing Mothers: It is not known whether beclomethasone dipropionate is excreted in human milk. Because other corticosteroids are excreted in human milk, caution should be exercised when BECONASE Nasal Inhaler is administered to nursing women.

Pediatric Use: Safety and effectiveness in children below the age of 12 years have not been established.

Adverse Reactions: In general, side effects in clinical studies have been primarily associated with the nasal mucous membranes.

Adverse reactions reported in controlled clinical trials and long term open studies in patients treated with BECONASE Nasal Inhaler are described below.

Sensations of irritation and burning in the nose (11 per 100 patients) following the use of BECONASE Nasal Inhaler have been reported. Also, occasional sneezing attacks (10 per 100 patients) have occurred immediately following the use of the intranasal inhaler.

Localized infections of the nose and pharynx with *Candida albicans* have occurred rarely. (see **Precautions**).

Less than 2 per 100 patients reported transient episodes of bloody discharge from the nose.

Ulceration of the nasal mucosa has been reported rarely. Systemic corticosteroid side effects were not reported during the controlled clinical trials. If recommended doses are exceeded, however, or if individuals are particularly sensitive, symptoms of hypercorticism, ie, Cushing's syndrome, could occur.

Dosage and Administration: *Adults and Children 12 years of age and over:* the usual dosage is one inhalation (42 mcg) in each nostril two to four times a day (total dose 168–336 mcg/day). Patients can often be maintained on a maximum dose of one inhalation in each nostril three times a day (252 mcg/day).

In patients who respond to BECONASE Nasal Inhaler, an improvement of the symptoms of seasonal or perennial rhinitis usually becomes apparent within a few days after the start of BECONASE Nasal Inhaler therapy.

The therapeutic effects of corticosteroids, unlike those of decongestants are not immediate. This should be explained to the patient in advance in order to ensure cooperation and continuation of treatment with the prescribed dosage regimen.

BECONASE Nasal Inhaler is *not* recommended for children below 12 years of age.

In the presence of excessive nasal mucus secretion or edema of the nasal mucosa, the drug may fail to reach the site of intended action. In such cases it is advisable to use a nasal vasoconstrictor during the first two to three days of BECONASE Nasal Inhaler therapy.

Continued on next page

Glaxo—Cont.

Directions for Use: Illustrated patient instructions for proper use accompany each package of BECONASE Nasal Inhaler.
CONTENTS UNDER PRESSURE. Do not puncture. Do not use or store near heat or open flame. Exposure to temperatures above 120°F may cause bursting. Never throw container into fire or incinerator. Keep out of reach of children.
Overdosage: When used at excessive doses, systemic corticosteroid effects such as hypercorticism and adrenal suppression may appear. If such symptoms appear, the dosage should be decreased. The oral LD$_{50}$ of beclomethasone dipropionate is greater than 1 g/kg in rodents. One canister of BECONASE Nasal Inhaler contains 8.4 mg. of beclomethasone dipropionate; therefore, acute overdosage is unlikely.
How Supplied: BECONASE Nasal Inhaler, 16.8 g canister; box of one. Supplied with nasal adapter and patient's instructions; (NDC 0173-0336-88).
Store between 2° and 30°C (36° and 86°F).
Shown in Product Identification Section, page 411

CORTICAINE® Cream
[cor′ tĭ-cāne]

Description: Corticaine Cream contains hydrocortisone acetate 0.5% and dibucaine 0.5% in a washable, non-greasy, mentholated, cream base composed of esters of mixed saturated fatty acids, stearyl alcohol, glycerin, polysorbate 40, BHA, BHT, disodium EDTA and purified water with methylparaben and propylparaben as preservatives. Corticaine Cream is an anti-inflammatory and local anesthetic cream for topical and intra-rectal use.
Clinical Pharmacology: Hydrocortisone acetate is a corticosteroid that acts to reduce swelling, itching, hyperemia and other manifestations of inflammation regardless of the cause. Dibucaine, an amide-type local anesthetic, provides relief from pain, itching and burning by reversibly blocking nerve conduction when applied topically. Because dibucaine is an amide, it can often be used in patients sensitive to ester-type local anesthetics such as procaine and tetracaine. The base has a soothing, lubricant action.
Indications and Usage: Corticaine Cream is indicated for the relief of the inflammatory manifestations of corticosteroid-responsive dermatosis. When combined with other recognized therapeutic measures, it is recommended for the symptomatic relief of itching, pain and irritation of certain anorectal, anogenital and dermatological conditions. On the skin, it offers symptomatic relief in atopic dermatitis, sumac or ivy dermatitis, mild sunburn, minor burns, insect bites, prickly heat, eczema, post-anal surgery, diaper rash and intertrigo. When introduced into the rectum, it helps to relieve the itching, pain and inflammation of internal hemorrhoids, as well as the anorectal discomfort of associated conditions such as proctitis, papillitis and cryptitis. When applied perianally, it can provide symptomatic relief from pruritus ani and external hemorrhoids.
Contraindications: Local tuberculosis, fungal and viral infections. Topical steroids and local anesthetics are contraindicated in those patients with a history of hypersensitivity to any of the components of the preparation. Not recommended for use in such diseases as pemphigus and discoid lupus erythematosus.
Precautions: GENERAL: Avoid use in the eyes. Do not apply to extensive areas for prolonged periods or with occlusive dressings as there may be increased systemic absorption of the ingredients. If irritation develops, the product should be discontinued and appropriate therapy instituted. In the presence of a secondary bacterial infection, the use of an appropriate antibacterial agent should be instituted; if a favorable response does not occur promptly, this preparation should be discontinued until the infection has been adequately controlled. Should not be used rectally without adequate proctologic examination. Not to be used with anorectal fistulas and abscesses.
USAGE IN PREGNANCY: Although topical steroids have not been reported to have an adverse effect on human pregnancy, the safety of their use in pregnant women has not been absolutely established. In laboratory animals, increases in incidence of fetal abnormalities have been associated with exposure of gestating females to topical corticosteroids—in some cases, at rather low dosage levels. Therefore, drugs of this class should not be used extensively on pregnant patients, in large amounts, or for prolonged periods of time.
Adverse Reactions: The following local adverse reactions have been reported with topical corticosteroids, especially under occlusive dressings: burning sensations, itching, irritation, dryness, folliculitis, hypertrichosis, acne-form eruptions, hypopigmentation, perioral dermatitis, allergic contact dermatitis, maceration of the skin, secondary infection, skin atrophy, striae and miliaria.
Dosage and Administration: FOR RECTAL USE—Cleanse the rectal area and dry thoroughly before use. Attach plastic applicator to tube, and squeeze tube lightly to fill applicator with cream. Lubricate applicator with cream, then gently insert into rectum and squeeze tube again lightly to extrude a similar applicator dose of cream into the rectum. Can also be applied topically to irritated anorectal tissues. Use morning and evening and after each bowel movement. Recommended duration of treatment: 2 to 6 days.
FOR TOPICAL USE—Apply to affected areas of the skin 2 to 4 times daily. Recommended duration of treatment: 2 weeks.
How Supplied: Corticaine Cream (hydrocortisone acetate 0.5% and dibucaine 0.5%) is supplied in a 1 oz tube with a rectal applicator (NDC 0173-0358-72). Keep container well-closed and store between 15° and 30° C. (59° and 86° F.).
Shown in Product Identification Section, page 412

CORTICAINE® SUPPOSITORIES
[cor′ tĭ-cāne]
Rectal Suppositories with Hydrocortisone

Description: CORTICAINE Suppositories contain hydrocortisone acetate, 10 mg, in a hydrogenated vegetable oil base with zinc oxide and menthol. CORTICAINE Suppositories are an anti-inflammatory for rectal use.
Clinical Pharmacology: Hydrocortisone is a corticosteroid that acts directly on the anorectal tissues to reduce swelling, itching, hyperemia and other manifestations of the tissue response to acute inflammation, regardless of the cause. The combination of hydrocortisone and the soothing ingredients of the base tends to reduce inflammation and edema.
Indications and Usage: When introduced into the rectum, CORTICAINE Suppositories help to relieve the symptoms of internal hemorrhoids and serve as an adjunct in the treatment of the discomfort associated with proctitis, papillitis, cryptitis and other inflammatory conditions of the anorectum.
Contraindications: CORTICAINE Suppositories are contraindicated in patients with local tuberculosis and viral infections and in those individuals with a history of hypersensitivity to any of the components of the preparation.
Precautions:
General—If irritation develops, the product should be discontinued and appropriate therapy instituted. In the presence of a secondary bacterial infection, the use of an appropriate antibacterial should be instituted; if a favorable response does not occur promptly, this preparation should be discontinued until the infection has been adequately controlled. Should not be used without adequate proctologic examination. Not to be used with anorectal fistulas and abscesses.
Use in Pregnancy—Although topical steroids have not been reported to have an adverse effect on human pregnancy, the safety of their use in pregnant women has not been absolutely established. In laboratory animals, increases in the incidence of fetal abnormalities have been associated with exposure of gestating females to topical steroids, in some cases at rather low dosage levels. Therefore, drugs of this class should not be used extensively on pregnant patients, in large amounts or for prolonged periods of time.
Pediatric Use—Safety and effectiveness in children have not been established.
Adverse Reactions: The following local adverse reactions have been reported with corticosteroid suppositories: burning, itching, irritation, dryness, folliculitis, hypopigmentation, allergic contact dermatitis and secondary infection.
Dosage and Administration: Insert one suppository in the rectum twice daily, morning and evening. Recommended duration of treatment, two to six days.
How Supplied: CORTICAINE Suppositories (hydrocortisone acetate, 10 mg) are supplied in white plastic containers of 12 (NDC 0173-0333-00). Keep at room temperature 15°–30°C (59°–86°F). May be refrigerated. Dispense in original plastic container.
Shown in Product Identification Section, page 412

ETHATAB® Tablets
[ĕth′ ă-tab]
(ethaverine hydrochloride)

Description: Each yellow ETHATAB Tablet contains ethaverine hydrochloride 100 mg.
Action: ETHATAB acts directly on the smooth muscle cells, without involving the autonomic nervous system or its receptors. It produces smooth muscle relaxation, particularly where spasm exists, affecting the larger blood vessels, especially systemic, peripheral and pulmonary vessels, smooth muscle of the intestines, biliary tree, and ureters.
Indications: In peripheral and cerebral vascular insufficiency associated with arterial spasm; also useful as a smooth muscle spasmolytic in spastic conditions of the gastrointestinal and genitourinary tracts.
Contraindications: The use of ETHATAB is contraindicated in the presence of complete atrioventricular dissociation.
Precautions: As with vasodilators, ETHATAB should be administered with caution to patients with glaucoma. The safety of ethaverine hydrochloride during pregnancy or lactation has not been established; therefore it should not be used in pregnant women or in women of childbearing age unless, in the judgment of the physician, its use is deemed essential to the welfare of the patient.
Side Effects: Even though the incidence of side effects as reported in the literature is very low, it is possible for a patient to evidence nausea, anorexia, abdominal distress, dryness of the throat, hypotension, malaise, lassitude, drowsiness, flushing, sweating, vertigo, respiratory depression, cardiac depression, cardiac arrhythmia and headache. If these side effects occur, reduce dosage or discontinue medication.
Dosage and Administration: In mild or moderate disease, the usual dose for adults is one tablet three times a day. In more difficult cases, dosage may be increased to two tablets three times a day. It is most effective given early in the course of the vascular disorder. Because of the chronic nature of the disease, long-term therapy is required.
Supplied: ETHATAB (ethaverine HCl) Tablets, yellow, oval, scored tablets, engraved with GLAXO and 281; bottles of 100 (NDC 0173-0281-43), 500 (NDC 0173-0281-44) and box of 100 (NDC 0173-0281-47) for unit-dose dispensing.

SEFFIN®
Cephalothin Sodium
for Injection, USP
Neutral

Description: SEFFIN® (cephalothin sodium for injection, USP, Glaxo) Neutral, is a semisynthetic cephalosporin antibiotic for parenteral use. It is the sodium salt of 7-(thiophene-2-acetamido) cephalosporanic acid. Sodium bicarbonate has been added to result in reconstituted solutions have a pH ranging between 6 and 8.5. The total sodium content is approximately 63mg (2.8mEq sodium ion) per g of SEFFIN.

Actions: Human Pharmacology—SEFFIN® is a broad-spectrum antibiotic for parenteral administration. After administration of a 500mg dose intramuscularly to normal volunteers, the average peak serum antibiotic level was 10mcg per ml at one-half hour; with a 1g dose, the average was about 20mcg per ml. Following a single 1g intravenous dose of cephalothin sodium, blood levels have been about 30mcg per ml at 15 minutes, have ranged from 3 to 12mcg at 1 hour, and have declined to about 1mcg at 4 hours. With continuous infusion, at the rate of 500mg per hour, levels have been from 14 to 20mcg per ml of serum. Dosages of 2g given intravenously over a 30 minute period have produced serum concentrations of 80 to 100mcg per ml one-half hour after the infusion; levels ranged from 10 to 40mcg per ml at 1 hour and from 3 to 6mcg per ml at 2 hours and were not assayable after 5 hours.

Sixty to 70 percent of an intramuscular dose is excreted by the kidneys in the first 6 hours; this results in high urine levels, e.g., 800mcg per ml of urine after a 500mg dose and 2500mcg per ml following 1g. Probenecid slows tubular excretion and almost doubles peak blood levels.

Spinal fluid levels have ranged from 0.4 to 1.4mcg per ml in a child and from 0.15 to 5mcg per ml in adults with meningeal inflammatory states. The antibiotic passes readily into other body fluids, eg, pleural, joint, and ascitic fluids. Studies of amniotic fluid and cord blood show prompt transfer of cephalothin sodium across the placenta. Secondary aqueous humor levels have averaged 0.5mcg per ml 30 minutes after a single 1g intravenous dose. The antibiotic has been detected in bile.

Microbiology—The *in vitro* bactericidal action of cephalothin results from inhibition of cell-wall synthesis.

SEFFIN is usually active against the following organisms *in vitro*:

Beta-hemolytic and other streptococci (many strains of enterococci, e.g., *Streptococcus faecalis*, are relatively resistant); staphylococci, including coagulase-positive, coagulase-negative and penicillinase-producing strains; *S. (Diplococcus) pneumoniae*; *Haemophilus influenzae*; *Escherichia coli* and other coliform bacteria; *Klebsiella*; *Proteus mirabilis*; *Salmonella* sp; *Shigella* sp.

Pseudomonas organisms are resistant to SEFFIN, as are most indole-producing *Proteus* species and motile *Enterobacter* species.

Susceptibility Plate Tests—If the Bauer-Kirby-Sherris-Turck method of disc susceptibility testing[1] is used, a disc containing 30mcg cephalothin should give a zone of over 17mm when tested against a cephalothin-susceptible bacterial strain, and a zone of over 14mm with an organism of intermediate susceptibility.

Indications: SEFFIN® is indicated for the treatment of serious infections caused by susceptible strains of the designated microorganisms in the diseases listed below. Culture and susceptibility studies should be performed. Therapy may be instituted before results of susceptibility studies are obtained.

Respiratory tract infections are caused by *S. pneumoniae*, staphylococci (penicillinase and non-penicillinase-producing), group A beta-hemolytic streptococci, *Klebsiella* and *H. influenzae*.

Skin and soft-tissue infections, including peritonitis, caused by staphylococci (penicillinase and non-penicillinase-producing), group A beta-hemolytic streptococci, *E. coli*, *P. mirabilis* and *Klebsiella*.

Genitourinary tract infections caused by *E. coli*, *P. mirabilis* and *Klebsiella*.

Septicemia, including endocarditis, caused by *S. pneumoniae*, staphylococci (penicillinase and non-penicillinase-producing), group A beta-hemolytic streptococci, *S. viridans*, *E. coli*, *P. mirabilis* and *Klebsiella*.

Gastrointestinal infections caused by *Salmonella* and *Shigella* species.

Meningitis caused by *S. pneumoniae*, group A beta-hemolytic streptococci, and staphylococci (penicillinase and non-penicillinase-producing).

NOTE: Inasmuch as only low levels of cephalothin sodium are found in the cerebrospinal fluid, the drug is not reliable in the treatment of meningitis and cannot be recommended for that purpose. Cephalothin sodium has, however, proved to be effective in a number of cases of meningitis and may be considered for unusual circumstances in which other, more reliably effective antibiotics cannot be used.

Bone and joint infections caused by staphylococci (penicillinase and non-penicillinase-producing).

The prophylactic administration of SEFFIN® (cephalothin sodium for injection, USP) preoperatively, intraoperatively and postoperatively may reduce the incidence of certain post-operative infections in patients undergoing surgical procedures (e.g., vaginal hysterectomy) that are classified as contaminated or potentially contaminated. The perioperative use of SEFFIN may also be effective in surgical patients in whom infection at the operative site would present a serious risk, e.g., during open-heart surgery and prosthetic arthroplasty.

The prophylactic administration of SEFFIN should be discontinued within a 24 hours period after the surgical procedure. If there are signs of infection, specimens for culture should be obtained for the identification of the causative organism so that appropriate therapy may be instituted (see **Dosage and Administration**).

NOTE: If the susceptibility tests show that the causative organism is resistant to SEFFIN, other appropriate antibiotic therapy should be instituted.

Contraindications: SEFFIN® is contraindicated in persons who have shown hypersensitivity to cephalosporin antibiotics.

Warnings: BEFORE CEPHALOTHIN THERAPY IS INSTITUTED, CAREFUL INQUIRY SHOULD BE MADE CONCERNING PREVIOUS HYPERSENSITIVITY REACTIONS TO CEPHALOSPORINS AND PENICILLIN. CEPHALOSPORIN C DERIVATIVES SHOULD BE GIVEN CAUTIOUSLY TO PENICILLIN-SENSITIVE PATIENTS.
SERIOUS ACUTE HYPERSENSITIVITY REACTIONS MAY REQUIRE EPINEPHRINE AND OTHER EMERGENCY MEASURES.

There is some clinical and laboratory evidence of partial cross-allergenicity of the penicillins and the cephalosporins. Patients have been reported to have had severe reactions (including anaphylaxis) to both drugs. Any patient who has demonstrated some form of allergy, particularly to drugs, should receive antibiotics cautiously and then only when absolutely necessary. No exceptions should be made with regard to SEFFIN.®

Usage in Pregnancy—Safety of this product for use during pregnancy has not been established.

Precautions: Patients should be followed carefully so that any side effects or unusual manifestations or drug idiosyncrasy may be detected. If an allergic reaction to SEFFIN® occurs, the drug should be discontinued and the patient treated with the usual agents (e.g., epinephrine or other pressor amines, antihistamines, or corticosteroids).

Although SEFFIN rarely produces alteration in kidney function, evaluation of renal status is recommended, especially in seriously ill patients receiving maximum doses. Patients with impaired renal function should be placed on the dosage schedule recommended under **Dosage and Administration**. Usual doses in such individuals may result in excessive serum concentrations.

When intravenous doses of cephalothin larger than 6g daily are given by infusion for periods longer than 3 days, they may be associated with thrombophlebitis, and the veins may have to be alternated. The addition of 10 to 25mg of hydrocortisone to intravenous solutions containing 4 to 6g of cephalothin may reduce the incidence of thrombophlebitis. The use of small IV needles in the larger available veins may be preferred.

Prolonged use of SEFFIN may result in the overgrowth of nonsusceptible organisms. Constant observation of the patient is essential. If superinfection occurs during therapy, appropriate measures should be taken.

A false-positive reaction for glucose in the urine may occur with Benedict's or Fehling's solution or with Clinitest® tablets but not with Tes-Tape® (Glucose Enzymatic Test Strip, USP, Lilly).

An increased incidence of nephrotoxicity has been reported following concomitant administration of cephalosporins and aminoglycoside antibiotics.

Adverse Reactions: **Hypersensitivity**—Maculopapular rash, urticaria, reactions resembling serum sickness, and anaphylaxis have been reported. Eosinophilia and drug fever have been observed to be associated with other allergic reactions. These reactions are most likely to occur in patients with a history of allergy, particularly to penicillin.

Blood—Neutropenia, thrombocytopenia and hemolytic anemia have been reported. Some individuals, particularly those with azotemia, have developed positive direct Coombs tests during cephalothin therapy.

Liver—Transient rise in SGOT and alkaline phosphatase has been noted.

Kidney—Rise in BUN and decreased creatinine clearance have been reported, particularly in patients with prior renal impairment. The role of SEFFIN® in renal changes is difficult to assess, because other factors predisposing to prerenal azotemia or to acute renal failure usually have been present.

Local Reactions—Pain, induration, tenderness, and elevation of temperature have been reported following repeated intramuscular injections. Thrombophlebitis has occurred and is usually associated with daily doses of more than 6g given by infusion for longer than three days.

Dosage and Administration: In adults, the usual dosage range is 500mg to 1g of cephalothin every 4 to 6 hours. A dosage of 500mg q.6h. is adequate in uncomplicated pneumonia, furunculosis with cellulitis, and most urinary tract infections. In severe infections, this may be increased by giving the injections q.4h. or, when the desired response is not obtained, by raising the dose to 1g. In life-threatening infections, doses up to 2g. q.4h. may be required.

For perioperative prophylactic use to prevent postoperative infections in contaminated or potentially contaminated surgery in adults, the following doses are recommended:

(a) 1 to 2g administered IV just prior to surgery (approximately one-half to 1 hour before the initial incision);
(b) 1 to 2g during surgery (administration modified according to the duration of the operative procedure); and
(c) 1 to 2g q.6h. postoperatively for 24 hours.

In children, 20 to 30mg per kg may be given at the times designated above.

Since SEFFIN® (cephalothin sodium for injection, USP) has a serum half-life of 30 to 50 minutes, it is important that:

(1) the preoperative dose be given just prior to the start of surgery so that adequate antibiotic levels are present in the serum and tissues at the time of initial surgical incision; and
(2) SEFFIN be administered, if necessary, at appropriate intervals during surgery to provide sufficient levels of the antibiotic at the anticipated moments of greatest exposure to infective organisms.

When renal function is reduced, an intravenous loading dose of 1 to 2g may be given. Continued dosage schedule should be determined by degree of renal impairment, severity of infection, and susceptibility of the causative organism. The maximum doses administered should be based on the following recommendations.

Dosage of SEFFIN®
when renal function is impaired

Status of Renal Function	Maximum Adult Dosage (Maintenance)
Mild impairment (C_{cr} = 80–50ml/min)	2g q.6h.

Continued on next page

Glaxo—Cont.

Moderate impairment (C_{cr} = 50–25ml/min)	1.5g q.6h.
Severe impairment (C_{cr} = 25–10ml/min)	1g q.6h
Marked impairment (C_{cr} = 10–2ml/min)	0.5g q.6h.
Essentially no function (C_{cr} = <2ml/min)	0.5g q.8h.

In infants and children, the dosage should be proportionately less in accordance with age, weight and severity of infection. Daily administration of 100 mg per kg (80 to 160mg per kg or 40 to 80mg per lb) in divided doses has been found effective for most infections susceptible to SEFFIN.

Antibiotic therapy in beta-hemolytic streptococcal infections should continue for at least 10 days. In staphylococcal infections, surgical procedures, such as incision and drainage, should be carried out in all cases when indicated.

SEFFIN may be given intravenously or by deep intramuscular injection into a large muscle mass, such as the gluteus or lateral aspect of the thigh, to minimize pain and induration.

Intramuscular—Each g of cephalothin should be diluted with 4ml of Sterile Water for Injection. If the vial contents do not completely dissolve, an additional small amount of diluent (e.g., 0.2 to 0.4ml) may be added and the contents warmed slightly.

Intravenous—The intravenous route may be preferable for patients with bacteremia, septicemia, or other severe or life-threatening infections who may be poor risks because of lowered resistance resulting from such debilitating conditions as malnutrition, trauma, surgery, diabetes, heart failure, or malignancy, particularly if shock is present, or impending. For these infections in patients with normal renal function, the intravenous dosage is 4 to 12g of cephalothin daily. In conditions such as septicemia, 6 to 8g per day may be given intravenously for several days at the beginning of therapy; then, depending on the clinical response and laboratory findings, the dosage may be gradually reduced.

For patients who are to receive cephalothin intravenously, it is convenient to use the 1 or 2g 100ml size vial (see **Precautions**).

For intermittent intravenous administration, a solution containing 1g cephalothin in 10ml of diluent may be slowly injected directly into the vein over a period of 3 to 5 minutes or may be given through the tubing when the patient is receiving parenteral solutions.

Intermittent intravenous infusion with a Y-type administration set can also be accomplished while bulk intravenous solutions are being infused. However, during infusion of the solution containing SEFFIN, it is desirable to discontinue the other solution. When this technique is employed, careful attention should be paid to the volume of the solution containing SEFFIN so that the calculated dose will be infused.

For continuous intravenous infusion, 1 or 2g of cephalothin, diluted and well mixed with at least 10ml of Sterile Water for Injection, may be added to an IV bottle containing one of the following intravenous solutions: Acetated Ringer's Injection, 5% Dextrose Injection, 5% Dextrose in Lactated Ringer's Injection, Ionosol® B in D5-W, Isolyte® M with 5% Dextrose, Lactated Ringer's Injection, Normosol® M in D5-W, Plasma-Lyte® Injection, Plasma-Lyte® M Injection in 5% Dextrose, Ringer's Injection, or 0.9% Sodium Chloride Injection. The choice of solution and the volume to be employed are dictated by fluid and electrolyte management.

Intraperitoneal—In peritoneal dialysis procedures, cephalothin has been added to dialysis fluid in concentrations up to 6mg per 100ml and instilled into the peritoneal space throughout an entire dialysis (16 to 30 hours). Careful assay procedures have shown that 44 percent of the administered drug was absorbed into the bloodstream. Serum levels of 10mcg per ml were reported, with no evidence of accumulation and no untoward local or systemic reactions.

The intraperitoneal administration of solutions containing 0.1% to 4% SEFFIN® (cephalothin sodium for injection, USP) in saline has been used in treating patients with peritonitis or contaminated peritoneal cavities. (The total daily dosage of SEFFIN should take into account the amount given by the intraperitoneal route.)

Stability: While stored under **refrigeration,** the solution has a satisfactory potency for 96 hours after reconstitution. Solutions may precipitate; they can be redissolved by being warmed to room temperature with constant agitation. Kept at **room temperature,** solutions for intramuscular injection should be given within 12 hours after being mixed. Intravenous infusions should be started within 12 hours and completed within 24 hours. For prolonged infusions, replace with a freshly prepared solution at least every 24 hours. The concentrated solution will darken, especially at room temperature. Slight discoloration of the solution is permissible.

Solutions of SEFFIN® in Sterile Water for Injection, 5% Dextrose Injection or 0.9% Sodium Chloride Injection that are frozen immediately after reconstitution in the original container are stable for as long as 12 weeks when stored at −20° C.

If the product is warmed, care should be taken to avoid heating it after the thawing is complete. Once thawed, the solution should not be refrozen. As with all glass containers freezing may induce cracks. Good Pharmaceutical Practice suggests inspection of vials prior to use.

How Supplied: SEFFIN® (cephalothin sodium for injection, USP) is supplied in rubber-stoppered vials, infusion bottles and pharmacy bulk packages.

NDC 0173-0366-31	*1g vials (Box of 25)
NDC 0173-0368-35	*2g vials (Box of 25)
NDC 0173-0367-32	*1g 100ml Infusion Pack (Box of 10)
NDC 0173-0369-32	*2g 100ml Infusion Pack (Box of 10)
NDC 0173-0370-37	*10g 100ml Pharmacy Bulk Package (Box of 6)

*Equivalent to Cephalothin

Reference[1] Bauer, A.W., Kirby, W.M.M., Sherris, J.C., and Turck, M.; Antibiotic Susceptibility Testing by a Standardized Single Disk Method, Am. J. Clin. Pathol., 45:493, 1966; Standardized Disc Susceptibility Test, Federal Register, 39:19182-19184, 1974.

THEOBID® and THEOBID® JR.
(theophylline anhydrous)
DURACAP® CAPSULES
(SUSTAINED RELEASE)

Description: Each sustained release capsule contains the labeled amount of theophylline anhydrous in a sustained release bead formulation.

Chemistry: Theophylline, a xanthine compound, is a white, odorless, crystalline powder having a bitter taste. It contains one molecule of water of hydration or is anhydrous. Structure is as follows: $C_7H_8N_4O_2 \cdot (H_2O)$

Clinical Pharmacology: Theophylline directly relaxes the smooth muscle of the bronchial airways and pulmonary blood vessels, thus acting mainly as a bronchodilator, pulmonary vasodilator and smooth muscle relaxant. The drug also possesses other actions typical of the xanthine derivatives: coronary vasodilator, diuretic, cardiac stimulant, cerebral stimulant, and skeletal muscle stimulant. The actions of theophylline may be mediated through inhibition of phosphodiesterase and a resultant increase in intracellular cyclic AMP which could mediate smooth muscle relaxation. At concentrations higher than attained *in vivo,* theophylline also inhibits the release of histamine mast cells.

In vitro, theophylline has been shown to react synergistically with beta agonists that increase intracellular cyclic AMP through the stimulation of adenyl cyclase (isoproterenol), but synergism has not been demonstrated in patient studies and more data is needed to determine if theophylline and beta agonists have a clinically important additive effect *in vivo.*

Apparently, no development of tolerance occurs with chronic use of theophylline.

The half-life is shortened with cigarette smoking. The half-life is prolonged in alcoholism, reduced hepatic or renal function, congestive heart failure, and in patients receiving antibiotics such as TAO (troleandomycin), erythromycin and clindamycin. High fever for prolonged periods may decrease theophylline elimination.

THEOPHYLLINE ELIMINATION CHARACTERISTICS

	Theophylline Clearance Rates (mean±S.D.)	Half-life Average (mean±S.D.)
Children (over six months of age)	1.45±0.58 ml/kg/min	3.7±1.1 hours
Adult nonsmokers with uncomplicated asthma	0.65±0.19 ml/kg/min	8.7±2.2 hours

Newborn infants have extremely slow clearances and half-lives exceeding 24 hours which approach those seen for older children after about 3-6 months.

Older adults with chronic obstructive pulmonary disease, any patients with cor pulmonale or other causes of heart failure, and patients with liver pathology may have much lower clearances with half-lives that may exceed 24 hours.

The half-life of theophylline in smokers (1 to 2 packs/day) averaged 4–5 hours among various studies, much shorter than the half-life in nonsmokers who averaged about 7-9 hours. The increase in theophylline clearance caused by smoking is probably the result of induction of drug-metabolizing enzymes that do not readily normalize after cessation of smoking. It appears that between 3 months and 2 years may be necessary for normalization of the effect of smoking on Theophylline Pharmacokinetics.

Indications: For relief and/or prevention of symptoms from asthma and reversible bronchospasm associated with chronic bronchitis and emphysema.

Contraindications: In individuals who have shown hypersensitivity to any of its components.

Warnings: Status asthmaticus is a medical emergency. Optimal therapy frequently requires additional medication including corticosteroids when the patient is not rapidly responsive to bronchodilators.

Excessive theophylline doses may be associated with toxicity thus serum theophylline levels are recommended to assure maximal benefit without excessive risk. Incidence of toxicity increases at levels greater than 20 mcg/ml. Morphine, curare, and stilbamidine should be used with caution in patients with airflow obstruction since they stimulate histamine release and can induce asthmatic attacks. They may also suppress respiration leading to respiratory failure. Alternative drugs should be chosen whenever possible.

There is an excellent correlation between high blood levels of theophylline resulting from conventional doses and associated clinical manifestations of toxicity in (1) patients with lowered body plasma clearances (due to transient cardiac decomposition), (2) patients with liver dysfunction or chronic obstructive lung disease, (3) patients who are older than 55 years of age, particularly males.

There are often no early signs of less serious theophylline toxicity such as nausea and restlessness, which may appear in up to 50 percent of patients prior to onset of convulsions. Ventricular arrhythmias or seizures may be the first signs of toxicity.

Many patients who have higher theophylline serum levels exhibit a tachycardia.

Theophylline products may worsen pre-existing arrhythmias.

Usage in Pregnancy: Safe use in pregnancy has not been established relative to possible adverse effects on fetal development, but neither have adverse effects on fetal development been established. This is, unfortunately, true for most antiasthmatic medications. Therefore, use of theophylline in pregnant women should be balanced against the risk of uncontrolled asthma.

Precautions: Mean half-life in smokers is shorter than in nonsmokers, therefore, smokers may require larger doses of theophylline. Theophylline should not be administered concurrently with other xanthine medications. Use with caution in patients with severe cardiac disease, severe hypoxemia, hypertension, hyperthyroidism, acute myocardial injury, cor pulmonale, congestive heart failure, liver disease, in the elderly (especially males) and in neonates. Great caution should especially be used in giving theophylline to patients with congestive heart failure. Such patients have markedly prolonged theophylline blood level curves with theophylline persisting in serum for long periods following discontinuation of the drug.

Use theophylline cautiously in patients with history of peptic ulcer. Theophylline may occasionally act as a local irritant to G.I. tract although gastrointestinal symptoms are more commonly central and associated with serum concentrations over 20 mcg/ml.

Adverse Reactions: The most consistent adverse reactions are usually due to overdose and are:
1. Gastrointestinal: nausea, vomiting, epigastric pain, hematemesis, diarrhea.
2. Central nervous system: headaches, irritability, restlessness, insomnia, reflex hyperexcitability, muscle twitching, clonic and tonic generalized convulsions.
3. Cardiovascular: palpitation, tachycardia, extra systoles, flushing, hypotension, circulatory failure, life threatening ventricular arrhythmias.
4. Respiratory: tachypnea.
5. Renal: albuminuria, increased excretion of renal tubular cells and red blood cells; potentiation of diuresis.
6. Other: hyperglycemia and inappropriate ADH syndrome.

Drug Interactions: Toxic synergism with ephedrine has been documented and may occur with some other sympathomimetic bronchodilators.

Recent controlled studies suggest that the addition of ephedrine to adequate dosage regimens of theophylline produces little or no increase in effectiveness over that of theophylline alone, but does produce a synergistic increase in toxic side effects.

DRUG	EFFECT
Aminophylline with Lithium Carbonate	Increased excretion of Lithium Carbonate
Aminophylline with Propranolol	Antagonism of Propranolol effect
Theophylline with Furosemide	Increased Diuresis of Furosemide
Theophylline with Hexamethonium	Decreased Hexamethonium - induced chromatropic effect
Theophylline with Reserpine	Reserpine-induced Tachycardia
Theophylline with Chlordiazepoxide	Chloridiazepoxide-induced fatty acid mobilization
Theophylline with Cyclamycin (TAO = Triacetyloleandomycin); erythromycin, lincomycin	Increased Theophylline plasma levels

Overdosage:
Management:
A. If potential oral overdose is established and seizure has not occurred:
1) Induce vomiting.
2) Administer a cathartic (this is particularly important when sustained-release preparations have been taken).
3) Administer activated charcoal.
B. If patient is having a seizure:
1) Establish an airway.
2) Administer O_2.
3) Treat the seizure with intravenous diazepam, 0.1 to 0.3 mg/kg up to 10 mg.
4) Monitor vital signs, maintain blood pressure and provide adequate hydration.
C. Post-Seizure Coma:
1) Maintain airway and oxygenation.
2) If a result of oral medication, follow above recommendations to prevent absorption of the drug, but intubation and lavage will have to be performed instead of inducing emesis, and the cathartic and charcoal will need to be introduced via a large bore gastric lavage tube.
3) Continue to provide full supportive care and adequate hydration while waiting for drug to be metabolized. In general, the drug is metabolized sufficiently rapid so as not to warrant consideration of dialysis.
D. Animal studies suggest that phenobarbital may decrease theophylline toxicity. There is as yet, however, insufficient data to recommend pre-treatment of an overdosage with phenobarbital.

NOTE: THIS PRODUCT IS NOT FOR TREATMENT OF ACUTE SYMPTOMS OF ASTHMA REQUIRING RAPID THEOPHYLLINIZATION

Dosage and Administration: Therapeutic serum levels associated with optimal likelihood for benefit and minimal risk of toxicity are considered to be between 10 mcg/ml and 20 mcg/ml. Levels above 20 mcg/ml may produce toxic effects. There is great variation from patient to patient in dosage needed in order to achieve a therapeutic blood levels because of variable rates of elimination. Because of this wide variation from patient to patient, and the relatively narrow therapeutic blood level range, dosage must be individualized and monitoring of therophylline serum levels is highly recommended.

Dosage should be calculated on the basis of lean (ideal) body weight where mg/kg doses are stated. Theophylline does not distribute into fatty tissue. Giving theophylline with food may prevent the rare case of stomach irritation; and though absorption may be slower, it is still complete.

When rapidly absorbed products such as solutions and uncoated tablets with rapid dissolution are used, dosing to maintain "around the clock" blood levels generally requires administration every 6 hours to obtain the greatest efficacy for clinical use in children; dosing intervals up to 8 hours may be satisfactory for adults because of their slower elimination. Children, and adults requiring higher than average doses, may benefit from products with slower absorption which may allow longer dosing intervals and/or less fluctuation in serum concentration over a dosing interval during chronic therapy.

Comments: To achieve optimal therapeutic theophylline dosage, it is recommended to monitor serum theophylline concentrations. However, it is not always possible or practical to obtain a serum theophylline level.

Patients should be closely monitored for signs of toxicity. The present data suggest that dosage recommendations will achieve therapeutic serum concentrations with minimal risk of toxicity for most patients. However, some risk of toxic serum concentrations is still present.

Adverse reactions to theophylline often occur when serum theophylline levels exceed 20 mcg/ml.

DOSAGE FOR PATIENT POPULATION
Chronic Asthma:
Theophyllinization is a treatment of first choice for the management of chronic asthma (to prevent symptoms and maintain patent airways). Slow clinical titration is generally preferred to assure acceptance and safety of the medicine.

Initial dose: 16 mg/kg/day or 520 mg/day (whichever is lower) in 1-2 divides doses at 12 hour intervals.

Increased dose: The above dosage may be increased in approximately 25 percent increments at 2-3 day intervals so long as no intolerance is observed, until the maximum indicated below is reached.

Maximum dose without measurement of serum concentrations:
Not to exceed the following: (WARNING: DO NOT ATTEMPT TO MAINTAIN ANY DOSE THAT IS NOT TOLERATED)
Age < 9 years—24 mg/kg/day
Age 9-12 years—20 mg/kg/day
Age 12-16 years—18 mg/kg/day
Age > 16 years—13 mg/kg/dayor 900 mg/day (WHICHEVER IS LESS)

Note: Use ideal weight for obese patients
Measurement of serum theophylline concentration during chronic therapy:
If the above maximum doses are to be maintained or exceeded, serum theophylline measurement is recommended. This should be obtained at the approximate time of peak absorption during chronic therapy for the product used (1-2 hours for liquids and plain uncoated tablets that undergo rapid dissolution, 3-5 hours for sustained release preparations). It is important that the patient will have missed no doses during the previous 48 hours and that dosing intervals will have been reasonably typical with no added doses during that period of time. DOSAGE ADJUSTMENT BASED ON SERUM THEOPHYLLINE MEASUREMENTS WHEN THESE INSTRUCTIONS HAVE NOT BEEN FOLLOWED MAY RESULT IN RECOMMENDATIONS THAT PRESENT RISK OF TOXICITY TO THE PATIENT.

Final dosage adjustment:
Caution should be exercised for younger children who cannot complain of minor side effects. Older adults, those with corpulmonale, congestive heart failure, and/or liver disease, may have unusually low dosage requirements and thus may experience toxicity at the maximal dosage recommended above.

It is important that no patient be maintained on any dosage that he is not tolerating. In instructing patients to increase dosage according to the schedule above, they should be instructed to not take a subsequent dose if apparent side effects occur and to resume therapy at a lower dose once adverse effects have disappeared.
[See table on next page].

Caution: Federal law prohibits dispensing without prescription.

How Supplied: The blue and clear Theobid® Duracap® 260 mg capsules are supplied in bottles of 60 (NDC 0173-0268-12) and 500 (NDC 0173-0268-14) and unit dose packs of 100 capsules (NDC 0173-0268-17). Each capsule is imprinted with "Glaxo" and "268."

The two-tone blue Theobid® Jr. Duracap® 130 mg capsules are supplied in bottles of 60 (NDC 0173-0295-12) and 500 (NDC 0173-0295-14). Each capsule is imprinted with "Glaxo" and "295."

Revised and Reissued January, 1982

82014247/4248

Shown in Product Identification Section, page 412

TRANDATE® ℞
(labetalol hydrochloride)
Tablets

Description: TRANDATE® (labetalol HCl) is an adrenergic receptor blocking agent that has both selective alpha$_1$- and nonselective beta-adrenergic receptor blocking actions in a single substance.

Labetalol HCl is 5-[1-hydroxy-2-[(1-methyl-3-phenylpropyl)amino]ethyl]salicylamide monohy-

Continued on next page

Glaxo—Cont.

drochloride, and has the following structure:

Labetalol HCl has the empirical formula $C_{19}H_{24}N_2O_3$ HCl and a molecular weight of 364.9. It has two asymmetric centers and therefore exists as a molecular complex of two diastereoisomeric pairs.

Labetalol HCl is a white or off-white crystalline powder, soluble in water.

TRANDATE Tablets contain 200 mg and 300 mg labetalol HCl and are taken orally.

Clinical Pharmacology: TRANDATE® combines both selective, competitive alpha$_1$-adrenergic blocking and nonselective, competitive beta-adrenergic blocking activity in a single substance. In man, the ratios of alpha- to beta- blockade have been estimated to be approximately 1:3 and 1:7 following oral and intravenous administration, respectively. Beta$_2$-agonist activity has been demonstrated in animals with minimal beta$_1$-agonist (ISA) activity detected. In animals, at doses greater than those required for alpha- or beta-adrenergic blockade, a membrane stabilizing effect has been demonstrated.

Pharmacodynamics: The capacity of labetalol HCl to block alpha receptors in man has been demonstrated by attenuation of the pressor effect of phenylephrine and by a significant reduction of the pressor response caused by immersing the hand in ice-cold water ("cold-pressor test"). Labetalol HCl's beta$_1$-receptor blockade in man was demonstrated by a small decrease in the resting heart rate, attenuation of tachycardia produced by isoproterenol or exercise, and by attenuation of the reflex tachycardia to the hypotension produced by amyl nitrite. Beta$_2$-receptor blockade was demonstrated by inhibition of the iso-proterenol-induced fall in diastolic blood pressure. Both the alpha- and beta-blocking actions of orally administered labetalol HCl contribute to a decrease in blood pressure in hypertensive patients. Labetalol HCl consistently, in dose-related fashion, blunted increases in exercise-induced blood pressure and heart rate, and in their double product. The pulmonary circulation during exercise was not affected by labetalol HCl dosing.

Single oral doses of labetalol HCl administered in patients with coronary artery disease had no significant effect on sinus rate, intraventricular conduction or QRS duration. The AV conduction time was modestly prolonged in 2 of 7 patients. In another study, intravenous labetalol HCl slightly prolonged AV nodal conduction time and atrial effective refractory period with only small changes in heart rate. The effects on AV nodal refractoriness were inconsistent.

Labetalol HCl produces dose-related falls in blood pressure without reflex tachycardia and without significant reduction in heart rate, presumably through a mixture of its alpha-blocking and beta-blocking effects. Hemodynamic effects are variable with small nonsignificant changes in cardiac output seen in some studies but not others, and small decreases in total peripheral resistance. Elevated plasma renins are reduced.

Doses of labetalol HCl that controlled hypertension did not affect renal function in mild to severe hypertensive patients with normal renal function. Due to the alpha$_1$-receptor blocking activity of labetalol HCl, blood pressure is lowered more in the standing than in the supine position, and symptoms of postural hypotension can occur. Following oral administration, when postural hypotension has occurred, it has been transient and is uncommon (2%) when the recommended starting dose and titration increments are closely followed (see **Dosage and Administration**). Symptomatic postural hypotension is most likely to occur 2 to 4 hours after a dose, especially following the use of large initial doses or upon large changes in dose. The peak effects of single oral doses of labetalol HCl occur within 2 to 4 hours. The duration of effect depends upon dose, lasting at least 8 hours following single oral doses of 100 mg and more than 12 hours following single oral doses of 300 mg. The maximum, steady-state blood pressure response upon oral, twice-a-day dosing occurs within 24 to 72 hours.

The antihypertensive effect of labetalol has a linear correlation with the logarithm of labetalol plasma concentration, and there is also a linear correlation between the reduction in exercise-induced tachycardia occurring at 2 hours after oral administration of labetalol HCl and the logarithm of the plasma concentration.

About 70% of the maximum beta-blocking effect is present for 5 hours after the administration of a single oral dose of 400 mg with suggestion that about 40% remains at 8 hours.

The anti-anginal efficacy of labetalol HCl has not been studied. In 37 patients with hypertension and coronary artery disease, labetalol HCl did not increase the incidence or severity of angina attacks. Exacerbation of angina and, in some cases, myocardial infarction and ventricular dysrhythmias have been reported after abrupt discontinuation of therapy with beta-adrenergic blocking agents in patients with coronary artery disease. Abrupt withdrawal of these agents in patients without coronary artery disease has resulted in transient symptoms, including tremulousness, sweating, palpitation, headache, and malaise. Several mechanisms have been proposed to explain these phenomena, among them increased sensitivity to catecholamines because of increased numbers of beta receptors.

Although beta-adrenergic receptor blockade is useful in the treatment of angina and hypertension, there are also situations in which sympathetic stimulation is vital. For example, in patients with severely damaged hearts, adequate ventricular function may depend on sympathetic drive. Beta-adrenergic blockade may worsen AV block by preventing the necessary facilitating effects of sympathetic activity on conduction. Beta$_2$-adrenergic blockade results in passive bronchial constriction by interfering with endogenous adrenergic bronchodilator activity in patients subject to bronchospasm and may also interfere with exogenous bronchodilators in such patients.

Pharmacokinetics and Metabolism: Labetalol HCl is completely absorbed from the gastrointestinal tract with peak plasma levels occurring 1 to 2 hours after oral administration. The relative bioavailability of labetalol HCl tablets compared to an oral solution is 100%. The absolute bioavailability (fraction of drug reaching systemic circulation) of labetalol when compared to an intravenous infusion is 25%; this is due to extensive "first-pass" metabolism. Despite "first-pass" metabolism there is a linear relationship between oral doses of 100 mg to 3000 mg and peak plasma levels. The absolute bioavailability of labetalol is increased when administered with food.

The plasma half-life of labetalol following oral administration is about 6 to 8 hours. Steady-state plasma levels of labetalol during repetitive dosing are reached by about the third day of dosing. In patients with decreased hepatic or renal function, the elimination half-life of labetalol is not altered; however, the relative bioavailability in hepatically impaired patients is increased due to decreased "first-pass" metabolism.

The metabolism of labetalol is mainly through conjugation to glucuronide metabolites. These metabolites are present in plasma and are excreted in the urine and, via the bile, into the feces. Approximately 55% to 60% of a dose appears in the urine as conjugates or unchanged labetalol within the first 24 hours of dosing.

Labetalol has been shown to cross the placental barrier in humans. Only negligible amounts of the drug crossed the blood-brain barrier in animal studies. Labetalol is approximately 50% protein bound.

Indications and Usage: TRANDATE® (labetalol HCl) Tablets are indicated in the management of hypertension. TRANDATE Tablets may be used alone or in combination with other antihypertensive agents, especially thiazide and loop diuretics.

Contraindications: TRANDATE® Tablets are contraindicated in bronchial asthma, overt cardiac failure, greater than first degree heart block, cardiogenic shock, and severe bradycardia (see **Warnings**).

Warnings: Cardiac Failure: Sympathetic stimulation is a vital component supporting circulatory function in congestive heart failure. Beta blockade carries a potential hazard of further depressing myocardial contractility and precipitating more severe failure. Although beta-blockers should be avoided in overt congestive heart failure, if necessary, labetalol HCl can be used with

Peak Theophylline Level mcg/ml	Adjustment in Total Daily Dose	Comment
< 5	100% increase	If patient is asymptomatic, consider trial off drug; repeat blood levels after adjustment.
5–7.5	50% increase	
8–10	20% increase	Even if patient is asymptomatic at this level, an increased serum concentration may prevent symptoms during a viral URI, or heavy exposure to an inhalent allergen.
11–13	cautious 10% increase if clinically indicated.	If patient is asymptomatic, no increase is necessary. If symptoms present during URI or exercise, increase as indicated.
	None	If "breakthrough" in asthmatic symptoms present, at end of dosing interval, change is sustained-release product and repeat blood level.
14–20	Occasional intolerance requires a 10% decrease	If side effects present, decrease total daily dose as indicated.
21–25	10% decrease	Even if side-effects are absent.
26–34	25–33% decrease	Even if side-effects are absent, omit next dose and decrease total daily dose as indicated. Repeat blood levels.
≥ 35	50% decrease	Omit next two doses, decrease as indicated and repeat blood levels.

caution in patients with a history of heart failure who are well-compensated. Congestive heart failure has been observed in patients receiving labetalol HCl. Labetalol HCl does not abolish the inotropic action of digitalis on heart muscle.

In Patients Without a History of Cardiac Failure: In patients with latent cardiac insufficiency, continued depression of the myocardium with beta-blocking agents over a period of time can in some cases lead to cardiac failure. At the first sign or symptom of impending cardiac failure, patients should be fully digitalized and/or be given a diuretic, and the response observed closely. If cardiac failure continues, despite adequate digitalization and diuretic, TRANDATE® (labetalol HCl) therapy should be withdrawn (gradually, if possible).

Exacerbation of Ischemic Heart Disease Following Abrupt Withdrawal: Angina pectoris has not been reported upon labetalol HCl discontinuation. However, hypersensitivity to catecholamines has been observed in patients withdrawn from beta-blocker therapy; exacerbation of angina and, in some cases, myocardial infarction have occurred after *abrupt* discontinuation of such therapy. When discontinuing chronically administered TRANDATE, particularly in patients with ischemic heart disease, the dosage should be gradually reduced over a period of 1 to 2 weeks and the patient should be carefully monitored. If angina markedly worsens or acute coronary insufficiency develops, TRANDATE administration should be reinstituted promptly, at least temporarily, and other measures appropriate for the management of unstable angina should be taken. Patients should be warned against interruption or discontinuation of therapy without the physician's advice. Because coronary artery disease is common and may be unrecognized, it may be prudent not to discontinue TRANDATE therapy abruptly even in patients treated only for hypertension.

Nonallergic Bronchospasm (eg, chronic bronchitis and emphysema): Patients with bronchospastic disease should, in general, not receive beta-blockers. TRANDATE may be used with caution, however, in patients who do not respond to, or cannot tolerate, other antihypertensive agents. It is prudent, if TRANDATE is used, to use the smallest effective dose, so that inhibition of endogenous or exogenous beta-agonists is minimized.

Pheochromocytoma: Labetalol HCl has been shown to be effective in lowering the blood pressure and relieving symptoms in patients with pheochromocytoma. However, paradoxical hypertensive responses have been reported in a few patients with this tumor; therefore, use caution when administering labetalol HCl to patients with pheochromocytoma.

Diabetes Mellitus and Hypoglycemia: Beta-adrenergic blockade may prevent the appearance of premonitory signs and symptoms (eg, tachycardia) of acute hypoglycemia. This is especially important with labile diabetics. Beta-blockade also reduces the release of insulin in response to hyperglycemia; it may therefore be necessary to adjust the dose of antidiabetic drugs.

Major Surgery: The necessity or desirability of withdrawing beta-blocking therapy prior to major surgery is controversial. Protracted severe hypotension and difficulty in restarting or maintaining a heart beat have been reported with beta-blockers. The effect of labetalol HCl's alpha-adrenergic activity has not been evaluated in this setting.

A synergism between labetalol HCl and halothane anesthesia has been shown (see **Drug Interactions**).

Precautions: General: *Impaired Hepatic Function:* TRANDATE® Tablets should be used with caution in patients with impaired hepatic function since metabolism of the drug may be diminished.

Jaundice or Hepatic Dysfunction: On rare occasions, labetalol HCl has been associated with jaundice (both hepatic and cholestatic). It is therefore recommended that treatment with labetalol HCl be stopped immediately should a patient develop jaundice or laboratory evidence of liver injury. Both have been shown to be reversible on stopping therapy.

Information for Patients: As with all drugs with beta-blocking activity, certain advice to patients being treated with labetalol HCl is warranted. This information is intended to aid in the safe and effective use of this medication. It is not a disclosure of all possible adverse or intended effects. While no incidence of the abrupt withdrawal phenomenon (exacerbation of angina pectoris) has been reported with labetalol HCl, dosing with TRANDATE Tablets should not be interrupted or discontinued without a physician's advice. Patients being treated with TRANDATE Tablets should consult a physician at any sign of impending cardiac failure. Also, transient scalp tingling may occur, usually when treatment with TRANDATE Tablets is initiated (see **Adverse Reactions**).

Laboratory Tests: As with any new drug given over prolonged periods, laboratory parameters should be observed over regular intervals. In patients with concomitant illnesses, such as impaired renal function, appropriate tests should be done to monitor these conditions.

Drug Interactions: In one survey, 2.3% of patients taking labetalol HCl in combination with tricyclic antidepressants experienced tremor as compared to 0.7% reported to occur with labetalol HCl alone. The contribution of each of the treatments to this adverse reaction is unknown, but the possibility of a drug interaction cannot be excluded.

Drugs possessing beta-blocking properties can blunt the bronchodilator effect of beta-receptor agonist drugs in patients with bronchospasm; therefore, doses greater than the normal anti-asthmatic dose of beta-agonist bronchodilator drugs may be required.

Cimetidine has been shown to increase the bioavailability of labetalol HCl. Since this could be explained either by enhanced absorption or by an alteration of hepatic metabolism of labetalol HCl, special care should be used in establishing the dose required for blood pressure control in such patients.

Synergism has been shown between halothane anesthesia and intravenously administered labetalol HCl. During controlled hypotensive anesthesia using labetalol HCl in association with halothane, high concentrations (3% or above) of halothane should not be used because the degree of hypotension will be increased and because of the possibility of a large reduction in cardiac output and an increase in central venous pressure. The anesthesiologist should be informed when a patient is receiving labetalol HCl.

Labetalol HCl blunts the reflex tachycardia produced by nitroglycerin without preventing its hypotensive effect. If labetalol HCl is used with nitroglycerin in patients with angina pectoris, additional antihypertensive effects may occur.

Drug/Laboratory Test Interactions: The presence of a metabolite of labetalol in the urine may result in falsely increased levels of urinary catecholamines when measured by a nonspecific trihydroxyindole (THI) reaction. In screening patients suspected of having a pheochromocytoma and being treated with labetalol HCl, specific radioenzymatic or high performance liquid chromatography assay techniques should be used to determine levels of catecholamines or their metabolites.

Carcinogenesis, Mutagenesis, Impairment of Fertility: Long-term oral dosing studies with labetalol HCl for 18 months in mice and for 2 years in rats showed no evidence of carcinogenesis. Studies with labetalol HCl, using dominant lethal assays in rats and mice, and exposing microorganisms according to modified Ames tests, showed no evidence of mutagenesis.

Pregnancy Category C: Teratogenic studies have been performed with labetalol in rats and rabbits at oral doses up to approximately 6 and 4 times the MRHD, respectively. No reproducible evidence of fetal malformations was observed. Increased fetal resorptions were seen in both species at doses approximating the MRHD. There are no adequate and well-controlled studies in pregnant women. Labetalol should be used during pregnancy only if the potential benefit justifies the potential risk to the fetus.

Nonteratogenic Effects: Infants of mothers who were treated with labetalol HCl during pregnancy did not appear to be adversely affected by the drug. Oral administration of labetalol to rats during late gestation through weaning at doses of 2 to 4 times the MRHD caused a decrease in neonatal survival.

Labor and Delivery: Labetalol HCl given to pregnant women with hypertension did not appear to affect the usual course of labor and delivery.

Nursing Mothers: Small amounts of labetalol (approximately 0.004% of the maternal dose) are excreted in human milk. Caution should be exercised when TRANDATE (labetalol HCl) Tablets are administered to a nursing mother.

Pediatric Use: Safety and effectiveness in children have not been established.

Adverse Reactions: Most adverse effects are mild, transient and occur early in the course of treatment. In controlled clinical trials of 3 to 4 months' duration, discontinuation of TRANDATE® Tablets due to one or more adverse effects was required in 7% of all patients. In these same trials, beta-blocker control agents led to discontinuation in 8% to 10% of patients, and a centrally acting alpha-agonist in 30% of patients.

The incidence rates of adverse reactions listed in the following table were derived from multicenter controlled clinical trials, comparing labetalol HCl, placebo, metoprolol and propranolol, over treatment periods of 3 and 4 months. Where the frequency of adverse effects for labetalol HCl and placebo is similar, causal relationship is uncertain. The rates are based on adverse reactions considered probably drug-related by the investigator. If all reports are considered, the rates are somewhat higher (eg, dizziness 20%, nausea 14%, fatigue 11%), but the overall conclusions are unchanged.

[See table on bottom next page].

The adverse effects were reported spontaneously and are representative of the incidence of adverse effects that may be observed in a properly selected hypertensive patient population, ie, a group excluding patients with bronchospastic disease, overt congestive heart failure, or other contraindications to beta-blocker therapy.

Clinical trials also included studies utilizing daily doses up to 2400 mg in more severely hypertensive patients. Certain of the side effects increased with increasing dose as shown in the table below which depicts the entire U.S. therapeutic trials data base for adverse reactions that are clearly or possibly dose-related.

[See table on top next page].

In addition, a number of other less common adverse events have been reported in clinical trials or the literature:

Central and Peripheral Nervous Systems: Paresthesias, most frequently described as scalp tingling. In most cases, it was mild, transient and usually occurred at the beginning of treatment.

Collagen Disorders: Systemic lupus erythematosus; positive antinuclear factor (ANF).

Eyes: Dry eyes.

Immunological System: Antimitochondrial antibodies.

Liver and Biliary System: Cholestasis with or without jaundice.

Musculo-Skeletal System: Muscle cramps; toxic myopathy.

Respiratory System: Bronchospasm.

Skin and Appendages: Rashes of various types, such as generalized maculopapular; lichenoid; urticarial; bullous lichen planus; psoriaform; facial erythema; Peyronie's disease; reversible alopecia.

Urinary System: Difficulty in micturition, including acute urinary bladder retention.

Following approval for marketing in the United Kingdom, a monitored release survey involving approximately 6,800 patients was conducted for further safety and efficacy evaluation of this product. Results of this survey indicate that the type,

Continued on next page

Glaxo—Cont.

severity, and incidence of adverse effects were comparable to those cited above.
Potential Adverse Effects: In addition, other adverse effects not listed above have been reported with other beta-adrenergic blocking agents.
Central Nervous System: Reversible mental depression progressing to catatonia; an acute reversible syndrome characterized by disorientation for time and place, short-term memory loss, emotional lability, slightly clouded sensorium, and decreased performance or neuropsychometrics.
Cardiovascular: Intensification of AV block (see **Contraindications**).
Allergic: Fever combined with aching and sore throat; laryngospasm; respiratory distress.
Hematologic: Agranulocytosis; thrombocytopenic or nonthrombocytopenic purpura.
Gastrointestinal: Mesenteric artery thrombosis; ischemic colitis.
The oculomucocutaneous syndrome associated with the beta-blocker practolol has not been reported with labetalol HCl.
Clinical Laboratory Tests: There have been reversible increases of serum transaminases in 4% of patients treated with labetalol HCl and tested, and more rarely, reversible increases in blood urea.
Overdosage: Overdosage with TRANDATE® (labetalol HCl) Tablets causes excessive hypotension which is posture sensitive, and sometimes, excessive bradycardia. Patients should be laid supine and their legs raised if necessary to improve the blood supply to the brain. The following additional measures should be employed if necessary: **Excessive bradycardia**—administer atropine (3.0 mg). If there is no response to vagal blockade, administer isoproterenol cautiously. **Cardiac failure**—administer a digitalis glycoside and a diuretic. **Hypotension**—administer vasopressors, eg, norepinephrine. There is pharmacological evidence that norepinephrine may be the drug of choice. **Bronchospasm**—administer a beta₂-stimulating agent and/or a theophylline preparation. Gastric lavage or pharmacologically induced emesis (using syrup of ipecac) is useful for removal of the drug shortly after ingestion. Labetalol HCl can be removed from the general circulation by hemodialysis.

The oral LD$_{50}$ value of labetalol HCl in the mouse is approximately 600 mg/kg and in the rat is greater than 2 g/kg. The intravenous LD$_{50}$ in these species is 50 to 60 mg/kg.

Dosage and Administration: DOSAGE MUST BE INDIVIDUALIZED. The recommended *initial* dose is 100 mg *twice* daily whether used alone or added to a diuretic regimen. After 2 or 3 days, using standing blood pressure as an indicator, dosage may be titrated in increments of 100 mg bid every 2 or 3 days. The usual *maintenance* dosage of labetalol HCl is between 200 and 400 mg *twice* daily.
Since the full antihypertensive effect of labetalol HCl is usually seen within the first 1 to 3 hours of the initial dose or dose increment, the assurance of a lack of an exaggerated hypotensive response can be clinically established in the office setting. The antihypertensive effects of continued dosing can be measured at subsequent visits, approximately 12 hours after a dose, to determine whether further titration is necessary.
Patients with severe hypertension may require from 1200 mg to 2400 mg per day, with or without thiazide diuretics. Should side effects (principally nausea or dizziness) occur with these doses administered bid, the same total daily dose administered tid may improve tolerability and facilitate further titration. Titration increments should not exceed 200 mg bid.

Labetalol HCl Daily Dose (mg)	200	300	400	600	800	900	1200	1600	2400
Number of Patients	522	181	606	608	503	117	411	242	175
Dizziness (%)	2	3	3	3	5	1	9	13	16
Fatigue	2	1	4	4	5	3	7	6	10
Nausea	<1	0	1	2	4	0	7	11	19
Vomiting	0	0	<1	<1	<1	0	1	2	3
Dyspepsia	1	0	2	1	1	0	2	2	4
Paresthesias	2	0	2	2	1	1	2	5	5
Nasal Stuffiness	1	1	2	2	2	0	4	5	6
Ejaculation Failure	0	2	1	2	3	0	4	3	5
Impotence	1	1	1	1	2	4	3	4	3
Edema	1	0	1	1	1	0	1	2	2

When a diuretic is added, an additive antihypertensive effect can be expected. In some cases this may necessitate a labetalol HCl dosage adjustment. As with most antihypertensive drugs, optimal dosages of TRANDATE® Tablets are usually lower in patients also receiving a diuretic.
When transferring patients from other antihypertensive drugs, TRANDATE Tablets should be introduced as recommended and the dosage of the existing therapy progressively decreased.
How Supplied: TRANDATE® Tablets, 200 mg, white, round, scored, film-coated tablets engraved on one side with "TRANDATE 200 GLAXO," bottles of 100 (NDC 0173-0347-43), bottles of 500 (NDC 0173-0347-44), and unit dose packs of 100 tablets (NDC 0173-0347-47).
TRANDATE Tablets, 300 mg, peach, round, film-coated tablets engraved on one side with "TRANDATE 300 GLAXO," bottles of 100 (NDC 0173-0348-43), bottles of 500 (NDC 0173-0348-44), and unit dose packs of 100 tablets (NDC 0173-0348-47).
TRANDATE Tablets should be stored between 2° and 30°C (36° and 86°F).
TRANDATE Tablets in the unit dose boxes should be protected from excessive moisture.
October 1984
Shown in Product Identification Section, page 412

TRI-CONE® Capsules

Composition: Each white and black capsule contains:
Amylase	10 mg
Prolase	10 mg
Lipase	10 mg
Simethicone	40 mg

Actions and Uses: Tri-cone is indicated for the symptomatic relief of functional digestive disorders characterized by functional gastric bloating, dyspepsia, and flatulence resulting from failure to chew food properly, inadequate digestive competency due to disease or age, or faulty dietary habits. Tri-Cone is also indicated as a supplement to normal enzyme activity of the body in absorptive and assimilative defects associated with surgery on the stomach, small bowel, or pancreas and associated with chronic pancreatitis and pancreatic insufficiency.
Simethicone acts to relieve or alleviate the pain and other symptoms of gaseousness produced by bacterial fermentation and aerophagia.
The enzymes, particularly the proteolytic enzyme, do not require acid conditions to be activated which may be of special benefit in aiding digestion in geriatric patients with insufficient gastric acidity due to hypochlorhydria.
Contraindications: Known allergy to an ingredient.
Dosage: Two or three capsules after meals as required to relieve the symptoms of gas and aid digestion of fats, starches and proteins.
How Supplied: Bottles of 60 and 500 capsules.

TRINSICON®
[trĭn'sĭ-cŏn]
Hematinic Concentrate
With Intrinsic Factor

A highly potent oral antianemia preparation
Description: Each capsule contains—
Special Liver-Stomach
 Concentrate (containing

	Labetalol HCl (N=227) %	Placebo (N=98) %	Propranolol (N=84) %	Metoprolol (N=49) %
Body as a whole				
fatigue	5	0	12	12
asthenia	1	1	1	0
headache	2	1	1	2
Gastrointestinal				
nausea	6	1	1	2
vomiting	<1	0	0	0
dyspepsia	3	1	1	0
abdominal pain	0	0	1	2
diarrhea	<1	0	2	0
taste distortion	1	0	0	0
Central and Peripheral Nervous Systems				
dizziness	11	3	4	4
paresthesias	<1	0	0	0
drowsiness	<1	2	2	2
Autonomic Nervous System				
nasal stuffiness	3	0	0	0
ejaculation failure	2	0	0	0
impotence	1	0	1	3
increased sweating	<1	0	0	0
Cardiovascular				
edema	1	0	0	0
postural hypotension	1	0	0	0
bradycardia	0	0	5	12
Respiratory				
dyspnea	2	0	1	2
Skin				
rash	1	0	0	0
Special Senses				
vision abnormality	1	0	0	0
vertigo	2	1	0	0

Intrinsic Factor) .... 240 mg.
Vitamin B$_{12}$ (activity equivalent) .... 15 mcg.
Iron, Elemental .... 110 mg.
(as Ferrous Fumarate)
Ascorbic Acid
(Vitamin C) .... 75 mg.
Folic Acid .... 0.5 mg.
with other factors of Vitamin B Complex present in the Liver-Stomach Concentrate.

Clinical Pharmacology: *Vitamin B$_{12}$ with Intrinsic Factor*—When secretion of intrinsic factor in gastric juice is inadequate or absent (e.g., in Addisonian pernicious anemia or after gastrectomy), vitamin B$_{12}$ in physiologic doses is absorbed poorly, if at all. The resulting deficiency of vitamin B$_{12}$ leads to the clinical manifestations of pernicious anemia. Similar megaloblastic anemias may develop in fish tapeworm *(Diphyllobothrium latum)* infection or after a surgically created small-bowel blind loop; in these situations, treatment requires freeing the host of the parasites or bacteria which appear to compete for the available vitamin B$_{12}$. Strict vegetarianism and malabsorption syndromes may also lead to vitamin B$_{12}$ deficiency. In the latter case, parenteral therapy, or oral therapy with so-called massive doses of vitamin B$_{12}$, may be necessary for adequate treatment of the patient.

Potency of intrinsic factor concentrates is determined physiologically, i.e., by their use in patients with pernicious anemia. The liver-stomach concentrate with intrinsic factor and the vitamin B$_{12}$ contained in 2 Trinsicon capsules provide 1½ times the minimum amount of therapeutic agent which, when given daily in an uncomplicated case of pernicious anemia, will produce a satisfactory reticulocyte response and relief of anemia and symptoms.

Concentrates of intrinsic factor derived from hog gastric, pyloric, and duodenal mucosa have been used successfully in patients who lack intrinsic factor. For example, Fouts *et al.* maintained patients with pernicious anemia in clinical remission with oral therapy (liver extracts or intrinsic factor concentrate with vitamin B$_{12}$) for as long as 29 years.

After total gastrectomy, Ficarra found multifactor preparations taken orally to be "just as effective in maintaining blood levels as any medication that has to be administered parenterally." His study was based on 24 patients who had survived for 5 years after total gastrectomy for cancer and who had been taking 2 Trinsicon capsules daily.

Folic Acid—Folic acid deficiency is the immediate cause of most, if not all, cases of nutritional megaloblastic anemia and of the megaloblastic anemias of pregnancy and infancy; usually, it is also at least partially responsible for the megaloblastic anemias of malabsorption syndromes, e.g., tropical and nontropical sprue.

It is apparent that in vitamin B$_{12}$ deficiency (e.g., pernicious anemia), lack of this vitamin results in impaired utilization of folic acid. There are other evidences of the close folic acid-vitamin B$_{12}$ interrelationship: (1) B$_{12}$ influences the storage, absorption, and utilization of folic acid, and (2), as a deficiency of B$_{12}$ progresses, the requirement for folic acid increases. However, folic acid does not change the requirement for vitamin B$_{12}$.

Iron—A very common anemia is that due to iron deficiency. In most cases, the response to iron salts is prompt, safe, and predictable. Within limits, the response is quicker and more certain to large doses of iron than to small doses.

Each Trinsicon capsule furnishes 110 mg. of elemental iron (as ferrous fumarate) to provide a maximum response.

Ascorbic Acid—Vitamin C plays a role in anemia therapy. It augments the conversion of folic acid to its active form, folinic acid. In addition, ascorbic acid promotes the reduction of ferric iron in food to the more readily absorbed ferrous form. Severe and prolonged vitamin C deficiency is associated with an anemia which is usually hypochromic but occasionally megaloblastic in type.

Indications and Usage: Trinsicon® (hematinic concentrate with intrinsic factor) is a multifactor preparation effective in the treatment of anemias that respond to oral hematinics, including pernicious anemia and other megaloblastic anemias and also iron-deficiency anemia. Therapeutic quantities of hematopoietic factors that are known to be important are present in the recommended daily dose.

Contraindications: Hemochromatosis and hemosiderosis are contraindications to iron therapy.

Precautions:
General Precautions—Anemia is a manifestation that requires appropriate investigation to determine its cause or causes.

Folic acid *alone* is unwarranted in the treatment of pure vitamin B$_{12}$ deficiency states, such as pernicious anemia. Folic acid may obscure pernicious anemia in that the blood picture may revert to normal while neurological manifestations remain progressive.

As with all preparations containing intrinsic factor, resistance may develop in some cases of pernicious anemia to the potentiation of absorption of physiologic doses of vitamin B$_{12}$. If resistance occurs, parenteral therapy, or oral therapy with so-called massive doses of vitamin B$_{12}$ may be necessary for adequate treatment of the patient. No single regimen fits all cases, and the status of the patient observed in follow-up is the final criterion for adequacy of therapy. Periodic clinical and laboratory studies are considered essential and are recommended.

Usage in Pregnancy—Pregnancy Category C—Animal reproduction studies have not been conducted with Trinsicon. It is also not known whether Trinsicon can cause fetal harm when administered to a pregnant woman or can affect reproduction capacity. Trinsicon should be given to a pregnant woman only if clearly needed.

Nursing Mothers—It is not known whether this drug is excreted in human milk. Because many drugs are excreted in human milk, caution should be exercised when Trinsicon is administered to a nursing woman.

Usage in Children—Safety and effectiveness in children below the age of 10 have not been established.

Adverse Reactions: Rarely, iron in therapeutic doses produces gastrointestinal reactions, such as diarrhea or constipation. Reducing the dose and administering it with meals will minimize these effects in the iron-sensitive patient.

In extremely rare instances, skin rash suggesting allergy has been noted following the oral administration of liver-stomach material. Allergic sensitization has been reported following both oral and parenteral administration of folic acid.

Overdosage:
Symptoms—Those of iron intoxication, which may include pallor and cyanosis, vomiting, hematemesis, diarrhea, melena, shock, drowsiness, and coma.

Treatment—For specific therapy, exchange transfusion and chelating agents. For general management, gastric and rectal lavage with sodium bicarbonate solution or milk, administration of intravenous fluids and electrolytes, and use of oxygen.

Dosage: One capsule twice a day. (Two capsules daily produce a standard response in the average uncomplicated case of pernicious anemia.)

How Supplied: Capsules, dark pink and dark red (No. 2). Bottles of 60 (NDC 0173-0364-22), bottles of 500 (NDC 0173-0364-24), and Unit Dose Packs of 100 capsules (NDC 0173-0364-27).

Shown in Product Identification Section, page 412

VENTOLIN® Inhaler   ℞
[ven′tō-lin″]
(albuterol)
Bronchodilator Aerosol
For Oral Inhalation Only

Description: The active component of VENTOLIN® Inhaler is albuterol (α′-[(*tert*-butylamino) methyl] - 4- hydroxy- *m*-xylene -α, α′-diol), a relatively selective beta$_2$-adrenergic bronchodilator having the chemical structure:
(See next column)

Albuterol is the official generic name in the United States. The international generic name for

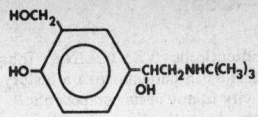

the drug is salbutamol. The molecular weight of albuterol is 239.3, and the empirical formula C$_{13}$H$_{21}$NO$_3$. Albuterol is a white to off-white crystalline solid. It is soluble in water, and very soluble in chloroform.

VENTOLIN Inhaler is a metered-dose aerosol unit for oral inhalation. It contains a microcrystalline suspension of albuterol in propellants (trichloromonofluoromethane and dichlorodifluoromethane) with oleic acid. Each actuation delivers from the mouthpiece 90 mcg of albuterol. Each canister provides at least 200 inhalations.

Clinical Pharmacology: The prime action of beta-adrenergic drugs is to stimulate adenyl cyclase, the enzyme which catalyzes the formation of cyclic-3′, 5′-adenosine monophosphate (cyclic AMP) from adenosine triphosphate (ATP). The cyclic AMP thus formed mediates the cellular responses. By virtue of its relatively selective action on beta$_2$-adrenoceptors, albuterol relaxes smooth muscle of the bronchi, uterus, and vascular supply to skeletal muscle, but may have less cardiac stimulant effects than does isoproterenol.

Albuterol is longer acting than isoproterenol by any route of administration in most patients because it is not a substrate for the cellular uptake processes for catecholamines nor for catechol-O-methyl transferase.

Because of its gradual absorption from the bronchi, systemic levels of albuterol are low after inhalation of recommended doses. Studies undertaken with four subjects administered tritiated albuterol resulted in maximum plasma concentrations occurring within two to four hours. Due to the sensitivity of the assay method, the metabolic rate and half-life of elimination of albuterol in plasma could not be determined. However, urinary excretion provided data indicating that albuterol has an elimination half-life of 3.8 hours. Approximately 72% of the inhaled dose is excreted within 24 hours in the urine, and consists of 28% of unchanged drug and 44% as metabolite.

Results of animal studies show that albuterol does not pass the blood-brain barrier.

The effects of rising doses of albuterol and isoproterenol aerosols were studied in volunteers and asthmatic patients. Results in normal volunteers indicated that albuterol is one-half to one-quarter as active as isoproterenol in producing increases in heart rate. In asthmatic patients similar cardiovascular differentiation between the two drugs was also seen.

Indications and Usage: VENTOLIN® (albuterol) Inhaler is indicated for the relief of bronchospasm in patients with reversible obstructive airway disease, and for the prevention of exercise-induced bronchospasm.

In controlled clinical trials the onset of improvement in pulmonary function was within 15 minutes, as determined by both maximal midexpiratory flow rate (MMEF) and FEV$_1$. MMEF measurements also showed that near maximum improvement in pulmonary function generally occurs within 60 to 90 minutes following 2 inhalations of albuterol and that clinically significant improvement generally continues for 3 to 4 hours in most patients. In clinical trials, some patients with asthma showed a therapeutic response (defined by maintaining FEV$_1$ values 15% or more above base line) which was still apparent at 6 hours. Continued effectiveness of albuterol was demonstrated over a 13-week period in these same trials.

In clinical studies, 2 inhalations of albuterol taken approximately 15 minutes prior to exercise prevented exercise-induced bronchospasm, as demonstrated by the maintenance of FEV$_1$ within 80% of baseline values in the majority, but not in all, of the patients studied.

Continued on next page

Glaxo—Cont.

Contraindications: VENTOLIN® Inhaler is contraindicated in patients with a history of hypersensitivity to any of its components.

Warnings: As with other adrenergic aerosols, the potential for paradoxical bronchospasm should be kept in mind. If it occurs, the preparation should be discontinued immediately and alternative therapy instituted.

Fatalities have been reported in association with excessive use of inhaled sympathomimetic drugs. The exact cause of death is unknown, but cardiac arrest following the unexpected development of a severe acute asthmatic crisis and subsequent hypoxia is suspected.

The contents of VENTOLIN® Inhaler are under pressure. Do not puncture. Do not use or store near heat or open flame. Exposure to temperatures above 120°F may cause bursting. Never throw container into fire or incinerator. Keep out of reach of children.

Precautions: Although it has less effect on the cardiovascular system than isoproterenol at recommended dosages, albuterol is a sympathomimetic amine and as such should be used with caution in patients with cardiovascular disorders, including coronary insufficiency and hypertension, in patients with hyperthyroidism or diabetes mellitus, and in patients who are unusually responsive to sympathomimetic amines.

Large doses of intravenous albuterol have been reported to aggravate preexisting diabetes and ketoacidosis. The relevance of this observation to the use of VENTOLIN® Inhaler is unknown, since the aerosol dose is much lower than the doses given intravenously.

Although there have been no reports concerning the use of VENTOLIN Inhaler during labor and delivery, it has been reported that high doses of albuterol administered intravenously inhibit uterine contractions. Although this effect is extremely unlikely as a consequence of aerosol use, it should be kept in mind.

Information For Patients: The action of VENTOLIN Inhaler may last up to six hours, and therefore it should not be used more frequently than recommended. Do not increase the number or frequency of doses without medical consultation. If symptoms get worse, medical consultation should be sought promptly. While taking VENTOLIN Inhaler, other inhaled medicines should not be used unless prescribed.

See Illustrated Patient's Instructions For Use.

Drug Interactions: Other sympathomimetic aerosol bronchodilators or epinephrine should not be used concomitantly with albuterol.

Albuterol should be administered with caution to patients being treated with monoamine oxidase inhibitors or tricyclic anti-depressants, since the action of albuterol on the vascular system may be potentiated.

Beta-receptor blocking agents and albuterol inhibit the effect of each other.

Carcinogenesis, Mutagenesis, Impairment of Fertility: In a 2-year study in the rat, albuterol sulfate caused a significant dose-related increase in the incidence of benign leiomyomata of the mesovarium at doses corresponding to 111, 555, and 2,800 times the maximum human inhalational dose. The relevance of these findings to humans is not known. An 18-month study in mice revealed no evidence of tumorigenicity. Studies with albuterol revealed no evidence of mutagenesis. Reproduction studies in rats revealed no evidence of impaired fertility.

Teratogenic Effects: *Pregnancy Category C:* Albuterol has been shown to be teratogenic in mice when given in doses corresponding to 14 times the human dose. There are no adequate and well-controlled studies in pregnant women. Albuterol should be used during pregnancy only if the potential benefit justifies the potential risk to the fetus. A reproduction study in CD-1 mice with albuterol (0.025, 0.25, and 2.5 mg/kg, corresponding to 1.4, 14, and 140 times the maximum human inhalational dose) showed a cleft palate formation in 5 of 111 (4.5%) fetuses at 0.25 mg/kg and in 10 of 108 (9.3%) fetuses at 2.5 mg/kg. None were observed at 0.025 mg/kg. Cleft palate also occurred in 22 of 72 (30.5%) fetuses treated with 2.5 mg/kg isoproterenol (positive control). A reproduction study in Stride Dutch rabbits revealed cranioschisis in 7 of 19 (37%) fetuses at 50 mg/kg, corresponding to 2,800 times the maximum human inhalational dose.

Nursing Mothers: It is not known whether this drug is excreted in human milk. Because of the potential for tumorigenicity shown for albuterol in animal studies, a decision should be made whether to discontinue nursing or to discontinue the drug, taking into account the importance of the drug to the mother.

Pediatric Use: Safety and effectiveness in children below the age of 12 years have not been established.

Adverse Reactions: The adverse reactions of albuterol are similar in nature to those of other sympathomimetic agents, although the incidence of certain cardiovascular effects is less with albuterol. A 13-week double-blind study compared albuterol and isoproterenol aerosols in 147 asthmatic patients. The results of this study showed that the incidence of cardiovascular effects was: palpitations, less than 10 per 100 with albuterol and less than 15 per 100 with isoproterenol. The incidences of tachycardia and increased blood pressure were 10 per 100 and less than 5 per 100, respectively, with both drugs. In the same study, both drugs caused tremor or nausea in less than 15 patients per 100, and dizziness or heartburn in less than 5 per 100 patients. Nervousness occurred in less than 10 per 100 patients receiving albuterol and in less than 15 per 100 patients receiving isoproterenol.

In addition, albuterol, like other sympathomimetic agents, can cause adverse reactions such as hypertension, angina, vomiting, vertigo, central stimulation, insomnia, headache, unusual taste, and drying or irritation of the oropharynx.

Overdosage: Exaggeration of the effects listed in **Adverse Reactions** can occur. Anginal pain and hypertension may result.

The oral LD_{50} in male and female rats and mice was greater than 2,000 mg/kg. The aerosol LD_{50} could not be determined.

Dialysis is not appropriate treatment for overdosage of VENTOLIN® (albuterol) Inhaler. The judicious use of a cardioselective beta-receptor blocker, such as a metoprolol tartrate, is suggested, bearing in mind the danger of inducing an asthmatic attack.

Dosage and Administration: The usual dosage for adults and children 12 years and older is 2 inhalations repeated every 4 to 6 hours; in some patients, 1 inhalation every 4 hours may be sufficient. More frequent administration or a larger number of inhalations is not recommended. The use of VENTOLIN® Inhaler can be continued as medically indicated to control recurring bouts of bronchospasm. During this time most patients gain optimal benefit from regular use of the inhaler. Safe usage for periods extending over several years has been documented.

If a previously effective dosage regimen fails to provide the usual relief, medical advice should be sought immediately as this is often a sign of seriously worsening asthma which would require reassessment of therapy.

Exercise-Induced Bronchospasm Prevention: The usual dosage for adults and children 12 years and older is 2 inhalations 15 minutes prior to exercise.

How Supplied: VENTOLIN® Inhaler, 17.0 g canister; box of one. Each actuation delivers 90 mcg of albuterol from the mouthpiece. It is supplied with an oral adapter and patient's instructions; (NDC 0173-0321-88). Also available, VENTOLIN Inhaler Refill, 17.0 g canister only with patient's instructions (NDC 0173-0321-98).

Store between 15° and 30°C (59° and 86°F).

Shown in Product Identification Section, page 412

VENTOLIN® Tablets ℞
[*ven′ tō-lin″*]
(albuterol sulfate)

Description: VENTOLIN Tablets contain albuterol sulfate, a relatively selective beta$_2$-adrenergic bronchodilator. Albuterol sulfate has the chemical name α^1-[(*tert*-Butylamino)methyl]-4-hydroxy-*m*-xylene-α,α′-diol sulfate (2:1)(salt).

Albuterol sulfate has a molecular weight of 576.7 and the empirical formula $(C_{13}H_{21}NO_3)_2 \cdot H_2SO_4$. Albuterol sulfate is a white crystalline powder, soluble in water and slightly soluble in ethanol. The international generic name for albuterol base is salbutamol.

Each VENTOLIN Tablet contains 2 or 4 mg of albuterol as 2.4 and 4.8 mg of albuterol sulfate, respectively.

Clinical Pharmacology: The prime action of beta-adrenergic drugs is to stimulate adenyl cyclase, the enzyme which catalyzes the formation of cyclic-3′,5′-adenosine monophosphate (cyclic AMP) from adenosine triphosphate (ATP). The cyclic AMP thus formed mediates the cellular responses. Based on pharmacologic studies in animals, albuterol appears to exert direct and preferential action on beta$_2$-adrenoceptors including those of the bronchial tree and uterus, and may have less cardiac stimulant effect than isoproterenol when given in the usual recommended dose.

Albuterol is longer acting than isoproterenol in most patients by any route of administration because it is not a substrate for the cellular uptake processes for catecholamines nor for catechol-O-methyl transferase.

In three normal volunteers given tablets containing 6 mg tritiated albuterol sulfate, the maximum plasma concentrations of albuterol occurred within 2.5 hours. In other studies, the analysis of peak plasma samples indicated that the metabolite of albuterol represented 80% of the radioactivity present. Albuterol was shown to have a plasma half-life ranging from 2.7 to 5.0 hours when administered orally. Analysis of urine samples showed that 76% of the dose was excreted over 3 days, with the majority of the dose being excreted within the first 24 hours. Sixty percent of this radioactivity was shown to be the metabolite. Feces collected over this period contained 4% of the administered dose.

Animal studies show that albuterol does not pass the blood-brain barrier.

Indications and Usage: VENTOLIN Tablets are indicated for the relief of bronchospasm in patients with reversible obstructive airway disease.

In controlled clinical trials in patients with asthma, the onset of improvement in pulmonary function, as measured by maximal midexpiratory flow rate, MMEF, was noted within 30 minutes after a dose of VENTOLIN Tablets with peak improvement occurring between 2 and 3 hours. In controlled clinical trials in which measurements were conducted for 6 hours, significant clinical improvement in pulmonary function (defined as maintaining a 15% or more increase in FEV$_1$ and a 20% or more increase in MMEF over baseline values) was observed in 60% of patients at 4 hours and in 40% at 6 hours. No decrease in the effectiveness of VENTOLIN Tablets has been reported in patients who received long-term treatment with the drug in uncontrolled studies for periods up to 6 months.

Contraindications: VENTOLIN Tablets are contraindicated in patients with a history of hypersensitivity to any of its components.

Precautions: General: Although albuterol usually has minimal effects on the beta$_1$-adrenoceptors of the cardiovascular system at the recommended dosage, occasionally the usual cardiovascular and CNS stimulatory effects common to all sympathomimetic agents have been seen with patients treated with albuterol necessitating discontinuation. Therefore, albuterol should be used with caution in patients with cardiovascular disorders, including coronary insufficiency and hypertension, in patients with hyperthyroidism or dia-

betes mellitus, and in patients who are unusually responsive to sympathomimetic amines.
Large doses of intravenous albuterol have been reported to aggravate preexisting diabetes mellitus and ketoacidosis. The relevance of this observation to the use of VENTOLIN Tablets is unknown.

Information for Patients: The action of VENTOLIN Tablets may last for six hours or longer and therefore it should not be taken more frequently than recommended. Do not increase the dose or frequency of medication without medical consultation. If symptoms get worse, medical consultation should be sought promptly.

Drug Interactions: The concomitant use of VENTOLIN Tablets and other oral sympathomimetic agents is not recommended since such combined use may lead to deleterious cardiovascular effects. This recommendation does not preclude the judicious use of an aerosol bronchodilator of the adrenergic stimulant type in patients receiving VENTOLIN Tablets. Such concomitant use, however, should be individualized and not given on a routine basis. If regular coadministration is required, then alternative therapy should be considered.
Albuterol should be administered with extreme caution to patients being treated with monoamine oxidase inhibitors or tricyclic antidepressants, since the action of albuterol on the vascular system may be potentiated.
Beta-receptor blocking agents and albuterol inhibit the effect of each other.

Carcinogenesis, Mutagenesis, Impairment of Fertility: Albuterol sulfate, like other agents in its class, caused a significant dose-related increase in the incidence of benign leiomyomas of the mesovarium in a 2-year study in the rat, at doses corresponding to 3, 16, and 78 times the maximum human oral dose. In another study this effect was blocked by the coadministration of propranolol. The relevance of these findings to humans is not known. An 18-month study in mice and a lifetime study in hamsters revealed no evidence of tumorigenicity. Studies with albuterol revealed no evidence of mutagenesis. Reproduction studies in rats revealed no evidence of impaired fertility.

Teratogenic Effects-Pregnancy Category C: Albuterol has been shown to be teratogenic in mice when given subcutaneously in doses corresponding to 0.4 times the maximum human oral dose. There are no adequate and well-controlled studies in pregnant women. Albuterol should be used during pregnancy only if the potential benefit justifies the potential risk to the fetus. A reproduction study in CD-1 mice with albuterol showed cleft palate formation in 5 of 111 (4.5%) fetuses at 0.25 mg/kg and in 10 of 108 (9.3%) fetuses at 2.5 mg/kg; none were observed at 0.025 mg/kg. Cleft palate also occurred in 22 of 72 (30.5%) fetuses treated with 2.5 mg/kg isoproterenol (positive control). A reproduction study in Stride Dutch rabbits revealed craniochisis in 7 of 19 (37%) fetuses at 50 mg/kg, corresponding to 78 times the maximum human oral dose of albuterol.

Labor and Delivery: Like other beta$_2$-adrenergic receptor stimulants, albuterol administered by the intravenous and oral routes, alone or concomitantly, has been reported to stop preterm labor; however, cessation of labor at term has not been reported with albuterol. Therefore, cautious use of VENTOLIN Tablets is required in pregnant patients when given for relief of bronchospasm so as to avoid interference with uterine contractility.

Nursing Mothers: It it not known whether this drug is excreted in human milk. Because of the potential for tumorigenicity shown for albuterol in animal studies, a decision should be made whether to discontinue nursing or to discontinue the drug, taking into account the importance of the drug to the mother.

Pediatric Use: Safety and effectiveness in children below the age of 12 years have not been established.

Adverse Reactions: The adverse reactions to albuterol are similar in nature to those to other sympathomimetic agents. The most frequent adverse reactions to VENTOLIN Tablets were nervousness and tremor, with each occurring in approximately 20 of 100 patients. Other reported reactions were headache, 7 of 100 patients; tachycardia and palpitations, 5 of 100 patients; muscle cramps, 3 of 100 patients; insomnia, nausea, weakness, and dizziness, each occurred in 2 of 100 patients. Drowsiness, flushing, restlessness, irritability, chest discomfort, and difficulty in micturition each occurred in less than 1 of 100 patients.
In addition, albuterol, like other sympathomimetic agents, can cause adverse reactions such as hypertension, angina, vomiting, vertigo, central stimulation, unusual taste, and drying or irritation of the oropharynx.
The reactions are generally transient in nature, and it is usually not necessary to discontinue treatment with VENTOLIN Tablets. In selected cases, however, dosage may be reduced temporarily; after the reaction has subsided, dosage should be increased in small increments to the optimal dosage.

Overdosage: Manifestations of overdosage include anginal pain, hypertension, hypokalemia, and exaggeration of the effects listed in **Adverse Reactions**.
The oral LD$_{50}$ in rats and mice was greater than 2,000 mg/kg.
Dialysis is not appropriate treatment for overdosage of VENTOLIN Tablets. The judicious use of a cardioselective beta-receptor blocker, such as metoprolol tartrate, is suggested, bearing in mind the danger of inducing an asthmatic attack.

Dosage and Administration: The following dosages of VENTOLIN Tablets are expressed in terms of albuterol base.

Usual Dose: The usual starting dosage for adults and children 12 years and over is 2 mg or 4 mg three or four times a day.

Dosage Adjustment: Doses above 4 mg four times a day should be used only when the patient fails to respond. If a favorable response does not occur with the 4 mg initial dosage, it should be cautiously increased step wise up to a maximum of 8 mg four times a day as tolerated.

Elderly Patients and Those Sensitive to Beta-Adrenergic Stimulators: An initial dosage of 2 mg three or four times a day is recommended for elderly patients and for those with a history of unusual sensitivity to beta-adrenergic stimulators. If adequate bronchodilatation is not obtained, dosage may be increased gradually to as much as 8 mg three or four times a day.
The total daily dose should not exceed 32 mg in adults and children 12 years and over.

How Supplied: VENTOLIN Tablets, 2 mg albuterol as the sulfate, white, round, compressed tablets, impressed with the product name (VENTOLIN) and the number 2 on one side, and scored on the other with "GLAXO" impressed on each side of the score; bottles of 100 (NDC 0173-0341-43) and 500 (NDC 0173-0341-44).
VENTOLIN Tablets, 4 mg albuterol as the sulfate, white, round, compressed tablets, impressed with the product name (VENTOLIN) and the number 4 on one side, and scored on the other with "GLAXO" impressed on each side of the score; bottles of 100 (NDC 0173-0342-43) and 500 (NDC 0173-0342-44).
Store between 2° and 30°C (36° and 86°F).
Shown in Product Identification Section, page 412

VICON–C® Capsules
[vi′cŏn]
(Therapeutic Vitamins and Minerals)

Composition: Each yellow and orange capsule contains:
Ascorbic Acid .... 300 mg.
Niacinamide .... 100 mg.
Thiamine Mononitrate .... 20 mg.
d-Calcium Pantothenate .... 20 mg.
Riboflavin .... 10 mg.
Pyridoxine Hydrochloride .... 5 mg.
Magnesium Sulfate USP* .... 70 mg.
Zinc Sulfate USP** .... 80 mg.
* As 50 mg. of dried Magnesium Sulfate
** As 50 mg. of dried Zinc Sulfate.

Actions and Uses: VICON-C® is indicated in the treatment of patients with deficiencies of, or increased requirements for, Vitamin C, B-Complex vitamins, zinc and/or magnesium. The components of Vicon-C® have important roles in nutrition, tissue growth and repair, and the prevention of hemorrhage. Tissue injury resulting from trauma, burns or surgery may rapidly deplete the body stores of Vitamin C, the B-Complex vitamins and zinc. Patients maintained on parenteral fluids for extended periods or patients with burns, wounds or diarrhea often develop deficiencies of Vitamin C, the B-Complex vitamins and zinc.
VICON-C® is recommended for deficiencies or the prevention of deficiencies of Vitamin C, the B-Complex vitamins, magnesium and/or zinc in conditions such as febrile diseases, chronic or acute infections, burns, fractures, surgery, toxic conditions, physiologic stress, alcoholism, pregnancy, lactation, geriatrics, gastritis, peptic ulcer, colitis and in conditions involving special diets and weight-reduction diets. It is also recommended in dentistry for these deficiencies in conditions such as herpetic stomatitis, aphthous stomatitis, cheilosis, herpangina, gingivitis and states involving oral surgery.

Administration and Dosage: One capsule 2 or 3 times daily or as directed by a physician for treatment of deficiencies.

How Supplied: Bottles of 60 and 500 Capsules and Unit Dose Pack of 100 Capsules.
Shown in Product Identification Section, page 412

VICON®–PLUS Capsules
[vi′con]
(Therapeutic Vitamins and Minerals)

Composition: Each red and beige capsule contains:
Vitamin A .... 4,000 I.U.
Vitamin E .... 50 I.U.
Ascorbic Acid .... 150 mg.
Zinc Sulfate USP* .... 80 mg.
Magnesium Sulfate USP** .... 70 mg.
Niacinamide .... 25 mg.
Thiamine Mononitrate .... 10 mg.
d-Calcium Pantothenate .... 10 mg.
Riboflavin .... 5 mg.
Manganese Chloride .... 4 mg.
Pyridoxine HCl .... 2 mg.
* As 50 mg. of Dried Zinc Sulfate
** As 50 mg. of Dried Magnesium Sulfate
Vicon-Plus is an extended range vitamin-mineral supplement formulated to aid patient recovery by helping to meet increased nutritional demands.

Indications: For nutritional supplementation of the patient undergoing physiologic stress due to surgery, burns, trauma, febrile illnesses, or poor nutrition.

Dosage: 1 capsule twice daily or as prescribed by a physician for treatment of deficiencies. Dosage should not exceed 8 capsules daily due to the possible toxicity of large dosages of vitamin A.

How Supplied: In bottles of 60 capsules and 500 capsules.
Shown in Product Identification Section, page 412

VICON FORTE® Capsules ℞
[vi′cŏn for′tā]
(Therapeutic Vitamin-Minerals)

Description: Each black and orange capsule for oral administration contains:
Vitamin A .... 8,000 I.U.
Vitamin E .... 50 I.U.
Ascorbic Acid .... 150 mg.
Zinc Sulfate USP* .... 80 mg.
Magnesium Sulfate USP** .... 70 mg.
Niacinamide .... 25 mg.
Thiamine Mononitrate .... 10 mg.
d-Calcium Pantothenate .... 10 mg.
Riboflavin .... 5 mg.
Manganese Chloride .... 4 mg.

Continued on next page

Glaxo—Cont.

Pyridoxine Hydrochloride ....2 mg.
Folic Acid ....1 mg.
Vitamin B$_{12}$(Cyanocobalamin) ....10 mcg.
* As 50 mg. of Dried Zinc Sulfate
** As 50 mg. of Dried Magnesium Sulfate
VICON FORTE® is a therapeutic vitamin-mineral preparation.
Indications and Usage: VICON FORTE® is indicated for the treatment and/or prevention of vitamin and mineral deficiencies associated with restricted diets, improper food intake, alcoholism, and decreased absorption. VICON FORTE® is also indicated in patients with increased requirements for vitamins and minerals due to chronic disease, infection, and burns and in persons using alcohol to excess. Pre- and post-operative use of VICON FORTE® can provide the increased amounts of vitamins and minerals necessary for optimal recovery from the stress of surgery.
Contraindications: None known.
Precautions: General—Folic acid in doses above 0.1 mg daily may obscure pernicious anemia in that hematologic remission can occur while neurological manifestations remain progressive.
Dosage and Administration: One capsule daily or as directed by the physician.
How Supplied: Capsules, orange and black imprinted with "Glaxo-316" in bottles of 60 (NDC 0173-0316-22) and 500 (NDC 0173-0316-24) capsules each and in unit dose packs of 100 (NDC 0173-0316-27) capsules.
Dispense in tight, light-resistant containers as defined in the National Formulary.
Shown in Product Identification Section, page 412

VI-ZAC® Capsules
[*vī-zăc'*]
(Therapeutic Vitamin-Mineral)
Composition: Each orange capsule contains:
Vitamin A .... 5000 I.U.
Ascorbic Acid .... 500 mg
Vitamin E .... 50 I.U.
Zinc Sulfate USP .... 80 mg
* as 50 mg Dried Zinc Sulfate.
Actions and Uses: VI-ZAC is indicated in the treatment of patients with deficiencies of, or increased requirements for, Vitamins A, C and E and zinc. The VI-ZAC formulation is a limited vitamin-mineral formulation designed to meet special needs. It is particularly indicated where there is no requirement for supplemental amounts of the B-Complex vitamins and their attendant appetite stimulation. The formulation is also designed for patients who cannot tolerate magnesium supplements but do need supplemental amounts of zinc.
Precautions: Although rarely encountered, vitamin A in large doses daily for several months or longer may cause toxicity.
Dosage: One or two capsules daily or as directed by the physician for the treatment of deficiencies.
How Supplied: In bottles of 60 and 500 capsules.
Shown in Product Identification Section, page 412

ZANTAC® INJECTION ℞
(ranitidine hydrochloride)
Description: The active ingredient in ZANTAC® Injection, ranitidine hydrochloride, is a histamine H$_2$ receptor antagonist. Chemically, it is N[2-[[[5-[(dimethylamino)-methyl]-2-furanyl]methyl]-thio]ethyl]-N'-methyl-2-nitro-1, 1-ethenediamine, hydrochloride. It has the following structure:

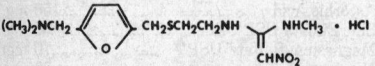

The empirical formula is C$_{13}$H$_{22}$N$_4$O$_3$S.HCl, representing a molecular weight of 350.87.
Ranitidine hydrochloride is a white to pale yellow granular substance which is soluble in water.
ZANTAC® Injection is a clear, colorless to yellow liquid which tends to darken slightly without adversely affecting potency. The pH of the injection solution is 6.7 to 7.3.
Sterile Injection for IM or IV Administration: *Single Dose Vials:* 2 ml (25 mg/ml): Each 1 ml of aqueous solution contains ranitidine 25 mg (as the hydrochloride); phenol 5 mg as preservative; 0.96 mg monobasic potassium phosphate and 2.4 mg dibasic sodium phosphate as buffers.
Multi-dose Vials: 10 ml (25 mg/ml): Each 1 ml of aqueous solution contains ranitidine 25 mg (as the hydrochloride); phenol 5 mg as preservative; 0.96 mg monobasic potassium phosphate and 2.4 mg dibasic sodium phosphate as buffers.
Clinical Pharmacology: ZANTAC® (ranitidine hydrochloride) is a competitive, reversible inhibitor of the action of histamine at the histamine H$_2$ receptors, including receptors on the gastric cells. ZANTAC does not lower serum Ca++ in hypercalcemic states. ZANTAC is not an anticholinergic agent.
Antisecretory Activity:
1. Effects on Acid Secretion: ZANTAC® Injection inhibits basal gastric acid secretion as well as gastric acid secretion stimulated by histamine and pentagastrin, as shown in the table below:
[See table below].
In a group of 10 known hypersecretors, ranitidine plasma levels of 71, 180 and 376 ng/ml inhibited basal acid secretion by 76%, 90% and 99.5%, respectively.
It appears that basal- and betazole-stimulated secretions are most sensitive to inhibition by ZANTAC, while pentagastrin-stimulated secretion is more difficult to suppress.
2. Effects on Other Gastrointestinal Secretions:
Pepsin: ZANTAC does not affect pepsin secretion. Total pepsin output is reduced in proportion to the decrease in volume of gastric juice.
Intrinsic Factor: ZANTAC has no significant effect on pentagastrin-stimulated intrinsic factor secretion.
Serum Gastrin: ZANTAC has little or no effect on fasting or postprandial serum gastrin.
Other Pharmacological Actions:
a. Gastric bacterial flora—increase in nitrate-reducing organisms, significance not known.
b. Prolactin levels—no effect in recommended oral or IV dosage, but small transient dose-related increases in serum prolactin have been reported after IV bolus injections of 100 mg or more.
c. Other pituitary hormones—no effect on serum gonadotropins, TSH, GH. Possible impairment of vasopressin release.
d. No change in cortisol, aldosterone, androgen or estrogen levels.
e. No anti-androgenic action.
f. No effect on count, motility or morphology of sperm.
Pharmacokinetics: Serum concentrations necessary to inhibit 50% of stimulated gastric acid secretion are estimated to be 36-94 ng/ml. Following single intravenous or intramuscular 50 mg doses, serum concentrations of ZANTAC are in this range for 6-8 hours.

Following intravenous injection approximately 70% of the dose is recovered in the urine as unchanged drug. Renal clearance averages 530 ml/min, with a total clearance of 760 ml/min. Volume of distribution is 1.4 L/kg; elimination half-life is 2-2.5 hours.
Four patients with clinically significant renal function impairment (creatinine clearance 25-35 ml/min) administered 50 mg ranitidine IV had an average plasma half-life of 4.8 hours, a ranitidine clearance of 29 ml/min and a volume of distribution of 1.76 L/kg. In general, these parameters appear to be altered in proportion to creatinine clearance (see **Dosage and Administration**).
ZANTAC is absorbed very rapidly after intramuscular injection. Mean peak levels of 576 ng/ml occur within 15 minutes or less following a 50 mg intramuscular dose. Absorption from intramuscular sites is virtually complete, with a bioavailability of 90% to 100% compared with intravenous administration. Following oral administration, the relative bioavailability of ZANTAC Tablets is 50%.
In man, the N-oxide is the principal metabolite in the urine; however, this amounts to less than 4% of the dose. Other metabolites are the S-oxide (1%) and the desmethyl ranitidine (1%). The remainder of the administered dose is found in the stool.
Studies in patients with hepatic dysfunction (compensated cirrhosis) indicate that there are minor, but clinically insignificant, alterations in ranitidine half-life, distribution, clearance and bioavailability.
Serum protein binding averages 15%.
Clinical Trials: *Duodenal Ulcer:* In a multicenter, double-blind controlled U.S. study of endoscopically diagnosed duodenal ulcers, earlier healing was seen in the patients treated with oral ZANTAC as shown above:
[See table above].
In these studies, patients treated with oral ZANTAC reported a reduction in both daytime and nocturnal pain, and they also consumed less antacid than the placebo-treated patients.
[See table on next page].
Pathological Hypersecretory Conditions (such as Zollinger-Ellison Syndrome): ZANTAC inhibits gastric acid secretion and reduces occurrence of diarrhea, anorexia, and pain in patients with pathological hypersecretion associated with Zollinger-Ellison Syndrome, systemic mastocytosis and other pathological hypersecretory conditions (eg, postoperative, "short-gut" syndrome, idiopathic). Use of oral ZANTAC was followed by healing of ulcers in 8 of 19 (42%) patients who were intractable to previous therapy.
Indications and Usage: ZANTAC® (ranitidine hydrochloride) Injection is indicated:
In some hospitalized patients with pathological hypersecretory conditions or intractable duodenal ulcers, or as an alternative to the oral dosage form for short-term use in patients who are unable to take oral medication.
Contraindications: ZANTAC® is contraindicated for patients known to have hypersensitivity to the drug.
Precautions: General:
1. Symptomatic response to ZANTAC® therapy does not preclude the presence of gastric malignancy.
2. Since ZANTAC is excreted primarily by the kidney, dosage should be adjusted in patients with impaired renal function (see **Dosage and Administration**). Caution should be observed in patients with hepatic dysfunction since ZANTAC is metabolized in the liver.

	Oral ZANTAC® *		Oral Placebo*	
	Number Entered	Healed/ Evaluable	Number Entered	Healed/ Evaluable
Outpatients Week 2	195	69/182 (38%)†	188	31/164 (19%)
Week 4		137/187 (73%)†		76/168 (45%)

*All patients were permitted prn antacids for relief of pain   †p < 0.0001

Effect of IV ZANTAC® on Gastric Acid Secretion

	Time after Dose, Hrs.	% Inhibition of Gastric Acid Output by IV Dose, mg		
		20 mg	60 mg	100 mg
Betazole	Up to 2	93	99	99
Pentagastrin	Up to 3	47	66	77

	Mean Daily Doses of Antacid	
	Ulcer Healed	Ulcer Not Healed
Oral ZANTAC®	0.06	0.71
Oral Placebo	0.71	1.43

3. In controlled studies in normal volunteers, elevations in SGPT have been observed when H_2 antagonists have been administered intravenously at greater than recommended doses for 5 days or longer. Therefore, it seems prudent in patients receiving IV ranitidine at doses greater than or equal to 100 mg q.i.d. for periods of 5 days or longer, to monitor SGPT daily (from day 5) for the remainder of IV therapy.

Laboratory Tests: False positive tests for urine protein with Multistix® may occur during ZANTAC therapy, and therefore testing with sulphosalicylic acid is recommended.

Drug Interactions: Although ZANTAC has been reported to bind weakly to cytochrome P-450 *in vitro*, recommended doses of the drug do not inhibit the action of the cytochrome P-450-linked oxygenase enzymes in the liver. However, there have been isolated reports of drug interactions which suggest that ZANTAC may affect the bioavailability of certain drugs by some mechanism as yet unidentified (eg, a pH-dependent effect on absorption or a change in volume of distribution).

Carcinogenesis, Mutagenesis, Impairment of Fertility: There is no indication of tumorigenic or carcinogenic effects in lifespan studies in mice and rats at oral doses up to 2000 mg/kg/day.
Ranitidine was not mutagenic in standard bacterial tests *(Salmonella, E coli)* for mutagenicity at concentrations up to the maximum recommended for these assays.
In a dominant lethal assay a single oral dose of 1000 mg/kg to male rats was without effect on the outcome of 2 matings per week for the next 9 weeks.

Usage in Pregnancy: *Pregnancy Category B:* Reproduction studies have been performed in rats and rabbits at oral doses up to 160 times the human oral dose and have revealed no evidence of impaired fertility or harm to the fetus due to ZANTAC. There are, however, no adequate and well-controlled studies in pregnant women. Because animal reproduction studies are not always predictive of human response, this drug should be used during pregnancy only if clearly needed.

Nursing Mothers: ZANTAC is secreted in human milk. Caution should be exercised when ZANTAC is administered to a nursing mother.

Pediatric Use: Safety and effectiveness in children have not been established.

Use in Elderly Patients: Ulcer healing rates in elderly patients (65-82 years) treated with oral ZANTAC were no different from those in younger age groups. The incidence rates for adverse events and laboratory abnormalities were also not different from those seen in other age groups.

Adverse Reactions: Transient pain at the site of intramuscular injections has been reported. Transient local burning or itching has been reported with intravenous administration of ZANTAC®.
The following have been reported as events in clinical trials or in the routine management of patients treated with oral ZANTAC. The relationship to ZANTAC therapy has been unclear in many cases. Headache, sometimes severe, seeems to be related to ZANTAC administration.

Central Nervous System: Rarely, malaise, dizziness, somnolence, insomnia and vertigo. Rare cases of reversible mental confusion, agitation, depression and hallucinations have been reported, predominantly in severely ill elderly patients.

Cardiovascular: Rare reports of tachycardia, bradycardia, premature ventricular beats.

Gastrointestinal: Constipation, diarrhea, nausea/vomiting, abdominal discomfort/pain.

Hepatic: In normal volunteers, SGPT values were increased to at least twice the pre-treatment levels in 6 of 12 subjects receiving 100 mg q.i.d. IV for 7 days, and in 4 of 24 subjects receiving 50 mg q.i.d. for 5 days. With oral administration there have been occasional reports of reversible hepatitis, hepatocellular or hepatocanalicular or mixed, with or without jaundice.

Musculoskeletal: Rare reports of arthralgias.

Hematologic: Rare reports of reversible leukopenia, granulocytopenia, thrombocytopenia and pancytopenia.

Endocrine: Controlled studies in animals and man have shown no stimulation of any pituitary hormone by ZANTAC, no anti-androgenic activity, and cimetidine-induced gynecomastia and impotence in hypersecretory patients have resolved when ZANTAC was substituted. However, occasional cases of gynecomastia, impotence and loss of libido have been reported in male patients receiving ZANTAC, but the incidence did not differ from that in the general population.

Integumental: Rash and, rarely, alopecia.

Other: Rare cases of hypersensitivity reactions (eg, bronchospasm, fever, rash, eosinophilia), small increases in serum creatinine.

Overdosage: There is no experience to date with deliberate overdosage. Clinical monitoring and supportive therapy should be employed.
Studies in dogs receiving doses of ZANTAC® in excess of 225 mg/kg/day have shown muscular tremors, vomiting, and rapid respiration. Single oral doses of 1000 mg/kg in mice and rats were not lethal. Intravenous LD_{50} values in rat and mouse were 83 mg/kg and 77 mg/kg, respectively.

Dosage and Administration: Parenteral Administration: In some hospitalized patients with pathological hypersecretory conditions or intractable duodenal ulcers, or in patients who are unable to take oral medication, ZANTAC® may be administered parenterally according to the following recommendations:

Intramuscular Injection: 50 mg (2 ml) every 6-8 hours. (No dilution necessary.)

Intravenous Injection: 50 mg (2 ml) every 6-8 hours. Dilute ZANTAC Injection, 50 mg, in 0.9% Sodium Chloride Injection or other compatible IV solution (see **Stability of ZANTAC Injection**) to a total volume of 20 ml and inject over a period of not less than 5 minutes.

Intermittent Intravenous Infusion: 50 mg (2 ml) every 6-8 hours. Dilute ZANTAC Injection, 50 mg, in 100 ml of 5% Dextrose Injection or other compatible IV solution (see **Stability of ZANTAC Injection**) and infuse over 15-20 minutes. In some patients it may be necessary to increase dosage. When this is necessary, the increases should be made by more frequent administration of a 50 mg dose, but generally should not exceed 400 mg per day.

Dosage Adjustment for Patients with Impaired Renal Function: On the basis of experience with a group of subjects with severely impaired renal function treated with ZANTAC, the recommended dose in patients with a creatinine clearance less than 50 ml/min is 50 mg every 18-24 hours. Should the patient's condition require, the frequency of dosing may be increased to every 12 hours or even further with caution. Hemodialysis reduces the level of circulating ranitidine. Ideally, the dosage schedule should be adjusted so that the timing of a scheduled dose coincides with the end of hemodialysis.

Stability of ZANTAC Injection: ZANTAC Injection is stable for 48 hours at room temperature when added to or diluted with most commonly used intravenous solutions, eg, 0.9% Sodium Chloride Injection, 5% Dextrose Injection, 10% Dextrose Injection, Lactated Ringer's Solution, or 5% Sodium Bicarbonate Injection.

Note: Parenteral drug products should be inspected visually for particulate matter and discoloration prior to administration wherever solution and container permit.

How Supplied: ZANTAC® Injection, 25 mg/ml, is available in 2 ml single dose vials in boxes of 10 (NDC 0173-0362-38) and in 10 ml multi-dose vials (NDC 0173-0363-39).
Store below 30°C (86°F). Protect from light.

ZANTAC® Tablets ℞
(ranitidine hydrochloride)

Description: The active ingredient in ZANTAC® Tablets, ranitidine hydrochloride, is a histamine H_2 receptor antagonist. Chemically it is N[2- [[[5- [(dimethylamino)methyl]-2-furanyl] methyl]thio]ethyl]- N'-methyl -2- nitro-1, 1-ethenediamine, hydrochloride.
The empirical formula is $C_{13}H_{22}N_4O_3S \cdot HCl$, representing a molecular weight of 350.87.
Ranitidine hydrochloride is a white to pale yellow granular substance which is soluble in water. It has a slightly bitter taste and sulphur-like odor. Each tablet for oral administration contains 168 mg of ranitidine hydrochloride, equivalent to 150 mg ranitidine.

Clinical Pharmacology: ZANTAC® (ranitidine hydrochloride) is a competitive, reversible inhibitor of the action of histamine at the histamine H_2 receptors, including receptors on the gastric cells. ZANTAC does not lower serum $Ca++$ in hypercalcemic states. ZANTAC is not an anticholinergic agent.

Antisecretory Activity:

1. Effects on Acid Secretion: ZANTAC inhibits both daytime and nocturnal basal gastric acid secretion as well as gastric acid secretion stimulated by food, histamine and pentagastrin, as shown in the table below.

It appears that basal-, nocturnal- and betazole-stimulated secretions are most sensitive to inhibition by ZANTAC, responding almost completely to doses of 100 mg or less, while pentagastrin and food-stimulated secretions are more difficult to suppress.

2. Effects on Other Gastrointestinal Secretions:
Pepsin: Oral ZANTAC 150 mg did not affect pepsin secretion. Total pepsin output was reduced in proportion to the decrease in volume of gastric juice.
Intrinsic factor: Oral ZANTAC 150 mg had no significant effect on pentagastrin-stimulated intrinsic factor secretion.
Serum gastrin: ZANTAC has little or no effect on fasting or postprandial serum gastrin.

Other Pharmacological Actions:
a. Gastric bacterial flora—increase in nitrate-reducing organisms, significance not known.
b. Prolactin levels—no effect in recommended oral or IV dosage, but small transient dose-related

Effect of Oral ZANTAC® on Gastric Acid Secretion

	Time After Dose, hrs.	% Inhibition of Gastric Acid Output by Dose, mg			
		75–80	100	150	200
Basal	Up to 4		99	95	
Nocturnal	Up to 13	95	96	92	
Betazole	Up to 3		97	99	
Pentagastrin	Up to 5	58	72	72	80
Meal	Up to 3		73	79	95

Continued on next page

Glaxo—Cont.

increases in serum prolactin have been reported after IV bolus injections of 100 mg or more.
c. Other pituitary hormones—no effect on serum gonadotropins, TSH, GH. Possible impairment of vasopressin release.
d. No change in cortisol, aldosterone, androgen or estrogen levels.
e. No anti-androgenic action.
f. No effect on count, motility or morphology of sperm.

Pharmacokinetics:
ZANTAC is 50% absorbed after oral administration compared to an IV injection with mean peak levels of 440–545 ng/ml occurring at 2–3 hours after a 150 mg dose. The elimination half-life is 2.5–3 hours.
Absorption is not significantly impaired by the administration of food or antacids. Propantheline slightly delays and increases peak blood levels of ZANTAC probably by delaying gastric emptying and transit time. In one study, simultaneous administration of high-potency antacid (150 m mol) in fasting subjects has been reported to decrease the absorption of ZANTAC.
Serum concentrations necessary to inhibit 50% of stimulated gastric acid secretion are estimated to be 36–94 ng/ml. Following a single oral dose of 150 mg, serum concentrations of ZANTAC are in this range up to 12 hours. However, blood levels bear no consistent relationship to dose or degree of acid inhibition.
The principal route of excretion is the urine, with approximately 30% of the orally administered dose collected in the urine as unchanged drug in 24 hours. Renal clearance is about 410 ml/min, indicating active tubular excretion.
In man, the N-oxide is the principal metabolite in the urine; however, this amounts to less than 4% of the dose. Other metabolites are the S-oxide (1%) and the desmethyl ranitidine (1%). The remainder of the administered dose is found in the stool.
The volume of distribution is about 1.4 L/kg. Serum protein binding averages 15%.

Clinical Trials: *Duodenal Ulcer:* In a multicenter, double-blind controlled U.S. study of endoscopically diagnosed duodenal ulcers, earlier healing was seen in the ZANTAC-treated patients as shown in Table I.
[See table below].
In these studies, ZANTAC-treated patients reported a reduction in both daytime and nocturnal pain, and they also consumed less antacid than the placebo-treated patients.
[See table above].
Studies have been limited to short-term treatment of acute duodenal ulcer. Patients whose ulcers healed during therapy had recurrences of ulcers at the usual rates. There have been no systematic studies to evaluate whether continued treatment with ZANTAC alters recurrence rates.

Pathological Hypersecretory Conditions (such as Zollinger-Ellison Syndrome):
ZANTAC inhibits gastric acid secretion and reduces occurrence of diarrhea, anorexia, and pain in patients with pathological hypersecretion associated with Zollinger-Ellison Syndrome, systemic mastocytosis and other pathological hypersecretory conditions (eg, postoperative, "short gut" syndrome, idiopathic). Use of ZANTAC was followed by healing of ulcers in 8 of 19 (42%) patients who were intractable to previous therapy.

Table II

	Mean Daily Doses of Antacid	
	Ulcer Healed	Ulcer Not Healed
ZANTAC®	0.06	0.71
Placebo	0.71	1.43

Indications and Usage: ZANTAC® (ranitidine hydrochloride) is indicated in:
1. Short-term treatment of active duodenal ulcer. Most patients heal within 4 weeks. Studies available to date have not assessed the safety of ranitidine in uncomplicated duodenal ulcer for periods of more than 8 weeks.
2. The treatment of pathological hypersecretory conditions (eg, Zollinger-Ellison Syndrome and systemic mastocytosis).
In active duodenal ulcer and hypersecretory states, antacids should be given as needed for relief of pain.

Contraindications: ZANTAC® is contraindicated for patients known to have hypersensitivity to the drug.

Precautions: General: 1. Symptomatic response to ZANTAC® therapy does not preclude the presence of gastric malignancy.
2. Since ZANTAC is excreted primarily by the kidney, dosage should be adjusted in patients with impaired renal function (see **Dosage and Administration**). Caution should be observed in patients with hepatic dysfunction; ZANTAC is metabolized in the liver.
Laboratory Tests: False positive tests for urine protein with Multistix® may occur during ZANTAC therapy and therefore testing with sulphosalicylic acid is recommended.
Drug Interactions: Although ZANTAC has been reported to bind weakly to cytochrome P-450 *in vitro*, recommended doses of the drug do not inhibit the action of the cytochrome P-450-linked oxygenase enzymes in the liver. However, there have been isolated reports of drug interactions which suggest that ZANTAC may affect the bioavailability of certain drugs by some mechanism as yet unidentified (eg, a pH-dependent effect on absorption or a change in volume of distribution).
Carcinogenesis, Mutagenesis, Impairment of Fertility: There was no indication of tumorigenic or carcinogenic effects in lifespan studies in mice and rats at doses up to 2000 mg/kg/day.
Ranitidine was not mutagenic in standard bacterial tests *(Salmonella, E Coli)* for mutagenicity at concentrations up to the maximum recommended for these assays.
In a dominant lethal assay a single oral dose of 1000 mg/kg to male rats was without effect on the outcome of 2 matings per week for the next 9 weeks.
Usage in Pregnancy: *Pregnancy Category B:* Reproduction studies have been performed in rats and rabbits at doses up to 160 times the human dose and have revealed no evidence of impaired fertility or harm to the fetus due to ZANTAC. There are, however, no adequate and well-controlled studies in pregnant women. Because animal reproduction studies are not always predictive of human response, this drug should be used during pregnancy only if clearly needed.
Nursing Mothers: ZANTAC is secreted in human milk. Caution should be exercised when ZANTAC is administered to a nursing mother.
Pediatric Use: Safety and effectiveness in children have not been established.

Use in Elderly Patients: Ulcer healing rates in elderly patients (65–82 years) were no different from those in younger age groups. The incidence rates for adverse events and laboratory abnormalities were also not different from those seen in other age groups.

Adverse Reactions: The following have been reported as events in clinical trials or in the routine management of patients treated with ZANTAC. The relationship to ZANTAC therapy has been unclear in many cases. Headache, sometimes severe, seems to be related to ZANTAC administration.
Central Nervous System: Rarely, malaise, dizziness, somnolence, insomnia and vertigo. Rare cases of reversible mental confusion, agitation, depression and hallucinations have been reported, predominantly in severely ill elderly patients.
Cardiovascular: Rare reports of tachycardia, bradycardia, premature ventricular beats.
Gastrointestinal: Constipation, diarrhea, nausea/vomiting, abdominal discomfort/pain.
Hepatic: In normal volunteers, SGPT values were increased to at least twice the pre-treatment levels in 6 of 12 subjects receiving 100 mg q.i.d. IV for 7 days, and in 4 of 24 subjects receiving 50 mg q.i.d. IV for 5 days. With oral administration there have been occasional reports of reversible hepatitis, heptocellular or heptocanalicular or mixed, with or without jaundice.
Musculoskeletal: Rare reports of arthralgias.
Hematologic: Rare reports of reversible leukopenia, granulocytopenia, thrombocytopenia and pancytopenia.
Endocrine: Controlled studies in animals and man have shown no stimulation of any pituitary hormone by ZANTAC, no anti-androgenic activity, and cimetidine-induced gynecomastia and impotence in hypersecretory patients have resolved when ZANTAC was substituted. However, occasional cases of gynecomastia, impotence and loss of libido have been reported in male patients receiving ZANTAC, but the incidence did not differ from that in the general population.
Integumental: Rash and, rarely, alopecia.
Other: Rare cases of hypersensitivity reactions (eg, bronchospasm, fever, rash, eosinophilia), small increases in serum creatinine.
Overdosage: There is no experience to date with deliberate overdosage. The usual measures to remove unabsorbed material from the gastrointestinal tract, clinical monitoring and supportive therapy should be employed.
Studies in animals receiving doses of ZANTAC® in excess of 225 mg/kg/day have shown muscular tremors, vomiting, and rapid respiration. Single oral doses of 1000 mg/kg in mice and rats were not lethal. Intravenous LD_{50} values in rat and mouse were 83 mg/kg and 77 mg/kg, respectively.

Dosage and Administration: *Duodenal Ulcer:* The current recommended adult oral dosage of ZANTAC® for duodenal ulcer is 150 mg twice daily, the only dose shown to speed healing of duodenal ulcer in U.S. clinical trials. Smaller doses have been shown to be equally effective in inhibiting gastric acid secretion in U.S. studies, and several foreign trials have shown that 100 mg b.i.d. is as effective as the 150 mg dose.
Since 38% of patients can be expected to show complete healing at the end of two weeks, documentation of healing at that time may make further treatment with ZANTAC unnecessary. Antacid should be given as needed for relief of pain (see **Pharmacokinetics** under **Clinical Pharmacology**).
Pathological Hypersecretory Conditions (such as Zollinger-Ellison Syndrome): Recommended adult oral dosage: 150 mg twice a day. In some patients it

Table I

	ZANTAC®*		Placebo*	
	Number Entered	Healed/ Evaluable	Number Entered	Healed/ Evaluable
Outpatients				
Week 2	195	69/182 (38%)†	188	31/164 (19%)
Week 4		137/187 (73%)†		76/168 (45%)

*All patients were permitted prn antacids for relief of pain. †p < 0.0001

may be necessary to administer ZANTAC 150 mg doses more frequently. Doses should be adjusted to individual patient needs, and should continue as long as clinically indicated. Doses up to 6 g/day have been employed in patients with severe disease.

Dosage Adjustment for Patients with Impaired Renal Function: On the basis of experience with a group of subjects with severely impaired renal function treated with ZANTAC, the recommended dose in patients with a creatinine clearance less than 50 ml/min is 150 mg every 24 hours. Should the patient's condition require, the frequency of dosing may be increased to every 12 hours or even further with caution. Hemodialysis reduces the level of circulating ranitidine. Ideally, the dosage schedule should be adjusted so that the timing of a scheduled dose coincides with the end of hemodialysis.

How Supplied: ZANTAC® Tablets (ranitidine hydrochloride equivalent to 150 mg ranitidine) are white tablets embossed with "ZANTAC 150" on one side and "Glaxo" on the other. They are available in bottles of 30 tablets (NDC 0173-0344-40), 60 tablets (NDC 0173-0344-42) and unit dose packs of 100 tablets (NDC 0173-0344-47).

Store at controlled room temperature in a dry place. Protect from light. Replace cap securely after each opening.

Shown in Product Identification Section, page 412

ZINACEF® ℞
[zin'ah-sef"]
(sterile cefuroxime sodium)

Description: ZINACEF® (sterile cefuroxime sodium, Glaxo) is a semisynthetic, broad-spectrum cephalosporin antibiotic for parenteral administration. It is the sodium salt of (6R, 7R)-3-carbamoyloxymethyl-7-[Z-2-methoxyimino-2-(fur-2-yl) acetamido] ceph-3-em-4-carboxylate. ZINACEF contains approximately 54.2 mg (2.4 mEq) of sodium per gram of cefuroxime activity. Solutions of ZINACEF range from light yellow to amber, depending on the concentration and diluent used. The pH of freshly constituted solutions usually ranges from 6.0 to 8.5.

Structural Formula:

Clinical Pharmacology: After intramuscular injection of a 750 mg dose of cefuroxime to normal volunteers, the mean peak serum concentration was 27 mcg/ml. The peak occurred at approximately 45 minutes (range 15–60 minutes). Following intravenous doses of 750 mg and 1.5 g, serum concentrations were approximately 50 mcg/ml and 100 mcg/ml, respectively, at 15 minutes. Therapeutic serum concentrations of approximately 2 mcg/ml or more were maintained for 5.3 hours and 8 hours or more, respectively. There was no evidence of accumulation of cefuroxime in the serum following intravenous administration of 1.5 g doses every 8 hours to normal volunteers. The serum half-life after either intramuscular or intravenous injections is approximately 80 minutes.

Approximatey 89% of a dose of cefuroxime is excreted by the kidneys over an 8-hour period, resulting in high urinary concentrations.

Following the intramuscular administration of a 750 mg single dose, urinary concentrations averaged 1300 mcg/ml during the first 8 hours. Intravenous doses of 750 mg and 1.5 g produced urinary levels averaging 1150 mcg/ml and 2500 mcg/ml, respectively, during the first 8-hour period.

The concomitant oral administration of probenecid with cefuroxime slows tubular secretion, decreases renal clearance by approximately 40%, increases the peak serum level by approximately 30%, and increases the serum half-life by approximately 30%. ZINACEF® is detectable in therapeutic concentrations in pleural fluid, joint fluid, bile, sputum, bone, cerebrospinal fluid (in patients with meningitis), and aqueous humor.

Cefuroxime is approximately 50% bound to serum protein.

Microbiology: Cefuroxime has *in vitro* activity against a wide range of gram-positive and gram-negative organisms, and it is highly stable in the presence of beta-lactamases of certain gram-negative bacteria. The bactericidal action of cefuroxime results from inhibition of cell-wall synthesis. Cefuroxime is usually active against the following organisms *in vitro*.

Gram-Negative: *Haemophilus influenzae* (including ampicillin-resistant strains); *Haemophilus parainfluenzae*; *Neisseria gonorrhoeae* (including penicillinase- and non-penicillinase-producing strains); *Neisseria meningitidis*; *Escherichia coli*; *Klebsiella* species (including *Klebsiella pneumoniae*); *Enterobacter* species; *Citrobacter* species; *Salmonella* species; *Shigella* species; *Proteus mirabilis*; *Proteus inconstans* (formerly *Providencia*); *Providencia rettgeri* (formerly *Proteus rettgeri*); *Morganella morganii* (formerly *Proteus morganii*).

Some strains of *M morganii*, *Enterobacter cloacae* and *Citrobacter* species have been shown by *in vitro* tests to be resistant to cefuroxime and other cephalosporins.

Gram-Positive: *Staphylococcus aureus* (including penicillinase- and non-penicillinase-producing strains); *Staphylococcus epidermidis*; *Streptococcus pyogenes* (and other streptococci); *Streptococcus pneumoniae* (formerly *Diplococcus pneumoniae*).

Certain strains of enterococci, eg, *Streptococcus faecalis*, are resistant.

Anaerobic Organisms: Gram-positive and gram-negative cocci (including *Peptococcus* and *Peptostreptococcus* species); gram-positive bacilli (including *Clostridium* species); gram-negative bacilli (including *Bacteroides* and *Fusobacterium* species). Most strains of *Bacteroides fragilis* are resistant.

Pseudomonas and *Campylobacter* species, *Acinetobacter calcoaceticus* (formerly *Mima* and *Herellea* species) and most strains of *Serratia* and *Proteus vulgaris* are resistant to cephalosporins. Methicillin-resistant staphylococci, *Clostridium difficile* and *Listeria monocytogenes* are resistant to cefuroxime.

Susceptibility Tests: Diffusion Techniques: Quantitative methods that require measurement of zone diameters give the most precise estimates of antibiotic susceptibility. One such procedure[1] has been recommended for use with disks to test susceptibility to cefuroxime. Interpretation involves correlation of the diameters obtained in the disk test with minimum inhibitory concentration (MIC) values for cefuroxime.

Reports from the laboratory giving results of the standardized single-disk susceptibility test[1] using a 30 mcg cefuroxime disk should be interpreted according to the following criteria:

Susceptible organisms produce zone sizes of 18 mm or greater, indicating that the tested organism is likely to respond to therapy.

Organisms that produce zones of 15 to 17 mm are expected to be susceptible if high dosage is used or if the infection is confined to tissues and fluids (eg, urine), in which high antibiotic levels are attained.

Resistant organisms produce zones of 14 mm or less, indicating that other therapy should be selected.

For gram-positive isolates, the test may be performed with either the cephalosporin-class disk (30 mcg cephalothin) or the cefuroxime disk (30 mcg cefuroxime) and a zone of 18 mm or greater indicates a cefuroxime-susceptible organism.

Gram-negative organisms should be tested with the cefuroxime disk (using the above criteria), since cefuroxime has been shown by *in vitro* tests to have activity against certain strains of enterobacteriaceae found resistant when tested with the cephalosporin-class disk. Gram-negative organisms having zones of less than 18 mm around the cephalothin disk are not necessarily of intermediate susceptibility or resistant to cefuroxime. The cefuroxime disk should not be used for testing susceptibility to other cephalosporins.

Standardized procedures require the use of laboratory control organisms. The 30 mcg cefuroxime disk should give zone diameters between 27 and 35 mm for *S aureus* ATCC 25923. For *E coli* ATCC 25922, the zone diameters should be between 20 and 26 mm.

Dilution Techniques: A bacterial isolate may be considered susceptible if the MIC value for cefuroxime is not more than 16 mcg/ml. Organisms are considered resistant if the MIC is greater than 32 mcg/ml.

As with standard diffusion methods, dilution procedures require the use of laboratory control organisms. Standard cefuroxime powder should give MIC values in the range of 0.5 mcg/ml and 2 mcg/ml for *S aureus* ATCC 25923. For *E coli* ATCC 25922, the MIC range should be between 2 mcg/ml and 8 mcg/ml.

Indications and Usage: ZINACEF® is indicated for the treatment of infections caused by susceptible strains of the designated microorganisms in the diseases listed below:

1. **Lower Respiratory Infections,** including pneumonia caused by *S pneumoniae* (formerly *D pneumoniae*), *H influenzae* (including ampicillin-resistant strains), *Klebsiella* species, *S aureus* (penicillinase- and non-penicillinase-producing), *S pyogenes,* and *E coli.*
2. **Urinary Tract Infections** caused by *E coli* and *Klebsiella* species.
3. **Skin and Skin Structure Infections** caused by *S aureus* (penicillinase- and non-penicillinase-producing) *S pyogenes, E coli, Klebsiella* species, and *Enterobacter* species.
4. **Septicemia** caused by *S aureus* (penicillinase- and non-penicillinase-producing), *S pneumoniae, E coli, H influenzae* (including ampicillin-resistant strains), and *Klebsiella* species.
5. **Meningitis** caused by *S pneumoniae, H influenzae* (including ampicillin-resistant strains), *N meningitidis,* and *S aureus* (penicillinase- and non-penicillinase-producing).
6. **Gonorrhea:** Uncomplicated and disseminated gonococcal infections due to *N gonorrhoeae* (penicillinase- and non-penicillinase-producing strains) in both males and females.

Clinical microbiological studies in skin and skin structure infections frequently reveal the growth of susceptible strains of both aerobic and anaerobic organisms. ZINACEF (sterile cefuroxime sodium, Glaxo) has been used successfully in these mixed infections in which several organisms have been isolated. Appropriate cultures and susceptibility studies should be performed to determine the susceptibility of the causative organisms to ZINACEF.

Therapy may be started while awaiting the results of these studies; however, once these results become available, the antibiotic treatment should be adjusted accordingly. In certain cases of confirmed or suspected gram-positive or gram-negative sepsis or in patients with other serious infections in which the causative organism has not been identified, ZINACEF may be used concomitantly with an aminoglycoside (see **Precautions**). The recommended doses of both antibiotics may be given depending on the severity of the infection and the patient's condition.

Prevention: The preoperative prophylactic administration of ZINACEF may prevent the growth of susceptible disease-causing bacteria and, thereby, may reduce the incidence of certain postoperative infections in patients undergoing surgical procedures (eg, vaginal hysterectomy) that are classified as clean-contaminated or potentially contaminated procedures. Effective prophylactic use of antibiotics in surgery depends on the time of administration. ZINACEF should usually be given one-half to 1 hour before the operation to allow sufficient time to achieve effective antibiotic con-

Continued on next page

Glaxo—Cont.

centrations in the wound tissues during the procedure. The dose should be repeated intraoperatively if the surgical procedure is lengthy. Prophylactic administration is usually not required after the surgical procedure ends and should be stopped within 24 hours. In the majority of surgical procedures, continuing prophylactic administration of any antibiotic does not reduce the incidence of subsequent infections but will increase the possibility of adverse reactions and the development of bacterial resistance. The perioperative use of ZINACEF has also been effective during open heart surgery for surgical patients in whom infections at the operative site would present a serious risk. For these patients it is recommended that ZINACEF therapy be continued for at least 48 hours after the surgical procedure ends. If an infection is present, specimens for culture should be obtained for the identification of the causative organism and appropriate antimicrobial therapy should be instituted.

Contraindications: ZINACEF® is contraindicated in patients with known allergy to the cephalosporin group of antibiotics.

Warnings: BEFORE THERAPY WITH ZINACEF® IS INSTITUTED, CAREFUL INQUIRY SHOULD BE MADE TO DETERMINE WHETHER THE PATIENT HAS HAD PREVIOUS HYPERSENSITIVITY REACTIONS TO CEPHALOSPORINS, PENICILLINS OR OTHER DRUGS. THIS PRODUCT SHOULD BE GIVEN CAUTIOUSLY TO PENICILLIN-SENSITIVE PATIENTS. ANTIBIOTICS SHOULD BE ADMINISTERED WITH CAUTION TO ANY PATIENT WHO HAS DEMONSTRATED SOME FORM OF ALLERGY, PARTICULARLY TO DRUGS. IF AN ALLERGIC REACTION TO ZINACEF OCCURS, DISCONTINUE THE DRUG. SERIOUS ACUTE HYPERSENSITIVITY REACTIONS MAY REQUIRE EPINEPHRINE AND OTHER EMERGENCY MEASURES.

Pseudomembranous colitis has been reported with the use of cephalosporins (and other broad-spectrum antibiotics); therefore, it is important to consider its diagnosis in patients who develop diarrhea in association with antibiotic use.

Treatment with broad-spectrum antibiotics alters normal flora of the colon and may permit overgrowth of clostridia. Studies indicate a toxin produced by *C difficile* is one primary cause of antibiotic-associated colitis. Cholestyramine and colestipol resins have been shown to bind the toxin *in vitro*.

Mild cases of colitis may respond to drug discontinuance alone. Moderate to severe cases should be managed with fluid, electrolyte, and protein supplementation as indicated.

When the colitis is not relieved by drug discontinuance or when it is severe, oral vancomycin is the treatment of choice for antibiotic-associated pseudomembranous colitis produced by *C difficile*. Other causes of colitis should also be considered.

Precautions: Although ZINACEF® rarely produces alterations in kidney function, evaluation of renal status during therapy is recommended, especially in seriously ill patients receiving the maximum doses. Cephalosporins should be given with caution to patients receiving concurrent treatment with potent diuretics as these regimens are suspected of adversely affecting renal function.

The total daily dose of ZINACEF should be reduced in patients with transient or persistent renal insufficiency (see **Dosage and Administration**), because high and prolonged serum antibiotic concentrations can occur in such individuals from usual doses.

As with other antibiotics, prolonged use of ZINACEF may result in overgrowth of non-susceptible organisms. Careful observation of the patient is essential. If superinfection does occur during therapy, appropriate measures should be taken. Broad-spectrum antibiotics should be prescribed with caution in individuals with a history of gastrointestinal disease, particularly colitis.

Nephrotoxicity has been reported following concomitant administration of aminoglycoside antibiotics and cephalosporins.

Interference with Laboratory Tests: A false positive reaction for glucose in the urine may occur with copper reduction tests (Benedict's or Fehling's solution or with Clinitest® tablets), but not with enzyme-based tests for glycosuria (eg, Tes-Tape®). As a false negative result may occur in the ferricyanide test, it is recommended that either the glucose oxidase or hexokinase method be used to determine blood plasma glucose levels in patients receiving ZINACEF.

Cefuroxime does not interfere with the assay of serum and urine creatinine by the alkaline picrate method.

Carcinogenesis, Mutagenesis, Impairment of Fertility: Although no long-term studies in animals have been performed to evaluate carcinogenic potential, no mutagenic potential of cefuroxime was found in standard laboratory tests.

Reproductive studies revealed no impairment of fertility in animals.

Usage in Pregnancy: *Pregnancy Category B:* Reproduction studies have been performed in mice and rabbits at doses up to 60 times the human dose and have revealed no evidence of impaired fertility or harm to the fetus due to cefuroxime. There are, however, no adequate, well-controlled studies in pregnant women. Because animal reproduction studies are not always predictive of human response, this drug should be used during pregnancy only if clearly needed.

Nursing Mothers: Since ZINACEF is excreted in human milk, caution should be exercised when ZINACEF is administered to a nursing woman.

Pediatric Use: Safety and effectiveness in children below the age of 3 months have not been established. Accumulation of other members of the cephalosporin class in newborn infants (with resulting prolongation of drug half-life) has been reported.

Adverse Reactions: ZINACEF® is generally well tolerated. The most common adverse effects have been local reactions following intravenous administration. Other adverse reactions have been encountered only rarely.

Local Reactions: Thrombophlebitis has occurred with intravenous administration in 1 in 60 patients.

Gastrointestinal: Gastrointestinal symptoms occurred in 1 in 150 patients and include diarrhea (1 in 220 patients) and nausea (1 in 440 patients). Symptoms of pseudomembranous colitis can appear during or after antibiotic treatment.

Hypersensitivity Reactions: Hypersensitivity reactions have been reported in less than 1% of the patients treated with ZINACEF and include rash (1 in 125). Pruritus and urticaria and positive Coombs' test each occurred in less than 1 in 250 patients.

Blood: A decrease in hemoglobin and hematocrit has been observed in 1 in 10 patients and transient eosinophilia in 1 in 14 patients. Less common reactions seen were transient neutropenia (less than 1 in 100 patients) and leukopenia (1 in 750 patients). A similar pattern and incidence was seen with other cephalosporins used in controlled studies.

Hepatic: Transient rise in SGOT and SGPT (1 in 25 patients), alkaline phosphatase (1 in 50 patients), LDH (1 in 75 patients) and bilirubin (1 in 500 patients) levels has been noted.

Kidney: Elevations in serum creatinine and/or blood urea nitrogen and a decreased creatinine clearance have been observed, but their relationship to cefuroxime is unknown.

Dosage and Administration: Adults: The usual adult dosage range for ZINACEF® (sterile cefuroxime sodium, Glaxo) is 750 mg to 1.5 g every 8 hours, usually for 5–10 days. In uncomplicated urinary tract infections, skin and skin structure infections, disseminated gonococcal infections, and uncomplicated pneumonia, a 750 mg dose every 8 hours is recommended. In severe or complicated infections, a 1.5 g dose every 8 hours is recommended. In life-threatening infections or infections due to less susceptible organisms, 1.5 g every 6 hours may be required. In bacterial meningitis, the dose should not exceed 3.0 g every 8 hours. The recommended dose for uncomplicated gonococcal infection is 1.5 g intramuscularly given as a single dose at two different sites together with 1.0 g of oral probenecid. For preventive use for clean-contaminated or potentially contaminated surgical procedures, a 1.5 g dose administered intravenously just prior to surgery (approximately one-half to 1 hour before the initial incision) is recommended. Thereafter, give 750 mg intravenously or intramuscularly every 8 hours when the procedure is prolonged.

For preventive use during open heart surgery, a 1.5 g dose administered intravenously at the induction of anesthesia and every 12 hours thereafter for a total of 6.0 g is recommended.

Impaired Renal Function: When renal function is impaired, a reduced dosage must be employed. Dosage should be determined by the degree of renal impairment and the susceptibility of the causative organism (see Table 1).

Table 1: Dosage of ZINACEF® in Adults with Reduced Renal Function

Creatinine Clearance ml/min	Dose	Frequency
> 20	750 mg–1.5 g	Every 8 hours
10–20	750 mg	Every 12 hours
< 10	750 mg	Every 24 hours*

* Since ZINACEF is dialyzable, patients on hemodialysis should be given a further dose at the end of the dialysis.

When only serum creatinine is available, the following formula (based on sex, weight, and age of the patient) may be used to convert this value into creatinine clearance. The serum creatinine should represent a steady state of renal function.

Males: $\dfrac{\text{Weight (kg)} \times (140-\text{age})}{72 \times \text{serum creatinine (mg/100 ml)}}$

Females: $0.85 \times$ above value

Note: As with antibiotic therapy in general, administration of ZINACEF should be continued for a minimum of 48 to 72 hours after the patient becomes asymptomatic or after evidence of bacterial eradication has been obtained; a minimum of 10 days of treatment is recommended in infections caused by *S pyogenes* in order to guard against the risk of rheumatic fever or glomerulonephritis; frequent bacteriologic and clinical appraisal is necessary during therapy of chronic urinary tract infection and may be required for several months after therapy has been completed; persistent infections may require treatment for several weeks; and doses smaller than those indicated above should not be used. In staphylococcal and other infections involving a collection of pus, surgical drainage should be carried out where indicated.

Infants and Children Above 3 Months of Age: Administration of 50–100 mg/kg/day in equally divided doses, every 6–8 hours, has been successful for most infections susceptible to cefuroxime. The higher dose of 100 mg/kg/day (not to exceed the maximum adult dose) should be used for the more severe or serious infections.

In cases of bacterial meningitis, larger doses of ZINACEF are recommended, 200–240 mg/kg/day intravenously in divided doses every 6–8 hours.

In children with renal insufficiency, the frequency of dosage should be modified consistent with the recommendations for adults.

Preparation of Solution and Suspension: The directions for preparing ZINACEF for both intravenous and intramuscular use are summarized in Table 2.

For Intramuscular Use: Each 750 mg vial of ZINACEF should be constituted with 3.6 ml of Sterile Water for Injection. Shake gently to disperse and withdraw 3.6 ml of the resulting suspension for injection.

For Intravenous Use: Each 750 mg vial should be constituted with 9.0 ml of Sterile Water for Injection. Withdraw 8.0 ml of the resulting solution for injection.

Each 1.5 g vial should be constituted with 16.0 ml of Sterile Water for Injection and the solution completely withdrawn for injection.

Each 750 mg and 1.5 g Infusion Pack should be constituted with 100 ml of Sterile Water for Injection, 5% Dextrose Injection, 0.9% Sodium Chloride Injection, or any of the solutions listed under the **Intravenous** portion of the **Compatibility and Stability** section.

[See table above].

Administration: After constitution, ZINACEF may be given intravenously or by deep intramuscular injection into a large muscle mass (such as the gluteus or lateral part of the thigh). Prior to injecting intramuscularly, aspiration is necessary to avoid inadvertent injection into a blood vessel.

Intravenous Administration: The intravenous route may be preferable for patients with bacterial septicemia or other severe or life-threatening infections or for patients who may be poor risks because of lowered resistance, particularly if shock is present or impending.

For Direct Intermittent Intravenous Administration: Slowly inject the solution into a vein over a period of 3-5 minutes or give it through the tubing system by which the patient is also receiving other intravenous solutions.

For Intermittent Intravenous Infusion with a Y-Type Administration Set: Dosing can be accomplished through the tubing system by which the patient may be receiving other intravenous solutions. However, during infusion of the solution containing ZINACEF, it is advisable to temporarily discontinue administration of any other solutions at the same site.

For Continuous Intravenous Infusion: A solution of ZINACEF may be added to an intravenous bottle containing one of the following fluids:

0.9% Sodium Chloride Injection; 5% Dextrose Injection; 10% Dextrose Injection; 5% Dextrose and 0.9% Sodium Chloride Injection; 5% Dextrose and 0.45% Sodium Chloride Injection; M/6 Sodium Lactate Injection.

Solutions of ZINACEF, like those of most beta-lactam antibiotics, should not be added to solutions of aminoglycoside antibiotics because of potential interaction.

However, if concurrent therapy with ZINACEF and an aminoglycoside is indicated, each of these antibiotics can be administered separately to the same patient.

Compatibility and Stability: Intramuscular: When constituted as directed with Sterile Water for Injection, suspensions of ZINACEF® for intramuscular injection maintain satisfactory potency for 24 hours at room temperature and for 48 hours under refrigeration (5°C).

After the periods mentiond above any unused suspensions should be discarded.

Intravenous: When the 750 mg and 1.5 g vials are constituted as directed with Sterile Water for Injection, the ZINACEF solutions for intravenous administration maintain satisfactory potency for 24 hours at room temperature and for 48 hours under refrigeration (5°C). More dilute solutions, such as 750 mg or 1.5 g plus 100 ml of Sterile Water for Injection, 5% Dextrose Injection or 0.9% Sodium Chloride Injection, maintain satisfactory potency for 24 hours at room temperature and for 7 days under refrigeration.

These solutions may be further diluted to concentrations of between 1 mg/ml and 30 mg/ml in the following solutions and will lose not more than 10% activity for 24 hours at room temperature or for at least 7 days under refrigeration: 0.9% Sodium Chloride Injection; M/6 Sodium Lactate Injection; Ringer's Injection USP; Lactated Ringer's Injection USP; 5% Dextrose and 0.9% Sodium Chloride Injection; 5% Dextrose Injection; 5% Dextrose and 0.45% Sodium Chloride Injection; 5% Dextrose and 0.225% Sodium Chloride Injection; 10% Dextrose Injection; 10% Invert Sugar in Water for Injection.

Unused solutions should be discarded after the time periods mentioned above.

Table 2: Preparation of Solution and Suspension

Strength	Amount of Diluent to be Added (ml)	Volume to be Withdrawn (ml)	Approximate Concentration (mg/ml)
750 mg Vial	3.6 (IM)	3.6*	208
750 mg Vial	9.0 (IV)	8.0	94
1.5 g Vial	16.0 (IV)	Total	90
750 mg Infusion Pack	100.0 (IV)	—	7.5
1.5 g Infusion Pack	100.0 (IV)	—	15

*Note: ZINACEF is a suspension at IM concentrations.

ZINACEF has also been found compatible for 24 hours at room temperature when admixed in intravenous infusion with: Heparin (10 and 50 units/ml) in 0.9% Sodium Chloride Injection; Potassium Chloride (10 and 40 mEq/L) in 0.9% Sodium Chloride Injection.

Frozen Stability: Constitute the 750 mg or 1.5 g vial as directed for IV administration in Table 2. Immediately withdraw either 8.0 ml (750 mg vial) or total contents (1.5 g vial) and add to a Travenol Viaflex® Minibag containing 50 ml or 100 ml of 0.9% Sodium Chloride Injection or 5% Dextrose Injection and freeze. Frozen solutions are stable for 6 months when stored at −20°C. Frozen solutions should be thawed at room temperature and not refrozen. Thawed solutions may be stored for 24 hours at room temperature or 7 days in a refrigerator.

Note: Parenteral drug products should be inspected visually for particulate matter and discoloration prior to administration whenever solution and container permit.

As with other cephalosporins, however, ZINACEF powder as well as solutions and suspensions tend to darken depending on storage conditions, without adversely affecting product potency.

How Supplied: ZINACEF® (sterile cefuroxime sodium, Glaxo) is a dry, white to off-white powder supplied in vials and infusion bottles.

Each vial contains cefuroxime sodium equivalent to 750 mg or 1.5 g cefuroxime. ZINACEF in the dry state should be stored at controlled room temperature and protected from light.

NDC 0173-0352-30 750 mg Vials (10 singles)
NDC 0173-0352-31 750 mg Vials (Tray of 25)
NDC 0173-0354-34 1.5 g Vials (10 singles)
NDC 0173-0354-35 1.5 g Vials (Tray of 25)
NDC 0173-0353-32 750 mg Infusion Pack (Tray of 10)
NDC 0173-0356-32 1.5 g Infusion Pack (Tray of 10)

Reference: 1. Bauer AW, Kirby WMM, Sherris JC, et al: Antibiotic susceptibility testing by a standardized single disc method, *Am J Clin Pathol* 1966; 45:493. Standardized disc susceptibility test, *Federal Register* 1974; 39 (May 30):19182-19184. National Committee for Clinical Laboratory Standards, Approved Standard: ASM-2, Performance Standards for Antimicrobial Disc Susceptibility Tests, July, 1975.

EDUCATIONAL MATERIAL

Booklets:
"Living With Hypertension"—A patient oriented booklet explains hypertension and is designed to enhance compliance. Free to physicians and pharmacists.

Samples:
Trandate® samples available upon request.

IDENTIFICATION PROBLEM?
Consult PDR's
Product Identification Section
where you'll find over 1200
products pictured actual size
and in full color.

Glenbrook Laboratories
Division of Sterling Drug Inc.
90 PARK AVENUE
NEW YORK, NY 10016

ARTHRITIS BAYER®
TIMED-RELEASE ASPIRIN
(aspirin)

Description: Each oblong white scored tablet contains 10 grains (650 mg.) of aspirin in microencapsulation form.

Indications: Bayer Timed-Release Aspirin is indicated for the temporary relief of low grade pain amenable to relief with salicylates, such as in rheumatoid arthritis, osteoarthritis, spondylitis, bursitis and other forms of rheumatism, as well as in many common musculoskeletal disorders. It possesses the same advantages for other types of prolonged aches and pains, such as minor injuries, dental pain and dysmenorrhea. Its long-lasting effectiveness should also make it valuable as an analgesic in simple headache, colds, grippe, flu and other similar conditions in which aspirin is indicated for symptomatic relief, either by itself or as an adjunct to specific therapy.

Dosage: Two Bayer Timed-Release Aspirin tablets q. 8 h. provide effective long-lasting pain relief. This two-tablet (20 grain or 1300 mg.) dose of timed-release aspirin promptly produces salicylate blood levels greater than those achieved by a 10-grain (650 mg.) dose of regular aspirin, and in the second 4 hour period produces a salicylate blood level curve which approximates that of two successive 10-grain (650 mg.) doses of regular aspirin at 4 hour intervals. The 10-grain (650 mg.) scored Bayer Timed-Release Aspirin tablets permit administration of aspirin in multiples of 5 grains (325 mg.) allowing individualization of dosage to meet the specific needs of the patient. For the convenience of patients on a regular aspirin dosage schedule, two 10-grain (650 mg.) Bayer Timed-Release Aspirin tablets may be administered with water every 8 hours. Whenever necessary, two tablets (20 grains or 1300 mg.) should be given before retiring to provide effective analgesic and anti-inflammatory action—for relief of pain throughout the night and lessening of stiffness upon arising. Do not exceed 6 tablets in 24 hours. Bayer Timed-Release Aspirin has been made in a special capsule-shaped tablet to permit easy swallowing. However, for patients who do have difficulty, Bayer Timed-Release Aspirin tablets may be gently crumbled in the mouth and swallowed with water without loss of timed-release effect. There is no bitter "aspirin" taste. For children under 12, per physician.

Side Effects: Side effects encountered with regular aspirin may be encountered with Bayer Timed-Release Aspirin. Tinnitus and dizziness are the ones most frequently encountered.

Contraindications and Precautions: Bayer Timed-Release Aspirin is contraindicated in patients with marked aspirin hypersensitivity, and should be given with extreme caution to any patient with a history of adverse reaction to salicylates. It may cautiously be tried in patients intolerant to aspirin because of gastric irritation, but the usual precautions for any form of aspirin should be observed in patients with gastric ulcers, bleeding tendencies, asthma, or hypoprothrombinemia.

Continued on next page

Glenbrook—Cont.

Supplied:
Tablets in Bottle of 30's   NDC-12843-191-72
Tablets in Bottle of 72's   NDC-12843-191-74
Tablets in Bottle of 125's   NDC-12843-191-76
All sizes packaged in child-resistant safety closure except 72's which is a size recommended for households without young children.
Samples available upon request.
Shown in Product Identification Section, page 412

BAYER® ASPIRIN AND BAYER® CHILDREN'S CHEWABLE ASPIRIN
Aspirin (Acetylsalicylic Acid)

Composition: Bayer Aspirin—Aspirin 5 grains. (325 mg.) contains a thin, inert, methyl-cellulose coating for easier swallowing. This is not an enteric coating and does not alter the onset of action of Bayer Aspirin.
Bayer Children's Chewable Aspirin—Aspirin 1¼ grains (81 mg.) per orange flavored chewable tablet.
Actions and Uses: Analgesic, antipyretic, anti-inflammatory, antiplatelet. For relief of headache; painful discomfort and fever of colds and flu; sore throats; muscular aches and pains; temporary relief of minor pains of arthritis, rheumatism, bursitis, lumbago, sciatica; toothache, teething pains, and pain following dental procedures; neuralgia and neuritic pain; functional menstrual pain; sleeplessness when caused by minor painful discomforts; painful discomfort and fever accompanying immunizations.
For antiplatelet use: In recurrent transient ischemic attacks or stroke in men. See below.
Administration and Dosage: The following dosages are those provided in the packaging, as appropriate for self-medication. Larger or more frequent dosage may be necessary as appropriate to the condition or needs of the patient.
The methyl-cellulose coating makes Bayer Aspirin particularly appropriate for those who must take frequent doses of aspirin and for those who have difficulty in swallowing uncoated tablets.
Bayer Aspirin—5 grain (325 mg.) tablets
Usual Adult Dose: One or two tablets with water. May be repeated every four hours as necessary up to 12 tablets a day.
Children's Dose: To be administered only under adult supervision.
Under 2 years .... per physician
2 to under 4 years.............................. ½ tablet
4 to under 6 years.............................. ¾ tablet
6 to under 9 years.............................. 1 tablet
9 to under 11 years........................... 1¼ tablets
11 to under 12 years.......................... 1½ tablets
Over 12 years..................................... same as adult
Indicated dosage may be repeated every 4 hours, up to but not more than five times a day.
For Antiplatelet Use: In recurrent TIA's or stroke in men. See below.
Larger dosage may be prescribed per physician.
Bayer Children's Chewable Aspirin—1¼ grain (81mg.) tablets.

Dosage
To be administered only under adult supervision.
For children under 2 consult physician.

Age (years)	Weight (lbs.)	Dosage
2 up to 4	27 to 35	2 tablets
4 up to 6	36 to 45	3 tablets
6 up to 9	46 to 65	4 tablets
9 up to 11	66 to 76	5 tablets
11 up to 12	77 to 83	6 tablets
12 and over	84 and over	8 tablets

Indicated dosage may be repeated every 4 hours, up to but not more than five times a day. Larger dosage may be prescribed per physician.
For Antiplatelet Use: In recurrent TIA's and stroke in men.
Indication: There is evidence that aspirin is safe and effective for reducing the risk of recurrent transient ischemic attacks or stroke in men who have had transient ischemia of the brain due to fibrin platelet emboli.

There is no evidence that aspirin is effective in reducing TIA's in women, or is of benefit in the treatment of completed strokes in men or women. Patients presenting with signs and symptoms of TIA's should have a complete medical and neurologic evaluation. Consideration should be given to other disorders which resemble TIA's.
It is important to evaluate and treat, if appropriate, other diseases associated with TIA's and stroke, such as hypertension and diabetes.
Dosage: The recommended dosage for this new indication is 1,300 mg/day (650 mg twice/day or 325 mg four times a day).
Precaution: A complete medical and neurologic examination should be performed on the male individual with recurrent TIA or stroke prior to instituting antiplatelet therapy with aspirin. The differential diagnosis should include consideration of disorders that resemble TIA's. An assessment of the presence and need for treatment of other diseases associated with TIA's or stroke, such as diabetes and hypertension, should be made.
The landmark studies which showed the effectiveness of aspirin in men with recurrent TIA's or stroke used a standard unbuffered aspirin preparation. It has been reported that concurrent administration of unabsorbable antacids may alter the available aspirin in plasma by decreasing the aspirin/salicylate ratio; the significance of this finding on recurrent TIA's has not been assessed clinically.
How Supplied:
Bayer Aspirin 5 grains (325 mg.)—
NDC-12843-101-10, packs of 12 tablets
NDC-12843-101-11, bottles of 24 tablets
NDC-12843-101-17, bottles of 50 tablets
NDC-12843-101-12, bottles of 100 tablets
NDC-12843-101-20, bottles of 200 tablets
NDC-12843-101-13, bottles of 300 tablets
Child-resistant safety closures on 12s, 24s, 50s, 200s, 300s. Bottle of 100s available without safety closure for households without small children.
Bayer Children's Chewable Aspirin 1¼ grains (81 mg.)—
NDC-12843-131-05, bottle of 36 tablets with child-resistant safety closure.
Samples available on request.
Shown in Product Identification Section, page 412

BAYER® CHILDREN'S COLD TABLETS
Composition: Each tablet contains phenylpropanolamine HCl 3.125 mg., aspirin 1¼ gr. (81 mg.); the tablets are orange flavored and chewable.
Action and Uses: Bayer Children's Cold Tablets combine two effective ingredients: a gentle decongestant to relieve nasal congestion and ease breathing, and genuine Bayer Aspirin to reduce fever and relieve minor aches and pains of colds and flu.
Administration and Dosage: The following dosage is provided in the packaging.
Under 3 years - consult physician
3 years - 1 tablet
4 to 5 years - 2 tablets
6 to 12 years - 4 tablets
Indicated dosage may be repeated every four hours up to but not more than four times a day. Larger or more frequent dosage may be necessary as appropriate to the condition or needs of the patient.
Contraindications: Side effects at higher doses may include nervousness, dizziness, sleeplessness. To be used with caution in presence of high blood pressure, heart disease, diabetes, asthma, or thyroid disease.
How Supplied: NDC-12843-181-01, bottles of 30 tablets with child-resistant safety closure.
Samples available on request.

BAYER® COUGH SYRUP FOR CHILDREN
Composition: Each 5 ml. (1 tsp.) contains phenylpropanolamine HCl 9 mg. and dextromethorphan hydrobromide 7.5 mg., alcohol 5% Cherry flavored.
Action and Uses: Bayer Cough Syrup for Children combines two effective ingredients in a syrup with a very appealing cherry flavor: a gentle nasal decongestant and a cough suppressant.
Administration and Dosage: The following dosage is provided on the packaging.
Under 2 years .... per physician
2–5 years: 1 teaspoon every 4 hours, not to exceed 4 teaspoons every 24 hours.
6–12 years: 2 teaspoons every 4 hours, not to exceed 8 teaspoons every 24 hours.
Contraindications and Precautions: To be used with caution in presence of high blood pressure, heart disease, diabetes, asthma, or thyroid disease.
How Supplied: NDC-12843-401-02, 3.0 oz. bottles. Samples available on request.

MAXIMUM BAYER® ASPIRIN
Aspirin (Acetylsalicylic Acid)

Composition: Maximum Bayer Aspirin — Aspirin 500 mg. (7.7 grains) contains a thin, inert, methylcellulose coating for easier swallowing. This is not an enteric coating and does not alter the onset of action of Bayer Aspirin.
Actions and Uses: Analgesic, antipyretic, anti-inflammatory. For relief of headache; painful discomfort and fever of colds and flu; sore throats; muscular aches and pains, temporary relief of minor pains of arthritis, rheumatism, bursitis, lumbago, sciatica, toothache, teething pains, and pain following dental prodecures; neuralgia and neurtic pain; functional menstrual pain; sleeplessness when caused by minor painful discomforts; painful discomfort and fever accompanying immunizations.
Administration and Dosage: The following dosages are those provided on the packaging, as appropriate for self-medication. Larger or more frequent dosage may be necessary as appropriate to the condition or needs of the patient.
The methyl-cellulose coating makes Maximum Bayer Aspirin particularly appropriate for those who must take frequent doses of aspirin and for those who have difficulty in swallowing uncoated tablets.
Maximum Bayer Aspirin — 500 mg. (7.7 grains) tablets.
Usual Adult Dose: One or two tablets with water. May be repeated every four hours as necessary up to 8 tablets a day.
How Supplied: Maximum Bayer Aspirin 500 mg (7.7 grains)
NDC-12843-161-53 bottles of 30 tablets
NDC-12483-161-56 bottles of 60 tablets
NDC-12843-161-58 bottles of 100 tablets
Child-resistant safety closures on 30's and 100's. Bottle of 60's available without safety closure for households without small children.
Samples available on request.
Shown in Product Identification Section, page 412

COSPRIN® 325
ENTERIC RELEASE ASPIRIN

Composition: 325 mg. of Bayer Aspirin in an enteric release formulation. This formulation is designed to allow the aspirin to pass through the stomach into the intestine, thus protecting against stomach upset.
Actions and Uses: Cosprin is indicated for temporary relief of the minor pain and inflammation of rheumatoid arthritis, osteoarthritis, spondylitis, bursitis and other forms of rheumatism, as well as many common musculoskeletal disorders. Cosprin is also effective in relieving backaches, muscle aches and other aches and pains.
Administration and Dosage: Adult recommended dosage is two tablets with liquid every four hours (or 3 tablets every 6 hours), not to exceed 12 tablets a day unless directed by a physician. Children—as recommended by physician.
Contraindications: To be used with caution in presence of gastric ulcer, allergies, asthma, or anticoagulant therapy.
How Supplied: Cosprin 325 mg. (5 grains)
NDC-12843-184-44 bottles of 60 tablets
NDC-12843-184-46 bottles of 125 tablets

COSPRIN® 650
ENTERIC RELEASE ASPIRIN

Composition: 650 mg. of Bayer Aspirin in an enteric release formulation. This formulation is designed to allow the aspirin to pass through the stomach into the intestine, thus protecting against stomach upset.

Actions and Uses: Cosprin is indicated for temporary relief of the minor pain and inflammation of rheumatoid arthritis, osteoarthritis, spondylitis, bursitis and other forms of rheumatism, as well as many common musculoskeletal disorders. Cosprin is also effective in relieving backaches, muscle aches and other aches and pains.

Administration and Dosage: Adult recommended dosage is one tablet with liquid every four hours, not to exceed 6 tablets a day unless directed by a physician.

Contraindications: To be used with caution in presence of gastric ulcer, allergies, asthma, or anticoagulant therapy.

How Supplied: Cosprin 650 mg. (10 grains)
NDC-12843-184-52 bottles of 36 tablets
NDC-12843-184-54 bottles of 72 tablets

MIDOL®
Original Formula

Composition: Each Caplet® contains Aspirin 454 mg (7 grains); Cinnamedrine Hydrochloride 14.9 mg; Caffeine 32.4 mg.

Action and Uses: Analgesic, antispasmodic. For fast relief of functional menstrual pain, cramps, irritability; headache, aches from swelling, and the irritability associated with premenstrual tension; headache, and low backache associated with menstruation. Inhibits the body's production of prostaglandins, known to be a major cause of menstrual cramps.

Usage Adult Dosage: Two Caplets with water. Repeat two Caplets every four hours as needed, up to eight Caplets per day.

How Supplied: White, capsule-shaped Caplets.
NDC-12843-151-29, professional dispenser, 250 2-Caplet Packets
NDC-12843-151-02, sample size bottle of 6 Caplets
NDC-12843-151-34, bottle of 12 Caplets
NDC-12843-151-36, bottles of 30 Caplets
NDC-12843-151-38, bottles of 60 Caplets
Child-resistant safety closures on bottles of 60 Caplets.

Samples Supplied: Available upon request.

MAXIMUM STRENGTH
MIDOL® PMS

Composition: Each capsule contains: Acetaminophen 500 mg.; Pamabrom 25 mg.; Pyrilamine Maleate 15 mg.

Action and Uses: Relieves the symptoms of Premenstrual Syndrome. For fast relief from premenstrual tension, irritability, bloating, water-weight gain, cramps, backache and headache.

Usual Adult Dosage: Two capsules with water. Repeat two capsules every four hours as needed, up to eight capsules per day.

How Supplied: Red and white capsules.
NDC 12843-151-34 bottles of 8 capsules
NDC 12843-151-36 bottles of 16 capsules
NDC 12843-151-38 bottles of 32 capsules

Samples Supplied: Available upon request.

MAXIMUM STRENGTH
MIDOL® FOR CRAMPS

Composition: Each Caplet® Contains: Aspirin 500 mg., Cinnamedrine Hydrochloride 14.9 mg., Caffeine 32.4 mg.

Action and Uses: Analgesic, antispasmodic. For fast relief of cramps, functional menstrual pain, headache, backache, leg aches, aches from swelling. Inhibits the body's production of prostaglandins, known to be a major cause of menstrual cramps.

Usual Adult Dosage:
Two Caplets with water. Repeat two Caplets every four hours as needed, up to eight Caplets per day.

How Supplied: White capsule shaped Caplets
NDC 12843-152-48 bottles of 8 Caplets
NDC 12843-152-49 bottles of 16 Caplets
NDC 12843-152-50 bottles of 32 Caplets

Samples Supplied: Available upon request.

CHILDREN'S PANADOL®
Acetaminophen Chewable Tablets, Liquid, Drops

Description: Each Children's PANADOL Chewable Tablet contains 80 mg. acetaminophen in a fruit flavored tablet. Children's PANADOL Acetaminophen Liquid is fruit flavored, red in color, and is both alcohol free and sugar free. Each ½ teaspoon contains 80 mg. of acetaminophen. Infant's PANADOL Drops are fruit flavored, red in color, and are both alcohol free and sugar free. Each 0.8 ml. (one calibrated dropper full) contains 80 mg. acetaminophen.

Actions and Indications: Acetaminophen, the active ingredient in PANADOL, is the analgesic/antipyretic most widely recommended by pediatricians for fast, effective relief of children's fevers. It also relieves the aches and pains of colds and flu, earaches, headaches, teething, immunizations, tonsillectomy, and childhood illnesses.

Precautions and Adverse Reactions: Children's PANADOL Tablets, Liquid, and Drops are aspirin free and contain no alcohol or sugar. The pleasant tasting formulations are not likely to upset to irritate children's stomachs.

Usual Dosage: Dosing is based on single doses in the range of 10–15 mg/kg body weight. Doses may be repeated every four hours up to 4 or 5 times daily, but not to exceed 5 doses in 24 hours. The package labeling states that for children under 2 years to "consult a physician".

Children's PANADOL Chewable Tablets: Children 2–3 years 2 tablets, 4–years 3 tablets, 6–8 years 4 tablets, 9–10 years 5 tablets, 11–12 years 6 tablets. For children under 2 consult your physician. Dosage may be repeated every four hours, no more than 5 times in 24 hours.

Children's PANADOL Liquid: (a special 3 teaspoon cup for accurate measurement is provided) Under 2 years consult a physician, 2–3 years 1 teaspoon, 4–5 years 1½ teaspoons, 6–8 teaspoons, 9–10 years 2½ teaspoons, 11 years 3 teaspoons. Repeat every 4 hours up to 5 times in a 24 hour period. Children's PANADOL Liquid may be administered alone or mixed with formula, milk, juice, cereal, etc.

Infant's PANADOL Drops: Under 2 years consult a physician, 2–3 years 1.6 ml. (2 droppers filled to 0.8 mark), 4–5 years 2.4 ml. (3 droppers filled to 0.8 mark). May be repeated every 4 hours, up to 5 times in a 24 hour period.

Warning: Since Children's PANADOL Acetaminophen Chewable Tablets, Liquid, and Drops are available without a prescription as an analgesic/antipyretic, the following appears on the package labels: "WARNING: Do not take this product for more than 5 days. If symptoms persist or new ones occur, consult physician. Keep this and all medicines out of the reach of children. In case of accidental overdose, consult a physician immediately. As with any drug, if you are pregnant or nursing a baby, seek the advice of a health professional before using the product. High fever, severe or persistent sore throat, heachache, nausea, or vomiting may be serious; consult a physician."

Tamper Resistent: Children's PANADOL Acetaminophen Chewable Tablets packaging provides tamper resistant features on both the outer carton and bottle. The following copy appears on the end flaps of this carton—"Purchase only if carton end flaps are sealed. Use only if printed neck seal over cap is intact." Children's PANADOL Liquid and Drops provide tamper resistant features on the bottle—"Use only if printed neck seal over cap is intact."

How Supplied: Chewable Tablets (colored pink and scored)—bottles of 30. Liquid (colored red)—bottles of 2 fl. oz. and 4 fl. oz. Drops (colored red)—bottles of ½ oz. (15 ml.).

All packages listed above have child resistant safety caps and tamper resistant features.

Shown in Product Identification Section, page 412

MAXIMUM STRENGTH
PANADOL®
Tablets and Capsules

Description: Each Maximum Strength PANADOL micro-thin coated Tablet and Capsule contains acetaminophen 500 mg.

Actions: PANADOL acetaminophen has been clinically proven as a fast, effective analgesic (pain reliever) and antipyretic (fever reducer). PANADOL acetaminophen is a non-aspirin product designed to provide relief without stomach upset. Its patented micro-thin coating makes each 500 mg. tablet easy to swallow.

Indications: For the temporary relief of minor aches, pain, headache, and fever when a maximum strength product is preferred over the usual doses of mild analgesic.

Precautions: If a rare sensitivity reaction occurs, the drug should be stopped. PANADOL acetaminophen has rarely been found to produce any side effects. It is usually well tolerated by aspirin sensitive patients.

Severe recurrent pain or high continued fever may indicate a serious condition. Under these circumstances consult a physician.

Warning: As with other products available without prescription, the following appears on the label of PANADOL acetaminophen: "Do not give to children 12 and under or use for more than 10 days unless directed by a physician. Keep this and all medication out of reach of children. In case of accidental overdose, contact a physician or poison control center immediately. If pregnant or nursing, consult a physician before using this or any other medication."

Usual Dosage: *Adults:* Two tablets or capsules every 4 hours as needed. Do not exceed eight tablets or capsules in 24 hours.

Overdosage: In massive overdosage acetaminophen may cause hepatic toxicity in some patients. Clinical and laboratory evidence of overdosage may be delayed up to 7 days. Under circumstances of suspected overdose, contact your regional poison control center immediately.

How Supplied: Tablets (white, micro-thin coated, imprinted "PANADOL" and "500"). Packaged in tamper-evident bottles of 10, 30, 60, and 100. Capsules (white, imprinted "PANADOL" and "500"). Packaged in tamper-evident bottles of 10, 24, 50, and 75.

Shown in Product Identification Section, page 412

PHILLIPS'® MILK OF MAGNESIA

Composition: A suspension of magnesium hydroxide, meeting all USP specifications.

Action and Uses: Phillips' Milk of Magnesia is a mild saline laxative and is indicated for the relief of constipation especially in patients with hemorrhoids, obstetric patients, cardiacs, and in geriatric patients where straining at stool is contraindicated. Phillips' also acts as an antacid, and is effective for the relief of symptoms associated with gastric hyperacidity.

Administration and Dosage: As a laxative, adults 2 to 4 tbsp. followed by a glass of water. Children-infants 1 tsp.; over one year ¼ to ½ adult dose, depending on age. As an antacid, 1 to 3 tsps. with a little water, up to four times a day. Children-1 to 12 years: ¼ to ½ adult dose up to four times a day.

Contraindications: Abdominal pain, nausea, vomiting or other symptoms of appendicitis.

How Supplied: Phillips' Milk of Magnesia is available in regular and mint in bottles of:

Regular
4 fl. oz.	NDC-12843-353-01
12 fl. oz.	NDC-12843-353-02
26 fl. oz.	NDC-12843-353-03

Mint
4 fl. oz.	NDC-12843-363-04
12 fl. oz.	NDC-12843-363-05
26 fl. oz.	NDC-12843-363-06

Also available in tablet form.

Continued on next page

Glenbrook—Cont.

VANQUISH®

Composition: Each Caplet contains aspirin 227 mg., acetaminophen 194 mg., caffeine 33 mg., dried aluminum hydroxide gel 25 mg.; magnesium hydroxide 50 mg.
Action and Uses: A buffered analgesic, antipyretic for relief of headache; muscular aches and pains; neuralgia and neuritic pain; pain following dental procedures; for painful discomforts and fever of colds and flu; functional menstrual pain, headache and pain due to cramps; temporary relief from minor pains of arthritis, rheumatism, bursitis, lumbago, sciatica.
Usual Adult Dosage: Two caplets with water. May be repeated every four hours if necessary up to 12 tablets per day. Larger or more frequent doses may be prescribed by physician if necessary.
Contraindications: Hypersensitivity to salicylates.
(To be used with caution during anticoagulant therapy or in asthmatic patients.)
How Supplied: White, capsule-shaped Caplets in bottles of:
 15 Caplets NDC 12843-171-42
 30 Caplets NDC 12843-171-44
 60 Caplets NDC 12843-171-46
 100 Caplets NDC 12843-171-48

Glenwood, Inc.
83 N. SUMMIT STREET
TENAFLY, NJ 07670

CALPHOSAN® ℞
(calcium glycerophosphate/calcium lactate)
calcium/phosphorus solution in metabolic disorders involving low calcium

Composition: CALPHOSAN is a specially processed solution containing calcium glycerophosphate and calcium lactate. CALPHOSAN is isotonic, with a pH of about 7 or somewhat above. (Other calcium solutions are usually quite acid, with pH values of 4.5 to 5.5). Each 10 ml. CALPHOSAN contains calcium glycerophosphate 50 mg. and calcium lactate 50 mg. in a physiological solution of sodium chloride, with 0.25% phenol as a preservative.
Advantages: Intramuscular injections of CALPHOSAN raise blood serum calcium levels, do not raise the calcium levels above normal.
Of conspicuous importance, intramuscular injections of CALPHOSAN are without pain, inflammatory reactions or sloughing.
Indications: Wherever calcium is indicated or in conditions associated with hypocalcemia.
Administration: One or two 10 ml. injections of CALPHOSAN each week for the first four or five weeks, and on a when-needed basis thereafter, is usually sufficient to raise blood calcium levels.
Contraindications: Hypercalcemia; and in view of the fact that hypercalcemia is associated with sarcoidosis and bone metastasis of neoplastic processes, it should not be used in those conditions. As there is a similarity in the actions of calcium and digitalis on the contractility and excitability of the heart muscle, CALPHOSAN is contraindicated in fully digitalized patients. **Do not use intramuscularly in infants and young children.**
Availability: 10 ml. ampuls in boxes of 10's—NDC 0516-0060-70 and 100's—NDC 0516-0060-01 and 60 ml. multiple dose vials—NDC 0516-0060-60.
Also Available: CALPHOSAN B-12: Calphosan plus 300 mcg. vitamin B$_{12}$ per 10 ml.—NDC 0516-0070-60.

MYOTONACHOL™ ℞
Bethanechol Chloride—Oral

Description: Bethanechol chloride is an ester of a choline-like compound.
Actions: Bethanechol chloride is a synthetic choline ester with postganglionic parasympathomimetic actions mediated via direct stimulation of cholinergic receptors. Its actions are similar to those of acetylcholine—the natural neurohormonal mediator of postganglionic parasympathetic receptors and of certain sympathetic nerves (sweat glands and some blood vessels)—which usually produce smooth muscle stimulation. However, unlike acetylcholine, bethanechol chloride is not inactivated by cholinesterases and therefore has more prolonged effects. Bethanechol chloride's principal effects are due predominately to its muscarinic action, i.e., stimulating micturition and gastrointestinal peristalsis while its nicotinic action is slight. Its cardiovascular effects when administered orally, are ordinarily inconspicious and constitute a slight transient fall in diastolic pressure with a minor reflex tachycardia. Other effects of bethanechol chloride's parasympathetic stimulating actions include contracted pupils, salivation, constricted bronchi, and dilated splanchnic vessels. The pharmacological actions of bethanechol chloride are more efficaciously produced following subcutaneous than with oral administration.
Indications: Acute postoperative and postpartum nonobstructive (functional) urinary retention, and neurogenic atony of the urinary bladder with retention.
Contraindications: Bethanechol chloride is contraindicated in the presence of mechanical obstruction of the gastrointestinal or urinary tracts and hollow viscera, or in conditions where the integrity of the gastrointestinal or bladder wall is questionable. Also, it is contraindicated in spastic, including peptic ulcer or acute in flammatory conditions of the gastrointestinal tract, or peritonitis.
Other major contraindications to the use of bethanechol chloride are latent or active asthma, hyperthyroidism, and coronary occlusion. Additional contraindications are bradycardia, atrio-ventricular conduction defects, vasomotor instability, hypotention, hypertention, coronary artery disease, epilepsy and parkinsonism.
Precautions: Special care and consideration are required when bethanechol chloride is administered to patients concomitantly being treated with other drugs with which pharmacologic interactions may occur. Examples of drugs with potentials for such interactions are: quinidine and procainamide, which may antagonize cholinergic effects; cholinergic drugs, particularly cholinesterase inhibitors, where additive effects may occur. When administered to patients receiving ganglionic blocking compounds a critical fall in blood pressure may occur which usually is preceeded by severe abdominal symptoms.
Adverse Reactions: Untoward effects are usually due to overdosage but occur infrequently with the oral administration of bethanechol chloride. Abdominal discomfort, salivation, flushing of the skin ("hot feeling"), sweating, nausea and vomiting are early signs of overdosage. Asthmatic attacks, especially in asthmatic individuals may be precipitated. Substernal pressure or pain may occur, however, it is uncertain whether this is due to bronchoconstriction, or spasm of the esophagus. Myocardial hypoxia must be considered if a marked fall in blood pressure occurs.
Transient syncope with cardiac arrest, transient complete heart block, dyspnea, and orthostatic hypotention may be associated with large doses. Patients with hypertention may react to the drug with a precipitious fall in blood pressure. Short periods of atrial fibrillation have been observed in hyperthyroid individuals following the administration of cholinergic drugs. Also, involuntary defecation and urinary urgency may occur after large doses.
Atropine sulfate is a specific antidote. A dose of 0.5 mg.—1.0 mg. ($^{1}/_{100}$ grain–$^{1}/_{50}$ grain), for intramuscular or intravenous administration, should be readily available to counteract severe toxic cardiovascular or bronconstrictor responses to bethanechol chloride.

Dosage and Administration: The usual adult oral dose is administered with 5, 10 or 25 mg. tablets, three or four times daily. The minimum effective dose is determined by giving 5 or 10 mg. initially and repeating in the same amounts at one or two hour intervals, to a maximum of 30 mg., until the desired response is obtained. The drug's effects appear within 60 to 90 minutes and persist for an hour.
How Supplied: Myotonachol.
 10 mg. tablets, flat, NDC 0516-0021-01 in bottles of 100s.
 25 mg. tablets, flat, NDC 0516-0022-01 in bottles of 100s.
Shown in Product Identification Section, page 413

POTABA® ℞
Potassium p-Aminobenzoate, Glenwood
Systemic ANTIFIBROSIS THERAPY

Formula: POTABA is chemically a pure potassium p-aminobenzoate, KPAB.

> **Indications:** Based on a review of this drug by the National Academy of Sciences-National Research Council and/or other information, FDA has classified the indications as follows:
> "Possibly" effective: Potassium aminobenzoate is possibly effective in the treatment of scleroderma, dermatomyositis, morphea, linear scleroderma, pemphigus, and Peyronie's disease.
> Final classification of the less-than-effective indications requires further investigation.

Advantages: POTABA offers a means of treatment of serious and often chronic entities involving fibrosis and nonsuppurative inflammation.
Pharmacology: P-Aminobenzoate is considered a member of the vitamin B complex. Small amounts are found in cereal, eggs, milk and meats. Detectable amounts are normally present in human blood, spinal fluid, urine, and sweat. PABA is a component of several biologically important systems, and it participates in a number of fundamental biological processes. It has been suggested that the antifibrosis action of POTABA is due to its mediation of increased oxygen uptake at the tissue level. Fibrosis is believed to occur from either too much serotonin or too little monoamine oxidase activity over a period of time. Monoamine oxidase requires an adequate supply of oxygen to function properly. By increasing oxygen supply at the tissue level POTABA may enhance MAO activity and prevent or bring about regression of fibrosis.
Clinical Uses:
PEYRONIE'S DISEASE: 21 patients with Peyronie's disease were placed on POTABA therapy for periods ranging from 3 months to 2 years. Pain disappeared from 16 of 16 cases in which it had been present. There was objective improvement in penile deformity in 10 of 17 patients, and decrease in plaque size in 16 of 21. The authors suggest that this medication offers no hazard of further local injury as may result from other therapy. There were no significant untoward effects encountered on long term POTABA therapy.
SCLERODERMA: Of 135 patients with diffuse systemic sclerosis treated with POTABA every patient but one has shown softening of the involved skin if treatment has been continued for 3 months or longer. The responses have been reported in a number of publications. The treatment program consists of systemic antifibrosis therapy with POTABA, physical therapy, including deep breathing exercises and dynamic traction splints where indicated, and bethanechol chloride (MYOCHOLINE, Glenwood) for relief of dysphagia as well as small doses of reserpine for amelioration of Raynaud's phenomena.
DERMATOMYOSITIS: Five patients with scleroderma and 2 with dermatomyositis were treated with POTABA. There was striking clinical improvement in each patient. Doses of 15-20 grams per day were well tolerated, and patients were easily able to take these doses.

MORPHEA and LINEAR SCLERODERMA:
All 14 patients with localized forms of scleroderma placed on long-term Potaba treatment showed softening of the sclerotic component of their disorder. Treatment is particularly indicated in patients where persistent compressive sclerosis may contribute even greater disfigurement or functional embarrassment from secondary pressure atrophy.

Dosage and Administration: The average adult daily dose of POTABA is 12 grams, usually given in four to six divided doses. Tablets and capsules 0.5 gram are given at the rate of 4 tablets or capsules 6 times daily, or 6 given four times daily, usually with meals, and at bed-time with a snack. Tablets must be dissolved in an adequate amount of liquid to prevent gastrointestinal upset.

POTABA Envules contain 2 grams pure drug each, and constitute the individual average dose. 6 Envules are given for a total of 12 grams POTABA daily.

POTABA Powder is used to prepare solutions, which are kept refrigerated, but for no longer than one week. 100 grams POTABA powder make 1 quart of 10% solution when dissolved in potable tap water. Children are given 1 gram POTABA daily in divided doses for each 10 lbs. of body weight.

Side Effects: Anorexia, nausea, fever and rash have occurred infrequently and subside with omission of the drug. Desensitization can be accomplished and treatment resumed.

Usage in Pregnancy: Safety for use in pregnancy or during lactation has not been established.

Precautions: Should anorexia or nausea occur, therapy is interrupted until the patient is eating normally again. This permits prompt subsidence of symptoms and also avoids the possible development of hypoglycemia. Give cautiously to patients with renal disease. If a hypersensitivity reaction should occur, Potaba should be stopped.

Contraindications: POTABA should not be administered to patients taking sulfonamides.

How Supplied: POTABA Capsules 0.5 gm. in 250's and 1,000's; POTABA Envules 2.0 gm. in boxes of 50's; POTABA Powder, pure, in 100 gm. and 1 lb.; POTABA Tablets 0.5 gm. in 100's and 1,000's.

Shown in Product Identification Section, page 412

PRIMER® Unna Boot

Composition: Zinc Oxide, Acacia, Glycerin, Castor Oil and White Petrolatum. No preservatives.

Actions and Uses: Treatment of venous insufficiency conditions such as stasis ulcers.

Administration and Dosage: The combination of PRIMER and TENSOPLAST elastic adhesive bandage produces a flexible cast boot. Apply the PRIMER over the entire lower leg, starting immediately behind the toes and continue up to the knee. Apply the elastic bandage over the PRIMER using firm evenly distributed pressure. Continue bandaging until the PRIMER is completely covered. The treatment is ambulatory and the patient should be encouraged to walk as much as possible. Change bandage at least once a week for the first two or three weeks, then every two or three weeks until healing is complete.

Precautions: If skin sensitivity or irritation develops discontinue use and consult a physician.

How Supplied: 3½" × 10 yards Unna Boot-List. No. 3000-1
NDC 0516-1410-30

RENOQUID® ℞
(Sulfacytine)

Description: Sulfacytine, a short-acting sulfonamide, is a white crystalline solid with a melting point in the range of 168.5° to 170°C. It is slightly soluable in pH 5 buffer (109 mg/100 ml). It can be dissolved in human urine to 500 mg/100 ml at pH 6.0. One gram in 5 ml hot 70% aqueous methanol makes a clear solution. Chemically, it is 1-ethyl-N-sulfanilylcytosine.

Actions: The systemic sulfonamides are bacteriostatic agents having a similar spectrum of activity. Sulfonamides competitively inhibit bacterial synthesis of folic acid (pteroylglutamic acid) from aminobenzoic acid. Resistant strains are capable of utilizing folic acid precursors or preformed folic acid.

Indications: Sulfacytine is indicated for the treatment of acute urinary tract infections only (primary pyelonephritis, pyelitis, and cystitis), in the absence of obstructive uropathy or foreign bodies when due to susceptible strains of the following microorganisms: *Escherichia coli, Klebsiella-Enterobacter, Staphylococcus aureus, Proteus mirabilis,* and *Proteus vulgaris.*

Important Note: *In vitro* sulfonamide sensitivity tests are not always reliable. The test must be carefully coordinated with bacteriologic and clinical response. When the patient is already taking sulfonamides, follow-up cultures should have aminobenzoic acid added to the culture media. Currently, the increasing frequency of resistant microorganisms is a limitation of the usefulness of antibacterial agents including the sulfonamides.

Contraindications: Hypersensitivity to sulfonamides. Infants less than two months of age. Pregnancy at term and during the nursing period because sulfanomides cross the placenta and are excreted in the breast milk and may cause kernicterus.

Warnings: Deaths associated with the administration of sulfonamides have been reported from hypersensitivity reactions, agranulocytosis, aplastic anemia, and other blood dyscrasias. The presence of clinical signs, such as sore throat, fever, palor, purpura, or jaundice, may be early indications of serious blood disorders.

Complete blood counts should be done frequently in patients receiving sulfanomides.

The frequency of renal complications is considerably lower in patients receiving the more soluble sulfanomides. Urinalysis with careful microscopic examination should be performed frequently for patients receiving sulfanomides.

Due to lack of clinical experience with sulfacytine in the pediatric age group, it is not recommended for use in children under age 14.

Precautions: Sulfanomides should be given with cation in patients with impaired renal or hepatic function and to those with severe allergies or bronchial asthma.

Adequate fluid intake must be maintained in order to prevent crystalluria and formation of calculi.

In glucose-6-phosphate dehydrogenase-deficient individuals, hemolysis may occur. This reaction is frquently dose-related.

Usage in Pregnancy: Reproduction studies have been performed in rats and rabbits and have revealed no evidence of impaired fertility or harm to the fetus due to sulfacytine. There are no well controlled studies in pregnant women. Therefore sulfacytine should be used in pregnant women only when clearly needed.

Adverse Reactions: The most common adverse reactions associated with sulfacytine are headache, gastrointestinal disturbances, and allergic reactions (rash).

The following have been associated with sulfanamide therapy.

Blood Dyscrasias: agranulocytosis, aplastic anemia, thrombocytopenia, leukopenia, hemolytic anemia, purpura, hypoprothrombinemia, methemoglobinemia.

Allergic reactions: erythema multiforme (including Stevens-Johnson syndrome), generalized skin eruptions, epidermal necrolysis, urticaria, serum sickness, pruritus, exfoliative dermatitis, anaphylactoid reactions, periorbital edema, conjunctival and scleral injection, photosensitization, arthralgia, and allergic myocarditis.

Gastrointestinal reactions: nausea, emasis, abdominal pains, hepatitis, diarrhea, anorexia, pancreatitis, and stomatitis.

CNS reactions: headache, peripheral neuritis, mental depression, convulsions, ataxoa, hallucinations, tinnitus, vertigo, and insomnia.

Miscellaneous reactions: drug fever, chills, and toxic nephrosis with oliguria and anuria. Periarteritis nodosum and lupus erythematosus phenomena have occured.

The sulfonamides bear certain chemical similarities to some goitrogens, diuretics (acetazolamide and the thiazides), and oral hypoglycemia agents. Goiter production, diuresis, and hypoglycemia have occured rarely in patients receiving sulfonamides. Cross-sensitivity may exist with these agents.

Rats appear to be especially susceptible to the goitrogenic effects of sulfonamides, and long-term administration has produced thyroid malignancies in the species.

Dosage and Administration: The usual adult dose is 500 mg initially as a loading dose, then 250 mg four times daily for 10 days.

Due to lack of clinical experience with sulfacytine in the pediatric group, it is not recommended for use in children under age 14.

How Supplied: Renoquid (sulfacytine) tablets—250 mg. NDC 0516-0081-01—bottle of 100.

Clinical Pharmacology: Sulfacytine is rapidly absorbed following single oral doses of 0.5, 1.0, 2.0, and 4.0 grams. Peak blood levels occur within two or three hours. The area under the blood level curve indicates essentially complete oral absorption. The plasma half-life is 4 hours.

A sulfacytine dose of 250 mg four times daily for seven days will produce a mean total sulfonamide plasma level of 16.8 mcg/ml, mean free plasma level of 16.5 mcg/ml for days 2 to 7.

Protein binding studies indicate that the unbound fraction of sulfacytine is 14%. The binding is readily reversible. Dialysis equilibrium studies with human plasma yielded a dissociation constant of 5×10^{-5} M for sulfacytine.

Sulfacytine is rapidly excreted by the kidneys. Following a single oral dose of 500 mg, 88% was recovered in the urine at the end of 24 hours, 95% at the end of five days. Following a dose of 250 mg four times daily for seven days, chromatographic analysis of the urine on the final day showed the following distribution: 79% free drug, 11% N-glucuronides, and 10% acetylated metabolite (inactive). The "free" form is considered to be the therapeutically active form.

Following administration of 500 mg initially, then 250 mg four times daily for seven days, the mean urinary concentration of free sulfacytine for all sampling periods was 419 mcg/ml. This over ten times the highest minimal inhibitory concentration (MIC) for sensitive strains of *Escherichia coli, Enterobacter,* and *Proteus* (31 mcg/ml).

YODOXIN® ℞
(iodoquinol Tablets, U.S.P.)
210 mg. and 650 mg. Tablets

Composition: Each tablet contains: Iodoquinol, U.S.P. 210 mg. or 650 mg.

Description: Iodoquinol is of a light yellowish to tan color, nearly odorless and stable in air. The compound is practically insoluble in water, and sparingly soluble in most other solvents. It contains 64 per cent organically bound iodine.

Action: Iodoquinol is amebicidal against Entamoeba histolytica and is considered effective against the trophozoite and cyst forms.

Indications: Iodoquinol is used in the treatment of intestinal amebiasis.

Contraindications: Known hypersensitivity to iodine and 8-hydroxyquinolines. Contraindicated in patients with hepatic damage.

Warnings: Optic neuritis, optic atrophy, and peripheral neuropathy have been reported following prolonged high dosage theraphy with halogenated 8-hydroxyquinolines. Long term use of this drug should be avoided.

Use in Pregnancy: Safety for use in pregnancy or during lactation has not been established.

Precautions: Iodoquinol should be used with caution in patients with thyroid disease.

Protein-bound serum iodine levels may be increased during treatment with iodoquinol and

Continued on next page

Glenwood—Cont.

therefore interfere with certain thyroid function tests. These effects may persist for as long as six months after discontinuation of therapy. Discontinue the drug if hypersensitivity reactions occur.

Adverse Reactions: Skin: various forms of skin eruptions (acneiform papular and pustular; ballae; vegetating of tuberous iododerma), urticaria and pruritus. Gastrointestinal: nausea, vomiting, abdominal cramps, diarrhea, and pruritus ani. Fever, chills, headache, vertigo and enlargement of thyroid have been reported. Optic neuritis, optic atrophy and peripheral neuropathy have been reported in association with prolonged high-dosage 8-hydroxyquinoline therapy.

Dosage and Administration: Usual adult dose: (210 mgm. each) 3 tablets three times daily, after meals for 20 days. Children 6 to 12 years: (210 mgm. each) 2 tablets, t.i.d. Children under 6: (210 mgm. each) one tablet per 15 pounds of body weight. Usual adult dose: (650 mgm. each) One tablet three times a day for twenty days, to be taken after meals. Children (650 mgm. each): For twenty days, 40 mg. per Kg. of body weight daily divided into 3 doses.

How Supplied: 210 mgm. NDC-00516-0092-01 bottle of 100 tablets and NDC-00516-0092-10 bottle of 1,000 tablets. 650 mgm. NDC-00516-0093-01 bottle of 100 tablets and NDC-00516-0093-10 bottle of 1,000 tablets.

Storage: Store at Controlled Room Temperature 15-30° C. (59-86°F.).

Caution: Federal law prohibits dispensing without prescription.

Mfg. for:
GLENWOOD INC.
Tenafly, New Jersey 07670
by VITARINE CO., Springfield Gardens, N.Y. 11413

5/82

Shown in Product Identification Section, page 412

Gray Pharmaceutical Co.
100 CONNECTICUT AVENUE
NORWALK, CT 06856

X-PREP® LIQUID
[ĕx′prep]
(standardized extract of senna fruit)

Action and Uses: An easy-to-administer, palatable, highly effective bowel evacuant for the preparation of the intestinal tract prior to G.I. and urological radiography as well as colonoscopy, sigmoidoscopy and other diagnostic bowel procedures. In addition, X-Prep Liquid may be used for preparation of the bowel prior to elective colon surgery. Permits excellent visualization without residual oil droplets. X-PREP Liquid is fully prepared in a single dose container—all the patient has to do is drink the contents of one small bottle (2½ fl. oz.). Good patient cooperation is ensured because of highly pleasant taste. Predictable effectiveness helps reduce or eliminate the need for enemas prior to radiography.

Contraindications: Acute surgical abdomen.

Caution: In diabetic patients, the physician should be aware of the sugar content of X-PREP Liquid (50 grams per 2½ fl. oz. dose).

Adverse Reactions: As with all potent purgatives, some patients may experience abdominal discomfort and nausea; vomiting is rare.

Administration and Dosage: For adults: X-PREP Liquid: entire contents of bottle should be taken between 2:00 and 4:00 p.m. on the day prior to diagnostic procedure or elective colon surgery. Patients should be advised to expect a thorough, strong bowel action to begin approximately six hours later. After X-PREP Liquid is taken, diet should be confined to clear fluids.

X-PREP Liquid has proved to be effective following the above regimen. However, at physician's discretion, X-PREP Liquid may be given in divided doses, particularly to elderly or debilitated patients. The following split dosage regimens are equally effective: (1) One-half (½) of the contents of the bottle is taken at bedtime two days prior to diagnostic procedure. On day prior to examination, remaining contents of bottle is taken, also at bedtime. OR (2) On the day prior to examination, one-half (½) contents of bottle is taken at noon and the remaining one-half (½) at 4:00 p.m.

Some physicians prefer the hydration method, with 24-hour liquid diet and consumption of several extra glasses of water during this period, prior to the administration of X-PREP Liquid. Morning enema is optional. X-PREP Liquid may be successfully combined with adjunctive laxative suppositories or citrate of magnesia.

How Supplied: 2½ fl. oz. bottles (alcohol 7% by volume), each providing a single, complete adult dose.

Now Available—Two X-PREP® Bowel Evacuant Kits.

Kit #1 contains: Two SENOKOT-S® Tablets (standardized senna concentrate and docusate sodium), one bottle of X-PREP Liquid 2½ fl. oz., and one RECTOLAX® Suppository (bisa-codyl 10 mg), plus easy-to-follow patient instructions for hydration, clear liquid diet, and the correct time-sequence for administering the above laxatives.

Kit #2 contains: One dose CITRALAX® Granules 1.06 oz. (effervescent citrate/sulfate of magnesia), one bottle of X-PREP Liquid 2½ fl. oz., and one RECTOLAX Suppository (bisacodyl 10 mg), plus easy-to-follow patient instructions.

Guardian Chemical
a division of United-Guardian, Inc.
P.O. Box 2500
SMITHTOWN, N.Y. 11787

CLORPACTIN® WCS-90
[klor-pak′tin]
(brand of sodium oxychlorosene)

Composition: Stabilized organic derivative of hypochlorous acid. A white, water soluble powder with a characteristic smell of hypochlorous acid. Active chlorine derived from calcium hypochlorite: 3–4%.

Action and Uses: For use as a topical antiseptic for treating localized infections, particularly when resistant organisms are present. Complete spectrum (bacteria, fungi, viruses, mold, yeast and spores); effective in cases of antibiotic resistance; nontoxic and non-allergenic in use concentrations.

Administration and Dosage: Applied by irrigation, instillations, spray, soaks or wet compresses, preferably thoroughly cleansing with gravity flow irrigation or syringe to provide copious quantities of fresh solution to remove the organic wastes and debris from the site of the involvement. Also for preoperative skin preparation and postoperative protection. Generally applied as the 0.4% solution in water, or isotonic saline, but as the 0.1% to 0.2% in Urology and Ophthalmology.

Contraindications: The use of this product is contraindicated where the site of the infection is not exposed to the direct contact with the solution. Not for systemic use.

How Supplied: In boxes containing 5 x 2 gram bottles.

LUBRASEPTIC® JELLY
[loo-bra″sep′tik]

Composition: Active ingredients: Aryl phenols, as phenyl phenol 0.1%, Alkyl phenols, as amyl phenol 0.02%, in water miscible form as an acid complex. Phenyl mercuric nitrate 0.007%.

Uses: For urethral instillation, prior to insertion of cystoscopes or sounds; for urethral dilations in the case of strictures. For proctologic use, in cases of hemorrhoids, or for post-hemorrhoidectomies, to provide increased comfort between and during the passage of stools. For endotracheal intubation. For use whenever a sterile water soluble lubricant is required: on cystoscopes and proctoscopes, in urological, rectal, and vaginal examinations or for use as a sterile dressing on burns, abrasions, and decubitus ulcers (bedsores).

Precautions and Side Effects: No serious side effects or contraindications are known. Urethral instillation, in some individuals, may cause a temporary burning or stinging sensation but this usually disappears in several minutes. Excessive pressure should be avoided when instilling where strictures may exist.

How Supplied: In boxes containing 24 sterile packets each with a 10 gram "bellows" shaped tube of jelly and a urethral Disposatip.

pHos-pHaid® ℞
[fos′făd]
(brand of urinary acidifier)

Composition: Each 0.5 Gm. tablet contains ammonium biphosphate, 190 mg., sodium biphosphate, 200 mg., and sodium acid pyrophosphate, 110 mg. pH: approximately 4.5. Sodium content: less than one grain per tablet.

Action and Uses: pHos-pHaid is a highly effective urinary acidifier which, in conjunction with an acid ash diet, can decrease the urinary pH to a 5-5.5 level. Useful in increasing the solubility of calcium in the urine to assist in preventing formation of calculi in the urinary tract.

Administration and Dosage: In conjunction with an acidifying diet, the recommended dosage is two 0.5 Gm. tablets, followed by a glass of water, t.i.d. Occasionally, higher dosage is required and may be employed when necessary.

Side Effects: Occasional hyperacidity, particularly where gastritis or ulceration exists, and/or occasional nausea have been observed in some patients on a high dosage level. This may be decreased or eliminated by the use of the Enteric-Coated tablets. Excessive doses may also act as a saline cathartic and cause diarrhea. In such cases dosage should be decreased until the symptoms disappear. In cases of severe or extensive renal damage, pHos-pHaid should be administered with caution.

How Supplied: In color-coded tablets, either regular or Enteric-Coated.

Size	Type	Packaged	Color
0.5 Gm.	Reg.	90 & 500	Blue
0.5 Gm.	Ent.-Coat	90 & 500	Orange
0.25 Gm.	Reg.	150	Pink
0.25 Gm.	Ent.-Coat	150	Green

Literature Available: Literature on pHospHaid and Acid Ash Diet Sheets are available to physicians on request.

RENACIDIN® ℞
[ren″a-sē′din]

Composition: Active Ingredients (in a 300 gram bottle): Citric acid, anhydrous, 156–171 grams; D-gluconic acid (primarily as the lactone), 21–30 grams. Inert Ingredients: Purified magnesium hydroxycarbonate, 75–87 grams; Magnesium Acid Citrate (MgHC$_6$H$_5$O$_7$), 9–15 grams; Calcium (as the carbonate), 2–6 grams; Water, combined and free, 17–21 grams.

Action and Uses: For use in preparing solutions for irrigating indwelling urethral catheters and the urinary bladder in order to dissolve or prevent formation of calcifications.

Administration and Dosage: As a 10% solution (sterile) in distilled water. Irrigation is carried out with 1-2 ounces, b.i.d. or t.i.d. by means of a small, sterile, rubber syringe.

Side Effects: Only occasionally will a patient complain of some temporary pain or burning sensation from this procedure, in which case use of the solution should be discontinued.

Contraindications: It is contraindicated for therapy or preventive therapy above the ureteral-vesical junction; therefore it is contraindicated for ureteral catheters, nephrostomy or pyelostomy tubes or renal lavage for dissolving calculi. Contraindicated for biliary calculi.

for possible revisions Product Information 1001

How Supplied: In bottles containing 300 grams; also in boxes containing six 25 gram bottles.

W. E. Hauck, Inc.
P.O. BOX 1065
ROSWELL, GA 30075

ANUJECT
Composition: Each ml. contains Procaine Base 1.25% in Almond Oil for protologic use only.
Supplied: 10 ml. multiple dose vials.

BESTA® CAPSULES   OTC
(Therapeutic Vitamins and Minerals)
Supplied: Bottles of 100.

CHLORAFED H.S. TIMECELLES*
Composition: Chlorpheniramine Maleate 4 mg.; Pseudoephedrine HCl 60 mg.
* In special time release beads.
Supplied: Bottles of 100.

CHLORAFED LIQUID   OTC
(Corn, Dye, Alcohol, Sugar Free)
Composition: Each 5 ml. of liquid contains: Chlorpheniramine Maleate 2 mg.; Pseudoephedrine HCl 30 mg.
Supplied: 4 oz. and pints.

CHLORAFED TIMECELLES*
Composition: Chlorpheniramine Maleate 8 mg.; Pseudoephedrine HCl-120 mg.;
*In special time release beads.
Supplied: Bottles of 100 and 500

DOLACET CAPSULES
Composition: Each imprinted teal green capsule contains Hydrocodone Bitartrate 5 mg. and Acetaminophen 500 mg.
Supplied: Imprinted capsules in bottles of 100 and 500.

ENTUSS TABLETS and LIQUID
(Sugar, Alcohol, Corn, Tartrazine Free)
Composition: Each tablet contains: Hydrocodone Bitartrate 5 mg., Guaifenesin 300 mg. Each 5 ml. of liquid contains: Hydrocodone Bitartrate 5 mg. Potassium Guaiacolsulfonate 300 mg.
Supplied: Tablets—bottles of 100. Liquid—pints.

ENTUSS-D LIQUID and TABLETS
Sugar, Dye, Corn, Alcohol Free
Composition: Each tablet or teaspoonful contains Hydrocodone Bitartrate 5 mg., Guaifenesin 300 mg. and Pseudoephedrine Hydrochloride 30 mg.
Supplied: Imprinted Tablets—Bottles of 100. Liquid—16 oz. bottles.

G-1® CAPSULES
G-2® CAPSULES
G-3® CAPSULES
Composition: Each G-1 Capsule contains: Acetaminophen 500 mg., Butalbital 50 mg., Caffeine 40 mg. Each G-2 Capsule contains: Acetaminophen 500 mg., Butalbital 50 mg., Codeine PO$_4$ 15 mg. Each G-3 Capsule contains: Acetaminophen 500 mg., Butalbital 50 mg., Codeine PO$_4$ 30 mg.
Supplied: Bottles of 100.

GERAVITE ELIXIR
Each 15 ml. contains: Lysine 150 mg.; Thiamine HCl 1 mg.; Riboflavin 1.2 mg.; Niacinamide 100 mg.; Cyanocobalamin 10 mcg.; Alcohol 15%
Supplied: Pints and gallons.

HISTOR-D® TIMECELLES*
Composition: Chlorpheniramine Maleate 8 mg.; Phenylephrine 20 mg.; Methscopolamine Nitrate 2.5 mg.
*In special time release beads.
Supplied: Bottles of 100 and 500.

ISOTRATE TIMECELLES
(Isosorbide Dinitrate)
Composition: Each Timecelle contains: 40 mg. Isosorbide Dinitrate in a microdialysis release base which lasts for 12 hours. Orange and clear capsules imprinted Isotrate T.C.
Supplied: Bottles of 100 and 500.

OTIC-H.C. EAR DROPS
Composition: Each ml. contains: Chloroxylenol 1 mg., Hydrocortisone 10 mg., Pramoxine 10 mg., in a non-aqueous Propylene Glycol vehicle with Acetic Acid and Benzalkonium Chloride.
Supplied: 10 ml. dropper tip bottle.

SINUFED TIMECELLES
Composition: Each imprinted capsule contains Pseudoephedrine hydrochloride 60 mg. in a special base to provide for prolonged action and Guaifenesin 300 mg. designed for immediate release for rapid action.
Supplied: Imprinted capsules in bottles of 100.

WEHLESS-105 TIMECELLES
Composition: Each capsule contains: Phendimetrazine Tartrate 105 mg. in a sustained release base which lasts for 10 hours. Black and clear capsule imprinted WEHLESS T.C. 105 mg.
Supplied: Bottles of 100.

Herbert Laboratories
Dermatology Division of Allergan Pharmaceuticals, Inc.
2525 DUPONT DRIVE
IRVINE, CA 92715

AEROSEB-DEX®
(dexamethasone)
Topical aerosol spray
Description: The topical corticosteroids constitute a class of primarily synthetic steroids used as anti-inflammatory and antipruritic agents.
Chemical Name: Pregna-1, 4-diene-3, 20-dione, 9-fluoro-11,17, 21-trihydroxy-16-methyl-, (11β, 16α)-.

Contains:
dexamethasone 0.01%
alcohol 68.5%
with: isopropyl myristate and propellant (butane).
Each 1 second of spray dispenses approximately 0.02 mg of dexamethasone.
Clinical Pharmacology: Topical corticosteroids share anti-inflammatory, antipruritic and vasoconstrictive actions.
The mechanism of anti-inflammatory activity of the topical corticosteroids is unclear. Various laboratory methods, including vasoconstrictor assays, are used to compare and predict potencies and/or clinical efficacies of the topical corticosteroids. There is some evidence to suggest that a recognizable correlation exists between vasoconstrictor potency and therapeutic efficacy in man.
Pharmacokinetics: The extent of percutaneous absorption of topical corticosteroids is determined by many factors including the vehicle, the integrity of the epidermal barrier and the use of occlusive dressings.
Topical corticosteroids can be absorbed from normal intact skin. Inflammation and/or other disease processes in the skin increase percutaneous absorption. Occlusive dressings substantially increase the percutaneous absorption of topical corticosteroids. Thus, occlusive dressings may be a valuable therapeutic adjunct for treatment of resistant dermatoses (see DOSAGE AND ADMINISTRATION).
Once absorbed through the skin, topical corticosteroids are handled through pharmacokinetic pathways similar to systemically administered corticosteroids. Corticosteroids are bound to plasma proteins in varying degrees. Corticosteroids are metabolized primarily in the liver and are then excreted by the kidneys. Some of the topical corticosteroids and their metabolites are also excreted into the bile.
Indications and Usage: Topical corticosteroids are indicated for the relief of the inflammatory and pruritic manifestations of corticosteroid-responsive dermatoses. Aeroseb-Dex® is particularly useful in treating conditions of the scalp such as seborrheic dermatitis.
Contraindications: Topical corticosteroids are contraindicated in those patients with a history of hypersensitivity to any of the components of the preparation.
Precautions:
General: Systemic absorption of topical corticosteroids has produced reversible hypothalamic-pituitary-adrenal (HPA) axis suppression, manifestations of Cushing's syndrome, hyperglycemia and glucosuria in some patients.
Conditions which augment systemic absorption include the application of more potent steroids, use over large surface areas, prolonged use and the addition of occlusive dressings.
Therefore, patients receiving a large dose of a potent topical steroid applied to a large surface area or under an occlusive dressing should be evaluated periodically for evidence of HPA axis suppression by using the urinary free cortisol and ACTH stimulation tests. If HPA axis suppression is noted, an attempt should be made to withdraw the drug, to reduce the frequency of application, or to substitute a less potent steroid.
Recovery of HPA axis function is generally prompt and complete upon discontinuation of the drug. Infrequently, signs and symptoms of steroid withdrawal may occur, requiring supplemental systemic corticosteroids.
Children may absorb proportionally larger amounts of topical corticosteroids and thus be more susceptible to systemic toxicity (see PRECAUTIONS—Pediatric Use).
This medication contains alcohol. It may produce irritation or burning sensations in open lesions. If irritation develops, topical corticosteroids should be discontinued and appropriate therapy instituted.
In the presence of dermatological infections, the use of an appropriate antifungal or antibacterial agent should be instituted. If a favorable response does not occur promptly, the corticosteroid should be discontinued until the infection has been adequately controlled.
Information for the Patient: Patients using topical corticosteroids should receive the following information and instructions:
1. This medication is to be used as directed by the physician. It is for external use only. Avoid contact with the eyes. When used about the face, the eyes should be covered and inhalation of the spray should be avoided.
2. Patients should be advised not to use this medication for any disorder other than for which it was prescribed.
3. The treated skin area should not be bandaged or otherwise covered or wrapped as to be occlusive unless directed by the physician.
4. Patients should report any signs of local adverse reactions especially under occlusive dressing.
5. Parents of pediatric patients should be advised not to use tight-fitting diapers or plastic pants on a child being treated in the diaper area, as these garments may constitute occlusive dressings.
Laboratory Tests. The urinary free cortisol test and the ACTH stimulation test may be helpful in evaluating the HPA axis suppression.

Continued on next page

Herbert—Cont.

Carcinogenesis, mutagenesis, impairment of fertility: Long-term animal studies have not been performed to evaluate the carcinogenic potential or the effect of topical corticosteroids on fertility. Studies to determine mutagenicity with prednisolone and hydrocortisone have revealed negative results.

Pregnancy Category C: Corticosteroids are generally teratogenic in laboratory animals when administered systemically at relatively low dosage levels. The more potent corticosteroids have been shown to be teratogenic after dermal application in laboratory animals. There are no adequate and well-controlled studies in pregnant women on teratogenic effects from topically applied corticosteroids. Therefore, topical corticosteroids should be used during pregnancy only if the potential benefit justifies the potential risk to the fetus. Drugs of this class should not be used extensively on pregnant patients, in large amounts, or for prolonged periods of time.

Nursing Mothers: It is not known whether topical administration of corticosteroids could result in sufficient systemic absorption to produce detectable quantities in breast milk. Systemically administered corticosteroids are secreted into breast milk in quantities not likely to have a deleterious effect on the infant. Nevertheless, caution should be exercised when topical corticosteroids are administered to a nursing woman.

Pediatric Use: Pediatric patients may demonstrate greater susceptibility to topical corticosteroid-induced HPA axis suppression and Cushing's syndrome than mature patients because of a larger skin surface area to body weight ratio. Hypothalamic-pituitary-adrenal (HPA) axis suppression, Cushing's syndrome and intracranial hypertension have been reported in children receiving topical corticosteroids. Manifestations of adrenal suppression in children include linear growth retardation, delayed weight gain, low plasma cortisol levels and absence of response to ACTH stimulation. Manifestations of intracranial hypertension include bulging fontanelles, headaches and bilateral papilledema.

Administration of topical corticosteroids to children should be limited to the least amount compatible with an effective therapeutic regimen. Chronic corticosteroid therapy may interfere with the growth and development of children.

Adverse Reactions: The following local adverse reactions are reported infrequently with topical corticosteroids, but may occur more frequently with the use of occlusive dressings. These reactions are listed in an approximate decreasing order of occurrence:

Burning	Perioral dermatitis
Itching	Allergic contact
Irritation	dermatitis
Dryness	Maceration of the skin
Folliculitis	Secondary infection
Hypertrichosis	Skin atrophy
Acneiform eruptions	Striae
Hypopigmentation	Miliaria

Overdosage: Topically applied corticosteroids can be absorbed in sufficient amounts to produce systemic effects (see PRECAUTIONS).

Dosage and Administration: Aeroseb-Dex® should be applied to the affected area two or three times daily depending on the severity of the condition.

Occlusive dressings may be used for management of psoriasis or recalcitrant conditions.

If an infection develops, the use of occlusive dressings should be discontinued and appropriate antimicrobial therapy instituted.

For use on the scalp: Apply to dry scalp after shampoo. Shake well before spraying.

1. Hold aerosol upright. Slide applicator tube under the hair so that it touches scalp.
   Spray while moving tube to all affected areas, keeping tube under hair and in contact with scalp throughout treatment. Spraying should take 1 to 2 seconds.
2. If some areas of the scalp are not covered adequately, they may be "spot" sprayed by sliding applicator tube through hair to touch scalp—press and immediately release spray button.
3. It is unnecessary to massage medication into the scalp.
4. Be sure that the tip of the applicator tube stops at the hairline so that forehead and eyes are not sprayed.

For other dermatoses: Remove applicator tube. Shake well before spraying. Hold the can upright, approximately six inches from the area to be treated. Spray each four-inch square of affected area for one or two seconds, two or three times a day.

Note: For best results and to avoid wasting medication, it is important to follow the application instructions carefully (application instructions appear on the carton; however, it is preferable that the physician demonstrate the proper application method to the patient).

Caution: Flammable. Do not spray near flame or heated surfaces. If medication accidentally gets in the eyes, wash thoroughly with water and contact physician immediately. Keep out of the reach of children. Contents under pressure. Do not puncture, incinerate, or expose to temperatures above 120°F.

How Supplied: In a 58 g aerosol with applicator tube.* On prescription only.

*U.S. Patent 3,730,182

AEROSEB–HC®
(hydrocortisone)
Topical aerosol spray

Description: The topical corticosteroids constitute a class of primarily synthetic steroids used as anti-inflammatory and antipruritic agents.

Chemical Name: Pregn-4-ene-3, 20-dione, 11, 17, 21-trihydroxy-, (11β)-.

Contains:
hydrocortisone 0.5%
alcohol 68%
with: isopropyl myristate and propellant (butane). Each 1 second of spray dispenses approximately 1 mg of hydrocortisone.

Clinical Pharmacology: Topical corticosteroids share anti-inflammatory, antipruritic and vasoconstrictive actions.

The mechanism of anti-inflammatory activity of the topical corticosteroids is unclear. Various laboratory methods, including vasoconstrictors assays, are used to compare and predict potencies and/or clinical efficacies of the topical corticosteroids. There is some evidence to suggest that a recognizable correlation exists between vasoconstrictor potency and therapeutic efficacy in man.

Pharmacokinetics: The extent of percutaneous absorption of topical corticosteroids is determined by many factors including the vehicle, the integrity of the epidermal barrier and the use of occlusive dressings.

Topical corticosteroids can be absorbed from normal intact skin. Inflammation and/or other disease processes in the skin increase percutaneous absorption. Occlusive dressings substantially increase the percutaneous absorption of topical corticosteroids. Thus, occlusive dressings may be a valuable therapeutic adjunct for treatment of resistant dermatoses (see DOSAGE AND ADMINISTRATION).

Once absorbed through the skin, topical corticosteroids are handled through pharmacokinetic pathways similar to systemically administered corticosteroids. Corticosteroids are bound to plasma proteins in varying degrees. Corticosteroids are metabolized primarily in the liver and are then excreted by the kidneys. Some of the topical corticosteroids and their metabolites are also excreted into the bile.

Indications and Usage: Topical corticosteroids are indicated for the relief of the inflammatory and pruritic manifestations of corticosteroid-responsive dermatoses. Aeroseb-HC® is particularly useful in treating conditions of the scalp such as seborrheic dermatitis.

Contraindications: Topical corticosteroids are contraindicated in those patients with a history of hypersensitivity to any of the components of the preparation.

Precautions:

General: Systemic absorption of topical corticosteroids has produced reversible hypothalamic-pituitary-adrenal (HPA) axis suppression, manifestations of Cushing's syndrome, hyperglycemia and glucosuria in some patients.

Conditions which augment systemic absorption include the application of more potent steroids, use over large surface areas, prolonged use and the addition of occlusive dressings.

Therefore, patients receiving a large dose of a potent topical steroid applied to a large surface area or under an occlusive dressing should be evaluated periodically for evidence of HPA axis suppression by using the urinary free cortisol and ACTH stimulation tests. If HPA axis suppression is noted, an attempt should be made to withdraw the drug, to reduce the frequency of application, or to substitute a less potent steroid.

Recovery of HPA axis function is generally prompt and complete upon discontinuation of the drug. Infrequently, signs and symptoms of steroid withdrawal may occur, requiring supplemental systemic corticosteroids.

Children may absorb proportionally larger amounts of topical corticosteroids and thus be more susceptible to systemic toxicity (see PRECAUTIONS - Pediatric Use).

This medication contains alcohol. It may produce irritation or burning sensations in open lesions. If irritation develops, topical corticosteroids should be discontinued and appropriate therapy instituted.

In the presence of dermatological infections, the use of an appropriate antifungal or antibacterial agent should be instituted. If a favorable response does not occur promptly, the corticosteroid should be discontinued until the infection has been adequately controlled.

Information for the Patient: Patients using topical corticosteroids should receive the following information and instructions:

1. This medication is to be used as directed by the physician. It is for external use only. Avoid contact with the eyes. When used about the face, the eyes should be covered and inhalation of the spray should be avoided.
2. Patients should be advised not to use this medication for any disorder other than for which it was prescribed.
3. The treated skin area should not be bandaged or otherwise covered or wrapped as to be occlusive unless directed by the physician.
4. Patients should report any signs of local adverse reactions especially under occlusive dressing.
5. Parents of pediatric patients should be advised not to use tight-fitting diapers or plastic pants on a child being treated in the diaper area, as these garments may constitute occlusive dressings.

Laboratory Tests: The urinary free cortisol test and the ACTH stimulation test may be helpful in evaluating the HPA axis suppression.

Carcinogenesis, mutagenesis, impairment of fertility: Long-term animal studies have not been performed to evaluate the carcinogenic potential or the effect of topical corticosteroids on fertility. Studies to determine mutagenicity with prednisolone and hydrocortisone have revealed negative results.

Pregnancy Category C: Corticosteroids are generally teratogenic in laboratory animals when administered systemically at relatively low dosage levels. The more potent corticosteroids have been shown to be teratogenic after dermal application in laboratory animals. There are no adequate and well-controlled studies in pregnant women on teratogenic effects from topically applied corticosteroids. Therefore, topical corticosteroids should be used during pregnancy only if the potential benefit justifies the potential risk to the fetus. Drugs of this class should not be used extensively on pregnant patients, in large amounts, or for prolonged periods of time.

Nursing Mothers: It is not known whether topical administration of corticosteroids could result in sufficient systemic absorption to produce detectable quantities in breast milk. Systemically administered corticosteroids are secreted into breast milk in quantities not likely to have a deleterious effect on the infant. Nevertheless, caution should be exercised when topical corticosteroids are administered to a nursing woman.

Pediatric Use: Pediatric patients may demonstrate greater susceptibility to topical corticosteroid-induced HPA axis suppression and Cushing's syndrome than mature patients because of a larger skin surface area to body weight ratio. Hypothalamic-pituitary-adrenal (HPA) axis suppression, Cushing's syndrome and intracranial hypertension have been reported in children receiving topical corticosteroids. Manifestations of adrenal suppression in children include linear growth retardation, delayed weight gain, low plasma cortisol levels and absence of response to ACTH stimulation. Manifestations of intracranial hypertension include bulging fontanelles, headaches and bilateral papilledema.

Administration of topical corticosteroids to children should be limited to the least amount compatible with an effective therapeutic regimen. Chronic corticosteroid therapy may interfere with the growth and development of children.

Adverse Reactions: The following local adverse reactions are reported infrequently with topical corticosteroids, but may occur more frequently with the use of occlusive dressings. These reactions are listed in an approximate decreasing order of occurrence:

Burning	Perioral dermatitis
Itching	Allergic contact dermatitis
Irritation	Maceration of the skin
Dryness	Secondary infection
Folliculitis	Skin atrophy
Hypertrichosis	Striae
Acneiform eruptions	Miliaria
Hypopigmentation	

Overdosage: Topically applied corticosteroids can be absorbed in sufficient amounts to produce systemic effects (see PRECAUTIONS).

Dosage and Administration: Aeroseb-HC® should be applied to the affected area from two or three times daily depending on the severity of the condition.

Occlusive dressings may be used for management of psoriasis or recalcitrant conditions.

If an infection develops, the use of occlusive dressings should be discontinued and appropriate antimicrobial therapy instituted.

For use on the scalp: Apply to dry scalp after shampoo. Shake well before spraying.
1. Hold aerosol upright. Slide applicator tube under the hair so that it touches scalp. Spray while moving tube to all affected areas, keeping tube under hair and in contact with scalp throughout treatment. Spraying should take 1 to 2 seconds.
2. If some areas of the scalp are not covered adequately, they may be "spot" sprayed by sliding applicator tube through hair to touch scalp—press and immediately release spray button.
3. It is unnecessary to massage medication into the scalp.
4. Be sure that the tip of the applicator tube stops at the hairline so that forehead and eyes are not sprayed.

For other dermatoses: Remove applicator tube. Shake well before spraying. Hold the can upright, approximately six inches from the area to be treated. Spray each four-inch square of affected area for one or two seconds, two or three times a day.

Note: For best results and to avoid wasting medication, it is important to follow the application instructions carefully (application instructions appear on the carton; however, it is preferable that the physician demonstrate the proper application method to the patient).

Caution: Flammable. Do not spray near flame or heated surfaces. If medication accidentally gets in the eyes, wash thoroughly with water and contact physician immediately. Keep out of the reach of children. Contents under pressure. Do not puncture, incinerate, or expose to temperatures above 120°F.

How Supplied: In a 58 g aerosol with applicator tube.* On prescription only.
*U.S. Patent 3,730,182

ERYMAX™ ℞
(erythromycin) 2% Topical Solution

Description: Erythromycin is an antibiotic produced from a strain of *Streptomyces erythraeus*. It is basic and readily forms salts with acids. Erymax™ (erythromycin) 2% Topical Solution contains 20 mg/ml erythromycin base in a clear solution vehicle of 66 percent alcohol and propylene glycol. May contain citric acid to adjust pH.

Action: Although the mechanism by which Erymax Solution acts in reducing inflammatory lesions of acne vulgaris is unknown, it is presumably due to its antibiotic action.

Indications: Erymax Solution is indicated for the topical control of acne vulgaris.

Contraindications: Erymax Solution is contraindicated in persons who have shown hypersensitivity to erythromycin or any of the other listed ingredients.

Warning: The safe use of Erymax Solution during pregnancy or lactation has not been established.

Precautions: Erymax Solution is recommended for external use only and should be kept away from the eyes, nose, mouth and other mucous membranes. Concomitant topical acne therapy should be used with caution because a cumulative irritancy effect may occur, especially with the use of peeling, desquamating or abrasive agents.

The use of antibiotic agents may be associated with the overgrowth of antibiotic-resistant organisms. If this occurs, administration of this drug should be discontinued and appropriate measures taken.

Adverse Reactions: Adverse conditions reported include dryness, tenderness, pruritus, desquamation, erythema, oiliness, and burning sensation. Irritation of the eyes has also been reported. A case of generalized urticarial reaction, possibly related to the drug, which required the use of systemic steroid therapy, has been reported.

Dosage and Administration: Erymax Solution should be applied to the affected area each morning and evening after the skin is thoroughly washed with warm water and soap and patted dry. Use enough solution to cover the affected area lightly. The hands should be washed after application.

Caution: Federal law prohibits dispensing without prescription.

Store at controlled room temperature (59°F–86°F).

How Supplied: Bottles of 4 fl oz (118 ml).
Manufactured by National Pharmaceutical Mfg. Co.
Baltimore, Maryland 21207
for
HERBERT LABORATORIES
Dermatology Division of
ALLERGAN PHARMACEUTICALS, INC.
Irvine, California 92713, U.S.A.

EXSEL® ℞
(selenium sulfide 2.5%)
Lotion

Description: Exsel® Lotion is an antiseborrheic dermatitis preparation for dermatological use.

Contains:
selenium sulfide 2.5%
with: edetate disodium; bentonite; sodium dodecylbenzene sulfonate; sodium C14-16 olefin sulfonate; glyceryl ricinoleate; dimethicone copolyol; titanium dioxide; citric acid monohydrate; sodium phosphate monobasic, monohydrate; perfume; and purified water.

Clinical Pharmacology: The mechanism of action of selenium sulfide in seborrheic dermatitis is unknown. Its antidandruff effectiveness is thought to result from its antimitotic activity and substantivity to the skin.

Indications and Usage: Selenium sulfide is indicated in the treatment of seborrheic dermatitis of the scalp, including dandruff.

Contraindications: This product should not be used by patients who are allergic to any of its components.

Warnings: Chemical conjunctivitis may result if this preparation comes in contact with the eyes.

Precautions:
General: This product should be used with caution when acute inflammation or exudation is present as an increase in absorption may occur.

Information for Patients: Avoid contact with eyes or eyelids. Do not take internally. Keep out of the reach of children.

Carcinogenesis, mutagenesis, impairment of fertility: Animal studies are in progress to evaluate the potential of these effects.

Pregnancy Category C: Animal reproduction studies have not been conducted with selenium sulfide. It is also not known whether selenium sulfide can cause fetal harm when administered to a pregnant woman or can affect reproduction capacity. Selenium sulfide should be given to a pregnant woman only if clearly needed.

Pediatric Use: Safety and effectiveness in children have not been established.

Adverse Reactions: Exact incidence figures are not available since no denominator of treated patients is available.
1. Hair loss has been reported with the use of selenium sulfide shampoos.
2. Discoloration of the hair may follow the use of selenium sulfide shampoo. This can be minimized by careful rinsing of the hair after treatment.
3. Oiliness of the hair and scalp may increase following the use of selenium sulfide shampoos.

Dosage and Administration:
1. Massage about 1 or 2 teaspoons of the medicated shampoo into the wet scalp. Avoid contact with the eyes.
2. Allow product to remain on the scalp for 2 to 3 minutes.
3. Rinse the scalp thoroughly.
4. Repeat application and rinse thoroughly.
5. After treatment, wash hands well.
6. Repeat treatments as directed by physician.

The preparation should not be applied more frequently than required to maintain control of symptoms.

Accidental Oral Ingestion: Selenium sulfide is highly toxic if ingested. Nausea and vomiting usually occur after oral ingestion. Treatment is to induce vomiting or if necessary perform gastric lavage, together with general supportive measures as required. Administer a purgative to hasten elimination.

How Supplied: In 4 oz plastic bottles. On prescription only. Protect from heat. For external use only. Keep out of reach of children.

FLUONID® ℞
(fluocinolone acetonide)
Ointment 0.025%
Cream 0.01%
Cream 0.025%
Topical Solution 0.01%

Description: The topical corticosteroids constitute a class of primarily synthetic steroids used as anti-inflammatory and antipruritic agents.

Chemical Name: Pregna-1, 4-diene-3, 20-dione, 6,9- difluoro- 11, 21-dihydroxy-16, 17-[(1-methylethylidene)bis (oxy)]-, (6α,11β,16α)-.

Fluonid® Cream contains:
fluocinolone acetonide 0.01%, 0.025%
with: methylparaben, propylparaben, stearic acid, propylene glycol, sorbitan monostearate, sorbitan monooleate, polyoxyethylene sorbitan monostearate, citric acid and purified water.

Fluonid® Ointment contains:
fluocinolone acetonide 0.025%
in white petrolatum.

Continued on next page

Herbert—Cont.

Fluonid® Topical Solution contains:
fluocinolone acetonide 0.01%
with: propylene glycol and citric acid.

Clinical Pharmacology: Topical corticosteroids share anti-inflammatory, antipruritic and vasoconstrictive actions.

The mechanism of anti-inflammatory activity of the topical corticosteroids is unclear. Various laboratory methods, including vasoconstrictor assays, are used to compare and predict potencies and/or clinical efficacies of the topical corticosteroids. There is some evidence to suggest that a recognizable correlation exists between vasoconstrictor potency and therapeutic efficacy in man.

Pharmacokinetics: The extent of percutaneous absorption of topical corticosteroids is determined by many factors including the vehicle, the integrity of the epidermal barrier and the use of occlusive dressings.

Topical corticosteroids can be absorbed from normal intact skin. Inflammation and/or other disease processes in the skin increase percutaneous absorption. Occlusive dressings substantially increase the percutaneous absorption of topical corticosteroids. Thus, occlusive dressings may be a valuable therapeutic adjunct for treatment of resistant dermatoses (see DOSAGE AND ADMINISTRATION).

Once absorbed through the skin, topical corticosteroids are handled through pharmacokinetic pathways similar to systemically administered corticosteroids. Corticosteroids are bound to plasma proteins in varying degrees. Corticosteroids are metabolized primarily in the liver and are then excreted by the kidneys. Some of the topical corticosteroids and their metabolites are also excreted into the bile.

Indications and Usage: Topical corticosteroids are indicated for the relief of the inflammatory and pruritic manifestations of corticosteroid-responsive dermatoses. Fluonid® Cream 0.01% and 0.025% are useful in corticosteroid-responsive dermatoses that require a mid-potency corticosteroid.

Fluonid® Ointment 0.025% is useful in such conditions as atopic dermatitis where an emollient effect is desired.

Fluonid® Topical Solution 0.01% is useful in hairy sites such as the scalp, particularly in treating seb- orrheic dermatitis.

Contraindications: Topical corticosteroids are contraindicated in those patients with a history of hypersensitivity to any of the components of the preparation.

Precautions:

General: Systemic absorption of topical corticosteroids has produced reversible hypothalamic-pituitary-adrenal (HPA) axis suppression, manifestations of Cushing's syndrome, hyperglycemia and glucosuria in some patients.

Conditions which augment systemic absorption include the application of more potent steroids, use over large surface areas, prolonged use and the addition of occlusive dressings.

Therefore, patients receiving a large dose of a potent topical steroid applied to a large surface area or under an occlusive dressing should be evaluated periodically for evidence of HPA axis suppression by using the urinary free cortisol and ACTH stimulation tests. If HPA axis suppression is noted, an attempt should be made to withdraw the drug, to reduce the frequency of application, or to substitute a less potent steroid.

Recovery of HPA axis function is generally prompt and complete upon discontinuation of the drug. Infrequently, signs and symptoms of steroid withdrawal may occur, requiring supplemental systemic corticosteroids.

Children may absorb proportionally larger amounts of topical corticosteroids and thus be more susceptible to systemic toxicity (see PRECAUTIONS—Pediatric Use).

If irritation develops, topical corticosteroids should be discontinued and appropriate therapy instituted.

In the presence of dermatological infections, the use of an appropriate antifungal or antibacterial agent should be instituted. If a favorable response does not occur promptly, the corticosteroid should be discontinued until the infection has been adequately controlled.

Information for the Patient: Patients using topical corticosteroids should receive the following information and instructions:

1. This medication is to be used as directed by the physician. It is for external use only. Avoid contact with the eyes.
2. Patients should be advised not to use this medication for any disorder other than for which it was prescribed.
3. The treated skin area should not be bandaged or otherwise covered or wrapped as to be occlusive unless directed by the physician.
4. Patients should report any signs of local adverse reactions especially under occlusive dressing.
5. Parents of pediatric patients should be advised not to use tight-fitting diapers or plastic pants on a child being treated in the diaper area, as these garments may constitute occlusive dressings.

Laboratory Tests: The urinary free cortisol test and the ACTH stimulation test may be helpful in evaluating the HPA axis suppression.

Carcinogenesis, mutagenesis, impairment of fertility: Long-term animal studies have not been performed to evaluate the carcinogenic potential or the effect of topical corticosteroids on fertility. Studies to determine mutagenicity with prednisolone and hydrocortisone have revealed negative results.

Pregnancy Category C: Corticosteroids are generally teratogenic in laboratory animals when administered systemically at relatively low dosage levels. The more potent corticosteroids have been shown to be teratogenic after dermal application in laboratory animals. There are no adequate and well-controlled studies in pregnant women on teratogenic effects from topically applied corticosteroids. Therefore, topical corticosteroids should be used during pregnancy only if the potential benefit justifies the potential risk to the fetus. Drugs of this class should not be used extensively on pregnant patients, in large amounts, or for prolonged periods of time.

Nursing Mothers: It is not known whether topical administration of corticosteroids could result in sufficient systemic absorption to produce detectable quantities in breast milk. Systemically administered corticosteroids are secreted into breast milk in quantities not likely to have a deleterious effect on the infant. Nevertheless, caution should be exercised when topical corticosteroids are administered to a nursing woman.

Pediatric Use: Pediatric patients may demonstrate greater susceptibility to topical corticosteroid-induced HPA axis suppression and Cushing's syndrome than mature patients because of a larger skin surface area to body weight ratio. Hypothalamic-pituitary-adrenal (HPA) axis suppression, Cushing's syndrome and intracranial hypertension have been reported in children receiving topical corticosteroids. Manifestations of adrenal suppression in children include linear growth retardation, delayed weight gain, low plasma cortisol levels and absence of response to ACTH stimulation. Manifestations of intracranial hypertension include bulging fontanelles, headaches and bilateral papilledema.

Administration of topical corticosteroids to children should be limited to the least amount compatible with an effective therapeutic regimen. Chronic corticosteroid therapy may interfere with the growth and development of children.

Adverse Reactions: The following local adverse reactions are reported infrequently with topical corticosteroids, but may occur more frequently with the use of occlusive dressings. These reactions are listed in an approximate decreasing order of occurrence:

Burning
Itching
Irritation
Dryness
Folliculitis
Hypertrichosis
Acneiform eruptions
Hypopigmentation
Perioral dermatitis
Allergic contact dermatitis
Maceration of the skin
Secondary infection
Skin atrophy
Striae
Miliaria

Overdosage: Topically applied corticosteroids can be absorbed in sufficient amounts to produce systemic effects (see PRECAUTIONS).

Dosage and Administration: Fluonid® (fluocinolone acetonide) should be applied to the affected area two to four times daily depending on the severity of the condition.

Fluonid® Cream 0.01% and 0.025% may be used over long periods of time in specific conditions when deemed necessary. Where an emollient effect is desired, as in atopic dermatitis, Fluonid® Ointment 0.025% may be preferred. When large areas are involved, Fluonid® Cream 0.01% is recommended. The cream should be massaged gently and thoroughly until it disappears.

Fluonid® Topical Solution should be applied directly on the lesion, taking note that small quantities are adequate. It should be rubbed in thoroughly but gently at each application. In hairy sites, the hair should be parted to allow direct contact with the lesion.

In some cases treated with Fluonid® Topical Solution, it has been observed that saprophytic or low-grade infections may clear spontaneously as the skin recovers its integrity under the influence of Fluonid® Topical Solution alone. This may be partially attributed to the inherent antimicrobial activity of the solution base, propylene glycol.

Occlusive dressings may be used for the management of psoriasis or recalcitrant conditions.

If an infection develops, the use of occlusive dressings should be discontinued and appropriate antimicrobial therapy instituted.

How Supplied: Fluonid® (fluocinolone acetonide)
Cream 0.01%—15 g and 60 g collapsible tubes and 425 g jars.
Cream 0.025%—15 g and 60 g collapsible tubes.
Ointment 0.025%—15 g and 60 g collapsible tubes.
Topical Solution 0.01%—20 ml and 60 ml plastic squeeze bottles.

These preparations are available on prescription only.

Manufactured by
Marion Laboratories, Inc.
Kansas City, Missouri 64137
for
Herbert Laboratories
Dermatology Division of
Allergan Pharmaceuticals, Inc.
Irvine, CA 92713, U.S.A.

FLUOROPLEX® ℞
(fluorouracil)
**1% Topical Solution
and 1% Topical Cream**

Description: Fluoroplex® (fluorouracil) 1% Topical Cream is a stable, standardized cream formulation of fluorouracil in an emulsion base with the following formula:
fluorouracil 1.0%
with: benzyl alcohol (0.5%), ethoxylated stearyl alcohol, mineral oil, isopropyl myristate, sodium hydroxide and purified water.

Fluoroplex® (fluorouracil) 1% Topical Solution is a stable, standardized solution of fluorouracil in a clear propylene glycol base with the following formula:
fluorouracil. 1.0%
with: propylene glycol, sodium hydroxide, hydrochloric acid to adjust to pH 9, and purified water.

Fluorouracil is a modified pyrimidine similar to uracil and thymine, with whose metabolism it competes. It is a white, crystalline substance with a melting point of $283 \pm 2°$ C., an empirical formula of $C_4H_3FN_2O_2$ and a molecular weight of 130.08. It has a characteristic ultraviolet absorption maximum at 266±1 millimicrons in 0.1N HCl.

Actions: There is evidence that fluorouracil (or its biological metabolites) blocks the methylation reaction of deoxyuridylic acid to thymidylic acid. In this fashion fluorouracil interferes with the synthesis of deoxyribonucleic acid (DNA) and to a lesser extent inhibits the formation of ribonucleic acid (RNA).

Indications: Fluoroplex® (fluorouracil) 1% Topical Solution and Fluoroplex® (fluorouracil) 1% Topical Cream are indicated for the topical treatment of multiple actinic (solar) keratoses.

Contraindications: Should not be used in patients with known hypersensitivity to any of the components of the drug.

Warnings:
1. If an occlusive dressing is used there may be an increase in the incidence of inflammatory reactions to the adjacent normal skin.
2. The patient should avoid prolonged exposure to sunlight or other forms of ultraviolet irradiation during treatment with Fluoroplex® as the intensity of the reaction may be increased.

Use in Pregnancy: Safety for use in pregnancy has not been established.

Precautions: The medication should be applied with care near the eyes, nose and mouth. Excessive reaction in these areas may occur due to irritation from accumulation of drug. To rule out the presence of a frank neoplasm, a biopsy should be made of those areas failing to respond to treatment or recurring after treatment.

Adverse Reactions: Pain, pruritus, burning, irritation, inflammation, dermatitis and telangiectasia have been reported. Occasionally, hyperpigmentation and scarring have also been reported.

Dosage and Administration: The patient should be instructed to apply sufficient medication to cover the entire face or other affected areas.

Apply medication twice daily with non-metallic applicator or fingertips and wash hands afterwards. A treatment period of 2-6 weeks is usually required.

Increasing frequency of application and a longer period of administration with Fluoroplex® may be required on areas other than the head and neck. When Fluoroplex® is applied to keratotic skin, a response occurs with the following sequence: erythema, usually followed by scaling, tenderness, erosion, ulceration, necrosis and re-epithelialization. When the inflammatory reaction reaches the erosion, necrosis and ulceration stage, the use of the drug should be terminated. Responses may sometimes occur in areas which appear clinically normal. These may be sites of subclinical actinic (solar) keratoses which the medication is affecting.

How Supplied: Fluoroplex® (fluorouracil) 1% Topical Solution is available in 30 ml plastic dropper bottles. On prescription only. Fluoroplex® (fluorouracil) 1% Topical Cream is available in 30 g tubes. On prescription only.

Avoid freezing.

Store at controlled room temperature (59°-86°F).

Gris–PEG® ℞
(griseofulvin ultramicrosize)
Tablets, USP
125 mg; 250 mg.

Description: Gris-PEG® Tablets contain ultramicrosize crystals of griseofulvin, an antibiotic derived from a species of *Penicillium*. Each Gris-PEG Tablet contains 125 mg or 250 mg griseofulvin ultramicrosize.

Action: *Microbiology*—Griseofulvin is fungistatic with *in vitro* activity against various species of *Microsporum, Epidermophyton* and *Trichophyton*. It has no effect on bacteria or other genera of fungi.

Human Pharmacology—Following oral administration, griseofulvin is deposited in the keratin precursor cells and has a greater affinity for diseased tissue. The drug is tightly bound to the new keratin which becomes highly resistant to fungal invasions.

The efficiency of gastrointestinal absorption of ultramicrocrystalline griseofulvin is approximately one and one-half times that of the conventional microsize griseofulvin. This factor permits the oral intake of two-thirds as much ultramicrocrystalline griseofulvin as the microsize form. However, there is currently no evidence that this lower dose confers any significant clinical differences with regard to safety and/or efficacy.

Indications: Gris-PEG (griseofulvin ultramicrosize) is indicated for the treatment of the following ringworm infections: *Tinea corporis* (ringworm of the body), *Tinea pedis* (athlete's foot), *Tinea cruris* (ringworm of the thigh), *Tinea barbae* (barber's itch), *Tinea capitis* (ringworm of the scalp), and *Tinea unguium* (onychomycosis, ringworm of the nails), when caused by one or more of the following genera of fungi: *Trichophyton rubrum, Trichophyton tonsurans, Trichophyton mentagrophytes, Trichophyton interdigitalis, Trichophyton verrucosum, Trichophyton megnini, Trichophyton gallinae, Trichophyton crateriform, Trichophyton sulphureum, Trichophyton schoenleini, Microsporum audouini, Microsporum canis, Microsporum gypseum* and *Epidermophyton floccosum*. Note: Prior to therapy, the type of fungi resposible for the infection should be identified. The use of the drug is not justified in minor or trivial infections which will respond to topical agents alone. Griseofulvin is *not* effective in the following: Bacterial infections, Candidiasis (Moniliasis), Histoplasmosis, Actinomycosis, Sporotrichosis, Chromoblastomycosis, Coccidioidomycosis, North American Blastomycosis, Cryptococcosis (Torulosis), *Tinea versicolor* and Nocardiosis.

Contraindications: This drug is contraindicated in patients with porphyria or hepatocellular failure and in individuals with a history of hypersensitivity to griseofulvin.

Warnings: *Prophylactic Usage*—Safety and efficacy of griseofulvin for prophylaxis of fungal infections has not been established. *Animal Toxicology*—Chronic feeding of griseofulvin, at levels ranging from 0.5%–2.5% of the diet resulted in the development of liver tumors in several strains of mice, particularly in males. Smaller particle sizes result in an enhanced effect. Lower oral dosage levels have not been tested. Subcutaneous administration of relatively small doses of griseofulvin once a week during the first three weeks of life has also been reported to induce hepatomata in mice. Thyroid tumors, mostly adenomas but some carcinomas, have been reported in male rats receiving griseofulvin at levels of 2.0%, 1.0% and 0.2% of the diet, and in female rats receiving the two higher dose levels. Although studies in other animal species have not yielded evidence of tumorigenicity, these studies were not of adequate design to form a basis for conclusion in this regard. In subacute toxicity studies, orally administered griseofulvin produced hepatocelular necrosis in mice, but this has not been seen in other species. Disturbances in porphyrin metabolism have been reported in griseofulvin-treated laboratory animals. Griseofulvin has been reported to have a colchicine-like effect on mitosis and cocarcinogenicity with methylcholanthrene in cutaneous tumor induction in laboratory animals. *Usage in Pregnancy*—The safety of this drug during pregnancy has not been established. *Animal Reproduction Studies*—It has been reported in the literature that griseofulvin was found to be embryotoxic and teratogenic on oral administration to pregnant rats. Pups with abnormalities have been reported in the litters of a few bitches treated with griseofulvin. Additional animal reproduction studies are in progress. Suppression of spermatogenesis has been reported to occur in rats, but investigation in man failed to confirm this.

Precautions: Patients on prolonged therapy with any potent medication should be under close observation. Periodic monitoring of organ system function, including renal, hepatic and hematopoietic, should be done. Since griseofulvin is derived from species of *Penicillium*, the possibility of cross sensitivity with penicillin exists; however, known penicillin-sensitive patients have been treated without difficulty. Since a photosensitivity reaction is occasionally associated with griseofulvin therapy, patients should be warned to avoid exposure to intense natural or artificial sunlight. Lupus erythematosus or lupus-like syndromes have been reported in patients receiving griseofulvin. Griseofulvin decreases the activity of warfarin-type anticoagulants so that patients receiving these drugs concomitantly may require dosage adjustment of the anticoagulant during and after griseofulvin therapy. Barbiturates usually depress griseofulvin activity and concomitant administration may require a dosage adjustment of the antifungal agent. The effect of alcohol may be potentiated by griseofulvin, producing such effects as tachycardia and flush.

Adverse Reactions: When adverse reactions occur, they are most commonly of the hypersensitivity type such as skin rashes, urticaria, and rarely, angioneurotic edema, and may necessitate withdrawal of therapy and appropriate countermeasures. Paresthesias of the hands and feet have been reported rarely after extended therapy. Other side effects reported occasionally are oral thrush, nausea, vomiting, epigastric distress, diarrhea, headache, fatigue, dizziness, insomnia, mental confusion, and impairment of performance of routine activities. Proteinuria and leukopenia have been reported rarely. Administration of the drug should be discontinued if granulocytopenia occurs. When rare, serious reactions occur with griseofulvin, they are usually associated with high dosages, long periods of therapy, or both.

Dosage and Administration: Accurate diagnosis of the infecting organism is essential. Identification should be made either by direct microscopic examination of a mounting of infected tissue in a solution of potassium hydroxide or by culture on an appropriate medium. Medication must be continued until the infecting organism is completely eradicated as indicated by appropriate clinical or laboratory examination. Representative treatment periods are *Tinea capitis*, 4 to 6 weeks; *Tinea corporis*, 2 to 4 weeks; *Tinea pedis*, 4 to 8 weeks; *Tinea unguium*—depending on rate of growth —fingernails, at least 4 months; toenails, at least 6 months.

General measures in regard to hygiene should be observed to control sources of infection or reinfection. Concomitant use of appropriate topical agents is usually required, particularly in treatment of *Tinea pedis*. In some forms of athlete's foot, yeasts and bacteria may be involved as well as fungi. Griseofulvin will not eradicate the bacterial or monillial infection.

Adults: Daily administration of 375 mg (as a single dose or in divided doses) will give a satisfactory response in most patients with *Tinea corporis, Tinea cruris,* and *Tinea capitis*. For those fungal infections more difficult to eradicate, such as *Tinea pedis* and *Tinea unguium*, a divided dose of 750 mg is recommended.

Children: Approximately 3.3 mg per pound of body weight per day of ultramicrosize griseofulvin is an effective dose for most children. On this basis, the following dosage schedule is suggested: Children weighing 35–60 pounds—125 mg to 187.5 mg daily. Children weighing over 60 pounds—187.5 mg to 375 mg daily. Children 2 years of age and younger—dosage has not been established.

Clinical experience with griseofulvin in children with *Tinea capitis* indicates that a single daily dose is effective. Clinical relapse will occur if the medication is not continued until the infecting organism is eradicated.

How Supplied: Gris-PEG® (griseofulvin ultramicrosize) Tablets, 125 mg, white, scored, elliptical-shaped, embossed "Gris-PEG on one side and "125" on the other. Gris-PEG (griseofulvin ultramicrosize) Tablets, 250 mg, white, scored, capsule-shaped, embossed "Gris-PEG" on one side and "250" on the other. The 125 mg strength is available in bottles of 100 and 500; the 250 mg strength is available in bottles of 100. Both strengths are film-coated.

Caution: Federal law prohibits dispensing without prescription.

Continued on next page

Herbert—Cont.

Manufactured by
SANDOZ, Inc.
East Hanover, N.J. 07936
for
Herbert Laboratories
Dermatology Division of
Allergan Pharmaceuticals, Inc.
Irvine, California 92713, U.S.A.
Revised January 1984

MAXIFLOR®   ℞
(diflorasone diacetate)
Cream 0.05%

Description: Each gram of Maxiflor® Cream (diflorasone diacetate) contains 0.5 mg diflorasone diacetate in a cream base.
Chemically, diflorasone diacetate is: $6\alpha,9\alpha$-Difluoro-11β, 17, 21-trihydroxy-16β-methylpregna-1, 4-diene-3,20-dione 17,21-diacetate.
Maxiflor® Cream contains diflorasone diacetate in an emulsified and hydrophilic cream base consisting of propylene glycol, stearic acid, polysorbate 60, sorbitan monostearate and monooleate, sorbic acid, citric acid and water. The corticosteroid is formulated as a solution in the vehicle using 15 percent propylene glycol to optimize drug delivery.

Clinical Pharmacology: Topical corticosteroids share anti-inflammatory, antipruritic and vasoconstrictive actions.
The mechanism of anti-inflammatory activity of the topical corticosteroids is unclear. Various laboratory methods, including vasoconstrictor assays, are used to compare and predict potencies and/or clinical efficacies of the topical corticosteroids. There is some evidence to suggest that a recognizable correlation exists between vasoconstrictor potency and therapeutic efficacy in man.

Pharmacokinetics
The extent of percutaneous absorption of topical corticosteroids is determined by many factors including the vehicle, the integrity of the epidermal barrier, and the use of occlusive dressings.
Topical corticosteroids can be absorbed from normal intact skin. Inflammation and/or other disease processes in the skin increase percutaneous absorption. Occlusive dressings substantially increase the percutaneous absorption of topical corticosteroids. Thus, occlusive dressings may be a valuable therapeutic adjunct for treatment of resistant dermatoses. (See DOSAGE AND ADMINISTRATION.)
Once absorbed through the skin, topical corticosteroids are handled through pharmacokinetic pathways similar to systemically administered corticosteroids. Corticosteroids are bound to plasma proteins in varying degrees. They are metabolized primarily in the liver and are then excreted by the kidneys. Some of the topical corticosteroids and their metabolites are also excreted into the bile.

Indications and Usage: Topical corticosteroids are indicated for relief of the inflammatory and pruritic manifestations of corticosteroid responsive dermatoses.

Contraindications: Topical steroids are contraindicated in those patients with a history of hypersensitivity to any of the components of the preparation.

Precautions:
General
Systemic absorption of topical corticosteroids has produced reversible hypothalamic-pituitary-adrenal (HPA) axis suppression, manifestations of Cushing's syndrome, hyperglycemia, and glucosuria in some patients.
Conditions which augment systemic absorption include the application of the more potent steroids, use over large surface areas, prolonged use, and the addition of occlusive dressings.
Therefore, patients receiving a large dose of a potent topical steroid applied to a large surface area or under an occlusive dressing should be evaluated periodically for evidence of HPA axis suppression by using the urinary free cortisol and ACTH stimulation tests. If HPA axis suppression is noted, an attempt should be made to withdraw the drug, to reduce the frequency of application, or to substitute a less potent steroid.
Recovery of HPA axis function is generally prompt and complete upon discontinuation of the drug. Infrequently, signs and symptoms of steroid withdrawal may occur, requiring supplemental systemic corticosteroids.
Children may absorb proportionally larger amounts of topical corticosteroids and thus be more susceptible to systemic toxicity. (See PRECAUTIONS—Pediatric Use.)
If irritation develops, topical corticosteroids should be discontinued and appropriate therapy instituted.
In the presence of dermatological infections, the use of an appropriate antifungal or antibacterial agent should be instituted. If a favorable response does not occur promptly, the corticosteroid should be discontinued until the infection has been adequately controlled.

Information for the Patient
Patients using topical corticosteroids should receive the following information and instructions:
1. This medication is to be used as directed by the physician. It is for external use only. Avoid contact with the eyes.
2. Patients should be advised not to use this medication for any disorder other than for which it was prescribed.
3. The treated skin area should not be bandaged or otherwise covered or wrapped as to be occlusive unless directed by the physician.
4. Patients should report any signs of local adverse reactions especially under occlusive dressing.
5. Parents of pediatric patients should be advised not to use tight-fitting diapers or plastic pants on a child being treated in the diaper area, as these garments may constitute occlusive dressings.

Laboratory Tests
The following tests may be helpful in evaluating the HPA axis suppression:
Urinary free cortisol test
ACTH stimulation test

Carcinogenesis, Mutagenesis, and Impairment of Fertility
Long-term animal studies have not been performed to evaluate the carcinogenic potential or the effect of topical corticosteroids on fertility.
Studies to determine mutagenicity with prednisolone and hydrocortisone have revealed negative results.

Pregnancy Category C
Corticosteroids are generally teratogenic in laboratory animals when administered systemically at relatively low dosage levels. The more potent corticosteroids have been shown to be teratogenic after dermal application in laboratory animals. There are no adequate and well-controlled studies in pregnant women on teratogenic effects from topically applied corticosteroids. Therefore, topical corticosteroids should be used during pregnancy only if the potential benefit justifies the potential risk to the fetus. Drugs of this class should not be used extensively on pregnant patients, in large amounts, or for prolonged periods of time.

Nursing Mothers
It is not known whether topical administration of corticosteroids could result in sufficient systemic absorption to produce detectable quantities in breast milk. Systemically administered corticosteroids are secreted into breast milk in quantities *not* likely to have a deleterious effect on the infant. Nevertheless, caution should be exercised when topical corticosteroids are administered to a nursing woman.

Pediatric Use
Pediatric patients may demonstrate greater susceptibility to topical corticosteroid-induced HPA axis suppression and Cushing's syndrome than mature patients because of a larger skin surface area to body weight ratio.
Hypothalamic-pituitary-adrenal (HPA) axis suppression, Cushing's syndrome, and intracranial hypertension have been reported in children receiving topical corticosteroids. Manifestations of adrenal suppression in children include linear growth retardation, delayed weight gain, low plasma cortisol levels, and absence of response to ACTH stimulation. Manifestations of intracranial hypertension include bulging fontanelles, headaches, and bilateral papilledema.
Administration of topical corticosteroids to children should be limited to the least amount compatible with an effective therapeutic regimen. Chronic corticosteroid therapy may interfere with the growth and development of children.

Adverse Reactions: The following local adverse reactions have been reported with topical corticosteroids, but may occur more frequently with the use of occlusive dressings. These reactions are listed in an approximate decreasing order of occurrence:

Burning	Allergic contact dermatitis
Itching	
Irritation	Maceration of the skin
Dryness	Secondary infection
Folliculitis	Skin atrophy
Hypertrichosis	Striae
Acneiform eruptions	Miliaria
Hypopigmentation	
Perioral dermatitis	

Overdosage: Topically applied corticosteroids can be absorbed in sufficient amounts to produce systemic effects. (See PRECAUTIONS.)

Dosage and Administration: Topical corticosteroids are generally applied to the affected area as a thin film from one to four times daily depending on the severity of the condition.
Occlusive dressings may be used for the management of psoriasis or recalcitrant conditions.
If an infection develops, the use of occlusive dressings should be discontinued and appropriate antimicrobial therapy instituted.

How Supplied: Maxiflor® (diflorasone diacetate) Cream 0.05% is available in collapsible tubes in the following sizes:
   15 gram NDC 0023-0766-15
   30 gram NDC 0023-0766-30
   60 gram NDC 0023-0766-60

Caution: Federal law prohibits dispensing without prescription.

Manufactured by
The Upjohn Company
Kalamazoo, Michigan 49001
For
Herbert Laboratories
Dermatology Division of
Allergan Pharmaceuticals, Inc.
Irvine, California 92713, U.S.A.

MAXIFLOR®   ℞
(diflorasone diacetate)
Ointment 0.05%

Description: Each gram of Maxiflor® Ointment (diflorasone diacetate) contains 0.5 mg diflorasone diacetate in a an ointment base.
Chemically, diflorasone diacetate is: $6\alpha,9\alpha$-Difluoro-11β, 17, 21-trihydroxy-16β-methylpregna-1, 4-diene-3,20-dione 17,21-diacetate.
Maxiflor® Cream contains 0.5 mg/gram of deflorasone diacetate in an emollient, occlusive base consisting of polyoxypropylene 15-stearyl ether, stearic acid, lanolin alcohol and white petrolatum.

Clinical Pharmacology: Topical corticosteroids share anti-inflammatory, antipruritic and vasoconstrictive actions.
The mechanism of anti-inflammatory activity of the topical corticosteroids is unclear. Various laboratory methods, including vasoconstrictor assays, are used to compare and predict potencies and/or clinical efficacies of the topical corticosteroids. There is some evidence to suggest that a recognizable correlation exists between vasoconstrictor potency and therapeutic efficacy in man.

Pharmacokinetics
The extent of percutaneous absorption of topical corticosteroids is determined by many factors including the vehicle, the integrity of the epidermal barrier, and the use of occlusive dressings.
Topical corticosteroids can be absorbed from normal intact skin. Inflammation and/or other dis-

ease processes in the skin increase percutaneous absorption. Occlusive dressings substantially increase the percutaneous absorption of topical corticosteroids. Thus, occlusive dressings may be a valuable therapeutic adjunct for treatment of resistant dermatoses. (See DOSAGE AND ADMINISTRATION.)

Once absorbed through the skin, topical corticosteroids are handled through pharmacokinetic pathways similar to systemically administered corticosteroids. Corticosteroids are bound to plasma proteins in varying degrees. They are metabolized primarily in the liver and are then excreted by the kidneys. Some of the topical corticosteroids and their metabolites are also excreted into the bile.

Indications and Usage: Topical corticosteroids are indicated for relief of the inflammatory and pruritic manifestations of corticosteroid responsive dermatoses.

Contraindications: Topical steroids are contraindicated in those patients with a history of hypersensitivity to any of the components of the preparation.

Precautions:
General
Systemic absorption of topical corticosteroids has produced reversible hypothalamic-pituitary-adrenal (HPA) axis suppression, manifestations of Cushing's syndrome, hyperglycemia, and glucosuria in some patients.

Conditions which augment systemic absorption include the application of the more potent steroids, use over large surface areas, prolonged use, and the addition of occlusive dressings.

Therefore, patients receiving a large dose of a potent topical steroid applied to a large surface area or under an occlusive dressing should be evaluated periodically for evidence of HPA axis suppression by using the urinary free cortisol and ACTH stimulation tests. If HPA axis suppression is noted, an attempt should be made to withdraw the drug, to reduce the frequency of application, or to substitute a less potent steroid.

Recovery of HPA axis function is generally prompt and complete upon discontinuation of the drug. Infrequently, signs and symptoms of steroid withdrawal may occur, requiring supplemental systemic corticosteroids.

Children may absorb proportionally larger amounts of topical corticosteroids and thus be more susceptible to systemic toxicity. (See PRECAUTIONS—Pediatric Use.)

If irritation develops, topical corticosteroids should be discontinued and appropriate therapy instituted.

In the presence of dermatological infections, the use of an appropriate antifungal or antibacterial agent should be instituted. If a favorable response does not occur promptly, the corticosteroid should be discontinued until the infection has been adequately controlled.

Information for the Patient
Patients using topical corticosteroids should receive the following information and instructions:
1. This medication is to be used as directed by the physician. It is for external use only. Avoid contact with the eyes.
2. Patients should be advised not to use this medication for any disorder other than for which it was prescribed.
3. The treated skin area should not be bandaged or otherwise covered or wrapped as to be occlusive unless directed by the physician.
4. Patients should report any signs of local adverse reactions especially under occlusive dressing.
5. Parents of pediatric patients should be advised not to use tight-fitting diapers or plastic pants on a child being treated in the diaper area, as these garments may constitute occlusive dressings.

Laboratory Tests
The following tests may be helpful in evaluating the HPA axis suppression:
   Urinary free cortisol test
   ACTH stimulation test

Carcinogenesis, Mutagenesis, and Impairment of Fertility
Long-term animal studies have not been performed to evaluate the carcinogenic potential or the effect of topical corticosteroids on fertility. Studies to determine mutagenicity with prednisolone and hydrocortisone have revealed negative results.

Pregnancy Category C
Corticosteroids are generally teratogenic in laboratory animals when administered systemically at relatively low dosage levels. The more potent corticosteroids have been shown to be teratogenic after dermal application in laboratory animals. There are no adequate and well-controlled studies in pregnant women on teratogenic effects from topically applied corticosteroids. Therefore, topical corticosteroids should be used during pregnancy only if the potential benefit justifies the potential risk to the fetus. Drugs of this class should not be used extensively on pregnant patients, in large amounts, or for prolonged periods of time.

Nursing Mothers
It is not known whether topical administration of corticosteroids could result in sufficient systemic absorption to produce detectable quantities in breast milk. Systemically administered corticosteroids are secreted into breast milk in quantities *not* likely to have a deleterious effect on the infant. Nevertheless, caution should be exercised when topical corticosteroids are administered to a nursing woman.

Pediatric Use
Pediatric patients may demonstrate greater susceptibility to topical corticosteroid-induced HPA axis suppression and Cushing's syndrome than mature patients because of a larger skin surface area to body weight ratio.

Hypothalamic-pituitary-adrenal (HPA) axis suppression, Cushing's syndrome, and intracranial hypertension have been reported in children receiving topical corticosteroids. Manifestations of adrenal suppression in children include linear growth retardation, delayed weight gain, low plasma cortisol levels, and absence of response to ACTH stimulation. Manifestations of intracranial hypertension include bulging fontanelles, headaches, and bilateral papilledema.

Administration of topical corticosteroids to children should be limited to the least amount compatible with an effective therapeutic regimen. Chronic corticosteroid therapy may interfere with the growth and development of children.

Adverse Reactions: The following local adverse reactions have been reported with topical corticosteroids, but may occur more frequently with the use of occlusive dressings. These reactions are listed in an approximate decreasing order of occurrence:

Burning	Allergic contact
Itching	dermatitis
Irritation	Maceration of the skin
Dryness	Secondary infection
Folliculitis	Skin atrophy
Hypertrichosis	Striae
Acneiform eruptions	Miliaria
Hypopigmentation	
Perioral dermatitis	

Overdosage: Topically applied corticosteroids can be absorbed in sufficient amounts to produce systemic effects. (See PRECAUTIONS.)

Dosage and Administration: Topical corticosteroids are generally applied to the affected area as a thin film from one to four times daily depending on the severity of the condition.

Occlusive dressings may be used for the management of psoriasis or recalcitrant conditions. If an infection develops, the use of occlusive dressings should be discontinued and appropriate antimicrobial therapy instituted.

How Supplied: Maxiflor® (diflorasone diacetate) Ointment 0.05% is available in collapsible tubes in the following sizes:
  15 gram NDC 0023-0770-15
  30 gram NDC 0023-0770-30
  60 gram NDC 0023-0770-60

Caution: Federal law prohibits dispensing without prescription.

Manufactured by
The Upjohn Company
Kalamazoo, Michigan 49001
For
Herbert Laboratories
Dermatology Division of
Allergan Pharmaceuticals, Inc.
Irvine, California 92713, U.S.A.

PENECORT™   R
(hydrocortisone)
Cream, USP, 1%
Topical Solution 1%

Description: The topical corticosteroids constitute a class of primarily synthetic steroids used as anti-inflammatory and anti-pruritic agents.

Structural Formula:

Chemical Name: Pregn-4-ene-3.20-dione, 11,17,21, trihydroxy-,(11β)-.

PENECORT™ Cream contains: hydrocortisone, USP 1% with: benzyl alcohol; petrolatum; stearyl alcohol; propylene glycol; isopropyl myristate; polyoxyl 40 stearate; carbomer 934; sodium lauryl sulfate; edetate disodium; sodium hydroxide to adjust the pH; and purified water.

PENECORT™ Topical Solution contains: hydrocortisone, USP, 1% with: alcohol (57%); propylene glycol; benzyl alcohol; and purified water.

Clinical Pharmacology: Topical corticosteroids share anti-inflammatory, anti-pruritic and vasoconstrictive actions.

The mechanism of anti-inflammatory activity of the topical corticosteroids is unclear. Various laboratory methods, including vasoconstrictor assays, are used to compare and predict potencies and/or clinical efficacies of the topical corticosteroids. There is some evidence to suggest that a recognizable correlation exists between vasoconstrictor potency and therapeutic efficacy in man.

Pharmacokinetics: The extent of percutaneous absorption of topical corticosteroids is determined by many factors, including the vehicle, the integrity of the epidermal barrier and the use of occlusive dressings.

Topical corticosteroids can be absorbed from normal intact skin. Inflammation and/or other disease processes in the skin increase percutaneous absorption. Occlusive dressings substantially increase the percutaneous absorption of topical corticosteroids. Thus, occlusive dressings may be a valuable therapeutic adjunct for treatment of resistant dermatoses. (See DOSAGE AND ADMINISTRATION.)

Once absorbed through the skin, topical corticosteroids are handled through pharmacokinetic pathways similar to systemically administered corticosteroids. Corticosteroids are bound to plasma proteins in varying degrees. Corticosteroids are metabolized primarily in the liver and are then excreted by the kidneys. Some of the topical corticosteroids and their metabolites are also excreted into the bile.

Indications and Usage: Topical corticosteroids are indicated for the relief of the inflammatory and pruritic manifestations of corticosteroids responsive dermatoses.

Contraindications: Topical corticosteroids are contraindicated in those patients with a history of hypersensitivity to any of the components of the preparation.

Precautions: General: Systemic absorption of topical corticosteroids has produced reversible hypothalamic-pituitary-adrenal (HPA) axis suppression, manifestations of Cushing's syndrome, hyperglycemia and glucosuria in some patients.

Continued on next page

Herbert—Cont.

Conditions which augment systemic absorption include the application of more potent steroids, use over large surface areas, prolonged use and the addition of occlusive dressings.

If HPA axis suppression is noted (by using the urinary tree cortisol and ACTH stimulation tests) an attempt should be made to withdraw the drug or to reduce the frequency of application.

Recovery of HPA axis function is generally prompt and complete upon discontinuation of the drug. Infrequently, signs and symptoms of steroid withdrawal may occur, requiring supplemental systemic corticosteroids.

Children may absorb proportionally larger amounts of topical corticosteroids and thus be more susceptible to systemic toxicity. (See PRECAUTIONS—Pediatric Use.)

If irritation develops, topical corticosteroids should be discontinued and appropriate therapy instituted.

In the presence of dermatological infections, the use of an appropriate antifungal or antibacterial agent should be instituted. If a favorable response does not occur promptly, the corticosteroid should be discontinued until the infection has been adequately controlled.

Information for the Patient: Patients using topical corticosteroids should receive the following information and instructions:
1. This medication is to be used as directed by the physician. It is for external use only. Avoid contact with the eyes.
2. Patients should be advised not to use this medication for any disorder other than that for which it was prescribed.
3. The treated skin area should not be bandaged or otherwise covered or wrapped as to be occlusive unless directed by the physician.
4. Patients should report any signs of local adverse reactions, especially under occlusive dressing.
5. Parents of pediatric patients should be advised not to use tight-fitting diapers or plastic pants on a child being treated in the diaper area, as these garments may constitute occlusive dressings.

Laboratory Tests: The urinary free cortisol test and the ACTH stimulation test may be helpful in evaluating the HPA axis suppression.

Carcinogenesis, mutagenesis, impairment of fertility: Long-term animal studies have not been performed to evaluate the carcinogenic potential or the effect of topical corticosteroids on fertility. Studies to determine mutagenicity with hydrocortisone have revealed negative results.

Pregnancy Category C: Corticosteroids are generally teratogenic in laboratory animals when administered systemically at relatively low dosage levels. The more potent corticosteroids have been shown to be teratogenic after dermal application in laboratory animals. There are no adequate and well-controlled studies in pregnant women on teratogenic effects from topically applied corticosteroids. Therefore, topical corticosteroids should be used during pregnancy only if the potential benefit justifies the potential risk to the fetus. Drugs of this class should not be used extensively on pregnant patients, in large amounts, or for prolonged periods of time.

Nursing Mothers: It is not known whether topical administration of corticosteroids could result in sufficient systemic absorption to produce detectable quantities in breast milk. Systemically administered corticosteroids are secreted into breast milk in quantities *not* likely to have a deleterious effect on the infant. Nevertheless, caution should be exercised when topical corticosteroids are administered to a nursing woman.

Pediatric Use: Pediatric patients may demonstrate greater susceptibility to topical corticosteroid-induced HPA axis suppression and Cushing's syndrome than mature patients because of a larger skin surface area to body weight ratio. Hypothalamic-pituitary-adrenal (HPA) axis suppression, Cushing's syndrome and intracranial hypertension have been reported in children receiving topical corticosteroids. Manifestations of adrenal suppression in children include linear growth retardation, delayed weight gain, low plasma cortisol levels and absence of response to ACTH stimulation. Manifestations of intracranial hypertension include bulging fontanelles, headaches and bilateral papilledema.

Administration of topical corticosteroids to children should be limited to the least amount compatible with an effective therapeutic regimen. Chronic corticosteroid therapy may interfere with the growth and development of children.

Adverse Reactions: The following local adverse reactions are reported infrequently with topical corticosteroids, but may occur more frequently with the use of occlusive dressings. These reactions are listed in an approximate decreasing order of occurrence:

Burning	Perioral dermatitis
Itching	Allergic contact
Irritation	dermatitis
Dryness	Maceration of the skin
Folliculitis	Secondary infection
Hypertrichosis	Skin atrophy
Acneiform eruptions	Striae
Hypopigmentation	Miliaria

Overdosage: Topically applied corticosteroids can be absorbed in sufficient amounts to produce systemic effects. (See PRECAUTIONS.)

Dosage And Administration: PENECORT™ (hydrocortisone) 1% should be applied to the affected area from two to four times daily depending on the severity of the condition.

Occlusive dressings may be used for the management of psoriasis or recalcitrant conditions. If an infection develops, the use of occlusive dressings should be discontinued and appropriate antimicrobial therapy instituted.

How Supplied:
PENECORT™ (hydrocortisone):
Cream, USP, 1%—30 g collapsible tubes, NDC 0023-0510-30.
Topical Solution 1%—30 ml plastic bottles, NDC 0023-0889-30.
Store away from heat. Protect cream from freezing.

These preparations are available on prescription only.

February 1984
Herbert Laboratories Dermatology Division of
Allergan Pharmaceuticals, Inc., Irvine, CA 92713, U.S.A.

PENECORT™ ℞
(hydrocortisone)
Cream, USP, 2.5%

Description: The topical corticosteroids constitute a class of primarily synthetic steroids used as anti-inflammatory and antipruritic agents.

Chemical Name: Pregn-4-ene-3,20-dione, 11,17,21, trihydroxy-,(11β)-.
Contains: hydrocortisone, USP ....2.5% with: benzyl alcohol; petrolatum; stearyl alcohol; propylene glycol; isopropyl myristate; polyoxyl 40 stearate; carbomer 934; sodium lauryl sulfate; edetate disodium; sodium hydroxide to adjust the pH; and purified water.

Clinical Pharmacology: Topical corticosteroids share anti-inflmmatory, anti-pruritic and vasoconstrictive actions.

The mechanism of anti-inflammatory activity of the topical corticosteroids is unclear. Various laboratory methods, including vasoconstrictor assays, are used to compare and predict potencies and/or clinical efficacies of the topical corticosteroids. There is some evidence to suggest that a recognizable correlation exists between vasoconstrictor potency and therapeutic efficacy in man.

Pharmacokinetics: The extent of percutaneous absorption of topical corticosteroids is determined by many factors, including the vehicle, the integrity of the epidermal barrier and the use of occlusive dressings.

Topical corticosteroids can be absorbed from normal intact skin. Inflammation and/or other disease processes in the skin increase percutaneous absorption. Occlusive dressings substantially increase the percutaneous absorption of topical corticosteroids. Thus, occlusive dressings may be a valuable therapeutic adjunct for treatment of resistant dermatoses. (See DOSAGE AND ADMINISTRATION.)

Once absorbed through the skin, topical corticosteroids are handled through pharmacokinetic pathways similar to systemically administered corticosteroids. Corticosteroids are bound to plasma proteins in varying degrees. Corticosteroids are metabolized primarily in the liver and are then excreted by the kidneys. Some of the topical corticosteroids and their metabolites are also excreted into the bile.

Indications and Usage: Topical corticosteroids are indicated for the relief of the inflammatory and pruritic manifestations of corticosteroid-responsive dermatoses.

Contraindications: Topical corticosteroids are contraindicated in those patients with a history of hypersensitivity to any of the components of the preparation.

Precautions: General: Systemic absorption of topical corticosteroids has produced reversible hypothalamic-pituitary-adrenal (HPA) axis suppression, manifestations of Cushing's syndrome, hyperglycemia and glucosuria in some patients. Conditions which augment systemic absorption include the application of more potent steroids, use over large surface areas, prolonged use and the addition of occlusive dressings.

If HPA axis suppression is noted (by using the urinary free cortisol and ACTH stimulation tests) an attempt should be made to withdraw the drug or to reduce the frequency of application.

Recovery of HPA axis function is generally prompt and complete upon discontinuation of the drug. Infrequently, signs and symptoms of steroid withdrawal may occur, requiring supplemental systemic corticosteroids.

Children may absorb proportionally larger amounts of topical corticosteroids and thus be more susceptible to systemic toxicity. (See PRECAUTIONS—Pediatric Use.)

If irritation develops, topical corticosteroids should be discontinued and appropriate therapy instituted.

In the presence of dermatological infections, the use of an appropriate antifungal or antibacterial agent should be instituted. If a favorable response does not occur promptly, the corticosteroid should be discontinued until the infection has been adequately controlled.

Information for the Patient: Patients using topical corticosteroids should receive the following information and instructions.
1. This medication is to be used as directed by the physician. It is for external use only. Avoid contact with the eyes.
2. Patients should be advised not to use this medication for any disorder other than that for which it was prescribed.
3. The treated skin area should not be bandaged or otherwise covered or wrapped as to be occlusive unless directed by the physician
4. Patients should report any signs of local adverse reactions, especially under occlusive dressing.
5. Parents of pediatric patients should be advised not to use tight-fitting diapers or plastic pants on a child being treated in the diaper area, as these garments may consitute occlusive dressings.

Laboratory Tests: The urinary free cortisol test and the ACTH stimulation test may be helpful in evaluating the HPA axis suppression.

Carcinogenesis, mutagenesis, impairment of fertility: Long-term animal studies have not been performed to evaluate the carcinogenic potential or the effect of topical corticosteroids on fertility. Studies to determine mutagenicity with hydrocortisone have revealed negative results.

Pregnancy Category C: Corticosteroids are generally teratogenic in laboratory animals when administered systemically at relatively low dosage levels. The more potent corticosteroids have been shown to be teratogenic after dermal application in laboratory animals. There are no adequate and well-controlled studies in pregnant women on teratogenic effects from topically applied corticosteroids. Therefore, topical corticosteroids should be used during pregnancy only if the potential benefit justifies the potential risk to the fetus. Drugs on this class should not be used extensively on pregnant patients, in large amounts, or for prolonged periods of time.

Nursing Mothers: It is not known whether topical administration of corticosteroids could result in sufficient systemic absorption to produce detectable quantities in breast milk. Systemically administered corticosteroids are secreted into breast milk in quantities not likely to have a deleterious effect on the infant. Nevertheless, caution should be exercised when topical corticosteroids are administered to a nursing woman.

Pediatric Use: Pediatric patients may demonstrate greater susceptibility to topical corticosteroid-induced HPA axis suppression and Cushing's syndrome than mature patients because of a larger skin surface area to body weight ratio. Hypothalamic-pituitary-adrenal (HPA) axis suppression, Cushing's syndrome and intracranial hypertension have been reported in children receiving topical corticosteroids. Manifestations of adrenal suppression in children include linear growth retardation, delayed weight gain, low plasma cortisol levels and absence of response to ACTH stimulation. Manifestations of intracranial hypertension include bulging fontanelles, headaches and bilateral papilledema.

Administration of topical corticosteroids to children should be limited to the least amount compatible with an effective therapeutic regimen. Chronic corticosteroid therapy may interfere with the growth and development of children.

Adverse Reactions: The following local adverse reactions are reported infrequently with topical corticosteroids, but may occur more frequently with the use of occlusive dressings. These reactions are listed in an approximate decreasing order of occurrence:

Burning	Perioral dermatitis
Itching	Allergic contact
Irritation	dermatitis
Dryness	Maceration of the skin
Folliculitis	Secondary infection
Hypertrichosis	Skin atrophy
Acneiform eruptions	Striae
Hypopigmentation	Miliaria

Overdosage: Topically applied corticosteroids can be absorbed in sufficient amounts to produce systemic effects. (See PRECAUTIONS.)

Dosage and Administration: PENECORT™ (hydrocortisone) Cream, USP, 2.5% should be applied to the affected area from two to four times daily depending on the severity of the condition. Occlusive dressings may be used for the management of psoriasis or recalcitrant conditions. If an infection develops, the use of occlusive dressings should be discontinued and appropriate antimicrobial therapy instituted.

How Supplied: PENECORT™ Cream, USP, 2.5% is supplied on prescription only in a 30 g collapsible tube, NDC 0023-0550-30. Store away from heat. Protect from freezing.

Herbert Laboratories Dermatology Division of **Allergan Pharmaceuticals, Inc.,** Irvine, CA 92713, U.S.A.

Dow B. Hickam, Inc.
P.O. BOX 2006
SUGAR LAND, TX 77487

GRANULEX ℞

Composition: Each 0.82 cc. of medication delivered to the wound site contains Trypsin crystallized 0.1 mg., Balsam Peru 72.5 mg., Castor Oil 650.0 mg., and an emulsifier.

Action: Trypsin is intended for debridement of eschar and other necrotic tissue. It appears that in many instances removal of wound debris strengthens humoral defense mechanisms sufficiently to retard proliferation of local pathogens. Balsam Peru is an effective capillary bed stimulant used to increase circulation in the wound site area. Also, Balsam Peru has a mildly bactericidal action. Castor Oil is used to improve epithelialization by reducing premature epithelial desiccation and cornification. Also, it can act as a protective covering and aids in the reduction of pain.

Indications: For the treatment of decubitus ulcers, varicose ulcers, debridement of eschar, dehiscent wounds and sunburn.

Uses: Granulex is in aerosol form which can be important to healing. It must be remembered, healing starts with a thin sheath of epithelium no more than a cell or two thick. Any rough movement or trauma can quickly destroy the healing tissue. Aerosols have the advantage of eliminating all extraneous physical contact with the wound. Granulex is easy to apply and quickly reduces odor frequently accompanying a decubitus ulcer. The wound may be left open or a wet bandage may be applied. As a suggestion; keep in mind wounds heal poorly in the presence of hemoglobin or zinc deficiency.

Warning: Do not spray on fresh arterial clots. Avoid spraying in eyes. Flammable, do not expose to fire or open flame. Contents under pressure. Do not puncture or incinerate. Do not store at temperature above 120°F. Keep out of reach of children. Use only as directed. Intentional misuse by deliberately concentrating and inhaling the contents can be harmful or fatal.

Dosage: Apply a minimum of twice daily or as often as necessary. Shake well, press the aerosol valve and coat the wound rapidly but not excessively.

How Supplied:
2 oz. Aerosol NDC 0514-0001-01
4 oz. Aerosol NDC 0514-0001-02

High Chemical Co.
Div. Day & Frick, Inc.
1760 N. HOWARD ST.
PHILADELPHIA, PA 19122

SARAPIN ℞

Composition: An aqueous distillate of Sarracenia purpurea, pitcher plant, prepared for parenteral administration.

Action and Uses: Local injection therapy for the relief of pain of neuro-muscular or neuralgic origin.

Administration and Dosage: Paravertebral nerve injection—2 to 10 cc. Local neuromuscular infiltration—5 to 10 cc.

Side Effects: None.

Precautions: Non-toxic.

Contraindications: Local inflammation.

How Supplied: One dozen 10 cc. ampuls and 50 cc. multi-dose vials.

Literature Available: Booklet "SARAPIN, Injection Technique in Pain Control."

Products are cross-indexed by generic and chemical names in the **YELLOW SECTION**

Hill Dermaceuticals, Inc.
P.O. BOX 19283
ORLANDO, FL 32814

DERMA CAS GEL ℞

Contains: Phenol 3%, Resorcinol 10%, in a fast-drying clear gel base.

DERMA-SMOOTHE/FS ℞

Contains: Fluocinolone Acetonide 0.01% in a blend of oils (NDC 28105 148-04).

DERMA-SONE® CREAM 1% ℞
Paraben Free

Contains: Hydrocortisone 1%, Pramoxine HCl 1% (NDC 28105-162-04).

HILL CORTAC® ℞

Contains: Hydrocortisone 0.5%, Sulfur 5%, Zinc Oxide 20%, Isopropyl Alcohol 5% (NDC 28105-149-02).

HILL-SHADE LOTION

Contains: Para-aminobenzoic Acid 5%, Alcohol 65% (NDC 28105-0160-04).

Hoechst-Roussel Pharmaceuticals Inc.
SOMERVILLE, NJ 08876

A/T/S® ℞
(erythromycin)
2% Acne Topical Solution

Description: A/T/S® (erythromycin) is an antibiotic produced from a strain of *Streptomyces erythraeus*. It is basic and readily forms salts with acids. Each mL of A/T/S (erythromycin) topical solution contains 20 mg of erythromycin base in a vehicle consisting of alcohol, propylene glycol, and citric acid. The alcohol content is 66%.

Actions: Although the mechanism by which A/T/S (erythromycin) acts in reducing inflammatory lesions of acne vulgaris is unknown, it is presumably due to its antibiotic action.

Indications: A/T/S (erythromycin) is indicated for the topical control of acne vulgaris.

Contraindications: A/T/S (erythromycin) is contraindicated in persons who have shown hypersensitivity to any of its ingredients.

Warning: The safe use of A/T/S (erythromycin) during pregnancy or lactation has not been established.

Precautions: A/T/S (erythromycin) is for external use only and should be kept away from the eyes, nose, mouth, and mucous membranes. Concomitant topical acne therapy should be used with caution because a cumulative irritant effect may occur, especially with the use of peeling, desquamating, or abrasive agents.

The use of antimicrobial agents may be associated with the overgrowth of antibiotic-resistant organisms; in such a case, antibiotic administration should be stopped and appropriate measures taken.

Adverse Reactions: Of a total of 90 patients exposed to the drug during clinical effectiveness studies, 17 experienced some type of adverse effect. These included dry skin, scaly skin, pruritus, irritation of the eye, and burning sensation.

Dosage and Administration: A/T/S (erythromycin) should be applied to the affected area twice a day after the skin is thoroughly washed with warm water and soap. Moisten the applicator or a pad with A/T/S (erythromycin), then rub over the entire facial area. Acne lesions on the neck, shoulder, chest, and back may also be treated in this manner.

Continued on next page

Hoechst-Roussel—Cont.

How Supplied: Topical Solution—60 mL. Store at controlled room temperature. 15° to 30°C (59°–86°F).

Shown in Product Identification Section, page 412

CLAFORAN® ℞
[kläf' or-an]
(cefotaxime sodium)
Sterile

Description: Sterile Claforan® (cefotaxime sodium) is a semisynthetic, broad spectrum cephalosporin antibiotic for parenteral administration. It is the sodium salt of 7-[2-(2-amino-4-thiazolyl) glyoxylamido]-3-(hydroxymethyl)-8-oxo-5-thia-1-azabicyclo [4.2.0] oct-2-ene-2-carboxylate 7^2-(Z)-(O-methyloxime), acetate (ester). Claforan contains approximately 50.5 mg (2.2 mEq) of sodium per gram of cefotaxime activity. Solutions of Claforan range from light yellow to amber depending on the concentration and the diluent used. The pH of freshly reconstituted solutions usually ranges from 4.5 to 6.5.

Clinical Pharmacology: Following IM administration of a single 500 mg or 1 g dose of Claforan to normal volunteers, mean peak serum concentrations of 11.7 and 20.5 μg/mL respectively were attained within 30 minutes and declined with an elimination half-life of approximately 1 hour. There was a dose-dependent increase in serum levels after the IV administration of 500 mg, 1 g and 2 g of Claforan (38.9, 101.7, and 214.4 μg/mL respectively) without alteration in the elimination half-life. There is no evidence of accumulation following repetitive IV infusion of 1 g doses every 6 hours for 14 days as there are no alterations of serum or renal clearance. About 60% of the administered dose was recovered from urine during the first 6 hours following the start of the infusion. Approximately 20–36% of an intravenously administered dose of ^{14}C-cefotaxime is excreted by the kidney as unchanged cefotaxime and 15–25% as the desacetyl derivative, the major metabolite. The desacetyl metabolite has been shown to contribute to the bactericidal activity. Two other urinary metabolites (M_2 and M_3) account for about 20–25%. They lack bactericidal activity.

A single 50 mg/kg dose of Claforan was administered as an intravenous infusion over a 10- to 15-minute period to 29 newborn infants grouped according to birth weight and age. The mean half-life of cefotaxime in infants with lower birth weights (≤ 1500 grams), regardless of age, was longer (4.6 hours) than the mean half-life (3.4 hours) in infants whose birth weight was greater than 1500 grams. Mean serum clearance was also smaller in the lower birth weight infants. Although the differences in mean half-life values are statistically significant for weight, they are not clinically important. Therefore, dosage should be based solely on age. (See **Dosage and Administration** section.)

Additionally, no disulfiram-like reactions were reported in a study conducted in 22 healthy volunteers administered Claforan and ethanol.

Microbiology
The bactericidal activity of cefotaxime sodium results from inhibition of cell wall synthesis. Cefotaxime sodium has *in vitro* activity against a wide range of gram-positive and gram-negative organisms. Claforan has a high degree of stability in the presence of beta-lactamases, both penicillinases and cephalosporinases, of gram-negative and gram-positive bacteria. Cefotaxime sodium has been shown to be a potent inhibitor of β-lactamases produced by certain gram-negative bacteria. Cefotaxime sodium is usually active against the following microorganisms both *in vitro* and in clinical infections (see **Indications and Usage**).

Aerobes, Gram-positive: *Staphylococcus aureus*, including penicillinase and non-penicillinase producing strains, *Staphylococcus epidermidis*, *Streptococcus pyogenes* (Group A beta-hemolytic streptococci), *Streptococcus agalactiae* (Group B streptococci), (NOTE: Most strains of enterococci, e.g., *S. faecalis* are resistant), *Streptococcus pneumoniae* (formerly *Diplococcus pneumoniae*).

Aerobes, Gram-negative: *Citrobacter* species, *Enterobacter* species, *Escherichia coli*, *Haemophilus influenzae* (including ampicillin-resistant *H. influenzae*), *Klebsiella* species (including *K. pneumoniae*), *Neisseria gonorrhoeae* (including penicillinase and non-penicillinase producing strains), *Neisseria meningitidis*, *Proteus mirabilis*, *Proteus morganii*, *Proteus rettgeri*, *Proteus vulgaris*, *Serratia* species.

NOTE: Many strains of the above organisms that are multiply resistant to other antibiotics, e.g., penicillins, cephalosporins, and aminoglycosides, are susceptible to cefotaxime sodium.

Cefotaxime sodium is active against some strains of *Pseudomonas aeruginosa*.

Anaerobes: *Bacteroides* species, including some strains of *B. fragilis*, *Clostridium* species (NOTE: Most strains of *C. difficile* are resistant), *Peptococcus* species, *Peptostreptococcus* species.

Cefotaxime sodium is highly stable *in vitro* to four of the five major classes of β-lactamases described by Richmond et al., including type IIIa (TEM) which is produced by many gram-negative bacteria. The drug is also stable to β-lactamase (penicillinase) produced by staphylococci. In addition, cefotaxime sodium shows high affinity for penicillin-binding proteins in the cell wall, including PBP, Ib and III.

Cefotaxime sodium also demonstrates *in vitro* activity against the following microorganisms although clinical significance is unknown: *Salmonella* species (including *S. typhi*), *Providencia* species, and *Shigella* species.

Cefotaxime sodium and aminoglycosides have been shown to be synergistic *in vitro* against some strains of *Pseudomonas aeruginosa*.

Susceptibility Tests
Quantitative methods that require measurement of zone diameters give the most precise estimate of antibiotic susceptibility. One such procedure[1] has been recommended for use with discs to test susceptibility to cefotaxime sodium. Interpretation involves correlation of the diameters obtained in the disc test with minimum inhibitory concentration (MIC) values for cefotaxime sodium.

Reports from the laboratory giving results of the standardized single-disc susceptibility test using a 30-μg cefotaxime sodium disc should be interpreted according to the following criteria:

Susceptible organisms produce zones of 20 mm or greater, indicating that the tested organism is likely to respond to therapy.

Organisms that produce zones of 15 to 19 mm are expected to be susceptible if high dosage is used or if the infection is confined to tissues and fluids (e.g., urine) in which high antibiotic levels are attained.

Resistant organisms produce zones of 14 mm or less, indicating that other therapy should be selected.

Organisms should be tested with the cefotaxime sodium disc, since cefotaxime sodium has been shown by *in vitro* tests to be active against certain strains found resistant when other beta lactam discs are used. The cefotaxime sodium disc should not be used for testing susceptibility to other cephalosporins. Organisms having zones of less than 18 mm around the cephalothin disc are not necessarily of intermediate susceptibility or resistant to cefotaxime sodium.

A bacterial isolate may be considered susceptible if the MIC value for cefotaxime sodium is not more than 16 μg/mL. Organisms are considered resistant to cefotaxime sodium if the MIC is equal to or greater than 64 μg/mL. Organisms having an MIC value of less than 64 μg/mL but greater than 16μg/mL are expected to be susceptible if high dosage is used or if the infection is confined to tissues and fluids (e.g., urine) in which high antibiotic levels are attained.

Indications and Usage:
Treatment
Claforan is indicated for the treatment of patients with serious infections caused by susceptible strains of the designated microorganisms in the diseases listed below.

(1) **Lower respiratory tract infections**, including pneumonia, caused by *Streptococcus pneumoniae* (formerly *Diplococcus pneumoniae*), *Streptococcus pyogenes* (Group A streptococci) and other streptococci (excluding enterococci, e.g., *Streptococcus faecalis*), *Staphylococcus aureus* (penicillinase and non-penicillinase producing), *Escherichia coli*, *Klebsiella* species, *Haemophilus influenzae* (including ampicillin resistant strains), *Proteus mirabilis*, *Serratia marcescens*, and *Enterobacter* species.

(2) **Genitourinary infections.** Urinary tract infections caused by *Enterococcus* species, *Staphylococcus epidermidis*, *Staphylococcus aureus* (penicillinase and non-penicillinase producing), *Citrobacter* species, *Enterobacter* species, *Escherichia coli*, *Klebsiella* species, *Proteus mirabilis*, indole positive *Proteus* (i.e., *Proteus morganii*, *Proteus rettgeri*, and *Proteus vulgaris*), and *Serratia marcescens*. Also, uncomplicated gonorrhea of single or multiple sites caused by *Neisseria gonorrhoeae*, including penicillinase producing strains.

(3) **Gynecologic infections**, including pelvic inflammatory disease, endometritis and pelvic cellulitis caused by *Staphylococcus epidermidis*, *Streptococcus* species, *Enterococcus* species, *Escherichia coli*, *Proteus mirabilis*, *Bacteroides* species (including *B. fragilis*), *Clostridium* species, and anaerobic cocci (including *Peptostreptococcus* species and *Peptococcus* species).

(4) **Bacteremia/Septicemia** caused by *Escherichia coli*, *Klebsiella* species, and *Serratia marcescens*.

(5) **Skin and skin structure infections** caused by *Staphylococcus aureus* (penicillinase and non-penicillinase producing), *Staphylococcus epidermidis*, *Streptococcus pyogenes* (Group A streptococci) and other streptococci, *Enterococcus* species, *Escherichia coli*, *Enterobacter* species, *Klebsiella* species, *Proteus mirabilis*, and indole positive *Proteus* (i.e., *Proteus morganii*, *Proteus rettgeri*, and *Proteus vulgaris*), *Pseudomonas* species, *Serratia marcescens*, *Bacteroides* species, and anaerobic cocci (including *Peptostreptococcus* species and *Peptococcus* species).

(6) **Intra-abdominal infections** including peritonitis caused by *Escherichia coli*, *Klebsiella* species, *Bacteroides* species, and anaerobic cocci (including *Peptostreptococcus* species and *Peptococcus species*).

(7) **Bone and/or joint infections** caused by *Staphylococcus aureus* (penicillinase and non-penicillinase producing strains).

(8) **Central nervous system infections**, e.g. meningitis and ventriculitis, caused by *Neisseria meningitidis*, *Haemophilus influenzae*, *Streptococcus pneumoniae*, *Klebsiella pneumoniae*, and *Escherichia coli*.

Although many strains of enterococci (e.g., *S. faecalis*) and *Pseudomonas* species are resistant to cefotaxime sodium *in vitro*, Claforan has been used successfully in treating patients with infections caused by susceptible organisms.

Specimens for bacteriologic culture should be obtained prior to therapy in order to isolate and identify causative organisms and to determine their susceptibilities to Claforan. Therapy may be instituted before results of susceptibility studies are known; however, once these results become available, the antibiotic treatment should be adjusted accordingly.

In certain cases of confirmed or suspected gram-positive or gram-negative sepsis or in patients with other serious infections in which the causative organism has not been identified, Claforan may be used concomitantly with an aminoglycoside. The dosage recommended in the labeling of both antibiotics may be given and depends on the severity of the infection and the patient's condition. Renal function should be carefully monitored, especially if higher dosages of the aminoglycosides are to be administered or if therapy is prolonged, because of the potential nephrotoxicity and ototoxicity of aminoglycoside antibiotics. Some β-lactam antibiotics also have a certain de-

Carcinogenesis, mutagenesis, impairment of fertility: Long-term animal studies have not been performed to evaluate the carcinogenic potential or the effect of topical corticosteroids on fertility. Studies to determine mutagenicity with hydrocortisone have revealed negative results.

Pregnancy Category C: Corticosteroids are generally teratogenic in laboratory animals when administered systemically at relatively low dosage levels. The more potent corticosteroids have been shown to be teratogenic after dermal application in laboratory animals. There are no adequate and well-controlled studies in pregnant women on teratogenic effects from topically applied corticosteroids. Therefore, topical corticosteroids should be used during pregnancy only if the potential benefit justifies the potential risk to the fetus. Drugs on this class should not be used extensively on pregnant patients, in large amounts, or for prolonged periods of time.

Nursing Mothers: It is not known whether topical administration of corticosteroids could result in sufficient systemic absorption to produce detectable quantities in breast milk. Systemically administered corticosteroids are secreted into breast milk in quantities not likely to have a deleterious effect on the infant. Nevertheless, caution should be exercised when topical corticosteroids are administered to a nursing woman.

Pediatric Use: Pediatric patients may demonstrate greater susceptibility to topical corticosteroid-induced HPA axis suppression and Cushing's syndrome than mature patients because of a larger skin surface area to body weight ratio. Hypothalamic-pituitary-adrenal (HPA) axis suppression, Cushing's syndrome and intracranial hypertension have been reported in children receiving topical corticosteroids. Manifestations of adrenal suppression in children include linear growth retardation, delayed weight gain, low plasma cortisol levels and absence of response to ACTH stimulation. Manifestations of intracranial hypertension include bulging fontanelles, headaches and bilateral papilledema.

Administration of topical corticosteroids to children should be limited to the least amount compatible with an effective therapeutic regimen. Chronic corticosteroid therapy may interfere with the growth and development of children.

Adverse Reactions: The following local adverse reactions are reported infrequently with topical corticosteroids, but may occur more frequently with the use of occlusive dressings. These reactions are listed in an approximate decreasing order of occurrence:

Burning	Perioral dermatitis
Itching	Allergic contact
Irritation	dermatitis
Dryness	Maceration of the skin
Folliculitis	Secondary infection
Hypertrichosis	Skin atrophy
Acneiform eruptions	Striae
Hypopigmentation	Miliaria

Overdosage: Topically applied corticosteroids can be absorbed in sufficient amounts to produce systemic effects. (See PRECAUTIONS.)

Dosage and Administration: PENECORT™ (hydrocortisone) Cream, USP, 2.5% should be applied to the affected area from two to four times daily depending on the severity of the condition. Occlusive dressings may be used for the management of psoriasis or recalcitrant conditions. If an infection develops, the use of occlusive dressings should be discontinued and appropriate antimicrobial therapy instituted.

How Supplied: PENECORT™ Cream, USP, 2.5% is supplied on prescription only in a 30 g collapsible tube, NDC 0023-0550-30. Store away from heat. Protect from freezing.

Herbert Laboratories Dermatology Division of Allergan Pharmaceuticals, Inc., Irvine, CA 92713, U.S.A.

Dow B. Hickam, Inc.
P.O. BOX 2006
SUGAR LAND, TX 77487

GRANULEX ℞

Composition: Each 0.82 cc. of medication delivered to the wound site contains Trypsin crystallized 0.1 mg., Balsam Peru 72.5 mg., Castor Oil 650.0 mg., and an emulsifier.

Action: Trypsin is intended for debridement of eschar and other necrotic tissue. It appears that in many instances removal of wound debris strengthens humoral defense mechanisms sufficiently to retard proliferation of local pathogens. Balsam Peru is an effective capillary bed stimulant used to increase circulation in the wound site area. Also, Balsam Peru has a mildly bactericidal action. Castor Oil is used to improve epithelialization by reducing premature epithelial desiccation and cornification. Also, it can act as a protective covering and aids in the reduction of pain.

Indications: For the treatment of decubitus ulcers, varicose ulcers, debridement of eschar, dehiscent wounds and sunburn.

Uses: Granulex is in aerosol form which can be important to healing. It must be remembered, healing starts with a thin sheath of epithelium no more than a cell or two thick. Any rough movement or trauma can quickly destroy the healing tissue. Aerosols have the advantage of eliminating all extraneous physical contact with the wound. Granulex is easy to apply and quickly reduces odor frequently accompanying a decubitus ulcer. The wound may be left open or a wet bandage may be applied. As a suggestion; keep in mind wounds heal poorly in the presence of hemoglobin or zinc deficiency.

Warning: Do not spray on fresh arterial clots. Avoid spraying in eyes. Flammable, do not expose to fire or open flame. Contents under pressure. Do not puncture or incinerate. Do not store at temperature above 120°F. Keep out of reach of children. Use only as directed. Intentional misuse by deliberately concentrating and inhaling the contents can be harmful or fatal.

Dosage: Apply a minimum of twice daily or as often as necessary. Shake well, press the aerosol valve and coat the wound rapidly but not excessively.

How Supplied:
2 oz. Aerosol NDC 0514-0001-01
4 oz. Aerosol NDC 0514-0001-02

High Chemical Co.
Div. Day & Frick, Inc.
1760 N. HOWARD ST.
PHILADELPHIA, PA 19122

SARAPIN ℞

Composition: An aqueous distillate of Sarracenia purpurea, pitcher plant, prepared for parenteral administration.

Action and Uses: Local injection therapy for the relief of pain of neuro-muscular or neuralgic origin.

Administration and Dosage: Paravertebral nerve injection—2 to 10 cc. Local neuromuscular infiltration—5 to 10 cc.

Side Effects: None.
Precautions: Non-toxic.
Contraindications: Local inflammation.
How Supplied: One dozen 10 cc. ampuls and 50 cc. multi-dose vials.
Literature Available: Booklet "SARAPIN, Injection Technique in Pain Control."

Products are cross-indexed by generic and chemical names in the
YELLOW SECTION

Hill Dermaceuticals, Inc.
P.O. BOX 19283
ORLANDO, FL 32814

DERMA CAS GEL ℞

Contains: Phenol 3%, Resorcinol 10%, in a fast-drying clear gel base.

DERMA-SMOOTHE/FS ℞

Contains: Fluocinolone Acetonide 0.01% in a blend of oils (NDC 28105 148-04).

DERMA-SONE® CREAM 1% ℞
Paraben Free

Contains: Hydrocortisone 1%, Pramoxine HCl 1% (NDC 28105-162-04).

HILL CORTAC® ℞

Contains: Hydrocortisone 0.5%, Sulfur 5%, Zinc Oxide 20%, Isopropyl Alcohol 5% (NDC 28105-149-02).

HILL-SHADE LOTION

Contains: Para-aminobenzoic Acid 5%, Alcohol 65% (NDC 28105-0160-04).

Hoechst-Roussel Pharmaceuticals Inc.
SOMERVILLE, NJ 08876

A/T/S® ℞
(erythromycin)
2% Acne Topical Solution

Description: A/T/S® (erythromycin) is an antibiotic produced from a strain of *Streptomyces erythraeus*. It is basic and readily forms salts with acids. Each mL of A/T/S (erythromycin) topical solution contains 20 mg of erythromycin base in a vehicle consisting of alcohol, propylene glycol, and citric acid. The alcohol content is 66%.

Actions: Although the mechanism by which A/T/S (erythromycin) acts in reducing inflammatory lesions of acne vulgaris is unknown, it is presumably due to its antibiotic action.

Indications: A/T/S (erythromycin) is indicated for the topical control of acne vulgaris.

Contraindications: A/T/S (erythromycin) is contraindicated in persons who have shown hypersensitivity to any of its ingredients.

Warning: The safe use of A/T/S (erythromycin) during pregnancy or lactation has not been established.

Precautions: A/T/S (erythromycin) is for external use only and should be kept away from the eyes, nose, mouth, and mucous membranes. Concomitant topical acne therapy should be used with caution because a cumulative irritant effect may occur, especially with the use of peeling, desquamating, or abrasive agents.

The use of antimicrobial agents may be associated with the overgrowth of antibiotic-resistant organisms; in such a case, antibiotic administration should be stopped and appropriate measures taken.

Adverse Reactions: Of a total of 90 patients exposed to the drug during clinical effectiveness studies, 17 experienced some type of adverse effect. These included dry skin, scaly skin, pruritus, irritation of the eye, and burning sensation.

Dosage and Administration: A/T/S (erythromycin) should be applied to the affected area twice a day after the skin is thoroughly washed with warm water and soap. Moisten the applicator or a pad with A/T/S (erythromycin), then rub over the entire facial area. Acne lesions on the neck, shoulder, chest, and back may also be treated in this manner.

Continued on next page

Hoechst-Roussel—Cont.

How Supplied: Topical Solution—60 mL. Store at controlled room temperature. 15° to 30°C (59°–86°F).

Shown in Product Identification Section, page 412

CLAFORAN® ℞
[klăf′or-an]
(cefotaxime sodium)
Sterile

Description: Sterile Claforan® (cefotaxime sodium) is a semisynthetic, broad spectrum cephalosporin antibiotic for parenteral administration. It is the sodium salt of 7-[2-(2-amino-4-thiazolyl) glyoxylamido]-3-(hydroxymethyl)-8-oxo-5-thia-1-azabicyclo [4.2.0] oct-2-ene-2-carboxylate 7^2-(Z)-(O-methyloxime), acetate (ester). Claforan contains approximately 50.5 mg (2.2 mEq) of sodium per gram of cefotaxime activity. Solutions of Claforan range from light yellow to amber depending on the concentration and the diluent used. The pH of freshly reconstituted solutions usually ranges from 4.5 to 6.5.

Clinical Pharmacology: Following IM administration of a single 500 mg or 1 g dose of Claforan to normal volunteers, mean peak serum concentrations of 11.7 and 20.5 µg/mL respectively were attained within 30 minutes and declined with an elimination half-life of approximately 1 hour. There was a dose-dependent increase in serum levels after the IV administration of 500 mg, 1 g and 2 g of Claforan (38.9, 101.7, and 214.4 µg/mL respectively) without alteration in the elimination half-life. There is no evidence of accumulation following repetitive IV infusion of 1 g doses every 6 hours for 14 days as there are no alterations of serum or renal clearance. About 60% of the administered dose was recovered from urine during the first 6 hours following the start of the infusion. Approximately 20–36% of an intravenously administered dose of ^{14}C-cefotaxime is excreted by the kidney as unchanged cefotaxime and 15–25% as the desacetyl derivative, the major metabolite. The desacetyl metabolite has been shown to contribute to the bactericidal activity. Two other urinary metabolites (M_2 and M_3) account for about 20–25%. They lack bactericidal activity.

A single 50 mg/kg dose of Claforan was administered as an intravenous infusion over a 10- to 15-minute period to 29 newborn infants grouped according to birth weight and age. The mean half-life of cefotaxime in infants with lower birth weights ($\leq$ 1500 grams), regardless of age, was longer (4.6 hours) than the mean half-life (3.4 hours) in infants whose birth weight was greater than 1500 grams. Mean serum clearance was also smaller in the lower birth weight infants. Although the differences in mean half-life values are statistically significant for weight, they are not clinically important. Therefore, dosage should be based solely on age. (See **Dosage and Administration** section.)

Additionally, no disulfiram-like reactions were reported in a study conducted in 22 healthy volunteers administered Claforan and ethanol.

Microbiology
The bactericidal activity of cefotaxime sodium results from inhibition of cell wall synthesis. Cefotaxime sodium has in vitro activity against a wide range of gram-positive and gram-negative organisms. Claforan has a high degree of stability in the presence of beta-lactamases, both penicillinases and cephalosporinases, of gram-negative and gram-positive bacteria. Cefotaxime sodium has been shown to be a potent inhibitor of β-lactamases produced by certain gram-negative bacteria. Cefotaxime sodium is usually active against the following microorganisms both in vitro and in clinical infections (see **Indications and Usage**).

Aerobes, Gram-positive: *Staphylococcus aureus*, including penicillinase and non-penicillinase producing strains, *Staphylococcus epidermidis*, *Streptococcus pyogenes* (Group A beta-hemolytic streptococci), *Streptococcus agalactiae* (Group B streptococci), (NOTE: Most strains of enterococci, e.g., *S. faecalis* are resistant), *Streptococcus pneumoniae* (formerly *Diplococcus pneumoniae*).

Aerobes, Gram-negative: *Citrobacter* species, *Enterobacter* species, *Escherichia coli*, *Haemophilus influenzae* (including ampicillin-resistant *H. influenzae*), *Klebsiella* species (including *K. pneumoniae*), *Neisseria gonorrhoeae* (including penicillinase and non-penicillinase producing strains), *Neisseria meningitidis*, *Proteus mirabilis*, *Proteus morganii*, *Proteus rettgeri*, *Proteus vulgaris*, *Serratia* species.
NOTE: Many strains of the above organisms that are multiply resistant to other antibiotics, e.g., penicillins, cephalosporins, and aminoglycosides, are susceptible to cefotaxime sodium.
Cefotaxime sodium is active against some strains of *Pseudomonas aeruginosa*.

Anaerobes: *Bacteroides* species, including some strains of *B. fragilis*, *Clostridium* species (NOTE: Most strains of *C. difficile* are resistant), *Peptococcus* species, *Peptostreptococcus* species.
Cefotaxime sodium is highly stable in vitro to four of the five major classes of β-lactamases described by Richmond et al., including type IIIa (TEM) which is produced by many gram-negative bacteria. The drug is also stable to β-lactamase (penicillinase) produced by staphylococci. In addition, cefotaxime sodium shows high affinity for penicillin-binding proteins in the cell wall, including PBP, Ib and III.
Cefotaxime sodium also demonstrates in vitro activity against the following microorganisms although clinical significance is unknown: *Salmonella* species (including *S. typhi*), *Providencia* species, and *Shigella* species.
Cefotaxime sodium and aminoglycosides have been shown to be synergistic in vitro against some strains of *Pseudomonas aeruginosa*.

Susceptibility Tests
Quantitative methods that require measurement of zone diameters give the most precise estimate of antibiotic susceptibility. One such procedure[1] has been recommended for use with discs to test susceptibility to cefotaxime sodium. Interpretation involves correlation of the diameters obtained in the disc test with minimum inhibitory concentration (MIC) values for cefotaxime sodium.
Reports from the laboratory giving results of the standardized single-disc susceptibility test using a 30-µg cefotaxime sodium disc should be interpreted according to the following criteria:
Susceptible organisms produce zones of 20 mm or greater, indicating that the tested organism is likely to respond to therapy.
Organisms that produce zones of 15 to 19 mm are expected to be susceptible if high dosage is used or if the infection is confined to tissues and fluids (e.g., urine) in which high antibiotic levels are attained.
Resistant organisms produce zones of 14 mm or less, indicating that other therapy should be selected.
Organisms should be tested with the cefotaxime sodium disc, since cefotaxime sodium has been shown by in vitro tests to be active against certain strains found resistant when other beta lactam discs are used. The cefotaxime sodium disc should not be used for testing susceptibility to other cephalosporins. Organisms having zones of less than 18 mm around the cephalothin disc are not necessarily of intermediate susceptibility or resistant to cefotaxime sodium.
A bacterial isolate may be considered susceptible if the MIC value for cefotaxime sodium is not more than 16 µg/mL. Organisms are considered resistant to cefotaxime sodium if the MIC is equal to or greater than 64 µg/mL. Organisms having an MIC value of less than 64 µg/mL but greater than 16µg/mL are expected to be susceptible if high dosage is used or if the infection is confined to tissues and fluids (e.g., urine) in which high antibiotic levels are attained.

Indications and Usage:
Treatment
Claforan is indicated for the treatment of patients with serious infections caused by susceptible strains of the designated microorganisms in the diseases listed below.

(1) **Lower respiratory tract infections**, including pneumonia, caused by *Streptococcus pneumoniae* (formerly *Diplococcus pneumoniae*), *Streptococcus pyogenes* (Group A streptococci) and other streptococci (excluding enterococci, e.g., *Streptococcus faecalis*), *Staphylococcus aureus* (penicillinase and non-penicillinase producing), *Escherichia coli*, *Klebsiella* species, *Haemophilus influenzae* (including ampicillin resistant strains), *Proteus mirabilis*, *Serratia marcescens*, and *Enterobacter* species.

(2) **Genitourinary infections.** Urinary tract infections caused by *Enterococcus* species, *Staphylococcus epidermidis*, *Staphylococcus aureus* (penicillinase and non-penicillinase producing), *Citrobacter* species, *Enterobacter* species, *Escherichia coli*, *Klebsiella* species, *Proteus mirabilis*, indole positive *Proteus* (i.e., *Proteus morganii*, *Proteus rettgeri*, and *Proteus vulgaris*), and *Serratia marcescens*. Also, uncomplicated gonorrhea of single or multiple sites caused by *Neisseria gonorrhoeae*, including penicillinase producing strains.

(3) **Gynecologic infections**, including pelvic inflammatory disease, endometritis and pelvic cellulitis caused by *Staphylococcus epidermidis*, *Streptococcus* species, *Enterococcus* species, *Escherichia coli*, *Proteus mirabilis*, *Bacteroides* species (including *B. fragilis*), *Clostridium* species, and anaerobic cocci (including *Peptostreptococcus* species and *Peptococcus* species).

(4) **Bacteremia/Septicemia** caused by *Escherichia coli*, *Klebsiella* species, and *Serratia marcescens*.

(5) **Skin and skin structure infections** caused by *Staphylococcus aureus* (penicillinase and non-penicillinase producing), *Staphylococcus epidermidis*, *Streptococcus pyogenes* (Group A streptococci) and other streptococci, *Enterococcus* species, *Escherichia coli*, *Enterobacter* species, *Klebsiella* species, *Proteus mirabilis*, and indole positive *Proteus* (i.e., *Proteus morganii*, *Proteus rettgeri*, and *Proteus vulgaris*), *Pseudomonas* species, *Serratia marcescens*, *Bacteroides* species, and anaerobic cocci (including *Peptostreptococcus* species and *Peptococcus* species).

(6) **Intra-abdominal infections** including peritonitis caused by *Escherichia coli*, *Klebsiella* species, *Bacteroides* species, and anaerobic cocci (including *Peptostreptococcus* species and *Peptococcus species*).

(7) **Bone and/or joint infections** caused by *Staphylococcus aureus* (penicillinase and non-penicillinase producing strains).

(8) **Central nervous system infections**, e.g. meningitis and ventriculitis, caused by *Neisseria meningitidis*, *Haemophilus influenzae*, *Streptococcus pneumoniae*, *Klebsiella pneumoniae*, and *Escherichia coli*.

Although many strains of enterococci (e.g., *S. faecalis*) and *Pseudomonas* species are resistant to cefotaxime sodium in vitro, Claforan has been used successfully in treating patients with infections caused by susceptible organisms.
Specimens for bacteriologic culture should be obtained prior to therapy in order to isolate and identify causative organisms and to determine their susceptibilities to Claforan. Therapy may be instituted before results of susceptibility studies are known; however, once these results become available, the antibiotic treatment should be adjusted accordingly.
In certain cases of confirmed or suspected gram-positive or gram-negative sepsis or in patients with other serious infections in which the causative organism has not been identified, Claforan may be used concomitantly with an aminoglycoside. The dosage recommended in the labeling of both antibiotics may be given and depends on the severity of the infection and the patient's condition. Renal function should be carefully monitored, especially if higher dosages of the aminoglycosides are to be administered or if therapy is prolonged, because of the potential nephrotoxicity and ototoxicity of aminoglycoside antibiotics. Some β-lactam antibiotics also have a certain de-

gree of nephrotoxicity. Although, to date, this has not been noted when Claforan was given alone, it is possible that nephrotoxicity may be potentiated if Claforan is used concomitantly with an aminoglycoside.

Prevention

The administration of Claforan preoperatively may reduce the incidence of certain infections in patients undergoing elective surgical procedures (e.g. abdominal or vaginal hysterectomy, gastrointestinal and genitourinary tract surgery) that may be classified as contaminated or potentially contaminated.

In patients undergoing cesarean section, intraoperative (after clamping the umbilical cord) and postoperative use of Claforan may also reduce the incidence of certain postoperative infections. See **Dosage and Administration** section.

Effective use for elective surgery depends on the time of administration. To achieve effective tissue levels, Claforan should be given ½ to 1½ hours before surgery. See **Dosage and Administration** section.

For patients undergoing gastrointestinal surgery, preoperative bowel preparation by mechanical cleansing as well as with a non-absorbable antibiotic (e.g., neomycin) is recommended.

If there are signs of infection, specimens for culture should be obtained for identification of the causative organism so that appropriate therapy may be instituted.

Contraindications: Claforan is contraindicated in patients who have shown hypersensitivity to cefotaxime sodium or the cephalosporin group of antibiotics.

Warnings: BEFORE THERAPY WITH CLAFORAN IS INSTITUTED, CAREFUL INQUIRY SHOULD BE MADE TO DETERMINE WHETHER THE PATIENT HAS HAD PREVIOUS HYPERSENSITIVITY REACTIONS TO CEFOTAXIME SODIUM, CEPHALOSPORINS, PENICILLINS, OR OTHER DRUGS. THIS PRODUCT SHOULD BE GIVEN WITH CAUTION TO PATIENTS WITH TYPE 1 HYPERSENSITIVITY REACTIONS TO PENICILLIN. ANTIBIOTICS SHOULD BE ADMINISTERED WITH CAUTION TO ANY PATIENT WHO HAS DEMONSTRATED SOME FORM OF ALLERGY, PARTICULARLY TO DRUGS. IF AN ALLERGIC REACTION TO CLAFORAN OCCURS, DISCONTINUE TREATMENT WITH THE DRUG. SERIOUS HYPERSENSITIVITY REACTIONS MAY REQUIRE EPINEPHRINE AND OTHER EMERGENCY MEASURES.

Pseudomembranous colitis has been reported with the use of cephalosporins (and other broad spectrum antibiotics); therefore, it is important to consider its diagnosis in patients who develop diarrhea in association with antibiotic use.

Treatment with broad spectrum antibiotics alters normal flora of the colon and may permit overgrowth of Clostridia. Studies indicate a toxin produced by *Clostridium difficile* is one primary cause of antibiotic-associated colitis. Cholestyramine and colestipol resins have been shown to bind the toxin *in vitro*.

Mild cases of colitis may respond to drug discontinuance alone.

Moderate to severe cases should be managed with fluid, electrolyte, and protein supplementation as indicated.

When the colitis is not relieved by drug discontinuance or when it is severe, oral vancomycin is the treatment of choice for antibiotic-associated pseudomembranous colitis produced by *C. difficile*. Other causes of colitis should also be considered.

Precautions: Claforan® (cefotaxime sodium) should be prescribed with caution in individuals with a history of gastrointestinal disease, particularly colitis.

Claforan has not been shown to be nephrotoxic; however, because high and prolonged serum antibiotic concentrations can occur from usual doses in patients with transient or persistent reduction of urinary output because of renal insufficiency, the total daily dosage should be reduced when Claforan is administered to such patients. Continued dosage should be determined by degree of renal impairment, severity of infection, and susceptibility of the causative organism.

Although there is no clinical evidence supporting the necessity of changing the dosage of cefotaxime sodium in patients with even profound renal dysfunction, it is suggested that, until further data are obtained, the dose of cefotaxime sodium be halved in patients with estimated creatinine clearances of less than 20 mL/min/1.73 m^2.

When only serum creatinine is available, the following formula^2 (based on sex, weight, and age of the patient) may be used to convert this value into creatinine clearance. The serum creatinine should represent a steady state of renal function.

$$\frac{\text{Weight (kg)} \times (140 - \text{age})}{72 \times \text{serum creatinine}}$$

Males
Females 0.85 × above value

As with other antibiotics, prolonged use of Claforan may result in overgrowth of nonsusceptible organisms. Repeated evaluation of the patient's condition is essential. If superinfection occurs during therapy, appropriate measures should be taken.

Drug Interactions: Increased nephrotoxicity has been reported following concomitant administration of cephalosporins and aminoglycoside antibiotics.

Carcinogenesis, Mutagenesis: Long-term studies in animals have not been performed to evaluate carcinogenic potential. Mutagenic tests included a micronucleus and an Ames test. Both tests were negative for mutagenic effects.

Pregnancy (Category B): Reproduction studies have been performed in mice and rats at doses up to 30 times the usual human dose and have revealed no evidence of impaired fertility or harm to the fetus because of cefotaxime sodium. However, there are no well-controlled studies in pregnant women. Because animal reproductive studies are not always predictive of human response, this drug should be used during pregnancy only if clearly needed.

Nonteratogenic Effects: Use of the drug in women of child-bearing potential requires that the anticipated benefit be weighed against the possible risks.

In perinatal and postnatal studies with rats, the pups in the group given 1200 mg/kg of Claforan were significantly lighter in weight at birth and remained smaller than pups in the control group during the 21 days of nursing.

Nursing Mothers: Claforan is excreted in human milk in low concentrations. Caution should be exercised when Claforan is administered to a nursing woman.

Adverse Reactions: Claforan is generally well tolerated. The most common adverse reactions have been local reactions following IM or IV injection. Other adverse reactions have been encountered infrequently.

The most frequent adverse reactions (greater than 1%) are:

Local (4.7%) - Injection site inflammation with IV administration. Pain, induration, and tenderness after IM injection.

Hypersensitivity (1.8%) - Rash, pruritus, and fever.

Gastrointestinal (1.7%) - Colitis, diarrhea, nausea, and vomiting.

Symptoms of pseudomembranous colitis can appear during or after antibiotic treatment.

Nausea and vomiting have been reported rarely.

Less frequent adverse reactions (less than 1%) are:

Hemic and Lymphatic System - Granulocytopenia, transient leukopenia, eosinophilia, and neutropenia have been reported. Some individuals have developed positive direct Coombs Tests during treatment with the cephalosporin antibiotics.

Genitourinary System - Moniliasis, vaginitis.

Central Nervous System - Headache.

Liver - Transient elevations in SGOT, SGPT, serum LDH, and serum alkaline phosphatase levels have been reported.

Kidney - As with some other cephalosporins, transient elevations of BUN have been occasionally observed with Claforan.

Dosage and Administration:

Adults

Dosage and route of administration should be determined by susceptibility of the causative organisms, severity of the infection, and the condition of the patient (see table for dosage guideline). Claforan may be administered IM or IV after reconstitution. The maximum daily dosage should not exceed 12 grams.

[See table above].

To prevent postoperative infection in contaminated or potentially contaminated surgery, the recommended dose is a single 1 gram IM or IV administered 30 to 90 minutes prior to start of surgery.

Cesarean Section Patients

The first dose of 1 gram is administered intravenously as soon as the umbilical cord is clamped. The second and third doses should be given as 1 gram intravenously or intramuscularly at 6 and 12 hours after the first dose.

Neonates, Infants and Children

The following dosage schedule is recommended:

Neonates (birth to 1 month):
0–1 week of age   50 mg/kg IV q 12 h
1–4 weeks of age   50 mg/kg IV q 8 h

It is not necessary to differentiate between premature and normal-gestational age infants.

Infants and Children (1 month to 12 years): For body weights less than 50 kg, the recommended daily dose is 50 to 180 mg/kg IV or IV of body weight divided into four to six equal doses. The higher dosages should be used for more severe or serious infections, including meningitis. For body weights 50 kg or more, the usual adult dosage should be used; the maximum daily dosage should not exceed 12 grams.

Impaired Renal Function - see **Precautions** section.

NOTE: As with antibiotic therapy in general, administration of Claforan should be continued for a minimum of 48 to 72 hours after the patient defervesces or after evidence of bacterial eradication has been obtained; a minimum of 10 days of treatment is recommended for infections caused by Group A beta-hemolytic streptococci in order to guard against the risk of rheumatic fever or glomerulonephritis; frequent bacteriologic and clinical appraisal is necessary during therapy of chronic urinary tract infection and may be required for several months after therapy has been completed; persistent infections may require treatment of several weeks and doses smaller than those indicated above should not be used.

Preparation of Solution: Claforan for IM or IV administration should be reconstituted as follows:

[See table on next page].

Shake to dissolve; inspect for particulate matter and discoloration prior to use. Solutions of Claforan range from light yellow to amber, depending

GUIDELINES FOR DOSAGE OF CLAFORAN

Type of Infection	Daily Dose (grams)	Frequency and Route
Gonorrhea	1	1 gram IM (single dose)
Uncomplicated infections	2	1 gram every 12 hours IM or IV
Moderate to severe infections	3–6	1–2 grams every 8 hours IM or IV
Infections commonly needing antibiotics in higher dosage (e.g., septicemia)	6–8	2 grams every 6–8 hours IV
Life-threatening infections	up to 12	2 grams every 4 hours IV

Continued on next page

Hoechst-Roussel—Cont.

on concentration, diluent used, and length and condition of storage.

For intramuscular use: Reconstitute with Sterile Water for Injection or Bacteriostatic Water for Injection as described above.

For intravenous use: Reconstitute the 1 g and 2 g strengths with at least 10 mL of Sterile Water for Injection. INFUSION BOTTLES may be reconstituted with 50 or 100 mL of 0.9% Sodium Chloride Injection or 5% Dextrose Injection. Reconstitute the 10g PHARMACY BULK PACKAGE with 47 mL of diluent for an approximate average concentration of 200 mg/mL or 97 mL of diluent for an approximate average concentration of 100 mg/mL. Stock solution may be further diluted for IV infusion. For other diluents see **Compatibility and Stability.**

NOTE: Solutions of Claforan must not be admixed with aminoglycoside solutions. If Claforan and aminoglycosides are to be administered to the same patient, they must be administered separately and not as mixed injection.

A SOLUTION OF 1 G CLAFORAN IN 14 ML OF STERILE WATER FOR INJECTION IS ISOTONIC.

IM Administration: As with all IM preparations, Claforan should be injected well within the body of a relatively large muscle such as the upper outer quadrant of the buttock (i.e., gluteus maximus); aspiration is necessary to avoid inadvertent injection into a blood vessel. Individual IM doses of 2 grams may be given if the dose is divided and is administered in different intramuscular sites.

IV Administration: The IV route is preferable for patients with bacteremia, bacterial septicemia, peritonitis, meningitis, or other severe or life-threatening infections, or for patients who may be poor risks because of lowered resistance resulting from such debilitating conditions as malnutrition, trauma, surgery, diabetes, heart failure, or malignancy, particularly if shock is present or impending.

For intermittent IV administration, a solution containing 1 gram or 2 grams in 10 mL of Sterile Water for Injection can be injected over a period of three to five minutes. With an infusion system, it may also be given over a longer period of time through the tubing system by which the patient may be receiving other IV solutions. However, during infusion of the solution containing Claforan, it is advisable to discontinue temporarily the administration of other solutions at the same site. For the administration of higher doses by continuous IV infusion, a solution of Claforan may be added to IV bottles containing the solutions discussed below.

Compatibility and Stability: Claforan reconstituted as described above (**Preparation of Solution**) maintains satisfactory potency for 24 hours at room temperature (at or below 22°C), for 10 days under refrigeration (below 5°C), and for at least 13 weeks in the frozen state.

After reconstitution Claforan may be stored in disposable glass or plastic syringes for 24 hours at room temperature (at or below 22°C), 5 days under refrigeration, and 13 weeks frozen.

Reconstituted solutions may be further diluted to 50 to 1000 mL with the following solutions and maintain potency for 24 hours at room temperature (at or below 22°C) and at least 5 days under refrigeration: 0.9% Sodium Chloride Injection; 5 or 10% Dextrose Injection; 5% Dextrose and 0.9% Sodium Chloride Injection; 5% Dextrose and 0.45% Sodium Chloride Injection; 5% Dextrose and 0.2% Sodium Chloride Injection; Lactated Ringers Solution; Sodium Lactate Injection (M/6); 10% Invert Sugar Injection, FREAMINE® II Injection.

Solutions of Claforan in 0.9% Sodium Chloride Injection and 5% Dextrose Injection in VIA-FLEX® intravenous bags are stable for 24 hours at room temperature (at or below 22°C), 5 days under refrigeration, and 13 weeks frozen.

Frozen samples should not be heated but should be thawed at room temperature before use. After the periods mentioned above, any unused solutions or frozen materials should be discarded. DO NOT REFREEZE. NOTE: Claforan solutions exhibit maximum stability in the pH 5–7 range. Solutions of Claforan should not be prepared with diluents having a pH above 7.5, such as Sodium Bicarbonate Injection.

How Supplied: Sterile Claforan is a dry white to off-white powder supplied in vials and bottles containing cefotaxime sodium as follows:

1 gram cefotaxime free acid equivalent in vials (NDC 0039 0018 01) and in infusion bottles (NDC 0039 0018 02)

2 gram cefotaxime free acid equivalent in vials (NDC 0039 0019 01) and in infusion bottles (NDC 0039 0019 02)

10 gram cefotaxime free acid equivalent in pharmacy bulk package bottles (NDC 0039 0020 01)

NOTE: Claforan in the dry state should be stored below 30°C. The dry material as well as solutions tend to darken depending on storage conditions and should be protected from elevated temperatures and excessive light.

References:
1) Bauer, A.W.; Kirby, W.M.M.; Sherris, J.C.; and Turck, M.: Antibiotic Susceptibility Testing by a Standardized Single Disk Method, Am. J. Clin. Pathol., 45:493, 1966; Standardized Disc Susceptibility Test, Federal Register, 39:19182-4, 1974. National Committee for Clinical Laboratory Standards, Approved Standard: ASM-2, Performance Standards for Antimicrobial Disc Susceptibility Tests, July, 1975.
2) Cockcroft, D.W. and Gault, M.H.: Prediction of Creatinine Clearance from Serum Creatinine. Nephron 16:31-41, 1976.

CLAFORAN® REG TM ROUSSEL-UCLAF
71789-2/84

DIAβETA® ℞
(glyburide)
Tablets 1.25, 2.5 and 5.0 mg

Description: Diaβeta® (glyburide) is an oral blood-glucose-lowering drug of the sulfonylurea class. It is a white, crystalline compound, formulated as tablets of 1.25 mg, 2.5 mg, and 5.0 mg strengths for oral administration.

Chemically, Diaβeta® (glyburide) is identified as 1-[[p-[2-(5-chloro-O-anisamido)ethyl] phenyl]-sulfonyl]-3-cyclohexylurea.

The molecular weight is 493.99. The aqueous solubility of Diaβeta® (glyburide) increases with pH as a result of salt formation.

Clinical Pharmacology: Diaβeta® (glyburide) appears to lower the blood glucose acutely by stimulating the release of insulin from the pancreas, an effect dependent upon functioning beta cells in the pancreatic islets. The mechanism by which Diaβeta® (glyburide) lowers blood glucose during long-term administration has not been clearly established.

With chronic administration in Type II diabetic patients, the blood glucose lowering effect persists despite a gradual decline in the insulin secretory response to the drug. Extrapancreatic effects may play a part in the mechanism of action of oral sulfonylurea hypoglycemic drugs.

In addition to its blood glucose lowering actions, Diaβeta® (glyburide) produces a mild diuresis by enhancement of renal free water clearance. Clinical experience to date indicates an extremely low incidence of disulfiram-like reactions in patients while taking Diaβeta® (glyburide).

Pharmacokinetics

Single-dose studies with Diaβeta® (glyburide) in normal subjects demonstrate significant absorption within one hour, peak drug levels at about four hours, and low but detectable levels at twenty-four hours. Mean serum levels of glyburide, as reflected by areas under the serum concentration-time curve, increase in proportion to corresponding increases in dose. Multiple-dose studies with Diaβeta® (glyburide) in diabetic patients demonstrate drug level concentration-time curves similar to single-dose studies, indicating no build-up of drug in tissue depots. The decrease of glyburide in the serum of normal healthy individuals is biphasic, the terminal half-life being about 10 hours. In single-dose studies in fasting normal subjects, the degree and duration of blood glucose lowering is proportional to the dose administered and to the area under the drug level concentration-time curve. The blood glucose lowering effect persists for 24 hours following single morning doses in non-fasting diabetic patients. Under conditions of repeated administration in diabetic patients, however, there is no reliable correlation between blood drug levels and fasting blood glucose levels. A one-year study of diabetic patients treated with Diaβeta® (glyburide) showed no reliable correlation between administered dose and serum drug level.

The major metabolite of Diaβeta® (glyburide) is the 4-trans-hydroxy derivative. A second metabolite, the 3-cis-hydroxy derivative, also occurs. These metabolites contribute no significant hypoglycemic action since they are only weakly active ($\frac{1}{400}$th and $\frac{1}{40}$th, respectively, as glyburide) in rabbits.

Diaβeta® (glyburide) is excreted as metabolites in the bile and urine, approximately 50% by each route. This dual excretory pathway is qualitatively different from that of other sulfonylureas, which are excreted primarily in the urine.

Sulfonylurea drugs are extensively bound to serum proteins. Displacement from protein binding sites by other drugs may lead to enhanced hypoglycemic action. *In vitro*, the protein binding exhibited by Diaβeta® (glyburide) is predominantly non-ionic, whereas that of other sulfonylureas (chlorpropamide, tolbutamide, tolazamide) is predominantly ionic. Acidic drugs such as phenylbutazone, warfarin, and salicylates displace the ionic-binding sulfonylureas from serum proteins to a far greater extent than the non-ionic binding Diaβeta® (glyburide). It has not been shown that this difference in protein binding will result in fewer drug-drug interactions with Diaβeta® (glyburide) in clinical use.

Indications and Usage: Diaβeta® (glyburide) is indicated as an adjunct to diet to lower the blood glucose in patients with non-insulin-dependent diabetes mellitus (Type II) whose hyperglycemia cannot be controlled by diet alone.

In initiating treatment for non-insulin-dependent diabetes, diet should be emphasized as the primary form of treatment. Caloric restriction and weight loss are essential in the obese diabetic patient. Proper dietary management alone may be effective in controlling the blood glucose and symptoms of hyperglycemia. The importance of regular physical activity should also be stressed, and cardiovascular risk factors should be identified and corrective measures taken where possible.

If this treatment program fails to reduce symptoms and/or blood glucose, the use of an oral sulfonylurea or insulin should be considered. Use of

Strength	Amount of Diluent To Be Added (mL)	Approximate Withdrawable Volume (mL)	Approximate Average Concentration (mg/mL)
Intramuscular			
1 g vial	3	3.4	300
2 g vial	5	6.0	330
Intravenous			
1 g vial	10	10.4	95
2 g vial	10	11.0	180
10 g bottle	47	52.0	200
10 g bottle	97	102.0	100

Diaβeta® (glyburide) must be viewed by both the physician and patient as a treatment in addition to diet, and not as a substitute for diet or as a convenient mechanism for avoiding dietary restraint. Furthermore, loss of blood glucose control on diet alone may be transient, thus requiring only short-term administration of Diaβeta® (glyburide).

During maintenance programs, Diaβeta® (glyburide) should be discontinued if satisfactory lowering of blood glucose is no longer achieved. Judgments should be based on regular clinical and laboratory evaluations.

In considering the use of Diaβeta® (glyburide) in asymptomatic patients, it should be recognized that controlling the blood glucose in non-insulin dependent diabetes has not been definitely established to be effective in preventing the long-term cardiovascular or neural complications of diabetes.

Contraindications: Diaβeta®[(glyburide) is contraindicated in patients with:
1. Known hypersensitivity to the drug.
2. Diabetic ketoacidosis, with or without coma. This condition should be treated with insulin.

WARNINGS:

SPECIAL WARNING ON INCREASED RISK OF CARDIOVASCULAR MORTALITY
The administration of oral hypoglycemic drugs has been reported to be associated with increased cardiovascular mortality as compared to treatment with diet alone or diet plus insulin. This warning is based on the study conducted by the University Group Diabetes Program (UGDP), a long-term prospective clinical trial designed to evaluate the effectiveness of glucose-lowering drugs in preventing or delaying vascular complications in patients with non-insulin-dependent diabetes. The study involved 823 patients who were randomly assigned to one of four treatment groups (Diabetes, 19 (supp. 2): 747-830, 1970).

UDGP reported that patients treated for 5 to 8 years with diet plus a fixed dose of tolbutamide (1.5 grams per day) had a rate of cardiovascular mortality approximately 2½ times that of patients treated with diet alone. A significant increase in total mortality was not observed, but the use of tolbutamide was discontinued based on the increase in cardiovascular mortality, thus limiting the opportunity for the study to show an increase in overall mortality. Despite controversy regarding the interpretation of these results, the findings of the UGDP study provide an adequate basis for this warning. The patient should be informed of the potential risks and advantages of Diaβeta® (glyburide) and of alternative modes of therapy. Although only one drug in the sulfonylurea class (tolbutamide) was included in this study, it is prudent from a safety standpoint to consider that this warning may also apply to other oral hypoglycemic drugs in this class, in view of their close similarities in mode of action and chemical structure.

Precautions:
General
Hypoglycemia: All sulfonylurea drugs are capable of producing severe hypoglycemia. Proper patient selection, dosage, and instructions are important to avoid hypoglycemic episodes. Renal or hepatic insufficiency may cause elevated blood levels of Diaβeta® (glyburide) and the latter may also diminish gluconeogenic capacity, both of which increase the risk of serious hypoglycemic reactions. Elderly, debilitated or malnourished patients, and those with adrenal or pituitary insufficiency are particularly susceptible to the hypoglycemic action of glucose-lowering drugs. Hypoglycemia may be difficult to recognize in the elderly, and in people who are taking beta-adrenergic blocking drugs. Hypoglycemia is more likely to occur when caloric intake is deficient, after severe or prolonged exercise, when alcohol is ingested, or when more than one glucose-lowering drug is used.

Loss of control of blood glucose: When a patient stabilized on any diabetic regimen is exposed to stress such as fever, trauma, infection, or surgery, a loss of control may occur. At such times, it may be necessary to discontinue Diaβeta® (glyburide) and administer insulin.

The effectiveness of any oral hypoglycemic drug, including Diaβeta® (glyburide), in lowering blood glucose to a desired level decreases in many patients over a period of time, which may be due to progression of the severity of the diabetes or to diminished responsiveness to the drug. This phenomenon is known as secondary failure, to distinguish it from primary failure in which the drug is ineffective in an individual patient when first given.

Information for Patients
Patients should be informed of the potential risks and advantages of Diaβeta® (glyburide) and of alternative modes of therapy. They should also be informed about the importance of adherence to dietary instructions, of a regular exercise program, and of regular testing of urine and/or blood glucose.

The risks of hypoglycemia, its symptoms and treatment, and conditions that predispose to its development should be explained to patients and responsible family members. Primary and secondary failure should also be explained.

Laboratory Tests
Blood and urine glucose should be monitored periodically. Measurement of glycosylated hemoglobin may be useful.

Drug Interactions
The hypoglycemic action of sulfonylureas may be potentiated by certain drugs including nonsteroidal anti-inflammatory agents and other drugs that are highly protein bound, salicylates, sulfonamides, chloramphenicol, probenecid, coumarins, monoamine oxidase inhibitors, and beta adrenergic blocking agents. When such drugs are administered to a patient receiving Diaβeta® (glyburide), the patient should be observed closely for hypoglycemia. When such drugs are withdrawn from a patient receiving Diaβeta® (glyburide), the patient should be observed closely for loss of control. Certain drugs tend to produce hyperglycemia and may lead to loss of control. These drugs include the thiazides and other diuretics, corticosteroids, phenothiazines, thyroid products, estrogens, oral contraceptives, phenytoin, nicotinic acid, sympathomimetics, calcium channel blocking drugs, and isoniazid. When such drugs are administered to a patient receiving Diaβeta® (glyburide), the patient should be closely observed for loss of control. When such drugs are withdrawn from a patient receiving Diaβeta® (glyburide), the patient should be observed closely for hypoglycemia.

Carcinogenesis, Mutagenesis, and Impairment of Fertility
Diaβeta® (glyburide) is non-mutagenic when studied in the Salmonella microsome test (Ames test) and in the DNA damage/alkaline elution assay. Studies in rats at doses up to 300 mg/kg/day for 18 months showed no carcinogenic effects.

Pregnancy
Teratogenic Effects: Pregnancy Category B
Reproduction studies have been performed in rats and rabbits at doses up to 500 times the human dose and have revealed no evidence of impaired fertility or harm to the fetus due to Diaβeta®(glyburide). There are, however, no adequate and well controlled studies in pregnant women. Because animal reproduction studies are not always predictive of human response, this drug should be used during pregnancy only if clearly needed.

Because recent information suggests that abnormal blood glucose levels during pregnancy are associated with a higher incidence of congenital abnormalities, many experts recommend that insulin be used during pregnancy to maintain blood glucose levels as close to normal as possible.

Nonteratogenic Effects
Prolonged severe hypoglycemia (4 to 10 days) has been reported in neonates born to mothers who were receiving a sulfonylurea drug at the time of delivery. This had been reported more frequently with the use of agents with prolonged half-lives. If Diaβeta® (glyburide) is used during pregnancy, it should be discontinued at least two weeks before the expected delivery date.

Nursing Mothers
Although it is not known whether Diaβeta® (glyburide) is excreted in human milk, some sulfonylureas are known to be excreted in human milk. Because the potential for hypoglycemia in nursing infants may exist, a decision should be made whether to discontinue nursing or to discontinue administering the drug, taking into account the importance of the drug to the mother. If Diaβeta® (glyburide) is discontinued and if diet alone is inadequate for controlling blood glucose, insulin therapy should be considered.

Pediatric Use: Safety and effectiveness in children have not been established.

Adverse Reactions:
Hypoglycemia: See **Precautions** and **Overdosage** Sections.

Gastrointestinal Reactions: Cholestatic jaundice may occur rarely; Diaβeta® (glyburide) should be discontinued if this occurs. Gastrointestinal disturbances, e.g., nausea, epigastric fullness, and heartburn, are the most common reactions and occur in 1.8% of treated patients. They tend to be dose-related and may disappear when dosage is reduced.

Dermatologic Reactions: Allergic skin reactions, e.g., pruritus, erythema, urticaria, and morbilliform or maculopapular eruptions, occur in 1.5% of treated patients. These may be transient and may disappear despite continued use of Diaβeta® (glyburide); if skin reactions persist, the drug should be discontinued.

Porphyria cutanea tarda and photosensitivity reactions have been reported with sulfonylureas.

Hematologic Reactions: Leukopenia, agranulocytosis, thrombocytopenia, hemolytic anemia, aplastic anemia, and pancytopenia have been reported with sulfonylureas.

Metabolic Reactions: Hepatic porphyria reactions have been reported with sulfonylureas; however, these have not been reported with Diaβeta® (glyburide). Disulfiram-like reactions have been reported very rarely with Diaβeta® (glyburide).

Overdosage: Overdosage of sulfonylureas, including Diaβeta® (glyburide), can produce hypoglycemia. Mild hypoglycemic symptoms without loss of consciousness or neurologic findings should be treated aggressively with oral glucose and adjustments in drug dosage and/or meal patterns. Close monitoring should continue until the physician is assured that the patient is out of danger. Severe hypoglycemic reactions with coma, seizure, or other neurological impairment occur infrequently, but constitute medical emergencies requiring immediate hospitalization. If hypoglycemic coma is diagnosed or suspected, the patient should be given a rapid intravenous injection of concentrated (50%) glucose solution. This should be followed by a continuous infusion of a more dilute (10%) glucose solution at a rate that will maintain the blood glucose at a level above 100 mg/dL. Patients should be closely monitored for a minimum of 24 to 48 hours, since hypoglycemia may recur after apparent clinical recovery.

Dosage and Administration: There is no fixed dosage regimen for the management of diabetes mellitus with Diaβeta® (glyburide) or any other hypoglycemic agent. In addition to the usual monitoring of urinary glucose, the patient's blood glucose must also be monitored periodically to determine the minimum effective dose for the patient; to detect primary failure, i.e., inadequate lowering of blood glucose at the maximum recommended dose of medication; and to detect secondary failure, i.e., loss of adequate blood glucose lowering response after an initial period of effectiveness. Glycosylated hemoglobin levels may also be of value in monitoring the patient's response to therapy.

Short-term administration of Diaβeta® (glyburide) may be sufficient during periods of transient loss of control in patients usually controlled well on diet.

Continued on next page

Hoechst-Roussel—Cont.

1. Usual Starting Dose
The usual starting dose of Diaβeta® (glyburide) as initial therapy is 2.5–5 mg daily, administered with breakfast or the first main meal. Those patients who may be more sensitive to hypoglycemic drugs should be started at 1.25 mg daily. (See **Precautions** Section for patients at increased risk). Failure to follow an appropriate dosage regimen may precipitate hypoglycemia. Patients who do not adhere to their prescribed dietary and drug regimen are more prone to exhibit unsatisfactory response to therapy.

Transfer of patients from other oral antidiabetic regimens to Diaβeta® (glyburide) should be done conservatively and the initial daily dose should be 2.5 to 5 mg. When transferring patients from oral hypoglycemic agents other than chlorpropamide to Diaβeta® (glyburide), no transition period and no initial or priming dose is necessary. When transferring patients from chlorpropamide, particular care should be exercised during the first two weeks because the prolonged retention of chlorpropamide in the body and subsequent overlapping drug effects may provoke hypoglycemia.

Some Type II diabetic patients being treated with insulin may respond satisfactorily to Diaβeta® (glyburide). If the insulin dose is less than 20 units daily, substitution of Diaβeta® (glyburide) 2.5 to 5 mg as a single daily dose may be tried. If the insulin dose is between 20 and 40 units daily, the patient may be placed directly on Diaβeta® (glyburide) 5 mg daily as a single dose. If the insulin dose is more than 40 units daily, a transition period is required for conversion to Diaβeta® (glyburide). In these patients, insulin dosage is decreased by 50% and Diaβeta® (glyburide) 5 mg daily is started. Please refer to Usual Maintenance Dose for further explanation.

2. Usual Maintenance Dose
The usual maintenance dose is in the range of 1.25 to 20 mg daily, which may be given as a single dose or in divided doses (See Dosage Interval Section). Dosage increases should be made in increments of no more than 2.5 mg at weekly intervals based upon the patient's blood glucose response.

No exact dosage relationship exists between Diaβeta® (glyburide) and the other oral hypoglycemic agents. Although patients may be transferred from the maximum dose of other sulfonylureas, the maximum starting dose of 5 mg of Diaβeta® (glyburide) should be observed. A maintenance dose of 5 mg Diaβeta® (glyburide) provides approximately the same degree of blood glucose control as 250 to 375 mg chlorpropamide, 250 to 375 mg tolazamide, 500 to 750 mg acetohexamide, or 1000 to 1500 mg tolbutamide. When transferring patients receiving more than 40 units of insulin daily, they may be started on a daily dose of Diaβeta® (glyburide) 5 mg concomitantly with a 50% reduction in insulin dose. Progressive withdrawal of insulin and increase of Diaβeta® (glyburide) in increments of 1.25 to 2.5 mg every 2 to 10 days is then carried out. During this conversion period when both insulin and Diaβeta® (glyburide) are being used, hypoglycemia may rarely occur. During insulin withdrawal, patients should test their urine for glucose and acetone at least three times daily and report results to their physician. The appearance of persistent acetonuria with glycosuria indicates that the patient is a Type I diabetic who requires insulin therapy.

3. Maximum Dose
Daily doses of more than 20 mg are not recommended.

4. Dosage Interval
Once-a-day therapy is usually satisfactory, based upon usual meal patterns and a 10 hour half-life of Diaβeta® (glyburide). Some patients, particularly those receiving more than 10 mg daily, may have a more satisfactory response with twice-a-day dosage.

In elderly patients, debilitated or malnourished patients, and patients with impaired renal or hepatic function, the initial and maintenance dosing should be conservative to avoid hypoglycemic reactions. (See **Precautions** Section.)

How Supplied: Diaβeta® (glyburide) tablets are supplied as white, oblong, monogrammed, scored tablets of 1.25 mg in bottles of 50 (NDC 0039-0050-05); pink, oblong, monogrammed, scored tablets of 2.5 mg in bottles of 100 (NDC 0039-0051-10); and light green, oblong, monogrammed, scored tablets of 5 mg in bottles of 100 (NDC 0039-0052-10) and 500 (NDC 0039-0052-50), and in Unit Dose Cartons of 100 (NDC 0039-0052-11).

Store at controlled room temperature (59°–86°F).
Dispense in well-closed containers with safety closures.
Caution: Federal law prohibits dispensing without a prescription.

75100-9/84
Shown in Product Identification Section, page 412

DOXIDAN®
[dox'i-dan"]

Composition: Doxidan is a combination of 60 mg docusate calcium USP, 50 mg danthron USP and up to 1.5% alcohol (w/w). This combination has a highly effective stool softener and a mild peristaltic stimulant that acts mainly in the lower bowel.

Action and Uses: Doxidan is a safe, gentle laxative for the relief and management of constipation. Due to the effectiveness of the stool softening component, Doxidan produces soft, formed, easily evacuated stools, with the least possible disturbance of normal body physiology. Doxidan has proved clinically effective in the management of constipation in geriatric or inactive patients, obstetric patients, and following surgery, particularly anorectal procedures. It may be used as a safe and effective evacuant prior to x-ray examination of the colon in preparing patients for barium enema.

Dosages: Adults and children over 12—one or two capsules daily. Children 6 to 12—one capsule daily. Give at bedtime for two or three days or until bowel movements are normal. For children under 6 consult a physician.

Warnings: Do not use when abdominal pain, nausea, or vomiting is present. Frequent or prolonged use of this preparation may result in dependence on laxatives. A harmless pink or orange discoloration may appear in urine. In some patients occasional cramping may occur. As with any drug, if you are pregnant or nursing a baby, seek the advice of a health professional before using this product.

How Supplied: Maroon, soft gelatin capsules in packages of 10 and 30, bottles of 100 and 1000, and Unit Dose 100's (10 × 10 strips).

Shown in Product Identification Section, page 412

FESTAL® II
[fes'tal]

Composition: Each enteric-coated tablet contains the following: Lipase 6,000 USP units, Amylase 30,000 USP units and Protease 20,000 USP units.

Action and Uses: Festal II provides a high degree of protected digestive activity in a formula of standardized enzymes. Enteric coating of the tablet prevents release of ingredients in the stomach so that high enzymatic potency is delivered to the site in the intestinal tract where digestion normally takes place.

Festal II is indicated in any condition where normal digestion is impaired by insufficiency of natural digestive enzymes, or when additional digestive enzymes may be beneficial. These conditions often manifest complaints of discomfort due to excess intestinal gas, such as bloating, cramps and flatulence. The following are conditions or situations where Festal II may be helpful: pancreatic insufficiency, chronic pancreatitis, pancreatic necrosis, removal of gas prior to x-ray examination.

Usual Dosage: *Adults*—one or two tablets with each meal, or as directed by a physician.
Contraindications: Festal II should not be given to patients sensitive to protein of porcine origin.
How Supplied: Bottles of 100 and 500 white, enteric-coated tablets for oral use.
Literature Available: Yes.
Shown in Product Identification Section, page 412

FESTALAN®
[fes' tah-lan"]

Description: A tablet consisting of digestive enzymes in an enteric-coated core with atropine methyl nitrate in the outer coating. In the outer layer: Atropine Methyl Nitrate 1 mg. In the enteric-coated core: Lipase 6,000 USP units, Amylase 30,000 USP units and Protease 20,000 USP units. The enzymes Lipase, Amylase and Protease in Festalan® are obtained from porcine pancreas. Although allergic reactions to the animal protein in this preparation occur only rarely, these enzymes should be used cautiously in patients with known sensitivity.

Clinical Pharmacology: Pharmacologic and biochemical effects of Lipase, Amylase and Protease are limited to their actions upon the contents of the gastrointestinal tract. None of these enzymes are known to exert systemic pharmacologic effects after oral administration.

Atropine, atropine methyl nitrate and related belladonna alkaloids block the parasympathomimetic (muscarinic) effects of acetylcholine. These drugs are variously known as anticholinergic, parasympatholytic or antispasmodic agents. They act distally on parasympathetic nerve endings to inhibit the action of acetylcholine on smooth muscle, exocrine glands and the heart. Atropine does not block transmission at the neuromuscular junction of skeletal muscle. Atropine is readily absorbed from the gastrointestinal tract and crosses the blood-brain barrier. Most is excreted in the urine within the first 12 hours.

It reduces both motility and secretory activity of the gastrointestinal system. Atropine does not cause CNS depression at usual oral clinical doses, but may decrease heart rate slightly without changing blood pressure. Most of the pharmacologic effects reported with atropine and its analogs are attributable to its cholinergic blockade of parasympathetic effectors.

Indications and Usage: Festalan® is indicated for the treatment of functional gastrointestinal disorders involving disturbed motor function, hypermotility and spasticity as in patients with irritable colon syndrome. Atropine methyl nitrate reduces gastrointestinal tone and spasm. The enzyme content is helpful in reducing symptoms of postprandial intestinal distress in conditions involving digestive enzyme insufficiency.

Contraindications: Festalan® should not be used in patients with glaucoma, reflux esophagitis (gastric retention), prostate hypertrophy, pyloric obstruction, obstruction of the bladder neck, congestive heart failure with tachycardia and achalasia (cardiospasm). Festalan® should not be given to patients sensitive to protein of porcine origin or to atropine.

Warnings: Serious adverse reactions to atropine usually occur at higher doses and are extensions of known pharmacologic effects such as signs of CNS stimulation followed by depression, orthostatic hypotension and respiratory arrest. Children are more susceptible to the toxic effects than adults.

Precautions:
General: Festalan® should be used with caution in patients with cardiac disease. Patients using Festalan® should be warned of signs of atropine intoxication, particularly with doses exceeding the usual recommended dose. These may include dry mouth, difficulty with speech and swallowing and marked thirst. Vision may be blurred and skin may feel hot, dry and flushed. Usage of the drug should be discontinued and a physician consulted if any of the above symptoms appear.

Drug Interactions: Antacids may interfere with absorption of atropine and should not be given with this drug.

Pregnancy: Pregnancy Category C. Animal reproduction studies have not been conducted with Festalan®. It is also not known whether Festalan® can cause fetal harm when administered to a pregnant woman or can effect reproduction capacity. Festalan® should be given to a pregnant woman only if clearly needed.

Atropine has negligible effects on the human uterus and the fetus is not adversely affected nor is respiration of the newborn depressed.*

Nursing Mothers: Traces of atropine are found in human milk. Caution should be observed when Festalan® is administered to a nursing woman.

Pediatric Use: The safety and effectiveness of Festalan® in children have not been established. See WARNINGS section.

Adverse Reactions: Adverse reactions associated with Festalan® may be of two main types: those due to allergic manifestations to pork proteins and those due to pharmacologic properties of atropine methyl nitrate. Allergic reactions occur only rarely and patients with known sensitivity should not be treated with Festalan®.

The most frequent adverse reactions seen after atropine are primarily due to the anticholinergic effects on various organs and systems. Dryness of the mouth, anhidrosis, mydriasis, cycloplegia, tachycardia (sometimes preceded by slowing), constipation, dysuria, and acute urinary retention may occur at clinical doses. At higher doses, marked dryness of the mouth, thirst, cardiac acceleration, blurring of vision, and speech difficulties may be encountered. Larger doses produce more marked development of symptoms, including CNS stimulation.

Overdosage: Symptoms of overdosage with atropine may comprise signs of CNS stimulation followed by depression, orthostatic hypotension and respiratory arrest. Children are more susceptible to the toxic effects than adults. Overdosage with atropine should be treated by gastric lavage to limit absorption. Physostigmine is an antidote for atropine poisoning and 1 to 4 mg (0.5 to 1.0 mg in children) may be given by slow intravenous injection to reduce or abolish delirium and coma caused by large doses of atropine. Phenothiazines should not be used for treatment of overdosage.

Dosage and Administration: Usual adult dose is one or two tablets with each meal. Pediatric dosage has not been established.

How Supplied: Festalan® is available in bottles of 100 and 1,000 orange, enteric-coated tablets. Store at controlled room temperature—59° to 86°F.

Reference: *Goodman and Gilman, *The Pharmacological Basis of Therapeutics*, 1980, 6th Edition, p. 126.
77307-5/83

Shown in Product Identification Section, page 413

LASIX® ℞
[la' siks]
(furosemide)
Oral Solution
Tablets/Injection
Diuretic

WARNING: Lasix (furosemide) is a potent diuretic which, if given in excessive amounts, can lead to a profound diuresis with water and electrolyte depletion. Therefore, careful medical supervision is required, and dose and dose schedule have to be adjusted to the individual patient's needs. (See under "DOSAGE AND ADMINISTRATION.")

Description: Lasix (furosemide) is an anthranilic acid derivative. Chemically, it is 4-chloro-N-furfuryl-5-sulfamoylanthranilic acid.

Actions: Investigations into the mode of action of Lasix (furosemide) have utilized micropuncture studies in rats, stop flow experiments in dogs, and various clearance studies in both humans and experimental animals. It has been demonstrated that Lasix (furosemide) inhibits primarily the reabsorption of sodium and chloride not only in the proximal and distal tubules but also in the loop of Henle. The high degree of efficacy is largely due to this unique site of action. The action on the distal tubule is independent of any inhibitory effect on carbonic anhydrase and aldosterone.

The onset of diuresis following oral administration is within 1 hour. The peak effect occurs within the first or second hour. The duration of diuretic effect is 6 to 8 hours.

The onset of diuresis following intravenous administration is within 5 minutes and somewhat later after intramuscular administration. The peak effect occurs within the first half hour. The duration of diuretic effect is approximately 2 hours.

Indications:

Edema—Lasix (furosemide) is indicated for the treatment of edema associated with congestive heart failure, cirrhosis of the liver, and renal disease, including the nephrotic syndrome. Lasix (furosemide) is particularly useful when an agent with greater diuretic potential than that of those commonly employed is desired.

Parenteral therapy should be reserved for patients unable to take oral medication or for patients in emergency clinical situations.

Lasix (furosemide) Injection is also indicated as adjunctive therapy in acute pulmonary edema. The intravenous administration of Lasix (furosemide) is indicated when a rapid onset of diuresis is desired, eg, in acute pulmonary edema.

If gastrointestinal absorption is impaired or oral medication is not practical for any reason, Lasix (furosemide) is indicated by the intravenous or intramuscular route. Parenteral use should be replaced with oral Lasix (furosemide) as soon as practical.

Hypertension—Oral Lasix (furosemide) may be used for the treatment of hypertension alone or in combination with other antihypertensive agents. Hypertensive patients who cannot be adequately controlled with thiazides will probably also not be adequately controlled with Lasix (furosemide) alone.

Contraindications: Lasix (furosemide) is contraindicated in anuria. It is contraindicated in patients with a history of hypersensitivity to this compound.

Warnings: Excessive diuresis may result in dehydration and reduction in blood volume with circulatory collapse and with the possibility of vascular thrombosis and embolism, particularly in elderly patients. Excessive loss of potassium in patients receiving digitalis glycosides may precipitate digitalis toxicity. Care should also be exercised in patients receiving potassium-depleting steroids.

Frequent serum electrolyte, CO_2, and BUN determinations should be performed during the first few months of therapy and periodically thereafter, and abnormalities corrected or the drug temporarily withdrawn.

In patients with hepatic cirrhosis and ascites, initiation of therapy with Lasix (furosemide) is best carried out in the hospital. In hepatic coma and in states of electrolyte depletion, therapy should not be instituted until the basic condition is improved. Sudden alterations of fluid and electrolyte balance in patients with cirrhosis may precipitate hepatic coma; therefore, strict observation is necessary during the period of diuresis. Supplemental potassium chloride and, if required, an aldosterone antagonist are helpful in preventing hypokalemia and metabolic alkalosis.

If increasing azotemia and oliguria occur during treatment of severe progressive renal disease, the drug should be discontinued.

As with many other drugs, patients should be observed regularly for the possible occurrence of blood dyscrasias, liver damage, or other idiosyncratic reactions.

Patients with known sulfonamide sensitivity may show allergic reactions to Lasix (furosemide).

Lasix (furosemide) may add to or potentiate the therapeutic effect of other antihypertensive drugs. Potentiation occurs with ganglionic or peripheral adrenergic blocking drugs.

The possibility exists of exacerbation or activation of systemic lupus erythematosus.

Lasix (furosemide) appears in breast milk. If use of the drug is deemed essential, the patient should stop nursing.

Parenterally administered Lasix (furosemide) may increase the ototoxic potential of aminoglycoside antibiotics. Especially in the presence of impaired renal function, the use of parenterally administered Lasix (furosemide) in patients to whom aminoglycoside antibiotics are also being given should be avoided, except in life-threatening situations.

When parenteral use of Lasix (furosemide) precedes its oral use, it should be kept in mind that cases of tinnitus and reversible hearing impairment have been reported. There have also been some reports of cases in which irreversible hearing impairment occurred. Usually, ototoxicity has been reported when Lasix (furosemide) was injected rapidly in patients with severe impairment of renal function at doses exceeding several times the usual recommended dose and in whom other drugs known to be ototoxic were given. If the physician elects to use high dose parenteral therapy in patients with severely impaired renal function, controlled intravenous infusion is advisable [for adults, an infusion rate not exceeding 4 mg Lasix (furosemide) per minute has been used].

Because of the amount of sorbitol present in the vehicle for Lasix (furosemide) Oral Solution, the possibility of diarrhea, especially in the pediatric population, exists when the formulation is given at higher doses.

Precautions: As with any effective diuretic, electrolyte depletion may occur during therapy with Lasix (furosemide), especially in patients receiving higher doses and a restricted salt intake. Periodic determinations of serum electrolytes to detect possible imbalance should be performed at appropriate intervals.

All patients receiving Lasix (furosemide) therapy should be observed for signs of fluid or electrolyte imbalance: namely, hyponatremia, hypochloremic alkalosis, and hypokalemia. Serum and urine electrolyte determinations are particularly important when the patient is vomiting excessively or receiving parenteral fluids. Medications such as digitalis may also influence serum electrolytes. Warning signs, irrespective of cause, are: dryness of mouth, thirst, weakness, lethargy, drowsiness, restlessness, muscle pains or cramps, muscular fatigue, hypotension, oliguria, tachycardia, arrhythmia, and gastrointestinal disturbances such as nausea and vomiting.

Hypokalemia may develop with Lasix (furosemide) as with any other potent diuretic, especially with brisk diuresis, when cirrhosis is present, or during concomitant use of corticosteroids or ACTH.

Interference with adequate oral electrolyte intake will also contribute to hypokalemia. Digitalis therapy may exaggerate metabolic effects of hypokalemia, especially with reference to myocardial activity.

Asymptomatic hyperuricemia can occur and gout may rarely be precipitated.

Periodic checks on urine and blood glucose should be made in diabetics and even those suspected of latent diabetes when receiving Lasix (furosemide). Increases in blood glucose and alterations in glucose tolerance tests with abnormalities of the fasting and 2-hour postprandial sugar have been observed, and rare cases of precipitation of diabetes mellitus have been reported.

Lasix (furosemide) may lower serum calcium levels, and rare cases of tetany have been reported. Accordingly, periodic serum calcium levels should be obtained.

Reversible elevations of BUN may be seen. These have been observed in association with dehydration, which should be avoided, particularly in patients with renal insufficiency.

Patients receiving high doses of salicylates, as in rheumatic disease, in conjunction with Lasix (furosemide) may experience salicylate toxicity at

Continued on next page

Hoechst-Roussel—Cont.

lower doses because of competitive renal excretory sites.

Lasix (furosemide) has a tendency to antagonize the skeletal muscle relaxing effect of tubocurarine and may potentiate the action of succinylcholine. Lithium generally should not be given with diuretics because they reduce its renal clearance and add a high risk of lithium toxicity.

It has been reported in the literature that diuretics such as furosemide may enhance the nephrotoxicity of cephaloridine. Therefore, Lasix (furosemide) and cephaloridine should not be administered simultaneously.

Lasix (furosemide) may decrease arterial responsiveness to norepinephrine. This diminution is not sufficient to preclude effectiveness of the pressor agent for therapeutic use.

It has been reported in the literature that coadministration of indomethacin may reduce the natriuretic and antihypertensive effects of Lasix (furosemide) in some patients. This effect has been attributed to inhibition of prostaglandin synthesis by indomethacin. Indomethacin may also affect plasma renin levels and aldosterone excretion; this should be borne in mind when a renin profile is evaluated in hypertensive patients. Patients receiving both indomethacin and Lasix (furosemide) should be observed closely to determine if the desired diuretic and/or antihypertensive effect of Lasix (furosemide) is achieved.

Renal calcifications (from barely visible on x-ray to staghorn) have occurred in some severely premature infants treated with intravenous Lasix® (furosemide) for edema due to patent ductus arteriosus and hyaline membrane disease. The concurrent use of chlorothiazide has been reported to decrease hypercalciuria and to dissolve some calculi.

Pregnancy

Pregnancy Category C. Furosemide has been shown to cause unexplained maternal deaths and abortions in rabbits at 2, 4 and 8 times the human dose. There are no adequate and well-controlled studies in pregnant women. Furosemide should be used during pregnancy only if the potential benefit justifies the potential risk to the fetus.

The effects of furosemide on embryonic and fetal development and on pregnant dams were studied in mice, rats and rabbits.

Furosemide caused unexplained maternal deaths and abortions in the rabbit when 50 mg/kg (4 times the maximal recommended human dose of 600 mg per day) was administered between days 12 and 17 of gestation. In a previous study the lowest dose of only 25 mg/kg (2 times the maximal recommended human dose of 600 mg per day) caused maternal deaths and abortions. In a third study, none of the pregnant rabbits survived a dose of 100 mg/kg. Data from the above studies indicate fetal lethality that can precede maternal deaths.

The results of the mouse study and one of the three rabbit studies also showed an increased incidence of hydronephrosis (distention of the renal pelvis and, in some cases, of the ureters) in fetuses derived from treated dams as compared to the incidence in fetuses from the control group.

Adverse Reactions

Gastrointestinal System Reactions
1. anorexia
2. oral and gastric irritation
3. nausea
4. vomiting
5. cramping
6. diarrhea
7. constipation
8. jaundice (intrahepatic cholestatic jaundice)
9. pancreatitis

Central Nervous System Reactions
1. dizziness
2. vertigo
3. paresthesias
4. headache
5. xanthopsia
6. blurred vision
7. tinnitus and hearing loss

Hematologic Reactions
1. anemia
2. leukopenia
3. agranulocytosis (rare)
4. thrombocytopenia
5. aplastic anemia (rare)

Dermatologic—Hypersensitivity Reactions
1. purpura
2. photosensitivity
3. rash
4. urticaria
5. necrotizing angiitis (vasculitis, cutaneous vasculitis)
6. exfoliative dermatitis
7. erythema multiforme
8. pruritus

Cardiovascular Reaction
Orthostatic hypotension may occur and be aggravated by alcohol, barbiturates, or narcotics.

Other
1. hyperglycemia
2. glycosuria
3. hyperuricemia
4. muscle spasm
5. weakness
6. restlessness
7. urinary bladder spasm
8. thrombophlebitis
9. transient pain at the injection site following intramuscular injection

Whenever adverse reactions are moderate or severe, Lasix (furosemide) dosage should be reduced or therapy withdrawn.

Dosage and Administration:

Oral Administration
Edema—Therapy should be individualized according to patient response. This therapy should be titrated to gain maximal therapeutic response as well as the minimal dose possible to maintain that therapeutic response.

ADULTS—The usual initial daily dose of oral Lasix (furosemide) is 20 to 80 mg given as a single dose. Ordinarily a prompt diuresis ensues. Depending on the patient's response, a second dose can be administered 6 to 8 hours later.

If the diuretic response to a single dose of 20 to 80 mg is not satisfactory, increase this dose by increments of 20 or 40 mg not sooner than 6 to 8 hours after the previous dose until the desired diuretic effect has been obtained. This individually determined single dose should then be given once or twice daily (eg, at 8:00 a.m. and 2:00 p.m.). The dose of Lasix (furosemide) may be carefully titrated up to 600 mg/day in those patients with severe clinical edematous states.

The mobilization of edema may be most efficiently and safely accomplished by utilizing an intermittent dosage schedule in which the diuretic is given for 2 to 4 consecutive days each week.

When doses exceeding 80 mg/day are given for prolonged periods, careful clinical and laboratory observations are particularly advisable.

INFANTS AND CHILDREN—The usual initial dose of oral Lasix (furosemide) in infants and children is 2 mg/kg body weight, given as a single dose. If the diuretic response is not satisfactory after the initial dose, dose may be increased by 1 or 2 mg/kg no sooner than 6 to 8 hours after the previous dose. Doses greater than 6 mg/kg body weight are not recommended.

For maintenance therapy in infants and children, the dose should be adjusted to the minimum effective level.

Hypertension—Therapy should be individualized according to the patient's response. This therapy should be titrated to gain maximal therapeutic response as well as the minimal dose possible to maintain that therapeutic response.

ADULTS—The usual initial daily dose of Lasix (furosemide) for antihypertensive therapy is 80 mg, usually divided into 40 mg twice a day. Dosage should then be adjusted according to response. If the patient does not respond, add other antihypertensive agents.

Careful observations for changes in blood pressure must be made when this compound is used with other antihypertensive drugs, especially during initial therapy. The dosage of other agents must be reduced by at least 50 percent as soon as Lasix (furosemide) is added to the regimen, to prevent excessive drop in blood pressure. As the blood pressure falls under the potentiating effect of Lasix (furosemide), a further reduction in dosage or even discontinuation of other antihypertensive drugs may be necessary.

Parenteral Administration
ADULTS—Parenteral therapy should be reserved for patients for whom oral medication is not practical or in emergency situations where prompt diuresis is desired. Parenteral therapy should be replaced by oral therapy as soon as this is practical for continued mobilization of edema.

Edema—The usual initial dose of Lasix (furosemide) is 20 to 40 mg given as a single dose, injected intramuscularly or intravenously. The intravenous injection should be given slowly (1 to 2 minutes). Ordinarily, a prompt diuresis ensues. Depending on the patient's response, a second dose can be administered 2 hours after the first dose or later.

If the diuretic response with a single dose of 20 to 40 mg is not satisfactory, increase this dose by increments of 20 mg not sooner than 2 hours after the previous dose until the desired diuretic effect has been obtained. This individually determined single dose should then be given once or twice daily.

If the physician elects to use high dose parenteral therapy it should be administered as a controlled infusion at a rate not exceeding 4 mg/min. Lasix (furosemide) Injection is a mildly buffered alkaline solution which should not be mixed with acidic solutions of pH below 5.5. To prepare infusion solutions, isotonic saline and lactated Ringer's injection and 5% dextrose injection have been used after pH has been adjusted when necessary. Therapy should be individualized according to patient response. This therapy should be titrated to gain maximal therapeutic response as well as the minimal dose possible to maintain that therapeutic response. Close medical supervision is necessary.

Acute Pulmonary Edema—The usual initial dose of Lasix (furosemide) is 40 mg injected intravenously. The injection should be given slowly (1 to 2 minutes). If 40 mg Lasix (furosemide) does not produce a satisfactory response within 1 hour the dose may be increased to 80 mg given intravenously (over 1 to 2 minutes).

If deemed necessary, additional therapy (eg, digitalis, oxygen) can be administered concomitantly.

INFANTS AND CHILDREN—Parenteral therapy should be reserved for patients for whom oral medication is not practical or in emergency situations where prompt diuresis is desired. Parenteral therapy should be replaced by oral therapy as soon as this is practical for continued mobilization of edema.

The usual initial dose of Lasix (furosemide) Injection (intravenously or intramuscularly) in infants and children is 1 mg/kg body weight and should be given slowly under close medical supervision. If the diuretic response after the initial dose is not satisfactory, dosage may be increased by 1 mg/kg not sooner than 2 hours after the previous dose, until the desired diuretic effect has been obtained. Doses greater than 6 mg/kg body weight are not recommended.

How Supplied: Lasix (furosemide) Tablets are supplied as white, round, monogrammed, scored tablets of 40 mg in amber bottles of 100, 500, and 1,000; unit dose 100s (20 strips of 5); and Unit of Use trays of 12 × 100, 25 × 30 and 25 × 60; white, oval, monogrammed tablets of 20 mg in amber bottles of 100, 500 and 1000, and unit dose 100s (10 strips of 10); and white, round, monogrammed, facetted-edge tablets of 80 mg in amber bottles of 50 and 500, and unit dose 100s (20 strips of 5).

Note: Dispense in well-closed, light-resistant containers. Exposure to light may cause slight discoloration. Discolored tablets should not be dispensed.

Lasix (furosemide) Oral Solution is supplied as an orange-flavored liquid containing furosemide 10 mg/mL in bottles of 60 mL (accompanied by graduated dropper) and bottles of 120 mL (accompanied by graduated dispensing spoon). The alcohol content is 11.5%.

Note: Store at controlled room temperature 59°–86°F). Dispense in light-resistant containers. Discard opened bottle after 60 days.

Lasix (furosemide) Injection is supplied as a sterile solution in 2 mL amber ampuls, boxes of 5 and 50;

4 mL amber ampuls, boxes of 5 and 25; 10 mL amber ampuls, boxes of 5 and 25; 2 mL prefilled syringes, boxes of 5; 4 mL prefilled syringes, boxes of 5; and 10 mL prefilled syringes, boxes of 5; 2mL, 4mL and 10mL single-use vials in cartons of 25. Each mL contains 10 mg furosemide. Syringes supplied with 22 gauge $\times$ 1¼"needle.

Note: Store at controlled room temperature. (59°–86°F). Do not use if solution is discolored. Protect syringes from light. Do not remove syringes from individual package until time of use.

Shown in Product Identification Section, page 413

LOPROX®
[lo' prahks]
(ciclopirox olamine) Cream 1%

Description: Loprox® (ciclopirox olamine) Cream 1% is for topical use.
Each gram of Loprox® (ciclopirox olamine) Cream 1% contains 10 mg ciclopirox olamine in a water miscible vanishing cream base consisting of 2-octyldodecanol, mineral oil, stearyl alcohol, cetyl alcohol, polysorbate 60, myristyl alcohol, cocamide DEA, sorbitan monostearate, lactic acid, purified water, and benzyl alcohol (1%).
Loprox® (ciclopirox olamine) Cream contains a synthetic broad-spectrum, antifungal agent ciclopirox olamine. The chemical name is 6-cyclohexyl-1- hydroxy-4-methyl- 2(1H)-pyridone, 2-aminoethanol salt.
Loprox® (ciclopirox olamine) Cream 1% has a pH of 7.

Clinical Pharmacology: Ciclopirox olamine is a broad-spectrum, antifungal agent that inhibits the growth of pathogenic dermatophytes, yeasts, and *Malassezia furfur.* Ciclopirox olamine exhibits fungicidal activity *in vitro* against isolates of *Trichophyton rubrum, Trichophyton mentagrophytes, Epidermophyton floccosum, Microsporum canis,* and *Candida albicans.*
Pharmacokinetic studies in men with tagged 1% ciclopirox olamine solution in polyethylene glycol 400 showed an average of 1.3% absorption of the dose when it was applied topically to 750 cm^2 on the back followed by occlusion for 6 hours. The biological half-life was 1.7 hours and excretion occurred via the kidney. Two days after application only 0.01% of the dose applied could be found in the urine. Fecal excretion was negligible.
Penetration studies in human cadaverous skin from the back, with Loprox® (ciclopirox olamine) Cream 1% with tagged ciclopirox olamine showed the presence of 0.8 to 1.6% of the dose in stratum corneum 1.5 to 6 hours after application. The levels in the dermis were still 10 to 15 times above the minimum inhibitory concentrations.
Autoradiographic studies with human cadaverous skin showed that ciclopirox olamine penetrates into the hair and through the epidermis and hair follicles into the sebaceous glands and dermis, while a portion of the drug remains in the stratum corneum.
Draize Human Sensitization Assay, 21-Day Cumulative Irritancy study, Phototoxicity study, and Photo-Draize study conducted in a total of 142 healthy male subjects showed no contact sensitization of the delayed hypersensitivity type, no irritation, no phototoxicity, and no photo-contact sensitization due to Loprox® (ciclopirox olamine) Cream 1%.

Indications and Usage: Loprox® (ciclopirox olamine) Cream 1% is indicated for the topical treatment of the following dermal infections: tinea pedis, tinea cruris and tinea corporis due to *Trichophyton rubrum, Trichophyton mentagrophytes, Epidermophyton floccosum,* and *Microsporum canis;* candidiasis (moniliasis) due to *Candida albicans;* and tinea (pityriasis) versicolor due to *Malassezia furfur.*

Contraindications: Loprox® (ciclopirox olamine) Cream 1% is contraindicated in individuals who have shown hypersensitivity to any of its components.

Warnings: General: Loprox® (ciclopirox olamine) Cream 1% is not for ophthalmic use.

Precautions: If a reaction suggesting sensitivity or chemical irritation should occur with the use of Loprox® (ciclopirox olamine) Cream 1%, treatment should be discontinued and appropriate therapy instituted.

Information for patients—
The patient should be told to:
1. Use the medication for the full treatment time even though symptoms may have improved and notify the physician if there is no improvement after four weeks.
2. Inform the physician if the area of application shows signs of increased irritation (redness, itching, burning, blistering, swelling, oozing) indicative of possible sensitization.
3. Avoid the use of occlusive wrappings or dressings.

Carcinogenesis, mutagenesis, impairment of fertility:
A carcinogenicity study in female mice dosed cutaneously twice per week for 50 weeks followed by a 6-month drug-free observation period prior to necropsy revealed no evidence of tumors at the application site. Several mutagenic tests indicated no potential for mutagenesis.

Pregnancy Category B:
Reproduction studies have been performed in the mouse, rat, rabbit, and monkey, (via various routes of administration) at doses 10 times or more the topical human dose and have revealed no significant evidence of impaired fertility or harm to the fetus due to ciclopirox olamine. There are, however, no adequate or well-controlled studies in pregnant women. Because animal reproduction studies are not always predictive of human response this drug should be used during pregnancy only if clearly needed.

Nursing mothers:
It is not known whether this drug is excreted in human milk. Because many drugs are excreted in human milk, caution should be exercised when Loprox® (ciclopirox olamine) Cream 1% is administered to a nursing woman.

Pediatric use:
Safety and effectiveness in children below the age of 10 years have not been established.

Adverse Reactions: In all controlled clinical studies with 514 patients using Loprox® (ciclopirox olamine) Cream 1% and in 296 patients using the vehicle cream, the incidence of adverse reactions was low. This included pruritus at the site of application in one patient and worsening of the clinical signs and symptoms in another patient using ciclopirox olamine cream 1% and burning in one patient and worsening of the clinical signs and symptoms in another patient using the vehicle cream.

Dosage and Administration: Gently massage Loprox® (ciclopirox olamine) Cream 1% into the affected and surrounding skin areas twice daily, in the morning and evening. Clinical improvement with relief of pruritus and other symptoms usually occurs within the first week of treatment. If a patient shows no clinical improvement after four weeks of treatment with Loprox® (ciclopirox olamine) Cream 1%, the diagnosis should be redetermined. Patients with tinea versicolor usually exhibit clinical and mycological clearing after two weeks of treatment.

How Supplied: Loprox® (ciclopirox olamine) Cream 1% is supplied in 15 gram and 30 gram tubes.
Store at controlled room temperature (59°– 86°F).
Loprox® REG TM HOECHST AG
70900-6/84

Shown in Product Identification Section, page 413

RELEFACT® TRH
(protirelin)
Injection IV

Description: Chemically, Relefact® TRH (protirelin) is identified as 5-oxo-L-prolyl-L-histidyl-L-proline amide. It is a synthetic tripeptide which is believed to be structurally identical with the naturally-occurring thyrotropin-releasing hormone produced by the hypothalamus.
Relefact TRH is supplied as 1 mL ampuls. Each ampul contains 500 mcg protirelin in a sterile non-pyrogenic isotonic saline solution having a pH of approximately 6.5. In addition, each ampul contains sodium chloride, 9.0 mg, Water for Injection, and hydrochloric acid as needed to adjust pH. Relefact TRH is intended for intravenous administration.

Clinical Pharmacology: Pharmacologically, Relefact TRH increases the release of the thyroid stimulating hormone (TSH) from the anterior pituitary. Prolactin release is also increased. It has recently been observed that approximately 65% of acromegalic patients tested respond with a rise in circulating growth hormone levels; the clinical significance is as yet not clear. Following intravenous administration, the mean plasma half-life of protirelin in normal subjects is approximately five minutes. TSH levels rise rapidly and reach a peak at 20 to 30 minutes. The decline in TSH levels takes place more slowly, approaching baseline levels after approximately three hours.

Indications and Usage: Relefact® TRH (protirelin) is indicated as an adjunctive agent in the diagnostic assessment of thyroid function. As an adjunct to other diagnostic procedures, testing with Relefact TRH may yield useful information in patients with pituitary or hypothalamic dysfunction.
Relefact TRH is indicated as an adjunct to evaluate the effectiveness of thyrotropin suppression with a particular dose of T4 in patients with nodular or diffuse goitre. A normal TSH baseline value and a minimal difference between the 30 minute and baseline response to Relefact TRH injection would indicate adequate suppression of the pituitary secretion of TSH.
Relefact TRH may be used, adjunctively, for adjustment of thyroid hormone dosage given to patients with primary hypothyroidism. A normal or slightly blunted TSH response, thirty minutes following Relefact TRH injection, would indicate adequate replacement therapy.

Warnings: Transient changes in blood pressure, either increases or decreases, frequently occur immediately following administration of Relefact TRH (protirelin). Blood pressure should therefore be measured before Relefact TRH is administered and at frequent intervals during the first 15 minutes after its administration.
Increases in systolic pressure (usually less than 30 mm Hg) and/or increases in diastolic pressure (usually less than 20 mm Hg) have been observed more frequently than decreases in pressure. These changes have not ordinarily persisted for more than 15 minutes nor have they required therapy. More severe degrees of hypertension or hypotension with or without syncope have been reported in a few patients. To minimize the incidence and /or severity of hypotension, the patient should be supine before, during, and after Relefact TRH administration. If a clinically important change in blood pressure occurs, monitoring of blood pressure should be continued until it returns to baseline levels.
Relefact® TRH (protirelin) should not be administered to patients in whom marked, rapid changes in blood pressure would be dangerous unless the potential benefit clearly outweighs the potential risk.

Precautions: Thyroid hormones reduce the TSH response to Relefact TRH. Accordingly, patients in whom Relefact TRH is to be used diagnostically should be taken off liothyronine (T3) approximately seven days prior to testing and should be taken off thyroid medications containing levothyroxine (T4), e.g., desiccated thyroid, thyroglobulin, or liatrix, at least 14 days before testing. Hormone therapy is NOT to be discontinued when the test is used to evaluate the effectiveness of thyroid suppression with a particular dose of T4 in patients with nodular or diffuse goitre, or for adjustment of thyroid hormone dosage given to patients with primary hypothyroidism.
Chronic administration of levodopa has been reported to inhibit the TSH response to Relefact TRH.

Continued on next page

Hoechst-Roussel—Cont.

It is not advisable to withdraw maintenance doses of adrenocortical drugs used in the therapy of known hypopituitarism. Several published reports have shown that prolonged treatment with glucocorticoids at physiologic doses has no significant effect of the TSH response to thyrotropin releasing hormone, but that the administration of pharmacologic doses of steroids reduces the TSH response. Therapeutic doses of acetylsalicylic acid (2 to 3.6 g/day) have been reported to inhibit the TSH response to protirelin. The ingestion of acetylsalicylic acid caused the peak level of TSH to decrease approximately 30% as compared to values obtained without acetylsalicylic acid administration. In both cases, the TSH peak occurred 30 minutes post-administration of protirelin.

Pregnancy: Reproduction studies have been performed in rats and rabbits. At doses 1½ and 6 times the human dose, there was an increase in the number of resorption sites in the pregnant rabbit. There are no studies in pregnant women which bear on the safety of Relefact® TRH (protirelin) for the human fetus. Relefact TRH should be used in pregnant women only when clearly needed.

Adverse Reactions: Side effects have been reported in about 50% of the patients tested with Relefact TRH. Generally, the side effects are minor, have occurred promptly, and have persisted for only a few minutes following injection.

Cardiovascular reactions:
Marked changes in blood pressure, including both hypertension and hypotension with or without syncope, have been reported in a small number of patients.

Endocrine reaction: Breast enlargement and leakage in lactating women for up to two or three days.

Other reactions: Headaches, sometimes severe, and transient amaurosis in patients with pituitary tumors.

Nausea; urge to urinate; flushed sensation; light-headedness; bad taste; abdominal discomfort; and dry mouth. Less frequently reported were: anxiety; sweating; tightness in the throat; pressure in the chest; tingling sensation; and drowsiness.

Dosage and Administration: Relefact TRH is intended for intravenous administration with the patient in the supine position. The drug is administered as a bolus over a period of 15 to 30 seconds, with the patient remaining supine until all scheduled postinjection blood samples have been taken. Blood pressure should be measured before Relefact TRH is administered and at frequent intervals during the first 15 minutes thereafter (see **Warnings**).

Dosage: Adults: 500 mcg. Doses between 200 and 500 mcg have been used. 500 mcg is considered the optimum dose to give the maximum response in the greatest number of patients. Doses greater than 500 mcg are unlikely to elicit a greater TSH response.

Children age 6 to 16 years: 7 mcg/kg body weight up to a dose of 500 mcg.

Infants and children up to 6 years: Experience is limited in this age group; doses of 7 mcg/kg have been administered.

One blood sample for TSH assay should be drawn immediately prior to the injection of Relefact® TRH (protirelin), and a second sample should be obtained 30 minutes after injection.

The TSH response to Relefact TRH is reduced by repetitive administration of the drug. Accordingly, if the Relefact TRH test is repeated, an interval of seven days before testing is recommended.

Elevated serum lipids may interfere with the TSH assay. Thus, fasting (except in patients with hypopituitarism) or a low-fat meal is recommended prior to the test.

Interpretation of Test Results: Interpretation of the TSH response to Relefact TRH requires an understanding of thyroid-pituitary-hypothalamic physiology and knowledge of the clinical status of the individual patient.

Because the TSH test results may vary with the laboratory, the physician should be familiar with the TSH assay method used and the normal range for the laboratory performing the assay.

TSH response 30 minutes after Relefact TRH administration in normal subjects and in patients with hyperthyroidism and hypothyroidism are presented in Figure 1. The diagnoses were established prior to the administration of Relefact TRH on the basis of the clinical history, physical examination, and the results of other thyroid and/or pituitary function tests.

Among the normal euthyroid subjects, women and children were found to have higher levels of TSH at 30 minutes than men. Among the patients with hyperthyroidism or primary (thyroidal), secondary (pituitary), or tertiary (hypothalamic) hypothyroidism, no significant differences in TSH levels by age or sex were found.

[See table below].

Normal: Baseline TSH levels of less than 10 microunits/mL (μU/mL) were observed in 97% of euthyroid normal subjects tested. Thirty minutes after Relefact® TRH (protirelin), the serum TSH increased by 2.0 μU/mL or more in 95% of euthyroid subjects.

Hyperthyroidism: All hyperthyroid patients tested had baseline TSH levels of less than 10 μU/mL and a rise of less than 2 μU/mL 30 minutes after Relefact TRH.

Primary (thyroidal) hypothyroidism: The diagnosis of primary hypothyroidism is frequently supported by finding clearly elevated baseline TSH levels; 93% of patients tested had levels above 10 μU/mL. Relefact TRH administration to these patients generally would not be expected to yield additional useful information. Ninety-four percent of patients with primary hypothyroidism given Relefact TRH in clinical trials responded with a rise in TSH of 2.0 μU/mL or greater, since this response is also found in normal subjects. Relefact TRH testing does not differentiate primary hypothyroidism from normal.

Table 1
Characterization Based on Serum TSH Levels at Baseline and 30 Minutes after Relefact TRH

	Baseline Serum TSH (μU/mL)	Change of Serum TSH (μU/mL) at 30 minutes
Euthyroidism (normal thyroid function)	10 or less (usually 6 or less; 20% have < 1.5 μU/mL)	2 or more (usually 6 to 30)
Hyperthyroidism	10 or less (usually 4 or less)	less than 2
Primary Hypothyroidism (thyroidal)	more than 10 (usually 15 to 100)	2 or more (usually 20 or more)
Secondary Hypothyroidism (pituitary)	10 or less (usually 6 or less)	less than 2 (59%) 2 to 50 (41%)
Tertiary Hypothyroidism (hypothalamic)	10 or less (often less than 2)	2 or more

Secondary (pituitary) and tertiary (hypothalamic) hypothyroidism: In the presence of clinical and other laboratory evidence of hypothyroidism, the finding of a baseline TSH level less than 10 μU/mL should suggest secondary or tertiary hypothyroidism. In this situation, a response to Relefact® TRH (protirelin) of less than 2 μU/mL suggests secondary hypothyroidism since this response was observed in about 60% of patients with secondary hypothyroidism and only approximately 5% of patients with tertiary hypothyroidism. A TSH response to Relefact TRH greater than 2 μU/mL is not helpful in differentiating between secondary and tertiary hypothyroidism since this response was noted in about 40% of the former and about 95% of the latter.

Establishing the diagnosis of secondary or tertiary hypothyroidism requires a careful history and physical examination along with appropriate tests of anterior pituitary and/or target gland function. The Relefact TRH test should not be used as the only laboratory determinant for establishing these diagnoses.

How Supplied: As 1 mL ampuls - boxes of 5 (NDC 0039-0081-08). Each mL contains Relefact TRH 0.50 mg (500 mcg), sodium chloride 9.0 mg for isotonicity, and hydrochloric acid for pH adjustment.

* RELEFACT® REG TM HOECHST AG
78100 - 1/83

Figure 1
Mean ± One Standard Deviation of TSH Levels (μU/mL) Observed at Baseline and 30 Minutes After Relefact® TRH (protirelin)

Number of Patients	Condition
73	Euthyroid Women
111	Euthyroid Men
56	Secondary Hypothyroid (pituitary)
21	Tertiary Hypothyroid (hypothalamic)
75	Hyperthyroid

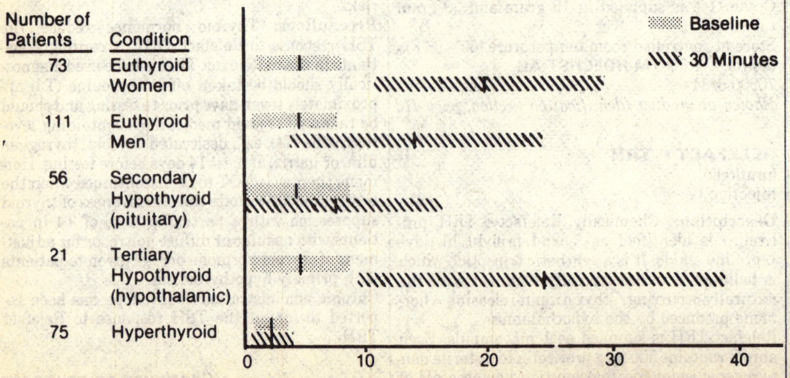

STREPTASE®
[strep' tās]
(streptokinase)

Description: Streptase® (streptokinase) is a sterile, purified preparation of a bacterial protein elaborated by group C β-hemolytic streptococci. It is supplied as a lyophilized white powder containing 25 mg cross-linked gelatin polypeptides, 25 mg sodium L-glutamate and 100 mg Normal Serum Albumin (Human) as stabilizers for intravenous and intracoronary administration.

Clinical Pharmacology: Streptase® (streptokinase) acts with plasminogen to produce an "activator complex" that converts plasminogen to the proteolytic enzyme plasmin. Plasmin degrades fibrin clots as well as fibrinogen and other plasma proteins (1). Intravenous infusion of streptokinase is followed by increased fibrinolytic activity. This hyperfibrinolytic effect disappears within a few hours after discontinuation, but a prolonged thrombin time, especially with prolonged administration, may persist for up to 24 hours due to a decrease in plasma levels of fibrinogen and an increase in the amount of circulating fibrin(ogen) degradation products (FDP). The thrombin time will usually decrease to less than two times normal control value within 4 hours.

Indications and Usage: STREPTASE® (STREPTOKINASE) IS INDICATED FOR THE LYSIS OF THROMBI IN SEVERAL CONDITIONS. THE ROUTE (METHOD) OF ADMINISTRATION, DURATION, AND DOSAGE VARY WITH EACH CONDITION (SEE DOSAGE AND ADMINISTRATION).

Pulmonary Embolism
With Streptase® (streptokinase) therapy, angiographic, lung scan and/or hemodynamic improvement is more rapid and complete than with heparin therapy (2-4).
Streptase® (streptokinase) is indicated in adults for:
- the lysis of acute pulmonary emboli, involving obstruction of blood flow to a lobe or multiple segments (5), or
- the lysis of pulmonary emboli accompanied by unstable hemodynamics, i.e., failure to maintain blood pressure without supportive measures.

The diagnosis should be confirmed by objective means, such as pulmonary angiography via an upper extremity vein, or noninvasive procedures such as lung scanning.

Deep Vein Thrombosis
Streptase® (streptokinase) is indicated in adults for lysis of acute, extensive thrombi of the deep veins, such as those involving the popliteal and more proximal vessels. Diagnosis should be confirmed by objective means, preferably ascending venography. Studies have demonstrated better salvage of valvular function and prevention of postphlebitic syndrome by streptokinase plus heparin than by heparin alone (6-8).
Should pulmonary embolism or recurrent pulmonary embolism occur during streptokinase therapy, the originally planned course of treatment should be completed in an attempt to lyse these emboli. While pulmonary embolism may occasionally occur during Streptase® (streptokinase) treatment of deep vein thrombosis, the incidence is no greater than when patients are treated with heparin alone (4,9-11).

Arterial Thrombosis and Embolism
Streptase® (streptokinase) is indicated in adults for the lysis of acute arterial thrombi and for the lysis of arterial emboli (12-14). However, the use of Streptase® (streptokinase) in arterial emboli originating from the left side of the heart (e.g., in mitral stenosis accompanied by atrial fibrillation) should be avoided due to the danger of new embolic phenomena, including those to cerebral vessels.

Arteriovenous Cannulae Occlusion
Streptase® (streptokinase) is indicated for clearing of totally or partially occluded arteriovenous cannulae as an alternative to surgical revision when acceptable flow cannot otherwise be achieved (15).

Coronary Artery Thrombosis
Streptase® (streptokinase) has been reported to lyse acute thrombi obstructing coronary arteries, associated with evolving transmural myocardial infarction. Diagnosis of acute myocardial infarction has been confirmed, and the site of coronary thrombosis identified by selective coronary angiography (16,17). Other studies (18-24) have demonstrated that (a) a thrombus is present in approximately 90% of patients evaluated within four hours of onset of symptoms; (b) when compared to concurrent or historical controls, the majority of patients who received intracoronary streptokinase within 6 hours of onset of symptoms, showed a more immediate recanalization (within a few minutes vs hours/days) of the involved vessel.
IT HAS NOT BEEN ESTABLISHED THAT INTRACORONARY ADMINISTRATION OF STREPTOKINASE DURING EVOLVING TRANSMURAL MYOCARDIAL INFARCTION RESULTS IN SALVAGE OF MYOCARDIAL TISSUE, NOR THAT IT REDUCES MORTALITY. CONTROLLED STUDIES ADDRESSING THESE PARAMETERS ARE IN PROGRESS (25) AND UNTIL COMPLETED,

THOSE PATIENTS WHO MIGHT BENEFIT FROM THIS THERAPY CANNOT BE DEFINED.

Contraindications: Because thrombolytic therapy increases the risk of bleeding, Streptase® (streptokinase) is contraindicated in the following situations:
- active internal bleeding
- recent (within 2 months) cerebrovascular accident, intracranial or intraspinal surgery (see **Warnings**)
- intracranial neoplasm

Warnings:
Bleeding
The aim of Streptase® (streptokinase) therapy is the production of sufficient amounts of plasmin for the lysis of intravascular deposits of fibrin; however, fibrin deposits which provide hemostasis, for example, at sites of needle punctures, are also lysed and bleeding from such sites may occur. Intramuscular injections and nonessential handling of the patient must be avoided during treatment with Streptase® (streptokinase). Venipunctures should be performed carefully and as infrequently as possible.
Should an arterial puncture be necessary during intravenous therapy, upper extremity vessels are preferable. Pressure should be applied for at least 30 minutes, a pressure dressing applied and the puncture site checked frequently for evidence of bleeding.
When internal bleeding occurs, it may be more difficult to manage than that which occurs with conventional anticoagulant therapy.
In the following conditions the risks of therapy may be increased and should be weighed against the anticipated benefits.
- Recent (within 10 days) major surgery, obstetrical delivery, organ biopsy, previous puncture of noncompressible vessels
- Recent serious gastrointestinal bleeding (within 10 days)
- Recent trauma including cardiopulmonary resuscitation
- Severe, uncontrolled arterial hypertension
- High likelihood of left heart thrombus, e.g., mitral stenosis with atrial fibrillation
- Subacute bacterial endocarditis
- Hemostatic defects including those secondary to severe hepatic or renal disease
- Pregnancy
- Cerebrovascular disease
- Diabetic hemorrhagic retinopathy
- Prior severe allergic reaction to streptokinase
- Septic thrombophlebitis or occluded AV cannula at seriously infected site
- Any other condition in which bleeding constitutes a significant hazard or would be particularly difficult to manage because of its location.

Should serious spontaneous bleeding (not controllable by local pressure) occur, the infusion of Streptase® (streptokinase) should be terminated immediately and treatment instituted as described under **Adverse Reactions**.

Use of Anticoagulants
Concurrent use of anticoagulants with intravenous administration of Streptase® (streptokinase) is not recommended. However, concurrent use of heparin may be required during intracoronary administration of Streptase® (streptokinase). Clinical studies with concurrent use of heparin and lower Streptase® (streptokinase) dosages employed during intracoronary administration have demonstrated no tendency toward increased bleeding that would not be attributable to the procedure or Streptase® (streptokinase) alone. Nevertheless, careful monitoring for excessive bleeding is advised.

Arrhythmias
Rapid lysis of coronary thrombi has been reported occasionally to cause reperfusion atrial or ventricular dysrhythmias requiring immediate treatment. During studies, careful monitoring for arrhythmia was maintained during and immediately following intracoronary administration of Streptase® (streptokinase).

Precautions:
General:
Non-cardiogenic pulmonary edema has been reported rarely in patients treated with streptokinase. The risk of this appears greatest in patients who have large myocardial infarctions and are undergoing thrombolytic therapy by the intracoronary route.

Use in Pregnancy and Children
Safety and effectiveness of Streptase® (streptokinase) therapy in children and during pregnancy has not been established. Therefore, treatment of such patients is not recommended.

Drug Interactions
The interaction of Streptase® (streptokinase) with other drugs has not been studied. Drugs that alter platelet function should not be used during therapy. Common examples are: aspirin, indomethacin, and phenylbutazone (6).

Patient Monitoring
Before commencing thrombolytic therapy, it is desirable to obtain a thrombin time (TT), activated partial thromboplastin time (APTT), prothrombin time (PT), hematocrit and platelet count to obtain hemostatic status of the patient.

Intracoronary Artery Infusion
During studies, laboratory monitoring of hemostatic parameters during intracoronary artery infusion showed minimal changes, if any. Heparin was continued during therapy or instituted following therapy and monitored accordingly.

Intravenous Infusion
If heparin has been given, it should be discontinued and the TT or APTT should be less than twice the normal control value before thrombolytic therapy is started.
During the infusion, decreases in the plasminogen and fibrinogen level and an increase in the level of FDP (the latter two serving to prolong the clotting times of coagulation tests) will generally confirm the existence of a lytic state. Therefore, therapy can be monitored by performing the TT or PT, approximately 4 hours after initiation of therapy. Following the infusion, **before (re)instituting heparin**, the TT should be less than twice the normal control value.

Adverse Reactions: The following adverse reactions have been frequently associated with intravenous therapy but may also occur with intracoronary artery infusion:

Bleeding
Minor bleeding occurs often with thrombolytic therapy mainly at invaded or disturbed sites. When lytic therapy is continued while local measures are used to control minor bleeding, do **not** reduce the dose as this will increase lytic activity since more plasminogen will be available for conversion to plasmin. Severe internal bleeding involving gastrointestinal, genitourinary, retroperitoneal or intracerebral sites, may occur. Several fatalities due to cerebral and other serious internal hemorrhage have occurred during intravenous thrombolytic therapy.
Should uncontrollable bleeding occur, Streptase® (streptokinase) infusion should be discontinued and, if necessary, blood loss and reversal of the bleeding tendency can be effectively managed with whole blood (fresh blood preferable), packed red blood cells and cryoprecipitate or fresh frozen plasma. Although the use of aminocaproic acid (ACA, AMICAR®) in humans as an antidote for streptokinase has not been documented, it may be considered in an emergency situation.

Allergic Reactions
Reactions attributed to possible anaphylaxis have been observed rarely in patients treated with Streptase® (streptokinase) intravenously. These ranged in severity from minor breathing difficulty to bronchospasm, periorbital swelling or angioneurotic edema. Other milder allergic effects such as urticaria, itching, flushing, nausea, headache and musculoskeletal pain have also been observed.
Mild or moderate reactions may be managed with concomitant antihistamine and/or corticosteroid therapy. Severe allergic reactions require immedi-

Continued on next page

Hoechst-Roussel—Cont.

ate discontinuation of Streptase® (streptokinase), with adrenergics, antihistamines, or corticosteroids administered intravenously as required.

Fever
Although Streptase® (streptokinase) is nonpyrogenic in standard animal tests, approximately one-third of patients treated with Streptase® (streptokinase) intravenously have shown increases in body temperature of $\geq 1.5°F$. Symptomatic treatment is usually sufficient to alleviate discomfort. The use of acetaminophen rather than aspirin is recommended.

Dosage and Administration:

A. Lysis of Coronary Artery Thrombi (18-23)
During clinical studies, Streptase® (streptokinase) was administered selectively into the thrombosed coronary artery via coronary catheter placed by the Judkins or Sones Technique. When administered within 6 hours of onset of symptoms of acute transmural myocardial infarction, at a bolus dose averaging 20,000 IU and a maintenance dose averaging 2,000 IU/min for 60 minutes, greater than 75% of occlusions were opened in less than 1 hour.

B. Treatment of Deep Vein Thrombosis, Pulmonary or Arterial Embolism or Arterial Thrombosis (26,27)
Streptokinase treatment should be instituted as soon as possible after onset of thrombotic event, preferably no later than seven days after onset. Any delay in instituting lytic therapy to evaluate the effect of heparin therapy decreases the potential for optimal efficacy (28). Reconstituted streptokinase solution may alter drop size which will influence the accuracy of drop counting infusion devices, either manually or instrument controlled. Use of volumetric or syringe infusion pumps is recommended.

Loading Dose
Since human exposure to streptococci is common, antibodies to streptokinase (streptokinase resistance) are found normally. Thus, a loading dose of Streptase® (streptokinase) sufficient to neutralize the resistance is required. A dose of 250,000 IU Streptase® (streptokinase) infused into a peripheral vein over 30 minutes has been found appropriate in over 90% of patients.

Maintenance Dose*
A maintenance dose infusion of 100,000 IU/hr is given following the loading dose. Administer this maintenance dose for 24 hours for the treatment of pulmonary embolism (up to 72 hours if concurrent deep vein thrombosis is suspected), 24-72 hours for the treatment of arterial thrombosis and arterial embolism, and 72 hours for the treatment of deep vein thrombosis.
If the thrombin time or any other parameter of lysis after 4 hours of therapy is less than approximately 1½ times the normal control value, discontinue Streptase® (streptokinase) as excessive resistance to streptokinase is present.

*A variable dosage of Streptase® (streptokinase) and frequent laboratory monitoring were recommended in the past (29). However, since experience shows that these do not increase the efficacy or safety of Streptase® (streptokinase) therapy, they are no longer recommended.

Anticoagulation after Terminating Intravenous Streptokinase Treatment
At the end of Streptase® (streptokinase) therapy, treatment with heparin by continuous intravenous infusion is recommended to prevent recurrent thrombosis (3). Heparin treatment (without a loading dose) should not begin until the thrombin time has decreased to **less than twice** the normal control value (approximately 3 to 4 hours). (See manufacturer's prescribing information for proper use of heparin.) This should be followed by oral anticoagulation in the conventional manner.

C. Treatment of Arteriovenous Cannula Occlusion:

1. Before Treatment:
Before using Streptase® (streptokinase), an attempt should be made to clear the cannula by careful syringe technique, using heparinized saline solution. If adequate flow is not reestablished, Streptase® (streptokinase) may be employed. Allow the effect of any pretreatment anticoagulants to diminish.

2. Streptase® (streptokinase) Administration: Instill 250,000 IU Streptase® (streptokinase) in 2 mL intravenous solution into each occluded limb of the cannula slowly. Clamp off cannula limb(s) for 2 hours. Observe the patient closely for possible adverse effects.

3. After Treatment:
Aspirate contents of infused cannula limb(s), flush with saline, reconnect cannula.

Reconstitution and Dilution:
For Intracoronary Artery and Intravenous Administration

Slight flocculation (described as thin translucent fibers) of reconstituted Streptase® (streptokinase) occurred occasionally during clinical trials but did not interfere with safe use of the solution. **Do not add any other medication to the container of Streptase® (streptokinase).**

The following reconstitution and dilution procedure will minimize flocculation.

1. Slowly add 5 mL Sodium Chloride Injection, USP or Dextrose (5%) Injection, USP, directing it at the side of the vacuum packed vial rather than into the Streptase® (streptokinase).

2. Roll and tilt the vial gently to reconstitute. **Avoid shaking.** (Shaking may cause foaming and/or increase flocculation.)

3. Further dilute the entire reconstituted contents of the vial slowly and carefully to a total volume of approximately 45 mL (see Table 1). Avoid shaking and agitation on dilution. (If necessary, total volume may be increased to a maximum of 500 mL with the infusion pump rate in Table 1 increased accordingly. To facilitate setting the infusion pump rate, a total volume of 45 mL, or multiple thereof, is recommended.)

4. The solution may be filtered through a 0.22 μm or a 0.45 μm filter.

5. Solutions containing **large amounts** of flocculation should be discarded.

6. If not used soon after reconstitution, store Streptase® (streptokinase) at 2-4°C. Discard reconstituted drug if not administered within 24 hours.

[See table below].

For Use in Arteriovenous Cannulae
Slowly reconstitute the contents of 250,000 IU Streptase® (streptokinase) vacuum packed vial with 2 mL Sodium Chloride Injection, USP or Dextrose (5%) Injection, USP.

How Supplied: Streptase® (streptokinase) is supplied as a lyophilized white powder in 6.5 mL vials (in packages of 10) with color-coded labels corresponding to the amount of purified Streptase® (streptokinase) in each vial as follows:
green-250,000 IU   blue-750,000 IU

Store unopened vials at controlled room temperature (15-30°C).

References:
1. McNicol, G.P.: The fibrinolytic system. Postgrad Med J 49 (Suppl): 10-2, 1973.
2. Brogden, R.N., Speight, T.M., Avery, G.S.: Streptokinase: A review of its clinical pharmacology, mechanism of action and therapeutic uses. Drugs 5:357-445, 1973.
3. Fratantoni, J.C., Ness, P., Simon, T.L.: Thrombolytic therapy: Current status. N Engl J Med 293:1073-8, 1975.
4. Urokinase Pulmonary Embolism Study Group: Urokinase-streptokinase embolism trial. JAMA 229:1606-13, 1974.
5. Sharma, G.V.R.K., Burleson, V.A., Sasahara, A.A.: Effect of thrombolytic therapy on pulmonary-capillary blood volume in patients with pulmonary embolism. N Engl J Med 303:842-5, 1980.
6. Common, H.H., Seaman, A.J., Rosch, J., et al: Deep vein thrombosis treated with streptokinase or heparin. Follow-up of a randomized study. Angiology 27:645-54, 1976.
7. Marder, V.J., Soulen, R.L., Atichartakarn, V., et al: Quantitative venographic assessment of deep vein thrombosis in the evaluation of streptokinase and heparin therapy. J Lab Clin Med 89:1018-29, 1977.
8. Johansson, L., Nylander, G., Hedner, U., et al: Comparison of streptokinase with heparin: Late results in the treatment of deep venous thrombosis. Acta Med Scand 206:93-8, 1979.
9. Urokinase pulmonary embolism trial study group: A urokinase pulmonary embolism trial. A national cooperative study. Circulation 47 (Suppl ll): 1-108, 1973.
10. Arnesen, H., Heilo, A., Jakobsen, E., et al: A prospective study of streptokinase and heparin in the treatment of venous thrombosis. Acta Med Scand 203: 457-463, 1978.
11. Elliot, M.S., Immelman, E.J., Jeffery, P., et al: A comparative randomized trial of heparin versus streptokinase in the treatment of acute proximal venous thrombosis. An interim report of a prospective trial. Br J Surg 66: 838-843, 1979.
12. Dotter, C.T., Rosch, J., Seaman, A.J., et al: Streptokinase treatment of thromboembolic disease. Radiology 102:283-90, 1972.
13. Persson, A.V., Thompson, J.E., Patman, R.D.: Acute arterial occlusions. Vasc Surg 11:359-63, 1977.
14. Reichle, F.A., Rao, N.A., Chang, K.H., et al: Thrombolysis of acute or subacute nonembolic arterial thrombosis. J Surg Res 22:202-208, 1977.
15. Data on File for Arteriovenous Cannulae Occlusion. Hoechst-Roussel Pharmaceuticals Inc.
16. Mathey, D.G., Kuck, K.H., Tilsner, V., et al: Nonsurgical coronary artery recanalization in acute transmural myocardial infarction. Circulation 63: 489-97, 1981.
17. Rentrop, P., Blanke H., Karsch, K.R., et al: Selective intracoronary thrombolysis in acute

TABLE I
Suggested Dilutions and Infusion Rates

Streptase® (streptokinase) Dosage/Infusion Rate	Streptase® (streptokinase) Vial Content Needed	Total Volume of Solution (mL)	Infusion Pump Rate
I. Intracoronary Artery Administration			
A. Bolus Injection 20,000 IU	1 vial, 250,000 IU*	125	Inject 10 mL
B. Maintenance Dose 2,000 IU/min			60 mL per hour
*sufficient for Bolus Injection and Maintenance Dose			
II. Intravenous Administration			
A. Loading Dose 250,000 IU/30 min	a) 1 vial, 250,000 IU or	45	90 mL per hour for 30 min
	b) 1 vial, 750,000 IU	45	30 mL per hour for 30 min
B. Maintenance Dose 100,000 IU/hr	1 vial, 750,000 IU	45**	6 mL per hour

** If necessary, total volume may be increased, in increments of 45 mL, to a maximum of 500 mL with the infusion pump rate increased accordingly. The total volume of 45 mL or multiple thereof is recommended.

myocardial infarction and unstable angina pectoris. Circulation 63: 307-17, 1981.
18. Cowley, M.J., Hastillo, A., Vetrovec, G.W., et al: Effects of intracoronary streptokinase in acute myocardial infarction. Am Heart J 102:1149-1158, 1981.
19. Mathey, D.G., Rodewald, G., Rentrop, P., et al: Intracoronary streptokinase thrombolytic recanalization and subsequent surgical bypass of remaining atherosclerotic stenosis in acute myocardial infarction: Complimentary combined approach effecting reduced infarct size, preventing reinfarction, and improving left ventricular function. Am Heart J 102:1194-1201, 1981.
20. Merx, W., Doerr, R., Rentrop, P., et al: Evaluation of the effectiveness of intracoronary streptokinase infusion in acute myocardial infarction: Postprocedure management and hospital course in 204 patients. Am Heart J 102:1181-1187, 1981.
21. Reduto, L.A., Freund, G.C., Gaeta, J.M., et al: Coronary artery reperfusion in acute myocardial infarction: Beneficial effects of intracoronary streptokinase on left ventricular salvage and performance. Am Heart J 102:1168-1177, 1981.
22. Rentrop, K.P., Karsch, K.R., Blanke H., et al: Changes in left ventricular function after intracoronary streptokinase infusion in clinically evolving myocardial infarction. Am Heart J 102:1188-1193, 1981.
23. Rutsch, W., Schartl, M., Mathey, D., et al: Percutaneous transluminal coronary recanalization: Procedure, results and acute complications. Am Heart J 102:1178-1180, 1981.
24. De Wood, M.A.; Spores J; Notske R; et al: Prevalence of total coronary occlusion during the early hours of transmural myocardial infarction. New Eng J. Med 303:897-902, 1980.
25. Workshop on Limitations of Infarct Size with Thrombolytic Agents. NIH, Bethesda, Maryland, 1981.
26. Marder, V.J.: The use of thrombolytic agents: Choice of patient, drug administration, laboratory monitoring. Ann Intern Med 90:802-8, 1979.
27. Bell, W.R., Meek, A.G.: Guidelines for the use of thrombolytic agents. N Eng J Med 301:1266-70, 1979.
28. Sherry, S., Bell, W.R., Duckert, F.H., et al: Thrombolytic Therapy in Thrombosis: A National Institutes of Health Consensus Development Conference. Ann Intern Med 93:141-4, 1980.
29. Porter, J.M., Seaman, A.J., Common, H.H., et al: Comparison of heparin and streptokinase in the treatment of venous thrombosis. Am Surg 40:511-19, 1975.
78500-1/84

SURFAK®
[ser' fak]
(docusate calcium USP)

Composition: Surfak is the stool softening agent, docusate calcium USP. Each 240 mg capsule contains 240 mg docusate calcium USP and up to 3% alcohol (w/w). Each 50 mg capsule contains 50 mg docusate calcium USP and up to 1.3% alcohol (w/w).
Action and Uses: Surfak is useful in patients where prevention of hard stools is essential to treatment, or in those conditions where laxative therapy is undesirable or contraindicated. Surfak is indicated for patients who require only fecal softening without propulsive action to accomplish defecation, such as obstetric, geriatric, surgical, and cardiac patients, those with anorectal conditions and after proctologic surgery. Surfak provides homogenization and formation of soft, easily evacuated stools without disturbance of body physiology, discomfort of bowel distention, oily leakage or interference with vitamin absorption.
Dosages: Adults—one red 240 mg capsule daily for several days or until bowel movements are normal. Children and adults with minimal needs —one to three orange 50 mg capsules daily. For use in children under 6, consult a physician.
Adverse Reactions: Surfak is non-habit forming. It has no known side effects or disadvantages, except for the unusual occurrence of mild, transitory cramping pains. Overdosage does not lead to systemic toxicity.
Warnings: If cramping pain occurs, discontinue the medication. As with any drug, if you are pregnant or nursing a baby, seek the advice of a health professional before using this product.
Contraindications: None.
How Supplied: 240 mg red, soft gelatin capsules - packages of 7 and 30, bottles of 100 and 500, and Unit Dose 100's (10 × 10 strips). 50 mg orange, soft gelatin capsules - bottles of 30 and 100.
Literature Available: Yes.
Shown in Product Identification Section, page 413

TOPICORT® R
[top' i-kort"]
(desoximetasone)
EMOLLIENT CREAM 0.25%
TOPICORT® LP
(desoximetasone)
EMOLLIENT CREAM 0.05%
TOPICORT® GEL
(desoximetasone) 0.05%
TOPICORT® OINTMENT
(desoximetasone) 0.25%

Description: Topicort® (desoximetasone) Emollient Cream 0.25%, Topicort® LP (desoximetasone) Emollient Cream 0.05%, Topicort® Gel (desoximetasone) 0.05%, and Topicort® Ointment (desoximetasone) 0.25% contain the active synthetic corticosteroid desoximetasone. The topical corticosteroids constitute a class of primarily synthetic steroids used as anti-inflammatory and antipruritic agents. Each gram of Topicort® (desoximetasone) Emollient Cream 0.25% contains 2.5 mg of desoximetasone in an emollient cream consisting of isopropyl myristate, cetylstearyl alcohol, white petrolatum, mineral oil, lanolin alcohol and purified water.
Each gram of Topicort® LP (desoximetasone) Emollient Cream 0.05% contains 0.5 mg of desoximetasone in an emollient cream consisting of isopropyl myristate, cetylstearyl alcohol, white petrolatum, mineral oil, lanolin alcohol, edetate disodium, lactic acid and purified water.
Each gram of Topicort® Gel (desoximetasone) 0.05% contains 0.5 mg desoximetasone in a gel consisting of purified water, SD alcohol 40 (20% w/w), isopropyl myristate, carbomer 940, trolamine, edetate disodium and docusate sodium.
Each gram of Topicort® Ointment (desoximetasone) 0.25% contains 2.5 mg of desoximetasone in a base of propylene glycol, sorbitan sesquioleate, fatty alcohol citrate, fatty acid pentaerythritol ester, beeswax, aluminum stearate, citric acid, butylated hydroxyanisole and white petrolatum.
The chemical name of desoximetasone is Pregna-1, 4-diene-3, 20-dione, 9-fluoro-11, 21-dihydroxy-16-methyl-, (11β,16α)-.
Desoximetasone has the empirical formula $C_{22}H_{29}FO_4$ and a molecular weight of 376.47. The CAS Registry Number is 382-67-2.
Clinical Pharmacology: Topical corticosteroids share anti-inflammatory, anti-pruritic and vasoconstrictive actions.
The mechanism of anti-inflammatory activity of the topical corticosteroids is unclear. Various laboratory methods, including vasoconstrictor assays, are used to compare and predict potencies and/or clinical efficacies of the topical corticosteroids. There is some evidence to suggest that a recognizable correlation exists between vasoconstrictor potency and therapeutic efficacy in man.
Pharmacokinetics
The extent of percutaneous absorption of topical corticosteroids is determined by many factors including the vehicle, the integrity of the epidermal barrier, and the use of occlusive dressings.
Topical corticosteroids can be absorbed from normal intact skin. Inflammation and/or other disease processes in the skin increase percutaneous absorption. Occlusive dressings substantially increase the percutaneous absorption of topical corticosteroids. Thus, occlusive dressings may be a valuable therapeutic adjunct for treatment of resistant dermatoses.
Once absorbed through the skin, topical corticosteroids are handled through pharmacokinetic pathways similar to systemically administered corticosteroids. Corticosteroids are bound to plasma proteins in varying degrees. Corticosteroids are metabolized primarily in the liver and are then excreted by the kidneys. Some of the topical corticosteroids and their metabolites are also excreted into the bile.
Pharmacokinetic studies in men with Topicort® (desoximetasone) Emollient Cream 0.25% with tagged desoximetasone showed a total of $5.2\% \pm 2.9\%$ excretion in urine ($4.1\% \pm 2.3\%$) and feces ($1.1\% \pm 0.6\%$) and no detectable level (limit of sensitivity: 0.005 μg/mL) in the blood when it was applied topically on the back followed by occlusion for 24 hours. Seven days after application, no further radioactivity was detected in urine or feces. The half-life of the material was 15 ± 2 hours (for urine) and 17 ± 2 hours (for feces) between the third and fifth trial day.
Pharmacokinetic studies in men with Topicort® Ointment (desoximetasone) 0.25% with tagged desoximetasone showed no detectable level (limit of sensitivity: 0.003 μg/mL) in 1 subject and 0.004 and 0.006 μg/mL in the remaining 2 subjects in the blood when it was applied topically on the back followed by occlusion for 24 hours. The extent of absorption for the ointment was 7% based on radioactivity recovered from urine and feces. Seven days after application, no further radioactivity was detected in urine or feces.
Studies with other similarly structured steroids have shown that predominant metabolite reaction occurs through conjugation to form the glucuronide and sulfate ester.
Indications and Usage: Topicort® (desoximetasone) Emollient Cream 0.25%, Topicort® LP (desoximetasone) Emollient Cream 0.05%, Topicort® Gel (desoximetasone) 0.05% and Topicort® Ointment (desoximetasone) 0.25% are indicated for the relief of the inflammatory and pruritic manifestations of corticosteroid-responsive dermatoses.
Contraindications: Topical corticosteroids are contraindicated in those patients with a history of hypersensitivity to any of the components of the preparation.
Precautions:
General
Systemic absorption of topical corticosteroids has produced reversible hypothalamic-pituitary-adrenal (HPA) axis suppression, manifestations of Cushing's syndrome, hyperglycemia, and glucosuria in some patients.
Conditions which augment systemic absorption include the application of the more potent steroids, use over large surface areas, prolonged use, and the addition of occlusive dressings.
Therefore, patients receiving a large dose of a potent topical steroid applied to a large surface area or under an occlusive dressing should be evaluated periodically for evidence of HPA axis suppression by using the urinary free cortisol and ACTH stimulation tests. If HPA axis suppression is noted, an attempt should be made to withdraw the drug, to reduce the frequency of application, or to substitute a less potent steroid.
Recovery of HPA axis function is generally prompt and complete upon discontinuation of the drug. Infrequently, signs and symptoms of steroid withdrawal may occur, requiring supplemental systemic corticosteroids.
Children may absorb proportionally larger amounts of topical corticosteroids and thus be more susceptible to systemic toxicity (See **Precautions—Pediatric Use**)
If irritation develops, topical corticosteroids should be discontinued and appropriate therapy instituted.

Continued on next page

Hoechst-Roussel—Cont.

In the presence of dermatological infections, the use of an appropriate antifungal or antibacterial agent should be instituted. If a favorable response does not occur promptly, the corticosteroid should be discontinued until the infection has been adequately controlled.

Information for the Patient
Patients using topical corticosteroids should receive the following information and instructions:
1. This medication is to be used as directed by the physician. It is for external use only. Avoid contact with the eyes.
2. Patients should be advised not to use this medication for any disorder other than for which it was prescribed.
3. The treated skin area should not be bandaged or otherwise covered or wrapped as to be occlusive unless directed by the physician.
4. Patients should report any signs of local adverse reactions especially under occlusive dressing.
5. Parents of pediatric patients should be advised not to use tight-fitting diapers or plastic pants on a child being treated in the diaper area, as these garments may constitute occlusive dressings.

Laboratory Tests
The following tests may be helpful in evaluating the HPA axis suppression:
    Urinary free cortisol test
    ACTH stimulation test

Carcinogenesis, Mutagenesis, and Impairment of Fertility
Long-term animal studies have not been performed to evaluate the carcinogenic potential or the effect on fertility of topical corticosteroids. Studies to determine mutagenicity with prednisolone and hydrocortisone have revealed negative results.

Pregnancy Category C
Corticosteroids are generally teratogenic in laboratory animals when administered systemically at relatively low dosage levels. The more potent corticosteroids have been shown to be teratogenic after dermal application in laboratory animals.
Desoximetasone has been shown to be teratogenic and embryotoxic in mice, rats, and rabbits when given in doses 3 to 30 times the human dose of Topicort® (desoximetasone) Emollient Cream 0.25% and Topicort Ointment (desoximetasone) 0.25%, or 15 to 150 times the human dose of Topicort® LP (desoximetasone) Emollient Cream 0.05% and Topicort® Gel (desoximetasone) 0.05%.
There are no adequate and well-controlled studies in pregnant women on teratogenic effects from topically applied corticosteroids. Therefore, Topicort® (desoximetasone) Emollient Cream 0.25%, Topicort® LP (desoximetasone) Emollient Cream 0.05%, Topicort® Gel (desoximetasone) 0.05% and Topicort® Ointment (desoximetasone) 0.25% should be used during pregnancy only if the potential benefit justifies the potential risk to the fetus. Drugs of this class should not be used extensively on pregnant patients, in large amounts, or for prolonged periods of time.

Nursing Mothers
It is not known whether topical administration of corticosteroids could result in sufficient systemic absorption to produce detectable quantities in breast milk. Systemically administered corticosteroids are secreted into breast milk in quantities not likely to have a deleterious effect on the infant. Nevertheless, caution should be exercised when topical corticosteroids are administered to a nursing woman.

Pediatric Use
Pediatric patients may demonstrate greater susceptibility to topical corticosteroid-induced HPA axis suppression and Cushing's syndrome than mature patients because of a larger skin surface area to body weight ratio.

Hypothalamic-pituitary-adrenal (HPA) axis suppression, Cushing's syndrome, and intracranial hypertension have been reported in children receiving topical corticosteroids. Manifestations of adrenal suppression in children include linear growth retardation, delayed weight gain, low plasma cortisol levels, and absence of response to ACTH stimulation. Manifestations of intracranial hypertension include bulging fontanelles, headaches, and bilateral papilledema.
Administration of topical corticosteroids to children should be limited to the least amount compatible with an effective therapeutic regimen. Chronic corticosteroid therapy may interfere with the growth and development of children. The safety and effectiveness of Topicort® Ointment (desoximetasone) 0.25% in children below the age of 10 have not been established.

Adverse Reactions: The following local adverse reactions are reported infrequently with topical corticosteroids, but may occur more frequently with the use of occlusive dressings. These reactions are listed in an approximate decreasing order of occurrence:

Burning	Perioral dermatitis
Itching	Allergic contact dermatitis
Irritation	Maceration of the skin
Dryness	Secondary infection
Folliculitis	Skin Atrophy
Hypertrichosis	Striae
Acneiform eruptions	Miliaria
Hypopigmentation	

In controlled clinical studies the incidence of adverse reactions was low (0.8%) for Topicort® (desoximetasone) Emollient Cream 0.25% and included burning, folliculitis and folliculo-pustular lesions. The incidence of adverse reactions was also 0.8% for Topicort® LP (desoximetasone) Emollient Cream 0.05% and included pruritus, erythema, vesiculation and burning sensation. In controlled clinical studies the incidence of adverse reactions was low (0.3%) for Topicort® Ointment (desoximetasone) 0.25% and consisted of development of comedones at the site of application.

Overdosage: Topically applied corticosteroids can be absorbed in sufficient amounts to produce systemic effects (See Precautions).

Dosage and Administration: Apply a thin film of Topicort® (desoximetasone) Emollient Cream 0.25%, Topicort® LP (desoximetasone) Emollient Cream 0.05%, Topicort® Gel (desoximetasone) 0.05% or Topicort® Ointment (desoximetasone) 0.25% to the affected skin areas twice daily. Rub in gently.

How Supplied: Topicort® (desoximetasone) Emollient Cream 0.25% is supplied in 15 gram, 60 gram, and 4 ounce tubes.
Topicort® LP (desoximetasone) Emollient Cream 0.05% is supplied in 15 gram and 60 gram tubes.
Topicort® Gel (desoximetasone) 0.05% is supplied in 15 gram and 60 gram tubes.
Topicort® Ointment (desoximetasone) 0.25% is supplied in 15 gram and 60 gram tubes.
Store at controlled room temperature (59°-86°F).
Topicort® REG TM Roussel Uclaf
Shown in Product Identification Section, page 413

TRENTAL® ℞
(pentoxifylline)
Tablets, 400 mg

Description: Trental® (pentoxifylline) tablets for oral administration contain 400 mg of the active drug in a controlled-release formulation. Trental® (pentoxifylline) is a trisubstituted xanthine derivative designated chemically as 1-(5-oxohexyl)-3, 7-dimethylxanthine that, unlike theophylline, is a hemorheologic agent, i.e. an agent that affects blood viscosity. Pentoxifylline is soluble in water and ethanol, and sparingly soluble in toluene.

Clinical Pharmacology:
Mode of Action
Pentoxifylline and its metabolites improve the flow properties of blood by decreasing its viscosity. In patients with chronic peripheral arterial disease, this increases blood flow to the affected microcirculation and enhances tissue oxygenation. The precise mode of action of pentoxifylline and the sequence of events leading to clinical improvement are still to be defined. Pentoxifylline administration has been shown to produce dose related hemorheologic effects, lowering blood viscosity, and improving erythrocyte flexibility. Tissue oxygen levels have been shown to be significantly increased by therapeutic doses of pentoxifylline in patients with peripheral arterial disease.

Pharmacokinetics and Metabolism
After oral administration in aqueous solution pentoxifylline is almost completely absorbed. It undergoes a first-pass effect and the various metabolites appear in plasma very soon after dosing. Peak plasma levels of the parent compound and its metabolites are reached within 1 hour. The major metabolites are Metabolite I (1-[5-hydroxyhexyl]-3,7-dimethylxanthine) and Metabolite V (1-[3-carboxypropyl]-3,-7-dimethylxanthine), and plasma levels of these metabolites are 5 and 8 times greater, respectively, than pentoxifylline. Following oral administration of aqueous solutions containing 100 to 400 mg of pentoxifylline, the pharmacokinetics of the parent compound and Metabolite I are dose-related and not proportional (non-linear), with half-life and area under the blood-level time curve (AUC) increasing with dose. The elimination kinetics of Metabolite V are not dose-dependent. The apparent plasma half-life of pentoxifylline varies from 0.4 to 0.8 hours and the apparent plasma half-lives of its metabolites vary from 1 to 1.6 hours. There is no evidence of accumulation or enzyme induction (Cytochrome P_{450}) following multiple oral doses.
Excretion is almost totally urinary; the main biotransformation product is Metabolite V. Essentially no parent drug is found in the urine. Despite large variations in plasma levels of parent compound and its metabolites, the urinary recovery of Metabolite V is consistent and shows dose proportionality. Less than 4% of the administered dose is recovered in feces. Food intake shortly before dosing delays absorption of an immediate release dosage form but does not affect total absorption. The pharmacokinetics and metabolism of Trental® (pentoxifylline) have not been studied in patients with renal and/or hepatic dysfunction, but AUC was increased and elimination rate decreased in an older population (60–68 years) compared to younger individuals (22–30 years).
After administration of the 400 mg controlled-release Trental® (pentoxifylline) tablet, plasma levels of the parent compound and its metabolites reach their maximum within 2 to 4 hours and remain constant over an extended period of time. The controlled release of pentoxifylline from the tablet eliminates peaks and troughs in plasma levels for improved gastrointestinal tolerance.

Indications and Usage: Trental® (pentoxifylline) is indicated for the treatment of patients with intermittent claudication on the basis of chronic occlusive arterial disease of the limbs. Trental® (pentoxifylline) can improve function and symptoms but is not intended to replace more definitive therapy, such as surgical bypass, or removal of arterial obstructions when treating peripheral vascular disease.

Contraindications: Trental® (pentoxifylline) should not be used in patients who have previously exhibited intolerance to this product or methylxanthines such as caffeine, theophylline, and theobromine.

Precautions:
General: Patients with chronic occlusive arterial disease of the limbs frequently show other manifestations of arteriosclerotic disease. Trental® (pentoxifylline) has been used safely for treatment of peripheral arterial disease in patients with concurrent coronary artery and cerebrovascular diseases, but there have been occasional reports of angina, hypotension, and arrhythmia. Controlled trials do not show that Trental® (pentoxifylline) causes such adverse effects more often than placebo, but, as it is a methylxanthine derivative, it is possible some individuals will experience such responses.

Drug Interactions: No drug interactions with Trental® (pentoxifylline) are known at this time. Although there have been no formal interaction studies, the drug has been used concurrently with antihypertensive drugs, beta blockers, digitalis, diuretics, antidiabetic agents, and antiarrhythmics, without observed problems. Small decreases in blood pressure have been observed in some patients treated with Tental® (pentoxifylline); periodic systemic blood pressure monitoring is recommended for patients receiving concomitant antihypertensive therapy. If indicated, dosage of the antihypertensive agents should be reduced.

Carcinogenesis, Mutagenesis and Impairment of Fertility: Long-term studies of the carcinogenic potential of pentoxifylline were conducted in mice and rats by dietary administration of the drug at doses up to approximately 24 times (570 mg/kg) the maximum recommended human daily dose (MRHD) of 24 mg/kg for 18 months in mice and 18 months in rats with an additional 6 months without drug exposure in the latter. No carcinogenic potential for pentoxifylline was noted in the mouse study. In the rat study, there was a statistically significant increase in benign mammary fibroadenomas in females in the high dose group (24 × MRHD). The relevance of this finding to human use is uncertain since this was only a marginal statistically significant increase for a tumor that is common in aged rats. Pentoxifylline was devoid of mutagenic activity in various strains of *Salmonella* (Ames test) when tested in the presence and absence of metabolic activation.

Pregnancy: Category C. Teratogenic studies have been performed in rats and rabbits at oral doses up to about 25 and 10 times the maximum recommended human daily dose (MRHD) of 24 mg/kg, respectively. No evidence of fetal malformation was observed. Increased resorption was seen in rats at 25 times MRHD. There are, however, no adequate and well controlled studies in pregnant women. Because animal reproduction studies are not always predictive of human response. Trental® (pentoxifylline) should be used during pregnancy only if clearly needed.

Nursing Mothers: It is not known whether this drug is excreted in human milk. Because many drugs are excreted in human milk and because of the potential for tumorigenicity shown for pentoxifyllin in rats, a decision should be made whether to discontinue nursing or discontinue the drug, taking into account the importance of the drug to the mother.

Pediatric Use: Safety and effectiveness in children below the age of 18 years have not been established.

Adverse Reactions: Clinical trials were conducted using either controlled-release Trental® (pentoxifylline) tablets for up to 60 weeks or immediate-release Trental® (pentoxifylline) capsules for up to 24 weeks. Dosage ranges in the tablet studies were 400 mg bid to tid and in the capsule studies, 200–400 mg tid.

The table summarizes the incidence (in percent) of adverse reactions considered drug related, as well as the numbers of patients who received controlled-release Trental® (pentoxifylline) tablets, immediate-release Trental® (pentoxifylline) capsules, or the corresponding placebos. The incidence of adverse reactions was higher in the capsule studies (where dose related increases were seen in digestive and nervous system side effects) than in the tablet studies. Studies with the capsule include domestic experience, whereas studies with the controlled-release tablets were conducted outside the U.S. The table indicates that in the tablet studies few patients discontinued because of adverse effects.
[See table above].

Trental® (pentoxifylline) has been marketed in Europe and elsewhere since 1972. In addition to the above symptoms, the following have been reported spontaneously since marketing or occurred in other clinical trials with an incidence of less than 1%; the causal relationship was uncertain: Cardiovascular—dyspnea, edema, hypotension; Digestive—anorexia, cholecystitis, constipation, dry mouth/thirst; Nervous—anxiety, confusion;

INCIDENCE (%) OF SIDE EFFECTS

	Controlled-Release Tablets		Immediate-Release Capsules	
	Trental®	Placebo	Trental®	Placebo
(Numbers of Patients at Risk)	(321)	(128)	(177)	(138)
Discontinued for Side Effect	3.1	0	9.6	7.2
CARDIOVASCULAR SYSTEM				
Angina/Chest pain	0.3	—	1.1	2.2
Arrhythmia/Palpitation	—	—	1.7	0.7
Flushing	—	—	2.3	0.7
DIGESTIVE SYSTEM				
Abdominal Discomfort	—	—	4.0	1.4
Belching/Flatus/Bloating	0.6	—	9.0	3.6
Diarrhea	—	—	3.4	2.9
Dyspepsia	2.8	4.7	9.6	2.9
Nausea	2.2	0.8	28.8	8.7
Vomiting	1.2	—	4.5	0.7
NERVOUS SYSTEM				
Agitation/Nervousness	—	—	1.7	0.7
Dizziness	1.9	3.1	11.9	4.3
Drowsiness	—	—	1.1	5.8
Headache	1.2	1.6	6.2	5.8
Insomnia	—	—	2.3	2.2
Tremor	0.3	0.8	—	—
Blurred Vision	—	—	2.3	1.4

Respiratory—epistaxis, flu-like symptoms, laryngitis, nasal congestion; Skin and Appendages—brittle fingernails, pruritus, rash, urticaria; Special Senses—blurred vision, conjunctivitis, earache, scotoma; and Miscellaneous—bad taste, excessive salivation, leukopenia, malaise, sore throat/swollen neck glands, weight change.

A few rare events have been reported spontaneously worldwide since marketing in 1972. Although they occurred under circumstances in which a causal relationship with pentoxifylline could not be established, they are listed to serve as information for physicians: Cardiovascular—angina, arrhythmia, tachycardia; Digestive—hepatitis, jaundice; and Hemic and Lymphatic—decreased serum fibrinogen, pancytopenia, purpura, thrombocytopenia.

Overdosage: Overdosage with Trental® (pentoxifylline) has been reported in children and adults. Symptoms appear to be dose related. A report from a poison control center on 44 patients taking overdoses of enteric-coated pentoxifylline tablets noted that symptoms usually occurred 4–5 hours after ingestion and lasted about 12 hours. The highest amount ingested was 80 mg/kg; flushing, hypotension, convulsions, somnolence, loss of consciousness, fever, and agitation occurred. All patients recovered.

In addition to symptomatic treatment and gastric lavage, special attention must be given to supporting respiration, maintaining systemic blood pressure, and controlling convulsions. Activated charcoal has been used to adsorb pentoxifylline in patients who have overdosed.

Dosage and Administration: The usual dosage of Trental® (pentoxifylline) in controlled-release tablet form is one tablet (400 mg) three times a day with meals.

While the effect of Trental® (pentoxifylline) may be seen within 2 to 4 weeks, it is recommended that treatment be continued for at least 8 weeks. Efficacy has been demonstrated in double-blind clinical studies of 6 months duration.

Digestive and central nervous system side effects are dose related. if patients develop these side effects it is recommended that the dosage be lowered to one tablet twice a day (800 mg/day). If side effects persist at this lower dosage, the administration of Trental® (pentoxifylline) should be discontinued.

How Supplied: Trental® (pentoxifylline) is available for oral administration as 400 mg pink sugar-coated oblong tablets imprinted Trental®; supplied in bottles of 100 (NDC 0039-0078-10).
Store at controlled room temperature (59°–86°F).
77800-8/84

Shown in Product Identification Section, page 413

Holland-Rantos Company, Inc.
P.O. BOX 385
865 CENTENNIAL AVE.
PISCATAWAY, NJ 08854

See YOUNGS DRUG PRODUCTS CORPORATION

Hoyt Laboratories
See Colgate-Hoyt Laboratories

Hyland Therapeutics Division
Travenol Laboratories, Inc.
444 W. GLENOAKS BLVD.
GLENDALE, CA 91202

AUTOPLEX™ ℞
Anti-Inhibitor Coagulant Complex

Supplied in single dose 30 ml vials (Factor VIII correctional activity is stated on label of each vial) with sterile diluent and needles for reconstitution and withdrawal.

BUMINATE® 5% ℞
Normal Serum Albumin (Human), U.S.P., 5% Solution

Supplied as a 5% solution in 250 ml and 500 ml bottles. For use with intravenous administration set.

BUMINATE® 25% ℞
Normal Serum Albumin (Human), U.S.P., 25% Solution

Supplied as a 25% solution in 20 ml, 50 ml, and 100 ml vials. For use with intravenous administration set.

HEMOFIL® ℞
**Antihemophilic Factor (Human), Factor VIII, AHF, AHG
Method Four, Dried**

Supplied in single dose 10 ml, 20 ml, and 30 ml vials (AHF activity is stated on label of each vial) with sterile diluent and needles for reconstitution and withdrawal.

Continued on next page

Hyland—Cont.

HEMOFIL® T ℞
**Antihemophilic Factor (Human), Factor VIII,
AHF, AHG
Method Four, Dried, Heat-Treated**

Supplied in single dose 10 ml, 20 ml, and 30 ml vials (AHF activity is stated on label of each vial) with sterile diluent double-ended needle, and a filter spike for reconstitution and withdrawal.

HU–TET® ℞
Tetanus Immune Globulin (Human), U.S.P.

Supplied in 250 units single dose vial or prefilled disposable syringe.

IMMUNE SERUM GLOBULIN ℞
**(HUMAN), U.S.P.
GAMMA GLOBULIN**

Supplied in 2 ml and 10 ml vials.

PROPLEX® ℞
**Factor IX Complex (Human)
(Factors II, VII, IX, and X), Dried**

Supplied in single dose 30 ml vials (Factor IX activity is stated on label of each vial) with sterile diluent and needles for reconstitution and withdrawal.

PROPLEX® SX ℞
**Factor IX Complex (Human)
(Factors II, VII, IX, and X), Dried**

Supplied in single dose 30 ml vials (Factor IX activity is stated on label of each vial) with sterile diluent and needles for reconstitution and withdrawal.

PROPLEX® SX-T ℞
**Factor IX Complex (Human)
Heat Treated**

Supplied in single dose 30 ml vials (Factor IX activity is stated on label of each vial) with sterile diluent and needles for reconstitution and withdrawal.

PROTENATE® 5% ℞
**Plasma Protein Fraction (Human),
U.S.P., 5% Solution**

Supplied as a 5% solution in 250 ml and 500 ml bottles. For use with intravenous administration set.

Hynson, Westcott & Dunning
**Division of Becton Dickinson and Co.
CHARLES & CHASE STS.
BALTIMORE, 21201**

BAL IN OIL AMPULES ℞
(Dimercaprol Injection, USP)

Description: Dimercaprol (2,3-dimercapto-1-propanol) is a colorless or almost colorless liquid, having a disagreeable, mercaptan-like odor. Each 1 ml sterile BAL in Oil contains 100 mg Dimercaprol in 200 mg benzyl benzoate and 700 mg peanut oil. The slight sediment which may be noticed in some ampules develops during sterilization. It is not an indication that the solution is deteriorating.
Action: Dimercaprol promotes the excretion of arsenic, gold and mercury in cases of poisoning. It is also used in combination with Edetate Calcium Disodium Injection, USP to promote the excretion of lead.
Indications: BAL in Oil (Dimercaprol Injection, USP) is indicated in the treatment of arsenic, gold and mercury poisoning. It is indicated in acute lead poisoning when used concomitantly with Edetate Calcium Disodium Injection, USP.
Dimercaprol Injection, USP is effective for use in acute poisoning by mercury salts if therapy is begun within one or two hours following ingestion. It is not very effective for chronic mercury poisoning. Dimercaprol Injection, USP is of questionable value in poisoning caused by other heavy metals such as antimony and bismuth. It should not be used in iron, cadmium, or selenium poisoning because the resulting dimercaprol-metal complexes are more toxic than the metal alone, especially to the kidneys.
Contraindications: BAL in Oil is contraindicated in most instances of hepatic insufficiency with the exception of postarsenical jaundice. The drug should be discontinued or used only with extreme caution if acute renal insufficiency develops during therapy.
Warnings: There may be local pain at the site of the injection. A reaction apparently peculiar to children is fever which may persist during therapy. It occurs in approximately 30% of children. A transient reduction of the percentage of polymorphonuclear leukocytes may also be observed.
Precautions: Because the dimercaprol-metal complex breaks down easily in an acid medium, production of an alkaline urine affords protection to the kidney during therapy. Medicinal iron should not be administered to patients under therapy with BAL. Data is not available regarding the use of dimercaprol during pregnancy and it should not be used unless judged by the physician to be necessary in the treatment of life threatening acute poisoning.
Adverse Reactions: One of the most consistent responses to Dimercaprol Injection, USP is a rise in blood pressure accompanied by tachycardia. This rise is roughly proportional to the dose administered. Doses larger than those recommended may cause other transitory signs and symptoms in approximate order of frequency as follows: (1) nausea and, in some instances, vomiting; (2) headache; (3) a burning sensation in the lips, mouth and throat; (4) a feeling of constriction, even pain, in the throat, chest, or hands; (5) conjunctivitis, lacrimation, blepharal spasm, rhinorrhea, and salivation; (6) tingling of the hands; (7) a burning sensation in the penis; (8) sweating of the forehead, hands and other areas; (9) abdominal pain; and (10) occasional appearance of painful sterile abscesses. Many of the above symptoms are accompanied by a feeling of anxiety, weakness, and unrest and often are relieved by administration of an antihistamine.
Dosage and Administration: By deep intramuscular injection only. For mild arsenic or gold poisoning, 2.5 mg/kg of body weight four times daily for two days, two times on the third day, and once daily thereafter for ten days; for severe arsenic or gold poisoning, 3 mg/kg every four hours for two days, four times on the third day, then twice daily thereafter for ten days. For mercury poisoning, 5 mg/kg initially, followed by 2.5 mg/kg one or two times daily for ten days. For acute lead encephalopathy 4 mg/kg body weight is given alone in the first dose and thereafter at four hour intervals in combination with Edetate Calcium Disodium Injection, USP administered at a separate site. For less severe poisoning the dose can be reduced to 3 mg/kg after the first dose. Treatment is maintained for two to seven days depending on clinical response. Successful treatment depends on beginning injections at the earliest possible moment and on the use of adequate amounts at frequent intervals. Other supportive measures should always be used in conjunction with BAL in Oil therapy.
How Supplied: 3 ml (100 mg/ml, ampules, box of 10, NDC 0011-8341-09).

LACTINEX® TABLETS AND GRANULES
(See PDR For Nonprescription Drugs)

Products are cross-indexed by generic and chemical names in the
YELLOW SECTION

Hyrex Pharmaceuticals
**3494 DEMOCRAT RD.
MEMPHIS, TN 38118**

BRONKOTUSS ℞
[brong′ ko-tus]
Cough Preparation—Non-Narcotic

How Supplied: 16 oz. and 128 oz.

GLUKOR INJECTION ℞
[glū′ kor]

Composition: When mixed, each ml contains: Chorionic Gonadotropin 200 U.S.P. units, Mannitol, Benzyl Alcohol 0.9%, Water for injection with Sodium Phosphate Dibasic and Sodium Phosphate Monobasic.
How Supplied: 10 ml and 25 ml vials with diluent.

HYREX-105 © ℞
[hī′ rex]

Composition: Phendimetrazine Tartrate 105 mg. In special slow release capsule.
How Supplied: Bottles of 100 capsules.

HYTINIC CAPSULES AND ELIXIR
[hī′ tin-ik]
(polysaccharide-iron complex)

Composition: HYTINIC is a highly water-soluble complex of iron and a low molecular weight polysaccharide. Each HYTINIC Capsule contains 150 mg. elemental iron. Each 5 ml. (teaspoonful) HYTINIC Elixir contains 100 mg. elemental iron, alcohol 10% (sugar free).
Action and Uses: HYTINIC is an easily assimilated source of iron for treatment of uncomplicated iron deficiency anemia. Because HYTINIC is a polysaccharide bound iron complex, it is relatively nontoxic and there are relatively few, if any, of the gastrointestinal side effects associated with iron therapy, thus permitting full therapeutic dosage (150 to 300 mg. elemental iron daily) in a single dose if desirable. There is no staining of teeth and no metallic aftertaste.
Indications: For treatment of uncomplicated iron deficiency anemia.
Contraindications: In patients with hemochromatosis and hemosiderosis, and in those with a known hypersensitivity to any of the ingredients.
Administration and Dosage: ADULTS: One or two HYTINIC Capsules daily, or one or two teaspoonfuls HYTINIC Elixir daily. CHILDREN 6 to 12 years of age: One teaspoonful HYTINIC Elixir daily; Children 2 to 6 years of age: ½ teaspoonful HYTINIC Elixir daily. For younger children, consult physician.
How Supplied: HYTINIC Capsules: (Green and white) Bottles of 50 and 500. HYTINIC Elixir: Bottles of 8 ounces.
Product Identification Mark: Hyrex.

HYTUSS TABLETS (100 mg)
[hī′ tus]
HYTUSS-2X CAPSULES (200 mg)
Brand of quaifenesin U.S.P. (formerly called glyceryl guaiacolate)

Composition: Each sugar-free Hytuss Tablet contains guaifenesin 100 mg. Each sugar-free Hytuss-2X Capsule contains guaifenesin 200 mg.
Action and Uses: This preparation utilizes the effective expectorant action of guaifenesin U.S.P. (formerly called glyceryl guaicolate) which significantly stimulates the secretion of respiratory tract fluid. The increased flow of less viscid fluid favors expectoration and has a demulcent effect on the tracheobronchial mucosa. The primary usefulness of Hytuss Tablets is to promote the change from a dry, unproductive cough to a productive cough. Hytuss is therefore useful in treating coughs due to the common cold, bronchitis, laryngitis, tracheitis, pharyngitis, influenza and the measles. The expectorant action of Hytuss may also provide symptomatic relief in some chronic respiratory

disorders when the patient experiences spasms of dry nonproductive coughing.
Precautions: Extremely large amounts may cause nausea and vomiting.
Dosage: HYTUSS TABLETS—*Adults*—1 or 2 tablets every 3 to 4 hours. Do not exceed 24 tablets in any 24 hour period.
Dosage: HYTUSS-2X CAPSULES—*Adults*—1 or 2 capsules 3 to 4 hours as needed. Do not exceed 12 capsules in any 24 hour period.
How Supplied: 100 mg. Tablet — White, scored, sugar-free, bottles of 100 — 1,000 — 5,000. Also 200 mg. Capsule, red and white, sugar-free, bottles of 100 — 1,000.
Product Identification Mark: Tablet—Hy. Capsule—Hyrex.
Shown in Product Identification Section, page 413

MEGATON ELIXIR   OTC
[*meg'ah-ton*]
Geriatric Vitamin Tonic

How Supplied: 16 oz.

TRAC TABS 2X   R
[*trak' tabs*]

Composition: TRAC TABS 2X: Each blue tablet coded Hy-408 contains Atropine Sulfate 0.06 mg, Hyoscyamine Sulfate 0.03 mg, Methenamine 120 mg, Methylene Blue 6 mg, Phenyl Salicylate 30 mg, Benzoic Acid 7.5 mg.
How Supplied: Bottles of 100 and 1,000. Trac 2X tablet coded Hy-408.
Shown in Product Identification Section, page 413

TWO-DYNE™   R
[*tō' dīn*]

Composition: Butalbital 50 mg, Caffeine 40 mg, Acetaminophen 325 mg.
How Supplied: Capsules—bottles of 100.

ICN Pharmaceuticals, Inc.
222 NORTH VINCENT AVENUE
COVINA, CA 91722

TESTRED®   R
brand of Methyltestosterone Capsules USP, 10 mg.

Description: The androgens are steroids that develop and maintain primary and secondary male sex characteristics. Methyltestosterone, a synthetic derivative of testosterone, is an androgenic preparation given by the oral route in a capsule form. Each capsule contains 10 mg. of USP Methyltestosterone, which has the following formula:

Methyltestosterone occurs as white or creamy white crystals or powder, which is soluble in various organic solvents but is practically insoluble in water.
Clinical Pharmacology: Endogenous androgens are responsible for the normal growth and development of the male sex organs and for maintenance of secondary sex characteristics. These effects include the growth and maturation of prostate, seminal vesicles, penis, and scrotum; the development of male hair distribution, such as beard, pubic, chest, and axillary hair; laryngeal enlargement, vocal chord thickening, alterations in body musculature, and fat distribution. Drugs in this class also cause retention of nitrogen, sodium, potassium, phosphorus, and decreased urinary excretion of calcium. Androgens have been reported to increase protein anabolism and decrease protein catabolism. Nitrogen balance is improved only when there is sufficient intake of calories and protein.

Androgens are responsible for the growth spurt of adolescence and for the eventual termination of linear growth which is brought about by fusion of the epiphyseal growth centers. In children, exogenous androgens accelerate linear growth rates, but may cause a disproportionate advancement in bone maturation. Use over long periods may result in fusion of the epiphyseal growth centers and termination of growth process. Androgens have been reported to stimulate the production of red blood cells by enhancing the production of erythropoietic stimulating factor.

During exogenous administration of androgens, endogenous testosterone release is inhibited through feedback inhibition of pituitary luteinizing hormone (LH). At large doses of exogenous androgens, spermatogenesis may also be suppressed through feedback inhibition of pituitary follicle stimulating hormone (FSH).

There is a lack of substantial evidence that androgens are effective in fractures, surgery, convalescence and functional uterine bleeding.

Pharmacokinetics
Testosterone given orally is metabolized by the gut and 44 percent is cleared by the liver in the first pass. Oral doses as high as 400 mg. per day are needed to achieve clinically effective blood levels for full replacement therapy. The synthetic androgen methyltestosterone is less extensively metabolized by the liver and has a longer half-life. It is more suitable than testosterone for oral administration.

Testosterone in plasma is 98 percent bound to a specific testosterone-estradiol binding globulin, and about 2 percent is free. Generally, the amount of this sex-hormone binding globulin in the plasma will determine the distribution of testosterone between free and bound forms, and the free testosterone concentration will determine its half-life.

About 90 percent of a dose of testosterone is excreted in the urine as glucuronic and sulfuric acid conjugates of testosterone and its metabolites; about 6 percent of a dose is excreted in the feces, mostly in the unconjugated form. Inactivation of testosterone occurs primarily in the liver. Testosterone is metabolized to various 17-keto steroids through two different pathways. There are considerable variations of the half-life of testosterone ranging from 10 to 100 minutes.

In many tissues the activity of testosterone appears to depend on reduction to dihydrotestosterone, which binds to cytosol receptor proteins. The steroid-receptor complex is transported to the nucleus where it initiates transcription events and cellular changes related to androgen action.

Indication and Usage:
1. Males
Androgens are indicated for replacement therapy in conditions associated with a deficiency or absence of endogenous testosterone;
  a. Primary hypogonadism (congenital or acquired)—testicular failure due to cryptorchidism, bilateral torsion, orchitis, vanishing testis syndrome; or orchidectomy.
  b. Hypogonadotropic hypogonadism (congenital or acquired)—idiopathic gonadotropin or LHRH deficiency, or pituitary-hypothalamic injury from tumors, trauma, or radiation.
If the above conditions occur prior to puberty, androgen therapy will be needed during the adolescent years for development of secondary sexual characteristics. Prolonged androgen treatment will be required to maintain sexual characteristics in these and other males who develop testosterone deficiency after puberty.
  c. Androgens may be used to stimulate puberty in carefully selected males with clearly delayed puberty. These patients usually have a familial pattern of delayed puberty that is not secondary to a pathological disorder; puberty is expected to occur spontaneously at a relatively late date. Brief treatment with conservative doses may occasionally be justified to these patients if they do not respond to psychological support. The potential adverse effect on bone maturation should be discussed with the patient and parents prior to androgen adminstration. An X-ray of the hand and wrist to determine bone age should be obtained every 6 months to assess the effect of treatment on the epiphyseal centers (see WARNINGS).

2. Females
Androgens may be used secondarily in women with advancing inoperable metastatic (skeletal) mammary cancer who are 1 to 5 years postmenopausal. Primary goals of therapy in these women include ablation of the ovaries. Other methods of counteracting estrogen activity are adrenalectomy, hypophysectomy, and/or antiestrogen therapy. This treatment has also been used in premenopausal women with breast cancer who have benefited from oophorectomy and are considered to have a hormone-responsive tumor. Judgment concerning androgen therapy should be made by an oncologist with expertise in this field.

Methyltestosterone has been used for the management of postpartum breast pain and engorgement.

Contraindications: Androgens are contraindicated in men with carcinomas of the breast or with known or suspected carcinomas of the prostate, and in women who are or may become pregnant. When administered to pregnant women, androgens cause virilization of the external genitalia of the female fetus. This virilization includes clitoromegaly, abnormal vaginal development, and fusion of genital folds to form a scrotal-like structure. The degree of masculinization is related to the amount of drug given and the age of the fetus, and is most likely to occur in the female fetus when the drugs are given in the first trimester. If the patient becomes pregnant while taking these drugs, she should be apprised of the potential hazard to the fetus.

Warnings: In patients with breast cancer, androgen therapy may cause hypercalcemia by stimulating osteolysis. In the case, the drug should be discontinued.

Prolonged use of high doses of androgens has been associated with the development of peliosis hepatis and hepatic neoplasms including hepatocellular carcinoma. (See PRECAUTIONS-Carcinogenesis). Peliosis hepatis can be a life-threatening or fatal complication.

Cholestatic hepatitis and jaundice occur with 17-alpha-alkylandrogens at a relatively low dose. If cholestatic hepatitis with jaundice appears or if liver function tests become abnormal, the androgen should be discontinued and the etiology should be determined. Drug-induced jaundice is reversible when the medication is discontinued.

Geriatric patients treated with androgens may be at an increased risk for the development of prostatic hypertrophy and prostatic carcinoma. Edema with or without congestive heart failure may be a serious complication in patients with preexisting cardiac, renal, or hepatic disease. In addition to discontinuation of the drug, diuretic therapy may be required.

Gynecomastia frequently develops and occasionally persists in patients being treated for hypogonadism.

Androgen therapy should be used cautiously in healthy males with delayed puberty. The effect on bone maturation should be monitored by assessing bone age of the wrist and hand every 6 months. In children, androgen treatment may accelerate bone maturation without producing compensatory gain in linear growth.

These adverse effects may result in compromised adult stature. The younger the child the greater the risk of compromising final mature height.

Precautions:
General
Women should be observed for signs of virilization (deepening of the voice, hirsutism, acne, clitoromegaly and menstrual irregularities). Discontinuation of drug therapy at the time of evidence of mild virilism is necessary to prevent irreversible virilization. Such virilization is usual following

Continued on next page

ICN Pharmaceuticals—Cont.

androgen use at high doses. A decision may be made by the patient and the physician that some virilization will be tolerated during treatment for breast carcinoma.

Information for the Patient
The physician should instruct patients to report any of the following side effects of androgens:

Adult or Adolescent Males:	Too frequent or persistent erections of the penis.
Women:	Hoarseness, acne, changes in menstrual periods, or more hair on the face.
All Patients:	Any nausea, vomiting, changes in skin color or ankle swelling.

Laboratory Tests
1. Women with disseminated breast carcinoma should have frequent determination of urine and serum calcium levels during the course of androgen therapy. (See WARNINGS).
2. Because of the hepatotoxicity associated with the use of 17-alpha-alkylated androgens, liver function tests should be obtained periodically.
3. Periodic (every 6 months) x-ray examinations of bone age should be made during treatment of prepubertal males to determine the rate of bone maturation and the effects of androgen therapy on the epiphyseal centers.
4. Hemoglobin and hematocrit should be checked periodically for polycythemia in patients who are receiving high doses of androgens.

Drug Interactions
1. **Anticoagulants:** C-17 substituted derivatives of testosterone, such as methandrostenolone, have been reported to decrease the anticoagulant requirements of patients receiving oral anticoagulants. Patients receiving oral anticoagulant therapy require close monitoring, especially when androgens are started or stopped.
2. **Oxyphenbutazone:** Concurrent administration of oxyphenbutazone and androgens may result in elevated serum levels of oxyphenbutazone.
3. **Insulin:** In diabetic patients the metabolic effects of androgens may decrease blood glucose and insulin requirements.

Drug/Laboratory Test Interferences
Androgens may decrease levels of thyroxine-binding globulin, resulting in decreased total T4 serum levels and increased resin uptake of T3 and T4. Free thyroid hormone levels remain unchanged, however, and there is no clinical evidence of thyroid dysfunction.

Carcinogenesis
Animal Data
Testosterone has been tested by subcutaneous injection and implantation in mice and rats. The implant induced cervical-uterine tumors in mice, which metastasized in some cases. There is suggestive evidence that injection of testosterone into some strains of female mice increases their susceptibility to hepatoma. Testosterone is also known to increase the number of tumors and decrease the degree of differentiation of chemically induced carcinomas of the liver in rats.

Human Data
There are rare reports of hepatocellular carcinoma in patients receiving long-term therapy with androgens in high doses. Withdrawal of the drugs did not lead to regression of the tumors in all cases. Geriatric patients treated with androgens may be at an increased risk for the development of prostatic hypertrophy and prostatic carcinoma.

Pregnancy
Teratogenic effects. Pregnancy Category X (See CONTRAINDICATIONS).

Nursing Mothers
It is not known whether androgens are excreted in human milk. Because many drugs are excreted in human milk and because of the potential for serious adverse reactions in nursing infants from androgens, a decision should be made whether to discontinue nursing or to discontinue the drug, taking into account the importance of the drug to the mother.

Pediatric Use
Androgen therapy should be used very cautiously in children and only by specialists who are aware of the adverse effects on bone maturation. Skeletal maturation must be monitored every six months by an x-ray of hand and wrist (See INDICATIONS AND USAGE and WARNINGS).

Adverse Reactions:
Endocrine and Urogenital
Female: The most common side effects of androgen therapy are amenorrhea and other menstrual irregularities, inhibition of gonadotropin secretion, and virilization, including deepening of the voice and clitoral enlargement. The latter usually is not reversible after androgens are discontinued. When administered to a pregnant woman androgens cause virilization of external genitalia of the female fetus.
Male: Gynecomastia, and excessive frequency and duration of penile erections. Oligospermia may occur at high dosages (see CLINICAL PHARMACOLOGY).
Skin and appendages: Hirsutism, male pattern of baldness, and acne.
Fluid and Electrolyte Disturbances: Retention of sodium, chloride, water, potassium, calcium, and inorganic phosphates.
Gastrointestinal: Nausea, cholestatic jaundice, alterations in liver function tests, rarely hepatocellular neoplasms and peliosis hepatis (see WARNINGS).
Hematologic: Suppression of clotting factors II, V, VII, and X, bleeding in patients on concomitant anticoagulant therapy, and polycythemia.
Nervous System: Increased or decreased libido, headache, anxiety, depression, and generalized paresthesia.
Metabolic: Increased serum cholesterol.
Miscellaneous: Inflammation and pain at the site of intramuscular injection or subcutaneous implantation of testosterone containing pellets, stomatitis with buccal preparation, and rarely anaphylactoid reactions.

Overdosage: There have been no reports of acute overdosage with the androgens.

Dosage and Administration: Androgens are administered as oral capsules. The suggested dosage for androgens varies depending on the age, sex, and diagnosis of the individual patient. Dosage is adjusted according to the patient's response and the appearance of adverse reactions. Replacement therapy in androgen-deficient males is 10–50 mg. of methyltestosterone daily. Various dosage regimens have been used to induce pubertal changes in hypogonadal males; some experts have advocated lower dosages initially, gradually increasing the dose as puberty progresses, with or without a decrease to maintenance levels. Other experts emphasize that higher dosages are needed to induce pubertal changes and lower dosages can be used for maintenance after puberty. The chronological and skeletal ages must be taken into consideration, both in determining the initial dose and in adjusting the dose.
Doses used in delayed puberty generally are in the range of 10 mg. of methyltestosterone daily, and for a limited duration, for example, 4 to 6 months.
Suggested dosages of oral methyltestosterone for use in the prevention of postpartum breast pain and engorgement is 80 mg. daily for 3 to 5 days after delivery.
Women with metastatic breast carcinoma must be followed closely because androgen therapy occasionally appears to accelerate the disease. Thus, many experts prefer to use the shorter acting androgen preparations rather than those with prolonged activity for treating breast carcinoma. The dosage of methyltestosterone for androgen therapy in breast carcinoma in females is from 50–200 mg. daily.

How Supplied: Red capsules branded on both sections ICN 0901 containing 10 mg. of methyltestosterone in bottles of 100, 500, and 1000.
CAUTION: Federal (U.S.A.) law prohibits dispensing without prescription.

Revision February 1983

Ives Laboratories Inc.
685 THIRD AVENUE
NEW YORK, NY 10017

CERUBIDINE®   ℞
[sīrew" bi" dēan]
(daunorubicin hydrochloride)
For injection

> **WARNINGS**
> 1. Cerubidine must be given into a rapidly flowing intravenous infusion. It must *never* be given by the intramuscular or subcutaneous route. Severe local tissue necrosis will occur if there is extravasation during administration.
> 2. Myocardial toxicity manifested in its most severe form by potentially fatal congestive heart failure may be encountered when total cumulative dosage exceeds 550 mg/m^2 in adults, 300 mg/m^2 in children more than 2 years of age, or 10 mg/kg in children less than two years of age.
> This may occur either during therapy or several months after termination of therapy. Treatment with digitalis, diuretics, sodium restriction, and bed-rest is indicated.
> 3. Severe myelosuppression occurs when used in therapeutic doses.
> 4. It is recommended that Cerubidine be administered only by physicians who are experienced in leukemia chemotherapy and in facilities with laboratory and supportive resources adequate to monitor drug tolerance and protect and maintain a patient compromised by drug toxicity. The physician and institution must be capable of responding rapidly and completely to severe hemorrhagic conditions, and/or overwhelming infection.
> 5. Dosage should be reduced in patients with impaired hepatic or renal function.

Description: Cerubidine (daunorubicin hydrochloride) is the hydrochloride salt of an anthracycline cytotoxic antibiotic produced by a strain of *Streptomyces coeruleorubidus*. It is provided as a sterile reddish lyophilized powder in vials for intravenous administration only. Each vial contains 20 mg of base activity (21.4 mg as the hydrochloride salt) and 100 mg of mannitol. It is soluble in water when adequately agitated and produces a reddish solution. It has the following structural formula which may be described with the chemical name of 7-(3-amino-2,3,6-trideoxy-L-lyxohexosyloxy) -9-acetyl-7,8,9,10-tetrahydro-6,9,11-trihydroxy-4-methoxy-5,12-naphthacenequinone hydrochloride. Its empirical formula is $C_{27}H_{29}NO_{10} \cdot HCl$ with a molecular weight of 563.99. It is a hygroscopic crystalline powder. The pH of a 5 mg/ml aqueous solution is 4.5–6.5.

STRUCTURAL FORMULA

Action: Cerubidine inhibits the synthesis of nucleic acids; its effect on deoxyribonucleic acid is particularly rapid and marked. Cerubidine has antimitotic and cytotoxic activity although the precise mode of action is unknown. Cerubidine displays an immuno-suppressive effect. It has been shown to inhibit the production of heterohemagglutinins in mice. *In vitro*, it inhibits blast cell transformation of canine lymphocytes at 0.01 mcg/ml.
Cerubidine possesses a potent antitumor effect against a wide spectrum of animal tumors either grafted or spontaneous.

Pharmacology: Following intravenous injection of Cerubidine, plasma levels of daunorubicin decline rapidly indicating rapid tissue uptake and concentration. Thereafter, plasma levels decline slowly with a half-life of 18.5 hours. By 1 hour after drug administration, the predominant plasma species is daunorubicinol, an active metabolite, which disappears with a half-life of 26.7 hours. Further metabolism via reduction cleavage of the glycosidic bond, 4-0 demethylation, and conjugation with both sulfate and glucuronide have been demonstrated. Simple glycosidic cleavage of daunorubicin or daunorubicinol is not a significant metabolic pathway in man. Twenty-five percent of an administered dose of Cerubidine is eliminated in an active form by urinary excretion, and an estimated 40% by biliary excretion.
There is no evidence that Cerubidine crosses the blood-brain barrier.

Indications and Usage: Cerubidine (daunorubicin hydrochloride) has been successfully used for remission induction in acute non-lymphocytic leukemia (myelogenous, monocytic, erythroid) of adults and as part of a remission induction program in acute lymphocytic leukemia of children.
In the treatment of acute non-lymphocytic leukemia, Cerubidine used as a single agent has produced complete remission rates of 40–50%, and in combination with cytarabine, has produced complete remission rates of 53–65%.
The addition of Cerubidine to the two drug induction regimen of vincristine-prednisone in the treatment of childhood acute lymphocytic leukemia does not increase the rate of complete remission. In children receiving only CNS prophylaxis and maintenance therapy (without consolidation) after induction, there is a prolongation of complete remission duration in those children induced with the three drug (Cerubidine-vincristine-prednisone) regimen as compared to two drugs (five-year disease-free survival 52% (three drugs) vs. 26% (two drugs), p < 0.02). There is no evidence of any impact of Cerubidine on the duration of complete remission when a consolidation (intensification) phase is employed as part of a total treatment program.

Warnings: Therapy with Cerubidine should not be started in patients with pre-existing drug-induced bone marrow suppression unless the benefit from such treatment warrants the risk.
Pre-existing heart disease and previous therapy with doxorubicin are co-factors of increased risk of Cerubidine-induced cardiac toxicity and the benefit to risk ratio of Cerubidine therapy in such patients should be weighed before starting Cerubidine.

Bone Marrow—Cerubidine is a potent bone marrow suppressant. Suppression will occur in all patients given a therapeutic dose of this drug.
Cardiac Effects[1-6]—Special attention must be given to the potential cardiac toxicity of Cerubidine, particularly in infants and children. *In adults* at total cumulative doses less than 550 mg/m^2, acute congestive heart failure is seldom encountered. However, rare instances of pericarditis-myocarditis, not dose-related, have been reported.
In adults, at cumulative doses exceeding 550 mg/m^2, there is an increased incidence of drug-induced congestive heart failure. Based on prior clinical experience with doxorubicin, this limit appears lower, namely 400 mg/m^2, in patients who received radiation therapy that encompassed the heart.
In infants and children, there appears to be a greater susceptibility to anthracycline-induced cardiotoxicity compared to that in adults, which is more clearly dose-related. However, there is very little risk for children over 2 years of age in developing Cerubidine-related cardiotoxicity below a cumulative dose of 300 mg/m^2 or in children less than 2 years of age (or < 0.5m^2 body surface area) below a cumulative dose of 10 mg/kg. In both children and adults, the total dose of Cerubidine administered should also take into account any previous or concomitant therapy with other potentially cardiotoxic agents or related compounds such as doxorubicin.

There is absolutely no reliable method of predicting the patients in whom acute congestive heart failure will develop as a result of the cardiac toxic effect of Cerubidine. However, certain changes in the electrocardiogram and a decrease in the systolic ejection fraction from pre-treatment baseline may help to recognize those patients at greatest risk to develop congestive heart failure. On the basis of the electrocardiogram, a decrease equal to or greater than 30% in limb lead QRS voltage has been associated with a significant risk of drug-induced cardiomyopathy. Therefore, an electrocardiogram and/or determination of systolic ejection fraction should be performed before each course of Cerubidine. In the event that one or the other of these predictive parameters should occur, the benefit of continued therapy must be weighed against the risk of producing cardiac damage.
Early clinical diagnosis of drug-induced congestive heart failure appears to be essential for successful treatment with digitalis, diuretics, sodium restriction, and bed rest.

Evaluation of Hepatic and Renal Function— Significant hepatic or renal impairment can enhance the toxicity of the recommended doses of Cerubidine (daunorubicin hydrochloride); therefore, prior to administration, evaluation of hepatic function and renal function using conventional clinical laboratory tests is recommended (see Dosage and Administration).

Pregnancy—Cerubidine can cause fetal harm when administered to a pregnant woman because of its teratogenic potential. If this drug is used during pregnancy, or if the patient becomes pregnant while taking this drug, the patient should be apprised of the potential hazard to the fetus.

Extravasation at Injection Site—Extravasation of Cerubidine at the site of intravenous administration can cause severe local tissue necrosis.

Precautions: Therapy with Cerubidine requires close observation of the patient and extensive chemical and laboratory monitoring.
Cerubidine may induce hyperuricemia secondary to rapid lysis of leukemic cells. Blood uric acid levels should be monitored and appropriate therapy initiated in the event that hyperuricemia develops.
Appropriate measures must be taken to control any systemic infection before beginning therapy with Cerubidine.
Cerubidine may transiently impart a red coloration to the urine after administration, and patients should be advised to expect this.

Carcinogenesis, Mutagenesis, Impairment of Fertility: Cerubidine, when injected subcutaneously into mice, causes fibrosarcomas to develop at the injection site. When administered to mice orally or intraperitoneally, no carcinogenic effect was noted after 22 months of observation.
In males dogs at a daily dose of 0.25 mg/kg administered intravenously, testicular atrophy was noted at autopsy. Histologic examination revealed total aplasia of the spermatocyte series in the seminiferous tubules with complete aspermatogenesis.

Pregnancy Category D. See Warnings Section.

Adverse Reactions: Dose-limiting toxicity includes myelosuppression and cardiotoxicity (see Warnings). Other reactions include:
Cutaneous—Reversible alopecia occurs in most patients.
Gastrointestinal—Acute nausea and vomiting occur but are usually mild. Antiemetic therapy may be of some help. Mucositis may occur three to seven days after administration. Diarrhea has occasionally been reported.
Local—If extravasation occurs during administration, tissue necrosis can result at the site.
Acute Reactions—Rarely fever, chills, and skin rash can occur.

Dosage and Administration:
Principles—In order to eradicate the leukemic cells and induce a complete remission, a profound suppression of the bone marrow is usually required. Evaluation of both the peripheral blood and bone marrow are mandatory in the formulation of appropriate treatment plans.

In the treatment of acute non-lymphocytic leukemia, Cerubidine is effective either alone or in combination with certain other antileukemic drugs. Combinations incorporating Cerubidine improve the complete remission frequency. Appropriate maintenance therapy should be instituted following the successful induction of a complete remission.
In the treatment of pediatric acute lymphocytic leukemia, induction of complete remission with Cerubidine-vincristine-prednisone (followed by maintenance therapy and appropriate central nervous system prophylaxis) increases the duration of continuous complete remission.
It is recommended that the dosage of Cerubidine be reduced in instances of hepatic or renal impairment. For example, using serum bilirubin and serum creatinine as indicators of liver and kidney function, the following dose modifications are recommended:

Serum Bilirubin	Serum Creatinine	Recommended Dose
1.2–3.0 mg%		¾ normal dose
> 3 mg%	> 3 mg%	½ normal dose

Representative dose schedules and combination for the approved indication of adult acute nonlymphocytic leukemia:
As a Single Agent[7]—Cerubidine (daunorubicin hydrochloride) 60 mg/m^2/day IV on days 1,2,3 every 3–4 weeks.
In Combination[8,9]—Cerubidine 45 mg/m^2/day IV on days 1,2,3 of the first course and on days 1,2 of subsequent courses **AND** cytosine arabinoside 100 mg/m^2/day IV infusion daily for 7 days for the first course and for 5 days for subsequent courses.
The attainment of a normal appearing bone marrow may require up to three courses of induction therapy. Evaluation of the bone marrow following recovery from the previous course of induction therapy determines whether a further course of induction treatment is required.

Representative dose schedule, in combination, for the approved indication of remission induction in pediatric acute lymphocytic leukemia.
In Combination[10,11]—Cerubidine 25 mg/m^2 IV on day 1 every week, vincristine 1.5 mg/m^2 IV on day 1 every week, prednisone 40 mg/m^2 PO daily. Generally, a complete remission will be obtained within four such courses of therapy; however, if after four courses the patient is in partial remission, an additional one or, if necessary, two courses may be given in an effort to obtain a complete remission.
In children less than 2 years of age or below 0.5 m^2 body surface area, calculation of dosage should be made on the basis of weight (mg/kg) instead of body surface area.[5]
The contents of a vial should be reconstituted with 4 ml of sterile water for injection, U.S.P., and agitated gently until the material has completely dissolved. The withdrawable vial contents provide 20 mg of daunorubicin activity, with 5 mg of daunorubicin activity per ml. The desired dose is withdrawn into a syringe containing 10–15 ml of normal saline and then injected into the tubing or sidearm of a rapidly flowing I.V. infusion of 5 percent glucose or normal saline solution. Cerubidine should not be administered mixed with other drugs or heparin. The reconstituted solution is stable for 24 hours at room temperature and 48 hours under refrigeration. It should be protected from exposure to sunlight.

How Supplied: Cerubidine (daunorubicin hydrochloride) for injection is available in butyl-stoppered vials, each containing 20 mg of base activity (21.4 mg as the hydrochloride salt) and 100 mg of mannitol as a sterile reddish lyophilized powder. When reconstituted with 4 ml of sterile water for injection, U.S.P., each ml contains 5 mg of daunorubicin activity. Each package contains 10 vials NDC 0082-4155-01.
Storage: (+15° to +25° C).

Continued on next page

Ives—Cont.

References:
1. Gilladoga AC, Manuel C Tan CTC, et al: The cardiotoxicity of adriamycin and daunomycin in children. Cancer 37:1070–1078, 1976.
2. Halzun JF, Wagner HR, Gaeta JF, et al: Daunorubicin cardiac toxicity in children with acute lymphocytic leukemia. Cancer 33:545–554, 1974.
3. Von Hoff DD, Rozenczweig M, Layard M, et al: Daunomycin-induced cardiotoxicity in children and adults: a review of 110 cases. Am J Med 62:200–208, 1977.
4. Goorin AM, Borow KM, Goldman A, Williams RG, Henderson IC, Sallan SE, Cohen H, Jaffe N: Congestive heart failure due to adriamycin cardiotoxicity: its natural history in children. Cancer 47:2810–2816, 1981.
5. Sallan SE; Personal communication, 1981.
6. Praga C, Bretta G, Vigo PL, et al: Adriamycin cardiotoxicity: A survey of 1273 patients. Cancer Treat Rep 63:827–834, 1979.
7. Wiernik PH, Schimpff SC, Schiffer CA et al: Randomized clinical comparison of daunorubicin (NSC-82151) alone with a combination of daunorubicin, cytosine arabinoside (NSC-63878), 6-Thioguanine (NSC-752) and pyrimethamine (NSC-3061) for the treatment of acute non-lymphocytic leukemia. Cancer Treat Rep 60:41–53, 1979.
8. Yates JW, Wallace JH, Ellison RR, Holland JF: Cytosine arabinoside (NSC-63878) and daunorubicin (NSC-83142) therapy in acute non-lymphocytic leukemia. Cancer Chemo Rep 57:485–488, 1973.
9. Rai KR, Holland JF, Glidewell O: Improvement in remission induction therapy of acute myelocytic leukemia. Proc. Am. Assoc. Cancer Res., Am Soc. Clin. Oncol. 16:265, 1975.
10. Aur RJA, Simone JV, Hustu HO, Verzosa MS: A comparative study of central nervous system irradiation and intensive chemotherapy early in remission of childhood acute lymphocytic leukemia. Cancer 29:381–391, 1972.
11. Mauer AM: Therapy for acute lymphoblastic leukemia of childhood: Blood 56:1–10, 1980.

[Cir. CI 3052-2 1/26/83]

CYCLOSPASMOL® ℞
[*cīclō″ spas″ mōl*]
(cyclandelate)
Capsules-Tablets

Composition: Each *blue* and *red* capsule contains 400 mg. of cyclandelate, and each *blue* capsule contains 200 mg. of cyclandelate. Each *orange* tablet contains 100 mg. cyclandelate.

Description: Cyclandelate is a white amorphous powder having a faint menthol-like odor. It is slightly soluble in water and highly soluble in ethyl alcohol and organic solvents. Cyclandelate has the following structural formula: 3,5,5,-trimethylcyclohexyl mandelate.

Actions: CYCLOSPASMOL is an orally acting vasodilator. The activity of this drug, as measured by pharmacological tests against various types of smooth-muscle spasm produced by acetylcholine, histamine, and barium chloride, exceeds that of papaverine, particularly in regard to the neurotropic component produced by the acetylcholine. Cyclandelate is musculotropic, acting directly on vascular smooth muscle, and has no significant adrenergic stimulating or blocking actions.

The drug is not intended to substitute for other appropriate medical or surgical programs in the treatment of peripheral or cerebral vascular disease.

Indications
Based on a review of this drug by the National Academy of Sciences—National Research Council and/or other information, FDA has classified the indications as follows:
"Possibly" effective: CYCLOSPASMOL is indicated for adjunctive therapy in intermittent claudication; arteriosclerosis obliterans; thrombophlebitis (to control associated vasospasm and muscular ischemia); nocturnal leg cramps; Raynaud's phenomenon; and for selected cases of ischemic cerebral vascular disease.
Final classification of the less-than-effective indications requires further investigation.

Contraindications: CYCLOSPASMOL is contraindicated in cases of known hypersensitivity to the drug.
Warnings: 1. Cyclandelate should be used with extreme caution in patients with severe obliterative coronary artery or cerebral-vascular disease, since there is a possibility that these diseased areas may be compromised by vasodilatory effects of the drug elsewhere. 2. **Use In Pregnancy:** The safety of cyclandelate for use during pregnancy or lactation has not been established; therefore, it should not be used in pregnant women or in women of childbearing age unless, in the judgment of the physician, its use is deemed absolutely essential to the welfare of the patient. 3. Although no prolongation of bleeding time has been demonstrated in humans in therapeutic dosages, it has been demonstrated in animals at very large doses. Therefore, the hazard of a prolonged bleeding time should be carefully considered when administering cyclandelate to a patient with active bleeding or a bleeding tendency.
Precautions: Since CYCLOSPASMOL (cyclandelate) is a vasodilator, it should be used with caution in patients having glaucoma.
Adverse Reactions: Gastrointestinal distress (pyrosis, pain, and eructation) may occur with CYCLOSPASMOL. These symptoms occur infrequently and are usually mild. Relief can often be obtained by taking the medication with meals or by the concomitant use of antacids.
Mild flush, headache, feeling of weakness, or tachycardia may occur, especially during the first weeks of administration.
Dosage and Administration: It is often advantageous to initiate therapy at higher dosage; e.g.: 1200-1600 mg. per day, given in divided doses before meals and at bedtime. When a clinical response is noted, the dosage can be decreased in 200-mg. decrements until the maintenance dosage is reached. The usual maintenance dosage of CYCLOSPASMOL (cyclandelate) is between 400 and 800 mg. per day given in two to four divided doses. Although objective signs of therapeutic benefit may be rapid and dramatic, more often, this improvement occurs gradually over weeks of therapy. It is strongly recommended that the patient be educated to the fact that prolonged use may be necessary. Short-term use of CYCLOSPASMOL is rarely beneficial, nor is it likely to be of any permanent value.
How Supplied: 400 mg. blue and red capsules in bottles of 100, and 500; and Clinipak®, Unit Dose Medication, 100 capsules (20 strips of 5). 200 mg. blue capsules in bottles of 100, 500, and 1000; and Clinipak®, Unit Dose Medication, 100 capsules (20 strips of 5); 100 mg. orange tablets in bottles of 100 and 500.
Literature Available: Yes.

[Cir. 3016-2 7/14/80]

Shown in Product Identification Section, page 413

ISORDIL® ℞
[*ī′ sore″ dil*]
(isosorbide dinitrate)
(1,4,3,6-dianhydro-sorbitol-2,5-dinitrate)

Description: Isordil has the following structural formula:

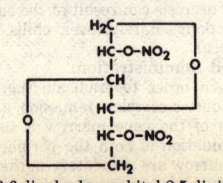

(1,4,3,6-dianhydro-sorbitol-2,5-dinitrate)

It is a white, crystalline, odorless compound, stable in air and in solution with a melting point of 70° C and optical rotation of + 134° (c = 1.0, alcohol, 20° C).

Actions: The basic action of Isordil is that of all nitrates, the relaxation of smooth muscle. How this relates to its clinical usefulness in the treatment of angina pectoris (pain of coronary-artery disease) is not clear, since the exact cause of this pain is also obscure.

The objective of therapy is a decrease in the frequency and severity of attacks of angina pectoris and a decrease in the need to use nitroglycerin. This is the only practical way to judge the effects of therapy, especially since there is a wide variation in symptomatic response to treatment. Isordil is widely accepted as a safe and useful therapeutic agent in the treatment of angina pectoris.

Indications
Based on a review of this drug by the National Academy of Sciences—National Research Council and/or other information, FDA has classified the indications as follows:
"Probably" effective: When taken by the sublingual or chewable route, Isordil Sublingual and Chewable Tablets are indicated for the treatment of acute anginal attacks and for prophylaxis in situations likely to provoke such attacks.

"Possibly" effective: When taken by the oral route, Isordil is indicated for the relief of angina pectoris (pain of coronary-artery disease). It is not intended to abort the acute anginal episode but is widely regarded as useful in the prophylactic treatment of angina pectoris.
Final classification of the less-than-effective indications requires further investigation.

Contraindication: Idiosyncrasy to this drug.
Warnings: Data supporting the use of nitrites and nitrates during the early days of the acute phase of myocardial infarction (the period during which clinical and laboratory findings are unstable) are insufficient to establish safety.
Precautions:
1. Tolerance to this drug and cross-tolerance to other nitrites and nitrates may occur.
2. In patients with functional or organic gastrointestinal hypermotility or malabsorption syndrome, it is suggested that either the Isordil 5 mg, 10 mg, 20 mg, or 30 mg Oral Titradose® tablets, Isordil 2.5 mg, 5 mg, or 10 mg Sublingual tablets, 10 mg Isordil Chewable tablets, or 40 mg Isordil Tembids® **capsules** be the preferred therapy. The reason for this is that a few patients have reported passing partially dissolved Isordil Tembids **tablets** in their stools. This phenomenon is believed to be on the basis of physiologic variability and to reflect rapid gastrointestinal transit of the tablet.

Adverse Reactions:
1. Cutaneous vasodilation with flushing.
2. Headache is common and may be severe and persistent.
3. Transient episodes of dizziness and weakness, as well as other signs of cerebral ischemia associated with postural hypotension, may occasionally develop.
4. This drug can act as a physiological antagonist to norepinephrine, acetylcholine, histamine, and many other agents.
5. An occasional individual exhibits marked sensitivity to the hypotensive effects of nitrite, and severe responses (nausea, vomiting, weakness, restlessness, pallor, perspiration, and collapse) can occur even with the usual therapeutic dose. Alcohol may enhance this effect.
6. Drug rash and/or exfoliative dermatitis may occasionally occur.

Dosage and Administration: Isordil (Isosorbide Dinitrate) 2.5 mg, 5 mg, and 10 mg Sublingual Tablets. The basic dosage is one 5 mg or 10 mg tablet every 2 to 3 hours. The 2.5 mg tablet facilitates adjustment of dosage in patients who may require it. All dosage forms are used sublingually for treatment of an angina pectoris attack (including angina decubitus) or prophylactically in situations likely to provoke such attacks.

Isordil 10 mg Chewable tablets. The smallest effective dose should be used. The initial dose should be no more than 5 mg ($\frac{1}{2}$ tablet) as an occasional severe hypotensive response may occur. The low dose may be effective in relieving the acute attack, but if no significant hypotension is seen, an increase in dose may permit more effective prevention of attacks. The chewable tablet is scored to permit dosage adjustment. For relief of the acute attack, the medication may be taken p.r.n. For prophylaxis, it may be taken every 2–3 hours.

Isordil 5 mg, 10 mg, 20 mg, or 30 mg Oral Titradose Tablets with E.Z. Split® scoring are administered orally. The dosage range is 5 mg to 30 mg q.i.d., with the usual dosage being 10 mg to 20 mg q.i.d., before meals and at bedtime.

The uniquely designed and patented **Titradose E.Z. Split** Oral Tablet dosage forms permit clean-cut splitting of the tablet into equal halves to simplify more accurate dosage titration. Thus, the physician may prescribe (or adjust) a dosage regimen to include half-tablet units for optimal relief. To break the tablet into two even halves, the patient has only to place the tablet on a hard, flat surface, scored side up, and then press the scored surface lightly with the index finger or thumb. Isordil Oral 5 mg, 10 mg, 20 mg, and 30 mg. **Titradose** Tablets replace the former, conventionally-scored tablets.

Isordil Tembids Tablets, 40 mg, and
Isordil Tembids Capsules, 40 mg.

These sustained-action medications are administered orally every 6 to 12 hours according to need. They are indicated for sustained prophylaxis against angina pectoris attacks including nocturnal angina. Although the latter condition is relatively infrequent, it is nonetheless angina, i.e., pain of coronary-artery disease. The drug is gradually released over a 6-hour period to provide 8–10 hours of sustained effect. Although experiencing a reduction in the number of anginal attacks while under Tembids therapy, patients may still have an attack under stressful conditions. In such cases, the therapy should be supplemented with Sublingual Isordil tablets or nitroglycerin. ISORDIL TEMBIDS SHOULD NOT BE CHEWED.

How Supplied:
Isordil Sublingual, 2.5 mg: Supplied in bottles of 100 and 500 yellow tablets.
Isordil Sublingual, 5 mg: Supplied in bottles of 100, 250, and 500 pink tablets.
Isordil® Sublingual, 10 mg: Supplied in bottles of 100 white tablets.
Isordil Chewable, 10 mg: Supplied in bottles of 100 scored, yellow tablets.
Isordil Oral Titradose®, 5 mg: Supplied in bottles of 100, 500, and 1000 scored, pink tablets.
Isordil Oral Titradose, 10 mg: Supplied in bottles of 100, 500, and 1000 scored, white tablets.
Isordil Oral Titradose, 20 mg: Supplied in bottles of 100 and 500 scored, green tablets.
Isordil Oral Titradose, 30 mg: Supplied in bottles of 100 and 500 scored, blue tablets.
Isordil Tembids® Tablets, 40 mg: Supplied in bottles of 100, 500, and 1000 scored, green, sustained-action tablets.
Isordil Tembids Capsules, 40 mg: Supplied in bottles of 100 and 500 sustained-action capsules (opaque blue cap and colorless, transparent body).
Clinipak® Unit Dose Medication, Boxes of 100 Tablets (20 strips of 5), is available as:
Isordil Sublingual Tablets, 2.5 mg
Isordil Sublingual Tablets, 5 mg
Isordil Sublingual Tablets, 10 mg
Isordil Chewable Tablets, 10 mg
Isordil Oral Titradose, 5 mg
Isordil Oral Titradose, 10 mg
Isordil Oral Titradose, 20 mg
Isordil Oral Titradose, 30 mg

Animal Pharmacology and Toxicology: Isordil (Isosorbide Dinitrate) has a solubility comparable to that of nitroglycerin. Its aqueous solubility is 1089 mcg/ml as compared to 1250 mcg/ml for nitroglycerin and 1.5 mcg/ml for pentaerythritol tetranitrate (PETN). The drug is also highly soluable in lipids.

The oral toxicity of isosorbide dinitrate was studied in rats and dogs. Following oral administration of the drug in rats, the acute oral LD_{50} was found to be approximately 1,100 mg/kg of body weight. Thus, the toxicity is low. These animal experiments indicate that approximately 500 times the usual therapeutic dose would be required to produce such toxic symptoms in humans.

Chronic oral toxicity was determined in rats and dogs. The following dosage levels were employed in the chronic toxicity studies:

Rats—control,
0.2%(weight of drug×100), 0.1%, and 0.05%. weight of food
Dogs—100 mg/kg, 50 mg/kg, and control.

Male rats and dogs at the highest dosage level showed a decrease in growth curve as compared to control animals and animals in the lower dosage groups. Histological examination of the tissues did not reveal evidence of toxic injury. There was no evidence of an effect on bone marrow, or the hematopoietic system nor the peripheral blood. Examination of blood samples in dogs for the presence of methemoglobin failed to reveal a significant level of the pigment. Studies in humans confirmed that the drug does not produce methemoglobinemia in the clinical doses.

Administration of the drug to anesthetized dogs via either the femoral vein or via the splenic vein produced comparable falls in blood pressure without markedly affecting respiration. This is in definite contrast to nitroglycerin which requires about 20 times more drug to lower blood pressure when injected into a vein which empties into the portal circulation, such as the splenic, than into a vein which bypasses the portal circulation, such as the femoral. These observations suggest thst isosorbide dinitrate, in contrast to nitroglycerin, is not rapidly inactivated by the liver.

The rate of inactivation of isosorbide dinitrate by fresh liver slices was determined, and the drug was found to be metabolized much more slowly than nitroglycerin. Another study of the enzymatic degradation of the organic nitrates confirmed that both isosorbide dinitrate and pentaerythritol tetranitrate were slowly inactivated by fresh liver enzymes.

The role of nitrates as "benign" coronary dilators has been questioned and the suggestion made that their effects are secondary to increased myocardial oxygen consumption. To clarify this relationship, an investigator prepared dogs so that coronary blood flow could be varied independently of aortic pressure. The left main coronary artery of the dog heart in situ was cannulated and perfused by a pump which delivered fixed rates of flow. Flow rates were selected that provided adequate perfusion to the normally beating heart. Flow was then decreased in stepwise decrements until a state of "coronary insufficiency" was produced. At this point there is an abrupt rise in left atrial pressure, maximal arterial-venous oxygen extraction, increased lactate production, and decreased coronary-vascular resistance. Intracoronary injection of isosorbide dinitrate or nitroglycerin caused a further decrease in coronary-vascular pressure and calculated coronary-vascular resistance without an accompanying change in coronary sinus pO_2. These effects were more marked at rates of adequate perfusion than at inadequate rates. Thus nitroglycerin or isosorbide dinitrate produces coronary vasodilation, without increased myocardial oxygen consumption, suggesting that the vasodilating action of these drugs is therefore not dependent upon this effect.

Clinical Studies: Isordil (Isosorbide Dinitrate) is widely regarded as an effective, long-acting coronary vasodilator for the management of angina pectoris associated with coronary insufficiency. It may significantly reduce the number, duration, and severity of angina attacks. Exercise tolerance may be increased in some patients with all forms of Isordil. The 5 mg sublingual tablet, however, provides greater benefit both in regard to the number of patients who respond to it and the amount of exercise tolerated. Clinical improvement has been customarily measured subjectively by reduction in number of angina attacks and by the change in nitroglycerin requirements.

The 5 mg Isordil Sublingual tablet has been evaluated clinically, and by employing exercise-tolerance tests, it has been found that this dosage has an onset of action within the range of 2 to 5 minutes, which in some instances is not as rapid as nitroglycerin (but almost equal in magnitude). Duration of action, however, ranges from 1 to 2 hours, which compares with a duration of action of 20 to 30 minutes in the case of nitroglycerin. Kinetocardiographic clinical studies indicate that the 10 mg oral tablets and 40 mg Tembids tablets are effective for prolonged periods. Exercise-tolerance tests have similarly shown that 40 mg Tembids capsules are effective for at least 6 hours.

In patients subjected to emotional or physical stress, the oral 5 mg, 10 mg, 20 mg, 30 mg, and 40 mg Isordil medications are of limited effectiveness. In situations where the patient may be exposed to unusual stress, it is suggested that the 2.5 mg, 5 mg, or 10 mg Isordil Sublingual tablets or 10 mg Chewable tablets be used supplementally as required.

Cinecoronary arteriographic studies have demonstrated that Isordil can produce a marked dilatation of the larger branches of the coronary arteries (larger than 200 microns). Dilatation of these coronary arteries and collateral coronary arteries persists for more than 2 hours after Sublingual Isordil, as demonstrated by cinecoronary arteriography. The correlation of this demonstrated dilation to increased coronary flow or improvement in clinical angina has not been established.

Bibliography: A bibliography on Isordil is available on request.

U S Pat Nos. 3883647 and
D224591 (Titradose®)
Manufactured for
IVES LABORATORIES INC.
NEW YORK, NY 10017
By WYETH LABORATORIES INC.
PHILA., PA 19101
Only Isordil Tembids Capsules manufactured by
K-V PHARMACEUTICAL CO.
ST. LOUIS, MO 63144
[Cir. CI3020-6]—Rev. July, 17, 1984]
Shown in Product Identification Section, pages 413

SURMONTIL®
[sir' mon" til]   ℞
(trimipramine maleate)
Description: Surmontil (trimipramine maleate) is 5-(3-dimethylamino-2-methylpropyl)-10,11-dihydro-5H-dibenz (b,f) azepine acid maleate (racemic form).

MOLECULAR FORMULA: $C_{20}H_{26}N_2 \cdot C_4H_4O_4$
MOLECULAR WEIGHT: 410.5

Trimipramine maleate is prepared as a racemic mixture which can be resolved into levorotatory and dextrorotatory isomers. The asymmetric center responsible for optical isomerism is marked in the formula by an asterisk. Trimipramine maleate is an almost odorless, white or slightly cream-colored, crystalline substance, melting at 140–144°C. It is very slightly soluble in ether and water, is slightly soluble in ethyl alcohol and acetone, and freely soluble in chloroform and methanol at 20°C.

Clinical Pharmacology: Surmontil is an antidepressant with an anxiety-reducing sedative component to its action. The mode of action of Surmontil on the central nervous system is not known. However, unlike amphetamine-type compounds it does not act primarily by stimulation of the central nervous system. It does not act by inhibition of the monoamine oxidase system.

Continued on next page

Ives—Cont.

Indications: Surmontil is indicated for the relief of symptoms of depression. Endogenous depression is more likely to be alleviated than other depressive states. In studies with neurotic outpatients, the drug appeared to be equivalent to amitriptyline in the less-depressed patients but somewhat less effective than amitriptyline in the more severely depressed patients. In hospitalized depressed patients, trimipramine and imipramine were equally effective in relieving depression.

Contraindications: Surmontil is contraindicated in cases of known hypersensitivity to the drug. The possibility of cross-sensitivity to other dibenzazepine compounds should be kept in mind. Surmontil should not be given in conjunction with drugs of the monoamine oxidase inhibitor class (e.g., tranylcypromine, isocarboxazid or phenelzine sulfate). The concomitant use of monoamine oxidase inhibitors (MAOI) and tricyclic compounds similar to Surmontil has caused severe hyperpyretic reactions, convulsive crises, and death in some patients. At least two weeks should elapse after cessation of therapy with MAOI before instituting therapy with Surmontil. Initial dosage should be low and increased gradually with caution and careful observation of the patient. The drug is contraindicated during the acute recovery period after a myocardial infarction.

Warnings:
Use in Children—This drug is not recommended for use in children, since safety and effectiveness in the pediatric age group have not been established.

General Consideration for Use—Extreme caution should be used when this drug is given to patients with any evidence of cardiovascular disease because of the possibility of conduction defects, arrhythmias, myocardial infarction, strokes, and tachycardia.

Caution is advised in patients with increased intraocular pressure, history of urinary retention, or history of narrow-angle glaucoma because of the drug's anticholinergic properties; hyperthyroid patients or those on thyroid medication because of the possibility of cardiovascular toxicity; patients with a history of seizure disorder, because this drug has been shown to lower the seizure threshold; patients receiving guanethidine or similar agents, since Surmontil may block the pharmacologic effects of these drugs.

Since the drug may impair the mental and/or physical abilities required for the performance of potentially hazardous tasks, such as operating an automobile or machinery, the patient should be cautioned accordingly.

Precautions: The possibility of suicide is inherent in any severely depressed patient and persists until a significant remission occurs. When a patient with a serious suicidal potential is not hospitalized, the prescription should be for the smallest amount feasible.

In schizophrenic patients activation of the psychosis may occur and require reduction of dosage or the addition of a major tranquilizer to the therapeutic regime.

Manic or hypomanic episodes may occur in some patients, in particular those with cyclic-type disorders. In some cases therapy with Surmontil must be discontinued until the episode is relieved, after which therapy may be reinstituted at lower dosages if still required.

Concurrent administration of Surmontil (trimipramine maleate) and electroshock therapy may increase the hazards of therapy. Such treatment should be limited to those patients for whom it is essential. When possible, discontinue the drug for several days prior to elective surgery.

Patients should be warned that the concomitant use of alcoholic beverages may be associated with exaggerated effects.

It has been reported that tricyclic antidepressants can potentiate the effects of catecholamines. Similarly, atropinelike effects may be more pronounced in patients receiving anticholinergic therapy. Therefore, particular care should be exercised when it is necessary to administer tricyclic antidepressants with sympathomimetic amines, local decongestants, local anesthetics containing epinephrine, atropine or drugs wih an anticholinergic effect. In resistant cases of depression in adults, a dose of 2.5 mg/kg/day may have to be exceeded. If a higher dose is needed, ECG monitoring should be maintained during the initiation of therapy and at appropriate intervals during stabilization of dose.

Usage in Pregnancy—Pregnancy Category C. Surmontil has shown evidence of embryotoxicity and/or increased incidence of major anomalies in rats or rabbits at doses 20 times the human dose. There are no adequate and well-controlled studies in pregnant women. Surmontil should be used during pregnancy only if the potential benefit justifies the potential risk to the fetus.

Semen studies in man (four schizophrenics and nine normal volunteers) revealed no significant changes in sperm morphology. It is recognized that drugs having a parasympathetic effect including tricyclic antidepressants, may alter the ejaculatory response.

Chronic animal studies showed occasional evidence of degeneration of seminiferous tubules at the highest dose of 60 mg/kg/day.

Surmontil should be used with caution in patients with impaired liver function.

Chronic animal studies showed occasional occurrence of hepatic congestion, fatty infiltration, or increased serum liver enzymes at the highest dose of 60 mg/kg/day.

Both elevation and lowering of blood sugar have been reported with tricyclic antidepressants.

Adverse Reactions:
Note: The pharmacological similarities among the tricyclic antidepressants require that each of the reactions be considered when Surmontil (trimipramine maleate) is administered. Some of the adverse reactions included in this listing have not in fact been reported with Surmontil.
Cardiovascular—Hypotension, hypertension, tachycardia, palpitation, myocardial infarction, arrhythmias, heart block, stroke.
Psychiatric—Confusional states (especially the elderly) with hallucinations, disorientation, delusions; anxiety, restlessness, agitation; insomnia and nightmares; hypomania; exacerbation of psychosis.
Neurological—Numbness, tingling, paresthesias of extremities; incoordination, ataxia, tremors, peripheral neuropathy; extrapyramidal symptoms; seizures, alterations in EEG patterns; tinnitus; syndrome of inappropriate ADH (antidiuretic hormone) secretion.
Anticholinergic—Dry mouth and, rarely, associated sublingual adenitis; blurred vision, disturbances of accommodation, mydriasis, constipation, paralytic ileus; urinary retention, delayed micturition, dilation of the urinary tract.
Allergic—Skin rash, petechiae, urticaria, itching, photosensitization, edema of face and tongue.
Hematologic—Bone-marrow depression including agranulocytosis, eosinophilia; purpura; thrombocytopenia. Leukocyte and differential counts should be performed in any patient who develops fever and sore throat during therapy; the drug should be discontinued if there is evidence of pathological neutrophil depression.
Gastrointestinal—Nausea and vomiting, anorexia, epigastric distress, diarrhea, peculiar taste, stomatitis, abdominal cramps, black tongue.
Endocrine—Gynecomastia in the male; breast enlargement and galactorrhea in the female; increased or decreased libido, impotence; testicular swelling; elevation or depression of blood-sugar levels.
Other—Jaundice (simulating obstructive); altered liver function; weight gain or loss; perspiration; flushing; urinary frequency; drowsiness, dizziness, weakness, and fatigue; headache; parotid swelling; alopecia.
Withdrawal Symptoms—Though not indicative of addiction, abrupt cessation of treatment after prolonged therapy may produce nausea, headache, and malaise.

Dosage and Administration: Dosage should be initiated at a low level and increased gradually, noting carefully the clinical response and any evidence of intolerance.

Lower dosages are recommended for elderly patients and adolescents. Lower dosages are also recommended for outpatients as compared to hospitalized patients who will be under close supervision. It is not possible to prescribe a single dosage schedule of Surmontil that will be therapeutically effective in all patients. The physical psychodynamic factors contributing to depressive symptomatology are very complex; spontaneous remissions or exacerbations of depressive symptoms may occur with or without drug therapy. Consequently, the recommended dosage regimens are furnished as a guide which may be modified by factors such as the age of the patient, chronicity and severity of the disease, medical condition of the patient, and degree of psychotherapeutic support.

Most antidepressant drugs have a lag period of ten days to four weeks before a therapeutic response is noted. Increasing the dose will not shorten this period but rather increase the incidence of adverse reactions.

Usual Adult Dose:
Outpatients and Office Patients—Initially, 75 mg/day in divided doses, increased to 150 mg/day. Dosages over 200 mg/day are not recommended. Maintenance therapy is in the range of 50–150 mg/day. For convenient therapy and to facilitate patient compliance, the total dosage requirement may be given at bedtime.
Hospitalized Patients—Initially, 100 mg/day in divided doses. This may be increased gradually in a few days to 200 mg/day, depending upon individual response and tolerance. If improvement does not occur in 2–3 weeks, the dose may be increased to the maximum recommended dose of 250–300 mg/day.
Adolescent and Geriatric Patients—Initially, a dose of 50 mg/day is recommended, with gradual increments up to 100 mg/day, depending upon patient response and tolerance.
Maintenance—Following remission, maintenance medication may be required for a longer period of time, at the lowest dose that will maintain remission. Maintenance therapy is preferably administered as a single dose at bedtime. To minimize relapse maintenance therapy should be continued for about three months.

Overdosage:
Signs and Symptoms—The response of the patient to toxic overdosage of tricyclic antidepressants may vary in severity and is conditioned by factors such as age, amount ingested, amount absorbed, interval between ingestion and start of treatment. Surmontil (trimipramine maleate) is not recommended for infants or young children. Should accidental ingestion occur in any amount, it should be regarded as serious and potentially fatal.

CNS abnormalities may include drowsiness, stupor, coma, ataxia, restlessness, agitation, hyperactive reflexes, muscle rigidity, athetoid and choreiform movements, and convulsions. Cardiac abnormalities may include arrhythmia, tachycardia, ECG evidence of impaired conduction, and signs of congestive failure. Other symptoms may include respiratory depression, cyanosis, hypotension, shock, vomiting, hyperpyrexia, mydriasis, and diaphoresis.

Treatment is supportive and symptomatic as no specific antidote is known. Depending upon need the following measures can be considered:

1. Surmontil is not recommended for use in infants and children. Hospitalization with continuous cardiac monitoring for up to 4 days is recommended for children who have ingested Surmontil in any amount. This is based on the reported greater sensitivity of children to acute overdosage with tricyclic antidepressants.
2. Blood and urine levels may not reflect the severity of the poisoning and are mostly of diagnostic value.

3. CNS involvement, respiratory depression, or cardiac arrhythmia can occur suddenly; hospitalization and close observation are necessary, even when the amount ingested is thought to be small or initial toxicity appears slight. Patients with any alteration of ECG should have continuous cardiac monitoring for at least 72 hours and be observed until well after the cardiac status has returned to normal; relapses may occur after apparent recovery.
4. The slow intravenous administration of physostigmine salicylate has been reported to reverse most of the cardiovascular and CNS effects of overdosage with tricyclic antidepressants. In adults, 1 to 3 mg has been reported to be effective. In children, start with 0.5 mg and repeat at 5-minute intervals to determine the minimum effective dose; do not exceed 2.0 mg. Avoid rapid injection, to reduce the possibility of physostigmine-induced convulsions. Because of the short duration of action of physostigmine, it may be necessary to repeat doses to 30- to 60-minute intervals as necessary.
5. In the alert patient, empty the stomach rapidly by induced emesis, followed by lavage. In the obtunded patient, secure the airway with a cuffed endotracheal tube before beginning lavage (do not induce emesis). Instillation of activated-charcoal slurry may help reduce absorption of trimipramine.
6. Minimize external stimulation to reduce the tendency to convulsions. If anticonvulsants are necessary, diazepam, short-acting barbiturates, paraldehyde, or methocarbamol may be useful. Do not use barbiturates if MAO inhibitors have been taken recently.
7. Maintain adequate respiratory exchange. Do not use respiratory stimulants.
8. Shock should be treated with supportive measures, such as intravenous fluids, oxygen, and corticosteroids. Digitalis may increase conduction abnormalities and further irritate an already sensitized myocardium. If congestive heart failure necessitates rapid digitalization, particular care must be exercised.
9. Hyperpyrexia should be controlled by whatever external means available, including ice packs and cooling sponge baths if necessary.
10. Hemodialysis, peritoneal dialysis, exchange transfusions, and forced diuresis have been generally reported as ineffective in tricyclic poisoning.

How Supplied: Surmontil® (trimipramine maleate) Capsules, Ives®, are available in the following dosage strengths:

25 mg, NDC 0082-4132, opaque blue and yellow capsule marked "Ives" and "4132" in bottles of 100 capsules and in Clinipak® cartons of 100 (20 strips of 5).

50 mg, NDC 0082-4133, opaque blue and orange capsule marked "Ives" and "4133" in bottles of 100 capsules and in Clinipak cartons of 100 (20 strips of 5).

100 mg, NDC 0082-4158, opaque, blue and white capsule marked "Ives" and "4158" in bottles of 100 capsules.

The appearance of these capsules is a trademark of Ives Laboratories.

Keep bottles tightly closed.
Dispense in tight containers.

Manufactured for
IVES LABORATORIES INC.
NEW YORK, NY 10017
By WYETH LABORATORIES INC.
PHILA., PA 19101

[Cir. C13407-1 Issued February 7, 1984]
Shown in Product Identification Section, page 413

SYNALGOS®-DC Capsules
[sĭn'ăl″gŏs]

Description: Each blue and gray capsule contains:
Drocode (dihydrocodeine)
bitartrate..16 mg
Warning—May be habit forming

Aspirin..356.4 mg
Caffeine ....30 mg

Actions: Dihydrocodeine is a semisynthetic narcotic analgesic, related to codeine, with multiple actions qualitatively similar to those of codeine; the most prominent of these involve the central nervous system and organs with smooth-muscle components. The principal action of therapeutic value is analgesia.
Synalgos-DC also contains the non-narcotic antipyretic-analgesic, aspirin.

Indications: For the relief of moderate to moderately severe pain.

Contraindications: Hypersensitivity to dihydrocodeine, codeine, or aspirin.

Warnings: Salicylates should be used with extreme caution in the presence of peptic ulcer or coagulation abnormalities.

Drug Dependence: Dihydrocodeine can produce drug dependence of the codeine type and therefore has the potential of being abused. Psychic dependence, physical dependence, and tolerance may develop upon repeated administration of dihydrocodeine, and it should be prescribed and administered with the same degree of caution appropriate to the use of other oral narcotic containing medications.
Like other narcotic-containing medications, dihydrocodeine is subject to the provisions of the Federal Controlled Substances Act.

Usage in Ambulatory Patients: Dihydrocodeine and may impair the mental and/or physical abilities required for the performance of potentially hazardous tasks such as driving a car or operating machinery. The patient using Synalgos-DC should be cautioned accordingly.

Interactions with other Central-Nervous-System Depressants: Patients receiving other narcotic analgesics, general anesthetics, tranquilizers, sedative-hypnotics or other CNS depressants (including alcohol) concomitantly with Synalgos-DC may exhibit an additive CNS depression. When such combined therapy is contemplated, the dose of one or both agents should be reduced.

Usage in Pregnancy: Reproduction studies have not been performed in animals. There is no adequate information on whether this drug may affect fertility in human males and females or has a teratogenic potential or other adverse effect on the fetus.

Usage in Children: Since there is no experience in children who have received this drug, safety and efficacy in children have not been established.

Precautions: Synalgos-DC should be given with caution to certain patients such as the elderly or debilitated.

Adverse Reactions: The most frequently observed reactions include light-headedness, dizziness, drowsiness, sedation, nausea, vomiting, constipation, pruritus, and skin reactions.

Dosage and Administration: Dosage should be adjusted according to the severity of the pain and the response of the patient. Synalgos-DC is given orally. The usual adult dose is two capsules every 4 hours as needed for pain.

Drug Interactions: The CNS depressant effects of Synalgos-DC may be additive with that of other CNS depressants.
See Warnings.
Aspirin may enhance the effects of anticoagulants and inhibit the uricosuric effects of uricosuric agents.

How Supplied: Synalgos®-DC Capsules, Ives®, are supplied in bottles of 100 and 500 capsules and in Clinipak® Unit Dose dispenser cartons of 25 capsules (DEA Schedule III):
NDC 0082-4191, blue and gray capsule marked "Ives" and "4191."
Store capsules below 25°C (77°F).
Keep bottles tightly closed.
Dispense in tight containers.

Manufactured for
IVES LABORATORIES INC.
NEW YORK, NY 10017
By WYETH LABORATORIES INC.
PHILA., PA 19101

CI 3347-1   Issued October 17, 1983

TRECATOR®-SC
[trek″ă'tōre]
(ethionamide)
Sugar-Coated Tablets

Description: Ethionamide is a yellow crystalline substance that is practically insoluble in water. It has a faint-to-moderate sulfide odor and is stable at all ordinary temperatures and levels of humidity.
Trecator has the following structural formula:

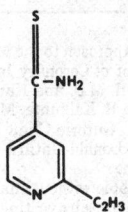

Action: Bacteriostatic against *Mycobacterium tuberculosis.*

Indications: Failure after adequate treatment with primary drugs (i.e. isoniazid, streptomycin, aminosalicylic acid) in any form of active tuberculosis. Ethionamide should only be given with other effective antituberculous agents.

Contraindications:
Severe hypersensitivity.
Severe hepatic damage.

Warning:
USE IN PREGNANCY: Teratogenic effects have been demonstrated in animals (rabbits, rats) receiving doses in excess of those recommended in humans. Use of the drug should be avoided during pregnancy or in women of childbearing potential, unless the benefits outweigh its possible hazard.
USE IN CHILDREN: Optimum dosage for children has not been established. This, however, does not preclude use of the drug when its use is crucial to therapy.

Precautions: Pretreatment examinations should include *in vitro* susceptibility tests of recent cultures of *M. tuberculosis* from the patient as measured against ethionomide and the usual primary antituberculous drugs.
Determinations of serum transaminase (SGOT, SGPT) should be made prior to and every 2 to 4 weeks during therapy.
In patients with diabetes mellitus, management may be more difficult and hepatitis occurs more frequently.
Ethionamide may intensify the adverse effects of the other antituberculous drugs administered concomitantly. Convulsions have been reported and special care should be taken, particularly when ethionamide is administered with cycloserine.

Adverse Reactions: The most common side effect is gastrointestinal intolerance.
Other adverse effects similar to those seen with isoniazid have been reported: peripheral neuritis, optic neuritis, psychic disturbances (including mental depression), postural hypotension, skin rashes, thrombocytopenia, pellagra-like syndrome, jaundice and/or hepatitis, increased difficulty in management of diabetes mellitus, stomatitis, gynecomastia, and impotence.

Dosage and Administration: Ethionamide should be administered with at least one other effective antituberculous drug.
Average adult dose: 0.5 gram to 1.0 gram/day in divided doses.
Concomitant administration of pyridoxine is recommended.

How Supplied: Trecator®-SC (ethionamide) Tablets, Ives®, are supplied as follows in bottles of 100 tablets:
250 mg, NDC 0082-4130, orange, sugar-coated tablet marked "Ives" and "4130."

Continued on next page

Ives—Cont.

Keep bottles tightly closed.
Dispense in tight containers.
Bibliography available upon request
[Cir. CI 3322-1—Revised June 7, 1983]

EDUCATIONAL MATERIAL

Film
"An Aggressive Approach to the Medical and Surgical Management of Coronary Insufficiency" by William H. Sewell, M.D. and Karlene V. Sewell, B.A. with Jagdish R. Kalkunte, M.D. and Edward V. Bennett, M.D., Guthrie Clinic and the Robert Packer Hospital, Donald Guthrie Foundation for Medical Research.
This film is available without charge for showing to physician audiences by writing to:

Ives Laboratories Inc.
685 Third Avenue
New York, N.Y. 10017

Jacobus Pharmaceutical Co., Inc.
P.O. BOX 5290
37 CLEVELAND LANE
PRINCETON, NJ 08540

DAPSONE USP ℞
[dap'sōne]
25 mg. & 100 mg.

Description: Dapsone-USP, 4-4' diaminodiphenylsulfone (DDS), is a primary treatment for Dermatitis herpetiformis. It is an effective antibacterial drug which has proved satisfactory in the treatment of leprosy. It is issued on prescription in tablets of 25 mg. and 100 mg. for oral administration.

Clinical Pharmacology:
Actions: The mechanism of action in Dermatitis herpetiformis has not been established.
By the kinetic method in mice, Dapsone is bactericidal as well as bacteriostatic against M. leprae.
Absorption and Excretion: Dapsone, when given orally, is rapidly and almost completely absorbed. About 85 percent of the daily intake is recoverable from the urine mainly in the form of water-soluble metabolites. Excretion of the drug is slow and a constant blood level can be maintained with the usual dosage.
Blood Levels: Detected a few minutes after ingestion, the drug reaches peak concentration in 4-8 hours. Daily administration for at least eight days is necessary to achieve a plateau level. With doses of 200 mg. daily, this level averaged 2.3 μgm/ml with a range of 0.1-7.0 μgm.
In man there are large individual differences in the rate of Dapsone clearance from the body. The half-life in the plasma in different individuals varies from ten hours to fifty hours and averages twenty eight hours. Repeat tests in the same individual show the clearance rate to be constant. Dapsone acetylation rates have been used to measure the acetylation phenotype. Daily administration (50-100 mg.) in leprosy patients will provide blood levels in excess of the usual minimum inhibitory concentration even for patients with a short Dapsone half-life.
Rifampicin lowers Dapsone levels 7 to 10 fold by accelerating plasma clearance.
Indications and Usage: Dermatitis herpetiformis (DH)
All forms of leprosy except for cases of proven Dapsone resistance.

Contraindication: Hypersensitivity to Dapsone and/or its derivatives.
Warnings: The patient should be warned to respond to the presence of clinical signs such as sore throat, fever, pallor, purpura or jaundice. Deaths associated with the administration of Dapsone have been reported from agranulocytosis, aplastic anemia and other blood dyscrasias.
Complete blood counts should be done frequently in patients receiving Dapsone. The FDA Dermatology Advisory Committee recommended that, when feasible, counts be done weekly for the first month, monthly for six months and semi-annually thereafter. If a significant reduction in leucocytes, platelets or hemopoiesis is noted, Dapsone should be discontinued and the patient followed intensively.
Severe anemia should be treated prior to initiation of therapy and hemoglobin monitored. Hemolysis and methemoglobin may be poorly tolerated by patients with severe cardio-pulmonary disease.
Dapsone has been found carcinogenic (sarcomagenic) for male rats and female mice causing mesenchymal tumors in the spleen and peritoneum, and thyroid carcinoma in female rats.
Cutaneous reactions, especially bullous, include exfoliative dermatitis and are probably one of the most serious, though rare, complications of sulfone therapy. They are directly due to drug sensitization. Such reactions include toxic erythema, erythema multiforme, toxic epidermal necrolysis, morbilliform and scarlatiniform reactions, urticaria and erythema nodosum. If new or toxic dermatologic reactions occur, sulfone therapy must be promptly discontinued and appropriate therapy instituted.
Leprosy reactional states, including cutaneous, are not hypersensitivity reactions to Dapsone and do not require discontinuation. See special section.
Precautions: Hemolysis and Heinz body formation may be exaggerated in individuals with glucose-6-phosphate dehydrogenase (G6PD) deficiency, or methemoglobin reductase deficiency, or hemoglobin M. This reaction is frequently dose-related. Dapsone should be given with caution to these patients or if the patient is exposed to other agents or conditions such as infection or diabetic ketosis capable of producing hemolysis. Drugs or chemicals which have produced significant hemolysis in G6PD or methemoglobin reductase deficient patients include Dapsone, sulfanilamide, nitrite, aniline, pheylhydrazine, naphthalene, niridazole, nitrofurantoin and 8-amino-antimalarials such as primaquine.
Toxic hepatitis and cholestatic jaundice have been reported early in therapy. Hyperbilirubinema may occur more often in G6PD deficient patients. When feasible, baseline and subsequent monitoring of liver function is recommended. If abnormal, Dapsone should be discontinued until the source of abnormality is established.
Pregnancy Category A: Extensive, but uncontrolled, experience and two published surveys on the use of Dapsone in pregnant women have not shown that Dapsone increases the risk of fetal abnormalities if administered during all trimesters of pregnancy. If this drug is used during pregnancy, the possibility of fetal harm appears remote. Because studies cannot rule out the possibility of harm, however, Dapsone should be used during pregnancy only if really needed. In general, for leprosy, USPHS at Carville recommends maintenance of Dapsone. Dapsone has been important for the management of some pregnant D.H. patients. Dapsone is generally not considered to have an effect on the later growth, development and functional maturation of the child. Because of the potential for tumorgenicity shown for Dapsone in animal studies, a decision should be made whether to discontinue nursing or discontinue the drug, taking into account the importance of the drug to the mother.
Adverse Reactions: In addition to the warnings listed above, the following syndromes and serious reactions have been reported in patients on Dapsone:
Dose-related hemolysis is the most common adverse effect and is seen in patients with or without G6PD deficiency. Almost all patients demonstrate the interrelated changes of a loss of a 1-2 gms. HB, an increase in the reticulocytes (2-12%), a shortened red cell life span and a rise in methemoglobin. G6PD deficient patients have greater responses.
Peripheral neuropathy is a definite but unusual complication of Dapsone therapy in non-leprosy patients. Motor loss is predominant. If muscle weakness appears, Dapsone should be withdrawn. Recovery on withdrawal is usually substantially complete. The mechanism of recovery is reportedly by axonal regeneration. In leprosy this complication has not been reported and may be difficult to distinguish from a leprosy reactional state.
In addition to the warnings and adverse effects reported above, additional adverse reactions include: nausea, vomiting, abdominal pains, vertigo, blurred vision, tinnitus, insomnia, fever, headache, psychosis, phototoxicity, hyperpigmented macules, tachycardia, albuminuria, the nephrotic syndrome, hypoalbuminemia without proteinuria, renal papillary necrosis, male infertility, drug-induced Lupus erythematosus and an infectious mononucleosis-like syndrome. In general, these adverse reactions have regressed off drug.
Dosage and Administration:
Dermatitis herpetiformis: The dosage should be individually titrated starting in adults with 50 mg. daily and correspondingly smaller doses in children. If full control is not achieved within the range of 50-300 mg. daily, higher doses may be tried. Dosage should be reduced to a minimum maintenance level as soon as possible. In responsive patients there is a prompt reduction in pruritus followed by clearance of skin lesions. There is no effect on the gastro-intestinal component of the disease.
Dapsone levels are influenced by acetylation rates. Patients with high acetylation rates or who are receiving treatment affecting acetylation may require an adjustment in dosage. Maintenance Dapsone dosage often can be reduced (approximately 50%) after six months on a gluten-free diet.
Leprosy: In order to reduce secondary Dapsone resistance the WHO Expert Committee on Leprosy has recommended that Dapsone should be commenced and maintained at full dosage without interruption. The recommended dosage is 6-10 mg/kg of body weight per week. This schedule amounts to 50-100 mg. daily in full-size adults with correspondingly smaller doses for children. In bacteriologically negative tuberculoid and indeterminate type leprosy patients, an adult dosage of 50 mg. daily is usually sufficient. After all signs of clinical activity are controlled, therapy should be continued a minimum of 3 years for tuberculoid and indeterminate patients.
In lepromatous and border line lepromatous patients, Dapsone therapy in full dosage should be administered for many years, perhaps for life. The WHO Committee recommends administration for <u>at least</u> 10 years after a patient is bacteriologically negative. More than five years of continuous therapy is required to render most patients with lepromatous leprosy bacteriologically negative.
Secondary Dapsone resistance should be suspected whenever a lepromatous or border-line lepromatous patient receiving Dapsone treatment relapses clinically and bacteriologically, solid staining bacilli being found in the smears taken from the new active lesions. If such cases show no response to regular and supervised Dapsone therapy within three to six months, Dapsone resistance should be considered confirmed clinically. Determination of drug sensitivity using the mouse footpad method is recommended and, after prior arrangement, is available without charge from the USPHS at Carville, LA. Patients with proven Dapsone resistance should be treated with other drugs.
Leprosy Reactional States: Abrupt changes in clinical activity occur in leprosy with any effective treatment and are known as reactional states. The majority can be classified into two groups.
Erythema nodosum leprosum (ENL) (lepromatous lepra reaction) (Type 2 reaction) occurs mainly in lepromatous patients and small numbers of borderline patients. Approximately 50 percent of

treated patients show this reaction in the first year. The principal clinical features are fever and tender erythematous skin nodules sometimes associated with malaise, neuritis, orchitis, albuminuria, joint swelling, iritis, epistaxis or depression. Skin lesions can become pustular and/or ulcerate. Histologically there is a vasculitis with an intense polymorphonuclear infiltrate. Elevated circulating immune complexes are considered to be the mechanism of the reaction. If severe, patients should be hospitalized. In general, anti-leprosy treatment is continued.

Analgesics, steroids and other agents available from USPHS Carville, LA, are used to suppress the reaction.

The "Reversal" reaction (Type 1) may occur in borderline or tuberculoid leprosy patients often soon after chemotherapy is started. The mechanism is presumed to result from a reduction in the antigenic load: the patient is able to mount an enhanced delayed hypersensitivity response to residual infection leading to swelling ("Reversal") of existing skin and nerve lesions. If severe, or if neuritis is present, large doses of steroids should always be used. If severe, the patient should be hospitalized. In general, anti-leprosy treatment is continued and therapy to suppress the reaction is indicated such as analgesics, steroids, or surgical decompression of swollen nerve trunks. USPHS at Carville, LA should be contacted for advice in management.

Overdosage: Symptoms of nausea, vomiting, hyperexcitability can appear a few minutes up to 24 hours after ingestion of an overdose. Methemoglobin induced depression, convulsions and severe cyanosis require prompt treatment. In normal and methemoglobin reductase deficient patients, methylene blue 1–2 mg/kg of body weight given slowly intravenously is the treatment of choice. The effect is complete in 30 minutes, but may have to be repeated if methemoglobin reaccumulates. For non-emergencies, if treatment is needed, methylene blue may be given orally in doses of 3–5 mg/kg every 4–6 hours.

Methylene blue reduction depends on G6PD and should not be given to fully expressed G6PD-deficient patients.

Properties: Dapsone is a white odorless crystalline powder, practically insoluble in water and insoluble in fixed and vegetable oils. The drug is not self-sterilizing but it may be sterilized by dry heat at 150°C for one hour.

How Supplied: Rx: 25 mg. and 100 mg. white scored tablets in light resistant, child proof bottles of 100. (25 mg. — NDC 49938-102-01) coded "Jacobus 102" and (100 mg. — NDC 49938-101-01) coded "Jacobus 101".

Distributed by: Jacobus Pharmaceutical Co., Inc., 37 Cleveland Lane, Princeton, NJ 08540.

Manufactured by: Rowell Laboratories, Inc., Baudette, MN 56623   2 E March, 1980

Jamol Laboratories Inc.
13 ACKERMAN AVENUE
EMERSON, NEW JERSEY 07630

PONARIS
Nasal Mucosal Emollient

Composition: Essential oils of cajeput, eucalyptus, and peppermint in a specially prepared iodized cottonseed oil. (Total Iodine 0.6%) Assimilable hence NON-lipoid potential.

Indications and Uses: Nasal emollient, for relief of nasal congestion due to colds, nasal irritations, atrophic rhinitis, (dry inflamed nasal passages), nasal mucosal encrustations and allergy manifestations.

Also nasal intubations and sterile gauze impregnated for epistaxis packing.

Administration and Dosage: 3 to 4 drops in each nostril 3 to 4 times daily. May be used in a compressed air nebulizer or a DeVilbiss nebulizer No. 33 or 40.

Childrens Dosage: As directed by physician.

How Supplied: One ounce bottle with dropper.

ROMA–NOL

Active Ingredient: An iodine solution for external use having none of the toxic, escharotic, or precipitating nature of usual iodine preparations.

Indications: For all skin and some mucous membrane infections.

Actions: By the J-R process the iodine is highly subdivided thus making **Roma-nol** the highest form of a water soluble iodine. The color density is increased by its high solubility. Hospital studies have proven unusual penetration qualities.

Dosage and Administration: The first 2 or 3 applications of **Roma-nol** act more like cleansers, the iodine color slowly disappearing as it combines with the infected organic matter, pus, mucous, etc. With the additional applications 2 to 4 times more, the impurities being eliminated, the iodine stain will remain. The infected parts have received the full compatible treatment with **Roma-nol** ending the treatment.

How Supplied: Bottles of 30 cc. each.

Janssen Pharmaceutica Inc.
40 KINGSBRIDGE ROAD
PISCATAWAY, NJ 08854

IMODIUM®   R
(loperamide HCl) Capsules
(loperamide HCl) Liquid

Description: IMODIUM (loperamide hydrochloride), 4-(p-chlorophenyl)-4-hydroxy-N, N-dimethyl-α,α-diphenyl-1-piperidinebutyramide monohydrochloride, is a synthetic antidiarrheal for oral use.

IMODIUM is available in 2 mg capsules and as a liquid containing 1 mg/5 ml.

Clinical Pharmacology: *In vitro* and animal studies show that IMODIUM acts by slowing intestinal motility and by affecting water and electrolyte movement through the bowel. IMODIUM inhibits peristaltic activity by a direct effect on the circular and longitudinal muscles of the intestinal wall.

In man, IMODIUM prolongs the transit time of the intestinal contents. It reduces the daily fecal volume, increases the viscosity and bulk density, and diminishes the loss of fluid and electrolytes. Tolerance to the antidiarrheal effect has not been observed.

Clinical studies have indicated that the apparent elimination half-life of loperamide in man is 10.8 hours with a range of 9.1–14.4 hours. Plasma levels of unchanged drug remain below 2 nanograms per ml after the intake of a 2 mg capsule of IMODIUM. Plasma levels are highest approximately five hours after administration of the capsule and 2.5 hours after the liquid. The peak plasma levels of loperamide were similar for both formulations. Of the total excreted in urine and feces, most of the administered drug was excreted in feces.

In those patients in whom biochemical and hematological parameters were monitored during clinical trials, no trends toward abnormality during IMODIUM therapy were noted. Similarly, urinalyses, EKG and clinical ophthalmological examinations did not show trends toward abnormality.

Indications and Usage: IMODIUM is indicated for the control and symptomatic relief of acute nonspecific diarrhea and of chronic diarrhea associated with inflammatory bowel disease. IMODIUM is also indicated for reducing the volume of discharge from ileostomies.

Contraindications: IMODIUM is contraindicated in patients with known hypersensitivity to the drug and in those in whom constipation must be avoided.

Warnings: Antiperistalic agents should not be used in acute diarrhea associated with organisms that penetrate the intestinal mucosa, e.g., enteroinvasive E. coli, salmonella, shigella, and in pseudomembranous colitis associated with broad-spectrum antibiotics.

Fluid and electrolyte depletion may occur in patients who have diarrhea. The use of IMODIUM does not preclude the administration of appropriate fluid and electrolyte therapy. In some patients with acute ulcerative colitis, agents which inhibit intestinal motility or delay intestinal transit time have been reported to induce toxic megacolon. IMODIUM therapy should be discontinued promptly if abdominal distention occurs or if other untoward symptoms develop in patients with acute ulcerative colitis.

IMODIUM should be used with special caution in young children because of the greater variability of response in this age group. Dehydration, particularly in younger children, may further influence the variability of response to IMODIUM.

Precautions

General: In acute diarrhea, if clinical improvement is not observed in 48 hours, the administration of IMODIUM should be discontinued.

Patients with hepatic dysfunction should be monitored closely for signs of CNS toxicity because of the apparent large first pass biotransformation.

Information for Patients: Patients should be advised to check with their physician if their diarrhea doesn't stop after a few days or if they develop a fever.

Drug Interactions: There was no evidence in clinical trials of drug interactions with concurrent medications.

Carcinogenesis, mutagenesis, impairment of fertility: In an 18-month rat study with doses up to 133 times the maximum human dose (on a mg/kg basis), there was no evidence of carcinogenesis. Mutagenicity studies were not conducted. Reproduction studies in rats indicated that high doses (150–200 times the human dose) could cause marked female infertility and reduced male fertility.

Pregnancy
Teratogenic Effects
Pregnancy Category B: Reproduction studies in rats and rabbits have revealed no evidence of impaired fertility or harm to the fetus at doses up to 30 times the human dose. Higher doses impaired the survival of mothers and nursing young. The studies offered no evidence of teratogenic activity. There are, however, no adequate and well-controlled studies in pregnant women. Because animal reproduction studies are not always predictive of human response, this drug should be used during pregnancy only if clearly needed.

Nursing Mothers: It is not known whether this drug is excreted in human milk. Because many drugs are excreted in human milk, caution should be exercised when IMODIUM is administered to a nursing woman.

Pediatric Use: See the "Warnings" Section for information on the greater variability of response in this age group.

In case of accidental overdosage of IMODIUM by children, see "Overdosage" Section for suggested treatment.

Adverse Reactions: The adverse effects reported during clinical investigations of IMODIUM are difficult to distinguish from symptoms associated with the diarrheal syndrome. Adverse experiences recorded during clinical studies with IMODIUM were generally of a minor and self-limiting nature. They were more commonly observed during the treatment of chronic diarrhea. The following patient complaints have been reported and are listed in decreasing order of frequency with the exception of hypersensitivity reactions which is listed first since it may be the most serious.

• Hypersensitivity reactions (including skin rash) have been reported with IMODIUM use.

Continued on next page

Janssen—Cont.

- Abdominal pain, distention or discomfort
- Nausea and vomiting
- Constipation
- Tiredness
- Drowsiness or dizziness
- Dry mouth

Drug Abuse and Dependence:

Abuse: A specific clinical study designed to assess the abuse potential of loperamide at high doses resulted in a finding of extremely low abuse potential. Additionally, after years of extensive use there has been no evidence of abuse or dependence.

Dependence: Physical dependence to IMODIUM in humans has not been observed. However, studies in morphine dependent monkeys demonstrated that loperamide hydrochloride at doses above those recommended for humans prevented signs of morphine withdrawal. However, in humans, the naloxone challenge pupil test, which when positive indicates opiate-like effects, performed after a single high dose, or after more than two years of therapeutic use of IMODIUM, was negative. Orally administered IMODIUM (loperamide formulated with magnesium stearate) is both highly insoluble and penetrates the CNS poorly.

Overdosage: Animal pharmacological and toxicological data indicate that overdosage in man may result in constipation, CNS depression, and gastrointestinal irritation. Clinical trials have demonstrated that a slurry of activated charcoal administered promptly after ingestion of loperamide hydrochloride can reduce the amount of drug which is absorbed into the systemic circulation by as much as ninefold. If vomiting occurs spontaneously upon ingestion, a slurry of 100 gms of activated charcoal should be administered orally as soon as fluids can be retained.

If vomiting has not occurred, gastric lavage should be performed followed by administration of 100 gms of the activated charcoal slurry through the gastric tube. In the event of overdosage, patients should be monitored for signs of CNS depression for at least 24 hours. Children may be more sensitive to central nervous system effects than adults. If CNS depression is observed, naloxone may be administered. If responsive to naloxone, vital signs must be monitored carefully for recurrence of symptoms of the overdose for at least 24 hours after the last dose of naloxone.

In view of the prolonged action of loperamide and the short duration (one to three hours) of naloxone, the patient must be monitored closely and treated repeatedly with naloxone as indicated. Since relatively little drug is excreted in urine, forced diuresis is not expected to be effective for IMODIUM overdosage.

In clinical trials an adult who took three 20 mg doses within a 24-hour period was nauseated after the second dose and vomited after the third dose. In studies designed to examine the potential for side-effects, intentional ingestion of up to 60 mg of loperamide hydrochloride in a single dose to healthy subjects resulted in no significant adverse effects.

Dosage and Administration: (1 teaspoonful = 1 mg.; 1 capsule = 2 mg.)

Acute diarrhea

Adults: The recommended initial dose is two IMODIUM Capsules or four teaspoonfuls of IMODIUM Liquid (4 mg) followed by one capsule or two teaspoonfuls of liquid (2 mg) after each unformed stool. Daily dosage should not exceed eight capsules or sixteen teaspoonfuls of liquid (16 mg). Clinical improvement is usually observed within 48 hours.

Children: IMODIUM use is not recommended for children under 2 years of age. In children 2 to 5 years of age (20 kg or less), IMODIUM liquid should be used; for ages 6 to 12, either IMODIUM liquid or capsules may be used. For children 2 to 12 years of age, the following schedule for capsules or liquid will usually fulfill initial dosage requirements:

Recommended First Day Dosage Schedule
Two to five years: 1 mg t.i.d.
(13 to 20 kg) (3 mg daily dose)
(1 teaspoonful t.i.d.)
Five to eight years: 2 mg b.i.d.
(20 to 30 kg) (4 mg daily dose)
(2 teaspoonfuls or 1 capsule b.i.d.)
Eight to twelve years: 2 mg t.i.d.
(greater than 30 kg) (6 mg daily dose)
(2 teaspoonfuls or 1 capsule t.i.d.)

Recommended Subsequent Daily Dosage
Following the first treatment day, it is recommended that subsequent IMODIUM doses (1 mg/10 kg body weight) be administered only after a loose stool. Total daily dosage should not exceed recommended dosages for the first day.

Chronic Diarrhea

Children: Although IMODIUM has been studied in a limited number of children with chronic diarrhea, the therapeutic dose for the treatment of chronic diarrhea in a pediatric population has not been established.

Adults: The recommended initial dose is two IMODIUM Capsules or four teaspoonfuls of IMODIUM Liquid (4 mg) followed by one capsule or two teaspoonfuls of liquid (2 mg) after each unformed stool until diarrhea is controlled, after which the dosage of IMODIUM should be reduced to meet individual requirements. When the optimal daily dosage has been established, this amount may then be administered as a single dose or in divided doses.

The average daily maintenance dosage in clinical trials was 4 to 8 mg (two to four capsules or four to eight teaspoonfuls of liquid). A dosage of 16 mg (eight capsules or sixteen teaspoonfuls of liquid) was rarely exceeded. If clinical improvement is not observed after treatment with 16 mg per day for at least 10 days, symptoms are unlikely to be controlled by further administration. IMODIUM administration may be continued if diarrhea cannot be adequately controlled with diet or specific treatment.

How Supplied: Liquid—containing 1 mg loperamide hydrochloride per 5 ml. Bottles of 4 oz.
Capsules—each capsule contains 2 mg of loperamide hydrochloride. The capsules have a light green body and a dark green cap with "JANSSEN" imprinted on one segment and "IMODIUM" on the other segment. IMODIUM capsules are supplied in bottles of 100 and 500 and in blister packs of 10 × 10 capsules.
NDC 50458-410-04
(4 oz. Liquid)
NDC 50458-400-01
(10 × 10 capsules—blister)
NDC 50458-400-10
(100 capsules)
NDC 50458-400-50
(500 capsules)
Date: June 1984, Sept. 1984
CAUTION: FEDERAL LAW PROHIBITS DISPENSING WITHOUT A PRESCRIPTION
An original product of
JANSSEN PHARMACEUTICA, n.v.
B-2340 Beerse
Belgium
JANSSEN PHARMACEUTICA INC.
Piscataway
New Jersey 08854
Printed in USA
U.S. Patent 3,714,159
Shown in Product Identification Section, page 413

INAPSINE® (droperidol) Injection ℞
[*in-ăp-sēn*]
(Protect from light—store at room temperature)
FOR INTRAVENOUS OR
INTRAMUSCULAR USE ONLY
Droperidol is a neuroleptic (tranquilizer) agent.

Description:
2 ml. and 5 ml. ampoules
Each ml. contains:
Droperidol .... 2.5 mg.
Lactic acid for pH adjustment to 3.4 ± 0.4.

10 ml. vials
Each ml. contains:
Droperidol .... 2.5 mg.
With 1.8 mg. methylparaben and 0.2 mg. propylparaben, and lactic acid for pH adjustment to 3.4 ± 0.4.

Actions: INAPSINE (droperidol) produces marked tranquilization and sedation. It also produces an antiemetic effect as evidenced by the antagonism of the emetic effect of apomorphine in dogs. It potentiates other CNS depressants. It also produces mild alpha-adrenergic blockade, peripheral vascular dilatation and reduction of the pressor effect of epinephrine. INAPSINE (droperidol) can produce hypotension and decreased peripheral vascular resistance. It may decrease pulmonary arterial pressure (particularly if it is abnormally high). It may reduce the incidence of epinephrine-induced arrhythmias but it does not prevent other cardiac arrhythmias. The onset of action is from three to ten minutes following intravenous or intramuscular administration. The full effect, however, may not be apparent for 30 minutes. The duration of the sedative and tranquilizing effects of INAPSINE (droperidol) generally is two to four hours. Alteration of consciousness may persist as long as 12 hours.

Indications: INAPSINE (droperidol) is indicated:
- to produce tranquilization and to reduce the incidence of nausea and vomiting in surgical and diagnostic procedures;
- for premedication, induction, and as an adjunct in the maintenance of general and regional anesthesia;
- in neuroleptanalgesia in which INAPSINE (droperidol) is given concurrently with a narcotic analgesic, such as SUBLIMAZE® (fentanyl) injection©, to aid in producing tranquility and decreasing anxiety and pain.

Contraindications: INAPSINE (droperidol) is contraindicated in patients with known intolerance to the drug.

Warnings: FLUIDS AND OTHER COUNTERMEASURES TO MANAGE HYPOTENSION SHOULD BE READILY AVAILABLE. As with other CNS depressant drugs, patients who have received INAPSINE (droperidol) should have appropriate surveillance.

If INAPSINE (droperidol) is administered with a narcotic analgesic such as SUBLIMAZE (fentanyl), the user should familiarize himself with the special properties of each drug, particularly the widely differing durations of action. In addition, when such a combination is used, *resuscitative equipment and a narcotic antagonist should be readily available to manage apnea*. See package insert for fentanyl before using.

Narcotic analgesics such as SUBLIMAZE (fentanyl) may cause muscle rigidity, particularly involving the muscles of respiration. This effect is related to the speed of injection. Its incidence can be reduced by the use of slow intravenous injection. Once this effect occurs, it is managed by the use of assisted or controlled respiration and, if necessary, by a neuromuscular blocking agent compatible with the patient's condition.

The respiratory depressant effect of narcotics persists longer than their measured analgesic effect. When used with INAPSINE (droperidol), the total dose of all narcotic analgesics administered should be considered by the practitioner before ordering narcotic analgesics during recovery from anesthesia. It is recommended that narcotics, when required, be used initially in reduced doses as low as ¼ to ⅓ those usually recommended.

Usage in Children—The safety of INAPSINE (droperidol) in children younger than two years of age has not been established.

Usage in Pregnancy—The safe use of INAPSINE (droperidol) has not been established with respect to possible adverse effects upon fetal development. Therefore, it should be used in women of childbearing potential only when, in the judgment of the physician, the potential benefits outweigh the possible hazards. There are insufficient data regarding placental transfer and fetal effects; therefore, safety for the infant in obstetrics has not been established.

Precautions: *The initial dose of INAPSINE (droperidol) should be appropriately reduced in elderly, debilitated and other poor-risk patients. The effect of the initial dose should be considered in determining incremental doses.*

Certain forms of conduction anesthesia, such as spinal anesthesia and some peridural anesthetics, can cause peripheral vasodilatation and hypotension because of sympathetic blockade. Through other mechanisms (see Actions), INAPSINE (droperidol) can also alter circulation. Therefore, when INAPSINE (droperidol) is used to supplement these forms of anesthesia, the anesthetist should be familiar with the physiological alterations involved, and be prepared to manage them in the patients selected for this form of anesthesia.

If hypotension occurs, the possibility of hypovolemia should be considered and managed with appropriate parenteral fluid therapy. Repositioning the patient to improve venous return to the heart should also be considered when operative conditions permit. It should be noted that in spinal and peridural anesthesia, tilting the patient into a head down position may result in a higher level of anesthesia than is desirable, as well as impair venous return to the heart. Care should be exercised in moving and positioning of patients because of the possibility of orthostatic hypotension. If volume expansion with fluids plus other countermeasures do not correct the hypotension, then the administration of pressor agents other than epinephrine should be considered. Epinephrine may paradoxically decrease the blood pressure in patients treated with INAPSINE (droperidol) due to the alpha-adrenergic blocking action of droperidol.

Since INAPSINE (droperidol) may decrease pulmonary arterial pressure, this fact should be considered by those who conduct diagnostic or surgical procedures where interpretation of pulmonary arterial pressure measurements might determine final management of the patient.

Vital signs should be monitored routinely.

Other CNS depressant drugs (e.g. barbiturates, tranquilizers, narcotics, and general anesthetics) have additive or potentiating effects with INAPSINE (droperidol). When patients have received such drugs, the dose of INAPSINE (droperidol) required will be less than usual. Likewise, following the administration of INAPSINE (droperidol), the dose of other CNS depressant drugs should be reduced. INAPSINE (droperidol) should be administered with caution to patients with liver and kidney dysfunction because of the importance of these organs in the metabolism and excretion of drugs.

When the EEG is used for postoperative monitoring, it may be found that the EEG pattern returns to normal slowly.

Since INAPSINE (droperidol) is frequently used with the narcotic analgesic SUBLIMAZE (fentanyl), it should be noted that fentanyl may produce bradycardia, which may be treated with atropine; however, fentanyl should be used with caution in patients with cardiac bradyarrhythmias.

Adverse Reactions: The most common adverse reactions reported to occur with INAPSINE (droperidol) are mild to moderate hypotension and occasionally tachycardia, but these effects usually subside without treatment. If hypotension occurs and is severe or persists, the possibility of hypovolemia should be considered and managed with appropriate parenteral fluid therapy. Postoperative drowsiness is also frequently reported.

Extrapyramidal symptoms (dystonia, akathisia, and oculogyric crisis) have been observed following administration of INAPSINE (droperidol). Restlessness, hyperactivity, and anxiety, which can be either the result of inadequate dosage of INAPSINE (droperidol) or a part of the symptom complex of akathisia, may occur. When extrapyramidal symptoms occur, they can usually be controlled with anti-parkinson agents.

Other adverse reactions that have been reported are dizziness, chills and/or shivering, laryngospasm, bronchospasm and postoperative hallucinatory episodes (sometimes associated with transient periods of mental depression).

When INAPSINE (droperidol) is used with a narcotic analgesic such as SUBLIMAZE (fentanyl), respiratory depression, apnea, and muscular rigidity can occur; if these remain untreated respiratory arrest could occur.

Elevated blood pressure, with or without preexisting hypertension has been reported following administration of INAPSINE (droperidol) combined with SUBLIMAZE (fentanyl) or other parenteral analgesics. This might be due to unexplained alterations in sympathetic activity following large doses; however, it is also frequently attributed to anesthetic or surgical stimulation during light anesthesia.

Dosage and Administration: *Dosage should be individualized.* Some of the factors to be considered in determining the dose are age, body weight, physical status, underlying pathological condition, use of other drugs, type of anesthesia to be used, and the surgical procedure involved.

Vital signs should be monitored routinely.

Usual Adult Dosage

I. *Premedication*—(to be appropriately modified in the elderly, debilitated, and those who have received other depressant drugs) 2.5 to 10 mg. (1 to 4 ml.) may be administered intramuscularly 30 to 60 minutes preoperatively.

II. *Adjunct to General Anesthesia*
Induction—2.5 mg. (1 ml.) per 20 to 25 pounds may be administered (usually intravenously) along with an analgesic and/or general anesthetic. Smaller doses may be adequate. The total amount of INAPSINE (droperidol) administered should be titrated to obtain the desired effect based on the individual patient's response.

Maintenance—1.25 to 2.5 mg. (0.5 to 1 ml.) usually intravenously (see warning regarding use with concomitant narcotic analgesic medication and the possibility of widely differing durations of action).

If INNOVAR® injection is administered in addition to INAPSINE (droperidol), the calculation of the recommended dose of INAPSINE (droperidol) should include the droperidol contained in the INNOVAR injection. See INNOVAR injection Package Insert for full prescribing information.

III. *Use Without A General Anesthetic In Diagnostic Procedures*—Administer the usual I.M. premedication 2.5 to 10 mg. (1 to 4 ml.) 30 to 60 minutes before the procedure. Additional 1.25 to 2.5 mg. (0.5 to 1 ml) amounts of INAPSINE (droperidol) may be administered, usually intravenously (see warning regarding use with concomitant narcotic analgesic medication and the possibility of widely differing durations of action).

Note: When INAPSINE (droperidol) is used in certain procedures, such as bronchoscopy, appropriate topical anesthesia is still necessary.

IV. *Adjunct to Regional Anesthesia*—2.5 to 5 mg. (1 to 2 ml.) may be administered intramuscularly or slowly intravenously when additional sedation is required.

Usual Children's Dosage

For children two to 12 years of age, a reduced dose as low as 1.0 to 1.5 mg. (0.4 to 0.6 ml.) per 20 to 25 pounds is recommended for premedication or for induction of anesthesia.

See Warnings and Precautions for use of INAPSINE (droperidol) with other CNS depressants, and in patients with altered response.

Overdosage:

Manifestations: The manifestations of INAPSINE (droperidol) overdosage are an extension of its pharmacologic actions.

Treatment: In the presence of hypoventilation or apnea, oxygen should be administered and respiration should be assisted or controlled as indicated. A patent airway must be maintained; an oropharyngeal airway or endotracheal tube might be indicated. The patient should be carefully observed for 24 hours; body warmth and adequate fluid intake should be maintained. If hypotension occurs and is severe or persists, the possibility of hypovolemia should be considered and managed with appropriate parenteral fluid therapy.

How Supplied: 2 ml. and 5 ml. ampoules—packages of 10; 10 ml. multiple-dose vials—packages of 10.
NDC 50458-010-02
NDC 50458-010-05
NDC 50458-010-10
U.S. Patent No. 3,161,645
Manufactured by McNEILAB, Inc. for
JANSSEN Pharmaceutica Inc.
Piscataway, NJ 08854
March 1980/Rev. June 1980

INNOVAR® Injection   © ℞
[in′ nō-văr]

FOR INTRAVENOUS OR INTRAMUSCULAR USE ONLY

(Protect from light–store at room temperature)

Description: Each ml. contains (in a 1:50 ratio):
Fentanyl .... 0.05 mg.
as the citrate
Warning: May be habit forming
Droperidol .... 2.5 mg.
Lactic acid for adjustment of pH to 3.5 ± 0.3

> The two components of INNOVAR injection, fentanyl and droperidol, have different pharmacologic actions. Before administering INNOVAR injection, the user should familiarize himself with the special properties of each drug, particularly the widely differing durations of action.

Actions: INNOVAR injection is a combination drug containing a narcotic analgesic, fentanyl, and a neuroleptic (major tranquilizer), droperidol. The combined effect, sometimes referred to as neuroleptanalgesia, is characterized by general quiescence, reduced motor activity, and profound analgesia; complete loss of consciousness usually does not occur from use of INNOVAR injection alone. The incidence of early postoperative pain and emesis may be reduced.

A. Fentanyl is a narcotic analgesic with actions qualitatively similar to those of morphine and meperidine. Fentanyl in a dose of 0.1 mg. (2.0 ml.) is approximately equivalent in analgesic activity to 10 mg. of morphine or 75 mg. of meperidine. The principal actions of therapeutic value are analgesia and sedation. Alterations in respiratory rate and alveolar ventilation, associated with narcotic analgesics, may last longer than the analgesic effect. As the dose of narcotic is increased, the decrease in pulmonary exchange becomes greater. Large doses may produce apnea. Fentanyl appears to have less emetic activity than other narcotic analgesics. Histamine assays, and skin wheal testing in man, as well as *in vivo* testing in dogs indicate that histamine release rarely occurs with fentanyl.

Fentanyl may cause muscle rigidity, particularly involving the muscles of respiration. It may also produce other signs and symptoms characteristic of narcotic analgesics including euphoria, miosis, bradycardia, and bronchoconstriction.

The onset of action of fentanyl is almost immediate when the drug is given intravenously; however, maximal analgesic and respiratory depressant effect may not be noted for several minutes. The usual duration of action of the analgesic effect is 30 to 60 minutes after a single I.V. dose of up to 0.1 mg. Following intramuscular administration, the onset of action is from seven to eight minutes, and the duration of action is from one to two hours.

As with longer-acting narcotic analgesics, the duration of the respiratory depressant effect of SUBLIMAZE® (fentanyl) may be longer than the analgesic effect. The following observations have been reported concerning altered respiratory response to CO_2 stimulation following administration of fentanyl to man:

Continued on next page

Janssen—Cont.

1. DIMINISHED SENSITIVITY TO CO_2 STIMULATION MAY PERSIST LONGER THAN DEPRESSION OF RESPIRATORY RATE. Fentanyl frequently slows the respiratory rate but this effect is seldom noted for over 30 minutes regardless of the dose administered.
2. Duration and degree of respiratory depression is dose related.
3. The peak respiratory depressant effect of a single intravenous dose of fentanyl is noted 5 to 15 minutes following injection.
4. Altered sensitivity to CO_2 stimulation has been demonstrated for up to four hours following a single intravenous dose of 0.6 mg. (12 ml.) fentanyl to healthy volunteers.

See also WARNINGS and PRECAUTIONS concerning respiratory depression.

B. Droperidol produces marked tranquilization and sedation. It also produces an antiemetic effect as evidenced by the antagonism of apomorphine in dogs. It potentiates other CNS depressants. It also produces mild alpha-adrenergic blockade, peripheral vascular dilatation and reduction of the pressor effect of epinephrine. Droperidol can produce hypotension and decreased peripheral vascular resistance. It may decrease pulmonary arterial pressure (particularly if it is abnormally high). It may reduce the incidence of epinephrine-induced arrhythmias but it does not prevent other cardiac arrhythmias. The onset of action is from three to ten minutes following intravenous or intramuscular administration. The full effect, however, may not be apparent for 30 minutes. The duration of the sedative and tranquilizing effects generally is two to four hours. Alteration of consciousness may persist as long as 12 hours. This is in contrast to the much shorter duration of fentanyl.

Indications: INNOVAR injection is indicated to produce tranquilization and analgesia for surgical and diagnostic procedures. It may be used as an anesthetic premedication, for the induction of anesthesia, and as an adjunct in the maintenance of general and regional anesthesia. If the supplementation of analgesia is necessary, SUBLIMAZE (fentanyl) injection alone rather than the combination drug INNOVAR injection, should usually be used; see Dosage and Administration Section.

Contraindications: INNOVAR injection is contraindicated in patients with known intolerance to either component.

Warnings: AS WITH OTHER CNS DEPRESSANTS, PATIENTS WHO HAVE RECEIVED *INNOVAR* INJECTION SHOULD HAVE APPROPRIATE SURVEILLANCE. RESUSCITATIVE EQUIPMENT AND A NARCOTIC ANTAGONIST SHOULD BE READILY AVAILABLE TO MANAGE APNEA.

See also discussion of narcotic antagonists in PRECAUTIONS and OVERDOSAGE.

FLUIDS AND OTHER COUNTERMEASURES TO MANAGE HYPOTENSION SHOULD ALSO BE AVAILABLE.

The respiratory depressant effect of narcotics persists longer than the measured analgesic effect. When used with INNOVAR *injection, the total dose of all narcotic analgesics administered should be considered by the practitioner before ordering narcotic analgesics during recovery from anesthesia. It is recommended that narcotics, when required, be used in reduced doses initially, as low as ¼ to ⅓ those usually recommended.*

INNOVAR *injection may cause muscle rigidity, particularly involving the muscles of respiration. This effect is due to the fentanyl component and is related to the speed of injection. Its incidence can be reduced by the use of slow intravenous injection. Once the effect occurs, it is managed by the use of assisted or controlled respiration and, if necessary, by a neuromuscular blocking agent compatible with the patient's condition.*

Drug Dependence: Fentanyl, the narcotic analgesic component, can produce drug dependence of the morphine type and therefore has the potential for being abused.

Severe and unpredictable potentiation by MAO inhibitors has been reported with narcotic analgesics. Since the safety of fentanyl in this regard has not been established, the use of INNOVAR injection or SUBLIMAZE (fentanyl) in patients who have received MAO inhibitors within 14 days is not recommended.

Head Injuries and Increased Intracranial Pressure: INNOVAR injection should be used with caution in patients who may be particularly susceptible to respiratory depression such as comatose patients who may have a head injury or brain tumor. In addition, INNOVAR injection may obscure the clinical course of patients with head injury.

Usage in Children: The safety of INNOVAR injection in children younger than two years of age has not been established.

Usage in Pregnancy: The safe use of INNOVAR injection has not been established with respect to possible adverse effects upon fetal development. Therefore, it should be used in women of childbearing potential only when, in the judgment of the physician, the potential benefits outweigh the possible hazards. There are insufficient data regarding placental transfer and fetal effects; therefore, safety for the infant in obstetrics has not been established.

Precautions: *The initial dose of* INNOVAR *injection should be appropriately reduced in elderly, debilitated and other poor-risk patients. The effect of the initial dose should be considered in determining incremental doses.*

Certain forms of conduction anesthesia, such as spinal anesthesia and some peridural anesthetics, can alter respiration by blocking intercostal nerves, and can cause peripheral vasodilation and hypotension because of sympathetic blockade. Through other mechanisms (see Actions), fentanyl and droperidol also depress respiration and blood pressure. Therefore, when INNOVAR injection is used to supplement these forms of anesthesia, the anesthetist must be familiar with the physiological alterations involved, and be prepared to manage them in the patients selected for this form of anesthesia.

If hypotension occurs, the possibility of hypovolemia should be considered and managed with appropriate parenteral fluid therapy. Repositioning the patient to improve venous return to the heart should be considered when operative conditions permit. It should be noted that in spinal and peridural anesthesia, tilting the patient into a head down position may result in a higher level of anesthesia than is desirable, as well as impair venous return to the heart. Care should be exercised in the moving and positioning of patients because of a possibility of orthostatic hypotension. If volume expansion with fluids plus these other countermeasures do not correct the hypotension, then the administration of pressor agents other than epinephrine should be considered. Epinephrine may paradoxically decrease the blood pressure in patients treated with INNOVAR injection due to the alpha-adrenergic blocking action of droperidol.

The droperidol component of INNOVAR injection may decrease pulmonary arterial pressure. This fact should be considered by those who conduct diagnostic or surgical procedures where interpretation of pulmonary arterial pressure measurements might determine final management of the patient.

Vital signs should be monitored routinely.

INNOVAR injection, and SUBLIMAZE (fentanyl), should be used with caution in patients with chronic obstructive pulmonary disease, patients with decreased respiratory reserve, and others with potentially compromised ventilation. In such patients narcotics may additionally decrease respiratory drive and increase airway resistance. During anesthesia this can be managed by assisted or controlled respiration. Postoperative respiratory depression caused by narcotic analgesics can be reversed by narcotic antagonists. Appropriate surveillance should be maintained because the duration of respiratory depression of doses of fentanyl (as SUBLIMAZE (fentanyl) or INNOVAR) employed during anesthesia may be longer than the duration of the narcotic antagonist action. Consult individual prescribing information (levallorphan, nalorphine and naloxone) before employing narcotic antagonists.

Should respiration be compromised by muscle rigidity, assisted or controlled respiration and possibly a neuromuscular blocking agent will be required. The occurrence of muscle rigidity is related to the speed of intravenous injection and the incidence can be reduced by slow intravenous injection.

Other CNS depressant drugs (e.g. barbiturates, tranquilizers, narcotics, and general anesthetics) have additive or potentiating effects with INNOVAR injection. When patients have received such drugs, the dose of INNOVAR injection required will be less than usual. Likewise, following the administration of INNOVAR injection, the dose of other CNS depressant drugs should be reduced.

INNOVAR injection should be administered with caution to patients with liver and kidney dysfunction because of the importance of these organs in the metabolism and excretion of drugs.

The fentanyl component may produce bradycardia, which may be treated with atropine; however, INNOVAR injection should be used with caution in patients with cardiac bradyarrhythmias.

When the EEG is used for postoperative monitoring, it may be found that the EEG pattern returns to normal slowly.

Adverse Reactions: The most common serious adverse reactions reported to occur with INNOVAR injection are respiratory depression, apnea, muscular rigidity, and hypotension; if these remain untreated, respiratory arrest, circulatory depression or cardiac arrest could occur.

Extrapyramidal symptoms (dystonia, akathisia, and oculogyric crisis) have been observed following administration of INNOVAR injection. Restlessness, hyperactivity and anxiety which can be either the result of inadequate tranquilization or part of the symptom complex of akathisia may occur. When extrapyramidal symptoms occur, they can usually be controlled with anti-Parkinson agents.

Elevated blood pressure, with and without preexisting hypertension, has been reported following administration of INNOVAR injection. This might be due to unexplained alterations of sympathetic activity following large doses; however, it is also frequently attributed to anesthetic or surgical stimulation during light anesthesia.

Other adverse reactions that have been reported are dizziness, chills and/or shivering, twitching, blurred vision, laryngospasm, bronchospasm, bradycardia, tachycardia, nausea and emesis, diaphoresis, emergence delirium, and postoperative hallucinatory episodes (sometimes associated with transient periods of mental depression).

Postoperative drowsiness is also frequently reported.

Dosage and Administration: *Dosage should be individualized.* Some of the factors to be considered in determining dose are age, body weight, physical status, underlying pathological condition, use of other drugs, the type of anesthesia to be used, and the surgical procedure involved.

Vital signs should be monitored routinely.

Most patients who have received INNOVAR injection do not require narcotic analgesics during the immediate postoperative period. It is recommended that narcotic analgesics, when required, be used initially in reduced doses, as low as ¼ to ⅓ those usually recommended.

Usual Adult Dosage:

I. *Premedication*—(to be appropriately modified in the elderly, debilitated, and those who have received other depressant drugs)—0.5 to 2.0 ml. may be administered *intramuscularly* 45 to 60 minutes prior to surgery with or without atropine.

II. *Adjunct to General Anesthesia*— *Induction*—1 ml. per 20 to 25 pounds of body weight may be administered slowly intravenously. Smaller doses may be adequate.

The total amount of INNOVAR injection administered should be carefully titrated to obtain the desired effect based on the individual patient's response.

There are several methods of administration of INNOVAR injection for induction of anesthesia.

A. Intravenous injection—To allow for the variable needs of patients INNOVAR injection may be administered intravenously in fractional parts of the calculated dose. With the onset of somnolence, the general anesthetic may be administered.

B. Intravenous drip—10 ml. of INNOVAR injection are added to 250 ml. of 5% dextrose in water and the drip given rapidly until the onset of somnolence. At that time, the drip may be either slowed or stopped and the general anesthetic administered.

Maintenance—INNOVAR injection is not indicated as the sole agent for the maintenance of surgical anesthesia. It is customarily used in combination with other measures such as nitrous oxide-oxygen, other inhalation anesthetics, and/or topical or regional anesthesia.

To prevent the possibility of excessive accumulation of the relatively long-acting droperidol component, SUBLIMAZE (fentanyl) alone should be used in increments of 0.025 to 0.05 mg. (0.5 to 1.0 ml.) for the maintenance of analgesia in patients initially given INNOVAR injection as an adjunct to general anesthesia. (See SUBLIMAZE (fentanyl) package insert for additional prescribing information.) However, in prolonged operations, additional 0.5 to 1.0 ml. amounts of INNOVAR injection may be administered with caution intravenously if changes in the patient's condition indicate lightening of tranquilization and analgesia.

III. *Use Without a General Anesthetic in Diagnostic Procedures*—Administer the usual I.M. premedication (0.5 to 2.0 ml.) 45 to 60 minutes before the procedure. To prevent the possibility of excessive accumulation of the relatively long-acting droperidol component, SUBLIMAZE (fentanyl) alone should be used in increments of 0.025 to 0.05 mg. (0.5 to 1.0 ml.) for the maintenance of analgesia in patients initially given INNOVAR injection. (See SUBLIMAZE (fentanyl) package insert for additional information). However, in prolonged operations, additional 0.5 to 1.0 ml. amounts of INNOVAR injection may be administered with caution intravenously if changes in the patient's condition indicate lightening of tranquilization and analgesia.

Note: When INNOVAR injection is used in certain procedures such as bronchoscopy, appropriate topical anesthesia is still necessary.

IV. *Adjunct to Regional Anesthesia*—1 to 2 ml. may be administered intramuscularly or slowly intravenously when additional sedation and analgesia are required.

Usual Children's Dosage:

I. *Premedication*—0.25 ml. per 20 lbs. body weight administered *intramuscularly* 45 to 60 minutes prior to surgery with or without atropine.

II. *Adjunct to General Anesthesia*—The total combined dose for induction and maintenance averages 0.5 ml. per 20 lbs. body weight. Following induction with INNOVAR injection, SUBLIMAZE (fentanyl) alone in a dose of $\frac{1}{4}$ to $\frac{1}{3}$ that recommended in the adult dosage section should usually be used when indicated to avoid the possibility of excessive accumulation of droperidol. However, in prolonged operations, additional increments of INNOVAR injection may be administered with caution when changes in the patient's condition indicate lightening of tranquilization and analgesia.

See Warnings and Precautions for use of INNOVAR injection with other CNS depressants, and in patients with altered response.

Overdosage: *Manifestations:* The manifestations of INNOVAR injection overdosage are an extension of its pharmacologic actions.

Treatment: In the presence of hypoventilation or apnea, oxygen should be administered and respiration should be assisted or controlled as indicated. A patent airway must be maintained; an oropharyngeal airway or endotracheal tube might be indicated. If depressed respiration is associated with muscular rigidity, an intravenous neuromuscular blocking agent might be required to facilitate assisted or controlled respiration. The patient should be carefully observed for 24 hours; body warmth and adequate fluid intake should be maintained. If hypotension occurs and is severe or persists, the possibility of hypovolemia should be considered and managed with appropriate parenteral fluid therapy. A specific narcotic antagonist such as nalorphine, levallorphan or naloxone should be available for use as indicated to manage respiratory depression caused by the narcotic component fentanyl. This does not preclude the use of more immediate countermeasures. The duration of respiratory depression following overdose of fentanyl may be longer than the duration of narcotic antagonist action. Consult the package inserts of the individual narcotic antagonists for details about use.

How Supplied: INNOVAR® injection is supplied in 2 ml. and 5 ml. ampoules, in packages of 10.
NDC 50458-020-02
NDC 50458-020-05
U.S. Patent No. 3,141,823
Manufactured by McNEILAB, Inc. for
JANSSEN Pharmaceutica Inc.
Piscataway, NJ 08854
March, 1980/Rev. October 1980

MONISTAT i.v.™   ℞
[mŏn-ĭ-stăt]
(miconazole)
**10mg/ml sterile solution
for intravenous infusion**

Description: MONISTAT i.v., (miconazole), 1-{2-(2,4-dichlorophenyl)-2-[(2,4-dichlorophenyl) methoxyl] ethyl}-1H-imidazole, is a synthetic antifungal supplied as a sterile solution for intravenous infusion. Each ml of this solution contains 10 mg of miconazole with 0.115 ml PEG 40 castor oil, 1.0 mg lactic acid USP, 0.5 mg methylparaben USP, 0.05 mg propylparaben USP in water for injection. Miconazole i.v. is a clear colorless to slightly yellow solution having a pH of 3.7 to 5.7.

Clinical Pharmacology: MONISTAT i.v. is rapidly metabolized in the liver and about 14% to 22% of the administered dose is excreted in the urine, mainly as inactive metabolites. The pharmacokinetic profile fits a three compartment open model with the following biologic half life: 0.4, 2.1, and 24.1 hours for each phase respectively. The pharmacokinetic profile of MONISTAT i.v. is unaltered in patients with renal insufficiency, including those patients on hemodialysis. The in vitro antifungal activity of MONISTAT i.v. is very broad. Clinical efficacy has been demonstrated in patients with the following species of fungi: *Coccidioides immitis*, *Candida albicans*, *Cryptococcus neoformans*, *Petriellidium boydii* (*Allescheria boydii*), and *Paracoccidioides brasiliensis*.

Recommended doses of MONISTAT i.v. produce serum concentrations of drug which exceed the in vitro MIC values for the fungal species noted above. Doses above 9 mg/kg of MONISTAT i.v. produce peak blood levels above 1µg/ml in most cases. The drug penetrates into joints.

Indications: MONISTAT i.v. is indicated for the treatment of the following severe systemic fungal infections: coccidioidomycosis, candidiasis, cryptococcosis, petriellidiosis (allescheriosis), paracoccidioidomycosis, and for the treatment of chronic mucocutaneous candidiasis.

However, in the treatment of fungal meningitis and urinary bladder infections an intravenous infusion alone is inadequate. It must be supplemented with intrathecal administration and bladder irrigation. Appropriate diagnostic procedures should be followed and MIC's should be determined.

MONISTAT i.v. should not be used to treat common trivial forms of fungal diseases.

Contraindications: MONISTAT i.v. is contraindicated in those patients who have shown hypersensitivity to it.

Warnings: Rapid injection of undiluted MONISTAT i.v. may produce transient tachycardia or arrhythmia.

Precautions: Before a treatment course of MONISTAT i.v. is started, the physician should make sure that the patient is not hypersensitive to the drug product. MONISTAT i.v. should be given by intravenous infusion. The treatment should be started under stringent conditions of hospitalization but subsequently may be given to suitable patients under ambulatory conditions with close clinical monitoring. It is recommended that an initial dose of 200 mg be given with the physician in attendance. It is also recommended that clinical laboratory monitoring including hemoglobin, hematocrit, electrolytes and lipids be performed.

It should be borne in mind that systemic fungal mycoses may be complications of chronic underlying conditions which in themselves may require appropriate measures.

Since *Petriellidium boydii* is difficult to histologically distinguish from species of *Aspergillus*, it is strongly recommended that cultures be grown.

Pregnancy: Reproductive studies with MONISTAT i.v. in rats and rabbits revealed no evidence of impaired fertility or harm to the fetus. There are no data, however, on the use of the drug in pregnant women.

Children: Since the safety of miconazole i.v. in children under one year of age has not been extensively studied, its benefits in this age group must be weighed against the possible risks involved.

Adverse Reactions: Adverse reactions which have been observed with MONISTAT i.v. therapy include phlebitis, pruritus, rash, nausea, vomiting, febrile reactions, drowsiness, diarrhea, anorexia and flushes. In the U.S. studies, 29% of 209 patients studied had phlebitis, 21% pruritus, 18% nausea, 10% fever and chills, 9% rash, and 7% emesis. Transient decreases in hematocrit and serum sodium values have been observed following infusion of MONISTAT i.v.

Thrombocytopenia has also been reported. No serious renal or hepatic toxicity has been reported. If pruritus and skin rashes are severe, discontinuation of treatment may be necessary. Nausea and vomiting can be mitigated with antihistaminic or antiemetic drugs given prior to MONISTAT i.v. infusion, or by reducing the dose, slowing the rate of infusion, or avoiding administration at mealtime.

Aggregation of erythrocytes or rouleau formation on blood smears has been reported. Hyperlipemia has occurred in patients and is reported to be due to the vehicle, Cremophor EL (PEG 40 castor oil).

Drug Interactions: Drugs containing cremophor type vehicles are known to cause electrophoretic abnormalities of the lipoprotein. These effects are reversible upon discontinuation of treatment but are usually not an indication that treatment should be discontinued.

Interaction with the coumarin drugs resulting in an enhancement of the anticoagulant effect has also been reported. In cases of simultaneous treatment with MONISTAT i.v. and coumarin drugs, the anticoagulant effect should be carefully titrated since reductions of the anticoagulant doses may be indicated.

A potential interaction between oral miconazole and oral hypoglycemic agents leading to severe hypoglycemia has been reported.

Since concomitant administration of rifampin and ketoconazole (an imidazole) reduces the blood levels of the latter, the concurrent administration of MONISTAT i.v. (an imidazole) and rifampin should be avoided.

Ketoconazole (an imidazole) increases the blood level of cyclosporin A; therefore, there is the possibility of a similar drug interaction involving cyclosporin A and MONISTAT i.v. (an imidazole).

Continued on next page

Janssen—Cont.

Blood levels of cyclosporin A should be monitored if the two drugs are given concomitantly.

Since concomitant administration of ketoconazole (an imidazole) with phenytoin may alter the metabolism of one or both of the drugs, it is also suggested that when MONISTAT i.v. (an imidazole) is used concurrently with phenytoin, consideration be given to the advisability of monitoring plasma levels of both drugs.

Dosage and Administration:
DOSAGE
Adults: The doses may vary with the diagnosis and with the infective agent, from 200 to 1200 mg per infusion. The following daily doses, which may be divided over 3 infusions, are recommended: [See table below].
*May be divided over 3 infusions.
Repeated courses may be necessitated by relapse or reinfection.
Children. A total daily dose of about 20 to 40 mg/kg is generally adequate. However, a dose of 15 mg/kg body weight per infusion should not be exceeded.
Administration: MONISTAT i.v. should be diluted by adding at least 200 ml of diluent. The diluent of choice is 0.9% sodium chloride or alternatively Dextrose 5% injectable solution. The intravenous infusion should be given over a period of 30 to 60 minutes.
Generally, treatment should be continued until all clinical and laboratory tests no longer indicate that active fungal infection is present. Inadequate periods of treatment may yield poor response and lead to early recurrence of clinical symptoms. The dosing intervals and sites and the duration of treatment vary from patient to patient and depend on the causative organism.
Other Modes of Administration:
Intrathecal: Administration of the undiluted injectable solution of MONISTAT i.v. by the various intrathecal routes (20 mg per dose) is indicated as an adjunct to intravenous treatment in fungal meningitis. Succeeding intrathecal injections may be alternated between lumbar, cervical, and cisternal punctures every 3 to 7 days. *Bladder installation:* 200 mg of miconazole in a diluted solution is indicated in the treatment of mycoses of the urinary bladder.
How Supplied: MONISTAT i.v. is supplied in 20 ml ampoules.
Store at controlled room temperatures (15° to 30°C/59° to 86°F).
NDC 50458-200-20
U.S. Patent No. 3,717,655; 3,839,574
Manufactured by TAYLOR PHARMACAL CO for JANSSEN PHARMACEUTICA Inc. March 1980
Piscataway, NJ 08854
Rev May 1981, Jan. 1982, Oct. 1984

NIZORAL®
[nī′ zōr-ăl]
(Ketoconazole)
Tablets

WARNING: Ketoconazole has been associated with hepatic toxicity, including some fatalities. Patients receiving this drug should be informed by the physician of the risk and should be closely monitored. See WARNINGS and PRECAUTIONS sections.

Description: NIZORAL® (ketoconazole) is a synthetic broad-spectrum antifungal agent available in scored white tablets, each containing 200 mg ketoconazole. Ketoconazole is *cis*-1- acetyl-4- [4-[[2-(2, 4-dichlorophenyl) -2- (1*H*-imidazol-1-ylmethyl) -1, 3-dioxolan-4-yl] methoxyl] phenyl] piperazine and has the following structural formula.

NIZORAL is a white to slightly beige, odorless powder, soluble in acids, with a molecular weight of 531.44.

Clinical Pharmacology: Mean peak plasma levels of approximately 3.5 µg/ml are reached within 1 to 2 hours, following oral administration of a single 200 mg dose taken with a meal. Subsequent plasma elimination is biphasic with a half life of 2 hours during the first 10 hours and 8 hours thereafter. Following absorption from the gastrointestinal tract, NIZORAL is converted into several inactive metabolites. The major identified metabolic pathways are: oxidation and degradation of the imidazole and piperazine rings, oxidative O-dealkylation and aromatic hydroxylation. About 13% of the dose is excreted in the urine, of which 2 to 4% is unchanged drug. The major route of excretion is through the bile into the intestinal tract. *In vitro*, the plasma protein binding is about 99%, mainly to the albumin fraction. Only a negligible proportion of NIZORAL reaches the cerebral-spinal fluid. NIZORAL is a weak dibasic agent and thus requires acidity for dissolution and absorption.
NIZORAL is active against clinical infections with *Blastomyces dermatitidis*, *Candida* spp., *Coccidioides immitis*, *Histoplasma capsulatum*, *Paracoccidioides brasiliensis*, and *Phialophora* spp. Development of resistance to NIZORAL has not yet been reported. NIZORAL is active *in vitro* against a variety of fungi and yeast. In animal models, activity has been demonstrated against *Candida* spp., *Blastomyces dermatitidis*, *Histoplasma capsulatum*, *Malassezia furfur*, *Coccidioides immitis*, and *Cryptococcus neoformans*. The clinical significance of preclinical *in vitro* and animal tests is unknown.
Mode of action: *In vitro* studies suggest that NIZORAL impairs the synthesis of ergosterol, which is a vital component of fungal cell membranes.
Indications and Usage: NIZORAL is indicated for the treatment of the following systemic fungal infections: candidiasis, chronic mucocutaneous candidiasis, oral thrush, candiduria, blastomycosis, coccidioidomycosis, histoplasmosis, chromomycosis, and paracoccidioidomycosis. NIZORAL should not be used for fungal meningitis because it penetrates poorly into the cerebral-spinal fluid.
For the initial diagnosis, the infective organism should be identified; however, therapy may be initiated prior to obtaining laboratory results.
Contraindications: NIZORAL is contraindicated in patients who have shown hypersensitivity to the drug.
Warnings: Hepatotoxicity, primarily of the hepatocellular type, has been associated with the use of NIZORAL. The reported incidence has been about 1:10,000 exposed patients, but this probably represents some degree of under-reporting, as is the case for most reported adverse reactions to drugs. The hepatic injury has usually been reversible upon discontinuation of NIZORAL treament, but in at least one case the hepatic necrosis was fatal. Several cases of hepatitis have been reported in children.
Prompt recognition of liver injury is essential. Liver function tests (such as SGGT, alkaline phosphatase, SGPT, SGOT and bilirubin) should be measured before starting treatment and at intervals (monthly or more frequently) during treatment. Patients receiving ketoconazole concurrently with other potentially hepatotoxic drugs should be carefully monitored, particularly those patients requiring prolonged therapy or those who have had a history of liver disease.
Transient minor elevations in liver enzymes have occurred during ketoconazole treatment, but the drug should be discontinued if even minor liver function test abnormalities persist, if abnormalities worsen, or if abnormalities become accompanied by symptoms of possible liver injury.
In rare cases anaphylaxis has been reported after the first dose. Several cases of hypersensitivity reactions including urticaria have also been reported.
In female rats treated three to six months with ketoconazole at dose levels of 80 mg/kg and higher, increased fragility of long bones, in some cases leading to fracture, was seen. The maximum "no-effect" dose level in these studies was 20 mg/kg (2.5 times the maximum recommended human dose). The mechanism responsible for this phenomenon is obscure. Limited studies in dogs failed to demonstrate such an effect on the metacarpals and ribs.
Precautions:
General: In four subjects with drug-induced achlorhydria, a marked reduction in NIZORAL absorption was observed. NIZORAL requires acidity for dissolution. If concomitant antacids, anticholinergics, and H_2-blockers are needed, they should be given at least two hours after NIZORAL administration. In cases of achlorhydria, the patients should be instructed to dissolve each tablet in 4 ml aqueous solution of 0.2 N HCl. For ingesting the resulting mixture, they should use a glass or plastic straw so as to avoid contact with the teeth. This administration should be followed with a cup of tap water.
Information for Patients: Patients should be instructed to report any signs and symptoms which may suggest liver dysfunction so that appropriate biochemical testing can be done. Such signs and symptoms may include unusual fatigue, anorexia, nausea and/or vomiting, jaundice, dark urine or pale stools (See WARNINGS).
Drug interactions: Imidazole compounds like ketoconazole may enhance the anticoagulant effect of coumarin-like drugs. In simultaneous treatment with imidazole drugs and coumarin drugs. The anticoagulant effect should be carefully titrated and monitored.
Concomitant administration of rifampin with ketoconazole reduces the blood levels of the latter. Both drugs should not be administered concomitantly.
Ketoconazole increases the blood level of cyclosporin A. Blood levels of cyclosporin A should be monitored if the two drugs are given concomitantly.
Concomitant administration of ketoconazole with phenytoin may alter the metabolism of one or both of the drugs. It is suggested to monitor both ketoconazole and phenytoin.
Because severe hypoglycemia has been reported in patients concomitantly receiving oral miconazole (an imidazole) and oral hypoglycemic agents, such a potential interaction involving the latter agents when used concomitantly with ketoconazole (an imidazole) can not be ruled out.
Carcinogenesis, Mutagenesis, Impairment of Fertility: The dominant lethal mutation test in male and female mice revealed that single oral doses of NIZORAL as high as 80 mg/kg produced no mutation in any stage of germ cell development. The *Ames Salmonella* microsomal activator assay was also negative. A long-term feeding study in Swiss Albino mice and in Wistar rats showed no evidence of oncogenic activity.

MONISTAT®

Organism	Dosage Range*	Duration of Successful Therapy (weeks)
Candidiasis	600 to 1800 mg per day	1 to > 20
Cryptococcosis	1200 to 2400 mg per day	3 to > 12
Coccidioidomycosis	1800 to 3600 mg per day	3 to > 20
Petriellidiosis (Allescheriosis)	600 to 3000 mg per day	5 to > 20
Paracoccidioidomycosis	200 to 1200 mg per day	2 to > 16

Pregnancy: Teratogenic effects: *Pregnancy Category C.* NIZORAL has been shown to be teratogenic (syndactylia and oligodactylia) in the rat when given in the diet at 80 mg/kg/day, (10 times the maximum recommended human dose). However, these effects may be related to maternal toxicity, evidence of which also was seen at this and higher dose levels.

There are no adequate and well controlled studies in pregnant women. NIZORAL should be used during pregnancy only if the potential benefit justifies the potential risk to the fetus.

Nonteratogenic effects: NIZORAL has also been found to be embryotoxic in the rat when given in the diet at doses higher than 80 mg/kg during the first trimester of gestation.

In addition, dystocia (difficult labor) was noted in rats administered NIZORAL during the third trimester of gestation. This occurred when NIZORAL was administered at doses higher than 10 mg/kg (higher than 1.25 times the maximum human dose).

It is likely that both the malformations and the embryotoxicity resulting from the administraiton of NIZORAL during gestation are a reflection of the particular sensitivity of the female rat to this drug. For example, the oral LD_{50} of NIZORAL given by gavage to the female rat is 166 mg/kg whereas in the male rat the oral LD_{50} is 287 mg/kg.

Nursing Mothers: Since NIZORAL is probably excreted in the milk, mothers who are under treatment should not breast feed.

Pediatric Use: Specific studies on children under 2 years have not been performed.

Adverse Reactions: In rare cases, anaphylaxis has been reported after the first dose. Several cases of hypersensitivity reactions including urticaria have also been reported. However, the most frequent adverse reactions were nausea and/or vomiting in approximately 3%, abdominal pain in 1.2%, pruritus in 1.5%, and the following in less than 1% of the patients: headache, dizziness, somnolence, fever and chills, photophobia, diarrhea, gynecomastia, impotence and thrombocytopenia. Oligospermia has been reported in investigational studies with the drug at dosages above those currently approved. Although oligospermia has not been reported at dosages up to 400 mg daily, sperm counts have been obtained infrequently in patients treated with these dosages. Most of these reactions were mild and transient and rarely required discontinuation of NIZORAL. In contrast, the rare occurrences of hepatic dysfunction require special attention (see WARNINGS).

Single-dose studies showed a decrease in testosterone and ACTH induced corticosteroid serum levels which returned to normal within 24 hours. No information on long-term studies is available.

Overdosage: In the event accidental overdosage, supportive measures, including gastric lavage with sodium bicarbonate, should be employed.

Dosage and Administration: *Adults:* The recommended starting dose of NIZORAL is a single daily administration of 200 mg (one tablet). In very serious infections or if clinical responsiveness is insufficient within the expected time, the dose of NIZORAL may be increased to 400 mg (two tablets) once daily.

Children: In children over 2 years the corresponding single daily dose is 3.3 to 6.6 mg/kg. In children of 2 years or less the daily dosage has not been established.

Generally, treatment should be continued until all clinical and laboratory tests indicate that active fungal infection has subsided. Inadequate periods of treatment may yield poor response and lead to early recurrence of clinical symptoms. Minimum treatment for candidasis is one or two weeks. Patients with chronic mucocutaneous candidiasis usually require maintenance therapy. Minimum treatment for the other indicated systemic mycoses is six months.

How Supplied: NIZORAL is available as white, scored tablets containing 200 mg of ketoconazole debossed "JANSSEN" and on the reverse side debossed "NIZORAL". They are supplied in bottles of 100 tablets and in blister packs of 10 × 10 tablets.
U.S. Patent 4,335,125
NDC 50458-220-01
(10 × 10 tablets—blister)
NDC 50458-220-10
(100 tablets)
Date: May 26, 1981
Rev: June 1983, Jan. 1984, Sept. 1984
Janssen Pharmaceutica Inc.
Piscataway
New Jersey 08854
USA
Shown in Product Identification Section, page 413

SUBLIMAZE®
[sa'blĭ-māz]
(fentanyl) as the citrate
INJECTION

Protect from light. Store at room temperature.
FOR INTRAVENOUS OR INTRAMUSCULAR USE ONLY

Description: Each ml. contains:
Fentanyl ....50 mcg. (0.05 mg.) as the citrate
Warning: May be habit forming.
Sodium hydroxide for adjustment of pH to 4.0–7.5.

Actions: SUBLIMAZE (fentanyl) is a narcotic analgesic. SUBLIMAZE (fentanyl) in a dose of 100 mcg. (0.1 mg.)(2.0 ml.) is approximately equivalent in analgesic activity to 10 mg. of morphine or 75 mg. of meperidine. The principal actions of therapeutic value are analgesia and sedation. Alterations in respiratory rate and alveolar ventilation, associated with narcotic analgesics, may last longer than the analgesic effect. As the dose of narcotic is increased, the decrease in pulmonary exchange becomes greater. Large doses may produce apnea. SUBLIMAZE (fentanyl) appears to have less emetic activity than other narcotic analgesics. Histamine assays and skin wheal testing in man, as well as in *in vivo* testing in dogs, indicate that clinically significant histamine release rarely occurs with SUBLIMAZE (fentanyl). Recent assays in man show no clinically significant histamine release in dosages up to 50 mcg./kg. (.05 mg./kg.)(1 ml./kg.). SUBLIMAZE (fentanyl) preserves cardiac stability, and obtunds stress-related hormonal changes at higher doses.

SUBLIMAZE (fentanyl) may cause muscle rigidity, particularly involving the muscles of respiration. It may also produce other signs and symptoms characteristic of narcotic analgesics including euphoria, miosis, bradycardia, and bronchoconstriction.

The onset of action of SUBLIMAZE (fentanyl) is almost immediate when the drug is given intravenously; however, the maximal analgesic and respiratory depressant effect may not be noted for several minutes. The usual duration of action of the analgesic effect is 30 to 60 minutes after a single I.V. dose of up to 100 mcg. (0.1 mg.)(2.0 ml.). Following intramuscular administration, the onset of action is from seven to eight minutes, and the duration of action is one to two hours. As with longer acting narcotic analgesics, the duration of the respiratory depressant effect of SUBLIMAZE (fentanyl) may be longer than the analgesic effect. The following observations have been reported concerning altered respiratory response to CO_2 stimulation following administration of fentanyl to man.

1. DIMINISHED SENSITIVITY TO CO_2 STIMULATION MAY PERSIST LONGER THAN DEPRESSION OF RESPIRATORY RATE. (Altered sensitivity to CO_2 stimulation has been demonstrated for up to four hours following a single intravenous dose of 600 mcg. (0.6 mg.)(12 ml.) fentanyl to healthy volunteers.) Fentanyl frequently slows the respiratory rate, duration and degree of respiratory depression being dose related.

2. The peak respiratory depressant effect of a single intravenous dose of fentanyl is noted 5 to 15 minutes following injection.

See also WARNINGS and PRECAUTIONS concerning respiratory depression.

Indications: SUBLIMAZE (fentanyl) is indicated:
— for analgesic action of short duration during the anesthetic periods, premedication, induction, and maintenance, and in the immediate postoperative period (recovery room) as the need arises.
— for use as a narcotic analgesic supplement in general or regional anesthesia.
— for administration with a neuroleptic such as *INAPSINE®* (droperidol) injection as an anesthetic premedication, for the induction of anesthesia and as an adjunct in the maintenance of general and regional anesthesia.
— for use as an anesthetic agent with oxygen in selected high risk patients, such as those undergoing open heart surgery or certain complicated neurological or orthopedic procedures.

Contraindications: SUBLIMAZE (fentanyl) is contraindicated in patients with known intolerance to the drug.

Warnings: AS WITH OTHER CNS DEPRESSANTS, PATIENTS WHO HAVE RECEIVED *SUBLIMAZE* (FENTANYL) SHOULD HAVE APPROPRIATE SURVEILLANCE. RESUSCITATION EQUIPMENT AND A NARCOTIC ANTAGONIST SHOULD BE READILY AVAILABLE TO MANAGE APNEA.

See also discussion of narcotic antagonists in Precautions and Overdosage.

If SUBLIMAZE (fentanyl) is administered with a tranquilizer such as *INAPSINE* (droperidol), the user should familiarize himself with the special properties of each drug, particularly the widely differing duration of action. In addition, when such a combination is used, *fluids and other countermeasures to manage hypotension should be available.*

As with other potent narcotics, the respiratory depressant effect of SUBLIMAZE (fentanyl) may persist longer than the measured analgesic effect. The total dose of all narcotic analgesics administered should be considered by the practitioner before ordering narcotic analgesics during recovery from anesthesia. It is recommended that narcotics, when required, should be used in reduced doses initially, as low as ¼ to ⅓ those usually recommended. SUBLIMAZE (fentanyl) may cause muscle rigidity, particularly involving the muscles of respiration. The effect is related to the speed of injection and its incidence can be reduced by the use of slow intravenous injection. Once the effect occurs, it is managed by the use of assisted or controlled respiration and, if necessary, by a neuromuscular blocking agent compatible with the patient's condition. Where moderate or high doses are used (above 10 mcg./kg.), there must be adequate facilities for postoperative observation, and ventilation if necessary, of patients who have received SUBLIMAZE (fentanyl). It is essential that these facilities be fully equipped to handle all degrees of respiratory depression.

Drug Dependence—SUBLIMAZE (fentanyl) can produce drug dependence of the morphine type and, therefore, has the potential for being abused. Severe and unpredictable potentiation by MAO inhibitors has been reported with narcotic analgesics. Since the safety of fentanyl in this regard has not been established, the use of SUBLIMAZE (fentanyl) in patients who have received MAO inhibitors within 14 days is not recommended.

Head Injuries and Increased Intracranial Pressure—SUBLIMAZE (fentanyl) should be used with caution in patients who may be particularly susceptible to respiratory depression, such as comatose patients who may have a head injury or brain tumor. In addition, SUBLIMAZE (fentanyl) may obscure the clinical course of patients with head injury.

Usage in Children—The safety of SUBLIMAZE (fentanyl) in children younger than two years of age has not been established.

Usage in Pregnancy—The safe use of SUBLIMAZE (fentanyl) has not been established with respect to possible adverse effects upon fetal devel-

Continued on next page

Janssen—Cont.

opment. Therefore, it should be used in women of childbearing potential only when, in the judgment of the physician, the potential benefits outweigh the possible hazards. There are insufficient data regarding placental transfer and fetal effects; therefore, safety for the infant in obstetrics has not been established.

Precautions: *The initial dose of SUBLIMAZE (fentanyl) should be appropriately reduced in elderly and debilitated patients. The effect of the initial dose should be considered in determining incremental doses. Nitrous oxide has been reported to produce cardiovascular depression when given with higher doses of fentanyl.*

Certain forms of conduction anesthesia, such as spinal anesthesia and some peridural anesthetics, can alter respiration by blocking intercostal nerves. Through other mechanisms (see Actions) SUBLIMAZE (fentanyl) can also alter respiration. Therefore, when SUBLIMAZE (fentanyl) is used to supplement these forms of anesthesia, the anesthetist should be familiar with the physiological alterations involved, and be prepared to manage them in the patients selected for these forms of anesthesia.

When used with a tranquilizer such as *INAPSINE* (droperidol), blood pressure may be altered and hypotension can occur.

Vital signs should be monitored routinely.

SUBLIMAZE (fentanyl) should be used with caution in patients with chronic obstructive pulmonary disease, patients with decreased respiratory reserve, and others with potentially compromised respiration. In such patients, narcotics may additionally decrease respiratory drive and increase airway resistance. During anesthesia, this can be managed by assisted or controlled respiration. Respiratory depression caused by narcotic analgesics can be reversed by narcotic antagonists. Appropriate surveillance should be maintained because the duration of respiratory depression of doses of fentanyl employed during anesthesia may be longer than the duration of the narcotic antagonist action. Consult individual prescribing information (levallorphan, nalorphine and naloxone) before employing narcotic antagonists.

When a tranquilizer such as *INAPSINE* (droperidol) is used with SUBLIMAZE (fentanyl) pulmonary arterial pressure may be decreased. This fact should be considered by those who conduct diagnostic and surgical procedures where interpretation of pulmonary arterial pressure measurements might determine final management of the patient. When high dose or anesthetic dosages of SUBLIMAZE (fentanyl) are employed, even relatively small dosages of diazepam may cause cardiovascular depression.

Other CNS depressant drugs (e.g. barbiturates, tranquilizers, narcotics, and general anesthetics) will have additive or potentiating effects with SUBLIMAZE (fentanyl). When patients have received such drugs, the dose of SUBLIMAZE (fentanyl) required will be less than usual. Likewise, following the administration of SUBLIMAZE (fentanyl), the dose of other CNS depressant drugs should be reduced.

SUBLIMAZE (fentanyl) should be administered with caution to patients with liver and kidney dysfunction because of the importance of these organs in the metabolism and excretion of drugs.

SUBLIMAZE (fentanyl) may produce bradycardia, which may be treated with atropine; however, SUBLIMAZE (fentanyl) should be used with caution in patients with cardiac bradyarrhythmias.

When SUBLIMAZE (fentanyl) is used with a tranquilizer such as *INAPSINE* (droperidol) hypotension can occur. If this occurs, the possibility of hypovolemia should also be considered and managed with appropriate parenteral fluid therapy. Repositioning the patient to improve venous return to the heart should be considered when operative conditions permit. Care should be exercised in moving and positioning of patients because of the possibility of orthostatic hypotension. If volume expansion with fluids plus other countermeasures do not correct hypotension, the administration of pressor agents other than epinephrine should be considered. Because of the alpha-adrenergic blocking action of *INAPSINE* (droperidol), epinephrine may pardoxically decrease the blood pressure in patients treated with *INAPSINE* (droperidol).

When *INAPSINE* (droperidol) is used with SUBLIMAZE (fentanyl) and the EEG is used for postoperative monitoring, it may be found that the EEG pattern returns to normal slowly.

Adverse Reactions: As with other narcotic analgesics, the most common serious adverse reactions reported to occur with SUBLIMAZE (fentanyl) are respiratory depression, apnea, muscular rigidity, and bradycardia; if these remain untreated, respiratory arrest, circulatory depression or cardiac arrest could occur. Other adverse reactions that have been reported are hypotension, dizziness, blurred vision, nausea, emesis, laryngospasm, and diaphoresis.

It has been reported that secondary rebound respiratory depression may occasionally occur postoperatively. Patients should be monitored for this possibility and appropriate countermeasures taken as necessary.

When a tranquilizer such as *INAPSINE* (droperidol) is used with SUBLIMAZE (fentanyl), the following adverse reactions can occur: chills and/or shivering, restlessness, and postoperative hallucinatory episodes (sometimes associated with transient periods of mental depression); extrapyramidal symptoms (dystonia, akathisia, and oculogyric crisis) have been observed up to 24 hours postoperatively. When they occur, extrapyramidal symptoms can usually be controlled with anti-parkinson agents. Postoperative drowsiness is also frequently reported following the use of *INAPSINE* (droperidol).

Elevated blood pressure, with and without preexisting hypertension, has been reported following administration of SUBLIMAZE (fentanyl) combined with *INAPSINE* (droperidol). This might be due to unexplained alterations in sympathetic activity following large doses; however, it is also frequently attributed to anesthetic and surgical stimulation during light anesthesia.

Dosage and Administration:

50 mcg. = .05 mg. = 1 ml.

Dosage should be individualized. Some of the factors to be considered in determining the dose are age, body weight, physical status, underlying pathological condition, use of other drugs, type of anesthesia to be used, and the surgical procedure involved. (See dosage range charts)

Vital signs should be monitored routinely.

I. *Premedication*—Premedication (to be appropriately modified in the elderly, debilitated, and those who have received other depressant drugs)—50 to 100 mcg. (0.05 to 0.1 mg.)(1 to 2 ml.) may be administered *intramuscularly* 30 to 60 minutes prior to surgery.

II. *Adjunct to General Anesthesia*—See Dosage Range Chart.

III. *Adjunct to Regional Anesthesia*—50 to 100 mcg. (0.05 to 0.1 mg.)(1 to 2 ml.) may be administered intramuscularly or slowly intravenously, over one to two minutes, when additional analgesia is required.

IV. *Postoperatively (recovery room)*—50 to 100 mcg. (0.05 to 0.1 mg.)(1 to 2 ml.) may be administered intramuscularly for the control of pain, tachypnea and emergence delirium. The dose may be repeated in one to two hours as needed.

Usual Children's Dosage: For induction and maintenance in children 2 to 12 years of age, a reduced dose as low as 20 to 30 mcg. (0.02 to 0.03 mg.)(0.4 to 0.6 ml.) per 20 to 25 pounds is recommended.

[See table on next page].

As a General Anesthetic

When attenuation of the responses to surgical stress is especially important, doses of 50 to 100 mcg./kg. (.05 to 0.1 mg./kg.)(1 to 2 ml./kg.) may be administered with oxygen and a muscle relaxant. This technique has been reported to provide anesthesia without the use of additional anesthetic agents. In certain cases, doses up to 150 mcg./kg. (.15 mg./kg.)(3 ml./kg.) may be necessary to produce this anesthetic effect. It has been used for open heart surgery and certain other major surgical procedures in patients for whom protection of the myocardium from excess oxygen demand is particularly indicated, and for certain complicated neurological and orthopedic procedures.

As noted above, it is essential that qualified personnel and adequate facilities be available for the management of respiratory depression.

See Warnings and Precautions for use of SUBLIMAZE (fentanyl) with other CNS depressants, and in patients with altered response.

Overdosage:

Manifestations: The manifestations of SUBLIMAZE (fentanyl) overdosage are an extension of its pharmacologic actions.

Treatment: In the presence of hypoventilation or apnea, oxygen should be administered and respiration should be assisted or controlled as indicated. A patent airway must be maintained; an oropharyngeal airway or endotracheal tube might be indicated. If depressed respiration is associated with muscular rigidity, an intravenous neuromuscular blocking agent might be required to facilitate assisted or controlled respiration. The patient should be carefully observed for 24 hours; body warmth and adequate fluid intake should be maintained. If hypotension occurs and is severe or persists, the possibility of hypovolemia should be considered and managed with appropriate parenteral fluid therapy. A specific narcotic antagonist such as nalorphine, levallorphan, or naloxone should be available for use as indicated to manage respiratory depression. This does not preclude the use of more immediate countermeasures. The duration of respiratory depression following overdosage of fentanyl may be longer than the duration of narcotic antagonist action. Consult the package insert of the individual narcotic antagonists for details about use.

How Supplied:

2 ml. and 5 ml. ampoules—packages of 10.

NDC 50458-030-02   NDC 50458-030-05

10 ml. and 20 ml. ampoules—packages of 5.

NDC 50458-030-10   NDC 50458-030-20

(FOR INTRAVENOUS USE BY HOSPITAL PERSONNEL SPECIFICALLY TRAINED IN THE USE OF NARCOTIC ANALGESICS)

U.S. Patent No. 3,164,600

Manufactured by McNEILAB, Inc. for JANSSEN Pharmaceutica Inc.

Piscataway, NJ 08854

March 1980/Rev. June 1980/Rev. Jan. 1981

Shown in Product Identification Section, page 413

SUFENTA®
(sufentanil citrate)
Injection

Caution: Federal Law Prohibits Dispensing Without Prescription

Description: SUFENTA (sufentanil citrate) is a potent opioid analgesic chemically designated as N-[4-(methoxymethyl)-1-[2-(2-thienyl)ethyl]-4-piperidinyl]-N-phenylpropanamide 2-hydroxy-1,2,3 -propanetricarboxylate (1:1).

SUFENTA is a sterile, preservative free, aqueous solution containing sufentanil citrate equivalent to 50 ug per ml of sufentanil base for intravenous injection. The solution has a pH range of 3.5-7.5.

Clinical Pharmacology: SUFENTA is an opioid analgesic. SUFENTA is approximately 5 to 7 times as potent as fentanyl. (Dosage requirements for equianalgesic effect will be $1/5$-$1/7$ those of fentanyl on a mg/kg basis. At doses of up to 8 ug/kg, SUFENTA provides profound analgesia; at doses ≥ 8 ug/kg, SUFENTA produces a deep level of anesthesia. SUFENTA produces a dose related attenuation of catecholamine release, particularly norepinephrine.

The pharmacokinetics of SUFENTA can be described as a three-compartment model, with a distribution time of 0.72 minutes, redistribution of 13.7 minutes and an elimination half-life of 148 minutes. The liver and small intestine are the major sites of biotransformation. Approximately 80% of the administered dose is excreted within 24

Product Information

SUBLIMAZE®

DOSAGE RANGE CHART

TOTAL DOSAGE

Low dose—2 mcg./kg. (.002 mg./kg.)(.04 ml./kg.) SUBLIMAZE® injection. Fentanyl in small doses is most useful for minor, but painful, surgical procedures. In addition to the analgesia during surgery, fentanyl may also provide some pain relief in the immediate post-operative period.

Maintenance: 2 mcg./kg. (.002 mg./kg.)(.04 ml./kg.) SUBLIMAZE® injection.

Additional dosages of SUBLIMAZE® injection are infrequently needed in these minor procedures.

Moderate dose—2–20 mcg./kg. (.002–.02 mg./kg.)(.04–0.4 ml./kg.) SUBLIMAZE® injection. Where surgery becomes more major, a larger dose is required. With this dose, in addition to adequate analgesia, one would expect to see some abolition of the stress response. However, respiratory depression will be such that artificial ventilation during anesthesia is necessary, and careful observation of ventilation post-operatively is essential.

Maintenance: 2–20 mcg./kg.)(.002–.02 mg./kg.)(.04–0.4 ml./kg.) SUBLIMAZE® injection

25 to 100 mcg. (0.025 to 0.1 mg.)(0.5 to 2.0 ml.) may be administered intravenously or intramuscularly when movement and/or changes in vital signs indicate surgical stress or lightening of analgesia.

High dose—20–50 mcg./kg. (.02–.05 mg./kg.)(0.4–1 ml./kg.) SUBLIMAZE® injection. During open heart surgery and certain more complicated neurosurgical and orthopedic procedures where surgery is more prolonged, and in the opinion of the anesthesiologist, the stress response to surgery would be detrimental to the well being of the patient, dosages of 20–50 mcg./kg. (.02–.05 mg.)(0.4–1 ml.) of SUBLIMAZE® injection with nitrous oxide oxygen have been shown to attenuate the stress response as defined by increased levels of circulating growth hormone, catecholamine, ADH, and prolactin.

When dosages in this range have been used during surgery, post-operative ventilation and observation are essential due to extended post-operative respiratory depression.

The main objective of this technique would be to produce "stress free" anesthesia.

Maintenance: 20–50 mcg./kg. (.02–.05 mg./kg.)(0.4–1 ml./kg.) SUBLIMAZE® injection.

Maintenance dosage (ranging from 25 mcg. (.025 mg.)(0.5 ml.) to one-half the initial loading dose) will be dictated by the changes in vital signs which indicate stress and lightening of analgesia. However, the additional dosage selected must be individualized especially if the anticipated remaining operative time is short.

---

hours and only 2% of the dose is eliminated as unchanged drug. Plasma protein binding of SUFENTA is approximately 92.5%.

SUFENTA has an immediate onset of action, with relatively limited accumulation. Rapid elimination from tissue storage sites allows for relatively more rapid recovery as compared with fentanyl. At dosages of SUFENTA of 1–2 ug/kg, recovery times are comparable to those observed with fentanyl; at dosages of > 2–6 ug/kg, recovery times are comparable to enflurane, isoflurane and fentanyl. Within the anesthetic dosage range of 8–30 ug/kg of SUFENTA, recovery times are more rapid compared to equipotent fentanyl dosages.

At dosages of ≥ 8 ug/kg, SUFENTA produces hypnosis and anesthesia without the use of additional anesthetic agents. A deep level of anesthesia is maintained at these dosages, as demonstrated by EEG patterns. Dosages of up to 25 ug/kg attenuate the sympathetic response to surgical stress. The catecholamine response, particularly norepinephrine, is further attenuated at doses of SUFENTA of 25–30 ug/kg, with hemodynamic stability and preservation of favorable myocardial oxygen balance.

The vagolytic effects of pancuronium may produce a dose dependent elevation in heart rate during SUFENTA-oxygen anesthesia. The vagolytic effect of pancuronium may be reduced in patients administered nitrous oxide with SUFENTA. The use of moderate doses of pancuronium or of a less vagolytic neuromuscular blocking agent may be used to maintain a stable lower heart rate and blood pressure during SUFENTA-oxygen anesthesia.

Preliminary data suggest that in patients administered high doses of SUFENTA, initial dosage requirements for nueromuscular blocking agents are generally lower as compared to patients given fentanyl or halothane, and comparable to patients given enflurane.

Bradycardia is infrequently seen in patients administered SUFENTA-oxygen anesthesia. The use of nitrous oxide with high doses of SUFENTA may decrease mean arterial pressure, heart rate and cardiac output.

Assays of histamine in patients administered SUFENTA have shown no elevation in plasma histamine levels and no indication of histamine release.

SUFENTA at 20 ug/kg has been shown to provide more adequate reduction in intracranial volume than equivalent doses of fentanyl, based upon requirements for furosemide and anesthesia supplementation in one study of patients undergoing craniotomy. During carotid endarterectomy, SUFENTA produced EEG patterns and reductions in cerebral blood flow and oxygen utilization comparable to those of fentanyl.

The intraoperative use of SUFENTA at anesthetic dosages maintains cardiac output, with a slight reduction in systemic vascular resistance during the initial postoperative period. The incidence of postoperative hypertension, need for vasoactive agents and requirements for postoperative analgesics are generally reduced in patients administered moderate or high doses of SUFENTA as compared to patients given inhalation agents.

Decreased respiratory drive and increased airway resistance occur with SUFENTA. The duration and degree of respiratory depression are dose related when SUFENTA is used at sub-anesthetic dosages. At high doses, a pronounced decrease in pulmonary exchange and apnea may be produced.

Indications and Usage: SUFENTA (sufentanil citrate) is indicated:

as an analgesic adjunct at dosages of up to 8 ug/kg in the maintenance of balanced general anesthesia.

as a primary anesthetic agent for the induction and maintenance of anesthesia with 100% oxygen in patients undergoing major surgical procedures, such as cardiovascular surgery or neurosurgical procedures in the sitting position, to provide favorable myocardial and cerebral oxygen balance or when extended postoperative ventilation is anticipated.

Contraindications: SUFENTA is contraindicated in patients with known hypersensitivity to the drug.

Warnings: SUFENTA should be administered only by persons specifically trained in the use of intravenous anesthetics and management of the respiratory effects of potent opioids.

An opioid antagonist, resuscitative and intubation equipment and oxygen should be readily available. SUFENTA may cause skeletal muscle rigidity, particularly of the truncal muscles. The incidence can be reduced by: 1) administration of up to ¼ of the full paralyzing dose of a non-depolarizing neuromuscular blocking agent just prior to administration of SUFENTA at dosages of up to 8 ug/kg, 2) administration of a full paralyzing dose of a neuromuscular blocking agent following loss of eyelash reflex when SUFENTA is used in anesthetic dosages (above 8 ug/kg) titrated by slow intravenous infusion, or, 3) simultaneous administration of SUFENTA and a full paralyzing dose of a neuromuscular blocking agent when SUFENTA is used in rapidly administrered anesthetic dosages (above 8 ug/kg).

The neuromuscular blocking agent used should be compatible with the patient's cardiovascular status. Adequate facilities should be available for postoperative monitoring and ventilation of patients administered anesthetic doses of SUFENTA. It is essential that these facilities be fully equipped to handle all degrees of respiratory depression.

Precautions: The initial dose of SUFENTA should be appropriately reduced in elderly and debilitated patients. The effect of the initial dose should be considered in determining supplemental doses.

Vital signs should be monitored routinely.

Nitrous oxide may produce cardiovascular depression when given with high doses of SUFENTA (see CLINICAL PHARMACOLOGY).

High doses of pancuronium may produce increases in heart rate during SUFENTA-oxygen anesthesia. Bradycardia has been reported infrequently with SUFENTA-oxygen anesthesia and has been responsive to atropine.

Head Injuries: SUFENTA may obscure the clinical course of patients with head injuries.

Continued on next page

Janssen—Cont.

Impaired Respiration: SUFENTA should be used with caution in patients with pulmonary disease, decreased respiratory reserve or potentially compromised respiration. In such patients, opioids may additionally decrease respiratory drive and increase airway resistance. During anesthesia, this can be managed by assisted or controlled respiration. Respiratory depression caused by opioid analgesics can be reversed by opioid antagonists such as naloxone. Because the duration of respiratory depression produced by SUFENTA may last longer than the duration of the opioid antagonist action, appropriate surveillance should be maintained.

Impaired Hepatic or Renal Function: In patients with liver or kidney dysfunction, SUFENTA should be administered with caution due to the importance of these organs in the metabolism and excretion of SUFENTA.

Drug Interactions: An additive effect with SUFENTA may be exhibited in patients receiving barbiturates, tranquilizers, other opioids, general anesthetics or other CNS depressants. In such cases of combined treatment, the dose of one or both agents should be reduced.

Carcinogenesis, Mutagenesis and Impairment of Fertility: No long-term animal studies of SUFENTA have been performed to evaluate carcinogenic potential. The micronucleus test in female rats revealed that single intravenous doses of SUFENTA as high as 80 ug/kg (approximately 2.5 times the upper human dose) produced no structural chromosome mutations. The Ames *Salmonella typhimurium* metabolic activating test also revealed no mutagenic activity. See ANIMAL TOXICOLOGY for reproduction studies in rats and rabbits.

Pregnancy Category C: SUFENTA has been shown to have an embryocidal effect in rats and rabbits when given in doses 2.5 times the upper human dose for a period of 10 days to over 30 days. These effects were most probably due to maternal toxicity (decreased food consumption with increased mortality) following prolonged administration of the drug.

No evidence of teratogenic effects have been observed after administration of SUFENTA in rats and rabbits.

There are no adequate and well-controlled studies in pregnant women. SUFENTA should be used during pregnancy only if the potential benefit justifies the potential risk to the fetus.

Labor and Delivery: There are insufficient data to support the use of SUFENTA in labor and delivery. Therefore, such use is not recommended.

Nursing Mothers: It is not known whether this drug is excreted in human milk. Because many drugs are excreted in human milk, caution should be exercised when SUFENTA is administered to a nursing woman.

Pediatric Use: The safety and effficacy of SUFENTA in children under two years of age undergoing cardiovascular surgery has been documented in a limited number of cases.

Animal Toxicology: The intravenous LD_{50} of SUFENTA is 16.8 to 18.0 mg/kg in mice, 11.8 to 13.0 mg/kg in guinea pigs and 10.1 to 19.5 mg/kg in dogs. Reproduction studies performed in rats and rabbits given doses of up to 2.5 times the upper human dose for a period of 10 to over 30 days revealed high maternal mortality rates due to decreased food consumption and anoxia, which preclude any meaningful interpretation of the results.

Adverse Reactions: The most common adverse reactions of opioids are respiratory depression and skeletal muscle rigidity. See CLINICAL PHARMACOLOGY, WARNINGS and PRECAUTIONS on the management of respiratory depression and skeletal muscle rigidity.

The most frequent adverse reactions in clinical trials involving 320 patients administered SUFENTA were: hypotension (7%), hypertension (3%), chest wall rigidity (3%) and bradycardia (3%).

Other adverse reactions with a reported incidence of less than 1% were:
Cardiovascular: tachycardia, arrhythmia
Gastrointestinal: nausea, vomiting
Respiratory: apnea, postoperative respiratory depression, bronchospasm
Dermatological: itching
Central Nervous System: chills
Miscellaneous: intraoperative muscle movement

Drug Abuse and Dependence: SUFENTA (sufentanil citrate) is a Schedule II controlled drug substance that can produce drug dependence of the morphine type and therefore has the potential for being abused.

Overdosage: Overdosage would be manifested by an extension of the pharmacological actions of SUFENTA (see CLINICAL PHARMACOLOGY) as with other potent opioid analgesics. However, no experiences of overdosage with SUFENTA have been established during clinical trials. The intravenous LD_{50} of SUFENTA in male rats is 9.34 to 12.5 mg/kg (see ANIMAL TOXICOLOGY for $LD_{50}s$ in other species. Intravenous administration of an opioid antagonist such as naloxone should be employed as a specific antidote to manage respiratory depression. The duration of respiratory depression following overdosage with SUFENTA may be longer than the duration of action of the opioid antagonist. Administration of an opioid antagonist should not preclude more immediate countermeasures. In the event of overdosage, oxygen should be administered and ventilation assisted or controlled as indicated for hypoventilation or apnea. A patent airway must be maintained, and a nasopharyngeal airway or endotracheal tube may be indicated. If depressed respiration is associated with muscular rigidity, a neuromuscular blocking agent may be required to facilitate assisted or controlled respiration. Intravenous fluids and vasopressors for the treatment of hypotension and other supportive measures may be employed.

Dosage and Administration: The dosage of SUFENTA should be individualized in each case according to body weight, physical status, underlying pathological condition, use of other drugs, and type of surgical procedure and anesthesia. In obese patients (more than 20% above ideal total body weight), the dosage of SUFENTA should be determined on the basis of lean body weight. Dosage should be reduced in elderly and debilitated patients (see PRECAUTIONS).

Vital signs should be monitored routinely.

See dosage range chart for the use of SUFENTA by intravenous injection 1) in doses of up to 8 ug/kg as an analgesic adjunct to general anesthesia, and 2) in doses ≥ 8 ug/kg as a primary anesthetic agent for induction and maintenance of anesthesia with 100% oxygen.

Usage in Children: For induction and maintenance of anesthesia in children less than 12 years of age undergoing cardiovascular surgery, an anesthetic dose of 10–25 ug/kg administered with 100% oxygen is generally recommended. Supplemental dosages of up to 25–50 ug are recommended for maintenance, based on response to initial dose and as determined by changes in vital signs indicating surgical stress or lightening of anesthesia.

Premedication: The selection of preanesthetic medications should be based upon the needs of the individual patient.

Neuromuscular Blocking Agents: The neuromuscular blocking agent selected should be compatible with the patient's condition, taking into account the hemodynamic effects of a particular muscle relaxant and the degree of skeletal muscle relaxation required (see CLINICAL PHARMACOLOGY, WARNINGS and PRECAUTIONS).
[See table left].

In patients administered high (anesthetic) doses of SUFENTA, it is essential that qualified personnel and adequate facilities are available for the management of postoperative respiratory depression. Also see WARNINGS and PRECAUTIONS sections.

Parenteral drug products should be inspected visually for particulate matter and discoloration prior to administration, whenever solution and container permit.

How Supplied: SUFENTA (sufentanil citrate) Injection for intravenous use is available as:
NDC 50458-050-01 50 ug/ml, 1 ml ampoules in packages of 10
NDC 50458-050-02 50 ug/ml, 2 ml ampoules in packages of 10
NDC 50458-050-05 50 ug/ml, 5 ml ampoules in packages of 10

SUFENTA® ADULT DOSAGE RANGE CHART

TOTAL DOAGE	MAINTENANCE DOSAGE
1–2 ug/kg: administered with nitrous oxide/oxygen in patients undergoing general surgery in which endotracheal intubation and mechanical ventilation are required.	**10–25 ug (0.2–0.5 ml):** as needed when movement and/or changes in vital signs indicate surgical stress or lightening of analgesia. Supplemental dosages should be individualized and adjusted to the remaining operative time anticipated.
2–8 ug/kg: administered with nitrous oxide/oxygen in patients undergoing more complicated major surgical procedures. At dosages in this range, SUFENTA has been shown to provide some attenuation of sympathetic reflex activity in response to surgical stimuli, provide hemodynamic stability and provide relatively rapid recovery.	**25–50 ug (0.5–1 ml):** as determined by changes in vital signs that indicate stress or lightening of analgesia. Supplemental dosages should be individualized, and adjustedto the remaining operative time anticipated .
8–30 ug/kg: (anesthetic doses) administered with 100% oxygen and a muscle relaxant. SUFENTA has been found to produce sleep at dosages ≥ 8 ug/kg and to maintain a deep level of anesthesia without the use of additional anesthetic agents. At dosages in this range of up to 25 ug/kg, catecholamine release is attenuated. Dosages of 25–30 ug/kg have been shown to block sympathetic responses including catecholamine release. High doses are indicated in patients undergoing major surgical procedures, such as cardiovascular surgery and neurosurgery in the sitting position with maintenance of favorable myocardial and cerebral oxygen balance. Postoperative mechanical ventilation and observation are essential at these dosages due to extended postoperative respiratory depression.	**25–50 ug (0.5–1 ml):** as determined by changes in vital signs that indicate stress and lightening of anesthesia.

SUBLIMAZE®

DOSAGE RANGE CHART

TOTAL DOSAGE

Low dose—2 mcg./kg. (.002 mg./kg.)(.04 ml./kg.) SUBLIMAZE® injection. Fentanyl in small doses is most useful for minor, but painful, surgical procedures. In addition to the analgesia during surgery, fentanyl may also provide some pain relief in the immediate post-operative period.
Maintenance: 2 mcg./kg. (.002 mg./kg.)(.04 ml./kg.) SUBLIMAZE® injection.

Additional dosages of SUBLIMAZE® injection are infrequently needed in these minor procedures.

Moderate dose—2–20 mcg./kg. (.002–.02 mg./kg.)(.04–0.4 ml./kg.) SUBLIMAZE® injection. Where surgery becomes more major, a larger dose is required. With this dose, in addition to adequate analgesia, one would expect to see some abolition of the stress response. However, respiratory depression will be such that artificial ventilation during anesthesia is necessary, and careful observation of ventilation post-operatively is essential.
Maintenance: 2–20 mcg./kg.)(.002–.02 mg./kg.)(.04–0.4 ml./kg.) SUBLIMAZE® injection

25 to 100 mcg. (0.025 to 0.1 mg.)(0.5 to 2.0 ml.) may be administered intravenously or intramuscularly when movement and/or changes in vital signs indicate surgical stress or lightening of analgesia.

High dose—20–50 mcg./kg. (.02–.05 mg./kg.)(0.4–1 ml./kg.) SUBLIMAZE® injection. During open heart surgery and certain more complicated neurosurgical and orthopedic procedures where surgery is more prolonged, and in the opinion of the anesthesiologist, the stress response to surgery would be detrimental to the well being of the patient, dosages of 20–50 mcg./kg. (.02–.05 mg.)(0.4–1 ml.) of SUBLIMAZE® injection with nitrous oxide oxygen have been shown to attenuate the stress response as defined by increased levels of circulating growth hormone, catecholamine, ADH, and prolactin.

When dosages in this range have been used during surgery, post-operative ventilation and observation are essential due to extended post-operative respiratory depression.

The main objective of this technique would be to produce "stress free" anesthesia.

Maintenance: 20–50 mcg./kg. (.02–.05 mg./kg.)(0.4–1 ml./kg.) SUBLIMAZE® injection.

Maintenance dosage (ranging from 25 mcg. (.025 mg.)(0.5 ml.) to one-half the initial loading dose) will be dictated by the changes in vital signs which indicate stress and lightening of analgesia. However, the additional dosage selected must be individualized especially if the anticipated remaining operative time is short.

---

hours and only 2% of the dose is eliminated as unchanged drug. Plasma protein binding of SUFENTA is approximately 92.5%.
SUFENTA has an immediate onset of action, with relatively limited accumulation. Rapid elimination from tissue storage sites allows for relatively more rapid recovery as compared with fentanyl. At dosages of SUFENTA of 1–2 ug/kg, recovery times are comparable to those observed with fentanyl; at dosages of > 2–6 ug/kg, recovery times are comparable to enflurane, isoflurane and fentanyl. Within the anesthetic dosage range of 8–30 ug/kg of SUFENTA, recovery times are more rapid compared to equipotent fentanyl dosages.
At dosages of ≥ 8 ug/kg, SUFENTA produces hypnosis and anesthesia without the use of additional anesthetic agents. A deep level of anesthesia is maintained at these dosages, as demonstrated by EEG patterns. Dosages of up to 25 ug/kg attenuate the sympathetic response to surgical stress. The catecholamine response, particularly norepinephrine, is further attenuated at doses of SUFENTA of 25–30 ug/kg, with hemodynamic stability and preservation of favorable myocardial oxygen balance.
The vagolytic effects of pancuronium may produce a dose dependent elevation in heart rate during SUFENTA-oxygen anesthesia. The vagolytic effect of pancuronium may be reduced in patients administered nitrous oxide with SUFENTA. The use of moderate doses of pancuronium or of a less vagolytic neuromuscular blocking agent may be used to maintain a stable lower heart rate and blood pressure during SUFENTA-oxygen anesthesia.
Preliminary data suggest that in patients administered high doses of SUFENTA, initial dosage requirements for nueromuscular blocking agents are generally lower as compared to patients given fentanyl or halothane, and comparable to patients given enflurane.
Bradycardia is infrequently seen in patients administered SUFENTA-oxygen anesthesia. The use of nitrous oxide with high doses of SUFENTA may decrease mean arterial pressure, heart rate and cardiac output.

Assays of histamine in patients administered SUFENTA have shown no elevation in plasma histamine levels and no indication of histamine release.
SUFENTA at 20 ug/kg has been shown to provide more adequate reduction in intracranial volume than equivalent doses of fentanyl, based upon requirements for furosemide and anesthesia supplementation in one study of patients undergoing craniotomy. During carotid endarterectomy, SUFENTA produced EEG patterns and reductions in cerebral blood flow and oxygen utilization comparable to those of fentanyl.
The intraoperative use of SUFENTA at anesthetic dosages maintains cardiac output, with a slight reduction in systemic vascular resistance during the initial postoperative period. The incidence of postoperative hypertension, need for vasoactive agents and requirements for postoperative analgesics are generally reduced in patients administered moderate or high doses of SUFENTA as compared to patients given inhalation agents.
Decreased respiratory drive and increased airway resistance occur with SUFENTA. The duration and degree of respiratory depression are dose related when SUFENTA is used at sub-anesthetic dosages. At high doses, a pronounced decrease in pulmonary exchange and apnea may be produced.
Indications and Usage: SUFENTA (sufentanil citrate) is indicated:
as an analgesic adjunct at dosages of up to 8 ug/kg in the maintenance of balanced general anesthesia.
as a primary anesthetic agent for the induction and maintenance of anesthesia with 100% oxygen in patients undergoing major surgical procedures, such as cardiovascular surgery or neurosurgical procedures in the sitting position, to provide favorable myocardial and cerebral oxygen balance or when extended postoperative ventilation is anticipated.
Contraindications: SUFENTA is contraindicated in patients with known hypersensitivity to the drug.
Warnings: SUFENTA should be administered only by persons specifically trained in the use of intravenous anesthetics and management of the respiratory effects of potent opioids.
An opioid antagonist, resuscitative and intubation equipment and oxygen should be readily available.
SUFENTA may cause skeletal muscle rigidity, particularly of the truncal muscles. The incidence can be reduced by: 1) administration of up to $\frac{1}{4}$ of the full paralyzing dose of a non-depolarizing neuromuscular blocking agent just prior to administration of SUFENTA at dosages of up to 8 ug/kg, 2) administration of a full paralyzing dose of a neuromuscular blocking agent following loss of eyelash reflex when SUFENTA is used in anesthetic dosages (above 8 ug/kg) titrated by slow intravenous infusion, or, 3) simultaneous administration of SUFENTA and a full paralyzing dose of a neuromuscular blocking agent when SUFENTA is used in rapidly administrered anesthetic dosages (above 8 ug/kg).
The neuromuscular blocking agent used should be compatible with the patient's cardiovascular status. Adequate facilities should be available for postoperative monitoring and ventilation of patients administered anesthetic doses of SUFENTA. It is essential that these facilities be fully equipped to handle all degrees of respiratory depression.
Precautions: The initial dose of SUFENTA should be appropriately reduced in elderly and debilitated patients. The effect of the initial dose should be considered in determining supplemental doses.
Vital signs should be monitored routinely.
Nitrous oxide may produce cardiovascular depression when given with high doses of SUFENTA (see CLINICAL PHARMACOLOGY).
High doses of pancuronium may produce increases in heart rate during SUFENTA-oxygen anesthesia. Bradycardia has been reported infrequently with SUFENTA-oxygen anesthesia and has been responsive to atropine.
Head Injuries: SUFENTA may obscure the clinical course of patients with head injuries.

Continued on next page

Janssen—Cont.

Impaired Respiration: SUFENTA should be used with caution in patients with pulmonary disease, decreased respiratory reserve or potentially compromised respiration. In such patients, opioids may additionally decrease respiratory drive and increase airway resistance. During anesthesia, this can be managed by assisted or controlled respiration. Respiratory depression caused by opioid analgesics can be reversed by opioid antagonists such as naloxone. Because the duration of respiratory depression produced by SUFENTA may last longer than the duration of the opioid antagonist action, appropriate surveillance should be maintained.

Impaired Hepatic or Renal Function: In patients with liver or kidney dysfunction, SUFENTA should be administered with caution due to the importance of these organs in the metabolism and excretion of SUFENTA.

Drug Interactions: An additive effect with SUFENTA may be exhibited in patients receiving barbiturates, tranquilizers, other opioids, general anesthetics or other CNS depressants. In such cases of combined treatment, the dose of one or both agents should be reduced.

Carcinogenesis, Mutagenesis and Impairment of Fertility: No long-term animal studies of SUFENTA have been performed to evaluate carcinogenic potential. The micronucleus test in female rats revealed that single intravenous doses of SUFENTA as high as 80 ug/kg (approximately 2.5 times the upper human dose) produced no structural chromosome mutations. The Ames *Salmonella typhimurium* metabolic activating test also revealed no mutagenic activity. See ANIMAL TOXICOLOGY for reproduction studies in rats and rabbits.

Pregnancy Category C: SUFENTA has been shown to have an embryocidal effect in rats and rabbits when given in doses 2.5 times the upper human dose for a period of 10 days to over 30 days. These effects were most probably due to maternal toxicity (decreased food consumption with increased mortality) following prolonged administration of the drug.

No evidence of teratogenic effects have been observed after administration of SUFENTA in rats and rabbits.

There are no adequate and well-controlled studies in pregnant women. SUFENTA should be used during pregnancy only if the potential benefit justifies the potential risk to the fetus.

Labor and Delivery: There are insufficient data to support the use of SUFENTA in labor and delivery. Therefore, such use is not recommended.

Nursing Mothers: It is not known whether this drug is excreted in human milk. Because many drugs are excreted in human milk, caution should be exercised when SUFENTA is administered to a nursing woman.

Pediatric Use: The safety and efficacy of SUFENTA in children under two years of age undergoing cardiovascular surgery has been documented in a limited number of cases.

Animal Toxicology: The intravenous LD_{50} of SUFENTA is 16.8 to 18.0 mg/kg in mice, 11.8 to 13.0 mg/kg in guinea pigs and 10.1 to 19.5 mg/kg in dogs. Reproduction studies performed in rats and rabbits given doses of up to 2.5 times the upper human dose for a period of 10 to over 30 days revealed high maternal mortality rates due to decreased food consumption and anoxia, which preclude any meaningful interpretation of the results.

Adverse Reactions: The most common adverse reactions of opioids are respiratory depression and skeletal muscle rigidity. See CLINICAL PHARMACOLOGY, WARNINGS and PRECAUTIONS on the management of respiratory depression and skeletal muscle rigidity.

The most frequent adverse reactions in clinical trials involving 320 patients administered SUFENTA were: hypotension (7%), hypertension (3%), chest wall rigidity (3%) and bradycardia (3%).

Other adverse reactions with a reported incidence of less than 1% were:
Cardiovascular: tachycardia, arrhythmia
Gastrointestinal: nausea, vomiting
Respiratory: apnea, postoperative respiratory depression, bronchospasm
Dermatological: itching
Central Nervous System: chills
Miscellaneous: intraoperative muscle movement

Drug Abuse and Dependence: SUFENTA (sufentanil citrate) is a Schedule II controlled drug substance that can produce drug dependence of the morphine type and therefore has the potential for being abused.

Overdosage: Overdosage would be manifested by an extension of the pharmacological actions of SUFENTA (see CLINICAL PHARMACOLOGY) as with other potent opioid analgesics. However, no experiences of overdosage with SUFENTA have been established during clinical trials. The intravenous LD_{50} of SUFENTA in male rats is 9.34 to 12.5 mg/kg (see ANIMAL TOXICOLOGY for LD_{50}s in other species). Intravenous administration of an opioid antagonist such as naloxone should be employed as a specific antidote to manage respiratory depression. The duration of respiratory depression following overdosage with SUFENTA may be longer than the duration of action of the opioid antagonist. Administration of an opioid antagonist should not preclude more immediate countermeasures. In the event of overdosage, oxygen should be administered and ventilation assisted or controlled as indicated for hypoventilation or apnea. A patent airway must be maintained, and a nasopharyngeal airway or endotracheal tube may be inserted. If depressed respiration is associated with muscular rigidity, a neuromuscular blocking agent may be required to facilitate assisted or controlled respiration. Intravenous fluids and vasopressors for the treatment of hypotension and other supportive measures may be employed.

Dosage and Administration: The dosage of SUFENTA should be individualized in each case according to body weight, physical status, underlying pathological condition, use of other drugs, and type of surgical procedure and anesthesia. In obese patients (more than 20% above ideal total body weight), the dosage of SUFENTA should be determined on the basis of lean body weight. Dosage should be reduced in elderly and debilitated patients (see PRECAUTIONS).

Vital signs should be monitored routinely.

See dosage range chart for the use of SUFENTA by intravenous injection 1) in doses of up to 8 ug/kg as an analgesic adjunct to general anesthesia, and 2) in doses ≥ 8 ug/kg as a primary anesthetic agent for induction and maintenance of anesthesia with 100% oxygen.

Usage in Children: For induction and maintenance of anesthesia in children less than 12 years of age undergoing cardiovascular surgery, an anesthetic dose of 10–25 ug/kg administered with 100% oxygen is generally recommended. Supplemental dosages of up to 25–50 ug are recommended for maintenance, based on response to initial dose and as determined by changes in vital signs indicating surgical stress or lightening of anesthesia.

Premedication: The selection of preanesthetic medications should be based upon the needs of the individual patient.

Neuromuscular Blocking Agents: The neuromuscular blocking agent selected should be compatible with the patient's condition, taking into account the hemodynamic effects of a particular muscle relaxant and the degree of skeletal muscle relaxation required (see CLINICAL PHARMACOLOGY, WARNINGS and PRECAUTIONS).
[See table left].

In patients administered high (anesthetic) doses of SUFENTA, it is essential that qualified personnel and adequate facilities are available for the management of postoperative respiratory depression. Also see WARNINGS and PRECAUTIONS sections.

Parenteral drug products should be inspected visually for particulate matter and discoloration prior to administration, whenever solution and container permit.

How Supplied: SUFENTA (sufentanil citrate) Injection for intravenous use is available as:
NDC 50458-050-01 50 ug/ml, 1 ml ampoules in packages of 10
NDC 50458-050-02 50 ug/ml, 2 ml ampoules in packages of 10
NDC 50458-050-05 50 ug/ml, 5 ml ampoules in packages of 10

SUFENTA® ADULT DOSAGE RANGE CHART

TOTAL DOSAGE	MAINTENANCE DOSAGE
1–2 ug/kg: administered with nitrous oxide/oxygen in patients undergoing general surgery in which endotracheal intubation and mechanical ventilation are required.	**10–25 ug (0.2–0.5 ml):** as needed when movement and/or changes in vital signs indicate surgical stress or lightening of analgesia. Supplemental dosages should be individualized and adjusted to the remaining operative time anticipated.
2–8 ug/kg: administered with nitrous oxide/oxygen in patients undergoing more complicated major surgical procedures. At dosages in this range, SUFENTA has been shown to provide some attenuation of sympathetic reflex activity in response to surgical stimuli, provide hemodynamic stability and provide relatively rapid recovery.	**25–50 ug (0.5–1 ml):** as determined by changes in vital signs that indicate stress or lightening of analgesia. Supplemental dosages should be individualized, and adjusted to the remaining operative time anticipated.
8–30 ug/kg: (anesthetic doses) administered with 100% oxygen and a muscle relaxant. SUFENTA has been found to produce sleep at dosages ≥ 8 ug/kg and to maintain a deep level of anesthesia without the use of additional anesthetic agents. At dosages in this range of up to 25 ug/kg, catecholamine release is attenuated. Dosages of 25–30 ug/kg have been shown to block sympathetic responses including catecholamine release. High doses are indicated in patients undergoing major surgical procedures, such as cardiovascular surgery and neurosurgery in the sitting position with maintenance of favorable myocardial and cerebral oxygen balance. Postoperative mechanical ventilation and observation are essential at these dosages due to extended postoperative respiratory depression.	**25–50 ug (0.5–1 ml):** as determined by changes in vital signs that indicate stress and lightening of anesthesia.

VERMOX®
[vĕr' mŏx]
(mebendazole)
Chewable Tablets

Description: VERMOX® (mebendazole) is a (synthetic) broad-spectrum anthelmintic available as chewable tablets, each containing 100 mg of mebendazole. Mebendazole is methyl 5-benzoyl-benzimidazole-2-carbamate and has the following structural formula:

Mebendazole is a white to slightly yellow powder with a molecular weight of 295.29. It is less than 0.05% soluable in water, dilute mineral acid solutions, alcohol, ether and chloroform, but is soluble in formic acid.

Clinical Pharmacology: Following administration of 100 mg twice daily for three consecutive days, plasma levels of VERMOX® and its primary metabolite, the 2-amine, do not exceed 0.03 $\mu g/ml$ and 0.09 $\mu g/ml$, respectively. All metabolites are devoid of anthelmintic activity. In man, approximately 2% of administered VERMOX® is excreted in urine and the remainder in the feces as unchanged drug or a primary metabolite.

Mode of Action: VERMOX® inhibits the formation of the worms' microtubules and causes the worms' glucose depletion.

Indications and Usage: VERMOX® is indicated for the treatment of *Enterobius vermicularis* (pinworm), *Trichuris trichiura* (whipworm), *Ascaris lumbricoides* (common roundworm), *Ancylostoma duodenale* (common hookworm), *Necator americanus* (American hookworm) in single or mixed infections.

Efficacy varies as a function of such factors as preexisting diarrhea and gastrointestinal transit time, degree of infection and helminth strains. Efficacy rates derived from various studies are shown in the table:
[See table above].

Contraindications: VERMOX® is contraindicated in in persons who have shown hypersensitivity to the drug.

Warnings: There is no evidence that VERMOX®, even at high doses, is effective for hydatid disease.

Precautions:
Information for Patients: Patients should be informed of the potential risk to the fetus in women taking VERMOX® during pregnancy, especially during the first trimester (see Use in Pregnancy). Patients should also be informed that cleanliness is important to prevent reinfection and transmission of the infection.

Carcinogenesis, Mutagenesis: In carcinogenicity tests of VERMOX® in mice and rats, no carcinogenic effects were seen at doses as high as 40 mg/kg given daily over two years. Dominant lethal mutation tests in mice showed no mutagenicity at single doses as high as 640 mg/kg. Neither the spermatocyte test, the F_1 translocation test, nor the Ames test indicated mutagenic properties.

Impairment of Fertility: Doses up to 40 mg/kg in mice, given to males for 60 days and to females for 14 days prior to gestation, had no effect upon fetuses and offspring, though there was slight maternal toxicity.

Use in Pregnancy: Pregnancy Category C. VERMOX® has shown embryotoxic and teratogenic activity in pregnant rats at single oral doses as low as 10 mg/kg. In view of these findings the use of VERMOX® is not recommended in pregnant women. In humans, a post-marketing survey has been done of a limited number of women who inadvertently had consumed VERMOX® during the first trimester of pregnancy. The incidence of spontaneous abortion and malformation did not exceed that in the general population. In 170 deliveries on term, no teratogenic risk of VERMOX® was identified. During pregnancy, especially during the first trimester, VERMOX® should be used only if the potential benefit justifies the potential risk to the fetus.

Nursing Mothers: It is not known whether VERMOX® is excreted in human milk. Because many drugs are excreted in human milk, caution should be exercised when VERMOX® is administered to a nursing woman.

Pediatric Use: The drug has not been extensively studied in children under two years; therefore, in the treatment of children under two years the relative benefit/risk should be considered.

Adverse Reactions: Transient symptoms of abdominal pain and diarrhea have occurred in cases of massive infection and expulsion of worms.

Overdosage: In the event of accidental overdosage gastrointestinal complaints lasting up to a few hours may occur. Vomiting and purging should be induced.

Dosage and Administration: The same dosage schedule applies to children and adults. The tablet may be chewed, swallowed, or crushed and mixed with food.
[See table below].
If the patient is not cured three weeks after treatment, a second course of treatment is advised. No special procedures, such as fasting or purging, are required.

How Supplied: VERMOX® is available as chewable tablets, each containing 100 mg of mebendazole, and is supplied in boxes of 36 tablets NDC 50458-110-30 (36 tablets-blister)
VERMOX® (mebendazole) is an original product of Janssen Pharmaceutica n.v. B-2340 Beerse, Belgium.

JANSSEN PHARMACEUTICA INC.
Piscataway, NJ 08854
©J.P.I. 1979, Rev. 9/83, 1/84, 8/84
U.S. Patent 3,657,267

Shown in Product Identification Section, page 413

Vermox®	Pinworm (enterobiasis)	Whipworm (trichuriasis)	Common Roundworm (ascariasis)	Hookworm
Cure rates mean	95%	68%	98%	96%
Egg reduction mean	—	93%	99%	99%

Vermox®	Pinworm (enterobiasis)	Whipworm (trichuriasis)	Common Roundworm (ascariasis)	Hookworm
Dose	1 tablet, once	1 tablet morning and evening for 3 consecutive days.	1 tablet morning and evening for 3 consecutive days.	1 tablet morning and evening for 3 consecutive days.

1044 Product Information Always consult Supplement

Johnson & Johnson Products Inc.
A Johnson & Johnson Company
PATIENT CARE DIVISION
501 GEORGE STREET
NEW BRUNSWICK, NJ 08903

DEBRISAN®
[deb'ri-san]
wound cleaning beads and paste.
Draws Exudate from Wet Ulcers and Wounds

Description: DEBRISAN® consists of spherical hydrophilic beads of dextranomer, 0.1–0.3mm in diameter; the paste is a mixture of the beads and polyethylene glycol. The beads are composed of a three dimensional network of macromolecular chains of cross-linked dextran which is large enough to allow substances with a molecular weight of less than 1000 to enter freely. Substances with a molecular weight of 1000–5000 enter the beads less freely, while those with a molecular weight greater than 5000 remain in the interspaces between the beads.

Characteristics: Because of its hydrophilic properties, each gram of DEBRISAN® beads absorbs approximately 4 ml. of fluid. The beads swell to approximately four times their original size. This swelling causes significant suction forces and capillary action in the spaces between the beads. This action is continuous as long as unsaturated beads or paste is in proximity to the ulcer or wound.
When DEBRISAN® beads or paste are applied to the surface of wet ulcers or wounds suction forces begin removing various exudates and particles that tend to impede tissue repair. For example, low molecular weight components of wound exudates are drawn up within the DEBRISAN® beads while higher molecular weight components, such as plasma proteins, and fibrinogen are found between the swollen beads. Removal of these latter components, particularly fibrin and fibrinogen, retards eschar formation. Additionally, there is *in vitro* evidence that the suction forces created by the beads remove bacteria and inflammatory exudates from the surface of the wound.
The use of DEBRISAN® beads or paste to remove exudates continuously from the surface of the wound results in a concomitant reduction of inflammation and edema.

Indications: DEBRISAN® beads and paste are indicated for use in cleaning wet ulcers and wounds such as venous stasis ulcers, decubitus ulcers, and infected traumatic and surgical wounds. DEBRISAN® beads are also indicated for use in cleaning infected burns.

Precautions: To minimize the possibility of cross-contamination, contents of a DEBRISAN® bead container should be limited to use in one patient.
When treating cratered decubitus ulcers, do not pack the wounds tightly. Allow for expansion of the beads. Do not use DEBRISAN® beads or paste in deep fistulas, sinus tracts, or any body cavity where complete removal is not assured.
Once the DEBRISAN® is saturated it should be removed. This avoids encrustation which makes removal more difficult. All DEBRISAN® must be removed before any surgical procedure to close the wound (*ie* graft or flap).
Wounds may appear larger during the first few days of treatment due to the reduction of edema. DEBRISAN® beads and paste are not effective in cleaning dry wounds.
Not all wounds require treatment with DEBRISAN® to complete healing. When the wound is no longer wet and a healthy granulation base has been established, the application of DEBRISAN® beads or paste should be discontinued. Treatment of the underlying condition (venous or arterial flow, pressure, etc.) should be addressed, in addition to using DEBRISAN® beads or paste.

Adverse Reactions: Upon application and/or removal of DEBRISAN® beads, transitory pain, bleeding, blistering and erythema have been reported in isolated cases.

Directions for Use:
Applying DEBRISAN®
Debride and wash the area in the usual manner. **DEBRISAN® beads and paste are not enzymes and will not debride.** Leave the area moist since this facilitates the action of DEBRISAN®.

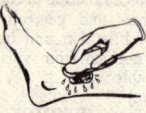

Apply DEBRISAN® beads or paste to at least ¼ inch (6mm) thickness. At least ¼ inch thickness is required to achieve desired suction effects.

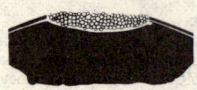

Apply a dressing. Close all four sides.

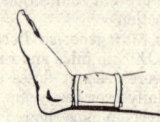

Use of paste
A paste mixture of DEBRISAN® beads may be used for application on irregular body surfaces or hard to reach areas. Three methods of application are possible:
1. DEBRISAN® may be purchased in a convenient, premixed paste form.
2. A paste mixture may be prepared by carefully pouring a small amount of glycerin on a dry dressing large enough to cover the wound and adding a sufficient amount of DEBRISAN® beads to make a layer at least ¼ inch thick.

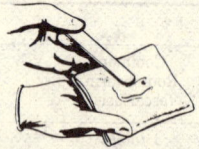

3. Or, DEBRISAN® beads (3 parts) may be mixed with glycerin (1 part) in a receptacle and applied directly to the wound with a spatula. Do not mix with any substance other than glycerin.
In any case, dress the wound in the usual manner. Use fresh paste for each application. Do not reuse.

Removing DEBRISAN®
When DEBRISAN® beads or paste become saturated, a color change will be noted indicating that they should be removed. Removal should be as complete as possible and is best achieved by irrigation. Occasionally vigorous irrigation, soaking, or whirlpool may be required to remove patches of DEBRISAN® that adhere to the wound.

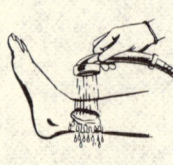

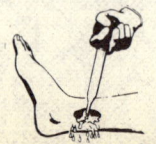

Reapply DEBRISAN® beads or paste every 12 hours, or more frequently if necessary. Reduce the number of applications as the exudate diminishes.
When to Discontinue:
When the area is free of exudate and edema.
When a healthy granulation base is present.
The patient should consult the physician if the condition worsens or persists beyond the expected length of treatment (normally 14–21 days).
How Supplied: DEBRISAN® beads are supplied sterile, in containers of 25, 60, 120 grams each and 4 gram packets in boxes of 7 or 14. DEBRISAN® paste is also available in a pre-mixed sterile form, in 10 gram foil packets, six per box. Store in a dry place below 85°F.
Avoid contact with eyes.
For external use only.
Spilling beads or paste onto the floor will result in a slippery surface.
Materials Available: Free samples and clinical literature available to physicians. Call 800-526-2459. In New Jersey, call 800-352-4845.
MANUFACTURED IN SWEDEN FOR
JOHNSON & JOHNSON
PRODUCTS INC.
A Johnson & Johnson company
NEW BRUNSWICK, NEW JERSEY 08903
©J&JPI83

SURGICEL® Absorbable Hemostat   B
[ser'ji-sel]
(oxidized regenerated cellulose)
For surgical use
(For dental application of this product, reference should be made to the package insert for dental use.)

Description: SURGICEL® Absorbable Hemostat is a sterile, absorbable knitted fabric prepared by the controlled oxidation of regenerated cellulose. The fabric is white with a pale yellow cast and has a faint, caramel-like aroma. It is strong and can be sutured or cut without fraying. It is stable and can be stored at controlled room temperature. A slight discoloration may occur with age, but this does not affect performance.
Actions: The mechanism of action whereby SURGICEL® Absorbable Hemostat accelerates clotting is not completely understood, but it appears to be a physical effect rather than any alteration of the normal physiologic clotting mechanism. After SURGICEL has been saturated with blood, it swells into a brownish or black gelatinous mass which aids in the formation of a clot, thereby serving as a hemostatic adjunct in the control of local hemorrhage. When used properly in minimal amounts, SURGICEL is absorbed from the sites of implantation with practically no tissue reaction. Absorption depends upon several factors including the amount used, degree of saturation with blood, and the tissue bed.
In addition to its local hemostatic properties, SURGICEL Absorbable Hemostat is bactericidal **in vitro** against a wide range of gram positive and gram negative organisms including aerobes and anaerobes. SURGICEL is bactericidal **in vitro** against strains of species including those of:
Staphylococcus aureus
Staphylococcus epidermidis
Micrococcus luteus
Streptococcus pyogenes Group A
Streptococcus pyogenes Group B
Bacillus subtilis
Proteus vulgaris
Corynebacterium serosis
Mycobacterium phlei
Clostridium tetani
Streptococcus salivarius
Branhamella catarrhalis
Escherichia coli
Klebsiella aerogenes
Lactobacillus sp.
Salmonella enteritidis
Shigella dysenteriae
Serratia marscescens
Clostridium perfringens

Bacteroides fragilis
Enterococcus
Enterobacter cloacae
Pseudomonas aeruginosa
Pseudomonas stutzeri
Proteus mirabilis

Studies conducted in animals show that SURGICEL in contrast to other hemostatic agents does not tend to enhance experimental infection.

Indications: SURGICEL® Absorbable Hemostat (oxidized regenerated cellulose) is used adjunctively in surgical procedures to assist in the control of capillary, venous, and small arterial hemorrhage when ligation or other conventional methods of control are impractical or ineffective.

Contraindications: Although packing or wadding sometimes is medically necessary, SURGICEL® Absorbable Hemostat should not be used in this manner unlss it is to be removed after hemostasis is achieved.

SURGICEL should not be used for implantation in bone defects, such as fractures, since there is a possibility of interference with callus formation and a theoretical chance of cyst formation.

When SURGICEL is used to help achieve hemostasis around the spinal cord in laminectomies, or around the optic nerve and chiasm, it must always be removed after hemostasis is achieved since it will swell and could exert unwanted pressure.

SURGICEL should not be used to control hemorrhage from large arteries.

SURGICEL should not be used on non-hemorrhagic serous oozing surfaces, since body fluids other than whole blood, such as serum, do not react with SURGICEL to produce satisfactory hemostatic effect.

Warnings: SURGICEL® Absorbable Hemostat is supplied sterile and should not be autoclaved because autoclaving causes physical breakdown of the product.

SURGICEL is not intended as a substitute for careful surgery and the proper use of sutures and ligatures.

Closing SURGICEL in a contaminated wound without drainage may lead to complications and should be avoided.

The hemostatic effect of SURGICEL is greater when it is applied dry; therefore it should not be moistened with water or saline.

SURGICEL should not be impregnated with anti-infective agents or with other materials such as buffering or hemostatic substances. Its hemostatic effect is not enhanced by the addition of thrombin, the activity of which is destroyed by the low pH of the product.

Although SURGICEL Absorbable Hemostat may be left in situ when necessary, it is advisable to remove it once hemostasis is achieved. It must always be removed from the site of application after use in laminectomy procedures and from foramina in bone when hemostasis is obtained. This is because SURGICEL, by swelling, may cause nerve damage by pressure in a bony confine. Paralysis has been reported when used around the spinal cord, particularly in surgery for herniated intervertebral disc.

Although SURGICEL is bactericidal against a wide range of pathogenic microorganisms, it is not intended as a substitute for systemically administered therapeutic or prophylactic antimicrobial agents to control or prevent post-operative infections.

Precautions: Use only as much SURGICEL® Absorbable Hemostat as is necessary for hemostasis, holding it in place until bleeding stops. Remove any excess before surgical closure in order to facilitate absorption and minimize the possibility of foreign body reaction.

SURGICEL should be applied loosely against the bleeding surface Wadding or packing should be avoided, especially within rigid cavities where swelling may intefere with normal function or possibly cause necrosis.

In urological procedures, minimal amounts of SURGICEL should be used and care must be exercised to prevent plugging of the urethra, ureter, or a catheter by dislodged portions of the product.

Since absorption of SURGICEL could be prevented in chemically cauterized areas, its use should not be preceded by application of silver nitrate or any other escharotic chemicals.

If SURGICEL is used temporarily to line the cavity of large open wounds, it should be placed so as not to overlap the skin edges. It should also be removed from open wounds by forceps or by irrigation with sterile water or saline solution after bleeding has stopped.

Precautions should be taken in otorhinolaryngologic surgery to assure that none of the material is aspirated by the patient. (Examples: controlling hemorrhage after tonsillectomy and controlling epistaxis.)

Care should be taken not to apply SURGICEL too tightly when it is used as a wrap during vascular surgery (See "ADVERSE REACTIONS" section).

Adverse Reactions: "Encapsulation" of fluid and foreign body reactions have been reported. There have been two reports of stenotic effect when SURGICEL® Absorbable Hemostat has been applied as a wrap during vascular surgery. Although it has not been established that the stenosis was directly related to the use of SURGICEL, it is important to be cautious and avoid applying the material tightly as a wrapping.

Possible prolongation of drainage in cholecystectomies and difficulty passing urine per urethra after prostatectomy have been reported. There has been one report of a blocked ureter after kidney resection, in which postoperative catheterization was required.

Occasional reports of "burning" and "stinging" sensations and sneezing when SURGICEL has been used as packing in epistaxis, are believed due to the low pH of the product.

Burning has been reported when SURGICEL was applied after nasal polyp removal and after hemorrhoidectomy. Headache, burning, stinging, and sneezing in epistaxis and other rhinological procedures, and stinging when SURGICEL was applied on surface wounds (varicose ulcerations, dermabrasions, and donor sites) also have been reported.

Dosage and Administration: Sterile technique should be observed in removing SURGICEL® Absorbable Hemostat from its envelope. Minimal amounts of SURGICEL in appropriate size are laid on the bleeding site or held firmly against the tissues until hemostasis is obtained. Opened, unused SURGICEL should be discarded, because it cannot be resterilized.

How Supplied: Sterile SURGICEL® Absorbable Hemostat (oxidized regenerated cellulose) is supplied as knitted fabric strips in envelopes in the following sizes.

2 in. × 14 in. (28 sq. in.) (5.1 × 35.6 cm. (180.6 sq. cm.))
4 in. × 8 in. (32 sq. in.) (10.2 × 20.3 cm. (206.5 sq. cm.))
2 in. × 3 in. (6 sq. in.) (5.1 × 7.6 cm. (38.7 sq. cm.))
½ in. × 2 in. (1 sq. in.) (1.3 × 5.1 cm. (6.5 sq. cm.))

Clinical Studies: SURGICEL® Absorbable Hemostat (oxidized regenerated cellulose) has been found useful in helping to control capillary or venous bleeding in a variety of surgical applications, including abdominal, thoracic, neurosurgical, and orthopedic, as well as in otorhinolaryngologic procedures. Examples include gallbladder surgery, partial hepatectomy, hemorrhoidectomy, resections or injuries of the pancreas, spleen, kidney, prostate, bowel, breast or thyroid, and in amputations. (1,3)

SURGICEL has been applied as a surface dressing on donor sites and superficial open wounds, controlling bleeding adequately, and causing no delay in healing or interference with epithelization (4,6). It also has been applied after dermabrasion, punch biopsy, excision biopsy, curettage, finger and toe-nail removal, and to traumatic wounds. In the foregoing applications, bleeding was controlled and the SURGICEL was absorbed from the sites where it was applied. (5)

In cardiovascular surgery, investigators have found SURGICEL useful in helping to control bleeding from implanted textile grafts, including those of the abdominal aorta. (2,7) Such grafts may leak or weep considerably, even when pre-clotted, but this seepage can be controlled by covering the graft with a layer or two of SURGICEL after the graft is in place and before releasing the proximal and distal clamps. When the flow has been reestablished and all the bleeding controlled, the fabric either can be removed or left in situ, since absorption of SURGICEL has been shown to occur without constriction of the graft or other untoward incident when proper wrapping technique is employed.

Otorhinolaryngologic experience with SURGICEL includes adjunctive use in controlling bleeding resulting from epistaxis, tonsillectomy, adenoidectomy, removal of nasal polyps, repair of deviated septum, tympanoplasty, stapes surgery, surgery for sinusitis, and removal of tumors. (8,9)

SURGICEL has been reported useful as a hemostatic adjunct in such gynecologic procedures as oophorectomy, hysterectomy, conization of the cervix, and repair of cystorectocele. (1,10)

Animal Pharmacology: The effects of SURGICEL® Absorbable Hemostat, absorbable gelatin sponge, and microfibrillar collagen hemostat were compared in a standardized infection model consisting of intra-abdominal and intrahepatic abscesses in mice. This infection mimics the common characteristics of human infection with nonspore-forming anaerobic bacteria, including a chronic and progressive course. SURGICEL did not increase the infectivity of normally subinfectious inocula of mixed anaerobic species in mice. With the other hemostatic agents, microfibrillar collagen hemostat and absorbable gelatin sponge, an enhancement of infectivity of anaerobic mixtures has been shown. SURGICEL Absorbable Hemostat, in contrast to these hemostatic agents, did not enhance or provide a site for bacterial growth.

It was also found that aerobic pathogens did not grow in the presence of SURGICEL Absorbable Hemostat. In these studies (11), SURGICEL® Absorbable Hemostat was placed in contaminated incisions of guinea pigs and markedly reduced bacterial growth of three different strains of common pathogens.

In a dog model (12), it was shown that bacterial contamination of implanted teflon patches in the aorta could be reduced by wrapping the area of the patch with SURGICEL prior to pathogen challenge. Also, in another study (13), SURGICEL® Absorbable Hemostat and an absorbable gelatin sponge were placed in two splenotomy sites in large mongrel dogs and the animals were then challenged intravenously and the number of organisms from the splenotomy sites were measured over a period of time. The number of organisms at the site of SURGICEL Absorbable Hemostat was significantly lower than that in the control, or the absorbable gelatin sponge site.

References:
1. Degenshein, G., Hurwitz, A., and S. Ribacoff: Experience with regenerated oxidized celluose. *New York State Journal of Medicine* 63(18):2639–2643, 1963.
2. Hurwitt, E.: A new absorbable hemostatic packing. *Bulletin de la Societe Internationale de Chirurgle XXI*(3):237–242, 1962.
3. Venn, R.: Reduction of postsurgical blood-replacement needs with SURGICEL hemostasis. *Medical Times* 93(10):1113–1116, 1965.
4. Miller, J., Ginsberg, M., McElfatrick, G., and H. Johnson: Clinical experience with oxidized regenerated cellulose. *Experimental Medicine and Surgery* 19(2–3):202–206, (June-Sept.) 1961.
5. Blau, S., Kanof, N., and L. Simonson: Absorbable hemostatic gauze SURGICEL in dermabrasions and dermatologic surgery. *Acta Dermato-Venerelogica* 40:358–361, 1960.
6. Shea, P., Jr.: Management of the donor site: a new dressing technic *Journal of the Medical Associaion of Georgia* 51(9):437–440, 1962.
7. Denck, H.: Use of resorbable oxycellulose in surgery. *Chirurg* 33(11):486–488, 1962.

Continued on next page

Johnson & Johnson—Cont.

8. Tibbels, E., Jr.: Evaluation of a new method of epistaxis management *Laryngoscope LXXIII*(3):306–314, 1963.

9. Huggins, S.: Control of hemorrhage in otorhinolaryngologic surgery with oxidized regenerated cellulose. *Eye, Ear, Nose and Throat Monthly 48*(7): (July) 1969.

10. Crisp, W.E., Shalauta, H., and W.A. Bennett: Shallow conization of the cervix. *Obstetrics and Gynecology 31*(6):755–758, 1968.

11. Dineen, P.: Antibacterial activity of oxidized regenerated cellulose. *Surgery, Gynecology and Obstetrics 142*:481–486, 1976.

12. Dineen, P.: The effect of oxidized regenerated cellulose on experimental intravascular infection. *Surgery 82*:576–579, 1977.

13. Dineen, P.: The effect of oxidized regenerated cellulose on experimental infected splenotomies. *Journal of Surgical Research 23*:114–116, 1977.

Materials Available: Free samples and clinical literature available to physicians. Call 800-526-2459. In New Jersey, call 800-352-4845.

Products are cross-indexed by generic and chemical names in the
YELLOW SECTION

Kenwood Laboratories, Inc.
490-A MAIN STREET
NEW ROCHELLE, NY 10801

GLUTOFAC Tablets™

Composition: Each tablet contains: Saccharomyces Siccum (a selected Brewer's Yeast)—390 mg. (contains Glucose Tolerance Factor—Chromium Complex)

		% U.S. RDA
Vitamin C (Ascorbic Acid)	250 mg.	416
Thiamine Hydrochloride (Vitamin B1)	15 mg.	1000
Riboflavin (Vitamin B2)	10 mg.	588
Niacinamide	50 mg.	250
Vitamin B6 (Pyridoxine Hydrochloride	50 mg.	2500
Calcium Pantothenate	20 mg.	200
Magnesium Sulfate*	70 mg.	17.5
Zinc Sulfate+	80 mg.	533

* AS 50 mg. Dried Magnesiium Sulfate
+ AS 50 mg. Dried Zinc Sulfate

Indication: For patients with nutritional deficiencies resulting from diabetes mellitus, physiologic stress, alcoholism and for other acute and chronic depletional states.

Dosage: Adults: One (1) tablet three (3) times daily or as directed by a physician.

Supplied: Green (film coated) tablets in bottles of 90 and 500.

I.L.X.™ B₁₂ Elixir Crystalline

Composition:
Each (15 cc) contain:
Elemental Iron (from Iron Ammonium Citrate, Brown) ....102 mg
Liver Fraction 1 ....98 mg
Thiamine Hydrochloride (Vitamin B1) ....5 mg
Riboflavin (Vitamin B2) ....2 mg
Nicotinamide ....10 mg
Vitamin B12 Crystalline (Cyanocobalamin) ....10 mcg
Alcohol 8% by Volume

Action and Uses: A readily assimilated elixir for oral therapy in the treatment of iron deficiency anemias.

Administration and Dosage: As a hematinic. One teaspoonful 3 times daily or as directed by physician.

How Supplied: 12 ounce bottles.

I.L.X.™ B₁₂ Tablets

Each tablet contains:
Elemental Iron (from Ferrous Gluconate) ....38 mg.
Vitamin C ....60 mg.
Cyanocobalamin USP (Vit. B12 Cryst.) ....10 mcg.
Liver (Desiccated) N.F. ....2 gr.
Thiamine Hydrochloride ....2 mg.
Riboflavin ....2 mg.
Niacinamide ....20 mg.

Indications: A readily assimilated oral hematinic for the treatment of nutritional and iron deficiency anemias such as those commonly seen in older patients, in convalescense from surgical procedures or medical diseases, and anemias of pregnancy.

Administration and Dosage: One tablet 3 times a day or as directed by physician.

How Supplied: I.L.X. B₁₂™ tablets are supplied in bottles of 100.

Memorandum

Key Pharmaceuticals, Inc.
18425 N.W. 2ND AVE.
MIAMI, FL 33169

AEROBID™ ℞
(flunisolide)
Inhaler system
For oral inhalation only

Description: Flunisolide, the active component of **AeroBid** Inhaler System, is an anti-inflamatory steroid having the chemical name 6α-fluoro-11β, 16α, 17, 21-tetrahydroxypregna-1, 4-diene-3, 20-dione cyclic-16, 17-acetal with acetone. It has the following structure:

Flunisolide is a white to creamy white crystalline powder with a molecular weight of 434.49. It is soluble in acetone, sparingly soluble in chloroform, slightly soluble in methanol, and practically insoluble in water. It has a melting point of about 245°C.

AeroBid Inhaler is delivered in a metered-dose aerosol system containing a microcrystalline suspension of flunisolide as the hemihydrate in propellants (trichloromonofluoromethane, dichlorodifluoromethane and dichlorotetrafluoroethane) with sorbitan trioleate as a dispersing agent. Each activation delivers approximately 250 mcg of flunisolide to the patient. One **AeroBid** Inhaler System is designed to deliver at least 100 metered inhalations.

Clinical Pharmacology: Flunisolide has demonstrated marked anti-inflammatory and anti-allergic activity in classical test systems. It is a corticosteroid that is several hundred times more potent in animal anti-inflammatory assays than the cortisol standard. The molar dose of each activation of flunisolide in this preparation is approximately 2½ to 7 times that of comparable inhaled corticosteroid products marketed for the same indication. The dose of flunisolide delivered per activation in this preparation is 10 times that per activation of Nasalide® (flunisolide) nasal solution. Clinical studies have shown therapeutic activity on bronchial mucosa with minimal evidence of systemic activity at recommended doses.

After oral inhalation of 1 mg flunisolide, total systemic availability was 40%. The flunisolide that is swallowed is rapidly and extensively converted to the 6β-OH metabolite and to water-soluble conjugates during the first pass through the liver. This offers a metabolic explanation for the low systemic activity of oral flunisolide itself since the metabolite has low corticosteroid potency (on the order of the cortisol standard). The inhaled flunisolide absorbed through the bronchial tree is converted to the same metabolites. Repeated inhalation of 2.0 mg of flunisolide per day (the maximum recommended dose) for 14 days did not show accumulation of the drug in plasma. The plasma half-life of flunisolide is approximately 1.8 hours.

The following observations relevant to systemic absorption were made in clinical studies. In one uncontrolled study a statistically significant decrease in responsiveness to metyrapone was noted in 15 adult steroid-independent patients treated with 2.0 mg of flunisolide per day (the maximum recommended dose) for 3 months. A small but statistically significant drop in eosinophils from 11.5% to 7.4% of total circulating leucocytes was noted in another study in children who were not taking oral corticosteroids simultaneously. A 5% incidence of menstrual disturbances was reported during open studies, in which there were no control groups for comparison.

Aerosol administration of flunisolide 2.0 mg twice daily for one week to 6 healthy male subjects revealed neither suppression of adrenal function as measured by early morning cortisol levels nor impairment of HPA axis function as determined by insulin hypoglycemia tests.

Controlled clinical studies have included over 500 patients with asthma, among them 150 children age 6 and over. More than 120 patients have been treated in open trials for two years or more. No significant adrenal suppression attributed to flunisolide was seen in these studies.

Significant decreases of systemic steroid dosages have been possible in flunisolide-treated patients. Asthma patients have had further symptomatic improvement with flunisolide treatment even while reducing concomitant medication.

Indications and Usage: **AeroBid** Inhaler is indicated only for patients who require chronic treatment with corticosteroids for control of the symptoms of bronchial asthma. Such patients would include those already receiving systemic corticosteroids, and selected patients who are inadequately controlled on a non-steroid regimen and in whom steroid therapy has been withheld because of concern over potential adverse effects. As with any topically applied medication, flunisolide is absorbed through the mucous membrane and is systemically available. For these reasons, **AeroBid** Inhaler should be used with caution for initial therapy and the recommended dosage should not be exceeded. When the drug is used chronically at 2 mg/day, patients should be monitored periodically for effects on the hypothalamic-pituitary-adrenal axis.

AeroBid Inhaler is NOT indicated:
1. For relief of asthma that can be controlled by bronchodilators and other non-steroid medications.
2. In patients who require systemic corticosteroid treatment infrequently.
3. In the treatment of non-asthmatic bronchitis.

Insufficient information is available to warrant use in children under the age of 6.

Contraindications: **AeroBid** Inhaler is contraindicated in the primary treamtent of status asthmaticus or other acute episodes of asthma where intensive measures are required.

Hypersensitivity to any of the ingredients on this preparation contraindicates its use.

Warnings:
Particular care is needed in patients who are transferred from systemically active corticosteroids to **AeroBid** Inhaler because deaths due to adrenal insufficiency have occurred in asthmatic patients during and after transfer from systemic corticosteroids to aerosol corticosteroids. After withdrawal from systemic corticosteroids, a number of months are required for recovery of hypothalamic-pituitary-adrenal (HPA) function. During this period of HPA suppression, patients may exhibit signs and symptoms of adrenal insufficiency when exposed to trauma, surgery or infections, particularly gastroenteritis. Although **AeroBid** Inhaler may provide control of asthmatic symptoms during these episodes, it does NOT provide the systemic steroid that is necessary for coping with these emergencies.

During periods of stress or a severe asthmatic attack, patients who have been withdrawn from systemic corticosteroids should be instructed to resume systemic steroids (in large doses) immediately and to contact their physician for further instruction. These patients should also be instructed to carry a warning card indicating that they may need supplementary systemic steroids during periods of stress or a severe asthma attack. To assess the risk of adrenal insufficiency in emergency situations, routine tests of adrenal cortical function, including measurement of early morning resting cortisol levels, should be performed periodically in all patients. An early morning resting cortisol level may be accepted as normal if it falls at or near the normal mean level.

Localized infections with *Candida albicans* or *Aspergillus niger* have occurred in the mouth and pharynx and occasionally in the larynx. Positive cultures for oral *Candida* may be present in up to 34% of patients. Although the frequency of clinically apparent infection is considerably lower, these infections may require treatment with appropriate antifungal therapy or discontinuance of treatment with **AeroBid** inhaler.

AeroBid Inhaler is not to be regarded as a bronchodilator and is not indicated for rapid relief of bronchospasm.

Patients should be instructed to contact their physician immediately when episodes of asthma that are not responsive to bronchodilators occur during the course of treatment. During such episodes, patients may require therapy with systemic corticosteroids.

There is no evidence that control of asthma can be achieved by administration of the drug in amounts greater than the recommended doses, which appear to be the therapeutic equivalent of approximately 10 mg/day of oral prednisone. Theoretically, the use of inhaled corticosteroids with alternate day prednisone systemic treatment should be accompanied by more HPA suppression than a therapeutically equivalent regimen of either alone.

Transfer of patients from systemic steroid therapy to **AeroBid** Inhaler may unmask allergic conditions previously suppressed by the systemic steroid therapy, e.g., rhinitis, conjunctivitis, and eczema.

Precautions:
General: Because of the relatively high molar dose of flunisolide per activation in this preparation, and because of the evidence suggesting higher levels of systemic absorption with flunisolide than with other comparable inhaled corticosteroids (see CLINICAL PHARMACOLOGY section), patients treated with **AeroBid** should be observed carefully for any evidence of systemic corticosteroid effect, including suppression of bone growth in children. Particular care should be taken in observing patients post-operatively or during periods of stress for evidence of a decrease in adrenal function. During withdrawal from oral steroids, some patients may experience symptoms of systemically active steroid withdrawal, e.g., joint and/or muscular pain, lassitude and depression, despite maintenance or even improvement of respiratory function (See DOSAGE AND ADMINISTRATION for details).

In responsive patients, flunisolide may permit control of asthmatic symptoms without suppression of HPA function. Since flunisolide is absorbed into the circulation and can be systemically active, the beneficial effects of **AeroBid** Inhaler in minimizing or preventing HPA dysfunction may be expected only when recommended dosages are not exceeded.

The long-term effects of the drug in human subjects are still unknown. In particular, the local effects of the agent on developmental or immunologic processes in the mouth, pharynx, trachea, and lung are unknown. There is also no information about the possible long-term systemic effects of the agent.

Continued on next page

Key—Cont.

INFORMATION FOR THE PATIENT
How to use your
AeroBid™
(flunisolide)
Inhaler System

Directions For Use: Before using your new **AeroBid** Inhaler System, it is important that you read over the following simple instructions and familiarize yourself with the inhaler and its metal cartridge.

As your doctor has probably told you, the **AeroBid** Inhaler System must be used for a few days before it begins working, and then should be used regularly to help reduce the frequency and severity of your asthma attacks. It is not a bronchodilator and will not provide relief during an actual asthmatic attack, but it can cut down the number of bad attacks if used regularly every day.

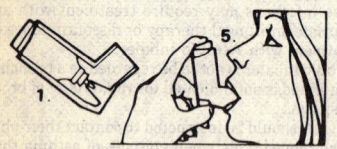

1. Before the first use, place the **AeroBid** metal cartridge inside the plastic container as shown.
2. Shake the inhaler system before each inhalation.
3. Remove cap from mouthpiece.
4. Breathe out as completely as possible.
5. Hold the inhaler system upright and put plastic mouthpiece in your mouth as shown, being sure to close your lips tightly around the mouthpiece.
6. Breathe in deeply and steadily through your mouth. At the same time firmly press down on the metal cartridge with your index finger.
7. Hold your breath as long as you can.
8. While holding your breath, stop pressing on the cartridge and remove mouthpiece from your mouth.
9. If your doctor has prescribed two or more inhalations at each use, wait a minute to allow pressure to build up again in the metal canister, then repeat steps two through eight (2–8). Be sure to shake the inhaler system *again* before each inhalation.
10. After the prescribed number of inhalations, rinse out your mouth thoroughly with water.
11. Clean the inhaler system every few days. To do so, remove the metal cartridge, then rinse the plastic inhaler and cap with briskly running warm water. Dry thoroughly. Replace the cartridge and cap.

Note: If your mouth becomes sore or develops a rash, be sure to mention this to your physician, but do not stop using your inhaler system unless he tells you.

Warning: The contents of the metal cartridge are under pressure. Do not puncture. Do not use or store near heat or open flame. Exposure to temperature above 120°F (49°C) may cause cartridge to explode. Never throw cartridge into fire or incinerator. Use by children should always be supervised by an adult.

The potential effects of the drug on acute, recurrent, or chronic pulmonary infections, including active or quiescent tuberculosis, are not known. Similarly, the potential effects of long-term administration of the drug on lung or other tissues are unknown.

Pulmonary infiltrates with eosinophilia may occur in patients on **AeroBid** Inhaler therapy. Although it is possible that in some patients this state may become manifest because of systemic steroid withdrawal when inhalational steroids are administered, a causative role for the drug and/or its vehicle cannot be ruled out.

Information for Patients:
There is no evidence that better control of asthma can be achieved by the administration of **AeroBid** Inhaler in amounts greater than the recommended doses; higher doses may induce adrenal suppression.

Since the relief from **AeroBid** Inhaler depends on its regular use and on proper inhalation technique, patients must be instructed to take inhalations at regular intervals. They should also be instructed in the correct method of use. (See Patient instruction Leaflet).

Patients receiving bronchodilators by inhalation should be advised to use the bronchodilator before **AeroBid** Inhaler in order to enhance penetration of flunisolide into the bronchial tree. After use of an aerosol bronchodilator, several minutes should elapse before using the **AeroBid** Inhaler.

Patients whose systemic corticosteroids have been reduced or withdrawn should be instructed to carry a warning card indicating they may need supplemental systemic steroids during periods of stress or a severe asthmatic attack that is not responsive to bronchodilators.

An illustrated leaflet of patient instructions for proper use accompanies each **AeroBid** Inhaler System.

CONTENTS UNDER PRESSURE
Do not puncture. Do not use or store near heat or open flame. Exposure to temperatures above 120°F (49°C) may cause container to explode. Never throw container into fire or incinerator. Keep out of reach of children.

Carcinogenesis: A 22-month study was conducted in Swiss derived mice to evaluate the carcinogenic potential of the drug. There was an increase in the incidence of pulmonary adenomas within the range of adenomas previously reported in the literature for untreated or control Swiss derived mice. An additional study is being conducted in a species with a lower incidence of spontaneous pulmonary tumors.

Impairment of fertility: Female rats receiving high doses of flunisolide (200 mcg/kg/day) showed some evidence of impaired fertility. Reproductive performance in the low (8 mcg/kg/day) and mid-dose (40 mcg/kg/day) groups was comparable to controls.

Pregnancy: Pregnancy Category C. As with other corticosteroids, flunisolide has been shown to be teratogenic in rabbits and rats at doses of 40 and 200 mcg/kg/day respectively. It was also fetotoxic in these animal reproductive studies. There are no adequate and well-controlled studies in pregnant women. Flunisolide should be used during pregnancy only if the potential benefit justifies the potential risk to the fetus.

Nursing Mothers: It is not known whether this drug is excreted in human milk. Because other corticosteroids are excreted in human milk, caution should be exercised when flunisolide is administered to nursing women.

Adverse Reactions: Adverse events reported in controlled clinical trials and long-term open studies in 514 patients treated with **AeroBid** are described below. Of those patients, 463 were treated for 3 months or longer, 407 for 6 months or longer, 287 for 1 year or longer, and 122 for 2 years or longer.

Musculoskeletal reactions were reported in 35% of steroid-dependent patients in whom the dose of oral steroid was being tapered. This is a well-known effect of steroid withdrawal.

Incidence 10% or greater:
Gastrointestinal: diarrhea (10%), nausea and/or vomiting (25%), upset stomach (10%)
General: flu (10%)
Mouth and Throat: sore throat (20%)
Nervous system: headache (25%)
Respiratory: cold symptoms (15%), nasal congestion (15%), upper respiratory infection (25%)
Special Senses: unpleasant taste (10%)

Incidence 3–9%
Cardiovascular: palpitations
Gastrointestinal: abdominal pain, heartburn
General: chest pain, decreased appetite, edema, fever
Mouth and Throat: *Candida* infection
Nervous System: dizziness, irritability, nervousness, shakiness
Reproductive: menstrual disturbances
Respiratory: chest congestion, cough*, hoarseness, rhinitis, runny nose, sinus congestion, sinus drainage, sinus infection, sinusitis, sneezing, sputum, wheezing*
Skin: eczema, itching (pruritus), rash
Special Senses: ear infection, loss of smell or taste

Incidence 1–3%
General: chills, increased appetite and weight gain, malaise, peripheral edema, sweating, weakness
Cardiovascular: hypertension, tachycardia
Gastrointestinal: constipation, dyspepsia, gas
Hemic/Lymph: capillary fragility, enlarged lymph nodes
Mouth and Throat: dry throat, glossitis, mouth irritation, pharyngitis, phlegm, throat irritation
Nervous System: anxiety, depression, faintness, fatigue, hyperactivity, hypoactivity, insomnia, moodiness, numbness, vertigo
Respiratory: bronchitis, chest tightness*, dyspnea, epistaxis, head stuffiness, laryngitis, nasal irritation, pleurisy, pneumonia, sinus discomfort
Skin: acne, hives, or urticaria
Special Senses: blurred vision, earache, eye discomfort, eye infection

Incidence less than 1%, judged by investigators as possibly or probably drug related: abdominal fullness, shortness of breath.

*The incidences as shown of cough, wheezing, and chest tightness were judged by investigators to be possibly or probably drug-related. In placebo-controlled trials, the *overall* incidences of these adverse events (regardless of investigators' judgment of drug relationship) were similar for drug and placebo-treated groups. They may be related to the vehicle or delivery system.

Dosage and Administration: The **AeroBid** Inhaler System is for oral inhalation only.
Adults: The recommended starting dose is 2 inhalations twice daily morning and evening for a total daily dose of 1 mg. The maximum daily dose should not exceed 4 inhalations twice a day for a total daily dose of 2 mg. When the drug is used chronically at 2 mg/day, patients should be monitored periodically for effects on the hypothalamic-pituitary-adrenal axis.
Children: For children 6–15 years of age, two inhalations may be administered twice daily for a total daily dose of 1 mg. Higher doses have not been studied. Insufficient information is available to warrant use in children under age 6. With chronic use, children should be monitored for growth as well as for effects on the HPA axis.
Rinsing the mouth after inhalation is advised. Patients receiving bronchodilators by inhalation should be advised to use the bronchodilator before **AeroBid** Inhaler in order to enhance penetration of flunisolide into the bronchial tree. After use of an aerosol bronchodilator, several minutes should elapse before use of the **AeroBid** inhaler to reduce the potential toxicity from the inhaled fluorocarbon propellants in the two aerosols.
*Different considerations must be given to the following groups of patients in order to obtain the full therapeutic benefit of **AeroBid** Inhaler.*
Patients not receiving systemic steroids: The use of **AeroBid** Inhaler is straightforward in patients

who are inadequately controlled with non-steroid medications but in whom systemic steroid therapy has been withheld because of concern over potential adverse reactions. In patients who respond to the drug, an improvement in pulmonary function is usually apparent within one to four weeks after the start of treatment.

Patients receiving systemic steroids: In those patients dependent on systemic steroids, transfer to **AeroBid** and subsequent management may be more difficult because recovery from impaired adrenal function is usually slow. Such suppression has been known to last for up to 12 months. Clinical studies, however, have demonstrated that **AeroBid** may be effective in the management of these asthmatic patients and may permit replacement or significant reduction in the dosage of systemic corticosteroids.

Inhaled corticosteroids generally are not recommended for chronic use with alternate day prednisone regimens (see WARNINGS).

The patient's asthma should be reasonably stable before treatment with **AeroBid** Inhaler is started. Initially, the aerosol should be used concurrently with the patient's usual maintenance dose of systemic steroid. After approximately one week, gradual withdrawal of the systemic steroid is started by reducing the daily or alternate daily dose. The next reduction is made after an interval of one or two weeks, depending on the response of the patient. Generally, these decrements should not exceed 2.5 mg of prednisone or its equivalent. A slow rate of withdrawal cannot be overemphasized. During withdrawal, some patients may experience symptoms of systemically active steroid withdrawal, e.g., joint and/or muscular pain, lassitude and depression, despite maintenance or even improvement of respiratory function. Such patients should be encouraged to continue with the Inhaler but should be watched carefully for objective signs of adrenal insufficiency, such as hypotension and weight loss. If evidence of adrenal insufficiency occurs, the systemic steroid dose should be boosted temporarily and thereafter further withdrawal should continue more slowly. *During periods of stress or a severe asthma attack, transfer patients will require supplementary treatment with systemic steroids.* Exacerbations of asthma that occur during the course of treatment with **AeroBid** Inhaler should be treated with a short course of systemic steroid that is gradually tapered as these symptoms subside. There is no evidence that control of asthma can be achieved by administration of the drug in amounts greater than the recommended doses.

How Supplied: **AeroBid** (flunisolide) Inhaler System is available in canisters of 100 metered inhalations.

(NDC 0369-3007-01)

Caution: Federal law prohibits dispensing without prescription.

Revised 0884
1300700

Mfd by: Riker Laboratories, Inc.
Northridge, California 91324
For: Key Pharmaceuticals, Inc.
Miami, Florida 33169

INSPIREASE™ ℞
Drug delivery system for metered dose inhalers

Description: InspirEase™ is an effective and easy-to-use portable drug delivery system for metered dose inhalers (MDIs). Its components are a replaceable reservoir bag and two mouthpieces adaptable to most of the MDIs currently available. The *light blue* mouthpiece is designed to be used with metered dose inhaler canisters that have a metal valve stem. The *darker blue* mouthpiece is designed to be used with inhaler canisters that have a white plastic valve stem. A carrying case is supplied for transporting and storing InspirEase and the MDI container.

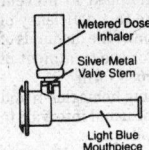 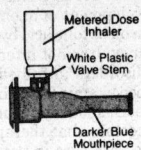

Indications: InspirEase improves the distribution and deposition in the lungs of aerosolized medications from MDIs. Therefore, the usual caution should be exercised in dosing medication and evaluating patient response.

1. Minimal patient skill is required for use.
   A significant number of patients fail to derive full benefit from their MDIs. This is sometimes due to inadequate instruction or to misuse of the device by anxious, breathless patients. The correct use of an MDI requires greater skill than is immediately apparent.[1–5]
   Studies have demonstrated that nearly 50% of patients had difficulty coordinating MDI activation with inspiration.[3–5] This is a major factor limiting aerosol delivery to the airways.[2] With MDIs alone, the patient has to carefully time each inspiration with activation of the inhaler. InspirEase eliminates the need for the patient to coordinate inspiration with activation of the MDI.

2. Medication is more effectively delivered to the airways.
   With InspirEase, medication is more effectively delivered to the airways—less is deposited on the oropharynx, because the aerosol particles are inhaled slowly and evenly. The reservoir bag acts as a collecting chamber for the medication emitted from MDIs. This permits the patient to calmly inhale medication and rebreathe with a second breath.

3. Proper breathing technique is encouraged.
   InspirEase has visual and auditory signals to help patients assess the rate and depth of each inhalation. Slow, deep inspiration results in deflation of the reservoir bag and *no* whistling sound. Rapid inspiration (greater than 0.3 L/s) produces a whistling sound from the flow rate monitor. This signals the patient to inhale more slowly. Patients can see and feel the bag collapsing.
   The volume of the fully extended reservoir bag is approximately 700 ml, which is approximately 1½ to 2 times the average adult tidal volume.

Directions for Use

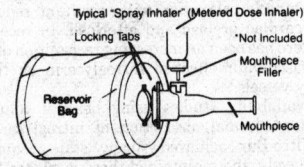

Your patient should:
1. Select the appropriate mouthpiece that fits his or her inhaler. Connect it to the reservoir bag by lining up *locking tabs*, pushing them into the bag and twisting clockwise to lock.

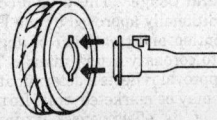

2. Untwist the reservoir bag gently to open it to its full size. Shake drug canister well before placing its stem into the *mouthpiece filler*. Make sure it fits snugly.

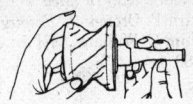

3. Place mouthpiece in mouth and close lips tightly around it.
4. Press down on drug canister to release one dose into the bag.
   NOTE: Patients should be reminded of the correct dosage schedule.

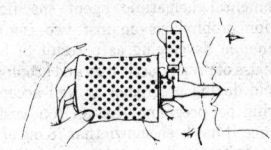

5. Breathe in slowly through the mouthpiece. If a whistling sound is produced, inhalation should be slowed until the sound stops.

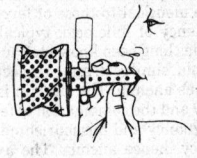

6. Breathe in the entire contents of the bag until further deflation is impossible and no more air can be taken in.
7. *Hold his or her breath while slowly counting to five.*
8. Breathe out slowly into the bag.

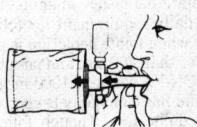

9. Repeat the inhale/exhale cycle (steps 5 through 8) a second time, keeping lips tightly closed around the mouthpiece.
10. Remove the mouthpiece from mouth. Take drug canister off the reservoir bag. Unlock mouthpiece from the bag and store all components in carrying case.

IMPORTANT CLEANING INSTRUCTIONS
Your patient should:
1. Clean only the mouthpiece thoroughly, with warm (not hot) running water *at least* once a day. *InspirEase is not dishwasher safe. Always clean by hand.*
2. Wait until mouthpiece is *completely dry* before placing in carrying case.
3. Replace reservoir bags every two to three weeks, or as needed, depending on the rate of use. However, if there is a hole or tear in it, replace immediately.
4. Replace mouthpiece every six to nine months, as needed.

Note: *InspirEase is designed for single-patient use and single-drug use.* Effectiveness in children below the age of 12 has not been established.

Caution: Federal law restricts this device to sale by or on the order of a physician.

References:
1. Sackner MA, Brown LK, Kim CS: *Chest* 80(suppl):915-918, 1981. 2. Tobin MJ, Jenouri G,

Continued on next page

Key—Cont.

Danta I, et al: *Am Rev Respir Dis* 126:670-675, 1982. **3.** Saunders KB: *Br Med J* 1:1037-1038, 1965. **4.** Gayrard P, Orehek J: *Respiration* 40:47-52, 1980. **5.** Shim C, Williams MH Jr: *Am J Med* 69:891-894, 1980.

IRCON®-FA
[ir′ kon] ℞

Description: IRCON-FA contains 1.0 mg of folic acid, and 250 mg of ferrous fumarate equivalent to 82 mg of elemental iron.

Clinical Pharmacology: IRCON-FA is a prenatal supplemental hematinic agent specifically intended for prophylaxis against two common types of anemia developing as a result of pregnancy. The use of prophylactic iron and prophylactic folic acid during pregnancy is well accepted. Child-bearing (per pregnancy) has an iron "cost" of about 725 mg. It has been shown that 78 mg of elemental iron, taken orally each day during the last half of pregnancy, will protect against iron deficiency anemia; half this dose is insufficient to maintain iron stores. Two hundred fifty mg of ferrous fumarate contain approximately 82 mg of iron. Absorption characteristics of ferrous fumarate are identical to those of ferrous sulfate.

A deficiency of folic acid, typically during pregnancy, has long been known to cause a megaloblastic anemia, similar in some respects to Addisonian pernicious anemia. The vitamin is not storable in the body and the combination of fetal demand during pregnancy and misnourishment can lead to a deficiency, hence anemia. The average daily requirement of folic acid during pregnancy is unknown. It has been found that a dosage of 20 mcg/day is inadequate. In other instances doses of 1000 mcg/day orally have been found to produce a prompt hematological response in megaloblastic anemia of pregnancy.

Daily doses of folic acid greater than 1.0 mg/day have not been shown to be necessary, even in cases of overt folate deficiency anemia. The estimated minimum daily requirement for folic acid in late pregnancy when folate depletion is present is said to be greater than 200 mcg and possibly 400 mcg or more. IRCON-FA contains 1000 mcg. Folic acid is nontoxic and has commonly been given in several times this daily dose. Though folic acid dietary deficiency in the United States is rare, prophylaxis during pregnancy is considered to be justified in view of the possibly serious consequences of its depletion, both for the mother (megaloblastic anemia) and the fetus.

Finally, it has been observed that the rapid production of red blood cells following treatment with iron alone may deplete the body of folate if there is inadequate intake; combining the two substances avoids this complication.

Indications and Usage: For maintenance of maternal hematopoiesis during pregnancy, particularly when diet is abnormal or substandard.

Contraindications:
1) Pernicious anemia. Although rare in the population likely to receive IRCON-FA this megaloblastic anemia must be borne in mind. It is due to faulty or blocked absorption of vitamin B_{12}, or extrinsic factor, on either a genetic, immunologic or surgical basis. The particular danger of missing a diagnosis of pernicious anemia—in relation to folic acid therapy—is that folic acid can mask PA by causing a hematologic remission while allowing the neurological complications of the disease to proceed apace. Thus, before IRCON-FA is prescribed for megaloblastic anemia in pregnancy, appropriate diagnostic exclusion of Addisonian pernicious anemia should be carried out.
2) Anemias other than those due to iron deficiency.

Warning: Folic acid alone is improper therapy in the treatment of pernicious anemia and other megaloblastic anemias where vitamin B_{12} is deficient.

Precautions:
1) If, at the time of initial examination, definite anemia is found, a diagnosis of its cause should be made.
2) IRCON-FA is primarily intended to prevent the development of anemia due to a deficiency of either iron or folic acid by reason of the demands of pregnancy. It is not intended for the treatment of these disorders in fully developed form.
3) Blood examinations including hemoglobin and hematocrit should be done at the usual intervals to make certain that therapy is adequate.
4) Use with care in the presence of peptic ulcer, regional enteritis and ulcerative colitis.
5) Folic acid especially in doses above 1.0 mg. daily may obscure pernicious anemia, in that hematologic remission may occur while neurological manifestations remain progressive.

Adverse Reactions:
1) Ferrous fumarate gastric distress, abdominal cramps, diarrhea.
2) Folic acid allergic sensitization has been reported following both oral and parenteral administration of folic acid.

Dosage and Administration: The usual dose in the second and third trimester of pregnancy is one tablet daily, taken in the morning between breakfast and lunch with a glass of water or milk. If hyperemesis gravidarum is a problem, the dose may be taken in mid-afternoon.

How Supplied: IRCON-FA tablets are available in bottles of 100.

Caution: FEDERAL LAW PROHIBITS DISPENSING WITHOUT PRESCRIPTION.

NITRO-DUR®
[ni′ tra-dur] ℞
(nitroglycerin)
Transdermal Infusion System

Description: The Nitro-Dur Transdermal Infusion System contains nitroglycerin in a gel-like matrix composed of glycerin, water (purified), lactose, polyvinyl alcohol, povidone and sodium citrate to provide a continuous source of the active ingredient. Nitro-Dur is available in dosage sizes $5cm^2$, $10cm^2$, $15cm^2$ and $20cm^2$, containing 26 mg, 51 mg, 77 mg and 104 mg of nitroglycerin, respectively, thereby providing a range of dosing levels of nitroglycerin. Nitro-Dur has a rated release in vivo of approximately $0.5mg/cm^2/24$ hours. Each unit is sealed in a polyester-foil-polyethylene laminate. The bandage portion consists of a medical grade non-woven, heat sealable, microporous tape.

Clinical Pharmacology: When the Nitro-Dur system is applied to the skin, nitroglycerin is absorbed continuously through the skin into the systemic circulation. This results in active drug reaching the target organs (heart, extremities) before deactivation by the liver. Nitroglycerin is a smooth muscle relaxant with vascular effects manifested predominantly by venous dilation and pooling. The major beneficial effect of nitroglycerin in angina pectoris is a reduction in myocardial oxygen consumption secondary to vascular smooth muscle relaxation with resultant reduction in cardiac preload and afterload. In recent years there has been an increasing recognition of a direct vasodilator effect of nitroglycerin on the coronary vessels.

In bioavailability studies using healthy volunteers[1], transdermal absorption of nitroglycerin from Nitro-Dur achieved steady state venous plasma levels, and maintained these levels for 24 hours. Detectable plasma levels were attained within 30 minutes after application of the system, and were still detectable 30 minutes after removal of the system. Precise definition of "therapeutic plasma level" is not known at this time.

Indications and Usage: This drug product has been conditionally approved by the FDA for the prevention and treatment of angina pectoris due to coronary artery disease. The conditional approval reflects a determination that the drug may be marketed while further investigation of its effectiveness is undertaken. A final evaluation of the effectiveness of the product will be announced by the FDA.

Contraindications: Intolerance of organic nitrate drugs, marked anemia.

Warnings: The Nitro-Dur system should be used under careful clinical and/or hemodynamic monitoring in patients with acute myocardial infarction or congestive heart failure.

In terminating treatment of anginal patients, both the dosage and frequency of application must be gradually reduced over a period of 4 to 6 weeks in order to prevent sudden withdrawal reactions, which are characteristic of all vasodilators in the nitroglycerin class.

Safe use in pregnancy has not been established relative to possible adverse effect on fetal development, but neither have adverse effects on fetal development been established. Therefore, use of nitroglycerin in pregnant women should be balanced against the risk of uncontrolled angina pectoris.

Precautions: Symptoms of hypotension, such as faintness, weakness or dizziness, particularly orthostatic hypotension, may be due to overdosage. If during the course of treatment these symptoms occur, the dosage should be reduced or use of the product discontinued.

Nitro-Dur is not intended for use in the treatment of acute anginal attacks. For this purpose, occasional use of sublingual nitroglycerin may be necessary.

Adverse Reactions: Transient headache is the most common side effect, especially when higher doses of the drug are administered. Headaches should be treated with mild analgesics while continuing Nitro-Dur therapy. If headache persists, the Nitro-Dur dosage should be reduced.

Adverse reactions reported less frequently include hypotension, increased heart rate, faintness, flushing, dizziness, nausea, vomiting, and dermatitis. Except for dermatitis, these symptoms are attributed to the pharmacologic effects of nitroglycerin. However, they may be symptoms of overdosage. When they persist, the Nitro-Dur dosage should be reduced or use of the product discontinued.

Dosage and Administration: To apply the Nitro-Dur system, tear away the printed foil surface, then peel away the sectioned release liner as you would an adhesive bandage. Apply the Nitro-Dur system firmly to the skin surface. The initial starting dose is a $5cm^2$ system. To achieve optimum therapeutic effect in some patients, it may be necessary to titrate to a higher dosing strength. Dosage should be titrated while monitoring clinical response, i.e., blood pressure, episodes of angina and subsequent use of sublingual nitroglycerin. The Nitro-Dur system may remain in place for periods of up to 24 hours as required to provide continuous prophylactic levels of nitroglycerin.

The Nitro-Dur system may be applied to any convenient skin area; a recommended site of application is the arm or chest. A suitable area may be shaved if necessary. Do not apply the Nitro-Dur system to the distal part of the extremities.

Storage Conditions: Store at controlled room temperature 15–30°C (59–86°F).

How Supplied: Nitro-Dur Transdermal Infusion System, $5cm^2$, $10cm^2$, $15cm^2$ and $20cm^2$, is available in unit dose packages of 28 and hospital unit dose packages of 100.

Caution: FEDERAL LAW PROHIBITS DISPENSING WITHOUT PRESCRIPTION.

Patient Instructions for Application: Patient Instructions are furnished with each unit dose package.

[1]Data on file: **KEY PHARMACEUTICALS, INC.**
Miami, Florida 33269—0670 (USA)

Shown in Product Identification Section, p. 413

NITROGLYN®
[nī′tra-glin]
(nitroglycerin)
Sustained Action Tablets

Description: NITROGLYN, formulated as sustained action tablets, contains nitroglycerin (glyceryl trinitrate). NITROGLYN is available in two strengths: 1/25 gr (2.6 mg) and 1/10 gr (6.5 mg).

Clinical Pharmacology: The principal action of nitroglycerin is to relax all smooth muscle, most prominently on vascular smooth muscle. The action on small post-capillary vessels dominates the hemodynamic picture. The resulting increase in cardiac output is transient, and followed by a moderate decrease due to reduced venous return, associated with peripheral vasodilation. The mean arterial pressure may not be affected, or may be decreased. The speed and magnitude of response depend on the dose, the rate of release from the tablet, the rate of absorption, and individual susceptibility. Availability of nitroglycerin at 2 dosage levels permits tailoring the required dose to the need of each patient with angina pectoris.

The release of nitroglycerin from NITROGLYN is gradual but the rate of absorption from the gastrointestinal tract in patients with angina pectoris has not been estabished. Dilation of the coronary arteries has been established in some anginal patients following sublingual administration but not in others. More often patients with coronary artery disease show no change or decrease in coronary flow. Nitroglycerin can act as physiological antagonist to norepinephrine, acetylcholine and histamine. While the mechanism of action of nitroglycerin in the treatment of patients with angina pectoris is still to be established, its use has been well documented for more than a century and is considered the drug of choice.

Indications and Usage:
Based on a review of this drug by the National Academy of Sciences-National Research Council and/or other information FDA has classified the indications as follows: "Possibly" Effective.
Sustained action tablets of nitroglycerin are possibly effective for indications relating to the management, prophylaxis or treatment of anginal attacks. This possibly effective classification applies also to conventional or extended action oral forms of all other organic nitrate antianginal drugs alone or in combination.

Contraindications: Data supporting the use of organic nitrates during the course of acute myocardial infarction are not sufficient to establish safety. Caution should be used in administration to anginal patients with postural hypotension or with closed-angle glaucoma.

Precautions: Use the smallest dose which proves effective. Tablets must be swallowed whole. FOR ORAL, NOT SUBLINGUAL USE. Store in cool, dry place and keep container tightly capped. Cross tolerance may develop to other organic nitrates. Continued treatment is not recommended unless the patient is benefited.

Adverse Reactions: Some patients exhibit hypersensitivity to the hypotensive effects of nitroglycerin, as shown by nausea, vomiting, restlessness, pallor, perspiration and collapse, from the usual dose. Other patients may develop severe and persistent headaches, cutaneous flushing, dizziness and weakness; occasionally drug rash or exfoliative dermatitis; these responses may disappear with decrease in dosage. Adverse effects are enhanced by ingestion of alcohol, which appears to increase absorption from the gastrointestinal tract.

Dosage and Administration: Administer the smallest effective dose 2 or 3 times daily unless clinical response suggests a different regimen. Discontinue if not effective.

How Supplied: NITROGLYN 1/25 gr (2.6 mg) and 1/10 gr (6.5 mg) sustained action tablets are available in bottles of 100.

Caution: FEDERAL LAW PROHIBITS DISPENSING WITHOUT PRESCRIPTION.

QUINORA®
[kwin-ō-ra]
(quinidine sulfate tablets U.S.P.)

Description: QUINORA tablets contain quinidine sulfate with no color additives in the base. QUINORA is available in two strengths, 200 mg and 300 mg.

Clinical Pharmacology: Quinidine is generally regarded as a myocardial depressant drug, because it depresses excitability, conduction velocity, and contractility of the myocardium. Besides these direct effects quinidine exerts some indirect effects on the heart through an anticholinergic action. Large oral doses may reduce the arterial pressure due to peripheral vasodilation. Hypotension of a serious degree is more likely with the parenteral use of the drug.

Quinidine is essentially completely absorbed after oral administration; maximal effects occur within 1 to 3 hours and persist for 6 to 8 or more hours. Blood levels of quinidine can be measured; the average therapeutic range is between 3 and 6 mg per liter of plasma; toxic reactions are almost certain to appear at levels above 8 mg per liter.

Indications and Usage: Quinidine sulfate is indicated in the treatment of premature atrial and ventricular contractions, paroxysmal atrial tachycardia, paroxysmal A-V junctional rhythm, atrial flutter, paroxysmal atrial fibrillation, established atrial fibrillation when therapy is appropriate, and paroxysmal ventricular tachycardia when not associated with complete heartblock, and for maintenance therapy after electrical conversion of atrial fibrillation and/or flutter.

Contraindications: Hypersensitivity or idiosyncrasy to the drug. History of thrombocytopenic purpura associated with previous quinidine administration. Digitalis intoxication manifested by A-V conduction disorders. Complete A-V block with an A-V nodal or idioventricular pacemaker. Ectopic impulses and rhythms due to escape mechanisms.

Warnings: In the treatment of atrial flutter, reversion to sinus rhythm may be preceded by a progressive reduction in the degree of A-V block to a 1:1 ratio resulting in extremely rapid ventricular rate. This possible hazard may be decreased by digitalization prior to giving quinidine. Evidence of quinidine cardiotoxicity (50% widening of QRS, frequent ventricular ectopic beats) mandates immediate discontinuation of the drug followed with close observation (ECG-monitoring) of the patient.

Usage in Pregnancy: The use of quinidine in pregnancy should be reserved only for those cases where the benefits outweigh the possible hazards to patient and fetus.

Precautions: Use quinidine with extreme caution in the presence of incomplete A-V block since complete block and asystole may result. Quinidine may cause unpredictable abnormalities of rhythm in digitalized hearts and it should be used with special caution in the presence of digitalis intoxication. **Note:** Quinidine effect is enhanced by potassium and reduced in the presence of hypokalemia.

The depressant actions of quinidine on cardiac contractility and arterial blood pressure limit its use in congestive heart failure and in hypotensive states unless these conditions are due to, or aggravated by, the arrhythmia. The potential disadvantage and benefits must be weighed. Continuous ECG-monitoring and determination of plasma quinidine levels are indicated when large doses, more than 2 g/day, are used.

Adverse Reactions:
Symptoms of cinchonism: (ringing in the ears, headache, nausea, disturbed vision) may appear (in sensitive patients) after a single dose of the drug.
Cardiovascular: widening of QRS-complex, cardiac asystole, ventricular ectopic beats, idioventricular rhythms including ventricular tachycardia and fibrillation, paradoxical tachycardia, arterial embolism.
Gastrointestinal: nausea, vomiting, abdominal pain, diarrhea.
Hematologic: acute hemalytic anemia, hypoprothrombinemia, thrombocytopenic purpura, agranulocytosis.
CNS: headache, fever, vertigo, apprehension, excitement, confusion, delirium and syncope, disturbed hearing (tinnitus, decreased auditory acuity), disturbed vision (mydriasis, blurred vision, disturbed color perception, photophobia, diplopia, night blindness, scotomata), optic neuritis.
Dermatologic: cutaneous flushing with intense pruritus.
Hypersensitivity reactions: Angioedema, acute asthmatic episode, vascular collapse, respiratory arrest.
Overdosage: Cardiotoxic effects of quinidine may be reversed in part by sodium lactate; the hypotension by vasoconstrictors and by catecholamines (since the vasodilation is partly due to α adrenergic blockade).

Dosage and Administration: A preliminary test dose of a single tablet of quinidine sulfate should be administered to determine whether the patient has an idiosyncrasy to it. Continuous ECG-monitoring is recommended in all cases where quinidine is used in large doses.
Usual Adult Dose: Premature atrial and ventricular contractions: 200 to 300 mg three or four times daily.
Paroxysmal supraventricular tachycardias: 400 to 600 mg every 2 or 3 hours until the paroxysm is terminated.
Atrial flutter: Quinidine should be administered after digitalization for this indication. Dosage is to be individualized.
Conversion of atrial fibrillation: Various schedules of quinidine administration have been in clinical use. A widely used technique is the administration of 200 mg of quinidine orally every 2 or 3 hours for 5 to 8 doses, with subsequent daily increase of the individual dose until sinus rhythm is restored or toxic effects occur. The total daily dose should not exceed 3 to 4 g, given by any schedule. Prior to quinidine administration the ventricular rate and congestive failure (if present) should be brought under control by digitalis therapy.
Maintenance therapy: 200 to 300 mg three or four times daily.

How Supplied: QUINORA 200 mg and 300 mg tablets are available in bottles of 100 and 1000.

Caution: FEDERAL LAW PROHIBITS DISPENSING WITHOUT PRESCRIPTION.

THEO-DUR®
[thē-a-dur]
(theophylline anhydrous sustained action tablets)

Description: THEO-DUR sustained action tablets contain anhydrous theophylline, a bronchodilator, in a sustained release formulation which allows a 12-hour dosing interval for a majority of patients and a 24-hour dosing interval for selected patients (see DOSAGE AND ADMINISTRATION section for description of appropriate patient populations). THEO-DUR contains no color additives and is available in three strengths: 100 mg, 200 mg and 300 mg.

The structural formula of theophylline, 1,3-dimethylxanthine is:

Anhydrous theophylline is a white, odorless, crystalline powder having a bitter taste.

Clinical Pharmacology: Theophylline directly relaxes the smooth muscle of the bronchial airways and pulmonary blood vessels, thus acting mainly as a bronchodilator and smooth muscle

Continued on next page

Key—Cont.

relaxant. The drug also produces other actions typical of the xanthine derivatives: coronary vasodilator, cardiac stimulant, diuretic, cerebral stimulant, and skeletal muscle stimulant. The actions of theophylline may be mediated through inhibition of phosphodiesterase and a resultant increase in intracellular cyclic AMP.

In-vitro theophylline has been shown to act synergistically with beta agonists that increase intracellular cyclic AMP through the stimulation of adenyl cyclase, but synergism has not been demonstrated in patient studies. More data are needed to determine if theophylline and beta agonists have a clinically important additive effect *in-vivo*. Apparently, no development of tolerance occurs with chronic use of theophylline.

Pharmacokinetics: The half-life of theophylline is influenced by a number of known variables. It is prolonged in patients suffering from chronic alcoholism, impaired hepatic or renal function, congestive heart failure, and in patients receiving macrolide antibiotics and cimetidine. Older adults (over age 55) and patients with chronic obstructive pulmonary disease, with or without cor pulmonale, may also have much slower clearance rates. For such patients, the theophylline half-life may exceed 24 hours.

Newborns and neonates have extremely slow clearance rates compared to older infants (over 6 months) and children, and may also have a theophylline half-life of over 24 hours. High fever for prolonged periods may also reduce the rate of theophylline elimination.

THEOPHYLLINE ELIMINATION CHARACTERISTICS

Theophylline Clearance Rates (mean ± S.D.)	Half-life Average (mean ± S.D.)
Children (over 6 months of age)	
1.45 ± 0.58 ml/kg/min	3.7 ± 1.1 hrs.
Adult non-smokers uncomplicated asthma	
0.65 ± 0.19 ml/kg/min	8.7 ± 2.2 hrs.

The half-life of theophylline in smokers (1 to 2 packs/day) averages 4–5 hours, much shorter than the half-life in non-smokers which averages 7–9 hours. The increase in theophylline clearance caused by smoking is probably the result of induction of drug-metabolizing enzymes that do not readily normalize after cessation of smoking. It appears that between 3 months and 2 years may be necessary for normalization of the effect of smoking on theophylline pharmacokinetics.

In single dose studies with 18 subjects, THEO-DUR, at 8 mg/kg body weight, produced mean peak theophylline blood levels of 7.5 ± 1.9 mcg/ml at 9.2 ± 1.9 hours following administration. In multiple dose, steady-state, 3 and 5 day studies with 12 subjects, THEO-DUR administered as 8mg/kg twice daily, achieved an average peak-trough difference of 4 mcg/ml. The Cmax and Cmin were 13.9 ± 6.9 and 9.9 ± 6.0, respectively. In a multiple dose (300–500 mg BID), steady-state, 5 day study involving 14 normal, nonfasting, subjects with theophylline half-lives between 5.8 and 12.3 hours (mean 8.0 ± 1.8 hours), THEO-DUR, dosed twice daily, produced mean Cmax and Cmin levels of 12.2 ± 2.0 and 10.2 ± 1.6 mcg/ml, respectively, over the a.m. dosing interval and Cmax and Cmin of 11.6 ± 1.6 and 8.7 ± 1.8 mcg/ml, respectively, over the p.m. dosing interval. In the same subjects, THEO-DUR given once daily, in the morning, in doses ranging from 600–1000 mg (same daily dose as for BID, above) produced a mean Cmax and Cmin of 14.4 ± 2.2 and 5.5 ± 2.0, respectively and a mean fraction of fluctuation of 0.63 ± 0.11 [Cmax -Cmin/ Cmax]. Average peak-trough differences over 24 hours were 8.9 ± 1.3 and 3.7 ± 2.2 mcg/ml when THEO-DUR was given once or twice daily, respectively. In both the twice daily and once daily dosing regimens, THEO-DUR exhibited complete bioavailability when compared to an immediate release product.

Indications: THEO-DUR is indicated for relief and/or prevention of symptoms of bronchial asthma and for reversible bronchospasm associated with chronic bronchitis and emphysema.

Contraindications: THEO-DUR is contraindicated in individuals who have shown hypersensitivity to theophylline or any of the tablet components.

Warnings: Status asthmaticus should be considered a medical emergency and is defined as that degree of bronchospasm which is not rapidly responsive to usual doses of conventional bronchodilators. Optimal therapy for such patients frequently requires both *additional medication*, parenterally administered, and *close monitoring*, preferably in an intensive care setting.

Although increasing the dose of theophylline may bring about relief, such treatment may be associated with toxicity. The likelihood of such toxicity developing increases significantly when the serum theophylline concentration exceeds 20 mcg/ml. Therefore, determination of serum theophylline levels is recommended to assure maximal benefit without excessive risk.

Serum levels above 20 mcg/ml are rarely found after appropriate administration of the recommended doses. However, in individuals in whom theophylline plasma clearance is reduced *for any reason*, even conventional doses may result in increased serum levels and potential toxicity. Reduced theophylline clearance has been documented in the following readily identifiable groups: 1) patients with impaired renal or liver function; 2) patients over 55 years of age, particularly males and those with chronic lung disease; 3) those with cardiac failure from any cause; 4) neonates; and 5) those patients taking certain drugs (macrolide antibiotics and cimetidine). Decreased clearance of theophylline may be associated with either influenza immunization or active infection with influenza.

Reduction of dosage and laboratory monitoring is especially appropriate in the above individuals. Less serious signs of theophylline toxicity, i.e. nausea and restlessness, may appear in up to 50% of patients. Unfortunately, however, serious side effects such as ventricular arrhythmias, convulsions or even death may appear as the first sign of toxicity without any previous warning. Stated differently; *serious toxicity is not reliably preceded by less severe side effects.*

Many patients who require theophylline may exhibit tachycardia due to their underlying disease process so that the cause/effect relationship to elevated serum theophylline concentrations may not be appreciated.

Theophylline products may cause dysrhythmia and/or worsen pre-existing arrhythmias and any significant change in rate and/or rhythm warrants monitoring and further investigation.

The occurrence of arrhythmias and sudden death (with histological evidence of necrosis of the myocardium) has been recorded in laboratory animals (minipigs, rodents and dogs) when theophylline and beta agonists were administered concomitantly, although not when either was administered alone. The significance of these findings when applied to human usage is currently unknown.

Precautions: THEO-DUR TABLETS SHOULD NOT BE CHEWED OR CRUSHED.

General: Theophylline half-life is shorter in smokers than in nonsmokers. Therefore, smokers may require larger or more frequent doses. Morphine and curare should be used with caution in patients with airway obstruction as they may suppress respiration and stimulate histamine release. Alternative drugs should be used when possible. Theophylline should not be administered concurrently with other xanthine medications. Use with caution in patients with severe cardiac disease, severe hypoxemia, hypertension, hyperthyroidism, acute myocardial injury, cor pulmonale, congestive heart failure, liver disease, in the elderly (especially males) and in neonates. In particular, great caution should be used in giving theophylline to patients with congestive heart failure. Frequently, such patients have markedly prolonged theophylline serum levels with theophylline persisting in serum for long periods following discontinuation of the drug. Individuals who are rapid metabolizers of theophylline, such as the young, smokers, and some non-smoking adults, may not be suitable candidates for once-daily dosing. These individuals will generally need to be dosed at 12 hourly or sometimes 8 hourly intervals. Such patients may exhibit symptoms of bronchospasm near the end of a dosing interval, or may have wider peak-to-trough differences than desired.

Use theophylline cautiously in patients with history of peptic ulcer. Theophylline may occasionally act as a local irritant to the G.I. tract although gastrointestinal symptoms are more commonly centrally mediated and associated with serum drug concentrations over 20 mcg/ml.

Information for Patients: The physician should reinforce the importance of taking only the prescribed dose and time interval between doses. THEO-DUR tablets should not be chewed or crushed. When dosing THEO-DUR on a once daily (q24h) basis, tablets should be taken whole and not split. As with any controlled-release theophylline product, the patient should alert the physician if symptoms occur repeatedly, especially near the end of the dosing interval.

Drug Interactions: Toxic synergism with ephedrine has been documented and may occur with some other sympathomimetic bronchodilators. In addition, the following drug interactions have been demonstrated:

Drug	Effect
Aminophylline with Lithium Carbonate	Increased excretion of Lithium Carbonate
Aminophylline with Propranolol	Antagonism of Propranolol effect
Theophylline with Cimetidine	Increased theophylline blood levels
Theophylline with troleandomycin, erythromycin	Increased theophylline blood levels

Drug-Laboratory Test Interactions: When plasma levels of theophylline are measured by spectrophotometric methods, coffee, tea, cola beverages, chocolate, and acetaminophen contribute falsely high values.

Carcinogenesis, Mutagenesis, and Impairment of Fertility: Long-term animal studies have not been performed to evaluate the carcinogenic potential, mutagenic potential, or the effect on fertility of xanthine compounds.

Pregnancy: Category C-Animal reproduction studies have not been conducted with theophylline. It is not known whether theophylline can cause fetal harm when administered to a pregnant woman or can affect reproduction capacity. Xanthines should be given to a pregnant woman only if clearly needed.

Nursing Mothers: It has been reported that theophylline distributes readily into breast milk and may cause adverse effects in the infant. Caution must be used if prescribing xanthine to a mother who is nursing, taking into account the risk-benefit of this therapy.

Pediatric Use: Safety and effectiveness of THEO-DUR administered:
1. Every 24 hours in children under 12 years of age, have not been established.
2. Every 12 hours in children under 6 years of age, have not been established.

Adverse Reactions: The most consistent adverse reactions are usually due to overdose and are:
1. *Gastrointestinal:* nausea, vomiting, epigastric pain, hematemesis, diarrhea.
2. *Central nervous system:* headaches, irritability, restlessness, insomnia, reflex hyperexcitability, muscle twitching, clonic and tonic generalized convulsions.
3. *Cardiovascular:* palpitation, tachycardia, extrasystoles, flushing, hypotension, circulatory failure, ventricular arrhythmias.

4. *Respiratory:* tachypnea.
5. *Renal:* albuminuria, increased excretion of renal tubular and red blood cells, potentiation of diuresis.
6. *Others:* rash, hyperglycemia and inappropriate ADH syndrome.

Overdosage:
Management:
If potential oral overdose is established and seizure has not occurred:
A. Induce vomiting.
B. Administer a cathartic (this is particularly important if sustained-release preparations have been taken).
C. Administer activated charcoal.

If patient is having a seizure:
A. Establish an airway.
B. Administer oxygen.
C. Treat the seizure with intravenous diazepam, 0.1 to 0.3 mg/kg up to 10 mg.
D. Monitor vital signs, maintain blood pressure and provide adequate hydration.

Post Seizure Coma:
A. Maintain airway and oxygenation.
B. If a result of oral medication, follow above recommendations to prevent absorption of the drug, but intubation and lavage will have to be performed instead of inducing emesis, and the cathartic and charcoal will need to be introduced via a large bore gastric lavage tube.
C. Continue to provide full supportive care and adequate hydration while waiting for drug to be metabolized. In general, the drug is metabolized sufficiently rapid so as not to warrant consideration of dialysis; however, if serum levels exceed 50 mcg/ml, charcoal hemoperfusion may be indicated.

Dosage and Administration: For most patients, *effective use* of theophylline, i.e. associated with optimal likelihood of benefit combined with minimal risk of toxicity, is considered to occur when serum levels are maintained between 10 and 20 mcg/ml. Levels above 20 mcg/ml may produce toxicity, and in a small number of patients, toxicity may even be seen with serum levels between 15–20 mcg/ml, particularly during initiation of therapy.

There is considerable variation from patient to patient in the dosage required to achieve and maintain therapeutic and safe levels, primarily due to variable rates of elimination. Therefore, it is essential that not only must dosage be individualized, but titration and monitoring of serum levels be utilized where available. When serum concentration cannot be obtained, restriction of dosage to the amounts and intervals recommended in the guidelines listed below becomes essential. Dosage should be calculated on the basis of lean (ideal) body weight where mg/kg doses are presented. Theophylline does not distribute into fatty tissue. Giving theophylline with food may prevent some local gastric irritation and though absorption is slower, it is still complete.

As a practical consideration, it is not always possible to obtain serum level determinations. Under such conditions, restriction of the daily dose (in otherwise healthy adults) to not greater than 16 mg/kg/day or up to 900 mg (of anhydrous theophylline) will result in relatively few patients exceeding serum levels of 20 mcg/ml and the resultant risk of toxicity. THEO-DUR is not intended for patients experiencing an acute episode of bronchospasm (associated with asthma, chronic bronchitis, or emphysema). Such patients require *rapid* relief of symptoms and should be treated with an immediate-release or intravenous theophylline preparation (or other bronchodilators) and not with controlled release products.

Dosage Guidelines:
WARNING: DO NOT ATTEMPT TO MAINTAIN ANY DOSE THAT IS NOT TOLERATED.
Dosage guidelines are approximations only, and the wide range of clearance of theophylline among individuals (particularly those with concomitant disease) makes indiscriminate usage hazardous. It is recommended that dosing be considered in two stages: initiation of therapy with THEO-DUR, and titration, adjustment, and chronic maintenance.

Initiation of therapy:
It is recommended that the appropriate dosage be established using an immediate-release preparation. Slow clinical titration is generally preferred to help assure acceptance and safety of the medication. Then, if the total 24 hour dose can be given by use of the available strengths of this product, the patient can usually be switched to THEO-DUR giving one-half of the daily dose at 12 hour intervals. However, certain patients, such as the young, smokers and some non-smoking adults are likely to metabolize theophylline rapidly and require dosing at 8 hour intervals. Such patients can generally be identified as having trough serum concentrations lower than desired or repeatedly exhibiting symptoms near the end of a dosing interval.

Alternatively, therapy can be initiated with THEO-DUR since it is available in dosage forms/strengths which permit titration and adjustment of dosage as outlined in the following dosing guidelines. It is recommended that for children under 25 kg, proper dosage be established with a liquid preparation to permit titration in small increments.
THE AVERAGE INITIAL ADULT AND CHILDREN'S (over 25 kg) DOSE IS ONE THEO-DUR 200 mg TABLET q12h.

Titration, Adjustment and Chronic Maintenance:
If the desired response is not achieved with the above AVERAGE INITIAL DOSE recommendations, there are no adverse reactions and the serum theophylline level cannot be measured, dosage adjustment should proceed by increasing the dose in approximately 25% increments at three day intervals. Following each adjustment, if the clinical reponse is satisfactory, then that dosage level should be maintained. Dosage increases may be made in this manner up to the following:

MAXIMUM DOSE WITHOUT MEASUREMENT OF SERUM CONCENTRATION

	Dose Per Interval
Children (25–35 kg)	250 mg q12h
Adults and Children (35–70 kg)	300 mg q12h
Adults (over 70 kg)	450 mg q12h

If an increased dose is not tolerated because of headaches or stomach upset (nausea, vomiting, diarrhea, etc.), decrease dose to previous tolerated level. Do not exceed the above recommended doses unless serum theophylline levels can be measured. If serum theophylline levels can be measured and the concentration is between 10 and 20 mcg/ml, maintain dose if tolerated. CHECK SERUM CONCENTRATION AT APPROXIMATELY 8 HOURS AFTER A DOSE WHEN NONE HAVE BEEN MISSED OR ADDED FOR AT LEAST 3 DAYS. RECHECK SERUM THEOPHYLLINE CONCENTRATION AT 6 TO 12 MONTH INTERVALS. THIS INTERVAL MAY NEED TO BE MORE FREQUENT IN SOME INDIVIDUALS.

Take the following action if the measured serum theophylline concentration is too high.
20 to 25 mcg/ml—Decrease dose by about 10% and serum theophylline levels should be rechecked after 3 days.*
25 to 30 mcg/ml—Skip next dose and decrease subsequent doses by 25% and serum theophylline levels should be rechecked after 3 days.
Over 30 mcg/ml—Skip next 2 doses and decrease subsequent doses by 50% and serum theophylline levels should be rechecked after 3 days.
Take the following action if the measured serum theophylline concentration is too low. 7.5 to 10 mcg/ml—Increase dose by 25%.**
5 to 7.5 mcg/ml—Increase dose by 25% RECHECK SERUM THEOPHYLLINE FOR GUIDANCE IN FURTHER DOSAGE ADJUSTMENT.
*Finer adjustments in dosage may be needed for some patients.

** Dividing the daily dosage into 3 doses administered at 8 hour intervals may be indicated if symptoms occur repeatedly at the end of a dosing interval.

Once-Daily Dosing:
The slow absorption rate of this preparation may allow once-daily administration in adult non-smokers with appropriate total body clearance and other patients with low dosage requirements. Once daily dosing should be considered only after the patient has been gradually and satisfactorily titrated to therapeutic levels with q12h dosing. Once-daily dosing should be based on twice the q12h dose and should be initiated at the end of the last q12h dosing interval. The trough concentration (Cmin) obtained following conversion to once-daily dosing may be lower (especially in high clearance patients) and the peak concentration (Cmax) may be higher (especially in low clearance patients) than that obtained with q12h dosing. If symptoms recur, or signs of toxicity appear during the once-daily dosing interval, dosing on the q12h basis should be reinstituted.

It is essential that serum theophylline concentrations be monitored before and after transfer to once-daily dosing.

Food and posture, along with changes associated with circadian rhythm, may influence the rate of absorption and/or clearance rates of theophylline from controlled-release dosage forms administered at night. The exact relationship of these and other factors to nighttime serum concentrations and the clinical significance of such findings require additional study. Therefore, it is not recommended that THEO-DUR, when used as a once-a-day product, be administered at night.

THEO-DUR, when used as a once-a-day product, must be taken whole and not broken. DOSAGE ADJUSTMENT BASED ON SERUM THEOPHYLLINE CONCENTRATION MEASUREMENTS WHEN THESE INSTRUCTIONS HAVE NOT BEEN FOLLOWED MAY RESULT IN RECOMMENDATIONS THAT PRESENT RISK OF TOXICITY TO THE PATIENT. Caution should be exercised for younger children who cannot complain of minor side effects. Older adults, those with cor pulmonale, congestive heart failure, and/or liver disease may have unusually low dosage requirements and thus may experience toxicity at the maximal dosage recommended above.

It is important that no patient be maintained on any dosage that is not tolerated. In instructing patients to increase dosage according to the schedule above, they should be instructed not to take a subsequent dose if apparent side effects occur and to resume therapy at a lower dose once adverse effects have disappeared.

How Supplied: THEO-DUR 100 mg, 200 mg and 300 mg sustained action tablets are available in bottles of 100, 500, 1000 and 5000, and in unit dose packages of 100.
100 mg tablet: NDC 0369-0804: round, white to off-white, debossed THEO-DUR 100 on one side and scored on the other side.
200 mg tablet: NDC 0369-0805: oval, white to off-white, debossed THEO-DUR 200 on one side and scored on the other side.
300 mg tablet: NDC 0369-0803: capsule shaped, white to off-white debossed THEO-DUR 300 on one side and scored on the other side.

Storage Conditions: Keep tightly closed. Store at controlled room temperature 15–30°C (59–86°F).
Caution: FEDERAL LAW PROHIBITS DISPENSING WITHOUT PRESCRIPTION.
KEY PHARMACEUTICALS, INC.
Miami, Florida 33269—0670 (U.S.A.)
Revised 12/83
Shown in Product Identification Section, p. 414

THEO-DUR® SPRINKLE ℞
[thē-a-dur]
(theophylline anhydrous sustained action capsules)

Description: THEO-DUR SPRINKLE sustained action capsules contain anhydrous theophylline, a

Continued on next page

Key—Cont.

bronchodilator, in a sustained release formulation with no color additives. THEO-DUR SPRINKLE is available in four strengths: 50, 75, 125 and 200 mg. THEO-DUR SPRINKLE capsules contain theophylline which has been microencapsulated in a proprietary coating of polymers to mask the bitter taste associated with the drug, while providing a prolonged therapeutic effect. THEO-DUR SPRINKLE capsules may be swallowed whole. In addition, the microencapsulation technique makes THEO-DUR SPRINKLE ideal for children 6 and over, and other patients who are unable to swallow a tablet or capsule. For these patients, the entire contents of a THEO-DUR SPRINKLE capsule should be sprinkled on a small amount of soft food immediately prior to ingestion. SUBDIVIDING THE CONTENTS OF A CAPSULE IS NOT RECOMMENDED. Each capsule is oversized to allow ease of opening.

Anhydrous theophylline, 1,3-dimethylxanthine, is a white, odorless, crystalline powder having a bitter taste. Its structural formula is:

[Structural formula of theophylline]

Clinical Pharmacology: Theophylline directly relaxes the smooth muscle of the bronchial airways and pulmonary blood vessels, thus acting mainly as a bronchodilator and smooth muscle relaxant. The drug also produces other actions typical of the xanthine derivatives: coronary vasodilation, cardiac stimulation, diuresis, cerebral stimulation, and skeletal muscle stimulation. The actions of theophylline may be mediated through inhibition of phosphodiesterase and a resultant increase in intracellular cyclic AMP.

In-vitro theophylline has been shown to act synergistically with beta agonists that increase intracellular cyclic AMP through the stimulation of adenyl cyclase, but synergism has not been demonstrated in patient studies. More data are needed to determine if theophylline and beta agonists have a clinically important additive effect *in vivo*. Apparently, no development of tolerance occurs with chronic use of theophylline.

Pharmacokinetics: The half-life of theophylline is influenced by a number of known variables. It is prolonged in patients suffering from chronic alcoholism, impaired hepatic or renal function, congestive heart failure, and in patients receiving macrolide antibiotics and cimetidine. Older adults (over age 55) and patients with chronic obstructive pulmonary disease, with or without cor pulmonale, may also have much slower clearance rates. For such patients, the theophylline half-life may exceed 24 hours.

Newborns and neonates have extremely slow clearance rates compared to older infants (over 6 months) and children, and may also have a theophylline half-life of over 24 hours. High fever for prolonged periods may also reduce the rate of theophylline elimination.

THEOPHYLLINE ELIMINATION CHARACTERISTICS

	Theophylline Clearance Rates (mean±S.D.)	Half-life Average (mean±S.D.)
Children (over 6 months of age)	1.45±0.58 ml/kg/min	3.7±1.1 hrs
Adult non-smokers uncomplicated asthma	0.65±0.19 ml/kg/min	8.7±2.2 hrs

The half-life of theophylline in smokers (1 to 2 packs/day) averages 4–5 hours, much shorter than the half-life in non-smokers which averages 7–9 hours. The increase in theophylline clearance caused by smoking is probably the result of induction of drug-metabolizing enzymes that do not readily normalize after cessation of smoking. It appears that between 3 months and 2 years may be necessary for normalization of the effect of smoking on theophylline pharmacokinetics.

In single dose studies the following bioavailability parameters were observed. THEO-DUR SPRINKLE administered in a 500 mg dose to 6 healthy adults produced mean peak theophylline blood levels of 9.03 ± 2.59 mcg/ml at 8.67 ± 1.03 hours following administration. Administration of two lots of THEO-DUR SPRINKLE in a 600 mg dose to 6 healthy adults produced mean peak theophylline blood levels of 9.08 ± 1.30 mcg/ml and 7.60 ± 0.95 mcg/ml at 8.33 ± 1.50 and 8.67 ± 3.01 hours after administration respectively. In these studies THEO-DUR SPRINKLE exhibited complete bioavailability when compared to an immediate release product.

Indications: THEO-DUR SPRINKLE is indicated for relief and/or prevention of symptoms of bronchial asthma and for reversible bronchospasm associated with chronic bronchitis and emphysema.

Contraindications: This product is contraindicated in individuals who have shown hypersensitivity to theophylline or any of the capsule components.

Warnings: Status asthmaticus should be considered a medical emergency and is defined as that degree of bronchospasm which is not rapidly responsive to usual doses of conventional bronchodilators. Optimal therapy for such patients frequently requires both *additional medication*, parenterally administered, and *close monitoring*, preferably in an intensive care setting.

Although increasing the dose of theophylline may bring about relief, such treatment may be associated with toxicity. The likelihood of such toxicity developing increases significantly when the serum theophylline concentration exceeds 20 mcg/ml. Therefore determination of serum theophylline levels is recommended to assure maximal benefit without excessive risk.

Serum levels above 20 mcg/ml are rarely found after appropriate administration of the recommended doses. However, in individuals in whom theophylline plasma clearance is reduced *for any reason*, even conventional doses may result in increased serum levels and potential toxicity. Reduced theophylline clearance has been documented in the following readily identifiable groups: 1) patients with impaired renal or liver function; 2) patients over 55 years of age, particularly males and those with chronic lung disease; 3) those with cardiac failure from any cause; 4) neonates; and 5) those patients taking certain drugs (macrolide antibiotics and cimetidine). Decreased clearance of theophylline may be associated with either influenza immunization or active infection with influenza.

Reduction of dosage and laboratory monitoring is especially appropriate in the above individuals. Less serious signs of theophylline toxicity, i.e. nausea and restlessness, may appear in up to 50% of patients. Unfortunately, however, serious side effects such as ventricular arrhythmias, convulsions or even death may appear as the first sign of toxicity without any previous warning. Stated differently; *serious toxicity is not reliably preceded by less severe side effects*.

Many patients who require theophylline may exhibit tachycardia due to their underlying disease process so that the cause/effect relationship to elevated serum theophylline concentrations may not be appreciated.

Theophylline products may cause dysrhythmia and/or worsen pre-existing arrhythmias and any significant change in rate and/or rhythm warrants monitoring and further investigation.

The occurence of arrhythmias and sudden death (with histological evidence of necrosis of the myocardium) has been recorded in laboratory animals (minipigs, rodents and dogs) when theophylline and beta agonists were administered concomitantly, although not when either was administered alone. The significance of these findings when applied to human usage is currently unknown.

Precautions: THE CONTENTS OF A THEO-DUR SPRINKLE CAPSULE SHOULD NOT BE CHEWED OR CRUSHED.

General: Theophylline half-life is shorter in smokers than in nonsmokers. Therefore, smokers may require larger or more frequent dose. Morphine and curare should be used with caution in patients with airway obstruction as they may suppress respiration and stimulate histamine release. Alternative drugs should be used when possible. Theophylline should not be administered concurrently with other xanthine medications. Use with caution in patients with severe cardiac disease, severe hypoxemia, hypertension, hyperthyroidism, acute myocardial injury, cor pulmonale, congestive heart failure, liver disease, in the elderly (especially males) and in neonates. In particular great caution should be used in giving theophylline to patients with congestive heart failure. Frequently, such patients have markedly prolonged theophylline serum levels with theophylline persisting in serum for long periods following discontinuation of the drug. Use theophylline cautiously in patients with history of peptic ulcer. Theophylline may occasionally act as a local irritant to the G.I. tract although gastrointestinal symptoms are more commonly centrally mediated and associated with serum drug concentrations over 20 mcg/ml.

Information for Patients: The physician should reinforce the importance of taking only the prescribed dose and time interval between doses. THEO-DUR SPRINKLE capsules may be swallowed whole. In addition, the microencapsulation technique makes THEO-DUR SPRINKLE ideal for children 6 years and over, and other patients who are unable to swallow a tablet or capsule. The entire contents of a THEO-DUR SPRINKLE capsule should be sprinkled on a small amount of soft food immediately prior to ingestion. SUBDIVIDING THE CONTENTS OF A CAPSULE IS NOT RECOMMENDED.

Drug Interactions: Toxic synergism with ephedrine has been documented and may occur with some other sympathomimetic bronchodilators. In addition, the following drug interactions have been demonstrated:

DRUG	EFFECT
Aminophylline with Lithium Carbonate	Increased excretion of Lithium Carbonate
Aminophylline with Propranolol	Antagonism of Propranolol effect
Theophylline with Cimetidine	Increased theophylline blood levels
Theophylline with troleandomycin, erythromycin	Increased theophylline blood levels

Drug-Laboratory Test Interactions: When plasma levels of theophylline are measured by spectrophotometric methods; coffee, tea, cola beverages, chocolate, and acetaminophen contribute falsely high values.

Carcinogenesis, Mutagenesis, and Impairment of Fertility: Long-term animal studies have not been performed to evaluate the carcinogenic potential, mutagenic potential, or the effect on fertility of xanthine compounds.

Pregnancy: Category C—Animal reproduction studies have not been conducted with theophylline. It is not known whether theophylline can cause fetal harm when administered to a pregnant woman or can affect reproduction capacity. Xanthines should be given to a pregnant woman only if clearly needed.

Nursing Mothers: It has been reported that theophylline distributes readily into breast milk and may cause adverse effects in the infant. Caution must be used if prescribing xanthines to a mother who is nursing, taking into account the risk-benefit of this therapy.

Pediatric Use: Safety and effectiveness of THEO-DUR SPRINKLE in children under 6 years of age has not been established.

Product Information

Adverse Reactions: The most consistent adverse reactions are usually due to overdose and are:
1. Gastrointestinal: nausea, vomiting, epigastric pain, hematemesis, diarrhea.
2. Central nervous system: headaches, irritability, restlessness, insomnia, reflex hyperexcitability, muscle twitching, clonic and tonic generalized convulsions.
3. Cardiovascular: palpitation, tachycardia, extrasystoles, flushing, hypotension, circulatory failure, ventricular arrhythmias.
4. Respiratory: tachypnea.
5. Renal: albuminuria, increased excretion of renal tubular and red blood cells, potentiation of diuresis.
6. Others: rash, hyperglycemia and inappropriate ADH syndrome.

Overdosage:
Management: If potential oral overdose is established and seizure has not occurred:
A. Induce vomiting.
B. Administer a cathartic (this is particularly important if sustained-release preparations have been taken).
C. Administer activated charcoal.

If patient is having a seizure:
A. Establish an airway.
B. Administer oxygen.
C. Treat the seizure with intravenous diazepam, 0.1 to 0.3 mg/kg up to 10 mg.
D. Monitor vital signs, maintain blood pressure and provide adequate hydration.

Post Seizure Coma:
A. Maintain airway and oxygenation.
B. If a result of oral medication, follow above recommendations to prevent absorption of the drug, but intubation and lavage will have to be performed instead of inducing emesis, and the cathartic and charcoal will need to be introduced via a large bore gastric lavage tube.
C. Continue to provide full supportive care and adequate hydration while waiting for drug to be metabolized. In general, the drug is metabolized sufficiently rapid so as not to warrant consideration of dialysis; however, if serum levels exceed 50 mcg/ml, charcoal hemoperfusion may be indicated.

Dosage and Administration: For most patients, *effective use* of theophylline, i.e. associated with optimal likelihood of benefit combined with minimal risk of toxicity, is considered to occur when serum levels are maintained between 10 and 20 mcg/ml. Levels above 20 mcg/ml may produce toxicity, and in a small number of patients, toxicity may even be seen with serum levels between 15–20 mcg/ml, particularly during initiation of therapy.

There is considerable variation from patient to patient in the dosage required to achieve and maintain therpeutic and safe levels, primarily due to variable rates of elimination. Therefore, it is essential that not only must dosage be individualized, but titration and monitoring of serum levels be utilized where available. When serum concentration cannot be obtained, restriction of dosage to the amounts and intervals recommended in the guidelines listed below becomes essential. Dosage should be calculated on the basis of lean (ideal) body weight where mg/kg doses are presented. Theophylline does not distribute into fatty tissue. Giving theophylline with food may prevent some local gastric irritation and though absorption may be slower, it is still complete.

As a practical consideration, it is not always possible to obtain serum level determinations. Under such conditions, restriction of the daily dose (in otherwise healthy adults) to not greater than 16 mg/kg/day (of anhydrous theophylline) in divided doses will result in relatively few patients exceeding serum levels of 20 mcg/ml and the resultant risk of toxicity.

THEO-DUR SPRINKLE is not intended for patients experiencing an acute episode of bronchospasm (associated with asthma, chronic bronchitis, or emphysema). Such patients require *rapid* relief of symptoms and should be treated with an immediate-release or intravenous theophylline preparation (or other bronchodilators) and not with controlled release products.

Dosage Guidelines:
WARNING: DO NOT ATTEMPT TO MAINTAIN ANY DOSE THAT IS NOT TOLERATED. Dosage guidelines are approximations only, and the wide range of clearance of theophylline among individuals (particularly those with concomitant disease) makes indiscriminate usage hazardous. It is recommended that dosing be considered in three stages: initiation of therapy with THEO-DUR SPRINKLE, titration and adjustment, and chronic maintenance.

Chronic Therapy: It is recommended that the appropriate dosage be established using an immediate-release preparation. Slow clinical titration is generally preferred to help assure acceptance and safety of the medication. Then, if the total 24 hour dose can be given by use of the available strengths of this product, the patient can usually be switched to THEO-DUR SPRINKLE giving one-half of the daily dose at 12 hour intervals. However, certain patients, such as the young, smokers and some nonsmoking adults are likely to metabolize theophylline rapidly and require dosing at 8 hour intervals. Such patients can generally be identified as having trough serum concentrations lower than desired or repeatedly exhibiting symptoms near the end of a dosing interval. Alternatively, therapy can be initiated with THEO-DUR SPRINKLE since it is available in dosage forms/strengths which permit titration and adjustment of dosage as outlined in the following dosing guidelines. It is recommended that for children under 25 kg, proper dosage be established with a liquid preparation to permit titration in small increments.

If the calculated dose falls between two available strengths of a capsule or combination of capsules, the lower strength should be utilized. If the calculated dose is less than 50 mg, alternate means of theophylline therapy should be considered.

The initial dose should be determined on the basis of body weight and patient history. The following guidelines may be used to determine an average initial dose.

AVERAGE INITIAL DOSE REQUIREMENTS
The recommended initial dose for children 6–9 years is 16 mg/kg/24 hours, for children 9–16 years is 12 mg/kg/24 hours and for adults is 9 mg/kg/24 hours; not to exceed 400 mg/24 hours of theophylline in divided doses at 12 hour intervals. If the desired response is not achieved with the above AVERAGE INITIAL DOSAGE recommendations and there are no adverse reactions the dose may be increased by approximately 25 percent increments at 2–3 day intervals.

Increase the dose *only until* the following MAXIMUM DOSE WITHOUT MEASUREMENT OF SERUM CONCENTRATION or maximum of 900 mg in any 24 hour period, WHICHEVER is less, is attained.

BODY WEIGHT* (Adults and children 6 to 9 years)	INITIAL DOSE q12h dose (daily dose)**	AFTER 3 DAYS, INCREASE THE DOSE TO: q12h dose (daily dose)**	MAXIMUM DOSE WITHOUT MEASUREMENT OF SERUM CONCENTRATION q12h dose (daily dose)**
Children 15 to 19 kg	125mg/12h (250 mg/24h)	150mg/12h (300mg/24h)	200mg/12h (400mg/24h)
Children 20 to 29 kg	150mg/12h (300mg/24h)	200mg/12h (400mg/24h)	250mg/12h (500mg/24h)
Children 30 to 34 kg	175mg/12h (350mg/24h)	250mg/12h (500mg/24h)	300mg/12h (600mg/24h)
Children 35 to 39 kg	200mg/12h (400mg/24h)	275mg/12h (550mg/24h)	350mg/12h (700mg/24h)
Adults and children over 40 kg	200mg/12h (400mg/24h)	300mg/12h (600mg/24h)	400mg/12h (800mg/24h)

* Use ideal body weight for obese patients.
**Some patients may require dosing every 8 hours, in which case the daily dose recommended above should be divided by 3.

WARNING: DO NOT ATTEMPT TO MAINTAIN ANY DOSE THAT IS NOT TOLERATED. [See table above].

If increased dose is not tolerated because of headaches or stomach upset (nausea, vomiting, diarrhea, etc.), decrease dose to AVERAGE INITIAL DOSE.

If serum theophylline concentration is between 10 and 20 mcg/ml, maintain dose if tolerated. CHECK SERUM CONCENTRATION BETWEEN 3 AND 8 HOURS AFTER A DOSE WHEN NONE HAVE BEEN MISSED OR ADDED FOR AT LEAST 3 DAYS. RECHECK SERUM THEOPHYLLINE CONCENTRATION AT 6 TO 12 MONTH INTERVALS.*

Take the following action if the serum theophylline concentration is too high.

20 to 25 mcg/ml—Decrease daily dose by about 10%. RECHECK SERUM THEOPHYLLINE CONCENTRATION AT 6 TO 12 MONTH INTERVALS.*

25 to 30 mcg/ml—Skip next dose and decrease subsequent doses by 25% to the nearest 50 mg q12h.

Over 30 mcg/ml—Skip next 2 doses and decrease subsequent doses by 50% to nearest 50 mg q12h. RECHECK SERUM THEOPHYLLINE CONCENTRATION.

Take the following action if the serum theophylline concentration is too low.

7.5 to 10 mcg/ml—Increase dose by 25% to nearest 50 mg.**

5 to 7.5 mcg/ml—Increase dose by 25% to the nearest 50 mg and RECHECK SERUM THEOPHYLLINE FOR GUIDANCE IN FURTHER DOSAGE ADJUSTMENT.

* Finer adjustments in dosage may be needed for some patients.
**Dividing the daily dosage into 3 doses administered at 8 hour intervals may be indicated if symptoms occur repeatedly at the end of a dosing interval.

DOSAGE ADJUSTMENT BASED ON SERUM THEOPHYLLINE CONCENTRATION MEASUREMENTS WHEN THESE INSTRUCTIONS HAVE NOT BEEN FOLLOWED MAY RESULT IN RECOMMENDATIONS THAT PRESENT RISK OF TOXICITY TO THE PATIENT.

Caution should be exercised for younger children who cannot complain of minor side effects. Older adults, those with cor pulmonale, congestive heart failure, and/or liver disease may have unusually low dosage requirements and thus may experience toxicity at the maximal dosage recommended above.

It is important that no patient be maintained on any dosage that is not tolerated. In instructing patients to increase dosage according to the schedule above, they should be instructed not to take a subsequent dose if apparent side effects occur and to resume therapy at a lower dose once adverse effects have disappeared.

Continued on next page

Key—Cont.

How Supplied: THEO-DUR SPRINKLE 50, 75, 125 and 200 mg sustained action capsules are available in bottles of 100.

50mg capsule: NDC 0369-0850: white opaque capsule body with clear cap embossed in black, THIS END UP THEO-DUR® SPRINKLE™ 50mg

75 mg capsule: NDC 0369-0875: white opaque capsule body with clear cap embossed in green, THIS END UP THEO-DUR® SPRINKLE™ 75 mg

125 mg capsule: NDC 0369-0812: white opaque capsule body with clear cap embossed in red, THIS END UP THEO-DUR® SPRINKLE™ 125mg

200 mg capsule: NDC 0369-0820: white opaque capsule body with clear cap embossed in blue, THIS END UP THEO-DUR® SPRINKLE™ 200 mg

Storage Conditions: Keep tightly closed. Store at controlled room temperature 15–30°C (59–86°F).

Caution: FEDERAL LAW PROHIBITS DISPENSING WITHOUT PRESCRIPTION.

KEY PHARMACEUTICALS, INC.
Miami, Florida 33269—0670 (USA)
Revised 0184

Shown in Product Identification Section, p. 414

TYZINE® ℞
[tī'zēn]
(tetrahydrozoline hydrochloride)
0.1% NASAL SOLUTION
and
0.05% PEDIATRIC NASAL DROPS

Clinical Pharmacology: Tyzine (tetrahydrozoline hydrochloride), a sympathomimetic amine, possesses vasoconstrictor and decongestant actions when applied to the nasal mucosa, resulting in constriction of the smaller arterioles of the nasal passages effecting a decongesting action. Tyzine administered systemically has a central depressant rather than stimulant effect.

Indications and Usage: For decongestion of nasal and nasopharyngeal mucosa.

Contraindications: Tyzine is contraindicated for patients who have shown previous hypersensitivity to its components. The 0.1% solution is contraindicated in children under six years of age. Tyzine is not to be used for infants under two years of age. Tyzine Pediatric Solution should be used for children between the ages of 2 and 6 years. (See "Dosage and Administration".) Tyzine should not be used by patients under treatment with MAO inhibitors.

Warnings: Clinical data in human beings are inadequate to establish conditions for safe use in pregnancy. Therefore, Tyzine Nasal Solution should not be used during pregnancy unless, in the judgement of the physician, the expected benefits outweigh the possible hazards.

Overdosage in children may produce profound sedation. This may be accompanied by profuse sweating. (See "Overdosage".)

Precautions: Avoid doses greater or more frequent than those recommended below. Excessive dosage in children may, on rare occasions, cause severe drowsiness. Profuse sweating may accompany this effect. Overdosage may also cause marked hypotension or even shock.

Use cautiously in patients with cardiovascular disease (e.g., coronary artery disease, hypertension), and metabolic-endocrine disease (e.g., hyperthyroidism, diabetes).

Adverse Reactions: The most frequent adverse reactions are burning, stinging, sneezing, dryness, headache, drowsiness, weakness, tremors, light-headedness, insomnia, and palpitations. Prolonged or excessive use may cause rebound congestion.

If adverse reactions occur, discontinue use.

Overdosage: The administration or ingestion of overdoses of Tyzine may result in oversedation in young children. Very occasionally in adults with very excessive overdoses, a shock-like syndrome with hypotension and bradycardia may occur. In either case, the treatment of overdosage is usually that of watchful expectancy and general supportive measures. The patient should be kept warm, fluid balance should be maintained orally, if possible, and parenterally, if necessary. If the respiratory rate drops to 10 or below, the patient should be given oxygen, and respiration assisted. Blood pressure should be watched carefully to prevent a hypotensive crisis.

There is no known antidote for Tyzine (tetrahydrozoline hydrochloride). The use of stimulants is contraindicated. To date, we have had no reports of fatalities resulting from overdosages of Tyzine and while the symptoms resulting from Tyzine overdosage may be alarming, they are self-limiting and the patient recovers with no sequelae.

Dosage and Administration:
Adults and Children 6 years and over:
It is recommended that 2 to 4 drops of Tyzine 0.1% Nasal Solution be instilled in each nostril as needed, never more often than every three hours. Less frequent administration is usually sufficient since relief is maintained for four hours or longer in most cases, and often for as long as eight hours. Bedtime instillation usually assures sleep undisturbed by the need for remedication before morning, or by insomnia from central stimulation.

Children 2 to 6 years of age:
It is recommended that 2 to 3 drops of Tyzine 0.05% Pediatric Nasal Drops be instilled in each nostril as needed and never more often than every three hours. Relief usually lasts for several hours so that instillations are usually needed only every four to six hours.

Instillation of nose drops can be most conveniently accomplished with the patient in the lateral headlow position.

How Supplied:
Tyzine
  Nasal Solution (0.1%)
  —1 fl. oz. (30 cc.) and 1 pint bottles
  —½ fl. oz. (15 cc.) plastic squeeze bottles
Pediatric Nasal Drops (0.05%)—½ fl. oz. (15 cc.) bottles

Caution: FEDERAL LAW PROHIBITS DISPENSING WITHOUT PRESCRIPTION.

Knoll Pharmaceutical Company
WHIPPANY, NJ 07981

AKINETON® TABLETS AND AMPULES ℞
(biperiden hydrochloride and biperiden lactate)

Description: Each AKINETON® Tablet for oral administration contains 2 mg biperiden hydrochloride. Each 1 ml AKINETON Ampule for intramuscular or intravenous administration contains 5 mg biperiden lactate in an aqueous 1.4 percent sodium lactate solution. No added preservative. AKINETON is an anticholinergic agent. Biperiden is α-5-Norbornen-2-yl-α-phenyl-1-piperidine-propanol. It is a white, crystalline, odorless powder, slightly soluble in water and alcohol. It is stable in air at normal temperatures.

Clinical Pharmacology: AKINETON is a weak visceral anticholinergic agent which is somewhat more potent than atropine on a dosage basis in terms of its ability to block nicotine-induced extensor spasm and death in mice. The mechanism of action of centrally acting anticholinergic drugs such as AKINETON in parkinsonism is thought to relate to their partial blocking effect on the striatal cholinergic receptors which predominate in parkinsonism, in which the inhibitory control by the nigrostriatal dopaminergic pathways is gradually lost. Thus, the balance of excitation and inhibition returns toward normal. Another possibility is that anticholinergic drugs block the re-uptake of dopamine by nerve terminals in the striatum, making more of the transmitter available to the receptors.

The parenteral form of AKINETON is an effective and reliable agent for the treatment of acute episodes of extrapyramidal disturbances during treatment with reserpine and the phenothiazines. Akathisia, akinesia, dyskinetic tremors, rigor, oculogyric crisis, spasmodic torticollis, and profuse sweating are markedly reduced or eliminated. With parenteral AKINETON, these drug-induced disturbances are rapidly brought under control. Subsequently, this can usually be maintained with oral doses which may be given with tranquilizer therapy in psychotic and other conditions requiring an uninterrupted program with phenothiazines or reserpine. This regimen can be particularly useful when drug-induced extrapyramidal disturbances interfere with indicated convulsant therapy.

The pharmacokinetics of AKINETON in humans have not been established. Six hours after an oral dose of 250 mg/kg in rats, 87% of the drug had been absorbed. Cardiovascular and respiratory studies in the dog and cat using large doses of biperiden hydrochloride reveal that the drug has only minor actions on these systems. When given subcutaneously its drying effect on the salivary glands of rabbits and its mydriatic effect on the mouse pupil are relatively weak compared with those of atropine. Biperiden lactate (10 mg/ml) was not irritating to the tissue of rabbits when injected intramuscularly (1.0 ml) into the sacrospinalis muscles and intradermally (0.25 ml) and subcutaneously (0.5 ml) into the shaved abdominal skin.

Indications and Usage: For use as an adjunct in the therapy of all forms of parkinsonism (postencephalitic, arteriosclerotic, idiopathic). Useful in the control of extrapyramidal disorders due to central nervous system drugs such as reserpine and phenothiazines.

Contraindications: Hypersensitivity to biperiden.

Warnings: Isolated instances of mental confusion, euphoria, agitation and disturbed behavior have been reported in susceptible patients. Also, the central anticholinergic syndrome can occur as an adverse reaction to properly prescribed anticholinergic medication, although it is more frequently due to overdosage. It may also result from concomitant administration of an anticholinergic agent and a drug that has secondary anticholinergic actions (see Drug Interactions and Overdosage sections). Caution should be observed in patients with manifest glaucoma, though no prohibitive rise in intraocular pressure has been noted following either oral or parenteral administration. Patients with prostatism or cardiac arrhythmia should be given this drug with caution.

Precautions

Drug Interactions: The central anticholinergic syndrome can occur when anticholinergic agents such as AKINETON are administered concomitantly with drugs that have secondary anticholinergic actions, e.g., certain narcotic analgesics such as meperidine, the phenothiazines and other antipsychotics, tricyclic antidepressants, certain antiarrhythmics such as the quinidine salts, and antihistamines. See Overdosage section for signs and symptoms of the central anticholinergic syndrome, and for treatment.

Pregnancy: Pregnancy Category C. Animal reproduction studies have not been conducted with AKINETON. It is also not known whether AKINETON can cause fetal harm when administered to a pregnant woman or can affect reproduction capacity. AKINETON should be given to a pregnant woman only if clearly needed.

Nursing Mothers: It is not known whether this drug is excreted in human milk. Because many drugs are excreted in human milk, caution should be exercised when AKINETON is administered to a nursing woman.

Pediatric Use: Safety and effectiveness in children have not been established.

Adverse Reactions: Dry mouth; blurred vision; drowsiness; euphoria or disorientation; urinary retention; postural hypotension; constipation; agitation; disturbed behavior. There have been no significant changes in blood pressure levels or pulse rate in patients who have been given the parenteral form of AKINETON although mild transient postural hypotension may occur. These side effects can be minimized or avoided by slow intravenous administration. No local tissue reactions have been reported following intramuscular injection. If gastric irritation occurs following oral administration, it can be avoided by administering the drug during or after meals.

The central anticholinergic syndrome can occur as an adverse reaction to properly prescribed anticholinergic medication. See Overdosage section for signs and symptoms of the central anticholinergic syndrome, and for treatment.

Overdosage
Signs and Symptoms: Overdosage with AKINETON produces typical central symptoms of atropine intoxication (the central anticholinergic syndrome). Correct diagnosis depends upon recognition of the peripheral signs of parasympathetic blockade including dilated and sluggish pupils; warm, dry skin; facial flushing; decreased secretions of the mouth, pharynx, nose, and bronchi; foul-smelling breath; elevated temperature, tachycardia, decreased bowel sounds, and urinary retention. Neuropsychiatric signs such as delirium, disorientation, anxiety, hallucinations, illusions, confusion, incoherence, agitation, hyperactivity, ataxia, loss of memory, paranoia, combativeness, and seizures may be present. The condition can progress to stupor, coma, and cardiac and respiratory arrest.

Treatment: If AKINETON was administered orally, gastric lavage or other measures to limit absorption should be instituted. A small dose of diazepam or a short acting barbiturate may be administered if CNS excitation is observed. Phenothiazines are contraindicated because the toxicity may be intensified due to their antimuscarinic action, causing coma. Respiratory support, artificial respiration or vasopressor agents may be necessary. Hyperpyrexia must be reversed, fluid volume replaced and acid-base balance maintained. Physostigmine salicylate may be administered to treat this syndrome. One mg (half this amount for the children or elderly) may be given intramuscularly or by slow intravenous infusion. If there is no response within 20 minutes, an additional 1 mg dose may be given; this may be repeated until a total of 4 mg has been administered or excessive cholinergic signs are seen. Frequent monitoring of clinical signs should be done. Since physostigmine is rapidly destroyed, additional injections may be required every one or two hours to maintain control. The relapse intervals tend to lengthen as the toxic anticholinergic agent is metabolized, so the patient should be carefully observed for 8 to 12 hours following the last relapse.

Toxicity in Animals: The acute subcutaneous toxicity (LD_{50}) of biperiden hydrochloride in mice was found to be 195 mg/kg and the intravenous toxicity (LD_{50}), 72 mg/kg. The acute oral toxicity (LD_{50}) in rats is 750 mg/kg. The intraperitoneal toxicity (LD_{50}) of biperiden lactate in rats was 270 mg/kg, and the intravenous toxicity (LD_{50}) in dogs was 222 mg/kg.

Dosage and Administration
Drug-Induced Extrapyramidal Symptoms:
Parenteral: The average adult dose is 2 mg intramuscularly or intravenously. May be repeated every half-hour until there is resolution of symptoms, but not more than four consecutive doses should be given in a 24-hour period.

Note: Parenteral drug products should be inspected visually for particulate matter and discoloration prior to administration, whenever solution and container permit.

Oral: One tablet one to three times daily.
Parkinson's Disease: Oral: One tablet three or four times daily.

How Supplied
AKINETON Tablets, 2 mg each, white, embossed on one face with a triangle, bisected on the reverse and imprinted with the number "11".
Bottles of 100—NDC #0044-0120-02.
Bottles of 1000—NDC #0044-0120-04.
Shown in Product Identification Section, page 414
AKINETON Ampules, 1 ml each containing 5 mg biperiden lactate per ml.
Boxes of 10—NDC #0044-0110-01.
Storage: All dosage forms of AKINETON should be stored at 59°–86°F, 15°–30°C.

DILAUDID®
(hydromorphone hydrochloride)

Description: DILAUDID (hydromorphone hydrochloride) (**WARNING:** May be habit forming), a hydrogenated ketone of morphine, is a narcotic analgesic. It is available in ampules (for parenteral administration) containing 1 mg, 2 mg, and 4 mg hydromorphone hydrochloride per ml with 0.2% sodium citrate, 0.2% citric acid solution; in a multiple dose vial (for parenteral administration), containing 20 ml of solution, each ml contains 2 mg hydromorphone hydrochloride and 0.5 mg edetate disodium with 1.8 mg methylparaben and 0.2 mg propylparaben as preservatives and pH adjusted with sodium hydroxide or hydrochloric acid; in color coded tablets (for oral administration) containing 1 mg, 2 mg, 3 mg and 4 mg hydromorphone hydrochloride; in suppositories (for rectal administration) containing 3 mg hydromorphone hydrochloride in cocoa butter base with 1% colloidal silica as an inactive ingredient; and in powder for prescription compounding. DILAUDID ampules and multiple dose vials are sterile.

Clinical Pharmacology: DILAUDID is a narcotic analgesic; its principal therapeutic effect is relief of pain. The precise mechanism of action of DILAUDID and other opiates is not known, although it is believed to relate to the existence of opiate receptors in the central nervous system. There is no intrinsic limit to the analgesic effect of DILAUDID; like morphine, adequate doses will relieve even the most severe pain. Clinically, however, dosage limitations are imposed by the adverse effects, primarily respiratory depression, nausea, and vomiting, which can result from high doses.

DILAUDID has diverse additional actions. It produces drowsiness, changes in mood and mental clouding, depresses the respiratory center and the cough center, stimulates the vomiting center, produces pinpoint constriction of the pupil, enhances parasympathetic activitiy, elevates cerebrospinal fluid pressure, increases biliary pressure, produces transient hyperglycemia.

Generally, the analgesic action of parenterally administered DILAUDID is apparent within 15 minutes and usually remains in effect for more than five hours. The onset of action of oral DILAUDID is somewhat slower, with measurable analgesia occurring within 30 minutes.

Radioimmunoassay techniques have recently been developed for the analysis of DILAUDID in human plasma. In humans the half-life of a DILAUDID 4 mg tablet is 2.6 hours. In a random crossover study in six subjects, 4mg of *oral* DILAUDID produced a mean concentration/time curve similar to that of 2mg DILAUDID I.V., after the first hour.

Indications and Usage: DILAUDID is indicated for the relief of moderate to severe pain such as that due to:
Surgery
Cancer
Trauma (soft tissue & bone)
Biliary Colic
Myocardial Infarction
Burns
Renal Colic

Contraindications: DILAUDID is contraindicated in patients with a known hypersensitivity to hydromorphone; in the presence of an intracranial lesion associated with increased intracranial pressure; and whenever ventilatory function is depressed (chronic obstructive pulmonary disease, cor pulmonale, emphysema, kyphoscoliosis, status asthmaticus).

Warnings
Respiratory Depression: DILAUDID produces dose-related respiratory depression by acting directly on brain stem respiratory centers. DILAUDID also affects centers that control respiratory rhythm, and may produce irregular and periodic breathing.

Head Injury and Increased Intracranial Pressure: The respiratory depressant effects of narcotics and their capacity to elevate cerebrospinal fluid pressure may be markedly exaggerated in the presence of head injury, other intracranial lesions or a pre-existing increase in intracranial pressure. Furthermore, narcotics produce adverse reactions which may obscure the clinical course of patients with head injuries.

Acute Abdominal Conditions: The administration of narcotics may obscure the diagnosis or clinical course of patients with acute abdominal conditions.

Precautions
Special Risk Patients: DILAUDID should be used with caution in elderly or debilitated patients and those with impaired renal or hepatic function, hypothyroidism, Addison's disease, prostatic hypertrophy or urethral stricture. As with any narcotic analgesic agent, the usual precautions should be observed and the possibility of respiratory depression should be kept in mind.

Cough Reflex: DILAUDID suppresses the cough reflex; as with all narcotics, caution should be exercised when DILAUDID is used postoperatively and in patients with pulmonary disease.

Usage in Ambulatory Patients: Narcotics may impair the mental and/or physical abilities required for the performance of potentially hazardous tasks such as driving a car or operating machinery; patients should be cautioned accordingly.

Drug Interactions: Patients receiving other narcotic analgesics, general anesthetics, phenothiazines, tranquilizers, sedative-hypnotics, tricyclic antidepressants or other CNS depressants (including alcohol) concomitantly with DILAUDID may exhibit an additive CNS depression. When such combined therapy is contemplated, the dose of one or both agents should be reduced.

Parenteral Administration: The parenteral form of DILAUDID may be given intravenously, but the injection should be given very slowly. Rapid intravenous injection of narcotic analgesics increases the possibility of side effects such as hypotension and respiratory depression.

Pregnancy: Pregnancy Category C. DILAUDID has been shown to be teratogenic in hamsters when given in doses 600 times the human dose. There are no adequate and well-controlled studies in pregnant women. DILAUDID should be used during pregnancy only if the potential benefit justifies the potential risk to the fetus.

Nonteratogenic effects: Babies born to mothers who have been taking opioids regularly prior to delivery will be physically dependent. The withdrawal signs include irritability and excessive crying, tremors, hyperactive reflexes, increased respiratory rate, increased stools, sneezing, yawning, vomiting, and fever. The intensity of the syndrome does not always correlate with the duration of maternal opioid use or dose. There is no consensus on the best method of managing withdrawal. Chlorpromazine 0.7 to 1.0 mg/kg q6h, phenobarbital 2 mg/kg q6h, and paregoric 2 to 4 drops/kg q4h, have been used to treat withdrawal symptoms in infants. The duration of therapy is 4 to 28 days, with the dosages decreased as tolerated.

Labor and Delivery: As with all narcotics, administration of DILAUDID to the mother shortly before delivery may result in some degree of respiratory depression in the newborn, especially if higher doses are used.

Nursing Mothers: It is not known whether this drug is excreted in human milk. Because many drugs are excreted in human milk and because of the potential for serious adverse reactions in nursing infants from DILAUDID, a decision should be made whether to discontinue nursing or to discontinue the drug, taking into account the importance of the drug to the mother.

Pediatric Use: Safety and effectiveness in children have not been established.

FD&C Yellow No. 5: DILAUDID 1 mg, 2 mg and 4 mg color coded tablets contain FD&C Yellow No. 5 (tartrazine) dye which may cause allergic-type reactions (including bronchial asthma) in certain susceptible individuals. Although the overall incidence of FD&C Yellow No. 5 (tartrazine) dye sensitivity in the general population is low, it is fre-

Continued on next page

Knoll—Cont.

quently seen in patients who also have aspirin hypersensitivity.

Adverse Reactions
Central Nervous System: Sedation, drowsiness, mental clouding, lethargy, impairment of mental and physical performance, anxiety, fear, dysphoria, dizziness, psychic dependence, mood changes.
Gastrointestinal System: Nausea and vomiting occur more frequently in ambulatory than in recumbent patients. The antiemetic phenothiazines are useful in suppressing these effects; however, some phenothiazine derivatives seem to be antianalgesic and to increase the amount of narcotic required to produce pain relief, while other phenothiazines reduce the amount of narcotic required to produce a given level of analgesia. Prolonged administration of DILAUDID may produce constipation.
Cardiovascular System: Circulatory depression, peripheral circulatory collapse and cardiac arrest have occurred after rapid intravenous injection. Orthostatic hypotension and fainting may occur if a patient stands up suddenly after receiving an injection of DILAUDID.
Genitourinary System: Ureteral spasm, spasm of vesical sphincters and urinary retention have been reported.
Respiratory Depression: DILAUDID produces dose-related respiratory depression by acting directly on brain stem respiratory centers. DILAUDID also affects centers that control respiratory rhythm, and may produce irregular and periodic breathing. If significant respiratory depression occurs, it may be antagonized by the use of naloxone hydrochloride. The usual adult dose of 0.4 to 0.8 mg given *intramuscularly* or *intravenously*, promptly reverses the effects of morphine-like opioid agonists such as DILAUDID. In patients who are physically dependent, small doses of naloxone may be sufficient not only to antagonize respiratory depression, but also to precipitate withdrawal phenomena. The dose of naloxone should therefore be adjusted accordingly in such patients. Since the duration of action of DILAUDID may exceed that of the antagonist, the patient should be kept under continued surveillance; repeated doses of the antagonist may be required to maintain adequate respiration. Apply other supportive measures when indicated.

Drug Abuse and Dependence: DILAUDID is a Schedule ⓒ narcotic. Psychic dependence, physical dependence, and tolerance may develop upon repeated administration of narcotics; therefore, DILAUDID should be prescribed and administered with caution. However, psychic dependence is unlikely to develop when DILAUDID is used for a short time for the treatment of pain. Physical dependence, the condition in which continued administration of the drug is required to prevent the appearance of a withdrawal syndrome, usually assumes clinically significant proportions only after several weeks of continued narcotic use, although some mild degree of physical dependence may develop after a few days of narcotic therapy. Tolerance, in which increasingly large doses are required in order to produce the same degree of analgesia, is manifested initially by a shortened duration of analgesic effect, and subsequently by decreases in the intensity of analgesia. The rate of development of tolerance varies among patients.

Overdosage
Signs and Symptoms: Serious overdosage with DILAUDID is characterized by respiratory depression (a decrease in respiratory rate and/or tidal volume, Cheyne-Stokes respiration, cyanosis), extreme somnolence progressing to stupor or coma, skeletal muscle flaccidity, cold and clammy skin, and sometimes bradycardia and hypotension. In severe overdosage, particularly by the intravenous route, apnea, circulatory collapse, cardiac arrest, and death may occur.
Treatment: Primary attention should be given to the reestablishment of adequate respiratory exchange through provision of a patent airway and institution of assisted or controlled ventilation. The narcotic antagonist naloxone hydrochloride is a specific antidote against respiratory depression which may result from overdosage or unusual sensitivity to narcotics, including DILAUDID. Therefore, naloxone hydrochloride should be administered as described under **Adverse Reactions** (see *Respiratory Depression*) in conjunction with ventilatory assistance.
Since the duration of action of DILAUDID may exceed that of the antagonist, the patient should be kept under continued surveillance; repeated doses of the antagonist may be required to maintain adequate respiration. An antagonist should not be administered in the absence of clinically significant respiratory or cardiovascular depression. Oxygen, intravenous fluids, vasopressors, and other supportive measures should be employed as indicated.
In cases of overdosage with oral DILAUDID, gastric lavage or induced emesis may be useful in removing unabsorbed drug from conscious patients.

Dosage and Administration
Parenteral The usual starting dose is 1–2 mg *subcutaneously* or *intramuscularly* every 4 to 6 hours as necessary for pain control. The dose should be adjusted according to the severity of pain, as well as the patient's underlying disease, age, and size. Patients with terminal cancer may be tolerant to narcotic analgesics and may, therefore, require higher doses for adequate pain relief.
Intravenous or subcutaneous administration is usually not painful. Should intravenous administration be necessary, the injection should be given *slowly*, over at least 2 to 3 minutes, depending on the dose. A gradual increase in dose may be required if analgesia is inadequate, tolerance occurs, or if pain severity increases. The first sign of tolerance is usually a reduced duration of effect.
NOTE: Parenteral drug products should be inspected visually for particulate matter and discoloration prior to administration, whenever solution and container permit. A slight yellowish discoloration may develop in DILAUDID ampules and multiple dose vials. No loss of potency has been demonstrated.
Oral: The usual oral dose is 2 mg every 4 to 6 hours as necessary. The dose must be individually adjusted according to severity of pain, patient response and patient size. More severe pain may require 4 mg or more every 4 to 6 hours. If the pain increases in severity, analgesia is not adequate or tolerance occurs, a gradual increase in dosage may be required. If pain is exceedingly severe, or if prompt response is desired, parenteral DILAUDID should be used initially in adequate amounts to control the pain.
Rectal: DILAUDID suppositories (3 mg) may provide longer duration of relief which could obviate additional medication during the sleeping hours. The usual adult dose is one (1) suppository inserted rectally every 6 to 8 hours or as directed by physician.

How Supplied
Ampules: 1 mg, 2 mg and 4 mg hydromorphone hydrochloride per ml with 0.2% sodium citrate, 0.2% citric acid solution. No added preservative.
1 mg/ml ampules—Boxes of 10—
  NDC# 0044-1011-01.
2 mg/ml ampules—Boxes of 10—
  NDC# 0044-1012-01.
  Boxes of 25—NDC# 0044-1012-09.
4 mg/ml ampules—Boxes of 10—
  NDC# 0044-1014-01.
Multiple Dose Vials: 20 ml sterile solution, each ml contains 2 mg hydromorphone hydrochloride and 0.5 mg edetate disodium with 1.8 mg methylparaben and 0.2 mg propylparaben as preservatives. pH adjusted with sodium hydroxide or hydrochloric acid.
2 mg/ml—20 ml multiple dose vial—
  NDC# 0044-1062-05.
Oral Color Coded Tablets: (NOT FOR INJECTION)
1 mg tablet (green)—Bottles of 100—
  NDC# 0044-1021-02.
2 mg tablet (orange)—Bottles of 100—
  NDC# 0044-1022-02.
Strip Pack of 100 (4 × 25)—
  NDC# 0044-1022-45
Bottles of 500—NDC# 0044-1022-03.
3 mg tablet (pink)—Bottles of 100—
  NDC# 0044-1023-02.
4 mg tablet (yellow)—Bottles of 100—
  NDC# 0044-1024-02.
Strip Pack of 100 (4 × 25)—
  NDC# 0044-1024-45
Bottles of 500—NDC# 0044-1024-03.
Rectal Suppositories: 3 mg hydromorphone hydrochloride in cocoa butter base with 1% colloidal silica as an inactive ingredient.
Boxes of 6—NDC# 0044-1053-01.
Powder: For prescription compounding.
15 grain vial—NDC# 0044-1040-01.
Storage: Parenteral and oral dosage forms of DILAUDID should be stored at 59°–86°F, 15°–30°C. Protect from light.
DILAUDID suppositories should be stored in a refrigerator.
DEA order form required.
A Schedule ⓒ Narcotic.
Shown in Product Identification Section, page 414

DILAUDID® COUGH SYRUP ⓒ ℞
(hydromorphone hydrochloride)

Description: Each 5 ml (1 teaspoonful) contains 1 mg DILAUDID (hydromorphone hydrochloride) (**WARNING:** May be habit forming) and 100 mg guaifenesin in a peach-flavored syrup containing 5% alcohol. DILAUDID is a hydrogenated ketone of morphine; it is a narcotic analgesic and antitussive.

Clinical Pharmacology: DILAUDID (hydromorphone hydrochloride) is a centrally acting narcotic antitussive which acts directly on the cough reflex center. DILAUDID is also an analgesic and has diverse additional actions. It may produce drowsiness, changes in mood and mental clouding, depress the respiratory center, stimulate the vomiting center, produce pinpoint constriction of the pupil, enhance parasympathetic activity, elevate cerebrospinal fluid pressure, increase biliary pressure, and produce transient hyperglycemia, depending on the amount administered and individual patient sensitivity.
Radioimmunoassay techniques have recently been developed for the analysis of DILAUDID in human plasma. In humans the half-life of a DILAUDID 4 mg tablet is 2.6 hours. In a random crossover study in six subjects, 4 mg of *oral* DILAUDID produced a mean concentration/time curve similar to that of 2 mg DILAUDID I.V., after the first hour.
Guaifenesin (glyceryl guaiacolate) reduces the viscosity of secretions, thereby increasing the efficiency of the cough reflex and of ciliary action in removing accumulated secretions from the trachea and bronchi. Unlike many other expectorants, guaifenesin rarely causes gastric irritation.

Indications and Usage: DILAUDID Cough Syrup is indicated for the control of persistent, exhausting cough or dry, non-productive cough.

Contraindications: DILAUDID Cough Syrup is contraindicated in patients with a known hypersensitivity to the drug; in the presence of an intracranial lesion associated with increased intracranial pressure; and whenever ventilatory function is depressed (chronic obstructive pulmonary disease, cor pulmonale, emphysema, kyphoscoliosis, status asthmaticus).

Warnings
Respiratory Depression: DILAUDID may produce dose-related respiratory depression by acting directly on brain stem respiratory centers in susceptible individuals or when used in excessive doses.
Head Injury and Increased Intracranial Pressure: The respiratory depressant effects of narcotics and their capacity to elevate cerebrospinal fluid pressure may be markedly exaggerated in the presence of head injury, other intracranial lesions or a preexisting increase in intracranial pressure. Furthermore, narcotics produce effects which may obscure the clinical course of patients with head injuries.
Acute Abdominal Conditions: The administration of narcotics may obscure the diagnosis or clin-

ical course of patients with acute abdominal conditions.

Precautions
Special Risk Patients: As with any narcotic, DILAUDID Cough Syrup should be used with caution in elderly or debilitated patients and those with impaired renal or hepatic function, hypothyroidism, Addison's disease, prostatic hypertrophy or urethral stricture. The usual precautions should be observed and the possibility of respiratory depression should be kept in mind.
Cough Reflex: DILAUDID Cough Syrup suppresses the cough reflex; as with all narcotics, caution should be exercised when DILAUDID Cough Syrup is used postoperatively and in patients with pulmonary disease.
Usage in Ambulatory Patients: Narcotics may impair the mental and/or physical abilities required for the performance of potentially hazardous tasks such as driving a car or operating machinery; patients should be cautioned accordingly.
Drug Interactions: Patients receiving other narcotics, general anesthetics, phenothiazines, tranquilizers, sedative-hypnotics, tricyclic antidepressants or other CNS depressants (including alcohol) concomitantly with DILAUDID Cough Syrup may exhibit an additive CNS depression. When such combined therapy is contemplated, the dose of one or both agents should be reduced.
Pregnancy: Pregnancy Category C. DILAUDID has been shown to be teratogenic in hamsters when given in doses 600 times the human dose. There are no adequate and well-controlled studies in pregnant women. DILAUDID Cough Syrup should be used during pregnancy only if the potential benefit justifies the potential risk to the fetus.
Nonteratogenic effects: Babies born to mothers who have been taking opioids regularly prior to delivery will be physically dependent. The withdrawal signs include irritability and excessive crying, tremors, hyperactive reflexes, increased respiratory rate, increased stools, sneezing, yawning, vomiting, and fever. The intensity of the syndrome does not always correlate with the duration of maternal opioid use or dose. There is no consensus on the best method of managing withdrawal. Chlorpromazine 0.7 to 1.0 mg/kg q6h, phenobarbital 2 mg/kg q6h, and paregoric 2 to 4 drops/kg q4h, have been used to treat withdrawal symptoms in infants. The duration of therapy is 4 to 28 days, with the dosage decreased as tolerated.
Labor and Delivery: As with all narcotics, administration of DILAUDID Cough Syrup to the mother shortly before delivery may result in some degree of respiratory depression in the newborn, especially if higher doses are used.
Nursing Mothers: It is not known whether this drug is excreted in human milk. Because many drugs are excreted in human milk and because of the potential for serious adverse reactions in nursing infants from DILAUDID Cough Syrup, a decision should be made whether to discontinue nursing or to discontinue the drug, taking into account the importance of the drug to the mother.
Pediatric Use: Safety and effectiveness in children have not been established.
FD&C Yellow No. 5: DILAUDID Cough Syrup contains FD&C Yellow No. 5 (tartrazine) dye which may cause allergic-type reactions (including bronchial asthma) in certain susceptible individuals. Although the overall incidence of FD&C Yellow No. 5 (tartrazine) dye sensitivity in the general population is low, it is frequently seen in patients who also have aspirin hypersensitivity.

Adverse Reactions
Central Nervous System: Sedation, drowsiness, mental clouding, lethargy, impairment of mental and physical performance, anxiety, fear, dysphoria, dizziness, psychic dependence, mood changes.
Gastrointestinal System: Nausea and vomiting occur more frequently in ambulatory than in recumbent patients. Some of the antiemetic phenothiazines are useful in suppressing these effects. Prolonged administration of DILAUDID Cough Syrup may produce constipation.
Genitourinary System: Ureteral spasm, spasm of vesical sphincters and urinary retention have been reported.

Respiratory Depression: DILAUDID may produce dose-related respiratory depression by acting directly on brain stem respiratory centers in susceptible individuals or when used in excessive doses. DILAUDID also affects centers that control respiratory rhythm, and may produce irregular and periodic breathing. If significant respiratory depression occurs, it can be antagonized by the use of naloxone hydrochloride, 0.005 mg/kg intravenously. Apply other supportive measures when indicated.
Drug Abuse and Dependence: DILAUDID is a Schedule ⓒ narcotic. Psychic dependence, physical dependence, and tolerance may develop upon repeated administration of narcotics; therefore, DILAUDID Cough Syrup should be prescribed and administered with caution.

Overdosage
Signs and Symptoms: Serious overdosage with DILAUDID Cough Syrup is characterized by respiratory depression (a decrease in respiratory rate and/or tidal volume, Cheyne-Stokes respiration, cyanosis), extreme somnolence progressing to stupor or coma, skeletal muscle flaccidity, cold and clammy skin, and sometimes bradycardia and hypotension. In severe overdosage, apnea, circulatory collapse, cardiac arrest and death may occur.
Treatment: Primary attention should be given to the reestablishment of adequate respiratory exchange through provision of a patent airway and the institution of assisted or controlled ventilation. The narcotic antagonist naloxone hydrochloride is a specific antidote against respiratory depression which may result from overdosage or unusual sensitivity to narcotics. Therefore, naloxone hydrochloride 0.005 mg/kg should be administered intravenously simultaneously with ventilatory assistance.
Since the duration of action of the narcotic may exceed that of the antagonist, the patient should be kept under continued surveillance and repeated doses of the antagonist should be administered as needed to maintain adequate respiratory function. An antagonist should not be administered in the absence of clinically significant respiratory or cardiovascular depression. Oxygen, intravenous fluids, vasopressors and other supportive measures should be employed as indicated. Gastric lavage or induced emesis may be useful in removing unabsorbed drug from conscious patients.

Dosage and Administration: The usual adult dose of DILAUDID Cough Syrup is one teaspoonful (5 ml) every 3 to 4 hours.
How Supplied: Bottles of 1 pint (473 ml)—NDC #0044-1080-01.
Storage: Store at 59°–86°F, 15°–30°C.
A Schedule ⓒ Narcotic.
DEA order form required.

DILAUDID–HP™ INJECTION   ⓒ ℞
10 mg/ml
(hydromorphone hydrochloride)

WARNING: DILAUDID-HP™ (HIGH POTENCY) IS A HIGHLY CONCENTRATED SOLUTION OF HYDROMORPHONE INTENDED FOR USE IN NARCOTIC-TOLERANT PATIENTS. DO NOT CONFUSE DILAUDID-HP WITH STANDARD PARENTERAL FORMULATIONS OF DILAUDID OR OTHER NARCOTICS. OVERDOSE AND DEATH COULD RESULT.
Description: DILAUDID (hydromorphone hydrochloride) (WARNING: May be habit forming), a hydrogenated ketone of morphine, is a narcotic analgesic, *HIGH POTENCY* DILAUDID is available in AMBER ampules for subcutaneous (SC) or intramuscular (IM) administration. Each 1 ml of sterile solution contains 10 mg hydromorphone hydrochloride with 0.2% sodium citrate, 0.2% citric acid solution.
The structural formula of DILAUDID (hydromorphone hydrochloride) is:

Clinical Pharmacology: Many of the effects described below are common to the class of narcotic analgesics. In some instances, data may not exist to demonstrate that DILAUDID-HP possesses similar or different effects than those observed with other narcotic analgesics. However, in the absence of data to the contrary, it is assumed that DILAUDID-HP would possess these effects.

Central Nervous System: Narcotic analgesics have multiple actions but exert their primary effects on the central nervous system and organs containing smooth muscle. The principal actions of therapeutic value are analgesia and sedation. A significant feature of the analgesia is that it occurs without loss of consciousness. Narcotic analgesics also suppress the cough reflex and cause respiratory depression, mood changes, mental clouding, euphoria, dysphoria, nausea, vomiting and electroencephalographic changes. The precise mode of analgesic action of narcotic analgesics is unknown. However, specific CNS opiate receptors have been identified. Narcotics are believed to express their pharmacological effects by combining with these receptors.
Narcotics depress the cough reflex by direct effect on the cough center in the medulla.
Narcotics produce respiratory depression by direct effect on brain stem respiratory centers. The mechanism of respiratory depression also involves a reduction in the responsiveness of the brain stem respiratory centers to increases in carbon dioxide tension.
Narcotics cause miosis. Pinpoint pupils are a common sign of narcotic overdose but are not pathognomonic (e.g., pontine lesions of hemorrhagic or ischemic origin may produce similar findings) and marked mydriasis occurs when asphyxia intervenes.

Gastrointestinal Tract and Other Smooth Muscle: Gastric, biliary and pancreatic secretions are decreased by narcotics. Narcotics cause a reduction in motility associated with an increase in tone in the antrum portion of the stomach and duodenum. Digestion of food in the small intestine is delayed and propulsive contractions are decreased. Propulsive peristaltic waves in the colon are decreased, and tone may be increased to the point of spasm. The end result is constipation. Narcotics can cause a marked increase in biliary tract pressure as a result of spasm of the sphincter of Oddi.

Cardiovascular System: Certain narcotics produce peripheral vasodilation which may result in orthostatic hypotension. Release of histamine may occur with narcotics and may contribute to narcotic-induced hypotension. Other manifestations of histamine release and/or peripheral vasodilation may include pruritis, flushing, and red eyes.
Effects on the myocardium after i.v. administration of narcotics are not significant in normal persons, vary with different narcotic analgesic agents and vary with the hemodynamic state of the patient, state of hydration and sympathetic drive.

Pharmacokinetics: In normal human volunteers hydromorphone is metabolized primarily in the liver. It is excreted primarily as the glucuronidated conjugate, with small amounts of parent drug and minor amounts of 6-hydroxy reduction metabolites.
Following intravenous administration of DILAUDID to normal volunteers, the mean half-life of elimination was 2.64 +/− 0.88 hours. The mean volume of distribution was 91.5 liters, suggesting extensive tissue uptake. DILAUDID is rapidly removed from the blood stream and distributed to skeletal muscle, kidneys, liver, intestinal tract, lungs, spleen and brain. DILAUDID also crosses the placental membranes.
In terms of area under the analgesic time-effect curve, hydromorphone is approximately 8 times more potent than morphine (i.e., 1.3 mg of hydromorphone produces analgesia equal to that pro-

Continued on next page

Knoll—Cont.

duced by 10 mg of morphine). After intramuscular administration, hydromorphone has a slightly more rapid onset and slightly shorter duration of action than morphine. The duration of DILAUDID analgesia in the non-tolerant patient with usual doses may be up to 4–5 hours. However, in tolerant subjects, duration will vary substantially depending on tolerance and dose. Dose should be adjusted so that 3–4 hours of pain relief may be achieved.

Indications and Usage: DILAUDID-HP (hydromorphone hydrochloride) is indicated for the relief of moderate-to-severe pain in narcotic-tolerant patients who require larger than usual doses of narcotics to provide adequate pain relief. Because DILAUDID-HP contains 10 mg of hydromorphone per ml, a smaller injection volume can be used than with other parenteral narcotic formulations. Discomfort associated with the intramuscular or subcutaneous injection of an unusually large volume of solution can therefore be avoided.

Contraindications: DILAUDID-HP is contraindicated in: patients who are not already receiving large amounts of parenteral narcotics, patients with known hypersensitivity to the drug, patients with respiratory depression in the absence of resuscitative equipment, and in patients with status asthmaticus. DILAUDID-HP is also contraindicated for use in obstetrical analgesia.

Warnings—Drug Dependence: DILAUDID-HP can produce drug dependence of the morphine type and therefore has the potential for being abused. Psychic dependence, physical dependence and tolerance may develop upon repeated administration of DILAUDID-HP, and it should be prescribed and administered with the same degree of caution appropriate for the use of morphine. Since DILAUDID-HP is indicated for use in patients who are already tolerant to and hence physically dependent on narcotics, abrupt discontinuance in the administration of DILAUDID-HP is likely to result in a withdrawal syndrome. (See *Drug Abuse and Dependence*).

Infants born to mothers physically dependent on DILAUDID-HP will also be physically dependent and may exhibit respiratory difficulties and withdrawal symptoms (see *Drug Abuse and Dependence*).

Impaired Respiration: Respiratory depression is the chief hazard of DILAUDID-HP. Respiratory depression occurs most frequently in the elderly, in the debilitated, and in those suffering from conditions accompanied by hypoxia or hypercapnia when even moderate therapeutic doses may dangerously decrease pulmonary ventilation.

DILAUDID-HP should be used with extreme caution in patients with chronic obstructive pulmonary disease or cor pulmonale, patients having a substantially decreased respiratory reserve, hypoxia, hypercapnia, or preexisting respiratory depression. In such patients even usual therapeutic doses of narcotic analgesics may decrease respiratory drive while simultaneously increasing airway resistance to the point of apnea.

Head Injury and Increased Intracranial Pressure: The respiratory depressant effects of DILAUDID-HP with carbon dioxide retention and secondary elevation of cerebrospinal fluid pressure may be markedly exaggerated in the presence of head injury, other intracranial lesions, or preexisting increase in intracranial pressure. Narcotic analgesics including DILAUDID-HP (hydromorphone hydrochloride) may produce effects which can obscure the clinical course and neurologic signs of further increase in pressure in patients with head injuries.

Hypotensive Effect: Narcotic analgesics, including DILAUDID-HP, may cause severe hypotension in an individual whose ability to maintain his blood pressure has already been compromised by a depleted blood volume, or a concurrent administration of drugs such as phenothiazines or general anesthetics (see also *Precautions—Drug Interactions*). DILAUDID-HP may produce orthostatic hypotension in ambulatory patients.

DILAUDID-HP should be administered with caution to patients in circulatory shock, since vasodilation produced by the drug may further reduce cardiac output and blood pressure.

Precautions:

General: Because of its high concentration, the delivery of precise doses of DILAUDID-HP may be difficult if low doses of hydromorphone are required. Therefore, DILAUDID-HP should be used only if the amount of hydromorphone required can be delivered accurately with this formulation.

In general, narcotics should be given with caution and the initial dose should be reduced in the elderly or debilitated and those with severe impairment of hepatic, pulmonary or renal function; myxedema or hypothyroidism; adrenocortical insufficiency (e.g., Addison's Disease); CNS depression or coma; toxic psychoses; prostatic hypertrophy or urethral stricture; gall bladder disease; acute alcoholism; delirium tremens; or kyphoscoliosis.

In the case of DILAUDID-HP, however, the patient is presumed to be receiving a narcotic to which he or she exhibits tolerance and the initial dose of DILAUDID-HP selected should be estimated based on the relative potency of hydromorphone and the narcotic previously used by the patient. See *Dosage and Administration* section.

The administration of narcotic analgesics including DILAUDID-HP may obscure the diagnosis or clinical course in patients with acute abdominal conditions and may aggravate preexisting convulsions in patients with convulsive disorders.

Narcotic analgesics including DILAUDID-HP (hydromorphone hydrochloride) should also be used with caution in patients about to undergo surgery of the biliary tract since it may cause spasm of the sphincter of Oddi.

Drug Interactions: The concomitant use of other central nervous system depressants including sedatives or hypnotics, general anesthetics, phenothiazines, tranquilizers and alcohol may produce additive depressant effects. Respiratory depression, hypotension and profound sedation or coma may occur. When such combined therapy is contemplated, the dose of one or both agents should be reduced. Narcotic analgesics, including DILAUDID-HP, may enhance the action of neuromuscular blocking agents and produce an increased degree of respiratory depression.

Pregnancy—Category C:

Human: Adequate animal studies on reproduction have not been performed to determine whether hydromorphone affects fertility in males or females. There are no well-controlled studies in women. Reports based on marketing experience do not identify any specific teratogenic risks following routine (short-term) clinical use. Although there is no clearly defined risk, such reports do not exclude the possibility of infrequent or subtle damage to the human fetus. DILAUDID-HP should be used in pregnant women only when clearly needed (see *Labor and Delivery* and *Drug Abuse and Dependence*).

Animal: Literature reports of hydromorphone hydrochloride administration to pregnant Syrian hamsters show that DILAUDID is teratogenic at a dose of 20 mg/kg which is 600 times the human dose. A maximal teratogenic effect (50% of fetuses affected) in the Syrian hamster was observed at a dose of 125 mg/kg.

Labor and Delivery: DILAUDID-HP is contraindicated in Labor and Delivery (see *Contraindications* section).

Nursing Mothers: Low levels of narcotic analgesics have been detected in human milk. As a general rule, nursing should not be undertaken while a patient is receiving DILAUDID-HP since it, and other drugs in this class, may be excreted in the milk.

Pediatric Use: Safety and effectiveness in children have not been established.

Adverse Reactions: The adverse effects of DILAUDID-HP are similar to those of other narcotic analgesics, and represent established pharmacological effects of the drug class. The major hazards include respiratory depression and apnea. To a lesser degree, circulatory depression, respiratory arrest, shock and cardiac arrest have occurred.

The most frequently observed adverse effects are lightheadedness, dizziness, sedation, nausea, vomiting, and sweating. These effects seem to be more prominent in ambulatory patients and in those not experiencing severe pain. Some adverse reactions in ambulatory patients may be alleviated if the patient lies down.

Less Frequently Observed With Narcotic Analgesics:

General and CNS: Dysphoria, euphoria, weakness, headache, agitation, tremor, uncoordinated muscle movements, alterations of mood (nervousness, apprehension, depression, floating feelings, dreams), muscle rigidity, paresthesia, muscle tremor, blurred vision, nystagmus, diplopia and miosis, transient hallucinations* and disorientation, visual disturbances, insomnia and increased intracranial pressure may occur.

* Hallucinations, although unusual with pure agonist narcotics, have been observed in one patient following both a 6 mg and a 4 mg DILAUDID-HP dose. However, the patient was receiving several concomitant medications during the second episode and a causal relationship cannot be established.

Cardiovascular: Flushing of the face, chills, tachycardia, bradycardia, palpitation, faintness, syncope, hypotension and hypertension have been reported.

Respiratory: Bronchospasm and laryngospasm have been known to occur.

Gastrointestinal: Dry mouth, constipation, biliary tract spasm, anorexia, diarrhea, cramps and taste alterations have been reported.

Genitourinary: Urinary retention or hesitancy, and antidiuretic effects have been reported.

Dermatologic: Pruritis, urticaria, other skin rashes, wheal and flare over the vein with intravenous injection, and diaphoresis have been reported with narcotic analgesics.

Other: In clinical trials, neither local tissue irritation nor induration was observed at the site of subcutaneous injection of DILAUDID-HP; pain at the injection site was rarely observed. However, local irritation and induration have been seen following parenteral injection of other narcotic drug products.

Drug Abuse and Dependence: Narcotic analgesics may cause psychological and physical dependence (see *Warnings*). Physical dependence results in withdrawal symptoms in patients who abruptly discontinue the drug. Withdrawal symptoms also may be precipitated in the patient with physical dependence by the administration of a drug with narcotic antagonist activity, e.g., naloxone (see also *Overdosage*). Physical dependence usually does not occur to a clinically significant degree until after several weeks of continued narcotic usage. Tolerance, in which increasingly large doses are required in order to produce the same degree of analgesia, is initially manifested by a shortened duration of analgesic effect, and subsequently, by decreases in the intensity of analgesia. In chronic pain patients, and in narcotic-tolerant cancer patients, the dose of DILAUDID-HP (hydromorphone hydrochloride) should be guided by the degree of tolerance manifested.

In chronic pain patients in whom narcotic analgesics including DILAUDID-HP are abruptly discontinued, a severe abstinence syndrome should be anticipated. This may be similar to the abstinence syndrome noted in patients who withdraw from heroin. The latter abstinence syndrome may be characterized by restlessness, lacrimation, rhinorrhea, yawning, perspiration, gooseflesh, restless sleep or "yen" and mydriasis during the first 24 hours. These symptoms may increase in severity and over the next 72 hours may be accompanied by increasing irritability, anxiety, weakness, twitching and spasms of muscles, kicking movements, severe backache, abdominal and leg pains, abdominal and muscle cramps, hot and cold flashes, insomnia, nausea, anorexia, vomiting, intestinal spasm, diarrhea, coryza and repetitive sneezing, increase in body temperature, blood pressure, respiratory rate and heart rate.

Because of excessive loss of fluids through sweating, or vomiting and diarrhea, there is usually marked weight loss, dehydration, ketosis, and disturbances in acid-base balance. Cardiovascular collapse can occur. Without treatment most observable symptoms disappear in 5–14 days; however, there appears to be a phase of secondary or chronic abstinence which may last for 2–6 months characterized by insomnia, irritability, muscular aches, and autonomic instability.

In the treatment of physical dependence on DILAUDID-HP, the patient may be detoxified by gradual reduction of the dosage, although this is unlikely to be necessary in the terminal cancer patient. If abstinence symptoms become severe, the patient may be given methadone. Temporary administration of tranquilizers and sedatives may aid in reducing patient anxiety. Gastrointestinal disturbances or dehydration should be treated accordingly.

Overdosage: Serious overdosage with DILAUDID-HP is characterized by respiratory depression, somnolence progressing to stupor or coma, skeletal muscle flaccidity, cold and clammy skin, constricted pupils, and sometimes bradycardia and hypotension. In serious overdosage, particularly following intravenous injection, apnea, circulatory collapse, cardiac arrest and death may occur.

In the treatment of overdosage primary attention should be given to the reestablishment of adequate respiratory exchange through provision of a patent airway and institution of assisted or controlled ventilation.

Narcotic-Tolerant Patient: Since tolerance to the respiratory and CNS depressant effects of narcotics develops concomitantly with tolerance to their analgesic effects, serious respiratory depression due to an acute overdose is unlikely to be seen in narcotic-tolerant patients receiving DILAUDID-HP for chronic pain.

NOTE: In such an individual who is physically dependent on narcotics, administration of the usual dose of the antagonist will precipitate an acute withdrawal syndrome. The severity will depend on the degree of physical dependence and the dose of the antagonist administered. Use of a narcotic antagonist in such a person should be avoided. If necessary to treat serious respiratory depression in the physically-dependent patient, the antagonist should be administered with extreme care and by titration with smaller than usual doses of the antagonist.

Non-Tolerant Patient: The narcotic antagonist, naloxone, is a specific antidote against respiratory depression which may result from overdosage, or unusual sensitivity to DILAUDID-HP. A dose of naloxone (usually 0.4 to 2.0 mg) should be administered intravenously, if possible, simultaneously with respiratory resuscitation. The dose can be repeated in 3 minutes. Naloxone should not be administered in the absence of clinically significant respiratory or circulatory depression. Naloxone should be administered cautiously to persons who are known, or suspected to be physically dependent on DILAUDID-HP. In such cases, an abrupt or complete reversal of narcotic effects may precipitate an acute abstinence syndrome.

Since the duration of action of DILAUDID may exceed that of the antagonist, the patient should be kept under continued surveillance; repeated doses of the antagonist may be required to maintain adequate respiration. Apply other supportive measures when indicated.

Supportive measures (including oxygen, vasopressors) should be employed in the management of circulatory shock and pulmonary edema accompanying overdose as indicated. Cardiac arrest or arrhythmias may require cardiac massage or defibrillation.

Dosage and Administration:
Parenteral: **DILAUDID-HP SHOULD BE GIVEN ONLY TO PATIENTS WHO ARE ALREADY RECEIVING LARGE DOSES OF NARCOTICS.** DILAUDID-HP is indicated for relief of moderate-to-severe pain in narcotic-tolerant patients. Thus, these patients will already have been treated with other narcotic analgesics. If the patient is being changed from regular DILAUDID to DILAUDID-HP, similar doses should be used, depending on the patient's clinical response to the drug. If DILAUDID-HP is substituted for a different narcotic analgesic, the following equivalency table should be used as a guide to determine the appropriate starting dose of DILAUDID-HP (hydromorphone hydrochloride).

[See table above].

* from Beaver WT
Management of cancer pain with parenteral medication
J. Am. Med. Assoc. 244:2653–2657 (1980)

† (in terms of the area under the analgesic time-effect curve.)

In open clinical trials with DILAUDID-HP in patients with terminal cancer, doses ranged from 1–14 mg subcutaneously or intramuscularly; one patient received 30 mg subcutaneously on two occasions. In these trials, both subcutaneous and intramuscular injections of DILAUDID-HP were well-tolerated, with minimal pain and/or burning at the injection site. Mild erythema was rarely noted after intramuscular injection. There was no induration after either intramuscular or subcutaneous administration of DILAUDID-HP. Subcutaneous injections of DILAUDID-HP (hydromorphone hydrochloride) were particularly well accepted when administered with a short, 30-gauge needle.

Experience with administration of DILAUDID-HP by the intravenous route is limited. Should intravenous administration be necessary, the injection should be given slowly, over at least 2 to 3 minutes. The intravenous route is usually painless.

A gradual increase in dose may be required if analgesia is inadequate, tolerance occurs, or if pain severity increases. The first sign of tolerance is usually a reduced duration of effect.

NOTE: Parenteral drug products should be inspected visually for particulate matter and discoloration prior to administration, whenever solution and container permit. A slight yellowish discoloration may develop in DILAUDID-HP ampules. No loss of potency has been demonstrated.

How Supplied: DILAUDID-HP *amber* ampules contain 10 mg hydromorphone hydrochloride per ml with 0.2% sodium citrate and 0.2% citric acid solution. No added preservative.

NOTE: DILAUDID-HP ampules are *amber* in color and marked with a distinctive violet-colored identification band.

HIGH POTENCY 10 mg/ml—Box of 10 ampules NDC 0044-1017-10

Storage: Parenteral forms of DILAUDID should be stored at 59°–86°F. (15–30°C). Protect from light.

DEA Order Form Required
A Schedule Ⓒ Narcotic.
January, 1984   6642
Shown in Product Identification Section, page 414

ISOPTIN® ℞
(verapamil hydrochloride)
for Intravenous Injection

Description: ISOPTIN (verapamil hydrochloride) is a slow-channel inhibitor or calcium antagonist. ISOPTIN is available in 5 mg per 2 ml and 10 mg per 4 ml ampules, 5 mg per 2 ml amd 10 mg per 4 ml syringes, 5 mg/2ml and 10mg/4ml single dose vials (for intravenous administration). Each 1 ml of solution contains 2.5 mg verapamil hydrochloride and 8.5 mg sodium chloride in water for injection. Hydrochloric acid is used for pH adjustment. The pH of the solution is between 4.1 and 6.0. Protect contents from light. Isoptin ampules, syringes and vials are sterile.

The structural formula of verapamil HCl is given below:

$C_{27}H_{38}N_2O_4 \cdot HCl$ M.W. = 491.08
Benzeneacetonitrile, α-[3-[[2-(3,4-dimethoxyphenyl) ethyl] methylamino] propyl] - 3,4-dimethoxy-α-(1-methylethyl) hydrochloride

Verapamil HCl is an almost white, crystalline powder, practically free of odor, with a bitter taste. It is soluble in water, chloroform and methanol. Verapamil HCl is not chemically related to other antiarrhythmic drugs.

Clinical Pharmacology
Mechanism of Action: ISOPTIN (verapamil HCl) inhibits the calcium ion (and possibly sodium ion) influx through slow channels into conductile and contractile myocardial cells and vascular smooth muscle cells. The antiarrhythmic effect of ISOPTIN appears to be due to its effect on the slow channel in cells of the cardiac conductile system. Electrical activity through the SA and AV nodes depends, to a significant degree, upon calcium influx through the slow channel. By inhibiting this influx, ISOPTIN slows AV conduction and prolongs the effective refractory period within the AV node in a rate-related manner, reducing elevated ventricular rate in patients with supraventricular tachycardia due to atrial flutter and/or atrial fi-

Continued on next page

STRONG ANALGESICS AND STRUCTURALLY RELATED DRUGS USED IN THE TREATMENT OF CANCER PAIN*

IM or SC Administration

Nonproprietary (Trade) Names	Dose, mg Equianalgesic to 10 mg of IM Morphine†	Duration Compared With Morphine
Morphine sulfate	10	Same
Papaveretum (Pantopon)	20	Same
Hydromorphone hydrochloride (DILAUDID)	1.3	Slightly shorter
Oxymorphone hydrochloride (Numorphan)	1.1	Slightly shorter
Nalbuphine hydrochloride (Nubain)	12	Same
Heroin, diamorphine hydrochloride (NA in U.S.)	4–5	Slightly shorter
Levorphanol tartrate (Levo-Dromoran)	2.3	Same
Butorphanol tartrate (Stadol)	1.5–2.5	Same
Pentazocine lactate or hydrochloride (Talwin)	60	Shorter
Meperidine, pethidine hydrochloride (Demerol)	80	Shorter
Methadone hydrochloride (Dolophine)	10	Same

Knoll—Cont.

brillation. By interrupting reentry at the AV node, ISOPTIN can restore normal sinus rhythm in patients with paroxysmal supraventricular tachycardias (PSVT), including Wolff-Parkinson-White syndrome. ISOPTIN has no effect on conduction across accessory bypass tracts. ISOPTIN does not alter the normal atrial action potential or intraventricular conduction time, but depresses amplitude, velocity of depolarization and conduction in depressed atrial fibers.

In the isolated rabbit heart, concentrations of ISOPTIN that markedly affect SA nodal fibers or fibers in the upper and middle regions of the AV node, have very little effect on fibers in the lower AV node (NH region) and no effect on atrial action potentials or HIS bundle fibers.

ISOPTIN does not induce peripheral arterial spasm.

ISOPTIN has a local anesthetic action that is 1.6 times that of procaine on an equimolar basis. It is not known whether this action is important at the doses used in man.

ISOPTIN does not alter total serum calcium levels.

Hemodynamics: In animals and man, ISOPTIN (verapamil HCl) reduces afterload and myocardial contractility. In most patients, including those with organic cardiac disease, the negative inotropic action of ISOPTIN is countered by reduction of afterload and cardiac index is usually not reduced, but in patients with moderately severe to severe cardiac dysfunction (pulmonary wedge pressure above 20 mm Hg, ejection fraction less than 30%), acute worsening of heart failure may be seen. Peak therapeutic effects occur within 3 to 5 minutes after a bolus injection. The commonly used intravenous doses of 5–10 mg ISOPTIN produce transient, usually asymptomatic, reduction in normal systemic arterial pressure, systemic vascular resistance and contractility; left ventricular filling pressure is slightly increased.

Pharmacokinetics: Intravenously administered ISOPTIN (verapamil HCl) has been shown to be rapidly metabolized in both humans and animals. Following intravenous infusion in man, verapamil is eliminated bi-exponentially, with a rapid early distribution phase (half-life about 4 minutes) and a slower terminal elimination phase (half-life 2–5 hours). In healthy men, orally administered ISOPTIN undergoes extensive metabolism in the liver with 12 metabolites having been identified, most in only trace amounts. The major metabolites have been identified as various N- and O-dealkylated products of ISOPTIN. Approximately 70% of an administered dose is excreted in the urine and 16% or more in the feces within 5 days. About 3–4% is excreted as unchanged drug.

Indications and Usage: ISOPTIN (verapamil HCl) is indicated for the treatment of supraventricular tachyarrhythmias, including:

- Rapid conversion to sinus rhythm of paroxysmal supraventricular tachycardias, including those associated with accessory bypass tracts (Wolff-Parkinson-White [W-P-W] and Lown-Ganong-Levine [L-G-L] syndromes). When clinically advisable, appropriate vagal maneuvers (e.g. Valsalva maneuver) should be attempted prior to ISOPTIN administration.
- Temporary control of rapid ventricular rate in atrial flutter or atrial fibrillation.

In controlled studies in the United States, about 60% of patients with supraventricular tachycardia converted to normal sinus rhythm within 10 minutes after intravenous ISOPTIN. Uncontrolled studies reported in the world literature describe a conversion rate of about 80%. About 70% of patients with atrial flutter and/or fibrillation with a fast ventricular rate respond with a decrease in heart rate of at least 20%. Conversion of atrial flutter or fibrillation to sinus rhythm is uncommon (about 10%) after ISOPTIN and may reflect the spontaneous conversion rate, since the conversion rate after placebo was similar. Slowing of the ventricular rate in patients with atrial fibrillation/flutter lasts 30–60 minutes after a single injection.

Because a small fraction (< 1.0%) of patients treated with ISOPTIN respond with life-threatening adverse responses (rapid ventricular rate in atrial flutter/fibrillation, marked hypotension, or extreme bradycardia/asystole—see Warnings), the initial use of intravenous ISOPTIN should, if possible, be in a treatment setting with monitoring and resuscitation facilities, including D.C.-cardioversion capability. As familiarity with the patient's response is gained, an office setting would be acceptable.

Contraindications: Verapamil HCl is contraindicated in:

1. Severe hypotension or cardiogenic shock
2. Second- or third-degree AV block
3. Sick sinus syndrome (except in patients with a functioning artificial ventricular pacemaker)
4. Severe congestive heart failure (unless secondary to a supraventricular tachycardia amenable to verapamil therapy)
5. Patients receiving **intravenous** beta adrenergic blocking drugs (e.g., propranolol). **Intravenous** verapamil and **intravenous** beta adrenergic blocking drugs should not be administered in close proximity to each other (within a few hours), since both may have a depressant effect on myocardial contractility and AV conduction.
6. Known hypersensitivity to verapamil hydrochloride.

Warnings: ISOPTIN SHOULD BE GIVEN AS A SLOW INTRAVENOUS INJECTION OVER AT LEAST A TWO MINUTE PERIOD OF TIME. (See Dosage and Administration)

Hypotension: Intravenous verapamil often produces a decrease in blood pressure below baseline levels that is usually transient and asymptomatic but may result in dizziness. Systolic pressure less than 90 mm Hg and/or diastolic pressure less than 60 mm Hg was seen in 5–10% of patients in controlled U.S. trials in supraventricular tachycardia and in about 10% of the patients with atrial flutter/fibrillation. The incidence of symptomatic hypotension observed in studies conducted in the U.S. was approximately 1.5%. Three of the five symptomatic patients required pharmacologic treatment (levarterenol bitartrate I.V., metaraminol bitartrate I.V., or 10% calcium gluconate I.V.). All recovered without sequelae.

Rapid Ventricular Response or Ventricular Fibrillation in Atrial Flutter/ Fibrillation: Patients with atrial flutter/fibrillation and an accessory AV pathway (e.g., Wolff-Parkinson-White or Lown-Ganong-Levine syndromes) may develop increased antegrade conduction across the aberrant pathway bypassing the AV node, producing a very rapid ventricular response after receiving verapamil (or digitalis). This has been reported in 1% of the patients treated in controlled double-blind trials in the United States. Treatment is usually D.C.-cardioversion. Cardioversion has been used safely and effectively after intravenous ISOPTIN. (See Adverse Reactions and Treatment of Adverse Reactions)

Extreme Bradycardia/Asystole: Verapamil slows conduction across the AV node and rarely may produce second- or third-degree AV block, bradycardia and, in extreme cases, asystole. This is more likely to occur in patients with a sick sinus syndrome (SA nodal disease), which is more common in older patients. Bradycardia associated with sick sinus syndrome was reported in 0.3% of the patients treated in controlled double-blind trials in the United States. The total incidence of bradycardia (ventricular rate less than 60 beats/min) was 1.2% in these studies. Asystole in patients other than those with sick sinus syndrome is usually of short duration (few seconds or less), with spontaneous return to AV nodal or normal sinus rhythm. If this does not occur promptly, appropriate treatment should be initiated immediately. (See Adverse Reactions and Treatment of Adverse Reactions)

Heart Failure: When heart failure is not severe or rate related, it should be controlled with optimum digitalization and diuretics, as appropriate, before ISOPTIN is used.

In patients with moderately severe to severe cardiac dysfunction (pulmonary wedge pressure above 20 mm Hg, ejection fraction less than 30%), acute worsening of heart failure may be seen.

Concomitant Antiarrhythmic Therapy:

Digitalis
Intravenous verapamil has been used concomitantly with digitalis preparations without the occurrence of serious adverse effects. However, since both drugs slow AV conduction, patients should be monitored for AV block or excessive bradycardia.

Quinidine—Procainamide
Intravenous verapamil has been administered to a small number of patients receiving oral quinidine and oral procainamide without the occurrence of serious adverse effects.

Beta Adrenergic Blocking Drugs
Intravenous verapamil has been administered to patients receiving **oral** beta blockers without the development of serious adverse effects. However, since both drugs may depress myocardial contractility or AV conduction, these possibilities should be considered. On rare occasions, the concomitant administration of **intravenous** beta blockers and **intravenous** verapamil has resulted in serious adverse reactions (see Contraindications), especially in patients with severe cardiomyopathy, congestive heart failure or recent myocardial infarction.

Disopyramide
Until data on possible interactions between verapamil and all forms of disopyramide phosphate are obtained, disopyramide should not be administered within 48 hours before or 24 hours after verapamil administration.

Heart Block: ISOPTIN prolongs AV conduction time. While high degree AV block has not been observed in controlled clinical trials in the U.S., a low percentage (less than 0.5%) has been reported in the world literature. Development of second- or third-degree AV block or unifascicular, bifascicular or trifascicular bundle branch block requires reduction in subsequent doses or discontinuation of verapamil and institution of appropriate therapy, if needed. (See Adverse Reactions and Concomitant Antiarrhythmic Therapy)

Hepatic and Renal Failure: Significant hepatic and renal failure should not increase the effects of a single intravenous dose of ISOPTIN but may prolong its duration. Repeated injections of intravenous ISOPTIN in such patients may lead to accumulation and an excessive pharmacologic effect of the drug. There is no experience to guide use of multiple doses in such patients and this generally should be avoided. If repeated injections are essential, blood pressure and PR interval should be closely monitored and smaller repeat doses should be utilized. Data on the clearance of verapamil by dialysis are not yet available.

Premature Ventricular Contractions: During conversion to normal sinus rhythm, or marked reduction in ventricular rate, a few benign complexes of unusual appearance (sometimes resembling premature ventricular contractions) may be seen after treatment with verapamil. Similar complexes are seen during spontaneous conversion of supraventricular tachycardias, after D.C.-cardioversion and other pharmacologic therapy. These complexes appear to have no clinical significance.

Precautions

Drug Interactions: (See Warnings: Concomitant Antiarrhythmic Therapy) Intravenous ISOPTIN (verapamil HCl) has been used concomitantly with other cardioactive drugs (especially digitalis and quinidine) without evidence of serious negative drug interactions, except, in rare instances, when patients with severe cardiomyopathy, congestive heart failure or recent myocardial infarction were given **intravenous** beta-adrenergic blocking agents or disopyramide. Drug interaction studies are ongoing. As verapamil is highly bound to plasma proteins, it should be administered with caution to patients receiving other highly protein bound drugs.

Product Information

Suggested Treatment of Acute Cardiovascular Adverse Reactions*
The frequency of these adverse reactions was quite low and experience with their treatment has been limited.

Adverse Reaction	Proven Effective Treatment	Treatment with Good Theoretical Rationale	Supportive Treatment
1. Symptomatic hypotension requiring treatment	Calcium chloride (I.V.) Levarterenol bitartrate (I.V.) Metaraminol bitartrate (I.V.) Isoproterenol HCl (I.V.) Dopamine (I.V.)	Dobutamine (I.V.)	Intravenous fluids Trendelenburg position
2. Bradycardia, AV block, Asystole	Isoproterenol HCl (I.V.) Calcium chloride (I.V.) Cardiac pacing Levarterenol bitartrate (I.V.) Atropine (I.V.)	———	Intravenous fluids (slow drip)
3. Rapid ventricular rate (due to antegrade conduction in flutter/fibrillation with W-P-W or L-G-L syndromes)	D.C.-cardioversion (high energy may be required) Procainamide (I.V.) Lidocaine (I.V.)		Intravenous fluids (slow drip)

* Actual treatment and dosage should depend on the severity of the clinical situation and the judgment and experience of the treating physician.

Pregnancy: Pregnancy Category B. Reproduction studies have been performed in rats and rabbits. At doses up to 2.5 and 1.5 times the human **oral** dose, respectively, no evidence of impaired fertility or harm to the fetus due to verapamil was revealed. There are, however, no adequate and well-controlled studies in pregnant women. Because animal reproduction studies are not always predictive of human response, this drug should be used during pregnancy only if clearly needed.

Labor and Delivery: There have been few controlled studies to determine whether the use of verapamil during labor or delivery has immediate or delayed adverse effects on the fetus, or whether it prolongs the duration of labor or increases the need for forceps delivery or other obstetric intervention. Such adverse experiences have not been reported in the literature, despite a long history of use of intravenous ISOPTIN in Europe in the treatment of cardiac side effects of beta-adrenergic agonist agents used to treat premature labor.

Nursing Mothers: It is not known whether this drug is excreted in human milk. Because many drugs are excreted in human milk and because of the potential for adverse reactions in nursing infants from verapamil, nursing should be discontinued while verapamil is administered.

Pediatrics: Controlled studies with verapamil have not been conducted in pediatric patients, but uncontrolled experience with intravenous administration in more than 250 patients, about half under 12 months of age and about 25% newborn, indicates that results of treatment are similar to those in adults. The most commonly used single doses in patients up to 12 months of age have ranged from 0.1 to 0.2 mg/kg of body weight, while in patients aged 1 to 15 years, the most commonly used single doses ranged from 0.1 to 0.3 mg/kg of body weight. Most of the patients received the lower dose of 0.1 mg/kg once, but in some cases, the dose was repeated once or twice every 10 to 30 minutes.

Adverse Reactions: The following reactions were reported with intravenous ISOPTIN use in controlled U.S. clinical trials involving 324 patients:

Cardiovascular: Symptomatic hypotension (1.5%); bradycardia (1.2%); severe tachycardia (1.0%). The worldwide experience in open clinical trials in more than 7,900 patients was similar.

Central Nervous System Effects: Dizziness (1.2%); headache (1.2%).

Gastrointestinal: Nausea (0.9%); abdominal discomfort (0.6%).

In rare cases of hypersensitive patients, broncho/laryngeal spasm accompanied by itch and urticaria have been reported.

The following reactions were reported in single patients: emotional depression, rotary nystagmus, sleepiness, vertigo, muscle fatigue or diaphoresis. [See table above]

Overdosage: Treatment of overdosage should be supportive. Beta-adrenergic stimulation or parenteral administration of calcium solutions (calcium chloride) may increase calcium ion flux across the slow channel. These pharmacologic interventions have been effectively used in treatment of deliberate overdosage with oral verapamil. Clinically significant hypotensive reactions or high degree AV block should be treated with vasopressor agents or cardiac pacing, respectively. Asystole should be handled by the usual measures including isoproterenol hydrochloride, other vasopressor agents or cardiopulmonary resuscitation. (See Treatment of Cardiovascular Adverse Reactions)

Dosage and Administration (For Intravenous Use Only)
ISOPTIN SHOULD BE GIVEN AS A SLOW INTRAVENOUS INJECTION OVER AT LEAST A TWO MINUTE PERIOD OF TIME.
The recommended intravenous doses of ISOPTIN are as follows:

ADULT: Initial dose: 5-10 mg (0.075—0.15 mg/kg body weight) given as an intravenous bolus over 2 minutes.

Repeat dose: 10 mg (0.15 mg/kg body weight) 30 minutes after the first dose if the initial response is not adequate. An optimal interval for subsequent I.V. doses has yet to be determined and should be individualized for each patient.

Older Patients: The dose should be administered over at least 3 minutes to minimize the risk of untoward drug effects.

PEDIATRIC: Initial dose
0—1 year: 0.1—0.2 mg/kg body weight (usual single dose range: 0.75—2 mg) should be administered as an intravenous bolus over 2 minutes under continuous ECG monitoring.
1—15 years: 0.1—0.3 mg/kg body weight (usual single dose range: 2—5 mg) should be administered as an intravenous bolus over 2 minutes. **Do not exceed 5 mg.**

Repeat dose
0—1 year: 0.1—0.2 mg/kg body weight (usual single dose range: 0.75—2 mg) 30 minutes after the first dose if the initial response is not adequate (under continuous ECG monitoring). An optimal interval for subsequent I.V. doses has yet to be determined and should be individualized for each patient.
1—15 years: 0.1—0.3 mg/kg body weight (usual single dose range: 2—5 mg) 30 minutes after the first dose if the initial response is not adequate. **Do not exceed 10 mg as a single dose.** An optimal interval for subsequent I.V. doses has yet to be determined and should be individualized for each patient.

Note: Parenteral drug products should be inspected visually for particulate matter and discoloration prior to administration, whenever solution and container permit.

How Supplied: Each 1 ml of sterile solution contains 2.5 mg verapamil hydrochloride and 8.5 mg sodium chloride. pH adjusted with hydrochloric acid.

5 mg/2 ml ampule—Individual unit carton—NDC 0044-1815-01
Space saver pack of 5 ampules—
NDC 0044-1815-05
*5 mg/2 ml syringe—Carton of 5 syringes
NDC 0044-1815-25
5mg/2ml vial—Single dose. No preservative. Individual unit carton—NDC 0044-1816-21
10 mg/4 ml ampule—Individual unit carton—NDC 0044-1815-11
Space saver pack of 5 ampules—NDC 0044-1815-15
*10 mg/4 ml syringe—Carton of 5 syringes
NDC 0044-1815-45
10mg/4ml vial—Single dose. No preservative. Individual unit carton—NDC 0044-1816-41
*Syringes manufactured for Knoll Pharmaceutical Company, Whippany, New Jersey 07981 by Taylor Pharmacal Company, Decatur, Illinois 62525.

Storage: 15°-30°C, 59°-86°F. Protect from light.
Shown in Product Identification Section, page 414

ISOPTIN®
(verapamil hydrochloride)
Oral Tablets

Description: ISOPTIN (verapamil hydrochloride) is a calcium ion influx inhibitor (slow channel blocker or calcium ion antagonist). ISOPTIN is available for oral administration as round, scored, film-coated tablets containing 80 mg or 120 mg verapamil hydrochloride.

The structural formula of verapamil HCl is given below:

$$CH_3O\text{-}\underset{CH_3O}{\bigcirc}\text{-}\underset{CH(CH_3)_2}{\overset{CN}{\underset{|}{C}}(CH_2)_3}\text{-}NCH_2CH_2\text{-}\underset{CH_3}{\bigcirc}\text{-}\underset{OCH_3}{OCH_3} \cdot HCl$$

Continued on next page

Knoll—Cont.

$C_{27}H_{38}N_2O_4 \cdot HCl$ M.W. = 491.08
Benzeneacetonitrile,
α-[3-[[2-(3,4-dimethoxyphenyl) ethyl]
methylamino]
propyl]-3,4-dimethoxy-α-(1-methylethyl)
hydrochloride

Verapamil HCl is an almost white, crystalline powder, practically free of odor, with a bitter taste. It is soluble in water, chloroform and methanol. Verapamil HCl is not chemically related to other cardioactive drugs.

Clinical Pharmacology: ISOPTIN is a calcium ion influx inhibitor (slow channel blocker or calcium ion antagonist) which exerts its pharmacologic effects by modulating the influx of ionic calcium across the cell membrane of the arterial smooth muscle as well as in conductile and contractile myocardial cells.

Mechanism of Action: The precise mechanism of action of ISOPTIN as an antianginal agent remains to be fully determined but includes the following mechanisms:

1. **Relaxation and prevention of coronary artery spasm**
   ISOPTIN dilates the main coronary arteries and coronary arterioles, both in normal and ischemic regions, and is a potent inhibitor of coronary artery spasm, whether spontaneous or ergonovine-induced. This property increases myocardial oxygen delivery in patients with coronary artery spasm, and is responsible for the effectiveness of ISOPTIN in vasospastic (Prinzmetal's or variant) as well as unstable angina at rest. Whether this effect plays any role in classical effort angina is not clear, but studies of exercise tolerance have not shown an increase in the maximum exercise rate-pressure product, a widely accepted measure of oxygen utilization. This suggests that, in general, relief of spasm or dilation of coronary arteries is not an important factor in classical angina.

2. **Reduction of oxygen utilization**
   ISOPTIN regularly reduces arterial pressure at rest and at a given level of exercise by dilating peripheral arterioles and reducing the total peripheral resistance (afterload) against which the heart works. This unloading of the heart reduces myocardial energy consumption and oxygen requirements and probably accounts for the effectiveness of ISOPTIN in chronic stable effort angina.

Electrical activity through the SA and AV nodes depends, to a significant degree, upon calcium influx through the slow channel. By inhibiting this influx, ISOPTIN slows AV conduction and prolongs the effective refractory period within the AV node in a rate-related manner. It can interfere with sinus node impulse generation and induce sinus arrest in patients with sick sinus syndrome and also can induce atrioventricular block, although this has been seen rarely in clinical use. ISOPTIN may shorten the antegrade effective refractory period of accessory bypass tracts. ISOPTIN does not alter the normal atrial action potential or intraventricular conduction time, but depresses amplitude, velocity of depolarization and conduction in depressed atrial fibers.
ISOPTIN has a local anesthetic action that is 1.6 times that of procaine on an equimolar basis. It is not known whether this action is important at the doses used in man.
ISOPTIN does not alter total serum calcium levels.

Pharmacokinetics and Metabolism: More than 90% of the orally administered dose of ISOPTIN is absorbed. Because of rapid biotransformation of verapamil during its first pass through the portal circulation, absolute bioavailability ranges from 20% to 35%. Peak plasma concentrations are reached between 1 and 2 hours after oral administration. Chronic oral administration of 120 mg of ISOPTIN every 6 hours resulted in plasma levels of verapamil ranging from 125 to 400 ng/ml with higher values reported occasionally. A close relationship exists between verapamil plasma concentration and prolongation of the PR interval. The mean elimination half-life in single dose studies ranged from 2.8 to 7.4 hours. In these same studies, after repetitive dosing, the half-life increased to a range from 4.5 to 12.0 hours (after less than 10 consecutive doses given 6 hours apart). Half-life may increase during titration due to saturation of hepatic enzyme systems as plasma verapamil levels rise.

In healthy men, orally administered ISOPTIN undergoes extensive metabolism in the liver. Twelve metabolites have been identified in plasma; all except norverapamil are present in trace amounts only. Norverapamil can reach steady-state plasma concentrations approximately equal to those of verapamil itself. The major metabolites of verapamil have been identified as various N- and O-dealkylated products of ISOPTIN. Approximately 70% of an administered dose is excreted as metabolites in the urine and 16% or more in the feces within 5 days. About 3% to 4% is excreted in the urine as unchanged drug. Approximately 90% is bound to plasma proteins. In patients with hepatic insufficiency, metabolism is delayed and elimination half-life prolonged up to 14 to 16 hours (see Precautions); the volume of distribution is increased and plasma clearance reduced to about 30% of normal. Verapamil clearance values suggest that patients with liver dysfunction may attain therapeutic verapamil plasma concentrations with one-third of the oral daily dose required for patients with normal liver function.

Hemodynamics and Myocardial Metabolism: In animals and man, ISOPTIN reduces afterload and myocardial contractility. In most patients, including those with organic cardiac disease, the negative inotropic action of ISOPTIN is countered by reduction of afterload and cardiac index is usually not reduced. In patients with severe left ventricular dysfunction however, (e.g., pulmonary wedge pressure above 20 mm Hg or ejection fraction lower than 30%), or in patients on beta-adrenergic blocking agents or other cardiodepressant drugs, deterioration of ventricular function may occur (see Drug Interactions).

Pulmonary Function: ISOPTIN does not induce bronchoconstriction and hence, does not impair ventilatory function.

Indications and Usage: ISOPTIN is indicated for the treatment of angina pectoris including:
1. Angina at rest including:
   • Vasospastic (Prinzmetal's variant) angina
   • Unstable (crescendo, pre-infarction) angina
2. Chronic stable angina (classic effort-associated angina)

Contraindications: Verapamil HCl is contraindicted in:
1. Severe left ventricular dysfunction (see Warnings)
2. Hypotension (less than 90 mm Hg systolic pressure) or cardiogenic shock
3. Sick sinus syndrome (except in patients with a functioning artificial ventricular pacemaker)
4. Second- or third-degree AV block

Warnings
Heart Failure: Verapamil has a negative inotropic effect which, in most patients, is compensated by its afterload reduction (decreased peripheral vascular resistance) properties without a net impairment of ventricular performance. In clinical experience with 1166 patients, 11 (0.9%) developed congestive heart failure or pulmonary edema. Congestive heart failure/pulmonary edema led to discontinuation or reduction in dosage of verapamil in 6 (0.5%) patients. Verapamil should be avoided in patients with severe left ventricular dysfunction (e.g., ejection fraction less than 30% or moderate to severe symptoms of cardiac failure) and in patients with any degree of ventricular dysfunction if they are receiving a beta blocker (see Drug Interactions). Patients with milder ventricular dysfunction should, if possible, be controlled with optimum doses of digitalis and/or diuretics before verapamil treatment (**Note interactions with digoxin under: Precautions**).

Hypotension: Occasionally, the pharmacologic action of verapamil may produce a decrease in blood pressure below normal levels which may result in dizziness or symptomatic hypotension. Hypotension is usually asymptomatic, orthostatic, mild and can be controlled by a decrease in the ISOPTIN dose. The incidence of hypotension observed in 1166 patients enrolled in clinical trials was 2.9%.

Elevated Liver Enzymes: Elevations of transaminases with and without concomitant elevations in alkaline phosphatase and bilirubin have been reported. Such elevations have sometimes been transient and may disappear even in the face of continued verapamil treatment; however, four cases of hepatocellular injury produced by verapamil have been proven by rechallenge. Two of these four cases had clinical symptoms of malaise, fever, and/or right upper quadrant pain in addition to elevations of SGOT, SGPT and alkaline phosphatase. Periodic monitoring of liver function in patients receiving verapamil is therefore prudent.

Atrial Flutter/Fibrillation with Accessory Bypass Tract: Patients with atrial flutter or fibrillation and an accessory AV pathway (e.g., Wolff-Parkinson-White or Lown-Ganong-Levine syndromes) may develop increased antegrade conduction across the aberrant pathway bypassing the AV node, producing a very rapid ventricular response after receiving verapamil (or digitalis). Treatment is usually D.C.-cardioversion. Cardioversion has been used safely and effectively after oral ISOPTIN.

Atrioventricular Block: The effect of verapamil on AV conduction and the SA node leads to first-degree AV block and transient bradycardia, sometimes accompanied by nodal escape rhythms, fairly commonly during the peaks of serum concentration. Higher degrees of AV block, however, were infrequently (0.8%) observed. Marked first-degree block or progressive development to second- or third-degree AV block requires a reduction in dosage or, in rare instances, discontinuation of verapamil HCl and institution of appropriate therapy depending upon the clinical situation.

Patients with Hypertrophic Cardiomyopathy (IHSS): In 120 patients with hypertrophic cardiomyopathy (most of them refractory or intolerant to propranolol) who received therapy with verapamil at doses up to 720 mg/day, a variety of serious adverse effects were seen. Three patients died in pulmonary edema; all had severe left ventricular outflow obstruction and a past history of left ventricular dysfunction. Eight other patients had pulmonary edema and/or severe hypotension; abnormally high (over 20 mm Hg) capillary wedge pressure and a marked left ventricular outflow obstruction were present in most of these patients. Concomitant administration of quinidine preceded the severe hypotension in 3 of the 8 patients (2 of whom developed pulmonary edema). Sinus bradycardia occurred in 11% of the patients, second-degree AV block in 4% and sinus arrest in 2%. It must be appreciated that this group of patients had a serious disease with a high mortality rate. Most adverse effects responded well to dose reduction and only rarely did verapamil have to be discontinued.

Precautions
General
Use in Patients with Impaired Hepatic Function: Since verapamil is highly metabolized by the liver, it should be administered cautiously to patients with impaired hepatic function. Severe liver dysfunction prolongs the elimination half-life of verapamil to about 14 to 16 hours; hence, approximately 30% of the dose given to patients with normal liver function should be administered to these patients. Careful monitoring for abnormal prolongation of the PR interval or other signs of excessive pharmacologic effects (See Overdosage) should be carried out.

Use in Patients with Impaired Renal Function: About 70% of an administered dose of verapamil is excreted as metabolites in the urine. Until further data are available, verapamil should be administered cautiously to patients with impaired renal function. These patients should be carefully monitored for abnormal prolongation of the PR interval or other signs of overdosage (see **Overdosage**).

Drug Interactions

Beta Blockers: Controlled studies in small numbers of patients suggest that the concomitant use of ISOPTIN and beta-blocking agents may be beneficial in patients with chronic stable angina but available information is not sufficient to predict with confidence the effects of concurrent treatment, especially in patients with left ventricular dysfunction or cardiac conduction abnormalities. The combination can have adverse effects on cardiac function. In one study of 15 patients treated with high doses of propranolol (median dose: 480 mg/day, range 160 to 1280 mg/day) for severe angina, with preserved left ventricular function (ejection fraction greater than 35%), the hemodynamic effects of additional therapy with ISOPTIN (verapamil HCl) were assessed using invasive methods. The addition of verapamil to high dose beta blockers induced modest negative inotropic and chronotropic effects which were not severe enough to limit short-term (48 hours) combination therapy in this study. These modest cardiodepressant effects persist for greater than 6, but less than 30 hours after abrupt withdrawal of beta blockers and were closely related to plasma levels of propranolol. The primary verapamil/beta-blocker interaction in this study appeared to be hemodynamic rather than electrophysiologic.

In three other studies involving 51 patients, verapamil did not induce negative inotropic or chronotropic effects in patients with preserved left ventricular function receiving low or moderate doses of propranolol (less than or equal to 320 mg/day). Because of the still limited experience with combination therapy verapamil should be used alone, if possible. If combined therapy is used, close surveillance of vital signs and clinical status should be carried out and the need for concomitant treatment with propranolol reassessed periodically. Combined therapy should usually be avoided in patients with atrioventricular conduction abnormalities and those with depressed left ventricular function.

Digitalis: Chronic verapamil treatment increases serum digoxin levels by 50% to 70% during the first week of therapy and this can result in digitalis toxicity. Maintenance digitalization doses should be reduced when verapamil is administered and the patient should be carefully monitored to avoid over- or underdigitalization. Whenever overdigitalization is suspected, the daily dose of digoxin should be reduced or temporarily discontinued. Upon discontinuation of ISOPTIN (verapamil HCl), the patient should be monitored to avoid underdigitalization.

Antihypertensive Agents: Verapamil administered concomitantly with oral antihypertensive agents (e.g., vasodilators, diuretics) may have an additive effect on lowering blood pressure. Patients receiving these combinations should be appropriately monitored. In patients who have recently received drugs such as methyldopa, which attenuate alpha-adrenergic response, combined therapy of verapamil and propranolol should probably be avoided (severe hypotension may occur).

Disopyramide: Until data on possible interactions between verapamil and disopyramide phosphate are obtained, disopyramide should not be administered within 48 hours before or 24 hours after verapamil administration.

Quinidine: In a small number of patients with hypertrophic cardiomyopathy (IHSS), concomitant use of verapamil and quinidine resulted in significant hypotension. Until further data are obtained, combined therapy of verapamil and quinidine in patients with hypertrophic cardiomyopathy should probably be avoided.

Nitrates: Verapamil has been given concomitantly with short- and long-acting nitrates without any undesirable drug interactions. The pharmacologic profile of both drugs and the clinical experience suggest beneficial interactions.

Carcinogenesis, Mutagenesis, Impairment of Fertility: Adequate animal carcinogenicity studies have not been performed with verapamil. An 18 month toxicity study in rats, at a low multiple (6 fold) of the maximum recommended human dose, and not the maximum tolerated dose, did not suggest a tumorigenic potential. A two year carcinogenicity study will be carried out in rats.

Verapamil was not mutagenic in the Ames test in 5 test strains at 3 mg per plate, with or without metabolic activation.

Studies in female rats at daily dietary doses up to 5.5 times (55 mg/kg/day) the maximum recommended human dose did not show impaired fertility. Effects on male fertility have not been determined.

Pregnancy: Pregnancy Category C. Reproduction studies have been performed in rabbits and rats at oral doses up to 1.5 (15 mg/kg/day) and 6 (60 mg/kg/day) times the human oral daily dose, respectively, and have revealed no evidence of teratogenicity. In the rat, however, this multiple of the human dose was embryocidal and retarded fetal growth and development, probably because of adverse maternal effects reflected in reduced weight gains of the dams. This oral dose has also been shown to cause hypotension in rats. There are no adequate and well-controlled studies in pregnant women. Because animal reproduction studies are not always predictive of human response, this drug should be used during pregnancy only if clearly needed.

Labor and Delivery: It is not known whether the use of verapamil during labor or delivery has immediate or delayed adverse effects on the fetus, or whether it prolongs the duration of labor or increases the need for forceps delivery or other obstetric intervention. Such adverse experiences have not been reported in the literature, despite a long history of use of ISOPTIN in Europe in the treatment of cardiac side effects of beta-adrenergic agonist agents used to treat premature labor.

Nursing Mothers: It is not known whether this drug is excreted in human milk. Because many drugs are excreted in human milk and because of the potential for adverse reactions in nursing infants from verapamil, nursing should be discontinued while verapamil is administered. Studies in rats at 2.5 times the maximum recommended human dose revealed no evidence of an effect of verapamil on lactation or weaning.

Animal Pharmacology and/or Animal Toxicology: Chronic animal toxicology studies indicate that verapamil causes lenticular and/or suture line changes at 30 mg/kg/day or greater and frank cataracts at 62.5 mg/kg/day or greater in the beagle dog but not the rat. These effects are thought to be species-specific. Development of cataracts due to verapamil has not been reported in man.

Adverse Reactions: Serious adverse reactions are rare when ISOPTIN therapy is initiated with upward dose titration within the recommended single and total daily dose. The following reactions to orally administered ISOPTIN were reported from clinical experience in 1166 patients with angina or arrhythmia. Adverse reactions occurred at a similar rate in controlled clinical trials and uncontrolled clinical experience.

Cardiovascular: Hypotension (2.9%), peripheral edema (1.7%), AV block (third-degree)(0.8%), bradycardia (HR <50/min, 1.1%), congestive heart failure or pulmonary edema (0.9%).

Central Nervous System: Dizziness (3.6%), headache (1.8%), fatigue (1.1%).

Gastrointestinal: Constipation (6.3%), nausea (1.6%). Elevations of liver enzymes have been reported (see **Warnings**).

The following reactions, reported in less than 0.5%, occurred under circumstances where a causal relationship is uncertain and are therefore mentioned to alert the physician to a possible relationship: ecchymosis, bruising, gynecomastia, psychotic symptoms, confusion, paresthesia, insomnia, somnolence, equilibrium disorder, blurred vision, syncope, muscle cramp, shakiness, claudication, hair loss, macules, spotty menstruation. In addition, more serious adverse events were observed, not readily distinguishable from the natural history of the disease in these patients. Of the 1166 patients evaluated 16 (1.4%) had myocardial infarctions. Nine of these 16 patients had myocardial infarctions while being treated for unstable angina, 4 of these were receiving placebo, the remaining 5 received verapamil.

The daily dose of verapamil was reduced in 6.3% and discontinued in 5.5% of the 1166 patients. In general, the highest incidence of adverse reactions was seen in the dose titration periods in all the studies.

Treatment of Acute Cardiovascular Adverse Reactions: The frequency of cardiovascular adverse reactions which require therapy is rare; hence, experience with their treatment is limited. Whenever severe hypotension or complete AV block occur following oral administration of verapamil, the appropriate emergency measures should be applied immediately, e.g., intravenously administered isoproterenol HCl, levarterenol bitartrate, atropine (all in the usual doses), or calcium gluconate (10% solution). In patients with hypertrophic cardiomyopathy (IHSS), alpha-adrenergic agents (phenylephrine, metaraminol bitartrate or methoxamine) should be used to maintain blood pressure and isoproterenol and levarterenol should be avoided. If further support is necessary, inotropic agents (dopamine or dobutamine) may be administered. Actual treatment and dosage should depend on the severity of the clinical situation and the judgment and experience of the treating physician.

Overdosage: Treatment of overdosage should be supportive. Beta-adrenergic stimulation or parenteral administration of calcium solutions may increase calcium ion flux across the slow channel, and have been used effectively in treatment of deliberate overdosage with verapamil. Clinically significant hypotensive reactions or fixed high degree AV block should be treated with vasopressor agents or cardiac pacing, respectively. Asystole should be handled by the usual measures including cardiopulmonary resuscitation.

Dosage and Administration: The dose of verapamil must be individualized by titration. ISOPTIN is available in 80 mg and 120 mg scored tablets. The usual initial dose is 80 mg three or four times a day. Dosage may be increased at daily (e.g., patients with unstable angina) or weekly intervals until optimum clinical response is obtained. In general, maximum effects of any given dosage would be apparent during the first 24 to 48 hours of therapy, but note that between 24 to 48 hours the half-life of verapamil increases, hence maximum response may be delayed. The total daily dose for most patients ranges from 320 to 480 mg. The usefulness and safety of dosages exceeding 480 mg per day in angina pectoris have not been established.

How Supplied: ISOPTIN tablets are supplied as round, scored, film-coated tablets containing either 80 mg or 120 mg of verapamil hydrochloride and embossed with "ISOPTIN 80" or "ISOPTIN 120" on one side and with "Knoll" on the reverse side.

80 mg (yellow)—
    Bottle of 100—NDC #0044-1822-02
    Bottle of 500—NDC #0044-1822-05
    Bottle of 1000—NDC #0044-1822-04
    Hospital Unit Dose (100 tablets—
    Strips of 10)—NDC #0044-1822-10
120 mg (white)—
    Bottle of 100—NDC #0044-1823-02
    Bottle of 500—NDC #0044-1823-05
    Bottle of 1000—NDC #0044-1823-04
    Hospital Unit Dose (100 tablets—
    Strips of 10)—NDC #0044-1823-10

Storage: 15° to 30°C, 59° to 86°F.

Shown in Product Identification Section, page 414

QUADRINAL™ Tablets and Suspension   ℞

Description: Each QUADRINAL™ Tablet contains ephedrine hydrochloride 24 mg; phenobarbital 24 mg [**Warning:** May be habit forming]; theophylline calcium salicylate 130 mg (equivalent to 65 mg anhydrous theophylline); potassium iodide

Continued on next page

Knoll—Cont.

320 mg. Each 5 ml (1 teaspoonful) of the fruit-flavored Suspension is equivalent to ½ tablet.

QUADRINAL contains two bronchodilators, theophylline and ephedrine. Phenobarbital serves as a mild sedative to help counteract central nervous system stimulation which may be caused by ephedrine. Wheezing and coughing are relieved by improved bronchodilation while the expectorant action of potassium iodide helps to remove secretions from the bronchial tree. Dyspnea is thus relieved or prevented and acute episodes of bronchospasm are often eliminated with consequent lessening of apprehension and distress.

Clinical Pharmacology: Theophylline directly relaxes the smooth muscle of the bronchial airways and pulmonary blood vessels, thus acting mainly as a bronchodilator, pulmonary vasodilator and smooth muscle relaxant. It also possesses other actions typical of the xanthine derivatives: coronary vasodilator, diuretic, and cardiac, cerebral, and skeletal muscle stimulant. The actions of theophylline may be mediated through inhibition of phosphodiesterase and a resultant increase in intracellular cyclic AMP which could mediate smooth muscle relaxation.

In vitro, theophylline has been shown to react synergistically with beta agonists (such as isoproterenol) that increase intracellular cyclic AMP through the stimulation of adenyl cyclase, but synergism has not been demonstrated in clinical studies and more data are needed to determine if theophylline and beta agonists have clinically important additive effects **in vivo.**

Apparently, tolerance does not develop with chronic use of theophylline.

The half-life is shortened with cigarette smoking. The half-life is prolonged in alcoholism, reduced hepatic or renal function, congestive heart failure, and in patients receiving cimetidine or antibiotics such as troleandomycin (TAO, Cyclamycin), erythromycin, lincomycin and clindamycin. High fever for prolonged periods may decrease theophylline elimination.

Theophylline Elimination Characteristics

	Theophylline Clearance Rates (mean ± S.D.)	Half-life Average (mean ± S.D.)
Children (over 6 months of age)	1.45 ± 0.58 ml/kg/min	3.7 ± 1.1 hrs.
Adult non-smokers with uncomplicated asthma	0.65 ± 0.19 ml/kg/min	8.7 ± 2.2 hrs.

Newborn infants have extremely slow clearances with half-lives exceeding 24 hours. These approach those seen for older children after about 3-6 months.

Older adults with chronic obstructive pulmonary disease, patients with cor pulmonale or other causes of heart failure, and patients with liver pathology may have much lower clearances with half-lives that may exceed 24 hours. The half-life is prolonged in alcoholism, reduced hepatic or renal function, congestive heart failure, and in patients receiving cimetidine or antibiotics such as troleandomycin (TAO, Cyclamycin), erythromycin, lincomycin and clindamycin. High fever for prolonged periods may decrease theophylline elimination.

The half-life of theophylline in smokers (1 to 2 packs/day) averaged 4 to 5 hours in various studies, much shorter than the 7 to 9 hour half-life in nonsmokers. The increase in theophylline clearance caused by smoking is probably the result of induction of drug-metabolizing enzymes that do not readily normalize after cessation of smoking. It appears that between 3 months and 2 years may be necessary for normalization of the effect of smoking on theophylline pharmacokinetics.

Indications: For chronic respiratory disease in which tenacious mucus and bronchospasm are dominant symptoms, such as bronchial asthma, chronic bronchitis and pulmonary emphysema.

Contraindications: Use of QUADRINAL is contraindicated in patients with enlarged thyroid or goiter or with known sensitivity to theophylline, potassium iodide, ephedrine or sympathomimetics, or barbiturates.

The iodide in QUADRINAL can cause fetal harm when administered to a pregnant woman. Development of goiter has been reported in infants whose mothers received iodide-containing medications during pregnancy. A few neonatal deaths resulting from tracheal obstruction due to congenital goiters have been reported. Use of barbiturates during pregnancy may cause physical dependence with resulting withdrawal symptoms in the neonate; may cause birth defects; may be associated with neonatal hemorrhage due to reduction in levels of vitamin K-dependent clotting factors in the neonate; may cause respiratory depression in the neonate.

QUADRINAL is contraindicated in women who are or may become pregnant. If this drug is used during pregnancy, or if the patient becomes pregnant while taking this drug, the patient should be apprised of the potential hazard to the fetus.

Warnings: Excessive theophylline doses may be associated with toxicity; determination of serum theophylline levels is recommended to assure maximal benefit without excessive risk. Incidence of toxicity increases at serum levels greater than 20 mcg/ml. Because of the theophylline content of QUADRINAL, it is unlikely that toxic levels of theophylline would be reached unless a serious overdosage occurs.

Morphine, curare, and stilbamidine should be used with caution in patients with airflow obstruction since they stimulate histamine release and can induce asthmatic attacks. They may also suppress respiration leading to respiratory failure. Alternative drugs should be chosen whenever possible.

There is an excellent correlation between clinical manifestations of toxicity and high blood levels of theophylline resulting from conventional doses in patients with lowered body plasma clearances (due to transient cardiac decompensation), patients with liver dysfunction or chronic obstructive lung disease, and patients who are older than 55 years of age, particularly males. In about 50% of patients, nausea and restlessness precede more severe manifestations of toxicity. In other patients, ventricular arrhythmias or seizures may be the first signs of toxicity. These more serious side effects are more likely to occur after intravenous administration of theophylline. Many patients who have high theophylline serum levels exhibit a tachycardia, and theophylline may worsen pre-existing arrhythmias.

Precautions: Mean half-life in smokers is shorter than in nonsmokers; therefore, smokers may require larger doses of theophylline. QUADRINAL, like all theophylline products, should not be administered concurrently with other xanthine medications. Use with caution in patients with severe cardiac disease, severe hypoxemia, hypertension, hyperthyroidism, acute myocardial injury, cor pulmonale, congestive heart failure, liver disease, peptic ulcer and in the elderly (especially males) and in neonates. Great caution should be used especially in giving theophylline to patients in congestive heart failure; such patients have shown markedly prolonged theophylline blood level curves with theophylline persisting in serum for long periods following discontinuation of the drug.

Theophylline may occasionally act as a local irritant to the G.I. tract although gastrointestinal symptoms are more commonly central in origin and associated with serum concentrations over 20 mcg/ml.

Ephedrine-containing medications should be used with caution in patients with cardiovascular disease, diabetes mellitus, predisposition to glaucoma, hypertension, hyperthyroidism, or prostatic hypertrophy.

Potassium iodide may aggravate acne in adolescents and adults.

Phenobarbital should be used with caution in patients with a history of drug abuse or dependence, impaired renal or hepatic function, hyperkinesis, uncontrolled pain, or history of porphyria.

Usage in Pregnancy: Pregnancy Category X. See "Contraindications" section.

Nursing Mothers: Because of the potential for serious adverse reactions in nursing infants from the potassium iodide, ephedrine and phenobarbital in QUADRINAL, a decision should be made whether to discontinue nursing or to discontinue the drug, taking into account the importance of the drug to the mother.

Pediatric Use: QUADRINAL is indicated for use in children on a short term basis. Chronic use should be reserved for patients in whom other expectorants have not been effective. If QUADRINAL is used chronically in children, the patient should be observed for signs of thyroid enlargement and worsening of acne.

Geriatric Patients: Geriatric patients may be more sensitive to the effects of ephedrine.

Adverse Reactions: The most frequent adverse reactions to theophylline are usually due to overdose (serum levels in excess of 20 mcg/ml) and are: nausea, vomiting, epigastric pain, hematemesis, diarrhea, headaches, irritability, restlessness, insomnia, reflex hyperexcitability, muscle twitching, clonic and tonic generalized convulsions, palpitations, tachycardia, extra systoles, flushing, hypotension, circulatory failure, ventricular arrhythmias, tachypnea, albuminuria, increased excretion of renal tubular cells and red blood cells, potentiation of diuresis, hyperglycemia and inappropriate ADH syndrome.

Thyroid adenoma, goiter and myxedema are possible side effects of potassium iodide.

Hypersensitivity to iodides may be manifested by angio-neurotic edema, cutaneous and mucosal hemorrhages, and symptoms resembling serum sickness, such as fever, arthralgia, lymph node enlargement and eosinophilia.

Chronic ingestion of iodides may result in chronic iodide poisoning, or iodism. Initial symptoms include an unpleasant brassy taste, burning in the mouth and throat, soreness of the teeth and gums, increased salivation, coryza, sneezing, irritation of the eyes with swelling of the eyelids, headache, cough, skin lesions, diarrhea, gastric irritation, anorexia, fever and depression. The symptoms of iodism disappear spontaneously within a few days after stopping the administration of iodide. Therefore, treatment consists of stopping QUADRINAL therapy and providing supportive measures as indicated by the symptoms. Abundant fluid and sodium chloride intake may hasten iodide elimination. In severe cases, the use of mannitol to establish an osmotic diuresis may be appropriate. Potassium iodide may produce hyperkalemia and, if ingested chronically, may lead to goiter.

Adverse reactions to ephedrine include nervousness, restlessness, trouble in sleeping, irregular heartbeat, difficult or painful urination, dizziness or light-headedness, headache, loss of appetite, nausea or vomiting, trembling, troubled breathing, unusual increase in sweating, unusual paleness, feeling of warmth, and weakness. Tolerance to ephedrine may develop with prolonged or excessive use.

Adverse reactions to phenobarbital include mental confusion or depression, shortness of breath or troubled breathing, skin rash, hives, swelling of eyelids, face or lips, wheezing or tightness in chest, sore throat and fever, unusual bleeding or bruising, unusual excitement, tiredness or weakness, unusually slow heartbeat, yellowing of eyes or skin.

Drug Interactions: Toxic synergism of theophylline with ephedrine has been documented and may occur with some other sympathomimetic bronchodilators.

[See table on next page].

Overdosage:

A. If potential overdose is established and seizure has not occurred and patient is conscious:
  1) Induce vomiting.
  2) Administer a cathartic.
  3) Administer activated charcoal.

B. If patient is having a seizure:
  1) Establish an airway.

2) Administer oxygen.
3) Treat the seizure with intravenous diazepam, 0.1 to 0.3 mg/kg up to 10 mg.
4) Monitor vital signs, maintain blood pressure and provide adequate hydration.

C. Post-seizure coma:
1) Maintain airway and oxygenation.
2) Following above recommendations to prevent absorption of drug, but intubation and lavage will have to be performed instead of inducing emesis, and introduce the cathartic and charcoal via a large bore gastric lavage tube.
3) Continue to provide full supportive care and adequate hydration while waiting for drug to be metabolized. In general, the drug is metabolized sufficiently rapidly so as not to require dialysis.

Dosage and Administration: When rapidly absorbed products such as solutions and uncoated tablets with rapid dissolution are used, dosing to maintain "around the clock" blood levels generally requires administration every 6 hours in children; dosing intervals up to 8 hours may be satisfactory for adults because of their slower elimination rate.

Pulmonary function measurements before and after a period of treatment permit an objective assessment of response to QUADRINAL.

Usual dose:
Adults—One tablet or two teaspoonfuls (10 ml) of the Suspension 3 or 4 times daily; if needed, an additional one tablet or two teaspoonfuls upon retiring for nighttime relief. In severe attacks, the usual dose may be increased by one half.
Children 6 to 12 years—one half tablet, or one teaspoonful (5 ml) of the Suspension three times daily.
Children under 6 years—dose is proportionately less.

How Supplied: QUADRINAL Tablets— white, round, bi-convex tablets, engraved with a triangle on one side, bisected on the other side and imprinted with the number "14".
Bottles of 100—NDC #0044-4520-02.
Bottles of 1000—NDC #0044-4520-04.
QUADRINAL Suspension—Reddish-pink in color, fruit-like flavor.
Bottles of 1 pint (473 ml)—NDC #0044-4580-01.
Storage: Store at 59°–86°F, 15°–30°C.
Shown in Product Identification Section, page 414

SANTYL® Ointment (collagenase) ℞

Description: SANTYL® OINTMENT is a sterile enzymatic debriding ointment which contains 250 collagenase units per gram of white petrolatum USP. The enzyme collagenase is derived from the fermentation by *Clostridium histolyticum*. It possesses the unique ability to digest native and denatured collagen in necrotic tissue.

Clinical Pharmacology: Since collagen accounts for 75% of the dry weight of skin tissue, the ability of collagenase to digest collagen in the physiological pH range and temperature makes it particularly effective in the removal of detritus.[1] Collagenase thus contributes towards the formation of granulation tissue and subsequent epithelization of dermal ulcers and severely burned areas.[2,3,4,5,6] Collagen in healthy tissue or in newly formed granulation tissue is not attacked.[2,3,4,5,6,7,8]

Indications: Santyl Ointment is indicated for debriding chronic dermal ulcers[2,3,4,5,6,8,9,10,11,12,13,14,15,16,17,18] and severely burned areas.[3,4,5,7,16,19,20,21]

Contraindications: Santyl Ointment is contraindicated in patients who have shown local or systemic hypersensitivity to collagenase.

Precautions: The optimal pH range of collagenase is 6 to 8. Higher or lower pH conditions will decrease the enzyme's activity and appropriate precautions should be taken. The enzymatic activity is also adversely affected by detergents, hexachlorophene and heavy metal ions such as mercury and silver which are used in some antiseptics. When it is suspected such materials have been used, the site should be carefully cleansed by repeated washings with normal saline before Santyl Ointment is applied. Soaks containing metal ions or acidic solutions such as Burow's solution should be avoided because of the metal ion and low pH. Cleansing materials such as hydrogen peroxide, Dakin's solution, and sterile saline are compatible with Santyl Ointment.

Debilitated patients should be closely monitored for systemic bacterial infections because of the theoretical possibility that debriding enzymes may increase the risk of bacteremia.

A slight transient erythema has been noted occasionally in the surrounding tissue, particularly when Santyl Ointment was not confined to the lesion. Therefore, the ointment should be applied carefully within the area of the lesion.

Adverse Reactions: No allergic sensitivity or toxic reactions have been noted in the recorded clinical investigations. However, one case of systemic manifestations of hypersensitivity to collagenase in a patient treated for more than one year with a combination of collagenase and cortisone has been reported to us.

Overdosage: Action of the enzyme may be stopped, should this be desired, by the application of Burow's solution USP (pH 3.6–4.4) to the lesion.

Dosage and Administration: Santyl Ointment should be applied once daily (or more frequently if the dressing becomes soiled, as from incontinence) in the following manner:
(1) Prior to application the lesion should be cleansed of debris and digested material by gently rubbing with a gauze pad saturated with hydrogen peroxide or Dakin's solution followed by sterile normal saline.
(2) Whenever infection is present it is desirable to use an appropriate topical antibacterial agent. Neomycin-Bacitracin-Polymyxin B (Neosporin) powder has been found to be compatible with Santyl Ointment. The antibiotic should be applied to the lesion prior to the application of Santyl Ointment. Should the infection not respond, therapy with Santyl Ointment should be discontinued until remission of the infection.
(3) Santyl Ointment should be applied directly to deep lesions with a wooden tongue depressor or spatula. For shallow lesions, Santyl Ointment may be applied to a sterile gauze pad which is then applied to the wound and properly secured.
(4) Crosshatching thick eschar with a #10 blade allows collagenase more surface contact with necrotic debris. It is also desirable to remove, with forceps and scissors, as much loosened detritus as can be done readily.
(5) All excess ointment should be removed each time dressing is changed.
(6) Use of Santyl Ointment should be terminated when debridement of necrotic tissue is complete and granulation tissue is well established.

How Supplied: Santyl Ointment contains 250 units of collagenase enzyme per gram of white petrolatum USP. The potency assay of collagenase is based on the digestion of undenatured collagen (from bovine Achilles tendon) at pH 7.2 and 37°C for 24 hours. The number of peptide bonds cleaved are measured by reaction with ninhydrin. Amino groups released by a trypsin digestion control are subtracted. One net collagenase unit will solubilize ninhydrin reactive material equivalent to 4 micromoles of leucine.

References:
1— Mandl, I., Adv. Enzymol. 23:163, 1961.
2— Boxer, A.M., Gottesman, N., Bernstein, H., & Mandl, I., Geriatrics 24:75, 1969.
3— Mazurek, I., Med. Welt 22:150, 1971.
4— Zimmerman, W.E., in "Collagenase," I. Mandl, ed., Gordon & Breach, Science Publishers, New York, 1971, p. 131, p. 185.
5— Vetra, H., & Whittaker, D., Geriatrics 30:53, 1975.
6— Rao, D.B., Sane, P.G., & Georgiev, E.L., J. Am. Geriatrics Soc. 23:22, 1975.
7— Vrabec, R., Moserova, J., Konickova, Z., Behounkova, E., & Blaha, J., J. Hyg.

Continued on next page

Drug	Effect
Aminophylline with lithium carbonate	Increased excretion of lithium carbonate
Potassium iodide with lithium	Increased hypothyroid and goiterogenic effects
Aminophylline with propranolol	Antagonism of propranolol effect
Theophylline with furosemide	Increased diuresis
Theophylline with hexamethonium	Decreased hexamethonium-induced chronotropic effect
Theophylline with reserpine	Reserpine-induced tachycardia
Theophylline with chlordiazepoxide	Chlordiazepoxide-induced fatty acid mobilization
Theophylline with troleandomycin (TAO, Cyclamycin), erythromycin, lincomycin, clindamycin	Increased theophylline plasma levels
Theophylline with phenytoin	Decreased phenytoin levels
Theophylline with cimetidine	Increased theophylline blood levels
Ephedrine with digitalis glycosides or anesthetics	May cause cardiac arrhythmias
Ephedrine with ergonovine, methylergonovine or oxytocin	Hypertension
Ephedrine with guanethidine	Decreased hypotensive effect
Ephedrine with MAO inhibitors	Potentiation of pressor effect of ephedrine
Ephedrine with reserpine	Decreased pressor effect of ephedrine
Ephedrine with other sympathomimetics	Increased effects of either medication
Ephedrine with tricyclic antidepressants	May antagonize the pressor action of ephedrine
Phenobarbital with alcohol, general anesthetics, other CNS depressants, or MAO inhibitors	Increased effects of either medication
Phenobarbital with oral anticoagulants	Decreased anticoagulant effects
Phenobarbital with corticosteroids, digitalis, digitoxin, doxycycline, tricyclic antidepressants, griseofulvin or phenytoin	Decreased effects of these drugs

Knoll—Cont.

Epidemiol. Microbiol. Immunol. 18:496, 1974.
8— Lippmann, H.I., Arch. Phys. Med. Rehabil. 54:588, 1973.
9— German, F.M., in "Collagenase," I. Mandl, ed. Gordon & Breach, Science Publishers, New York, 1971, p. 165.
10— Haimovici, H. & Strauch, B., in "Collagenase," I. Mandl, ed., Gordon & Breach, Science Publishers, New York, 1971, p. 177.
11— Lee, L.K., & Ambrus, J.L., Geriatrics 30:91, 1975.
12— Locke, R.K., & Heifitz, N.M., J. Am. Pod. Assoc. 65:242, 1975.
13— Varma, A.O., Bugatch, E., & German, F.M., Surg. Gynecol. Obstet. 136:281, 1973.
14— Barrett, D., Jr., & Klibanski, A., Am. J. Nurs. 73:849, 1973.
15— Bardfeld, L.A., J. Pod. Ed. 1:41, 1970.
16— Blum, G., Schweiz. Rundschau Med. Praxis 62:820, 1973. Abstr. in Dermatology Digest, Feb. 1974, p. 36.
17— Zaruba, F., Lettl, A., Brozkova, L., Skrdlantova, H., & Krs, V., J. Hyg. Epidemiol. Microbiol. Immunol. 18:499, 1974.
18— Altman, M.I., Goldstein, L., Horowitz, S., J. Am. Pod. Assoc. 68:11, 1978.
19— Rehn, V.J., Med. Klin. 58:799, 1963.
20— Krauss, H., Koslowski, L., & Zimmermann, W.E., Langenbecks Arch. Klin. Chir. 303:23, 1963.
21— Gruenagel, H.H., Med. Klin. 58:442, 1963.

Shown in Product Identification Section, page 414

VICODIN® TABLETS

Description: Each VICODIN® tablet contains:
hydrocodone bitartrate .... 5 mg
 (**WARNING:** May be habit forming.)
acetaminophen .... 500 mg
Hydrocodone bitartrate is an opioid analgesic and antitussive and occurs as fine, white crystals or as a crystalline powder. It is affected by light. The structural formula of hydrocodone bitartrate is:

Acetaminophen is a nonopiate, nonsalicylate analgesic and antipyretic which occurs as a white, odorless, crystalline powder possessing a slightly bitter taste. It may be represented by the following structural formula:

Clinical Pharmacology: Hydrocodone is a semisynthetic narcotic analgesic and antitussive with multiple actions qualitatively similar to those of codeine. Most of these involve the central nervous system and smooth muscle. The precise mechanism of action of hydrocodone and other opiates is not known, although it is believed to relate to the existence of opiate receptors in the central nervous system. In addition to analgesia, narcotics may produce drowsiness, changes in mood and mental clouding.
Radioimmunoassay techniques have recently been developed for the analysis of hydrocodone in human plasma. After a 10 mg oral dose of hydrocodone bitartrate, a mean peak serum drug level of 23.6 ng/ml and an elimination half-life of 3.8 hours were found.
The analgesic action of acetaminophen involves peripheral and central influences, but the specific mechanism is as yet undetermined. Antipyretic activity is mediated through hypothalamic heat regulating centers. Acetaminophen inhibits prostaglandin synthetase. Therapeutic doses of acetaminophen have negligible effects on the cardiovascular or respiratory systems; however, toxic doses may cause circulatory failure and rapid, shallow breathing. Acetaminophen is rapidly and almost completely absorbed from the gastrointestinal tract, producing maximum serum concentrations within 30 minutes to one hour. The plasma half-life in adults and children ranges from 0.90 hours to 3.25 hours with an average of approximately 2 hours. The drug distributes uniformly in most body fluids and is approximately 25% protein bound. Acetaminophen is conjugated in the liver, with less than 3% of the dose excreted unchanged in 24 hours. The primary metabolic pathway is conjugation to sulfate and glucuronide by-products. A minor oxidative pathway forms cysteine and mercapturic acid. These compounds are subsequently excreted by the kidneys into the urine.

Indications and Usage: For the relief of moderate to moderately severe pain.

Contraindications: Hypersensitivity to acetaminophen or hydrocodone.

Warnings

Respiratory Depression: At high doses or in sensitive patients, hydrocodone may produce dose-related respiratory depression by acting directly on brain stem respiratory centers. Hydrocodone also affects centers that control respiratory rhythm, and may produce irregular and periodic breathing. If significant respiratory depression occurs, it may be antagonized by the use of naloxone hydrochloride, 0.005 mg/kg intravenously. Since the duration of action of hydrocodone may exceed that of the antagonist, the patient should be kept under continued surveillance and repeated doses of the antagonist should be administered as needed to maintain adequate respiration. Apply other supportive measures when indicated.

Head Injury and Increased Intracranial Pressure: The respiratory depressant effects of narcotics and their capacity to elevate cerebrospinal fluid pressure may be markedly exaggerated in the presence of head injury, other intracranial lesions or a preexisting increase in intracranial pressure. Furthermore, narcotics produce adverse reactions which may obscure the clinical course of patients with head injuries.

Acute Abdominal Conditions: The administration of narcotics may obscure the diagnosis or clinical course of patients with acute abdominal conditions.

Precautions

Special Risk Patients: As with any narcotic analgesic agent, VICODIN should be used with caution in elderly or debilitated patients and those with severe impairment of hepatic or renal function, hypothyroidism, Addison's disease, prostatic hypertrophy or urethral stricture. The usual precautions should be observed and the possibility of respiratory depression should be kept in mind.

Information for Patients: VICODIN, like all narcotics, may impair the mental and/or physical abilities required for the performance of potentially hazardous tasks such as driving a car or operating machinery; patients should be cautioned accordingly.

Cough Reflex: Hydrocodone suppresses the cough reflex; as with all narcotics, caution should be exercised when VICODIN is used postoperatively and in patients with pulmonary disease.

Drug Interactions: Patients receiving other narcotic analgesics, antipsychotics, antianxiety agents, or other CNS depressants (including alcohol) concomitantly with VICODIN may exhibit an additive CNS depression. When combined therapy is contemplated, the dose of one or both agents should be reduced.
The use of MAO inhibitors or tricyclic antidepressants with hydrocodone preparations may increase the effect of either the antidepressant or hydrocodone.
The concurrent use of anticholinergics with hydrocodone may produce paralytic ileus.

Usage in Pregnancy: Pregnancy Category C. Hydrocodone has been shown to be teratogenic in hamsters when given in doses 700 times the human dose. There are no adequate and well-controlled studies in pregnant women. VICODIN should be used during pregnancy only if the potential benefit justifies the potential risk to the fetus.

Nonteratogenic effects: Babies born to mothers who have been taking opioids regularly prior to delivery will be physically dependent. The withdrawal signs include irritability and excessive crying, tremors, hyperactive reflexes, increased respiratory rate, increased stools, sneezing, yawning, vomiting, and fever. The intensity of the syndrome does not always correlate with the duration of maternal opioid use or dose. There is no consensus on the best method of managing withdrawal. Chlorpromazine 0.7 to 1.0 mg/kg q6h, and paregoric 2 to 4 drops/kg q4h, have been used to treat withdrawal symptoms in infants. The duration of therapy is 4 to 28 days, with the dosage decreased as tolerated.

Labor and Delivery: As with all narcotics, administration of VICODIN to the mother shortly before delivery may result in some degree of respiratory depression in the newborn, especially if higher doses are used.

Nursing Mothers: It is not known whether this drug is excreted in human milk. Because many drugs are excreted in human milk and because of the potential for serious adverse reactions in nursing infants from VICODIN, a decision should be made whether to discontinue nursing or to discontinue the drug, taking into account the importance of the drug to the mother.

Pediatric Use: Safety and effectiveness in children have not been established.

Adverse Reactions

Central Nervous System: Sedation, drowsiness, mental clouding, lethargy, impairment of mental and physical performance, anxiety, fear, dysphoria, dizziness, psychic dependence, mood changes.

Gastrointestinal System: Nausea and vomiting may occur; they are more frequent in ambulatory than in recumbent patients. The antiemetic phenothiazines are useful in suppressing these effects; however, some phenothiazine derivatives seem to be antianalgesic and to increase the amount of narcotic required to produce pain relief, while other phenothiazines reduce the amount of narcotic required to produce a given level of analgesia. Prolonged administration of VICODIN may produce constipation.

Genitourinary System: Ureteral spasm, spasm of vesical sphincters and urinary retention have been reported.

Respiratory Depression: VICODIN may produce dose-related respiratory depression by acting directly on brain stem respiratory centers. Hydrocodone also affects centers that control respiratory rhythm, and may produce irregular and periodic breathing. If significant respiratory depression occurs, it may be antagonized by the use of naloxone hydrochloride, 0.005 mg/kg intravenously. Since the duration of action of hydrocodone may exceed that of the antagonist, the patient should be kept under continued surveillance and repeated doses of the antagonist should be administered as needed to maintain adequate respiration. Apply other supportive measures when indicated.

Drug Abuse and Dependence: VICODIN is subject to the Federal Controlled Substances Act (Schedule ⓒ).
Psychic dependence, physical dependence, and tolerance may develop upon repeated administration of narcotics; therefore, VICODIN should be prescribed and administered with caution. However, psychic dependence is unlikely to develop when VICODIN is used for a short time for the treatment of pain. Physical dependence, the condition in which continued administration of the drug is required to prevent the appearance of a withdrawal syndrome, assumes clinically significant proportions only after several weeks of continued narcotic use, although some mild degree of physical dependence may develop after a few days of narcotic therapy. Tolerance, in which increasingly large doses are required in order to produce the same degree of analgesia, is manifested initially by a shortened duration of analgesic effect, and subse-

quently by decreases in the intensity of analgesia. The rate of development of tolerance varies among patients.

Overdosage
Hydrocodone
Signs and Symptoms: Serious overdose with hydrocodone is characterized by respiratory depression (a decrease in respiratory rate and/or tidal volume, Cheyne-Stokes respiration, cyanosis), extreme somnolence progressing to stupor or coma, skeletal muscle flaccidity, cold and clammy skin, and sometimes bradycardia and hypotension. In severe overdosage, apnea, circulatory collapse, cardiac arrest and death may occur.

Treatment: Primary attention should be given to the reestablishment of adequate respiratory exchange through provision of a patent airway and the institution of assisted or controlled ventilation. The narcotic antagonist naloxone is a specific antidote against respiratory depression which may result from overdosage or unusual sensitivity to narcotics, including hydrocodone. Therefore, 0.005 mg/kg of naloxone should be administered, preferably by the intravenous route, and simultaneously with efforts at respiratory resuscitation. Since the duration of action of hydrocodone may exceed that of the antagonist, the patient should be kept under continued surveillance and repeated doses of the antagonist should be administered as needed to maintain adequate respiration.

An antagonist should not be administered in the absence of clinically significant respiratory or cardiovascular depression. Oxygen, intravenous fluids, vasopressors and other supportive measures should be employed as indicated.

Gastric emptying may be useful in removing unabsorbed drug.

Acetaminophen
Signs and Symptoms: Acetaminophen in massive overdosage may cause hepatic toxicity in some patients. In all cases of suspected overdose, immediately call your Regional Poison Center or the Rocky Mountain Poison Center's toll free number (800/525-6115) for assistance in diagnosis and for directions in the use of N-acetylcysteine as an antidote, a use currently restricted to investigational status.

In adults, hepatic toxicity has rarely been reported with acute overdoses of less than 10 grams and fatalities with less than 15 grams. Importantly, young children seem to be more resistant than adults to the hepatotoxic effect of an acetaminophen overdose. Despite this, the measures outlined below should be initiated in any adult or child suspected of having ingested an acetaminophen overdose.

Early symptoms following a potentially hepatotoxic overdose may include: nausea, vomiting, diaphoresis and general malaise. Clinical and laboratory evidence of hepatic toxicity may not be apparent until 48 to 72 hours post-ingestion.

Treatment: The stomach should be emptied promptly by lavage or by induction of emesis with syrup of ipecac. Patients' estimates of the quantity of a drug ingested are notoriously unreliable. Therefore, if an acetaminophen overdose is suspected, a serum acetaminophen assay should be obtained as early as possible, but no sooner than four hours following ingestion. Liver function studies should be obtained initially and repeated at 24-hour intervals.

The antidote, N-acetylcysteine, should be administered as early as possible, and within 16 hours of the overdose ingestion for optimal results. Following recovery, there are no residual, structural or functional hepatic abnormalities.

Dosage and Administration: Dosage should be adjusted according to the severity of the pain and the response of the patient. However, tolerance to hydrocodone can develop with continued use and the incidence of untoward effects is dose related. The usual dose is one tablet every six hours as needed for pain. If necessary, this dose may be repeated at four hour intervals. In cases of more severe pain, two tablets every six hours (up to 8 tablets in 24 hours) may be required.

How Supplied: White, flat, capsule shaped, bisected tablets inscribed with a double K logo on one side and the number "24" on the other side. Bottles of 100—NDC #0044-0727-02.
Hospital Unit Dose Package—100 tablets (4×25 tablets)—NDC #0044-0727-41.
Storage: VICODIN should be stored at 59°–86°F, 15°–30°C.
A Schedule Ⓒ Narcotic.
Shown in Product Identification Section, page 414

EDUCATIONAL MATERIAL

Continuing Education Booklets
"Calcium in Cardiac Metabolism" (3 credits)
  Home Study Module, $5.00 - Pharmacists
"Cardiac Arrhythmias" (2 credits)
  Home Study Module, $5.00 - Pharmacists
"Treatment of Cardiac Arrhythmias" (3 credits)
  Home Study Module, $5.00 - Pharmacists
"Angina Pectoris" (2 credits)
  Home Study Module, $5.00 - Pharmacists
"Management of Angina Pectoris" (3 credits)
  Home Study Module, $5.00 - Pharmacists

Kramer Pharmacal, Inc.
8778 S.W. 8TH STREET
MIAMI, FL 33174

BANQUIN™ ℞
[ban'kwin]
Skin Bleaching Cream

Composition: Hydroquinone 4% and Octyldimethyl PABA 3%.
Indications: For the g radual fading of discolorations in the skin such as: freckles, age and liver spots or pigmentations in the skin that may occur in pregnancy or from the use of oral contraceptives.
Warnings: Some users of this product may experience a mild skin irritation. If skin irritation becomes severe, stop its use and consult a physician. Avoid contact with eyes.
This product contains a sunscreen to help darkening from reoccurring. It is not, however, for use in the prevention of sunburn. Do not use on children under 12 years of age.
Adverse Reactions: No systemic adverse reactions have been reported. Occasional hypersensitivity (localized contact dermatitis) may occur in which cases the medications should be discontinued and the physician notified immediately.
Drug Dosage and Administration: Apply a small amount of Banquin as a thin layer on the affected area twice daily or as directed by physician. If no improvement is seen after three months of treatment, use of this product should be discontinued. Lightening effects of this product may not be noticeable on very dark skin.
Sun exposure should be limited by using a sunscreen agent, as in Banquin, sun blocking agent, or protective clothing to prevent darkening form recurring.
How Supplied: Banquin Skin Bleaching Cream is supplied in 1 ounce tubes. (NDC 52083-522-01)

FUNGI-NAIL™ ℞
[fun'gi-nāl]
Tineture

Composition: Resorcinol 1%; Salicylic Acid 2%; Parachlorometaxilenol 2%; Benzocaine 0.5%; Acetic Acid 2.5%; Propylene glycol, Hydroxypropylmethyl Cellulose, Alcohol 50%.
Indications: For topical treatment of ringworm infections of the nails tinea unguum (onychomycosis), and other fungus and bacterial infections of the skin.
Precautions: Avoid contact with eyes and mucous membranes. Do not use on broken skin or irritated areas.

Dosage and Administration: Apply to affected nails and other affected areas of the skin twice daily.
How Supplied: 1 oz. bottle with brush applicator. (NDC 52083-529-26)

OTIPYRIN™ OTIC SOLUTION ℞
[o"ti-pi'rin]

Composition: Each ml. contains: Antipyrine 54 mg; Benzocaine 14 mg; Glacial Acetic Acid 20 mg; Glycerin Anhydrous q.s. 1 ml. (Also contains Oxyquinoline Sulfate).
Clinical Pharmacology: OTIPYRIN Otic Solution combines the hygroscopic property of anhydrous glycerin with the analgesic action of antipyrine and benzocaine to relieve pressure, reduce inflammation and congestion, and to alleviate pain and discomfort in acute otitis media. OTIPYRIN Otic Solution also combines the bactericide and fungicide properties of the acetic acid. OTIPYRIN Otic Solution does not blanch the tympanic membrane or mask the landmarks and therefore, does not distort the otoscopic picture.
Indications and Usage: Acute otitis media of various etiologies.
—Prompt relief of pain and reduction of inflammation in the congestive serous stages.
—Adjuvant therapy during systemic antibiotic administration for resolution of the infection. Because of the close anatomical relationship of the eustachian tube to the nasal cavity, otitis media is a frequent problem, especially in children in whom the tube is shorter, wider and more horizontal than in adults.
—Removal of cerumen- Facilitates the removal of excessive or impacted cerumen.
Contraindications: Hypersensitivity to any of the components or substances related to them. In the presence of spontaneous perforation or discharge.
Precautions:
Carcinogenesis, Mutagenesis, Impairment of Fertility: No long term studies in animals or humans have been conducted.
Pregnancy Category C. Animal reproduction studies have not been conducted with Otipyrin Otic Solution. It is also not known whether this product can cause harm when administered to a pregnant woman, or can affect reproduction capacity. Therefore, this product should be given to a pregnant woman only if clearly needed.
Nursing Mothers: It is not known whether this drug is excreted in human milk; caution should be exercised when this product is administered to a nursing mother.
Dosage and Administration: Acute otitis media: Instill Otipyrin, permitting the solution to run along the wall of the canal until it is filled. Avoid touching the ear with the tip of the container. Then moisten a cotton pledget with the solution and insert into meatus. Repeat every one or two hours until pain and congestion are relieved.
Removal of Cerumen: Before: Instill Otipyrin Otic Solution three times daily for 2 or 3 days to help detach cerumen from wall of canal and facilitate removal. After: Otipyrin is useful in drying out the canal or relieving discomfort. Before and after removal of cerumen, a cotton pledget with the solution should be inserted into the meatus following instillation.
How Supplied: Otipyrin Otic Solution is supplied in 15 ml (½ fl. oz.) plastic squeeze bottle with otic tip (NDC 52083-021-15).

YOHIMEX™ Tablets ℞
[yō-him'eks]

Description: Yohimbine is an indoalkylamine alkaloid with chemical similarity to reserpine. It is a 3α-15α-20β-17α hydroxy Yohimbine-16α- carboxylic acid methylester. The alkaloid is found in Rubaceae and related trees and in Rauwolfia Serpentina(L) Benth.

Continued on next page

Kramer—Cont.

Each pink tablet contains: Yohimbine Hydrochloride 5 mg ($1/12$ grain).
Actions: Yohimbine blocks presynaptic alpha-2 adrenergic receptors.
Its action on peripheral blood vessels is similar to that of reserpine, though its of short duration and weaker. Yohimbine's peripheral autonomic nervous system effect is to increase parasympathetic (cholinergic) and decrease sympathetic (adrenergic) activity. It is to be noted that in males sexual performance, erection is linked to cholinergic activity and to alpha-2—adrenergic blockade which may theoretically result in increased enile inflow, decreased penile outflow, or both. Yohimbine exerts a stimulating action on mood and can increase anxiety. These actions have not been adequately studied or related to dosage although it appears to require high doses of Yohimbine. Yohimbine has a mild antidiuretic action, probably via hypothalamus stimulation and release of posterior pituitary hormone. As reported, Yohimbine exerts no significant influence on cardiac stimulation and other effects mediated by β-adrenergic receptors. Its effect on blood pressure, if any, would be to lower it; however, no adequate studies are at hand to quantitate this terms of Yohimbine dosage.
Indications: No claims are made by the manufacturer for effectiveness in any indications. At present time, there is growing interest among urologists to use Yohimbine experimentally for the treatment and the diagnostic classification of certain types of mle erectile impotence.
Contraindications: Sensitivity to the drug and renal diseases. No additional contraindications can be offered due to the limited and inadequate information available.
Warning: Generally, Yohimex is not proposed for use in females and certainly must not be used during pregnancy. This drug is not proposed for use in pediatric, cardio-renal patients with gastric or duodenal history, nor geriatric patients. It should not be used in conjunction with mood modifying agents such as antidepressants, nor in psychiatric patients.
Adverse Reactions: Yohimbine HCl readily penetrates the CNS and produces a complex patterns of responses in lower doses than required to produce peripheral adrenergic blockade. These includes: antidiuresis, a general picture of central excitation including elevation of blood pressure and heart rate increased motor activity, tremor and irritability. Dizziness, headache, and skin flushing reactions have been reported following oral administration of Yohimbine HCl.
Dosage: Experimental dosage reported in the treatment of erectile impotence is of 1 tablet (5 mg of Yohimbine HCl) three times a day, to adult males taken orally. The occasional side effects reported with this dosage are nausea, dizziness, or nervousness. If side effects occurs, the dosage is to be reduced to $1/2$ tablet 3 times a day followed by gradual increases to 1 tablet 3 times a day. The therapy reported is not more than 10 weeks.
How Supplied: Yohimex Tablets in bottles of 100's (NDC 52083-848-10).
Revised: 7/84

Important Notice
Before prescribing or administering any product described in PHYSICIANS' DESK REFERENCE always consult the PDR Supplement for possible new or revised information

---

Kremers-Urban Company
Please refer to William H. Rorer, Inc. for product information.

LactAid Inc.
600 FIRE ROAD
P.O. BOX 111
PLEASANTVILLE, NJ 08232-0111

LACTAID®
[lăkt′ād]
LactAid liquid drops
and
LactAid Tablets
(lactase enzyme)

Description:
LIQUID: Each 5 drop dosage contains not less than 1000 NLU (Neutral Lactase Units) of Beta-D-galactosidase derived from Kluyveromyces lactis yeast. The enzyme is in a liquid carrier of glycerol (50%), water (30%), and inert yeast dry matter (20%). 4-5 drops hydrolyzes approximately 70% of the lactose in 1 quart of milk at refrigerator temperature, @ 42°F–6°C in 24 hours, or will do the same in 2 hours @ 85°F–30°C. Additional time and/or enzyme required for 100% lactose conversion. 1 U.S. quart of milk will contain approximately 50 gm lactose prior to lactose hydrolysis and will contain 15 gm or less, after.
Action: Hydrolysis converts the lactose into its simple sugar components: glucose and galactose.
Indications: Lactase insufficiency in the patient, suspected from g.i. disturbances after consumption of milk or milk content products: e.g., bloat, distension, flatulence, diarrhea; or identified by a lactose tolerance test.
Usage: Added to milk. 4–10 drops per quart of milk depending on level of lactose conversion desired.
Toxicity: Animal studies @ 4% of enzyme by body weight (equivalent of 24,000-5 drop dosages in a 50-kilo adult) showed no effects. LD_{50} not achievable. LactAid is not a drug but a food which modifies another food to make it more digestible.
Other Uses: In vivo activity has been demonstrated, indicating usage in tube feedings and other lactose-content solid and liquid foods, with addition at time of consumption.
How Supplied: Lactase enzyme in a stable liquid form, in sales units of 4, 12, 30 and 75 one-quart dosages at 4 drops per dose.
TABLETS: Each tablet contains not less than 3300 FCC lactase units of Beta-D-Galactosidase from Aspergillis oryzae. 1 to 2 tablets taken with a meal will normally handle a lactose challenge equal to 1 glass of milk. In severe cases, 3 tablets may be required.
Precautions: Diabetics should be aware that the milk sugar will now be metabolically available and must be taken into account (25 gm glucose and 25 gm galactose per quart). No reports received of any diabetics' reactions. Galactosemics may not have milk in any form, lactase enzyme modified or not.
How Supplied: In bottles of 100 and boxes of 12. Also in most areas of the U.S.: Fresh hydrolyzed lowfat milk from dairies, ready to drink, sold in food markets. Lactose hydrolysis level: 70%. If desired, further conversion of the dairy-treated milk can be done at home or institution with the LactAid liquid enzyme. Also in some areas: LactAid lactose reduced cottage cheese, American process cheese, ice cream.
Any person or institution unable to locate LactAid enzyme locally can order direct from LactAid Inc. at retail or wholesale. Sample and full product information to doctors, institutions and nutritionists on request. Call toll-free 800-257-8650.

Shown in Product Identification Section, page 414

Lafayette Pharmacal, Inc.
4200 SOUTH HULEN STREET
FORT WORTH, TX 76109

SUGAR-FREE
KONSYL®
[kon-sil']
Refined Psyllium Hydrophilic Mucilloid

Konsyl is an effective non-irritating, all-natural fiber. Its lubricating action helps normalize elimination functions. Konsyl can be used in the treatment of constipation or nonspecific diarrhea as directed by physician.
All-natural Konsyl contains less than 4 mg. of sodium per dose and has no added sugar, medication or drugs.
Konsyl is made from the highly refined coating of the plantago ovata variety of the psyllium seed, a medically recognized ingredient in the regulation of elimination functions.
Dosage: Adults: One rounded teaspoon in a full glass of liquid one to three times daily, before or after meals, at bedtime, or as directed by physician. **Children, 6 years or older:** $1/2$ the adult dose or less as directed by physician. **Note:** Several days' use may be needed to establish regularity.
Caution: Drink at least eight glasses of liquids daily unless advised otherwise by physician.
KEEP ALL MEDICATIONS OUT OF THE REACH OF CHILDREN. Store below 86°F (30°C). Protect contents from humidity; keep tightly closed.
How Supplied: Canisters of 300 grams (NDC #0224-1801-06), 450 grams (NDC #0224-1801-07), and carton of 25, 6 gram packets (NDC #0224-1801-05).

KONSYL®-D
[kon-sil'-d]
(FORMERLY L.A. FORMULA)
Refined Psyllium Hydrophilic Mucilloid With Dextrose Added

Konsyl-D contains refined psyllium hydrophilic mucilloid, an effective non-irritating, all-natural fiber. Its lubricating action helps normalize elimination functions. Konsyl-D can be used in the treatment of constipation or nonspecific diarrhea as directed by physician.
Konsyl-D contains less than 4 mg. of sodium per dose and has no added medication or drugs.
Konsyl-D is made from the highly refined coating of the plantago ovata variety of the psyllium seed, a medically recognized ingredient in the regulation of elimination functions.
Dosage: Adults: One rounded teaspoon in a full glass of liquid one to three times daily, before or after meals, at bedtime, or as directed by physician. **Children, 6 years or older:** $1/2$ the adult dose or less as directed by physician. **Note:** Several days' use may be needed to establish regularity.
Caution: Drink at least eight glasses of liquids daily unless advised otherwise by physician.
KEEP ALL MEDICATIONS OUT OF THE REACH OF CHILDREN. Store below 86°F (30°C). Protect contents from humidity; keep tightly closed.
How Supplied: Canisters of 325 grams (NDC #0224-1802-06), 500 grams (NDC #0224-1802-07), and carton of 25, 6 gram packets (NDC #0224-1802-08).

Products are cross-indexed
by product classifications
in the
BLUE SECTION

Lambda Pharmacal Corporation
Subsidiary of A. J. Bart, Inc.
GURABO INDUSTRIAL PARK
POST OFFICE BOX 813
GURABO, PUERTO RICO 00658

MIGRALAM™ CAPSULES

Description: Each white MIGRALAM capsule contains: Isometheptene Mucate 65 mg., Caffeine 100 mg., Acetaminophen 325 mg.
Actions: Isometheptene Mucate, a sympathomimetic amine, acts by constricting dilated cranial and cerebral arterioles, thus reducing the stimuli that lead to vascular headaches. It is particularly desirable in patients predisposed to nausea and vomiting and where ergotamines are precluded. Its action is similar to ergotamine but possessed of a low order of toxicity. Caffeine, also a cranial vasoconstrictor, is added to further enhance the vasoconstrictor effect. Acetaminophen, an effective non-narcotic analgesic, reduces the perception of pain impulses originating from dilated cerebral vessels. It is unlikely to produce many of the side effects associated with aspirin.
Indications: For relief of vascular and tension headaches.

Based on a review for this drug (isometheptene mucate), The National Academy of Sciences-National Research Council and/ or other information, FDA has classified the other indications as "Possibly" effective in the treatment of migraine headache.
Final classification of the less-than-effective indication requires further investigation.

Contraindications: MIGRALAN is contraindicated in Glaucoma and/or severe cases of renal disease, hypertension, organic heart disease, hepatic disease and in those patients who are on monoamine-oxidase (MAO) inhibitor therapy.
Precautions: Caution should be observed in hypertension, peripheral vascular disease and after recent cardiovascular attacks.
Adverse Reactions: Transient dizziness and skin rash may appear in hypersensitive patients. This can usually be eliminated by reducing the dose.
Dosage and Administration: FOR RELIEF OF MIGRAINE HEADACHE. The usual adult dosage is two capsules at once, followed by one capsule every hour until relieved, up to 5 capsules within a twelve hour period.
FOR RELIEF OF TENSION HEADACHE. The usual adult dose is one or two capsules every four hours up to 8 capsules a day.
How Supplied: Bottles of 100 capsules (NDC 49326-116-90) and 500 capsules (NDC 49326-116-75).

NEURO™ B-12 INJECTABLE
(B-12, B-1)

Description: Each cc in NEURO B-12 contains: Cyanocobalamin (Vitamin B-12) 1000 mcg., Thiamine HCl. (Vitamin B-1) 100 mg., Benzyl Alcohol 1.5% and Disodium E.D.T.A. 0.5 mg. in a sterile aqueous solution.
How Supplied: NEURO B-12 Injectable is supplied in a 10 cc multidose vial (NDC 49326-114-10).

NEURO™ B-12 FORTE INJECTABLE
(B-12, B-1, B-6)

Description: Each cc in NEURO B-12 FORTE contains: Cyanocobalamin 1000 mcg., Thiamine HCl 100 mg., Pyridoxine HCl 100 mg., Benzyl Alcohol 1.5% in a physiological salt solution q.s.
How Supplied: NEURO B-12 FORTE Injectable is supplied in 10 cc multidose vials (NDC 49326-115-10).

VITA-NUMONYL INJECTABLE
(Expectorant and Antiseptic)

Description: Each ml. contains:
Vitamin A Palmitate ....2,500 I.U.
Vitamin D$_2$ (Ergocalciferol) ....250 I.U.
Eucaliptol ....75 mg.
Oil of Niaouli ....15 mg.
Oil of Arachis ....C.s.h. 1.0 ml.
Pharmacological Use and Action: The balsamics exert and expectorant and antiseptic action of the respiratory tracks. The prophylactic properties of Vitamins "A" and "D" are added to this action.
Dosage: Adults: 2 ml. intramuscular daily for 5 days or according to physician.
Children: 1 ml. intramuscular daily for 5 days.
How Supplied: In 1 ml. and 2 ml. ampoules, boxes of 25.

The Lannett Company, Inc.
9000 STATE ROAD
PHILADELPHIA, PA 19136

ACNEDERM™ LOTION
(See PDR For Nonprescription Drugs)

CODALAN™

Composition: Each tablet contains: Codeine Phosphate* 8 mg. in No. 1; 15 mg. in No. 2; 30 mg. in No. 3; Acetaminophen 500 mg.; and caffeine 30 mg.
*Warning: May be habit-forming.
Action and Uses: Analgesic, antitussive. Indicated for the relief of pain of all degrees of severity up to that which requires morphine.
Administration and Dosage: One (No. 1, No. 2 or No. 3) as required to relieve pain.
How Supplied: No. 1 orange color, No. 2 white color, No. 3 green color; all strengths in bottles of 100 and 500. No. 2 and No. 3 also available in bottles of 1000.
Literature Available: Complete Data Card.

DISONATE™ Capsules and Liquid
(dioctyl sodium sulfosuccinate)

Composition: Docusate Sodium, U.S.P. (Dioctyl sodium sulfosuccinate), an effective stool-softener.
Action and Uses: Disonate keeps stools soft for easy passage. It is not a laxative and does not irritate the intestinal tract. Useful in treating constipation due to hard stools, in painful anorectal conditions, in cardiac and other patients who must avoid straining at stool.
Dosage: Adults and older children 60 to 240 mg. daily. Children 6 to 12 years of age 40 to 120 mg. daily. Higher doses are recommended for initial therapy and the effect on stools is usually apparent one to three days after the initial dose. Divided dosage may be used and dosage should be adjusted to individual response.
How Supplied: Capsules of 60 mg., 100 mg., and 240 mg. Bottles of 100, 500 and 1000 capsules. Solution, 10 mg/cc Pint Bottle. Syrup, 20 mg/5 cc Pint and Gallon Bottle.
Literature Available: Yes.

MAGNATRIL™ SUSPENSION AND TABLETS
(See PDR For Nonprescription Drugs)

Products are cross-indexed by generic and chemical names in the **YELLOW SECTION**

LaSalle Laboratories, Inc.
Subsidiary of Mallard, Inc.
3021 WABASH AVENUE
DETROIT, MI 48216

DYTUSS
Antihistaminic Expectorant

Description: Each 30 ml (fl. oz.) contains:
Diphenhydramine HCl .... 80 mg.
Ammonium Chloride ....778 mg.
Sodium Citrate ....324 mg.
Menthol ....6.4 mg.
Alcohol ....5% U.S.P.
How Supplied: Available in 16 fl. oz. (1 pint) bottles.
Literature: Available upon request.

FETRIN
Hematinic with Vitamins B-12 & C

Description: Each sustained release capsule contains:
Ferrous Fumarate (equivalent to 66
  mg. elemental Iron) ....200 mg.
Ascorbic Acid .... 60 mg.
Cyanocobalamin ....5 mcg.
With Intrinsic Factor
How Supplied: Bottles of 100 capsules.
Literature: Available on request.

HYCO-PAP

Description: Each tablet contains:
Hydrocodone Bitartrate ....5 mg.
  (Warning—May be habit forming)
Aspirin ....230 mg.
Acetaminophen ....150 mg.
Caffeine ....30 mg.
How Supplied: Available in bottles of 100 tablets.
Literature: Available on request.

ORABEX-TF
Therapeutic B-Complex Vitamins with Vitamin C and Folic Acid.

Description: Each coated tablet contains:
Vitamin A (Acetate) .... 6000 I.U.
Vitamin D (Ergocalciferol) .... 400 I.U.
Vitamin E (as 25 mg. d-Alpha
  Tocopherol Succinate) .... 30 I.U.
Folic Acid .... 1.0 mg.
Ascorbic Acid .... 60 mg.
Thiamine Mononitrate .... 1.1 mg.
Riboflavin .... 1.8 mg.
Pyridoxine Hydrochloride .... 2.5 mg.
Vitamin B-12 (Cyanocobalamin) .... 5 mcg.
Niacin (as Niacinamide) .... 15 mg.
Calcium (as Calcium Carbonate) .... 125 mg.
Iron (as Ferrous Fumarate) .... 65 mg.
How Supplied: Bottle of 100 tablets.
Literature: Available on request.

PACAPS

Description: Each capsule contains:
Butalbital ....50 mg.
  (May be habit forming)
Caffeine ....40 mg.
Acetaminophen ....325 mg.
How Supplied: Available in bottles of 100 capsules.
Literature: Available on request.

PROTID, Improved Formula

Description: Each timed release tablet contains:
Acetaminophen ....500 mg.
Chlorpheniramine Maleate ....8 mg.
Phenylephrine HCl ....40 mg.
How Supplied: Bottles of 100 tablets.
Literature: Available on request.

Laser, Inc.
2000 N. MAIN ST.
P.O. BOX 905
POINT, IN 46307

DALLERGY® Syrup, Tablets and Sustained-Release Capsules ℞

Composition: Each 5 ml. (teaspoonful) of purple, grape flavored syrup contains: chlorpheniramine maleate 2 mg., phenylephrine hydrochloride 10 mg., methscopolamine nitrate 0.625 mg. Each white scored tablet contains: chlorpheniramine maleate 4 mg., phenylephrine hydrochloride 10 mg., methscopolamine nitrate 1.25 mg. Each pink and white sustained-release capsule contains: chlorpheniramine maleate 8 mg., phenylephrine hydrochloride 20 mg., methscopolamine nitrate 2.5 mg.

DONATUSSIN DC SYRUP ⓒ ℞

Composition: Each 5 ml. (teaspoonful) of red syrup contains: hydrocodone bitartrate 2.5 mg. (WARNING: May be habit forming), phenylephrine hydrochloride 7.5 mg., guaifenesin 50 mg.

DONATUSSIN DROPS ℞

Composition: Each ml. of orange syrup contains: chlorpheniramine maleate 1 mg., phenylephrine hydrochloride 2 mg., guaifenesin 20 mg.

LACTOCAL–F TABLETS ℞

Multivitamin, Multimineral supplement for pregnant or lactating women. Orange, film-coated tablets embossed Laser, 173.

RESPAIRE®–60 SR CAPSULES ℞
RESPAIRE®–120 SR CAPSULES ℞

Composition: Each Sustained-Release RESPAIRE-60 SR Capsule (opaque green and clear capsule with white pellets) contains pseudoephedrine hydrochloride 60 mg. and guaifenesin 200 mg. Each Sustained-Release RESPAIRE-120 SR Capsule (opaque orange and clear capsule with white and orange pellets) contains pseudoephrine hydrochloride 120 mg. and guaifenesin 250 mg.

THEOSPAN® –SR CAPSULES 130 mg. ℞
(theophylline anhydrous USP)

THEOSPAN® –SR CAPSULES 260 mg. ℞
(theophylline anhydrous USP)

Composition: Each sustained-release THEOSPAN-SR Capsule 130 mg. (white and clear capsule with orange and white pellets) contains theophylline anhydrous USP 130 mg. Each sustained-release THEOSPAN-SR Capsule 260 mg. (dye-free, white and clear capsule with white pellets) contains theophylline anhydrous USP 260 mg.

THEOSTAT® 80 SYRUP ℞
(theophylline anhydrous USP)

Composition: Each 15 ml. (tablespoonful) of dye-free THEOSTAT Syrup contains theophylline anhydrous USP 80 mg., alcohol 1%.

TRIMSTAT® TABLETS ⓒ ℞
(phendimetrazine tartrate)

Composition: Each tan tablet contains: phendimetra ine tartrate 35 mg.

Products are listed alphabetically in the **PINK SECTION.**

Lederle Laboratories
A Division of American Cyanamid Co.
ONE CYANAMID PLAZA
WAYNE, NJ 07470

Lederle Parenterals, Inc.
CAROLINA, PUERTO RICO 00630

Lederle Piperacillin, Inc.
CAROLINA, PUERTO RICO 00630

LEDERMARK® Product Identification Code

To provide quick and positive identification of Lederle products, we have imprinted an alphanumeric code on the tablet and capsule products. In order that you may quickly identify a product by its code, following is an alphanumeric list of LEDERMARK codes with their corresponding product names.

Code	Product
A1	ARISTOCORT® Tabs., 1 mg.
A2	ARISTOCORT® Tabs., 2 mg.
A3	ACHROMYCIN® V Caps., 250 mg.
A4	ARISTOCORT® Tabs., 4 mg.
A4	ARISTO-PAK® Tabs., 4 mg.
A5	ACHROMYCIN® V Caps., 500 mg.
A8	ARISTOCORT® Tabs., 8 mg.
A9	ARTANE® SEQUELS® 5 mg.
A10	AMICAR® Tabs., 500 mg.
A11	ARTANE® Tabs., 2 mg.
A12	ARTANE® Tabs., 5 mg.
A13	ASENDIN® Tabs., 25 mg.
A15	ASENDIN® Tabs., 50 mg.
A16	ARISTOCORT® Tabs., 16 mg.
A17	ASENDIN® Tabs., 100 mg.
A18	ASENDIN® Tabs., 150 mg.
A19	Acetaminophen Tabs., 500 mg.
A20	Acetaminophen Caps., 500 mg.
A21	Acetaminophen Tabs., USP, 325 mg.
A23	Acetaminophen w/Codeine Tabs., 30 mg.
A24	Amitriptyline HCl Tabs., USP, 10 mg.
A25	Amitriptyline HCl Tabs., USP, 25 mg.
A26	Amitriptyline HCl Tabs., USP, 50 mg.
A27	Amitriptyline HCl Tabs., USP, 75 mg.
A28	Amitriptyline HCl Tabs., USP, 100 mg.
A31	Ampicillin Trihydrate Caps., USP, 250 mg.
A32	Ampicillin Trihydrate Caps., USP, 500 mg.
A33	Amoxicillin Capsules, USP, 250 mg.
A34	Amoxicillin Capsules, USP, 500 mg.
A36	Ascorbic Acid Tabs., USP, 250 mg.
A37	Ascorbic Acid Tabs., USP, 500 mg.
A38	Ascorbic Acid Tabs., USP, 1000 mg.
A39	Acetaminophen w/Codeine Tablets, 60 mg.
B6	Butalbital with APC Tabs.
C600	CALTRATE™ 600 Tabs.
C40	CALTRATE™ 600 + D
C1	CENTRUM®, Advanced Formula
C2	CENTRUM® JR.
C39	CENTRUM, JR® + C
C7	Chlorthalidone Tabs., USP, 25 mg.
C9	Chlordiazepoxide HCl Caps., USP, 5 mg.
C10	Chlordiazepoxide HCl Caps., USP, 10 mg.
C11	Chlordiazepoxide HCl Caps., USP, 25 mg.
C13	Chlorothiazide Tabs., USP, 250 mg.
C14	Chlorothiazide Tabs., USP, 500 mg.
C15	Chlorthalidone Tabs., USP, 50 mg.
C16	Chlorpheniramine Maleate Tabs., USP, 4 mg.
C17	Chlorpheniramine Maleate T.D. Caps., 8 mg.
C18	Chlorpheniramine Maleate T.D. Caps., 12 mg.
C19	Chlorzoxazone w/Acetaminophen Tabs., 250 mg./300 mg.
C22	Chlorpromazine HCl Tabs., USP, 25 mg.
C23	Chlorpromazine HCl Tabs., USP, 50 mg.
C24	Chlorpromazine HCl Tabs., USP, 100 mg.
C25	Chlorpromazine HCl Tabs., USP, 200 mg.
C30	Cloxacillin Sodium Caps., USP, 250 mg.
C31	Cloxacillin Sodium Caps., USP, 500 mg.
C37	Chlorpropamide Tablets, USP, 100 mg.
C38	Chlorpropamide Tablets, USP, 250 mg.
D1	DIAMOX® Tabs., 125 mg.
D2	DIAMOX® Tabs., 250 mg.
D3	DIAMOX® SEQUELS® 500 mg.
D9	DECLOMYCIN® Caps., 150 mg.
D11	DECLOMYCIN® Tabs., 150 mg.
D12	DECLOMYCIN® Tabs., 300 mg.
D16	Dicloxacillin Sodium Capsules, USP, 250 mg.
D17	Dicloxacillin Sodium Capsules, USP, 500 mg.
D22	Doxycycline Hyclate Caps., USP, 50 mg.
D23	Dicyclomine HCl Caps., USP, 10 mg.
D24	Dicyclomine HCl Tabs., USP, 20 mg.
D25	Doxycycline Hyclate Caps., USP, 100 mg.
D27	Ergoloid Mesylates Sublingual Tabs., 0.5 mg. (Dihydroergotoxine Methanesulfonate)
D28	Ergoloid Mesylates Sublingual Tabs., 1.0 mg. (Dihydroergotoxine Methanesulfonate)
D31	Diphenoxylate HCl 2.5 mg. and Atropine Sulfate 0.025 mg. Tabs., USP
D32	Docusate Sodium (DSS), USP, Caps., 100 mg.
D33	Docusate Sodium (DSS), USP, Caps., 250 mg.
D34	Docusate Sodium (DSS), 100 mg., USP, w/Casanthranol 30 mg., Caps.
D35	DOLENE® AP-65 Tabs.
D36	DOLENE® Caps., USP, 65 mg.
D37	DOLENE® Compound-65 Caps.
D38	Diphenhydramine HCl Caps., USP, 25 mg.
D39	Diphenhydramine HCl Caps., USP, 50 mg.
D41	Doxycycline Hyclate Tabs., 100 mg.
D44	Dipyridamole Tabs., 25 mg.
D45	Dipyridamole Tabs., 50 mg.
D46	Dipyridamole Tabs., 75 mg.
E2	Erythromycin Stearate Tabs., USP, 250 mg.
E3	Ergoloid Mesylates Tabs., oral, 1.0 mg.
E5	Erythromycin Stearate Tabs., USP, 500 mg.
F1	FOLVITE® Tabs., 1 mg.
F2	FERRO-SEQUELS®
F4	FILIBON® Tabs.
F5	FILIBON® F.A. Tabs.
F6	FILIBON® FORTE Tabs.
F10	FOLVRON® Caps.
F11	Furosemide Tabs., USP, 20 mg.
F12	Furosemide Tabs., USP, 40 mg.
F13	Furosemide Tablets, USP, 80 mg.
F20	Ferrous Sulfate Tabs., USP, 300 mg.
F21	Ferrous Gluconate Iron Supplnt Tabs., USP, 300 mg.
G1	GEVRAL® Tabs.
G2	GEVRAL® T Tabs.
G4	GEVRITE® Tabs.
H1	HYDROMOX® Tabs., 50 mg.
H2	HYDROMOX® R Tabs.
H11	Hydralazine HCl Tabs., USP, 25 mg.
H12	Hydralazine HCl Tabs., USP, 50 mg.
H14	Hydrochlorothiazide Tabs., USP, 25 mg.
H15	Hydrochlorothiazide Tabs., USP, 50 mg.
H17	Hydroxyzine HCl Tabs., 10 mg.
H18	Hydroxyzine HCl Tabs., 25 mg.
H22	Reserpine 0.1 mg. Hydrochlorothiazide 15 mg. Hydralazine HCl 25 mg. (Formerly R-HCTZ-H™)
I11	Imipramine HCl Tabs., USP, 10 mg.
I12	Imipramine HCl Tabs., USP, 25 mg.
I13	Imipramine HCl Tabs., USP, 50 mg.
I15	Isosorbide Dinitrate Tabs., 5 mg.
I16	Isosorbide Dinitrate Tabs., 10 mg.
I17	Isosorbide Dinitrate Tab., 2.5 mg. Sublingual
I18	Isosorbide Dinitrate Tabs., USP, 5 mg. Sublingual
I19	Indomethacin Capsules, USP, 25 mg.
I20	Indomethacin Capsules, USP, 50 mg.
I21	Isoxsuprine HCl Tabs., USP, 10 mg.
I22	Isoxsuprine HCl Tabs., USP, 20 mg.
I23	Isosorbide Dinitrate T.D. Tablets, USP, 40 mg.
L1	LOXITANE® Caps., 5 mg.
L2	LOXITANE® Caps., 10 mg.
L3	LOXITANE® Caps., 25 mg.
L4	LOXITANE® Caps., 50 mg.
L6	LEDERPLEX® Caps.
L7	LEDERPLEX® Tabs.
L9	LEDERCILLIN® VK Tabs., USP, 500 mg.

for possible revisions **Product Information** 1073

Code	Product
L10	LEDERCILLIN® VK Tabs., USP, 250 mg.
L11	Levothyroxine Sodium Tabs., USP, 0.1 mg.
L12	Levothyroxine Sodium Tabs., USP, 0.2 mg.
L13	Levothyroxine Sodium Tabs., USP, 0.3 mg.
L15	Brompheniramine maleate 12 mg., phenylephrine HCl 15 mg., and phenylpropanolamine 15 mg. SEQUELS® Sustained Release Tablets (Formerly LEDER-BP™ SEQUELS®)
M1	Methotrexate Tabs., 2.5 mg.
M2	MINOCIN® Caps, 50 mg.
M3	MINOCIN® Tabs., 50 mg.
M4	MINOCIN® Caps, 100 mg.
M5	MINOCIN® Tabs., 100 mg.
M6	MYAMBUTOL® Tabs., 100 mg.
M7	MYAMBUTOL® Tabs., 400 mg.
M8	MAXIDE™ Tabs.
M10	MATERNA® Tabs.
M12	Meclizine HCl Tabs., USP, 12.5 mg.
M13	Meclizine HCl Tabs., USP, 25 mg.
M19	Methocarbamol Tabs., USP, 500 mg.
M20	Methocarbamol Tabs., USP, 750 mg.
M21	Methyldopa Tablets, USP, 125 mg.
M22	Methyldopa Tablets, USP, 250 mg.
M23	Methyldopa Tablets, USP, 500 mg.
M24	Methyclothiazide Tabs., 2.5 mg.
M25	Methyclothiazide Tabs., 5 mg.
M26	Metronidazole Tabs., 250 mg.
N1	NEPTAZANE® Tabs., 50 mg.
N5	NILSTAT® Oral Tabs.
N6	NILSTAT® Vaginal Tabs.
N10	Neomycin Sulfate Tabs., USP, 500 mg.
N20	Nitroglycerin T.D. Caps., 2.5 mg.
N21	Nitroglycerin T.D. Caps., 6.5 mg.
N23	Nylidrin HCl Tabs., USP, 6 mg.
N24	Nylidrin HCl Tabs., USP, 12 mg.
P1	PATHIBAMATE® 200 Tabs.
P2	PATHIBAMATE® 400 Tabs.
P4	PATHILON® Tabs., 25 mg.
P7	PERIHEMIN® Caps.
P8	PERITINIC® Tabs.
P9	PRONEMIA® Caps.
P11	Papaverine HCl Time Release Caps., 150 mg.
P13	Papaverine HCl Tabs., USP, 100 mg.
P17	Penicillin G Potassium Tabs., USP, 400,000 Units
P21	Phenobarbital Tabs., USP, 30 mg.
P24	Prednisone Tabs., USP, 5 mg.
P25	Probenecid Tabs., USP, 500 mg.
P26	Probenecid with Colchicine Tabs., 500 mg./0.5 mg.
P29	Procainamide HCl Caps., USP, 250 mg.
P30	Procainamide HCl Caps., USP, 375 mg.
P31	Procainamide HCl Caps., USP, 500 mg.
P32	Propantheline Bromide Tabs., USP, 15 mg.
P33	Propylthiouracil Tabs., USP, 50 mg.
P34	Pseudoephedrine HCl Tabs., USP, 60 mg.
P35	Pseudoephedrine HCl Tabs., USP, 30 mg.
P36	Pyrazinamide Tabs., 500 mg.
P37	Pyridoxine HCl (Vitamin B-6) Tabs., USP, 25 mg.
P38	Pyridoxine HCl (Vitamin B-6) Tabs., USP, 50 mg.
Q11	Quinidine Sulfate Tabs., USP, 200 mg.
Q13	Quinidine Sulfate Tabs., USP, 200 mg.
Q15	Quinine Sulfate Caps., USP, 200 mg.
S1	STRESSTABS® 600, Advanced Formula
S2	STRESSTABS® 600 w/Iron, Advanced Formula
S3	STRESSTABS® 600 w/Zinc, Advanced Formula
S5	STRESSCAPS®
S12	Spironolactone with Hydrochlorothiazide Tabs., 25 mg/25 mg.
S13	Spironolactone Tabs., USP, 25 mg.
S14	Sulfasalazine Tabs., 0.5 Gram
S15	Sulfisoxazole Tabs., USP, 500 mg.
S22	SPARTUS® High Potency Vitamins & Minerals plus Electrolytes Tablets.
S23	SPARTUS® +Iron Vitamins & Minerals plus Electrolytes Tablets
T1	TriHEMIC® 600 Tabs.
T10	Thioridazine HCl USP, 10 mg.
T11	Thiamine HCl (Vitamin B-1) Tabs., 50 mg.
T12	Thiamine HCl (Vitamin B-1) Tabs., 100 mg.
T13	Sulfamethoxazole & Trimethoprim Tablets, 400 mg./80 mg.
T14	Thyroid Tabs., USP, 60 mg.
T16	Sulfamethoxazole & Trimethoprim Tablets, 800 mg./160 mg.
T17	Tolbutamide Tabs., USP, 500 mg.
T21	Triple Sulfas (Trisulfapyrimidines USP) Tabs.
T23	Triprolidine HCl and Pseudoephedrine HCl Tabs., 2.5 mg./60 mg.
T25	Thioridazine HCl Tabs., USP, 25 mg.
T27	Thioridazine HCl Tabs., USP, 50 mg.
V11	Vitamin A Caps., Natural USP, 25,000 I.U.
V14	Vitamin C Chewable Tabs., 250 mg.
V15	Vitamin C Chewable Tabs., 500 mg.
V19	Vitamin E Caps., Natural, USP, 400 I.U.
V21	Vitamin E Caps., USP., 200 I.U.
V22	Vitamin E Caps., USP., 400 I.U.
V23	Vitamin E Caps., USP, 600 I.U.
V24	Vitamin E Caps., USP, 1,000 I.U.

LEDERLE STANDARD PRODUCTS

PRODUCT IDENTITY CODE NO.	PRODUCT
—	Acetaminophen Elixir, USP, 160mg/5ml
A19	Acetaminophen Tablets, 500mg
A20	Acetaminophen Capsules, USP, 500mg
A21	Acetaminophen Tablets, USP, 325mg
A23	Acetaminophen w/Codeine Tablets, 30mg
A39	Acetaminophen w/Codeine Tablets, 60 mg
A24	Amitriptyline HCl Tablets, USP, 10mg
A25	Amitriptyline HCl Tablets, USP, 25mg
A26	Amitriptyline HCl Tablets, USP, 50mg
A27	Amitriptyline HCl Tablets, USP, 75mg
A28	Amitriptyline HCl Tablets, USP, 100mg
A31	Ampicillin Trihydrate Capsules, USP, 250mg
A32	Ampicillin Trihydrate Capsules, USP, 500mg
—	Ampicillin Trihydrate for Oral Suspension, USP, 125mg/5ml
—	Ampicillin Trihydrate for Oral Suspension, USP, 250mg/5ml
A33	Amoxicillin Capsules, USP, 250 mg
A34	Amoxicillin Capsules, USP, 500 mg
—	Amoxicillin Suspension 125 mg/5 ml
—	Amoxicillin Suspension 250 mg/5 ml
A36	Ascorbic Acid Tablets, USP, 250mg
A37	Ascorbic Acid Tablets, USP, 500mg
A38	Ascorbic Acid Tablets, USP, 1,000mg
—	Brompheniramine Compound Elixir
L15	Brompheniramine Maleate, N.F., 12mg, Phenylephrine HCl 15mg, and Phenylpropanolamine HCl 15mg Sustained Release Tablets (Formerly LEDER-BP™ SEQUELS®)
—	Brompheniramine Maleate With Codeine, D.C., Expectorant
C 9	Chlordiazepoxide HCl Capsules, USP, 5mg
C10	Chlordiazepoxide HCl Capsules, USP, 10mg
C11	Chlordiazepoxide HCl Capsules, USP, 25mg
C13	Chlorothiazide Tablets, USP 250mg
C14	Chlorothiazide Tablets, USP 500mg
C16	Chlorpheniramine Maleate Tablets, USP, 4mg
C17	Chlorpheniramine Maleate T.D. Capsules, 8mg
C18	Chlorpheniramine Maleate T.D. Capsules, 12mg
C22	Chlorpromazine HCl Tablets, USP, 25mg
C23	Chlorpromazine HCl Tablets, USP, 50mg
C24	Chlorpromazine HCl Tablets, USP, 100mg
C25	Chlorpromazine HCl Tablets, USP, 200mg
—	Chlorpromazine HCl Liquid Concentrate 100mg/ml
C37	Chlorpropamide Tablets, USP, 100 mg
C38	Chlorpropamide Tablets, USP, 250 mg
C 7	Chlorthalidone Tablets, USP, 25mg
C15	Chlorthalidone Tablets, USP, 50mg
C19	Chlorzoxazone w/Acetaminophen Tablets 250mg/300mg
C30	Cloxacillin Sodium Capsules, USP, 250mg
C31	Cloxacillin Sodium Capsules, USP, 500mg
D16	Dicloxacillin Sodium Capsules, USP, 250 mg
D17	Dicloxacillin Sodium Capsules, USP, 500 mg
D23	Dicyclomine HCl Capsules, USP, 10mg
D24	Dicyclomine HCl Tablets, USP, 20mg
—	Diphenhydramine HCl Elixir, USP, 12.5mg/5ml
—	Diphenhydramine HCl Cough Syrup, 12.5mg/5ml
D31	Diphenoxylate HCl 2.5mg + Atropine Sulfate 0.025mg Tablets, USP
D44	Dipyridamole Tablets, 25mg
D45	Dipyridamole Tablets, 50mg
D46	Dipyridamole Tablets, 75mg
D32	Docusate Sodium, (DSS) USP, Capsules, 100mg
D33	Docusate Sodium, (DSS) USP, Capsules, 250mg
D34	Docusate Sodium, (DSS) USP, 100mg, w/Casanthranol, 30mg, Capsules
—	Docusate Sodium (DSS) Syrup, USP, 20mg/5ml
—	Docusate Sodium (DSS), 60 mg/15 ml, w/Casanthranol, 30 mg/15 ml syrup
D36	DOLENE® Capsules, Propoxyphene HCl, Plain, 65mg
D35	DOLENE® AP-65 Tablets, Propoxyphene HCl, Acetaminophen
D42	DOLENE® Compound-65 Capsules, Propoxyphene HCl, Aspirin, and Caffeine
D22	Doxycycline Hyclate Capsules, USP, 50mg
D25	Doxycycline Hyclate Capsules, USP, 100mg
D41	Doxycycline Hyclate Tablets, USP, 100mg
E 3	Ergoloid Mesylates Tablets, Oral 1mg
D27	Ergoloid Mesylates Tablets, Sublingual, 0.5mg
D28	Ergoloid Mesylates Tablets, Sublingual, 1.0mg
—	Erythromycin Ethylsuccinate Oral Suspension, 200mg/5ml
—	Erythromycin Ethylsuccinate Oral Suspension, 400mg/5ml
E 2	Erythromycin Stearate Tablets, USP, 250mg
E 5	Erythromycin Stearate Tablets, USP, 500mg
—	Erythromycin Estolate Oral Suspension, 125mg/5ml
—	Erythromycin Estolate Oral Suspension, 250mg/5ml
—	Ferrous Gluconate Iron Supplement Tablets, USP, 300mg
—	Ferrous Sulfate Elixir, 220mg/5ml
F20	Ferrous Sulfate Tablets, USP, 300mg
F11	Furosemide Tablets, USP, 20mg
F12	Furosemide Tablets, USP, 40mg
F13	Furosemide Tablets, USP, 80mg
—	Guaifenesin Syrup, USP, 100mg/5ml
—	Guaifenesin, 100mg, w/D-Methorphan Hydrobromide Syrup, 15mg/5ml
H11	Hydralazine HCl Tablets, USP, 25mg
H12	Hydralazine HCl Tablets, USP, 50mg
H14	Hydrochlorothiazide Tablets, USP, 25mg
H15	Hydrochlorothiazide Tablets, USP, 50mg
H17	Hydroxyzine HCl Tablets, USP, 10mg

Continued on next page

Lederle—Cont.

H18	Hydroxyzine HCl Tablets, 25mg	
I11	Imipramine HCl Tablets, USP, 10mg	
I12	Imipramine HCl Tablets, USP, 25mg	
I13	Imipramine HCl Tablets, USP, 50mg	
I19	Indomethacin Capsules, USP 25, mg	
I20	Indomethacin Capsules, USP 50, mg	
I15	Isosorbide Dinitrate Tablets, oral, 5mg	
I16	Isosorbide Dinitrate Tablets, oral, 10mg	
I17	Isosorbide Dinitrate Tablets, Sublingual, 2.5mg	
I18	Isosorbide Dinitrate Tablets, USP, Sublingual, 5.0mg	
I23	Isosorbide Dinitrate T.D. Tablets, USP, 40 mg	
I21	Isoxsuprine HCl Tablets, USP, 10mg	
I22	Isoxsuprine HCl Tablets, USP, 20mg	
—	LEDERCILLIN® VK, for Oral Solution, 125mg/5ml	
—	LEDERCILLIN® VK, for Oral Solution, 250mg/5ml	
L10	LEDERCILLIN® VK, USP, Tablets, 250mg	
L 9	LEDERCILLIN® VK, USP, Tablets, 500mg	
L11	Levothyroxine Sodium Tabs., USP, 0.1mg	
L12	Levothyroxine Sodium Tabs., USP, 0.2mg	
L13	Levothyroxine Sodium Tabs., USP, 0.3mg	
M12	Meclizine HCl Tablets, USP, 12.5mg	
M13	Meclizine HCl Tablets, USP, 25mg	
—	Methenamine Mandelate Suspension, 500mg/5ml	
M19	Methocarbamol Tablets, USP, 500mg	
M20	Methocarbamol Tablets, USP, 750mg	
M24	Methyclothiazide Tablets, 2.5mg	
M25	Methyclothiazide Tablets, 5mg	
M21	Methyldopa Tablets, USP, 125 mg	
M22	Methyldopa Tablets, USP, 250 mg	
M23	Methyldopa Tablets, USP, 500 mg	
M26	Metronidazole Tablets, USP, 250mg	
M27	Metronidazole Tablets, USP, 500mg	
N10	Neomycin Sulfate Tablets, USP, 500mg	
N20	Nitroglycerin T.D. Capsules, 2.5mg	
N21	Nitroglycerin T.D. Capsules, 6.5mg	
N23	Nylidrin HCl Tablets, N.F., 6mg	
N24	Nylidrin HCl Tablets, N.F., 12mg	
P11	Papaverine HCl T.R. Capsules, 150mg	
P13	Papaverine HCl Tablets, USP, 100mg	
P17	Penicillin G Potassium Tablets, USP, 400,000 Units	
P21	Phenobarbital Tablets, USP, 30mg (½ gr)	
—	Potassium Chloride Liquid 10%	
—	Potassium Chloride Liquid 20%	
—	Potassium Gluconate Elixir, USP, 4.68gm/15ml	
P24	Prednisone Tablets, USP, 5mg	
P25	Probenecid Tablets, USP, 500mg	
P26	Probenecid w/Colchicine Tablets, 500mg/0.5mg	
P29	Procainamide HCl Capsules, USP, 250mg	
P30	Procainamide HCl Capsules, USP, 375mg	
P31	Procainamide HCl Capsules, USP, 500mg	
—	Promethazine HCl Expectorant, Plain, 5mg/5ml	
—	Promethazine HCl Expectorant w/Codeine, 10mg/5ml	
—	Promethazine HCl Expectorant VC w/Codeine, 10mg/5ml	
—	Promethazine HCl Expectorant VC, Plain	
P33	Propylthiouracil Tablets, USP, 50mg	
—	Pseudoephedrine HCl USP, Syrup, 30mg/5ml	
P35	Pseudoephedrine HCl Tablets, USP, 30mg	
P34	Pseudoephedrine HCl Tablets, USP, 60mg	
P36	Pyrazinamide Tablets, 500mg	
P37	Pyridoxine HCl (Vitamin B-6) Tablets, USP, 25mg	
P38	Pyridoxine HCl (Vitamin B-6) Tablets, USP, 50mg	
Q13	Quinidine Gluconate Sustained Release Tablets, 324mg	
Q11	Quinidine Sulfate Tablets, USP, 200mg	
Q15	Quinine Sulfate Capsules, USP, 325mg	
H22	Reserpine 0.1mg, Hydrochlorthiazide 15mg and Hydralazine HCl 25mg Combination Tablets	
S13	Spironolactone Tablets, USP, 25mg	
S12	Spironolactone w/Hydrochlorothiazide Tablets, 25mg/25mg	
	Sulfamethoxazole and Trimethoprim Pediatric Suspension, 200 mg/40 mg per 5 ml	
T13	Sulfamethoxazole and Trimethoprim Tablets 400 mg/80 mg	
T16	Sulfamethoxazole and Trimethoprim Tablets, 800 mg/160 mg	
S14	Sulfasalazine Tablets, 0.5gm	
T11	Thiamine HCl (Vitamin B-1) Tablets, 50mg	
T12	Thiamine HCl (Vitamin B-1) Tablets, 100mg	
T10	Thioridazine HCl Tablets, USP, 10mg	
T25	Thioridazine HCl Tablets, USP, 25mg	
T27	Thioridazine HCl Tablets, USP, 50mg	
T28	Thioridazine HCl Tablets, USP, 100mg	
T14	Thyroid Tablets, USP, 60mg	
T17	Tolbutamide Tablets, USP, 500mg	
—	Triprolidine HCl with Pseudoephedrine HCl Syrup 1.25mg/30mg per 5ml	
T23	Triprolidine HCl with Pseudoephedrine HCl Tablets 2.5mg/60mg	
V11	Vitamin A Capsules, Natural, USP, 25,000 I.U.	
V14	Vitamin C Chewable Tablets, 250mg	
V15	Vitamin C Chewable Tablets, 500mg	
V19	Vitamin E Capsules, Natural, USP, 400 I.U.	
V21	Vitamin E Capsules, USP, 200 I.U.	
V22	Vitamin E Capsules, USP, 400 I.U.	
V23	Vitamin E Capsules, USP, 600 I.U.	
V24	Vitamin E Capsules, USP, 1000 I.U.	

ACHROMYCIN®
[a-krō-mī-cin]
Sterile Tetracycline Hydrochloride
Intramuscular/Intravenous

ACHROMYCIN tetracycline hydrochloride is an antibiotic isolated from *Streptomyces aureofaciens*. Chemically it is the hydrochloride of 4-dimethylamino-1,4,4a,5,5a,6,11,12a-octahydro-3, 6, 10, 12, 12a-pentahydroxy-6-methyl-1,11-dioxo-2-naphthacenecarboxamide.

Actions: The tetracyclines are primarily bacteriostatic and are thought to exert their antimicrobial effect by the inhibition of protein synthesis. Tetracyclines are active against a wide range of gram-negative and gram-positive organisms. The drugs in the tetracycline class have closely similar antimicrobial spectra, and cross-resistance among them is common. Microorganisms may be considered susceptible if the M.I.C. (minimum inhibitory concentration) is not more than 4.0 mcg/ml and intermediate if the M.I.C. is 4.0 to 12.5 mcg/ml. Susceptibility plate testing: A tetracycline disc may be used to determine microbial susceptibility to drugs in the tetracycline class. If the Kirby-Bauer method of disc susceptibility testing is used, a 30 mcg tetracycline disc should give a zone of at least 19 mm, when tested against a tetracycline-susceptible bacterial strain.

Tetracyclines are readily absorbed and are bound to plasma proteins in varying degree. They are concentrated by the liver in the bile and excreted in the urine and feces at high concentrations and in a biologically active form.

Indications: ACHROMYCIN tetracycline HCl is indicated infections caused by the following microorganisms:

Rickettsiae: (Rocky Mountain spotted fever, typhus fever and the typhus group, Q fever, rickettsial pox and tick fevers).

Mycoplasma pneumoniae (PPLO, Eaton Agent)
Agents of psittacosis and ornithosis,
Agents of lymphogranuloma venereum and granuloma inguinale,
The spirochetal agent of relapsing fever (*Borrelia recurrentis*).
The following gram-negative microorganisms:
Haemophilus ducreyi (chancroid),
Pasteurella pestis and *Pasteurella tularensis*,
Bartonella bacilliformis,
Bacteroides species,
Vibrio comma and Vibrio fetus,
Brucella species (in conjunction with streptomycin).

Because many strains of the following groups of microorganisms have been shown to be resistant to tetracyclines, culture and susceptibility testing are recommended.

Tetracycline is indicated for treatment of infections caused by the following gram-negative microorganisms, when bacteriologic testing indicates appropriate susceptibility to the drug:
Escherichia coli,
Enterobacter aerogenes (formerly *Aerobacter aerogenes*),
Shigella species,
Mima species and *Herellea* species,
Haemophilus influenzae (respiratory infections),
Klebsiella species (respiratory and urinary infections).

Tetracycline is indicated for treatment of infections caused by the following gram-positive microorganisms when bacteriologic testing indicates appropriate susceptibility to the drug:
Streptococcus species:
Up to 44 percent of strains of *Streptococcus pyogenes* and 74 percent of *Streptococcus faecalis* have been found to be resistant to tetracycline drugs. Therefore, tetracyclines should not be used for streptococcal disease unless the organism has been demonstrated to be sensitive.

For upper respiratory infections due to group A beta-hemolytic streptococci, penicillin is the usual drug of choice, including prophylaxis of rheumatic fever.

Diplococcus pneumoniae,
Staphylococcus aureus, skin and soft tissue infections. Tetracyclines are not the drug of choice in the treatment of any type of staphylococcal infection.

When penicillin is contraindicated, tetracyclines are alternative drugs in the treatment of infections due to:
Neisseria gonorrhoeae and (Neisseria meningitidis*)
Treponema pallidum and *Treponema pertenue* (syphillis and yaws),
Listeria monocytogenes,
Clostridium species,
Bacillus anthracis,
Fusobacterium fusiforme (Vincent's infection),
Actinomyces species.
*Intravenous only

In acute intestinal amebiasis, the tetracyclines may be a useful adjunct to amebicides. ACHROMYCIN tetracycline HCl is indicated in the treatment of trachoma, although the infectious agent is not always eliminated, as judged by immunofluorescence.

Inclusion conjunctivitis may be treated with oral tetracyclines or with a combination of oral and topical agents.

Contraindications: This drug is contraindicated in persons who have shown hypersensitivity to any of the tetracyclines.

Warnings: THE USE OF DRUGS OF THE TETRACYCINE CLASS DURING TOOTH DEVELOPMENT (LAST HALF OF PREGNANCY, INFANCY AND CHILDHOOD TO THE AGE OF 8 YEARS) MAY CAUSE PERMANENT DISCOLORATION OF THE TEETH (YELLOW-GRAY-BROWN). This adverse reaction is more common during long-term use of the drugs but has been observed following repeated short-term courses. Enamel hypoplasia has also been reported. TETRACYCLINES, THEREFORE, SHOULD NOT BE USED IN THIS AGE GROUP UNLESS OTHER

DRUGS ARE NOT LIKELY TO BE EFFECTIVE OR ARE CONTRAINDICATED.

If renal impairment exists, even usual oral or parenteral doses may lead to excessive systemic accumulation of the drug and possible liver toxicity. Under such conditions, lower than usual total doses are indicated and, if therapy is prolonged, serum level determinations of the drug may be advisable. This hazard is of particular importance in the parenteral administration of tetracyclines to pregnant or postpartum patients with pyelonephritis. When used under these circumstances, the blood level should not exceed 15 micrograms/ml and liver function tests should be made at frequent intervals. Other potentially hepatotoxic drugs should not be prescribed concomitantly.

(In the presence of renal dysfunction, particularly in pregnancy, intravenous tetracycline therapy in daily doses exceeding 2 grams has been associated with deaths due to liver failure.)

Photosensitivity manifested by an exaggerated sunburn reaction has been observed in some individuals taking tetracyclines. Patients apt to be exposed to direct sunlight or ultraviolet light should be advised that this reaction can occur with tetracycline drugs, and treatment should be discontinued at the first evidence of skin erythema.

The antianabolic action of the tetracyclines may cause in increase in BUN. While this is not a problem in those with normal renal function, in patients with significantly impaired function, higher serum levels of tetracycline may lead to azotemia, hyperphosphatemia, and acidosis.

Usage in Pregnancy: (See above "Warnings" about use during tooth development). Results of animal studies indicate that tetracyclines cross the placenta, are found in fetal tissues and can have toxic effects on the developing fetus (often related to retardation of skeletal development). Evidence of embryotoxicity has also been noted in animals treated early in pregnancy.

Usage in newborns, infants, and children (See above "Warnings" about use during tooth development).

All tetracyclines form a stable calcium complex in any bone-forming tissue.

A decrease in the fibula growth rate has been observed in prematures given oral tetracycline in doses of 25 mg/kg every 6 hours. This reaction was shown to be reversible when the drug was discontinued.

Tetracyclines are present in the milk of lactating women who are taking a drug in this class.

Precautions: As with other antibiotic preparations, use of this drug may result in overgrowth of nonsusceptible organisms, including fungi. If superinfection occurs, the antibiotic should be discontinued and appropriate therapy should be instituted.

In venereal diseases when coexistent syphilis is suspected, darkfield examination should be done before treatment is started and the blood serology repeated monthly for at least 4 months.

Because tetracyclines have shown to depress plasma prothrombin activity, patients who are on anticoagulant therapy may require downward adjustment of their anticoagulant dosage.

In long-term therapy, period laboratory evaluation of organ systems, including hematopoietic, renal and hepatic studies should be performed.

All infections due to Group A beta-hemolytic streptococci should be treated for at least 10 days.

Since bacteriostatic drugs may interfere with the bactericidal action of penicillin, it is advisable to avoid giving tetracycline in conjunction with penicillin.

Adverse Reactions: Local irritation may be present after intramuscular injection. The injection should be deep, with care taken not to injure the sciatic nerve nor inject intravascularly.

Gastrointestinal: Anorexia, nausea, vomiting, diarrhea, glossitis, dysphagia, enterocolitis, and inflammatory lesions (with monilial overgrowth) in the anogenital region. These reactions have been caused by both the oral and parenteral administration of tetracyclines.

Skin: Maculopapular and erythematous rashes. Exfoliative dermatitis has been reported but is uncommon. Photosensitivity is discussed above. (See "Warnings")

Renal toxicity: Rise in BUN has been reported and apparently dose related. (See "Warnings")

Hypersensitivity reactions: Urticaria, angioneurotic edema, anaphylaxis, anaphylactoid purpura, pericarditis and exacerbation of systemic lupus erythematosus.

Bulging fontanels have been reported in young infants following full therapeutic dosage. This sign disappeared rapidly when the drug was discontinued.

Blood: Hemolytic anemia, thrombocytopenia, neutropenia, and eosinophilia have been reported. When given over prolonged periods, tetracyclines have been reported to produced brown-black microscopic discoloration of thyroid glands. No abnormalities of thyroid function studies are known to occur.

Preparation of Solution:
Intravenous
Vials of ACHROMYCIN sterile tetracycline hydrochloride, intravenous should be initially reconstituted by adding 5 ml of Sterile Water for Injection to 250 mg vial and 10 ml of Sterile Water for Injection to the 500 mg vial, and then further diluted prior to administration to at least 100 ml (up to 1000 ml) with any of the following diluents:
Ringer's Injection, USP
Sodium Chloride Injection, USP
Dextrose Injection, USP
 (5% Dextrose in Sterile Water for Injection, USP)
Dextrose and Sodium Chloride
 Injection, USP (5% in Sodium Chloride Injection, USP)
Lactated Ringer's Injection, USP
Protein Hydrolysate Injection,
 Low Sodium, USP 5%
 5% with Dextrose 5%
 5% with Invert Sugar 10%

The initial reconstituted solutions are stable at room temperature for twelve hours without significant loss of potency. The final dilution for administration should be administered immediately.

Note: The use of solutions containing calcium should be avoided as these tend to form precipitates (especially in neutral to alkaline solution) and, therefore, should not be used unless necessary. However, Ringer's Injection, USP and Lactated Ringer's Injection, USP can be used with caution since the calcium ion content in these diluents does not normally precipitate tetracycline in an acid media.

Intramuscular
Add 2 ml of Sterile Water for Injection USP (or Sodium Chloride Injection USP) to the 100 mg or 250 mg vial. The resulting solution may be stored at room temperature and should not be used after 24 hours.

Dosage and Administration:
Intravenous: **Note:** Rapid administration is to be avoided. Parenteral therapy is indicated only when oral therapy is not adequate or tolerated. Oral therapy should be instituted as soon as possible. If intravenous therapy is given over prolonged periods of time, thrombophlebitis may result.

ADULTS: The usual adult dose: 250 to 500 mg every 12 hours and should not exceed 500 mg every 6 hours. The drug may be dissolved and then diluted in 100–1,000 ml of Dextrose 5 percent in water, Isotonic Sodium Chloride Solution or Ringer's solution, but not in other solutions containing calcium (a precipitate may form). For children above eight years of age: The usual dose: 12mg/kg/day, divided into 2 doses, but from 10 to 20 mg/kg/day may be given, depending on the severity of the infection.

Gonorrhea patients sensitive to penicillin may be treated with tetracycline administered as an initial oral dose of 1.5 grams followed by 0.5 grams every 6 hours for 4 days, a total dosage of 9 grams. Intravenous therapy should be reserved for situations in which oral therapy is not feasible.

In patients with renal impairment: (See "Warnings").

Total dosage should be decreased by reduction of recommended individual doses and/or by extending time intervals between doses.

Intramuscular administration, Adults: The usual daily dose is 250 mg administered once every 24 hours or 300 mg given in divided doses at 8- to 12-hour intervals.

For children above eight years of age: 15–25 mg/kg body weight up to a maximum of 250 mg per single daily injection. Dosage may be divided and given to 8- to 12-hour intervals.

Gonorrhea patients sensitive to penicillin may be treated with tetracycline administered as an initial oral dose of 1.5 grams followed by 0.5 grams every 6 hours for 4 days, a total dosage of 9 grams. Intramuscular therapy should be reserved for situations in which oral therapy is not feasible.

In patients with renal impairment: (See "Warnings").

Total dosage should be decreased by reduction of recommended individual doses and/or extending time intervals between doses.

The intramuscular administration of ACHROMYCIN sterile tetracycline hydrochloride produces lower blood levels than oral administration in the recommended dosages. Patients placed on intramuscular tetracyclines should be changed to the oral dosage form as soon as possible. If rapid, high blood levels are needed, ACHROMYCIN should be administered intravenously.

ACHROMYCIN intramuscular should be injected deeply into a large muscle mass such as the gluteal region. Inadvertent injection into the subcutaneous or fat layers may cause pain and induration, which can be relieved by applying an ice pack.

How Supplied:
Intramuscular:
Sterile Tetracycline Hydrochloride
 100 mg/vial   250 mg/vial
 NDC 0005-4772-94   NDC 0005-5357-95
Procaine HCl
 40 mg/vial   40 mg/vial
Magnesium Chloride
 46.84 mg/vial   46.84 mg/vial
Ascorbic Acid
 250 mg/vial   275 mg/vial
 packages of 1   packages of 1
 and 100 vials   and 100 vials

Intravenous:
Sterile Tetracycline Hydrochloride 250 mg with 625 mg ascorbic acid/vial NDC 0005-5352-95
Sterile Tetracycline Hydrochloride 500 mg with 1250 mg ascorbic acid/vial NDC 0005-4771-96
500 mg vial: Military: NSN 6505-00-660-0138

ACHROMYCIN® ℞
[a-krō-mī-cin]
tetracycline hydrochloride
Ophthalmic Suspension 1.0%
Sterile

Description: ACHROMYCIN *tetracycline hydrochloride* OPHTHALMIC SUSPENSION, STERILE contains 10 mg. of Tetracycline Hydrochloride per ml with Plastibase 50W and Light Mineral Oil as inactive ingredients.

Chemically, Achromycin tetracycline hydrochloride is: [4S-(4α,4aα,5aα,6β,12aα,)]-4-(Diethylamino)-1,4,4a,5,5a,6,11,12a-octahydro-3,6,10,12,12a,-pentahydroxy-6-methyl-1,11-dioxo-z-naphthacene carboxamide hydrochloride.

Indications: For the treatment of superficial ocular infections susceptible to ACHROMYCIN *tetracycline hydrochloride*.

For prophylaxis of ophthalmia neonatorum due to *Neisseria gonorrhoeae* or *Chlamydia trachomatis*. The Center for Disease Control (U.S.P.H.S.) and the Committee on Drugs, the Committee on Fetus

Continued on next page

The information on each product appearing here is based on labelling effective in August, 1984 and is either the entire official brochure or an accurate condensation therefrom. Information concerning all Lederle products may be obtained from the Professional Services Department, Lederle Laboratories, Pearl River, New York, 10965.

Lederle—Cont.

and Newborn, and the Committee on Infectious Diseases of the American Academy of Pediatrics recommend 1 percent silver nitrate solution in single-dose ampoules or single-use tubes of an ophthalmic ointment containing 0.5 percent erythromycin or 1 percent tetracycline as "effective and acceptable regimens for prophylaxis of gonococcal ophthalmia neonatorum."[1] (For infants born to mothers with clinically apparent gonorrhea, intravenous or intramuscular injections of aqueous crystalline penicillin G should be given: a single dose of 50,000 units for term infants or 20,000 units for infants of low birth weight. Topical prophylaxis alone is inadequate for these infants.[1])
The following organisms have demonstrated susceptibility to ACHROMYCIN:
Staphylococcus aureus,
Streptococci including *Streptococcus pneumoniae,*
E. coli,
Neisseria species
Chlamydia trachomatis
When treating trachoma a concomitant oral tetracycline is helpful.
Other organisms, not known to cause superficial eye infections, but with demonstrated susceptibility to ACHROMYCIN, have bee omitted from the above list.
ACHROMYCIN does not provide adequate coverage against:
Haemophilus influenzae
Klebsiella/Enterobacter species
Pseudomonas aeruginosa
Serratia marcescens
Contraindications: This product is contraindicated in persons who have shown hypersensitivity to any of the tetracyclines.
Precautions: The use of antibiotics occasionally may result in overgrowth of nonsusceptible organisms. Constant observation of the patient is essential. If new infections appear during therapy, appropriate measures should be taken.
Adverse Reactions: Dermatitis and allied symptomatology have been reported.
If adverse reaction or idiosyncrasy occurs, discontinue medication and institute appropriate therapy.
Dosage and Administration: For most susceptible bacterial infections shake well, then gently squeeze the plastic dropper bottle to instill 1 or 2 drops in the affected eye, or if neccessary, in both eyes, 2 or 4 times daily, or more frequently, depending upon the severity of the infection. Very severe infections may require days of treatment, whereas other cases may be cured by instillation with much less frequency for 48 hours.
In acute and chronic trachoma instill 2 drops in each eye 2 to 4 times daily. This treatment should be continued for 1 to 2 months except that certain individual or complicated cases may require a longer duration. A concomitant oral tetracycline is helpful.
How Supplied: 4 ml plastic dropper-type bottle (NDC 0005-3505-18).
Store at Controlled Room Temperature 15–30° C (59–86° F).
Reference: 1. American Academy of Pediatrics: Prophylaxis and Treatment of Neonatal Gonococcal Infections, Pediatrics, 65:1047, 1980.
A.H.F.S. 52:04:04

ACHROMYCIN® V
[a-krō-mī-cin]
tetracycline HCl
for ORAL USE

Description: ACHROMYCIN V *tetracycline HCl* is an antibiotic isolated from *Streptomyces aureofaciens*. Chemically it is the monohydrochloride of [4S-(4, 4a, 5a, 6β, 12a,)]-4-(Dimethylamino)-1, 4, 4a, 5, 5a, 6, 11, 12a-octahydro-3, 6, 10, 12, 12a-pentahydroxy-6-methyl-1,11-dioxo-2-naphthacenecarboxamide.
Actions: The tetracyclines are primarily bacteriostatic and are thought to exert their antimicrobial effect by the inhibition of protein synthesis. Tetracyclines are active against a wide range of gram-negative and gram-positive organisms.
The drugs in the tetracycline class have closely similar antimicrobial spectra, and cross-resistance among them is common. Microorganisms may be considered susceptible if the M.I.C. (minimum inhibitory concentration) is not more than 4.0 mcg/ml and intermediate if the M.I.C. is 4.0 to 12.5 mcg/ml.
Susceptibility plate testing: A tetracycline disc may be used to determine microbial susceptibility to drugs in the tetracycline class. If the Kirby-Bauer method of disc susceptibility testing is used, a 30 mcg tetracycline HCl disc should give a zone of at least 19 mm. when tested against a tetracycline-susceptible bacterial strain.
Tetracyclines are readily absorbed and are bound to plasma proteins in varying degree. They are concentrated by the liver in the bile and excreted in the urine and feces at high concentrations and in a biologically active form.
Indications: ACHROMYCIN V *tetracycline HCl* is indicated in infections caused by the following microorganisms.
Rickettsiae: (Rocky Mountain spotted fever, typhus fever and the typhus group, Q fever, rickettsialpox, tick fevers).
Mycoplasma pneumoniae (PPLO, Eaton agent).
Agents of psittacosis and ornithosis.
Agents of lymphogranuloma venereum and granuloma inguinale.
The spirochetal agent of relapsing fever (*Borrelia recurrentis*).
The following gram-negative microorganisms:
Haemophilus ducreyi (chancroid),
Pasteurella pestis and *Pasteurella tularensis,*
Bartonella bacilliformis,
Bacteroides species,
Vibrio comma and *Vibrio fetus.*
Brucella species (in conjunction with streptomycin).
Because many strains of the following groups of microorganisms have been shown to be resistant to tetracyclines, culture and susceptibility testing are recommended.
Tetracycline is indicated for treatment of infections caused by the following gram-negative microorganisms, when bacteriologic testing indicates appropriate susceptibility to the drug:
Escherichia coli,
Enterobacter aerogenes (formerly *Aerobacter aerogenes*),
Shigella species,
Mima species and *Herellea* species,
Haemophilus influenzae (respiratory infections),
Klebsiella species (respiratory and urinary infections).
Tetracycline is indicated for treatment of infections caused by the following gram-positive microorganisms when bacteriologic testing indicates appropriate susceptibility to the drug:
Streptococcus species:
Up to 44 percent of strains of *Streptococcus pyogenes* and 74 percent of *Streptococcus faecalis* have been found to be resistant to tetracycline drugs. Therefore, tetracyclines should not be used for streptococcal disease unless the organism has been demonstrated to be sensitive.
For upper respiratory infections due to group A beta-hemolytic streptococci, penicillin is the usual drug of choice, including prophylaxis of rheumatic fever.
Diplococcus pneumoniae,
Staphylococcus aureus, skin and soft tissue infections. Tetracyclines are not the drug of choice in the treatment of any type of staphylococcal infection.
When penicillin is contraindicated, tetracyclines are alternative drugs in the treatment of infections due to:
Neisseria gonorrhoeae,
Treponema pallidum and *Treponema pertenue* (syphilis and yaws),
Listeria monocytogenes,
Clostridium species,
Bacillus anthracis,
Fusobacterium fusiforme (Vincent's infection)
Actinomyces species.
In acute intestinal amebiasis, the tetracyclines may be a useful adjunct to amebicides.
In severe acne, the tetracyclines may be useful adjunctive therapy.
ACHROMYCIN V *tetracycline HCl* is indicated in the treatment of trachoma, although the infectious agent is not always eliminated, as judged by immunofluorescence.
Inclusion conjunctivitis may be treated with oral tetracyclines or with a combination of oral and topical agents.
Tetracycline hydrochloride is indicated for the treatment of uncomplicated urethral, endocervical or rectal infections in adults caused by *Chlamydia trachomatis.*[1]
Contraindications: This drug is contraindicated in persons who have shown hypersensitivity to any of the tetracyclines.
Warnings: THE USE OF DRUGS OF THE TETRACYCLINE CLASS DURING TOOTH DEVELOPMENT (LAST HALF OF PREGNANCY, INFANCY AND CHILDHOOD TO THE AGE OF 8 YEARS) MAY CAUSE PERMANENT DISCOLORATION OF THE TEETH (YELLOW-GRAY-BROWN). This adverse reaction is more common during long-term use of the drugs but has been observed following repeated short-term courses. Enamel hypoplasia has also been reported. TETRACYCLINES DRUGS, THEREFORE, SHOULD NOT BE USED IN THIS AGE GROUP UNLESS OTHER DRUGS ARE NOT LIKELY TO BE EFFECTIVE OR ARE CONTRAINDICATED.
If renal impairment exists, even usual oral or parental doses may lead to excessive systemic accumulation of the drug and possible liver toxicity. Under such conditions, lower than usual total doses are indicated and, if therapy is prolonged, serum level determinations of the drug may be advisable.
Photosensitivity manifested by an exaggerated sunburn reaction has been observed in some individuals taking tetracyclines. Patients apt to be exposed to direct sunlight or ultraviolet light should be advised that this reaction can occur with tetracycline drugs, and treatment should be discontinued at the first evidence of skin erythema.
The anti-anabolic action of the tetracyclines may cause an increase in BUN. While this is not a problem in those with normal renal function, in patients with significantly impaired function, higher serum levels of tetracycline may lead to azotemia, hyperphosphatemia, and acidosis.
Usage in pregnancy (See above "Warnings" about use during tooth development). Results of animal studies indicate that tetracyclines cross the placenta, are found in fetal tissues and can have toxic effects on the developing fetus (often related to retardation of skeletal development). Evidence of embryotoxicity has also been noted in animals treated early in pregnancy.
Usage in newborns, infants, and children (See above "Warnings" about use during tooth development).
All tetracyclines form a stable calcium complex in any bone forming tissue. A decrease in the fibula growth rate has been observed in prematures given oral tetracyclines in doses of 25 mg/kg every 6 hours. This reaction was shown to be reversible when the drug was discontinued.
Tetracyclines are present in the milk of lactating women who are taking the drug in this class.
Precautions: As with other antibiotics preparations, use of this drug may result in over-growth of non-susceptible organisms, including fungi. If superinfection occurs, the antibiotic should be discontinued and appropriate therapy should be instituted.
In veneral diseases when coexistent syphilis is suspected, darkfield examination should be done before treatment is started and the blood serology repeated monthly for at least 4 months.
Because tetracyclines have been shown to depress plasma prothrombin activity, patients who are on anticoagulant therapy may require downward adjustment of their anticoagulant dosage.

In long-term therapy, periodic laboratory evaluation of organ systems, including hematopoietic, renal and hepatic studies should be performed. All infections due to Group A beta-hemolytic streptococci should be treated for at least 10 days. Since bacteriostatic drugs may interfere with the bactericidal action of penicillin, it is advisable to avoid giving tetracycline in conjunction with penicillin.

Adverse Reactions:
Gastrointestinal: Anorexia, nausea, vomiting, diarrhea, glossitis, dysphagia, enterocolitis, and inflammatory lesions (with monilial overgrowth) in the anogenital region. These reactions have been caused by both the oral and parenteral administration of tetracyclines.
Skin: Maculopapular and erythematous rashes. Exfoliative dermatitis has been reported but is uncommon. Photosensitivity is discussed above. (See "Warnings").
Renal toxicity: Rise in BUN has been reported and is apparently dose related (See "Warnings"). Hypersensitivity reactions: Urticaria, angioneurotic edema, anaphylaxis, anaphylactoid purpura, pericarditis and exacerbation of systemic lupus erythematosus.
Bulging fontanels have been reported in young infants following full therapeutic dosage. This sign disappeared rapidly when the drug was discontinued.
Blood: Hemolytic anemia, thrombocytopenia, neutropenia and eosinophilia have been reported.

When given over prolonged periods, tetracyclines have been reported to produce brown-black microscopic discoloration of thyroid glands. No abnormalities of thyroid function studies are known to occur.
Dosage and Administration: Therapy should be continued for at least 24–48 hours after symptoms and fever have subsided.
Concomitant therapy: Antacids containing aluminum, calcium, or magnesium impair absorption and should not be given to patients taking oral tetracycline.
Foods and some dairy products also interfere with absorption. Oral forms of tetracycline should be given 1 hour before or 2 hours after meals.
In patients with renal impairment: (See "Warnings"). Total dosage should be decreased by reduction of recommended individual doses and/or by extending time intervals between doses.
In the treatment of streptococcal infections, a therapeutic dose of tetracycline should be administered for at least 10 days.
Adults: Usual daily dose, 1–2 Grams divided in two or four equal doses, depending on the severity of the infection.
For children above eight years of age: usual daily dose, 10–20 mg (25–50 mg/kg) per pound of body weight divided in two or four equal doses.
For treatment of brucellosis, 500 mg tetracycline four times daily for 3 weeks should be accompanied by streptomycin, 1 gram intramuscularly twice daily the first week and once daily the second week.
For treatment of syphilis, a total of 30–40 grams in equally divided doses over a period of 10–15 days should be given. Close followup, including laboratory tests, is recommended.
Gonorrhea patients sensitive to pencillin may be treated with tetracycline, administered as an initial oral dose of 1.5 grams followed by 0.5 grams every 6 hours for 4 days to a total dosage of 9 grams.
Uncomplicated urethral, endocervical, or rectal infection in adults caused by *Chlamydia trachomatis:* 500 mg, by mouth, 4 times a day for at least 7 days.
How Supplied: ACHROMYCIN® V *Tetracycline HCl* is available as follows:
CAPSULES
500 mg - Two-piece, hard shell, elongated No. 0, opaque capsules with a blue cap and a yellow body, printed with Lederle over A5 on one half and Lederle over 500 mg on the other in gray ink, supplied as follows:

NDC 0005-4875-23—Bottles of 100
NDC 0005-4875-34—Bottles of 1,000
NDC 0005-4875-59—Unit of Issue 12 × 20's
NDC 0005-4875-60—Unit Dose 10 × 10's
NDC 0005-4875-64—Unit of Issue 50 × 20's
250 mg - Two-piece, hard shell, No. 1, opaque capsules with a blue cap and yellow body, printed with Lederle over A3 on one half and Lederle over 250 mg on the other in gray ink, are supplied as follows:
NDC 0005-4880-23—Bottles of 100
NDC 0005-4880-34—Bottles of 1,000
NDC 0005-4880-59—Unit of Issue 12 × 20's
NDC 0005-4880-60—Unit Dose 10 × 10's
NDC 0005-4880-61—Unit of Issue 12 × 40's
NDC 0005-4880-63—Unit of Issue 12 × 28's
NDC 0005-4880-65—Unit of Issue 12 × 100's
NDC 0005-4880-66—Unit of Issue 50 × 28's
Store at Controlled Room Temperature 15–30°C (59–86°F)
ORAL SUSPENSION
Tetracycline equivalent to 125 mg Tetracycline HCl per teaspoonful (5 ml). Preserved with Methylparaben 0.12% and Propylparaben 0.03%, cherry-flavored, is supplied as follows:
NDC 0005-5410-56—Bottles of 2 Fl. Oz. (60 ml)
NDC 0005-5410-65—Bottles of 16 Fl. Oz. (473 ml)
Store at Controlled Room Temperature 15–30°C (59–86°F)

DO NOT FREEZE
Reference: 1. CDC Sexually Transmitted Diseases Treatment Guidelines 1982.
Military Depots:
NSN 6505-01-059-8997–250 mg.—40's
NSN 6505-00-655-8355–250 mg.—100's
NSN 6505-00-963-4924–250 mg.—1000's
Shown in Product Identification Section, page 414

ACHROMYCIN®
tetracycline

is also supplied in a number of other dosage forms and combinations for special purposes (for details of indications, dosage, administration and precautions, see circular in package.)

ACHROMYCIN ℞
tetracycline HCl
Ophthalmic Ointment 1% (sterile)
⅛ oz. tube NDC 0005-3501-51.

ACHROMYCIN
tetracycline HCl
3% Ointment (For topical use)
½ oz. tube– NDC 0005-4796-56
1 oz. tube– NDC 0005-4796-55.
℞ not required

AMICAR® ℞
[ă-mĭ-car]
Aminocaproic Acid
Intravenous, Syrup, and Tablets

Description: AMICAR *aminocaproic acid Lederle* is a monoaminocarboxylic acid which acts as an effective inhibitor of fibrinolysis.
The chemical structure is $NH_2CH_2(CH_2)_3CH_2COOHC_6H_{13}NO_2$ MW 131.17
Actions: The beneficial fibrinolysis-inhibitory effects of AMICAR appear to be principally via inhibition of plasminogen activator substances and, to a lesser degree, through antiplasmin activity. The drug is absorbed rapidly following oral administration. Whether administered by the oral or intravenous route, a major portion of the compound is recovered unmetabolized in the urine. The renal clearance of AMICAR is high (about 75 percent of the creatinine clearance). Thus the drug is excreted rapidly. After prolonged administration, AMICAR distributes throughout both the extravascular and intravascular compartments of the body and readily penetrates human red blood and other tissue cells.
Indications: AMICAR is useful in enhancing hemostasis when fibrinolysis contributes to bleeding. In life-threatening situations, fresh whole blood transfusions, fibrinogen infusions, and other emergency measures may be required.

Fibrinolytic bleeding may frequently be associated with *surgical complications* following heart surgery (with or without cardiac bypass procedures) and portacaval shunt; *hematological disorders* such as aplastic anemia, *abruptio placentae, hepatic cirrhosis, neoplastic disease* such as carcinoma of the prostate, lung, stomach, and cervix. Urinary fibrinolysis, usually a normal physiological phenomenon, may frequently be associated with life-threatening complications following severe trauma, anoxia and shock. Symptomatic of such complications is *surgical hematuria* (following prostatectomy and nephrectomy) or *non-surgical hematuria* (accompanying polycystic or neoplastic diseases of the genitourinary system). (See *WARNINGS*)
Contraindications: AMICAR should not be used when there is evidence of an active intravascular clotting process.
When there is uncertainty as to whether the cause of bleeding is primary fibrinolysis or disseminated intravascular coagulation (DIC), this distinction must be made before administering AMICAR. The following tests can be applied to differentiate the two conditions:
• Platelet count is usuallly decreased in DIC but normal in primary fibrinolysis.
• Protamine Paracoagulation test is positive in DIC; a precipitate forms when protamine sulphate is dropped into citrated plasma. The test is negative in the presence of primary fibrinolysis.
• The euglobulin clot lysis test is abnormal in primary fibrinolysis, but normal in DIC.
AMICAR must not be used in the presence of DIC without concomitant heparin.
Warnings: Safe use of AMICAR has not been established with respect to adverse effects upon fetal development. Therefore, it should not be used in women of child-bearing potential and particularly during early pregnancy, unless in the judgement of the physician the potential benefits outweigh the possible hazards. Antifertility effects, consistent with the drug's antifibrinolytic activity, have been suggested in some rodent studies.
In patients with upper urinary tract bleeding, AMICAR administration has been known to cause intrarenal obstruction in the form of glomerular capillary thrombosis, or clots in the renal pelvis and ureters. For this reason, AMICAR should not be used in hematuria of upper urinary tract origin, unless the possible benefits outweight the risk.
Precautions: AMICAR *aminocaproic acid* has a very specific action in that it inhibits both plasminogen activator substances and, to a lesser degree, plasmin activity. The drug should NOT be administered without a definite diagnosis, and/or laboratory findings indicative of hyperfibrinolysis (hyperplasminemia).*
*Stefanini, M. and Dameshek, W.: The Hemorrhagic Disorder, Ed. 2, New York, Grune and Stratton, pp. 510–514, 1962.
The use of AMICAR should be accompanied by tests designed to determine the amount of fibrinolysis present. There are presently available (a) general tests, such as those for the determination of the lysis of a clot of blood or plasma and (b) more specific tests for the study of various phases of fibrinolytic mechanisms. These latter tests include both semi-quantitative and quantitative techniques for the determination of profibrinolysin, fibrinolysin, and antifibrinolysin.
Animal experiments indicate particular caution should be taken in administering AMICAR to patients with cardiac, hepatic or renal diseases. Demonstrable animal pathology in some cases has shown endocardial hemorrhages and myocardial

Continued on next page

The information on each product appearing here is based on labelling effective in August, 1984 and is either the entire official brochure or an accurate condensation therefrom. Information concerning all Lederle products may be obtained from the Professional Services Department, Lederle Laboratories, Pearl River, New York, 10965.

Lederle—Cont.

fat degeneration. Rarely, skeletal muscle weakness with necrosis of muscle fibers has been reported clinically; the possibility of cardiac muscle damage should be considered also when skeletal myopathy occurs. The use of this drug should thus be restricted to patients in whom the benefit expected would outweight the potential hazard. Physicians are cautioned in the use of this product because of animal data showing rat teratogenicity and kidney concretions.

Rapid intravenous administration of the drug should be avoided since this may induce hypotension, bradycardia and/or arrhythmia.

One case of *cardiac* and *hepatic lesions* observed in man has been reported. The patient received 2 grams of aminocaproic acid every 6 hours for a total dose of 26 grams. Death was due to continued cerebrovascular hemorrhage. Necrotic changes in the heart and liver were noted at autopsy.

Fibrinolysis is a normal process, presumably active at all times to ensure the fluidity of blood. Inhibition of fibrinolysis by aminocaproic acid *may* theoretically result in clotting or thrombosis. However, there is no definite evidence that administration of aminocaproic acid has been responsible for the few reported cases of *intravascular clotting* which followed this treatment. Rather, it appears that such intravascular clotting was most likely due to the patient's pre-existing clinical condition, e.g., the presence of DIC.

It has been postulated that *extravascular clots* formed *in vivo* may not undergo spontaneous lysis as do normal clots.

Adverse Reactions: Occasionally nausea, cramps, diarrhea, hypotension, dizziness, tinnitus, malaise, conjunctival suffusion, nasal stuffiness, headache, myopathy, and skin rash have been reported as results of the administration of aminocaproic acid. The myopathy may be accompanied with general weakness, fatigue, and elevated serum enzymes. Rarely, rhabdomyolysis with myoglobinuria and renal failure may occur. Only rarely has it been necessary to discontinue or reduce medication because of one or more of these effects.

There have also been some reports of dry ejaculation during the period of AMICAR treatment. These have been reported to date only in hemophilia patients who received the drug after undergoing dental surgical procedures. However, this symptom resolved in all patients within 24 to 48 hours of completion of therapy.

Two cases of convulsions occurring following intravenous administration of AMICAR have been reported. However, definite associations between the seizures and the drug have not been established.

Thrombophlebitis, a possibility with all intravenous therapy, should be guarded against by strict attention to the proper insertion of the needle and the fixing of its position.

Dosage and Administration: *Initial Therapy:* An initial priming dose of 5 grams of AMICAR administered either orally or intravenously followed by 1.0 to 1.25 gram doses at hourly intervals thereafter should achieve and sustain plasma levels of 0.130 mg/ml of the drug. This is the concentration apparently necessary for the inhibition of fibrinolysis. Administration of more than 30 grams in any 24-hour period is not recommended.

Intravenous: AMICAR *aminocaproic acid* Intravenous is administered by infusion, utilizing the usual compatible intravenous vehicles (e.g., Sterile Water for Injection, physiologic saline, 5% dextrose or Ringer's Solution). RAPID INJECTION OF AMICAR INTRAVENOUS UNDILUTED INTO A VEIN IS NOT RECOMMENDED.

For the treatment of *acute* bleeding syndromes due to elevated fibrinolytic activity, it is suggested that 16 to 20 ml (4.0 to 5.0 grams) of AMICAR Intravenous in 250 ml of diluent be administered by infusion during the first hour of treatment, followed by a continuing infusion at the rate of 4 ml (1.0 gram) per hour in 50 ml of diluent. This method of treatment would ordinarily be continued for about 8 hours or until the bleeding situation has been controlled.

Oral Therapy: If the patient is able to take medication by mouth, an identical dosage regimen may be followed by administering AMICAR Tablets or 25% Syrup as follows: For the treatment of *acute* bleeding syndromes due to elevated fibrinolytic activity, it is suggested that 10 tablets (5.0 grams) or 4 teaspoonfuls of syrup (5.0 grams) of AMICAR be administered during the first hour of treatment, followed by a continuing rate of 2 tablets (1.0 grams) or 1 teaspoonful of syrup (1.25 grams) per hour. This method of treatment would ordinarily be continued for about 8 hours or until the bleeding situation has been controlled.

How Supplied: *AMICAR *Lederle Intravenous:* Each 20 ml vial contains 5.0 Grams of Aminocaproic Acid (250 mg per ml) as an aqueous solution, with 0.9% benzyl alcohol as a preservative. The pH is adjusted to approx. 6.8 with Hydrochloric Acid. 20 ml vials, Product No. NDC 0205-4668-37. Each 96 ml vial contains 24 grams of Aminocaproic Acid (250 mg per ml) as an aqueous solution, with 0.9% benzyl alcohol as a preservative. The pH is adjusted to approx. 6.8 with Hydrochloric Acid. 96 ml vials, Product No. NDC 0205-4668-73.

AMICAR *Lederle 25% Syrup:* Each ml of raspberry flavored syrup contains 250 mg of Aminocaproic Acid with 0.1% Sodium Benzoate and 0.2% Potassium Sorbate as preservative. 16 Fl. Oz. bottles, Product No. NDC 0005-4667-65.

AMICAR *Lederle Tablets:* Each tablet round, white, engraved with LL on one side and scored on the other with A to the left of the score and 10 on the right, contains 500 mg of Aminocaproic Acid. Bottles of 100, Product No. NDC 0005-4665-23.

Store at Controlled Room Temperature 15–30°C (59–86°F).

Intravenous 250 mg/ml 20 ml vial
Military: NSN 6505-00-926-1442
VA: NSN 6505-00-926-1442A
*Manufactured for
LEDERLE LABORATORIES DIVISION
American Cyanamid Company
Pearl River, NY 10965
by
LEDERLE PARENTERALS INC.
Carolina, Puerto Rico 00630
Shown in Product Identification Section, page 414

ARISTOCORT® ℞
[*a-ris-tō- cort*]
triamcinolone
TABLETS
ARISTOCORT®
triamcinolone diacetate
SYRUP

Description: ARISTOCORT *triamcinolone* is a synthetic adrenocorticosteroid. The tablets contain Triamcinolone, 9α-fluoro-16α-hydroxyprednisolone, Syrup contains Triamcinolone Diacetate, 9α-fluoro-16α-hydroxyprednisolone diacetate. It is readily absorbed from the gastrointestinal tract.

Action: ARISTOCORT is primarily glucocorticoid in action and has potent anti-inflammatory, hormonal and metabolic effects common to cortisone-like drugs. It is essentially devoid of mineralocorticoid activity when administered in therapeutic doses, causing little or no sodium retention, with potassium excretion minimal or absent. The body's immune responses to diverse stimuli is also modified by its action.

Indications:
1. Endocrine Disorders:
Primary or secondary adrenocortical insufficiency (hydrocortisone or cortisone is the first choice; synthetic analogs may be used in conjunction with mineralocorticoids where applicable. In infancy mineralocorticoid supplementation is of particular importance).
Congenital adrenal hyperplasia.
Nonsuppurative thyroiditis.
Hypercalcemia associated with cancer.
2. Rheumatic Disorders:
As adjunctive therapy for short-term administration (to tide the patient over an acute episode or exacerbation) in:
Psoriatic arthritis.
Rheumatoid arthritis including juvenile rheumatoid arthritis (selected cases may require low-dose maintenance therapy).
Ankylosing spondylitis.
Acute and subacute bursitis.
Acute nonspecific tenosynovitis.
Acute gouty arthritis.
Post-traumatic osteoarthritis.
Synovitis of osteoarthritis.
Epicondylitis.
3. Collagen Diseases:
During an exacerbation or as maintenance therapy in selected cases of—
Systemic lupus erythematosus.
Acute rheumatic carditis.
4. Dermatologic Diseases:
Pemphigus.
Bullous dermatitis herpetiformis.
Severe erythema multiforme (Stevens-Johnson syndrome).
Exfoliative dermatitis.
Mycosis fungoides.
Severe psoriasis.
Severe seborrheic dermatitis.
5. Allergic States:
Control of severe or incapacitating allergic conditions intractable to adequate trials of conventional treatment:
Seasonal or perennial allergic rhinitis.
Bronchial asthma.
Contact dermatitis.
Atopic dermatitis.
Serum sickness.
Drug hypersensitivity reactions.
6. Ophthalmic Diseases:
Severe acute and chronic allergic and inflammatory processes involving the eye and its adnexa such as—
Allergic conjunctivitis.
Keratitis.
Allergic corneal marginal ulcers.
Herpes zoster ophthalmicus.
Iritis and iridocyclitis.
Chorioretinitis.
Anterior segment inflammation.
Diffuse posterior uveitis and choroiditis.
Optic neuritis.
Sympathetic ophthalmia.
7. Respiratory Diseases:
Symptomatic sarcoidosis.
Loeffler's syndrome not manageable by other means.
Berylliosis.
Fulminating or disseminated pulmonary tuberculosis when used concurrently with appropriate antituberculous chemotherapy.
Aspiration pneumonitis.
8. Hematologic Disorders:
Idiopathic thrombocytopenic purpura in adults.
Secondary thrombocytopenia in adults.
Acquired (autoimmune) hemolytic anemia.
Erythroblastopenia (RBC anemia).
Congenital (erythroid) hypoplastic anemia.
9. Neoplastic Diseases:
For palliative management of:
Leukemias and lymphomas in adults.
Acute leukemia of childhood.
10. Edematous States:
To induce a diuresis or remission of proteinuria in the nephrotic syndrome, without uremia, of the idiopathic type or that due to lupus erythematosus.
11. Gastrointestinal Diseases:
To tide the patient over a critical period of the disease in:
Ulcerative Colitis.
Regional enteritis.
12. Nervous System:
Acute exacerbations of multiple sclerosis.

13. Miscellaneous:
Tuberculous meningitis with subarachnoid block or impending block when used concurrently with appropriate antituberculous chemotherapy.

Trichinosis with neurologic or myocardial involvement.

Contraindications:
Systemic fungal infections.
Sensitivity to the drug or any of its components.

Warnings: In patients on corticosteroid therapy subjected to unusual stress, increased dosage of rapidly acting corticosteroids before, during, and after the stressful situation is indicated.

Corticosteroids may mask some signs of infection, and new infections may appear during their use. There may be decreased resistance and inability to localize infection when corticosteroids are used.

Prolonged use of corticosteroids may produce posterior subcapsular cataracts, glaucoma with possible damage to the optic nerves, and may enhance the establishment of secondary ocular infections due to fungi or viruses.

Usage in pregnancy: Since adequate human reproduction studies have not been done with corticosteroids, the use of these drugs in pregnancy, nursing mothers or women of childbearing potential requires that the possible benefits of the drug be weighed against the potential hazards to the mother and embryo or fetus. Infants born of mothers who have received substantial doses of corticosteroids during pregnancy should be carefully observed for signs of hypoadrenalism.

Average and large doses of hydrocortisone or cortisone can cause elevation of blood pressure, salt and water retention, and increased excretion of potassium. These effects are less likely to occur with ARISTOCORT *triamcinolone* except when used in large doses. Dietary salt restriction and potassium supplementation may be necessary. All corticosteroids increase calcium excretion.

While on Corticosteroid Therapy Patients Should Not Be Vaccinated Against Smallpox. Other Immunization Procedures Should Not Be Undertaken in Patients Who are on Corticosteroids, Especially on High Dose, Because of Possible Hazards of Neurological Complications and a Lack of Antibody Response.

The use of Triamcinolone in active tuberculosis should be restricted to those cases of fulminating or disseminated tuberculosis in which the corticosteroid is used for the management of the disease in conjunction with an appropriate antituberculous regimen.

If corticosteroids are indicated in patients with latent tuberculosis or tuberculin reactivity, close observation is necessary as reactivation of the disease may occur. During prolonged corticosteroid therapy, these patients should receive chemoprophylaxis.

Precautions: Drug-induced secondary adrenocortical insufficiency may be minimized by gradual reduction of dosage. This type of relative insufficiency may persist for months after discontinuation of therapy; therefore, in any situation of stress occurring during that period, hormone therapy should be reinstituted. Since mineralocorticoid secretion may be impaired, salt and/or a mineralocorticoid should be administered concurrently.

There is an enhanced effect of corticosteroids on patients with hypothyroidism and in those with cirrhosis.

Corticosteroids should be used cautiously in patients with ocular herpes simplex because of possible corneal perforation.

The lowest possible dose of corticosteroid should be used to control the condition under treatment, and when reduction in dosage is possible, the reduction should be gradual.

Psychic derangements may appear when corticosteroids are used, ranging from euphoria, insomnia, mood swings, personality changes, and severe depression, to frank psychotic manifestations. Also, existing emotional instability or psychotic tendencies may be aggravated by corticosteroids.

Aspirin should be used cautiously in conjunction with corticosteroids in hypoprothrombinemia.

Steroids should be used with caution in nonspecific ulcerative colitis if there is a probability of impending perforation, abscess or other pyogenic infection; diverticulitis; fresh intestinal anastomoses; active or latent peptic ulcer; renal insufficiency; hypertension; osteoporosis; and myasthenia gravis.

Growth and development of infants and children on prolonged corticosteroid therapy should be carefully observed.

Although controlled clinical trials have shown corticosteroids to be effective in speeding the resolution of acute exacerbations of multiple sclerosis they do not show that they affect the ultimate outcome or natural history of the disease. The studies do show relatively high doses of corticosteroids are necessary to demonstrate a significant effect. (See Dosage and Administration).

Since complications of treatment with glucocorticoid are dependent on the size of the dose and the duration of treatment a risk/benefit decision must be made in each individual case as to dose and duration of treatment and as to whether daily or intermittent therapy should be used.

Adverse Reactions:
Fluid and Electrolyte Disturbances.
Sodium retention.
Fluid retention.
Congestive heart failure in susceptible patients.
Potassium loss.
Hypokalemic alkalosis.
Hypertension.
Musculoskeletal.
Muscle weakness.
Steroid myopathy.
Loss of muscle mass.
Osteoporosis.
Vertebral compression fractures.
Aseptic necrosis of femoral and humeral heads.
Pathologic fracture of long bones.
Gastrointestinal.
Peptic ulcer with possible perforation and hemorrhage.
Pancreatitis.
Abdominal distention.
Ulcerative esophagitis.
Dermatologic.
Impaired wound healing.
Thin fragile skin.
Petechiae and ecchymoses.
Facial erythema.
Increased sweating.
May suppress reactions to skin tests.
Neurological.
Convulsions.
Increased intracranial pressure with papilledema (pseudotumor cerebri) usually after treatment.
Vertigo.
Headache.
Endocrine.
Menstrual irregularities.
Development of Cushingoid state.
Suppression of growth in children.
Secondary adrenocortical and pituitary unresponsiveness, particularly in times of stress, as in trauma, surgery or illness.
Decreased carbohydrate tolerance.
Manifestations of latent diabetes mellitus.
Increased requirements for insulin or oral hypoglycemic agents in diabetics.
Ophthalmic.
Posterior subcapsular cataracts.
Increased intraocular pressure.
Glaucoma.
Exophthalmos.
Metabolic.
Negative nitrogen balance due to protein catabolism.

Dosage and Administration:
General Principles:
1. The initial dosage of ARISTOCORT *triamcinolone* may vary from 4 mg. to 48 mg. per day depending on the specific disease entity being treated. In situations of less severity lower doses will generally suffice while in selected patients higher initial doses may be required. The initial dosage should be maintained or adjusted until a satisfactory response is noted. If after a reasonable period of time there is a lack of satisfactory clinical response, the drug should be discontinued and the patient transferred to other appropriate therapy. *IT SHOULD BE EMPHASIZED THAT DOSAGE REQUIREMENTS ARE VARIABLE AND MUST BE INDIVIDUALIZED ON THE BASIS OF THE DISEASE UNDER TREATMENT AND THE RESPONSE OF THE PATIENT.* After a favorable response is noted, the proper maintenance dosage should be determined by decreasing the initial drug dosage in small increments at appropriate time intervals until the lowest dosage which will maintain an adequate clinical response is reached. It should be kept in mind that constant monitoring is needed in regard to drug dosage. Included in the situations which may make dosage adjustments necessary are changes in clinical status secondary to remissions or exacerbations in the disease process, the patient's individual drug responsiveness, and the effect of patient exposure to stressful situations not directly related to the disease entity under treatment; in this latter situation it may be necessary to increase the dosage of ARISTOCORT for a period of time consistent with the patient's condition. If after long-term therapy the drug is to be stopped, it is recommended that it be withdrawn gradually rather than abruptly.

2. Dosage should be individualized according to the severity of the disease and the response of the patient. For infants and children, the recommended dosage should be governed by the same considerations rather than by strict adherence to the ratio indicated by age or body weight.

3. Hormone therapy is an adjunct to, and not a replacement for, conventional therapy.

4. The severity, prognosis and expected duration of the disease and the reaction of the patient to medication are primary factors in determining dosage.

5. If a period of spontaneous remission occurs in a chronic condition, treatment should be discontinued.

6. Blood pressure, body weight, routine laboratory studies, including 2-hour postprandial blood glucose and serum potassium, and a chest X-ray should be obtained at regular intervals during prolonged therapy. Upper GI X-rays are desirable in patients with known or suspected peptic ulcer disease.

7. Suppression of autogenous pituitary function, a common effect of exogenous corticosteroid administration, may be reduced, modified or minimized by revision of dose schedules. The time of maximum corticoid effect is from midnight to 8 a.m. and minimal during the intervening hours. Use of a single daily dose beginning at or after 8 a.m. will be effective in most conditions, will lower corticoid overload and will cause the least interference with the diurnal system of endogenous secretion and hypothalamopituitary-adrenal function; alternate-day dosage in some conditions and intermittent administration in certain severe disorders requiring long-term and/or high dose maintenance levels have proven both clinically effective and less likely to produce adverse reactions. The maximum daily morning dose not associated with lasting adrenocorticoid suppression is 8 mg.

8. *Alternate-Day Therapy.* After the conventional dose has been established, some patients may be maintained on alternate day therapy. It has been shown that the activity of the adrenal cortex varies throughout the day, being greatest from about midnight to 8:00 a.m. Exogenous corticoid suppresses this activity least when given at the time of maximum activity. A 48-hour interval appears to be necessary since shorter intervals are

Continued on next page

The information on each product appearing here is based on labelling effective in August, 1984 and is either the entire official brochure or an accurate condensation therefrom. Information concerning all Lederle products may be obtained from the Professional Services Department, Lederle Laboratories, Pearl River, New York, 10965.

Lederle—Cont.

accompanied by adrenal suppression similar to that of conventional daily divided doses. Therefore, with the alternate day dose plan, a total 48-hour requirement is given every other day at 8:00 a.m. As with other regimens, the minimum effective dose level should be sought.

9.* *Intermittent-Type Therapy.* An additional modification of corticosteroid usage has been recommended and used for treatment of disorders often requiring long-term-administration of medium or high dose range. It is generally recommended that treatment be initiated with a single calculated dose of ARISTOCORT given once daily and continued daily until clinical response is adequate or appropriate. The time of maximum corticoid effect is from midnight to 8 a.m. and minimal during the intervening hours. Therefore, dosage beginning at or after 8 a.m. will offer good effect and lower corticoid overload. Thereafter, the patient is maintained on a calculated single daily dose given each morning for 3-4 consecutive days, followed by a "rest period" of 3 days, during which no corticosteroid is administered. This schedule is continued for as long as therapeutically indicated.
*For syrup only.

Specific Dosage Recommendations:

1. *Endocrine Disorders:* Wide variation in dosage requirements for the endocrine disorders such as *congenital adrenal hyperplasia, non-suppurative thyroiditis,* and *hypercalcemia associated* with *cancer* precludes specific recommendation except for *adrenocortical insufficiency* where the dose is usually 4-12 mg. daily in addition to mineralocorticoid therapy.

2. *Rheumatic Disorders: Rheumatoid arthritis; acute gouty arthritis; ankylosing spondylitis;* and *selected cases of psoriatic arthritis;* in *acute* and *subacute bursitis;* and in *acute nonspecific tenosynovitis.* The initial suppressive dose of ARISTOCORT in these conditions ranges from 8 mg. to 16 mg. per day, although the occasional patient may require higher doses. Patients may show an early or a delayed effect, characterized by a reduction in the inflammatory reaction and in joint swelling, together with alleviation of pain and stiffness, resulting in an increased range of motion of the affected joints or tissues. Maintenance doses are adjusted to keep symptoms at a level tolerable to the patient. Rapid reduction of the steroid or its abrupt discontinuance may result in recurrence or even exacerbation of signs and symptoms. Short-term administration is desirable as a rule. ARISTOCORT *triamcinolone* is ordinarily administered as a single morning dose daily or on alternate days, depending on the need of the patient. Occasional patients may secure more effective relief on divided daily doses, either 2 to 4 times daily.

3. *Collagen Diseases: Systemic Lupus Erythematosus:* The initial dose is usually 20 mg. to 32 mg. daily continued until the desired response is obtained, when reduced maintenance levels are sought. Patients with more severe symptoms may require higher initial doses, 48 mg. or more daily, and higher maintenance doses. Although some patients with systemic lupus erythematosus appear to have spontaneous remissions or to tolerate the disorder in its milder forms for prolonged periods of time, adjustment of dosage scheduling to reduce adverse suppression of the pituitary-adrenal axis may be useful.

Acute Rheumatic Carditis: In severely ill patients with carditis, pericardial effusion and/or congestive heart failure, corticosteroid therapy is effective in the control of the acute and severe inflammatory changes and may be lifesaving. Initial doses of ARISTOCORT may be from 20 mg. to 60 mg. daily, and clinical response is usually rapid and the drug can then be reduced. Maintenance therapy should be continued for at least 6 to 8 weeks and is seldom required beyond a period of 3 months. Corticosteroid therapy does not preclude conventional treatment, including antibiotics and salicylization.

4. *Dermatological Disorders: Pemphigus; bullous dermatitis herpetiformis, severe erythema multiforme* (Stevens-Johnson Syndrome); *exfoliative dermatitis;* and *mycosis fungoides.* The initial dose is 8 mg. to 16 mg. daily. In these conditions, as well as in certain allergic dermatoses, *alternate-day* administration has been found effective and apparently less likely to produce adverse side effects. *Severe psoriasis:* ARISTOCORT may produce reduction or remission of the disabling skin manifestations following initial doses of 8 mg. to 16 mg. daily. The period of maintenance is dependent on the clinical response. Corticosteroid reduction or discontinuation of therapy should be attempted with caution since relapse may occur and may appear in a more aggravated form, the so-called "rebound phenomenon".

5. *Allergic States:* ARISTOCORT *triamcinolone* is administered in doses of 8 mg. to 12 mg. daily in acute seasonal or perennial *allergic rhinitis.* Intractable cases may require high initial and maintenance doses. In *bronchial asthma,* 8 mg. to 16 mg. daily are usually effective. The usual therapeutic measures for control of bronchial asthma should be carried out in addition to ARISTOCORT therapy. In both allergic rhinitis and bronchial asthma, therapy is directed at alleviation of acute distress and chronic long-term use of corticosteroids is neither desirable nor often essential. Some patients may be maintained on alternate day therapy. In such conditions as *contact dermatitis* and *atopic dermatitis,* topical therapy may be supplemented with short courses of ARISTOCORT by mouth in doses of 8 mg. to 16 mg. daily. In severely ill patients with *serum sickness,* epinephrine may be the drug of choice for immediate therapy, often supplemented by antihistamines. ARISTOCORT is frequently useful as adjunctive treatment in such cases, with the dosage determined by the severity of the disorder, the speed with which therapeutic response is desired and the response of the patient to initial therapy.

6. *Ophthalmological Disease: Allergic conjunctivitis; keratitis; allergic corneal marginal ulcers, iritis* and *iridocyclitis; chorioretinitis; anterior segment inflammation; diffuse posterior uveitis* and *choroiditis; optic neuritis* and *sympathetic ophthalmia.* Initial doses range from 12 mg. to 40 mg. daily depending on the severity of the condition, the nature and degree of involvement of ocular structure, but response is usually rapid and therapy of short-term duration.

7. *Respiratory Diseases: Symptomatic sarcoidosis; Loeffler's Syndrome; berylliosis;* and in certain cases of *fulminating* or *disseminated pulmonary tuberculosis* when concurrently accompanied by appropriate antituberculous chemotherapy. Initial doses are usually in the range of 16 mg. to 48 mg. daily.

8. *Hematologic Disorders: Idiopathic* and *secondary thrombocytopenia* in *adults, acquired (autoimmune) hemolytic anemia; erythroblastopenia (RBC anemia); congenital (erythroid) hypoplastic anemia.* ARISTOCORT is used to produce a remission of symptoms and may, in some instances, produce an apparent regression of abnormal cellular blood elements to normal states, temporary or permanent. The recommended dose varies between 16 mg. and 60 mg. daily, with reduction after adequate clinical response.

9. *Neoplastic Diseases: Acute leukemia in childhood.* The usual dose of ARISTOCORT is 1 mg. per kilogram of body weight daily, although as much as 2 mg. per kilogram may be necessary. Initial response is usually seen within 6 to 21 days and therapy continued from 4 to 6 weeks.
Acute leukemia and *lymphoma in adults.* The usual dose of ARISTOCORT is 16 mg. to 40 mg. daily, although it may be necessary to give as much as 100 mg. daily in leukemia. ARISTOCORT therapy in these neoplasias is only palliative and not curative. Other therapeutic and supportive measures must be used when appropriate.

10. *Edematous States: Nephrotic Syndrome:* ARISTOCORT may be used to induce a diuresis or remission of proteinuria in the *nephrotic syndrome,* without uremia, of the idiopathic type or that due to *lupus erythematosus.* The average dose is 16 to 20 mg. (up to 48 mg.) daily until diuresis occurs. The diuresis may be massive and usually occurs by the 14th day, but occasionally may be delayed. After diuresis begins it is advisable to continue treatment until maximal or complete chemical and clinical remission occurs, at which time the dosage should be reduced gradually and then discontinued. In less severe cases maintenance dosages of as little as 4 mg. daily may be adequate. Alternatively and when maintenance therapy may be prolonged, ARISTOCORT may be administered on alternate-day dose schedules.

11. *Miscellaneous: Tuberculous meningitis:* ARISTOCORT may be useful when accompanied by appropriate antituberculous therapy when there is subarachnoid block or impending block. The average dosage is 32 to 48 mg. daily in either single or divided doses.
[See table below].

How Supplied:
1 mg. Tablets-Scored yellow; Engraved LL A1 bottles of 50 NDC 0005-4409-18.
2 mg. Tablets-Scored pink; Engraved LL A2 bottles of 100 NDC 0005-4405-23.
4 mg. Tablets-Scored white; Engraved LL A4 Bottle of 30 NDC 0005-4406-13; Bottle of 100 NDC-0005-4406-23; Bottle of 500 NDC 0005-4406-31 ARISTO-PAK® 16's Engraved LL 4 (for 6 days' therapy) NDC 0005-4406-07.
8 mg. Tablets-Scored yellow; Engraved LL A8 bottles of 50 NDC 005-4444-18.
16 mg. Tablets-Scored white: Engraved LL A16 bottles of 30 NDC 0005-4416-13.
Syrup 2 mg./5 ml. triamcinolone diacetate; cherry flavored; bottles of 4 fl. oz. Preservatives: Methylparaben 0.08% and Propylparaben 0.02% NDC 0005-4421-58.
A.H.F.S. 68:04
Tablets and ARISTO-PAK 4 mg.
Shown in Product Identification Section, page 414

ARISTOCORT®   R
[a-ris-tō-cort]
triamcinolone acetonide
Topical Products

[See table on next page].
The topical corticosteroids constitute a class of primarily synthetic steroids used as anti-inflammatory and anti-pruritic agents.

Clinical Pharmacology: Topical corticosteroids share anti-inflammatory, anti-pruritic and vasoconstrictive actions.
The mechanism of anti-inflammatory activity of the topical corticosteroids is unclear. Various laboratory methods, including vasoconstrictor assays, are used to compare and predict potencies and/or clinical efficacies of the topical corticosteroids. There is some evidence to suggest that a recognizable correlation exists between vasoconstrictor potency and therapeutic efficacy in man.

Pharmacokinetics
The extent of percutaneous absorption of topical corticosteroids is determined by many factors including the vehicle, the integrity of the epidermal barrier, and the use of occlusive dressings.

Equivalence Table

	Anti-inflammatory Relative Potency		Frequently Used Tablet Strength (mg)		Tablet × Potency Equivalent Value
Hydrocortisone	1	×	20	=	20
Prednisolone	4	×	5	=	20
ARISTOCORT® Triamcinolone	5	×	4	=	20
Dexamethasone	25	×	0.75	=	18.75

Topical corticosteroids can be absorbed from normal intact skin, inflammation and/or other disease processes in the skin increase percutaneous absorption. Occlusive dressings substantially increase the percutaneous absorption of topical corticosteroids. Thus, occlusive dressings may be a valuable therapeutic adjunct for treatment of resistant dermatoses. (See **DOSAGE AND ADMINISTRATION**). Once absorbed through the skin, topical corticosteroids are handled through pharmacokinetic pathways similar to systemically administered corticosteroids. Corticosteroids are bound to plasma proteins in varying degrees. Corticosteroids are metabolized primarily in the liver and are then excreted by the kidneys. Some of the topical corticosteroids and their metabolites are also excreted into the bile.

Indications and Usage: Topical corticosteroids are indicated for the relief of the inflammatory and pruritic manifestations of corticosteroid-responsive dermatoses.

Contraindications: Topical corticosteroids are contraindicated in those patients with a history of hypersensitivity to any of the components of the preparation.

Precautions:
General
Systemic absorption of topical corticosteroids has produced reversible hypothalamic-pituitary-adrenal (HPA) axis suppression, manifestations of Cushing's syndrome, hyperglycemia, and glucosuria in some patients

Conditions which augment systemic absorption include the application of the more potent steroids, use over large surface areas, prolonged use, and the addition of occlusive dressings.

Therefore, patients receiving a large dose of a potent topical steroid applied to a large surface area or under an occlusive dressing should be evaluated periodically for evidence of HPA axis suppression by using the urinary free cortisol and ACTH stimulation tests. If HPA axis suppression is noted, an attempt should be made to withdraw the drug, to reduce the frequency of application, or to substitute a less potent steroid.

Recovery of HPA axis function is generally prompt and complete upon discontinuation of the drug. Infrequently, signs and symptoms of steroid withdrawal may occur, requiring supplemental systemic corticosteroids.

Children may absorb proportionally larger amounts of topical corticosteroids and thus be more susceptible to systemic toxicity. (See **PRECAUTIONS-Pediatric Use**).

If irritation develops, topical corticosteroids should be discontinued and appropriate therapy instituted.

In the presence of dermatological infections, the use of an appropriate antifungal or antibacterial agent should be instituted. If a favorable response does not occur promptly, the corticosteroid should be discontinued until the infection has been adequately controlled.

Information for the Patient
Patients using topical corticosteroids should receive the following information and instructions:
1. This medication is to be used as directed by the physician. It is for external use only. Avoid contact with the eyes.
2. Patients should be advised not to use this medication for any disorder other than for which it was prescribed.
3. The treated skin area should not be bandaged or otherwise covered or wrapped as to be occlusive unless directed by the physician.
4. Patients should report any signs of local adverse reactions especially upon occlusive dressing.
5. Parents of pediatric patients should be advised not to use tight-fitting diapers or plastic pants on a child being treated in the diaper area, as these garments may constitute occlusive dressings.

Laboratory Tests
The following tests may be helpful in evaluating the HPA axis suppression:

Urinary free cortisol test
ACTH stimulation test

Carcinogenesis, Mutagenesis, and Impairment of Fertility
Long-term animal studies have not been performed to evaluate the carcinogenic potential or the effect on fertility of topical corticosteroids. Studies to determine mutagenicity with prednisolone and hydrocortisone have revealed negative results.

Pregnancy Category C
Corticosteroids are generally teratogenic in laboratory animals when administered systemically at relatively low dosage levels. The more potent corticosteroids have been shown to be teratogenic after dermal application in laboratory animals. There are no adequate and well-controlled studies in pregnant women on teratogenic effects from topically applied corticosteroids. Therefore, topical corticosteroids should be used during pregnancy only if the potential benefit justifies the potential risk to the fetus. Drugs of this class should not be used extensively on pregnant patients, in large amounts, or for prolonged periods of time.

Nursing Mothers
It is not known whether topical administration of corticosteroids could result in sufficient systemic absorption to produce detectable quantities in breast milk. Systemically administered corticosteroids are secreted into breast milk in quantities *not* likely to have a deleterious effect on the infant. Nevertheless, caution should be exercised when topical corticosteroids are administered to a nursing woman.

Pediatric Use
Pediatric patients may demonstrate greater susceptibility to topical corticosteroid-induced HPA axis suppression and Cushing's syndrome than mature patients because of a larger skin surface area to body weight ratio. Hypothalamic-pituitary-adrenal (HPA) axis suppression, Cushing's syndrome, and intracranial hypertension have been reported in children receiving topical corticosteroids. Manifestations of adrenal suppression in children include linear growth retardation, delayed weight gain, low plasma cortiso levels, and absence of response to ACTH stimulation. Manifestations of intracranial hypertension include bulging fontanelles, headaches, and bilateral papilledema.

Administration of topical corticosteroids to children should be limited to the least amount compatible with an effective therapeutic regimen. Chronic corticosteroid therapy may interfere with the growth and development of children.

Adverse Reactions: The following local adverse reactions are reported infrequently with topical corticosteroids, but may occur more frequently with the use of occlusive dressings. These reactions are listed in an approximate decreasing order of occurrence:

Burning
Itching
Irritation
Dryness
Folliculitis
Hypertrichosis
Acneiform eruptions
Hypopigmentation

Perioral dermatitis
Allergic contact dermatitis
Maceration of the skin
Secondary infection
Skin Atrophy
Striae
Miliaria

Overdosage: Topically applied corticosteroids can be absorbed in sufficient amounts to produce systemic effects (See **PRECAUTIONS**).

How Supplied:
Cream 0.025%
15 gram tubes—NDC 0005-5130-09
60 gram tubes—NDC 0005-5130-40
240 gram jars—NDC 0005-5130-57
5.25 lb. jars—NDC 0005-5130-54
Cream 0.1%
15 gram tubes—NDC 0005-5131-09
60 gram tubes—NDC 0005-5131-40
240 gram jars—NDC 0005-5131-57
5.25 lb. jars—NDC 0005-5131-54
Cream 0.5%
15 gram tubes—NDC 0005-5132-09
240 gram jars—NDC 0005-5132-57
Ointment 0.1%
15 gram tubes—NDC 0005-5175-09
60 gram tubes—NDC 0005-5175-40
240 gram jars—NDC 0005-5175-57
5 lb. jars—NDC 0005-5175-70
Ointment 0.5%
15 gram tubes—NDC 0005-5178-09
240 gram jars—NDC 00055-5178-57
Store at Controlled Room Temperature 15–30° C (59–86°F)
Shown in Product Identification Section, page 414

Suspensions
ARISTOCORT®   ℞
[*a-ris-tō-cort*]
triamcinolone diacetate
Forte parenteral
Intralesional

NOT FOR INTRAVENOUS USE

FORTE PARENTERAL:
Description: A suspension of 40 mg./ml. of *triamcinolone diacetate* micronized in:

Continued on next page

The information on each product appearing here is based on labelling effective in August, 1984 and is either the entire official brochure or an accurate condensation therefrom. Information concerning all Lederle products may be obtained from the Professional Services Department, Lederle Laboratories, Pearl River, New York, 10965.

ARISTOCORT® Triamcinolone Acetonide TOPICAL PRODUCTS

	Cream 0.025%	Cream 0.1%	Cream 0.5%	Ointment 0.1%	Ointment 0.5%
Each gram contains Triamcinolone Acetonide	0.25 mg.	1 mg.	5 mg.	1 mg.	5 mg.
Preservatives: Sorbic Acid	0.1%	0.1%	0.1%		
Potassium Sorbate	0.1%	0.1%	0.1%		
Inactive Ingredients:	In a water base: Mono and Diglycerides, Squalane NF, Polysorbate 80 Cetyl Esters Wax, Polysorbate 60, Stearyl Alcohol, Tenox II, and Sorbitol Solution USP			white Petrolatum	
Dosage and Administration	Apply to the affected areas 3 or 4 times daily. The cream should be rubbed in gently and thoroughly until it disappears.			Apply to the affected areas 3 or 4 times daily.	

Lederle—Cont.

Polysorbate 80 NF 0.20%
Polyethylene Glycol 4000 NF 3%
Sodium Chloride..0.85%
Benzyl Alcohol...0.90%
Water for Injection q.s.....................................100%
Hydrochloric Acid and Sodium Hydroxide to approx. pH 6

This preparation is a slightly soluble suspension suitable for parenteral administration through a 24-gauge needle (or larger), but NOT suitable for intravenous use. It may be administered by the intramuscular, intra-articular, or intrasynovial routes, depending upon the situation. The response to each glucocorticoid varies considerably with each type of disease indication and each corticosteroid prescribed. Irreversible clumping occurs when product is frozen.

Chemically Triamcinolone Diacetate NF is Pregna -1, 4-diene-3, 20-dione, 16, 21-bis-(acetyloxy)-9 fluoro-11, 17-dihydroxy-, $(11\beta, 16\alpha)$ - 9 - Fluoro-11β, 16α, 17,21-tetrahydroxy- pregna-1, 4-diene-3, 20-dione 16, 21-diacetate. Molecular weight is 478.51.

Action: ARISTOCORT is primarily glucocorticoid in action and has potent anti-inflammatory, hormonal and metabolic effects common to cortisone-like drugs. It is essentially devoid of mineralocorticoid activity when administered in therapeutic doses, causing little or no sodium retention, with potassium excretion minimal or absent. The body's immune responses to diverse stimuli is also modified by its action.

Indications: Where oral therapy is not feasible or temporarily desirable in the judgment of the physician, ARISTOCORT *triamcinolone diacetate* FORTE 40 mg./ml. is indicated for intramuscular use as follows:

1. Endocrine disorders.
   Primary or secondary adrenocortical insufficiency (hydrocortisone or cortisone is the drug of choice; synthetic analogs may be used in conjunction with mineralocorticoids where applicable; in infancy, mineralocorticoid supplementation is of particular importance).
   Preoperatively and in the event of serious trauma or illness, in patients with known adrenal insufficiency or when adrenocortical reserve is doubtful.
   Congenital adrenal hyperplasia.
   Nonsuppurative thyroiditis.
   Hypercalcemia associated with cancer.
2. Rheumatic disorders. As adjunctive therapy for short-term administration to tide the patient over an acute episode or exacerbation) in:
   Post-traumatic osteoarthritis.
   Synovitis of osteoarthritis.
   Rheumatoid arthritis including juvenile rheumatoid arthritis (selected cases may require low-dose maintenance therapy).
   Acute and subacute bursitis.
   Epicondylitis.
   Acute nonspecific tenosynovitis.
   Acute gouty arthritis.
   Psoriatic arthritis.
   Ankylosing spondylitis.
3. Collagen diseases. During an exacerbation or as maintenance therapy in selected cases of:
   Systemic lupus erythematosus.
   Acute rheumatic carditis.
4. Dermatologic diseases. Pemphigus.
   Severe erythema multiforme (Stevens-Johnson syndrome).
   Exfoliative dermatitis.
   Bullous dermatitis herpetiformis.
   Severe seborrheic dermatitis.
   Severe psoriasis.
   Mycosis fungoides.
5. Allergic states. Control of severe or incapacitating allergic conditions intractable to adequate trials of conventional treatment in:
   Bronchial asthma.
   Contact dermatitis.
   Seasonal or perennial allergic rhinitis.
   Drug hypersensitivity reactions.
   Urticarial transfusion reactions.
   Atopic dermatitis.
   Serum sickness.
   Acute noninfectious laryngeal edema (epinephrine is the drug of first choice).
6. Ophthalmic diseases. Severe acute and chronic allergic and inflammatory processes involving the eye, such as:
   Herpes zoster ophthalmicus.
   Iritis, iridocyclitis.
   Chorioretinitis.
   Sympathetic ophthalmia.
   Diffuse posterior uveitis and choroiditis.
   Optic neuritis.
   Keratitis.
   Allergic conjunctivitis.
   Allergic corneal marginal ulcers.
7. Gastrointestinal diseases. To tide the patient over a critical period of disease in:
   Ulcerative colitis - (Systemic therapy).
   Regional enteritis - (Systemic therapy).
8. Respiratory diseases.
   Symptomatic sarcoidosis.
   Berylliosis.
   Fulminating or disseminated pulmonary tuberculosis when used concurrently with appropriate antituberculous chemotherapy.
   Aspiration pneumonitis.
   Loeffler's syndrome not manageable by other means.
9. Hematologic disorders.
   Acquired (autoimmune) hemolytic anemia.
   Secondary thrombocytopenia in adults.
   Erythroblastopenia (RBC anemia).
   Congenital (erythroid) hypoplastic anemia.
10. Neoplastic diseases. For palliative management of:
    Leukemias and lymphomas in adults.
    Acute leukemia of childhood.
11. Edematous state. To induce diuresis or remission of proteinuria in the nephrotic syndrome, without uremia, of the idiopathic type or that due to lupus erythematosus.
12. Nervous System.
    Acute exacerbations of multiple sclerosis.
13. Miscellaneous. Tuberculosis meningitis with subarachnoid block or impending block when used concurrently with appropriate antituberculous chemotherapy.
    Trichinosis with neurologic or myocardial involvement.

ARISTOCORT *triamcinolone diacetate* FORTE 40 mg./ml. is indicated for intra-articular or soft tissue use as follows:

As adjunctive therapy for short-term administration (to tide the patient over an acute episode or exacerbation) in:
   Synovitis of osteoarthritis.
   Rheumatoid arthritis.
   Acute and subacute bursitis.
   Acute gouty arthritis.
   Epicondylitis.
   Acute nonspecific tenosynovitis.
   Post-traumatic osteoarthritis.

ARISTOCORT FORTE is indicated for intralesional use as follows:
   Keloids
   Localized hypertrophic, infiltrated, inflammatory lesions of: lichen planus, psoriatic plaques, granuloma annulare and lichen simplex chronicus (neurodermatitis).
   Discoid lupus erythematosus.
   Necrobiosis lipoidica diabeticorum.
   Alopecia areata.
   It may also be useful in cystic tumors of an aponeurosis or tendon (ganglia).

INTRALESIONAL:
Description: ARISTOCORT *triamcinolone diacetate*, 9α fluoro 16α hydroxy prednisolone diacetate possesses glucocorticoid properties while being essentially devoid of mineralocorticoid activity thus causing little or no sodium retention.

A suspension of 25 mg./ml. micronized in:
Polysorbate 80 USP 0.20%
Polyethylene Glycol 4000 USP 3%
Sodium Chloride..0.85%
Benzyl Alcohol...0.90%
Water for Injection q.s.....................................100%
Hydrochloric Acid to approx. pH 6

Chemically triamcinolone diacetate NF is Pregna 1, 4 - diene - 3, 20 - dione, 16, 21 - bis - (acetyloxy) - 9 fluoro - 11, 17-dihydroxy-,$(11\beta, 16\alpha)$- or 9-Fluoro-11β, 16α, 17, 21-tetrahydro- xypregna-1, 4-diene-3,20-dione 16,21-diacetate. Molecular weight is 478.51.

Actions: Naturally occurring glucocorticoids (hydrocortisone), which also have salt-retaining properties, are used as replacement therapy in adrenocortical deficiency states. Their synthetic analogs are primarily used for their potent anti-inflammatory effects in disorders of many organ systems. Glucocorticoids cause profound and varied metabolic effects. In addition, they modify the body's immune responses to diverse stimuli.

Indications: ARISTOCORT INTRALESION- AL is indicated by the intralesional route for:
   Keloids
   Localized hypertrophic, infiltrated, inflammatory lesions of:
   lichen planus, psoriatic plaques, granuloma annulare and lichen simplex chronicus (neurodermatitis).
   Discoid lupus erythematosus.
   Necrobiosis lipoidica diabeticorum.
   Alopecia areata.
It may also be useful in cystic tumors of an aponeurosis or tendon (ganglia).

When used intra-articularly it is also indicated for: Adjunctive therapy for short-term administration (to tide the patient over an acute episode or exacerbation) in:
   Synovitis of osteoarthritis.
   Rheumatoid arthritis.
   Acute and subacute bursitis.
   Acute gouty arthritis.
   Epicondylitis.
   Acute nonspecific tenosynovitis.
   Post-traumatic osteoarthritis.

FORTE AND INTRALESIONAL:
Contraindications: Systemic fungal infections.
Warnings: In patients on corticosteroid therapy subjected to any unusual stress, increased dosage of rapidly acting corticosteroids before, during, and after the stressful situation is indicated. Corticosteroids may mask some signs of infection, and new infections may appear during their use. There may be decreased resistance and inability to localize infection when corticosteroids are used. Prolonged use of corticosteroids may produce posterior subcapsular cataracts, glaucoma with possible damage to the optic nerves, and may enhance the establishment of secondary ocular infections due to fungi or viruses.

Usage in pregnancy
Since adequate human reproduction studies have not been done with corticosteroids, the use of these drugs in pregnancy, nursing mothers, or women of childbearing potential requires that the possible benefits of the drug be weighed against the potential hazards to the mother and embryo or fetus. Infants born of mothers who have received substantial doses of corticosteroids during pregnancy should be carefully observed for signs of hypoadrenalism.

Average and large doses of cortisone or hydrocortisone can cause elevation of blood pressure, salt and water retention, and increased excretion of potassium. These effects are less likely to occur with the synthetic derivatives except when used in large doses. Dietary salt restriction and potassium supplementation may be necessary. All corticosteroids increase calcium excretion.

While on Corticosteroid Therapy Patients Should Not Be Vaccinated Against Smallpox. Other Immunization Procedures Should Not Be Undertaken in Patients Who Are on Corticosteroids, Especially in High Doses, Because of Possible Hazards of Neurological Complications and Lack of Antibody Response.

The use of ARISTOCORT *triamcinolone diacetate* in active tuberculosis should be restricted to those cases of fulminating or disseminated tuberculosis in which the corticosteroid is used for the management of the disease in conjunction with appropriate antituberculous regimen.

If corticosteroids are indicated in patients with latent tuberculosis or tuberculin reactivity, close observation is necessary as reactivation of the disease may occur. During prolonged corticosteroid therapy, these patients should receive chemoprophylaxis.

Because rare instances of anaphylactoid reactions have occurred in patients receiving parenteral corticosteroid therapy, appropriate precautionary measures should be taken prior to administration, especially when the patient has a history of allergy to any drug.

Postinjection flare (following intra-articular) and Charcot-like arthropathy have been associated with parenteral corticosteroid therapy.

Intralesional or Sublesional injection of excessive dosage whether by single or multiple injection into any given area may cause cutaneous or subcutaneous atrophy.

Precautions: Drug-induced secondary adrenocortical insufficiency may be minimized by gradual reduction of dosage. This type of relative insufficiency may persist for months after discontinuation of therapy; therefore, in any situation of stress occurring during that period, hormone therapy should be reinstituted. Since mineralocorticoid secretion may be impaired, salt and/or a mineralocorticoid should be administered concurrently.

There is an enhanced effect of corticosteroids in patients with hypothyroidism and in those with cirrhosis.

Corticosteroids should be used cautiously in patients with ocular herpes simplex for fear of corneal perforation.

The lowest possible dose of corticosteroid should be used to control the condition under treatment, and when reduction in dosage is possible, the reduction must be gradual.

Psychic derangements may appear when corticosteroids are used, ranging from euphoria, insomnia, mood swings, personality changes, and severe depression to frank psychotic manifestations. Also, existing emotional instability or psychotic tendencies may be aggravated by corticosteroids.

Aspirin should be used cautiously in conjunction with corticosteroids in hypoprothrombinemia.

Steroids should be used with caution in nonspecific ulcerative colitis, if there is a probability of impending perforation, abscess or other pyogenic infection, also in diverticulitis, fresh intestinal anastomoses, active or latent peptic ulcer, renal insufficiency, hypertension, osteoporosis, and myasthenia gravis.

Growth and development of infants and children on prolonged corticosteroid therapy should be carefully followed.

The following additional precautions apply for parenteral corticosteroids. Intra-articular injection of a corticosteroid may produce systemic as well as local effects.

Appropriate examination of any joint fluid present is necessary to exclude a septic process.

A marked increase in pain accompanied by local swelling, further restriction of joint motion, fever, and malaise are suggestive of septic arthritis. If this complication occurs and the diagnosis of sepsis is confirmed, appropriate antimicrobial therapy should be instituted.

Local injection of a steroid into a previously infected joint is to be avoided.

Corticosteroids should not be injected into unstable joints.

The slower rate of absorption by intramuscular administration should be recognized.

Routine laboratory studies, such as urinalysis, two-hour postprandial blood sugar, determination of blood pressure and body weight, and a chest x-ray should be made at regular intervals during prolonged therapy. Upper GI x-rays are desirable in patients with an ulcer history or significant dyspepsia.

Accidental injection into soft tissue during intra-articular administration decreases local effectiveness in the joint and, by increasing rate of absorption, may produce systemic effects.

Although controlled clinical trials have shown corticosteroids to be effective in speeding the resolution of acute exacerbations of multiple sclerosis they do not show that they affect the ultimate outcome or natural history of the disease. The studies do show that relatively high doses of corticosteroids are necessary to demonstrate a significant effect. (See Dosage and Administration).

Since complications of treatment with glucocorticoid are dependent on the size of the dose and the duration of treatment a risk/benefit decision must be made in each individual case as to dose and duration of treatment and as to whether daily or intermittent therapy should be used.

Adverse Reactions:
Fluid and electrolyte disturbances:
  Sodium retention.
  Fluid retention.
  Congestive heart failure in susceptible patients.
  Potassium loss.
  Hypokalemic alkalosis.
  Hypertension.
Musculoskeletal:
  Muscle weakness.
  Steroid myopathy.
  Loss of muscle mass.
  Osteoporosis.
  Vertebral compression fractures.
  Aseptic necrosis of femoral and humeral heads.
  Pathologic fracture of long bones.
Gastrointestinal:
  Peptic ulcer with possible subsequent perforation and hemorrhage.
  Pancreatitis.
  Abdominal distention.
  Ulcerative esophagitis.
Dermatologic:
  Impaired wound healing.
  Thin fragile skin.
  Petechiae and ecchymoses.
  Facial erythema.
  Increased sweating.
  May suppress reactions to skin tests.
Neurological:
  Increased intracranial pressure with papilledema (pseudotumor cerebri) usually after treatment.
  Convulsions.
  Vertigo.
  Headache.
Endocrine:
  Menstrual irregularities.
  Development of Cushingoid state.
  Suppression of growth in children.
  Secondary adrenocortical and pituitary unresponsiveness, particularly in times of stress, as in trauma, surgery, or illness.
  Decreased carbohydrate tolerance.
  Manifestations of latent diabetes mellitus.
  Increased requirements for insulin or oral hypoglycemic agents in diabetics.
Ophthalmic:
  Posterior subcapsular cataracts.
  Increased intraocular pressure.
  Glaucoma.
  Exophthalmos.
Metabolic:
  Negative nitrogen balance due to protein catabolism.

The following additional adverse reactions are related to parenteral and intralesional corticosteroid therapy:
  Rare instances of blindness associated with intralesional therapy around the orbit or intranasally.
  Hyperpigmentation or hypopigmentation.
  Subcutaneous and cutaneous atrophy.
  Sterile abscess.

Dosage and Administration:
General
The initial dosage of ARISTOCORT *triamcinolone diacetate* may vary from 3 to 48 mg. per day depending on the specific disease entity being treated. In situations of less severity, lower doses will generally suffice while in selected patients higher initial doses may be required. Usually the parenteral dosage ranges are one-third to one-half the oral dose given every 12 hours. However, in certain overwhelming, acute, life-threatening situations, administration in dosages exceeding the usual dosages may be justified and may be in multiples of the oral dosages.

The initial dosage should be maintained or adjusted until a satisfactory response is noted. If after a reasonable period of time there is a lack of satisfactory clinical response, ARISTOCORT *triamcinolone diacetate* should be discontinued and the patient transferred to other appropriate therapy. It Should Be Emphasized That Dosage Requirements Are Variable and Must Be Individualized on the Basis of the Disease Under Treatment and the Response of the Patient. After a favorable response is noted, the proper maintenance dosage should be determined by decreasing the initial drug dosage in small increments at appropriate time intervals until the lowest dosage which will maintain an adequate clinical response is reached. It should be kept in mind that constant monitoring is needed in regard to drug dosage. Included in the situations which may make dosage adjustments necessary are changes in clinical status secondary to remissions or exacerbations in the disease process, the patient's individual drug responsiveness, and the effect of patient exposure to stressful situations not directly related to the disease entity under treatment; in this latter situation, it may be necessary to increase the dosage of ARISTOCORT *triamcinolone diacetate* for a period of time consistent with the patient's condition. If after long-term therapy the drug is to be stopped, it is recommended that it be withdrawn gradually rather than abruptly.

For intra-articular, intralesional and soft tissue use, a lesser initial dosage range of Triamcinolone Diacetate may produce the desired effect when the drug is administered to provide a localized concentration. The site of the injection and the volume of the injection should be carefully considered when Triamcinolone Diacetate is administered for this purpose.

Specific
Forte:
ARISTOCORT FORTE Parenteral is a suspension of 40 mg./ml. of *triamcinolone diacetate*. The full-strength suspension may be employed. If preferred, the suspension may be diluted with normal saline or water. The diluent may also be prepared by mixing equal parts of normal saline and 1% procaine hydrochloride or other similar local anesthetics. The use of diluents containing preservatives such as methylparaben, propylparaben, phenol, etc. must be avoided as these preparations tend to cause flocculation of the steroid. These dilutions retain full potency for at least one week. Topical ethyl chloride spray may be used locally prior to injection.

Intramuscular: Although ARISTOCORT FORTE Parenteral may be administered intramuscularly for initial therapy, most physicians prefer to adjust the dose orally until adequate control is attained. Intramuscular administration provides a sustained or depot action which can be used to supplement or replace initial oral therapy. With intramuscular therapy, greater supervision of the amount of steroid used is made possible in the patient who is inconsistent in following an oral dosage schedule. In maintenance therapy, the patient-to-patient response is not uniform and, therefore, the dose must be individualized for optimal control.

Although triamcinolone diacetate may possess greater anti-inflammatory potency than many glucocorticoids, this is only dose-related since side effects, such as osteoporosis, peptic ulcer, etc. related to glucocorticoid activity, have not been diminished.

Continued on next page

The information on each product appearing here is based on labelling effective in August, 1984 and is either the entire official brochure or an accurate condensation therefrom. Information concerning all Lederle products may be obtained from the Professional Services Department, Lederle Laboratories, Pearl River, New York, 10965.

Lederle—Cont.

The average dose is 40 mg. (1 ml.) administered intramuscularly once a week for conditions in which anti-inflammatory action is desired.
In general, a single parenteral dose 4 to 7 times the oral daily dose may be expected to control the patient from 4 to 7 days up to 3 to 4 weeks. Dosage should be adjusted to the point where adequate but not necessarily complete relief of symptoms is obtained.
Intra-Articular and Intrasynovial: The usual dose varies from 5 to 40 mg. The average for the knee, for example, is 25 mg. The duration of effect varies from one week to 2 months. However, acutely inflamed joints may require more frequent injections.
A lesser initial dosage range of Triamcinolone Diacetate may produce the desired effect when the drug is administered to provide a localized concentration. The site of the injection and the volume of the injection should be carefully considered when Triamcinolone Diacetate is administered for this purpose.
A specific dose depends largely on the size of the joint.
Strict surgical asepsis is mandatory. The physician should be familiar with anatomical relationships as described in standard text books. ARISTOCORT FORTE Parenteral may be used in any accessible joint except the intervertebrals. In general, intrasynovial therapy is suggested under the following circumstances:
1. When systemic steroid therapy is contraindicated because of side effects such as peptic ulcer.
2. When it is desirable to secure relief in one or two specific joints.
3. When good systemic maintenance fails to control flare-ups in a few joints and it is desirable to secure relief without increasing oral therapy.

Such treatment should not be considered to constitute a cure; although this method will ameliorate the joint symptoms, it does not preclude the need for the conventional measures usually employed.
It is suggested that infiltration of the soft tissue by local anesthetic precede intra-articular injection. A 24-gauge or larger needle on a dry syringe may be inserted into the joint and excess fluid aspirated. For the first few hours following injection, there may be local discomfort in the joint but this is usually followed rapidly by effective relief of pain and improvement in local function.
[See table below].
Intralesional
When ARISTOCORT INTRALESIONAL is administered by injection strict aseptic technique is mandatory. Full strength suspensions may be employed, or if preferred, the suspension may be diluted, either to a 1:1 or 1:10 concentration, thus obtaining a working concentration of 12.5 mg./ml. or approximately 2.5 mg./ml. respectively. Normal (isotonic) saline solution alone or equal parts of normal (isotonic) saline solution and 1% procaine or other local anesthetics, may be used as diluents. These dilutions usually retain full potency for at least one week. Topical ethyl chloride spray may be used as a local anesthetic. The use of diluents containing preservatives such as methylparaben, propylparaben, phenol, etc. must be avoided as these preparations tend to cause flocculations of the steroid.
Intralesional or Sublesional: For small lesions, injection is usually well tolerated and a local anesthetic is not necessary. The location and type of lesion will determine the route of injection: intralesional, sublesional, intradermal, subdermal, intracutaneous, or subcutaneous. The size of the lesion will determine: the total amount of drug needed, the concentration used, and the number and pattern of injection sites utilized (e.g. from a total of 5 mg. ARISTOCORT INTRALESIONAL in a 2 ml. volume divided over several locations in small lesions, ranging up to 48 mg. total ARISTOCORT INTRALESIONAL for large psoriatic plaques). Avoid injecting too superficially. In general, no more than 12.5 mg. per injection site should be used. An average of 25 mg. is the usual limit for any one lesion. Large areas require multiple injections with smaller doses per injection.
For a majority of conditions, sublesional injection directly through the lesion into the deep dermal tissue is suggested. In cases where it is difficult to inject intradermally, the suspension may be introduced subcutaneously, as superficially as possible.
Two or three injections at one to two week intervals may suffice as an average course of treatment for many conditions. Within 5-7 days after initial injection involution of the lesion can usually be seen, with pronounced clearing towards normal tissue after 12-14 days. Multiple injections of small amounts of equal strength may be convenient in alopecia areata and in psoriasis where there are large or confluent lesions. This is best accomplished by a series of fan-like injections ½ to 1 inch apart.
Alopecia areata and totalis require an average dose of 25 mg. to 30 mg. in a concentration of 10 mg./ml. subcutaneously 1 to 2 times a week, to stimulate hair regrowth. Results may be expected in 3 to 6 weeks on this dosage, and hair growth may last 3-6 months after initial injection. No more than 0.5 ml. should be given in any one site, because excessive deposition may produce local skin atrophy. Continued periodic local injections may be necessary to maintain response and continued hair growth. Use of more dilute solutions diminish the incidence and degree of local atrophy in the injection site.
In keloids and similar dense scars, injections are usually made directly into the lesion.
Injections may be repeated as required, but probably a total of no more than 75 mg. of ARISTOCORT *triamcinolone* a week should be given to any one patient. The need for repeated injections is best determined by clinical response. Remissions may be expected to last from a few weeks up to eleven months.
Intra-articular or Intrasynovial: Strict surgical asepsis is mandatory. The physician should be familiar with anatomical relationships as described in standard text books. A recent paper details the anatomy and the technical approach in arthrocentesis.
It is usually recommended that infiltration by local anesthetic of the soft tissue precede intra-articular injection. A 22-gauge or larger needle on a dry syringe should be inserted into the joint and excess fluid if present should be aspirated. The specific dose depends primarily on the size of the joint. The usual dose varies from 5 mg. to 40 mg. with the average for the knee being 25 mg. Smaller joints as in the fingers require 2 mg. to 5 mg. The duration of effect varies from one week to two months. However, acutely inflamed joints may require more frequent injections. Accidental injection into soft tissue is usually not harmful but decreases the local effectiveness and, because the drug is more rapidly absorbed, may produce a systemic effect. Injection into subcutaneous lipoid tissue may produce "pseudo-atrophy" with a persistent depression of the overlying dermis, lasting several weeks or months.
Administration and dosage of ARISTOCORT INTRALESIONAL must be individualized according to the nature, severity and chronicity of the disease or disorder treated, and should be undertaken with a view of the patient's entire clinical condition. Corticosteroid therapy is considered an adjunct to and not usually a replacement for conventional therapy. Therapy with ARISTOCORT INTRALESIONAL, as with all steroids, is of the suppressive type, related to its anti-inflammatory effect. The dose should be regulated during therapy according to the degree of therapeutic response, and should be reduced gradually to maintenance levels, whereby the patient obtains adequate or acceptable control of symptoms. When such control occurs, consideration should be given to gradual decrease in dosage and eventual cessation of therapy. Remission of symptoms may be due to therapy or may be spontaneous and a therapeutic test of gradual withdrawal of steroid treatment is usually indicated.
How Supplied:
*Intralesional: (25 mg./ml.); 5 ml. Vials NDC 0005-4422-31.
*Forte: (40 mg./ml.); 1 ml. and 5 ml. Vials NDC 0005-4450-24, NDC 0005-4450-31.
*Manufactured for
LEDERLE LABORATORIES DIVISION
American Cyanamid Company
Pearl River, NY 10965
by
LEDERLE PARENTERALS INC.
Carolina, Puerto Rico 00630

ARISTOCORT A® ℞
[a-ris-tō-cort]
Triamcinolone Acetonide Cream
ARISTOCORT A® ℞
Triamcinolone Acetonide Ointment

Description: Each gram of 0.025% Cream contains 0.25 mg of the highly active steroid, Triamcinolone Acetonide (a derivative of triamcinolone); each gram of 0.1% Cream contains 1 mg Triamcinolone Acetonide; each gram of 0.5% Cream contains 5 mg of Triamcinolone Acetonide; all in AQUATAIN™, a specially formulated cream base composed of emulsifying wax NF, isopropyl palmitate, glycerin USP, sorbitol solution USP, lactic acid, 2% benzyl alcohol, and purified water. AQUATAIN is non-staining, water-washable, paraben-free, spermaceti-free, and has a light texture and consistency.
Each gram of 0.1% Ointment contains 1 mg Triamcinolone Acetonide; each gram of 0.5% Ointment contains 5 mg Triamcinolone Acetonide; both in a specially formulated ointment base composed of emulsifying wax NF, white petrolatum, and propylene glycol, Tenox II (butylated hydroxyanisole, propyl gallate, citric acid, propylene glycol) and lactic acid.
The topical corticosteroids constitute a class of primarily synthetic steroids used as anti-inflammatory and anti-pruritic agents.
Clinical Pharmacology: Topical corticosteroids share anti-inflammatory, anti-pruritic and vasoconstrictive actions.
The mechanism of anti-inflammatory activity of the topical corticosteroids is unclear. Various laboratory methods, including vasoconstrictor assays, are used to compare and predict potencies and/or clinical efficacies of the topical corticosteroids. There is some evidence to suggest that a recognizable correlation exists between vasoconstrictor potency and therapeutic efficacy in man.
Pharmacokinetics: The extent of percutaneous absorption of topical corticosteroids is determined by many factors including the vehicle, the integrity of the epidermal barrier, and the use of occlusive dressings.
Topical corticosteroids can be absorbed from normal intact skin. Inflammation and/or other disease processes in the skin increase percutaneous absorption. Occlusive dressings substantially increase the percutaneous absorption of topical corticosteroids. Thus, occlusive dressings may be a

Equivalence Table

	Anti-inflammatory Relative Potency		Frequently Used Tablet Strength (mg)		Tablet × Potency Equivalent Value
Hydrocortisone	1	×	20	=	20
Prednisolone	4	×	5	=	20
ARISTOCORT® triamcinolone	5	×	4	=	20
Dexamethasone	25	×	0.75	=	18.75

valuable therapeutic adjunct for treatment of resistant dermatoses. (See *DOSAGE AND ADMINISTRATION*).

Once absorbed through the skin, topical corticosteroids are handled through pharmacokinetic pathways similar to systemically administered corticosteroids. Corticosteroids are bound to plasma proteins in varying degrees.

Corticosteroids are metabolized primarily in the liver and are then excreted by the kidneys. Some of the topical corticosteroids and their metabolites are also excreted into the bile.

Indications and Usage: Topical corticosteroids are indicated for the relief of the inflammatory and pruritic manifestations of corticosteroids-responsive dermatoses.

Contraindications: Topical corticosteroids are contraindicated in those patients with a history of hypersensitivity to any of the components of the preparation.

Precautions: *General:* Systemic absorption of topical corticosteroids has produced reversible hypothalamic-pituitary-adrenal (HPA) axis suppression, manifestations of Cushing's syndrome, hyperglycemia, and glucosuria in some patients. Conditions which augment systemic absorption include the application of the more potent steroids, use over large surface areas, prolonged use, and the addition of occlusive dressings.

Therefore, patients receiving a large dose of a potent topical steroid applied to a large surface area or under an occlusive dressing should be evaluated periodically for evidence of HPA axis suppression by using the urinary free cortisol and ACTH stimulation tests. If HPA axis suppression is noted, an attempt should be made to withdraw the drug, to reduce the frequency of application, or to substitute a less potent steroid.

Recovery of HPA axis function is generally prompt and complete upon discontinuation of the drug. Infrequently, signs and symptoms of steroid withdrawal may occur, requiring supplemental systemic corticosteroids.

Children may absorb proportionally larger amounts of topical corticosteroids and thus be more susceptible to systemic toxicity. (See *PRECAUTIONS—Pediatric Use*).

If irritation develops, topical corticosteroids should be discontinued and appropriate therapy instituted.

In the presence of dermatological infections, the use of an appropriate antifungal or antibacterial agent should be instituted. If a favorable response does not occur promptly, the corticosteroid should be discontinued until the infection has been adequately controlled.

Information for the Patient: Patients using topical corticosteroids should receive the following information and instructions:

1. This medication is to be used as directed by the physician. It is for external use only. Avoid contact with the eyes.
2. Patients should be advised not to use the medication for any disorder other than for which it was prescribed.
3. The treated skin area should not be bandaged or otherwise covered or wrapped as to be occlusive unless directed by the physician.
4. Patients should report any signs of local adverse reactions especially under occlusive dressing.
5. Parents of pediatric patients should be advised not to use tight-fitting diapers or plastic pants on a child being treated in the diaper area, as these garments may constitute occlusive dressings.

Laboratory Tests: The following tests may be helpful in evaluating the HPA axis suppression:
Urinary free cortisol test
ACTH stimulation test

Carcinogenesis, Mutagenesis, and Impairment of Fertility: Long-term animal studies have not been performed to evaluate the carcinogenic potential or the effect on fertility of topical corticosteroids.

Studies to determine mutagenicity with prednisolone and hydrocortisone have revealed negative results.

Pregnancy Category C: Corticosteroids are generally teratogenic in laboratory animals when administered systemically at relatively low dosage levels. The more potent corticosteroids have been shown to be teratogenic after dermal application in laboratory animals. There are no adequate and well-controlled studies in pregnant women on teratogenic effects from topically applied corticosteroids. Therefore, topical corticosteroids should be used during pregnancy only if the potential benefit justifies the potential risk to the fetus. Drugs of this class should not be used extensively on pregnant patients, in large amounts, or for prolonged periods of time.

Nursing Mothers: It is not known whether topical administration of corticosteroids could result in sufficient systemic absorption to produce detectable quantities in breast milk. Systemically administered corticosteroids are secreted into breast milk in quantities *not* likely to have a deleterious effect on the infant. Nevertheless, caution should be exercised when topical corticosteroids are administered to a nursing woman.

Pediatric Use: Pediatric patients may demonstrate greater susceptibility to topical corticosteroid-induced HPA axis suppression and Cushing's syndrome than mature patients because of a larger skin surface area to body weight ratio.

Hypothalamic-pituitary-adrenal (HPA) axis suppression, Cushing's syndrome, and intracranial hypertension have been reported in children receiving topical corticosteroids. Manifestations of adrenal suppression in children include linear growth retardation, delayed weight gain, low plasma cortisol levels, and absence of response to ACTH stimulation. Manifestations of intracranial hypertension include bulging fontanelles, headaches, and bilateral papilledema.

Administration of topical corticosteroids to children should be limited to the least amount compatible with an effective therapeutic regimen. Chronic corticosteroid therapy may interfere with the growth and development of children.

Adverse Reactions: The following local adverse reactions are reported infrequently with topical corticosteroids, but may occur more frequently with the use of occlusive dressings. These reactions are listed in an approximate decreasing order of occurrence:
Burning
Itching
Irritation
Dryness
Folliculitis
Hypertrichosis
Acneform eruptions
Hypopigmentation
Perioral dermatitis
Allergic contact dermatitis
Maceration of the skin
Secondary infection
Skin Atrophy
Striae
Miliaria

Overdosage: Topically applied corticosteroids can be absorbed in sufficient amounts to produce systemic effects (See *PRECAUTIONS*).

Dosage and Administration: Topical corticosteroids are generally applied to the affected area as a thin film from three to four times daily depending on the severity of the condition.

Occlusive dressings may be used for the management of psoriasis or recalcitrant conditions.

If an infection develops, the use of occlusive dressings should be discontinued and appropriate antimicrobial therapy instituted.

How Supplied:
0.025% Cream:
 15 gram tubes—NDC 0005-5169-09
 60 gram tubes—NDC 0005-5169-40
0.1% Cream:
 15 gram tubes—NDC 0005-5191-09
 60 gram tubes—NDC 0005-5191-40
 240 gram jars—NDC 0005-5191-57
0.5% Cream:
 15 gram tubes—NDC 0005-5192-09
 240 gram jars—NDC 0005-5192-57
0.1% Ointment:
 15 gram tubes—NDC 0005-5468-09
 60 gram tubes—NDC 0005-5468-40
0.5% Ointment:
 15 gram tubes—NDC 0005-5194-09
Store at Controlled Room Temperature 15–30°C (59–86°F)
Do Not Freeze
60 gm tube VA: NSN 6505-01-107-1731A
60 gm tube Military: NSN 6505-01-107-1731
Shown in Product Identification Section, pages 414, 415

ARISTOSPAN® R
[*a-ris-tō-span*]
Sterile Triamcinolone Hexacetonide
Suspension, USP
For Intralesional Administration
5 mg./ml.—Parenteral
For Intra-articular Administration
20 mg./ml.—Parenteral
NOT FOR INTRAVENOUS USE

Description:
Intralesional:
A sterile suspension containing 5 mg./ml. of micronized triamcinolone hexacetonide in the following inactive ingredients:
 Polysorbate 80 NF ....0.20% w/v
 Sorbitol Solution USP........................50.00% v/v
 Water for Injection qs ad.................100.00% V
  Preservative:
 Benzyl Alcohol ....0.90% w/v
Intra-articular:
A sterile suspension containing 20 mg./ml. of micronized triamcinolone hexacetonide in the following inactive ingredients:
 Polysorbate 80 NF ....0.40% w/v
 Sorbitol Solution USP........................50.00% v/v
 Water for Injection qs ad ....100.00% V
  Preservative:
 Benzyl Alcohol ....0.90% w/v

The hexacetonide ester of the potent glucocorticoid triamcinolone is relatively insoluble (0.0002% at 25° C. in water). When injected intralesionally, sublesionally, or intra-articularly, it can be expected to be absorbed slowly from the injection site.

Chemically triamcinolone hexacetonide USP is 9-Fluoro-11β, 16α, 17,21-tetrahydroxypregna-1,4-diene-3,20-dione cyclic 16,17-acetal with acetone 21-(3,3-dimethylbutyrate). Molecular weight 532.65.

Actions: Naturally occurring glucocorticoids (hydrocortisone), which also have salt-retaining properties, are used as replacement therapy in adrenocortical deficiency states. Their synthetic analogs are primarily used for their potent anti-inflammatory effects in disorders of many organ systems.

Glucocorticoids cause profound and varied metabolic effects. In addition, they modify the body's immune responses to diverse stimuli.

Indications:
Intralesional or sublesional ARISTOSPAN *sterile triamcinolone hexacetonide suspension* is indicated for the following:
Keloids
Localized hypertrophic, infiltrated, inflammatory lesions of: lichen planus, psoriatic plaques, granuloma annulare and lichen simplex chronicus (neurodermatitis).
Discoid lupus erythematosus.
Necrobiosis lipoidica diabeticorum.
Alopecia areata.
They may also be useful in cystic tumors of an aponeurosis or tendon (ganglia).

Continued on next page

The information on each product appearing here is based on labelling effective in August, 1984 and is either the entire official brochure or an accurate condensation therefrom. Information concerning all Lederle products may be obtained from the Professional Services Department, Lederle Laboratories, Pearl River, New York. 10965.

Lederle—Cont.

Intra-articular:
As adjunctive therapy for short-term administration (to tide the patient over an acute episode or exacerbation) in:
- Synovitis of osteoarthritis
- Acute and subacute bursitis
- Epicondylitis
- Posttraumatic osteoarthritis
- Rheumatoid arthritis
- Acute gouty arthritis
- Acute nonspecific tenosynovitis

Contraindications: Systemic fungal infections.

Warnings: In patients on corticosteroid therapy subjected to any unusual stress, increased dosage of rapidly acting corticosteroids before, during, and after the stressful situation is indicated.

Corticosteroids may mask some signs of infection, and new infections may appear during their use. There may be decreased resistance and inability to localize infection when corticosteroids are used.

Prolonged use of corticosteroids may produce posterior subcapsular cataracts, glaucoma with possible damage to the optic nerves and may enhance the establishment of secondary ocular infections due to fungi or viruses.

Usage in pregnancy
Since adequate human reproduction studies have not been done with corticosteroids, the use of these drugs in pregnancy, nursing mothers, or women of childbearing potential requires that the possible benefits of the drug be weighed against the potential hazards to the mother and embryo or fetus. Infants born of mothers who have received substantial doses of corticosteroids during pregnancy should be carefully observed for signs of hypoadrenalism.

Average and large doses of cortisone or hydrocortisone can cause elevation of blood pressure, salt and water retention, and increased excretion of potassium. These effects are less likely to occur with the synthetic derivatives except when used in large doses. Dietary salt restriction and potassium supplementation may be necessary. All corticosteroids increase calcium excretion.

While on Corticosteroid Therapy Patients Should Not Be Vaccinated Against Smallpox. Other Immunization Procedures Should Not Be Undertaken in Patients Who Are on Corticosteroids, Especially in High Doses, Because of Possible Hazards of Neurological Complications and Lack of Antibody Response.

The use of ARISTOSPAN *sterile triamcinolone hexacetonide suspension* in active tuberculosis should be restricted to those cases of fulminating or disseminated tuberculosis in which the corticosteroid is used for the management of the disease in conjunction with appropriate antituberculous regimen.

If corticosteroids are indicated in patients with latent tuberculosis or tuberculin reactivity, close observation is necessary as reactivation of the disease may occur. During prolonged corticosteroid therapy, these patients should receive chemoprophylaxis.

Because rare instances of anaphylactoid reactions have occurred in patients receiving parenteral corticosteroid therapy, appropriate precautionary measures should be taken prior to administration, especially when the patient has a history of allergy to any drug.

Intralesional or sublesional injection of excessive dosage whether by single or multiple injection into any given area may cause cutaneous or subcutaneous atrophy.

Post-injection flare (following intra-articular use) and charcot-like arthropathy have been associated with parenteral corticosteroid therapy.

Precautions: Drug-induced secondary adrenocortical insufficiency may be minimized by gradual reduction of dosage. This type of relative insufficiency may persist for months after discontinuation of therapy; therefore, in any situation of stress occurring during that period, hormone therapy should be reinstituted. Since mineralocorticoid secretion may be impaired, salt and/or a mineralocorticoid should be administered concurrently.

There is an enhanced effect of corticosteroids in patients with hypothyroidism and in those with cirrhosis.

Corticosteroids should be used cautiously in patients with ocular herpes simplex for fear of corneal perforation.

The lowest possible dose of corticosteroid should be used to control the condition under treatment, and when reduction in dosage is possible, the reduction must be gradual.

Psychic derangements may appear when corticosteroids are used, ranging from euphoria, insomnia, mood swings, personality changes, and severe depression to frank psychotic manifestations. Also, existing emotional instability or psychotic tendencies may be aggravated by corticosteroids.

Aspirin should be used cautiously in conjunction with corticosteroids in hypoprothrombinemia.

Steroids should be used with caution in nonspecific ulcerative colitis, if there is a probability of impending perforation, abscess or other pyogenic infection, also in diverticulitis, fresh intestinal anastomoses, active or latent peptic ulcer, renal insufficiency, hypertension, osteoporosis, and myasthenia gravis.

Growth and development of infants and children on prolonged corticosteroid therapy should be carefully followed.

The following additional precautions apply for parenteral corticosteroids.

Intra-articular injection of a corticosteroid may produce systemic as well as local effects.

Appropriate examination of any joint fluid present is necessary to exclude a septic process.

A marked increase in pain accompanied by local swelling, further restriction of joint motion, fever, and malaise are suggestive of septic arthritis. If this complication occurs and the diagnosis of sepsis is confirmed, appropriate antimicrobial therapy should be instituted.

Local injection of a steroid into a previously infected joint is to be avoided.

Corticosteroids should not be injected into unstable joints.

The slower rate of absorption by intramuscular administration should be recognized.

Routine laboratory studies, such as urinalysis, two-hour postprandial blood sugar, determination of blood pressure and body weight, and a chest X-ray should be made at regular intervals during prolonged therapy. Upper GI X-rays are desirable in patients with an ulcer history or significant dyspepsia.

Adverse Reactions:
Fluid and electrolyte disturbances:
- Sodium retention.
- Fluid retention.
- Congestive heart failure in susceptible patients.
- Potassium loss.
- Hypokalemic alkalosis.
- Hypertension.

Musculoskeletal:
- Muscle weakness.
- Steroid myopathy.
- Loss of muscle mass.
- Osteoporosis.
- Vertebral compression fractures.
- Aseptic necrosis of femoral and humeral heads.
- Pathologic fracture of long bones.

Gastrointestinal:
- Peptic ulcer with possible subsequent perforation and hemorrhage.
- Pancreatitis.
- Abdominal distention.
- Ulcerative esophagitis.

Dermatologic:
- Impaired wound healing.
- Thin fragile skin.
- Petechiae and ecchymoses.
- Facial erythema.
- Increased sweating.
- May suppress reactions to skin tests.

Neurological:
- Convulsions
- Increased intracranial pressure with papilledema (pseudotumor cerebri) usually after treatment.
- Vertigo.
- Headache.

Endocrine:
- Menstrual irregularities.
- Development of Cushingoid state.
- Suppression of growth in children.
- Secondary adrenocortical and pituitary unresponsiveness, particularly in times of stress, as in trauma, surgery, or illness.
- Decreased carbohydrate tolerance.
- Manifestations of latent diabetes mellitus.
- Increased requirements for insulin or oral hypoglycemic agents in diabetics.

Ophthalmic:
- Posterior subcapsular cataracts.
- Increased intraocular pressure.
- Glaucoma.
- Exophthalmos.

Metabolic:
- Negative nitrogen balance due to protein catabolism.

The following additional adverse reactions are related to parenteral and intralesional corticosteroid therapy:
- Rare instances of blindness associated with intralesional therapy around the orbit or intranasally.
- Hyperpigmentation or hypopigmentation.
- Sterile abscess.
- Subcutaneous and cutaneous atrophy.

Dosage and Administration:
General
The initial dosage of ARISTOSPAN *sterile triamcinolone hexacetonide suspension* may vary from 2 to 48 mg. per day depending on the specific disease entity being treated. In situations of less severity, lower doses will generally suffice while in selected patients higher initial doses may be required. Usually the parenteral dosage ranges are one-third to one-half the oral dose given every 12 hours. However, in certain overwhelming, acute, life-threatening situations, administration in dosages exceeding the usual dosages may be justified and may be in multiples of the oral dosages.

The initial dosage should be maintained or adjusted until a satisfactory response is noted. If after a reasonable period of time there is a lack of satisfactory clinical response, ARISTOSPAN should be discontinued and the patient transferred to other appropriate therapy. It Should Be Emphasized That Dosage Requirements Are Variable and Must Be Individualized on the Basis of the Disease Under Treatment and the Response of the Patient. After a favorable response is noted, the proper maintenance dosage should be determined by decreasing the initial drug dosage in small increments at appropriate time intervals until the lowest dosage which will maintain an adequate clinical response is reached. It should be kept in mind that constant monitoring is needed in regard to drug dosage. Included in the situations which may make dosage adjustments necessary are changes in clinical status secondary to remissions or exacerbations in the disease process, the patient's individual drug responsiveness, and the effect of patient exposure to stressful situations not directly related to the disease entity under treatment; in this latter situation it may be necessary to increase the dosage of ARISTOSPAN for a period of time consistent with the patient's condition. If after long-term therapy the drug is to be stopped, it is recommended that it be withdrawn gradually rather than abruptly.

Directions for Use
Strict aseptic administration technique is mandatory. Topical ethyl chloride spray may be used locally before injection.

The syringe should be gently agitated to achieve uniform suspension before use. Since ARISTOSPAN suspension has been designed for ease of administration, a small bore needle not smaller than 24 gauge may be used.

Dilution—Intralesional 5 mg./ml.
ARISTOSPAN suspension may be diluted, if desired, with Dextrose and Sodium Chloride Injection USP, (5% and 10% Dextrose), Sodium Chloride Injection USP, or Sterile Water for Injection USP.

The optimum dilution, i.e., 1:1, 1:2, 1:4, should be determined by the nature of the lesion, its size, the depth of injection, the volume needed, and location of the lesion. In general, more superficial injections should be performed with greater dilution. Certain conditions, such as keloids, require a less dilute suspension such as 5 mg./ml., with variation in dose and dilution as dictated by the condition of the individual patient. Subsequent dosage, dilution, and frequency of injections are best judged by the clinical response.

The suspension may also be mixed with 1% or 2% Lidocaine Hydrochloride, using the formulations which do not contain parabens. Similar local anesthetics may also be used. Diluents containing methylparaben, propylparaben, phenol, etc., should be avoided since these compounds may cause flocculation of the steroid. These dilutions will retain full potency for one week, but care should be exercised to avoid contamination of the vial's contents and the dilutions should be discarded after 7 days.

Intralesional or Sublesional
Average Dose—up to 0.5 mg. per square inch of affected skin injected intralesionally or sub- lesionally. The frequency of subsequent injections is best determined by the clinical response. If desired, the vial may be diluted as indicated under DIRECTIONS FOR USE.

A lesser initial dosage range of ARISTOSPAN may produce the desired effect when the drug is administered to provide a localized concentration. The site of the injection and the volume of the injection should be carefully considered when ARISTOSPAN is administered for this purpose.

Dilution—Intra-articular 20 mg./ml.
ARISTOSPAN suspension may be mixed with 1% or 2% Lidocaine Hydrochloride, using the formulations which do not contain parabens. Similar local anesthetics may also be used. Diluents containing methylparaben, propylparaben, phenol, etc., should be avoided since these compounds may cause flocculation of the steroid. These dilutions will retain full potency for one week, but care should be exercised to avoid contamination.

Intra-articular
Average dose—2 to 20 mg. (0.1 ml. to 1.0 ml.)
The dose depends on the size of the joint to be injected, the degree of inflammation, and the amount of fluid present. In general, large joints (such as knee, hip, shoulder) require 10 to 20 mg. For small joints (such as interphalangeal, metacarpophalangeal), 2 to 6 mg, may be employed. When the amount of synovial fluid is increased, aspiration may be performed before administering ARISTOSPAN. Subsequent dosage and frequency of injections can best be judged by clinical response.

The usual frequency of injection into a single joint is every three or four weeks, and injection more frequently than that is generally not advisable. To avoid possible joint destruction from repeated use of intra-articular corticosteroids, injection should be as infrequent as possible, consistent with adequate patient care. Attention should be paid to avoiding deposition of drug along the needle path which might produce atrophy.

How Supplied:
*Intralesional, 5 ml. (in a 12.5 ml. vial) NDC 0205-4502-31.
*Intra-articular, 1 ml. vial and 5 ml. vial NDC 0205-4505-24, NDC 0205-4505-31.
A.H.F.S. 68:04
Military Depots: NSN-6505-00-148-6985, 5 ml vial
*Manufactured for
LEDERLE LABORATORIES DIVISION
American Cyanamid Company
Pearl River, NY 10965
by
LEDERLE PARENTERALS INC.
Carolina, Puerto Rico 00630

ARTANE® ℞
[ar-tāne]
trihexyphenidyl HCl
Tablets, Elixir, and SEQUELS—Sustained Release Capsules

Description: ARTANE *trihexyphenidyl HCl* is a synthetic antispasmodic drug available in the following forms:
TABLETS: 2 mg—round, flat, scored, white tablets; engraved ARTANE above 2 on one side and LL above A11 below the score on the other side. 5 mg—round, flat, scored, white tablets; engraved ARTANE above 5 on one side and LL above A12 below the score on the other side.
ELIXIR: 2 mg/5ml in a clear, colorless, lime-mint flavored preparation with 0.08% methylparaben, 0.02% propylparaben, and 5% alcohol as preservatives.
SEQUELS: The 5 mg Sustained Release Capsules are soft shelled, oval shaped, clear blue, printed A9L.
Actions: ARTANE *trihexyphenidyl HCl Lederle* is the substituted piperidine salt, 3-(1-piperidyl)-1-phenyl-cyclohexyl-1-propanol hydrochloride, which exerts a direct inhibitory effect upon the parasympathetic nervous system. It also has a relaxing effect on smooth musculature; exerted both directly upon the muscle tissue itself and indirectly through an inhibitory effect upon the parasympathetic nervous system. Its therapeutic properties are similar to those of atropine, although undesirable side effects are ordinarily less frequent and severe than with the latter.
Indications:
This drug is indicated as an adjunct in the treatment of all forms of parkinsonism (postencephalitic, arteriosclerotic, and idiopathic). It is often useful as adjuvant therapy when treating these forms of parkinsonism with levodopa. Additionally, it is indicated for the control of extrapyramidal disorders caused by central nervous system drugs such as the dibenzoxazepines, phenothiazines, thioxanthenes, and butyrophenones.
SEQUELS—For maintenance therapy after patients have been stabilized on trihexyphenidyl hydrochloride in conventional dosage forms (tablets or elixir).
Warning: Patients to be treated with ARTANE should have a gonioscope evaluation and close monitoring of intraocular pressures at regular periodic intervals.
Precautions: Although trihexyphenidyl HCl is *not* contraindicated for patients with cardiac, liver, or kidney disorders, or with hypertension, such patients should be maintained under close observation.
Since the use of trihexyphenidyl HCl may, in some cases, continue indefinitely and since it has atropine-like properties, patients should be subjected to constant and careful long-term observation to avoid allergic and other untoward reactions. Inasmuch as trihexyphenidyl HCl possesses some parasympatholytic activity, it should be used with caution in patients with glaucoma, obstructive disease of the gastrointestinal or genitourinary tracts, and in elderly males with possible prostatic hypertrophy. Geriatric patients, particularly over the age of 60, frequently develop increased sensitivity to the actions of drugs of this type, and hence, require strict dosage regulation. Incipient glaucoma may be precipitated by parasympatholytic drugs such as trihexyphenidyl HCl.
Adverse Reactions: Minor side effects, such as dryness of the mouth, blurring of vision, dizziness, mild nausea or nervousness, will be experienced by 30 to 50 per cent of all patients. These sensations, however, are much less troublesome with ARTANE *trihexyphenidyl HCl* than with belladonna alkaloids and are usually less disturbing than unalleviated parkinsonism. Such reactions tend to become less pronounced, and even to disappear, as treatment continues. Even before these reactions have remitted spontaneously, they may often be controlled by careful adjustment of dosage form, amount of drug, or interval between doses.

Isolated instances of suppurative parotitis secondary to excessive dryness of the mouth, skin rashes, dilatation of the colon, paralytic ileus, and certain psychiatric manifestations such as delusions and hallucinations, plus one doubtful case of paranoia all of which may occur with any of the atropine-like drugs, have been rarely reported with ARTANE.
Patients with arteriosclerosis or with a history of idiosyncrasy to other drugs may exhibit reactions of mental confusion, agitation, disturbed behavior, or nausea and vomiting. Such patients should be allowed to develop a tolerance through the initial administration of a small dose and gradual increase in dose until an effective level is reached. If a severe reaction should occur, administration of the drug should be discontinued for a few days and then resumed at a lower dosage. Psychiatric disturbances can result from indiscriminate use (leading to overdosage) to sustain continued euphoria.
Potential side effects associated with the use of any atropine-like drugs include constipation, drowsiness, urinary hesitancy or retention, tachycardia, dilation of the pupil, increased intraocular tension, weakness, vomiting, and headache.
The occurrence of angle-closure glaucoma due to long-term treatment with trihexyphenidyl hydrochloride has been reported.
Dosage and Administration: Dosage should be individualized. The initial dose should be low and then increased gradually, especially in patients over 60 years of age. Whether ARTANE *trihexyphenidyl HCl* may best be given before or after meals should be determined by the way the patient reacts. Postencephalitic patients, who are usually more prone to excessive salivation, may prefer to take it after meals and may, in addition, require small amounts of atropine which, under such circumstances, is sometimes an effective adjuvant. If ARTANE tends to dry the mouth excessively, it may be better to take it before meals, unless it causes nausea. If taken after meals, the thirst sometimes induced can be allayed by mint candies, chewing gum or water.
ARTANE Trihexyphenidyl HCl in Idiopathic Parkinsonism
As initial therapy for parkinsonism, 1 mg of ARTANE in tablet or elixir form may be administered the first day. The dose may then be increased by 2 mg increments at intervals of three to five days, until a total of 6 to 10 mg is given daily. The total daily dose will depend upon what is found to be the optimal level. Many patients derive maximum benefit from this daily total of 6 to 10 mg, but some patients, chiefly those in the postencephalitic group, may require a total daily dose of 12 to 15 mg.
ARTANE Trihexyphenidyl HCl in Drug-Induced Parkinsonism
The size and frequency of dose of ARTANE needed to control extrapyramidal reactions to commonly employed tranquilizers, notably the phenothiazines, thioxanthenes, and butyrophenones, must be determined empirically. The total daily dosage usually ranges between 5 and 15 mg although, in some cases, these reactions have been satisfactorily controlled on as little as 1 mg daily. It may be advisable to commence therapy with a single 1 mg dose. If the extrapyramidal manifestations are not controlled in a few hours, the subsequent doses may be progressively increased until satisfactory control is achieved. Satisfactory control may sometimes be more rapidly achieved by temporarily reducing the dosage of the tranquilizer on instituting ARTANE trihexyphenidyl HCl therapy and then adjusting dosage of both drugs until the de-

Continued on next page

The information on each product appearing here is based on labelling effective in August, 1984 and is either the entire official brochure or an accurate condensation therefrom. Information concerning all Lederle products may be obtained from the Professional Services Department, Lederle Laboratories, Pearl River, New York, 10965.

Lederle—Cont.

sired ataractic effect is retained without onset of extrapyramidal reactions.

It is sometimes possible to maintain the patient on a reduced ARTANE dosage after the reactions have remained under control for several days. Instances have been reported in which these reactions have remained in remission for long periods after ARTANE therapy was discontinued.

Concomitant Use of ARTANE Trihexyphenidyl HCl with Levodopa

When ARTANE is used concomitantly with levodopa, the usual dose of each may need to be reduced. Careful adjustment is necessary, depending on side effects and degree of symptom control. ARTANE dosage of 3 to 6 mg daily, in divided doses, is usually adequate.

Concomitant Use of ARTANE Trihexyphenidyl HCl with Other Parasympathetic Inhibitors

ARTANE *trihexyphenidyl HCl* may be substituted, in whole or in part, for other parasympathetic inhibitors. The usual technique is partial substitution initially, with progressive reduction in the other medication as the dose of trihexyphenidyl HCl is increased.

ARTANE TABLETS and ELIXIR—The total daily intake of ARTANE tablets or elixir is tolerated best if divided into 3 doses and taken at mealtimes. High doses (> 10 mg daily) may be divided into 4 parts, with 3 doses administered at mealtimes and the fourth at bedtime.

ARTANE SEQUELS—Because of the relatively high dosage in each controlled release capsule, this dosage form should not be used for initial therapy. After patients are stabilized on trihexyphenidyl HCl in conventional dosage forms (tablet or elixir), for convenience of administration they may be switched to the controlled release capsules on a milligram per milligram total daily dose basis, as a single dose after breakfast or in two divided doses 12 hours apart. Most patients will be adequately maintained on the controlled release form, but some may develop an exacerbation of parkinsonism and have to be returned to the conventional form.

How Supplied:

ARTANE® Trihexyphenidyl HCl is available as follows:

TABLETS: 2 mg—round, flat, scored, white tablets; engraved ARTANE above 2 on one side and LL above A11 below the score on the other side, are supplied as follows:

NDC 0005-4434-23—Bottles of 100
NDC 0005-4434-34—Bottles of 1000
NDC 0005-4434-60—Unit Dose 10 × 10's

5 mg—round, flat, scored, white tablets; engraved ARTANE above 5 on one side and LL above A12 below the score on the other side, are supplied as follows:

NDC 0005-4436-23—Bottles of 100
NDC 0005-4436-34—Bottles of 1000
NDC 0005-4436-60—Unit Dose 10 × 10's

Store at Controlled Room Temperature 15–30° C (59–86° F)

ELIXIR: 2 mg/5ml—NDC 0005-4440-65—Bottles of 16 Fl. Oz.

Store at Controlled Room Temperature 15–30° C (59–86°F) DO NOT FREEZE

SEQUELS SUSTAINED RELEASE CAPSULES: 5 mg—soft shell, oval shaped, clear blue, printed A9L, are supplied as follows:

NDC 0005-4438-32—Unit-of-Issue 60's with CRC
NDC 0005-4438-31—Bottles of 500

Store at Controlled Room Temperature 15–30° C (59–86° F)

VA depot NSN 6505-00-890-1378A—16 oz.

Shown in Product Identification Section, page 415

ASENDIN®
[a-sen-din]
amoxapine

Description: ASENDIN *amoxapine* is an antidepressant of the dibenzoxazepine class, chemically distinct from the dibenzazepines, dibenzocycloheptenes, and dibenzoxepines.

It is designated chemically as 2-chloro-11-(1-piperazinyl)dibenz-[b,f][1,4] oxazepine. The molecular weight is 313.8. The empirical formula is $C_{17}H_{16}ClN_3O$.

ASENDIN is supplied for oral administration as 25 mg, 50 mg, 100 mg, and 150 mg tablets.

Clinical Pharmacology: ASENDIN is an antidepressant with a mild sedative component to its action. The mechanism of its clinical action in man is not well understood. In animals, amoxapine reduced the uptake of norepinephrine and serotonin and blocked the response of dopamine receptors to dopamine. Amoxapine is not a monoamine oxidase inhibitor.

ASENDIN is absorbed rapidly and reaches peak blood levels approximately 90 minutes after ingestion. It is almost completely metabolized. The main route of excretion is the kidney. *In vitro* tests show that amoxapine binding to human serum is approximately 90%.

In man, amoxapine serum concentration declines with a half-life of 8 hours. However, the major metabolite, 8-hydroxyamoxapine, has a biologic half-life of 30 hours. Metabolites are excreted in the urine in conjugated form as glucuronides.

Clinical studies have demonstrated that ASENDIN has a more rapid onset of action than either amitriptyline or imipramine. The initial clinical effect may occur within four to seven days and occurs within two weeks in over 80% of responders.

Indications and Usage: ASENDIN is indicated for the relief of symptoms of depression in patients with neurotic or reactive depressive disorders as well as endogenous and psychotic depressions. It is indicated for depression accompanied by anxiety or agitation.

Contraindications: ASENDIN is contraindicated in patients who have shown prior hypersensitivity to dibenzoxazepine compounds. It should not be given concomitantly with monoamine oxidase inhibitors. Hyperpyretic crises, severe convulsions, and deaths have occurred in patients receiving tricyclic antidepressants and monoamine oxidase inhibitors simultaneously. When it is desired to replace a monoamine oxidase inhibitor with ASENDIN, a minimum of 14 days should be allowed to elapse after the former is discontinued. ASENDIN should then be initiated cautiously with gradual increase in dosage until optimum response is achieved. The drug is not recommended for use during the acute recovery phase following myocardial infarction.

Warnings: ASENDIN should be used with caution in patients with a history of urinary retention, angle-closure glaucoma or increased intraocular pressure. Patients with cardiovascular disorders should be watched closely. Tricyclic antidepressant drugs, particularly when given in high doses, can induce sinus tachycardia, changes in conduction time, and arrhythmias. Myocardial infarction and stroke have been reported with drugs of this class.

Extreme caution should be used in treating patients with a history of convulsive disorder or those with overt or latent seizure disorders.

Precautions:

General:

In prescribing the drug it should be borne in mind that the possibility of suicide is inherent in any severely depressed patient, and persists until a significant remission occurs; the drug should be dispensed in the smallest suitable amount. Manic depressive patients may experience a shift to the manic phase. Schizophrenic patients may develop increased symptoms of psychosis; patients with paranoid symptomatology may have an exaggeration of such symptoms. This may require reduction of dosage or the addition of a major tranquilizer to the therapeutic regimen. Antidepressant drugs can cause skin rashes and/or "drug fever" in susceptible individuals. These allergic reactions may, in rare cases, be severe. They are more likely to occur during the first few days of treatment, but may also occur later. ASENDIN should be discontinued if rash and/or fever develop. Amoxapine possesses a degree of dopamine-blocking activity which may cause extrapyramidal symptoms in <1% of patients. Rarely, symptoms indicative of tardive dyskinesia have been reported, possibly related to treatment with amoxapine.

Information for the patient:

Patients should be warned of the possibility of drowsiness that may impair performance of potentially hazardous tasks such as driving an automobile or operating machinery.

Drug interactions:

See "Contraindications" about concurrent usage of tricyclic antidepressants and monoamine oxidase inhibitors. Paralytic ileus may occur in patients taking tricyclic antidepressants in combination with anticholenergic drugs. ASENDIN may enhance the response to alcohol and the effects of barbiturates and other CNS depressants.

Therapeutic interactions:

Concurrent administration with electroshock therapy may increase the hazards associated with such therapy.

Carcinogenesis, impairment of fertility:

In a 21-month toxicity study at 3 dose levels in rats, pancreatic islet cell hyperplasia occurred with slightly increased incidence at doses 5–10 times the human dose. Pancreatic adenocarcinoma was detected in low incidence in the mid-dose group only, and may possibly have resulted from endocrine-mediated organ hyperfunction. The significance of these findings to man is not known.

Treatment of male rats with 5–10 times the human dose resulted in a slight decrease in the number of fertile matings. Female rats receiving oral doses within the therapeutic range displayed a reversible increase in estrous cycle length.

Pregnancy. Pregnancy category C:

Studies performed in mice, rats and rabbits have demonstrated no evidence of teratogenic effect due to ASENDIN. Embryotoxicity was seen in rats and rabbits given oral doses approximating the human dose. Fetotoxic effects (intrauterine death, stillbirth, decreased birth weight) were seen in animal studies at oral doses 3–10 times the human dose. Decreased postnatal survival (between days 0–4) was demonstrated in the offspring of rats at 5–10 times the human dose. There are no adequate and well-controlled studies in pregnant women. ASENDIN should be used during pregnancy only if the potential benefit justifies the potential risk to the fetus.

Nursing mothers:

ASENDIN, like many other systemic drugs, is excreted in human milk. Because effects of the drug on infants are unknown, caution should be exercised when ASENDIN is administered to nursing women.

Pediatric use:

Safety and effectiveness in children below the age of 16 have not been established.

Adverse Reactions: Adverse reactions reported in controlled studies in the United States are categorized with respect to incidence below. Following this is a listing of reactions known to occur with other antidepressant drugs of this class but not reported to date with ASENDIN.

INCIDENCE GREATER THAN 1%

The most frequent types of adverse reactions occurring with ASENDIN in controlled clinical trials were sedative and anticholinergic: these included drowsiness (14%), dry mouth (14%), constipation (12%), and blurred vision (7%).

Less frequently reported reactions were:

CNS and Neuromuscular—anxiety, insomnia, restlessness, nervousness, palpitations, tremors, confusion, excitement, nightmares, ataxia, alterations in EEG patterns.

Allergic—edema.

Gastrointenstinal—Nausea.

Other—dizziness, headache, fatigue, weakness, excessive appetite, increased perspiration.

INCIDENCE LESS THAN 1%

Anticholinergic—disturbances of accommodation, mydriasis, delayed micturition, urinary retention, nasal stuffiness.

Cardiovascular—hypotension, hypertension, syncope, tachycardia.

Allergic—drug fever with skin rash, photosensitization, pruritus, rarely vasculitis.

CNS and Neuromuscular—tingling, paresthesias of the extremities, tinnitus, disorientation, seizures, hypomania, numbness, incoordination, disturbed concentration, hyperthermia, extrapyramidal symptoms, including, rarely, tardive dyskinesia.
Hematologic—Leukopenia.
Gastrointestinal—epigastric distress, vomiting, flatulence, abdominal pain, peculiar taste, diarrhea.
Endocrine—increased or decreased libido, impotence, menstrual irregularity, breast enlargement and galactorrhea in the female.
Other—lacrimation, weight gain or loss, altered liver function.
DRUG RELATIONSHIP UNKNOWN
The following reactions have been reported very rarely, and occurred under controlled circumstances where a drug relationship was difficult to assess. These observations are listed to serve as alerting information to physicians.
Allergic—urticaria and petechiae.
Anticholinergic—paralytic ileus.
Cardiovascular—atrial arrhythmias (including atrial fibrillation), myocardial infarction, stroke, heart block.
CNS *and Neuromuscular*—hallucinations, nightmares.
Hematologic—thrombocytopenia, purpura.
Gastrointestinal—parotid swelling.
Endocrine—change in blood glucose levels.
Other—pancreatitis, hepatitis, jaundice, urinary frequency, testicular swelling, anorexia.
ADDITIONAL ADVERSE REACTIONS
The following reactions have been reported with other antidepressant drugs, but not with ASENDIN.
Anticholinergic—sublingual adenitis, dilation of the urinary tract.
CNS *and Neuromuscular*—delusions, syndrome of inappropriate ADH secretion.
Hematologic—agranulocytosis, eosinophilia.
Gastrointestinal—stomatitis, black tongue.
Endocrine—gynecomastia.
Other—alopecia.
Overdosage:
Signs and Symptoms
Initial toxic manifestations of ASENDIN overdosage typically are CNS effects: delirium, lethargy with diminished deep tendon reflexes, and/or seizures. Cardiovascular effects, when they occur, are usually limited to sinus tachycardia and transient minor EKG changes. Serious hypotension, hypertension, or cardiac arrhythmias are rare. Respiratory acidosis may develop following repeated seizures, and metabolic acidosis has been reported.
Important
Renal impairment may develop three to five days after substantial overdosage in patients who may appear otherwise recovered. Oliguria, hematuria, and renal failure have been reported. Tubular necrosis and rhabdomyolysis with myoglobinuria may also occur in such cases. Treatment is the same as that for non-drug-induced renal dysfunction. In a limited series of cases of renal failure following overdosage, 70% have recovered with appropriate treatment.
In general, treatment of overdosage must be symptomatic and supportive. If the patient is conscious, induced emesis followed by gastric lavage with appropriate precautions to prevent pulmonary aspiration should be accomplished as soon as possible. Following lavage, activated charcoal may be administered to reduce absorption. An adequate airway should be established in comatose patients and assisted ventilation instituted if necessary. Convulsions, should they occur, may respond to standard anticonvulsant therapy; however, barbiturates may potentiate any respiratory depression. Specific treatment should be guided by the predominant symptoms which may suggest use of a particular pharmacologic agent. For example, the slow intravenous administration of physostigmine salicylate has been reported to reverse most of the serious cardiovascular and CNS effects of overdosage with tricyclic antidepressants, such as cardiac arrythmias and convulsions. (Avoid rapid injection to reduce the possibility of physostigmin induced convulsions.) Convulsions may also be treated with intravenous diazepam. Acidosis may be treated by cautious intravenous administration of sodium bicarbonate.

A patient who has ingested a toxic overdose of a tricyclic antidepressant may remain medically and psychiatrically unstable for several days due to sustained excessive drug levels. Unexpected cardiac deaths have occurred up to six days post overdose with other antidepressants. The QRS interval of the electocardiogram appears a reliable correlate of the severity of overdosage. If the QRS interval exceeds 100 milliseconds anytime during the first 24 hours after overdose, cardiac function should be continuously monitored for five or six days. (Prolongation of the QRS interval beyond 100 milliseconds has not been reported with ASENDIN overdosage, and there have been no deaths due to primary cardiac toxicity.)

The smallest estimated lethal overdose reported has been 2.6 grams. On the other hand, some patients have survived much larger overdoses. Age and physical condition of the patient, concomitant ingestion of other drugs, and especially the interval between drug ingestion and initiation of emergency treatment, are important determining factors in the probability of survival.

Dosage and Administration: Effective dosage of ASENDIN may vary from one patient to another. Usual effective dosage is 200 mg to 300 mg daily. Three weeks constitutes an adequate period of trial providing dosage has reached 300 mg daily (or a lower level of tolerance) for at least two weeks. If no response is seen at 300 mg, dosage may be increased, depending upon tolerance, up to 400 mg daily. Hospitalized patients who have been refractory to antidepressant therapy and who have no history of convulsive seizures may have dosage raised cautiously up to 600 mg daily in divided doses.

ASENDIN may be given in a single daily dose, not to exceed 300 mg, preferably at bedtime. If the total daily dosage exceeds 300 mg, it should be given in divided doses.

Initial Dosage for Adults—Usual starting dosage is 50 mg three times daily. Depending upon tolerance, dosage may be increased to 100 mg three times daily on the third day of treatment. (Initial dosage of 300 mg daily may be given, but notable sedation may occur in some patients during the first few days of therapy at this level.) Increases above 300 mg daily should be made only if 300 mg daily has been ineffective during a trial period of at least two weeks. When effective dosage is established, the drug may be given in a single dose (not to exceed 300 mg) at bedtime.

Elderly Patients—In general, lower dosages of the tricyclic antidepressants are recommended for these patients. Recommended starting dosage of ASENDIN is 25 mg three times daily. If no intolerance is observed, dosage may be increased after three days to 50 mg three times daily. Although 100–150 mg daily may be adequate for many elderly patients, some may require higher dosage. Careful increases up to 300 mg daily are indicated in such cases.

Once an effective dosage is established, ASENDIN may conveniently be given in a single bedtime dose, not to exceed 300 mg.

Maintenance—Recommended maintenance dosage of ASENDIN is the lowest dose that will maintain remission. If symptoms reappear, dosage should be increased to the earlier level until they are controlled.

For maintenance therapy at dosage of 300 mg or less, a single dose at bedtime is recommended.

How Supplied: ASENDIN *Amoxapine* Tablets are supplied as follows:

25 mg—white, heptagon-shaped tablets, engraved on one side with LL above 25 and with A13 on the other scored side.
 (Product No. NDC 0005-5389-23)—bottles of 100
50 mg—orange, heptagon-shaped tablets, engraved on one side with LL above 50 and with A15 on the other scored side.
 (Product No. NDC 0005-5390-23)—bottles of 100
 (Product No. NDC 0005-5390-31)—bottles of 500
 (Product No. NDC 0005-5390-60)—10 × 10 Unit Dose
100 mg—Blue, heptagon-shaped tablets, engraved on one side with LL above 100 and with A17 on the other scored side.
 (Product No. NDC 0005-5391-23)—bottles of 100
 (Product No. NDC 0005-5391-60)—10 × 10 Unit Dose
150 mg—Peach, heptagon-shaped tablets, engraved on one side with LL above 150 and with A18 on the other scored side.
 (Product No. NDC 0005-5392-38)—bottles of 30 with CRC
Store at Controlled Room Temperature 15–30°C (59–86°F)
VA Depot: NSN 6505-01-111-3195A 50 mg-100's
NSN 6505-01-111-3194A 100 mg-100's
Military Depots: NSN 6505-01-111-3195 50 mg-100's
NSN 6505-01-111-3194 100 mg-100's
Shown in Product Identification Section, page 415

AUREOMYCIN®
[*or-ḗo-mī-cin*]
chlortetracycline HCl 3%
OINTMENT

How Supplied: ½ and 1 oz. tubes. Rx not required NDC 0005-4442-56, NDC 0005-4442-55.

CALTRATE™ 600
High Potency Calcium Supplement

(See PDR For Nonprescription Drugs)

CALTRATE™ 600 + D
High Potency Calcium Supplement

(See PDR For Nonprescription Drugs)

Advanced Formula
CENTRUM®
[*sĕn-trŭm*]
High Potency
Multivitamin-Multimineral Formula

(See PDR For Nonprescription Drugs)

Children's Chewable
CENTRUM, Jr.®
[*sĕn-trŭm*]
Vitamin/Mineral Formula + Iron

(See PDR For Nonprescription Drugs)

CHOLERA VACCINE   ℞
[*kŏl-ĕra*]
(India Strains)

How Supplied: 1 ml. vial (1 immunization) NDC 0005-1976-24
COMPLETE INFORMATION FURNISHED IN THE PACKAGE.

CYCLOCORT®   ℞
[*sī-clō-cŏrt*]
Amcinonide Topical Cream 0.1%
with AQUATAIN™ hydrophilic base
CYCLOCORT®   ℞
Amcinonide Ointment 0.1%

Description: 0.1% topical cream.
Each gram of CYCLOCORT Topical Cream contains 1 mg of the active steroid Amcinonide in AQUATAIN, a specially formulated cream base composed of emulsifying wax NF, isopropyl palmitate, glycerin USP, sorbitol solution USP, lactic

Continued on next page

The information on each product appearing here is based on labelling effective in August, 1984 and is either the entire official brochure or an accurate condensation therefrom. Information concerning all Lederle products may be obtained from the Professional Services Department, Lederle Laboratories, Pearl River, New York, 10965.

Lederle—Cont.

acid, 2% benzyl alcohol and purified water. AQUATAIN is non-staining, water-washable, paraben-free, spermaceti-free and has a light texture and consistency. Amcinonide is (11β, 16α)-21-(acetyloxy)-16, 17-[cyclopentylid-enebis(oxy)]-9-fluoro-11-hydroxypregna-1,4-diene-3, 20-dione.

0.1% topical ointment.
Each gram of CYCLOCORT Ointment contains 1 mg of the active steroid amcinonide in a specially formulated base composed of petrolatum, white USP; benzyl alcohol NF, emulsifying wax NF; and Tenox II (butylated hydroxyanisole, propyl gallate, citric acid, propylene glycol).

The topical corticosteroids constitute a class of primarily synthetic steroids used as anti-inflammatory and anti-pruritic agents.

Clinical Pharmacology: Topical corticosteroids share anti-inflammatory, antipruritic and vasoconstrictive actions.

The mechanism of anti-inflammatory activity of the topical corticosteroids is unclear. Various laboratory methods, including vasoconstrictor assays, are used to compare and predict potencies and/or clinical efficacies of the topical corticosteroids. There is some evidence to suggest that a recognizable correlation exists between vasoconstrictor potency and therapeutic efficacy in man.

Pharmacokinetics: The extent of percutaneous absorption of topical corticosteroids is determined by many factors including the vehicle, the integrity of the epidermal barrier, and the use of occlusive dressings.

Topical corticosteroids can be absorbed from normal intact skin. Inflammation and/or other disease processes in the skin increase percutaneous absorption. Occlusive dressings substantially increase the percutaneous absorption of topical corticosteroids. Thus, occlusive dressings may be a valuable therapeutic adjunct for treatment of resistant dermatoses. (See *DOSAGE AND ADMINISTRATION*).

Once absorbed through the skin, topical corticosteroids are handled through pharmacokinetic pathways similar to systemically administered corticosteroids. Corticosteroids are bound to plasma proteins in varying degrees. Corticosteroids are metabolized primarily in the liver and are then excreted by the kidneys. Some of the topical corticosteroids and their metabolites are also excreted into the bile.

Indications and Usage: Topical corticosteroids are indicated for the relief of the inflammatory and pruritic manifestations of corticosteroid-responsive dermatoses.

Contraindications: Topical corticosteroids are contraindicated in those patients with a history of hypersensitivity to any of the components of the preparation.

Precautions: *General:* Systemic absorption of topical corticosteroids has produced reversible hypothalamic-pituitary-adrenal (HPA) axis suppression, manifestations of Cushing's syndrome, hyperglycemia, and glucosuria in some patients. Conditions which augment systemic absorption include the application of the more potent steroids, use over large surface areas, prolonged use, and the addition of occlusive dressings.

Therefore, patients receiving a large dose of a potent topical steroid applied to a large surface area or under an occlusive dressing should be evaluated periodically for evidence of HPA axis suppression by using the urinary free cortisol and ACTH stimulation tests. If HPA axis suppression is noted, an attempt should be made to withdraw the drug, to reduce the frequency of application, or to substitute a less potent steroid.

Recovery of HPA axis function is generally prompt and complete upon discontinuation of the drug. Infrequently, signs and symptoms of steroid withdrawal may occur, requiring supplemental systemic corticosteroids.

Children may absorb proportionally larger amounts of topical corticosteroids and thus be more susceptible to system toxicity. (See *PRECAUTIONS—Pediatric Use*). If irritation develops, topical corticosteroids should be discontinued and appropriate therapy instituted.

In the presence of dermatological infections, the use of an appropriate antifungal or antibacterial agent should be instituted. If a favorable response does not occur promptly, the corticosteroid should be discontinued until the infection has been adequately controlled.

The product is not for ophthalmic use.

Information for the Patient: Patients using topical corticosteroids should receive the following information and instructions:
1. This medication is to be used as directed by the physician. It is for external use only. Avoid contact with the eyes.
2. Patients should be advised not to use this medication for any disorder other than for which it was prescribed.
3. The treated skin area should not be bandaged or otherwise covered or wrapped as to be occlusive unless directed by the physician.
4. Patients should report any signs of local adverse reactions especially under occlusive dressing.
5. Parents of pediatric patients should be advised not to use tight-fitting diapers or plastic pants on a child being treated in the diaper area, as these garments may constitute occlusive dressings.

Laboratory Tests: The following tests may be helpful in evaluating the HPA axis suppression:
Urinary free cortisol test.
ACTH stimulation test.

Carcinogenesis, Mutagenesis, and Impairment of Fertility: Long-term animal studies have not been performed to evaluate the carcinogenic potential or the effect on fertility of topical corticosteroids.
Studies to determine mutagenicity with prednisolone and hydrocortisone have revealed negative results.

Pregnancy Category C: Corticosteroids are generally teratogenic in laboratory animals when administered systemically at relatively low dosage levels. The more potent corticosteroids have been shown to be teratogenic after dermal application in laboratory animals. There are no adequate and well-controlled studies in pregnant women on teratogenic effects from topically applied corticosteroids. Therefore, topical corticosteroids should be used during pregnancy only if the potential benefit justifies the potential risk to the fetus. Drugs of this class should not be used extensively on pregnant patients, in large amounts, or for prolonged periods of time.

Nursing Mothers: It is not known whether topical administration of corticosteroids could result in sufficient systemic absorption to produce detectable quantities in breast milk. Systemically administered corticosteroids are secreted into breast milk in quantities *not* likely to have a deleterious effect on the infant. Nevertheless, caution should be exercised when topical corticosteroids are administered to a nursing woman.

Pediatric Use: Pediatric patients *may demonstrate greater susceptibility to topical corticosteroid-induced HPA axis suppression and Cushing's syndrome than mature patients because of a larger skin surface area to body weight ratio.*
Hypothalamic-pituitary-adrenal (HPA) axis suppression, Cushing's syndrome, and intracranial hypertension have been reported in children receiving topical corticosteroids. Manifestations of adrenal suppression in children include linear growth retardation, delayed weight gain, low plasma cortisol levels, and absence of response to ACTH stimulation. Manifestations of intracranial hypertension include bulging fontanelles, headaches, and bilateral papilledema.

Administration of topical corticosteroids to children should be limited to the least amount compatible with an effective therapeutic regimen. Chronic corticosteroid therapy may interfere with the growth and development of children.

Adverse Reactions: The following local adverse reactions are reported infrequently with topical corticosteroids, but may occur more frequently with the use of occlusive dressings. These reactions are listed in an approximate decreasing order of occurrence: burning, itching, irritation, dryness, folliculitis, hypertrichosis, acneiform eruptions, hypopigmentation, perioral dermatitis, allergic contact dermatitis, maceration of the skin, secondary infection, skin atrophy, striae, miliaria.

Overdosage: Topically applied corticosteroids can be absorbed in sufficient amounts to produce systemic effects (See *PRECAUTIONS*).

Dosage and Administration: CYCLOCORT Cream 0.1% should be applied to the affected area as a thin film from two to three times daily, depending on the severity of the condition. CYCLOCORT Ointment 0.1% should be applied to the affected area as a thin film twice daily, depending on the severity of the condition.

Occlusive dressings may be used for the management of psoriasis or recalcitrant conditions.
If an infection develops, the use of occlusive dressings should be discontinued and appropriate antimicrobial therapy instituted.

How Supplied: CYCLOCORT® Amcinonide Cream 0.1% (1 mg/gm) with AQUATAIN hydrophilic base is available as follows:
15 gram tubes—NDC 0005-9183-09
30 gram tubes—NDC 0005-9183-32
60 gram tubes—NDC 0005-9183-40
CYCLOCORT® Amcinonide Topical Ointment 0.1% (1 mg/gm) is available as follows:
15 gram tubes—NDC 0005-9345-09
30 gram tubes—NDC 0005-9345-32
60 gram tubes—NDC 0005-9345-40
Store at Controlled Room Temperature 15–30°C (59–86°F)
60 gram tube VA NSN 6505-01-093-7968A
Military Depot: NSN 6505-01-139-5001, 15 gm tube NSN 6505-01-093-7968, 60 gm tube
Shown in Product Identification Section, page 415

DECLOMYCIN®   R
[dĕk-lō-mī-sĭn]
Demeclocycline Hydrochloride
For Oral Use

Description: DECLOMYCIN *demeclocycline hydrochloride* is an antibiotic isolated from a mutant strain of *Streptomyces aureofaciens*. Chemically it is [4S-(4α,4aα,5aα,6β,12aα)]-7-Chloro-4-dimethylamino)-1,4,4a,5,5a,6,11,12a-octahydro-3,6,10,12,12a-pentahydroxy-1,11-dioxo-2-naphthacenecarboxamide monohydrochloride.

Actions: The tetracyclines are primarily bacteriostatic and are thought to exert their antimicrobial effect by the inhibition of protein synthesis. Tetracyclines are active against a wide range of gram-negative and gram-positive organisms.

The drugs in the tetracycline class have closely similar antimicrobial spectra, and cross-resistance among them is common. Micro-organisms may be considered susceptible if the M.I.C. (minimum inhibitory concentration) is not more than 4.0 mcg./ml. and intermediate if the M.I.C. is 4.0 to 12.5 mcg./ml.

Susceptibility plate testing: A tetracycline disc may be used to determine microbial susceptibility to drugs in the tetracycline class. If the Kirby-Bauer method of disc susceptibility testing is used, a 30 mcg. tetracycline disc should give a zone of at least 19 mm. when tested against a tetracycline-susceptible bacterial strain.

Tetracyclines are readily absorbed and are bound to plasma proteins in varying degree. They are concentrated by the liver in the bile and excreted in the urine and feces at high concentrations and in a biologically active form.

Indications: DECLOMYCIN *demeclocycline hydrochloride* is indicated in infections caused by the following micro-organisms:
Rickettsiae: (Rocky Mountain spotted fever, typhus fever and the typhus group, Q fever, rickettsialpox, tick fevers.)
Mycoplasma pneumoniae (PPLO, Eaton agent).
Agents of psittacosis and ornithosis.
Agents of lymphogranuloma venereum and granuloma inguinale.
The spirochetal agent of relapsing fever (*Borrelia recurrentis*).
The following gram-negative micro-organisms:
Haemophilus ducreyi (chancroid),
Pasteurella pestis and *Pasteurella tularensis*,

Bartonella bacilliformis,
Bacteroides species,
Vibrio comma and *Vibrio fetus.*
Brucella species (in conjunction with streptomycin).

Because many strains of the following groups of micro-organisms have been shown to be resistant to tetracyclines, culture and susceptibility testing are recommended.

Demeclocycline is indicated for treatment of infections caused by the following gram-negative micro-organisms, when bacteriologic testing indicates appropriate susceptibility to the drug:

Escherichia coli,
Enterobacter aerogenes (formerly *Aerobacter aerogenes*),
Shigella species,
Mima species and *Herellea* species,
Haemophilus influenzae (respiratory infections),
Klebsiella species (respiratory and urinary infections).

Demeclocycline is indicated for treatment of infections caused by the following gram-positive micro-organisms when bacteriologic testing indicates appropriate susceptibility to the drug:
Streptococcus species:
Up to 44 percent of strains of *Streptococcus pyogenes* and 74 percent of *Streptococcus faecalis* have been found to be resistant to tetracycline drugs. Therefore, tetracyclines should not be used for streptococcal disease unless the organism has been demonstrated to be sensitive.

For upper respiratory infections due to group A beta-hemolytic streptococci, penicillin is the usual drug of choice, including prophyaxis of rheumatic fever.

Diplococcus pneumoniae,
Staphylococcus aureus, skin and soft tissue infections. Tetracyclines are not the drugs of choice in the treatment of any type of staphylococcal infection.

When penicillin is contraindicated, tetracyclines are alternative drugs in the treatment of infections due to:

Neisseria gonorrhoeae,
Treponema pallidum and *Treponema pertenue* (syphilis and yaws),
Listeria monocytogenes,
Clostridium species,
Bacillus anthracis,
Fusobacterium fusiforme (Vincent's infection),
Actinomyces species.

In acute intestinal amebiasis, the tetracyclines may be a useful adjunct to amebicides.

DECLOMYCIN *demeclocycline hydrochloride* is indicated in the treatment of trachoma, although the infectious agent is not always eliminated, as judged by immunofluorescence.

Inclusion conjunctivitis may be treated with oral tetracyclines or with a combination of oral and topical agents.

Contraindications: This drug is contraindicated in persons who have shown hypersensitivity to any of the tetracyclines.

Warnings: THE USE OF DRUGS OF THE TETRACYCLINE CLASS DURING TOOTH DEVELOPMENT (LAST HALF OF PREGNANCY, INFANCY AND CHILDHOOD TO THE AGE OF 8 YEARS) MAY CAUSE PERMANENT DISCOLORATION OF THE TEETH (YELLOW-GRAY-BROWN).

This adverse reaction is more common during long-term use of the drugs but has been observed following repeated short-term courses. Enamel hypoplasia has also been reported. TETRACYCLINE DRUGS, THEREFORE, SHOULD NOT BE USED IN THIS AGE GROUP UNLESS OTHER DRUGS ARE NOT LIKELY TO BE EFFECTIVE OR ARE CONTRAINDICATED.

If renal impairment exists, even usual oral or parenteral doses may lead to excessive systemic accumulation of the drug and possible liver toxicity. Under such conditions, lower than usual total doses are indicated and, if therapy is prolonged, serum level determinations of the drug may be advisable.

Phototoxic reactions can occur in individuals taking demeclocycline, and are characterized by severe burns of exposed surfaces resulting from direct exposure of patients to sunlight during therapy with moderate or large doses of demeclocycline. Patients apt to be exposed to direct sunlight or ultraviolet light should be advised that this reaction can occur, and treatment should be discontinued at the first evidence of skin erythema. The anti-anabolic action of the tetracyclines may cause an increase in BUN. While this is not a problem in those with normal renal function, in patients with significantly impaired function, higher serum levels of tetracycline may lead to azotemia, hyperphosphatemia, and acidosis.

Administration of demeclocycline has resulted in appearance of the diabetes insipidus syndrome (polyuria, polydipsia and weakness) in some patients on long term therapy. The syndrome has been shown to be nephrogenic, dose-dependent and reversible on discontinuance of therapy.

Usage in pregnancy (See above "Warnings" about use during tooth development.)

Results of animal studies indicate that tetracyclines cross the placenta, are found in fetal tissues and can have toxic effects on the developing fetus (often related to retardation of skeletal development). Evidence of embryotoxicity has also been noted in animals treated early in pregnancy.

Usage in newborns, infants, and children (See above "Warnings" about use during tooth development.)

All tetracyclines form a stable calcium complex in any bone forming tissue. A decrease in the fibula growth rate has been observed in prematures given oral tetracycline in doses of 25 mg./kg. every 6 hours. This reaction was shown to be reversible when the drug was discontinued.

Tetracyclines are present in the milk of lactating women who are taking a drug in this class.

Precautions: As with other antibiotic preparations, use of this drug may result in overgrowth of nonsusceptible organisms, including fungi. If superinfection occurs, the antibiotic should be discontinued and appropriate therapy should be instituted.

In venereal diseases when coexistent syphilis is suspected, darkfield examination should be done before treatment is started and the blood serology repeated monthly for at least 4 months.

Because the tetracyclines have been shown to depress plasma prothrombin activity, patients who are on anticoagulant therapy may require downward adjustment of their anticoagulant dosage.

In long-term therapy, periodic laboratory evaluation of organ systems, including hematopoietic, renal and hepatic studies should be performed.

All infections due to Group A beta-hemolytic streptococci should be treated for at least 10 days. Since bacteriostatic drugs may interfere with the bactericidal action of penicillin, it is advisable to avoid giving demeclocycline in conjunction with penicillin.

Interpretation of Bacteriologic Studies: Following a course of therapy, persistence for several days in both urine and blood of bacterio-suppressive levels of demeclocycline may interfere with culture studies. These levels should not be considered therapeutic.

Adverse Reactions: Gastrointestinal: Anorexia, nausea, vomiting, diarrhea, glossitis, dysphagia, enterocolitis, and inflammatory lesions (with monilial overgrowth) in the anogenital region. These reactions have been caused by both the oral and parenteral administration of tetracyclines.

Skin: Maculopapular and erythematous rashes. Exfoliative dermatitis has been reported but is uncommon. Photosensitivity is discussed above. (See "Warnings").

Renal toxicity: Rise in BUN has been reported and is apparently dose related. Nephrogenic diabetes insipidus. (See "'Warnings").

Hypersensitivity reactions: Urticaria, angioneurotic edema, anaphylaxis, anaphylactoid purpura, pericarditis and exacerbation of systemic lupus erythematosus.

Bulging fontanels have been reported in young infants following full therapeutic dosage. This sign disappeared rapidly when the drug was discontinued.

Blood: Hemolytic anemia, thrombocytopenia, neutropenia and eosinophilia have been reported.

When given over prolonged periods, tetracyclines have been reported to produce brown-black microscopic discoloration of thyroid glands. No abnormalities of thyroid function studies are known to occur.

Dosage and Administration: Therapy should be continued for at least 24-48 hours after symptoms and fever have subsided.

Concomitant therapy: Antacids containing aluminum, calcium, or magnesium impair absorption and should not be given to patients taking oral tetracycline.

Foods and some dairy products also interfere with absorption. Oral forms of tetracycline should be given 1 hour before or 2 hours after meals.

In patients with renal impairment: (See "Warnings"). Total dosage should be decreased by reduction of recommended individual doses and/or by extending time intervals between doses.

In the treatment of streptococcal infections, a therapeutic dose of demeclocycline should be administered for at least 10 days.

Adults: Usual daily dose—Four divided doses of 150 mg. each or two divided doses of 300 mg. each. For children above eight years of age: Usual daily dose, 3–6 mg.. per pound body weight per day, depending upon the severity of the disease, divided into 2 or 4 doses.

Gonorrhea patients sensitive to penicillin may be treated with demeclocycline administered as an initial oral dose of 600 mg. followed by 300 mg. every 12 hours for 4 days to a total of 3 grams.

How Supplied:
Capsules: 150 mg.. *demeclocycline hydrochloride* (soft shell two tone coral) printed Lederle D9 bottles of 100. NDC 005-9208-23
Tablets: 150 mg.. *demeclocycline hydrochloride* (Film Coated Red) D11 bottles of 100. NDC 005-9218-23
300 mg.. *demeclocycline hydrochloride* (Film Coated Red) engraved LL D12 bottles of 48. NDC 005-9270-29
A.H.F.S. 8:12.24
Shown in Product Identification Section, page 415

DIAMOX® ℞
[*dīa-mŏx*]
acetazolamide
TABLETS, PARENTERAL AND SEQUELS®
Sustained Release Capsules

Description: Tablets: 125 mg of acetazolamide, round, flat-faced, beveled, white tablets engraved with DIAMOX and 125 on one side and scored in half on the other side. Engraved with LL on the right of the score and D1 on the left. 250 mg of acetazolamide, round, convex, white tablets engraved with DIAMOX and 250 on one side and scored in quarters on the other side. Engraved with LL in the upper right quadrant and D2 in the lower left quadrant.

Parenteral: *Each vial contains acetazolamide 500 mg (as sodium salt) and pH adjusted to approximately 9.2 with sodium hydroxide and, if necessary, hydrochloric acid.

SEQUELS: DIAMOX *acetazolamide* SEQUELS Lederle are sustained-release capsules each containing 500 mg. of acetazolamide.

Actions: DIAMOX is a potent carbonic anhydrase inhibitor, effective in the control of fluid secretion (e.g. some types of glaucoma), in the treatment of certain convulsive disorders (e.g. epilepsy) and in the promotion of diuresis in instances of abnormal fluid retention (e.g. cardiac edema).

Continued on next page

The information on each product appearing here is based on labelling effective in August, 1984 and is either the entire official brochure or an accurate condensation therefrom. Information concerning all Lederle products may be obtained from the Professional Services Department, Lederle Laboratories, Pearl River, New York, 10965.

Lederle—Cont.

DIAMOX is not a mercurial diuretic. Rather it is a nonbacteriostatic sulfonamide possessing a chemical structure and pharmacological activity distinctly different from the bacteriostatic sulfonamides.

DIAMOX is an enzyme inhibitor which acts specifically on carbonic anhydrase, the enzyme which catalyzes the reversible reaction involving the hydration of carbon dioxide and the dehydration of carbonic acid. In the eye, this inhibitory action of acetazolamide decreases the secretion of aqueous humor and results in a drop in intraocular pressure, a reaction considered desirable in cases of glaucoma and even in certain non-glaucomatous conditions. Evidence seems to indicate that DIAMOX has utility as an adjuvant in the treatment of certain dysfunctions of the central nervous system (e.g. epilepsy). Inhibition of carbonic anhydrase in this area appears to retard abnormal, paroxysmal, excessive discharge from central nervous system neurons. The diuretic effect of DIAMOX *acetazolamide* is due to its action in the kidney on the reversible reaction involving hydration of carbon dioxide and dehydration of carbonic acid. The result is renal loss of HCO_3 ion, which carries out sodium, water, and potassium. Alkalinization of the urine and promotion of diuresis are thus effected.

SEQUELS: DIAMOX Acetazolamide SEQUELS Sustained Release Capsules provide prolonged action to inhibit aqueous humor secretion for 18 to 24 hours after each dose, whereas tablets act for only 8 to 12 hours. The prolonged/continuous effect of SEQUELS permits a reduction in dosage frequency.

Blood level concentrations of acetazolamide peak between 8 to 12 hours after administration of DIAMOX SEQUELS, compared to 2 to 4 hours with tablets.

Indications—Tablets and Parenteral: For adjunctive treatment of: edema due to congestive heart failure; drug-induced edema; centrencephalic epilepsies (petit mal, unlocalized seizures); chronic simple (open angle) glaucoma, secondary glaucoma, and preoperatively in acute angle closure glaucoma where delay of surgery is desired in order to lower intraocular pressure.

Indications—SEQUELS: For adjunctive treatment of: chronic simple (open angle) glaucoma, secondary glaucoma, and preoperatively in acute angle closure glaucoma where delay of surgery is desired in order to lower intraocular pressure.

Contraindications: Acetazolamide therapy is contraindicated in situations in which sodium and/or potassium blood serum levels are depressed, in cases of marked kidney and liver disease or dysfunction, suprarenal gland failure, and hyperchloremic acidosis.

Long-term administration of DIAMOX *acetazolamide* is contraindicated in patients with chronic noncongestive angle closure glaucoma since it may permit organic closure of the angle to occur while the worsening glaucoma is masked by lowered intraocular pressure.

Warning: Studies of acetazolamide in rats and mice have demonstrated teratogenic and embryocidal effects at doses in excess of ten times those recommended in human beings. There is no evidence of these effects in human beings, however acetazolamide should not be used in pregnancy, especially during the first trimester, unless the benefits to be expected outweigh these potential adverse effects.

Precautions: Increasing the dose does not increase the diuresis and may increase the incidence of drowsiness and/or paresthesia. Increasing the dose often results in a decrease in diuresis. Under certain circumstances, however, very large doses have been given in conjunction with other diuretics in order to secure diuresis in complete refractory failure.

Adverse reactions common to all sulfonamide derivatives may occur: fever, rash, crystalluria, renal calculus, bone marrow depression, thrombocytopenic purpura, hemolytic anemia, leukopenia, pancytopenia and agranulocytosis. Precaution is advised for early detection of such reactions and the drug should be discontinued and appropriate therapy instituted. To monitor for hematologic reactions common to all sulfonamides, it is recommended that a baseline CBC and platelet count be obtained on patients prior to initiating DIAMOX therapy and at regular intervals during therapy. If significant changes occur, early discontinuance and institution of appropriate therapy are important.

In patients with pulmonary obstruction or emphysema where alveolar ventilation may be impaired, DIAMOX acetazolamide which may precipitate or aggravate acidosis, should be used with caution. Precaution is advised for patients receiving concomitant high-dose aspirin and DIAMOX acetazolamide, as anorexia, tachypnea, lethargy and coma have been rarely reported due to a possible drug interaction.

Adverse Reactions: Adverse reactions during short-term therapy are minimal. Those effects which have been noted include: paresthesias, particularly a "tingling" feeling in the extremities; some loss of appetite; polyuria and occasional instances of drowsiness and confusion.

During long-term therapy, an acidotic state may occasionally supervene. This can usually be corrected by the administration of bicarbonate.

Transient myopia has been reported. This condition invariably subsides upon diminution or discontinuance of the medication.

Other occasional adverse reactions include: urticaria; melena; hematuria; glycosuria; hepatic insufficiency; flaccid paralysis; and convulsions.

Dosage and Administration:
Preparation and Storage of Parenteral Solution:
Each 500 mg. vial containing DIAMOX *sterile acetazolamide sodium* Parenteral should be reconstituted with at least 5 ml. of Sterile Water for Injection prior to use. Reconstituted solutions retain potency for one week if refrigerated. Since this product contains no preservative, use within 24 hours of reconstitution is strongly recommended. The direct intravenous route of administration is preferred. Intramuscular administration may be employed but is painful, due to the alkaline pH of the solution.

Glaucoma: DIAMOX *acetazolamide* should be used as an adjunct to the usual therapy. The dosage employed in the treatment of *chronic simple (open-angle) glaucoma* ranges from 250 mg. to 1 Gram of DIAMOX per 24 hours, usually in divided doses for amounts over 250 mg. It has usually been found that a dosage in excess of 1 Gram per 24 hours does not produce an increased effect. In all cases, the dosage should be adjusted with careful individual attention both to symptomatology and ocular tension. Continuous supervision by a physician is advisable.

In the treatment of secondary glaucoma and in the preoperative treatment of some cases of *acute congestive (closed-angle) glaucoma*, the preferred dosage is 250 mg. every 4 hours, although some cases have responded to 250 mg. twice daily on short-term therapy. In some acute cases, it may be more satisfactory to administer an initial dose of 500 mg. followed by 125 or 250 mg. every 4 hours depending on the individual case. Intravenous therapy may be used for rapid relief of ocular tension in acute cases. A complementary effect has been noted when DIAMOX has been used in conjunction with miotics or mydriatics as the case demanded.

Epilepsy: It is not clearly known whether the beneficial effects observed in epilepsy are due to direct inhibition of carbonic anhydrase in the central nervous system or whether they are due to the slight degree of acidosis produced by the divided dosage. The best results to date have been seen in petit mal in children. Good results, however, have been seen in patients, both children and adult, in other types of seizures such as grand mal, mixed seizure patterns, myoclonic jerk patterns, etc. The suggested total daily dose is 8 to 30 mg. per Kg. in divided doses. Although some patients respond to a low dose, the optimum range appears to be from 375 to 1000 mg. daily. However, some investigators feel that daily doses in excess of 1 Gram do not produce any better results than a 1 Gram dose. When DIAMOX is given in combination with other anti-convulsants, it is suggested that the starting dose should be 250 mg. once daily in addition to the existing medications. This can be increased to levels as indicated above.

The change from other medication to DIAMOX should be gradual in accordance with usual practice in epilepsy therapy.

Congestive Heart Failure: For diuresis in congestive heart failure, the starting dose is usually 250 to 375 mg. once daily in the morning (5 mg./Kg.). If after an initial response, the patient fails to continue to lose edema fluid, do not increase the dose but allow for kidney recovery by skipping medication for a day. DIAMOX *acetazolamide* yields best diuretic results when given on alternate days, or for 2 days alternating with a day of rest.

Failures in therapy may be due to overdosage or too frequent dosage. The use of DIAMOX does not eliminate the need for other therapy such as digitalis, bed rest, and salt restriction.

Drug-Induced Edema: Recommended dosage is 250 mg. to 375 mg. of DIAMOX once a day for 1 or 2 days, alternating with a day of rest.

Note: The dosage recommendations for glaucoma and epilepsy differ considerably from those for congestive heart failure, since the first two conditions are not dependent upon carbonic anhydrase inhibition in the kidney which requires intermittent dosage if it is to recover from the inhibitory effect of the therapeutic agent.

SEQUELS: The recommended dose is 1 capsule (500 mg.) 2 times a day. Usually 1 capsule is administered in the morning and 1 capsule in the evening. It may be necessary to adjust the dose but it has usually been found that dosage in excess of 2 capsules (1 Gram) does not produce an increased effect. The dosage should be adjusted with careful individual attention both to symptomatology and intraocular tension. In all cases, continuous supervision by a physician is advisable.

In those unusual instances where adequate control is not obtained by the twice-a-day administration of DIAMOX *acetazolamide* SEQUELS, sustained release capsules, the desired control may be established by means of DIAMOX (Tablets or Parenteral). Use tablets or parenteral in accordance with the more frequent dosage schedules recommended for these items, such as 250 mg. every 4 hours, or an initial dose of 500 mg. followed by 250 mg. or 125 mg. every 4 hours; depending on the case in question.

How Supplied: Tablets 125 mg—Round, flat-faced, beveled, white tablets engraved with DIAMOX and 125 on one side and scored in half on the other side. Engraved with LL on the right of the score and D1 on the left.
Bottles of 100—Product Number NDC 0005-4398-23

Tablets 250 mg—Round, convex, white tablets engraved with DIAMOX and 250 on one side and scored in quarters on the other side. Engraved with LL in the upper right quadrant and D2 in the lower left quadrant.
Bottle of 100—NDC 0005-4469-23
Bottle of 1,000 NDC 0005-4469-34
Unit of Issue, 50 × 100's—NDC 0005-4469-73
Unit Dose Pkg. 10-10's—NDC 0005-4469-60
Parenteral—500 mg vials of cryodesiccated powder—Product Number NDC 0005-4466-96 SEQUELS® sustained release capsules (soft shell, orange) printed with "DIAMOX" over D3, 500 mg.—bottles of 30 NDC 0005-4465-13 and 100 NDC 0005-4465-23.
Store at controlled room temperature 15–30°C (59–86°F).

Lederle Laboratories Division
American Cyanamid Company
Pearl River, N.Y.
NSN 6505-00-064-8724, 500 mg vial
A.H.F.S. 40:28
SEQUELS, 500 mg
Military Depot: NSN 6505-00-880-4949, 100's
VA Depot: NSN 6505-00-880-4949A, 100's

Product Information

LEDERLE PARENTERALS INC.
Carolina, Puerto Rico 00630
Tablets and SEQUELS
Shown in Product Identification Section, page 415

DIPHTHERIA AND TETANUS TOXOIDS ADSORBED PUROGENATED®
NDC 0005-1858-31

How Supplied: 5 ml. vials (5 immunizations). COMPLETE INFORMATION FURNISHED IN THE PACKAGE.

FERRO–SEQUELS®
[fĕrrō sē-quls]
Sustained Release
Iron Capsules

Composition: Each capsule contains 150 mg of ferrous fumarate, equivalent to approximately 50 mg of elemental iron, and 100 mg of docusate sodium (DSS).
Indications: For the treatment of iron-deficiency anemias.
Warning: As with any drug, if you are pregnant or nursing a baby, seek the advice of a health professional before using this product. Keep this and all medications out of the reach of children. In case of accidental overdose, seek professional assistance or contact a Poison Control Center immediately.
Dosage: 1 capsule, once or twice daily or as prescribed by the physician.
How Supplied: Bottles of 30 capsules, NDC 0005-4612-13
Bottles of 100 capsules, NDC 0005-4612-23 Unit Dose Pkg., 10-10's
20 × Pkg. 10-10's, Per Pkg. NDC 0005-4612-60
Bottles of 1,000, NDC 0005-4612-34
Store at Controlled Room Temperature 15-30° C (59-86° F).
Capsules (light green) Printed Lederle FERRO-SEQUELS F2
Military Depots
30's..NSN 6505-00-149-0103
Individually sealed 100's (Unit Dose) NSN 6505-00-131-8870
1000's.....................................NSN 6505-00-074-2981
Shown in Product Identification Section, page 415

FILIBON®
[fĭl-ă-bŏn]
prenatal tablets

Each tablet contains: For Pregnant or Lactating Women Percentage of U.S. Recommended Daily Allowance (U.S. RDA)

Vitamin A (as Acetate)	5000 I.U. (63%)
Vitamin D$_2$	400 I.U. (100%)
Vitamin E (as dl-Alpha Tocopheryl Acetate)	30 I.U. (100%)
Vitamin C (Ascorbic Acid)	60 mg (100%)
Folic Acid (Folacin)	0.4 mg (50%)
Vitamin B$_1$ (as Thiamine Mononitrate)	1.5 mg (88%)
Vitamin B$_2$ (as Riboflavin)	1.7 mg (85%)
Niacinamide	20 mg (100%)
Vitamin B$_6$ (as Pyridoxine Hydrochloride)	2 mg (80%)
Vitamin B$_{12}$ (as Cyanocobalamin)	6 mcg (75%)
Calcium (as Calcium Carbonate)	125 mg (10%)
Iodine (as Potassium Iodide)	150 mcg (100%)
Iron (as Ferrous Fumarate)	18 mg (100%)
Magnesium (as Magnesium Oxide)	100 mg (22%)

A phosphorus-free vitamin and mineral dietary supplement for use in prenatal care and lactation.
Recommended Intake: 1 daily, or as prescribed by the physician.
How Supplied: Capsule-shaped tablets (film-coated, pink) engraved LL-F4—bottles of 100 NDC 0005-4294-23.
Shown in Product Identification Section, page 415

FILIBON® F.A.
[fĭl-ă-bŏn]
prenatal tablets

Each tablet contains: Percentage of U.S. Recommended Daily Allowance (U.S. RDA)

Vitamin A (as Acetate)	8000 I.U. (100%)
Vitamin D$_2$	400 I.U. (100%)
Vitamin E (as dl-Alpha Tocopheryl Acetate)	30 I.U. (100%)
Vitamin C (as Ascorbic Acid)	60 mg (100%)
Folic Acid (as Folacin)	1 mg (125%)
Vitamin B$_1$ (as Thiamine Mononitrate)	1.7 mg (100%)
Vitamin B$_2$ (as Riboflavin)	2 mg (100%)
Niacinamide	20 mg (100%)
Vitamin B$_6$ (as Pyridoxine Hydrochloride)	4.0 mg (160%)
Vitamin B$_{12}$ (as Cyanocobalamin)	8 mcg (100%)
Calcium (as Calcium Carbonate)	250 mg (19%)
Iodine (as Potassium Iodide)	150 mcg (100%)
Iron (as Ferrous Fumarate)	45 mg (250%)
Magnesium (as Magnesium Oxide)	100 mg (22%)

Precaution: Folic acid may obscure pernicious anemia in that the peripheral blood picture may revert to normal while neurological manifestations remain progressive.
How Supplied: Capsule-shaped tablets (film-coated, pink) engraved LL-F5—bottles of 100 NDC 0005-4225-23.
Shown in Product Identification Section, page 415

FILIBON® FORTE
[fĭl-ă-bŏn for-tā]
prenatal tablets

Each tablet contains: Percentage of U.S. Recommended Daily Allowance (U.S. RDA)

Vitamin A (as Acetate)	8000 I.U. (100%)
Vitamin D$_2$	400 I.U. (100%)
Vitamin E (as dl-Alpha Tocopheryl Acetate)	45 I.U. (150%)
Vitamin C (Ascorbic Acid)	90 mg (150%)
Folic Acid (Folacin)	1 mg (125%)
Vitamin B$_1$ (as Thiamine Mononitrate)	2 mg (118%)
Vitamin B$_2$ (as Riboflavin)	2.5 mg (125%)
Niacinamide	30 mg (150%)
Vitamin B$_6$ as Pyridoxine Hydrochloride)	3 mg (120%)
Vitamin B$_{12}$ (as Cyanocobalamin)	12 mcg (150%)
Calcium (as Calcium Carbonate)	300 mg (23%)
Iodine (as Potassium Iodide)	200 mg (133%)
Iron (as Ferrous Fumarate)	45 mg (250%)
Magnesium (as Magnesium Oxide)	100 mg (22%)

Recommended Intake: 1 tablet daily. This dosage provides 23% and 22% the Recommended Daily Allowance of calcium and magnesium respectively, therefore, supplementation of the diet by milk or other sources of calcium may be advisable.
Precaution: Folic Acid may obscure pernicious anemia in that the peripheral blood picture may revert to normal while neurological manifestations remain progressive.
How Supplied: Tablets—film coated (pink) scored LL-F6—bottles of 100 NDC 0005-4226-23.
Shown in Product Identification Section, page 415

FOLVITE®
[fōl-vīt]
folic acid
Tablets—Parenteral Solution

Description: Folic Acid, N-[p[[(2-Amino-4-hydroxy-6-pteridinyl)-methyl]Amino]benzoyl] glutamic acid, is a complex organic compound present in liver, yeast, and other substances, which may be prepared synthetically.
Tablets
1 mg Folic Acid
Parenteral
Each ml of FOLVITE *folic acid*-Solution contains sodium folate equivalent to 5 mg of FOLIC ACID.
Inactive Ingredients: Sequestrene Sodium 0.2% and Water for Injection q.s. 100%, Sodium Hydroxide to approx. pH 9, Preservative: Benzyl Alcohol 1.5%.
Actions: In man, an exogenous source of folate is required for nucleoprotein synthesis and maintenance of normal erythropoiesis. Folic Acid, whether given by mouth or parenterally, stimulates specifically the production of red blood cells, white blood cells, and platelets in persons suffering from certain megaloblastic anemias.
Indications: Folic Acid is effective in the treatment of megaloblastic anemias due to a deficiency of Folic Acid as may be seen in tropical or nontropical sprue, in anemias of nutritional origin, pregnancy, infancy, or childhood.
Warnings: Folic Acid alone is improper therapy in the treatment of pernicious anemia and other megaloblastic anemias where Vitamin B$_{12}$ is deficient.
Precautions: Folic acid in doses above 0.1 mg daily may obscure pernicious anemia in that hematologic remission can occur while neurological manifestations remain progressive.
Adverse Reactions: Allergic sensitization has been reported following both oral and parenteral administration of Folic Acid.
Dosage and Administration:
Oral administration: Folic Acid is well absorbed and may be administered orally with satisfactory results except in severe instances of intestinal malabsorption.
Parenteral administration: Intramuscular, intravenous, and subcutaneous routes may be used if the disease is exceptionally severe or if gastrointestinal absorption may be, or is known to be, impaired.
Usual therapeutic dosage—In adults and children (regardless of age): up to 1.0 mg daily. Resistant cases may require larger doses.
Maintenance level: When clinical symptoms have subsided and the blood picture has become normal, a maintenance level should be used, i.e., 0.1 mg for infants and up to 0.3 mg for children under four years of age, 0.4 mg for adults and children four or more years of age, and 0.8 mg for pregnant and lactating women, per day, but never less than 0.1 mg per day. Patients should be kept under close supervision and adjustment of the maintenance level made if relapse appears imminent.
In the presence of alcoholism, hemolytic anemia, anticonvulsant therapy, or chronic infection, the maintenance level may need to be increased.
How Supplied: Tablets (Scored, orange) engraved LL F1—1 mg.—bottles of 100 NDC 0005-4165-23 and 1,000 NDC 0005-4165-34; Unit-dose 10 x 10's NDC 0005-4165-60. *Parenteral Solution, 5 mg./ml.—10 ml. vials NDC 0205-4154-34.
A.H.F.S. 88:08
*Manufactured for
LEDERLE LABORATORIES DIVISION
American Cyanamid Company
Pearl River, NY 10965
by
LEDERLE PARENTERALS INC.
Carolina, Puerto Rico 00630

FOOTWORK™
Athlete's Foot Remedy
(See PDR For Nonprescription Drugs)

GEVRABON®
[jĕv-ra-bŏn]
(vitamin-mineral supplement)
(See PDR for Nonprescription Drugs)

Continued on next page

Lederle—Cont.

GEVRAL®
[jĕv-ral]
Multivitamin and Multimineral Supplement for Adults and Children 4 or More Years of Age
TABLETS

(See PDR For Nonprescription Drugs)

GEVRAL® T
[jĕv-ral]
High Potency Multivitamin and Multimineral Supplement for Adults and Children 4 or More Years of Age
TABLETS

(See PDR For Nonprescription Drugs)

HYDROMOX® ℞
[hū-drō-mŏx]
quinethazone
Tablets

Description: Chemistry: HYDROMOX is a quinazoline derivative, in which a cyclic carbamyl group replaces the cyclic sulfamyl group present in the thiazide derivatives.

Chemical name: 7-Chloro-2-ethyl-1,2,3,4-tetrahydro-4-oxo-6-sulfamyl-quinazoline
Tablet Size: 50 mg. scored

Actions: HYDROMOX produces urinary excretion of sodium and chloride in approximately equivalent amounts (saluresis), while potassium is excreted to a much lesser degree. The saluretic effect of HYDROMOX is rapid and relatively prolonged, beginning within 2 hours after administration, reaching a peak at 6 hours, and lasting for 18 to 24 hours. While HYDROMOX is chemically different, it is pharmacologically genetic to the benzothiadiazine group of drugs.

The dominant action of quinethazone is to increase the renal excretion of sodium and chloride and an accompanying volume of water. This results from inhibition of the tubular mechanism of electrolyte reabsorption. The renal effect is virtually independent of alterations in acid-base balance.

Quinethazone, like other drugs in this class, inhibits the proximal reabsorption of sodium and chloride. The excretion of potassium results from increased potassium secretion by the distal tubule where potassium is exchanged for sodium.

Quinethazone may exert its antihypertensive effect by diuresis and sodium loss and/or on vascular function to reduce peripheral resistance.

Indications: HYDROMOX *quinethazone* Lederle, a nonmercurial oral diuretic agent is indicated as adjunctive therapy in edema associated with congestive heart failure, hepatic cirrhosis and corticosteroid and estrogen therapy.

HYDROMOX has also been found useful in edema due to various forms of renal dysfunction such as: nephrotic syndrome; acute glomerulonephritis; and chronic renal failure.

HYDROMOX is indicated in the management of hypertension either as the sole therapeutic agent or to enhance the effectiveness of other antihypertensive drugs in the more severe forms of hypertension.

Usage in Pregnancy: The routine use of diuretics in an otherwise healthy woman is inappropriate and exposes mother and fetus to unnecessary hazard. Diuretics do not prevent development of toxemia of pregnancy, and there is no satisfactory evidence that they are useful in the treatment of developed toxemia.

Edema during pregnancy may arise from pathological causes or from the physiologic and mechanical consequences of pregnancy. Diuretics are indicated in pregnancy when edema is due to pathologic causes, just as they are in the absence of pregnancy (however, see Warnings, below). Dependent edema in pregnancy, resulting from restriction of venous return by the expanded uterus, is properly treated through elevation of the lower extremities and use of support hose; use of diuretics to lower intravascular volume in this case is illogical and unnecessary. There is hypervolemia during normal pregnancy which is harmful to neither the fetus nor the mother (in the absence of cardiovascular disease), but which is associated with edema, including generalized edema, in the majority of pregnant women. If this edema produces discomfort, increased recumbency will often provide relief. In rare instances, this edema may cause extreme discomfort which is not relieved by rest. In these cases, a short course of diuretics may provide relief and may be appropriate.

Contraindications:
A. Anuria
B. Hypersensitivity to this or other sulfonamide derived drugs.

Warnings: Diuretics should be used with caution in severe renal disease. In patients with renal disease, diuretics may precipitate azotemia. Cumulative effects of the drug may develop in patients with impaired renal function.

Diuretics should be used with caution in patients with impaired hepatic function or progressive liver disease, since minor alterations of fluid and electrolyte balance may precipitate hepatic coma. Quinethazone may add to or potentiate the action of other antihypertensive drugs. Potentiation occurs with ganglionic or peripheral adrenergic blocking drugs.

Sensitivity reactions may occur in patients with a history of allergy or bronchial asthma.

The possibility of exacerbation or activation of systemic lupus erythematosus has been reported.

Usage in Pregnancy: Quinethazone crosses the placental barrier and appears in cord blood. The use of quinethazone in pregnant women requires that the anticipated benefit be weighed against possible hazards to the fetus. These hazards include fetal or neonatal jaundice, thrombocytopenia, and possible other adverse reactions which have occurred in the adult.

Nursing Mothers: Quinethazone appears in breast milk. If use of the drug is deemed essential, the patient should stop nursing.

Precautions: (1) Quinethazone should be used with caution in patients with impaired hepatic function or progressive liver disease, since minor alterations of fluid and electrolyte balance may precipitate hepatic coma. (2) Whereas electrolyte abnormalities are often present in such conditions as heart failure and cirrhosis as a result of underlying disease process, they may also be aggravated or may be produced independently by any potent diuretic affecting electrolyte excretion. Caution is especially important during prolonged or intensive therapy and when salt intake is restricted or during concomitant use of steroids or ACTH. Hypokalemia attributable to HYDROMOX *quinethazone* therapy has been mild and infrequent, and other electrolyte abnormalities have been rare. The possibility of potassium depletion and its toxic sequelae must be kept in mind, particularly in cirrhotics and patients receiving digitalis. As a preventive measure the use of foods rich in potassium, such as orange juice, or supplements of potassium chloride may be desirable. (3) In patients with impaired renal function, azotemia and/or excessive drug accumulation may develop. (4) As with other potent diuretics, when HYDROMOX is added to a regimen that includes ganglionic-blocking agents, the dosage of these latter preparations should be reduced to avoid a sudden drop in blood pressure. Reduction of dosage is also necessary when one or more of these antihypertensive agents is added to an established HYDROMOX regimen. (5) As with the thiazide diuretics, increases of serum uric acid may occur but precipitation of gout has been rare. (6) A decreased glucose tolerance as evidenced by hyperglycemia and glycosuria thus aggravating or provoking diabetes mellitus has occurred. (7) Quinethazone may decrease arterial responsiveness to norepinephrine and therefore should be withdrawn 48 hours before elective surgery. If emergency surgery is indicated, pre-anesthetic and anesthetic agents should be administered in reduced dosage. Quinethazone may also increase the responsiveness to tubocurarine. The antihypertensive effects of the drug may be enhanced in the post-sympathectomy patient. (8) Sensitivity reactions may be more likely to occur in patients with a history of allergy or bronchial asthma. (9) The possibility of exacerbation or activation of systemic lupus erythematosus has been suggested for sulfonamide derived drugs.

Adverse Reactions: The following adverse reactions have been reported with the diuretic drugs some of which may be expected to occur with quinethazone:
A. *Gastrointestinal System reactions:* 1. anorexia, 2. gastric irritation, 3. nausea, 4. vomiting, 5. cramping, 6. diarrhea, 7. constipation, 8. jaundice (intrahepatic cholestatic jaundice), 9. pancreatitis, 10. hyperglycemia, 11. glycosuria.
B. *Central Nervous System reactions:* 1. dizziness, 2. vertigo, 3. paresthesias, 4. headache, 5. xanthopsia.
C. *Hematologic Reactions:* 1. leukopenia, 2. thrombocytopenia, 3. agranulocytosis, 4. aplastic anemia.
D. *Dermatologic—hypersensitivity reactions:* 1. purpura, 2. photosensitivity, 3. rash, 4. urticaria, 5. necrotizing angiitis (vasculitis) (cutaneous vasculitis).
E. *Cardiovascular Reactions:* 1. orthostatic hypotension may occur and may be potentiated by alcohol, barbiturates or narcotics.
F. *Miscellaneous:* 1. muscle spasm, 2. weakness, 3. restlessness. Whenever adverse reactions are moderate or severe, thiazide dosage should be reduced or therapy withdrawn.

Dosage: Average Adult Dosage: One or two 50 mg. tablets, orally, once a day. Because of its relatively prolonged duration of activity, a single daily dose is generally sufficient. Occasionally, 1 tablet (50 mg.) is administered twice a day. Infrequently, a total daily dose of 3 to 4 tablets (150 to 200 mg.) may be necessary. The dosage employed depends upon the severity of the condition being treated and the responsiveness of the patient, and often must be adjusted at the beginning or during the course of therapy. When HYDROMOX *quinethazone* is used in combination with other antihypertensive agents, the dosage of each drug may often be reduced because of potentiation. (See under Precautions concerning the necessity for dosage adjustment when one or more of these drugs is added to an already established therapeutic regime.)

How Supplied: 50 mg. tablets (scored) engraved LL H1—bottles of 100 NDC 0005-4458-23 and 500 NDC 0005-4458-31.

Shown in Product Identification Section, page 415

HYDROMOX® R ℞
[hī-drō-mŏx]
Quinethazone with Reserpine
TABLETS

Warnings:

> This fixed combination drug is not indicated for initial therapy of hypertension. Hypertension requires therapy titrated to the individual patient. If the fixed combination represents the dosage so determined, its use may be more convenient in patient management. The treatment of hypertension is not static, but must be reevaluated as conditions in each patient warrant.

Description: HYDROMOX R tablets each contain 50 mg quinethazone and 0.125 mg reserpine. HYDROMOX® *quinethazone* Lederle is a nonmercurial oral diuretic agent, effective in the treatment of edema and hypertension. It is chemically distinct from the benzothiadiazine series of compounds. Reserpine, an antihypertensive agent, has been combined with quinethazone in a dosage form designed to be useful in the treatment of hypertension with or without edema.

Chemistry: HYDROMOX is a quinazoline derivative, in which a cyclic carbamyl group replaces the

cyclic sulfamyl group present in the thiazide derivatives.
Quinethazone is 7-Chloro-2-ethyl-1,2,3,4-tetrahydro-4-oxo-6-quinazolinesulfonamide.
Reserpine is $3\beta, 16\beta, 17\alpha, 18\beta, 20\alpha$)-11,17-Dimethoxy-18-[(3,4,5-trimethoxybenxoyl)oxy]-yohimban-16-carboxylic acid methyl ester.

Actions: HYDROMOX produces urinary excretion of sodium and chloride in approximately equivalent amounts (saluresis), while potassium is excreted to a much lesser degree. The saluretic effect of HYDROMOX is rapid and relatively prolonged, beginning within 2 hours after administration, reaching a peak at 6 hours, and lasting for 18 to 24 hours. While HYDROMOX is chemically different, it is pharmacologically genetic to the benzothiadiazine group of drugs.

The dominant action of quinethazone is to increase the renal excretion of sodium and chloride and an accompanying volume of water. This results from inhibition of the tubular mechanism of electrolyte reabsorption. The renal effect is virtually independent of alterations in acid-base balance.

Quinethazone, like other drugs in this class, inhibits the proximal reabsorption of sodium and chloride. The excretion of potassium results from increased potassium secretion by the distal tubule where potassium is exchanged for sodium.

Quinethazone may exert its antihypertensive effect by diuresis and sodium loss and/or on vascular function to reduce peripheral resistance.

Reserpine is an antihypertensive agent which produces a mild type of sedation that is tranquilizing rather than hypnotic. The most prominent actions of reserpine are upon the cardiovascular and central nervous systems. In clinical hypertension, reserpine produces a gradual and moderate fall in both systolic and diastolic blood pressures after oral administration for several days to 2-3 weeks. Its effects persist about 3-4 weeks after medication is withdrawn. With an increase in dose, a prolongation of hypotensive effect, rather than an intensification of blood pressure fall, tends to occur. The doses employed in the therapy of hypertension are smaller than those used in psychiatric disorders.

The dosage form combining quinethazone with reserpine is designed to provide effective antihypertensive action upon patients who have failed to show satisfactory response to the use of quinethazone or reserpine alone. This combination of quinethazone and reserpine frequently permits use of a lower dosage of each agent and hence tends to produce the desired antihypertensive effect while eliminating, or at least minimizing, adverse reactions. Blood pressure reductions averaging about -30/-15 have been demonstrated within the first 2 weeks of treatment. Continuation of therapy beyond 2 weeks may be expected to produce further *small* drops in blood pressure. The enhanced reduction in blood pressure produced by quinethazone with reserpine appears to be an additive rather than a potentiating effect.

Indications: HYDROMOX R is indicated in the management of hypertension (see box warnings) either as the sole therapeutic agent or to enhance the effectiveness of other antihypertensive drugs in the more severe forms of hypertension.

Usage in Pregnancy
The routine use of diuretics in an otherwise healthy woman is inappropriate and exposes mother and fetus to unnecessary hazard. Diuretics do not prevent development of toxemia of pregnancy, and there is no satisfactory evidence that they are useful in the treatment of developed toxemia.

Edema during pregnancy may arise from pathological causes or from the physiologic and mechanical consequences of pregnancy. Diuretics are indicated in pregnancy when edema is due to pathologic causes, just as they are in the absence of pregnancy (however, see WARNINGS, below). Dependent edema in pregnancy, resulting from restriction of venous return by the expanded uterus, is properly treated through elevation of the lower extremities and use of support hose; use of diuretics to lower intravascular volume in this case is illogical and unnecessary. There is hypervolemia during normal pregnancy which is harmful to neither the fetus nor the mother (in the absence of cardiovascular disease), but which is associated with edema, including generalized edema, in the majority of pregnant women. If this edema produces discomfort, increased recumbency will often provide relief. In rare instances, this edema may cause extreme discomfort which is not relieved by rest. In these cases, a short course of diuretics may provide relief and may be appropriate.

Contraindications:
A. Anuria
B. Hypersensitivity to this or other sulfonamide derived drugs.
C. Progressively impaired renal function. Since reserpine may increase gastric secretion and motility, its use alone or in combination requires caution and is sometimes contraindicated in patients with a history of peptic or duodenal ulcer or other gastrointestinal disorders.
D. HYDROMOX R should not be administered to patients with severe hepatic dysfunction. The use of the drug should be avoided in patients with a history of mental depression or psychosis. HYDROMOX R should not be used by patients who are known to be hypersensitive to either agent.

Warnings: Diuretics should be used with caution in severe renal disease. In patients with renal disease, diuretics may precipitate azotemia. Cumulative effects of the drug may develop in patients with impaired renal function.

Diuretics should be used with caution in patients with impaired hepatic function or progressive liver disease, since minor alterations of fluid and electrolyte balance may precipitate hepatic coma. HYDROMOX R may add to or potentiate the action of other antihypertensive drugs. Potentiation occurs with ganglionic or peripheral adrenergic blocking drugs.

Sensitivity reactions may occur in patients with a history of allergy or bronchial asthma.

The possibility of exacerbation or activation of systemic lupus erythematosus has been reported with sulfonamide-derived drugs.

Usage in Pregnancy
HYDROMOX R crosses the placental barrier and appears in cord blood. The use of HYDROMOX R in pregnant women requires that the anticipated benefit be weighed against possible hazards to the fetus. These hazards include fetal or neonatal jaundice, thrombocytopenia, and possibly other adverse reactions which have occurred in the adult.

Nursing Mothers
HYDROMOX R appears in breast milk. If use of the drug is deemed essential, the patient should stop nursing.

Reserpine has been reported to cause central nervous system depression of the newborn infant when given to the mother in the immediate ante partum period.

HYDROMOX R should be discontinued promptly if any symptoms of mental depression occur with the use of the drug.

Precautions:
Quinethazone:
(1) Quinethazone should be used with caution in patients with impaired hepatic function or progressive liver disease, since minor alterations of fluid and electrolyte balance may precipitate hepatic coma.
(2) Whereas electrolyte abnormalities are often present in such conditions as heart failure and cirrhosis as a result of underlying disease process, they may also be aggravated or may be produced independently by any potent diuretic affecting electrolyte excretion. Caution is especially important during prolonged or intensive therapy and when salt intake is restricted or during concomitant use of steroids or ACTH. Hypokalemia attributable to HYDROMOX *quinethazone* therapy has been mild and infrequent, and other electrolyte abnormalities have been rare. The possibility of potassium depletion and its toxic sequelae must be kept in mind, particularly in cirrhotics and patients receiving digitalis. As a preventive measure the use of foods rich in potassium, such as orange juice, or supplements of potassium chloride may be desirable.
(3) In patients with impaired renal function, azotemia and/or excessive drug accumulation may develop.
(4) As with other potent diuretics, when HYDROMOX is added to a regimen that includes ganglionic-blocking agents, the dosage of these latter preparations should be reduced to avoid a sudden drop in blood pressure. Reduction of dosage is also necessary when one or more of these antihypertensive agents is added to an established HYDROMOX regimen.
(5) As with the thiazide diuretics, increases of serum uric acid may occur but precipitation of gout has been rare.
(6) A decreased glucose tolerance as evidenced by hyperglycemia and glycosuria thus aggravating or provoking diabetes mellitus has occurred.
(7) Quinethazone may decrease arterial responsiveness to norepinephrine and therefore should be withdrawn 48 hours before elective surgery. If emergency surgery is indicated, preanesthetic and anesthetic agents should be administered in reduced dosage. Quinethazone may also increase the responsiveness to tubocurarine. The antihypertensive effects of the drug may be enhanced in the post-sympathectomy patient.
(8) Sensitivity reactions may be more likely to occur in patients with a history of allergy or bronchial asthma.
(9) The possibility of exacerbation or activation of systemic lupus erythematosus has been suggested for sulfonamide derived drugs.

Reserpine:
Reserpine may precipitate biliary colic in patients with gallstones, or bronchial asthma in susceptible patients. Reserpine preparations should be used with caution in patients with a history of peptic ulcer, ulcerative colitis and other gastrointestinal disorders. It may cause severe depression and suicidal risk and may produce pseudoparkinsonism (a paralysis agitans-like syndrome). Administration of reserpine should be discontinued 2 weeks or more before electroconvulsant therapy if possible to preclude severe, even fatal, reactions.

Reserpine may cause cardiotoxic effects, e.g. premature ventricular contractions and other arrhythmias, possible sensitization to digitalis (which might be further complicated by any hypokalemic effects of quinethazone), fluid retention, and congestive failure.

Animal tumorigenicity: rodent studies have shown that reserpine is an animal tumorigen, causing an increased incidence of mammary fibroadenomas in female mice, malignant tumors of the seminal vesicles in male mice, and malignant adrenal medullary tumors in male rats. These findings arose in 2 year studies in which the drug was administered in the feed at concentrations of 5 and 10 ppm-about 100 to 300 times the usual human dose. The breast neoplasms are thought to be related to reserpine's prolactin-elevating effect. Several other prolactin-elevating drugs have also been associated with an increased incidence of mammary neoplasis in rodents.

The extent to which these findings indicate a risk to humans is uncertain. Tissue culture experiments show that about one-third of human breast

Continued on next page

The information on each product appearing here is based on labelling effective in August, 1984 and is either the entire official brochure or an accurate condensation therefrom. Information concerning all Lederle products may be obtained from the Professional Services Department, Lederle Laboratories, Pearl River, New York, 10965.

Lederle—Cont.

tumors are prolactin-dependent *in vitro,* a factor of considerable importance if the use of the drug is contemplated in a patient with previously detected breast cancer. The possibility of an increased risk of breast cancer in reserpine users has been studied extensively; however, no firm conclusion has emerged. Although a few epidemiologic studies have suggested a slightly increased risk (less than twofold in all studies except one) in women who have used reserpine, other studies of generally similar design have not confirmed this. Epidemiologic studies conducted using other drugs (neuroleptic agents) that, like reserpine, increase prolactin levels, and therefore would be considered rodent mammary carcinogens, have not shown an association between chronic administration of the drug and human mammary tumorigenesis. While long-term clinical observation has not suggested such an association, the available evidence is considered too limited to be conclusive at this time. An association of reserpine intake with pheochromocytoma or tumors of the seminal vesicles has not been explored.

Adverse Reactions: The following adverse reactions have been reported with the diuretic drugs some of which may be expected to occur with quinethazone:
  A. Gastrointestinal System reactions
   1. anorexia
   2. gastric irritation
   3. nausea
   4. vomiting
   5. cramping
   6. diarrhea
   7. constipation
   8. jaundice (intrahepatic cholestatic jaundice)
   9. pancreatitis
   10. hyperglycemia
   11. glycosuria
  B. Central Nervous System reactions
   1. dizziness
   2. vertigo
   3. paresthesias
   4. headache
   5. xanthopsia
  C. Hematologic reactions
   1. leukopenia
   2. thrombocytopenia
   3. agranulocytosis
   4. asplastic anemia
  D. Dermatologic—hypersensitivity reactions
   1. purpura
   2. photosensitivity
   3. rash
   4. urticaria
   5. necrotizing angiitis (vasculitis) (cutaneous vasculitis)
  E. Cardiovascular reactions
   1. orthostatic hypotension may occur and may be potentiated by alcohol, barbiturates or narcotics.
  F. Miscellaneous
   1. muscle spasm
   2. weakness
   3. restlessness

Reserpine:
With reserpine, nasal congestion, weight gain, and diarrhea are the most frequently noted side effects. The drug may reactivate old peptic ulcers because it increases hydrochloric acid secretion by the stomach. More serious reactions are excessive drowsiness, fatigue, weakness, insomnia, nightmares, excitement, irrational behavior, and incipient parkinsonism. Sodium retention edema may occur when reserpine is used.
Whenever adverse reactions are moderate or severe, thiazide dosage should be reduced or therapy withdrawn.

Dosage and Administration:
Dosage: As determined by individual titration (see box warning).
Usual Initial Adult Loading Dosage: If considered necessary, 3 to 4 HYDROMOX R Tablets (150 mg quinethazone with 0.375 mg reserpine to 200 mg quinethazone with 0.5 mg reserpine) may be administered orally, once a day, for not more than 2 weeks.
Average (or Maintenance) Adult Dosage: 1 to 2 HYDROMOX R Tablets (50 mg quinethazone with 0.125 mg reserpine to 100 mg quinethazone with 0.25 mg reserpine) administered orally, once a day. Because of the relatively prolonged effect of HYDROMOX R, a single daily dose is usually sufficient. Occasionally 1 tablet is administered twice a day, but ordinarily medication is administered only in the morning to avoid the inconvenience of nocturia.
With the exception of the initial loading phase, a total dose of 3 to 4 tablets of HYDROMOX R Quinethazone with Reserpine is not recommended since the 0.375 mg to 0.5 mg of reserpine thus provided is more than is routinely necessary for a hypotensive effect and serves to increase the risk of adverse reactions. If more than 100 mg of quinethazone per day is desired, it is recommended that HYDROMOX Quinethazone Tablets be used to supplement HYDROMOX R.
The dosage of HYDROMOX R to be employed depends upon the severity of the condition being treated and the responsiveness of the individual patient and often must be adjusted at the beginning of, or during the course of, therapy. Reduction of dosage is often possible after 2 weeks, when as little as 1 tablet a day may be sufficient for maintenance.
When HYDROMOX R Tablets are used in combination with other antihypertensive drugs, the dosage of each drug may often be reduced because of potentiation. (See under Precautions concerning the necessity for dosage adjustment when one or more of these drugs is added to an already established therapeutic regimen.)

How Supplied: HYDROMOX® R Quinethazone with Reserpine Tablets are round, yellow, scored tablets engraved with LL on one side and H above and 2 below the score on the other side, supplied as follows:
NDC 0005-4457-23—bottles of 100
NDC 0005-4457-31—bottles of 500
Store at Controlled Room Temperature 15–30° C (59–86° F).
Shown in Product Identification Section, page 415

INCREMIN®
[*ĭn-cre-mĭn*]
WITH IRON • SYRUP
(vitamins B₁, B₆, B₁₂-lysine-iron)
Dietary Supplement
(See PDR for Nonprescription Drugs)

LEDERPLEX®
[*lĕder-plĕx*]
Dietary Supplement of B-Complex Vitamins for Adults and Children 4 or More Years of Age
Capsules—Liquid
(See PDR For Nonprescription Drugs)

LEUCOVORIN CALCIUM INJECTION ℞
[*lu-cō-vor-ĭn*]

Description: Each 1 ml ampul of Leucovorin Calcium *Lederle* contains Leucovorin 3 mg as the calcium salt which is the form preferred for intramuscular injection. Preservative: Benzyl Alcohol 0.9% w/v. The inactive ingredients are Sodium Chloride 0.56% w/v, Water for Injection q.s. 100% and sodium hydroxide or hydrochloric acid is used to adjust the pH to approximately 7.7.
Each 50 mg vial of Leucovorin Calcium cryodesiccated powder when reconstituted with 5 ml of sterile diluent contains Leucovorin 10 mg per ml as the calcium salt which is the form preferred for intramuscular injection.
Contains no preservative. Dilute only with Bacteriostatic Water for Injection USP which contains benzyl alcohol. The inactive ingredients are sodium chloride 40 mg/vial, and sodium hydroxide or hydrochloric acid qs to pH approximately 8.1. When reconstituted as directed, the resulting solution must be used within 7 days. If the product is reconstituted with Water for Injection USP, use immediately.

Actions: Leucovorin (folinic acid) is the formyl derivative and active form of folic acid.
Leucovorin Calcium is useful clinically in circumventing the action of folate reductase. There is no evidence that intramuscular doses of greater than 1 mg have greater efficacy than those of 1 mg.

Indications: Indicated (a) to diminish the toxicity and counteract the effect of inadvertently administered overdosages of folic acid antagonists. (See Warnings). (b) In the treatment of the megaloblastic anemias due to sprue, nutritional deficiency, pregnancy, and infancy when oral therapy is not feasible.

Contraindications: Not to be administered for the treatment of pernicious anemia or other megaloblastic anemias where Vitamin B₁₂ is deficient.

Warnings: Leucovorin is improper therapy for pernicious anemia and other megaloblastic anemias secondary to lack of vitamin B₁₂. A hematologic remission may occur while neurologic manifestations remain progressive.
In the treatment of overdosage of folic acid antagonists, leucovorin must be administered within 1 hour, if possible, and is usually ineffective if administered after a delay of 4 hours.

Precautions: In the presence of pernicious anemia a hematologic remission may occur while neurologic manifestations remain progressive.

Adverse Reactions: Allergic sensitization has been reported following both oral and parenteral administration of folic acid.

Dosage: Megaloblastic anemia: No more than or up to 1 mg daily. There is no evidence that intramuscular doses greater than 1 mg daily have greater efficacy than those of 1 mg; additionally, loss of folate in the urine becomes roughly logarithmic as the amount administered exceeds 1 mg. For the treatment of overdosage of folic acid antagonists: To be given in amounts equal to the weight of the antagonist given.

How Supplied:
6 — 1 ml ampuls NDC 0205-4004-51.
50 mg vials of cryodesiccated powder NDC 0205-5330-92.
Military Depot
NSN 6505-01-054-7008, 50 mg/vial
VA Depots
NSN 6505-01-054-7008A, 50 mg/vial for IM use
Manufactured for
LEDERLE LABORATORIES DIVISION
American Cyanamid Company
Pearl River, NY 10965
by
LEDERLE PARENTERALS INC.
Carolina, Puerto Rico 00630
Shown in Product Identification Section, page 415

LOXITANE® ℞
[*lŏks-ĭ-tāne*]
Loxapine Succinate
Capsules
LOXITANE® C ℞
Loxapine Hydrochloride
Oral Concentrate
LOXITANE® IM ℞
Loxapine Hydrochloride
For Intramuscular Use Only

Description: LOXITANE *loxapine*, a dibenzoxazepine compound, represents a new subclass of tricyclic antipsychotic agent, chemically distinct from the thioxanthenes, butyrophenones, and phenothiazines. Chemically, it is 2-chloro-11-(4-methyl-1-piperazinyl)dibenz[b,f]-[1,4]oxazepine. It is present in capsules as the succinate salt, and in the concentrate and parenteral primarily as the HCl.
CAPSULES—Each capsule contains loxapine succinate equivalent to 5, 10, 25 or 50 mg of loxapine base.
ORAL CONCENTRATE—Each ml contains loxapine hydrochloride equivalent to 25 mg of loxapine base.

INTRAMUSCULAR—(Sterile)—Not for Intravenous Use—Each ml contains loxapine hydrochloride equivalent to 50 mg of loxapine base. Inactive Ingredients: polysorbate 80 NF 5% w/v; propylene glycol 70% v/v; and water for injection qs ad 100% v. Hydrochloric acid or Sodium hydroxide qs pH approx. 5.8.

Clinical Pharmacology: Pharmacologically, loxapine is a tranquilizer for which the exact mode of action has not been established. However, changes in the level of excitability of subcortical inhibitory areas have been observed in several animal species in association with such manifestations of tranquilization as calming effects and suppression of aggressive behavior.

In normal human volunteers, signs of sedation were seen within 20 to 30 minutes after administration, were most pronounced within 1½ to 3 hours, and lasted through 12 hours. Similar timing of primary pharmacologic effects was seen in animals.

Absorption of loxapine following oral or parenteral administration is virtually complete. The drug is removed rapidly from the plasma and distributed in tissues. Animal studies suggest an initial preferential distribution in lungs, brain, spleen, heart, and kidney. Loxapine is metabolized extensively and is excreted mainly in the first 24 hours. Metabolites are excreted in the urine in the form of conjugates and in the feces unconjugated.

Indications: LOXITANE is indicated for the management of the manifestations of psychotic disorders. The antipsychotic efficacy of LOXITANE was established in clinical studies which enrolled newly hospitalized and chronically hospitalized acutely ill schizophrenic patients as subjects.

Contraindications: LOXITANE is contraindicated in comatose or severe drug-induced depressed states (alcohol, barbiturates, narcotics, etc.).

LOXITANE is contraindicated in individuals with known hypersensitivity to dibenzoxazepines.

Warnings:
Usage in Pregnancy: Safe use of LOXITANE during pregnancy or lactation has not been established; therefore, its use in pregnancy, in nursing mothers, or in women of childbearing potential requires that the benefits of treatment be weighed against the possible risks to mother and child. No embryotoxicity or teratogenicity was observed in studies in rats, rabbits or dogs although, with the exception of one rabbit study, the highest dosage was only two times the maximum recommended human dose and in some studies it was below this dose. Perinatal studies have shown renal papillary abnormalities in offspring of rats treated from mid-pregnancy with doses of 0.6 and 1.8 mg/kg, doses which approximate the usual human dose but which are considerably below the maximum recommended human dose.

Pediatric Use: Studies have not been performed in children; therefore, this drug is not recommended for use in children below the age of 16.

LOXITANE, like other tranquilizers, may impair mental and/or physical abilities, especially during the first few days of therapy. Therefore, ambulatory patients should be warned about activities requiring alertness (e.g., operating vehicles or machinery) and about concomitant use of alcohol and other CNS depressants.

LOXITANE has not been evaluated for the management of behavioral complications in patients with mental retardation, and therefore, it cannot be recommended.

Precautions:
General: LOXITANE should be used with extreme caution in patients with a history of convulsive disorders since it lowers the convulsive threshold. Seizures have been reported in patients receiving LOXITANE at antipsychotic dose levels, and may occur even with maintenance of routine anticonvulsant drug therapy.

Loxapine has an antiemetic effect in animals. Since this effect may also occur in man, loxapine may mask signs of overdosage of toxic drugs and may obscure conditions such as intestinal obstruction and brain tumor.

LOXITANE should be used with caution in patients with cardiovascular disease. Increased pulse rates have been reported in the majority of patients receiving antipsychotic doses; transient hypotension has been reported. In the presence of severe hypotension requiring vasopressor therapy, the preferred drugs may be norepinephrine or angiotensin. Usual doses of epinephrine may be ineffective because of inhibition of its vasopressor effect by loxapine.

The possibility of ocular toxicity from loxapine cannot be excluded at this time. Therefore, careful observation should be made for pigmentary retinopathy and lenticular pigmentation since these have been observed in some patients receiving certain other antipsychotic drugs for prolonged periods.

Because of possible anticholinergic action, the drug should be used cautiously in patients with glaucoma or a tendency to urinary retention, particularly with concomitant administration of anticholinergic-type antiparkinson medication.

Experience to date indicates the possibility of a slightly higher incidence of extrapyramidal effects following intramuscular administration than normally anticipated with oral formulations. The increase may be attributable to higher plasma levels following intramuscular injection.

Neuroleptic drugs elevate prolactin levels; the elevation persists during chronic administration. Tissue culture experiments indicate that approximately one-third of human breast cancers are prolactin dependent *in vitro*, a factor of potential importance if the prescription of these drugs is contemplated in a patient with a previously detected breast cancer. Although disturbances such as galactorrhea, amenorrhea, gynecomastia, and impotence have been reported, the clinical significance of elevated serum prolactin levels is unknown for most patients. An increase in mammary neoplasms has been found in rodents after chronic administration of neuroleptic drugs. Neither clinical studies nor epidemiologic studies conducted to date, however, have shown an association between chronic administration of these drugs and mammary tumorigenesis; the available evidence is considered too limited to be conclusive at this time.

Drug Interactions: Neuroleptic drugs may significantly increase blood levels of antidepressants administered concomitantly. If LOXITANE is co-administered with an antidepressant, dosage of the antidepressant drug may require reduction.

Carcinogenesis, mutagenesis, impairment of fertility
LOXITANE did not induce neoplastic changes in rats after chronic administration in the diet at doses up to twice the human dose. LOXITANE was negative in microbial mutagenicity tests and in the mouse micronucleus test.

Neuroleptic drugs elevate prolactin levels; the elevation persists during chronic administration. Tissue culture experiments indicate that approximately one-third of human breast cancers are prolactin dependent *in vitro*, a factor of potential importance if the prescription of these drugs is contemplated in a patient with a previously detected breast cancer. Although disturbances such as galactorrhea, amenorrhea, gynecomastia, and impotence have been reported, the clinical significance of elevated serum prolactin levels is unknown for most patients. An increase in mammary neoplasms has been found in rodents after chronic administration of neuroleptic drugs. Neither clinical studies nor epidemiologic studies conducted to date, however, have shown an association between chronic administration of these drugs and mammary tumorigenesis; the available evidence is considered too limited to be conclusive at this time.

No antifertility effects were seen in rabbits or dogs given LOXITANE in oral or intramuscular doses up to twice the human dose. Male rats treated prior to mating with oral doses within the human therapeutic range did not demonstrate impaired fertility. Female rats similarly treated showed persistent diestrus and failure to copulate. Reduced numbers of pregnancies were apparent in female mice given twice the human dose orally from 5 days after copulation until late gestation. These effects in rodents are consistent with those of a variety of potent neuroleptic agents, and occurred at doses at least 40 times the pharmacologically effective dose in these species.

Pregnancy
Pregnancy Category C: LOXITANE was not teratogenic when given orally or intramuscularly to mice, rats, rabbits or dogs at doses up to two times the maximum recommended human dose. Oral or intramuscular doses up to twice the human dose were not fetotoxic to rabbits or dogs. Fetotoxic effects (increased resorptions, decreased fetal weight) were seen in rats and mice given doses within the range of the human therapeutic dose. These effects in rodents are consistent with those of a variety of neuroleptic agents, and occurred at doses at least 50 times the pharmacologically effective dose in these species. There are no adequate and well controlled studies in pregnant women. LOXITANE should be used during pregnancy only if the potential benefit justifies the potential risk to the fetus.

Nursing mothers
It is not known whether this drug is excreted in human milk, but LOXITANE and its metabolites have been shown to be transported into milk of lactating dogs. Caution should be exercised when LOXITANE is administered to a nursing woman.

Adverse Reactions: Adverse reactions reported in controlled studies in the United States are categorized with respect to incidence as follows:
INCIDENCE GREATER THAN 1%
The most frequent types of adverse reactions occurring with LOXITANE in controlled clinical trials were extrapyramidal and sedative effects. These included rigidity (27%), tremor (22%), akathisia (20%), dystonic reactions (7%), and drowsiness (11%). Both extrapyramidal effects and sedation are most common during the first few days of treatment or following dosage increases.
Less frequently reported reactions were:
Anticholinergic—blurred vision, dry mouth.
Behavioral—insomnia, confusion.
CNS and Neuromuscular—excessive salivation, dizziness, parkinsonism.
Gastrointestinal—nausea.
Cardiovascular—tachycardia.
INCIDENCE LESS THAN 1%
Anticholinergic—paralytic ileus, urinary retention, constipation, nasal congestion.
Behavioral—agitation, tension.
Cardiovascular—hypotension, hypertension, orthostatic hypotension, syncope.
CNS and Neuromuscular—seizures, akinesia, dyskinesia, slurred speech, shuffling gait, weakness, paresthesia, numbness, rarely neuroleptic malignant syndrome (NMS).
Endocrine—galactorrhea, amenorrhea, gynecomastia.
Gastrointestinal—vomiting.
Hematologic—rarely, agranulocytosis, thrombocytopenia, leukopenia.
Hepatic—elevation of liver enzymes, rarely, jaundice and/or hepatitis questionably related to LOXITANE treatment.
Skin—rarely, rash, alopecia.
Other—hyperpyrexia, weight gain, weight loss, dyspnea, ptosis, flushing, headache, polydipsia.
Persistent Tardive Dyskinesia—As with all antipsychotic agents, tardive dyskinesia may appear in some patients on long-term therapy or may appear after drug therapy has been discontinued. The risk appears to be greater in elderly patients on high-dose therapy, especially females. The symptoms are persistent and in some patients appear to be irreversible. The syndrome is characterized by rhythmical involuntary movement of the tongue, face, mouth, or jaw (e.g., protrusion of

Continued on next page

The information on each product appearing here is based on labelling effective in August, 1984 and is either the entire official brochure or an accurate condensation therefrom. Information concerning all Lederle products may be obtained from the Professional Services Department, Lederle Laboratories. Pearl River, New York. 10965.

Lederle—Cont.

tongue, puffing of cheeks, puckering of mouth, chewing movements). Sometimes these may be accompanied by involuntary movements of extremities.

There is no known effective treatment for tardive dyskinesia; antiparkinson agents usually do not alleviate the symptoms of this syndrome. It is suggested that all antipsychotic agents be discontinued if these symptoms appear. Should it be necessary to reinstitute treatment, or increase the dosage of the agent, or switch to a different antipsychotic agent, the syndrome may be masked. It has been suggested that fine vermicular movements of the tongue may be an early sign of the syndrome, and if the medication is stopped at that time the syndrome may not develop.

Dosage and Administration: LOXITANE is administered, usually in divided doses, two to four times a day. Daily dosage (in terms of base equivalents) should be adjusted to the individual patient's needs as assessed by the severity of symptoms and previous history of response to antipsychotic drugs.

Oral Administration

Initial dosage of 10 mg twice daily is recommended, although in severely disturbed patients initial dosage up to a total of 50 mg daily may be desirable. Dosage should then be increased fairly rapidly over the first seven to ten days until there is effective control of psychotic symptoms. The usual therapeutic and maintenance range is 60 mg to 100 mg daily. However, as with other antipsychotic drugs, some patients respond to lower dosage and others require higher dosage for optimal benefit. Daily dosage higher than 250 mg is not recommended.

LOXITANE C Oral Concentrate should be mixed with orange or grapefruit juice shortly before administration. Use only the enclosed calibrated (10 mg, 15 mg, 25 mg, 50 mg) dropper for dosage.

Maintenance Therapy

For maintenance therapy, dosage should be reduced to the lowest level compatible with symptom control; many patients have been maintained satisfactorily at dosages in the range of 20 mg to 60 mg daily.

Intramuscular Administration

LOXITANE IM is utilized for prompt symptomatic control in the acutely agitated patient and in patients whose symptoms render oral medication temporarily impractical. During clinical trial there were no reports of significant local tissue reaction.

LOXITANE IM is administered by intramuscular (not intravenous) injection in doses of 12.5 mg (¼ ml) to 50 mg (1 ml) at intervals of four to six hours or longer, both dose and interval depending on patient response. Many patients have responded satisfactorily to twice-daily dosage. As described above for oral administration, attention is directed to the necessity for dosage adjustment on an individual basis over the early days of loxapine administration.

Once the desired symptomatic control is achieved and the patient is able to take medication orally, loxapine should be administered in capsule or oral concentrate form. Usually this should occur within five days.

Overdosage: Signs and symptoms of overdosage will depend on the amount ingested and individual patient tolerance. As would be expected from the pharmacologic actions of the drug, the clinical findings may range from mild depression of the CNS and cardiovascular systems to profound hypotension, respiratory depression, and unconsciousness. The possibility of occurrence of extrapyramidal symptoms and/or convulsive seizures should be kept in mind. Renal failure following loxapine overdosage has also been reported.

The treatment of overdosage is essentially symptomatic and supportive. Early gastric lavage and extended dialysis might be expected to be beneficial. Centrally acting emetics may have little effect because of the antiemetic action of loxapine. In addition, emesis should be avoided because of the possibility of aspiration of vomitus. Avoid analeptics, such as pentylenetetrazol, which may cause convulsions. Severe hypotension might be expected to respond to the administration of levarterenol or phenylephrine. EPINEPHRINE SHOULD NOT BE USED SINCE ITS USE IN A PATIENT WITH PARTIAL ADRENERGIC BLOCKADE MAY FURTHER LOWER THE BLOOD PRESSURE. Severe extrapyramidal reactions should be treated with anticholinergic antiparkinson agents or diphenhydramine hydrochloride, and anticonvulsant therapy should be initiated as indicated. Additional measures include oxygen and intravenous fluids.

How Supplied: LOXITANE *loxapine succinate* capsules are supplied in the following base equivalent strengths:

5 mg—Hard Shell, opaque, dark green capsules printed with Lederle over L1 on one half and 5 mg on the other, are supplied as follows:
NDC 0005-5359-23—Bottles of 100's
NDC 0005-5359-60—Unit Dose 10 × 10's

10 mg—Hard Shell, opaque, with yellow body and a dark green cap, printed with Lederle over L2 on one half and 10 mg on the other, are supplied as follows:
NDC 0005-5360-23—Bottles of 100's
NDC 0005-5360-34—Bottles of 1000's
NDC 0005-5360-60—Unit Dose 10 × 10's

25 mg—Hard Shell, opaque, with a light green body and a dark green cap, printed with Lederle over L3 on one half and 25 mg on the other, are supplied as follows:
NDC 0005-5361-23—Bottles of 100's
NDC 0005-5361-34—Bottles of 1000's
NDC 0005-5361-60—Unit Dose 10 × 10's

50 mg—Hard Shell, opaque with a blue body and a dark green cap, printed with Lederle over L4 on one half and 50 mg on the other, are supplied as follows:
NDC 0005-5362-23—Bottles of 100's
NDC 0005-5362-34—Bottles of 1000's
NDC 0005-5362-60—Unit Dose 10 × 10's

Store at Controlled Room Temperature 15-30° C (59-86° F).

LOXITANE C *loxapine hydrochloride* Oral Concentrate is supplied as follows:
NDC 0005-5387-58—4 Fl. Oz. (120 ml) with calibrated dropper. Each ml contains loxitane HCl equivalent to 25 mg loxapine base.
Store at Controlled Room Temperature 15-30° C (59-86° F).
DO NOT FREEZE

*LOXITANE IM *loxapine hydrochloride* for Intramuscular use only is supplied as follows:
NDC 0205-5385-55—sterile 10—1 ml ampuls
NDC 0205-5385-34—10 ml multi-dose vials
Each ml contains loxapine HCl equivalent to 50 mg of loxapine base.
Keep package closed to protect from light. Intensification of the straw color to a light amber will not alter potency or therapeutic efficacy; if noticeably discolored, ampul or vial should not be used.
Store at Controlled Room Temperature 15-30° C (59-86° F).
DO NOT FREEZE
VA Depots
LOXITANE loxapine succinate capsules
NSN-6505-01-048-3719A-25 mg—1000's
NSN-6505-01-048-3718A-50 mg—1000's
LOXITANE C loxapine HCl
NSN 6505-01-026-0101A Oral Concentrate, 25 mg—4 oz.
*Manufactured for
LEDERLE LABORATORIES DIVISION
American Cyanamid Company
Pearl River, NY 10965
by
LEDERLE PARENTERALS INC.
Carolina, Puerto Rico 00630

Shown in Product Identification Section, page 415

MATERNA® 1·60
[ma-ter-na]
Prenatal Vitamin and Mineral Tablets
For the woman full of life™

Each tablet contains:		For Pregnant or Lactating Women % of U.S. RDA
Vitamin A Acetate	8,000 I.U.	(100%)
Vitamin D	400 I.U.	(100%)
Vitamin E (as dl-Alpha Tocopheryl Acetate)	30 I.U.	(100%)
Vitamin C (Ascorbic Acid)	100 mg	(167%)
Folic Acid	1 mg	(125%)
Thiamine (as Thiamine Mononitrate Vitamin B_1)	3 mg	(224%)
Riboflavin (Vitamin B_2)	3.4 mg	(170%)
Vitamin B_6 (as Pyridoxine Hydrochloride)	4 mg	(160%)
Niacinamide	20 mg	(100%)
Vitamin B_{12} (Cyanocobalamin)	12 mcg	(150%)
Calcium (as Calcium Carbonate)	250 mg	(19%)
Iodine (as Potassium Iodide)	0.3 mg	(200%)
Iron (as Ferrous Fumarate)	60 mg	(333%)
Magnesium (as Magnesium Oxide)	25 mg	(6%)
Copper (as Cupric Oxide)	2 mg	(100%)
Zinc (as Zinc Sulfate)	25 mg	(167%)

Caution: Federal law prohibits dispensing without prescription.

A PHOSPHORUS-FREE VITAMIN AND MINERAL DIETARY SUPPLEMENT FOR USE DURING PREGNANCY AND LACTATION. RECOMMENDED INTAKE: 1 daily or as prescribed by physician. WARNING: Keep out of the reach of children.

Precaution: Folic acid may obscure pernicious anemia in that the peripheral blood picture may revert to normal while neurological manifestations remain progressive.

Allergic sensitization has been reported following both oral and parenteral administration of Folic Acid.

Store at Controlled Room Temperature 15-30°C (59-86°F).

How Supplied: Light pink, film coated engraved MATERNA and M10—Bottles of 100.
NDC 0005-5536-23
Control No.
PATENTED
U.S. Pat. No. 4,431,634
©1984

Shown in Product Indentification Section, page 415

MAXZIDE™ TABLETS
triamterene 75 mg
hydrochlorothiazide 50 mg

Description: Each yellow, scored MAXZIDE™ triamterene 75 mg/hydrochlorothiazide 50 mg tablet for oral use contains 75 mg of triamterene, a potassium-conserving diuretic and 50 mg of hydrochlorothiazide, a natriuretic agent.

Triamterene is 2,4,7-triamino-6-phenylpteridine. Triamterene is practically insoluble in water, benzene, chloroform, ether and dilute alkali hydroxides. It is soluble in formic acid and sparingly soluble in methoxyethanol. Triamterene is very slightly soluble in acetic acid, alcohol and dilute mineral acids. Its molecular weight is 253.27.
Hydrochlorothiazide is 6-chloro-3,4-dihydro-2H-1,2,4, benzothiadiazine-7-sulfonamide 1, 1-dioxide. Hydrochlorothiazide is slightly soluble in water and freely soluble in sodium hydroxide solution, n-butylamine and dimethylformamide. It is sparingly soluble in methanol and insoluble in ether, chloroform and dilute mineral acids. Its molecular weight is 297.73.

Clinical Pharmacology: MAXZIDE is a diuretic antihypertensive drug product, principally due to its hydrochlorothiazide component; the triamterene component of MAXZIDE reduces the excessive potassium loss which may occur with

Hydrochlorothiazide
Hydrochlorothiazide is a diuretic and antihypertensive agent. It blocks the renal tubular absorption of sodium and chloride ions. This natriuresis and diuresis is accompanied by a secondary loss of potassium and bicarbonate. Onset of hydrochlorothiazide's diuretic effect occurs within two hours and the peak action takes place in four hours. Diuretic activity persists for approximately six to twelve hours.

The exact mechanism of hydrochlorothiazide's antihypertensive action is not known although it may relate to the excretion and redistribution of body sodium. Hydrochlorothiazide does not affect normal blood pressure.

Following oral administration, peak hydrochlorothiazide plasma levels are attained in approximately two hours. It is excreted rapidly and unchanged in the urine.

Triamterene
Triamterene is a potassium conserving (antikaliuretic) diuretic with relatively weak natriuretic properties. It exerts its diuretic effect on the distal renal tubule to inhibit the reabsorption of sodium in exchange for potassium and hydrogen. With this action, triamterene increases sodium excretion and reduces the excessive loss of potassium and hydrogen associated with hydrochlorothiazide. Triamterene is not a competitive antagonist of the mineralocorticoids and its potassium-conserving effect is observed in patients with Addison's disease, i.e., without aldosterone. Triamterene's onset and duration of activity is similar to hydrochlorothiazide. No predictable antihypertensive effect has been demonstrated with triamterene.

Triamterene is rapidly absorbed following oral administration. Peak plasma levels are achieved within one hour after dosing. Triamterene is primarily metabolized to the sulfate conjugate of hydroxytriamterene. Both the plasma and urine levels of this metabolite greatly exceed triamterene levels.

The amount of triamterene added to 50 mg of hydrochlorothiazide in MAXZIDE tablets was determined from steady-state dose response evaluations in which various doses of liquid preparations of triamterene were administered to hypertensive persons who developed hypokalemia with hydrochlorothiazide (50 mg/day). Daily doses of 75 mg triamterene produced maximal increases in serum potassium levels. Doses exceeding 75 mg daily provided no additional elevations in serum potassium levels. Ordinarily, triamterene does not entirely reverse the kaliuretic effect of hydrochlorothiazide. In some individuals, however, it may induce hyperkalemia (see WARNINGS).

The triamterene and hydrochlorothiazide components of MAXZIDE™ triamterene 75 mg/hydrochlorothiazide 50 mg are well absorbed and are bioequivalent to liquid preparations of the individual components administered orally. The hydrochlorothiazide component of MAXZIDE™ is bioequivalent to single entity hydrochlorothiazide tablet formulations.

Indications and Usage:
1. MAXZIDE is indicated for the treatment of hypertension or edema in patients who develop hypokalemia on hydrochlorothiazide alone.
2. MAXZIDE™ (triamterene and hydrochlorothiazide) is also indicated for those patients who require a thiazide diuretic and in whom the development of hypokalemia cannot be risked (e.g., patients on concomitant digitalis preparations, or with a history of cardiac arrhythmias, etc.).

This fixed combination drug is not indicated for the initial therapy of edema or hypertension except in individuals in whom the development of hypokalemia cannot be risked.

MAXZIDE™ may be used alone or in combination with other antihypertensive drugs such as beta-blockers. Since MAXZIDE may enhance the actions of these drugs, dosage adjustments may be necessary.

Usage in Pregnancy
The routine use of diuretics in an otherwise healthy woman is inappropriate and exposes mother and fetus to unnecessary hazard. Diuretics do not prevent development of toxemia in pregnancy, and there is no satisfactory evidence that they are useful in the treatment of developed toxemia.

Edema during pregnancy may arise from pathological causes or from the physiologic and mechanical consequences of pregnancy. Thiazides are indicated in pregnancy when edema is due to pathologic causes, just as they are in absence of pregnancy. Dependent edema in pregnancy, resulting from restriction of venous return by the expanded uterus, is properly treated through elevation of the lower extremities and use of support hose; use of diuretics to lower intravascular volume in this case is illogical and unnecessary. There is hypervolemia during normal pregnancy which is harmful to neither the fetus nor the mother (in the absence of cardiovascular disease), but which is associated with edema, including generalized edema, in the majority of pregnant women. If this edema produces discomfort, increased recumbency will often provide relief. In rare instances, this edema may cause extreme discomfort which is not relieved by rest. In these cases, a short course of diuretics may provide relief and may be appropriate.

Contraindications:
Hyperkalemia
MAXZIDE should not be used in the presence of elevated serum potassium levels (greater than 5.5 mEq/liter). If hyperkalemia develops, this drug should be discontinued and a thiazide alone should be substituted.

Antikaliuretic Therapy or Potassium Supplementation
MAXZIDE™ should not be given to patients receiving other potassium conserving agents such as spironolactone, amiloride HCl or other formulations containing triamterene. Concomitant potassium supplementation in the form of medication, potassium-containing salt substitute or potassium-enriched diets should also not be used.

Impaired Renal Function
MAXZIDE is contraindicated in patients with anuria, acute and chronic renal insufficiency or significant renal impairment.

Hypersensitivity
MAXZIDE should not be used in patients who are hypersensitive to triamterene or hydrochlorothiazide or other sulfonamide-derived drugs.

Warnings:
Hyperkalemia

> Abnormal elevation of serum potassium levels (greater than or equal to 5.5 mEq/liter) can occur with all potassium-conserving diuretic combinations, including MAXZIDE. Hyperkalemia is more likely to occur in patients with renal impairment, diabetes (even without evidence of renal impairment), or elderly or severely ill patients. Since uncorrected hyperkalemia may be fatal, serum potassium levels must be monitored at frequent intervals especially in patients first receiving MAXZIDE™, when dosages are changed or with any illness that may influence renal function.

If hyperkalemia is suspected, (warning signs include paresthesias, muscular weakness, fatigue, flaccid paralysis of the extremities, bradycardia and shock) an electrocardiogram (ECG) should be obtained. However, it is important to monitor serum potassium levels because mild hyperkalemia may not be associated with ECG changes.

If hyperkalemia is present, MAXZIDE™ triamterene 75 mg/hydrochlorothiazide 50 mg should be discontinued immediately and a thiazide only should be substituted. If the serum potassium exceed 6.5 mEq/liter, more vigorous therapy is required. The clinical situation dictates the procedures to be employed. These include the intravenous administration of calcium chloride solution, sodium bicarbonate solution and/or the oral or parenteral administration of glucose with a rapid-acting insulin preparation. Cationic exchange resins such as sodium polystyrene sulfonate may be orally or rectally administered. Persistent hyperkalemia may require dialysis.

The development of hyperkalemia associated with potassium-sparing diuretics is accentuated in the presence of renal impairment (see CONTRAINDICATIONS). Patients with mild renal function impairment should not receive this drug without frequent and continuing monitoring of serum electrolytes. Cumulative drug effects may be observed in patients with impaired renal function. The renal clearances of hydrochlorothiazide and the pharmacologically active metabolite of triamterene, the sulfate ester of hydroxytriamterene, have been shown to be reduced and the plasma levels increased following MAXZIDE administration to elderly patients and patients with impaired renal function.

Hyperkalemia has been reported in diabetic patients with the use of potassium conserving agents even in the absence of apparent renal impairment. Accordingly, MAXZIDE should be avoided in diabetic patients. If it is employed, serum electrolytes must be frequently monitored.

Metabolic or Respiratory Acidosis
Potassium conserving therapy should also be avoided in severely ill patients in whom respiratory or metabolic acidosis may occur. Acidosis may be associated with rapid elevations in serum potassium levels. If MAXZIDE is employed, frequent evaluations of acid/base balance and serum electrolytes are necessary.

Precautions:
General
Electrolyte Imbalance and BUN Increases
Patients receiving MAXZIDE should be carefully monitored for fluid or electrolyte imbalances, i.e., hyponatremia, hypochloremic alkalosis, hypokalemia and hypomagnesemia. Serum and urine electrolyte determinations should be frequently performed and are especially important when the patient is vomiting or receiving parenteral fluids. Warning signs or symptoms of fluid and electrolyte imbalance include: dryness of mouth, thirst, weakness, lethargy, drowsiness, restlessness, muscle pains or cramps, muscular fatigue, hypotension, oliguria, tachycardia and gastrointestinal disturbances such as nausea and vomiting.

Any chloride deficit thiazide therapy is generally mild and usually does not require any specific treatment except under extraordinary circumstances (as in liver disease or renal disease). Dilutional hyponatremia may occur in edematous patients in hot weather; appropriate therapy is water restriction, rather than administration of salt, except in rare instances when the hyponatremia is life threatening. In actual salt depletion, appropriate replacement is the therapy of choice.

Hypokalemia may develop with thiazide therapy, especially with brisk diuresis, when severe cirrhosis is present, or during concomitant use of corticosteroids, ACTH, amphotericin B or after prolonged thiazide therapy. However, hypokalemia of this type is usually prevented by the triamterene component of MAXZIDE™ triamterene 75 mg/hydrochlorothiazide 50 mg.

Interference with adequate oral electrolyte intake will also contribute to hypokalemia. Hypokalemia can sensitize or exaggerate the response of the heart to the toxic effects of digitalis (e.g., increased ventricular irritability).

MAXZIDE may produce an elevated blood urea nitrogen level (BUN), creatinine level or both. This is probably not the result of renal toxicity but is secondary to a reversible reduction of the glomerular filtration rate or a depletion of the intravascular fluid volume. Periodic BUN and creatinine determinations should be made especially in elderly patients, patients with suspected or confirmed hepatic disease or renal insufficiencies. If azotemia increases, MAXZIDE™ should be discontinued.

Hepatic Coma
MAXZIDE™ should be used with caution in patients with impaired hepatic function or progressive liver disease, since minor alterations of fluid and electrolyte balance may precipitate hepatic

Continued on next page

Lederle—Cont.

coma.
Renal Stones
Triamterene has been reported in renal stones in association with other calculus components. MAXZIDE should be used with caution in patients with histories or renal lithiasis.
Folic Acid Deficiency
Triamterene is a weak folic acid antagonist and may contribute to the appearance of megaloblastosis in instances where folic acid stores are decreased. In such patients, periodic blood evaluations are recommended.
Hyperuricemia
Hyperuricemia may occur or acute gout may be precipitated in certain patients receiving thiazide therapy.
Metabolic and Endocrine Effects
The thiazides may decrease serum PBI levels without signs of thyroid disturbance.
Calcium excretion is decreased by thiazides. Pathological changes in the parathyroid gland with hypercalcemia and hypophosphatemia have been observed in a few patients on prolonged thiazide therapy. The common complications of hyperparathyroidism such as renal lithiasis, bone resorption, and peptic ulceration have not been seen. Thiazides should be discontinued before carrying out tests for parathyroid function.
Insulin requirements in diabetic patients may be increased, decreased or unchanged. Diabetes mellitus which has been latent may become manifest during thiazide administration.
Hypersensitivity
Sensitivity reactions to thiazides may occur in patients with or without a history of allergy or bronchial asthma.
Possible exacerbation or activation of systemic lupus erythematosus by thiazides has been reported.
Drug Interactions
Thiazides may add to or potentiate the action of other antihypertensive drugs.
The thiazides may decrease arterial responsiveness to norepinephrine. This diminution is not sufficient to preclude effectiveness of the pressor agent for therapeutic use. Thiazides have also been shown to increase responsiveness to tubocurarine.
Lithium generally should not be given with diuretics because they reduce its renal clearance and add a high risk of lithium toxicity. Refer to the package insert on lithium before use of such concomitant therapy.
Acute renal failure has been reported in a few patients receiving indomethacin and other formulations containing triamterene and hydrochlorothiazide. Caution is therefore advised when administering nonsteroidal anti-inflammatory agents with MAXZIDE™ triamterene 75 mg/hydrochlorothiazide 50 mg.
Drug/Laboratory Test Interactions
Triamterene and quinidine have similar fluorescence spectra; thus MAXZIDE may interfere with the measurement of quinidine.
Pregnancy Category C
The safe use of MAXZIDE in pregnancy has not been established. Animal reproduction studies have not been conductd with MAXZIDE. It is also not known if MAXZIDE™ can cause fetal harm when administered to a pregnant woman or can affect reproductive capacity. Thiazides cross the placental barrier and appear in cord blood. The use of thiazides in pregnant women requires that the anticipated benefit be weighed against possible hazards to the fetus. These hazards include fetal or neonatal jaundice, thrombocytopenia, pancreatitis and possibly other adverse reactions which have occurred in the adult. MAXZIDE should be given to a pregnant woman only if clearly needed.
Nursing Mothers
Thiazides appear in breast milk. If the use of MAXZIDE™ is deemed essential, the patient should stop nursing.
Pediatric Use
The safety and effectiveness of MAXZIDE™ in children has not been established.
Adverse Reactions:
Side effects observed in association with the use of MAXZIDE include drowsiness and fatigue, insomnia, muscle cramps and weakness, headache, nausea, appetite disturbance, vomiting, diarrhea, constipation, dizziness, decreased sexual performance, shortness of breath and chest pain, dry mouth, depression and anxiety. These adverse reactions are common to other triamterene and hydrochlorothiazide containing products. Other adverse reactions which have been reported with the individual active drugs include:
Hydrochlorothiazide
Gastrointestinal: anorexia, gastric irritation, cramping, jaundice (intrahepatic cholestatic jaundice), pancreatitis, sialadenitis.
Central Nervous System: vertigo, paresthesias, xanthopsia.
Hematologic: leukopenia, agranulocytosis, thrombocytopenia, aplastic anemia, hemolytic anemia, megaloblastosis.
Cardiovascular: orthostatic hypotension (may be aggravated by alcohol, barbiturates, or narcotics).
Hypersensitivity: anaphylaxis, purpura, photosensitivity, rash, urticaria, necrotizing angiitis (vasculitis, cutaneous vasculitis), fever, respiratory distress including pneumonitis.
Other: hyperglycemia, glycosuria, hyperuricemia, restlessness, transient blurred vision.
Triamterene
Hypersensitivity: anaphylaxis, photosensitivity and rash.
Other: Triamterene has been reported in renal stones in association with other calculus materials. Triamterene has been associated with blood dyscrasias.
Whenever adverse reactions are moderate to severe, therapy should be reduced or withdrawn.
Overdosage:
No specific data are available regarding MAXZIDE™ triamterene 75 mg/hydrochlorothiazide 50 mg overdosage in humans and no specific antidote is available.
Fluid and electrolyte imbalances are the most important concern. Excessive doses of the triamterene component may elicit hyperkalemia, dehydration, nausea, vomiting and weakness and possibly hypotension. Overdosing with hydrochlorothiazide has been associated with hypokalemia, hypochloremia, hyponatremia, dehydration, lethargy (may progress to coma) and gastrointestinal irritation. Treatment is symptomatic and supportive. Therapy with MAXZIDE™ should be discontinued. Induce emesis or institute gastric lavage. Monitor serum electrolyte levels and fluid balance. Institute supportive measures as required to maintain hydration, electrolyte balance, respiratory, cardiovascular and renal function.
Dosage and Administration:
The recommended dosage of MAXZIDE™ is one tablet daily with appropriate monitoring of serum potassium levels (see WARNINGS). Patients receiving 50 mg of hydrochlorothiazide who become hypokalemic may be transferred to MAXZIDE™ directly. In patients requiring 50 mg of hydrochlorothiazide in whom hypokalemia cannot be risked, therapy may be initiated with MAXZIDE™. There is no clinical experience with doses exceeding one tablet daily.
Clinical studies have shown that patients already taking less bioavailable formulations of triamterene and hydrochlorothiazide (totaling 50–100 mg of hydrochlorothiazide and 100–200 mg of triamterene) may be safely changed to one MAXZIDE™ tablet per day; these patients should be monitored clinically and with serum potassium after the transfer.
How Supplied:
MAXZIDE™ triamterene 75 mg/hydrochlorothiazide 50 mg tablets are bow-tie shaped, flat-faced beveled, light yellow tablets, engraved with MAXZIDE on one side and scored on the other with LL on left and M8 on right of the score. Each tablet contains 75 mg of triamterene, USP and 50 mg of hydrochlorothiazide, USP. They are supplied as follows:
NDC 0005-4460-43—Bottles of 100 with CRC
NDC 0005-4460-60—Unit Dose 10 × 10's
Store at Controlled Room Temperature 15–30° C (59–86° F).
Protect from light.
Dispense in a tight, light-resistant, child-resistant container.
Manufactured for
LEDERLE LABORATORIES DIVISION
American Cyanamid Company, Pearl River, N.Y. 10965
by
MYLAN PHARMACEUTICALS, INC.
Morgantown, West Virginia 26505
Shown in Product Identification Section, page 415

METHOTREXATE ℞
[meth-ō-trĕx-āte]
Tablets and Parenteral

> **WARNING**
> METHOTREXATE MUST BE USED ONLY BY PHYSICIANS EXPERIENCED IN ANTIMETABOLITE CHEMOTHERAPY.
> BECAUSE OF THE POSSIBILITY OF FATAL OR SEVERE TOXIC REACTIONS THE PATIENT SHOULD BE FULLY INFORMED BY THE PHYSICIAN OF THE RISKS INVOLVED AND SHOULD BE UNDER HIS CONSTANT SUPERVISION.
> DEATHS HAVE BEEN REPORTED WITH THE USE OF METHOTREXATE IN THE TREATMENT OF PSORIASIS.
> IN THE TREATMENT OF PSORIASIS METHOTREXATE SHOULD BE RESTRICTED TO SEVERE, RECALCITRANT, DISABLING, PSORIASIS WHICH IS NOT ADEQUATELY RESPONSIVE TO OTHER FORMS OF THERAPY, BUT ONLY WHEN THE DIAGNOSIS HAS BEEN ESTABLISHED, AS BY BIOPSY AND/OR AFTER DERMATOLOGIC CONSULTATION.
> 1. Methotrexate may produce marked depression of bone marrow, anemia, leukopenia, thrombocytopenia and bleeding.
> 2. Methotrexate may be hepatotoxic, particularly at high dosage or with prolonged therapy. Liver atrophy, necrosis, cirrhosis, fatty changes, and periportal fibrosis have been reported. Since changes may occur without previous signs of gastrointestinal or hematologic toxicity, it is imperative that hepatic function be determined prior to initiation of treatment and monitored regularly throughout therapy. Special caution is indicated in the presence of preexisting liver damage or impaired hepatic function. Concomitant use of other drugs with hepatotoxic potential (including alcohol) should be avoided.
> 3. Methotrexate has caused fetal death and/or congenital anomalies, therefore, it is not recommended in women of childbearing potential unless there is appropriate medical evidence that the benefits can be expected to outweigh the considered risks. Pregnant psoriatic patients should not receive Methotrexate.
> 4. Impaired renal function is usually a contraindication.
> 5. Diarrhea and ulcerative stomatitis are frequent toxic effects and require interruption of therapy; otherwise hemorrhagic enteritis and death from intestinal perforation may occur.
> METHOTREXATE HAS BEEN ADMINISTERED IN VERY HIGH DOSAGE FOLLOWED BY LEUCOVORIN RESCUE IN EXPERIMENTAL TREATMENT OF CERTAIN NEOPLASTIC DISEASES. THIS PROCEDURE IS INVESTIGATIONAL AND HAZARDOUS.

Description:
Methotrexate Lederle (formerly A-methopterin) is an antimetabolite used in the treatment of certain neoplastic diseases. Chemically methotrexate is N-[4-[[(2,4-Diamino-6-Pteridinyl) methyl]-Methylamino]benzoyl]-L-glutamic acid.
Methotrexate Tablets contain 2.5 mg of Methotrexate.

Methotrexate Sodium Parenteral, preserved, is available both in 2.5 mg/ml and 25 mg/ml strengths each available in 2 ml vials.

Each 2.5 mg/ml (5.0 mg) vial contains per 2 ml: Methotrexate Sodium equivalent to 5 mg Methotrexate, 0.90% w/v of benzyl alcohol as a preservative, and the following Inactive Ingredients. Sodium Chloride 0.630% w/v and Water for Injection qs ad 100% V. Sodium Hydroxide and if necessary, Hydrochloric Acid to adjust pH to approx. 8.5.

Each 25 mg/ml (50 mg) vial contains per 2 ml: Methotrexate Sodium equivalent to 50 mg Methotrexate, 0.90% w/v of benzyl alcohol as a preservative, and the following Inactive Ingredients: Sodium Chloride 0.260% w/v and Water for Injection qs ad 100% V. Sodium Hydroxide and, if necessary, Hydrochloric Acid to adjust pH to approx. 8.5.

If desired, the solution may be further diluted with a compatible medium such as Sodium Chloride Injection USP. Storage for 24 hours at a temperature of 21° to 25° C results in a product which is within 90% of label potency.

Methotrexate LPF® Sodium Parenteral, Isotonic, preservative free, single use only, is available in 2 ml (50 mg), 4 ml (100 mg), and 8 ml (200 mg) vials.

Each 25 mg/ml, 2 ml (50 mg) vial contains: Methotrexate Sodium equivalent to 50 mg Methotrexate, and the following Inactive Ingredients: Sodium Chloride 0.490% w/v and Water for Injection qs ad 100% V. Sodium Hydroxide and, if necessary, Hydrochloric Acid to adjust pH to approx. 8.5. Contains approximately 0.43 milliequivalents of sodium per vial and is an isotonic solution.

Each 25 mg/ml, 4 ml (100 mg) vial contains: Methotrexate Sodium equivalent to 100 mg Methotrexate, and the following Inactive Ingredients: Sodium Chloride 0.490% w/v and Water for Injection qs ad 100% V. Sodium Hydroxide and, if necessary, Hydrochloric Acid to adjust pH to approx. 8.5. Contains approximately 0.86 milliequivalents of sodium per vial and is an isotonic solution.

Each 25 mg/ml, 8 ml (200 mg) vial contains: Methotrexate Sodium equivalent to 200 mg Methotrexate, and the following Inactive Ingredients: Sodium Chloride 0.490% w/v and Water for Injection qs ad 100% V. Sodium Hydroxide and, if necessary, Hydrochloric Acid to adjust pH to approx. 8.5. Contains approximately 1.72 milliequivalents of sodium per vial and is an isotonic solution.

If desired, the solution may be further diluted immediately prior to use with an appropriate sterile, preservative free medium such as 5% Dextrose Solution USP or Sodium Chloride Injection, USP.

Each Low Sodium 20 mg vial of sterile cryodesiccated powder, for single use only, contains: Methotrexate Sodium equivalent to 20 mg Methotrexate. Contains no preservative. Sodium Hydroxide and, if necessary, Hydrochloric Acid added during manufacture to adjust pH. Contains approximately 0.14 milliequivalents of sodium per vial. Each Low Sodium 50 mg vial of sterile cryodesiccated powder, for single use only, contains: Methotrexate Sodium equivalent to 50 mg Methotrexate. Contains no preservative. Sodium Hydroxide and, if necessary, Hydrochloric Acid added during manufacture to adjust pH. Contains approximately 0.33 milliequivalents of sodium per vial.

Each Low Sodium 100 mg vial of sterile cryodesiccated powder, for single use only, contains: Methotrexate Sodium equivalent to 100 mg Methotrexate. Contains no preservative. Sodium Hydroxide and, if necessary, Hydrochloric Acid added to manufacture to adjust pH. Contains approximately 0.65 milliequivalents of sodium per vial.

Action: Methotrexate has as its principal mechanism of action the competitive inhibition of the enzyme folic acid reductase. Folic acid must be reduced to tetrahydrofolic acid by this enzyme in the process of DNA synthesis and cellular replication. Methotrexate inhibits the reduction of the folic acid and interferes with tissue-cell reproduction.

Actively proliferating tissues such as malignant cells, bone marrow, fetal cells, dermal epithelium, buccal and intestinal mucosa and cells of the urinary bladder are in general more sensitive to the effect of Methotrexate. Cellular proliferation in malignant tissue is greater than in most normal tissue and thus Methotrexate may impair malignant growth without irreversible damage to normal tissues.

Orally administered Methotrexate is absorbed rapidly in most, but not all patients, and reaches peak serum levels in 1–2 hours. After parenteral injection, peak serum levels are seen in about one-half this period. Approximately one-half the absorbed Methotrexate is reversibly bound to serum protein, but exchanges with body fluids easily and diffuses into the body tissue cells.

Excretion of single daily doses occurs through the kidneys in amounts from 55% to 88% or higher within 24 hours. Repeated doses daily result in more sustained serum levels and some retention of Methotrexate over each 24 hour period which may result in accumulation of the drug within the tissues. The liver cells appear to retain certain amounts of the drug for prolonged periods even after a single therapeutic dose. Methotrexate is retained in the presence of impaired renal function and may increase rapidly in the serum and in the tissue cells under such conditions. Methotrexate does not penetrate the blood cerebrospinal fluid barrier in therapeutic amounts when given orally or parenterally. High concentrations of the drug when needed may be attained by direct intrathecal administration.

In psoriasis, the rate of production of epithelial cells in the skin is greatly increased over normal skin. This differential in reproductive rates is the basis for the use of Methotrexate to control the psoriatic process.

Indications:
Anti-neoplastic Chemotherapy
Methotrexate is indicated for the treatment of gestational choriocarcinoma, and in patients with chorioadenoma destruens and hydatidiform mole. Methotrexate is indicated for the palliation of acute lymphocytic leukemia. It is also indicated in the treatment and prophylaxis of meningeal leukemia. Greatest effect has been observed in palliation of acute lymphoblastic (stem-cell) leukemias in children. In combination with other anticancer drugs or suitable agents Methotrexate may be used for induction of remission, but it is most commonly used, as described in the literature, in the maintenance of induced remissions.

Methotrexate may be used alone or in combination with other anticancer agents in the management of breast cancer, epidermoid cancers of the head and neck, and lung cancer, particularly squamous cell and small cell types.

Methotrexate is also effective in the treatment of the advanced stages (III and IV, Peters Staging System) of lymphosarcoma, particularly in those cases in children; and in advanced cases of mycosis fungoides.

Psoriasis Chemotherapy **[See box warnings at top of Insert]** Because of high risk attending its use, Methotrexate is only indicated in the symptomatic control of severe, recalcitrant, disabling psoriasis which is not adequately responsive to other forms of therapy, *but only when the diagnosis has been established, as by biopsy and/or after dermatologic consultation.*

Contraindications: Pregnant psoriatic patients should not receive Methotrexate. Psoriatic patients with severe renal or hepatic disorders should not receive Methotrexate.

Psoriatic patients with pre-existing blood dyscrasias, such as bone marrow hypoplasia, leukopenia, thrombocytopenia or anemia, should not receive Methotrexate.

Warnings: See Box Warnings
Precautions: Methotrexate has a high potential toxicity, usually dose-related. The physician should be familiar with the various characteristics of the drug and its established clinical usage. Patients undergoing therapy should be subject to appropriate supervision so that signs or symptoms of possible toxic effects or adverse reactions may be detected and evaluated with minimal delay. Pretreatment and periodic hematologic studies are essential to the use of Methotrexate in chemotherapy because of its common effect of hematopoietic suppression. This may occur abruptly and on apparent safe dosage, and any profound drop in blood-cell count indicates immediate stopping of the drug and appropriate therapy. In patients with malignant disease who have pre-existing bone marrow aplasia, leukopenia, thrombocytopenia or anemia, the drug should be used with caution, if at all.

Methotrexate is excreted principally by the kidneys. Its use in the presence of impaired renal function may result in accumulation of toxic amounts or even additional renal damage. The patient's renal status should be determined prior to and during Methotrexate therapy and proper caution exercised should significant renal impairment be disclosed. Drug dosage should be reduced or discontinued until renal function is improved or restored.

In general, the following laboratory tests are recommended as part of essential clinical evaluation and appropriate monitoring of patients chosen for or receiving Methotrexate therapy: complete hemogram; hematocrit; urinalysis; renal function tests; and liver function tests. A chest x-ray is also recommended. The purpose is to determine any existing organ dysfunction or system impairment. The tests should be performed prior to therapy, at appropriate periods during therapy and after termination of therapy. It may be useful or important to perform liver biopsy or bone marrow aspiration studies where high dose or long-term therapy is being followed.

Methotrexate is bound in part to serum albumin after absorption and toxicity may be increased because of displacement by certain drugs such as salicylates, sulfonamides, phenytoin, phenylbutazone, and some antibacterials as tetracycline, chloramphenicol and para-amino-benzoic acid. These drugs, especially salicylates, phenylbutazone, and sulfonamides, whether antibacterial, hypoglycemic or diuretic, should not be given concurrently until the significance of these findings is established.

Vitamin preparations containing folic acid or its derviatives may alter responses to Methotrexate. Methotrexate should be used with extreme caution in the presence of infection, peptic ulcer, ulcerative colitis, debility, and in extreme youth and old age.

If profound leukopenia occurs during therapy, bacterial infection may occur or become a threat. Cessation of the drug and appropriate antibiotic therapy is usually indicated. In severe bone marrow depression, blood or platelet transfusions may be necessary.

Since it is reported that Methotrexate may have an immunosuppressive action, this factor must be taken into consideration in evaluating the use of the drug where immune responses in a patient may be important or essential.

In all instances where the use of Methotrexate is considered for chemotherapy, the physician must evaluate the need and usefulness of the drug against the risks of toxic effects or adverse reaction. Most such adverse reactions are reversible if detected early. When such effects or reactions do occur, the drug should be reduced in dosage or discontinued and appropriate corrective measures should be taken, according to the clinical judgment of the physician. Reinstitution of Methotrexate therapy should be carried out with caution, with adequate consideration of further need for the drug and alertness as to possible recurrence of toxicity.

Adverse Reactions: The most common adverse reactions include ulcerative stomatitis, leukopenia, nausea and abdominal distress. Others re-

Continued on next page

The information on each product appearing here is based on labelling effective in August, 1984 and is either the entire official brochure or an accurate condensation therefrom. Information concerning all Lederle products may be obtained from the Professional Services Department, Lederle Laboratories, Pearl River, New York, 10965.

Lederle—Cont.

ported are malaise, undue fatigue, chills and fever, dizziness and decreased resistance to infection. In general, the incidence and severity of side effects are considered to be dose-related. Adverse reactions as reported for the various systems are as follows:

Skin: erythematous rashes, pruritus, urticaria, photosensitivity, depigmentation, alopecia, ecchymosis, telangiectasia, acne, furunculosis. Lesions of psoriasis may be aggravated by concomitant exposure to ultraviolet radiation.

Blood: bone marrow depression, leukopenia, thrombocytopenia, anemia, hypogammaglobulinemia, hemorrhage from various sites, septicemia.

Alimentary System: gingivitis, pharyngitis, stomatitis, anorexia, vomiting, diarrhea, hematemesis, melena, gastrointestinal ulceration and bleeding, enteritis, hepatic toxicity resulting in acute liver atrophy, necrosis, fatty metamorphosis, periportal fibrosis, or hepatic cirrhosis.

Urogenital System: renal failure, azotemia, cystitis, hematuria; defective oogenesis or spermatogenesis, transient oligospermia, menstrual dysfunction; infertility, abortion, fetal defects, severe nephropathy.

Pulmonary System: Interstitial Pneumonitis. Deaths have been reported and chronic interstitial obstructive pulmonary disease has occasionally occurred.

Central Nervous System: Headaches, drowsiness, blurred vision. Aphasia, hemiparesis, paresis and convulsions have also occurred following administration of Methotrexate.

There have been reports of leucoencephalopathy following intravenous administration of Methotrexate to patients who have had craniospinal irradiation.

After the intrathecal use of Methotrexate, the central nervous system toxicity which may occur can be classified as follows: (1) chemical arachnoiditis manifested by such symptoms as headache, back pain, nuchal rigidity, and fever; (2) paresis, usually transient, manifested by paraplegia associated with involvement with one or more spinal nerve roots; (3) leucoencephalopathy manifested by confusion, irritability, somnolence, ataxia, dementia, and occasionally major convulsions.

Other reactions related to or attributed to the use of Methotrexate such as metabolic changes, precipitating diabetes; osteoporotic effects, abnormal tissue cell changes, and even sudden death have been reported.

Dosage and Administration:
Anti-neoplastic chemotherapy

Oral administration in tablet form is often preferred since absorption is rapid and effective serum levels are obtained. Methotrexate sodium parenteral may be given by intramuscular, intravenous, intraarterial or intrathecal route. Initial treatment is usually undertaken with the patient under hospital care.

For conversion of mg/kg b.w. to mg/M^2 of body surface or the reverse, a ratio of 1:30 is given as a guideline. The conversion factor varies between 1:20 and 1:40 depending on age and body build.

Choriocarcinoma and similar trophoblastic diseases: Methotrexate is administered orally or intramuscularly in doses of 15 to 30 mg daily for a 5 day course. Such courses are usually repeated for 3 to 5 times as required, with rest periods of one or more weeks interposed between courses, until any manifesting toxic symptoms subside. The effectiveness of therapy is ordinarily evaluated by 24 hour quantitative analysis of urinary chorionic gonadotropin hormone (CGH), which should return to normal or less than 50 IU/24 hr. usually after the 3rd or 4th course and usually be followed by a complete resolution of measurable lesions in 4 to 6 weeks. One to two courses of Methotrexate after normalization of CGH is usually recommended. Before each course of the drug careful clinical assessment is essential. Cyclic combination therapy of Methotrexate with other antitumor drugs has been reported as being useful. Since hydatidiform mole may precede or be followed by choriocarcinoma, prophylactic chemotherapy with Methotrexate has been recommended. Chorioadenoma destruens is considered to be an invasive form of hydatidiform mole. Methotrexate is administered in these disease states in doses similar to those recommended for choriocarcinoma.

Leukemia: acute lymphatic (lymphoblastic) leukemia in children and young adolescents is the most responsive to present day chemotherapy. In young adults and older patients, clinical remission is more difficult to obtain and early relapse is more common. In chronic lymphatic leukemia, the prognosis for adequate response is less encouraging. Methotrexate alone or in combination with steroids was used initially for induction of remission of lymphoblastic leukemias. More recently corticosteroid therapy in combination with other antileukemic drugs or in cyclic combinations with Methotrexate included appear to produce rapid and effective remissions. When used for induction, Methotrexate in doses of 3.3 mg/M^2 in combination with prednisone 60 mg/M^2, given daily, produced remission in 50% of patients treated, usually within a period of 4 to 6 weeks. Methotrexate alone or in combination with other agents appears to be the drug of choice for securing maintenance of drug-induced remissions. When remission is achieved and supportive care has produced general clinical improvement, maintenance therapy is initiated, as follows: Methotrexate is administered 2 times weekly either by mouth or intramuscularly in doses of 30 mg/M^2. It has also been given in doses of 2.5 mg/kg intravenously every 14 days. If and when relapse does occur, reinduction of remission can again usually be obtained by repeating the initial induction regimen. Various experts have recently introduced a variety of dosage schedules for both induction and maintenance of remission with various combinations of alkylating and antifolic agents. Multiple drug therapy with several agents, including Methotrexate given concomitantly is gaining increasing support in both the acute and chronic forms of leukemia. The physician should familiarize himself with the new advances in antileukemic therapy.

Acute granulocytic leukemia is rare in children but common in adults. This form of leukemia responds poorly to chemotherapy and remissions are short with relapses common, and resistance to therapy develops rapidly.

Meningeal leukemia: Patients with leukemia are subject to leukemic invasion of the central nervous system. This may manifest characteristic signs or symptoms or may remain silent and be diagnosed only by examination of the cerebrospinal fluid which contains leukemic cells in such cases. Therefore, the CSF should be examined in all leukemic patients. Since passage of Methotrexate from blood serum to the cerebrospinal fluid is minimal, for adequate therapy the drug is administered intrathecally. It is now common practice because of the noted increased frequency of meningeal leukemia to administer Methotrexate intrathecally as prophylaxis in all cases of lymphocytic leukemia.

By intrathecal injection, the sodium salt of Methotrexate is administered in solution in doses of 12 mg per square meter of body surface or in an empirical dose of 15 mg. The solution is made in a strength of 1 mg per ml with an appropriate, sterile, preservative-free medium such as Sodium Chloride Injection, USP. For the treatment of meningeal leukemia, Methotrexate is given at intervals of 2 to 5 days. Methotrexate is administered until the cell count of the cerebrospinal fluid returns to normal. At this point one additional dose is advisable.

For prophylaxis against meningeal leukemia, the dosage is the same as for treatment except for the intervals of administration.

On this subject, it is advisable for the physician to consult the medical literature.

Large doses may cause convulsions. Untoward side effects may occur with any given intrathecal injection and are commonly neurological in character. Methotrexate given by intrathecal route appears significantly in the systemic circulation and may cause systemic Methotrexate toxicity. Therefore, systemic antileukemic therapy with the drug should be appropriately adjusted, reduced or discontinued. Focal leukemic involvement of the central nervous system may not respond to intrathecal chemotherapy and is best treated with radiotherapy.

Lymphomas: in Burkitt's Tumor, Stages I-II, Methotrexate has produced prolonged remissions in some cases. Recommended dosage is 10 to 25 mg per day orally for 4 to 8 days. In stage III, Methotrexate is commonly given concomitantly with other antitumor agents. Treatment in all stages usually consists of several courses of the drug interposed with 7 to 10 day rest periods. Lymphosarcomas in Stage III may respond to combined drug therapy with Methotrexate given in doses of 0.625 mg to 2.5 mg/kg daily. Hodgkin's Disease responds poorly to Methotrexate and to most types of chemotherapy.

Mycosis fungoides: therapy with Methotrexate appears to produce clinical remissions in one half of the cases treated. Dosage is usually 2.5 to 10 mg daily by mouth for weeks or months. Dose levels of drug and adjustment of dose regimen by reduction or cessation of drug are guided by patient response and hematologic monitoring. Methotrexate has also been given intramuscularly in doses of 50 mg once weekly or 25 mg 2 times weekly.

Psoriasis Chemotherapy

The patient should be fully informed of the risks involved and should be under constant supervision of the physician.

Assessment of renal function, liver function, and blood elements should be made by history, physical examination, and laboratory tests (such as CBC, urinalysis, serum creatinine, liver function studies, and liver biopsy if indicated) before beginning Methotrexate, periodically during Methotrexate therapy, and before reinstituting Methotrexate therapy after a rest period. Appropriate steps should be taken to avoid conception during and for at least eight weeks following Methotrexate therapy.

There are three commonly used general types of dosage schedules:
1) weekly oral or parenteral intermittent large doses
2) divided dose intermittent oral schedule over a 36 hour period
3) daily oral with a rest period

All schedules should be continually tailored to the individual patient. Dose schedules cited below pertain to an average 70 Kg adult. An initial test dose one week prior to initiation of therapy is recommended to detect any idiosyncrasy. A suggested dose range is 5–10 mg parenterally.

Recommended starting dose schedules:
1. Weekly single oral, IM or IV dose schedule: 10–25 mg per week until adequate response is achieved. With this dosage schedule, 50 mg per week should ordinarily not be exceeded.
2. Divided oral dose schedule: 2.5 mg at 12 hour intervals for three doses or at 8 hour intervals for four doses each week. With this dosage schedule, 30 mg per week should not be exceeded.
3. Daily oral dose schedule: 2.5 mg daily for five days followed by at least a two day rest period. With this dosage schedule, 6.25 mg per day should not be exceeded.

SPECIAL NOTE: Available data suggest that schedule 3 may carry an increased risk of serious liver pathology.

Dosages in each schedule may be gradually adjusted to achieve optimal clinical response, but not to exceed the maximum stated for each schedule. Once optimal clinical response has been achieved, each dosage schedule should be reduced to the lowest possible amount of drug and to the longest possible rest period. The use of Methotrexate may permit the return to conventional topical therapy, which should be encouraged.

Antidote for Overdosage: Leucovorin (citrovorum factor) is a potent agent for neutralizing the immediate toxic effects of Methotrexate on the hematopoietic system. Where large doses or overdoses are given, Calcium Leucovorin may be ad-

for possible revisions — **Product Information** — **1103**

ministered by intravenous infusion in doses up to 75 mg within 12 hours, followed by 12 mg intramuscularly every 6 hours for 4 doses. Where average doses of Methotrexate appear to have an adverse effect, 2 to 4 ml (6 to 12 mg) of Calcium Leucovorin may be given intramuscularly every 6 hours for 4 doses. In general, where overdosage is suspected, the dose of Leucovorin should be equal to or higher than the offending dose of Methotrexate and should best be administered within the first hour. Use of Calcium Leucovorin after an hour delay is much less effective.

CAUTION: Pharmacist: Because of its potential to cause severe toxicity, Methotrexate therapy requires close supervision of the patient by the physician. Pharmacists should dispense no more than a seven (7) day supply of the drug at one time. Refill of such prescriptions should be by direct order (written or oral) of the physician only.

Reconstitution of Low Sodium Cryodesiccated Powders

Dilute immediately prior to use.

For IV or IM administration, reconstitute to a concentration of no greater than 25 mg/ml with an appropriate sterile, preservative-free medium such as Sodium Chloride USP (IM) or 5% Dextrose Solution USP (IV).

For intrathecal injection, reconstitute to a concentration of 1 mg/ml with an appropriate sterile, preservative-free medium such as Sodium Chloride Injection USP.

How Supplied:

*Parenterals:

Low Sodium Cryodesiccated Powders—Pre- servative Free, Single Use Only

20 mg Vial—Product No. NDC 0205-4654-90 (Dark Blue Cap)

50 mg Vial—Product No. NDC 0205-9337-92 (Violet Cap)

100 mg Vial—Product No. NDC 0205-9338-94 (Green Cap)

Store at Controlled Room Temperature 15–30° C (59–86°F)

Isotonic Liquids—Preservative Free, Single Use Only Methotrexate LPF Sodium

25 mg/ml—2 ml (50 mg) Vials—Product No. NDC 0205-5325-26 (Brown Cap)

25 mg/ml—4 ml (100 mg) Vials—Product No. NDC 0205-5326-18 (Light Blue Cap)

25 mg/ml—8 ml (200 mg) Vials—Product No. NDC 0205-5327-30 (Orange Cap)

Store at Controlled Room Temperature 15–30° C (50–86°F)

Isotonic Liquids—Preserved

25 mg per ml—2 ml Vials—Product NDC 0205-4556-26 (Red Cap)

Store at Controlled Room Temperature 15–30° C (59–86°F)

*Parenterals:

Isotonic Liquid—Preserved

2.5 mg per ml—2 ml Vials—Product No. NDC 0005-4554-26 (White Cap)

Store at Controlled Room Temperature 15–30° C (50–86°F)

*Lederle Parenterals, Inc.

Carlina, Puerto Rico 00630

Oral:

Description

Methotrexate tablets contain 2.5 mg of Methotrexate and are round, convex, yellow tablets, engraved with LL on one side, scored in half on the other side, and engraved with M above the score, and 1 below. 2.5 mg Tablets—Bottles of 100—Product No. NDC 0005-4507-23

Store at Controlled Room Temperature 15–30° C (59–86°F)

Lederle Laboratories Division
American Cyanamid Company,
Pearl River, N.Y. 10965

Military Depot:

Tablets, 2.5 mg, 100's, NSN 6505-00-963-5353
Sodium Injection, 25 mg/ml, 2 ml, NSN 6505-01-020-2367

Methotrexate LPF®
Sodium Parenteral
25 mg/ml, 8 ml vial—200 mg
NSN 6505-01-125-6505

VA Depots:

Methotrexate LPF®
Sodium Parenteral
25 mg/ml 2 ml, NSN 6505-01-125-6503A
25 mg/ml 4 ml, NSN 6505-01-125-6504A
25 mg/ml 8 ml, NSN 01-125-6505A
Shown in Product Identification Section, page 415

MINOCIN® ℞
[mī-nō-sĭn]
Sterile
minocycline hydrochloride
Intravenous
100 mg/Vial

Description: MINOCIN *minocycline hydrochloride*, a semi-synthetic derivative of tetracycline, is named [4S-(4α, 4aα, 5aα, 12aα)]-4,7-bis(dimethylamino) -1,4,4a,5,5a,6,11,12a-octahydro-3,10,12,12a -tetrahydroxy -1, 11- dioxo -2- naphthacenecarboxamide monohydrochloride.

Each vial, dried by cryodesiccation, contains Sterile Minocycline Hydrochloride equivalent to 100 mg Minocycline. When reconstituted with 5 ml of Sterile Water For Injection the pH ranges from 2.0 to 2.8.

Actions: Microbiology—The tetracyclines are primarily bacteriostatic and are thought to exert their antimicrobial effect by the inhibition of protein synthesis. Minocycline HCl is a tetracycline with antibacterial activity comparable to other tetracyclines with activity against a wide range of gram-negative and gram-positive organisms.

Tube dilution testing: Microorganisms may be considered susceptible (likely to respond to minocycline therapy) if the minimum inhibitory concentration (M.I.C.) is not more than 4.0 mcg/ml. Microorganisms may be considered intermediate (harboring partial resistance) if the M.I.C. is 4.0 to 12.5 mcg/ml and resistant (not likely to respond to minocycline therapy) if the M.I.C. is greater than 12.5 mcg/ml.

Susceptibility plate testing: If the Kirby-Bauer method of susceptibility testing (using a 30 mcg tetracycline disc) gives a zone of 18 mm. or greater, the bacterial strain is considered to be susceptible to any tetracycline. Minocycline shows moderate *in vitro* activity against certain strains of staphylococci which have been found resistant to other tetracyclines. For such strains, minocycline susceptibility powder may be used for additional susceptibility testing.

Human Pharmacology—Following a single dose of 200 mg administered to 10 healthy male volunteers, serum levels ranged from 2.52 to 6.63 mcg/ml (average 4.18), after 12 hours they ranged from 0.82 to 2.64 mcg/ml (average 1.38). In a group of 5 healthy male volunteers serum levels of 1.4–1.8 mcg/ml were maintained at 12 and 24 hours with doses of 100 mg every 12 hours for three days. When given 200 mg once daily for three days the serum levels had fallen to approximately 1 mcg/ml at 24 hours. The serum half-life following I.V. doses of 100 mg every 12 hours or 200 mg once daily did not differ significantly and ranged from 15 to 23 hours. The serum half-life following a single 200 mg oral dose in 12 essentially normal volunteers ranged from 11 to 17 hours, in 7 patients with hepatic dysfunction ranged from 11 to 16 hours, and in 5 patients with renal dysfunction from 18 to 69 hours.

Intravenously administered Minocycline appears similar to oral doses in excretion. The urinary and fecal recovery of oral minocycline when administered to 12 normal volunteers is one-half to one-third that of other tetracyclines.

Indications: MINOCIN *minocycline HCl* is indicated in infections caused by the following microorganisms:

Rickettsiae: (Rocky Mountain spotted fever, typhus fever and the typhus group, Q fever, rickettsialpox, tick fevers).

Mycoplasma pneumoniae (PPLO, Eaton agent).

Agents of psittacosis and ornithosis.

Agents of lymphogranuloma venereum and granuloma inguinale.

The spirochetal agent of relapsing fever (*Borrelia recurrentis*).

The following gram-negative microorganisms:
Hemophilus ducreyi (chancroid),
Pasteurella pestis and *Pasteurella tularensis*,
Bartonella bacilliformis,
Bacteroides species,
Vibrio comma and *Vibrio fetus*,
Brucella species (in conjunction with streptomycin).

Because many strains of the following groups of microorganisms have been shown to be resistant to tetracyclines, culture and susceptibility testing are recommended.

MINOCIN *minocycline HCl* is indicated for treatment of infections caused by the following gram-negative microorganisms, when bacteriologic testing indicates appropriate susceptibility to the drug:

Escherichia coli,
Enterobacter aerogenes (formerly *Aerobacter aerogenes*),
Shigella species,
Mima species and *Herellea* species,
Haemophilus influenzae (respiratory infections),
Klebsiella species (respiratory and urinary infections).

MINOCIN is indicated for treatment of infections caused by the following gram-positive microorganisms when bacteriologic testing indicates appropriate susceptibility to the drug:

Streptococcus species:

Up to 44 percent of strains of *Streptococcus pyogenes* and 74 percent of *Streptococcus faecalis* have been found to be resistant to tetracycline drugs. Therefore, tetracyclines should not be used for streptococcal disease unless the organism has been demonstrated to be sensitive.

For upper respiratory infections due to group A beta-hemolytic streptococci, penicillin is the usual drug of choice, including prophylaxis of rheumatic fever.

Diplococcus pneumoniae,
Staphylococcus aureus, skin and soft tissue infections.

Tetracyclines are not the drug of choice in the treatment of any type of staphylococcal infection.

When penicillin is contraindicated, tetracyclines are alternative drugs in the treatment of infections due to:

Neisseria gonorrhoeae, and *Neisseria meningitidis*,
Treponema pallidum and *Treponema pertenue* (syphilis and yaws),
Listeria monocytogenes,
Clostridium species,
Bacillus anthracis,
Fusobacterium fusiforme (Vincent's infection),
Actinomyces species.

In acute intestinal amebiasis, the tetracyclines may be a useful adjunct to amebicides.

MINOCIN is indicated in the treatment of trachoma, although the infectious agent is not always eliminated as judged by immunofluorescence.

Inclusion conjunctivitis may be treated with oral tetracyclines or with a combination of oral and topical agents.

Contraindications: This drug is contraindicated in persons who have shown hypersensitivity to any of the tetracyclines.

Warnings: In the presence of renal dysfunction, particularly in pregnancy, intravenous tetracycline therapy in daily doses exceeding 2 grams has been associated with deaths through liver failure. When the need for intensive treatment outweighs its potential dangers (mostly during pregnancy or in individuals with known or suspected renal or liver impairment), it is advisable to perform renal

Continued on next page

The information on each product appearing here is based on labelling effective in August, 1984 and is either the entire official brochure or an accurate condensation thereform. Information concerning all Lederle products may be obtained from the Professional Services Department, Lederle Laboratories, Pearl River, New York. 10965.

Lederle—Cont.

and liver function tests before and during therapy. Also tetracycline serum concentrations should be followed.

If renal impairment exists, even usual oral or parenteral doses may lead to excessive systemic accumulation of the drug and possible liver toxicity. Under such conditions, lower than usual total doses are indicated, and if therapy is prolonged, serum level determinations of the drug may be advisable. This hazard is of particular importance in the parenteral administration of tetracyclines to pregnant or postpartum patients with pyelonephritis. When used under these circumstances, the blood level should not exceed 15 micrograms/ml and liver function tests should be made at frequent intervals. Other potentially hepatotoxic drugs should not be prescribed concomitantly.

THE USE OF TETRACYCLINES DURING TOOTH DEVELOPMENT (LAST HALF OF PREGNANCY, INFANCY AND CHILDHOOD TO THE AGE OF 8 YEARS) MAY CAUSE PERMANENT DISCOLORATION OF THE TEETH (YELLOW-GRAY-BROWN). This adverse reaction is more common during long-term use of the drugs but has been observed following repeated short-term courses. Enamel hypoplasia has also been reported. TETRACYCLINES, THEREFORE, SHOULD NOT BE USED IN THIS AGE GROUP UNLESS OTHER DRUGS ARE NOT LIKELY TO BE EFFECTIVE OR ARE CONTRAINDICATED.

Photosensitivity manifested by an exaggerated sunburn reaction has been observed in some individuals taking tetracyclines. Patients apt to be exposed to direct sunlight or ultraviolet light should be advised that this reaction can occur with tetracycline drugs, and treatment should be discontinued at the first evidence of skin erythema. Studies to date indicate that photosensitivity does not occur with MINOCIN *minocycline HCl*.

The antianabolic action of the tetracyclines may cause an increase in BUN. While this is not a problem in those with normal renal function, in patients with significantly impaired function, higher serum levels of tetracyclines may lead to azotemia, hyperphosphatemia, and acidosis.

CNS side effects including lightheadedness, dizziness or vertigo have been reported. Patients who experience these symptoms should be cautioned about driving vehicles or using hazardous machinery while on minocycline therapy. These symptoms may disappear during therapy and always disappear rapidly when the drug is discontinued.

Usage in Pregnancy—(See above "Warnings" about use during tooth development.)

Results of animal studies indicate that tetracyclines cross the placenta, are found in fetal tissues and can have toxic effects on the developing fetus (often related to retardation of skeletal development). Evidence of embryotoxicity has also been noted in animals treated early in pregnancy. The safety of minocycline HCl for use during pregnancy has not been established.

Usage in newborns, infants, and children—(See above "Warnings" about use during tooth development.)

All tetracyclines form a stable calcium complex in any bone forming tissue. A decrease in the fibula growth rate has been observed in prematures given oral tetracycline in doses of 25 mg/kg every 6 hours. This reaction was shown to be reversible when the drug was discontinued.

Tetracyclines are present in the milk of lactating women who are taking a drug in this class.

Precautions: As with other antibiotic preparations, use of this drug may result in overgrowth of nonsusceptible organisms, including fungi. If superinfection occurs, the antibiotic should be discontinued and appropriate therapy should be instituted.

In venereal diseases when coexistent syphilis is suspected, darkfield examination should be done before treatment is started and the blood serology repeated monthly for at least 4 months.

Because tetracyclines have been shown to depress plasma prothrombin activity, patients who are on anticoagulant therapy may require downward adjustment of their anticoagulant dosage.

In long-term therapy, periodic laboratory evaluation of organ systems, including hematopoietic, renal and hepatic studies should be performed.

All infections due to Group A beta-hemolytic streptococci should be treated for at least 10 days. Since bacteriostatic drugs may interfere with the bactericidal action of penicillin, it is advisable to avoid giving tetracycline in conjunction with penicillin.

Adverse Reactions: Gastrointestinal: Anorexia, nausea, vomiting, diarrhea, glossitis, dysphagia, enterocolitis, and inflammatory lesions (with monilial overgrowth) in the anogenital region.

These reactions have been caused by both the oral and parenteral administration of tetracyclines.

Skin: Maculopapular and erythematous rashes. Exfoliative dermatitis has been reported but is uncommon. Photosensitivity is discussed above. (See "Warnings".)

Tooth discoloration has been reported rarely in adults.

Renal toxicity: Rise in BUN has been reported and is apparently dose related (See "Warnings".)

Hypersensitivity reactions: Urticaria, angioneurotic edema, anaphylaxis, anaphylactoid purpura, pericarditis and exacerbation of systemic lupus erythematosus.

Bulging fontanels have been reported in young infants following full therapeutic dosage. Pseudotumor Cerebri has been very rarely been reported in adults. These signs disappeared rapidly when the drug was discontinued.

Blood: Hemolytic anemia, thrombocytopenia, neutropenia and eosinophilia have been reported.

CNS: (See "Warnings".)

When given over prolonged periods, tetracyclines have been reported to produce brown-black microscopic discoloration of thyroid glands. No abnormalities of thyroid function studies are known to occur.

Dosage and Administration: Note: Rapid administration is to be avoided. Parenteral therapy is indicated only when oral therapy is not adequate or tolerated. Oral therapy should be instituted as soon as possible. If intravenous therapy is given over prolonged periods of time, thrombophlebitis may result.

Adults: Usual adult dose: 200 mg followed by 100 mg every 12 hours and should not exceed 400 mg in 24 hours. The drug should be initially dissolved and then further diluted to 500–1,000 ml with either Sodium Chloride Injection USP, Dextrose Injection USP, Dextrose and Sodium Chloride Injection USP, Ringer's Injection USP, or Lactated Ringer's Injection USP but not in other solutions containing calcium (a precipitate may form).

The reconstituted solutions are stable at room temperature for 24 hours without significant loss of potency. Any unused portions must be discarded after that period. The final dilution for administration should be administered immediately.

For children above eight years of age: Usual pediatric dose: 4 mg/kg followed by 2 mg/kg every 12 hours.

In patients with renal impairment: (See "Warnings").

Total dosage should be decreased by reduction of recommended individual doses and/or by extending time intervals between doses.

How Supplied: 100 mg vials of sterile cryodesiccated powder

Product No. NDC 0205-5305-94

Store at Controlled Room Temperature 15–30°C (59–86°F)

Military Depot: Intravenous—100 mg vial—NSN 6505-00-149-0574

*Manufactured for
LEDERLE LABORATORIES DIVISION
American Cyanamid Company
Pearl River, NY 10965
by
LEDERLE PARENTERALS, INC.
Carolina, Puerto Rico 00630

MINOCIN®
[mī-nō-sĭn]
Minocycline Hydrochloride for Oral Use

Description: MINOCIN minocycline hydrochloride, a semi-synthetic derivative of tetracycline, is named [4S-(4α, 4aα, 5aα, 12aα)]-4,7-bis(dimethylamino) -1,4,4a,5,5a,6,11,12a-octahydro-3,10,12,12a-tetrahydroxy -1, 11- dioxo -2- naphthacenecarboxamide monohydrochloride.

Actions: Microbiology—The tetracyclines are primarily bacteriostatic and are thought to exert their antimicrobial effect by the inhibition of protein synthesis. Minocycline HCl is a tetracycline with antibacterial activity comparable to other tetracyclines with activity against a wide range of gram-negative and gram-positive organisms.

Tube dilution testing: Microorganisms may be considered susceptible (likely to respond to minocycline therapy) if the minimum inhibitory concentration (M.I.C.) is not more than 4.0 mcg/ml. Microorganisms may be considered intermediate (harboring partial resistance) if the M.I.C. is 4.0 to 12.5 mcg/ml and resistant (not likely to respond to minocycline therapy) if the M.I.C. is greater than 12.5 mcg/ml.

Susceptibility plate testing: If the Kirby-Bauer method of susceptibility testing (using a 30 mcg tetracycline disc) gives a zone of 18 mm or greater, the bacterial strain is considered to be susceptible to any tetracycline. Minocycline shows moderate *in vitro* activity against certain strains of staphylococci which have been found resistant to other tetracyclines. For such strains minocycline susceptibility powder may be used for additional susceptibility testing.

Human Pharmacology—Following a single dose of two 100 mg of minocycline HCl capsules administered to ten normal adult volunteers, serum levels ranged from 0.74 to 4.45 mcg/ml in one hour (average 2.24), after 12 hours, they ranged from 0.34 to 2.36 mcg/ml (average 1.25). The serum half-life following a single 200 mg dose in 12 essentially normal volunteers ranged from 11 to 17 hours, in 7 patients with hepatic dysfunction ranged from 11 to 16 hours, and in 5 patients with renal dysfunction from 18 to 69 hours. The urinary and fecal recovery of minocycline when administered to 12 normal volunteers is one-half to one-third that of other tetracyclines.

Indications: MINOCIN *minocycline HCl* is indicated in infections caused by the following microorganisms:

Rickettsiae: (Rocky Mountain spotted fever, typhus fever and the typhus group, Q fever, rickettsialpox, tick fevers).

Mycoplasma pneumoniae (PPLO, Eaton agent).

Agents of psittacosis and ornithosis.

Agents of lymphogranuloma venereum and granuloma inguinale.

The spirochetal agent of relapsing fever (*Borrelia recurrentis*).

The following gram-negative micro-organisms:

Hemophilus ducreyi (chancroid),
Pasteurella pestis and *Pasteurella tularensis*,
Bartonella bacilliformis,
Bacteroides species,
Vibrio comma and *Vibrio fetus*,
Brucella species (in conjunction with streptomycin).

Because many strains of the following groups of micro-organisms have been shown to be resistant to tetracyclines, culture and susceptibility testing are recommended.

MINOCIN *minocycline hydrochloride* is indicated for treatment of infections caused by the following gram-negative microorganisms when bacteriologic testing indicates appropriate susceptibility to the drug:

Escherichia coli,
Enterobacter aerogenes (formerly *Aerobacter aerogenes*),
Shigella species,
Acinetobacter calcoaceticus (syn. *Herellea*, *Mima*),

Haemophilus influenzae (respiratory infections), *Klebsiella* species (respiratory and urinary infections).

MINOCIN is indicated for treatment of infections caused by the following gram-positive microorganisms when bacteriologic testing indicates appropriate susceptibility to the drug:

Streptococcus species:

Up to 44 percent of strains of *Streptococcus pyogenes* and 74 percent of *Streptococcus faecalis* have been found to be resistant to tetracycline drugs. Therefore, tetracyclines should not be used for streptococcal disease unless the organism has been demonstrated to be sensitive.

For upper respiratory infections due to group A beta-hemolytic streptococci, penicillin is the usual drug of choice, including prophylaxis of rheumatic fever.

Diplococcus pneumoniae,
Staphylococcus aureus, skin and soft tissue infections.

Tetracyclines are not the drugs of choice in the treatment of any type of staphylococcal infection.
MINOCIN is indicated for the treatment of uncomplicated gonococcal urethritis in men due to *Neisseria gonorrhoeae.*

When penicillin is contraindicated, tetracyclines are alternative drugs in the treatment of infections due to:

Neisseria gonorrhoeae (in women),
Treponema pallidum and *Treponema pertenue* (syphilis and yaws),
Listeria monocytogenes,
Clostridium species,
Bacillus anthracis,
Fusobacterium fusiforme (Vincent's infection),
Actinomyces species.

In acute intestinal amebiasis, the tetracyclines may be a useful adjunct to amebicides.

In severe acne, the tetracyclines may be useful adjunctive therapy.

MINOCIN is indicated in the treatment of trachoma, alhtough the infectious agent is not always eliminated, as judged by immunofluorescence.
Minocycline hydrochloride is indicated for the treatment of uncomplicated urethral, endocervical or rectal infections in adults caused by *Chlamydia trachomatis* or *Ureaplasma urealyticum*.[1]
Inclusion conjunctivitis may be treated with oral tetracyclines or with a combination of oral and topical agents.

Minocycline is indicated in the treatment of asymptomatic carriers of *N. meningitidis* to eliminate meningococci from the nasopharynx.

In order to preserve the usefulness of MINOCIN *minocycline HCl* in the treatment of asymtomatic meningococcal carriers, diagnostic laboratory procedures, including serotyping and susceptibility testing, should be performed to establish the carrier state and the correct treatment. It is recommended that the drug be reserved for situations in which the risk of meningococcal meningitis is high.

Minocycline by oral administration is not indicated for the treatment of meningococcal infection.

Although no controlled clinical efficacy studies have been conducted, limited clinical data show that oral minocycline hydrochloride has been used successfully in the treatment of infections caused by Mycobacterium marinum.

Contraindications: This drug is contraindicated in persons who have shown hypersensitivity to any of the tetracyclines.

Warnings: THE USE OF DRUGS OF THE TETRACYCLINE CLASS DURING TOOTH DEVELOPMENT (LAST HALF OF PREGNANCY, INFANCY, AND CHILDHOOD TO THE AGE OF 8 YEARS) MAY CAUSE PERMANENT DISCOLORATION OF THE TEETH (YELLOW-GRAY-BROWN). This adverse reaction is more common during long-term use of the drugs but has been observed following repeated short-term courses. Enamel hypoplasia has also been reported. TETRACYCLINE DRUGS, THEREFORE, SHOULD NOT BE USED IN THIS AGE GROUP UNLESS OTHER DRUGS ARE NOT LIKELY TO BE EFFECTIVE OR ARE CONTRAINDICATED.

If renal impairment exists, even usual oral or parenteral doses may lead to excessive systemic accumulations of the drug and possible liver toxicity. Under such conditions, lower than usual total doses are indicated, and if therapy is prolonged, serum level determinations of the drug may be advisable.

Photosensitivity manifested by an exaggerated sunburn reaction has been observed in some individuals taking tetracyclines. Patients apt to be exposed to direct sunlight or ultraviolet light should be advised that this reaction can occur with tetracycline drugs, and treatment should be discontinued at the first evidence of skin erythema. Studies to date indicate that photosensitivity is rarely reported with MINOCIN *minocycline HCl.*
The anti-anabolic action of the tetracyclines may cause an increase in BUN. While this is not a problem in those with normal renal function, in patients with significantly impaired function, higher serum levels of tetracycline may lead to azotemia, hyperphosphatemia, and acidosis.

CNS side effects including lightheadedness, dizziness, or vertigo have been reported. Patients who experience these symptoms should be cautioned about driving vehicles or using hazardous machinery while on minocycline therapy. These symptoms may disappear during therapy and always disappear rapidly when the drug is discontinued.

Usage in pregnancy (See above "Warnings" about use during tooth development). Results of animal studies indicate that tetracyclines cross the placenta, are found in fetal tissues and can have toxic effects on the developing fetus (often related to retardation of skeletal development). Evidence of embryotoxicity has also been noted in animals treated early in pregnancy.

The safety of minocycline HCl for use during pregnancy has not been established.

Usage in newborns, infants, and children (See above "Warnings" about use during tooth development).

All tetracyclines form a stable calcium complex in any bone forming tissue. A decrease in the fibula growth rate has been observed in prematures given oral tetracycline in doses of 25 mg/kg every 6 hours. This reaction was shown to be reversible when the drug was discontinued.

Tetracyclines are present in the milk of lactating women who are taking a drug in this class.

Precautions: As with other antibiotic preparations, use of this drug may result in overgrowth of nonsusceptible organisms, including fungi. If superinfection occurs, the antibiotic should be discontinued and appropriate therapy should be instituted.

In venereal diseases when coexistent syphilis is suspected, darkfield examination should be done before treatment is started and the blood serology repeated monthly for at least 4 months.

Because tetracyclines have been shown to depress plasma prothrombin activity, patients who are on anticoagulant therapy may require downward adjustment of their anticoagulant dosage.

In long-term therapy, periodic laboratory evaluation of organ systems, including hematopoietic, renal and hepatic studies should be performed.
All infections due to Group A beta-hemolytic streptococci should be treated for at least 10 days.
Since bacteriostatic drugs may interfere with the bactericidal action of penicillin, it is advisable to avoid giving tetracycline in conjunction with penicillin.

Adverse Reactions: Gastrointestinal: Anorexia, nausea, vomiting, diarrhea, glossitis, dysphagia, enterocolitis, and inflammatory lesions (with monilial overgrowth) in the anogenital region.
These reactions have been caused by both the oral and parenteral administration of tetracyclines.

Skin: Maculopapular and erythematous rashes. Exfoliative dermatitis has been reported but is uncommon. Photosensitivity is discussed above. (See "Warnings").

Pigmentation of the skin and mucous membranes has been reported.

Tooth discoloration has been reported rarely in adults.

Renal toxicity: Rise in BUN has been reported and is apparently dose related (See "Warnings").
Hypersensitivity reactions: Urticaria, angioneurotic edema, anaphylaxis, anaphylactoid purpura, pericarditis and exacerbation of systemic lupus erythematosus.

Bulging fontanels have been reported in young infants following full therapeutic dosage. Pseudotumor Cerebri has very rarely been reported in adults. These signs disappeared rapidly when the drug was discontinued.

Blood: Hemolytic anemia, thrombocytopenia, neutropenia and eosinophilia have been reported.
CNS: (See "Warnings").

When given over prolonged periods, tetracyclines have been reported to produce brown-black microscopic discoloration of thyroid glands. No abnormalities of thyroid function studies are known to occur.

Dosage and Administration: Therapy should be continued for at least 24-48 hours after symptoms and fever have subsided.

Concomitant therapy: Antacids containing aluminum, calcium, or magnesium impair absorption and should not be given to patients taking oral tetracycline.

Studies to date have indicated that the absorption of MINOCIN is not notably influenced by foods and dairy products.

In patients with renal impairment: (See "Warnings"). Total dosage should be decreased by reduction of recommended individual doses and/or extending time intervals between doses.

In the treatment of streptococcal infections, a therapeutic dose of tetracycline should be administered for at least 10 days.

ADULTS: The usual dosage of MINOCIN *minocycline HCl* is 200 mg initially followed by 100 mg every 12 hours. Alternatively, if more frequent doses are preferred, two or four 50 mg capsules or tablets may be given initially followed by one 50 mg capsule or tablet four times daily.

For children above eight years of age: The usual dosage of MINOCIN *minocycline HCl* is 4 mg/kg initially followed by 2 mg/kg every 12 hours.

For treatment of syphilis, the usual dosage of MINOCIN should be administered over a period of 10-15 days. Close followup, including laboratory tests, is recommended.

Gonorrhea patients sensitive to penicillin may be treated with MINOCIN, administered as 200 mg initially followed by 100 mg every twelve hours for a minimum of 4 days, with post-therapy cultures within 2-3 days.

In the treatment of meningococcal carrier state recommended dose is 100 mg every 12 hours for five days.

Mycobacterium marinum infections: Although optimal doses have not been established, 100 mg twice a day for 6-8 weeks have been used successfully in a limited number of cases.

Uncomplicated urethral, endocervical, or rectal infection in adults caused by *Chlamydia trachomatis* or *Ureaplasma urealyticum:* 100 mg, by mouth, 2 times a day for at least 7 days.[1]

In the treatment of uncomplicated gonococcal urethritis in men, 100 mg twice a day orally for 5 days is recommended.

How Supplied:
CAPSULES
Minocycline hydrochloride equivalent to 100 mg minocycline.

Hardshell orange and purple with Lederle over M4 printed on one half and MINOCIN over 100 mg on the other.

Continued on next page

The information on each product appearing here is based on labelling effective in August, 1984 and is either the entire official brochure or an accurate condensation therefrom. Information concerning all Lederle products may be obtained from the Professional Services Department, Lederle Laboratories, Pearl River, New York, 10965.

Lederle—Cont.

NDC 0005-5301-18 Bottle of 50's
NDC 0005-5301-23 Bottle of 100's
NDC 0005-5301-60 Unit Dose (strips) 10×10's
Store at Controlled Room Temperature 15–30° C (59–86° F)
Minocycline hydrochloride equivalent to 50 mg minocycline.
Hardshell orange with Lederle over M2 printed on one half and MINOCIN over 50 mg on the other.
NDC 0005-5300-23 Bottle of 100's
NDC 0005-5300-60 Unit Dose (strips) 10×10's
Store at Controlled Room Temperature 15–30° C (59–86° F)

ORAL SUSPENSION
Minocycline hydrochloride equivalent to 50 mg minocycline per teaspoonful (5 ml). Preserved with propylparaben 0.10% and butylparaben 0.06% with Alcohol USP 5% v/v, Custard-flavored.
NDC 0005-5313-56 Bottle 2 fl. oz. (60 ml)
Store at Controlled Room Temperature 15–30° C (59–86° F)

DO NOT FREEZE

TABLETS
Minocycline hydrochloride equivalent to 100 mg minocycline. Round, convex, orange film-coated tablet engraved with M over bisect and 5 under bisect on one side of the tablet and LL on the other.
NDC 0005-9376-18 Bottle of 50's
Store at Controlled Room Temperature 15–30° C (59–86° F)
Minocycline hydrochloride equivalent to 50 mg minocycline. Round, convex, orange film-coated tablet engraved with M3 on one side and LL on other.
NDC 0005-9375-23 Bottle of 100's
Store at Controlled Room Temperature 15–30° C (59–86° F)

Animal Pharmacology and Toxicology: MINOCIN *minocycline HCl* has been found to produce high blood concentrations following oral dosage to various animal species and to be extensively distributed to all tissues examined in ^{14}C-labeled drug studies in dogs. MINOCIN has been found experimentally to produce discoloration of the thyroid glands. This finding has been observed in rats and dogs. Changes in thyroid function have also been found in these animal species. However, no change in thyroid function has been observed in humans.

Reference: 1. CDC Sexually Transmitted Diseases Treatment Guidelines 1982.

Military Depot:
Capsules, 50 mg—100's
NSN 6505-01-015-4147
Capsules 100 mg—50's
NSN 6505-00-003-5112
Capsules, 100 mg individually, sealed 100's (unit dose)
NSN 6505-01-153-3577
VA Depots:
Capsules, 50 mg 100's—NSN 6505-01-015-4147A
Capsules, 100 mg, 100's—NSN 6505-01-108-9040A

Lederle Laboratories Division
American Cyanamid Company
Pearl River, N.Y. 10965

Shown in Product Identification Section, page 415

MYAMBUTOL®
[mī-am-bū-tŏl]
ethambutol hydrochloride
Tablets

Description: MYAMBUTOL *ethambutol hydrochloride Lederle* is an oral chemotherapeutic agent which is specifically effective against actively growing microorganisms of the genus *Mycobacterium*, including *M. tuberculosis*.

Action: MYAMBUTOL, following a single oral dose of 25 mg./Kg. of body weight, attains a peak of 2 to 5 micrograms/ml. in serum 2 to 4 hours after administration. When the drug is administered daily for longer periods of time at this dose, serum levels are similar. The serum level of MYAMBUTOL falls to undetectable levels by 24 hours after the last dose except in some patients with abnormal renal function. The intracellular concentrations of erythrocytes reach peak values approximately twice those of plasma and maintain this ratio throughout the 24 hours.

During the 24-hour period following oral administration of MYAMBUTOL, approximately 50 percent of the initial dose is excreted unchanged in the urine, while an additional 8 to 15 percent appears in the form of metabolites. The main path of metabolism appears to be an initial oxidation of the alcohol to an aldehydic intermediate, followed by conversion to a dicarboxylic acid. From 20 to 22 percent of the initial dose is excreted in the feces as unchanged drug. No drug accumulation has been observed with consecutive single daily doses of 25 mg./Kg. in patients with normal kidney function, although marked accumulation has been demonstrated in patients with renal insufficiency.

MYAMBUTOL diffuses into actively growing *mycobacterium* cells such as tubercle bacilli. MYAMBUTOL appears to inhibit the synthesis of one or more metabolites, thus causing impairment of cell metabolism, arrest of multiplication, and cell death. No cross resistance with other available antimycobacterial agents has been demonstrated. MYAMBUTOL has been shown to be effective against strains of *Mycobacterium tuberculosis* but does not seem to be active against fungi, viruses, or other bacteria.

Mycobacterium tuberculosis strains previously unexposed to MYAMBUTOL have been uniformly sensitive to concentrations of 8 or less micrograms/ml., depending on the nature of the culture media. When MYAMBUTOL has been used alone for treatment of tuberculosis, tubercle bacilli from these patients have developed resistance to MYAMBUTOL by *in vitro* susceptibility tests; the development of resistance has been unpredictable and appears to occur in a step-like manner. No cross resistance between MYAMBUTOL and other antituberculous drugs has been reported. MYAMBUTOL has reduced the incidence of the emergence of mycobacterial resistance to isoniazid when both drugs have been used concurrently.

An agar diffusion microbiologic assay, based upon inhibition of *Mycobacterium smegmatis* (ATCC 607) may be used to determine concentrations of MYAMBUTOL in serum and urine. This technique has not been published, but further information can be obtained upon inquiry to Lederle Laboratories.

Animal Pharmacology: Toxicological studies in dogs on high prolonged doses produced evidence of myocardial damage and failure, and depigmentation of the tapetum lucidum of the eyes, the significance of which is not known. Degenerative changes in the central nervous system, apparently not dose-related, have also been noted in dogs receiving ethambutol hydrochloride over a prolonged period.

In the rhesus monkey, neurological signs appeared after treatment with high doses given daily over a period of several months. These were correlated with specific serum levels of ethambutol hydrochloride and with definite neuro-anatomical changes in the central nervous system. Focal interstitial carditis was also noted in monkeys which received ethambutol hydrochloride in high doses for a prolonged period.

When pregnant mice or rabbits were treated with high doses of ethambutol hydrochloride, fetal mortality was slightly but not significantly ($P > 0.05$) increased. Female rats treated with ethambutol hydrochloride displayed slight but insignificant ($P > 0.05$) decreases in fertility and litter size.

In fetuses born of mice treated with high doses of ethambutol hydrochloride during pregnancy, a low incidence of cleft palate, exencephaly and abnormality of the vertebral column were observed. Minor abnormalities of the cervical vertebra were seen in the newborn of rats treated with high doses of ethambutol hydrochloride during pregnancy. Rabbits receiving high doses of ethambutol hydrochloride during pregnancy gave birth to two fetuses with monophthalmia, one with a shortened right forearm accompanied by bilateral wrist-joint contracture and one with hare lip and cleft palate.

Indications: MYAMBUTOL *ethambutol hydrochloride* is indicated for the treatment of pulmonary tuberculosis. It should not be used as the sole antituberculous drug, but should be used in conjunction with at least one other antituberculous drug. Selection of the companion drug should be based on clinical experience, considerations of comparative safety and appropriate *in vitro* susceptibility studies.

In patients who have not received previous antituberculous therapy, i.e. initial treatment, the most frequently used regimens have been the following:
MYAMBUTOL plus isoniazid
MYAMBUTOL plus isoniazid plus streptomycin.

In patients who have received previous antituberculous therapy, mycobacterial resistance to other drugs used in initial therapy is frequent. Consequently, in such retreatment patients, MYAMBUTOL should be combined with at least one of the second line drugs not previously administered to the patient and to which bacterial susceptibility has been indicated by appropriate *in vitro* studies. Antituberculous drugs used with MYAMBUTOL have included cycloserine, ethionamide, pyrazinamide, viomycin and other drugs. Isoniazid, aminosalicylic acid, and streptomycin have also been used in multiple drug regimens. Alternating drug regimens have also been utilized.

Contraindications: MYAMBUTOL is contraindicated in patients who are known to be hypersensitive to this drug. It is also contraindicated in patients with known optic neuritis unless clinical judgment determines that it may be used.

Precautions: The effects of combinations of ethambutol hydrochloride with other antituberculous drugs on the fetus is not known. While administration of this drug to pregnant human patients has produced no detectable effect upon the fetus, the possible teratogenic potential in women capable of bearing children should be weighed carefully against the benefits of therapy. There are published reports of five women who received the drug during pregnancy without apparent adverse effect upon the fetus.

MYAMBUTOL is not recommended for use in children under thirteen years of age since safe conditions for use have not been established.

Patients with decreased renal function need the dosage reduced as determined by serum levels of MYAMBUTOL, since the main path of excretion of this drug is by the kidneys.

Because this drug may have adverse effects on vision, physical examination should include ophthalmoscopy, finger perimetry and testing of color discrimination. In patients with visual defects such as cataracts, recurrent inflammatory conditions of the eye, optic neuritis, and diabetic retinopathy, the evaluation of changes in visual acuity is more difficult, and care should be taken to be sure the variations in vision are not due to the underlying disease conditions. In such patients, consideration should be given to relationship between benefits expected and possible visual deterioration since evaluation of visual changes is difficult. (For recommended procedures, see next paragraphs under Adverse Reactions.)

As with any potent drug, periodic assessment of organ system functions, including renal, hepatic, and hematopoietic, should be made during long-term therapy.

Adverse Reactions: MYAMBUTOL may produce decreases in visual acuity which appear to be due to optic neuritis and to be related to dose and duration of treatment. The effects are generally reversible when administration of the drug is discontinued promptly.

In rare cases recovery may be delayed for up to one year or more and the effect may possibly be irreversible in these cases.

Patients should be advised to report promptly to their physician any change of visual acuity. The change in visual acuity may be unilateral or bilateral and hence *each eye must be tested separately and both eyes tested together.* Testing of visual acuity should be performed before beginning MYAM-

BUTOL ethambutol hydrochloride therapy and periodically during drug administration, except that it should be done monthly when a patient is on a dosage of more than 15 mg. per Kilogram per day. Snellen eye charts are recommended for testing of visual acuity. Studies have shown that there are definite fluctuations of one or two lines of the Snellen chart in the visual acuity of many tuberculous patients *not* receiving MYAMBUTOL.

The table may be useful in interpreting possible changes in visual acuity attributable to MYAMBUTOL. [See table above].

In general, changes in visual acuity less than those indicated under "Significant Number of Lines" and "Decreases-Number of Points", may be due to chance variation, limitations of the testing method or physiologic variability. Conversely, changes in visual acuity equaling or exceeding those under "Significant Number of Lines" and "Decreases-Number of Points" indicate need for retesting and careful evaluation of the patient's visual status. If careful evaluation confirms the magnitude of visual change and fails to reveal another cause, MYAMBUTOL should be discontinued and the patient reevaluated at frequent intervals. Progressive decreases in visual acuity during therapy must be considered to be due to MYAMBUTOL. If corrective glasses are used prior to treatment, these must be worn during visual acuity testing. During 1 to 2 years of therapy, a refractive error may develop which must be corrected in order to obtain accurate test results. Testing the visual acuity through a pinhole eliminates refractive error. Patients developing visual abnormality during MYAMBUTOL treatment may show subjective visual symptoms before, or simultaneously with, the demonstration of decreases in visual acuity, and all patients receiving MYAMBUTOL should be questioned periodically about blurred vision and other subjective eye symptoms.

Recovery of visual acuity generally occurs over a period of weeks to months after the drug has been discontinued. Patients have then received MYAMBUTOL again without recurrence of loss of visual acuity.

Other adverse reactions reported include: anaphylactoid reactions, dermatitis, pruritus and joint pain; anorexia, nausea, vomiting, gastrointestinal upset, abdominal pain; fever, malaise, headache, and dizziness; mental confusion, disorientation and possible hallucinations. Numbness and tingling of the extremities due to peripheral neuritis have been reported infrequently.

Elevated serum uric acid levels occur and precipitation of acute gout has been reported. Transient impairment of liver function as indicated by abnormal liver function tests is not an unusual finding. Since MYAMBUTOL is recommended for therapy in conjunction with one or more other antituberculous drugs, these changes may be related to the concurrent therapy.

Dosage and Administration: MYAMBUTOL should not be used alone, in initial treatment or in retreatment. MYAMBUTOL should be administered on a once every 24-hour basis only. Absorption is not significantly altered by administration with food. Therapy, in general, should be continued until bacteriological conversion has become permanent and maximal clinical improvement has occurred.

MYAMBUTOL is not recommended for use in children under thirteen years of age since safe conditions for use have not been established.

Initial Treatment: In patients who have not received previous antituberculous therapy, administer MYAMBUTOL 15 mg. per Kilogram (7 mg. per pound) of body weight, as a single oral dose once every 24 hours. In the more recent studies, isoniazid has been administered concurrently in a single, daily, oral dose.

Retreatment: In patients who have received previous antituberculous therapy, administer MYAMBUTOL 25 mg. per Kilogram (11 mg. per pound) of body weight, as a single oral dose once every 24 hours. Concurrently administer at least one other antituberculous drug to which the organisms have been demonstrated to be susceptible by appropriate *in vitro* tests. Suitable drugs usually consist of those not previously used in the treatment of the patient. After 60 days of MYAMBUTOL (ethambutol hydrochloride) administration, decrease the dose to 15 mg. per Kilogram (7 mg. per pound) of body weight, and administer as a single oral dose once every 24 hours.

During the period when a patient is on a daily dose of 25 mg./kg., monthly eye examinations are advised.

See Table for easy selection of proper weight-dose tablet(s).

MYAMBUTOL VISUAL ACUITY TABLE

Initial Snellen Reading	Reading Indicating Significant Decrease	Significant Number of Lines	Decreases Number of Points
20/13	20/25	3	12
20/15	20/25	2	10
20/20	20/30	2	10
20/25	20/40	2	15
20/30	20/50	2	20
20/40	20/70	2	30
20/50	20/70	1	20

Weight-Dose Table
15 mg./Kg. (7 mg./lb.) Schedule

Weight Range Pounds	Kilograms	Daily Dose In mg.
Under 85 lbs.	Under 37 Kg	500
85–94.5	37–43	600
95–109.5	43–50	700
110–124.5	50–57	800
125–139.5	57–64	900
140–154.5	64–71	1000
155–169.5	71–79	1100
170–184.5	79–84	1200
185–199.5	84–90	1300
200–214.5	90–97	1400
215 and Over	Over 97	1500

25 mg./Kg. (11 mg./lb.) Schedule

Weight Range Pounds	Kilograms	Daily Dose In mg.
Under 85 lbs.	Under 38 Kg.	900
85–92.5	38–42	1000
93–101.5	42–45.5	1100
102–109.5	45.5–50	1200
110–118.5	50–54	1300
119–128.5	54–58	1400
129–136.5	58–62	1500
137–146.5	62–67	1600
147–155.5	67–71	1700
156–164.5	71–75	1800
165–173.5	75–79	1900
174–182.5	79–83	2000
183–191.5	83–87	2100
192–199.5	87–91	2200
200–209.5	91–95	2300
210–218.5	95–99	2400
219 and Over	Over 99	2500

How Supplied: Tablets 100 mg round, convex, white, coated tablets engraved M6 on one side and LL on the other, are supplied as follows:
NDC 0005-5015-23 - bottles of 100
NDC 0005-5015-34 bottles of 1000
400 mg round, convex, white scored, film coated tablets engraved with LL on one side and M to the left and 7 to the right of the score on the other side, are supplied as follows:
NDC 0005-5084-62 Unit-of-Issue 100's with CRC
NDC 0005-5084-34 bottles of 1000
NDC 0005-5084-60 - Unit Dose 10 × 10's
Store at Controlled Room Temperature 15–30°C (59–86°F)
A.H.F.S. 8:16
Tablets, 100 mg.
Military Depot NSN 6505-00-403-7645, 100's
Tablets 400 mg.
Military Depot NSN 6505-00-812-2579, 100's
VA Depot NSN 6505-00-812-2543A, 1000's

NEOLOID®
[nēo-loid]
EMULSIFIED CASTOR OIL
For the treatment of isolated bouts of constipation
PEPPERMINT FLAVORED - SHAKE WELL

Contains: Castor Oil USP 36.4% (w/w) with 0.1% (w/w) Sodium Benzoate and 0.2% (w/w) Potassium Sorbate added as preservatives, emulsifying and flavoring agents in water. NEOLOID is an emulsion with an exceptionally bland, pleasant taste.

Dosage: Infants ½ to 1½ teaspoonfuls; children, adjust between infant and adult dose. Average adult dose, 2 to 4 tablespoonfuls, or as prescribed by the physician. Not to be used when abdominal pain, nausea, vomiting, or other symptoms of appendicitis are present. Frequent or continued use of this preparation may result in dependence on laxatives. Do not use during pregnancy except on a physician's advice. Keep this and all drugs out of the reach of children.

Warning: As with any drug, if you are pregnant or nursing a baby, seek the advice of a health professional before using this product. In case of accidental overdose, seek professional assistance or contact a Poison Control Center immediately.
Store at Controlled Room Temperature 15-30° C (59-86° F)
DO NOT FREEZE
NET 4 Fl. Oz. (118 ml) NDC 0005-5442-58.

NEPTAZANE® ℞
[nĕp-ta-zāne]
methazolamide

Description: NEPTAZANE *methazolamide* is a white crystalline powder, weakly acid, slightly soluble in water, and is a complex sulfonamide derivative. It is available as a 50 mg white convex scored tablet.

Action: NEPTAZANE is a potent inhibitor of the enzyme carbonic anhydrase. It is absorbed somewhat slowly from the gastrointestinal tract and disappears more slowly from the plasma than does acetazolamide, which may account for the delay in onset and duration of its activity. It is distributed throughout the body, and can be assayed in the blood plasma, the cerebrospinal fluid, the aqueous humor of the eye, the red blood cell, in the bile and the extra-cellular fluid. Urinary excretion accounts for only 15% of NEPTAZANE in man. It is not cumulative in its concentration. The drug is considered nonbactericidal. Although concentration in the cerebrospinal fluid is high, it is not considered an effective anticonvulsant.

Methazolamide does have a diuretic effect, resulting in increase in urinary volume, with excretion of sodium and potassium and chloride, but it is less active than acetazolamide. This effect is transient and of low degree and the drug is not used as a diuretic. Serum electrolyte changes in sodium, potassium and chloride are minimal and return to pretreatment levels after daily administration for three to four days. Inhibition of renal bicarbonate reabsorption produces an alkaline urine. Plasma bicarbonate decreases temporarily and a relative and transient metabolic acidosis may occur due to a disequilibrium in CO_2 transport in the red cell. This is quickly restored to balance by the initiation of compensatory mechanisms. Urinary citrate excretion is decreased by 40% on doses of 100 mgs every 8 hours with variations in urinary volume output. Uric acid output was decreased 36% in the first 24 hour period and varied thereafter. The oral administration of the drug by inhibition of car-

Continued on next page

The information on each product appearing here is based on labelling effective in August, 1984 and is either the entire official brochure or an accurate condensation therefrom. Information concerning all Lederle products may be obtained from the Professional Services Department, Lederle Laboratories, Pearl River, New York, 10965.

Lederle—Cont.

bonic anhydrase in the various tissues of the eye causes a decrease in the rate of aqueous humor formation. Various authors differ somewhat as to the time of onset of intraocular pressure fall, of the peak of activity and the duration of the effect on the pressure, of a 24 hour period of ingestion, but on the average, th onset of fall in intraocular pressure occurs within 2-4 hours, with peak of fall in 6-8 hours, the effect lasting from 10-18 hours.

Indications: For adjunctive treatment of: chronic simple (open angle) glaucoma, secondary glaucoma, and preoperatively in acute angle closure glaucoma where delay of surgery is desired in order to lower intraocular pressure.

Contraindications: Severe or absolute glaucoma and chronic noncongestive angle closure glaucoma. It is of doubtful use in glaucoma due to severe peripheral anterior synechiae or hemorrhagic glaucoma.

NEPTAZANE *methazolamide* is contraindicated in patients with adrenocortical insufficiency, hepatic insufficiency, renal insufficiency, or an electrolyte imbalance state such as hyperchloremic acidosis, and sodium and potassium depletion states.

Warning: Studies in rats have demonstrated teratogenic effects (skeletal anomalies) at high doses. There is no evidence of these effects in human beings and no fetal defects have been reported. However, methazolamide should not be used in women of childbearing potential or in pregnancy, especially in the first trimester, unless the benefits to be gained in the control of glaucoma outweigh potential adverse effects.

Precautions: Potassium excretion is increased initially, upon administration of methazolamide and in patients with cirrhosis or hepatic insufficiency could precipitate an hepatic coma. It should be used with caution in patients on steroid therapy because of the potentiality of hypokalemic state. Adequate and balanced electrolyte intake is essential in all patients whose concomitant clinical condition may occasion electrolyte imbalance.

In patients with pulmonary obstruction or emphysema where alveolar ventilation may be impaired, methazolamide, which may precipitate or aggravate acidosis, should be used with caution.

Adverse reactions common to all sulfonamide derivatives may occur: fever, rash, crystalluria, renal calculus, bone marrow depression, thrombocytopenic purpura, hemolytic anemia, leukopenia, pancytopenia and agranulocytosis. Precaution is advised for early detection of such reactions and the drug should be discontinued and appropriate therapy instituted.

Adverse Reactions: Most adverse reactions to methazolamide have been relatively mild in character and disappear upon withdrawal of the drug or adjustment of dosage. They are as follows: anorexia, nausea, vomiting; malaise, fatigue or drowsiness, headache; vertigo, mental confusion, depression, and paresthesias of fingers, toes, hands or feet and occasionally at the mucocutaneous junction of the lips, mouth and anus.

Urinary citrate excretion is decreased during the administration of NEPTAZANE *methazolamide* as is uric acid output, but urinary calculi clearly due to the drug have not been reported. The effect on citrate excretion is less than that reported from the administration of acetazolamide.

Dosage and Administration: The effective therapeutic dose administered in tablet form varies from 50 mg to 100 mg 2-3 times daily. The drug may be used concomitantly with miotic and osmotic agents. It is not available for parenteral use.

How Supplied: Tablets, 50 mg (scored white) embossed LL on one side and N on the left of a bisect and 1 on the right on the other side.—Bottles of 100 NDC 0005-4570-23.

Military Depots:
Tablets, 50 mg—100's
NSN 6505-00-065-4205

Shown in Product Identification Section, page 415

NILSTAT® ℞
[*nĭl-stăt*]
Nystatin Oral Suspension

Description: This antifungal agent is obtained from *Streptomyces noursei*. It is a polyene antibiotic of undetermined structural formula.

Nystatin is an antibiotic with antifungal activity produced by a strain of *Streptomyces noursei*. NILSTAT *nystatin* Oral Suspension, Lederle is a cherry flavored, ready-to-use suspension containing 100,000 units of nystatin per ml.-with methylparaben (0.12%) and propylparaben (0.03%) as preservatives.

Actions: Nystatin probably acts by binding to sterols in the cell membrane of the fungus with a resultant change in membrane permeability allowing leakage of intracellular components. It is absorbed very sparingly following oral administration, with no detectable blood levels when given in the recommended doses.

Indications: For the treatment of infections of the oral cavity caused by *Candida* (Monilia) *albicans*.

Contraindications: Hypersensitivity to the drug.

Adverse Reactions:
Nausea and vomiting, Gastrointestinal distress, Diarrhea.

Dosage and Administration:
Infants: 2 ml. (200,000 units) four times daily (1 ml. in each side of mouth).
Children and adults: 4-6 ml. (400,000 to 600,000 units) four times daily (one-half of dose in each side of mouth).
Note: Limited clinical studies in prematures and low birth weight infants indicate that 1 ml. four times daily is effective.

Local treatment should be continued at least 48 hours after perioral symptoms have disappeared and cultures returned to normal.

It is recommended that the drug be retained in the mouth as long as possible before swallowing.

How Supplied: 60 ml bottle with dropper NDC 0005-5429-18 and 16 fl. oz. NDC 0005-5429-65.

NILSTAT® ℞
[*nĭl-stăl*]
Nystatin, USP
For Extemporaneous Preparation of Oral Suspension

Description: Nystatin, USP is an antifungal antibiotic which is both fungistatic and fungicidal *in vitro* against a wide variety of yeasts and yeast-like fungi. It is a polyene antibiotic of undetermined structural formula that is obtained from *Streptomyces noursei*. Nystatin, USP, which contains no excipients or preservatives, is a ready-to-use non-sterile powder for oral administration available in bottles of one billion and two billion units.

Clinical Pharmacology: Nystatin probably acts by binding to sterols in the cell membrane of the fungus with a resultant change in membrane permeability allowing leakage of intracellular components. It is absorbed very sparingly following oral administration, with no detectable blood levels when given in the recommended doses. Most of the orally administered nystatin is passed unchanged in the stool.

Indications and Usage: For treatment of infections of the oral cavity caused by *Candida albicans* (monilia).

Contraindications: Hypersensitivity to the drug.

Adverse Reactions: Large oral doses of nystatin have occasionally produced diarrhea, gastrointestinal distress, nausea and vomiting.

Dosage and Administration: Adults and older children: add ⅛ tsp. (500,000 units) of Nystatin, USP to approximately ½ to 1 cup (120 to 240 ml, or 4 to 8 oz.) of water and stir well. The entire dose should then be used to thoroughly rinse the mouth and the dose should be retained in the mouth as long as possible before swallowing. This dose should be given orally four times daily, and should be continued for at least 48 hours after perioral symptoms have disappeared and cultures have returned to normal. One-eighth tsp. of nystatin, USP is equivalent to the recommended dose for adults and children of NILSTAT® Oral Suspension (4 to 6 ml, or 400,000 to 600,000 units). This product contains no preservative and therefore should be used immediately after mixing and should not be stored.

How Supplied: Bottles containing one billion units and bottles containing two billion units—(one billion units is approximately 170–200 grams, depending on potency of powder).

NDC 0005-5421-10—One Billion Units
NDC 0005-5421-11—Two Billion Units

Store under refrigeration 2–8° C (36–46° F) in tight, light resistant containers.

Note: The potency of this product cannot be assured for longer than 90 days after the container is first opened.

NILSTAT® ℞
[*nĭl-stăt*]
Nystatin Vaginal Tablets U.S.P.

Description: NILSTAT *nystatin* Vaginal Tablets, USP are oblong shaped vaginal tablets, each containing 100,000 units Nystatin, USP.

Nystatin is a polyene antibiotic of undetermined structural formula that is obtained from *streptomyces noursei*.

Clinical Pharmacology: Nystatin is an antifungal antibiotic which is both fungistatic and fungicidal *in vitro* against a wide variety of yeasts and yeast-like fungi. It probably acts by binding to sterols in the cell membrane of the fungus with a resultant change in membrane permeability allowing leakage of intracellular components. It exhibits no appreciable activity against bacteria or trichomonads.

Indications and Usage: NILSTAT *nystatin* Vaginal Tablets, USP are effective for the local treatment of vulvovaginal candidiasis (moniliasis). The diagnosis should be confirmed, prior to therapy, by KOH smears and/or cultures. Other pathogens commonly associated with vulvovaginitis (Trichomonas and *Haemophilus vaginalis*) do not respond to nystatin and should be ruled out by appropriate laboratory methods.

Contraindications: This preparation is contraindicated in patients with a history of hypersensitivity to any of its components.

Precautions:
General
Discontinue treatment if sensitization or irritation is reported during use.
Laboratory Tests:
If there is a lack of response to NILSTAT *nystatin* Vaginal Tablets, USP, appropriate microbiological studies should be repeated to confirm the diagnosis and rule out other pathogens, before instituting another course of antimycotic therapy.
Usage in Pregnancy:
No adverse effects or complications have been attributed to nystatin in infants born to women treated with nystatin vaginal tablets.

Adverse Reactions: Nystatin is virtually nontoxic and nonsensitizing and is well tolerated by all age groups, even on prolonged administration. Rarely, irritation or sensitization may occur (see PRECAUTIONS).

Dosage and Administration: The usual dosage is one tablet (100,000 units nystatin) daily for two weeks. The tablets should be deposited high in the vagina by means of the applicator. "Instructions for the Patient" are enclosed in each package. Even though symptomatic relief may occur within a few days, treatment should be continued for the full course.

It is important that therapy be continued during menstruation. Adjunctive measures such as therapeutic douches are unnecessary and sometimes inadvisable. Cleansing douches may be used by nonpregnant women, if desired, for esthetic purposes.

How Supplied: Oblong shaped—pale yellow—engraved LL and N6 in packages of 15 and 30 Vaginal Tablets with Applicator. 15 tablets: NDC 0005-5428-06; 30 tablets: NDC 0005-5428-08.

NILSTAT ℞
[nĭl-stăt]
nystatin
Oral Tablets (film-coated) pink—engraved LL and N5

500,000 Units per tablet, bottles of 100 NDC-0005-5426-23; unit-dose 10 x 10's NDC-0005-5426-60.

NILSTAT ℞
nystatin
Topical Cream, 100,000 Units per Gm.

Inactive ingredients in a vanishing cream water base: Emulsifying Wax NF, Isopropyl Myristate, Glycerin, Lactic Acid and Sodium Hydroxide. Preservative: Sorbic Acid 0.2%.

How Supplied: 15 gm tube NDC-0005-5433-09, 240 gm jar NDC-0005-5433-57.

Military Depot
NSN 6505-01-063-1141, 240 gm jar

NILSTAT ℞
nystatin
Topical Ointment, 100,000 Units per Gm.

Inactive Ingredients: Light Mineral Oil and Plastibase 50 W.

15 Gm. tubes NDC-0005-5432-09.

ORIMUNE® ℞
[or-ĭ-mune]
POLIOVIRUS VACCINE,
LIVE, ORAL, TRIVALENT
0.5 ml Dose Contains Sorbitol
SABIN STRAINS TYPES 1, 2 and 3
FOR ORAL ADMINISTRATION—NOT FOR INJECTION

Description:
Manufacture and Composition: ORIMUNE® TRIVALENT VACCINE is a mixture of three types of attenuated polioviruses which have been propagated in cercopithecus monkey kidney cell culture. The cells are grown in the presence of Eagle's Basal Medium consisting of Earle's Balanced Salt Solution containing amino acids, antibiotics and calf serum. After cell growth, the medium is removed and replaced with fresh medium containing the inoculating virus but no calf serum. The final vaccine is diluted with a modified cell culture maintenance medium containing sorbitol. Each dose (0.5 ml) contains less than 25 micrograms of each of the antibiotics, streptomycin and neomycin.

The potency is expressed in terms of the amount of virus contained in the recommended dose as tissue culture infective doses ($TCID_{50}$). The human dose of vaccine containing all three virus types shall be constituted to have infectivity titers in the final container material of $10^{5.4}$ to $10^{6.4}$ for Type 1, $10^{4.5}$ to $10^{5.5}$ for Type 2 and $10^{5.2}$ to $10^{6.2}$ for Type 3.[1]

Color Change: This vaccine contains phenol red as a pH indicator. The usual color of the vaccine is pink, although some containers of vaccine, shipped or stored in dry ice, may exhibit a yellow coloration due to the very low temperature or possible absorption of carbon dioxide. The color of the vaccine prior to use (red-pink-yellow) has no effect on the virus or efficacy of the vaccine.

Indications and Usage: The purpose of administering any attenuated, live, virus vaccine is to stimulate the body mechanism to produce an active immunity by simulating the natural infection without producing untoward symptoms of the disease. To accomplish this with live poliovirus vaccine, it is necessary for the virus to multiply in the intestinal tract. A primary series of this vaccine is designed to produce an antibody response to poliovirus Types 1, 2 and 3. This response is comparable to the immunity induced by the natural disease. The antibodies thus formed help protect the individual against clinical poliomyelitis infection by any of the three types of poliovirus. When used in the prescribed manner for primary immunization, type specific neutralizing antibodies will be induced in 90% or more of susceptibles.

This vaccine is indicated for use in the prevention of poliomyelitis caused by Poliovirus Types 1, 2 and 3. Infants starting at six to twelve weeks of age, *all unimmunized children* and *adolescents* through age 18 are the usual candidates for routine prophylaxis.

The Immunization Practices Advisory Committee of the Public Health Service states that trivalent oral poliovirus vaccine (TOPV) and inactivated poliovirus vaccine (IPV) are both effective in preventing poliomyelitis. TOPV is the vaccine of choice for primary immunization of children in the United States when the benefits and risks for the entire population are considered. TOPV is preferred because it induces intestinal immunity, is simple to administer, is well accepted by patients, results in immunization of some contacts of vaccinated persons, and has a record of having essentially eliminated disease associated with wild poliovirus in this country.[2] The choice of TOPV as the preferred poliovirus vaccine in the United States has also been made by the Committee on Infectious Diseases of the American Academy of Pediatrics and a special expert committee of the Institute of Medicine, National Academy of Science.[3,4] TOPV is also recommended for control of epidemic poliomyelitis.[2,3]

Past history of clinical poliomyelitis or prior vaccination with IPV in otherwise healthy individuals does not preclude the administration of TOPV when otherwise indicated.

Serologic evidence indicates that measles and rubella vaccines or combinations (measles-mumps-rubella vaccine) given simultaneously with trivalent oral poliovirus vaccine can be expected to give adequate antibody response.[5]

Routine poliomyelitis immunization for adults residing in the continental United States is not necessary because of extreme unlikelihood of exposure. However, primary immunization with IPV is recommended whenever feasible for those unimmunized adults subject to *increased risk* of exposure, as by travel to or contact with epidemic or endemic areas and for those employed in hospitals, medical laboratories, clinics or sanitation facilities. If less than 4 weeks are available before protection is needed, a single dose of TOPV is recommended, with IPV given later if the person remains at increased risk. Immunization with IPV may be indicated for unimmunized parents and those in other special situations where, in the judgment of the attending physician, protection may be needed.[2] (See CONTRAINDICATIONS and ADVERSE REACTIONS.)

Contraindications: *Under no circumstances should this vaccine be administered parenterally.* Administration of the vaccine should be postponed or avoided in those experiencing any acute illness and in those with any advanced debilitated condition or persistent vomiting or diarrhea.

ORIMUNE *must not* be administered to patients with immune deficiency diseases such as combined immunodeficiency, hypogammaglobulinemia and agammaglobulinemia. It would also be prudent to withhold ORIMUNE from siblings of a child known to have an immunodeficiency syndrome. Further, ORIMUNE *must not* be administered to patients with altered immune states such as those occurring in thymic abnormalities, leukemia, lymphoma or generalized malignancy or by lowered resistance from therapy with corticosteroids, alkylating drugs, antimetabolites or radiation. All persons with altered immune status should avoid close household-type contact with recipients of the vaccine for at least 6-8 weeks. IPV is preferred for immunizing all persons in this setting.[2,3,4,6,7]

Precautions: Other viruses (including poliovirus and other enterovirus) may interfere with the desired response to this vaccine, since their presence in the intestinal tract may interfere with the replication of the attenuated strains of poliovirus in the vaccine.

It would seem prudent not to administer TOPV shortly after Immune Serum Globulin (ISG) unless such a procedure is unavoidable, for example, with unexpected travel to or contact with epidemic areas or endemic areas. If TOPV is given with or shortly after ISG, the dose probably should be repeated after three months, if immunization is still indicated.[8] However, ISG may not interfere with immunization with TOPV.[9]

The vaccine is not effective in modifying or preventing cases of existing and/or incubating poliomyelitis.

Use in Pregnancy: Although there is no convincing evidence documenting adverse effects of either TOPV or IPV on the developing fetus or pregnant woman, it is prudent on theoretical grounds to avoid vaccinating pregnant women. However, if immediate protection against poliomyelitis is needed, TOPV is recommended.[2] (See CONTRAINDICATIONS and ADVERSE REACTIONS.)

Adverse Reactions: Paralytic disease following the ingestion of live poliovirus vaccines has been, on rare occasion, reported in individuals receiving the vaccine, (see for example CONTRAINDICATIONS) and in persons who were in close contact with vaccinees.[2,3,4,10,11,12,13] The vaccine viruses are shed in the vaccinee's stools for at least 6 to 8 weeks as well as via the pharyngeal route. Most reports of paralytic disease following ingestion of the vaccine or contact with a recent vaccinee are based on epidemiological analysis and temporal association between vaccination or contact and the onset of symptoms. Most authorities believe that a causal relationship exists.[2,10,14,15]

The risk of vaccine-associated paralysis is extremely small for vaccinees, susceptible family members and other close personal contacts.[2] However, prior to administration of the vaccine, the attending physician should warn or specifically direct personnel acting under his authority to convey the warnings to the vaccinee, parent, guardian or other responsible person of the possibility of vaccine-associated paralysis. The Centers for Disease Control report that during the years 1969 through 1980 approximately 290 million doses of TOPV were distributed in the United States. In the same 12 years, 25 "vaccine-associated" and 55 "contact vaccine-associated" paralytic cases were reported. Twelve other "vaccine-associated" cases have been reported in persons (recipients or contacts) with immune deficiency conditions.[2] These statistics do not provide a satisfactory basis for estimating these risks on a per person basis.[14]

When the attenuated vaccine strains are to be introduced into a household with adults who have not been adequately vaccinated or whose immune status cannot be determined, the risk of vaccine-associated paralysis can be minimized by giving these adults three doses of IPV a month apart before the children receive ORIMUNE.[2] The CDC reports that no paralytic reactions to IPV are known to have occurred since the 1955 cluster of poliomyelitis cases caused by vaccine that contained live polioviruses that had escaped inactivation.[2]

The Immunization Practices Advisory Committee of the U.S. Public Health Service states:

"Because of the overriding importance of ensuring prompt and complete immunization of the child and the extreme rarity of OPV-associated disease in contacts, the Committee recommends the administration of OPV to a child regardless of the poliovirus-vaccine status of adult household contacts. This is the usual practice in the United States. The responsible adult should be informed of the small risk involved. An acceptable alternative, if there is strong assurance that ultimate, full immunization of the child will not be jeopardized or unduly delayed, is to immunize adults according to the schedule outlined above before giving OPV to the child."[2]

The Immunization Practices Advisory Committee has concluded that "Oral polio vaccine remains the vaccine of choice for primary immunization of Children."[2]

Continued on next page

The information on each product appearing here is based on labelling effective in August, 1984 and is either the entire official brochure or an accurate condensation therefrom. Information concerning all Lederle products may be obtained from the Professional Services Department, Lederle Laboratories, Pearl River, New York, 10965.

Lederle—Cont.

Administration: ORIMUNE is to be administered *orally, under the supervision of a physician. Under no circumstances should this vaccine be administered parenterally.* For convenience, the vaccine is supplied in a disposable pipette containing a single dose of 0.5 ml. The vaccine can be administered directly or mixed with distilled water, tap water free of chlorine, simple syrup USP or milk. Alternatively, it may be adsorbed on any one of a number of foods such as bread, cake or cube sugar.

Community Programs
Poliovirus Vaccine, Live, Oral, Trivalent has been recommended for epidemic control. Within an epidemic area, TOPV should be provided for all persons over 6 weeks of age who have not been completely immunized or whose immunization status is unknown, with the exceptions noted under immunodeficiency.[2,3]

Dosage:
Dose: Each single dose consists of 0.5 ml of Poliovirus Vaccine, Live, Oral, Trivalent ORIMUNE.

Initial Administration (Primary Series)
Infants: The primary series is three doses. The Immunization Practices Advisory Committee (Public Health Service) recommends that the three dose immunization series be started at 6 to 12 weeks of age, commonly with the first DTP inoculation. The second dose should be given not less than 6 and preferably 8 weeks later. The third dose is an integral part of the primary immunization and should be administered 8 to 12 months after the second dose.[2]

The American Academy of Pediatrics recommends that the vaccine be administered at 2 months, 4 months, and at approximately 18 months of age. An optional dose of TOPV may be given at 6 months in areas where poliomyelitis is endemic.[3] Administration to the newborn (under 6 weeks) is not generally recommended because of the varying persistence of maternal antibodies. However, in certain tropical endemic areas, where poliomyelitis has been increasing in recent years, the physician may wish to administer TOPV to the infant at birth, and complete the basic course during the first six months of life.[3] If the physician chooses to immunize the infant at birth, it may be wise to wait until the child is three days old, and it may be prudent to recommend abstention from breast-feeding for two to three hours before and after oral vaccination to permit establishment of the vaccine viruses in the gut.[16]

Older Children and Adolescents (through age 18): Two doses, given not less than 6 and preferably 8 weeks apart and the third dose 6 to 12 months after the second dose.[2,3]

Adults: See INDICATIONS and ADVERSE REACTIONS. Where ORIMUNE is given to unimmunized adults, the dosage is as indicated for children and adolescents.

Booster Doses—School Entrance: On entering elementary school, all children who have completed the primary series should be given a single follow-up dose of trivalent oral poliovirus vaccine.[2,3] All other should complete the primary series.

The Public Health Service Advisory Committee does not recommend routine booster doses of vaccine on the basis of current information, beyond that given at the time of entering school.[2] Recent data indicates that over 95% of children studied five years after full immunization with oral poliovirus vaccine had protective antibodies to all three types of poliovirus.[17]

Increased risk: If an individual who has completed a primary series is subjected to a substantially increased risk by virtue of contact, travel or occupation, a single dose of TOPV has been suggested.[2]

Storage:
To maintain potency it is necessary to store this vaccine at a temperature which will maintain ice continuously in a solid state. This vaccine may remain fluid at temperatures above −14°C (+7°F) because of its sorbitol content. If frozen, the vaccine must be completely thawed prior to use. An *unopened* container of vaccine that has been frozen and then is thawed may be carried through a maximum of 10 freeze-thaw cycles, provided the temperature does not exceed 8°C (46°F) during the periods of thaw, and provided the total cumulative duration of thaw does not exceed 24 hours. If the 24-hour period is exceeded, the vaccine then must be used within 30 days, during which time it must be stored at a temperature between 2-8°C (36-46°F).

Disclaimer of Representations and Warranties:
This vaccine has been produced and tested in accordance with the regulations of the United States Food and Drug Administration for the production of Poliovirus Vaccine, Live, Oral, Trivalent. The Manufacturer makes no representation or warranty, expressed or implied, with respect to the merchantability or fitness for use of this vaccine other than that the vaccine has been produced in accordance with the standards for its production prescribed by the United States Food and Drug Administration and applicable thereto at the time of its release by the manufacturer. While the use of this preparation and other measures described herein as consistent with accepted standards of medical practice, their use as described cannot be expected necessarily to assure a specific result.

How Supplied:
NDC 0005-2084-08—10 (0.5 ml) DISPETTES® Disposable Pipettes
NDC 0005-2084-12—50 (0.5 ml) DISPETTES®
Military Depot: 10-1 dose DISPETTE® - NSN 6505-01-127-0046.

References:
1. *Code of Federal Regulations. 21 CFR:* 630.17[c], page 84, Revised April 1, 1982.
2. Recommendations of the Public Health Service Immunization Practices Advisory Committee [ACIP]. *Morbidity and Mortality Weekly Report* 31[3]: 22-34 [Jan. 29] 1982.
3. *Report of the Committee on the Control of Infectious Diseases. Amer. Acad. of Ped.* 19th Edition, 207–211, 1982.
4. Nightingale, E.O.: Recommendations for a National Policy on Poliomyelitis Vaccination. *N. Engl. J. Med.* 297[5]: 249–253, 1977.
5. Recommendations of ACIP Simultaneous Administration of Certain Live Virus Vaccines. *Morbidity and Mortality Weekly Report* 21[47]:403 [Nov. 25] 1972.
6. Feigin, R.D. *et. al.:* Vaccine-Related Paralytic Poliomyelitis in an Immunodeficient Child. *J. Pediatr.* 79[4]:642–647, 1971.
7. Riker, J.B. *et al.:* Vaccine-Associated Poliomyelitis in a Child With Thymic Abnormality. *Pediatrics* 48[6] 923-929, 1971.
8. Immunization Practices Advisory Committee [ACIP], General Recommendations on Immunization. *Morbidity and Mortality Weekly Report* 29[7]:75–83 [Feb. 22] 1980.
9. Melnick, J.L.: Advantages and Disadvantages of Killed and Live Poliomyelitis Vaccines. *Bull. W.H.O.* 56[1], 21–38 (1978).
10. Henderson, D.A. *et al.:* Paralytic Disease Associated with Oral Polio Vaccines. *JAMA* 190[1]: 41–48 [Oct. 5] 1964.
11. Morse, L.J. *et. al.:* Vaccine-Acquired Paralytic Poliomyelitis in an Unvaccinated Mother. *JAMA* 197:[12]: 1034–1035 [Sept. 19] 1966.
12. Swanson, P.D. *et al.:* Poliomyelitis Associated with Type 2 Virus. *JAMA* 201[10]: 771–773 [Sept. 4] 1967.
13. Balduzzi, P. *et al.:* Paralytic Poliomyelitis in a Contact of a Vaccinated Child. *N. Engl. J. Med.* 276[14]: 796–797, 1967.
14. Center for Disease Control: *Neurotropic Diseases Surveillance Annual Poliomyelitis Summary 1971.* [March 1973].
15. Evidence on the Safety and Efficacy of Live Poliomyelitis Vaccines Currently in Use, with Special Reference to Type 3 Poliovirus, *Bull. W.H.O.* 40[6]: 925–945, 1969.
16. Welsh, J.K. *et. al.:* Anti-infective Properties of Breast Milk. *J. Pediatr.* 94 [1] 1–9, 1979.
17. Krugman, R.D. *et al.:* Antibody Persistence After Primary Immunization With Trivalent Oral Poliovirus Vaccine. *Pediatrics* 60[1]:80–82, 1977.

PATHIBAMATE®-200 ℞
[path-ĭ-bă-māte]
tridihexethyl chloride-meprobamate
PATHIBAMATE®-400 ℞
tridihexethyl chloride-meprobamate
Tablets

Description: PATHILON® *tridihexethyl chloride* is a synthetic quaternary ammonium compound. Meprobamate is 2-methyl-2-propyltrimethylene dicarbamate.

Actions: *PATHIBAMATE tridihexethyl chloride-meprobamate* combines tridihexethyl chloride, an anticholinergic agent with meprobamate, a tranquilizing agent.

Tridihexethyl chloride
Tridihexethyl chloride possesses antimuscarinic actions. Gastrointestinal actions include reduction in both gastric secretion and gastrointestinal motility.

Meprobamate
Meprobamate is a carbamate derivative which has been shown in animal studies to have effects at multiple sites in the central nervous system, including the thalamus and limbic system.

> **INDICATIONS**
> Based on a review of this drug by the National Academy of Sciences-National Research Council and/or other information, FDA has classified the indications as follows:
> Possibly Effective: as adjunctive therapy in peptic ulcer and in the irritable bowel syndrome (irritable colon, spastic colon, mucous colitis, and functional gastrointestinal disorders), especially when accompanied by anxiety or tension. It should be used as an adjunct to other appropriate measures such as proper diet and antacids.

Contraindications:
Tridihexethyl chloride
Allergic or idiosyncratic reactions to tridihexethyl chloride or related compounds; glaucoma; obstructive uropathy (e.g., bladder neck obstruction due to prostatic hypertrophy); obstructive disease of the gastrointestinal tract (as in achalasia, paralytic ileus, pyloroduodenal stenosis, etc.); intestinal atony of the elderly or debilitated patient; unstable cardiovascular status in acute hemorrhage; severe ulcerative colitis; toxic megacolon complicating ulcerative colitis; myasthenia gravis.

Meprobamate
Acute intermittent porphyria as well as allergic or idiosyncratic reactions to meprobamate or related compounds such as carisoprodol, mebutamate, tybamate, or carbromal.

Warnings:
Tridihexethyl chloride
In the presence of a high environment temperature, heat prostration can occur with drug use (fever and heat stroke due to decreased sweating). Diarrhea may be an early symptom of incomplete intestinal obstruction, especially in patients with ileostomy or colostomy. In this instance treatment with this drug would be inappropriate and possibly harmful.

This drug may produce drowsiness or blurred vision. In this event, the patient should be warned not to engage in activities requiring mental alertness such as operating a motor vehicle or other machinery or perform hazardous work while taking this drug.

Meprobamate
Drug Dependence—Physical dependence, psychological dependence, and abuse have occurred. When chronic intoxication from prolonged use occurs, it usually involves ingestion of greater than recommended doses and is manifested by ataxia, slurred speech, and vertigo. Therefore, careful supervision of dose and amounts prescribed is advised, as well as avoidance of prolonged administration, especially for alcoholics and other patients with a known propensity for

taking excessive quantities of drugs. Sudden withdrawal of the drug after prolonged and excessive use may precipitate recurrence of pre-existing symptoms, such as anxiety, anorexia, or insomnia, or withdrawal reactions, such as vomiting, ataxia, tremors, muscle twitching, confusional states, hallucinosis, and, rarely, convulsive seizures. Such seizures are more likely to occur in persons with central nervous system damage or pre-existent or latent convulsive disorders. Onset of withdrawal symptoms occurs usually within 12 to 48 hours after discontinuation of meprobamate; symptoms usually cease within the next 12 to 48 hours.

When excessive dosage has continued for weeks or months, dosage should be reduced gradually over a period of one or two weeks rather than abruptly stopped. Alternatively, a short-acting barbiturate may be substituted, then gradually withdrawn.

Potentially Hazardous Tasks—Patients should be warned that this drug may impair the mental and/or physical abilities required for the performance of potentially hazardous tasks such as driving a motor vehicle or operating machinery.

Additive Effects—Since the effects of meprobamate and alcohol or meprobamate and other CNS depressants or psychotropic drugs may be additive, appropriate caution should be exercised with patients who take more than one of these agents simultaneously.

Usage in Pregnancy and Lactation—An increased risk of congenital malformations associated with the use of minor tranquilizers (meprobamate, chlordiazepoxide, and diazepam) during the first trimester of pregnancy has been suggested in several studies. Because use of these drugs is rarely a matter of urgency, their use during this period should also always be avoided. The possibility that a woman of childbearing potential may be pregnant at the time of institution of therapy should be considered. Patients should be advised that if they become pregnant during therapy or intend to become pregnant, they should communicate with their physicians about the desirability of discontinuing the drug.

Meprobamate passes the placental barrier. It is present both in umbilical cord blood at or near maternal plasma levels and in breast milk of lactating mothers at concentrations two to four times that of maternal plasma. When use of meprobamate is contemplated in breast-feeding patients, the drug's higher concentrations in breast milk as compared to maternal plasma levels should be considered.

Precautions:
Tridihexethyl chloride
Use with caution in patients with:
 Autonomic neuropathy.
 Hepatic or renal disease.
 Early evidence of ileus as in peritonitis.
 Ulcerative colitis-large doses may suppress intestinal motility to the point of producing a paralytic ileus and the use of this drug may precipitate or aggravate the serious complication of toxic megacolon.
 Hyperthyroidism, coronary heart disease, congestive heart failure, cardiac arrhythmias, hypertension and non-obstructing prostatic hypertrophy.
 Hiatal hernia associated with reflux esophagitis since anticholinergic drugs may aggravate this condition.
 It should be noted that the use of anticholinergic drugs in the treatment of gastric ulcer may produce a delay in gastric emptying time and may complicate such therapy (antral stasis).
 Do not rely on the use of the drug in the presence of complication of biliary tract disease.
 Investigate any tachycardia before giving anticholinergic (atropine-like) drugs since they may increase the heart rate.
 With overdosage, a curare-like action may occur.

Meprobamate
The lowest effective dose should be administered, particularly to elderly and/or debilitated patients, in order to preclude oversedation.

The possibility of suicide attempts should be considered and the least amount of drug feasible should be dispensed at any one time.

Meprobamate is metabolized in the liver and excreted by the kidney; to avoid its excess accumulation, caution should be exercised in administration to patients with compromised liver or kidney function.

Meprobamate occasionally may precipitate seizures in epileptic patients.

Adverse Reactions: In evaluating adverse reactions to this combination, consider the possibility of adverse reactions that can occur with either component, as listed below:

Tridihexethyl chloride
Adverse reactions may be physiologic or toxic, depending upon the individual patient's response, and may include xerostomia; urinary hesitancy and retention; tachycardia; palpitations; blurred vision; mydriasis; cycloplegia; increased ocular tension; loss of taste; headaches; nervousness; drowsiness; weakness; dizziness; insomnia; nausea; vomiting; impotence; suppression of lactation; constipation; bloated feeling; severe allergic reaction or drug idiosyncrasies including anaphylaxis; urticaria and other dermal manifestations; decreased sweating; some degree of mental confusion and/or excitement especially in elderly persons.

Meprobamate
Central Nervous System—Drowsiness, ataxia, dizziness, slurred speech, headache, vertigo, weakness, paresthesias, impairment of visual accommodation, euphoria, overstimulation, paradoxical excitement, fast EEG activity.

Gastrointestinal—Nausea, vomiting, diarrhea.

Cardiovascular—Palpitations, tachycardia, various forms of arrhythmia, transient ECG changes, syncope; also, hypotensive crises (including one fatal case).

Allergic or Idiosyncratic—Allergic or idiosyncratic reactions are usually seen within the period of the first to fourth dose in patients having had no previous contact with the drug. Milder reactions are characterized by an itchy, urticarial, or erythematous maculopapular rash which may be generalized or confined to the groin. Other reactions have included leukopenia, acute nonthrombocytopenic purpura, petechiae, ecchymoses, eosinophilia, peripheral edema, adenopathy, fever, fixed drug eruption with cross reaction to carisoprodol, and cross sensitivity between meprobamate/mebutamate and meprobamate/carbromal.

More severe hypersensitivity reactions, rarely reported, include hyperpyrexia, chills, angioneurotic edema, bronchospasm, oliguria, and anuria. Also, anaphylaxis, erythema multiforme, exfoliative dermatitis, stomatitis, proctitis, Stevens-Johnson syndrome, and bullous dermatitis, including one fatal case of the latter following administration of meprobamate in combination with prednisolone.

In case of allergic or idiosyncratic reactions to meprobamate, discontinue the drug and initiate appropriate symptomatic therapy, which may include epinephrine, antihistamines, and in severe cases, corticosteroids. In evaluating possible allergic reactions, also consider allergy to excipients (information on excipients is available to physicians on request).

Hematologic (See also *Allergic or Idiosyncratic*.) —Agranulocytosis and aplastic anemia have been reported, although no causal relationship has been established. These cases rarely were fatal. Rare cases of thrombocytopenic purpura have been reported.

Other—Exacerbation of porphyric symptoms.

Dosage and Administration: The usual adult dose of PATHIBAMATE *tridihexethyl chloride-meprobamate*-400 (meprobamate 400 mg. + tridihexethyl chloride 25 mg.) is one tablet three times a day at mealtimes, and two tablets at bedtime. If a greater anticholinergic effect is desired, the usual adult dose is two PATHIBAMATE *tridihexethyl chloride-meprobamate*-200 (meprobamate 200 mg. + tridihexethyl chloride 25 mg.) tablets three times a day at mealtimes, and two tablets at bedtime. Doses of meprobamate above 2400 mg. daily are not recommended.

Not for use in children under age 12.

Overdosage: Overdosage information on this combination is lacking. However, consider the possibility of signs and symptoms that can occur with either component, as listed below:

Tridihexethyl chloride
Acute overdosage of anticholinergic agents can produce dry mouth, difficulty in swallowing, marked thirst; blurred vision, photophobia; flushed, hot, dry skin; rash; hyperthermia; palpitations, tachycardia with weak pulse, elevated blood pressure; urinary urgency with difficulty in micturition; abdominal distention; restlessness, confusion, delirium and other signs suggestive of an acute organic psychosis. Treatment should include removal of remaining drug from stomach after administration of Universal Antidote, and supportive and symptomatic therapy as indicated. Universal Antidote is a mixture of 2 parts activated charcoal, 1 part magnesium oxide, and 1 part tannic acid, given as ½ ounce in a half glass of warm water.

Meprobamate
Suicidal attempts with meprobamate have resulted in drowsiness, lethargy, stupor, ataxia, coma, shock, vasomotor and respiratory collapse. Some suicidal attempts have been fatal.

The following data on meprobamate tablets have been reported in the literature and from other sources. These data are not expected to correlate with each case (considering factors such as individual susceptibility and length of time from ingestion to treatment), but represent the *usual ranges* reported.

Acute simple overdose (meprobamate alone): Death has been reported with ingestion of as little as 12 Grams meprobamate and survival with as much as 40 Grams.

Blood Levels:
0.5-2.0 mg.% represents the usual blood level range of meprobamate after therapeutic doses. The level may occasionally be as high as 3.0 mg.%. 3-10 mg.% usually corresponds to findings of mild to moderate symptoms of overdosage, such as stupor or light coma.

10-20 mg.% usually corresponds to deeper coma, requiring more intensive treatment. Some fatalities occur.

At levels greater than 20 mg.%, more fatalities than survivals can be expected.

Acute combined overdose (meprobamate with alcohol or other CNS depressants or psychotropic drugs): Since effects can be additive, a history of ingestion of a low dose of meprobamate plus any of these compounds (or of a relatively low blood or tissue level) cannot be used as a prognostic indicator.

In cases where excessive doses have been taken, sleep ensues rapidly; and blood pressure, pulse, and respiratory rates are reduced to basal levels. Any drug remaining in the stomach should be removed and symptomatic therapy given. Should respiration or blood pressure become compromised, respiratory assistance, central nervous system stimulants, and pressor agents should be administered cautiously as indicated. Meprobamate is metabolized in the liver and excreted by the kidney. Diuresis, osmotic (mannitol) diuresis, peritoneal dialysis, and hemodialysis have been used successfully. Careful monitoring of urinary output is necessary and caution should be taken to avoid overhydration. Relapse and death, after initial recovery, have been attributed to incomplete gastric emptying and delayed absorption. Meprobamate can be measured in biological fluids by two methods: colorimetric (Hoffman, A.J. and Ludwig, B.J.: *J Amer Pharm Assn 48:*740,1959) and gas chromatographic (Douglas, J.F. et al: *Anal Chem 39:*956, 1967).

Continued on next page

The information on each product appearing here is based on labelling effective in August, 1984 and is either the entire official brochure or an accurate condensation therefrom. Information concerning all Lederle products may be obtained from the Professional Services Department, Lederle Laboratories, Pearl River, New York, 10965.

Lederle—Cont.

How Supplied: PATHIBAMATE *tridihexethyl chloride-meprobamate* is available in two formulations:
PATHIBAMATE-400: Yellow embossed Lederle P2
Each tablet contains:
  meprobamate .... 400 mg.
  tridihexethyl chloride .... 25 mg.
400 Tablets
Bottle of 100 - NDC 0005-5071-23
Bottle of 1,000 - NDC 0005-5071-34
PATHIBAMATE-200: Yellow, coated tablets. Printed LL above P1
Each tablet contains:
  meprobamate .... 200 mg.
  tridihexethyl chloride .... 25 mg.
200 Tablets
Bottle of 100 - NDC-0005-5070-23
Bottle of 1,000 - NDC-0005-5070-34
A.H.F.S. 12:08
Shown in Product Identification Section, page 415

PATHILON® ℞
[păth-ĭ-lon]
Tridihexethyl Chloride
Tablets

Description: PATHILON *tridihexethyl chloride* is a synthetic anticholinergic quaternary ammonium compound.

Actions: PATHILON relieves pain by reducing spasm of the gastrointestinal tract.

Indications: Effective for use as adjunctive therapy in the treatment of peptic ulcer.

Contraindications: Glaucoma; obstructive uropathy (for example, bladder neck obstruction due to prostatic hypertrophy); obstructive disease of the gastrointestinal tract (as in achalasia, paralytic ileus, pyloroduodenal stenosis, etc.); intestinal atony of the elderly or debilitated patient; unstable cardiovascular status in acute hemorrhage; severe ulcerative colitis; toxic megacolon complicating ulcerative colitis; myasthenia gravis.

Warnings: USE IN PREGNANCY—The use of any drug in pregnancy, lactation, or in women of child-bearing potential requires that the potential benefit of the drug be weighed against its possible hazards to the mother and child. As with all anticholinergic drugs, an inhibiting effect on lactation may occur.
In the presence of a high environmental temperature, heat prostration can occur with drug use (fever and heat stroke due to decreased sweating). Diarrhea may be an early symptom of incomplete intestinal obstruction, especially in patients with ileostomy or colostomy. In this instance, treatment with this drug would be inappropriate and possibly harmful.
PATHILON *tridihexethyl chloride* may produce drowsiness or blurred vision. In this event, the patient should be warned not to engage in activities requiring mental alertness such as operating a motor vehicle or other machinery or perform hazardous work while taking this drug.

Precautions: Use with caution in patients with:
Autonomic neuropathy.
Hepatic or renal disease.
Early evidence of ileus as in peritonitis.
Ulcerative colitis—large doses may suppress intestinal motility to the point of producing a paralytic ileus and the use of this drug may precipitate or aggravate the serious complication of toxic megacolon.
Hyperthyroidism, coronary heart disease, congestive heart failure, cardiac arrhythmias, hypertension and non-obstructing prostatic hypertrophy.
Hiatal hernia associated with reflux esophagitis since anticholinergic drugs may aggravate this condition.
It should be noted that the use of anticholinergic drugs in the treatment of gastric ulcer may produce a delay in gastric emptying time and may complicate such therapy (antral stasis).
Do not rely on the use of the drug in the presence of complication of biliary tract disease.
Investigate any tachycardia before giving anticholinergic (atropine-like) drugs since they may increase the heart rate.
With overdosage, a curare-like action may occur.

Adverse Reactions: Anticholinergics produce certain effects which may be physiologic or toxic, depending upon the individual patient's response. The physician must delineate these.
Adverse reactions may include xerostomia; urinary hesitancy and retention; blurred vision and tachycardia; palpitations; mydriasis; dilatation of the pupil; cycloplegia; increased ocular tension; loss of taste; headaches; nervousness; drowsiness; weakness; dizziness; insomnia; nausea; vomiting; impotence; suppression of lactation; constipation; bloated feeling; severe allergic reaction or drug idiosyncrasies including anaphylaxis; urticaria and other dermal manifestation; some degree of mental confusion and/or excitement, especially in elderly persons.
Decreased sweating is another adverse reaction that may occur. It should be noted that adrenergic innervation of the eccrine sweat glands on the palms and soles make complete control of sweating impossible. An end point of complete anhidrosis cannot occur because large doses of drug would be required, and this would produce severe side effects from parasympathetic paralysis.

Dosage and Administration: For effective therapeutic results, in particular with anticholinergic drugs, it is absolutely necessary to titrate dosage against the patient's individual needs and response.
The average oral adult dose is 25 to 50 mg. of PATHILON *tridihexethyl chloride*, 3 to 4 times per day. The usual bedtime dose has been 50 mg. A few patients are well controlled on as little as 10 mg 3 times per day, while some require as much as 75 mg 4 times per day. The suggested initial dose is 25 mg 3 times per day before meals and 50 mg at bedtime.

Overdosage:
Tridihexethyl chloride
Acute overdosage of anticholinergic agents can produce dry mouth, difficulty swallowing, marked thirst; blurred vision, photophobia; flushed, hot, dry skin; rash; hyperthermia; palpitations, tachycardia with weak pulse, elevated blood pressure; urinary urgency with difficulty in micturition; abdominal distention; restlessness, confusion, delirium and other signs suggestive of an acute organic psychosis. Treatment should include removal of remaining drug from stomach after administration of Universal Antidote, and supportive and symptomatic therapy as indicated. Universal Antidote is a mixture of 2 parts activated charcoal, 1 part magnesium oxide, and 1 part tannic acid, given as ½ ounce in a half glass of warm water.

How Suppled:
Tablets 25 mg—Pink, coated P4 Bottles of 100 NDC-0005-5079-23.
Store at Controlled Room Temperature 15–30°C (59–86°F)
Shown in Product Identification Section, page 415

PERIHEMIN® ℞
[perĭ-hĭm-ĭn]
hematinic Capsules

Description: PERIHEMIN *hematinic* Capsules for children over 12 and adults.
Each capsule contains: Vitamin B_{12} (as Cyanocobalamin U.S.P.) 5 mcg.; Intrinsic Factor Concentrate 25 mg.; Ferrous Fumarate 168 mg., (Elemental Iron 55 mg.); Folic Acid 0.33 mg.; Ascorbic Acid (C) 50 mg.

Actions: PERIHEMIN *Lederle* is a general hematinic for the oral treatment of the common anemias. They contain the common substances used in the prevention and treatment of anemic conditions produced or aggravated by insufficient food intake.

Indications: PERIHEMIN is primarily indicated in the hypochromic, microcytic anemias due to insufficient iron intake or absorption. It is also useful in the treatment of macrocytic hyperchromic anemias where an increased intake of oral B_{12} or folic acid is desirable.

Warnings: Folic Acid alone is improper therapy in the treatment of pernicious anemia and other megaloblastic anemias where vitamin B_{12} is deficient.

Precautions: Some patients affected with pernicious anemia may not respond to orally administered Vitamin B_{12} with intrinsic factor concentrate and there is no known way to predict which patients will respond or which patients may cease to respond. Periodic examinations and laboratory studies of pernicious anemia patients are essential and recommended.
Folic acid especially in doses above 1.0 mg. daily may obscure pernicious anemia, in that hematologic remission may occur while neurological manifestations remain progressive.
Overdosage or accidental overingestion of iron-containing compounds may lead to gastrointestinal hemorrhage in children. If symptoms of intolerance develop, the drug should be temporarily or permanently discontinued.
PERIHEMIN *hematinic* preparations should not be relied on to correct the serious folic acid deficiency characterizing sprue or the malabsorption syndromes. In these conditions therapeutic amounts of folic acid should be administered.

Adverse Reactions: Allergic sensitization has been reported following both oral and parenteral administration of Folic Acid.

Dosage: PERIHEMIN Capsules for children over 12 and adults.
1 capsule 3 times daily with or after meals.

How Supplied: Capsules—soft shell red printed P7—Bottles of 100 NDC 0005-5121-23.

PERITINIC
[perĭ-tĭn-ĭk]
Hematinic with Vitamins and Fecal Softener Tablets (Film Coated)

In the prevention of nutritional anemias, certain vitamin deficiencies and iron-deficiency anemias.
Recommended Intake: Adults, 1 or 2 tablets daily.
Warning: As with any drug, if you are pregnant or nursing a baby, seek the advice of a health professional before using this product.
Keep out of the reach of children.
In case of accidental overdose, seek professional assistance or contact a Poison Control Center immediately.
60 TABLETS
Each tablet contains:
Elemental Iron .... 100 mg
  (as Ferrous Fumarate)
Docusate Sodium U.S.P. .. 100 mg
  (DSS) (to counteract the constipating effect of iron)
Vitamin B_1 .... 7.5 mg (7½ MDR)
  (as Thiamine Mononitrate)
Vitamin B_2 .... 7.5 mg (6¼ MDR)
  (Riboflavin)
Vitamin B_6 .... 7.5 mg
  (Pyridoxine Hydrochloride)
Vitamin B_{12} .... 50 mcg
  (Cyanocobalamin)
Vitamin C .... 200 mg (6⅔ MDR)
  (Ascorbic Acid)
Niacinamide .... 30 mg (3 MDR)
Folic Acid .... 0.05 mg
Pantothenic Acid .... 15 mg
  (as D-Pantothenyl Alcohol)
MDR—Adult Minimum Daily Requirement
Tablets (maroon capsule-shaped, film coated) embossed LL and P8
NDC 0005-5124-19

PIPERACILLIN SERUM LEVELS IN ADULTS (mcg/ml) after a 2-3 minute IV INJECTION										
DOSE	0	10 min	20 min	30 min	1 hr	1.5 hr	2 hr	3 hr	4 hr	6 hr	8 hr
2	305 (159-615)	202 (164-225)	156 (52-165)	67 (41-88)	40 (25-57)	24 (18-31)	20 (14-24)	8 (3-11)	3 (2-4)	2 (<0.6-3)	—
4	412 (389-484)	344 (315-379)	295 (269-330)	117 (98-138)	93 (78-110)	60 (50-67)	36 (26-51)	20 (17-24)	8 (7-11)	4 (3.7-4.1)	0.9 (0.7-1)
6	775 (695-849)	609 (530-670)	563 (492-630)	325 (292-363)	208 (180-239)	138 (115-175)	90 (71-113)	38 (29-53)	33 (25-44)	8 (3-19)	3.2 (<2-6)

PIPERACILLIN SERUM LEVELS IN ADULTS (mcg/ml) after a 30 minute IV INFUSION										
DOSE	0	5 min	10 min	15 min	30 min	45 min	1 hr	1.5 hr	2 hr	4 hr	6 hr	7.5 hr
4	244 (155-298)	215 (169-247)	186 (140-209)	177 (142-213)	141 (122-156)	146 (110-265)	105 (85-133)	72 (53-105)	53 (36-69)	15 (6-24)	4 (1-9)	2 (0.5-3)
6	353 (324-371)	298 (242-339)	298 (232-331)	272 (219-314)	229 (185-249)	180 (144-209)	149 (117-171)	104 (89-113)	73 (66-94)	22 (12-39)	16 (5-49)	—

PIPRACIL®
[pip-ra-sil] ℞

sterile piperacillin sodium
For Intravenous and Intramuscular Use

Description: PIPRACIL® sterile piperacillin sodium is a semisynthetic broad spectrum penicillin for parenteral use derived from d (-) α-aminobenzylpenicillin. The chemical name of piperacillin sodium is sodium [2S-[2α,5α,6β(S*)]]-6-[[[[(4-ethyl-2,3-dioxo-1-piperazinyl) carbonyl]amino]phenylacetyl]amino]-3,3-dimethyl-7-oxo-4-thia-1-azabicyclo[3.2.0]heptane-2-carboxylate.

PIPRACIL is a white to off-white hygroscopic cryodesiccated crystalline powder which is readily soluble in water and gives a colorless to pale-yellow solution. The pH of the aqueous solution is 5.5 to 7.5. One gram contains 1.85 mEq (42.5 mg) of sodium (Na+).

Clinical Pharmacology:

Intravenous Administration. In healthy adult volunteers, mean serum levels immediately after a 2 to 3 minute intravenous injection of 2, 4 or 6 grams were 305, 412, and 775 mcg/ml. Serum levels lack dose proportionality.
[See table above].

A 30 minute infusion of 6 grams every 6 hours gave, on the fourth day, a mean peak serum concentration of 420 mcg/ml.

Intramuscular Administration. PIPRACIL® is rapidly absorbed after intramuscular injection. In healthy volunteers, the mean peak serum concentration occurs approximately 30 minutes after a single dose of 2 g and is about 36 mcg/ml. The oral administration of 1 g probenecid before injection produces an increase in piperacillin peak serum level of about 30%. The area under the curve (AUC) is increased by approximately 60%.

General. PIPRACIL is not absorbed when given orally. Peak serum concentrations are attained approximately 30 minutes after intramuscular injections and immediately after completion of intravenous injection or infusion. The serum half-life in healthy volunteers ranges from 36 minutes to 1 hour and 12 minutes. The mean elimination half-life of PIPRACIL in healthy adult volunteers is 54 minutes following administration of 2 grams and 63 minutes following 6 grams. As with other penicillins, PIPRACIL is eliminated primarily by glomerular filtration and tubular secretion; it is excreted rapidly as unchanged drug in high concentrations in the urine. Approximately 60 to 80% of the administered dose is excreted in the urine in the first 24 hours. Piperacillin urine concentrations, determined by microbioassay, were as high as 14,100 mcg/ml following a 6 g intravenous dose and 8,500 mcg/ml following a 4 g intravenous dose. These urine drug concentrations remained well above 1,000 mcg/ml throughout the dosing interval. The elimination half-life is increased two-fold in mild to moderate renal impairment and five- to six-fold in severe impairment.

PIPRACIL® binding to human serum proteins is 16%. The drug is widely distributed in human tissues and body fluids, including bone, prostate, and heart and reaches high concentrations in bile. After a 4 gram bolus, maximum biliary concentrations averaged 3205 mcg/ml. It penetrates into the cerebral spinal fluid in the presence of inflamed meninges. Because PIPRACIL is excreted by the biliary route, as well as by the renal route, it can be used safely in appropriate dosage (see DOSAGE AND ADMINISTRATION) in patients with severely restricted kidney function, and can be used effectively in treatment of hepatobiliary infections.

Microbiology:
PIPRACIL is an antibiotic which exerts its bactericidal activity by inhibiting both septum and cell wall synthesis. It is active against a variety of gram-positive and gram-negative aerobic and anaerobic bacteria. *In vitro*, piperacillin is active against most strains of clinical isolates of the following micro-organisms:

Aerobic and facultatively anaerobic organisms
Gram-negative bacteria
Escherichia coli
Proteus mirabilis
Proteus vulgaris
Morganella morganii (formerly *Proteus morganii*)
Providencia rettgerii (formerly *Proteus rettgerii*)
Serratia species including *S. marcescens* and *S. liquefaciens*
Klebsiella pneumoniae
Klebsiella species
Enterobacter species including *E. aerogenes* and *E. cloacae*
Citrobacter species including *C. freundii* and *C. diversus*
Salmonella species*
Shigella species*
Pseudomonas aeruginosa
Pseudomonas species including *P. cepacia*,* *P. maltophilia** and *P fluorescens*
Acinetobacter species (formerly *Mima-Herellea*)
Haemophilus influenzae (non-β-lactamase-producing strains)
Neisseria gonorrhoeae
*Neisseria meningitidis**
Moraxella species*
Yersinia species* (formerly *Pasteurella*)

Gram-positive bacteria
Group D streptococci including
  Enterococci *(Streptococcus faecalis, S. faecium)*
  Non-enterococci*
Beta-hemolytic streptococci including
  Streptococcus Group A *(S. pyogenes)*
  Streptococcus Group B *(S. agalactiae)*
Streptococcus pneumoniae
Streptococcus viridans
Staphylococcus aureus (non-penicillinase-producing)*
Staphylococcus epidermidis (non-penicillinase-producing)*

Anaerobic bacteria
Actinomyces species*
Bacteroides species including
  B. fragilis group *(B. fragilis, B. vulgatus)*
  Non-*B. fragilis* *(B. melaninogenicus)*
  *B. asaccharolyticus**
Clostridium species including
  C. perfringens and *C. difficile**
Eubacterium species
Fusobacterium species including
  F. nucleatum and *F. necrophorum*
Peptococcus species
Peptostreptococcus species
Veillonella species

*Piperacillin has been shown to be active *in vitro* against these organisms; however, clinical efficacy has not yet been established.

In vitro, PIPRACIL® sterile piperacillin sodium is inactivated by staphylococcal β-lactamases, and β-lactamases produced by gram-negative bacteria. However, it is active against β-lactamase-producing gonococci.
Many strains of gram-negative organisms resistant to certain antibiotics have been found to be susceptible to PIPRACIL.
PIPRACIL has excellent activity against gram-positive organisms, including enterococci *(S. faecalis)*. It is active against obligate anaerobes such as *Bacteroides* and also against *Clostridium difficile* (which has been associated with pseudomembranous colitis).
Piperacillin is active against many gram-negative bacteria including *Enterobacteriaceae, Klebsiella, Serratia, Pseudomonas, E coli, Proteus,* and *Citrobacter,* and in addition it is active against anaerobes and enterococci. *In vitro* tests show PIPRACIL to act synergistically with aminoglycoside antibiotics against most isolates of *Pseudomonas aeruginosa.*

Susceptibility Testing:
The use of antibiotic disc susceptibility test methods which measure zone diameter gives an accurate estimation of susceptibility of organisms to PIPRACIL. The following standard procedure** has been recommended for use with discs for testing antimicrobials. Piperacillin 100 mcg discs should be used for the determination of the susceptibility of organisms to piperacillin.

**NCCLS Approved Standard; M2-A2 (Formerly ASM-2) Performance Standards for Antimicrobic Disk Susceptibility Tests, Second Edition, available from the National Committee of Clinical Laboratory Standards.

With this type of procedure, a report of "susceptible" from the laboratory indicates that the infect-

Continued on next page

The information on each product appearing here is based on labelling effective in August, 1984 and is either the entire official brochure or an accurate condensation therefrom. Information concerning all Lederle products may be obtained from the Professional Services Department, Lederle Laboratories, Pearl River, New York. 10965.

Lederle—Cont.

ing organism is likely to respond to therapy. A report of "intermediate susceptibility" suggests that the organism would be susceptible if high dosage is used or if the infection is confined to tissue and fluids (e.g., urine) in which high antibiotic levels are obtained. A report of "resistant" indicates that the infecting organism is not likely to respond to therapy. With the piperacillin disc, a zone of 18 mm or greater indicates susceptibility, zone sizes of 14 mm or less indicate resistance, and zone sizes of 15 to 17 mm indicate intermediate susceptibility.

Haemophilus and *Neisseria* species which give zones of ≥ 29 mm are susceptible; resistant strains give zones of ≤ 28 mm. The above interpretive criteria are based on the use of the standardized procedure. Antibiotic susceptibility testing requires carefully prescribed procedures. Susceptibility tests are biased to a considerable degree when different methods are used.

The standardized procedure requires the use of control organisms. The 100 mcg piperacillin disc should give zone diameters between 24 and 30 mm for *E coli* ATCC No. 25922 and between 25 and 33 mm for *Pseudomonas aeruginosa* ATCC No. 27853. Dilution methods such as those described in the International Collaborative Study† have been used to determine susceptibility of the following organisms to PIPRACIL:

†Acta Pathol Microbiol Scand (B) Suppl. 217 (1971).

Enterobacteriaceae, Pseudomonas species and *Acinetobacter* spp. are considered susceptible if the minimal inhibitory concentration (MIC) of piperacillin is no greater than 64 mcg/ml and are considered resistant if the MIC is greater than 128 mcg/ml.

Haemophilus and *Neisseria* species are considered susceptible if the MIC of PIPRACIL is less than or equal to 1 mcg/ml.

When anaerobic organisms are isolated from infection sites, it is recommended that other tests such as the modified Broth-Disk Method* be used to determine the antibiotic susceptibility of these slow-growing organisms.

*Wilkins TD, Thiel T: *Antimicrob Agents Chemother* 3:350-356, March 1973.

Indications and Usage:

Therapeutic: PIPRACIL is indicated for the treatment of serious infections caused by susceptible strains of the designated organisms in the conditions as listed below.

Intra-abdominal Infections including hepatobiliary and surgical infections caused by *Escherichia coli, Pseudomonas aeruginosa*, enterococci, *Clostridium* spp., anaerobic cocci, and *Bacteroides* spp., including *B. fragilis*.

Urinary Tract Infections caused by *E coli, Klebsiella* spp., *P. aeruginosa, Proteus* spp. including *P. mirabilis* and enterococci.

Gynecologic Infections including endometritis, pelvic inflammatory disease, pelvic cellulitis caused by *Bacteroides* spp. including *B. fragilis*, anaerobic cocci, *Neisseria gonorrhoeae*, and enterococci *(Streptococcus faecalis)*.

Septicemia, including bacteremia caused by *E coli, Klebsiella* spp., *Enterobacter* spp., *Serratia* spp., *P. mirabilis, S. pneumoniae*, enterococci, *Pseudomonas aeruginosa, Bacteroides* spp., and anaerobic cocci.

Lower Respiratory Tract Infections caused by *Escherichia coli, Klebsiella* spp., *Enterobacter* spp., *Pseudomonas aeruginosa, Serratia* spp., *Haemophilus influenzae, Bacteroides* species, and anaerobic cocci. Although improvement has been noted in patients with cystic fibrosis, lasting bacterial eradication may not necessarily be achieved.

Skin and Skin Structure Infections caused by *E coli, Klebsiella* spp., *Serratia* spp., *Acinetobacter* spp., *Enterobacter* spp., *Pseudomonas aeruginosa*, indolepositive *Proteus* spp., *Proteus mirabilis, Bacteroides* spp. including *B. fragilis*, anaerobic cocci, and enterococci.

Bone and Joint Infections caused by *P. aeruginosa*, enterococci, *Bacteroides* spp., and anaerobic cocci.

Gonococcal Infections PIPRACIL has been effective in the treatment of uncomplicated gonococcal urethritis.

PIPRACIL® sterile piperacillin sodium has also been shown to be clinically effective for the treatment of infections at various sites caused by *Streptococcus* species including Group A β-hemolytic *Streptococcus* and *Streptococcus pneumoniae*; however, infections caused by these organisms are ordinarily treated with more narrow spectrum penicillins. Because of its broad spectrum of bactericidal activity against gram-positive and gram-negative aerobic and anaerobic bacteria, PIPRACIL is particularly useful for the treatment of mixed infections and presumptive therapy prior to the identification of the causative organisms. Also, PIPRACIL may be administered as single drug therapy in some situations where normally two antibiotics might be employed.

PIPRACIL has been successfully used with aminoglycosides, especially in patients with impaired host defenses. Both drugs should be used in full therapeutic doses.

Appropriate cultures should be made for susceptibility testing before initiating therapy and therapy adjusted, if appropriate, once the results are known.

Prophylaxis: PIPRACIL is indicated for prophylactic use in surgery including intra-abdominal (gastrointestinal and biliary) procedures, vaginal hysterectomy, abdominal hysterectomy, and cesarean section. Effective prophylactic use depends on the time of administration and PIPRACIL should be given ½ to 1 hour before the operation so that effective levels can be achieved in the wound prior to the procedure.

The prophylactic use of piperacillin should be stopped within 24 hours, since continuing administration of any antibiotic increases the possibility of adverse reactions, but in the majority of surgical procedures, does not reduce the incidence of subsequent infections. If there are signs of infection, specimens for culture should be obtained for identification of the causative organism so that appropriate therapy can be instituted.

Contraindications: A history of allergic reactions to any of the penicillins and/or cephalosporins.

Warnings: Serious and occasionally fatal hypersensitivity (anaphylactic) reactions have been reported in patients receiving therapy with penicillins. These reactions are more apt to occur in persons with a history of sensitivity to multiple allergens.

There have been reports of patients with a history of penicillin hypersensitivity who have experienced severe hypersensitivity reactions when treated with a cephalosporin. Before initiating therapy with PIPRACIL, careful inquiry should be made concerning previous hypersensitivity reactions to penicillins, cephalosporins, and other allergens. If an allergic reactions occurs during therapy with PIPRACIL, the antibiotic should be discontinued. The usual agents (antihistamines, pressor amines, and corticosteroids) should be readily available. SERIOUS ANAPHYLACTOID REACTIONS REQUIRE IMMEDIATE EMERGENCY TREATMENT WITH EPINEPHRINE. OXYGEN AND INTRAVENOUS CORTICOSTEROIDS AND AIRWAY MANAGEMENT INCLUDING INTUBATION SHOULD ALSO BE ADMINISTERED AS NECESSARY.

Precautions:

General. While PIPRACIL possesses the characteristic low toxicity of the penicillin group of antibiotics, periodic assessment of organ system functions, including renal, hepatic, and hematopoietic, during prolonged therapy is advisable.

Bleeding manifestations have occurred in some patients receiving beta-lactam antibiotics including piperacillin. These reactions have sometimes been associated with abnormalities of coagulation tests such as clotting time, platelet aggregation and prothrombin time and are more likely to occur in patients with renal failure.

If bleeding manifestations occur, the antibiotic should be discontinued and appropriate therapy instituted.

The possibility of the emergence of resistant organisms which might cause superinfections should be kept in mind, particularly during prolonged treatment. If this occurs, appropriate measures should be taken.

As with other penicillins, patients may experience neuromuscular excitability or convulsions if higher than recommended doses are given intravenously.

PIPRACIL® is a monosodium compound containing 1.85 milliequivalents of Na+ per gram. This should be considered when treating patients requiring restricted salt intake. Periodic electrolyte determinations should be made in patients with low potassium reserves, and the possibility of hypokalemia should be kept in mind with patients who have potentially low potassium reserves and who are receiving cytotoxic therapy or diuretics. Antimicrobials used in high doses for short periods to treat gonorrhea may mask or delay the symptoms of incubating syphilis. Therefore, prior to treatment, patients with gonorrhea should also be evaluated for syphilis. Specimens for darkfield examination should be obtained from patients with any suspected primary lesion, and serologic tests should be performed. In all cases where concomitant syphilis is suspected, monthly serological tests should be made for a minimum of 4 months. As with other semisynthetic penicillins PIPRACIL therapy has been associated with an increased incidence of fever and rash in cystic fibrosis patients.

Drug Interactions. The mixing of PIPRACIL® with an aminoglycoside *in vitro* can result in substantial inactivation of the aminoglycosides.

Pregnancy—Pregnancy Category B. Although reproduction studies in mice and rats performed at doses up to 4 times the human dose have shown no evidence of impaired fertility or harm to the fetus, safety of PIPRACIL use in pregnant women has not been determined by adequate and well-controlled studies. Because animal reproduction studies are not always predictive of human response, this drug should be used during pregnancy only if clearly needed. It has been found to cross the placenta in rats.

Nursing Mothers. Caution should be exercised when PIPRACIL is administered to nursing mothers. It is excreted in low concentrations in milk.

Pediatric Use. Dosages for children under the age of 12 have not been established. The safety of PIPRACIL® in neonates is not known. In dog neonates dilated renal tubules and peri-tubular hyalinization occurred following administration of PIPRACIL.

Adverse Effects: PIPRACIL is generally well tolerated. The most common adverse reactions have been local in nature, following intravenous or intramuscular injection. The following adverse reactions may occur.

Local Reactions. In clinical trials thrombophlebitis was noted in 4% of patients. Pain, erythema, and/or induration at the injection site occurred in 2% of patients. Less frequent reactions including ecchymosis, deep vein thrombosis and hematomas have also occurred.

Gastrointestinal. Diarrhea and loose stools were noted in 2% of patients. Other less frequent reactions included vomiting, nausea, increases in liver enzymes (LDH, SGOT, SGPT), hyperbilirubinemia, cholestatic hepatitis, bloody diarrhea.

Hypersensitivity Reactions. Anaphylactoid Reactions, see WARNINGS.

Rash was noted in 1% of patients. Other less frequent findings included pruritus, vesicular eruptions, positive Coombs' test.

Renal. Elevations of creatinine or BUN.

Central Nervous System. Headache, dizziness, fatigue.

Hemic and Lymphatic. Reversible leukopenia, neutropenia, thrombocytopenia and/or eosinophilia have been reported. As with other β-lactam antibiotics, reversible leukopenia (neutropenia) is more apt to occur in patients receiving prolonged therapy at high dosages or in association with drugs known to cause this reaction.

Serum Electrolytes. Individuals with liver disease or individuals receiving cytotoxic therapy or diuretics were reported rarely to demonstrate a decrease in serum potassium concentrations with high doses of PIPRACIL.®

Skeletal. Rarely, prolonged muscle relaxation.

Other. Superinfection, including candidiasis. Hemorrhagic manifestations.

Dosage and Administration: PIPRACIL may be administered by the intramuscular route or intravenously. It can be administered in a 3 to 5 minute intravenous injection. The usual dosage of PIPRACIL for serious infections is 3 to 4 grams given every 4 to 6 hours as a 20 to 30 minute infusion. For serious infections, the intravenous route of administration should be used.

PIPRACIL should not be mixed with an aminoglycoside in a syringe or infusion bottle since this can result in inactivation of the aminoglycoside. The maximum daily dose for adults is usually 24 g/day, although higher doses have been used. Intramuscular injections should be limited to 2 g per injection site. This route of administration has been used primarily in the treatment of patients with uncomplicated gonorrhea and urinary tract infections.
[See table right].
[See table below].

Infants and Children. Dosages in infants and children under 12 years of age have not been established.

Intravenous Administration

Directions. Reconstitute each gram of PIPRACIL with at least 5 ml of a suitable diluent such as Bacteriostatic Water for Injection, Bacteriostatic Sodium Chloride Injection, or diluents listed below. Shake well until dissolved. It may be further diluted to the desired volume.

Intravenous Injection—Following reconstitution in order to help avoid vein irritation, the solution should be administered slowly over a 3- to 5-minute period.

Intermittent Intravenous Infusion—Reconstitute as described above, using a suitable intravenous solution listed below, dilute the total content of the vial or infusion bottle, and then further dilute to the desired volume (at least 50 ml). Administer by infusion over a period of about 30 minutes. During infusion it is desirable to discontinue the primary intravenous solution.

Stability of PIPRACIL® Following Reconstitution. PIPRACIL is stable in both glass and plastic containers when reconstituted with recommended diluents and diluted with the indicated intravenous solutions and intravenous admixtures.
Extensive stability studies have demonstrated chemical stability (potency, pH, and clarity) through 24 hours at room temperature, up to one week refrigerated, and up to one month frozen ($-10°$ to $-20°C$). Appropriate consideration of aseptic technique and individual hospital policy, however, may recommend the more conservative label instructions to discard unused portions after storage for 24 hours at room temperature or for 48 hours when refrigerated.

PIPRACIL DOSAGE RECOMMENDATIONS

Type of Infections	Usual Total Daily Dosage	Frequency of Administration
Serious infections such as septicemia nosocomial pneumonia, intra-abdominal infections, aerobic and anaerobic gynecologic infections, and skin and soft-tissue infections	12–18 g IV (200–300 mg/kg)	Every four to six hours
Complicated urinary tract infections	8–16 g IV (125–200 mg/kg)	Every six to eight hours
Uncomplicated urinary tract infections and most community-acquired pneumonia	6–8 g IM or IV (100–125 mg/kg)	Every six to twelve hours
Uncomplicated gonorrhea infections	2 g IM*	Single dose

*One gram of probenecid given orally $\frac{1}{2}$ hour prior to injection.

The average duration of PIPRACIL treatment is from 7 to 10 days, except in the treatment of gynecologic infections, in which it is from 3 to 10 days; the duration should be guided by the patient's clinical and bacteriological progress. For most acute infections, treatment should be continued for at least 48 to 72 hours after the patient becomes asymptomatic. Antibiotic therapy for Group A beta-hemolytic streptococcal infections should be maintained for at leat 10 days to reduce the risk of rheumatic fever or glomerulonephritis.
When PIPRACIL is given concurrently with aminoglycosides, both drugs should be used in full therapeutic doses.

Dosage in renal impairment

Renal Impairment Creatinine Clearance ml/min	Urinary Tract Infection (uncomplicated)	Urinary Tract Infection (complicated)	Serious Systemic Infection
>40	No dosage adjustment necessary		
20–40	No dosage adjustment necessary	9 g/day (3 g every 8 hr)	12 g/day (4 g every 8 hr)
<20	6 g/day (3 g every 12 hr)	6 g/day (3 g every 12 hr)	8 g/day (4 g every 12 hr)

For patients on hemodialysis the maximum daily dose is 6 g day (2 g every 8 hr.). In addition because hemodialysis removes 30–50% of piperacillin in 4 hours, 1 g additional dose should be administered following each dialysis period.

For patients with renal failure and hepatic insufficiency, measurement of serum levels of PIPRACIL® sterile piperacillin sodium will provide additional guidance for adjusting dosage.

Diluents for Reconstitution.
Sterile Water for Injection, USP
†Bacteriostatic Water for Injection, USP
Sodium Chloride Injection, USP
†Bacteriostatic Sodium Chloride Injection, USP
**Lidocaine HCl 0.5-1% (without epinephrine)
**For Intramuscular Use Only
†Either Parabens or Benzyl Alcohol

Intravenous Solutions.
Dextrose 5% in Water.
0.9% Sodium Chloride
Dextrose 5% and 0.9% Sodium Chloride
Lactated Ringer's Injection, USP
Dextran 6% in 0.9% Sodium Chloride

Intravenous Admixtures.
Normal Saline [+ KCl 40 mEq]
5% Dextrose/Water D₅W [+ KCl 40 mEq]
5% Dextrose/Normal Saline D₅NS [+ KCl 40 mEq]
Ringer's Injection, USP [+ KCl 40 mEq]
Lactated Ringer's Injection, USP [+ KCl 40 mEq]

Intramuscular Administration

When indicated by clinical and bacteriological findings, intramuscular administration of 6 to 8 grams daily of PIPRACIL,® in divided doses, may be utilized for initiation of therapy. In addition, intramuscular administration of the drug may be considered for maintenance therapy after clinical and bacteriologic improvement has been obtained with intravenous piperacillin sodium treatment. Intramuscular administration should not exceed 2 grams per injection at any one site.
The preferred site is the upper outer quadrant of the buttock (i.e., gluteus maximus).
The deltoid area should be used only if well-developed, and then only with caution to avoid radial nerve injury. Intramuscular injections should not be made into the lower or mid-third of the upper arm.

Reconstitution for Intramuscular Use
Directions. Recommended diluents for 2 g, 3 g and 4 g standard vials are listed below.
Each gram of PIPRACIL® should be reconstituted with a minimum of 2 ml using one of the following diluents:

Continued on next page

Prophylaxis

INDICATION	1st Dose	2nd Dose	3rd Dose
Intra-abdominal Surgery	2 g IV just prior to surgery	2 g during surgery	2 g every 6 hr. Post-Op for no more than 24 hours
Vaginal Hysterectomy	2 g IV just prior to surgery	2 g 6 hr. after 1st dose	2 g 12 hr. after 1st dose
Cesarean Section	2 g IV after cord is clamped	2 g 4 hr. after 1st dose	2 g 8 hr. after 1st dose
Abdominal Hysterectomy	2 g IV just prior to surgery	2 g on return to recovery room	2 g after 6 hours

The information on each product appearing here is based on labelling effective in August, 1984 and is either the entire official brochure or an accurate condensation therefrom. Information concerning all Lederle products may be obtained from the Professional Services Department, Lederle Laboratories, Pearl River, New York, 10965.

Lederle—Cont.

1. Sterile Water for Injection, USP
2. Bacteriostatic Water for Injection, USP
3. Sodium Chloride Injection, USP
4. Bacteriostatic Sodium Chloride Injection, USP
5. Sterile Lidocaine HCl Injection, USP, 0.5–1.0% for Intramuscular Use Only (without epinephrine). Lidocaine HCl is contraindicated in patients with a known history of hypersensitivity to local anesthetics of the amide type.

Dilution Table for IM Use

Volume of Diluent for the Following Vial Size			Volume to be Withdrawn for a
2g	3g	4g	1g Dose
4.0 ml	6.0 ml	7.8 ml	2.5 ml

To expedite reconstitution, the vial contents should be shaken immediately after adding the diluent.

How Supplied: PIPRACIL® sterile cryodesiccated piperacillin sodium is available in vials containing sterile freeze-dried piperacillin sodium powder equivalent to two, three and four grams of piperacillin. One gram of piperacillin (as a monosodium salt) contains approximately 1.85 mEq (42.5 mg) of sodium.

Product Numbers:
2 gram/vial—NDC 0206-3879-14
2 gram/vial—10 per box—NDC 0206-3879-16
3 gram/vial—NDC 0206-3882-06
3 gram/vial—25 per box—NDC 0206-3882-21
4 gram/vial—NDC 0206-3880-18
4 gram/vial—25 per box—NDC 0206-3880-22
2 gram infusion bottle in box—NDC 0206-3879-45
2 gram infusion bottle—10 per box—NDC 0206-3879-47
3 gram infusion bottle in box—NDC 0206-3882-68
3 gram infusion bottle—10 per box—NDC 0206-3882-65
4 gram infusion bottle in box—NDC 0206-3880-69
4 gram infusion bottle—10 per box—NDC 0206-3880-66
3 gm vial (25's)
MILITARY NSN 6505-01-130-4451
4 gm vial (25's)
MILITARY NSN 6505-01-130-4452
2 gm (10's)
VA NSN 6505-01-148-5040A
3 gm vial (25's)
VA NSN 6505-01-130-4451A
3 gm—infusion bottle (10's)
VA NSN 6505-01-137-0039
4 gm vial (25's)
VA NSN 6505-01-130-4452A

This product should be stored at controlled room temperature, 15–30°C (59–86°F).

LEDERLE PIPERACILLIN, INC.
Carolina, Puerto Rico 00630
Shown in Product Identification Section, page 416

PNU-IMUNE® 23   ℞
[new-ĭ-mune]
Pneumococcal Vaccine, Polyvalent

Description: Pneumococcal Vaccine Polyvalent, PNU-IMUNE 23 is a sterile liquid vaccine for intramuscular or subcutaneous use, consisting of a mixture of purified capsular polysaccharides from 23 pneumococcal types:
[See table below].
It is indicated for immunization against infections caused by the 23 most prevalent types of pneumococci responsible for approximately 90 percent of serious pneumococcal disease in the United States and the rest of the world.[1-5] Each of the pneumococcal polysaccharide types is produced separately by Lederle Laboratories to give a high degree of purity. After an individual pneumococcal type is grown, the polysaccharide is separated from the cell and purified by a series of steps including ethanol fractionation. The resultant 23 purified polysaccharides are combined in amounts to give 25 micrograms of each type per dose (0.5 ml) in the final vaccine. Thimerosal (a mercury derivative) at a final concentration of 0.01% is added as a preservative.

Clinical Pharmacology: Pneumococci are the etiologic agents for a significant number of the pneumonias occurring throughout the world. The emergence of strains of pneumococci with increased resistance to one or more of the common antibiotics[4] and recent isolations of pneumococci with multiple-antibiotic resistance[6] emphasize the importance of vaccine prophylaxis against pneumococcal disease.

Based on projections from limited observations in the United States, it has been estimated that 150,000 to 570,000 cases of pneumococcal pneumonia may occur annually. The overall case fatality rate ranges from 5–7%.[2] As many as 60 percent of all deaths among patients with pneumococcal bacteremia treated with penicillin or tetracycline occur within five days of onset of the illness.[6] Thus vaccination offers an effective means for further reducing the mortality and morbidity of this disease. Populations at high risk are the elderly,[7,8] individuals with immune deficiencies, asplenics and patients with splenic deficiencies including sickle cell anemia and other severe hemoglobinopathies, alcoholics and patients with the following disease conditions: chronic respiratory illness, the nephrotic syndrome, multiple myeloma, Hodgkin's Disease and cirrhosis.[2] Antibiotics have only been partially effective in reducing the mortality of pneumococcal pneumonia. The pneumococcus is also a major infectious agent in meningitis[9] and otitis media. Other illnesses caused by pneumococci include sinus infection, arthritis and conjunctivitis. The annual incidence of pneumococcal meningitis is approximately 1.5 to 2.5 per 100,000 population. One-half of the cases occur in children in whom the fatality rate is about 40%.[1,8]

The polysaccharide capsules of pneumococci endow these organisms with resistance to the phagocytic action of polymorphonuclear leukocytes and monocytes. The opsonin activity of type-specific antibody facilitates their destruction in the body by complement-mediated activities.

The protection induced by the vaccine is of long duration but its extent is not yet known. Elevated antibody levels have been shown to persist for at least 5 years after immunization with other pneumococcal vaccines.[10]

Children under 2 years of age do not respond adequately to some of the important polysaccharide types.[12]

PNU-IMUNE 23 has not been studied in children under 2 years of age. Recipients of polyvalent vaccines acquired less nasopharyngeal carriage of pneumococcal types included in the vaccine.[2,11]

A repeat (booster) injection of pneumococcal vaccine *should not be given* to previously vaccinated subjects regardless of the time interval from the previous injection. Available data indicate that revaccination may result in more frequent and severe local reactions at the site of injection, especially in persons who have retained high antibody titers. Such adverse reactions have occurred with booster doses given after long intervals from the initial vaccination. There is also evidence that booster doses do not result in increased antibody titers.[2]

In clinical studies with PNU-IMUNE 23, more than 90% of all adults showed a 2-fold or greater increase in geometric mean antibody titer for each vaccine capsular type.[13]

Patients over the age of 2 years with anatomical or functional asplenia and otherwise intact lymphoid function responded to PNU-IMUNE® 23 *pneumococcal vaccine, polyvalent* and other comparable pneumococcal vaccines with a serological conversion comparable to that observed in healthy individuals of the same age.[14]

Polyvalent pneumococcal vaccines, from other sources, were shown to be effective in preventing pneumococcal disease. Controlled field trials in South Africa involving 12,000 gold miners have shown a 6-valent and a 13-valent pneumococcal vaccine to be 78.5% effective in preventing type-specific pneumococcal pneumonia and 82.3% effective in preventing pneumococcal bacteremia with the types in the vaccine.[15] In a preliminary study of an 8-valent polysaccharide vaccine in a group consisting of 77 patients with sickle cell disease and 19 asplenic persons, there were no pneumococcal infections in the immunized patients within two years of immunization. There were eight cases of pneumococcal infection in 106 unimmunized, age-matched patients with sickle cell disease. Antibody response of the asplenic patients was comparable to normal controls.[16]
In a study carried out by Austrian et al.[15] with 13-valent pneumococcal vaccines prepared for the National Institute of Allergy and Infectious Disease, the reduction in pneumonias caused by the capsular types in the vaccines was 79%. Reduction in type-specific pneumococcal bacteremia was 82%.

In a double-blind study of a 14-valent pneumococcal vaccine carried out in Papua, New Guinea, pneumococcal infection was less in the vaccinated group by 84%. Mortality from pneumonia was less by 44%.[17]

Pneumococcal polysaccharide vaccine was found to significantly reduce clinical cases of pneumococcal otitis media in a six-month post-vaccination period of observation. In a controlled study there were 455 children ages two to six years with a history of prior episodes of otitis media. Two hundred seventy four of these patients received 14 valent pneumococcal vaccine. Overall, there was a 73% reduction in frequency of cases caused by serotypes in the pneumococcal vaccine, other than type 6 for which no protection was found. These Finnish otitis studies revealed a marked fall-off protective efficacy later than 6 months after immunization.[18]

Indications and Usage: PNU-IMUNE® 23 is indicated for immunization against pneumococcal disease caused by those pneumococcal types included in the vaccine.

Use in preventing pneumococcal otitis media. Children two years or older who, in the judgment of the physician, are clearly in need of protection due to a risk of developing otitis media. (See "CLINICAL PHARMACOLOGY" for clinical data.)

Use in Selected Individuals: Persons over 2 years of age as follows: (1) who have anatomical asplenia or who have splenic dysfunction due to sickle cell disease or other causes; (2) persons with chronic illnesses in which there is an increased risk of pneumococcal disease, such as diabetes mellitus, functional impairment of cardiorespiratory, hepatic and renal systems; (3) persons 50 years of age or older, and (4) patients about to undergo immunosuppressive therapy.[2] It is reasonable to assume that patients on immunosuppressive therapy are at increased risk of pneumococcal disease. When possible, vaccination should be given at least 10 days and preferably more than 14 days prior to initiation of such immunosuppressive therapy. Impairment of antibody response in Hodgkin's Disease patients receiving radiotherapy, chemotherapy or both, was demonstrated.[20]

Use in Communities. Persons over 2 years of age as follows: (1) closed groups such as those in residential schools, nursing homes and other institutions; (2) groups epidemiologically at risk in the community when there is a generalized outbreak in the population due to a single pneumococcal type included in the vaccine, and (3) patients at high risk of influenza complications, particularly pneumonia.[11]

Simultaneous administration of pneumococcal polysaccharide vaccine and whole-virus influenza vaccine has been found to give satisfactory antibody response without increasing the incidence of side effects. Although not yet studied, simultaneous administration of the pneumococcal vaccine

Nomenclature	Pneumococcal Types
Danish	1 2 3 4 5 6B 7F 8 9N 9V 10A 11A 12F 14 15B 17F 18C 19A 19F 20 22F 23F 33F
U.S.	1 2 3 4 5 26 51 8 9 68 34 43 12 14 54 17 56 57 19 20 22 23 70

and split-virus influenza vaccine may also be expected to yield satisfactory results.[2,19]

Contraindications: *Children below 2 years of age.* While pneumococcal polysaccharide vaccines have been shown to be highly immunogenic and effective in adults, their usefulness in children is still being evaluated. Although some pneumococcal polysaccharides have been reported to be immunogenic from the age of three months (particularly serotype 3), serum antibody responses to most of the polysaccharides present in the 14-valent vaccine have been shown to be poor in children under two years of age.[22]

Hypersensitivity. Known hypersensitivity to any component of the vaccine including hypersensitivity to thimerosal. Remedial measures for anaphylactoid reactions, including epinephrine injection (1:1000), must be available for immediate use.

Patients on Immunosuppressive Therapy. Immunization of patients should not be attempted less than 10 days prior to or during treatment with immunosuppressive drugs or irradiation. Administration of vaccine to patients on such therapy for Hodgkin's Disease resulted in reduction of preexisting antibody levels.[20]

Previously vaccinated subjects. The use of PNU-IMUNE 23 is contraindicated in persons who have been immunized with any polyvalent pneumococcal vaccine.

Warnings: *PNU-IMUNE 23 is not an effective agent for prophylaxis against pneumococcal disease caused by types not present in the vaccine.* The vaccine may not be effective in patients undergoing treatment causing therapeutic suppression of the immune-response system.

Patients who have received extensive chemotherapy and/or splenectomy for the treatment of Hodgkin's Disease have been shown to have an impaired serum antibody response to pneumococcal vaccine.[20]

A repeat (booster) injection of pneumococcal vaccine *should not be given* to previously vaccinated subjects regardless of the time interval from the previous injection. Available data indicate that revaccination may result in more frequent and severe local reactions at the site of injection, especially in persons who have retained high antibody titers. Such adverse reactions have occurred with booster doses given after long intervals from the initial vaccination. There is also evidence that booster doses do not result in increased antibody titers.[2]

Intradermal administration may cause severe local reactions.

Precautions: *General.* The vaccine should be injected subcutaneously or intramuscularly. *Do not inject intravenously.*

In the presence of any febrile respiratory illness or other active infection, the vaccine should not be used.

The parenteral administration of any biological product should be surrounded by every known precaution for the prevention and arrest of allergic and other untoward reactions. (See CONTRAINDICATIONS).

When administering this vaccine, a separate heat-sterilized syringe and needle or a new disposable equivalent should be used for each patient to prevent transmission of hepatitis B (homologous serum hepatitis) or other infectious agents.

Patients who have had episodes of pneumococcal pneumonia or other pneumococcal infection may have high levels of preexisting pneumococcal antibodies which may result in increased reactions to PNU-IMUNE 23, mostly local, but occasionlly systemic.[21] Caution should be exercised if such patients are considered for vaccination with PNU-IMUNE 23.

Pregnancy Category C: Animal reproduction studies have not been conducted with PNU-IMUNE 23. It is also not known whether PNU-IMUNE 23 can cause fetal harm when administered to a pregnant woman or can affect reproduction capacity. PNU-IMUNE 23 is not recommended for use in pregnant women.

It is not known whether the drug is excreted in human milk. Because many drugs are excreted in human milk, caution should be exercised when PNU-IMUNE 23 is administered to a nursing woman.

Pediatric Use. PNU-IMUNE® 23 has not been studied in children under two years of age. While pneumococcal polysaccharide vaccines have been shown to be highly immunogenic and effective in adults, their usefulness in children is still being evaluated. Although some pneumococcal polysaccharides have been reported to be immunogenic from the age three months (particularly serotype 3), serum antibody responses to most of the polysaccharides present in the 14-valent vaccine have been shown to be poor in children under two years of age.[22]

Adverse Reactions: PNU-IMUNE® 23 *pneumococcal vaccine, polyvalent* is associated with a relatively low incidence of adverse reactions. The adverse reactivity observed in clinical studies was not serious and of short duration.

In a study of 32 individuals who received PNU-IMUNE 23, 23 (72%) experienced local reaction characterized by local soreness at the injection site within 3 days after vaccination.

Low grade fever (less than 100°F) and mild myalgia occur occasionally with PNU-IMUNE 23 and are usually confined to the 24-hour period following vaccination. Rash and arthralgia have been reported rarely.

Although rare, fever over 102° and marked local swelling has been reported with pneumococcal polysaccharide vaccine.

Patients with otherwise stabilized idiopathic thrombocytopenic purpura have, on rare occasions, experienced a relapse in their thrombocytopenia, occurring 2 to 14 days after vaccination, and lasting up to 2 weeks.[23]

Reactions of greater severity, or extent are unusual. Rarely, anaphylactoid reactions have been reported.

A repeat (booster) injection of pneumococcal vaccine *should not be given* to previously vaccinated subjects regardless of the time interval from the previous injection. Available data indicate that revaccination may result in more frequent and severe local reactions at the site of injection, especially in persons who have retained high antibody titers. Such adverse reactions have occurred with booster doses given after long intervals from the initial vaccination. There is also evidence that booster doses do not result in increased antibody titers.[2]

Temporal association of neurological disorders have been reported following parenteral injections of biological products.

Dosage and Administration: *Do not inject intravenously.* The immunization schedule consists of a single 0.5 ml dose given subcutaneously or intramuscularly.

Parenteral drug products should be inspected visually for particulate matter and discoloration prior to administration, whenever solution and container permit.

PNU-IMUNE 23 *must not* be administered to persons who have been immunized previously with any polyvalent pneumococcal vaccine.

A repeat (booster) injection of pneumococcal vaccine *should not be given* to previously vaccinated subjects regardless of the time interval from the previous injection. Available data indicate that revaccination may result in more frequent and severe local reactions at the site of injection, especially in persons who have retained high antibody titers. Such adverse reactions have occurred with booster doses given after long intervals from the initial vaccination. There is also evidence that booster doses do not result in increased antibody titers.[2]

Directions for Use of the LEDERJECT® Disposable Syringe.

1. Twist the plunger rod clockwise to be sure that rod is secure to rubber plunger base.
2. Hold needle shield in place with index finger and thumb of one hand while with the other thumb exert light pressure on plunger rod until the plunger base has been freed and demonstrates slight movement when pressure is applied.
3. Grasp the rubber needle shield at its base; twist and pull to remove.
4. Pull back plunger rod slowly and carefully to insure smooth plunger operation.
5. Expel the air bubble.

Storage and Use: Store syringes and unopened or opened vials at 2-8°C (35-46°F).

The vaccine is used directly as supplied. No dilution or reconstitution is necessary. Thimerosal (a mercury derivative) is present in the vaccine as a preservative at a final concentration of 0.01%. Discard unused vials beyond expiration date.

How Supplied: PNU-IMUNE 23 is supplied as follows:

NDC 0005-2309-31 5 dose vial, for use with syringe only.

NDC 0005-2309-33 5 × One dose LEDERJECT® Disposable Syringes.

References:

1. Austrian, R. "Surveillance of Pneumococcal Infection for Field Trials of Polyvalent Vaccines." Annual Contract Prog. Report to the Nat. Inst. of Allerg. and Inf. Dis. (1975) Updated to Dec. 1977, personal communication.
2. Recommendation of the Immunization Practices Advisory Committee, Morb. Mort. Weekly Report 30 (33):410–419 August 28, 1981.
3. Lund, E. "Distribution of Pneumococcal Types at Different Times and Different Areas" in *Bayer Symposium III. Bacterial Infections.* "Changes in Their Causative Agents, Trends and Possible Basis." M. Finland, W. Marget and K. Bartman (eds.) Berlin, Springer-Verlag:49, (1971).
4. Mufson, M. A., Kruss, D.M., Wasil, R.E. and Metzger, W.I. "Capsular Types and Outcome of Bacteremic Pneumococcal Disease in the Antibiotic Era." Arch. Int. Med., 134:505, (1974).
5. Robbins, J.B., Austrian, R., Lee, C.J., Rastogi, S.C., Schiffman, G., Henrichsen, J., Mäkelä, P.H., Broome, C.V., Facklam, R.R., Tiesjema, R.H., and Parke, J.C., Jr. "Consideration for Formulating the Second Generation Pneumococcal Capsule Polysaccharide Vaccine with Emphasis on the Cross-Reactive Types Within Groups." J. Infec. Dis. 1983 (In press).
6. Epidemiologic Notes and Reports, Multiple-Antibiotic Resistance of Pneumococci—South Africa Morb. Mort. Weekly Report 26 (35):285–286 September 2, 1977.
7. Austrian, R., and Gold, J. "Pneumococcal Bacteremia with Especial Reference to Bacteremic Pneumococcal Pneumonia." Ann. Int. Med., 60:759, (1964).
8. Valenti, W.M., Jenzer, M. and Bently, W. "Type-Specific Pneumococcal Respiratory Disease in the Elderly and Chronically Ill." Am. Rev. Resp. Dis., 117:233, (1978).
9. Fraser, D.W., Geil, C.C., and Feldman, R.A. "Meningitis in Bernalillo County, New Mexico. A Comparison with Three Other American Populations." Am. J. Epidemiol., 100:29, (1974).
10. Mufson, M.A., Krause, H.E. and Schiffman, G. "Long Term Persistence of Antibody Following Immunization with Pneumococcal Polysaccharide Vaccine." Proc. Soc. Exptl. Biol. & Med. In press. June 1983.
11. Mufson, M.A. and Drause, H.E. "Role of Antibody in Prevention of Acquisition of Pneumococcal Carriage Among Vaccinees." Clin. Res., 24:577A, (1976).
12. Report of the Committee on Infectious Diseases. Pneumococcal Infections. Amer. Acad. of Ped. 19th Edition: 205–206, 1982.

Continued on next page

The information on each product appearing here is based on labelling effective in August, 1984 and is either the entire official brochure or an accurate condensation therefrom. Information concerning all Lederle products may be obtained from the Professional Services Department, Lederle Laboratories, Pearl River, New York, 10965.

Lederle—Cont.

13. Data on File, Lederle Laboratories.
14. Sullivan, J.L., Ochs, H.D., Schiffman, G., Hammerschlag, M.R., Miser, J., Vichinsky, E., and Wedgwood, R.J. "Immune Response After Splenectomy." Lancet, 178, (1978).
15. Austrian, R., Douglas, R.M., Schiffman, G., Coetzee, A.M., Koornhof, H.J., Hayden-Smith, S. and Reid, R.D.W. "Prevention of Pneumococcal Pneumonia by Vaccination." Trans. Asc. Am. Physicians, 89:184, (1976).
16. Amman, A.J., Addiego, K., Wara, D.W., Lubin, B., Smith, W.B. and Mentzer, W.C. "Polyvalent Pneumococcal-Polysaccharide Immunization of Patients with Sickle-Cell Anemia and Patients with Splenectomy." New Eng. J. Med., 297:897, (1977).
17. Riley, I.D., Andrews, M., Howard, R., Tarr, P.I., Pfeiffer, M., Challands, P. and Jennison, G. "Immunization with Polyvalent Pneumococcal Vaccine." Lancet, 1338, (1977).
18. Makela, P.H., Sibakov, M., Herva, E., Henrichsen, J., Luotonen, J., Timonen, M., Lienonen, M., Koskela, M., Pukander, J., Pontynen, S., Gronroos, P., Karma, P. Pneumococcal Vaccine and Otitis Media. Lancet 547-551, 1980.
19. DeStefano, F., Goodman, R.A., Noble, G.R., McClary, G.D., Smith, S.J. and Broome, C.V. "Simultaneous Administration of Influenza and Pneumococcal Vaccines" JAMA 247:2551–2554, (1982).
20. Siber, G.R., Weitzman, S.A., Aisenberg, A.C., Weinstein, H.J., and Schiffman, G. "Impaired Antibody Response to Pneumococcal Vaccine After Treatment for Hodgkin's Disease." New Eng. J. Med., 299:442, (1978).
21. Pönkä, A. and Leinonen, M. "Adverse Reactions to Polyvalent Pneumococcal Vaccine." Scand. J. Infect. Dis., 14:67–71, (1982).
22. Douglas, R.M., Paton, J.C., Duncan, S.J., and Hansman, D.J. "Antibody Response to Pneumococcal Vaccination in Children Younger than Five Years of Age." J. Infec. Dis., (1):13-137, (1983).
23. Kelton, J.G. "Vaccination-Associated Relapse of Immune Thrombocytopenia." J. Am. Med. Assoc., 245(4):369-371, 1981.

Rev. 1/84

LEDERLE LABORATORIES DIVISION
American Cyanamid Company, Pearl River, N.Y. 10965

PRONEMIA® ℞
[prō-nēēm-ēa]
hematinic
Capsules

Composition: Each capsule contains: Vitamin B_{12} (as Cobalamin Concentrate) 15 mcg.; Intrinsic Factor Concentrate 75 mg.; Ferrous Fumarate 350 mg. (Elemental Iron 115 mg.); Ascorbic Acid (Vitamin C) 150 mg. and Folic Acid 1 mg.

Indications: Indicated for treatment and maintenance in common anemias, including iron-deficiency anemia, megaloblastic anemias of pregnancy, and those of nutritional origin. All of the other means that are recognized as suited to the treatment of these anemias should also be employed. If cases prove resistant to this form of therapy, further exploration of the etiology and additional therapeutic measures should be instituted.

Warnings: Folic Acid alone is improper therapy in the treatment of pernicious anemia and other megaloblastic anemias where vitamin B_{12} is deficient.

Precautions: Some patients affected with pernicious anemia may not respond to orally administered Vitamin B_{12} with intrinsic factor concentrate and there is no known way to predict which patients will respond or which patients may cease to respond. Periodic examinations and laboratory studies of pernicious anemia patients are essential and recommended.

If any symptoms of intolerance occur, the drug should be temporarily or permanently discontinued.
Folic acid in doses above 0.1 mg. daily may obscure pernicious anemia, in that hematologic remission can occur while neurological manifestations remain progressive.

Adverse Reactions: Allergic sensitization has been reported following both oral and parenteral administration of Folic Acid.

Administration and Dosage: One capsule daily with or after meals to treat and maintain the average uncomplicated case of anemia.

How Supplied: Capsules (red)—P9 bottles of 100 NDC 0005-5150-23.

SPARTUS®
[spar-tus]
High Potency Vitamins & Minerals plus Electrolytes

(See PDR For Nonprescription Drugs)

SPARTUS® + Iron
[spar-tus]
High Potency Vitamins & Minerals plus Electrolytes

(See PDR For Nonprescription Drugs)

STRESSCAPS®
[strĕs-caps]
stress formula B + C vitamins

(See PDR For Nonprescription Drugs)

STRESSTABS® 600, Advanced Formula
[strĕs-tabs]
High Potency
Stress Formula Vitamins

(See PDR For Nonprescription Drugs)

STRESSTABS® 600 with IRON,
[strĕs-tabs]
Advanced Formula
High Potency
Stress Formula Vitamins

(See PDR For Nonprescription Drugs)

STRESSTABS® 600 with ZINC,
[strĕs-tabs]
Advanced Formula
High Potency
Stress Formula Vitamins

(See PDR For Nonprescription Drugs)

TETANUS AND DIPHTHERIA ℞ TOXOIDS, ADSORBED PUROGENATED®

How Supplied: 5 ml. vial; 10 x 0.5 ml. LEDERJECT® Disposable Syringe.
COMPLETE INFORMATION FURNISHED IN THE PACKAGE.

TETANUS TOXOID, ADSORBED ℞ PUROGENATED®

How Supplied: 5 ml. vial (5 immunizations); 10 x 0.5 ml. and 100 x 0.5 ml. LEDERJECT® Disposable Syringe.
COMPLETE INFORMATION FURNISHED IN THE PACKAGE.

TETANUS TOXOID® ℞ PUROGENATED®
(Tetanus Toxoid fluid)

How Supplied: 7.5 ml. vial (5 immunizations); 10 x 0.5 ml. and 100 x 0.5 ml. LEDERJECT® Disposable Syringe.
COMPLETE INFORMATION FURNISHED IN THE PACKAGE.

THIOTEPA ℞
[thī̄o-tēpa]
N,N',N''-triethylenethiophosphoramide parenteral Sterile

THIOTEPA Lederle is a polyfunctional alkylating agent used in the chemotherapy of certain neoplastic diseases.

Description: Thiotepa is the ethylenimine-type compound N, N', N''-Triethylenethiophosphoramide and is available in powder form in vials which contain a sterile mixture of 15 mg. Thiotepa, 80 mg. NaCl, and 50 mg. $NaHCO_3$. Thiotepa has also been known as TESPA and TSPA and is not the same as TEPA. Thiotepa is stable in alkaline medium and unstable in acid medium. When reconstituted with Sterile Water for Injection, the resulting solution has a pH of approximately 7.6.

Action: Thiotepa is a cytotoxic agent of the polyfunctional alkylating type (more than one reactive ethylenimine group) related chemically and pharmacologically to nitrogen mustard. Its radiomimetic action is believed to occur through the release of ethylenimine radicals which, like irradiation, disrupt the bonds of DNA. One of the principal bond disruptions is initiated by alkylation of guanine at the N-7 position, which severs the linkage between the purine base and the sugar and liberates alkylated guanines. On the basis of tissue concentration studies, it is reported that Thiotepa has no differential affinity for neoplasms. Most of the drug appears to be excreted unchanged in the urine.

Indications: Thiotepa has been tried with varying results in the palliation of a wide variety of neoplastic diseases. However, the most consistent results have been seen in the following tumors:
1. Adenocarcinoma of the breast.
2. Adenocarcinoma of the ovary.
3. For controlling intracavitary effusions secondary to diffuse or localized neoplastic disease of various serosal cavities.
4. For the treatment of superficial papillary carcinoma of the urinary bladder.

While now largely superseded by other treatments, Thiotepa has been effective against other lymphomas, such as lymphosarcoma and Hodgkin's disease.

Contraindications: Therapy is probably contraindicated in cases of existing hepatic, renal, or bone-marrow damage. However, if the need overweighs the risk in such patients, Thiotepa may be used in low dosage, and accompanied by hepatic, renal, and hemopoietic function tests.
Thiotepa is contraindicated in patients with a known hypersensitivity (allergy) to this preparation.

Warnings: The administration of Thiotepa to pregnant women is not recommended except in cases where the benefit to be gained outweighs the risk of teratogenicity involved.
Thiotepa is highly toxic to the hematopoietic system. A rapidly falling white blood cell or platelet count indicates the necessity for discontinuing or reducing the dosage of Thiotepa. Weekly blood and platelet counts are recommended during therapy and for at least three weeks after therapy has been discontinued.
Thiotepa is a polyfunctional alkylating agent, capable of cross-linking the DNA within a cell and changing its nature. The replication of the cell is, therefore, altered, and Thiotepa may be described as mutagenic. An in vitro study has shown that it causes chromosomal aberrations of the chromatid type and that the frequency of induced aberrations increases with the age of the subject.
Like all alkylating agents, Thiotepa is carcinogenic. Carcinogenicity is shown most clearly in mouse studies, but there is strong circumstantial evidence of carcinogenicity in man.

Precautions: The serious complication of excessive Thiotepa therapy, or sensitivity to the effects of Thiotepa, is bone-marrow depression. If proper precautions are not observed Thiotepa may cause leukopenia, thrombocytopenia, and anemia. Death from septicemia and hemorrhage has occurred as a direct result of hematopoietic depression by Thiotepa.

It is not advisable to combine simultaneously or sequentially cancer chemotherapeutic agents or a cancer chemotherapeutic agent and a therapeutic modality having the same mechanism of action. Therefore, Thiotepa combined with other alkylating agents such as nitrogen mustard or cyclophosphamide or Thiotepa combined with irradiation would serve to intensify toxicity rather than to enhance therapeutic response. If these agents must follow each other, it is important that recovery from the first agent, as indicated by white blood cell count, be complete before therapy with the second agent is instituted.

The most reliable guide to Thiotepa toxicity is the white blood cell count. If this falls to 3000 or less, the dose should be discontinued. Another good index of Thiotepa toxicity is the platelet count; if this falls to 150,000, therapy should be discontinued. Red blood cell count is a less accurate indicator of Thiotepa toxicity.

Other drugs which are known to produce bone-marrow depression should be avoided.

There is no known antidote for overdosage with Thiotepa. Transfusions of whole blood or platelets or leukocytes have proved beneficial to the patient in combatting hematopoietic toxicity.

Adverse Reactions: Apart from its effect on the blood-forming elements, Thiotepa may cause other adverse reactions. These include pain at the site of injection, nausea, vomiting, anorexia, dizziness, headache, amenorrhea, and interference with spermatogenesis.

Febrile reaction and weeping from a subcutaneous lesion may occur as the result of breakdown of tumor tissue.

Allergic reactions are rare, but hives and skin rash have been noted occasionally. One case of alopecia has been reported. In addition, a patient who had received Thiotepa and other anticancer agents experienced prolonged apnea after succinylcholine administered prior to surgery. It was theorized that this was caused by decrease of pseudocholinesterase activity caused by the anticancer drugs.

Dosage: Parenteral routes of administration are most reliable since absorption of Thiotepa from the gastrointestinal tract is variable.

Since Thiotepa is nonvesicant, intravenous doses may be given directly and rapidly without need for slow drip or large volumes of diluent. Some physicians prefer to give Thiotepa directly into the tumor mass. This may be effected transrectally, transvaginally, or intracerebrally. The technique is discussed in the appropriate section which follows. For the control of malignant effusions, Thiotepa is instilled directly into the cavity involved. Dosage must be carefully individualized. A slow response to Thiotepa may be deceptive and may occasion unwarranted frequency of administration with subsequent signs of toxicity. After maximum benefit is obtained by initial therapy, it is necessary to continue patient on maintenance therapy (1 to 4 week intervals). In order to continue optimal effect, maintenance doses should be no more frequent than weekly in order to preserve correlation between dose and blood counts.

Initial and Maintenance Doses: Initially the higher dose in the given range is commonly administered. The maintenance dose should be adjusted weekly on the basis of pretreatment control blood counts and subsequent blood counts.

Intravenous Administration: Thiotepa may be given by rapid intravenous administration in doses of 0.3–0.4 mg/kg. Doses should be given at 1–4 week intervals.

For conversion of mg/kg of body weight to mg/M² of body surface or the reverse, a ratio of 1:30 is given as a guideline. The conversion factor varies between 1:20 and 1:40 depending on age and body build.

Intratumor Administration: Thiotepa in initial doses of 0.6–0.8 mg/kg may be injected directly into a tumor by means of a 22-gauge needle. A small amount of local anesthetic is injected first; then the syringe is removed and the Thiotepa solution is injected through the same needle. The drug is diluted in Sterile Water for injection, 10 mg per 1 ml. Maintenance doses at one to four week intervals range from 0.07 mg/kg to 0.8 mg/kg depending on the condition of the patient.

Intracavitary Administration: The dosage recommended is 0.6–0.8 mg/kg. Administration is usually effected through the same tubing which is used to remove the fluid from the cavity involved.

Intravesical Administration: Patients with papillary carcinoma of the bladder are dehydrated for 8 to 12 hours prior to treatment. Then 60 mg of Thiotepa in 30–60 ml of Sterile Water for Injection is instilled into the bladder by catheter. For maximum effect, the solution should be retained for 2 hours. If the patient finds it impossible to retain 60 ml for 2 hours, the dose may be given in a volume of 30 ml. If desired, the patient may be positioned every 15 minutes for maximum area contact. The usual course of treatment is once a week for 4 weeks. The course may be repeated if necessary, but second and third courses must be given with caution since bone-marrow depression may be increased. Deaths have occurred after intravesical administration, caused by bone-marrow depression from systemically absorbed drug.

Preparation of Solution: The powder should be reconstituted preferably in Sterile Water for Injection. The amount of diluent most often used is 1.5 ml. resulting in a drug concentration of 5 mg. in each 0.5 ml. of solution. Larger volumes are usually employed for intracavity use, intravenous drip, or perfusion therapy. The 1.5 ml. reconstituted preparation may be added to larger volumes of other diluents: Sodium Chloride Injection USP, Dextrose Injection USP, Dextrose and Sodium Chloride Injection USP, Ringer's Injection USP, or Lactated Ringer's Injection USP. Reconstituted solutions should be clear to slightly opaque but solutions that are grossly opaque or precipitated should not be used.

Since the original powder form contains 15 mg. Thiotepa, 80 mg. NaCl, 50 mg. NaHCO₃, the addition of Sterile Water for Injection produces an isotonic solution. The addition of other diluents may result in hypertonic solutions, which may cause mild to moderate discomfort on injection.

For local use into single or multiple sites, Thiotepa may be mixed with procaine HCl 2%, epinephrine HCl 1:1000, or both.

Whether in its original powder form or in reconstituted solution, Thiotepa must be stored in the refrigerator at 2°–8° C. (35–46° F.).

Reconstituted solutions may be kept for 5 days in a refrigerator without substantial loss of potency.

How Supplied: 15 mg. vials, sterile NDC 0005-4650-91.

A.H.F.S. 10:00

Shown in Product Identification Section, page 416

TriHEMIC® 600 ℞
[trī-hĕm-ĭk]
hematinic
Tablets

Description:
Each tablet contains:
Vitamin C (Ascorbic Acid) ....600 mg.
Vitamin B₁₂ (Cyanocobalamin) ....25 mcg.
Intrinsic Factor Concentrate ....75 mg.
Folic Acid (Folacin) ....1 mg.
Vitamin E (dl-Alpha
 Tocopheryl Acetate) ....30 Int. Units
Elemental Iron (as 350 mg. of
 Ferrous Fumarate) ....115 mg.
Docusate Sodium USP (DSS) ....50 mg.

Actions: TriHEMIC 600 *hematinic* is a preparation containing those ingredients essential to normal erythropoiesis, plus a stool softener to counteract the constipating effects of iron.

Indications: TriHEMIC 600 is a multiphasic preparation for use in the treatment of most megaloblastic, macrocytic and iron-deficiency anemias, in the anemias of pregnancy, in those anemias occurring in a variety of malabsorption syndromes, and those of nutritional origin. It is a useful adjuvant in patients in whom erythropoiesis is suppressed due to severe infections, malignancies or to the toxic effects of certain chemotherapeutic agents. A deficiency of Vitamin E may increase the fragility of red blood cells, with resultant enhanced hemolysis. Vitamin C is present to aid in the absorption of iron.

Warnings: Folic Acid alone is improper therapy in the treatment of pernicious anemia and other megaloblastic anemias where Vitamin B₁₂ is deficient.

Precautions: Some patients affected with pernicious anemia may not respond to orally administered Vitamin B₁₂ with intrinsic factor concentrate and there is no known way to predict which patients will respond or which patients may cease to respond. Periodic examinations and laboratory studies of pernicious anemia patients are essential and recommended.

If any symptoms of intolerance occur, the drug should be temporarily or permanently discontinued.

Folic Acid in doses above 0.1 mg. daily may obscure pernicious anemia, in that hematologic remission can occur while neurological manifestations remain progressive.

Adverse Reactions: Gastrointestinal intolerance may develop and be manifest by nausea, vomiting, diarrhea or abdominal pain. Skin rashes of various types may occur. Such reactions can necessitate temporary or permanent changes in dosage or usage.

Allergic sensitization has been reported following both oral and parenteral administration of Folic Acid.

Dosage and Administration: One tablet daily. Adjustment of dosage is dependent on patient response and the physician's clinical judgment.

How Supplied: Film coated, red; engraved LL T1 bottles of 30 tablets NDC-0005-4590-13, and 500 tablets NDC-0005-4590-31.

Shown in Product Identification Section, page 416

TRI-IMMUNOL® ℞
[trī-ĭm-u-nōl]
diphtheria and tetanus toxoids and pertussis vaccine adsorbed

How Supplied: 7.5 ml. vials. (15 immunizations).
COMPLETE INFORMATION FURNISHED IN THE PACKAGE.

ZINCON®, Improved Richer, Thicker
[zink'on]
Formula Dandruff Shampoo

(See PDR For Nonprescription Drugs)

Leeming Division
Pfizer, Inc. 100
JEFFERSON ROAD
PARSIPPANY, NJ 07054

BEN–GAY® EXTERNAL
[ben-gā']
ANALGESIC PRODUCTS

(See PDR For Nonprescription Drugs)

DESITIN® OINTMENT
[des"i-tin']

(See PDR For Nonprescription Drugs)

UNISOM® NIGHTTIME OTC
[yu'na-som]
SLEEP–AID
(doxylamine succinate)

Description: Pale blue oval scored tablets containing 25 mg. of doxylamine succinate, 2-(α-(2-dimethylaminoethoxy)α-methylbenzyl) pyridine succinate.

Action and Uses: Doxylamine succinate is an antihistamine of the ethanolamine class, which characteristically shows a high incidence of sedation. In a comparative clinical study of over 20 antihistamines on more than 3000 subjects, doxylamine succinate 25 mg. was one of the three most sedating antihistamines, producing a significantly

Continued on next page

Leeming—Cont.

reduced latency to end of wakefulness and comparing favorably with established hypnotic drugs such as secobarbital and pentobarbital in sedation activity. It was chosen as the antihistamine, based on dosage, causing the earliest onset of sleep. In another clinical study, doxylamine succinate 25 mg. scored better than secobarbital 100 mg. as a nighttime hypnotic. Two additional, identical clinical studies, involving a total of 121 subjects demonstrated that doxylamine succinate 25 mg. reduced the sleep latency period by a third, compared to placebo. Duration of sleep was 26.6% longer with doxylamine succinate, and the quality of sleep was rated higher with the drug than with placebo. An EEG study on 6 subjects confirmed the results of these studies. In yet another study, no statistically significant difference was found between doxylamine succinate and flurazepam in the average time required for 200 patients with mild to moderate insomnia to fall asleep over 5 nights following a nightly dose of doxylamine succinate 25 mg. or flurazepam 30 mg., nor was any statistically significant difference found in the total time the 200 patients slept. Patients on doxylamine succinate awoke an average of 1.2 times per night while those on flurazepam awoke an average of 0.9 times per night. In either case the patients awoke rested the following morning. On a rating scale of 1 to 5, doxylamine succinate was given a 3.0, flurazepam a 3.4 by patients rating the degree of restfulness provided by their medication (5 represents "very well rested"). Although statistically significant, the difference between doxylamine succinate 25 mg. and flurazepam 30 mg. in the number of awakenings and degree of restfulness are clinically insignificant.

Administration and Dosage: One tablet 30 minutes before retiring. Not for children under 12 years of age.

Side Effects: Occasional anticholinergic effects may be seen.

Precautions: Unisom® should be taken only at bedtime.

Contraindications: Asthma, glaucoma, enlargement of the prostate gland. This product should not be taken by pregnant women or those who are nursing a baby.

Warnings: Should be taken with caution if alcohol is being consumed. Product should not be taken if patient is concurrently on any other drug, without prior consultation with physician. Should not be taken for longer than two weeks unless approved by physician.

How Supplied: Boxes of 8, 16, 32 or 48 tablets.

Legere Pharmaceuticals, Inc.
7326 E. EVANS ROAD
SCOTTSDALE, AZ 85260

Product Number	Product Name		
1038	ACE + Z Tablets	OTC	
	Vitamin A	5000 I.U.	
	Vitamin C	1000 mg.	
	Vitamin E (Succinate)	50 I.U.	
	Magnesium (oxide)	100 mg.	
	Zinc Sulfate	100 mg.	
1066	ACETACO Tablets	℞ ⓒ	
	Acetaminophen	300 mg.	
	Codeine Phosphate	30 mg.	
046	ALLERDRYL 50 10 ml.	℞	
	Diphenhydramine HCL.	50 mg.	
005	B-COMPLEX 100 30 ml.	℞	
	Thiamine HCl	100 mg.	
	Riboflavin	5 mg.	
	Sodium Phosphate	2 mg.	
069	BROSEMA 10 ml.	℞	
	Dyphylline	250 mg.	
095	B–S–P 5 ml.	℞	
	Betamethasone Sodium Phosphate	4 mg.	
086	CEE-500 50 ml.	℞	
	Ascorbic Acid	500 mg.	
1073	CEE-1000 T.D. Tablets	OTC	
	Ascorbic Acid	1000 mg.	
055	CINALONE 40 5 ml.	℞	
	Triamcinolone Diacetate	40 mg.	
101	CINONIDE 40 5 ml.	℞	
	Triamcinolone Acetonide	40 mg.	
004	COBOLIN-M 30 ml.	℞	
	Cyanocobalamin	1000 mcg.	
062	DEPO-PREDATE 80 10 ml.	℞	
	Methylprednisolone Acetate	80 mg.	
121	DEPO-PREDATE 40 10 ml.	℞	
	Methylprednisolone Acetate	40 mg.	
010	DEXASONE 4 5 ml.	℞	
	Dexamethasone Phosphate	4 mg.	
011	DEXASONE LA 5 ml.	℞	
	Dexamethasone Acetate	8 mg.	
113	DEXASONE 10 5 ml.	℞	
	Dexamethasone Sodium Phosphate	10 mg.	
1058	DEXOL T.D. Tablets	OTC	
	Pantothenic Acid	1000 mg.	
074	DEXOL 300 30 ml.	℞	
	Dexpanthenol	300 mg.	
065	DEXTRARON-50 10 ml.	℞	
	Iron Dextran	50 mg.	
1111	DI-ATRO Tablets	℞ ⓒ	
	Diphenoxylate HCl	2.5 mg.	
	Atropine Sulfate	0.025 mg.	
1130	DIEUTRIM Capsules	℞	
	Phenylpropanolamine HCl	75 mg.	
	Benzocaine	9 mg.	
	Carboxymethylcellulose	75 mg.	
0122	DI-HYDROTIC 10 ml.	℞	
	Polymyxin B Sulfate	10,000 units	
	Neomycin Sulfate (Equiv. to Neomycin base)	3.5 mg.	
	Hydrocortisone 1%	10 mg.	
015	E-CYPIONATE 10 ml.	℞	
	Estradiol Cypionate	5 mg.	
019	ESTRONE 10 ml.	℞	
	Estrone	2 mg.	
114	KABOLIN 2 ml.	℞	
	Nandrolone Decanoate	50 mg.	
026	LIDOCAINE 1% 50 ml.	℞	
	Lidocaine Hydrochloride	10 mg.	
027	LIDOCAINE 2%	℞	
	Lidocaine Hydrochloride	20 mg.	
059	LIVOLEX 30 ml.	℞	
	Liver Vitamins and Iron		
119	MEGAPLEX I.M.	℞	
	Multi-Vitamin Injection		
117	MENAVAL 20 10 ml.	℞	
	Estradiol Valerate	20 mg.	
023	MENAVAL 40 10 ml.	℞	
	Estradiol Valerate	40 mg.	
028	MERSALYL-THEOPHYLLINE 30 ml.	℞	
	Sodium Mersalyl	100 mg.	
	Theophylline	50 mg.	
018	NATURAL ESTROGENIC SUBSTANCE	℞	
	Each ml.—2 ml. Estrone Suspension	2 mg.	
049	NEUCALM 50 10 ml.	℞	
	Hydroxyzine HCl	50 mg.	
1063	O.B. THERA Tablets	OTC	
	Pre-natal Vitamins		
031	PREDATE 50 10 ml.	℞	
	Prednisolone Acetate Suspension	50 mg.	
032	PREDATE S 10 ml.	℞	
	Prednisolone Sodium Phosphate	20 mg.	
033	PREDATE TBA 10 ml.	℞	
	Prednisolone Tebutate Suspension	20 mg.	
088	PRODROX 250 5 ml.	℞	
	Hydroxyprogesterone Caproate	250 mg.	
081	PROGESTERONE 50 10 ml.	℞	
	Progesterone	50 mg.	
034	PROMET 50 10 ml.	℞	
	Promethazine Hydrochloride	50 mg.	
1133	PT 105 Capsules	℞ ⓒ	
	Phendimetrazine	105 mg.	
1022	PHENAZINE Tablets and Capsules	℞ ⓒ	
	Phendimetrazine Tartrate	35 mg.	
1132	PROBAHIST Capsules	℞	
	Pseudoephedrine	120 mg.	
	Chlorpheniramine	8 mg.	
073	RODEX 30 ml.	℞	
	Pyridoxine HCl	100 mg.	
1037	RODEX T.D. Capsules	OTC	
	Pyridoxine	150 mg.	
054	STEMETIC 20 ml.	℞	
	Trimethobenzamide HCl	100 mg.	
039	T-CYPIONATE 10 ml.	℞	
	Testosterone Cypionate	200 mg.	
1025	TERAMINE Capsules	℞ ⓒ	
	Phentermine HCl	30 mg.	
050	TESTAVAL 90/4 10 ml.	℞	
	Testosterone Enanthate	90 mg.	
	Estradiol Valerate	4 mg.	
030	TESTOSTERONE SUSPENSION 10 ml.	℞	
	Testosterone 100 Aqueous	100 mg.	
1120	THERA-RON Tablets	OTC	
	Multi-Vitamins		
2001	VAGIMIDE CREAM 4 oz.	℞	
	Sulfanilamide	15%	
	Allantoin	2.0%	
	Aminacrine HCl	0.2%	
1044	VITABESE Capsules	OTC	
	Multi-Vitamins		

KATO® ℞
[kay'tō]
(potassium chloride for oral solution)
20 mEq. (1.5 g. KCl)

Description: KATO® (potassium chloride for oral solution) is a pleasantly flavored spray-dried tomato powder containing 20 mEq potassium (equivalent to 1.5 g KCl) per 5.7 grams of powder (one dose). KATO® is a potassium replacement product. Each daily dose (2 packets) contains approximately 0.5 mEq sodium.

Clinical Pharmacology: As the principal intracellular cation of most body tissues, potassium is instrumental in physiological processes such as maintenance of intracellular tonicity, contractility of cardiac, skeletal, and smooth muscles, maintenance of renal function, and transmission of nervous impulses.

Poassium depletion may occur when potassium intake is insufficient to compensate for potassium loss from the G.I. tract or via renal excretion. Such loss may slowly develop during prolonged oral diuretic therapy, in hyperaldosteronism, diabetic ketoacidosis, severe diarrhea, or where potassium intake is inadequate in patients receiving prolonged parenteral nutrition.

The potassium deficit is usually accompanied by chloride depletion and is manifested by hypokalemia and a hypochloremic metabolic alkalosis. Clinical symptoms and signs include weakness, fatigue, disturbances of cardiac rhythmicity (primarily ectopic beats), EKG changes (prominent U waves) and, in severe cases, flaccid paralysis and/or impaired urinary concentration.

Potassium chloride is therefore regarded as the appropriate potassium salt for use in correcting potassium depletion states associated with metabolic alkalosis.

Indications and Usage: KATO® is indicated for the treatment or prevention of potassium deficit, particularly when accompanied by hypochloremic alkalosis in conjunction with thiazide diuretic therapy, in digitalis intoxication, or as a result of long-term corticosteroid therapy, low dietary intake of potassium, or excessive vomiting or diarrhea.

Contraindication: Potassium is contraindicated in patients with: severe renal impairment involving oliguria, anuria or azotemia; untreated Addison's disease; familial periodic paralysis; acute dehydration; heat cramps; and hyperkalemia from any cause.

Warnings: Potassium intoxication may result from overdosage or from the usual therapeutic dose in patients for whom the drug is contraindicated. Hyperkalemia, when detected, must be treated immediately because lethal levels can be reached in a few hours. (See Overdosage for treatment of hyperkalemia).

Precautions

General: Patients receiving potassium supplementation should be monitored with periodic checks of plasma potassium levels.

A high plasma concentration of potassium ion may cause death through cardiac depression, arrhythmias or arrest. Therefore, the drug should be used with caution in patients with cardiac disease. The drug should not be used in patients with low urinary output or renal decompensation because of the heightened likelihood of overdosage.

In rare circumstances (e.g. patients with renal tubular acidosis) potassium depletion may be associated with a hyperchloremic metabolic acidosis. In such patients, potassium depletion is appropriately corrected using potassium salts other than the chloride.

As with other concentrated potassium supplements, KATO® must be reconstituted with the proper amount of water (2 oz. for 1 packet) to avoid the possibility of gastrointestinal irritation.

Drug Interactions: Concomitant administration of potassium chloride and a potassium-sparing diuretic (e.g. aldosterone antagonists or triamterene) can lead to severe hyperkalemia.

Adverse Reactions: Adverse reactions are related to the gastrointestinal system. Vomiting, diarrhea, nausea and abdominal discomfort may occur.

Overdosage: The symptoms and signs of potassium intoxication include paresthesias of the extremities, flaccid paralysis, listlessness, mental confusion, weakness and heaviness of the legs, fall in blood pressure, cardiac arrhythmias and heart block. Hyperkalemia may be associated with the following electrocardiographic abnormalities: disappearance of the P wave, widening and slurring of QRS complex, changes of the S-T segment and tall peaked T waves.

The drug is dialyzable.

Treatment of hyperkalemia includes: 1. Elimination of potassium-containing foods and medicaments. 2. Dextrose solution 10% or 25% containing 10 units of crystalline insulin per 20 g dextrose, given i.v. with a dose of 300 cc to 500 cc in an hour. 3. Adsorption and exchange of potassium using sodium or ammonium cycle cation exchange resin, orally or as retention enema. 4. Hemodialysis or peritoneal dialysis.

Warning: Digitalis toxicity can be precipitated by lowering the plasma potassium concentration too rapidly in digitalized patients.

Dosage and Administration: The usual adult dose is 1 packet of KATO® (20 mEq potassium) mixed with 2 ounces of cold water twice daily. If possible it should stand for 15 minutes to allow the tomato powder to absorb moisture. The preparation should be taken with meals, if convenient. If not, drink ½ glass of water immediately after taking the medication. Larger doses may be required, but should be administered under close supervision because of the possibility of potassium intoxication.

The appropriate dosage of potassium for pediatric use may be calculated from the adult dosage according to relative total body weight.

How Supplied: KATO® is available in cartons of 30 (NDC 25332-112-03) and 120 (NDC 25332-112-12) 5.7-gram unit dose packets (20 mEq potassium each). Store away from heat.

02-112-30   Rev. 3/83

Products are cross-indexed
by product classifications
in the
BLUE SECTION

Lemmon Ethical Division
Lemmon Company
SELLERSVILLE, PA 18960

ADIPEX-P® Tablets
[ăd′ĭ-pĕx]
(phentermine hydrochloride)

Description: Each tablet contains:
Phentermine Hydrochloride, 37.5 mg. (equivalent to 30 mg. of Phentermine base)

Phentermine hydrochloride is designated chemically as phenyl-tert-butylamine hydrochloride. It is a white crystalline powder, very soluble in water and alcohol.

Actions: Phentermine hydrochloride is a sympathomimetic amine with pharmacologic activity similar to the prototype drugs of this class used in obesity, the amphetamines. Actions include central nervous system stimulation and elevation of blood pressure. Tachyphylaxis and tolerance have been demonstrated with all drugs of this class in which these phenomena have been looked for.

Drugs of this class used in obesity are commonly known as "anorectics" or "anorexigenics". It has not been established, however, that the action of such drugs in treating obesity is primarily one of appetite suppression. Other central nervous system actions, or metabolic effects, may be involved, for example.

Adult obese subjects instructed in dietary management and treated with "anorectic" drugs, lose more weight on the average than those treated with placebo and diet, as determined in relatively short-term clinical trials. The magnitude of increased weight loss of drug-treated patients over placebo-treated patients is only a fraction of a pound a week. The rate of weight loss is greatest in the first weeks of therapy for both drug and placebo subjects and tends to decrease in succeeding weeks. The possible origins of the increased weight loss due to the various drug effects are not established. The amount of weight loss associated with the use of an "anorectic" drug varies from trial to trial, and the increased weight loss appears to be related in part to variables other than the drug prescribed, such as the physician-investigator, the population treated, and the diet prescribed. Studies do not permit conclusions as to the relative importance of the drug and non-drug factors on weight loss.

The natural history of obesity is measured in years, whereas, the studies cited are restricted to a few weeks duration; thus, the total impact of drug-induced weight loss over that of diet alone must be considered clinically limited.

Indications: Phentermine hydrochloride is indicated in the management of exogenous obesity as a short term adjunct (a few weeks) in a regimen of weight reduction based on caloric restriction.

The limited usefulness of agents of this class (see ACTIONS) should be measured against possible risk factors inherent in their use such as those described below.

Contraindications: Advanced arteriosclerosis, symptomatic cardiovascular disease, moderate to severe hypertension, hyperthyroidism, known hypersensitivity or idiosyncrasy to the sympathomimetic amines, glaucoma.

Agitated states.

Patients with a history of drug abuse.

During or within 14 days following the administration of monoamine oxidase inhibitors (hypertensive crisis may result).

Warnings: Tolerance to the anorectic effect usually develops within a few weeks. When this occurs, the recommended dose should not be exceeded in an attempt to increase the effect; rather, the drug should be discontinued. Phentermine hydrochloride may impair the ability of the patient to engage in potentially hazardous activities such as operating machinery or driving a motor vehicle; the patient should therefore be cautioned accordingly.

Drug Dependence: Phentermine hydrochloride is related chemically and pharmacologically to the amphetamines. Amphetamines and related stimulant drugs have been extensively abused, and the possibility of abuse of phentermine hydrochloride should be kept in mind when evaluating the desirability of including a drug as part of a weight reduction program. Abuse of amphetamines and related drugs may be associated with intense psychological dependence and severe social dysfunction. There are reports of patients who have increased the dosage to many times that recommended. Abrupt cessation following prolonged high dosage administration results in extreme fatigue and mental depression; changes are also noted in the sleep EEG. Manifestations of chronic intoxication with anorectic drugs include severe dermatoses, marked insomnia, irritability, hyperactivity, and personality changes. The most severe manifestation of chronic intoxications is psychosis, often clinically indistinguishable from schizophrenia.

Usage in Pregnancy: No reproduction studies or teratology studies of phentermine hydrochloride, in animals or humans, have been published. Therefore, use of phentermine hydrochloride by women who are or may become pregnant, requires that the potential benefit be weighed against the possible hazard to mother and infant.

Usage In Children: Phentermine hydrochloride is not recommended for use in children under 12 years of age.

Precautions: Caution is to be exercised in prescribing phentermine hydrochloride for patients with even mild hypertension.

Insulin requirements in diabetes mellitus may be altered in association with the use of phentermine hydrochloride and the concomitant dietary regimen.

Phentermine hydrochloride may decrease the hypotensive effect of guanethidine.

The least amount feasible should be prescribed or dispensed at one time in order to minimize the possibility of overdosage.

Adverse Reactions:

Cardiovascular: Palpitation, tachycardia, elevation of blood pressure.

Central Nervous System: Overstimulation, restlessness, dizziness, insomnia, euphoria, dysphoria, tremor, headache; rarely psychotic episodes at recommended doses.

Gastrointestinal: Dryness of the mouth, unpleasant taste, diarrhea, constipation, other gastrointestinal disturbances.

Allergic: Urticaria.

Endocrine: Impotence, changes in libido.

Dosage and Administration: The usual adult dose is one tablet daily, administered before breakfast or 1-2 hours after breakfast. Dosage may be adjusted to the patient's need. For some patients ½ tablet daily may be adequate, while in some cases it may be desirable to give ½ tablet two times a day.

Phentermine hydrochloride is not recommended for use in children under 12 years of age.

Overdosage: Manifestations of acute overdosage with phentermine hydrochloride include restlessness, tremor, hyperreflexia, rapid respiration, confusion, assaultive behavior hallucinations, panic states.

Fatigue and depression usually follow the central stimulation.

Cardiovascular effects include arrhythmias, hypertension or hypotension and circulatory collapse. Gastrointestinal symptoms include nausea, vomiting, diarrhea, and abdominal cramps. In fatal poisoning, death is usually preceded by convulsions and coma.

Management of acute phentermine hydrochloride intoxication is largely symptomatic and includes lavage and sedation with a barbiturate. Experience with hemodialysis or peritoneal dialysis is inadequate to permit recommendation in this regard. Acidification of the urine increases phentermine hydrochloride excretion. Intravenous phentolamine (Regitine) has been suggested for possible acute, severe hypertension, if this complicates phentermine hydrochloride overdosage.

Continued on next page

Lemmon—Cont.

How Supplied: Tablets (white with blue specks, oblong, $^{13}/_{32}''$ length, scored, engraved Lemmon /9) in bottles of 100, 400, and 1000 (NDC 0093-0009).
Also available: Capsules (blue and white, imprinted 93-019) in bottles of 100 and 400 (NDC 0093-0019).
Shown in Product Identification Section, page 417

POTAGE™   ℞
[pō-tage¹]
(potassium chloride for oral solution)
20 mEq (1.5g KCl)

Description: POTAGE is an oral potassium (K+) and chloride (Cl⁻) supplement offered as a powder for reconstitution in individual packets. Each packet contains Potassium Chloride 1.5 g (20 mEq) in a pleasant tasting Beef or Chicken flavored base. When reconstituted as directed, makes a delicious broth which is low in sodium.
How Supplied: POTAGE™ (Potassium Chloride for Oral Solution). Each 5 g packet in solution provides 20 mEq of potassium and chloride. NDC 0093-0243-56 Beef Flavor. Boxes of 30 Unit-Dose Packets. NDC 0093-0242-56 Chicken Flavor. Boxes of 30 Unit-Dose Packets.

RHUS TOX ANTIGEN™   ℞
[rūs tŏx ant-ĭ-jen]
(poison ivy extract)

Composition: Each ml. of sterile solution contains 40 mg. poison ivy extract in a 35 per cent aqueous-alcoholic menstruum, with 4 per cent benzyl alcohol to reduce pain of injection; pH adjusted with lactic acid.
Indications: For prophylaxis and treatment of rhus dermatitis.
Precautions: Attention is directed to reports that renal complications may follow extensive dermatitis of various types, and that with severe rhus dermatitis there may be an aggravation of symptoms following administration of poison ivy extract.
Dosage and Administration: Specific Treatment of Rhus Dermatitis—1 ml. intramuscularly every 12 to 24 hours until symptoms are controlled. A minimum of four injections is recommended even if symptoms are alleviated within a few hours; the tendency to future attacks will be lessened. Children usually tolerate the same dose as adults.
Prophylactic Treatment—Susceptible persons can usually be protected against attacks of rhus dermatitis for a season or longer by preseasonal injections of RHUS TOX ANTIGEN. Dose: 1 ml. intramuscularly every 4 to 7 days for four or more injections. In very sensitive individuals it may be advisable to start with a smaller dose—0.25 to 0.5 ml.—and increase the dose gradually to 1 ml., giving a total of 4 ml. or more.
Note: The patient usually complains of a burning sensation at site of the injection. This is due to the alcohol and disappears in a few seconds. In some individuals, localized soreness or a dull ache may be noted for 24 to 48 hours.
How Supplied: Boxes of four 1 ml. vials. Refrigeration not required. Full prescribing information is available on request (NDC 0093-0401).

These fine products are also available:
Acetaminophen w/Codeine   ℞ ⓒ
Capsules #3	100	NDC 0093-0152-01
	500	NDC 0093-0152-05
Capsules #4	100	NDC 0093-0172-01
Tablets #2	100	NDC 0093-0050-01
	1000	NDC 0093-0050-10
Tablets #3	100	NDC 0093-0150-01
	1000	NDC 0093-0150-10
Tablets #4	100	NDC 0093-0350-01
	1000	NDC 0093-0350-10

Beta-Val™   ℞
(betamethasone valerate)
Cream 0.1%	15 gm‡	NDC 0093-0673-15
	45 gm‡	NDC 0093-0673-95

*Cotrim™   ℞
(sulfamethoxazole with trimethoprim)
Tablets	100	NDC 0093-0188-01
	500	NDC 0093-0188-05
Double Strength Tablets	100	NDC 0093-0189-01
	500	NDC 0093-0189-05
Pediatric Suspension	16 oz	NDC 0093-0190-16

*Doxy-Lemmon™   ℞
(doxycycline hyclate)
100 mg Capsules	50	NDC 0093-0743-53
	500	NDC 0093-0743-05
50 mg Capsules	50	NDC 0093-0742-53
100 mg Tablets	50	NDC 0093-0485-53

Glucamide™
(chlorpropamide)
100 mg Tablets	100	NDC 0093-0010-01
	500	NDC 0093-0010-05
250 mg Tablets	100	NDC 0093-0007-01
	250	NDC 0093-0007-52

Indo-Lemmon™
(indomethacin)
25 mg Capsules	100	NDC 0093-0585-01
	500	NDC 0093-0585-05
50 mg Capsules	100	NDC 0093-0587-01
	500	NDC 0093-0587-05

*Metryl™
(metronidazole)
250 mg Tablets	100	NDC 0093-0551-01
	250	NDC 0093-0551-52
	500	NDC 0093-0551-05
500 mg Tablets	50	NDC 0093-0500-53

Myco-Triacet™
(nystatin, neomycin sulfate, gramicidin, triamcinolone acetonide)
Cream	15 gm‡	NDC 0093-0941-15
	30 gm‡	NDC 0093-0941-30
	60 gm‡	NDC 0093-0941-92
Ointment	15 gm‡	NDC 0093-0677-15
	30 gm	NDC 0093-0677-30

Nystatin   ℞
Oral Tablets (500,000 Units)	100	NDC 0093-0983-01
	1000	NDC 0093-0983-10
Vaginal Tablets (100,000 Units)	15	NDC 0093-0943-51
	30	NDC 0093-0943-56
Cream (100,000 Units)	15 gm‡	NDC 0093-0955-15

Otocort® Sterile Ear Drops   ℞
(neomycin sulfate, polymyxin B sulfate, hydrocortisone)
Solution	10 ml‡	NDC 0093-0047-43
Suspension	10 ml‡	NDC 0093-0363-43

* Literature available
‡ Minimum quantity shipped in shelf cartons of 12

IDENTIFICATION PROBLEM?
Consult PDR's
Product Identification Section
where you'll find over 1200
products pictured actual size
and in full color.

Eli Lilly and Company
307 E. McCARTY ST.
INDIANAPOLIS, IN 46285

LEGEND

Aspirol®—*Inhalant in an Ampoule, Lilly*
Disket®—*Dispersible Tablet, Lilly*
Enseal®—*Enteric-Release Tablet, Lilly*
Faspak™—*Flexible Plastic Bag, Lilly*
Gelseal®—*Filled Elastic Capsule, Lilly*
Identi-Code®—*Formula Identification Code, Lilly*
Identi-Dose®—*Unit Dose Medication, Lilly*
Pulvule®—*Filled Gelatin Capsule, Lilly*
Redi Vial®—*Dual Compartment Vial, Lilly*
℞Pak—*Prescription Package, Lilly*
Solvet®—*Soluble Tablet, Lilly*
Traypak™—*Multivial Carton, Lilly*

IDENTI-CODE® Index

Illustrations of examples of products bearing Identi-Code® appear in Product Identification Section.

Identi-Code®	Product Name
A01-A36 (Enseals®)	
A01	**Ammonium Chloride** Composition (Each Enseal®): Ammonium Chloride, USP, 7½ grs (486 mg)
A02	**Ferrous Sulfate** Composition (Each Enseal®): Ferrous Sulfate, USP, 5 grs (324 mg) (equiv. to 65 mg elemental iron), Red
A04	**Pancreatin** Composition (Each Enseal®): Pancreatin, Triple Strength, equivalent to 1 g Pancreatin, USP
A05	**Potassium Chloride** Composition (Each Enseal®): Potassium chloride, 300 mg
A06	**Potassium Iodide** Composition (Each Enseal®): Potassium Iodide, USP, 300 mg
A09	**Sodium Chloride** Composition (Each Enseal®): Sodium Chloride, USP, 15½ grs (1.004 g)
A10	**Sodium Salicylate** Composition (Each Enseal®): Sodium Salicylate, USP, 5 grs (324 mg)
A11	**Sodium Salicylate** Composition (Each Enseal®): Sodium Salicylate, USP, 10 grs (648 mg)
A12	**Ammonium Chloride** Composition (Each Enseal®): Ammonium Chloride, USP, 15 grs (972 mg)
A14	**Thyroid** Composition (Each Enseal®): Thyroid, USP, 30 mg
A15	**Thyroid** Composition (Each Enseal®): Thyroid, USP, 60 mg
A16	**Thyroid** Composition (Each Enseal®): Thyroid, USP, 120 mg
A17	**Thyroid** Composition (Each Enseal®): Thyroid, USP, 200 mg
A19	**Diethylstilbestrol** Composition (Each Enseal®): Diethylstilbestrol, USP, 0.1 mg
A20	**Diethylstilbestrol** Composition (Each Enseal®): Diethylstilbestrol, USP, 0.25 mg
A21	**Diethylstilbestrol** Composition (Each Enseal®): Diethylstilbestrol, USP, 0.5 mg
A22	**Diethylstilbestrol** Composition (Each Enseal®): Diethylstilbestrol, USP, 1 mg
A24	**Seconal® Sodium** Composition (Each Enseal®): Secobarbital sodium, 100 mg

for possible revisions — Product Information

- **A25** A.S.A.®
  Composition (Each Enseal®): Aspirin, USP, 5 grs (324 mg)
- **A26** Ox Bile Extract
  Composition (Each Enseal®): Ox bile extract, 5 grs (324 mg)
- **A30** Aminosalicylic Acid
  Composition (Each Enseal®): Aminosalicylic Acid, USP, 500 mg
- **A31** Potassium Chloride
  Composition (Each Enseal®): Potassium chloride, 1 g
- **A32** A.S.A.®
  Composition (Each Enseal®): Aspirin, USP, 10 grs (648 mg)
- **A33** Diethylstilbestrol
  Composition (Each Enseal®): Diethylstilbestrol, USP, 5 mg
- **A36** Ferrous Sulfate
  Composition (Each Enseal®): Ferrous Sulfate, USP, 5 grs (324 mg) (equiv. to 65 mg elemental iron), Green

C06-C71 (Coated Tablets)

- **C06** Cascara
  Composition (Each Coated Tablet): Cascara, USP, 5 grs (324 mg)
- **C07** Cascara Compound
  Composition (Each Coated Tablet): Ext. cascara, 16 mg; aloin, 16 mg; podophyllum resin, 10 mg; ext. belladonna, 8 mg (total alkaloids, 0.1 mg); oleoresin ginger, 4 mg
- **C09** Digiglusin®
  Composition (Each Coated Tablet): Digitalis glucosides, 1 USP digitalis unit
- **C11** Rhinitis, Full Strength
  Composition (Each Coated Tablet): Camphor, 32.5 mg; quinine sulfate, 32.5 mg; ext. belladonna leaf, 5.8 mg (total alkaloids, 1/960 gr)
- **C13** Ferrous Sulfate
  Composition (Each Coated Tablet): Ferrous Sulfate, USP, 5 grs (324 mg) (equiv. to 65 mg elemental iron)
- **C15** Menadione
  Composition (Each Coated Tablet): Menadione, USP, 5 mg
- **C16** Pagitane® Hydrochloride
  Composition (Each Coated Tablet): Cycrimine Hydrochloride, USP, 1.25 mg
- **C17** Pagitane® Hydrochloride
  Composition (Each Coated Tablet): Cycrimine Hydrochloride, USP, 2.5 mg
- **C27** V-Cillin K®
  Composition (Each Coated Tablet): Penicillin V Potassium, USP, 125 mg
- **C29** V-Cillin K®
  Composition (Each Coated Tablet): Penicillin V Potassium, USP, 250 mg
- **C36** Quinine Sulfate
  Composition (Each Coated Tablet): Quinine Sulfate, USP, 5 grs (324 mg)
- **C46** V-Cillin K®
  Composition (Each Coated Tablet): Penicillin V Potassium, USP, 500 mg
- **C47** Hepicebrin®
  Composition (Each Coated Tablet): Vitamin A acetate, 5000 IU (1.5 mg); vitamin D (as ergocalciferol), 400 IU (10 mcg); ascorbic acid (vitamin C), 75 mg; thiamine mononitrate (vitamin B_1), 2 mg; riboflavin (vitamin B_2), 3 mg; niacinamide, 20 mg (USP)
- **C51** Darvocet-N® 50
  Composition (Each Coated Tablet): Propoxyphene napsylate, 50 mg; acetaminophen, 325 mg (USP)
- **C53** Darvon-N®
  Composition (Each Coated Tablet): Propoxyphene Napsylate, USP, 100 mg
- **C54** Darvon-N® with A.S.A.®
  Composition (Each Coated Tablet): Propoxyphene napsylate, 100 mg; aspirin, 325 mg (USP)
- **C63** Darvocet-N® 100
  Composition (Each Coated Tablet): Propoxyphene napsylate, 100 mg; acetaminophen, 650 mg (USP)
- **C71** Multicebrin®
  Composition (Each Coated Tablet): Thiamine (vitamin B_1), 3 mg; riboflavin (vitamin B_2), 3 mg; pyridoxine (vitamin B_6), 1.2 mg; pantothenic acid, 5 mg; niacinamide, 25 mg; vitamin B_{12} (activity equivalent), 3 mcg; ascorbic acid (vitamin C), 75 mg; dl-alpha tocopheryl acetate (vitamin E), 6.6 IU (6.6 mg); vitamin A, 10,000 IU (3 mg); vitamin D, 400 IU (10 mcg)

F03-H72 (Pulvules®)

- **F03** Zentinic®
  Composition (Each Pulvule®): Iron, elemental (as ferrous fumarate), 100 mg; folic acid, 0.05 mg; thiamine mononitrate (vitamin B_1), 7.5 mg; riboflavin (vitamin B_2), 7.5 mg; pyridoxine hydrochloride (vitamin B_6), 7.5 mg; vitamin B_{12} (activity equivalent), 50 mcg; pantothenic acid (as calcium pantothenate), 15 mg; niacinamide, 30 mg; ascorbic acid (vitamin C), 200 mg
- **F04** Seromycin®
  Composition (Each Pulvule®): Cycloserine, USP, 250 mg
- **F11** A.S.A.®
  Composition (Each Pulvule®): Aspirin, USP, 5 grs (324 mg), Clear
- **F12** A.S.A.®
  Composition (Each Pulvule®): Aspirin, USP, 5 grs (324 mg), Pink
- **F13** A.S.A.® Compound
  Composition (Each Pulvule®): Aspirin, 227 mg; phenacetin, 160 mg; caffeine, 32.5 mg; White Opaque
- **F14** Ephedrine and Amytal®
  Composition (Each Pulvule®): Ephedrine sulfate, 25 mg; amobarbital, 50 mg
- **F15** Lextron®
  Composition (Each Pulvule®): Liver-stomach concentrate (as intrinsic powder), 50 mg; iron, elemental (as iron and ammonium citrates green), 30 mg; vitamin B_{12} (activity equivalent), 2 mcg; thiamine hydrochloride (vitamin B_1), 1 mg; riboflavin (vitamin B_2), 0.25 mg; with other factors of vitamin B complex present in the liver-stomach concentrate
- **F16** Lextron® Ferrous
  Composition (Each Pulvule®): Liver-stomach concentrate (as intrinsic powder), 50 mg; iron, elemental (as ferrous sulfate), 35 mg; vitamin B_{12} (activity equivalent), 2 mcg; thiamine hydrochloride (vitamin B_1), 1 mg; riboflavin (vitamin B_2), 0.25 mg; with other factors of vitamin B complex present in the liver-stomach concentrate
- **F19** Extralin®
  Composition (Each Pulvule®): Liver-stomach concentrate (as intrinsic powder), 50 mg
- **F20** Ephedrine and Seconal® Sodium
  Composition (Each Pulvule®): Ephedrine sulfate, 25 mg; secobarbital sodium, 50 mg
- **F21** Extralin® B
  Composition (Each Pulvule®): Liver-stomach concentrate (as intrinsic powder), 67 mg; vitamin B_{12} (activity equivalent), 3 mcg; thiamine hydrochloride (vitamin B_1), 1 mg; riboflavin (vitamin B_2), 0.25 mg; with other factors of vitamin B complex present in the liver-stomach concentrate
- **F22** Lextron® F. G.
  Composition (Each Pulvule®): Liver-stomach concentrate (as intrinsic powder), 50 mg; iron, elemental (as ferrous gluconate), 20 mg; vitamin B_{12} (activity equivalent), 2 mcg; thiamine hydrochloride (vitamin B_1), 1 mg; riboflavin (vitamin B_2), 0.25 mg; with other factors of vitamin B complex present in the liver-stomach concentrate
- **F23** Amytal® Sodium
  Composition (Each Pulvule®): Amobarbital Sodium, USP, 65 mg
- **F24** Ephedrine Sulfate
  Composition (Each Pulvule®): Ephedrine Sulfate, USP, 25 mg
- **F25** Ephedrine Sulfate
  Composition (Each Pulvule®): Ephedrine Sulfate, USP, 50 mg
- **F26** Quinine Sulfate
  Composition (Each Pulvule®): Quinine Sulfate, USP, 2 grs (130 mg)
- **F27** Quinine Sulfate
  Composition (Each Pulvule®): Quinine Sulfate, USP, 3 grs (194 mg)
- **F29** Quinine Sulfate
  Composition (Each Pulvule®): Quinine Sulfate, USP, 5 grs (324 mg)
- **F30** A.S.A.® Compound
  Composition (Each Pulvule®): Aspirin, 227 mg; phenacetin, 160 mg; caffeine, 32.5 mg; Pink
- **F31** Acidulin®
  Composition (Each Pulvule®): Glutamic acid hydrochloride, 340 mg
- **F32** Digitalis
  Composition (Each Pulvule®): Digitalis, USP, 100 mg
- **F33** Amytal® Sodium
  Composition (Each Pulvule®): Amobarbital Sodium, USP, 200 mg
- **F34** Carbarsone
  Composition (Each Pulvule®): Carbarsone, USP, 250 mg
- **F36** Copavin®
  Composition (Each Pulvule®): Codeine sulfate, 15 mg; papaverine hydrochloride, 15 mg
- **F39** Quinidine Sulfate
  Composition (Each Pulvule®): Quinidine Sulfate, USP, 200 mg
- **F40** Seconal® Sodium
  Composition (Each Pulvule®): Secobarbital Sodium, USP, 100 mg
- **F41** Bilron®
  Composition (Each Pulvule®): Iron bile salts, 300 mg
- **F42** Seconal® Sodium
  Composition (Each Pulvule®): Secobarbital Sodium, USP, 50 mg
- **F43** Vitamin B Complex (Betalin® Compound)
  Composition (Each Pulvule®): Thiamine (vitamin B_1), 1 mg; riboflavin (vitamin B_2), 2 mg; pyridoxine (vitamin B_6), 0.4 mg; pantothenic acid, 3.333 mg; niacinamide, 10 mg; vitamin B_{12} (activity equivalent), 1 mcg
- **F44** Ferrous Gluconate
  Composition (Each Pulvule®): Ferrous Gluconate, USP, 5 grs (324 mg)
- **F50** A.S.A.® and Codeine Compound, No. 2
  Composition (Each Pulvule®): Codeine phosphate, 15 mg; phenacetin, 150 mg; aspirin, 230 mg; caffeine, 30 mg
- **F51** A.S.A.® and Codeine Compound, No. 3
  Composition (Each Pulvule®): Codeine phosphate, 30 mg; aspirin, 380 mg; caffeine, 30 mg
- **F52** Dibasic Calcium Phosphate with Vitamin D
  Composition (Each Pulvule®): Dibasic calcium phosphate, anhydrous, equivalent to 500 mg of dibasic calcium

Continued on next page

* Identi-Code® symbol.

Lilly—Cont.

phosphate dihydrate; vitamin D synthetic, 33 IU (0.825 mcg)

F54 Dicumarol
Composition (Each Pulvule®): Dicumarol, USP, 50 mg

F56 Calcium Gluconate with Vitamin D
Composition (Each Pulvule®): Calcium gluconate, 325 mg; vitamin D synthetic, 0.825 mcg

F61 Bilron®
Composition (Each Pulvule®): Iron bile salts, 150 mg

F63 Dibasic Calcium Phosphate with Vitamin D and Iron
Composition (Each Pulvule®): Dibasic calcium phosphate, anhydrous, equivalent to 500 mg of dibasic calcium phosphate dihydrate; vitamin D, 33 IU (0.825 mcg); iron (as iron pyrophosphate), 10 mg

F64 Tuinal®
Composition (Each Pulvule®): Secobarbital sodium, 25 mg; amobarbital sodium, 25 mg (USP)

F65 Tuinal®
Composition (Each Pulvule®): Secobarbital sodium, 50 mg; amobarbital sodium, 50 mg (USP)

F66 Tuinal®
Composition (Each Pulvule®): Secobarbital sodium, 100 mg; amobarbital sodium, 100 mg (USP)

F67 A.S.A.® and Codeine Compound, No. 4
Composition (Each Pulvule®): Codeine phosphate, 60 mg; phenacetin, 150 mg; aspirin, 230 mg; caffeine, 30 mg

F71 Dicumarol
Composition (Each Pulvule®): Dicumarol, USP, 25 mg

F72 Seconal® Sodium
Composition (Each Pulvule®): Secobarbital Sodium, USP, 30 mg

F74 Tycopan®
Composition: Three Pulvules® contain thiamine mononitrate (vitamin B_1), 10 mg; riboflavin (vitamin B_2), 8 mg; pyridoxine hydrochloride (vitamin B_6), 10 mg; pantothenic acid (as calcium pantothenate), 60 mg; niacinamide, 60 mg; vitamin B_{12} (activity equivalent), 15 mcg; ascorbic acid (vitamin C), 200 mg; dl-alpha tocopheryl acetate (vitamin E), 22 IU (22 mg); biotin, 0.16 mg; folic acid, 0.45 mg; aminobenzoic acid, 33 mg; inositol, 160 mg; choline (as choline bitartrate), 160 mg; lipoic acid, 0.3 mg; vitamin A synthetic, 20,000 IU (6 mg); vitamin D synthetic, 1000 IU (25 mcg)

F92 Extralin® F
Composition (Each Pulvule®): Special Liver-Stomach Concentrate, Lilly (containing intrinsic factor), 390 mg; Cobalamin Concentrate, USP, equivalent to cobalamin, 15 mcg (the total vitamin B_{12} activity in the Special Liver-Stomach Concentrate, Lilly, and the Cobalamin Concentrate, USP, is 30 mcg); folic acid, 1 mg

F96 Reticulex®
Composition (Each Pulvule®): Liver-stomach concentrate (as intrinsic powder), 222 mg; vitamin B_{12} (activity equivalent), 10 mcg; iron, elemental (as ferrous sulfate), 75 mg; ascorbic acid (vitamin C), 50 mg; folic acid, 0.3 mg

G01 Vitamin A (Alphalin®)
Composition (Each Pulvule®): Vitamin A synthetic (palmitate), 10,000 IU (3 mg)

H02 Darvon®
Composition (Each Pulvule®): Propoxyphene Hydrochloride, USP, 32 mg

H03 Darvon®
Composition (Each Pulvule®): Propoxyphene Hydrochloride, USP, 65 mg

H04 Darvon® with A.S.A.®
Composition (Each Pulvule®): Propoxyphene hydrochloride, 65 mg; aspirin, 325 mg

H05 Darvon® Compound
Composition (Each Pulvule®): Propoxyphene hydrochloride, 32 mg; aspirin, 389 mg; caffeine, 32.4 mg

H06 Darvon® Compound-65
Composition (Each Pulvule®): Propoxyphene hydrochloride, 65 mg; aspirin, 389 mg; caffeine, 32.4 mg

H10 En-Cebrin® F
Composition (Each Pulvule®): Vitamin A synthetic, 4000 IU (1.2 mg); thiamine mononitrate (vitamin B_1), 3 mg; riboflavin (vitamin B_2), 2 mg; niacinamide, 10 mg; pyridoxine hydrochloride (vitamin B_6), 2 mg; folic acid, 1 mg; vitamin B_{12} (activity equivalent), 5 mcg; pantothenic acid (as calcium pantothenate), 5 mg; ascorbic acid (vitamin C), 50 mg; vitamin D synthetic, 400 IU (10 mcg); calcium (as the carbonate), 250 mg; iron (as ferrous fumarate), 30 mg; iodine (as potassium iodide), 0.15 mg; copper (as the sulfate), 1 mg; magnesium (as the hydroxide), 5 mg; manganese (as the glycerophosphate), 1 mg; zinc (as the chloride), 1.5 mg

H12 En-Cebrin®
Composition (Each Pulvule®): Vitamin A, 4000 IU (1.2 mg); thiamine mononitrate (vitamin B_1), 3 mg; riboflavin (vitamin B_2), 2 mg; niacinamide, 10 mg; pyridoxine (vitamin B_6), 1.7 mg; vitamin B_{12} (activity equivalent), 5 mcg; pantothenic acid, 5 mg; ascorbic acid (vitamin C), 50 mg; vitamin D, 400 IU (10 mcg); calcium (as the carbonate), 250 mg; iron (as ferrous fumarate), 30 mg; iodine (as potassium iodide), 0.15 mg; copper (as the sulfate), 1 mg; magnesium (as the hydroxide), 5 mg; manganese (as the glycerophosphate), 1 mg; zinc (as the chloride), 1.5 mg

H17 Aventyl® HCl
Composition (Each Pulvule®): Nortriptyline Hydrochloride, USP, 10 mg (equiv. to base)

H19 Aventyl® HCl
Composition (Each Pulvule®): Nortriptyline Hydrochloride, USP, 25 mg (equiv. to base)

H72 Theracebrin®
Composition (Each Pulvule®): Thiamine (as the mononitrate) (vitamin B_1), 15 mg; riboflavin (vitamin B_2), 10 mg; pyridoxine (as the hydrochloride) (vitamin B_6), 2.5 mg; pantothenic acid (as d-calcium pantothenate), 20 mg; niacinamide, 150 mg; vitamin B_{12} (activity equivalent), 10 mcg; ascorbic acid (vitamin C), 150 mg; dl-alpha tocopheryl acetate (vitamin E), 18.5 IU (18.5 mg); vitamin A synthetic, 25,000 IU (7.5 mg); vitamin D synthetic, 1500 IU (37.5 mcg)

3061 Ceclor®
Composition (Each Pulvule®): Cefaclor, USP, 250 mg

3062 Ceclor®
Composition (Each Pulvule®): Cefaclor, USP, 500 mg

3074 Hista-Clopane®
Composition (Each Pulvule®): Chlorpheniramine maleate, 4 mg; cyclopentamine hydrochloride, 12.5 mg

3075 Histadyl® and A.S.A.®
Composition (Each Pulvule®): Chlorpheniramine maleate, 4 mg; aspirin, 325 mg

---

J02-J99 (Compressed Tablets)

J02 Atropine Sulfate
Composition (Each Compressed Tablet): Atropine Sulfate, USP, 0.4 mg

J03 Belladonna Extract
Composition (Each Compressed Tablet): Belladonna Extract, USP, 15 mg ($\frac{1}{4}$ gr) (total alkaloids, 0.187 mg)

J04 Bismuth Subcarbonate
Composition (Each Compressed Tablet): Bismuth subcarbonate, 5 grs (324 mg)

J05 Citrated Caffeine
Composition (Each Compressed Tablet): Citrated caffeine, 1 gr (64.8 mg)

J09 Codeine Sulfate
Composition (Each Compressed Tablet): Codeine Sulfate, USP, 15 mg

J10 Codeine Sulfate
Composition (Each Compressed Tablet): Codeine Sulfate, USP, 30 mg

J11 Codeine Sulfate
Composition (Each Compressed Tablet): Codeine Sulfate, USP, 60 mg

J13 Colchicine
Composition (Each Compressed Tablet): Colchicine, USP, 0.6 mg

J20 Quinidine Sulfate
Composition (Each Compressed Tablet): Quinidine Sulfate, USP, 200 mg

J23 Soda Mint
Composition (Each Compressed Tablet): Sodium bicarbonate, 5 grs; oil peppermint

J24 Sodium Bicarbonate
Composition (Each Compressed Tablet): Sodium Bicarbonate, USP, 5 grs (324 mg)

J25 Thyroid
Composition (Each Compressed Tablet): Thyroid, USP, 60 mg

J26 Thyroid
Composition (Each Compressed Tablet): Thyroid, USP, 120 mg

J29 Thyroid
Composition (Each Compressed Tablet): Thyroid, USP, 30 mg

J30 Thyroid
Composition (Each Compressed Tablet): Thyroid, USP, 15 mg

J31 Phenobarbital
Composition (Each Compressed Tablet): Phenobarbital, USP, 15 mg

J32 Phenobarbital
Composition (Each Compressed Tablet): Phenobarbital, USP, 30 mg

J33 Phenobarbital
Composition (Each Compressed Tablet): Phenobarbital, USP, 100 mg

J36 Ergotrate® Maleate
Composition (Each Compressed Tablet): Ergonovine Maleate, USP, 0.2 mg

J37 Phenobarbital
Composition (Each Compressed Tablet): Phenobarbital, USP, 60 mg

J41 Niacin
Composition (Each Compressed Tablet): Niacin, USP, 20 mg

J42 Niacin
Composition (Each Compressed Tablet): Niacin, USP, 100 mg

J43 Niacin
Composition (Each Compressed Tablet): Niacin, USP, 50 mg

J45 Pyridoxine Hydrochloride (Hexa-Betalin®)
Composition (Each Compressed Tablet): Pyridoxine Hydrochloride, USP, 25 mg

Product Information

J46 Niacinamide
Composition (Each Compressed Tablet): Niacinamide, USP, 50 mg

J47 Riboflavin
Composition (Each Compressed Tablet): Riboflavin, USP, 5 mg

J49 Diethylstilbestrol
Composition (Each Compressed Tablet): Diethylstilbestrol, USP, 0.1 mg

J50 Diethylstilbestrol
Composition (Each Compressed Tablet): Diethylstilbestrol, USP, 0.25 mg

J51 Diethylstilbestrol
Composition (Each Compressed Tablet): Diethylstilbestrol, USP, 0.5 mg

J52 Diethylstilbestrol
Composition (Each Compressed Tablet): Diethylstilbestrol, USP, 1 mg

J53 Pantholin®
Composition (Each Compressed Tablet): Calcium Pantothenate, USP, 10 mg

J54 Diethylstilbestrol
Composition (Each Compressed Tablet): Diethylstilbestrol, USP, 5 mg

J56 Pyridoxine Hydrochloride (Hexa-Betalin®)
Composition (Each Compressed Tablet): Pyridoxine Hydrochloride, USP, 10 mg

J57 Crystodigin®
Composition (Each Compressed Tablet): Digitoxin, USP, 0.2 mg

J60 Crystodigin®
Composition (Each Compressed Tablet): Digitoxin, USP, 0.1 mg

J61 Papaverine Hydrochloride
Composition (Each Compressed Tablet): Papaverine Hydrochloride, USP, 30 mg

J62 Papaverine Hydrochloride
Composition (Each Compressed Tablet): Papaverine Hydrochloride, USP, 60 mg

J63 Riboflavin
Composition (Each Compressed Tablet): Riboflavin, USP, 10 mg

J64 Dolophine® Hydrochloride
Composition (Each Compressed Tablet): Methadone Hydrochloride, USP, 5 mg

J69 Propylthiouracil
Composition (Each Compressed Tablet): Propylthiouracil, USP, 50 mg

J72 Dolophine® Hydrochloride
Composition (Each Compressed Tablet): Methadone Hydrochloride, USP, 10 mg

J73 Methyltestosterone
Composition (Each Compressed Tablet): Methyltestosterone, USP, 10 mg

J74 Methyltestosterone
Composition (Each Compressed Tablet): Methyltestosterone, USP, 25 mg

J75 Crystodigin®
Composition (Each Compressed Tablet): Digitoxin, USP, 0.05 mg

J76 Crystodigin®
Composition (Each Compressed Tablet): Digitoxin, USP, 0.15 mg

J94 Tapazole®
Composition (Each Compressed Tablet): Methimazole, USP, 5 mg

J95 Tapazole®
Composition (Each Compressed Tablet): Methimazole, USP, 10 mg

J96 Tylosterone®
Composition (Each Compressed Tablet): Diethylstilbestrol, 0.25 mg; methyltestosterone, 5 mg

J97 Paveril® Phosphate
Composition (Each Compressed Tablet): Dioxyline phosphate, 100 mg

J99 Sandril®
Composition (Each Compressed Tablet): Reserpine, USP, 0.1 mg

S05-S17 (Suppositories)

S05 Seconal® Sodium
Composition (Each Suppository): Secobarbital sodium, 120 mg

S07 Diethylstilbestrol
Composition (Each Suppository): Diethylstilbestrol, USP, 0.1 mg

S09 Diethylstilbestrol
Composition (Each Suppository): Diethylstilbestrol, USP, 0.5 mg

S11 Seconal® Sodium
Composition (Each Suppository): Secobarbital sodium, 200 mg

S13 Surfacaine®
Composition (Each Suppository): Cyclomethycaine Sulfate, USP, 10 mg

S14 Seconal® Sodium
Composition (Each Suppository): Secobarbital sodium, 60 mg

S15 A.S.A.®
Composition (Each Suppository): Aspirin, USP, 5 grs (324 mg)

S16 A.S.A.®
Composition (Each Suppository): Aspirin, USP, 10 grs (648 mg)

S17 Seconal® Sodium
Composition (Each Suppository): Secobarbital sodium, 30 mg

T01-U56 (Compressed Tablets)

T01 Zentron® Chewable
Composition (Each Compressed Tablet): Iron, elemental (as ferrous fumarate), 20 mg; thiamine mononitrate (vitamin B_1), 1 mg; riboflavin (vitamin B_2), 1 mg; pyridoxine hydrochloride (vitamin B_6), 1 mg; cyanocobalamin (vitamin B_{12} crystalline), 5 mcg; pantothenic acid (as panthenol), 1 mg; niacinamide, 5 mg; ascorbic acid (vitamin C), 100 mg

T05 A.S.A.®
Composition (Each Compressed Tablet): Aspirin, USP, 5 grs (324 mg)

T06 A.S.A.®
Composition (Each Compressed Tablet): Aspirin, USP, 5 grs (324 mg), Pink

T07 A.S.A.® Compound
Composition (Each Compressed Tablet): Aspirin, 227 mg; phenacetin, 160 mg; caffeine, 32.5 mg

T13 Calcium Lactate
Composition (Each Compressed Tablet): Calcium Lactate, USP, 5 grs (324 mg)

T14 Calcium Lactate
Composition (Each Compressed Tablet): Calcium Lactate, USP, 10 grs (648 mg)

T20 Methenamine
Composition (Each Compressed Tablet): Methenamine, USP, 7½ grs (500 mg)

T21 Methenamine and Sodium Biphosphate
Composition (Each Compressed Tablet): Methenamine, 325 mg; sodium biphosphate, 325 mg (USP)

T23 Sodium Chloride
Composition (Each Compressed Tablet): Sodium Chloride, USP, 2.25 g

T24 Sodium Chloride
Composition (Each Compressed Tablet): Sodium Chloride, USP, 1 g

T26 Pancreatin
Composition (Each Compressed Tablet): Pancreatin, Single Strength, equivalent to 325 mg Pancreatin, USP

T29 Sodium Bicarbonate
Composition (Each Compressed Tablet): Sodium Bicarbonate, USP, 10 grs (648 mg)

T32 Amytal®
Composition (Each Compressed Tablet): Amobarbital, USP, 100 mg

T35 Calcium Carbonate
Composition (Each Compressed Tablet): Calcium Carbonate, USP, Aromatic, 10 grs (648 mg)

T36 Calcium Gluconate
Composition (Each Compressed Tablet): Calcium Gluconate, USP, 1 g

T37 Amytal®
Composition (Each Compressed Tablet): Amobarbital, USP, 50 mg

T39 Calcium Gluconate
Composition (Each Compressed Tablet): Calcium Gluconate, USP, 7½ grs (486 mg)

T40 Amytal®
Composition (Each Compressed Tablet): Amobarbital, USP, 15 mg

T42 A.S.A.® and Codeine Compound, No. 2
Composition (Each Compressed Tablet): Codeine phosphate, 15 mg; aspirin, 230 mg; phenacetin, 150 mg; caffeine, 30 mg

T44 Calcium Gluconate with Vitamin D
Composition (Each Compressed Tablet): Calcium gluconate, 1 g; vitamin D synthetic, 1.65 mcg

T45 Vitamin C (Cevalin®)
Composition (Each Compressed Tablet): Ascorbic Acid, USP, 100 mg

T46 Sulfapyridine
Composition (Each Compressed Tablet): Sulfapyridine, USP, 0.5 g

T49 A.S.A.® and Codeine Compound, No. 3
Composition (Each Compressed Tablet): Codeine phosphate, 30 mg; aspirin, 380 mg; caffeine, 30 mg

T50 A.S.A.® Compound
Composition (Each Compressed Tablet): Aspirin, 227 mg; phenacetin, 160 mg; caffeine, 32.5 mg; Pink

T52 Thiamine Hydrochloride (Betalin® S)
Composition (Each Compressed Tablet): Thiamine Hydrochloride, USP, 10 mg

T53 Niacinamide
Composition (Each Compressed Tablet): Niacinamide, USP, 100 mg

T54 Sulfadiazine
Composition (Each Compressed Tablet): Sulfadiazine, USP, 0.5 g

T55 Papaverine Hydrochloride
Composition (Each Compressed Tablet): Papaverine Hydrochloride, USP, 100 mg

T56 Amytal®
Composition (Each Compressed Tablet): Amobarbital, USP, 30 mg

T59 Thiamine Hydrochloride (Betalin® S)
Composition (Each Compressed Tablet): Thiamine Hydrochloride, USP, 25 mg

T60 Vitamin C (Cevalin®)
Composition (Each Compressed Tablet): Ascorbic Acid, USP, 250 mg

T61 Dibasic Calcium Phosphate
Composition (Each Compressed Tablet): Dibasic calcium phosphate, anhydrous, equivalent to 7½ grs (486 mg) of dibasic calcium phosphate dihydrate (USP)

T62 Thiamine Hydrochloride (Betalin® S)
Composition (Each Compressed Tablet): Thiamine Hydrochloride, USP, 50 mg

Continued on next page

* Identi-Code® symbol.

Lilly—Cont.

T63 **Thiamine Hydrochloride (Betalin® S)**
Composition (Each Compressed Tablet): Thiamine Hydrochloride, USP, 100 mg

T67 **Vitamin C (Cevalin®)**
Composition (Each Compressed Tablet): Ascorbic Acid, USP, 500 mg

T72 **Pyridoxine Hydrochloride (Hexa-Betalin®)**
Composition (Each Compressed Tablet): Pyridoxine Hydrochloride, USP, 50 mg

T73 **Papaverine Hydrochloride**
Composition (Each Compressed Tablet): Papaverine Hydrochloride, USP, 200 mg

T75 **Neotrizine®**
Composition (Each Compressed Tablet): Sulfadiazine, 167 mg; sulfamerazine, 167 mg sulfamethazine, 167 mg (USP)

T91 **Paveril® Phosphate**
Composition (Each Compressed Tablet): Dioxyline phosphate, 200 mg

T93 **Isoniazid**
Composition (Each Compressed Tablet): Isoniazid, USP, 100 mg

T96 **Neomycin Sulfate**
Composition (Each Compressed Tablet): Neomycin Sulfate, USP, 500 mg (equiv. to 350 mg base)

T99 **Haldrone®**
Composition (Each Compressed Tablet): Paramethasone Acetate, USP, 1 mg

---

U01 **Haldrone®**
Composition (Each Compressed Tablet): Paramethasone Acetate, USP, 2 mg

U03 **Dymelor®**
Composition (Each Compressed Tablet): Acetohexamide, USP, 250 mg

U07 **Dymelor®**
Composition (Each Compressed Tablet): Acetohexamide, USP, 500 mg

U09 **Anhydron®**
Composition (Each Compressed Tablet): Cyclothiazide, USP, 2 mg

U23 **Isoniazid**
Composition (Each Compressed Tablet): Isoniazid, USP, 300 mg

U29 **Reserpine (Sandril®)**
Composition (Each Compressed Tablet): Reserpine, USP, 0.25 mg

U53 **Methadone Hydrochloride**
Composition (Each Disket®): Methadone Hydrochloride, USP, 40 mg

U56 **Folic Acid**
Composition (Each Compressed Tablet): Folic Acid, USP, 1 mg

W07-W16 (Miscellaneous)

W07 **V-Cillin K®, for Oral Solution**
Composition (When Mixed as Directed): Each 5 ml contain penicillin V potassium equivalent to penicillin V, 125 mg (USP).

W16 **V-Cillin K®, for Oral Solution**
Composition (When Mixed as Directed): Each 5 ml contain penicillin V potassium equivalent to penicillin V, 250 mg (USP).

5057 **Ceclor®, for Oral Suspension**
Composition (When Mixed as Directed): Each 5 ml contain cefaclor, 125 mg (USP).

5058 **Ceclor®, for Oral Suspension**
Composition (When Mixed as Directed): Each 5 ml contain cefaclor, 250 mg (USP).

UNIT-DOSE PACKAGING

Dispenser Strip
Identi-Dose® (unit dose medication, Lilly)
Reverse-Numbered Package
Closed-circuit control of medication from pharmacy to nurse to patient and return. Simplifies counting and dispensing whether in single-unit or prescription-size quantities. Fits into any dispensing system for ready identification and legibility, better inventory control, protection from contamination, easier handling and recording under Medicare, prevention of drug loss through pilferage or spilling, better control of Federal Controlled Substances, and less chance of medication errors.
The following products are available through normal channels of supply:

Dispenser Strip
Pulvules®
No.
ⓒ 303 Tuinal®, 100 mg
Identi-Dose® (ID100)
Pulvules®
No.
ⓒ 240 Seconal® Sodium, 100 mg
ⓒ 303 Tuinal®, 100 mg
ⓒ 304 Tuinal®, 200 mg
ⓒ 364 Darvon®, 32 mg
ⓒ 365 Darvon®, 65 mg
ⓒ 369 Darvon® Compound-65
387 Aventyl® HCl, 10 mg
389 Aventyl® HCl, 25 mg
3061 Ceclor®, 250 mg
3062 Ceclor®, 500 mg
Tablets
No.
55 Hepicebrin®
100 Multicebrin®
186 A.S.A.®, 5 grs
ⓒ 558 Codeine Sulfate, USP, 30 mg
1125 Quinidine Sulfate, USP, 200 mg
ⓒ 1544 Phenobarbital, USP, 15 mg
ⓒ 1545 Phenobarbital, USP, 30 mg
ⓒ 1546 Phenobarbital, USP, 100 mg
1572 Ergotrate® Maleate, 0.2 mg
ⓒ 1574 Phenobarbital, USP, 60 mg
1671 Papaverine Hydrochloride, USP, 100 mg
1703 Crystodigin®, 0.1 mg, Pink
1803 Neomycin Sulfate, USP, 500 mg
1842 Dymelor®, 250 mg
1843 Dymelor®, 500 mg, Yellow
ⓒ 1883 Darvon-N®, 100 mg
ⓒ 1890 Darvocet-N® 50
ⓒ 1893 Darvocet-N® 100
Miscellaneous
M-126 V-Cillin K®, for Oral Solution, 125 mg
M-142 V-Cillin K®, for Oral Solution, 250 mg
Reverse-Numbered Package (RN500)
Pulvules®
No.
ⓒ 365 Darvon®, 65 mg
Tablets
No.
ⓒ 1893 Darvocet-N® 100
Single-Cut Identi-Dose® (ID500)
Tablets
No.
ⓒ 1893 Darvocet-N® 100

ⓒ, ⓒ, ⓒ Federal Controlled Substances.

ACIDULIN®   OTC
[ă-sĭd'ū-lĭn]
(glutamic acid hydrochloride)

Description: Each Pulvule® contains 340 mg glutamic acid hydrochloride and is equivalent to about 10 minims of Diluted Hydrochloric Acid, USP, or to about 16.8 ml of 0.1 N hydrochloric acid.
Hydrochloric acid deficiency can be corrected easily and safely with Pulvules Acidulin. The Pulvule form, unlike solutions, is tasteless, cannot injure mucous membranes or teeth, and is safe and convenient for the patient to carry when traveling or dining out.
Indications: Acidulin is administered to counterbalance deficiency of hydrochloric acid in the gastric juice and to destroy or inhibit the growth of putrefactive microorganisms in ingested food. A deficiency of hydrochloric acid is often associated with pernicious anemia, gastric carcinoma, congenital achlorhydria, and allergy.
Contraindications: Should not be used if gastric hyperacidity or peptic ulcers are present.
Dosage: 1 to 3 Pulvules three times daily before meals, or as directed by the physician.
Overdosage: *Symptoms*—Massive overdosage may produce systemic acidosis. *Treatment*—Alkalies, such as sodium bicarbonate or sodium r-lactate solution, one molar (to be diluted).
How Supplied: Pulvules No. 213, Acidulin® (glutamic acid hydrochloride, Lilly), F31,*340 mg (No. 1, Pink), in bottles of 100 (NDC 0002-0631-02) and 1000 (NDC 0002-0631-04).

[101582]

AEROLONE® SOLUTION   ℞
[ār'ō-lōn sō-lū'shŭn]
(isoproterenol hydrochloride inhalation)
(Not USP)

Description: Aerolone® Solution (isoproterenol hydrochloride inhalation, Lilly) is a bronchodilator. Each 100 ml contain isoproterenol hydrochloride, 0.25 g, with propylene glycol, ascorbic acid, coloring, and purified water, q.s. Sodium hydroxide is added during manufacture to adjust the p_H.
This product differs from the USP Inhalation in that it contains 80 percent propylene glycol by volume instead of purified water and it is not isotonic.
Actions: Isoproterenol is an adrenergic (sympathomimetic) agent and relieves bronchospasm by relaxing the smooth muscle of the bronchioles.
Indications: Aerolone® Solution (isoproterenol hydrochloride inhalation, Lilly) is indicated for the treatment of bronchospasm associated with acute and chronic bronchial asthma, pulmonary emphysema, bronchitis, and bronchiectasis.
Contraindications: Aerolone® Solution (isoproterenol hydrochloride inhalation, Lilly) is contraindicated in patients with (1) known hypersensitivity to isoproterenol or (2) cardiac arrhythmia associated with tachycardia.
Warnings: Occasional patients have been reported to develop severe paradoxical airway resistance with repeated excessive use of isoproterenol inhalation preparations. The cause of this refractory state is unknown. It is advisable that, in such instances, the use of this preparation be discontinued immediately and alternative therapy instituted, since in the reported cases the patients did not respond to other forms of therapy until the drug was withdrawn.
Deaths have been reported following excessive use of isoproterenol inhalation preparations, and the exact cause is unknown. Cardiac arrest was noted in several instances.
Usage in Pregnancy—Safe use during pregnancy has not been established relative to possible adverse effects on fetal development. Therefore, Aerolone Solution should not be used in pregnant women unless, in the judgment of the physician, the potential benefits outweigh the possible hazards.
Precautions: Aerolone® Solution (isoproterenol hydrochloride inhalation, Lilly) should be used with caution in patients having serious cardiac disease, hypertension, or hyperthy- roidism.
Adverse Reactions: Rarely, insomnia, nervousness, vertigo, tachycardia, and palpitation may occur.
Dosage and Administration: For use by aerosol only. The technique is the same as that for administering epinephrine, 1:100. A nebulizer which produces a fine mist is necessary. The mist is inhaled through the mouth, and the breath is held in momentarily. Usually, 6 to 12 inhalations will bring adequate relief. Mild cases may require only one treatment per day; severe cases may need the treatment repeatedly at intervals of 15 minutes. If relief is not noticeable after three such treatments at 15-minute intervals, consult a physician. Ordinarily, the number of such treatments for re-

peated attacks should not exceed eight per 24 hours.

Physicians prescribing isoproterenol for use in inhalation therapy equipment should bear in mind the fact that different dosages of medication are delivered into the patient's airways depending on the proficiency of the therapist and the type of inhalator used.

Proficiency in the use of any of these devices can be gained only by firsthand experience. Furthermore, some equipment can deliver 100 percent of the medication deep into the airways, whereas other inhalators may deliver considerably less than the prescribed dose. The number of inhalations per treatment and the frequency of re-treatment should, therefore, be titrated to the patient's response.

Overdosage: *Symptoms*—Insomnia, nervousness, vertigo, tachycardia, and palpitation resulting from CNS stimulation.

Treatment—No specific treatment; general management consists in controlling symptoms of CNS stimulation by the use of sedatives, such as the barbiturates.

How Supplied: (℞) *Solution No. 50, Aerolone* Solution (isoproterenol hydrochloride inhalation, Lilly), in 1-fl-oz bottles (NDC 0002-2605-67).

[090783]

AMYTAL®
[ăm′ ĭ-tăl]
(amobarbital)

WARNING: MAY BE HABIT-FORMING

Description: Amytal® (amobarbital, Lilly) is a white, crystalline powder that is odorless, has a bitter taste, and is hygroscopic. It is very slightly soluble in water, soluble in alcohol, ether, and chloroform. Amytal is 5-ethyl-5-isopentylbarbiturate and has the empirical formula $C_{11}H_{18}N_2O_3$. Amytal is available as tablets and elixir for oral administration. The scored tablets contain 15 mg, 30 mg, 50 mg, or 100 mg amobarbital, and the elixir, 880 mg/100 ml.

Clinical Pharmacology: Amobarbital, a short-acting barbiturate, is a central-nervous-system depressant. It is a rapid-acting sedative and hypnotic, with a duration of effect ranging from eight to 11 hours. It is detoxified in the liver.

Indications and Usage: Amytal® (amobarbital, Lilly) is indicated in any conditions that require degrees of sedation ranging from minimum doses for the relief of anxiety and tension to hypnotic doses for preanesthetic medication.

Contraindications: Amytal® (amobarbital, Lilly) is contraindicated in patients who are hypersensitive to barbiturates. It is also contraindicated in patients with a history of manifest or latent porphyria, marked impairment of liver function, or respiratory disease in which dyspnea or obstruction is evident. It should not be administered to persons with known previous addiction to sedative/hypnotics, since ordinary doses may be ineffectual and may contribute to further addiction. Amytal should not be administered in the presence of acute or chronic pain, because paradoxical excitement may be induced or important symptoms may be masked.

Precautions: *General Precautions* — Barbiturates induce liver microsomal enzyme activity. This accelerates the biotransformation of various drugs and is probably part of the mechanism of the tolerance encountered with barbiturates. Amytal® (amobarbital, Lilly) should, therefore, be used with caution in patients with decreased liver function. This drug should also be administered cautiously to patients with a history of drug dependence or abuse (see Drug Abuse and Dependence). Amytal may decrease the potency of coumarin anticoagulants; therefore, patients receiving such concomitant therapy should have more frequent prothrombin determinations.

As with other sedatives and hypnotics, elderly or debilitated patients may react to barbiturates with marked excitement or depression.

The systemic effects of exogenous hydrocortisone and endogenous hydrocortisone (cortisol) may be diminished by Amytal. Thus, this product should be administered with caution to patients with borderline hypoadrenal function, regardless of whether it is of pituitary or of primary adrenal origin.

Information for Patients—Amytal may impair the mental and/or physical abilities required for the performance of potentially hazardous tasks, such as driving a car or operating machinery. The patient should be cautioned accordingly.

Drug Interactions—Amytal in combination with alcohol, tranquilizers, and other central-nervous-system depressants has additive depressant effects, and the patient should be so advised. Patients taking this drug should be warned not to exceed the dosage recommended by their physician. Toxic effects and fatalities have occurred following overdoses of Amytal alone and in combination with other central-nervous-system depressants. Caution should be exercised in prescribing unnecessarily large amounts of Amytal for patients who have a history of emotional disturbances or suicidal ideation or who have misused alcohol and other CNS drugs (see Overdosage).

Usage in Pregnancy—*Pregnancy Category B*—Reproduction studies have been performed in animals and have revealed no evidence of impaired fertility or harm to the fetus due to Amytal. There are, however, no adequate and well-controlled studies in pregnant women. Because animal reproduction studies are not always predictive of human response, this drug should be used during pregnancy only if clearly needed.

Nursing Mothers—Caution should be exercised when Amytal is administered to a nursing woman.

Usage in Children—Safety and effectiveness have not been established in children below the age of six years.

Adverse Reactions: Idiosyncrasy, in the form of excitement, hangover, or pain, may appear. Hypersensitivity reactions occur in some patients, especially in those with asthma, urticaria, or angioneurotic edema.

Drug Abuse and Dependence: *Controlled Substance*—Amytal® (amobarbital, Lilly) is a Schedule II drug.

Dependence—Prolonged, uninterrupted use of barbiturates (particularly the short-acting drugs), even in therapeutic doses, may result in psychic and physical dependence. Withdrawal symptoms due to physical dependence following chronic use of large doses of barbiturates may include delirium, convulsions, and death.

Overdosage: *Symptoms*— The manifestations of overdosage are early hypothermia followed by fever, sluggish or absent reflexes, respiratory depression, gradual appearance of circulatory collapse, pulmonary edema, and coma.

Treatment—General management should consist in symptomatic and supportive therapy, including gastric lavage, administration of intravenous fluids, and maintenance of blood pressure, body temperature, and adequate respiratory exchange. Dialysis will increase the rate of removal of barbiturates from the body fluids. Antibiotics may be required to control pulmonary complications.

Dosage and Administration: Because of the wide variation in individual response to the barbiturates, the dosage range is relatively great, and doses must be individualized for each patient. The adult dosage range for daytime sedation may be from 15 to 120 mg two to four times a day. However, the usual adult dosage for daytime sedation is 30 to 50 mg two or three times a day. Dosage may be adjusted to relieve tension and anxiety without significant loss of mental acuity. The usual adult hypnotic dose is 100 to 200 mg. On occasion, a larger dose may be necessary to produce the desired degree of hypnosis.

How Supplied: ⓒ *Elixir No. 237, Amytal®* (amobarbital, Lilly), 880 mg/100 ml (Not USP), in 16-fl-oz bottles (NDC 0002-2441-05). Alcohol, 34 percent. This product differs from the USP elixir in that it contains a greater proportion of alcohol than the USP drug.

(ⓒ) *Tablets Amytal®* (Amobarbital Tablets, USP) (scored): *No. 1678, T56,* *30 mg, Yellow, in bottles of 100 (NDC 0002-2056-02); *No. 1550, T37,* *50 mg, Orange, in bottles of 100 (NDC 0002-2037-02); *No. 1462, T32,* *100 mg, Pink, in bottles of 100 (NDC 0002-2032-02).

[012083]

Shown in Product Identification Section, page 417

AMYTAL® SODIUM   ⓒ
[ăm′ ĭ-tăl sō′ dĭ-ŭm]
(amobarbital sodium)
Sterile, USP
VIALS

WARNING: MAY BE HABIT-FORMING

Caution: These products are to be used by the physician or under his direction. The intravenous administration of Amytal Sodium carries with it the potential dangers inherent in the intravenous use of any potent hypnotic.

Description: Amytal Sodium is a white, friable, granular powder that is odorless, has a bitter taste, and is hygroscopic. It is very soluble in water, soluble in alcohol, and practically insoluble in ether and chloroform. Amytal Sodium is sodium-5-ethyl-5-isopentylbarbiturate and has the empirical formula $C_{11}H_{17}N_2NaO_3$.

Vials Amytal® Sodium (Sterile Amobarbital Sodium, USP, Lilly) are for parenteral administration. The vials contain 250 mg or 0.5 g sterile amobarbital sodium.

Clinical Pharmacology: Amobarbital sodium, a short-acting barbiturate, is a central-nervous-system depressant. It is a rapid-acting sedative and hypnotic, with a duration of effect ranging from eight to 11 hours. It is detoxified in the liver.

Indications and Usage: Amytal® Sodium (amobarbital sodium, Lilly) may be used intravenously or intramuscularly for the control of convulsive seizures such as may be due to chorea, eclampsia, meningitis, tetanus, procaine or cocaine reactions, or poisoning from such drugs as strychnine or picrotoxin. It may be administered for the management of catatonic and negativistic reactions, manic reactions, and epileptiform seizures. It is also useful in narcoanalysis and narcotherapy and as a diagnostic aid in schizophrenia.

Contraindications: Amytal® Sodium (amobarbital sodium, Lilly) is contraindicated in patients who are hypersensitive to barbiturates. It is also contraindicated in patients with a history of manifest or latent porphyria, marked impairment of liver function, or respiratory disease in which dyspnea or obstruction is evident. It should not be administered to persons with known previous addiction to the sedative/hypnotic group, since ordinary doses may be ineffectual and may contribute to further addiction. Amytal Sodium should not be administered in the presence of acute or chronic pain, because paradoxical excitement may be induced or important symptoms may be masked.

Warnings: The rate of intravenous injection must not exceed 1 ml/minute.

Either too-rapid injection or relative overdosage may cause apnea or hypotension. Respiratory depression is more likely to occur if other central-nervous-system agents have been used concurrently.

The maximum single dose should not exceed 1 g in adult patients. The maximum intramuscular dose should not exceed 0.5 g. No greater volume than 5 ml, irrespective of drug concentration, should be injected intramuscularly at any one site.

Several minutes may be required for the drug to dissolve completely, but under no circumstances should a solution be injected if it has not become absolutely clear within five min- utes' time. Also, a solution that forms a precipitate after clearing should not be used. Amytal Sodium hydrolyzes in solution or upon exposure to air. Not more than 30 minutes should elapse from the time the vial is opened until its contents are injected. Amytal Sodium supplied in capsules should not be used for injection purposes.

Continued on next page

* Identi-Code® symbol.

Lilly—Cont.

Precautions: *General Precautions*—Barbiturates induce liver microsomal enzyme activity. This accelerates the biotransformation of various drugs and is probably part of the mechanism of the tolerance encountered with barbiturates. Amytal Sodium should, therefore, be used with caution in patients with decreased liver function. This drug should also be administered cautiously to patients with a history of drug dependence or abuse (*see* Drug Abuse and Dependence). Amytal Sodium may decrease the potency of coumarin anticoagulants; therefore, patients receiving such concomitant therapy should have more frequent prothrombin determinations.

As with other sedatives and hypnotics, elderly or debilitated patients may react to barbiturates with marked excitement or depression.

The systemic effects of exogenous hydrocortisone and endogenous hydrocortisone (cortisol) may be diminished by Amytal® Sodium (amobarbital sodium, Lilly). Thus, this product should be administered with caution to patients with borderline hypoadrenal function, regardless of whether it is of pituitary or of primary adrenal origin.

Information for the Patients—Amytal Sodium may impair the mental and/or physical abilities required for the performance of potentially hazardous tasks, such as driving a car or operating machinery. The patient should be cautioned accordingly.

Drug Interactions—Amytal Sodium in combination with alcohol, tranquilizers, and other central-nervous-system depressants has additive depressant effects, and the patient should be so advised. Patients taking this drug should be warned not to exceed the dosage recommended by their physician. Toxic effects and fatalities have occurred following overdoses of Amytal Sodium alone and in combination with other central-nervous-system depressants. Caution should be exercised in prescribing unnecessarily large amounts of Amytal Sodium for patients who have a history of emotional disturbances or suicidal ideation or who have misused alcohol and other CNS drugs (*see* Overdosage).

Usage in Pregnancy—Pregnancy Category B—Reproduction studies have been performed in animals and have revealed no evidence of impaired fertility or harm to the fetus due to Amytal Sodium. There are, however, no adequate and well-controlled studies in pregnant women. Because animal reproduction studies are not always predictive of human response, this drug should be used during pregnancy only if clearly needed.

Labor and Delivery—Depression has been noted in infants born following the use of Amytal Sodium during labor.

Nursing Mothers—Caution should be exercised when Amytal Sodium is administered to a nursing woman.

Usage in Children—Safety and effectiveness have not been established in children below the age of six years.

Adverse Reactions: In the general use of barbiturates by the intravenous route, respiratory depression is the most serious side effect.

Idiosyncrasy, in the form of excitement, hangover, or pain, may appear. Hypersensitivity reactions occur in some patients, especially in those with asthma, urticaria, or angioneurotic edema. Laryngospasm may develop during normal induction or as a result of improper dosage. Rapid intravenous administration may also induce vasodilation and some fall in blood pressure.

Nausea and vomiting, postoperative atelectasis, and circulatory disturbances are uncommon. When they occur, they are usually due to overdosage or extraneous factors. Embolism has not been reported following intravenous use of Amytal® Sodium (amobarbital sodium, Lilly).

Drug Abuse and Dependence: *Controlled Substance*—Amytal® Sodium (amobarbital sodium, Lilly) is a Schedule II drug.

Dependence—Prolonged, uninterrupted use of barbiturates (particularly the short-acting drugs), even in therapeutic doses, may result in psychic and physical dependence. Withdrawal symptoms due to physical dependence following chronic use of large doses of barbiturates may include delirium, convulsions, and death.

Overdosage: *Symptoms*—The manifestations of overdosage are early hypothermia followed by fever, sluggish or absent reflexes, respiratory depression, gradual appearance of circulatory collapse, pulmonary edema, and coma. *Treatment*—General management should consist in symptomatic and supportive therapy, including gastric lavage, administration of intravenous fluids, and maintenance of blood pressure, body temperature, and adequate respiratory exchange. Dialysis will increase the rate of removal of barbiturates from the body fluids. Antibiotics may be required to control pulmonary complications.

Dosage and Administration: Solutions of Amytal® Sodium (amobarbital sodium, Lilly) should be made up aseptically with Sterile Water for Injection. The accompanying table will aid in preparing solutions of various concentrations. Ordinarily, a 10 percent solution is used; the maximum single dose for an adult is 1 g. After Sterile Water for Injection is added, the vial should be rotated to facilitate solution of the powder. **Do not shake the vial.**

[See table below].

Intramuscular Use—No more than 5 ml should be injected at any one site. Depositions should be made deeply in large muscles, such as the gluteus maximus. Superficial intramuscular or subcutaneous injections may be painful and may produce sterile abscesses or sloughs.

The average intramuscular dose ranges from 65 mg to 0.5 g. Twenty percent solutions may be used so that a small volume can contain a large dose.

Intravenous Use—The rate of intravenous injection should not exceed 1 ml/minute. When the 10 percent solution is used, faster rates of administration may precipitate serious respiratory depression. Because of their higher metabolic rate, children tolerate comparatively larger doses. The final dosage is determined to a great extent by the patient's reaction to the slow administration of the drug. Ordinarily, 65 mg to 0.5 g may be given to a child six to 12 years of age.

How Supplied: ℞ *Vials Amytal® Sodium (Sterile Amobarbital Sodium, USP)* (Dry Powder): *No. 386*, 250 mg, in Traypak™ (multivial carton, Lilly) of 10 (NDC 0002-7214-10) and 25 (NDC 0002-7214-25); *No. 387*, 0.5 g, in Traypak of 10 (NDC 0002-7215-10) and 25 (NDC 0002-7215-25).

[020982]

AMYTAL® SODIUM

[ăm′ ĭ-tăl sō′ dĭ-ŭm]
(amobarbital sodium)
PULVULES®
Capsules, USP

WARNING: MAY BE HABIT-FORMING

Description: Amytal® Sodium (Amobarbital Sodium, USP, Lilly) is a white, friable, granular powder that is odorless, has a bitter taste, and is hygroscopic. It is very soluble in water, soluble in alcohol, and practically insoluble in ether and chloroform. Amytal Sodium is sodium-5-ethyl-5-isopentylbarbiturate and has the empirical formula $C_{11}H_{17}N_2NaO_3$.

Each Pulvule contains 65 or 200 mg of amobarbital sodium for oral administration.

Clinical Pharmacology: Amobarbital sodium, a short-acting barbiturate, is a central-nervous-system depressant. It is a rapid-acting sedative and hypnotic, with a duration of effect ranging from eight to 11 hours. It is detoxified in the liver.

Indications and Usage: Amytal® Sodium (amobarbital sodium, Lilly) is indicated for sedation and relief of anxiety (in minimum doses); for hypnotic effects; as preanesthetic medication; and to control convulsive disorders. The prolonged administration of Amytal Sodium is not recommended, since it has not been shown to be effective for a period of more than 14 days. If insomnia persists, drug-free intervals of one or more weeks should elapse before re-treatment is considered. Attempts should be made to find alternative non-drug therapy for chronic insomnia.

Contraindications: Amytal® Sodium (amobarbital sodium, Lilly) is contraindicated in patients who are hypersensitive to barbiturates. It is also contraindicated in patients with a history of manifest or latent porphyria, marked impairment of liver function, or respiratory disease in which dyspnea or obstruction is evident. It should not be administered to persons with known previous addiction to the sedative/hypnotic group, since ordinary doses may be ineffectual and may contribute to further addiction. Amytal Sodium should not be administered in the presence of acute or chronic pain, because paradoxical excitement may be induced or important symptoms may be masked.

Precautions: *General Precautions*—Barbiturates induce liver microsomal enzyme activity. This accelerates the biotransformation of various drugs and is probably part of the mechanism of the tolerance encountered with barbiturates. Amytal® Sodium (amobarbital sodium, Lilly) should, therefore, be used with caution in patients with decreased liver function. This drug should also be administered cautiously to patients with a history of drug dependence or abuse (*see* Drug Abuse and Dependence). Amytal Sodium may decrease the potency of coumarin anticoagulants; therefore, patients receiving such concomitant therapy should have more frequent prothrombin determinations.

As with other sedatives and hypnotics, elderly or debilitated patients may react to barbiturates with marked excitement or depression.

The systemic effects of exogenous hydrocortisone and endogenous hydrocortisone (cortisol) may be diminished by Amytal Sodium. Thus, this product should be administered with caution to patients with borderline hypoadrenal function, regardless of whether it is of pituitary or of primary adrenal origin.

Information for the Patients—Amytal Sodium may impair the mental and/or physical abilities required for the performance of potentially hazardous tasks, such as driving a car or operating machinery. The patient should be cautioned accordingly.

Drug Interactions—Amytal Sodium in combination with alcohol, tranquilizers, and other central-nervous-system depressants has additive depressant effects, and the patient should be so advised. Patients taking this drug should be warned not to exceed the dosage recommended by their physician. Toxic effects and fatalities have occurred following overdoses of Amytal Sodium alone and in combination with other central-nervous-system

---

Quantity of Sterile Water for Injection Required to Dilute the Contents of a Given Vial of Amytal Sodium to Obtain the Percentages Listed. Solutions Derived Will Be in Weight/Volume.

AMYTAL® SODIUM (amobarbital sodium, Lilly)

Vial Number	Content in Weight	1 Percent	2.5 Percent	5 Percent	10 Percent	20 Percent
386	250 mg	25 ml	10 ml	5 ml	2.5 ml	1.25 ml
387	0.5 g	50 ml	20 ml	10 ml	5 ml	2.5 ml

depressants. Caution should be exercised in prescribing unnecessarily large amounts of Amytal Sodium for patients who have a history of emotional disturbances or suicidal ideation or who have misused alcohol and other CNS drugs (see Overdosage).

Usage in Pregnancy—Pregnancy Category B—Reproduction studies have been performed in animals and have revealed no evidence of impaired fertility or harm to the fetus due to Amytal Sodium. There are, however, no adequate and well-controlled studies in pregnant women. Because animal reproduction studies are not always predictive of human response, this drug should be used during pregnancy only if clearly needed.

Labor and Delivery—Depression has been noted in infants born following the use of Amytal® Sodium (amobarbital sodium, Lilly) during labor.

Nursing Mothers—Caution should be exercised when Amytal Sodium is administered to a nursing woman.

Usage in Children—Safety and effectiveness in children have not been established.

Adverse Reactions: The following adverse reactions have been reported:

CNS Depression—Residual sedation or "hangover," drowsiness, lethargy.

Respiratory/Circulatory—Respiratory depression, apnea, circulatory collapse.

Allergic—Hypersensitivity reactions, especially in individuals with asthma, urticaria, angioneurotic edema, or similar conditions; skin eruptions.

Other—Nausea and vomiting; headache.

Drug Abuse and Dependence: *Controlled Substance*—Amytal® Sodium (amobarbital sodium, Lilly) is a Schedule II drug.

Dependence—Prolonged, uninterrupted use of barbiturates (particularly the short-acting drugs), even in therapeutic doses, may result in psychic and physical dependence. Withdrawal symptoms due to physical dependence following chronic use of large doses of barbiturates may include delirium, convulsions, and death.

Overdosage: *Symptoms* — The manifestations of overdosage are early hypothermia followed by fever, sluggish or absent reflexes, respiratory depression, gradual appearance of circulatory collapse, pulmonary edema, and coma.

Treatment— General management should consist in symptomatic and supportive therapy, including gastric lavage, administration of intravenous fluids, and maintenance of blood pressure, body temperature, and adequate respiratory exchange. Dialysis will increase the rate of removal of barbiturates from the body fluids. Antibiotics may be required to control pulmonary complications.

Dosage and Administration: Because of the wide variation in individual response to the barbiturates, the dosage range is relatively great. For insomnia, 65 to 200 mg by mouth at bedtime. For preanesthetic sedation, 200 mg one or two hours before surgery. In labor, the initial dose is 200 to 400 mg, and additional quantities of 200 to 400 mg may be given at one to three-hour intervals for a total dose of not more than 1 g.

How Supplied: (Ⓒ) *Pulvules Amytal® Sodium (Amobarbital Sodium Capsules, USP): No. 111, F23,* 65 mg* (No. 4, Blue), in bottles of 100 (NDC 0002-0623-02) and 500 (NDC 0002-0623-03); *No. 222, F33,* 200 mg* (No. 2, Blue), in bottles of 100 (NDC 0002-0633-02).

[090882]

Shown in Product Identification Section, page 417

ANHYDRON® R
[ăn-hī'drŏn]
(cyclothiazide)
Tablets, USP

Description: Anhydron® (cyclothiazide, Lilly) is 6-chloro-3,4-dihydro-3-(5-norbornen-2-yl) -7- sulfamoyl - 1,2,4 - benzothiadiazine-1,1-dioxide. Cyclothiazide is a white crystalline solid with a melting point of approximately 220°C. It is moderately soluble in hot ethyl alcohol and hot dilute alcohol, very soluble in cold ethyl acetate (an ethyl acetate solvate is formed), and relatively insoluble in ether, benzene, or chloroform.

Action: The action of Anhydron® (cyclothiazide, Lilly) results in interference with electrolyte reabsorption by the renal tubules. At maximum therapeutic dosage, all thiazides have approximately equal diuretic potency. The mechanism by which thiazides function in the control of hypertension is unknown.

Indications: Anhydron® (cyclothiazide, Lilly) is indicated as adjunctive therapy in edema associated with congestive heart failure, hepatic cirrhosis, and corticosteroid and estrogen therapy.

Anhydron has also been found useful in edema due to various forms of renal dysfunction, such as nephrotic syndrome, acute glomerulonephritis, and chronic renal failure.

Anhydron is indicated in the management of hypertension either as the sole therapeutic agent or to enhance the effectiveness of other antihypertensive drugs in the more severe forms of hypertension.

Usage in Pregnancy—The routine use of diuretics in an otherwise healthy woman is inappropriate and exposes mother and fetus to unnecessary hazard. Diuretics do not prevent development of toxemia of pregnancy, and there is no satisfactory evidence that they are useful in the treatment of developed toxemia.

Edema during pregnancy may arise from pathologic causes or from the physiologic and mechanical consequences of pregnancy. Thiazides are indicated in pregnancy when edema is due to pathologic causes, just as they are in the absence of pregnancy (however, see Warnings below). Dependent edema in pregnancy, resulting from restriction of venous return by the expanded uterus, is properly treated through elevation of the lower extremities and use of support hose; use of diuretics to lower intravascular volume in this case is illogical and unnecessary. There is hypervolemia during normal pregnancy which is harmful to neither the fetus nor the mother (in the absence of cardiovascular disease) but which is associated with edema, including generalized edema, in the majority of pregnant women. If this edema produces discomfort, increased recumbency will often provide relief. In rare instances, such edema may cause extreme discomfort that is not relieved by rest. In these cases, a short course of diuretics may provide relief and may be appropriate.

Contraindications: Anhydron® (cyclothiazide, Lilly) is contraindicated in anuria and in patients who are hypersensitive to cyclothiazide or other sulfonamide-derived drugs.

Warnings: Thiazides should be used with caution in severe renal disease. In patients with renal disease, thiazides may precipitate azotemia. Cumulative effects of the drug may develop in patients with impaired renal function.

Thiazides should be used with caution in patients with impaired hepatic function or progressive liver disease, since minor alterations of fluid and electrolyte balance may precipitate hepatic coma.

Thiazides may add to or potentiate the action of other antihypertensive drugs. Potentiation occurs with ganglionic or peripheral adrenergic blocking drugs.

Sensitivity reactions may occur in patients with a history of allergy or bronchial asthma.

The possibility of exacerbation or activation of systemic lupus erythematosus has been reported.

Usage in Pregnancy—Thiazides cross the placental barrier and appear in cord blood. The use of thiazides in pregnant women requires that the anticipated benefit be weighed against possible hazards to the fetus. These hazards include fetal or neonatal jaundice, thrombocytopenia, and possibly other adverse reactions which have occurred in the adult.

Nursing Mothers—Thiazides appear in breast milk. If use of the drug is deemed essential, the patient should stop nursing.

Precautions: Determination of serum electrolytes to detect possible imbalance should be performed at appropriate intervals.

All patients receiving thiazides should be observed for clinical signs of fluid or electrolyte imbalance, e.g., hyponatremia, hypochloremic alkalosis, and hypokalemia. Serum and urine electrolyte determinations are particularly important when the patient is vomiting excessively or receiving parenteral fluids. Medication such as digitalis may also influence serum electrolytes. Warning signs, irrespective of cause, are dryness of mouth, thirst, weakness, lethargy, drowsiness, restlessness, muscle pains or cramps, muscular fatigue, hypotension, oliguria, tachycardia, and gastrointestinal disturbances, such as nausea and vomiting.

Hypokalemia may develop with use of thiazides as with any other potent diuretic, especially with brisk diuresis, in the presence of severe cirrhosis, or during concomitant use of corticosteroids or ACTH. Interference with adequate oral electrolyte intake will also contribute to hypokalemia. Digitalis therapy may exaggerate metabolic effects of hypokalemia, especially in regard to myocardial activity.

Any chloride deficit is generally mild and usually does not require specific treatment except under extraordinary circumstances (as in liver or renal disease). Dilutional hyponatremia may occur in edematous patients in hot weather. Appropriate therapy is water restriction instead of administration of salt (except in rare instances when the hyponatremia is life threatening). In actual salt depletion, appropriate replacement is the therapy of choice.

Hyperuricemia may occur or frank gout may be precipitated in certain patients receiving thiazide therapy.

Insulin requirements in diabetic patients may be increased, decreased, or unchanged. Latent diabetes mellitus may become manifest during thiazide administration.

Thiazide drugs may increase the responsiveness to tubocurarine.

The antihypertensive effects of the drug may be enhanced in postsympathectomy patients.

Thiazides may decrease arterial responsiveness to norepinephrine. This diminution is not sufficient to preclude effectiveness of the pressor agent for therapeutic use.

If progressive renal impairment becomes evident, as indicated by a rising nonprotein nitrogen or blood urea nitrogen, therapy should be carefully reappraised, because it may be necessary to withhold or discontinue diuretic therapy.

Thiazides may decrease serum PBI levels without signs of thyroid disturbance.

Adverse Reactions: *Gastrointestinal*—Anorexia, gastric irritation, nausea, vomiting, cramping, diarrhea, constipation, jaundice (intrahepatic cholestatic jaundice), pancreatitis

Central Nervous System—Dizziness, vertigo, paresthesias, headache, xanthopsia

Hematologic—Leukopenia, agranulocytosis, thrombocytopenia, aplastic anemia

Dermatologic and Hypersensitivity—Purpura, photosensitivity, rash, urticaria, necrotizing angiitis (vasculitis or cutaneous vasculitis)

Cardiovascular—Orthostatic hypotension may occur and may be aggravated by alcohol, barbiturates, or narcotics.

Other—Hyperglycemia, glycosuria, hyperuricemia, muscle spasm, weakness, restlessness

Whenever adverse reactions are moderate or severe, thiazide dosage should be reduced or therapy withdrawn.

Dosage and Administration: Therapy should be individualized according to patient response. This therapy should be titrated to gain maximum therapeutic response as well as the minimum dose possible to maintain that therapeutic response.

For Diuretic Effect—The usual adult dosage of Anhydron® (cyclothiazide, Lilly) is ½ or 1 tablet (1 or 2 mg) once a day, preferably given early in the morning in order to obtain diuresis predominantly during the day and avoid disturbing the patient's rest at night. After the edema is eliminated, the dosage should be reduced according to the patient's need; body weight is usually a very helpful

---

Continued on next page

* Identi-Code® symbol.

Lilly—Cont.

guide. For maintenance therapy, ½ or 1 tablet given on alternate days or two or three times a week frequently may be sufficient. Such an intermittent dosage schedule reduces the possibility of excessive depletion of body sodium and chloride or of potassium deficiency.

For Antihypertensive Effect—The dosage of Anhydron, like that of other thiazides, is often greater than that required for diuresis. The usual dosage of Anhydron is 1 tablet (2 mg) once a day; in some cases, it may be necessary to give 1 tablet two or three times a day.

Since Anhydron augments the action of other antihypertensive drugs, dosage of the latter should be reduced—perhaps to 50 percent of the usually recommended dosage—at the start of treatment and carefully readjusted upward or downward according to the patient's response and need.

How Supplied: (R) Tablets No. 1850, Anhydron® (Cyclothiazide Tablets, USP), U09,* 2 mg, Pink (capsule-shaped, scored), in bottles of 100 (NDC 0002-2109-02) and 1000 (NDC 0002-2109-04).

[051983]

AVENTYL® HCL R
[ăv'ĕn-tĭl ăch'sē-ĕl]
(nortriptyline hydrochloride)
USP

Description: Aventyl® HCl (nortriptyline hydrochloride, Lilly) is 5-(3-methylaminopropylidene)-10,11-dihydro-5H-dibenzo [a,d] cycloheptene hydrochloride. Its molecular weight is 299.8, and its empirical formula is $C_{19}H_{21}N \cdot HCl$.

Actions: The mechanism of mood elevation by tricyclic antidepressant is at present unknown. Aventyl® HCl (nortriptyline hydrochloride, Lilly) is not a monoamine oxidase inhibitor. It inhibits the activity of such diverse agents as histamine, 5-hydroxytryptamine, and acetylcholine. It increases the pressor effect of norepinephrine but blocks the pressor response of phenethylamine. Studies suggest that Aventyl HCl interferes with the transport, release, and storage of catecholamines. Operant conditioning techniques in rats and pigeons suggest that Aventyl HCl has a combination of stimulant and depressant properties.

Indications: Aventyl® HCl (nortriptyline hydrochloride, Lilly) is indicated for the relief of symptoms of depression. Endogenous depressions are more likely to be alleviated than are other depressive states.

Contraindications: The use of Aventyl® HCl (nortriptyline hydrochloride, Lilly) or other tricyclic antidepressants concurrently with a monoamine oxidase (MAO) inhibitor is contraindicated. Hyperpyretic crises, severe convulsions, and fatalities have occurred when similar tricyclic antidepressants were used in such combinations. It is advisable to have discontinued the MAO inhibitor for at least two weeks before treatment with Aventyl HCl is started. Patients hypersensitive to Aventyl HCl should not be given the drug.

Cross-sensitivity between Aventyl HCl and other dibenzazepines is a possibility.

Aventyl HCl is contraindicated during the acute recovery period after myocardial infarction.

Warnings: Patients with cardiovascular disease should be given Aventyl® HCl (nortriptyline hydrochloride, Lilly) only under close supervision because of the tendency of the drug to produce sinus tachycardia and to prolong the conduction time. Myocardial infarction, arrhythmia, and strokes have occurred. The antihypertensive action of guanethidine and similar agents may be blocked. Because of its anticholinergic activity, Aventyl HCl should be used with great caution in patients who have glaucoma or a history of urinary retention. Patients with a history of seizures should be followed closely when Aventyl HCl is administered, inasmuch as this drug is known to lower the convulsive threshold. Great care is required if Aventyl HCl is given to hyperthyroid patients or to those receiving thyroid medication, since cardiac arrhythmias may develop.

Aventyl HCl may impair the mental and/or physical abilities required for the performance of hazardous tasks, such as operating machinery or driving a car; therefore, the patient should be warned accordingly.

Excessive consumption of alcohol in combination with nortriptyline therapy may have a potentiating effect, which may lead to the danger of increased suicidal attempts or overdosage, especially in patients with histories of emotional disturbances or suicidal ideation.

Use in Pregnancy—Safe use of Aventyl HCl during pregnancy and lactation has not been established; therefore, when the drug is administered to pregnant patients, nursing mothers, or women of childbearing potential, the potential benefits must be weighed against the possible hazards. Animal reproduction studies have yielded inconclusive results.

Use in Children—This drug is not recommended for use in children, since safety and effectiveness in the pediatric age group have not been established.

Precautions: *General*—The use of Aventyl® HCl (nortriptyline hydrochloride, Lilly) in schizophrenic patients may result in an exacerbation of the psychosis or may activate latent schizophrenic symptoms. If the drug is given to overactive or agitated patients, increased anxiety and agitation may occur. In manic-depressive patients, Aventyl HCl may cause symptoms of the manic phase to emerge.

Troublesome patient hostility may be aroused by the use of Aventyl HCl. Epileptiform seizures may accompany its administration, as is true of other drugs of its class.

When it is essential, the drug may be administered with electroconvulsive therapy, although the hazards may be increased. Discontinue the drug for several days, if possible, prior to elective surgery.

The possibility of a suicidal attempt by a depressed patient remains after the initiation of treatment; in this regard, it is important that the least possible quantity of drug be dispensed at any given time.

Both elevation and lowering of blood sugar levels have been reported.

Drug Interactions: Steady-state serum concentrations of the tricyclic antidepressants are reported to fluctuate significantly as cimetidine is either added or deleted from the drug regimen. Serious anticholinergic symptoms (severe dry mouth, urinary retention, blurred vision) have been associated with elevations in the serum levels of the tricyclic antidepressant when cimetidine is added to the drug regimen. In addition, higher than expected steady-state serum concentrations of the tricyclic antidepressant have been observed when therapy is initiated in patients already taking cimetidine.

Alternatively, decreases in the steady-state serum concentration of the tricyclic antidepressant have been reported in well-controlled patients on concurrent therapy, upon discontinuance of the cimetidine. The therapeutic efficacy of the tricyclic antidepressant may be compromised in these patients as the cimetidine is discontinued. Several of the tricyclic antidepressants have been cited in these reports.

Administration of reserpine during therapy with a tricyclic antidepressant has been shown to produce a "stimulating" effect in some depressed patients.

Close supervision and careful adjustment of the dosage are required when Aventyl HCl is used with other anticholinergic drugs and sympathomimetic drugs.

The patient should be informed that the reponse to alcohol may be exaggerated.

Adverse Reactions: Note—Included in the following list are a few adverse reactions that have not been reported with this specific drug. However, the pharmacologic similarities among the tricyclic antidepressant drugs require that each of the reactions be considered when nortriptyline is administered.

Cardiovascular—Hypotension, hypertension, tachycardia, palpitation, myocardial infarction, arrhythmias, heart block, stroke.

Psychiatric—Confusional states (especially in the elderly) with hallucinations, disorientation, delusions; anxiety, restlessness, agitation; insomnia, panic, nightmares; hypomania; exacerbation of psychosis.

Neurologic—Numbness, tingling, paresthesias of extremities; incoordination, ataxia, tremors; peripheral neuropathy; extrapyramidal symptoms; seizures, alteration in EEG patterns; tinnitus.

Anticholinergic—Dry mouth and, rarely, associated sublingual adenitis; blurred vision, disturbance of accommodation, mydriasis; constipation, paralytic ileus; urinary retention, delayed micturition, dilation of the urinary tract.

Allergic—Skin rash, petechiae, urticaria, itching, photosensitization (avoid excessive exposure to sunlight); edema (general or of face and tongue), drug fever, cross-sensitivity with other tricyclic drugs.

Hematologic—Bone-marrow depression, including agranulocytosis; eosinophilia; purpura; thrombocytopenia.

Gastrointestinal—Nausea and vomiting, anorexia, epigastric distress, diarrhea; peculiar taste, stomatitis, abdominal cramps, black-tongue.

Endocrine—Gynecomastia in the male; breast enlargement and galactorrhea in the female; increased or decreased libido, impotence; testicular swelling; elevation or depression of blood sugar levels; syndrome of inappropriate ADH (antidiuretic hormone) secretion.

Other—Jaundice (simulating obstructive); altered liver function; weight gain or loss; perspiration; flushing; urinary frequency, nocturia; drowsiness, dizziness, weakness, fatigue; headache; parotid swelling; alopecia.

Withdrawal Symptoms—Though these are not indicative of addiction, abrupt cessation of treatment after prolonged therapy may produce nausea, headache, and malaise.

Dosage and Administration: Aventyl® HCl (nortriptyline hydrochloride, Lilly) is not recommended for children.

Aventyl HCl is administered orally in the form of Pulvules® or liquid. Lower than usual dosages are recommended for elderly patients and adolescents. Lower dosages are also recommended for outpatients than for hospitalized patients who will be under close supervision. The physician should initiate dosage at a low level and increase it gradually, noting carefully the clinical response and any evidence of intolerance. Following remission, maintenance medication may be required for a longer period of time at the lowest dose that will maintain remission.

If a patient develops minor side effects, the dosage should be reduced. The drug should be discontinued promptly if adverse effects of a serious nature or allergic manifestations occur.

Usual Adult Dose—25 mg three or four times daily; dosage should begin at a low level and be increased as required. Doses above 100 mg/day are not recommended.

Elderly and Adolescent Patients—30 to 50 mg/day, in divided doses.

Overdosage: Toxic overdosage may result in confusion, restlessness, agitation, vomiting, hyperpyrexia, muscle rigidity, hyperactive reflexes, tachycardia, ECG evidence of impaired conduction, shock, congestive heart failure, stupor, coma, and CNS stimulation with convulsions followed by respiratory depression. Deaths have occurred following overdosage with drugs of this class.

No specific antidote is known. General supportive measures are indicated, with gastric lavage. Respiratory assistance is apparently the most effective measure when indicated. The use of CNS depressants may worsen the prognosis.

The administration of barbiturates for control of convulsions alleviates an increase in the cardiac workload but should be undertaken with caution to avoid potentiation of respiratory depression. Intramuscular paraldehyde or diazepam provides anticonvulsant activity with less respiratory depression than do the barbiturates; diazepam seems to be preferred.

The use of digitalis and/or physostigmine may be considered in case of serious cardiovascular abnormalities or cardiac failure.

The value of dialysis has not been established.

How Supplied: (℞) *Liquid No. 38, Aventyl® HCl (Nortriptyline Hydrochloride Oral Solution, USP),* 10 mg (equivalent to base) per 5 ml, in 16-fl-oz bottles (NDC 0002-2468-05). Alcohol, 4 percent.

(℞) *Pulvules Aventyl® HCl (Nortriptyline Hydrochloride Capsules, USP): No. 387, H17** (No. 3, White Opaque Body, Yellow Opaque Cap), 10 mg (equivalent to base), and *No. 389, H19** (No. 1, White Opaque Body, Yellow Opaque Cap), 25 mg (equivalent to base), in bottles of 100 (NDC 0002-0817-02 and 0819-02) and 500 (NDC 0002-0817-03 and 0819-03) and in 10 strips of 10 individually labeled blisters each containing 1 Pulvule (ID100) (NDC 0002-0817-33 and 0819-33).

[073084]

Shown in Product Identification Section, page 417

BREVITAL® SODIUM ℮
[brĕv′ĭ-tăl sō′dĭ-ŭm]
(methohexital sodium)
For Injection, USP
For Intravenous Use

> **WARNING**
> This drug should be administered by persons qualified in the use of intravenous anesthetics and with the ready availability of appropriate resuscitative equipment for prevention and treatment of anesthetic emergencies.

Description: Brevital® Sodium (Methohexital Sodium for Injection, USP, Lilly) is sodium α-dl-1-methyl-5-allyl-5-(1-methyl-2-pentynyl) barbiturate. It differs chemically from the established barbiturate anesthetics in that it contains no sulfur.

Action: Methohexital sodium is a rapid, ultrashort-acting barbiturate anesthetic agent.

Indications: For induction of anesthesia, for supplementing other anesthetic agents, as intravenous anesthesia for short surgical procedures with minimum painful stimuli, or as an agent for inducing a hypnotic state.

Contraindications: Methohexital sodium is contraindicated when general anesthesia is contraindicated, in patients with latent or manifest porphyria, or in patients with a known hypersensitivity to barbiturates.

Warnings: May be habit-forming.

Repeated or continuous infusion may cause cumulative effects resulting in prolonged somnolence and respiratory and circulatory depression.

Usage in Pregnancy—Safe use of methohexital sodium has not been established with respect to possible adverse effects on human fetal development. Therefore, if methohexital sodium is to be given to women who are pregnant, the benefits to the mother should be weighed against possible risks to the fetus. When administered to pregnant rabbits and rats at four and seven times the human dose respectively, methohexital sodium produced no evidence of teratogenicity and no fetal abnormalities.

Precautions: Respiratory depression, apnea, or hypotension may occur owing to variations in tolerance from individual to individual or to the physical status of the patient. Caution should be exercised in debilitated patients or in those with impaired function of respiratory, circulatory, renal, hepatic, or endocrine systems.

Methohexital sodium should be used with extreme caution in patients in status asthmaticus.

Extravascular injection may cause pain, swelling, ulceration, and necrosis. Intra-arterial injection is dangerous and may produce gangrene of an extremity. The central-nervous-system (CNS) depressant effect of methohexital sodium may be additive with that of other CNS depressants, including alcohol.

Preparation of Solutions of Brevital® Sodium (methohexital sodium)
Preparation of Solution—FOLLOW DILUTING INSTRUCTIONS EXACTLY.
Diluents—DO NOT USE DILUENTS CONTAINING BACTERIOSTATS.
Sterile Water for Injection is the preferred diluent.
Dextrose Injection (5%) or Sodium Chloride Injection (0.9%) may be used.
(Brevital Sodium is not compatible with Lactated Ringer's Injection.)
Dilution Instructions—For a 1% solution (10 mg/ml), contents of vials should be diluted as follows:
Vials No. 660 (500 mg)—add 50 ml of diluent
Vials No. 760 (500 mg)—add 50 ml of accompanying diluent
Vials No. 664 (2.5 g)—add 250 ml of diluent
Vials No. 662 (5 g)—add 500 ml of diluent

Vial No.	Amount of Diluent to Be Added to the Vial	For 1% Solution Dilute to
663 (2.5 g)	15 ml	250 ml
659 (5 g)	30 ml	500 ml

When the first dilution is made with Vials No. 663 or No. 659, the solution in the vial will be yellow. When further diluted to make a 1% solution, it must be *clear and colorless* or should not be used.

Adverse Reactions: The following reactions have been reported:
Circulatory depression
Thrombophlebitis
Pain at injection site
Respiratory depression, including apnea
Laryngospasm
Bronchospasm
Salivation
Hiccups
Skeletal-muscle hyperactivity (twitching to convulsive-like movements)
Emergence delirium
Headache
Injury to nerves adjacent to injection site
Nausea
Emesis

Acute allergic reactions, such as erythema, pruritus, urticaria, rhinitis, dyspnea, hypotension, restlessness, anxiety, abdominal pain, and peripheral vascular collapse, have been reported with the use of Brevital® Sodium (methohexital sodium, Lilly).

Dosage and Administration: Preanesthetic medication is generally advisable. Brevital® Sodium (methohexital sodium, Lilly) may be used with any of the recognized preanesthetic medications, but the phenothiazines are less satisfactory than the combination of an opiate and a belladonna derivative.

Facilities for assisting respirations and administering oxygen are necessary adjuncts for intravenous anesthesia.

[See table above].

For continuous drip anesthesia, prepare a 0.2% solution by adding 500 mg of Brevital Sodium to 250 ml of diluent. For this dilution, we recommend as solvents either 5% glucose solution or isotonic (0.9%) sodium chloride solution instead of distilled water in order to avoid extreme hypotonicity.

Administration—A 1% solution is recommended for induction of anesthesia and for maintenance by intermittent injection. Dosage of all intravenous barbiturates must be individualized according to the patient's response. The usual range for Brevital® Sodium (methohexital sodium, Lilly) is 5 to 12 ml of a 1% solution (50 to 120 mg). This induction dose will provide anesthesia for five to seven minutes. The rate of injection is not fixed, but it is usually found to be about 1 ml of the 1% solution (10 mg) in five seconds. If intermittent injection of a 1% solution is used for maintenance, additional amounts of about 2 to 4 ml (20 to 40 mg) will be required every four to seven minutes.

Some anesthesiologists have preferred the continuous drip method of maintenance with a 0.2% solution. The rate of flow must be individualized for each patient. As a guide, 1 drop per second may be used.

Storage—Brevital Sodium is stable in Sterile Water for Injection at room temperature (25°C or below) for at least *six weeks.* Dextrose Injection (5%) or isotonic (0.9%) sodium chloride injection may be used as diluents, but these solutions are not stable for much more than *24 hours.* Solutions may be stored and used as long as they remain clear and colorless.

Compatibility Information: Solutions of Brevital® Sodium (methohexital sodium, Lilly) should not be mixed with acid solutions such as atropine sulfate, Metubine® Iodide (Metocurine Iodide Injection, USP, Lilly), and succinylcholine chloride. However, because of numerous requests from anesthesiologists for information regarding the chemical compatibility of these mixtures, the following is provided.

The soluble sodium salts of barbiturates are the forms used for intravenous administration. Solubility is maintained only at a relatively high (basic) pH. The accompanying chart contains information obtained from compatibility studies in which a 1% solution of Brevital Sodium was mixed with therapeutic amounts of agents whose solutions have a low (acid) pH.

Solutions of Brevital Sodium are incompatible with silicone and should not be allowed to come in contact with rubber stoppers or parts of disposable syringes that have been treated with silicone. [See table on next page].

How Supplied: *Vials Brevital® Sodium (Methohexital Sodium for Injection, USP)* are supplied as follows:

(℮) *No. 660,* 500 mg, 50-ml size, multiple dose, rubber-stoppered (Dry Powder), in singles (10 per carton) (NDC 0002-1446-01) and in packages of 25 (NDC 0002-1446-25).
Each vial contains—
Brevital® Sodium (methohexital sodium, Lilly)..500 mg
Anhydrous Sodium Carbonate.................... 30 mg
Contains no preservative.

(℮) *No. 760,* 500 mg, 50-ml size, multiple dose, rubber-stoppered (Dry Powder), in singles (10 per carton) (NDC 0002-1465-01). Each package contains one 50-ml vial of Sterile Water for Injection.
Each vial contains—
Brevital® Sodium (methohexital sodium, Lilly)..500 mg
Anhydrous Sodium Carbonate.................... 30 mg
Contains no preservative.

(℮) *No. 663,* 2.5 g, rubber-stoppered (Dry Powder), in singles (10 per carton) (NDC 0002-1448-01) and in packages of 25 (NDC 0002-1448-25).
Each vial contains—
Brevital® Sodium (methohexital sodium, Lilly)..2.5 g
Anhydrous Sodium Carbonate....................150 mg
Contains no preservative.

(℮) *No. 664,* 2.5 g, 250-ml size, multiple dose, rubber-stoppered (Dry Powder), in singles (NDC 0002-1449-01) and in packages of 25 (NDC 0002-1449-25).
Each vial contains—
Brevital® Sodium (methohexital sodium, Lilly)..2.5 g

Continued on next page

* Identi-Code® symbol.

Lilly—Cont.

Anhydrous Sodium Carbonate......................150 mg
 Contains no preservative.
(ⓒ) *No. 659*, 5 g, rubber-stoppered (Dry Powder), in singles (10 per carton) (NDC 0002-1445-01).
Each vial contains—
Brevital® Sodium (methohexital
 sodium, Lilly)..5 g
Anhydrous Sodium Carbonate......................300 mg
 Contains no preservative.
(ⓒ) *No. 662*, 5 g, 500-ml size, multiple dose, rubber-stoppered (Dry Powder), in singles (NDC 0002-1447-01) and in packages of 25 (NDC 0002-1447-25).
Each vial contains—
Brevital® Sodium (methohexital
 sodium, Lilly)..5 g
Anhydrous Sodium Carbonate......................300 mg
 Contains no preservative.   [102582]

CAPASTAT® SULFATE ℞
[kăp′a-stăt sŭl′fāt]
(capreomycin sulfate)
Sterile, USP
Not for Pediatric Use

Warnings

The use of capreomycin in patients with renal insufficiency or preexisting auditory impairment must be undertaken with great caution, and the risk of additional eighth-nerve impairment or renal injury should be weighed against the benefits to be derived from therapy.
Refer to animal pharmacology section for additional information.
Since other parenteral antituberculosis agents (streptomycin, viomycin) also have similar and sometimes irreversible toxic effects, particularly on eighth-cranial-nerve and renal function, simultaneous administration of these agents with capreomycin is not recommended. Use with nonantituberculosis drugs (polymyxin, colistin sulfate, gentamicin, tobramycin, vancomycin, kanamycin, and neomycin) having ototoxic or nephrotoxic potential should be undertaken only with great caution.
Usage in Pregnancy—The safety of the use of capreomycin in *pregnancy* has not been determined.
Pediatric Usage—Safety of the use of capreomycin in infants and children has not been established.

Description: Capastat® Sulfate (capreomycin sulfate, Lilly) is a polypeptide antibiotic isolated from *Streptomyces capreolus*. It is a complex of four microbiologically active components which have been characterized in part; however, complete structural determination of all the components has not been established.
Capreomycin is supplied as the disulfate salt and is soluble in water. In complete solution, it is almost colorless.

Actions: *Human Pharmacology*—Capastat®Sulfate (capreomycin sulfate, Lilly) is not absorbed in significant quantities from the gastrointestinal tract and must be administered parenterally. In two studies of ten patients each, peak serum concentrations following 1 g of capreomycin given intramuscularly were achieved one to two hours after administration, and average peak levels reached were 28 and 32 mcg/ml respectively (range, 20 to 47 mcg/ml). Low serum concentrations were present at 24 hours. However, 1 g of capreomycin daily for 30 days or more produced no significant accumulation in subjects with normal renal function. Two patients with marked reduction of renal function had high serum concentrations 24 hours after administration of the drug. When a 1-g dose of capreomycin was given intramuscularly to normal volunteers, 52 percent was excreted in the urine within 12 hours.
Paper chromatographic studies indicated that capreomycin is excreted essentially unaltered. Urine concentrations averaged 1.68 mg/ml (average urine volume, 228 ml) during the six hours following a 1-g dose.
Microbiology—Capreomycin is active against human strains of *Mycobacterium tuberculosis*.
The susceptibility of strains of *M. tuberculosis* in vitro varies with the media and techniques employed. In general, the minimum inhibitory concentrations for *M. tuberculosis* are lowest in liquid media that are free of egg protein (7H10 or Dubos) and range from 1 to 5 mcg/ml when the indirect method is used. Comparable inhibitory concentrations are obtained when 7H10 agar is used for direct susceptibility testing. When indirect susceptibility tests are performed on standard tube slants with 7H10 media, susceptible strains are inhibited by 10 to 25 mcg/ml. Egg-containing media, such as Löwenstein-Jensen or ATS, require concentrations of 25 to 50 mcg/ml to inhibit susceptible strains.
Cross-Resistance—Frequent cross-resistance occurs between capreomycin and viomycin. Varying degrees of cross-resistance between capreomycin and kanamycin and neomycin have been reported. No cross-resistance has been observed between capreomycin and isoniazid, aminosalicylic acid, cycloserine, streptomycin, ethionamide, or ethambutol.
Indications: Capreomycin, which is to be used concomitantly with other appropriate antituberculosis agents, is indicated in pulmonary infections caused by capreomycin-susceptible strains of *M. tuberculosis* when the primary agents (isoniazid, aminosalicylic acid, and streptomycin) have been ineffective or cannot be used because of toxicity or the presence of resistant tubercle bacilli.
Susceptibility studies should be performed to determine the presence of a capreomycin-susceptible strain of *M. tuberculosis*.
Contraindication: Capreomycin is contraindicated in those patients who are hypersensitive to it.
Precautions: Audiometric measurements and assessment of vestibular function should be performed prior to initiation of therapy with capreomycin and at regular intervals during treatment. Regular tests of renal function should be made throughout the period of treatment, and reduced dosage should be employed in patients with known or suspected renal impairment.
Renal injury, with tubular necrosis, elevation of the blood urea nitrogen (BUN) or nonprotein nitrogen (NPN), and abnormal urinary sediment, has been noted. Renal function studies should be made both before capreomycin therapy is started and on a weekly basis during treatment. Slight elevation of the BUN or NPN has been observed in a significant number of patients receiving prolonged therapy. The appearance of casts, red cells, and white cells in the urine has been noted in a high percentage of these cases. Elevation of the BUN above 30 mg/100 ml or any other evidence of decreasing renal function with or without a rise in BUN levels calls for careful evaluation of the patient, and the dosage should be reduced or the drug completely withdrawn. The clinical significance of abnormal urine sediment and slight elevation in the BUN (or total NPN) observed during long-term capreomycin therapy has not been established.
Since hypokalemia may occur during capreomycin therapy, serum potassium levels should be determined frequently.
The peripheral neuromuscular blocking action that has been attributed to other polypeptide antibiotics (colistin sulfate, polymyxin A sulfate, paromomycin, and viomycin) and aminoglycoside antibiotics (streptomycin, dihydrostreptomycin, neomycin, and kanamycin) has been studied with capreomycin. A partial neuromuscular block was demonstrated after large intravenous doses of capreomycin. This action was enhanced by ether anesthesia (as has been reported for neomycin) and was antagonized by neostigmine.
Caution should be exercised in the administration of antibiotics, including capreomycin, to any patient who has demonstrated some form of allergy, particularly to drugs.
Adverse Reactions: *Nephrotoxicity*—In 36 percent of 722 patients treated with capreomycin, elevation of the BUN above 20 mg/100 ml and of the NPN above 35 mg/100 ml has been observed. In many instances, there was also depression of PSP excretion and abnormal urine sediment. In 10 percent of this series, the BUN elevation exceeded 30 mg/100 ml or the NPN exceeded 50 mg/100 ml. Toxic nephritis was reported in one patient with tuberculosis and portal cirrhosis who was treated with capreomycin (1 g) and aminosalicylic acid daily for one month. This patient developed renal insufficiency and oliguria and died. Autopsy showed subsiding acute tubular necrosis.
Ototoxicity—Subclinical auditory loss was noted in approximately 11 percent of patients undergoing treatment with capreomycin. This has been a 5 to 10-decibel loss in the 4000 to 8000-CPS range. Clinically apparent hearing loss occurred in 3 percent of 722 subjects. Some audiometric changes were reversible. Other cases with permanent loss were not progressive following withdrawal of capreomycin.
Tinnitus and vertigo have occurred.
Liver—Serial tests of liver function have demonstrated a decrease in BSP excretion without change in SGOT or SGPT in the presence of preexisting liver disease. Abnormal results in liver function tests have occurred in many persons receiving capreomycin in combination with other antituberculosis agents which also are known to cause changes in hepatic function. The role of capreomycin in producing these abnormalities is not clear; however, periodic determinations of liver function are recommended.
Blood—Leukocytosis and leukopenia have been observed. The majority of patients treated have had eosinophilia exceeding 5 percent while receiving daily injections of capreomycin. This has subsided with reduction of the capreomycin dosage to 2 or 3 g weekly.
Pain and induration at the injection sites have been observed. Excessive bleeding at the injection site has been reported. Sterile abscesses have been noted.
Hypersensitivity—Urticaria and maculopapular skin rashes associated in some cases with febrile reactions have been reported when cap- reomycin

Compatibility of Brevital® Sodium (methohexital sodium) with Solutions Having a Low pH

Active Ingredient	Potency per ml	Volume Used	Imme-diate	Physical Change 15 min	30 min	1 hr
BREVITAL SODIUM	10 mg	10 ml		CONTROL		
Atropine sulfate	1/150 gr	1 ml	None	Haze		
Atropine sulfate	1/100 gr	1 ml	None	Ppt.	Ppt.	
Succinylcholine chloride	0.5 mg	4 ml	None	None	Haze	
Succinylcholine chloride	1 mg	4 ml	None	None	Haze	
Metocurine iodide	0.5 mg	4 ml	None	None	Ppt.	
Metocurine iodide	1 mg	4 ml	None	None	Ppt.	
Scopolamine hydrobromide	1/120 gr	1 ml	None	None	None	Haze
Tubocurarine chloride	3 mg	4 ml	None	Haze		

and other antituberculosis drugs were given concomitantly.

Dosage and Administration: Capastat® Sulfate (capreomycin sulfate, Lilly) should be dissolved in 2 ml of 0.9% Sodium Chloride Injection or Sterile Water for Injection. Two to three minutes should be allowed for complete solution. For administration of a 1-g dose, the entire contents of the vial should be given. For dosages less than 1 g, the accompanying dilution table may be used.
[See table above].

The solution may acquire a pale straw color and darken with time, but this is not associated with loss of potency or the development of toxicity. After reconstitution, solutions of Capastat Sulfate may be stored for 48 hours at room temperature and up to 14 days under refrigeration.

Capastat Sulfate should be given by deep intramuscular injection into a large muscle mass, since superficial injections may be associated with increased pain and the development of sterile abscesses.

Capreomycin is always administered in combination with at least one other antituberculosis agent to which the patient's strain of tubercle bacilli is susceptible. The usual dose is 1 g daily (not to exceed 20 mg/kg/day) given intramuscularly for 60 to 120 days, followed by 1 g intramuscularly two or three times weekly. (*Note*—Therapy for tuberculosis should be maintained for 18 to 24 months. If facilities for administering injectable medication are not available, a change to appropriate oral therapy is indicated on the patient's release from the hospital.)

Animal Pharmacology: In addition to renal and eighth-cranial-nerve toxicity demonstrated in animal toxicology studies, two dogs have developed cataracts while on doses of 62 mg/kg and 100 mg/kg for prolonged periods.

In teratology studies, a low incidence of "wavy ribs" was noted in litters of female rats treated with daily doses of 50 mg/kg or more of capreomycin.

How Supplied: (℞) *Vials No. 718, Capastat® Sulfate (Sterile Capreomycin Sulfate, USP)*, equivalent to 1 g capreomycin activity, 10-ml size, rubber-stoppered (Dry Powder), in singles (NDC 0002-1485-01) (10 per carton).

[102682]

CECLOR® ℞
[sē' klôr]
(cefaclor)

Description: Ceclor® (cefaclor, Lilly) is a semisynthetic cephalosporin antibiotic for oral administration. It is chemically designated as 3-chloro-7-D- (2-phenylglycinamido)-3-cephem-4-carboxylic acid. Ceclor is available in 250-mg and 500-mg Pulvules® and in a powder for oral suspension containing 125 or 250 mg/5 ml.

Clinical Pharmacology: Cefaclor is well absorbed after oral administration to fasting subjects. Total absorption is the same whether the drug is given with or without food; however, when it is taken with food, the peak concentration achieved is 50 to 75 percent of that observed when the drug is administered to fasting subjects and generally appears from three-fourths to one hour later. Following administration of 250-mg, 500-mg, and 1-g doses to fasting subjects, average peak serum levels of approximately 7, 13, and 23 mcg/ml respectively were obtained within 30 to 60 minutes. Approximately 60 to 85 percent of the drug is excreted unchanged in the urine within eight hours, the greater portion being excreted within the first two hours. During this eight-hour period, peak urine concentrations following the 250-mg, 500-mg, and 1-g doses were approximately 600, 900, and 1900 mcg/ml respectively. The serum half-life in normal subjects is 0.6 to 0.9 hour. In patients with reduced renal function, the serum half-life of cefaclor is slightly prolonged. In those with complete absence of renal function, the biologic half-life of the intact molecule is 2.3 to 2.8 hours. Excretion pathways in patients with markedly impaired renal function have not been deter-

DILUTION TABLE FOR CAPASTAT® SULFATE (capreomycin sulfate)

Diluent Added to 1-g Vial	Volume of Capastat Sulfate Solution	Concentration* (Approx.)
2.15 ml	2.85 ml	350 mg/ml
2.63 ml	3.33 ml	300 mg/ml
3.3 ml	4 ml	250 mg/ml
4.3 ml	5 ml	200 mg/ml

*Stated in terms of mg of capreomycin activity.

---

mined. Hemodialysis shortens the half-life by 25 to 30 percent.

Microbiology—In vitro tests demonstrate that the bactericidal action of the cephalosporins results from inhibition of cell-wall synthesis. Cefaclor is usually active against the following organisms in vitro and in clinical infections:

Staphylococci, including coagulase-positive, coagulase-negative, and penicillinase-producing strains
Streptococcus pyogenes (group A beta-hemolytic streptococci)
S. pneumoniae (formerly *Diplococcus pneumoniae*)
Escherichia coli
Proteus mirabilis
Klebsiella species
Haemophilus influenzae, including some beta-lactamase-producing ampicillin-resistant strains

Note: *Pseudomonas* species, *Acinetobacter calcoaceticus* (formerly *Mima* and *Herellea* species), and most strains of enterococci (*S. faecalis*, group D streptococci), *Enterobacter* species, indole-positive *Proteus*, and *Serratia* species are resistant to cefaclor. When tested by in vitro methods, staphylococci exhibit cross-resistance between cefaclor and methicillin-type antibiotics.

Disc Susceptibility Tests—Quantitative methods that require measurement of zone diameters give the most precise estimates of antibiotic susceptibility. One such procedure* has been recommended for use with discs for testing susceptibility to cephalothin. The currently accepted zone diameter interpretative criteria for the cephalothin disc are appropriate for determining bacterial susceptibility to cefaclor. With this procedure, a report from the laboratory of "resistant" indicates that the infecting organism is not likely to respond to therapy. A report of "intermediate susceptibility" suggests that the organism would be susceptible if the infection is confined to tissues and fluids (e.g., urine) in which high antibiotic levels can be obtained or if high dosage is used.

Indications and Usage: Ceclor® (cefaclor, Lilly) is indicated in the treatment of the following infections when caused by susceptible strains of the designated microorganisms:

Otitis media caused by *S. pneumoniae (D. pneumoniae), H. influenzae*, staphylococci, and *S. pyogenes* (group A beta-hemolytic streptococci)

Lower respiratory infections, including pneumonia caused by *S. pneumoniae (D. pneumoniae), H. influenzae*, and *S. pyogenes* (group A beta-hemolytic streptococci)

Upper respiratory infections, including pharyngitis and tonsillitis caused by *S. pyogenes* (group A beta-hemolytic streptococci)
Note: Penicillin is the usual drug of choice in the treatment and prevention of streptococcal infections, including the prophylaxis of rheumatic fever. Ceclor is generally effective in the eradication of streptococci from the nasopharynx; however, substantial data establishing the efficacy of Ceclor in the subsequent prevention of rheumatic fever are not available at present.

Urinary tract infections, including pyelonephritis and cystitis caused by *E. coli, P. mirabilis, Klebsiella* species, and coagulase-negative staphylococci

Skin and skin-structure infections caused by *Staphylococcus aureus* and *S. pyogenes* (group A beta-hemolytic streptococci)

Appropriate culture and susceptibility studies should be performed to determine susceptibility of the causative organism to Ceclor.

Contraindication: Ceclor® (cefaclor, Lilly) is contraindicated in patients with known allergy to the cephalosporin group of antibiotics.

Warnings: IN PENICILLIN-SENSITIVE PATIENTS, CEPHALOSPORIN ANTIBIOTICS SHOULD BE ADMINISTERED CAUTIOUSLY. THERE IS CLINICAL AND LABORATORY EVIDENCE OF PARTIAL CROSS-ALLERGENICITY OF THE PENICILLINS AND THE CEPHALOSPORINS, AND THERE ARE INSTANCES IN WHICH PATIENTS HAVE HAD REACTIONS, INCLUDING ANAPHYLAXIS, TO BOTH DRUG CLASSES.

Antibiotics, including Ceclor® (cefaclor, Lilly), should be administered cautiously to any patient who has demonstrated some form of allergy, particularly to drugs.

Pseudomembranous colitis has been reported with virtually all broad-spectrum antibiotics (including macrolides, semisynthetic penicillins, and cephalosporins); therefore, it is important to consider its diagnosis in patients who develop diarrhea in association with the use of antibiotics. Such colitis may range in severity from mild to life-threatening. Treatment with broad-spectrum antibiotics alters the normal flora of the colon and may permit overgrowth of clostridia. Studies indicate that a toxin produced by *Clostridium difficile* is one primary cause of antibiotic-associated colitis.

Mild cases of pseudomembranous colitis usually respond to drug discontinuance alone. In moderate to severe cases, management should include sigmoidoscopy, appropriate bacteriologic studies, and fluid, electrolyte, and protein supplementation. When the colitis does not improve after the drug has been discontinued, or when it is severe, oral vancomycin is the drug of choice for antibiotic-associated pseudomembranous colitis produced by *C. difficile*. Other causes of colitis should be ruled out.

Precautions: *General Precautions*—If an allergic reaction to cefaclor occurs, the drug should be discontinued, and, if necessary, the patient should be treated with appropriate agents, e.g., pressor amines, antihistamines, or corticosteroids.

Prolonged use of Ceclor® (cefaclor, Lilly) may result in the overgrowth of nonsusceptible organisms. Careful observation of the patient is essential. If superinfection occurs during therapy, appropriate measures should be taken.

Positive direct Coombs' tests have been reported during treatment with the cephalosporin antibiotics. In hematologic studies or in transfusion cross-matching procedures when antiglobulin tests are performed on the minor side or in Coombs' testing of newborns whose mothers have received cephalosporin antibiotics before parturition, it should be recognized that a positive Coombs' test may be due to the drug.

Ceclor should be administered with caution in the presence of markedly impaired renal function. Under such conditions, careful clinical observation and laboratory studies should be made because safe dosage may be lower than that usually recommended.

As a result of administration of Ceclor, a false-positive reaction for glucose in the urine may oc-

Continued on next page

* Identi-Code® symbol.

Lilly—Cont.

cur. This has been observed with Benedict's and Fehling's solutions and also with Clinitest® tablets but not with Tes-Tape® (Glucose Enzymatic Test Strip, USP, Lilly).

Broad-spectrum antibiotics should be prescribed with caution in individuals with a history of gastrointestinal disease, particularly colitis.

Usage in Pregnancy—Pregnancy Category B—Reproduction studies have been performed in mice and rats at doses up to 12 times the human dose and in ferrets given three times the maximum human dose and have revealed no evidence of impaired fertility or harm to the fetus due to Ceclor. There are, however, no adequate and well-controlled studies in pregnant women. Because animal reproduction studies are not always predictive of human response, this drug should be used during pregnancy only if clearly needed.

Nursing Mothers—Small amounts of Ceclor have been detected in mother's milk following administration of single 500-mg doses. Average levels were 0.18, 0.20, 0.21, and 0.16 mcg/ml at two, three, four, and five hours respectively. Trace amounts were detected at one hour. The effect on nursing infants is not known. Caution should be exercised when Ceclor is administered to a nursing woman.

Usage in Children—Safety and effectiveness of this product for use in infants less than one month of age have not been established.

Adverse Reactions: Adverse effects considered related to therapy with Ceclor® (cefaclor, Lilly) are uncommon and are listed below:

Gastrointestinal symptoms occur in about 2.5 percent of patients and include diarrhea (1 in 70).

Symptoms of pseudomembranous colitis may appear either during or after antibiotic treatment. Nausea and vomiting have been reported rarely.

Hypersensitivity reactions have been reported in about 1.5 percent of patients and include morbilliform eruptions (1 in 100). Pruritus, urticaria, and positive Coombs' tests each occur in less than 1 in 200 patients. Cases of serum-sickness-like reactions (erythema multiforme or the above skin manifestations accompanied by arthritis/arthralgia and, frequently, fever) have been reported. These reactions are apparently due to hypersensitivity and have usually occurred during or following a second course of therapy with Ceclor. Such reactions have been reported more frequently in children than in adults. Signs and symptoms usually occur a few days after initiation of therapy and subside within a few days after cessation of therapy. No serious sequelae have been reported. Antihistamines and corticosteroids appear to enhance resolution of the syndrome.

Cases of anaphylaxis have been reported, half of which have occurred in patients with a history of penicillin allergy.

Other effects considered related to therapy include eosinophilia (1 in 50 patients) and genital pruritus or vaginitis (less than 1 in 100 patients).

Causal Relationship Uncertain—Transitory abnormalities in clinical laboratory test results have been reported. Although they were of uncertain etiology, they are listed below to serve as alerting information for the physician.

Hepatic—Slight elevations in SGOT, SGPT, or alkaline phosphatase values (1 in 40).

Hematopoietic—Transient fluctuations in leukocyte count, predominantly lymphocytosis occurring in infants and young children (1 in 40).

Renal—Slight elevations in BUN or serum creatinine (less than 1 in 500) or abnormal urinalysis (1 in 200).

Dosage and Administration: Ceclor® (cefaclor, Lilly) is administered orally.

Adults—The usual adult dosage is 250 mg every eight hours. For more severe infections (such as pneumonia) or those caused by less susceptible organisms, doses may be doubled. Doses of 4 g/day have been administered safely to normal subjects for 28 days, but the total daily dosage should not exceed this amount.

Children—The usual recommended daily dosage for children is 20 mg/kg/day in divided doses every eight hours, as indicated:

Child's Weight	Ceclor Suspension 125 mg/5 ml	250 mg/5 ml
9 kg	½ tsp t.i.d.	
18 kg	1 tsp t.i.d.	½ tsp t.i.d.

In more serious infections, otitis media, and infections caused by less susceptible organisms, 40 mg/kg/day are recommended, with a maximum dosage of 1 g/day.

Ceclor may be administered in the presence of impaired renal function. Under such a condition, the dosage usually is unchanged (*see* Precautions). In the treatment of beta-hemolytic streptococcal infections, a therapeutic dosage of Ceclor should be administered for at least ten days.

How Supplied: (℞) *Ceclor® (Cefaclor, USP), for Oral Suspension*, M-5057, 125 mg/5 ml (strawberry flavor) and M-5058, 250 mg/5 ml (strawberry flavor), in 75 (NDC 0002-5057-18 and NDC 0002-5058-18) and 150-ml-size (NDC 0002-5057-68 and NDC 0002-5058-68) packages.

Directions for mixing are included on the label. After mixing, store in a refrigerator. Shake well before using. Keep tightly closed. The mixture may be kept for 14 days without significant loss of potency. Discard unused portion after 14 days.

(℞) *Pulvules® Ceclor® (Cefaclor, USP): No. 3061*, 250 mg (White Opaque Body, Purple Opaque Cap), and *No. 3062*, 500 mg (Gray Opaque Body, Purple Opaque Cap), in bottles of 15 (NDC 0002-3061-15 and NDC 0002-3062-15) and 100 (NDC 0002-3061-02 and NDC 0002-3062-02) in 10 strips of 10 individually labeled blisters each containing one Pulvule (ID100) (NDC 0002-3061-33 and NDC 0002-3062-33).

Shown in Product Identification Section, page 417

* Bauer, A. W., Kirby, W. M. M., Sherris, J. C., and Turck, M.: Antibiotic Susceptibility Testing by a Standardized Single Disk Method, Am. J. Clin. Pathol, *45:* 493, 1966; Standardized Disc Susceptibility Test, Federal Register, *39:* 19182–19184, 1974.

[051884]

CEFACLOR, see Ceclor® (cefaclor, Lilly).

CEFAMANDOLE NAFATE, see Mandol® (cefamandole nafate, Lilly).

CEFAZOLIN SODIUM, see Kefzol® (cefazolin sodium, Lilly).

CEPHALOTHIN SODIUM, see Keflin® (cephalothin sodium, Lilly).

COLCHICINE ℞
[käl′ chĭ-sēn]
Injection, USP

This product to be used by the physician or under his direction.

Description: A phenanthrene derivative, colchicine is the active alkaloidal principle derived from various species of *Colchicum;* it appears as pale-yellow amorphorus scales or powder that darkens on exposure to light.

The empirical formula is $C_{22}H_{25}NO_6$ (399.45).

One g dissolves in 25 ml of water and in 220 ml of ether. Colchicine is freely soluble in alcohol and chloroform.

Colchicine, an acetyltrimethylcolchicinic acid, is hydrolyzed in the presence of dilute acids or alkalies, with cleavage of a methyl group as methanol and formation of *colchiceine*, which has very little therapeutic activity. On hydrolysis with strong acids, colchicine is converted to trimethylcolchicinic acid.

Ampoules Colchicine Injection, USP, provide an aqueous solution of colchicine for intravenous use. Each ampoule contains 1 mg of colchicine in 2 ml of solution. Sodium hydroxide may have been added during manufacture to adjust the pH.

Clinical Pharmacology: The mechanism of the relief afforded by colchicine in acute attacks of gouty arthritis is not completely known, but studies on the processes involved in precipitation of an acute attack have helped elucidate how this drug may exert its effects. The drug is not an analgesic, does not relieve other types of pain or inflammation, and is of no value in other types of arthritis. It is not a diuretic and does not influence the renal excretion of uric acid or its level in the blood or the magnitude of the "miscible pool" of uric acid. It also does not alter the solubility of urate in the plasma.

Colchicine is not a uricosuric agent. An acute attack of gout apparently occurs as a result of an inflammatory reaction to crystals of monosodium urate that are deposited in the joint tissue from hyperuric body fluids; the reaction is aggravated as more urate crystals accumulate. The initial inflammatory response involves local infiltration of granulocytes that phagocytize the urate crystals. Interference with these processes will prevent the development of an acute attack. Colchicine apparently exerts its effect by reducing the inflammatory response to the deposited crystals and also by diminishing phagocytosis. The deposition of uric acid is favored by an acid pH. In synovial tissues and in leukocytes associated with inflammatory processes, lactic acid production is high, and this favors a local decrease in pH that enhances uric acid deposition. Colchicine diminishes lactic acid production by leukocytes directly and by diminishing phagocytosis and thereby interrupts the cycle of urate crystal deposition and inflammatory response that sustains the acute attack. The oxidation of glucose in phagocytizing as well as in nonphagocytizing leukocytes in vitro is suppressed by colchicine; this suppression may explain the diminished lactic acid production. The precise biochemical step that is affected by colchicine is not yet known. That the antimitotic activity of colchicine is unrelated to its effectiveness in the treatment of acute gout is indicated by the fact that trimethylcolchicinic acid, an analog of colchicine, has no antimitotic activity except in extremely high doses.

Indications and Usage: Colchicine is indicated for the treatment of gout. It is effective in relieving the pain of acute attacks, especially if therapy is begun early in the attack and in adequate dosage. Many therapists use colchicine as interval therapy to prevent acute attacks of gout. It has no effect on nongouty arthritis or on uric acid metabolism.

The intravenous use of colchicine is advantageous when a rapid response is desired or when gastrointestinal side effects interfere with oral administration of the medication. Occasionally, intravenous colchicine is effective when the oral preparation is not. After the acute attack has subsided, the patient can usually be given colchicine tablets by mouth.

Contraindications: Colchicine is contraindicated in patients with gout who also have serious gastrointestinal, renal, or cardiac disorders.

Warnings: Colchicine can cause fetal harm when administered to a pregnant woman. If this drug is used during pregnancy, or if the patient becomes pregnant while taking it, the woman should be apprised of the potential hazard to the fetus.

Precautions: *General Precautions*—Colchicine should be administered with great caution to aged and debilitated patients, especially those with renal, gastrointestinal, or heart disease. Reduction in dosage is indicated if weakness, anorexia, nausea, vomiting, or diarrhea appears. Rarely, thrombophlebitis occurs at the site of injection.

Drug Interactions—Colchicine has been shown to induce reversible malabsorption of vitamin B_{12}, apparently by altering the function of ileal mucosa. The possibility that colchicine may increase response to central-nervous-system depressants and to sympathomimetic agents is suggested by the results of experiments on animals.

Usage in Pregnancy—Pregnancy Category D—See Warnings.

Nursing Mothers—It is not known whether this drug is excreted in human milk. Because many drugs are excreted in human milk, caution should be exercised when colchicine is administered to a nursing woman.

Usage in Children—Safety and effectiveness in children have not been established.

Adverse Reactions: These are usually gastrointestinal in nature and consist of abdominal pain, nausea, vomiting, and diarrhea. The diarrhea may be severe. The gastrointestinal symptoms may occur even though the drug is given intravenously; however, such symptoms are unusual unless the recommended dose is exceeded.

Prolonged administration may cause bone-marrow depression, with agranulocytosis, thrombocytopenia, and aplastic anemia. Peripheral neuritis and depilation have also been reported.

Overdosage: There is usually a latent period between overdosage and the onset of symptoms, regardless of the route of administration. The lethal dose of colchicine has been estimated to be 65 mg. However, deaths have been reported with as little as 8 mg, although higher doses have been taken without fatal results. The first symptoms to appear are gastrointestinal—nausea, vomiting, abdominal pain, and diarrhea. The diarrhea may be severe and bloody owing to hemorrhagic gastroenteritis. To control the diarrhea and cramps, paregoric is usually administered. Burning sensations in the throat, stomach, and skin may also occur. Extensive vascular damage may result in shock. The kidney may show evidence of damage by hematuria and oliguria, since it is an excretory site. Severe dehydration and hypotension develop. Muscular weakness is marked, and an ascending paralysis of the central nervous system may develop. The patient usually remains conscious. However, delirium and convulsions may occur. Death usually is the result of respiratory depression.

Recent studies[1,2] appear to support the use of hemodialysis or peritoneal dialysis as part of the treatment of acute overdosage. Shock must be combated. Atropine and morphine may relieve the abdominal pain. Respiratory assistance may be needed to insure proper oxygenation and ventilation.

Dosage and Administration: Colchicine Injection is for intravenous use only. Severe local irritation occurs if it is administered subcutaneously or intramuscularly.

It is extremely important that the needle be properly positioned in the vein before colchicine is injected. If leakage into surrounding tissue or outside the vein along its course should occur during intravenous administration, considerable irritation may follow. There is no specific antidote for the prevention of this irritation. Local application of heat or cold, as well as administration of analgesics, may afford relief.

The injection should take two to five minutes for completion. Colchicine Injection should not be diluted with 5% Dextrose in Water. If a decrease in concentration of colchicine in solution is required, 0.9% Sodium Chloride Injection, which does not contain a bacteriostatic agent, should be used. Solutions which thereafter become turbid should not be injected.

In the treatment of acute gouty arthritis, the average initial dose of Colchicine Injection is 2 mg (4 ml). This may be followed by 0.5 mg (1 ml) every six hours until a satisfactory response is achieved. In general, the total dosage for the first 24-hour period should not exceed 4 mg (8 ml). The total dose for one course of treatment should not exceed 4 mg. Some clinicians recommend a single intravenous dose of 3 mg, whereas others recommend not more than 1 mg of colchicine intravenously for the initial dose, followed by 0.5 mg once or twice daily if needed.

If pain recurs, it may be necessary to administer a daily dose of 1 to 2 mg (2 to 4 ml) for several days. Many patients can be transferred to the oral colchicine in a similar dosage to that being given intravenously.

In the prophylactic or maintenance therapy of recurrent or chronic gouty arthritis, a dosage of 0.5 to 1 mg (1 to 2 ml) once or twice daily may be used. However, in these cases, oral administration of colchicine is preferable, usually in conjunction with a uricosuric agent.

How Supplied: (℞) *Ampoules No. 656, Colchicine Injection, USP*, 1 mg, 2 ml, in packages of 6 (NDC 0002-1443-16).

[061083]

1. Donigian, D. W., and Owellen, R. J.: Interaction of Vinblastine, Vincristine, and Colchicine with Serum Proteins, Biochem. Pharmacol., 22:2113, 1973.
2. Wolen, R. L.: Unpublished data, Lilly Research Laboratories, 1975.

COLCHICINE ℞
[*kăl′ chĭ-sēn*]
Tablets, USP

Description and Clinical Pharmacology: See under Colchicine Injection, USP.

Indications and Usage: Colchicine is indicated for the treatment of gout. It is effective in relieving the pain of acute attacks, especially if therapy is begun early in the attack and in adequate dosage. Many therapists use colchicine as interval therapy to prevent acute attacks of gout. It has no effect on nongouty arthritis or on uric acid metabolism.

Contraindications, Warnings, and Precautions: See under Colchicine Injection, USP.

Adverse Reactions: In full dosage, colchicine produces nausea, vomiting, or diarrhea. However, it is generally necessary to reach such dose levels for an adequate therapeutic effect. Paregoric may be given either concurrently or when diarrhea develops.

Prolonged administration may cause bone-marrow depression, with agranulocytosis, thrombocytopenia, and aplastic anemia. Peripheral neuritis and depilation have also been reported.

Overdosage: See under Colchicine Injection, USP.

Recent studies[1,2] would appear to support the use of hemodialysis or peritoneal dialysis as part of the treatment of acute overdosage in addition to gastric lavage. Shock must be combated. Atropine and morphine may relieve the abdominal pain. Respiratory assistance may be needed to insure proper oxygenation and ventilation.

Dosage and Administration: Colchicine should be started at the first warning of an acute attack; a delay of a few hours impairs its effectiveness. The usual adult dose is 1 or 2 tablets initially, followed by 1 tablet every one to two hours until pain is relieved or nausea, vomiting, or diarrhea develops. Some physicians use 2 tablets every two hours. Since the number of doses required may range from six to 16, the total dose is variable. As interval treatment, 1 tablet may be taken one to four times a week for the mild or moderate case, once or twice daily for the severe case.

How Supplied: (℞) *Tablets No. 560, Colchicine Tablets, USP, J13,** 0.6 mg, in bottles of 100 (NDC 0002-1013-02) and 1000 (NDC 0002-1013-04).

[080883]

1. Donigian, D. W., and Owellen, R. J.: Interaction of Vinblastine, Vincristine, and Colchicine with Serum Proteins, Biochem. Pharmacol., 22:2113, 1973.
2. Wolen, R. L.: Unpublished data, Lilly Research Laboratories, 1975.

CRYSTODIGIN® ℞
[*krĭs-tō-dĭj′ ĭn*]
(digitoxin)
Tablets, USP

Description: Crystodigin® (digitoxin, Lilly) is a crystalline-pure single cardiac glycoside obtained from *Digitalis purpurea* and is identical in pharmacologic action with whole-leaf digitalis.

Digitoxin is the most slowly excreted of all digitalis compounds (excretion time is 14 to 21 days). It is most useful in patients with impaired renal function, since excretion and metabolism are independent of renal function.

Crystodigin is noted for its uniform potency, complete absorption, and lack of gastrointestinal irritation. It permits accurate dosage adjustments to produce maximum therapeutic effect smoothly and dependably.

Crystodigin, for oral administration, is available in tablets containing 0.05, 0.1, 0.15, or 0.2 mg crystalline digitoxin.

Digitoxin is a cardiotonic glycoside. The chemical name is card-20 (22) - enolide,3-[(O-2,6-dideoxy-β-D-*ribo*-hexopyranosyl-(1→4)-O-2,6 - dideoxy-β-D-*ribo*-hexopyranosyl- (1→4) -2,6- dideoxy- β-D-*ribo*-hexopyranosyl) oxy]-14-hydroxy,(3β,5β) -. The empirical formula of digitoxin is $C_{41}H_{64}O_{13}$.

Clinical Pharmacology: The cellular basis for the inotropic effects of digitalis is probably enhancement of excitation-contraction coupling, that process by which chemical energy is converted into mechanical energy when triggered by membrane depolarization. Most evidence relates this process to the entry of calcium ions into the cell during depolarization of the membrane and /or to the release of calcium from intracellular binding sites on the sarcoplasmic reticulum. The free calcium ion mediates the interaction of actin and myosin, resulting in contraction.

The amount of glycoside absorbed depends largely on its polarity, which is a function of the net electronic charge on the molecule. The more nonpolar or lipid soluble, the better is the absorption, because of the greater permeability of lipid membrane of the intestinal mucosa for lipid-soluble substances. The nonpolar, lipophilic digitoxin is completely absorbed; the oral dose, therefore, is the same as the intravenous dose. Other glycosides are not as well absorbed.

Nonpolar digitoxin is over 90 percent bound to tissue proteins. The firm binding of digitoxin to protein is responsible for its long half-life (seven to nine days).

Digitoxin differs from other commonly used glycosides not only in its firm binding to protein but also because it is metabolized in the liver, with the only active metabolite being digoxin, which represents only a small fraction of the total metabolites. All other metabolites are inert and are probably excreted as such in the urine. The portion of digitoxin that is not metabolized is excreted in the bile to the intestines and recycled to the liver until it is completely metabolized. The portion of digitoxin that is bound to protein is in equilibrium with free digitoxin in the serum. Thus, as more and more of the free digitoxin is metabolized after a single dose, there is proportionately less bound digitoxin.

Indications and Usage: Crystodigin® (digitoxin, Lilly) is indicated in the treatment of heart failure, atrial flutter, atrial fibrillation, and supraventricular tachycardia. Parenteral administration of Crystodigin is indicated for neonates and immature infants.

Contraindications: If the indications are carefully observed, there are few contraindications to digitalis therapy except toxic response to digitalis or idiosyncrasy, ventricular tachycardia, beriberi heart disease, and some instances of the hypersensitive carotid sinus syndrome.

Patients already taking digitalis preparations must not be given the rapid digitalizing dose of Crystodigin® (digitoxin, Lilly) or parenteral calcium.

Warnings: Many of the arrhythmias for which digitalis is advised are identical with those reflecting digitalis intoxication. When the possibility of digitalis intoxication cannot be excluded, cardiac glycosides should be withheld temporarily if the clinical situation permits.

The patient with congestive heart failure may complain of nausea and vomiting. Since these symptoms may also be associated with digitalis intoxication, a clinical determination of their

Continued on next page

* Identi-Code® symbol.

Lilly—Cont.

cause must be attempted before further administration of the drug.

Cases of idiopathic hypertrophic subaortic stenosis must be managed with extreme care. Unless cardiac failure is severe, it is doubtful whether digitalis should be employed.

Children—During the first month of life, infants have a sharply defined tolerance to digitalis. Impaired renal function must also be considered. Premature and immature infants are particularly sensitive, and reduction in dosage may be necessary.

The presence of acute glomerulonephritis accompanied by congestive failure requires extreme care in digitalization. A relatively low total dose, administered in divided doses, and concomitant use of reserpine or other antihypertensive agents have been recommended. Constant ECG monitoring is essential. Digitalis should be discontinued as soon as possible.

Patients with rheumatic carditis, especially when severe, are unusually sensitive to digitalis and prone to disturbances of rhythm. If heart failure develops, digitalization may be tried with relatively low doses; these must be cautiously increased until a beneficial effect is obtained. If a therapeutic trial does not result in improvement, the drug should be discontinued.

NOTE: Digitalis glycosides are an important cause of accidental poisoning in children.

Precautions: *General Precautions*—When the risk of digitalis intoxication is great, the use of a short-acting, rapidly eliminated glycoside, such as digoxin, is advisable. Although intoxication cannot always be prevented by the selection of one glycoside over another, certain glycosides may be preferred in patients who have fixed disabilities (e.g., liver impairment, drug intolerance). However, digitoxin can be used in patients with impaired renal function.

Newborn infants with heart disease, especially prematures, are particularly susceptible to digitalis intoxication, and frequent electrocardiographic monitoring is essential in these patients. Special care must likewise be exercised in elderly patients receiving digitalis because their body mass tends to be small and renal clearance is likely to be reduced. In addition, digitalis must be used cautiously in the presence of active heart disease, such as acute myocardial infarction or acute myocarditis. In patients with acute or unstable chronic atrial fibrillation, digitalis may not normalize the ventricular rate even when the serum concentration exceeds the usual therapeutic level. Although these patients may be less sensitive to the toxic effects of digitalis than are patients with normal sinus rhythm, dosage should not be increased to potentially toxic levels.

Hypokalemia predisposes to digitalis toxicity, and even a moderate decrease in the concentration of serum potassium can precipitate serious arrhythmias.

Impaired liver function may necessitate reduction in dosage of any digitalis preparation, including digitoxin.

Sensitive radioimmunoassay techniques have been developed for measuring serum levels of digitoxin, and these procedures can be instituted in almost any hospital. Serum levels must, however, be evaluated in conjunction with clinical history and the results of the electrocardiogram and other laboratory tests. A therapeutic serum level for one patient may be excessive or inadequate for another patient.

Drug Interactions—The synthesis of microsomal enzymes that metabolize digitoxin in the liver is subject to stimulation by a number of drugs, such as antihistamines, anticonvulsants, barbiturates, oral hypoglycemic agents, and others.

When digitoxin is the glycoside used for digitalis maintenance, drugs that are liver-microsomal-enzyme inducers should not be used at the same time. Phenobarbital, phenylbutazone, and diphenylhydantoin will increase the rate of metabolism of digitoxin. In patients receiving 60 mg of phenobarbital three times a day for 12 weeks, the steady-state concentration of digitoxin in plasma fell approximately 50 percent when the drugs were administered concurrently and returned to previous levels when phenobarbital was discontinued.

When drugs that increase the rate of metabolism of digitoxin in the liver are discontinued, toxicity may occur.

Hypokalemia is most frequently encountered in patients receiving concomitant diuretic therapy, because the most widely used and most effective diuretics (i.e., thiazides and furosemide) increase the urinary loss of potassium. Prescribing a potassium-sparing agent (spironolactone or triamterene) together with the potassium-wasting diuretic is a reliable means for maintaining the serum potassium level. Alternatively, potassium chloride supplements may be prescribed.

Mineralocorticoids (e.g., prednisone) and, rarely, certain antibiotics (e.g., amphotericin B) may also cause increased excretion of potassium.

Usage in Pregnancy—*Pregnancy Category C*—Animal reproduction studies have not been conducted with Crystodigin. It is also not known whether this drug can cause fetal harm when administered to a pregnant woman or can affect reproduction capacity. Crystodigin should be given to a pregnant woman only if clearly needed.

Labor and Delivery—No information is available concerning the use of Crystodigin in labor and delivery.

Nursing Mothers—It is not known whether this drug is excreted in human milk. Because many drugs are excreted in human milk, caution should be exercised when Crystodigin is administered to a nursing woman.

Adverse Reactions: Anorexia, nausea, and vomiting have been reported. These effects are central in origin, but following large oral doses, there is also a local emetic action. Abdominal discomfort or pain and diarrhea may also occur.

Overdosage: Overdosage causes side effects, such as mental depression, anorexia, nausea, vomiting, premature beats, complete heart block, AV dissociation, ventricular tachycardia, ventricular fibrillation, restlessness, yellow vision, mental confusion, disorientation, and delirium.

Alterations in cardiac rate and rhythm occurring in digitalis poisoning may simulate almost any known type of arrhythmia seen clinically. Extrasystoles are probably the most frequent effect. An electrocardiogram is necessary in the clinical management of the patient to aid in the differentiation of arrhythmia due to digitalis poisoning from that due to heart disease. Older patients and particularly those with disease of the coronary arteries and impaired myocardial blood supply are more susceptible to these untoward effects. Sinus arrhythmia may occur early as a minor toxic effect. Paroxysmal atrial and ventricular tachycardia call for immediate cessation of the drug. Atrial fibrillation can occur following large doses of digitalis. Ventricular fibrillation is the most common cause of death from digitalis poisoning.

Potassium ion is probably the best agent for prompt suppression of digitalis arrhythmias. It can be administered intravenously in the form of potassium chloride at a rate of 0.5 mEq/minute in sodium chloride (isotonic) or dextrose (5 percent) solution containing 50 to 100 mEq of potassium per liter. Administration of the potassium salt in normal saline is preferred. Constant electrocardiographic monitoring is essential during injection of the solution. Since the action of potassium ion lasts only minutes after infusion is discontinued, oral therapy with potassium chloride may be given for prolonged suppression of arrhythmias. Potassium is contraindicated in the presence of renal failure. Diphenylhydantoin may be used if potassium fails or is contraindicated. If both potassium and diphenylhydantoin fail, procainamide and quinidine can be used. Disodium edetate has been used for terminating digitalis-induced ventricular arrhythmias and abnormalities of atrioventricular conduction.

Dosage and Administration: *Adults: Slow Digitalization*—0.2 mg twice daily for a period of four days, followed by maintenance dosage. *Rapid Digitalization*—Preferably 0.6 mg initially, followed by 0.4 mg and then 0.2 mg at intervals of four to six hours. *Maintenance Dosage*—Ranges from 0.05 to 0.3 mg daily, the most common dose being 0.15 mg daily.

Children: Digitalization must be individualized. Generally, premature and immature infants are particularly sensitive and require reduced parenteral dosage of Crystodigin that must be determined by careful titration.

After the neonatal period, the dose is as follows:
Under one year of age—0.045 mg/kg
One to two years of age—0.04 mg/kg
Over two years of age—0.03 mg/kg (0.75 mg/m^2)

The total dose should be divided into three, four, or more portions, with six hours or more between doses.

For a maintenance dose, the patient should be given one-tenth of the digitalizing dose.

How Supplied: (℞) *Tablets Crystodigin®* (*Digitoxin Tablets, USP*) (scored): *No. 1736, J75,* * 0.05 mg, Orange, in bottles of 100 (NDC 0002-1075-02); *No. 1703, J60,* *0.1 mg, Pink, in bottles of 100 (NDC 0002-1060-02), 500 (NDC 0002-1060-03), and 5000 (NDC 0002-1060-31) and in 10 strips of 10 individually labeled blisters each containing 1 tablet (ID100) (NDC 0002-1060-33); *No. 1737, J76,* * 0.15 mg, Yellow, in bottles of 100 (NDC 0002-1076-02); *No. 1694, J57,* * 0.2 mg, White, in bottles of 100 (NDC 0002-1057-02) and 500 (NDC 0002-1057-03).

[030984]

Shown in Product Identification Section, page 417

CYCLOMETHYCAINE SULFATE, *see* Surfacaine® (cyclomethycaine sulfate, Lilly)

CYCLOSERINE, *see* Seromycin® (cycloserine, Lilly).

CYCLOTHIAZIDE, *see* Anhydron® (cyclothiazide, Lilly).

DARVOCET-N® 50
[där' vō-sĕt ĕn]
and
DARVOCET-N® 100
(propoxyphene napsylate and acetaminophen)
USP

DARVON-N®
[där' vŏn ĕn]
(propoxyphene napsylate)
USP

DARVON-N® WITH A.S.A.®
[där' vŏn ĕn with ā' ĕs-ā]
(propoxyphene napsylate and aspirin)
USP

Description: Propoxyphene napsylate (Darvon-N®) is an odorless white crystalline solid with a bitter taste. It is very slightly soluble in water and soluble in methanol, ethanol, chloroform, and acetone. Chemically, it is α-(+)- 4- (Dimethylamino)-3-methyl-1,2-diphenyl-2-butanol Propionate (ester) 2-Naphthalene-sulfonate (salt) Hydrate.

Propoxyphene napsylate differs from propoxyphene hydrochloride in that it allows more stable liquid dosage forms and tablet formulations. Because of differences in molecular weight, a dose of 100 mg of propoxyphene napsylate is required to supply an amount of propoxyphene equivalent to that present in 65 mg of propoxyphene hydrochloride.

Each tablet of Darvocet-N 50 contains 50 mg propoxyphene napsylate and 325 mg acetaminophen.
Each tablet of Darvocet-N 100 contains 100 mg propoxyphene napsylate and 650 mg acetaminophen.
Each 5 ml of Suspension Darvon-N contain 50 mg propoxyphene napsylate.
Each tablet of Darvon-N contains 100 mg propoxyphene napsylate.
Each tablet of Darvon-N with A.S.A. contains 100 mg propoxyphene napsylate and 325 mg aspirin.

Clinical Pharmacology: Propoxyphene is a centrally acting narcotic analgesic agent. Equimolar doses of propoxyphene hydrochloride or napsylate provide similar plasma concentrations. Following administration of 65, 130, or 195 mg of propoxyphene hydrochloride, the bioavailability of propoxyphene is equivalent to that of 100, 200, or 300 mg respectively of propoxyphene napsylate. Peak plasma concentrations of propoxyphene are reached in two to two and one-half hours. After a 100-mg oral dose of propoxyphene napsylate, peak plasma levels of 0.05 to 0.1 mcg/ml are achieved. As shown in Figure 1, the napsylate salt tends to be absorbed more slowly than the hydrochloride. At or near therapeutic doses, this difference is small when compared with that among subjects and among doses. (See Figure 1)

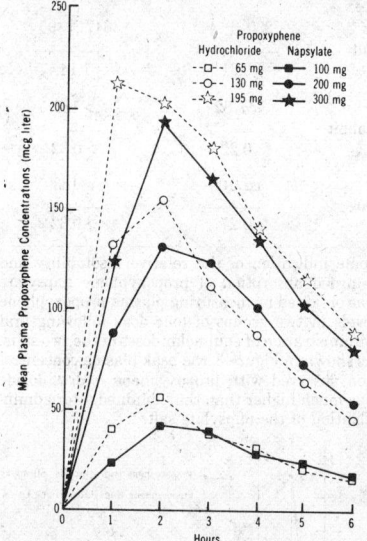

Figure 1. Mean plasma concentrations of propoxyphene in eight human subjects following oral administration of 65 and 130 mg of the hydrochloride salt and 100 and 200 mg of the napsylate salt and in seven given 195 mg of the hydrochloride and 300 mg of the napsylate salt

Because of this several hundredfold difference in solubility, the absorption rate of very large doses of the napsylate salt is significantly lower than that of equimolar doses of the hydrochloride.

Repeated doses of propoxyphene at six-hour intervals lead to increasing plasma concentrations, with a plateau after the ninth dose at 48 hours. Propoxyphene is metabolized in the liver to yield norpropoxyphene. Propoxyphene has a half-life of six to 12 hours, whereas that of norpropoxyphene is 30 to 36 hours.

Norpropoxyphene has substantially less central-nervous-system-depressant effect than propoxyphene but a greater local anesthetic effect, which is similar to that of amitriptyline and antiarrhythmic agents, such as lidocaine and quinidine.

In animal studies in which propoxyphene and norpropoxyphene were continuously infused in large amounts, intracardiac conduction time (PR and QRS intervals) was prolonged. Any intracardiac conduction delay attributable to high concentrations of norpropoxyphene may be of relatively long duration.

Actions: Propoxyphene is a mild narcotic analgesic structurally related to methadone. The potency of propoxyphene napsylate is from two-thirds to equal that of codeine.

Darvocet-N 50 and Darvocet-N 100 provide the analgesic activity of propoxyphene napsylate and the antipyretic-analgesic activity of acetaminophen.

The combination of propoxyphene and acetaminophen produces greater analgesia than that produced by either propoxyphene or acetaminophen administered alone.

The combination of propoxyphene with aspirin produces greater analgesia than that produced by either drug administered alone.

Indications: Darvocet-N 50, Darvocet-N 100, and Darvon-N with A.S.A. are indicated for the relief of mild to moderate pain, either when pain is present alone or when it is accompanied by fever. Darvon-N® (propoxyphene napsylate, Lilly) is indicated for the relief of mild to moderate pain.

Contraindications: Hypersensitivity to propoxyphene, acetaminophen, or aspirin.

WARNINGS

- Do not prescribe propoxyphene for patients who are suicidal or addiction-prone.
- Prescribe propoxyphene with caution for patients taking tranquilizers or antidepressant drugs and patients who use alcohol in excess.
- Tell your patients not to exceed the recommended dose and to limit their intake of alcohol.

Propoxyphene products in excessive doses, either alone or in combination with other CNS depressants, including alcohol, are a major cause of drug-related deaths. Fatalities within the first hour of overdosage are not uncommon. In a survey of deaths due to overdosage conducted in 1975, in approximately 20 percent of the fatal cases, death occurred within the first hour (5 percent occurred within 15 minutes). Propoxyphene should not be taken in doses higher than those recommended by the physician. The judicious prescribing of propoxyphene is essential to the safe use of this drug. With patients who are depressed or suicidal, consideration should be given to the use of non-narcotic analgesics. Patients should be cautioned about the concomitant use of propoxyphene products and alcohol because of potentially serious CNS-additive effects of these agents. Because of its added depressant effects, propoxyphene should be prescribed with caution for those patients whose medical condition requires the concomitant administration of sedatives, tranquilizers, muscle relaxants, antidepressants, or other CNS-depressant drugs. Patients should be advised of the additive depressant effects of these combinations.

Many of the propoxyphene-related deaths have occurred in patients with previous histories of emotional disturbances or suicidal ideation or attempts as well as histories of misuse of tranquilizers, alcohol, and other CNS-active drugs. Some deaths have occurred as a consequence of the accidental ingestion of excessive quantities of propoxyphene alone or in combination with other drugs. Patients taking propoxyphene should be warned not to exceed the dosage recommended by the physician.

Drug Dependence—Propoxyphene, when taken in higher-than-recommended doses over long periods of time, can produce drug dependence characterized by psychic dependence and, less frequently, physical dependence and tolerance. Propoxyphene will only partially suppress the withdrawal syndrome in individuals physically dependent on morphine or other narcotics. The abuse liability of propoxyphene is qualitatively similar to that of codeine although quantitatively less, and propoxyphene should be prescribed with the same degree of caution appropriate to the use of codeine.

Usage in Ambulatory Patients—Propoxyphene may impair the mental and/or physical abilities required for the performance of potentially hazardous tasks, such as driving a car or operating machinery. The patient should be cautioned accordingly.

Precautions: *General*—Propoxyphene should be administered with caution to patients with hepatic or renal impariment, since higher serum concentrations or delayed elimination may occur.

Salicylates should be used with extreme caution in the presence of peptic ulcer or coagulation abnormalities.

Drug Interactions—The CNS-depressant effect of propoxyphene is additive with that of other CNS depressants, including alcohol.

As is the case with many medicinal agents, propoxyphene may slow the metabolism of a concomitantly administered drug. Should this occur, the higher serum concentrations of that drug may result in increased phamacologic or adverse effects of that drug. Such occurrences have been reported when propoxyphene was administered to patients on antidepressants, anticonvulsants, or warfarin-like drugs.

Salicylates may enhance the effect of anticoagulants and inhibit the uricosuric effect of uricosuric agents.

Usage in Pregnancy—Safe use in pregnancy has not been established relative to possible adverse effects on fetal development. Instances of withdrawal symptoms in the neonate have been reported following usage during pregnancy. Therefore, propoxyphene should not be used in pregnant women unless, in the judgment of the physician, the potential benefits outweigh the possible hazards.

Usage in Nursing Mothers—Low levels of propoxyphene have been detected in human milk. In postpartum studies involving nursing mothers who were given propoxyphene, no adverse effects were noted in infants receiving mother's milk.

Usage in Children—Propoxyphene is not recommended for use in children, because documented clinical experience has been insufficient to establish safety and a suitable dosage regimen in the pediatric age group.

A Patient Information Sheet is available for these products. See text following "How Supplied" section below.

Adverse Reactions: In a survey conducted in hospitalized patients, less than 1 percent of patients taking propoxyphene hydrochloride at recommended doses experienced side effects. The most frequently reported have been dizziness, sedation, nausea, and vomiting. Some of these adverse reactions may be alleviated if the patient lies down.

Other adverse reactions include constipation, abdominal pain, skin rashes, lightheadedness, headache, weakness, euphoria, dysphoria, and minor visual disturbances.

Cases of liver dysfunction have been reported.

Dosage and Administration: These products are given orally. The usual dose of Darvocet-N 50 or Darvocet-N 100 is 100 mg propoxyphene napsylate and 650 mg acetaminophen every four hours as needed for pain.

The usual dose of Darvon-N® (propoxyphene napsylate, Lilly) is 100 mg every four hours as needed for pain.

The usual dose of Darvon-N with A.S.A. is 100 mg propoxyphene napsylate and 325 mg aspirin every four hours as needed for pain.

The maximum recommended dose of propoxyphene napsylate is 600 mg per day.

Consideration should be given to a reduced total daily dosage in patients with hepatic or renal impairment.

Management of Overdosage: In all cases of suspected overdosage, call your regional Poison Control Center to obtain the most up-to-date information about the treatment of overdosage. This recommendation is made because, in general, information regarding the treatment of overdosage may change more rapidly than do package inserts. Initial consideration should be given to the management of the CNS effects of propoxyphene overdosage. Resuscitative measures should be initiated promptly.

Symptoms of Propoxyphene Overdosage—The manifestations of acute overdosage with propoxy-

Continued on next page

* Identi-Code® symbol.

Lilly—Cont.

phene are those of narcotic overdosage. The patient is usually somnolent but may be stuporous or comatose and convulsing. Respiratory depression is characteristic. The ventilatory rate and/or tidal volume is decreased, which results in cyanosis and hypoxia. Pupils, initially pinpoint, may become dilated as hypoxia increases. Cheyne-Stokes respiration and apnea may occur. Blood pressure and heart rate are usually normal initially, but blood pressure falls and cardiac performance deteriorates, which ultimately results in pulmonary edema and circulatory collapse, unless the respiratory depression is corrected and adequate ventilation is restored promptly. Cardiac arrhythmias and conduction delay may be present. A combined respiratory-metabolic acidosis occurs owing to retained CO_2 (hypercapnea) and to lactic acid formed during anaerobic glycolysis. Acidosis may be severe if large amounts of salicylates have also been ingested. Death may occur.

Treatment of Propoxyphene Overdosage — Attention should be directed first to establishing a patent airway and to restoring ventilation. Mechanically assisted ventilation, with or without oxygen, may be required, and positive pressure respiration may be desirable if pulmonary edema is present. The narcotic antagonist naloxone will markedly reduce the degree of respiratory depression, and 0.4 to 2 mg should be administered promptly, preferably intravenously. If the desired degree of counteraction with improvement in respiratory functions is not obtained, naloxone should be repeated at two to three-minute intervals. The duration of action of the antagonist may be brief. If no response is observed after 10 mg of naloxone have been administered, the diagnosis of propoxyphene toxicity should be questioned. (Nalorphine and levallorphan may be used if naloxone is not available, but these agents are not as satisfactory as naloxone.)

Treatment of Propoxyphene Overdosage in Children—The usual inital dose of naloxone in children is 0.01 mg/kg body weight given intravenously. If this dose does not result in the desired degree of clinical improvement, a subsequent increased dose of 0.1 mg/kg body weight may be administered. If an IV route of administration is not available, naloxone may be administered IM or subcutaneously in divided doses. If necessary, naloxone can be diluted with sterile water for injection.

Blood gases, pH, and electrolytes should be monitored in order that acidosis and any electrolyte disturbance present may be corrected promptly. Acidosis, hypoxia, and generalized CNS depression predispose to the development of cardiac arrhythmias. Ventricular fibrillation or cardiac arrest may occur and necessitate the full complement of cardiopulmonary resuscitation (CPR) measures. Respiratory acidosis rapidly subsides as ventilation is restored and hypercapnea eliminated, but lactic acidosis may require intravenous bicarbonate for prompt correction.

Electrocardiographic monitoring is essential. Prompt correction of hypoxia, acidosis, and electrolyte disturbance (when present) will help prevent these cardiac complications and will increase the effectiveness of agents administered to restore normal cardiac function.

In addition to the use of a narcotic antagonist, the patient may require careful titration with an anticonvulsant to control convulsions. Analeptic drugs (for example, caffeine or amphetamine) should not be used because of their tendency to precipitate convulsions.

General supportive measures, in addition to oxygen, include, when necessary, intravenous fluids, vasopressor-inotropic compounds, and, when infection is likely, anti-infective agents. Gastric lavage may be useful, and activated charcoal can adsorb a significant amount of ingested propoxyphene. Dialysis is of little value in poisoning due to propoxyphene. Efforts should be made to determine whether other agents, such as alcohol, barbiturates, tranquilizers, or other CNS depressants, were also ingested, since these increase CNS depression as well as cause specific toxic effects.

Symptoms of Acetaminophen Overdosage— Shortly after oral ingestion of an overdose of acetaminophen and for the next 24 hours, anorexia, nausea, vomiting, and abdominal pain have been noted. The patient may then present no symptoms, but evidence of liver dysfunction may be apparent during the next 24 to 48 hours, with elevated serum transaminase and lactic dehydrogenase levels, an increase in serum bilirubin concentrations, and a prolonged prothrombin time. Death from hepatic failure may result three to seven days after overdosage.

Treatment of Acetaminophen Overdosage— Acetaminophen in massive overdosage may cause hepatic toxicity in some patients. *In all cases of suspected overdose, immediately call your regional poison center or the Rocky Mountain Poison Center's toll-free number* (800-525-6115) for assistance in diagnosis and for directions in the use of N-acetylcysteine as an antidote, a use currently restricted to investigational status.

In adults, hepatic toxicity has rarely been reported with acute overdoses of less than 10 g and fatalities with less than 15 g. Importantly, young children seem to be more resistant than adults to the hepatotoxic effect of an acetaminophen overdose. Despite this, the measures outlined below should be initiated in any adult or child suspected of having ingested an acetaminophen overdose.

Clinical and laboratory evidence of hepatic toxicty may not be apparent until 48 to 72 hours postingestion. Early symptoms following a potentially hepatotoxic overdose may include: nausea, vomiting, diaphoresis, and general malaise.

The stomach should be emptied promptly by lavage or by induction of emesis with syrup of ipecac. Patients' estimates of the quantity of a drug ingested are notoriously unreliable. Therefore, if an acetaminophen overdose is suspected, a serum acetaminophen assay should be obtained as early as possible, but no sooner than four hours following ingestion. Liver function studies should be obtained initially and repeated at 24-hour intervals. The antidote, N-acetylcysteine, should be administered as early as possible, and within 16 hours of the overdose ingestion for optimal results. Following recovery, there are no residual, structural, or functional hepatic abnormalities.

Symptoms of Salicylate Overdosage—Such symptoms include central nausea and vomiting, tinnitus and deafness, vertigo and headaches, mental dullness and confusion, diaphoresis, rapid pulse, and increased respiration and respiratory alkalosis.

Treatment of Salicylate Overdosage—When Darvon-N with A.S.A. has been ingested, the clinical picture may be complicated by salicylism.

The treatment of acute salicylate intoxication includes minimizing drug absorption, promoting elimination through the kidneys, and correcting metabolic derangements affecting body temperature, hydration, acid-base balance, and electrolyte balance. The technique to be employed for eliminating salicylate from the bloodstream depends on the degree of drug intoxication.

If the patient is seen within four hours of ingestion, the stomach should be emptied by inducing vomiting or by gastric lavage as soon as possible. The nomogram of Done is a useful prognostic guide in which the expected severity of salicylate intoxication is based on serum salicylate levels and the time interval between ingestion and taking the blood sample.

Exchange transfusion is most feasible for a small infant. Intermittent peritoneal dialysis is useful for cases of moderate severity in adults. Intravenous fluids alkalinized by the addition of sodium bicarbonate or potassium citrate are helpful. Hemodialysis with the artificial kidney is the most effective means of removing salicylate and is indicated for the very severe cases of salicylate intoxication.

Animal Toxicology: The acute lethal doses of the hydrochloride and napsylate salts of propoxyphene were determined in four species. The results shown in Figure 2 indicate that, on a molar basis, the napsylate salt is less toxic than the hydrochloride. This may be due to the relative insolubility and retarded absorption of propoxyphene napsylate.

Figure 2. Acute oral toxicity of propoxyphene

	LD_{50} (mg/kg) $\pm$ SE	
	LD_{50} (mmole/kg)	
Species	Propoxyphene Hydrochloride	Propoxyphene Napsylate
Mouse	282 $\pm$ 39	915 $\pm$ 163
	0.75	1.62
Rat	230 $\pm$ 44	647 $\pm$ 95
	0.61	1.14
Rabbit	ca. 82	> 183
	0.22	> 0.32
Dog	ca. 100	> 183
	0.27	> 0.32

Some indication of the relative insolubility and retarded absorption of propoxyphene napsylate was obtained by measuring plasma propoxyphene levels in two groups of four dogs following oral administration of equimolar doses of the two salts. As shown in Figure 3, the peak plasma concentration observed with propoxyphene hydrochloride was much higher than that obtained after administration of the napsylate salt.

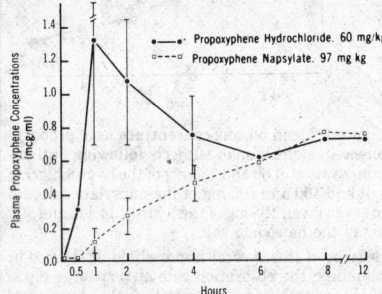

Figure 3. Plasma propoxyphene concentrations in dogs following large doses of the hydrochloride and napsylate salts

Although none of the animals in this experiment died, three of the four dogs given propoxyphene hydrochloride exhibited convulsive seizures during the time interval corresponding to the peak plasma levels. The four animals receiving the napsylate salt were mildly ataxic but not acutely ill.

How Supplied: ℂ *Darvocet-N®* 50 *(Propoxyphene Napsylate and Acetaminophen, USP), Tablets No. 1890, C51,* Specially Coated, Dark-Orange, in bottles of 500 (NDC 0002-0351-03), in 10 strips of 10 individually labeled blisters each containing 1 tablet (ID100) (NDC 0002-0351-33), and in ℞Paks (prescription packages, Lilly) in bottles of 100 (NDC 0002-0351-02). All ℞Paks have safety closures.

500's—6505-00-279-7469A.

ℂ *Darvocet-N®* 100 *(Propoxyphene Napsylate and Acetaminophen, USP), Tablets No. 1893, C63,* Specially Coated, Dark-Orange, in bottles of 500 (NDC 0002-0363-03), in 10 strips of 10 individually labeled blisters each containing 1 tablet (ID100) (NDC 0002-0363-33), in 500 single-cut individually labeled blisters each containing 1 tablet (ID500) (NDC 0002-0363-43), in 20 rolls, each consisting of 25 tablets in individual unit-dose packets, reverse-numbered (RN500) (NDC 0002-0363-46), and in ℞Paks in bottles of 100 (NDC 0002-0363-02). All ℞Paks have safety closures.

ID100—6505-00-111-8373; 500's—6505-00-111-8359

℞ Darvon-N® (Propoxyphene Napsylate Oral Suspension, USP), Suspension No. M-135, 50 mg per 5 ml, in 16-fl-oz (473-ml) bottles (NDC 0002-2371-05). Avoid freezing.

℞ Darvon-N® (Propoxyphene Napsylate Tablets, USP), Tablets No. 1883, C53,* 100 mg, Specially Coated, Buff, in bottles of 100 (℞Pak) (NDC 0002-0353-02) and 500 (NDC 0002-0353-03), in 10 strips of 10 individually labeled blisters each containing 1 tablet (ID100) (NDC 0002-0353-33), and in ℞Paks in 20 packages of 50 (NDC 0002-0353-51). All ℞Paks have safety closures.

ID100—6505-00-197-9201A; 500's—6505-00-111-8383

℞ Darvon-N® with A.S.A.® (Propoxyphene Napsylate and Aspirin, USP), Tablets No. 1884, C54,* Specially Coated, Orange, in bottles of 100 (℞Pak) (NDC 0002-0354-02) and 500 (NDC 0002-0354-03). All ℞Paks have safety closures.

500's—6505-00-212-6109A

*Identi-Code® symbol.

Shown in Product Identification Section, page 417
The following information, including illustrations of dosage forms and the maximum daily dosage of each, is available to patients receiving Darvon products.

Patient Information Sheet
YOUR PRESCRIPTION FOR A DARVON® (PROPOXYPHENE) PRODUCT ℞

Summary: Products containing Darvon are used to relieve pain.
LIMIT YOUR INTAKE OF ALCOHOL WHILE TAKING THIS DRUG. Make sure your doctor knows that you are taking tranquilizers, sleep aids, antidepressants, antihistamines, or any other drugs that make you sleepy. Combining propoxyphene with alcohol or these drugs in excessive doses is dangerous.
Use care while driving a car or using machines until you see how the drug affects you because propoxyphene can make you sleepy. Do not take more of the drug than your doctor prescribed. Dependence has occurred when patients have taken propoxyphene for a long period of time at doses greater than recommended.
The rest of this leaflet gives you more information about propoxyphene. Please read it and keep it for future use.
Uses of Darvon: Products containing Darvon are used for the relief of mild to moderate pain. Products which contain Darvon plus aspirin or acetaminophen are prescribed for the relief of pain or pain associated with fever.
Before Taking Darvon: Make sure your doctor knows if you have ever had an allergic reaction to propoxyphene, aspirin, or acetaminophen. Some forms of propoxyphene products contain aspirin to help relieve the pain. Your doctor should be advised if you have a history of ulcers or if you are taking an anticoagulant ("blood thinner"). The aspirin may irritate the stomach lining and may cause bleeding, particularly if an ulcer is present. Also, bleeding may occur if you are taking an anticoagulant. In a small group of people, aspirin may cause an asthma attack. If you are one of these people, be sure your drug does not contain aspirin. The effect of propoxyphene in children under 12 has not been studied. Therefore, use of the drug in this age group is not recommended.
How to Take Darvon: Follow your doctor's directions exactly. Do not increase the amount you take without your doctor's approval. If you miss a dose of the drug, do not take twice as much the next time.
Pregnancy: Do not take propoxyphene during pregnancy unless your doctor knows you are pregnant and specifically recommends its use. Cases of temporary dependence in the newborn have occurred when the mother has taken propoxyphene consistently in the weeks before delivery. As a general principle, no drug should be taken during pregnancy unless it is clearly necessary.
General Cautions: Heavy use of alcohol with propoxyphene is hazardous and may lead to overdosage symptoms (see "Overdose" below). THEREFORE, LIMIT YOUR INTAKE OF ALCOHOL WHILE TAKING PROPOXYPHENE.
Combinations of excessive doses of propoxyphene, alcohol, and tranquilizers are dangerous. Make sure your doctor knows you are taking tranquilizers, sleep aids, antidepressant drugs, antihistamines, or any other drugs that make you sleepy. The use of these drugs with propoxyphene increases their sedative effects and may lead to overdosage symptoms, including death (see "Overdose" below).
Propoxyphene may cause drowsiness or impair your mental and/or physical abilities; therefore, use caution when driving a vehicle or operating dangerous machinery. DO NOT perform any hazardous task until you have seen your response to this drug.
Propoxyphene may increase the concentration in the body of medications such as anticoagulants ("blood thinners"), antidepressants, or drugs used for epilepsy. The result may be excessive or adverse effects of these medications. Make sure your doctor knows if you are taking any of these medications.
Dependence: You can become dependent on propoxyphene if you take it in higher than recommended doses over a long period of time. Dependence is a feeling of need for the drug and a feeling that you cannot perform normally without it.
Overdose: An overdose of Darvon, alone or in combination with other drugs, including alcohol, may cause weakness, difficulty in breathing, confusion, anxiety, and more severe drowsiness and dizziness. Extreme overdosage may lead to unconsciousness and death.
If the propoxyphene product contains acetaminophen, the overdosage symptoms include nausea, vomiting, lack of appetite, and abdominal pain. Liver damage may occur.
When the propoxyphene product contains aspirin, symptoms of taking too much of the drug are headache, dizziness, ringing in the ears, difficulty in hearing, dim vision, confusion, drowsiness, sweating, thirst, rapid breathing, nausea, vomiting, and, occasionally, diarrhea.
In any suspected overdosage situation, contact your doctor or nearest hospital emergency room. GET EMERGENCY HELP IMMEDIATELY.
KEEP THIS DRUG AND ALL DRUGS OUT OF THE REACH OF CHILDREN.
Possible Side Effects: When propoxyphene is taken as directed, side effects are infrequent. Among those reported are drowsiness, dizziness, nausea, and vomiting. If these effects occur, it may help if you lie down and rest.
Less frequently reported side effects are constipation, abdominal pain, skin rashes, lightheadedness, headache, weakness, minor visual disturbances, and feelings of elation or discomfort.
If side effects occur and concern you, contact your doctor.
Other Information: The safe and effective use of propoxyphene depends on your taking it exactly as directed. This drug has been prescribed specifically for you and your present condition. Do not give this drug to others who may have similar symptoms. Do not use it for any other reason.
If you would like more information about propoxyphene, ask your doctor or pharmacist. They have a more technical leaflet (professional labeling) you may read.

Prescription Vial Sticker
Tell your doctor if you are taking tranquilizers, antidepressant drugs, or sleep aids. LIMIT alcohol use with Darvon-N® (propoxyphene napsylate) and Darvon® (propoxyphene hydrochloride) products.

[072384]

DARVON® ℞
[där'von]
(propoxyphene hydrochloride)
Capsules, USP

DARVON® COMPOUND and
[där'von käm'pound]
DARVON® COMPOUND-65
(propoxyphene hydrochloride, aspirin, and caffeine)

DARVON® WITH A.S.A.®
[där'von with ā'es-ā]
(propoxyphene hydrochloride and aspirin)

Description: Darvon® (propoxyphene hydrochloride, Lilly) is an odorless white crystalline powder with a bitter taste. It is freely soluble in water. Chemically, it is alpha-(+)-4-(Dimethylamino)-3-methyl- 1,2-diphenyl-2-butanol Propionate Hydrochloride.
Each Pulvule® Darvon contains 32 or 65 mg propoxyphene hydrochloride.

Pulvules No. 368 Darvon® Compound	Pulvules No. 369 Darvon® Compound-65
32 mg .... Darvon® .... 65 mg
(propoxyphene hydrochloride, Lilly)
389 mg .... A.S.A.® .... 389 mg
(aspirin, Lilly)
32.4 mg .... Caffeine .... 32.4 mg

Each Pulvule Darvon with A.S.A. contains 65 mg propoxyphene hydrochloride and 325 mg aspirin.
Clinical Pharmacology: Propoxyphene is a centrally acting narcotic analgesic agent. Equimolar doses of propoxyphene hydrochloride or napsylate provide similar plasma concentrations. Following administration of 65, 130, or 195 mg of propoxyphene hydrochloride, the bioavailability of propoxyphene is equivalent to that of 100, 200, or 300 mg respectively of propoxyphene napsylate. Peak plasma concentrations of propoxyphene are reached in two to two and one-half hours. After a 65-mg oral dose of propoxyphene hydrochloride, peak plasma levels of 0.05 to 0.1 mcg/ml are achieved.
Repeated doses of propoxyphene at six-hour intervals lead to increasing plasma concentrations, with a plateau after the ninth dose at 48 hours.
Propoxyphene is metabolized in the liver to yield norpropoxyphene. Propoxyphene has a half-life of six to 12 hours, whereas that of norpropoxyphene is 30 to 36 hours.
Norpropoxyphene has substantially less central-nervous-system-depressant effect than propoxyphene but a greater local anesthetic effect, which is similar to that of amitriptyline and antiarrhythmic agents, such as lidocaine and quinidine.
In animal studies in which propoxyphene and norpropoxyphene were continuously infused in large amounts, intracardiac conduction time (PR and QRS intervals) was prolonged. Any intracardiac conduction delay attributable to high concentrations of norpropoxyphene may be of relatively long duration.
Actions: Propoxyphene is a mild narcotic analgesic structurally related to methadone. The potency of propoxyphene hydrochloride is from two-thirds to equal that of codeine.
The combination of propoxyphene with a mixture of aspirin and caffeine produces greater analgesia than that produced by either propoxyphene or aspirin and caffeine administered alone.
Indications: Darvon® (propoxyphene hydrochloride, Lilly) is indicated for the relief of mild to moderate pain.
Darvon Compound, Darvon Compound-65, and Darvon with A.S.A. are indicated for the relief of mild to moderate pain, either when pain is present alone or when it is accompanied by fever.

Continued on next page

* Identi-Code® symbol.

Lilly—Cont.

Contraindication: Hypersensitivity to propoxyphene, aspirin, or caffeine.

WARNINGS
- Do not prescribe propoxyphene for patients who are suicidal or addiction-prone.
- Prescribe propoxyphene with caution for patients taking tranquilizers or antidepressant drugs and patients who use alcohol in excess.
- Tell your patients not to exceed the recommended dose and to limit their intake of alcohol.

Propoxyphene products in excessive doses, either alone or in combination with other CNS depressants, including alcohol, are a major cause of drug-related deaths. Fatalities within the first hour of overdosage are not uncommon. In a survey of deaths due to overdosage conducted in 1975, in approximately 20 percent of the fatal cases, death occurred within the first hour (5 percent occurred within 15 minutes). Propoxyphene should not be taken in doses higher than those recommended by the physician. The judicious prescribing of propoxyphene is essential to the safe use of this drug. With patients who are depressed or suicidal, consideration should be given to the use of non-narcotic analgesics. Patients should be cautioned about the concomitant use of propoxyphene products and alcohol because of potentially serious CNS-additive effects of these agents. Because of its added depressant effects, propoxyphene should be prescribed with caution for those patients whose medical condition requires the concomitant administration of sedatives, tranquilizers, muscle relaxants, antidepressants, or other CNS-depressant drugs. Patients should be advised of the additive depressant effects of these combinations.

Many of the propoxyphene-related deaths have occurred in patients with previous histories of emotional disturbances or suicidal ideation or attempts as well as histories of misuse of tranquilizers, alcohol, and other CNS-active drugs. Some deaths have occurred as a consequence of the accidental ingestion of excessive quantities of propoxyphene alone or in combination with other drugs. Patients taking propoxyphene should be warned not to exceed the dosage recommended by the physician.

Drug Dependence—Propoxyphene, when taken in higher-than-recommended doses over long periods of time, can produce drug dependence characterized by psychic dependence and, less frequently, physical dependence and tolerance. Propoxyphene will only partially suppress the withdrawal syndrome in individuals physically dependent on morphine or other narcotics. The abuse liability of propoxyphene is qualitatively similar to that of codeine although quantitatively less, and propoxyphene should be prescribed with the same degree of caution appropriate to the use of codeine.

Usage in Ambulatory Patients—Propoxyphene may impair the mental and/or physical abilities required for the performance of potentially hazardous tasks, such as driving a car or operating machinery. The patient should be cautioned accordingly.

Precautions: *General Precautions*—Salicylates should be used with extreme caution in the presence of peptic ulcer or coagulation abnormalities.

Drug Interactions—The CNS-depressant effect of propoxyphene is additive with that of other CNS depressants, including alcohol.

Salicylates may enhance the effect of anticoagulants and inhibit the uricosuric effect of uricosuric agents.

Usage in Pregnancy—Safe use in pregnancy has not been established relative to possible adverse effects on fetal development. Instances of withdrawal symptoms in the neonate have been reported following usage during pregnancy. Therefore, propoxyphene should not be used in pregnant women unless, in the judgment of the physician, the potential benefits outweigh the possible hazards.

Usage in Nursing Mothers—Low levels of propoxyphene have been detected in human milk. In postpartum studies involving nursing mothers who were given propoxyphene, no adverse effects were noted in infants receiving mother's milk.

Usage in Children—Propoxyphene is not recommended for use in children, because documented clinical experience has been insufficient to establish safety and a suitable dosage regimen in the pediatric age group.

A Patient Information Sheet is available for these products. See text following "How Supplied" section below.

Adverse Reactions: In a survey conducted in hospitalized patients, less than 1 percent of patients taking propoxyphene hydrochloride at recommended doses experienced side effects. The most frequently reported have been dizziness, sedation, nausea, and vomiting. Some of these adverse reactions may be alleviated if the patient lies down.

Other adverse reactions include constipation, abdominal pain, skin rashes, lightheadedness, headache, weakness, euphoria, dysphoria, and minor visual disturbances.

Cases of liver dysfunction have been reported.

Dosage and Administration: These products are given orally. The usual dosage of Darvon® (propoxyphene hydrochloride, Lilly) is 65 mg every four hours as needed for pain.

The usual dosage of Darvon Compound and Darvon Compound-65 is 32 or 65 mg propoxyphene hydrochloride, 389 mg aspirin, and 32.4 mg caffeine every four hours as needed for pain.

The usual dosage of Darvon with A.S.A. is 65 mg propoxyphene hydrochloride and 325 mg aspirin every four hours as needed for pain.

The maximum recommended dose of propoxyphene hydrochloride is 390 mg per day.

Management of Overdosage: Initial consideration should be given to the management of the CNS effects of propoxyphene overdosage. Resuscitative measures should be initiated promptly.

Symptoms of Propoxyphene Overdosage—The manifestations of acute overdosage with propoxyphene are those of narcotic overdosage. The patient is usually somnolent but may be stuporous or comatose and convulsing. Respiratory depression is characteristic. The ventilatory rate and/or tidal volume is decreased, which results in cyanosis and hypoxia. Pupils, initially pinpoint, may become dilated as hypoxia increases. Cheyne-Stokes respiration and apnea may occur. Blood pressure and heart rate are usually normal initially, but blood pressure falls and cardiac performance deteriorates, which ultimately results in pulmonary edema and circulatory collapse, unless the respiratory depression is corrected and adequate ventilation is restored promptly. Cardiac arrhythmias and conduction delay may be present. A combined respiratory-metabolic acidosis occurs owing to retained CO_2 (hypercapnea) and to lactic acid formed during anaerobic glycolysis. Acidosis may be severe if large amounts of salicylates have also been ingested. Death may occur.

Treatment of Propoxyphene Overdosage—Attention should be directed first to establishing a patent airway and to restoring ventilation. Mechanically assisted ventilation, with or without oxygen, may be required, and positive pressure respiration may be desirable if pulmonary edema is present. The narcotic antagonist naloxone will markedly reduce the effect of respiratory depression and should be administered promptly, preferably intravenously, 0.4 to 0.8 mg, and carefully repeated, as necessary, at 20 to 30-minute intervals. The duration of action of the antagonist may be brief. If no response is observed after 10 mg of naloxone have been administered, the diagnosis of propoxyphene toxicity should be questioned. (Nalorphine and levallorphan may be used if naloxone is not available, but these agents are not as satisfactory as naloxone.)

Blood gases, pH, and electrolytes should be monitored in order that acidosis and any electrolyte disturbance present may be corrected promptly. Acidosis, hypoxia, and generalized CNS depression predispose to the development of cardiac arrhythmias. Ventricular fibrillation or cardiac arrest may occur and necessitate the full complement of cardiopulmonary resuscitation (CPR) measures. Respiratory acidosis rapidly subsides as ventilation is restored and hypercapnea eliminated, but lactic acidosis may require intravenous bicarbonate for prompt correction.

Electrocardiographic monitoring is essential. Prompt correction of hypoxia, acidosis, and electrolyte disturbance (when present) will help prevent these cardiac complications and will increase the effectiveness of agents administered to restore normal cardiac function.

In addition to the use of a narcotic antagonist, the patient may require careful titration with an anticonvulsant to control convulsions. Analeptic drugs (for example, caffeine or amphetamine) should not be used because of their tendency to precipitate convulsions.

General supportive measures, in addition to oxygen, include, when necessary, intravenous fluids, vasopressor-inotropic compounds, and, when infection is likely, anti-infective agents. Gastric lavage may be useful, and activated charcoal can adsorb a significant amount of ingested propoxyphene. Dialysis is of little value in poisoning due to propoxyphene. Efforts should be made to determine whether other agents, such as alcohol, barbiturates, tranquilizers, or other CNS depressants, were also ingested, since these increase CNS depression as well as cause specific toxic effects.

Symptoms of Salicylate Overdosage—Such symptoms include central nausea and vomiting, tinnitus and deafness, vertigo and headaches, mental dullness and confusion, diaphoresis, rapid pulse, and increased respiration and respiratory alkalosis.

Treatment of Salicylate Overdosage—When Darvon Compound, Darvon Compound-65, or Darvon with A.S.A. has been ingested, the clinical picture may be complicated by salicylism.

The treatment of acute salicylate intoxication includes minimizing drug absorption, promoting elimination through the kidneys, and correcting metabolic derangements affecting body temperature, hydration, acid-base balance, and electrolyte balance. The technique to be employed for eliminating salicylate from the bloodstream depends on the degree of drug intoxication.

If the patient is seen within four hours of ingestion, the stomach should be emptied by inducing vomiting or by gastric lavage as soon as possible. The nomogram of Done is a useful prognostic guide in which the expected severity of salicylate intoxication is based on serum salicylate levels and the time interval between ingestion and taking the blood sample.

Exchange transfusion is most feasible for a small infant. Intermittent peritoneal dialysis is useful for cases of moderate severity in adults. Intravenous fluids alkalinized by the addition of sodium bicarbonate or potassium citrate are helpful. Hemodialysis with the artificial kidney is the most effective means of removing salicylate and is indicated for the very severe cases of salicylate intoxication.

How Supplied: ℞ *Pulvules Darvon®* (*Propoxyphene Hydrochloride Capsules, USP*): *No. 364, HO2,* *32 mg (No. 4, Light-Pink Opaque), in bottles of 100 (℞Pak) (NDC 0002-0802-02) and 500 (NDC 0002-0802-03) and in 10 strips of 10 individually labeled blisters each containing 1 Pulvule (ID100) (NDC 0002-0802-33); *No. 365, HO3,* *65 mg (No. 3, Light-Pink Opaque), in bottles of 100 (℞Pak) (NDC 0002-0803-02) and 500 (NDC 0002-0803-03), and in 10 strips of 10 individually labeled blisters each containing 1 Pulvule (ID100) (NDC 0002-0803-33), and in 20 rolls, each consisting of 25 Pulvules in individual unit-dose packets, reverse-numbered (RN500) (NDC 0002-0803-46). All ℞Paks have safety closures.

℞ *Darvon Compound, Pulvules No. 368, USP, HO5** (No. 0, Light-Pink Opaque Body, Light-Gray Opaque Cap), in bottles of 100 (℞Pak) (NDC 0002-3110-02) and 500 (NDC 0002-3110-03). All ℞Paks have safety closures.

℞ *Darvon Compound-65, Pulvules No. 369, USP, HO6** (No. 0, Red Opaque Body, Light-Gray Opaque Cap), in bottles of 100 (℞Pak) (NDC 0002-3111-02) and 500 (NDC 0002-3111-03), and in 10 strips of 10 individually labeled blisters each containing 1 Pulvule (ID100) (NDC 0002-3111-33). All ℞Paks have safety closures.

℞ *Darvon with A.S.A., Pulvules No. 366, HO4**(No. 0, Red Opaque Body, Light-Pink Opaque Cap), in bottles of 100 (℞Pak) (NDC 0002-0804-02) and 500 (NDC 0002-0804-03). All ℞Paks have safety closures.

Shown in Product Identification Section, page 417

*Identi-Code® symbol.
The following information, including illustrations of dosage forms and the maximum daily dosage of each, is available to patients receiving Darvon products.

Patient Information Sheet
YOUR PRESCRIPTION FOR A DARVON® (PROPOXYPHENE) PRODUCT ℞

Summary: Products containing Darvon are used to relieve pain.
LIMIT YOUR INTAKE OF ALCOHOL WHILE TAKING THIS DRUG. Make sure your doctor knows that you are taking tranquilizers, sleep aids, antidepressants, antihistamines, or any other drugs that make you sleepy. Combining propoxyphene with alcohol or these drugs in excessive doses is dangerous.
Use care while driving a car or using machines until you see how the drug affects you because propoxyphene can make you sleepy. Do not take more of the drug than your doctor prescribed. Dependence has occurred when patients have taken propoxyphene for a long period of time at doses greater than recommended.
The rest of this leaflet gives you more information about propoxyphene. Please read it and keep it for future use.
Uses of Darvon: Products containing Darvon are used for the relief of mild to moderate pain. Products which contain Darvon plus aspirin or acetaminophen are prescribed for the relief of pain or pain associated with fever.
Before Taking Darvon: Make sure your doctor knows if you have ever had an allergic reaction to propoxyphene, aspirin, or acetaminophen. Some forms of propoxyphene products contain aspirin to help relieve the pain. Your doctor should be advised if you have a history of ulcers or if you are taking an anticoagulant ("blood thinner"). The aspirin may irritate the stomach lining and may cause bleeding, particularly if an ulcer is present. Also, bleeding may occur if you are taking an anticoagulant. In a small group of people, aspirin may cause an asthma attack. If you are one of these people, be sure your drug does not contain aspirin. The effect of propoxyphene in children under 12 has not been studied. Therefore, use of the drug in this age group is not recommended.
How to Take Darvon: Follow your doctor's directions exactly. Do not increase the amount you take without your doctor's approval. If you miss a dose of the drug, do not take twice as much the next time.
Pregnancy: Do not take propoxyphene during pregnancy unless your doctor knows you are pregnant and specifically recommends its use. Cases of temporary dependence in the newborn have occurred when the mother has taken propoxyphene consistently in the weeks before delivery. As a general principle, no drug should be taken during pregnancy unless it is clearly necessary.
General Cautions: Heavy use of alcohol with propoxyphene is hazardous and may lead to overdosage symptoms (see "Overdose" below). THEREFORE, LIMIT YOUR INTAKE OF ALCOHOL WHILE TAKING PROPOXYPHENE.
Combinations of excessive doses of propoxyphene, alcohol, and tranquilizers are dangerous. Make sure your doctor knows you are taking tranquilizers, sleep aids, antidepressant drugs, antihistamines, or any other drugs that make you sleepy. The use of these drugs with propoxyphene increases their sedative effects and may lead to overdosage symptoms, including death (see "Overdose" below).
Propoxyphene may cause drowsiness or impair your mental and/or physical abilities: therefore, use caution when driving a vehicle or operating dangerous machinery. DO NOT perform any hazardous task until you have seen your response to this drug.
Dependence: You can become dependent on propoxyphene if you take it in higher than recommended doses over a long period of time. Dependence is a feeling of need for the drug and a feeling that you cannot perform normally without it.
Overdose: An overdose of Darvon, alone or in combination with other drugs, including alcohol, may cause weakness, difficulty in breathing, confusion, anxiety, and more severe drowsiness and dizziness. Extreme overdosage may lead to unconsciousness and death.
If the propoxyphene product contains acetaminophen, the overdosage symptoms include nausea, vomiting, lack of appetite, and abdominal pain. Liver damage may occur.
When the propoxyphene product contains aspirin, symptoms of taking too much of the drug are headache, dizziness, ringing in the ears, difficulty in hearing, dim vision, confusion, drowsiness, sweating, thirst, rapid breathing, nausea, vomiting, and, occasionally, diarrhea.
In any suspected overdosage situation, contact your doctor or nearest hospital emergency room. GET EMERGENCY HELP IMMEDIATELY.
KEEP THIS DRUG AND ALL DRUGS OUT OF THE REACH OF CHILDREN.
Possible Side Effects: When propoxyphene is taken as directed, side effects are infrequent. Among those reported are drowsiness, dizziness, nausea, and vomiting. If these effects occur, it may help if you lie down and rest.
Less frequently reported side effects are constipation, abdominal pain, skin rashes, lightheadedness, headache, weakness, minor visual disturbances, and feelings of elation or discomfort.
If side effects occur and concern you, contact your doctor.
Other Information: The safe and effective use of propoxyphene depends on your taking it exactly as directed. This drug has been prescribed specifically for you and your present condition. Do not give this drug to others who may have similar symptoms. Do not use it for any other reason.
If you would like more information about propoxyphene, ask your doctor or pharmacist. They have a more technical leaflet (professional labeling) you may read.

Prescription Vial Sticker
Tell your doctor if you are taking tranquilizers, antidepressant drugs, or sleep aids. LIMIT alcohol use with Darvon-N® (propoxyphene napsylate) and Darvon® (propoxyphene hydrochloride) products.

[050784]

DIETHYLSTILBESTROL ℞
[dī-eth′ĭl-stĭl-bĕs′trōl]
USP

1. USE OF ESTROGENS HAS BEEN REPORTED TO INCREASE THE RISK OF ENDOMETRIAL CARCINOMA
Three independent case-control studies have reported an increased risk of endometrial cancer in postmenopausal women exposed to exogenous estrogens for more than one year. This risk was independent of other known risk factors for endometrial cancer. These studies are further supported by the finding that, since 1969, the incidence rate of endometrial cancer has increased sharply in eight different areas of the United States which have population-based cancer reporting systems.
The three case-control studies reported that the risk of endometrial cancer in estrogen users was about 4.5 to 13.9 times greater than in nonusers. The risk appears to depend on both the duration of treatment and the dose of estrogen. In view of these findings, the lowest dose that will control symptoms should be utilized when estrogens are used for the treatment of menopausal symptoms, and medication should be discontinued as soon as possible. When prolonged treatment is medically indicated, a reassessment should be made on at least a semiannual basis to determine the need for continued therapy. Although the evidence must be considered preliminary, one study suggests that cyclic administration of low doses of estrogen may carry less risk than does continuous administration; it therefore appears prudent to utilize such a regimen.
Close clinical surveillance of all women taking estrogens is important. In all cases of undiagnosed persistent or recurring abnormal vaginal bleeding, adequate diagnostic measures should be undertaken to rule out malignancy.
At present, there is no evidence that "natural" estrogens are more or less hazardous than "synthetic" estrogens at equivalent estrogenic doses.

2. ESTROGENS SHOULD NOT BE USED DURING PREGNANCY
The use of female sex hormones, both estrogens and progestogens, during early pregnancy may affect the offspring. It has been reported that females exposed *in utero* to diethylstilbestrol, a nonsteroidal estrogen, may have an increased risk of developing later in life a rare form of vaginal or cervical cancer. This risk has been estimated to be 0.14 to 1.4 per 1000 exposures. Furthermore, from 30 to 90 percent of such exposed women have been found to have vaginal adenosis and epithelial changes of the vagina and cervix. Although these changes are histologically benign, it is not known whether they are precursors of malignancy. Even though similar data are not available with the use of other estrogens, it cannot be presumed that they would not induce similar changes.
Several reports suggest that there is an association between intrauterine exposure to female sex hormones and congenital anomalies, including congenital heart defects and limb-reduction defects. One case-control study estimated a 4.7-fold increased risk of limb-reduction defects in infants exposed *in utero* to sex hormones (oral contraceptives, hormone withdrawal tests for pregnancy, or attempted treatment for threatened abortion). Some of these exposures were very short and involved only a few days of treatment. The data suggest that the risk of limb-reduction defects in exposed fetuses is somewhat less than 1 per 1000.
In the past, female sex hormones have been used during pregnancy in an attempt to treat threatened or habitual abortion; however, their efficacy was never conclusively proved or disproved.
If diethylstilbestrol is administered during pregnancy, or if the patient becomes pregnant while taking this drug, she should be apprised of the potential risks to the fetus and of the advisability of pregnancy continuation.

THIS DRUG PRODUCT SHOULD NOT BE USED AS A POSTCOITAL CONTRACEPTIVE
Description: Diethylstilbestrol is a crystalline synthetic estrogenic substance capable of produc-

Continued on next page

* Identi-Code® symbol.

Lilly—Cont.

ing all the pharmacologic and therapeutic responses attributed to natural estrogens. Diethylstilbestrol may be administered orally (in the form of Enseals® [enteric-release tablets, Lilly] and tablets) or vaginally (in the form of suppositories). Chemically, diethylstilbestrol is α,α'-diethyl-4,4'-stilbenediol.

Indications: Diethylstilbestrol is indicated in the treatment of:
1. Moderate to severe *vasomotor* symptoms associated with the menopause (There is no evidence that estrogens are effective for nervous symptoms or depression which might occur during menopause, and they should not be used to treat these conditions.)
2. Atrophic vaginitis
3. Kraurosis vulvae
4. Female hypogonadism
5. Female castration
6. Primary ovarian failure
7. Breast cancer (for palliation only) in appropriately selected women and men with metastatic disease
8. Prostatic carcinoma—palliative therapy of advanced disease

DIETHYLSTILBESTROL SHOULD NOT BE USED FOR ANY PURPOSE DURING PREGNANCY. ITS USE MAY CAUSE SEVERE HARM TO THE FETUS (SEE BOXED WARNING).

Contraindications: Estrogens should not be used in women (or men) with any of the following conditions:
1. Known or suspected cancer of the breast, except in appropriately selected patients being treated for metastatic disease
2. Known or suspected estrogen-dependent neoplasia
3. Known or suspected pregnancy (see boxed warning)
4. Undiagnosed abnormal genital bleeding
5. Active thrombophlebitis or thromboembolic disorders
6. A past history of thrombophlebitis, thrombosis, or thromboembolic disorders associated with previous use of estrogen (except when used in treatment of breast or prostatic malignancy)

Warnings: 1. *Induction of Malignant Neoplasms* —In certain animal species, long-term continuous administration of natural and synthetic estrogens increases the frequency of carcinomas of the breast, cervix, vagina, kidney, and liver. There are now reports that prolonged use of estrogens increases the risk of carcinoma of the endometrium in humans (see boxed warning).

At the present time, there is no satisfactory evidence that administration of estrogens to postmenopausal women increases the risk of cancer of the breast. This possibility, however, has been raised by a recent long-term follow-up of one physician's practice. Because of the animal data, there is a need for caution in prescribing estrogens for women with a family history of breast cancer or for women who have breast nodules, fibrocystic disease, or abnormal mammograms.

2. *Gallbladder Disease*—A recent study reported a two-to-threefold increase in the risk of gallbladder disease occurring in women receiving postmenopausal estrogen therapy, similar to the twofold increased risk previously noted in women using oral contraceptives. In the case of oral contraceptives, this increased risk appeared after two years of use.

3. *Effects Similar to Those Caused by Estrogen-Progestogen Oral Contraceptives*—There are several serious adverse effects associated with the use of oral contraceptives; however, most of these adverse effects have not as yet been documented as consequences of postmenopausal estrogen therapy. This may reflect the comparatively low doses of estrogen used in postmenopausal women. It would be expected that these adverse effects are more likely to occur following administration of the larger doses of estrogen used for treating prostatic or breast cancer. It has, in fact, been shown that there is an increased risk of thrombosis with the administration of estrogens for prostatic cancer in men and for postpartum breast engorgement in women.

a. *Thromboembolic Disease*—It is now well established that women taking oral contraceptives run an increased risk of various thromboembolic and thrombotic vascular diseases, such as thrombophlebitis, pulmonary embolism, stroke, and myocardial infarction. Cases of retinal thrombosis, mesenteric thrombosis, and optic neuritis have been reported in users of oral contraceptives. There is evidence that the risk of several of these adverse reactions is related to the dose of the drug. An increased risk of postsurgical thromboembolic complications has also been reported in users of oral contraceptives. If feasible, estrogen therapy should be discontinued at least four weeks before any surgery that may be associated with an increased risk of thromboembolism or that may require periods of prolonged immobilization.

Although an increased rate of thromboembolic and thrombotic disease has not been noted in postmenopausal users of estrogen, this does not rule out the possiblity that such an increase may be present or that it exists in subgroups of women who have underlying risk factors or who are receiving relatively large doses of estrogens. Therefore, estrogens should not be used in persons with active thrombophlebitis or thromboembolic disorders, nor should they be used (except in treatment of malignancy) in persons with a history of such disorders associated with estrogen therapy. Estrogens should be administered cautiously to patients with cerebral vascular or coronary artery disease and only when such therapy is clearly needed.

In a large prospective clinical trial in men, large doses of estrogen (5 mg of conjugated estrogens per day), comparable to those used to treat cancer of the prostate and breast, have been shown to increase the risk of nonfatal myocardial infarction, pulmonary embolism, and thrombophlebitis. When such large doses of estrogen are used, any of the thromboembolic and thrombotic adverse effects associated with the use of oral contraceptives should be considered a clear risk.

b. *Hepatic Adenoma*—Benign hepatic adenomas appear to be associated with the use of oral contraceptives. Although these adenomas are benign and rare, they may rupture and may cause death by intra-abdominal hemorrhage. Such lesions have not yet been reported in association with the administration of other estrogen or progestogen preparations, but they should be considered when abdominal pain and tenderness, abdominal mass, or hypovolemic shock occurs in persons receiving estrogen therapy. Hepatocellular carcinoma has also been reported in women taking estrogen-containing oral contraceptives. The relationship of this malignancy to such drugs is not known at this time.

c. *Elevated Blood Pressure*—Increased blood pressure is not uncommon in women taking oral contraceptives. There is now one report that this may occur with use of estrogens in the menopause, and blood pressure should be monitored during estrogen therapy, especially if high doses are used.

d. *Glucose Tolerance*—A decrease in glucose tolerance has been observed in a significant percentage of patients on estrogen-containing oral contraceptives. For this reason, diabetic patients should be carefully observed while receiving estrogen.

4. *Hypercalcemia*—Administration of estrogens may lead to severe hypercalcemia in patients with breast cancer and bone metastases. If this occurs, the drug should be stopped and appropriate measures taken to reduce the serum calcium level.

Precautions: A. General Precautions.
1. A complete medical and family history should be taken prior to initiation of any estrogen therapy. In the pretreatment and periodic physical examinations, special consideration should be given to blood pressure, breasts, abdomen, and pelvic organs, and a Papanicolaou smear should be performed. As a general rule, estrogen should not be prescribed for over a year without another physical examination.

2. Fluid retention—Because estrogens may cause some degree of fluid retention, conditions which might be influenced by this factor, such as epilepsy, migraine, and cardiac or renal dysfunction, require careful observation.

3. Certain patients may develop undesirable manifestations of excessive estrogenic stimulation, such as abnormal or excessive uterine bleeding, mastodynia, etc.

4. Oral contraceptives appear to be associated with an increased incidence of mental depression. Although it is not clear whether this is due to the estrogenic or progestogenic component of the contraceptive agent, patients with a history of depression should be carefully observed.

5. Preexisting uterine leiomyomata may increase in size with administration of estrogens.

6. The pathologist should be advised of estrogen therapy when relevant specimens are submitted.

7. Patients with a past history of jaundice during pregnancy run an increased risk of recurrence of jaundice while receiving estrogen-containing oral contraceptive therapy. If jaundice develops in any patient receiving estrogen, the medication should be discontinued while the cause is investigated.

8. Estrogens may be poorly metabolized in patients with impaired liver function, and they should therefore be administered with caution in such patients.

9. Because estrogens influence the metabolism of calcium and phosphorus, they should be used with caution in patients with metabolic bone diseases associated with hypercalcemia or in patients with renal insufficiency.

10. Because of the effects of estrogens on epiphyseal closure, they should be used judiciously in young patients in whom bone growth is not complete.

11. Certain endocrine and liver function tests may be affected by estrogen-containing oral contraceptives. The following similar changes may be expected with larger doses of estrogen:
  a. Increased sulfobromophthalein retention
  b. Increased prothrombin and factors VII, VIII, IX, and X; decreased antithrombin 3; increased norepinephrine-induced platelet aggregability
  c. Increased thyroid-binding globulin (TBG) leading to increased circulating total thyroid hormone, as measured by PBI, T^4 by column, or T^4 by radioimmunoassay. Free T^3 resin uptake is decreased, reflecting the elevated TBG; free T^4 concentration is unaltered
  d. Impaired glucose tolerance
  e. Decreased pregnanediol excretion
  f. Reduced response to metyrapone test
  g. Reduced serum folate concentration
  h. Increased serum triglyceride and phospholipid concentration

B. Information for the Patient. *See* text of Patient Package Insert.

C. Pregnancy Category X. *See* Contraindications and boxed warning.

D. Nursing Mothers. As a general principle, any drug should be administered to nursing mothers only when clearly necessary, since many drugs are excreted in human milk.

Adverse Reactions: (*See* Warnings regarding induction of neoplasia, adverse effects on the fetus, increased incidence of gallbladder disease, and adverse effects similar to those of oral contraceptives, including thromboembolism.) The following additional adverse reactions have been reported with estrogenic therapy, including oral contraceptives:

1. *Genitourinary System*
  Breakthrough bleeding, spotting, change in menstrual flow
  Dysmenorrhea
  Premenstrual-like syndrome
  Amenorrhea during and after treatment

Increase in size of uterine fibromyomata
Vaginal candidiasis
Change in cervical eversion and in degree of cervical secretion
Cystitis-like syndrome
2. *Breasts*
Tenderness, enlargement, secretion
3. *Gastrointestinal*
Nausea, vomiting
Abdominal cramps, bloating
Cholestatic jaundice
4. *Skin*
Chloasma or melasma which may persist when drug is discontinued
Erythema multiforme
Erythema nodosum
Hemorrhagic eruption
Loss of scalp hair
Hirsutism
5. *Eyes*
Steepening of corneal curvature
Intolerance to contact lenses
6. *CNS*
Headache, migraine, dizziness
Mental depression
Chorea
7. *Miscellaneous*
Increase or decrease in weight
Reduced carbohydrate tolerance
Aggravation of porphyria
Edema
Changes in libido

Acute Overdosage: Numerous reports indicate that serious ill effects do not occur when large doses of estrogen-containing oral contraceptives are ingested by young children. Overdosage of estrogen may cause nausea, and withdrawal bleeding may occur in females.

Dosage and Administration: 1. *Given Cyclically for Short-Term Use Only:*
For treatment of moderate to severe *vasomotor* symptoms, atrophic vaginitis, or kraurosis vulvae associated with the menopause.
The lowest dose that will control symptoms should be chosen, and medication should be discontinued as promptly as possible.
Administration should be cyclic (e.g., three weeks on and one week off).
Attempts to discontinue or taper medication should be made at three to six-month intervals. The usual dosage range is 0.2 to 0.5 mg daily. Patients with atrophic vaginitis may require up to 2 mg daily, and cyclic administration may be necessary for several years. Patients with atrophic vaginitis may notice relief of symptoms sooner if up to 1 mg of the suppository form is administered daily for ten to 14 days concomitantly with oral diethylstilbestrol. Consideration should also be given to prescribing the suppository form as the only means of estrogenic therapy for patients with atrophic vaginitis or kraurosis vulvae, in which case the dosage may be increased to 5 to 7 mg weekly.
2. *Given Cyclically:*
Female hypogonadism
Female castration
Primary ovarian failure
0.2 to 0.5 mg daily
3. *Given Chronically:*
Inoperable progressing prostatic cancer
1 to 3 mg daily initially, increased in advanced cases; the dosage may later be reduced to an average of 1 mg daily.
Inoperable progressing breast cancer in appropriately selected men and postmenopausal women (*see* Indications)
15 mg daily
Patients with an intact uterus should be closely monitored for signs of endometrial cancer, and appropriate diagnostic measures should be taken to rule out malignancy in the event of persistent or recurring abnormal vaginal bleeding.

How Supplied: (℞) *Enseals—Diethylstilbestrol Tablets, USP (Enteric: No. 46, A19,* 0.1 mg, in bottles of 100 (NDC 0002-0119-02); *No. 47, A20,* 0.25 mg, in bottles of 100 (NDC 0002-0120-02); *No. 48, A21,* 0.5 mg, in bottles of 100 (NDC 0002-0121-02); *No. 49, A22,* 1 mg, in bottles of 100 (NDC 0002-0122-02) and 1000 (NDC 0002-0122-04); and *No. 85, A33,* 5 mg, in bottles of 100 (NDC 0002-0133-02).
(℞) *Diethylstilbestrol Suppositories, USP* (Vaginal): *No. 14, SO7,* *0.1 mg, in packages of 6 (NDC 0002-1907-16) and *No. 15, SO9,* *0.5 mg, in packages of 6 (NDC 0002-1909-16). In addition to the diethylstilbestrol, the suppositories also contain glycerin, gelatin, polysorbate 20, and propylene glycol. *Refrigerate.*
(℞) *Tablets—Diethylstilbestrol Tablets, USP: No. 1649, J52,* 1 mg, in bottles of 100 (NDC 0002-1052-02) and 1000 (NDC 0002-1052-04); *No. 1685, J54,* 5 mg, in bottles of 100) (NDC 0002-1054-02) and 1000 (NDC 0002-1054-04). [061384]

*Identi-Code® symbol.

DOBUTREX®   ℞
[dō′ bū-trĕks]
(dobutamine hydrochloride)
For Injection
USP

Description: Dobutrex® (dobutamine hydrochloride, Lilly) is ($\pm$)-4-[2-[[3-(p-hydroxyphenyl)-1-methylpropyl]amino]-ethyl] -pyro- catechol hydrochloride. It is a synthetic catecholamine.
The clinical formulation is supplied in a sterile lyophilized form for intravenous use only. Each vial contains 250 mg of dobutamine and 250 mg of mannitol. Hydrochloric acid is used to adjust the pH. The pH of the reconstituted solution is between 2.5 and 5.5.

Clinical Pharmacology: Dobutrex® (dobutamine hydrochloride, Lilly) is a direct-acting inotropic agent whose primary activity results from stimulation of the beta receptors of the heart while producing comparatively mild chronotropic, hypertensive, arrhythmogenic, and vasodilative effects. It does not cause the release of endogenous norepinephrine, as does dopamine. In animal studies, dobutamine produces less increase in heart rate and less decrease in peripheral vascular resistance for a given inotropic effect than does isoproterenol.
In patients with depressed cardiac function, both dobutamine and isoproterenol increase the cardiac output to a similar degree. In the case of dobutamine, this increase is usually not accompanied by marked increases in heart rate (although tachycardia is occasionally observed), and the cardiac stroke volume is usually increased. In contrast, isoproterenol increases the cardiac index primarily by increasing the heart rate while stroke volume changes little or declines.
Facilitation of atrioventricular conduction has been observed in human electrophysiologic studies and in patients with atrial fibrillation.
Systemic vascular resistance is usually decreased with administration of dobutamine. Occasionally, minimum vasoconstriction has been observed.
Most clinical experience with dobutamine is short-term—up to several hours in duration. In the limited number of patients who were studied for 24, 48, and 72 hours, a persistent increase in cardiac output occurred in some, whereas the output of others returned toward base-line values.
The onset of action of Dobutrex is within one to two minutes; however, as much as ten minutes may be required to obtain the peak effect of a particular infusion rate.
The plasma half-life of dobutamine in humans is two minutes. The principal routes of metabolism are methylation of the catechol and conjugation. In human urine, the major excretion products are the conjugates of dobutamine and 3-O-methyl dobutamine. The 3-O-methyl derivative of dobutamine is inactive.
Alteration of synaptic concentrations of catecholamines with either reserpine or tricyclic antidepressants does not alter the actions of dobutamine in animals, which indicates that the actions of dobutamine are not dependent on presynaptic mechanisms.

Indications and Usage: Dobutrex® (dobutamine hydrochloride, Lilly) is indicated when parenteral therapy is necessary for inotropic support in the short-term treatment of adults with cardiac decompensation due to depressed contractility resulting either from organic heart disease or from cardiac surgical procedures.
In patients who have atrial fibrillation with rapid ventricular response, a digitalis preparation should be used prior to institution of therapy with Dobutrex.

Contraindication: Dobutrex® (dobutamine hydrochloride, Lilly) is contraindicated in patients with idiopathic hypertrophic subaortic stenosis.

Warnings: 1. *Increase in Heart Rate or Blood Pressure*—Dobutrex® (dobutamine hydrochloride, Lilly) may cause a marked increase in heart rate or blood pressure, especially systolic pressure. Approximately 10 percent of patients in clinical studies have had rate increases of 30 beats/minute or more, and about 7.5 percent have had a 50-mm Hg or greater increase in systolic pressure. Reduction of dosage usually reverses these effects promptly. Because dobutamine facilitates atrioventricular conduction, patients with atrial fibrillation are at risk of developing rapid ventricular response. Patients with preexisting hypertension appear to face an increased risk of developing an exaggerated pressor response.
2. *Ectopic Activity*—Dobutrex may precipitate or exacerbate ventricular ectopic activity, but it rarely has caused ventricular tachycardia.

Precautions: 1. During the administration of Dobutrex® (dobutamine hydrochloride, Lilly), as with any adrenergic agent, ECG and blood pressure should be continuously monitored. In addition, pulmonary wedge pressure and cardiac output should be monitored whenever possible to aid in the safe and effective infusion of Dobutrex.
2. Hypovolemia should be corrected with suitable volume expanders before treatment with Dobutrex is instituted.
3. Animal studies indicate that Dobutrex may be ineffective if the patient has recently received a beta-blocking drug. In such a case, the peripheral vascular resistance may increase.
4. No improvement may be observed in the presence of marked mechanical obstruction, such as severe valvular aortic stenosis.
Usage Following Acute Myocardial Infarction—Clinical experience with Dobutrex following myocardial infarction has been insufficient to establish the safety of the drug for this use. There is concern that any agent which increases contractile force and heart rate may increase the size of an infarction by intensifying ischemia, but it is not known whether dobutamine does so.
Usage in Pregnancy—Reproduction studies performed in rats and rabbits have revealed no evidence of impaired fertility, harm to the fetus, or teratogenic effects due to dobutamine. However, the drug has not been administered to pregnant women and should be used only when the expected benefits clearly outweigh the potential risks to the fetus.
Pediatric Use—The safety and effectiveness of Dobutrex for use in children have not been studied.
Drug Interactions—There was no evidence of drug interactions in clinical studies in which Dobutrex was administered concurrently with other drugs, including digitalis preparations, furosemide, spironolactone, lidocaine, glyceryl trinitrate, isosorbide dinitrate, morphine, atropine, heparin, protamine, potassium chloride, folic acid, and acetaminophen. Preliminary studies indicate that the concomitant use of dobutamine and nitroprusside results in a higher cardiac output and, usually, a lower pulmonary wedge pressure than when either drug is used alone.

Adverse Reactions: *Increased Heart Rate, Blood Pressure, and Ventricular Ectopic Activity*—A 10 to 20-mm increase in systolic blood pressure and an increase in heart rate of five to 15 beats/minute have been noted in most patients.

Continued on next page

* Identi-Code® symbol.

Lilly—Cont.

(*See* Warnings regarding exaggerated chronotropic and pressor effects.) Approximately 5 percent of patients have had increased premature ventricular beats during infusions. These effects are dose related.

Miscellaneous Uncommon Effects—The following adverse effects have been reported in 1 to 3 percent of patients: nausea, headache, anginal pain, nonspecific chest pain, palpitations, and shortness of breath.

No abnormal laboratory values attributable to Dobutrex® (dobutamine hydrochloride, Lilly) have been observed.

Longer-Term Safety—Infusions of up to 72 hours have revealed no adverse effects other than those seen with shorter infusions.

Overdosage: In case of overdosage, as evidenced by excessive alteration of blood pressure or by tachycardia, reduce the rate of administration or temporarily discontinue Dobutrex® (dobutamine hydrochloride, Lilly) until the patient's condition stabilizes. Because the duration of action of Dobutrex is short, usually no additional remedial measures are necessary.

Dosage and Administration: *Reconstitution and Stability*—Dobutrex® (dobutamine hydrochloride, Lilly) is incompatible with alkaline solutions and should not be mixed with products such as 5% Sodium Bicarbonate Injection.

Dobutrex may be reconstituted with Sterile Water for Injection or 5% Dextrose Injection. To reconstitute, add 10 ml of diluent to Vial No. 7051, Dobutrex, 250 mg. If the material is not completely dissolved, add another 10 ml of diluent. The reconstituted solution may be stored under refrigeration for 48 hours or at room temperature for six hours.

Reconstituted Dobutrex must be further diluted to at least 50 ml prior to administration in 5% Dextrose Injection, 0.9% Sodium Chloride Injection, or Sodium Lactate Injection. Intravenous solutions should be used within 24 hours.

Solutions containing Dobutrex may exhibit a color that, if present, will increase with time. This color change is due to slight oxidation of the drug, but there is no significant loss of potency during the reconstituted time periods stated above.

Recommended Dosage—The rate of infusion needed to increase cardiac output usually ranges from 2.5 to 10 mcg/kg/min (see table). On rare occasions, infusion rates up to 40 mcg/kg/min have been required to obtain the desired effect. [See table below].

The rate of administration and the duration of therapy should be adjusted according to the patient's response, as determined by heart rate, presence of ectopic activity, blood pressure, urine flow, and, whenever possible, measurement of central venous or pulmonary wedge pressure and cardiac output.

Concentrations up to 5000 mcg/ml have been administered to humans (250 mg/50 ml). The final volume administered should be determined by the fluid requirements of the patient.

How Supplied: (℞) *Vials No. 7051, Dobutrex® (Dobutamine Hydrochloride for Injection, USP), for Injection* (lyophilized), equivalent to 250 mg dobutamine, 20-ml size, rubber-stoppered, in singles (10/carton) (NDC 0002-7051-01). [012282]

DOLOPHINE® HYDROCHLORIDE
[*dō′ lō-fēn hī-drō-klō′ rīd*]
(methadone hydrochloride)
Injection, USP

AMPOULES AND VIALS

CONDITIONS FOR DISTRIBUTION
AND USE OF METHADONE PRODUCTS:
Code of Federal Regulations,
Title 21, Sec. 291.505

METHADONE PRODUCTS, WHEN USED FOR THE TREATMENT OF NARCOTIC ADDICTION IN DETOXIFICATION OR MAINTENANCE PROGRAMS, SHALL BE DISPENSED ONLY BY APPROVED HOSPITAL PHARMACIES, APPROVED COMMUNITY PHARMACIES, AND MAINTENANCE PROGRAMS APPROVED BY THE FOOD AND DRUG ADMINISTRATION AND THE DESIGNATED STATE AUTHORITY.

APPROVED MAINTENANCE PROGRAMS SHALL DISPENSE AND USE METHADONE IN ORAL FORM ONLY AND ACCORDING TO THE TREATMENT REQUIREMENTS STIPULATED IN THE FEDERAL METHADONE REGULATIONS (21 CFR 291.505).

FAILURE TO ABIDE BY THE REQUIREMENTS IN THESE REGULATIONS MAY RESULT IN CRIMINAL PROSECUTION, SEIZURE OF THE DRUG SUPPLY, REVOCATION OF THE PROGRAM APPROVAL, AND INJUNCTION PRECLUDING OPERATION OF THE PROGRAM.

A METHADONE PRODUCT, WHEN USED AS AN ANALGESIC, MAY BE DISPENSED IN ANY LICENSED PHARMACY.

Description: Dolophine® Hydrochloride (Methadone Hydrochloride, USP, Lilly) (4,4-diphenyl-6-dimethylamino-heptanone-3 hydrochloride) is a white crystalline material which is water soluble.

Each ml contains methadone hydrochloride, 10 mg, and sodium chloride, 0.9 percent. Sodium hydroxide and/or hydrochloric acid may have been added during manufacture to adjust the pH. The 20-ml vials also contain chlorobutanol (chloroform derivative), 0.5 percent, as a preservative.

Actions: Methadone hydrochloride is a synthetic narcotic analgesic with multiple actions quantitatively similar to those of morphine, the most prominent of which involve the central nervous system and organs composed of smooth muscle. The principal actions of therapeutic value are analgesia and sedation and detoxification or temporary maintenance in narcotic addiction. The methadone abstinence syndrome, although qualitatively similar to that of morphine, differs in that the onset is slower, the course is more prolonged, and the symptoms are less severe.

A parenteral dose of 8 to 10 mg of methadone is approximately equivalent in analgesic effect to 10 mg of morphine. With single-dose administration, the onset and duration of analgesic action of the two drugs are similar.

When administered orally, methadone is approximately one-half as potent as when given parenterally. Oral administration results in a delay of the onset, a lowering of the peak, and an increase in the duration of analgesic effect.

Indications: (See Note below.)
For relief of severe pain.
For detoxification treatment of narcotic addiction.
For temporary maintenance treatment of narcotic addiction.

NOTE

If methadone is administered for treatment of heroin dependence for more than three weeks, the procedure passes from treatment of the acute withdrawal syndrome (detoxification) to maintenance therapy. Maintenance treatment is permitted to be undertaken only by approved methadone programs. This does not preclude the maintenance treatment of an addict who is hospitalized for medical conditions other than addiction and who requires temporary maintenance during the critical period of his stay or whose enrollment has been verified in a program which has approval for maintenance treatment with methadone.

Contraindication: Hypersensitivity to methadone.

Warnings: Methadone hydrochloride, a narcotic, is a Schedule II controlled substance under the Federal Controlled Substances Act. Appropriate security measures should be taken to safeguard stocks of methadone against diversion.

DRUG DEPENDENCE—METHADONE CAN PRODUCE DRUG DEPENDENCE OF THE MORPHINE TYPE AND, THEREFORE, HAS THE POTENTIAL FOR BEING ABUSED. PSYCHIC DEPENDENCE, PHYSICAL DEPENDENCE, AND TOLERANCE MAY DEVELOP UPON REPEATED ADMINISTRATION OF METHADONE, AND IT SHOULD BE PRESCRIBED AND ADMINISTERED WITH THE SAME DEGREE OF CAUTION APPROPRIATE TO THE USE OF MORPHINE.

Interaction with Other Central-Nervous-System Depressants—Methadone should be used with caution and in reduced dosage in patients who are concurrently receiving other narcotic analgesics, general anesthetics, phenothiazines, other tranquilizers, sedative-hypnotics, tricyclic antidepressants, and other CNS depressants (including alcohol). Respiratory depression, hypotension, and profound sedation or coma may result.

Anxiety—Since methadone, as used by tolerant subjects at a constant maintenance dosage, is not a tranquilizer, patients who are maintained on this drug will react to life problems and stresses with the same symptoms of anxiety as do other individuals. The physician should not confuse such symptoms with those of narcotic abstinence and should not attempt to treat anxiety by increasing the dosage of methadone. The action of methadone in maintenance treatment is limited to the control of narcotic symptoms and is ineffective for relief of general anxiety.

Head Injury and Increased Intracranial Pressure—The respiratory depressant effects of methadone and its capacity to elevate cerebrospinal-fluid pressure may be markedly exaggerated in the presence of increased intracranial pressure. Furthermore, narcotics produce side effects that may obscure the clinical course of patients with head injuries. In such patients, methadone must be used with caution and only if it is deemed essential.

Asthma and Other Respiratory Conditions— Methadone should be used with caution in patients having an acute asthmatic attack, in those with chronic obstructive pulmonary disease or cor pulmonale, and in individuals with a substantially

Dobutrex® (dobutamine hydrochloride)—Rates of Infusion
for Concentrations of 250, 500, and 1000 mcg/ml
Infusion Delivery Rate

Drug Delivery Rate (mcg/kg/min)	250 mcg/ml* (ml/kg/min)	500 mcg/ml† (ml/kg/min)	1000 mcg/ml‡ (ml/kg/min)
2.5	0.01	0.005	0.0025
5	0.02	0.01	0.005
7.5	0.03	0.015	0.0075
10	0.04	0.02	0.01
12.5	0.05	0.025	0.0125
15	0.06	0.03	0.015

*250 mg/liter of diluent
†500 mg/liter or 250 mg/500 ml of diluent
‡1000 mg/liter or 250 mg/250 ml of diluent

decreased respiratory reserve, preexisting respiratory depression, hypoxia, or hypercapnia. In such patients, even usual therapeutic doses of narcotics may decrease respiratory drive while simultaneously increasing airway resistance to the point of apnea.

Hypotensive Effect—The administration of methadone may result in severe hypotension in an individual whose ability to maintain his blood pressure has already been compromised by a depleted blood volume or concurrent administration of such drugs as the phenothiazines or certain anesthetics.

Use in Ambulatory Patients—Methadone may impair the mental and/or physical abilities required for the performance of potentially hazardous tasks, such as driving a car or operating machinery. The patient should be cautioned accordingly. Methadone, like other narcotics, may produce orthostatic hypotension in ambulatory patients.

Use in Pregnancy—Safe use in pregnancy has not been established in relation to possible adverse effects on fetal development. Therefore, methadone should not be used in pregnant women unless, in the judgment of the physician, the potential benefits outweigh the possible hazards. Methadone is not recommended for obstetric analgesia because its long duration of action increases the probability of respiratory depression in the newborn.

Use in Children—Methadone is not recommended for use as an analgesic in children, since documented clinical experience has been insufficient to establish a suitable dosage regimen for the pediatric age group.

Precautions: Interaction with Penta- zocine—Patients who are addicted to heroin or who are on the methadone maintenance program may experience withdrawal symptoms when given pentazocine.

Interaction with Rifampin—The concurrent administration of rifampin may possibly reduce the blood concentration of methadone to a degree sufficient to produce withdrawal symptoms. The mechanism by which rifampin may decrease blood concentrations of methadone is not fully understood, although enhanced microsomal drug-metabolized enzymes may influence drug disposition.

Acute Abdominal Conditions—The administration of methadone or other narcotics may obscure the diagnosis or clinical course in patients with acute abdominal conditions.

Interaction with Monoamine Oxidase (MAO) Inhibitors—Therapeutic doses of meperidine have precipitated severe reactions in patients concurrently receiving monoamine oxidase inhibitors or those who have received such agents within 14 days. Similar reactions thus far have not been reported with methadone; but if the use of methadone is necessary in such patients, a sensitivity test should be performed in which repeated small incremental doses are administered over the course of several hours while the patient's condition and vital signs are under careful observation.

Special-Risk Patients—Methadone should be given with caution and the initial dose should be reduced in certain patients, such as the elderly or debilitated and those with severe impairment of hepatic or renal function, hypothyroidism, Addison's disease, prostatic hypertrophy, or urethral stricture.

Adverse Reactions: THE MAJOR HAZARDS OF METHADONE, AS OF OTHER NARCOTIC ANALGESICS, ARE RESPIRATORY DEPRESSION AND, TO A LESSER DEGREE, CIRCULATORY DEPRESSION. RESPIRATORY ARREST, SHOCK, AND CARDIAC ARREST HAVE OCCURRED.

The most frequently observed adverse reactions include lightheadedness, dizziness, sedation, nausea, vomiting, and sweating. These effects seem to be more prominent in ambulatory patients and in those who are not suffering severe pain. In such individuals, lower doses are advisable. Some adverse reactions may be alleviated in the ambulatory patient if he lies down.

Other adverse reactions include the following:
Central Nervous System—Euphoria, dysphoria, weakness, headache, insomnia, agitation, disorientation, and visual disturbances.

Gastrointestinal—Dry mouth, anorexia, constipation, and biliary tract spasm.
Cardiovascular—Flushing of the face, bradycardia, palpitation, faintness, and syncope.
Genitourinary—Urinary retention or hesitancy, antidiuretic effect, and reduced libido and/or potency.
Allergic—Pruritus, urticaria, other skin rashes, edema, and, rarely, hemorrhagic urticaria.

In addition, pain at injection site; local tissue irritation and induration following subcutaneous injection, particularly when repeated.

Dosage and Administration: *For Relief of Pain*—Dosage should be adjusted according to the severity of the pain and the response of the patient. Occasionally it may be necessary to exceed the usual dosage recommended in cases of exceptionally severe pain or in those patients who have become tolerant to the analgesic effect of narcotics.

Although subcutaneous administration is suitable for occasional use, intramuscular injection is preferred when repeated doses are required.

The usual adult dosage is 2.5 to 10 mg intramuscularly or subcutaneously every three or four hours as necessary.

For Detoxification Treatment—THE DRUG SHALL BE ADMINISTERED DAILY UNDER CLOSE SUPERVISION AS FOLLOWS:

A detoxification treatment course shall not exceed 21 days and may not be repeated earlier than four weeks after completion of the preceding course.

The oral form of administration is preferred. However, if the patient is unable to ingest oral medication, he may be started on the parenteral form initially.

In detoxification, the patient may receive methadone when there are significant symptoms of withdrawal. The dosage schedules indicated below are recommended but could be varied in accordance with clinical judgment. Initially, a single dose of 15 to 20 mg of methadone will often be sufficient to suppress withdrawal symptoms. Additional methadone may be provided if withdrawal symptoms are not suppressed or if symptoms reappear. When patients are physically dependent on high doses, it may be necessary to exceed these levels. Forty mg/day in single or divided doses will usually constitute an adequate stabilizing dosage level. Stabilization can be continued for two to three days, and then the amount of methadone normally will be gradually decreased. The rate at which methadone is decreased will be determined separately for each patient. The dose of methadone can be decreased on a daily basis or at two-day intervals, but the amount of intake shall always be sufficient to keep withdrawal symptoms at a tolerable level. In hospitalized patients, a daily reduction of 20 percent of the total daily dose may be tolerated and may cause little discomfort. In ambulatory patients, a somewhat slower schedule may be needed. If methadone is administered for more than three weeks, the procedure is considered to have progressed from detoxification or treatment of the acute withdrawal syndrome to maintenance treatment, even though the goal and intent may be eventual total withdrawal.

Overdosage: *Symptoms*—Serious overdosage of methadone is characterized by respiratory depression (a decrease in respiratory rate and/or tidal volume, Cheyne-Stokes respiration, cyanosis), extreme somnolence progressing to stupor or coma, maximally constricted pupils, skeletal-muscle flaccidity, cold and clammy skin, and, sometimes, bradycardia and hypotension. In severe overdosage, particularly by the intravenous route, apnea, circulatory collapse, cardiac arrest, and death may occur.

Treatment—Primary attention should be given to the reestablishment of adequate respiratory exchange through provision of a patent airway and institution of assisted or controlled ventilation. If a nontolerant person, especially a child, takes a large dose of methadone, effective narcotic antagonists are available to counteract the potentially lethal respiratory depression. The physician must remember, however, that methadone is a long-acting depressant (36 to 48 hours), whereas the antagonists act for much shorter periods (one to three hours). The patient must, therefore, be monitored continuously for recurrence of respiratory depression and treated repeatedly with the narcotic antagonist as needed. If the diagnosis is correct and respiratory depression is due only to overdosage of methadone, the use of other respiratory stimulants is not indicated.

An antagonist should not be administered in the absence of clinically significant respiratory or cardiovascular depression. Intravenously administered narcotic antagonists (naloxone, nalorphine, and levallorphan) are the drugs of choice to reverse signs of intoxication. These agents should be given repeatedly until the patient's status remains satisfactory. The hazard that the narcotic antagonist will further depress respiration is less likely with the use of naloxone.

Oxygen, intravenous fluids, vasopressors, and other supportive measures should be employed as indicated.

> NOTE: IN AN INDIVIDUAL PHYSICALLY DEPENDENT ON NARCOTICS, THE ADMINISTRATION OF THE USUAL DOSE OF A NARCOTIC ANTAGONIST WILL PRECIPITATE AN ACUTE WITHDRAWAL SYNDROME. THE SEVERITY OF THIS SYNDROME WILL DEPEND ON THE DEGREE OF PHYSICAL DEPENDENCE AND THE DOSE OF THE ANTAGONIST ADMINISTERED. THE USE OF A NARCOTIC ANTAGONIST IN SUCH A PERSON SHOULD BE AVOIDED IF POSSIBLE. IF IT MUST BE USED TO TREAT SERIOUS RESPIRATORY DEPRESSION IN THE PHYSICALLY DEPENDENT PATIENT, THE ANTAGONIST SHOULD BE ADMINISTERED WITH EXTREME CARE AND BY TITRATION WITH SMALLER THAN USUAL DOSES OF THE ANTAGONIST.

How Supplied: (ⓒ) *Dolophine® Hydrochloride (Methadone Hydrochloride Injection, USP): Ampoules No. 456,* 10 mg, 1 ml, in packages of 12 (NDC 0002-1687-12) and 100 (NDC 0002-1687-02). *Vials No. 435,* 10 mg per ml, 20 ml, multiple dose, rubber-stoppered, in singles (10/carton) (NDC 0002-1682-01) and in packages of 25 (NDC 0002-1682-25). [071884]

DOLOPHINE® HYDROCHLORIDE ⓒ
[dō′lō-fēn hī-drō-klō′rīd]
(methadone hydrochloride)
Tablets, USP

CONDITIONS FOR DISTRIBUTION AND USE OF METHADONE PRODUCTS: *See under* Ampoules Dolophine Hydrochloride.

Description, Actions, Indications, and Contraindication: *See under* Ampoules Dolophine Hydrochloride.

Warnings:

> Tablets Dolophine® Hydrochloride (methadone hydrochloride, Lilly) are for oral administration only and *must not* be used for injection. It is recommended that Tablets Dolophine Hydrochloride, if dispensed, be packaged in child-resistant containers and kept out of the reach of children to prevent accidental ingestion.

See also under Ampoules Dolophine Hydrochloride.

Precautions and Adverse Reactions: *See under* Ampoules Dolophine Hydrochloride.

Dosage and Administration: *For Relief of Pain*—Dosage should be adjusted according to the severity of the pain and the response of the pa-

Continued on next page

* Identi-Code® symbol.

Lilly—Cont.

tient. Occasionally it may be necessary to exceed the usual dosage recommended in cases of exceptionally severe pain or in those patients who have become tolerant to the analgesic effect of narcotics.
The usual adult dosage is 2.5 to 10 mg every three or four hours as necessary.
See also under Ampoules Dolophine Hydrochloride.
If the patient cannot ingest methadone orally, parenteral administration may be substituted.
Overdosage: *See under* Ampoules Dolophine Hydrochloride.
How Supplied: (©) *Tablets Dolophine® Hydrochloride (Methadone Hydrochloride Tablets, USP):* No. 1712, J64,* 5 mg, in bottles of 100 (NDC 0002-1064-02); *No.* 1730, J72,*10 mg, in bottles of 100 (NDC 0002-1072-02).
[031284]

DURACILLIN® A.S.
[dū-ra-sĭl'-ĭn ā-ĕs']
see Penicillin G Procaine Suspension, Sterile.

DYMELOR®   ℞
[dĭ' mĕ-lōr]
(acetohexamide)
Tablets, USP

Description: Dymelor® (acetohexamide, Lilly) is a sulfonylurea characterized by the presence of an acetyl group in the para position of the phenyl ring and the incorporation of a cyclohexyl group on the urea moiety. Chemically, it is N-(p-acetylphenylsulfonyl)-N'-cyclohexylurea.
Action: Dymelor® (acetohexamide, Lilly) is an oral antidiabetic agent which is effective in controlling the blood glucose in properly selected patients with maturity-onset diabetes.
The mode of action of Dymelor is stimulation of release of insulin from the beta cells of the pancreas. In addition, a number of extrapancreatic actions of this class of drug have been elucidated; the most important of these is a reduction in glucose output from the liver.
Indications: The principal clinical indication for Dymelor® (acetohexamide, Lilly) is diabetes mellitus of the stable type (without such complications as ketosis or acidosis), variously described as relatively mild adult, maturity-onset, or nonketotic type.
The use of Dymelor in insulin-dependent patients may reduce the insulin requirements.
Contraindications: Dymelor® (acetohexamide, Lilly) is contraindicated in patients with hyperglycemia and glycosuria which may be associated with primary renal disease. If reduction of the blood sugar becomes essential in these cases, insulin is indicated.
Warnings: *Use in Pregnancy*—Safe use in pregnancy *has not been* established at this time, from the standpoint of either the mother or the fetus. Therefore, the use of Dymelor® (acetohexamide, Lilly) is not recommended for the management of diabetes when complicated by pregnancy. The advisability of administering Dymelor to women of childbearing age should be considered with caution.
Dymelor is of no value in diabetes complicated by acidosis and coma. These conditions require insulin.
In times of stress to the patient, such as fever of any cause, trauma, infection, or surgical procedures, it may be necessary to return the patient to insulin therapy or to use insulin in addition to Dymelor.
Precautions: The principles of management of diabetes mellitus are necessary to insure optimum control with Dymelor® (acetohexamide, Lilly) and are the same as for patients requiring insulin.
In patients with impaired hepatic and/or renal function and in debilitated or malnourished individuals, careful observation of the patient and adjustment of dosage are mandatory to prevent the occurrence of hypoglycemia.
Thiazide-type diuretics may aggravate the diabetic state and alter the dosage of Dymelor required.
Preparations containing phenylbutazone interfere with the excretion of the active metabolite hydroxyhexamide; as a result, increased sulfonylurea levels depress the blood glucose. This may also be true of probenecid and the absorbed antimicrobial sulfas.
Nonsteroidal anti-inflammatory agents have an affinity for albumin and may displace other albumin-bound drugs from their binding sites; this may lead to drug interaction. Patients receiving both Dymelor and nonsteroidal anti-inflammatory agents should be observed for signs of toxicity to these drugs.
Sulfonylurea compounds, like antimicrobial sulfa drugs and barbiturates, may aggravate hepatic porphyria.
Patients receiving sulfonylureas may experience peculiar symptoms, referred to as the "disulfiram reaction," following the ingestion of alcohol.
Secondary failures and the spontaneous tendency of diabetes to fluctuate in severity may occur. Therefore, patients should be seen by their physicians at regular intervals and their diabetes evaluated in order to avoid hyperglycemic and hypoglycemic episodes.
Adverse Reactions: Hypoglycemia may occur in those patients who do not eat regularly or who exercise without caloric supplementation. It is most likely to appear during the period of transition from insulin to Dymelor® (acetohexamide, Lilly) and should be considered in patients who have hepatic or renal disease as well as those who are debilitated or malnourished. Other untoward reactions consist principally in gastrointestinal disturbances (nausea, epigastric fullness, heartburn) and headache, appear to be dose related, and may disappear when dosage is reduced.
Allergic skin manifestations (pruritus, erythema, urticaria, morbilliform or maculopapular eruptions) occur but are usually transient and may disappear with continued dosage. If the skin reactions persist, the drug should be stopped. Photosensitivity reactions may be noted. Jaundice of both the cholestatic and mixed hepatic types has been observed with Dymelor.
As with other sulfonylurea drugs, leukopenia, thrombocytopenia, pancytopenia, agranulocytosis, aplastic anemia, and hemolytic anemia may occur with Dymelor.
Dosage and Administration: Since diabetes may be of various degrees of severity, there can be no fixed dosage of either Dymelor® (acetohexamide, Lilly) or insulin. Daily oral dosage of Dymelor may range between 250 mg and 1.5 g. No loading dose is required. Patients who do not respond to 1.5 g daily usually will not respond to a higher dose. For this reason, doses in excess of 1.5 g daily are not recommended.
The majority of patients receiving 1 g or less per day can be controlled on a convenient once-daily dosage. Patients who need 1.5 g per day usually benefit from twice-daily dosage, given before the morning and evening meals.
Dymelor may be used in combination with insulin. Various measures have been employed to establish patients on Dymelor, and the following procedures are suggested.
Patients Not Previously Receiving Insulin or Drug Therapy—In mild, stable diabetes (after dietary regulation), therapy may be initiated with 250 mg daily before breakfast; subsequent adjustment of the dosage may be made by increments of 250 to 500 mg every five to seven days as necessary. The 250-mg or the 500-mg tablet (scored and easily broken in half) may be used.
Because of reports of hyperresponsiveness of some elderly diabetics to Dymelor® (acetohexamide, Lilly), patients in this group should be started with a single dose of 250 mg before breakfast, and their blood and urine sugars should be checked during the first 24 hours of therapy. If control appears to be satisfactory, this dose may be continued on a daily basis or, if necessary, gradually increased. If, however, there appears to be a tendency toward hypoglycemia, this dose should be reduced or the drug should be discontinued.
Patients Receiving Other Oral Agents—When transfer is made from tolbutamide, the initial dose of Dymelor® (acetohexamide, Lilly) should be about half the tolbutamide dose (e.g., 250 mg of Dymelor in place of 500 mg of tolbutamide), up to a maximum of 1.5 g of Dymelor.
When transfer is made from chlorpropamide, the initial dose of Dymelor should be about double the chlorpropamide dose (e.g., 500 mg of Dymelor in place of 250 mg of chlorpropamide).
No transition period is required. Subsequent adjustment of dosage should be made according to clinical response. The maximum recommended dose of Dymelor is 1.5 g.
Clinical reports on the efficacy of once-daily dosage of Dymelor indicate that its effect on the blood sugar is better sustained than that of tolbutamide. However, patients requiring more than 1 g of Dymelor daily should be treated with divided doses.
Patients Receiving Insulin—In general, patients who were previously maintained on insulin in small dosage (e.g., up to 20 units per day) may be placed on Dymelor® (acetohexamide, Lilly) directly and their insulin administration abruptly discontinued. Patients requiring larger doses of insulin, such as 20 to 40 units or more per day, should have an initial reduction of insulin dosage by 25 to 30 percent daily or every other day and subsequent further reduction depending on the response to Dymelor. An initial dose of 250 mg of Dymelor can be used, with readjustment depending on response to therapy. Because of the potential hazards of hypoglycemia in the elderly, patients in this age group should be carefully observed during the transition from insulin to Dymelor.
During the period of insulin withdrawal, the patient should test his urine for sugar and acetone at least three times a day and report the results frequently to his physician so that appropriate adjustments of therapy may be made. In some cases, it may be advisable to consider hospitalization during the transition period from insulin to Dymelor.
It should be noted that, as with other sulfonylureas, primary and secondary failures may occur with Dymelor.
Overdosage: Hypoglycemia may appear in those patients who do not eat regularly or who exercise without caloric supplementation. This is treated in the usual manner, by supplying carbohydrate in various forms, dependent on the clinical status.
In patients with protracted hypoglycemia, treatment with 10 to 50 percent dextrose in water is advisable until the tendency toward hypoglycemia has subsided.
How Supplied: (℞) *Tablets Dymelor® (Acetohexamide Tablets, USP)* (capsule-shaped, scored): *No. 1842, U03,* 250 mg, White, and *No. 1843, U07,* 500 mg, Yellow, in bottles of 50 (NDC 0002-2103-50 and 2107-50), 200 (NDC 0002-2103-22 and 2107-22), and 500 (NDC 0002-2103-03 and 2107-03) and in 10 strips of 10 individually labeled blisters each containing 1 tablet (ID100) (NDC 0002-2103-33 and 2107-33).
[012484]
Shown in Product Identification Section, page 417
Tablets No. 1843, 500 mg—50's—6505-00-765-0589; 500's—6505-00-765-2068A

ERGOTRATE® MALEATE   ℞
[ŭr'gō-trāt măl' ē-āt]
(ergonovine maleate)
Injection, USP
AMPOULES

Description: Ergonovine is the hydroxyisopropylamide of lysergic acid. It is somewhat soluble in water, and its salts are readily soluble. It is obtained from ergot and has been shown to possess all of the desirable oxytocic activity of ergot itself. Each ampoule contains 0.2 mg of the active ingredient, ergonovine maleate, with ethyl lactate, 0.1

percent, lactic acid, 0.1 percent, and phenol, 0.25 percent, as a preservative.

The empirical formula of ergonovine maleate is $C_{19}H_{23}N_3O_2 \cdot C_4H_4O_4$. Chemically, it is 9,10-didehydro-N-[(S)-2-hydroxy-1-methylethyl]-6-methylergoline-8β-carboxamide maleate (1:1) (salt).

Clinical Pharmacology: Injection Ergotrate® Maleate (Ergonovine Maleate Injection, USP, Lilly) produces a firm contraction of the uterus. Upon the initial tetanic contraction is superimposed a succession of minor relaxations and contractions. The extent of relaxation gradually increases over a period of about one and one-half hours, but vigorous rhythmic contractions continue for a period of three or more hours after injection. The prolonged initial contraction is the type necessary to control uterine hemorrhage.

Indications and Usage: Ergotrate® Maleate (ergonovine maleate, Lilly) is indicated for the prevention and treatment of postpartum and postabortal hemorrhage and of puerperal morbidity.

Contraindications: Ergotrate® Maleate (ergonovine maleate, Lilly) is contraindicated for the induction of labor and in cases of threatened spontaneous abortion. It should not be administered to those patients who have shown allergic or idiosyncratic reactions to it.

Warnings: All oxytocic agents are potentially dangerous. Mothers and infants have been injured, and some have died because of their injudicious use. Hyperstimulation of the uterus during labor may lead to uterine tetany with marked impairment of the uteroplacental blood flow, uterine rupture, cervical and perineal lacerations, amniotic fluid embolism, and trauma to the infant (e.g., hypoxia, intracranial hemorrhage). Because of these hazards which result from overdosage, oxytocic agents must be administered under conditions of meticulous observation.

Precautions: *General Precautions*—Because of the high uterine tone produced, Ergotrate® Maleate (ergonovine maleate, Lilly) is not recommended for routine use prior to the delivery of the placenta unless the operator is versed in the technique described by Davis and others and has adequate facilities and personnel at his disposal.

As is the case with all ergot preparations, prolonged use of Ergotrate Maleate is to be avoided. Discontinue Ergotrate Maleate if symptoms of ergotism appear.

Ergotrate Maleate should be used cautiously in patients with hypertension, heart disease, venoatrial shunts, mitral-valve stenosis, obliterative vascular disease, sepsis, or hepatic or renal impairment.

The character and amount of vaginal bleeding should be observed. Hypocalcemia may affect patient response to the drug. If the patient is not also taking digitalis, cautious administration of calcium gluconate IV may produce the desired oxytocic action.

Laboratory Tests—Blood pressure, pulse, and uterine response should be monitored. Sudden changes in vital signs or frequent periods of uterine relaxation should be noted.

Adverse Reactions: Nausea and vomiting may occur, but they are uncommon. Allergic phenomena, including shock, have been reported. Ergotism has also been reported. Elevation of blood pressure (sometimes extreme) may appear in a small percentage of patients, most frequently in association with regional anesthesia (caudal or spinal), previous administration of a vasoconstrictor, and the intravenous route of administration of the oxytocic. The mechanism of such hypertension is obscure, since it may occur in the absence of anesthesia, vasoconstrictors, and oxytocics. These elevations are no more frequent with Ergotrate® Maleate (ergonovine maleate, Lilly) than with other oxytocics. They usually subside promptly following intravenous administration of 15 mg of chlorpromazine.

Overdosage: *Symptoms*—The principal manifestations of serious overdosage are convulsions and gangrene. Symptoms of overdosage include the following: vomiting, diarrhea, dizziness, rise or fall in blood pressure, weak pulse, dyspnea, loss of consciousness, numbness and coldness of the extremities, tingling, pain in the chest, gangrene of the fingers and toes, and hypercoagulability.

Treatment—Treat convulsions. Control hypercoagulability by the administration of heparin, and maintain blood-clotting time at approximately three times the normal. Give a vasodilator such as tolazine as an antidote; the rate of administration may be controlled by monitoring pulse rate and blood pressure. For emergency measures, delay absorption of ingested Ergotrate® Maleate (ergonovine maleate, Lilly) by giving tap water, milk, or activated charcoal and then removing by gastric lavage or emesis followed by catharsis. Gangrene will require surgical amputation.

Dosage and Administration: Ergotrate® Maleate (ergonovine maleate, Lilly) is intended primarily for routine intramuscular injection in obstetric practice. By this route, it usually produces a firm contraction of the uterus within a few minutes. Intravenous administration leads to a quicker response. However, because of the higher incidence of nausea and other side effects, it is recommended that the intravenous route be confined to emergencies such as excessive uterine bleeding. The usual intramuscular (or emergency intravenous) dose of Ergotrate Maleate is 0.2 mg, one ampoule. Severe uterine bleeding may call for repeated doses, but injection will rarely be required more often than once in two to four hours.

In some calcium-deficient patients, the uterus may fail to respond to Ergotrate Maleate. In such instances, responsiveness can be immediately restored by the cautious intravenous injection of calcium salts. Calcium should not be given intravenously to patients under the influence of digitalis. Tablets Ergotrate Maleate are available for oral administration.

Storage—Ampoules Ergotrate Maleate should be stored in a cold place (below 46°F). However, delivery-room stock may be kept at room temperature (although periods of more than 60 days at room temperature prior to use are not recommended).

How Supplied: (℞) *Ampoules No. 302, Ergotrate® Maleate (Ergonovine Maleate Injection, USP),* 0.2 mg, 1 ml, in packages of 6 (NDC 0002-1629-16) and 100 (NDC 0002-1629-02).

[031284]

ERGOTRATE® MALEATE ℞
[ûr′gō-trāt māl′ē-āt]
(ergonovine maleate)
Tablets, USP

Description: Ergonovine is the hydroxyisopropylamide of lysergic acid. It is somewhat soluble in water, and its salts are readily soluble. It is obtained from ergot and has been shown to possess all of the desirable oxytocic activity of ergot itself. The empirical formula of ergonovine maleate is $C_{19}H_{23}N_3O_2 \cdot C_4H_4O_4$.

Clinical Pharmacology: Within six to 15 minutes, Ergotrate® Maleate (ergonovine maleate, Lilly) produces a firm tetanic contraction of the postpartum uterus which, in the course of about 90 minutes, gradually changes to a series of clonic contractions that persist for another 90 minutes or more.

Indications and Usage: Ergotrate® Maleate (ergonovine maleate, Lilly) is indicated for the prevention and treatment of postpartum and postabortal hemorrhage due to uterine atony.

Contraindications, Warnings, Precautions, Adverse Reactions, and Overdosage: *See under Ergotrate Maleate, Injection, USP.*

Dosage and Administration: The immediate postpartum dose of Ergotrate® Maleate (ergonovine maleate, Lilly) is usually 0.2 mg. It is ordinarily administered parenterally. To minimize late postpartum bleeding, 1 or 2 tablets may be given orally two to four times daily (every six to 12 hours) until the danger of uterine atony has passed—usually 48 hours. Severe cramping is evidence of effectiveness but may justify reduction in dosage. Tablets Ergotrate Maleate may also be administered sublingually.

How Supplied: (℞) *Tablets No. 1572, Ergotrate® Maleate (Ergonovine Maleate Tablets, USP), J36,** 0.2 mg, in bottles of 100 (NDC 0002-1036-02) and 1000 (NDC 0002-1036-04) and in 10 strips of 10 individually labeled blisters each containing 1 tablet (ID100) (NDC 0002-1036-33).

[042484]

FOLIC ACID ℞
[fō′lĭk ăs′ĭd]
Tablets, USP

Description: Folic acid is a member of the vitamin B complex.

Action: Folic acid acts on megaloblastic bone marrow to produce a normoblastic marrow.

Indications: It is effective in the treatment of megaloblastic anemias due to a deficiency of folic acid (as may be seen in tropical or nontropical sprue) and in anemias of nutritional origin, pregnancy, infancy, or childhood.

Warning: Administration of folic acid alone is improper therapy for pernicious anemia and other megaloblastic anemias in which vitamin B_{12} is deficient.

Precaution: Folic acid in doses above 0.1 mg daily may obscure pernicious anemia in that hematologic remission can occur while neurologic manifestations remain progressive.

Adverse Reaction: Allergic sensitization has been reported following both oral and parenteral administration of folic acid.

Dosage and Administration: Folic acid is well absorbed and may be administered orally with satisfactory results except in severe instances of intestinal malabsorption.

The usual therapeutic dosage in adults and children (regardless of age) is up to 1 mg daily. Resistant cases may require larger doses.

When clinical symptoms have subsided and the blood picture has become normal, a daily maintenance level should be used, i.e., 0.1 mg for infants and up to 0.3 mg for children under four years of age, 0.4 mg for adults and children four or more years of age, and 0.8 mg for pregnant and lactating women, but never less than 0.1 mg/day. Patients should be kept under close supervision and adjustment of the maintenance level made if relapse appears imminent.

In the presence of alcoholism, hemolytic anemia, anticonvulsant therapy, or chronic infection, the maintenance level may need to be increased.

How Supplied: (℞) *Tablets No. 1897, Folic Acid, USP, U56,*1 mg,* in bottles of 100 (NDC 0002-2156-02).

[082283]

GLUCAGON FOR INJECTION ℞
[gloō′ka-gŏn]
USP

Description: Glucagon is produced in the pancreas (alpha cells of the islands of Langerhans). Purified and crystallized by scientists at the Lilly Research Laboratories, it is used in the treatment of hypoglycemic states and is effective in small doses.

Chemically unrelated to insulin, glucagon is a single-chain polypeptide containing 29 amino acid residues and having a molecular weight of 3483. The empirical formula is $C_{153}H_{225}N_{43}O_{49}S$.

Crystalline glucagon is a white powder containing less than 0.01 percent zinc. It is relatively insoluble in water but is soluble at a pH of less than 3 or more than 9.5. Glucagon is stable in lyophilized form at room temperatures. It will remain potent in solution for as long as three months if kept under refrigeration.

Vials No. 666, Glucagon for Injection, USP, contain 1 unit (1 mg) of glucagon as the hydrochloride with 49 mg of lactose. (Vials No. 667, Diluting Solution for Glucagon for Injection, USP, 1 ml, contain glycerin, 1.6%, with 0.2% phenol added as a preservative. Sodium hydroxide and/or hydrochloric acid may have been added during manufacture to adjust the pH.)

Continued on next page

* Identi-Code® symbol.

Lilly—Cont.

Vials No. 668, Glucagon for Injection, USP, contain 10 units (10 mg) of glucagon as the hydrochloride with 140 mg of lactose. (Vials No. 669, Diluting Solution for Glucagon for Injection, USP, 10 ml, contain glycerin, 1.6%, with 0.2% phenol added as a preservative. Sodium hydroxide and/or hydrochloric acid may have been added during manufacture to adjust the pH.) If properly refrigerated, Vials No. 668 may be used up to three months after reconstitution.

Clinical Pharmacology: Glucagon causes an increase in blood glucose concentration and is used in the treatment of hypoglycemic states. It is effective in small doses, and no evidence of toxicity has been reported with its use. Glucagon acts only on liver glycogen, converting it to glucose.
Parenteral administration of glucagon produces relaxation of the smooth muscle of the stomach, duodenum, small bowel, and colon.
The half-life of glucagon in plasma is approximately three to six minutes, which is similar to that of insulin.

Indications and Usage: *For the treatment of hypoglycemia:* Glucagon is useful in counteracting severe hypoglycemic reactions in diabetic patients or during insulin shock therapy in psychiatric patients. Glucagon is helpful in hypoglycemia only if liver glycogen is available. It is of little or no help in states of starvation, adrenal insufficiency, or chronic hypoglycemia.
The patient with juvenile-type diabetes does not have as great a response in blood glucose levels as does the adult-type stable diabetic. Therefore, supplementary carbohydrate should be given as soon as possible to the juvenile patient especially.
For use as a diagnostic aid: Glucagon is indicated as a diagnostic aid in the radiologic examination of the stomach, duodenum, small bowel, and colon when a hypotonic state would be advantageous. Glucagon is as effective for this examination as are the anticholinergic drugs, but it has fewer side effects. When glucagon is administered concomitantly with an anticholinergic agent, the response is not significantly greater than when either drug is used alone. However, the addition of the anticholinergic agent results in increased side effects.

Contraindication: Since glucagon is a protein, hypersensitivity is a possibility.

Warnings: Glucagon should be administered cautiously to patients with a history of insulinoma and/or pheochromocytoma. In patients with insulinoma, intravenous administration of glucagon will produce an initial increase in blood glucose but, because of its insulin-releasing effect, may cause the insulinoma to release its insulin and thus, may subsequently cause hypoglycemia. A patient developing symptoms of hypoglycemia after a dose of glucagon should be given glucose orally, intravenously, or by gavage, whichever is more appropriate.
Exogenous glucagon also stimulates the release of catecholamines. In the presence of pheochromocytoma, glucagon can cause the tumor to release catecholamines, which results in a sudden and marked increase in blood pressure. If a patient suddenly develops a marked increase in blood pressure, 5 to 10 mg of phentolamine mesylate may be administered intravenously in an attempt to control the blood pressure.
Generalized allergic reactions, including urticaria, respiratory distress, and hypotension, have been reported in patients who received glucagon injection.

Precautions: *General Precautions*—In the treatment of hypoglycemic shock with glucagon, liver glycogen must be available. Glucose by the intravenous route or by gavage should be considered in the hypoglycemic patient.
Laboratory Tests—Blood glucose determinations may be obtained to follow the patient in hypoglycemic shock until he or she is asymptomatic.
Carcinogenesis, Mutagenesis, Impairment of Fertility—Glucagon is administered in one or two doses to patients in hypoglycemic shock or for diagnostic radiology. The drug has a half-life of approximately three to six minutes. Because glucagon is usually given in a single dose and has a very short half-life, no studies have been done regarding carcinogenesis.
Reproduction studies have been performed in rats at doses up to 2 mg/kg b.i.d., or 90 to 120 times the human dose) and have revealed no evidence of impaired fertility.
Usage in Pregnancy—Pregnancy Category B—Reproduction studies have been performed in rats at doses up to 2 mg/kg b.i.d., or 90 to 120 times the human dose, and have revealed no evidence of harm to the fetus due to glucagon. There are, however, no adequate and well-controlled studies in pregnant women. Because animal reproduction studies are not always predictive of human response, this drug should be used during pregnancy only if clearly needed.
Nursing Mothers—It is not known whether this drug is excreted in human milk. Because many drugs are excreted in human milk, caution should be exercised when glucagon is administered to a nursing woman. The plasma half-life of glucagon is approximately three to six minutes. If the drug is excreted in human milk during this short period, it will be handled like any other polypeptide, i.e., it will be hydrolyzed and absorbed. Glucagon is not active when taken orally because it is destroyed in the gastrointestinal tract before it is absorbed.

Adverse Reactions: Glucagon is relatively free of adverse reactions except for occasional nausea and vomiting, which may also occur with hypoglycemia.

Overdosage: *Symptoms and Treatment*—The LD_{50} for glucagon in rats is approximately 300 mg/kg. To date, there have been no reported cases of human overdosage of glucagon. When glucagon was given in large doses to cardiac patients, investigators reported a positive inotropic effect. These investigators administered glucagon in doses of 0.5 to 16 mg/hour by continuous infusion for periods of five to 166 hours. Total doses ranged from 25 to 996 mg, and a 21-month-old child received approximately 8.25 mg in 165 hours. Side effects included nausea, vomiting, and decreasing serum potassium. The serum potassium could be maintained within normal limits with supplemental potassium.
In view of the extremely short half-life of glucagon and its prompt destruction and excretion, the treatment of overdosage is symptomatic, primarily for nausea, vomiting, and possible hypokalemia.

Dosage and Administration: *For the treatment of hypoglycemia:* The diluent is provided for use only in the preparation of glucagon for *intermittent* parenteral injection and for no other use.
Directions for Use of Glucagon—1. Dissolve the lyophilized glucagon in the accompanying solvent.

2. Give 0.5 to 1 unit of glucagon by subcutaneous, intramuscular, or intravenous injection.
3. The patient will usually awaken in five to 20 minutes. If the response is delayed, there is no contraindication to the administration of one or two additional doses of glucagon; however, in view of the deleterious effects of cerebral hypoglycemia and depending on the duration and depth of coma, the use of parenteral glucose *must* be considered by the physician.
4. Intravenous glucose *must* be given if the patient fails to respond to glucagon.
5. When the patient responds, give supplemental carbohydrate to restore the liver glycogen and prevent secondary hypoglycemia.
General Management of Hypoglycemia—The following are helpful measures in the prevention of hypoglycemic reactions due to insulin:
1. Reasonable uniformity from day to day with regard to diet, insulin, and exercise.
2. Careful adjustment of the insulin program so that the type (or types) of insulin, dose, and time (or times) of administration are suited to the individual patient.
3. Frequent testing of the urine so that a change in insulin requirements can be foreseen.
4. Routine carrying of sugar, candy, or other readily absorbable carbohydrate by the patient so that it may be taken at the first warning of an oncoming reaction.
If the patient is unaware of the symptoms of hypoglycemia, he may lapse into insulin shock; therefore, the physician should instruct the patient in this regard when feasible.
It is important that the patient be aroused as quickly as possible, for prolonged hypoglycemic reactions may result in cortical damage. Glucagon or intravenous glucose will awaken the patient sufficiently so that oral carbohydrates may be taken.
Instructions to the Family—Instructions describing the method of using this preparation are included in the literature which accompanies the patient's package. It is advisable for the patient to become familiar with the technique of preparing glucagon for injection before an emergency arises. CAUTION—Although glucagon may be used for the treatment of hypoglycemia by the patient during an emergency, the physician must still be notified when hypoglycemic reactions occur so that the dose of insulin may be adjusted more accurately.
Insulin Shock Therapy—Dissolve the lyophilized glucagon in the accompanying diluting solution. After one hour of coma, inject 0.5 to 1 unit of glucagon by the subcutaneous, intramuscular, or intravenous route. Larger doses may be employed if desired.
The patient will usually awaken in ten to 25 minutes. If no response occurs within the desired interval, the dose may be repeated. Upon awakening, the patient should be fed orally as soon as possible and the usual dietary regimen followed.
In a very deep state of coma, such as Stage IV or Stage V of Himwich, intravenous glucose should be given in addition to glucagon for a more immediate response. Glucagon and glucose may be used together without decreasing the efficacy of glucose administration.
For use as a diagnostic aid: Dissolve the lyophilized glucagon in the accompanying diluting solution.
The doses in the accompanying chart may be administered for relaxation of the stomach, duodenum, and small bowel, depending on the time of onset of action and the duration of effect required for the examination. Since the stomach is less sensitive to the effect of glucagon, ½ unit IV or 2 units IM are recommended.
[See table left].
For examination of the colon, it is recommended that a 2-unit dose (2 mg) be administered intramuscularly approximately ten minutes prior to initiation of the procedure. Relaxation of the colon and reduction of discomfort to the patient will allow the radiologist to perform a more satisfactory examination.

How Supplied: (℞) *Vials Glucagon for Injection, USP:* are supplied in lyophilized form with accom-

Dosage of Glucagon as a Diagnostic Aid

Dose	Route of Administration	Time of Onset of Action	Approximate Duration of Effect
¼–½ unit (0.25–0.5 mg)	IV	1 minute	9–17 minutes
1 unit (1 mg)*	IM	8–10 minutes	12–27 minutes
2 units (2 mg)*	IV	1 minute	22–25 minutes
2 units (2 mg)*	IM	4–7 minutes	21–32 minutes

*Administration of 2-unit doses produces a higher incidence of nausea and vomiting than do lower doses.

panying diluting solution: *No. 666*, 1 unit (1 mg), rubber-stoppered (Dry Powder), with 49 mg of lactose, in single packages (10 per carton) (NDC 0002-1450-01); *No. 668*, 10 units (10 mg), rubber-stoppered (Dry Powder), multiple dose, with 140 mg of lactose, in single packages (10 per carton) (NDC 0002-1451-01).

Prior to reconstitution, the vials may be stored at controlled room temperature, 59° to 86°F (15° to 30°C). After reconstitution, if storage is desired, the vials should be refrigerated and used within three months.

[052984]

HEPARIN SODIUM ℞
[hĕp′a-rĭn]
Injection, USP

WARNING—This is a potent drug, and serious consequences may result if used other than under constant medical supervision.

Description: Heparin Sodium Injection, USP, is a sterile solution of heparin sodium derived from porcine intestinal mucosa, standardized for use as an anticoagulant. Its potency is determined by biological assay with a USP reference standard based on units of heparin activity/milligram.

Each ml of Vial No. 405 contains 1000 USP heparin units (derived from porcine intestinal mucosa) and sodium chloride, 0.5%.

Each ml of Vial No. 520 contains 10,000 USP heparin units (derived from porcine intestinal mucosa) and sodium chloride, 0.1%.

Each ml of Vial No. 642 contains 20,000 USP heparin units (derived from porcine intestinal mucosa).

Each ml of Vial No. 622 contains 20,000 USP heparin units (derived from porcine intestinal mucosa). During manufacture, 1% benzyl alcohol has been added as a preservative to each vial of heparin sodium. Sodium hydroxide and/or hydrochloric acid may have been added during manufacture to adjust the *p*H.

Actions: Heparin sodium inhibits reactions that lead to the clotting of blood and the formation of fibrin clots both in vitro and in vivo. Heparin acts at multiple sites in the normal coagulation system. Small amounts of heparin in combination with antithrombin III (heparin cofactor) can prevent the development of a hypercoagulable state by inactivating activated Factor X and inhibiting the conversion of prothrombin to thrombin. Once a hypercoagulable state exists, larger amounts of heparin in combination with antithrombin III can inhibit the coagulation process by inactivating thrombin and earlier clotting intermediates and thus prevent the conversion of fibrinogen to fibrin. Heparin also prevents the formation of a stable fibrin clot by inhibiting the activation of the fibrin stabilizing factor.

Bleeding time is usually unaffected by heparin. Clotting time is prolonged by full therapeutic doses of heparin; in most cases, it is not measurably affected by low doses of heparin.

Heparin does not have fibrinolytic activity; therefore, it will not lyse existing clots.

Indications: Heparin sodium is indicated for:
Anticoagulant therapy in prophylaxis and treatment of venous thrombosis and its extension

Low-dose regimen for prevention of postoperative deep venous thrombosis and pulmonary embolism in patients undergoing major abdominothoracic surgery who are at risk of developing thromboembolic disease (*see* Dosage and Administration)

Prophylaxis and treatment of pulmonary embolism

Atrial fibrillation with embolization

Diagnosis and treatment of acute and chronic consumption coagulopathies (disseminated intravascular coagulation)

Prevention of clotting in arterial and heart surgery

Prevention of cerebral thrombosis in evolving stroke

Heparin sodium is indicated as an adjunct both in treating coronary occlusion with acute myocardial infarction and in the prophylaxis and treatment of peripheral arterial embolism.

Heparin sodium may also be employed as an anticoagulant in blood transfusions, extracorporeal circulation, and dialysis procedures and in blood samples for laboratory purposes.

Contraindications: Heparin sodium is contraindicated in patients known to have a hypersensitivity to heparin.

It is also contraindicated when suitable blood coagulation tests—e.g., the whole-blood clotting time, partial thromboplastin time, etc.— cannot be performed at the required intervals. (There is usually no need to monitor the effect of low-dose heparin in patients with normal coagulation parameters.) The drug is contraindicated during any uncontrollable active bleeding state (*see* Warnings).

Warnings:

> Heparin sodium should be used with extreme caution in disease states in which there is increased danger of hemorrhage.

When heparin sodium is administered in therapeutic amounts, its dosage should be regulated by frequent blood coagulation tests. If the coagulation test is unduly prolonged or if hemorrhage occurs, heparin sodium should be discontinued promptly (*see* Overdosage).

Some of the conditions in which increased danger of hemorrhage exists are as follows:

Cardiovascular—Subacute bacterial endocarditis; arterial sclerosis; increased capillary permeability; during and immediately following (a) spinal tap or spinal anesthesia or (b) major surgery, especially involving the brain, spinal cord, or eye.

Hematologic—Conditions associated with increased bleeding tendencies, such as hemophilia, some purpuras, and thrombocytopenia.

Gastrointestinal—Inaccessible ulcerative lesions and continuous tube drainage of the stomach or small intestine.

Heparin sodium may prolong the one-stage prothrombin time. Therefore, when heparin sodium is given with dicumarol or warfarin sodium, a period of at least five hours after the last intravenous dose or 24 hours after the last subcutaneous (intrafat, i.e., above the iliac crest or abdominal fat layer) dose should elapse before blood is drawn if a valid prothrombin time is to be obtained.

Drugs (such as acetylsalicylic acid, dextran, phenylbutazone, ibuprofen, indomethacin, dipyridamole, and hydroxychloroquine) that interfere with platelet-aggregation reactions (the main hemostatic defense of heparinized patients) may induce bleeding and should be used with caution in patients receiving heparin sodium.

Although there is experimental evidence that heparin sodium may antagonize the action of ACTH, insulin, or corticoids, this effect has not been clearly defined.

There is also evidence in experimental animals that heparin sodium may modify or inhibit allergic reactions. However, the application of these findings to human patients has not been fully defined.

It may be necessary to increase doses of heparin sodium in the febrile state.

Digitalis, tetracyclines, nicotine, or antihistamines may partially counteract the anticoagulant action of heparin sodium. An increased resistance to the drug is frequently encountered in thrombosis, thrombophlebitis, infections with thrombosing tendencies, myocardial infarction, cancer, and postsurgical patients.

Usage in Pregnancy—Heparin sodium injection should be used with caution during pregnancy, especially during the last trimester and in the immediate postpartum period.

There is no adequate information as to whether heparin may affect human fertility or have a teratogenic potential or other adverse effect on the fetus.

Heparin does not cross the placental barrier; it is not excreted in human milk.

Precautions: Because heparin sodium is derived from animal tissue, it should be used with caution in any patient with a history of allergy.

Before a therapeutic dose is given to such a patient, a trial dose of 1000 units may be advisable. Heparin sodium should be used with caution in the presence of hepatic or renal disease, in hypertension, during menstruation, or in patients with indwelling catheters.

A higher incidence of bleeding may be seen in women over 60 years of age.

Caution should be exercised when administering ACD-converted blood (i.e., blood collected in heparin sodium and later converted to ACD blood), since the anticoagulant activity of its heparin sodium content persists without loss for 22 days. ACD-converted blood may alter the coagulation system of the recipient, especially if it is given in multiple transfusions.

Adverse Reactions: Hemorrhage is the chief complication that may result from heparin sodium therapy. An overly prolonged clotting time or minor bleeding during therapy can usually be controlled by withdrawing the drug (*see* Overdosage). The occurrence of significant gastrointestinal or urinary tract bleeding during anticoagulant therapy may indicate the presence of an underlying occult lesion.

Adrenal hemorrhage, with resultant acute adrenal insufficiency, has occurred during anticoagulant therapy. Therefore, such treatment should be discontinued in patients who develop signs and symptoms of acute adrenal hemorrhage and insufficiency. Plasma cortisol levels should be measured immediately, and vigorous therapy with intravenous corticosteroids should be instituted promptly. Initiation of therapy should not depend on laboratory confirmation of the diagnosis, since any delay in an acute situation may result in the patient's death.

Intramuscular injection of heparin sodium frequently causes local irritation, mild pain, or hematoma and, for these reasons, should be avoided. These effects are less often seen following deep subcutaneous (intrafat) injection. Histamine-like reactions have also been observed at the site of injection.

Hypersensitivity reactions have been reported, with chills, fever, and urticaria as the most usual manifestations. Asthma, rhinitis, lacrimation, and anaphylactoid reactions have also been reported. Vasospastic reactions may develop, independent of the origin of heparin, six to ten days after the initiation of therapy and may last for four to six hours. The affected limb is painful, ischemic, and cyanosed. An artery to this limb may have been recently catheterized. After repeated injections, the reaction may gradually increase to include generalized vasospasm, with cyanosis, tachypnea, feeling of oppression, and headache. Protamine sulfate treatment has no marked therapeutic effect. Itching and burning, especially on the plantar side of the feet, is possibly caused by a similar allergic vasospastic reaction. Chest pain, elevated blood pressure, arthralgias, and/or headache have also been reported in the absence of definite peripheral vasospasm. Anaphylactic shock has been reported rarely following the intravenous administration of heparin sodium.

Acute reversible thrombocytopenia has been reported following the intravenous administration of heparin sodium. Osteoporosis and suppression of renal function following long-term administration of high doses, suppression of aldosterone synthesis, delayed transient alopecia, priapism, and rebound hyperlipemia on discontinuation of heparin sodium have also been reported.

Dosage and Administration: Heparin sodium is not effective by oral administration and should be given by intermittent intravenous injection, intravenous infusion, or deep subcutaneous (intrafat) injection. The intramuscular route of administration should be avoided because of the frequent occurrence of hematoma at the injection site.

Continued on next page

* Identi-Code® symbol.

Lilly—Cont.

The dosage of heparin sodium should be adjusted according to the patient's coagulation test results, which, during the first day of treatment, should be determined just prior to each injection. (There is usually no need to monitor the effect of low-dose heparin in patients with normal coagulation parameters.) Dosage is considered adequate when the whole-blood clotting time is elevated approximately two and one-half to three times the control value.

When heparin sodium is given by continuous intravenous infusion, the coagulation time should be determined approximately every four hours in the early stages of treatment.

When the drug is administered intermittently by intravenous or deep subcutaneous (intrafat) injection, coagulation tests should be performed before each injection during the early stages of treatment and daily thereafter.

When an oral anticoagulant of the coumadin or similar type is administered with heparin sodium, coagulation tests and prothrombin activity should be determined at the start of therapy. For an immediate anticoagulant effect, give heparin sodium in the usual therapeutic dosage. When the results of the initial prothrombin tests are known, administer the first dose of an oral anticoagulant in the usual initial amount. Thereafter, perform a coagulation test and determine the prothrombin activity at appropriate intervals. A period of at least five hours after the last intravenous dose or 24 hours after the last subcutaneous (intrafat) dose of heparin sodium should elapse before blood is drawn if a valid prothrombin time is to be obtained. When the oral anticoagulant shows its full effect and prothrombin activity is in the desired therapeutic range, heparin sodium may be discontinued and therapy continued with the oral anticoagulant.

Therapeutic Anticoagulant Effect with Full-Dose Heparin—Although dosage must be adjusted for the individual patient according to the results of suitable laboratory tests, the dosage schedules in the accompanying chart may be used as guidelines.

1. *Deep Subcutaneous (Intrafat) Injection*—After an initial intravenous injection of 5000 units, inject 10,000 to 20,000 units of a concentrated heparin sodium solution subcutaneously, followed by 8000 to 10,000 units every eight hours or 15,000 to 20,000 units every 12 hours. A different site should be used for each injection to prevent the development of a massive hematoma.

2. *Intermittent Intravenous Injection*—Initially, 10,000 units; then, 5000 to 10,000 units every four to six hours. These amounts may be given undiluted or diluted with 50 to 100 ml of isotonic Sodium Chloride Injection.

3. *Continuous Intravenous Infusion*—After an initial intravenous injection of 5000 units, add 20,000 to 40,000 units of heparin sodium to 1000 ml of isotonic Sodium Chloride Injection for infusion. For most patients, the rate of flow should be adjusted to deliver approximately 20,000 to 40,000 units in 24 hours.
[See table below].

Surgery of the Heart and Blood Vessels—Patients undergoing total body perfusion for open-heart surgery should receive an initial dose of not less than 150 units of heparin sodium/kg of body weight. Frequently, a dose of 300 units/kg is used for procedures estimated to last less than 60 minutes or 400 units/kg for those estimated to last longer than 60 minutes.

Low-Dose Prophylaxis of Postoperative Thromboembolism—A number of well-controlled clinical trials have demonstrated that low-dose heparin prophylaxis, given just prior to and after surgery, will reduce the incidence of postoperative deep-vein thrombosis in the legs (as measured by the I-125 fibrinogen technique and venography) and of clinical pulmonary embolism. The most widely used dosage has been 5000 units two hours before surgery and 5000 units every eight to 12 hours thereafter for seven days or until the patient is fully ambulatory, whichever is longer. The heparin is given by deep subcutaneous (intrafat) injection in the arm or abdomen with a fine (25 to 26-gauge) needle to minimize tissue trauma. A concentrated solution of heparin sodium is recommended. Such prophylaxis should be reserved for patients over the age of 40 who are undergoing major surgery. Patients with bleeding disorders and those having neurosurgery, spinal anesthesia, eye surgery, or potentially sanguineous operations should be excluded, as should patients receiving oral anticoagulants or platelet-active drugs (*see* Warnings). The value of such prophylaxis in hip surgery has not been established. The possibility of increased bleeding during surgery or postoperatively should be borne in mind. If such bleeding occurs, discontinuance of heparin and neutralization with protamine sulfate are advisable. If clinical evidence of thromboembolism develops despite low-dose prophylaxis, full therapeutic doses of anticoagulants should be given unless contraindicated. All patients should be screened prior to heparinization to rule out bleeding disorders, and monitoring with appropriate coagulation tests should be performed just prior to surgery. Coagulation test values should be normal or only slightly elevated. There is usually no need for daily monitoring of the effect of low-dose heparin in patients with normal coagulation parameters.

Extracorporeal Dialysis—Follow equipment manufacturers' operating directions carefully.

Blood Transfusion—Addition of 400 to 600 USP units/100 ml of whole blood. Usually, 7500 USP units of heparin sodium are added to 100 ml of Sterile Sodium Chloride Injection (or 75,000 USP units/1000 ml of Sterile Sodium Chloride Injection) and mixed; from this sterile solution, 6 to 8 ml are added/100 ml of whole blood. Leukocyte counts should be performed on heparinized blood within two hours after addition of the heparin. Heparinized blood should not be used for isoagglutinin, complement, or erythrocyte fragility tests or platelet counts.

Laboratory Samples—Addition of 70 to 150 units of heparin sodium per 10 to 20-ml sample of whole blood is usually employed to prevent coagulation of the sample. See comments under *Blood Transfusion*.

Overdosage: Protamine sulfate (1 percent solution) given by *slow infusion* will neutralize heparin sodium. *No more than 50 mg* should be administered, *very slowly*, in any ten-minute period. Each mg of protamine sulfate neutralizes approximately 100 USP heparin units (or injection of 1 to 1.5 mg neutralizes approximately 1 mg of heparin sodium). Heparins derived from various animal sources require different amounts of protamine sulfate for neutralization. This fact is of most importance during procedures of regional heparinization, including dialysis.

The amount of protamine required decreases as the time interval since the last heparin injection increases. Thirty minutes after a dose of heparin sodium, approximately 0.5 mg of protamine is sufficient to neutralize each 100 units of administered heparin. In some cases, blood or plasma transfusions may be necessary; these dilute but do not neutralize heparin sodium.

How Supplied: (℞) Vials (Multiple Dose) Heparin Sodium Injection, USP: No. 405, 1000 USP units/ml, 10 ml (NDC 0002-7216-01); No. 520, 10,000 USP units/ml, 5 ml (NDC 0002-7217-01); No. 622, 20,000 USP units/ml, 1 ml (NDC 0002-7218-01); and No. 642, 20,000 USP units/ml, 2 ml, rubber-stoppered, in singles (10 per carton) (NDC 0002-7219-01).

[090782]

HUMULIN® N   OTC
[hū' mū-lĭn ĕn]
(NPH human insulin [recombinant DNA origin])
Isophane Suspension

INFORMATION FOR THE PATIENT
WARNINGS
THIS LILLY HUMAN INSULIN PRODUCT DIFFERS FROM ANIMAL-SOURCE INSULINS BECAUSE IT IS STRUCTURALLY IDENTICAL TO THE INSULIN PRODUCED BY YOUR BODY'S PANCREAS AND BECAUSE OF ITS UNIQUE MANUFACTURING PROCESS.
ANY CHANGE OF INSULIN SHOULD BE MADE CAUTIOUSLY AND ONLY UNDER MEDICAL SUPERVISION. CHANGES IN REFINEMENT, PURITY, STRENGTH, BRAND (MANUFACTURER), TYPE (REGULAR, NPH, LENTE®, ETC.), AND/OR METHOD OF MANUFACTURE (RECOMBINANT DNA VERSUS ANIMAL-SOURCE INSULIN) MAY RESULT IN THE NEED FOR A CHANGE IN DOSAGE.
SOME PATIENTS TAKING HUMULIN® (HUMAN INSULIN, RECOMBINANT DNA ORIGIN, LILLY) WILL REQUIRE A CHANGE IN DOSAGE FROM THAT USED WITH ANIMAL-SOURCE INSULINS. IF AN ADJUSTMENT IS NEEDED, IT MAY OCCUR WITH THE FIRST DOSE OR OVER A PERIOD OF SEVERAL WEEKS.

Insulin and Diabetes: Your doctor has explained that you have diabetes. You have learned that the treatment of your diabetes requires injections of insulin.

Dosage Schedule Guidelines for Administration of Heparin Sodium

Method of Administration	Frequency	Recommended Dose*
Deep Subcutaneous (Intrafat) Injection	Initial dose	5000 units by IV injection, followed by 10,000–20,000 units of a concentrated solution, subcutaneously
	Every 8 hours	8000–10,000 units of a concentrated solution
	or Every 12 hours	15,000–20,000 units of a concentrated solution
Intermittent Intravenous Injection	Initial dose	10,000 units, either undiluted or in 50–100 ml of isotonic Sodium Chloride Injection
	Every 4 to 6 hours	5000–10,000 units, either undiluted or in 50–100 ml of isotonic Sodium Chloride Injection
Intravenous Infusion	Initial dose Continuous	5000 units by IV injection 20,000–40,000 units/day in 1000 ml of isotonic Sodium Chloride Injection for infusion

*Based on 150-lb (68-kg) patient.

Product Information

Insulin is a hormone produced by the pancreas, a large gland that lies near the stomach. This hormone is necessary for the body's correct use of food, especially sugar. Diabetes occurs when the pancreas does not make enough insulin to meet your body's needs.

To control your diabetes, your doctor has prescribed injections of insulin to keep your blood sugar at a nearly normal level and to keep your urine as free of sugar as possible. Each case of diabetes is different. Your doctor has told you which insulin to use, how much, and when and how often to inject it. This schedule has been individualized for you. Proper control of your diabetes requires close and constant cooperation with your doctor. In spite of diabetes, you can lead an active, healthy, and useful life if you eat a balanced diet daily, exercise regularly, and take your insulin injections exactly as prescribed by your doctor.

You have been instructed to test your urine and/or your blood regularly for sugar. If your urine tests consistently show the presence of sugar or your blood tests consistently show above-normal sugar levels, your diabetes is not properly controlled and you must let your doctor know.

Use the Proper Type of Insulin: This insulin, manufactured by Eli Lilly and Company, has the trademark Humulin and is available in two formulations—Regular and NPH. These products can be identified by a large letter that appears on the carton and vial (bottle) label following the name Humulin: Humulin R (regular) or Humulin N (NPH).

These types of insulin differ mainly in the time they require to take effect and in the length of time their action lasts. Your doctor has prescribed the type of insulin that he/she believes is best for you. **DO NOT USE ANY OTHER INSULIN EXCEPT ON HIS/HER ADVICE AND DIRECTION.**

If your physician has directed you to take Humulin, when your receive your insulin from the pharmacy, always check to see that:
1. The name Humulin appears on the carton and bottle label and is followed by the proper letter designation and name for the insulin formulation: R-Regular; N-NPH.
2. The carton and bottle label are correct for your type of insulin.
3. The human insulin is of recombinant DNA origin.
4. The insulin strength is U-100.
5. The expiration date on the package will allow you to use the insulin before that date.

NPH Human Insulin: Humulin® N (NPH Human Insulin, Recombinant DNA Origin, Lilly) is synthesized in a non-disease-producing special laboratory strain of *Escherichia coli* bacteria which has been genetically altered by the addition of the human gene for insulin production. This product is a modification of a solution of zinc-insulin crystals providing a different duration of action than regular insulin. The result is an intermediate-acting insulin with a slower onset of action than regular insulin and a longer duration of activity (slightly less than 24 hours).

Humulin N should look uniformly cloudy, or milky. If the insulin substance (the cloudy material) settles at the bottom of the bottle, the bottle must be carefully rotated before the injection so that the contents are uniformly mixed (see instructions under Preparing the Dose). Do not use a vial of insulin if you see lumps that float or stick to the sides. Also, the insulin should not be used if it is clear and remains clear after the bottle is rotated.

Storage: Insulin should be stored in a cold place, preferably in a refrigerator, but not in the freezing compartment. Do not let it freeze or leave it in direct sunlight. If refrigeration is not possible, the bottle of insulin which you are currently using can be kept unrefrigerated as long as it is kept as cool as possible and away from heat and sunlight. Do not use a bottle of insulin after the expiration date stamped on the label.

Use the Correct Syringe: Doses of insulin are measured in **units**. The number of units in each milliliter (ml) is clearly stated on the package. It is important to use a syringe which is marked for an insulin preparation with 100 units per ml. Failure to use the proper syringe can lead to a mistake in dosage, and you may receive too little or too much insulin. This can cause serious problems for you, ranging from a blood sugar level that is too low or too high, to coma (unconsciousness) or, rarely, death.

IMPORTANT: TO HELP AVOID CONTAMINATION AND POSSIBLE INFECTION, FOLLOW THESE INSTRUCTIONS EXACTLY.

Disposable Syringes: Disposable syringes and needles require no sterilization; they should be used only once and then discarded.

Sterilizing and Assembling Reusable Syringes: Your reusable syringe and needle must be sterilized before each injection—**follow the package directions supplied with your syringe.** Boiling, as described below, is the best method of sterilizing.
1. Put syringe, plunger, and needle in strainer, place in saucepan, and cover with water. Boil for five minutes.
2. Remove articles from water. When they have cooled, insert plunger into barrel, and fasten needle to syringe with a slight twist.
3. Push plunger in and out several times until water is completely removed. (If the syringe, plunger, and needle cannot be boiled, as when you are traveling, they may be sterilized by immersion for at least five minutes in Isopropyl Alcohol, 91%. Do not use bathing, rubbing, or medicated alcohol for this sterilization. If the syringe is sterilized with alcohol, it must be absolutely dry before use.)

Preparing the Dose:
1. Wash your hands.
2. Gently roll the insulin bottle several times to mix the insulin. Be sure it is completely mixed. Do not shake bottle. Flip off the colored protective cap on the bottle, but **do not** remove the rubber stopper.

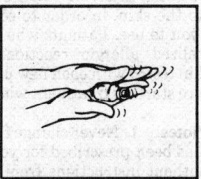

3. Wipe top of bottle with alcohol swab.

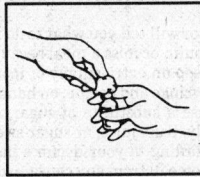

4. Draw air into the syringe by pulling back on the plunger. The amount of air should be equal to your insulin dose.

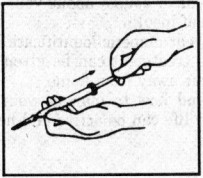

5. Remove the needle cover. Put the needle through rubber top of insulin bottle.

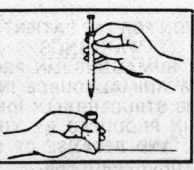

6. Push plunger in. The air injected into the bottle will allow insulin to be easily withdrawn into syringe.

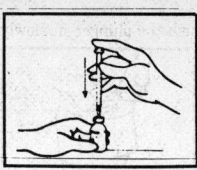

7. Turn bottle and syringe upside down in one hand. Be sure tip of needle is in insulin. Your other hand will be free to move the plunger. Draw back on plunger slowly to draw the correct dose of insulin into syringe.

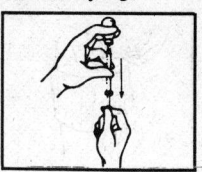

8. Check for air bubbles. The air is harmless, but too large an air bubble will reduce the insulin dose. To remove air bubbles, push insulin back into the bottle and measure your correct dose of insulin.

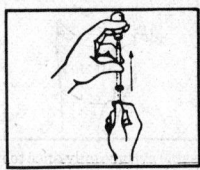

9. Double check your dose. Remove needle from bottle. Cover needle with guard or lay syringe down so that needle does not touch anything.

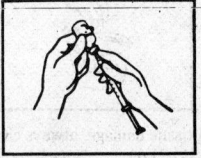

Injecting the Dose:
1. Cleanse the skin where the injection is to be made.

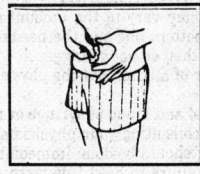

2. With one hand, stabilize the skin by spreading it or pinching up a large area of skin.

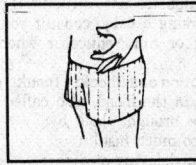

3. Pick up syringe with other hand, and hold it as you would a pencil. Insert needle straight into the skin (90° angle). After the needle is in, pull back the plunger very slightly. If blood comes into the syringe, the needle has entered a blood vessel. Remove the needle and put it in at another location. If blood does not appear in the

Continued on next page

* Identi-Code® symbol.

Lilly—Cont.

syringe, push the plunger in slowly as far as it will go.

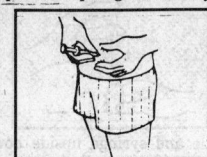

4. To inject the insulin, push plunger all the way down, using less than five seconds to inject the dose.

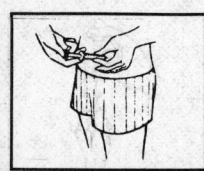

5. Hold alcohol swab near the needle and pull needle straight out of skin. Press alcohol swab over injection site for several seconds.

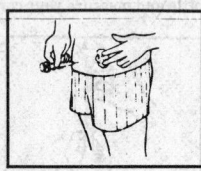

6. Use disposable syringe only once to insure sterility of syringe and needle and accuracy of dose. Destroy syringes as directed.

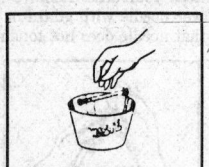

7. To avoid tissue damage, always change the site for each injection.

Warnings—See Additional Warnings Above: Patients who have been directed by their physicians to mix two types of insulin should be aware that insulin hypodermic syringes of different manufacturers may vary in the amount of space between the bottom line and the needle.
Because of this, do not change:
1. The order of mixing that the physician has prescribed or
2. The model and brand of syringe or needle without first consulting your physician.
The mixing should be done immediately prior to injection. Failure to heed this warning could result in a dosage error.

Usage in Pregnancy: Pregnancy may make managing your diabetes more difficult. If you are pregnant or nursing a baby, consult your physician, pharmacist, or nurse-educator when using this product.

Insulin Reaction and Shock: Insulin reaction (too little sugar in the blood, also called "hypoglycemia") can be brought about by:
1. Taking too much insulin
2. Missing or delaying meals
3. Exercising or working too hard just before a meal
4. An infection or illness (especially with diarrhea or vomiting)
5. A change in the body's need for insulin

The first symptoms of insulin reaction usually come on suddenly and may include fatigue, nervousness or "shakiness," headache, rapid heartbeat, nausea, and a cold sweat.
A few patients who experienced hypoglycemic reactions after being transferred to Humulin have reported that these early warning symptoms were less pronounced than they were with animal-source insulin.
Eating sugar or a sugar-sweetened product will often correct the condition and prevent more serious symptoms.
If the reaction becomes more severe, breathing will be shallow and the skin pale. Contact a doctor at once if you develop any of these symptoms.

Diabetic Acidosis and Coma: Diabetic acidosis may develop if your body has too little insulin. (This is the opposite of insulin reaction, which is the result of too much insulin in the blood.) Diabetic acidosis may be brought on if you omit your insulin or take less than the doctor has prescribed, eat significantly more than your diet calls for, or develop a fever or infection. With acidosis, urine tests show a large amount of sugar and acetone. The first symptoms of diabetic acidosis usually come on gradually, over a period of hours or days, and include a drowsy feeling, flushed face, thirst, and loss of appetite. Heavy breathing and a rapid pulse are more severe symptoms. It is important that you notify your doctor immediately, because diabetic coma (unconsciousness) can follow.

Allergy to Insulin: Patients occasionally experience redness, swelling, and itching at the site of injection of insulin. This condition, called local allergy, usually clears up in a few days to a few weeks. If you have local reactions, contact your physician, who may recommend a change in the type or species source of insulin.
Less common, but potentially more serious, is generalized allergy to insulin, which may cause rash over the whole body, shortness of breath, wheezing, reduction in blood pressure, fast pulse, or sweating. Severe cases of generalized allergy may be life-threatening. If you think you are having a generalized allergic reaction to insulin, notify a physician immediately. Your doctor may recommend skin testing, injecting small doses of other insulins into the skin, in order to select the best insulin for you to use. Patients who have had severe generalized allergic reactions to insulin should be skin tested with each new preparation to be used before starting treatment with that preparation.

Important Notes: 1. Never change from the insulin that has been prescribed for you to another insulin without instructions from your doctor. Changing the type, strength, species, or manufacturer of insulin can cause problems with your diabetes.
2. Your doctor will tell you what to do if you miss a dose of insulin or miss a meal because of illness. Always keep an extra supply of insulin, as well as spare syringe and needle, on hand. If you miss a meal, use a substitute of sugar, sugar-sweetened candy, fruit juice, or sugar-sweetened beverage according to your doctor's instructions.
3. If you become ill from any cause, especially with nausea and vomiting, your insulin requirements may change. Test your urine and/or blood and notify your doctor at once.
4. Consult your doctor if you notice anything unusual or have doubts about your condition or your use of insulin.
5. Always wear diabetic identification so that appropriate treatment can be given if complications occur away from home.
6. Understand how to manage your diabetes so that your life can be active and healthy.
[031584]

HUMULIN® R OTC
[hū'mŭ-lĭn är]
(regular human insulin [recombinant DNA origin])
Injection

INFORMATION FOR THE PATIENT
WARNINGS
THIS LILLY HUMAN INSULIN PRODUCT DIFFERS FROM ANIMAL-SOURCE INSULINS BECAUSE IT IS STRUCTURALLY IDENTICAL TO THE INSULIN PRODUCED BY YOUR BODY'S PANCREAS, AND BECAUSE OF ITS UNIQUE MANUFACTURING PROCESS.
ANY CHANGE OF INSULIN SHOULD BE MADE CAUTIOUSLY AND ONLY UNDER MEDICAL SUPERVISION. CHANGES IN REFINEMENT, PURITY, STRENGTH, BRAND (MANUFACTURER), TYPE (REGULAR, NPH, LENTE®, ETC.), AND/OR METHOD OF MANUFACTURE (RECOMBINANT DNA VERSUS ANIMAL-SOURCE INSULIN) MAY RESULT IN THE NEED FOR A CHANGE IN DOSAGE.
SOME PATIENTS TAKING HUMULIN® (HUMAN INSULIN, RECOMBINANT DNA ORIGIN, LILLY) WILL REQUIRE A CHANGE IN DOSAGE FROM THAT USED WITH ANIMAL-SOURCE INSULINS. IF AN ADJUSTMENT IS NEEDED, IT MAY OCCUR WITH THE FIRST DOSE OR OVER A PERIOD OF SEVERAL WEEKS.

Insulin and Diabetes: Your doctor has explained that you have diabetes. You have learned that the treatment of your diabetes requires injections of insulin.
Insulin is a hormone produced by the pancreas, a large gland that lies near the stomach. This hormone is necessary for the body's correct use of food, especially sugar. Diabetes occurs when the pancreas does not make enough insulin to meet your body's needs.
To control your diabetes, your doctor has prescribed injections of insulin to keep your blood sugar at a nearly normal level and to keep your urine as free of sugar as possible. Each case of diabetes is different. Your doctor has told you which insulin to use, how much, and when and how often to inject it. This schedule has been individualized for you. Proper control of your diabetes requires close and constant cooperation with your doctor.
In spite of diabetes, you can lead an active, healthy, and useful life if you eat a balanced diet daily, exercise regularly, and take your insulin injections exactly as prescribed by your doctor.
You have been instructed to test your urine and/or your blood regularly for sugar. If your urine tests consistently show the presence of sugar or your blood tests consistently show above-normal sugar levels, your diabetes is not properly controlled and you must let your doctor know.

Use the Proper Type of Insulin: This insulin, manufactured by Eli Lilly and Company, has the trademark Humulin and is available in two formulations—Regular and NPH. These products can be identified by a large letter that appears on the carton and vial (bottle) label following the name Humulin: Humulin R (regular) or Humulin N (NPH).
These types of insulin differ mainly in the time they require to take effect and in the length of time their action lasts. Your doctor has prescribed the type of insulin that he/she believes is best for you. DO NOT USE ANY OTHER INSULIN EXCEPT ON HIS/HER ADVICE AND DIRECTION.
If your physician has directed you to take Humulin, when you receive your insulin from the pharmacy, always check to see that:
1. The name Humulin appears on the carton and bottle label and is followed by the proper letter designation and the name for the insulin formulation: R-Regular; N-NPH.
2. The carton and bottle label are correct for your type of insulin.
3. The human insulin is of recombinant DNA origin.
4. The insulin strength is U-100.
5. The expiration date on the package will allow you to use the insulin before that date.

Neutral Regular Human Insulin: Humulin® R (Human Insulin, Recombinant DNA Origin, Injection, Lilly) is synthesized in a non-disease-producing special laboratory strain of *Escherichia coli* bacteria which has been genetically altered by the addition of the human gene for insulin production. This product consists of zinc-insulin crystals dissolved in a clear fluid. Humulin R has had nothing added to change the speed or length of its action. It takes effect rapidly and has a relatively short duration of activity (six to eight hours) as compared with other insulins.
Humulin R should be clear and colorless. Do not use it if it is cloudy, unusually viscous, precipitated, or even slightly colored.

Storage: Insulin should be stored in a cold place, preferably in a refrigerator, but not in the freezing

for possible revisions — **Product Information** — 1153

compartment. Do not let it freeze or leave it in direct sunlight. If refrigeration is not possible, the bottle of insulin which you are currently using can be kept unrefrigerated as long as it is kept as cool as possible and away from heat and sunlight. Do not use a bottle of insulin after the expiration date stamped on the label.

Use the Correct Syringe: Doses of insulin are measured in **units**. The number of units in each milliliter (ml) is clearly stated on the package. It is important to use a syringe which is marked for an insulin preparation with 100 units per ml. Failure to use the proper syringe can lead to a mistake in dosage, and you may receive too little or too much insulin. This can cause serious problems for you, ranging from a blood sugar level that is too low or too high, to coma (unconsciousness) or, rarely, death.

IMPORTANT: TO HELP AVOID CONTAMINATION AND POSSIBLE INFECTION, FOLLOW THESE INSTRUCTIONS EXACTLY.

Disposable Syringes: Disposable syringes and needles require no sterilization; they should be used only once and then discarded.

Sterilizing and Assembling Reusable Syringes: Your reusable syringe and needle must be sterilized before each injection—**follow the package directions supplied with your syringe.** Boiling, as described below, is the best method of sterilizing.

1. Put syringe, plunger, and needle in strainer, place in saucepan, and cover with water. Boil for five minutes.
2. Remove articles from water. When they have cooled, insert plunger into barrel, and fasten needle to syringe with a slight twist.
3. Push plunger in and out several times until water is completely removed. (If the syringe, plunger, and needle cannot be boiled, as when you are traveling, they may be sterilized by immersion for at least five minutes in Isopropyl Alcohol, 91%. Do not use bathing, rubbing, or medicated alcohol for this sterilization. If the syringe is sterilized with alcohol, it must be absolutely dry before use.)

Preparing the Dose:
1. Wash your hands.
2. Flip off the colored protective cap on the bottle, but **do not** remove the rubber stopper.
3. Wipe top of bottle with alcohol swab.

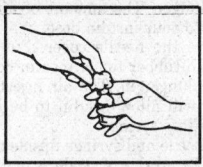

4. Draw air into the syringe by pulling back on the plunger. The amount of air should be equal to your insulin dose.

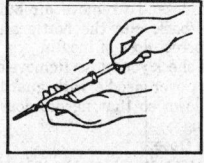

5. Remove the needle cover. Put the needle through rubber top of insulin bottle.

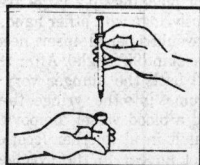

6. Push plunger in. The air injected into the bottle will allow insulin to be easily withdrawn into syringe.

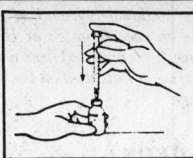

7. Turn bottle and syringe upside down in one hand. Be sure tip of needle is in insulin. Your other hand will be free to move the plunger. Draw back on plunger slowly to draw the correct dose of insulin into syringe.

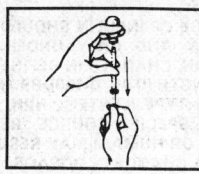

8. Check for air bubbles. The air is harmless, but too large an air bubble will reduce the insulin dose. To remove air bubbles, push insulin back into the bottle and measure your correct dose of insulin.

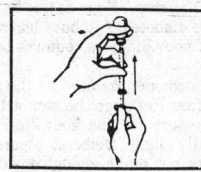

9. Double check your dose. Remove needle from bottle. Cover needle with guard or lay syringe down so that needle does not touch anything.

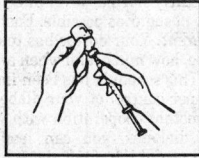

Injecting the Dose:
1. Cleanse the skin where the injection is to be made.

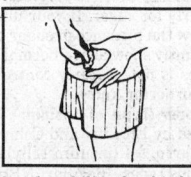

2. With one hand, stabilize the skin by spreading it or pinching up a large area of skin.

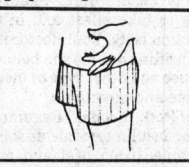

3. Pick up syringe with other hand, and hold it as you would a pencil. Insert needle straight into the skin (90° angle). After the needle is in, pull back the plunger very slightly. If blood comes into the syringe, the needle has entered a blood vessel. Remove the needle and put it in at another location. If blood does not appear in the syringe, push the plunger in slowly as far as it will go.

4. To inject the insulin, push plunger all the way down, using less than 5 seconds to inject the dose.

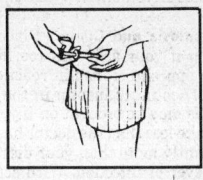

5. Hold alcohol swab near the needle and pull needle straight out of skin. Press alcohol swab over injection site for several seconds.

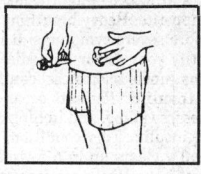

6. Use disposable syringe only once to insure sterility of syringe and needle and accuracy of dose. Destroy syringes as directed.

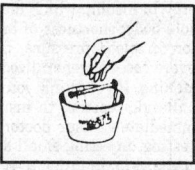

7. To avoid tissue damage, always change the site for each injection.

Warnings—See Additional Warnings Above: Patients who have been directed by their physicians to mix two types of insulin should be aware that insulin hypodermic syringes of different manufacturers may vary in the amount of space between the bottom line and the needle. Because of this, do not change:

1. The order of mixing that the physician has prescribed or
2. The model and brand of syringe or needle without first consulting your physician.

The mixing should be done immediately prior to injection. Failure to heed this warning could result in a dosage error.

Usage in Pregnancy: Pregnancy may make managing your diabetes more difficult. If you are pregnant or nursing a baby, consult your physician, pharmacist, or nurse-educator when using this product.

Insulin Reaction and Shock: Insulin reaction (too little sugar in the blood, also called "hypoglycemia") can be brought about by:

1. Taking too much insulin
2. Missing or delaying meals
3. Exercising or working too hard just before a meal
4. An infection or illness (especially with diarrhea or vomiting)
5. A change in the body's need for insulin

The first symptoms of insulin reaction usually come on suddenly and may include fatigue, nervousness or "shakiness," headache, rapid heartbeat, nausea, and a cold sweat.

A few patients who experienced hypoglycemic reactions after being transferred to Humulin have reported that these early warning symptoms were less pronounced than they were with animal-source insulin.

Eating sugar or a sugar-sweetened product will often correct the condition and prevent more serious symptoms.

If the reaction becomes more severe, breathing will be shallow and the skin pale. Contact your

Continued on next page

* Identi-Code® symbol.

Lilly—Cont.

doctor at once if you develop any of these symptoms.

Diabetic Acidosis and Coma: Diabetic acidosis may develop if your body has too little insulin. (This is the opposite of insulin reaction, which is the result of too much insulin in the blood.) Diabetic acidosis may be brought on if you omit your insulin or take less than the doctor has prescribed, eat significantly more than your diet calls for, or develop a fever or infection. With acidosis, urine tests show a large amount of sugar and acetone. The first symptoms of diabetic acidosis usually come on gradually, over a period of hours or days, and include a drowsy feeling, flushed face, thirst, and loss of appetite. Heavy breathing and a rapid pulse are more severe symptoms. It is important that you notify your doctor immediately, because diabetic coma (unconsciousness) can follow.

Allergy to Insulin: Patients occasionally experience redness, swelling, and itching at the site of injection of insulin. This condition, called local allergy, usually clears up in a few days to a few weeks. If you have local reactions, contact your physician, who may recommended a change in the type or species source of insulin.

Less common, but potentially more serious, is generalized allergy to insulin, which may cause rash over the whole body, shortness of breath, wheezing, reduction in blood pressure, fast pulse, or sweating. Severe cases of generalized allergy may be life-threatening. If you think you are having a generalized allergic reaction to insulin, notify a physician immediately. Your doctor may recommend skin testing, injecting small doses of other insulins into the skin, in order to select the best insulin for you to use. Patients who have had severe generalized allergic reactions to insulin should be skin tested with each new preparation to be used before starting treatment with that preparation.

Important Notes: 1. Never change from the insulin that has been prescribed for you to another insulin without instructions from your doctor. Changing the type, strength, species, or manufacturer of insulin can cause problems with your diabetes.

2. Your doctor will tell you what to do if you miss a dose of insulin or miss a meal because of illness. Always keep an extra supply of insulin, as well as a spare syringe and needle, on hand. If you miss a meal, use a substitute of sugar, sugar-sweetened candy, fruit juice, or sugar-sweetened beverage according to your doctor's instructions.

3. If you become ill from any cause, especially with nausea and vomiting, your insulin requirements may change. Test your urine and/or blood and notify your doctor at once.

4. Consult your doctor if you notice anything unusual or have doubts about your condition or your use of insulin.

5. Always wear diabetic identification so that appropriate treatment can be given if complications occur away from home.

6. Understand how to manage your diabetes so that your life can be active and healthy.

[031584]

ILETIN® (INSULIN, LILLY)—
[ī' lĕ-tĭn]
REGULAR AND MODIFIED INSULIN PRODUCTS

All of the insulins listed below are prepared from a mixture of insulin crystals extracted from beef and pork pancreas, except for Regular (Concentrated) Iletin® II (purified pork insulin injection, Lilly), U-500, which is prepared from pork insulin only. Regular Iletin® II (purified insulin injection, Lilly), Lente® Iletin® II (purified insulin zinc suspension, Lilly), NPH Iletin® II (isophane purified insulin suspension, Lilly), and Protamine, Zinc & Iletin® II (protamine zinc purified insulin suspension, Lilly) made solely from beef or pork source are available on special order in U-100 strength only. When insulin is prepared from a single animal source, the species is indicated on the vial label and on the package.

REGULAR ILETIN® I
[rĕg' ū-lĕr ī' lĕ-tĭn wŭn]
(Beef-Pork)
(insulin injection)
USP

INFORMATION FOR THE PATIENT
WARNINGS:
ANY CHANGE OF INSULIN SHOULD BE MADE CAUTIOUSLY AND ONLY UNDER MEDICAL SUPERVISION. CHANGES IN REFINEMENT, PURITY, STRENGTH (U-40, U-100), BRAND (MANUFACTURER), TYPE (LENTE®, NPH, REGULAR, ETC.), AND SPECIES SOURCE (BEEF, PORK, BEEF-PORK, OR HUMAN) MAY RESULT IN THE NEED FOR A CHANGE IN DOSAGE.
SOME PATIENTS TAKING THIS BEEF-PORK INSULIN WILL REQUIRE SUCH A CHANGE IN DOSAGE. IF AN ADJUSTMENT IS NEEDED, IT MAY OCCUR WITH THE FIRST DOSE OR OVER A PERIOD OF SEVERAL WEEKS.

Insulin and Diabetes: Your doctor has explained that you have diabetes. You have learned that the treatment of your diabetes requires injections of insulin.

Insulin is a hormone produced by the pancreas, a large gland that lies near the stomach. This hormone is necessary for the body's correct use of food, especially sugar. Diabetes occurs when the pancreas does not make enough insulin to meet the body's needs.

To control your diabetes, your doctor has prescribed injections of insulin to keep your blood sugar at a nearly normal level and to keep your urine as free of sugar as possible. Each case of diabetes is different. Your doctor has told you which insulin to use, how much, and when and how often to inject it. This schedule has been individualized for you. Proper control of your diabetes requires close and constant cooperation with your doctor. In spite of diabetes, you can lead an active, healthy, and useful life if you eat a balanced diet daily, exercise regularly, and take your insulin injections exactly as prescribed by your doctor. You have been instructed to test your urine and/or blood regularly for sugar. If your urine tests consistently show the presence of sugar or your blood tests consistently show above-normal sugar levels, your diabetes is not properly controlled and you must let your doctor know.

Use the Proper Type of Insulin: This insulin, manufactured by Eli Lilly and Company, has the trademark Iletin® I (insulin, Lilly) and is available in various types—Regular, NPH, Protamine Zinc, Lente, Semilente®, and Ultralente®.

These types of insulin differ mainly in the time they require to take effect and in the length of time their action lasts. Your doctor has prescribed the type of insulin that he/she believes is best for you. **Do not use any other type of insulin except on his/her advice and direction.**

Regular Beef-Pork Insulin: Regular Iletin I, consisting of zinc-insulin crystals dissolved in a clear fluid, is obtained from beef and pork pancreas. Regular beef-pork insulin is "unmodified" (that is, nothing has been added to change the speed or length of its action). It takes effect rapidly and has a relatively short duration of activity (six to eight hours) as compared with other insulins.

Regular beef-pork insulin should be clear and colorless. Do not use it if it is cloudy, unusually viscous, precipitated, or even slightly colored.

Storage: Insulin should be stored in a cold place, preferably in a refrigerator, but not in the freezing compartment. Do not let it freeze or leave it in direct sunlight. If refrigeration is not possible, the bottle of insulin which you are currently using can be kept unrefrigerated as long as it is kept as cool as possible and away from heat and sunlight. Do not use a bottle of insulin after the expiration date stamped on the label.

Use the Correct Syringe: Doses of insulin are measured in **units**. The number of units in each cubic centimeter (cc) is clearly stated on the package. Two strengths are available for each type of insulin: U-40 (40 units per cc) and U-100 (100 units per cc). It is important that you understand the markings on your syringe, because the volume of insulin you inject depends on the strength, that is, the number of units per cc. For this reason, you should always use a syringe marked for the strength of insulin you are injecting. Failure to use the proper syringe can lead to a mistake in dosage, and you may receive too little or too much insulin. This can cause serious problems for you, ranging from a blood sugar that is too low or too high to coma (unconsciousness) or, rarely, death.
IMPORTANT: TO HELP AVOID CONTAMINATION AND POSSIBLE INFECTION, FOLLOW THESE INSTRUCTIONS EXACTLY.

Disposable Syringes: Disposable syringes and needles require no sterilization; they should be used only once and then discarded.

Sterilizing and Assembling Reusable Syringes: Your reusable syringe and needle must be sterilized before each injection—**follow the package directions supplied with your syringe.** Boiling, as described below, is the best method of sterilizing.

1. Put syringe, plunger, and needle in strainer, place in saucepan, and cover with water. Boil for five minutes.
2. Remove articles from water. When they have cooled, insert plunger into barrel, and fasten needle to syringe with a slight twist.
3. Push plunger in and out several times until water is completely removed. (If the syringe, plunger, and needle cannot be boiled, as when you are traveling, they may be sterilized by immersion for at least five minutes in Isopropyl Alcohol, 91%. Do not use bathing, rubbing, or medicated alcohol for this sterilization. If the syringe is sterilized with alcohol, it must be absolutely dry before use.)

Preparing the Dose:
1. Wash your hands.
2. Flip off the colored protective cap on the bottle, but **do not** remove rubber stopper.
3. Wipe top of bottle with alcohol swab.
4. Draw air into the syringe by pulling back on the plunger. The amount of air should be equal to your insulin dose.
5. Remove the needle cover. Put the needle through rubber top of insulin bottle.
6. Push plunger in. The air injected into the bottle will allow insulin to be easily withdrawn into syringe.
7. Turn bottle and syringe upside down in one hand. Be sure tip of needle is in insulin. Your other hand will be free to move the plunger. Draw back on plunger slowly to draw the correct dose of insulin into syringe.
8. Check for air bubbles. The air is harmless, but too large an air bubble will reduce the insulin dose. To remove air bubbles, push insulin back into the bottle and measure your correct dose of insulin.
9. Double check your dose. Remove needle from bottle. Cover needle with guard or lay syringe down so that needle does not touch anything.

Injecting the Dose:
1. Clean the skin where the injection is to be made.
2. With one hand, stabilize the skin by spreading it or pinching up a large area of skin.
3. Pick up syringe with other hand, and hold it as you would a pencil. Insert needle straight into the skin (90° angle). After the needle is in, pull back the plunger very slightly. If blood comes into the syringe, the needle has entered a blood vessel. Remove the needle and put it in at another location. If blood does not appear in the syringe, push the plunger in slowly as far as it will go.
4. To inject the insulin, push plunger all the way down, using less than five seconds to inject the dose.

5. Hold alcohol swab near the needle and pull needle straight out of skin. Press alcohol swab over injection site for several seconds.
6. Use disposable syringe only once to insure sterility of syringe and needle and accuracy of dose. Destroy syringes as directed.
7. To avoid tissue damage, always change the site for each injection.

Warnings—See Additional Warnings Above: Patients who have been directed by their physicians to mix two types of insulin should be aware that insulin hypodermic syringes of different manufacturers may vary in the amount of space between the bottom line and the needle.
Because of this, do not change:
1. The order of mixing that the physician has prescribed or
2. The model and brand of syringe or needle without first consulting your physician.

The mixing should be done immediately prior to injection. Failure to heed this warning could result in a dosage error.

Usage in Pregnancy: Pregnancy may make managing your diabetes more difficult. If you are pregnant or nursing a baby, consult your physician, pharmacist, or nurse-educator when using this product.

Insulin Reaction and Shock: Insulin reaction (too little sugar in the blood, also called "hypoglycemia") can be brought about by:
1. Taking too much insulin
2. Missing or delaying meals
3. Exercising or working too hard just before a meal
4. An infection or illness (especially with diarrhea or vomiting)
5. A change in the body's need for insulin

The first symptoms of insulin reaction usually come on suddenly and may include fatigue, nervousness or "shakiness," headache, rapid heartbeat, nausea, and a cold sweat. Eating sugar or a sugar-sweetened product will often correct the condition and prevent more serious symptoms. If the reaction becomes more severe, breathing will be shallow and the skin pale. Contact your doctor at once if you develop any of these symptoms.

Diabetic Acidosis and Coma: Diabetic acidosis may develop if your body has too little insulin. (This is the opposite of insulin reaction, which is the result of too much insulin in the blood.) Diabetic acidosis may be brought on if you omit your insulin or take less than the doctor has prescribed, eat significantly more than your diet calls for, or develop a fever or infection. With acidosis, urine tests show a large amount of sugar and acetone. The first symptoms of diabetic acidosis usually come on gradually, over a period of hours or days, and include a drowsy feeling, flushed face, thirst, and loss of appetite. Heavy breathing and a rapid pulse are more severe symptoms. It is important that you notify your doctor immediately, because diabetic coma (unconsciousness) can follow.

Allergy to Insulin: Patients occasionally experience redness, swelling, and itching at the site of injection of insulin. This condition, called local allergy, usually clears up in a few days to a few weeks. If you have local reactions, contact your physician, who may recommend a change in the type or species source of insulin.

Less common, but potentially more serious, is generalized allergy to insulin, which may cause rash over the whole body, shortness of breath, wheezing, reduction in blood pressure, fast pulse, or sweating. Severe cases of generalized allergy may be life-threatening. If you think you are having a generalized allergic reaction to insulin, notify a physician immediately. Your doctor may recommend skin testing, injecting small doses of other insulins into the skin, in order to select the best insulin for you to use. Patients who have had severe generalized allergic reactions to insulin should be skin tested with each new preparation to be used before starting treatment with that preparation.

Important Notes:
1. Never change from the insulin that has been prescribed by you to another insulin without instructions from your doctor. Changing the type, strength, species, or manufacturer of insulin can cause problems with your diabetes.
2. Your doctor will tell you what to do if you miss a dose of insulin or miss a meal because of illness. Always keep an extra supply of insulin, as well as spare syringe and needle, on hand. If you miss a meal, use a substitute of sugar, sugar-sweetened candy, fruit juice, or sugar-sweetened beverage according to your doctor's instructions.
3. If you become ill from any cause, especially with nausea and vomiting, your insulin requirement may change. Test your urine and/or blood and notify your doctor at once.
4. Consult your doctor if you notice anything unusual or have doubts about your condition or your use of insulin.
5. Always wear diabetic identification so that appropriate treatment can be given if complications occur away from home.
6. Understand how to manage your diabetes so that your life can be active and healthy.

How Supplied: *Regular Iletin ® I (Insulin Injection, USP) (Beef-Pork)* is supplied in rubber-stoppered vials as follows:
CP-240, U-40, 40 units/cc, 10 cc (400 units) (NDC 0002-8240-01).
CP-210, U-100, 100 units/cc, 10 cc (1000 units) (NDC 0002-8210-01). The above products are supplied 10 per carton. *Refrigerate. Avoid freezing.*
[031584]

REGULAR (CONCENTRATED) ℞
ILETIN® II, U-500
[rĕg-ū-lĕr ī′ lĕ-tĭn]
(purified pork insulin injection)

WARNINGS: ANY CHANGE OF INSULIN SHOULD BE MADE CAUTIOUSLY AND ONLY UNDER MEDICAL SUPERVISION. CHANGES IN PURITY, STRENGTH (U-40, U-100), BRAND (MANUFACTURER), TYPE (LENTE®, NPH, REGULAR, ETC.), AND/OR SPECIES SOURCE (BEEF, PORK, BEEF-PORK, OR HUMAN) MAY RESULT IN THE NEED FOR A CHANGE IN DOSAGE. SEE BELOW.
IT IS NOT POSSIBLE TO IDENTIFY WHICH PATIENTS WILL REQUIRE A REDUCTION IN DOSE TO AVOID HYPOGLYCEMIA WHEN USING THIS INSULIN. HOWEVER, IT IS KNOWN THAT A SMALL NUMBER OF PATIENTS MAY REQUIRE A SIGNIFICANT CHANGE.
ADJUSTMENT MAY BE NEEDED WITH THE FIRST DOSE OR OCCUR OVER A PERIOD OF SEVERAL WEEKS. BE AWARE OF THE POSSIBILITY OF SYMPTOMS OF EITHER HYPOGLYCEMIA OR HYPERGLYCEMIA. (SEE SECTIONS ENTITLED INSULIN REACTION AND SHOCK and DIABETIC ACIDOSIS AND COMA .)
This insulin is prepared from pork pancreas only. The dose of pork insulin for patients with insulin resistance due to antibodies to beef insulin may be only a fraction of that of beef insulin.
This insulin preparation contains 500 units of insulin in each milliliter. Extreme caution must be observed in the measurement of dosage because inadvertent overdose may result in irreversible insulin shock. Serious consequences may result if it is used other than under constant medical supervision.
Description: This Lilly pork insulin product differs from previous pork insulin preparations because it has undergone additional steps of chromatographic purification.
Regular (Concentrated) Iletin® II (purified pork insulin injection, Lilly), U-500, is an aqueous solution made from the antidiabetic principle of pork pancreas as stated on the label. Each milliliter contains 500 units of regular (unmodified) insulin and approximately 1.6 percent glycerin (w/v), with approximately 0.25 percent m-cresol (w/v) as a preservative. Sodium hydroxide and hydrochloric acid are added during manufacture to adjust the pH. All preparations of Iletin® II (purified pork insulin, Lilly) are made from zinc-insulin crystals. Adequate insulin dosage permits the diabetic patient to utilize carbohydrates and fats in a comparatively satisfactory manner. Regardless of concentration, the action of insulin is basically the same: to enable carbohydrate metabolism to occur and thus to prevent the production of ketone bodies by the liver. Although, under usual circumstances, diabetes can be controlled with doses in the vicinity of 40 to 60 units or less, an occasional patient develops such resistance or becomes so unresponsive to the effect of insulin that daily doses of several hundred, or even several thousand, units are required. Fortunately, there seems to be no condition of absolute resistance; all resistant patients will apparently respond to some dose, if it is large enough.
Occasionally, a cause of the insulin resistance can be found (such as hemochromatosis, cirrhosis of the liver, some complicating disease of the endocrine glands other than the pancreas, allergy, or infection), but in other cases, no cause of the high insulin requirement can be determined.
Iletin II, U-500, is unmodified by any agent that might prolong its action; however, clinical experience has shown that it frequently has a time action similar to a repository insulin preparation and that a single dose may show activity over a 24-hour period. This effect has been credited to the high concentration of the preparation.
Indications: Iletin® II (purified pork insulin injection, Lilly), U-500, is especially useful for the treatment of diabetic patients with marked insulin resistance (daily requirements more than 200 units), since a large dose may be administered subcutaneously in a reasonable volume.
Precautions: Every patient exhibiting insulin resistance who requires Iletin® II (purified pork insulin injection, Lilly), U-500, for the control of diabetes should be held under close observation until dosage is established. The response will vary among patients. Some can be controlled with a single dose daily; others may require two or three injections per day.
Most patients will show a "tolerance" to insulin, so that minor variations in dosage can occur without the development of untoward symptoms of insulin shock.
Insulin resistance is frequently self-limited; after several weeks or months during which high dosage is required, responsiveness to the pharmacologic effect of insulin may be regained and dosage can be reduced.
Insulin should be kept in a cold place, preferably in a refrigerator. Do not inject insulin that is not water-clear. Discoloration, turbidity, or unusual viscosity indicates deterioration or contamination. Use of a package of insulin should not be started after the expiration date stamped on it.
Adverse Reactions: As with other insulin preparations, hypoglycemic reactions may be associated with the administration of Iletin® II (purified pork insulin injection, Lilly), U-500. However, deep secondary hypoglycemic reactions may develop 18 to 24 hours after the original injection of Iletin II, U-500. Consequently, patients should be carefully observed, and prompt treatment of such reactions should be initiated with glucagon injections and/or with glucose by intravenous injection or gavage.
Allergic Reactions: Erythema, swelling, or pruritus may occur at injection sites. Such localized allergic manifestations usually resolve within a few days to a few weeks.
Less common, but potentially more serious, is systemic allergy to insulin, which may cause generalized urticaria, dyspnea, wheezing, which may, upon continued administration of the insulin, progress to anaphylaxis.
If a severe allergic reaction occurs, the drug should be discontinued and the patient treated with the usual agents (e.g., epinephrine, antihistamines, or corticosteroids).
Patients who have experienced severe systemic allergic symptoms should be skin tested with an-

Continued on next page

* Identi-Code® symbol.

Lilly—Cont.

other insulin preparation before its initiation. Desensitization procedures may permit resumption of insulin administration.

Dosage and Administration: Iletin® II (purified pork insulin injection, Lilly), U-500, can be administered by both the subcutaneous and the intramuscular routes. It is inadvisable to inject Iletin II, U-500, intravenously because of the possible development of allergic or anaphylactoid reactions.

It is recommended that a tuberculin type of syringe be utilized for the measurement of dosage. Variations in dosage are frequently possible in the insulin-resistant patient, since the individual is unresponsive to the pharmacologic effect of the insulin. Nevertheless, accuracy of measurement is to be encouraged because of the potential danger of the preparation.

How Supplied: (℞) *CP-2500, Regular (Concentrated) Iletin® II (purified pork insulin injection, Lilly), U-500,* 500 units/cc, 20 cc, rubber-stoppered vials (10,000 units) (10 per carton) (NDC 0002-8500-01). *Refrigerate. Avoid freezing.*

[120583]

LENTE® ILETIN® I
[lĕn-ta i′lĕ-tĭn]
(Beef-Pork)
(insulin zinc suspension)
USP

SEMILENTE® ILETIN® I
[sĕm′ĭ-lĕn′la ĭ′lĕ-tĭn]
(Beef-Pork)
(prompt insulin zinc suspension)
USP

ULTRALENTE® ILETIN® I
[ŭl′tra-lĕn′ta ĭ′lĕ-tĭn]
(Beef-Pork)
(extended insulin zinc suspension)
USP

INFORMATION FOR THE PATIENT

WARNINGS, Insulin and Diabetes, and Use of Proper Type of Insulin: *See under* Regular Iletin® I.

Lente Beef-Pork Insulin: Lente beef-pork insulin is obtained from beef and pork pancreas. Insulin has been combined with zinc to form small crystals. Lente beef-pork insulin has an intermediate time of activity. Its action starts more slowly than does that of regular beef-pork insulin and lasts somewhat longer (slightly over 24 hours).

Lente beef-pork insulin should look uniformly cloudy or milky. If the insulin substance (the cloudy material) settles at the bottom of the vial, the vial must be carefully rotated before the injection so that the contents are uniformly mixed (see instructions under Preparing the Dose). Do not use a vial of insulin if you see lumps that float or stick to the sides. Also, the insulin should not be used if it is clear and remains clear after the vial is rotated.

Semilente Beef-Pork Insulin: Semilente beef-pork insulin comes from beef and pork pancreas. Insulin has been combined with zinc to form small crystals. Semilente beef-pork insulin has a short period of activity. Its action starts nearly as rapidly as that of regular insulin and lasts slightly longer (approximately 12 to 16 hours). This type of insulin will shorten the action time of Lente insulin (an intermediate-acting form) when they are mixed. Semilente beef-pork insulin should look uniformly cloudy or milky. If the insulin substance (the cloudy material) settles at the bottom of the vial, the vial must be carefully rotated before the injection so that the contents are uniformly mixed (see instructions under Preparing the Dose). Do not use a vial of insulin if you see lumps that float or stick to the sides. Also, the insulin should not be used if it is clear and remains clear after the vial is rotated.

Ultralente Beef-Pork Insulin: Ultralente beef-pork insulin comes from beef and pork pancreas. Insulin has been combined with zinc to form small crystals. Ultralente beef-pork insulin takes effect very gradually and, in comparison with regular insulin, has a long period of activity (more than 36 hours). This type of insulin will lengthen the action time of Lente insulin (an intermediate-acting form) when they are mixed.

Ultralente beef-pork insulin should look uniformly cloudy or milky. If the insulin substance (the cloudy material) settles at the bottom of the vial, the vial must be carefully rotated before the injection so that the contents are uniformly mixed (see instructions under Preparing the Dose). Do not use a vial of insulin if you see lumps that float or stick to the sides. Also, the insulin should not be used if it is clear and remains clear after the vial is rotated.

Storage, Use the Correct Syringe, Disposable Syringes, and Sterilizing and Assembling Reusable Syringes: *See under* Regular Iletin® I.

Preparing the Dose:
1. Wash your hands.
2. Gently roll the insulin bottle several times to mix the insulin. Be sure it is completely mixed. Do not shake bottle. Flip off the colored protective cap on the bottle, but **do not** remove the rubber stopper. *See also under* Regular Iletin® I.

Injecting the Dose, Warnings, Usage in Pregnancy, Insulin Reaction and Shock, Diabetic Acidosis and Coma, Allergy to Insulin, and Important Notes: *See under* Regular Iletin® I.

How Supplied: *Lente® Iletin® I (Insulin Zinc Suspension, USP)* is supplied in rubber-stoppered vials as follows:

CP-440, U-40, 40 units/cc, 10 cc (400 units) (NDC 0002-8440-01).

CP-410, U-100, 100 units/cc, 10 cc (1000 units) (NDC 0002-8410-01).

Semilente® Iletin® I (Prompt Insulin Zinc Suspension, USP) is supplied in rubber-stoppered vials as follows:

CP-540, U-40, 40 units/cc, 10 cc (400 units) (NDC 0002-8540-01).

CP-510, U-100, 100 units/cc, 10 cc (1000 units) (NDC 0002-8510-01).

Ultralente® Iletin® I (Extended Insulin Zinc Suspension, USP) is supplied in rubber-stoppered vials as follows:

CP-640, U-40, 40 units/cc, 10 cc (400 units) (NDC 0002-8640-01).

CP-610, U-100, 100 units/cc, 10 cc (1000 units) (NDC 0002-8610-01).

The above products are supplied 10/carton. *Refrigerate. Avoid freezing.*

[031484]

NPH ILETIN® I
[ĕn′pē-āch ĭ′lĕ-tĭn]
(Beef-Pork)
(isophane insulin suspension)
USP

INFORMATION FOR THE PATIENT

WARNINGS, Insulin and Diabetes, and Use of Proper Type of Insulin: *See under* Regular Iletin® I.

NPH Beef-Pork Insulin: NPH beef-pork insulin is obtained from beef and pork pancreas. Insulin has been combined with protamine and zinc so that its action is similar to that of a mixture of Regular and Protamine Zinc insulins. The result is an intermediate-acting insulin with a slower speed of action than Regular insulin and a shorter time of activity than Protamine Zinc insulin. The effect of NPH beef-pork insulin lasts slightly more than 24 hours.

NPH beef-pork insulin should look uniformly cloudy or milky. If the insulin substance (the cloudy material) settles at the bottom of the vial, the vial must be carefully rotated before the injection so that the contents are uniformly mixed (see instructions under Preparing the Dose). Do not use a vial of insulin if you see lumps that float or stick to the sides. Also, the insulin should not be used if it is clear and remains clear after the vial is rotated.

Storage, Use the Correct Syringe, Disposable Syringes, and Sterilizing and Assembling Reusable Syringes: *See under* Regular Iletin® I.

Preparing the Dose: *See under* Lente® Iletin® I and Regular Iletin® I.

Injecting the Dose, Warnings, Usage in Pregnancy, Insulin Reaction and Shock, Diabetic Acidosis and Coma, Allergy to Insulin, and Important Notes: *See under* Regular Iletin® I.

How Supplied: *NPH Iletin® I (Isophane Insulin Suspension, USP)* is supplied in rubber-stoppered vials as follows:

CP-340, U-40, 40 units/cc, 10 cc (400 units) (NDC 0002-8340-01).

CP-310, U-100, 100 units/cc, 10 cc (1000 units) (NDC 0002-8310-01).

The above products are supplied 10/carton. *Refrigerate. Avoid freezing.*

[031484]

PROTAMINE, ZINC & ILETIN® I
[prō′ta-mēn zĭngk ănd ĭ′lĕ-tĭn]
(Beef-Pork)
(protamine zinc insulin suspension)
USP

INFORMATION FOR THE PATIENT

WARNINGS, Insulin and Diabetes, and Use of Proper Type of Insulin: *See under* Regular Iletin® I.

Protamine Zinc Beef-Pork Insulin: Protamine zinc beef-pork insulin is obtained from beef and pork pancreas. Protamine and zinc have been added to lengthen the time of action. Protamine zinc beef-pork insulin takes effect gradually and, in comparison with regular beef-pork insulin, has a long period of activity (well over 24 hours).

Protamine zinc beef-pork insulin should look uniformly cloudy or milky. If the insulin substance (the cloudy material) settles at the bottom of the vial, the vial must be carefully rotated before the injection so that the contents are uniformly mixed (see instructions under Preparing the Dose). Do not use a vial of insulin if you see lumps that float or stick to the sides. Also, the insulin should not be used if it is clear and remains clear after the vial is rotated.

Storage, Use the Correct Syringe, Disposable Syringes, and Sterilizing and Assembling Reusable Syringes: *See under* Regular Iletin® I.

Preparing the Dose: *See under* Lente® Iletin® I and Regular Iletin® I.

Injecting the Dose, Warnings, Usage in Pregnancy, Insulin Reaction and Shock, Diabetic Acidosis and Coma, Allergy to Insulin, and **Important Notes:** *See under* Regular Iletin® I.

How Supplied: *Protamine, Zinc & Iletin® I (Protamine Zinc Insulin Suspension, USP)* is supplied in rubber-stoppered vials as follows:

CP-140, U-40, 40 units/cc, 10 cc (400 units) (NDC 0002-8140-01).

CP-110, U-100, 100 units/cc, 10 cc (1000 units) (NDC 0002-8110-01).

The above products are supplied 10/carton. *Refrigerate. Avoid freezing.*

[031484]

IPECAC ℞
[ĭp′ĕ-kăk]
Syrup, USP

Description: Ipecac Syrup contains 7 g of ipecac/100 ml (32 grs/fl oz). Contains alcohol, 2 percent.

Ipecac syrup is an emetic for oral use.

Ipecac consists of the dried rhizome and roots of *Cephaelis ipecacuanha* (Brotero) A. Richard, known in commerce as Rio or Brazilian ipecac, or of *Cephaelis acuminata* Karsten, known in commerce as Cartagena, Nicaragua, or Panama ipecac (Fam. *Rubiaceae*). Ipecac yields not less than 2 percent of the ether-soluble alkaloids of ipecac. Ipecac contains *emetine* (methylcephaeline) [$C_{29}H_{40}N_2O_4$], *cephaeline*, [$C_{28}H_{38}N_2O_4$], *psychotrine* [$C_{28}H_{36}N_2O_4$], *emetamine* [$C_{29}H_{36}$-N_2O_4], *ipecamine*, also *ipecacuanhic acid*, pectin, starch, resin, sugar, etc. All of the alkaloids are interrelated and may be synthesized from one another. Brazilian roots yield as much as 2.5 percent of total alkaloids and Cartagena root, 2 percent.

Ipecac syrup is a clear amber hydroalcoholic syrup with a characteristic odor.

Clinical Pharmacology: Ipecac alkaloids act both locally on the gastric mucosa and centrally on the chemoreceptor trigger zone to induce vomiting. An adequate dose causes vomiting within 30 minutes in more than 90 percent of patients; the average time is usually less than 20 minutes. The emetic action is increased if 200 to 300 ml of water are taken immediately after administration of the syrup. In young and frightened children, giving water prior to the ipecac syrup may be more successful.

It should be recognized that an episode of vomiting does not necessarily completely empty the stomach.

Indications and Usage: Ipecac syrup is useful as an emetic (inducing vomiting) for emergency use in the treatment of drug overdosage and in certain cases of poisoning.

Contraindications: This drug should not be given to unconscious patients. It should not be used if strychnine, corrosives such as alkalies (lye) and strong acids, or petroleum distillates such as kerosene, gasoline, coal oil, fuel oil, paint thinner, or cleaning fluid have been ingested. (Some authorities consider emesis with ipecac syrup to be appropriate in certain instances of hydrocarbon ingestion.)

Warnings: IPECAC SYRUP SHOULD NOT BE CONFUSED WITH IPECAC FLUID EXTRACT, WHICH IS 14 TIMES STRONGER AND HAS CAUSED SOME DEATHS.

If ipecac syrup is not vomited, the alkaloid emetine may be absorbed; this has been associated with cardiotoxic effects in the long-term treatment of amebiasis.

Precautions:
Note to the Pharmacist:
The Food and Drug Administration has determined that, in the interest of public health, ipecac syrup should be available for sale without prescription provided it is packaged in a quantity of 1 fl oz (30 ml) and, in addition to other required labeling, containing the following:

1. A statement, conspicuously boxed and in red letters, to the effect: "For emergency use to cause vomiting in poisoning. Before using, call physician, the Poison Control Center, or hospital emergency room immediately for advice."
2. A warning to the effect: "Warning—Keep out of reach of children. Do not use in unconscious persons. Ordinarily, this drug should not be used if strychnine, corrosives such as alkalies (lye) and strong acids, or petroleum distillates such as kerosene, gasoline, coal oil, fuel oil, paint thinner, or cleaning fluid have been ingested."
3. Usual dosage: 1 tablespoonful (15 ml) in persons over one year of age.

Information for Patients—See Precautions.
Drug Interactions—Activated charcoal should not be given with ipecac syrup, because the charcoal adsorbs the ipecac and nullifies its emetic effect; however, it may be given after vomiting has occurred.

Usage in Pregnancy—Pregnancy Category C—Animal reproduction studies have not been conducted with ipecac syrup. It is not known whether the drug can cause harm when administered to a pregnant woman or can affect reproductive capacity. Minimal systemic absorption would be expected when ipecac syrup is used as directed (see Dosage and Administration). (The alkaloid emetine, obtained from ipecac, is used by injection for systemic treatment of disease, e.g., amebiasis. This use of emetine may be associated with significant toxicity and is not recommended in pregnancy.)

Nursing Mothers—It is not known whether the alkaloids of ipecac are excreted in human milk. Caution should be exercised if ipecac syrup is used for treatment of a nursing woman. (The alkaloid emetine, when used for treatment of systemic disease, is detoxicated and excreted from the body very slowly, over a period of several weeks.)

Adverse Reactions: When ipecac syrup does not cause emesis, absorption of the alkaloid emetine may occur. (In the treatment of amebiasis, emetine may cause heart conduction disturbances, atrial fibrillation, or fatal myocarditis.)

Overdosage: See **Warnings.**
Dosage and Administration: Children less than one year of age, 1 to 2 teaspoonfuls; children over one year of age and adults, 3 teaspoonfuls.

If vomiting does not occur within 20 minutes, a similar dose is repeated once. Then, if the patient does not vomit within 30 minutes, the dosage should be recovered (lavage).

How Supplied: (B) *Syrup No. 37, Ipecac, USP,* in 16-fl-oz bottles (NDC 0002-2520-05).

[041382]

ISOPROTERENOL HYDROCHLORIDE INHALATION,
[ī′ sō-prō-těr-ē′ nōl]

see Aerolone® Solution.

KEFLIN® B
[kĕf′ lĭn]
(cephalothin sodium)
For Injection, USP
Neutral

Description: Keflin® (cephalothin sodium, Lilly), Neutral, is a semisynthetic cephalosporin antibiotic for parenteral use. It is the sodium salt of 7-(thiophene-2-acetamido) cephalosporanic acid. Sodium bicarbonate has been added to result in reconstituted solutions having a pH ranging between 6 and 8.5. The total sodium content is approximately 63 mg (2.8 mEq sodium ion) per g of Keflin.

Cephalothin was synthesized in the Lilly Research Laboratories by the reaction of thiophene-2-acetic acid with 7-aminocephalosporanic acid. The cephalosporanic acid nucleus is obtained from cephalosporin C, which is produced by the fungus *Cephalosporium*. Cephalothin is supplied as the sodium salt of 7-(thiophene-2-acetamido) cephalosporanic acid.

Cephalothin is a cream-colored crystalline solid which is stable in the dry state and moderately soluble in distilled water (250 to 300 mg/ml).

Keflin, Neutral, contains 30 mg of sodium bicarbonate/g of cephalothin sodium. Free cephalothin acid does not form within this range, and the solubility and freezability are thereby enhanced.

The molecular weight of cephalothin sodium is 418.4.

Clinical Pharmacology: *Human Pharmacology*—Keflin® (cephalothin sodium, Lilly) is a broad-spectrum antibiotic for parenteral administration. After administration of a 500-mg dose intramuscularly to normal volunteers, the average peak serum antibiotic level was 10 mcg/ml at one-half hour; with a 1-g dose, the average was about 20 mcg/ml. Following a single 1-g intravenous dose of Keflin, blood levels have been about 30 mcg/ml at 15 minutes, have ranged from 3 to 12 mcg at one hour, and have declined to about 1 mcg at four hours. With continuous infusion, at the rate of 500 mg/hour, levels have been from 14 to 20 mcg/ml of serum. Dosages of 2 g given intravenously over a 30-minute period have produced serum concentrations of 80 to 100 mcg/ml one-half hour after the infusion; levels ranged from 10 to 40 mcg/ml at one hour and from 3 to 6 mcg/ml at two hours and were not assayable after five hours.

Sixty to 70 percent of an intramuscular dose is excreted by the kidneys in the first six hours; this results in high urine levels, e.g., 800 mcg/ml of urine after a 500-mg dose and 2500 mcg/ml following 1 g. Probenecid slows tubular excretion and almost doubles peak blood levels.

Spinal-fluid levels have ranged from 0.4 to 1.4 mcg/ml in a child and from 0.15 to 5 mcg/ml in adults with meningeal inflammatory states. The antibiotic passes readily into other body fluids, e.g., pleural, joint, and ascitic fluids. Studies of amniotic fluid and cord blood show prompt transfer of Keflin across the placenta.

Following single 1-g intramuscular doses of cephalothin, peak maternal levels were reached between 31 and 45 minutes after injection; the peak levels in the infants occurred about 15 minutes later. All plasma levels in the infants were far below those of the mothers.

Secondary aqueous-humor levels have averaged 0.5 mcg/ml 30 minutes after a single 1-g intravenous dose. The antibiotic has been detected in bile.

Microbiology—The in vitro bactericidal action of cephalothin results from inhibition of cell-wall synthesis.

Keflin is usually active against the following organisms in vitro:

Beta-hemolytic and other streptococci (many strains of enterococci, e.g., *Streptococcus faecalis*, are relatively resistant)

Staphylococci, including coagulase-positive, coagulase-negative, and penicillinase-producing strains

S. (Diplococcus) pneumoniae
Haemophilus influenzae
Escherichia coli and other coliform bacteria
Klebsiella
Proteus mirabilis
Salmonella sp.
Shigella sp.

Pseudomonas organisms are resistant to Keflin, as are most indole-producing *Proteus* species and motile *Enterobacter* species.

Susceptibility Plate Tests—If the Bauer-Kirby-Sherris-Turck method of disc susceptibility testing is used (*Am. J. Clin. Pathol., 45:* 493, 1966; *Federal Register, 39:* 19182-19184, 1974), a disc containing 30 mcg cephalothin should give a zone of over 17 mm when tested against a cephalothin-susceptible bacterial strain and a zone of over 14 mm with an organism of intermediate susceptibility.

Indications and Usage: Keflin® (cephalothin sodium, Lilly) is indicated for the treatment of serious infections caused by susceptible strains of the designated microorganisms in the diseases listed below. Culture and susceptibility studies should be performed. Therapy may be instituted before results of susceptibility studies are obtained.

Respiratory tract infections caused by *S. pneumoniae*, staphylococci (penicillinase and non-penicillinase-producing), group A beta-hemolytic streptococci, *Klebsiella*, and *H. influenzae*

Skin and soft-tissue infections, including peritonitis, caused by staphylococci (penicillinase and non-penicillinase-producing), group A beta-hemolytic streptococci, *E. coli, P. mirabilis,* and *Klebsiella*

Genitourinary tract infections caused by *E. coli, P. mirabilis,* and *Klebsiella*

Septicemia, including endocarditis, caused by *S. pneumoniae*, staphylococci (penicillinase and non-penicillinase-producing), group A beta-hemolytic streptococci, *S. viridans, E. coli, P. mirabilis,* and *Klebsiella*

Gastrointestinal infections caused by *Salmonella* and *Shigella* species

Meningitis caused by *S. pneumoniae*, group A beta-hemolytic streptococci, and staphylococci (penicillinase and non-penicillinase-producing)

NOTE: Inasmuch as only low levels of Keflin are found in the cerebrospinal fluid, the drug is not reliable in the treatment of meningitis and cannot be recommended for that purpose. Keflin has, however, proved to be effective in a number of cases of meningitis and may be considered for unusual circumstances in which other, more reliably effective antibiotics cannot be used.

Bone and joint infections caused by staphylococci (penicillinase and non-penicillinase-producing)

The prophylactic administration of Keflin preoperatively, intraoperatively, and postoperatively may reduce the incidence of certain postoperative infections in patients undergoing surgical proce-

Continued on next page

* Identi-Code® symbol.

Lilly—Cont.

dures (e.g., vaginal hysterectomy) that are classified as contaminated or potentially contaminated. The perioperative use of Keflin also may be effective in surgical patients in whom infection at the operative site would present a serious risk, e.g., during open-heart surgery and prosthetic arthroplasty.

The prophylactic administration of Keflin should be discontinued within a 24-hour period after the surgical procedure. If there are signs of infection, specimens for culture should be obtained for the identification of the causative organism so that appropriate therapy may be instituted. (*See* Dosage and Administration.)

NOTE: If the susceptibility tests show that the causative organism is resistant to Keflin, other appropriate antibiotic therapy should be instituted.

Contraindication: Keflin® (cephalothin sodium, Lilly) is contraindicated in persons who have shown hypersensitivity to cephalosporin antibiotics.

Warnings: BEFORE CEPHALOTHIN THERAPY IS INSTITUTED, CAREFUL INQUIRY SHOULD BE MADE CONCERNING PREVIOUS HYPERSENSITIVITY REACTIONS TO CEPHALOSPORINS AND PENICILLIN. CEPHALOSPORIN C DERIVATIVES SHOULD BE GIVEN CAUTIOUSLY TO PENICILLIN-SENSITIVE PATIENTS.

SERIOUS ACUTE HYPERSENSITIVITY REACTIONS MAY REQUIRE EPINEPHRINE AND OTHER EMERGENCY MEASURES.

There is some clinical and laboratory evidence of partial cross-allergenicity of the penicillins and the cephalosporins. Patients have been reported to have had severe reactions (including anaphylaxis) to both drugs.

Any patient who has demonstrated some form of allergy, particularly to drugs, should receive antibiotics cautiously and then only when absolutely necessary. No exception should be made with regard to Keflin® (cephalothin sodium, Lilly).

Pseudomembranous colitis has been reported with virtually all broad-spectrum antibiotics (including macrolides, semisynthetic penicillins, and cephalosporins); therefore, it is important to consider its diagnosis in patients who develop diarrhea in association with the use of antibiotics. Such colitis may range in severity from mild to life-threatening. Treatment with broad-spectrum antibiotics alters the normal flora of the colon and may permit overgrowth of clostridia. Studies indicate that a toxin produced by *Clostridium difficile* is one primary cause of antibiotic-associated colitis.

Mild cases of pseudomembranous colitis usually respond to drug discontinuance alone. In moderate to severe cases, management should include sigmoidoscopy, appropriate bacteriologic studies, and fluid, electrolyte, and protein supplementation. When the colitis does not improve after the drug has been discontinued, or when it is severe, oral vancomycin is the drug of choice for antibiotic-associated pseudomembranous colitis produced by *C. difficile*. Other causes of colitis should be ruled out.

Precautions: *General Precautions*—Patients should be followed carefully so that any side effects or unusual manifestations of drug idiosyncrasy may be detected. If an allergic reaction to Keflin® (cephalothin sodium, Lilly) occurs, the drug should be discontinued and the patient treated with the usual agents (e.g., epinephrine or other pressor amines, antihistamines, or corticosteroids).

Although Keflin rarely produces alteration in kidney function, evaluation of renal status is recommended, especially in seriously ill patients receiving maximum doses. Patients with impaired renal function should be placed on the dosage schedule recommended under Dosage and Administration. Usual doses in such individuals may result in excessive serum concentrations.

When intravenous doses of cephalothin larger than 6 g daily are given by infusion for periods longer than three days, they may be associated with thrombophlebitis, and the veins may have to be alternated. The addition of 10 to 25 mg of hydrocortisone to intravenous solutions containing 4 to 6 g of cephalothin may reduce the incidence of thrombophlebitis. The use of small IV needles in the larger available veins may be preferred.

Prolonged use of Keflin may result in the overgrowth of nonsusceptible organisms. Constant observation of the patient is essential. If superinfection occurs during therapy, appropriate measures should be taken.

A false-positive reaction for glucose in the urine may occur with Benedict's or Fehling's solution or with Clinitest® tablets but not with Tes-Tape® (Glucose Enzymatic Test Strip, USP, Lilly).

An increased incidence of nephrotoxicity has been reported following concomitant administration of cephalosporins and aminoglycoside antibiotics.

Broad-spectrum antibiotics should be prescribed with caution in individuals with a history of gastrointestinal disease, particularly colitis.

*Usage in Pregnancy—Pregnancy Category B—*Reproduction studies have been performed in rabbits given doses of 200 mg/kg and have revealed no evidence of impaired fertility or harm to the fetus due to Keflin. There are, however, no adequate and well-controlled studies in pregnant women. Because animal reproduction studies are not always predictive of human response, this drug should be used during pregnancy only if clearly needed.

*Nursing Mothers—*Caution should be exercised when Keflin is administered to a nursing woman.

Adverse Reactions: *Hypersensitivity—*Maculopapular rash, urticaria, reactions resembling serum sickness, and anaphylaxis have been reported. Eosinophilia and drug fever have been observed to be associated with other allergic reactions. These reactions are most likely to occur in patients with a history of allergy, particularly to penicillin.

*Blood—*Neutropenia, thrombocytopenia, and hemolytic anemia have been reported. Some individuals, particularly those with azotemia, have developed positive direct Coombs' tests during cephalothin therapy.

*Liver—*Transient rise in SGOT and alkaline phosphatase has been noted.

*Kidney—*Rise in BUN and decreased creatinine clearance have been reported, particularly in patients with prior renal impairment. The role of Keflin® (cephalothin sodium, Lilly) in renal changes is difficult to assess, because other factors predisposing to prerenal azotemia or to acute renal failure usually have been present.

*Local Reactions—*Pain, induration, tenderness, and elevation of temperature have been reported following repeated intramuscular injections. Thrombophlebitis has occurred and is usually associated with daily doses of more than 6 g given by infusion for longer than three days.

*Gastrointestinal—*Symptoms of pseudomembranous colitis may appear either during or after antibiotic treatment. Nausea and vomiting have been reported rarely.

Dosage and Administration: *In adults,* the usual dosage range is 500 mg to 1 g of cephalothin every four to six hours. A dosage of 500 mg every six hours is adequate in uncomplicated pneumonia, furunculosis with cellulitis, and most urinary tract infections. In severe infections, this may be increased by giving the injections every four hours or, when the desired response is not obtained, by raising the dose to 1 g. In life-threatening infections, doses up to 2 g every four hours may be required.

For perioperative prophylactic use to prevent postoperative infection in contaminated or potentially contaminated surgery in adults, the following doses are recommended:

(a) 1 to 2 g administered IV just prior to surgery (approximately one-half to one hour before the initial incision);
(b) 1 to 2 g during surgery (administration modified according to the duration of the operative procedure); and
(c) 1 to 2 g every six hours postoperatively for 24 hours.

In children, 20 to 30 mg/kg may be given at the times designated above.

Since Keflin has a serum half-life of 30 to 50 minutes, it is important that (1) the preoperative dose be given just prior to the start of surgery so that adequate antibiotic levels are present in the serum and tissues at the time of initial surgical incision; and (2) Keflin be administered, if necessary, at appropriate intervals during surgery to provide sufficient levels of the antibiotic at the anticipated moments of greatest exposure to infective organisms.

When renal function is reduced, an intravenous loading dose of 1 to 2 g may be given. Continued dosage schedule should be determined by degree of renal impairment, severity of infection, and susceptibility of the causative organism. The maximum doses administered should be based on the following recommendations.

DOSAGE OF KEFLIN® (CEPHALOTHIN SODIUM, LILLY) WHEN RENAL FUNCTION IS IMPAIRED

STATUS OF RENAL FUNCTION	MAXIMUM ADULT DOSAGE (Maintenance)
Mild Impairment (C_{cr} = 80–50 ml/min)	2 g q. 6 h.
Moderate Impairment (C_{cr} = 50–25 ml/min)	1.5 g q. 6 h.
Severe Impairment (C_{cr} = 25–10 ml/min)	1 g q. 6 h.
Marked Impairment (C_{cr} = 10–2 ml/min)	0.5 g q. 6 h.
Essentially No Function (C_{cr} = < 2 ml/min)	0.5 g q. 8 h.

In infants and children, the dosage should be proportionately less in accordance with age, weight, and severity of infection. Daily administration of 100 mg/kg (80 to 160 mg/kg or 40 to 80 mg/lb) in divided doses has been found effective for most infections susceptible to Keflin® (cephalothin sodium, Lilly).

Antibiotic therapy in beta-hemolytic streptococcal infections should continue for at least ten days. In staphylococcal infections, surgical procedures, such as incision and drainage, should be carried out in all cases when indicated.

Keflin may be given intravenously or by deep intramuscular injection into a large muscle mass, such as the gluteus or lateral aspect of the thigh, to minimize pain and induration.

*Intramuscular—*Each g of cephalothin should be diluted with 4 ml of Sterile Water for Injection. If the vial contents do not completely dissolve, an additional small amount of diluent (e.g., 0.2 to 0.4 ml) may be added and the contents warmed slightly.

*Intravenous—*The intravenous route may be preferable for patients with bacteremia, septicemia, or other severe or life-threatening infections who may be poor risks because of lowered resistance resulting from such debilitating conditions as malnutrition, trauma, surgery, diabetes, heart failure, or malignancy, particularly if shock is present or impending. For these infections in patients with normal renal function, the intravenous dosage is 4 to 12 g of cephalothin daily. In conditions such as septicemia, 6 to 8 g/day may be given intravenously for several days at the beginning of therapy; then, depending on the clinical response and laboratory findings, the dosage may gradually be reduced.

For patients who are to receive cephalothin intravenously, it is convenient to use the 1 or 2-g 100-ml-size vial (*see* Precautions).

For intermittent intravenous administration, a solution containing 1 g cephalothin in 10 ml of diluent may be slowly injected directly into the vein over a period of three to five minutes or may be given through the tubing when the patient is receiving parenteral solutions.

Intermittent intravenous infusion with a Y-type administration set can also be accomplished while bulk intravenous solutions are being infused. However, during infusion of the solution containing Keflin® (cephalothin sodium, Lilly), it is desirable to discontinue the other solution. When this technique is employed, careful attention should be paid to the volume of the solution containing Keflin so that the calculated dose will be infused.

For continuous intravenous infusion, 1 or 2 g of cephalothin, diluted and well mixed with at least 10 ml of Sterile Water for Injection, may be added to an IV bottle containing one of the following intravenous solutions: Acetated Ringer's Injection, 5% Dextrose Injection, 5% Dextrose in Lactated Ringer's Injection, Ionosol® B in D5-W, Isolyte® M with 5% Dextrose, Lactated Ringer's Injection, Normosol®-M in D5-W, Plasma-Lyte® Injection, Plasma-Lyte®-M Injection in 5% Dextrose, Ringer's Injection, or 0.9% Sodium Chloride Injection. The choice of solution and the volume to be employed are dictated by fluid and electrolyte management.

Intraperitoneal—In peritoneal dialysis procedures, cephalothin has been added to dialysis fluid in concentrations up to 6 mg/100 ml and instilled into the peritoneal space throughout an entire dialysis (16 to 30 hours). Careful assay procedures have shown that 44 percent of the administered drug was absorbed into the bloodstream. Serum levels of 10 mcg/ml were reported, with no evidence of accumulation and no untoward local or systemic reactions.

The intraperitoneal administration of solutions containing 0.1 to 4 percent Keflin in saline has been used in treating patients with peritonitis or contaminated peritoneal cavities. (The total daily dosage of Keflin should take into account the amount given by the intraperitoneal route.)

Stability: While stored under *refrigeration*, the solution has a satisfactory potency for 96 hours after reconstitution. Solutions may precipitate; they can be redissolved by being warmed to room temperature with constant agitation. Kept at *room temperature*, solutions for intramuscular injection should be given within 12 hours after being mixed. Intravenous infusions should be started within 12 hours and completed within 24 hours. For prolonged infusions, replace with a freshly prepared solution at least every 24 hours.

The concentrated solution will darken, especially at room temperature. Slight discoloration of the solution is permissible.

Solutions of Keflin® (cephalothin sodium, Lilly) in Sterile Water for Injection, 5% Dextrose Injection, or 0.9% Sodium Chloride Injection that are frozen immediately after reconstitution in the original container are stable for as long as 12 weeks when stored at −20°C. **If the product is warmed, care should be taken to avoid heating it after the thawing is complete. Once thawed, the solution should not be refrozen.**

How Supplied: (℞) *Vials Keflin® (Cephalothin Sodium for Injection, USP), Neutral*, rubber-stoppered (Dry Powder): *No. 7001*, 1 g (equivalent to cephalothin), 10-ml size, in singles (NDC 0002-7001-01) (10/carton) and Traypak™ (multivial carton, Lilly) of 25 (NDC 0002-7001-25); *No. 7000*, 1 g (equivalent to cephalothin), 100-ml size (NDC 0002-7000-10). *No. 7003*, 2 g (equivalent to cephalothin), 20-ml size (NDC 0002-7003-10); *No. 7002*, 2 g (equivalent to cephalothin), 100-ml size (NDC 0002-7002-10), and *No. 7004*, 4 g (equivalent to cephalothin), 50-ml size (NDC 0002-7004-10), in Traypak of 10; *No. 7020*, 20 g (equivalent to cephalothin), 200-ml size, in Traypak of 6 (NDC 0002-7020-16). *Faspak™ (flexible plastic bag, Lilly) No. 7190*, 1 g (equivalent to cephalothin), in Faspak of 96 (NDC 0002-7190-74); *No. 7191*, 2 g, in Faspak of 96 (NDC 0002-7191-74). [052184]

No. 7001, 1 g—1's—6505-00-000-0072

KEFZOL® ℞
[kĕf'zōl]
(cefazolin sodium)
Sterile, USP

Description: Kefzol® (cefazolin sodium, Lilly) is a semisynthetic cephalosporin for parenteral administration. It is the sodium salt of 3- [[(5-methyl-1,3,4-thiadiazol-2-yl) -thio]methyl]-7-[2-(1H-tetrazol-1-yl) acetamido] -3- cephem- 4-carboxylic acid. The sodium content is 48.3 mg/g of cefazolin sodium. In addition to cefazolin sodium, the Faspak™ (flexible plastic bag, Lilly) also contains 0.04% polysorbate 80.

The molecular formula is $C_{14}H_{14}N_8O_4S_3$ (sodium salt). The molecular weight is 476.5.

The dry crystalline powder is stable for at least two years when stored at room temperature (25°C). After reconstitution, the solution should be stored in a refrigerator and used within 96 hours. If kept at room temperature, the solution should be used within 24 hours.

The pH of the reconstituted solution is between 4.5 and 6.

Clinical Pharmacology: *Microbiology*—In vitro tests demonstrate that the bactericidal action of cephalosporins results from inhibition of cell-wall synthesis. Kefzol® (cefazolin sodium, Lilly) is active against the following organisms in vitro:
  Staphylococcus aureus (penicillin-sensitive and penicillin-resistant)
  Group A beta-hemolytic streptococci and other strains of streptococci (many strains of enterococci are resistant)
  Streptococcus (Diplococcus) pneumoniae
  Escherichia coli
  Proteus mirabilis
  Klebsiella species
  Enterobacter aerogenes
  Haemophilus influenzae

Most strains of *E. cloacae* and indole-positive *Proteus* (*P. vulgaris, P. morganii, P. rettgeri*) are resistant. Methicillin-resistant staphylococci, *Serratia, Pseudomonas, Mima*, and *Herellea* species are almost uniformly resistant to cefazolin.

Human Pharmacology—Table 1 demonstrates the blood levels and duration of cefazolin following intramuscular administration.

TABLE 1. SERUM CONCENTRATIONS AFTER INTRAMUSCULAR ADMINISTRATION

Dose	½ hr	1 hr	2 hr	4 hr	6 hr	8 hr
250 mg	15.5	17	13	5.1	2.5	
500 mg	36.2	36.8	37.9	15.5	6.3	3
1 g*	60.1	63.8	54.3	29.3	13.2	7.1

*Average of two studies

Clinical pharmacology studies in patients hospitalized with infections indicate that cefazolin produces mean peak serum levels approximately equivalent to those seen in normal volunteers.

In a study (using normal volunteers) of constant intravenous infusion with dosages of 3.5 mg/kg for one hour (approximately 250 mg) and 1.5 mg/kg the next two hours (approximately 100 mg), cefazolin produced a steady serum level at the third hour of approximately 28 mcg/ml. Table 2 shows the average serum concentrations after IV injection of a single 1-g dose; average half-life was 1.4 hours.

TABLE 2. SERUM CONCENTRATIONS AFTER 1-G INTRAVENOUS DOSE

5 min	15 min	30 min	1 hr	2 hr	4 hr
188.4	135.8	106.8	73.7	45.6	16.5

Controlled studies on adult normal volunteers receiving 1 g four times a day for ten days, monitoring CBC, SGOT, SGPT, bilirubin, alkaline phosphatase, BUN, creatinine, and urinalysis, indicated no clinically significant changes attributed to cefazolin.

Cefazolin is excreted unchanged in the urine primarily by glomerular filtration and, to a lesser degree, by tubular secretion. Following intramuscular injection of 500 mg, 56 to 89 percent of the administered dose is recovered within six hours and 80 to nearly 100 percent in 24 hours. Cefazolin achieves peak urine concentrations greater than 1000 mcg/ml and 4000 mcg/ml respectively following 500-mg and 1-g intramuscular doses.

When cefazolin is administered to patients with unobstructed biliary tracts, high concentrations well over serum levels occur in the gallbladder tissue and bile. In the presence of obstruction, however, concentration of the antibiotic is considerably lower in bile than in serum.

Cefazolin readily crosses an inflamed synovial membrane, and the concentration of the antibiotic achieved in the joint space is comparable to levels measured in the serum.

Cefazolin readily crosses the placental barrier into the cord blood and amniotic fluid. It is present in very low concentrations in the milk of nursing mothers.

Disc Susceptibility Tests—Quantitative methods that require measurement of zone diameters give the most precise estimates of antibiotic susceptibility. One such procedure *(Am. J. Clin. Pathol., 45:493, 1966; Federal Register, 39:19182-19184, 1974)* has been recommended for use with discs for testing susceptibility to cephalosporin-class antibiotics. Interpretations correlate diameters of the disc test with MIC values for Kefzol® (cefazolin sodium, Lilly). With this procedure, a report from the laboratory of "susceptible" indicates that the infecting organism is likely to respond to therapy. A report of "resistant" indicates that the infecting organism is not likely to respond to therapy. A report of "intermediate susceptibility" suggests that the organism would be susceptible if high dosage is used or if the infection is confined to tissues and fluids (e.g., urine) in which high antibiotic levels are attained.

Indications and Usage: Kefzol® (cefazolin sodium, Lilly) is indicated in the treatment of the following serious infections due to susceptible organisms:

Respiratory tract infections due to *S. pneumoniae, Klebsiella* species, *H. influenzae, S. aureus* (penicillin-sensitive and penicillin-resistant), and group A beta-hemolytic streptococci

Injectable penicillin G benzathine is considered to be the drug of choice in the treatment and prevention of streptococcal infections, including the prophylaxis of rheumatic fever.

Kefzol is effective in the eradication of streptococci from the nasopharynx; however, data establishing the efficacy of Kefzol in the subsequent prevention of rheumatic fever are not available at present.

Genitourinary tract infections due to *E. coli, P. mirabilis, Klebsiella* species, and some strains of *Enterobacter* and enterococci

Skin and soft-tissue infections due to *S. aureus* (penicillin-sensitive and penicillin-resistant) and group A beta-hemolytic streptococci and other strains of streptococci

Biliary tract infections due to *E. coli*, various strains of streptococci, *P. mirabilis, Klebsiella* species, and *S. aureus*

Bone and joint infections due to *S. aureus*

Septicemia due to *S. pneumoniae, S. aureus* (penicillin-sensitive and penicillin-resistant), *P. mirabilis, E. coli,* and *Klebsiella* species

Endocarditis due to *S. aureus* (penicillin-sensitive and penicillin-resistant) and group A beta-hemolytic streptococci

Appropriate culture and susceptibility studies should be performed to determine susceptibility of the causative organism to Kefzol.

Perioperative Prophylaxis—The prophylactic administration of Kefzol preoperatively, intraopera-

Continued on next page

* Identi-Code® symbol.

Lilly—Cont.

tively, and postoperatively may reduce the incidence of certain postoperative infections in patients undergoing surgical procedures that are classified as contaminated or potentially contaminated (e.g., vaginal hysterectomy or cholecystectomy in high-risk patients such as those over 70 years of age, with acute cholecystitis, obstructive jaundice, or common-bile-duct stones).

The perioperative use of Kefzol also may be effective in surgical patients in whom infection at the operative site would present a serious risk (e.g., during open-heart surgery and prosthetic arthroplasty).

The prophylactic administration of Kefzol should usually be discontinued within a 24-hour period after the surgical procedure. In surgery in which the occurrence of infection may be particularly devastating (e.g., open-heart surgery and prosthetic arthroplasty), the prophylactic administration of Kefzol may be continued for three to five days following the completion of surgery. If there are signs of infection, specimens for culture should be obtained for the identification of the causative organism so that appropriate therapy may be instituted. (*See* Dosage and Administration.)

Contraindication: Kefzol® (cefazolin sodium, Lilly) is contraindicated in patients with known allergy to the cephalosporin group of antibiotics.

Warnings: BEFORE CEFAZOLIN THERAPY IS INSTITUTED, CAREFUL INQUIRY SHOULD BE MADE CONCERNING PREVIOUS HYPERSENSITIVITY REACTIONS TO CEPHALOSPORINS AND PENICILLINS. CEPHALOSPORIN C DERIVATIVES SHOULD BE GIVEN CAUTIOUSLY TO PENICILLIN-SENSITIVE PATIENTS.

SERIOUS ACUTE HYPERSENSITIVITY REACTIONS MAY REQUIRE EPINEPHRINE AND OTHER EMERGENCY MEASURES.

There is some clinical and laboratory evidence of partial cross-allergenicity of the penicillins and the cephalosporins. Patients have been reported to have had severe reactions (including anaphylaxis) to both drugs.

Antibiotics, including Kefzol® (cefazolin sodium, Lilly), should be administered cautiously to any patient who has demonstrated some form of allergy, particularly to drugs.

Pseudomembranous colitis has been reported with virtually all broad-spectrum antibiotics (including macrolides, semisynthetic penicillins, and cephalosporins); therefore, it is important to consider its diagnosis in patients who develop diarrhea in association with the use of antibiotics. Such colitis may range in severity from mild to life-threatening.

Treatment with broad-spectrum antibiotics alters the normal flora of the colon and may permit overgrowth of clostridia. Studies indicate that a toxin produced by *Clostridium difficile* is one primary cause of antibiotic-associated colitis.

Mild cases of pseudomembranous colitis usually respond to drug discontinuance alone. In moderate to severe cases, management should include sigmoidoscopy, appropriate bacteriologic studies, and fluid, electrolyte, and protein supplementation. When the colitis does not improve after the drug has been discontinued, or when it is severe, oral vancomycin is the drug of choice for antibiotic-associated pseudomembranous colitis produced by *C. difficile*. Other causes of colitis should be ruled out.

Usage in Infants—Safety for use in prematures and infants under one month of age has not been established.

Precautions: *General Precautions*—If an allergic reaction to Kefzol® (cefazolin sodium, Lilly) occurs, the drug should be discontinued and the patient treated with the usual agents (e.g., epinephrine or other pressor amines, antihistamines, or corticosteroids).

Prolonged use of Kefzol may result in the overgrowth of nonsusceptible organisms. Careful clinical observation of the patient is essential. If superinfection occurs during therapy, appropriate measures should be taken.

When Kefzol is administered to patients with low urinary output because of impaired renal function, lower daily dosage is required (see dosage instructions).

A false-positive reaction for glucose in the urine may occur with Benedict's or Fehling's solution or with Clinitest® tablets but not with Tes-Tape® (Glucose Enzymatic Test Strip, USP, Lilly).

An increased incidence of nephrotoxicity has been reported following concomitant administration of cephalosporins and aminoglycoside antibiotics.

Broad-spectrum antibiotics should be prescribed with caution in individuals with a history of gastrointestinal disease, particularly colitis.

Usage in Pregnancy—Pregnancy Category B—Reproduction studies have been performed in rats given doses of 500 mg or 1 g of cefazolin/kg and have revealed no evidence of impaired fertility or harm to the fetus due to Kefzol. There are, however, no adequate and well-controlled studies in pregnant women. Because animal reproduction studies are not always predictive of human response, this drug should be used during pregnancy only if clearly needed.

Nursing Mothers—The concentration of cefazolin in mothers' milk was very low. Levels of less than 0.9 mcg/ml were found only in isolated milk samples after intramuscular administration of 500 mg three times daily for two days.

Caution should be exercised when Kefzol is administered to a nursing woman.

Adverse Reactions: The following reactions have been reported:

Hypersensitivity—Drug fever, skin rash, vulvar pruritus, and eosinophilia have occurred.

Blood—Neutropenia, leukopenia, thrombocythemia, and positive direct and indirect Coombs' tests have occurred.

Hepatic and Renal—Transient rise in SGOT, SGPT, BUN, and alkaline phosphatase levels has been observed without clinical evidence of renal or hepatic impairment.

Gastrointestinal—Symptoms of pseudomembranous colitis may appear either during or after antibiotic treatment. Nausea and vomiting have been reported rarely. Anorexia, diarrhea, and oral candidiasis (oral thrush) have been reported.

Other—Pain on intramuscular injection, sometimes with induration, has occurred infrequently. Phlebitis at the site of injection has been noted. Other reactions have included genital and anal pruritus, genital moniliasis, and vaginitis.

Dosage and Administration: Kefzol® (cefazolin sodium, Lilly) may be administered intramuscularly or intravenously after reconstitution.

Intramuscular Administration—Reconstitute with 0.9% Sodium Chloride Injection, Sterile Water for Injection, or Bacteriostatic Water for Injection according to Table 3. Shake well until dissolved.

Kefzol should be injected into a large muscle mass. Pain on injection is infrequent with Kefzol. [See table below].

Intravenous Administration—Kefzol® (cefazolin sodium, Lilly) may be administered by intravenous injection or by continuous or intermittent infusion. Total daily dosages are the same as with intramuscular injection.

Intermittent intravenous infusion: Kefzol can be administered along with primary intravenous fluid management programs in a volume control set or in a separate, secondary IV bottle. Reconstituted 500 mg or 1 g of Kefzol may be diluted in 50 to 100 ml of one of the following intravenous solutions: 0.9% Sodium Chloride Injection, 5% or 10% Dextrose Injection, 5% Dextrose in Lactated Ringer's Injection, 5% Dextrose and 0.9% Sodium Chloride Injection (also may be used with 5% Dextrose and 0.45% or 0.2% Sodium Chloride Injection), Lactated Ringer's Injection, 5% or 10% Invert Sugar in Sterile Water for Injection, Ringer's Injection, Normosol®-M in D5-W, Ionosol® B with Dextrose 5%, or Plasma-Lyte® with 5% Dextrose.

Direct intravenous injection: Dilute the reconstituted 500 mg or 1 g of Kefzol in a minimum of 10 ml of Sterile Water for Injection. Inject solution slowly over three to five minutes. It may be administered directly into a vein or through the tubing for a patient receiving the above parenteral fluids.

Dosage—The usual adult dosages are given in Table 4.

TABLE 4. USUAL ADULT DOSAGE OF KEFZOL® (CEFAZOLIN SODIUM)

Type of Infection	Dose	Frequency
Pneumococcal pneumonia	500 mg	q. 12 h.
Mild infections caused by susceptible gram-positive cocci	250 to 500 mg	q. 8 h.
Acute uncomplicated urinary tract infections	1 g	q. 12 h.
Moderate to severe infections	500 mg to 1 g	q. 6 to 8 h.

Cefazolin has been administered in dosages of 6 to 12 g/day in life-threatening infections such as endocarditis and septicemia.

In adults with renal impairment, cefazolin is not readily excreted. After a loading dose of 500 mg, the following recommendations for *maintenance dosage* (Table 5) may be used as a guide. [See table on next page].

Perioperative Prophylactic Use—To prevent postoperative infection in contaminated or potentially contaminated surgery, the recommended doses are as follows:

a. 1 g IV or IM administered one-half to one hour prior to the start of surgery.
b. For lengthy operative procedures (e.g., two hours or more), 0.5 to 1 g IV or IM during surgery (administration modified according to the duration of the operative procedure).
c. 0.5 to 1 g IV or IM every six to eight hours postoperatively.

It is important that (1) the preoperative dose be given just (one-half to one hour) prior to the start of surgery so that adequate antibiotic levels are present in the serum and tissues at the time of the initial surgical incision and (2) Kefzol be administered, if necessary, at appropriate intervals during surgery to provide sufficient levels of the antibiotic at the anticipated moments of greatest exposure to infective organisms.

In surgery in which the occurrence of infection may be particularly devastating (e.g., open-heart surgery and prosthetic arthroplasty), the prophylactic administration of Kefzol may be continued

TABLE 3. DILUTION TABLE FOR KEFZOL® (CEFAZOLIN SODIUM)

Vial Size	Diluent to Be Added	Approximate Available Volume	Approximate Average Concentration
250 mg	2 ml	2 ml	125 mg/ml
500 mg	2 ml	2.2 ml	225 mg/ml
1 g	2.5 ml	3 ml	330 mg/ml

for three to five days following the completion of surgery.

In children, a total daily dosage of 25 to 50 mg/kg (approximately 10 to 20 mg/lb) of body weight, divided into three or four equal doses, is effective for most mild to moderately severe infections (Table 6). Total daily dosage may be increased to 100 mg/kg (45 mg/lb) of body weight for severe infections.

TABLE 6. PEDIATRIC DOSAGE GUIDE FOR KEFZOL® (CEFAZOLIN SODIUM)

Weight		25 mg/kg/Day Divided into 3 Doses		25 mg/kg/Day Divided into 4 Doses	
lb	kg	Approximate Single Dose (mg q. 8 h.)	Vol. (ml) Needed with Dilution of 125 mg/ml	Approximate Single Dose (mg q. 6 h.)	Vol. (ml) Needed with Dilution of 125 mg/ml
10	4.5	40 mg	0.35 ml	30 mg	0.25 ml
20	9	75 mg	0.6 ml	55 mg	0.45 ml
30	13.6	115 mg	0.9 ml	85 mg	0.7 ml
40	18.1	150 mg	1.2 ml	115 mg	0.9 ml
50	22.7	190 mg	1.5 ml	140 mg	1.1 ml

Weight		50 mg/kg/Day Divided into 3 Doses		50 mg/kg/Day Divided into 4 Doses	
lb	kg	Approximate Single Dose (mg q. 8 h.)	Vol. (ml) Needed with Dilution of 225 mg/ml	Approximate Single Dose (mg q. 6 h.)	Vol. (ml) Needed with Dilution of 225 mg/ml
10	4.5	75 mg	0.35 ml	55 mg	0.25 ml
20	9	150 mg	0.7 ml	110 mg	0.5 ml
30	13.6	225 mg	1 ml	170 mg	0.75 ml
40	18.1	300 mg	1.35 ml	225 mg	1 ml
50	22.7	375 mg	1.7 ml	285 mg	1.25 ml

In children with mild to moderate renal impairment (creatinine clearance of 70 to 40 ml/min), 60 percent of the normal daily dose given in divided doses every 12 hours should be sufficient. In patients with moderate impairment (creatinine clearance of 40 to 20 ml/min), 25 percent of the normal daily dose given in divided doses every 12 hours should be sufficient. In children with severe impairment (creatinine clearance of 20 to 5 ml/min), 10 percent of the normal daily dose given every 24 hours should be adequate. All dosage recommendations apply after an initial loading dose. Since safety for use in premature infants and in infants under one month of age has not been established, the use of Kefzol in these patients is not recommended.

Stability: Reconstituted Kefzol® (cefazolin sodium, Lilly) and dilutions of Kefzol in the recommended intravenous fluids are stable for 24 hours at room temperature and for 96 hours if stored under refrigeration (5°C).

Solutions of Kefzol in Sterile Water for Injection, 5% Dextrose Injection, or 0.9% Sodium Chloride Injection that are frozen immediately after reconstitution in the original container are stable for as long as 12 weeks when stored at −20°C. **If the product is warmed, care should be taken to avoid heating it after the thawing is complete. Once thawed, the solution should not be refrozen.**

How Supplied: (℞) *Vials Kefzol® (Sterile Cefazolin Sodium, USP)*, rubber-stoppered (Dry Powder): *No. 766*, 250 mg (equivalent to cefazolin), 10-ml size (NDC 0002-1496-01), in singles (10/carton); *No. 767*, 500 mg (equivalent to cefazolin), and *No. 768*, 1 g (equivalent to cefazolin), 10-ml size, in singles (NDC 0002-1497-01 and NDC 0002-1498-01) (10/carton) and in Traypak™ (multivial carton, Lilly) of 25 (NDC 0002-1497-25 and NDC 0002-1498-25); *No. 7018*, 500 mg (equivalent to cefazolin) (NDC 0002-7018-10), and *No. 7011*, 1 g (equivalent

TABLE 5. MAINTENANCE DOSAGE OF KEFZOL® (CEFAZOLIN SODIUM) IN ADULTS WITH REDUCED RENAL FUNCTION

Renal Function	BUN* (mg %)	Creatinine Clearance (ml/min)	Dosage Mild to Moderate Infection	Dosage Moderate to Severe Infection	Serum Half-Life (Hours)
Mild impairment	20–34	70–40	250 to 500 mg q. 12 h.	500 mg to 1.25 g q. 12 h.	3–5
Moderate impairment	35–49	40–20	125 to 250 mg q. 12 h.	250 to 600 mg q. 12 h.	6–12
Severe impairment	50–75	20–5	75 to 150 mg q. 24 h.	150 to 400 mg q. 24 h.	15–30
Essentially no function	>75	<5	37.5 to 75 mg q. 24 h.	75 to 200 mg q. 24 h.	30–40

*If used to estimate degree of renal impairment, BUN concentrations should reflect a steady state of renal azotemia.

to cefazolin) (NDC 0002-7011-10), 100-ml size, in Traypak of 10; *No. 7014*, 10 g (equivalent to cefazolin), 100-ml size, in Traypak of 6 (NDC 0002-7014-16).

(℞) *Redi Vial® (dual compartment vial, Lilly) Kefzol® (Sterile Cefazolin Sodium, USP): No. 7082*, 500 mg (equivalent to cefazolin), and *No. 7083*, 1 g (equivalent to cefazolin), in singles (NDC 0002-7082-01 and NDC 0002-7083-01) (10/carton) and in Traypak of 10 (NDC 0002-7082-10 and NDC 0002-7083-10).

(℞) *Faspak™ (flexible plastic bag, Lilly) Kefzol® (Sterile Cefazolin Sodium, USP), No. 7201*, 500 mg (equivalent to cefazolin), and *No. 7202*, 1 g (equivalent to cefazolin), in Faspak of 96 (NDC 0002-7201-74 and NDC 0002-7202-74). [031584]

LENTE® ILETIN® I
[lĕn'tā' ī lĕ-tĭn]
(insulin zinc suspension, Lilly), see under Iletin® (insulin, Lilly).

MANDOL® ℞
[măn'dŏl]
(cefamandole nafate) For Injection USP

Description: Mandol® (cefamandole nafate, Lilly) is a semisynthetic broad-spectrum cephalosporin antibiotic for parenteral administration. It is the sodium salt of 7-D-mandelamido-3-[[(1-methyl-1H-tetrazol-5-yl)-thio]methyl]-3-cephem-4-carboxylic acid, formate (ester). Mandol also contains 63 mg sodium carbonate/g of cefamandole activity. The total sodium content is approximately 77 mg (3.3 mEq sodium ion) per g of cefamandole activity. After addition of diluent, cefamandole nafate rapidly hydrolyzes to cefamandole, and both compounds have microbiologic activity in vivo. Solutions of Mandol range from light-yellow to amber, depending on concentration and diluent used. The pH of freshly reconstituted solutions usually ranges from 6.0 to 8.5.

Clinical Pharmacology: After intramuscular administration of a 500-mg dose of cefamandole to normal volunteers, the mean peak serum concentration was 13 mcg/ml. After a 1-g dose, the mean peak concentration was 25 mcg/ml. These peaks occurred at 30 to 120 minutes. Following intravenous doses of 1, 2, and 3 g, serum concentrations were 139, 240, and 533 mcg/ml respectively at ten minutes. These concentrations declined to 0.8, 2.2, and 2.9 mcg/ml at four hours. Intravenous administration of 4-g doses every six hours produced no evidence of accumulation in the serum. The half-life after an intravenous dose is 32 minutes; after intramuscular administration, the half-life is 60 minutes.

Sixty-five to 85 percent of cefamandole is excreted by the kidneys over an eight-hour period, resulting in high urinary concentrations. Following intramuscular doses of 500 mg and 1 g, urinary concentrations averaged 254 and 1357 mcg/ml respectively. Intravenous doses of 1 and 2 g produced urinary levels averaging 750 and 1380 mcg/ml respectively. Probenecid slows tubular excretion and doubles the peak serum level and the duration of measurable serum concentrations.

The antibiotic reaches therapeutic levels in pleural and joint fluids and in bile and bone.

Microbiology—The bactericidal action of cefamandole results from inhibition of cell-wall synthesis. Cephalosporins have in vitro activity against a wide range of gram-positive and gram-negative organisms. Cefamandole is usually active against the following organisms in vitro and in clinical infections:

Gram-positive
  Staphylococcus aureus, including penicillinase and non-penicillinase-producing strains
  S. epidermidis
  Beta-hemolytic and other streptococci (Most strains of enterococci, e.g., *Streptococcus faecalis*, are resistant.)
  S. pneumoniae (formerly *Diplococcus pneumoniae*)

Gram-negative
  Escherichia coli
  Klebsiella species
  Enterobacter species (Initially susceptible organisms occasionally may become resistant during therapy.)
  Haemophilus influenzae
  Proteus mirabilis
  P. rettgeri
  P. morganii
  P. vulgaris (Some strains of *P. vulgaris* have been shown by in vitro tests to be resistant to cefamandole and other cephalosporins.)

Anaerobic organisms
  Gram-positive and gram-negative cocci (including *Peptococcus* and *Peptostreptococcus* species)
  Gram-positive bacilli (including *Clostridium* species)
  Gram-negative bacilli (including *Bacteroides* and *Fusobacterium* species). Most strains of *Bacteroides fragilis* are resistant.

Pseudomonas, Acinetobacter calcoaceticus (formerly *Mima* and *Herellea* species), and most *Serratia* strains are resistant to cephalosporins. Cefamandole is resistant to degradation by beta-lactamases from certain members of the *Enterobacteriaceae*.

Susceptibility Tests—Quantitative methods that require measurement of zone diameters give the most precise estimates of antibiotic susceptibility. One such procedure[1] has been recommended for

Continued on next page

* Identi-Code® symbol.

Lilly—Cont.

use with discs to test susceptibility to cefamandole. Interpretation involves correlation of the diameters obtained in the disc test with minimum inhibitory concentration (MIC) values for cefamandole. Reports from the laboratory giving results of the standardized single-disc susceptibility test[1] using a 30-mcg cefamandole disc should be interpreted according to the following criteria:

Susceptible organisms produce zones of 18 mm or greater, indicating that the tested organism is likely to respond to therapy.

Organisms of intermediate susceptibility produce zones of 15 to 17 mm, indicating that the tested organism would be susceptible if high dosage is used or if the infection is confined to tissues and fluids (e.g., urine), in which high antibiotic levels are attained.

Resistant organisms produce zones of 14 mm or less, indicating that other therapy should be selected.

For gram-positive isolates, the test may be performed with either the cephalosporin-class disc (30 mcg cephalothin) or the cefamandole disc (30 mcg cefamandole), and a zone of 18 mm is indicative of a cefamandole-susceptible organism.

Gram-negative organisms should be tested with the cefamandole disc (using the above criteria), since cefamandole has been shown by in vitro tests to have activity against certain strains of *Enterobacteriaceae* found resistant when tested with the cephalosporin-class disc. Gram-negative organisms having zones of less than 18 mm around the cephalothin disc are not necessarily of intermediate susceptibility or resistant to cefamandole. The cefamandole disc should not be used for testing susceptibility to other cephalosporins.

A bacterial isolate may be considered susceptible if the MIC value for cefamandole[2] is not more than 16 mcg/ml. Organisms are considered resistant if the MIC is greater than 32 mcg/ml.

Indications and Usage: Mandol® (cefamandole nafate, Lilly) is indicated for the treatment of serious infections caused by susceptible strains of the designated microorganisms in the diseases listed below:

Lower respiratory infections, including pneumonia caused by *S. pneumoniae (D. pneumoniae), H. influenzae, Klebsiella* species, *S. aureus* (penicillinase and non-penicillinase-producing), beta-hemolytic streptococci, and *P. mirabilis*

Urinary tract infections caused by *E. coli*, *Proteus* species (both indole-negative and indole-positive), *Enterobacter* species, *Klebsiella* species, group D streptococci (*Note:* Most enterococci, e.g., *S. faecalis*, are resistant), and *S. epidermidis*

Peritonitis caused by *E. coli* and *Enterobacter* species

Septicemia caused by *E. coli*, *S. aureus* (penicillinase and non-penicillinase-producing), *S. pneumoniae*, *S. pyogenes* (group A beta-hemolytic streptococci), *H. influenzae*, and *Klebsiella* species

Skin and skin-structure infections caused by *S. aureus* (penicillinase and non-penicillinase-producing), *S. pyogenes* (group A beta-hemolytic streptococci), *H. influenzae*, *E. coli*, *Enterobacter* species, and *P. mirabilis*

Bone and joint infections caused by *S. aureus* (penicillinase and non-penicillinase-producing)

Clinical microbiologic studies in nongonococcal pelvic inflammatory disease in females, lower respiratory infections, and skin infections frequently reveal the growth of susceptible strains of both aerobic and anaerobic organisms. Mandol has been used successfully in these infections in which several organisms have been isolated. Most strains of *B. fragilis* are resistant in vitro; however, infections caused by susceptible strains have been treated successfully.

Specimens for bacteriologic cultures should be obtained in order to isolate and identify causative organisms and to determine their susceptibilities to cefamandole. Therapy may be instituted before results of susceptibility studies are known; however, once these results become available, the antibiotic treatment should be adjusted accordingly.

In certain cases of confirmed or suspected gram-positive or gram-negative sepsis or in patients with other serious infections in which the causative organism has not been identified, Mandol may be used concomitantly with an aminoglycoside (see Precautions). The recommended doses of both antibiotics may be given, depending on the severity of the infection and the patient's condition. The renal function of the patient should be carefully monitored, especially if higher dosages of the antibiotics are to be administered.

Antibiotic therapy of beta-hemolytic streptococcal infections should continue for at least ten days.

Preventive Therapy—The administration of Mandol preoperatively, intraoperatively, and postoperatively may reduce the incidence of certain postoperative infections in patients undergoing surgical procedures that are classified as contaminated or potentially contaminated (e.g., gastrointestinal surgery, cesarean section, vaginal hysterectomy, or cholecystectomy in high-risk patients such as those with acute cholecystitis, obstructive jaundice, or common-bile-duct stones).

In major surgery in which the risk of postoperative infection is low but serious (cardiovascular surgery, neurosurgery, or prosthetic arthroplasty), Mandol may be effective in preventing such infections.

The perioperative use of Mandol should be discontinued after 24 hours; however, in prosthetic arthroplasty, it is recommended that administration be continued for 72 hours. If signs of infection occur, specimens for culture should be obtained for identification of the causative organism so that appropriate antibiotic therapy may be instituted.

Contraindication: Mandol® (cefamandole nafate, Lilly) is contraindicated in patients with known allergy to the cephalosporin group of antibiotics.

Warnings: BEFORE THERAPY WITH MANDOL® (cefamandole nafate, Lilly) IS INSTITUTED, CAREFUL INQUIRY SHOULD BE MADE TO DETERMINE WHETHER THE PATIENT HAS HAD PREVIOUS HYPERSENSITIVITY REACTIONS TO CEPHALOSPORINS, PENICILLINS, OR OTHER DRUGS. THIS PRODUCT SHOULD BE GIVEN CAUTIOUSLY TO PENICILLIN-SENSITIVE PATIENTS. ANTIBIOTICS SHOULD BE ADMINISTERED WITH CAUTION TO ANY PATIENT WHO HAS DEMONSTRATED SOME FORM OF ALLERGY, PARTICULARLY TO DRUGS. SERIOUS ACUTE HYPERSENSITIVITY REACTIONS MAY REQUIRE EPINEPHRINE AND OTHER EMERGENCY MEASURES.

In newborn infants, accumulation of other cephalosporin-class antibiotics (with resulting prolongation of drug half-life) has been reported.

Pseudomembranous colitis has been reported with virtually all broad-spectrum antibiotics (including macrolides, semisynthetic penicillins, and cephalosporins); therefore, it is important to consider its diagnosis in patients who develop diarrhea in association with the use of antibiotics. Such colitis may range in severity from mild to life-threatening. Treatment with broad-spectrum antibiotics alters the normal flora of the colon and may permit overgrowth of clostridia. Studies indicate that a toxin produced by *Clostridium difficile* is one primary cause of antibiotic-associated colitis.

Mild cases of pseudomembranous colitis usually respond to drug discontinuance alone. In moderate to severe cases, management should include sigmoidoscopy, appropriate bacteriologic studies, and fluid, electrolyte, and protein supplementation. When the colitis does not improve after the drug has been discontinued, or when it is severe, oral vancomycin is the drug of choice for antibiotic-associated pseudomembranous colitis produced by *C. difficile*. Other causes of colitis should be ruled out.

Precautions: *General Precautions*—Although Mandol® (cefamandole nafate, Lilly) rarely produces alteration in kidney function, evaluation of renal status is recommended, especially in seriously ill patients receiving maximum doses.

Prolonged use of Mandol may result in the overgrowth of nonsusceptible organisms. Careful observation of the patient is essential. If superinfection occurs during therapy, appropriate measures should be taken.

Nephrotoxicity has been reported following concomitant administration of aminoglycoside antibiotics and cephalosporins.

A false-positive reaction for glucose in the urine may occur with Benedict's or Fehling's solution or with Clinitest® tablets but not with Tes-Tape® (Glucose Enzymatic Test Strip, USP, Lilly). There may be a false-positive test for proteinuria with acid and denaturization-precipitation tests.

As with other broad-spectrum antibiotics, hypoprothrombinemia, with or without bleeding, has been reported rarely, but it has been promptly reversed by administration of vitamin K. Such episodes usually have occurred in elderly, debilitated, or otherwise compromised patients with deficient stores of vitamin K. Treatment of such individuals with antibiotics possessing significant gram-negative and/or anaerobic activity is thought to alter the number and/or type of intestinal bacterial flora, with consequent reduction in synthesis of vitamin K. Prophylactic administration of vitamin K may be indicated in such patients, especially when intestinal sterilization and surgical procedures are performed.

In a few patients receiving Mandol, nausea, vomiting, and vasomotor instability with hypotension and peripheral vasodilatation occurred following the ingestion of ethanol.

Cefamandole inhibits the enzyme acetaldehyde dehydrogenase in laboratory animals. This causes accumulation of acetaldehyde when ethanol is administered concomitantly.

Broad-spectrum antibiotics should be prescribed with caution in individuals with a history of gastrointestinal disease, particularly colitis.

Usage in Pregnancy—Pregnancy Category B—Reproduction studies have been performed in rats given doses of 500 or 1000 mg/kg/day and have revealed no evidence of impaired fertility or harm to the fetus due to Mandol. There are, however, no adequate and well-controlled studies in pregnant women. Because animal reproduction studies are not always predictive of human response, this drug should be used during pregnancy only if clearly needed.

Nursing Mothers—Caution should be exercised when Mandol is administered to a nursing woman.

Usage in Infancy—Mandol has been effectively used in this age group, but all laboratory parameters have not been extensively studied in infants between one and six months of age; safety of this product has not been established in prematures and infants under one month of age. Therefore, if Mandol is administered to infants, the physician should determine whether the potential benefits outweigh the possible risks involved.

Adverse Reactions: *Gastrointestinal*—Symptoms of pseudomembranous colitis may appear either during or after antibiotic treatment. Nausea and vomiting have been reported rarely.

Hypersensitivity—Maculopapular rash, urticaria, eosinophilia, and drug fever have been reported. These reactions are more likely to occur in patients with a history of allergy, particularly to penicillin.

Blood—Thrombocytopenia has been reported rarely. Neutropenia has been reported, especially in long courses of treatment. Some individuals have developed positive direct Coombs' tests during treatment with the cephalosporin antibiotics.

Liver—Transient rise in SGOT, SGPT, and alkaline phosphatase levels has been noted.

Kidney—Decreased creatinine clearance has been reported in patients with prior renal impairment. As with some other cephalosporins, transitory elevations of BUN have occasionally been observed with Mandol® (cefamandole nafate, Lilly); their frequency increases in patients over 50 years of age. In some of these cases, there was also a mild increase in serum creatinine.

Local Reactions—Pain on intramuscular injection is infrequent. Thrombophlebitis occurs rarely.

Dosage and Administration: *Dosage—Adults:* The usual dosage range for cefamandole is 500 mg to 1 g every four to eight hours.

In infections of skin structures and in uncomplicated pneumonia, a dosage of 500 mg every six hours is adequate.

In uncomplicated urinary tract infections, a dosage of 500 mg every eight hours is sufficient. In more serious urinary tract infections, a dosage of 1 g every eight hours may be needed.

In severe infections, 1-g doses may be given at four to six-hour intervals.

In life-threatening infections or infections due to less susceptible organisms, doses up to 2 g every four hours (i.e., 12 g/day) may be needed.

Infants and Children: Administration of 50 to 100 mg/kg/day in equally divided doses every four to eight hours has been effective for most infections susceptible to Mandol® (cefamandole nafate, Lilly). This may be increased to a total daily dose of 150 mg/kg (not to exceed the maximum adult dose) for severe infections. (*See* Warnings and Precautions for this age group.)

Note: As with antibiotic therapy in general, administration of Mandol should be continued for a minimum of 48 to 72 hours after the patient becomes asymptomatic or after evidence of bacterial eradication has been obtained; a minimum of ten days of treatment is recommended in infections caused by group A beta-hemolytic streptococci in order to guard against the risk of rheumatic fever or glomerulonephritis; frequent bacteriologic and clinical appraisal is necessary during therapy of chronic urinary tract infection and may be required for several months after therapy has been completed; persistent infections may require treatment for several weeks; and doses smaller than those indicated above should not be used.

For perioperative use of Mandol, the following dosages are recommended:

Adults—1 or 2 g intravenously or intramuscularly one-half to one hour prior to the surgical incision followed by 1 or 2 g every six hours for 24 to 48 hours.

Children (three months of age and older)—50 to 100 mg/kg/day in equally divided doses by the routes and schedule designated above.

Note: In patients undergoing prosthetic arthroplasty, administration is recommended for as long as 72 hours.

In patients undergoing cesarean section, the initial dose may be administered just prior to surgery or immediately after the cord has been clamped.

Impaired Renal Function—When renal function is impaired, a reduced dosage must be employed and the serum levels closely monitored. After an initial dose of 1 to 2 g (depending on the severity of infection), a maintenance dosage schedule should be followed (see chart). Continued dosage should be determined by degree of renal impairment, severity of infection, and susceptibility of the causative organism.

[See table above].

When only serum creatinine is available, the following formula (based on sex, weight, and age of the patient) may be used to convert this value into creatinine clearance. The serum creatinine should represent a steady state of renal function.

Males: $\dfrac{\text{Weight (kg)} \times (140 - \text{age})}{72 \times \text{serum creatinine}}$

Females: 0.9 × above value

Modes of Administration—Mandol® (cefamandole nafate, Lilly) may be given intravenously or by deep intramuscular injection into a large muscle mass (such as the gluteus or lateral part of the thigh) to minimize pain.

Intramuscular Administration—Each g of Mandol should be diluted with 3 ml of one of the following diluents: Sterile Water for Injection, Bacteriostatic Water for Injection, 0.9% Sodium Chloride Injection, or Bacteriostatic Sodium Chloride Injection. Shake well until dissolved.

MANDOL® (CEFAMANDOLE NAFATE)—MAINTENANCE DOSAGE GUIDE FOR PATIENTS WITH RENAL IMPAIRMENT

Creatinine Clearance (ml/min/1.73 m^2)	Renal Function	Life-Threatening Infections— Maximum Dosage	Less Severe Infections
>80	Normal	2 g q. 4 h.	1–2 g q. 6 h.
80–50	Mild Impairment	1.5 g q. 4 h. OR 2 g q. 6 h.	0.75–1.5 g q. 6 h.
50–25	Moderate Impairment	1.5 g q. 6 h. OR 2 g q. 8 h.	0.75–1.5 g q. 8 h.
25–10	Severe Impairment	1 g q. 6 h. OR 1.25 g q. 8 h.	0.5–1 g q. 8 h.
10–2	Marked Impairment	0.67 g q. 8 h. OR 1 g q. 12 h.	0.5–0.75 g q. 12 h.
<2	None	0.5 g q. 8 h. OR 0.75 g q. 12 h.	0.25–0.5 g q. 12 h.

Intravenous Administration—The intravenous route may be preferable for patients with bacterial septicemia, localized parenchymal abscesses (such as intra-abdominal abscess), peritonitis, or other severe or life-threatening infections when they may be poor risks because of lowered resistance. In those with normal renal function, the intravenous dosage for such infections is 3 to 12 g of Mandol daily. In conditions such as bacterial septicemia, 6 to 12 g/day may be given initially by the intravenous route for several days, and dosage may then be gradually reduced according to clinical response and laboratory findings.

If combination therapy with Mandol and an aminoglycoside is indicated, each of these antibiotics should be administered in different sites. *Do not mix an aminoglycoside with Mandol in the same intravenous fluid container.*

A SOLUTION OF 1 G MANDOL IN 22 ML OF STERILE WATER FOR INJECTION IS ISOTONIC.

The choice of saline, dextrose, or electrolyte solution and the volume to be employed are dictated by fluid and electrolyte management.

For direct intermittent intravenous administration, each g of cefamandole should be reconstituted with 10 ml of Sterile Water for Injection, 5% Dextrose Injection, or 0.9% Sodium Chloride Injection. Slowly inject the solution into the vein over a period of three to five minutes, or give it through the tubing of an administration set while the patient is also receiving one of the following intravenous fluids: 0.9% Sodium Chloride Injection; 5% Dextrose Injection; 10% Dextrose Injection; 5% Dextrose and 0.9% Sodium Chloride Injection; 5% Dextrose and 0.45% Sodium Chloride Injection; 5% Dextrose and 0.2% Sodium Chloride Injection; or Sodium Lactate Injection (M/6).

Intermittent intravenous infusion with a Y-type administration set or volume control set can also be accomplished while any of the above-mentioned intravenous fluids are being infused. However, during infusion of the solution containing Mandol® (cefamandole nafate, Lilly), it is desirable to discontinue the other solution. When this technique is employed, careful attention should be paid to the volume of the solution containing Mandol so that the calculated dose will be infused. When a Y-tube hookup is used, 100 ml of the appropriate diluent should be added to the 1 or 2-g piggyback (100-ml) vial. If Sterile Water for Injection is used as the diluent, reconstitute with approximately 20 ml/g to avoid a hypotonic solution.

For continuous intravenous infusion, each g of cefamandole should be diluted with 10 ml of Sterile Water for Injection. An appropriate quantity of the resulting solution may be added to an IV bottle containing one of the following fluids: 0.9% Sodium Chloride Injection; 5% Dextrose Injection; 10% Dextrose Injection; 5% Dextrose and 0.9% Sodium Chloride Injection; 5% Dextrose and 0.45% Sodium Chloride Injection; 5% Dextrose and 0.2% Sodium Chloride Injection; or Sodium Lactate Injection (M/6).

Stability: Reconstituted Mandol® (cefamandole nafate, Lilly) is stable for 24 hours at room temperature (25°C) and for 96 hours if stored under refrigeration (5°C). *During storage at room temperature, carbon dioxide develops inside the vial after reconstitution. This pressure may be dissipated prior to withdrawal of the vial contents, or it may be used to aid withdrawal if the vial is inverted over the syringe needle and the contents are allowed to flow into the syringe.*

Solutions of Mandol in Sterile Water for Injection, 5% Dextrose Injection, or 0.9% Sodium Chloride Injection that are frozen immediately after reconstitution in the original container are stable for six months when stored at −20°C. If the product is warmed (to a maximum of 37°C), care should be taken to avoid heating it after the thawing is complete. Once thawed, the solution should not be refrozen.

How Supplied: (℞) *Vials Mandol® (Cefamandole Nafate for Injection, USP),* rubber-stoppered (Dry Powder): *No. 7060,* 500 mg (equivalent to cefamandole activity) (NDC 0002-7060-25), and *No. 7061,* 1 g (equivalent to cefamandole activity) (NDC 0002-7061-25), 10-ml size, in Traypak™ (multivial carton, Lilly) of 25; *No. 7068,* 1 g (equivalent to cefamandole activity), 100-ml size (NDC 0002-7068-10), *No. 7064,* 2 g (equivalent to cefamandole activity), 20-ml size (NDC 0002-7064-10), and *No. 7069,* 2 g (equivalent to cefamandole activity), 100-ml size (NDC 0002-7069-10), in Traypak of 10; *No. 7072,* 10 g (equivalent to cefamandole activity), 100-ml size (NDC 0002-7072-16), in Traypak of 6.

(℞) *Faspak™ (flexible plastic bag, Lilly) Mandol® (Cefamandole Nafate for Injection, USP): No. 7208,* 1 g (equivalent to cefamandole activity) (NDC 0002-7208-74), and *No. 7209,* 2 g (equivalent to cefamandole activity) (NDC 0002-7209-74), in packages of 96.

[062084]

---

1. Bauer, A. W., Kirby, W. M. M., Sherris, J. C., and Turck, M.: Antibiotic Susceptibility Testing by a Standardized Single Disk Method, Am. J. Clin. Pathol., 45:493, 1966; Standardized Disc Susceptibility Test, Fed-

Continued on next page

* Identi-Code® symbol.

Lilly—Cont.

eral Register, 39:19182-19184, 1974. National Committee for Clinical Laboratory Standards. Approved Standard: ASM-2, Performance Standards for Antimicrobial Disc Susceptibility Tests, July, 1975.

2. Determined by the ICS agar-dilution method (Ericsson, H. M., and Sherris, J. C.: Acta Pathol. Microbiol. Scand. [B], Supplement No. 217, 1971) or any other method that has been shown to give equivalent results.

METHADONE HYDROCHLORIDE
[měth'a-dōn hī-drō- klō-rīd]
DISKETS® (dispersible tablets, Lilly)
Tablets, USP
(*See also* Dolophine® Hydrochloride)

CONDITIONS FOR DISTRIBUTION AND USE OF METHADONE PRODUCTS:

Code of Federal Regulations, Title 21, Sec. 291.505

METHADONE PRODUCTS, WHEN USED FOR THE TREATMENT OF NARCOTIC ADDICTION IN DETOXIFICATION OR MAINTENANCE PROGRAMS, SHALL BE DISPENSED ONLY BY APPROVED HOSPITAL PHARMACIES, APPROVED COMMUNITY PHARMACIES, AND MAINTENANCE PROGRAMS APPROVED BY THE FOOD AND DRUG ADMINISTRATION AND THE DESIGNATED STATE AUTHORITY.

APPROVED MAINTENANCE PROGRAMS SHALL DISPENSE AND USE METHADONE IN ORAL FORM ONLY AND ACCORDING TO THE TREATMENT REQUIREMENTS STIPULATED IN THE FEDERAL METHADONE REGULATIONS (21 CFR 291.505).

FAILURE TO ABIDE BY THE REQUIREMENTS IN THESE REGULATIONS MAY RESULT IN CRIMINAL PROSECUTION, SEIZURE OF THE DRUG SUPPLY, REVOCATION OF THE PROGRAM APPROVAL, AND INJUNCTION PRECLUDING OPERATION OF THE PROGRAM.

Description: Methadone Hydrochloride, USP (4, 4- diphenyl -6- dimethylamino - heptanone-3 hydrochloride), is a white crystalline material which is water soluble. However, the Disket preparation of methadone hydrochloride has been specially formulated with insoluble excipients to deter the use of this drug by injection.

Actions: Methadone hydrochloride is a synthetic narcotic analgesic with multiple actions quantitatively similar to those of morphine, the most prominent of which involve the central nervous system and organs composed of smooth muscle. The principal actions of therapeutic value are analgesia and sedation and detoxification or maintenance in narcotic addiction. The methadone abstinence syndrome, although qualitatively similar to that of morphine, differs in that the onset is slower, the course is more prolonged, and the symptoms are less severe.

When administered orally, methadone is approximately one-half as potent as when given parenterally. Oral administration results in a delay of the onset, a lowering of the peak, and an increase in the duration of analgesic effect.

Indications: 1. Detoxification treatment of narcotic addiction (heroin or other morphine-like drugs).
2. Maintenance treatment of narcotic addiction (heroin or other morphine-like drugs), in conjunction with appropriate social and medical services.

NOTE
If methadone is administered for treatment of heroin dependence for more than three weeks, the procedure passes from treatment of the acute withdrawal syndrome (detoxification) to maintenance therapy. Maintenance treatment is permitted to be undertaken only by approved methadone programs. This does not preclude the maintenance treatment of an addict who is hospitalized for medical conditions other than addiction and who requires temporary maintenance during the critical period of his stay or whose enrollment has been verified in a program which has approval for maintenance treatment with methadone.

Contraindication: Hypersensitivity to methadone.

Warnings:

Diskets Methadone Hydrochloride are for oral administration only. This preparation contains insoluble excipients and therefore *must not* be injected. It is recommended that Diskets Methadone Hydrochloride, if dispensed, be packaged in child-resistant containers to prevent accidental ingestion.

Methadone hydrochloride, a narcotic, is a Schedule II controlled substance under the Federal Controlled Substances Act. Appropriate security measures should be taken to safeguard stocks of methadone against diversion.

DRUG DEPENDENCE—METHADONE CAN PRODUCE DRUG DEPENDENCE OF THE MORPHINE TYPE AND, THEREFORE, HAS THE POTENTIAL FOR BEING ABUSED. PSYCHIC DEPENDENCE, PHYSICAL DEPENDENCE, AND TOLERANCE MAY DEVELOP UPON REPEATED ADMINISTRATION OF METHADONE, AND IT SHOULD BE PRESCRIBED AND ADMINISTERED WITH THE SAME DEGREE OF CAUTION APPROPRIATE TO THE USE OF MORPHINE.

Interaction with Other Central-Nervous-System Depressants—Methadone should be used with caution and in reduced dosage in patients who are concurrently receiving other narcotic analgesics, general anesthetics, phenothiazines, other tranquilizers, sedative-hypnotics, tricyclic antidepressants, and other CNS depressants (including alcohol). Respiratory depression, hypotension, and profound sedation or coma may result.

Anxiety—Since methadone, as used by tolerant subjects at a constant maintenance dosage, is not a tranquilizer, patients who are maintained on this drug will react to life problems and stresses with the same symptoms of anxiety as do other individuals. The physician should not confuse such symptoms with those of narcotic abstinence and should not attempt to treat anxiety by increasing the dosage of methadone. The action of methadone in maintenance treatment is limited to the control of narcotic symptoms and is ineffective for relief of general anxiety.

Head Injury and Increased Intracranial Pressure—The respiratory depressant effects of methadone and its capacity to elevate cerebrospinal-fluid pressure may be markedly exaggerated in the presence of increased intracranial pressure. Furthermore, narcotics produce side effects that may obscure the clinical course of patients with head injuries. In such patients, methadone must be used with caution and only if it is deemed essential.

Asthma and Other Respiratory Conditions—Methadone should be used with caution in patients having an acute asthmatic attack, in those with chronic obstructive pulmonary disease or cor pulmonale, and in individuals with a substantially decreased respiratory reserve, preexisting respiratory depression, hypoxia, or hypercapnia. In such patients, even usual therapeutic doses of narcotics may decrease respiratory drive while simultaneously increasing airway resistance to the point of apnea.

Hypotensive Effect—The administration of methadone may result in severe hypotension in an individual whose ability to maintain his blood pressure has already been compromised by a depleted blood volume or concurrent administration of such drugs as the phenothiazines or certain anesthetics.

Use in Ambulatory Patients—Methadone may impair the mental and/or physical abilities required for the performance of potentially hazardous tasks, such as driving a car or operating machinery. The patient should be cautioned accordingly.

Methadone, like other narcotics, may produce orthostatic hypotension in ambulatory patients.

Use in Pregnancy—Safe use in pregnancy has not been established in relation to possible adverse effects on fetal development. Therefore, methadone should not be used in pregnant women unless, in the judgment of the physician, the potential benefits outweigh the possible hazards.

Precautions: *Interaction with Pentazocine*—Patients who are addicted to heroin or who are on the methadone maintenance program may experience withdrawal symptoms when given pentazocine.

Interaction with Rifampin—The concurrent administration of rifampin may possibly reduce the blood concentration of methadone to a degree sufficient to produce withdrawal symptoms. The mechanism by which rifampin may decrease blood concentrations of methadone is not fully understood, although enhanced microsomal drug-metabolized enzymes may influence drug disposition.

Acute Abdominal Conditions—The administration of methadone or other narcotics may obscure the diagnosis or clinical course in patients with acute abdominal conditions.

Interaction with Monoamine Oxidase (MAO) Inhibitors—Therapeutic doses of meperidine have precipitated severe reactions in patients concurrently receiving monoamine oxidase inhibitors or those who have received such agents within 14 days. Similar reactions thus far have not been reported with methadone; but if the use of methadone is necessary in such patients, a sensitivity test should be performed in which repeated small incremental doses are administered over the course of several hours while the patient's condition and vital signs are under careful observation.

Special-Risk Patients—Methadone should be given with caution and the initial dose should be reduced in certain patients, such as the elderly or debilitated and those with severe impairment of hepatic or renal function, hypothyroidism, Addison's disease, prostatic hypertrophy, or urethral stricture.

Adverse Reactions: *Heroin Withdrawal*—During the induction phase of methadone maintenance treatment, patients are being withdrawn from heroin and may therefore show typical withdrawal symptoms, which should be differentiated from methadone-induced side effects. They may exhibit some or all of the following symptoms associated with acute withdrawal from heroin or other opiates: lacrimation, rhinorrhea, sneezing, yawning, excessive perspiration, gooseflesh, fever, chilliness alternating with flushing, restlessness, irritability, "sleepy yen," weakness, anxiety, depression, dilated pupils, tremors, tachycardia, abdominal cramps, body aches, involuntary twitching and kicking movements, anorexia, nausea, vomiting, diarrhea, intestinal spasms, and weight loss.

Initial Administration—Initially, the dosage of methadone should be carefully titrated to the individual. Induction too rapid for the patient's sensitivity is more likely to produce the following effects.

THE MAJOR HAZARDS OF METHADONE, AS OF OTHER NARCOTIC ANALGESICS, ARE RESPIRATORY DEPRESSION AND, TO A LESSER DEGREE, CIRCULATORY DEPRESSION. RESPIRATORY ARREST, SHOCK, AND CARDIAC ARREST HAVE OCCURRED.

The most frequently observed adverse reactions include lightheadedness, dizziness, sedation, nausea, vomiting, and sweating. These effects seem to be more prominent in ambulatory patients and in those who are not suffering severe pain. In such individuals, lower doses are advisable. Some adverse reactions may be alleviated in the ambulatory patient if he lies down.

Other adverse reactions include the following:
Central Nervous System—Euphoria, dysphoria, weakness, headache, insomnia, agitation, disorientation, and visual disturbances.
Gastrointestinal—Dry mouth, anorexia, constipation, and biliary tract spasm.
Cardiovascular—Flushing of the face, bradycardia, palpitation, faintness, and syncope.
Genitourinary—Urinary retention or hesitancy, antidiuretic effect, and reduced libido and/or potency.
Allergic—Pruritus, urticaria, other skin rashes, edema, and, rarely, hemorrhagic urticaria.
Maintenance on a Stabilized Dose—During prolonged administration of methadone, as in a methadone maintenance treatment program, there is a gradual, yet progressive, disappearance of side effects over a period of several weeks. However, constipation and sweating often persist.

Dosage and Administration: *For Detoxification Treatment*—THE DRUG SHALL BE ADMINISTERED DAILY UNDER CLOSE SUPERVISION AS FOLLOWS:
A detoxification treatment course shall not exceed 21 days and may not be repeated earlier than four weeks after completion of the preceding course. In detoxification, the patient may receive methadone when there are significant symptoms of withdrawal. The dosage schedules indicated below are recommended but could be varied in accordance with clinical judgment. Initially, a single oral dose of 15 to 20 mg of methadone will often be sufficient to suppress withdrawal symptoms. Additional methadone may be provided if withdrawal symptoms are not suppressed or if symptoms reappear. When patients are physically dependent on high doses, it may be necessary to exceed these levels. Forty mg/day in single or divided doses will usually constitute an adequate stabilizing dosage level. Stabilization can be continued for two to three days, and then the amount of methadone normally will be gradually decreased. The rate at which methadone is decreased will be determined separately for each patient. The dose of methadone can be decreased on a daily basis or at two-day intervals, but the amount of intake shall always be sufficient to keep withdrawal symptoms at a tolerable level. In hospitalized patients, a daily reduction of 20 percent of the total daily dose may be tolerated and may cause little discomfort. In ambulatory patients, a somewhat slower schedule may be needed. If methadone is administered for more than three weeks, the procedure is considered to have progressed from detoxification or treatment of the acute withdrawal syndrome to maintenance treatment, even though the goal and intent may be eventual total withdrawal.

For Maintenance Treatment—In maintenance treatment, the initial dosage of methadone should control the abstinence symptoms that follow withdrawal of narcotic drugs but should not be so great as to cause sedation, respiratory depression, or other effects of acute intoxication. It is important that the initial dosage be adjusted on an individual basis to the narcotic tolerance of the new patient. If such a patient has been a heavy user of heroin up to the day of admission, he may be given 20 mg four to eight hours later or 40 mg in a single oral dose. If he enters treatment with little or no narcotic tolerance (e.g., if he has recently been released from jail or other confinement), the initial dosage may be one-half these quantities. When there is any doubt, the smaller dose should be used initially. The patient should then be kept under observation, and, if symptoms of abstinence are distressing, additional 10-mg doses may be administered as needed. Subsequently, the dosage should be adjusted individually, as tolerated and required, up to a level of 120 mg daily. The patient will initially ingest the drug under observation daily, or at least six days a week, for the first three months. After demonstrating satisfactory adherence to the program regulations for at least three months, the patient may be permitted to reduce to three times weekly the occasions when he must ingest the drug under observation. He shall receive no more than a two-day take-home supply. With continuing adherence to the program's requirements for at least two years, he may then be permitted twice-weekly visits to the program for drug ingestion under observation, with a three-day take-home supply. A daily dose of 120 mg or more shall be justified in the medical record. Prior approval from state authority and the Food and Drug Administration is required for any dose above 120 mg administered at the clinic and for any dose above 100 mg to be taken at home. A regular review of dosage level should be made by the responsible physician, with careful consideration given to reduction of dosage as indicated on an individual basis. A new dosage level is only a test level until stability is achieved.

Special Considerations for a Pregnant Patient—Caution shall be taken in the maintenance treatment of pregnant patients. Dosage levels shall be kept as low as possible if continued methadone treatment is deemed necessary. It is the responsibility of the program sponsor to assure that each female patient be fully informed concerning the possible risks to a pregnant woman or her unborn child from the use of methadone.

Special Limitations—
Treatment of Patients under Age 18
1. The safety and effectiveness of methadone for use in the treatment of adolescents have not been proved by adequate clinical study. Special procedures are therefore necessary to assure that patients under age 16 will not be admitted to a program and that patients between 16 and 18 years of age will be admitted to maintenance treatment only under limited conditions.
2. Patients between 16 and 18 years of age who were enrolled and under treatment in approved programs on December 15, 1972, may continue in maintenance treatment. No new patients between 16 and 18 years of age may be admitted to a maintenance treatment program after March 15, 1973, unless a parent, legal guardian, or responsible adult designated by the state authority completes and signs Form FD 2635, "Consent for Methadone Treatment."
Methadone treatment of new patients between the ages of 16 and 18 years will be permitted after December 15, 1972, only with a documented history of two or more unsuccessful attempts at detoxification and a documented history of dependence on heroin or other morphine-like drugs beginning two years or more prior to application for treatment. No patient under age 16 may be continued or started on methadone treatment after December 15, 1972, but these patients may be detoxified and retained in the program in a drug-free state for follow-up and aftercare.
3. Patients under age 18 who are not placed on maintenance treatment may be detoxified. Detoxification may not exceed three weeks. A repeat episode of detoxification may not be initiated until four weeks after the completion of the previous detoxification.

Overdosage: *Symptoms*—Serious overdosage of methadone is characterized by respiratory depression (a decrease in respiratory rate and/or tidal volume, Cheyne-Stokes respiration, cyanosis), extreme somnolence progressing to stupor or coma, maximally constricted pupils, skeletal-muscle flaccidity, cold and clammy skin, and, sometimes, bradycardia and hypotension. In severe overdosage, particularly by the intravenous route, apnea, circulatory collapse, cardiac arrest, and death may occur.
Treatment—Primary attention should be given to the reestablishment of adequate respiratory exchange through provision of a patent airway and institution of assisted or controlled ventilation. If a nontolerant person, especially a child, takes a large dose of methadone, effective narcotic antagonists are available to counteract the potentially lethal respiratory depression. **The physician must remember, however, that methadone is a long-acting depressant (36 to 48 hours), whereas the antagonists act for much shorter periods (one to three hours).** The patient must, therefore, be monitored continuously for recurrence of respiratory depression and treated repeatedly with the narcotic antagonist as needed. If the diagnosis is correct and respiratory depression is due only to overdosage of methadone, the use of respiratory stimulants is not indicated.
An antagonist should not be administered in the absence of clinically significant respiratory or cardiovascular depression. Intravenously administered narcotic antagonists (naloxone, nalorphine, and levallorphan) are the drugs of choice to reverse signs of intoxication. These agents should be given repeatedly until the patient's status remains satisfactory. The hazard that the narcotic antagonist will further depress respiration is less likely with the use of naloxone.
Oxygen, intravenous fluids, vasopressors, and other supportive measures should be employed as indicated.

NOTE: IN AN INDIVIDUAL PHYSICALLY DEPENDENT ON NARCOTICS, THE ADMINISTRATION OF THE USUAL DOSE OF A NARCOTIC ANTAGONIST WILL PRECIPITATE AN ACUTE WITHDRAWAL SYNDROME. THE SEVERITY OF THIS SYNDROME WILL DEPEND ON THE DEGREE OF PHYSICAL DEPENDENCE AND THE DOSE OF THE ANTAGONIST ADMINISTERED. THE USE OF A NARCOTIC ANTAGONIST IN SUCH A PERSON SHOULD BE AVOIDED IF POSSIBLE. IF IT MUST BE USED TO TREAT SERIOUS RESPIRATORY DEPRESSION IN THE PHYSICALLY DEPENDENT PATIENT, THE ANTAGONIST SHOULD BE ADMINISTERED WITH EXTREME CARE AND BY TITRATION WITH SMALLER THAN USUAL DOSES OF THE ANTAGONIST.

How Supplied: (Ⓒ) Diskets No. 1, Methadone Hydrochloride Tablets, USP, U53,* 40 mg, Peach-Colored (cross-scored), in bottles of 100 (NDC 0002-2153-02). [011184]
Shown in Product Identification Section, page 417

METUBINE® IODIDE ℞
[mĕ-tū' bĕn ī-ō-dīd]
(metocurine iodide)
Injection, USP

THIS DRUG SHOULD BE ADMINISTERED ONLY BY ADEQUATELY TRAINED INDIVIDUALS WHO ARE FAMILIAR WITH ITS ACTIONS, CHARACTERISTICS, AND HAZARDS.

Description: Metubine® Iodide (metocurine iodide, Lilly) is a nondepolarizing muscle relaxant and is presented as a sterile isotonic solution for intravenous injection.
Each ml contains 2 mg metocurine iodide and sodium chloride, 0.9 percent, with 0.5 percent phenol as a preservative. Sodium carbonate and/or hydrochloric acid may have been added during manufacture to adjust the pH in the range of 4 to 4.3.
The empirical formula is $C_{40}H_{48}I_2N_2O_6$, and the molecular weight is 906.64.
Clinical Pharmacology: Metubine® Iodide (metocurine iodide, Lilly) is a methyl analogue of tubocurarine which produces nondepolarizing (competitive) neuromuscular blockade at the myoneural junction. Recent animal studies suggest that Metubine Iodide does not produce the autonomic ganglionic blockade seen with other nondepolarizing muscle relaxants. Recent clinical findings suggest that Metubine Iodide reaches the neuromuscular junction more rapidly than does tubocurarine. After intravenous injection, there is rapid onset (one to four minutes) of muscle relaxation with maximum twitch inhibition (96 percent) in 1.5 to ten minutes. The maximum effect lasts 35 to 60 minutes. The time for recovery to 50 percent of control twitch response is in excess of three hours.
Following bolus injection of 0.05 mg/kg, the mean terminal half-life of Metubine Iodide was 3.6 hours (217 minutes). Approximately 50 percent of the

Continued on next page

* Identi-Code® symbol.

Lilly—Cont.

dose was excreted as unchanged drug in the urine over 48 hours, and 2 percent was excreted unchanged in the bile. Approximately 35 percent is protein bound, mainly to the beta and gamma globulins.

The use of repeated doses may be accompanied by a cumulative effect. The duration of action and degree of muscle relaxation may be altered by dehydration, body temperature changes, hypocalcemia, excess magnesium, or acid-base imbalance. Concurrently administered general anesthetics, certain antibiotics, and neuromuscular disease may potentiate the neuromuscular blocking action of Metubine Iodide.

Histamine release with Metubine Iodide occurs less frequently than d-tubocurarine and is related to dosage and rapidity of administration. Effects on the cardiovascular system (e.g., changes in pulse rate, hypotension) are less than those reported with equipotent doses of d-tubocurarine and gallamine.

Because the main excretory pathway for Metubine Iodide is through the kidneys, severe renal disease or conditions associated with poor renal perfusion (shock states) may result in prolonged neuromuscular blockade.

Following intravenous injection in the mother, placental transfer of Metubine Iodide occurs rapidly, and, after six minutes, the fetal plasma concentration is approximately one-tenth the maternal level.

Indications and Usage: Metubine® Iodide (metocurine iodide, Lilly) is indicated as an adjunct to anesthesia to induce skeletal-muscle relaxation. It may be employed to reduce the intensity of muscle contractions in pharmacologically or electrically induced convulsions. It may also be employed to facilitate the management of patients undergoing mechanical ventilation.

Contraindications: Metubine® Iodide (metocurine iodide, Lilly) is contraindicated in those persons with known hypersensitivity to the drug or to its iodide content.

Warnings: METUBINE® IODIDE (METOCURINE IODIDE, LILLY) SHOULD BE ADMINISTERED IN CAREFULLY ADJUSTED DOSES BY OR UNDER THE SUPERVISION OF EXPERIENCED CLINICIANS WHO ARE FAMILIAR WITH THE COMPLICATIONS WHICH MAY OCCUR WITH THE USE OF THIS DRUG. Metubine Iodide should not be administered unless facilities for intubation, artificial ventilation, oxygen therapy, and reversal agents are immediately available. The clinician must be prepared to assist or control respiration.

Metubine Iodide should be used with extreme caution in patients with myasthenia gravis. In such patients, a peripheral nerve stimulator may be valuable in assessing the effects of administration.

Precautions: *General Precautions*—Metubine® Iodide (metocurine iodide, Lilly) should be used with caution in patients with poor renal perfusion or severe renal disease (*see* Clinical Pharmacology).

Rapid administration of large doses of Metubine Iodide may produce changes in blood pressure or heart rate or signs of histamine release.

Metubine Iodide has no effect on consciousness, pain threshold, or cerebration; therefore, it should be used with adequate anesthesia.

Drug Interactions—Synergistic or antagonistic effects may result when depolarizing and nondepolarizing muscle relaxants are administered simultaneously or sequentially.

Parenteral administration of high doses of certain antibiotics may intensify or resemble the neuroblocking action of muscle relaxants. These include neomycin, streptomycin, bacitracin, kanamycin, gentamicin, dihydrostreptomycin, polymyxin B, colistin, sodium colistimethate, and tetracyclines. If muscle relaxants and antibiotics must be administered simultaneously, the patient should be observed closely for any unexpected prolongation of respiratory depression.

Certain general anesthetics have a synergistic action with neuromuscular blocking agents. Diethyl ether, halothane, and isoflurane potentiate the neuromuscular blocking action of other nondepolarizing agents and may be presumed to do so with Metubine Iodide.

Administration of quinidine shortly after recovery may produce recurrent paralysis.

The effect of diazepam on neuromuscular blockade by Metubine Iodide is not clear. Until more information is available, patients should be carefully monitored for unexpected drug response and prolongation of action.

The use of magnesium sulfate in preeclamptic patients potentiates the effects of both depolarizing and nondepolarizing muscle relaxants.

Usage in Pregnancy—Pregnancy Category C—Intrauterine growth retardation and limb deformities resembling clubfoot were produced by d-tubocurarine chloride and succinylcholine chloride when administered to the rat fetus between the sixteenth and nineteenth days of gestation or when injected in chick embryos from the fifth to the fifteenth day of incubation. When d-tubocurarine was injected intramuscularly into the interscapular region of the fetuses on the sixteenth to the nineteenth day of gestation, the incidence of growth retardation and limb deformity ranged from 21 to 23 percent and 7 to 8 percent respectively.

There are no adequate and well-controlled studies of Metubine Iodide in pregnant women. Metubine Iodide should be used during pregnancy only if the potential benefit justifies the risk to the fetus.

Labor and Delivery—It is not known whether the use of muscle relaxants during labor or delivery has immediate or delayed adverse effects on the fetus, prolongs the duration of labor, or increases the likelihood that forceps delivery, obstetric intervention, or resuscitation of the newborn will be necessary.

Nursing Mothers—It is not known whether Metubine Iodide is excreted in human milk. Because many drugs are excreted in human milk, caution should be excercised when Metubine Iodide is administered to a nursing woman.

Usage in Children—A clinical study has shown that Metubine Iodide is twice as potent as d-tubocurarine in children, but the rate of recovery is the same. There may be a slight increase in heart rate, but no change occurs in blood pressure or ECG. Doses calculated on the basis of body weight or body surface area may be applicable when the advantages of nondepolarizing neuromuscular blockade are desired.

Adverse Reactions: The most frequently noted adverse reaction is prolongation of the drug's pharmacologic action. Neuromuscular effects may range from skeletal-muscle weakness to a profound relaxation that produces respiratory insufficiency or apnea.

Possible adverse reactions include allergic or hypersensitivity reactions to the drug or its iodide content and histamine release when large doses are administered rapidly. Signs of histamine release include erythema, edema, flushing, tachycardia, arterial hypotension, bronchospasm, and circulatory collapse.

Prolonged apnea and respiratory depression have occurred following the use of muscle relaxants. Many physiologic factors, drug interactions, and individual sensitivities may contribute to the development of respiratory paralysis (*see* Clinical Pharmacology and Precautions).

Overdosage: An overdose of Metubine® Iodide (metocurine iodide, Lilly) may result in prolonged apnea, cardiovascular collapse, and sudden release of histamine.

Massive doses of metocurarine are not reversible by the antagonists edrophonium or neostigmine and atropine.

Overdosage may be avoided by the careful monitoring of response by means of a peripheral nerve stimulator.

The primary treatment for residual neuromuscular blockade with respiratory paralysis or inadequate ventilation is maintenance of the patient's airway and manual or mechanical ventilation. Accompanying derangements of blood pressure, electrolyte imbalance, or circulating blood volume should be determined and corrected by appropriate fluid and electrolyte therapy.

Residual neuromuscular blockade following surgery may be reversed by the use of anticholinesterase inhibitors such as neostigmine or pyridostigmine bromide and atropine. Prescribing information should be consulted for the appropriate drug selection based on dosage and desired duration of action.

Dosage and Administration: Metubine® Iodide (metocurine iodide, Lilly) should be administered intravenously as a sustained injection over a period of 30 to 60 seconds. INTRAMUSCULAR ADMINISTRATION OF METUBINE IODIDE IS NOT RECOMMENDED. Care must be taken to avoid overdosage. The use of a peripheral nerve stimulator to monitor response will minimize the risk of overdosage. The type of anesthetic used and nature of the surgical procedure will influence the amount of Metubine Iodide required. Doses of 0.2 to 0.4 mg/kg have been found satisfactory for endotracheal intubation. Relaxation following the initial dose may be expected to be effective for periods of 25 to 90 minutes, with an average of approximately 60 minutes. Supplemental administration may be made as indicated to provide needed surgical relaxation. Supplemental doses average 0.5 to 1 mg. The use of strong anesthetics that potentiate the effect of neuromuscular blocking drugs such as halothane, diethyl ether, isoflurane, or enflurane reduces the requirement for Metubine Iodide. Incremental doses should be reduced by approximately one-third to one-half.

Recommended Doses for Use during Electroshock Therapy—Doses required for satisfactory relaxation range from 1.75 to 5.5 mg. When the patient is treated for the first time, the drug is administered slowly by the intravenous route as a sustained injection until a head-drop response ensues. After dosage has been established, subsequent injections are completed in 15 to 50 seconds. The average dose ranges from 2 to 3 mg.

Drug Incompatibilities—Metubine Iodide is unstable in alkaline solutions. When it is combined with barbiturate solutions, precipitation may occur. Solutions of barbiturates, meperidine, and morphine sulfate should not be administered from the same syringe.

How Supplied: (℞) Vials (Multiple Dose) No. 586, *Metubine® Iodide (Metocurine Iodide Injection, USP)*, 2 mg/ml, 20 ml, rubber-stoppered, in singles (10/carton) (NDC 0002-1421-01). Store at controlled room temperature, 59° to 86°F (15° to 30°C).

[032984]

MOXAM®   ℞
[*mŏks'ăm*]
(moxalactam disodium)

Description: Moxam® (moxalactam disodium, Lilly) is a semisynthetic broad-spectrum β-lactam antibiotic for parenteral administration. It is the disodium salt of (6R, 7R)-7-[[(carboxy (4-hydroxyphenyl) acetyl] amino] -7-methoxy-3-[[(1-methyl-1H -tetrazol-5-yl)thio] methyl]-8-oxo-5-oxa-1-azabicyclo[4.2.0] oct-2- ene-2-carboxylic acid.

Moxam is a sterile dry powder which contains 150 mg mannitol/g of moxalactam activity. The total sodium content is approximately 88 mg (3.8 mEq sodium ion)/g of moxalactam activity. Sodium bicarbonate and/or sodium hydroxide may have been added during manufacture for neutralization. The pH of freshly reconstituted solutions usually ranges from 5.5 to 6.5.

Clinical Pharmacology: After rapid intravenous infusion (two minutes) of 500-mg and 1-g doses of moxalactam in normal adult volunteers, mean peak serum levels of 57 mcg/ml and 94 mcg/ml respectively were achieved.

Average serum concentrations following intravenous doses of 0.25, 0.5, 1, 2, 3, and 4 g infused over a 20-minute period in adult volunteers are listed in Table 1. Intravenous administration of 4-g doses every eight hours for seven doses produced no evidence of accumulation in the serum. The half-life after an intravenous dose is approximately 1.9 hours (114 minutes).

TABLE 1. MOXALACTAM SERUM LEVELS IN ADULTS (MCG/ML)

IV Dose	20 Minutes*	4 Hours*	8 Hours*
0.25 g	24	4	1
0.5 g	48	7	2
1 g	101	13	3
2 g	204	31	8
3 g	262	40	9
4 g	443	61	13

* Time after beginning of infusion.

Following intramuscular administration of 250-mg, 500-mg, and 1-g doses of moxalactam to normal adult volunteers, the mean peak serum concentrations were 10, 16, and 27 mcg/ml respectively. These peaks occurred at 60 to 120 minutes. After intramuscular administration, the half-life is approximately 2.1 hours (126 minutes).

Sixty to 90 percent of an intramuscular or intravenous dose is excreted by the kidneys over a 24-hour period, which results in high urinary concentrations. No metabolite of moxalactam has been detected in the urine. Following intravenous doses of 250 mg, 500 mg, 1 g, and 2 g, urinary concentrations were highest during the first two hours and were 170, 446, 1820, and 4220 mcg/ml respectively. These levels decreased at ten to 12 hours to 14, 59, 96, and 156 mcg/ml respectively.

The mean renal clearance of moxalactam was approximately 78 ml/min, with a calculated mean total body clearance of 99.3 ml/min for a man weighing 70 kg.

In patients with reduced renal function, the serum half-life of moxalactam is significantly prolonged. Although serum concentrations in patients with normal renal function declined to 0 within 24 to 48 hours after a 1-g intravenous dose, serum concentrations in patients with severe renal impairment were approximately 25 and 10 percent of peak levels at 24 and 48 hours respectively.

Therapeutic levels of moxalactam are achieved in the following fluids: pleural fluid, interstitial fluid, aqueous humor, and the cerebrospinal fluid of patients with normal and inflamed meninges.

Microbiology—The bactericidal activity of moxalactam results from inhibition of cell-wall synthesis. Moxalactam has in vitro activity against a wide range of gram-negative and certain gram-positive organisms. Moxalactam has a high degree of stability in the presence of β-lactamases, both penicillinases and cephalosporinases produced by gram-negative and gram-positive bacteria. Because of its unique chemical structure, moxalactam is also a potent inhibitor of β-lactamases from certain gram-negative bacteria, e.g., *Enterobacter cloacae* and *Pseudomonas aeruginosa*. Moxalactam is usually active against the following microorganisms in vitro and in clinical infections (see Indications and Usage).

Aerobes, gram-negative: *Haemophilus influenzae*, including ampicillin-resistant strains; *Escherichia coli*; *Klebsiella* species, including *Klebsiella pneumoniae*; *Proteus mirabilis*; *P. vulgaris*; *Providencia rettgeri* (formerly *Proteus rettgeri*); *Morganella morganii* (formerly *Proteus morganii*); *Enterobacter* species; *P. aeruginosa* (some strains are resistant); *Serratia* species.

Note.: Many strains of the above organisms that are multiply resistant to other antibiotics, e.g., penicillins, cephalosporins, and aminoglycosides, are susceptible to moxalactam.

Aerobes, gram-positive: staphylococci, including penicillinase-producing strains (*Note:* Methicillin-resistant staphylococci as well as some strains of *Staphylococcus epidermidis* are resistant to moxalactam); *Streptococcus pyogenes* (group A β-hemolytic streptococci); *S. agalactiae* (group B streptococci); *S. pneumoniae* (formerly *Diplococcus pneumoniae*) (*Note:* Most strains of enterococci, e.g., *S. faecalis*, are resistant).

Anaerobes: *Bacteroides* species, including *Bacteroides fragilis*; *Fusobacterium* species; *Clostridium* species (*Note:* Most strains of *Clostridium difficile* are resistant); *Eubacterium* species; *Peptococcus* species; *Peptostreptococcus* species; *Veillonella* species.

Moxalactam also demonstrates in vitro activity against the following microorganisms, although its clinical significance is unknown: *Neisseria gonorrhoeae*; *N. meningitidis*; *Providencia* species; *Salmonella* species, including *Salmonella typhi*; *Shigella* species.

Moxalactam is highly resistant to hydrolysis by β-lactamases of Richmond Types I, II, III, IV, and V. These enzymes are frequently produced by strains of *Enterobacteriaceae*, *P. aeruginosa*, *Acinetobacter* species, *H. influenzae*, and *Neisseria* species. Furthermore, moxalactam is stable to some β-lactamases not classified as Richmond types, such as those produced by strains of *S. aureus* and *B. fragilis*.

Moxalactam and aminoglycosides have been shown to be synergistic in vitro against some strains of *Enterobacteriaceae* and *P. aeruginosa*.

Disc Susceptibility Tests—Quantitative methods that require measurement of zone diameters give the most precise estimate of antibiotic susceptibility. One such procedure[1] has been recommended for use with discs to test suceptibility to moxalactam.

Reports from the laboratory giving results of the standard single-disc susceptibility test with a 30-mcg moxalactam disc should be interpreted according to the following criteria:

Susceptible organisms produce zones of 20 mm or greater, indicating that the test organism is likely to respond to therapy.

Organisms that produce zones of 15 to 19 mm are expected to be susceptible if high dosage is used or if the infection is confined to tissues and fluids (e.g., urine) in which high antibiotic levels are attained.

Resistant organisms produce zones of 14 mm or less, indicating that other therapy should be selected.

Organisms should be tested with the moxalactam disc, since moxalactam has been shown by in vitro tests to be active against certain strains found resistant when other β-lactam discs are used.

In other susceptibility testing procedures, e.g., ICS agar dilution[2] or the equivalent, a bacterial isolate may be considered susceptible if the MIC value for moxalactam is not more than 16 mcg/ml. Organisms are considered resistant to moxalactam if the MIC is equal to or greater than 64 mcg/ml. Organisms having an MIC value of less than 64 mcg/ml but greater than 16 mcg/ml are expected to be susceptible if high dosage is used or if the infection is confined to tissues and fluids (e.g., urine) in which high antibiotic levels are attained.

Indications and Usage: Moxam® (moxalactam disodium, Lilly) is indicated for the treatment of infections caused by susceptible strains of the designated microorganisms in the diseases listed below:

Lower respiratory infections, including pneumonia, caused by *S. pneumoniae*, *H. influenzae*, *Klebsiella* species, *Enterobacter* species, *S. aureus* (penicillin-sensitive and penicillin-resistant strains), *E. coli*, and *P. mirabilis*.

Urinary tract infections caused by *E. coli*, *Klebsiella* species, *Enterobacter* species, *Proteus* species (indole-positive and indole-negative), and *Serratia* species.

Intra-abdominal infections, such as peritonitis, endometritis, and pelvic cellulitis, caused by *E. coli*; *Peptostreptococcus* species; *Bacteroides* species, including *B. fragilis*, mixed aerobic and anaerobic organisms, such as *K. pneumoniae*, *S. agalactiae* (group B streptococci), *P. mirabilis*, *Enterobacter* species, *P. aeruginosa*, *Peptococcus* species, *Clostridium* species, *Fusobacterium* species, and *Eubacterium* species.

Bacterial septicemia caused by *S. aureus*, *E. coli*, *S. pneumoniae*, *Klebsiella* species, *Serratia* species, *Pseudomonas* species, and *B. fragilis*.

Central-nervous-system infections, e.g., meningitis and ventriculitis, caused by *E. coli* and *Klebsiella* species. Moxam has been used successfully in the treatment of a limited number of patients with meningitis and ventriculitis caused by other *Enterobacteriaceae* and *H. influenzae*.

Skin and skin-structure infections caused by *S. aureus* (penicillinase and non-penicillinase-producing); *S. pyogenes* (group A β-hemolytic streptococci); *E. coli*; *Serratia* species; mixed aerobic and anaerobic organisms, such as *Proteus* species, *Klebsiella* species, *Enterobacter* species, *Peptococcus* species, *Peptostreptococcus* species, *Bacteroides* species, and *Clostridium* species.

Bone and joint infections caused by *S. aureus* (penicillinase and non-penicillinase-producing), *P. aeruginosa*, and *Serratia* species.

Because of the serious nature of infections due to *P. aeruginosa* and because many strains of *Pseudomonas* species are moderately susceptible to moxalactam, higher dosage is recommended in serious systemic infections caused by this organism (see Dosage and Administration). Moxam has been used successfully in the treatment of some patients with serious lower-respiratory tract infections caused by *P. aeruginosa* and *Serratia* species. In such cases, higher dosage is recommended, and other therapy should be instituted if the response is not prompt.

Moxam has been used successfully in surgical infections in cases where concomitant therapy with other antibiotics may be used.

Specimens for bacteriologic cultures should be obtained in order to isolate and identify causative organisms and to determine their susceptibilities to moxalactam. Therapy may be instituted before results of susceptibility studies are known; however, once these results become available, the antibiotic treatment should be adjusted accordingly.

In certain cases of confirmed or suspected gram-positive or gram-negative sepsis or in patients with other serious infections in which the causative organism has not been identified, Moxam may be used concomitantly with an aminoglycoside. The dosage recommended in the labeling of both antibiotics may be given and depends on the severity of the infection and the patient's condition. Renal function should be carefully monitored, especially if higher dosages of the aminoglycosides are to be administered or if therapy is prolonged, because of the potential nephrotoxicity and ototoxicity of aminoglycosidic antibiotics. Some β-lactam antibiotics also have a certain degree of nephrotoxicity. Although, to date, this has not been noted when Moxam was given alone, it is possible that nephrotoxicity may be potentiated if Moxam is used concomitantly with an aminoglycoside.

Contraindication: Moxam® (moxalactam disodium, Lilly) is contraindicated in patients with known allergy to the drug.

Warnings

Moxalactam can interfere with hemostasis through three different mechanisms: hypoprothrombinemia, platelet dysfunction, and very rarely, immune-mediated thrombocytopenia. Bleeding can be associated with these induced abnormalities. A total of 2.5 percent of clinical trial patients treated for four or more days experienced a bleeding event, most of which were serious.

Bleeding associated with hypoprothrombinemia can be prevented by the use of vitamin K. It is recommended that patients who receive moxalactam be given 10 mg of vitamin K per week prophylactically. The inhibition of platelet function, which may be accompanied by a prolonged bleeding time, is dose-dependent and can generally be avoided by limiting dosage to 4 g per day. It is recommended that the bleeding time be monitored in patients with normal renal function who receive more than 4 g of moxalactam per day for more than three days. All patients with significantly impaired renal function should have appropriate dosage reduction (see Dosage and Administration) and should be monitored periodically with bleeding times. If the bleeding

Continued on next page

* Identi-Code® symbol.

Lilly—Cont.

time becomes unduly prolonged, moxalactam should be discontinued.

If bleeding occurs in a patient receiving moxalactam and if the prothrombin time is prolonged, vitamin K should be given. Administration of fresh frozen plasma, packed red cells, and platelet concentrates may be indicated. Moxalactam should be discontinued if bleeding is due to platelet dysfunction. If moxalactam is discontinued because of platelet dysfunction, other beta-lactam antibiotics that are known to be associated with this phenomenon should be used with caution. See current prescribing information for alternative therapy.

Bleeding during moxalactam therapy may also be related to complications of underlying diseases (e.g., sepsis, malignancy, renal and hepatic dysfunction) or may result from the combined effects of underlying diseases and moxalactam therapy. When bleeding occurs, it is important to rule out disseminated intravascular coagulation (DIC) through appropriate laboratory tests since DIC occurs frequently in patients with sepsis, malignancy, or hepatic disease.

Hepatic and renal dysfunction, poor alimentation, thrombocytopenia, and the concomitant use of "high dose" heparin (more than 20,000 units/day), oral anticoagulants, and other drugs that affect hemostasis (e.g., aspirin) are factors that may increase the risk of bleeding during moxalactam therapy.

BEFORE THERAPY WITH MOXAM® (MOXALACTAM DISODIUM, LILLY) IS INSTITUTED, CAREFUL INQUIRY SHOULD BE MADE FOR A HISTORY OF HYPERSENSITIVITY REACTIONS TO MOXALACTAM DISODIUM, CEPHALOSPORINS, PENICILLINS, OR OTHER DRUGS. THIS PRODUCT SHOULD BE GIVEN WITH CAUTION TO PATIENTS WITH TYPE 1 HYPERSENSITIVITY REACTIONS TO PENICILLIN. ANTIBIOTICS SHOULD BE GIVEN WITH CAUTION TO ANY PATIENT WHO HAS HAD SOME FORM OF ALLERGY, PARTICULARLY TO DRUGS. IF AN ALLERGIC REACTION TO MOXALACTAM OCCURS, DISCONTINUE THE DRUG. SERIOUS HYPERSENSITIVITY REACTIONS MAY REQUIRE EPINEPHRINE AND OTHER EMERGENCY MEASURES.

Pseudomembranous colitis has been reported with virtually all broad-spectrum antibiotics (including macrolides, semisynthetic penicillins, and cephalosporins); therefore, it is important to consider its diagnosis in patients who develop diarrhea in association with the use of antibiotics. Such colitis may range in severity from mild to life-threatening. Treatment with broad-spectrum antibiotics alters the normal flora of the colon and may permit overgrowth of clostridia. Studies indicate that a toxin produced by *Clostridium difficile* is one primary cause of antibiotic-associated colitis.

Mild cases of pseudomembranous colitis usually respond to drug discontinuance alone. In moderate to severe cases, management should include sigmoidoscopy, appropriate bacteriologic studies, and fluid, electrolyte, and protein supplementation. When the colitis does not improve after the drug has been discontinued, or when it is severe, oral vancomycin is the drug of choice for antibiotic-associated pseudomembranous colitis produced by *C. difficile*. Other causes of colitis should be ruled out.

Precautions: A disulfiram-like reaction, i.e., nausea, vomiting, and vasomotor instability with hypotension and peripheral vasodilatation, has occurred following the ingestion of ethanol. The timing of the ingestion of alcohol is an important factor. When alcohol was ingested prior to the first dose of Moxam® (moxalactam disodium, Lilly), this syndrome was not observed. It has been reported only when ethanol ingestion followed the administration of Moxam. This has been observed as late as 48 hours after the last dose of Moxam. Moxalactam inhibits the enzyme acetaldehyde dehydrogenase in laboratory animals. This causes accumulation of acetaldehyde when ethanol is administered concomitantly.

Prolonged use of Moxam may result in the overgrowth of nonsusceptible organisms (e.g., enterococci). Careful observation of the patient is essential. If superinfection occurs during therapy, appropriate measures should be taken.

Broad-spectrum antibiotics should be prescribed with caution in individuals with a history of gastrointestinal disease, particularly colitis.

Usage in Pregnancy—Pregnancy Category C—Reproduction studies have been performed in mice, rats, rabbits, and ferrets. Administration of Moxam at ten to 20 times the usual human dose has resulted in an increased incidence of birth defects or embryotoxicity in the ferret. Since the incidence of birth defects and embryotoxicity in control ferrets was high and variable, its significance in ferrets after the administration of Moxam is unknown. Studies in mice and rats at doses up to 20 times the usual human dose (eight times the maximum dose) have revealed no evidence of impaired fertility or teratogenicity. A decrease in offspring viability was noted in rats, perhaps due to drug-related growth depression and decrease in food consumption by the pregnant dams. There are no adequate and well-controlled studies in pregnant women. Moxam should be used during pregnancy only if the potential benefit justifies the potential risk to the fetus.

Nursing Mothers—It is not known whether this drug is excreted in human milk. Studies have shown that it is excreted in the milk of rats. Because many drugs are excreted in human milk, caution should be exercised when Moxam is administered to a nursing woman.

Adverse Reactions: In clinical studies, adverse effects considered related to moxalactam therapy or of uncertain etiology are listed below:

Hematopoietic abnormalities, half of which were of uncertain etiology, occurred in about 5 percent of patients and included eosinophilia (1 in 35), disturbances in vitamin K-dependent clotting function (decreased prothrombin), increased bleeding time, thrombocytopenia (1 in 276) (*see* Precautions), and reversible leukopenia (1 in 145). Reversible neutropenia has been reported in children who were three years of age or younger (1 in 23).

Local effects were reported in less than 4 percent of patients and included pain at the site of injection (1 in 70) and phlebitis (1 in 50).

Hypersensitivity reactions were reported in about 3 percent of patients and included morbilliform eruptions (1 in 60), fever (1 in 155), and positive Coombs' test (1 in 180). Two-thirds of the occurrences were considered related to therapy. Anaphylaxis occurred in one patient.

Gastrointestinal symptoms occurred in less than 3 percent of patients, the most frequent being diarrhea (1 in 60).

Symptoms of pseudomembranous colitis may appear either during or after antibiotic treatment. Nausea and vomiting have been reported rarely.

Hepatic enzyme elevations (SGOT, SGPT, alkaline phosphatase) occurred in about 1 in 25 patients. Ninety percent of the abnormalities were of uncertain etiology.

Causal Relationship Uncertain—Although of uncertain etiology, the following transient abnormalities in clinical laboratory renal function test results are listed to serve as alerting information for the physician:

Elevated BUN (1 in 150), pyuria and hematuria (1 of each in 250), and elevated serum creatinine (1 in 300).

Dosage and Administration: *Dosage: Adults*—The usual daily dose of Moxam® (moxalactam disodium, Lilly) is 2 to 4 g administered in divided doses every eight to 12 hours for five to ten days or up to 14 days. Most mild to moderate infections can be expected to respond to a dosage of 500 mg to 2 g every 12 hours.

In mild skin and skin-structure infections and in uncomplicated pneumonia, a dosage of 500 mg every eight hours is recommended.

In mild, uncomplicated urinary tract infections, a dosage of 250 mg every 12 hours is adequate. In urinary tract infections that are more difficult to treat, a dosage of 500 mg every 12 hours may be needed. In serious urinary tract infections, the dosage frequency may be increased to every eight hours.

In life-threatening infections or infections due to less susceptible organisms (e.g., *P. aeruginosa*), doses up to 4 g every eight hours (i.e., 12 g/day) may be needed. It is recommended that the bleeding time should be monitored in patients who receive more than 4 g of moxalactam/day for more than three days.

Prophylactic vitamin K, 10 mg/week, should be given to patients treated with Moxam.

Neonates, Infants, and Children—The following dosage schedule is recommended:

PEDIATRIC DOSAGE SCHEDULE

Neonates
- 0–1 week of age 50 mg/kg q. 12 h.
- 1–4 weeks of age 50 mg/kg q. 8 h.

Infants 50 mg/kg q. 8 h.
Children 50 mg/kg q. 6 h. or q. 8 h.

This may be increased to a total daily dose of 200 mg/kg (not to exceed the maximum adult dose) for serious infections.

In pediatric gram-negative meningitis, an initial loading dose of 100 mg/kg is recommended prior to the utilization of the above dosage schedule.

Impaired Renal Function—When renal function is impaired, a reduced dose must be employed and the serum levels closely monitored. After an intial dose of 1 to 2 g (depending on the severity of the infection), a maintenance dosage schedule should be followed. Continued dosage should be determined by the degree of renal impairment, the severity of infection, and the susceptibility of the causative organism.

When only serum creatinine is available, the following formula (based on sex, weight, and age of the patient) may be used to convert this value into creatinine clearance. The serum creatinine should represent a steady state of renal function.

$$\frac{\text{Weight (kg)} \times (140 - \text{age})}{\text{serum creatinine}}$$

Males: $72 \times$ serum creatinine
Females: $0.9 \times$ male value

[See table on top next page].

The serum half-life of moxalactam during hemodialysis has ranged from two to five hours. Maintenance doses of Moxam should be repeated following regular hemodialysis.

Administration: Moxam® (moxalactam disodium, Lilly) may be given intravenously or by deep intramuscular injection into a large muscle mass (such as the upper outer quadrant of the gluteus maximus or lateral part of the thigh).

Intramuscular Administration—Moxam should be diluted with one of the following diluents according to the table below: Sterile Water for Injection, Bacteriostatic Water for Injection, 0.9% Sodium Chloride Injection, Bacteriostatic Sodium Chloride Injection, or 0.5% or 1% Lidocaine Hydrochloride Injection.

[See table on bottom next page].

Individual IM doses of 2 g or more of Moxam at one site are not recommended.

Intravenous Administration—The intravenous route may be preferable for patients with bacterial septicemia, localized parenchymal abscesses (such as intra-abdominal abscess), peritonitis, meningitis, or other severe or life-threatening infections. In those with normal renal function, the intravenous dosage for such infections is 3 to 12 g of Moxam daily. In conditions such as septicemia, 6 to 12 g/day may be given initially by the intravenous route for several days, and the dosage may then be gradually reduced according to clinical response and laboratory findings.

A solution of 1 g of Moxam in 20 ml of Sterile Water for Injection is isotonic.

Solutions of Moxam, like those of most β-lactam antibiotics should not be added directly to aminoglycoside solutions (e.g., tobramycin sulfate, gentamicin sulfate, amikacin sulfate) because of potential interaction. However, Moxam and aminoglycosides may be administered sequentially by intermittent intravenous infusion to the same patient. After the administration of one of the two drugs, flush the tubing with an approved diluent and then administer the other drug solution.

For direct intermittent intravenous administration, add 10 ml of Sterile Water for Injection, 5% Dextrose Injection, or 0.9% Sodium Chloride Injection/g of moxalactam. Slowly inject directly into the vein over a period of three to five minutes or give through the tubing of an administration set while the patient is also receiving one of the approved *intravenous* diluents outlined in the Compatibility and Stability section.

Intravenous solutions containing alcohol should be avoided (*see* Precautions).

Intermittent intravenous infusion with a Y-type administration set or volume control set can also be accomplished while any of the approved intravenous fluids are being infused. However, during infusion of the solution containing Moxam, it is desirable to discontinue the other solution. When this technique is employed, careful attention should be paid to the volume of the solution containing moxalactam so that the calculated dose will be infused. When a Y-tube hookup is used, 50 to 100 ml of an appropriate intravenous diluent should be added to the 1 or 2-g piggyback (100-ml) vial. If Sterile Water for Injection is used as the diluent, reconstitute with approximately 20 ml to avoid a hypotonic solution.

For continuous intravenous infusion, each g of moxalactam should be diluted with 10 ml of Sterile Water for Injection. An appropriate quantity of the resulting solution may be added to an IV bottle containing one of the approved intravenous diluents outlined below under Compatibility and Stability.

Compatibility and Stability: *Intramuscular*—One g of Moxam® (moxalactam disodium, Lilly) reconstituted with 3 ml of Sterile Water for Injection, Bacteriostatic Water for Injection, 0.9% Sodium Chloride Injection, Bacteriostatic Sodium Chloride Injection, or 0.5% or 1% Lidocaine Hydrochloride Injection (without epinephrine) maintains satisfactory potency for 24 hours at room temperature (25°C) or for 96 hours under refrigeration (5°C) when stored in the original glass containers.

One g of Moxam reconstituted with 3 ml of Sterile Water for Injection, 0.9% Sodium Chloride Injection, or 5% Dextrose Injection maintains potency for at least six months in the frozen state at −20°C when stored in the original glass containers.

Intravenous—The following diluents as constituted with Moxam to 1 g with 50 ml maintain potency for 24 hours at room temperature (25°C) or 96 hours under refrigeration (5°C) when stored in the original glass container: 5% Dextrose Injection, 10% Dextrose Injection, 0.9% Sodium Chloride Injection, 5% Dextrose and 0.2% Sodium Chloride Injection, 5% Dextrose and 0.45% Sodium Chloride Injection, 5% Dextrose and 0.9% Sodium Chloride Injection, Ringer's Injection, Lactated Ringer's Injection, Lactated Ringer's and 5% Dextrose Injection, Acetated Ringer's Injection, 5% Dextrose and 0.15% (20 mEq/L) Potassium Chloride Injection, 5% Dextrose and 0.2% Sodium Bicarbonate Injection, 10% Fructose Injection, Sodium Lactate Injection (M/6 Sodium Lactate), Plasma-Lyte® M in 5% Dextrose Injection, 5% Osmitrol® in Water for Injection, 6% Gentran® 75 Injection and 10% Travert®, Normosol®-M in D5-W Injection, and Ionosol®-B in D5-W Injection.

The following diluents as constituted with Moxam to 1 g with 50 ml and stored in Viaflex® intravenous containers maintain potency for 24 hours at room temperature (25°C) or 96 hours under refrigeration: 5% Dextrose Injection, 0.9% Sodium Chloride Injection, and Lactated Ringer's and 5% Dextrose Injection.

MOXAM® (MOXALACTAM DISODIUM)— MAINTENANCE DOSAGE GUIDE FOR PATIENTS WITH RENAL IMPAIRMENT

Creatinine Clearance (ml/min/1.73 m^2)	Renal Function	Life-Threatening Infections— Maximum Dosage	Less Severe Infections
>80	Normal	4 g q. 8 h.	0.5–2 g q. 8–12 h.
50–80	Mild Impairment	3 g q. 8 h.	0.5–1 g q. 8 h.
25–50	Moderate Impairment	2 g q. 8 h. OR 3 g q. 12 h.	0.25–1 g q. 12 h.
2–25	Severe Impairment	1 g q. 8 h. OR 1.25 g q. 12 h.	0.25–0.5 g q. 8 h.
<2	0	1 g q. 24 h.	0.25–0.5 g q. 12 h.

One g of Moxam reconstituted with 50 ml 5% Dextrose Injection or 0.9% Sodium Chloride Injection maintains potency for at least six months when stored in the frozen state at −20°C in either the original glass or Viaflex plastic containers.

Note: After the reconstitution periods mentioned above, any unused solutions or frozen material should be discarded. Do not refreeze.

Moxam in the dry state should be stored below 78°F (26°C). The dry material as well as solutions tend to darken with age, depending on storage conditions. Product potency, however, is not adversely affected.

How Supplied: (℞) *Vials Moxam® (moxalactam disodium, Lilly): No. 7152,* 1 g (equivalent to moxalactam activity), 10-ml size (NDC 0002-7152-10), and *No. 7154,* 2 g (equivalent to moxalactam activity), 20-ml size (NDC 0002-7154-10), in Traypak™ (multivial carton, Lilly) of 10; *No. 7162,* 10 g (equivalent to moxalactam activity), 100-ml size (NDC 0002-7162-16), in Traypak of 6.

[071483]

1. *Am. J. Clin. Pathol., 45:* 493, 1966; Federal Register, *39:* 19182–19184, 1974.
2. Ericsson, H. M., and Sherris, J. C.: Acta Pathol. Microbiol. Scand. [B], Supplement No. 217, 1971.

MULTICEBRIN®   OTC
[mŭl-tĭ-sē′ brĭn]
(pan-vitamins)

Description: Each tablet contains—
Thiamine (Vitamin B$_1$)..................3 mg
Riboflavin (Vitamin B$_2$)..................3 mg
Pyridoxine (Vitamin B$_6$)..................1.2 mg
Pantothenic Acid..............................5 mg
Niacinamide....................................25 mg
Vitamin B$_{12}$ (Activity Equivalent)...........3 mcg
Ascorbic Acid (Vitamin C)...............75 mg
dl-Alpha Tocopheryl Acetate
(Vitamin E)................................6.6 IU (6.6 mg)
Vitamin A......................................10,000 IU (3 mg)
Vitamin D......................................400 IU (10 mcg)

Indications: One tablet supplies the optimum requirements of six essential vitamins and significant amounts of other important factors for which optimum requirements have not been established. Tablets Multicebrin are indicated in the prophylaxis or treatment of multiple vitamin deficiencies, in patients on restricted diets, in pregnancy, in wasting diseases, and in any situation characterized by improper food intake, utilization, or absorption.

Dosage: 1 tablet a day, or as directed by the physician.

How Supplied: *Tablets No. 100, Multicebrin® (pan-vitamins, Lilly), C71,** Coated, Red, in bottles of 100 (NDC 0002-0371-02) and in 10 strips of 10 individually labeled blisters each containing 1 tablet (ID100) (NDC 0002-0371-33).   [082384]

ONCOVIN®   ℞
[ŏn′ kō-vĭn]
(vincristine sulfate injection)
Solution

Description: Oncovin® (vincristine sulfate, Lilly) is the salt of an alkaloid obtained from a common flowering herb, the periwinkle plant (*Vinca rosea* Linn.). Originally known as leurocristine, it has also been referred to as LCR and VCR. The empirical formula for vincristine sulfate is $C_{46}H_{56}N_4O_{10} \cdot H_2SO_4$.

Each ml contains vincristine sulfate, 1 mg; mannitol, 100 mg; methylparaben, 1.3 mg; propylparaben, 0.2 mg; water for injection, q.s. Acetic acid and sodium acetate have been added for *p*H control. The *p*H of Oncovin Solution ranges from 3.5 to 5.5.

Action: The mode of action of Oncovin® (vincristine sulfate, Lilly) is unknown but is under investigation. Treatment of neoplastic cells in vitro with Oncovin demonstrated that it may cause an arrest of mitotic division at the stage of metaphase.

Central-nervous-system leukemia has been reported in patients undergoing otherwise successful therapy with Oncovin. This suggests that Oncovin does not penetrate well into the cerebrospinal fluid.

Indications: Oncovin® (vincristine sulfate, Lilly) is indicated in acute leukemia.

It has also been shown to be useful in combination with other oncolytic agents in Hodgkin's disease, lymphosarcoma, reticulum-cell sarcoma, rhabdomyosarcoma, neuroblastoma, and Wilms' tumor.

Contraindications: There are no contraindications to the use of Oncovin® (vincristine sulfate, Lilly), but careful attention should be given to those conditions listed under Warnings and Precautions.

Warnings: This preparation is for intravenous use only. The intrathecal administration of Oncovin® (vincristine sulfate, Lilly) is uniformly fatal.

Since reproduction studies have not been performed in animals, there is insufficient information as to whether this drug may affect fertility in men and women or have teratogenic or other adverse effects on the fetus. The physician should weigh the benefits in relation to the risks when using this and other chemotherapeutic agents in populations in which reproduction may be a factor.

Precautions: Acute uric acid nephropathy, which may occur after the administration of oncolytic agents, has also been reported with Oncovin® (vincristine sulfate, Lilly). In the presence of

Continued on next page

IM Dilution Table

Vial Size	Volume Diluent to Be Added (ml)	Approximate Available Volume (ml)	Approximate Average Concentration (mg/ml)
1 g	3	3.7	270

Shake well until dissolved.

* Identi-Code® symbol.

Lilly—Cont.

leukopenia or a complicating infection, administration of the next dose of Oncovin warrants careful consideration.

If central-nervous-system leukemia is diagnosed, additional agents may be required, since Oncovin does not appear to cross the blood-brain barrier in adequate amounts.

Particular attention should be given to dosage and neurologic side effects if Oncovin is administered to patients with preexisting neuromuscular disease and also when other drugs with neurotoxic potential are being used.

Acute shortness of breath and severe bronchospasm have been reported following the administration of vinca alkaloids. These reactions have been encountered most frequently when the vinca alkaloid was used in combination with mitomycin-C. The onset may be in minutes or several hours after the vinca is injected.

Adverse Reactions: In general, adverse reactions are reversible and are related to dosage. The most common adverse reaction is hair loss; the most troublesome are neuromuscular in origin. When single weekly doses of the drug are employed, the adverse reactions of leukopenia, neuritic pain, constipation, and difficulty in walking are usually of short duration (i.e., less than seven days). When the dosage is reduced, these reactions may lessen or disappear. They seem to be increased when the calculated amount of drug is given in divided doses. Other adverse reactions, such as hair loss, sensory loss, paresthesia, slapping gait, loss of deep-tendon reflexes, and muscle wasting, may persist for at least as long as therapy is continued. In most instances, they have disappeared by about the sixth week after discontinuance of treatment, but in some patients the neuromuscular difficulties may persist for prolonged periods.

In addition to constipation (mentioned below), paralytic ileus may occur, particularly in young children. The ileus will reverse itself upon temporary discontinuance of Oncovin® (vincristine sulfate, Lilly) and with symptomatic care. It mimics the "surgical abdomen."

Frequently, there is a sequence in the development of neuromuscular side effects. Initially, only sensory impairment and paresthesias may be encountered. With continued treatment, neuritic pain may appear and, later, motor difficulties. No reports have yet been made of any agent that can reverse the neuromuscular manifestations accompanyng therapy with Oncovin.

Convulsions, frequently with hypertension, have been reported in a few patients receiving Oncovin. Rare occurrences of the syndrome attributed to inappropriate antidiuretic hormone secretion have been observed in patients treated with Oncovin. The syndrome has been described in association with several disease states. There is high urinary sodium excretion in the presence of hyponatremia; renal or adrenal disease, hypotension, dehydration, azotemia, and clinical edema are absent. With fluid deprivation, improvement occurs in the hyponatremia and in the renal loss of sodium.

Constipation may take the form of upper-colon impaction, and, on physical examination, the rectum may be found to be empty. Colicky abdominal pain coupled with an empty rectum may mislead the physician. A flat film of the abdomen is useful in demonstrating this condition. All cases have responded to high enemas and laxatives. A routine prophylatic regimen against constipation is recommended for all patients receiving Oncovin. Other adverse reactions that have been reported are abdominal cramps, ataxia, foot drop, weight loss, optic atrophy with blindness, transient cortical blindness, fever, cranial nerve manifestations, paresthesia and numbness of the digits, polyuria, dysuria, oral ulceration, headache, vomiting, diarrhea, and intestinal necrosis and/or perforation. Oncovin does not appear to have any constant or significant effect on the platelets or the red blood cells. Thrombocytopenia, if present when therapy with Oncovin is begun, may actually improve before the appearance of marrow remission.

Dosage and Administration: This preparation is for intravenous use only (see **Warnings**).

Extreme care must be used in calculating and administering the dose of Oncovin® (vincristine sulfate, Lilly) since overdosage may have a very serious or fatal outcome.

The drug is administered intravenously *at weekly intervals*. The usual dose of Oncovin for children is 2 mg/m^2; for adults, 1.4 mg/m^2. Various dosage schedules have been used (see the package insert for references).

The solution may be injected either directly into a vein or into the tubing of a running intravenous infusion. Injection of the Oncovin may be completed in about one minute.

Caution—It is extremely important that the needle be properly positioned in the vein before any vincristine is injected. If leakage into surrounding tissue should occur during intravenous administration of Oncovin, it may cause considerable irritation. The injection should be discontinued immediately, and any remaining portion of the dose should then be introduced into another vein. Local injection of hyaluronidase and the application of moderate heat to the area of leakage help disperse the drug and are thought to minimize discomfort and the possibility of cellulitis.

Parenteral drug products should be inspected visually for particulate matter and discoloration prior to administration, whenever solution and container permit.

Overdosage: Side effects following the use of Oncovin® (vincristine sulfate, Lilly) are dose related. Therefore, following administration of an overdose, patients can be expected to experience side effects in an exaggerated fashion. Supportive care should include the following: (1) prevention of side effects resulting from the syndrome of inappropriate secretion of antidiuretic hormone (this would include restriction of fluid intake and perhaps the administration of a diuretic affecting the function of the loop of Henle and the distal tubule); (2) administration of anticonvulsant doses of phenobarbital; (3) use of enemas to prevent ileus (in some instances, decompression of gastrointestinal tract may be necessary); (4) monitoring the cardiovascular system; and (5) determining daily blood counts for guidance in transfusion requirements. Folinic acid has been observed to have a protective effect in normal mice which were administered lethal doses of Oncovin (Cancer Res., 23:1390, 1963). Isolated case reports suggest that folinic acid may be helpful in treating humans who have received an overdose of Oncovin. A suggested schedule is to administer 15 mg of folinic acid intravenously every three hours for 24 hours and then every six hours for at least 48 hours. Theoretical tissue levels of Oncovin derived from pharmacokinetic data are predicted to remain significantly elevated for at least 72 hours. Treatment with folinic acid does not eliminate the need for the above-mentioned supportive measures.

How Supplied: (℞) Vials Oncovin® (vincristine sulfate injection, Lilly), Solution: No. 7194, 1 mg/1 ml (NDC 0002-7194-01), No. 7195, 2 mg/2 ml (NDC 0002-7195-01), and No. 7196, 5 mg/5 ml (NDC 0002-7196-01), in single packages. *Refrigerate.*

[031684]

**PENICILLIN G PROCAINE ℞
SUSPENSION, STERILE, USP**
Duracillin® A.S.
[dū-ra-sĭl-ĭn ā-ĕs']

Description: Duracillin® A.S. (Sterile Penicillin G Procaine Suspension, USP, Lilly) is a ready-to-use aqueous suspension of Duracillin® (Penicillin G Procaine, USP, Lilly), the original penicillin G procaine, which was developed in the Lilly laboratories to fill a need for a long-acting parenteral penicillin preparation. Penicillin G procaine is a stable crystalline salt which is only slightly soluble in water. When combined with certain dispersing agents and suspended in water, it is slowly absorbed (because of its low solubility in body fluids) from the injection site in the muscle.

Each vial contains 300,000 units crystalline penicillin G procaine; sodium citrate, 4%; lecithin, 1%; povidone, 0.1%; with methylparaben, 0.15%, propylparaben, 0.02%, benzyl alcohol, 1%, as preservatives; water for injection, q.s, 1 ml.

Actions and Pharmacology: Penicillin G is bactericidal against penicillin-susceptible microorganisms during the stage of active multiplication. It produces its effect by inhibiting biosynthesis of cell-wall mucopeptide. It is not active against the penicillinase-producing bacteria, which include many strains of staphylococci. Penicillin G exerts high in vitro activity against staphylococci (except penicillinase-producing strains), streptococci (groups A, C, G, H, L, and M), and pneumococci. Other organisms susceptible to penicillin G are *Neisseria gonorrhoeae, Corynebacterium diphtheriae, Bacillus anthracis, Clostridium, Actinomyces bovis, Streptobacillus moniliformis, Listeria monocytogenes,* and *Leptospira. Treponema pallidum* is extremely susceptible to the bactericidal action of penicillin G.

Disc Susceptibility Tests—Quantitative methods that require measurement of zone diameters give the most precise estimates of antibiotic susceptibility. One such procedure (*Am. J. Clin. Pathol., 45*:493, 1966; *Federal Register, 39*:19182–19184, 1974) has been recommended for use with discs for testing susceptibility to penicillin.

Penicillin G procaine is an equimolecular compound of procaine and penicillin G administered intramuscularly as a suspension. It dissolves slowly at the site of injection and gives a plateau type of blood level at about four hours, which falls slowly over a period of the next 15 to 20 hours. Approximately 60 percent of penicillin G is bound to serum protein. The drug is distributed throughout the body tissues in widely varying amounts. Highest levels are found in the kidneys, and lesser amounts appear in the liver, skin, and intestines. Small concentrations are found in all other body tissues and the cerebrospinal fluid. With normal kidney function, the drug is excreted rapidly by tubular excretion. In neonates, young infants, and individuals with impaired kidney function, excretion is considerably delayed. Approximately 60 to 90 percent of a dose of parenteral penicillin G is excreted in the urine within 24 to 36 hours.

Indications: Penicillin G procaine is indicated in the treatment of moderately severe infections due to penicillin-G-susceptible microorganisms that are sensitive to the low and persistent serum levels common to this particular dosage form. Therapy should be guided by bacteriologic studies (including susceptibility tests) and by clinical response.

NOTE: When high, sustained serum levels are required, aqueous penicillin G should be used either intramuscularly or intravenously.

The following infections will usually respond to adequate dosages of intramuscular penicillin G procaine:

Streptococcal Infections (Group A) (without Bacteremia)—Moderately severe to severe infections of the upper respiratory tract, skin and soft-tissue infections, scarlet fever, and erysipelas.

NOTE: Streptococci in groups A, C, G, H, L, and M are very susceptible to penicillin G. Other groups, including group D (enterococcus), are resistant. Aqueous penicillin G is recommended for streptococcal infections with bacteremia.

Pneumococcal Infections—Moderately severe infections of the respiratory tract.

NOTE: Severe pneumonia, empyema, bacteremia, pericarditis, meningitis, peritonitis, and arthritis of pneumococcal etiology are better treated with aqueous penicillin G during the acute stage.

Staphylococcal Infections Susceptible to Penicillin G—Moderately severe infections of the skin and soft tissues.

NOTE: Reports indicate an increasing number of strains of staphylococci resistant to penicillin G, which emphasizes the need for culture and susceptibility studies in treating suspected staphylococcal infections.

for possible revisions

Indicated surgical procedures should be performed.
Fusospirochetosis (Vincent's Gingivitis and Pharyngitis)—Moderately severe infections of the oropharynx respond to therapy with penicillin G procaine.
NOTE: Necessary dental care should be accomplished in infections involving the gum tissue.
Syphilis (T. pallidum)—All stages
Acute and Chronic Gonorrhea (without Bacteremia) (N. gonorrhoeae)
Yaws, Bejel, Pinta
Diphtheria (C. diphtheriae)—Penicillin G procaine as an adjunct to antitoxin for prevention of the carrier stage.
Anthrax
Rat-Bite Fever (S. moniliformis and *Spirillum minus)*
Erysipeloid
Subacute Bacterial Endocarditis (Group A Streptococci)—Limited to extremely susceptible strains.
Although no controlled clinical efficacy studies have been conducted, aqueous crystalline penicillin G for injection and penicillin G procaine suspension have been suggested by the American Heart Association and the American Dental Association for use as part of a combined parenteral-/oral regimen for prophylaxis against bacterial endocarditis in patients with congenital heart disease or rheumatic or other acquired valvular heart disease when they undergo dental procedures and surgical procedures of the upper respiratory tract.[1] Since alpha-hemolytic streptococci relatively resistant to penicillin may be found when patients are receiving continuous oral penicillin for secondary prevention of rheumatic fever, prophylactic agents other than penicillin may be chosen for these patients and prescribed in addition to their continuous prophylactic regimen for rheumatic fever.
NOTE: When selecting antibiotics for the prevention of bacterial endocarditis, the physician or dentist should read the full joint statement of the American Heart Association and the American Dental Association.[1]
Contraindication: A previous hypersensitivity reaction to any penicillin is a contraindication.
Warnings: Serious and occasionally fatal hypersensitivity (anaphylactoid) reactions have been reported in patients receiving penicillin therapy. Although anaphylaxis is more frequent following parenteral therapy, it has occurred in patients given oral penicillins. These reactions are more likely in individuals with a history of sensitivity to multiple allergens.
There have been well-documented reports of individuals with a history of penicillin hypersensitivity who have experienced severe reactions when treated with a cephalosporin. Before therapy with a penicillin, careful inquiry should be made concerning previous hypersensitivity reactions to penicillins, cephalosporins, and other allergens. If an allergic reaction occurs, the drug should be discontinued and the patient treated with the usual agents (e.g., epinephrine or other pressor amines, antihistamines, or corticosteroids).
Immediate toxic reactions to procaine may occur in some individuals, particularly when a large single dose is administered in the treatment of gonorrhea (4,800,000 units). These reactions may be manifested by mental disturbances, including anxiety, confusion, agitation, depression, weakness, seizures, hallucinations, combativeness, and expressed "fear of impending death." The reactions noted in carefully controlled studies occurred in approximately one of 500 patients treated for gonorrhea. Reactions are transient and last from 15 to 30 minutes.
Precautions: Penicillin should be used with caution in individuals having histories of significant allergies and/or asthma.
In intramuscular therapy, care should be taken to avoid accidental intravenous administration.
In suspected staphylococcal infections, proper laboratory studies, including susceptibility tests, should be performed.

A small percentage of patients are sensitive to procaine. If there is a history of sensitivity, make the usual test: Inject 0.1 ml of a 1 to 2 percent procaine solution intradermally. Development of an erythema, wheal, flare, or eruption indicates procaine sensitivity. Sensitivity should be treated by the usual methods, including barbiturates, and penicillin procaine preparations should not be used. Antihistamines appear beneficial in treatment of procaine reactions.
The use of antibiotics may result in overgrowth of nonsusceptible organisms. Constant observation of the patient is essential. If new infections due to bacteria or fungi appear during therapy, the drug should be discontinued and appropriate measures taken. Whenever allergic reactions occur, penicillin should be withdrawn unless, in the opinion of the physician, the condition being treated is life threatening and amenable only to penicillin therapy.
In prolonged therapy with penicillin, and particularly with high dosage schedules, periodic evaluation of the renal and hematopoietic systems is recommended.
When gonococcal infections are treated in which primary or secondary syphilis may be suspected, proper diagnostic procedures, including darkfield examinations, should be performed. In all cases in which concomitant syphilis is suspected, monthly serologic tests should be made for at least four months.
Adverse Reactions: Penicillin is a substance of low toxicity but does have a significant index of sensitization. The following hypersensitivity reactions have been reported: skin rashes ranging from maculopapular eruptions to exfoliative dermatitis; urticaria; and reactions resembling serum sickness, including chills, fever, edema, arthralgia, and prostration. Severe and often fatal anaphylaxis has occurred (*see* Warnings). As with other treatments for syphilis, the Jarisch-Herxheimer reaction has been reported.
Procaine toxicity manifestations have been reported (*see* Warnings). Procaine hypersensitivity reactions have not been reported with this drug.
Dosage and Administration: Penicillin G procaine (aqueous) is for intramuscular injection only.
Recommended dosage is as follows:
Pneumonia (Pneumococcus)—Moderately severe (uncomplicated): 600,000 to 1,000,000 units daily.
Streptococcal Infections (Group A)—Moderately severe to severe tonsillitis, erysipelas, scarlet fever, and upper respiratory tract, skin, and soft-tissue infections: 600,000 to 1,000,000 units daily for a minimum of ten days.
Staphylococcal Infections—Moderately severe to severe: 600,000 to 1,000,000 units daily.
For prophylaxis against bacterial endocarditis[1] in patients with congenital heart disease or rheumatic or other acquired valvular heart disease when undergoing dental procedures or surgical procedures of the upper respiratory tract, use a combined parenteral/oral regimen. One million units of aqueous crystalline penicillin G (30,000 units/kg in children) mixed with 600,000 units of procaine penicillin G (600,000 units for children) should be given intramuscularly one-half to one hour before the procedure. Oral penicillin V (phenoxymethyl penicillin), 500 mg for adults or 250 mg for children weighing less than 30 kg, should be given every six hours for eight doses. Doses for children should not exceed the recommendations for adults for a single dose or for a 24-hour period.
Syphilis—Primary, secondary, and latent with a negative spinal fluid in adults and children over 12 years of age: 600,000 units daily for eight days (total, 4,800,000 units).
Late (tertiary and latent syphilis and neurosyphilis with positive spinal-fluid examination or no spinal fluid examination): 600,000 units daily for ten to 15 days (total, 6,000,000 to 9,000,000 units).
Congenital syphilis in a patient weighing less than 70 pounds: 10,000 units/kg/day for ten days.
Syphilis in pregnancy: Treatment should correspond to the stage of the disease.
Yaws, Bejel, and Pinta—Same treatment as for syphilis in corresponding stage of disease.

Gonorrheal Infections (Uncomplicated)—Men or women: 4,800,000 units intramuscularly, divided into at least two doses and injected at different sites during one visit, together with 1 g of oral probenecid, preferably given at least 30 minutes prior to the injection.
NOTE: Gonorrheal endocarditis should be treated intensively with aqueous penicillin G.
Diphtheria—Adjunctive therapy with antitoxin: 300,000 to 600,000 units daily.
Diphtheria Carrier State—300,000 units daily for ten days.
Anthrax (Cutaneous)—600,000 to 1,000,000 units/day.
Vincent's Infection (Fusospirochetosis)—600,000 to 1,000,000 units/day.
Erysipeloid—600,000 to 1,000,000 units/day.
Rat-Bite Fever (S. moniliformis and *S. minus)*—600,000 to 1,000,000 units/day.
Reference: 1. American Heart Association: Prevention of Bacterial Endocarditis, Circulation, 56:139A, 1977.
How Supplied: (℞) *Vials (Multiple Dose) No. 554, Sterile Penicillin G Procaine Suspension, USP,* 300,000 units/ml, 10 ml, rubber-stoppered, in singles (10/carton) (NDC 0002-7185-01) and in Traypak™ (multivial carton, Lilly) of 100 (NDC 0002-7185-02).
Refrigerate. Avoid freezing.

[031682]

PENICILLIN V POTASSIUM PRODUCTS
[vĕ-sĭl' ĭn kā]
see V-Cillin K® (penicillin V potassium, Lilly).

PROTAMINE SULFATE ℞
[prō' tạ-mĕn sŭl' fāt]
Injection, USP

Description: Protamines are simple proteins of low molecular weight that are rich in arginine and strongly basic. They occur in the sperm of salmon and certain other species of fish.
Each 5-ml ampoule of Protamine Sulfate Injection, USP, contains protamine sulfate equivalent to 50 mg of activity, and each 25-ml vial contains protamine sulfate equivalent to 250 mg of activity. Both products also contain 0.9 percent sodium chloride. Sodium phosphate and/or sulfuric acid may have been added during manufacture to adjust the pH. Contains no preservative.
Actions: When administered alone, protamine has an anticoagulant effect. However, when it is given in the presence of heparin (which is strongly acidic), a stable salt is formed which results in the loss of anticoagulant activity of both drugs.
Indication: Protamine sulfate is indicated in the treatment of heparin overdosage.
Warnings: Hyperheparinemia or bleeding has been reported in experimental animals and in some patients 30 minutes to 18 hours after cardiac surgery (under cardiopulmonary bypass) in spite of complete neutralization of heparin by adequate doses of protamine sulfate at the end of the operation.
Therefore, it is important to keep the patient under close observation after cardiac surgery. Additional doses of protamine sulfate should be administered if indicated by coagulation studies, such as the heparin titration test with protamine and the determination of plasma thrombin time.
Too rapid administration of protamine sulfate can cause severe hypotension and anaphylactoid-like reactions. Facilities to treat shock should be available. (*See* **Dosage and Administration**).
Usage in Pregnancy—Reproduction studies have not been performed in animals. There is no adequate information as to whether this drug may affect fertility in human males or females or have a teratogenic potential or other adverse effect on the fetus.

Continued on next page

• Identi-Code® symbol.

Lilly—Cont.

Precautions: Because of the anticoagulant effect of protamine, it is unwise to give more than 100 mg over a short period unless there is certain knowledge of a larger requirement.

Patients with a history of allergy to fish may develop hypersensitivity reactions to protamine, although to date no relationship has been established between allergic reactions to protamine and fish allergy. A number of individuals hypersensitive to fish have received protamine sulfate without developing allergic reactions.

Adverse Reactions: Intravenous injections of protamine may cause a sudden fall in blood pressure, bradycardia, dyspnea, or transitory flushing and a feeling of warmth. There have been reports of anaphylaxis that resulted in respiratory embarrassment (see Precautions).

Because fatal reactions often resembling anaphylaxis have been reported after administration of protamine sulfate, the drug should be given only when resuscitation techniques and treatment of anaphylactoid shock are readily available.

Dosage and Administration: Each mg of protamine sulfate neutralizes approximately 90 USP units of heparin activity derived from lung tissue or about 115 USP units of heparin activity derived from intestinal mucosa.

Protamine Sulfate Injection, USP, should be given by very slow intravenous injection in doses not to exceed 50 mg of protamine sulfate in any ten-minute period (see Warnings).

Protamine sulfate is intended for injection without further dilution; however, if further dilution is desired, D5-W or normal saline may be used. Diluted solutions should not be stored since they contain no preservative.

Protamine sulfate should not be mixed with other drugs without knowledge of their compatibility, because protamine sulfate has been shown to be incompatible with certain antibiotics, including several of the cephalosporins and penicillins.

Because heparin disappears rapidly from the circulation, the dose of protamine sulfate required also decreases rapidly with the time elapsed following intravenous injection of heparin. For example, if the protamine sulfate is administered 30 minutes after the heparin, one-half the usual dose may be sufficient.

The dosage of protamine sulfate should be guided by blood coagulation studies (see Warnings).

How Supplied: (℞) *Protamine Sulfate Injection, USP: Ampoules No. 473*, 5 ml (equivalent to 50 mg of activity), in packages of 6 (NDC 0002-1691-16) and 25 (NDC 0002-1691-25); *Vials No. 735*, 25 ml (equivalent to 250 mg of activity), rubber-stoppered, in singles (10/carton) (NDC 0002-1462-01). *Refrigerate. Avoid freezing.*

Both products should be stored in the refrigerator above freezing and below 50°F.

CAUTION—The total dose of protamine sulfate contained in Vials No. 735 (250 mg of activity in 25 ml) is five times greater than that in Ampoules No. 473 (50 mg of activity in 5 ml).

The large-size vials (No. 735) are designed only for antiheparin treatment in certain cases in which large doses of heparin have been given during surgery and are to be neutralized by large doses of protamine sulfate after surgical procedures.

[040984]

Ampoules No. 473, 5 ml—6's—6505-00-299-9667

REGULAR ILETIN® I

[rĕg′ ū-lẽr ī′ lĕ-tĭn]
(insulin injection, Lilly), see under Iletin® (insulin, Lilly).

SECONAL® SODIUM

[sĕk′ o′ năl sō′ dĭ-ŭm]
(secobarbital sodium)
Capsules, USP

WARNING: MAY BE HABIT-FORMING

Description: The barbiturates are nonselective central-nervous-system (CNS) depressants that are primarily used as sedative-hypnotics. In subhypnotic doses, they are also used as anticonvulsants. The barbiturates and their sodium salts are subject to control under the Federal Controlled Substances Act. Seconal® Sodium (Secobarbital Sodium, USP, Lilly) is a barbituric acid derivative and occurs as a white, odorless, bitter powder that is very soluble in water, soluble in alcohol, and practically insoluble in ether.

Each Pulvule® contains 50 or 100 mg of secobarbital sodium.

Chemically, the drug is sodium 5-allyl-5-(1-methylbutyl)barbiturate, with the empirical formula $C_{12}H_{17}N_2NaO_3$.

Clinical Pharmacology: Seconal® Sodium (secobarbital sodium, Lilly), a short-acting barbiturate, is a CNS depressant. In ordinary doses, the drug acts as a sedative and hypnotic.

Barbiturates are capable of producing all levels of CNS mood alteration, from excitation to mild sedation, hypnosis, and deep coma. Overdosage can produce death. Barbiturates depress the sensory cortex, decrease motor activity, alter cerebellar function, and produce drowsiness, sedation, and hypnosis.

Barbiturate-induced sleep differs from physiologic sleep. Sleep laboratory studies have demonstrated that barbiturates reduce the amount of time spent in the rapid eye movement (REM) phase of sleep, or dreaming state. Also, Stages III and IV sleep are decreased. Following abrupt cessation of barbiturates used regularly, patients may experience markedly increased dreaming, nightmares, and /or insomnia. Therefore, withdrawal of a single therapeutic dose over five or six days has been recommended to lessen the REM rebound and disturbed sleep which contribute to drug withdrawal syndrome (for example, decrease the dose from three to two doses a day for one week).

Seconal Sodium has been found to lose most of its effectiveness for both inducing and maintaining sleep by the end of 14 days of continued drug administration, even with the use of multiple doses.

Barbiturates have little analgesic action at subanesthetic doses. Rather, in subanesthetic doses these drugs may increase the reaction to painful stimuli. All barbiturates exhibit anticonvulsant activity in anesthetic doses. However, of the drugs in this class, only phenobarbital, mephobarbital, and metharbital are effective as oral anticonvulsants in subhypnotic doses.

Barbiturates are respiratory depressants, and the degree of depression is dependent on the dose. With hypnotic doses, respiratory depression is similar to that which occurs during physiologic sleep accompanied by a slight decrease in blood pressure and heart rate.

Barbiturates do not impair normal hepatic function but have been shown to induce liver microsomal enzymes, thus increasing and/or altering the metabolism of barbiturates and other drugs. (See PRECAUTIONS—*Drug Interactions*.)

Pharmacokinetics—Barbiturates are weak acids that are absorbed and rapidly distributed to all tissues and fluids, with high concentrations in the brain, liver, and kidneys. Lipid solubility of the barbiturates is the dominant factor in their distribution within the body. Barbiturates are bound to plasma and tissue proteins; the degree of binding increases as a function of lipid solubility. The onset of action of Seconal Sodium is from ten to 15 minutes, and the duration of action ranges from three to four hours. The plasma half-life of Seconal Sodium is 15 to 40 hours.

Secobarbital has a high lipid solubility, plasma protein binding, brain protein binding, a short delay in onset of activity, and a short duration of action.

Seconal Sodium is metabolized primarily by the hepatic microsomal enzyme system, and the metabolic products are excreted in the urine and, less commonly, in the feces. Seconal Sodium is detoxified in the liver.

Indications and Usage: Seconal® Sodium (secobarbital sodium, Lilly) is indicated for use as a hypnotic, for the short-term treatment of insomnia, since barbiturates appear to lose their effectiveness for sleep induction and sleep maintenance after two weeks (see Clinical Pharmacology above). It is also indicated for use as a preanesthetic agent.

Contraindications: Seconal® Sodium (secobarbital sodium, Lilly) is contraindicated in patients who are hypersensitive to barbiturates. It is also contraindicated in patients with a history of manifest or latent porphyria, marked impairment of liver function, or respiratory disease in which dyspnea or obstruction is evident. It should not be administered to persons with known previous addiction to the sedative/hypnotic group, since ordinary doses may be ineffectual and may contribute to further addiction. Seconal Sodium should not be administered in the presence of acute or chronic pain, because paradoxical excitement may be induced or important symptoms may be masked.

Warnings: 1. *Habit-Forming*—Seconal® Sodium (secobarbital sodium, Lilly) may be habit-forming. Tolerance and psychologic and physical dependence may occur with continued use (see Drug Abuse and Dependence). Patients who have psychologic dependence on barbiturates may increase the dosage or decrease the dosage interval without consulting a physician and subsequently may develop a physical dependence on barbiturates. To minimize the possibility of overdosage or development of dependence, the prescribing and dispensing of Seconal Sodium should be limited to the amount required for the interval until the next appointment. The abrupt cessation after prolonged use of Seconal Sodium in a person who is dependent on the drug may result in withdrawal symptoms, including delirium, convulsions, and possibly death. Seconal Sodium should be withdrawn gradually from any patient known to be taking excessive doses over long periods (see Drug Abuse and Dependence).

2. *Usage in Pregnancy*—Barbiturates may cause fetal damage when administered to a pregnant woman. Retrospective, case-controlled studies have suggested that there may be a relationship between the maternal consumption of barbiturates and a higher than expected incidence of fetal abnormalities. Seconal Sodium readily crosses the placental barrier and is distributed throughout fetal tissues; the highest concentrations are found in the placenta, liver, and brain.

Withdrawal symptoms occur in infants born to women who receive Seconal Sodium throughout the last trimester of pregnancy (see Drug Abuse and Dependence). If Seconal Sodium is used during pregnancy or if the patient becomes pregnant while taking this drug, the patient should be apprised of the potential hazard to the fetus.

3. *Synergistic Effects*—The concomitant use of alcohol or other CNS depressants may produce additive CNS depressant effects.

Precautions: *General Precautions*—Barbiturates may be habit-forming. Tolerance and psychologic and physical dependence may occur with continuing use (see Drug Abuse and Dependence below). Barbiturates should be administered with caution, if at all, to patients who are mentally depressed, have suicidal tendencies, or have a history of drug abuse.

Elderly or debilitated patients may react to barbiturates with marked excitement, depression, or confusion. In some persons, barbiturates repeatedly produce excitement rather than depression. Barbiturates induce liver microsomal enzyme activity. This accelerates the biotransformation of various drugs and is probably part of the mechanism of the tolerance encountered with barbiturates. Seconal® Sodium (secobarbital sodium, Lilly) should, therefore, be used with caution in patients with decreased liver function. Seconal Sodium may decrease the potency of coumarin anticoagulants; therefore, patients receiving such concomitant therapy should have more frequent prothrombin determinations.

The systemic effects of exogenous hydrocortisone and endogenous hydrocortisone (cortisol) may be diminished by Seconal Sodium. Thus, this product should be administered with caution to patients with borderline hypoadrenal function, regardless of whether it is of pituitary or primary adrenal origin.

Information for Patients—The following information should be given to patients receiving Seconal Sodium:
1. The use of Seconal Sodium carries with it an associated risk of psychologic and/or physical dependence. The patient should be warned against increasing the dose of the drug without consulting a physician.
2. Seconal Sodium may impair the mental and/or physical abilities required for the performance of potentially hazardous tasks, such as driving a car or operating machinery. The patient should be cautioned accordingly.
3. Alcohol should not be consumed while taking Seconal Sodium. The concurrent use of Seconal Sodium with other CNS depressants (e.g., alcohol, narcotics, tranquilizers, and antihistamines) may result in additional CNS depressant effects.

Laboratory Tests—Prolonged therapy with barbiturates should be accompanied by periodic evaluation of organic systems, including hematopoietic, renal and hepatic systems (*see General Precautions* and Adverse Reactions).

Drug Interactions—Seconal Sodium in combination with alcohol, tranquilizers, and other CNS depressants has additive depressant effects, and the patient should be so advised. Toxic effects and fatalities have occurred following overdoses of Seconal Sodium alone and in combination with other CNS depressants. Caution should be exercised in prescribing unnecessarily large amounts of Seconal Sodium for patients who have a history of emotional disturbances or suicidal ideation or who have misused alcohol and other CNS drugs (*see* Overdosage).

For information regarding concomitant administration of Seconal Sodium and coumarin anticoagulants or corticosteroids, see *General Precautions*. Monoamine oxidase inhibitors prolong the effects of barbiturates, probably because the metabolism of the barbiturate is inhibited.

Usage in Pregnancy—1. *Teratogenic Effects. Pregnancy Category D. See* Warnings section—*Usage in Pregnancy.*

2. *Nonteratogenic Effects.* Reports of infants suffering from long-term barbiturate exposure in utero included the acute withdrawal syndrome of seizures and hyperirritability from birth to a delayed onset of up to 14 days (*see* Drug Abuse and Dependence).

Labor and Delivery—Hypnotic doses of barbiturates do not appear to impair uterine activity significantly during labor. Full anesthetic doses of barbiturates decrease the force and frequency of uterine contractions. Administration of sedative/hypnotic barbiturates to the mother during labor may result in respiratory depression in the newborn. Premature infants are particularly susceptible to the depressant effects of barbiturates. If barbiturates are used during labor and delivery, resuscitation equipment should be available.

Data are not available to evaluate the effect of barbiturates when forceps delivery or other intervention is necessary or to determine the effect of barbiturates on the later growth, development, and functional maturity of the child.

Nursing Mothers—Caution should be exercised when Seconal Sodium is administered to a nursing woman, because small amounts of barbiturates are excreted in the milk.

Adverse Reactions: The following adverse reactions and their incidences were compiled from surveillance of thousands of hospitalized patients who received barbiturates. Because such patients may be less aware of certain of the milder adverse effects of barbiturates, the incidence of these reactions may be somewhat higher in fully ambulatory patients.

More than 1 in 100 Patients
The most common adverse reaction estimated to occur at a rate of one to three patients per 100 is the following:
Nervous System: Somnolence

Less than 1 in 100 Patients
Adverse reactions estimated to occur at a rate of less than one in 100 patients are listed below, grouped by organ system and by decreasing order of occurrence:

Nervous System: Agitation, confusion, hyperkinesia, ataxia, CNS depression, nightmares, nervousness, psychiatric disturbance, hallucinations, insomnia, anxiety, dizziness, abnormality in thinking
Respiratory System: Hypoventilation, apnea
Cardiovascular System: Bradycardia, hypotension, syncope
Digestive System: Nausea, vomiting, constipation
Other Reported Reactions: Headache, injection site reactions, hypersensitivity reactions (angioedema, skin rashes, exfoliative dermatitis), fever, liver damage

Drug Abuse and Dependence: *Controlled Substance*—Seconal Sodium® (secobarbital sodium, Lilly) is a Schedule II drug.

Dependence—Barbiturates may be habit-forming; tolerance, psychologic dependence, and physical dependence may occur, especially following prolonged use of high doses of barbiturates. Daily administration in excess of 400 mg of secobarbital for approximately 90 days is likely to produce some degree of physical dependence. A dosage of 600 to 800 mg for at least 35 days is sufficient to produce withdrawal seizures. The average daily dose for the barbiturate addict is usually about 1.5 g. As tolerance to barbiturates develops, the amount needed to maintain the same level of intoxication increases; tolerance to a fatal dosage, however, does not increase more than twofold. As this occurs, the margin between intoxicating dosage and fatal dosage becomes smaller.

Symptoms of acute intoxication with barbiturates include unsteady gait, slurred speech, and sustained nystagmus. Mental signs of chronic intoxication include confusion, poor judgment, irritability, insomnia, and somatic complaints.

Symptoms of barbiturate dependence are similar to those of chronic alcoholism. If an individual appears to be intoxicated with alcohol to a degree that is radically disproportionate to the amount of alcohol in his or her blood, the use of barbiturates should be suspected. The lethal dose of a barbiturate is far less if alcohol is also ingested.

The symptoms of barbiturate withdrawal can be severe and may cause death. Minor withdrawal symptoms may appear eight to 12 hours after the last dose of a barbiturate. These symptoms usually appear in the following order: anxiety, muscle twitching, tremor of hands and fingers, progressive weakness, dizziness, distortion in visual perception, nausea, vomiting, insomnia, and orthostatic hypotension. Major withdrawal symptoms (convulsions and delirium) may occur within 16 hours and last up to five days after abrupt cessation of barbiturates. Intensity of withdrawal symptoms gradually declines over a period of approximately 15 days. Individuals susceptible to barbiturate abuse and dependence include alcoholics and opiate abusers as well as other sedative-hypnotic and amphetamine abusers.

Drug dependence on barbiturates arises from repeated administration on a continuous basis, generally in amounts exceeding therapeutic dose levels. The characteristics of drug dependence on barbiturates include the following: (a) a strong desire or need to continue taking the drug; (b) a tendency to increase the dose; (c) a psychic dependence on the effects of the drug related to subjective and individual appreciation of those effects; and (d) a physical dependence on the effects of the drug, requiring its presence for maintenance of homeostasis and resulting in a definite, characteristic, and self-limited abstinence syndrome when the drug is withdrawn.

Treatment of barbiturate dependence consists of cautious and gradual withdrawal of the drug. Barbiturate-dependent patients can be withdrawn by using a number of different withdrawal regimens. In all cases, withdrawal takes an extended period. One method involves substituting a 30-mg dose of phenobarbital for each 100 to 200-mg dose of barbiturate that the patient has been taking. The total daily amount of phenobarbital is then administered in three or four divided doses, not to exceed 600 mg daily. Should signs of withdrawal occur on the first day of treatment, a loading dose of 200 to 300 mg of phenobarbital may be administered IM in addition to the oral dose. After stabilization on phenobarbital, the total daily dose is decreased by 30 mg a day as long as withdrawal is proceeding smoothly. A modification of this regimen involves initiating treatment at the patient's regular dosage level and decreasing the daily dosage by 10 percent if tolerated by the patient.

Infants that are physically dependent on barbiturates may be given phenobarbital, 3 to 10 mg/kg/day. After withdrawal symptoms (hyperactivity, disturbed sleep, tremors, and hyperreflexia) are relieved, the dosage of phenobarbital should be gradually decreased and completely withdrawn over a two-week period.

Overdosage: The toxic dose of barbiturates varies considerably. In general, an oral dose of 1 g of most barbiturates produces serious poisoning in an adult. Death commonly occurs after 2 to 10 g of ingested barbiturate. Barbiturate intoxication may be confused with alcoholism, bromide intoxication, and various neurologic disorders.

Symptoms—Acute overdosage with barbiturates is manifested by CNS and respiratory depression, which may progress to Cheyne-Stokes respiration, areflexia, constriction of the pupils to a slight degree (although in severe poisoning they may show paralytic dilation), oliguria, tachycardia, hypotension, lowered body temperature, and coma. Typical shock syndrome (apnea, circulatory collapse, respiratory arrest, and death) may occur.

In extreme overdose, all electrical activity in the brain may cease, in which case a "flat" EEG normally equated with clinical death cannot be accepted. This effect is fully reversible unless hypoxic damage occurs. Consideration should be given to the possibility of barbiturate intoxication even in situations that appear to involve trauma.

Complications such as pneumonia, pulmonary edema, cardiac arrhythmias, congestive heart failure, and renal failure may occur. Uremia may increase CNS sensitivity to barbiturates if renal function is impaired. Differential diagnosis should include hypoglycemia, head trauma, cerebrovascular accidents, convulsive states, and diabetic coma.

The sedated, therapeutic blood levels of secobarbital range between 0.5 to 5 mcg/ml; the usual lethal blood level ranges from 15 to 40 mcg/ml.

Treatment—Treatment of overdosage is mainly supportive and consists of the following:
1. Maintenance of an adequate airway, with assisted respiration and oxygen administration as necessary.
2. Monitoring of vital signs and fluid balance.
3. If the patient is conscious and has not lost the gag reflex, emesis may be induced with ipecac. Care should be taken to prevent pulmonary aspiration of vomitus. After completion of vomiting, 30 grams activated charcoal in a glass of water may be administered.
4. If emesis is contraindicated, gastric lavage may be performed with a cuffed endotracheal tube in place with the patient in the face down position. Activated charcoal may be left in the emptied stomach and a saline cathartic administered.
5. Fluid therapy and other standard treatment for shock, if needed.
6. If renal function is normal, forced diuresis may aid in the elimination of the barbiturate. Alkalinization of the urine increases renal excretion of some barbiturates, especially phenobarbital, also aprobarbital, and mephobarbital (which is metabolized to phenobarbital).
7. Although not recommended as a routine procedure, hemodialysis may be used in severe barbiturate intoxications or if the patient is anuric or in shock.
8. Patient should be rolled from side to side every 30 minutes.
9. Antibiotics should be given if pneumonia is suspected.

Continued on next page

• Identi-Code® symbol.

Lilly—Cont.

10. Appropriate nursing care to prevent hypostatic pneumonia, decubiti, aspiration, and other complications of patients with altered states of consciousness.

Dosage and Administration: Dosages of barbiturates must be individualized with full knowledge of their particular characteristics. Factors of consideration are the patient's age, weight, and condition.

Special Patient Population—Dosage should be reduced in the elderly or debilitated because these patients may be more sensitive to barbiturates. Dosage should be reduced for patients with impaired renal function or hepatic disease.

Adults—As a hypnotic, 100 mg at bedtime. Preoperatively, 200 to 300 mg one to two hours before surgery.

Children—Preoperatively, 2 to 6 mg/kg, with a maximum dosage of 100 mg.

How Supplied: (C) Pulvules® Seconal® Sodium (Secobarbital Sodium Capsules, USP): No. 243, F42, *50 mg (No. 4, Orange), in bottles of 100 (NDC 0002-0642-02); No. 240, F40, *100 mg (No. 3, Orange), in bottles of 100 (NDC 0002-0640-02) and 500 (NDC 0002-0640-03), and in 10 strips of 10 individually labeled blisters each containing 1 Pulvule (ID100) (NDC 0002-0640-33).

[031684]

Shown in Product Identification Section, page 417

SECONAL® SODIUM
[sĕk'ō-năl sō'dĭ-ŭm]
(secobarbital sodium, Lilly) and
AMYTAL® SODIUM
[ăm'ĭ-tăl sō'dĭ-ŭm]
(amobarbital sodium, Lilly), see Tuinal® (secobarbital sodium and amobarbital sodium, Lilly).

SEMILENTE® ILETIN® I
[sĕm'ĭ-lĕn'tā ī'lĕ-tĭn]
(prompt insulin zinc suspension, Lilly), see under Iletin® (insulin, Lilly).

SEROMYCIN® ℞
[sĕr-ō-mī'sĭn]
(cycloserine)
Capsules, USP

Description: Seromycin® (cycloserine, Lilly), D-4-amino-3-isoxazolidinone, is a broad-spectrum antibiotic which is produced by a strain of *Streptomyces orchidaceus* and has also been synthesized. A white powder that is soluble in water and stable in alkaline solution, it is rapidly destroyed at neutral or acid pH.

Actions: Cycloserine inhibits cell-wall synthesis in susceptible strains of gram-positive and gram-negative bacteria and in *Mycobacterium tuberculosis*.

Indications: Seromycin® (cycloserine, Lilly) is indicated in the treatment of active pulmonary and extrapulmonary tuberculosis (including renal disease) when the organisms are susceptible to this drug and after failure of adequate treatment with the primary medications (streptomycin, isoniazid, and ethambutol). Like all antituberculosis drugs, Seromycin should be administered in conjunction with other effective chemotherapy and not as the sole therapeutic agent.

Seromycin may be effective in the treatment of acute urinary tract infections caused by susceptible strains of gram-positive and gram-negative bacteria, especially *Enterobacter* and *Escherichia coli*. It is generally no more and is usually less effective than other antimicrobial agents in the treatment of urinary tract infections caused by bacteria other than mycobacteria. Use of Seromycin in these infections should be considered only when the more conventional therapy has failed and when the organism has been demonstrated to be sensitive to the drug.

Contraindications: Administration is contraindicated in patients with any of the following:

Hypersensitivity to cycloserine
Epilepsy
Depression, severe anxiety, or psychosis
Severe renal insufficiency
Excessive concurrent use of alcoholic beverages

Warnings: Administration of Seromycin® (cycloserine, Lilly) should be discontinued or the dosage reduced if the patient develops allergic dermatitis or symptoms of central-nervous-system toxicity, such as convulsions, psychosis, somnolence, depression, confusion, hyperreflexia, headache, tremor, vertigo, paresis, or dysarthria.

The toxicity of Seromycin is closely related to excessive blood levels (above 30 mcg/ml), which are determined by high dosage or inadequate renal clearance. The ratio of toxic dose to effective dose in tuberculosis is small.

The risk of convulsions is increased in chronic alcoholics.

Patients should be monitored by hematologic, renal excretion, blood level, and liver function studies.

Usage in Pregnancy—The safety of the use of Seromycin during pregnancy has not been established.
Usage in Children—Safety and dosage have not been established for pediatric use.

Precautions: Before treatment with Seromycin® (cycloserine, Lilly) is initiated, cultures should be taken and the organism's susceptibility to the drug should be established. In tuberculous infections, its sensitivity to the other antituberculosis agents in the regimen should also be demonstrated.

Blood levels should be determined at least weekly for patients having reduced renal function, for individuals receiving a daily dosage of more than 500 mg, and for those showing signs and symptoms suggestive of toxicity. The dosage should be adjusted to keep the blood level below 30 mcg/ml.

Anticonvulsant drugs or sedatives may be effective in controlling symptoms of central-nervous-system toxicity, such as convulsions, anxiety, and tremor. Patients receiving more than 500 mg of Seromycin daily should be closely observed for such symptoms. The value of pyridoxine in preventing CNS toxicity from cycloserine has not been proved.

Administration of Seromycin and other antituberculosis drugs has been associated in a few instances with vitamin B_{12} and/or folic acid deficiency, megaloblastic anemia, and sideroblastic anemia. If evidence of anemia develops during treatment, appropriate studies and therapy should be instituted.

Adverse Reactions: Most adverse reactions occurring during therapy with Seromycin® (cycloserine, Lilly) involve the nervous system or are manifestations of drug hypersensitivity. The following side effects have been observed in patients receiving Seromycin:

Nervous system symptoms (which appear to be related to higher dosages of drug, i.e., more than 500 mg daily)
  Convulsions
  Drowsiness and somnolence
  Headache
  Tremor
  Dysarthria
  Vertigo
  Confusion and disorientation with loss of memory
  Psychoses, possibly with suicidal tendencies
    Character changes
    Hyperirritability
    Aggression
  Paresis
  Hyperreflexia
  Paresthesias
  Major and minor (localized)
    clonic seizures
  Coma
Allergic (apparently not related to dosage)
  Skin rash
Miscellaneous
  Elevated serum transaminase, especially in patients with preexisting liver disease

Dosage and Administration: Seromycin® (cycloserine, Lilly) is effective orally and is currently administered only by this route. The usual dosage is 500 mg to 1 g daily in divided doses monitored by blood levels. The initial adult dosage most frequently given is 250 mg twice daily at 12-hour intervals for the first two weeks. The daily dosage of 1 g should not be exceeded.

How Supplied: (℞) Pulvules® No. 12, Seromycin® (Cycloserine Capsules, USP), F04,* 250 mg (No. 1, Light-Gray Opaque Body, Red Opaque Cap), in bottles of 40 (NDC 0002-0604-40).

[022084]

SILVER NITRATE ℞
[sĭl'vĕr nī'trāt]
Ophthalmic Solution, USP
One Percent (Buffered)
Wax Ampoules

This product is to be used by the physician or under his direction.

Description: Silver nitrate ophthalmic solution is a 1% solution of silver nitrate in a water medium. It contains not less than 0.95% and not more than 1.05% of $AgNO_3$. The solution may be buffered by the addition of sodium acetate.

Silver nitrate ophthalmic solution is an anti-infective (ophthalmic).

Clinical Pharmacology: Silver nitrate in weak solutions is used as a germicide and astringent to mucous membranes. The germicidal action is due to precipitation of bacterial proteins by liberated silver ions.

Indications and Usage: Silver nitrate ophthalmic solution is indicated for the prevention of gonorrheal ophthalmia neonatorum.

It has not been effective for prevention of neonatal chlamydial conjunctivitis.[1]

Contraindications: None known.

Warnings: A 1% solution is considered optimal; however, it must be used with caution, since cauterization of the cornea and blindness may result, especially with repeated applications.

When ingested, silver nitrate is highly toxic to the gastrointestinal tract and central nervous system. Swallowing can cause severe gastroenteritis that may end fatally. Sodium chloride may be used by gastric lavage to remove the chemical.

Silver nitrate is caustic and irritating to the skin and mucous membranes.

Precautions: *General Precautions*—Solutions of silver nitrate must be handled carefully, since they tend to stain skin and utensils. Silver nitrate stains may be removed from linen by applications of iodine tincture followed by sodium thiosulfate solution.

Adverse Reactions: A mild chemical conjunctivitis should result from a properly performed Credé prophylaxis using silver nitrate. With the 1% solution of silver nitrate, chemical conjunctivitis occurs in 20 percent or less of cases.

Overdosage: When a solution of 2% or higher silver nitrate concentration is used in the eye, conjunctivitis may be produced. The eye should be irrigated with an isotonic solution of sodium chloride after solutions of silver nitrate stronger than 1% are instilled.

Dosage and Administration: Immediately after the child is born, the eyelids should be cleaned with sterile absorbent cotton or gauze and sterile water. A separate pledget should be used for each eye, and the lids, without being opened, should be washed from the nose outward until quite free of all blood, mucus, or meconium.

Next, the lids should be separated, and two drops of 1% silver nitrate solution should be dropped into the eye. The lids should be separated and elevated away from the eyeball so that a lake of silver nitrate may lie for a half minute or longer between them, coming in contact with every portion of the conjunctival sac.

The American Academy of Pediatrics has endorsed a statement of the Committee on Ophthalmia Neonatorum of the National Society for the Prevention of Blindness which does not recommend irrigation of the eyes following instillation of the silver nitrate.

Method of Use: *See* the package literature for illustrations. Pierce the end of the ampoule with a needle, making sure that its entry into the interior of the ampoule is accomplished.

To express the contents of the ampoule, press between the thumb and first finger.

The ampoule should be kept at controlled room temperature, 59° to 86°F (15° to 30°C). Do not freeze. It should not be used when cold. Protect from light.

How Supplied: (℞) *Wax Ampoules No. 146, Silver Nitrate Ophthalmic Solution, USP, 1% (Buffered),* in packages of 100 (NDC 0002-1608-02). Sodium acetate and acetic acid are contained as buffers.

1. Schachter, J., et al.: Prospective Study of Chlamydial Infection in Neonates, Lancet, 2:377-379, August 25, 1979.

[061482]

TAPAZOLE® ℞
[tăp′ a-zōl]
(methimazole)
Tablets, USP

Description: Tapazole® (methimazole, Lilly) (1-methyl-2-mercaptoimidazole) is a white crystalline substance that is freely soluble in water. It differs chemically from the drugs of the thiouracil series primarily in that it has a five instead of a six-membered ring.

Each tablet contains 5 or 10 mg methimazole, an orally administered antithyroid drug. The molecular weight is 114.16, and the empirical formula is $C_4H_6N_2S$.

Clinical Pharmacology: Methimazole inhibits the synthesis of thyroid hormones and thus is effective in the treatment of hyperthyroidism. The drug does not inactivate existing thyroxine and triiodothyronine which is stored in the thyroid or is circulating in the blood, nor does it interfere with the effectiveness of thyroid hormones given by mouth or by injection.

The actions and use of methimazole are similar to those of propylthiouracil. On a weight basis, the drug is at least ten times as potent as propylthiouracil, but methimazole may be less consistent in action.

Methimazole is readily absorbed from the gastrointestinal tract. It is metabolized rapidly and requires frequent administration. Methimazole is excreted in the urine.

Indications and Usage: Tapazole® (methimazole, Lilly) is indicated in the medical treatment of hyperthyroidism. Long-term therapy may lead to remission of the disease. Tapazole may also be used to ameliorate hyperthyroidism in preparation for subtotal thyroidectomy or radioactive iodine therapy. Tapazole is also used when thyroidectomy is contraindicated or not advisable.

Contraindications: Tapazole® (methimazole, Lilly) is contraindicated in the presence of hypersensitivity to the drug and in nursing mothers, since the drug is excreted in milk.

Warnings: Agranulocytosis is potentially the most serious side effect of therapy with Tapazole® (methimazole, Lilly). Leukopenia and thrombocytopenia may also occur. Patients should be instructed to report any symptoms of agranulocytosis, such as fever or sore throat.

Precautions: *General Precautions*—Patients who receive Tapazole® (methimazole, Lilly) should be under close surveillance and should be impressed with the necessity of reporting immediately any evidence of illness, particularly sore throat, skin eruptions, fever, headache, or general malaise. In such cases, white-blood-cell and differential counts should be made to determine whether agranulocytosis has developed. Particular care should be exercised with patients who are receiving additional drugs known to cause agranulocytosis.

Laboratory Tests—Because Tapazole may cause hypoprothrombinemia and bleeding, prothrombin time should be monitored during therapy with the drug, especially before surgical procedures. *See General Precautions.*

Drug Interactions—The activity of anticoagulants may be potentiated by anti-vitamin-K activity attributed to Tapazole.

Carcinogenesis, Mutagenesis, Impairment of Fertility—Such effects have not been observed or reported.

Usage in Pregnancy—Pregnancy Category D—Tapazole, used judiciously, is an effective drug in hyperthyroidism complicated by pregnancy. Because the drug readily crosses the placental membranes and can induce goiter and even cretinism in the developing fetus, it is important that a sufficient, but not excessive, dose be given. In many pregnant women, the thyroid dysfunction diminishes as the pregnancy proceeds; consequently, a reduction in dosage may be possible. In some instances, Tapazole can be withdrawn two or three weeks before delivery.

The administration of thyroid along with Tapazole to the pregnant hyperthyroid woman is also recommended in order to prevent hypothyroidism in the mother and her fetus. Administration should continue throughout the pregnancy and after delivery.

If this drug is used during pregnancy, or if the patient becomes pregnant while taking this drug, the patient should be apprised of the potential hazard to the fetus.

Nursing Mothers—The drug appears in human milk and is contraindicated in nursing mothers.

Usage in Children—See Dosage and Administration.

Adverse Reactions: Adverse reactions probably occur in less than 3 percent of patients.

Major adverse reactions (much less common than the minor adverse reactions) include inhibition of myelopoiesis (agranulocytosis, granulopenia, and thrombocytopenia), drug fever, a lupuslike syndrome, hepatitis (jaundice may persist for several weeks after discontinuation of the drug), periarteritis, and hypoprothrombinemia. Nephritis is very rare.

Minor adverse reactions include skin rash, urticaria, nausea, vomiting, epigastric distress, arthralgia, paresthesia, loss of taste, abnormal loss of hair, myalgia, headache, pruritus, drowsiness, neuritis, edema, vertigo, skin pigmentation, jaundice, sialadenopathy, and lymphadenopathy.

It should be noted that about 10 percent of patients with untreated hyperthyroidism have leukopenia (white-blood-cell count of less than 4000/mm³), often with relative granulopenia.

Overdosage: Agranulocytosis is the most serious effect. Rarely, exfoliative dermatitis, hepatitis, neuropathies, or CNS stimulation or depression may occur.

Symptoms—Nausea, vomiting, epigastric distress, headache, fever, arthralgia, pruritus, edema, and pancytopenia. Prolonged therapy may result in hypothyroidism.

Treatment—For specific therapy, the drug should be discontinued in the presence of agranulocytosis, pancytopenia, hepatitis, fever, or exfoliative dermatitis.

For bone-marrow depression, use of an antibiotic and transfusions of fresh whole blood should be considered.

For hepatitis, rest and adequate diet may be indicated.

General management may consist in symptomatic and supportive therapy, including rest, analgesics, gastric lavage, intravenous fluids, and mild sedation.

Dosage and Administration: Tapazole® (methimazole, Lilly) is administered orally. It is usually given in three equal doses at approximately eight-hour intervals.

Adult—The initial daily dosage is 15 mg for mild hyperthyroidism, 30 to 40 mg for moderately severe hyperthyroidism, and 60 mg for severe hyperthyroidism, divided into three doses at eight-hour intervals. The maintenance dosage is 5 to 15 mg daily.

Pediatric—Initially, the daily dosage is 0.4 mg/kg of body weight divided into three doses and given at eight-hour intervals. The maintenance dosage is approximately one-half of the initial dose.

How Supplied: (℞) *Tablets Tapazole® (Methimazole Tablets, USP)* (scored): *No. 1765, J94,** 5 mg (NDC 0002-1094-02), and *No. 1770, J95,** 10 mg (NDC 0002-1095-02), in bottles of 100. [090282]

TUBOCURARINE CHLORIDE ℞
[tōō′ bō-kyū-rär′ ēn klō′ rīd]
Injection, USP
See also Metubine® Iodide (metocurine iodide, Lilly)

> THIS DRUG SHOULD BE ADMINISTERED ONLY BY ADEQUATELY TRAINED INDIVIDUALS WHO ARE FAMILIAR WITH ITS ACTIONS, CHARACTERISTICS, AND HAZARDS.

Description: Tubocurarine Chloride Injection, USP, is a sterile isotonic solution for intravenous use. Each ml of the solution contains 3 mg (20 units) tubocurarine chloride, sodium bisulfite, 0.1 percent, and sodium chloride, 0.7 percent, with chlorobutanol (chloroform derivative), 0.5 percent, as a preservative. Sodium hydroxide and/or hydrochloric acid are sometimes added during manufacture to adjust the pH.

Actions: Tubocurarine chloride blocks nerve impulses to skeletal muscles at the myoneural junction. This is a nondepolarizing neuromuscular blockade. When it is administered intravenously (intramuscular injection is unpredictable), the onset of flaccid paralysis occurs within a few minutes.

Muscle paralysis may be expected for periods of 25 to 90 minutes. The use of repeated doses may be accompanied by a cumulative effect. Since tubocurarine chloride is excreted by the kidneys, severe renal disease or hypotension may result in a more prolonged action of this drug.

Concurrently administered general anesthetics, certain antibiotics, abnormal states (e.g., acidosis), electrolyte imbalance, and neuromuscular disease have been reported to cause a potentiation of this drug's activity.

Rapid intravenous injection may produce increased release of histamine with resultant decreased respiratory capacity due to bronchospasm and paralysis of the respiratory muscles. Hypotension may occur owing to ganglionic blockade, or it may be a complication of positive pressure respiration.

Tubocurarine chloride does not affect consciousness or cerebration, and it does not relieve pain. A patient in severe pain may not be able to communicate this to the anesthesiologist.

Indications: Tubocurarine chloride is indicated as an adjunct to anesthesia to induce skeletal-muscle relaxation. It may be employed to reduce the intensity of muscle contractions in pharmacologically or electrically induced convulsions. It may be used as a diagnostic agent for myasthenia gravis when the results of tests with neostigmine or edrophonium are inconclusive. It may also be employed to facilitate the management of patients undergoing mechanical ventilation.

Contraindications: Tubocurarine chloride is contraindicated in those persons who have shown an allergic reaction or hypersensitivity to the drug and in patients in whom histamine release is a definite hazard.

Warnings: TUBOCURARINE CHLORIDE IS A POTENT DRUG WHICH MAY CAUSE RESPIRATORY DEPRESSION. THEREFORE, IT SHOULD BE USED ONLY BY THOSE EXPERIENCED IN THE TECHNIQUE OF ARTIFICIAL RESPIRATION AND THE ADMINISTRATION OF OXYGEN UNDER POSITIVE PRESSURE. FACILITIES FOR THESE PROCEDURES SHOULD BE IMMEDIATELY AVAILABLE AT ALL TIMES.

Prolonged apnea with its attendant hazards due to hypoxia may result from overdosages of this preparation.

It should be employed with extreme caution in patients with known myasthenia gravis.

The administration of quinidine during postoperative recovery to patients who have received tubo-

Continued on next page

* Identi-Code® symbol.

Lilly—Cont.

curarine chloride may result in recurarization leading to respiratory paralysis.

Usage in Pregnancy—The safe use of tubocurarine chloride has not been established with respect to the possible adverse effects upon child development. Therefore, it should not be administered to women of childbearing potential and especially not during early pregnancy unless, in the judgment of the physician, the potential benefits outweigh the possible hazards.

Precautions: When sufficiently excessive dosage of curare has been administered, there is no antidote. It is again emphasized that dosage should be controlled so that emergency measures need not be instituted.

Tubocurarine chloride should be used with caution in patients with respiratory depression or with renal, hepatic, or pulmonary diseases.

Hypotension can follow the administration of large doses.

Adverse Reactions: Adverse reactions consist primarily in extension of the drug's pharmacologic actions. Profound and prolonged muscle relaxation may occur, with consequent respiratory depression to the point of apnea.

Hypersensitivity to the drug may exist in rare instances.

Idiosyncrasy, interference with physical signs of anesthesia, circulatory depression, ganglionic blockade, and release of histamine are complications that can result from the use of this medication.

Drug Interaction: The intensity of blockade and duration of action of tubocurarine chloride are increased in patients receiving patent inhalational anesthetics such as halothane, diethyl ether, methoxyflurane, and enflurane. No increased intensity of blockade or duration of action is noted from the use of thiobarbiturates, narcotic analgesics, nitrous oxide, or droperidol.

Prior administration of succinylcholine chloride, such as that used for endotracheal intubation, may enhance the relaxant effect of tubocurarine chloride. If succinylcholine chloride is used before tubocurarine, the administration of tubocurarine should be delayed until the succinylcholine shows signs of wearing off.

Dosage and Administration:

Conversion Table for Calculating Dosage
20 units are contained in each ml
1 mg equals 7 units
1 unit is contained in 0.05 ml of this solution

Tubocurarine chloride is administered intravenously as a sustained injection over a period of 1 to 1½ minutes. As a precaution, the initial dose should be reduced to 20 units below the calculated amount. The speed of injection of the drug influences the amount administered. Although rapid injection may be dangerous, curarization can be accomplished with a smaller dose than that mentioned above if this is given more rapidly.

Tubocurarine chloride should be administered only by or under the supervision of experienced clinicians. The dosage must be individualized in each case after evaluation of the patient and consideration of factors that might alter the action of the drug in a particular case. If inhalational anesthetics known to enhance the action of curariform drugs are being used, the initial dose should be reduced and the response noted as a guide to incremental doses. If enhanced sensitivity is suspected, fractional dosage is advised initially to avoid overdosage. The following doses are for average patients without altered sensitivity.

Surgery—In the patient of average weight, 40 to 60 units of Tubocurarine Chloride Injection are administered intravenously at the time the skin incision is made, and 20 to 30 units in three to five minutes if required for further relaxation. For long operations, supplemental doses of 20 units may be given as required. As a general rule, dosage may be calculated on the basis of ½ unit/lb of body weight.

Electroshock Therapy—Tubocurarine chloride is administered just before electroshock therapy in the treatment of mental diseases. It reduces the severity of the convulsions and is useful as a means of preventing fractures. The patient should be observed closely until consciousness is regained in case respiratory failure should develop. A dose of ½ unit/lb of body weight is given intravenously and slowly as a sustained 1 to 1 ½-minute injection. Rapid administration is dangerous. The initial dose is 20 units less than this.

Diagnosis of Myasthenia Gravis—Tubocurarine chloride has been useful as a diagnostic agent in patients suspected of having myasthenia gravis. When small doses are given, a profound exaggeration of this syndrome occurs. The dosage is $1/15$ to $1/5$ of the average adult electroshock-therapy dose administered intravenously.

Every effort should be made to control dosage to the end that emergencies do not arise. It is important that physicians familiarize themselves with the dangers involved in using the drug and that preparations be made in advance for treating the patient if unwarranted side effects occur (see Contraindications and Adverse Reactions).

Tubocurarine chloride is adjusted to a pH sufficiently low to assure full stability for indefinite periods without the need for refrigeration; therefore, because of the high pH of barbiturate solutions, a precipitate will form when tubocurarine chloride is combined with such agents as Brevital® Sodium (Methohexital Sodium for Injection, USP, Lilly) and Thiopental Sodium.

It is recommended that each component be given from a separate syringe to assure more uniform and predictable results with each of the drugs. A single needle and tube attached to a three-way stopcock apparatus can readily be adapted to this method if it is desirable to utilize as few of the patient's veins as possible.

Management of Adverse Reactions: If hypotension occurs, the etiology should be determined. When it is due to ganglionic blockade, hypotension may be treated with fluid and vasopressors which act as the adrenergic receptors as required. Apnea or prolonged curarization should be treated with controlled respiration. Edrophonium or neostigmine may antagonize the skeletal-muscle-relaxant action of tubocurarine chloride. Neostigmine injection should be accompanied or preceded by an injection of atropine sulfate or its equivalent. A nerve stimulator may be used to assess the nature and degree of the neuromuscular blockade. The optimum time to administer the antagonist is when the patient is being hyperventilated and the carbon-dioxide level of the blood is low. The effects of neostigmine given intravenously last from 30 to 90 minutes; the effects of edrophonium are usually dissipated within five minutes. The antagonists are merely adjuncts. Before they are used, the package inserts of these drugs should be consulted for prescribing information.

Pharmacology: Tubocurarine chloride blocks nervous impulses to skeletal muscles at the myoneural junction.

Renal excretion occurs fairly rapidly; therefore, the physiologic effect is of relatively short duration.

How Supplied: (℞) Vials (Multiple Dose) No. 449, Tubocurarine Chloride Injection, USP, 3 mg/ml, 10 ml, rubber-stoppered, in singles (10/carton) (NDC 0002-1685-01). [011282]

TUINAL®
[too' i-nǎl]
(secobarbital sodium and amobarbital sodium)
Capsules, USP

WARNING: MAY BE HABIT-FORMING

Description: Tuinal is a combination of equal parts of Seconal® Sodium (secobarbital sodium, Lilly) and Amytal® Sodium (amobarbital sodium, Lilly), barbituric acid derivatives that occur as white, odorless, bitter powders. They are very soluble in water, soluble in alcohol, and practically insoluble in ether and in chloroform.

Each Pulvule No. 302 contains 25 mg Seconal Sodium and 25 mg Amytal Sodium.
Each Pulvule No. 303 contains 50 mg Seconal Sodium and 50 mg Amytal Sodium.
Each Pulvule No. 304 contains 100 mg Seconal Sodium and 100 mg Amytal Sodium.

Chemically, Seconal Sodium is sodium 5-allyl-5-(1-methylbutyl)barbiturate, with the empirical formula $C_{12}H_{17}N_2NaO_3$.

Amytal Sodium is sodium 5-ethyl-5-isopentylbarbiturate, with the empirical formula $C_{11}H_{17}N_2NaO_3$.

Clinical Pharmacology: Tuinal, a moderately long-acting barbiturate, is a central-nervous system depressant. In ordinary doses, the drug acts as a hypnotic. Its onset of action occurs in 15 to 30 minutes, and the duration of action ranges from three to 11 hours. It is detoxified in the liver.

Indications and Usage: For use whenever prompt and moderately sustained hypnotic effect is required. Not suitable for continuous daytime sedation. The prolonged administration of Tuinal is not recommended, since it has not been shown to be effective for a period of more than 14 days. If insomnia persists, drug-free intervals of one or more weeks should elapse before re-treatment is considered.

Attempts should be made to find alternative non-drug therapy for chronic insomnia.

Contraindications: Tuinal is contraindicated in patients who are hypersensitive to barbiturates. It is also contraindicated in patients with a history of manifest or latent porphyria, marked impairment of liver function, or respiratory disease in which dyspnea or obstruction is evident. It should not be administered to persons with known previous addiction to the sedative/hypnotic group, since ordinary doses may be ineffectual and may contribute to further addiction. Tuinal should not be administered in the presence of acute or chronic pain, because paradoxical excitement may be induced or important symptoms may be masked.

Warnings: Prolonged, uninterrupted use of barbiturates (particularly the short-acting drugs), even in therapeutic doses, may result in psychic and physical dependence.

The central-nervous-system-depressant effect of secobarbital and amobarbital may be additive with that of other CNS depressants, including alcohol.

Precautions: *General Precautions*—Barbiturates induce liver microsomal enzyme activity. This accelerates the biotransformation of various drugs and is probably part of the mechanism of the tolerance encountered with barbiturates. Tuinal should, therefore, be used with caution in patients with decreased liver function. This drug should also be administered cautiously to patients with a history of drug dependence or abuse (see Drug Abuse and Dependence). Tuinal may decrease the potency of coumarin anticoagulants; therefore, patients receiving such concomitant therapy should have more frequent prothrombin determinations.

As with other sedatives and hypnotics, elderly or debilitated patients may react to barbiturates with marked excitement or depression.

The systemic effects of exogenous hydrocortisone and endogenous hydrocortisone (cortisol) may be diminished by Tuinal. Thus, this product should be administered with caution to patients with borderline hypoadrenal function, regardless of whether it is of pituitary or of primary adrenal origin.

Information for Patients—Tuinal may impair the mental and/or physical abilities required for the performance of potentially hazardous tasks, such as driving a car or operating machinery. The patient should be cautioned accordingly.

Drug Interactions—Tuinal in combination with alcohol, tranquilizers, and other central-nervous-system depressants has additive depressant effects, and the patient should be so advised. Patients taking this drug should be warned not to exceed the dosage recommended by their physician. Toxic effects and fatalities have occurred following overdoses of Tuinal alone and in combination with other central-nervous-system depressants. Caution should be exercised in prescribing

for possible revisions

unnecessarily large amounts of Tuinal for patients who have a history of emotional disturbances or suicidal ideation or who have misused alcohol and other CNS drugs (see Overdosage).

Usage in Pregnancy—Pregnancy Category B—Reproduction studies have been performed in animals and have revealed no evidence of impaired fertility or harm to the fetus due to Tuinal. There are, however, no adequate and well-controlled studies in pregnant women. Because animal reproduction studies are not always predictive of human response, this drug should be used during pregnancy only if clearly needed.

Labor and Delivery—Depression has been noted in infants born following the use of Tuinal during labor.

Nursing Mothers—Caution should be exercised when Tuinal is administered to a nursing woman.

Usage in Children—Safety and effectiveness in children have not been established.

Adverse Reactions: The following adverse reactions have been reported:

CNS Depression—Residual sedation or "hangover," drowsiness, and lethargy.

Respiratory/Circulatory—Respiratory depression, apnea, circulatory collapse.

Allergic—Hypersensitivity reactions, especially in individuals with asthma, urticaria, angioneurotic edema, or similar conditions; skin eruptions.

Other—Nausea and vomiting; headache.

Drug Abuse and Dependence: *Controlled Substance*—Tuinal is a Schedule II drug.

Dependence—Prolonged, uninterrupted use of barbiturates (particularly the short-acting drugs), even in therapeutic doses, may result in psychic and physical dependence. Withdrawal symptoms due to physical dependence following chronic use of large doses of barbiturates may include delirium, convulsions, and death (see Contraindications).

Overdosage: *Symptoms*—The manifestations of overdosage are early hypothermia followed by fever, sluggish or absent reflexes, respiratory depression, gradual appearance of circulatory collapse, pulmonary edema, and coma.

Treatment—General management should consist in symptomatic and supportive therapy, including gastric lavage, administration of intravenous fluids, and maintenance of blood pressure, body temperature, and adequate respiratory exchange. Dialysis will increase the rate of removal of barbiturates from the body fluids. Antibiotics may be required to control pulmonary complications.

Dosage and Administration: 50 to 200 mg at bedtime or one hour preoperatively.

How Supplied: (©) *Pulvules® Tuinal®* (Secobarbital Sodium and Amobarbital Sodium Capsules, USP), *No. 302, F64,* *50 mg (No. 4, Blue Body, Orange Cap), in bottles of 100 (NDC 0002-0664-02); *No. 303, F65,* *100 mg (No. 3, Blue Body, Orange Cap), in bottles of 100 (NDC 0002-0665-02) and 1000 (NDC 0002-0665-04), in 10 strips of 10 individually labeled blisters each containing 1 Pulvule (ID100) (NDC 0002-0665-33), and in strip packages of individually sealed Pulvules (DS1000) (NDC 0002-0665-35); *No. 304, F66,* *200 mg (No. 2, Blue Body, Orange Cap), in bottles of 100 (NDC 0002-0666-02) and 1000 (NDC 0002-0666-04) and in 10 strips of 10 individually labeled blisters each containing 1 Pulvule (ID100) (NDC 0002-0666-33).

[042182]

Shown in Product Identification Section, page 417

ULTRALENTE® ILETIN® I
[ŭl' trá-lĕn' tā ĭ' lĕ-tĭn]
(extended insulin zinc suspension, Lilly), see under Iletin® (insulin, Lilly).

VANCOCIN® HCL
[văn' kō-sĭn ăch' sē-ĕl]
(vancomycin hydrochloride)
Sterile, USP
IntraVenous

Description: Vancocin® HCl (vancomycin hydrochloride, Lilly), IntraVenous, is a glycopeptide antibiotic derived from *Streptomyces orientalis* which is bactericidal against many gram-positive bacteria. It should be administered intravenously, in dilute solution (see Dosage and Administration).

Actions: Vancocin® HCl (vancomycin hydrochloride, Lilly) is poorly absorbed by mouth, but an intravenous dose of 1 g produces serum levels averaging 25 mcg/ml at two hours. Its half-life in the circulation is about six hours. Many strains of streptococci, staphylococci, *Clostridium difficile*, and other gram-positive bacteria are susceptible in vitro to concentrations of 0.5 to 5 mcg/ml. Staphylococci are generally susceptible to less than 5 mcg of Vancocin HCl/ml, but a small proportion of *Staphylococcus aureus* strains require 10 or 20 mcg/ml for inhibition. If the Bauer-Kirby method of disc susceptibility testing is used, a 30-mcg disc of Vancocin HCl should produce a zone of more than 11 mm when tested against a vancomycin-susceptible bacterial strain.

Clinically effective concentrations of this antibiotic in the blood are usually achieved and maintained by its intravenous administration; moreover, inhibitory concentrations can be demonstrated in pleural, pericardial, ascitic, and synovial fluids and in urine. This antibiotic does not readily diffuse across normal meninges into the spinal fluid. However, when the meninges are inflamed as a result of infection, Vancocin HCl penetrates into the spinal fluid.

About 80 percent of injected Vancocin HCl is excreted by the kidneys. Concentrations are high in the urine. Impairment of renal function results in delayed excretion and in high blood levels associated with an increase in drug toxicity.

Indications: Vancocin® HCl (vancomycin hydrochloride, Lilly) is indicated in potentially life-threatening infections which cannot be treated with another effective, less toxic antimicrobial drug, including the penicillins and cephalosporins. Vancocin HCl is useful in therapy of severe staphylococcal (including methicillin-resistant staphylococci) infections in patients who cannot receive or who have failed to respond to the penicillins and cephalosporins or who have infections with staphylococci that are resistant to other antibiotics, including methicillin. Vancocin HCl has been used successfully alone in the treatment of staphylococcal (including methicillin-resistant staphylococci) endocarditis. Its effectiveness has been documented in other infections due to staphylococci (including methicillin-resistant staphylococci), including osteomyelitis, pneumonia, septicemia, and soft-tissue infections. When staphylococcal infections are localized and purulent, antibiotics are used as adjuncts to appropriate surgical measures.

The parenteral form may be administered orally for treatment of staphylococcal enterocolitis and antiobiotic-associated pseudomembranous colitis produced by *C. difficile*. Parenteral antibiotic administration may be used concomitantly. Vancomycin is *not* effective by the oral route for other types of infection.

Contraindication: Vancocin® HCl (vancomycin hydrochloride, Lilly) is contraindicated in patients with known hypersensitivity to this antibiotic.

Warnings: Because of its ototoxicity and nephrotoxicity, Vancocin® HCl (vancomycin hydrochloride, Lilly) should be used with care in patients with renal insufficiency. The risk of toxicity is appreciably increased by high blood concentrations or prolonged therapy.

Vancocin HCl should be avoided in patients with previous hearing loss. If it is used in such patients, the dose of Vancocin HCl should be regulated, if possible, by periodic determination of the drug level in the blood. Deafness may be preceded by tinnitus. The elderly are more susceptible to auditory damage. Experience with other antibiotics suggests that deafness may be progressive despite cessation of treatment.

Concurrent and sequential use of other neurotoxic and/or nephrotoxic antibiotics, particularly streptomycin, neomycin, kanamycin, gentamicin, cephaloridine, paromomycin, viomycin, polymyxin B, colistin, tobramycin, and amikacin, requires careful monitoring.

Precautions: Patients with borderline renal function and individuals over the age of 60 should be given serial tests of auditory function and of vancomycin blood levels. All patients receiving the drug should have periodic hematologic studies, urinalyses, and liver and renal function tests.

Vancocin® HCl (vancomycin hydrochloride, Lilly) is very irritating to tissue and causes necrosis when injected intramuscularly; it must be administered intravenously. Pain and thrombophlebitis occur in many patients receiving Vancocin HCl and are occasionally severe. The frequency and severity of thrombophlebitis can be minimized if the drug is administered in a volume of at least 200 ml of glucose or saline solution and if the sites of injection are rotated.

Adverse Reactions: Nausea, chills, fever, urticaria, and macular rashes have been associated with the administration of Vancocin® HCl (vancomycin hydrochloride, Lilly). It may also produce eosinophilia and anaphylactoid reactions.

A throbbing type of pain in the muscles of the back and neck has been described. This pain can usually be minimized or avoided by slower administration (see Dosage and Administration section). Hypotension has been reported and is more apt to occur with rapid administration. Flushing of the skin over the neck and shoulder area with transitory fine rash, including urticaria, has been observed during rapid administration.

Neutropenia has been reported and appears to be reversible promptly when the drug is discontinued.

The use of Vancocin HCl may result in overgrowth of nonsusceptible organisms. If new infections due to bacteria or fungi appear during therapy with this product, appropriate measures should be taken.

Dosage and Administration: *Adults*—The usual intravenous dose is 500 mg (in 0.9% Sodium Chloride Injection or 5% glucose in Sterile Water for Injection) every six hours or 1 g every 12 hours. The majority of patients with infections caused by organisms susceptible to the antibiotic show a therapeutic response by 48 to 72 hours. The total duration of therapy is determined by the type and severity of the infection and the clinical response of the patient. In staphylococcal endocarditis, therapy for three weeks or longer is recommended.

Children—The total daily dosage of Vancocin® HCl (vancomycin hydrochloride, Lilly), calculated on the basis of 20 mg/lb of body weight, can be divided and figured in with the child's 24-hour requirement of fluid.

Patients with Impaired Renal Function—Dosage adjustment must be made in patients with impaired renal function to avoid toxic serum levels. Serum levels should be checked regularly, since accumulation in such patients has been reported to occur over several weeks of treatment. Vancomycin serum levels may be determined by use of microbiologic assay, a commercially available radioimmunoassay kit, or a commercial fluorescence polarization immunoassay.

For most patients with renal impairment, the dosage calculation may be made by using the accompanying nomogram[1] if the creatinine clearance value is known.

[See table on next page].

1. Moellering, R. C., Jr., *et al:* Vancomycin Therapy in Patients with Impaired Renal Function: A Nomogram for Dosage, Ann. Intern. Med., 94:343, 1981.

The nomogram is not valid for functionally anephric patients on dialysis. For such patients, a loading dose of 15 mg/kg of body weight should be given in order to achieve therapeutic serum levels promptly, and the dose required to maintain stable levels is 1.9 mg/kg/24 h.

When only serum creatinine is available, the following formula (based on sex, weight, and age of the patient) may be used to convert this value into

Continued on next page

* Identi-Code® symbol.

Lilly—Cont.

estimated creatinine clearance. The serum creatinine should represent a steady state of renal function.

Males: $\dfrac{\text{Weight (kg)} \times (140 - \text{age})}{72 \times \text{serum creatinine}}$

Females: $0.85 \times$ above value

PREPARATION OF SOLUTION:
At the time of use, add 10 ml of Sterile Water for Injection to the vial of dry, sterile Vancocin HCl powder.
FURTHER DILUTION IS REQUIRED. READ INSTRUCTIONS WHICH FOLLOW:
1. Intermittent Infusion (the preferred method of administration)
   The above solution (containing 500 mg Vancocin HCl) can be added to 100–200 ml of 0.9% Sodium Chloride Injection or 5% glucose in Serile Water for Injection. This intravenous infusion should be given over a period of at least 60 minutes every six hours.
2. Continuous Infusion (should be used only when intermittent infusion is not feasible)
   Two to four vials of the above (1 to 2 g) can be added to a sufficiently large volume of 0.9% Sodium Chloride Injection or 5% glucose in Sterile Water for Injection to permit the desired daily dose to be administered slowly by intravenous drip over a 24-hour period.

For Oral Administration—The contents of one vial (500 mg) may be diluted in 1 oz of water and given to the patient to drink, or the diluted material may be administered via nasogastric tube. The usual adult dosage for antibiotic-associated pseudomembranous colitis produced by *C. difficile* is 500 mg to 2 g of Vancocin HCl orally per day in three or four divided doses for seven to ten days. For convenience of oral administration, Vancocin HCl is also available in screw-cap containers (No. M-206 and No. M-5105).

Stability of Prepared Solution: After reconstitution, the solution may be stored in a refrigerator for 96 hours without significant loss of potency.
How Supplied: (℞) *Vials No. 657, Vancocin® HCl (Sterile Vancomycin Hydrochloride, USP), IntraVenous,* equivalent to 500 mg vancomycin, 10-ml size, rubber-stoppered (Dry Powder), in singles (10/carton) (NDC 0002-1444-01).

[081684]

VANCOCIN® HCl   ℞
[văn'kō-sĭn ăch'sē-ĕl]
(vancomycin hydrochloride)
For Oral Solution, USP

> This preparation is for oral use only. If parenteral vancomycin therapy is desired, use Vancocin® HCl (Sterile Vancomycin Hydrochloride, USP), IntraVenous, and consult package insert accompanying that preparation.

Description: Vancocin® HCl (vancomycin hydrochloride, Lilly) is a glycopeptide antibiotic derived from *Streptomyces orientalis* which is bactericidal against many gram-positive bacteria.
Actions: Vancocin® HCl (vancomycin hydrochloride, Lilly) is poorly absorbed by mouth. Many strains of streptococci, staphylococci, *Clostridium difficile,* and other gram-positive bacteria are susceptible in vitro to concentrations of 0.5 to 5 mcg/ml. Staphylococci are generally susceptible to less than 5 mcg of Vancocin HCl per ml, but a small proportion of *Staphylococcus aureus* strains require 10 or 20 mcg/ml for inhibition. If the Bauer-Kirby method of disc susceptibility testing is used, a 30-mcg disc of Vancocin HCl should produce a zone of more than 11 mm when tested against a vancomycin-susceptible bacterial strain.
Indications: Vancocin® HCl (vancomycin hydrochloride, Lilly) may be administered orally for treatment of staphylococcal enterocolitis and antibiotic-associated pseudomembranous colitis produced by *C. difficile.* Parenteral antibiotic administration may be used concomitantly. Vancomycin is *not* effective by the oral route for other types of infection.
Contraindication: Vancocin® HCl (vancomycin hydrochloride, Lilly) is contraindicated in patients with known hypersensitivity to this antibiotic.
Warnings: Because of its ototoxicity and nephrotoxicity, Vancocin® HCl (vancomycin hydrochloride, Lilly) should be used with care in patients with renal insufficiency. During parenteral therapy, the risk of toxicity is appreciably increased by high blood concentrations or prolonged treatment. If it is necessary to use Vancocin HCl parenterally in such patients, doses of less than 2 g/day usually will provide satisfactory blood levels.
Vancomycin HCl should also be avoided in patients with previous hearing loss. If it is used in such patients, the dose of Vancocin HCl should be regulated, if possible, by periodic determination of the drug level in the blood. Deafness may be preceded by tinnitus. The elderly are more susceptible to auditory damage. Experience with other antibiotics suggests that deafness may be progressive despite cessation of treatment.
Concurrent and sequential use of other neurotoxic and/or nephrotoxic antibiotics, particularly streptomycin, neomycin, kanamycin, gentamicin, cephaloridine, paromomycin, viomycin, polymyxin B, colistin, tobramycin, and amikacin, requires careful monitoring.
Precautions: Patients with borderline renal function and individuals over the age of 60 should be given serial tests of auditory function and of vancomycin blood levels. All patients receiving the drug should have periodic hematologic studies, urinalyses, and liver and renal function tests.
Adverse Reactions: Nausea, chills, fever, urticaria, and macular rashes have been associated with the administration of Vancocin HCl. It may also produce eosinophilia and anaphylactoid reactions.
The use of Vancocin® HCl (vancomycin hydrochloride, Lilly) may result in overgrowth of non-susceptible organisms. If new infections due to bacteria or fungi appear during therapy with this product, appropriate measures should be taken.
Dosage and Administration: The contents of the 10-g vial may be mixed with distilled or deionized water (115 ml) for oral administration. When mixed with 115 ml of water, each 6 ml provide approximately 500 mg of vancomycin. The contents of the 1-g vial may be mixed with distilled or deionized water (20 ml). When reconstituted with 20 ml, each 5 ml contains approximately 250 mg of vancomycin. Mix thoroughly to dissolve. These mixtures may be kept for two weeks in a refrigerator without significant loss of potency.
Adults—The usual dose is 500 mg every six hours or 1 g every 12 hours.
The usual adult dosage for antibiotic-associated pseudomembranous colitis produced by *C. difficile* is 500 mg to 2 g of vancomycin orally/day in three or four divided doses administered for seven to ten days.
Children—The total daily dose is 20 mg/lb of body weight in divided doses.
How Supplied: (℞) *Vancocin® HCl (Vancomycin Hydrochloride for Oral Solution, USP): M-5105,* 1 g (equivalent to vancomycin), in a Traypak™ (multivial carton, Lilly) of 6 (NDC 0002-5105-16); *M-206,* 10 g (equivalent to vancomycin), in a screw-cap container (NDC 0002-2372-37).

[072183]

VANCOMYCIN HYDROCHLORIDE,
[văn'kō-sĭn ăch'sē-ĕl]
see Vancocin® HCl (vancomycin hydrochloride, Lilly).

V-CILLIN K®   ℞
[vē-sĭl'ĭn kā]
(penicillin V potassium)
USP

Description: V-Cillin K® (Penicillin V Potassium, USP, Lilly) is the potassium salt of V-Cillin® (Penicillin V, USP, Lilly). This chemically improved form combines acid stability with immediate solubility and rapid absorption.
Actions and Pharmacology: V-Cillin K® (penicillin V potassium, Lilly) is bactericidal against penicillin-sensitive microorganisms during the stage of active multiplication. It produces its effect by inhibiting biosynthesis of cell-wall mucopeptide. It is not active against the penicillinase-producing bacteria, which include many strains of staphylococci. The drug exerts high in vitro activity against staphylococci (except penicillinase-producing strains), streptococci (groups A, C, G, H, L, and M), and pneumococci. Other organisms sensitive in vitro to penicillin V are *Corynebacterium diphtheriae, Bacillus anthracis,* clostridia, *Actinomyces bovis, Streptobacillus moniliformis, Listeria monocytogenes, Leptospira,* and *Neisseria gonorrhoeae. Treponema pallidum* is extremely sensitive.
V-Cillin K has the distinct advantage over penicillin G in being resistant to inactivation by gastric acid. It may be given with meals; however, blood levels are slightly higher when the drug is given on an empty stomach. Average blood levels are two to five times higher than those following the same dose of oral penicillin G and also show much less individual variation.
Once absorbed, about 80 percent of V-Cillin K is bound to serum protein. Tissue levels are highest in the kidneys, and lesser amounts appear in the liver, skin, and intestines. Small concentrations are found in all other body tissues and the cerebrospinal fluid. The drug is excreted as rapidly as it is absorbed in individuals with normal kidney function; however, recovery of the drug from the urine indicates that only about 25 percent of the dose given is absorbed. In neonates, young infants, and individuals with impaired kidney function, excretion is considerably delayed.
Indications: V-Cillin K® (penicillin V potassium, Lilly) is indicated in the treatment of mild to moderately severe infections due to microorganisms whose sensitivity to penicillin G is within the range of serum levels common to this particular dosage form. Therapy should be guided by bacteri-

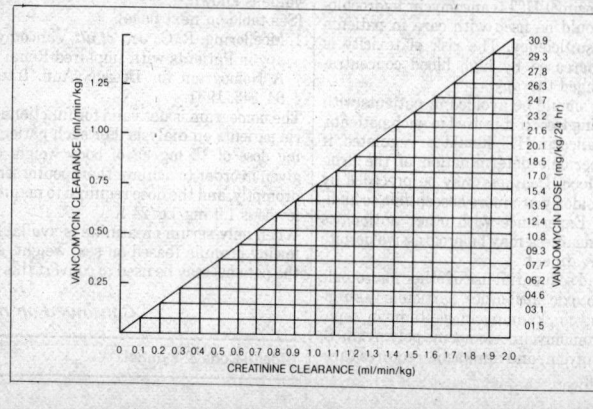

ologic studies (including susceptibility tests) and by clinical response.

NOTE: Severe pneumonia, empyema, bacteremia, pericarditis, meningitis, and arthritis should not be treated with penicillin V during the acute stage. Indicated surgical procedures should be performed.

The following infections will usually respond to adequate dosage of penicillin V:

Streptococcal Infections (without Bacteremia)—Mild to moderate infections of the upper respiratory tract, scarlet fever, and mild erysipelas.

NOTE: Streptococci in groups A, C, G, H, L, and M are very sensitive to penicillin. Other groups, including group D (enterococcus), are resistant.

Pneumococcal Infections—Mild to moderately severe infections of the respiratory tract.

Staphylococcal Infections Sensitive to Penicillin G—Mild infections of the skin and soft tissues.

NOTE: Reports indicate an increasing number of strains of staphylococci resistant to penicillin G, which emphasizes the need for culture and susceptibility studies in treating suspected staphylococcal infections.

Fusospirochetosis (Vincent's Gingivitis and Pharyngitis)—Mild to moderately severe infections of the oropharynx usually respond to therapy with oral penicillin.

NOTE: Necessary dental care should be accomplished in infections involving the gum tissue.

Medical Conditions in Which Oral Penicillin Therapy Is Indicated as Prophylaxis—To prevent recurrence following rheumatic fever and/or chorea. Prophylaxis with oral penicillin on a continuing basis has proved effective in preventing recurrence of these conditions.

Although no controlled clinical efficacy studies have been conducted, penicillin V has been suggested by the American Heart Association and the American Dental Association for use as part of a parenteral/oral regimen and as an alternative oral regimen for prophylaxis against bacterial endocarditis in patients with congenital heart disease or rheumatic or other acquired valvular heart disease when they undergo dental procedures and surgical procedures of the respiratory tract.[1] Since alpha-hemolytic streptococci relatively resistant to penicillin may be found when patients are receiving continuous oral penicillin for secondary prevention of rheumatic fever, prophylactic agents other than penicillin may be chosen for these patients and prescribed in addition to their continuous prophylactic regimen for rheumatic fever. Oral penicillin should not be used as adjunctive prophylaxis for genitourinary instrumentation or surgery, lower intestinal tract surgery, sigmoidoscopy, and childbirth.

Note: When selecting antibiotics for the prevention of bacterial endocarditis, the physician or dentist should read the full joint statement of the American Heart Association and the American Dental Association.[1]

Contraindication: A previous hypersensitivity reaction to any penicillin is a contraindication.

Warnings: Serious and occasionally fatal hypersensitivity (anaphylactoid) reactions have been reported in patients receiving penicillin therapy. Although anaphylaxis is more frequent following parenteral therapy, it has occurred in patients given oral penicillins. These reactions are more likely in individuals with a history of sensitivity to multiple allergens.

There have been well-documented reports of individuals with a history of penicillin hypersensitivity who have experienced severe reactions when treated with a cephalosporin. Before therapy with a penicillin, careful inquiry should be made concerning previous hypersensitivity reactions to penicillins, cephalosporins, and other allergens. If an allergic reaction occurs, the drug should be discontinued and the patient treated with the usual agents (e.g., epinephrine or other pressor amines, antihistamines, or corticosteroids).

Precautions: Penicillin should be used with caution in individuals with histories of significant allergies and/or asthma.

The oral route of administration should not be relied on in patients with severe illness or with nausea, vomiting, gastric dilatation, cardiospasm, or intestinal hypermotility.

Occasional patients will not absorb therapeutic amounts of orally administered penicillin. In streptococcal infections, therapy must be sufficient to eliminate the organism (a minimum of ten days); otherwise, the sequelae of streptococcal disease may occur. Cultures should be taken following completion of treatment to determine whether streptococci have been eradicated.

Prolonged use of antibiotics may promote the overgrowth of nonsusceptible organisms, including fungi. If superinfection occurs, appropriate measures should be taken.

Adverse Reactions: Although reactions have been reported much less frequently after oral than after parenteral penicillin therapy, it should be remembered that all degrees of hypersensitivity, including fatal anaphylaxis, have been observed with oral penicillin.

The most common reactions to oral penicillin are nausea, vomiting, epigastric distress, diarrhea, and black, hairy tongue. The hypersensitivity reactions noted are skin eruptions (ranging from maculopapular to exfoliative dermatitis); urticaria; reactions resembling serum sickness, including chills, fever, edema, arthralgia, and prostration; laryngeal edema; and anaphylaxis. Fever and eosinophilia may frequently be the only reactions observed. Hemolytic anemia, leukopenia, thrombocytopenia, neuropathy, and nephropathy are infrequent reactions and are usually associated with high doses of parenteral penicillin.

Dosage and Administration: The dosage of V-Cillin K® (penicillin V potassium, Lilly) should be determined according to the sensitivity of the causative microorganism and the severity of infection and should be adjusted to the clinical response of the patient.

The usual dosage recommendations for adults and children 12 years and over are as follows:

Streptococcal Infections—Mild to moderately severe infections of the upper respiratory tract, including scarlet fever and mild erysipelas: 200,000 to 500,000 units every six to eight hours for ten days.

Pneumococcal Infections—Mild to moderately severe infections of the respiratory tract, including otitis media: 400,000 to 500,000 units every six hours until the patient has been afebrile for at least two days.

Staphylococcal Infections—Mild infections of skin and soft tissue (culture and susceptibility tests should be performed): 400,000 to 500,000 units every six to eight hours.

Fusospirochetosis (Vincent's Infection) of the Oropharynx—Mild to moderately severe infections: 400,000 to 500,000 units every six to eight hours.

Prophylaxis in the Following Conditions—To prevent recurrence following rheumatic fever and/or chorea: 200,000 to 250,000 units twice daily on a continuing basis.

For prophylaxis against bacterial endocarditis[1] in patients with congenital heart disease or rheumatic or other acquired valvular heart disease when undergoing dental procedures or surgical procedures of the upper respiratory tract, one of two regimens may be selected:

(1) For the oral regimen, the usual adult dosage is 2 g of penicillin V (1 g for children under 30 kg) one-half to one hour before the procedure and then 500 mg (250 mg for children under 30 kg) every six hours for eight doses; or

(2) For the combined parenteral/oral regimen, the dosage schedule is 1,000,000 units of aqueous crystalline penicillin G (30,000 units/kg for children) intramuscularly mixed with 600,000 units procaine penicillin G (600,000 units for children) one-half to one hour before the procedure and then oral penicillin V, 500 mg for adults or 250 mg for children less than 30 kg, every six hours for eight doses. Doses for children should not exceed recommendations for adults for a single dose or for a 24-hour period.

NOTE: Therapy for children under 12 years of age is calculated on the basis of body weight. For infants and small children, the suggested daily dose is 25,000 to 90,000 units (15 to 50 mg)/kg in three to six divided doses.

How Supplied: (℞) *For Oral Solution, V-Cillin K® (Penicillin V Potassium for Oral Solution, USP): M-126, W07,* *125 mg (200,000 units) (equivalent to penicillin V) per 5 ml of solution, in 100 (NDC 0002-2307-48), 150 (NDC 0002-2307-68), and 200-ml-size (NDC 0002-2307-89) packages and in unit-dose bottles of 100 (ID100) (NDC 0002-2307-33); *M-142, W16,* *250 mg (400,000 units) (equivalent to penicillin V) per 5 ml of solution, in 100 (NDC 0002-2316-48), 150 (NDC 0002-2316-68), and 200-ml-size (NDC 0002-2316-89) packages and in unit-dose bottles of 100 (ID100) (NDC 0002-2316-33)

Each package consists of a bottle containing penicillin V potassium equivalent to penicillin V in a dry, pleasantly flavored mixture, buffered with sodium citrate and citric acid.

After being mixed, the solution should be stored in a refrigerator. It may be kept for 14 days without significant loss of potency. *Shake well before using. Keep tightly closed.*

(℞) *Tablets V-Cillin K® (Penicillin V Potassium Tablets, USP),* Specially Coated: *No. 1830, C27,* * 125 mg (200,000 units) (equivalent to penicillin V), in bottles of 100 (NDC 0002-0327-02); *No. 1831, C29,* *250 mg (400,000 units) (equivalent to penicillin V), in 100 (NDC 0002-0329-02), and 500 (NDC 0002-0329-03); and *No. 1832, C46,* *500 mg (800,000 units) (equivalent to penicillin V) in bottles of 24 (NDC 0002-0346-24), 100 (NDC 0002-0346-02), and 500 (NDC 0002-0346-03).

[072484]

Reference: 1. American Heart Association: Prevention of Bacterial Endocarditis, Circulation, 56:139A, 1977.

VELBAN® ℞
[vĕl' băn]
(vinblastine sulfate)
Sterile, USP

Description: Velban® (Vinblastine Sulfate, USP, Lilly) is the salt of an alkaloid extracted from *Vinca rosea* Linn., a common flowering herb known as the periwinkle (more properly known as *Catharanthus roseus* G. Don). Previously, the generic name was vincaleukoblastine, abbreviated VLB.

Chemical and physical evidence indicates that Velban has the empirical formula $C_{46}H_{58}O_9N_4 \cdot H_2SO_4$ and that it is a dimeric alkaloid containing both indole and dihydroindole moieties.

Vials of Velban contain 10 mg of vinblastine sulfate, in the form of a lyophilized plug, without excipients. When sodium chloride solution is added prior to injection, the pH of the resulting solution lies in the range of 3.5 to 5.

Actions: Velban® (vinblastine sulfate, Lilly) has been used for the palliative treatment of a variety of malignant neoplastic conditions. In susceptible clinical cases, Velban has produced temporary reduction in the size or temporary disappearance of some tumors. It has relieved pain and other symptoms and allowed some patients to regain appetite and weight.

Experimental data indicate that the action of Velban is different from that of other recognized antineoplastic agents. Tissue-culture studies suggest an interference with metabolic pathways of amino acids leading from glutamic acid to the citric acid cycle and to urea. In vivo experiments tend to confirm the in vitro results. A number of studies in vitro and in vivo have demonstrated that Velban produces a stathmokinetic effect and various atypical mitotic figures. The therapeutic responses, however, are not fully explained by the cytologic changes, since these changes are sometimes observed clinically and experimentally in the absence of any oncolytic effects.

Continued on next page

* Identi-Code® symbol.

Lilly—Cont.

Reversal of the antitumor effect of Velban by glutamic acid or tryptophan has been observed. In addition, glutamic acid and aspartic acid have protected mice from lethal doses of Velban. Aspartic acid was relatively ineffective in reversing the antitumor effect.

Other studies indicate that Velban has an effect on cell-energy production required for mitosis and interferes with nucleic acid synthesis.

Hematologic Effects—Clinically, leukopenia is an expected effect of Velban® (vinblastine sulfate, Lilly), and the level of the leukocyte count is an important guide to therapy with this drug. In general, the larger the dose employed, the more profound and longer lasting the leukopenia will be. The fact that the white-blood-cell count returns to normal levels after drug-induced leukopenia is an indication that the white-cell-producing mechanism is not permanently depressed. Usually, the white count has completely returned to normal after the virtual disappearance of white cells from the peripheral blood.

Following therapy with Velban, the nadir in white-blood-cell count may be expected to occur five to ten days after the last day of drug administration. Recovery of the white blood count is fairly rapid thereafter and is usually complete within another seven to 14 days. With the smaller doses employed for maintenance therapy, leukopenia may not be a problem.

Although the thrombocyte count ordinarily is not significantly lowered by therapy with Velban, patients whose bone marrow has been recently impaired by prior therapy with radiation or with other oncolytic drugs may show thrombocytopenia (less than 200,000 platelets/mm^3). When other chemotherapy or radiation has not been employed previously, thrombocyte reduction below the level of 200,000/mm^3 is rarely encountered, even when Velban may be causing significant leukopenia. Rapid recovery from thrombocytopenia within a few days is the rule.

The effect of Velban upon the red-cell count and hemoglobin is usually insignificant when other therapy does not complicate the picture. It should be remembered, however, that patients with malignant disease may exhibit anemia even in the absence of any therapy.

Indications: Vinblastine sulfate is indicated in the palliative treatment of the following:

I. Frequently Responsive Malignancies—
  Generalized Hodgkin's disease (Stages III and IV, Ann Arbor modification of Rye staging system)
  Lymphocytic lymphoma (nodular and diffuse, poorly and well differentiated)
  Histiocytic lymphoma
  Mycosis fungoides (advanced stages)
  Advanced carcinoma of the testis
  Kaposi's sarcoma
  Letterer-Siwe disease (histiocytosis X)

II. Less Frequently Responsive Malignancies—
  Choriocarcinoma resistant to other chemotherapeutic agents
  Carcinoma of the breast, unresponsive to appropriate endocrine surgery and hormonal therapy

Current principles of chemotherapy for many types of cancer include the concurrent administration of several antineoplastic agents. For enhanced therapeutic effect without additive toxicity, agents with different dose-limiting clinical toxicities and different mechanisms of action are generally selected. Therefore, although Velban® (vinblastine sulfate, Lilly) is effective as a single agent in the aforementioned indications, it is usually administered in combination with other antineoplastic drugs. Such combination therapy produces a greater percentage of response than does a single-agent regimen. These principles have been applied, for example, in the chemotherapy of Hodgkin's disease.

Hodgkin's Disease—Velban has been shown to be one of the most effective single agents for the treatment of Hodgkin's disease. Advanced Hodgkin's disease has also been successfully treated with several multiple-drug regimens that included Velban. Patients who had relapses after treatment with the MOPP program—mechlorethamine hydrochloride (nitrogen mustard), vincristine sulfate (Oncovin® [vincristine sulfate, Lilly]), prednisone, and procarbazine—have likewise responded to combination-drug therapy that included Velban. A protocol using cyclophosphamide in place of nitrogen mustard and Velban instead of Oncovin is an alternative therapy for previously untreated patients with advanced Hodgkin's disease. Advanced testicular germinal-cell cancers (embryonal carcinoma, teratocarcinoma, and choriocarcinoma) are sensitive to Velban alone, but better clinical results are achieved when Velban is administered concomitantly with other antineoplastic agents. The effect of bleomycin is significantly enhanced if Velban is administered six to eight hours prior to the administration of bleomycin; this schedule permits more cells to be arrested during metaphase, the stage of the cell cycle in which bleomycin is active.

Contraindications: Velban® (vinblastine sulfate, Lilly) is contraindicated in patients who are leukopenic. It should not be used in the presence of bacterial infection. Such infections must be brought under control prior to the initiation of therapy with Velban.

Warnings: *Usage in Pregnancy*—Caution is necessary with the administration of all oncolytic drugs during pregnancy. Information on the use of Velban® (vinblastine sulfate, Lilly) during pregnancy is very limited. Although no abnormalities of the human fetus have been reported thus far, animal studies with Velban suggest that teratogenic effects may occur.

Aspermia has been reported in man. Animal studies show metaphase arrest and degenerative changes in germ cells.

Precautions: If leukopenia with less than 2000 white blood cells/mm^3 occurs following a dose of Velban® (vinblastine sulfate, Lilly), the patient should be watched carefully for evidence of infection until the white-blood-cell count has returned to a safe level.

When cachexia or ulcerated areas of the skin surface are present, there may be a more profound leukopenic response to the drug; therefore, its use should be avoided in older persons suffering from either of these conditions.

In patients with malignant-cell infiltration of the bone marrow, the leukocyte and platelet counts have sometimes fallen precipitously after moderate doses of Velban. Further use of the drug in such patients is inadvisable.

Acute shortness of breath and severe bronchospasm have been reported following the administration of vinca alkaloids. These reactions have been encountered most frequently when vinca alkaloid was used in combination with mitomycin-C. The onset may be within minutes or several hours after the vinca is injected.

The use of small amounts of Velban daily for long periods is not advised, even though the resulting total weekly dosage may be similar to that recommended. Little or no added therapeutic effect has been demonstrated when such regimens have been used. *Strict adherence to the recommended dosage schedule is very important.* When amounts equal to several times the recommended weekly dosage were given in seven daily installments for long periods, convulsions, severe and permanent central-nervous-system damage, and even death occurred.

Care must be taken to avoid contamination of the eye with concentrations of Velban used clinically. If accidental contamination occurs, severe irritation (or, if the drug was delivered under pressure, even corneal ulceration) may result. The eye should be washed with water immediately and thoroughly.

Adverse Reactions: *Prior to the use of the drug, patients should be advised of the possibility of untoward symptoms.*

In general, the incidence of adverse reactions attending the use of Velban® (vinblastine sulfate, Lilly) appears to be related to the size of the dose employed. With the exception of epilation, leukopenia, and neurologic side effects, adverse reactions generally have not persisted for longer than 24 hours. Neurologic side effects are not common; but when they do occur, they often last for more than 24 hours. Leukopenia, the most common adverse reaction, is usually the dose-limiting factor. The following are manifestations which have been reported as adverse reactions:

Gastrointestinal—Nausea, vomiting, constipation, vesiculation of the mouth, ileus, diarrhea, anorexia, abdominal pain, rectal bleeding, pharyngitis, hemorrhagic enterocolitis, bleeding from an old peptic ulcer

Neurologic—Numbness, paresthesias, peripheral neuritis, mental depression, loss of deep-tendon reflexes, headache, convulsions

Miscellaneous—Malaise, weakness, dizziness, pain in tumor site, vesiculation of the skin

Nausea and vomiting usually may be controlled with ease by antiemetic agents. When epilation develops, it frequently is not total; and, in some cases, hair regrows while maintenance therapy continues.

Extravasation during intravenous injection may lead to cellulitis and phlebitis. If the amount of extravasation is great, sloughing may occur.

Dosage and Administration: There are variations in the depth of the leukopenic response which follows therapy with Velban® (vinblastine sulfate, Lilly). For this reason, it is recommended that the drug be given no more frequently than *once every seven days.* It is wise to initiate therapy for adults by administering a single intravenous dose of 3.7 mg/m^2 of body surface area (bsa). Thereafter, white-blood-cell counts should be made to determine the patient's sensitivity to Velban.

A simplified and conservative incremental approach to dosage *at weekly intervals* may be outlined as follows:

	Adults	Children
First dose	3.7 mg/m^2 bsa	2.5 mg/m^2 bsa
Second dose	5.5 mg/m^2 bsa	3.75 mg/m^2 bsa
Third dose	7.4 mg/m^2 bsa	5.0 mg/m^2 bsa
Fourth dose	9.25 mg/m^2 bsa	6.25 mg/m^2 bsa
Fifth dose	11.1 mg/m^2 bsa	7.5 mg/m^2 bsa

The above-mentioned increases may be used until a maximum dose (not exceeding 18.5 mg/m^2 bsa for adults and 12.5 mg/m^2 bsa for children) is reached. The dose should not be increased after that dose which reduces the white-cell count to approximately 3000 cells/mm^3. In some adults, 3.7 mg/m^2 bsa may produce this leukopenia; other adults may require more than 11.1 mg/m^2 bsa; and, very rarely, as much as 18.5 mg/m^2 bsa may be necessary. For most adult patients, however, the weekly dosage will prove to be 5.5 to 7.4 mg/m^2 bsa.

When the dose of Velban which will produce the above degree of leukopenia has been established, a dose *one increment smaller* than this should be administered at weekly intervals for maintenance. Thus, the patient is receiving the maximum dose that does not cause leukopenia. *It should be emphasized that, even though seven days have elapsed, the next dose of Velban should not be given until the white-cell count has returned to at least 4000/mm^3.*

In some cases, oncolytic activity may be encountered before leukopenic effect. When this occurs, there is no need to increase the size of subsequent doses.

The duration of maintenance therapy varies according to the disease being treated and the combination of antineoplastic agents being used. There are differences of opinion regarding the duration of maintenance therapy with the same protocol for a particular disease; for example, various durations have been used with the MOPP program in treating Hodgkin's disease. Prolonged chemotherapy for maintaining remissions involves several risks, among which are life-threatening infectious diseases, sterility, and possibly the appearance of other cancers through suppression of immune surveillance. In some disorders, survival following complete remission may not be as prolonged as that achieved with shorter periods of maintenance therapy. On the other hand, failure to provide maintenance therapy in some patients may lead to unnecessary relapse; complete remissions in patients with testicular cancer, unless maintained for at least two years, often result in early relapse. To prepare a solution containing 1 mg of Velban/ml, add 10 ml of Sodium Chloride Injection (preserved with phenol or benzyl alcohol) to the 10 mg of Velban in the sterile vial. Other solutions are not recommended. The drug dissolves instantly to give a clear solution. After a solution has been made in this way and a portion of it has been removed from a vial, the remainder of the vial's contents may be stored in a refrigerator for future use for 30 days without significant loss of potency. The dose of Velban (calculated to provide the desired amount) may be injected either into the tubing of a running intravenous infusion or directly into a vein. The latter procedure is readily adaptable to outpatient therapy. In either case, the injection may be completed in about one minute. If care is taken to insure that the needle is securely within the vein and that no solution containing Velban is spilled extravascularly, cellulitis and/or phlebitis will not occur. To minimize further the possibility of extravascular spillage, it is suggested that the syringe and needle be rinsed with venous blood before withdrawal of the needle. The dose should not be diluted in large volumes of diluent (i.e., 100 to 250 ml) or given intravenously for prolonged periods (ranging from 30 to 60 minutes or more), since this frequently results in irritation of the vein and increases the chance of extravasation.

Because of the enhanced possibility of thrombosis, it is considered inadvisable to inject a solution of Velban into an extremity in which the circulation is impaired or potentially impaired by such conditions as compressing or invading neoplasm, phlebitis, or varicosity.

Caution—If leakage into surrounding tissue should occur during intravenous administration of Velban® (vinblastine sulfate, Lilly), it may cause considerable irritation. The injection should be discontinued immediately, and any remaining portion of the dose should then be introduced into another vein. Local injection of hyaluronidase and the application of moderate heat to the area of leakage help disperse the drug and are thought to minimize discomfort and the possibility of cellulitis.

How Supplied: (℞) Vials No. 687, Velban® (Sterile Vinblastine Sulfate, USP), 10 mg, 10-ml size, rubber-stoppered (Dry Powder), in singles (10 per carton) (NDC 0002-1452-01). *The vials should be stored in a refrigerator (2° to 8°C, or 36° to 46°F) to assure extended stability.*

[110283]

ZINC-INSULIN CRYSTALS
[ī' lĕ-tĭn]
see under Iletin® (insulin, Lilly).

LyphoMed, Inc.
2020 RUBY STREET
MELROSE PARK, IL 60160

PENTAM™ 300   ℞
(Sterile Pentamidine Isethionate)

Description: PENTAM™ 300 (Sterile Pentamidine Isethionate), an antiprotozoal agent, is a nonpyrogenic lyophilized product. After reconstitution, it should be administered by parenteral (IM or IV) routes. For full prescribing information see package insert.

How Supplied:
Product No.
113-15   PENTAM™ 300 (Sterile Pentamidine Isethionate) 300 mg, lyophilized product in single dose vials, packaged in boxes of 7's. (NDC 0469-1130-90)

Store the dry product between 2° and 8°C. Protect the dry product from light. Discard unused portion.

Macsil, Inc.
1326 FRANKFORD AVENUE
PHILADELPHIA, PA 19125

BALMEX® BABY POWDER
(See PDR For Nonprescription Drugs)

BALMEX® EMOLLIENT LOTION
(See PDR For Nonprescription Drugs)

BALMEX® OINTMENT
(See PDR For Nonprescription Drugs)

Mallard Incorporated
3021 WABASH AVE.
DETROIT, MI 48216

ALLERSONE OINTMENT   ℞
[ăl'er-sōne]
Composition:
Hydrocortisone 0.5%
Diperodon Hydrochloride 0.5%
Zinc Oxide 5.0%
How Supplied: 15 gm. tubes and 1 lb. jars.

ANOQUAN   ℞
[an'o-kwan]
Description—Each capsule contains:
Butalbital .... 50 mg.
Caffeine .... 40 mg.
Acetaminophen .... 325 mg.
How Supplied: Bottles of 1000's and 100's.

ENZOBILE Improved Formula   OTC
[en-zo-bile]
Each enteric coated tablet contains:
Outer coating (Gastro soluble)
Pepsin .... 150 mg.
Enteric coated inner core:
Pancreatic Enzyme Concentrate ...... 100 mg.
Oxbile Extract .... 100 mg.
Cellulase .... 10 mg.
How Supplied: Bottles of 500's and 100's.

HYSONE OINTMENT   ℞
[hi-sōn]
Composition:
Iodochlorhydroxyquin 3%
Hydrocortisone 1%
How Supplied: 15 gm. tubes.

PHENATE   ℞
[fē' nate]
Description: Each timed release tablet contains:
Acetaminophen .... 325 mg.
Chlorpheniramine Maleate .... 4 mg.
Phenylpropanolamine HCl .... 40 mg.
How Supplied: Bottles of 1000's and 100's.

SALETO   OTC
[să-lē-tō]
Description: Each tablet contains:
Aspirin .... 210 mg.
Acetaminophen .... 115 mg.
Salicylamide .... 65 mg.
Caffeine Anhydrous .... 16 mg.
How Supplied: Bottles of 50, 100, and 1000.

Marion Laboratories, Inc.
Pharmaceutical Products Division
MARION INDUSTRIAL PARK
MARION PARK DRIVE
KANSAS CITY, MO 64137

PRODUCT IDENTIFICATION NUMERICAL SUMMARY SOLID ORAL DOSAGE FORMS

Marion Laboratories, Inc.
Kansas City, MO 64137
To provide quick and positive identification of Marion Laboratories prescription drug products, we have imprinted an identifying number and the name MARION on the following tablets or capsules.

1375	DITROPAN® Tablets (oxybutynin chloride)
1525	DUOTRATE® Capsules, 30 mg (pentaerythritol tetranitrate)
1530	DUOTRATE® Capsules, 45 mg (pentaerythritol tetranitrate)
1550	NITRO-BID® Capsules, 2.5 mg (nitroglycerin)
1551	NITRO-BID® Capsules, 6.5 mg (nitroglycerin)
1553	NITRO-BID® Capsules, 9 mg (nitroglycerin)
1555	PAVABID® Capsules, 150 mg (papaverine hydrochloride)*
1712	CARAFATE® Tablets, 1 gm (sucralfate)
1771	CARDIZEM® Tablets, 30 mg (diltiazem hydrochloride)
1772	CARDIZEM® Tablets, 60 mg (diltiazem hydrochloride)

PAVABID® HP Capsulets, 300 mg (papaverine hydrochloride) is identified by the name MARION on one side and PAVABID HP on the reverse side.
* PAVABID Capsules, 150 mg (papaverine hydrochloride) also bear the brand name PAVABID.
Marion THYROID and THYROID STRONG Tablets bear the following identification numbers.

ML 626	THYROID STRONG Tablets (Coated), ½ grain
ML 627	THYROID STRONG Tablets (Coated), 1 grain
ML 628	THYROID STRONG Tablets (Coated), 2 grain
ML 629	THYROID STRONG Tablets (Coated), 3 grain
ML 674	THYROID STRONG Tablets (Plain), 1 grain
ML 675	THYROID STRONG Tablets (Plain), 2 grain
ML 686	THYROID STRONG Tablets (Plain), ½ grain
ML 777	THYROID Tablets, USP (Plain), 60 mg
ML 778	THYROID Tablets, USP (Plain), 120 mg

AMBENYL® Cough Syrup   C ℞
[ăm' bĕ-nĭl]
Description: Each 5 ml of AMBENYL Cough Syrup contains:
Codeine phosphate (Warning—May be habit-forming) .... 10 mg
Bromodiphenhydramine hydrochloride ...... 12.5 mg
Alcohol, 5%

Chemically codeine phosphate is morphinan-6-ol,7,8-didehydro-4,5-epoxy-3-methoxy-17-methyl-,(5α,6α)-,phosphate(1:1)(salt),hemihydrate and bromodiphenhydramine hydrochloride is ethanamine,2-[(4-bromophenyl) phenyl-methoxy]-N,N-dimethyl-, hydrochloride.
AMBENYL Cough Syrup is for oral administration.

Clinical Pharmacology: AMBENYL is a combination of an antihistaminic agent, along with a well-recognized agent exhibiting antitussive properties.

Indications and Usage: AMBENYL is indicated for relief of upper respiratory symptoms and

Continued on next page

Marion—Cont.

coughs associated with allergies or the common cold.

Contraindications: Use in Newborn or Premature Infants: This drug should *not* be used in newborn or premature infants.

Use in Nursing Mothers: Because of the higher risk of antihistamines for infants generally and for newborns and prematures in particular, antihistamine therapy is contraindicated in nursing mothers.

Use in Lower Respiratory Disease: Antihistamines *should NOT* be used to treat lower respiratory tract symptoms including asthma.

Antihistamines are also contraindicated in the following conditions: Hypersensitivity to bromodiphenhydramine and other antihistamines of similar chemical structure.

Monoamine oxidase inhibitor therapy (see Drug Interactions Section).

Warnings: Antihistamines should be used with considerable caution in patients with:
  Narrow angle glaucoma
  Stenosing peptic ulcer
  Pyloroduodenal obstruction
  Symptomatic prostatic hypertrophy
  Bladder neck obstruction

Use in Children: In infants and children, especially, antihistamines in *overdosage* may cause hallucinations, convulsions, or death. As in adults, antihistamines may diminish mental alertness in children. In the young child, particularly, they may produce excitation.

Use in Pregnancy: Experience with this drug in pregnant women is inadequate to determine whether there exists a potential for harm to the developing fetus.

Use with CNS Depressants: AMBENYL Cough Syrup has additive effects with alcohol and other CNS depressants (hypnotics, sedatives, tranquilizers, etc.).

Use in Activities Requiring Mental Alertness: Patients should be warned about engaging in activities requiring mental alertness such as driving a car or operating appliances, machinery, etc.

Use in the Elderly (approximately 60 years or older): Antihistamines are more likely to cause dizziness, sedation, and hypotension in elderly patients.

Precautions: Bromodiphenhydramine has an atropine-like action and, therefore, should be used with caution in patients with:
  History of bronchial asthma
  Increased intraocular pressure
  Hyperthyroidism
  Cardiovascular disease
  Hypertension

Drug Interactions: Codeine may potentiate the effects of other narcotics, general anesthetics, tranquilizers, sedatives and hypnotics, tricyclic antidepressants, MAO inhibitors, alcohol, and other CNS depressants.

Adverse Reactions: The following side effects may occur in patients taking AMBENYL:

drowsiness	tingling, heaviness,
confusion	weakness of hands
nervousness	nasal stuffiness
restlessness	vertigo
nausea	palpitation
vomiting	headache
diarrhea	insomnia
blurring of vision	urticaria
diplopia	drug rash
difficulty in urination	photosensitivity
constipation	hemolytic anemia
tightness of the chest and wheezing	hypotension epigastric distress
thickening of bronchial secretions	
dryness of mouth, nose, and throat	

Drug Abuse and Dependence: Codeine can produce drug dependence of the morphine type and, therefore, has the potential for being abused. Psychic dependence, physical dependence, and tolerance may develop upon repeated administration of this drug, and it should be prescribed and administered with the same degree of caution appropriate to the user of other oral narcotic-containing medications. Like other narcotic-containing medications, the drug is subject to the Federal Controlled Substances Act.

Overdosage: Antihistamine overdosage reactions may vary from central nervous system depression to stimulation. Stimulation is particularly likely in children. Atropine-like signs and symptoms—dry mouth; fixed, dilated pupils; flushing; and gastrointestinal symptoms may also occur.

If vomiting has not occurred spontaneously, the patient should be induced to vomit. This is best done by having him drink a glass of water or milk after which he should be made to gag. Precautions against aspiration must be taken, especially in infants and children.

If vomiting is unsuccessful, gastric lavage is indicated within three hours after ingestion and even later if large amounts of milk or cream were given beforehand. Isotonic and ½ isotonic saline is the lavage solution of choice.

Saline cathartics, as milk of magnesia, by osmosis draw water into the bowel and, therefore, are valuable for their action in rapid dilution of bowel content.

Stimulants should *not* be used.

Vasopressors may be used to treat hypotension.

Dosage and Administration: DOSAGE SHOULD BE INDIVIDUALIZED ACCORDING TO THE NEEDS AND THE RESPONSE OF THE PATIENT.

Adults—one or two teaspoonfuls every four to six hours, not to exceed 12 teaspoonfuls in 24 hours. Children (total intake of codeine phosphate should not exceed 1 mg/kg/24 hours)—Six to under 12 years of age—one-half to one teaspoonful every six hours.

Not recommended for use in children under six years of age.

How Supplied: AMBENYL Cough Syrup is red and is supplied in 4-fl-oz (NDC 0088-1240-11), 1-pt (NDC 0088-1240-18), and 1-gal (NDC 0088-1240-99) bottles. Store at controlled room temperature (59°–86° F).

Issued 1/84

AMBENYL®-D   OTC
[ăm′ bĕ-nĭl]
Decongestant Cough Formula

Antitussive-Expectorant-Nasal Decongestant

Two teaspoonfuls (10 ml) contain the following active ingredients:
Guaifenesin (glyceryl guaiacolate) .... 200 mg
Pseudoephedrine hydrochloride .... 60 mg
Dextromethorphan hydrobromide .... 30 mg
Also contains 9.5% alcohol.

Indications: AMBENYL®-D is for temporary relief of nasal congestion due to the common cold or associated with sinusitis, helps loosen phlegm, calms cough impulses without narcotics, and temporarily helps you cough less.

Directions for Use: Adult Dose (12 years and over)—Two teaspoonfuls every six hours. Child Dose (6–12 years)—One teaspoonful every six hours. (2–6 years)—One-half teaspoonful every six hours.

No more than four doses per day.

Warnings: Do not give this product to children under two years except under the advice and supervision of a physician. Do not take this product for persistent or chronic cough such as occurs with smoking, asthma, or emphysema, or where cough is accompanied by excessive secretions, except under the advice and supervision of a physician. Do not exceed recommended dosage because at higher doses nervousness, dizziness, or sleeplessness may occur.

Caution: A persistent cough may be a sign of a serious condition. If cough persists for more than one week, tends to recur, or is accompanied by high fever, rash, or persistent headache, consult a physician.

If symptoms do not improve within seven days or are accompanied by high fever, consult a physician before continuing use. Do not take this product if you have high blood pressure, heart disease, diabetes, or thyroid disease, except under the advice and supervision of a physician.

If pregnant or nursing a baby, consult your physician or pharmacist before using this product.

Drug Interaction Precaution: Do not take this product if you are presently taking a prescription antihypertensive or antidepressant drug containing a monoamine oxidase inhibitor except under the advice and supervision of a physician.

Store at a controlled room temperature (59°–86°F).

Keep this and all drugs out of reach of children.

In case of accidental overdose, seek professional assistance or contact a poison control center immediately.

How Supplied: Ambenyl-D Decongestant Cough Formula is supplied in a 4-fl-oz bottle.

Issued 5/84

CARAFATE® Tablets   ℞
[kăr′ ă-fāt]
(sucralfate) 1 gm

Description: CARAFATE® (sucralfate) is α-D-Glucopyranoside, β-D-fructofuranosyl-, octakis-(hydrogen sulfate) aluminum complex. Tablets for oral administration contain 1 gm of sucralfate.

Therapeutic category: antiulcer

Clinical Pharmacology: Sucralfate is only minimally absorbed from the gastrointestinal tract. The small amounts of the sulfated disaccharide that are absorbed are excreted primarily in the urine.

Although the mechanism of sucralfate's ability to accelerate healing of duodenal ulcers remains to be fully defined, it is known that it exerts its effect through a local, rather than systemic, action. The following observations also appear pertinent:

1. Studies in human subjects and with animal models of ulcer disease have shown that sucralfate forms an ulcer-adherent complex with proteinaceous exudate at the ulcer site.
2. In vitro, a sucralfate-albumin film provides a barrier to diffusion of hydrogen ions.
3. In human subjects, sucralfate given in doses recommended for ulcer therapy inhibits pepsin activity in gastric juice by 32%.
4. In vitro, sucralfate adsorbs bile salts.

These observations suggest that sucralfate's antiulcer activity is the result of formation of an ulcer-adherent complex that covers the ulcer site and protects it against further attack by acid, pepsin, and bile salts. Sucralfate has negligible acid-neutralizing capacity, and its antiulcer effects cannot be attributed to neutralization of gastric acid.

Clinical Trials: Over 600 patients have participated in well-controlled clinical trials worldwide. Multicenter trials conducted in the United States, both of them placebo-controlled studies with endoscopic evaluation at 2 and 4 weeks, showed: [See table on left].

The sucralfate-placebo differences were statistically significant in both studies at 4 weeks but not at 2 weeks. The poorer result in the first study may have occurred because sucralfate was given two

---

CARAFATE

	Treatment Groups	Ulcer Healing/No. Patients	
		2 wk.	4 wk. (Overall)
Study 1	Sucralfate	37/105 (35.2%)	82/109 (75.2%)
	Placebo	26/106 (24.5%)	68/107 (63.6%)
		2 wk.	4 wk. (Overall)
Study 2	Sucralfate	8/24 (33%)	22/24 (92%)
	Placebo	4/31 (13%)	18/31 (58%)

hours after meals and at bedtime rather than one hour before meals and at bedtime, the regimen used in international studies and in the second United States study. In addition, in the first study liquid antacid was utilized as needed, whereas in the second study antacid tablets were used.

Indications and Usage: CARAFATE (sucralfate) is indicated in the short-term (up to 8 weeks) treatment of duodenal ulcer.

Antacids may be prescribed as needed for relief of pain.

Contraindications: There are no known contraindications to the use of sucralfate.

Precautions: Duodenal ulcer is a chronic, recurrent disease. While short-term treatment with sucralfate can result in complete healing of the ulcer, a successful course of treatment with sucralfate should not be expected to alter the post-healing frequency or severity of duodenal ulceration.

Drug Interactions: Animal studies have shown that the simultaneous administration of CARAFATE with tetracycline, phenytoin, or cimetidine will result in a statistically significant reduction in the bioavailability of these agents. This interaction appears to be nonsystemic in origin, presumably resulting from these agents being bound by the CARAFATE in the gastrointestinal tract. The bioavailability of these agents may be restored simply by separating the administration of these agents from that of CARAFATE by two hours. The clinical significance of these animal studies is yet to be defined.

Carcinogenesis, Mutagenesis, Impairment of Fertility: Chronic oral toxicity studies of 24 months' duration were conducted in mice and rats at doses up to 1 gm/kg (12 times the human dose). There was no evidence of drug-related tumorigenicity. A reproduction study in rats at doses up to 38 times the human dose did not reveal any indication of fertility impairment. Mutagenicity studies were not conducted.

Pregnancy: Teratogenic effects. Pregnancy Category B. Teratogenicity studies have been performed in mice, rats, and rabbits at doses up to 50 times the human dose and have revealed no evidence of harm to the fetus due to sucralfate. There are, however, no adequate and well-controlled studies in pregnant women. Because animal reproduction studies are not always predictive of human response, this drug should be used during pregnancy only if clearly needed.

Nursing Mothers: It is not known whether this drug is excreted in human milk. Because many drugs are excreted in human milk, caution should be exercised when sucralfate is administered to a nursing woman.

Pediatric Use: Safety and effectiveness in children have not been established.

Adverse Reactions: Adverse reactions to sucralfate in clinical trials were minor and only rarely led to discontinuation of the drug. In studies involving over 2,500 patients treated with sucralfate, adverse effects were reported in 121 (4.7%). Constipation was the most frequent complaint (2.2%). Other adverse effects, reported in no more than one of every 350 patients, were diarrhea, nausea, gastric discomfort, indigestion, dry mouth, rash, pruritus, back pain, dizziness, sleepiness, and vertigo.

Overdosage: There is no experience in humans with overdosage. Acute oral toxicity studies in animals, however, using doses up to 12 gm/kg body weight, could not find a lethal dose. Risks associated with overdosage should, therefore, be minimal.

Dosage and Administration: The recommended adult oral dosage for duodenal ulcer is 1 gm four times a day on an empty stomach.

Antacids may be prescribed as needed for relief of pain but should not be taken within one-half hour before or after sucralfate.

While healing with sucralfate may occur during the first week or two, treatment should be continued for 4 to 8 weeks unless healing has been demonstrated by x-ray or endoscopic examination.

How Supplied: CARAFATE (sucralfate) 1-gm tablets are supplied in bottles of 100 (NDC 0088-1712-47) and in Unit Dose Identification Paks of 100 (NDC 0088-1712-49). Light pink 1-gm tablets are embossed with MARION/1712.

Issued 3/84
Shown in Product Identification Section, page 417

CARDIZEM® Tablets ℞
[kăr'dĭ-zĕm]
(diltiazem HCl)
30 mg and 60 mg

Description: CARDIZEM® (diltiazem hydrochloride) is a calcium ion influx inhibitor (slow channel blocker or calcium antagonist). Chemically, diltiazem hydrochloride is 1,5-Benzothiazepin-4(5H)one, 3-(acetyloxy)-5-[2-(dimethylamino)ethyl]-2, 3-dihydro-2-(4-methoxyphenyl)-,monohydrochloride,(+)-cis-.

Diltiazem hydrochloride is a white to off-white crystalline powder with a bitter taste. It is soluble in water, methanol, and chloroform. It has a molecular weight of 450.98. Each tablet of CARDIZEM contains either 30 mg or 60 mg diltiazem hydrochloride for oral administration.

Clinical Pharmacology: The therapeutic benefits achieved with CARDIZEM are believed to be related to its ability to inhibit the influx of calcium ions during membrane depolarization of cardiac and vascular smooth muscle.

Mechanisms of Action. Although precise mechanisms of its antianginal actions are still being delineated, CARDIZEM is believed to act in the following ways:

1. Angina Due to Coronary Artery Spasm: CARDIZEM has been shown to be a potent dilator of coronary arteries both epicardial and subendocardial. Spontaneous and ergonovine-induced coronary artery spasm are inhibited by CARDIZEM.
2. Exertional Angina: CARDIZEM has been shown to produce increases in exercise tolerance, probably due to its ability to reduce myocardial oxygen demand. This is accomplished via reductions in heart rate and systemic blood pressure at submaximal and maximal exercise work loads.

In animal models, diltiazem interferes with the slow inward (depolarizing) current in excitable tissue. It causes excitation-contraction uncoupling in various myocardial tissues without changes in the configuration of the action potential. Diltiazem produces relaxation of coronary vascular smooth muscle and dilation of both large and small coronary arteries at drug levels which cause little or no negative inotropic effect. The resultant increases in coronary blood flow (epicardial and subendocardial) occur in ischemic and nonischemic models and are accompanied by dose-dependent decreases in systemic blood pressure and decreases in peripheral resistance.

Hemodynamic and Electrophysiologic Effects. Like other calcium antagonists, diltiazem decreases sinoatrial and atrioventricular conduction in isolated tissues and has a negative inotropic effect in isolated preparations. In the intact animal, prolongation of the AH interval can be seen at higher doses.

In man, diltiazem prevents spontaneous and ergonovine-provoked coronary artery spasm. It causes a decrease in peripheral vascular resistance and a modest fall in blood pressure and, in exercise tolerance studies in patients with ischemic heart disease, reduces the heart rate-blood pressure product for any given work load. Studies to date, primarily in patients with good ventricular function, have not revealed evidence of a negative inotropic effect; cardiac output, ejection fraction, and left ventricular end diastolic pressure have not been affected. There are as yet few data on the interaction of diltiazem and beta-blockers. Resting heart rate is usually unchanged or slightly reduced by diltiazem.

Intravenous diltiazem in doses of 20 mg prolongs AH conduction time and AV node functional and effective refractory periods approximately 20%. In a study involving single oral doses of 300 mg of CARDIZEM in six normal volunteers, the average maximum PR prolongation was 14% with no instances of greater than first-degree AV block. Diltiazem-associated prolongation of the AH interval is not more pronounced in patients with first-degree heart block. In patients with sick sinus syndrome, diltiazem significantly prolongs sinus cycle length (up to 50% in some cases).

Chronic oral administration of CARDIZEM in doses of up to 240 mg/day has resulted in small increases in PR interval, but has not usually produced abnormal prolongation. There were, however, three instances of second-degree AV block and one instance of third-degree AV block in a group of 959 chronically treated patients.

Pharmacokinetics and Metabolism. Diltiazem is absorbed from the tablet formulation to about 80% of a reference capsule and is subject to an extensive first-pass effect, giving an absolute bioavailability (compared to intravenous dosing) of about 40%. CARDIZEM undergoes extensive hepatic metabolism in which 2% to 4% of the unchanged drug appears in the urine. In vitro binding studies show CARDIZEM is 70% to 80% bound to plasma proteins. Competitive ligand binding studies have also shown CARDIZEM binding is not altered by therapeutic concentrations of digoxin, hydrochlorothiazide, phenylbutazone, propranolol, salicylic acid, or warfarin. Single oral doses of 30 to 120 mg of CARDIZEM result in detectable plasma levels within 30 to 60 minutes and peak plasma levels two to three hours after drug administration. The plasma elimination half-life following single or multiple drug administration is approximately 3.5 hours. Desacetyl diltiazem is also present in the plasma at levels of 10% to 20% of the parent drug and is 25% to 50% as potent a coronary vasodilator as diltiazem. Therapeutic blood levels of CARDIZEM appear to be in the range of 50 to 200 ng/ml. There is a departure from dose-linearity when single doses above 60 mg are given; a 120-mg dose gave blood levels three times that of the 60-mg dose. There is no information about the effect of renal or hepatic impairment on excretion or metabolism of diltiazem.

Indications and Usage:
1. **Angina Pectoris Due to Coronary Artery Spasm.** CARDIZEM is indicated in the treatment of angina pectoris due to coronary artery spasm. CARDIZEM has been shown effective in the treatment of spontaneous coronary artery spasm presenting as Prinzmetal's variant angina (resting angina with ST-segment elevation occurring during attacks).
2. **Chronic Stable Angina (Classic Effort-Associated Angina).** CARDIZEM is indicated in the management of chronic stable angina. CARDIZEM has been effective in controlled trials in reducing angina frequency and increasing exercise tolerance.

There are no controlled studies of the effectiveness of the concomitant use of diltiazem and beta-blockers or of the safety of this combination in patients with impaired ventricular function or conduction abnormalities.

Contraindications: CARDIZEM is contraindicated in (1) patients with sick sinus syndrome except in the presence of a functioning ventricular pacemaker, (2) patients with second- or third-degree AV block except in the presence of a functioning ventricular pacemaker, and (3) patients with hypotension (less than 90 mm Hg systolic).

Warnings:
1. **Cardiac Conduction.** CARDIZEM prolongs AV node refractory periods without significantly prolonging sinus node recovery time, except in patients with sick sinus syndrome. This effect may rarely result in abnormally slow heart rates (particularly in patients with sick sinus syndrome) or second- or third-degree AV block (six of 1243 patients for 0.48%). Concomitant use of diltiazem with beta-blockers or digitalis may result in additive effects on cardiac conduction. A patient with Prinzmetal's angina developed periods of asystole (2 to 5 seconds) after a single dose of 60 mg diltiazem.
2. **Congestive Heart Failure.** Although diltiazem has a negative inotropic effect in isolated ani-

Continued on next page

Marion—Cont.

mal tissue preparations, hemodynamic studies in humans with normal ventricular function have not shown a reduction in cardiac index nor consistent negative effects on contractility (dp/dt). Experience with the use of CARDIZEM alone or in combination with beta-blockers in patients with impaired ventricular function is very limited. Caution should be exercised when using the drug in such patients.

3. **Hypotension.** Decreases in blood pressure associated with CARDIZEM therapy may occasionally result in symptomatic hypotension.
4. **Acute Hepatic Injury.** In rare instances, patients receiving CARDIZEM have exhibited reversible acute hepatic injury as evidenced by moderate to extreme elevations of liver enzymes. (See **Precautions** and **Adverse Reactions**).

Precautions:
General. CARDIZEM (diltiazem hydrochloride) is extensively metabolized by the liver and excreted by the kidneys and in bile. As with any new drug given over prolonged periods, laboratory parameters should be monitored at regular intervals. The drug should be used with caution in patients with impaired renal or hepatic function. In subacute and chronic dog and rat studies designed to produce toxicity, high doses of diltiazem were associated with hepatic damage. In special subacute hepatic studies, oral doses of 125 mg/kg and higher in rats were associated with histological changes in the liver which were reversible when the drug was discontinued. In dogs, doses of 20 mg/kg were also associated with hepatic changes; however, these changes were reversible with continued dosing.

Drug Interaction. Pharmacologic studies indicate that there may be additive effects in prolonging AV conduction when using beta-blockers or digitalis concomitantly with CARDIZEM. (See Warnings.)

Controlled and uncontrolled domestic studies suggest that concomitant use of CARDIZEM and beta-blockers or digitalis is usually well tolerated. Available data are not sufficient, however, to predict the effects of concomitant treatment, particularly in patients with left ventricular dysfunction or cardiac conduction abnormalities. In healthy volunteers, diltiazem has been shown to increase serum digoxin levels up to 20%.

Carcinogenesis, Mutagenesis, Impairment of Fertility. A 24-month study in rats and a 21-month study in mice showed no evidence of carcinogenicity. There was also no mutagenic response in in vitro bacterial tests. No intrinsic effect on fertility was observed in rats.

Pregnancy. Category C. Reproduction studies have been conducted in mice, rats, and rabbits. Administration of doses ranging from five to ten times greater (on a mg/kg basis) than the daily recommended therapeutic dose has resulted in embryo and fetal lethality. These doses, in some studies, have been reported to cause skeletal abnormalities. In the perinatal/postnatal studies, there was some reduction in early individual pup weights and survival rates. There was an increased incidence of stillbirths at doses of 20 times the human dose or greater.

There are no well-controlled studies in pregnant women; therefore, use CARDIZEM in pregnant women only if the potential benefit justifies the potential risk to the fetus.

Nursing Mothers. It is not known whether this drug is excreted in human milk. Because many drugs are excreted in human milk, exercise caution when CARDIZEM is administered to a nursing woman if the drug's benefits are thought to outweigh its potential risks in this situation.

Pediatric Use. Safety and effectiveness in children have not been established.

Adverse Reactions: Serious adverse reactions have been rare in studies carried out to date, but it should be recognized that patients with impaired ventricular function and cardiac conduction abnormalities have usually been excluded.

In domestic placebo-controlled trials, the incidence of adverse reactions reported during CARDIZEM therapy was not greater than that reported during placebo therapy.

The following represent occurrences observed in clinical studies which can be at least reasonably associated with the pharmacology of calcium influx inhibition. In many cases, the relationship to CARDIZEM has not been established. The most common occurrences, as well as their frequency of presentation, are: edema (2.4%), headache (2.1%), nausea (1.9%), dizziness (1.5%), rash (1.3%), asthenia (1.2%), AV block (1.1%). In addition, the following events were reported infrequently (less than 1%) with the order of presentation corresponding to the relative frequency of occurrence.
Cardiovascular: Flushing, arrhythmia, hypotension, bradycardia, palpitations, congestive heart failure, syncope.
Nervous System: Paresthesia, nervousness, somnolence, tremor, insomnia, hallucinations, and amnesia.
Gastrointestinal: Constipation, dyspepsia, diarrhea, vomiting, mild elevations of alkaline phosphatase, SGOT, SGPT, and LDH.
Dermatologic: Pruritus, petechiae, urticaria, photosensitivity.
Other: Polyuria, nocturia.

The following additional experiences have been noted:
A patient with Prinzmetal's angina experiencing episodes of vasospastic angina developed periods of transient asymptomatic asystole approximately five hours after receiving a single 60-mg dose of CARDIZEM.

The following postmarketing events have been reported infrequently in patients receiving CARDIZEM: erythema multiforme; leukopenia; and extreme elevations of alkaline phosphatase, SGOT, SGPT, LDH, and CPK. However, a definitive cause and effect between these events and CARDIZEM therapy is yet to be established.

Overdosage or Exaggerated Response: Overdosage experience with oral diltiazem has been limited. Single oral doses of 300 mg of CARDIZEM have been well tolerated by healthy volunteers. In the event of overdosage or exaggerated response, appropriate supportive measures should be employed in addition to gastric lavage. The following measures may be considered:
Bradycardia: Administer atropine (0.60 to 1.0 mg). If there is no response to vagal blockade, administer isoproterenol cautiously.
High-Degree AV Block: Treat as for bradycardia above. Fixed high-degree AV block should be treated with cardiac pacing.
Cardiac Failure: Administer inotropic agents (isoproterenol, dopamine, or dobutamine) and diuretics.
Hypotension: Vasopressors (eg, dopamine or levarterenol bitartrate).

Actual treatment and dosage should depend on the severity of the clinical situation and the judgment and experience of the treating physician.

The oral LD_{50}'s in mice and rats range from 415 to 740 mg/kg and from 560 to 810 mg/kg, respectively. The intravenous LD_{50}'s in these species were 60 and 38 mg/kg, respectively. The oral LD_{50} in dogs is considered to be in excess of 50 mg/kg, while lethality was seen in monkeys at 360 mg/kg. The toxic dose in man is not known, but blood levels in excess of 800 ng/ml have not been associated with toxicity.

Dosage and Administration: Exertional Angina Pectoris Due to Atherosclerotic Coronary Artery Disease or Angina Pectoris at Rest Due to Coronary Artery Spasm. Dosage must be adjusted to each patient's needs. Starting with 30 mg four times daily, before meals and at bedtime, dosage should be increased gradually (given in divided doses three or four times daily) at one- to two-day intervals until optimum response is obtained. Although individual patients may respond to any dosage level, the average optimum dosage range appears to be 180 to 240 mg/day. There are no available data concerning dosage requirements in patients with impaired renal or hepatic function. If the drug must be used in such patients, titration should be carried out with particular caution.

Concomitant Use With Other Antianginal Agents:
1. **Sublingual NTG** may be taken as required to abort acute anginal attacks during CARDIZEM therapy.
2. **Prophylactic Nitrate Therapy**—CARDIZEM may be safely coadministered with short- and long-acting nitrates, but there have been no controlled studies to evaluate the antianginal effectiveness of this combination.
3. **Beta-blockers.** (See **Warnings** and **Precautions**.)

How Supplied: CARDIZEM 30-mg tablets are supplied in bottles of 100 (NDC 0088-1771-47) and in Unit Dose Identification Paks of 100 (NDC 0088-1771-49). Each green tablet is engraved with MARION on one side and 1771 engraved on the other. CARDIZEM 60-mg scored tablets are supplied in bottles of 100 (NDC 0088-1772-47) and in Unit Dose Identification Paks of 100 (NDC 0088-1772-49). Each yellow tablet is engraved with MARION on one side and 1772 on the other.

Issued 4/1/84
Shown in Product Identification Section, page 417

DEBROX® Drops   OTC
[dē' brŏx]

Description: Carbamide peroxide 6.5% in a specially prepared anhydrous glycerol.

Actions: DEBROX® penetrates, softens, and facilitates removal of earwax. DEBROX Drops foam on contact with earwax due to the release of oxygen.

Indications: DEBROX Drops provides a safe, nonirritating method of softening and removing earwax.

Directions: Use directly from bottle. Tilt head sideways and squeeze bottle gently so that 5 to 10 drops flow into ear. Tip of bottle should not enter ear canal. Keep drops in ear for several minutes while head remains tilted or by inserting cotton. Repeat twice daily for up to four days if needed or as directed by physician. Any remaining wax may be removed by flushing with warm water, using a soft rubber bulb ear syringe. Avoid excessive pressure.

Warnings: Do not use if you have ear drainage or discharge, ear pain, irritation or rash in the ear, or are dizzy, unless directed by a physician. Do not use if you have an injury or perforation (hole) of the eardrum or after ear surgery, unless directed by a physician. Do not use for more than four consecutive days. If excessive earwax remains after use of this product, consult a physician. Consult a physician prior to use in children under 12.

Cautions: Avoid exposing bottle to excessive heat and direct sunlight. Keep color tip on bottle when not in use. **AVOID CONTACT WITH EYES. KEEP THIS AND ALL DRUGS OUT OF THE REACH OF CHILDREN. IN CASE OF ACCIDENTAL INGESTION, SEEK PROFESSIONAL ASSISTANCE OR CONTACT A POISON CONTROL CENTER IMMEDIATELY.**

How Supplied: DEBROX Drops in ½- or 1-fl-oz plastic squeeze bottles with applicator spouts.

Issued 8/83

DITROPAN® Tablets and Syrup   ℞
[dī' trō"păn]
(oxybutynin chloride)

Description: Each scored biconvex, engraved blue DITROPAN® Tablet contains 5 mg of oxybutynin chloride. Each 5 ml of DITROPAN® Syrup contains 5 mg of oxybutynin chloride. Chemically, oxybutynin chloride is the dl(racemic) form of 4-diethylamino-2-butynyl phenylcyclohexylglycolate hydrochloride. The empirical formula of oxybutynin chloride is $C_{22}H_{32}Cl\ NO_3$.

Oxybutynin chloride is a white crystalline solid with a molecular weight of 393.9. It is readily soluble in water and acids, but relatively insoluble in alkalis.

Action: DITROPAN® (oxybutynin chloride) exerts direct antispasmodic effect on smooth muscle and inhibits the muscarinic action of acetylcholine on smooth muscle. DITROPAN exhibits only one-fifth of the anticholinergic activity of atropine on the rabbit detrusor muscle, but four to ten times the antispasmodic activity. No blocking effects occur at skeletal neuromuscular junctions or autonomic ganglia (antinicotinic effects).

In patients with uninhibited neurogenic and reflex neurogenic bladder, cystometric studies have demonstrated that DITROPAN increases vesical capacity, diminishes the frequency of uninhibited contractions of the detrusor muscle, and delays the initial desire to void. These effects are more consistently improved in patients with uninhibited neurogenic bladder.

DITROPAN was well tolerated in patients administered the drug in controlled studies of 30 days' duration and in uncontrolled studies in which some of the patients received the drug for two years.

Indications: DITROPAN® (oxybutynin chloride) is indicated for the relief of symptoms associated with voiding in patients with uninhibited neurogenic and reflex neurogenic bladder.

Pretreatment examination should include cystometry and other appropriate diagnostic procedures. Cystometry should be repeated at appropriate intervals to evaluate response to therapy. The appropriate antimicrobial therapy should be instituted in the presence of infection.

Contraindications: DITROPAN® (oxybutynin chloride) is contraindicated in patients with glaucoma. It is also contraindicated in partial or complete obstruction of the gastrointestinal tract, paralytic ileus, intestinal atony of the elderly or debilitated patient, megacolon, toxic megacolon complicating ulcerative colitis, severe colitis, and myasthenia gravis. It is contraindicated in patients with obstructive uropathy and in patients with unstable cardiovascular status in acute hemorrhage.

Warnings: DITROPAN® (oxybutynin chloride), when administered in the presence of high environmental temperature, can cause heat prostration (fever and heat stroke due to decreased sweating).

Diarrhea may be an early symptom of incomplete intestinal obstruction, especially in patients with ileostomy or colostomy. In this instance treatment with DITROPAN would be inappropriate and possibly harmful.

DITROPAN may produce drowsiness or blurred vision. The patient should be cautioned regarding activities requiring mental alertness such as operating a motor vehicle or other machinery or performing hazardous work while taking this drug.

PREGNANCY: Reproduction studies in the hamster, rabbit, rat, and mouse have shown no definite evidence of impaired fertility or harm to the animal fetus. The safety of DITROPAN administered to women who are or who may become pregnant has not been established. Therefore, DITROPAN should not be given to pregnant women unless, in the judgment of the physician, the probable clinical benefits outweigh the possible hazards.

USAGE IN CHILDREN: The safety and efficacy of DITROPAN administration have been demonstrated for children five years of age and older (see **Dosage and Administration**). However, as there is insufficient clinical data for children under age five, DITROPAN is not recommended for this age group.

Precautions: DITROPAN® (oxybutynin chloride) should be used with caution in the elderly and in all patients with autonomic neuropathy, hepatic or renal disease. Administration of DITROPAN in large doses to patients with ulcerative colitis may suppress intestinal motility to the point of producing a paralytic ileus and precipitate or aggravate toxic megacolon, a serious complication of the disease.

The symptoms of hyperthyroidism, coronary heart disease, congestive heart failure, cardiac arrhythmias, tachycardia, hypertension, and prostatic hypertrophy may be aggravated following administration of DITROPAN. DITROPAN should be administered with caution to patients with hiatal hernia associated with reflux esophagitis, since anticholinergic drugs may aggravate this condition.

Adverse Reactions: Following administration of DITROPAN® (oxybutynin chloride), the symptoms that can be associated with the use of other anticholinergic drugs may occur: dry mouth, decreased sweating, urinary hesitance and retention, blurred vision, tachycardia, palpitations, dilatation of the pupil, cycloplegia, increased ocular tension, drowsiness, weakness, dizziness, insomnia, nausea, vomiting, constipation, bloated feeling, impotence, suppression of lactation, severe allergic reactions or drug idiosyncrasies including urticaria and other dermal manifestations.

Dosage and Administration: Tablet —Adult: The usual dose is one 5-mg tablet two to three times a day. The maximum recommended dose is one 5-mg tablet four times a day.

Children over 5 years of age: The usual dose is one 5-mg tablet two times a day. The maximum recommended dose is one 5-mg tablet three times a day.

Syrup—Adults: The usual dose is one teaspoon (5 mg/5 ml) syrup two to three times a day. The maximum recommended dose is one teaspoon (5 mg/5 ml) syrup four times a day.

Children over 5 years of age: The usual dose is one teaspoon (5 mg/5 ml) two times a day. The maximum recommended dose is one teaspoon (5 mg/5 ml) three times a day.

Overdosage: The symptoms of overdosage with DITROPAN® (oxybutynin chloride) progress from an intensification of the usual side effects of CNS disturbance (from restlessness and excitement to psychotic behavior), circulatory changes (flushing, fall in blood pressure, circulatory failure), respiratory failure, paralysis, and coma.

Measures to be taken are (1) immediate lavage of the stomach and (2) injection of physostigmine 0.5 to 2.0 mg intravenously, and repeated as necessary up to a total of 5.0 mg. Fever may be treated symptomatically (alcohol sponging, ice packs). Excitement of a degree which demands attention may be managed with sodium thiopental 2% solution given slowly intravenously or chloral hydrate (100 to 200 ml of a 2% solution) by rectal infusion. In the event of progression of the curare-like effect to paralysis of the respiratory muscles, artificial respiration is required.

How Supplied: DITROPAN® (oxybutynin chloride) Tablets are supplied in bottles of 100 tablets (NDC 0088-1375-47) and 1,000 tablets (NDC 0088-1375-58) and in Unit Dose Identification Paks of 100 tablets (NDC 0088-1375-49). Blue scored tablets are engraved with MARION on one side and 1375 on the other side.

Shown in Product Identification Section, page 417

DITROPAN® Syrup is supplied in bottles of 16 fluid ounces (473 ml) (NDC 0088-1373-18).

Pharmacist: Dispense in tight, light-resistant container as defined in the USP.

Store at controlled room temperature (59°–86°F).

U.S. Patent 3,176,019

Issued 1/84

DUOTRATE® and DUOTRATE® 45   ℞
[dū′ō-trāt]
Plateau CAPS®
(pentaerythritol tetranitrate)

Each sustained-release capsule contains:
DUOTRATE® (pentaerythritol
 tetranitrate) .... 30 mg
White pellets in a black and clear capsule imprinted with MARION/1525.
DUOTRATE® 45 (pentaerythritol
 tetranitrate) .... 45 mg
White pellets in a black and light blue capsule imprinted with MARION/1530.

DUOTRATE® and DUOTRATE® 45 (pentaerythritol tetranitrate) are 2,2-Bishydroxymethyl-1,3-propanediol tetranitrate.

Action: The mechanism of action in the relief of angina pectoris is unknown at this time, although the basic pharmacologic action is to relax smooth muscle. The effect of pentaerythritol tetranitrate is usually measured by its ability to reduce the frequency, duration and severity of anginal attacks and reduce the need for sublingual nitroglycerin.

Indications:
Based on a review of this drug by the National Academy of Sciences-National Research Council and/or other information, FDA has classified the indications as follows:
Possibly effective: For the management, prophylaxis, or treatment of anginal attacks.
Final classification of the less-than-effective indications requires further investigation.

Contraindication: Idiosyncrasy to this drug.

Warnings: Data supporting the use of DUOTRATE® and DUOTRATE® 45 (pentaerythritol tetranitrate) during the early days of the acute phase of myocardial infarction (the period during which clinical and laboratory findings are unstable) are insufficient to establish safety.

Precautions: Intraocular pressure is increased; therefore, caution is required in administering to patients with glaucoma. Tolerance to this drug and cross-tolerance to other nitrites and nitrates may occur.

Adverse Reactions: Cutaneous vasodilation with flushing. Headache is common and may be severe and persistent. Transient episodes of dizziness and weakness, as well as other signs of cerebral ischemia associated with postural hypotension, may occasionally develop. This drug can act as a physiological antagonist to norepinephrine, acetylcholine, histamine, and many other agents. An occasional individual exhibits marked sensitivity to the hypotensive effects of nitrite and severe responses (nausea, vomiting, weakness, restlessness, pallor, perspiration and collapse) can occur, even with the usual therapeutic dose. Alcohol may enhance this effect. Drug rash and/or exfoliative dermatitis may occasionally occur.

Dosage and Administration: One capsule every 12 hours on an empty stomach. One capsule should be taken with an adequate amount of water before breakfast, and a second capsule approximately 12 hours later on an empty stomach. When medication is started, there is a delay from one to two hours before a significant change in pain level occurs. The selection of DUOTRATE® should be based on the patient's need for approximately 30 mg of pentaerythritol tetranitrate during a 12-hour period. The selection of DUOTRATE® 45 should be based on the patient's need for approximately 45 mg of pentaerythritol tetranitrate during a 12-hour period. Use the smallest dose that proves effective.

How Supplied: Each of the products described is available in bottles of 100 capsules. DUOTRATE® Capsules are imprinted with MARION/1525. DUOTRATE® 45 Capsules are imprinted with MARION/1530.

Caution: Federal law prohibits dispensing without a prescription.

Mfd. by:
KV Pharmaceutical Co.
St. Louis, MO 63144

Dist. by:
Marion Laboratories, Inc.
Kansas City, MO 64137

Issued 1/81

Shown in Product Identification Section, pages 417, 418

GAVISCON® Antacid Tablets   OTC
[gāv′ĭs-kŏn]

Composition: Each chewable tablet contains the following active ingredients:
Aluminum hydroxide dried gel .... 80 mg
Magnesium trisilicate .... 20 mg
and the following inactive ingredients: sucrose, alginic acid, sodium bicarbonate, starch, calcium stearate, and flavoring.

Continued on next page

Marion—Cont.

Indications: GAVISCON is specifically formulated for the temporary relief of heartburn (acid indigestion) due to acid reflux. GAVISCON is not indicated for the treatment of peptic ulcers.
Directions: Chew two to four tablets four times a day or as directed by a physician. Tablets should be taken after meals and at bedtime or as needed. For best results follow by a half glass of water or other liquid. DO NOT SWALLOW WHOLE.
Warnings: Do not take more than 16 tablets in a 24-hour period or 16 tablets daily for more than 2 weeks, except under the advice and supervision of a physician. Do not use this product except under the advice and supervision of a physician if you are on a sodium-restricted diet. Each GAVISCON Tablet contains approximately 0.8 mEq sodium.
Drug Interaction Precautions: Do not take this product if you are presently taking a prescription antibiotic drug containing any form of tetracycline.
STORE AT A CONTROLLED ROOM TEMPERATURE IN A DRY PLACE.
KEEP THIS AND ALL DRUGS OUT OF THE REACH OF CHILDREN.
In case of accidental overdose, seek professional assistance or contact a poison control center immediately.
How Supplied: Available in bottle of 100 tablets and in foil-wrapped 2's in box of 30 tablets.

Issued 12/83
Shown in Product Identification Section, page 418

GAVISCON® Liquid Antacid OTC
[găv'ĭs-kŏn]

Composition: Each tablespoonful (15 ml) contains the following active ingredients:
Aluminum hydroxide .... 95 mg
Magnesium carbonate .... 412 mg
and the following inactive ingredients: water, sorbitol solution, glycerin, sodium alginate, xanthan gum, edetate disodium, preservatives, flavorings, and colors.
Indications: For the relief of heartburn, sour stomach, and/or acid indigestion and upset stomach associated with heartburn, sour stomach, and/or indigestion*.
Directions: Shake well before using. Take one to two tablespoonfuls four times a day or as directed by a physician. GAVISCON Liquid should be taken after meals and at bedtime, followed by half a glass of water.
Warnings: Except under the advice and supervision of a physician: do not take more than 8 tablespoonfuls in a 24-hour period or 8 tablespoonfuls daily for more than two weeks. May have laxative effect. Do not use this product if you have a kidney disease; do not use this product if you are on a sodium-restricted diet. Each tablespoonful of GAVISCON Liquid contains approximately 1.7 mEq sodium.
Drug Interaction Precautions: Do not take this product if you are presently taking a prescription antibiotic drug containing any form of tetracycline.
KEEP TIGHTLY CLOSED. AVOID FREEZING. STORE AT A CONTROLLED ROOM TEMPERATURE.
KEEP THIS AND ALL DRUGS OUT OF THE REACH OF CHILDREN.
In case of accidental overdose, seek professional assistance or contact a poison control center immediately.
How Supplied: Bottles of 12 fluid ounces (355 ml) and 6 fluid ounces (177 ml).

Issued 5/84
*GAVISCON is not indicated for the treatment of peptic ulcers.

GAVISCON®-2 Antacid Tablets OTC
[găv'ĭs-kŏn]

Composition: Each chewable tablet contains the following active ingredients:
Aluminum hydroxide dried gel .... 160 mg
Magnesium trisilicate .... 40 mg
and the following inactive ingredients: sucrose, alginic acid, sodium bicarbonate, starch, calcium stearate and flavoring.
Indications: GAVISCON is specifically formulated for the temporary relief of heartburn (acid indigestion) due to acid reflux. GAVISCON is not indicated for the treatment of peptic ulcers.
Directions: Chew one to two tablets four times a day or as directed by a physician. Tablets should be taken after meals and at bedtime or as needed. For best results follow by a half glass of water or other liquid. DO NOT SWALLOW WHOLE.
Warnings: Do not take more than 8 tablets in a 24-hour period or 8 tablets daily for more than 2 weeks, except under the advice and supervision of a physician. Do not use this product except under the advice and supervision of a physician if you are on a sodium-restricted diet. Each GAVISCON-2 Tablet contains approximately 1.6 mEq sodium.
Drug Interaction Precautions: Do not take this product if you are presently taking a prescription antibiotic drug containing any form of tetracycline.
STORE AT A CONTROLLED ROOM TEMPERATURE IN A DRY PLACE.
KEEP THIS AND ALL DRUGS OUT OF THE REACH OF CHILDREN.
In case of accidental overdose, seek professional assistance or contact a poison control center immediately.
How Supplied: Box of 48 foil-wrapped tablets.

Issued 12/83
Shown in Product Identification Section, page 418

GLY-OXIDE® Liquid OTC
[glī-ăk'sīd]

Description: Carbamide peroxide 10% in specially prepared anhydrous glycerol. Artificial flavor added.
Actions: GLY-OXIDE® is a safe, stabilized oxygenating agent. Specifically formulated for topical oral administration, it provides unique chemomechanical cleansing and debriding action which allows normal healing to occur.
Indications: Local treatment and hygienic prevention (as an aid to professional care) of minor oral inflammation such as canker sores, denture irritation, and postdental procedure irritation. GLY-OXIDE Liquid provides effective aid to oral hygiene when normal cleansing measures are inadequate or impossible (eg, total-care geriatric patients). As an adjunct to oral hygiene (orthodontics, dental appliances) after regular brushing.
Precautions: Severe or persistent oral inflammation or denture irritation may be serious. If these or unexpected effects occur, consult physician or dentist promptly.
Dosage and Administration: DO NOT DILUTE—use directly from the bottle. Apply four times daily after meals and at bedtime, or as directed by a dentist or physician. Place several drops on affected area; expectorate after two to three minutes, or place 10 drops onto tongue, mix with saliva, swish for several minutes, expectorate. Do not rinse. Foams on contact with saliva. AVOID CONTACT WITH EYES. Protect from heat and direct sunlight. Keep this and all drugs out of the reach of children. In case of accidental ingestion, seek professional assistance or contact a poison control center immediately.
How Supplied: GLY-OXIDE Liquid is available in ½-fl-oz and 2-fl-oz non-spill plastic squeeze bottles with applicator spouts.

Issued 3/84

NICO-400® OTC
[nī'kō]
(nicotinic acid)

A dietary supplement for 12-year-olds and older. Each capsule contains:
Nicotinic acid (niacin) .... 400 mg
equivalent to 20 times the Recommended Daily Allowance of niacin.
Directions: Take one capsule daily, as a dietary supplement for 12-year-olds and older.
Ingredients: Niacin, sugar, starch, povidone, pharmaceutical glaze, calcium stearate, talc.
Keep tightly closed.
Store between 59°–86°F.
Keep out of reach of children.
How Supplied: NICO-400 is available in bottles of 100 capsules. Capsules are imprinted with MARION/1575.
Dist. by:
Marion Laboratories, Inc.
Kansas City, MO 64137

Issued 3/83
Shown in Product Identification Section, page 418

NITRO-BID® Plateau CAPS® R
[nī'trō-bĭd]
(nitroglycerin) 2.5 mg, 6.5 mg, and 9 mg

Description: Each NITRO-BID® Controlled-Release Capsule contains:
2.5 mg nitroglycerin: Light purple and clear capsule with white beads; identification imprint MARION/1550.
6.5 mg nitroglycerin: Dark blue and yellow capsule with white beads; identification imprint MARION/1551.
9 mg nitroglycerin: Green and yellow capsule with white beads; identification imprint MARION/1553.
Action: The mechanism of action of nitroglycerin in the relief of angina pectoris is not as yet known. However, its main pharmacologic action is to relax smooth muscle, principally in the smaller blood vessels, thus dilating arterioles and capillaries, especially in the coronary circulation. In therapeutic doses, nitroglycerin is thought to increase the blood supply to the myocardium which may, in turn, relieve myocardial ischemia, the possible functional basis for the pain of angina pectoris. The sublingual administration of nitroglycerin is normally rapid and transient, but nitroglycerin in controlled-release NITRO-BID® 2.5, NITRO-BID® 6.5, and NITRO-BID® 9 produces a prolonged action.

> **Indications:**
> Based on a review of this drug and a related drug by the National Academy of Sciences-National Research Council and/or other information, FDA has classified the indications as follows:
> "Possibly" effective:
> For the management, prophylaxis or treatment of anginal attacks.
> Final classification of the less-than-effective indications requires further investigation.

Contraindications: Acute or recent myocardial infarction, severe anemia, closed-angle glaucoma, postural hypotension, increased intracranial pressure, and idiosyncrasy to the drug.
Warnings: Capsules must be swallowed. FOR ORAL, NOT SUBLINGUAL, USE. NITRO-BID® 2.5, NITRO-BID® 6.5, and NITRO-BID® 9 Controlled-Release Capsules are not intended for immediate relief of anginal attacks.
Precautions: Intraocular pressure may be increased; therefore, caution is required in administering to patients with glaucoma. Tolerance to this drug and cross-tolerance to other organic nitrites and nitrates may occur. If blurring of vision, dryness of mouth, or lack of benefit occurs, the drug should be discontinued.
Adverse Reactions: Severe and persistent headaches, cutaneous flushing, dizziness, and weakness. Occasionally, drug rash or exfoliative dermatitis and nausea and vomiting may occur; these responses may disappear with a decrease in dosage. Adverse effects are enhanced by ingestion of alcohol, which appears to increase absorption from the gastrointestinal tract.
Dosage and Administration: Administer the smallest effective dose two or three times daily at 8- to 12-hour intervals, unless clinical response suggests a different regimen. Patient should be

titrated to anginal relief or hemodynamic response. Hemodynamic response can be measured by drop in systolic blood pressure. Discontinue if not effective.

How Supplied: NITRO-BID® (nitroglycerin) 2.5, 6.5, and 9 Controlled-Release Capsules are available in 60- and 100-count bottles.

Caution: Federal law prohibits dispensing without a prescription.

Storage: STORE AT A CONTROLLED ROOM TEMPERATURE. Dispense only in the original unopened container.

Issued 3/83

Shown in Product Identification Section, page 418

NITRO–BID® IV ℞
[*ni' trō-bid"*]
(nitroglycerin)
FOR INTRAVENOUS USE ONLY

NOT FOR DIRECT INTRAVENOUS INJECTION. NITRO-BID IV MUST BE DILUTED IN DEXTROSE (5.0%) INJECTION, USP OR SODIUM CHLORIDE (0.9%) INJECTION, USP BEFORE INTRAVENOUS ADMINISTRATION. THE ADMINISTRATION SET USED FOR INFUSION MAY AFFECT THE AMOUNT OF NITRO-BID IV DELIVERED TO THE PATIENT. (SEE **Warnings** AND **Dosage and Administration** SECTIONS.)

CAUTION: SEVERAL PREPARATIONS OF NITROGLYCERIN FOR INJECTION ARE AVAILABLE. THEY DIFFER IN CONCENTRATION AND/OR VOLUME PER VIAL. WHEN SWITCHING FROM ONE PRODUCT TO ANOTHER, ATTENTION MUST BE PAID TO THE DILUTION AND DOSAGE AND ADMINISTRATION INSTRUCTIONS.

Description: NITRO-BID IV (nitroglycerin) is a clear, practically colorless additive solution for intravenous infusion after dilution. Each milliliter contains 5 mg nitroglycerin and 45 mg propylene glycol dissolved in 70% ethanol.

The solution is sterile, nonpyrogenic, and nonexplosive. NITRO-BID IV, an organic nitrate, is a vasodilator. The chemical name for nitroglycerin is 1,2,3 propanetriol trinitrate.

Clinical Pharmacology: Relaxation of vascular smooth muscle is the principal pharmacologic action of NITRO-BID IV (nitroglycerin). Although venous effects predominate, nitroglycerin produces, in a dose-related manner, dilation of both arterial and venous beds. Dilation of the postcapillary vessels, including large veins, promotes peripheral pooling of blood and decreases venous return to the heart, reducing left ventricular end-diastolic pressure (preload). Arteriolar relaxation reduces systemic vascular resistance and arterial pressure (afterload). Myocardial oxygen consumption or demand (as measured by the pressure-rate product, tension-time index, and stroke-work index) is decreased by both the arterial and venous effects of nitroglycerin, and a more favorable supply-demand ratio can be achieved.

Therapeutic doses of intravenous nitroglycerin reduce systolic, diastolic, and mean arterial blood pressures. Effective coronary perfusion pressure is usually maintained, but can be compromised if blood pressure falls excessively or increased heart rate decreases diastolic filling time.

Elevated central venous and pulmonary capillary wedge pressures, pulmonary vascular resistance, and systemic vascular resistance are also reduced by nitroglycerin therapy. Heart rate is usually slightly increased, presumably a reflex response to the fall in blood pressure. Cardiac index may be increased, decreased, or unchanged. Patients with elevated left ventricular filling pressure and systemic vascular resistance values in conjunction with a depressed cardiac index are likely to experience an improvement in cardiac index. On the other hand, when filling pressures and cardiac index are normal, cardiac index may be slightly reduced by intravenous nitroglycerin.

Nitroglycerin is widely distributed in the body with an apparent volume of distribution of approximately 200 liters in adult male subjects, and is rapidly metabolized to dinitrates and mononitrates, with a short half-life, estimated at one to four minutes. This results in a low plasma concentration after intravenous infusion. At plasma concentrations of between 50 and 100 ng/ml, the binding of nitroglycerin to plasma proteins is approximately 60%, while that of 1,2 dinitroglycerin and 1,3 dinitroglycerin is 60% and 30%, respectively. The activity and half-life of the dinitroglycerins are not well characterized. The mononitrate is not active.

Indications and Usage: NITRO-BID IV (nitroglycerin) is indicated for:

1. **Control of blood pressure in perioperative hypertension,** ie, hypertension associated with surgical procedures, especially cardiovascular procedures, such as the hypertension seen during intratracheal intubation, anesthesia, skin incision, sternotomy, cardiac bypass, and in the immediate postsurgical period.
2. **Congestive heart failure associated with acute myocardial infarction.**
3. **Treatment of angina pectoris** in patients who have not responded to recommended doses of organic nitrates and/or a beta-blocker.
4. **Production of controlled hypotension during surgical procedures.**

Contraindications: NITRO-BID IV (nitroglycerin) should not be administered to individuals with:

1. A known hypersensitivity to nitroglycerin or a known idiosyncratic reaction to organic nitrates.
2. Hypotension or uncorrected hypovolemia, as the use of NITRO-BID IV in such states could produce severe hypotension or shock.
3. Increased intracranial pressure (eg, head trauma or cerebral hemorrhage).
4. Inadequate cerebral circulation, constrictive pericarditis, and pericardial tamponade.

Warnings:

1. Nitroglycerin readily migrates into many plastics. To avoid absorption of nitroglycerin into plastic parenteral solution containers, the dilution and storage of nitroglycerin for intravenous infusion should be made only in glass parenteral solution bottles.
2. Some filters also absorb nitroglycerin; they should be avoided.
3. Forty percent to 80% of the total amount of nitroglycerin in the final diluted solution for infusion is absorbed by the polyvinyl chloride (PVC) tubing of the intravenous administration sets currently in general use. The higher rates of absorption occur when flow rates are low, nitroglycerin concentrations are high, and tubing is long. Although the rate of loss is highest during the early phase of administration (when flow rates are lowest), the loss is neither constant nor self-limiting; consequently, no simple calculation or correction can be performed to convert the theoretical infusion rate (based on the concentration of the infusion solution) to the actual delivery rate. Because of this problem, Marion Laboratories recommends the use of the least absorptive infusion tubing available for infusions of NITRO-BID IV. DOSING INSTRUCTIONS MUST BE FOLLOWED WITH CARE. IT SHOULD BE NOTED THAT WHEN THESE INFUSION SETS ARE USED, THE CALCULATED DOSE WILL BE DELIVERED TO THE PATIENT DEPENDENT UPON THE LOSS OF NITROGLYCERIN DUE TO ABSORPTIVE TUBING. NOTE THAT THE DOSAGES COMMONLY USED IN PUBLISHED STUDIES UTILIZED GENERAL-USE PVC TUBING, AND RECOMMENDED DOSES BASED ON THIS EXPERIENCE ARE TOO HIGH IF NEW, LESS ABSORPTIVE INFUSION TUBING IS USED.
4. PROTECT FROM LIGHT UNTIL READY FOR USE.
5. NITRO-BID IV AMPULES AND VIALS ARE INTENDED FOR SINGLE-DOSE ONLY. PROPERLY DISCARD ANY UNUSED PORTION.

Precautions: NITRO-BID IV (nitroglycerin) should be used with caution in patients who have severe hepatic or renal disease.

Excessive hypotension, especially for prolonged periods of time, must be avoided because of possible deleterious effects on the brain, heart, liver, and kidney from poor perfusion and the attendant risk of ischemia, thrombosis, and altered function of these organs. Patients with normal or low pulmonary capillary wedge pressure are especially sensitive to the hypotensive effects of NITRO-BID IV. If pulmonary capillary wedge pressure is being monitored, it will be noted that a fall in wedge pressure precedes the onset of arterial hypotension, and the pulmonary capillary wedge pressure is thus a useful guide to safe titration of the drug.

Carcinogenesis, Mutagenesis, Impairment of Fertility: No long-term studies in animals were performed to evaluate carcinogenic potential of NITRO-BID IV (nitroglycerin).

Pregnancy: Category C. Animal reproduction studies have not been conducted with NITRO-BID IV. It is also not known whether NITRO-BID IV can cause fetal harm when administered to a pregnant woman or can affect reproduction capacity. NITRO-BID IV should be given to a pregnant woman only if clearly needed.

Nursing Mothers: It is not known whether nitroglycerin is excreted in human milk. Because many drugs are excreted in human milk, caution should be exercised when NITRO-BID IV is administered to a nursing woman.

Pediatric Use: The safety and effectiveness of NITRO-BID IV in children have not been established.

NITRO-BID IV contains alcohol and propylene glycol; safety for intracoronary injection has not been shown.

Adverse Reactions: The most frequent adverse reaction in patients treated with nitroglycerin is headache, which occurs in approximately 2% of patients. Other adverse reactions occurring in less than 1% of patients are the following: tachycardia, nausea, vomiting, apprehension, restlessness, muscle twitching, retrosternal discomfort, palpitations, dizziness, and abdominal pain. Paradoxical bradycardia and increased angina pectoris may accompany nitroglycerin-induced hypotension. The following additional adverse reactions have been reported with the oral and/or topical use of nitroglycerin: cutaneous flushing, weakness, and, occasionally, drug rash or exfoliative dermatitis.

Overdosage: Accidental overdosage of nitroglycerin may result in severe hypotension and reflex tachycardia which can be treated by elevating the legs and decreasing or temporarily terminating the infusion until the patient's condition stabilizes. Since the duration of the hemodynamic effects following nitroglycerin administration is quite short, additional corrective measures are usually not required. However, if further therapy is indicated, administration of an intravenous alpha-adrenergic agonist (eg, methoxamine or phenylephrine) should be considered.

Dosage and Administration:
NOT FOR DIRECT INTRAVENOUS INJECTION. NITRO-BID IV (NITROGLYCERIN) IS A CONCENTRATED, POTENT DRUG WHICH MUST BE DILUTED IN DEXTROSE (5.0%) INJECTION, USP OR SODIUM CHLORIDE (0.9%) INJECTION, USP PRIOR TO ITS INFUSION. NITRO-BID IV SHOULD NOT BE ADMIXED WITH OTHER DRUGS.

Dilution: It is important to consider the fluid requirements of the patient as well as the expected duration of infusion in selecting the appropriate dilution of NITRO-BID IV.

[See table on next page].

Dosage: Dosage is affected by the type of infusion set used (see **Warnings**). Although the usual starting adult dose range reported in clinical studies was 25 mcg/min or more, those studies used PVC TUBING. The use of nonabsorbing tubing will result in the need to use reduced doses.

The dosage for NITRO-BID IV (nitroglycerin) infusion should initially be 5 mcg/min delivered through an infusion pump capable of exact and constant delivery of the drug. Subsequent titration

Continued on next page

Marion—Cont.

must be adjusted to the clinical situation, with dose increments becoming more cautious as partial response is seen. Initial titration should be in 5-mcg/min increments, with increases every three to five minutes until some response is noted. If no response is seen at 20 mcg/min, increments of 10 and later 20 mcg/min can be used. Once a partial blood pressure response is observed, the dose increase should be reduced and the interval between increments should be lengthened. Patients with normal or low left ventricular filling pressure or pulmonary capillary wedge pressure (eg, angina patients without other complications) may be hypersensitive to the effects of NITRO-BID IV and may respond fully to doses as small as 5 mcg/min. These patients require especially careful titration and monitoring.

There is no fixed optimum dose of NITRO-BID IV. Due to variations in the responsiveness of individual patients to the drug, each patient must be titrated to the desired level of hemodynamic function. Therefore, continuous monitoring of physiologic parameters (eg, blood pressure, heart rate, and pulmonary capillary wedge pressure) MUST BE PERFORMED to achieve the correct dose. Adequate systemic blood pressure and coronary perfusion pressure must be maintained.

How Supplied:
AMPULES
NITRO-BID® IV is supplied in boxes of ten 1-ml ampules (NDC 0088-1800-07), each ampule containing 5 mg nitroglycerin (5 mg/ml); ten 5-ml ampules (NDC 0088-1800-08), each ampule containing 25 mg nitroglycerin (5 mg/ml); and five 10-ml ampules (NDC 0088-1800-13), each ampule containing 50 mg nitroglycerin (5 mg/ml).

VIALS
NITRO-BID® IV is supplied in boxes of ten 1-ml vials (NDC 0088-1800-31), each vial containing 5mg of nitroglycerin (5 mg/ml); ten 5-ml vials (NDC 0088-1800-32), each vial containing 25 mg nitroglycerin (5 mg/ml); and five 10-ml vials (NDC 0088-1800-33), each vial containing 50 mg nitroglycerin (5 mg/ml).

Mfd. for
Marion Laboratories, Inc.
Mfd. by
Taylor Pharmacal Co.
Decatur, IL 62525

Issued 6/84

NITRO–BID® Ointment ℞
[nī′trō-bid″]
(nitroglycerin 2%)

Description: NITRO-BID® Ointment contains 2% nitroglycerin and lactose in a special absorptive lanolin and white petrolatum base formulated to provide a controlled release of the active ingredient. Each inch, as squeezed from the tube, or the contents squeezed from the pouch, contains approximately 15 mg nitroglycerin.

Actions: When the ointment is spread on the skin, nitroglycerin is absorbed continuously into the systemic circulation. Nitroglycerin ointment reduces the work load of the heart by virtue of its smooth-muscle relaxation. This results predominantly in peripheral venous dilatation which reduces preload, but also to a lesser degree in peripheral arteriolar dilatation which reduces afterload. These hemodynamic effects have been advanced as explanations for the beneficial actions of nitroglycerin ointment in angina pectoris.

Computerized digital plethysmographic studies have shown the duration of action of nitroglycerin ointment (2 inches applied to the chest) to be eight hours in comparison to placebo; the onset of action occurred within 30 minutes of administration. Controlled clinical studies have demonstrated that nitroglycerin ointment increased measured exercise tolerance in patients with angina pectoris up to three hours after application (the maximal time interval studied).

Indications: This drug product has been conditionally approved by the FDA for the prevention and treatment of angina pectoris due to coronary artery disease. The conditional approval reflects a determination that the drug may be marketed while further investigation of its effectiveness is undertaken. A final evaluation of the effectiveness of the product will be announced by the FDA.

Contraindications: In patients known to be intolerant of the organic nitrate drugs.

Warnings: In acute myocardial infarction or congestive heart failure, nitroglycerin ointment should be used under careful clinical and/or hemodynamic monitoring.

Precautions: Nitroglycerin ointment should not be used for treatment of acute anginal attacks. Symptoms of hypotension, particularly when suddenly arising from the recumbent position, are signs of overdosage. When they occur, the dosage should be reduced.

Adverse Reactions: Transient headaches are the most common side effect, especially at higher dosages. Headaches should be treated with mild analgesics, and nitroglycerin ointment continued. Only with untreatable headaches should the dosage be reduced. Although uncommon, hypotension, an increase in heart rate, faintness, flushing, dizziness, and nausea may occur. These all are attributable to the pharmacologic effects of nitroglycerin on the cardiovascular system, but are symptoms of overdosage. When they occur and persist, the dosage should be reduced.

Occasionally, contact dermatitis has been reported with continuous use of topical nitroglycerin. Such incidence may be reduced by changing the site of application or by using topical corticosteroids.

Dosage and Administration: When applying the ointment, place the specially designed Dose Measuring Applicator, supplied with the package, printed side down and squeeze the necessary amount of ointment from the tube or pouch onto the applicator. Then place the applicator with the ointment side down onto the desired area of the skin, usually the chest (although other areas can be used). Spread the ointment over a 6x6-inch (150x150-mm) area in a thin, uniform layer using the applicator. Cover the area with plastic wrap which can be held in place by adhesive tape. The applicator allows the patient to measure the necessary amount of ointment and to spread it without its being absorbed through the fingers while applying it to the skin surface.

The usual therapeutic dose is 2 inches (50 mm) applied every eight hours, although some patients may require as much as 4 to 5 inches (100 to 125 mm) and/or application every four hours.

Tube: Start at 1/2 inch (12.5 mm) every eight hours and increase the dose by 1/2 inch (12.5 mm) with each successive application to achieve the desired clinical effects. The optimal dosage should be selected based upon the clinical response, side effects, and the effects of therapy upon blood pressure. The greatest attainable decrease in resting blood pressure which is not associated with clinical symptoms of hypotension, especially during orthostasis, indicates the optimal dosage. To decrease adverse reactions, the dose and frequency of application should be tailored to the individual patient's needs.

Keep the tube tightly closed and store at room temperature 59° to 86°F (15° to 30° C).

Foil Pouch: The 1-gram foil pouch is approximately equivalent to one inch as squeezed from a tube and is designed to be used in increments of one inch. Apply the ointment by squeezing the contents of the pouch onto a specially designed Dose Measuring Applicator, supplied with the package, printed side down.

Patient Instructions for Application: Information furnished with Dose Measuring Applicators.

How Supplied: NITRO-BID® Ointment is available in 20-gram and 60-gram UNI-Rx® Paks (six tubes per pack); in individual 20-gram, 60-gram, and 100-gram tubes; and in Unit Dose Identification Paks of 100 1-gram foil pouches.

Issued 7/83

OS–CAL® 250 Tablets OTC
[ăhs′kăl]
calcium supplement with vitamin D

Each tablet contains: 625 mg of calcium carbonate from oyster shell which provides:
Elemental calcium.............................. 250 mg
Vitamin D .... 125 USP Units

Indications: OS-CAL® 250 Tablets provide a source of calcium when it is desired to increase the dietary intake of this mineral. OS-CAL 250 also contains Vitamin D to aid in the absorption of calcium.

Directions: Take one tablet three times a day at mealtime. Three tablets daily provide:

	Quantity	%U.S.RDA* for Adults
Calcium	750 mg	75%
Vitamin D	375 units	94%

*Percent U.S. Recommended Daily Allowance.
STORE AT ROOM TEMPERATURE.
Keep out of reach of children.

How Supplied: Bottles of 100, 240, 500, and 1000 tablets.

Issued 11/83
Shown in Product Identification Section, page 418

OS–CAL® 500 Tablets OTC
[ăhs′kăl]
calcium supplement

Each tablet contains:
1,250 mg of calcium carbonate from oyster shell which provides:
Elemental calcium .... 500 mg

Indications: OS-CAL 500 Tablets provide a source of calcium when it is desired or recommended by a physician to increase the dietary intake of this mineral.

Directions: Take one tablet two or three times a day at mealtime or as directed. Two tablets daily provide:

	Quantity	%U.S.RDA†
Calcium	1,000 mg	100%* / 77%**

NITRO-BID IV Administration Table

Each 1-ml ampule or vial = 5 mg nitroglycerin
Each 5-ml ampule or vial = 25 mg nitroglycerin
Each 10-ml ampule or vial = 50 mg nitroglycerin

Mixing Instructions	1 ml in 100 ml 5 ml in 500 ml 10 ml in 1000 ml	1 ml in 50 ml 5 ml in 250 ml 10 ml in 500 ml 20 ml in 1000 ml	2 ml in 50 ml 10 ml in 250 ml 20 ml in 500 ml 40 ml in 1000 ml	FLOW RATE milliliters/hour microdrops/minute
Concentration	50 mcg/ml	100 mcg/ml	200 mcg/ml	
Dosage	mcg/min	mcg/min	mcg/min	microdrops/min
	2.5	5	10	3
	5	10	20	6
	10	20	40	12
	20	40	80	24
	40	80	160	48
	60	120	240	72
	80	160	320	96

for possible revisions

Three tablets daily provide:

	Quantity	%U.S.RDA†
Calcium	1,500 mg	150%*
		115%**

†Percent U.S. Recommended Daily Allowance.
*For adults and children 12 or more years of age.
**For pregnant and lactating women.

STORE AT ROOM TEMPERATURE.
Keep out of reach of children.

How Supplied: Bottles of 60 and 120 tablets.

Issued 5/84

Shown in Product Identification Section, page 418

OS–CAL FORTE® Tablets   OTC
[ăhs′kăl]
multivitamin and mineral supplement

Each tablet contains:
Vitamin A (palmitate)............... 1668 USP Units
Vitamin D .... 125 USP Units
Thiamine mononitrate (vitamin B$_1$)......... 1.7 mg
Riboflavin (vitamin B$_2$)................... 1.7 mg
Pyridoxine hydrochloride
 (vitamin B$_6$) .... 2.0 mg
Cyanocobalamin (vitamin B$_{12}$)................ 1.6 mcg
Ascorbic acid (vitamin C)................... 50 mg
dl-alpha-tocopherol acetate
 (vitamin E) .... 0.8 IU
Niacinamide .... 15 mg
Calcium (from oyster shell)................ 250 mg
Iron (as ferrous fumarate) .... 5 mg
Copper (as sulfate) .... 0.3 mg
Iodine (as potassium iodide) .... 0.05 mg
Magnesium (as oxide) .... 1.6 mg
Manganese (as sulfate).................... 0.3 mg
Zinc (as sulfate) .... 0.5 mg

Indication: Multivitamin and mineral supplement.

Dosage: One tablet three times daily or as directed by physician.

How Supplied: Bottles of 100 tablets.
Keep out of reach of children.
Store at room temperature.

Issued 11/83

Shown in Product Identification Section, page 418

OS–CAL–GESIC® Tablets   OTC
[ăhs′kăl-jē″zĭk]
antiarthritic

Each tablet contains:
Salicylamide .... 400 mg
Calcium (from oyster shell)................ 100 mg
Vitamin D .... 50 USP Units

Indication: For temporary relief of symptoms associated with arthritis.

Dosage: Initially–2 tablets hourly for 3 or 4 doses.
Maintenance–1 or 2 tablets four times daily.

How Supplied: Available in bottles of 100 tablets.
Keep this and all drugs out of reach of children. In case of accidental overdose, seek professional assistance or contact a poison control center immediately.
Store at room temperature.

Issued 11/83

Shown in Product Identification Section, page 418

OS–CAL® Plus Tablets   OTC
[ăhs′kăl]
multivitamin and multimineral supplement

Each tablet contains:
Calcium (from oyster shell) .... 250 mg
Vitamin D.................................. 125 USP Units
Plus:
Vitamin A (palmitate)................. 1666 USP Units
Vitamin C (ascorbic acid)................. 33 mg
Vitamin B$_2$ (riboflavin) .... 0.66 mg
Vitamin B$_1$ (thiamine mononitrate)......... 0.5 mg
Vitamin B$_6$ (pyridoxine HCl) .... 0.5 mg
Niacinamide .... 3.33 mg
Iron (as ferrous fumarate) .... 16.6 mg
Zinc (as the sulfate) .... 0.75 mg
Manganese (as the sulfate).................. 0.75 mg
Copper (as the sulfate) .... 0.036 mg
Iodine (as potassium iodide) .... 0.036 mg

Indications: As a multivitamin and multimineral supplement.

Product Information

Dosage: One tablet three times a day before meals or as directed by a physician. For children under four years of age, consult a physician.
Store at room temperature.
Keep out of reach of children.

How Supplied: Bottles of 100 tablets.

Issued 11/83

Shown in Product Identification Section, page 418

PAVABID® Plateau CAPS®   ℞
[păv′ŭh-bĭd]
(papaverine hydrochloride) 150 mg

Composition:
Each capsule contains:
Papaverine hydrochloride.......................... 150 mg
in a specially prepared base to provide prolonged activity.

Action and Uses: The main actions of papaverine are exerted on cardiac and smooth muscle. Like quinidine, papaverine acts directly on the heart muscle to depress conduction and prolong the refractory period. Papaverine relaxes various smooth muscles. This relaxation may be prominent if spasm exists. The muscle cell is not paralyzed by papaverine, and still responds to drugs and other stimuli causing contraction. The antispasmodic effect is a direct one, and unrelated to muscle innervation. Papaverine is practically devoid of effects on the central nervous system. Papaverine relaxes the smooth musculature of the larger blood vessels, especially coronary, systemic peripheral, and pulmonary arteries. Perhaps by its direct vasodilating action on cerebral blood vessels, papaverine increases cerebral blood flow and decreases cerebral vascular resistance in normal subjects; oxygen consumption is unaltered. These effects may explain the benefit reported from the drug in cerebral vascular encephalopathy.

The direct actions of papaverine on the heart to depress conduction and irritability and to prolong the refractory period of the myocardium provide the basis for its clinical trial in abrogating atrial and ventricular premature systoles and ominous ventricular arrhythmias. The coronary vasodilator action could be an additional factor of therapeutic value when such rhythms are secondary to insufficiency or occlusion of the coronary arteries. In patients with acute coronary thrombosis, the occurrence of ventricular rhythms is serious and requires measures designed to decrease myocardial irritability. Papaverine may have advantages over quinidine, used for a similar purpose, in that it may be given in an emergency by the intravenous route, does not depress myocardial contraction or cause cinchonism, and produces coronary vasodilation.

Indications: For the relief of cerebral and peripheral ischemia associated with arterial spasm and myocardial ischemia complicated by arrhythmias.

Precautions: Use with caution in patients with glaucoma. Hepatic hypersensitivity has been reported with gastrointestinal symptoms, jaundice, eosinophilia, and altered liver function tests. Discontinue medication if these occur.

Adverse Reactions: Although occurring rarely, the reported side effects of papaverine include nausea, abdominal distress, anorexia, constipation, malaise, drowsiness, vertigo, sweating, headache, diarrhea, and skin rash.

Dosage and Administration: One capsule every 12 hours. In difficult cases administration may be increased to one capsule every 8 hours, or two capsules every 12 hours.

How Supplied: Pavabid® (papaverine hydrochloride) Capsules are available in bottles of 60, 100, 250, 1000, 5000, and in Unit Dose Identification Paks of 100 capsules. Capsules are imprinted with MARION/1555.

Caution: Federal law prohibits dispensing without prescription.

Issued 6/84

Shown in Product Identification Section, page 418

PAVABID® HP Capsulets   ℞
[păv′ŭh-bĭd]
(papaverine hydrochloride) 300 mg

Composition: Each capsule contains:
Papaverine hydrochloride........................... 300 mg

Action and Uses: The main actions of papaverine are exerted on cardiac and smooth muscle. Like quinidine, papaverine acts directly on the heart muscle to depress conduction and prolong the refractory period. Papaverine relaxes various smooth muscles. This relaxation may be prominent if spasm exists. The muscle cell is not paralyzed by papaverine, and still responds to drugs and other stimuli causing contraction. The antispasmodic effect is a direct one, and unrelated to muscle innervation. Papaverine is practically devoid of effects on the central nervous system. Papaverine relaxes the smooth musculature of the larger blood vessels, especially coronary, systemic peripheral, and pulmonary arteries. Perhaps by its direct vasodilating action on cerebral blood vessels, papaverine increases cerebral blood flow and decreases cerebral vascular resistance in normal subjects; oxygen consumption is unaltered. These effects may explain the benefit reported from the drug in cerebral vascular encephalopathy.

The direct actions of papaverine on the heart to depress conduction and irritability and to prolong the refractory period of the myocardium provide the basis for its clinical trial in abrogating atrial and ventricular premature systoles and ominous ventricular arrhythmias. The coronary vasodilator action could be an additional factor of therapeutic value when such rhythms are secondary to insufficiency or occlusion of the coronary arteries. In patients with acute coronary thrombosis, the occurrence of ventricular rhythms is serious and requires measures designed to decrease myocardial irritability. Papaverine may have advantages over quinidine, used for a similar purpose, in that it may be given in an emergency by the intravenous route, does not depress myocardial contraction or cause cinchonism, and produces coronary vasodilation.

Indications: For the relief of cerebral and peripheral ischemia associated with arterial spasm and myocardial ischemia complicated by arrhythmias.

Precautions: Use with caution in patients with glaucoma. Hepatic hypersensitivity has been reported with gastrointestinal symptoms, jaundice, eosinophilia, and altered liver function tests. Discontinue medication if these occur.

Adverse Reactions: Although occurring rarely, the reported side effects of papaverine include nausea, abdominal distress, anorexia, constipation, malaise, drowsiness, vertigo, sweating, headache, diarrhea, and skin rash.

Dosage and Administration: Dosage should be started at 150 mg (one-half capsule) two to three times daily and titrated upward to the desired level. The 300-mg capsule breaks into two separate half capsules. To break: place capsule on a hard surface with the embossed MARION M facing up, press down on the embossed M.

How Supplied: PAVABID® (papaverine hydrochloride) HP Capsulets are available in 60-count bottles. Each light-orange capsulet is embossed with a raised M stamped MARION on one side and PAVABID HP on the other side.

Caution: Federal law prohibits dispensing without prescription.

Issued 6/84

Shown in Product Identification Section, page 418

SILVADENE® Cream   ℞
[sĭl′vă-dēn]
(1% silver sulfadiazine)

Description: SILVADENE Cream is a soft, white, water-miscible cream containing the antimicrobial agent, silver sulfadiazine in micronized form. Each gram of SILVADENE Cream contains 10 mg of micronized silver sulfadiazine. The cream

Continued on next page

Marion—Cont.

vehicle consists of white petrolatum, stearyl alcohol, isopropyl myristate, sorbitan monooleate, polyoxyl 40 stearate, propylene glycol, and water, with methylparaben 0.3% as a preservative.

Actions: SILVADENE Cream (silver sulfadiazine) spreads easily and can be washed off readily with water.

Silver sulfadiazine has broad antimicrobial activity. It is bactericidal for many gram-negative and gram-positive bacteria as well as being effective against yeast. Results from in vitro testing are listed below. Sufficient data have been obtained to demonstrate that silver sulfadiazine will inhibit bacteria that are resistant to other antimicrobial agents and that the compound is superior to sulfadiazine.

No. of Sensitive Strains/Total Strains Tested Concentration of silver sulfadiazine

Genus & Species	50 µg/ml	100 µg/ml
Pseudomonas aeruginosa	130/130	130/130
Pseudomonas maltophilia	7/7	7/7
Enterobacter species	48/50	50/50
Enterobacter cloacae	24/24	24/24
Klebsiella	53/54	54/54
Escherichia coli	63/63	63/63
Serratia	27/28	28/28
Proteus mirabilis	53/53	53/53
Proteus morganii	10/10	10/10
Proteus rettgeri	2/2	2/2
Proteus vulgaris	2/2	2/2
Providencia	1/1	1/1
Citrobacter	10/10	10/10
Herellea	8/9	9/9
Mima	2/2	2/2
Staphylococcus aureus	100/101	101/101
Staphylococcus epidermidis	51/51	51/51
β-hemolytic Streptococcus	4/4	4/4
Enterococcus (Group D Streptococcus)	52/53	53/53
Corynebacterium diphtheriae	2/2	2/2
Clostridium perfringens	0/2	2/2
Candida albicans	43/50	50/50

Studies utilizing radioactive micronized silver sulfadiazine, electron microscopy, and elaborate biochemical techniques have revealed that the mechanism of action of silver sulfadiazine on bacteria differs from silver nitrate and sodium sulfadiazine. SILVADENE Cream (silver sulfadiazine) acts only on the cell membrane and cell wall to produce its bactericidal effect.

Silver sulfadiazine by its chemical nature is not a carbonic anhydrase inhibitor. **Acidosis in patients treated with SILVADENE Cream has not been reported.** Since it is not a carbonic anhydrase inhibitor, SILVADENE Cream may be particularly of value in treating pediatric burn patients.

Indications: SILVADENE Cream (silver sulfadiazine) is a topical antimicrobial drug indicated as an adjunct for the prevention and treatment of wound sepsis in patients with second- and third-degree burns.

Contraindications: Because sulfonamide therapy is known to increase the possibility of kernicterus, SILVADENE Cream should not be used at term pregnancy, on premature infants, or on newborn infants during the first month of life.

Warnings: SILVADENE Cream should be administered with great caution to patients with history of hypersensitivity to SILVADENE Cream. It is not known whether there is cross-sensitivity to other sulfonamides. If allergic reactions attributable to treatment with SILVADENE Cream occur, discontinuation of SILVADENE Cream must be considered. The use of SILVADENE Cream in some cases of glucose-6-phosphate dehydrogenase deficient individuals may be hazardous, as hemolysis may occur.

Use in Pregnancy: Safe use of SILVADENE Cream during pregnancy has not been established. Therefore, the preparation is not recommended for the treatment of women of childbearing potential, unless the burned area covers more than 20 percent of the total body surface area or the need for therapeutic benefit of SILVADENE Cream is, in the physician's judgment, greater than the possible risk to the fetus.

Fungal colonization in and below the eschar may occur concomitantly with reduction of bacterial growth in the burn wound. However, fungal dissemination is rare.

In the treatment of burn wounds involving extensive areas of the body, the serum sulfa concentration may approach adult therapeutic levels (8 to 12 mg%). Therefore, in these patients it would be advisable to monitor serum sulfa concentrations. Renal function should be carefully monitored and the urine should be checked for sulfa crystals.

Precautions: If hepatic and renal functions become impaired and elimination of drug decreases, accumulation may occur and discontinuation of SILVADENE Cream should be weighed against the therapeutic benefit being achieved.

In considering the use of topical proteolytic enzymes in conjunction with SILVADENE Cream, the possibility should be noted that silver may inactivate such enzymes.

Adverse Reactions: It is frequently difficult to distinguish between an adverse reaction due to SILVADENE Cream (silver sulfadiazine) and reactions that may occur due to the concomitant use of other therapeutic agents used in the treatment of a patient having a severe burn wound. In the aggregate of 2,297 patients treated with SILVADENE Cream, there were 59 drug-related reactions (2.5%). Of these there were 51 cases of burning, 5 of rash, 2 of itching, and 1 of interstitial nephritis. However, SILVADENE Cream therapy was discontinued in only 0.9% of the patient population.

Since significant quantities of silver sulfadiazine are absorbed, it is possible that any of the adverse reactions attributable to sulfonamides may occur.

Dosage and Administration: Prompt institution of appropriate regimens for care of the burned patient is of prime importance and includes the control of shock and pain. The burn wounds are then cleansed and debrided and SILVADENE Cream (silver sulfadiazine) is applied with sterile, gloved hand. The burn areas should be covered with SILVADENE Cream at all times. The cream should be applied once to twice daily to a thickness of approximately 1/16 inch. Whenever necessary, the cream should be reapplied to any areas from which it has been removed by patient activity. Administration may be accomplished in minimal time because dressings are not required. However, if individual patient requirements make dressings necessary, they may be used.

When feasible, the patient should be bathed daily. This is an aid in debridement. A whirlpool bath is particularly helpful, but the patient may be bathed in bed or in a shower.

Reduction in bacterial growth after application of topical antibacterial agents has been reported to permit spontaneous healing of deep partial-thickness burns by preventing conversion of the partial thickness to full thickness by sepsis. However, reduction in bacterial colonization has caused delayed separation, in some cases necessitating escharotomy in order to prevent contracture.

Treatment with SILVADENE Cream should be continued until satisfactory healing has occurred or the burn site is ready for grafting. **The drug should not be withdrawn from the therapeutic regimen while there remains the possibility of infection except if a significant adverse reaction occurs.**

How Supplied: SILVADENE Cream (silver sulfadiazine) is available in 50-gm, 400-gm, and 1000-gm jars, and 20-gm tubes.
U.S. Patent 3,761,590.

Issued 3/82

THROAT DISCS®   OTC
Throat Lozenges

Description: Each lozenge contains capsicum, peppermint, anise, cubeb, glycyrrhiza extract (licorice), and linseed.

Indications: Effective for soothing, temporary relief of minor throat irritations from hoarseness and coughs due to colds.

Precautions: For severe or persistent cough or sore throat, or sore throat accompanied by high fever, headache, nausea, and vomiting, consult physician promptly. Not recommended for children under 3 years of age.

Dosage: Allow lozenge to dissolve slowly in mouth. One or two should give the desired relief. Do not use more than four lozenges per hour.

How Supplied: Box of 60 lozenges.

Issued 2/83

THYROID STRONG TABLETS   ℞
THYROID TABLETS, USP   ℞
[thī′roid]

Description: Thyroid hormone drugs are natural or synthetic preparations containing tetraiodothyronine (T_4, levothyroxine) sodium or triiodothyronine (T_3, liothyronine) sodium or both. T_4 and T_3 are produced in the human thyroid gland by the iodination and coupling of the amino acid tyrosine. T_4 contains four iodine atoms and is formed by the coupling of two molecules of diiodotyrosine (DIT). T_3 contains three atoms of iodine and is formed by the coupling of one molecule of DIT with one molecule of monoiodotyrosine (MIT). Both hormones are stored in the thyroid colloid as thyroglobulin. Thyroid hormone preparations belong to two categories: (1) natural hormonal preparations derived from animal thyroid, and (2) synthetic preparations. Natural preparations include desiccated thyroid and thyroglobulin. Desiccated thyroid is derived from domesticated animals that are used for food by man (either beef or hog thyroid), and thyroglobulin is derived from thyroid glands of the hog. The United States Pharmacopeia (USP) has standardized the total iodine content of natural preparations. Thyroid, USP contains not less than (NLT) 0.17% and not more than (NMT) 0.23% iodine and thyroglobulin contains not less than (NLT) 0.7% of organically bound iodine. Iodine content is only an indirect indicator of true hormonal biologic activity.

There are five preparations in the USP. They are (1) Thyroid Tablets, (2) Thyroglobulin Tablets, (3) Levothyroxine Sodium Tablets, (4) Liothyronine Sodium Tablets, and (5) Liotrix Tablets (a ratio, by weight, of 4 to 1, of the sodium salts of T_4 and T_3, respectively).

Thyroid tablets are prepared from defatted, desiccated thyroid glands of edible animals. Thyroid, USP is standardized to contain 0.2% iodine. Thyroid Strong is standardized to contain 0.3% iodine. The standard of 0.3% iodine was adopted before the USP Standard was established and is 50% stronger than the USP specification. Each grain of Thyroid Strong is equivalent to 1-½ grains of Thyroid, USP. Thyroid is assayed both chemically and biologically to assure uniform potency. In this preparation the active thyroid hormones, thyroxine and liothyronine, are available in their natural state.

[See table on next page]

Clinical Pharmacology: The steps in the synthesis of the thyroid hormones are controlled by thyrotropin (Thyroid Stimulating Hormone, TSH) secreted by the anterior pituitary. This hormone's secretion is in turn controlled by a feedback mechanism affected by the thyroid hormones themselves and by thyrotropin-releasing hormone

(TRH), a tripeptide of hypothalamic origin. Endogenous thyroid hormone secretion is suppressed when exogenous thyroid hormones are administered to euthyroid individuals in excess of the normal gland's secretion.

The mechanisms by which thyroid hormones exert their physiologic action are not well understood. These hormones enhance oxygen consumption by most tissues of the body, increase the basal metabolic rate, and the metabolism of carbohydrates, lipids, and proteins. Thus, they exert a profound influence on every organ system in the body and are of particular importance in the development of the central nervous system.

The normal thyroid gland contains approximately 200 mcg of levothyroxine (T_4) per gram of gland, and 15 mcg of triiodothyronine (T_3) per gram. The ratio of these two hormones in the circulation does not represent the ratio in the thyroid gland, since about 80% of peripheral triiodothyronine comes from monodeiodination of levothyroxine. Peripheral monodeiodination of levothyroxine at the 5 position (inner ring) also results in the formation of reverse triiodothyronine (rT_3), which is calorigenically inactive. These facts would seem to advocate levothyroxine as the treatment of choice for the hypothyroid patient and to militate against the administration of hormone combinations which, while normalizing thyroxine levels, may produce triiodothyronine levels in the thyrotoxic range.

Triiodothyronine (T_3) level is low in the fetus and newborn, in old age, in chronic caloric deprivation, hepatic cirrhosis, renal failure, surgical stress, and chronic illnesses representing what has been called the "low triiodothyronine syndrome."

Pharmacokinetics: Animal studies have shown that T_4 is only partially absorbed from the gastrointestinal tract. The degree of absorption is dependent on the vehicle used for its administration and by the character of the intestinal contents, including the intestinal flora, plasma protein, and soluble dietary factors, all of which bind thyroid and thereby make it unavailable for diffusion. Only 41% is absorbed when given in a gelatin capsule as opposed to a 74% absorption when given with an albumin carrier.

Depending on other factors, absorption has varied from 48 to 79% of the administered dose. Fasting increases absorption. Malabsorption syndromes, as well as dietary factors (children's soybean formula, concomitant use of anionic exchange resins such as cholestyramine) cause excessive fecal loss. T_3 is almost totally absorbed, 95% in four hours. The hormones contained in the natural preparations are absorbed in a manner similar to the synthetic hormones.

More than 99% of circulating hormones are bound to serum proteins, including thyroid-binding globulin (TBg), thyroid-binding prealbumin (TBPA), and albumin (TBa), whose capacities and affinities vary for the hormones. The higher affinity of levothyroxine (T_4) for both TBg and TBPA as compared to triiodothyronine (T_3) partially explains the higher serum levels and longer half-life of the former hormone. Both protein-bound hormones exist in reverse equilibrium with minute amounts of free hormone, the latter accounting for the metabolic activity.

Deiodination of levothyroxine (T_4) occurs at a number of sites, including liver, kidney, and other tissues. The conjugated hormone, in the form of glucuronide or sulfate, is found in the bile and gut where it may complete an enterohepatic circulation. Eighty-five percent of levothyroxine (T_4) metabolized daily is deiodinated.

Indications and Usage: Thyroid hormone drugs are indicated:
1. As replacement of supplemental therapy in patients with hypothyroidism of any etiology, except transient hypothyroidism during the recovery phase of subacute thyroiditis. This category includes cretinism, myxedema, and ordinary hypothyroidism in patients of any age (children, adults, the elderly) or state (including pregnancy); primary hypothyroidism resulting from functional deficiency, primary atrophy, partial or total absence of thyroid gland, or the effects of surgery, radiation, or drugs, with or without the presence of goiter; and secondary (pituitary), or tertiary (hypothalamic) hypothyroidism (See Warnings).
2. As pituitary TSH suppressants in the treatment or prevention of various types of euthyroid goiters, including thyroid nodules, subacute or chronic (Hashimoto's) lymphocytic thyroiditis, multinodular goiter, and in the management of thyroid cancer.
3. As diagnostic agents in suppression tests to differentiate suspected mild hyperthyroidism or thyroid gland autonomy.

Contraindications: Thyroid hormone preparations are generally contraindicated in patients with diagnosed but as yet uncorrected adrenal cortical insufficiency, untreated thyrotoxicosis, and apparent hypersensitivity to any of their active or extraneous constituents. There is no well-documented evidence from the literature, however, of true allergic or idiosyncratic reactions to thyroid hormone.

Warnings:

> Drugs with thyroid hormone activity, alone or together with other therapeutic agents, have been used for the treatment of obesity. In euthyroid patients, doses within the range of daily hormonal requirements are ineffective for weight reduction. Larger doses may produce serious or even life-threatening manifestations of toxicity, particularly when given in association with sympathomimetic amines such as those used for their anorectic effects.

The use of thyroid hormones in the therapy of obesity, alone or combined with other drugs, is unjustified and has been shown to be ineffective. Neither is their use justified for the treatment of male or female infertility unless this condition is accompanied by hypothyroidism.

Precautions:
General: Thyroid hormones should be used with great caution in a number of circumstances where the integrity of the cardiovascular system, particularly the coronary arteries, is suspected. These include patients with angina pectoris or the elderly, in whom there is a greater likelihood of occult cardiac disease. In these patients, therapy should be initiated with low doses, ie, 25 to 50 mcg levothyroxine (T_4) or its isocaloric equivalents. When, in such patients, a euthyroid state can only be reached at the expense of an aggravation of the cardiovascular disease, thyroid hormone dosage should be reduced.

Thyroid hormone therapy in patients with concomitant diabetes mellitus or insipidus or adrenal cortical insufficiency aggravates the intensity of their symptoms. Appropriate adjustments of the various therapeutic measures directed at these concomitant endocrine diseases are required. The therapy of myxedema coma requires simultaneous administration of glucocorticoids (see **Dosage and Administration**).

Hypothyroidism decreases and hyperthyroidism increases the sensitivity to oral anticoagulants. Prothrombin time should be closely monitored in thyroid-treated patients on oral anticoagulants and dosage of the latter agents adjusted on the basis of frequent prothrombin time determinations. In infants, excessive doses of thyroid hormone preparations may produce craniosynostosis.

Information for the Patient: Patients on thyroid hormone preparations and parents of children on thyroid therapy should be informed that:
1. Replacement therapy is to be taken essentially for life, with the exception of cases of transient hypothyroidism, usually associated with thyroiditis, and in those patients receiving a therapeutic trial of the drug.
2. They should immediately report during the course of therapy any signs or symptoms of thyroid hormone toxicity, eg, chest pain, increased pulse rate, palpitations, excessive sweating, heat intolerance, nervousness, or any other unusual event.
3. In case of concomitant diabetes mellitus, the daily dosage of antidiabetic medication may need readjustment as thyroid hormone replacement is achieved. If thyroid medication is stopped, a downward readjustment of the dosage of insulin or oral hypoglycemic agent may be necessary to avoid hypoglycemia. At all times, close monitoring of urinary glucose levels is mandatory in such patients.
4. In case of concomitant oral anticoagulant therapy, the prothrombin time should be measured frequently to determine if the dosage of oral anticoagulants is to be readjusted.
5. Partial loss of hair may be experienced by children in the first few months of thyroid therapy, but this is usually a transient phenomenon and later recovery is usually the rule.

Laboratory Tests: Treatment of patients with thyroid hormones requires the periodic assessment of thyroid status by means of appropriate laboratory tests besides the full clinical evaluation. The TSH suppression test can be used to test the effectiveness of any thyroid preparation, bearing in mind the relative insensitivity of the infant pituitary to the negative feedback effect of thyroid hormones. Serum T_4 levels can be used to test the effectiveness of all thyroid medications except T_3. When the total serum T_4 is low but TSH is normal, a test specific to assess unbound (free) T_4 levels is warranted. Specific measurements of T_4 and T_3 by competitive protein binding or radioimmunoassay are not influenced by blood levels of organic or inorganic iodine and have essentially replaced older tests of thyroid hormone measurements, ie, PBI, BEI, and T_4 by column.

Drug Interactions:
ORAL ANTICOAGULANTS—Thyroid hormones appear to increase catabolism of vitamin K-dependent clotting factors. If oral anticoagulants are also being given, compensatory increases in clotting-factor synthesis are impaired. Patients stabilized on oral anticoagulants who are found to require thyroid replacement therapy should be watched very closely when thyroid is started. If a patient is truly hypothyroid, it is likely that a reduction in anticoagulant therapy is begun in a patient already stabilized on maintenance thyroid replacement therapy.

INSULIN OR ORAL HYPOGLYCEMICS —Initiating thyroid replacement therapy may cause increases in insulin or oral hypoglycemic requirements. The effects seen are poorly understood and depend upon a variety of factors such

Continued on next page

TABLE I
AMOUNTS OF T_3 AND T_4 IN MARION'S THYROID PRODUCTS

Product	Strength	T_3	T_4
Thyroid Strong and Thyroid Strong (Sugar-Coated)	½ gr	9.25 mg	28.75 mg
	1 gr	18.5 mg	57.5 mg
	2 gr	37 mg	115 mg
Thyroid Strong (Sugar-Coated)	3 gr	55.5 mg	172.5 mg
Thyroid, USP	1 gr	12.3 mg	38.3 mg
	2 gr	24.6 mg	76.6 mg

Marion—Cont.

as dose and type of thyroid preparations and endocrine status of the patient. Patients receiving insulin or oral hypoglycemics should be closely watched during initiation of thyroid replacement therapy.

CHOLESTYRAMINE—Cholestyramine binds both T_4 and T_3 in the intestine, thus impairing absorption of these thyroid hormones. In vitro studies indicate that the binding is not easily removed. Therefore, four to five hours should elapse between administration of cholestyramine and thyroid hormones.

ESTROGEN, ORAL CONTRACEPTIVES—Estrogens tend to increase serum thyroxine-binding globulin (TBg). In a patient with a nonfunctioning thyroid gland who is receiving thyroid replacement therapy, free levothyroxine may be decreased when estrogens are started, thus increasing thyroid requirements. However, if the patient's thyroid gland has sufficient function, the decreased free thyroxine will result in a compensatory increase in thyroxine output by the thyroid. Therefore, patients without a functioning thyroid gland who are on thyroid replacement therapy may need to increase their thyroid dose if estrogens or estrogen-containing oral contraceptives are given.

Drug/Laboratory Test Interactions: The following drugs or moieties are known to interfere with laboratory tests performed in patients on thyroid hormone therapy: androgens, corticosteroids, estrogens, oral contraceptives containing estrogens, iodine-containing preparations, and the numerous preparations containing salicylates.

1. Changes in TBg concentration should be taken into consideration in the interpretation of T_4 and T_3 values. In such cases, the unbound (free) hormone should be measured. Pregnancy, estrogens, and estrogen-containing oral contraceptives increase TBg concentrations. TBg may also be increased during infectious hepatitis. Decreases in TBg concentrations are observed in nephrosis, acromegaly, and after androgen or corticosteroid therapy. Familial hyperthyroxine- or hypothyroxine-binding globulinemias have been described. The incidence of TBg deficiency approximates 1 in 9,000. The binding of thyroxine by TBPA is inhibited by salicylates.
2. Medicinal or dietary iodine interferes with all in vivo tests of radioiodine uptake, producing low uptakes which may not be reflective of a true decrease in hormone synthesis.
3. The persistence of clinical and laboratory evidence of hypothyroidism in spite of adequate dosage replacement indicates either poor patient compliance, poor absorption, excessive fecal loss, or inactivity of the preparation. Intracellular resistance to thyroid hormone is quite rare.

Carcinogenesis, Mutagenesis, and Impairment of Fertility: A reportedly apparent association between prolonged thyroid therapy and breast cancer has not been confirmed, and patients on thyroid for established indications should not discontinue therapy. No confirmatory long-term studies in animals have been performed to evaluate carcinogenic potential, mutagenicity, or impairment of fertility in either males or females.

Pregnancy-Category A: Thyroid hormones do not readily cross the placental barrier. The clinical experience to date does not indicate any adverse effect on fetuses when thyroid hormones are administered to pregnant women. On the basis of current knowledge, thyroid replacement therapy to hypothyroid women should not be discontinued during pregnancy.

Nursing Mothers: Minimal amounts of thyroid hormones are excreted in human milk. Thyroid is not associated with serious adverse reactions and does not have a known tumorigenic potential. However, caution should be exercised when thyroid is administered to a nursing woman.

Pediatric Use: Pregnant mothers provide little or no thyroid hormone to the fetus. The incidence of congenital hypothyroidism is relatively high (1 in 4,000) and the hypothyroid fetus would not derive any benefit from the small amounts of hormone crossing the placental barrier. Routine determinations of serum (T_4) and/or TSH is strongly advised in neonates in view of the deleterious effects of thyroid deficiency on growth and development. Treatment should be initiated immediately upon diagnosis, and maintained for life, unless transient hypothyroidism is suspected; in which case, therapy may be interrupted for 2 to 8 weeks after the age of 3 years to reassess the condition. Cessation of therapy is justified in patients who have maintained a normal TSH during those 2 to 8 weeks.

Adverse Reactions: Adverse reactions other than those indicative of hyperthyroidism because of therapeutic overdosage, either initially or during the maintenance period, are rare (see **Overdosage**).

Overdosage:

Signs and Symptoms: Excessive doses of thyroid result in a hypermetabolic state resembling in every respect the condition of endogenous origin. The condition may be self-induced.

Treatment of Overdosage: Dosage should be reduced or therapy temporarily discontinued if signs and symptoms of overdosage appear. Treatment may be reinstituted at a lower dosage. In normal individuals, normal hypothalamic-pituitary-thyroid axis function is restored in 6 to 8 weeks after thyroid suppression.

Treatment of acute massive thyroid hormone overdosage is aimed at reducing gastrointestinal absorption of the drugs and counteracting central and peripheral effects, mainly those of increased sympathetic activity. Vomiting may be induced initially if further gastrointestinal absorption can reasonably be prevented and barring contraindications such as coma, convulsions, or loss of the gagging reflex. Treatment is symptomatic and supportive. Oxygen may be administered and ventilation maintained.

Cardiac glycosides may be indicated if congestive heart failure develops. Measures to control fever, hypoglycemia, or fluid loss should be instituted if needed. Antiadrenergic agents, particularly propranolol, have been used advantageously in the treatment of increased sympathetic activity. Propranolol may be administered intravenously at a dosage of 1 to 3 mg over a 10-minute period or orally, 80 to 160 mg per day, especially when no contraindications exist for its use.

Dosage and Administration: The dosage of thyroid hormones is determined by the indication and must in every case be individualized according to patient response and laboratory findings.

Thyroid hormones are given orally. In acute, emergency conditions, injectable sodium levothyroxine may be given intravenously when oral administration is not feasible or desirable, as in the treatment of myxedema coma, or during total parenteral nutrition. Injectable sodium liothyronine is also available upon request from the manufacturer, under investigational status, for the treatment of myxedema coma. Intramuscular administration of these two preparations is not advisable because of reported poor absorption.

Hypothyroidism: Therapy is usually instituted using low doses, with increments which depend on the cardiovascular status of the patient. The usual starting dose is 50 mcg of levothyroxine (T_4) or its isocaloric equivalent, with increments of 25 mcg every 2 to 3 weeks.

A lower starting dosage, 25 mcg per day, is recommended in patients with long-standing myxedema, particularly if cardiovascular impairment is suspected, in which case extreme caution is recommended. The appearance of angina is an indication for the reduction in dosage. The 200 to 400 mcg of levothyroxine (T_4) recommended in the early trials are now considered excessive and most patients require 100 to 200 mcg per day or the caloric equivalent. Failure to respond to doses of 300 mcg suggests lack of compliance or malabsorption. Maintenance dosages of 100 to 200 mcg per day usually result in normal serum levothyroxine (T_4) and triiodothyronine (T_3) levels. Adequate therapy usually results in normal TSH and T_4 levels after 2 to 3 weeks of therapy.

Readjustment of thyroid hormone dosage should be made within the first four weeks of therapy, after proper clinical and laboratory evaluations, including serum levels of T_4, bound and free, and TSH.

The rapid onset and dissipation of action of sodium liothyronine (T_3), as compared with sodium levothyroxine (T_4), has led some clinicians to prefer its use in patients who might be more susceptible to the untoward effects of thyroid medication. However, the wide swings in serum T_3 levels that follow its administration and the possibility of more pronounced cardiovascular side effects tend to counterbalance the stated advantages.

T_3 may be used in preference to levothyroxine (T_4) during radioisotope scanning procedures, since induction of hypothyroidism in those cases is more abrupt and can be of shorter duration. It may also be preferred when impairment of peripheral conversion of T_4 and T_3 is suspected.

Myxedema Coma: Myxedema coma is usually precipitated in the hypothyroid patient of long standing by intercurrent illness or drugs such as sedatives and anesthetics and should be considered a medical emergency. Therapy should be directed at the correction of electrolyte disturbances and possible infection besides the administration of thyroid hormones.

Corticosteroids should be administered routinely. T_4 and T_3 may be administered via a nasogastric tube, but the preferred route of administration of both hormones is intravenous. Sodium levothyroxine (T_4) is given at a starting dose of 400 mcg (100 mcg/ml) given rapidly, and is usually well tolerated, even in the elderly. This initial dose is followed by daily supplements of 100 to 200 mcg given intravenously. Normal T_4 levels are achieved in 24 hours followed in three days by threefold elevation of T_3. Triiodothyronine (T_3)—which is obtained only by special request from the manufacturer—is given at doses of 200 mcg intravenously followed by 25-mcg supplements at eight-hour intervals. Oral therapy with either hormone should be resumed as soon as the clinical situation has been stabilized and the patient is able to take oral medication.

Thyroid Cancer: Exogenous thyroid hormone may produce regression of metastases from follicular and papillary carcinoma of the thyroid and is used as ancillary therapy of these conditions with radioactive iodine. TSH should be suppressed to low or undetectable levels; therefore, larger amounts of thyroid hormone than those used for replacement therapy are required. Medullary carcinoma of the thyroid is usually unresponsive to this therapy.

Thyroid Suppression Therapy: Administration of thyroid hormone in doses higher than those produced physiologically by the gland results in suppression of the production of endogenous hormone. This is the basis for the thyroid suppression test and is used as an aid in the diagnosis of patients with signs of mild hyperthyroidism in whom baseline laboratory tests appear normal, or to demonstrate thyroid gland autonomy in patients with Grave's ophthalmopathy. Iodine 131 uptake is determined before and after the administration of the exogenous hormone. A 50% or greater suppression of uptake indicates a normal thyroid-pituitary axis and thus rules out thyroid gland autonomy.

For adults, the usual suppressive dose of levothyroxine (T_4) is 2.6 mcg/kg of body weight per day given for seven to ten days. These doses usually yield normal serum T_4 and T_3 levels and lack of response to TSH.

T_3 is given in doses of 75 to 100 mcg per day for seven days and radioactive iodine uptake is determined before and after administration of the hormone. If thyroid function is under normal control, the radioactive iodine uptake will drop significantly after treatment with either hormone.

Both hormones should be administered cautiously to patients in whom there is a strong suspicion of thyroid gland autonomy, in view of the fact that

Product Information

TABLE II RECOMMENDED PEDIATRIC DOSAGE FOR CONGENITAL HYPOTHYROIDISM

Tetraiodothyronine (T$_4$, levothyroxine) sodium

Age	Doses per day	Daily doses per kg of body weight
0–6 mos	25–50 mcg	8–10 mcg
6–12 mos	50–75 mcg	6– 8 mcg
1–5 yrs	75–100 mcg	5– 6 mcg
6–12 yrs	100 –150 mcg	4– 5 mcg
over 12 yrs	over 150 mcg	2– 3 mcg

the exogenous hormone effects will be additive to the endogenous source.
Pediatric Dosage: Pediatric dosage should follow the recommendations summarized in Table II. In infants with congenital hypothyroidism, therapy with full doses should be instituted as soon as the diagnosis has been made.
[See table above].
How Supplied: Thyroid Tablets, USP are supplied as:
Compressed Tablets (plain)

| NDC 0088-0777-58 | 1 gr (60 mg) | 1000's |
| NDC 0088-0778-58 | 2 gr (120 mg) | 1000's |

Thyroid Strong Tablets are supplied as:
Compressed Tablets (plain)

NDC 0088-0686-47	½ gr (30 mg)	100's
NDC 0088-0686-58	½ gr (30 mg)	1000's
NDC 0088-0674-47	1 gr (60 mg)	100's
NDC 0088-0674-58	1 gr (60 mg)	1000's
NDC 0088-0675-47	2 gr (120 mg)	100's
NDC 0088-0675-58	2 gr (120 mg)	1000's

Compressed Tablets (sugar-coated)

NDC 0088-0626-47	½ gr (30 mg)	100's
NDC 0088-0627-47	1 gr (60 mg)	100's
NDC 0088-0627-58	1 gr (60 mg)	1000's
NDC 0088-0628-47	2 gr (120 mg)	100's
NDC 0088-0629-47	3 gr (180 mg)	100's

Caution: Federal law prohibits dispensing without prescription.
Mfd for
Pharmaceutical Division
Marion Laboratories, Inc.
Kansas City, Missouri 64137
By
Pharmaceutical
Basics, Incorporated
Denver, CO 80123

Issued 5/84
Shown in Product Identification Section, page 418

Marlyn Company, Inc.
350 PAUMA PLACE
ESCONDIDO, CA 92025

HEP-FORTE®
[hep-for'tay]

Description: Hep Forte is a comprehensive formulation of protein, B factors and other nutritional factors which can be important in maintenance and support of normal hepatic function.
Composition: Each capsule contains:

Vitamin A (Palmitate)	1,200 I.U.
Vitamin E (d-Alpha Tocopherol)	10 I.U.
Vitamin C (Ascorbic Acid)	10 mg.
Folic Acid	0.06 mg.
Vitamin B1 (Thiamine Mononitrate)	1 mg.
Vitamin B2 (Riboflavin)	1 mg.
Niacinamide	10 mg.
Vitamin B6 (Pyridoxine HCl)	0.5 mg.
Vitamin B12 (Cobalamin)	1 mcg.
Biotin	3.3 mg.
Pantothenic Acid	2 mg.
Choline Bitartrate	21 mg.
Zinc (Zinc Sulfate)	2 mg.
Desiccated Liver	194.4 mg.
Liver Concentrate	64.8 mg.
Liver Fraction Number 2	64.8 mg.
Yeast (Dried)	64.8 mg.
dl-Methionine	10 mg.
Inositol	10 mg.

Indications: Hep Forte is of value as supportive or adjunctive treatment in cases of: alcoholism, hepatic dysfunction due to hepatotoxic drugs and liver poisons, male and female infertility due to hormonal imbalance caused by hepatic dysfunction.
Contraindications: There are no known contraindications to Hep Forte.
Dosage: Three to six capsules daily.
How Supplied: Bottles of 100, 300 or 500 capsules.
Literature Available.

MARLYN® FORMULA 50®

Composition: Each capsule contains:
Amino Acids .... 0.3 Gm*
Vitamin B6 (pyridoxine HCl) .... 1.0 mg.
*Approximate analysis of the amino acids: indispensable amino acids (lysine, tryptophan, phenylalanine, methionine, threonine, leucine, isoleucine, valine), 35.30%; semi-dispensable amino acids (arginine, histidine, tyrosine, cystine, glycine), 19.18%; dispensable amino acids (glutamic acid, alanine, aspartic acid, serine, proline), 45.56%.
Amino acids: Protein "building blocks" important to growth and development of all protein containing tissue including nails, hair, and skin.
Dosage and Administration: The recommended daily dose is 6 capsules daily.
Supply: Bottles of 100, 250 and 1000 capsules.

MARLYN® PMS™
(See PDR For Nonprescription Drugs)

Mason Pharmaceuticals, Inc.
1201 DOVE STREET
SUITE #520
NEWPORT BEACH, CA 92660

DAMACET-P®
[dā″mă-set-p]

Description: Each blue tablet contains:
Hydrocodone Bitartrate* .... 5 mg.
*WARNING: May be habit forming.
Acetaminophen .... 500 mg.
Hydrocodone is a hydrogenated ketone of codeine available as bitartrate salt. Hydrocodone bitartrate is an opioid analgesic and antitussive and occurs as fine, white crystals or as a crystalline powder. It is affected by light. Acetaminophen is a non-opiate, non-salicylate analgesic and antipyretic which occurs as a white, odorless, crystalline powder possessing a slightly bitter taste.
Clinical Pharmacology: Hydrocodone is a semisynthetic narcotic analgesic and antitussive with multiple actions similar to those of codeine. Most of these actions involve the central nervous system and smooth muscle. The precise action of hydrocodone and other opiates is not known, although it is believed to relate to the existence of opiate receptors in the central nervous system. In addition to analgesia, narcotics may produce drowsiness, changes in mood and mental clouding.
Radioimmunoassay techniques have recently been developed for the analysis of hydrocodone in human plasma. After a 10 mg. oral dose of hydrocodone bitartrate, a mean peak serum drug level of 23.6 ng/ml and an elimination half-life of 3.8 hours were found.
The analgesic action of acetaminophen involves both the peripheral and central nervous system, but the specific mechanism is as yet unknown. Acetaminophen inhibits prostaglandin synthetase. Antipyretic activity is mediated through heat regulating centers. Therapeutic doses of acetaminophen have minimal effects on the cardiovascular or respiratory systems; however, toxic doses may cause circulatory failure and rapid, shallow breathing. Acetaminophen is rapidly and almost completely absorbed from the gastro-intestinal tract, producing maximum serum concentrations within 30 minutes to one hour. The plasma half-life in adults and children ranges from 0.90 hours to 3.25 hours with an average of approximately 2 hours. The drug distributes uniformly in most body fluids and is approximately 25% protein bound. Acetaminophen is conjugated in the liver, with less than 3% of the dose excreted unchanged in 24 hours. The primary metabolic pathway is conjugation to sulfate and glucuronide by-products. A minor oxidative pathway forms cysteine and mercapturic acid. These compounds are subsequently excreted by the kidneys into the urine.
Indications and Usage: For the relief of moderate to moderately severe pain.
Contraindications: Hypersensitivity to acetaminophen or hydrocodone.
Warnings:
Acute Abdominal Conditions: The administration of narcotics may obscure the diagnosis or clinical course of patients with acute abdominal conditions.
Head Injury and Increased Intracranial Pressure: The respiratory depressant effects of narcotics and their capacity to elevate cerebrospinal fluid pressure may be markedly exaggerated in the presence of head injury, other intracranial lesions or a preexisting increase in intracranial pressure. Furthermore, narcotics produce adverse reactions which may obscure the clinical course of patients with head injuries.
Respiratory Depression: At high doses or in sensitive patients, hydrocodone may produce dose-related respiratory depression by acting directly on brain stem respiratory centers. Hydrocodone also affects centers that control respiratory rhythm, and may produce irregular and periodic breathing.
Precautions:
Special Risk Patients: As with any narcotic analgesic agent, DAMACET-P should be used with caution in elderly or debilitated patients and those with severe impairment of hepatic or renal function, Addison's disease, hypothyroidism, prostatic hypertrophy or urethral stricture. The usual precautions should be observed and the possibility of respiratory depression should be considered. DAMACET-P should be used with caution on patients allergic to codeine.
Information for Patients: DAMACET-P, like all narcotics, may impair the mental and/or physical abilities required for the performance of potentially hazardous tasks such as driving a car or operating machinery; patients should be cautioned accordingly. DAMACET-P should be taken after meals or with a full glass of water.
Cough Reflex: Hydrocodone supresses the cough reflex; as with all narcotics, caution should be exercised when Acetaminophen and Hydrocodone Bitartrate Tablets are used postoperatively and in patients with pulmonary disease.
Drug Interactions: Patients receiving other narcotic analgesics, antipsychotics, antianxiety agents, or other CNS depressants (including alcohol) concommitantly with acetaminophen and hydrocodone tablets may exhibit an additive CNS depression. When combined therapy is contemplated, the dose of one or both agents should be reduced.
The concurrent use of anticholinergics with hydrocodone may produce paralytic ileus.
The use of MAO inhibitors or tricyclic antidepressants with hydrocodone preparations may in-

Continued on next page

Mason—Cont.

crease the effect of either the antidepressant or hydrocodone.

Usage in Pregnancy: Pregnancy Category C. Hydrocodone has been shown to be teratogenic in hamsters when given in doses 700 times the human dose. There are no adequate and well-controlled studies in pregnant women. DAMACET-P should be used during pregnancy only if the potential benefit justifies the potential risk to the fetus.

Nonteratogenic Effects: Babies born to mothers who have been taking opioids regularly prior to delivery will be physically dependent. The withdrawal signs incude irritability and excessive crying, tremors, hyperactive reflexes, increased respiratory rate, increased stools, sneezing, yawning, vomiting, and fever. The intensity of the syndrome does not always correlate with the duration of maternal opioid use or dose. There is no consensus on the best method of managing withdrawal. Chlorpromazine 0.7 to 1.0 mg/kg q6h, and paregoric 2 to 4 drops/kg q4h, have been used to treat withdrawal symptoms in infants. The duration of therapy is 4 to 28 days, with the dosage decreased as tolerated.

Labor and Delivery: As with all narcotics, administration of DAMACET-P to the mother shortly before delivery may result in some degree of respiratory depression in the newborn, especially if higher doses are used.

Nursing Mothers: It is not known whether this drug is excreted in human milk. Because many drugs are excreted in human milk and because of the potential for serious adverse reactions in nursing infants from Acetaminophen and Hydrocodone Bitartrate Tablets, a decision should be made whether to discontinue nursing or to discontinue the drug, taking into account the importance of the drug to the mother. Hydrocodone is almost completely excreted within 72 hours.

Pediatric Use: Safety and efficacy in children have not been established.

Adverse Reactions:
Central Nervous System: Sedation, drowsiness, mental clouding, lethargy, impairment of mental and physical performance, anxiety, fear, dysphoria, dizziness, psychic dependence or mood changes may occur.

Gastrointestinal System: Nausea and vomiting occur infrequently; they are more frequent in ambulatory than in recumbent patients. The antiemetic phenothiazines are useful in suppressing these effects; however, some phenothiazine derivatives seem to be antianalgesic and to increase the amount of narcotic required to produce a given level of analgesia. Prolonged administration of Acetaminophen and Hydrocodone Bitartrate Tablets may produce constipation.

Genitourinary System: Ureteral spasm, spasm of vesical sphincters and urinary retention have been reported with codeine and its derivatives.

Drug Abuse and Dependence: DAMACET-P is subject to the Federal Controlled Substance Act (Schedule III). Psychic dependence, physical dependence, and tolerance may develop upon repeated administration of narcotics; therefore, Acetaminophen and Hydrocodone Bitartrate Tablets should be prescribed and administered with caution. However, psychic dependence is unlikely to develop when Acetaminophen and Hydrocodone Bitartrate Tablets are used for a short time for the treatment of pain.

Physical dependence, the condition in which continued administration of the drug is required to prevent the appearance of a withdrawal syndrome, assumes clinically significant proportions only after several weeks of continued narcotic use, although some mild degree of physical dependence may develop after a few days of narcotic therapy. Tolerance, in which increasingly larger doses are required in order to produce the same degree of analgesia, is manifested initially by a shortened duration of analgesic effect, and subsequently by decreases in the intensity of analgesia. The rate of development of tolerance varies among patients.

Overdosage:
Acetaminophen:
Signs and Symptoms: Acetaminophen in massive overdosage may cause hepatic toxicity in some patients. In all cases of suspected overdose, immediately call your regional poison center or the Rocky Mountain Poison Center's toll-free number (800-525-5115) for assistance in diagnosis and for directions in the use of N-acetylcysteine as an antidote, a use currently restricted to investigational status.

In adults, hepatic toxicity has rarely been reported with acute overdose of less than 10 grams and fatalities with less than 15 grams. Importantly, young children seem to be more resistant than adults to the hepatotoxic effect of an acetaminophen overdose. Despite this, the measures outlined below should be initiated in any adult or child suspected of having ingested an acetaminophen overdose.

Early symptoms following a potentially hepatotoxic overdose may include: nausea, vomiting, diaphoresis and general malaise. Clinical and laboratory evidence of hepatic toxicity may not be apparent until 48 to 72 hours post-ingestion.
Treatment: The stomach should be emptied promptly by lavage or by induction of emesis with syrup of ipecac. Patients' estimates of the quantity of a drug ingested are notoriously unreliable. Therefore, if an acetaminophen overdose is suspected, a serum acetaminophen assay should be obtained as early as possible, but no sooner than four hours following ingestion. Liver function studies should be obtained initially and repeated at 24-hour intervals.

The antidote, N-acetylcysteine, should be administered as early as possible, and within 16 hours of the overdose ingestion for optimal results. Following recovery, there are no residual, structural or functional hepatic abnormalities.

Hydrocodone:
Signs and Symptoms: Serious overdose with hydrocodone is characterized by respiratory depression (a decrease in respiratory rate and/or tidal volume, Cheyne-Stokes respiration, cyanosis), extreme somnolence progressing to stupor or coma, skeletal muscle flaccidity, cold and clammy skin, and sometimes bradycardia and hypotension. In severe overdosage, apnea circulatory collapse, cardiac arrest and death may occur.

Treatment: Primary attention should be given to the reestablishment of adequate respiratory exchange through provision of a patent airway and the institution of assisted or controlled ventilation. The narcotic antagonist naloxone hydrochloride is a specific antidote against respiratory depression which may result from overdosage or unusual sensitivity to narcotics, including hydrocodone. Therefore, an appropriate dose of naloxone hydrochloride, 0.55 mg/kgm, should be administered intravenously, (see package insert), simultaneously with efforts at respiratory resuscitation. Since the duration of action of hydrocodone may exceed that of the antagonist, the patient should be kept under continued surveillance and repeated doses of the antagonist should be administered as needed to maintain adequate respiration.

An antagonist should not be administered in the absence of clinically significant respiratory or cardiovascular depression. Oxygen, intravenous fluids, vasopressors and other supportive measures should be employed as indicated.

Gastric emptying may be useful in removing unabsorbed drug.

Dosage and Administration: Dosage should be adjusted according to the severity of the pain and the response of the patient. However, it should be kept in mind that tolerance to hydrocodone can develop with continued use and that the incidence of untoward effects may be dose-related.

The usual dose is one tablet every six hours as needed for pain. If necessary, this dose may be repeated at four hour intervals. In cases of more severe pain, two tablets every six hours (up to 8 tablets in 24 hours) may be required.

Caution: Federal Law prohibits dispensing without prescription.

DAMACET-P has a schedule III classification which permits prescription refill up to six months or five times on physician's specification.
How Supplied: DAMACET-P is supplied as 7/16", round, blue mottled tablets with an "M" logo on one side and "D-C" on the other.
Supplied in bottles of 100, NDC 12758-066-01
          bottles of 500, NDC 12758-066-05
Storage: DAMACET-P should be stored at 59°–86°F, 15°–30°C.
Manufactured by:
Anabolic, Inc., Irvine, CA 92714
Manufactured expressly for
Mason Pharmaceuticals, Inc.
Newport Beach, CA 92660
Shown in Product Identification Section, page 418

DAMASON-P
[dā″mā″son-p]

Description: Each pink tablet of DAMASON-P contains:
Hydrocodone Bitartrate .... 5 mg
  (Warning: May be habit forming)
Aspirin .... 224 mg
Caffeine .... 32 mg
Hydrocodone is a hydrogenated ketone of codeine available as bitartrate salt. Hydrocodone bitartrate is an opioid analgesic and antitussive and occurs as fine, white crystals or as a crystalline powder. It is affected by light.

Clinical Pharmacology: Hydrocodone is a semisynthetic narcotic analgesic with multiple actions similar to those of codeine. Most of these actions involve the central nervous system and smooth muscle. The precise mechanism of action of hydrocodone and other opiates is not known, although it is believed to relate to the existence of opiate receptors in the central nervous system. In addition to analgesia, narcotics may produce drowsiness, changes in mood and mental clouding. Radioimmunoassay techniques have recently been developed for the analysis of hydrocodone in human plasma. After a 10 mg. oral dose of hydrocodone bitartrate, a mean peak serum drug level of 23.6 ng/ml and an elimination half-life of 3.8 hours were found. DAMASON-P also contains the non-narcotic, anti-inflammatory, antipyretic analgesic, aspirin and caffeine.

Indications and Usage: For the relief of moderate to moderately severe pain.

Contraindications: Hypersensitivity to aspirin, caffeine or hydrocodone.

Warnings:
Acute Abdominal Conditions: The administration of narcotics may obscure the diagnosis or clinical course of patients with acute abdominal conditions.

Head Injury and Increased Intracranial Pressure: The respiratory depressant effects of narcotics and their capacity to elevate cerebrospinal fluid pressure may be markedly exaggerated in the presence of head injury, other intracranial lesions or a preexisting increase in intracranial pressure. Furthermore, narcotics produce adverse reactions which may obscure the clinical course of patients with head injuries.

Respiratory Depression: At high doses or in sensitive patients, hydrocodone may produce dose-related respiratory depression by acting directly on brain stem respiratory centers. Hydrocodone also affects centers that control respiratory rhythm, and may produce irregular and periodic breathing.

Other: Salicylates should be used with extreme caution in the presence of peptic ulcer or coagulation abnormalities.

Precautions:
Special Risk Patients: As with any narcotic analgesic agent, DAMASON-P should be used with caution in elderly or debilitated patients and those with severe impairment of hepatic or renal functions, hypothyroidism, Addison's disease, prostatic hypertrophy or urethral stricture. The usual precautions should be observed and the possibility of respiratory depression should be kept in mind.
Information for Patients: DAMASON-P, like all narcotics, may impair the mental and/or physical

abilities required for the performance of potentially hazardous tasks such as driving a car or operating machinery; patients should be cautioned accordingly. DAMASON-P should be taken after meals or with a full glass of water.
Cough Reflex: Hydrocodone suppresses the cough reflex; as with all narcotics, caution should be exercised when DAMASON-P is used postoperatively and in patients with pulmonary disease.
Drug Interactions: Patients receiving other narcotic analgesics, general anesthetics, phenothiazines, other tranquilizers, sedative-hypnotics or other CNS depressants (including alcohol) concomitantly with DAMASON-P may exhibit an additive CNS depression. When such combined therapy is contemplated, the dose of one or both agents should be reduced. Aspirin may enhance the effects of anti-coagulants and inhibit the uricosuric effects of uricosuric agents.
The concurrent use of anticholinergics with hydrocodone may produce paralytic ileus.
The use of MAO inhibitors or tricyclic antidepressants with hydrocodone preparations may increase the effect of either the antidepressant or hydrocodone.
Usage In Pregnancy: Pregnancy Category C. Hydrocodone has been shown to be teratogenic in hamsters when given in doses 700 times the human dose. There are no adequate and well-controlled studies in pregnant women. DAMASON-P should be used during pregnancy only if the potential benefit justifies the potential risk to the fetus.
Nonteratogenic Effects: Babies born to mothers who have been taking opioids regularly prior to delivery will be physically dependent. The withdrawal signs include irritability and excessive crying, tremors, hyperactive reflexes, increased respiratory rate, increased stools, sneezing, yawning, vomiting, and fever. The intensity of the syndrome does not always correlate with the duration of maternal opioid use or dose. There is no consensus on the best method of managing withdrawal. Chlorpromazine 0.7 to 1.0 mg/kg q6h, and paregoric 2 to 4 drops/kg q4h, have been used to treat withdrawal symptoms in infants. The duration of therapy is 4 to 28 days, with the dosage decreased as tolerated.
Labor and Delivery: As with all narcotics, administration of DAMASON-P to the mother shortly before delivery may result in some degree of respiratory depression in the newborn, especially if higher doses are used.
Nursing Mothers: It is not known whether this drug is excreted in human milk. Because many drugs are excreted in human milk and because of the potential for serious adverse reactions in nursing infants from DAMASON-P, a decision should be made whether to discontinue nursing or to discontinue the drug, taking into account the importance of the drug to the mother. Hydrocodone is almost completely excreted within 72 hours.
Pediatric Use: Safety and efficacy in children have not been established.
Adverse Reactions:
Central Nervous System: As with all narcotics, sedation, drowsiness, mental clouding, lethargy, impairment of mental and physical performance, anxiety, fear, dysphoria, dizziness, psychic dependence and mood changes may occur.
Gastrointestinal System: Nausea and vomiting occur infrequently; they are more frequent in ambulatory than in recumbent patients. Administration with meals may help reduce this problem. The antiemetic phenothiazines are useful in suppressing these effects; however, some phenothiazine derivatives seem to be antianalgesic and to increase the amount of narcotic required to produce a given level of analgesia. Prolonged administration of DAMASON-P may produce constipation.
Genitourinary System: Ureteral spasm, spasm of vesical sphincters and urinary retention have been reported with codeine and its derivatives.
Drug Abuse and Dependence: DAMASON-P is subject to the Federal Controlled Substance Act (Schedule III). Psychic dependence, physical dependence, and tolerance may develop upon repeated administration of narcotics; therefore, DAMASON-P Tablets should be prescribed and administered with caution. However, psychic dependence is unlikely to develop when DAMASON-P Tablets are used for a short time for the treatment of pain.
Physical dependence, the condition in which continued administration of the drug is required to prevent the appearance of a withdrawal syndrome, assumes clinically significant proportions only after several weeks of continued narcotic use, although some mild degree of physical dependence may develop after a few days of narcotic therapy. Tolerance, in which increasingly larger doses are required in order to produce the same degree of analgesia, is manifested initially by a shortened duration of analgesic effect, and subsequently by decreases in the intensity of analgesia. The rate of development of tolerance varies among patients.
Overdosage:
Aspirin:
Signs and Symptoms: Respiratory alkalosis is characteristic of the early phase in intoxication with aspirin while hyperventilation is occurring, and is quickly followed by metabolic acidosis in most people with severe intoxication. This occurs more readily in children. Hypoglycemia may occur in children who have taken large overdoses. Other laboratory findings associated with aspirin intoxication include ketonuria, hyponatremia, hypokalemia, and occasionally protein-uria. A slight rise in lactic dehydrogenase and hydroxybutyric dehydrogenase may occur.
Methemoglobin and sulfhemoglobin formation are seldom clinically significant in adults but may contribute to general toxicity. When prominent, they appear as a grayish cyanosis seen most clearly in the lips and nailbeds. Definitive diagnosis is made by spectroscopic analysis of water-diluted (1:100) blood specimen, which shows an abnormal band at 630 nm for methamoglobin and at 618 nm for sulfhemoglobin.
Concentrations of aspirin in plasma above 30 mg/100 ml are associated with toxicity. The single lethal dose of aspirin in adults is probably about 25-30 gm, but is not known with certainty.
Hydrocodone:
Signs and Symptoms: Serious overdose with hydrocodone is characterized by respiratory depression (a decrease in respiratory rate and/or tidal volume, Cheyne-Stokes respiration, cyanosis), extreme somnolence progressing to stupor or coma, skeletal muscle flaccidity, cold and clammy skin, and sometimes bradycardia and hypotension. In severe overdosage, apnea, circulatory collapse, cardiac arrest and death may occur.
Treatment: Primary attention should be given to the reestablishment of adequate respiratory exchange through provision of a patent airway and the institution of assisted or controlled ventilation. The narcotic antagonist naloxone hydrochloride is a specific antidote against respiratory depression which may result from overdosage or unusual sensitivity to narcotics, including hydrocodone. Therefore, an appropriate dose of naloxone hydrochloride, 0.55 mg/kgm, should be administered intravenously, (see package insert), simultaneously with efforts at respiratory resuscitation. Since the duration of action of hydrocodone may exceed that of the antagonist, the patient should be kept under continued surveillance and repeated doses of the antagonist should be administered as needed to maintain adequate respiration.
An antagonist should not be administered in the absence of clinically significant respiratory or cardiovascular depression. Oxygen, intravenous fluids, vasopressors and other supportive measures should be employed as indicated.
Gastric emptying may be useful in removing unabsorbed drug.
Dosage and Administration: Dosage should be adjusted according to the severity of the pain and the response of the patient. However, it should be kept in mind that tolerance to hydrocodone can develop with continued use and that the incidence of untoward effects may be dose-related.
The usual dose is one tablet every six hours as needed for pain, with water or other liquids. If necessary, this dose may be repeated at four hour intervals. In cases of more severe pain, two tablets every six hours (up to 8 tablets in 24 hours) may be required.
Caution: Federal Law prohibits dispensing without prescription.
DAMASON-P has a schedule III classification which permits prescription refill up to six months or five times on physician's specification.
How Supplied: DAMASON-P is supplied as 7/16", round, pink mottled tablets with an "M" logo on one side and "D-P" on the other. Supplied in bottles of 100, NDC 12758-055-01, bottles of 500, NDC 12758-055-05, and in hospital packs of 100, NDC 12758-055-25.
Storage: DAMASON-P should be stored at 59°-86°F, 15°-30°C.
Manufactured by:
Anabolic Inc.
Irvine, CA 92712
Manufactured expressly for:
Mason Pharmaceuticals, Inc.
Newport Beach, CA 92660
5815E-Revised May, 1984
Shown in Product Identification Section, page 418

Products are

listed alphabetically

in the

PINK SECTION.

Products are crossed-indexed

by product classifications

in the

BLUE SECTION

Products are crossed-indexed by

generic and chemical names

in the

YELLOW SECTION

IDENTIFICATION PROBLEM?
Consult PDR's
Product Identification Section
where you'll find over 1200
products pictured actual size
and in full color.

Mayrand, Inc.
P. O. BOX 8869
FOUR DUNDAS CIRCLE
GREENSBORO, NC 27419

ANAMINE T.D.* Caps ℞
ANAMINE Syrup
Sugar-Free/Alcohol-Free/Dye-Free

Description:
ANAMINE T.D. Caps
Each Capsule Contains:
Chlorpheniramine Maleate ....8 mg.
Pseudoephedrine Hydrochloride ....120 mg.
ANAMINE Syrup
Each 5 ml (teaspoonful) contains:
Chlorpheniramine Maleate ....2 mg.
Pseudoephedrine Hydrochloride ....30 mg.
*Mayrand brand of sustained release capsules.
How Supplied: ANAMINE T.D. Caps in bottles of 100. ANAMINE Syrup in bottles of 473 ml. (1 pint).

BUFF-A COMP Tablets ℞
Buffered Analgesic-Relaxant

Description: Each tablet contains:
Aspirin ....(10 gr.) 650 mg.
Caffeine .... 40 mg.
Butalbital .... 50 mg.
(Warning: May be habit forming.)
Buffered with calcium carbonate.
Indication and Usage: Buff-A Comp Tablets are indicated for the symptom complex of muscle contraction (tension headache). Buff-A Comp provides an effective analgesic/relaxant with caffeine to relieve tension headache. Aspirin helps alleviate pain while butalbital reduces the tension component of the muscle contraction headache syndrome.
Contraindications: Hypersensitivity to any of the components.
Warnings:
Use In Pregnancy: Adequate studies have not been performed to establish the safety of the drug during pregnancy. Therefore, Buff-A Comp should be used cautiously and only when absolutely necessary in pregnant women.
Drug Dependency: Prolonged use of barbituates can produce drug dependence.
Precautions: Salicylates should be used with caution in the presence of peptic ulcer or coagulation abnormalities.
Adverse Reactions: Drowsiness, dizziness, lightheadedness, gastro-intestinal disturbances; ie. nausea, vomiting and flatulence may occur.
Dosage and Administration: The usual adult dose is one tablet 3 or 4 times daily.
How Supplied: Buff-A Comp Tablets are supplied in bottles of 100.

BUFF-A COMP #3 Tablets ©

Description: Each tablet contains:
Aspirin ....(5 gr.) 325 mg.
Butalbital ....50 mg
(Warning: May be habit forming.)
Caffeine ....40 mg.
Codeine Phosphate ....30 mg.
(Warning: May be habit forming.)
How Supplied: Buff-A Comp #3 Tablets are supplied in bottles of 100.

ELDERCAPS ℞

Description: Each capsule contains:
Vitamin A Acetate ....4,000 I.U.
Vitamin D₂ ....400 I.U.
Vitamin E ....25 I.U.
Ascorbic Acid ....200 mg.
Thiamine Mononitrate ....10 mg.
Riboflavin ....5 mg.
Pyridoxine HCl ....2 mg.
Niacinamide ....25 mg.
d-Calcium Pantothenate ....10 mg.
Zinc Sulfate ....110 mg.
Magnesium Sulfate ....70 mg.
Manganese Sulfate ....5 mg.
Folic Acid ....1 mg.
Indications: ELDERCAPS are indicated for the prophylaxis or treatment of vitamin and mineral deficiencies associated with restricted diets, improper food intake, and decreased absorption or utilization. ELDERCAPS are also indicated in patients with increased requirements for vitamins and minerals due to chronic disease, infection or the stress of surgery.
Warnings: Folic acid alone is improper therapy in the treatment of pernicious anemia and other megaloblastic anemias where vitamin B₁₂ is deficient.
Precautions: Folic acid, especially in doses above 1 mg. daily, may obscure pernicious anemia, that is, hematological remission may occur while neurologic manifestations remain progressive.
Dosage: One capsule daily or as directed by the physician.
How Supplied: Bottles of 100 capsules.

ELDERTONIC

Description: Each 45 ml. contains:
Thiamine HCl ....1.5 mg.
Riboflavin ....1.7 mg.
Pyridoxine HCl ....2.0 mg.
Vitamin B-12 ....6.0 mcg.
Dexpanthenol ....10.0 mg.
Niacinamide ....20.0 mg.
Zinc (elemental) ....15 mg.
  (as zinc sulfate)
Manganese ....2.0 mg.
  (as manganese sulfate)
Magnesium* ....2.0 mg.
  (as magnesium sulfate)
Alcohol 13.5%
In special sherry wine base.
*Minimum magnesium content based on added magnesium.
How Supplied: 8 oz, pints, gallons.

NU-IRON 150 Caps
NU-IRON Elixir (polysaccharide-iron complex)
Sugar Free

Description: NU-IRON is a highly water soluble complex of iron and a low molecular weight polysaccharide.
Each NU-IRON 150 Capsule contains:
Iron (elemental) ....150 mg.
  (as polysaccharide Iron Complex)
Each 5 ml. of NU-IRON Elixir contains:
Iron (elemental) ....100 mg.
  (as Polysaccharide Iron Complex)
Action and Uses: NU-IRON is a non-ionic, easily assimilated, relatively non-toxic form of iron. Full therapeutic doses may be achieved with virtually no gastrointestinal side effects. There is no metallic aftertaste and no staining of teeth.
Indications: For treatment of uncomplicated iron deficiency anemia.
Contraindications: Hemochromatosis, hemosiderosis or a known hypersensitivity to any of the ingredients.
Dosage: ADULTS; One or two NU-IRON 150 Caps daily, or one or two teaspoonfuls NU-IRON Elixir daily. CHILDREN; 6 to 12 years old; one teaspoonful NU-IRON Elixir daily; 2 to 6 years old: ½ teaspoonful daily; under 2 years: ¼ teaspoonful daily.
How Supplied: NU-IRON 150 Caps in bottles of 100. NU-IRON Elixir in 8 fl. oz. bottles.

NU-IRON-PLUS Elixir ℞
Composition: Each 5 ml (teaspoonful) contains:
Iron (Elemental) ....100 mg.
  (as Polysaccharide Iron Complex)
Folic Acid ....1 mg.
Vitamin B₁₂ ....25 mcg.
Alcohol 10%
How Supplied: Bottles of 8 fl. oz.

NU-IRON-V Tablets ℞
Description: Each film-coated tablet contains:
Iron (Elemental) ....60 mg.
  (as Polysaccharide Iron Complex)
Folic Acid ....1 mg.
Ascorbic Acid ....50 mg.
  (as sodium ascorbate)
Cyancobalamin ....3 mcg.
  (Vitamin B-12)
Vitamin A ....4000 I.U.
Vitamin D-2 ....400 I.U.
Thiamine Mononitrate ....3 mg.
Riboflavin ....3 mg.
Pyridoxine HCl ....2 mg.
Niacinamide ....10 mg.
Calcium Carbonate ....312 mg.
Indications: For the prevention and/or treatment of dietary vitamin and iron deficiencies.
Dosage: Prophylactic—one tablet daily or as directed by a physician.
Contraindications: Sensitivity to any of the ingredients.
Precautions: The use of folic acid in patients having or who may develop pernicious anemia involves the hazard of treating the anemia characteristic of the disease while permitting progressive development of combined system disease of the spinal cord.
Parenteral Vitamin B₁₂ is the drug of choice in pernicious anemia and should be used in patients receiving folic acid unless pernicious anemia has been ruled out.
How Supplied: Bottles of 100 tablets.

SEDAPAP-10 Tablets ℞

Description: Each white oblong tablet contains:
Acetaminophen .... 650 mg.
                                                         (10 gr.)
Butalbital .... 50 mg.
(Warning: May be habit forming)
Indications and Usage: Sedapap-10 Tablets are indicated for the symptom complex of muscle contraction (tension headache). Sedapap-10 provides an effective analgesic/relaxant to relieve tension headache. Acetaminophen helps alleviate pain while butalbital reduces the tension component of the muscle contraction headache syndrome.
Contraindications: In patients with hepatic disease and in patients sensitive to either component.
Warnings:
Use in Pregnancy: Adequate studies have not been performed to establish the safety of the drug during pregnancy. Therefore, Sedapap-10 should be used cautiously and only when absolutely necessary in pregnant women.
Drug Dependency: Prolonged use of barbituates can produce drug dependence.
Adverse Reactions: Drowsiness, dizziness, lightheadedness, gastrointestinal disturbances; ie. nausea, vomiting and flatulence may occur.
Dosage and Administration: The usual adult dose is one tablet 3 or 4 times daily.
How Supplied: Sedapap-10 Tablets are supplied in bottles of 100.

SORBIDE ℞
(Isosorbide Dinitrate)

Available as:
SORBIDE T.D. * Capsules 40 mg.
*MAYRAND brand of sustained release Capsules.
How Supplied: Bottles of 100.

STERAPRED UNI-PAK ℞
(Prednisone 5 mg.)

Prednisone in convenient decremental dosage, for unit dispensing.
How Supplied: Box of 21 tablets.

TRIMCAPS © ℞
(Phendimetrazine Tartrate 105 mg.)
Slow Release Capsule

How Supplied: Bottles of 30 and 100.

TRIMTABS
(Phendimetrazine Tartrate 35 mg.)
How Supplied: Bottles of 100 and 500.

McGregor Pharmaceuticals
32580 GRAND RIVER AVENUE
FARMINGTON, MI 48024

ALL McGREGOR PRODUCTS ARE COMPLETELY DYE FREE.

Full prescribing information for all McGregor Pharmaceuticals products is available from your McGregor Pharmaceuticals representative.

Product Identification Codes
To provide quick and positive identification of McGregor Pharmaceuticals products, we have had imprinted the product identification number on our capsules. In order that you may quickly identify a product by its code number, we provide the following list of code numbers:

Product	Code Number
Rhindecon™ (Phenylpropanolamine HCl, 75 mg) Sustained Release Capsules ℞	MCG 215
Rhinolar™ (Phenylpropanolamine HCl 75 mg, Chlorpheniramine Maleate 8 mg, Methscopolamine Nitrate 2.5 mg) Sustained Release Capsule ℞	MCG 219
Rhinolar-EX™ (Phenylpropanolamine HCl 75 mg, Chlorpheniramine Maleate 8 mg) Sustained Release Capsule ℞	MCG 210
Rhinolar-EX 12™ (Phenylpropanolamine HCl 75 mg, Chlorpheniramine Maleate 12 mg) Sustained Release Capsule ℞	MCG 211

EDUCATIONAL MATERIAL

Samples: Starter samples on above products available upon request.

McNeil Consumer Products Company
McNEILAB, INC.
FORT WASHINGTON, PA 19034

CoTYLENOL® Cold Medication Tablets and Capsules — OTC

Description: Each CoTYLENOL Tablet or Capsule contains acetaminophen 325 mg., chlorpheniramine maleate 2 mg., pseudoephedrine hydrochloride 30 mg. and dextromethorphan hydrobromide 15 mg.

Actions: CoTYLENOL Cold Medication Tablets and Capsules contain a clinically proven analgesic-antipyretic, decongestant, cough suppressant and antihistamine. Acetaminophen produces analgesia by elevation of the pain threshold and antipyresis through action on the hypothalamic heat-regulating center. Pseudoephedrine hydrochloride is a sympathomimetic amine which provides temporary relief of nasal congestion. Dextromethorphan is a cough suppressant which provides temporary relief of coughs due to minor throat irritations that may occur with the common cold. Chlorpheniramine is an antihistamine which helps provide temporary relief of runny nose and sneezing due to the common cold.

Indications: CoTYLENOL provides effective symptomatic relief of fever, aches, pains and general discomfort associated with colds and other upper respiratory infections.

Adverse Reactions: While the acetaminophen component is equal to aspirin in analgesic and antipyretic effectiveness, it is unlikely to produce many of the side effects associated with aspirin and aspirin-containing products. Although pseudoephedrine is virtually without pressor effect in normotensive patients, it should be used with caution in hypertensives.

Usual Dosage: Adults: Two tablets or capsules every 6 hours, not to exceed 8 tablets or capsules in 24 hours. Children (6–12 years): One capsule or tablet every 6 hours, not to exceed 4 tablets or capsules in 24 hours.

Note: Since CoTYLENOL Cold Medication Tablets and Capsules are available without prescription, the following appears on the package label: "WARNING: Do not administer to children under 6 or exceed the recommended dosage because nervousness, dizziness, or sleeplessness may result. Do not take if you have asthma, glaucoma, high blood pressure, heart disease, diabetes, thyroid disease, enlargement of the prostate gland, persistent cough due to smoking or emphysema, or are presently taking a prescription drug for the treatment of high blood pressure or emotional disorders, without advice and supervision of a doctor. This preparation may cause drowsiness. Do not drive, operate machinery or drink alcoholic beverages while taking. Persistent cough may indicate a serious condition. Consult a doctor after 3 days if fever persists, or after 7 days if symptoms do not improve or cough persists, tends to recur or is accompanied by high fever, rash, or persistent headaches. Do not use if carton is opened, or if printed green neck wrap or printed foil inner seal is broken (for Capsules). Do not use if carton is opened or printed foil inner seal is broken (for Tablets). Keep this and all medication out of the reach of children. As with any drug, if you are pregnant or nursing a baby, seek the advice of a health professional before using this product. In case of accidental overdosage, contact a physician or poison control center immediately."

Overdosage: Acetaminophen in massive overdosage may cause hepatic toxicity in some patients. In all cases of suspected overdose, immediately call your regional poison center or the Rocky Mountain Poison Center's toll-free number (800-525-6115) for assistance in diagnosis and for directions in the use of N-acetylcysteine as an antidote, a use currently restricted to investigational status. In adults, hepatic toxicity has rarely been reported with acute overdoses of less than 10 grams and fatalities with less than 15 grams. Importantly, young children seem to be more resistant than adults to the hepatotoxic effect of an acetaminophen overdose. Despite this, the measures outlined below should be initiated in any adult or child suspected of having ingested an acetaminophen overdose.

Early symptoms following a potentially hepatotoxic overdose may include: nausea, vomiting, diaphoresis and general malaise. Clinical and laboratory evidence of hepatic toxicity may not be apparent until 48 to 72 hours postingestion. The stomach should be emptied promptly by lavage or by induction of emesis with syrup of ipecac. Patients' estimates of the quantity of a drug ingested are notoriously unreliable. Therefore, if an acetaminophen overdose is suspected, a serum acetaminophen assay should be obtained as early as possible, but no sooner than four hours following ingestion. Liver function studies should be obtained initially and repeated at 24 hour intervals. The antidote, N-acetylcysteine, should be administered as early as possible, and within 16 hours of the overdose ingestion for optimal results. Following recovery, there are no residual, structural or functional hepatic abnormalities.

Chlorpheniramine toxicity should be treated as you would an antihistamine/anticholinergic overdose and is likely to be present within a few hours after acute ingestion.

Symptoms from pseudoephedrine overdose consist most often of mild anxiety, tachycardia and/or mild hypertension. Symptoms usually appear within 4 to 8 hours of ingestion and are transient, usually requiring no treatment.

Acute dextromethorphan overdose usually does not result in serious signs and symptoms unless massive amounts have been ingested. Signs and symptoms of a substantial overdose may include nausea and vomiting, visual disturbances, CNS disturbances, and urinary retention.

How Supplied: Tablets (colored yellow, imprinted "CoTYLENOL")—blister packs of 24, tamper-resistant bottles of 50 and 100. Capsules (colored dark green and light yellow, imprinted "CoTYLENOL")—blister packs of 20 and tamper-resistant bottles of 40.

Shown in Product Identification Section, page 418

CoTYLENOL® Cold Medication Liquid — OTC

Description: Each 30 ml (1 fl. oz.) contains acetaminophen 650 mg., chlorpheniramine maleate 4 mg., pseudoephedrine hydrochloride 60 mg., and dextromethorphan hydrobromide 30 mg. (alcohol 7.5%).

Actions: CoTYLENOL Liquid Cold Medication contains a clinically proven analgesic-antipyretic, decongestant, cough suppressant and antihistamine. Acetaminophen produces analgesia by elevation of the pain threshold and antipyresis through action on the hypothalamic heat-regulating center. Pseudoephedrine hydrochloride is a sympathomimetic amine which provides temporary relief of nasal congestion. Dextromethorphan is a cough suppressant which provides temporary relief of coughs due to minor throat irritations that may occur with the common cold. Chlorpheniramine is an antihistamine which helps provide temporary relief of runny nose and sneezing due to the common cold.

Indications: CoTYLENOL provides effective symptomatic relief of fever, aches, pains and general discomfort associated with colds and other upper respiratory infections.

Adverse Reactions: While the acetaminophen component is equal to aspirin in analgesic and antipyretic effectiveness, it is unlikely to produce many of the side effects associated with aspirin and aspirin-containing products. Although pseudoephedrine is virtually without pressor effect in normotensive patients, it should be used with caution in hypertensives.

Usual Dosage: Measuring cup is provided and marked for accurate dosing. Adults: 1 fluid ounce (2 tbsp.) every 6 hours as needed, not to exceed 4 doses in 24 hours. Children (6–12 yrs): ½ the adult dose (1 tbsp.) as indicated on the measuring cup provided, not to exceed 4 doses in 24 hours.

Note: Since CoTYLENOL Liquid Cold Medication is available without a prescription, the following appears on the package label: "WARNING: Do not administer to children under 6 or exceed the recommended dosage because nervousness, dizziness or sleeplessness may result. Do not take if you have asthma, glaucoma, high blood pressure, heart disease, diabetes, thyroid disease, enlargement of the prostate gland, persistent cough due to smoking or emphysema, or are presently taking a prescription drug for the treatment of high blood pressure or emotional disorders, without advice and supervision of a doctor. This product may cause drowsiness. Do not drive, operate machinery or drink alcoholic beverages while taking. Persistent cough may indicate a serious condition. Consult a doctor after 3 days if fever persists, or after 7 days if symptoms do not improve or cough persists, tends to recur or is accompanied by high fever, rash, or persistent headaches. Do not use if carton is opened, or if printed plastic overwrap or printed foil inner seal is broken. Keep this and all medication out of the reach of children. As with any drug, if you are pregnant or nursing a baby, seek the advice of a health professional before using this product. In case of accidental overdosage, contact a physician or poison control center immediately."

Continued on next page

McNeil Consumer—Cont.

Overdosage: Acetaminophen in massive overdosage may cause hepatic toxicity in some patients. In all cases of suspected overdose, immediately call your regional poison center or the Rocky Mountain Poison Center's toll-free number (800-525-6115) for assistance in diagnosis and for directions in the use of N-acetylcysteine as an antidote, a use currently restricted to investigational status. In adults, hepatic toxicity has rarely been reported with acute overdoses of less than 10 grams and fatalities with less than 15 grams. Importantly, young children seem to be more resistant than adults to the hepatotoxic effect of an acetaminophen overdose. Despite this, the measures outlined below should be initiated in any adult or child suspected of having ingested an acetaminophen overdose.

Early symptoms following a potentially hepatotoxic overdose may include: nausea, vomiting, diaphoresis and general malaise. Clinical and laboratory evidence of hepatic toxicity may not be apparent until 48 to 72 hours postingestion. The stomach should be emptied promptly by lavage or by induction of emesis with syrup of ipecac. Patients' estimates of the quantity of a drug ingested are notoriously unreliable. Therefore, if an acetaminophen overdose is suspected, a serum acetaminophen assay should be obtained as early as possible, but no sooner than four hours following ingestion. Liver function studies should be obtained initially and repeated at 24-hour intervals. The antidote, N-acetylcysteine, should be administered as early as possible, and within 16 hours of overdose ingestion for optimal results. Following recovery, there are no residual, structural or functional hepatic abnormalities.

Chlorpheniramine toxicity should be treated as you would an antihistamine/anticholinergic overdose and is likely to be present within a few hours after acute ingestion.

Symptoms from pseudoephedrine overdose consist most often of mild anxiety, tachycardia and/or mild hypertension. Symptoms usually appear within 4 to 8 hours of ingestion and are transient, usually requiring no treatment.

Acute dextromethorphan overdose usually does not result in serious signs and symptoms unless massive ammounts have be ingested. Signs and symptoms of a substantial overdose may include nausea and vomiting, visual disturbances, CNS disturbances, and urinary retention.

How Supplied: Cherry/mint mentholated flavored (colored amber) in 5 oz. bottles with child-resistant safety cap, special dosage cup graded in ounces and tablespoons, and tamper-resistant packaging.

CHILDREN'S CoTYLENOL®   OTC
Chewable Cold Tablets and Liquid Cold Formula

Description: Each Children's CoTYLENOL Chewable Cold Tablet contains acetaminophen 80 mg, chlorpheniramine maleate 0.5 mg and phenylpropanolamine hydrochloride 3.125 mg. Children's CoTYLENOL Liquid Cold Formula is stable, cherry-flavored, red in color and contains 8.5% alcohol. Each teaspoon (5 ml) contains acetaminophen 160 mg, chlorpheniramine maleate 1 mg, and phenylpropanolamine hydrochloride 6.25 mg.

Actions and Indications: Children's CoTYLENOL Chewable Cold Tablets and Liquid Cold Formula combine the nonsalicylate analgesic-antipyretic acetaminophen with the decongestant phenylpropanolamine hydrochloride and the antihistamine chlorpheniramine maleate to help relieve nasal congestion, dry runny noses and prevent sneezing as well as to relieve the fever, aches, pains and general discomfort associated with colds and upper respiratory infections.

While the acetaminophen component is equal to aspirin in analgesic and antipyretic effectiveness, it is unlikely to produce the following side effects often associated with aspirin or aspirin-containing products: allergic reactions, even in aspirin-sensitive children or those with a history of allergy in general; "therapeutic toxicity" in feverish children, since electrolyte imbalance and acid-base changes are not likely to occur; gastric irritation even in children with an already upset stomach.

Dosage: Children's CoTYLENOL Chewable Cold Tablets: 2–5 years—2 tablets, 6–11 years—4 tablets.
Children's CoTYLENOL Liquid Cold Formula: Measuring Cup is provided and marked for accurate dosing. 2–5 years—1 teaspoonful; 6–11 years—2 teaspoonsful.
Doses may be repeated every 4 hours as needed, not to exceed 5 doses in 24 hours.

Note: Since Children's CoTYLENOL Chewable Cold Tablets and Liquid Cold Formula are available without prescription, the following information appears on the package labels: "WARNING: Do not exceed the recommended dosage. Reduce dosage if nervousness, restlessness or sleeplessness occurs. Do not use if glaucoma, high blood pressure, heart disease, diabetes, or thyroid disease is present. This preparation may cause drowsiness, or in some instances, excitability. If presently taking a prescription drug for the treatment of high blood pressure or emotional disorders, or if you have asthma, do not use except under advice and supervision of a physician. Do not drive or operate machinery while taking this medication. If symptoms do not improve within seven days, or are accompanied by high fever or persistent cough, consult a physician before continuing use.

Do not use if carton is opened, or if printed plastic bottle wrap or printed foil inner seal is broken. Keep this and all medicine out of the reach of children. In case of accidental overdosage, contact a physician or poison control center immediately.

Overdosage: Acetaminophen in massive overdosage may cause hepatic toxicity in some patients. In all cases of suspected overdose, immediately call your regional poison center or the Rocky Mountain Poison Center's toll-free number (800-525-6115) for assistance in diagnosis and for directions in the use of N-acetylcysteine as an antidote, a use currently restricted to investigational status. The occurence of acetaminophen overdose toxicity is uncommon in the pediatric age group. Even with large overdoses, children appear to be less vulnerable than adults to developing hepatotoxicity. This may be due to age-related differences that have been demonstrated in the metabolism of acetaminophen. Despite these differences, the measures outlined below should be immediately initiated in any child suspected of having ingested an acetaminophen overdose.

Early symptoms following a potentially hepatotoxic overdose may include: nausea, vomiting, diaphoresis and general malaise. Clinical and laboratory evidence of hepatic toxicity may not be apparent until 48 to 72 hours post-ingestion. The stomach should be emptied promptly by lavage or by induction of emesis with syrup of ipecac. If an acute dose of 150 mg/kg body weight or greater was ingested, or if the dose cannot be accurately determined, a serum acetaminophen assay should be obtained as early as possible, but no sooner than four hours following ingestion. If in the toxic range, liver function studies should be obtained at 24-hour intervals. The antidote, N-acetylcysteine, should be administered as early as possible, and within 16 hours of the overdose ingestion for optimal results. Following recovery, there are no residual, structural or functional hepatic abnormalities.

Chlorpheniramine toxicity should be treated as you would an antihistamine/anticholinergic overdose and is likely to be present within a few hours after acute ingestion.

Phenylpropanolamine may produce central nervous system stimulation and sympathomimetic effects on the cardiovascular system which are likely to be manifested within a few hours following ingestion. Hypertension is the most likely manifestation.

How Supplied: Chewable Tablets (colored orange, scored, imprinted "CoTYLENOL")—bottles of 24. Cold Formula—bottles (colored red) of 4 fl. oz.
Shown in Product Identification Section, page 418

SINE-AID®   OTC
Sinus Headache Tablets

Description: Each SINE-AID® Tablet contains acetaminophen 325 mg and pseudoephedrine hydrochloride 30 mg.

Actions: SINE-AID® Tablets contain a clinically proven analgesic-antipyretic and a decongestant. Acetaminophen produces analgesia by elevation of the pain threshold and antipyresis through action on the hypothalamic heat-regulating center. Pseudoephedrine hydrochloride is a sympathomimetic amine which promotes sinus cavity drainage by reducing nasopharyngeal mucosal congestion.

Indications: SINE-AID® Tablets provide effective symptomatic relief from sinus headache pain and pressure caused by sinusitis.

Adverse Reactions: While the acetaminophen component is equal to aspirin in analgesic and antipyretic effectiveness, it is unlikely to produce many of the side effects associated with aspirin and aspirin-containing products. Since the product contains no antihistamine, SINE-AID® Tablets will not produce the drowsiness that may interfere with work, driving an automobile or operating dangerous machinery. SINE-AID® is particularly well-suited in patients with aspirin allergy, hemostatic disturbances (including anticoagulant therapy), and bleeding diatheses (e.g. hemophilia) and upper gastrointestinal disease (e.g. ulcer, gastritis, hiatus hernia). If a rare sensitivity occurs, the drug should be discontinued. Although pseudoephedrine is virtually without pressor effect in normotensive patients, it should be used with caution in hypertensives.

Usual Dosage: Adult dosage: Two tablets every four to six hours. Do not exceed eight tablets in any 24 hour period. **Note:** Since SINE-AID® tablets are available without a prescription, the following appears on the package labels: "WARNING: Do not exceed the recommended dosage or administer to children under 12. Reduce dosage if nervousness or sleeplessness occurs. If you have high blood pressure, heart disease, diabetes, or thyroid disease, or are presently taking a prescription drug for the treatment of high blood pressure or emotional disorders, do not take except under the advice and supervision of a physician. If symptoms persist for 7 days or are accompanied by high fever, consult a physician. **Do not use if carton is opened, or if printed foil inner seal is broken. Keep this and all medication out of the reach of children. As with any drug, if you are pregnant or nursing a baby, seek the advice of a health professional before using this product. In case of accidental overdosage, contact a physician or poison control center.**

Overdosage: Acetaminophen in massive overdosage may cause hepatic toxicity in some patients. In all cases of suspected overdose, immediately call your regional poison center or the Rocky Mountain Poison Center's toll-free number (800-525-6115) for assistance in diagnosis and for directions in the use of N-acetylcysteine as an antidote, a use currently restricted to investigational status. In adults, hepatic toxicity has rarely been reported with acute overdoses of less than 10 grams and fatalities with less than 15 grams. Importantly, young children seem to be more resistant than adults to the hepatotoxic effect of an acetaminophen overdose. Despite this, the measures outlined below should be initiated in any adult or child suspected of having ingested an acetaminophen overdose.

Early symptoms following a potentially hepatotoxic overdose may include: nausea, vomiting, diaphoresis and general malaise. Clinical and laboratory evidence of hepatic toxicity may not be apparent until 48 to 72 hours postingestion. The stomach should be emptied promptly by lavage or by induction of emesis with syrup of ipecac. Patients' estimates of the quantity of a drug ingested are notoriously unreliable. Therefore, if an acetaminophen overdose is suspected, a serum acetaminophen assay should be obtained as early as possible, but no sooner than four hours following ingestion. Liver function studies should be obtained initially and repeated at 24-hour intervals. The antidote, N-acetylcysteine, should be administered as early as possible, and within 16 hours of the overdose ingestion for optimal results. Following recovery, there are no residual structural or functional hepatic abnormalities.

Symptoms from pseudoephedrine overdose consist most often of mild anxiety, tachycardia and/or mild hypertension. Symptoms usually appear within 4 to 8 hours of ingestion and are transient, usually requiring no treatment.

How Supplied: Tablets (colored white, imprinted "SINE-AID®")—tamper-resistant bottles of 24, 50 and 100.

EXTRA STRENGTH SINE-AID®   OTC
Sinus Headache Capsules

Description: Each EXTRA STRENGTH SINE-AID® Capsule contains acetaminophen 500 mg and pseudoephedrine hydrochloride 30 mg.

Actions: EXTRA-STRENGTH SINE-AID® Capsules contain a clinically proven analgesic-antipyretic and a decongestant. Maximum allowable non-prescription levels of acetaminophen and pseudoephedrine provide temporary relief of sinus congestion and pain. Acetaminophen produces analgesia by elevation of the pain threshold and antipyresis through action on the hypothalamic heat-regulating center. Pseudoephedrine hydrochloride is a sympathomimetic amine which promotes sinus cavity drainage by reducing nasopharyngeal mucosal congestion.

Indications: EXTRA STRENGTH SINE-AID® Capsules provide effective symptomatic relief from sinus headache pain and pressure caused by sinusitis.

Adverse Reactions: While the acetaminophen component is equal to aspirin in analgesic and antipyretic effectiveness, it is unlikely to produce many of the side effects associated with aspirin and aspirin-containing products. Since the product contains no antihistamine, EXTRA-STRENGTH SINE-AID® Capsules will not produce the drowsiness that may interfere with work, driving an automobile or operating dangerous machinery. SINE-AID® is particularly well-suited in patients with aspirin allergy, hemostatic disturbances (including anticoagulant therapy), and bleeding diatheses (e.g. hemophilia) and upper gastrointestinal disease (e.g. ulcer, gastritis, hiatus hernia). If a rare sensitivity occurs, the drug should be discontinued. Although pseudoephedrine is virtually without pressor effect in normotensive patients, it should be used with caution in hypertensives.

Usual Dosage: Adult dosage: Two capsules every four to six hours. Do not exceed eight capsules in any 24 hour period. **Note:** Since EXTRA STRENGTH SINE-AID® Capsules are available without a prescription, the following appears on the package labels: "WARNING: Do not exceed the recommended dosage or administer to children under 12. Reduce dosage if nervousness or sleeplessness occurs. If you have high blood pressure, heart diease, diabetes, or thyroid disease or are presently taking a prescription drug for the treatment of high blood pressure or emotional disorders, do not take except under the advise and supervision of a physician. If symptoms persist for 7 days or are accompanied by high fever, consult a physician. **Do not use if carton is opened, or if printed red-neck wrap or printed foil inner seal is broken. Keep this and all medication out of the reach of children. As with any drug, if you are pregnant or nursing a baby, seek the advise of a health professional before using this product. In case of accidental overdosage, contact a physician or poison control center.**

Overdosage: Acetaminophen in massive overdosage may cause hepatic toxicity in some patients. In all cases of suspected overdose, immediately call your regional poison center or the Rocky Mountain Center's toll-free number (800-525-6115) for assistance in diagnosis and for directions in the use of N-acetylcysteine as an antidote, a use currently restricted to investigational status. In adults hepatic toxicity has rarely been reported with acute overdoses of less than 10 grams and fatalities with less than 15 grams. Importantly, young children seem to be more resistant than adults to the hepatotoxic effect of an acetaminophen overdose. Despite this, the measures outlined below should be initiated in any adult or child suspected of having ingested an acetaminophen overdose.

Early symptoms following a potentially hepatotoxic overdose may include: nausea, vomiting, diaphoresis and general malaise. Clinical and laboratory evidence of hepatic toxicity may not be apparent until 48 to 72 hours postingestion. The stomach should be emptied promptly by lavage or by induction of emesis with syrup of ipecac. Patients' estimates of the quantity of a drug ingested are notoriously unreliable. Therefore, if an acetaminophen overdose is suspected, a serum acetaminophen assay should be obtained as early as possible, but no sooner than four hours following ingestion. Liver function studies should be obtained initially and repeated at 24-hour intervals. The antidote, N-acetylcysteine, should be administered as early as possible, and within 16 hours of the overdose ingestion for optimal results. Following recovery, there are no residual structural or functional hepatic abnormalities.

Symptoms from pseudoephedrine overdose consist most often of mild anxiety, tachycardia and/or mild hypertension. Symptoms usually appear within 4 to 8 hours of ingestion and are transient, usually requiring no treatment.

How Supplied: Capsules (colored yellow and white imprinted "EXTRA STRENGTH SINE-AID®") - tamper-resistant bottles of 20.

CHILDREN'S TYLENOL®   OTC
acetaminophen
Chewable Tablets, Elixir, Drops

Description: Each Children's TYLENOL Chewable Tablet contains 80 mg. acetaminophen in a fruit flavored tablet. Children's TYLENOL acetaminophen Elixir is stable, cherry flavored, red in color and is alcohol free. Infants' TYLENOL Drops are stable, fruit flavored, orange in color and are alcohol free.

Children's TYLENOL Elixir: Each 5 ml. contains 160 mg. acetaminophen.

Infant's TYLENOL Drops: Each 0.8 ml. (one calibrated dropperful) contains 80 mg. acetaminophen.

Actions: TYLENOL acetaminophen is an effective antipyretic/analgesic. It produces antipyresis through action on the hypothalamic heat-regulating center and analgesia by elevation of the pain threshold.

Indications: Children's TYLENOL Chewable Tablets, Elixir and Drops are designed for treatment of infants and children with conditions requiring reduction of fever or relief of pain—such as mild upper respiratory infections (tonsillitis, common cold, "grippe"), headache, myalgia, post-immunization reactions, post-tonsillectomy discomfort and gastroenteritis. TYLENOL acetaminophen is useful as an analgesic and antipyretic in many bacterial or viral infections, such as bronchitis, pharyngitis, tracheobronchitis, sinusitis, pneumonia, otitis media, and cervical adenitis.

Precautions and Adverse Reactions: TYLENOL acetaminophen has rarely been found to produce any side effects. If a rare sensitivity reaction occurs, the drug should be stopped. It is usually well tolerated by aspirin-sensitive patients.

Usual Dosage: Doses may be repeated 4 or 5 times daily, but not to exceed 5 doses in 24 hours. Children's TYLENOL Chewable Tablets: 1-2 years: one and one half tablets. 2-3 years: two tablets. 4-5 years: three tablets. 6-8 years: four tablets. 9-10 years: five tablets. 11-12 years: six tablets.

Children's TYLENOL Elixir: (special cup for measuring dosage is provided) 4-11 months: one-half teaspoon. 12-23 months: three-quarters teaspoon, 2-3 years: one teaspoon. 4-5 years: one and one-half teaspoons. 6-8 years: 2 teaspoons. 9-10 years: two and one-half teaspoons. 11-12 years: three teaspoons.

Infants' TYLENOL Drops: 0-3 months: 0.4 ml. 4-11 months: 0.8 ml. 12-23 months: 1.2 ml. 2-3 years: 1.6 ml. 4-5 years: 2.4 ml.

Note: Since Children's TYLENOL acetaminophen Chewable Tablets, Elixir and Drops are available without prescription as an analgesic, the following appears on the package labels: "WARNING: Consult your physician if fever persists for more than three days or if pain continues for more than five days. **Do not use if safety seals are broken. Keep this and all medication out of the reach of children. In cases of accidental overdosage, contact a physician or poison control center immediately.**"

Overdosage: Acetaminophen in massive overdosage may cause hepatic toxicity in some patients. In all cases of suspected overdose, immediately call your regional poison center or the Rocky Mountain Poison Center's toll-free number (800-525-6115) for assistance in diagnosis and for directions in the use of N-acetylcysteine as an antidote, a use currently restricted to investigational status. The occurrence of acetaminophen overdose toxicity is uncommon in the pediatric age group. Even with large overdoses, children appear to be less vulnerable than adults to developing hepatotoxicity. This may be due to age-related differences that have been demonstrated in the metabolism of acetaminophen. Despite these differences, the measures outlined below should be immediately initiated in any child suspected of having ingested an overdose of acetaminophen.

Early symptoms following a potentially hepatotoxic overdose may include: nausea, vomiting, diaphoresis and general malaise. Clinical and laboratory evidence of hepatic toxicity may not be apparent until 48 to 72 hours post-ingestion. The stomach should be emptied promptly by lavage or by induction of emesis with syrup of ipecac. If an acute dose of 150 mg/kg body weight or greater was ingested, or if the dose cannot be accurately determined, a serum acetaminophen assay should be obtained as early as possible, but no sooner than four hours following ingestion. If in the toxic range, liver function studies should be obtained and repeated at 24-hour intervals. The antidote, N-acetylcysteine, should be administered as early as possible, and within 16 hours of the overdose ingestion for optimal results. Following recovery, there are no residual, structural or functional hepatic abnormalities.

How Supplied: Chewable Tablets (colored pink, scored, imprinted "TYLENOL")—Bottles of 30. Elixir (colored red)—bottles of 2 and 4 fl. oz. Drops (colored orange)—bottles of ½ oz. (15 ml.) with calibrated plastic dropper.

All packages listed above have child-resistant safety caps.

Shown in Product Identification Section, page 418

Regular Strength
TYLENOL® acetaminophen Tablets   OTC
and Capsules

Description: Each Regular Strength TYLENOL Tablet or Capsule contains acetaminophen 325 mg.

Actions: TYLENOL acetaminophen is a clinically proven analgesic and antipyretic. TYLENOL acetaminophen produces analgesia by elevation of the pain threshold and antipyresis through action on the hypothalamic heat-regulating center.

Indications: TYLENOL acetaminophen provides effective analgesia in a wide variety of arthritic and rheumatic conditions involving musculoskeletal pain, as well as in other painful disorders such as headache, dysmenorrhea, myalgias and neuralgias. In addition, TYLENOL acetaminophen is indicated as an analgesic and antipyretic in diseases accompanied by discomfort and fever, such as the common cold and other viral infections. TYLENOL acetaminophen is particularly well suited as an analgesic-antipyretic in the presence

Continued on next page

McNeil Consumer—Cont.

of aspirin allergy, hemostatic disturbances (including anticoagulant therapy), and bleeding diatheses (e.g., hemophilia) and upper gastrointestinal disease (e.g., ulcer, gastritis, hiatus hernia).

Precautions and Adverse Reactions: If a rare sensitivity reaction occurs, the drug should be stopped. TYLENOL acetaminophen has rarely been found to produce any side effects. It is usually well tolerated by aspirin-sensitive patients.

Usual Dosage: Adults: One to two tablets or capsules every 4–6 hours. Not to exceed 12 tablets or capsules per day. Children (6 to 12): One-half to one tablet 3 or 4 times daily. (TYLENOL acetaminophen Chewable Tablets, Elixir and Drops are available for greater convenience in younger patients).

Note: Since TYLENOL acetaminophen tablets and capsules are available without prescription as an analgesic, the following appears on the package labels: "Caution: If pain persists for more than 10 days, or redness is present, or in arthritic or rheumatic conditions affecting children under 12 years, consult a physician immediately." **WARNING: Do not use if printed red neck wrap or printed foil inner seal is broken. Keep this and all medications out of the reach of children. As with any drug, if you are pregnant or nursing a baby, seek the advice of a health professional before using this product. In case of accidental overdosage, contact a physician or poison control center immediately."**

Overdosage: Acetaminophen in massive overdosage may cause hepatic toxicity in some patients. In all cases of suspected overdose, immediately call your regional poison center or the Rocky Mountain Poison Center's toll-free number (800-525-6115) for assistance in diagnosis and for directions in the use of N-acetylcysteine as an antidote, a use currently restricted to investigational status. In adults, hepatic toxicity has rarely been reported with acute overdoses of less than 10 grams and fatalities with less than 15 grams. Importantly, young children seem to be more resistant than adults to the hepatotoxic effect of an acetaminophen overdose. Despite this, the measures outlined below should be initiated in any adult or child suspected of having ingested an acetaminophen overdose.

Early symptoms following a potentially hepatotoxic overdose may include: nausea, vomiting, diaphoresis and general malaise. Clinical and laboratory evidence of hepatic toxicity may not be apparent until 48 to 72 hours postingestion.

The stomach should be emptied promptly by lavage or by induction of emesis with syrup of ipecac. Patients' estimates of the quantity of a drug ingested are notoriously unreliable. Therefore, if an acetaminophen overdose is suspected, a serum acetaminophen assay should be obtained as early as possible, but no sooner than four hours following ingestion. Liver function studies should be obtained initially and repeated at 24-hour intervals. The antidote, N-acetylcysteine, should be administered as early as possible, and within 16 hours of the overdose ingestion for optimal results. Following recovery, there are no residual, structural or functional hepatic abnormalities.

How Supplied: Tablets (colored white, scored, imprinted "TYLENOL")—tins and vials of 12, and tamper-resistant bottles of 24, 50, 100 and 200. Capsules (colored gray and white, imprinted "TYLENOL 325 mg.")—tamper-resistant bottles of 24, 50 and 100.

Also Available: For additional pain relief, Extra-Strength TYLENOL® Tablets and Capsules, 500 mg, and Extra-Strength TYLENOL® Adult Liquid Pain Reliever (colored green; 1 fl. oz. = 1000 mg.).

Shown in Product Identification Section, page 418

Extra-Strength TYLENOL® acetaminophen OTC
Tablets, Capsules and Caplets

Description: Each Extra-Strength TYLENOL Tablet, Capsule or Caplet contains acetaminophen 500 mg.

Actions: TYLENOL acetaminophen is a clinically proven analgesic and antipyretic. Acetaminophen produces analgesia by elevation of the pain threshold and antipyresis through action on the hypothalamic heat-regulating center.

Indications: For relief of pain and fever. Extra-Strength TYLENOL acetaminophen Tablets and Capsules provide increased analgesic strength for minor conditions when the usual doses of mild analgesics are insufficient.

Precautions and Adverse Reactions: If a rare sensitivity reaction occurs, the drug should be stopped. TYLENOL acetaminophen has rarely been found to produce any side effects. It is usually well tolerated by aspirin-sensitive patients.

Usual Dosage: Adults: Two tablets or capsules 3 or 4 times daily. No more than a total of eight tablets or capsules in any 24-hour period.

Note: Since Extra-Strength TYLENOL acetaminophen Tablets or Capsules are available without a prescription, the following appears on the package labels: "Severe or recurrent pain or high or continued fever may be indicative of serious illness. Under these conditions, consult a physician. **WARNING: Do not use if printed red neck wrap or printed foil inner seal is broken. Keep this and all medication out of the reach of children. As with any drug, if you are pregnant or nursing a baby, seek the advice of a health professional before using this product. In case of accidental overdosage, contact a physician or poison control center immediately."**

Overdosage: Acetaminophen in massive overdosage may cause hepatic toxicity in some patients. In all cases of suspected overdose, immediately call your regional poison center or the Rocky Mountain Poison Center's toll-free number (800-525-6115) for assistance in diagnosis and for directions in the use of N-acetylcysteine as an antidote, a use currently restricted to investigational status. In adults, hepatic toxicity has rarely been reported with acute overdoses of less than 10 grams and fatalities with less than 15 grams. Importantly, young children seem to be more resistant than adults to the hepatotoxic effect of an acetaminophen overdose. Despite this, the measures outlined below should be initiated in any adult or child suspected of having ingested an acetaminophen overdose.

Early symptoms following a potentially hepatotoxic overdose may include: nausea, vomiting, diaphoresis and general malaise. Clinical and laboratory evidence of hepatic toxicity may not be apparent until 48 to 72 hours postingestion.

The stomach should be emptied promptly by lavage or by induction of emesis with syrup of ipecac. Patients' estimates of the quantity of a drug ingested are notoriously unreliable. Therefore, if an acetaminophen overdose is suspected, a serum acetaminophen assay should be obtained as early as possible, but no sooner than four hours following ingestion. Liver function studies should be obtained initially and repeated at 24-hour intervals. The antidote, N-acetylcysteine, should be administered as early as possible, and within 16 hours of the overdose ingestion for optimal results. Following recovery, there are no residual, structural or functional hepatic abnormalities.

How Supplied: Tablets (colored white, imprinted "TYLENOL" and "500")—vials of 10 and tamper-resistant bottles of 30, 60, 100, and 200; Capsules (colored red and white, imprinted "TYLENOL 500 mg.")—vial of 8, tamper-resistant bottles of 24, 50, 100 and 165.

Also Available: For adults who prefer liquids or can't swallow solid medication, Extra-Strength TYLENOL® Adult Liquid Pain Reliever (colored green; 1 fl. oz. = 1000 mg.).

Shown in Product Identification Section, page 418

Extra-Strength TYLENOL® acetaminophen OTC
Adult Liquid Pain Reliever

Description: Each 15 ml. (½ fl. oz. or one tablespoonful) contains 500 mg. acetaminophen (alcohol 8 ½%).

Actions: TYLENOL acetaminophen is a clinically proven analgesic and antipyretic. Acetaminophen produces analgesia by elevation of the pain threshold and antipyresis through action on the hypothalamic heat-regulating center.

Indications: TYLENOL acetaminophen provides fast, effective relief of pain and/or fever for adults who prefer liquids or can't swallow solid medication, e.g., the aged, patients with easily triggered gag reflexes, extremely sore throats, or those on liquid diets.

Precautions and Adverse Reactions: If a rare sensitivity reaction occurs, the drug should be stopped. TYLENOL acetaminophen has rarely been found to produce any side effects. It is usually well tolerated by aspirin-sensitive patients.

Usual Dosage: Extra-Strength TYLENOL Adult Liquid Pain Reliever is an adult preparation. Not for use in children under 12. Measuring cup is marked for accurate dosage. Extra-Strength Dose—1 fl. oz. (30 ml or 2 tablespoonsful, 1000 mg), which is equivalent to two 500 mg Extra-Strength TYLENOL Tablets, Capsules or Caplets. Take every 4–6 hours, no more than 4 doses in any 24-hour period.

Note: Since Extra-Strength TYLENOL Adult Liquid Pain Reliever is available without a prescription, the following appears on the package labels: "Severe or recurrent pain or high or continued fever may be indicative of serious illness. Under these conditions, consult a physician. **WARNING: Do not use if printed plastic overwrap or printed foil inner seal is broken. Keep this and all medication out of the reach of children. As with any drug, if you are pregnant or nursing a baby, seek the advice of a health professional before using this product. In case of accidental overdosage, contact a physician or poison control center immediately."**

Overdosage: Acetaminophen in massive overdosage may cause hepatic toxicity in some patients. In all cases of suspected overdose, immediately call your regional poison center or the Rocky Mountain Poison Center's toll-free number (800-525-6115) for assistance in diagnosis and for directions in the use of N-acetylcysteine as an antidote, a use currently restricted to investigational status. In adults, hepatic toxicity has rarely been reported with acute overdoses of less than 10 grams and fatalitites with less than 15 grams. Importantly, young children seem to be more resistant than adults to the hepatotoxic effect of an acetaminophen overdose. Despite this, the measures outlined below should be initiated in any adult or child suspected of having ingested an acetaminophen overdose.

Early symptoms following a potentially hepatotoxic overdose may include: nausea, vomiting, diaphoresis and general malaise. Clinical and laboratory evidence of hepatic toxicity may not be apparent until 48 to 72 hours post-ingestion.

The stomach should be emptied promptly by lavage or by induction of emesis with syrup of ipecac. Patients' estimates of the quantity of a drug ingested are notoriously unreliable. Therefore, if an acetaminophen overdose is suspected, a serum acetaminophen assay should be obtained as early as possible, but no sooner than four hours following ingestion. Liver function studies should be obtained initially and repeated at 24-hour intervals.

The antidote, N-acetylcysteine, should be administered as early as possible, and within 16 hours of the overdose ingestion for optimal results. Following recovery, there are no residual, structural or functional hepatic abnormalities.

How Supplied: Mint-flavored liquid (colored green), 8 fl. oz. tamper-resistant bottle with child resistant safety cap and special dosage cup.

Maximum-Strength TYLENOL® Sinus Medication OTC
Tablets and Capsules

Description: Each Maximum-Strength TYLENOL® Sinus Medication tablet or capsule contains acetaminophen 500 mg and pseudoephedrine hydrochloride 30 mg.

Actions: TYLENOL Sinus Medication contains a clinically proven analgesic-antipyretic and a decongestant. Maximum allowable non-prescription levels of acetaminophen and pseudoephedrine provide temporary relief of sinus congestion and pain.

TYLENOL® Acetaminophen produces analgesia by elevation of the pain threshold and antipyresis through action on the hypothalamic heat-regulating center. Pseudoephedrine hydrochloride is a sympathomimetic amine which promotes sinus cavity drainage by reducing nasopharyngeal mucosal congestion.

Indications: Maximum-Strength TYLENOL Sinus Medication provides effective symptomatic relief from sinus headache pain and pressure caused by sinusitis.

Adverse Reactions: While Maximum-Strength TYLENOL Sinus Medication's acetaminophen component is equal to aspirin in analgesic and antipyretic effectiveness, it is unlikely to produce many of the side effects associated with aspirin and aspirin-containing products. Since it contains no antihistamine, TYLENOL Sinus Medication will not produce the drowsiness that may interfere with work, driving an automobile or operating dangerous machinery. Maximim-Strength TYLENOL Sinus Medication is particularly well-suited in patients with aspirin allergy, hemostatic disturbances (including anticoagulant therapy), and bleeding diatheses (e.g. hemophilia) and upper gastrointestinal disease (e.g. ulcer, gastritis, hiatus hernia). If a rare sensitivity occurs, the drug should be discontinued. Although pseudoephedrine is virtually without pressor effect in normotensive patients, it should be used with caution in hypertensives.

Usual Dosage: Adult dosage: Two tablets or capsules every four to six hours. Do not exceed eight tablets or capsules in any 24 hour period.
Note: Since TYLENOL Sinus Medication tablets and capsules are available without a prescription, the following appears on the package labels: "WARNING: Do not exceed the recommended dosage or administer to children under 12. Reduce dosage if nervousness, or sleeplessness occurs. If you have high blood pressure, heart disease, diabetes, or thyroid disease, or are presently taking a prescription drug for the treatment of high blood pressure or emotional disorders, do not take except under the advice and supervision of a physician. If symptoms persist for 7 days or are accompanied by high fever, consult a physician." **Do not use tablets if carton is opened or if printed foil inner seal is broken. Do not use capsules if carton is opened or if printed green neck wrap or printed foil inner seal is broken. Keep this and all medication out of the reach of children. As with any drug, if you are pregnant or nursing a baby, seek the advice of a health professional before using this product. In case of accidental overdosage, contact a physician or poison control center.**

Overdosage: Acetaminophen in massive overdosage may cause hepatic toxicity in some patients. In all cases of suspected overdose, immediately call your regional poison center or the Rocky Mountain Center's toll-free number (800-525-6115) for assistance in diagnosis and for directions in the use of N-acetylcysteine as an antidote, a use currently restricted to investigational status. In adults hepatic toxicity has rarely been reported with acute overdoses of less than 10 grams and fatalities with less than 15 grams. Importantly, young children seem to be more resistant than adults to the hepatotoxic effect of an acetaminophen overdose. Despite this, the measures outlined below should be initiated in any adult or child suspected of having ingested an acetaminophen overdose.

Early symptoms following a potentially hepatotoxic overdose may include: nausea, vomiting, diaphoresis and general malaise. Clinical and laboratory evidence of hepatic toxicity may not be apparent until 48 to 72 hours postingestion.
The stomach should be emptied promptly by lavage or by induction of emesis with syrup of ipecac. Patients' estimates of the quantity of a drug ingested are notoriously unreliable. Therefore, if an acetaminophen overdose is suspected, a serum acetaminophen assay should be obtained as early as possible, but no sooner than four hours following ingestion. Liver function studies should be obtained initially and repeated at 24-hour intervals. The antidote, N-acetylcysteine, should be administered as early as possible, and within 16 hours of the overdose ingestion for optimal results. Following recovery, there are no residual structuring. Symptoms from pseudoephedrine overdose consist most often of mild anxiety, tachycardia and/or mild hypertension. Symptoms usually appear within 4 to 8 hours of ingestion and are transient, usually requiring no treatment.

How Supplied: Tablets (colored light green, imprinted "Maximum-Strength TYLENOL Sinus")—tamper-resistant bottles of 24 and 50. Capsules (colored green and white, imprinted "Maximum-Strength TYLENOL Sinus")—tamper-resistant bottles of 20 and 40.

Shown in Product Identification Section, page 418

McNeil Pharmaceutical
McNEILAB, INC.
SPRING HOUSE, PA 19477

HALDOL® brand of haloperidol ℞
[hal-dole']
tablets, concentrate, injection
1 mg (1000's):
Military NSN 6505-01-003-2415
VA NSN 6505-01-003-2415A
2 mg (1000's):
Military NSN 6505-00-876-7239
VA NSN 6505-00-876-7239A
5 mg (1000's):
Military NSN 6505-01-003-2416
VA NSN 6505-01-003-2416A
10 mg (1000's):
Military NSN 6505-01-003-2417
VA NSN 6505-01-003-2417A
Concentrate 120 ml:
Military NSN 6505-01-003-5341
VA NSN 6505-01-003-5341A
Injection 1 ml:
VA NSN 6505-00-268-8530A

Description: Haloperidol is the first of the butyrophenone series of major tranquilizers. The chemical designation is 4-[4-(p-chlorophenyl)-4-hydroxypiperidino] -4'-fluorobutyrophenone.
HALDOL haloperidol dosage forms include: tablets (½, 1*, 2, 5*, 10* mg and 20 mg); a concentrate with 2 mg per ml haloperidol (as the lactate); and a sterile parenteral form for intramuscular injection. The injection provides 5 mg haloperidol (as the lactate) with 1.8 mg methylparaben and 0.2 mg propylparaben per ml, and lactic acid for pH adjustment between 3.0–3.6.
* Contains FD&C Yellow No. 5 (see Precautions)
Actions: The precise mechanism of action has not been clearly established.
Indications: HALDOL haloperidol is indicated for use in the management of manifestations of psychotic disorders.
HALDOL is indicated for the control of tics and vocal utterances of Tourette's disorder in children and adults.
HALDOL is effective for the treatment of severe behavior problems in children of combative, explosive hyperexcitability (which cannot be accounted for by immediate provocation).
HALDOL is effective in the short-term treatment of hyperactive children who show excessive motor activity with accompanying conduct disorders consisting of some or all of the following symptoms: impulsivity, difficulty sustaining attention, aggressivity, mood lability, and poor frustration tolerance.

Contraindications: HALDOL haloperidol is contraindicated in severe toxic central nervous system depression or comatose states from any cause and in individuals who are hypersensitive to this drug or have Parkinson's disease.

Warnings: *Usage in Pregnancy:* Rodents given 2 to 20 times the usual maximum human dose of haloperidol by oral or parenteral routes showed an increase in incidence of resorption, reduced fertility, delayed delivery and pup mortality. No teratogenic effect has been reported in rats, rabbits or dogs at dosages within this range, but cleft palate has been observed in mice given 15 times the usual maximum human dose. Cleft palate in mice appears to be a non-specific response to stress or nutritional imbalance as well as to a variety of drugs, and there is no evidence to relate this phenomenon to predictable human risk for most of these agents. There are no well controlled studies with HALDOL haloperidol in pregnant women. There are reports, however, of two cases of limb malformations observed following maternal use of HALDOL along with other drugs which have suspected teratogenic potential during the first trimester of pregnancy. Causal relationships were not established in either case. Since such experience does not exclude the possibility of fetal damage due to HALDOL, this drug should be used during pregnancy or in women likely to become pregnant only if the benefit clearly justifies a potential risk to the fetus. Infants should not be nursed during drug treatment.

Combined Use of HALDOL and Lithium: An encephalopathic syndrome (characterized by weakness, lethargy, fever, tremulousness and confusion, extrapyramidal symptoms, leukocytosis, elevated serum enzymes, BUN, and FBS) followed by irreversible brain damage has occurred in a few patients treated with lithium plus HALDOL. A causal relationship between these events and the concomitant administration of lithium and HALDOL has not been established; however, patients receiving such combined therapy should be monitored closely for early evidence of neurological toxicity and treatment discontinued promptly if such signs appear.

General: A number of cases of bronchopneumonia, some fatal, have followed the use of major tranquilizers, including HALDOL. It has been postulated that lethargy and decreased sensation of thirst due to central inhibition may lead to dehydration, hemoconcentration and reduced pulmonary ventilation. Therefore, if the above signs and symptoms appear, especially in the elderly, the physician should institute remedial therapy promptly.
Although not reported with HALDOL, decreased serum cholesterol and/or cutaneous and ocular changes have been reported in patients receiving chemically-related drugs.

HALDOL may impair the mental and/or physical abilities required for the performance of hazardous tasks such as operating machinery or driving a motor vehicle. The ambulatory patient should be warned accordingly.
The use of alcohol with this drug should be avoided due to possible additive effects and hypotension.

Precautions: HALDOL haloperidol should be administered cautiously to patients:
—with severe cardiovascular disorders, because of the possibility of transient hypotension and/or precipitation of anginal pain. Should hypotension occur and a vasopressor be required, epinephrine should not be used since HALDOL may block its vasopressor activity and paradoxical further lowering of the blood pressure may occur.
—receiving anticonvulsant medication, because HALDOL may lower the convulsive threshold. Adequate anticonvulsant therapy should be maintained concomitantly.
—with known allergies, or with a history of allergic reactions to drugs.

Continued on next page

McNeil Pharm.—Cont.

—receiving anticoagulants, since an isolated instance of interference occurred with the effects of one anticoagulant (phenindione).

If concomitant antiparkinson medication is required, it may have to be continued after HALDOL is discontinued because of the difference in excretion rates. If both are discontinued simultaneously, extrapyramidal symptoms may occur. The physician should keep in mind the possible increase in intraocular pressure when anticholinergic drugs, including antiparkinson agents, are administered concomitantly with HALDOL.

When HALDOL is used to control mania in cyclic disorders, there may be a rapid mood swing to depression.

Severe neurotoxicity (rigidity, inability to walk or talk) may occur in patients with thyrotoxicosis who are also receiving antipsychotic medication, including HALDOL.

Neuroleptic drugs elevate prolactin levels; the elevation persists during chronic administration. Tissue culture experiments indicate that approximately one-third of human breast cancers are prolactin dependent *in vitro*, a factor of potential importance if the prescription of these drugs is contemplated in a patient with a previously detected breast cancer. Although disturbances such as galactorrhea, amenorrhea, gynecomastia, and impotence have been reported, the clinical significance of elevated serum prolactin levels is unknown for most patients. An increase in mammary neoplasms has been found in rodents after chronic administration of neuroleptic drugs. Neither clinical studies nor epidemiologic studies conducted to date, however, have shown an association between chronic administration of these drugs and mammary tumorigenesis: the available evidence is considered too limited to be conclusive at this time.

FD&C Yellow No. 5 (tartrazine) may cause allergic-type reactions (including bronchial asthma) in certain susceptible individuals. Although the overall incidence of FD&C Yellow No. 5 (tartrazine) sensitivity in the general population is low, it is frequently seen in patients who also have aspirin hypersensitivity.

Adverse Reactions: *CNS Effects: Extrapyramidal Reactions*—Neuromuscular (extrapyramidal) reactions during the administration of HALDOL haloperidol have been reported frequently, often during the first few days of treatment. In most patients, these reactions involved Parkinson-like symptoms which, when first observed, were usually mild to moderately severe and usually reversible. Other types of neuromuscular reactions (motor restlessness, dystonia, akathisia, hyperreflexia, opisthotonos, oculogyric crises) have been reported far less frequently, but were often more severe. Severe extrapyramidal reactions have been reported to occur at relatively low doses. Generally the occurrence and severity of most extrapyramidal symptoms are dose related since they occur at relatively high doses and have been shown to disappear or become less severe when the dose is reduced. Administration of antiparkinson drugs such as benztropine mesylate U.S.P. or trihexyphenidyl hydrochloride U.S.P. may be required for control of such reactions. It should be noted that persistent extrapyramidal reactions have been reported and that the drug may have to be discontinued in such cases.

Withdrawal Emergent Neurological Signs— Generally, patients receiving short term therapy experience no problems with abrupt discontinuation of antipsychotic drugs. However, some patients on maintenance treatment experience transient dyskinetic signs after abrupt withdrawal. In certain of these cases the dyskinetic movements are indistinguishable from the syndrome described below under "Persistent Tardive Dyskinesia" except for duration. It is not known whether gradual withdrawal of antipsychotic drugs will reduce the rate of occurrence of withdrawal emergent neurological signs but until further evidence becomes available, it seems reasonable to gradually withdraw use of HALDOL.

Persistent Tardive Dyskinesia—As with all antipsychotic agents HALDOL has been associated with persistent dyskinesias. Tardive dyskinesia may appear in some patients on long-term therapy or may occur after drug therapy has been discontinued. The risk appears to be greater in elderly patients on high-dose therapy, especially females. The symptoms are persistent and in some patients appear irreversible. The syndrome is characterized by rhythmical involuntary movements of tongue, face, mouth or jaw (e.g., protrusion of tongue, puffing of cheeks, puckering of mouth, chewing movements). Sometimes these may be accompanied by involuntary movements of extremities.

There is no known effective treatment for tardive dyskinesia; antiparkinson agents usually do not alleviate the symptoms of this syndrome. It is suggested that all antipsychotic agents be discontinued if these symptoms appear. Should it be necessary to reinstitute treatment, or increase the dosage of the agent, or switch to a different antipsychotic agent, this syndrome may be masked.

It has been reported that fine vermicular movement of the tongue may be an early sign of the syndrome and if the medication is stopped at that time the syndrome may not develop.

Other CNS Effects—Insomnia, restlessness, anxiety, euphoria, agitation, drowsiness, depression, lethargy, headache, confusion, vertigo, grand mal seizures, exacerbation of psychotic symptoms including hallucinations and catatonic-like behavioral states which may be responsive to drug withdrawal and/or treatment with anticholinergic drugs.

Body as a Whole: As with other neuroleptic drugs, hyperpyrexia has been reported, sometimes alone and sometimes in association with muscle rigidity, elevated CPK or myoglobinuria (rhabdomyolysis), evidence of autonomic instability (irregular pulse or blood pressure) and/or acute renal failure. This symptom complex is sometimes referred to as neuroleptic malignant syndrome.

Cardiovascular Effects: Tachycardia, hypotension, hypertension and ECG changes.

Hematologic Effects: Reports have appeared citing the occurrence of mild and usually transient leukopenia and leukocytosis, minimal decreases in red blood cell counts, anemia, or a tendency toward lymphomonocytosis. Agranulocytosis has rarely been reported to have occurred with the use of HALDOL and then only in association with other medication.

Liver Effects: Impaired liver function and/or jaundice have been reported.

Dermatologic Reactions: Maculopapular and acneiform skin reactions and isolated cases of photosensitivity and loss of hair.

Endocrine Disorders: Lactation, breast engorgement, mastalgia, menstrual irregularities, gynecomastia, impotence, increased libido, hyperglycemia, hypoglycemia and hyponatremia.

Gastrointestinal Effects: Anorexia, constipation, diarrhea, hypersalivation, dyspepsia, nausea and vomiting.

Autonomic Reactions: Dry mouth, blurred vision, urinary retention and diaphoresis.

Respiratory Effects: Laryngospasm, bronchospasm and increased depth of respiration.

Other: Cases of sudden and unexpected death have been reported in association with the administration of HALDOL. The nature of the evidence makes it impossible to determine definitively what role, if any, HALDOL played in the outcome of the reported cases. The possibility that HALDOL caused death cannot, of course, be excluded, but it is to be kept in mind that sudden and unexpected death may occur in psychotic patients when they go untreated or when they are treated with other neuroleptic drugs.

Overdosage: *Manifestations:* In general, the symptoms of overdosage would be an exaggeration of known pharmacologic effects and adverse reactions, the most prominent of which would be: 1) severe extrapyramidal reactions, 2) hypotension, or 3) sedation. The patient would appear comatose with respiratory depression and hypotension which could be severe enough to produce a shock-like state. The extrapyramidal reaction would be manifest by muscular weakness or rigidity and a generalized or localized tremor as demonstrated by the akinetic or agitans types respectively. With accidental overdosage, hypertension rather than hypotension occurred in a two-year old child.

Treatment: Gastric lavage or induction of emesis should be carried out immediately followed by administration of activated charcoal. Since there is no specific antidote, treatment is primarily supportive. A patent airway must be established by use of an oropharyngeal airway or endotracheal tube or, in prolonged cases of coma, by tracheostomy. Respiratory depression may be counteracted by artificial respiration and mechanical respirators. Hypotension and circulatory collapse may be counteracted by use of intravenous fluids, plasma, or concentrated albumin, and vasopressor agents such as norepinephrine. Epinephrine should not be used. In case of severe extrapyramidal reactions, antiparkinson medication should be administered.

Dosage and Administration: There is considerable variation from patient to patient in the amount of medication required for treatment. As with all neuroleptic drugs, dosage should be individualized according to the needs and response of each patient. Dosage adjustments, either upward or downward, should be carried out as rapidly as practicable to achieve optimum therapeutic control.

To determine the initial dosage, consideration should be given to the patient's age, severity of illness, previous response to other neuroleptic drugs, and any concomitant medication or disease state. Children, debilitated or geriatric patients, as well as those with a history of adverse reactions to neuroleptic drugs may require less HALDOL haloperidol. The optimal response in such patients is usually obtained with more gradual dosage adjustments and at lower dosage levels, as recommended below.

Clinical experience suggests the following recommendations:

Oral Administration
Initial Dosage Range
Adults

Moderate Symptomatology	0.5 mg to 2.0 mg b.i.d. or t.i.d.
Severe Symptomatology	3.0 mg to 5.0 mg b.i.d. or t.i.d.
To achieve prompt control, higher doses may be required in some cases.	
Geriatric or Debilitated Patients	0.5 mg to 2.0 mg b.i.d. or t.i.d.
Chronic or Resistant Patients	3.0 mg to 5.0 mg b.i.d. or t.i.d.

Patients who remain severely disturbed or inadequately controlled may require dosage adjustment. Daily dosages up to 100 mg may be necessary in some cases to achieve an optimal response. Infrequently, HALDOL has been used in doses above 100 mg for severely resistant patients; however, the limited clinical usage has not demonstrated the safety of prolonged administration of such doses.

Children
The following recommendations apply to children between the ages of 3 and 12 years (weight range 15 to 40 kg). HALDOL is not intended for children under 3 years old. Therapy should begin at the lowest dose possible (0.5 mg per day). If required, the dose should be increased by an increment of 0.5 mg at 5 to 7 day intervals until the desired therapeutic effect is obtained. (See chart next page)

The total dose may be divided, to be given b.i.d. or t.i.d.

Psychotic Disorders
0.05 mg/kg/day to 0.15 mg/kg/day

Non-Psychotic Behavior
0.05 mg/kg/day to 0.075 mg/kg/day
Disorders and Tourette's Disorder

Severely disturbed psychotic children may require higher doses. In severely disturbed, non-psychotic children or in hyperactive children with accompanying conduct disorders, it should be noted that since these behaviors may be short-lived, short-term administration of HALDOL may suffice. There is no evidence establishing a maximum effective dosage. There is little evidence that behavior improvement is further enhanced in dosages beyond 6 mg per day.

Maintenance Dosage
Upon achieving a satisfactory therapeutic response, dosage should then be gradually reduced to the lowest effective maintenance level.

Intramuscular Administration
Adults
Parenteral medication, administered intramuscularly in doses of 2 to 5 mg, is utilized for prompt control of the acutely agitated patient with moderately severe to very severe symptoms. Depending on the response of the patient, subsequent doses may be given, administered as often as every hour, although 4 to 8 hour intervals may be satisfactory. Controlled trials to establish the safety and effectiveness of intramuscular administration in children have not been conducted.

Switchover Procedure
The oral form should supplant the injectable as soon as practicable. In the absence of bioavailability studies establishing bioequivalence between these two dosage forms the following guidelines for dosage are suggested. For an initial approximation of the total daily dose required, the parenteral dose administered in the preceeding 24 hours may be used. Since this dose is only an initial estimate, it is recommended that careful monitoring of clinical signs and symptoms, including clinical efficacy, sedation, and adverse effects, be carried out periodically for the first several days following the initiation of switchover. In this way, dosage adjustments, either upward or downward, can be quickly accomplished. Depending on the patient's clinical status, the first oral dose should be given within 12-24 hours following the last parenteral dose.
[See table below].

HALDOL® brand of haloperidol Concentrate 2 mg per ml (as the lactate) Colorless, Odorless, and Tasteless Solution—NDC 0045-0250-15, bottles of 15 ml and NDC 0045-0250-04, bottles of 120 ml.
HALDOL® brand of haloperidol Injection 5 mg per ml (as the lactate)—**NDC 0045-0255-01**, units of 10 × 1 ml ampuls; **NDC 0045-0255-49**, 10 ml multiple-dose vial; **NDC 0045-0255-31** units of 10 × 1 ml disposable Pre-filled Syringe.
Dispense HALDOL haloperidol tablets and concentrate in a tight, light-resistant container as defined in the official compendium.

8/30/84
Shown in Product Identification Section, page 418

ORAP®
[or'ap]
(pimozide)
Tablets

Description: ORAP (pimozide) is an orally active neuroleptic agent of the diphenyl-butylpiperidine series. The structural formula of pimozide, 1-(1-(4,4- bis(4-fluorophenyl)-butyl)-4-piperidinyl)-1,3-dihydro-2H-benzimidazol-2-one is:

The solubility of pimozide in water is less than 0.01 mg/ml; it is slightly soluble in most organic solvents.
Each white ORAP tablet contains 2 mg of pimozide.

Clinical Pharmacology:
Pharmacodynamic Actions: ORAP (pimozide) is an orally active neuroleptic drug product which shares with other neuroleptics the ability to blockade dopaminergic receptors on neurons in the central nervous system. Although its exact mode of action has not been established, the ability of pimozide to suppress motor and phonic tics in Tourette's Disorder is thought to be a function of its dopaminergic blocking activity. However, receptor blockade is often accompanied by a series of secondary alterations in central dopamine metabolism and function which may contribute to both pimozide's therapeutic and untoward effects. In addition, pimozide, in common with other neuroleptic drugs, has various effects on other central nervous system receptor systems which are not fully characterized.

Metabolism and Pharmacokinetics: More than 50% of a dose of pimozide is absorbed after oral administration. Based on the pharmacokinetic and metabolic profile, pimozide appears to undergo significant first pass metabolism. Peak serum levels occur generally six to eight hours (range 4–12 hours) after dosing. Pimozide is extensively metabolized, primarily by N-dealkylation in the liver. Two major metabolites have been identified, 1-(4-piperidyl)-2-benzimidazolinone and 4,4-bis(4-fluorophenyl) butyric acid. The neuroleptic activity of these metabolites is undetermined. The major route of elimination of pimozide and its metabolites is through the kidney.
The mean serum elimination half-life of pimozide in schizophrenic patients was approximately 55 hours. There was a 13-fold interindividual difference in the area under the serum pimozide level-time curve and an equivalent degree of variation in peak serum levels among patients studied. The significance of this is unclear since there are few correlations between plasma levels and clinical findings.
Effects of food, disease or concomitant medication upon the absorption, distribution, metabolism and elimination of pimozide are not known.

Indications and Usage: ORAP (pimozide) is indicated for the suppression of motor and phonic tics in patients with Tourette's Disorder who have failed to respond satisfactorily to standard treatment. ORAP is not intended as a treatment of first choice nor is it intended for the treatment for tics that are merely annoying or cosmetically troublesome. ORAP should be reserved for use in Tourette's Disorder patients whose development and/or daily life function is severely compromised by the presence of motor and phonic tics.
Evidence supporting approval of pimozide for use in Tourette's Disorder was obtained in two controlled clinical investigations which enrolled patients between the ages of 8 and 53 years. Most subjects in the two trials were 12 or older.

Contraindications:
1. ORAP (pimozide) is contraindicated in the treatment of simple tics or tics other than those associated with Tourette's Disorder.
2. ORAP should not be used in patients taking drugs that may, themselves, cause motor and phonic tics (e.g., pemoline, methylphenidate and amphetamines) until such patients have been withdrawn from these drugs to determine whether or not the drugs, rather than Tourette's Disorder, are responsible for the tics.
3. Because ORAP prolongs the QT interval of the electrocardiogram it is contraindicated in patients with congenital long QT syndrome, patients with a history of cardiac arrhythmias, or patients taking other drugs which prolong the QT interval of the electrocardiogram (see DRUG INTERACTIONS).
4. ORAP is contraindicated in patients with severe toxic central nervous system depression or comatose states from any cause.
5. ORAP is contraindicated in patients with hypersensitivity to it. As it is not known whether cross-sensitivity exists among the neuroleptics, pimozide should be used with appropriate caution in patients who have demonstrated hypersensitivity to other neuroleptic drugs.

Warnings: The use of ORAP (pimozide) in the treatment of Tourette's Disorder involves different risk/benefit considerations than when neuroleptic drugs are used to treat other conditions. Consequently, a decision to use ORAP should take into consideration the following (see also PRECAUTIONS—Information for Patients).

Tardive Dyskinesia: A syndrome of potentially irreversible, involuntary movement develops over time in some of the patients treated with neuroleptic drugs. The likelihood of developing the movements and the associated likelihood of their proving irreversible is believed to increase with chronicity of treatment and the total cumulative dose of neuroleptic administered. See ADVERSE REACTIONS section for a description of the syndrome and additional details.

Other: Sudden, unexpected deaths have occurred in experimental studies of conditions other than Tourette's Disorder. These deaths occurred while patients were receiving dosages in the range of 1 mg per kg. One possible mechanism for such deaths is prolongation of the QT interval predisposing patients to ventricular arrhythmia. An electrocardiogram should be performed before ORAP treatment is initiated and periodically thereafter, especially during the period of dose adjustment.
ORAP may have a tumorigenic potential. Based on studies conducted in mice, it is known that pimozide can produce a dose related increase in pituitary tumors. The full significance of this finding is not known, but should be taken into consideration in the physician's and patient's decisions to use this drug product. This finding should be given special consideration when the patient is young and chronic use of pimozide is anticipated. (see PRECAUTIIONS—Carcinogenesis, Mutagenesis. Impairment of Fertility).

Precautions:
General: ORAP (pimozide) may impair the mental and/or physical abilities required for the performance of potentially hazardous tasks, such as driving a car or operating machinery, especially during the first few days of therapy.

Continued on next page

How Supplied: HALDOL* brand of haloperidol Tablets Scored, Imprinted "McNEIL" and "HALDOL"

		Bottles containing 100	1000	Unit Dose Blister Pack 10 × 10
1/2mg white	NDC 0045-0240	x	x	x
1mg yellow	NDC 0045-0241	x	x	x
2mg pink	NDC 0045-0242	x	x	x
5mg green	NDC 0045-0245	x	x	x
10mg aqua	NDC 0045-0246	x	x	x
20mg salmon	NDC 0045-0248	x		x

McNeil Pharm.—Cont.

ORAP produces anticholinergic side effects and should be used with caution in individuals whose conditions may be aggravated by anticholinergic activity.

ORAP should be administered cautiously to patients with impairment of liver or kidney function, because it is metabolized by the liver and excreted by the kidneys.

Neuroleptics should be administered with caution to patients receiving anticonvulsant medication, because they may lower the convulsive threshold. Adequate anticonvulsant therapy should be maintained concomitantly.

Information for Patients: Treatment with ORAP exposes the patient to serious risks. A decision to use ORAP chronically in Tourette's Disorder is one that deserves full consideration by the patient (or patient's family) as well as by the treating physician. Because the goal of treatment is symptomatic improvement, the patient's view of the need for treatment and assessment of response are critical in evaluating the impact of therapy and weighing its benefits against the risks. Since the physician is the primary source of information about the use of a drug in any disease, it is recommended that the following information be discussed with patients and/or their families.

ORAP is intended only for use in patients with Tourette's Disorder whose symptoms are severe and who cannot tolerate, or who do not respond to HALDOL® (haloperidol).

Given the likelihood that a proportion of patients exposed chronically to neuroleptics will develop tardive dyskinesia, it is advised that all patients in whom chronic use is contemplated be given, if possible, full information about this risk. The decision to inform patients and/or their guardians must obviously take into account the clinical circumstances and the competency of the patient to understand the information provided.

There is *very* little information available on the use of ORAP in children under 12 years of age.

The information available on ORAP from foreign marketing experience and from U.S. clinical trials indicate that ORAP has a side effect profile similar to that of other neuroleptic drugs. Patients should be informed that all types of side effects associated with the use of neuroleptics may be associated with the use of ORAP.

In addition, sudden, unexpected deaths have occurred in patients taking high doses of ORAP for conditions other than Tourette's Disorder. These deaths may have been the result of an effect of ORAP upon the heart. Therefore, patients should be instructed not to exceed the prescribed dose of ORAP and they should realize the need for the initial ECG and for follow-up ECGs during treatment.

Also, pimozide, at a dose about 15 times that given humans, caused an increase in the number of benign tumors of the pituitary gland in female mice. It is not possible to say how important this is. Similar tumors were not seen in rats given pimozide, nor at lower doses in mice, which is reassuring. However, any such finding must be considered to suggest a possible risk of long term use of the drug.

Laboratory tests: An ECG should be done at baseline and periodically thereafter throughout the period of dose adjustment. Any indication of prolongation of the QT, interval beyond an absolute limit of 0.47 seconds (children) or 0.52 seconds (adults), or more than 25% above the patient's original baseline should be considered a basis for stopping further dose increase (see CONTRAINDICATIONS) and considering a lower dose.

Since hypokalemia has been associated with ventricular arrhythmias, potassium insufficiency, secondary to diuretics, diarrhea, or other cause, should be corrected before ORAP therapy is initiated and normal potassium maintained during therapy.

Drug Interactions: Because ORAP prolongs the QT interval of the electrocardiogram, an additive effect on QT interval would be anticipated if administered with other drugs, such as phenothiazines, tricyclic antidepressants or antiarrhythmic agents, which prolong the QT interval. Such concomitant administration should not be undertaken (see CONTRAINDICATIONS).

ORAP may be capable of potentiating CNS depressants, including analgesics, sedatives, anxiolytics, and alcohol.

Carcinogenesis, Mutagenesis, Impairment of Fertility: Carcinogenicity studies were conducted in mice and rats. In mice, pimozide causes a dose-related increase in pituitary and mammary tumors.

When mice were treated for up to 18 monthss with pimozide, pituitary gland changes developed in females only. These changes were characterized as hyperplasia at doses approximating the human dose and adenoma at doses about fifteen times the maximum recommended human dose on a mg per kg basis. The mechanism for the induction of pituitary tumors in mice is not known.

Mammary gland tumors in female mice were also increased, but these tumors are expected in rodents treated with neuroleptic drugs which elevate prolactin levels. Chonic administration of a neuroleptic also causes elevated prolactin levels in humans. Tissue culture experiments indicate that approximately one-third of human breast cancers are prolactin-dependent *in vitro*, a factor of potential importance if the prescription of these drugs is contemplated in a patient with a previously detected breast cancer. Although disturbances such as galactorrhea, amenorrhea, gynecomastia, and impotence have been reported with neuroleptic drugs, the clinical significance of elevated serum prolactin levels is unknown for most patients. Neither clinical studies nor epidemiologic studies conducted to date have shown an association between chronic administration of these drugs and mammary tumorigenesis. The available evidence, however, is considered too limited to be conclusive at this time.

In a 24 month carcinogenicity study in rats, animals received up to 50 times the maximum recommended human dose. No increased incidence of overall tumors or tumors at any site was observed in either sex. Because of the limited number of animals surviving this study, the meaning of these results is unclear.

Pimozide did not have mutagenic activity in the Ames test with four bacterial test strains, in the mouse dominant lethal test or in the micronucleus test in rats.

Reproduction studies in animals were not adequate to assess all aspects of fertility. Nevertheless, female rats administered pimozide had prolonged estrus cycles, an effect also produced by other neuroleptic drugs.

Pregnancy: *Category C.* Reproduction studies performed in rats and rabbits at oral doses up to 8 times the maximum human dose did not reveal evidence of teratogenicity. In the rat, however, this multiple of the human dose resulted in decreased pregnancies and in the retarded development of fetuses. These effects are thought to be due to an inhibition or delay in implantation which is also observed in rodents administered other neuroleptic drugs. In the rabbit, maternal toxicity, mortality, decreased weight gain, and embryotoxicity including increased resorptions were dose related. Because animal reproduction studies are not always predictive of human response, pimozide should be given to a pregnant woman only if the potential benefits of treatment clearly outweight the potential risks.

Labor and Delivery: This drug has no recognized use in labor or delivery.

Nursing Mothers: It is not known whether pimozide is excreted in human milk. Because many drugs are excreted in human milk and because of the potential for tumorigenicity and unknown cardiovascular effects in the infant, a decision should be made whether to discontinue nursing or to discontinue the drug, taking into account the importance of the drug to the mother.

Pediatric Use: Although Tourette's Disorder most often has its onset between the ages of 2 and 15 years, information on the use and efficacy of ORAP in patients less than 12 years of age is limited. Because its use and safety have not been evaluated in other childhood disorders, ORAP is not recommended for use in any condition other than Tourette's Disorder.

Adverse Reactions:

General: Extrapyramidal reactions: Neuromuscular (extrapyramidal) reactions during the administration of ORAP (pimozide) have been reported frequently, often during the first few days of treatment. In most patients, these reactions involved Parkinson-like symptoms which, when first observed, were usually mild to moderately severe and usually reversible.

Other types of neuromuscular reactions (motor restlessness, dystonia, akathisia, hyperreflexia, opisthotonos, oculogyric crises) have been reported far less frequently. Severe extrapyramidal reactions have been reported to occur at relatively low doses. Generally the occurrence and severity of most extrapyramidal symptoms are dose related since they occur at relatively high doses and have been shown to disappear or become less severe when the dose is reduced. Administration of anti-parkinson drugs such as benztropine mesylate or trihexyphenidyl hydrochloride may be required for control of such reactions. It should be noted that persistent extrapyramidal reactions have been reported and that the drug may have to be discontinued in such cases.

Withdrawal Emergent Neurological Signs: Generally, patients receiving short term therapy experience no problems with abrupt discontinuation of neuroleptic drugs. However, some patients on maintenance treatment experience transient dyskinetic signs after abrupt withdrawal. In certain of these cases the dyskinetic movements are indistinguishable from the syndrome described below under "Persistent Tardive Dyskinesia" except for duration. It is not known whether gradual withdrawal of neuroleptic drugs will reduce the rate of occurrence of withdrawal emergent neurological signs but until further evidence becomes available, it seems reasonable to gradually withdraw use of ORAP.

Persistent Tardive Dyskinesia: ORAP may be associated with persistent dyskinesias. Tardive dyskinesia may appear in some patients on long-term therapy or may occur after drug therapy has been discontinued. The risk appears to be greater in elderly patients on high-dose therapy, especially females. The symptoms are persistent and in some patients appear irreversible. The syndrome is characterized by rhythmical involuntary movements of tongue, face, mouth or jaw (e.g., protrusion of tongue, puffing of cheeks, puckering of mouth, chewing movements). Sometimes these may be accompanied by involuntary movements of extremities.

There is no known effective treatment for tardive dyskinesia; antiparkinson agents usually do not alleviate the symptoms of this syndrome. It is suggested that all neuroleptic agents be discontinued if these symptoms appear. Should it be necessary to reinstitute treatment, or increase the dosage of the agent, or switch to a different neuroleptic agent, this syndrome may be masked.

It has been reported that fine vermicular movement of the tongue may be an early sign of the syndrome and if the medication is stopped at that time the syndrome may not develop.

Electrocardiographic Changes: Electrocardiographic changes have been observed in clinical trials of ORAP In Tourette's Disorder and schizophrenia. These have included prolongation of the QT interval, flattening, notching and inversion of the T wave and the appearance of U waves. Sudden, unexpected deaths and grand mal seizure have occurred at doses above 20 mg/day.

Hyperpyrexia: Hyperpyrexia has been reported with other neuroleptic drugs, sometimes alone, and sometimes in association with muscle rigidity, elevated CPK or myoglobinuria (rhabdomyolysis), evidence of autonomic instability (irregular pulse or blood pressure) and/or acute renal failure. This symptom complex is sometimes referred to as neuroleptic malignant syndrome.

Clinical Trials: The following adverse reaction tabulation was derived from 20 patients in a 6 week long placebo controlled clinical trial of ORAP in Tourette's Disorder.

Body System/ Adverse Reaction	Pimozide (N = 20)	Placebo N = 20
Body as a Whole		
Headache	1	2
Gastrointestinal		
Dry mouth	5	1
Diarrhea	1	0
Nausea	0	2
Vomiting	0	1
Constipation	4	2
Eructations	0	1
Thirsty	1	0
Appetite increase	1	0
Endocrine		
Menstrual disorder	0	1
Breast secretions	0	1
Musculoskeletal		
Muscle cramps	0	1
Muscle tightness	3	0
Stooped posture	2	0
CNS		
Drowsiness	7	3
Sedation	14	5
Insomnia	2	2
Dizziness	0	1
Akathisia	8	0
Rigidity	2	0
Speech disorder	2	0
Handwriting change	1	0
Akinesia	8	0
Psychiatric		
Depression	2	3
Excitement	0	1
Nervous	1	0
Adverse behavior effect	5	0
Special Senses		
Visual disturbance	4	0
Taste change	1	0
Sensitivity of eyes to light	1	0
Decreased accommodation	4	1
Spots before eyes	0	1
Urogenital		
Impotence	3	0

Because clinical investigational experience with ORAP in Tourette's Disorder is limited, uncommon adverse reactions may not have been detected. The physician should consider that other adverse reactions associated with neuroleptics may occur.

Other Adverse Reactions: In addition to the adverse reactions listed above, those listed below have been reported in U.S. clinical trials of ORAP in conditions other than Tourette's Disorder.
Body as a Whole: Asthenia, chest pain, periorbital edema
Cardiovascular/Respiratory: Postural hypotension, hypotension, hypertension, tachycardia, palpitations
Gastrointestinal: Increased salivation, nausea, vomiting, anorexis, GI distress
Endocrine: Loss of libido
Metabolic/Nutritional: Weight gain, weight loss
Central Nervous System: Dizziness, tremor, parkinsonism, fainting, dyskinesia
Psychiatric: Excitement
Skin: Rash, sweating, skin irritation
Special Senses: Blurred vision, cataracts
Urogenital: Nocturia, urinary frequency
Overdosage: In general, the signs and symptoms of overdosage with ORAP (pimozide) would be an exaggeration of known pharmacologic effects and adverse reactions, the most prominent of which would be: 1) electrocardiographic abnormalities, 2) severe extrapyramidal reactions, 3) hypotension, 4) a comatose state with respiratory depression.
In the event of overdosage, gastric lavage, establishment of a patent airway and, if necessary, mechanically-assisted respiration are advised. Electrocardiographic monitoring should commence immediately and continue until the ECG parameters are within the normal range. Hypotension and circlatory collapse may be counteracted by use of intravenous fluids, plasma, or concentrated albumin, and vasopressor agents such as norepinephrine. Epinephrine should not be used. In case of severe extrapyramidal reactions, antiparkinson medication should be administered. Because of the long half-life of pimozide, patients who take an overdose should be observed for at least 4 days. As with all drugs, the physician should consider contacting a poison control center for additional information on the treatment of overdose.
Dosage and Administration: Reliable dose response data for the effects of ORAP (pimozide) on tic manifestations in Tourette's Disorder patients below the age of twelve are not available. Consequently, the suppression of tics by ORAP requires a slow and gradual introduction of the drug. The patient's dose should be carefully adjusted to a point where the suppression of tics and the relief afforded is balanced against the untoward side effects of the drug.
An ECG should be done at baseline and periodically thereafter especially during the period of dose adjustment (see WARNINGS and PRECAUTIONS-Laboratory Tests).
In general, treatment with ORAP should be initiated with a dose of 1 to 2 mg a day in divided doses. The dose may be increased thereafter every other day. Most patients are maintained at less than 0.2 mg/kg per day, or 10 mg/day, whichever is less. In no case should a dose of 0.3 mg/kg/day or 20 mg/day be exceeded.
Periodic attempts should be made to reduce the dosage of ORAP to see whether or not tics persist at the level and extent first identified. In attempts to reduce the dosage of ORAP, consideration should be given to the possibility that increases of tic intensity and frequency may represent a transient, withdrawal related phenomenon rather than a return of disease symptoms. Specifically, one to two weeks should be allowed to elapse before one concludes that an increase in tic manifestations is a function of the underlying disease syndrome rather than a response to drug withdrawal. A gradual withdrawal is recommended in any case.
Animal Pharmacology: A chronic study in dogs indicated that pimozide caused gingival hyperplasia when administered for several months at about 5 times the maximum recommended human dose. This condition was reversible after withdrawal. This condition has not been observed following chronic administration of ORAP to man.
How Supplied: ORAP® pimozide tablets, scored, imprinted "McNeil" and "ORAP"—2 mg (white) NDC 0045-0352-60, bottles of 100.
Dispense in tight, light-resistant containers as defined in the official compendium.
10/26/84

PANCREASE® ℞
[pan' kre-ace]
(pancrelipase) capsules
ENTERIC COATED MICROSPHERES

Description: PANCREASE pancrelipase is a white, dye-free, orally administered capsule containing enteric coated microspheres of porcine pancreatic enzyme concentrate, predominately steapsin (pancreatic lipase), amylase and protease. Each capsule contains no less than:

Lipase	4,000 U.S.P. Units
Amylase	20,000 U.S.P. Units
Protease	25,000 U.S.P. Units

Clinical Pharmacology: PANCREASE pancrelipase capsules resist gastric inactivation and deliver predictable, high levels of biologically active enzymes into the duodenum. The enzymes catalyze the hydrolysis of fats into glycerol and fatty acids, protein into proteoses and derived substances, and starch into dextrins and sugars. PANCREASE capsules are effective in controlling steatorrhea and its consequences at low daily dosage levels.

Indications and Usage: PANCREASE pancrelipase capsules are indicated for patients with exocrine pancreatic enzyme deficiency as in but not limited to:
- cystic fibrosis
- chronic pancreatitis
- post-pancreatectomy
- post-gastrointestinal bypass surgery (e.g. Billroth II gastroenterostomy)
- ductal obstruction from neoplasm (e.g. of the pancreas or common bile duct).

Contraindications: PANCREASE pancrelipase capsules are contraindicated in patients known to be hypersensitive to pork protein.
Warnings: Should hypersensitivity occur, discontinue medication and treat symptomatically.
Precautions: TO PROTECT ENTERIC COATING, MICROSPHERES SHOULD NOT BE CRUSHED OR CHEWED.
Where swallowing of capsules is difficult, they may be opened and the microspheres shaken onto a small quantity of a soft food (e.g. applesause, gelatin, etc.), which does not require chewing, and swallowed immediately. Contact of the microspheres with foods having a pH greater than 5.5 can dissolve the protective enteric shell.
Pregnancy Category C. Diethylphthalate, an enteric coating component of PANCREASE pancrelipase capsules has been shown with high intraperitoneal dosing to be tetratogenic in rats. However, when this coating was administered orally to rats up to 100 times the human dose, no teratogenic or embryocidal effects were observed. There were no adequate and well-controlled studies in pregnant women. PANCREASE capsules should be used in pregnancy only if the potential benefit justifies the potential risk to the fetus.
Adverse Reactions: Few adverse reactions, including gastrointestinal distress, have been reported with PANCREASE pancrelipase capsules. Extremely high doses of exogenous pancreatic enzymes have been associated with hyperuricosuria and hyperuricemia.
Dosage and Administration: Usual dosage: One or two capsules during each meal and one capsule with snacks. Occasionally a third capsule with meals may be required depending upon individual requirements for control of steatorrhea.
How Supplied: PANCREASE® pancrelipase capsules (white, dye-free, imprinted "McNeil" and "Pancrease") in bottles of:
100 ....NDC 0045-0095-60
250 ....NDC 0045-0095-69
Keep bottle tightly closed and store in a dry place at controlled room temperature (59°- 86°F). Do not refrigerate.
Manufactured by:
McNEIL PHARMACEUTICAL
McNEILAB, INC.
SPRING HOUSE, PA 19477
11/21/84
Shown in Product Identification Section, page 418

PARAFLEX® (chlorzoxazone) tablets ℞
[par-a-flex']
Description: Each tablet contains chlorzoxazone *250 mg. *5-chlorobenzoxazolinone
Actions: Chlorzoxazone is a centrally-acting agent for painful musculoskeletal conditions. Data available from animal experiments as well as human study indicate that chlorzoxazone acts primarily at the level of the spinal cord and subcortical areas of the brain where it inhibits multisynaptic reflex arcs involved in producing and maintaining skeletal muscle spasm of varied etiology. The clinical result is a reduction of the skeletal muscle spasm with relief of pain and increased mobility of the involved muscles. Blood levels of chlorzoxazone can be detected in man during the first hour after administration and reach peak levels in the third and fourth hours. Chlorzoxazone is rapidly metabolized and is excreted in the urine, primarily in a conjugated form as the glucuronide. Less than one percent of a dose of chlorzoxazone is excreted unchanged in the urine in 24 hours.

Continued on next page

McNeil Pharm.—Cont.

Indications: PARAFLEX chlorzoxazone is indicated as an adjunct to rest, physical therapy, and other measures for the relief of discomfort associated with acute, painful musculoskeletal conditions. The mode of action of this drug has not been clearly identified, but may be related to its sedative properties. Chlorzoxazone does not directly relax tense skeletal muscles in man.

Contraindications: PARAFLEX chlorzoxazone is contraindicated in patients with known intolerance to the drug.

Warnings: The concomitant use of alcohol or other central nervous system depressants may have an additive effect.

Usage in Pregnancy: The safe use of PARAFLEX chlorzoxazone has not been established with respect to the possible adverse effects upon fetal development. Therefore, it should be used in women of childbearing potential only when, in the judgment of the physician, the potential benefits outweigh the possible risks.

Precautions: PARAFLEX chlorzoxazone should be used with caution in patients with known allergies or with a history of allergic reactions to drugs. If a sensitivity reaction occurs such as urticaria, redness, or itching of the skin, the drug should be stopped.

If any symptoms suggestive of liver dysfunction are observed, the drug should be discontinued.

Adverse Reactions: After more than twenty-two years of extensive clinical use of PARAFLEX chlorzoxazone and other chlorzoxazone-containing products in an estimated twenty-seven million patients, it is apparent that the drug is well tolerated and seldom produces undesirable side effects. Occasional patients may develop gastrointestinal disturbances. It is possible in rare instances that PARAFLEX chlorzoxazone may have been associated with gastrointestinal bleeding. Drowsiness, dizziness, lightheadedness, malaise, or overstimulation may be noted by an occasional patient. Rarely, allergic-type skin rashes, petechiae, or ecchymoses may develop during treatment. Angioneurotic edema or anaphylactic reactions are extremely rare. There is no evidence that the drug will cause renal damage. Rarely, a patient may note discoloration of the urine resulting from a phenolic metabolite of chlorzoxazone. This finding is of no known clinical significance.

Approximately twenty-seven patients have been reported in whom the administration of PARAFLEX chlorzoxazone or other chlorzoxazone-containing products was suspected as being the cause of liver damage. In one case, the jaundice was subsequently considered to be due to a carcinoma of the head of the pancreas rather than to the drug. In a second case, there was no jaundice but an elevated alkaline phosphatase and BSP retention. In this patient there was a malignancy with bony and liver metastases. The role of the drug was difficult to determine. A third and fourth case had cholelithiasis. Diagnosis in a fifth case was submassive hepatic necrosis possibly due to abusive use of the drug for approximately one year. The remaining cases had a clinical picture compatible with either a viral hepatitis or a drug-induced hepatitis. In all these latter cases the drug was stopped, and, with one exception, the patients recovered. It is not possible to state that the hepatitis in these patients was or was not drug-induced.

Dosage and Administration: *Usual Adult Dosage:* One tablet (250 mg) three or four times daily. Initial dosage for *painful musculoskeletal conditions* should be two tablets (500 mg) three or four times daily. If adequate response is not obtained with this dose, it may be increased to three tablets (750 mg) three or four times daily. As improvement occurs dosage can usually be reduced.

Usual Child's Dosage: One-half to two tablets (125 mg to 500 mg) three or four times daily given according to age and weight. The tablets may be crushed and mixed with food or a suitable vehicle for administration to children.

Overdosage:
Symptoms: Initially, gastrointestinal disturbances such as nausea, vomiting, or diarrhea together with drowsiness, dizziness, lightheadedness or headache may occur. Early in the course there may be malaise or sluggishness followed by marked loss of muscle tone, making voluntary movement impossible. The deep tendon reflexes may be decreased or absent. The sensorium remains intact, and there is no peripheral loss of sensation. Respiratory depression may occur with rapid, irregular respiration and intercostal and substernal retraction. The blood pressure is lowered, but shock has not been observed.

Treatment: Gastric lavage or induction of emesis should be carried out, followed by administration of activated charcoal. Thereafter, treatment is entirely supportive. If respirations are depressed, oxygen and artificial respiration should be employed and a patent airway assured by use of an oropharyngeal airway or endotracheal tube. Hypotension may be counteracted by use of dextran, plasma, concentrated albumin or a vasopressor agent such as norepinephrine. Cholinergic drugs or analeptic drugs are of no value and should not be used.

How Supplied: PARAFLEX® (chlorzoxazone) 250 mg tablets (colored orange, scored, imprinted "PARAFLEX" "McNEIL")—bottles of 100 NDC 0045-0317-60.

Dispense in tight container as defined in the official compendium. 3/18/81

PARAFON FORTE® ℞
[par-a-fon for-ta']
(chlorzoxazone and acetaminophen)
tablets

Description: Each tablet contains chlorzoxazone 250 mg and acetaminophen 300 mg.

Actions: PARAFON FORTE tablets provide symptomatic relief of pain, stiffness, and limitation of motion associated with most musculoskeletal disorders through (a) relaxation of muscle spasm by chlorzoxazone, an effective and well-tolerated centrally-acting agent; and (b) analgesia by acetaminophen, a nonsalicylate analgesic useful in skeletal muscle pain.

Data available from animal experiments, as well as human study, indicate that chlorzoxazone acts primarily at the level of the spinal cord and subcortical areas of the brain where it inhibits multisynaptic reflex arcs involved in producing and maintaining skeletal muscle spasm of varied etiology. Blood levels of chlorzoxazone can be detected in man during the first hour after administration and reach peak levels by the third to fourth hour. Chlorzoxazone is rapidly metabolized and is excreted in the urine, primarily in a conjugated form as the glucuronide. Less than one percent of a dose of chlorzoxazone is excreted unchanged in the urine in 24 hours.

Acetaminophen provides analgesic action to supplement that which results secondarily from muscle relaxation. Acetaminophen is rapidly absorbed after oral administration, with peak plasma levels occurring in one to two hours. After eight hours, only negligible amounts remain in the blood. Only 4 percent is excreted unchanged; 85 percent of the ingested dose is recovered in the urine in conjugated form as the glucuronide.

Indications: Based on a review of this drug by the National Academy of Sciences-National Research Council and/or other information, FDA has classified the indications as follows:

"Probably" effective as an adjunct to the rest and physical therapy for the relief of the discomfort associated with acute, painful musculoskeletal conditions. The mode of action of this drug has not been clearly identified, but may be related to its sedative properties. Chlorzoxazone does not directly relax tense skeletal muscles in man.

Contraindications: PARAFON FORTE tablets are contraindicated in patients sensitive to either component.

Warnings: The concomitant use of alcohol or other central nervous system depressants may have an additive effect.

Usage in Pregnancy: The safe use of PARAFON FORTE tablets has not been established with respect to the possible adverse effects upon fetal development. Therefore, it should be used in women of childbearing potential only when, in the judgment of the physician, the potential benefits outweigh the possible risks.

Precautions: PARAFON FORTE tablets should be used with caution in patients with known allergies or with a history of allergic reactions to drugs. If a sensitivity reaction occurs such as urticaria, redness, or itching of the skin, the drug should be stopped.

If any signs or symptoms suggestive of liver dysfunction are observed, the drug should be discontinued.

This product contains FD&C Yellow No. 5 (tartrazine) which may cause allergic-type reactions (including bronchial asthma) in certain susceptible individuals. Although the overall incidence of FD&C Yellow No. 5 (tartrazine) sensitivity in the general population is low, it is frequently seen in patients who also have aspirin hypersensitivity.

Adverse Reactions: After more than twenty-two years of extensive clinical use of PARAFLEX® (chlorzoxazone) tablets and other chlorzoxazone-containing products in an estimated twenty-seven million patients, it is apparent that the drug is well tolerated and seldom produces undesirable side effects. Occasional patients may develop gastrointestinal disturbances. It is possible in rare instances that chlorzoxazone may have been associated with gastrointestinal bleeding. Drowsiness, dizziness, lightheadedness, malaise, or overstimulation may be noted by an occasional patient. Rarely, allergic-type skin rashes, petechiae, or ecchymoses may develop during treatment. Angioneurotic edema or anaphylactic reactions are extremely rare. There is no evidence that the drug will cause renal damage. Rarely, a patient may note discoloration of the urine resulting from a phenolic metabolite of chlorzoxazone. This finding is of no known clinical significance.

Approximately twenty-seven patients have been reported in whom the administration of PARAFLEX chlorzoxazone or other chlorzoxazone-containing products was suspected as being the cause of liver damage. In one case, the jaundice was subsequently considered to be due to a carcinoma of the head of the pancreas rather than to the drug. In a second case, there was no jaundice but an elevated alkaline phosphatase and BSP retention. In this patient there was a malignancy with bony and liver metastases. The role of the drug was difficult to determine. A third and fourth case had cholelithiasis. Diagnosis in a fifth case was submassive hepatic necrosis possibly due to abusive use of the drug for approximately one year. The remaining cases had a clinical picture compatible with either a viral hepatitis or a drug-induced hepatitis. In all these latter cases the drug was stopped, and, with one exception, the patients recovered. It is not possible to state that the hepatitis in these patients was or was not drug induced.

Acetaminophen has rarely been found to produce any side effects.

Dosage and Administration *Usual Adult Dosage:* Two tablets 4 times daily.

Overdosage:
Acetaminophen
Acetaminophen in massive overdosage may cause hepatic toxicity in some patients. In adults, hepatic toxicity has rarely been reported with less than 10 grams and fatalities with less than 15 grams, taken as single, massive overdoses. Importantly, for reasons not fully understood, young children seem to be more resistant than adults to the hepatotoxic effect of acetaminophen overdose. Early symptoms following a potentially hepatotoxic overdose may include: nausea, vomiting, diaphoresis and general malaise. Clinical and laboratory evidence of hepatic toxicity usually are not apparent until 48 to 72 hours post-ingestion. Following recovery there are no residual, structural or functional hepatic abnormalities.

Since patients' estimates of the quantity of a drug ingested are notoriously unreliable, if an acetaminophen overdose is suspected a serum acetaminophen assay should be obtained as early as possible, but no sooner than four hours following ingestion. Liver function studies should be obtained initially and repeated at 24 hour intervals.

Antidotal therapy with N-acetylcysteine appears effective in preventing and/or minimizing the toxic effects of acetaminophen. For optimal results, the antidote should be administered within 16 hours of ingestion of the overdose.

The Rocky Mountain Poison Center (800-525-6115) should be contacted for assistance in interpreting plasma levels and for directions on the administration of N-acetylcysteine as an antidote, a use currently restricted to investigational status.

Chlorzoxazone

Symptoms: Initially, gastrointestinal disturbances such as nausea, vomiting, or diarrhea together with drowsiness, dizziness, lightheadedness or headache may occur. Early in the course there may be malaise or sluggishness followed by marked loss of muscle tone, making voluntary movement impossible. The deep tendon reflexes may be decreased or absent. The sensorium remains intact, and there is no peripheral loss of sensation. Respiratory depression may occur with rapid, irregular respiration and intercostal and substernal retraction. The blood pressure is lowered, but shock has not been observed.

Treatment: Gastric lavage or induction of emesis should be carried out, followed by administration of activated charcoal. Thereafter, treatment is entirely supportive. If respirations are depressed, oxygen and artificial respiration should be employed and a patent airway assured by use of an oropharyngeal airway or endotracheal tube. Hypotension may be counteracted by use of dextran, plasma, concentrated albumin or a vasopressor agent such as norepinephrine. Cholinergic drugs or analeptic drugs are of no value and should not be used.

How Supplied: PARAFON FORTE® Tablets (colored green, imprinted "McNEIL"and "PARAFON FORTE")—bottles of 100 **NDC** 0045-0322-60 and 500 **NDC** 0045-0322-70; Unit dose of 200 **NDC** 0045-0322-58.

Dispense in a tight container as defined in the official compendium.

Tablets manufactured by McNeil Pharmaceutical Co., Dorado, PR 00646.

2/25/83

Shown in Product Identification Section, page 419

THEOPHYL® ℞
[the′a-fil]
(anhydrous theophylline)
CHEWABLE TABLETS
for oral use

Description: Each double-scored white tablet contains not less than 94.0 percent and not more than 106.0 percent of 100 mg anhydrous theophylline USP. Theophylline ($C_7H_8N_4O_2$), a xanthine compound, is a white odorless crystalline powder having a bitter taste. The scoring of THEOPHYL® Chewable Tablets allows for titration in 25 mg (¼ tablet) increments.

Clinical Pharmacology: Theophylline directly relaxes the smooth muscle of the bronchial airways and pulmonary blood vessels, thus acting mainly as a bronchodilator, pulmonary vasodilator and smooth muscle relaxant. It also possesses other actions typical of the xanthine derivatives: coronary vasodilator, diuretic, and cardiac, cerebral, and skeletal muscle stimulant. The actions of theophylline may be mediated through inhibition of phosphodiesterase and a resultant increase in intracellular cyclic AMP which could mediate smooth muscle relaxation.

In vitro, theophylline has been shown to react synergistically with beta agonists (such as isoproterenol) that increase intracellular cyclic AMP through the stimulation of adenyl cyclase, but synergism has not been demonstrated in clinical studies and more data are needed to determine if theophylline and beta agonists have clinically important additive effects **in vivo.**

Apparently, tolerance does not develop with chronic use of theophylline.

The half-life is shortened with cigarette smoking. The half-life is prolonged in alcoholism, reduced hepatic or renal function, congestive heart failure, and in patients receiving cimetidine or certain antibiotics such as troleandomycin, (TAO, cyclamycin) erythromycin, lincomycin and clindamycin. High fever for prolonged periods may decrease theophylline elimination.

Theophylline Elimination Characteristics:

	Theophylline Clearance Rates (mean ± S.D.)	Half-Life Average (mean ± S.D.)
Children (over 6 months of age)	1.45 ± 0.58 ml/kg/min	3.7 ± 1.1 hours
Adult nonsmokers with uncomplicated asthma	0.65 ± 0.19 ml/kg/min	8.7 ± 2.2 hours

Newborn infants have extremely slow clearances with half-lives exceeding 24 hours. These approach those seen for older children after about 3–6 months.

Older adults with chronic obstructive pulmonary disease, patients with cor pulmonale or other causes of heart failure, and patients with liver pathology may have much lower clearances with half-lives that may exceed 24 hours. The half-life is prolonged in alcoholism, reduced hepatic or renal function, congestive heart failure, and in patients receiving cimetidine or certain antibiotics such as TAO (troleandomycin), erythromycin, and clindamycin. High fever for prolonged periods may decrease theophylline elimination.

The half-life of theophylline in smokers (1 to 2 packs/day) averaged 4 to 5 hours in various studies, much shorter than the 7 to 9 hour half-life in nonsmokers. The increase in theophylline clearance caused by smoking is probably the result of induction of drug-metabolizing enzymes that do not readily normalize after cessation of smoking. It appears that between 3 months and 2 years may be necessary for normalization of the effect of smoking on theophylline pharmacokinetics.

THEOPHYL Chewable Tablets are a rapidly releasing form of theophylline. Bioavailability of these tablets has been shown to be 98% ± 5% when chewed and 101% ± 4% when swallowed whole.

Indications: For relief and/or prevention of symptoms of asthma and reversible bronchospasm associated with chronic bronchitis and emphysema.

Contraindications: Avoid using THEOPHYL Chewable Tablets in individuals who have shown hypersensitivity to any of its components.

Warnings: Status asthmaticus should be considered a medical emergency and is defined as the degree of bronchospasm which is not rapidly responsive to usual doses of conventional bronchodilators. Optimal therapy for such patients frequently requires both **additional medication,** parenterally administered, and **close monitoring,** preferably in an intensive care setting.

Although increasing the dose of theophylline may bring about relief, such treatment may be associated with toxicity. The likelihood of such toxicity developing increases significantly when the serum theophylline concentration exceeds 20 µg/ml. Therefore, determination of serum theophylline levels is recommended to assure maximal benefit without excessive risk.

Serum levels above 20 µg/ml are rarely found after appropriate administration of the recommended doses. However, in individuals in whom theophylline plasma clearance is reduced **for any reason,** even conventional doses may result in increased serum levels and potential toxicity. Reduced theophylline clearance has been documented in the following readily identifiable groups: 1) patients with impaired renal or liver function; 2) patients over 55 years of age, particularly males and those with chronic lung disease; 3) those with cardiac failure from any cause; 4) neonates; and 5) those patients taking certain drugs (macrolide antibiotics and cimetidine). Decreased clearance of theophylline may be associated with either influenza immunization or active infection with influenza.

Reduction of dosage and laboratory monitoring is especially appropriate in the above individuals. Less serious signs of theophylline toxicity, i.e. nausea and restlessness, may appear in up to 50% of patients. Unfortunately however, serious side effects such as ventricular arrhythmias, convulsions or even death may appear as the first sign of toxicity without any previous warning. Stated differently: **serious toxicity is not reliably preceeded by less severe side effects.**

Many patients who require theophylline may exhibit tachycardia due to their underlying disease process so that the cause/effect relationship to elevated serum theophylline concentrations may not be appreciated.

Theophylline products may cause dysrhythmia and/or worsen pre-existing arrythmias and any significant change in rate and/or rhythm warrants monitoring and further investigation.

The occurrence of arrhythmias and sudden death (with histological evidence of necrosis of the myocardium) has been recorded in laboratory animals (minipigs, rodents and dogs) when theophylline and beta agonists were administered concomitantly, although not when either was administered alone. The significance of these findings when applied to human usage is currently unknown.

Usage in Pregnancy: Safe use in pregnancy has not been established relative to possible adverse effects on fetal development, but neither have adverse effects on fetal development been established. This is, unfortunately, true for most antiasthmatic medications. Therefore, use of theophylline in pregnant women should be balanced against the risk of uncontrolled asthma.

Precautions: Mean half-life in smokers is shorter than in nonsmokers; therefore, smokers may require larger doses of theophylline. THEOPHYL Chewable Tablets, like all theophylline products, should not be administered concurrently with other xanthine medications. Use with caution in patients with severe cardiac disease, severe hypoxemia, hypertension, hyperthyroidism, acute myocardial injury, cor pulmonale, congestive heart failure, liver disease, peptic ulcer and in the elderly (especially males) and in neonates. Great caution should be used especially in giving theophylline to patients in congestive heart failure; such patients have shown markedly prolonged theophylline blood level curves with theophylline persisting in serum for long periods following discontinuation of the drug.

Theophylline may occasionally act as a local irritant to the GI tract although gastrointestinal symptoms are more commonly central in origin and associated with serum concentrations over 20 mcg/ml.

It has been reported that theophylline distributes readily into breast milk and may cause adverse effects in the infant. Caution must be used if prescribing xanthines to a mother who is nursing, taking into account the risk-benefit of this therapy.

Due to the marked variation in theophylline metabolism in infants under 6 months of age, this drug is not recommended for this age group.

Adverse Reactions: The most frequent adverse reactions to theophylline are usually due to overdose (serum levels in excess of 20 µg/ml) and are:

Gastrointestinal: nausea, vomiting, epigastric pain, hematemesis, diarrhea.

Central nervous system: headaches, irritability, restlessness, insomnia, reflex hyperexcitability, muscle twitching, clonic and tonic generalized convulsions.

Continued on next page

McNeil Pharm.—Cont.

Cardiovascular: palpitations, tachycardia, extra systoles, flushing, hypotension, circulatory failure, ventricular arrhythmias.
Respiratory: tachypnea.
Renal: albuminuria, increased excretion of renal tubular cells and red blood cells, potentiation of diuresis.
Others: hyperglycemia and inappropriate ADH syndrome.

Drug Interactions: Toxic synergism with ephedrine has been documented and may occur with some other sympathomimetic bronchodilators.

DRUG	EFFECT
Aminophylline with lithium carbonate	Increased excretion of lithium carbonate
Aminophylline with propranolol	Antagonism of propranolol effect
Theophylline with furosemide	Increased diuresis
Theophylline with hexamethonium	Decreased hexamethonium-induced chronotropic effect
Theophylline with reserpine	Reserpine-induced tachycardia
Theophylline with chlordiazepoxide	Chlordiazepoxide-induced fatty acid mobilization
Theophylline with cimetidine, troleandomycin, (TAO) erythromycin, cyclamycin) lincomycin, clindamycin	Increased theophylline plasma levels
Theophylline with phenytoin	Decreased phenytoin levels

Management of Overdose:
A. If potential overdose is established and seizure has not occurred:
   1. Induce vomiting.
   2. Administer a cathartic.
   3. Administer activated charcoal.
B. If patient is having a seizure:
   1. Establish an airway.
   2. Administer O_2.
   3. Treat the seizure with intravenous diazepam, 0.1 to 0.3 mg/kg up to 10 mg.
   4. Monitor vital signs, maintain blood pressure and provide adequate hydration.
C. Post-seizure coma:
   1. Maintain airway and oxygenation.
   2. Follow above recommendations to prevent absorption of drug, but intubation and lavage will have to be performed instead of inducing emesis, and introduce the cathartic and charcoal via a large bore gastric lavage tube.
   3. Continue to provide full supportive care and adequate hydration while waiting for drug to be metabolized. In general, the drug is metabolized sufficiently rapidly so as not to require dialysis, however, if serum levels exceed 50 µg/ml, charcoal hemoperfusion may be indicated.

Dosage and Administration: Therapeutic serum levels associated with optimal likelihood for benefit and minimal risk of toxicity are considered to be between 10 µg/ml and 20 µg/ml. Levels above 20 µg/ml may produce toxic effects. There is great variation from patient to patient in dosage needed to achieve a therapeutic blood level because of variable rates of elimination. Therefore, dosage must be individualized and monitoring of theophylline serum levels is highly recommended. Serum theophylline measurement should be obtained at the time of peak absorption, which has been shown to be 2.0 ± 0.3 hours for THEOPHYL Chewable Tablets when chewed and 2.2 ± 0.3 hours when swallowed whole. Samples for serum theophylline measurement should be taken after a patient has been on a given dose for at least 3 days and has missed no doses during the previous 48 hours. **Unless the above instructions with regard to serum theophylline measurement are followed, the results may be misleading and dosage adjustments based on these results may be incorrect, possibly increasing the risk of toxicity.**

As theophylline does not distribute into fatty tissue, dosage should be calculated on the basis of lean (ideal) body weight.

Giving theophylline with food may prevent the rare case of stomach irritation; though absorption may be slower, it is still complete.

When rapidly absorbed products such as solutions and uncoated tablets with rapid dissolution are used, dosing to maintain "around the clock" blood levels generally requires administration every 6 hours in children; dosing intervals up to 8 hours may be satisfactory for adults because of their slower elimination rate.

Children, and adults requiring higher than average doses, may benefit from products with slower absorption, such as THEOPHYL® SR Capsules, which may allow longer dosing intervals and/or less fluctuation in serum concentration over a dosing interval during chronic therapy.

Once a patient is stabilized on a particular dose of theophylline, his blood levels tend to remain constant with that dose.

Pulmonary function measurements before and after a period of treatment permit an objective assessment of response to THEOPHYL Chewable Tablets.

As a practical consideration, it is not always possible to obtain serum level determinations. Under such conditions, restriction of the daily dose (in otherwise healthy adults) to not greater than 16 mg/kg/day in divided doses will result in relatively few patients exceeding serum levels of 20 µg/ml and the resultant risk of toxicity.

I. Dosage of THEOPHYL® Chewable Tablets for Patients Exhibiting Acute Symptoms of Asthma Requiring Rapid Theophyllinization and Not Currently Receiving Theophylline Products.
[See table below].
II. Dosage for Patients Currently Receiving Theophylline Therapy.

Determine, where possible, the time, amount, route of administration and form of the patient's last dose. Ideally, the loading dose should be deferred if a serum theophylline determination can be rapidly obtained. If this is not possible, the clinician must exercise his judgment in selecting a dose based on the principle that each 0.5 mg/kg of theophylline administered as a loading dose will result in a .1 µg/ml increase in serum theophylline concentration. When there is sufficient respiratory distress to warrant a small risk, 2.5 mg/kg of theophylline is likely to increase the serum concentration by only about 5 µg/ml when administered as a loading dose. If the patient is not already experiencing theophylline toxicity, this is unlikely to result in dangerous adverse effects. Subsequent maintenance dosage recommendations are the same as those described above.

III. Dosage for Chronic Asthma.
Theophyllinization is a treatment of first choice for the management of chronic asthma (to prevent symptoms and maintain patent airways). Slow clinical titration is generally preferred to assure acceptance and safety of the medication.

Initial Dose: 16 mg/kg/day or 450 mg/day (whichever is lower) in 3–4 divided doses at 6–8 hour intervals.

Increased Dose: The above dosage may be increased in approximately 25 percent increments at 2–3 day intervals so long as no intolerance is observed, until a maximum indicated below is reached.

Maximum Dose Without Measurement of Serum Concentration:
Not to exceed the following: **(WARNING: DO NOT ATTEMPT TO MAINTAIN ANY DOSE THAT IS NOT TOLERATED)**

Age Less than 9 years	–24 mg/kg/day
Age 9–12 years	–20 mg/kg/day
Age 12–16 years	–18 mg/kg/day
Age Greater than 16 years	–13 mg/kg/day or 900 mg/day (WHICHEVER IS LESS)

NOTE: Use ideal body weight for obese patients.

How Supplied: THEOPHYL® chewable tablets (white, round, double bisected one side, imprinted "THEOPHYL 100") contains 100mg of anhydrous theophylline-bottles of 100-NDC 0045-0420-60.

Store at 59°–86°F (15°–30°C). Protect from moisture. Dispense in a tight, light-resistant container as defined in the official compendium.

Manufactured by Knoll Pharmaceutical, Whippany, N.J. 07961 for:
McNeil PHARMACEUTICAL
McNEILAB, INC.
SPRING HOUSE, PA 19477

11/17/82

THEOPHYL®-SR   R

[the'ō-fil]
(anhydrous theophylline)
CAPSULES
for oral use

Description: Each sustained release capsule contains not less than 94.0 percent and not more than 106.0 percent of 125 mg (yellow and clear capsules) or 250 mg (green and clear capsules) anhydrous theophylline in a coated bead timed-release formulation. Theophylline anhydrous, a xanthine bronchodilator, is a white odorless crystalline powder having a bitter taste.

Clinical Pharmacology: Theophylline directly relaxes the smooth muscle of the bronchial airways and pulmonary blood vessels, thus acting mainly as a bronchodilator and smooth muscle relaxant. The drug also produces other actions typical of the xanthine derivatives: coronary vasodilator, cardiac stimulant, diuretic, cerebral stimulant, and skeletal muscle stimulant. The actions of theophylline may be mediated through inhibition of phosphodiesterase and a resultant increase in intracellular cyclic AMP.

In vitro, theophylline has been shown to act synergistically with beta agonists that increase intracellular cyclic AMP through the stimulation of adenyl cyclase, but synergism has not been demonstrated in patient studies. More data are needed to determine if theophylline and beta agonists have a clinically important additive effect in vivo.
Apparently, no development of tolerance occurs with chronic use of theophylline.

Pharmacokinetics: The half-life of theophylline is influenced by a number of known variables. It is prolonged in patients suffering from chronic alcoholism, impaired hepatic or renal function,

THEOPHYL	Loading Dose	Maintenance Dose For Next 12 Hours	Maintenance Dose Beyond 12 Hours
1. Children 6 months to 9 years	6 mg/kg	4 mg/kg q4h	4 mg/kg q6h
2. Children age 9–16 and young adult smokers	6 mg/kg	3 mg/kg q4h	3 mg/kg q6h
3. Otherwise healthy nonsmoking adults	6 mg/kg	3 mg/kg q6h	3 mg/kg q8h
4. Older patients and patients with cor pulmonale	6 mg/kg	2 mg/kg q6h	2 mg/kg q8h
5. Patients with congestive heart failure, liver failure	6 mg/kg	2 mg/kg q8h	1–2 mg/kg q12h

congestive heart failure, and in patients receiving macrolide antibiotics and cimetidine. Older adults (over age 55) and patients with chronic obstructive pulmonary disease, with or without cor pulmonale, may also have much slower clearance rates. For such patients, the theophylline half-life may exceed 24 hours.

Theophylline Elimination Characteristics:

	Theophylline Clearance Rates (mean ± S.D.)	Half-Life Average (mean ± S.D.)
Children (over 6 months of age)	1.45 ± 0.58 ml/kg/min	3.7 ± 1.1 hours
Adult nonsmokers uncomplicated asthma	0.65 ± 0.19 ml/kg/min	8.7 ± 2.2 hours

Newborns and neonates have extremely slow clearance rates compared to older infants (over 6 months) and children, and may also have a theophylline half-life of over 24 hours. High fever for prolonged periods may also reduce the rate of theophylline elimination.

The half-life of theophylline in smokers (1 to 2 packs/day) averages 4–5 hours, much shorter than the half-life in nonsmokers (7–9 hours). The increase in theophylline clearance caused by smoking is probably the result of induction of drug-metabolizing enzymes that do not readily normalize after cessation of smoking. It appears that between 3 months and 2 years may be necessary for normalization of the effect of smoking on theophylline pharmacokinetics.

Following single doses of 500 to 625 mg of THEOPHYL SR capsules to 15 fasted patients, who continued to fast 4 hours after the study dose, a peak serum theophylline concentration (C max) of 12.2 ± 3.6 µg/ml (mean ± sd) was reached at 4.7 ± 1.5 hours. Following administration of a single 250 mg THEOPHYL SR capsule every eight hours to 12 (normal subjects, who fasted 12 hours before and 2 hours after the test dose, a steady state peak serum concentration (C max) of 10.5 ± 2.5 µg/ml was reached at 3.7 ± 1.0 hours. The pre-dose minimum serum concentration (C min) at steady state was 8.2 ± 2.1 µg/ml. The data for the 125 mg capsule are equivalent.

Indications: For relief and/or prevention of symptoms from asthma and reversible bronchospasm associated with chronic bronchitis and emphysema.

Contraindications: THEOPHYL SR capsules are contraindicated in individuals who have shown hypersensitivity to any of its components. THEOPHYL SR, as a sustained release preparation, is not recommended in the initial treatment of patients requiring emergency theophyllinization.

Warnings:
Status asthmaticus should be considered a medical emergency and is defined as the degree of bronchospasm which is not rapidly responsive to usual doses of conventional bronchodilators. Optimal therapy for such patients frequently requires both **additional medication**, parenterally administered, and **close monitoring**, preferably in an intensive care setting.

Although increasing the dose of theophylline may bring about relief, such treatment may be associated with toxicity. The likelihood of such toxicity developing increases significantly when the serum theophylline concentration exceeds 20 µg/ml. Therefore, determination of serum theophylline levels is recommended to assure maximal benefit without excessive risk.

Serum levels above 20 µg/ml are rarely found after appropriate administration of the recommended doses. However, in individuals in whom theophylline plasma clearance is reduced **fo any reason**, even conventional doses may result in increased serum levels and potential toxicity. Reduced theophylline clearance has been documented in the following readily identifiable groups: 1) patients with impaired renal or liver function; 2) patients over 55 years of age, particularly males and those with chronic lung disease; 3) those with cardiac failure from any cause; 4) neonates; and 5) those patients taking certain drugs (macrolide antibiotics and cimetidine). Decreased clearance of theophylline may be associated with either influenza immunization or active infection with influenza.

Reduction of dosage and laboratory monitoring is especially appropriate in the above individuals.

Less serious signs of theophylline toxicity, i.e. nausea and restlessness, may appear in up to 50% of patients. Unfortunately however, serious side effects such as ventricular arrhythmias, convulsions or even death may appear as the first sign of toxicity without any previous warning. Stated differently; **serious toxicity is not reliably preceded by less severe side effects.**

Many patients who require theophylline may exhibit tachycardia due to their underlying disease process so that the cause/effect relationship to elevated serum theophylline concentrations may not be appreciated.

Theophylline products may cause dysrhythmia and/or worsen pre-existing arrhythmias and any significant change in rate and/or rhythm warrants monitoring and further investigation.

The occurrence of arrhythmias and sudden death (with histological evidence of necrosis of the myocardium) has been recorded in laboratory animals (minipigs, rodents and dogs) when theophylline and beta agonists were administered concomitantly, although not when either was administered alone. The significance of these findings when applied to human usage is currently unknown.

Precautions:
General: Theophylline half-life is shorter in smokers than in nonsmokers. Therefore, smokers may require larger or more frequent doses. Morphine and curare should be used with caution in patients with airway obstruction as they may suppress respiration and stimulate histamine release. Alternative drugs should be used when possible. THEOPHYL SR should not be administered concurrently with other xanthine medications. Use with caution in patients with severe cardiac disease, severe hypoxemia, hypertension, hyperthyroidism, acute myocardial injury, cor pulmonale, congestive heart failure, liver disease, and in the elderly (especially males) and in neonates. In particular, great caution should be used in giving theophylline to patients with congestive heart failure. Frequently such patients have markedly prolonged theophylline serum levels with theophylline persisting in serum for long periods following discontinuation of the drug.

Use THEOPHYL SR cautiously in patients with history of peptic ulcer. Theophylline may occasionally act as a local irritant to G.I. tract although gastrointestinal symptoms are more commonly centrally mediated and associated with serum drug concentrations over 20 µg/ml.

Information for Patients: The physician should reinforce the importance of taking only the prescribed dose and time interval between doses.

The patient should alert the physician if symptoms occur repeatedly, especially near the end of a dosing interval.

Drug Interactions: Toxic synergism with ephedrine has been documented and may occur with some other sympathomimetic bronchodilators. In addition, the following drug interactions have been demonstrated:

DRUG	EFFECT
Lithium Carbonate	Increased excretion of lithium carbonate
Propranolol	Antagonism of propranolol effect
Cimetidine	Increased theophylline blood levels
Troleandomycin, erythromycin	Increased theophylline blood levels

Drug-Food Interaction: THEOPHYL SR has not been adequately studied to determine whether its bioavailability is altered when it is given with food.

Available data suggest that drug administration at the time of food ingestion may influence the absorption characteristics of theophylline controlled-release products, resulting in serum values different from those found after administration in the fasting state.

A drug-food effect, if any, would likely have its greatest clinical significance when high theophylline serum levels are being maintained and/or when large single doses (greater than 13 mg/kg or 900 mg) of a controlled-release theophylline product are given. The influence of the type and amount of food on performance of controlled-release theophylline products is under study at this time.

Drug-Laboratory Test Interactions: When plasma levels of theophylline are measured by spectrophotometric methods; coffee, tea, cola beverages, chocolate, and acetaminophen contribute falsely high values.

Carcinogenesis, Mutagenesis, and Impairment of Fertility: Long-term animal studies have not been performed to evaluate the carcinogenic potential, mutagenic potential, or the effect on fertility of xanthine compounds.

Pregnancy: Category C—Animal reproduction studies have not been conducted with theophylline. It is not known whether theophylline can cause fetal harm when administered to a pregnant woman or can affect reproduction capacity. Xanthines should be given to a pregnant woman only if clearly needed.

Nursing Mothers: It has been reported that theophylline distributes readily into breast milk and may cause adverse effects in the infant. Caution must be used if prescribing xanthines to a mother who is nursing, taking into account the risk-benefit of this therapy.

Pediatric Use: Safety and effectiveness in children under six years of age have not been established with this product.

Adverse Reactions: The most consistent adverse reactions to theophylline are usually due to overdose and are:

Gastrointestinal: nausea, vomiting, epigastric pain, hematemesis, diarrhea.

Central nervous system: headaches, irritability, restlessness, insomnia, reflex hyperexcitability, muscle twitching, clonic and tonic generalized convulsions.

Cardiovascular: palpitation, tachycardia, extra systoles, flushing, hypotension, circulatory failure, ventricular arrhythmias.

Respiratory: tachypnea.

Renal: albuminuria, increased excretion of renal tubular, rash and red blood cells, potentiation of diuresis.

Others: hyperglycemia and inappropriate ADH syndrome.

Overdosage
Management:
If potential overdose is established and seizure has not occurred:
a. Induce vomiting.
b. Administer a cathartic (This is particularly important if sustained release preparations have been taken).
c. Administer activated charcoal.

If patient is having a seizure:
a. Establish an airway.
b. Administer oxygen.
c. Treat the seizure with intravenous diazepam, 0.1 to 0.3 mg/kg up to 10 mg.
d. Monitor vital signs, maintain blood pressure and provide adequate hydration.

Post-seizure coma:
a. Maintain airway and oxygenation.
b. In addition to the above recommendations to prevent absorption of the drug, intubation and lavage will have to be performed instead of inducing emesis, and the cathartic and charcoal will need to be introduced via a large bore gastric lavage tube.
c. Continue to provide full supportive care and adequate hydration while waiting for drug to be metabolized. In general, the drug is metabolized sufficiently rapidly so as not to warrant consideration of dialysis, however, if serum levels exceed 50 µg/ml, charcoal hemoperfusion may be indicated.

Continued on next page

McNeil Pharm.—Cont.

Dosage and Administration: THEOPHYL SR has not been adequately studied for its bioavailability when administered with food. (See PRECAUTIONS, Drug-Food Interactions.)

For most patients, effective use of theophylline, i.e. associated with optimal likelihood of benefit combined with minimal risk of toxicity, is considered to occur when serum levels are maintained between 10 and 20 μg/ml. Levels above 20 μg/ml may produce toxicity, and in a small number of patients, toxicity may even be seen with serum levels between 15–20 μg/ml, particularly during initiation of therapy.

There is considerable variation from patient to patient in the dosage required to achieve and maintain therapeutic and safe levels, primarily due to variable rates of elimination. Therefore, it is essential that not only must dosage be individualized, but titration and monitoring of serum levels be utilized where available. When serum concentration cannot be obtained, restriction of dosage to the amounts and intervals recommended in the guidelines listed below becomes essential. As theophylline does not distribute into fatty tissue, dosage should be calculated on the basis of lean (ideal) body weight.

Dosage Guidelines:

I. Acute Symptoms
THEOPHYL SR is not intended for patients experiencing an acute episode of bronchospasm (associated with asthma, chronic bronchitis, or emphysema). Such patients require *rapid* relief of symptoms and should be treated with an immediate-release or intravenous theophylline preparation (or other bronchodilators) and not with controlled release products.

II. Chronic Therapy
Therapy with THEOPHYL SR capsules should be initiated at the patient's current total daily dosage, with one third of the total daily dose administered every 8 hours. Certain patients, such as the young, smokers, and some non-smoking adults are likely to metabolize theophylline rapidly and may require dosing at more frequent intervals. Such patients can generally be identified as having trough serum concentrations lower than desired or repeatedly exhibiting symptoms near the end of a dosing interval.

III. Maximum Dose of Theophylline Where the Serum Concentration is Not Measured.

Not to exceed the following:
Age < 9 years	24 mg/kg/day
Age 9–12 years	20 mg/kg/day
Age 12–16 years	18 mg/kg/day
Age > 16 years	13 mg/kg/day
	OR 900 mg/day (WHICHEVER IS LESS)

WARNING: DO NOT ATTEMPT TO MAINTAIN ANY DOSE THAT IS NOT TOLERATED.

IV. Measurement of Serum Theophylline Concentrations During Chronic Therapy:
If the above maximum doses are to be maintained or exceeded, serum theophylline measurement is recommended. The serum sample should be obtained at the time of peak absorption, which has been shown to be 3.7 ± 1.0 hours (mean ± standard deviation) for THEOPHYL SR capsules. It is important that the patient will have missed no doses during the previous 48 hours and that dosing intervals will have been reasonably typical with no added doses during that period of time. DOSAGE ADJUSTMENT BASED ON SERUM THEOPHYLLINE MEASUREMENTS WHEN THESE INSTRUCTIONS HAVE NOT BEEN FOLLOWED MAY RESULT IN RECOMMENDATIONS THAT PRESENT RISK OF TOXICITY TO THE PATIENT.

V. Final adjustment of Dosage:
Dosage adjustment after serum theophylline measurement

If serum theophylline is:		Directions:
Within normal	10 to 20 μg/ml	Maintain dosage if tolerated. Recheck serum theophylline concentration at 6- to 12-month intervals.*
Too high	20 to 25 μg/ml	Decrease doses about 10%. Recheck serum theophylline concentration at 6- to 12-month intervals.*
	25 to 30 μg/ml	Skip next dose and decrease subsequent doses about 25%. Recheck serum theophylline.
	Over 30 μg/ml	Skip next 2 doses and decrease subsequent doses by 50%. Recheck serum theophylline.
Too low	7.5 to 10 μg/ml	Increase dose by about 25%.** Recheck serum theophylline concentration at 6- to 12-month intervals.*
	5 to 7.5 μg/ml	Increase dose by about 25% to the nearest dose increment and recheck serum theophylline for guidance in further dosage adjustment (another increase will probably be needed, but this provides a safety check).

* Finer adjustments in dosage may be needed for some patients
** The total drug dose may need to be administered at more frequent intervals if symptoms occur repeatedly at the end of the dosing interval.

Caution should be exercised for younger children who cannot complain of minor side effects. Older adults, those with cor pulmonale, congestive heart failure, and/or liver disease may have unusually low dosage requirements and thus may experience toxicity at the maximal dosage recommended above.

It is important that no patient be maintained on any dosage that is not tolerated. In instructing patients to increase dosage according to the schedule above, they should be instructed not to take a subsequent dose if apparent side effects occur and to resume therapy at a lower dose once adverse effects have disappeared.

How Supplied:
THEOPHYL®-SR (anhydrous theophylline) 125 mg capsules (yellow and clear, imprinted "Theophyl" and "125"), NDC 0045-0422, bottles of 100.
THEOPHYL®-SR (anhydrous theophylline) 250 mg capsules (green and clear, imprinted "Theophyl" and "250"), NDC 0045-0423, bottles of 100.
Store at controlled room temperature (15°—30°C, 59°—86°F). Protect from moisture.
Dispense in tight, light-resistant container as defined in the official compendium.
Manufactured by:
CORD LABORATORIES, INC.
BROOMFIELD, CO 80020
Marketed by:
McNEIL PHARMACEUTICAL
McNEILAB, Inc.
SPRING HOUSE, PA 19477
11/21/84

THEOPHYL®-225
[thē-a-fil]
(anhydrous theophylline)
TABLETS and ELIXIR
for oral use

Description: Each scored, white tablet contains not less than 94.0 percent and not more than 106.0 percent of 225 mg anhydrous theophylline USP. Each 30 ml (two TABLESPOONFULS) of banana-mint flavored THEOPHYL elixir contains not less than 94.0 percent and not more than 106.0 percent of 225 mg anhydrous theophylline, USP, and 225 mg calcium salicylate as a solubilizing agent, with 5% alcohol.

Theophylline anhydrous, a xanthine bronchodilator, is a white, odorless crystalline powder having a bitter taste.

Clinical Pharmacology: Theophylline directly relaxes the smooth muscle of the bronchial airways and pulmonary blood vessels, thus acting mainly as a bronchodilator and smooth muscle relaxant. The drug also produces other actions typical of the xanthine derivatives: coronary vasodilator, cardiac stimulant, diuretic, cerebral stimulant, and skeletal muscle stimulant. The actions of theophylline may be mediated through inhibition of phosphodiesterase and a resultant increase in intracellular cyclic AMP.

In vitro, theophylline has been shown to act synergistically with beta agonists that increase intracellular cyclic AMP through the stimulation of adenyl cyclase, but synergism has not been demonstrated in patient studies. More data are needed to determine if theophylline and beta agonists have a clinically important additive effects *in vivo.* Apparently, no development of tolerance occurs with chronic use of theophylline.

Pharmacokinetics: The half-life of theophylline is influenced by a number of variables. It is prolonged in patients suffering from chronic alcoholism, impaired hepatic or renal function, congestive heart failure, and in patients receiving macrolide antibiotics and cimetidine. Older adults (over age 55) and patients with chronic obstructive pulmonary disease, with or without cor pulmonale, may also have much slower clearance rates. For such patients, the theophylline half-life may exceed 24 hours.

THEOPHYLLINE ELIMINATION CHARACTERISTICS:

	Theophylline Clearance Rates (mean ± S.D.)	Half-Life Average (mean ± S.D.)
Children (over 6 months of age)	1.45 ± 0.58 ml/kg/min	3.7 ± 1.1 hours
Adult nonsmokers uncomplicated asthma	0.65 ± 0.19 ml/kg/min	8.7 ± 2.2 hours

Newborns and neonates have extremely slow clearance rates compared to older infants (over 6 months) and children, and may also have a theophylline half-life of over 24 hours. High fever for prolonged periods may also reduce the rate of theophylline elimination.

The half-life of theophylline in smokers (1 to 2 packs/day) averaged 4 to 5 hours, much shorter than the 7 to 9 hour half-life in nonsmokers. The increase in theophylline clearance caused by smoking is probably the result of induction of drug-metabolizing enzymes that do not readily normalize after cessation of smoking. It appears that between 3 months and 2 years may be necessary for normalization of the effect of smoking on theophylline pharmacokinetics.

Indications: For relief and/or prevention of symptoms from asthma and reversible bronchospasm associated with chronic bronchitis and emphysema.

Contraindications: THEOPHYL tablets and elixir are contraindicated in individuals who have shown hypersensitivity to any of their components.

Warnings: Status asthmaticus should be considered a medical emergency and is defined as the degree of bronchospasm which is not rapidly responsive to usual doses of conventional bronchodilators. Optimal therapy for such patients frequently requires both **additional medication,** parenterally administered, and **close monitoring,** preferably in an intensive care setting.

Although increasing the dose of theophylline may bring about relief, such treatment may be associated with toxicity. The likelihood of such toxicity developing increases significantly when the serum theophylline concentration exceeds 20 μg/ml. Therefore, determination of serum theophylline levels is recommended to assure maximal benefit without excessive risk.

Serum levels above 20 μg/ml are rarely found after appropriate administration of the recommended doses. However, in individuals in whom theophylline plasma clearance is reduced **for any reason**, even conventional doses may result in increased serum levels and potential toxicity. Reduced theophylline clearance has been documented in the following readily identifiable groups: 1) patients with impaired renal or liver funtion; 2) patients over 55 years of age, particularly males and those with chronic lung disease; 3) those with cardiac failure from any cause; 4) neonates; and 5) those patients taking certain drugs (macrolide antibiotics and cimetidine). Decreased clearance of theophylline may be associated with either influenza immunization or active infection with influenza.

Reduction of dosage and laboratory monitoring is especially appropriate in the above individuals. Less serious signs of theophylline toxicity, i.e. nausea and restlessness, may appear in up to 50% of patients. Unfortunately however, serious side effects such as ventricular arrhythmias, convulsions or even death may appear as the first sign of toxicity without any previous warning. Stated differently; **serious toxicity is not reliably preceded by less severe side effects.**

Many patients who require theophylline may exhibit tachycardia due to their underlying disease process so that the cause/effect relationship to elevated serum theophylline concentrations may not be appreciated.

Theophylline products may cause dysrhythmia and/or worsen pre-existing arrhythmias and any significant change in rate and/or rhythm warrants monitoring and further investigation.

The occurence of arrhythmias and sudden death (with histological evidence of necrosis of the myocardium) has been recorded in laboratory animals (minipigs, rodents and dogs) when theophylline and beta agonists were administered concomitantly, although not when either was administered alone. The significance of these findings when applied to human usage is currently unknown.

THEOPHYL elixir contains 37.5 mg of calcium salicylate per cc as a solubilizing agent. Therefore, concomitant use of aspirin should either be avoided (by use of acetaminophen for analgesia and antipyresis) or should be confined to a dose that provides a total (aspirin and calcium salicylate) of no more than 15 mg/kg at intervals of 6 hours or longer.

Intolerance to aspirin is not intolerance to salicylates generally; aspirin-sensitive patients are not more likely to react to other salicylates such as calcium salicylate than to unrelated materials.

Precautions:
General: Theophylline half-life is shorter in smokers than in nonsmokers. Therefore, smokers may require larger or more frequent doses. Morphine and curare should be used with caution in patients with airway obstruction as they may suppress respiration and stimulate histamine release. Alternative drugs should be used when possible. THEOPHYL-225 should not be administered concurrently with other xanthine medications. Use with caution in patients with severe cardiac disease, severe hypoxemia, hypertension, hyperthyroidism, acute myocardial injury, cor pulmonale, congestive heart failure, liver disease in the elderly (especially males) and in neonates. In particular, great caution should be used in giving theophylline to patients in congestive heart failure. Frequently, such patients have markedly prolonged theophylline serum levels with theophylline persisting in serum for long periods following discontinuation of the drug.

Use THEOPHYL-225 cautiously in patients with history of peptic ulcer. Theophylline may occasionally act as a local irritant to G.I. tract although gastrointestinal symptoms are more commonly centrally mediated and associated with serum drug concentrations over 20 μg/ml.

Information for Patients: The physician should reinforce the importance of taking only the prescribed dose and the time interval between doses. If necessary, taking the drug with food will help avoid local irritation of the G.I. tract.

Drug Interactions: Toxic synergism with ephedrine has been documented and may occur with some other sympathomimetic bronchodilators. In addition, the following drug interactions have been demonstrated:

DRUG	EFFECT
Lithium Carbonate	Increased excretion of lithium carbonate
Propranolol	Antagonism of propranolol effect
Cimetidine	Increases theophylline blood levels
Troleandomycin, erythromycin	Increased theophylline blood levels

Drug—Laboratory Test Interactions: When plasma levels of theophylline are measured by spectrophotometric methods; coffee, tea, cola beverages, chocolate, and acetaminophen contribute falsely high values.

Carcinogenesis, Mutagenesis, and Impairment of Fertility: Long-term animal studies have not been performed to evaluate the carcinogenic potential, mutagenic potential, or the effect on fertility of xanthine compounds.

Pregnancy: Category C—Animal reproduction studies have not been conducted with theophylline. It is not known whether theophylline can cause fetal harm when administered to a pregnant woman or can affect reproduction capacity. Xanthines should be given to a pregnant woman only if clearly needed.

Nursing Mothers: It has been reported that theophylline distributes readily into breast milk and may cause adverse effects in the infant. Caution must be used if prescribing xanthines to a mother who is nursing, taking into account the risk-benefit of this therapy.

Pediatric Use: Due to the marked variation in theophylline metabolism in infants under 6 months of age, this drug is not recommended for this age group.

Adverse Reactions: The most consistent adverse reactions to theophylline are usually due to overdose and are:
Gastrointestinal: nausea, vomiting, epigastric pain, hematemesis, diarrhea.
Central nervous system: headaches, irritability, restlessness, insomnia, reflex hyperexcitability, muscle twitching, clonic and tonic generalized convulsions.
Cardiovascular: palpitation, tachycardia, extrasystoles, flushing, hypotension, circulatory failure, ventricular arrhythmias.
Respiratory: tachypnea.
Renal: albuminuria, increased excretion of renal tubular cells and red blood cells, potentiation of diuresis.
Others: hyperglycemia and inappropriate ADH syndrome, rash.

Overdosage:
Management: If potential overdose is established and seizure has not occurred:
 a. Induce vomiting.
 b. Administer a cathartic.
 c. Administer activated charcoal.
If patient is having a seizure:
 a. Establish an airway.
 b. Administer oxygen.
 c. Treat the seizure with intravenous diazepam, 0.1 to 0.3 mg/kg up to 10 mg.
 d. Monitor vital signs, maintain blood pressure and provide adequate hydration.
Post seizure coma:
 a. Maintain airway and oxygenation.
 b. In addition to the above recommendations to prevent absorption of drug, intubation and lavage will have to be performed instead of inducing emesis, and the cathartic and charcoal will need to be introduced via a large bore gastric lavage tube.
 c. Continue to provide full supportive care and adequate hydration while waiting for drug to be metabolized. In general, the drug is metabolized sufficiently rapidly so as not to warrant consideration of dialysis; however, if serum levels exceed 50μg/ml, charcoal hemoperfusion may be indicated.

Dosage and Administration: For most patients, effective use of theophylline, i.e. associated with optimal likelihood for benefit combined with minimal risk of toxicity, is considered to occur when serum levels are maintained between 10 and 20 μg/ml. Levels above 20 μg/ml may produce toxicity, and in a small number of patients, toxicity may even be seen with serum levels between 15–20 μg/ml, particularly during initiation of therapy.

There is considerable variation from patient to patient in dosage required to achieve and maintain therapeutic and safe levels, primarily due to variable rates of elimination. Therefore, it is essential that not only must dosage be individualized, but titration and monitoring of serum levels be utilized where available. When serum concentration cannot be obtained, restriction of dosage to the amounts and intervals recommended in the guidelines listed below becomes essential. As theophylline does not distribute into fatty tissue, dosage should be calculated on the basis of lean (ideal) weight. Giving THEOPHYL-225 with food may prevent some local gastric irritation and though absorption may be slower, it is still complete.

Frequency of Dosing: When immediate release products with rapid absorption (such as tablets or liquid) are used, dosing to maintain serum levels generally requires administration every 6 hours. This is particularly true in children, but dosing intervals up to 8 hours may be satisfactory in adults since they eliminate the drug at a slower rate. Some children, and adults requiring higher than average doses (those having rapid rates of clearance, e.g. half-lives of under 6 hours) may benefit and be more effectively controlled during chronic therapy when given products with sustained-release characteristics, such as THEOPHYL®-SR capsules, since these provide longer dosing intervals and/or less fluctuation in serum concentration between dosing. Those sustained release products which provide flexibility in dosage through formulations of varying strengths are also helpful in controlling serum levels.

Dosage guidelines are approximations only. and the wide range of theophylline clearance between individuals (particularly those with concomitant disease) makes indiscriminate usage hazardous. As a practical consideration, it is not always possible to obtain serum level determinations. Under such conditions, restriction of the daily dose (in otherwise healthy adults) to not greater than 16 mg/kg/day (anhydrous theophylline) in divided doses will result in relatively few patients exceeding serum levels of 20 μg/ml and the resultant risk of toxicity.

Dosage Guidelines: I. Acute Symptoms of Asthma Requiring Rapid Theophyllinization
A. Dosage of THEOPHYL-225 tablets and elixir for Patients Exhibiting Acute Symptoms of Asthma Requiring Rapid Theophyllinization and **not** Currently Receiving Theophylline Products.

Loading Dose	Maintenance Dose For Next 12 Hours	Maintenance Dose Beyond 12 Hours
Children 6 months to 9 years		
6 mg/kg	4 mg/kg q4h	4 mg/kg q6h
Children age 9–16 and young adult smokers		
6 mg/kg	3 mg/kg q4h	3 mg/kg q6h
Otherwise healthy nonsmoking adults		
6 mg/kg	3 mg/kg q6h	3 mg/kg q8h
Older patients and patients with cor pulmonale		
6 mg/kg	2 mg/kg q6h	2 mg/kg q8h
Patients with congestive heart failure, liver failure		
6 mg/kg	2 mg/kg q8h	1–2 mg/kg q12h

B.Dosage for Patients Currently Receiving Theophylline Therapy.
Determine, where possible, the time, amount, route of administration and form of the patient's last dose. Ideally, the loading dose should be de-

Continued on next page

McNeil Pharm.—Cont.

ferred if a serum theophylline determination can be rapidly obtained. If this is not possible, the clinician must exercise his judgment in selecting a dose based on the potential for benefit and risk. The loading dose of theophylline is based on the principle that each 0.5 mg/kg of theophylline administered as a loading dose will result in a 1 µg/ml increase in serum theophylline concentration. When there is sufficient respiratory distress to warrant a small risk, 2.5 mg/kg of theophylline is likely to increase the serum concentration by only about 5 µg/ml when administered as a loading dose. If the patient is not already experiencing theophylline toxicity, this is unlikely to result in dangerous adverse effects. Subsequent maintenance dosage recommendations are the same as those described above.

II. Dosage for Chronic Asthma.

Theophyllinization is a treatment of first choice for the management of chronic asthma (to prevent symptoms and maintain patent airways). Slow clinical titration is generally preferred to assure acceptance and safety of the medication.

Initial Dosage: 16 mg/kg/day or 400 mg/day (whichever is lower) in the 3–4 divided doses at 6–8 hour intervals.

Increasing Dosage: The above dosage may be increased in approximately 25 percent increments at 2–3 day intervals so long as no intolerance is observed, until a maximum indicated below (III.) is reached.

III. Maximum Dose of Theophylline Where the Serum Concentration is Not Measured.

Not to exceed the following:

Age < 9 years	24 mg/kg/day
Age 9–12 years	20 mg/kg/day
Age 12–16 years	18 mg/kg/day
Age > 16 years	13 mg/kg/day
	OR 900 mg/day
	(WHICHEVER IS LESS)

WARNING: DO NOT ATTEMPT TO MAINTAIN ANY DOSE THAT IS NOT TOLERATED.

IV. Measurement of Serum Theophylline Concentrations During Chronic Therapy:

If the above maximum doses are to be maintained or exceeded, serum theophylline measurement is recommended. The serum sample should be obtained at the time of peak absorption, which has been shown to be 2.0 ± 0.3 hours for THEOPHYL-225 tablets and 1.4 ± 0.3 hours for THEOPHYL-225 elixir. It is important that the patient will have missed no doses during the previous 48 hours and that dosing intervals will have been reasonably typical with no added doses during that period of time. DOSAGE ADJUSTMENT BASED ON SERUM THEOPHYLLINE MEASUREMENTS WHEN THESE INSTRUCTIONS HAVE NOT BEEN FOLLOWED MAY RESULT IN RECOMMENDATIONS THAT PRESENT RISK OF TOXICITY TO THE PATIENT.

V. Final adjustment of Dosage:

Dosage adjustment after serum theophylline measurement.

If serum theophylline is:		Directions:
Within normal	10 to 20 µg/ml	Maintain dosage if tolerated. Recheck serum theophylline concentration at 6- to 12-month intervals.*
Too high	20 to 25 µg/ml	Decrease doses about 10%. Recheck serum theophylline concentrations at 6- to 12-month intervals.*
	25 to 30 µg/ml	Skip next dose and decrease subsequent doses about 25%. Recheck serum theophylline.
	Over 30 µg/ml	Skip next 2 doses and decrease subsequent doses by 50%. Recheck serum theophylline.
Too low	7.5 to 10 µg/ml	Increase dose by about 25%.** Recheck serum theophylline concentration at 6- to 12-month intervals.*
	5 to 7.5 µg/ml	Increase dose by about 25% to the nearest dose increment and recheck serum theophylline for guidance in further dosage adjustment (another increase will probably be needed, but this provides a safety check).

*Finer adjustments in dosage may be needed for some patients

**The total daily dose may need to be administered at more frequent intervals if symptoms occur repeatedly at the end of a dosing intervals.

Caution should be exercised for younger children who cannot complain of minor side effects. Older adults, those with cor pulmonale, congestive heart failure, and/or liver disease may have unusually low dosage requirements and thus may experience toxicity at the maximal dosage recommended above.

It is important that no patient be maintained on any dosage that is not tolerated. In instructing patients to increase dosage according to the schedule above, they should be instructed not to take a subsequent dose if apparent side effects occur and to resume therapy at a lower dose once adverse effects have disappeared.

How Supplied: THEOPHYL®-225 tablets (anhydrous theophylline) 225 mg (white, triangle shaped, bisected, imprinted "THEOPHYL 225") NDC 0045-0424, bottles of 100.

THEOPHYL®-225 elixir (anhydrous theophylline) 225 mg per 30 ml (2 TABLESPOONFULS) (colored orange yellow, banana-mint flavored), NDC 0045-0421, pint bottles (473 ml).

Store at 59°–86° F (15°–30° C).

Dispense in tight, light-resistant container as defined in the official compendium.

Manufactured by:
KNOLL PHARMACEUTICAL
WHIPPANY, NJ 07981

Marketed by:
McNEIL PHARMACEUTICAL
McNEILAB, Inc.
SPRING HOUSE, PA 19477

7612800A   Revised 3/21/84

TOLECTIN® DS (tolmetin sodium) ℞
[tōl-ek-tin]
capsules
TOLECTIN® (tolmetin sodium) tablets
200 mg tablets—100's:
Military NSN 6505-01-038-7460
VA NSN 6505-01-038-7460A
400 mg capsules—100's:
VA NSN 6505-01-091-9624A

Description: TOLECTIN DS (tolmetin sodium) capsules for oral administration contain tolmetin sodium as the dihydrate in an amount equivalent to 400 mg of tolmetin. Each capsule contains 36 mg (1.568 mEq) of sodium.

TOLECTIN (tolmetin sodium) tablets for oral administration contain tolmetin sodium as the dihydrate in an amount equivalent to 200 mg of tolmetin (scored for 100 mg). Each tablet contains 18 mg (0.784 mEq) of sodium.

Tolmetin sodium is a non-steroidal anti-inflammatory agent.

Clinical Pharmacology: Studies in animals have shown TOLECTIN (tolmetin sodium) to possess anti-inflammatory, analgesic and antipyretic activity. In the rat, TOLECTIN prevents the development of experimentally induced polyarthritis and also decreases established inflammation.

The mode of action of TOLECTIN is not known. However, studies in laboratory animals and man have demonstrated that the anti-inflammatory action of TOLECTIN is *not* due to pituitary-adrenal stimulation. TOLECTIN inhibits prostaglandin synthetase *in vitro* and lowers the plasma level of prostaglandin E in man. This reduction in prostaglandin synthesis may be responsible for the anti-inflammatory action. TOLECTIN does not appear to alter the course of the underlying disease in man.

In patients with rheumatoid arthritis and in normal volunteers, TOLECTIN is rapidly and almost completely absorbed with peak plasma levels being reached within 30–60 minutes after an oral therapeutic dose. The drug is eliminated from the plasma with a mean half-life of one hour. Peak plasma levels of approximately 40 µg/ml are obtained with a 400 mg oral dose. Essentially all of the administered dose is recovered in the urine in 24 hours either as an inactive oxidative metabolite or as conjugates of TOLECTIN.

In two fecal blood loss studies of 4 to 6 days duration involving 15 subjects each, TOLECTIN did not induce an increase in blood loss over that observed during a 4-day drug-free control period. In the same studies, aspirin produced a greater blood loss than occurred during the drug-free control period, and a greater blood loss than occurred during the TOLECTIN treatment period. In one of the two studies, indomethacin produced a greater fecal blood loss than occurred during the drug-free control period; in the second study, indomethacin did not induce a significant increase in blood loss.

TOLECTIN does not interfere with the clinical assessment of the tuberculin skin test or the immediate-type hypersensitivity skin test. It appears that the drug does not interfere with the immune mechanism as measured by skin testing.

Indications and Usage: TOLECTIN (tolmetin sodium) is indicated for the relief of signs and symptoms of rheumatoid arthritis and osteoarthritis. TOLECTIN is indicated in the treatment of acute flares and the long-term management of the chronic disease. TOLECTIN is also indicated for treatment of juvenile rheumatoid arthritis.

The safety and effectiveness of TOLECTIN have not been established in those patients with rheumatoid arthritis who are designated by the American Rheumatism Association as Functional Class IV (incapacitated, largely or wholly bedridden or confined to a wheelchair; little or no self-care).

Improvement in patients treated with TOLECTIN for rheumatoid arthritis has been demonstrated by a reduction in joint swelling, a reduction in pain, a reduction in the number of inflamed joints, a reduction in the duration of morning stiffness, a decrease in disease activity as assessed by both the investigator and the patient, and improved functional capability as demonstrated by an increase in grip strength, a delay in the time to onset of fatigue and a decrease in the time to walk 50 feet.

Improvement in patients treated with TOLECTIN for osteoarthritis has been demonstrated by a reduction of pain at rest and pain on motion, a reduction of swelling, redness and tenderness, a reduction in the duration of morning stiffness and in the inflammation of Heberden's Nodes, a decrease in disease activity as assessed by both the investigator and patient, an increase in range of motion of affected joints, a decrease in the time to walk 50 feet and an improved functional capability as demonstrated by an increase in grip strength and performance of daily activities.

In clinical studies in patients with either rheumatoid arthritis or osteoarthritis, TOLECTIN has been shown to be comparable to aspirin and to indomethacin in controlling disease activity but the frequency of the milder gastrointestinal adverse effects and tinnitus was less than in aspirin-treated patients, and the incidence of central nervous system adverse effects was less than in indomethacin-treated patients. It is not known whether TOLECTIN causes less peptic ulceration than aspirin or indomethacin.

Clinical studies have shown that, when added to a regimen of gold salts or corticosteroids, TOLECTIN has produced additional therapeutic benefit, although this effect was somewhat less when patients were receiving gold salts than when they were receiving corticosteroids. The use of TOLECTIN in conjunction with salicylates is not recommended since there does not appear to be any greater benefit from the combination over that achieved with aspirin alone, and the potential for adverse reactions is increased.

In clinical studies in patients with juvenile rheumatoid arthritis, TOLECTIN has been shown to be comparable to aspirin in controlling disease activity, with a similar incidence of adverse reactions. In liver function tests, mean SGOT values, initially elevated in patients on previous aspirin therapy, remained elevated in the aspirin group and decreased in the TOLECTIN group. The safety and effectiveness of TOLECTIN have not been established in infants under 2 years of age.

Contraindications: TOLECTIN (tolmetin sodium) should not be used in patients who have previously exhibited intolerance to it. Because the potential exists for cross-sensitivity to aspirin and other non-steroidal anti-inflammatory drugs, TOLECTIN should not be given to patients in whom aspirin and other non-steroidal anti-inflammatory drugs induce symptoms of asthma, rhinitis or urticaria.

Warnings: TOLECTIN (tolmetin sodium) should be given under close supervision to patients with a history of upper gastrointestinal tract disease and only after consulting the "Adverse Reactions" section. Peptic ulceration and gastrointestinal bleeding, sometimes severe, have been reported in patients receiving TOLECTIN.

In patients with active peptic ulcer, attempts should be made to treat the arthritis with non-ulcerogenic drugs, such as gold. If TOLECTIN must be given, the patient should be under close supervision for signs of ulcer perforation or severe gastrointestinal bleeding.

Precautions: *General:* Clinical studies of up to two years duration have shown no changes in the eyes attributable to TOLECTIN (tolmetin sodium) administration; however, because of microscopic changes in the lens in rats receiving TOLECTIN at doses about twice the maximum recommended dose in man and because of ocular changes observed clinically with other non-steroidal anti-inflammatory drugs, it is recommended that ophthalmologic examinations be carried out within a reasonable time after starting chronic therapy and at periodic intervals thereafter.

In a chronic study in rats, lesions of the renal papillae were observed at doses of TOLECTIN approximately twice the maximum recommended human dose. In a chronic study in mice, chronic nephritis and glomerular sclerosis occurred in animals receiving doses of one and a half times the human dose. In a chronic study in monkeys a single instance (one in eight) of renal papillary necrosis was observed at a dose more than three times the maximum recommended human dosage.

There has been no evidence of renal toxicity in clinical studies; however, renal failure, sometimes acutely associated with nephrotic syndrome, has been reported.

Since TOLECTIN is eliminated by the kidneys, patients with impaired renal function should be closely monitored, and they may require lower doses.

TOLECTIN prolongs bleeding time. Patients who may be adversely affected by prolongation of bleeding time should be carefully observed when TOLECTIN is administered.

In patients receiving concomitant TOLECTIN-steroid therapy, any reduction in steroid dosage should be gradual to avoid the possible complications of sudden steroid withdrawal.

TOLECTIN has been shown to cause some retention of water and sodium, and mild peripheral edema has been reported in about 7% of patients receiving TOLECTIN. Therefore, TOLECTIN should be used with caution in patients with compromised cardiac function.

The metabolites of tolmetin in urine have been found to give positive tests for proteinuria using tests which rely on acid precipitation as their endpoint (e.g. sulfosalicylic acid). No interference is seen in the tests for proteinuria using dye-impregnated commercially available reagent strips (e.g. Albustix®, Uristix®, etc.).

As with other nonsteroidal anti-inflammatory drugs, anaphylactoid reactions have been reported. Because of the possibility of cross-sensitivity due to structural relationships which exist among nonsteroidal anti-inflammatory drugs, anaphylactoid reactions may be more likely to occur in patients who have exhibited allergic reactions to these compounds, particularly zomepirac sodium. Patients who have had anaphylactoid reactions on TOLECTIN should be treated with conventional therapy, such as epinephrine, antihistamines, and/or steroids.

As with other nonsteroidal anti-inflammatory drugs, borderline elevations of one or more liver tests may occur in up to 15% of patients. These abnormalities may progress, may remain essentially unchanged, or may be transient with continued therapy. The SGPT (ALT) test is probably the most sensitive indicator of liver dysfunction. Meaningful (3 times the upper limit of normal) elevations of SGPT or SGOT (AST) occurred in controlled clinical trials in less than 1% of patients. A patient with symptoms and/or signs suggesting liver dysfunction, or in whom an abnormal liver test has occurred, should be evaluated for evidence of the development of more severe hepatic reaction while on therapy with TOLECTIN. Severe hepatic reactions, including jaundice and fatal hepatitis, have been reported with TOLECTIN as with other nonsteroidal anti-inflammatory drugs. Although such reactions are rare, if abnormal liver tests persist or worsen, if clinical signs and symptoms consistent with liver disease develop, or if systemic manifestations occur (e.g. eosinophilia, rash, etc.), TOLECTIN should be discontinued.

Usage in Pregnancy: Since TOLECTIN has not been studied in pregnant women, the use of TOLECTIN during pregnancy is not recommended. Reproduction studies in rats and rabbits at doses up to 1.7 times the maximum clinical dose revealed no evidence of impaired fertility or teratogenesis due to TOLECTIN. However, as with other non-steroidal anti-inflammatory drugs known to inhibit prostaglandin synthesis, an increased incidence of dystocia and delayed parturition occurs in rats. These effects were absent when TOLECTIN was discontinued 24 hours prior to expected delivery.

Nursing Mothers: It is not known whether TOLECTIN is secreted in human milk; however, it is secreted in the milk of lactating rats. As a general rule nursing should not be undertaken while a patient is on TOLECTIN since it may be excreted in human milk.

Drug Interactions: The *in vitro* binding of warfarin to human plasma proteins is unaffected by tolmetin, and tolmetin does not alter the prothrombin time of normal volunteers. However, in patients there have been rare reports that prothrombin time may increase and bleeding may occur.

In adult diabetic patients under treatment with either sulfonylureas or insulin there is no change in the clinical effects of either TOLECTIN or the hypoglycemic agents.

Adverse Reactions: The adverse reactions which have been observed in clinical trials encompass observations in about 4370 patients treated with TOLECTIN (tolmetin sodium), over 800 of whom have undergone at least one year of therapy. These adverse reactions, reported below by body system, are among those typical of nonsteroidal anti-inflammatory drugs and, as expected, gastrointestinal complaints were most frequent. In clinical trials with TOLECTIN, about 10% of patients dropped out because of adverse reactions, mostly gastrointestinal in nature.

Incidence Greater Than 1%

The following adverse reactions which occurred more frequently than 1 in 100 were reported in controlled clinical trials.

Gastrointestinal: Nausea (11%), dyspepsia,* gastrointestinal distress,* abdominal pain,* diarrhea,* flatulence,* vomiting,* constipation, gastritis, and peptic ulcer. Forty percent of the ulcer patients had a prior history of peptic ulcer disease and/or were receiving concomitant anti-inflammatory drugs including corticosteroids, which are known to produce peptic ulceration.

Body as a Whole: Headache,* asthenia,* chest pain
Cardiovascular: Elevated blood pressure,* edema*
Central Nervous System: Dizziness,* drowsiness, depression
Metabolic/Nutritional: Weight gain,* weight loss*
Dermatologic: Skin irritation
Special Senses: Tinnitus, visual disturbance
Hematologic: Small and transient decreases in hemoglobin and hematocrit not associated with gastrointestinal bleeding have occurred. These are similar to changes reported with other nonsteroidal anti-inflammatory drugs.
Urogenital: Elevated BUN, urinary tract infection

* Reactions occurring in 3% to 9% of patients treated with TOLECTIN. Reactions occurring in fewer than 3% of the patients are unmarked.

Incidence Less Than 1%
(Causal Relationship Probable)

The following adverse reactions were reported less frequently than 1 in 100 in controlled clinical trials or were reported since marketing. The probability exists that there is a causal relationship between TOLECTIN and these adverse reactions.
Gastrointestinal: Gastrointestinal bleeding with or without evidence of peptic ulcer, glossitis, stomatitis, hepatitis, liver function abnormalities
Body as a Whole: Anaphylactoid reactions, fever, lymphadenopathy
Hematologic: Hemolytic anemia, thrombocytopenia, granulocytopenia, agranulocytosis
Cardiovascular: Congestive heart failure in patients with marginal cardiac function
Dermatologic: Urticaria, purpura, erythema multiforme, toxic epidermal necrolysis
Urogenital: Hematuria, proteinuria, dysuria, renal failure

Incidence Less Than 1%
(Causal Relationship Unknown)

Other adverse reactions were reported less frequently than 1 in 100 in controlled clinical trials or were reported since marketing, but a causal relationship between TOLECTIN and the reaction could not be determined. These rarely reported reactions are being listed as alerting information for the physician since the possibility of a causal relationship cannot be excluded.
Body as Whole: Epistaxis

Management of Overdosage: In the event of overdosage, the stomach should be emptied by inducing vomiting or by gastric lavage followed by the administration of activated charcoal.

Dosage and Administration: In adults, the recommended starting dose is 400 mg three times daily (1200 mg daily), preferably including a dose on arising and a dose at bedtime. To achieve optimal therapeutic effect the dose should be adjusted according to the patient's response. For rheumatoid arthritis control is usually achieved at doses of 600–1800 mg daily in divided doses (t.i.d. or q.i.d.). For osteoarthritis control is usually achieved at doses of 600–1600 mg daily in divided doses (t.i.d. or q.i.d.). Doses larger than 2000 mg/day for rheumatoid arthritis and 1600 mg/day for osteoarthritis have not been studied and therefore are not recommended.

The recommended starting dose for children (two years and older) is 20 mg/kg/day in divided doses (t.i.d. or q.i.d.). When control has been achieved the usual dose ranges from 15 to 30 mg/kg/day. Doses higher than 30 mg/kg/day have not been studied and therefore are not recommended.

A therapeutic response to TOLECTIN (tolmetin sodium) can be expected in a few days to a week. Progressive improvement can be anticipated during succeeding weeks of therapy. If gastrointestinal symptoms occur, administer TOLECTIN with meals, milk or antacids, other than sodium bicarbonate.

How Supplied:
TOLECTIN® DS (tolmetin sodium) capsules 400 mg (colored orange opaque, with contrasting parallel bands imprinted "McNEIL" and "TOLECTIN

Continued on next page

McNeil Pharm.—Cont.

DS"), **NDC** 0045-0414, bottles of 100; and unit dose of 100's.

TOLECTIN® (tolmetin sodium) tablets 200 mg (colored white, scored, imprinted "200", "McNeil" and "TOLECTIN"), bottles of 100 (**NDC** 0045-0412); and 500.

Dispense in tight container as defined in the official compendium.

8/17/83

Shown in Product Identification Section, page 419

TYLENOL® with Codeine tablets ©,
[ti' len-awl co' děn]
capsules © and elixir ©   ℞

Description:
Each TYLENOL with Codeine tablet contains:
No. 1 Codeine Phosphate* .... 7.5 mg (⅛ gr)
  Acetaminophen .... 300 mg
No. 2 Codeine Phosphate* .... 15 mg (¼ gr)
  Acetaminophen .... 300 mg
No. 3 Codeine Phosphate* .... 30 mg (½ gr)
  Acetaminophen .... 300 mg
No. 4 Codeine Phosphate* .... 60 mg (1 gr)
  Acetaminophen .... 300 mg
Each TYLENOL with Codeine capsule contains:
No. 3 Codeine Phosphate* .... 30 mg (½ gr)
  Acetaminophen .... 300 mg
No. 4 Codeine Phosphate* .... 60 mg (1 gr)
  Acetaminophen .... 300 mg
Each 5 ml TYLENOL with Codeine elixir contains:
  Codeine Phosphate* .... 12 mg
  Acetaminophen .... 120 mg
    Alcohol 7%

*Warning—May be habit forming.

Acetaminophen is a non-salicylate analgesic-antipyretic which occurs as a white, odorless crystalline powder, possessing a slightly bitter taste.
Codeine is an opioid analgesic-antitussive. Codeine is an alkaloid obtained from opium or prepared from morphine by methylation. Codeine occurs as colorless or white crystals, effloresces slowly in dry air and is affected by light.

Clinical Pharmacology: TYLENOL with Codeine tablets, capsules and elixir combine the analgesic effects of a centrally acting analgesic, codeine, with a peripherally acting analgesic, acetaminophen. Both ingredients of TYLENOL with Codeine are well absorbed orally. Following oral administration of two TYLENOL with Codeine No. 3 tablets, a peak plasma codeine concentration of 173 ng/ml is reached at 75 minutes. After 6 hours, 27 percent of this remains in plasma. A peak plasma acetaminophen concentration of 7.3 μg/ml is reached 42 minutes after administration of two TYLENOL with Codeine No. 3 tablets. After 6 hours, 16 percent of the acetaminophen remains in plasma. The plasma elimination half-life is 2.3 hours for acetaminophen and 2.5 hours for codeine.

Codeine retains at least one-half of its analgesic activity when administered orally. A reduced first-pass metabolism of codeine by the liver accounts for the greater oral efficacy of codeine when compared to most other morphine-like narcotics. Following absorption, codeine is metabolized by the liver and metabolic products are excreted in the urine. Approximately 10 percent of the administered codeine is demethylated to morphine, which may account for its analgesic activity.

Acetaminophen is distributed throughout most tissues of the body. Acetaminophen is metabolized primarily in the liver. Little unchanged drug is excreted in the urine, but most metabolic products appear in the urine within 24 hours.

Indications and Usage: TYLENOL with Codeine No. 1, No. 2 (one or two), and No. 3 (one) are indicated for the relief of mild to moderate pain; two TYLENOL with Codeine No. 3 and one No. 4 are indicated for the relief of moderate to severe pain.
TYLENOL with Codeine elixir is indicated for the relief of mild to moderate pain.

Contraindications: TYLENOL with Codeine tablets, capsules or elixir should not be administered to patients who have previously exhibited hypersensitivity to codeine or acetaminophen.

Warnings:
Drug Dependence: Codeine can produce drug dependence of the morphine type, and therefore has the potential for being abused. Psychic dependence, physical dependence and tolerance may develop upon repeated administration of this drug, and it should be prescribed and administered with the same degree of caution appropriate to the use of other oral narcotic-containing medications. Like other narcotic-containing medications, this drug is subject to the Federal Controlled Substances Act.

Precautions:
General
Head Injury and Increased Intracranial Pressure: The respiratory depressant effects of narcotics and their capacity to elevate cerebrospinal fluid pressure may be markedly exaggerated in the presence of head injury, other intracranial lesions or a pre-existing increase in intracranial pressure. Furthermore, narcotics produce adverse reactions which may obscure the clinical course of patients with head injuries.
Acute Abdominal Conditions: The administration of this product or other narcotics may obscure the diagnosis or clinical course of patients with acute abdominal conditions.
Special Risk Patients: This drug should be given with caution to certain patients such as the elderly or debilitated, and those with severe impairment of hepatic or renal function, hypothyroidism, Addison's disease, and prostatic hypertrophy or urethral stricture.

Information for Patients
Codeine may impair the mental and/or physical abilities required for the performance of potentially hazardous tasks such as driving a car or operating machinery. The patient using this drug should be cautioned accordingly.

Drug Interactions
Patients receiving other narcotic analgesics, antipsychotics, anti-anxiety agents, or other CNS depressants (including alcohol) concomitantly with this drug may exhibit an additive CNS depression. When such combined therapy is contemplated, the dose of one or both agents should be reduced.
The use of MAO inhibitors or tricyclic antidepressants with codeine preparations may increase the effect of either the antidepressant or codeine.
The concurrent use of anticholinergics with codeine may produce paralytic ileus.

Carcinogenesis, Mutagenesis, Impairment of Fertility
No long-term studies in animals have been performed with acetaminophen or codeine to determine carcinogenic potential or effects on fertility. Acetaminophen and codeine have been found to have no mutagenic potential using the Ames Salmonella-Microsomal Activation test, the Basc test on Drosophila germ cells, and the Micronucleus test on mouse bone marrow.

Teratogenic Effects
Pregnancy Category C. Codeine has been shown to be teratogenic in mice when given in doses 17 times the maximum human daily dose. There are no adequate and well controlled studies in pregnant women. TYLENOL with Codeine should be used during pregnancy only if the potential benefit justifies the potential risk to the fetus.

Nursing Mothers
It is not known whether the components of this drug are excreted in human milk. Because many drugs are excreted in human milk, caution should be exercised when TYLENOL with Codeine is administered to a nursing woman.

Pediatric Use
Safe dosage of the elixir has not been established in children below the age of three; tablets and capsules should not be administered to children under 12.

Adverse Reactions: The most frequently observed adverse reactions include lightheadedness, dizziness, sedation, shortness of breath, nausea and vomiting. These effects seem to be more prominent in ambulatory than in non-ambulatory patients, and some of these adverse reactions may be alleviated if the patient lies down. Other adverse reactions include euphoria, dysphoria, constipation, and pruritus.
At higher doses codeine has most of the disadvantages of morphine including respiratory depression.

Drug Abuse and Dependence: TYLENOL with Codeine tablets and capsules are Schedule III controlled substances.
TYLENOL with Codeine elixir is a Schedule V controlled substance.
Codeine can produce drug dependence and has the potential for being abused (see WARNINGS).

Overdosage:
Acetaminophen
Signs and Symptoms: Acetaminophen in massive overdosage may cause hepatic toxicity in some patients. **In all cases of suspected overdose, immediately call your regional poison center or the Rocky Mountain Poison Center's toll-free number** (800-525-6115) for assistance in diagnosis and for directions in the use of N-acetylcysteine as an antidote, a use currently restricted to investigational status.
In adults, hepatic toxicity has rarely been reported with acute overdoses of less than 10 grams and fatalities with less than 15 grams. Importantly, young children seem to be more resistant than adults to the hepatotoxic effect of an acetaminophen overdose. Despite this, the measures outlined below should be initiated in any adult or child suspected of having ingested an acetaminophen overdose.
Early symptoms following a potentially hepatotoxic overdose may include: nausea, vomiting, diaphoresis and general malaise. Clinical and laboratory evidence of hepatic toxicity may not be apparent until 48 to 72 hours post-ingestion.
Treatment: The stomach should be emptied promptly by lavage or by induction of emesis with syrup of ipecac. Patients' estimates of the quantity of a drug ingested are notoriously unreliable. Therefore, if an acetaminophen overdose is suspected, a serum acetaminophen assay should be obtained as early as possible, but no sooner than four hours following ingestion. Liver function studies should be obtained initially and repeated at 24 hour intervals.
The antidote, N-acetylcysteine, should be administered as early as possible, and within 16 hours of the overdose ingestion for optimal results. Following recovery, there are no residual, structural or functional hepatic abnormalities.
Codeine
Signs and Symptoms: Serious overdose with codeine is characterized by respiratory depression (a decrease in respiratory rate and/or tidal volume, Cheyne-Stokes respiration, cyanosis), extreme somnolence progressing to stupor or coma, skeletal muscle flaccidity, cold and clammy skin, and sometimes bradycardia and hypotension. In severe overdosage, apnea, circulatory collapse, cardiac arrest and death may occur.
Treatment: Primary attention should be given to the reestablishment of adequate respiratory exchange through provision of a patent airway and the institution of assisted or controlled ventilation. The narcotic antagonist naloxone is a specific antidote against respiratory depression which may result from overdosage or unusual sensitivity to narcotics, including codeine. Therefore, an appropriate dose of naloxone (see package insert) should be administered, preferably by the intravenous route, and simultaneously with efforts at respiratory resuscitation. Since the duration of action of codeine may exceed that of the antagonist, the patient should be kept under continued surveillance and repeated doses of the antagonist should be administered as needed to maintain adequate respiration.
An antagonist should not be administered in the absence of clinically significant respiratory or cardiovascular depression. Oxygen, intravenous fluids, vasopressors and other supportive measures should be employed as indicated.
Gastric emptying may be useful in removing unabsorbed drug.

Dosage and Administration: Dosage should be adjusted according to severity of pain and response of the patient.

TYLENOL with Codeine tablets and capsules are given orally. The usual adult dose is: Tablets No. 1, No. 2, and No. 3 and Capsules No. 3: One or two every four hours as required. Tablets and Capsules No. 4: One every four hours as required.

The recommended dose of codeine in children is 0.5 mg/kg body weight.

TYLENOL with Codeine elixir contains 12 mg of codeine/5 ml teaspoon and is given orally. The usual doses are:

Children (3 to 6 years): 1 teaspoonful (5 ml) 3 or 4 times daily; *(7 to 12 years):* 2 teaspoonsful (10 ml) 3 or 4 times daily; *(under 3 years):* safe dosage has not been established.

Adults: 1 tablespoonful (15 ml) every 4 hours as needed.

How Supplied: TYLENOL® with Codeine tablets (white, imprinted "McNEIL," "TYLENOL CODEINE" and either "1", "2", "3", "4") No. 1—NDC 0045-0510-60, bottles of 100; No. 2—NDC 0045-0511, bottles of 100 and 500; No. 3—NDC 0045-0513, bottles of 100, 500, and 1000; and No. 4—NDC 0045-0515—bottles of 100 and 500. No. 2, No. 3, and No. 4 also available in a Unit Dose Dispensit (20 × 25).

TYLENOL® with Codeine capsules No. 3 (colored white with red bands, imprinted "McNeil"/ "TYLENOL 3 CODEINE")—NDC 0045-0521, bottles of 100 and unit dose of 100's; TYLENOL® with Codeine capsules No. 4 (colored red with white bands, imprinted "McNeil" and "TYLENOL 4 CODEINE")—NDC 0045-0522, bottles of 100 and unit dose of 100's.

TYLENOL® with Codeine elixir (colored amber, cherry flavored)—NDC 0045-0508-16, bottles of 1 pint.

Dispense in tight, light-resistant container as defined in the official compendium.

Manufactured by McNeil Pharmaceutical Co., Dorado, PR 00646.

9/15/82

Shown in Product Identification Section, page 419

TYLOX® capsules ⓒ ℞
[ti' lox]
(oxycodone and acetaminophen)
100's
Military NSN 6505-01-053-8621
Unit Dose (100's) 6505-01-053-8622

Description: Each capsule contains:
Oxycodone Hydrocholoride .... 4.5 mg.
  Warning—May be habit forming.
Oxycodone Terephthalate .... 0.38 mg
  Warning—May be habit forming.
Acetaminophen .... 500 mg

Oxycodone, a semisynthetic narcotic, is a white, odorless crystalline powder which is derived from the opium alkaloid, thebaine.

TYLOX capsules also contain the nonsalicylate analgesic-antipyretic acetaminophen.

Acetaminophen occurs as a white, odorless crystalline powder possessing a slightly bitter taste.

Clinical Pharmacology: TYLOX capsules combine the analgesic effects of a potent centrally acting analgesic, oxycodone, with a peripherally acting analgesic, acetaminophen. This combination is well absorbed orally. Following oral administration of one TYLOX capsule, a peak oxycodone plasma level of 11.0 ng/ml is reached after 120 minutes. After 6 hours, 19% of this level remains in plasma. The plasma elimination half-life of oxycodone is 132 minutes. A peak plasma acetaminophen concentration of 5.8 μg/ml is reached 65 minutes following the administration of one TYLOX capsule. After 6 hours, 16% of this level of acetaminophen remains in plasma. The plasma elimination half-life of acetaminophen is 116 minutes.

TYLOX capsules have been shown in well-controlled clinical studies to significantly relieve pain as early as one-half hour after administration. This pain relief lasted for as long as six hours.

Acetaminophen is distributed throughout most tissues of the body. Acetaminophen is metabolized primarily in the liver. Little unchanged drug is excreted in the urine, but most metabolic products appear in the urine within 24 hours.

Indications and Usage: TYLOX capsules are indicated for the relief of moderate to moderately severe pain.

Contraindications: TYLOX capsules should not be administered to patients who have previously exhibited hypersensitivity to oxycodone or acetaminophen.

Warnings:

Drug dependence: Oxycodone can produce drug dependence of the morphine type and, therefore, has the potential for being abused. Psychic dependence, physical dependence, and tolerance may develop upon repeated administration of TYLOX capsules, and they should be prescribed and administered with the same degree of caution appropriate to the use of other oral narcotic-containing medications. Like other narcotic-containing medications, TYLOX capsules are subject to the Federal Controlled Substances Act.

Precautions:
General
Head Injury and Increased Intracranial Pressure: The respiratory depressant effects of narcotics and their capacity to elevate cerebrospinal fluid pressure may be markedly exaggerated in the presence of head injury, other intracranial lesions, or a preexisting increase in intracranial pressure. Furthermore, narcotics produce adverse reactions which may obscure the clinical course of patients with head injuries.

Acute Abdominal Conditions: The administration of TYLOX capsules or other narcotics may obscure the diagnosis or clinical course in patients with acute abdominal conditions.

Special Risk Patients: TYLOX capsules should be given with caution to certain patients such as the elderly or debilitated, and those with severe impairment of hepatic or renal function, hypothyroidism, Addison's disease, and prostatic hypertrophy or urethral stricture.

Information for Patients
Oxycodone may impair the mental and/or physical abilities required for the performance of potentially hazardous tasks such as driving a car or operating machinery. The patient using TYLOX capsules should be cautioned accordingly.

Drug Interactions
Patients receiving other narcotic analgesics, antipsychotics, antianxiety agents, or other CNS depressants, including alcohol, concomitantly with TYLOX capsules, may exhibit additive CNS depression due to the oxycodone component. When such combined therapy is contemplated, the dose of one or both agents should be reduced.

The use of MAO inhibitors or tricyclic antidepressants with oxycodone preparations may increase the effect of either the antidepressant or oxycodone.

The concurrent use of anticholinergics with oxycodone may produce paralytic ileus.

Carcinogenesis, Mutagenesis, Impairment of Fertility
No long-term studies in animals have been performed with oxycodone to determine carcinogenic and mutagenic potential, or effects on fertility. Acetaminophen has been found to have no mutagenic potential using the Ames Salmonella-Microsomal Activation test, the Basc test on Drosophila germ cells, and the Micronucleus test on mouse bone marrow. In animals, acetaminophen has not been evaluated for carcinogenic potential or for effects on fertility.

Teratogenic Effects
Pregnancy Category C. Animal reproductive studies have not been conducted with TYLOX. It is also not known whether TYLOX can cause fetal harm when administered to a pregnant woman or can affect reproductive capacity. TYLOX should be given to a pregnant woman only if clearly needed.

Nursing Mothers
It is not known whether the components of this drug are excreted in human milk. Because many drugs are excreted in human milk, caution should be exercised when TYLOX is administered to a nursing woman.

Pediatric Use
TYLOX capsules should not be administered to children.

Adverse Reactions: The most frequently observed adverse reactions include lightheadedness, dizziness, sedation, nausea, and vomiting. These effects seem to be more prominent in ambulatory patients than in non-ambulatory patients, and some of these adverse reactions may be alleviated if the patient lies down.

Other adverse reactions include euphoria, dysphoria, constipation, skin rash, and pruritus.

At higher doses oxycodone has most of the disadvantages of morphine including respiratory depression.

Drug Abuse and Dependence: TYLOX capsules are a Schedule II controlled substance.

Oxycodone can produce drug dependence and has the potential for being abused. (see WARNINGS)

Overdosage:
Acetaminophen
Signs and Symptoms: Acetaminophen in massive overdosage may cause hepatic toxicity in some patients. In all cases of suspected overdose, immediately call your regional poison center or the Rocky Mountain Poison Center's toll-free number (800-525-6115) for assistance in diagnosis and for directions in the use of N-acetylcysteine as an antidote, a use currently restricted to investigational status.

In adults, hepatic toxicity has rarely been reported with acute overdoses of less than 10 grams and fatalities with less than 15 grams. Importantly, young children seem to be more resistant than adults to the hepatotoxic effect of an acetaminophen overdose. Despite this, the measures outlined below should be initiated in any adult or child suspected of having ingested an acetaminophen overdose.

Early symptoms following a potentially hepatotoxic overdose may include: nausea, vomiting, diaphoresis, and general malaise. Clinical and laboratory evidence of hepatic toxicity may not be apparent until 48 to 72 hours post-ingestion.

Treatment: The stomach should be emptied promptly by lavage or by induction of emesis with syrup of ipecac. Patients' estimates of the quantity of a drug ingested are notoriously unreliable. Therefore, if an acetaminophen overdose is suspected, a serum acetaminophen assay should be obtained as early as possible, but no sooner than four hours following ingestion. Liver function studies should be obtained initially and repeated at 24-hour intervals.

The antidote, N-acetylcysteine, should be administered as early as possible, and within 16 hours of the overdose ingestion for optimal results. Following recovery, there are no residual, structural, or functional hepatic abnormalities.

Oxycodone
Signs and symptoms: Serious overdosage with oxycodone is characterized by respiratory depression (a decrease in respiratory rate and/or tidal volume, Cheyne-Stokes respiration, cyanosis), extreme somnolence progressing to stupor or coma, skeletal muscle flaccidity, cold and clammy skin, and sometimes bradycardia and hypotension. In severe overdosage, apnea, circulatory collapse, cardiac arrest, and death may occur.

Treatment: Primary attention should be given to the reestablishment of adequate respiratory exchange through provision of a patent airway and the institution of assisted or controlled ventilation. The narcotic antagonist naloxone is a specific antidote against respiratory depression which may result from overdosage or unusual sensitivity to narcotics, including oxycodone. Therefore, an appropriate dose of naloxone should be administered (see package insert) preferably by the intravenous route and simultaneously with efforts at respiratory resuscitation. Since the duration of action of oxycodone may exceed that of the antagonist, the patient should be kept under continued

Continued on next page

McNeil Pharm.—Cont.

surveillance, and repeated doses of the antagonist should be administered as needed to maintain adequate respiration.

An antagonist should not be administered in the absence of clinically significant respiratory or cardiovascular depression.

Oxygen, intravenous fluids, vasopressors, and other supportive measures should be employed as indicated.

Gastric emptying may be useful in removing unabsorbed drug.

Dosage and Administration: Dosage should be adjusted according to the severity of the pain and the response of the patient.

TYLOX capsules are given orally. The usual adult dose is one TYLOX capsule every 6 hours as needed for pain.

How Supplied: TYLOX® capsules (colored red, imprinted "TYLOX McNEIL") NDC 0045-0525—bottles of 100 and unit dose 25's.

Dispense in tight container as defined in the official compendium.

2/17/82

Shown in Product Identification Section, page 419

Mead Johnson Laboratories
Mead Johnson & Company
2404 W. PENNSYLVANIA ST.
EVANSVILLE, INDIANA 47721

ESTRACE®
[es' trās]
(Estradiol)

WARNING
1. ESTROGENS HAVE BEEN REPORTED TO INCREASE THE RISK OF ENDOMETRIAL CARCINOMA.

Three independent case control studies have shown an increased risk of endometrial cancer in postmenopausal women exposed to exogenous estrogens for prolonged periods.[1-3] This risk was independent of the other known risk factors for endometrial cancer. These studies are further supported by the finding that incidence rates of endometrial cancer have increased sharply since 1969 in eight different areas of the United States with population based cancer reporting systems, an increase which may be related to the rapidly expanding use of estrogens during the last decade.[4]

The three case control studies reported that the risk of endometrial cancer in estrogen users was about 4.5 to 13.9 times greater than in nonusers. The risk appears to depend on both duration of treatment[1] and on estrogen dose.[3] In view of these findings, when estrogens are used for the treatment of menopausal symptoms, the lowest dose that will control symptoms should be utilized and medication should be discontinued as soon as possible. When prolonged treatment is medically indicated, the patient should be reassessed on at least a semiannual basis to determine the need for continued therapy. Although the evidence must be considered preliminary, one study suggests that cyclic administration of low doses of estrogen may carry less risk than continuous administration;[3] it therefore appears prudent to utilize such a regimen.

Close clinical surveillance of all women taking estrogens is important. In all cases of undiagnosed persistent or recurring abnormal vaginal bleeding, adequate diagnostic measures should be undertaken to rule out malignancy.

There is no evidence at present that "natural" estrogens are more or less hazardous than "synthetic" estrogens at equiestrogenic doses.

2. ESTROGENS SHOULD NOT BE USED DURING PREGNANCY.

The use of female sex hormones, both estrogens and progestogens, during early pregnancy may seriously damage the offspring. It has been shown that females exposed *in utero* to diethylstilbestrol, a non-steroidal estrogen, have an increased risk of developing in later life a form of vaginal or cervical cancer that is ordinarily extremely rare.[5,6] This risk has been estimated as not greater than 4 per 1000 exposures.[7] Furthermore, a high percentage of such exposed women (from 30 to 90 percent) have been found to have vaginal adenosis,[8-12] epithelial changes of the vagina and cervix. Although these changes are histologically benign, it is not known whether they are precursors of malignancy. Although similar data are not available with the use of other estrogens, it cannot be presumed they would not induce similar changes.

Several reports suggest an association between intrauterine exposure to female sex hormones and congenital anomalies, including congenital heart defects and limb reduction defects.[13-16] One case control study[16] estimated a 4.7-fold increased risk of limb reduction defects in infants exposed *in utero* to sex hormones (oral contraceptives, hormone withdrawal tests for pregnancy, or attempted treatment for threatened abortion). Some of these exposures were very short and involved only a few days of treatment. The data suggest that the risk of limb reduction defects in exposed fetuses is somewhat less than 1 per 1000.

In the past, female sex hormones have been used during pregnancy in an attempt to treat threatened or habitual abortion. There is considerable evidence that estrogens are ineffective for these indications, and there is no evidence from well controlled studies that progestogens are effective for these uses.

If Estrace® is used during pregnancy, or if the patient becomes pregnant while taking this drug, she should be apprised of the potential risks to the fetus and the advisability of pregnancy continuation.

Description: Estrace® oral tablets contain 1 or 2 mg. of micronized estradiol. Estradiol (17β-estradiol) is a white, crystalline solid, chemically described as estra-1,3,5(10)-triene-3,17β-diol. Estrace® oral tablets provide estrogen replacement therapy. The structural formula is:

Clinical Pharmacology

17β-Estradiol is the most potent physiologic estrogen and, in fact, is the major estrogenic hormone secreted by the human. Estradiol in Estrace® has been micronized and demonstrated to be rapidly and effectively absorbed from the gastrointestinal tract.[17]

Indications: Estrace® affords effective treatment of:

1. Moderate to severe *vasomotor* symptoms associated with the menopause. (There is no evidence that estrogens are effective for nervous symptoms or depression which might occur during menopause, and they should not be used to treat these conditions.) **2.** Atrophic vaginitis. **3.** Kraurosis vulvae. **4.** Female hypogonadism. **5.** Female castration. **6.** Primary ovarian failure. **7.** Breast cancer (for palliation only) in appropriately selected women and men with metastatic disease. **8.** Prostatic carcinoma—palliative therapy of advanced disease.

ESTRACE® HAS NOT BEEN SHOWN TO BE EFFECTIVE FOR ANY PURPOSE DURING PREGNANCY AND ITS USE MAY CAUSE SEVERE HARM TO THE FETUS (SEE BOXED WARNING).

Contraindications: Estrogens should not be used in women (or men) with any of the following conditions: **1.** Known or suspected cancer of the breast except in appropriately selected patients being treated for metastatic disease. **2.** Known or suspected estrogen-dependent neoplasia. **3.** Known or suspected pregnancy (See Boxed Warning). **4.** Undiagnosed abnormal genital bleeding. **5.** Active thrombophlebitis or thromboembolic disorders. **6.** A past history of thrombophlebitis, thrombosis or thromboembolic disorders associated with previous estrogen use (except when used in treatment of breast or prostatic malignancy).

Warnings:

1. Induction of malignant neoplasms. Long term continuous administration of natural and synthetic estrogens in certain animal species increases the frequency of carcinomas of the breast, cervix, vagina, and liver. There is now evidence that estrogens increase the risk of carcinoma of the endometrium in humans. (See Boxed Warning).

At the present time there is no satisfactory evidence that estrogens given to postmenopausal women increase the risk of cancer of the breast,[18] although a recent long-term followup of a single physician's practice has raised this possibility.[19] Because of the animal data there is a need for caution in prescribing estrogens for women with a strong family history of breast cancer or who have breast nodules, fibrocystic disease, or abnormal mammograms.

2. Gall bladder disease. A recent study has reported a 2 to 3-fold increase in the risk of surgically confirmed gall bladder disease in women receiving postmenopausal estrogens,[18] similar to the 2-fold increase previously noted in users of oral contraceptives. In the case of oral contraceptives,[20,34] the increased risk appeared after two years of use.[34]

3. Effects similar to those caused by estrogen-progestogen oral contraceptives. There are several serious adverse effects of oral contraceptives, most of which have not, up to now, been documented as consequences of postmenopausal estrogen therapy. This may reflect the comparatively low doses of estrogen used in postmenopausal women. It would be expected that the larger doses of estrogen used to treat prostatic or breast cancer or postpartum breast engorgement are more likely to result in these adverse effects, and, in fact, it has been shown that there is an increased risk of thrombosis in men receiving estrogens for prostatic cancer and women for postpartum breast engorgement.[21-24]

a. **Thromboembolic disease.** It is now well established that users of oral contraceptives have an increased risk of various thromboembolic and thrombotic vascular diseases, such as thrombophlebitis, pulmonary embolism, stroke, and myocardial infarction.[25-32] Cases of retinal thrombosis, xmesenteric thrombosis, and optic neuritis have been reported in oral contraceptive users. There is evidence that the risk of several of these adverse reactions is related to the dose of the drug.[33,34] An increased risk of post-surgery thromboembolic complications has also been reported in users of oral contraceptives.[35-36] If feasible, estrogen should be discontinued at least 4 weeks before surgery of the type associated with an increased risk of thromboembolism, or during periods of prolonged immobilization.

While an increased rate of thromboembolic and thrombotic disease in postmenopausal users of estrogens has not been found,[19,37] this does not rule out the possibility that such an increase may be present or that subgroups of women who have underlying risk factors or who are receiving relatively large doses of estrogens may have increased risk. Therefore estrogens should not be used in persons with active thrombophlebitis or thromboembolic disorders, and they should not be used (except in treatment of malignancy) in persons with a history of such disorders in association with estrogen use. They should be used with caution in patients with cerebral vascular or coronary artery disease and only for those in whom estrogens are clearly needed.

Large doses of estrogen (5 mg conjugated estrogens per day), comparable to those used to treat cancer of the prostate and breast, have been shown in a large prospective clinical trial in men[38] to increase the risk of nonfatal myocardial infarction, pulmonary embolism and thrombophlebitis. When estrogen doses of this size are used, any of the thromboembolic and thrombotic adverse effects associated with oral contraceptive use should be considered a clear risk.

    b. **Hepatic adenoma.** Hepatic adenomas appear to be associated with the use of oral contraceptives.[39-41] Although rare, these may rupture and may cause death through intraabdominal hemorrhage. Such lesions have not yet been reported in association with other estrogen or progestogen preparations but should be considered in estrogen users having abdominal pain and tenderness, abdominal mass, or hypovolemic shock. Hepatocellular carcinoma has also been reported in women taking estrogen-containing oral contraceptives.[40] The relationship of this malignancy to these drugs is not known at this time.

    c. **Elevated blood pressure.** Increased blood pressure is not uncommon in women using oral contraceptives. There is now a report that this may occur with use of estrogens in the menopause[42] and blood pressure should be monitored with estrogen use, especially if high doses are used.

    d. **Glucose tolerance.** A worsening of glucose tolerance has been observed in a significant percentage of patients on estrogen-containing oral contraceptives. For this reason, diabetic patients should be carefully observed while receiving estrogen.

4. **Hypercalcemia.** Administration of estrogens may lead to severe hypercalcemia in patients with breast cancer and bone metastases. If this occurs, the drug should be stopped and appropriate measures taken to reduce the serum calcium level.

Precautions:
A. General Precautions.
1. A complete medical and family history should be taken prior to the initiation of any estrogen therapy. The pretreatment and periodic physical examinations should include special reference to blood pressure, breasts, abdomen, and pelvic organs, and should include a Papanicolaou smear. As a general rule, estrogen should not be prescribed for longer than one year without another physical examination being performed.
2. Fluid retention—Because estrogens may cause some degree of fluid retention, conditions which might be influenced by this factor such as epilepsy, migraine, and cardiac or renal dysfunction, require careful observation.
3. Certain patients may develop undesirable manifestations of excessive estrogenic stimulation, such as abnormal or excessive uterine bleeding, mastodynia, etc.
4. Oral contraceptives appear to be associated with an increased incidence of mental depression. Although it is not clear whether this is due to the estrogenic or progestogenic component of the contraceptive, patients with a history of depression should be carefully observed.
5. Preexisting uterine leiomyomata may increase in size during estrogen use.
6. The pathologist should be advised of estrogen therapy when relevant specimens are submitted.
7. Patients with a past history of jaundice during pregnancy have an increased risk of recurrence of jaundice while receiving estrogen-containing oral contraceptive therapy. If jaundice develops in any patient receiving estrogen, the medication should be discontinued while the cause is investigated.
8. Estrogens may be poorly metabolized in patients with impaired liver function and they should be administered with caution in such patients.
9. Because estrogens influence the metabolism of calcium and phosphorus, they should be used with caution in patients with metabolic bone diseases that are associated with hypercalcemia or in patients with renal insufficiency.
10. Because of the effects of estrogens on epiphyseal closure, they should be used judiciously in young patients in whom bone growth is not complete.
11. Certain endocrine and liver function tests may be affected by estrogen-containing oral contraceptives. The following similar changes may be expected with larger doses of estrogen:
    a. Increased sulfobromophthalein retention.
    b. Increased prothrombin and factors VII and VIII, IX, and X; decreased antithrombin 3; increased norepinephrine-induced platelet aggregability.
    c. Increased thyroid binding globulin (TBG) leading to increased circulating total thyroid hormone, as measured by PBI, T4 by column, or T4 by radioimmunoassay. Free T3 resin uptake is decreased, reflecting the elevated TBG; free T4 concentration is unaltered.
    d. Impaired glucose tolerance.
    e. Decreased pregnanediol excretion.
    f. Reduced response to metyrapone test.
    g. Reduced serum folate concentration.
    h. Increased serum triglyceride and phospholipid concentration.
B. Information for the Patient. See text of Patient Package Insert.
C. Pregnancy Category X. See Contraindications and Boxed Warning.
D. Nursing Mothers. As a general principle, the administration of any drug to nursing mothers should be done only when clearly necessary since many drugs are excreted in human milk.

Estrace 2 mg tablets contain FD&C Yellow No. 5 (tartrazine) which may cause allergic-type reactions (including bronchial asthma) in certain susceptible individuals. Although the overall incidence of FD&C Yellow No. 5 (tartrazine) sensitivity in the general population is low, it is frequently seen in patients who also have aspirin hypersensitivity.

Adverse Reactions: (See Warnings regarding induction of neoplasia, adverse effects on the fetus, increased incidence of gall bladder disease, and adverse effects similar to those of oral contraceptives, including thromboembolism.) The following additional adverse reactions have been reported with estrogenic therapy, including oral contraceptives:
1. **Genitourinary system.**
Breakthrough bleeding, spotting, change in menstrual flow.
Dysmenorrhea.
Premenstrual-like syndrome.
Amenorrhea during and after treatment.
Increase in size of uterine fibromyomata.
Vaginal candidiasis.
Change in cervical eversion and in degree of cervical secretion.
Cystitis-like syndrome.
2. **Breast.**
Tenderness, enlargement, secretion.
3. **Gastrointestinal.**
Nausea, vomiting.
Abdominal cramps, bloating.
Cholestatic jaundice.
4. **Skin.**
Chloasma or melasma which may persist when drug is discontinued.
Erythema multiforme.
Erythema nodosum.
Hemorrhagic eruption.
Loss of scalp hair.
Hirsutism.
5. **Eyes.**
Steepening of corneal curvature.
Intolerance to contact lenses.
6. **CNS.**
Headache, migraine, dizziness.
Mental depression.
Chorea.
7. **Miscellaneous.**
Increase or decrease in weight.
Reduced carbohydrate tolerance.
Aggravation of porphyria.
Edema.
Changes in libido.

Acute Overdosage: Numerous reports of ingestion of large doses of estrogen-containing oral contraceptives by young children indicate that serious ill effects do not occur. Overdosage of estrogen may cause nausea, and withdrawal bleeding may occur in females.

Dosage and Administration:
1. **Given cyclically for short term use only:**
For treatment of moderate to severe **vasomotor** symptoms, atrophic vaginitis, or kraurosis vulvae associated with the menopause.
The lowest dose that will control symptoms should be chosen and medication should be discontinued as promptly as possible.
Administration should be cyclic (e.g., 3 weeks on and 1 week off).
Attempts to discontinue or taper medication should be made at 3 to 6 month intervals.
The usual initial dosage range is 1 or 2 mg. daily of micronized estradiol adjusted as necessary to control presenting symptoms. The minimal effective dose for maintenance therapy should be determined by titration.
2. **Given cyclically:**
Female hypogonadism.
Female castration.
Primary ovarian failure.
Treatment is usually initiated with a dose of 1 or 2 mg. daily of micronized estradiol, adjusted as necessary to control presenting symptoms; the minimal effective dose for maintenance therapy should be determined by titration.
3. Given chronically:
Inoperable progressing prostatic cancer—Suggested dosage is 1 to 2 mg. three times daily. The effectiveness of therapy can be judged by phosphatase determinations as well as by symptomatic improvement of the patient.
Inoperable progressing breast cancer in appropriately selected men and postmenopausal women (see INDICATIONS)—Suggested dosage is 10 mg. three times daily for a period of at least three months.
Treated patients with an intact uterus should be monitored closely for signs of endometrial cancer and appropriate diagnostic measures should be taken to rule out malignancy in the event of persistent or recurring abnormal vaginal bleeding.

How Supplied:
Estrace 1 mg; lavender scored tablets
NDC 0087-0755-01   Bottles of 100
Estrace 2 mg; turquoise scored tablets
NDC 0087-0756-01   Bottles of 100

PATIENT LABELING
What You Should Know About Estrogens: Estrogens are female hormones produced principally by the ovaries. The ovaries make several different kinds of estrogens. In addition, scientists have been able to make a variety of synthetic estrogens. As far as we know, all these estrogens have the same properties and therefore much the same usefulness, side effects, and risks. This leaflet is intended to help you understand what estrogens are used for, the risks involved in their use, and how to use them as safely as possible.

This leaflet includes important information about Estrace® (estradiol) and estrogens in general, but not all the information. If you want to know more you can ask your doctor or pharmacist to let you read the professional package insert.

Uses of Estrogen: Estrogens are prescribed by doctors for a number of purposes, including:
1. To provide estrogen during a period of adjustment when a woman's ovaries no longer produce it, in order to prevent certain uncomfortable symptoms of estrogen deficiency. (All women normally experience a decrease in the production of estrogens, generally between 45-55; this is called the menopause.)
2. To prevent symptoms of estrogen deficiency when a woman's ovaries have been removed surgically before the natural menopause.

Continued on next page

Mead Johnson Labs.—Cont.

3. To prevent pregnancy. (Some estrogens are given along with a progestogen, another female hormone; these combinations are called oral contraceptives or birth control pills. They will not be discussed in this leaflet.) However, Estrace is not intended for this use.
4. To treat certain cancers in women and men.
5. To prevent painful swelling of the breasts after pregnancy in women who choose not to nurse their babies.

THERE IS NO PROPER USE OF ESTROGENS IN A PREGNANT WOMAN.

Estrogens in The Menopause: In the natural course of their lives, all women eventually experience a decrease in estrogen production. This usually occurs between ages 45 and 55 but may occur earlier or later. Sometimes the ovaries may need to be removed before natural menopause by an operation, producing a "surgical menopause." When the amount of estrogen in the blood begins to decrease, many women may develop typical symptoms: feelings of warmth in the face, neck, and chest or sudden intense episodes of heat and sweating throughout the body (called "hot flashes" or "hot flushes"). These symptoms are sometimes very uncomfortable. A few women eventually develop changes in the vagina (called "atrophic vaginitis") which cause discomfort, especially during and after intercourse.

Estrogens can be prescribed to treat these symptoms of the menopause. It is estimated that considerably more than half of all women undergoing the menopause have only mild symptoms or no symptoms at all and therefore do not need estrogens. Other women may need estrogens for a few months, while their bodies adjust to lower estrogen levels. Sometimes the need will be for periods longer than six months. In an attempt to avoid over-stimulation of the uterus (womb), estrogens are usually given cyclically during each month of use, that is three weeks of pills followed by one week without pills.

Sometimes women experience nervous symptoms or depression during menopause. There is no evidence that estrogens are effective for such symptoms and they should not be used to treat them, although other treatment may be needed.

You may have heard that taking estrogens for long periods (years) after the menopause will keep your skin soft and supple and keep you feeling young. There is no evidence that this is so, however, and such long-term treatment carries additional risks.

Estrogens To Prevent Swelling of The Breasts After Pregnancy: If you do not breast feed your baby after delivery, your breasts may fill up with milk and become painful and engorged. This usually begins about three to four days after delivery and may last for a few days to up to a week or more. Sometimes the discomfort is severe, but usually it is not and can be controlled by pain-relieving drugs such as aspirin and by binding the breasts up tightly. Estrogens can sometimes be used successfully to try to prevent the breasts from filling up. While this treatment is sometimes successful, in many cases the breasts fill up to some degree in spite of treatment. The dose of estrogens needed to prevent pain and swelling of the breasts is much larger than the dose needed to treat symptoms of the menopause and this may increase your chances of developing blood clots in the legs or lungs or other parts of the body (see below, 4. Abnormal Blood Clotting). Therefore, it is important that you discuss the benefits and the risks of estrogen use with your doctor, before using estrogen, if you have decided not to breast feed your baby.

The Dangers of Estrogens:
1. **Cancer of the uterus.** If estrogens are used in the postmenopausal period for more than a year, there is an increased risk of **cancer of the endometrium** (uterine lining). Women taking estrogens have roughly 5 to 15 times as great a chance of getting this cancer as women who take no estrogens. To put this another way, while a postmenopausal woman not taking estrogens has one chance in 1,000 each year of getting cancer of the uterus, a woman taking estrogens has 5 to 15 chances in 1,000 each year. For this reason **it is important to take estrogens only when you really need them.**

The risk of this cancer is greater the longer estrogens are used and also seems to be greater when larger doses are taken. For this reason **it is important to take the lowest dose of estrogen that will control symptoms and to take it only as long as it is needed.** If estrogens are needed for longer periods of time, your doctor will want to reevaluate your need for estrogens at least every six months.

Women using estrogens should report any irregular vaginal bleeding to their doctors; such bleeding may be of no importance, but it can be an early warning of cancer of the uterus. If you have undiagnosed vaginal bleeding, you should not use estrogens until a diagnosis is made and you are certain there is no cancer of the uterus. If you have had your uterus completely removed (total hysterectomy), there is no danger of developing cancer of the uterus.

2. **Other possible cancers.** Estrogens can cause development of other tumors in animals, such as tumors of the breast, cervix, vagina, or liver, when given for a long time. At present there is no satisfactory evidence that women using estrogens in the menopause have an increased risk of such tumors, but there is no way yet to be sure they do not; and one study raises the possibility that use of estrogens in the menopause may increase the risk of breast cancer many years later. This is a further reason to use estrogens only when clearly needed. While you are taking estrogens, it is important that you go to your doctor at least once a year for a physical examination. Also, if members of your family have had breast cancer or if you have breast nodules or abnormal mammograms (breast x-rays), your doctor may wish to carry out more frequent examinations.

3. **Gall bladder disease.** Women who use estrogens after menopause are two or three times more likely to develop gall bladder disease needing surgery than women who do not use estrogens. Birth control pills have a similar effect.

4. **Abnormal blood clotting.** Oral contraceptives increase the risk of blood clotting in various parts of the body. This can occur in different parts of the circulatory system causing thrombophlebitis (clot in the legs or pelvis), retinal thrombosis or optic neuritis (clots affecting vision, including blindness), mesenteric thrombosis (clots in the intestinal blood vessels), stroke (clot in the brain), heart attack (clot in a vessel of the heart) or a pulmonary embolism (clot which eventually lodges in the lungs). These can be fatal.

At this time use of estrogens in the menopause is not known to cause increased blood clotting, this has not been fully studied and there could still prove to be such a risk. It is recommended that if you have had clotting in the legs or lungs or a heart attack or stroke while you were using estrogens or birth control pills, you should not use estrogens (unless they are being used to treat cancer of the breast or prostate). If you have had a stroke or heart attack or if you have angina pectoris, estrogens should be used with great caution and only if clearly needed (for example, if you have severe symptoms of the menopause).

The larger doses of estrogen used to prevent swelling of the breasts after pregnancy have been reported to cause abnormal blood clotting **as indicated above.**

Special Warning About Pregnancy: You should not receive estrogen if you are pregnant. If this should occur, there is a greater than usual chance that the developing child will be born with a birth defect, although the possibility remains fairly small. A female child may have an increased risk of developing cancer of the vagina or cervix later in life (in the teens or twenties). Every possible effort should be made to avoid exposure to estrogens during pregnancy. If exposure occurs, see your doctor.

Other Effects of Estrogens: In addition to the serious known risks of estrogens described above, estrogens may have the following side effects and potential risks which, if occurring, should be discussed promptly with your doctor.

1. **Nausea and vomiting.** The most common side effect of estrogen therapy is nausea. Vomiting is less common.
2. **Effects on breasts.** Estrogens may cause breast tenderness or enlargement and may cause the breasts to secrete a liquid.
3. **Effects on the uterus.** Estrogens may cause benign fibroid tumors of the uterus to get larger. Some women will have menstrual bleeding when estrogens are stopped. But if the bleeding occurs on days you are still taking estrogens, you should report this to your doctor.
4. **Effects on liver.** Women taking oral contraceptives develop on rare occasions a tumor of the liver which can rupture, bleed into the abdomen, and cause death. So far, these tumors have not been reported in women using estrogens in the menopause, but you should report any swelling or unusual pain or tenderness in the abdomen to your doctor immediately.

Women with a past history of jaundice (yellowing of the skin and white parts of the eyes) may get jaundice again during estrogen use. If this occurs, stop taking estrogens and see your doctor.

5. **Other effects.** Estrogens may cause excess fluid to be retained in the body. This may make some conditions worse, such as epilepsy, migraine, heart disease, or kidney disease. Mental depression or high blood pressure may occur. A spotty darkening of the skin, particularly of the face, is possible and may persist.

Summary: Estrogens have important uses, and they may have serious risks as well. You must decide, with your doctor, whether the risks are acceptable to you in view of the benefits of treatment. Except where your doctor has prescribed estrogens for use in special cases of cancer of the breast or prostate, you should not use estrogens if you have cancer of the breast or uterus, are pregnant, have undiagnosed abnormal vaginal bleeding, clotting in the legs or lungs or have had a stroke, heart attack or angina, or clotting in the legs or lungs in the past while you were taking estrogens.

You can use estrogens as safely as possible by understanding that your doctor will require regular physical examinations while you are taking them and will try to discontinue the drug as soon as possible and use the smallest dose possible. Be alert for signs of trouble including:

1. Abnormal bleeding from the vagina.
2. Pains in the calves or chest or sudden shortness of breath, or coughing blood (indicating possible clots in the legs, heart, or lungs).
3. Severe headache, dizziness, faintness, or changes in vision (indicating possible developing clots in the brain or eye).
4. Breast lumps (you should ask your doctor how to examine your own breasts).
5. Jaundice (yellowing of the skin).
6. Mental depression.

Based on his or her assessment of your medical needs, your doctor has prescribed this drug for you. Do not give the drug to anyone else.

References:
1. Ziel HK, Finkel WD: Increased risk of endometrial carcinoma among users of conjugated estrogens. New Eng J Med 293:1167–1170, 1975.
2. Smith DC, Prentice R, Thompson DJ, Herrmann WL: Association of exogenous estrogen and endometrial carcinoma. New Eng J Med 293:1164–1167, 1975.
3. Mack TM, Pike MC, Henderson BE, et al: Estrogens and endometrial cancer in a retirement community. New Eng J Med 294:1262–1267, 1976.
4. Weiss NS, Szekely DR, Austin DF: Increasing incidence of endometrial cancer in the United States. New Eng J Med 294:1259–1262, 1976.

5. Herbst AL, Ulfelder H, Poskanzer DC: Adenocarcinoma of vagina. New Eng J Med 284:878–881, 1971.
6. Greenwald P, Barlow J, Nasca P, Burnett W: Vaginal cancer after maternal treatment with synthetic estrogens. New Eng J Med 285:390–392, 1971.
7. Lanier A, Noller K, Decker D, et al: Cancer and stilbestrol. A follow-up of 1719 persons exposed to estrogens in utero and born 1943–1959. Mayo Clin Proceedings 48:793–799, 1973.
8. Herbst A, Kurman R, Scully R: Vaginal and cervical abnormalities after exposure to stilbestrol in utero. Obstet and Gynec 40:287–298, 1972.
9. Herbst A, Robboy S, Macdonald G, Scully R: The effects of local progesterone on stilbestrol-associated vaginal adenosis. Am J Obstet Gynec 118:607–615, 1974.
10. Herbst A, Poskanzer D, Robboy S, et al: Prenatal exposure to stilbestrol, a prospective comparison of exposed female offspring with unexposed controls. New Eng J Med 292:334–339, 1975.
11. Stafl A, Mattingly R, Foley D, Fetherston W: Clinical diagnosis of vaginal adenosis. Obstet and Gynec 43:118–128, 1974.
12. Sherman Al, Goldrath M, Berlin A, et al: Cervical-vaginal adenosis after in utero exposure to synthetic estrogens. Obstet Gynec 44:531–545, 1974.
13. Gal I, Kirman B, Stern J: Hormone pregnancy tests and congenital malformation. Nature 216:83, 1967.
14. Levy EP, Cohen A, Fraser FC: Hormone treatment during pregnancy and congenital heart defects. Lancet 1:611, 1973.
15. Nora J, Nora A: Birth defects and oral contraceptives. Lancet 1:941–942, 1973.
16. Janerich DT, Piper JM, Glebatis DM: Oral contraceptives and congenital limb-reduction defects. New Eng J Med 291:697–700, 1974.
17. Yen SSC, Martin PL, Burnier AM, et al: Circulating estradiol, estrone and gonadotropin levels following the administration of orally active 17β-estradiol in postmenopausal women. J Clin Endocrinol Metab 40:518–521, 1975.
18. Boston Collaborative Drug Surveillance Program: Surgically confirmed gall bladder disease, venous thromboembolism and breast tumors in relation to post-menopausal estrogen therapy. New Eng J Med 290:15–19, 1974.
19. Hoover R, Gray LA Sr, Cole P, MacMahon B: Menopausal estrogens and breast cancer. New Eng J Med 295:15–19, 1974.
20. Boston Collaborative Drug Surveillance Program: Oral contraceptives and venous thromboembolic disease, surgically confirmed gall bladder disease, and breast tumors. Lancet 1:1399–1404, 1973.
21. Daniel DG, Campbell H, Turnbull AC: Puerperal thromboembolism and suppression of lactation. Lancet 2:287–289, 1967.
22. The Veterans Administration Cooperative Urological Research Group: Carcinoma of the prostate: treatment comparisons. J Urol 98:516–522, 1967.
23. Bailar JC: Thromboembolism and oestrogen therapy. Lancet 2:560, 1967.
24. Blackard C, Doe R, Mellinger G, Byar D: Incidence of cardiovascular disease and death in patients receiving diethylstilbestrol for carcinoma of the prostate. Cancer 26:249–256, 1970.
25. Royal College of General Practitioners: Oral contraception and thromboembolic disease. J Roy Coll Gen Pract 13:267–279, 1967.
26. Inman WHW, Vessey MP: Investigation of deaths from pulmonary, coronary, and cerebral thrombosis and embolism in women of child-bearing age. Brit M J 2:193–199, 1968.
27. Vessey MP, Doll R: Investigation of relation between use of oral contraceptives and thromboembolic disease. A further report. Brit M J 2:651–657, 1969.
28. Sartwell PE, Masi AT, Arthes FG, et al: Thromboembolism and oral contraceptives: an epidemiological case control study. Am J Epidemiol 90:365–380, 1969.
29. Collaborative Group for the Study of Stroke in Young Women: Oral contraception and increased risk of cerebral ischemia or thrombosis. New Eng J Med 288:871–878, 1973.
30. Collaborative Group for the Study of Stroke in Young Women: Oral contraceptives and stroke in young women: Associated risk factors. JAMA 231:718–722, 1975.
31. Mann JI, Inman WHW: Oral contraceptives and death from myocardial infarction. Brit M J 2:245–248, 1975.
32. Mann JI, Vessey MP, Thorogood M, Doll R: Myocardial infarction in young women with special reference to oral contraceptive practice. Brit M J 2:241–245, 1975.
33. Inman WHW, Vessey VP, Westerholm B, Engelund A: Thromboembolic disease and the steroidal content of oral contraceptives. Brit M J 2:203–209, 1970.
34. Stolley PD, Tonascia JA, Tockman MS, et al: Thrombosis with low-estrogen oral contraceptives. Am J Epidemiol 102:197–208, 1975.
35. Vessey MP, Doll R, Fairbairn AS, Glober G: Post-operative thromboembolism and the use of the oral contraceptives. Brit M J 3:123–126, 1970.
36. Greene GR, Sartwell PE: Oral contraceptive use in patients with thromboembolism following surgery, trauma or infection. Am J Pub Health 62:680–685, 1972.
37. Rosenberg L, Armstrong MB, Jick H: Myocardial infarction and estrogen therapy in postmenopausal women. New Eng J Med 294:1256–1259, 1976.
38. Coronary Drug Project Research Group: The coronary drug project: initial findings leading to modifications of its research protocol. JAMA 214:1303–1313, 1970.
39. Baum J, Holtz F, Bookstein JJ, Klein EW: Possible association between benign hepatomas and oral contraceptives. Lancet 2:926–928, 1973.
40. Mays ET, Christopherson WM, Mahr MM, Williams HC: Hepatic changes in young women ingesting contraceptive steroids, hepatic hemorrhage and primary hepatic tumors. JAMA 235:730–732, 1976.
41. Edmondson HA, Henderson B, Benton B: Liver cell adenomas associated with the use of oral contraceptives. New Eng J Med 294:470–472, 1976.
42. Pfeffer RI, Van Den Noort S: Estrogen use and stroke risk in postmenopausal women. Am J Epidemiol 103:445–456, 1976.

Shown in Product Identification Section, page 419

ESTRACE®
[ĕs′ trace]
(Estradiol Vaginal Cream 0.01%)

WARNING
1. ESTROGENS HAVE BEEN REPORTED TO INCREASE THE RISK OF ENDOMETRIAL CARCINOMA.

Three independent case control studies have shown an increased risk of endometrial cancer in postmenopausal women exposed to exogenous estrogens for prolonged periods.[1–3] This risk was independent of the other known risk factors for endometrial cancer. These studies are further supported by the finding that incidence rates of endometrial cancer have increased sharply since 1969 in eight different areas of the United States with population-based cancer reporting systems, an increase which may be related to the rapidly expanding use of estrogens during the last decade.[4]

The three case control studies reported that the risk of endometrial cancer in estrogen users was about 4.5 to 13.9 times greater than in nonusers. The risk appears to depend on both duration of treatment[1] and on estrogen dose.[3] In view of these findings, when estrogens are used for the treatment of menopausal symptoms, the lowest dose that will control symptoms should be utilized and medication should be discontinued as soon as possible. When prolonged treatment is medically indicated, the patient should be reassessed on at least a semiannual basis to determine the need for continued therapy. Although the evidence must be considered preliminary, one study suggests that cyclic administration of low doses of estrogen may carry less risk than continuous administration,[3] it therefore appears prudent to utilize such a regimen.

Close clinical surveillance of all women taking estrogens is important. In all cases of undiagnosed persistent or recurring abnormal vaginal bleeding, adequate diagnostic measures should be undertaken to rule out malignancy.

There is no evidence at present that "natural" estrogens are more or less hazardous than "synthetic" estrogens at equiestrogenic doses.

2. ESTROGENS SHOULD NOT BE USED DURING PREGNANCY.

The use of female sex hormones, both estrogens and progestogens, during early pregnancy may seriously damage the offspring. It has been shown that females exposed *in utero* to diethylstilbestrol, a non-steroidal estrogen, have an increased risk of developing in later life a form of vaginal or cervical cancer that is ordinarily extremely rare.[5,6] This risk has been estimated as not greater than 4 per 1,000 exposures.[7] Furthermore, a high percentage of such exposed women (from 30 to 90 percent) have been found to have vaginal adenosis,[9–12] epithelial changes of the vagina and cervix. Although these changes are histologically benign, it is not known whether they are precursors of malignancy. Although similar data are not available with the use of other estrogens, it cannot be presumed they would not induce similar changes.

Several reports suggest an association between intrauterine exposure to female sex hormones and congenital anomalies, including congenital heart defects and limb reduction defects.[13–16] One case control study[16] estimated a 4.7-fold increased risk of limb reduction defects in infants exposed *in utero* to sex hormones (oral contraceptives, hormone withdrawal tests for pregnancy, or attempted treatment for threatened abortion). Some of these exposures were very short and involved only a few days of treatment. The data suggest that the risk of limb reduction defects in exposed fetuses is somewhat less than 1 per 1,000.

In the past, female sex hormones have been used during pregnancy in an attempt to treat threatened or habitual abortion. There is considerable evidence that estrogens are ineffective for these indications, and there is no evidence from well controlled studies that progestogens are effective for these uses.

If Estrace® is used during pregnancy, or if the patient becomes pregnant while taking this drug, she should be apprised of the potential risks to the fetus and the advisability of pregnancy continuation.

Description: Each gram of Estrace® (17β-estradiol) Vaginal Cream contains 0.1 mg 17β-estradiol in a nonliquefying base containing purified water, propylene glycol, stearyl alcohol, white ceresin wax, glyceryl monostearate, hydroxypropyl methylcellulose, sodium lauryl sulfate, methylparaben, disodium edetate and tertiary-butylhydroquinone. Estradiol is chemically described as estra-1, 3, 5(10)-triene-3, 17β-diol. The structural formula is:

Clinical Pharmacology: Estrogens are important in the development and maintenance of the female reproductive system and secondary sex characteristics. They promote growth and develop-

Continued on next page

Mead Johnson Labs.—Cont.

ment of the vagina, uterus, and fallopian tubes, and enlargement of the breasts. Indirectly, they contribute to the shaping of the skeleton, maintenance of tone and elasticity or urogenital structures, changes in the epiphyses of the long bones that allow for the pubertal growth spurt and its termination, growth of axillary and pubic hair, and pigmentation of the nipples and genitals. Decline of estrogenic activity at the end of the menstrual cycle can bring on menstruation, although the cessation of progesterone secretion is the most important factor in the mature ovulatory cycle. However, in the preovulatory or non-ovulatory cycle, estrogen is the primary determinant in the onset of menstruation. Estrogens also affect the release of pituitary gonadotropins.

Micronized 17β-estradiol achieves its pharmacologic effect in estrogen-responsive target tissues via anabolic stimulus at the cellular level. Micronized 17β-estradiol in Estrace Vaginal Cream is readily absorbed from mucosal surfaces.

In responsive tissues (female genital organs, breasts, hypothalamus, pituitary) estrogens enter the cell and are transported into the nucleus. As a result of estrogen action, specific RNA and protein synthesis occurs.

Metabolism and inactivation occur primarily in the liver. Some estrogens are excreted into the bile; however, they are reabsorbed from the intestine and returned to the liver through the portal venous system. Water-soluble estrogen conjugates are strongly acidic and are ionized in body fluids, which favor excretion through the kidneys since tubular reabsorption is minimal.

Indications: Estrace Vaginal Cream is indicated in the treatment of atrophic vaginitis and kraurosis vulvae.

ESTRACE® HAS NOT BEEN SHOWN TO BE EFFECTIVE FOR ANY PURPOSE DURING PREGNANCY AND ITS USE MAY CAUSE SEVERE HARM TO THE FETUS (SEE BOXED WARNING).

Contraindications: Estrogens should not be used in women (or men) with any of the following conditions:

1. Known or suspected cancer of the breast, except in appropriately selected patients being treated for metastatic disease. 2. Known or suspected estrogen-dependent neoplasia. 3. Known or suspected pregnancy (See Boxed Warning). 4. Undiagnosed abnormal genital bleeding. 5. Active thrombophlebitis or thromboembolic disorders. 6. A past history of thrombophlebitis, thrombosis or thromboembolic disorders associated with previous estrogen use (except when used in treatment of breast or prostatic malignancy).

Warnings: 1. **Induction of malignant neoplasms.** Long-term continuous administration of natural and synthetic estrogens in certain animal species increases the frequency of carcinomas of the breast, cervix, vagina, and liver. There is now evidence that estrogens increase the risk of carcinoma of the endometrium in humans. (See Boxed Warning).

At the present time there is no satisfactory evidence that estrogens given to postmenopausal women increase the risk of cancer of the breast,[17] although a recent long-term follow-up of a single physician's practice has raised this possibility.[18] Because of the animal data there is a need for caution in prescribing estrogens for women with a strong family history of breast cancer or who have breast nodules, fibrocystic disease, or abnormal mammograms.

2. **Gallbladder disease.** A recent study has reported a 2- to 3-fold increase in the risk of surgically confirmed gallbladder disease in women receiving postmenopausal estrogens,[17] similar to the 2-fold increase previously noted in users of oral contraceptives.[18,24a]

3. **Effects similar to those caused by estrogen-progestogen oral contraceptives.** There are several serious adverse effects of oral contraceptives, most of which have not, up to now, been docu-

mented as consequences of postmenopausal estrogen therapy. This may reflect the comparatively low doses of estrogen used in postmenopausal women. It would be expected that the larger doses of estrogen used to treat prostatic or breast cancer or postpartum breast engorgement are more likely to result in these adverse effects, and, in fact, it has been shown that there is an increased risk of thrombosis in men receiving estrogens for prostatic cancer and women for postpartum breast engorgement.[20-23]

a. **Thromboembolic disease.** It is now well established that users of oral contraceptives have an increased risk of various thromboembolic and thrombotic vascular diseases, such as thrombophlebitis, pulmonary embolism, stroke, and myocardial infarction.[24-31] Cases of retinal thrombosis, mesenteric thrombosis, and optic neuritis have been reported in oral contraceptive users. There is evidence that the risk of several of these adverse reactions is related to the dose of the drug.[32,33] An increased risk of post-surgery thromboembolic complications has also been reported in users of oral contraceptives.[34,35] If feasible, estrogen should be discontinued at least 4 weeks before surgery of the type associated with an increased risk of thromboembolism, or during periods of prolonged immobilization.

While an increased rate of thromboembolic and thrombotic disease in postmenopausal users of estrogens has not been found,[17-34] this does not rule out the possibility that such an increase may be present or that subgroups of women who have underlying risk factors or who are receiving relatively large doses of estrogens may have increased risk. Therefore, estrogens should not be used in persons with active thrombophlebitis or thromboembolic disorders, and they should not be used (except in treatment of malignancy) in persons with a history of such disorders in association with estrogen use. They should be used with caution in patients with cerebral vascular or coronary artery disease and only for those in whom estrogens are clearly needed.

Large doses of estrogen (5 mg conjugated estrogens per day), comparable to those used to treat cancer of the prostate and breast, have been shown in a large prospective clinical trial in men[37] to increase the risk of nonfatal myocardial infarction, pulmonary embolism and thrombophlebitis. When estrogen doses of this size are used, any of the thromboembolic and thrombotic adverse effects associated with oral contraceptive use should be considered a clear risk.

b. **Hepatic adenoma.** Hepatic adenomas appear to be associated with the use of oral contraceptives.[38-40] Although rare, these may rupture and may cause death through intraabdominal hemorrhage. Such lesions have not yet been reported in association with other estrogen or progestogen preparations but should be considered in estrogen users having abdominal pain and tenderness, abdominal mass, or hypovolemic shock. Hepatocellular carcinoma has also been reported in women taking estrogen-containing oral contraceptives.[36] The relationship of this malignancy to these drugs is not known at this time.

c. **Elevated blood pressure.** Increased blood pressure is not uncommon in women using oral contraceptives. There is now a report that this may occur with use of estrogens in the menopause[41] and blood pressure should be monitored with estrogen use, especially if high doses are used.

d. **Glucose tolerance.** A worsening of glucose tolerance has been observed in a significant percentage of patients on estrogen-containing oral contraceptives. For this reason, diabetic patients should be carefully observed while receiving estrogen.

4. **Hypercalcemia.** Administration of estrogens may lead to severe hypercalcemia in patients with breast cancer and bone metastases. If this occurs, the drug should be stopped and appropriate measures taken to reduce the serum calcium level.

Precautions: A. General Precautions.

1. A complete medical and family history should be taken prior to the initiation of any estrogen therapy. The pretreatment and periodic physical examinations should include special reference to blood pressure, breasts, abdomen, and pelvic organs, and should include a Papanicolaou smear. As a general rule, estrogen should not be prescribed for longer than one year without another physical examination being performed.

2. Fluid retention — Because estrogens may cause some degree of fluid retention, conditions which might be influenced by this factor such as epilepsy, migraine, and cardiac or renal dysfunction, require careful observation.

3. Certain patients may develop undesirable manifestations of excessive estrogenic stimulation, such as abnormal or excessive uterine bleeding, mastodynia, etc.

4. Oral contraceptives appear to be associated with an increased incidence of mental depression.[24a] Although it is not clear whether this is due to the estrogenic or progestogenic component of the contraceptive, patients with a history of depression should be carefully observed.

5. Pre-existing uterine leiomyomata may increase in size during estrogen use.

6. The pathologist should be advised of estrogen therapy when relevant specimens are submitted.

7. Patients with a past history of jaundice during pregnancy have an increased risk of recurrence of jaundice while receiving estrogen-containing oral contraceptive therapy. If jaundice develops in any patient receiving estrogen, the medication should be discontinued while the cause is investigated.

8. Estrogens may be poorly metabolized in patients with impaired liver function and they should be administered with caution in such patients.

9. Because estrogens influence the metabolism of calcium and phosphorus, they should be used with caution in patients with metabolic bone diseases that are associated with hypercalcemia or in patients with renal insufficiency.

10. Because of the effects of estrogens on epiphyseal closure, they should be used judiciously in young patients in whom bone growth is not complete.

11. Certain endocrine and liver function tests may be affected by estrogen-containing oral contraceptives. The following similar changes may be expected with larger doses of estrogen:

a. Increased sulfobromophthalein retention.

b. Increased prothrombin and factors VII and VIII, IX, and X; decreased antithyrombin 3; increased norepinephrine-induced platelet aggregability.

c. Increased thyroid binding globulin (TBG) leading to increased circulating total thyroid hormone, as measured by PBI, T4 by volume, or T4 by radioimmunoassay, free T3 resin uptake is decreased, reflecting the elevated TBG; free T4 concentration is unaltered.

d. Impaired glucose tolerance.

e. Decreased pregnanediol excretion.

f. Reduced response to metyrapone test.

g. Reduced serum folate concentration.

h. Increased serum triglyceride and phospholipid concentration.

B. Information for the Patient. See text which appears after the physician References.

C. Pregnancy Category X. See Contraindications and Boxed Warning.

D. Nursing Mothers. As a general principle, the administration of any drug to nursing mothers should be done only when clearly necessary since many drugs are excreted in human milk.

Adverse Reactions: (See Warnings regarding induction of neoplasia, adverse effects on the fetus, increased incidence of gall bladder disease, and adverse effects similar to those of oral contraceptives, including thromboembolism.) The following additional adverse reactions have been reported with estrogenic therapy, including oral contraceptives:

1. **Genitourinary system.**

Breakthrough bleeding, spotting, change in menstrual flow.

Dysmenorrhea.
Premenstrual-like syndrome.
Amenorrhea during and after treatment.
Increase in size of uterine fibromyomata.
Vaginal candidiasis.
Change in cervical eversion and in degree of cervical secretion.
Cystitis-like syndrome.
2. **Breast.**
Tenderness, enlargement, secretion.
3. **Gastrointestinal.**
Nausea, vomiting.
Abdominal cramps, bloating.
Cholestatic jaundice.
4. **Skin.**
Chloasma or melasma which may persist when drug is discontinued.
Erythema multiforme   Erythema nodosum
Hemorrhagic eruption   Loss of scalp hair
Hirsutism
5. **Eyes.**
Steepening of corneal curvature.
Intolerance to contact lenses.
6. **CNS.**
Headache, migraine, dizziness.
Mental depression.
Chorea.
7. **Miscellaneous.**
Increase or decrease in weight.
Reduced carbohydrate tolerance.
Aggravation of porphyria.
Edema.
Changes in libido.

Overdosage: Numerous reports of ingestion of large doses of estrogen-containing oral contraceptives by young children indicate that serious ill effects do not occur. Overdosage of estrogen may cause nausea, and withdrawal bleeding may occur in females.

Dosage and Administration: Given cyclically for short term use only.
For treatment of atrophic vaginitis or kraurosis vulvae.
The lowest dose that will control symptoms should be chosen and medication should be discontinued as promptly as possible. Administration should be cyclic (e.g., 3 weeks on and 1 week off).
Attempts to discontinue or taper medication should be made at 3 to 6 month intervals.
Usual Dosage: The usual dosage range is 2 to 4 g (marked on the applicator) daily for one or two weeks, then gradually reduced to one half initial dosage for a similar period. A maintenance dosage of 1 g. one to three times a week, may be used after restoration of the vaginal mucosa has been achieved.
Patients with an intact uterus should be monitored closely for signs of endometrial cancer and appropriate diagnostic measures should be taken to rule out malignancy in eventual persistent or recurring abnormal vaginal bleeding.

How Supplied: Estrace (estradiol) Vaginal Cream.
Each gram contains 0.1 mg 17β-estradiol in a nonliquefying base containing purified water, propylene glycol, stearyl alcohol, white ceresin wax, glyceryl monostearate, hydroxypropyl methylcellulose, sodium lauryl sulfate, methylparaben, disodium edetate, and t-butylhydroquinone.
Combination Package: Each contains Net Wt. 1½ oz. (42.5 g) tube with one calibrated plastic applicator for delivery of 1, 2, 3 or 4 g.
Also available — Refill Package. Each contains Net Wt. 1½ oz. (42.5 g) tube.

INFORMATION FOR THE PATIENT
What You Should Know About Estrogens: Estrogens are female hormones produced principally by the ovaries. The ovaries make several different kinds of estrogens. In addition, scientists have been able to make a variety of synthetic estrogens. As far as we know, all these estrogens have the same properties and therefore much the same usefulness, side effects, and risks. This leaflet is intended to help you understand what estrogens are used for, the risks involved in their use, and how to use them as safely as possible.
This leaflet includes important information about Estrace® (estradiol) and estrogens in general, but not all the information. If you want to know more, you can ask your doctor or pharmacist to let you read the professional package insert.

Uses of Estrogen: Estrogens are prescribed by doctors for a number of purposes, including:
1. To provide estrogen during a period of adjustment when a woman's ovaries no longer produce it, in order to prevent certain uncomfortable symptoms of estrogen deficiency. (All women normally experience a decrease in the production of estrogens, generally between 45–55; this is called the menopause.)
2. To prevent symptoms of estrogen deficiency when a woman's ovaries have been removed surgically before the natural menopause.
3. To prevent pregnancy. (Some estrogens are given along with a progestogen, another female hormone; these combinations are called oral contraceptives or birth control pills. They will not be discussed in this leaflet.) However, Estrace is not intended for this use.
4. To treat certain cancers in women and men.
5. To prevent painful swelling of the breasts after pregnancy in women who choose not to nurse their babies.

THERE IS NO PROPER USE OF ESTROGENS IN A PREGNANT WOMAN.

Estrogens in the Menopause: In the natural course of their lives, all women eventually experience a decrease in estrogen production. This usually occurs between ages 45 and 55 but may occur earlier or later. Sometimes the ovaries may need to be removed before natural menopause by an operation, producing a "surgical menopause."
When the amount of estrogen in the blood begins to decrease, many women may develop typical symptoms: feelings of warmth in the face, neck, and chest or sudden intense episodes of heat and sweating throughout the body (called "hot flashes" or "hot flushes"). These symptoms are sometimes very uncomfortable. A few women eventually develop changes in the vagina (called "atrophic vaginitis") which cause discomfort, especially during and after intercourse.
Estrogens can be prescribed to treat these symptoms of the menopause. It is estimated that considerably more than half of all women undergoing the menopause have only mild symptoms or no symptoms at all and therefore do not need estrogens. Other women may need estrogens for a few months, while their bodies adjust to lower estrogen levels. Sometimes the need will be for periods longer than six months. In an attempt to avoid over-stimulation of the uterus (womb), estrogens are usually given cyclically during each month of use, that is three weeks of therapy followed by one week without therapy.
Sometimes women experience nervous symptoms or depression during menopause. There is no evidence that estrogens are effective for such symptoms and they should not be used to treat them, although other treatment may be needed.
You may have heard that taking estrogens for long periods (years) after the menopause will keep your skin soft and supple and keep you feeling young. There is no evidence that this is so, however, and such long-term treatment carries additional risks.

Estrogens To Prevent Swelling of The Breasts After Pregnancy: If you do not breast feed your baby after delivery, your breasts may fill up with milk and become painful and engorged. This usually begins about three to four days after delivery and may last for a few days to up to a week or more. Sometimes the discomfort is severe, but usually it is not and can be controlled by pain-relieving drugs such as aspirin and by binding the breasts up tightly. Estrogens can sometimes be used successfully to try to prevent the breasts from filling up. While this treatment is sometimes successful, in many cases the breasts fill up to some degree in spite of treatment. The dose of estrogens needed to prevent pain and swelling of the breasts is much larger than the dose needed to treat symptoms of the menopause and this may increase your chances of developing blood clots in the legs or lungs or other parts of the body (see below, 4. **Abnormal Blood Clotting**). Therefore, it is important that you discuss the benefits and the risks of estrogen use with your doctor, before using estrogen, if you have decided not to breast feed your baby.

The Dangers of Estrogens:
1. **Cancer of the uterus.** If estrogens are used in the postmenopausal period for more than a year, there is an increased risk of cancer of the endometrium (uterine lining). Women taking estrogens have roughly 5 to 15 times as great a chance of getting this cancer as women who take no estrogens. To put this another way, while a postmenopausal woman not taking estrogens has one chance in 1,000 each year of getting cancer of the uterus, a woman taking estrogens has 5 to 15 chances in 1,000 each year. For this reason **it is important to take estrogens only when you really need them.**
The risk of this cancer is greater the longer estrogens are used and also seems to be greater when larger doses are taken. For this reason **it is important to take the lowest dose of estrogen that will control symptoms and to take it only as long as it is needed.** If estrogens are needed for longer periods of time, your doctor will want to reevaluate your need for estrogens at least every six months.
Women using estrogens should report any irregular vaginal bleeding to their doctors; such bleeding may be of no importance, but it can be an early warning of cancer of the uterus. If you have undiagnosed vaginal bleeding, you should not use estrogens until a diagnosis is made and you are certain there is no cancer of the uterus.
NOTE: If you have had your uterus completely removed (total hysterectomy), there is no danger of developing cancer of the uterus.
2. **Other possible cancers.** Estrogens can cause development of other tumors in animals, such as tumors of the breast, cervix, vagina, or liver, when given for a long time. At present, there is no satisfactory evidence that women using estrogens in the menopause have an increased risk of such tumors, but there is no way yet to be sure they do not; and one study raises the possibility that use of estrogens in the menopause may increase the risk of breast cancer many years later. This is a further reason to use estrogens only when clearly needed. While you are taking estrogens, it is important that you go to your doctor at least once a year for a physical examination. Also, if members of your family have had breast cancer or if you have breast nodules or abnormal mammograms (breast x-rays), your doctor may wish to carry out more frequent examinations.
3. **Gall bladder disease.** Women who use estrogens after menopause are two or three times more likely to develop gall bladder disease needing surgery than women who do not use estrogens. Birth control pills have a similar effect.
4. **Abnormal blood clotting.** Oral contraceptives increase the risk of blood clotting in various parts of the body. This can occur in different parts of the circulatory system causing thrombophlebitis (clot in the legs or pelvis), retinal thrombosis or optic neuritis (clots affecting vision, including blindness), mesenteric thrombosis (clots in the intestinal blood vessels), stroke (clot in the brain), heart attack (clot in a vessel of the heart) or a pulmonary embolism (clot which eventually lodges in the lungs). These can be fatal.
At this time, use of estrogens in the menopause is not known to cause increased blood clotting; this has not been fully studied and there could still prove to be such a risk. It is recommended that if you have had clotting in the legs or lungs or a heart attack or stroke while you were using estrogens or birth control pills, you should not use estrogens (unless they are being used to treat cancer of the breast or prostate). If you have had a stroke or heart attack or if you have angina pectoris, estrogens should be used with great caution and only if clearly needed (for example, if you have severe symptoms of the menopause).

Continued on next page

Mead Johnson Labs.—Cont.

The larger doses of estrogen used to prevent swelling of the breasts after pregnancy have been reported to cause abnormal blood clotting as indicated above.

Special Warning About Pregnancy: You should not receive estrogen if you are pregnant. If this should occur, there is a greater than usual chance that the developing child will be born with a birth defect, although the possibility remains fairly small. A female child may have an increased risk of developing cancer of the vagina or cervix later in life (in the teens or twenties). Every possible effort should be made to avoid exposure to estrogens during pregnancy. If exposure occurs, see your doctor.

Other Effects of Estrogens: In addition to the serious known risks of estrogens described above, estrogens have the following side effects and potential risks which, if occurring, should be discussed promptly with your doctor.
1. **Nausea and vomiting.** The most common side effect of estrogen therapy is nausea. Vomiting is less common.
2. **Effects on breasts.** Estrogens may cause breast tenderness or enlargement and may cause the breasts to secrete a liquid.
3. **Effects on the uterus.** Estrogens may cause benign fibroid tumors of the uterus to get larger. Some women will have menstrual bleeding when estrogens are stopped. But if the bleeding occurs on days you are still taking estrogens, you should report this to your doctor.
4. **Effects on liver.** Women taking oral contraceptives develop on rare occasions a tumor of the liver which can rupture, bleed into the abdomen, and cause death. So far, these tumors have not been reported in women using estrogens in the menopause, but you should report any swelling or unusual pain or tenderness in the abdomen to your doctor immediately.
Women with a past history of jaundice (yellowing of the skin and white parts of the eyes) may get jaundice again during estrogen use. If this occurs, stop taking estrogens and see your doctor.
5. **Other effects.** Estrogens may cause excess fluid to be retained in the body. This may make some conditions worse, such as epilepsy, migraine, heart disease, or kidney disease. Mental depression or high blood pressure may occur. A spotty darkening of the skin, particularly of the face, is possible and may persist.

Summary: Estrogens have important uses, and they may have serious risks as well. You must decide, with your doctor, whether the risks are acceptable to you in view of the benefits of treatment. Except where your doctor has prescribed estrogens for use in special cases of cancer of the breast or prostate, you should not use estrogens if you have cancer of the breast or uterus, are pregnant, have undiagnosed abnormal vaginal bleeding, clotting in the legs or lungs or have had a stroke, heart attack or angina, or clotting in the legs or lungs in the past while you were taking estrogens.

You can use estrogens as safely as possible by understanding that your doctor will require regular physical examinations while you are taking them and will try to discontinue the drug as soon as possible and use the smallest dose possible. Be alert for signs of trouble including:
1. Abnormal bleeding from the vagina.
2. Pains in the calves or chest or sudden shortness of breath, or coughing blood (indicating possible clots in the legs, heart, or lungs).
3. Severe headache, dizziness, faintness, or changes in vision (indicating possible developing clots in the brain or eye).
4. Breast lumps (you should ask your doctor how to examine your own breasts).
5. Jaundice (yellowing of the skin).
6. Mental depression.

Your doctor has prescribed this drug for you. Do not give this drug to anyone else.

How Supplied: Estrace® Vaginal Cream—Estrace in a nonliquefying base, designed for vaginal use with a calibrated plastic applicator for delivery of 1, 2, 3 or 4 g.

References:
1. Ziel HK, Finkel WD: Increased risk of endometrial carcinoma among users of conjugated estrogens. New Eng J Med 293:1167–1170, 1975.
2. Smith, DC, Prentice R, Thompson DJ, Herrmann WL: Association of exogenous estrogen and endometrial carcinoma. New Eng J Med 293:1164–1167, 1975.
3. Mack TM, Pike MC, Henderson BE, et al: Estrogens and the endometrial cancer in a retirement community. New Eng J Med 294:1262–1267, 1976.
4. Weiss, NS, Szekely DR, Austin DF: Increasing incidence of endometrial cancer in the United States. New Eng J Med 294:1259–1262, 1976.
5. Herbst AL, Ulfelder H, Poskanzer DC: Adenocarcinoma of vagina. New Eng J Med 284:878–881, 1971.
6. Greenwald P, Barlow J, Nasca P, Burnett W: Vaginal cancer after maternal treatment with synthetic estrogens. New Eng J Med 285:390–392, 1971.
7. Lanier A, Noller K, Decker D, et al: Cancer and stilbestrol. A follow-up of 1719 persons exposed to estrogens in utero and born 1943–1959. Mayo Clin Proceedings 48:793–799, 1973.
8. Herbst A, Kurman R, Scully R: Vaginal and cervical abnormalities after exposure to stilbestrol in utero. Obstet and Gynec 40:287–298, 1972.
9. Herbst A, Robboy S, MacDonald G, Scully R: The effects of local progesterone on stilbestrol-associated vaginal adenosis. Am J Obstet Gynec 118:607–615, 1974.
10. Herbst A, Poskanzer D, Robboy S, et al: Prenatal exposure to stilbestrol, a prospective comparison of exposed female offspring with unexposed controls. New Eng J Med 292:334–339, 1975.
11. Stafl A, Mattingly R, Foley D, Fetherston W: Clinical diagnosis of vaginal adenosis. Obstet and Gynec 43:118–128, 1974.
12. Sherman Al, Goldrath M, Berlin A, et al: Cervical-vaginal adenosis after in utero exposure to synthetic estrogens. Obstet Gynec 44:531–545, 1974.
13. Gal I, Kirman B, Stern J: Hormone pregnancy tests and congenital malformation. Nature 216:83, 1967.
14. Levy EP, Cohen A, Fraser FC: Hormone treatment during pregnancy and congenital heart defects. Lancet 1:611, 1973.
15. Nora J, Nora A: Birth defects and oral contraceptives. Lancet 1:941–942, 1973.
16. Janerich DT, Piper JM, Glebatis DM: Oral contraceptives and congenital limb-reduction defects. New Engl J Med 291:697–700, 1974.
17. Boston Collaborative Drug Surveillance Program: Surgically confirmed gall bladder disease venous thromboembolism and breast tumors in relation to post-menopausal estrogen therapy. New Eng J Med 290:15–19, 1974.
18. Hoover R, Gray LA Sr, Cole P, MacMahon B: Menopausal estrogens and breast cancer. New Eng J Med 295:15–19, 1974.
19. Boston Collaborative Drug Surveillance Program: Oral contraceptives and venous thromboembolic disease, surgically confirmed gall bladder disease, and breast tumors. Lancet 1:1399–1404, 1973.
20. Daniel DG, Campbell H, Turnbull AC: Puerperal thromboemboism and suppression of lactation. Lancet 2:287–289, 1967.
21. The Veterans Administration Cooperative Urological Research Group: Carcinoma of the prostate; treatment comparisons. J Urol 98:516–522, 1967.
22. Bailar JC: Thromboembolism and oestrogen therapy. Lancet 2:560, 1967.
23. Blackard C, Doe R, Mellinger G, Byar D: Incidence of cardiovascular disease and death in patients receiving diethylstilbestrol for carcinoma of the prostate. Cancer 26:249–256, 1970.
24. Royal College of General Practitioners: Oral contraception and thromboembolic disease. J Roy Coll Gen Pract 13:267–279, 1967.
24a. Royal College of General Practitioners: Oral Contraceptives and Health, New York, Pitman Corp, 1974.
25. Inman WHW, Vessey MP: Investigation of deaths from pulmonary, coronary, and cerebral thrombosis and embolism in women of childbearing age. Brit M J 2:193–199, 1968.
26. Vessey MP, Doll R: Investigation of relation between use of oral contraceptives and thromboembolic disease. A further report. Brit M J 2:651–657, 1969.
27. Sartwell PE, Masi AT, Arthes FG, et al: Thromboembolism and oral contraceptives: an epidemiological case control study. Am J Epidemiol 90:365–380, 1969.
28. Collaborative Group for the Study of Stroke in Young Women: Oral contraception and increased risk of cerebral ischemia or thrombosis. New Eng J Med 288:871–878, 1973.
29. Collaborative Group for the Study of Stroke in Young Women: Oral contraceptives and stroke in young women: Associated risk factors. JAMA 231:718–722, 1975.
30. Mann JI, Inman WHW: Oral contraceptives and death from myocardial infarction. Brit M J 2:245–248, 1975.
31. Mann JI, Vessey MP, Thorogood M, Doll R: Myocardial infarction in young women with special reference to oral contraceptive practice. Brit M J 2:241–245, 1975.
32. Inman WHW, Vessey MP, Westerholm B, Engelund A: Thromboembolic disease and the steroidal content of oral contraceptives. Brit M J 2:203–209, 1970.
33. Stolley PD, Tonascia JA, Tockman MS, et al: Thrombosis with low-estrogen oral contraceptives. Am J Epidemiol 102:197–208, 1975.
34. Vessey MP, Doll R, Fairbairn AS, Glober G: Post-operative thromboembolism and the use of the oral contraceptives. Brit M J 3:123–126, 1970.
35. Greene GR, Sartwell PE: Oral contraceptive use in patients with thromboembolism following surgery, trauma or infection. Am J Pub Health 62:680–685, 1972.
36. Rosenberg L, Armstrong MB, Jick H: Myocardial infarction and estrogen therapy in postmenopausal women. New Eng J Med 294:1256–1259, 1976.
37. Coronary Drug Project Research Group: The coronary drug project: initial findings leading to modifications of its research protocol. JAMA 214:1303–1313, 1970.
38. Baum J, Holtz F, Bookstein JJ, Klein EW: Possible association between benign hepatomas and oral contraceptives. Lancet 2:926–928, 1973.
39. Mays ET, Christopherson WM, Mahr MM, Williams HC: Hepatic changes in young women ingesting contraceptive steroids, hepatic hemorrhage and primary hepatic tumors. JAMA 235:730–732, 1976.
40. Edmondson HA, Henderson B, Benton B: Liver cell adenomas associated with the use of oral contraceptives. New Eng J Med 294:470–472, 1976.
41. Pfeffer RI, Van Den Noort S: Estrogen use and stroke risk in postmenopausal women. Am J Epidemiol 103:445–456, 1976.

Shown in Product Identification Section, page 419

K-LYTE®
[k′ līt]
Effervescent Tablets

Each tablet in solution provides 25 mEq (978 mg) potassium as bicarbonate and citrate.

K-LYTE® DS
Effervescent Tablets

Each tablet in solution provides 50 mEq (1955 mg) potassium as bicarbonate and citrate.

K-LYTE/CL®
Effervescent Tablets and Powder

Each tablet in solution and each dose of powder in solution provide the equivalent of 25 mEq (1865 mg) potassium chloride.

K-LYTE/CL® 50
Effervescent Tablets

Each tablet in solution provides the equivalent of 50 mEq (3730 mg) potassium chloride.

Description:
[See table right].

	K-LYTE	K-LYTE DS	K-LYTE/CL	K-LYTE/CL POWDER	K-LYTE/CL 50
Potassium Chloride	—	—	1.5 gm	1.86 gm	2.24 gm
Potassium Bicarbonate	2.5 gm	2.5 gm	0.5 gm	—	2.0 gm
Potassium Citrate	—	2.7 gm	—	—	—
L-lysine Monohydrochloride	—	—	0.91 gm	—	3.65 gm
Citric Acid	2.1 gm	2.1 gm	0.55 gm	—	1.0 gm

Clinical Pharmacology: Potassium ion is the principal intracellular cation of most body tissues and participates in a number of essential physiological processes. These include numerous enzymatic reactions in intermediary metabolism, the maintenance of intracellular tonicity, the transmission of nerve impulses, and the function of cardiac, skeletal, and smooth muscle. Disturbances in potassium metabolism may, therefore, elicit a broad range of clinical disorders. The normal serum potassium level is maintained principally by close renal regulation of potassium balance.

Potassium depletion may occur whenever potassium loss through renal excretion and/or loss from the gastrointestinal tract exceeds the potassium intake. Such depletion usually develops slowly as a consequence of prolonged therapy with oral diuretics, primary or secondary hyperaldosteronism, diabetic ketoacidosis, severe vomiting and diarrhea, or inadequate replacement of potassium in patients on prolonged parenteral nutrition. Potassium depletion may be accompanied by hypokalemia as well as hypochloremia and metabolic alkalosis.

Potassium deficiency may be manifested by generalized weakness, drowsiness, anorexia, and nausea; oliguria, edema, and chronic ileus with distention; shallow and infrequent respirations; low blood pressure, altered cardiac rhythms, and systolic murmurs; hypokalemia and such ECG changes as prominent U wave, lengthening of the Q-T interval, depression of the S-T segment, and depression or inversion of the T wave.

Indications and Usage: All K-LYTE® products are used for therapy or prophylaxis of potassium deficiency. They are useful when thiazide diuretics, corticosteroids, or vomiting and diarrhea cause excessive potassium loss; and when dietary potassium is low. These products may also be useful when potassium therapy is indicated in digitalis intoxication. K-LYTE/Cl and K-LYTE/Cl 50 are recommended in the management of hypokalemia accompanied by metabolic alkalosis and hypochloremia, e.g. as induced by vomiting.

Contraindications: Potassium supplements are contraindicated in patients with hyperkalemia since a further increase in serum potassium concentration in such patients can produce cardiac arrest. Hyperkalemia may complicate any of the following conditions: chronic renal impairment, metabolic acidosis such as diabetic acidosis, acute dehydration, extensive tissue breakdown as in severe burns or adrenal insufficiency. Hypokalemia should not be treated by the concomitant administration of potassium salts and a potassium-sparing diuretic (e.g., spironolactone or triamterene), since the simultaneous administration of these agents can produce severe hyperkalemia.

Warnings: In patients with impaired mechanisms for excreting potassium, the administration of potassium salts can produce hyperkalemia and cardiac arrest. This occurs most commonly in patients given potassium by the intravenous route but may also occur in patients given potassium orally. Potentially fatal hyperkalemia can develop rapidly and may be asymptomatic. The use of potassium salts in patients with chronic renal disease, or any other condition which impairs potassium excretion, requires particularly careful monitoring of the serum potassium concentration and appropriate dosage adjustment.

Precautions: General precautions—The diagnosis of potassium depletion is ordinarily made by demonstrating hypokalemia in a patient with a clinical history suggesting some cause for potassium depletion. When interpreting the serum potassium level, the physician should bear in mind that acute alkalosis *per se* can produce hypokalemia in the absence of a deficit in total body potassium, while acute acidosis *per se* can increase the serum potassium concentration into the normal range even in the presence of a reduced total body potassium. Therefore, the treatment of potassium depletion requires careful attention to acid-base balance and appropriate monitoring of serum electrolytes, the ECG, and the clinical status of the patient.

Information for patients—To minimize the possibility of gastrointestinal irritation associated with the oral ingestion of concentrated potassium salt preparations, patients should be carefully directed to dissolve each dose completely in the stated amount of water.

Laboratory tests—Frequent clinical evaluation of the patient should include ECG and serum potassium determinations.

Drug interactions—The simultaneous administration of potassium supplements and a potassium-sparing diuretic can produce severe hyperkalemia (see Contraindications). Potassium supplements should be used cautiously in patients who are using salt substitutes because most of the latter contain substantial amounts of potassium. Such concomitant use could result in hyperkalemia.

Usage in Pregnancy—Pregnancy Category C—Animal reproduction studies have not been conducted with any of the K-LYTE products. It is also not known whether these products can cause fetal harm when administered to a pregnant woman or can affect reproduction capacity. They should be given to a pregnant woman only if clearly needed.

Nursing Mothers—Many drugs are excreted in human milk and because of the potential for serious adverse reactions in nursing infants from oral potassium supplements, a decision should be made whether to discontinue nursing or discontinue the drug, taking into account the importance of the drug to the mother.

Usage in Children—Safety and effectiveness in children have not been established.

Adverse Reactions: The most common adverse reactions to oral potassium supplements are nausea, vomiting, diarrhea and abdominal discomfort. These side effects occur more frequently when the medication is not taken with food or is not diluted properly or dissolved completely.

Hyperkalemia occurs only rarely in patients with normal renal function receiving potassium supplements orally. Signs and symptoms of hyperkalemia are cardiac arrhythmias, mental confusion, unexplained anxiety, numbness or tingling in hands, feet or lips, shortness of breath or difficult breathing, unusual tiredness or weakness and weakness or heaviness of legs (see Contraindications, Warnings and Overdosage).

Overdosage: The administration of oral potassium salts to persons with normal renal function rarely causes serious hyperkalemia. However, in patients with chronic renal disease, or any other condition which impairs potassium excretion or if potassium is administered too rapidly intravenously, potentially fatal hyperkalemia can result (see Contraindications and Warnings). The earliest clinical manifestations of this condition may be only increased serum potassium levels and characteristic ECG changes such as peaking of T-waves, loss of P-wave, depression of S-T segment and prolongation of the QT interval. These changes in the ECG usually appear when serum potassium concentration reaches 7 to 8 mEq per liter. Other clinical manifestations occurring at a concentration of 9 to 10 mEq per liter may include muscle paralysis and death from cardiac arrest.

The treatment of severe hyperkalemia should focus on reducing the serum potassium concentration by promoting the transfer of potassium from the extracellular to the intracellular space. The measures taken may include the following: a) intravenous administration of 1 liter of a 10 percent glucose solution containing 30-40 units of insulin; b) in the acidotic patient, intravenous administration of 150 mEq to 300 mEq of sodium bicarbonate. Other measures should include the elimination of potassium-containing medications and potassium-sparing diuretics and frequently the oral administration of a cation exchange resin (such as sodium polystyrene sulfonate) to remove gastrointestinal potassium. To assure rapid movement of the resin through the gastrointestinal tract, a nonabsorbable polyhydric alcohol (e.g., sorbitol) should be given in quantities sufficient to induce a soft to semiliquid bowel movement every few hours.

Hemodialysis is an effective alternative means of removing excess potassium.

Dosage and Administration: Adults—One (1) K-LYTE/Cl 50 tablet (50 mEq potassium and chloride) or K-LYTE DS tablet (50 mEq potassium) completely dissolved in 6 to 8 ounces of cold or ice water, 1 to 2 times daily, depending on the requirements of the patient. One (1) K-LYTE/Cl tablet (25 mEq potassium and chloride) or one (1) K-LYTE tablet (25 mEq potassium) completely dissolved in 3 to 4 ounces of cold or ice water, 2 to 4 times daily, depending on the requirements of the patient. One dose (25 mEq potassium chloride) of K-LYTE/Cl powder completely dissolved in 6 ounces of cold or ice water, 2 to 4 times daily, depending on the requirements of the patient.

Note: It is suggested that all K-LYTE products be taken with meals and sipped slowly over a 5 to 10 minute period.

How Supplied:
K-LYTE® Effervescent Tablets. Each tablet in solution provides 25 mEq (978 mg) potassium.
NDC 0087-0760-01 Lime flavor, Boxes of 30
NDC 0087-0760-43 Lime flavor, Boxes of 100
NDC 0087-0760-02 Lime flavor, Boxes of 250
NDC 0087-0761-01 Orange flavor, Boxes of 30
NDC 0087-0761-43 Orange flavor, Boxes of 100
NDC 0087-0761-02 Orange flavor, Boxes of 250
VA 6505-00-934-3477A (Box of 30) Lime
VA 6505-00-934-3477 (Box of 30) Defense
K-LYTE® DS Effervescent Tablets. Each tablet provides 50 mEq (1955 mg) potassium.
NDC 0087-0772-41 Lime flavor, Boxes of 30
NDC 0087-0772-42 Lime flavor, Boxes of 100
NDC 0087-0771-41 Orange flavor, Boxes of 30
NDC 0087-0771-42 Orange flavor, Boxes of 100
K-LYTE/CL® Effervescent Tablets. Each tablet in solution provides the equivalent of 25 mEq (1865 mg) potassium chloride.
NDC 0087-0766-41 Citrus flavor, Boxes of 30
NDC 0087-0766-43 Citrus flavor, Boxes of 100
NDC 0087-0766-42 Citrus flavor, Boxes of 250
NDC 0087-0767-41 Fruit Punch flavor, Boxes of 30
NDC 0087-0767-43 Fruit Punch flavor, Boxes of 100

Continued on next page

Mead Johnson Labs.—Cont.

NDC 0087-0767-42 Fruit Punch flavor, Boxes of 250

K-LYTE/CL® Powder. Each dose in solution provides the equivalent of 25 mEq (1865 mg) potassium chloride.

NDC 0087-0763-01 Fruit Punch flavor, 225 g can (30 measured doses with scoop)

K-LYTE/CL® 50 mEq Effervescent Tablets. Each tablet in solution provides the equivalent of 50 mEq (3730 mg) potassium chloride.

NDC 0087-0757-41 Fruit Punch flavor, Boxes of 30
NDC 0087-0757-42 Fruit Punch flavor, Boxes of 100
NDC 0087-0758-41 Citrus flavor, Boxes of 30
NDC 0087-0758-42 Citrus flavor, Boxes of 100
Store Below 86°F (30°C).

Shown in Product Identification Section, page 419

NATALINS® tablets
[nă-tă-lins]
Multivitamin and multimineral supplement

Composition: Each Natalins tablet supplies:

		% U.S. RDA Pregnant or Lactating Women
Vitamins		
Vitamin A, IU	8,000	100
Vitamin D, IU	400	100
Vitamin E, IU	30	100
Vitamin C (Ascorbic acid), mg	90	150
Folic acid, mg	0.8	100
Thiamine (Vitamin B_1), mg	1.7	100
Riboflavin (Vitamin B_2), mg	2	100
Niacin, mg	20	100
Vitamin B_6, mg	4	160
Vitamin B_{12}, mcg	8	100
Minerals		
Calcium, mg	200	15
Iodine, mcg	150	100
Iron, mg	45	250
Magnesium, mg	100	22

Ingredients: Calcium carbonate, magnesium hydroxide, polyvinylpyrrolidone USP, gum arabic, ion exchange resin, methyl cellulose, magnesium stearate, ethyl cellulose, silicon dioxide, glycerin, titanium dioxide (color), vitamin A acetate, cholecalciferol, dl-alpha-tocopheryl acetate, sodium ascorbate, folic acid, thiamine mononitrate, riboflavin (color), niacinamide, pyridoxine hydrochloride, cyanocobalamin, calcium iodate and ferrous fumarate.

Indications and Usage: Diet supplementation during pregnancy or lactation.

Dosage and Administration: One tablet a day or as indicated.

How Supplied:
Natalins® tablets
NDC 0087-0700-01 Bottles of 100
NDC 0087-0700-06 Bottles of 1000

Shown in Product Identification Section, page 419

NATALINS® RX ℞
[nă-tă-lins]
Multivitamin and Multimineral Supplement Tablets with 1 mg folic acid and 60 mg Iron

Natalins Rx tablets provide twelve vitamins and six minerals to supplement the diet during pregnancy or lactation.

Composition: Each Natalins Rx tablet supplies:

		% U.S. RDA Pregnant Or Lactating Women
Vitamins		
Vitamin A, IU	8,000	100
Vitamin D, IU	400	100
Vitamin E, IU	30	100
Vitamin C (Ascorbic acid), mg	90	150
Folic acid (Folacin), mg	1	125
Thiamine (Vitamin B_1), mg	2.55	150
Riboflavin (Vitamin B_2), mg	3	150
Niacin, mg	20	100
Vitamin B_6, mg	10	400
Vitamin B_{12}, mcg	8	100
Biotin, mg	0.05	16
Pantothenic acid, mg	15	150
Minerals		
Calcium, mg	200	15
Iodine, mcg	150	100
Iron, mg	60	333
Magnesium, mg	100	22
Copper, mg	2	100
Zinc, mg	15	100

Ingredients: Vitamin A acetate, cholecalciferol, dl-alpha-tocopheryl acetate, sodium ascorbate, folic acid, thiamine mononitrate, riboflavin, niacinamide, pyridoxine hydrochloride, cyanocobalamin, biotin, calcium pantothenate, calcium carbonate, calcium iodate, ferrous fumarate, magnesium hydroxide, cupric oxide and zinc oxide.

Indications and Usage: Natalins Rx tablets help assure an adequate intake of the vitamins and minerals listed above.
Folic acid helps prevent the development of megaloblastic anemia during pregnancy.

Contraindications: Supplemental vitamins and minerals should not be prescribed for patients with hemochromatosis or Wilson's disease.

Warning: Keep Natalins Rx tablets out of the reach of children.

Precautions:
General—pernicious anemia should be excluded before using this product since folic acid may mask the symptoms of pernicious anemia. The calcium content should be considered before prescribing for patients with kidney stones. Do not exceed the recommended dose.

Adverse Reactions: No adverse reactions or undesirable side effects have been attributed to the use of Natalins Rx tablets.

Dosage and Administration: One tablet daily, or as prescribed.

How Supplied:
Natalins® Rx Tablets: (Available on prescription.)
NDC 0087-0702-01 Bottles of 100
NDC 0087-0702-02 Bottles of 1000

Shown in Product Identification Section, page 419

OVCON®-50 ℞
[ŏv'kăn]

21 tablets of norethindrone 1 mg and ethinyl estradiol 0.05 mg. Each green tablet in the 28 day regimen contains inert ingredients.

OVCON®-35 ℞
21 tablets of norethindrone 0.4 mg and ethinyl estradiol 0.035 mg. Each green tablet in the 28 day regimen contains inert ingredients.

Oral contraceptives

Description: 28-Day OVCON®-50 and OVCON®-35 tablets provide a continuous regimen for oral contraception derived from 21 tablets composed of norethindrone and ethinyl estradiol to be followed by 7 green tablets of inert ingredients.
21-Day OVCON®-50 and OVCON®-35 tablets provide a regimen for oral contraception derived from 21 tablets composed of norethindrone and ethinyl estradiol. The chemical name for norethindrone is 17-hydroxy-19-nor-17α-pregn-4-en-20-yn-3-one and for ethinyl estradiol the chemical name is 19-nor-17α-pregna-1,3,5 (10)-trien-20-yne-3, 17-diol. The structural formulas are:

NORETHINDRONE

ETHINYL ESTRADIOL

The active OVCON-50 tablets contain 1 mg norethindrone and 50 mcg ethinyl estradiol. The active OVCON-35 tablets contain 0.4 mg norethindrone and 35 mcg ethinyl estradiol.
The green tablets contain inert ingredients.

Clinical Pharmacology: Combination oral contraceptives act primarily through the mechanism of gonadotropin suppression due to the estrogenic and progestational activity of the ingredients. Although the primary mechanism of action is inhibition of ovulation, alterations in the genital tract including changes in the cervical mucus (which increase the difficulty of sperm penetration) and the endometrium (which reduce the likelihood of implantation) may also contribute to contraceptive effectiveness.

Indications and Usage: OVCON is indicated for the prevention of pregnancy in women who elect to use oral contraceptives as a method of contraception.
Oral contraceptives are highly effective. The pregnancy rate in women using conventional combination oral contraceptives (containing 35 mcg or more of ethinyl estradiol or 50 mcg or more of mestranol) is generally reported as less than one pregnancy per 100 woman-years of use. Slightly higher rates (somewhat more than 1 pregnancy per 100 woman-years of use) are reported for some combination products containing 35 mcg or less of ethinyl estradiol, and rates on the order of 3 pregnancies per 100 woman-years are reported for the progestin-only oral contraceptives.
These rates are derived from separate studies conducted by different investigators in several population groups and cannot be compared precisely. Furthermore, pregnancy rates tend to be lower as clinical studies are continued, possibly due to selective retention in the longer studies of those patients who accept the treatment regimen and do not discontinue as a result of adverse reactions, pregnancy, or other reasons.
In clinical trials with OVCON-50, 1,126 patients completed 9,558 cycles and a total of 7 pregnancies were reported. This represents a pregnancy rate of 0.88 per 100 woman-years.
In clinical trials with OVCON-35, 2493 patients completed 35,881 cycles and a total of 33 pregnancies were reported. This represents a pregnancy rate of 1.10 per 100 woman-years.
The following table gives ranges of pregnancy rates reported in a standard textbook[1] for other means of contraception. An individual patient may achieve higher or lower rates with any given method (except the IUD), depending upon the degree of adherence to the method.

Pregnancies per 100 Woman-Years: IUD, less than 1-6; Diaphragm with spermicidal product (creams or jellies), 2-20; Condom, 3-36; Aerosol foams, 2-29; Jellies and creams, 4-36; Rhythm (all types), less than 1-47: 1. Calendar method, 14-47; 2. Temperature method, 1-20; 3. Temperature method—intercourse only in post-ovulatory phase, less than 1-7; 4. Mucus method, 1-25; No contraception, 60-80.

Dose-Related Risk of Thromboembolism from Oral Contraceptives: Two studies have shown a positive association between the dose of estrogens in oral contraceptives and the risk of thromboembolism.[2,3] For this reason, it is prudent and in keeping with good principles of therapeutics to minimize exposure to estrogen. The oral contraceptive product prescribed for any given patient should be that product which contains the least amount of estrogen that is compatible with an acceptable pregnancy rate and patient acceptance. It is recommended that new acceptors of oral contraceptives be started on preparations containing 50 mcg or less of estrogen.

Contraindications: Oral contraceptives should not be used in women with any of the following conditions:

for possible revisions   **Product Information**   1225

1. Thrombophlebitis or thromboembolic disorders.
2. A past history of deep vein thrombophlebitis or thromboembolic disorders.
3. Cerebral vascular or coronary artery disease.
4. Known or suspected carcinoma of the breast.
5. Known or suspected estrogen dependent neoplasia.
6. Undiagnosed abnormal genital bleeding.
7. Known or suspected pregnancy (see warning No. 5).
8. Benign or malignant liver tumor which developed during the use of oral contraceptives or other estrogen containing products.

Warnings:

> Cigarette smoking increases the risk of serious cardiovascular side effects from oral contraceptive use. This risk increases with age and with heavy smoking (15 or more cigarettes per day) and is quite marked in women over 35 years of age. Women who use oral contraceptives should be strongly advised not to smoke.
>
> The use of oral contraceptives is associated with increased risk of several serious conditions including thromboembolism, stroke, myocardial infarction, hepatic adenoma, gall bladder disease, hypertension. Practitioners prescribing oral contraceptives should be familiar with the following information relating to these risks.

1. Thromboembolic Disorders and Other Vascular Problems An increased risk of thromboembolic and thrombotic disease associated with the use of oral contraceptives is well established. Three principal studies in Great Britain[4-6] and three in the United States[7-10] have demonstrated an increased risk of fatal and nonfatal venous thromboembolism and stroke, both hemorrhagic and thrombotic. These studies estimate that users of oral contraceptives are 4 to 11 times more likely than nonusers to develop these diseases without evident cause (Table 2).

Cerebrovascular Disorders: In a collaborative American study[9,10] of cerebrovascular disorders in women with and without predisposing causes, it was estimated that the risk of hemorrhagic stroke was 2.0 times greater in users than nonusers and the risk of thrombotic stroke was 4 to 9.5 times greater in users than in nonusers (Table 2).

TABLE 2
SUMMARY OF RELATIVE RISK OF THROMBOEMBOLIC DISORDERS AND OTHER VASCULAR PROBLEMS IN ORAL CONTRACEPTIVE USERS COMPARED TO NONUSERS

	Relative risk, times greater
Idiopathic thromboembolic disease	4–11
Post surgery thromboembolic complications	4–6
Thrombotic stroke	4–9.5
Hemorrhagic stroke	2
Myocardial infarction	2–12

Myocardial Infarction: An increased risk of myocardial infarction associated with the use of oral contraceptives has been reported[11-13] confirming a previously suspected association. These studies, conducted in the United Kingdom, found, as expected, that the greater the number of underlying risk factors for coronary artery disease (cigarette smoking, hypertension, hypercholesterolemia, obesity, diabetes, history of preeclamptic toxemia) the higher the risk of developing myocardial infarction, regardless of whether the patient was an oral contraceptive user or not. Oral contraceptives, however, were found to be a clear additional risk factor.

In terms of relative risk, it has been estimated[52] that oral contraceptive users who do not smoke (smoking is considered a major predisposing condition to myocardial infarction) are about twice as likely to have a fatal myocardial infarction as nonusers who do not smoke. Oral contraceptive users who are also smokers have about a 5-fold increased risk of fatal infarction compared to users who do not smoke, but about a 10- to 12-fold increased risk compared to nonusers who do not smoke. Furthermore, the amount of smoking is also an important factor. In determining the importance of these relative risks, however, the baseline rates for various age groups, as shown in Table 3, must be given serious consideration. The importance of other predisposing conditions mentioned above in determining relative and absolute risks has not as yet been quantified; it is quite likely that the same synergistic action exists, but perhaps to a lesser extent.

TABLE 3
ESTIMATED ANNUAL MORTALITY RATE PER 100,000 WOMEN FROM MYOCARDIAL INFARCTION BY USE OF ORAL CONTRACEPTIVES, SMOKING HABITS, AND AGE (IN YEARS)

	Myocardial infarction			
	Women aged 30–39		Women aged 40–44	
Smoking habits	Users	Non Users	Users	Non Users
All smokers	10.2	2.6	62.0	15.9
Heavy[1]	13.0	5.1	78.7	31.3
Light	4.7	.9	28.6	5.7
Nonsmokers	1.8	1.2	10.7	7.4
Smokers and nonsmokers	5.4	1.9	32.8	11.7

[1]Heavy smoker: 15 or more cigarettes per day. From Jain, A.K., Studies in Family Planning, 8:50, 1977.

	Interim Report	Later Report	Most Recent Report
Statistically Significant Findings			
• Royal College of Gen. Practitioners		Higher rate of reporting of cerebrovascular accidents in users[26]	Increased incidence of cerebrovascular disease among users[56]
• British Family Planning Association		Association between O.C. user and occurrence stroke[58]	
• Walnut Creek Study			
Degree of Risk			
• Royal College of Gen. Practitioners			4-fold increase in mortality from circulatory disease in users[54]
• British Family Planning Association			4-fold increase (associated with age and smoking) in venous thrombosis and pulmonary embolism in users[58]
• Walnut Creek Study			Risk of subarachnoid hemorrhage associated with O.C. use, heavy smoking and age.[57,59]
Persistence of Risk			
• Royal College of Gen. Practitioners		Rate of circulatory disease increased with duration of use, may persist after discontinuation[53]	Cerebrovascular disease significantly greater in former users (up to six years) than in controls[56]
• Walnut Creek Study			Significant association between past O.C. use and risk of subarachnoid hemorrhage[57]
• U S Hospital-Based Study			2–3 fold increase in rate of myocardial infarction in former users of more than 10 years[55]

Risk of Dose: In an analysis of data derived from several national adverse reaction reporting systems,[2] British investigators concluded that the risk of thromboembolism including coronary thrombosis is directly related to the dose of estrogen used in oral contraceptives. Preparations containing 100 mcg or more of estrogen were associated with a higher risk of thromboembolism than those containing 50–80 mcg of estrogen. Their analysis did suggest, however, that the quantity of estrogen may not be the sole factor involved. This finding has been confirmed in the United States.[3] Careful epidemiological studies to determine the degree of thromboembolic risk associated with progestogen-only oral contraceptives have not been performed. Cases of thromboembolic disease have been reported in women using these products, and they should not be presumed to be free of excess risk.

Persistence of Risk: Persistence of risk after discontinuation of oral contraceptive use has been reported for circulatory disease in general,[53,54] for non-rheumatic heart disease[54,55] and for cerebrovascular disease[54,56] including subarachnoid hemorrhage,[53,54,57] cerebral thrombosis,[56] and transient ischemic attacks.[56]

[See table above].

Estimate of Excess Mortality from Circulatory Diseases: A large prospective study[53] carried out in the U.K. estimated the mortality rate per 100,000 women per year from diseases of the circulatory system for users and nonusers of oral contraceptives according to age, smoking habits, and duration of use. The overall excess death rate annually from circulatory diseases for oral contraceptive users was estimated to be 20 per 100,000 (ages 15–34—5/100,000; ages 35–44—33/100,000; ages 45–49—140/100,000), the risk being concentrated in older women, in those with a long duration of use, and in cigarette smokers. It was not possible, however, to examine the interrelationships of age, smoking and duration of use, nor to

Continued on next page

Mead Johnson Labs.—Cont.

compare the effects of continuous versus intermittent use. Although the study showed a 10-fold increase in death due to circulatory diseases in users for 5 or more years, all of these deaths occurred in women 35 or older. Until larger numbers of women under 35 with continuous use for 5 or more years are available, it is not possible to assess the magnitude of the relative risk for this younger age group.

The available data from a variety of sources have been analyzed[14] to estimate the risk of death associated with various methods of contraception. The estimates of risk of death for each method include the combined risk of the contraceptive method (e.g., thromboembolic and thrombotic disease in the case of oral contraceptives) plus the risk attributable to pregnancy or abortion in the event of method failure. This latter risk varies with the effectiveness of the contraceptive method. The findings of this analysis are shown in Figure 1 below.[14] The study concluded that the mortality associated with all methods of birth control is low and below that associated with childbirth, with the exception of oral contraceptives in women over 40 who smoke. (The rates given for pill only/smokers for each age group are for smokers as a class. For "heavy" smokers [more than 15 cigarettes a day], the rates given would be about double; for "light" smokers [less than 15 cigarettes a day], about 50 percent.) The lowest mortality is associated with the condom or diaphragm backed up by early abortion.

OVCON-50, -35

The risk of thromboembolic and thrombotic disease associated with oral contraceptives increases with age after approximately age 30 and, for myocardial infarction, is further increased by hypertension, hypercholesterolemia, obesity, diabetes, or history of preeclamptic toxemia and especially by cigarette smoking.

Based on the data currently available, the following chart gives a gross estimate of the risk of death from circulatory disorders associated with the use of oral contraceptives:

SMOKING HABITS AND OTHER PREDISPOSING CONDITIONS—RISK ASSOCIATED WITH USE OF ORAL CONTRACEPTIVES

Age	Below 30	30–39	40+
Heavy smokers	C	B	A
Light smokers	D	C	B
Nonsmokers (no predisposing conditions)	D	C,D	C
Nonsmokers (other predisposing conditions)	C	C,B	B,A

A—Use associated with very high risk.
B—Use associated with high risk.
C—Use associated with moderate risk.
D—Use associated with low risk.

The physician and the patient should be alert to the earliest manifestations of thromboembolic and thrombotic disorders (e.g., thrombophlebitis, pulmonary embolism, cerebrovascular insufficiency, coronary occlusion, retinal thrombosis, and mesenteric thrombosis). Should any of these occur or be suspected, the drug should be discontinued immediately.

A four- to six-fold increased risk of post surgery thromboembolic complications has been reported in oral contraceptive users.[15,16] If feasible, oral contraceptives should be discontinued at least 4 weeks before surgery of a type associated with an increased risk of thromboembolism or prolonged immobilization.

2. *Ocular Lesions.* There have been reports of neuro-ocular lesions such as optic neuritis or retinal thrombosis associated with the use of oral contraceptives. Discontinue oral contraceptive medication if there is unexplained, sudden or gradual, partial or complete loss of vision; onset of proptosis or diplopia; papilledema; or retinal vascular lesions and institute appropriate diagnostic and therapeutic measures.

3. *Carcinoma.* Long-term continuous administration of either natural or synthetic estrogen in certain animal species increases the frequency of carcinoma of the breast, cervix, vagina, and liver. Certain synthetic progestogens, none currently contained in oral contraceptives, have been noted to increase the incidence of mammary nodules, benign and malignant, in dogs.

In humans, three case control studies have reported an increased risk of endometrial carcinoma associated with the prolonged use of exogenous estrogen in post menopausal women.[17-19] One publication[20] reported on the first 21 cases submitted by physicians to a registry of cases of adenocarcinoma of the endometrium in women under 40 on oral contraceptives. Of the cases found in women without predisposing risk factors for adenocarcinoma of the endometrium (e.g., irregular bleeding at the time oral contraceptives were first given, polycystic ovaries), nearly all occurred in women who had used a sequential oral contraceptive. These products are no longer marketed. No evidence has been reported suggesting an increased risk of endometrial cancer in users of conventional combination or progestogen-only oral contraceptives.

Several studies[8,21-24] have found no increase in breast cancer in women taking oral contraceptives or estrogens. One study[25] however, while also noting no overall increased risk of breast cancer in women treated with oral contraceptives, found an excess risk in the subgroups of oral contraceptive users with documented benign breast disease. A reduced occurrence of benign breast tumors in users of oral contraceptives has been well-documented.[8,21,25-27]

In summary, there is at present no confirmed evidence from human studies of an increased risk of cancer associated with oral contraceptives. Close clinical surveillance of all women taking oral contraceptives is, nevertheless, essential. In all cases of undiagnosed persistent or recurrent abnormal vaginal bleeding, appropriate diagnostic measures should be taken to rule out malignancy. Women with a strong family history of breast cancer or who have breast nodules, fibrocystic disease or abnormal mammograms should be monitored with particular care if they elect to use oral contraceptives instead of other methods of contraception.

4. *Hepatic Tumors.* Benign hepatic adenomas have been found to be associated with the use of oral contraceptives.[28-30,46] One study[46] showed that oral contraceptive formulations with high hormonal potency were associated with a higher risk than lower potency formulations. Although benign, hepatic adenomas may rupture and may cause death through intra-abdominal hemorrhage. This has been reported in short-term as well as long-term users of oral contraceptives. Two studies relate risk with duration of use of the contraceptive, the risk being much greater after 4 or more years of oral contraceptive use.[30,46] While hepatic adenoma is a rare lesion, it should be considered in women presenting abdominal pain and tenderness, abdominal mass or shock.

A few cases of hepatocellular carcinoma have been reported in women taking oral contraceptives. The relationship of these drugs to this type of malignancy is not known at this time.

5. *Use in or Immediately Preceding Pregnancy, Birth Defects in Offspring, and Malignancy in Female Offspring.*

The use of female sex hormones—both estrogenic and progestational agents—during early pregnancy may seriously damage the offspring. It has been shown that females exposed in utero to diethylstilbestrol, a nonsteroidal estrogen, have an increased risk of developing in later life a form of vaginal or cervical cancer that is ordinarily extremely rare.[31,32] This risk has been estimated to be of the order of 1 in 1,000 exposures or less.[33,47] Although there is no evidence at the present time that oral contraceptives further enhance the risk of developing this type of malignancy, such patients should be monitored with particular care if they elect to use oral contraceptives instead of other methods of contraception. Furthermore, a high percentage of such exposed women (from 30 to 90%) have been found to have epithelial changes of the vagina and cervix.[34-38] Although these changes are histologically benign, it is not known whether this condition is a precursor of vaginal malignancy. Male children so exposed may develop abnormalities of the urogenital tract.[48-50] Although similar data are not available

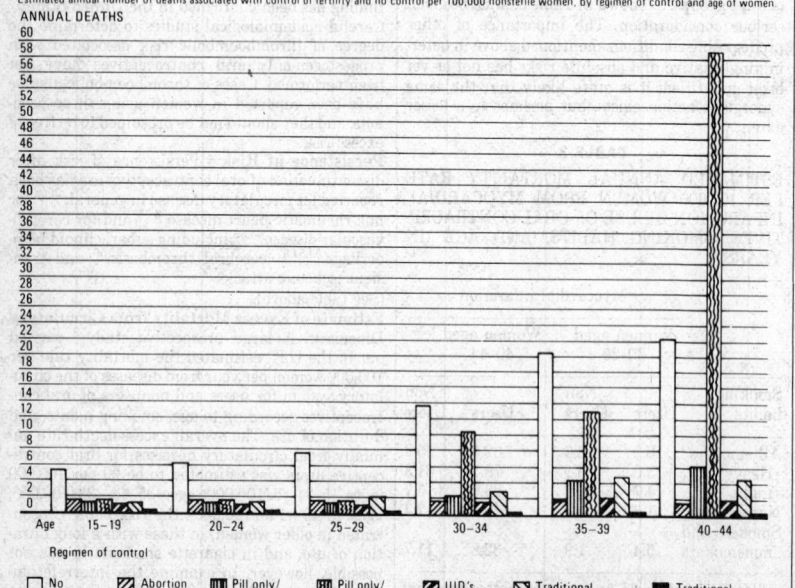

Figure 1
Estimated annual number of deaths associated with control of fertility and no control per 100,000 nonsterile women, by regimen of control and age of women.

with the use of other estrogens, it cannot be presumed that they would not induce similar changes. An increased risk of congenital anomalies, including heart defects and limb defects, has been reported with the use of sex hormones, including oral contraceptives, in pregnancy.[39-42,51] One case control study[42] has estimated a 4.7-fold increase in risk of limb-reduction defects in infants exposed in utero to sex hormones (oral contraceptives, hormonal withdrawal tests for pregnancy or attempted treatment for threatened abortion). Some of these exposures were very short and involved only a few days of treatment. The data suggest that the risk of limb-reduction defects in exposed fetuses is somewhat less than one in 1,000 live births.

In the past, female sex hormones have been used during pregnancy in an attempt to treat threatened or habitual abortion. There is considerable evidence that estrogens are ineffective for these indications, and there is no evidence from well controlled studies that progestogens are effective for these uses.

There is some evidence that triploidy and possibly other types of polyploidy are increased among abortuses from women who become pregnant soon after ceasing oral contraceptives.[43] Embryos with these anomalies are virtually always aborted spontaneously. Whether there is an overall increase in spontaneous abortion of pregnancies conceived soon after stopping oral contraceptives is unknown.

It is recommended that for any patient who has missed two consecutive periods, pregnancy should be ruled out before continuing the contraceptive regimen. If the patient has not adhered to the prescribed schedule, the possibility of pregnancy should be considered at the time of the first missed period (or after 45 days from the last menstrual period if the progestogen-only oral contraceptives are used), and further use of oral contraceptives should be withheld until pregnancy has been ruled out. If pregnancy is confirmed, the patient should be apprised of the potential risks to the fetus and the advisability of continuation of the pregnancy should be discussed in the light of these risks.

It is also recommended that women who discontinue oral contraceptives with the intent of becoming pregnant use an alternate form of contraception for a period of time before attempting to conceive. Many clinicians recommend 3 months although no precise information is available on which to base this recommendation.

The administration of progestogen-only or progestogen-estrogen combinations to induce withdrawal bleeding should not be used as a test of pregnancy.

6. Gallbladder Disease.
Studies[8,23,26] report an increased risk of surgically confirmed gallbladder disease in users of oral contraceptives and estrogens. In one study, an increased risk appeared after 2 years of use and doubled after 4 or 5 years of use. In one of the other studies, an increased risk was apparent between 6 and 12 months of use.

7. Carbohydrate and Lipid Metabolic Effects.
A decrease in glucose tolerance has been observed in a significant percentage of patients on oral contraceptives. For this reason, prediabetic and diabetic patients should be carefully observed while receiving oral contraceptives.

An increase in triglycerides and total phospholipids has been observed in patients receiving oral contraceptives.[44] The clinical significance of this finding remains to be defined.

8. Elevated Blood Pressure.
An increase in blood pressure has been reported in patients receiving oral contraceptives.[26] In some women, hypertension may occur within a few months of beginning oral contraceptive use. In the first year of use, the prevalence of women with hypertension is low in users and may be no higher than that of a comparable group of nonusers. The prevalence in users increases, however, with longer exposure, and in the fifth year of use is two and a half to three times the reported prevalence in the first year. Age is also strongly correlated with the development of hypertension in oral contraceptive users. Women who previously have had hypertension during pregnancy may be more likely to develop elevation of blood pressure when given oral contraceptives. Hypertension that develops as a result of taking oral contraceptives usually returns to normal after discontinuing the drug.

9. Headache.
The onset or exacerbation of migraine or development of headache of a new pattern which is recurrent, persistent, or severe, requires discontinuation of oral contraceptives and evaluation of the cause.

10. Bleeding Irregularities.
Breakthrough bleeding, spotting, and amenorrhea are frequent reasons for patients discontinuing oral contraceptives. In breakthrough bleeding, as in all cases of irregular bleeding from the vagina, nonfunctional causes should be borne in mind. In undiagnosed persistent or recurrent abnormal bleeding from the vagina, adequate diagnostic measures are indicated to rule out pregnancy or malignancy. If pathology has been excluded, time or a change to another formulation may solve the problem. Changing to an oral contraceptive with a higher estrogen content, while potentially useful in minimizing menstrual irregularity, should be done only if necessary since this may increase the risk of thromboembolic disease.

Women with a past history of oligomenorrhea or secondary amenorrhea or young women without regular cycles may have a tendency to remain anovulatory or to become amenorrheic after discontinuation of oral contraceptives. Women with these pre-existing problems should be advised of this possibility and encouraged to use other contraceptive methods. Post-use anovulation, possibly prolonged, may also occur in women without previous irregularities.

11. Ectopic Pregnancy.
Ectopic as well as intrauterine pregnancy may occur in contraceptive failures. However, in progestogen-only oral contraceptive failures, the ratio of ectopic to intrauterine pregnancies is higher than in women who are not receiving oral contraceptives, since the drugs are more effective in preventing intrauterine than ectopic pregnancies.

12. Breast Feeding.
Oral contraceptives given in the postpartum period may interfere with lactation. There may be a decrease in the quantity and quality of the breast milk. Furthermore, a small fraction of the hormonal agents in oral contraceptives has been identified in the milk of mothers receiving these drugs.[45] The effects, if any, on the breast-fed child have not been determined. If feasible, the use of oral contraceptives should be deferred until the infant has been weaned.

Precautions:
General

1. A complete medical and family history should be taken prior to the initiation of oral contraceptives. The pretreatment and periodic physical examinations should include special reference to blood pressure, breasts, abdomen and pelvic organs, including Papanicolaou smear and relevant laboratory tests. As a general rule, oral contraceptives should not be prescribed for longer than 1 year without another physical examination being performed.

2. Under the influence of estrogen-progestogen preparations, pre-existing uterine leiomyomata may increase in size.

3. Patients with a history of psychic depression should be carefully observed and the drug discontinued if depression recurs to a serious degree. Patients becoming significantly depressed while taking oral contraceptives should stop the medication and use an alternate method of contraception in an attempt to determine whether the symptom is drug related.

4. Oral contraceptives may cause some degree of fluid retention. They should be prescribed with caution, and only with careful monitoring, in patients with conditions which might be aggravated by fluid retention, such as convulsive disorders, migraine syndrome, asthma, or cardiac or renal insufficiency.

5. Patients with a past history of jaundice during pregnancy have an increased risk of recurrence of jaundice while receiving oral contraceptive therapy. If jaundice develops in any patient receiving such drugs, the medication should be discontinued.

6. Steroid hormones may be poorly metabolized in patients with impaired liver function and should be administered with caution in such patients.

7. Oral contraceptive users may have disturbances in normal tryptophan metabolism which may result from a relative pyridoxine deficiency. The clinical significance of this is yet to be determined.

8. Serum folate levels may be depressed by oral contraceptive therapy. Since the pregnant woman is predisposed to the development of folate deficiency and the incidence of folate deficiency increases with increasing gestation, it is possible that if a woman becomes pregnant shortly after stopping oral contraceptives, she may have a greater chance of developing folate deficiency, and complications attributed to this deficiency.

9. The pathologist should be advised of oral contraceptive therapy when relevant specimens are submitted.

10. Certain endocrine and liver function tests and blood components may be affected by estrogen-containing oral contraceptives:
   a. Increased sulfobromophthalein-retention.
   b. Increased prothrombin and factors VII, VIII, IX, and X; decreased antithrombin 3; increased norepinephrine-induced platelet aggregability.
   c. Increased thyroid binding globulin (TBG) leading to increased circulating total thyroid hormone, as measured by protein-bound iodine (PBI), T4 by column, or T4 by radioimmunoassay. Free T3 resin uptake is decreased, reflecting the elevated TBG, free T4 concentration is unaltered.
   d. Decreased pregnanediol excretion.
   e. Reduced response to metyrapone test.

11. The active yellow tablets and the inert green tablets in OVCON-50 (21 and 28 day regimens) and the inert green tablets in the 28 day regimen of OVCON-35 contain FD&C Yellow No. 5 (tartrazine) which may cause allergic-type reactions (including bronchial asthma) in certain susceptible individuals. Although the overall incidence of FD&C Yellow No. 5 (tartrazine) sensitivity in the general population is low, it is frequently seen in patients who also have aspirin hypersensitivity.

Information for the Patient: See Patient Labeling Printed below

Drug Interactions: Reduced efficacy and increased incidence of breakthrough bleeding have been associated with concomitant use of rifampin. A similar association has been suggested with barbiturates, phenylbutazone, phenytoin sodium, ampicillin, and tetracycline.

Carcinogenesis: See Warning section for information on the carcinogenic potential of oral contraceptives.

Pregnancy: Pregnancy category X. See Contraindications and Warnings.

Nursing Mothers: See Warnings.

Adverse Reactions: An increased risk of the following serious adverse reactions has been associated with the use of oral contraceptives (see Warnings):

    Thrombophlebitis.
    Pulmonary embolism.
    Coronary thrombosis.
    Cerebral thrombosis.
    Cerebral hemorrhage.
    Hypertension.
    Gallbladder disease.
    Benign hepatomas.
    Congenital anomalies.

There is evidence of an association between the following conditions and the use of oral contraceptives, although additional confirmatory studies are needed:

Continued on next page

Mead Johnson Labs.—Cont.

Mesenteric thrombosis.
Neuro-ocular lesions, e.g., retinal thrombosis and optic neuritis.

The following adverse reactions have been reported in patients receiving oral contraceptives and are believed to be drug related:

Nausea and/or vomiting, usually the most common adverse reactions, occur in approximately 10% or less of patients during the first cycle. Other reactions, as a general rule, are seen much less frequently or only occasionally.

Gastrointestinal symptoms (such as abdominal cramps and bloating).
Breakthrough bleeding.
Spotting.
Change in menstrual flow.
Dysmenorrhea.
Amenorrhea during and after treatment.
Temporary infertility after discontinuance of treatment.
Edema.
Chloasma or melasma which may persist.
Breast changes: tenderness, enlargement, and secretion.
Change in weight (increase or decrease).
Change in cervical erosion and cervical secretion.
Possible diminution in lactation when given immediately postpartum.
Cholestatic jaundice.
Migraine.
Increase in size of uterine leiomyomata.
Rash (allergic).
Mental depression.
Reduced tolerance to carbohydrates.
Vaginal candidiasis.
Change in corneal curvature (steepening).
Intolerance to contact lenses.

The following adverse reactions have been reported in users of oral contraceptives, and the association has been neither confirmed nor refuted:

Premenstrual-like syndrome.
Cataracts.
Changes in libido.
Chorea.
Changes in appetite.
Cystitis-like syndrome.
Headache.
Nervousness.
Dizziness.
Hirsutism.
Loss of scalp hair.
Erythema multiforme.
Erythema nodosum.
Hemorrhagic Eruption.
Vaginitis.
Porphyria.

Acute Overdose: Serious ill effects have not been reported following acute ingestion of large doses of oral contraceptives by young children. Overdosage may cause nausea, and withdrawal bleeding may occur in females.

Dosage and Administration: To achieve maximum contraceptive effectiveness, OVCON-50 or OVCON-35 must be taken exactly as directed and at intervals not exceeding 24 hours.

28-DAY REGIMEN

The patient takes one tablet daily from a convenient package as follows: (yellow or peach tablet containing active ingredients, green tablet containing inert ingredients)

For the first cycle of use only, the first yellow or peach tablet is taken on day 5 of the menstrual cycle, counting the first day of bleeding as day 1. One tablet is taken daily in the same sequence as in the package—first the yellow or peach, then the green tablets. After the last green tablet is taken, the first yellow or peach tablet from a new package is taken **the following day**. Withdrawal bleeding will usually begin while the patient is taking the green tablets and may continue during the first few tablets from the next package.

21-DAY REGIMEN

The patient takes one tablet daily from a convenient package as follows: (yellow or peach)

For the first cycle of use only, the first yellow or peach tablet is taken on day 5 of the menstrual cycle, counting the first day of bleeding as day 1. Continue taking one tablet daily from the 5th through the 25th day of the menstrual cycle. If the first tablet is taken later than the fifth day of the first menstrual cycle an additional form of contraception should be used for at least one week. Withdrawal bleeding will normally begin within 2–3 days after taking the last tablet. The first tablet of the next package should be taken on the eighth day after the last tablet, even if menstrual bleeding has not ceased. The dosage regimen then continues with one tablet daily for 21 days followed by 7 days of no medication, thus a cycle of three-weeks-on and one-week-off.

Patients should be cautioned to follow the dosage schedule strictly.

Evening administration is suggested. If the regimen is interrupted, an additional contraceptive method is recommended for the rest of the cycle. Should spotting or breakthrough bleeding occur, it is recommended that the patient continue medication. If bleeding is persistent or recurrent, the patient should consult her physician.

Use of oral contraceptives in the event of a missed menstrual period:

1. If the patient has not adhered to the prescribed dosage regimen, the possibility of pregnancy should be considered after the first missed period and oral contraceptives should be withheld until pregnancy has been ruled out.

2. If the patient has adhered to the prescribed regimen and misses two consecutive periods, pregnancy should be ruled out before continuing the contraceptive regimen.

How Supplied:
OVCON®-50 is available in 21 and 28 day regimens. Each package contains 21 yellow tablets of 1.0 mg. norethindrone and 0.05 mg. ethinyl estradiol. Each green tablet in the 28 day regimen contains inert ingredients.

NDC 0087-0584-40	Package of 21 tablets
NDC 0087-0584-42	Carton of 6 packages
NDC 0087-0579-40	Package of 28 tablets
NDC 0087-0579-41	Carton of 6 packages

OVCON®-35 is available in 21 and 28 day regimens. Each package contains 21 peach tablets of 0.4 mg. norethindrone and 0.035 mg. ethinyl estradiol. Each green tablet in the 28 day regimen contains inert ingredients.

NDC 0087-0583-40	Package of 21 tablets
NDC 0087-0583-42	Carton of 6 packages
NDC 0087-0578-40	Package of 28 tablets
NDC 0087-0578-41	Carton of 6 packages

References:

1. "Population Reports," Series H, Number 2, May 1974; Series I, Number 1, June 1974; Series B, Number 2, Jan 1975; Series H, Number 3, 1975; Series H, Number 4, Jan 1976 (published by the Population Information Program, The George Washington University Medical Center, 2001 S St. NW Washington, DC).
2. Inman WHW, et al.: Brit M J 2:203, 1970.
3. Stolley PD, et al.: Am J Epidemiol 102:197, 1975.
4. Royal College of General Practitioners, J Coll Gen Pract 13:267, 1967.
5. Inman WHW, et al.: Brit M J 2:193, 1968.
6. Vessey MP, Doll R: Brit M J 2:651, 1969.
7. Sartwell PE, et al.: Am J Epidemiol 90:365, 1969.
8. Boston Collaborative Drug Surveillance Program: Lancet 1:1399, 1973.
9. Collaborative Group for the Study of Stroke in Young Women: N Eng J Med 288:871, 1973.
10. Collaborative Group for the Study of Stroke in Young Women: JAMA 231:871, 1975.
11. Mann JI, Inman WHW: Brit M J 2:245, 1975.
12. Mann JI, et al.: Brit M J 2:445, 1976.
13. Mann JI, et al.: Brit M J 2:241, 1975.
14. Tietze C: Family Planning Perspectives 9:74, 1977.
15. Vessey MP, et al.: Brit M J 3:123, 1970.
16. Greene GR, Sartwell PE: Am J Pub Health 62:680, 1972.
17. Smith DC, et al.: N Eng J Med 293:1164, 1975.
18. Ziel HK, Finkle WD: N Eng J Med 293:1167, 1975.
19. Mack TN, et al.: New Eng J Med 294:1262, 1976.
20. Silverberg SG, Makowski EL: Ob Gyn 46:503, 1975.
21. Vessey MP, et al.: Brit M J 3:719, 1972.
22. Vessey MP, et al.: Lancet 1:941, 1975.
23. Boston Collaborative Drug Surveillance Program: New Eng J Med 290:15, 1974.
24. Arthes FG, et al.: Cancer 28:1391, 1971.
25. Fasal E, Paffenbarger RS: J Natl Cancer Inst 55:767, 1975.
26. Royal College of General Practitioners: Oral Contraceptives and Health, London, Pitman, 1974.
27. Ory H, et al.:, New Eng J Med 294:419, 1976.
28. Baum J, et al.: Lancet 2:926, 1973.
29. Mays ET, et al.: JAMA 235:730, 1976.
30. Edmondson HA, et al.: New Eng J Med 294:470, 1976.
31. Herbst AL, et al.: New Eng J Med 284:878, 1971.
32. Greenwald P, et al.: New Eng J Med 285:390, 1971.
33. Lanier AP, et al.: Mayo Clin Proc 48:793, 1973.
34. Herbst AL: Ob Gyn 40:287, 1972.
35. Herbst AL, et al.: Am J Ob Gyn 118:607, 1974.
36. Herbst AL, et al.: New Eng J Med 292:334, 1975.
37. Stafl A, et al.: Ob Gyn 43:118, 1974.
38. Sherman AI, et al.: Ob Gyn 44:531, 1974.
39. Gal I, et al.: Nature 216:83, 1967.
40. Levy EP, et al.: Lancet 1:611, 1973.
41. Nora JJ, Nora AH: Lancet 1:941, 1973.
42. Janerich DT, et al.: New Eng J Med 291:697, 1974.

43. Carr DH: Canadian Med Assoc J 103:343, 1970.
44. Wynn V, et al.: Lancet 2:720, 1966.
45. Laumas KR, et al.: Am J Ob Gyn 98:411, 1967.
46. Center for Disease Control, Morbidity and Mortality Weekly Report, 26:293, 1977.
47. Herbst AL, et al.: Am J Ob Gyn 128:43, 1977.
48. Bibbo M, et al.: J Reprod Med 15:29, 1975.
49. Gill WB, et al.: J Reprod Med 16:147, 1976.
50. Henderson BE, et al.: Pediatrics 58:505, 1976.
51. Heinonen OP, et al.: New Eng J Med 296:67, 1977.
52. Jain AK: Studies in Family Planning 8:50, 1977.
53. Beral V: Lancet 2:727, 1977.
54. Layde PM, et al.: Lancet 1:541, 1981
55. Slone D, et al.: N Eng J Med 305:420, 1981.
56. Layde PM, et al.: J R Coll Gen Pract 33:75, 1983.
57. Petitti DB, et al.: Lancet 2:234, 1978.
58. Vessey M, et al.: J Biosoc Sci 8:373, 1976.
59. Ramcharan S, et al.: The Walnut Creek Contraceptive Drug Study, Vol. 3, US. Govt. Ptg. Off. J Reprod Med 25:346, 1980.

The Patient Labeling for oral contraceptive drug products is set forth below:

BRIEF SUMMARY
PATIENT PACKAGE INSERT

Warning:

> Cigarette smoking increases the risk of serious adverse effects on the heart and blood vessels from oral contraceptive use. This risk increases with age and with heavy smoking (15 or more cigarettes per day) and is quite marked in women over 35 years of age. Women who use oral contraceptives should not smoke.

Oral contraceptives taken as directed are about 99% effective in preventing pregnancy. (The mini-pill, however, is somewhat less effective.) Forgetting to take your pills increases the chance of pregnancy. Various drugs, such as antibiotics, may also decrease the effectiveness of oral contraceptives. Women who have or have had clotting disorders, cancer of the breast or sex organs, unexplained vaginal bleeding, a stroke, heart attack, angina pectoris, or who suspect they may be pregnant should not use oral contraceptives.
Most side effects of the pill are not serious. The most common side effects are nausea, vomiting, bleeding between menstrual periods, weight gain, and breast tenderness. However, proper use of oral contraceptives requires that they be taken under your doctor's continuous supervision, because they can be associated with serious side effects which may be fatal. Fortunately, these occur very infrequently. The serious side effects are:

1. Blood clots in the legs, lungs, brain, heart or other organs and hemorrhage into the brain due to bursting of a blood vessel.
2. Liver tumors, which may rupture and cause severe bleeding.
3. Birth defects if the pill is taken while you are pregnant.
4. High blood pressure.
5. Gallbladder disease.

The symptoms associated with these serious side effects are discussed in the detailed leaflet given you with your supply of pills. Notify your doctor if you notice any unusual physical disturbance while taking the pill.
The estrogen in oral contraceptives has been found to cause breast cancer and other cancers in certain animals. These findings suggest that oral contraceptives may also cause cancer in humans. However, studies to date in women taking currently marketed oral contraceptives have not confirmed that oral contraceptives cause cancer in humans.
The detailed leaflet describes more completely the benefits and risks of oral contraceptives. It also provides information on other forms of contraception. Read it carefully. If you have any questions, consult your doctor.
Caution: Oral contraceptives are of no value in the prevention or treatment of venereal disease.

Detailed Patient Labeling

What You Should Know About Oral Contraceptives: Oral contraceptives ("the pill") are the most effective way (except for sterilization) to prevent pregnancy. They are also convenient and, for most women, free of serious or unpleasant side effects. Oral contraceptives must always be taken under the continuous supervision of a physician. It is important that any woman who considers using an oral contraceptive understand the risks involved. Although the oral contraceptives have important advantages over other methods of contraception, they have certain risks that no other method has. Only you can decide whether the advantages are worth these risks. This leaflet will tell you about the most important risks. It will explain how you can help your doctor prescribe the pill as safely as possible by telling him about yourself and being alert for the earliest signs of trouble. And it will tell you how to use the pill properly, so that it will be as effective as possible. There is more detailed information available in the leaflet prepared for doctors. Your pharmacist can show you a copy; you may need your doctor's help in understanding parts of it.

Who Should Not Use Oral Contraceptives:
A. If you have any of the following conditions you should not use the pill:
 1. Clots in the legs or lungs.
 2. Angina pectoris.
 3. Known or suspected cancer of the breast or sex organs.
 4. Unusual vaginal bleeding that has not yet been diagnosed.
 5. Known or suspected pregnancy.
B. If you have had any of the following conditions you should not use the pill:
 1. Heart attack or stroke.
 2. Clots in the legs or lungs.

Warning:

> C. Cigarette smoking increases the risk of serious adverse effects on the heart and blood vessels from oral contraceptive use. This risk increases with age and with heavy smoking (15 or more cigarettes per day) and is quite marked in women over 35 years of age. Women who use oral contraceptives should not smoke.

D. If you have scanty or irregular periods or are a young woman without a regular cycle, you should use another method of contraception because, if you use the pill, you may have difficulty becoming pregnant or may fail to have menstrual periods after discontinuing the pill.

Deciding to Use Oral Contraceptives: If you do not have any of the conditions listed above and are thinking about using oral contraceptives, to help you decide, you need information about the advantages and risks of oral contraceptives and of other contraceptive methods as well. This leaflet describes the advantages and risks of oral contraceptives. Except for sterilization, the IUD and abortion, which have their own exclusive risks, the only serious risks of other methods of contraception are those due to pregnancy should the method fail. Your doctor can answer questions you may have with respect to other methods of contraception. He can also answer any questions you may have after reading this leaflet on oral contraceptives.

1. What Oral Contraceptives Are and How They Work. Oral Contraceptives are of two types. The most common, often simply called "the pill" is a combination of an estrogen and a progestogen, the two kinds of female hormones. The amount of estrogen and progestogen can vary, but the amount of estrogen is most important because both the effectiveness and some of the dangers of oral contraceptives are related to the amount of estrogen. This kind of oral contraceptive works principally by preventing release of an egg from the ovary. When the amount of estrogen is 50 micrograms or more of mestranol or 35 micrograms or more of ethinyl estradiol and the pill is taken as directed, oral contraceptives are more than 99% effective (i.e., there would be less than one pregnancy if 100 women used the pill for 1 year). Pills that contain 20 to 35 micrograms of estrogen vary slightly in effectiveness, ranging from 98% to more than 99% effective.
The second type of oral contraceptive, often called the "mini-pill", contains only a progestogen. It works in part by preventing release of an egg from the ovary but also by keeping sperm from reaching the egg and by making the uterus (womb) less receptive to any fertilized egg that reaches it. The mini-pill is less effective than the combination oral contraceptive, about 97% effective. In addition, the progestogen-only pill has a tendency to cause irregular bleeding which may be quite inconvenient, or cessation of bleeding entirely. The progestogen-only pill is used despite its lower effectiveness in the hope that it will prove not to have some of the serious side effects of the estrogen-containing pill (see below) but it is not yet certain that the mini-pill does in fact have fewer serious side effects. The discussion below, while based mainly on information about the combination pills, should be considered to apply as well to the mini-pill.

2. Other Nonsurgical Ways to Prevent Pregnancy. As this leaflet will explain, oral contraceptives have several serious risks. Other methods of contraception have lesser risks or none at all. They are also less effective than oral contraceptives, but, used properly, may be effective enough for many women. The following table gives reported pregnancy rates (the number of women out of 100 who would become pregnant in 1 year) for these methods:

Pregnancies per 100 Women per year:
Intrauterine device (IUD), less than 1–6;
Diaphragm with spermicidal products (creams or jellies), 2–20;
Condom (rubber), 3–36;
Aerosol foams, 2–29;
Jellies and creams, 4–36;
Periodic abstinence (rhythm) all types, less than 1–47;
 1. Calendar method, 14–47;
 2. Temperature method, 1–20;
 3. Temperature method—intercourse only in post-ovulatory phase, less than 1–7;
 4. Mucus method, 1–25;
No contraception, 60–80.
The figures (except for the IUD) vary widely because people differ in how well they use each

Continued on next page

Mead Johnson Labs.—Cont.

method. Very faithful users of the various methods obtain very good results, except for users of the calendar method of periodic abstinence (rhythm). Except for the IUD, effective use of these methods requires somewhat more effort than simply taking a single pill every morning, but it is an effort that many couples undertake successfully. Your doctor can tell you a great deal more about these methods of contraception.

3. The Dangers of Oral Contraceptives.

a. Circulatory disorders (abnormal blood clotting and stroke due to hemorrhage). Blood clots (in various blood vessels of the body) are the most common of the serious side effects of oral contraceptives. A clot can result in a stroke (if the clot is in the brain), a heart attack (if the clot is in a blood vessel of the heart), or a pulmonary embolus (a clot which forms in the legs or pelvis, then breaks off and travels to the lungs). Any of these can be fatal. Clots also occur rarely in the blood vessels of the eye, resulting in blindness or impairment of vision in that eye. There is evidence that the risk of clotting increases with higher estrogen doses. It is therefore important to keep the dose of estrogen as low as possible, so long as the oral contraceptive used has an acceptable pregnancy rate and doesn't cause unacceptable changes in the menstrual pattern. Furthermore, cigarette smoking by oral contraceptive users increases the risk of serious adverse effects on the heart and blood vessels. This risk increases with age and with heavy smoking (15 or more cigarettes per day) and begins to become quite marked in women over 35 years of age. For this reason women who use oral contraceptives should not smoke.

The risk of abnormal clotting increases with age in both users and nonusers of oral contraceptives, but the increased risk from the contraceptive appears to be present at all ages. For oral contraceptive users in general, it has been estimated that in women between the ages of 15 and 34 the risk of death due to a circulatory disorder is about 1 in 12,000 per year, whereas for nonusers the rate is about 1 in 50,000 per year. In the age group 35 to 44, the risk is estimated to be about 1 in 2,500 per year for oral contraceptive users and about 1 in 10,000 per year for nonusers.

Even without the pill the risk of having a heart attack increases with age and is also increased by such heart attack risk factors as high blood pressure, high cholesterol, obesity, diabetes, and cigarette smoking. Without any risk factors present, the use of oral contraceptives alone may double the risk of heart attack. However, the combination of cigarette smoking, especially heavy smoking, and oral contraceptive use greatly increases the risk of heart attack. Oral contraceptive users who smoke are about 5 times more likely to have a heart attack than users who do not smoke and about 10 times more likely to have a heart attack than nonusers who do not smoke. It has been estimated that users between the ages of 30 and 39 who smoke have about a 1 in 10,000 chance each year of having a fatal heart attack compared to about a 1 in 50,000 chance in users who do not smoke, and about a 1 in 100,000 chance in nonusers who do not smoke. In the age group 40 to 44, the risk is about 1 in 1,700 per year for users who smoke compared to about 1 in 10,000 for users who do not smoke and to about 1 in 14,000 per year for nonusers who do not smoke. Heavy smoking (about 15 cigarettes or more a day) further increases the risk. If you do not smoke and have none of the other heart attack risk factors described above, you will have a smaller risk than listed. If you have several heart attack risk factors, the risk may be considerably greater than listed.

In addition to blood-clotting disorders, it has been estimated that women taking oral contraceptives are twice as likely as nonusers to have a stroke due to rupture of a blood vessel in the brain.

b. Formation of tumors. Studies have found that when certain animals are given the female sex hormone estrogen, which is an ingredient of oral contraceptives, continuously for long periods, cancers may develop in the breast, cervix, vagina, and liver.

These findings suggest that oral contraceptives may cause cancer in humans. However, studies to date in women taking currently marketed oral contraceptives have not confirmed that oral contraceptives cause cancer in humans. Several studies have found no increase in breast cancer in users, although one study suggested oral contraceptives might cause an increase in breast cancer in women who already have benign breast disease. Women with a strong family history of breast cancer or who have breast nodules, fibrocystic disease, or abnormal mammograms or who were exposed to DES (diethylstilbestrol), an estrogen, during their mother's pregnancy must be followed very closely by their doctors if they choose to use oral contraceptives instead of another method of contraception. Many studies have shown that women taking oral contraceptives have less risk of getting benign breast disease than those who have not used oral contraceptives. Recently, strong evidence has emerged that estrogens (one component of oral contraceptives), when given for periods of more than one year to women after the menopause, increase the risk of cancer of the uterus (womb). There is also some evidence that a kind of oral contraceptive which is no longer marketed, the sequential oral contraceptive, may increase the risk of cancer of the uterus. There remains no evidence, however, that the oral contraceptives now available increase the risk of this cancer.

Oral contraceptives do cause, although rarely, a benign (non-malignant) tumor of the liver. These tumors do not spread, but they may rupture and cause internal bleeding, which may be fatal. A few cases of cancer of the liver have been reported in women using oral contraceptives, but it is not yet known whether the drug caused them.

c. Dangers to a developing child if oral contraceptives are used in or immediately preceding pregnancy. Oral contraceptives should not be taken by pregnant women because they may damage the developing child. An increased risk of birth defects, including heart defects and limb defects, has been associated with the use of sex hormones, including oral contraceptives, in pregnancy. In addition, the developing female child whose mother has received DES (diethylstilbestrol), an estrogen, during pregnancy has a risk of getting cancer of the vagina or cervix in her teens or young adulthood. This risk is estimated to be about 1 in 1,000 exposures or less. Abnormalities of the urinary and sex organs have been reported in male offspring so exposed. It is possible that other estrogens, such as the estrogens in oral contraceptives, could have the same effect in the child if the mother takes them during pregnancy.

If you stop taking oral contraceptives to become pregnant, your doctor may recommend that you use another method of contraception for a short while. The reason for this is that there is evidence from studies in women who have had "miscarriages" soon after stopping the pill that the lost fetuses are more likely to be abnormal. Whether there is an overall increase in "miscarriage" in women who become pregnant soon after stopping the pill as compared with women who do not use the pill is not known, but it is possible that there may be. If, however, you do become pregnant soon after stopping oral contraceptives, and do not have a miscarriage, there is no evidence that the baby has an increased risk of being abnormal.

d. Gallbladder disease. Women who use oral contraceptives have a greater risk than nonusers of having gallbladder disease requiring surgery. The increased risk may first appear within 1 year of use and may double after 4 or 5 years of use.

e. Other side effects of oral contraceptives. Some women using oral contraceptives experience unpleasant side effects that are not dangerous and are not likely to damage their health. Some of these may be temporary. Your breasts may feel tender, nausea and vomiting may occur, you may gain or lose weight and your ankles may swell. A spotty darkening of the skin, particularly of the face, is possible and may persist. You may notice unexpected vaginal bleeding or changes in your menstrual period. Irregular bleeding is frequently seen when using the mini-pill or combination oral contraceptives containing less than 50 micrograms of estrogen.

More serious side effects include worsening of migraine, asthma, epilepsy, and kidney or heart disease because of a tendency for water to be retained in the body when oral contraceptives are used. Other side effects are growth of pre-existing fibroid tumors of the uterus; mental depression; and liver problems with jaundice (yellowing of the skin). Your doctor may find that levels of sugar and fatty substances in your blood are elevated; the long-term effects of these changes are not known. While taking oral contraceptives some women develop high blood pressure which may persist after discontinuation.

Other reactions, although not proved to be caused by oral contraceptives, are occasionally reported. These include more frequent urination and some discomfort when urinating, nervousness, dizziness, some loss of scalp hair, an increase in body hair, an increase or decrease in sex drive, appetite changes, cataracts, and a need for a change in contact lens prescription or inability to use contact lenses.

After you stop using oral contraceptives there may be a delay before you are able to become pregnant or before you resume having menstrual periods. This is especially true of women who had irregular menstrual cycles prior to the use of oral contraceptives. As discussed previously, your doctor may recommend that you wait a short while after stopping the pill before you try to become pregnant. During this time, use another form of contraception. You should consult your physician before resuming use of oral contraceptives after childbirth, especially if you plan to nurse your baby. Drugs in oral contraceptives are known to appear in the milk, and the long-range effects on infants is not known at this time. Furthermore, oral contraceptives may cause a decrease in your milk supply as well as in the quality of the milk.

4. Comparison of the Risks of Oral Contraceptives and Other Contraceptive Methods. The many studies on the risks and effectiveness of oral contraceptives and other methods of contraception have been analyzed to estimate the risk of death associated with various methods of contraception. This risk has two parts: (a) the risk of the method itself (e.g., the risk that oral contraceptives will cause death due to abnormal clotting), and (b) the risk of death due to pregnancy or abortion in the event the method fails. The results of this analysis are shown in the bar graph below. The height of the bars is the number of deaths per 100,000 women each year. There are six sets of bars, each set referring to specific age groups of women. Within each set of bars there is a single bar for each of the different contraceptive methods. For oral contraceptives, there are two bars—one for smokers and the other for nonsmokers. The analysis is based on present knowledge and new information could, of course, alter it. The analysis shows that the risk of death from all methods of birth control is low and below that associated with child birth, except for oral contraceptives in women over 40 who smoke. It shows that the lowest risk of death is associated with the condom or diaphragm (traditional contraception) backed up by early abortion in case of failure of the condom or diaphragm to prevent pregnancy. Also, at any age the risk of death (due to unexpected pregnancy) from the use of traditional contraception, even without a backup of abortion, is generally the same as or less than that from use of oral contraceptives. (See Figure 1)

Product Information

OVCON-50, -35

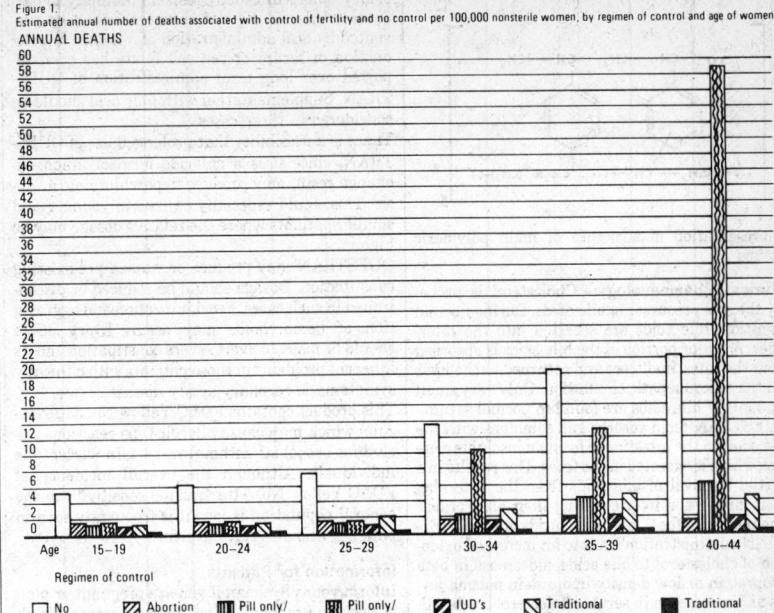

Figure 1.
Estimated annual number of deaths associated with control of fertility and no control per 100,000 nonsterile women, by regimen of control and age of women.

How to Use Oral Contraceptives as Safely and Effectively as Possible, Once You Have Decided to Use Them:

NOTE:
Reduced effectiveness and an increased incidence of breakthrough bleeding have been associated with the use of oral contraceptives with antibiotics such as rifampicin, ampicillin, and tetracycline or with certain other drugs, such as barbiturates, phenylbutazone or phenytoin sodium. You should use an additional means of contraception during any cycle in which any of these drugs are taken.

1. What to Tell your Doctor.
You can make use of the pill as safe as possible by telling your doctor if you have any of the following:

 a. Conditions that mean you should not use oral contraceptives:
 Clots in the legs or lungs.
 Clots in the legs or lungs in the past.
 A stroke, heart attack, or angina pectoris.
 Known or suspected cancer of the breast or sex organs.
 Unusual vaginal bleeding that has not yet been diagnosed.
 Known or suspected pregnancy.

 b. Conditions that your doctor will want to watch closely or which might cause him to suggest another method of contraception:
 A family history of breast cancer.
 Breast nodules, fibrocystic disease of the breast, or an abnormal mammogram.
 Diabetes.
 High blood pressure.
 High cholesterol.
 Cigarette smoking.
 Migraine headaches.
 Heart or kidney disease.
 Epilepsy.
 Mental depression.
 Fibroid tumors of the uterus.
 Gallbladder disease.

 c. Once you are using oral contraceptives, you should be alert for signs of a serious adverse effect and call your doctor if they occur:
 Sharp pain in the chest, coughing blood, or sudden shortness of breath (indicating possible clots in the lungs).
 Pain in the calf (possible clot in the leg).
 Crushing chest pain or heaviness (indicating possible heart attack).
 Sudden severe headache or vomiting, dizziness or fainting, disturbance of vision or speech or weakness or numbness in an arm or leg (indicating a possible stroke).
 Sudden partial or complete loss of vision (indicating a possible clot in the eye).
 Breast lumps (you should ask your doctor to show you how to examine your own breasts).
 Severe pain in the abdomen (indicating a possible ruptured tumor of the liver).
 Severe depression.
 Yellowing of the skin (jaundice).

2. How to Take the Pill So That It Is Most Effective. To achieve maximum contraceptive effectiveness, OVCON-50 or OVCON-35 must be taken exactly as directed and at intervals not exceeding 24 hours.

28-DAY REGIMEN

The patient takes one tablet daily from a convenient package as follows: (yellow or peach tablet containing active ingredients, green tablet containing inert ingredients)

For the first cycle of use only, the first yellow or peach tablet is taken on day 5 of the menstrual cycle, counting the first day of bleeding as day 1. One tablet is taken daily in the same sequence as in the package—first the yellow or peach, and then the green tablets. After the last green tablet is taken, the first yellow or peach tablet from a new package is taken **the following day**. Withdrawal bleeding will usually begin while the patient is taking the green tablets and may continue during the first few tablets from the next package.

21-DAY REGIMEN

The patient takes one tablet daily from a convenient package as follows: (yellow or peach)

For the first cycle of use only, the first yellow or peach tablet is taken on day 5 of the menstrual cycle, counting the first day of bleeding as day 1. Continue taking one tablet daily from the 5th through the 25th day of the menstrual cycle. If the first tablet is taken later than the fifth day of the first menstrual cycle an additional form of contraception should be used for at least one week. Withdrawal bleeding will normally begin within 2-3 days after taking the last tablet. The first tablet of the next package should be taken on the eighth day after the last tablet even if menstrual bleeding has not ceased. The dosage regimen then continues with one tablet daily for 21 days followed by 7 days of no medication, thus a cycle of three-weeks-on and one-week-off.

Patients should be cautioned to follow the dosage schedule strictly.
Evening administration is suggested. If the regimen is interrupted, an additional contraceptive method is recommended for the rest of the cycle. Should spotting or breakthrough bleeding occur, it is recommended that the patient continue medication. If bleeding is persistent or recurrent, the patient should consult her physician.

3. Use of oral contraceptives in the event of a missed menstrual period:

 a. If the patient has not adhered to the prescribed dosage regimen, the possibility of pregnancy should be considered after the first missed period and oral contraceptives should be withheld until pregnancy has been ruled out.

 b. If the patient has adhered to the prescribed regimen and misses two consecutive periods, pregnancy should be ruled out before continuing the contraceptive regimen.

 c. At times there may be no menstrual period after a cycle of pills. Therefore, if you miss one menstrual period but have taken the pills **exactly as you were supposed to**, continue as usual into the next cycle. If you have not taken the pills correctly and miss a menstrual period, you may be pregnant and should stop taking oral contraceptives until your doctor determines whether or not you are pregnant. Until you can get to your doctor, use another form of contraception. If two consecutive menstrual periods are missed, you should stop taking pills until it is determined whether you are pregnant. If you do become pregnant while using oral contraceptives, you should discuss the risks to the developing child with your doctor.

4. Periodic Examination.
Your doctor will take a complete medical and family history before prescribing oral contraceptives. At that time and about once a year thereafter, he will generally examine your blood pressure, breasts, abdomen, and pelvic organs (including a Papanicolaou smear, i.e., test for cancer).

5. Note.
Each Ovcon-50 tablet (both yellow and green tablets) and the green tablets in the 28-day Ovcon-35 contain FD&C Yellow No. 5 (tartrazine) which may cause allergic type reactions (such as asthma symptoms) in a small number of women. Although the overall incidence of this allergy is very low, it may occur in persons who are also allergic to aspirin.

Summary: Oral contraceptives are the most effective method, except sterilization, for preventing pregnancy. Other methods, when used conscientiously, are also very effective and have fewer risks. The serious risks of oral contraceptives are uncommon and the "pill" is a very convenient method of preventing pregnancy.

If you have certain conditions or have had these conditions in the past, you should not use oral contraceptives because the risk is too great. These conditions are listed in the leaflet. If you do not have these conditions, and decide to use the "pill," please read the leaflet carefully so that you can use the "pill" most safely and effectively.

Based on his or her assessment of your medical needs, your doctor has prescribed this drug for you. Do not give the drug to anyone else.

Shown in Product Identification Section, page 419

QUESTRAN® Powder ℞
[kwest′ răn]
(Cholestyramine Resin Powder)

Description: QUESTRAN Powder (cholestyramine resin powder), the chloride salt of a basic anion exchange resin, a cholesterol lowering agent, is intended for oral administration. Cholestyramine resin is quite hydrophilic, but insoluble in water. The cholestyramine resin in QUESTRAN is not absorbed from the digestive tract. Nine grams of QUESTRAN Powder contain 4 grams of anhydrous cholestyramine resin. It is represented by the following structural formula:

Continued on next page

Mead Johnson Labs.—Cont.

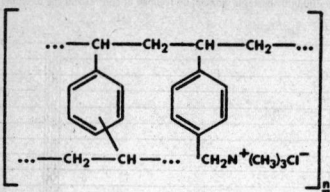

Representation of structure of main polymeric groups

Clinical Pharmacology: Cholesterol is probably the sole precursor of bile acids. During normal digestion, bile acids are secreted into the intestines. A major portion of the bile acids is absorbed from the intestinal tract and returned to the liver via the enterohepatic circulation. Only very small amounts of bile acids are found in normal serum. QUESTRAN resin adsorbs and combines with the bile acids in the intestine to form an insoluble complex which is excreted in the feces. This results in a partial removal of the bile acids from the enterohepatic circulation by preventing their absorption. The increased fecal loss of bile acids due to QUESTRAN administration leads to an increased oxidation of cholesterol to bile acids, a decrease in beta lipoprotein or low density lipoprotein plasma levels and a decrease in serum cholesterol levels. Although in man QUESTRAN (cholestyramine resin) produces an increase in hepatic synthesis of cholesterol, plasma cholesterol levels fall.

In patients with partial biliary obstruction, the reduction of serum bile acid levels by QUESTRAN reduces excess bile acids deposited in the dermal tissue with resultant decrease in pruritus.

Indications and Usage: Since no drug is innocuous, strict attention should be paid to the indications and contraindications, particularly when selecting drugs for chronic long term use.

1) *QUESTRAN is indicated as adjunctive therapy to diet for the reduction of elevated serum cholesterol in patients with primary hypercholesterolemia (elevated low density lipoproteins). QUESTRAN may be useful to lower elevated cholesterol that occurs in patients with combined hypercholesterolemia and hypertriglyceridemia, but it is not indicated where hypertriglyceridemia is the abnormality of most concern.*

It has not been established whether the drug-induced lowering of serum cholesterol or triglyceride levels has a beneficial effect, no effect, or a detrimental effect on the morbidity due to atherosclerosis including coronary heart disease. Current investigations now in progress may yield an answer to this question.

2) QUESTRAN is indicated for the relief of pruritus associated with partial biliary obstruction. QUESTRAN has been shown to have a variable effect on serum cholesterol in these patients. Patients with primary biliary cirrhosis may exhibit an elevated cholesterol as part of their disease.

Contraindications: QUESTRAN is contraindicated in patients with complete biliary obstruction where bile is not secreted into the intestine and in those individuals who have shown hypersensitivity to any of its components.

Precautions:
General
Before instituting therapy with QUESTRAN (cholestyramine resin) an attempt should be made to control serum cholesterol by appropriate dietary regimen, weight reduction, and the treatment of any underlying disorder which might be the cause of the hypercholesterolemia. A favorable trend in cholesterol reduction should occur during the first month of QUESTRAN therapy. The therapy should be continued to sustain cholesterol reduction.

Chronic use of QUESTRAN may be associated with increased bleeding tendency due to hypoprothrombinemia associated with Vitamin K deficiency. This will usually respond promptly to parenteral Vitamin K_1 and recurrences can be prevented by oral administration of Vitamin K_1. Reduction of serum or red cell folate has been reported over long term administration of QUESTRAN. Supplementation with folic acid should be considered in these cases.

There is a possibility that prolonged use of QUESTRAN, since it is a chloride form of anion exchange resin, may produce hyperchloremic acidosis. This would especially be true in younger and smaller patients where the relative dosage may be higher.

QUESTRAN may produce or worsen pre-existing constipation. Dosage should be reduced or discontinued in such cases. Fecal impaction and aggravation of hemorrhoids may occur. Every effort should be made to avert severe constipation and its inherent problems in those patients with clinically symptomatic coronary artery disease.

This product contains FD&C Yellow No. 5 (tartrazine) which may cause allergic-type reactions (including bronchial asthma) in certain susceptible individuals. Although the overall incidence of FD&C Yellow No. 5 (tartrazine) sensitivity in the general population is low, it is frequently seen in patients who also have aspirin hypersensitivity.

Information for Patients
Inform your physician if you are pregnant or plan to become pregnant or are breast feeding. Drink plenty of fluids and mix each 9-gram dose of QUESTRAN Powder in at least 4 to 6 ounces of fluid before taking.

Laboratory Tests
Serum cholesterol levels should be determined frequently during the first few months of therapy and periodically thereafter. Serum triglyceride levels should be measured periodically to detect whether significant changes have occurred.

Drug Interactions
QUESTRAN may delay or reduce the absorption of concomitant oral medication such as phenylbutazone, warfarin, chlorothiazide (acidic), as well as tetracycline, penicillin G, phenobarbital, thyroid and thyroxine preparations, and digitalis. The discontinuance of QUESTRAN (cholestyramine resin) could pose a hazard to health if a potentially toxic drug such as digitalis has been titrated to a maintenance level while the patient was taking QUESTRAN.

Because cholestyramine binds bile acids, QUESTRAN may interfere with normal fat digestion and absorption and thus may prevent absorption of fat soluble vitamins such as A, D and K. When QUESTRAN is given for long periods of time, concomitant supplementation with water-miscible (or parenteral) form of vitamins A and D should be considered.)

SINCE QUESTRAN MAY BIND OTHER DRUGS GIVEN CONCURRENTLY, PATIENTS SHOULD TAKE OTHER DRUGS AT LEAST ONE HOUR BEFORE OR 4-6 HOURS AFTER QUESTRAN (OR AT AS GREAT AN INTERVAL AS POSSIBLE) TO AVOID IMPEDING THEIR ABSORPTION.

Carcinogenesis, Mutagenesis and Impairment of Fertility
In studies conducted in rats in which cholestyramine resin was used as a tool to investigate the role of various intestinal factors, such as fat, bile salts and microbial flora, in the development of intestinal tumors induced by potent carcinogens, the incidence of such tumors was observed to be greater in cholestyramine resin treated rats than in control rats.

The relevance of this laboratory observation from studies in rats to the clinical use of QUESTRAN is not known. Large-scale, long-term human studies have shown no evidence of any difference relating to toxicity, including the incidence of cancer, between subjects taking QUESTRAN Powder and those receiving a placebo.

Pregnancy
Since QUESTRAN is not absorbed systemically, it is not expected to cause fetal harm when administered during pregnancy in recommended dosages. There are, however, no adequate and well controlled studies in pregnant women and, the known interference with absorption of fat soluble vitamins may be detrimental even in the presence of supplementation.

Nursing Mothers
Caution should be exercised when QUESTRAN is administered to a nursing mother. The possible lack of proper vitamin absorption described in the "Pregnancy" section may have an effect on nursing infants.

Pediatric Use
As experience in infants and children is limited, a practical dosage schedule has not been established.

In calculating pediatric dosage, 44.4 mg of anhydrous cholestyramine resin are contained in 100 mg of QUESTRAN.

The effects of long term drug administration, as well as its effects in maintaining lowered cholesterol levels in pediatric patients, are unknown.

Adverse Reactions: The most common adverse reaction is constipation. When used as a cholesterol lowering agent predisposing factors for most complaints of constipation are high dose and increased age (more than 60 years old). Most instances of constipation are mild, transient, and controlled with conventional therapy. Some patients require a temporary decrease in dosage or discontinuation of therapy.

Less Frequent Adverse Reactions: Abdominal discomfort, flatulence, nausea, vomiting, diarrhea, heartburn, anorexia, indigestive feeling and steatorrhea, bleeding tendencies due to hypoprothrombinemia (Vitamin K deficiency) as well as Vitamin A (one case of night blindness reported) and D deficiencies, hyperchloremic acidosis in children, osteoporosis, rash and irritation of the skin, tongue and perianal area. One ten month old baby with biliary atresia had an impaction presumed to be due to QUESTRAN (cholestyramine resin) after three days administration of 9 grams daily. She developed acute intestinal sepsis and died.

Occasional calcified material has been observed in the biliary tree, including calcification of the gall bladder, in patients to whom cholestyramine resin has been given. However, this may be a manifestation of the liver disease and not drug related.

One patient experienced biliary colic on each of three occasions on which he took QUESTRAN. One patient diagnosed as acute abdominal symptom complex was found to have a "pasty mass" in the transverse colon on x-ray.

Other events (not necessarily drug-related) reported in patients taking QUESTRAN include:
Gastrointestinal—GI-rectal bleeding, black stools, hemorrhoidal bleeding, bleeding from known duodenal ulcer, dysphagia, hiccups, ulcer attack, sour taste, pancreatitis, rectal pain, diverticulitis.
Hematologic—Decreased prothrombin time, ecchymosis, anemia.
Hypersensitivity—Urticaria, asthma, wheezing, shortness of breath.
Musculoskeletal—Backache, muscle and joint pains, arthritis.
Neurologic—Headache, anxiety, vertigo, dizziness, fatigue, tinnitus, syncope, drowsiness, femoral nerve pain, paresthesia.
Eye—Uveitis.
Renal—Hematuria, dysuria, burnt odor to urine, diuresis.
Miscellaneous—Weight loss, weight gain, increased libido, swollen glands, edema, dental bleeding.

Overdosage: Overdosage of QUESTRAN has not been reported. Should overdosage occur, however, the chief potential harm would be obstruction of the gastrointestinal tract. The location of such potential obstruction, the degree of obstruction, and the presence or absence of normal gut motility would determine treatment.

Dosage and Administration: The recommended adult dose is one packet or one scoopful (9 grams of QUESTRAN Powder contain 4 grams of anhydrous cholestyramine resin) one to six times daily. Dosage may be adjusted as required to meet the patient's needs.

QUESTRAN should not be taken in its dry form. Always mix QUESTRAN Powder with water or other fluids before ingesting. See Preparation Instructions.

Preparation: The color of QUESTRAN (cholestyramine resin) may vary somewhat from batch to batch, but this variation does not affect the performance of the product. Mix contents of one packet or one level scoopful of QUESTRAN with 4 to 6 fluid ounces of the preferred beverage (water, milk, fruit juice or other noncarbonated beverage). QUESTRAN may also be mixed with highly fluid soups or pulpy fruits with a high moisture content, such as applesauce or crushed pineapple.

How Supplied: QUESTRAN is available in cartons of fifty 9-gram packets and in cans containing 378 grams. Nine grams of QUESTRAN Powder contain 4 grams of anhydrous cholestyramine resin.
NDC 0087-0580-01 Cartons of 50 packets
NDC 0087-0580-05 Cans, 378 gm
6505-00-105-0372 (Cartons of 50 packets)
Defense
VA6505-00-105-0372A (Cartons of 50 packets)

QUIBRON®
[kwi¹ bron]
(Theophylline-Guaifenesin)

Description: Each Quibron® soft gelatin capsule or tablespoon (15 ml) of liquid contains 150 mg of theophylline (anhydrous) and 90 mg of guaifenesin, as an oral bronchodilator-expectorant.
Quibron Liquid contains no alcohol and is dye-free.

QUIBRON®-300
(Theophylline-Guaifenesin)

Description: Each Quibron®-300 soft gelatin capsule contains 300 mg of theophylline (anhydrous) and 180 mg of guaifenesin, as an oral bronchodilator-expectorant. The structural formulae for the active ingredients of Quibron and Quibron-300 are presented below:

Theophylline
[1.3 Dimethylxanthine]

Guaifenesin (Glyceryl Guaiacolate)
[3-(o-Methoxy phenoxy)-1,2-propanediol]

Theophylline, a xanthine compound, is a white, odorless crystalline powder, having a bitter taste. Guaifenesin, a guaiacol compound, is a white to slightly yellow crystalline powder with a bitter, aromatic taste.

Clinical Pharmacology:
Theophylline
Mode of Action
Theophylline acts as a bronchodilator by direct relaxation of bronchial smooth muscle. Theophylline is a competitive inhibitor of cyclic nucleotide phosphodiesterase resulting in increased intracellular levels of cAMP which mediates smooth muscle relaxation. Like some other xanthines, theophylline acts as a coronary vasodilator, cardiac stimulant, skeletal muscle stimulant, central nervous system stimulant and diuretic.

Pharmacokinetics
As theophylline is released from the formulation it is, under usual conditions, absorbed completely and fairly rapidly. Excretion, principally as inactive metabolites, occurs primarily via the kidney. The half-life of theophylline varies among individuals with a wide range having been documented. Theophylline half-life is shortened in cigarette smokers. Half-life is prolonged in alcoholism, reduced hepatic or renal function, congestive heart failure and in patients receiving antibiotics such as troleandomycin or erythromycin. High fever for prolonged periods may decrease theophylline elimination. The theophylline half-life is generally shorter in children.

Representative Theophylline Serum Half-lives
Half-life (hours)

	Mean	Range
Adults		
non-smokers	8.7	6.1–12.8
smokers	5.5	4.0– 7.7
congestive heart failure	22.9	3.1–82.0
Children (6–16 yrs)	3.7	1.4– 7.9

Therapeutic serum theophylline levels are usually 10–20 µg/ml.
Binding to plasma proteins is not extensive and theophylline is not preferentially taken up by any particular organ.
Theophylline-containing products may increase the plasma levels of free fatty acids and the urinary levels of epinephrine and norepinephrine.
Apparently no development of tolerance occurs with chronic use of theophylline.

Clinical Pharmacology:
Guaifenesin
Mode of Action
Guaifenesin increases respiratory tract secretions, possibly by stimulating the goblet cells.
Pharmacokinetics
Guaifenesin appears to be well absorbed, but its pharmacokinetics has not been well studied.

Indications and Usage:
Quibron and Quibron-300 are indicated for the symptomatic treatment of bronchospasm associated with such conditions as bronchial asthma, chronic bronchitis and pulmonary emphysema.

Contraindications:
Quibron products are contraindicated in individuals who have shown hypersensitivity to any of their components or xanthine derivatives.

Warnings:
Excessive theophylline doses may be associated with toxicity; thus serum theophylline levels should be monitored to assure maximal benefit without excessive risk.
Serum levels of theophylline above the accepted therapeutic range (10–20 µg/ml) are associated with an increased incidence of toxicity. Such levels may be reached with customary doses in individuals who metabolize the drug slowly, especially patients (1) with lowered body plasma clearance (2) with liver dysfunction or chronic obstructive pulmonary disease or (3) older than 55 years of age, particularly males.
Serious toxicity, such as seizure or ventricular arrhythmias, is not necessarily preceded by less serious side-effects such as nausea, irritability or restlessness.
Many patients who have higher (greater than 20 µg/ml) theophylline serum levels exhibit tachycardia. Theophylline products may exacerbate pre-existing arrhythmias.

Precautions:
General
Use with caution in patients with severe cardiac disease, hypertension, acute myocardial injury, congestive heart failure, cor pulmonale, severe hypoxemia, hyperthyroidism, hepatic impairment, history of peptic ulcer, alcoholism and in the elderly. Concurrent administration with certain antibiotics (see DRUG INTERACTIONS section) may result in increased serum theophylline levels. A decrease in serum half-life is seen in smokers (see Clinical Pharmacology/Pharmacokinetics). Particular caution should be used in administering theophylline to patients in congestive heart failure. Reduced theophylline clearance in these patients may cause theophylline blood levels to persist long after discontinuing the drug.
Theophylline should not be administered concurrently with other xanthine medications.

Usage in Pregnancy
Teratogenic effects: Pregnancy Category C. Animal reproduction studies have not been conducted with Quibron products. It is also not known whether Quibron products can cause fetal harm when administered to a pregnant woman or can affect reproduction capacity. Quibron products should be given to a pregnant woman only if clearly indicated.
Nonteratogenic effects: It is not known whether use of this drug during labor or delivery has immediate or delayed adverse effects on the fetus, or whether it prolongs the duration of labor or increases the possibility of forceps delivery or other obstetrical intervention.

Nursing Mothers
Theophylline has been reported to be excreted in human milk and to have caused irritability in a nursing infant. Because of the potential for serious adverse reactions, a decision should be made whether to discontinue nursing or to discontinue Quibron or Quibron-300, taking into account the importance of this drug to the mother.

Drug Interactions

Drug	Effect
Theophylline with lithium carbonate	Increased renal excretion of lithium
Theophylline with propranolol	Mutual antagonism of therapeutic effects
Theophylline with cimetidine	Increased serum theophylline levels
Theophylline with clindamycin	Increased serum theophylline levels
Theophylline with lincomycin	Increased serum theophylline levels
Theophylline with troleandomycin or erythromycin	Increased serum theophylline levels

Drug/Laboratory Test Interactions
Theophylline may interfere with the assay of uric acid, especially the phosphotungstate method. Thus, serum uric acid levels may be overestimated. Metabolites of guaifenesin may contribute to increased 5-hydroxyindoleacetic acid readings when determined with nitrosonaphthol reagent.

Adverse Reactions: The frequency of adverse reactions is related to serum theophylline levels and is usually not a problem at levels below 20 µg/ml. The most consistent adverse reactions are usually due to overdosage and, while all have not been reported with Quibron or Quibron-300, the following reactions may be considered when theophylline is administered. Central nervous system: clonic and tonic generalized convulsions, muscle twitching, reflex hyperexcitability, headaches, insomnia, restlessness, and irritability. Cardiovascular: circulatory failure, ventricular arrhythmias, hypotension, extrasystoles, tachycardia, palpitation, and flushing. Gastrointestinal: hematemesis, vomiting, diarrhea, epigas-

Continued on next page

Mead Johnson Labs.—Cont.

tric pain, and nausea. Renal: increased excretion of renal tubular cells and red blood cells, albuminuria, and diuresis. Respiratory: tachypnea. Others: hyperglycemia and inappropriate ADH syndrome.

Overdosage:
Symptoms
Nervousness, agitation, headache, insomnia, vomiting, tachycardia, extrasystoles, hypcrreflexia, fasciculations and clonic and tonic convulsions. Children may be particularly prone to restlessness and hyperactivity that can proceed to convulsions.

Management
If potential oral overdose is established and seizure has **not** occurred.
1. Induce vomiting.
2. Administer a cathartic (this is particularly important if sustained release preparations have been taken).
3. Administer activated charcoal.
4. Monitor vital signs, maintain blood pressure and provide adequate hydration.

If patient is having seizure
1. Establish an airway.
2. Administer O_2.
3. Treat the seizure with intravenous diazepam 0.1 to 0.3 mg/kg up to 10 mg.
4. Monitor vital signs, maintain blood pressure and provide adequate hydration.

Post-Seizure Coma
1. Maintain airway and oxygenation.
2. If a result of oral medication, follow above recommendations to prevent absorption of drug, but intubation and lavage will have to be performed instead of inducing emesis and the cathartic and charcoal will need to be introduced via a large bore gastric lavage tube.
3. Continue to provide full supportive care and adequate hydration while waiting for drug to be metabolized. In general, the drug is metabolized rapidly enough so as to not warrant consideration of dialysis.

General
The oral LD_{50} of theophylline in mice is 350 mg/kg. The oral LD_{50} of guaifenesin in mice is 1725 mg/kg. In humans, adverse reactions often occur when serum theophylline levels exceed 20 μg/ml. Information on physiological variables which influence excretion of theophylline can be found under the heading "Clinical Pharmacology."

Dosage and Administration:
General
Therapeutic serum levels associated with optimal likelihood for benefit and minimal risk of toxicity are considered to be between 10 and 20 μg/ml, although levels of 5-10 μg/ml are reported to be effective for some patients. Levels above 20 μg/ml may produce toxic effects. There is great variation from patient to patient and dosage must be individualized because there is a relatively narrow range between therapeutic and toxic levels of theophylline. Monitoring of serum theophylline levels is highly recommended. Since theophylline does not distribute into fatty tissue, dosage should be calculated on the basis of ideal body weight.
Giving theophylline with food may prevent the rare case of stomach irritation and, although absorption may be slower, it is still complete.

Quibron
Treatment should be *initiated* at a dose of 16 mg/kg/day or 400 mg/day, whichever is smaller. The usual adjusted dosages are—Adults: 1-2 capsules or 1-2 tablespoons (15 ml) liquid every 6-8 hours. Children 9 to 12: 4-5 mg theophylline/kg body weight every 6-8 hours. Children under 9: 4-6 mg theophylline/kg body weight every 6-8 hours.
Approximate mg/kg dosage by TEASPOON (5 ml) of Quibron Liquid may be determined from the following table:

BODY WEIGHT		AVERAGE DOSAGE IN TEASPOONS (5 ml) TO PROVIDE THE FOLLOWING MG OF THEOPHYLLINE/ KG BODY WEIGHT/DOSE		
Lbs	Kgs	4 mg/kg	5 mg/kg	6 mg/kg
20	9	3/4	1	1
30	14	1	1 1/2	1 3/4
40	18	1 1/2	2	2 1/4
50	23	1 3/4	2 1/4	2 3/4
60	27	2	2 3/4	3 1/4
70	32	2 1/2	3	3 3/4
80	36	3	3 1/2	4 1/4
90	41	3 1/4	4	5
100	46	3 1/2	4 1/2	5 1/2

If the desired response is not achieved with the recommended initial dose, and there are no adverse reactions, the dose may be cautiously adjusted upward in increments of no more than 25 percent at 2–3 day intervals until the following MAXIMUM DOSE WITHOUT MEASUREMENT OF SERUM CONCENTRATION or a maximum of 900 mg in any 24 hour period (whichever is less) is attained:

MAXIMUM DAILY DOSE WITHOUT MEASUREMENT OF SERUM CONCENTRATION

	mg per kg Body Weight*
Children (under 9)	24
Children (9–12)	20
Adolescents (12–16)	18
Adults	13

*Use ideal body weight for obese patients

Do not attempt to maintain any dose that is not tolerated. If doses higher than those contained in the above MAXIMUM DOSE WITHOUT MEASUREMENT OF SERUM CONCENTRATION are necessary, it is recommended that serum theophylline levels be monitored. For therapeutic levels, draw blood sample just before next dose is due; for toxic levels, draw blood sample when last dose peaks (~2 hours after dosing). It is important that the patient has missed no doses during the previous 72 hours and that dosing intervals have been reasonably typical with no added doses during that period of time. DOSAGE ADJUSTMENT BASED ON SERUM THEOPHYLLINE MEASUREMENTS WHEN THESE INSTRUCTIONS HAVE **NOT** BEEN FOLLOWED, MAY RESULT IN RECOMMENDATIONS THAT PRESENT RISK OF TOXICITY TO THE PATIENT.

Quibron-300 Capsules
Quibron–300 is appropriate therapy when higher theophylline dosages are required. The usual recommended dosages for Quibron–300 are **Adults:** 1 capsule every 6–8 hours for patients whose dosage has been adjusted upward to achieve therapeutic serum levels.

How Supplied:
Quibron® Capsules (yellow) in bottles of 100 (NDC 0087-0516-01); and 1000 (NDC 0087-0516-02, 6505-00-764-3366 Defense); Unit Dose 100's (NDC 0087-0516-03).
Quibron® Liquid in 1 pint (NDC 0087-0510-03) and 1 gallon (NDC 0087-0510-01).
Quibron®–300 Capsules (yellow and white) in bottles of 100 (NDC 0087-0515-41).
Store at controlled room temperature of 59°–86°F (15°–30°C).

Shown in Product Identification Section, page 419

QUIBRON PLUS®
[kwi' bron]
(Theophylline, Guaifenesin, Ephedrine and Butabarbital)

Description: Each Quibron Plus capsule or tablespoon (15 ml) of elixir contains theophylline (anhydrous) 150 mg, guaifenesin 100 mg, ephedrine HCl 25 mg, and butabarbital 20 mg (Warning: may be habit-forming) as an oral bronchodilator-expectorant. Elixir contains alcohol 15%.
Theophylline (1,3 dimethylxanthine) is a xanthine bronchodilator with the following structure:

[Chemical structure of theophylline]

Guaifenesin (glyceryl guaiacolate or 3-(o-methoxy phenoxy)-1,2-propanediol) is an expectorant with the following structure:

[Chemical structure of guaifenesin]

Ephedrine (α-[1-(methylamino)ethyl]benzenemethanol) is an adrenergic bronchodilator with the following structure:

[Chemical structure of ephedrine]

Butabarbital (5-sec-butyl-5-ethyl-barbituric acid) is a sedative with the following structure:

[Chemical structure of butabarbital]

Clinical Pharmacology:
Theophylline:
Mode of Action
Theophylline acts as a bronchodilator by direct relaxation of bronchial smooth muscle. Theophylline is a competitive inhibitor of cyclic nucleotide phosphodiesterase resulting in increased intracellular levels of cAMP which mediates smooth muscle relaxation. Like some other xanthines, theophylline acts as a coronary vasodilator, cardiac stimulant, skeletal muscle stimulant, central nervous system stimulant and diuretic.

Pharmacokinetics
Theophylline is, under usual conditions, absorbed completely and fairly rapidly. Excretion, principally as inactive metabolites, occurs primarily via the kidney. The half-life of theophylline varies among individuals with a wide range having been documented. Theophylline half-life is shortened in cigarette smokers. Half-life is prolonged in alcoholism, reduced hepatic or renal function, congestive heart failure and patients receiving antibiotics such as troleandomycin or erythromycin. High fever for prolonged periods may decrease theophylline elimination. The theophylline half-life is generally shorter in children.

Representative Theophylline Serum Half-Lives

	Half-life (hours)	
	Mean	Range
Adults		
non-smokers	8.7	6.1 – 12.8
smokers	5.5	4.0 – 7.7
congestive heart failure	22.9	3.1 – 82.0
Children (6–16 yrs.)	3.7	1.4 – 7.9

Therapeutic serum theophylline levels are usually 10–20 μg/ml when theophylline is administered as the sole bronchodilator agent. Binding to plasma proteins is not extensive and theophylline is not preferentially taken up by any particular organ.

Theophylline-containing products may increase the plasma levels of free fatty acids and the urinary levels of epinephrine and norepinephrine. Apparently no development of tolerance occurs with chronic use of theophylline.

Guaifenesin:
Mode of Action
Guaifenesin increases respiratory tract secretions, possibly by stimulating the goblet cells.

Pharmacokinetics
Guaifenesin appears to be well absorbed, but its pharmacokinetics has not been well studied.

Ephedrine:
Mode of Action
Ephedrine acts as a bronchodilator by stimulating β-adrenergic receptors with a resulting increase in intracellular cAMP which mediates smooth muscle relaxation. Ephedrine stimulates both α- and β-adrenergic receptors and acts as a cardiac and CNS stimulant and a vasoconstrictor.

Pharmacokinetics
Ephedrine appears to be well-absorbed and has a reasonably long duration of action, but its pharmacokinetics has not been well-studied.

Butabarbital:
Mode of Action
Butabarbital reversibly depresses the activity of all excitable tissues probably by interfering with the chemical transmission across neuronal and neuroeffector junctions.

Pharmacokinetics
Barbiturates in general appear to be well-absorbed. The rate-limiting step in absorption is usually the dissolution and dispersal of the drug in the gastrointestinal contents. Food may decrease the rate of absorption, but not the amount absorbed. Otherwise, the specific pharmacokinetics of butabarbital has not been well studied.

Indications and Usage:

Indications
Based on a review of a similar drug by the National Academy of Sciences-National Research Council and/or other information, FDA has classified the indications as follows: "Possibly" effective: bronchial asthma; bronchitis, bronchiectasis, and emphysema in which bronchospasm is present, or for the relief of bronchospasm. Final classification of the less-than-effective indications requires further investigation.

Contraindications: Quibron Plus is contraindicated in individuals who have shown hypersensitivity to any of its components or xanthine derivatives. Because of its ephedrine content Quibron Plus should not be administered within 14 days following administration of monoamine oxidase (MAO) inhibitors.

Warnings: Serum levels of theophylline above the accepted therapeutic range (10–20 $\mu g/ml$) are associated with an increased incidence of toxicity. Such levels may be reached with customary doses in individuals who metabolize the drug slowly, especially patients (1) with lowered body plasma clearance, (2) with liver dysfunction or chronic obstructive pulmonary disease, or (3) older than 55 years of age, particularly males.
Serious toxicity, such as a seizure or ventricular arrhythmia, is not necessarily preceded by less serious side effects such as nausea, irritability, or restlessness. Many patients who have higher (greater than 20 $\mu g/ml$) theophylline serum levels exhibit tachycardia. Theophylline products may exacerbate pre-existing arrhythmias.
Use cautiously in patients with degenerative heart disease (anginal pain may be induced in patients with angina pectoris) and in hyperthyroid or hypertensive individuals who are particularly susceptible to the pressor response to ephedrine. Butabarbital may be habit-forming.

Precautions:
General
Use with caution in patients with severe cardiac disease (including angina pectoris, cardiac arrhythmias and coronary insufficiency), hypertension, acute myocardial injury, congestive heart failure, cor pulmonale, severe hypoxemia, hyperthyroidism, hepatic impairment, history of peptic ulcer, alcoholism, drug-dependence or abuse, pain, porphyria, hyperkinesis, diabetes mellitus, prostatic hypertrophy, angle-closure glaucoma (or predisposition to it) and in the elderly.
Concurrent administration of barbiturates with several drugs (see DRUG INTERACTIONS) is known to decrease the effect of the principal drug because they induce the formation of drug-metabolizing, hepatic microsomal enzymes.
Concurrent administration with certain antibiotics (see DRUG INTERACTIONS section) may result in increased serum theophylline levels.
The incidence of side effects has been reported to be increased in patients receiving both theophylline and ephedrine.
A decrease in serum half-life is seen in smokers (see Clinical Pharmacology/Pharmacokinetics).
Particular caution should be used in administering theophylline to patients in congestive heart failure. Reduced theophylline clearance in these patients may cause theophylline blood levels to persist long after discontinuing the drug. Theophylline should not be administered concurrently with other xanthine medications.

Drug Interactions

Drug	Effect
Theophylline with lithium carbonate	Increased renal excretion of lithium
Theophylline with propranolol	Mutual antagonism of therapeutic effects
Theophylline with cimetidine	Increased serum theophylline levels
Theophylline with clindamycin	Increased serum theophylline levels
Theophylline with lincomycin	Increased serum theophylline levels
Theophylline with troleandomycin or erythromycin	Increased serum theophylline levels
Ephedrine with general anesthetics or digitalis glycosides	Cardiac arrhythmias
Ephedrine with ergonovine or methylergonovine or oxytocin	Severe hypertension
Ephedrine with guanethidine	Decreased hypotensive effect
Ephedrine with monoamine oxidase inhibitors	Potentiated pressor effect with hypertensive crisis
Ephedrine with other sympathomimetics	Increased sympathetic stimulation and potential for side effects
Butabarbital with alcohol, general anesthetics, CNS depressants, or monoamine oxidase inhibitors	Increased therapeutic effects
Butabarbital with oral anticoagulants, corticosteroid, digitalis, digitoxin or doxycycline or tricyclic antidepressants	Decreased therapeutic effects due to increased metabolism resulting from induction of hepatic microsomal enzymes
Butabarbital with griseofulvin	Decreased therapeutic effects due to impaired absorption

Drug/Laboratory Test Interactions
Theophylline may interfere with the assay of uric acid, especially the phosphotungstate method. Thus, serum uric acid levels may be overestimated. Metabolites of guaifenesin may contribute to increased 5-hydroxy-indoleacetic acid readings when determined with nitrosonaphthol reagent.

Carcinogenesis, Mutagenesis, Impairment of Fertility
Long-term animal studies have not been conducted to evaluate the carcinogenic potential of Quibron Plus.

Use in Pregnancy
Teratogenic effects: Pregnancy Category C. Animal reproduction studies have not been conducted with Quibron Plus. It is also not known whether Quibron Plus can cause fetal harm when administered to a pregnant woman or can affect reproduction capacity. Quibron Plus should be given to a pregnant woman only if clearly indicated.
Nonteratogenic Effects: Barbiturates such as butabarbital cross the placental barrier and may cause respiratory depression in the neonate or neonatal hemorrhage due to a reduced level of vitamin-K-dependent clotting factors. Chronic use may cause physical dependence in the neonate with resulting withdrawal symptoms.
Since barbiturates are known to cross the placenta, chronic use of one of this class of drugs during pregnancy may cause physical dependence with resulting withdrawal symptoms in the neonate. Use during late pregnancy or labor may cause respiratory depression in the neonate (especially the premature neonate) because of immature hepatic function.

Nursing Mothers: Theophylline, ephedrine, and barbiturates such as butabarbital have been reported to be excreted in human milk. Because of the potential for serious adverse reactions in nursing infants from Quibron Plus, a decision should be made whether to discontinue nursing or to discontinue the drug, taking into account the importance of the drug to the mother.

Adverse Reactions: The frequency of adverse reactions due to theophylline is related to serum levels and is usually not a problem at levels below 20 $\mu g/ml$. The most consistent adverse reactions are usually due to overdosage and, while all have not been reported with Quibron Plus, the following reactions may be considered when theophylline is administered. Central nervous system: clonic and tonic generalized convulsions, muscle twitching, reflex hyperexcitability, headaches, insomnia, restlessness, and irritability. Cardiovascular: circulatory failure, ventricular arrhythmias, hypotension, extrasystoles, tachycardia, palpitation, and flushing. Gastrointestinal: hermatemesis, vomiting, diarrhea, epigastric pain, and nausea. Renal: increased excretion of renal tubular cells and red blood cells, albuminuria, and diuresis. Respiratory: tachypnea. Others: hyperglycemia and inappropriate ADH syndrome.

The following reactions may be considered when ephedrine is administered. Central nervous system: dizziness or lightheadedness, headache, nervousness, restlessness, trembling, trouble in sleeping, weakness. Cardiovascular: palpitation, chest pain, tachycardia, peripheral vasoconstriction, flushing. Gastrointestinal: epigastric pain, nausea, vomiting. Renal: difficulty of micturition. Respiratory: troubled breathing. Others: unusual increase in sweating.

The following reactions may be considered when butabarbital is administered: Central nervous system: mental confusion or depression, unusual excitement, clumsiness, unsteadiness, dizziness or lightheadedness, drowsiness, headache, joint or muscle pain, slurred speech, possible withdrawal symptoms including convulsions or seizures, feeling faint, hallucinations, increased dreaming, nightmares, trembling, trouble in sleeping, unusual restlessness, unusual weakness. Cardiovascular: unusually slow heart beat. Gastrointestinal: diarrhea, nausea, vomiting. Respiratory: shortness of breath, wheezing or tightness in chest. Other: Skin rash or hives or swelling of eyelids, face or lips, sore throat and fever, unusual bleeding or bruising, yellowing of eyes or skin, joint or muscle pain.

Continued on next page

Mead Johnson Labs.—Cont.

Overdosage:
Symptoms
Overdosage due to theophylline and ephedrine: nervousness, agitation, headache, insomnia, vomiting, tachycardia, extrasystoles, hyperreflexia, fasciculations and clonic and tonic convulsions. Overdosage due to butabarbital: coma, early hypothermia, late fever, sluggish or absent reflexes, respiratory depression, gradual appearance of circulatory collapse and pulmonary edema.

Management
If potential overdosage is established and the patient is conscious:
1. Induce vomiting
2. Administer a cathartic
3. Administer activated charcoal
4. Monitor vital signs, maintain blood pressure and provide adequate hydration.

If the patient is having a seizure:
1. Establish an airway.
2. Administer O_2.
3. Treat seizure with intravenous diazepam 0.1 to 0.3 mk/kg up to 10 mg.
4. Monitor vital signs, maintain blood pressure and provide adequate hydration.

If the patient is in a coma:
1. Maintain airway and oxygenation.
2. Aspirate stomach contents, taking care to avoid pulmonary aspiration. Administer a cathartic and charcoal via a large bore gastric lavage tube.
3. Monitor vital signs and provide full supportive care and adequate hydration.
4. If renal function is normal, forced diuresis may aid in the elimination of the barbiturate.

General
The oral LD_{50} of theophylline in mice is 350 mg/kg. In humans, adverse reactions often occur when serum theophylline levels exceed 20 μg/ml. The oral LD_{50} of ephedrine in mice is 283 mg/kg. The oral LD_{50} of butabarbital in mice is 204 mg/kg, and the oral LD_{50} of guaifenesin in mice is 1725 mg/kg.

Dosage and Administration
Dosage should be adjusted on an individual basis. Administration with food may prevent the rare case of stomach irritation and absorption, although it may be slower, should still be complete.

Dosage:
Adults: 1–2 capsules or 1–2 tablespoons (15–30 ml) elixir 2–3 times daily.
Children 8–12: 1 capsule or 1 tablespoon (15 ml) elixir 2–3 times daily.
Children under 8: Up to ½ teaspoon (2–5 ml) elixir per 10 lb body weight 2–3 times daily.

How Supplied:
QUIBRON PLUS Capsules (green) in bottles of 100 (NDC-0087-0518-01).
QUIBRON PLUS Elixir in 1 pint bottles (NDC-0087-0511-01).
Store at controlled room temperature of 59°–86°F (15°–30°C).
Shown in Product Identification Section, page 419

QUIBRON®-T ℞
[kwi¹ bron-t]
(Theophylline Anhydrous)
DIVIDOSE® TABLETS

IMMEDIATE RELEASE BRONCHODILATOR
Description: Quibron®-T tablets provide 300 mg of anhydrous theophylline as an oral bronchodilator in an immediate release formulation combined with the convenience of the unique Dividose® tablet design. With functional trisects and bisects, Quibron-T tablets can be conveniently and accurately divided into 100, 150, and 200 mg segments to provide a variety of dosing increments, as required.

QUIBRON-T tablets
One-third tablet	= 100 mg
One-half tablet	= 150 mg
Two-thirds tablet	= 200 mg
One tablet	= 300 mg

QUIBRON®-T/SR ℞
(Theophylline Anhydrous)
DIVIDOSE® TABLETS

SUSTAINED RELEASE BRONCHODILATOR
Description: Quibron®-T/SR tablets provide 300 mg of anhydrous theophylline as an oral bronchodilator in a sustained release formulation combined with the convenience of the unique Dividose® tablet design. With functional trisects and bisects, Quibron-T/SR tablets can be conveniently and accurately divided into 100, 150, and 200 mg segments to provide a variety of dosing increments, as required.

QUIBRON-T/SR tablets
One-third tablet	= 100 mg
One-half tablet	= 150 mg
Two-thirds tablet	= 200 mg
One tablet	= 300 mg

Theophylline is a white odorless crystalline powder which has a bitter taste. It is chemically related to caffeine and its structure is shown below:

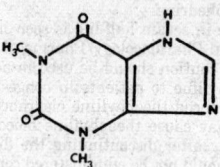

Theophylline
(1,3 Dimethylxanthine)

Clinical Pharmacology:
Mode of Action
Theophylline acts as a bronchodilator by direct relaxation of bronchial smooth muscle. Theophylline is a competitive inhibitor of cyclic nucleotide phosphodiesterase resulting in increased intracellular levels of cAMP which mediates smooth muscle relaxation. Like some other xanthines, theophylline acts as a coronary vasodilator, cardiac stimulant, skeletal muscle stimulant, central nervous system stimulant and diuretic.

Pharmacokinetics
Theophylline is, under usual conditions, absorbed completely and fairly rapidly. Excretion, principally as inactive metabolites, occurs primarily via the kidney. The half-life of theophylline varies among individuals with a wide range having been documented. Theophylline half-life is shorter in cigarette smokers. Half-life is prolonged in alcoholism, reduced hepatic or renal function, congestive heart failure and in patients receiving antibiotics such as troleandomycin or erythromycin. High fever for prolonged periods may decrease theophylline elimination. The theophylline half-life is generally shorter in children.

Representative Theophylline Serum Half-Lives
	Half-life (hours)	
	Mean	Range
Adults		
non-smokers	8.7	6.1–12.8
smokers	5.5	4.0–7.7
congestive heart failure	22.9	3.1–82.0
Children (6–16 yrs)	3.7	1.4–7.9

Therapeutic serum theophylline levels are usually 10–20 μg/ml.
Binding to plasma proteins is not extensive and theophylline is not preferentially taken up by any particular organ.
Theophylline-containing products may increase the plasma levels of free fatty acids and the urinary levels of epinephrine and norepinephrine. Apparently no development of tolerance occurs with chronic use of theophylline.

Indications and Usage: Quibron-T tablets and Quibron-T/SR tablets are indicated for the symptomatic treatment of bronchospasm associated with such conditions as bronchial asthma, chronic bronchitis and pulmonary emphysema.

Contraindications: Quibron-T tablets and Quibron-T/SR tablets are contraindicated in individuals who have shown hypersensitivity to any of its components or xanthine derivatives.

Warnings: Excessive theophylline doses may be associated with toxicity; thus serum theophylline levels should be monitored to assure maximal benefit without excessive risk. Serum levels of theophylline above the accepted therapeutic range (10–20 μg/ml) are associated with an increased incidence of toxicity. Such levels may be reached with customary doses in individuals who metabolize the drug slowly, especially patients (1) with lowered body plasma clearance, (2) with liver dysfunction or chronic obstructive pulmonary disease, or (3) older than 55 years of age, particularly males.

Serious toxicity, such as seizure or ventricular arrhythmias, is not necessarily preceded by less serious side effects such as nausea, irritability or restlessness. Many patients who have higher (greater than 20 μg/ml) theophylline serum levels exhibit tachycardia. Theophylline products may exacerbate pre-existing arrhythmias.

Precautions:
General
Quibron-T/SR tablets should not be chewed or crushed.
Use with caution in patients with severe cardiac disease, hypertension, acute myocardial injury, congestive heart failure, cor pulmonale, severe hypoxemia, hyperthyroidism, hepatic impairment, history of peptic ulcer, alcoholism and in the elderly. Concurrent administration with certain antibiotics (see DRUG INTERACTIONS section) may result in increased serum theophylline levels. A decrease in serum half-life is seen in smokers (see Clinical Pharmacology/Pharmacokinetics).

Particular caution should be used in administering theophylline to patients in congestive heart failure. Reduced theophylline clearance in these patients may cause theophylline blood levels to persist long after discontinuing the drug.

Theophylline should not be administered concurrently with other xanthine medications.

Patients should be instructed carefully on how to divide Quibron-T tablets and Quibron-T/SR tablets along the appropriate tablet score.

Sustained release theophylline is not useful in status asthmaticus.

Usage in Pregnancy
Teratogenic effects: Pregnancy Category C. Animal reproduction studies have not been conducted with Quibron-T tablets and Quibron-T/SR tablets. It is also not known whether Quibron-T tablets and Quibron-T/SR tablets can cause fetal harm when administered to a pregnant woman or can affect reproduction capacity. Quibron-T tablets and Quibron-T/SR tablets should be given to a pregnant woman only if clearly indicated.

Nonteratogenic effects: it is not known whether use of this drug during labor or delivery has immediate or delayed adverse effects on the fetus, or whether it prolongs the duration of labor or increases the possibility of forceps delivery or other obstetrical intervention.

Nursing Mothers
Theophylline has been reported to be excreted in human milk and to have caused irritability in a nursing infant. Because of the potential for serious adverse reactions, a decision should be made whether to discontinue nursing or to discontinue Quibron-T tablets and Quibron-T/SR tablets, taking into account the importance of these drugs to the mother.

Drug Interactions

Drug	Effect
Theophylline with lithium carbonate	Increased renal excretion of lithium
Theophylline with propranolol	Mutual antagonism of therapeutic effects
Theophylline with cimetidine	Increased serum theophylline levels
Theophylline with clindamycin	Increased serum theophylline levels
Theophylline with lincomycin	Increased serum theophylline levels
Theophylline with troleandomycin or erythromycin	Increased serum theophylline levels

Drug/Laboratory Test Interactions
Theophylline may interfere with the assay of uric acid, especially the phosphotungstate method. Thus, serum uric acid levels may be overestimated.

Adverse Reactions: The frequency of adverse reactions is related to serum theophylline levels and is usually not a problem at levels below 20 $\mu g/ml$. The most consistent adverse reactions are usually due to overdosage and, while not all have been reported with Quibron-T tablets and/or with Quibron-T/SR tablets, the following reactions may be considered when theophylline is administered. Central nervous system: clonic and tonic generalized convulsions, muscle twitching, reflex hyperexcitability, headaches, insomnia, restlessness, and irritability. Cardiovascular: circulatory failure, ventricular arrhythmias, hypotension, extrasystoles, tachycardia, palpitation, and flushing. Gastrointestinal: hematemesis, vomiting, diarrhea, epigastric pain, and nausea. Renal: increased excretion of renal tubular cells and red blood cells, albuminuria, and diuresis. Respiratory: tachypnea. Others: hyperglycemia and inappropriate ADH syndrome.

Overdosage:
Symptoms
Nervousness, agitation, headache, insomnia, nausea, vomiting, tachycardia, extrasystoles, hyperreflexia, fasciculations and clonic and tonic convulsions. Children may be particularly prone to restlessness and hyperactivity that can proceed to convulsions.

Management
If potential oral overdose is established and seizure has **not** occurred.
1. Induce vomiting.
2. Administer a cathartic (this is particularly important if a sustained release preparation has been taken).
3. Administer activated charcoal.
4. Monitor vital signs, maintain blood pressure and provide adequate hydration.

If patient is having a seizure.
1. Establish an airway.
2. Administer O_2.
3. Treat the seizure with intravenous diazepam 0.1 to 0.3 mg/kg up to total dose of 10 mg.
4. Monitor vital signs, maintain blood pressure and provide adequate hydration.

Post-seizure Coma.
1. Maintain airway and oxygenation.
2. If the reaction occurred after oral medication, follow above recommendations to prevent absorption of drug, but intubation and lavage will have to be performed instead of inducing emesis and the cathartic and charcoal will need to be introduced via a large bore gastric lavage tube.
3. Continue to provide full supportive care and adequate hydration while waiting for drug to be metabolized. In general, the drug is metabolized rapidly enough so as to not warrant consideration of dialysis.

General
The oral LD_{50} of theophylline in mice is 350 mg/kg. In humans, adverse reactions often occur when serum theophylline levels exceed 20 $\mu g/ml$. Information on physiological variables which influence excretion of theophylline can be found under the heading "Clinical Pharmacology."

Quibron-T
Quibron-T/SR

DOSAGE FOR PATIENT POPULATION
ACUTE ASTHMA REQUIRING RAPID THEOPHYLLINIZATION

I. Patients not currently receiving a theophylline product:

Group	Oral Loading Dose (Theophylline)	Maintenance Dose for Next 12 Hours (Theophylline)	Maintenance Dose Beyond 12 Hours (Theophylline)
1. Children 6 months to 9 years	6 mg/kg	4 mg/kg q4h	4 mg/kg q6h
2. Children age 9–16 and young adult	6 mg/kg	3 mg/kg q4h	3 mg/kg q6h
3. Otherwise healthy non-smoking adults	6 mg/kg	3 mg/kg q6h	3 mg/kg q8h
4. Older patients and patients with cor pulmonale	6 mg/kg	2 mg/kg q6h	2 mg/kg q8h
5. Patients with congestive heart failure, liver failure	6 mg/kg	2 mg/kg q8h	1–2 mg/kg q12h

Dosage and Administration:
General
Therapeutic serum levels associated with optimal likelihood for benefit and minimal risk of toxicity are considered to be between 10 $\mu g/ml$ and 20 $\mu g/ml$, although levels of 5–10 $\mu g/ml$ have been reported to be effective for some patients. Levels above 20 $\mu g/ml$ may produce toxic effects. Because of the variable rates of theophylline elimination among patients the dose necessary to achieve the desired serum level of 10–20 μg theophylline per ml varies from patient to patient. Thus, dosage must be individualized (see CLINICAL PHARMACOLOGY and WARNINGS sections) because there is a relatively narrow range between therapeutic and toxic levels of theophylline. Monitoring of serum theophylline levels is highly recommended.

Since theophylline does not distribute into fatty tissue, dosage should be calculated on the basis of ideal body weight. Giving theophylline with food may prevent the rare case of stomach irritation and, although absorption may be slower, it is still complete.

Quibron-T Tablets
To maintain the desired serum level of theophylline generally requires dosing every six hours to obtain the optimal clinical benefit in children and some adult patients (e.g., heavy smokers) because of their rapid clearance of the drug. However, dosing intervals of eight hours may be satisfactory for most adults because of their slower elimination rate.
[See table above].

Note: Due to their slower rate of absorption, sustained-release theophylline products are *not* designed for use in conditions requiring rapid theophyllinization.

II. Patients currently receiving a theophylline product:
Determine, where possible, the time, amount, route of administration and form of the patient's last dose.

The loading dose for theophylline should be based on the principle that each 1 mg/kg of theophylline administered as a loading dose will result in a 2 mcg/ml increase in serum theophylline concentration. Ideally, then, the loading dose should be deferred if a serum theophylline concentration can be rapidly obtained. If this is not possible, the clinician should exercise his/her judgment in selecting a dose based on the potential for benefit and risk. When there is sufficient respiratory distress to warrant a small risk, 2.5 mg/kg of theophylline is likely to increase the serum concentration when administered as a loading dose in rapidly absorbed form by only about 5 mcg/ml. If the patient is not already experiencing theophylline toxicity, this is unlikely to result in dangerous adverse effects.

Subsequent to the modified decision regarding a loading dose in this group of patients, the subsequent maintenance dosage recommendations are the same as those described above.
Comments: To achieve optimal therapeutic theophylline dosage, it is recommended to monitor serum theophylline concentrations. However, it is not always possible or practical to obtain a serum theophylline level.

Patients should be closely monitored for signs of toxicity. The present data suggest that the above dosage recommendations will achieve therapeutic serum concentrations with minimal risk of toxicity for most patients. However, some risk of toxic serum concentrations is still present. Adverse reactions to theophylline often occur when serum theophylline levels exceed 20 mcg/ml.

CHRONIC ASTHMA
Theophyllinization is a treatment of first choice for the management of chronic asthma (to prevent symptoms and maintain patent airways). Slow clinical titration is generally preferred to assure acceptance and safety of the medication. Initial Dose: 16 mg/kg/day or 400 mg/day (whichever is less) in 3 or 4 divided doses at 6 to 8 hour intervals. If the desired response is not achieved with the recommended initial dose, and there are no adverse reactions, the dose may be cautiously adjusted upward in increments of no more than 25 percent at 2-3 day intervals until the following MAXIMUM DOSE WITHOUT MEASUREMENT OF SERUM CONCENTRATION or, in the case of adults, a maximum of 900 mg in any 24 hour period (whichever is less) is attained:

MAXIMUM DAILY DOSE WITHOUT MEASUREMENT OF SERUM CONCENTRATION

	mg per kg Body Weight* per day
Children (under 9)	24
Children (9–12)	20
Adolescents (12–16)	18
Adults	13

*Use ideal body weight for obese patients.
Do not attempt to maintain any dose that is not tolerated. If doses higher than those contained in the above MAXIMUM DOSE WITHOUT MEASUREMENT OF SERUM CONCENTRATION are necessary, it is recommended that serum theophylline levels be monitored. For therapeutic levels, draw blood sample when last dose peaks ($\simeq$ 2 hours after dosing). It is important that the patient has missed no doses during the previous 72 hours

Continued on next page

Mead Johnson Labs.—Cont.

and that dosing intervals have been reasonably typical with no doses added during that period of time. DOSE ADJUSTMENT BASED ON SERUM THEOPHYLLINE MEASUREMENTS MADE WHEN THESE INSTRUCTIONS HAVE NOT BEEN FOLLOWED MAY RESULT IN RECOMMENDATIONS THAT PRESENT RISK OF TOXICITY TO THE PATIENT.

Quibron-T/SR Tablets

The average initial dose for children (under 9 years of age) is one third (100 mg) of a Quibron-T/SR Tablet q 12 h.

The average initial dose for children (ages 9–12) is one half (150 mg) of a Quibron-T/SR Tablet q 12 h.

The average initial dose for adolescents (ages 12–16) is two thirds (200 mg) of a Quibron-T/SR Tablet q 12 h.

The average initial dose for adults is two thirds (200 mg) Quibron-T/SR Tablet q 12 h.

If the desired response is not achieved with the recommended initial dose, and there are no adverse reactions, the dose may be cautiously adjusted upward in increments of no more than 25 percent at 2–3 day intervals until the following MAXIMUM DOSE WITHOUT MEASUREMENT OF SERUM CONCENTRATION or, in the case of adults, a maximum of 900 mg in any 24 hour period (whichever is less) is attained:

MAXIMUM DOSE WITHOUT MEASUREMENT OF SERUM CONCENTRATION

	mg per kg Body Weight* per day**
Children (under 9)	24
Children (9–12)	20
Adolescents (12–16)	18
Adults	13

* Use ideal body weight for obese patients.
** Some patients who clear theophylline more rapidly (e.g., children and heavy smokers) may require dosing at intervals more frequent than 12 hours.

Do not attempt to maintain any dose that is not tolerated. If doses higher than those contained in the above MAXIMUM DOSE WITHOUT MEASUREMENT OF SERUM CONCENTRATION are necessary, it is recommended that serum theophylline levels be monitored. For therapeutic levels, draw blood sample when last dose peaks (4–5 hours after dosing). It is important that the patient has missed no doses during the previous 72 hours and that dosing intervals have been reasonably typical with no doses added during that period of time. DOSE ADJUSTMENT BASED ON SERUM THEOPHYLLINE MEASUREMENTS MADE WHEN THESE INSTRUCTIONS HAVE NOT BEEN FOLLOWED MAY RESULT IN RECOMMENDATIONS THAT PRESENT RISK OF TOXICITY TO THE PATIENT.

How Supplied:
QUIBRON®-T tablets (ivory, in the Dividose® tablet design) containing 300 mg anhydrous theophylline.

NDC 0087-0512-41   Bottles of 100

QUIBRON®-T/SR tablets (white, in the Dividose® tablet design) containing 300 mg anhydrous theophylline.

NDC 0087-0519-41   Bottles of 100
Store below 86°F (30°C).

Shown in Product Identification Section, page 419

Memorandum

Mead Johnson Nutritional Division follows on the opposite page which is 1243.

Mead Johnson Nutritional Division

Mead Johnson & Company
2404 W. PENNSYLVANIA ST.
EVANSVILLE, INDIANA 47721

CASEC® powder
[kā'sek]
Calcium caseinate
Protein modifier
(See PDR For Nonprescription Drugs)

CE-VI-SOL®
[se'vi-sahl"]
Vitamin C supplement drops
(See PDR For Nonprescription Drugs)

CRITICARE HN®
[cri'tĭ-care"]
Ready to Use High Nitrogen Elemental Diet
(See PDR for Nonprescription Drugs)

ENFAMIL® concentrated liquid • powder
[en'fah-mĭl"]
Infant formula
(See PDR For Nonprescription Drugs)

ENFAMIL® with Iron
[en'fah-mĭl"]
concentrated liquid • powder
Infant formula
(See PDR For Nonprescription Drugs)

ENFAMIL NURSETTE®
[en'fah-mĭl"]
Infant formula
(See PDR For Nonprescription Drugs)

ENFAMIL® ready-to-use
[en'fah-mĭl"]
Infant formula
(See PDR For Nonprescription Drugs)

ENFAMIL® with Iron ready-to-use
[en'fah-mĭl"]
Infant formula
(See PDR For Nonprescription Drugs)

FER-IN-SOL®
[fair'ĭn-sahl"]
Iron supplement
• drops
• syrup
• capsules
Ferrous sulfate, Mead Johnson
(See PDR For Nonprescription Drugs)

ISOCAL®
[ī'sō-cal"]
Complete liquid diet
(See PDR For Nonprescription Drugs)

ISOCAL® HCN
[ī'sō-cal"]
High Calorie and Nitrogen Nutritionally Complete Liquid Tube Feeding Formula
(See PDR For Nonprescription Drugs)

	Poly-Vi-Flor chewable tablets		Percentage of U.S. Recommended Daily Allowance	
Each tablet supplies:	1.0mg	0.5mg	Children 2–4	Adults & Children 4 or More
Vitamin A, IU	2500	2500	100	50
Vitamin D, IU	400	400	100	100
Vitamin E, IU	15	15	150	50
Vitamin C, mg	60	60	150	100
Folic acid, mg	0.3	0.3	150	75
Thiamine, mg	1.05	1.05	150	70
Riboflavin, mg	1.2	1.2	150	70
Niacin, mg	13.5	13.5	150	68
Vitamin B_6, mg	1.05	1.05	150	53
Vitamin B_{12}, mcg	4.5	4.5	150	75
Fluoride, mg	1	0.5	*	*

* U.S. Recommended Daily Allowance has not been established.

LOFENALAC® powder
[lō-fen'ah-lak"]
Low phenylalanine food
(See PDR For Nonprescription Drugs)

LONALAC® powder
[lŏn'ah-lak"]
Low sodium, high protein beverage mix
(See PDR For Nonprescription Drugs)

LYTREN®
[lī'tren]
Oral electrolyte solution
(See PDR For Nonprescription Drugs)

MODUCAL® Dietary Carbohydrate
[mah'dju-cal"]
(See PDR For Nonprescription Drugs)

NATURACIL®
[natch'er-ah-sil"]
A natural-fiber laxative

Description: Naturacil is a unique non-powdered, chewable form of bulk laxative. It is a safe and effective natural-fiber bulking agent that promotes evacuation through normal physiological mechanisms.

The active ingredient in Naturacil is ground and purified psyllium seed husks, widely recognized as an excellent source of dietary fiber. Each adult dose of Naturacil (two pieces) contains: 3.4 g of psyllium seed husks, and also contains artificial chocolate flavor and color, corn syrup, glycerin, nonfat milk, partially hydrogenated vegetable oil (soybean and cottonseed oil), sugar, 0.011 g (11 mg) of sodium, 54 Calories, and 9.6 g of available carbohydrate.

Clinical Pharmacology: One of the most important causes of constipation is lack of adequate fiber in the diet. The psyllium seed husks in Naturacil provide an excellent source of dietary fiber because they contain a mucilage which has a high water-holding capacity. Known chemically as an arabinoxylan, this mucilage, when mixed with intestinal fluid, forms a gel which increases the bulk and water content of the stool. Because of this action, Naturacil, when taken with liquid, promotes the gentle, natural evacuation of the sigmoid colon and rectum.

Indications and Usage: Naturacil is indicated for the relief and prevention of simple constipation, for restoring regularity, and for the bowel management of patients with:
• Functional Constipation
• Diverticulosis
• Hemorrhoids
• Irritable Bowel Syndrome/Spastic Colon
• Postsurgical Bowel Requirements

Naturacil is a non-habit-forming bulking agent that may be used when long-term therapy is indicated. Diabetic patients should take into consideration that Naturacil contains 38.4 Calories from carbohydrates per dose.

Clinical Studies: One hundred forty adults who occasionally use bulk producing agents to promote bowel regularity were subjects in two randomized, crossover studies to evaluate the efficacy, organoleptic properties, and convenience of new Naturacil and the most widely used form of Metamucil® (regular-flavor powder). The properties of both products were rated independently on a numerical scale and the two products were then compared. Naturacil was found to be as safe and effective as Metamucil for the bowel management of patients with functional constipation, diverticulosis, hemorrhoids, irritable bowel syndrome/spastic colon, and postsurgical bowel requirements.

No significant differences were found between the two products in mean number of daily bowel movements, stool consistency, gastrointestinal symptoms, and the patients' perceived effectiveness. No significant differences were found between Naturacil and Metamucil in gastrointestinal symptoms or side effects.

Comparing the two products for taste and convenience, a significantly greater number of subjects considered Naturacil to be better-tasting and more convenient to take than Metamucil among those who reported a preference.

Contraindications: Naturacil or any bulk-forming laxative is contraindicated in cases of intestinal obstruction or fecal impaction.

Dosage and Administration: The usual adult dosage is two pieces, one to three times daily; the dosage for children 6 to 12 years of age is one piece, one to three times daily. Doses should be accompanied by 8 fluid ounces of any liquid the patient prefers. Results may occur within 24 hours, but continued use for two to three days may be necessary for optimal effect.

Storage: Store at room temperature.

How Supplied: Cartons of 24 pieces (12 adult doses) and 40 pieces (20 adult doses). Each piece is individually wrapped in foil.

Naturacil 24's: NDC #0087-0444-01
Naturacil 40's: NDC #0087-0444-02

Is This Product OTC: Yes. See also PDR for Nonprescription Drugs.

NUTRAMIGEN®
[nū-tram'ĭ-jen"]
Protein hydrolysate formula
• powder
• ready-to-feed, 8 fl oz
   Nursette® bottles
(See PDR For Nonprescription Drugs)

POLY-VI-FLOR®   B
[pahl-ē-vī'flōr"]
• 1.0 mg
• 0.5 mg
Multivitamin and fluoride supplement chewable tablets

Description:
[See table above].
Ingredients: Vitamin A acetate, ergocalciferol, dl-alpha-tocopheryl acetate, ascorbic acid, sodium ascorbate, folic acid, thiamine mononitrate, riboflavin, niacinamide, pyridoxine hydrochloride, cyanocobalamin, and sodium fluoride.

Continued on next page

Mead Johnson Nutr.—Cont.

Made with natural sweeteners.

Clinical Pharmacology: It is well established that fluoridation of the water supply (1 ppm fluoride) during the period of tooth development leads to a significant decrease in the incidence of dental caries.

Poly-Vi-Flor 1.0 mg and 0.5 mg chewable tablets provide sodium fluoride, and ten essential vitamins in a chewable tablet. Because the tablets are chewable, they provide a *topical* as well as *systemic* source of fluoride.[1,2]

Hydroxyapatite is the principal crystal for all calcified tissue in the human body. The fluoride ion reacts with the *hydroxyapatite* in the tooth as it is formed to produce the more caries-resistant crystal, *fluorapatite*. The reaction may be expressed by the equation:[3]

$$Ca_{10}(PO_4)_6(OH)_2 + 2F^- \rightarrow Ca_{10}(PO_4)_6F_2 + 2OH^-$$
(Hydroxyapatite) (Fluorapatite)

Three stages of fluoride deposition in tooth enamel can be distinguished.[3]

1. Small amounts (reflecting the low levels of fluoride in tissue fluids) are incorporated into the enamel crystals while they are being formed.
2. After enamel has been laid down, fluoride deposition continues in the surface enamel. Diffusion of fluoride from the surface inward is apparently restricted.
3. After eruption, the surface enamel acquires fluoride from water, food, supplementary fluoride and smaller amounts from saliva.

Indications and Usage: Supplementation of the diet with ten essential vitamins.

Supplementation of the diet with the fluoride for caries prophylaxis.

Poly-Vi-Flor 1.0 mg chewable tablets provide fluoride in tablet form for children over 3 years in areas where the water fluoride level is less than 0.3 ppm.[4]

Poly-Vi-Flor 0.5 mg chewable tablets provide fluoride in tablet form for children 2-3 years of age where the drinking water has a fluoride content of 0.3 ppm or less, and for children 3 years of age and above where the drinking water has a fluoride level greater than 0.3 ppm and not more than 0.7 ppm.[4]

Poly-Vi-Flor chewable tablets supply significant amounts of vitamins A, D, E, C, thiamine, riboflavin, niacin, pyridoxine, cyanocobalamin and folic acid to supplement the diet, and to help assure that nutritional deficiencies of these vitamins will not develop. Thus, in a single easy-to-use preparation, children over three years of age obtain ten essential vitamins and the important mineral, fluoride.

The American Academy of Pediatrics recommends that children up to age 16, in areas where drinking water contains less than optimal levels of fluoride, receive daily fluoride supplementation.

Children using Poly-Vi-Flor chewable tablets regularly should receive semiannual dental examinations. The regular brushing of teeth and attention to good oral hygiene practices are also essential.

Warnings: As in the case of all medications, keep out of the reach of children.

Precautions: The suggested dose *should not be exceeded*, since dental fluorosis may result from continued ingestion of large amounts of fluoride. Before prescribing Vi-Flor® products, the physician should:

1. determine the fluoride content of the drinking water.
2. make sure the child is not receiving significant amounts of fluoride from other medications.
3. periodically check to make sure that the child does not develop significant dental fluorosis.

Adverse Reactions: Allergic rash and other idiosyncrasies have been rarely reported.

Dosage and Administration: One tablet daily or as prescribed by the physician.

How Supplied: Poly-Vi-Flor 1.0 mg (multivitamin and fluoride supplement) chewable tablets are available on prescription only in 100- and 1000-tablet bottles.
NDC 0087-0474-02 Bottles of 100
NDC 0087-0474-03 Bottles of 1000
Poly-Vi-Flor 0.5 mg (multivitamin and fluoride supplement) chewable tablets are available on prescription only in 100 tablet bottles.
NDC 0087-0468-41 Bottles of 100

Literature Available: Yes.

References:
1. Hennon, D.K.; Stookey, G.K., and Muhler, J.C.: The Clinical Anticariogenic Effectiveness of Supplementary Fluoride-Vitamin Preparations—Results at the End of Three Years, J. Dentistry for Children 33:3–12 (Jan.) 1966.
2. Hennon, D.K.; Stookey, G.K., and Muhler, J.C.: The Clinical Anticariogenic Effectiveness of Supplementary Fluoride-Vitamin Preparations—Results at the End of Four Years, J. Dentistry for Children 34:439–443 (Nov.) 1967.
3. Brudevold, F., and McCann, H.G.: Fluoride and Caries Control—Mechanism of Action, in Nizel, A.E.: The Science of Nutrition and Its Application in Clinical Dentistry, Philadelphia, W.B. Saunders Company, 1966, pp. 331–347.
4. American Academy of Pediatrics Committee on Nutrition: Fluoride Supplementation: Revised Dosage Schedule. Pediatrics 63:150, 1979.

POLY–VI–FLOR® R
[*pahl-ē-vī' flōr"*]
● 0.5 mg
● 0.25 mg
Multivitamin and fluoride supplement drops

Description:
[See table below].
See INDICATIONS AND USAGE section below for use by infants and children under two years of age.
This product does not contain the essential vitamin folic acid.

Ingredients: Vitamin A palmitate, ergocalciferol, D-alpha-tocopheryl succinate, ascorbic acid, thiamine hydrochloride, riboflavin-5-phosphate sodium, niacinamide, pyridoxine hydrochloride, cyanocobalamin, and sodium fluoride.
Made with natural sweeteners.

Clinical Pharmacology: For information on fluoridation see Poly-Vi-Flor 1.0mg and 0.5mg chewable tablets.

Indications and Usage: Supplementation of the diet with nine essential vitamins.
Supplementation of the diet with fluoride for caries prophylaxis.
The American Academy of Pediatrics recommends that children up to age 16, in areas where drinking water contains less than optimal levels of fluoride, receive daily fluoride supplementation.
Poly-Vi-Flor 0.5 mg (multivitamin and fluoride supplement) drops provide fluoride in drop form for children ages 2–3 years in areas where the drinking water contains less than 0.3 ppm fluoride; and for children over 3 years in areas where the drinking water contains 0.3 thru 0.7 ppm of fluoride.[2] Each 1.0 ml provides sodium fluoride (0.5 mg fluoride) plus nine essential vitamins.
Poly-Vi-Flor 0.25 mg (multivitamin and fluoride supplement) drops provide fluoride in drop form for infants and young children from birth to 2 years of age in areas where the drinking water contains less than 0.3 ppm of fluoride and for children ages 2–3 years in areas where the drinking water contains 0.3 thru 0.7 ppm of fluoride. Each 1.0 ml supplies sodium fluoride (0.25 mg fluoride) plus nine essential vitamins.
The American Academy of Pediatrics[2] and the American Dental Association[3] currently recommend that infants and children under 2 years of age, in areas where drinking water contains less than 0.3 ppm of fluoride, and children 2-3, in areas where the drinking water contains 0.3 through 0.7 ppm of fluoride, receive 0.25 mg of supplemental fluoride daily which is provided in a full dose (1 ml) of Poly-Vi-Flor® 0.25 mg drops. A half dose (0.5 ml) of Poly-Vi-Flor 0.5 mg drops could also provide a daily fluoride intake of 0.25 mg; however, this dosage reduces vitamin supplementation by half.
Poly-Vi-Flor 0.5 mg drops and 0.25 mg drops supply significant amounts of vitamins A, D, E, C, thiamine, riboflavin, niacin, pyridoxine, and cyanocobalamin to supplement the diet, and to help assure that nutritional deficiencies of these vitamins will not develop. Thus in a single easy-to-use preparation, infants and children obtain nine essential vitamins and fluoride.
A comprehensive 5½ year series of studies of the effectiveness of Tri-Vi-Flor® and Poly-Vi-Flor® products in caries protection has been published.[4-7] Children in this continuing study lived in an area where the water supply contained only 0.05 ppm fluoride. The subjects were divided into two groups, one which used only nonfluoridated Vi-Sol® vitamin products and the other Tri-Vi-Flor and Poly-Vi-Flor vitamin-fluoride products. The three-year interim report showed 63% fewer carious surfaces in primary teeth and 43% fewer carious surfaces in permanent teeth of the children taking Vi-Flor® vitamin-fluoride products.[4] After four years the studies continued to support the effectiveness of Tri-Vi-Flor and Poly-Vi-Flor, showing a reduction in carious surfaces of 68% in primary teeth and 46% in permanent teeth.[5] Results at the end of 5½ years further confirmed the previous findings and indicated that significant reductions in dental caries are apparent with the continued use of Vi-Flor vitamin-fluoride products.[6]

Warnings: As in the case of all medications, keep out of the reach of children.

Precautions: The suggested dose should not be exceeded since dental fluorosis may result from continued ingestion of large amounts of fluoride. When prescribing Vi-Flor products, the physician should:

1. determine the fluoride content of the drinking water.
2. make sure the child is not receiving significant amounts of fluoride from other medications.
3. periodically check to make sure that the child does not develop significant dental fluorosis.

Poly-Vi-Flor 0.5 mg drops and 0.25 mg drops should be dispensed in the original plastic container, since contact with glass leads to instability and precipitation. (The amount of sodium fluoride in both the 30- and 50-ml sizes (0.5 mg drops) and in the 50 ml size (0.25 mg drops) is well below the maximum to be dispensed at one time according to

	Poly-Vi-Flor drops		Percentage of U.S. Recommended Daily Allowance	
Each 1.0 ml supplies:	0.5mg	0.25mg	Infants	Children Under 4
Vitamin A, IU	1500	1500	100	60
Vitamin D, IU	400	400	100	100
Vitamin E, IU	5	5	100	50
Vitamin C, mg	35	35	100	88
Thiamine, mg	0.5	0.5	100	71
Riboflavin, mg	0.6	0.6	100	75
Niacin, mg	8	8	100	89
Vitamin B$_6$, mg	0.4	0.4	100	57
Vitamin B$_{12}$, mcg	2	2	100	67
Fluoride, mg	0.5	0.25	*	*

* U.S. Recommended Daily Allowance has not been established.

for possible revisions — **Product Information** — 1245

recommendations of the American Dental Association.)
Adverse Reactions: Allergic rash and other idiosyncrasies have been rarely reported.
Dosage and Administration: Poly-Vi-Flor 0.5 mg drops: 1.0 ml daily for children 2 years of age or older, or as prescribed by the physician. Poly-Vi-Flor 0.25 mg drops: 1.0 ml daily or as prescribed by the physician.
Drops may be dropped directly into mouth with 'Safti-Dropper,' or mixed with cereal, fruit juice or other food.
How Supplied: Poly-Vi-Flor 0.5 mg (multivitamin and fluoride supplement) drops are available on prescription only in bottles of 30 and 50 ml.
NDC 0087-0472-01 Bottles of 1 fl oz (30 ml)
NDC 0087-0472-02 Bottles of 1⅔ fl oz (50 ml)
FSN 6505-080-0967 (50 ml)
Poly-Vi-Flor 0.25 mg (multivitamin and fluoride supplement) drops are available on prescription only in bottles of 50 ml.
NDC 0087-0451-41 Bottles of 50 ml.
Literature Available: Yes.
References:
1. Brudevold, F., and McCann, H.G.: Fluoride and Caries Control—Mechanism of Action, in Nizel, A.E.: The Science of Nutrition and its Application in Clinical Dentistry, Philadelphia, W. B. Saunders Company, 1966, pp. 331–347.
2. American Academy of Pediatrics, Committee on Nutrition: Fluoride Supplementation: Revised Dosage Schedule, Pediatrics 63:150, 1979.
3. Accepted Dental Therapeutics, Ed. 38, Chicago, American Dental Association, 1979, p. 321.
4. Hennon, D.K.; Stookey, G.K., and Muhler, J.C.: The Clinical Anticariogenic Effectiveness of Supplementary Fluoride-Vitamin Preparations—Results at the End of Three Years, J. Dentistry for Children 33:3–12 (Jan.) 1966.
5. Hennon, D.K.; Stookey, G.K., and Muhler, J.C.: The Clinical Anticariogenic Effectiveness of Supplementary Fluoride-Vitamin Preparations—Results at the End of Four Years, J. Dentistry for Children 24:439–443 (Nov.) 1967.
6. Hennon, D.K.; Stookey, G.K., and Muhler, J.C.: The Clinical Anticariogenic Effectiveness of Supplementary Fluoride-Vitamin Preparations—Results at the End of Five and a Half Years, Phar. and Ther. in Dent. 1:1, 1970.
7. Hennon, D.K.; Stookey, G.K., and Beiswanger, B.B.: Fluoride vitamin supplements: Effects on dental caries and fluorosis when used in areas with suboptimum fluoride in the water supply. J.Am.Dent.Assoc. 95:965, 1977.

POLY-VI-FLOR® with Iron ℞
[pahl-ē-vī' flōr'']
● 1.0 mg
● 0.5 mg
Multivitamin, iron and fluoride supplement chewable tablets

Description:
[See table above].
Ingredients: Vitamin A acetate, ergocalciferol, dl-alpha-tocopheryl acetate, ascorbic acid, sodium ascorbate, folic acid, thiamine mononitrate, riboflavin, niacinamide, pyridoxine hydrochloride, cyanocobalamin, ferrous fumarate, cupric oxide, zinc oxide, and sodium fluoride.

	Poly-Vi-Flor chewable tablets		Percentage of U.S. Recommended Daily Allowance	
	1.0 mg w/Iron	0.5 mg w/Iron	Children 2-4	Adults & Children 4 or More
Each tablet supplies:				
Vitamin A, IU	2500	2500	100	50
Vitamin D, IU	400	400	100	100
Vitamin E, IU	15	15	150	50
Vitamin C, mg	60	60	150	100
Folic acid, mg	0.3	0.3	150	75
Thiamine, mg	1.05	1.05	150	70
Riboflavin, mg	1.2	1.2	150	70
Niacin, mg	13.5	13.5	150	68
Vitamin B_6, mg	1.05	1.05	150	53
Vitamin B_{12}, mcg	4.5	4.5	150	75
Iron, mg	12	12	120	67
Copper, mg	1	1	100	50
Zinc, mg	10	10	125	67
Fluoride, mg	1	0.5	*	*

*U.S. Recommended Daily Allowance has not been established.

Made with natural sweeteners.
Clinical Pharmacology: For information on fluoridation see Poly-Vi-Flor 1.0 mg and 0.5 mg chewable tablets.
Poly-Vi-Flor with Iron chewable tablets provide sodium fluoride, iron, copper, zinc and ten essential vitamins in a chewable tablet. Because the tablets are chewable, they provide a *topical* as well as *systemic* source of fluoride.[1,2]
Indications and Usage: Supplementation of the diet with ten essential vitamins, iron, copper and zinc.
Supplementation of the diet with fluoride, for caries prophylaxis.
The American Academy of Pediatrics recommends that children up to age 16, in areas where drinking water contains less than optimal levels of fluoride, receive daily fluoride supplementation.
Poly-Vi-Flor 1.0 mg chewable tablets with Iron were developed to provide fluoride in tablet form for children over 3 years in areas where the water fluoride level is less than 0.3 ppm.[3]
Poly-Vi-Flor 0.5 mg with Iron chewable tablets provides fluoride for children 2–3 years of age where the drinking water has fluoride content of 0.3 ppm or less, and for children 3 years of age and above where the drinking water has a fluoride level greater than 0.3 ppm and not more than 0.7 ppm.[3]
Poly-Vi-Flor with Iron chewable tablets supply significant amounts of vitamins A, D, E, C, thiamine, riboflavin, niacin, pyridoxine, cyanocobalamin, folic acid, iron, copper and zinc to supplement the diet, and to help assure that deficiencies of these nutrients will not develop. Thus, in a single easy-to-use preparation, children over three years of age obtain ten essential vitamins, iron, and fluoride.
Children using Poly-Vi-Flor with Iron chewable tablets regularly should receive semiannual dental examinations. The regular brushing of teeth and attention to good oral hygiene practices are also essential.
Warnings: As in the case of all medications, keep out of the reach of children.
Precautions: The suggested dose of Poly-Vi-Flor with Iron chewable tablets *should not be exceeded*, since dental fluorosis may result from continued ingestion of large amounts of fluoride.
Before prescribing Vi-Flor® products, the physician should:
1. determine the fluoride content of the drinking water.
2. make sure the child is not receiving significant amounts of fluoride from other medications.
3. periodically check to make sure that the child does not develop significant dental fluorosis.

The toxicity of ferrous fumarate is not established. However, to prevent possible serious harmful effects in the event of accidental overdosage, it is recommended that no more than 100 tablets be dispensed at one time.
Adverse Reactions: Allergic rash and other idiosyncrasies have been rarely reported.
Dosage and Administration: One tablet daily or as prescribed by the physician.
How Supplied: Poly-Vi-Flor 1.0 mg with Iron (multivitamin, mineral and fluoride supplement) chewable tablets are available by prescription only in 100- and 1000-tablet bottles.
Poly-Vi-Flor 0.5 mg with Iron (multivitamin, mineral and iron supplement) chewable tablets are available on prescription only in 100-tablet bottles.
NDC 0087-0476-03 Bottles of 100
NDC 0087-0476-04 Bottles of 1000
Literature Available: Yes.
References:
1. Hennon, D.K.; Stookey, G.K., and Muhler, J.C.: The Clinical Anticariogenic Effectiveness of Supplementary Fluoride-Vitamin Preparations—Results at the End of Three Years, J. Dentistry for Children 33:3–12 (Jan.) 1966.
2. Hennon, D.K.; Stookey, G.K., and Muhler, J.C.: The Clinical Anticariogenic Effectiveness of Supplementary Fluoride-Vitamin Preparations—Results at the End of Four Years, J. Dentistry for Children 34:439–443 (Nov.) 1967.
3. American Academy of Pediatrics Committee on Nutrition: Fluoride Supplementation: Revised Dosage Schedule. Pediatrics 63:150, 1979.

POLY-VI-FLOR® with Iron ℞
[pahl-ē-vī' flōr'']
● 0.5 mg
● 0.25 mg
Multivitamin, iron and fluoride supplement drops

Description:
(See table left.)
*U.S. Recommended Daily Allowance has not been established.
See INDICATIONS AND USAGE section below for use by infants and children under two years of age.
This product does not contain the essential vitamins folic acid and B_{12}.

	Poly-Vi-Flor drops		Percentage of U.S. Recommended Daily Allowance	
	0.5 mg w/Iron	0.25 mg w/Iron	Infants	Children Under 4
Each 1.0 ml supplies:				
Vitamin A, IU	1500	1500	100	60
Vitamin D, IU	400	400	100	100
Vitamin E, IU	5	5	100	50
Vitamin C, mg	35	35	100	88
Thiamine, mg	0.5	0.5	100	71
Riboflavin, mg	0.6	0.6	100	75
Niacin, mg	8	8	100	89
Vitamin B_6, mg	0.4	0.4	100	57
Iron, mg	10	10	67	100
Fluoride, mg	0.5	0.25	*	*

Continued on next page

Mead Johnson Nutr.—Cont.

Ingredients: Vitamin A palmitate, ergocalciferol, D-alpha-tocopheryl succinate, ascorbic acid, thiamine hydrochloride, riboflavin-5-phosphate sodium, niacinamide, pyridoxine hydrochloride, ferrous sulfate and sodium fluoride. Made with natural sweeteners.

Clinical Pharmacology: For information on fluoridation see Poly-Vi-Flor 1.0 mg and 0.5 mg chewable tablets.

Indications and Usage: Supplementation of the diet with eight essential vitamins and iron. Supplementation of the diet with fluoride for caries prophylaxis.

The American Academy of Pediatrics recommends that children up to age 16, in areas where drinking water contains less than optimal levels of fluoride, receive daily fluoride supplementation.

Poly-Vi-Flor 0.5 mg with Iron (multivitamin, iron, and fluoride supplement) drops provide fluoride in drop form for children ages 2–3 years in areas where the drinking water contains less than 0.3 ppm fluoride; and for children over 3 years in areas where the drinking water contains 0.3 thru 0.7 ppm of fluoride.[1] Each 1.0 ml provides sodium fluoride (0.5 mg fluoride) plus eight essential vitamins and iron.

Poly-Vi-Flor 0.25 mg with Iron drops provide fluoride in drop form for infants and young children from birth to 2 years of age in areas where the drinking water contains less than 0.3 ppm of fluoride and for children ages 2-3 years in areas where the drinking water contains 0.3 thru 0.7 ppm of fluoride. Each 1.0 ml supplies sodium fluoride (0.25 mg fluoride) plus eight essential vitamins and iron.

The American Academy of Pediatrics[1] and the American Dental Association[2] currently recommend that infants and children under 2 years of age, in areas where drinking water contains less than 0.3 ppm of fluoride, and children 2-3, in areas where the drinking water contains 0.3 through 0.7 ppm of fluoride, receive 0.25 mg of supplemental fluoride daily which is provided in a full dose (1 ml) of Poly-Vi-Flor® 0.25 mg with Iron drops. A half dose (0.5 ml) of Poly-Vi-Flor 0.5 mg with Iron drops could also provide a daily fluoride intake of 0.25 mg; however, this dosage reduces vitamin supplementation by half.

Poly-Vi-Flor with Iron drops supply significant amounts of vitamins A, D, E, C, thiamine, riboflavin, niacin, pyridoxine, and ferrous sulfate to supplement the diet, and to help assure that deficiencies of these nutrients will not develop. Thus, in a single easy-to-use preparation, infants and children obtain eight essential vitamins and iron, plus fluoride.

A comprehensive 5½ year series of studies of the effectiveness of Tri-Vi-Flor® and Poly-Vi-Flor® products in caries protection has been published.[3, 6] Children in this continuing study lived in an area where the water supply contained only 0.05 ppm fluoride. The subjects were divided into two groups, one which used only nonfluoridated Vi-Sol® vitamin products and the other Tri-Vi-Flor and Poly-Vi-Flor vitamin-fluoride products.

The three-year interim report showed 63% fewer carious surfaces in primary teeth and 43% fewer carious surfaces in permanent teeth of the children taking Vi-Flor® vitamin-fluoride products.[3] After four years the studies continued to support the effectiveness of Tri-Vi-Flor and Poly-Vi-Flor, showing a reduction in carious surfaces of 68% in primary teeth and 46% in permanent teeth.[4] Results at the end of 5½ years further confirmed the previous findings and indicated that significant reductions in dental caries are apparent with the continued use of Vi-Flor vitamin-fluoride products.[5]

Warnings: As in the case of all medications, keep out of the reach of children.

Precautions: The suggested dose should not be exceeded since dental fluorosis may result from continued ingestion of large amounts of fluoride.

When prescribing Vi-Flor products, the physician should:
1. determine the fluoride content of the drinking water.
2. make sure the child is not receiving significant amounts of fluoride from other medications.
3. periodically check to make sure that the child does not develop significant dental fluorosis.

Poly-Vi-Flor with Iron drops should be dispensed in the original plastic container, since contact with glass leads to instability and precipitation. (The amount of sodium fluoride in the 50-ml. size is well below the maximum to be dispensed at one time according to recommendations of the American Dental Association.)

Adverse Reactions: Allergic rash and other idiosyncrasies have been reported rarely.

Dosage and Administration: Poly-Vi-Flor 0.5 mg with Iron drops: 1.0 ml daily for children 2 years of age and older, or as prescribed by the physician.

Poly-Vi-Flor 0.25 mg with Iron drops: 1.0 ml daily or as prescribed by the physician.

May be dropped directly into mouth with 'Safti-Dropper,' or mixed with cereal, fruit juice or other foods.

How Supplied: Poly-Vi-Flor 0.5 mg (multivitamin, fluoride and iron supplement) with Iron drops are available on prescription only in bottles of 50 ml.

Poly-Vi-Flor 0.25 mg (multivitamin, fluoride and iron supplement) with Iron drops are available on prescription only in bottles of 50 ml.

NDC 0087-0469-41 Bottles of 1⅔ fl oz (50 ml)

Literature Available: Yes.

References:
1. American Academy of Pediatrics, Committee on Nutrition: Fluoride Supplementation: Revised Dosage Schedule, Pediatrics 63:150, 1979.
2. Accepted Dental Therapeutics, Ed. 38, Chicago, American Dental Association, 1979, p. 321.
3. Hennon, D.K.; Stookey, G.K., and Muhler, J.C.: The Clinical Anticariogenic Effectiveness of Supplementary Fluoride-Vitamin Preparations—Results at the End of Three Years, J. Dentistry for Children 33:3–12 (Jan.) 1966.
4. Hennon, D.K.; Stookey, G.K., and Muhler, J.C.: The Clinical Anticariogenic Effectiveness of Supplementary Fluoride-Vitamin Preparations—Results at the End of Four Years, J. Dentistry for Children 34:439–443 (Nov.) 1967.
5. Hennon, D.K.; Stookey, G.K., and Muhler, J.C.: The Clinical Anticariogenic Effectiveness of Supplementary Fluoride-Vitamin Preparations—Results at the End of Five and a Half Years, Phar. and Ther. In Dent. 1:1, 1970.
6. Hennon, D.K.; Stookey, G.K., and Beiswanger, B.B.: Fluoride-vitamin supplements: Effects on Dental Caries and Fluorosis When Used in Areas With Suboptimum Fluoride in the Water Supply. J. Am. Dent. Assoc. 95:965, 1977.

POLY-VI-SOL®
[pahl-ē-vī'sahl″]
Vitamins
drops • chewable tablets

(See PDR For Nonprescription Drugs)

POLY-VI-SOL® with Iron
[pahl-ē-vī'sahl″]
Chewable vitamins with iron and zinc

(See PDR For Nonprescription Drugs)

POLY-VI-SOL® with Iron
[pahl-ē-vī'sahl″]
Multivitamin and Iron supplement drops

(See PDR For Nonprescription Drugs)

PORTAGEN®
[port'ă-jen]
Nutritionally complete dietary powder with Medium Chain Triglycerides
U.S. Patent No. 3,450,819

(See PDR For Nonprescription Drugs)

PREGESTIMIL®
[prĕ-jest'ĭ-mĭl″]
Protein hydrolysate formula with medium chain triglycerides and added amino acids

(See PDR For Nonprescription Drugs)

PROSOBEE® concentrated liquid • ready-to-use • powder
[prō-sō'be]
Milk-free, sucrose-free formula with soy protein isolate

(See PDR For Nonprescription Drugs)

SUSTACAL®
[sŭs'tă-cal″]
• liquid (ready to use)
• powder (mix with milk)
• pudding (ready-to-eat)
Nutritionally complete food

(See PDR For Nonprescription Drugs)

SUSTACAL® HC
[sŭs'tă-cal″]
High Calorie Nutritionally Complete Food

(See PDR for Nonprescription Drugs)

SUSTAGEN® powder
[sus'tă-jen]
Nutritional supplement

(See PDR For Nonprescription Drugs)

TEMPRA® drops, syrup, and chewable tablets
[tem'prah]
Acetaminophen

(See PDR For Nonprescription Drugs)

TRAUMACAL™
[tră'mă-cal″]
Nutritionally Complete Liquid for Traumatized Patients

(See PDR For Nonprescription Drugs)

TRIND® liquid
[trĭnd]
nasal decongestant • antihistamine

(See PDR For Nonprescription Drugs)

TRIND–DM® liquid
[trĭnd]
antitussive • nasal
decongestant • antihistamine

(See PDR For Nonprescription Drugs)

TRI–VI–FLOR® 1.0 mg ℞
[tri'vĭ-flōr″]
Vitamins A, D, C and fluoride
chewable tablets

Description:
[See table on top next page].
Ingredients: Vitamin A acetate, ergocalciferol, sodium ascorbate, ascorbic acid and sodium fluoride.
Made with natural sweeteners.
Clinical Pharmacology: For information of fluoridation see Poly-Vi-Flor® 1.0 mg and 0.5 mg chewable tablets.
Tri-Vi-Flor tablets provide sodium fluoride (1 mg fluoride) and three basic vitamins in a chewable tablet. Because the tablets are chewable, they provide a *topical* as well as *systemic* source of fluoride.[1,2]
Indications and Usage: Supplementation of the diet with vitamins A, D, and C.

Supplementation of the diet with fluoride for caries prophylaxis.
The American Academy of Pediatrics recommends that children up to age 16, in areas where drinking water contains less than optimal levels of fluoride, receive daily fluoride supplementation.
Tri-Vi-Flor 1.0 mg (vitamins A, D, C and fluoride) chewable tablets provide fluoride in tablet form for children 3 years of age and older where the drinking water contains less than 0.3 ppm of fluoride.[3]
Tri-Vi-Flor 1.0 mg chewable tablets supply vitamins A, D and C to help assure that nutritional deficiencies of these vitamins will not develop.
Tri-Vi-Flor 1.0 mg chewable tablets also provide the important mineral fluoride for caries prophylaxis. Thus in a single easy-to-use preparation, children over 3 years of age obtain three basic vitamins and the important mineral fluoride.
A study of fluoride tablets given to 121 children revealed the efficacy of sodium fluoride in tablet form. The authors concluded that the caries reduction was comparable to that previously reported for children drinking fluoridated water.[4]
A comprehensive 5½ year series of studies of the effectiveness of Tri-Vi-Flor® and Poly-Vi-Flor® products in caries protection has been published.[1,2,5] Children in this continuing study lived in an area where the water supply contained only 0.05 ppm fluoride. The subjects were divided into two groups, one which used only non-fluoridated Vi-Sol® vitamin products and the other Tri-Vi-Flor and Poly-Vi-Flor vitamin-fluoride products.
The three-year interim report showed 63% fewer carious surfaces in primary teeth and 43% fewer carious surfaces in permanent teeth of the children taking Vi-Flor® vitamin-fluoride products.[1]
After four years the studies continued to support the effectiveness of Tri-Vi-Flor and Poly-Vi-Flor, showing a reduction in carious surfaces of 68% in primary teeth and 46% in permanent teeth.[2]
Results at the end of 5½ years further confirmed the previous findings and indicated that significant reductions in dental caries are apparent with the continued use of Vi-Flor vitamin-fluoride products.[5]
Warnings: As in the case of all medications, keep out of the reach of children.
Precautions: The suggested dose of Tri-Vi-Flor 1.0 mg chewable tablets *should not be exceeded,* since dental fluorosis may result from continued ingestion of large amounts of fluoride.
When prescribing Vi-Flor products, the physician should:
1. determine the fluoride content of the drinking water.
2. make sure the child is not receiving significant amounts of fluoride from other medications.
3. periodically check to make sure that the child does not develop significant dental fluorosis.
Adverse Reactions: Allergic rash and other idiosyncrasies have been rarely reported.
Dosage and Administration: One chewable tablet daily or as prescribed by the physician.
How Supplied: Tri-Vi-Flor 1.0 mg (vitamins A, D, C and fluoride) chewable tablets are available on prescription only in 100- and 1000-tablet bottles.
NDC 0087-0477-01 Bottles of 100
NDC 0087-0477-02 Bottles of 1000
Literature Available: Yes.
References:
1. Hennon, D.K., Stookey, G.K. and Muhler, J.C.: The Clinical Anticariogenic Effectiveness of Supplementary Fluoride-Vitamin Preparations—Results at the End of Three Years. J Dent for Children 33:3–12 (Jan.) 1966.
2. Hennon, D.K., Stookey, G.K. and Muhler, J.C.: The Clinical Anticariogenic Effectiveness of Supplementary Fluoride-Vitamin Preparations—Results at the End of Four Years, J Dent for Children 34:439–443 (Nov.) 1967.
3. American Academy of Pediatrics, Committee on Nutrition: Fluoride supplementation: Revised Dosage Schedule. Pediatrics 63:150, 1979.
4. Arnold, F.A., Jr., McClure, F.J. and White, C.L.: Sodium Fluoride Tablets for Children, Dental Progress 1:12–16 (Oct.) 1960.
5. Hennon, D.K., Stookey, G.K. and Muhler, J.C.: The Clinical Anticariogenic Effectiveness of Supplementary Fluoride-Vitamin Preparations—Results at the End of Five and a Half Years, Phar. and Ther. in Dent. 1:1, 1970.

TRI–VI–FLOR® ℞
[*trī' vĭ-flōr"*]
● 0.5 mg
● 0.25 mg
Vitamins A, D, C and fluoride drops
Description:
[See table below].
*U.S. Recommended Daily Allowance has not been established.
See INDICATIONS AND USAGE section below for use by infants and children under two years of age.
Ingredients: Vitamin A palmitate, ergocalciferol, ascorbic acid and sodium fluoride. Made with natural sweeteners.
Clinical Pharmacology: For information on fluoridation see Poly-Vi-Flor® 1.0 mg and 0.5 mg chewable tablets.
Indications and Usage: Supplementation of the diet with vitamins A, D and C.
Tri-Vi-Flor drops also provide fluoride for caries prophylaxis.
The American Academy of Pediatrics recommends that children up to age 16, in areas where drinking water contains less than optimal levels of fluoride, receive daily fluoride supplementation.
Tri-Vi-Flor 0.5 mg (vitamins A, D, C and fluoride) drops provide fluoride in drop form for children ages 2-3 years in areas where the drinking water contains less than 0.3 ppm fluoride; and for children over 3 years in areas where the drinking water contains 0.3 thru 0.7 ppm of fluoride.[1] Each 1.0 ml provides sodium fluoride (0.5 mg fluoride) plus three basic vitamins.
Tri-Vi-Flor 0.25 mg (vitamins A, D, C and fluoride) drops provide fluoride in drop form for infants and young children from birth to 2 years of age in areas where the drinking water contains less than 0.3 ppm of fluoride; and for children ages 2-3 years in areas where the drinking water contains 0.3 thru 0.7 ppm of fluoride. Each 1.0 ml supplies sodium fluoride (0.25 mg fluoride) plus three basic vitamins.
The American Academy of Pediatrics[1] and the American Dental Association[6] currently recommend that infants and children under 2 years of age, in areas where drinking water contains less than 0.3 ppm of fluoride, and children 2-3, in areas where the drinking water contains 0.3 through 0.7 ppm of fluoride, receive 0.25 mg of supplemental fluoride daily which is provided in a full dose (1 ml) of Tri-Vi-Flor® 0.25 mg drops. A half dose (0.5 ml) of Tri-Vi-Flor 0.5 mg drops could also provide a daily fluoride intake of 0.25 mg; however, this dosage reduces vitamin supplementation by half.
A comprehensive 5½ year series of studies of the effectiveness of Tri-Vi-Flor® and Poly-Vi-Flor® products in caries protection has been published.[2-5] Children in this continuing study lived in an area where the water supply contained only 0.05 ppm fluoride. The subjects were divided into two groups, one which used only nonfluoridated Vi-Sol® vitamin products and the other Tri-Vi-Flor and Poly-Vi-Flor vitamin-fluoride products.
The three-year interim report showed 63% fewer carious surfaces in primary teeth and 43% fewer carious surfaces in permanent teeth of the children taking Vi-Flor® vitamin-fluoride products.[2]
After four years the studies continued to support the effectiveness of Tri-Vi-Flor and Poly-Vi-Flor, showing a reduction in carious surfaces of 68% in primary teeth and 46% in permanent teeth.[3]
Results at the end of 5½ years further confirmed the previous findings and indicated that significant reductions in dental caries are apparent with the continued use of Vi-Flor vitamin-fluoride products.[4]
Warnings: As in the case of all medications, keep out of the reach of children.
Precautions: The suggested dose should not be exceeded since dental fluorosis may result from continued ingestion of large amounts of fluoride.
When prescribing Vi-Flor products, the physician should:
1. determine the fluoride content of the drinking water.
2. make sure the child is not receiving significant amounts of fluoride from other medications.
3. periodically check to make sure that the child does not develop significant dental fluorosis.
Tri-Vi-Flor drops should be dispensed in the original plastic container, since contact with glass leads to instability and precipitation. (The amount of sodium fluoride in both the 30- and 50-ml sizes is well below the maximum to be dispensed at one time acccording to recommendations of the American Dental Association.)
Adverse Reactions: Allergic rash and other idiosyncrasies have been rarely reported.
Dosage and Administration: Tri-Vi-Flor 0.5 mg drops: 1.0 ml daily for children 2 years of age and older, or as prescribed by the physician. Tri-Vi-Flor 0.25 mg drops: 1.0 ml daily, or as prescribed by the physician.
May be dropped directly into mouth with 'Safti-Dropper,' or mixed with cereal, fruit juice or other food.
How Supplied: Tri-Vi-Flor 0.5 mg (vitamins A,D,C, and fluoride) drops are available on prescription only in bottles of 30 and 50 ml.
NDC 0087-0473-01 Bottles of 1 fl oz (30 ml)
NDC 0087-0473-02 Bottles of 1⅔ fl oz (50 ml)
Tri-Vi-Flor 0.25 mg (vitamins A, D, C and fluoride) drops are available on prescription only in bottles of 50 ml.

	Tri-Vi-Flor Chewable tablets 1.0 mg	Percentage of U.S. Recommended Daily Allowance Children 2-4	Percentage of U.S. Recommended Daily Allowance Adults & Children 4 or More
Each tablet supplies:			
Vitamin A, IU	2500	100	50
Vitamin D, IU	400	100	100
Vitamin C, mg	60	150	100
Fluoride, mg	1.0	*	*

*U.S. Recommended Daily Allowance has not been established.

	Tri-Vi-Flor Drops 0.5mg	Tri-Vi-Flor Drops 0.25mg	Percentage of U.S. Recommended Daily Allowance Infants	Percentage of U.S. Recommended Daily Allowance Children Under 4
Each 1.0 ml supplies:				
Vitamin A, IU	1500	1500	100	60
Vitamin D, IU	400	400	100	100
Vitamin C, mg	35	35	100	100
Fluoride, mg	0.5	0.25	*	*

Continued on next page

Mead Johnson Nutr.—Cont.

NDC 0087-0452-41 Bottles of 50 ml.
Literature Available: Yes.
References:
1. American Academy of Pediatrics, Committee on Nutrition: Fluoride Supplementation: Revised Dosage Schedule, Pediatrics 63:150, 1979.
2. Hennon, D.K.; Stookey, G.K., and Muhler, J.C.: The Clinical Anticariogenic Effectiveness of Supplementary Fluoride-Vitamin Preparations—Results at the End of Three Years, J. Dentistry for Children 33:3–12 (Jan.) 1966.
3. Hennon, D.K.; Stookey, G.K., and Muhler, J.C.: The Clinical Anticariogenic Effectiveness of Supplementary Fluoride-Vitamin Preparations—Results at the End of Four Years, J. Dentistry for Children 34:439–443 (Nov.) 1967.
4. Hennon, D.K.; Stookey, G.K., and Muhler, J.C.: The Clinical Anticariogenic Effectiveness of Supplementary Fluoride-Vitamin Preparations—Results at the End of Five and a Half Years, Phar. and Ther. in Dent. 1:1, 1970.
5. Hennon, D.K.; Stookey, G.K., and Beiswanger, B.B.: Fluoride-vitamin supplements: Effects on dental caries and fluorosis when used in areas with suboptimal fluoride in the water supply. J. Am. Dent. Assoc. 95:965, 1977.
6. Accepted Dental Therapeutics, Ed. 38, Chicago, American Dental Association, 1979, p. 321.

TRI–VI–FLOR® 0.25 mg with Iron ℞
[trī' vī-flōr'']
Vitamins A, D, C, iron and fluoride drops

Description:

	Percentage of U.S. Recommended Daily Allowance	
Each 1.0 ml supplies	Infants	Children Under 4
Vitamin A, IU	1500	100	60
Vitamin D, IU	400	100	100
Vitamin C, mg	35	100	88
Iron, mg	10	67	100
Fluoride, mg	0.25	*	*

* U.S. Recommended Daily Allowance has not been established.
Ingredients: Vitamin A palmitate, ergocalciferol, ascorbic acid, ferrous sulfate and sodium fluoride. Made with natural sweeteners.
Clinical Pharmacology: For information on fluoridation see Poly-Vi-Flor® 1.0 mg and 0.5 mg chewable tablets.
Indications and Usage: Supplementation of the diet with vitamins A, D, C and iron.
Supplementation of the diet with fluoride for caries prophylaxis.
The American Academy of Pediatrics recommends that children up to age 16, in areas where drinking water contains less than optimal levels of fluoride, receive daily fluoride supplementation.
Tri-Vi-Flor 0.25 mg with Iron (vitamins A, D, C, iron and fluoride) drops provide fluoride in drop form for infants and young children from birth to 2 years of age in areas where the drinking water contains less than 0.3 ppm of fluoride; and for children ages 2-3 years in areas where the drinking water contains 0.3 thru 0.7 ppm of fluoride.[2] Each 1.0 ml supplies sodium fluoride (0.25 mg fluoride) plus three basic vitamins and iron.
Warnings: As in the case of all medications, keep out of the reach of children.
Precautions: The suggested dose should not be exceeded since dental fluorosis may result from continued ingestion of large amounts of fluoride. When prescribing Vi-Flor® products, the physician should:
1. determine the fluoride content of the drinking water.
2. make sure the child is not receiving significant amounts of fluoride from other medications.
3. periodically check to make sure that the child does not develop significant dental fluorosis.

TRI-VI-FLOR 0.25 mg with Iron drops should be dispensed in the original plastic container, since contact with glass leads to instability and precipitation. (The amount of sodium fluoride in the 50-ml size is well below the maximum to be dispensed at one time according to recommendations of the American Dental Association.)
Adverse Reactions: Allergic rash and other idiosyncrasies have been rarely reported.
Dosage and Administration: 1.0 ml daily, or as prescribed by the physician. May be dropped directly into mouth with 'Safti-Dropper', or mixed with cereal, fruit juice or other food.
USE FULL DOSAGE.
How Supplied: Tri-Vi-Flor 0.25 mg with Iron (vitamins A, D, C, iron and fluoride) drops are available on prescription only in bottles of 50 ml.
References:
1. Brudevold, F. and McCann, H.G.: Fluoride and caries control—mechanism of action, in Nizel, A.E.: The Science of Nutrition and its Application in Clinical Dentistry, Philadelphia, WB Saunders Company, 1966, pp 332–347.
2. American Academy of Pediatrics, Committee on Nutrition: Fluoride Supplementation: Revised Dosage Schedule, Pediatrics 63:150, 1979.

TRI-VI-SOL®
[trī' vī-sahl'']
Vitamin A, D and C Supplement drops

(See PDR For Nonprescription Drugs)

TRI-VI-SOL® with Iron
[trī' vī-sahl'']
Vitamins A, D, C and Iron Drops

(See PDR For Nonprescription Drugs)

Mead Johnson Pharmaceutical Division
Mead Johnson & Company
2404 W. PENNSYLVANIA ST.
EVANSVILLE, INDIANA 47721

COLACE®
[kō' lās]
Docusate sodium, Mead Johnson
capsules • syrup • liquid (drops)

Description: Colace (Docusate sodium) is a stool softener.
Actions and Uses: Colace, a surface-active agent, helps to keep stools soft for easy, natural passage. Not a laxative, thus not habit forming. Useful in constipation due to hard stools, in painful anorectal conditions, in cardiac and other conditions in which maximum ease of passage is desirable to avoid difficult or painful defecation, and when peristaltic stimulants are contraindicated. *Note:* When peristaltic stimulation is needed due to inadequate bowel motility, see Peri-Colace® (laxative and stool softener).
Contraindications: There are no known contraindications to Colace.
Side Effects: The incidence of side effects—none of a serious nature—is exceedingly small. Bitter taste, throat irritation, and nausea (primarily associated with the use of the syrup and liquid) are the main side effects reported. Rash has occurred.
Administration and Dosage: *Orally*—Suggested daily Dosage: *Adults and older children:* 50 to 200 mg. *Children 6 to 12:* 40 to 120 mg. *Children 3 to 6:* 20 to 60 mg. *Infants and children under 3:* 10 to 40 mg. The higher doses are recommended for initial therapy. Dosage should be adjusted to individual response. The effect on stools is usually apparent one to three days after the first dose. Give Colace liquid in half a glass of milk or fruit juice or in infant formula, to mask bitter taste. *In enemas*—Add 50 to 100 mg. Colace (5 to 10 ml. Colace liquid) to a retention or flushing enema.

Warning: As with any drug, if you are pregnant or nursing a baby, seek the advice of a health professional before using this product.
How Supplied: Colace® capsules, 50 mg.
 NDC 0087-0713-01 Bottles of 30
 NDC 0087-0713-02 Bottles of 60
 NDC 0087-0713-03 Bottles of 250
 NDC 0087-0713-05 Bottles of 1000
 NDC 0087-0713-07 Cartons of 100 single unit packs
Colace® capsules, 100 mg.
 NDC 0087-0714-43 Cartons of 10 single unit packs
 NDC 0087-0714-01 Bottles of 30
 NDC 0087-0714-02 Bottles of 60
 NDC 0087-0714-03 Bottles of 250
 NDC 0087-0714-05 Bottles of 1000
 NDC 0087-0714-07 Cartons of 100 single unit packs
Note: Colace capsules should be stored at controlled room temperature (59°–86°F. or 15°–30°C.)
Colace® liquid, 1% solution; 10 mg./ml. (with calibrated dropper)
 NDC 0087-0717-04 Bottles of 16 fl. oz.
 NDC 0087-0717-02 Bottles of 30 ml.
 6505-00-045-7786 (Bottle of 30 ml) Defense
Colace® syrup, 20 mg./5-ml. teaspoon; contains not more than 1% alcohol
 NDC 0087-0720-01 Bottles of 8 fl. oz.
 NDC 0087-0720-02 Bottles of 16 fl. oz.
Shown in Product Identification Section, page 419

DEAPRIL–ST® ℞
[dē' uh-pral]
(ergoloid mesylates)
SUBLINGUAL TABLETS

Description:
Each Deapril-ST **1.0 mg.** Sublingual Tablet contains dihydroergocornine 0.333 mg., dihydroergocristine 0.333 mg., and dihydroergocryptine 0.333 mg. (dihydro-alpha-ergocryptine and dihydro-beta-ergocryptine in the proportion of 2:1) as the methanesulfonates (mesylates), representing a total of 1.0 mg.
Actions: There is no specific evidence which clearly establishes the mechanism by which an ergoloid mesylates preparation such as Deapril-ST produces mental effects, nor is there conclusive evidence that it particularly affects cerebral arteriosclerosis or cerebrovascular insufficiency.
Indications: A proportion of individuals over sixty years of age who manifest signs and symptoms of an idiopathic decline in mental capacity (e.g., cognitive and interpersonal skills, mood, self-care, apparent motivation) can experience some symptomatic relief upon treatment with ergoloid mesylates preparations. The identity of the specific trait(s) or condition(s), if any, which would usefully predict a response to ergoloid mesylates therapy is not known. It appears, however, that those individuals who do respond come from groups of patients who may suffer from a disorder related in a poorly defined manner to the aging process or who have some underlying condition which compromises mental capacity (e.g., primary progressive dementia, Alzheimer's dementia, senile onset, or multi-infarct dementia).
Before prescribing ergoloid mesylates therapy, the physician should exclude the possibility that the patient's signs and symptoms arise from a potentially reversible and treatable condition. Particular care should be taken to exclude delirium and dementiform illness secondary to systemic disease, primary neurological disease or primary disturbance of mood.
Ergoloid mesylates preparations are not indicated in the treatment of acute or chronic psychosis, regardless of etiology (see CONTRAINDICATIONS section).
The decision to use ergoloid mesylates therapy in the treatment of an individual with a symptomatic decline in mental capacity of unknown etiology should be continually reviewed since the presenting clinical picture may subsequently evolve sufficiently to allow a specific diagnosis and a specific alternative treatment. In addition, continued clinical evaluation is required to determine whether

any initial benefit conferred by ergoloid mesylates therapy persists with time.

The efficacy of ergoloid mesylates therapy was evaluated using a special rating scale. The specific items on this scale on which modest but statistically significant changes were observed at the end of twelve weeks concerned mental alertness, confusion, recent memory, orientation, emotional lability, self-care, depression, anxiety/fears, cooperation, sociability, appetite, dizziness, fatigue, bothersome(ness), and an overall impression of clinical status.

Contraindications: Deapril-ST Sublingual Tablets are contraindicated in individuals who have previously shown hypersensitivity to the drug. Ergoloid mesylates preparations are also contraindicated in patients who have psychosis, acute or chronic, regardless of etiology.

Precautions: *Practitioners are advised that because the target symptoms are of unknown etiology careful diagnosis should be attempted before prescribing ergoloid mesylates sublingual tablets.*

This product contains FD&C Yellow No. 5 (tartrazine) which may cause allergic-type reactions (including bronchial asthma) in certain susceptible individuals. Although the overall incidence of FD&C Yellow No. 5 (tartrazine) sensitivity in the general population is low, it is frequently seen in patients who also have aspirin hypersensitivity.

Adverse Reactions: Deapril-ST Sublingual Tablets have not been found to produce serious side effects. Some sublingual irritation, transient nausea, and gastric disturbances have been reported. Ergoloid mesylates sublingual tablets do not possess the vasoconstrictor properties of the natural ergot alkaloids.

Dosage and Administration: One Deapril-ST 1.0 mg. Sublingual Tablet three times a day. Alleviation of symptoms is usually gradual and results may not be observed for 3–4 weeks.

How Supplied: Deapril-ST 1.0 mg, Sublingual Tablets

NDC 0087-0555-41 Bottles of 100
Shown in Product Identification Section, page 419

DESYREL®
[des'ĕ-rel]
(Trazodone HCl)

Description: DESYREL®, trazodone hydrochloride, is an antidepressant chemically unrelated to tricyclic, tetracyclic, or other known antidepressant agents. It is a triazolopyridine derivative designated as 2-[3-[4-(3-chlorophenyl)-1-piperazinyl] propyl]-1,2,4-triazolo[4, 3-a]pyridin-3(2H)-one hydrochloride. DESYREL is a white odorless crystalline powder which is freely soluble in water. Its molecular weight is 408.3. The empirical formula is $C_{19}H_{22}ClN_5O \cdot HCl$ and the structural formula is represented as follows:

DESYREL is supplied for oral administration in 50 mg and 100 mg tablets.

Clinical Pharmacology: The mechanism of DESYREL's antidepressant action in man is not fully understood. In animals, DESYREL selectively inhibits serotonin uptake by brain synaptosomes and potentiates the behavioral changes induced by the serotonin precursor, 5-hydroxytryptophan. Cardiac conduction effects of DESYREL in the anesthetized dog are qualitatively dissimilar and quantitatively less pronounced than those seen with tricyclic antidepressants. DESYREL is not a monoamine oxidase inhibitor and, unlike amphetamine-type drugs, does not stimulate the central nervous system.

In man, DESYREL is well absorbed after oral administration without selective localization in any tissue. When DESYREL is taken shortly after ingestion of food, there may be an increase in the amount of drug absorbed, a decrease in maximum concentration and a lengthening in the time to maximum concentration. Peak plasma levels occur approximately one hour after dosing when DESYREL is taken on an empty stomach or two hours after dosing when taken with food. Elimination of DESYREL is biphasic, consisting of an initial phase (half-life 3–6 hours) followed by a slower phase (half-life 5–9 hours), and is unaffected by the presence or absence of food. Since the clearance of DESYREL from the body is sufficiently variable, in some patients DESYREL may accumulate in the plasma.

For those patients who responded to DESYREL, one-third of the inpatients and one-half of the outpatients had a significant therapeutic response by the end of the first week of treatment. Three-fourths of all responders demonstrated a significant therapeutic effect by the end of the second week. One-fourth of responders required 2–4 weeks for a significant therapeutic response.

Indications and Usage: DESYREL is indicated for the treatment of depression. The efficacy of DESYREL has been demonstrated in both inpatient and outpatient settings and for depressed patients with and without prominent anxiety. The depressive illness of patients studied corresponds to the Major Depressive Episode criteria of the American Psychiatric Association's Diagnostic and Statistical Manual, III.[a]

Major Depressive Episode implies a prominent and relatively persistent (nearly every day for at least two weeks) depressed or dysphoric mood that usually interferes with daily functioning, and includes at least four of the following eight symptoms: change in appetite, change in sleep, psychomotor agitation or retardation, loss of interest in usual activities or decrease in sexual drive, increased fatigability, feelings of guilt or worthlessness, slowed thinking or impaired concentration, and suicidal ideation or attempts.

Contraindications: DESYREL is contraindicated in patients hypersensitive to DESYREL.

Warnings: Recent clinical studies in patients with pre-existing cardiac disease indicate that DESYREL may be arrhythmogenic in some patients in that population. Arrhythmias identified include isolated PVC's, ventricular couplets, and in two patients short episodes (3–4 beats) of ventricular tachycardia. Until the results of prospective studies are available, patients with pre-existing cardiac disease should be closely monitored particularly for cardiac arrhythmias. There have also been post-introduction reports of arrhythmias in DESYREL-treated patients, some of whom did not have pre-existing cardiac disease.

DESYREL is not recommended for use during the initial recovery phase of myocardial infarction.

Precautions:
General: The possibility of suicide in seriously depressed patients is inherent in the illness and may persist until significant remission occurs. Therefore, prescriptions should be written for the smallest number of tablets consistent with good patient management.

Hypotension, including orthostatic hypotension and syncope, has been reported to occur in patients receiving DESYREL. Concomitant administration of antihypertensive therapy with DESYREL may require a reduction in the dose of the antihypertensive drug.

Little is known about the interaction between DESYREL and general anesthetics; therefore, prior to elective surgery, DESYREL should be discontinued for as long as clinically feasible.

Information for Patients: Because priapism has been reported to occur in patients receiving DESYREL, patients with prolonged or inappropriate penile erection should immediately discontinue the drug and consult with the physician.

Antidepressants may impair the mental and/or physical abilities required for the performance of potentially hazardous tasks, such as operating an automobile or machinery; the patient should be cautioned accordingly.

DESYREL may enhance the response to alcohol, barbiturates, and other CNS depressants.

DESYREL should be given shortly after a meal or light snack. Within any individual patient, total drug absorption may be up to 20% higher when the drug is taken with food rather than on an empty stomach. The risk of dizziness/lightheadedness may increase under fasting conditions.

Laboratory Tests: Occasional low white blood cell and neutrophil counts have been noted in patients receiving DESYREL. These were not considered clinically significant and did not necessitate discontinuation of the drug; however, the drug should be discontinued in any patient whose white blood cell count or absolute neutrophil count falls below normal levels. White blood cell and differential counts are recommended for patients who develop fever and sore throat (or other signs of infection) during therapy.

Drug Interactions: Increased serum digoxin or phenytoin levels have been reported to occur in patients receiving DESYREL concurrently with either of those two drugs.

It is not known whether interactions will occur between monoamine oxidase (MAO) inhibitors and DESYREL. Due to the absence of clinical experience, if MAO inhibitors are discontinued shortly before or are to be given concomitantly with DESYREL, therapy should be initiated cautiously with gradual increase in dosage until optimum response is achieved.

Therapeutic Interactions: Concurrent administration with electroshock therapy should be avoided because of the absence of experience in this area.

Carcinogenesis, Mutagenesis, Impairment of Fertility: No drug- or dose-related occurrence of carcinogenesis was evident in rats receiving DESYREL in daily oral doses up to 300 mg/kg for 18 months.

Pregnancy Category C: DESYREL has been shown to cause increased fetal resorption and other adverse effects on the fetus in two studies using the rat when given at dose levels approximately 30–50 times the proposed maximum human dose. There was also an increase in congenital anomalies in one of three rabbit studies at approximately 15–50 times the maximum human dose. There are no adequate and well-controlled studies in pregnant women. DESYREL should be used during pregnancy only if the potential benefit justifies the potential risk to the fetus.

Nursing Mothers: DESYREL and/or its metabolites have been found in the milk of lactating rats, suggesting that the drug may be secreted in human milk. Caution should be exercised when DESYREL is administered to a nursing woman.

Pediatric Use: Safety and effectiveness in children below the age of 18 have not been established.

Adverse Reactions: Because the frequency of adverse drug effects is affected by diverse factors (e.g., drug dose, method of detection, physician judgment, disease under treatment, etc.) a single meaningful estimate of adverse event incidence is difficult to obtain. This problem is illustrated by the variation in adverse event incidence observed and reported from the inpatients and outpatients treated with DESYREL. It is impossible to determine precisely what accounts for the differences observed.

Clinical Trial Reports: The table below is presented solely to indicate the relative frequency of adverse events reported in representative controlled clinical studies conducted to evaluate the safety and efficacy of DESYREL.
[See table on next page].

The figures cited cannot be used to predict precisely the incidence of untoward events in the course of usual medical practice where patient characteristics and other factors often differ from those which prevailed in the clinical trials. These incidence figures, also, cannot be compared with those obtained from other clinical studies involving related drug products and placebo as each group of drug trials is conducted under a different set of conditions.

Occasional sinus bradycardia has occurred in long-term studies.

Continued on next page

Mead Johnson Pharm.—Cont.

In addition to the relatively common (i.e., greater than 1%) untoward events enumerated above, the following adverse events have been reported to occur in association with the use of DESYREL in the controlled clinical studies: akathisia, allergic reaction, anemia, chest pain, delayed urine flow, early menses, flatulence, hallucinations/delusions, hematuria, hypersalivation, hypomania, impaired speech, impotence, increased appetite, increased libido, increased urinary frequency, missed periods, muscle twitches, numbness, and retrograde ejaculation.

Post Introduction Reports: Voluntary reports received since market introduction include the following: agitation, apnea, diplopia, edema, grand mal seizures, hallucinations, hemolytic anemia, liver enzyme alterations, methemoglobinemia, nausea/vomiting (most frequently), paresthesia, priapism (see PRECAUTIONS, Information for Patients; some patients have required surgical intervention), rash, and weakness.

Cardiovascular system effects which have been reported are the following: Orthostatic hypotension and syncope, palpitations, bradycardia, atrial fibrillation, myocardial infarction, cardiac arrest, arrhythmia, and ventricular ectopic activity, including ventricular tachycardia (see WARNINGS).

Overdose:
Animal Oral LD$_{50}$
The oral LD$_{50}$ of the drug is 610 mg/kg in mice, 486 mg/kg in rats, and 560 mg/kg in rabbits.

Signs and Symptoms: Death from overdose has occurred in patients ingesting DESYREL and other drugs concurrently (namely, alcohol; alcohol + chloral hydrate + diazepam; amobarbital, chlordiazepoxide; or meprobamate).

The most severe reactions reported to have occurred with overdose of DESYREL alone have been priapism, respiratory arrest, seizures, and EKG changes. The reactions reported most frequently have been drowsiness and vomiting. Overdosage may cause an increase in incidence or severity of any of the reported adverse reactions (see ADVERSE REACTIONS).

Treatment: There is no specific antidote for DESYREL. Treatment should be symptomatic and supportive in the case of hypotension or excessive sedation. Any patient suspected of having taken an overdose should have the stomach emptied by gastric lavage. Forced diuresis may be useful in facilitating elimination of the drug.

Dosage and Administration: The dosage should be initiated at a low level and increased gradually, noting the clinical response and any evidence of intolerance. Occurrence of drowsiness may require the administration of a major portion of the daily dose at bedtime or a reduction of dosage. DESYREL should be taken shortly after a meal or light snack. Symptomatic relief may be seen during the first week, with optimal antidepressant effects typically evident within two weeks. Twenty-five percent of those who respond to DESYREL require more than two weeks (up to four weeks) of drug administration.

Usual Adult Dosage: An initial dose of 150 mg/day in divided doses is suggested. The dose may be increased by 50 mg/day every three to four days. The maximum dose for outpatients usually should not exceed 400 mg/day in divided doses. Inpatients (i.e. more severely depressed patients) may be given up to but not in excess of 600 mg/day in divided doses.

Maintenance: Dosage during prolonged maintenance therapy should be kept at the lowest effective level. Once an adequate response has been achieved, dosage may be gradually reduced, with subsequent adjustment depending on therapeutic response.

How Supplied: DESYREL® (trazodone hydrochloride)
Tablets, 50 mg—round, orange/scored, film-sealed (imprinted with MJ logo)
NDC 0087-0775-41   Bottles of 100
NDC 0087-0775-43   Bottles of 1000
NDC 0087-0775-42   Cartons of 100 Unit Doses
Tablets, 100 mg—round, white/scored, film-sealed (imprinted with MJ logo)
NDC 0087-0776-41   Bottles of 100
NDC 0087-0776-43   Bottles of 1000
NDC 0087-0776-42   Cartons of 100 Unit Doses
Store at room temperature. Protect from temperatures above 104°F (40°C).
Dispense in tight, light-resistant container (USP).

References:
a. Williams JBW, Ed: Diagnostic and Statistical Manual of Mental Disorders-III, American Psychiatric Association, May, 1980.
U.S. Pat. No. 3,381,009
Shown in Product Identification Section, page 419

Treatment Emergent Symptom Incidence

	Inpts. D	Inpts. P	Outpts. D	Outpts. P
Number of Patients	142	95	157	158
% of Patients Reporting				
Allergic				
Skin Condition/Edema	2.8	1.1	7.0	1.3
Autonomic				
Blurred Vision	6.3	4.2	14.7	3.8
Constipation	7.0	4.2	7.6	5.7
Dry Mouth	14.8	8.4	33.8	20.3
Cardiovascular				
Hypertension	2.1	1.1	1.3	*
Hypotension	7.0	1.1	3.8	0.0
Shortness of Breath	*	1.1	1.3	0.0
Syncope	2.8	2.1	4.5	1.3
Tachycardia/Palpitations	0.0	0.0	7.0	7.0
CNS				
Anger/Hostility	3.5	6.3	1.3	2.5
Confusion	4.9	0.0	5.7	7.6
Decreased Concentration	2.8	2.1	1.3	0.0
Disorientation	2.1	0.0	*	0.0
Dizziness/Lightheadedness	19.7	5.3	28.0	15.2
Drowsiness	23.9	6.3	40.8	19.6
Excitement	1.4	1.1	5.1	5.7
Fatigue	11.3	4.2	5.7	2.5
Headache	9.9	5.3	19.8	15.8
Insomnia	9.9	10.5	6.4	12.0
Impaired Memory	1.4	0.0	*	*
Nervousness	14.8	10.5	6.4	8.2
Gastrointestinal				
Abdominal/Gastric Disorder	3.5	4.2	5.7	4.4
Bad Taste in Mouth	1.4	0.0	0.0	0.0
Diarrhea	0.0	1.1	4.5	1.9
Nausea/Vomiting	9.9	1.1	12.7	9.5
Musculoskeletal				
Musculoskeletal Aches/Pains	5.6	3.2	5.1	2.5
Neurological				
Incoordination	4.9	0.0	1.9	0.0
Paresthesia	1.4	0.0	0.0	*
Tremors	2.8	1.1	5.1	3.8
Sexual Function				
Decreased Libido	*	1.1	1.3	*
Other				
Decreased Appetite	3.5	5.3	0.0	*
Eyes Red/Tired/Itching	2.8	0.0	0.0	0.0
Head Full-Heavy	2.8	0.0	0.0	0.0
Malaise	2.8	0.0	0.0	0.0
Nasal/Sinus Congestion	2.8	0.0	5.7	3.2
Nightmares/Vivid Dreams	*	1.1	5.1	5.7
Sweating/Clamminess	1.4	1.1	*	*
Tinnitus	1.4	0.0	0.0	*
Weight Gain	1.4	0.0	4.5	1.9
Weight Loss	*	3.2	5.7	2.5

*Incidence less than 1%.

D = DESYREL   P = Placebo

DURICEF® ℞
[dur' ĭ-sef]
(Cefadroxil)

Description: DURICEF® (cefadroxil) is a semi-synthetic cephalosporin antibiotic intended for oral administration. It is a white to yellowish-white crystalline powder. It is soluble in water and it is acid-stable. It is chemically designated as 7-[[D-2-amino-2-(4-hydroxyphenyl) acetyl] amino]-3-methyl-8-oxo -5- thia-1-azabicyclo [4.2.0] oct-2- ene-2-carboxylic acid monohydrate. It has the following structural formula:

Clinical Pharmacology—DURICEF (cefadroxil) is rapidly absorbed after oral administration. Following single doses of 500 and 1000 mg., average peak serum concentrations were approximately 16 and 28 mcg./ml., respectively. Measurable levels were present 12 hours after administration. Over 90 percent of the drug is excreted unchanged in the urine within twenty-four hours. Peak urine concentrations are approximately 1800 mcg./ml. during the period following a single 500 mg. oral dose. Increases in dosage generally produce a proportionate increase in DURICEF urinary concentration. The urine antibiotic concentration, following a 1 gm. dose, was maintained well above the MIC of susceptible urinary pathogens for 20 to 22 hours.

Microbiology: *In vitro* tests demonstrate that the cephalosporins are bactericidal because of their inhibition of cell-wall synthesis. DURICEF is active against the following organisms *in vitro*:

Beta-hemolytic streptococci
Staphylococci, including coagulase-positive, coagulase-negative, and penicillinase-producing strains
Streptococcus (Diplococcus) pneumoniae
Escherichia coli.
Proteus mirabilis
Klebsiella species

Note:—Most strains of *Enterococci (Streptococcus faecalis* and *S. faecium)* are resistant to DURICEF. It is not active against most strains of *Enterobacter* species, *P. morganii,* and *P. vulgaris,* It has no activity against *Pseudomonas* sp. and *Acinetobacter calcoaceticus* (formerly *Mima* and *Herellea* sp.)

Disc Susceptibility Tests.—Quantitative methods that require measurement of zone diameters give the most precise estimates of antibiotic susceptibility. One recommended procedure (CFR Section 460.1) uses cephalosporin class disc for testing susceptibility; interpretations correlate zone diameters of this disc test with MIC values for DURICEF. With this procedure, a report from the laboratory of "resistant" indicates that the infecting organism is not likely to respond to therapy. A report of "intermediate susceptibility" suggests that the organism would be susceptible if the infection is confined to the urinary tract, as DURICEF produces high antibiotic levels in the urine.

Indications: DURICEF (cefadroxil) is indicated for the treatment of the following infections when caused by susceptible strains of the designated microorganisms:

Urinary tract infections caused by *E. coli, P. mirabilis,* and *Klebsiella* species

Skin and skin structure infections caused by staphylococci and/or streptococci

Pharyngitis and tonsillitis caused by Group A beta-hemolytic streptococci (Penicillin is the usual drug of choice in the treatment and prevention of streptococcal infections, including the prophylaxis of rheumatic fever. DURICEF is generally effective in the eradication of streptococci from the nasopharynx; however substantial data establishing the efficacy of DURICEF in the subsequent prevention of rheumatic fever are not available at present.)

Note: Culture and susceptibility tests should be initiated prior to and during therapy. Renal function studies should be performed when indicated.

Contraindications: DURICEF (cefadroxil) is contraindicated in patients with known allergy to the cephalosporin group of antibiotics.

WARNING: IN PENICILLIN-ALLERGIC PATIENTS, CEPHALOSPORIN ANTIBIOTICS SHOULD BE USED WITH GREAT CAUTION. THERE IS CLINICAL AND LABORATORY EVIDENCE OF PARTIAL CROSS-ALLERGENICITY OF THE PENICILLINS AND THE CEPHALOSPORINS, AND THERE ARE INSTANCES OF PATIENTS WHO HAVE HAD REACTIONS TO BOTH DRUGS (INCLUDING FATAL ANAPHYLAXIS AFTER PARENTERAL USE).

Any patient who has demonstrated a history of some form of allergy, particularly to drugs, should receive antibiotics cautiously and then only when absolutely necessary. No exception should be made with regard to DURICEF (cefadroxil).

Pseudomembranous colitis has been reported with the use of cephalosporins (and other broad spectrum antibiotics); therefore, it is important to consider its diagnosis in patients who develop diarrhea in association with antibiotic use.

Treatment with broad spectrum antibiotics alters normal flora of the colon and may permit overgrowth of clostridia. Studies indicate a toxin produced by *Clostridium difficile* is one primary cause of antibiotic-associated colitis. Cholestyramine and colestipol resins have been shown to bind the toxin *in vitro*.

Duricef Suspension

Child's Weight				
lbs	kg	125 mg/5 ml	250 mg/5 ml	500 mg/5 ml
10	4.5	½ tsp b.i.d.		
20	9.1	1 tsp b.i.d.	½ tsp b.i.d.	
30	13.6	1½ tsp b.i.d.	¾ tsp b.i.d.	
40	18.2	2 tsp b.i.d.	1 tsp b.i.d.	½ tsp b.i.d.
50	22.7	2½ tsp b.i.d.	1¼ tsp b.i.d.	¾ tsp b.i.d.

Mild cases of colitis may respond to drug discontinuance alone.

Moderate to severe cases should be managed with fluid, electrolyte and protein supplementation as indicated.

When the colitis is not relieved by drug discontinuance or when it is severe, oral vancomycin is the treatment of choice for antibiotic-associated pseudomembranous colitis produced by *C. difficile*. Other causes of colitis should also be considered.

Precautions: Patients should be followed carefully so that any side-effects or unusual manifestations of drug idiosyncrasy may be detected. If a hypersensitivity reaction occurs, the drug should be discontinued and the patient treated with the usual agents (e.g., epinephrine or other pressor amines, antihistamines, or corticosteroids).

DURICEF (cefadroxil) should be used with caution in the presence of markedly impaired renal function (creatinine clearance rate of less than 50 ml/min/1.73 M^2). (See Dosage and Administration.) In patients with known or suspected renal impairment, careful clinical observation and appropriate laboratory studies should be made prior to and during therapy.

Prolonged use of DURICEF may result in the overgrowth of nonsusceptible organisms. Careful observation of the patient is essential. If superinfection occurs during therapy, appropriate measures should be taken.

Positive direct Coombs tests have been reported during treatment with the cephalosporin antibiotics. In hematologic studies or in transfusion cross-matching procedures when antiglobulin tests are performed on the minor side or in Coombs testing of newborns whose mothers have received cephalosporin antibiotics before parturition, it should be recognized that a positive Coombs test may be due to the drug.

DURICEF should be prescribed with caution in individuals with a history of gastrointestinal disease, particularly colitis.

Usage in Pregnancy: Pregnancy Category B: Reproduction studies have been performed in mice and rats at doses up to 11 times the human dose and have revealed no evidence of impaired fertility or harm to the fetus due to cefadroxil. There are, however, no adequate and well controlled studies in pregnant women. Because animal reproduction studies are not always predictive of human response, this drug should be used during pregnancy only if clearly needed.

Nursing Mothers: Caution should be exercised when cefadroxil is administered to a nursing mother.

Adverse Reactions: Gastrointestinal—Symptoms of pseudomembranous colitis can appear during antibiotic treatment. Nausea and vomiting have been reported rarely.

Hypersensitivity—Allergies (in the form of rash, urticaria, and angioedema) have been observed. These reactions usually subsided upon discontinuation of the drug.

Other reactions have included genital pruritus, genital moniliasis, vaginitis, and moderate transient neutropenia.

Dosage and Administration: DURICEF (cefadroxil) is acid stable and may be administered orally without regard to meals. Administration with food may be helpful in diminishing potential gastrointestinal complaints occasionally associated with oral cephalosporin therapy.

Adults—

Urinary Tract Infections

For uncomplicated lower urinary tract infections (i.e. cystitis) the usual dosage is one or two grams per day in single (q.d.) or divided doses (b.i.d.).

For all other urinary tract infections the usual dosage is two grams per day in divided doses (b.i.d.).

Skin and Skin Structure Infections

For skin and skin structure infections the usual dosage is one gram per day in single (q.d.) or divided doses (b.i.d.).

Pharyngitis and Tonsillitis

Treatment of Group A beta hemolytic streptococcal pharyngitis and tonsillitis—One gram per day in divided doses (b.i.d.) for ten days.

Children—

The recommended daily dosage for children is 30 mg/kg/day in divided doses every 12 hours as indicated:

[See table above].

In the treatment of beta-hemolytic streptococcal infections, a therapeutic dosage of Duricef should be administered for at least ten days.

In patients with renal impairment, the dosage of cefadroxil should be adjusted according to creatinine clearance rates to prevent drug accumulation. The following schedule is suggested. In adults, the initial dose is 1000 mg of DURICEF (cefadroxil) and the maintenance dose (based on the creatinine clearance rate [ml/min/1.73M^2]) is 500 mg at the time intervals listed below.

Creatinine Clearances	Dosage Interval
0/10 ml/min	36 hours
10–25 ml/min	24 hours
25–50 ml/min	12 hours

Patients with creatinine clearance rates over 50 ml/min may be treated as if they were patients having normal renal function.

How Supplied:

DURICEF® (cefadroxil) for Oral Suspension
125 mg/5 ml   50 ml size (NDC 0087-0786-42)
                  100 ml size (NDC 0087-0786-41)
250 mg/5 ml   50 ml size (NDC 0087-0782-42)
                  100 ml size (NDC 0087-0782-41)
500 mg/5 ml 100 ml size (NDC 0087-0783-41)

All with orange-pineapple flavor. Directions for mixing are included on the label. Shake well before using. Keep container tightly closed. After mixing, store in refrigerator. Discard unused portion after 14 days.

DURICEF (cefadroxil) capsules, 500 mg, in bottles of 24 (NDC 0087-0784-41), 100 (NDC 0087-0784-42) and in 10 strips of 10 individually labeled blisters each containing 1 capsule (NDC 0087-0784-04).

DURICEF (cefadroxil) tablets, 1 gm, in bottles of 24 (NDC 0087-0785-41), 100 (NDC 0087-0785-42) and in 10 strips of 10 individually labeled blisters each containing 1 tablet (NDC 0087-0785-44).

U.S. Patent Re. 29,164

Shown in Product Identification Section, page 419

KLOTRIX®   ℞
[klō′ trix]
(Potassium Chloride)
Slow-Release Tablets 10 mEq

Description: KLOTRIX is a film-coated (not enteric-coated) tablet containing 750 mg potassium chloride (equivalent to 10 mEq) in a wax matrix. This formulation is intended to provide a controlled release of potassium from the matrix to minimize the likelihood of producing high localized concentrations of potassium within the gastrointestinal tract.

Actions: Potassium ion is the principal intracellular cation of most body tissues. Potassium ions participate in a number of essential physiological

Continued on next page

Mead Johnson Pharm.—Cont.

processes, including the maintenance of intracellular tonicity, the transmission of nerve impulses, the contraction of cardiac, skeletal, and smooth muscle and the maintenance of normal renal function.

Potassium depletion may occur whenever the rate of potassium loss through renal excretion and/or loss from the gastrointestinal tract exceeds the rate of potassium intake. Such depletion usually develops slowly as a consequence of prolonged therapy with oral diuretics, primary or secondary hyperaldosteronism, diabetic ketoacidosis, severe diarrhea, or inadequate replacement of potassium in patients on prolonged parenteral nutrition.

Potassium depletion due to these causes is usually accompanied by a concomitant deficiency of chloride and is manifested by hypokalemia and metabolic alkalosis. Potassium depletion may produce weakness, fatigue, disturbances of cardiac rhythm (primarily ectopic beats), prominent U-waves in the electrocardiogram, and in advanced cases flaccid paralysis and/or impaired ability to concentrate urine.

Potassium depletion associated with metabolic alkalosis is managed by correcting the fundamental causes of the deficiency whenever possible and administering supplemental potassium chloride, in the form of high potassium food or potassium chloride solution or tablets.

In rare circumstances (e.g., patients with renal tubular acidosis) potassium depletion may be associated with metabolic acidosis and hyperchloremia. In such patients potassium replacement should be accomplished with potassium salts other than the chloride, such as potassium bicarbonate, potassium citrate, or potassium acetate.

Indications: BECAUSE OF REPORTS OF INTESTINAL AND GASTRIC ULCERATION AND BLEEDING WITH SLOW RELEASE POTASSIUM CHLORIDE PREPARATIONS, THESE DRUGS SHOULD BE RESERVED FOR THOSE PATIENTS WHO CANNOT TOLERATE OR REFUSE TO TAKE LIQUID OR EFFERVESCENT POTASSIUM PREPARATIONS OR FOR PATIENTS IN WHOM THERE IS A PROBLEM OF COMPLIANCE WITH THESE PREPARATIONS.

1. For therapeutic use in patients with hypokalemia with or without metabolic alkalosis; in digitalis intoxication and in patients with hypokalemic familial periodic paralysis.
2. For prevention of potassium depletion when the dietary intake of potassium is inadequate in the following conditions: Patients receiving digitalis and diuretics for congestive heart failure; hepatic cirrhosis with ascites; states of aldosterone excess with normal renal function; potassium-losing nephropathy, and certain diarrheal states.
3. The use of potassium salts in patients receiving diuretics for uncomplicated essential hypertension is often unnecessary when such patients have a normal dietary pattern. Serum potassium should be checked periodically, however, and, if hypokalemia occurs, dietary supplementation with potassium-containing foods may be adequate to control milder cases. In more severe cases supplementation with potassium salts may be indicated.

Contraindications: Potassium supplements are contraindicated in patients with hyperkalemia since a further increase in serum potassium concentration in such patients can produce cardiac arrest. Hyperkalemia may complicate any of the following conditions: chronic renal failure, systemic acidosis such as diabetic acidosis, acute dehydration, extensive tissue breakdown as in severe burns, adrenal insufficiency, or the administration of a potassium-sparing diuretic (e.g., spironolactone, triamterene).

Wax-matrix potassium chloride preparations have produced esophageal ulceration in certain cardiac patients with esophageal compression due to an enlarged left atrium.

All solid forms of potassium supplements are contraindicated in any patient in whom there is cause for arrest or delay in tablet passage through the gastrointestinal tract. In these instances, potassium supplementation should be with a liquid preparation.

Warnings:
Hyperkalemia
In patients with impaired mechanisms for excreting potassium, the administration of potassium salts can produce hyperkalemia and cardiac arrest. This occurs most commonly in patients given potassium by the intravenous route but may also occur in patients given potassium orally. Potentially fatal hyperkalemia can develop rapidly and be asymptomatic.

The use of potassium salts in patients with chronic renal disease, or any other condition which impairs potassium excretion, requires particularly careful monitoring of the serum potassium concentration and appropriate dosage adjustment.

Interaction with Potassium-Sparing Diuretics
Hypokalemia should not be treated by the concomitant administration of potassium salts and a potassium-sparing diuretic (e.g., spironolactone or triamterene), since the simultaneous administration of these agents can produce severe hyperkalemia.

Gastrointestinal lesions
Potassium chloride tablets have produced stenotic and/or ulcerative lesions of the small bowel and deaths. These lesions are caused by a high localized concentration of potassium ion in the region of a rapidly dissolving tablet, which injures the bowel wall and thereby produces obstruction, hemorrhage, or perforation. Klotrix is a wax-matrix tablet formulated to provide a controlled rate of release of potassium chloride and thus to minimize the possibility of a high local concentration of potassium ion near the bowel wall. While the reported frequency of small-bowel lesions is much less with wax-matrix tablets (less than one per 100,000 patient-years) than with enteric-coated potassium chloride tablets (40–50 per 100,000 patient-years) cases associated with wax-matrix tablets have been reported both in foreign countries and in the United States. In addition, perhaps because the wax-matrix preparations are not enteric-coated and release potassium in the stomach, there have been reports of upper gastrointestinal bleeding associated with these products. The total number of gastrointestinal lesions remains less than one per 100,000 patient-years. Klotrix should be discontinued immediately and the possibility of bowel obstruction or perforation considered if severe vomiting, abdominal pain, distention, or gastrointestinal bleeding occurs.

Metabolic acidosis
Hypokalemia in patients with metabolic acidosis should be treated with an alkalinizing potassium salt such as potassium bicarbonate, potassium citrate, or potassium acetate.

Precautions: The diagnosis of potassium depletion is ordinarily made by demonstrating hypokalemia in a patient with a clinical history suggesting some cause for potassium depletion. In interpreting the serum potassium level, the physician should bear in mind that acute alkalosis *per se* can produce hypokalemia in the absence of a deficit in total body potassium, while acute acidosis *per se* can increase the serum potassium concentration into the normal range even in the presence of a reduced total body potassium. The treatment of potassium depletion, particularly in the presence of cardiac disease, renal disease, or acidosis, requires careful attention to acid-base balance and appropriate monitoring of serum electrolytes, the electrocardiogram, and the clinical status of the patient.

Adverse Reactions: The most common adverse reactions to oral potassium salts are nausea, vomiting, abdominal discomfort, and diarrhea. These symptoms are due to irritation of the gastrointestinal tract and are best managed by diluting the preparation further, taking the dose with meals, or reducing the dose.

One of the most severe adverse effects is hyperkalemia (see Contraindications, Warnings and Overdosage). There also have been reports of upper and lower gastrointestinal conditions including obstruction, bleeding, ulceration and perforation (see Contraindications and Warnings); other factors known to be associated with such conditions were present in many of these patients. Skin rash has been reported rarely.

Overdosage: The administration of oral potassium salts to persons with normal excretory mechanisms for potassium rarely causes serious hyperkalemia. However, if excretory mechanisms are impaired or if potassium is administered too rapidly intravenously, potentially fatal hyperkalemia can result (see Contraindications and Warnings). It is important to recognize that hyperkalemia is usually asymptomatic and may be manifested only by an increased serum potassium concentration and characteristic electrocardiographic changes (peaking of T-waves, loss of P-wave, depression of S-T segment, and prolongation of the QT interval). Late manifestations include muscle paralysis and cardiovascular collapse from cardiac arrest. Treatment measures for hyperkalemia include the following: (1) elimination of foods and medications containing potassium and of potassium-sparing diuretics; (2) intravenous administration of 300 to 500 ml/hr of 10% dextrose solution containing 10–20 units of insulin per 1,000 ml; (3) correction of acidosis, if present, with intravenous sodium bicarbonate; (4) use of exchange resins, hemodialysis, or peritoneal dialysis.

In treating hyperkalemia, it should be recalled that in patients who have been stabilized on digitalis, too rapid a lowering of the serum potassium concentration can produce digitalis toxicity.

Dosage and Administration: The usual dietary intake of potassium by the average adult is 40 to 80 mEq per day. Potassium depletion sufficient to cause hypokalemia usually requires the loss of 200 or more mEq of potassium from the total body store. Dosage must be adjusted to the individual needs of each patient but is typically in the range of 20 mEq per day for the prevention of hypokalemia to 40–100 mEq per day or more for the treatment of potassium depletion.

Note: Klotrix slow-release tablets must be swallowed whole and never crushed or chewed.

Following release of the potassium chloride, the expended wax matrix, which is not absorbed, may be observed in the stool.

How Supplied: Tablets (light orange, film-coated) each containing 750 mg potassium chloride (equivalent to 10 mEq each of potassium and chloride).

NDC 0087-0770-41	Bottles of 100
NDC 0087-0770-42	Bottles of 1000
NDC 0087-0770-43	Unit Dose Cartons of 100
VA6505-01-103-0211B	(1000's)

U.S. Pat. No. 4,140,756
Shown in Product Identification Section, page 419

MUCOMYST® ℞
[*mū'co-mist*]
(Acetylcysteine)

Description: Mucomyst® is a solution of the sodium salt of acetylcysteine, and is used as a mucolytic agent. Acetylcysteine is the N-acetyl derivative of the naturally occurring amino acid, cysteine. The compound is a white crystalline powder with the molecular formula $C_5H_9NO_3S$, a molecular weight of 163.2, and chemical name of N-acetyl-L-cysteine. Acetylcysteine has the following structural formula.

$$\begin{array}{c} HSCH_2CHCOOH \\ | \\ NHCOCH_3 \end{array}$$

Clinical Pharmacology: The viscosity of pulmonary mucous secretions depends on the concentrations of mucoprotein and to a lesser extent deoxyribonucleic acid (DNA). The latter increases with increasing purulence owing to the presence of cellular debris. The mucolytic action of acetylcysteine is related to the sulfhydryl group in the molecule. This group probably "opens" disulfide link-

BRONCHODILATORS				
Isoproterenol HCl[2]		Compatible	3.0%	0.5%
Isoproterenol HCl[2]		Compatible	10%	0.05%
Isoproterenol HCl[2]		Compatible	20%	0.05%
Isoproterenol HCl	Winthrop (Isuprel 1%)	Compatible	13.3% (2 parts)	.33% (1 part)
Aerolone Compound	Lilly	Compatible	13.3% (2 parts)	(1 part)
Bronkosol	Breon	Compatible	13.3% (2 parts)	(1 part)
Epinephrine HCl	Parke, Davis (Adrenalin HCl 1:100)	Compatible	13.3% (2 parts)	.33% (1 part)
CONTRAST MEDIA				
Iodized Oil U.S.P.	Fougera (Lipiodol)	Incompatible	20%/20 ml	40%/10 ml
DECONGESTANTS				
Phenylephrine HCl[2]		Compatible	3.0%	.25%
Phenylephrine HCl	Winthrop (Neo-Synephrine HCl Nasal Solution, 0.5%)	Compatible	13.3% (2 parts)	.17% (1 part)
ENZYMES				
Pancreatic Dornase (mix and use at once)	Merck (Dornavac)	Compatible	16.7%	8,000 U/ml
Chymotrypsin	Armour	Incompatible	5%	400 γ/ml
Trypsin	Armour	Incompatible	5%	400 γ/ml
SOLVENTS				
Alcohol		Compatible	12%	10–20%
Propylene Glycol		Compatible	3%	10%
STEROIDS				
Dexamethasone 21-Phosphate	Merck (Decadron Phosphate)	Compatible	16%	0.8 mg/ml
Prednisolone 21-Phosphate[5]	Merck (Hydeltrasol)	Compatible	16.7%	3.3 mg/ml
OTHER AGENTS				
Hydrogen Peroxide		Incompatible	(All ratios)	
Sodium Bicarbonate, U.S.P.		Compatible	20% (1 part)	4.2% (1 part)

ages in mucus thereby lowering the viscosity. The mucolytic activity of acetylcysteine is unaltered by the presence of DNA, and increases with increasing pH. Significant mucolysis occurs between pH 7 and 9.

Acetylcysteine undergoes rapid deacetylation *in vivo* to yield cysteine or oxidation to yield diacetylcystine.

Occasionally, patients exposed to the inhalation of an acetylcysteine aerosol respond with the development of increased airways obstruction of varying and unpredictable severity. Those patients who are reactors cannot be identified *a priori* from a random patient population. Even when patients are known to have reacted previously to the inhalation of an acetylcysteine aerosol, they may not react during a subsequent treatment. The converse is also true; patients who have had inhalation treatments of acetylcysteine without incident may still react to a subsequent inhalation with increased airways obstruction. Most patients with bronchospasm are quickly relieved by the use of a bronchodilator given by nebulization. If bronchospasm progresses, the medication should be discontinued immediately.

Indications and Usage: Mucomyst is indicated as adjuvant therapy for patients with abnormal, viscid, or inspissated mucous secretions in such conditions as:

Chronic bronchopulmonary disease (chronic emphysema, emphysema with bronchitis, chronic asthmatic bronchitis, tuberculosis, bronchiectasis and primary amyloidosis of the lung)
Acute bronchopulmonary disease (pneumonia, bronchitis, tracheobronchitis)
Pulmonary complications of cystic fibrosis
Tracheostomy care
Pulmonary complications associated with surgery
Use during anesthesia
Post-traumatic chest conditions
Atelectasis due to mucous obstruction
Diagnostic bronchial studies (bronchograms, bronchospirometry, and bronchial wedge catheterization)

Contraindications: Mucomyst is contraindicated in those patients who are sensitive to it.

Warnings: After proper administration of Mucomyst, an increased volume of liquefied bronchial secretions may occur. When cough is inadequate, the airway must be maintained open by mechanical suction if necessary. When there is a mechanical block due to foreign body or local accumulation, the airway should be cleared by endotracheal aspiration, with or without bronchoscopy. Asthmatics under treatment with Mucomyst should be watched carefully. Most patients with bronchospasm are quickly relieved by the use of a bronchodilator given by nebulization. If bronchospasm progresses, the medication should be discontinued immediately.

Precautions: With the administration of Mucomyst, the patient may observe initially a slight disagreeable odor that is soon not noticeable. With a face mask there may be stickiness on the face after nebulization. This is easily removed by washing with water.

Under certain conditions, a color change may occur in Mucomyst in the opened bottle. The light purple color is the result of a chemical reaction which does not significantly affect safety or mucolytic effectiveness of Mucomyst.

Continued nebulization of Mucomyst solution with a dry gas will result in an increased concentration of the drug in the nebulizer because of evaporation of the solvent. Extreme concentration may impede nebulization and efficient delivery of the drug. Dilution of the nebulizing solution with appropriate amounts of Sterile Water for Injection, USP, as concentration occurs, will obviate this problem. (See table above)

Usage in Pregnancy: Pregnancy Category B. Reproduction studies have been performed in rats and rabbits at doses up to 17 times the human dose and have revealed no evidence of impaired fertility or harm to the fetus due to acetylcysteine. There are, however, no adequate and well-controlled studies in pregnant women. Because animal reproduction studies may not always be predictive of human responses, this drug should be used during pregnancy only if clearly needed.

Nursing Mothers
It is not known whether this drug is excreted in human milk. Because many drugs are excreted in human milk, caution should be exercised when Mucomyst is administered to a nursing woman.

Adverse Reactions: Adverse effects have included stomatitis, nausea, vomiting, fever, rhinorrhea, drowsiness, clamminess, chest tightness, and bronchoconstriction. Clinically overt acetylcysteine induced bronchospasm occurs infrequently and unpredictably even in patients with asthmatic bronchitis or bronchitis complicating bronchial asthma. Acquired sensitization to acetylcysteine has been reported rarely. Reports of sensitization in patients have not been confirmed by patch testing. Sensitization has been confirmed in several inhalation therapists who reported a history of dermal eruptions after frequent and extended exposure to acetylcysteine. Reports of irritation to the tracheal and bronchial tracts have been received and although hemoptysis has occurred in patients receiving acetylcysteine such findings are not uncommon in patients with bronchopulmonary disease and a causal relationship has not been established.

Dosage and Administration: Adults and Children: Mucomyst is available in plastic stoppered glass vials containing 4, 10, or 30 ml. The 20% solution may be diluted to a lesser concentration with either Sodium Chloride for Injection, USP, Sodium Chloride for Inhalation, USP, Sterile Water for Injection, USP, or Sterile Water for Inhalation, USP. The 10% solution may be used undiluted.

Nebulization—face mask, mouth piece, tracheostomy:
When nebulized into a face mask, mouth piece, or tracheostomy, 1 to 10 ml of the 20% solution or 2 to 20 ml of the 10% solution may be given every 2 to 6 hours; the recommended doses for most patients is 3 to 5 ml of the 20% solution or 6 to 10 ml of the 10% solution 3 to 4 times a day.

Nebulization-tent, Croupette:
In special circumstances it may be necessary to nebulize into a tent or Croupette, and this method of use must be individualized to take into account the available equipment and the patient's particular needs. This form of administration requires

Continued on next page

Mead Johnson Pharm.—Cont.

IN VITRO COMPATIBILITY[1] TESTS OF MUCOMYST

PRODUCT AND/OR AGENTS	MANUFACTURER (TRADEMARK)	COMPATIBILITY RATING	RATIO TESTED[6] ACETYLCYSTEINE	RATIO TESTED[6] PRODUCT OR AGENT
ANESTHETIC, GAS				
Halothane U.S.P.	Ayerst (Halothane)	Compatible	20%	Infinite
Nitrous Oxide U.S.P.	National Cylinder Gas Company	Compatible	20%	Infinite
ANESTHETIC LOCAL				
Cocaine HCl	Merck	Compatible	10%	5%
Lidocaine HCl	Astra (Xylocaine HCl)	Compatible	10%	2%
Tetracaine HCl	Winthrop (Pontocaine HCl)	Compatible	10%	1%
ANTIBACTERIALS (A parenteral form of each antibiotic was used)				
Bacitracin[2,3] (mix and use at once)	Upjohn	Compatible	10%	5,000 U/ml
Cephaloridine[2,4]	Lilly (Loridine)	Compatible	10%	46 mg/ml
Chloramphenicol Sodium Succinate	Parke, Davis (Chloromycetin)	Compatible	20%	20 mg/ml
Disodium Carbenicillin[2] (mix and use at once)	Roerig (Geopen)	Compatible	10%	125 mg/ml
Gentamicin Sulfate[2]	Schering (Garamycin)	Compatible	10%	20 mg/ml
Kanamycin Sulfate[2] (mix and use at once)	Bristol (Kantrex)	Compatible	10%	167 mg/ml
		Compatible	17%	85 mg/ml
Lincomycin HCl[2]	Upjohn (Lincocin)	Compatible	10%	150 mg/ml
Neomycin Sulfate[2]	Upjohn (Mycifradin Sulfate)	Compatible	10%	100 mg/ml
Novobiocin Sodium[2]	Upjohn (Albamycin)	Compatible	10%	25 mg/ml
Penicillin G Potassium[2] (mix and use at once)	Lilly (Buffered Potassium Penicillin G)	Compatible	10%	25,000 U/ml
Polymyxin B Sulfate[2]	Burroughs Wellcome (Aerosporin)	Compatible	10%	100,000 U/ml
Rolitetracycline[2] (mix and use at once)	Bristol (Syntetrin-IM)	Compatible	10%	50,000 U/ml
Sodium Cephalothin	Lilly (Keflin)	Compatible	10%	87.5 mg/ml
Sodium Colistimethate[2] (mix and use at once)	Warner-Chilcott (Coly-Mycin M)	Compatible	10%	110 mg/ml
Vancomycin HCl[2]	Lilly (Vancocin HCl)	Compatible	10%	37.5 mg/ml
Amphotericin B	Squibb (Fungizone Intravenous)	Incompatible	4–15%	25 mg/ml
Chlortetracycline HCl[2]	Lederle (Aureomycin HCl)	Incompatible	10%	1.0–4.0 mg/ml
Erythromycin Lactobionate	Abbott (Erythrocin Lactobionate-IV)	Incompatible	10%	12.5 mg/ml
Oxytetracycline HCl	Pfizer (Terramycin IV)	Incompatible	10%	15 mg/ml
Sodium Ampicillin	Bristol (Polycillin-N)	Incompatible	10%	12.5 mg/ml
Tetracycline HCl	Lederle (Achromycin)	Incompatible	10%	50 mg/ml
				12.5 mg/ml

[1]The rating, **Incompatible**, is based on the formation of a precipitate, a change in clarity, immiscibility, or a rapid loss of potency of acetylcysteine or the active ingredient of the PRODUCT AND/OR AGENT in the admixture.

The rating **Compatible**, means that there was no significant physical change in the admixture when compared with a control solution of the PRODUCT AND/OR AGENT, and that there was no predicted chemical incompatibility. All of the admixtures have been tested for short-term chemical compatibility by assaying for the concentration of acetylcysteine after mixing.

[2]The active ingredient in the PRODUCT AND/OR AGENT was also assayed after mixing. Some of the admixtures developed minor physical changes which were considered to be insufficient to rate the admixture **Incompatible**. These are listed in footnotes 3, 4, and 5.

[3]A strong odor developed after storage for 24 hours at room temperature.

[4]The admixture was a slightly darker shade of yellow than a control solution of the PRODUCT AND/OR AGENT.

[5]A light tan color developed after storage for 24 hours at room temperature.

[6]Entries are final concentrations. Values in parentheses relate volumes of Mucomyst® solutions to volumes of test solutions.

very large volumes of the solution, occasionally as much as 300 ml during a single treatment period. If a tent or Croupette must be used, the recommended dose is the volume of Mucomyst (using 10% or 20%) that will maintain a very heavy mist in the tent or Croupette for the desired period. Administration for intermittent or continuous prolonged periods, including overnight, may be desirable.

Direct Instillation:
When used by direct instillation, 1 to 2 ml of a 10 to 20% solution may be given as often as every hour. When used for the routine nursing care of patients with tracheostomy, 1 to 2 ml of a 10 to 20% solution may be given every 1 to 4 hours by instillation into the tracheostomy.

Mucomyst may be introduced directly into a particular segment of the bronchopulmonary tree by inserting (under local anesthesia and direct vision) a small plastic catheter into the trachea. Two to 5 ml of the 20% solution may then be instilled by means of a syringe connected to the catheter.

Mucomyst may also be given through a percutaneous intratracheal catheter. One to 2 ml of the 20% or 2 to 4 ml of the 10% solution every 1 to 4 hours may then be given by a syringe attached to the catheter.

Diagnostic Bronchograms:
For diagnostic bronchial studies, 2 or 3 administrations of 1 to 2 ml of the 20% solution or 2 to 4 ml of the 10% solution should be given by nebulization or by instillation intratracheally, prior to the procedure.

Administration of Aerosol:
Materials:
Mucomyst may be administered using conventional nebulizers made of plastic or glass. Certain materials used in nebulization equipment react with acetylcysteine. The most reactive of these are certain metals (notably iron and copper) and rubber. Where materials may come into contact with Mucomyst solution, parts made of the following acceptable materials should be used: glass, plastic, aluminum, anodized aluminum, chromed metal, tantalum, sterling silver, or stainless steel. Silver may become tarnished after exposure, but this is not harmful to the drug action or the patient.

Nebulizing Gases:
Compressed tank gas (air) or an air compressor should be used to provide pressure for nebulizing the solution. Oxygen may also be used but should be used with the usual precautions in patients with severe respiratory disease and CO_2 retention.

Apparatus
Mucomyst is usually administered as a fine nebula and the nebulizer used should be capable of providing optimal quantities of a suitable range of particle sizes.
Commercially available nebulizers will produce nebulae of Mucomyst satisfactory for retention in the respiratory tract. Most of the nebulizers tested will supply a high proportion of the drug solution as particles of less than 10 micrometers in diameter. Mitchell[a] has shown that particles less than 10 micrometers should be retained in the respiratory tract satisfactorily.
Units that nebulized this solution with satisfactory efficiency were the Maxi-Myst® Nebulizer (Mead Johnson Pharmaceutical Division, Evansville, Indiana), Hand-E-Vent intermittent positive pressure breathing device (Ohio Medical Products, 3030 Airco Drive, Madison, Wisconsin), and various other intermittent positive pressure breathing devices, No. 40 De Vilbiss (The De Vilbiss Co., Somerset, Pennsylvania), Bennett Twin-Jet Nebulizer (Puritan Bennett Corp. Oak at 13th St., Kansas City, Missouri).
The nebulized solution may be inhaled directly from the nebulizer. Nebulizers may also be attached to plastic face masks or plastic mouthpieces. Suitable nebulizers may also be fitted for use with the various intermittent positive pressure breathing (IPPB) machines. The nebulizing equipment should be cleaned immediately after use because the residues may clog the smaller orifices or corrode metal parts.
Hand bulbs are not recommended for routine use for nebulizing Mucomyst because their output is generally too small. Also, some hand-operated nebulizers deliver particles that are larger than optimum for inhalation therapy.
Mucomyst should not be placed directly into the chamber of a heated (hot pot) nebulizer. A heated nebulizer may be part of the nebulization assembly to provide a warm saturated atmosphere if the

Mucomyst aerosol is introduced by means of a separate unheated nebulizer. Usual precautions for administration of warm saturated nebulae should be observed.

The nebulized solution may be breathed directly from the nebulizer. Nebulizers may also be attached to plastic face masks, plastic face tents, plastic mouth pieces, conventional plastic oxygen tents, or head tents. Suitable nebulizers may also be fitted for use with the various intermittent positive pressure breathing (IPPB) machines.

The nebulizing equipment should be cleaned immediately after use, otherwise the residues may occlude the fine orifices or corrode metal parts.

Prolonged Nebulization:
When three-fourths of the initial volume of Mucomyst solution have been nebulized, a quantity of Sterile Water for Injection, USP (approximately equal to the volume of solution remaining) should be added to the nebulizer. This obviates any concentration of the agent in the residual solvent remaining after prolonged nebulization.

Storage of Opened Vials: Mucomyst does not contain an antimicrobial agent and care must be taken to minimize contamination of the sterile solution. If only a portion of the solution in a vial is used, store the remainder in a refrigerator and use within 96 hours.

Storage of Unopened Vials: Store unopened vials at controlled room temperature, 59° to 86°F (15° to 30°C).
[See table on preceding page].

Compatibility: The physical and chemical compatibility of Mucomyst solutions with certain other drugs that might be concomitantly administered by nebulization, direct instillation, or topical application, has been studied.

Mucomyst should not be mixed with certain antibiotics. For example, the antibiotics tetracycline hydrochloride, oxytetracycline hydrochloride, and erythromycin lactobionate were found to be incompatible when mixed in the same solution. These agents may be administered from separate solutions if administration of these agents is desirable.

The supplying of these data should not be interpreted as a recommendation for combining Mucomyst with other drugs. The table is not presented as positive assurance that no incompatibility will be present, since these data are based only on short-term compatibility studies done in the Mead Johnson Research Center. Manufacturers of drug products may change formulations. This could alter compatibilities. These data are intended **to serve only as a guide** for predicting compounding problems.

If it is deemed advisable to prepare an admixture, it should be administered as soon as possible after preparation. Do not store unused mixtures.

How Supplied:
Mucomyst® 20% acetylcysteine solution (200 mg Acetylcysteine per ml). Sterile, Not for injection

NDC 0087-0570-03	Cartons of three 10 ml vials, 1 plastic dropper
VA 6505-00-767-9111A	
6505-00-767-9111	Defense
NDC 0087-0570-09	Cartons of three 30 ml vials
VA 6505-00-782-2688A	
6505-00-782-2688	Defense
NDC 0087-0570-07	Cartons of twelve 4 ml vials

Mucomyst®-10, 10% acetylcysteine solution. (100 mg Acetylcysteine per ml). Sterile, Not for injection

NDC 0087-0572-01	Cartons of three 10 ml vials, 1 plastic dropper
NDC 0087-0572-02	Cartons of three 30 ml vials
NDC 0087-0572-03	Cartons of twelve 4 ml vials

[a]Amer. Rev. Resp. Dis. 82: 627–639, 1960.

PERI–COLACE® capsules • syrup
[peri-kō'lās]
Casanthranol and docusate sodium

Description: Peri-Colace is a combination of the mild stimulant laxative Peristim (casanthranol, Mead Johnson) and the stool-softener Colace (docusate sodium, Mead Johnson). Each capsule contains 30 mg of Peristim and 100 mg of Colace; the syrup contains 30 mg of Peristim and 60 mg of Colace per 15-ml tablespoon (10 mg of Peristim and 20 mg of Colace per 5-ml teaspoon) and 10% alcohol.

Action and Uses: Peri-Colace provides gentle peristaltic stimulation and helps to keep stools soft for easier passage. Bowel movement is induced gently—usually overnight or in 8 to 12 hours. Nausea, griping, abnormally loose stools, and constipation rebound are minimized. Useful in management of chronic or temporary constipation.

Note: To prevent hard stools when laxative stimulation is not needed or undesirable, see Colace (stool softener).

Side Effects: The incidence of side effects—none of a serious nature—is exceedingly small. Nausea, abdominal cramping or discomfort, diarrhea, and rash are the main side effects reported.

Administration and Dosage: *Adults*—1 or 2 capsules, or 1 or 2 tablespoons syrup at bedtime, or as indicated. In severe cases, dosage may be increased to 2 capsules or 2 tablespoons twice daily, or 3 capsules at bedtime. *Children*—1 to 3 teaspoons of syrup at bedtime, or as indicated.

Warnings: Do not use when abdominal pain, nausea, or vomiting are present. Frequent or prolonged use of this preparation may result in dependence on laxatives.

As with any drug, if you are pregnant or nursing a baby, seek the advice of a health professional before using this product.

Overdosage: In addition to symptomatic treatment, gastric lavage, if timely, is recommended in cases of large overdosage.

How Supplied: Peri-Colace® Capsules
NDC 0087-0715-43 Cartons of 10 single unit packs
NDC 0087-0715-01 Bottles of 30
NDC 0087-0715-02 Bottles of 60
NDC 0087-0715-03 Bottles of 250
NDC 0087-0715-05 Bottles of 1000
NDC 0087-0715-07 Cartons of 100 single unit packs

Note: Peri-Colace capsules should be stored at controlled room temperatures (59°–86°F or 15°–30°C).
Peri-Colace® Syrup
NDC 0087-0721-01 Bottles of 8 fl. oz.
NDC 0087-0721-02 Bottles of 16 fl. oz.
Shown in Product Identification Section, page 419

VASODILAN® ℞
[vasō-dī'lăn]
(Isoxsuprine HCl)
tablets • injection

Indications
Based on a review of this drug by the National Academy of Sciences—National Research Council and/or other information, the FDA has classified the indications as follows:
Possibly Effective:
1. For the relief of symptoms associated with cerebral vascular insufficiency.
2. In peripheral vascular disease of arteriosclerosis obliterans, thromboangiitis obliterans (Buerger's Disease) and Raynaud's disease.

Final classification of the less-than-effective indications requires further investigation.

Composition:
Vasodilan tablets, isoxsuprine HCl, 10 mg. and 20 mg.

Vasodilan injection, each ml. contains 5 mg. isoxsuprine hydrochloride and 2.5% Glycerin U.S.P., in Water for Injection U.S.P. pH adjusted with hydrochloric acid or sodium hydroxide.

Dosage and Administration:
Oral: 10 to 20 mg., three or four times daily.
Intramuscular: 5 to 10 mg. (1 to 2 ml.) two or three times daily. Intramuscular administration may be used initially in severe or acute conditions.

Contraindications and Cautions:
Oral
There are no known contraindications to oral use when administered in recommended doses. Should not be given immediately postpartum or in the presence of arterial bleeding.

Parenteral
Parenteral administration is not recommended in the presence of hypotension or tachycardia.
Intravenous administration should not be given because of increased likelihood of side effects.
Should not be given immediately postpartum or in the presence of arterial bleeding.

Adverse Reactions: On rare occasions oral administration of the drug has been associated in time with the occurrence of hypotension, tachycardia, chest pain, nausea, vomiting, dizziness, abdominal distress, and severe rash. If rash appears the drug should be discontinued.

Although available evidence suggests a temporal association of these reactions with isoxsuprine, a causal relationship can be neither confirmed nor refuted.

Single doses of 10 mg intramuscularly may result in transient hypotension and tachycardia. These symptoms are more pronounced in higher doses. For these reasons single intramuscular doses exceeding 10 mg are not recommended. Repeated administration of 5 to 10 mg intramuscularly at suitable intervals may be employed.

β-Adrenergic receptor stimulants such as isoxsuprine hydrochloride have been used to inhibit preterm labor. Maternal and fetal tachycardia may occur under such use. Hypocalcemia, hypoglycemia, hypotension and ileus have been reported to occur in infants whose mothers received isoxsuprine. Pulmonary edema has been reported in mothers treated with β-stimulants. Vasodilan is neither approved nor recommended for use in the treatment of premature labor.

How Supplied: Tablets, 10 mg.
NDC 0087-0543-01 Bottles of 100
NDC 0087-0543-02 Bottles of 1000
NDC 0087-0543-07 Bottles of 5000
NDC 0087-0543-05 Unit Dose
Tablets, 20 mg.
NDC 0087-0544-01 Bottles of 100
NDC 0087-0544-02 Bottles of 500
NDC 0087-0544-06 Bottles of 1000
NDC 0087-0544-47 Bottles of 5000
NDC 0087-0544-03 Unit Dose
Injection, 10 mg. per 2 ml. ampul
NDC 0087-0540-01 Boxes of six 2 ml. ampuls
Shown in Product Identification Section, page 419

IDENTIFICATION PROBLEM?

Consult PDR's

Product Identification Section

where you'll find over 1200

products pictured actual size

and in full color.

Medical Products Panamericana, Inc.
P.O. BOX 771
CORAL GABLES, FL 33134

VG CAPSULES™ ℞

Composition: Each capsule contains: Vitamin C (Ascorbic Acid) 500 mg.; Vitamin B1 (Thiamine) 15 mg.; Vitamin B2 (Riboflavin) 15 mg.; Niacinamide 100 mg.; Vitamin B6 (Pyridoxine) 5 mg.; Vitamin B12 5 mcg.; Calcium Pantothenate 20 mg.; Folic Acid 0.5 mg.; Vitamin E (d-alpha tocopheryl acetate) 30 I.U.; 1-lysine Hydrochloride (need in human nutrition established, but no U.S. RDA established) 25 mg.; Manganese Sulfate 4 mg.; Magnesium Sulfate 35 mg. (equivalent to 25 mg. dried $MgSO_4$); Zinc Sulfate 80 mg. (equivalent to 25 mg. dried $ZnSO_4$).

Indications: Indicated in the treatment of patients with deficiencies of, or increased requirements for Vitamin C and/or B-Complex Vitamins including Folic Acid, Zinc, Magnesium and/or Manganese.

Administration and Dosage: One Capsule Daily or as directed by a physician.

Precautions: Folic Acid may obscure pernicious anemia; the peripheral blood picture may revert to normal while neurological manifestations remain progressive.

Caution: Federal Law prohibits dispensing without prescription.

Supplied: NDC 0576-0506-30 Bottle of 30 Capsules.

Medicone Company
225 VARICK ST.
NEW YORK, NY 10014

DERMA MEDICONE® Ointment
(See PDR For Nonprescription Drugs)

DERMA MEDICONE®-HC Ointment ℞

Composition: Each gram contains:
Hydrocortisone acetate .... 10.0 mg.
Benzocaine .... 19.8 mg.
8-Hydroxyquinoline sulfate .... 10.4 mg.
Ephedrine hydrochloride .... 1.1 mg.
Menthol .... 4.8 mg.
Ichthammol .... 9.9 mg.
Zinc oxide .... 135.8 mg.
Petrolatum, Lanolin, perfume ....

Action and Uses: Offers the advantage of quick, lasting comfort during treatment of severely inflamed dermatoses by affording prompt temporary local anesthetic action, inhibiting pain, burning, itching and controlling the scratch reflex. The hydrocortisone acetate reduces inflammation and swelling, aiding the normal healing process. The non-drying base will not disintegrate or liquefy at body temperature and is not washed off by exudate, perspiration or urine. Effectively suppresses inflammation, pain, swelling, burning and itching in contact dermatitis, eczematoid dermatitis, atopic dermatitis, neurodermatitis, seborrheic dermatitis, allergic dermatitis, rhus dermatitis, pruritus ani and pruritus vulvae.

Administration and Dosage: Apply to affected area 2 to 4 times daily. When adequate improvement is noted, reduce frequency of application or continue maintenance control with regular Derma Medicone ointment.

Precautions: Observe the usual adrenocorticosteroid precautions. Exercise care if the patient is on other corticosteroid therapy or if infection is present or if rash or irritation develops. Do not use in the eyes.

Contraindications: Do not use in the presence of tuberculosis of the skin.

How Supplied: 7 gram and 20 gram tubes.

MEDICONE® DRESSING Cream
(See PDR For Nonprescription Drugs)

MEDICONET®
(medicated rectal wipes)
(See PDR For Nonprescription Drugs)

RECTAL MEDICONE® SUPPOSITORIES
(See PDR For Nonprescription Drugs)

RECTAL MEDICONE®-HC SUPPOSITORIES ℞

Composition: Each suppository contains:
Hydrocortisone acetate .... 10 mg.
Benzocaine .... 2 gr.
8-Hydroxyquinoline sulfate .... ¼ gr.
Zinc oxide .... 3 gr.
Menthol .... ⅐ gr.
Balsam Peru .... 1 gr.
Cocoa butter—vegetable & petroleum
  oil base, Certified color added .... q.s.

Action and Uses: The hydrocortisone acetate reduces and controls severe anorectal inflammation and swelling, effecting better management of the basic condition. Provides prompt, temporary relief from pain, burning and itching. Soothes, lubricates and protects; makes bowel evacuation more comfortable while accelerating the normal healing process. Useful as initial therapy in hemorrhoids, acute and chronic proctitis, post-operative edema, cryptitis, pruritus ani and inflamed post-operative scar tissue.

ANESTHETIC—ANTI-INFLAMMATORY
ANTIPRURITIC—ANTIBACTERIAL

Administration and Dosage: Start therapy with one Rectal Medicone-HC Suppository twice daily for a recommended period of three to six days. Continue maintenance control against recurring symptoms with regular Rectal Medicone Suppositories and/or Unguent as required.

Precautions: A thorough proctologic diagnosis should be made when use of hydrocortisone is considered. Care should be exercised if the patient is on other corticosteroid therapy or if infection is present or if rash or irritation develops.

Contraindications: Do not use in the presence of tuberculosis of the rectum.

How Supplied: Boxes of 12 individually foil-wrapped pink suppositories.
Shown in Product Identification Section, page 420

RECTAL MEDICONE® UNGUENT
(See PDR For Nonprescription Drugs)

Important Notice

Before prescribing or administering
any product described in
PHYSICIANS' DESK REFERENCE
always consult the PDR Supplement for
possible new or revised information

Merck Sharp & Dohme
DIVISION OF MERCK & CO., INC.
WEST POINT, PA 19486
Product Identification Codes

To provide quick and positive identification of Merck Sharp & Dohme products, we have imprinted a code number on tablet and capsule products. In order that you may identify a product by its code number, we have compiled below a numerical list of code numbers with their corresponding product names. We are also listing the code numbers by alphabetical listing of products as a cross reference.

The code number as it appears on tablets and capsules bears the letters MSD plus the numerical code. Decadron® (Dexamethasone, MSD) tablets 0.25 mg is identified MSD 20.

Numerical Listing

MSD Code No.	Product	Product No.
20	Decadron® (Dexamethasone, MSD) Tablets 0.25 mg.	7592
21	Cogentin® (Benztropine Mesylate, MSD) Tablets 0.5 mg.	3297
23	Elavil® (Amitriptyline HCl, MSD) Tablets 10 mg.	3287
25	Indocin® (Indomethacin, MSD) Capsules 25 mg.	3316
26	Vivactil® (Protriptyline HCl, MSD) Tablets 5 mg.	3313
41	Decadron® (Dexamethasone, MSD) Tablets 0.5 mg.	7598
42	HydroDIURIL® (Hydrochlorothiazide, MSD) Tablets 25 mg.	3263
43	Mephyton® (Phytonadione, MSD) Tablets 5 mg.	7776
45	Elavil® (Amitriptyline HCl, MSD) Tablets 25 mg.	3288
47	Vivactil® (Protriptyline HCl, MSD) Tablets 10 mg.	3314
49	Daranide® (Dichlorphenamide, MSD) Tablets 50 mg.	3256
50	Indocin® (Indomethacin, MSD) Capsules 50 mg.	3317
52	Inversine® (Mecamylamine HCl, MSD) Tablets 2.5 mg.	3219
53	Hydropres® 25 (Reserpine-Hydrochlorothiazide, MSD) Tablets	3265
59	Blocadren® (Timolol Maleate, MSD) Tablets 5 mg.	3343
60	Cogentin® (Benztropine Mesylate, MSD) Tablets 2 mg.	3172
62	Periactin® (Cyproheptadine HCl, MSD) Tablets 4 mg.	3276
63	Decadron® (Dexamethasone, MSD) Tablets 0.75 mg.	7601
65	Edecrin® (Ethacrynic Acid, MSD) Tablets 25 mg.	3321
67	Timolide® 10-25 (Timolol Maleate-Hydrochlorothiazide, MSD) Tablets	3373
90	Edecrin® (Ethacrynic Acid, MSD) Tablets 50 mg.	3322
92	Midamor® (Amiloride HCl, MSD) Tablets 5 mg.	3381
95	Decadron® (Dexamethasone, MSD) Tablets 1.5 mg.	7638
97	Decadron® (Dexamethasone, MSD) Tablets 4 mg.	7645
102	Elavil® (Amitriptyline HCl, MSD) Tablets 50 mg.	3320
105	HydroDIURIL® (Hydrochlorothiazide, MSD) Tablets 50 mg.	3264
127	Hydropres® 50 (Reserpine-Hydrochlorothiazide, MSD) Tablets	3266
135	Aldomet® (Methyldopa, MSD) Tablets 125 mg.	3341
136	Blocadren® (Timolol Maleate, MSD) Tablets 10 mg.	3344
147	Decadron® (Dexamethasone, MSD) Tablets 6 mg.	7648
214	Diuril® (Chlorothiazide, MSD) Tablets 250 mg.	3244

Product Information

MSD Code No.	Product	Product No.
219	Cortone® (Cortisone Acetate, MSD) Tablets 25 mg.	7063
230	Diupres 250® Tablets	3261
401	Aldomet® (Methyldopa, MSD) Tablets 250 mg.	3290
403	Urecholine® (Bethanechol Chloride, MSD) Tablets 5 mg.	7785
405	Diupres 500® Tablets	3262
410	HydroDIURIL® (Hydrochlorothiazide, MSD) Tablets 100 mg.	3340
412	Urecholine® (Bethanechol Chloride, MSD) Tablets 10 mg.	7787
423	Aldoril® 15 (Methyldopa-Hydrochlorothiazide, MSD) Tablets	3294
430	Elavil® (Amitriptyline HCl, MSD) Tablets 75 mg.	3348
432	Diuril® (Chlorothiazide, MSD) Tablets 500 mg.	3245
435	Elavil® (Amitriptyline HCl, MSD) Tablets 100 mg.	3349
437	Blocadren® (Timolol Maleate, MSD) Tablets 20 mg.	3371
456	Aldoril® 25 (Methyldopa-Hydrochlorothiazide, MSD) Tablets	3295
457	Urecholine® (Bethanechol Chloride, MSD) Tablets 25 mg.	7788
460	Urecholine® (Bethanechol Chloride, MSD) Tablets 50 mg.	7790
501	Benemid® (Probenecid, MSD) Tablets 0.5 g.	3337
516	Aldomet® (Methyldopa, MSD) Tablets 500 mg.	3292
517	Triavil® 4-50 Tablets	3364
602	Cuprimine® (Penicillamine, MSD) Capsules 250 mg.	3299
612	Aldoclor® 150, Tablets	3318
613	Propadrine® (Phenylpropanolamine HCl, MSD) Capsules 50 mg.	2198
614	ColBENEMID® (Probenecid-Colchicine, MSD) Tablets	3283
619	Hydrocortone® (Hydrocortisone, MSD) Tablets 10 mg.	7604
625	Hydrocortone® (Hydrocortisone, MSD) Tablets 20 mg.	7602
634	Aldoclor® 250, Tablets	3319
635	Cogentin® (Benztropine Mesylate, MSD) Tablets 1 mg.	3334
647	Sinemet® 10-100 (Carbidopa-Levodopa, MSD) Tablets	3346
650	Sinemet® 25-100 (Carbidopa-Levodopa, MSD) Tablets	3365
654	Sinemet® 25-250 (Carbidopa-Levodopa, MSD) Tablets	3347
672	Cuprimine® (Penicillamine, MSD) Capsules 125 mg.	3350
673	Elavil® (Amitriptyline HCl, MSD) Tablets 150 mg.	3351
675	Dolobid® (Diflunisal, MSD) Tablets 250 mg.	3390
690	Demser® (Metyrosine, MSD) Capsules 250 mg.	3355
693	Indocin® SR (Indomethacin, MSD) Capsules 75 mg.	3370
694	Aldoril® D30 (Methyldopa-Hydrochlorothiazide, MSD) Tablets	3362
697	Dolobid® (Diflunisal, MSD) Tablets 500 mg.	3392
707	Tonocard® (Tocainide HCl, MSD) Tablets 400 mg.	3409
709	Tonocard® (Tocainide HCl, MSD) Tablets 600 mg.	3410
907	Mintezol® (Thiabendazole, MSD) Chewable Tablets 500 mg.	3332
914	Triavil® 2-10 Tablets	3328
917	Moduretic® (Amiloride HCl-Hydrochlorothiazide, MSD) Tablets	3385
921	Triavil® 2-25 Tablets	3311
931	Flexeril® (Cyclobenzaprine HCl, MSD) Tablets 10 mg.	3358
934	Triavil® 4-10 Tablets	3310
935	Aldoril® D50 (Methyldopa-Hydrochlorothiazide, MSD) Tablets	3363
941	Clinoril® (Sulindac, MSD) Tablets 150 mg.	3360
942	Clinoril® (Sulindac, MSD) Tablets 200 mg.	3353
946	Triavil® 4-25 Tablets	3312

Alphabetical Listing

MSD Code No.	Product	Product No.
612	Aldoclor® 150, Tablets	3318
634	Aldoclor® 250, Tablets	3319
135	Aldomet® (Methyldopa, MSD) Tablets 125 mg.	3341
401	Aldomet® (Methyldopa, MSD) Tablets 250 mg.	3290
516	Aldomet® (Methyldopa, MSD) Tablets 500 mg.	3292
423	Aldoril® 15 (Methyldopa-Hydrochlorothiazide, MSD) Tablets	3294
456	Aldoril® 25 (Methyldopa-Hydrochlorothiazide, MSD) Tablets	3295
694	Aldoril® D30 (Methyldopa-Hydrochlorothiazide, MSD) Tablets	3362
935	Aldoril® D50 (Methyldopa-Hydrochlorothiazide, MSD) Tablets	3363
501	Benemid® (Probenecid, MSD) Tablets 0.5 g.	3337
59	Blocadren® (Timolol Maleate, MSD) Tablets 5 mg.	3343
136	Blocadren® (Timolol Maleate, MSD) Tablets 10 mg.	3344
437	Blocadren® (Timolol Maleate, MSD) Tablets 20 mg.	3371
941	Clinoril® (Sulindac, MSD) Tablets 150 mg.	3360
942	Clinoril® (Sulindac, MSD) Tablets 200 mg.	3353
21	Cogentin® (Benztropine Mesylate, MSD) Tablets 0.5 mg.	3297
635	Cogentin® (Benztropine Mesylate, MSD) Tablets 1 mg.	3334
60	Cogentin® (Benztropine Mesylate, MSD) Tablets 2 mg.	3172
614	ColBENEMID® (Probenecid-Colchicine, MSD) Tablets	3283
219	Cortone® (Cortisone Acetate, MSD) Tablets 25 mg.	7063
672	Cuprimine® (Penicillamine, MSD) Capsules 125 mg.	3350
602	Cuprimine® (Penicillamine, MSD) Capsules 250 mg.	3299
49	Daranide® (Dichlorphenamide, MSD) Tablets 50 mg.	3256
20	Decadron® (Dexamethasone, MSD) Tablets 0.25 mg.	7592
41	Decadron® (Dexamethasone, MSD) Tablets 0.5 mg.	7598
63	Decadron® (Dexamethasone, MSD) Tablets 0.75 mg.	7601
95	Decadron® (Dexamethasone, MSD) Tablets 1.5 mg.	7638
97	Decadron® (Dexamethasone, MSD) Tablets 4 mg.	7645
147	Decadron® (Dexamethasone, MSD) Tablets 6 mg.	7648
690	Demser® (Metyrosine, MSD) Capsules 250 mg.	3355
230	Diupres 250® Tablets	3261
405	Diupres 500® Tablets	3262
214	Diuril® (Chlorothiazide, MSD) Tablets 250 mg.	3244
432	Diuril® (Chlorothiazide, MSD) Tablets 500 mg.	3245
675	Dolobid® (Diflunisal, MSD) Tablets 250 mg.	3390
697	Dolobid® (Diflunisal, MSD) Tablets 500 mg.	3392
65	Edecrin® (Ethacrynic Acid, MSD) Tablets 25 mg.	3321
90	Edecrin® (Ethacrynic Acid, MSD) Tablets 50 mg.	3322
23	Elavil® (Amitriptyline HCl, MSD) Tablets 10 mg.	3287
45	Elavil® (Amitriptyline HCl, MSD) Tablets 25 mg.	3288
102	Elavil® (Amitriptyline HCl, MSD) Tablets 50 mg.	3320
430	Elavil® (Amitriptyline HCl, MSD) Tablets 75 mg.	3348
435	Elavil® (Amitriptyline HCl, MSD) Tablets 100 mg.	3349
673	Elavil® (Amitriptyline HCl, MSD) Tablets 150 mg.	3351
931	Flexeril® (Cyclobenzaprine HCl, MSD) Tablets 10 mg.	3358
619	Hydrocortone® (Hydrocortisone, MSD) Tablets 10 mg.	7604
625	Hydrocortone® (Hydrocortisone, MSD) Tablets 20 mg.	7602
42	HydroDIURIL® (Hydrochlorothiazide, MSD) Tablets 25 mg.	3263
105	HydroDIURIL® (Hydrochlorothiazide, MSD) Tablets 50 mg.	3264
410	HydroDIURIL® (Hydrochlorothiazide, MSD) Tablets 100 mg.	3340
53	Hydropres® 25 (Reserpine-Hydrochlorothiazide, MSD) Tablets	3265
127	Hydropres® 50 (Reserpine-Hydrochlorothiazide, MSD) Tablets	3266
25	Indocin® (Indomethacin, MSD) Capsules 25 mg.	3316
50	Indocin® (Indomethacin, MSD) Capsules 50 mg.	3317
693	Indocin® SR (Indomethacin, MSD) Capsules 75 mg.	3370
52	Inversine® (Mecamylamine HCl, MSD) Tablets 2.5 mg.	3219
43	Mephyton® (Phytonadione, MSD) Tablets 5 mg.	7776
92	Midamor® (Amiloride HCl, MSD) Tablets 5 mg.	3381
907	Mintezol® (Thiabendazole, MSD) Chewable Tablets 500 mg.	3332
917	Moduretic® (Amiloride HCl-Hydrochlorothiazide, MSD) Tablets	3385
62	Periactin® (Cyproheptadine HCl, MSD) Tablets 4 mg.	3276
613	Propadrine® (Phenylpropanolamine HCl, MSD) Capsules 50 mg.	2198
647	Sinemet® 10-100 (Carbidopa-Levodopa, MSD) Tablets	3346
650	Sinemet® 25-100 (Carbidopa-Levodopa, MSD) Tablets	3365
654	Sinemet® 25-250 (Carbidopa-Levodopa, MSD) Tablets	3347
67	Timolide® 10-25 (Timolol Maleate-Hydrochlorothiazide, MSD) Tablets	3373
707	Tonocard® (Tocainide HCl, MSD) Tablets 400 mg.	3409
709	Tonocard® (Tocainide HCl, MSD) Tablets 600 mg.	3410
914	Triavil® 2-10 Tablets	3328
921	Triavil® 2-25 Tablets	3311
934	Triavil® 4-10 Tablets	3310
946	Triavil® 4-25 Tablets	3312
517	Triavil® 4-50 Tablets	3364
403	Urecholine® (Bethanechol Chloride, MSD) Tablets 5 mg.	7785
412	Urecholine® (Bethanechol Chloride, MSD) Tablets 10 mg.	7787
457	Urecholine® (Bethanechol Chloride, MSD) Tablets 25 mg.	7788
460	Urecholine® (Bethanechol Chloride, MSD) Tablets 50 mg.	7790
26	Vivactil® (Protriptyline HCl, MSD) Tablets 5 mg.	3313
47	Vivactil® (Protriptyline HCl, MSD) Tablets 10 mg.	3314

Continued on next page

Information on the Merck Sharp & Dohme products listed on these pages is the full prescribing information from product circulars in use November 1, 1984.

Merck Sharp & Dohme—Cont.

ALDOCLOR® Tablets ℞
Antihypertensive

> **WARNING**
>
> This fixed combination drug is not indicated for initial therapy of hypertension. Hypertension requires therapy titrated to the individual patient. If the fixed combination represents the dosage so determined, its use may be more convenient in patient management. The treatment of hypertension is not static, but must be reevaluated as conditions in each patient warrant.

Description

ALDOCLOR® is a combination of methyldopa and chlorothiazide. The chemical name for methyldopa is levo-3-(3,4-dihydroxyphenyl)-2-methylalanine. Chlorothiazide is 6-chloro-$2H$-1, 2, 4-benzothiadiazine-7-sulfonamide 1, 1-dioxide.

Actions

ALDOMET® (Methyldopa, MSD)
Methyldopa, a unique antihypertensive, is an aromatic-amino-acid decarboxylase inhibitor in animals and in man. Although the mechanism of action has yet to be conclusively demonstrated, the antihypertensive effect of methyldopa probably is due to its metabolism to alpha-methylnorepinephrine, which then lowers arterial pressure by stimulation of central inhibitory alpha-adrenergic receptors, false neurotransmission, and/or reduction of plasma renin activity. Methyldopa has been shown to cause a net reduction in the tissue concentration of serotonin, dopamine, norepinephrine, and epinephrine.

Only methyldopa, the *L*-isomer of alpha-methyldopa, has the ability to inhibit dopa decarboxylase and to deplete animal tissues of norepinephrine. In man, the antihypertensive activity appears to be due solely to the *L*-isomer. About twice the dose of the racemate (*DL*-alpha-methyldopa) is required for equal antihypertensive effect.

Methyldopa has no direct effect on cardiac function and usually does not reduce glomerular filtration rate, renal blood flow, or filtration fraction. Cardiac output usually is maintained without cardiac acceleration. In some patients the heart rate is slowed.

Normal or elevated plasma renin activity may decrease in the course of methyldopa therapy.

Methyldopa reduces both supine and standing blood pressure. It usually produces highly effective lowering of the supine pressure with infrequent symptomatic postural hypotension. Exercise hypotension and diurnal blood pressure variations rarely occur.

DIURIL® (Chlorothiazide, MSD)
Chlorothiazide is a diuretic and antihypertensive. It affects the renal tubular mechanism of electrolyte reabsorption. At maximal therapeutic dosage all thiazides are approximately equal in their diuretic efficacy.

Chlorothiazide increases excretion of sodium and chloride in approximately equivalent amounts. Natriuresis may be accompanied by some loss of potassium and bicarbonate.

The mechanism of the antihypertensive effect of thiazides is unknown. Chlorothiazide does not affect normal blood pressure.

Chlorothiazide is eliminated rapidly by the kidney.

ALDOCLOR
The concomitant use of methyldopa and chlorothiazide, as provided in ALDOCLOR, frequently produces a more pronounced antihypertensive response than when either compound is the sole therapeutic agent. Particularly in those cases of hypertensive vascular disease where sodium and water retention is a problem, the coadministration of these two drugs in the form of ALDOCLOR will help control the fluid imbalance.

In severe essential hypertension and in malignant hypertension, ALDOCLOR may achieve effective lowering of blood pressure with fewer side effects than occur with other compounds used for this purpose.

ALDOCLOR reduces both supine and standing blood pressure; more effective lowering of the supine pressure with less frequent symptomatic postural hypotension can be obtained with ALDOCLOR than with most other antihypertensive agents. In patients treated with ALDOCLOR, exercise hypotension and diurnal blood pressure variations rarely occur.

Indication

Hypertension (see box warning).

Contraindications

Active hepatic disease, such as acute hepatitis and active cirrhosis.
If previous methyldopa therapy has been associated with liver disorders (see WARNINGS).
Anuria.
Hypersensitivity to methyldopa, or to chlorothiazide or other sulfonamide-derived drugs.

Warnings

Methyldopa
It is important to recognize that a positive Coombs test, hemolytic anemia, and liver disorders may occur with methyldopa therapy. The rare occurrences of hemolytic anemia or liver disorders could lead to potentially fatal complications unless properly recognized and managed. Read this section carefully to understand these reactions.

With prolonged methyldopa therapy, 10 to 20 percent of patients develop a positive direct Coombs test which usually occurs between 6 and 12 months of methyldopa therapy. Lowest incidence is at daily dosage of 1 g or less. This on rare occasions may be associated with hemolytic anemia, which could lead to potentially fatal complications. One cannot predict which patients with a positive direct Coombs test may develop hemolytic anemia.

Prior existence or development of a positive direct Coombs test is not in itself a contraindication to use of methyldopa. If a positive Coombs test develops during methyldopa therapy, the physician should determine whether hemolytic anemia exists and whether the positive Coombs test may be a problem. For example, in addition to a positive direct Coombs test there is less often a positive indirect Coombs test which may interfere with cross matching of blood.

At the start of methyldopa therapy, it is desirable to do a blood count (hematocrit, hemoglobin, or red cell count) for a baseline or to establish whether there is anemia. Periodic blood counts should be done during therapy to detect hemolytic anemia. It may be useful to do a direct Coombs test before therapy and at 6 and 12 months after the start of therapy.

If Coombs-positive hemolytic anemia occurs, the cause may be methyldopa and the drug should be discontinued. Usually the anemia remits promptly. If not, corticosteroids may be given and other causes of anemia should be considered. If the hemolytic anemia is related to methyldopa, the drug should not be reinstituted.

When methyldopa causes Coombs positivity alone or with hemolytic anemia, the red cell is usually coated with gamma globulin of the IgG (gamma G) class only. The positive Coombs test may not revert to normal until weeks to months after methyldopa is stopped.

Should the need for transfusion arise in a patient receiving methyldopa, both a direct and an indirect Coombs test should be performed on his blood. In the absence of hemolytic anemia, usually only the direct Coombs test will be positive. A positive direct Coombs test alone will not interfere with typing or cross matching. If the indirect Coombs test is also positive, problems may arise in the major cross match and the assistance of a hematologist or transfusion expert will be needed.

Occasionally, fever has occurred within the first three weeks of methyldopa therapy, associated in some cases with eosinophilia or abnormalities in one or more liver function tests, such as serum alkaline phosphatase, serum transaminases (SGOT, SGPT), bilirubin, cephalin cholesterol flocculation, prothrombin time, and bromsulphalein retention. Jaundice, with or without fever, may occur with onset usually within the first two to three months of therapy. In some patients the findings are consistent with those of cholestasis. Rarely fatal hepatic necrosis has been reported after use of methyldopa. These hepatic changes may represent hypersensitivity reactions. Periodic determination of hepatic function should be done particularly during the first 6 to 12 weeks of therapy or whenever an unexplained fever occurs. If fever, abnormalities in liver function tests, or jaundice appear, stop therapy with methyldopa. If caused by methyldopa, the temperature and abnormalities in liver function characteristically have reverted to normal when the drug was discontinued. Methyldopa should not be reinstituted in such patients.

Rarely, a reversible reduction of the white blood cell count with a primary effect on the granulocytes has been seen. The granulocyte count returned promptly to normal on discontinuance of the drug. Rare cases of granulocytopenia have been reported. In each instance, upon stopping the drug, the white cell count returned to normal. Reversible thrombocytopenia has occurred rarely. When methyldopa is used with other antihypertensive drugs, potentiation of antihypertensive effect may occur. Patients should be followed carefully to detect side reactions or unusual manifestations of drug idiosyncrasy.

Chlorothiazide
Use with caution in severe renal disease. In patients with renal disease, thiazides may precipitate azotemia. Cumulative effects of the drug may develop in patients with impaired renal function. Thiazides should be used with caution in patients with impaired hepatic function or progressive liver disease, since minor alterations of fluid and electrolyte balance may precipitate hepatic coma. Thiazides may add to or potentiate the action of other antihypertensive drugs.

Sensitivity reactions may occur in patients with or without a history of allergy or bronchial asthma. The possibility of exacerbation or activation of systemic lupus erythematosus has been reported. Lithium generally should not be given with diuretics because they reduce its renal clearance and add a high risk of lithium toxicity. Read circulars for lithium preparations before use of such concomitant therapy.

Pregnancy and Nursing

Use of any drug in women who are or may become pregnant requires that anticipated benefits be weighed against possible risks.

Methyldopa crosses the placental barrier and appears in cord blood. No unusual adverse reactions have been reported in association with the use of methyldopa during pregnancy. Though no obvious teratogenic effects have been reported, the possibility of fetal injury cannot be excluded.

Thiazides also cross the placental barrier and appear in cord blood. Hazards include fetal or neonatal jaundice, thrombocytopenia, and possibly other adverse reactions which have occurred in the adult.

Methyldopa and thiazides appear in breast milk. Patients taking ALDOCLOR should not nurse.

Precautions

Methyldopa
Methyldopa should be used with caution in patients with a history of previous liver disease or dysfunction (see WARNINGS).

Methyldopa may interfere with measurement of: urinary uric acid by the phosphotungstate method, serum creatinine by the alkaline picrate method, and SGOT by colorimetric methods. Interference with spectrophotometric methods for SGOT analysis has not been reported.

Since methyldopa causes fluorescence in urine samples at the same wave lengths as catecholamines, falsely high levels of urinary catecholamines may be reported. This will interfere with the diagnosis of pheochromocytoma. It is important to recognize this phenomenon before a patient with a possible pheochromocytoma is subjected to surgery. Methyldopa does not interfere with measurement of VMA (vanillylmandelic acid), a test for pheochromocytoma, by those methods which convert VMA to vanillin. Methyldopa is not recommended for the treatment of patients with pheochromocytoma. Rarely, when urine is exposed to air after voiding, it may darken because of breakdown of methyldopa or its metabolites.

Rarely, involuntary choreoathetotic movements have been observed during therapy with methyldopa in patients with severe bilateral cerebrovascular disease. Should these movements occur, stop therapy.

Patients may require reduced doses of anesthetics when on methyldopa. If hypotension does occur during anesthesia, it usually can be controlled by vasopressors. The adrenergic receptors remain sensitive during treatment with methyldopa.

Hypertension has recurred occasionally after dialysis in patients given methyldopa because the drug is removed by this procedure.

Chlorothiazide

Periodic determination of serum electrolytes to detect possible electrolyte imbalance should be performed at appropriate intervals.

All patients receiving diuretic therapy should be observed for evidence of fluid or electrolyte imbalance: namely, hyponatremia, hypochloremic alkalosis, and hypokalemia. Serum and urine electrolyte determinations are particularly important when the patient is vomiting excessively or receiving parenteral fluids. Warning signs or symptoms of fluid and electrolyte imbalance include dryness of mouth, thirst, weakness, lethargy, drowsiness, restlessness, muscle pains or cramps, muscular fatigue, hypotension, oliguria, tachycardia, and gastrointestinal disturbances such as nausea and vomiting.

Hypokalemia may develop, especially with brisk diuresis, when severe cirrhosis is present, during concomitant use of corticosteroids or ACTH, or after prolonged therapy.

Interference with adequate oral electrolyte intake will also contribute to hypokalemia. Hypokalemia can sensitize or exaggerate the response of the heart to the toxic effects of digitalis (e.g., increased ventricular irritability). Hypokalemia may be avoided or treated by use of potassium supplements such as foods with a high potassium content.

Although any chloride deficit is generally mild and usually does not require specific treatment except under extraordinary circumstances (as in liver disease or renal disease), chloride replacement may be required in the treatment of metabolic alkalosis.

Dilutional hyponatremia may occur in edematous patients in hot weather; appropriate therapy is water restriction, rather than administration of salt, except in rare instances when the hyponatremia is life threatening. In actual salt depletion, appropriate replacement is the therapy of choice.

Hyperuricemia may occur or acute gout may be precipitated in certain patients receiving thiazides.

Insulin requirements in diabetic patients may be increased, decreased, or unchanged. Latent diabetes mellitus may become manifest during thiazide therapy.

Thiazides may increase the responsiveness to tubocurarine.

The antihypertensive effects of the drug may be enhanced in the postsympathectomy patient. Thiazides may decrease arterial responsiveness to norepinephrine. This diminution is not sufficient to preclude effectiveness of the pressor agent for therapeutic use.

If progressive renal impairment becomes evident, consider withholding or discontinuing diuretic therapy.

Thiazides may decrease serum PBI levels without signs of thyroid disturbance.

Thiazides may decrease urinary calcium excretion. Thiazides may cause intermittent and slight elevation of serum calcium in the absence of known disorders of calcium metabolism. Marked hypercalcemia may be evidence of hidden hyperparathyroidism. Thiazides should be discontinued before carrying out tests for parathyroid function.

Adverse Reactions

Methyldopa

Sedation, usually transient, may occur during the initial period of therapy or whenever the dose is increased. Headache, asthenia, or weakness may be noted as early and transient symptoms. However, significant adverse effects due to methyldopa have been infrequent and this agent usually is well tolerated.

Nervous System/Psychiatric: Sedation, headache, asthenia or weakness, dizziness, lightheadedness, symptoms of cerebrovascular insufficiency, paresthesias, parkinsonism, Bell's palsy, decreased mental acuity, involuntary choreoathetotic movements. Psychic disturbances including nightmares and reversible mild psychoses or depression.

Cardiovascular: Bradycardia, prolonged carotid sinus hypersensitivity, aggravation of angina pectoris. Orthostatic hypotension (decrease daily dosage). Edema (and weight gain) usually relieved by use of a diuretic. (Discontinue methyldopa if edema progresses or signs of heart failure appear.)

Digestive: Nausea, vomiting, distention, constipation, flatus, diarrhea, colitis, mild dryness of mouth, sore or "black" tongue, pancreatitis, sialadenitis.

Hepatic: Abnormal liver function tests, jaundice, liver disorders.

Hematologic: Positive Coombs test, hemolytic anemia. Bone marrow depression, leukopenia, granulocytopenia, thrombocytopenia. Positive tests for antinuclear antibody, LE cells, and rheumatoid factor.

Allergic: Drug-related fever, lupus-like syndrome, myocarditis, pericarditis.

Skin: Rash as in eczema or lichenoid eruption; toxic epidermal necrolysis.

Respiratory: Nasal stuffiness.

Metabolic: Rise in BUN.

Urogenital: Breast enlargement, gynecomastia, lactation, amenorrhea, impotence, decreased libido.

Endocrine: Hyperprolactinemia.

Musculoskeletal: Mild arthralgia, with or without joint swelling; myalgia.

Chlorothiazide

Body as a Whole: Weakness.

Cardiovascular: Orthostatic hypotension (may be aggravated by alcohol, barbiturates, or narcotics).

Digestive: Anorexia, gastric irritation, nausea, vomiting, cramping, diarrhea, constipation, jaundice (intrahepatic cholestatic jaundice), pancreatitis, sialadenitis.

Hematologic: Leukopenia, agranulocytosis, thrombocytopenia, aplastic anemia, hemolytic anemia.

Metabolic: Hyperglycemia, glycosuria, hyperuricemia, electrolyte imbalance (see PRECAUTIONS).

Musculoskeletal: Muscle spasm.

Nervous System/Psychiatric: Dizziness, vertigo, paresthesias, headache, restlessness.

Special Senses: Transient blurred vision, xanthopsia.

Hypersensitivity: Purpura, photosensitivity, rash, urticaria, necrotizing angiitis (vasculitis and cutaneous vasculitis), fever, respiratory distress including pneumonitis and pulmonary edema, anaphylactic reactions.

Whenever adverse reactions are moderate or severe, thiazide dosage should be reduced or therapy withdrawn.

Dosage and Administration

Dosage: As determined by individual titration (see box warning).

The usual starting dosage is 1 tablet of ALDOCLOR 150 or 1 tablet of ALDOCLOR 250 two or three times a day in the first 48 hours. The daily dosage then may be increased or decreased, preferably at intervals of not less than two days, until an adequate response is achieved. To minimize the sedation associated with methyldopa, start dosage increases in the evening. By adjustment of dosage, morning hypotension may be prevented without sacrificing control of afternoon blood pressure.

When ALDOCLOR is given to patients on other antihypertensives, the dose of these agents may need to be adjusted to effect a smooth transition. When ALDOCLOR is given with antihypertensives other than thiazides, the initial dosage of methyldopa should be limited to 500 mg daily in divided doses.

Although occasional patients have responded to higher doses, the maximum recommended daily dosage is 3.0 g of methyldopa and 1.0 to 2.0 g of chlorothiazide. Once an effective dosage range is attained, a smooth blood pressure response occurs in most patients in 12 to 24 hours. If ALDOCLOR alone does not adequately control blood pressure, additional methyldopa may be given separately to obtain the maximum blood pressure response.

Since both components of ALDOCLOR have a relatively short duration of action, withdrawal is followed by return of hypertension usually within 48 hours. This is not complicated by an overshoot of blood pressure.

Occasionally tolerance may occur, usually between the second and third month of therapy. Increasing the dosage of either methyldopa or chlorothiazide separately or together frequently will restore effective control of blood pressure.

Methyldopa is largely excreted by the kidney and patients with impaired renal function may respond to smaller doses of ALDOCLOR. Syncope in older patients may be related to an increased sensitivity and advanced arteriosclerotic vascular disease. This may be avoided by lower doses.

How Supplied

No. 3318—Tablets ALDOCLOR 150 are beige, oval, film coated tablets coded MSD 612. Each tablet contains 250 mg of methyldopa and 150 mg of chlorothiazide. They are supplied as follows:
NDC 0006-0612-68 bottles of 100.
Shown in Product Identification Section, page 420
No. 3319—Tablets ALDOCLOR 250 are green, oval, film coated tablets coded MSD 634. Each tablet contains 250 mg of methyldopa and 250 mg of chlorothiazide. They are supplied as follows:
NDC 0006-0634-68 bottles of 100.
Shown in Product Identification Section, page 420
A.H.F.S. Category: 24:08
DC 6078624 Issued November 1983
COPYRIGHT © MERCK & CO., INC., 1983
All rights reserved

ALDOMET® Tablets ℞
(methyldopa, MSD), U.S.P.

ALDOMET® Oral Suspension ℞
(methyldopa, MSD), U.S.P.

Description

Methyldopa is the *L*-isomer of alpha-methyldopa. Its chemical name is levo-3-(3,4-dihydroxyphenyl)-2-methylalanine.

ALDOMET is supplied as tablets, in three strengths, each containing 125 mg, 250 mg, or 500 mg of methyldopa per tablet. Oral suspension ALDOMET is supplied as a white to off-white preparation; each 5 ml contains 250 mg of methyldopa

Continued on next page

Information on the Merck Sharp & Dohme products listed on these pages is the full prescribing information from product circulars in use November 1, 1984.

Merck Sharp & Dohme—Cont.

and alcohol 1 percent, with benzoic acid 0.1 percent and sodium bisulfite 0.2 percent added as preservatives.

Actions

ALDOMET® (Methyldopa, MSD), a unique antihypertensive, is an aromatic-amino-acid decarboxylase inhibitor in animals and in man. Although the mechanism of action has yet to be conclusively demonstrated, the antihypertensive effect of methyldopa probably is due to its metabolism to alpha-methylnorepinephrine, which then lowers arterial pressure by stimulation of central inhibitory alpha-adrenergic receptors, false neurotransmission, and/or reduction of plasma renin activity. Methyldopa has been shown to cause a net reduction in the tissue concentration of serotonin, dopamine, norepinephrine, and epinephrine.

Only methyldopa, the *L*-isomer of alpha-methyldopa, has the ability to inhibit dopa decarboxylase and to deplete animal tissues of norepinephrine. In man the antihypertensive activity appears to be due solely to the *L*-isomer. About twice the dose of the racemate (*DL*-alpha-methyldopa) is required for equal antihypertensive effect.

Methyldopa has no direct effect on cardiac function and usually does not reduce glomerular filtration rate, renal blood flow, or filtration fraction. Cardiac output usually is maintained without cardiac acceleration. In some patients the heart rate is slowed.

Normal or elevated plasma renin activity may decrease in the course of methyldopa therapy.

ALDOMET reduces both supine and standing blood pressure. Methyldopa usually produces highly effective lowering of the supine pressure with infrequent symptomatic postural hypotension. Exercise hypotension and diurnal blood pressure variations rarely occur.

Indication

Hypertension.

Contraindications

Active hepatic disease, such as acute hepatitis and active cirrhosis.
If previous methyldopa therapy has been associated with liver disorders (see WARNINGS).
Hypersensitivity.

Warnings

It is important to recognize that a positive Coombs test, hemolytic anemia, and liver disorders may occur with methyldopa therapy. The rare occurrences of hemolytic anemia or liver disorders could lead to potentially fatal complications unless properly recognized and managed. Read this section carefully to understand these reactions.

With prolonged methyldopa therapy, 10 to 20 percent of patients develop a positive direct Coombs test which usually occurs between 6 and 12 months of methyldopa therapy. Lowest incidence is at daily dosage of 1 g or less. This on rare occasions may be associated with hemolytic anemia, which could lead to potentially fatal complications. One cannot predict which patients with a positive direct Coombs test may develop hemolytic anemia.

Prior existence or development of a positive direct Coombs test is not in itself a contraindication to use of methyldopa. If a positive Coombs test develops during methyldopa therapy, the physician should determine whether hemolytic anemia exists and whether the positive Coombs test may be a problem. For example, in addition to a positive direct Coombs test there is less often a positive indirect Coombs test which may interfere with cross matching of blood.

At the start of methyldopa therapy, it is desirable to do a blood count (hematocrit, hemoglobin, or red cell count) for a baseline or to establish whether there is anemia. Periodic blood counts should be done during therapy to detect hemolytic anemia. It may be useful to do a direct Coombs test before therapy and at 6 and 12 months after the start of therapy.

If Coombs-positive hemolytic anemia occurs, the cause may be methyldopa and the drug should be discontinued. Usually the anemia remits promptly. If not, corticosteroids may be given and other causes of anemia should be considered. If the hemolytic anemia is related to methyldopa, the drug should not be reinstituted.

When methyldopa causes Coombs positivity alone or with hemolytic anemia, the red cell is usually coated with gamma globulin of the IgG (gamma G) class only. The positive Coombs test may not revert to normal until weeks to months after methyldopa is stopped.

Should the need for transfusion arise in a patient receiving methyldopa, both a direct and an indirect Coombs test should be performed on his blood. In the absence of hemolytic anemia, usually only the direct Coombs test will be positive. A positive direct Coombs test alone will not interfere with typing or cross matching. If the indirect Coombs test is also positive, problems may arise in the major cross match and the assistance of a hematologist or transfusion expert will be needed.

Occasionally, fever has occurred within the first 3 weeks of methyldopa therapy, associated in some cases with eosinophilia or abnormalities in one or more liver function tests, such as serum alkaline phosphatase, serum transaminases (SGOT, SGPT), bilirubin, cephalin cholesterol flocculation, prothrombin time, and bromsulphalein retention. Jaundice, with or without fever, may occur with onset usually within the first 2 to 3 months of therapy. In some patients the findings are consistent with those of cholestasis.

Rarely fatal hepatic necrosis has been reported after use of methyldopa. These hepatic changes may represent hypersensitivity reactions. Periodic determinations of hepatic function should be done particularly during the first 6 to 12 weeks of therapy or whenever an unexplained fever occurs. If fever, abnormalities in liver function tests, or jaundice appear, stop therapy with methyldopa. If caused by methyldopa, the temperature and abnormalities in liver function characteristically have reverted to normal when the drug was discontinued. Methyldopa should not be reinstituted in such patients.

Rarely, a reversible reduction of the white blood cell count with a primary effect on the granulocytes has been seen. The granulocyte count returned promptly to normal on discontinuance of the drug. Rare cases of granulocytopenia have been reported. In each instance, upon stopping the drug, the white cell count returned to normal. Reversible thrombocytopenia has occurred rarely.

When methyldopa is used with other antihypertensive drugs, potentiation of antihypertensive effect may occur. Patients should be followed carefully to detect side reactions or unusual manifestations of drug idiosyncrasy.

Pregnancy and Nursing

Use of any drug in women who are or may become pregnant or intend to nurse requires that anticipated benefits be weighed against possible risks. Methyldopa crosses the placental barrier, appears in cord blood, and appears in breast milk.

No unusual adverse reactions have been reported in association with the use of methyldopa during pregnancy. Though no obvious teratogenic effects have been reported, the possibility of fetal injury cannot be excluded. Also, the possibility of injury to a nursing infant cannot be excluded.

Precautions

Methyldopa should be used with caution in patients with a history of previous liver disease or dysfunction (see WARNINGS).

Methyldopa may interfere with measurement of: urinary uric acid by the phosphotungstate method, serum creatinine by the alkaline picrate method, and SGOT by colorimetric methods. Interference with spectrophotometric methods for SGOT analysis has not been reported.

Since methyldopa causes fluorescence in urine samples at the same wave lengths as catecholamines, falsely high levels of urinary catecholamines may be reported. This will interfere with the diagnosis of pheochromocytoma. It is important to recognize this phenomenon before a patient with a possible pheochromocytoma is subjected to surgery. Methyldopa does not interfere with measurement of VMA (vanillylmandelic acid), a test for pheochromocytoma, by those methods which convert VMA to vanillin. Methyldopa is not recommended for the treatment of patients with pheochromocytoma. Rarely, when urine is exposed to air after voiding, it may darken because of breakdown of methyldopa or its metabolites.

Rarely involuntary choreoathetotic movements have been observed during therapy with methyldopa in patients with severe bilateral cerebrovascular disease. Should these movements occur, stop therapy.

Patients may require reduced doses of anesthetics when on methyldopa. If hypotension does occur during anesthesia, it usually can be controlled by vasopressors. The adrenergic receptors remain sensitive during treatment with methyldopa.

Hypertension has recurred occasionally after dialysis in patients given methyldopa because the drug is removed by this procedure.

Adverse Reactions

Sedation, usually transient, may occur during the initial period of therapy or whenever the dose is increased. Headache, asthenia, or weakness may be noted as early and transient symptoms. However, significant adverse effects due to ALDOMET have been infrequent and this agent usually is well tolerated.

Nervous System/Psychiatric: Sedation, headache, asthenia or weakness, dizziness, lightheadedness, symptoms of cerebrovascular insufficiency, paresthesias, parkinsonism, Bell's palsy, decreased mental acuity, involuntary choreoathetotic movements. Psychic disturbances including nightmares and reversible mild psychoses or depression.

Cardiovascular: Bradycardia, prolonged carotid sinus hypersensitivity, aggravation of angina pectoris. Orthostatic hypotension (decrease daily dosage). Edema (and weight gain) usually relieved by use of a diuretic. (Discontinue methyldopa if edema progresses or signs of heart failure appear.)

Digestive: Nausea, vomiting, distention, constipation, flatus, diarrhea, colitis, mild dryness of mouth, sore or "black" tongue, pancreatitis, sialadenitis.

Hepatic: Abnormal liver function tests, jaundice, liver disorders.

Hematologic: Positive Coombs test, hemolytic anemia. Bone marrow depression, leukopenia, granulocytopenia, thrombocytopenia. Positive tests for antinuclear antibody, LE cells, and rheumatoid factor.

Allergic: Drug-related fever, lupus-like syndrome, myocarditis, pericarditis.

Skin: Rash as in eczema or lichenoid eruption; toxic epidermal necrolysis.

Respiratory: Nasal stuffiness.

Metabolic: Rise in BUN.

Urogenital: Breast enlargement, gynecomastia, lactation, amenorrhea, impotence, decreased libido.

Endocrine: Hyperprolactinemia.

Musculoskeletal: Mild arthralgia, with or without joint swelling; myalgia.

Dosage and Administration

ADULTS

Initiation of Therapy

The usual starting dosage of ALDOMET is 250 mg two or three times a day in the first 48 hours. The daily dosage then may be increased or decreased, preferably at intervals of not less than two days, until an adequate response is achieved. To minimize the sedation, start dosage increases in the evening. By adjustment of dosage, morning hypotension may be prevented without sacrificing control of afternoon blood pressure.

When methyldopa is given to patients on other antihypertensives, the dose of these agents may need to be adjusted to effect a smooth transition. When ALDOMET is given with antihypertensives other than thiazides, the initial dosage of ALDOMET should be limited to 500 mg daily in divided doses; when ALDOMET is added to a thiazide, the dosage of thiazide need not be changed.

Maintenance Therapy
The usual daily dosage of ALDOMET is 500 mg to 2.0 g in two to four doses. Although occasional patients have responded to higher doses, the maximum recommended daily dosage is 3.0 g. Once an effective dosage range is attained, a smooth blood pressure response occurs in most patients in 12 to 24 hours. Since methyldopa has a relatively short duration of action, withdrawal is followed by return of hypertension usually within 48 hours. This is not complicated by an overshoot of blood pressure.

Occasionally tolerance may occur, usually between the second and third month of therapy. Adding a diuretic or increasing the dosage of methyldopa frequently will restore effective control of blood pressure. A thiazide may be added at any time during methyldopa therapy and is recommended if therapy has not been started with a thiazide or if effective control of blood pressure cannot be maintained on 2.0 g of methyldopa daily. Methyldopa is largely excreted by the kidney and patients with impaired renal function may respond to smaller doses. Syncope in older patients may be related to an increased sensitivity and advanced arteriosclerotic vascular disease. This may be avoided by lower doses.

CHILDREN
Initial dosage is based on 10 mg/kg of body weight daily in two to four doses. The daily dosage then is increased or decreased until an adequate response is achieved. The maximum dosage is 65 mg/kg or 3.0 g daily, whichever is less.

How Supplied

No. 3341—Tablets ALDOMET, 125 mg, are yellow, film coated, round tablets, coded MSD 135. They are supplied as follows:
NDC 0006-0135-68 bottles of 100.
Shown in Product Identification Section, page 420
No. 3290—Tablets ALDOMET, 250 mg, are yellow, film coated, round tablets, coded MSD 401. They are supplied as follows:
NDC 0006-0401-68 bottles of 100
(6505-00-890-1856, 250 mg 100's)
NDC 0006-0401-28 unit dose packages of 100
(6505-00-149-0090, 250 mg individually sealed 100's)
NDC 0006-0401-78 unit of use bottles of 100
NDC 0006-0401-82 bottles of 1000
(6505-00-931-6646, 250 mg 1000's).
Shown in Product Identification Section, page 420
No. 3292—Tablets ALDOMET, 500 mg, are yellow, film coated, round tablets, coded MSD 516. They are supplied as follows:
NDC 0006-0516-54 unit of use bottles of 60
NDC 0006-0516-68 bottles of 100
NDC 0006-0516-28 unit dose packages of 100
NDC 0006-0516-78 unit of use bottles of 100
NDC 0006-0516-74 bottles of 500.
Shown in Product Identification Section, page 420
No. 3382—Oral Suspension ALDOMET, 250 mg per 5 ml, is an off-white, creamy suspension with a citric orange-pineapple flavor, and is supplied as follows:
NDC 0006-3382-74 bottles of 473 ml.

A.H.F.S. Category: 24:08
DC 6649717 Issued November 1983
COPYRIGHT © MERCK & CO., INC., 1983
All rights reserved

ALDOMET® Ester HCl Injection   ℞
(methyldopate hydrochloride, MSD), U.S.P.

Description

Injection ALDOMET® ester hydrochloride (Methyldopate Hydrochloride, MSD) is an antihypertensive agent for intravenous use, each 5 ml of which contains:
Methyldopate
hydrochloride .... 250.0 mg
Inactive ingredients:
  Citric acid anhydrous .... 25.0 mg
  Disodium edetate .... 2.5 mg
  Monothioglycerol .... 10.0 mg
Sodium hydroxide to adjust pH
Water for Injection, q.s. to .... 5.0 ml
Methylparaben 7.5 mg, propylparaben 1.0 mg, and sodium bisulfite 16.0 mg added as preservatives. Methyldopate hydrochloride [levo-3-(3,4-dihydroxyphenyl)-2-methylalanine, ethyl ester hydrochloride] is the ethyl ester of methyldopa, supplied as the hydrochloride salt. Methyldopate hydrochloride is more soluble and stable in solution than methyldopa and is the preferred form for intravenous use.

Actions

ALDOMET® (Methyldopa, MSD), a unique antihypertensive, is an aromatic-amino-acid decarboxylase inhibitor in animals and in man. Although the mechanism of action has yet to be conclusively demonstrated, the antihypertensive effect of methyldopa probably is due to its metabolism to alpha-methylnorepinephrine, which then lowers arterial pressure by stimulation of central inhibitory alpha-adrenergic receptors, false neurotransmission, and/or reduction of plasma renin activity. Methyldopa has been shown to cause a net reduction in the tissue concentration of serotonin, dopamine, norepinephrine, and epinephrine.

Only methyldopa, the *L*-isomer of alpha-methyldopa, has the ability to inhibit dopa decarboxylase and to deplete animal tissues of norepinephrine. In man the antihypertensive activity appears to be due solely to the *L*-isomer. About twice the dose of the racemate (*DL*-alpha-methyldopa) is required for equal antihypertensive effect.

Methyldopa has no direct effect on cardiac function and usually does not reduce glomerular filtration rate, renal blood flow, or filtration fraction. Cardiac output usually is maintained without cardiac acceleration. In some patients the heart rate is slowed.

Normal or elevated plasma renin activity may decrease in the course of methyldopa therapy.

Methyldopa reduces both supine and standing blood pressure. It usually produces highly effective lowering of the supine pressure with infrequent symptomatic postural hypotension. Exercise hypotension and diurnal blood pressure variations rarely occur.

Methyldopate hydrochloride is the ethyl ester of methyldopa hydrochloride and possesses the same pharmacologic attributes.

Indication

Hypertension, when parenteral medication is indicated.

The treatment of hypertensive crises may be initiated with injection ALDOMET ester hydrochloride.

Contraindications

Active hepatic disease, such as acute hepatitis and active cirrhosis.

If previous methyldopa therapy has been associated with liver disorders (see WARNINGS).

Hypersensitivity to any component of this product.

Warnings

It is important to recognize that a positive Coombs test, hemolytic anemia, and liver disorders may occur with methyldopa therapy. The rare occurrences of hemolytic anemia or liver disorders could lead to potentially fatal complications unless properly recognized and managed. Read this section carefully to understand these reactions.

With prolonged methyldopa therapy, 10 to 20 percent of patients develop a positive direct Coombs test which usually occurs between 6 and 12 months of methyldopa therapy. Lowest incidence is at daily dosage of 1 g or less. This on rare occasions may be associated with hemolytic anemia, which could lead to potentially fatal complications. One cannot predict which patients with a positive direct Coombs test may develop hemolytic anemia.

Prior existence or development of a positive direct Coombs test is not in itself a contraindication to use of methyldopa. If a positive Coombs test develops during methyldopa therapy, the physician should determine whether hemolytic anemia exists and whether the positive Coombs test may be a problem. For example, in addition to a positive direct Coombs test there is less often a positive indirect Coombs test which may interfere with cross matching of blood.

At the start of methyldopa therapy, it is desirable to do a blood count (hematocrit, hemoglobin, or red cell count) for a baseline or to establish whether there is anemia. Periodic blood counts should be done during therapy to detect hemolytic anemia. It may be useful to do a direct Coombs test before therapy and at 6 and 12 months after the start of therapy.

If Coombs-positive hemolytic anemia occurs, the cause may be methyldopa and the drug should be discontinued. Usually the anemia remits promptly. If not, corticosteroids may be given and other causes of anemia should be considered. If the hemolytic anemia is related to methyldopa, the drug should not be reinstituted.

When methyldopa causes Coombs positivity alone or with hemolytic anemia, the red cell is usually coated with gamma globulin of the IgG (gamma G) class only. The positive Coombs test may not revert to normal until weeks to months after methyldopa is stopped.

Should the need for transfusion arise in a patient receiving methyldopa, both a direct and an indirect Coombs test should be performed on his blood. In the absence of hemolytic anemia, usually only the direct Coombs test will be positive. A positive direct Coombs test alone will not interfere with typing or cross matching. If the indirect Coombs test is also positive, problems may arise in the major cross match and the assistance of a hematologist or transfusion expert will be needed.

Occasionally, fever has occurred within the first three weeks of methyldopa therapy, associated in some cases with eosinophilia or abnormalities in one or more liver function tests, such as serum alkaline phosphatase, serum transaminases (SGOT, SGPT), bilirubin, cephalin cholesterol flocculation, prothrombin time, and bromsulphalein retention. Jaundice, with or without fever, may occur with onset usually within the first two to three months of therapy. In some patients the findings are consistent with those of cholestasis. Rarely fatal hepatic necrosis has been reported after use of methyldopa. These hepatic changes may represent hypersensitivity reactions. Periodic determination of hepatic function should be done particularly during the first 6 to 12 weeks of therapy or whenever an unexplained fever occurs. If fever, abnormalities in liver function tests, or jaundice appear, stop therapy with methyldopa. If caused by methyldopa, the temperature and abnormalities in liver function characteristically have reverted to normal when the drug was discontinued. Methyldopa should not be reinstituted in such patients.

Rarely, a reversible reduction of the white blood cell count with a primary effect on the granulocytes has been seen. The granulocyte count returned promptly to normal on discontinuance of the drug. Rare cases of granulocytopenia have been reported. In each instance, upon stopping the

Continued on next page

Information on the Merck Sharp & Dohme products listed on these pages is the full prescribing information from product circulars in use November 1, 1984.

Merck Sharp & Dohme—Cont.

drug, the white cell count returned to normal. Reversible thrombocytopenia has occurred rarely. When methyldopa is used with other antihypertensive drugs, potentiation of antihypertensive effect may occur. Patients should be followed carefully to detect side reactions or unusual manifestations of drug idiosyncrasy.

Pregnancy and Nursing
Use of any drug in women who are or may become pregnant or intend to nurse requires that anticipated benefits be weighed against possible risks. Methyldopa crosses the placental barrier, appears in cord blood, and appears in breast milk.
No unusual adverse reactions have been reported in association with the use of methyldopa during pregnancy. Though no obvious teratogenic effects have been reported, the possibility of fetal injury cannot be excluded. Also, the possibility of injury to a nursing infant cannot be excluded.

Precautions

Methyldopa should be used with caution in patients with a history of previous liver disease or dysfunction (see WARNINGS).
Methyldopa may interfere with measurement of: urinary uric acid by the phosphotungstate method, serum creatinine by the alkaline picrate method, and SGOT by colorimetric methods. Interference with spectrophotometric methods for SGOT analysis has not been reported.
A paradoxical pressor response has been reported with intravenous administration of ALDOMET ester hydrochloride.
Since methyldopa causes fluorescence in urine samples at the same wave lengths as catecholamines, falsely high levels of urinary catecholamines may be reported. This will interfere with the diagnosis of pheochromocytoma. It is important to recognize this phenomenon before a patient with a possible pheochromocytoma is subjected to surgery. Methyldopa does not interfere with measurement of VMA (vanillylmandelic acid), a test for pheochromocytoma, by those methods which convert VMA to vanillin. Methyldopa is not recommended for the treatment of patients with pheochromocytoma. Rarely, when urine is exposed to air after voiding, it may darken because of breakdown of methyldopa or its metabolites.
Rarely involuntary choreoathetotic movements have been observed during therapy with methyldopa in patients with severe bilateral cerebrovascular disease. Should these movements occur, stop therapy.
Patients may require reduced doses of anesthetics when on methyldopa. If hypotension does occur during anesthesia, it usually can be controlled by vasopressors. The adrenergic receptors remain sensitive during treatment with methyldopa. Hypertension has recurred occasionally after dialysis in patients given methyldopa because the drug is removed by this procedure.

Adverse Reactions

Sedation, usually transient, may occur during the initial period of therapy or whenever the dose is increased. Headache, asthenia, or weakness may be noted as early and transient symptoms. However, significant adverse effects due to methyldopa have been infrequent and this agent usually is well tolerated.
Nervous System/Psychiatric: Sedation, headache, asthenia or weakness, dizziness, lightheadedness, symptoms of cerebrovascular insufficiency, paresthesias, parkinsonism, Bell's palsy, decreased mental acuity, involuntary choreoathetotic movements. Psychic disturbances including nightmares and reversible mild psychoses or depression.
Cardiovascular: Bradycardia, prolonged carotid sinus hypersensitivity, aggravation of angina pectoris. Paradoxical pressor response with intravenous use. Orthostatic hypotension (decrease daily dosage). Edema (and weight gain) usually relieved by use of a diuretic. (Discontinue methyldopa if edema progresses or signs of heart failure appear.)
Digestive: Nausea, vomiting, distention, constipation, flatus, diarrhea, colitis, mild dryness of mouth, sore or "black" tongue, pancreatitis, sialadenitis.
Hepatic: Abnormal liver function tests, jaundice, liver disorders.
Hematologic: Positive Coombs test, hemolytic anemia. Bone marrow depression, leukopenia, granulocytopenia, thrombocytopenia. Positive tests for antinuclear antibody, LE cells, and rheumatoid factor.
Allergic: Drug-related fever, lupus-like syndrome, myocarditis, pericarditis.
Skin: Rash as in eczema or lichenoid eruption; toxic epidermal necrolysis.
Respiratory: Nasal stuffiness.
Metabolic: Rise in BUN.
Urogenital: Breast enlargement, gynecomastia, lactation, amenorrhea, impotence, decreased libido.
Endocrine: Hyperprolactinemia.
Musculoskeletal: Mild arthralgia, with or without joint swelling; myalgia.

Dosage and Administration

Injection ALDOMET ester hydrochloride, when given intravenously in effective doses, causes a decline in blood pressure that may begin in four to six hours and last 10 to 16 hours after injection. Add the desired dose of injection ALDOMET ester hydrochloride to 100 ml of 5 percent Dextrose Injection U.S.P. Alternatively the desired dose may be given in 5% dextrose in water in a concentration of 100 mg/10 ml. Give this intravenous infusion slowly over a period of 30 to 60 minutes.

ADULTS
The usual adult dosage intravenously is 250 to 500 mg at six hour intervals as required. The maximum recommended intravenous dose is 1.0 g every six hours.
When control has been obtained, oral therapy with tablets ALDOMET (Methyldopa, MSD) may be substituted for intravenous therapy, starting with the same dosage schedule used for the parenteral route. The effectiveness and anticipated responses are described in the circular for tablets ALDOMET (Methyldopa, MSD).
Since methyldopa has a relatively short duration of action, withdrawal is followed by return of hypertension usually within 48 hours. This is not complicated by an overshoot of blood pressure. Occasionally tolerance may occur, usually between the second and third month of therapy. Adding a diuretic or increasing the dosage of methyldopa frequently will restore effective control of blood pressure. A thiazide may be added at any time during methyldopa therapy and is recommended if therapy has not been started with a thiazide or if effective control of blood pressure cannot be maintained on 2.0 g of methyldopa daily. Methyldopa is largely excreted by the kidney and patients with impaired renal function may respond to smaller doses. Syncope in older patients may be related to an increased sensitivity and advanced arteriosclerotic vascular disease. This may be avoided by lower doses.

CHILDREN
The recommended daily dosage is 20 to 40 mg/kg of body weight in divided doses every six hours. The maximum dosage is 65 mg/kg or 3.0 g daily, whichever is less. When the blood pressure is under control, continue with oral therapy using tablets ALDOMET (Methyldopa, MSD) in the same dosage as for the parenteral route.

How Supplied
No. 3293—Injection ALDOMET ester hydrochloride, 250 mg per 5 ml, is a clear, colorless solution and is supplied as follows:
NDC 0006-3293-05 in 5 ml vials.
A.H.F.S. Category: 24:08
DC 6112026 Issued November 1983
COPYRIGHT © MERCK & CO., INC., 1983
All rights reserved

ALDORIL® Tablets
(methyldopa-hydrochlorothiazide, MDS)   ℞

> **WARNING**
>
> This fixed combination drug is not indicated for initial therapy of hypertension. Hypertension requires therapy titrated to the individual patient. If the fixed combination represents the dosage so determined, its use may be more convenient in patient management. The treatment of hypertension is not static, but must be reevaluated as conditions in each patient warrant.

Description

ALDORIL® (Methyldopa-Hydrochlorothiazide, MSD) is a combination of two antihypertensive agents methyldopa and hydrochlorothiazide. The chemical name for methyldopa is levo-3-(3,4-dihydroxyphenyl)-2-methylalanine. Hydrochlorothiazide is 6-chloro-3,4-dihydro-2*H*-1,2,4-benzothiadiazine-7- sulfonamide 1,1-dioxide.

Actions

ALDOMET® (Methyldopa, MSD)
Methyldopa, a unique antihypertensive, is an aromatic-amino-acid decarboxylase inhibitor in animals and in man. Although the mechanism of action has yet to be conclusively demonstrated, the antihypertensive effect of methyldopa probably is due to its metabolism to alpha-methylnorepinephrine, which then lowers arterial pressure by stimulation of central inhibitory alpha-adrenergic receptors, false neurotransmission, and/or reduction of plasma renin activity. Methyldopa has been shown to cause a net reduction in the tissue concentration of serotonin, dopamine, norepinephrine, and epinephrine.
Only methyldopa, the *L*-isomer of alpha-methyldopa, has the ability to inhibit dopa decarboxylase and to deplete animal tissues of norepinephrine. In man, the antihypertensive activity appears to be due solely to the *L*-isomer. About twice the dose of the racemate (*DL*-alpha-methyldopa) is required for equal antihypertensive effect.
Methyldopa has no direct effect on cardiac function and usually does not reduce glomerular filtration rate, renal blood flow, or filtration fraction. Cardiac output usually is maintained without cardiac acceleration. In some patients the heart rate is slowed.
Normal or elevated plasma renin activity may decrease in the course of methyldopa therapy. Methyldopa reduces both supine and standing blood pressure. It usually produces highly effective lowering of the supine pressure with infrequent symptomatic postural hypotension. Exercise hypotension and diurnal blood pressure variations rarely occur.

HydroDIURIL®
(Hydrochlorothiazide, MSD)
Hydrochlorothiazide is a diuretic and antihypertensive. It affects the renal tubular mechanism of electrolyte reabsorption. At maximal therapeutic dosage all thiazides are approximately equal in their diuretic efficacy.
Hydrochlorothiazide increases excretion of sodium and chloride in approximately equivalent amounts. Natriuresis may be accompanied by some loss of potassium and bicarbonate.
The mechanism of the antihypertensive effect of thiazides is unknown. Hydrochlorothiazide does not affect normal blood pressure.
Hydrochlorothiazide is eliminated rapidly by the kidney.

ALDORIL (Methyldopa-Hydrochlorothiazide, MSD)
The concomitant use of methyldopa and hydrochlorothiazide, as provided in ALDORIL, frequently produces a more pronounced antihypertensive response than when either compound is the sole therapeutic agent. Particularly in those cases of hypertensive vascular disease where so-

dium and water retention is a problem, the coadministration of these two drugs in the form of ALDORIL will help control the fluid imbalance.
In severe essential hypertension and in malignant hypertension ALDORIL may achieve effective lowering of blood pressure with fewer side effects than occur with other compounds used for this purpose.
ALDORIL reduces both supine and standing blood pressure; more effective lowering of the supine pressure with less frequent symptomatic postural hypotension can be obtained with ALDORIL than with most other antihypertensive agents. In patients treated with ALDORIL, exercise hypotension and diurnal blood pressure variations rarely occur.

Indication

Hypertension (see box warning).

Contraindications

Active hepatic disease, such as acute hepatitis and active cirrhosis.
If previous methyldopa therapy has been associated with liver disorders (see WARNINGS).
Anuria.
Hypersensitivity to methyldopa, or to hydrochlorothiazide or other sulfonamide-derived drugs.

Warnings

Methyldopa
It is important to recognize that a positive Coombs test, hemolytic anemia, and liver disorders may occur with methyldopa therapy. The rare occurrences of hemolytic anemia or liver disorders could lead to potentially fatal complications unless properly recognized and managed. Read this section carefully to understand these reactions.
With prolonged methyldopa therapy, 10 to 20 percent of patients develop a positive direct Coombs test which usually occurs between 6 and 12 months of methyldopa therapy. Lowest incidence is at daily dosage of 1 g or less. This on rare occasions may be associated with hemolytic anemia, which could lead to potentially fatal complications. One cannot predict which patients with a positive direct Coombs test may develop hemolytic anemia.
Prior existence or development of a positive direct Coombs test is not in itself a contraindication to use of methyldopa. If a positive Coombs test develops during methyldopa therapy, the physician should determine whether hemolytic anemia exists and whether the positive Coombs test may be a problem. For example, in addition to a positive direct Coombs test there is less often a positive indirect Coombs test which may interfere with cross matching of blood.
At the start of methyldopa therapy, it is desirable to do a blood count (hematocrit, hemoglobin, or red cell count) for a baseline or to establish whether there is anemia. Periodic blood counts should be done during therapy to detect hemolytic anemia. It may be useful to do a direct Coombs test before therapy and at 6 and 12 months after the start of therapy.
If Coombs-positive hemolytic anemia occurs, the cause may be methyldopa and the drug should be discontinued. Usually the anemia remits promptly. If not, corticosteroids may be given and other causes of anemia should be considered. If the hemolytic anemia is related to methyldopa, the drug should not be reinstituted.
When methyldopa causes Coombs positivity alone or with hemolytic anemia, the red cell is usually coated with gamma globulin of the IgG (gamma G) class only. The positive Coombs test may not revert to normal until weeks to months after methyldopa is stopped.
Should the need for transfusion arise in a patient receiving methyldopa, both a direct and an indirect Coombs test should be performed on his blood. In the absence of hemolytic anemia, usually only the direct Coombs test will be positive. A positive direct Coombs test alone will not interfere with typing or cross matching. If the indirect Coombs test is also positive, problems may arise in the major cross match and the assistance of a hematologist or transfusion expert will be needed.
Occasionally, fever has occurred within the first three weeks of methyldopa therapy, associated in some cases with eosinophilia or abnormalities in one or more liver function tests, such as serum alkaline phosphatase, serum transaminases (SGOT, SGPT), bilirubin, cephalin cholesterol flocculation, prothrombin time, and bromsulphalein retention. Jaundice, with or without fever, may occur with onset usually within the first two to three months of therapy. In some patients the findings are consistent with those of cholestasis. Rarely fatal hepatic necrosis has been reported after use of methyldopa. These hepatic changes may represent hypersensitivity reactions. Periodic determination of hepatic function should be done particularly during the first 6 to 12 weeks of therapy or whenever an unexplained fever occurs. If fever, abnormalities in liver function tests, or jaundice appear, stop therapy with methyldopa. If caused by methyldopa, the temperature and abnormalities in liver function characteristically have reverted to normal when the drug was discontinued. Methyldopa should not be reinstituted in such patients.
Rarely, a reversible reduction of the white blood cell count with a primary effect on the granulocytes has been seen. The granulocyte count returned promptly to normal on discontinuance of the drug. Rare cases of granulocytopenia have been reported. In each instance, upon stopping the drug, the white cell count returned to normal. Reversible thrombocytopenia has occurred rarely. When methyldopa is used with other antihypertensive drugs, potentiation of antihypertensive effect may occur. Patients should be followed carefully to detect side reactions or unusual manifestations of drug idiosyncrasy.
Hydrochlorothiazide
Use with caution in severe renal disease. In patients with renal disease, thiazides may precipitate azotemia. Cumulative effects of the drug may develop in patients with impaired renal function.
Thiazides should be used with caution in patients with impaired hepatic function or progressive liver disease, since minor alterations of fluid and electrolyte balance may precipitate hepatic coma.
Thiazides may add to or potentiate the action of other antihypertensive drugs.
Sensitivity reactions may occur in patients with or without a history of allergy or bronchial asthma. The possibility of exacerbation or activation of systemic lupus erythematosus has been reported.
Lithium generally should not be given with diuretics because they reduce its renal clearance and add a high risk of lithium toxicity. Read circulars for lithium preparations before use of such concomitant therapy.

Pregnancy and Nursing

Use of any drug in women who are or may become pregnant requires that anticipated benefits be weighed against possible risks.
Methyldopa crosses the placental barrier and appears in cord blood. No unusual adverse reactions have been reported in association with the use of methyldopa during pregnancy. Though no obvious teratogenic effects have been reported, the possibility of fetal injury cannot be excluded.
Thiazides also cross the placental barrier and appear in cord blood. Hazards include fetal or neonatal jaundice, thrombocytopenia, and possibly other adverse reactions which have occurred in the adult.
Methyldopa and thiazides appear in breast milk. Patients taking ALDORIL should not nurse.

Precautions

Methyldopa
Methyldopa should be used with caution in patients with a history of previous liver disease or dysfunction (see WARNINGS).
Methyldopa may interfere with measurement of: urinary uric acid by the phosphotungstate method, serum creatinine by the alkaline picrate method, and SGOT by colorimetric methods. Interference with spectrophotometric methods for SGOT analysis has not been reported.
Since methyldopa causes fluorescence in urine samples at the same wave lengths as catecholamines, falsely high levels of urinary catecholamines may be reported. This will interfere with the diagnosis of pheochromocytoma. It is important to recognize this phenomenon before a patient with a possible pheochromocytoma is subjected to surgery. Methyldopa does not interfere with measurement of VMA (vanillylmandelic acid), a test for pheochromocytoma, by those methods which convert VMA to vanillin. Methyldopa is not recommended for the treatment of patients with pheochromocytoma. Rarely, when urine is exposed to air after voiding, it may darken because of breakdown of methyldopa or its metabolites.
Rarely, involuntary choreoathetotic movements have been observed during therapy with methyldopa in patients with severe bilateral cerebrovascular disease. Should these movements occur, stop therapy.
Patients may require reduced doses of anesthetics when on methyldopa. If hypotension does occur during anesthesia, it usually can be controlled by vasopressors. The adrenergic receptors remain sensitive during treatment with methyldopa.
Hypertension has recurred occasionally after dialysis in patients given methyldopa because the drug is removed by this procedure.
Hydrochlorothiazide
Periodic determination of serum electrolytes to detect possible electrolyte imbalance should be performed at appropriate intervals.
All patients receiving diuretic therapy should be observed for evidence of fluid or electrolyte imbalance: namely, hyponatremia, hypochloremic alkalosis, and hypokalemia. Serum and urine electrolyte determinations are particularly important when the patient is vomiting excessively or receiving parenteral fluids. Warning signs or symptoms of fluid and electrolyte imbalance include dryness of mouth, thirst, weakness, lethargy, drowsiness, restlessness, muscle pains or cramps, muscular fatigue, hypotension, oliguria, tachycardia, and gastrointestinal disturbances such as nausea and vomiting.
Hypokalemia may develop, especially with brisk diuresis, when severe cirrhosis is present, during concomitant use of corticosteroids or ACTH, or after prolonged therapy.
Interference with adequate oral electrolyte intake will also contribute to hypokalemia. Hypokalemia can sensitize or exaggerate the response of the heart to the toxic effects of digitalis (e.g., increased ventricular irritability). Hypokalemia may be avoided or treated by use of potassium supplements such as foods with a high potassium content.
Although any chloride deficit is generally mild and usually does not require specific treatment except under extraordinary circumstances (as in liver disease or renal disease), chloride replacement may be required in the treatment of metabolic alkalosis.
Dilutional hyponatremia may occur in edematous patients in hot weather; appropriate therapy is water restriction, rather than administration of salt, except in rare instances when the hyponatremia is life threatening. In actual salt depletion, appropriate replacement is the therapy of choice.
Hyperuricemia may occur or acute gout may be precipitated in certain patients receiving thiazides.

Continued on next page

Information on the Merck Sharp & Dohme products listed on these pages is the full prescribing information from product circulars in use November 1, 1984.

Merck Sharp & Dohme—Cont.

Insulin requirements in diabetic patients may be increased, decreased, or unchanged. Latent diabetes mellitus may become manifest during thiazide therapy.

Thiazides may increase the responsiveness to tubocurarine.

The antihypertensive effects of the drug may be enhanced in the postsympathectomy patient. Thiazides may decrease arterial responsiveness to norepinephrine. This diminution is not sufficient to preclude effectiveness of the pressor agent for therapeutic use.

If progressive renal impairment becomes evident, consider withholding or discontinuing diuretic therapy.

Thiazides may decrease serum PBI levels without signs of thyroid disturbance.

Thiazides have been shown to increase the urinary excretion of magnesium; this may result in hypomagnesemia.

Thiazides may decrease urinary calcium excretion. Thiazides may cause intermittent and slight elevation of serum calcium in the absence of known disorders of calcium metabolism. Marked hypercalcemia may be evidence of hidden hyperparathyroidism. Thiazides should be discontinued before carrying out tests for parathyroid function.

Adverse Reactions

Methyldopa
Sedation, usually transient, may occur during the initial period of therapy or whenever the dose is increased. Headache, asthenia, or weakness may be noted as early and transient symptoms. However, significant adverse effects due to methyldopa have been infrequent and this agent usually is well tolerated.
Nervous System/Psychiatric: Sedation, headache, asthenia or weakness, dizziness, lightheadedness, symptoms of cerebrovascular insufficiency, paresthesias, parkinsonism, Bell's palsy, decreased mental acuity, involuntary choreoathetotic movements. Psychic disturbances including nightmares and reversible mild psychoses or depression.
Cardiovascular: Bradycardia, prolonged carotid sinus hypersensitivity, aggravation of angina pectoris. Orthostatic hypotension (decrease daily dosage). Edema (and weight gain) usually relieved by use of a diuretic. (Discontinue methyldopa if edema progresses or signs of heart failure appear.)
Digestive: Nausea, vomiting, distention, constipation, flatus, diarrhea, colitis, mild dryness of mouth, sore or "black" tongue, pancreatitis, sialadenitis.
Hepatic: Abnormal liver function tests, jaundice, liver disorders.
Hematologic: Positive Coombs test, hemolytic anemia. Bone marrow depression, leukopenia, granulocytopenia, thrombocytopenia. Positive tests for antinuclear antibody, LE cells, and rheumatoid factor.
Allergic: Drug-related fever, lupus-like syndrome, myocarditis, pericarditis.
Skin: Rash as in eczema or lichenoid eruption; toxic epidermal necrolysis.
Respiratory: Nasal stuffiness.
Metabolic: Rise in BUN.
Urogenital: breast enlargement, gynecomastia, lactation, amenorrhea, impotence, decreased libido.
Endocrine: Hyperprolactinemia.
Musculoskeletal: Mild arthralgia, with or without joint swelling; myalgia.
Hydrochlorothiazide
Body as a Whole: Weakness.
Cardiovascular: Orthostatic hypotension (may be aggravated by alcohol, barbiturates, or narcotics).
Digestive: Anorexia, gastric irritation, nausea, vomiting, cramping, diarrhea, constipation, jaundice (intrahepatic cholestatic jaundice), pancreatitis, sialadenitis.
Hematologic: Leukopenia, agranulocytosis, thrombocytopenia, aplastic anemia, hemolytic anemia.
Metabolic: Hyperglycemia, glycosuria, hyperuricemia, electrolyte imbalance (See PRECAUTIONS).
Musculoskeletal: Muscle spasm.
Nervous System/Psychiatric: Dizziness, vertigo, paresthesias, headache, restlessness.
Special Senses: Transient blurred vision, xanthopsia.
Hypersensitivity: Purpura, photosensitivity, rash, urticaria, necrotizing angiitis (vasculitis and cutaneous vasculitis), fever, respiratory distress including pneumonitis and pulmonary edema, anaphylactic reactions.
Whenever adverse reactions are moderate or severe, thiazide dosage should be reduced or therapy withdrawn.

Dosage and Administration

Dosage: As determined by individual titration (see box warning).
The usual dosage is 1 tablet of ALDORIL 15, ALDORIL 25, ALDORIL D30, or ALDORIL D50 two or three times a day in the first 48 hours. The daily dosage then may be increased or decreased, preferably at intervals of not less than two days, until an adequate response is achieved. To minimize the sedation associated with methyldopa, start dosage increases in the evening. By adjustment of dosage, morning hypotension may be prevented without sacrificing control of afternoon blood pressure.
When ALDORIL is given to patients on other antihypertensives, the dose of these agents may need to be adjusted to effect a smooth transition. When ALDORIL is given with antihypertensives other than thiazides, the initial dosage of methyldopa should be limited to 500 mg daily in divided doses.
Although occasional patients have responded to higher doses, the maximum recommended daily dosage is 3.0 g of methyldopa and 100 to 200 mg of hydrochlorothiazide. Once an effective dosage range is attained, a smooth blood pressure response occurs in most patients in 12 to 24 hours. If ALDORIL alone does not adequately control blood pressure, additional methyldopa may be given separately to obtain the maximum blood pressure response.
Since both components of ALDORIL have a relatively short duration of action, withdrawal is followed by return of hypertension usually within 48 hours. This is not complicated by an overshoot of blood pressure.
Occasionally tolerance may occur, usually between the second and third month of therapy. Increasing the dosage of either methyldopa or hydrochlorothiazide separately or together frequently will restore effective control of blood pressure.
Methyldopa is largely excreted by the kidney and patients with impaired renal function may respond to smaller doses of ALDORIL. Syncope in older patients may be related to an increased sensitivity and advanced arteriosclerotic vascular disease. This may be avoided by lower doses.

How Supplied

No. 3294—Tablets ALDORIL 15 are salmon, round, film coated tablets, coded MSD 423. Each tablet contains 250 mg of methyldopa and 15 mg of hydrochlorothiazide. They are supplied as follows:
NDC 0006-0423-68 bottles of 100
NDC 0006-0423-28 unit dose packages of 100
NDC 0006-0423-82 bottles of 1000.
Shown in Product Identification Section, page 420
No. 3295—Tablets ALDORIL 25 are white, round, film coated tablets, coded MSD 456. Each tablet contains 250 mg of methyldopa and 25 mg of hydrochlorothiazide. They are supplied as follows:
NDC 0006-0456-68 bottles of 100
NDC 0006-0456-28 unit dose packages of 100
NDC 0006-0456-82 bottles of 1000.
Shown in Product Identification Section, page 420
No. 3362—Tablets ALDORIL D30 are salmon, oval, film coated tablets, coded MSD 694. Each tablet contains 500 mg of methyldopa and 30 mg of hydrochlorothiazide. They are supplied as follows:
NDC 0006-0694-68 bottles of 100.
Shown in Product Identification Section, page 420
No. 3363—Tablets ALDORIL D50 are white, oval, film coated tablets, coded MSD 935. Each tablet contains 500 mg of methyldopa and 50 mg of hydrochlorothiazide. They are supplied as follows:
NDC 0006-0935-68 bottles of 100.
Shown in Product Identification Section, page 420
A.H.F.S. Category: 24:08
DC 6086032   Issued May 1984
COPYRIGHT © MERCK & CO., INC., 1984
All rights reserved

ANTIVENIN   R
(latrodectus mactans), MSD, U.S.P.
Black Widow Spider Antivenin
Equine Origin

Indications

Antivenin (Latrodectus mactans), MSD is used to treat patients with symptoms due to bites by the black widow spider (Latrodectus mactans). Early use of the Antivenin is emphasized for prompt relief.
Local muscular cramps begin from 15 minutes to several hours after the bite which usually produces a sharp pain similar to that caused by puncture with a needle. The exact sequence of symptoms depends somewhat on the location of the bite. The venom acts on the myoneural junctions or on the nerve endings, causing an ascending motor paralysis or destruction of the peripheral nerve endings. The groups of muscles most frequently affected at first are those of the thigh, shoulder, and back. After a varying length of time, the pain becomes more severe, spreading to the abdomen, and weakness and tremor usually develop. The abdominal muscles assume a boardlike rigidity, but tenderness is slight. Respiration is thoracic. The patient is restless and anxious. Feeble pulse, cold, clammy skin, labored breathing and speech, light stupor, and delirium may occur. Convulsions also may occur, particularly in small children. The temperature may be normal or slightly elevated. Urinary retention, shock, cyanosis, nausea and vomiting, insomnia, and cold sweats also have been reported. The syndrome following the bite of the black widow spider may be confused easily with any medical or surgical condition with acute abdominal symptoms.
The symptoms of black widow spider bite increase in severity for several hours, perhaps a day, and then very slowly become less severe, gradually passing off in the course of two or three days except in fatal cases. Residual symptoms such as general weakness, tingling, nervousness, and transient muscle spasm may persist for weeks or months after recovery from the acute stage.
If possible, the patient should be hospitalized. Other additional measures giving greatest relief are prolonged warm baths and intravenous injection of 10 ml of 10 percent solution of calcium gluconate repeated as necessary to control muscle pain. Morphine also may be required to control pain. Barbiturates may be used for extreme restlessness. However, as the venom is a neurotoxin, it can cause respiratory paralysis. This must be borne in mind when considering use of morphine or a barbiturate. Adrenocorticosteroids have been used with varying degrees of success. Supportive therapy is indicated by the condition of the patient. Local treatment of the site of the bite is of no value. Nothing is gained by applying a tourniquet or by attempting to remove venom from the site of the bite by incision and suction.
In otherwise healthy individuals between the ages of 16 and 60, the use of Antivenin may be deferred and treatment with muscle relaxants may be considered.

Precautions

Prior to treatment with any product prepared from horse serum, a careful review of the patient's history should be taken emphasizing prior exposure to horse serum or any allergies. Serious sickness and even death could result from the use of horse serum in a sensitive patient. A skin or conjunctival test should be performed prior to administration of Antivenin.

Skin test: Inject into (not under) the skin not more than 0.02 ml of the test material (1:10 dilution of normal horse serum in physiologic saline). Evaluate result in 10 minutes. A positive reaction is an urticarial wheal surrounded by a zone of erythema. A control test using Sodium Chloride Injection facilitates interpretation of the results.

Conjunctival test: For adults instill into the conjunctival sac one drop of a 1:10 dilution of horse serum and for children one drop of 1:100 dilution. Itching of the eye and reddening of the conjunctiva indicate a positive reaction, usually within 10 minutes.

Patients should be observed for serum sickness for an average of 8 to 12 days following administration of Antivenin.

Desensitization should be attempted only when the administration of Antivenin is considered necessary to save life. Epinephrine must be available in case of untoward reaction.

Desensitization: If the history is positive or the results of the sensitivity tests are mildly or questionably positive, Antivenin should be administered as follows to reduce the risk of an immediate severe allergic reaction:

1. In separate sterile vials or syringes prepare 1:10 or 1:100 dilutions of Antivenin in Sodium Chloride for Injection.
2. Allow at least 15 but preferably 30 minutes between injections and only proceed with the next dose if no reactions occurred following the previous dose.
3. Using a tuberculin syringe, inject subcutaneously 0.1, 0.2 and 0.5 ml of the 1:100 dilution at 15 or 30 minute intervals; repeat with the 1:10 dilution, and finally the undiluted Antivenin.
4. If there is a reaction after any of the injections, place a tourniquet proximal to the sites of injection and administer epinephrine, 1:1000 (0.3 to 1.0 ml subcutaneously, 0.05 to 0.1 ml intravenously), proximal to the tourniquet or into another extremity. Wait at least 30 minutes before giving another injection of Antivenin, the amount of which should be the same as the last one not evoking a reaction.
5. If no reaction has occurred after 0.5 ml of undiluted Antivenin has been given, it is probably safe to continue the dose at 15 minute intervals until the entire dose has been injected.

Method of Preparation

Antivenin (Latrodectus mactans), MSD is prepared from the blood serum of horses immunized against the venom of the black widow spider.

Each vial contains not less than 6000 Antivenin units. One unit of Antivenin will neutralize one average mouse lethal dose of black widow spider venom when the Antivenin and the venom are injected simultaneously in mice under suitable conditions.

Using a sterile syringe, remove from the accompanying vial 2.5 ml of Sterile Diluent for Antivenin and inject into the vial of Antivenin. With the needle still in the rubber stopper, shake the vial to dissolve the contents completely.

Dosage and Administration

The dose for adults and children is the entire contents of a restored vial (2.5 ml) of Antivenin. It may be given intramuscularly, preferably in the region of the anterolateral thigh so that a tourniquet may be applied in the event of a systemic reaction. Symptoms usually subside in 1 to 3 hours. Although one dose of Antivenin usually is adequate, a second dose may be necessary in some cases. Antivenin also may be given intravenously in 10 to 50 ml of saline solution over a 15 minute period. It is the preferred route in severe cases, or when the patient is under 12, or in shock. One restored vial usually is enough.

How Supplied

No. 4084—Antivenin (Latrodectus mactans), MSD equine origin is supplied in a vial containing not less than 6000 Antivenin units. Thimerosal (mercury derivative) 1:10,000 is added as preservative, NDC 0006-4084-00. A 2.5 ml vial of Sterile Diluent for Antivenin is included. Also supplied is a 1 ml vial of normal horse serum (1:10 dilution) for sensitivity testing. Thimerosal (mercury derivative) 1:10,000 is added as preservative.

A.H.F.S. Category: 80:04
DC 6145211   Issued April 1975

AQUAMEPHYTON® Injection   ℞
(phytonadione, MSD), U.S.P.
Aqueous Colloidal Solution of Vitamin K_1

WARNING—INTRAVENOUS USE

Severe reactions, including fatalities, have occurred during and immediately after INTRAVENOUS injection of AquaMEPHYTON® (Phytonadione, MSD), even when precautions have been taken to dilute the AquaMEPHYTON and to avoid rapid infusion. Typically these severe reactions have resembled hypersensitivity or anaphylaxis, including shock and cardiac and/or respiratory arrest. Some patients have exhibited these severe reactions on receiving AquaMEPHYTON for the first time. Therefore the INTRAVENOUS route should be restricted to those situations where other routes are not feasible and the serious risk involved is considered justified.

Description

AquaMEPHYTON injection is a yellow, sterile, aqueous colloidal solution of vitamin K_1, available for injection by the intravenous, intramuscular, and subcutaneous routes. Each milliliter contains:
Phytonadione ....2 mg or 10 mg
Inactive ingredients:
  Polyoxyethylated fatty acid
  derivative ....70 mg
  Dextrose ....37.5 mg
  Water for Injection, q.s. ....1 ml
Added as preservative:
  Benzyl alcohol 0.9%

Actions

AquaMEPHYTON aqueous colloidal solution of vitamin K_1 for parenteral injection, possesses the same type and degree of activity as does naturally-occurring vitamin K, which is necessary for the production via the liver of active prothrombin (factor II), proconvertin (factor VII), plasma thromboplastin component (factor IX), and Stuart factor (factor X). The prothrombin test is sensitive to the levels of three of these four factors—II, VII, and X. The mechanism by which vitamin K promotes formation of these clotting factors in the liver is not known.

The action of the aqueous colloidal solution, when administered intravenously, is generally detectable within an hour or two and hemorrhage is usually controlled within 3 to 6 hours. A normal prothrombin level may often be obtained in 12 to 14 hours.

In the prophylaxis and treatment of hemorrhagic disease of the newborn, phytonadione has demonstrated a greater margin of safety than that of the water-soluble vitamin K analogues.

Indications

AquaMEPHYTON is indicated in the following coagulation disorders which are due to faulty formation of factors II, VII, IX and X when caused by vitamin K deficiency or interference with vitamin K activity.

AquaMEPHYTON injection is indicated in:
— anticoagulant-induced prothrombin deficiency;
— prophylaxis and therapy of hemorrhagic disease of the newborn;
— hypoprothrombinemia due to antibacterial therapy;
— hypoprothrombinemia secondary to factors limiting absorption or synthesis of vitamin K, e.g., obstructive jaundice, biliary fistula, sprue, ulcerative colitis, celiac disease, intestinal resection, cystic fibrosis of the pancreas, and regional enteritis;
— other drug-induced hypoprothrombinemia where it is definitely shown that the result is due to interference with vitamin K metabolism, e.g., salicylates.

Contraindication

Hypersensitivity to any component of this medication.

Warnings

Benzyl alcohol as a preservative in Bacteriostatic Sodium Chloride Injection has been associated with toxicity in newborns. Data are unavailable on the toxicity of other preservatives in this age group. There is no evidence to suggest that the small amount of benzyl alcohol contained in AquaMEPHYTON, when used as recommended, is associated with toxicity.

An immediate coagulant effect should not be expected after administration of phytonadione. It takes a minimum of 1 to 2 hours for measurable improvement in the prothrombin time. Whole blood or component therapy may also be necessary if bleeding is severe.

Phytonadione will not counteract the anticoagulant action of heparin.

When vitamin K_1 is used to correct excessive anticoagulant-induced hypoprothrombinemia, anticoagulant therapy still being indicated, the patient is again faced with the clotting hazards existing prior to starting the anticoagulant therapy. Phytonadione is not a clotting agent, but overzealous therapy with vitamin K_1 may restore conditions which originally permitted thromboembolic phenomena. Dosage should be kept as low as possible, and prothrombin time should be checked regularly as clinical conditions indicate.

Repeated large doses of vitamin K are not warranted in liver disease if the response to initial use of the vitamin is unsatisfactory. Failure to respond to vitamin K may indicate that the condition being treated is inherently unresponsive to vitamin K. Reproduction studies have not been performed in animals. There is no adequate information of whether this drug may affect fertility in human males or females or have a teratogenic potential or other adverse effect on the fetus.

Precautions

Protect from light at all times.
Temporary resistance to prothrombin-depressing anticoagulants may result, especially when larger doses of phytonadione are used. If relatively large doses have been employed, it may be necessary when reinstituting anticoagulant therapy to use somewhat larger doses of the prothrombin-depressing anticoagulant, or to use one which acts on a different principle, such as heparin sodium.

Adverse Reactions

Deaths have occurred after intravenous administration. (See Box Warning at beginning of circular.)

Transient "flushing sensations" and "peculiar" sensations of taste have been observed, as well as rare instances of dizziness, rapid and weak pulse,

Continued on next page

Information on the Merck Sharp & Dohme products listed on these pages is the full prescribing information from product circulars in use November 1, 1984.

Merck Sharp & Dohme—Cont.

profuse sweating, brief hypotension, dyspnea, and cyanosis.

Pain, swelling, and tenderness at the injection site may occur. The possibility of allergic sensitivity, including an anaphylactoid reaction, should be kept in mind.

Rarely, after repeated injections, reactions resembling erythema perstans have been reported.

Hyperbilirubinemia has been observed in the newborn following administration of phytonadione. This has occurred rarely and primarily with doses above those recommended.

Dosage and Administration

Whenever possible, AquaMEPHYTON should be given by the subcutaneous or intramuscular route. When intravenous administration is considered unavoidable, the drug should be injected very slowly, not exceeding 1 mg per minute.

The human minimum daily requirements for vitamin K have not been established officially but they have been estimated to be 1 to 5 mcg/kg of body weight for infants and 0.03 mcg/kg for adults. Usually, the dietary abundance of vitamin K will satisfy these requirements, except during the first five to eight days of the neonatal period.

Anticoagulant-Induced
Prothrombin Deficiency

To correct excessively prolonged prothrombin time caused by oral anticoagulant therapy—2.5 to 10 mg or up to 25 mg initially is recommended. In rare instances 50 mg may be required. Frequency and amount of subsequent doses should be determined by prothrombin time response or clinical condition. If in 6 to 8 hours after parenteral administration the prothrombin time has not been shortened satisfactorily, the dose should be repeated.

In the event of shock or excessive blood loss, the use of whole blood or component therapy is indicated.

Smaller doses are recommended for patients being treated with the shorter-acting anticoagulants, and for those in need of continued anticoagulant therapy. The smallest effective dose should be sought to obviate the possibility of temporary refractoriness to further anticoagulant therapy, and to avoid lowering the prothrombin time too far below that indicating an effective level of anticoagulant activity.

Larger doses are recommended for patients on the longer-acting anticoagulants, for those with severe bleeding, and for those not needing further anticoagulant therapy. Although more than 25 mg may be necessary and a dose may need to be repeated, these courses of action are indicated *only rarely*.

Prophylaxis and Treatment
of Hemorrhagic Disease of the Newborn
Prophylaxis

The Committee on Nutrition of the American Academy of Pediatrics recommends that vitamin K_1 be given to the newborn. A single intramuscular dose of AquaMEPHYTON 0.5 to 1.0 mg is recommended. Although less desirable, AquaMEPHYTON 1 to 5 mg may be given to the mother 12 to 24 hours before delivery.

Treatment

AquaMEPHYTON 1.0 mg should be given either subcutaneously or intramuscularly. Higher doses may be necessary if the mother has been receiving oral anticoagulants.

Empiric administration of vitamin K_1 should not replace proper laboratory evaluation of the coagulation mechanism. A prompt response (shortening of the prothrombin time in 2 to 4 hours) following administration of vitamin K_1 is usually diagnostic of hemorrhagic disease of the newborn, and failure to respond indicates another diagnosis or coagulation disorder.

Whole blood or component therapy may be indicated if bleeding is excessive. This therapy, however, does not correct the underlying disorder and AquaMEPHYTON should be given concurrently.

Hypoprothrombinemia Due to
Other Causes

A dosage of 2.5 to 25 mg or more (rarely up to 50 mg) is recommended, the amount and route of administration depending upon the severity of the condition and response obtained.

If possible, discontinuation or reduction of the dosage of drugs interfering with coagulation mechanisms (such as salicylates, antibiotics) is suggested as an alternative to administering concurrent AquaMEPHYTON. The severity of the coagulation disorder should determine whether the immediate administration of AquaMEPHYTON is required in addition to discontinuation or reduction of interfering drugs.

Directions for Dilution

AquaMEPHYTON may be diluted with 0.9% Sodium Chloride Injection, 5% Dextrose Injection, or 5% Dextrose and Sodium Chloride Injection. Benzyl alcohol as a preservative has been associated with toxicity in newborns. *Therefore, all of the above diluents should be preservative-free* (See WARNINGS). *Other diluents should not be used.* When dilutions are indicated, administration should be started immediately after mixture with the diluent, and unused portions of the dilution should be discarded, as well as unused contents of the ampul.

How Supplied

Injection AquaMEPHYTON is a yellow, sterile, aqueous colloidal solution and is supplied in the following concentrations:

No. 7780—10 mg of vitamin K_1 per ml
NDC 0006-7780-64 boxes of 6–1 ml ampuls (6505-00-854-2499 10 mg 1.0 ml 6's)
NDC 0006-7780-66 boxes of 25–1 ml ampuls.
No. 7782—10 mg of vitamin K_1 per ml
NDC 0006-7782-30 in 2.5 ml multiple dose vials.
NDC 0006-7782-03 in 5 ml multiple dose vials.
No. 7784—1 mg of vitamin K_1 per 0.5 ml
NDC 0006-7784-33 boxes of 25–0.5 ml ampuls (6505-00-180-6372 1 mg 0.5 ml 25's).
A.H.F.S. Category: 88:24
DC 6136713   Issued June 1982

ARAMINE® Injection   ℞
(metaraminol bitartrate, MSD), U.S.P.

Description

Injection ARAMINE® (Metaraminol Bitartrate, MSD) is a sterile solution, each ml of which contains:

Metaraminol bitartrate equivalent to metaraminol..............................10.0 mg
Inactive ingredients:
Sodium chloride..............................4.4 mg
Water for Injection q.s. ad.......................1.0 ml
Methylparaben 0.15%, propylparaben 0.02%, and sodium bisulfite 0.2% added as preservatives.

Metaraminol bitartrate is the generic name for levo-1-(m-hydroxyphenyl)-2-amino-1-propanol hydrogen D-tartrate. Metaraminol bitartrate is a white, crystalline powder, freely soluble in water, slightly soluble in alcohol, and practically insoluble in chloroform and in ether.

Actions

ARAMINE is a potent sympathomimetic amine that increases both systolic and diastolic blood pressure.

The pressor effect of ARAMINE begins in 1 to 2 minutes after intravenous infusion, in about 10 minutes after intramuscular injection, and in 5 to 20 minutes after subcutaneous injection. The effect lasts from about 20 minutes to one hour. ARAMINE has a positive inotropic effect on the heart and a peripheral vasoconstrictor action.

Renal, coronary, and cerebral blood flow are a function of perfusion pressure and regional resistance. In most instances of cardiogenic shock, the beneficial effect of sympathomimetic amines is attributable to their positive inotropic effect. In patients with insufficient or failing vasoconstriction, there is additional advantage to the peripheral action of ARAMINE, but in most patients with shock, vasoconstriction is adequate and any further increase is unnecessary. Therefore, blood flow to vital organs may decrease with ARAMINE if regional resistance increases excessively.

The pressor effect of ARAMINE is decreased but not reversed by alpha-adrenergic blocking agents. Primary or secondary fall in blood pressure and tachyphylactic response to repeated use are uncommon.

INDICATIONS

Based on a review of this drug by the National Academy of Sciences-National Research Council and/or other information, FDA has classified the indications as follows:

Effective: ARAMINE is indicated for prevention and treatment of the acute hypotensive state occurring with spinal anesthesia. Adjunctive treatment of hypotension due to hemorrhage; reactions to medications; surgical complications; and shock associated with brain damage due to trauma or tumor.

"Probably" effective: It may also be useful as an adjunct in the treatment of hypotension due to cardiogenic shock or septicemia.

Final classification of the less-than-effective indications requires further investigation.

Contraindications

Use of ARAMINE with cyclopropane or halothane anesthesia should be avoided, unless clinical circumstances demand such use.

Hypersensitivity to any component of this product.

Precautions

Caution should be used to avoid excessive blood pressure response. Rapidly induced hypertensive responses have been reported to cause acute pulmonary edema, arrhythmias, and cardiac arrest. ARAMINE should be used with caution in digitalized patients, since the combination of digitalis and sympathomimetic amines is capable of causing ectopic arrhythmic activity.

Patients with cirrhosis should be treated with caution, with adequate restoration of electrolytes if diuresis ensues. Fatal ventricular arrhythmia has been reported in one patient with Laennec's cirrhosis while receiving metaraminol bitartrate. In several instances, ventricular extrasystoles that appeared during infusion of this vasopressor subsided promptly when the rate of infusion was reduced.

With the prolonged action of ARAMINE, a cumulative effect is possible, and with an excessive vasopressor response there may be a prolonged elevation of blood pressure even with discontinuation of therapy. Monoamine oxidase inhibitors have been reported to potentiate the action of sympathomimetic amines.

When vasopressor amines are used for long periods, the resulting vasoconstriction may prevent adequate expansion of circulating volume and may cause perpetuation of the shock state. There is evidence that plasma volume may be reduced in all types of shock, and that the measurement of central venous pressure is useful in assessing the adequacy of the circulating blood volume. Therefore, blood or plasma volume expanders should be employed when the principal reason for hypotension or shock is decreased circulating volume.

Because of its vasoconstrictor effect ARAMINE should be given with caution in heart or thyroid disease, hypertension, or diabetes. Sympathomimetic amines may provoke a relapse in patients with a history of malaria.

Adverse Reactions

Sympathomimetic amines, including ARAMINE, may cause sinus or ventricular tachycardia, or other arrhythmias, especially in patients with myocardial infarction. See also PRECAUTIONS. Also, in patients with a history of malaria, these compounds may provoke a relapse.

Abscess formation, tissue necrosis, or sloughing rarely may follow the use of ARAMINE. In choosing the site of injection, it is important to avoid those areas recognized as *not* suitable for use of any pressor agent and to discontinue the infusion immediately if infiltration or thrombosis occurs. Although the physician may be forced by the urgent nature of the patient's condition to choose injection sites that are not recognized as suitable, he should, when possible, use the preferred areas of injection. The larger veins of the antecubital fossa or the thigh are preferred to veins in the dorsum of the hand or ankle veins, particularly in patients with peripheral vascular disease, diabetes mellitus, Buerger's disease, or conditions with coexistent hypercoagulability.

Dosage and Administration

ARAMINE may be given intramuscularly, subcutaneously, or intravenously, the route depending on the nature and severity of the indication.

Allow at least 10 minutes to elapse before increasing the dose because the maximum effect is not immediately apparent. When the vasopressor is discontinued, observe the patient carefully as the effect of the drug tapers off, so that therapy can be reinitiated promptly if the blood pressure falls too rapidly. The response to vasopressors may be poor in patients with coexistent shock and acidosis. Established methods of shock management, such as blood or fluid replacement when indicated, and other measures directed to the specific cause of the shock state also should be used.

Intramuscular or Subcutaneous Injection (for prevention of hypotension—see INDICATIONS):
The recommended dose is 2 to 10 mg (0.2 to 1 ml). As with other agents given subcutaneously, only the preferred sites of injection, as set forth in standard texts, should be used.

Intravenous Infusion (for adjunctive treatment of hypotension—see INDICATIONS):
The recommended dose is 15 to 100 mg (1.5 to 10 ml) in 500 ml of Sodium Chloride Injection or 5% Dextrose Injection, adjusting the rate of infusion to maintain the blood pressure at the desired level. Higher concentrations of ARAMINE, 150 to 500 mg per 500 ml of infusion fluid, have been used. If the patient needs more saline or dextrose solution at a rate of flow that would provide an excessive dose of the vasopressor, the recommended volume of infusion fluid (500 ml) should be increased accordingly. ARAMINE may also be added to *less* than 500 ml of infusion fluid if a smaller volume is desired.

Compatibility Information
In addition to Sodium Chloride Injection* and Dextrose Injection 5%*, the following infusion solutions were found physically and chemically compatible with injection ARAMINE when 5 ml of injection ARAMINE, 10 mg/ml (metaraminol equivalent), was added to 500 ml of infusion solution: Ringer's Injection*, Lactated Ringer's Injection*, Dextran 6% in Saline†, Normosol®-R pH 7.4†, and Normosol®-M in D5-W†.

When injection ARAMINE is mixed with an infusion solution, sterile precautions should be observed. Since infusion solutions generally do not contain preservatives, mixtures should be used within 24 hours.

Direct Intravenous Injection: In severe shock, where time is of great importance, this agent should be given by direct intravenous injection. The suggested dose is 0.5 to 5 mg (0.05 to 0.5 ml), followed by an infusion of 15 to 100 mg (1.5 to 10 ml) in 500 ml of infusion fluid as described previously.

If necessary, vials may be sterilized by autoclaving or by immersion in a sterilizing solution.

How Supplied

No. 3222X—Injection ARAMINE 1%, containing metaraminol bitartrate equivalent to 10 mg of metaraminol per ml, is a clear, colorless solution and is supplied as follows:
NDC 0006-3222-10 in 10 ml vials (6505-00-753-9601 10 ml vial)
NDC 0006-3222-17 in 12 × 1 ml vials.

*U.S.P.
†Product of Abbott Laboratories
A.H.F.S. Category: 12:12
DC 6019019   Issued December 1977

ATTENUVAX®
(measles virus vaccine, live, attenuated, MSD), U.S.P.
(More Attenuated Enders' Line)
Prepared in Cell Cultures of Chick Embryo

Description

ATTENUVAX® (Measles Virus Vaccine, Live, Attenuated, MSD) is a live virus vaccine for immunization against measles (rubeola).

ATTENUVAX is a lyophilized preparation of a more attenuated line of measles virus derived from Enders' attenuated Edmonston strain. The further modification of the virus in ATTENUVAX was achieved in the Merck Institute for Therapeutic Research by multiple passage of Edmonston virus in cell cultures of chick embryo at low temperature.

When reconstituted as directed, the dose for injection contains not less than the equivalent of 1,000 TCID$_{50}$ (tissue culture infectious doses) of measles virus vaccine expressed in terms of the assigned titer of the FDA Reference Measles Virus. Each dose also contains approximately 25 mcg of neomycin.

Actions

ATTENUVAX produces a modified measles infection in susceptible persons. Fever and rash may appear. Extensive clinical trials have demonstrated that ATTENUVAX is highly immunogenic and generally well tolerated. A single injection of the vaccine has been shown to induce measles hemagglutination-inhibiting (HI) antibodies in 97 percent or more of susceptible persons. Vaccine-induced antibody levels have been shown to persist for at least eight years without substantial decline. If the present pattern continues, it will provide a basis for the expectation that immunity following the vaccine will be permanent. However, continued surveillance will be required to demonstrate this point.

Indications

ATTENUVAX is recommended for active immunization of children 15 months of age or older against measles (rubeola). A booster is not needed. Infants who are less than 15 months of age may fail to respond to the vaccine due to presence in the circulation of residual measles antibody of maternal origin; the younger the infant, the lower the likelihood of seroconversion. In geographically isolated or other relatively inaccessible populations for whom immunization programs are logistically difficult, and in population groups in which natural measles infection may occur in a significant proportion of infants before 15 months of age, it may be desirable to give the vaccine to infants at an earlier age. The advantage of early protection must be weighed against the chance for failure of response; infants vaccinated under these conditions should be revaccinated after reaching 15 months of age.

Children for whom ATTENUVAX is strongly recommended include those living in schools, orphanages, and similar institutions. It is also recommended for children with inactive tuberculosis or active tuberculosis under treatment, as well as for those with chronic diseases such as cystic fibrosis, heart disease, asthma, and other chronic pulmonary diseases, to minimize the risk of serious complications of natural measles.

ATTENUVAX given immediately after exposure to natural measles may provide some protection. If, however, the vaccine is given a few days before exposure, substantial protection may be provided. Ordinarily, adults need not be immunized, since most are immune to measles. However, vaccination may be advisable for high school and college persons in epidemic situations and for adults in isolated communities where measles is not endemic.

Revaccination: Children vaccinated before 12 months of age—particularly if vaccine was administered with immune serum globulin or measles immune globulin, a standardized globulin preparation—should be revaccinated with live measles vaccine at about 15 months of age for optimal protection.

Based on available evidence, there is no reason to routinely revaccinate children originally vaccinated when 12 months of age or older. The decision to revaccinate should be based on evaluation of each individual case.

Despite the risk of local reaction (see ADVERSE REACTIONS), children who have previously been given inactivated vaccine alone or followed by live vaccine within 3 months should be revaccinated with live vaccine to avoid the severe atypical form of natural measles that may occur.

Use with Other Live Virus Vaccines

There are no data available concerning simultaneous use of ATTENUVAX with monovalent or trivalent poliovirus vaccine, live, oral, or with killed poliovirus vaccines. However, serologic evidence shows that when M-M-R® (Measles, Mumps and Rubella Virus Vaccine, Live, MSD), containing the HPV-77 rubella strain, is given simultaneously with trivalent poliovirus vaccine, live, oral, antibody responses can be expected to be comparable to those which follow administration of the vaccines at different times. From this it follows that when ATTENUVAX is given simultaneously with either monovalent or trivalent poliovirus vaccine, live, oral, MERUVAX® II (Rubella Virus Vaccine, Live, MSD) and/or MUMPSVAX® (Mumps Virus Vaccine, Live, MSD), antibody responses can be expected to be comparable to those which follow administration of the vaccines at different times.

Contraindications

ATTENUVAX is contraindicated in the following conditions:

Hypersensitivity to neomycin (each dose of reconstituted vaccine contains approximately 25 mcg of neomycin).

Any febrile respiratory illness, or other active febrile infection.

Active untreated tuberculosis.

Patients receiving therapy with ACTH, corticosteroids, irradiation, alkylating agents or antimetabolites.

This contraindication does not apply to patients who are receiving corticosteroids as replacement therapy, e.g., for Addison's disease.

Individuals with blood dyscrasias, leukemia, lymphomas of any type, or other malignant neoplasms affecting the bone marrow or lymphatic systems.

Primary immuno-deficiency states, including cellular immune deficiencies, hypogammaglobulinemic and dysgammaglobulinemic states.

Hypersensitivity to Eggs, Chicken, or Chicken Feathers

This vaccine is essentially devoid of potentially allergenic substances derived from host tissues (chick embryo).* However, because the attenuated virus in this vaccine is propagated in cell cultures of chick embryo, there is a potential risk of hyper-

Continued on next page

Information on the Merck Sharp & Dohme products listed on these pages is the full prescribing information from product circulars in use November 1, 1984.

Merck Sharp & Dohme—Cont.

sensitivity reactions in patients allergic to eggs, chicken, or chicken feathers. Widespread use of the vaccine for more than a decade has resulted in only rare, isolated reports of minor allergic reactions attributed to allergens of this kind, possibly related to the vaccine. Significantly, when children with known allergies to eggs, chicken, and chicken feathers were given a similarly prepared vaccine in a clinical study, none experienced reactions other than those reactions previously observed in nonallergic children.

Pregnancy

The effects of ATTENUVAX on fetal development are unknown at this time. Therefore, live attenuated measles virus vaccine should not be given to persons known to be pregnant; furthermore, pregnancy should be avoided for three months following vaccination.

Reports have indicated that contracting of natural measles during pregnancy enhances fetal risk. Increased rates of spontaneous abortion, stillbirth, congenital defects and prematurity have been observed subsequent to natural measles during pregnancy. There are no adequate studies of the attenuated (vaccine) strain of measles virus in pregnancy. However, it would be prudent to assume that the vaccine strain of virus is also capable of inducing adverse fetal effects for up to three months following vaccination.

Vaccine administration to post-pubertal females entails a potential for inadvertent immunization during pregnancy. Theoretical risks involved should be weighed against the risks that measles poses to the unimmunized adolescent or adult. Advisory committees reviewing this matter have recommended vaccination of post-pubertal females who are presumed to be susceptible to measles and not known to be pregnant. If a measles exposure occurs during pregnancy, one should consider the possibility of providing temporary passive immunity through the administration of immune serum globulin (human).

Precautions

For subcutaneous administration; *do not give intravenously.*
Epinephrine should be available for immediate use should an anaphylactoid reaction occur.
ATTENUVAX may be given simultaneously with monovalent or trivalent poliovirus vaccine, live, oral, with MERUVAX$_{II}$ (Rubella Virus Vaccine, Live, MSD) and/or MUMPSVAX (Mumps Virus Vaccine, Live, MSD). ATTENUVAX should not be given less than one month before or after administration of other live virus vaccines.
Due caution should be employed in administration of measles vaccine to children with a history of febrile convulsions, or cerebral injury, or of any other condition in which stress due to fever should be avoided. The physician should be alert to the temperature elevation which may occur following vaccination.
The occurrence of thrombocytopenia and purpura associated with live virus measles vaccines has been extremely rare.
Vaccination should be deferred for at least 3 months following blood or plasma transfusions, or administration of human immune serum globulin.
It has been reported that attenuated measles virus vaccine, live, may result in a temporary depression of tuberculin skin sensitivity. Therefore, if a tuberculin test is to be done, it should be administered either before or simultaneously with ATTENUVAX.
Children under treatment for tuberculosis have not experienced exacerbation of the disease when immunized with live measles virus vaccine; no studies have been reported to date of the effect of measles virus vaccines on untreated tuberculous children.

Adverse Reactions

Because of the slightly acidic pH (6.2-6.6) of the vaccine, patients may complain of burning and/or stinging of short duration at the injection site.
Occasional
Moderate fever [101-102.9°F (38.3-39.4°C)] may occur during the month after vaccination. Generally, fever, rash, or both appear between the 5th and the 12th days. Rash, when it occurs, is usually minimal, but rarely may be generalized.
Less Common
High fever [over 103°F (39.4°C)].
Rare
Reactions at injection site. Allergic reactions such as wheal and flare at the injection site or urticaria have been reported.
Children developing fever may, on rare occasions, exhibit febrile convulsions.
Experience from more than 80 million doses of all live measles vaccines given in the U.S. through 1975 indicates that significant central nervous system reactions such as encephalitis and encephalopathy, occurring within 30 days after vaccination, have been temporally associated with measles vaccine approximately once for every million doses. In no case has it been shown that reactions were actually caused by vaccine. The Center for Disease Control has pointed out that "a certain number of cases of encephalitis may be expected to occur in a large childhood population in a defined period of time even when no vaccines are administered." However, the data suggest the possibility that some of these cases may have been caused by measles vaccines. The risk of such serious neurological disorders following live measles virus vaccine administration remains far less than that for encephalitis and encephalopathy with natural measles (one per thousand reported cases).
There have been isolated reports of ocular palsies and Guillain-Barre syndrome occurring after immunization with vaccines containing live attenuated measles virus. The ocular palsies have occurred approximately 3–24 days following vaccination. No definite causal relationship has been established between either of these events and vaccination.
There have been reports of subacute sclerosing panencephalitis (SSPE) in children who did not have a history of natural measles but did receive measles vaccine. Some of these cases may have resulted from unrecognized measles in the first year of life or possibly from the measles vaccination. Based on estimated nationwide measles vaccine distribution, the association of SSPE cases to measles vaccination is about one case per million vaccine doses distributed. This is far less than the association with natural measles, 5–10 cases of SSPE per million cases of measles. The results of a retrospective case-controlled study conducted by the Center for Disease Control suggest that the overall effect of measles vaccine has been to protect against SSPE by preventing measles with its inherent higher risk of SSPE.
Local reactions characterized by marked swelling, redness and vesiculation at the injection site of attenuated live virus measles vaccines have occurred in children who have previously received killed measles vaccine.

Dosage and Administration

After suitable cleansing of the immunization site, inject the total volume of reconstituted vaccine subcutaneously, preferably into the outer aspect of the upper arm. Do not inject intravenously.
The dosage of vaccine is the same for all patients.
Do not give immune serum globulin (ISG) concurrently with ATTENUVAX.
CAUTION: A sterile syringe free of preservatives, antiseptics, and detergents should be used for each injection of the vaccine because these substances may inactivate the live virus vaccine. A 25 gauge, ⅝″ needle is recommended.

Shipment, Storage and Reconstitution

During shipment, to insure that there is no loss of potency, the vaccine must be maintained at a temperature of 10°C (50°F) or less.
Prior to reconstitution, store the vaccine in a refrigerator at 2–8° C (35.6–46.4° F). *Protect from light.*
The reconstituted vaccine should be protected from light, since such exposure may inactivate the virus.
To reconstitute, withdraw the entire volume of diluent into the syringe to be used for reconstitution. Inject all the diluent in the syringe into the vial of lyophilized vaccine. Agitate to ensure thorough mixing. Draw the entire volume of reconstituted vaccine into a syringe. Each dose of ATTENUVAX contains not less than 1,000 TCID$_{50}$ (tissue culture infectious doses) of measles virus vaccine expressed in terms of the assigned titer of the FDA Reference Measles Virus.
It is important to use a separate sterile syringe and needle for each individual patient to prevent transmission of hepatitis B virus and other infectious agents from one person to another.
Use only the diluent supplied and reconstitute ATTENUVAX just before using. Protect the vaccine from light at all times. If not used immediately, return the reconstituted vaccine to a dark place at 2–8° C (35.6–46.4° F). Discard if not used within eight hours.
Color: The color of the vaccine when reconstituted is yellow. It is acceptable for use only if clear.

How Supplied

No. 4709—ATTENUVAX is supplied as a single-dose vial of lyophilized vaccine, NDC 0006-4709-00, and a vial of diluent.
No. 4589X/4309—ATTENUVAX is supplied as follows: (1) a box of 10 single-dose vials of lyophilized vaccine (package A), NDC 0006-4589-00; and (2) a box of 10 vials of diluent (package B). To conserve refrigerator space, the diluent may be stored separately at room temperature.

A.H.F.S. Category: 80:12
DC 7075505   Issued February 1983
COPYRIGHT © MERCK & CO., INC., 1983
All rights reserved

BENEMID® Tablets ℞
(probenecid, MSD), U.S.P.

Description

Probenecid is the generic name for 4-[(dipropylamino)sulfonyl] benzoic acid (molecular weight 285.36).
Probenecid is a white or nearly white, fine, crystalline powder. Probenecid is soluble in dilute alkali, in alcohol, in chloroform, and in acetone; it is practically insoluble in water and in dilute acids.

Actions

BENEMID® (Probenecid, MSD) is a uricosuric and renal tubular blocking agent. It inhibits the tubular reabsorption of urate, thus increasing the urinary excretion of uric acid and decreasing serum urate levels. Effective uricosuria reduces the miscible urate pool, retards urate deposition, and promotes resorption of urate deposits.
BENEMID inhibits the tubular secretion of penicillin and usually increases penicillin plasma levels by any route the antibiotic is given. A 2-fold to 4-fold elevation has been demonstrated for various penicillins.
BENEMID also has been reported to inhibit the renal transport of many other compounds including aminohippuric acid (PAH), aminosalicylic acid (PAS), indomethacin, sodium iodomethamate and related iodinated organic acids, 17-ketosteroids, pantothenic acid, phenolsulfonphthalein (PSP), sulfonamides, and sulfonylureas. See also DRUG INTERACTIONS.
BENEMID decreases both hepatic and renal excretion of sulfobromophthalein (BSP). The tubular reabsorption of phosphorus is inhibited in

---

*Morbidity and Mortality Weekly Report 25 (44): 350, Nov. 12, 1976.

hypoparathyroid but not in euparathyroid individuals.
BENEMID does not influence plasma concentrations of salicylates, nor the excretion of streptomycin, chloramphenicol, chlortetracycline, oxytetracycline, or neomycin.

Indications

For treatment of the hyperuricemia associated with gout and gouty arthritis.
As an adjuvant to therapy with penicillin or with ampicillin, methicillin, oxacillin, cloxacillin, or nafcillin, for elevation and prolongation of plasma levels by whatever route the antibiotic is given.

Contraindications

Hypersensitivity to this product.
Children under 2 years of age.
Not recommended in persons with known blood dyscrasias or uric acid kidney stones.
Therapy with BENEMID should not be started until an acute gouty attack has subsided.

Warnings

Exacerbation of gout following therapy with BENEMID may occur; in such cases colchicine or other appropriate therapy is advisable.
BENEMID increases plasma concentrations of methotrexate in both animals and humans. In animal studies, increased methotrexate toxicity has been reported. If BENEMID is given with methotrexate, the dosage of methotrexate should be reduced and serum levels may need to be monitored.
In patients on BENEMID the use of salicylates in either small or large doses is contraindicated because it antagonizes the uricosuric action of BENEMID. The biphasic action of salicylates in the renal tubules accounts for the so-called "paradoxical effect" of uricosuric agents. In patients on BENEMID who require a mild analgesic agent the use of acetaminophen rather than small doses of salicylates would be preferred.
The appearance of hypersensitivity reactions requires cessation of therapy with BENEMID.
Use in Pregnancy: BENEMID crosses the placental barrier and appears in cord blood. The use of any drug in women of childbearing potential requires that the anticipated benefit be weighed against possible hazards.

Precautions

Hematuria, renal colic, costovertebral pain, and formation of uric acid stones associated with the use of BENEMID in gouty patients may be prevented by alkalization of the urine and a liberal fluid intake (*see* DOSAGE AND ADMINISTRATION). In these cases when alkali is administered, the acid-base balance of the patient should be watched.
Use with caution in patients with a history of peptic ulcer.
BENEMID has been used in patients with some renal impairment but dosage requirements may be increased. BENEMID may not be effective in chronic renal insufficiency particularly when the glomerular filtration rate is 30 ml/minute or less. Because of its mechanism of action, BENEMID is not recommended in conjunction with a penicillin in the presence of *known* renal impairment.
A reducing substance may appear in the urine of patients receiving BENEMID. This disappears with discontinuance of therapy. Suspected glycosuria should be confirmed by using a test specific for glucose.

Adverse Reactions

Headache, gastrointestinal symptoms (e.g., anorexia, nausea, vomiting), urinary frequency, hypersensitivity reactions (including anaphylaxis, dermatitis, pruritus, and fever), sore gums, flushing, dizziness, and anemia have occurred.

In gouty patients exacerbation of gout, and uric acid stones with or without hematuria, renal colic, or costovertebral pain, have been observed. Nephrotic syndrome, hepatic necrosis, and aplastic anemia occur rarely. Hemolytic anemia which in some instances could be related to genetic deficiency of glucose-6-phosphate dehydrogenase in red blood cells has been reported.

Drug Interactions

The use of salicylates antagonizes the uricosuric action of BENEMID (*see* WARNINGS). The uricosuric action of BENEMID is also antagonized by pyrazinamide.
BENEMID produces an insignificant increase in free sulfonamide plasma concentrations but a significant increase in total sulfonamide plasma levels. Since BENEMID decreases the renal excretion of conjugated sulfonamides, plasma concentrations of the latter should be determined from time to time when a sulfonamide and BENEMID are coadministered for prolonged periods. BENEMID may prolong or enhance the action of oral sulfonylureas and thereby increase the risk of hypoglycemia.
When BENEMID is given to patients receiving indomethacin, the plasma levels of indomethacin are likely to be increased. Therefore, a lower dosage of indomethacin may be required to produce a therapeutic effect, and increases in the dosage of indomethacin should be made cautiously and in small increments. BENEMID may increase plasma levels of rifampin. The clinical significance of this is not known.
In animals and in humans, BENEMID has been reported to increase plasma concentrations of methotrexate (*see* WARNINGS).
Falsely high readings for theophylline have been reported in an *in vitro* study, using the Schack and Waxler technic, when therapeutic concentrations of theophylline and BENEMID were added to human plasma.

Dosage and Administration

Gout
Therapy with BENEMID should not be *started* until an acute gouty attack has subsided. However, if an acute attack is precipitated *during* therapy, BENEMID may be continued without changing the dosage, and full therapeutic dosage of colchicine or other appropriate therapy should be given to control the acute attack.
The recommended adult dosage is 0.25 g (½ tablet of BENEMID) twice a day for one week, followed by 0.5 g (1 tablet) twice a day thereafter.
Some degree of renal impairment may be present in patients with gout. A daily dosage of 1 g may be adequate. However, if necessary, the daily dosage may be increased by 0.5 g increments every 4 weeks within tolerance (and usually not above 2 g per day) if symptoms of gouty arthritis are not controlled or the 24 hour uric acid excretion is not above 700 mg. As noted, BENEMID may not be effective in chronic renal insufficiency particularly when the glomerular filtration rate is 30 ml/minute or less.
Gastric intolerance may be indicative of overdosage, and may be corrected by decreasing the dosage.
As uric acid tends to crystallize out of an acid urine, a liberal fluid intake is recommended, as well as sufficient sodium bicarbonate (3 to 7.5 g daily) or potassium citrate (7.5 g daily) to maintain an alkaline urine (*see* PRECAUTIONS).
Alkalization of the urine is recommended until the serum urate level returns to normal limits and tophaceous deposits disappear, i.e., during the period when urinary excretion of uric acid is at a high level. Thereafter, alkalization of the urine and the usual restriction of purine-producing foods may be somewhat relaxed.
BENEMID should be continued at the dosage that will maintain normal serum urate levels. When acute attacks have been absent for 6 months or more and serum urate levels remain within normal limits, the daily dosage may be decreased by

0.5 g every 6 months. The maintenance dosage should not be reduced to the point where serum urate levels tend to rise.

BENEMID and Penicillin Therapy (General)
Adults:
The recommended dosage is 2 g (4 tablets of BENEMID) daily in divided doses. This dosage should be reduced in older patients in whom renal impairment may be present.
Children 2-14 years of age:
Initial dose: 25 mg/kg body weight (*or* 0.7 g/square meter body surface).
Maintenance dose: 40 mg/kg body weight (*or* 1.2 g/square meter body surface) per day, divided into 4 doses.
For children weighing more than 50 kg (110 lb) the adult dosage is recommended.
BENEMID is contraindicated in children under 2 years of age.
The PSP excretion test may be used to determine the effectiveness of BENEMID in retarding penicillin excretion and maintaining therapeutic levels. The renal clearance of PSP is reduced to about one-fifth the normal rate when dosage of BENEMID is adequate.
Penicillin Therapy (Gonorrhea)
[See table on next page].

How Supplied

No. 3337—Tablets BENEMID, 0.5 g, are yellow, capsule shaped, scored, film coated tablets, coded MSD 501. They are supplied as follows:
NDC 0006-0501-68 bottles of 100
(6505-00-104-9735 100's)
NDC 0006-0501-28 unit dose packages of 100.
NDC 0006-0501-82 bottles of 1000.
(6505-00-181-8387 1000's)
Shown in Product Identification Section, page 420
A.H.F.S. Category: 40:40
DC 6103916 Issued September 1978

BIAVAX® II ℞
(rubella and mumps virus vaccine, live, MSD), U.S.P.

Description

BIAVAX® II (Rubella and Mumps Virus Vaccine, Live, MSD) is a live virus vaccine for immunization against rubella (German measles) and mumps.
BIAVAX II is a lyophilized preparation of MERUVAX® II (Rubella Virus Vaccine, Live, MSD), the Wistar RA 27/3 strain of live attenuated rubella virus grown in human diploid cell (WI-38) culture; and MUMPSVAX® (Mumps Virus Vaccine, Live, MSD), the Jeryl Lynn (B level) mumps strain grown in cell cultures of chick embryo. The two viruses are mixed before being lyophilized. The product contains no preservative.
When reconstituted as directed, the dose for injection is 0.5 ml and contains not less than 1,000 $TCID_{50}$ (tissue culture infectious doses) of Rubella Virus Vaccine, Live, and 5,000 $TCID_{50}$ of Mumps Virus Vaccine, Live, expressed in terms of the assigned titer of the FDA Reference Rubella and Mumps Viruses. Each dose contains approximately 25 mcg of neomycin.

Actions

Clinical studies of 73 double seronegative children 12 months to 2 years of age demonstrated that BIAVAX II is highly immunogenic and generally well tolerated. In these studies, a single injection of the vaccine induced rubella hemagglutination inhibition (HI) antibodies in 100 percent, and

Continued on next page

Information on the Merck Sharp & Dohme products listed on these pages is the full prescribing information from product circulars in use November 1, 1984.

Merck Sharp & Dohme—Cont.

mumps neutralizing antibodies in 97 percent of the susceptible children.

The RA 27/3 rubella strain in BIAVAX II elicits higher immediate post-vaccination HI, complement-fixing and neutralizing antibody levels than other strains of rubella vaccine and has been shown to induce a broader profile of circulating antibodies including anti-theta and anti-iota precipitating antibodies. The RA 27/3 rubella strain immunologically simulates natural infection more closely than other rubella vaccine viruses. The increased levels and broader profile of antibodies produced by RA 27/3 strain rubella virus vaccine appear to correlate with greater resistance to subclinical reinfection with the wild virus, and provide greater confidence for lasting immunity.

Data relating to persistence of vaccine-induced antibodies are not available for BIAVAX II at this time; however, it is expected that the antibodies against rubella and mumps will be just as durable following administration of BIAVAX II as after the single vaccines given separately. Antibody levels after immunization with RA 27/3 strain rubella virus vaccine have persisted for at least six years without substantial decline, and for ten years after MUMPSVAX (Mumps Virus Vaccine, Live, MSD).

Indications

BIAVAX II is indicated for simultaneous immunization against rubella and mumps in children 12 months of age or older, and adults.

The vaccine is not recommended for infants younger than 12 months because they may retain maternal rubella and mumps neutralizing antibodies which may interfere with the immune response. Previously unimmunized children of susceptible pregnant women should receive live attenuated rubella vaccine, because an immunized child will be less likely to acquire natural rubella and introduce the virus into the household.

Non-Pregnant Adolescent and Adult Females
Immunization of susceptible non-pregnant adolescent and adult females of child-bearing age with live attenuated rubella virus vaccine is indicated if certain precautions are observed (see below). Vaccinating susceptible postpubertal females confers individual protection against subsequently acquiring rubella infection during pregnancy, which in turn prevents infection of the fetus and consequent congenital rubella injury.

Pregnant females *must not* be given live attenuated rubella virus vaccine. It is not known to what extent infection of the fetus with attenuated virus might occur following vaccination, or whether damage to the fetus could result. Subjects should be considered for vaccination only if they agree that they will not become pregnant within three months following vaccination, and if they are informed of the reason for this precaution.* If a pregnant woman is inadvertently vaccinated or if she becomes pregnant within three months of vaccination, she should be counseled on the possible risks to the fetus.

It is recommended that rubella susceptibility be determined by serologic testing prior to immunization.** If immune, as evidenced by a specific rubella antibody titer of 1:8 or greater (hemagglutination inhibition test), vaccination is unnecessary. Congenital malformations do occur in up to seven percent of all live births. Their chance appearance after vaccination could lead to misinterpretation of the cause, particularly if the prior rubella-immune status of vaccinees is unknown.

BENEMID® (Probenecid, MSD) Penicillin Therapy (Gonorrhea)*

	Recommended Regimens**	Remarks
Uncomplicated gonococcal infection in men and women (urethral, cervical, rectal)	4.8 million units of aqueous procaine penicillin G† I.M., in at least 2 doses injected at different sites at one visit + 1 g of BENEMID (Probenecid, MSD) orally just before injections or 3.5 g of ampicillin† orally + 1 g of BENEMID orally given simultaneously.	Follow-up: Obtain urethral and other appropriate cultures from men, and cervical, anal, and other appropriate cultures from women, 7 to 14 days after completion of treatment. Treatment of sexual partners: Persons with known recent exposure to gonorrhea should receive same treatment as those known to have gonorrhea. Examination and treatment of male sex partners of persons with gonorrhea are essential because of high prevalence of nonsymptomatic urethral gonococcal infection in such men.
Pharyngeal gonococcal infection in men and women	4.8 million units of aqueous procaine penicillin G† I.M., in at least 2 doses injected at different sites at one visit + 1 g of BENEMID orally just before injections	Pharyngeal gonococcal infections may be more difficult to treat than anogenital gonorrhea. Posttreatment cultures are essential.
Uncomplicated gonorrhea in pregnant patients	4.8 million units of aqueous procaine penicillin G† I.M., in at least 2 doses injected at different sites at one visit *or* 3.5 g of ampicillin† orally + 1 g of BENEMID orally given simultaneously	
Acute gonococcal salpingitis	*Outpatients:* Aqueous procaine penicillin G† or ampicillin† with BENEMID as for gonorrhea in pregnancy, followed by 500 mg of ampicillin 4 times a day for 10 days *Hospitalized patients:* See details in CDC recommendations	Follow-up of patients with acute salpingitis is essential. All patients should receive repeat pelvic examinations and cultures for *Neisseria gonorrhoeae* after treatment. Examination and appropriate treatment of male sex partners are essential because of high prevalence of nonsymptomatic urethral gonorrhea in such men.
Disseminated gonococcal infection (arthritis-dermatitis syndrome)	10 million units of aqueous crystalline penicillin G† I.V. a day for 3 days or till significant clinical improvement occurs. May be followed with 500 mg of ampicillin† 4 times a day orally to complete 7 days of treatment or 3.5 g of ampicillin† orally with 1 g of BENEMID, followed by 500 mg of ampicillin† 4 times a day for at least 7 days	
Gonococcal infection in children	For postpubertal children and/or those weighing over 45 kg (100 lb) use the dosage regimens given above for adults Uncomplicated vulvovaginitis and urethritis: aqueous procaine penicillin G† 75,000—100,000 units/kg I.M., with BENEMID 23 mg/kg orally	See CDC recommendations for detailed information about prevention and treatment of neonatal gonococcal infection and gonococcal ophthalmia.

Note: Before treating gonococcal infections in patients with suspected primary or secondary syphilis, perform proper diagnostic procedures including darkfield examinations. If concomitant syphilis is suspected, perform monthly serological tests for at least 4 months.
* Recommended by Venereal Disease Control Advisory Committee, Center for Disease Control, U.S. Department of Health, Education, and Welfare, Public Health Service (Morbidity and Mortality Weekly Report, Vol. 23: 341, 342, 347, 348, Oct. 11, 1974).
** See CDC recommendations for definition of regimens of choice, alternative regimens, treatment of hypersensitive patients, and other aspects of therapy.
† See package circulars of manufacturers for detailed information about contraindications, warnings, precautions, and adverse reactions.

Postpubertal females should be informed of the frequent occurrence of self-limited arthralgia and possible arthritis beginning 2 to 4 weeks after vaccination (See ADVERSE REACTIONS).

It has been found convenient in many instances to vaccinate rubella-susceptible women in the immediate postpartum period.

Revaccination: Based on available evidence, there is no reason to routinely revaccinate children originally vaccinated when 12 months of age or older; however, children vaccinated when younger than 12 months of age should be revaccinated. The decision to revaccinate should be based on evaluation of each individual case.

Use with Other Live Virus Vaccines

There are no data available concerning simultaneous use of BIAVAX II with monovalent or trivalent poliovirus vaccine, live, oral, or with killed poliovirus vaccines. However, serologic evidence shows that when M-M-R® (Measles, Mumps and Rubella Virus Vaccine, Live, MSD), containing the HPV-77 rubella strain, is given simultaneously with trivalent poliovirus vaccine, live, oral, antibody responses can be expected to be comparable to those which follow administration of the vaccines at different times. From this it follows that when BIAVAX II is given simultaneously with either monovalent or trivalent poliovirus vaccine, live, oral and/or ATTENUVAX® (Measles Virus Vaccine, Live, Attenuated, MSD), antibody responses can be expected to be comparable to those which follow administration of the vaccines at different times.

Contraindications

Do not give BIAVAX II to pregnant females; the possible effects of the vaccine on fetal development are unknown at this time. If vaccination of postpubertal females is undertaken, pregnancy must be avoided for three months following vaccination.
Hypersensitivity to neomycin (each dose of reconstituted vaccine contains approximately 25 mcg of neomycin).
Any febrile respiratory illness or other active febrile infection.
Patients receiving therapy with ACTH, corticosteroids, irradiation, alkylating agents or antimetabolites. This contraindication does not apply to patients who are receiving corticosteroids as replacement therapy, e.g., for Addison's disease.
Individuals with blood dyscrasias, leukemia, lymphomas of any type, or other malignant neoplasms affecting the bone marrow or lymphatic systems.
Primary immuno-deficiency states, including cellular immune deficiencies, hypogammaglobulinemic and dysgammaglobulinemic states.

Hypersensitivity to Eggs, Chicken, or Chicken Feathers

This vaccine is essentially devoid of potentially allergenic substances derived from host tissues (chick embryos).* However, because the attenuated mumps virus in this vaccine is propagated in cell cultures of chick embryo, there is a potential risk of hypersensitivity reactions in patients allergic to eggs, chicken, or chicken feathers. Widespread use of the vaccine for more than a decade has resulted in only rare, isolated reports of minor allergic reactions attributed to allergens of this kind, possibly related to the vaccine. Significantly when children with known allergies to eggs, chicken, and chicken feathers were given a similarly prepared vaccine in a clinical study, none experienced reactions other than those reactions previously observed in nonallergic children.

Precautions

Administer BIAVAX II subcutaneously; *do not give intravenously.*
Epinephrine should be available for immediate use in case an anaphylactoid reaction occurs.
BIAVAX II may be given simultaneously with monovalent or trivalent poliovirus vaccine, live, oral and/or with ATTENUVAX (Measles Virus Vaccine, Live, Attenuated, MSD). BIAVAX II should not be given less than one month before or after administration of other live virus vaccines.
Vaccination should be deferred for at least 3 months following blood or plasma transfusions, or administration of human immune serum globulin.
Excretion of small amounts of the live attenuated rubella virus from the nose and throat has occurred in the majority of susceptible individuals 7–28 days after vaccination. There is no confirmed evidence to indicate that such virus is transmitted to susceptible persons who are in contact with the vaccinated individuals. Consequently, transmission, while accepted as a theoretical possibility, is not regarded as a significant risk.**
There are no reports of transmission of live attenuated mumps virus from vaccinees to susceptible contacts.
It has been reported that live attenuated rubella and mumps virus vaccines given individually may result in a temporary depression of tuberculin skin sensitivity. Therefore, if a tuberculin test is to be done, it should be administered either before or simultaneously with BIAVAX II.
As for any vaccine, vaccination with BIAVAX II may not result in seroconversion in 100% of susceptible subjects given the vaccine.

Adverse Reactions

Because of the slightly acidic pH (6.2–6.6) of the vaccine, patients may complain of burning and/or stinging of short duration at the injection site.
The adverse clinical reactions associated with the use of BIAVAX II are those expected to follow administration of the monovalent vaccines given separately. These may include malaise, sore throat, headache, fever, and rash; mild local reactions such as erythema, induration, tenderness and regional lymphadenopathy; parotitis; orchitis; thrombocytopenia and purpura; allergic reactions such as wheal and flare at the injection site or urticaria; and arthritis, arthralgia and polyneuritis.
Moderate fever [101–102.9°F (38.3–39.4°C)] occurs occasionally, and high fever [above 103°F (39.4°C)] occurs less commonly. On rare occasions, children developing fever may exhibit febrile convulsions. Rash occurs infrequently and is usually minimal, but rarely may be generalized.
Clinical experience with live attenuated rubella and mumps virus vaccines given individually indicates that encephalitis and other nervous system reactions have occurred very rarely. These might occur also with BIAVAX II.
Transient arthritis, arthralgia and polyneuritis are features of natural rubella and vary in frequency and severity with age and sex, being greatest in adult females and least in prepubertal children. This type of involvement has also been reported following administration of MERUVAX II (Rubella Virus Vaccine, Live, MSD). In children, joint reactions are rare and of brief duration if they do occur. In women, incidence rates for arthritis and arthralgia are generally higher than those seen in children (children: 0–3%; women: 12–20%), and the reactions tend to be more marked and of longer duration. Rarely, symptoms may persist for a matter of months. In adolescent girls, the reactions appear to be intermediate in incidence between those seen in children and in adult women. Even in older women (35–45 years), these reactions are generally well tolerated and rarely interfere with normal activities.

Dosage and Administration

After suitably cleansing the immunization site, inject the total volume of reconstituted vaccine subcutaneously, preferably into the outer aspect of the upper arm. Do not inject BIAVAX II intravenously. *Do not give immune serum globulin (ISG) concurrently with BIAVAX II.*
CAUTION: A sterile syringe free of preservatives, antiseptics, and detergents should be used for each injection of the vaccine because these substances may inactivate the live virus vaccine. A 25 gauge, 5/8" needle is recommended.

Shipment, Storage, and Reconstitution

During shipment, to insure that there is no loss of potency, the vaccine must be maintained at a temperature of 10°C (50°F) or less.
Before reconstitution, store BIAVAX II at 2–8°C (35.6–46.4°F). *Protect from light.*
To reconstitute, use only the diluent supplied, since it is free of preservatives or other antiviral substances which might inactivate the vaccine. First withdraw the entire volume of diluent into the syringe to be used for reconstitution. Inject all the diluent in the syringe into the vial of lyophilized vaccine, and agitate to mix thoroughly. Withdraw the entire contents into a syringe and inject the total volume of restored vaccine subcutaneously.
It is important to use a separate sterile syringe and needle for each individual patient to prevent transmission of hepatitis B and other infectious agents from one person to another.
The color of the vaccine when reconstituted is yellow.
It is recommended that the vaccine be used as soon as possible after reconstitution. Protect the vaccine from light at all times. Store reconstituted vaccine in a dark place at 2–8°C (35.6–46.4°F) and discard if not used within eight hours.

How Supplied

No. 4746—BIAVAX II is supplied as a single-dose vial of lyophilized vaccine, NDC 0006-4746-00, and a vial of diluent.
No. 4669/4309—BIAVAX II is supplied as follows: (1) a box of 10 single-dose vials of lyophilized vaccine (package A), NDC 0006-4669-00; and (2) a box of 10 vials of diluent (package B). To conserve refrigerator space, the diluent may be stored separately at room temperature.

A.H.F.S. Category: 80:12
DC 7032306   Issued February 1983
COPYRIGHT © MERCK & CO., INC., 1983
All rights reserved

BLOCADREN® Tablets
(timolol maleate, MSD), U.S.P.

Description

BLOCADREN® (Timolol Maleate, MSD) is a non-

Continued on next page

---

* NOTE: The Immunization Practices Advisory Committee (ACIP) has recommended "In view of the importance of protecting this age group against rubella, asking females if they are pregnant, excluding those who say they are, and explaining the theoretical risks to the others are reasonable precautions in a rubella immunization program."

** NOTE: The Immunization Practices Advisory Committee (ACIP) has stated "When practical, and when reliable laboratory services are available, potential vaccinees of childbearing age can have serologic tests to determine susceptibility to rubella.... However, routinely performing serologic tests for all females of childbearing age to determine susceptibility so that vaccine is given only to proven susceptibles is expensive and has been ineffective in some areas. Accordingly, the ACIP believes that rubella vaccination of a woman who is not known to be pregnant and has no history of vaccination is justifiable without serologic testing."

* Morbidity and Mortality Weekly Report 25(44): 350, Nov. 12, 1976.

** Recommendation of the Immunization Practices Advisory Committee (ACIP), Morbidity and Mortality Weekly Report 30(4): 37–42, 47, Feb. 6, 1981.

Information on the Merck Sharp & Dohme products listed on these pages is the full prescribing information from product circulars in use November 1, 1984.

Merck Sharp & Dohme—Cont.

selective beta-adrenergic receptor blocking agent. The chemical name for timolol maleate is (S)-1-[(1, 1-dimethylethyl) amino] -3- [[4-(4-morpholinyl)-1, 2, 5-thiadiazol-3-yl]oxy]-2-propanol, (Z)-butenedioate (1:1) salt. It possesses an asymmetric carbon atom in its structure and is provided as the levoisomer. Its empirical formula is $C_{13}H_{24}N_4O_3S \cdot C_4H_4O_4$.

Timolol maleate has a molecular weight of 432.49. It is a water-soluble, white, crystalline solid. It is supplied as 5 mg, 10 mg and 20 mg tablets for oral administration.

Clinical Pharmacology

BLOCADREN is a beta$_1$ and beta$_2$ (non-selective) adrenergic receptor blocking agent that does not have significant intrinsic sympathomimetic, direct myocardial depressant, or local anesthetic activity.

Pharmacodynamics

Clinical pharmacology studies have confirmed the beta-adrenergic blocking activity as shown by (1) changes in resting heart rate and response of heart rate to changes in posture; (2) inhibition of isoproterenol-induced tachycardia; (3) alteration of the response to the Valsalva maneuver and amyl nitrite administration; and (4) reduction of heart rate and blood pressure changes on exercise.

BLOCADREN decreases the positive chronotropic, positive inotropic, bronchodilator, and vasodilator responses caused by beta-adrenergic receptor agonists. The magnitude of this decreased response is proportional to the existing sympathetic tone and the concentration of BLOCADREN at receptor sites.

In normal volunteers, the reduction in heart rate response to a standard exercise was dose dependent over the test range of 0.5 to 20 mg, with a peak reduction at 2 hours of approximately 30% at higher doses.

Beta-adrenergic receptor blockade reduces cardiac output in both healthy subjects and patients with heart disease. In patients with severe impairment of myocardial function beta-adrenergic receptor blockade may inhibit the stimulatory effect of the sympathetic nervous system necessary to maintain adequate cardiac function.

Beta-adrenergic receptor blockade in the bronchi and bronchioles results in increased airway resistance from unopposed parasympathetic activity. Such an effect in patients with asthma or other bronchospastic conditions is potentially dangerous.

Clinical studies indicate that BLOCADREN at a dosage of 20–60 mg/day reduces blood pressure without causing postural hypotension in most patients with essential hypertension. Administration of BLOCADREN to patients with hypertension results initially in a decrease in cardiac output, little immediate change in blood pressure, and an increase in calculated peripheral resistance. With continued administration of BLOCADREN blood pressure decreases within a few days, cardiac output usually remains reduced, and peripheral resistance falls toward pretreatment levels. Plasma volume may decrease or remain unchanged during therapy with BLOCADREN. In the majority of patients with hypertension BLOCADREN also decreases plasma renin activity. Dosage adjustment to achieve optimal antihypertensive effect may require a few weeks. When therapy with BLOCADREN is discontinued, the blood pressure tends to return to pretreatment levels gradually. In most patients the antihypertensive activity of BLOCADREN is maintained with long-term therapy and is well tolerated.

The mechanism of the antihypertensive effects of beta-adrenergic receptor blocking agents is not established at this time. Possible mechanisms of action include reduction in cardiac output, reduction in plasma renin activity, and a central nervous system sympatholytic action.

A Norwegian multi-center, double-blind study compared the effects of timolol maleate with placebo in 1,884 patients who had survived the acute phase of a myocardial infarction. Patients with systolic blood pressure below 100 mm Hg, sick sinus syndrome and contraindications to beta blockers, including uncontrolled heart failure, second or third degree AV block and bradycardia (<50 beats per minute), were excluded from the multi-center trial. Therapy with BLOCADREN, begun 7 to 28 days following infarction, was shown to reduce overall mortality; this was primarily attributable to a reduction in cardiovascular mortality. BLOCADREN significantly reduced the incidence of sudden deaths (deaths occurring without symptoms or within 24 hours of the onset of symptoms), including those occurring within one hour, and particularly instantaneous deaths (those occurring without preceding symptoms). The protective effect of BLOCADREN was consistent regardless of age, sex or site of infarction. The effect was clearest in patients with a first infarction who were considered at a high risk of dying, defined as those with one or more of the following characteristics during the acute phase: transient left ventricular failure, cardiomegaly, newly appearing atrial fibrillation or flutter, systolic hypotension, or SGOT (ASAT) levels greater than four times the upper limit of normal. Therapy with BLOCADREN also reduced the incidence of non-fatal reinfarction. The mechanism of the protective effect of BLOCADREN is unknown.

Pharmacokinetics and Metabolism

BLOCADREN is rapidly and nearly completely absorbed (about 90%) following oral ingestion. Detectable plasma levels of timolol occur within one-half hour and peak plasma levels occur in about one to two hours. The drug half-life in plasma is approximately 4 hours and this is essentially unchanged in patients with moderate renal insufficiency. Timolol is partially metabolized by the liver and timolol and its metabolites are excreted by the kidney. Timolol is not extensively bound to plasma proteins; i.e., <10% by equilibrium dialysis and approximately 60% by ultrafiltration. An *in vitro* hemodialysis study, using ^{14}C timolol added to human plasma or whole blood, showed that timolol was readily dialyzed from these fluids; however, a study of patients with renal failure showed that timolol did not dialyze readily. Plasma levels following oral administration are about half those following intravenous administration indicating approximately 50% first pass metabolism. The level of beta sympathetic activity varies widely among individuals, and no single correlation exists between the dose or plasma level of timolol maleate and its therapeutic activity. Therefore, objective clinical measurements such as reduction of heart rate and/or blood pressure should be used as guides in determining the optimal dosage for each patient.

Indications and Usage

Hypertension

BLOCADREN is indicated for the treatment of hypertension. It may be used alone or in combination with other antihypertensive agents, especially thiazide-type diuretics.

Myocardial Infarction

BLOCADREN is indicated in patients who have survived the acute phase of a myocardial infarction, and are clinically stable, to reduce cardiovascular mortality and the risk of reinfarction. It is recommended that treatment should be initiated within 1 to 4 weeks after infarction. Data are not available as to whether benefit would ensue if initiated later.

Contraindications

BLOCADREN is contraindicated in patients with bronchial asthma or with a history of bronchial asthma, or severe chronic obstructive pulmonary disease (see WARNINGS); sinus bradycardia; second and third degree atrioventricular block; overt cardiac failure (see WARNINGS); cardiogenic shock; hypersensitivity to this product.

Warnings

Cardiac Failure

Sympathetic stimulation may be essential for support of the circulation in individuals with diminished myocardial contractility, and its inhibition by beta-adrenergic receptor blockade may precipitate more severe failure. Although beta-blockers should be avoided in overt congestive heart failure, they can be used, if necessary, with caution in patients with a history of failure who are well-compensated, usually with digitalis and diuretics. Both digitalis and timolol maleate slow AV conduction. If cardiac failure persists, therapy with BLOCADREN should be withdrawn.

In Patients Without a History of Cardiac Failure continued depression of the myocardium with beta-blocking agents over a period of time can, in some cases, lead to cardiac failure. At the first sign or symptom of cardiac failure, patients receiving BLOCADREN should be digitalized and/or be given a diuretic, and the response observed closely. If cardiac failure continues, despite adequate digitalization and diuretic therapy, BLOCADREN should be withdrawn.

> *Exacerbation of Ischemic Heart Disease Following Abrupt Withdrawal*—Hypersensitivity to catecholamines has been observed in patients withdrawn from beta blocker therapy; exacerbation of angina and, in some cases, myocardial infarction have occurred after *abrupt* discontinuation of such therapy. When discontinuing chronically administered timolol maleate, particularly in patients with ischemic heart disease, the dosage should be gradually reduced over a period of one to two weeks and the patient should be carefully monitored. If angina markedly worsens or acute coronary insufficiency develops, timolol maleate administration should be reinstituted promptly, at least temporarily, and other measures appropriate for the management of unstable angina should be taken. Patients should be warned against interruption or discontinuation of therapy without the physician's advice. Because coronary artery disease is common and may be unrecognized, it may be prudent not to discontinue timolol maleate therapy abruptly even in patients treated only for hypertension.

Non-Allergic Bronchospasm

In patients with non-allergic bronchospasm or with a history of non-allergic bronchospasm (e.g., chronic bronchitis, emphysema), BLOCADREN should be administered with caution since it may block bronchodilation produced by endogenous and exogenous catecholamine stimulation of beta$_2$ receptors.

Major Surgery

The necessity or desirability of withdrawal of beta-blocking therapy prior to major surgery is controversial. Beta-adrenergic receptor blockade impairs the ability of the heart to respond to beta-adrenergically mediated reflex stimuli. This may augment the risk of general anesthesia in surgical procedures. Some patients receiving beta-adrenergic receptor blocking agents have been subject to protracted severe hypotension during anesthesia. Difficulty in restarting and maintaining the heartbeat has also been reported. For these reasons, in patients undergoing elective surgery, some authorities recommend gradual withdrawal of beta-adrenergic receptor blocking agents.

If necessary during surgery, the effects of beta-adrenergic blocking agents may be reversed by sufficient doses of such agonists as isoproterenol, dopamine, dobutamine or levarterenol (see OVERDOSAGE).

Diabetes Mellitus

BLOCADREN should be administered with caution in patients subject to spontaneous hypoglycemia or to diabetic patients (especially those with labile diabetes) who are receiving insulin or oral hypoglycemic agents. Beta-adrenergic receptor blocking agents may mask the signs and symptoms of acute hypoglycemia.

Thyrotoxicosis
Beta-adrenergic blockade may mask certain clinical signs (e.g., tachycardia) of hyperthyroidism. Patients suspected of developing thyrotoxicosis should be managed carefully to avoid abrupt withdrawal of beta blockade which might precipitate a thyroid storm.

Precautions

General
Impaired Hepatic or Renal Function: Since BLOCADREN is partially metabolized in the liver and excreted mainly by the kidneys, dosage reductions may be necessary when hepatic and/or renal insufficiency is present.
Dosing in the Presence of Marked Renal Failure: Although the pharmacokinetics of BLOCADREN are not greatly altered by renal impairment, marked hypotensive responses have been seen in patients with marked renal impairment undergoing dialysis after 20 mg doses. Dosing in such patients should therefore be especially cautious.
Muscle Weakness: Beta-adrenergic blockade has been reported to potentiate muscle weakness consistent with certain myasthenic symptoms (e.g., diplopia, ptosis, and generalized weakness). Timolol has been reported rarely to increase muscle weakness in some patients with myasthenic symptoms.

Drug Interactions
Close observation of the patient is recommended when BLOCADREN is administered to patients receiving catecholamine-depleting drugs such as reserpine, because of possible additive effects and the production of hypotension and/or marked bradycardia, which may produce vertigo, syncope, or postural hypotension.
Blunting of the antihypertensive effect of beta-adrenoceptor blocking agents by non-steroidal anti-inflammatory drugs has been reported. When using these agents concomitantly, patients should be observed carefully to confirm that the desired therapeutic effect has been obtained.

Carcinogenesis, Mutagenesis, Impairment of Fertility
In a two-year study of timolol maleate in rats, there was a statistically significant ($P \le 0.05$) increase in the incidence of adrenal pheochromocytomas in male rats administered 300 times the maximum recommended human dose (1 mg/kg/day). Similar differences were not observed in rats administered doses equivalent to 25 or 100 times the maximum recommended human dose. In a lifetime study in mice, there were statistically significant ($P \le 0.05$) increases in the incidence of benign and malignant pulmonary tumors and benign uterine polyps in female mice at 500 mg/kg/day, but not at 5 or 50 mg/kg/day. There was also a significant increase in mammary adenocarcinomas at the 500 mg/kg/day dose. This was associated with elevations in serum prolactin which occurred in female mice administered timolol at 500 mg/kg, but not at doses of 5 or 50 mg/kg/day. An increased incidence of mammary adenocarcinomas in rodents has been associated with administration of several other therapeutic agents which elevate serum prolactin, but no correlation between serum prolactin levels and mammary tumors has been established in man. Furthermore, in adult human male subjects who received oral dosages of up to 60 mg of timolol maleate, the maximum recommended human oral dosage, there were no clinically meaningful changes in serum prolactin.
There was a statistically significant increase ($P \le 0.05$) in the overall incidence of neoplasms in female mice at the 500 mg/kg/day dosage level. Timolol maleate was devoid of mutagenic potential when evaluated *in vivo* (mouse) in the micronucleus test and cytogenetic assay (doses up to 800 mg/kg) and *in vitro* in a neoplastic cell transformation assay (up to 100 µg/ml). In Ames tests the highest concentrations of timolol employed, 5000 or 10,000 µg/plate, were associated with statistically significant elevations ($P \le 0.05$) of revertants observed with tester strain TA100 (in seven replicate assays), but not in the remaining three strains. In the assays with tester strain TA100, no consistent dose response relationship was observed, nor did the ratio of test to control revertants reach 2. A ratio of 2 is usually considered the criterion for a positive Ames test.
Reproduction and fertility studies in rats showed no adverse effect on male or female fertility at doses up to 150 times the maximum recommended human dose.

Pregnancy
Pregnancy Category C. Teratogenic studies with timolol in mice and rabbits at doses up to 50 mg/kg/day (50 times the maximum recommended human dose) showed no evidence of fetal malformations. Although delayed fetal ossification was observed at this dose in rats, there were no adverse effects on postnatal development of offspring. Doses of 1000 mg/kg/day (1,000 times the maximum recommended human dose) were maternotoxic in mice and resulted in an increased number of fetal resorptions. Increased fetal resorptions were also seen in rabbits at doses of 100 times the maximum recommended human dose, in this case without apparent maternotoxicity. There are no adequate and well-controlled studies in pregnant women. BLOCADREN should be used during pregnancy only if the potential benefit justifies the potential risk to the fetus.

Nursing Mothers
Because of the potential for serious adverse reactions from timolol in nursing infants, a decision should be made whether to discontinue nursing or to discontinue the drug, taking into account the importance of the drug to the mother.

Pediatric Use
Safety and effectiveness in children have not been established.

Adverse Reactions

BLOCADREN is usually well tolerated in properly selected patients. Most adverse effects have been mild and transient.
In a multicenter (12-week) clinical trial comparing timolol maleate and placebo, the following adverse reactions were reported spontaneously and considered to be causally related to timolol maleate:

	Timolol Maleate (n = 176) %	Placebo (n = 168) %
BODY AS A WHOLE		
fatigue/tiredness	3.4	0.6
headache	1.7	1.8
chest pain	0.6	0
asthenia	0.6	0
CARDIOVASCULAR		
bradycardia	9.1	0
arrhythmia	1.1	0.6
syncope	0.6	0
edema	0.6	1.2
DIGESTIVE		
dyspepsia	0.6	0.6
nausea	0.6	0
SKIN		
pruritus	1.1	0
NERVOUS SYSTEM		
dizziness	2.3	1.2
vertigo	0.6	0
paresthesia	0.6	0
PSYCHIATRIC		
decreased libido	0.6	0
RESPIRATORY		
dyspnea	1.7	0.6
bronchial spasm	0.6	0
rales	0.6	0
SPECIAL SENSES		
eye irritation	1.1	0.6
tinnitus	0.6	0

These data are representative of the incidence of adverse effects that may be observed in a properly selected hypertensive patient population, e.g., a group excluding patients with bronchospastic disease, congestive heart failure or other contraindications to beta blocker therapy. These adverse reactions can also occur in patients with coronary artery disease.
In a different population, the coronary artery disease population, studied in the Norwegian multicenter trial (see CLINICAL PHARMACOLOGY), the frequency of the principal adverse reactions and the frequency with which these resulted in discontinuation of therapy in the timolol and placebo groups were:
[See table above]:

BLOCADREN	Adverse Reaction†		Withdrawal‡	
	Timolol (n = 945) %	Placebo (n = 939) %	Timolol (n = 945) %	Placebo (n = 939) %
Asthenia or Fatigue	5	1	<1	<1
Heart Rate <40 beats/minute	5	<1	4	<1
Cardiac Failure-Nonfatal	8	7	3	2
Hypotension	3	2	3	1
Pulmonary Edema-Nonfatal	2	<1	<1	<1
Claudication	3	3	1	<1
AV Block 2nd or 3rd degree	<1	<1	<1	<1
Sinoatrial Block	<1	<1	<1	<1
Cold Hands and Feet	8	<1	<1	0
Nausea or Digestive Disorders	8	6	1	<1
Dizziness	6	4	1	0
Bronchial Obstruction	2	<1	1	<1

† When an adverse reaction recurred in a patient, it is listed only once.
‡ Only principal reason for withdrawal in each patient is listed.

These adverse reactions can also occur in patients treated for hypertension.
The following additional adverse effects have been reported in clinical experience with the drug: *Body as a Whole:* extremity pain, decreased exercise tolerance, weight loss; *Cardiovascular:* cardiac failure, cerebral vascular accident, worsening of angina pectoris, worsening of arterial insufficiency, Raynaud's phenomenon, palpitations, vasodilatation; *Digestive:* gastrointestinal pain, hepatomegaly, vomiting, diarrhea, dyspepsia; *Hematologic:* nonthrombocytopenic purpura; *Endocrine:* hyperglycemia, hypoglycemia; *Skin:* rash, skin irritation, increased pigmentation, sweating; *Musculoskeletal:* arthralgia; *Nervous System:* local weakness; *Psychiatric:* depression, nightmares, somnolence, insomnia, nervousness, diminished concentration, hallucinations; *Respiratory:* cough; *Special Senses:* visual disturbances, diplopia, ptosis, dry eyes; *Urogenital:* impotence, urination difficulties.
There have been reports of retroperitoneal fibrosis in patients receiving timolol maleate and in patients receiving other beta-adrenergic blocking agents. A causal relationship between this condi-

Continued on next page

Information on the Merck Sharp & Dohme products listed on these pages is the full prescribing information from product circulars in use November 1, 1984.

Merck Sharp & Dohme—Cont.

tion and therapy with beta-adrenergic blocking agents has not been established.

Potential Adverse Effects: In addition, a variety of adverse effects not observed in clinical trials with BLOCADREN, but reported with other beta-adrenergic blocking agents, should be considered potential adverse effects of BLOCADREN: *Nervous System:* Reversible mental depression progressing to catatonia; an acute reversible syndrome characterized by disorientation for time and place, short-term memory loss, emotional lability, slightly clouded sensorium, and decreased performance on neuropsychometrics; *Cardiovascular:* Intensification of AV block (see CONTRAINDICATIONS); *Digestive:* Mesenteric arterial thrombosis, ischemic colitis; *Hematologic:* Agranulocytosis, thrombocytopenic purpura; *Allergic:* Erythematous rash, fever combined with aching and sore throat, laryngospasm and respiratory distress; *Miscellaneous:* Reversible alopecia, Peyronie's disease.

There have been reports of a syndrome comprising psoriasiform skin rash, conjunctivitis sicca, otitis, and sclerosing serositis attributed to the beta-adrenergic receptor blocking agent, practolol. This syndrome has not been reported with BLOCADREN.

Clinical Laboratory Test Findings: Clinically important changes in standard laboratory parameters were rarely associated with the administration of BLOCADREN. Slight increases in blood urea nitrogen, serum potassium, and serum uric acid, and slight decreases in hemoglobin and hematocrit occurred, but were not progressive or associated with clinical manifestations.

Overdosage

No data are available in regard to overdosage in humans.

The oral LD_{50} of the drug is 1190 and 900 mg/kg in female mice and female rats, respectively.

An *in vitro* hemodialysis study, using ^{14}C timolol added to human plasma or whole blood, showed that timolol was readily dialyzed from these fluids; however, a study of patients with renal failure showed that timolol did not dialyze readily.

The most common signs and symptoms to be expected with overdosage with a beta-adrenergic receptor blocking agent are symptomatic bradycardia, hypotension, bronchospasm, and acute cardiac failure. Therapy with BLOCADREN should be discontinued and the patient observed closely. The following additional therapeutic measures should be considered:

(1) *Gastric lavage*

(2) *Symptomatic bradycardia:* Use atropine sulfate intravenously in a dosage of 0.25 mg to 2 mg to induce vagal blockade. If bradycardia persists, intravenous isoproterenol hydrochloride should be administered cautiously. In refractory cases the use of a transvenous cardiac pacemaker may be considered.

(3) *Hypotension:* Use sympathomimetic pressor drug therapy, such as dopamine, dobutamine or levarterenol. In refractory cases the use of glucagon hydrochloride has been reported to be useful.

(4) *Bronchospasm:* Use isoproterenol hydrochloride. Additional therapy with aminophylline may be considered.

(5) *Acute cardiac failure:* Conventional therapy with digitalis, diuretics, and oxygen should be instituted immediately. In refractory cases the use of intravenous aminophylline is suggested. This may be followed if necessary by glucagon hydrochloride which has been reported to be useful.

(6) *Heart block (second or third degree):* Use isoproterenol hydrochloride or a transvenous cardiac pacemaker.

Dosage and Administration

Hypertension

The usual initial dosage of BLOCADREN is 10 mg twice a day, whether used alone or added to diuretic therapy. The usual total maintenance dosage is 20–40 mg per day. Depending on blood pressure and pulse rate, increases in dosage to a maximum of 60 mg per day divided into two doses may be necessary. There should be an interval of at least seven days between increases in dosages.

BLOCADREN may be used with a thiazide diuretic or with other antihypertensive agents. Patients should be observed carefully during initiation of such concomitant therapy.

Myocardial Infarction

The recommended dosage for long-term prophylactic use in patients who have survived the acute phase of a myocardial infarction is 10 mg given twice daily.

How Supplied

No. 3343—Tablets BLOCADREN, 5 mg, are light blue, round, compressed tablets, with code MSD 59 on one side and BLOCADREN on the other. They are supplied as follows:
  NDC 0006-0059-68 bottles of 100.
No. 3344—Tablets BLOCADREN, 10 mg, are light blue, round, scored, compressed tablets, with code MSD 136 on one side and BLOCADREN on the other. They are supplied as follows:
  NDC 0006-0136-68 bottles of 100
  NDC 0006-0136-28 single unit packages of 100.
Shown in Product Identification Section, page 420
No. 3371—Tablets BLOCADREN, 20 mg, are light blue, capsule shaped, scored, compressed tablets, with code MSD 437 on one side and BLOCADREN on the other. They are supplied as follows:
  NDC 0006-0437-68 bottles of 100.
Shown in Product Identification Section, page 420
A.H.F.S. Category: 24:04, 24:08
DC 7117616 Issued July 1983
COPYRIGHT © MERCK & CO., INC., 1983
All rights reserved

CLINORIL® Tablets ℞
(sulindac, MSD), U.S.P.

Description

Sulindac is a non-steroidal, anti-inflammatory indene derivative designated chemically as (Z)-5-fluoro-2-methyl - 1 - [[*p*- (methylsulfinyl) phenyl]methylene]-1*H*-indene-3-acetic acid. It is not a salicylate, pyrazolone or propionic acid derivative. Its empirical formula is $C_{20}H_{17}FO_3S$, with a molecular weight of 356.42. Sulindac, a yellow crystalline compound, is a weak organic acid practically insoluble in water below pH 4.5, but very soluble as the sodium salt or in buffers of pH 6 or higher. Following absorption, sulindac undergoes two major biotransformations—reversible reduction to the sulfide metabolite, and irreversible oxidation to the sulfone metabolite. Available evidence indicates that the biological activity resides with the sulfide metabolite.

Clinical Pharmacology

CLINORIL® (Sulindac, MSD) is a non-steroidal anti-inflammatory drug, also possessing analgesic and antipyretic activities. Its mode of action, like that of other non-steroidal, anti-inflammatory agents, is not known; however, its therapeutic action is not due to pituitary-adrenal stimulation. Inhibition of prostaglandin synthesis by the sulfide metabolite may be involved in the anti-inflammatory action of CLINORIL.

Sulindac is approximately 90% absorbed in man after oral administration. The peak plasma concentrations of the biologically active sulfide metabolite are achieved in about two hours when sulindac is administered in the fasting state, and in about three to four hours when sulindac is administered with food. The mean half-life of sulindac is 7.8 hours while the mean half-life of the sulfide metabolite is 16.4 hours. Sustained plasma levels of the sulfide metabolite are consistent with a prolonged anti-inflammatory action which is the rationale for a twice per day dosage schedule.

Sulindac and its sulfone metabolite undergo extensive enterohepatic circulation relative to the sulfide metabolite in animals. Similar enterohepatic circulation together with the reversible metabolism are probably major contributors to sustained plasma levels of the active drug in man.

The primary route of excretion in man is via the urine as both sulindac and its sulfone metabolite (free and glucuronide conjugates). Approximately 50% of the administered dose is excreted in the urine, with the conjugated sulfone metabolite accounting for the major portion. Less than 1% of the administered dose of sulindac appears in the urine as the sulfide metabolite. Approximately 25% is found in the feces, primarily as the sulfone and sulfide metabolites.

The bioavailability of sulindac, as assessed by urinary excretion, was not changed by concomitant administration of an antacid containing magnesium and aluminum hydroxides (MAALOX®, William H. Rorer, Inc.).

In healthy men, the average fecal blood loss, measured over a two-week period during administration of 400 mg per day of CLINORIL, was similar to that for placebo, and was statistically significantly less than that resulting from 4800 mg per day of aspirin.

In controlled clinical studies CLINORIL was evaluated in the following five conditions:
1. *Osteoarthritis*

In patients with osteoarthritis of the hip and knee, the anti-inflammatory and analgesic activity of CLINORIL was demonstrated by clinical measurements that included: assessments by both patient and investigator of overall response; decrease in disease activity as assessed by both patient and investigator; improvement in ARA Functional Class; relief of night pain; improvement in overall evaluation of pain, including pain on weight bearing and pain on active and passive motion; improvement in joint mobility, range of motion, and functional activities; decreased swelling and tenderness; and decreased duration of stiffness following prolonged inactivity.

In clinical studies in which dosages were adjusted according to patient needs, CLINORIL 200 to 400 mg daily was shown to be comparable in effectiveness to aspirin 2400 to 4800 mg daily. CLINORIL was generally well tolerated, and patients on it had a lower overall incidence of total adverse effects, of milder gastrointestinal reactions, and of tinnitus than did patients on aspirin. (See ADVERSE REACTIONS.)

2. *Rheumatoid Arthritis*

In patients with rheumatoid arthritis, the anti-inflammatory and analgesic activity of CLINORIL was demonstrated by clinical measurements that included: assessments by both patient and investigator of overall response; decrease in disease activity as assessed by both patient and investigator; reduction in overall joint pain; reduction in duration and severity of morning stiffness; reduction in day and night pain; decrease in time required to walk 50 feet; decrease in general pain as measured on a visual analog scale; improvement in the Ritchie articular index; decrease in proximal interphalangeal joint size; improvement in ARA Functional Class; increase in grip strength; reduction in painful joint count and score; reduction in swollen joint count and score; and increased flexion and extension of the wrist.

In clinical studies in which dosages were adjusted according to patient needs, CLINORIL 300 to 400 mg daily was shown to be comparable in effectiveness to aspirin 3600 to 4800 mg daily. CLINORIL was generally well tolerated, and patients on it had a lower overall incidence of total adverse effects, of milder gastrointestinal reactions, and of tinnitus than did patients on aspirin. (See ADVERSE REACTIONS.)

In patients with rheumatoid arthritis, CLINORIL may be used in combination with gold salts at usual dosage levels. In clinical studies, CLINORIL added to the regimen of gold salts usually resulted in additional symptomatic relief but did not alter the course of the underlying disease.

3. *Ankylosing spondylitis*

In patients with ankylosing spondylitis, the anti-inflammatory and analgesic activity of CLINORIL was demonstrated by clinical measurements that included: assessments by both patient and investigator of overall response; decrease in disease activity as assessed by both patient and investigator; improvement in ARA Functional Class; improvement in patient and investigator evaluation of spinal pain, tenderness and/or spasm; reduction in the duration of morning stiffness; increase in the time to onset of fatigue; relief of night pain; increase in chest expansion; increase in spinal mobility evaluated by fingers-to-floor distance, occiput to wall distance, the Schober Test, and the Wright Modification of the Schober Test. In a clinical study in which dosages were adjusted according to patient need, CLINORIL 200 to 400 mg daily was as effective as indomethacin 75 to 150 mg daily. In a second study, CLINORIL 300 to 400 mg daily was comparable in effectiveness to phenylbutazone 400 to 600 mg daily. CLINORIL was better tolerated than phenylbutazone. (See ADVERSE REACTIONS.)

4. *Acute painful shoulder (Acute subacromial bursitis/supraspinatus tendinitis)*
In patients with acute painful shoulder (acute subacromial bursitis/supraspinatus tendinitis), the anti-inflammatory and analgesic activity of CLINORIL was demonstrated by clinical measurements that included: assessments by both patient and investigator of overall response; relief of night pain, spontaneous pain, and pain on active motion; decrease in local tenderness; and improvement in range of motion measured by abduction, and internal and external rotation. In clinical studies in acute painful shoulder, CLINORIL 300 to 400 mg daily and oxyphenbutazone 400 to 600 mg daily were shown to be equally effective and well tolerated.

5. *Acute gouty arthritis*
In patients with acute gouty arthritis, the anti-inflammatory and analgesic activity of CLINORIL was demonstrated by clinical measurements that included: assessments by both the patient and investigator of overall response; relief of weight-bearing pain; relief of pain at rest and on active and passive motion; decrease in tenderness; reduction in warmth and swelling; increase in range of motion; and improvement in ability to function. In clinical studies, CLINORIL at 400 mg daily and phenylbutazone at 600 mg daily were shown to be equally effective. In these short-term studies in which reduction of dosage was permitted according to response, both drugs were equally well tolerated.

Indications and Usage

CLINORIL is indicated for acute or long-term use in the relief of signs and symptoms of the following:
1. Osteoarthritis
2. Rheumatoid arthritis*
3. Ankylosing spondylitis
4. Acute painful shoulder (Acute subacromial bursitis/supraspinatus tendinitis)
5. Acute gouty arthritis

Contraindications

CLINORIL should not be used in:
Patients who are hypersensitive to this product.
Patients in whom acute asthmatic attacks, urticaria, or rhinitis are precipitated by aspirin or other non-steroidal anti-inflammatory agents.

Warnings

Peptic ulceration and gastrointestinal bleeding have been reported in patients receiving CLINORIL. In patients with active gastrointestinal bleeding or an active peptic ulcer, an appropriate ulcer regimen should be instituted, and the physician

---
* The safety and effectiveness of CLINORIL have not been established in rheumatoid arthritis patients who are designated in the American Rheumatism Association classification as Functional Class IV (incapacitated, largely or wholly bedridden, or confined to wheelchair; little or no self-care).

---

must weigh the benefits of therapy with CLINORIL against possible hazards, and carefully monitor the patient's progress. When CLINORIL is given to patients with a history of upper gastrointestinal tract disease, it should be given under close supervision and only after consulting the ADVERSE REACTIONS section.

Rarely, fever and other evidence of hypersensitivity (see ADVERSE REACTIONS) including abnormalities in one or more liver function tests and severe skin reactions have occurred during therapy with CLINORIL. Fatalities have occurred in these patients. Hepatitis, jaundice, or both, with or without fever, may occur usually within the first one to three months of therapy. Determinations of liver function should be considered whenever a patient on therapy with CLINORIL develops unexplained fever, rash or other dermatologic reactions or constitutional symptoms. If unexplained fever or other evidence of hypersensitivity occurs, therapy with CLINORIL should be discontinued. The elevated temperature and abnormalities in liver function caused by CLINORIL characteristically have reverted to normal after discontinuation of therapy. Administration of CLINORIL should not be reinstituted in such patients.

In addition to hypersensitivity reactions involving the liver, in some patients the findings are consistent with those of cholestatic hepatitis. As with other non-steroidal anti-inflammatory drugs, borderline elevations of one or more liver tests without any other signs and symptoms may occur in up to 15% of patients. These abnormalities may progress, may remain essentially unchanged, or may be transient with continued therapy. The SGPT (ALT) test is probably the most sensitive indicator of liver dysfunction. Meaningful (3 times the upper limit of normal) elevations of SGPT or SGOT (AST) occurred in controlled clinical trials in less than 1% of patients. A patient with symptoms and/or signs suggesting liver dysfunction, or in whom an abnormal liver test has occurred, should be evaluated for evidence of the development of more severe hepatic reaction while on therapy with CLINORIL. Although such reactions as described above are rare, if abnormal liver tests persist or worsen, if clinical signs and symptoms consistent with liver disease develop, or if systemic manifestations occur (e.g. eosinophilia, rash, etc.), CLINORIL should be discontinued.

Precautions

General
Although CLINORIL has less effect on platelet function and bleeding time than aspirin, it is an inhibitor of platelet function; therefore, patients who may be adversely affected should be carefully observed when CLINORIL is administered.

Because of reports of adverse eye findings with non-steroidal anti-inflammatory agents, it is recommended that patients who develop eye complaints during treatment with CLINORIL have ophthalmologic studies.

Since CLINORIL is eliminated primarily by the kidneys, patients with significantly impaired renal function should be closely monitored and a reduction of daily dosage may be anticipated to avoid excessive drug accumulation.

In chronic studies in mice, rats and monkeys at high dosages, there were occasional occurrences of mild renal toxicity as evidenced by papillary edema or mild interstitial nephritis in some animals. Papillary necrosis occurred infrequently in mice and rats.

Edema has been observed in some patients taking CLINORIL. Therefore, as with other non-steroidal anti-inflammatory drugs, CLINORIL should be used with caution in patients with compromised cardiac function, hypertension, or other conditions predisposing to fluid retention.

CLINORIL may allow a reduction in dosage or the elimination of chronic corticosteroid therapy in some patients with rheumatoid arthritis. However, it is generally necessary to reduce corticosteroids gradually over several months in order to avoid an exacerbation of disease or signs and symptoms of adrenal insufficiency. Abrupt withdrawal of chronic corticosteroid treatment is generally not recommended even when patients have had a serious complication of chronic corticosteroid therapy.

Use in Pregnancy
CLINORIL is not recommended for use in pregnant women, since safety for use has not been established, and because of the known effect of drugs of this class on the human fetal cardiovascular system (closure of the ductus arteriosus) during the third trimester of pregnancy. In reproduction studies in the rat, a decrease in average fetal weight and an increase in numbers of dead pups were observed on the first day of the postpartum period at dosage levels of 20 and 40 mg/kg/day (2½ and 5 times the usual maximum daily dose in humans), although there was no adverse effect on the survival and growth during the remainder of the postpartum period. CLINORIL prolongs the duration of gestation in rats, as do other compounds of this class which also may cause dystocia and delayed parturition in pregnant animals. Visceral and skeletal malformations observed in low incidence among rabbits in some teratology studies did not occur at the same dosage levels in repeat studies, nor at a higher dosage level in the same species.

Nursing Mothers
Nursing should not be undertaken while a patient is on CLINORIL. It is not known whether sulindac is secreted in human milk; however, it is secreted in the milk of lactating rats.

Use in Children
Pediatric indications and dosage have not been established, but studies in juvenile rheumatoid arthritis are in progress.

Drug Interactions
DMSO should not be used with sulindac. Concomitant administration has been reported to reduce the plasma levels of the active sulfide metabolite and potentially reduce efficacy. In addition, this combination has been reported to cause peripheral neuropathy.

Although sulindac and its sulfide metabolite are highly bound to protein, studies, in which CLINORIL was given at a dose of 400 mg daily, have shown no clinically significant interaction with oral anticoagulants or oral hypoglycemic agents. However, patients should be monitored carefully until it is certain that no change in their anticoagulant or hypoglycemic dosage is required. Special attention should be paid to patients taking higher doses than those recommended and to patients with renal impairment or other metabolic defects that might increase sulindac blood levels.

The concomitant administration of aspirin with sulindac significantly depressed the plasma levels of the active sulfide metabolite. A double-blind study compared the safety and efficacy of CLINORIL 300 or 400 mg daily given alone or with aspirin 2.4 g/day for the treatment of osteoarthritis. The addition of aspirin did not alter the types of clinical or laboratory adverse experiences for CLINORIL; however, the combination showed an increase in the incidence of gastrointestinal adverse experiences. Since the addition of aspirin did not have a favorable effect on the therapeutic response to CLINORIL, the combination is not recommended.

The concomitant administration of CLINORIL and diflunisal in normal volunteers resulted in lowering of the plasma levels of the active sulindac sulfide metabolite by approximately one-third.

Probenecid given concomitantly with sulindac had only a slight effect on plasma sulfide levels, while plasma levels of sulindac and sulfone were increased. Sulindac was shown to produce a modest reduction in the uricosuric action of probenecid,

Continued on next page

Information on the Merck Sharp & Dohme products listed on these pages is the full prescribing information from product circulars in use November 1, 1984.

Merck Sharp & Dohme—Cont.

which probably is not significant under most circumstances.
Neither propoxyphene hydrochloride nor acetaminophen had any effect on the plasma levels of sulindac or its sulfide metabolite.

Adverse Reactions

The following adverse reactions were reported in clinical trials or have been reported since the drug was marketed. The probability exists of a causal relationship between CLINORIL and these adverse reactions. The adverse reactions which have been observed in clinical trials encompass observations in 1,865 patients, including 232 observed for at least 48 weeks.

Incidence Greater Than 1%
Gastrointestinal
The most frequent types of adverse reactions occurring with CLINORIL are gastrointestinal; these include gastrointestinal pain (10%), dyspepsia*, nausea* with or without vomiting, diarrhea*, constipation*, flatulence, anorexia and gastrointestinal cramps.
Dermatologic
Rash*, pruritus.
Central Nervous System
Dizziness*, headache*, nervousness.
Special Senses
Tinnitus.
Miscellaneous
Edema (see PRECAUTIONS).

* Incidence between 3% and 9%. Those reactions occurring in 1 to 3% of patients are not marked with an asterisk.

Incidence Less Than 1 in 100
Gastrointestinal
Gastritis or gastroenteritis. Peptic ulcer and gastrointestinal bleeding have been reported. GI perforation has been reported rarely.
Liver function abnormalities; jaundice, sometimes with fever; cholestasis; hepatitis.
Pancreatitis.
Dermatologic
Stomatitis, sore or dry mucous membranes, alopecia.
Erythema multiforme, toxic epidermal necrolysis, Stevens-Johnson syndrome, and exfoliative dermatitis have been reported.
Cardiovascular
Congestive heart failure, especially in patients with marginal cardiac function; palpitation; hypertension.
Hematologic
Thrombocytopenia; ecchymosis; purpura; leukopenia; agranulocytosis; neutropenia; bone marrow depression, including aplastic anemia; increased prothrombin time in patients on oral anticoagulants (see PRECAUTIONS).
Genitourinary
Urine discoloration; vaginal bleeding; hematuria; renal impairment, including renal failure; interstitial nephritis; nephrotic syndrome.
Psychiatric
Depression; psychic disturbances including acute psychosis.
Nervous System
Vertigo; insomnia; paresthesia; convulsions; syncope.
Special Senses
Blurred vision; decreased hearing.
Respiratory
Epistaxis.
Hypersensitivity Reactions
Anaphylaxis and angioneurotic edema.
A potentially fatal apparent hypersensitivity syndrome has been reported. This has consisted of some or all of the following findings: fever, chills, skin rash or other dermatologic reactions (see above), changes in liver function, jaundice, pancreatitis, pneumonitis, leukopenia, eosinophilia, anemia, adenitis, and renal impairment, including renal failure.

Causal Relationship Unknown
Other reactions have been reported in clinical trials or since the drug was marketed, but occurred under circumstances where a causal relationship could not be established. However, in these rarely reported events, that possibility cannot be excluded. Therefore, these observations are listed to serve as alerting information to physicians.
Hematologic
Hemolytic anemia.
Nervous System
Neuritis.
Special Senses
Transient visual disturbances.

Management of Overdosage

In the event of overdosage, the stomach should be emptied by inducing vomiting or by gastric lavage, and the patient carefully observed and given symptomatic and supportive treatment.
Animal studies show that absorption is decreased by the prompt administration of activated charcoal and excretion is enhanced by alkalinization of the urine.

Dosage and Administration

CLINORIL should be administered orally twice a day with food. In clinical studies to date, the usual maximum dosage was 400 mg per day. Although a few patients have received higher dosages, until further clinical experience is obtained, dosages above 400 mg per day are not recommended.
In osteoarthritis, rheumatoid arthritis, and ankylosing spondylitis, the recommended starting dosage is 150 mg twice a day. The dosage may be lowered or raised depending on the response.
A prompt response (within one week) can be expected in about one-half of patients with osteoarthritis, ankylosing spondylitis, and rheumatoid arthritis. Others may require longer to respond.
In acute painful shoulder (acute subacromial bursitis/supraspinatus tendinitis) and acute gouty arthritis, the recommended dosage is 200 mg twice a day. After a satisfactory response has been achieved, the dosage may be reduced according to the response. In acute painful shoulder, therapy for 7–14 days is usually adequate. In acute gouty arthritis, therapy for 7 days is usually adequate.

How Supplied

CLINORIL is available for oral administration as 150 mg yellow tablets, and as 200 mg scored yellow tablets.
No. 3360—Tablets CLINORIL 150 mg are yellow, hexagon-shaped, compressed tablets, coded MSD 941. They are supplied as follows:
NDC 0006-0941-54 unit of use bottles of 60
NDC 0006-0941-68 in bottles of 100
NDC 0006-0941-78 unit of use bottles of 100
NDC 0006-0941-28 single unit packages of 100.
Shown in Product Identification Section, page 420
No. 3353—Tablets CLINORIL 200 mg are yellow, hexagon-shaped, scored, compressed tablets, coded MSD 942. They are supplied as follows:
NDC 0006-0942-54 unit of use bottles of 60
NDC 0006-0942-68 in bottles of 100
NDC 0006-0942-78 unit of use bottles of 100
NDC 0006-0942-28 single unit packages of 100.
Shown in Product Identification Section, page 420
A.H.F.S. Category: 28:08
DC 7020018   Issued August 1983
COPYRIGHT© MERCK & CO., INC., 1982
All rights reserved

COGENTIN® Tablets ℞
(benztropine mesylate, MSD), U.S.P.
COGENTIN® Injection ℞
(benztropine mesylate, MSD), U.S.P.

Description

Benztropine mesylate is a synthetic compound resulting from the combination of the active portions of atropine and diphenhydramine.
It is a crystalline white powder, very soluble in water.
COGENTIN® (Benztropine Mesylate, MSD) is supplied as tablets in three strengths (0.5 mg, 1 mg, and 2 mg per tablet), and as an injection for intravenous and intramuscular use.
Each milliliter of the injection contains:
Benztropine mesylate ....1.0 mg
Sodium chloride ....9.0 mg
Water for injection q.s.....................................1.0 ml

Actions

COGENTIN possesses both anticholinergic and antihistaminic effects, although only the former have been established as therapeutically significant in the management of parkinsonism.
In the isolated guinea pig ileum, the anticholinergic activity of this drug is about equal to that of atropine; however, when administered orally to unanesthetized cats, it is only about half as active as atropine.
In laboratory animals, its antihistaminic activity and duration of action approach those of pyrilamine maleate.

Indications

For use as an adjunct in the therapy of all forms of parkinsonism.
Useful also in the control of extrapyramidal disorders (except tardive dyskinesia—see PRECAUTIONS) due to neuroleptic drugs (e.g., phenothiazines).

Contraindications

Hypersensitivity to COGENTIN tablets or to any component of COGENTIN injection.
Because of its atropine-like side effects, this drug is contraindicated in children under three years of age, and should be used with caution in older children.

Warnings

Safe use in pregnancy has not been established.
COGENTIN may impair mental and/or physical abilities required for performance of hazardous tasks, such as operating machinery or driving a motor vehicle.
When COGENTIN is given concomitantly with phenothiazines or other drugs with anticholinergic activity, patients should be advised to report gastrointestinal complaints promptly. Paralytic ileus, sometimes fatal, has occurred in patients taking anticholinergic-type antiparkinsonism drugs, including COGENTIN, in combination with phenothiazines and/or tricyclic antidepressants.
Since COGENTIN contains structural features of atropine, it may produce anhidrosis. For this reason, it should be administered with caution during hot weather, especially when given concomitantly with other atropine-like drugs to the chronically ill, the alcoholic, those who have central nervous system disease, and those who do manual labor in a hot environment. Anhidrosis may occur more readily when some disturbance of sweating already exists. If there is evidence of anhidrosis, the possibility of hyperthermia should be considered. Dosage should be decreased at the discretion of the physician so that the ability to maintain body heat equilibrium by perspiration is not impaired. Severe anhidrosis and fatal hyperthermia have occurred.

Precautions

Since COGENTIN has cumulative action, continued supervision is advisable. Patients with a tendency to tachycardia and patients with prostatic hypertrophy should be observed closely during treatment.
Dysuria may occur, but rarely becomes a problem.
In large doses, the drug may cause complaints of weakness and inability to move particular muscle

groups. For example, if the neck has been rigid and suddenly relaxes, it may feel weak, causing some concern. In this event, dosage adjustment is required.

Mental confusion and excitement may occur with large doses, or in susceptible patients. Visual hallucinations have been reported occasionally. Furthermore, in the treatment of extrapyramidal disorders due to neuroleptic drugs (e.g., phenothiazines), in patients with mental disorders, occasionally there may be intensification of mental symptoms. In such cases, at times, increased doses of antiparkinsonian drugs can precipitate a toxic psychosis. These patients should be kept under careful observation, especially at the beginning of treatment or if dosage is increased.

Tardive dyskinesia may appear in some patients on long-term therapy with phenothiazines and related agents, or may occur after therapy with these drugs has been discontinued. Antiparkinsonism agents do not alleviate the symptoms of tardive dyskinesia, and in some instances may aggravate them. COGENTIN is not recommended for use in patients with tardive dyskinesia.

The physician should be aware of the possible occurrence of glaucoma. Although the drug does not appear to have any adverse effect on simple glaucoma, it probably should not be used in angle-closure glaucoma.

Adverse Reactions

Adverse reactions may be anticholinergic or antihistaminic in nature.

Dry mouth, blurred vision, nausea, and nervousness may develop. Adjustment of dosage or time of administration sometimes helps to control these reactions. If dry mouth is so severe that there is difficulty in swallowing or speaking, or loss of appetite and weight, reduce dosage, or discontinue the drug temporarily.

Vomiting occurs infrequently. Nausea unaccompanied by vomiting usually can be disregarded. Slight reduction in dosage may control the nausea and still give sufficient relief of symptoms. Vomiting may be controlled by temporary discontinuation, followed by resumption at a lower dosage.

Other adverse reactions include constipation, numbness of the fingers, listlessness and depression.

Occasionally, an allergic reaction, e.g., skin rash, develops. Sometimes this can be controlled by reducing dosage, but occasionally medication has to be discontinued.

Dosage and Administration

COGENTIN tablets should be used when patients are able to take oral medication.

The injection is especially useful for psychotic patients with acute dystonic reactions or other reactions that make oral medication difficult or impossible. It is recommended also when a more rapid response is desired than can be obtained with the tablets.

Since there is no significant difference in onset of effect after intravenous or intramuscular injection, usually there is no need to use the intravenous route. The drug is quickly effective after either route, with improvement sometimes noticeable a few minutes after injection. In emergency situations, when the condition of the patient is alarming, 1 to 2 ml of the injection normally will provide quick relief. If the parkinsonian effect begins to return, the dose can be repeated.

Because of cumulative action, therapy should be initiated with a low dose which is increased gradually at five or six-day intervals to the smallest amount necessary for optimal relief. Increases should be made in increments of 0.5 mg, to a maximum of 6 mg, or until optimal results are obtained without excessive adverse reactions.

Postencephalitic and Idiopathic Parkinsonism—

The usual daily dose is 1 to 2 mg, with a range of 0.5 to 6 mg orally or parenterally.

As with any agent used in parkinsonism, dosage must be individualized according to age and weight, and the type of parkinsonism being treated. Generally, older patients and thin patients cannot tolerate large doses. Most patients with postencephalitic parkinsonism need fairly large doses and tolerate them well. Patients with a poor mental outlook are usually poor candidates for therapy.

In idiopathic parkinsonism, therapy may be initiated with a single daily dose of 0.5 to 1 mg at bedtime. In some patients, this will be adequate; in others 4 to 6 mg a day may be required.

In postencephalitic parkinsonism, therapy may be initiated in most patients with 2 mg a day in one or more doses. In highly sensitive patients, therapy may be initiated with 0.5 mg at bedtime, and increased as necessary.

Some patients experience greatest relief by taking the entire dose at bedtime; others react more favorably to divided doses, two to four times a day. Frequently, one dose a day is sufficient, and divided doses may be unnecessary or undesirable. The long duration of action of this drug makes it particularly suitable for bedtime medication when its effects may last throughout the night, enabling patients to turn in bed during the night more easily, and to rise in the morning.

When COGENTIN is started, do not terminate therapy with other antiparkinsonian agents abruptly. If the other agents are to be reduced or discontinued, it must be done gradually. Many patients obtain greatest relief with combination therapy.

COGENTIN may be used concomitantly with SINEMET® (Carbidopa-Levodopa, MSD), or with levodopa, in which case periodic dosage adjustment may be required in order to maintain optimum response.

Drug-Induced Extrapyramidal Disorders—In treating extrapyramidal disorders due to neuroleptic drugs (e.g., phenothiazines), the recommended dosage is 1 to 4 mg once or twice a day orally or parenterally. Dosage must be individualized according to the need of the patient. Some patients require more than recommended; others do not need as much.

In acute dystonic reactions, 1 to 2 ml of the injection usually relieves the condition quickly. After that, the tablets, 1 to 2 mg twice a day, usually prevent recurrence.

When extrapyramidal disorders develop soon after initiation of treatment with neuroleptic drugs (e.g., phenothiazines), they are likely to be transient. One to 2 mg of COGENTIN tablets two or three times a day usually provides relief within one or two days. After one or two weeks, the drug should be withdrawn to determine the continued need for it. If such disorders recur, COGENTIN can be reinstituted.

Certain drug-induced extrapyramidal disorders that develop slowly may not respond to COGENTIN.

Overdosage

Manifestations—May be any of those seen in atropine poisoning or antihistamine overdosage: CNS depression, preceded or followed by stimulation; confusion; nervousness; listlessness; intensification of mental symptoms or toxic psychosis in patients with mental illness being treated with neuroleptic drugs (e.g., phenothiazines); hallucinations (especially visual); dizziness; muscle weakness; ataxia; dry mouth; mydriasis; blurred vision; palpitations; nausea; vomiting; dysuria; numbness of fingers; dysphagia; allergic reactions, e.g., skin rash; headache; hot, dry, flushed skin; delirium; coma; shock; convulsions; respiratory arrest; anhidrosis; hyperthermia; glaucoma; constipation.

Treatment—Physostigmine salicylate, 1 to 2 mg, sc or iv, reportedly will reverse symptoms of anticholinergic intoxication (Duvoisin, R.C.; Katz, R.: J. Amer. Med. Ass. 206:1963-1965, Nov. 25, 1968). A second injection may be given after 2 hours if required. Otherwise treatment is symptomatic and supportive. Induce emesis or perform gastric lavage (contraindicated in precomatose, convulsive, or psychotic states). Maintain respiration. A short-acting barbiturate may be used for CNS excitement, but with caution to avoid subsequent depression; supportive care for depression (avoid convulsant stimulants such as picrotoxin, pentylenetetrazol, or bemegride); artificial respiration for severe respiratory depression; a local miotic for mydriasis and cycloplegia; ice bags or other cold applications and alcohol sponges for hyperpyrexia, a vasopressor and fluids for circulatory collapse. Darken room for photophobia.

How Supplied

No. 3297—Tablets COGENTIN, 0.5 mg, are white, round, scored, compressed tablets, coded MSD 21. They are supplied as follows:
NDC 0006-0021-68 in bottles of 100.
Shown in Product Identification Section, page 420
No. 3334—Tablets COGENTIN, 1 mg, are white, oval shaped, scored, compressed tablets, coded MSD 635. They are supplied as follows:
NDC 0006-0635-68 in bottles of 100.
NDC 0006-0635-28 unit dose packages of 100.
Shown in Product Identification Section, page 420
No. 3172—Tablets COGENTIN, 2 mg, are white, round, scored, compressed tablets, coded MSD 60. They are supplied as follows:
NDC 0006-0060-68 in bottles of 100.
(6505-00-680-1907 2 mg 100's)
NDC 0006-0060-28 unit dose packages of 100.
NDC 0006-0060-82 in bottles of 1000.
Shown in Product Identification Section, page 420
No. 3275—Injection COGENTIN, 1 mg per ml, is a clear, colorless solution and is supplied as follows:
NDC 0006-3275-16 in boxes of 6×2 ml ampuls.
A.H.F.S. Category: 12:08
DC 6460714 Issued September 1978

ColBENEMID® Tablets
(probenecid-colchicine, MSD), U.S.P.

Description

ColBENEMID® (Probenecid-Colchicine, MSD) contains BENEMID® (Probenecid, MSD) and colchicine.

Probenecid is the generic name for 4-[(dipropylamino) sulfonyl] benzoic acid (molecular weight 285.36).

Probenecid is a white or nearly white, fine, crystalline powder. It is soluble in dilute alkali, in alcohol, in chloroform, and in acetone; it is practically insoluble in water and in dilute acids.

Colchicine is an alkaloid obtained from various species of Colchicum. The chemical name for colchicine is (S)-N-(5,6,7,9-tetrahydro-1,2,3,10-tetramethoxy-9-oxobenzo [a] heptalen-7-yl) acetamide (molecular weight 399.43).

Colchicine consists of pale yellow scales or powder; it darkens on exposure to light. Colchicine is soluble in water, freely soluble in alcohol and in chloroform, and slightly soluble in ether.

Actions

Probenecid is a uricosuric and renal tubular blocking agent. It inhibits the tubular reabsorption of urate, thus increasing the urinary excretion of uric acid and decreasing serum urate levels. Effective uricosuria reduces the miscible urate pool, retards urate deposition, and promotes resorption of urate deposits.

Probenecid inhibits the tubular secretion of penicillin and usually increases penicillin plasma levels by any route the antibiotic is given. A 2-fold to 4-fold elevation has been demonstrated for various penicillins.

Probenecid also has been reported to inhibit the renal transport of many other compounds including aminohippuric acid (PAH), aminosalicylic acid (PAS), indomethacin, sodium iodomethamate and related iodinated organic acids, 17-ketosteroids,

Continued on next page

Information on the Merck Sharp & Dohme products listed on these pages is the full prescribing information from product circulars in use November 1, 1984.

Merck Sharp & Dohme—Cont.

pantothenic acid, phenolsulfonphthalein (PSP), sulfonamides, and sulfonylureas. See also DRUG INTERACTIONS.
Probenecid decreases both hepatic and renal excretion of sulfobromophthalein (BSP). The tubular reabsorption of phosphorus is inhibited in hypoparathyroid but not in euparathyroid individuals.
Probenecid does not influence plasma concentrations of salicylates, nor the excretion of streptomycin, chloramphenicol, chlortetracycline, oxytetracycline, or neomycin.
The mode of action of colchicine in gout is unknown. It is not an analgesic, though it relieves pain in acute attacks of gout. It is not a uricosuric agent and will not prevent progression of gout to chronic gouty arthritis. It does have a prophylactic, suppressive effect that helps to reduce the incidence of acute attacks and to relieve the residual pain and mild discomfort that patients with gout occasionally feel.
In man and certain other animals, colchicine can produce a temporary leukopenia that is followed by leukocytosis.
Colchicine has other pharmacologic actions in animals: It alters neuromuscular function, intensifies gastrointestinal activity by neurogenic stimulation, increases sensitivity to central depressants, heightens response to sympathomimetic compounds, depresses the respiratory center, constricts blood vessels, causes hypertension by central vasomotor stimulation, and lowers body temperature.

Indications

For the treatment of chronic gouty arthritis when complicated by frequent, recurrent acute attacks of gout.

Contraindications

Hypersensitivity to this product or to probenecid or colchicine.
Children under 2 years of age.
Not recommended in persons with known blood dyscrasias or uric acid kidney stones.
Therapy with ColBENEMID should not be started until an acute gouty attack has subsided.
Pregnancy: Probenecid crosses the placental barrier and appears in cord blood. Colchicine can arrest cell division in animals and plants. In certain species of animal under certain conditions, colchicine has produced teratogenic effects. The possibility of such effects in humans also has been reported. Because of the colchicine component, ColBENEMID is contraindicated in pregnant patients. The use of any drug in women of childbearing potential requires that the anticipated benefit be weighed against possible hazards.

Warnings

Exacerbation of gout following therapy with ColBENEMID may occur; in such cases additional colchicine or other appropriate therapy is advisable.
Probenecid increases plasma concentrations of methotrexate in both animals and humans. In animal studies, increased methotrexate toxicity has been reported. If ColBENEMID is given with methotrexate, the dosage of methotrexate should be reduced and serum levels may need to be monitored.
In patients on ColBENEMID the use of salicylates in either small or large doses is contraindicated because it antagonizes the uricosuric action of probenecid. The biphasic action of salicylates in the renal tubules accounts for the so-called "paradoxical effect" of uricosuric agents. In patients on ColBENEMID who require a mild analgesic agent the use of acetaminophen rather than small doses of salicylates would be preferred.
The appearance of hypersensitivity reactions requires cessation of therapy with ColBENEMID.
Colchicine has been reported to adversely affect spermatogenesis in animals. Reversible azoospermia has been reported in one patient.

Precautions

Hematuria, renal colic, costovertebral pain, and formation of uric acid stones associated with the use of ColBENEMID in gouty patients may be prevented by alkalization of the urine and a liberal fluid intake (*see* DOSAGE AND ADMINISTRATION). In these cases when alkali is administered, the acid-base balance of the patient should be watched.
Use with caution in patients with a history of peptic ulcer.
ColBENEMID has been used in patients with some renal impairment but dosage requirements may be increased. ColBENEMID may not be effective in chronic renal insufficiency particularly when the glomerular filtration rate is 30 ml/minute or less.
A reducing substance may appear in the urine of patients receiving probenecid. This disappears with discontinuance of therapy. Suspected glycosuria should be confirmed by using a test specific for glucose.
Adequate animal studies have not been conducted to determine the carcinogenicity potential of probenecid or this drug combination. Since colchicine is an established mutagen, its ability to act as a carcinogen must be suspected and administration of ColBENEMID should involve a weighing of the benefit-vs-risk when long-term administration is contemplated.

Adverse Reactions

Headache, gastrointestinal symptoms (e.g., anorexia, nausea, vomiting), urinary frequency, hypersensitivity reactions (including anaphylaxis, dermatitis, pruritus, and fever), sore gums, flushing, dizziness, and anemia have occurred following the use of probenecid. In gouty patients exacerbation of gout, and uric acid stones with or without hematuria, renal colic, or costovertebral pain, have been observed. Nephrotic syndrome, hepatic necrosis, and aplastic anemia occur rarely. Hemolytic anemia which in some instances could be related to genetic deficiency of glucose-6-phosphate dehydrogenase in red blood cells has been reported.
Side effects due to colchicine appear to be a function of dosage. The most prominent symptoms are referable to the gastrointestinal tract (e.g., nausea, vomiting, abdominal pain, diarrhea) and may be particularly troublesome in the presence of peptic ulcer or spastic colon. At toxic doses colchicine may cause severe diarrhea, generalized vascular damage, and renal damage with hematuria and oliguria. Muscular weakness, which disappears with discontinuance of therapy, urticaria, dermatitis, and purpura have also been reported. Hypersensitivity to colchicine is a very rare occurrence, but should be borne in mind. The appearance of any of the aforementioned symptoms may require reduction of dosage or discontinuance of the drug.
When given for prolonged periods, colchicine may cause agranulocytosis, aplastic anemia, and peripheral neuritis. Loss of hair attributable to colchicine therapy has been reported. The possibility of increased colchicine toxicity in the presence of hepatic dysfunction should be considered.

Drug Interactions

The use of salicylates antagonizes the uricosuric action of probenecid (*see* WARNINGS). The uricosuric action of probenecid is also antagonized by pyrazinamide.
Probenecid produces an insignificant increase in free sulfonamide plasma concentrations but a significant increase in total sulfonamide plasma levels. Since probenecid decreases the renal excretion of conjugated sulfonamides, plasma concentrations of the latter should be determined from time to time when a sulfonamide and ColBENEMID are coadministered for prolonged periods. Probenecid may prolong or enhance the action of oral sulfonylureas and thereby increase the risk of hypoglycemia.
When probenecid is given to patients receiving indomethacin, the plasma levels of indomethacin are likely to be increased. Therefore, a lower dosage of indomethacin may be required to produce a therapeutic effect, and increases in the dosage of indomethacin should be made cautiously and in small increments. Probenecid may increase plasma levels of rifampin. The clinical significance of this is not known.
In animals and in humans, probenecid has been reported to increase plasma concentrations of methotrexate (*see* WARNINGS).
Falsely high readings for theophylline have been reported in an *in vitro* study, using the Schack and Waxler technic, when therapeutic concentrations of theophylline and probenecid were added to human plasma.

Dosage and Administration

Therapy with ColBENEMID should not be *started* until an acute gouty attack has subsided. However, if an acute attack is precipitated *during* therapy, ColBENEMID may be continued without changing the dosage, and additional colchicine or other appropriate therapy should be given to control the acute attack.
The recommended adult dosage is 1 tablet of ColBENEMID daily for one week, followed by 1 tablet twice a day thereafter.
Some degree of renal impairment may be present in patients with gout. A daily dosage of 2 tablets may be adequate. However, if necessary, the daily dosage may be increased by 1 tablet every four weeks within tolerance (and usually not above 4 tablets per day) if symptoms of gouty arthritis are not controlled or the 24 hour uric acid excretion is not above 700 mg. As noted, probenecid may not be effective in chronic renal insufficiency particularly when the glomerular filtration rate is 30 ml/minute or less.
Gastric intolerance may be indicative of overdosage, and may be corrected by decreasing the dosage.
As uric acid tends to crystallize out of an acid urine, a liberal fluid intake is recommended, as well as sufficient sodium bicarbonate (3 to 7.5 g daily) or potassium citrate (7.5 g daily) to maintain an alkaline urine (*see* PRECAUTIONS).
Alkalization of the urine is recommended until the serum urate level returns to normal limits and tophaceous deposits disappear, i.e., during the period when urinary excretion of uric acid is at a high level. Thereafter, alkalization of the urine and the usual restriction of purine-producing foods may be somewhat relaxed.
ColBENEMID (or probenecid) should be continued at the dosage that will maintain normal serum urate levels. When acute attacks have been absent for six months or more and serum urate levels remain within normal limits, the daily dosage of ColBENEMID may be decreased by 1 tablet every six months. The maintenance dosage should not be reduced to the point where serum urate levels tend to rise.

How Supplied

No. 3283—Tablets ColBENEMID are white to off-white, capsule-shaped, scored tablets, coded MSD 614. Each tablet contains 0.5 g of probenecid and 0.5 mg of colchicine. They are supplied as follows:
NDC 0006-0614-68 bottles of 100.
Shown in Product Identification Section, page 420
A.H.F.S. Category: 40:40
DC 6213021 Issued December 1979

COSMEGEN® Injection ℞
(dactinomycin, MSD), U.S.P.

WARNING

Dactinomycin is extremely corrosive to soft tissue. If extravasation occurs during intravenous use, severe damage to soft tissues will occur. In at least one instance, this has led to contracture of the arms.

DOSAGE

The dosage of COSMEGEN® (Dactinomycin, MSD) is calculated in micrograms (mcg). The usual adult dosage is 500 micrograms (0.5 mg) daily intravenously for a maximum of five days. The dosage for adults or children should not exceed 15 mcg/kg or 400-600 mcg/square meter of body surface daily intravenously for five days. Calculation of the dosage for obese or edematous patients should be on the basis of surface area in an effort to relate dosage to lean body mass.

Description

Dactinomycin is one of the actinomycins, a group of antibiotics produced by various species of *Streptomyces*. Dactinomycin is the principal component of the mixture of actinomycins produced by *Streptomyces parvullus*. Unlike other species of *Streptomyces*, this organism yields an essentially pure substance that contains only traces of similar compounds differing in the amino acid content of the peptide side chains. The empirical formula is $C_{62}H_{86}N_{12}O_{16}$.

COSMEGEN is a sterile, yellow lyophilized powder for injection by the intravenous route or by regional perfusion after reconstitution. Each vial contains 0.5 mg (500 mcg) of dactinomycin and 20.0 mg of mannitol.

Clinical Pharmacology
Action

Generally, the actinomycins exert an inhibitory effect on gram-positive and gram-negative bacteria and on some fungi. However, the toxic properties of the actinomycins (including dactinomycin) in relation to antibacterial activity are such as to preclude their use as antibiotics in the treatment of infectious diseases.

Because the actinomycins are cytotoxic, they have an antineoplastic effect which has been demonstrated in experimental animals with various types of tumor implant. This cytotoxic action is the basis for their use in the palliative treatment of certain types of cancer.

Pharmacokinetics and Metabolism

Results of a study in patients with malignant melanoma indicate that dactinomycin (^3H actinomycin D) is minimally metabolized, is concentrated in nucleated cells, and does not penetrate the blood brain barrier. Approximately 30% of the dose was recovered in urine and feces in one week. The terminal plasma half-life for radioactivity was approximately 36 hours.

Indications and Usage

Wilms' Tumor

The neoplasm responding most frequently to COSMEGEN is Wilms' tumor. With low doses of both dactinomycin and radiotherapy, temporary objective improvement may be as good as and may last longer than with higher doses of each given alone. In the National Wilms' Tumor study, combination therapy with dactinomycin and vincristine together with surgery and radiotherapy, was shown to have significantly improved the prognosis of patients in groups II and III. Dactinomycin and vincristine were given for a total of seven cycles, so that maintenance therapy continued for approximately 15 months.

Postoperative radiotherapy in group I patients and optimal combination chemotherapy for those in group IV are unsettled issues. About 70 percent of lung metastases have disappeared with an appropriate combination of radiation, dactinomycin and vincristine.

Rhabdomyosarcoma

Temporary regression of the tumor and beneficial subjective results have occurred with dactinomycin in rhabdomyosarcoma which, like most soft tissue sarcomas, is comparatively radio-resistant.

Several groups have reported successful use of cyclophosphamide, vincristine, dactinomycin and doxorubicin hydrochloride in various combinations. Effective combinations have included vincristine and dactinomycin; vincristine, dactinomycin and cyclophosphamide (VAC therapy) and all four drugs in sequence. At present, the most effective treatment for children with inoperable or metastatic rhabdomyosarcoma has been VAC chemotherapy. Two thirds of these children were doing well without evidence of disease at a median time of three years after diagnosis.

Carcinoma of Testis and Uterus

The sequential use of dactinomycin and methotrexate, along with meticulous monitoring of human chorionic gonadotropin levels until normal, has resulted in survival in the majority of women with metastatic choriocarcinoma. Sequential therapy is used if there is:
1. Stability in gonadotropin titers following two successive courses of an agent.
2. Rising gonadotropin titers during treatment.
3. Severe toxicity preventing adequate therapy.

In patients with nonmetastatic choriocarcinoma, dactinomycin or methotrexate or both, have been used successfully, with or without surgery.

Dactinomycin has been beneficial as a single agent in the treatment of metastatic nonseminomatour testicular carcinoma when used in cycles of 500 mcg/day for five consecutive days, every 6-8 weeks for periods of four months or longer.

Other Neoplasms

Dactinomycin has been given intravenously or by regional perfusion, either alone or with other antineoplastic compounds or x-ray therapy, in the palliative treatment of Ewing's sarcoma and sarcoma botryoides. For nonmetastatic Ewing's sarcoma, promising results were obtained when dactinomycin (45 mcg/m^2) and cyclophosphamide (1200 mg/m^2) were given sequentially and with radiotherapy, over an 18 month period. Those with metastatic disease remain the subject of continued investigation with a more aggressive chemotherapeutic regimen employed initially.

Temporary objective improvement and relief of pain and discomfort have followed the use of dactinomycin usually in conjunction with radiotherapy for sarcoma botryoides. This palliative effect ranges from transitory inhibition of tumor growth to a considerable but temporary regression in tumor size.

COSMEGEN (Dactinomycin, MSD) and Radiation Therapy

Much evidence suggests that dactinomycin potentiates the effects of x-ray therapy. The converse also appears likely; i.e., dactinomycin may be more effective when radiation therapy also is given. With combined dactinomycin-radiation therapy, the normal skin, as well as the buccal and pharyngeal mucosa, show early erythema. A smaller than usual x-ray dose when given with dactinomycin causes erythema and vesiculation, which progress more rapidly through the stages of tanning and desquamation. Healing may occur in four to six weeks rather than two to three months. Erythema from previous x-ray therapy may be reactivated by dactinomycin alone, even when irradiation occurred many months earlier, and especially when the interval between the two forms of therapy is brief. This potentiation of radiation effect represents a special problem when the irradiation treatment area includes the mucous membrane. When irradiation is directed toward the nasopharynx, the combination may produce severe oropharyngeal mucositis. *Severe reactions may ensue if high doses of both dactinomycin and radiation therapy are used or if the patient is particularly sensitive to such combined therapy.*

Because of this potentiating effect, dactinomycin may be tried in radio-sensitive tumors not responding to doses of x-ray therapy that can be tolerated. Objective improvement in tumor size and activity may be observed when lower, better tolerated doses of both types of therapy are employed.

COSMEGEN (Dactinomycin, MSD) and Perfusion Technic

Dactinomycin alone or with other antineoplastic agents has also been given by the isolation-perfusion technic, either as palliative treatment or as an adjunct to resection of a tumor. Some tumors considered resistant to chemotherapy and radiation therapy may respond when the drug is given by the perfusion technic. Neoplasms in which dactinomycin has been tried by this technic include various types of sarcoma, carcinoma, and adenocarcinoma.

In some instances tumors regressed, pain was relieved for variable periods, and surgery made possible. On other occasions, however, the outcome has been less favorable. Nevertheless, in selected cases, the drug by perfusion may provide more effective palliation than when given systemically. Dactinomycin by the isolation-perfusion technic offers certain advantages, provided leakage of the drug through the general circulation into other areas of the body is minimal. By this technic the drug is in continuous contact with the tumor for the duration of treatment. The dose may be increased well over that used by the systemic route, usually without adding to the danger of toxic effects. If the agent is confined to an isolated part, it should not interfere with the patient's defense mechanism. Systemic absorption of toxic products from neoplastic tissue can be minimized by removing the perfusate when the procedure is finished.

Contraindications

If dactinomycin is given at or about the time of infection with chicken pox or herpes zoster, a severe generalized disease, which may result in death, may occur.

Precautions

General

COSMEGEN should be administered only under the supervision of a physician who is experienced in the use of cancer chemotherapeutic agents.

This drug is highly toxic and both powder and solution must be handled and administered with care. Inhalation of dust or vapors and contact with skin or mucous membranes, especially those of the eyes, must be avoided. Should accidental eye contact occur, copious irrigation with water should be instituted immediately, followed by prompt ophthalmologic consultation. Should accidental skin contact occur, the affected part must be irrigated immediately with copious amounts of water for at least 15 minutes.

As with all antineoplastic agents, dactinomycin is a toxic drug and very careful and frequent observation of the patient for adverse reactions is necessary. These reactions may involve any tissue of the body. The possibility of an anaphylactoid reaction should be borne in mind.

Increased incidence of gastrointestinal toxicity and marrow suppression has been reported when dactinomycin was given with x-ray therapy.

Particular caution is necessary when administering dactinomycin in the first two months after irradiation for the treatment of right-sided Wilms' tumor, since hepatomegaly and elevated SGOT levels have been noted.

Nausea and vomiting due to dactinomycin make it necessary to give this drug intermittently. It is extremely important to observe the patient daily for toxic side effects when multiple chemotherapy is employed, since a full course of therapy occasionally is not tolerated. If stomatitis, diarrhea, or severe hemopoietic depression appear during therapy, these drugs should be discontinued until the patient has recovered.

Continued on next page

Information on the Merck Sharp & Dohme products listed on these pages is the full prescribing information from product circulars in use November 1, 1984.

Merck Sharp & Dohme—Cont.

Recent reports indicate an increased incidence of second primary tumors following treatment with radiation and anti-neoplastic agents, such as dactinomycin. Multi-modal therapy creates the need for careful, long-term observation of cancer survivors.

Laboratory Tests
Many abnormalities of renal, hepatic, and bone marrow function have been reported in patients with neoplastic disease and receiving dactinomycin. It is advisable to check renal, hepatic, and bone marrow functions frequently.

Drug/Laboratory Test Interactions
It has been reported that dactinomycin may interfere with bioassay procedures for the determination of antibacterial drug levels.

Carcinogenesis, Mutagenesis, Impairment of Fertility
The International Agency on Research on Cancer has judged that dactinomycin is a positive carcinogen in animals. Local sarcomas were produced in mice and rats after repeated subcutaneous or intraperitoneal injection. Mesenchymal tumors occurred in male F344 rats given intraperitoneal injections of 0.05 mg/kg, 2 to 5 times per week for 18 weeks. The first tumor appeared at 23 weeks. Dactinomycin has been shown to be mutagenic in a number of test systems *in vitro* and *in vivo* including human fibroblasts and leucocytes, and HELA cells. DNA damage and cytogenetic effects have been demonstrated in the mouse and the rat. Adequate fertility studies have not been reported.

Pregnancy
Pregnancy Category C. COSMEGEN has been shown to cause malformations and embryotoxicity in the rat, rabbit and hamster when given in doses of 50–100 mcg/kg intravenously (3–7 times the maximum recommended human dose). There are no adequate and well-controlled studies in pregnant women. COSMEGEN should be used during pregnancy only if the potential benefit justifies the potential risk to the fetus.

Nursing Mothers
It is not known whether this drug is excreted in human milk. Because many drugs are excreted in human milk and because of the potential for serious adverse reactions in nursing infants from COSMEGEN, a decision should be made whether to discontinue nursing or to discontinue the drug, taking into account the importance of the drug to the mother.

Pediatric Use
The greater frequency of toxic effects of dactinomycin in infants suggest that this drug should be given to infants only over the age of 6 to 12 months.

Adverse Reactions

Toxic effects (excepting nausea and vomiting) usually do not become apparent until two to four days after a course of therapy is stopped, and may not be maximal before one to two weeks have elapsed. Deaths have been reported. However, adverse reactions are usually reversible on discontinuance of therapy. They include the following:
Miscellaneous (malaise, fatigue, lethargy, fever, myalgia, proctitis, hypocalcemia).
Oral (cheilitis, dysphagia, esophagitis, ulcerative stomatitis, pharyngitis).
Gastrointestinal (anorexia, nausea, vomiting, abdominal pain, diarrhea, gastrointestinal ulceration). Nausea and vomiting, which occur early during the first few hours after administration, may be alleviated by giving antiemetics.
Hematologic (anemia, even to the point of aplastic anemia, agranulocytosis, leukopenia, thrombopenia, pancytopenia, reticulopenia). Platelet and white cell counts should be done *daily* to detect severe hemopoietic depression. If either count markedly decreases, the drug should be withheld to allow marrow recovery. This often takes up to three weeks.

Dermatologic (alopecia, skin eruptions, acne, flare-up of erythema or increased pigmentation of previously irradiated skin).
Soft tissues. Dactinomycin is extremely corrosive. If extravasation occurs during intravenous use, severe damage to soft tissues will occur. In at least one instance, this has led to contracture of the arms.

Overdosage

The intravenous LD_{50} of COSMEGEN in the rat is 460 mcg/kg.

Dosage and Administration

Toxic reactions due to dactinomycin are frequent and may be severe (see ADVERSE REACTIONS), thus limiting in many instances the amount that may be given. However, the severity of toxicity varies markedly and is only partly dependent on the dose employed. The drug must be given in short courses.

Intravenous Use
The dosage of dactinomycin varies depending on the tolerance of the patient, the size and location of the neoplasm, and the use of other forms of therapy. It may be necessary to decrease the usual dosages suggested below when other chemotherapy or x-ray therapy is used concomitantly or has been used previously.
The dosage for adults or children should not exceed 15 mcg/kg or 400–600 mcg/square meter of body surface daily intravenously for five days. Calculation of the dosage for obese or edematous patients should be on the basis of surface area in an effort to relate dosage to lean body mass.
Adults: The usual adult dosage is 500 mcg (0.5 mg) daily intravenously for a maximum of five days.
Children: In children 15 mcg (0.015 mg) per kilogram of body weight is given intravenously daily for five days. An alternative schedule is a total dosage of 2500 mcg (2.5 mg) per square meter of body surface given intravenously over a one week period.
In both adults and children, a second course may be given after at least three weeks have elapsed, provided all signs of toxicity have disappeared.
Reconstitute COSMEGEN by adding 1.1 ml of **Sterile Water for Injection (without preservative)** using aseptic precautions. The resulting solution of dactinomycin will contain approximately 500 mcg or 0.5 mg per ml.
Parenteral drug products should be inspected visually for particulate matter and discoloration prior to administration, whenever solution and container permit. When reconstituted, COSMEGEN is a clear, gold-colored solution.
Once reconstituted, the solution of dactinomycin can be added to infusion solutions of Dextrose Injection 5 percent or Sodium Chloride Injection either directly or to the tubing of a running intravenous infusion.
Although reconstituted COSMEGEN is chemically stable, the product does not contain a preservative and accidental microbial contamination might result. Any unused portion should be discarded. Use of water containing preservatives (benzyl alcohol or parabens) to reconstitute COSMEGEN for injection, results in the formation of a precipitate.
Partial removal of dactinomycin from intravenous solutions by cellulose ester membrane filters used in some intravenous in-line filters has been reported.
Since dactinomycin is extremely corrosive to soft tissue, precautions for materials of this nature should be observed.
If the drug is given directly into the vein without the use of an infusion, the "two-needle technic" should be used. Reconstitute and withdraw the calculated dose from the vial with one sterile needle. Use another sterile needle for direct injection into the vein.
Discard any unused portion of the dactinomycin solution.

Isolation-Perfusion Technic
The dosage schedules and the technic itself vary from one investigator to another; the published literature, therefore, should be consulted for details. In general, the following doses are suggested:
50 mcg (0.05 mg) per kilogram of body weight for lower extremity or pelvis.
35 mcg (0.035 mg) per kilogram of body weight for upper extremity.
It may be advisable to use lower doses in obese patients, or when previous chemotherapy or radiation therapy has been employed.
Complications of the perfusion technic are related mainly to the amount of drug that escapes into the systemic circulation and may consist of hemopoietic depression, absorption of toxic products from massive destruction of neoplastic tissue, increased susceptibility to infection, impaired wound healing, and superficial ulceration of the gastric mucosa. Other side effects may include edema of the extremity involved, damage to soft tissues of the perfused area, and (potentially) venous thrombosis.

How Supplied

No. 3298—Injection COSMEGEN is a lyophilized powder and is supplied as follows: **NDC 0006-3298-22** in vials containing 0.5 mg (500 micrograms) of dactinomycin and 20.0 mg of mannitol. In the dry form the compound is an amorphous yellow powder. The solution is clear and gold-colored.

Special Handling
Due to the drug's toxic and mutagenic properties, appropriate precautions including the use of appropriate safety equipment are recommended for the preparation of COSMEGEN for parenteral administration. The National Institutes of Health presently recommends that the preparation of injectable antineoplastic drugs should be performed in a Class II laminar flow biological safety cabinet and that personnel preparing drugs of this class should wear surgical gloves and a closed front surgical-type gown with knit cuffs.
A.H.F.S. Category: 10:00
DC 6059221   Issued September 1983
COPYRIGHT © MERCK & CO., INC., 1983
All rights reserved

CUPRIMINE® Capsules ℞
(penicillamine, MSD), U.S.P.

> Physicians planning to use penicillamine should thoroughly familiarize themselves with its toxicity, special dosage considerations, and therapeutic benefits. Penicillamine should never be used casually. Each patient should remain constantly under the close supervision of the physician. Patients should be warned to report promptly any symptoms suggesting toxicity.

Description

Penicillamine is 3-mercapto-D-valine. It is a white or practically white, crystalline powder, freely soluble in water, slightly soluble in alcohol, and insoluble in ether, acetone, benzene, and carbon tetrachloride. Although its configuration is D, it is levorotatory as usually measured:
$$[\alpha]25° = -63° \pm 5° (C = 1, 1\underline{N} \text{ NaOH})\cdot$$
D
The empirical formula is $C_5H_{11}NO_2S$, giving it a molecular weight of 149.21.
It reacts readily with formaldehyde or acetone to form a thiazolidine-carboxylic acid.

Clinical Pharmacology

Penicillamine is a chelating agent recommended for the removal of excess copper in patients with Wilson's disease. From *in vitro* studies which indicate that one atom of copper combines with two molecules of penicillamine, it would appear that one gram of penicillamine should be followed by the excretion of about 200 milligrams of copper;

however, the actual amount excreted is about one percent of this.

Penicillamine also reduces excess cystine excretion in cystinuria. This is done, at least in part, by disulfide interchange between penicillamine and cystine, resulting in formation of penicillamine-cysteine disulfide, a substance that is much more soluble than cystine and is excreted readily.

Penicillamine interferes with the formation of cross-links between tropocollagen molecules and cleaves them when newly formed.

The mechanism of action of penicillamine in rheumatoid arthritis is unknown although it appears to suppress disease activity. Unlike cytotoxic immunosuppressants, penicillamine markedly lowers IgM rheumatoid factor but produces no significant depression in absolute levels of serum immunoglobulins. Also unlike cytotoxic immunosuppressants which act on both, penicillamine *in vitro* depresses T-cell activity but not B-cell activity.

In vitro, penicillamine dissociates macroglobulins (rheumatoid factor) although the relationship of the activity to its effect in rheumatoid arthritis is not known.

In rheumatoid arthritis, the onset of therapeutic response to CUPRIMINE® (Penicillamine, MSD) may not be seen for two or three months. In those patients who respond, however, the first evidence of suppression of symptoms such as pain, tenderness, and swelling is generally apparent within three months. The optimum duration of therapy has not been determined. If remissions occur, they may last from months to years, but usually require continued treatment (see DOSAGE AND ADMINISTRATION).

In patients with rheumatoid arthritis, it is important that CUPRIMINE be given on an empty stomach, at least one hour before meals and at least one hour apart from any other drug, food, or milk. This permits maximum absorption and reduces the likelihood of inactivation by metal binding.

Methodology for determining the bioavailability of penicillamine is not available; however, penicillamine is known to be a very soluble substance.

Indications

CUPRIMINE is indicated in the treatment of Wilson's disease, cystinuria, and in patients with severe, active rheumatoid arthritis who have failed to respond to an adequate trial of conventional therapy. Available evidence suggests that CUPRIMINE is not of value in ankylosing spondylitis.

Wilson's Disease—Wilson's disease (hepatolenticular degeneration) results from the interaction of an inherited defect and an abnormality in copper metabolism. The metabolic defect, which is the consequence of the autosomal inheritance of one abnormal gene from each parent, manifests itself in a greater positive copper balance than normal. As a result, copper is deposited in several organs and appears eventually to produce pathologic effects most prominently seen in the brain, where degeneration is widespread; in the liver, where fatty infiltration, inflammation, and hepatocellular damage progress to postnecrotic cirrhosis; in the kidney, where tubular and glomerular dysfunction results; and in the eye, where characteristic corneal copper deposits are known as Kayser-Fleischer rings.

Two classes of patients require treatment for Wilson's disease: (1) the symptomatic, and (2) the asymptomatic in whom it can be assumed the disease will develop in the future if the patient is not treated.

Diagnosis, suspected on the basis of family or individual history, physical examination, or a low serum concentration of ceruloplasmin*, is confirmed by the demonstration of Kayser-Fleischer rings or, particularly in the asymptomatic patient, by the quantitative demonstration in a liver biopsy specimen of a concentration of copper in excess of 250 mcg/g dry weight.

---

*For quantitative test for serum ceruloplasmin see: Morell, A.G.; Windsor, J.; Sternlieb, I.; Scheinberg, I.H.: Measurement of the concentration of ceruloplasmin in serum by determination of its oxidase activity, in "Laboratory Diagnosis of Liver Disease", F.W. Sunderman; F.W. Sunderman, Jr. (eds.), St. Louis, Warren H. Green, Inc., 1968, pp. 193-195.

Treatment has two objectives:
 (1) to minimize dietary intake and absorption of copper.
 (2) to promote excretion of copper deposited in tissues.

The first objective is attained by a daily diet that contains no more than one or two milligrams of copper. Such a diet should exclude, most importantly, chocolate, nuts, shellfish, mushrooms, liver, molasses, broccoli, and cereals enriched with copper, and be composed to as great an extent as possible of foods with a low copper content. Distilled or demineralized water should be used if the patient's drinking water contains more than 0.1 mg of copper per liter.

For the second objective, a copper chelating agent is used. Penicillamine is the only one of these agents that is orally effective.

In symptomatic patients this treatment usually produces marked neurologic improvement, fading of Kayser-Fleischer rings, and gradual amelioration of hepatic dysfunction and psychic disturbances.

Clinical experience to date suggests that life is prolonged with the above regimen.

Noticeable improvement may not occur for one to three months. Occasionally, neurologic symptoms become worse during initiation of therapy with CUPRIMINE. Despite this, the drug should not be discontinued permanently, although temporary interruption may result in clinical improvement of the neurological symptoms but it carries an increased risk of developing a sensitivity reaction upon resumption of therapy (see WARNINGS).

Treatment of asymptomatic patients has been carried out for over ten years. Symptoms and signs of the disease appear to be prevented indefinitely if daily treatment with CUPRIMINE can be continued.

Cystinuria—Cystinuria is characterized by excessive urinary excretion of the dibasic amino acids, arginine, lysine, ornithine, and cystine, and the mixed disulfide of cysteine and homocysteine. The metabolic defect that leads to cystinuria is inherited as an autosomal, recessive trait. Metabolism of the affected amino acids is influenced by at least two abnormal factors: (1) defective gastrointestinal absorption and (2) renal tubular dysfunction. Arginine, lysine, ornithine, and cysteine are soluble substances, readily excreted. There is no apparent pathology connected with their excretion in excessive quantities.

Cystine, however, is so slightly soluble at the usual range of urinary pH that it is not excreted readily, and so crystallizes and forms stones in the urinary tract. Stone formation is the only known pathology in cystinuria.

Normal daily output of cystine is 40 to 80 mg. In cystinuria, output is greatly increased and may exceed 1 g/day. At 500 to 600 mg/day, stone formation is almost certain. When it is more than 300 mg/day, treatment is indicated.

Conventional treatment is directed at keeping urinary cystine diluted enough to prevent stone formation, keeping the urine alkaline enough to dissolve as much cystine as possible, and minimizing cystine production by a diet low in methionine (the major dietary precursor of cystine). Patients must drink enough fluid to keep urine specific gravity below 1.010, take enough alkali to keep urinary pH at 7.5 to 8, and maintain a diet low in methionine. This diet is not recommended in growing children and probably is contraindicated in pregnancy because of its low protein content (see PRECAUTIONS).

When these measures are inadequate to control recurrent stone formation, CUPRIMINE may be used as additional therapy. When patients refuse to adhere to conventional treatment, CUPRIMINE may be a useful substitute. It is capable of keeping cystine excretion to near normal values, thereby hindering stone formation and the serious consequences of pyelonephritis and impaired renal function that develop in some patients.

Bartter and colleagues depict the process by which penicillamine interacts with cystine to form penicillamine-cysteine mixed disulfide as:

CSSC + PS' $\rightleftharpoons$ CS' + CSSP
PSSP + CS' $\rightleftharpoons$ PS' + CSSP
CSSC + PSSP $\rightleftharpoons$ 2 CSSP
CSSC = cystine
CS' = deprotonated cysteine
PSSP = penicillamine
PS' = deprotonated penicillamine sulfhydryl
CSSP = penicillamine-cysteine mixed disulfide

In this process, it is assumed that the deprotonated form of penicillamine, PS', is the active factor in bringing about the disulfide interchange.

Rheumatoid Arthritis—Because CUPRIMINE can cause severe adverse reactions, its use in rheumatoid arthritis should be restricted to patients who have severe, active disease and who have failed to respond to an adequate trial of conventional therapy. Even then, benefit-to-risk ratio should be carefully considered. Other measures, such as rest, physiotherapy, salicylates, and corticosteroids should be used, when indicated, in conjunction with CUPRIMINE (see PRECAUTIONS).

Contraindications

Penicillamine should not be administered to patients with rheumatoid arthritis who are pregnant (see PRECAUTIONS).

Patients with a history of penicillamine-related aplastic anemia or agranulocytosis should not be restarted on penicillamine (see WARNINGS and ADVERSE REACTIONS). Because of its potential for causing renal damage, penicillamine should not be administered to rheumatoid arthritis patients with a history or other evidence of renal insufficiency.

Warnings

The use of penicillamine has been associated with fatalities due to certain diseases such as aplastic anemia, agranulocytosis, thrombocytopenia, Goodpasture's syndrome, and myasthenia gravis. Because of the potential for serious hematological and renal adverse reactions to occur at any time, routine urinalysis, white and differential blood cell count, hemoglobin determination, and direct platelet count must be done every two weeks for at least the first six months of penicillamine therapy and monthly thereafter. Patients should be instructed to report promptly the development of signs and symptoms of granulocytopenia and/or thrombocytopenia such as fever, sore throat, chills, bruising or bleeding. The above laboratory studies should then be promptly repeated.

Leukopenia and thrombocytopenia have been reported to occur in up to five percent of patients during penicillamine therapy. Leukopenia is of the granulocytic series and may or may not be associated with an increase in eosinophils. A confirmed reduction in WBC below 3500 per cubic ml mandates discontinuance of penicillamine therapy. Thrombocytopenia may be on an idiosyncratic basis, with decreased or absent megakaryocytes in the marrow, when it is part of an aplastic anemia. In other cases the thrombocytopenia is presumably on an immune basis since the number of megakaryocytes in the marrow has been reported to be normal or sometimes increased. The development of a platelet count below 100,000 per cubic ml, even in the absence of clinical bleeding, requires at least temporary cessation of penicillamine therapy. A progressive fall in either platelet count or WBC in three successive determina-

Continued on next page

Information on the Merck Sharp & Dohme products listed on these pages is the full prescribing information from product circulars in use November 1, 1984.

Merck Sharp & Dohme—Cont.

tions, even though values are still within the normal range, likewise requires at least temporary cessation.

Proteinuria and/or hematuria may develop during therapy and may be warning signs of membranous glomerulopathy which can progress to a nephrotic syndrome. Close observation of these patients is essential. In some patients the proteinuria disappears with continued therapy; in others, penicillamine must be discontinued. When a patient develops proteinuria or hematuria the physician must ascertain whether it is a sign of drug-induced glomerulopathy or is unrelated to penicillamine. Rheumatoid arthritis patients who develop moderate degrees of proteinuria may be continued cautiously on penicillamine therapy, provided that quantitative 24-hour urinary protein determinations are obtained at intervals of one to two weeks. Penicillamine dosage should not be increased under these circumstances. Proteinuria which exceeds 1 g/24 hours, or proteinuria which is progressively increasing, requires either discontinuance of the drug or a reduction in the dosage. In some patients, proteinuria has been reported to clear following reduction in dosage.

In rheumatoid arthritis patients, penicillamine should be discontinued if unexplained gross hematuria or persistent microscopic hematuria develops.

In patients with Wilson's disease or cystinuria the risks of continued penicillamine therapy in patients manifesting potentially serious urinary abnormalities must be weighed against the expected therapeutic benefits.

When penicillamine is used in cystinuria, an annual x-ray for renal stones is advised. Cystine stones form rapidly, sometimes in six months.

Up to one year or more may be required for any urinary abnormalities to disappear after penicillamine has been discontinued.

Because of rare reports of intrahepatic cholestasis and toxic hepatitis, liver function tests are recommended every six months for the duration of therapy.

Goodpasture's syndrome has occurred rarely. The development of abnormal urinary findings associated with hemoptysis and pulmonary infiltrates on x-ray requires immediate cessation of penicillamine.

Obliterative bronchiolitis has been reported rarely. The patient should be cautioned to report immediately pulmonary symptoms such as exertional dyspnea, unexplained cough or wheezing. Pulmonary function studies should be considered at that time.

Myasthenic syndrome sometimes progressing to myasthenia gravis has been reported. In the majority of cases, symptoms of myasthenia have receded after withdrawal of penicillamine.

Pemphigoid-type reactions characterized by bullous lesions clinically indistinguishable from pemphigus have occurred and have required discontinuation of penicillamine and treatment with corticosteroids.

Once instituted for Wilson's disease or cystinuria, treatment with penicillamine should, as a rule, be continued on a daily basis. Interruptions for even a few days have been followed by sensitivity reactions after reinstitution of therapy.

Precautions

Some patients may experience drug fever, a marked febrile response to penicillamine, usually in the second to third week following initiation of therapy. Drug fever may sometimes be accompanied by a macular cutaneous eruption.

In the case of drug fever in patients with Wilson's disease or cystinuria, because no alternative treatment is available, penicillamine should be temporarily discontinued until the reaction subsides. Then penicillamine should be reinstituted with a small dose that is gradually increased until the desired dosage is attained. Systemic steroid therapy may be necessary, and is usually helpful, in such patients in whom toxic reactions develop a second or third time.

In the case of drug fever in rheumatoid arthritis patients, because other treatments are available, penicillamine should be discontinued and another therapeutic alternative tried since experience indicates that the febrile reaction will recur in a very high percentage of patients upon readministration of penicillamine.

The skin and mucous membranes should be observed for allergic reactions. Early and late rashes have occurred. Early rash occurs during the first few months of treatment and is more common. It is usually a generalized pruritic, erythematous, maculopapular or morbilliform rash and resembles the allergic rash seen with other drugs. Early rash usually disappears within days after stopping penicillamine and seldom recurs when the drug is restarted at a lower dosage. Pruritus and early rash may often be controlled by the concomitant administration of antihistamines. Less commonly, a late rash may be seen, usually after six months or more of treatment, and requires discontinuation of penicillamine. It is usually on the trunk, is accompanied by intense pruritus, and is usually unresponsive to topical corticosteroid therapy. Late rash may take weeks to disappear after penicillamine is stopped and usually recurs if the drug is restarted.

The appearance of a drug eruption accompanied by fever, arthralgia, lymphadenopathy or other allergic manifestations usually requires discontinuation of penicillamine.

Certain patients will develop a positive antinuclear antibody (ANA) test and some of these may show a lupus erythematosus-like syndrome similar to drug-induced lupus associated with other drugs. The lupus erythematosus-like syndrome is not associated with hypocomplementemia and may be present without nephropathy. The development of a positive ANA test does not mandate discontinuance of the drug; however, the physician should be alerted to the possibility that a lupus erythematosus-like syndrome may develop in the future.

Some patients may develop oral ulcerations which in some cases have the appearance of aphthous stomatitis. The stomatitis usually recurs on rechallenge but often clears on a lower dosage. Although rare, cheilosis, glossitis and gingivostomatitis have also been reported. These oral lesions are frequently dose-related and may preclude further increase in penicillamine dosage or require discontinuation of the drug.

Hypogeusia (a blunting or diminution in taste perception) has occurred in some patients. This may last two to three months or more and may develop into a total loss of taste; however, it is usually self-limited despite continued penicillamine treatment. Such taste impairment is rare in patients with Wilson's disease.

Penicillamine should not be used in patients who are receiving concurrently gold therapy, antimalarial or cytotoxic drugs, oxyphenbutazone or phenylbutazone because these drugs are also associated with similar serious hematologic and renal adverse reactions. Patients who have had gold salt therapy discontinued due to a major toxic reaction may be at greater risk of serious adverse reactions with penicillamine but not necessarily of the same type.

Patients who are allergic to penicillin may theoretically have cross-sensitivity to penicillamine. The possibility of reactions from contamination of penicillamine by trace amounts of penicillin has been eliminated now that penicillamine is being produced synthetically rather than as a degradation product of penicillin.

Because of their dietary restrictions, patients with Wilson's disease and cystinuria should be given 25 mg/day of pyridoxine during therapy, since penicillamine increases the requirement for this vitamin. Patients also may receive benefit from a multivitamin preparation, although there is no evidence that deficiency of any vitamin other than pyridoxine is associated with penicillamine. In Wilson's disease, multivitamin preparations must be copper-free.

Rheumatoid arthritis patients whose nutrition is impaired should also be given a daily supplement of pyridoxine. Mineral supplements should not be given, since they may block the response to penicillamine.

Iron deficiency may develop, especially in children and in menstruating women. In Wilson's disease, this may be a result of adding the effects of the low copper diet, which is probably also low in iron, and the penicillamine to the effects of blood loss or growth. In cystinuria, a low methionine diet may contribute to iron deficiency, since it is necessarily low in protein. If necessary, iron may be given in short courses, but a period of two hours should elapse between administration of penicillamine and iron, since orally administered iron has been shown to reduce the effects of penicillamine.

Penicillamine causes an increase in the amount of soluble collagen. In the rat this results in inhibition of normal healing and also a decrease in tensile strength of intact skin. In man this may be the cause of increased skin friability at sites especially subject to pressure or trauma, such as shoulders, elbows, knees, toes, and buttocks. Extravasations of blood may occur and may appear as purpuric areas, with external bleeding if the skin is broken, or as vesicles containing dark blood. Neither type is progressive. There is no apparent association with bleeding elsewhere in the body and no associated coagulation defect has been found. Therapy with penicillamine may be continued in the presence of these lesions. They may not recur if dosage is reduced. Other reported effects probably due to the action of penicillamine on collagen are excessive wrinkling of the skin and development of small, white papules at venipuncture and surgical sites.

The effects of penicillamine on collagen and elastin make it advisable to consider a reduction in dosage to 250 mg/day, when surgery is contemplated. Reinstitution of full therapy should be delayed until wound healing is complete.

Carcinogenesis—Long-term animal carcinogenicity studies have not been done with penicillamine. There is a report that five of ten autoimmune disease-prone NZB hybrid mice developed lymphocytic leukemia after 6 months' intraperitoneal treatment with a dose of 400 mg/kg penicillamine 5 days per week.

Use in Pregnancy—Penicillamine has been shown to be teratogenic in rats when given in doses several times higher than the highest dose recommended for human use. Skeletal defects, cleft palates and fetal toxicity (resorptions) have been reported.

Wilson's Disease—There are no controlled studies in pregnant women with Wilson's disease, but experience does not include any positive evidence of adverse effects on the fetus. Reported experience* shows that continued treatment with penicillamine throughout pregnancy protects the mother against relapse of the Wilson's disease, and that discontinuation of penicillamine has deleterious effects on the mother. It indicates that the drug does not increase the risks of fetal abnormalities, but it does not exclude the possibility of infrequent or subtle damage to the fetus.

If penicillamine is administered during pregnancy to patients with Wilson's disease, it is recommended that the daily dosage be limited to 1 g. If cesarean section is planned, the daily dosage should be limited to 250 mg during the last six weeks of pregnancy and postoperatively until wound healing is complete.

Cystinuria—If possible, penicillamine should not be given during pregnancy to women with cystinuria. There is a report of a woman with cystinuria treated with 2 g/day of penicillamine during pregnancy who gave birth to a child with a generalized connective tissue defect that may have been caused by penicillamine. If stones continue to form in these patients, the benefits of therapy to the

---

*Scheinberg, I.H., Sternlieb, I.: N. Engl. J. Med. 293: 1300-1302, Dec. 18, 1975.

mother must be evaluated against the risk to the fetus.

Rheumatoid Arthritis—Penicillamine should not be administered to rheumatoid arthritis patients who are pregnant (see CONTRAINDICATIONS) and should be discontinued promptly in patients in whom pregnancy is suspected or diagnosed. Penicillamine should be used in women of childbearing potential only when the expected benefits outweigh possible hazards. Women of childbearing potential should be informed of the possible hazards of penicillamine to the developing fetus and should be advised to report promptly any missed menstrual periods or other indications of possible pregnancy.

There is a report that a woman with rheumatoid arthritis treated with less than one gram a day of penicillamine during pregnancy gave birth (cesarean delivery) to an infant with growth retardation, flattened face with broad nasal bridge, low set ears, short neck with loose skin folds, and unusually lax body skin.

Usage in Children—The efficacy of CUPRIMINE in juvenile rheumatoid arthritis has not been established.

Adverse Reactions

Penicillamine is a drug with a high incidence of untoward reactions, some of which are potentially fatal. Therefore, it is mandatory that patients receiving penicillamine therapy remain under close medical supervision throughout the period of drug administration (see WARNINGS and PRECAUTIONS).

Reported incidences (%) for the most commonly occurring adverse reactions in rheumatoid arthritis patients are noted, based on 17 representative clinical trials reported in the literature (1270 patients).

Allergic—Generalized pruritus, early and late rashes (5%), pemphigoid-type reactions, and drug eruptions which may be accompanied by fever, arthralgia, or lymphadenopathy have occurred (see WARNINGS and PRECAUTIONS). Some patients may show a lupus erythematosus-like syndrome similar to drug-induced lupus produced by other pharmacological agents (see PRECAUTIONS).

Urticaria and exfoliative dermatitis have occurred.

Thyroiditis has been reported but is extremely rare.

Some patients may develop a migratory polyarthralgia, often with objective synovitis (see DOSAGE AND ADMINISTRATION).

Gastrointestinal—Anorexia, epigastric pain, nausea, vomiting, or occasional diarrhea may occur (17%).

Isolated cases of reactivated peptic ulcer have occurred, as have hepatic dysfunction and pancreatitis. Intrahepatic cholestasis and toxic hepatitis have been reported rarely. There have been a few reports of increased serum alkaline phosphatase, lactic dehydrogenase, and positive cephalin flocculation and thymol turbidity tests.

Some patients may report a blunting, diminution, or total loss of taste perception (12%), or may develop oral ulcerations. Although rare, cheilosis, glossitis, and gingivostomatitis have been reported (see PRECAUTIONS).

Gastrointestinal side effects are usually reversible following cessation of therapy.

Hematological—Penicillamine can cause bone marrow depression (see WARNINGS). Leukopenia (2%) and thrombocytopenia (4%) have occurred. Fatalities have been reported as a result of thrombocytopenia, agranulocytosis, and aplastic anemia.

Thrombotic thrombocytopenic purpura, hemolytic anemia, red cell aplasia, monocytosis, leukocytosis, eosinophilia, and thrombocytosis have also been reported.

Renal—Patients on penicillamine therapy may develop proteinuria (6%) and/or hematuria which, in some, may progress to the development of the nephrotic syndrome as a result of an immune complex membranous glomerulopathy (see WARNINGS).

Central Nervous System—Tinnitus has been reported. Reversible optic neuritis has been reported following administration of penicillamine.

Neuromuscular—Myasthenia gravis (see WARNINGS).

Other—Adverse reactions that have been reported rarely include thrombophlebitis; hyperpyrexia (see PRECAUTIONS); falling hair or alopecia; lichen planus; polymyositis; dermatomyositis; mammary hyperplasia; elastosis perforans serpiginosa; toxic epidermal necrolysis; anetoderma (cutaneous macular atrophy); and Goodpasture's syndrome, a severe and ultimately fatal glomerulonephritis associated with intra-alveolar hemorrhage (see WARNINGS). Fatal renal vasculitis has also been reported. Allergic alveolitis, obliterative bronchiolitis, interstitial pneumonitis and pulmonary fibrosis have been reported in patients with severe rheumatoid arthritis, some of whom were receiving penicillamine. Bronchial asthma also has been reported.

Increased skin friability, excessive wrinkling of skin, and development of small white papules at venipuncture and surgical sites have been reported (see PRECAUTIONS).

The chelating action of the drug may cause increased excretion of other heavy metals such as zinc, mercury and lead.

There have been reports associating penicillamine with leukemia. However, circumstances involved in these reports are such that a cause and effect relationship to the drug has not been established.

Dosage and Administration

Wilson's Disease—CUPRIMINE capsules should be given on an empty stomach, four times a day; one-half to one hour before meals and at bedtime—at least two hours after the evening meal. Optimal dosage can be determined only by measurement of urinary copper excretion. The urine must be collected in copper-free glassware, and should be quantitatively analyzed for copper before and soon after initiation of therapy with CUPRIMINE. Continued therapy should be monitored by doing a 24-hour urinary copper analysis every three months or so for the duration of therapy. Since a low copper diet should keep copper absorption down to less than one milligram a day, the patient probably will be in negative copper balance if 0.5 to one milligram of copper is present in a 24-hour collection of urine.

To achieve this, the suggested initial dosage of CUPRIMINE in the treatment of Wilson's disease is 1 g/day for children or adults. This may be increased, as indicated by the urinary copper analyses, but it is seldom necessary to exceed a dosage of 2 g/day.

In patients who cannot tolerate as much as 1 g/day initially, initiating dosage with 250 mg/day, and increasing gradually to the requisite amount, gives closer control of the effects of the drug and may help to reduce the incidence of adverse reactions.

Cystinuria—It is recommended that CUPRIMINE be used along with conventional therapy. By reducing urinary cystine, it decreases crystalluria and stone formation. In some instances, it has been reported to decrease the size of, and even to dissolve, stones already formed.

The usual dosage of CUPRIMINE in the treatment of cystinuria is 2 g/day for adults, with a range of 1 to 4 g/day. For children, dosage can be based on 30 mg/kg/day. The total daily amount should be divided into four doses. If four equal doses are not feasible, give the larger portion at bedtime. If adverse reactions necessitate a reduction in dosage, it is important to retain the bedtime dose.

Initiating dosage with 250 mg/day, and increasing gradually to the requisite amount, gives closer control of the effects of the drug and may help to reduce the incidence of adverse reactions.

In addition to taking CUPRIMINE, patients should drink copiously. It is especially important to drink about a pint of fluid at bedtime and another pint once during the night when urine is more concentrated and more acid than during the day. The greater the fluid intake, the lower the required dosage of CUPRIMINE.

Dosage must be individualized to an amount that limits cystine excretion to 100–200 mg/day in those with no history of stones, and below 100 mg/day in those who have had stone formation and/or pain. Thus, in determining dosage, the inherent tubular defect, the patient's size, age, and rate of growth, and his diet and water intake all must be taken into consideration.

The standard nitroprusside cyanide test has been reported useful as a qualitative measure of the effective dose*: Add 2 ml of freshly prepared 5 percent sodium cyanide to 5 ml of a 24-hour aliquot of protein-free urine and let stand ten minutes. Add 5 drops of freshly prepared 5 percent sodium nitroprusside and mix. Cystine will turn the mixture magenta. If the result is negative, it can be assumed that cystine excretion is less than 100 mg/g creatinine.

Although penicillamine is rarely excreted unchanged, it also will turn the mixture magenta. If there is any question as to which substance is causing the reaction, a ferric chloride test can be done to eliminate doubt: Add 3 percent ferric chloride dropwise to the urine. Penicillamine will turn the urine an immediate and quickly fading blue. Cystine will not produce any change in appearance.

Rheumatoid Arthritis—The principal rule of treatment with CUPRIMINE in rheumatoid arthritis is patience. The onset of therapeutic response is typically delayed. Two or three months may be required before the first evidence of a clinical response is noted (see CLINICAL PHARMACOLOGY).

When treatment with CUPRIMINE has been interrupted because of adverse reactions or other reasons, the drug should be reintroduced cautiously by starting with a lower dosage and increasing slowly.

Initial Therapy—The currently recommended dosage regimen in rheumatoid arthritis begins with a single daily dose of 125 mg or 250 mg which is thereafter increased at one to three month intervals, by 125 mg or 250 mg/day, as patient response and tolerance indicate. If a satisfactory remission of symptoms is achieved, the dose associated with the remission should be continued (see *Maintenance Therapy*). If there is no improvement and there are no signs of potentially serious toxicity after two to three months of treatment with doses of 500–750 mg/day, increases of 250 mg/day at two to three month intervals may be continued until a satisfactory remission occurs (see *Maintenance Therapy*) or signs of toxicity develop (see WARNINGS and PRECAUTIONS). If there is no discernible improvement after three to four months of treatment with 1000 to 1500 mg of penicillamine/day, it may be assumed the patient will not respond and CUPRIMINE should be discontinued.

It is important that CUPRIMINE be given on an empty stomach at least one hour before meals and at least one hour apart from any other drug, food or milk (see CLINICAL PHARMACOLOGY).

Maintenance Therapy—The maintenance dosage of CUPRIMINE must be individualized, and may require adjustment during the course of treatment. Many patients respond satisfactorily to a dosage within the 500–750 mg/day range. Some need less.

Changes in maintenance dosage levels may not be reflected clinically or in the erythrocyte sedimentation rate for two to three months after each dosage adjustment.

---

*Lotz, M., Potts, J.T. and Bartter, F.C.: Brit. Med. J. *2*:521, Aug. 28, 1965 (in Medical Memoranda).

Continued on next page

Information on the Merck Sharp & Dohme products listed on these pages is the full prescribing information from product circulars in use November 1, 1984.

Merck Sharp & Dohme—Cont.

Some patients will subsequently require an increase in the maintenance dosage to achieve maximal disease suppression. In those patients who do respond, but who evidence incomplete suppression of their disease after the first six to nine months of treatment, the daily dosage of CUPRIMINE may be increased by 125 mg or 250 mg/day at three-month intervals. It is unusual in current practice to employ a dosage in excess of 1 g/day, but up to 1.5 g/day has sometimes been required.

Management of Exacerbations—During the course of treatment some patients may experience an exacerbation of disease activity following an initial good response. These may be self-limited and can subside within twelve weeks. They are usually controlled by the addition of nonsteroidal anti-inflammatory drugs, and only if the patient has demonstrated a true "escape" phenomenon (as evidenced by failure of the flare to subside within this time period) should an increase in the maintenance dose ordinarily be considered.

In the rheumatoid patient, migratory polyarthralgia due to penicillamine is extremely difficult to differentiate from an exacerbation of the rheumatoid arthritis. Discontinuance or a substantial reduction in dosage of CUPRIMINE for up to several weeks will usually determine which of these processes is responsible for the arthralgia.

Duration of Therapy—The optimum duration of therapy with CUPRIMINE in rheumatoid arthritis has not been determined. If the patient has been in remission for six months or more, a gradual, stepwise dosage reduction in decrements of 125 mg or 250 mg/day at approximately three month intervals may be attempted.

Concomitant Drug Therapy—CUPRIMINE should not be used in patients who are receiving gold therapy, antimalarial or cytotoxic drugs, oxyphenbutazone, or phenylbutazone (see PRECAUTIONS). Other measures, such as salicylates, other nonsteroidal anti-inflammatory drugs, or systemic corticosteroids, may be continued when penicillamine is initiated. After improvement commences, analgesic and anti-inflammatory drugs may be slowly discontinued as symptoms permit. Steroid withdrawal must be done gradually, and many months of treatment with CUPRIMINE may be required before steroids can be completely eliminated.

Dosage Frequency—Based on clinical experience dosages up to 500 mg/day can be given as a single daily dose. Dosages in excess of 500 mg/day should be administered in divided doses.

How Supplied

No. 3299—Capsules CUPRIMINE, 250 mg, are ivory-colored capsules containing a white or nearly white powder, and are coded MSD 602. They are supplied as follows:
NDC 0006-0602-68 in bottles of 100.
Shown in Product Identification Section, page 420
No. 3350—Capsules CUPRIMINE, 125 mg, are opaque yellow and gray capsules containing a white or nearly white powder, and are coded MSD 672. They are supplied as follows:
NDC 0006-0672-68 in bottles of 100.
Shown in Product Identification Section, page 420
A.H.F.S. Category: 64:00
DC 6177830   Issued November 1982
COPYRIGHT © MERCK & CO., INC., 1982
All rights reserved

DECADRON® Elixir   ℞
(dexamethasone, MSD), U.S.P.

Description

Glucocorticoids are adrenocortical steroids, both naturally occurring and synthetic, which are readily absorbed from the gastrointestinal tract. Dexamethasone, a synthetic adrenocortical steroid, is a white to practically white, odorless, crystalline powder. It is stable in air. It is practically insoluble in water. The molecular weight is 392.47. It is designated chemically as 9-fluoro-11β, 17, 21-trihydroxy-16α-methylpregna -1, 4- diene-3,20-dione. The empirical formula is $C_{22}H_{29}FO_5$.

DECADRON® (Dexamethasone, MSD) elixir contains 0.5 mg of dexamethasone in each 5 ml. Benzoic acid, 0.1%, is added as a preservative. It also contains alcohol 5%.

Actions

Naturally occurring glucocorticoids (hydrocortisone and cortisone), which also have salt-retaining properties, are used as replacement therapy in adrenocortical deficiency states. Their synthetic analogs, including dexamethasone, are primarily used for their potent anti-inflammatory effects in disorders of many organ systems.

Glucocorticoids cause profound and varied metabolic effects. In addition, they modify the body's immune responses to diverse stimuli.

At equipotent anti-inflammatory doses, dexamethasone almost completely lacks the sodium-retaining property of hydrocortisone and closely related derivatives of hydrocortisone.

Indications

1. *Endocrine Disorders*
   Primary or secondary adrenocortical insufficiency (hydrocortisone or cortisone is the first choice; synthetic analogs may be used in conjunction with mineralocorticoids where applicable; in infancy mineralocorticoid supplementation is of particular importance)
   Congenital adrenal hyperplasia
   Nonsuppurative thyroiditis
   Hypercalcemia associated with cancer
2. *Rheumatic Disorders*
   As adjunctive therapy for short-term administration (to tide the patient over an acute episode or exacerbation) in:
   Psoriatic arthritis
   Rheumatoid arthritis, including juvenile rheumatoid arthritis (selected cases may require low-dose maintenance therapy)
   Ankylosing spondylitis
   Acute and subacute bursitis
   Acute nonspecific tenosynovitis
   Acute gouty arthritis
   Post-traumatic osteoarthritis
   Synovitis of osteoarthritis
   Epicondylitis
3. *Collagen Diseases*
   During an exacerbation or as maintenance therapy in selected cases of—
   Systemic lupus erythematosus
   Acute rheumatic carditis
4. *Dermatologic Diseases*
   Pemphigus
   Bullous dermatitis herpetiformis
   Severe erythema multiforme (Stevens-Johnson syndrome)
   Exfoliative dermatitis
   Mycosis fungoides
   Severe psoriasis
   Severe seborrheic dermatitis
5. *Allergic States*
   Control of severe or incapacitating allergic conditions intractable to adequate trials of conventional treatment:
   Seasonal or perennial allergic rhinitis
   Bronchial asthma
   Contact dermatitis
   Atopic dermatitis
   Serum sickness
   Drug hypersensitivity reactions
6. *Ophthalmic Diseases*
   Severe acute and chronic allergic and inflammatory processes involving the eye and its adnexa, such as—
   Allergic conjunctivitis
   Keratitis
   Allergic corneal marginal ulcers
   Herpes zoster ophthalmicus
   Iritis and iridocyclitis
   Chorioretinitis
   Anterior segment inflammation
   Diffuse posterior uveitis and choroiditis
   Optic neuritis
   Sympathetic ophthalmia
7. *Respiratory Diseases*
   Symptomatic sarcoidosis
   Loeffler's syndrome not manageable by other means
   Berylliosis
   Fulminating or disseminated pulmonary tuberculosis when used concurrently with appropriate antituberculous chemotherapy
   Aspiration pneumonitis
8. *Hematologic Disorders*
   Idiopathic thrombocytopenic purpura in adults
   Secondary thrombocytopenia in adults
   Acquired (autoimmune) hemolytic anemia
   Erythroblastopenia (RBC anemia)
   Congenital (erythroid) hypoplastic anemia
9. *Neoplastic Diseases*
   For palliative management of:
   Leukemias and lymphomas in adults
   Acute leukemia of childhood
10. *Edematous States*
    To induce a diuresis or remission of proteinuria in the nephrotic syndrome, without uremia, of the idiopathic type or that due to lupus erythematosus
11. *Gastrointestinal Diseases*
    To tide the patient over a critical period of the disease in:
    Ulcerative colitis
    Regional enteritis
12. *Miscellaneous*
    Tuberculous meningitis with subarachnoid block or impending block when used concurrently with appropriate antituberculous chemotherapy
    Trichinosis with neurologic or myocardial involvement
13. *Diagnostic testing of adrenocortical hyperfunction.*

Contraindications

Systemic fungal infections
Hypersensitivity to this product

Warnings

In patients on corticosteroid therapy subjected to unusual stress, increased dosage of rapidly acting corticosteroids before, during, and after the stressful situation is indicated.

Drug-induced secondary adrenocortical insufficiency may result from too rapid withdrawal of corticosteroids and may be minimized by gradual reduction of dosage. This type of relative insufficiency may persist for months after discontinuation of therapy; therefore, in any situation of stress occurring during that period, hormone therapy should be reinstituted. If the patient is receiving steroids already, dosage may have to be increased. Since mineralocorticoid secretion may be impaired, salt and/or a mineralocorticoid should be administered concurrently.

Corticosteroids may mask some signs of infection, and new infections may appear during their use. There may be decreased resistance and inability to localize infection when corticosteroids are used. Moreover, corticosteroids may affect the nitro-blue-tetrazolium test for bacterial infection and produce false negative results.

In cerebral malaria, a double-blind trial has shown that the use of corticosteroids is associated with prolongation of coma and a higher incidence of pneumonia and gastrointestinal bleeding.

Corticosteroids may activate latent amebiasis. Therefore, it is recommended that latent or active amebiasis be ruled out before initiating corticosteroid therapy in any patient who has spent time in the tropics or any patient with unexplained diarrhea.

Prolonged use of corticosteroids may produce posterior subcapsular cataracts, glaucoma with possible damage to the optic nerves, and may enhance the establishment of secondary ocular infections due to fungi or viruses.

Usage in pregnancy: Since adequate human reproduction studies have not been done with corticosteroids, use of these drugs in pregnancy or in women of childbearing potential requires that the anticipated benefits be weighed against the possible hazards to the mother and embryo or fetus. Infants born of mothers who have received substantial doses of corticosteroids during pregnancy should be carefully observed for signs of hypoadrenalism.

Corticosteroids appear in breast milk and could suppress growth, interfere with endogenous corticosteroid production, or cause other unwanted effects. Mothers taking pharmacologic doses of corticosteroids should be advised not to nurse.

Average and large doses of hydrocortisone or cortisone can cause elevation of blood pressure, salt and water retention, and increased excretion of potassium. These effects are less likely to occur with the synthetic derivatives except when used in large doses. Dietary salt restriction and potassium supplementation may be necessary. All corticosteroids increase calcium excretion.

Administration of live virus vaccines, including smallpox, is contraindicated in individuals receiving immunosuppressive doses of corticosteroids. If inactivated viral or bacterial vaccines are administered to individuals receiving immunosuppressive doses of corticosteroids, the expected serum antibody response may not be obtained. However, immunization procedures may be undertaken in patients who are receiving corticosteroids as replacement therapy, e.g., for Addison's disease.

The use of DECADRON elixir in active tuberculosis should be restricted to those cases of fulminating or disseminated tuberculosis in which the corticosteroid is used for the management of the disease in conjunction with an appropriate antituberculous regimen.

If corticosteroids are indicated in patients with latent tuberculosis or tuberculin reactivity, close observation is necessary as reactivation of the disease may occur. During prolonged corticosteroid therapy, these patients should receive chemoprophylaxis.

Precautions

Following prolonged therapy, withdrawal of corticosteroids may result in symptoms of the corticosteroid withdrawal syndrome including fever, myalgia, arthralgia, and malaise. This may occur in patients even without evidence of adrenal insufficiency.

There is an enhanced effect of corticosteroids in patients with hypothyroidism and in those with cirrhosis.

Corticosteroids should be used cautiously in patients with ocular herpes simplex because of possible corneal perforation.

The lowest possible dose of corticosteroid should be used to control the condition under treatment, and when reduction in dosage is possible, the reduction should be gradual.

Psychic derangements may appear when corticosteroids are used, ranging from euphoria, insomnia, mood swings, personality changes, and severe depression, to frank psychotic manifestations. Also, existing emotional instability or psychotic tendencies may be aggravated by corticosteroids.

Aspirin should be used cautiously in conjunction with corticosteroids in hypoprothrombinemia.

Steroids should be used with caution in nonspecific ulcerative colitis, if there is a probability of impending perforation, abscess, or other pyogenic infection; diverticulitis; fresh intestinal anastomoses; active or latent peptic ulcer; renal insufficiency; hypertension; osteoporosis; and myasthenia gravis. Signs of peritoneal irritation following gastrointestinal perforation in patients receiving large doses of corticosteroids may be minimal or absent. Fat embolism has been reported as a possible complication of hypercortisonism.

When large doses are given, some authorities advise that corticosteroids be taken with meals and antacids taken between meals to help to prevent peptic ulcer.

Growth and development of infants and children on prolonged corticosteroid therapy should be carefully observed.

Steroids may increase or decrease motility and number of spermatozoa in some patients.

Phenytoin, phenobarbital, ephedrine, and rifampin may enhance the metabolic clearance of corticosteroids, resulting in decreased blood levels and lessened physiologic activity, thus requiring adjustment in corticosteroid dosage. These interactions may interfere with dexamethasone suppression tests which should be interpreted with caution during administration of these drugs.

The prothrombin time should be checked frequently in patients who are receiving corticosteroids and coumarin anticoagulants at the same time because of reports that corticosteroids have altered the response to these anticoagulants. Studies have shown that the usual effect produced by adding corticosteroids is inhibition of response to coumarins, although there have been some conflicting reports of potentiation not substantiated by studies.

When corticosteroids are administered concomitantly with potassium-depleting diuretics, patients should be observed closely for development of hypokalemia.

Adverse Reactions

Fluid and Electrolyte Disturbances
  Sodium retention
  Fluid retention
  Congestive heart failure in susceptible patients
  Potassium loss
  Hypokalemic alkalosis
  Hypertension

Musculoskeletal
  Muscle weakness
  Steroid myopathy
  Loss of muscle mass
  Osteoporosis
  Vertebral compression fractures
  Aseptic necrosis of femoral and humeral heads
  Pathologic fracture of long bones
  Tendon rupture

Gastrointestinal
  Peptic ulcer with possible perforation and hemorrhage
  Perforation of the small and large bowel, particularly in patients with inflammatory bowel disease
  Pancreatitis
  Abdominal distention
  Ulcerative esophagitis

Dermatologic
  Impaired wound healing
  Thin fragile skin
  Petechiae and ecchymoses
  Erythema
  Increased sweating
  May suppress reactions to skin tests
  Other cutaneous reactions, such as allergic dermatitis, urticaria, angioneurotic edema

Neurologic
  Convulsions
  Increased intracranial pressure with papilledema (pseudotumor cerebri) usually after treatment
  Vertigo
  Headache

Endocrine
  Menstrual irregularities
  Development of cushingoid state
  Suppression of growth in children
  Secondary adrenocortical and pituitary unresponsiveness, particularly in times of stress, as in trauma, surgery, or illness
  Decreased carbohydrate tolerance
  Manifestations of latent diabetes mellitus
  Increased requirements for insulin or oral hypoglycemic agents in diabetics
  Hirsutism

Ophthalmic
  Posterior subcapsular cataracts
  Increased intraocular pressure
  Glaucoma
  Exophthalmos

Metabolic
  Negative nitrogen balance due to protein catabolism

Other
  Hypersensitivity
  Thromboembolism
  Weight gain
  Increased appetite
  Nausea
  Malaise

Dosage and Administration

For oral administration
DOSAGE REQUIREMENTS ARE VARIABLE AND MUST BE INDIVIDUALIZED ON THE BASIS OF THE DISEASE AND THE RESPONSE OF THE PATIENT.

The initial dosage varies from 0.75 to 9 mg a day depending on the disease being treated. In less severe diseases doses lower than 0.75 mg may suffice, while in severe diseases doses higher than 9 mg may be required. The initial dosage should be maintained or adjusted until the patient's response is satisfactory. If satisfactory clinical response does not occur after a reasonable period of time, discontinue DECADRON elixir and transfer the patient to other therapy.

After a favorable initial response, the proper maintenance dosage should be determined by decreasing the initial dosage in small amounts to the lowest dosage that maintains an adequate clinical response.

Patients should be observed closely for signs that might require dosage adjustment, including changes in clinical status resulting from remissions or exacerbations of the disease, individual drug responsiveness, and the effect of stress (e.g., surgery, infection, trauma). During stress it may be necessary to increase dosage temporarily.

If the drug is to be stopped after more than a few days of treatment, it usually should be withdrawn gradually.

The following milligram equivalents facilitate changing to DECADRON from other glucocorticoids:

DECADRON	Methylprednisolone and Triamcinolone	Prednisolone and Prednisone	Hydrocortisone	Cortisone
0.75 mg =	4 mg =	5 mg =	20 mg =	25 mg

Dexamethasone suppression tests
1. Tests for Cushing's syndrome
   Give 1.0 mg of DECADRON orally at 11:00 p.m. Blood is drawn for plasma cortisol determination at 8:00 a.m. the following morning. For greater accuracy, give 0.5 mg of DECADRON orally every 6 hours for 48 hours. Twenty-four hour urine collections are made for determination of 17-hydroxycorticosteroid excretion.
2. Test to distinguish Cushing's syndrome due to pituitary ACTH excess from Cushing's syndrome due to other causes
   Give 2.0 mg of DECADRON orally every 6 hours for 48 hours. Twenty-four hour urine collections are made for determination of 17-hydroxycorticosteroid excretion.

Continued on next page

Information on the Merck Sharp & Dohme products listed on these pages is the full prescribing information from product circulars in use November 1, 1984.

Merck Sharp & Dohme—Cont.

How Supplied

No. 7622—Elixir DECADRON, 0.5 mg dexamethasone per 5 ml, is a clear, red liquid and is supplied as follows:
NDC 0006-7622-55 bottles of 100 ml with calibrated dropper assembly.
NDC 0006-7622-66 bottles of 237 ml without dropper assembly.

A.H.F.S. Category: 68:04
DC 6030724   Issued April 1983

DECADRON® Tablets ℞
(dexamethasone, MSD), U.S.P.

Description

Glucocorticoids are adrenocortical steroids, both naturally occurring and synthetic, which are readily absorbed from the gastrointestinal tract. Dexamethasone, a synthetic adrenocortical steroid, is a practically white, odorless, crystalline powder. It is stable in air. It is practically insoluble in water. The molecular weight is 392.47. It is designated chemically as 9-fluoro-11β,17,21-trihydroxy-16α-methylpregna-1, 4-diene-3,20-dione. The empirical formula is $C_{22}H_{29}FO_5$.
DECADRON® (Dexamethasone, MSD) tablets are supplied in six potencies, 0.25 mg, 0.5 mg, 0.75 mg, 1.5 mg, 4 mg, and 6 mg.

Actions

Naturally occurring glucocorticoids (hydrocortisone and cortisone), which also have salt-retaining properties, are used as replacement therapy in adrenocortical deficiency states. Their synthetic analogs including dexamethasone are primarily used for their potent anti-inflammatory effects in disorders of many organ systems.
Glucocorticoids cause profound and varied metabolic effects. In addition, they modify the body's immune responses to diverse stimuli.
At equipotent anti-inflammatory doses, dexamethasone almost completely lacks the sodium retaining property of hydrocortisone and closely related derivatives of hydrocortisone.

Indications

1. *Endocrine Disorders*
   Primary or secondary adrenocortical insufficiency (hydrocortisone or cortisone is the first choice; synthetic analogs may be used in conjunction with mineralocorticoids where applicable; in infancy mineralocorticoid supplementation is of particular importance).
   Congenital adrenal hyperplasia
   Nonsuppurative thyroiditis
   Hypercalcemia associated with cancer
2. *Rheumatic Disorders*
   As adjunctive therapy for short-term administration (to tide the patient over an acute episode or exacerbation) in:
   Psoriatic arthritis
   Rheumatoid arthritis, including juvenile rheumatoid arthritis (selected cases may require low-dose maintenance therapy)
   Ankylosing spondylitis
   Acute and subacute bursitis
   Acute nonspecific tenosynovitis
   Acute gouty arthritis
   Post-traumatic osteoarthritis
   Synovitis of osteoarthritis
   Epicondylitis
3. *Collagen Diseases*
   During an exacerbation or as maintenance therapy in selected cases of—
   Systemic lupus erythematosus
   Acute rheumatic carditis
4. *Dermatologic Diseases*
   Pemphigus
   Bullous dermatitis herpetiformis
   Severe erythema multiforme (Stevens-Johnson syndrome)
   Exfoliative dermatitis
   Mycosis fungoides
   Severe psoriasis
   Severe seborrheic dermatitis
5. *Allergic States*
   Control of severe or incapacitating allergic conditions intractable to adequate trials of conventional treatment:
   Seasonal or perennial allergic rhinitis
   Bronchial asthma
   Contact dermatitis
   Atopic dermatitis
   Serum sickness
   Drug hypersensitivity reactions
6. *Ophthalmic Diseases*
   Severe acute and chronic allergic and inflammatory processes involving the eye and its adnexa, such as—
   Allergic conjunctivitis
   Keratitis
   Allergic corneal marginal ulcers
   Herpes zoster ophthalmicus
   Iritis and iridocyclitis
   Chorioretinitis
   Anterior segment inflammation
   Diffuse posterior uveitis and choroiditis
   Optic neuritis
   Sympathetic ophthalmia
7. *Respiratory Diseases*
   Symptomatic sarcoidosis
   Loeffler's syndrome not manageable by other means
   Berylliosis
   Fulminating or disseminated pulmonary tuberculosis when used concurrently with appropriate antituberculous chemotherapy
   Aspiration pneumonitis
8. *Hematologic Disorders*
   Idiopathic thrombocytopenic purpura in adults
   Secondary thrombocytopenia in adults
   Acquired (autoimmune) hemolytic anemia
   Erythroblastopenia (RBC anemia)
   Congenital (erythroid) hypoplastic anemia
9. *Neoplastic Diseases*
   For palliative management of:
   Leukemias and lymphomas in adults
   Acute leukemia of childhood
10. *Edematous States*
    To induce a diuresis or remission of proteinuria in the nephrotic syndrome, without uremia, of the idiopathic type or that due to lupus erythematosus
11. *Gastrointestinal Diseases*
    To tide the patient over a critical period of the disease in:
    Ulcerative colitis
    Regional enteritis
12. *Cerebral Edema* associated with primary or metastatic brain tumor, craniotomy, or head injury. Use in cerebral edema is not a substitute for careful neurosurgical evaluation and definitive management such as neurosurgery or other specific therapy.
13. *Miscellaneous*
    Tuberculous meningitis with subarachnoid block or impending block when used concurrently with appropriate antituberculous chemotherapy
    Trichinosis with neurologic or myocardial involvement
14. *Diagnostic testing of adrenocortical hyperfunction.*

Contraindications

Systemic fungal infections
Hypersensitivity to this drug

Warnings

In patients on corticosteroid therapy subjected to unusual stress, increased dosage of rapidly acting corticosteroids before, during, and after the stressful situation is indicated.
Drug-induced secondary adrenocortical insufficiency may result from too rapid withdrawal of corticosteroids and may be minimized by gradual reduction of dosage. This type of relative insufficiency may persist for months after discontinuation of therapy; therefore, in any situation of stress occurring during that period, hormone therapy should be reinstituted. If the patient is receiving steroids already, dosage may have to be increased. Since mineralocorticoid secretion may be impaired, salt and/or a mineralocorticoid should be administered concurrently.
Corticosteroids may mask some signs of infection, and new infections may appear during their use. There may be decreased resistance and inability to localize infection when corticosteroids are used. Moreover, corticosteroids may affect the nitro-blue-tetrazolium test for bacterial infection and produce false negative results.
In cerebral malaria, a double-blind trial has shown that the use of corticosteroids is associated with prolongation of coma and a higher incidence of pneumonia and gastrointestinal bleeding.
Corticosteroids may activate latent amebiasis. Therefore, it is recommended that latent or active amebiasis be ruled out before initiating corticosteroid therapy in any patient who has spent time in the tropics or any patient with unexplained diarrhea.
Prolonged use of corticosteroids may produce posterior subcapsular cataracts and glaucoma with possible damage to the optic nerves, and may enhance the establishment of secondary ocular infections due to fungi or viruses.
Usage in pregnancy: Since adequate human reproduction studies have not been done with corticosteroids, use of these drugs in pregnancy or in women of childbearing potential requires that the anticipated benefits be weighed against the possible hazards to the mother and embryo or fetus. Infants born of mothers who have received substantial doses of corticosteroids during pregnancy should be carefully observed for signs of hypoadrenalism.
Corticosteroids appear in breast milk and could suppress growth, interfere with endogenous corticosteroid production, or cause other unwanted effects. Mothers taking pharmacologic doses of corticosteroids should be advised not to nurse.
Average and large doses of hydrocortisone or cortisone can cause elevation of blood pressure, salt and water retention, and increased excretion of potassium. These effects are less likely to occur with the synthetic derivatives except when used in large doses. Dietary salt restriction and potassium supplementation may be necessary. All corticosteroids increase calcium excretion.
Administration of live virus vaccines, including smallpox, is contraindicated in individuals receiving immunosuppressive doses of corticosteroids. If inactivated viral or bacterial vaccines are administered to individuals receiving immunosuppressive doses of corticosteroids, the expected serum antibody response may not be obtained. However, immunization procedures may be undertaken in patients who are receiving corticosteroids as replacement therapy, e.g., for Addison's disease.
The use of DECADRON tablets in active tuberculosis should be restricted to those cases of fulminating or disseminated tuberculosis in which the corticosteroid is used for the management of the disease in conjunction with an appropriate antituberculous regimen.
If corticosteroids are indicated in patients with latent tuberculosis or tuberculin reactivity, close observation is necessary as reactivation of the disease may occur. During prolonged corticosteroid therapy, these patients should receive chemoprophylaxis.

Precautions

Following prolonged therapy, withdrawal of corticosteroids may result in symptoms of the corticosteroid withdrawal syndrome including fever, myalgia, arthralgia, and malaise. This may occur in patients even without evidence of adrenal insufficiency.
There is an enhanced effect of corticosteroids in patients with hypothyroidism and in those with cirrhosis.
Corticosteroids should be used cautiously in patients with ocular herpes simplex because of possible corneal perforation.

The lowest possible dose of corticosteroid should be used to control the condition under treatment, and when reduction in dosage is possible, the reduction should be gradual.

Psychic derangements may appear when corticosteroids are used, ranging from euphoria, insomnia, mood swings, personality changes, and severe depression, to frank psychotic manifestations. Also, existing emotional instability or psychotic tendencies may be aggravated by corticosteroids.

Aspirin should be used cautiously in conjunction with corticosteroids in hypoprothrombinemia.

Steroids should be used with caution in nonspecific ulcerative colitis, if there is a probability of impending perforation, abscess, or other pyogenic infection, diverticulitis, fresh intestinal anastomoses, active or latent peptic ulcer, renal insufficiency, hypertension, osteoporosis, and myasthenia gravis. Signs of peritoneal irritation following gastrointestinal perforation in patients receiving large doses of corticosteroids may be minimal or absent. Fat embolism has been reported as a possible complication of hypercortisonism.

When large doses are given, some authorities advise that corticosteroids be taken with meals and antacids taken between meals to help to prevent peptic ulcer.

Growth and development of infants and children on prolonged corticosteroid therapy should be carefully observed.

Steroids may increase or decrease motility and number of spermatozoa in some patients.

Phenytoin, phenobarbital, ephedrine, and rifampin may enhance the metabolic clearance of corticosteroids, resulting in decreased blood levels and lessened physiologic activity, thus requiring adjustment in corticosteroid dosage. These interactions may interfere with dexamethasone suppression tests which should be interpreted with caution during administration of these drugs.

The prothrombin time should be checked frequently in patients who are receiving corticosteroids and coumarin anticoagulants at the same time because of reports that corticosteroids have altered the response to these anticoagulants. Studies have shown that the usual effect produced by adding corticosteroids is inhibition of response to coumarins, although there have been some conflicting reports of potentiation not substantiated by studies.

When corticosteroids are administered concomitantly with potassium-depleting diuretics, patients should be observed closely for development of hypokalemia.

Adverse Reactions

Fluid and Electrolyte Disturbances
Sodium retention
Fluid retention
Congestive heart failure in susceptible patients
Potassium loss
Hypokalemic alkalosis
Hypertension
Musculoskeletal
Muscle weakness
Steroid myopathy
Loss of muscle mass
Osteoporosis
Vertebral compression fractures
Aseptic necrosis of femoral and humeral heads
Pathologic fracture of long bones
Tendon rupture
Gastrointestinal
Peptic ulcer with possible perforation and hemorrhage
Perforation of the small and large bowel, particularly in patients with inflammatory bowel disease
Pancreatitis
Abdominal distention
Ulcerative esophagitis
Dermatologic
Impaired wound healing
Thin fragile skin
Petechiae and ecchymoses
Erythema
Increased sweating
May suppress reactions to skin tests
Other cutaneous reactions, such as allergic dermatitis, urticaria, angioneurotic edema
Neurologic
Convulsions
Increased intracranial pressure with papilledema (pseudotumor cerebri) usually after treatment
Vertigo
Headache
Endocrine
Menstrual irregularities
Development of cushingoid state
Suppression of growth in children
Secondary adrenocortical and pituitary unresponsiveness, particularly in times of stress, as in trauma, surgery, or illness
Decreased carbohydrate tolerance
Manifestations of latent diabetes mellitus
Increased requirements for insulin or oral hypoglycemic agents in diabetics
Hirsutism
Ophthalmic
Posterior subcapsular cataracts
Increased intraocular pressure
Glaucoma
Exophthalmos
Metabolic
Negative nitrogen balance due to protein catabolism
Other
Hypersensitivity
Thromboembolism
Weight gain
Increased appetite
Nausea
Malaise

Dosage and Administration

For oral administration
DOSAGE REQUIREMENTS ARE VARIABLE AND MUST BE INDIVIDUALIZED ON THE BASIS OF THE DISEASE AND THE RESPONSE OF THE PATIENT.

The initial dosage varies from 0.75 to 9 mg a day depending on the disease being treated. In less severe diseases doses lower than 0.75 mg may suffice, while in severe diseases doses higher than 9 mg may be required. The initial dosage should be maintained or adjusted until the patient's response is satisfactory. If satisfactory clinical response does not occur after a reasonable period of time, discontinue DECADRON tablets and transfer the patient to other therapy.

After a favorable initial response, the proper maintenance dosage should be determined by decreasing the initial dosage in small amounts to the lowest dosage that maintains an adequate clinical response.

Patients should be observed closely for signs that might require dosage adjustment, including changes in clinical status resulting from remissions or exacerbations of the disease, individual drug responsiveness, and the effect of stress (e.g., surgery, infection, trauma). During stress it may be necessary to increase dosage temporarily.

If the drug is to be stopped after more than a few days of treatment, it usually should be withdrawn gradually.

The following milligram equivalents facilitate changing to DECADRON from other glucocorticoids:

DECADRON	Methylprednisolone and Triamcinolone	Prednisolone and Prednisone	Hydrocortisone	Cortisone
0.75 mg =	4 mg =	5 mg =	20 mg =	25 mg

In *acute, self-limited allergic disorders or acute exacerbations of chronic allergic disorders*, the following dosage schedule combining parenteral and oral therapy is suggested:
DECADRON® phosphate (Dexamethasone Sodium Phosphate, MSD) injection, 4 mg per ml:
First Day
  1 or 2 ml, intramuscularly
DECADRON tablets, 0.75 mg:
Second Day
  4 tablets in two divided doses
Third Day
  4 tablets in two divided doses
Fourth Day
  2 tablets in two divided doses
Fifth Day
  1 tablet
Sixth Day
  1 tablet
Seventh Day
  No treatment
Eighth Day
  Follow-up visit

This schedule is designed to ensure adequate therapy during acute episodes, while minimizing the risk of overdosage in chronic cases.

In *cerebral edema*, DECADRON phosphate (Dexamethasone Sodium Phosphate, MSD) injection is generally administered initially in a dosage of 10 mg intravenously followed by 4 mg every six hours intramuscularly until the symptoms of cerebral edema subside. Response is usually noted within 12 to 24 hours and dosage may be reduced after two to four days and gradually discontinued over a period of five to seven days. For palliative management of patients with recurrent or inoperable brain tumors, maintenance therapy with either DECADRON phosphate (Dexamethasone Sodium Phosphate, MSD) injection or DECADRON tablets in a dosage of two mg two or three times daily may be effective.

Dexamethasone suppression tests

1. Tests for Cushing's syndrome
   Give 1.0 mg of DECADRON orally at 11:00 p.m. Blood is drawn for plasma cortisol determination at 8:00 a.m. the following morning. For greater accuracy, give 0.5 mg of DECADRON orally every 6 hours for 48 hours. Twenty-four hour urine collections are made for determination of 17-hydroxycorticosteroid excretion.
2. Test to distinguish Cushing's syndrome due to pituitary ACTH excess from Cushing's syndrome due to other causes
   Give 2.0 mg of DECADRON orally every 6 hours for 48 hours. Twenty-four hour urine collections are made for determination of 17-hydroxycorticosteroid excretion.

How Supplied

Tablets DECADRON are compressed, pentagonal-shaped tablets, colored to distinguish potency. They are scored and coded on one side and are available as follows:
No. 7648—6 mg, green in color and coded MSD 147.
NDC 0006-0147-50 bottles of 50.
NDC 0006-0147-28 single unit packages of 100.
Shown in Product Identification Section, page 420
No. 7645—4 mg, white in color and coded MSD 97.
NDC 0006-0097-50 bottles of 50.
NDC 0006-0097-28 single unit packages of 100.
Shown in Product Identification Section, page 420
No. 7638—1.5 mg, pink in color and coded MSD 95.
NDC 0006-0095-50 bottles of 50.

Continued on next page

Information on the Merck Sharp & Dohme products listed on these pages is the full prescribing information from product circulars in use November 1, 1984.

Merck Sharp & Dohme—Cont.

NDC 0006-0095-28 single unit packages of 100.
Shown in Product Identification Section, page 420
No. 7601—0.75 mg, bluish-green in color and coded MSD 63.
NDC 0006-0063-12 5-12 PAK® (package of 12).
NDC 0006-0063-68 bottles of 100.
NDC 0006-0063-28 single unit packages of 100.
NDC 0006-0063-82 bottles of 1000.
Shown in Product Identification Section, page 420
No. 7598—0.5 mg, yellow in color and coded MSD 41.
NDC 0006-0041-68 bottles of 100.
(6505-00-687-8482 0.5 mg 100's).
NDC 0006-0041-28 single unit packages of 100.
NDC 0006-0041-82 bottles of 1000.
Shown in Product Identification Section, page 420
No. 7592—0.25 mg, orange in color and coded MSD 20.
NDC 0006-0020-68 bottles of 100.
Shown in Product Identification Section, page 420
A.H.F.S. Category: 68:04
DC 6025241   Issued April 1983

DECADRON® Phosphate Injection   R
(dexamethasone sodium phosphate, MSD), U.S.P.

Description

Dexamethasone sodium phosphate, a synthetic adrenocortical steroid, is a white or slightly yellow, crystalline powder. It is freely soluble in water and is exceedingly hygroscopic. The molecular weight is 516.14. It is designated chemically as 9-fluoro-11β, 17-dihydroxy-16α-methyl-21-(phosphonooxy)pregna-1, 4-diene-3, 20-dione disodium salt. The empirical formula is $C_{22}H_{28}FNa_2O_8P$.
DECADRON® Phosphate (Dexamethasone Sodium Phosphate, MSD) injection is a sterile solution (pH 7.0 to 8.5) of dexamethasone sodium phosphate, and is supplied in two concentrations: 4 mg/ml and 24 mg/ml. The 24 mg/ml concentration offers the advantage of less volume in indications where high doses of corticosteroids by the intravenous route are needed.
Each milliliter of DECADRON Phosphate injection, 4 mg/ml, contains dexamethasone sodium phosphate equivalent to 4 mg dexamethasone phosphate or 3.33 mg dexamethasone. Inactive ingredients per ml: 8 mg creatinine, 10 mg sodium citrate, sodium hydroxide to adjust pH, and Water for Injection q.s., with 1 mg sodium bisulfite, 1.5 mg methylparaben, and 0.2 mg propylparaben added as preservatives.
Each milliliter of DECADRON Phosphate injection, 24 mg/ml, contains dexamethasone sodium phosphate equivalent to 24 mg dexamethasone phosphate or 20 mg dexamethasone. Inactive ingredients per ml: 8 mg creatinine, 10 mg sodium citrate, 0.5 mg disodium edetate, sodium hydroxide to adjust pH, and Water for Injection q.s., with 1 mg sodium bisulfite, 1.5 mg methylparaben, and 0.2 mg propylparaben added as preservatives.

Actions

DECADRON Phosphate injection has a rapid onset but short duration of action when compared with less soluble preparations. Because of this, it is suitable for the treatment of acute disorders responsive to adrenocortical steroid therapy.
Naturally occurring glucocorticoids (hydrocortisone and cortisone), which also have salt-retaining properties, are used as replacement therapy in adrenocortical deficiency states. Their synthetic analogs, including dexamethasone, are primarily used for their potent anti-inflammatory effects in disorders of many organ systems.
Glucocorticoids cause profound and varied metabolic effects. In addition, they modify the body's immune responses to diverse stimuli.
At equipotent anti-inflammatory doses, dexamethasone almost completely lacks the sodium-retaining property of hydrocortisone and closely related derivatives of hydrocortisone.

Indications

A. By intravenous or intramuscular injection when oral therapy is not feasible:
 1. *Endocrine disorders*
Primary or secondary adrenocortical insufficiency (hydrocortisone or cortisone is the drug of choice; synthetic analogs may be used in conjunction with mineralocorticoids where applicable; in infancy, mineralocorticoid supplementation is of particular importance)
Acute adrenocortical insufficiency (hydrocortisone or cortisone is the drug of choice; mineralocorticoid supplementation may be necessary, particularly when synthetic analogs are used)
Preoperatively, and in the event of serious trauma or illness, in patients with known adrenal insufficiency or when adrenocortical reserve is doubtful
Shock unresponsive to conventional therapy if adrenocortical insufficiency exists or is suspected
Congenital adrenal hyperplasia
Nonsuppurative thyroiditis
Hypercalcemia associated with cancer
 2. *Rheumatic disorders*
As adjunctive therapy for short-term administration (to tide the patient over an acute episode or exacerbation) in:
Post-traumatic osteoarthritis
Synovitis of osteoarthritis
Rheumatoid arthritis, including juvenile rheumatoid arthritis (selected cases may require low-dose maintenance therapy)
Acute and subacute bursitis
Epicondylitis
Acute nonspecific tenosynovitis
Acute gouty arthritis
Psoriatic arthritis
Ankylosing spondylitis
 3. *Collagen diseases*
During an exacerbation or as maintenance therapy in selected cases of:
Systemic lupus erythematosus
Acute rheumatic carditis
 4. *Dermatologic diseases*
Pemphigus
Severe erythema multiforme (Stevens-Johnson syndrome)
Exfoliative dermatitis
Bullous dermatitis herpetiformis
Severe seborrheic dermatitis
Severe psoriasis
Mycosis fungoides
 5. *Allergic states*
Control of severe or incapacitating allergic conditions intractable to adequate trials of conventional treatment in:
Bronchial asthma
Contact dermatitis
Atopic dermatitis
Serum sickness
Seasonal or perennial allergic rhinitis
Drug hypersensitivity reactions
Urticarial transfusion reactions
Acute noninfectious laryngeal edema (epinephrine is the drug of first choice)
 6. *Ophthalmic diseases*
Severe acute and chronic allergic and inflammatory processes involving the eye, such as:
Herpes zoster ophthalmicus
Iritis, iridocyclitis
Chorioretinitis
Diffuse posterior uveitis and choroiditis
Optic neuritis
Sympathetic ophthalmia
Anterior segment inflammation
Allergic conjunctivitis
Keratitis
Allergic corneal marginal ulcers
 7. *Gastrointestinal diseases*
To tide the patient over a critical period of the disease in:
Ulcerative colitis (Systemic therapy)
Regional enteritis (Systemic therapy)
 8. *Respiratory diseases*
Symptomatic sarcoidosis
Berylliosis
Fulminating or disseminated pulmonary tuberculosis when used concurrently with appropriate antituberculous chemotherapy
Loeffler's syndrome not manageable by other means
Aspiration pneumonitis
 9. *Hematologic disorders*
Acquired (autoimmune) hemolytic anemia
Idiopathic thrombocytopenic purpura in adults (I.V. only; I.M. administration is contraindicated)
Secondary thrombocytopenia in adults
Erythroblastopenia (RBC anemia)
Congenital (erythroid) hypoplastic anemia
 10. *Neoplastic diseases*
For palliative management of:
Leukemias and lymphomas in adults
Acute leukemia of childhood
 11. *Edematous states*
To induce diuresis or remission of proteinuria in the nephrotic syndrome, without uremia, of the idiopathic type, or that due to lupus erythematosus
 12. *Miscellaneous*
Tuberculous meningitis with subarachnoid block or impending block when used concurrently with appropriate antituberculous chemotherapy
Trichinosis with neurologic or myocardial involvement
 13. *Diagnostic testing of adrenocortical hyperfunction*
 14. *Cerebral Edema* associated with primary or metastatic brain tumor, craniotomy, or head injury. Use in cerebral edema is not a substitute for careful neurosurgical evaluation and definitive management such as neurosurgery or other specific therapy.
B. By intra-articular or soft tissue injection:
As adjunctive therapy for short-term administration (to tide the patient over an acute episode or exacerbation) in:
Synovitis of osteoarthritis
Rheumatoid arthritis
Acute and subacute bursitis
Acute gouty arthritis
Epicondylitis
Acute nonspecific tenosynovitis
Post-traumatic osteoarthritis
C. By intralesional injection:
Keloids
Localized hypertrophic, infiltrated, inflammatory lesions of: lichen planus, psoriatic plaques, granuloma annulare, and lichen simplex chronicus (neurodermatitis)
Discoid lupus erythematosus
Necrobiosis lipoidica diabeticorum
Alopecia areata
May also be useful in cystic tumors of an aponeurosis or tendon (ganglia)

Contraindications

Systemic fungal infections (See WARNINGS re amphotericin B)
Hypersensitivity to any component of this product

Warnings

Corticosteroids may exacerbate systemic fungal infections and therefore should not be used in the presence of such infections unless they are needed to control drug reactions due to amphotericin B. Moreover, there have been cases reported in which concomitant use of amphotericin B and hydrocortisone was followed by cardiac enlargement and congestive failure.
In patients on corticosteroid therapy subjected to any unusual stress, increased dosage of rapidly acting corticosteroids before, during, and after the stressful situation is indicated.
Drug-induced secondary adrenocortical insufficiency may result from too rapid withdrawal of corticosteroids and may be minimized by gradual reduction of dosage. This type of relative insufficiency may persist for months after discontinua-

tion of therapy; therefore, in any situation of stress occurring during that period, hormone therapy should be reinstituted. If the patient is receiving steroids already, dosage may have to be increased. Since mineralocorticoid secretion may be impaired, salt and/or a mineralocorticoid should be administered concurrently.

Corticosteroids may mask some signs of infection, and new infections may appear during their use. There may be decreased resistance and inability to localize infection when corticosteroids are used. Moreover, corticosteroids may affect the nitro-blue-tetrazolium test for bacterial infection and produce false negative results.

In cerebral malaria, a double-blind trial has shown that the use of corticosteroids is associated with prolongation of coma and a higher incidence of pneumonia and gastrointestinal bleeding.

Corticosteroids may activate latent amebiasis. Therefore, it is recommended that latent or active amebiasis be ruled out before initiating corticosteroid therapy in any patient who has spent time in the tropics or any patient with unexplained diarrhea.

Prolonged use of corticosteroids may produce posterior subcapsular cataracts, glaucoma with possible damage to the optic nerves, and may enhance the establishment of secondary ocular infections due to fungi or viruses.

Usage in pregnancy. Since adequate human reproduction studies have not been done with corticosteroids, use of these drugs in pregnancy or in women of childbearing potential requires that the anticipated benefits be weighed against the possible hazards to the mother and embryo or fetus. Infants born of mothers who have received substantial doses of corticosteroids during pregnancy should be carefully observed for signs of hypoadrenalism.

Corticosteroids appear in breast milk and could suppress growth, interfere with endogenous corticosteroid production, or cause other unwanted effects. Mothers taking pharmacologic doses of corticosteroids should be advised not to nurse.

Average and large doses of cortisone or hydrocortisone can cause elevation of blood pressure, salt and water retention, and increased excretion of potassium. These effects are less likely to occur with the synthetic derivatives except when used in large doses. Dietary salt restriction and potassium supplementation may be necessary. All corticosteroids increase calcium excretion.

Administration of live virus vaccines, including smallpox, is contraindicated in individuals receiving immunosuppressive doses of corticosteroids. If inactivated viral or bacterial vaccines are administered to individuals receiving immunosuppressive doses of corticosteroids, the expected serum antibody response may not be obtained. However, immunization procedures may be undertaken in patients who are receiving corticosteroids as replacement therapy, e.g., for Addison's disease.

The use of DECADRON Phosphate injection in active tuberculosis should be restricted to those cases of fulminating or disseminated tuberculosis in which the corticosteroid is used for the management of the disease in conjunction with an appropriate antituberculous regimen.

If corticosteroids are indicated in patients with latent tuberculosis or tuberculin reactivity, close observation is necessary as reactivation of the disease may occur. During prolonged corticosteroid therapy, these patients should receive chemoprophylaxis.

Because rare instances of anaphylactoid reactions have occurred in patients receiving parenteral corticosteroid therapy, appropriate precautionary measures should be taken prior to administration, especially when the patient has a history of allergy to any drug.

Precautions

This product, like many other steroid formulations, is sensitive to heat. Therefore, it should not be autoclaved when it is desirable to sterilize the exterior of the vial.

Following prolonged therapy, withdrawal of corticosteroids may result in symptoms of the corticosteroid withdrawal syndrome including fever, myalgia, arthralgia, and malaise. This may occur in patients even without evidence of adrenal insufficiency.

There is an enhanced effect of corticosteroids in patients with hypothyroidism and in those with cirrhosis.

Corticosteroids should be used cautiously in patients with ocular herpes simplex for fear of corneal perforation.

The lowest possible dose of corticosteroid should be used to control the condition under treatment, and when reduction in dosage is possible, the reduction must be gradual.

Psychic derangements may appear when corticosteroids are used, ranging from euphoria, insomnia, mood swings, personality changes, and severe depression to frank psychotic manifestations. Also, existing emotional instability or psychotic tendencies may be aggravated by corticosteroids.

Aspirin should be used cautiously in conjunction with corticosteroids in hypoprothrombinemia.

Steroids should be used with caution in nonspecific ulcerative colitis, if there is a probability of impending perforation, abscess, or other pyogenic infection, also in diverticulitis, fresh intestinal anastomoses, active or latent peptic ulcer, renal insufficiency, hypertension, osteoporosis, and myasthenia gravis. Signs of peritoneal irritation following gastrointestinal perforation in patients receiving large doses of corticosteroids may be minimal or absent. Fat embolism has been reported as a possible complication of hypercortisonism.

When large doses are given, some authorities advise that antacids be administered between meals to help to prevent peptic ulcer.

Growth and development of infants and children on prolonged corticosteroid therapy should be carefully followed.

Steroids may increase or decrease motility and number of spermatozoa in some patients.

Phenytoin, phenobarbital, ephedrine, and rifampin may enhance the metabolic clearance of corticosteroids, resulting in decreased blood levels and lessened physiologic activity, thus requiring adjustment in corticosteroid dosage. These interactions may interfere with dexamethasone suppression tests which should be interpreted with caution during administration of these drugs.

The prothrombin time should be checked frequently in patients who are receiving corticosteroids and coumarin anticoagulants at the same time because of reports that corticosteroids have altered the response to these anticoagulants. Studies have shown that the usual effect produced by adding corticosteroids is inhibition of response to coumarins, although there have been some conflicting reports of potentiation not substantiated by studies.

When corticosteroids are administered concomitantly with potassium-depleting diuretics, patients should be observed closely for development of hypokalemia.

Intra-articular injection of a corticosteroid may produce systemic as well as local effects.

Appropriate examination of any joint fluid present is necessary to exclude a septic process.

A marked increase in pain accompanied by local swelling, further restriction of joint motion, fever, and malaise is suggestive of septic arthritis. If this complication occurs and the diagnosis of sepsis is confirmed, appropriate antimicrobial therapy should be instituted.

Injection of a steroid into an infected site is to be avoided.

Corticosteroids should not be injected into unstable joints.

Patients should be impressed strongly with the importance of not overusing joints in which symptomatic benefit has been obtained as long as the inflammatory process remains active.

Frequent intra-articular injection may result in damage to joint tissues.

The slower rate of absorption by intramuscular administration should be recognized.

Adverse Reactions

Fluid and electrolyte disturbances
Sodium retention
Fluid retention
Congestive heart failure in susceptible patients
Potassium loss
Hypokalemic alkalosis
Hypertension
  Musculoskeletal
Muscle weakness
Steroid myopathy
Loss of muscle mass
Osteoporosis
Vertebral compression fractures
Aseptic necrosis of femoral and humeral heads
Pathologic fracture of long bones
Tendon rupture
  Gastrointestinal
Peptic ulcer with possible subsequent perforation and hemorrhage
Perforation of the small and large bowel, particularly in patients with inflammatory bowel disease
Pancreatitis
Abdominal distention
Ulcerative esophagitis
  Dermatologic
Impaired wound healing
Thin fragile skin
Petechiae and ecchymoses
Erythema
Increased sweating
May suppress reactions to skin tests
Burning or tingling, especially in the perineal area (after I.V. injection)
Other cutaneous reactions, such as allergic dermatitis, urticaria, angioneurotic edema
  Neurologic
Convulsions
Increased intracranial pressure with papilledema (pseudotumor cerebri) usually after treatment
Vertigo
Headache
  Endocrine
Menstrual irregularities
Development of cushingoid state
Suppression of growth in children
Secondary adrenocortical and pituitary unresponsiveness, particularly in times of stress, as in trauma, surgery, or illness
Decreased carbohydrate tolerance
Manifestations of latent diabetes mellitus
Increased requirements for insulin or oral hypoglycemic agents in diabetics
Hirsutism
  Ophthalmic
Posterior subcapsular cataracts
Increased intraocular pressure
Glaucoma
Exophthalmos
  Metabolic
Negative nitrogen balance due to protein catabolism
  Other
Anaphylactoid or hypersensitivity reactions
Thromboembolism
Weight gain
Increased appetite
Nausea
Malaise

The following *additional* adverse reactions are related to parenteral corticosteroid therapy:

Rare instances of blindness associated with intralesional therapy around the face and head

Continued on next page

Information on the Merck Sharp & Dohme products listed on these pages is the full prescribing information from product circulars in use November 1, 1984.

Merck Sharp & Dohme—Cont.

Hyperpigmentation or hypopigmentation
Subcutaneous and cutaneous atrophy
Sterile abscess
Postinjection flare (following intra-articular use)
Charcot-like arthropathy

Dosage and Administration

DECADRON Phosphate injection, 4 mg/ml—*For intravenous, intramuscular, intra-articular, intralesional, and soft tissue injection.*
DECADRON Phosphate injection, 24 mg/ml—*For intravenous injection only.*
DECADRON Phosphate injection can be given directly from the vial or the disposable syringe, or it can be added to Sodium Chloride Injection or Dextrose Injection and administered by intravenous drip.
Solutions used for intravenous administration or further dilution of this product should be preservative-free when used in the neonate, especially the premature infant.
When it is mixed with an infusion solution, sterile precautions should be observed. Since infusion solutions generally do not contain preservatives, mixtures should be used within 24 hours.
DOSAGE REQUIREMENTS ARE VARIABLE AND MUST BE INDIVIDUALIZED ON THE BASIS OF THE DISEASE AND THE RESPONSE OF THE PATIENT.

Intravenous and Intramuscular Injection
The initial dosage of DECADRON Phosphate injection varies from 0.5 to 9 mg a day depending on the disease being treated. In less severe diseases doses lower than 0.5 mg may suffice, while in severe diseases doses higher than 9 mg may be required.
The initial dosage should be maintained or adjusted until the patient's response is satisfactory. If a satisfactory clinical response does not occur after a reasonable period of time, discontinue DECADRON Phosphate injection and transfer the patient to other therapy.
After a favorable initial response, the proper maintenance dosage should be determined by decreasing the initial dosage in small amounts to the lowest dosage that maintains an adequate clinical response.
Patients should be observed closely for signs that might require dosage adjustment, including changes in clinical status resulting from remissions or exacerbations of the disease, individual drug responsiveness, and the effect of stress (e.g., surgery, infection, trauma). During stress it may be necessary to increase dosage temporarily.
If the drug is to be stopped after more than a few days of treatment, it usually should be withdrawn gradually.
When the intravenous route of administration is used, dosage usually should be the same as the oral dosage. In certain overwhelming, acute, life-threatening situations, however, administration in dosages exceeding the usual dosages may be justified and may be in multiples of the oral dosages. The slower rate of absorption by intramuscular administration should be recognized.

Shock
There is a tendency in current medical practice to use high (pharmacologic) doses of corticosteroids for the treatment of unresponsive shock. The following dosages of DECADRON phosphate injection have been suggested by various authors:

Author*	Dosage
Cavanagh[1]	3 mg/kg of body weight per 24 hours by constant intravenous infusion after an initial intravenous injection of 20 mg
Dietzman[2]	2 to 6 mg/kg of body weight as a single intravenous injection
Frank[3]	40 mg initially followed by repeat intravenous injection every 4 to 6 hours while shock persists
Oaks[4]	40 mg initially followed by repeat intravenous injection every 2 to 6 hours while shock persists
Schumer[5]	1 mg/kg of body weight as a single intravenous injection

Administration of high dose corticosteroid therapy should be continued only until the patient's condition has stabilized and usually not longer than 48 to 72 hours.
Although adverse reactions associated with high dose, short term corticosteroid therapy are uncommon, peptic ulceration may occur.

---

*1. Cavanagh, D.; Singh, K. B.: Endotoxin shock in pregnancy and abortion, in "Corticosteroids in the Treatment of Shock", Schumer, W.; Nyhus, L. M., Editors, Urbana, University of Illinois Press, 1970, pp. 86-96.
2. Dietzman, R. H.; Ersek, R. A.; Bloch, J. M.; Lillehei, R. C.: High-output, low-resistance gram-negative septic shock in man, Angiology 20: 691-700, Dec. 1969.
3. Frank, E.: Clinical observations in shock and management (In: Shields, T. F., ed.: Symposium on current concepts and management of shock), J. Maine Med. Ass. 59: 195-200, Oct. 1968.
4. Oaks, W. W.; Cohen, H. E.: Endotoxin shock in the geriatric patient, Geriat. 22: 120-130, Mar. 1967.
5. Schumer, W.; Nyhus, L. M.: Corticosteroid effect on biochemical parameters of human oligemic shock, Arch. Surg. 100: 405-408, Apr. 1970.

Cerebral Edema
DECADRON Phosphate injection is generally administered initially in a dosage of 10 mg intravenously followed by 4 mg every six hours intramuscularly until the symptoms of cerebral edema subside. Response is usually noted within 12 to 24 hours and dosage may be reduced after two to four days and gradually discontinued over a period of five to seven days. For palliative management of patients with recurrent or inoperable brain tumors, maintenance therapy with two mg two or three times a day may be effective.

Acute Allergic Disorders
In acute, self-limited allergic disorders or acute exacerbations of chronic allergic disorders, the following dosage schedule combining parenteral and oral therapy is suggested:
DECADRON Phosphate injection, 4 mg/ml: *first day*, 1 or 2 ml (4 or 8 mg), intramuscularly.
DECADRON® (Dexamethasone, MSD) tablets, 0.75 mg: *second and third days*, 4 tablets in two divided doses each day; *fourth day*, 2 tablets in two divided doses; *fifth and sixth days*, 1 tablet each day; *seventh day*, no treatment; *eighth day*, follow-up visit.
This schedule is designed to ensure adequate therapy during acute episodes, while minimizing the risk of overdosage in chronic cases.

Intra-articular, Intralesional, and Soft Tissue Injection
Intra-articular, intralesional, and soft tissue injections are generally employed when the affected joints or areas are limited to one or two sites. Dosage and frequency of injection varies depending on the condition and the site of injection. The usual dose is from 0.2 to 6 mg. The frequency usually ranges from once every three to five days to once every two to three weeks. Frequent intra-articular injection may result in damage to joint tissues. Some of the usual single doses are:

Site of Injection	Amount of Dexamethasone Phosphate (mg)
Large Joints (e.g., Knee)	2 to 4
Small Joints (e.g., Interphalangeal, Temporomandibular)	0.8 to 1
Bursae	2 to 3
Tendon Sheaths	0.4 to 1
Soft Tissue Infiltration	2 to 6
Ganglia	1 to 2

DECADRON Phosphate injection is particularly recommended for use in conjunction with one of the less soluble, longer-acting steroids for intra-articular and soft tissue injection.

How Supplied

No. 7628X—Injection DECADRON Phosphate, 4 mg per ml, is a clear, colorless solution, and is available in 1 ml and 2.5 ml disposable syringes and in 1 ml, 5 ml, and 25 ml vials as follows:
NDC 0006-7628-01, 1 ml single dose disposable syringe
(6505-00-935-4117, 1 ml syringe)
NDC 0006-7628-66, boxes of 25 × 1 ml vials
NDC 0006-7628-30, 2.5 ml single dose disposable syringe
NDC 0006-7628-03, 5 ml vial
(6505-00-963-5355, 5 ml vial)
NDC 0006-7628-25, 25 ml vial
FOR INTRAVENOUS USE ONLY:
No. 7646—Injection DECADRON Phosphate, 24 mg per ml, is a clear, colorless to light yellow solution and is available in 5 ml and 10 ml vials as follows:
NDC 0006-7646-03, 5 ml vial
NDC 0006-7646-10, 10 ml vial.
A.H.F.S. Category: 68:04
DC 6597120   Issued April 1983

DECADRON® Phosphate ℞
(dexamethasone sodium phosphate, MSD), U.S.P.
0.05% Dexamethasone Phosphate Equivalent
Sterile Ophthalmic Ointment

Description

Sterile Ophthalmic Ointment DECADRON® Phosphate (Dexamethasone Sodium Phosphate, MSD) is a topical steroid ointment containing dexamethasone sodium phosphate equivalent to 0.5 mg (0.05%) dexamethasone phosphate in each gram. Inactive ingredients: white petrolatum and mineral oil.
Dexamethasone sodium phosphate is an inorganic ester of dexamethasone.

Action

Inhibition of inflammatory response to inciting agents of mechanical, chemical or immunological nature. No generally accepted explanation of this steroid property has been advanced.

Indications

For the treatment of the following conditions:
Steroid responsive inflammatory conditions of the palpebral and bulbar conjunctiva, cornea, and anterior segment of the globe, such as allergic conjunctivitis, acne rosacea, superficial punctate keratitis, herpes zoster keratitis, iritis, cyclitis, selected infective conjunctivitis when the inherent hazard of steroid use is accepted to obtain an advisable diminution in edema and inflammation; corneal injury from chemical or thermal burns, or penetration of foreign bodies.

Contraindications

Acute superficial herpes simplex keratitis.
Fungal diseases of ocular structures.
Acute infectious stages of vaccinia, varicella and most other viral diseases of the cornea and conjunctiva.

Tuberculosis of the eye.
Hypersensitivity to a component of this medication.

Warnings

Employment of steroid medication in the treatment of stromal herpes simplex requires great caution; frequent slit-lamp microscopy is mandatory.
Prolonged use may result in elevated intraocular pressure and/or glaucoma, damage to the optic nerve, defects in visual acuity and fields of vision, posterior subcapsular cataract formation, or may result in secondary ocular infections.
Viral, bacterial, and fungal infections of the cornea may be exacerbated by the application of steroids.
Acute purulent untreated infection of the eye may be masked or activity enhanced by the presence of steroid medication.
In those diseases causing thinning of the cornea or sclera, perforation has been known to occur with the use of topical steroids.

Usage in Pregnancy
Safety of intensive or protracted use of topical steroids during pregnancy has not been substantiated.

Precautions

As fungal infections of the cornea are particularly prone to develop coincidentally with long-term local steroid applications, fungus invasion must be considered in any persistent corneal ulceration where a steroid has been used or is in use.
Intraocular pressure should be checked frequently.

Adverse Reactions

Glaucoma with optic nerve damage, visual acuity and field defects, posterior subcapsular cataract formation, secondary ocular infection from pathogens including herpes simplex, perforation of the globe.
Rarely, filtering blebs have been reported when topical steroids have been used following cataract surgery.
Rarely, stinging or burning may occur.

Dosage and Administration

The duration of treatment will vary with the type of lesion and may extend from a few days to several weeks, according to therapeutic response. Relapses, more common in chronic active lesions than in self-limited conditions, usually respond to retreatment.
Apply a thin coating of ointment three or four times a day. When a favorable response is observed, reduce the number of daily applications to two, and later to one a day as a maintenance dose if this is sufficient to control symptoms.
Ophthalmic ointment DECADRON phosphate is particularly convenient when an eye pad is used. It may also be the preparation of choice for patients in whom therapeutic benefit depends on prolonged contact of the active ingredients with ocular tissues.

How Supplied

No. 7615—0.05% Sterile Ophthalmic Ointment DECADRON phosphate is a clear unctuous ointment and is supplied as follows:
NDC 0006-7615-04 in 3.5 g tubes.
A.H.F.S. Category: 52:08
DC 6033125 Issued May 1981

DECADRON® Phosphate ℞
(dexamethasone sodium phosphate, MSD), U.S.P.
0.1% Dexamethasone Phosphate Equivalent
Sterile Ophthalmic Solution

Description

Ophthalmic Solution DECADRON® Phosphate (Dexamethasone Sodium Phosphate, MSD) in the 5 ml OCUMETER® ophthalmic dispenser is a topical steroid solution containing dexamethasone sodium phosphate equivalent to 1 mg (0.1%) dexamethasone phosphate in each milliliter of buffered solution. Inactive ingredients: creatinine, sodium citrate, sodium borate, polysorbate 80, disodium edetate, hydrochloric acid to adjust pH, and water for injection. Sodium bisulfite 0.1%, phenylethanol 0.25% and benzalkonium chloride 0.02% added as preservatives.
Dexamethasone sodium phosphate is a water soluble, inorganic ester of dexamethasone. It is approximately three thousand times more soluble in water at 25°C than hydrocortisone.

Action

Inhibition of inflammatory response to inciting agents of mechanical, chemical or immunological nature. No generally accepted explanation of this steroid property has been advanced.

Indications

For the treatment of the following conditions:
Ophthalmic:
Steroid responsive inflammatory conditions of the palpebral and bulbar conjunctiva, cornea, and anterior segment of the globe, such as allergic conjunctivitis, acne rosacea, superficial punctate keratitis, herpes zoster keratitis, iritis, cyclitis, selected infective conjunctivitis when the inherent hazard of steroid use is accepted to obtain an advisable diminution in edema and inflammation; corneal injury from chemical or thermal burns, or penetration of foreign bodies.
Otic:
Steroid responsive inflammatory conditions of the external auditory meatus, such as allergic otitis externa, selected purulent and nonpurulent infective otitis externa when the hazard of steroid use is accepted to obtain an advisable diminution in edema and inflammation.

Contraindications

Acute superficial herpes simplex keratitis.
Fungal diseases of ocular or auricular structures.
Acute infectious stages of vaccinia, varicella and most other viral diseases of the cornea and conjunctiva.
Tuberculosis of the eye.
Hypersensitivity to a component of this medication.
Perforation of a drum membrane.

Warnings

Employment of steroid medication in the treatment of stromal herpes simplex requires great caution; frequent slit-lamp microscopy is mandatory.
Prolonged use may result in elevated intraocular pressure and/or glaucoma, damage to the optic nerve, defects in visual acuity and fields of vision, posterior subcapsular cataract formation, or may result in secondary ocular infections.
Viral, bacterial, and fungal infections of the cornea may be exacerbated by the application of steroids.
Acute purulent untreated infection of the eye or ear may be masked or activity enhanced by the presence of steroid medication.
In those diseases causing thinning of the cornea or sclera, perforation has been known to occur with the use of topical steroids.

Usage in Pregnancy
Safety of intensive or protracted use of topical steroids during pregnancy has not been substantiated.

Precautions

As fungal infections of the cornea are particularly prone to develop coincidentally with long-term local steroid applications, fungus invasion must be considered in any persistent corneal ulceration where a steroid has been used or is in use.
Intraocular pressure should be checked frequently.

Adverse Reactions

Glaucoma with optic nerve damage, visual acuity and field defects, posterior subcapsular cataract formation, secondary ocular infection from pathogens including herpes simplex, perforation of the globe.
Rarely, filtering blebs have been reported when topical steroids have been used following cataract surgery.
Rarely, stinging or burning may occur.

Dosage and Administration

The duration of treatment will vary with the type of lesion and may extend from a few days to several weeks, according to therapeutic response. Relapses, more common in chronic active lesions than in self-limited conditions, usually respond to retreatment.
Eye—Instill one or two drops of solution into the conjunctival sac every hour during the day and every two hours during the night as initial therapy. When a favorable response is observed, reduce dosage to one drop every four hours. Later, further reduction in dosage to one drop three or four times daily may suffice to control symptoms.
Ear—Clean the aural canal thoroughly and sponge dry. Instill the solution directly into the aural canal. A suggested initial dosage is three or four drops two or three times a day. When a favorable response is obtained, reduce dosage gradually and eventually discontinue.
If preferred, the aural canal may be packed with a gauze wick saturated with solution. Keep the wick moist with the preparation and remove from the ear after 12 to 24 hours. Treatment may be repeated as often as necessary at the discretion of the physician.

How Supplied

Sterile ophthalmic solution DECADRON Phosphate is a clear, colorless to pale yellow solution.
No. 7643—Ophthalmic solution DECADRON Phosphate is supplied as follows:
NDC 0006-7643-03 in 5 ml white, opaque, plastic OCUMETER ophthalmic dispenser with a controlled drop tip.
(6505-00-007-4536 0.1% 5 ml)
A.H.F.S. Category: 52:08
DC 6460012 Issued May 1981

DECADRON® Phosphate ℞
RESPIHALER®
(dexamethasone sodium phosphate, MSD), U.S.P.

Description

RESPIHALER® DECADRON® Phosphate (Dexamethasone Sodium Phosphate, MSD) is an aerosol for oral inhalation which contains dexamethasone sodium phosphate, an inorganic ester of dexamethasone, a synthetic adrenocortical steroid with basic glucocorticoid actions and effects.
Each RESPIHALER DECADRON Phosphate contains an amount sufficient to deliver at least 170 sprays. The metering valve of the aerosol-mechanism of the RESPIHALER dispenses dexamethasone sodium phosphate equivalent to approximately 0.1 mg of dexamethasone phosphate or approximately 0.084 mg of dexamethasone with each activation. On a regimen of 12 inhalations daily, it has been determined that the patient absorbs approximately 0.4-0.6 mg of dexamethasone.

Continued on next page

Information on the Merck Sharp & Dohme products listed on these pages is the full prescribing information from product circulars in use November 1, 1984.

Merck Sharp & Dohme—Cont.

The inactive ingredients are fluorochlorohydrocarbons included as propellants. Alcohol 2%.
Dexamethasone sodium phosphate, a synthetic adrenocortical steroid, is a white or slightly yellow, crystalline powder. It is freely soluble in water and is exceedingly hygroscopic. It is prepared by a special process to produce particles in the range of 0.5 to 4 microns in size. The molecular weight is 516.41. It is designated chemically as 9-fluoro-11β, 17-dihydroxy-16α-methyl-21-(phosphono-oxy)pregna-1, 4-diene-3, 20-dione disodium salt. The empirical formula is $C_{22}H_{28}FNa_2O_8P$.

Actions

Because of the high water solubility of dexamethasone sodium phosphate, the aerosolized particles dissolve readily in the secretions of the bronchial and bronchiolar mucous membrane.

Indications

RESPIHALER DECADRON Phosphate is indicated for the treatment of bronchial asthma and related corticosteroid responsive bronchospastic states intractable to adequate trial of conventional therapy.

Contraindications

Systemic fungal infections.
Hypersensitivity to any component of this medication.
Persistently positive cultures of the sputum for *Candida albicans*.

Warnings

Rare instances of laryngeal and pharyngeal fungal infections have been observed in patients using RESPIHALER DECADRON Phosphate. These have usually responded promptly to discontinuation of therapy and institution of antifungal treatment.
In patients on therapy with RESPIHALER DECADRON Phosphate subjected to unusual stress, increased dosage of rapidly acting corticosteroids before, during, and after the stressful situation is indicated.
Drug-induced secondary adrenocortical insufficiency may result from too rapid withdrawal of corticosteroids and may be minimized by gradual reduction of dosage. This type of relative insufficiency may persist for months after discontinuation of therapy; therefore, in any situation of stress occurring during that period, hormone therapy should be reinstituted. If the patient is receiving steroids already, dosage may have to be increased. Since mineralocorticoid secretion may be impaired, salt and/or a mineralocorticoid should be administered concurrently.
Dexamethasone may mask some signs of infection, and new infections may appear during its use. There may be decreased resistance and inability to localize infection when corticosteroids are used. Moreover, dexamethasone may affect the nitroblue-tetrazolium test for bacterial infection and produce false negative results.
Corticosteroids may activate latent amebiasis. Therefore, it is recommended that latent or active amebiasis be ruled out before initiating corticosteroid therapy in any patient who has spent time in the tropics or any patient with unexplained diarrhea.
Prolonged use of RESPIHALER DECADRON Phosphate may produce posterior subcapsular cataracts, glaucoma with possible damage to the optic nerves, and may enhance the establishment of secondary ocular infections due to fungi or viruses.
Usage in pregnancy: Since adequate human reproduction studies have not been done with RESPIHALER DECADRON Phosphate, use of this drug in pregnancy or in women of childbearing potential requires that the anticipated benefits be weighed against the possible hazards to the mother and embryo or fetus. Infants born of mothers who have received substantial doses of dexamethasone during pregnancy, should be carefully observed for signs of hypoadrenalism.
Dexamethasone appears in breast milk and could suppress growth, interfere with endogenous corticosteroid production, or cause other unwanted effects. Mothers taking pharmacologic doses of dexamethasone should be advised not to nurse.
Average and large doses of hydrocortisone or cortisone can cause elevation of blood pressure, salt and water retention, and increased excretion of potassium. These effects are less likely to occur with the synthetic derivatives and with RESPIHALER DECADRON Phosphate, except when used in large doses. Dietary salt restriction and potassium supplementation may be necessary. All corticosteroids increase calcium excretion.
Administration of live virus vaccines, including smallpox, is contraindicated in individuals receiving immunosuppressive doses of corticosteroids. If inactivated viral or bacterial vaccines are administered to individuals receiving immunosuppressive doses of corticosteroids, the expected serum antibody response may not be obtained.
If RESPIHALER DECADRON Phosphate is indicated in patients with latent tuberculosis or tuberculin reactivity, close observation is necessary as reactivation of the disease may occur. During prolonged therapy with RESPIHALER DECADRON Phosphate, these patients should receive chemoprophylaxis.

Precautions

RESPIHALER DECADRON Phosphate is *not* indicated for relief of the occasional mild and isolated attack of asthma which is readily responsive to the immediate, though short-lived, action of epinephrine, isoproterenol, aminophylline, etc. Nor should it be employed for the treatment of severe status asthmaticus where intensive measures are required. RESPIHALER DECADRON should be considered only for the following classes of patients: patients not on corticosteroid therapy who have not responded adequately to other treatment; patients already on systemic corticosteroid therapy—in an attempt to reduce or eliminate systemic administration.
Although systemic absorption is low when RESPIHALER DECADRON Phosphate is used in the recommended dosage, adrenal suppression may occur. In addition, other systemic effects of steroid administration must be considered as a possibility.
Following prolonged therapy, withdrawal of corticosteroids may result in symptoms of the corticosteroid withdrawal syndrome including fever, myalgia, arthralgia, and malaise. This may occur in patients even without evidence of adrenal insufficiency.
There is an enhanced effect of dexamethasone in patients with hypothyroidism and in those with cirrhosis.
RESPIHALER DECADRON Phosphate should be used cautiously in patients with ocular herpes simplex for fear of corneal perforation.
The lowest possible dose of RESPIHALER DECADRON Phosphate should be used to control the condition under treatment, and when reduction in dosage is possible, the reduction must be gradual.
Psychic derangements may appear when dexamethasone is used, ranging from euphoria, insomnia, mood swings, personality changes, and severe depression, to frank psychotic manifestations. Also, existing emotional instability or psychotic tendencies may be aggravated.
Aspirin should be used cautiously in conjunction with RESPIHALER DECADRON Phosphate in hypoprothrombinemia.
RESPIHALER DECADRON Phosphate should be used with caution in nonspecific ulcerative colitis, if there is a probability of impending perforation, abscess or other pyogenic infection; also in diverticulitis; fresh intestinal anastomoses; active or latent peptic ulcer; renal insufficiency; hypertension; osteoporosis; and myasthenia gravis. Signs of peritoneal irritation following gastrointestinal perforation in patients receiving large doses of corticosteroids may be minimal or absent. Fat embolism has been reported as a possible complication of hypercortisonism.
Growth and development of infants and children on prolonged therapy with RESPIHALER DECADRON Phosphate should be carefully followed.
Dexamethasone may increase or decrease motility and number of spermatozoa in some patients.
Phenytoin, phenobarbital, ephedrine and rifampin may enhance the metabolic clearance of dexamethasone, resulting in decreased blood levels and lessened physiologic activity, thus requiring adjustment in dexamethasone dosage.
The prothrombin time should be checked frequently in patients who are receiving RESPIHALER DECADRON Phosphate and coumarin anticoagulants at the same time because of reports that corticosteroids have altered the response to these anticoagulants. Studies have shown that the usual effect produced by adding corticosteroids is inhibition of response to coumarins, although there have been some conflicting reports of potentiation, not substantiated by studies.
When RESPIHALER DECADRON Phosphate is used concomitantly with potassium-depleting diuretics, patients should be observed closely for development of hypokalemia.
Since the contents of RESPIHALER DECADRON Phosphate are under pressure, the container should not be broken, stored in extreme heat, or incinerated. It should be stored at a temperature below 120°F.

Adverse Reactions

Side effects which may occur in patients treated with RESPIHALER DECADRON Phosphate include throat irritation, hoarseness, coughing, and laryngeal and pharyngeal fungal infections.
Patients should be observed for the hormonal effects described below:

Fluid and Electrolyte Disturbances
   Sodium retention
   Fluid retention
   Congestive heart failure in susceptible patients
   Potassium loss
   Hypokalemic alkalosis
   Hypertension

Musculoskeletal
   Muscle weakness
   Steroid myopathy
   Loss of muscle mass
   Osteoporosis
   Vertebral compression fractures
   Aseptic necrosis of femoral and humeral heads
   Pathologic fracture of long bones
   Tendon rupture

Gastrointestinal
   Peptic ulcer with possible subsequent perforation and hemorrhage
   Perforation of the small and large bowel, particularly in patients with inflammatory bowel disease
   Pancreatitis
   Abdominal distention
   Ulcerative esophagitis

Dermatologic
   Impaired wound healing
   Thin fragile skin
   Petechiae and ecchymoses
   Erythema
   Increased sweating
   May suppress reactions to skin tests
   Other cutaneous reactions, such as allergic dermatitis, urticaria, angioneurotic edema

Neurologic
   Convulsions
   Increased intracranial pressure with papilledema (pseudotumor cerebri) usually after treatment
   Vertigo
   Headache

Endocrine
   Menstrual irregularities

oids. Therefore, topical corticosteroids should be used during pregnancy only if the potential benefit justifies the potential risk to the fetus. Drugs of this class should not be used extensively on pregnant patients, in large amounts, or for prolonged periods of time.

Nursing Mothers
It is not known whether topical administration of corticosteroids could result in sufficient systemic absorption to produce detectable quantities in breast milk. Systemically administered corticosteroids are secreted into breast milk in quantities *not* likely to have a deleterious effect on the infant. Nevertheless, caution should be exercised when topical corticosteroids are administered to a nursing woman.

Pediatric Use
Pediatric patients may demonstrate greater susceptibility to topical corticosteroid-induced HPA axis suppression and Cushing's syndrome than mature patients because of a larger skin surface area to body weight ratio.

Hypothalamic-pituitary-adrenal (HPA) axis suppression, Cushing's syndrome, and intracranial hypertension have been reported in children receiving topical corticosteroids. Manifestations of adrenal suppression in children include linear growth retardation, delayed weight gain, low plasma cortisol levels, and absence of response to ACTH stimulation. Manifestations of intracranial hypertension include bulging fontanelles, headaches, and bilateral papilledema.

Administration of topical corticosteroids to children should be limited to the least amount compatible with an effective therapeutic regimen. Chronic corticosteroid therapy may interfere with the growth and development of children.

Adverse Reactions

The following adverse reactions are reported infrequently with topical corticosteroids, but may occur more frequently with the use of occlusive dressings. These reactions are listed in an approximate decreasing order of occurrence:

  Burning
  Itching
  Irritation
  Dryness
  Folliculitis
  Hypertrichosis
  Acneiform eruptions
  Hypopigmentation
  Perioral dermatitis
  Allergic contact dermatitis
  Maceration of the skin
  Secondary infection
  Skin atrophy
  Striae
  Miliaria

Overdosage

Topically applied corticosteroids can be absorbed in sufficient amounts to produce systemic effects (See PRECAUTIONS).

Dosage and Administration

Patients should be instructed in the correct way to use DECASPRAY. The preparation is readily applied, even on hairy areas. It does not have to be rubbed into the skin.
Optimal effects will be obtained with DECASPRAY when these directions are followed:
1. Keep the affected area clean to reduce the possibility of infection.
2. Shake the container *gently* once or twice each time before using. Hold it about six inches from the area to be treated. Effective medication may be obtained with the container held either upright or inverted, since it is fitted with a special valve that dispenses approximately the same dosage in either position.
3. Spray each four inch square of affected area for one or two seconds three or four times a day, depending on the nature of the condition and the response to therapy.
4. When a favorable response is obtained, reduce dosage gradually and eventually discontinue.
5. Occlusive dressings may be used for the management of psoriasis or recalcitrant conditions.

How Supplied

No. 7623X—DECASPRAY is supplied as follows:
NDC 0006-7623-25 in a 25 g pressurized container.
A.H.F.S. Category: 84:06
DC 6005318   Issued April 1983
COPYRIGHT © MERCK & CO., INC., 1983
All rights reserved

DEMSER® Capsules   ℞
(metyrosine, MSD), U.S.P.

Description

DEMSER® (Metyrosine, MSD) is (—)-α-methyl-*L*-tyrosine.
Metyrosine [(—)-α-methyl-*L*-tyrosine](α-MPT) is a white, crystalline compound of molecular weight 195. It is very slightly soluble in water, acetone, and methanol, and insoluble in chloroform and benzene. It is soluble in acidic aqueous solutions. It is also soluble in alkaline aqueous solutions, but is subject to oxidative degradation under these conditions.
Each capsule of DEMSER contains 250 mg metyrosine.

Clinical Pharmacology

DEMSER inhibits tyrosine hydroxylase, which catalyzes the first transformation in catecholamine biosynthesis, i.e., the conversion of tyrosine to dihydroxyphenylalanine (DOPA). Because the first step is also the rate-limiting step, blockade of tyrosine hydroxylase activity results in decreased endogenous levels of catecholamines, usually measured as decreased urinary excretion of catecholamines and their metabolites.
In patients with pheochromocytoma, who produce excessive amounts of norepinephrine and epinephrine, administration of one to four grams of DEMSER per day has reduced catecholamine biosynthesis from about 35 to 80 percent as measured by the total excretion of catecholamines and their metabolites (metanephrine and vanillylmandelic acid). The maximum biochemical effect usually occurs within two to three days, and the urinary concentration of catecholamines and their metabolites usually returns to pretreatment levels within three to four days after DEMSER is discontinued. In some patients the total excretion of catecholamines and catecholamine metabolites may be lowered to normal or near normal levels (less than 10 mg/24 hours). In most patients the duration of treatment has been two to eight weeks, but several patients have received DEMSER for periods of one to 10 years.
Most patients with pheochromocytoma treated with DEMSER experience decreased frequency and severity of hypertensive attacks with their associated headache, nausea, sweating, and tachycardia. In patients who respond, blood pressure decreases progressively during the first two days of therapy with DEMSER; after withdrawal, blood pressure usually increases gradually to pretreatment values within two to three days.
Metyrosine is well absorbed from the gastrointestinal tract in animals and in man. In the dog, about 70 percent of an oral dose was recovered unchanged in the urine within 24 hours after administration. In man, from 53 to 88 percent (mean 69 percent) was recovered in the urine as unchanged drug following maintenance oral dosages of 600 to 4000 mg/24 hours. A very small percentage of administered drug was recovered as catechol metabolites, consisting of alpha-methyldopa, alpha-methyldopamine, and alpha-methylnorepinephrine. Although it is estimated that the sum of all catechol metabolites of metyrosine accounts for less than 0.5 percent of the administered dose, this is sufficient to interfere with accurate determination of urinary catecholamines in normal individuals. The catechol metabolites probably are not present in sufficient amounts to contribute to the biochemical effects of metyrosine.
For further information refer to: Sjoerdsma, A.; Engelman, K.; Waldman, T. A.; Cooperman, L. H.; Hammond, W. G.: Pheochromocytoma: Current concepts of diagnosis and treatment, Ann. Intern. Med. 65:1302–1326, Dec. 1966.

Indications

DEMSER is indicated in the treatment of patients with pheochromocytoma for:
1. preoperative preparation of patients for surgery
2. management of patients when surgery is contraindicated
3. chronic treatment of patients with malignant pheochromocytoma.

DEMSER is not recommended for the control of essential hypertension.

Contraindications

DEMSER is contraindicated in persons known to be hypersensitive to this compound.

Warnings

1. *Maintain fluid volume during and after surgery*
When DEMSER is used preoperatively, alone or especially in combination with alpha-adrenergic blocking drugs, adequate intravascular volume must be maintained intraoperatively (especially after tumor removal) and postoperatively to avoid hypotension and decreased perfusion of vital organs resulting from vasodilatation and expanded volume capacity. Following tumor removal, large volumes of plasma may be needed to maintain blood pressure and central venous pressure within the normal range.
In addition, life-threatening arrhythmias may occur during anesthesia and surgery, and may require treatment with a beta blocker or lidocaine. During surgery, patients should have continuous monitoring of blood pressure and electrocardiogram.
2. *Intraoperative Effects*
While the preoperative use of DEMSER in patients with pheochromocytoma is thought to decrease intraoperative problems with blood pressure control, DEMSER does not eliminate the danger of hypertensive crises or arrhythmias during manipulation of the tumor, and the alpha-adrenergic blocking drug, phentolamine, may be needed.

Precautions

1. *Metyrosine Crystalluria*
Crystalluria and urolithiasis have been found in dogs treated with DEMSER (Metyrosine, MSD) at doses similar to those used in humans, and crystalluria has also been observed in a few patients. To minimize the risk of crystalluria, patients should be urged to maintain water intake sufficient to achieve a daily urine volume of 2000 ml or more, particularly when doses greater than 2 g per day are given. Routine examination of the urine should be carried out. Metyrosine will crystallize as needles or rods. If metyrosine crystalluria occurs, fluid intake should be increased further. If crystalluria persists, the dosage should be reduced or the drug discontinued.
2. *Interaction with phenothiazines or butyrophenones*
Caution should be observed in administering DEMSER to patients receiving phenothiazines or haloperidol because the extrapyramidal effects of these drugs can be expected to be potentiated by inhibition of catecholamine synthesis; this has been documented to date only for haloperidol.

Continued on next page

Information on the Merck Sharp & Dohme products listed on these pages is the full prescribing information from product circulars in use November 1, 1984.

Merck Sharp & Dohme—Cont.

3. Relatively little data regarding long-term use
Although no evidence of adverse effects on hepatic, hematologic, or other functions, except for a few instances of increased SGOT levels, has been noted during clinical trials of DEMSER, the total human experience with the drug is quite limited (approximately 300 patients as of 1979) and few patients have been studied long-term. Chronic animal studies have not been carried out. Therefore, suitable laboratory tests should be carried out periodically in patients requiring prolonged use of DEMSER and caution should be observed in patients with impaired hepatic or renal function.

4. Interference with urinary catecholamine measurements
Spurious increases in urinary catecholamines may be observed in patients receiving DEMSER due to the presence of metabolites of the drug.

5. Usage in Pregnancy
Complete reproduction studies have not been performed in animals to determine whether DEMSER affects fertility in males or females, has teratogenic potential, or has other adverse effects on the fetus. There are no well-controlled studies of DEMSER in pregnant women. The use of DEMSER in pregnant women should be avoided, if possible, but may be appropriate when anticipated benefits outweigh the potential risks.

6. Nursing Mothers
It is not known whether DEMSER is excreted in human milk. If use of this drug is necessary, nursing should be discontinued.

Adverse Reactions

Central Nervous System
1. Sedation
The most common adverse reaction to DEMSER is moderate to severe sedation, which has been observed in almost all patients. It occurs at both low and high dosages. Sedative effects begin within the first 24 hours of therapy, are maximal after two to three days, and tend to wane during the next few days. Sedation usually is not obvious after one week unless the dosage is increased, but at dosages greater than 2000 mg/day some degree of sedation or fatigue may persist.
When receiving DEMSER, patients should be warned about engaging in activities requiring mental alertness and motor coordination, such as driving a motor vehicle or operating machinery. DEMSER may have additive effects with alcohol and other CNS depressants, e.g., hypnotics, sedatives, tranquilizers, antianxiety agents.
In most patients who experience sedation, temporary changes in sleep pattern occur following withdrawal of the drug. Changes consist of insomnia that may last for two or three days and feelings of increased alertness and ambition. Even patients who do not experience sedation while on DEMSER may report symptoms of psychic stimulation when the drug is discontinued.

2. Extrapyramidal Signs
Extrapyramidal signs such as drooling, speech difficulty, and tremor have been reported in approximately 10 percent of patients. These occasionally have been accompanied by trismus and frank parkinsonism.

3. Anxiety and Psychic Disturbances
Anxiety and psychic disturbances such as depression, hallucinations, disorientation, and confusion may occur. These effects seem to be dose-dependent and may disappear with reduction of dosage.

Diarrhea
Diarrhea occurs in about 10 percent of patients and may be severe. Antidiarrheal agents may be required if continuation of DEMSER is necessary.

Miscellaneous
Infrequently, slight swelling of the breast, galactorrhea, nasal stuffiness, decreased salivation, dry mouth, headache, nausea, vomiting, abdominal pain, and impotence or failure of ejaculation may occur. Crystalluria (see PRECAUTIONS) and transient dysuria and hematuria have been observed in a few patients. Eosinophilia, increased SGOT levels, peripheral edema, and hypersensitivity reactions such as urticaria and pharyngeal edema have been reported rarely.

Dosage and Administration

The recommended initial dosage of DEMSER for adults and children 12 years of age and older is 250 mg orally four times daily. This may be increased by 250 mg to 500 mg every day to a maximum of 4.0 g/day in divided doses. When used for preoperative preparation, the optimally effective dosage of DEMSER should be given for at least five to seven days.
Optimally effective dosages of DEMSER usually are between 2.0 and 3.0 g/day, and the dose should be titrated by monitoring clinical symptoms and catecholamine excretion. In patients who are hypertensive, dosage should be titrated to achieve normalization of blood pressure and control of clinical symptoms. In patients who are usually normotensive, dosage should be titrated to the amount that will reduce urinary metanephrines and/or vanillylmandelic acid by 50 percent or more.
If patients are not adequately controlled by the use of DEMSER, an alpha-adrenergic blocking agent (phenoxybenzamine) should be added.
Use of DEMSER in children under 12 years of age has been limited and a dosage schedule for this age group cannot be given.

How Supplied

No. 3355—Capsules DEMSER, 250 mg, are opaque, two-toned blue capsules coded MSD 690 on one side and DEMSER on the other. They are supplied as follows:
NDC 0006-0690-68 bottles of 100.
Shown in Product Identification Section, page 420
A.H.F.S. Category: 92:00
DC 7111501 Issued May 1979
COPYRIGHT© MERCK & CO., INC., 1979
All rights reserved

DIUPRES® Tablets ℞
Antihypertensive

> **WARNING**
> This fixed combination drug is not indicated for initial therapy of hypertension. Hypertension requires therapy titrated to the individual patient. If the fixed combination represents the dosage so determined, its use may be more convenient in patient management. The treatment of hypertension is not static, but must be reevaluated as conditions in each patient warrant.

Description

DIUPRES® combines two antihypertensive agents: DIURIL® (Chlorothiazide, MSD) and reserpine. The chemical name for chlorothiazide is 6-chloro-2H-1,2,4-benzothiadiazine-7-sulfonamide 1,1-dioxide. Reserpine (11,17α-dimethoxy-18β-[(3,4,5-trimethoxybenzoyl)oxy]-3β, 20α-yohimban-16β-carboxylic acid methyl ester) is a crystalline alkaloid derived from Rauwolfia serpentina.

Actions

Chlorothiazide
Chlorothiazide is a diuretic and antihypertensive. It affects the renal tubular mechanism of electrolyte reabsorption. At maximal therapeutic dosage all thiazides are approximately equal in their diuretic efficacy.
Chlorothiazide increases excretion of sodium and chloride in approximately equivalent amounts. Natriuresis may be accompanied by some loss of potassium and bicarbonate.
The mechanism of the antihypertensive effect of thiazides is unknown. Chlorothiazide does not affect normal blood pressure.
Chlorothiazide is eliminated rapidly by the kidney.

Reserpine
Reserpine has antihypertensive, bradycardic, and tranquilizing properties. It lowers arterial blood pressure by depletion of catecholamines. Reserpine is beneficial in relieving anxiety, tension, and headache in the hypertensive patient. It acts at the hypothalamic level of the central nervous system to promote relaxation without hypnosis or analgesia. The sleep pattern shown by the electroencephalogram following barbiturates does not occur with this drug. In laboratory animals spontaneous activity and response to external stimuli are decreased, but confusion or difficulty of movement is not evident.
The bradycardic action of reserpine promotes relaxation and may eliminate sinus tachycardia. It is most pronounced in subjects with sinus tachycardia and usually is not prominent in persons with a normal pulse rate.
Miosis, relaxation of the nictitating membrane, ptosis, hypothermia, and increased gastrointestinal activity are noted in animals given reserpine, sometimes in subclinical doses. None of these effects, except increased gastrointestinal activity, has been found to be clinically significant in man with therapeutic doses.

Indication

Hypertension (see box warning)

Contraindications

Chlorothiazide is contraindicated in anuria.
DIUPRES is contraindicated in hypersensitivity to chlorothiazide or other sulfonamide-derived drugs or to reserpine.
Electroshock therapy should not be given to patients while on reserpine, as severe and even fatal reactions have been reported with minimal convulsive electroshock dosage. After discontinuing reserpine, allow at least seven days before starting electroshock therapy.
Active peptic ulcer, ulcerative colitis, and active mental depression, especially suicidal tendencies, are contraindications to reserpine therapy.

Warnings

Chlorothiazide
Use with caution in severe renal disease. In patients with renal disease, thiazides may precipitate azotemia. Cumulative effects of the drug may develop in patients with impaired renal function. Thiazides should be used with caution in patients with impaired hepatic function or progressive liver disease, since minor alterations of fluid and electrolyte balance may precipitate hepatic coma.
Thiazides may add to or potentiate the action of other antihypertensive drugs.
Sensitivity reactions may occur in patients with or without a history of allergy or bronchial asthma.
The possibility of exacerbation or activation of systemic lupus erythematosus has been reported.
Lithium generally should not be given with diuretics because they reduce its renal clearance and add a high risk of lithium toxicity. Read circulars for lithium preparations before use of such concomitant therapy.

Reserpine
The occurrence of mental depression due to reserpine in doses of 0.25 mg daily or less is unusual. In any event, DIUPRES should be discontinued at the first sign of depression.

Use in Pregnancy
Reserpine has been demonstrated to cross the placental barrier in guinea pigs with depression of adrenal catecholamine stores in the newborn. There is some evidence that side effects such as nasal congestion, lethargy, depressed Moro reflex, and bradycardia may appear in infants born of reserpine-treated mothers.
Thiazides cross the placental barrier and appear in cord blood. The use of thiazides in pregnancy requires that the anticipated benefit be weighed against possible hazards to the fetus. These hazards include fetal or neonatal jaundice, thrombo-

cytopenia, and possibly other adverse reactions which have occurred in the adult.

Nursing Mothers
Thiazides and reserpine appear in breast milk. If use of the drug is deemed essential, the patient should stop nursing.

Precautions

Chlorothiazide
Periodic determination of serum electrolytes to detect possible electrolyte imbalance should be performed at appropriate intervals.

All patients receiving diuretic therapy should be observed for evidence of fluid or electrolyte imbalance: namely, hyponatremia, hypochloremic alkalosis, and hypokalemia. Serum and urine electrolyte determinations are particularly important when the patient is vomiting excessively or receiving parenteral fluids. Warning signs or symptoms of fluid and electrolyte imbalance include dryness of mouth, thirst, weakness, lethargy, drowsiness, restlessness, muscle pains or cramps, muscular fatigue, hypotension, oliguria, tachycardia, and gastrointestinal disturbances such as nausea and vomiting.

Hypokalemia may develop, especially with brisk diuresis, when severe cirrhosis is present, during concomitant use of corticosteroids or ACTH, or after prolonged therapy.

Interference with adequate oral electrolyte intake will contribute to hypokalemia. Hypokalemia can sensitize or exaggerate the response of the heart to the toxic effects of digitalis (e.g., increased ventricular irritability). Hypokalemia may be avoided or treated by use of potassium supplements such as foods with a high potassium content.

Although any chloride deficit is generally mild and usually does not require specific treatment except under extraordinary circumstances (as in liver disease or renal disease), chloride replacement may be required in the treatment of metabolic alkalosis.

Dilutional hyponatremia may occur in edematous patients in hot weather. Appropriate therapy is water restriction, rather than administration of salt, except in rare instances when the hyponatremia is life threatening. In actual salt depletion, appropriate replacement is the therapy of choice. Hyperuricemia may occur or acute gout may be precipitated in certain patients receiving thiazides.

Insulin requirements in diabetic patients may be increased, decreased, or unchanged. Latent diabetes mellitus may become manifest during thiazide therapy.

Thiazides may increase the responsiveness to tubocurarine.

The antihypertensive effect of the drug may be enhanced in the postsympathectomy patient. Thiazides may decrease arterial responsiveness to norepinephrine. This diminution is not sufficient to preclude effectiveness of the pressor agent for therapeutic use.

If progressive renal impairment becomes evident, consider withholding or discontinuing diuretic therapy.

Thiazides may decrease serum PBI levels without signs of thyroid disturbance.

Thiazides may decrease urinary calcium excretion. Thiazides may cause intermittent and slight elevation of serum calcium in the absence of known disorders of calcium metabolism. Marked hypercalcemia may be evidence of hidden hyperparathyroidism. Thiazides should be discontinued before carrying out tests for parathyroid function.

Reserpine
Since reserpine may increase gastric secretion and motility, it should be used cautiously in patients with a history of peptic ulcer, ulcerative colitis, or other gastrointestinal disorder. This compound may precipitate biliary colic in patients with gallstones, or bronchial asthma in susceptible persons. Reserpine may cause hypotension including orthostatic hypotension.

In hypertensive patients on reserpine therapy significant hypotension and bradycardia may develop during surgical anesthesia. The anesthesiologist should be aware that reserpine has been taken, since it may be necessary to give vagal blocking agents parenterally to prevent or reverse hypotension and/or bradycardia.

Anxiety or depression, as well as psychosis, may develop during reserpine therapy. If depression is present when therapy is begun, it may be aggravated. Mental depression is unusual with reserpine doses of 0.25 mg daily or less. In any case, DIUPRES should be discontinued at the first sign of depression. Extreme caution should be used in treating patients with a history of mental depression, and the possibility of suicide should be kept in mind.

As with most antihypertensive therapy, caution should be exercised when treating hypertensive patients with renal insufficiency, since they adjust poorly to lowered blood pressure levels. Use reserpine cautiously with digitalis and quinidine; cardiac arrhythmias have occurred with reserpine preparations.

When two or more antihypertensives are given, the individual dosages may have to be reduced to prevent excessive drop in blood pressure. In hypertensive patients with coronary artery disease, it is important to avoid a precipitous drop in blood pressure.

Animal tumorigenicity: Rodent studies have shown that reserpine is an animal tumorigen, causing an increased incidence of mammary fibroadenomas in female mice, malignant tumors of the seminal vesicles in male mice, and malignant adrenal medullary tumors in male rats. These findings arose in 2 year studies in which the drug was administered in the feed at concentrations of 5 and 10 ppm-about 100 to 300 times the usual human dose. The breast neoplasms are thought to be related to reserpine's prolactin-elevating effect. Several other prolactin-elevating drugs have also been associated with an increased incidence of mammary neoplasia in rodents.

The extent to which these findings indicate a risk to humans is uncertain. Tissue culture experiments show that about one-third of human breast tumors are prolactin-dependent *in vitro*, a factor of considerable importance if the use of the drug is contemplated in a patient with previously detected breast cancer. The possibility of an increased risk of breast cancer in reserpine users has been studied extensively; however, no firm conclusion has emerged. Although a few epidemiologic studies have suggested a slightly increased risk (less than twofold in all studies except one) in women who have used reserpine, other studies of generally similar design have not confirmed this. Epidemiologic studies conducted using other drugs (neuroleptic agents) that, like reserpine, increase prolactin levels and therefore would be considered rodent mammary carcinogens, have not shown an association between chronic administration of the drug and human mammary tumorigenesis. While long-term clinical observation has not suggested such an association, the available evidence is considered too limited to be conclusive at this time. An association of reserpine intake with pheochromocytoma or tumors of the seminal vesicles has not been explored.

Adverse Reactions

Chlorothiazide
Body as a Whole: Weakness.
Cardiovascular: Orthostatic hypotension (may be aggravated by alcohol, barbiturates, or narcotics).
Digestive: Anorexia, gastric irritation, nausea, vomiting, cramping, diarrhea, constipation, jaundice (intrahepatic cholestatic jaundice), pancreatitis, sialadenitis.
Hematologic: Leukopenia, agranulocytosis, thrombocytopenia, aplastic anemia, hemolytic anemia.
Metabolic: Hyperglycemia, glycosuria, hyperuricemia, electrolyte imbalance (see PRECAUTIONS).
Musculoskeletal: Muscle spasm.
Nervous System/Psychiatric: Dizziness, vertigo, paresthesias, headache, restlessness.
Special Senses: Transient blurred vision, xanthopsia.
Hypersensitivity: Purpura, photosensitivity, rash, urticaria, necrotizing angiitis (vasculitis and cutaneous vasculitis), fever, respiratory distress including pneumonitis and pulmonary edema, anaphylactic reactions.

Whenever adverse reactions are moderate or severe, thiazide dosage should be reduced or therapy withdrawn.

Reserpine
Cardiovascular: Bradycardia, angina pectoris, arrhythmia, premature ventricular contractions, and other direct cardiac effects (e.g., fluid retention, congestive failure).
Digestive: Hypersecretion and increased motility, nausea, vomiting, anorexia, diarrhea, dryness of mouth, increased salivation.
Hematologic: Excessive bleeding following prostatic surgery, thrombocytopenic purpura.
Metabolic: Weight gain.
Musculoskeletal: Muscular aches.
Nervous System/Psychiatric: Excessive sedation, mental depression, nightmares, headache, dizziness, syncope, nervousness, paradoxical anxiety, central nervous system sensitization (dull sensorium, deafness, glaucoma, uveitis, optic atrophy), parkinsonism (usually reversible with decreased dosage or discontinuance of therapy).
Respiratory: Nasal congestion, dyspnea, epistaxis, enhanced susceptibility to colds.
Hypersensitivity: Flushing of skin, pruritus, rash.
Urogenital: Dysuria, nonpuerperal lactation, impotence, decreased libido.

Dosage and Administration

The initial dosage of DIUPRES should conform to the dosages of the individual components established during titration (see box warning).

The usual adult dosage of DIUPRES 250 is 1 or 2 tablets once or twice a day; that of DIUPRES 500 is 1 tablet once or twice a day. Dosage may require adjustment according to the blood pressure response of the patient.

Careful observations for changes in blood pressure must be made when DIUPRES is used with other antihypertensive drugs.

How Supplied

No. 3261—Tablets DIUPRES 250 are pink, round, scored, compressed tablets, coded MSD 230. Each tablet contains 250 mg of chlorothiazide and 0.125 mg of reserpine. They are supplied as follows:
NDC 0006-0230-68 in bottles of 100
NDC 0006-0230-82 in bottles of 1000.
Shown in Product Identification Section, page 420
No. 3262—Tablets DIUPRES 500 are pink, round, scored, compressed tablets, coded MSD 405. Each tablet contains 500 mg of chlorothiazide and 0.125 mg of reserpine. They are supplied as follows:
NDC 0006-0405-68 in bottles of 100
NDC 0006-0405-82 in bottles of 1000.
Shown in Product Identification Section, page 420
A.H.F.S. Category: 24:08
DC 6053130   Issued November 1983
COPYRIGHT © MERCK & CO., INC., 1983
All rights reserved

DIURIL® Intravenous Sodium   ℞
(chlorothiazide sodium, MSD), U.S.P.

Description

DIURIL® (Chlorothiazide, MSD) is 6-chloro-2H-1,2,4-benzothiadiazine-7-sulfonamide 1,1- dioxide. It is a white, or practically white, crystalline compound very slightly soluble in water, but readily soluble in dilute aqueous sodium hydroxide. It is

Continued on next page

Information on the Merck Sharp & Dohme products listed on these pages is the full prescribing information from product circulars in use November 1, 1984.

Merck Sharp & Dohme—Cont.

soluble in urine to the extent of about 150 mg per 100 ml at pH 7.
Intravenous Sodium DIURIL® (Chlorothiazide Sodium, MSD) is supplied in a vial containing:
Chlorothiazide sodium equivalent
  to chlorothiazide..0.5 g
Inactive ingredients:
  Mannitol ....0.25 g
Sodium hydroxide to adjust pH, with 0.4 mg thimerosal (mercury derivative) added as preservative.

Actions

DIURIL is a diuretic and antihypertensive.
DIURIL affects the renal tubular mechanism of electrolyte reabsorption. At maximal therapeutic dosage all thiazides are approximately equal in their diuretic efficacy.
DIURIL increases excretion of sodium and chloride in approximately equivalent amounts. Natriuresis may be accompanied by some loss of potassium and bicarbonate.
After oral use diuresis begins within 2 hours, peaks in about 4 hours and lasts about 6 to 12 hours. Following intravenous use of Sodium DIURIL, onset of the diuretic action occurs in 15 minutes and the maximal action in 30 minutes. DIURIL is eliminated rapidly by the kidney.
The mechanism of the antihypertensive effect of thiazides is unknown. DIURIL does not affect normal blood pressure.

Indications

Intravenous Sodium DIURIL is indicated as adjunctive therapy in edema associated with congestive heart failure, hepatic cirrhosis, and corticosteroid and estrogen therapy.
Intravenous Sodium DIURIL has also been found useful in edema due to various forms of renal dysfunction such as nephrotic syndrome, acute glomerulonephritis, and chronic renal failure.
Use in Pregnancy. Routine use of diuretics during normal pregnancy is inappropriate and exposes mother and fetus to unnecessary hazard. Diuretics do not prevent development of toxemia of pregnancy and there is no satisfactory evidence that they are useful in the treatment of toxemia.
Edema during pregnancy may arise from pathologic causes or from the physiologic and mechanical consequences of pregnancy. Thiazides are indicated in pregnancy when edema is due to pathologic causes, just as they are in the absence of pregnancy (however, see WARNINGS). Dependent edema in pregnancy, resulting from restriction of venous return by the gravid uterus, is properly treated through elevation of the lower extremities and use of support stockings. Use of diuretics to lower intravascular volume in this instance is illogical and unnecessary. During normal pregnancy there is hypervolemia which is not harmful to the fetus or the mother in the absence of cardiovascular disease. However, it may be associated with edema, rarely generalized edema. If such edema causes discomfort, increased recumbency will often provide relief. Rarely this edema may cause extreme discomfort which is not relieved by rest. In these instances, a short course of diuretic therapy may provide relief and be appropriate.

Contraindications

Anuria.
Hypersensitivity to any component of this product or to other sulfonamide-derived drugs.

Warnings

Intravenous use in infants and children has been limited and is not generally recommended.
Use with caution in severe renal disease. In patients with renal disease, thiazides may precipitate azotemia. Cumulative effects of the drug may develop in patients with impaired renal function.
Thiazides should be used with caution in patients with impaired hepatic function or progressive liver disease, since minor alterations of fluid and electrolyte balance may precipitate hepatic coma.
Thiazides may add to or potentiate the action of other antihypertensive drugs.
Sensitivity reactions may occur in patients with or without a history of allergy or bronchial asthma. The possibility of exacerbation or activation of systemic lupus erythematosus has been reported.
Lithium generally should not be given with diuretics because they reduce its renal clearance and add a high risk of lithium toxicity. Read circulars for lithium preparations before use of such concomitant therapy.
Use in Pregnancy. Thiazides cross the placental barrier and appear in cord blood. The use of thiazides in pregnancy requires that the anticipated benefit be weighed against possible hazards to the fetus. These hazards include fetal or neonatal jaundice, thrombocytopenia, and possibly other adverse reactions which have occurred in the adult.
Nursing Mothers. Thiazides appear in breast milk. If use of the drug is deemed essential, the patient should stop nursing.

Precautions

Periodic determination of serum electrolytes to detect possible electrolyte imbalance should be performed at appropriate intervals.
All patients receiving diuretic therapy should be observed for evidence of fluid or electrolyte imbalance: namely, hyponatremia, hypochloremic alkalosis, and hypokalemia. Serum and urine electrolyte determinations are particularly important when the patient is vomiting excessively or receiving parenteral fluids. Warning signs or symptoms of fluid and electrolyte imbalance include dryness of mouth, thirst, weakness, lethargy, drowsiness, restlessness, muscle pains or cramps, muscular fatigue, hypotension, oliguria, tachycardia, and gastrointestinal disturbances such as nausea and vomiting.
Hypokalemia may develop especially with brisk diuresis, when severe cirrhosis is present, during concomitant use of corticosteroids or ACTH, or after prolonged therapy.
Interference with adequate oral electrolyte intake will also contribute to hypokalemia. Hypokalemia can sensitize or exaggerate the response of the heart to the toxic effects of digitalis (e.g., increased ventricular irritability). Hypokalemia may be avoided or treated by use of potassium supplements such as foods with a high potassium content.
Although any chloride deficit is generally mild and usually does not require specific treatment except under extraordinary circumstances (as in liver disease or renal disease), chloride replacement may be required in the treatment of metabolic alkalosis.
Dilutional hyponatremia may occur in edematous patients in hot weather; appropriate therapy is water restriction, rather than administration of salt, except in rare instances when the hyponatremia is life threatening. In actual salt depletion, appropriate replacement is the therapy of choice.
Hyperuricemia may occur or acute gout may be precipitated in certain patients receiving thiazides.
Insulin requirements in diabetic patients may be increased, decreased, or unchanged. Latent diabetes mellitus may become manifest during thiazide therapy.
Thiazides may increase the responsiveness to tubocurarine.
The antihypertensive effects of the drug may be enhanced in the postsympathectomy patient.
Thiazides may decrease arterial responsiveness to norepinephrine. This diminution is not sufficient to preclude effectiveness of the pressor agent for therapeutic use.
If progressive renal impairment becomes evident, consider withholding or discontinuing diuretic therapy.
Thiazides may decrease serum PBI levels without signs of thyroid disturbance.
Thiazides may decrease urinary calcium excretion. Thiazides may cause intermittent and slight elevation of serum calcium in the absence of known disorders of calcium metabolism. Marked hypercalcemia may be evidence of hidden hyperparathyroidism. Thiazides should be discontinued before carrying out tests for parathyroid function.

Adverse Reactions

Body as a Whole: Weakness.
Cardiovascular: Orthostatic hypotension (may be aggravated by alcohol, barbiturates, or narcotics).
Digestive: Anorexia, gastric irritation, nausea, vomiting, cramping, diarrhea, constipation, jaundice (intrahepatic cholestatic jaundice), pancreatitis, sialadenitis.
Hematologic: Leukopenia, agranulocytosis, thrombocytopenia, aplastic anemia, hemolytic anemia.
Metabolic: Hyperglycemia, glycosuria, hyperuricemia, electrolyte imbalance (see PRECAUTIONS).
Musculoskeletal: Muscle spasm.
Nervous System/Psychiatric: Dizziness, vertigo, paresthesias, headache, restlessness.
Special Senses: Transient blurred vision, xanthopsia.
Urogenital: Hematuria (one case following intravenous use).
Hypersensitivity: Purpura, photosensitivity, rash, urticaria, necrotizing angiitis (vasculitis and cutaneous vasculitis), fever, respiratory distress including pneumonitis and pulmonary edema, anaphylactic reactions.
Whenever adverse reactions are moderate or severe, thiazide dosage should be reduced or therapy withdrawn.

Dosage and Administration

Intravenous Sodium DIURIL should be reserved for patients unable to take oral medication or for emergency situations.
Therapy should be individualized according to patient response. Use the smallest dosage necessary to achieve the required response.
Intravenous use in infants and children has been limited and is not generally recommended.
When medication can be taken orally, therapy with DIURIL tablets or oral suspension may be substituted for intravenous therapy, using the same dosage schedule as for the parenteral route.
Add 18 ml of Sterile Water for Injection to the vial to form an isotonic solution for intravenous injection. Never add less than 18 ml. Unused solution may be stored at room temperature for 24 hours, after which it must be discarded. The solution is compatible with dextrose or sodium chloride solutions for intravenous infusion. Avoid simultaneous administration of solutions of chlorothiazide with whole blood or its derivatives.
Extravasation must be rigidly avoided. Do not give subcutaneously or intramuscularly.
The usual adult dosage is 0.5 to 1.0 g once or twice a day. Many patients with edema respond to intermittent therapy, i.e., administration on alternate days or on three to five days each week. With an intermittent schedule, excessive response and the resulting undesirable electrolyte imbalance are less likely to occur.

How Supplied

No. 3250—Intravenous Sodium DIURIL is a dry, white powder usually in plug form, supplied in vials containing chlorothiazide sodium equivalent to 0.5 g of chlorothiazide. **NDC 0006-3250-32.**
A.H.F.S. Category: 40:28
DC 6435019   Issued November 1983
COPYRIGHT © MERCK & CO., INC. 1983
All rights reserved

DIURIL® Tablets ℞
(chlorothiazide, MSD), U.S.P.
DIURIL® Oral Suspension ℞
(chlorothiazide, MSD), U.S.P.

Description

DIURIL® (Chlorothiazide, MSD) is 6-chloro-2H-1,2,4-benzothiadiazine-7-sulfonamide 1,1-dioxide. It is a white, or practically white, crystalline compound very slightly soluble in water, but readily soluble in dilute aqueous sodium hydroxide. It is soluble in urine to the extent of about 150 mg per 100 ml at pH 7.

DIURIL is supplied as 250 mg and 500 mg tablets, and as an oral suspension containing 250 mg per 5 ml, alcohol 0.5 percent, with methylparaben 0.12 percent, propylparaben 0.02 percent, and benzoic acid 0.1 percent added as preservatives.

Actions

DIURIL is a diuretic and antihypertensive.
DIURIL affects the renal tubular mechanism of electrolyte reabsorption. At maximal therapeutic dosage all thiazides are approximately equal in their diuretic efficacy.
DIURIL increases excretion of sodium and chloride in approximately equivalent amounts. Natriuresis may be accompanied by some loss of potassium and bicarbonate.
After oral use diuresis begins within 2 hours, peaks in about 4 hours and lasts about 6 to 12 hours. DIURIL is eliminated rapidly by the kidney.
The mechanism of the antihypertensive effect of thiazides is unknown. DIURIL does not affect normal blood pressure.

Indications

DIURIL is indicated as adjunctive therapy in edema associated with congestive heart failure, hepatic cirrhosis, and corticosteroid and estrogen therapy.
DIURIL has also been found useful in edema due to various forms of renal dysfunction such as nephrotic syndrome, acute glomerulonephritis, and chronic renal failure.
DIURIL is indicated in the management of hypertension either as the sole therapeutic agent or to enhance the effectiveness of other antihypertensive drugs in the more severe forms of hypertension.
Use in Pregnancy. Routine use of diuretics during normal pregnancy is inappropriate and exposes mother and fetus to unnecessary hazard. Diuretics do not prevent development of toxemia of pregnancy and there is no satisfactory evidence that they are useful in the treatment of toxemia.
Edema during pregnancy may arise from pathologic causes or from the physiologic and mechanical consequences of pregnancy. Thiazides are indicated in pregnancy when edema is due to pathologic causes, just as they are in the absence of pregnancy (however, see WARNINGS, below). Dependent edema in pregnancy, resulting from restriction of venous return by the gravid uterus, is properly treated through elevation of the lower extremities and use of support stockings. Use of diuretics to lower intravascular volume in this instance is illogical and unnecessary. During normal pregnancy there is hypervolemia which is not harmful to the fetus or the mother in the absence of cardiovascular disease. However, it may be associated with edema, rarely generalized edema. If such edema causes discomfort, increased recumbency will often provide relief. Rarely this edema may cause extreme discomfort which is not relieved by rest. In these instances, a short course of diuretic therapy may provide relief and be appropriate.

Contraindications

Anuria.
Hypersensitivity to this product or to other sulfonamide-derived drugs.

Warnings

Use with caution in severe renal disease. In patients with renal disease, thiazides may precipitate azotemia. Cumulative effects of the drug may develop in patients with impaired renal function. Thiazides should be used with caution in patients with impaired hepatic function or progressive liver disease, since minor alterations of fluid and electrolyte balance may precipitate hepatic coma.
Thiazides may add to or potentiate the action of other antihypertensive drugs.
Sensitivity reactions may occur in patients with or without a history of allergy or bronchial asthma. The possibility of exacerbation or activation of systemic lupus erythematosus has been reported.
Lithium generally should not be given with diuretics because they reduce its renal clearance and add a high risk of lithium toxicity. Read circulars for lithium preparations before use of such concomitant therapy.
Use in Pregnancy. Thiazides cross the placental barrier and appear in cord blood. The use of thiazides in pregnancy requires that the anticipated benefit be weighed against possible hazards to the fetus. These hazards include fetal or neonatal jaundice, thrombocytopenia, and possibly other adverse reactions which have occurred in the adult.
Nursing Mothers. Thiazides appear in breast milk. If use of the drug is deemed essential, the patient should stop nursing.

Precautions

Periodic determination of serum electrolytes to detect possible electrolyte imbalance should be performed at appropriate intervals.
All patients receiving diuretic therapy should be observed for evidence of fluid or electrolyte imbalance: namely, hyponatremia, hypochloremic alkalosis, and hypokalemia. Serum and urine electrolyte determinations are particularly important when the patient is vomiting excessively or receiving parenteral fluids. Warning signs or symptoms of fluid and electrolyte imbalance include dryness of mouth, thirst, weakness, lethargy, drowsiness, restlessness, muscle pains or cramps, muscular fatigue, hypotension, oliguria, tachycardia, and gastrointestinal disturbances such as nausea and vomiting.
Hypokalemia may develop, especially with brisk diuresis, when severe cirrhosis is present, during concomitant use of corticosteroids or ACTH, or after prolonged therapy.
Interference with adequate oral electrolyte intake will also contribute to hypokalemia. Hypokalemia can sensitize or exaggerate the response of the heart to the toxic effects of digitalis (e.g., increased ventricular irritability). Hypokalemia may be avoided or treated by use of potassium supplements such as foods with a high potassium content.
Although any chloride deficit is generally mild and usually does not require specific treatment except under extraordinary circumstances (as in liver disease or renal disease), chloride replacement may be required in the treatment of metabolic alkalosis.
Dilutional hyponatremia may occur in edematous patients in hot weather; appropriate therapy is water restriction, rather than administration of salt, except in rare instances when the hyponatremia is life threatening. In actual salt depletion, appropriate replacement is the therapy of choice.
Hyperuricemia may occur or acute gout may be precipitated in certain patients receiving thiazides.
Insulin requirements in diabetic patients may be increased, decreased, or unchanged. Latent diabetes mellitus may become manifest during thiazide therapy.
Thiazides may increase the responsiveness to tubocurarine.
The antihypertensive effects of the drug may be enhanced in the postsympathectomy patient.
Thiazides may decrease arterial responsiveness to norepinephrine. This diminution is not sufficient to preclude effectiveness of the pressor agent for therapeutic use.
If progressive renal impairment becomes evident, consider withholding or discontinuing diuretic therapy.
Thiazides may decrease serum PBI levels without signs of thyroid disturbance.
Thiazides may decrease urinary calcium excretion. Thiazides may cause intermittent and slight elevation of serum calcium in the absence of known disorders of calcium metabolism. Marked hypercalcemia may be evidence of hidden hyperparathyroidism. Thiazides should be discontinued before carrying out tests for parathyroid function.

Adverse Reactions

Body as a Whole: Weakness.
Cardiovascular: Orthostatic hypotension (may be aggravated by alcohol, barbiturates, or narcotics).
Digestive: Anorexia, gastric irritation, nausea, vomiting, cramping, diarrhea, constipation, jaundice (intrahepatic cholestatic jaundice), pancreatitis, sialadenitis.
Hematologic: Leukopenia, agranulocytosis, thrombocytopenia, aplastic anemia, hemolytic anemia.
Metabolic: Hyperglycemia, glycosuria, hyperuricemia, electrolyte imbalance (see PRECAUTIONS).
Musculoskeletal: Muscle spasm.
Nervous System/Psychiatric: Dizziness, vertigo, paresthesias, headache, restlessness.
Special Senses: Transient blurred vision, xanthopsia.
Hypersensitivity: Purpura, photosensitivity, rash, urticaria, necrotizing angiitis (vasculitis and cutaneous vasculitis), fever, respiratory distress including pneumonitis and pulmonary edema, anaphylactic reactions.
Whenever adverse reactions are moderate or severe, thiazide dosage should be reduced or therapy withdrawn.

Dosage and Administration

Therapy should be individualized according to patient response. Use the smallest dosage necessary to achieve the required response.
Adults
For Diuresis
The usual adult dosage is 0.5 to 1.0 g once or twice a day. Many patients with edema respond to intermittent therapy, i.e., administration on alternate days or on three to five days each week. With an intermittent schedule, excessive response and the resulting undesirable electrolyte imbalance are less likely to occur.
For Control of Hypertension
The usual adult starting dosage is 0.5 or 1.0 g a day as a single or divided dose. Dosage is increased or decreased according to blood pressure response. Rarely some patients may require up to 2.0 g a day in divided doses.
When thiazides are used with other antihypertensives, the dose of the latter may need to be reduced to prevent excessive decrease in blood pressure.
Infants and Children
The usual oral pediatric dosage is based on 10 mg of DIURIL per pound of body weight per day in two doses. Infants under 6 months of age may require up to 15 mg per pound per day in two doses.
On this basis, infants up to 2 years of age may be given 125 to 375 mg daily in two doses (2.5 to 7.5 ml, or ½ to 1½ teaspoonfuls of the oral suspension daily). Children from 2 to 12 years of age may be given 375 mg to 1.0 g daily in two doses (7.5 to 20 ml, or 1½ to 4 teaspoonfuls of oral suspension daily). Dosage in both age groups should be based on body weight.

Continued on next page

Information on the Merck Sharp & Dohme products listed on these pages is the full prescribing information from product circulars in use November 1, 1984.

Merck Sharp & Dohme—Cont.

How Supplied

No. 3244—Tablets DIURIL, 250 mg, are white, round, scored, compressed tablets, coded MSD 214. They are supplied as follows:
NDC 0006-0214-68 bottles of 100
NDC 0006-0214-28 unit dose packages of 100
NDC 0006-0214-82 bottles of 1000.
Shown in Product Identification Section, page 420
No. 3245—Tablets DIURIL, 500 mg, are white, round, scored, compressed tablets, coded MSD 432. They are supplied as follows:
NDC 0006-0432-68 bottles of 100
NDC 0006-0432-28 unit dose packages of 100
NDC 0006-0432-82 bottles of 1000
NDC 0006-0432-86 bottles of 5000.
Shown in Product Identification Section, page 420
No. 3239—Oral Suspension DIURIL, 250 mg per 5 ml, is a yellow, creamy suspension, and is supplied as follows:
NDC 0006-3239-66 bottles of 237 ml.
A.H.F.S. Category: 40:28
DC 6020742 Issued November 1983
COPYRIGHT © MERCK & CO., INC., 1983
All rights reserved

DOLOBID® Tablets ℞
(diflunisal, MSD)

Description

Diflunisal is 2′, 4′-difluoro-4-hydroxy-3-biphenylcarboxylic acid. Its empirical formula is $C_{13}H_8F_2O_3$.
Diflunisal has a molecular weight of 250.20. It is a stable, white, crystalline compound with a melting point of 211–213°C. It is practically insoluble in water at neutral or acidic pH. Because it is an organic acid, it dissolves readily in dilute alkali to give a moderately stable solution at room temperature. It is soluble in most organic solvents including ethanol, methanol, and acetone.
DOLOBID® (Diflunisal, MSD) is available in 250 and 500 mg tablets for oral administration.

Clinical Pharmacology

Action
DOLOBID is a non-steroidal drug with analgesic, anti-inflammatory and antipyretic properties. It is a peripherally-acting non-narcotic analgesic drug. Habituation, tolerance and addiction have not been reported.
Diflunisal is a difluorophenyl derivative of salicylic acid. Chemically, diflunisal differs from aspirin (acetylsalicylic acid) in two respects. The first of these two is the presence of a difluorophenyl substituent at carbon 1. The second difference is the removal of the 0-acetyl group from the carbon 4 position. Diflunisal is not metabolized to salicylic acid, and the fluorine atoms are not displaced from the difluorophenyl ring structure.
The precise mechanism of the analgesic and anti-inflammatory actions of diflunisal is not known. Diflunisal is a prostaglandin synthetase inhibitor. In animals, prostaglandins sensitize afferent nerves and potentiate the action of bradykinin in inducing pain. Since prostaglandins are known to be among the mediators of pain and inflammation, the mode of action of diflunisal may be due to a decrease of prostaglandins in peripheral tissues.
Pharmacokinetics and Metabolism
DOLOBID is rapidly and completely absorbed following oral administration with peak plasma concentrations occurring between 2 to 3 hours. The drug is excreted in the urine as two soluble glucuronide conjugates accounting for about 90% of the administered dose. Little or no diflunisal is excreted in the feces. Diflunisal appears in human milk in concentrations of 2–7% of those in plasma. More than 99% of diflunisal in plasma is bound to proteins.
As is the case with salicylic acid, concentration-dependent pharmacokinetics prevail when DOLOBID is administered; a doubling of dosage produces a greater than doubling of drug accumulation. The effect becomes more apparent with repetitive doses. Following single doses, peak plasma concentrations of 41 ± 11 μg/ml (mean $\pm$ S.D.) were observed following 250 mg doses, 87 ± 17 μg/ml were observed following 500 mg and 124 ± 11 μg/ml following single 1,000 mg doses. However, following administration of 250 mg b.i.d., a mean peak level of 56 ± 14 μg/ml was observed on day 8, while the mean peak level after 500 mg b.i.d. for 11 days was 190 ± 33 μg/ml. In contrast to salicylic acid which has a plasma half-life of 2½ hours, the plasma half-life of diflunisal is 3 to 4 times longer (8 to 12 hours), because of a difluorophenyl substituent at carbon 1. Because of its long half-life and nonlinear pharmacokinetics, several days are required for diflunisal plasma levels to reach steady state following multiple doses. For this reason, an initial loading dose is necessary to shorten the time to reach steady state levels, and 2 to 3 days of observation are necessary for evaluating changes in treatment regimens if a loading dose is not used.
Studies in baboons to determine passage across the blood brain barrier have shown that only small quantities of diflunisal, under normal or acidotic conditions are transported into the cerebrospinal fluid (CSF). The ratio of blood/CSF concentrations after intravenous doses of 50 mg/kg or oral doses of 100 mg/kg of diflunisal was 100:1. In contrast, oral doses of 500 mg/kg of aspirin resulted in a blood/CSF ratio of 5:1.
Mild to Moderate Pain
DOLOBID is a peripherally-acting analgesic agent with a long duration of action. DOLOBID produces significant analgesia within 1 hour and maximum analgesia within 2 to 3 hours.
Consistent with its long half-life, clinical effects of DOLOBID mirror its pharmacokinetic behavior, which is the basis for recommending a loading dose when instituting therapy. Patients treated with DOLOBID, on the first dose, tend to have a slower onset of pain relief when compared with drugs achieving comparable peak effects. However, DOLOBID produces longer-lasting responses than the comparative agents.
Comparative single dose clinical studies have established the analgesic efficacy of DOLOBID at various dose levels relative to other analgesics. Analgesic effect measurements were derived from hourly evaluations by patients during eight and twelve-hour postdosing observation periods. The following information may serve as a guide for prescribing DOLOBID.
DOLOBID 500 mg was comparable in analgesic efficacy to aspirin 650 mg, acetaminophen 600 mg or 650 mg, and acetaminophen 650 mg with propoxyphene napsylate 100 mg. Patients treated with DOLOBID had longer lasting responses than the patients treated with the comparative analgesics.
DOLOBID 1000 mg was comparable in analgesic efficacy to acetaminophen 600 mg with codeine 60 mg. Patients treated with DOLOBID had longer lasting responses than the patients who received acetaminophen with codeine.
A loading dose of 1000 mg provides faster onset of pain relief, shorter time to peak analgesic effect, and greater peak analgesic effect than an initial 500 mg dose.
In contrast to the comparative analgesics, a significantly greater proportion of patients treated with DOLOBID did not remedicate and continued to have a good analgesic effect eight to twelve hours after dosing. Seventy-five percent (75%) of patients treated with DOLOBID continued to have a good analgesic response at four hours. When patients having a good analgesic response at four hours were followed, 78% of these patients continued to have a good analgesic response at eight hours and 64% at twelve hours.
Osteoarthritis
The effectiveness of DOLOBID for the treatment of osteoarthritis was studied in patients with osteoarthritis of the hip and/or knee. The activity of DOLOBID was demonstrated by clinical improvement in the signs and symptoms of disease activity.
In a double-blind multicenter study of 12 weeks' duration in which dosages were adjusted according to patient response, DOLOBID, 500 or 750 mg daily, was shown to be comparable in effectiveness to aspirin, 2,000 or 3,000 mg daily. Patients treated with DOLOBID had a lower overall incidence of digestive system adverse experiences, and of dizziness, edema, and tinnitus. In open-label extensions of this study to 24 or 48 weeks, DOLOBID continued to show similar effectiveness and generally was well tolerated.
Rheumatoid Arthritis
In controlled clinical trials, the effectiveness of DOLOBID was established for both acute exacerbations and long-term management of rheumatoid arthritis. The activity of DOLOBID was demonstrated by clinical improvement in the signs and symptoms of disease activity.
In a double-blind multicenter study of 12 weeks' duration in which dosages were adjusted according to patient response, DOLOBID 500 or 750 mg daily was comparable in effectiveness to aspirin 2,600 or 3,900 mg daily. Patients on DOLOBID had a lower incidence of dyspepsia, gastrointestinal pain and tinnitus. In open-label extensions of this study to 52 weeks, DOLOBID continued to be effective and was generally well tolerated. Patients treated with DOLOBID had a lower incidence of tinnitus and a lower overall incidence of gastrointestinal adverse experiences.
DOLOBID 500, 750, or 1,000 mg daily was compared with aspirin 2,000, 3,000, or 4,000 mg daily in a multicenter study of 8 weeks' duration in which dosages were adjusted according to patient response. In this study, DOLOBID was comparable in efficacy to aspirin. Patients receiving DOLOBID had a lower incidence of gastrointestinal adverse effects than did patients treated with aspirin. Patients treated with DOLOBID also had a lower incidence of tinnitus and hearing loss.
In a double-blind multicenter study of 12 weeks' duration in which dosages were adjusted according to patient needs, DOLOBID 500 or 750 mg daily and ibuprofen 1,600 or 2,400 mg daily were comparable in effectiveness and tolerability.
In a double-blind multicenter study of 12 weeks' duration, DOLOBID 750 mg daily was comparable in efficacy to naproxen 750 mg daily. The incidence of gastrointestinal adverse effects and tinnitus was comparable for both drugs. This study was extended to 48 weeks on an open-label basis. DOLOBID continued to be effective and generally well tolerated.
In patients with rheumatoid arthritis, DOLOBID and gold salts may be used in combination at their usual dosage levels. In clinical studies, DOLOBID added to the regimen of gold salts usually resulted in additional symptomatic relief but did not alter the course of the underlying disease.
Antipyretic Activity
DOLOBID is not recommended for use as an antipyretic agent. In single 250 mg, 500 mg, or 750 mg doses, DOLOBID produced measurable but not clinically useful decreases in temperature in patients with fever; however, the possibility that it may mask fever in some patients, particularly with chronic or high doses, should be considered.
Uricosuric Effect
In normal volunteers, an increase in the renal clearance of uric acid and a decrease in serum uric acid was observed when DOLOBID was administered at 500 mg or 750 mg daily in divided doses. Patients on long-term therapy taking DOLOBID at 500 mg to 1000 mg daily in divided doses showed a prompt and consistent reduction across studies in mean serum uric acid levels, which were lowered as much as 1.4 mg%. It is not known whether DOLOBID interferes with the activity of other uricosuric agents.
Effect on Platelet Function
As an inhibitor of prostaglandin synthetase, DOLOBID has a dose-related effect on platelet function and bleeding time. In normal volunteers, 250 mg b.i.d. for 8 days had no effect on platelet function, and 500 mg b.i.d., the usual recommended dose, had a slight effect. At 1000 mg b.i.d., which exceeds the maximum recommended dosage, however, DOLOBID inhibited platelet func-

Merck Sharp & Dohme—Cont.

uretics, patients should be observed closely for development of hypokalemia.
Since the contents of TURBINAIRE DECADRON Phosphate are under pressure, the container should not be broken, stored in extreme heat, or incinerated. It should be stored at a temperature below 120°F.

Adverse Reactions

Nasal irritation and dryness are the most common adverse reactions. The following have been reported: headache, lightheadedness, urticaria, nausea, epistaxis, rebound congestion, bronchial asthma, perforation of the nasal septum, and anosmia. Signs of adrenal hypercorticism may occur in some patients, especially with overdosage.
Systemic effects from therapy with TURBINAIRE DECADRON Phosphate are less likely to occur than with oral or parenteral corticosteroid therapy because of a lower total dose administered. Nevertheless, patients should be observed for the hormonal effects described below because of absorption of dexamethasone from the nasal mucosa.
Fluid and Electrolyte Disturbances
  Sodium retention
  Fluid retention
  Congestive heart failure in susceptible patients
  Potassium loss
  Hypokalemic alkalosis
  Hypertension
Musculoskeletal
  Muscle weakness
  Steroid myopathy
  Loss of muscle mass
  Osteoporosis
  Vertebral compression fractures
  Aseptic necrosis of femoral and humeral heads
  Pathologic fracture of long bones
  Tendon rupture
Gastrointestinal
  Peptic ulcer with possible subsequent perforation and hemorrhage
  Perforation of the small and large bowel, particularly in patients with inflammatory bowel disease
  Pancreatitis
  Abdominal distention
  Ulcerative esophagitis
Dermatologic
  Impaired wound healing
  Thin fragile skin
  Petechiae and ecchymoses
  Erythema
  Increased sweating
  May suppress reactions to skin tests
Other cutaneous reactions, such as allergic dermatitis, urticaria, angioneurotic edema.
Neurologic
  Convulsions
  Increased intracranial pressure with papilledema (pseudotumor cerebri) usually after treatment
  Vertigo
  Headache
Endocrine
  Menstrual irregularities
  Development of cushingoid state
  Suppression of growth in children
  Secondary adrenocortical and pituitary unresponsiveness, particularly in times of stress, as in trauma, surgery, or illness
  Decreased carbohydrate tolerance
  Manifestations of latent diabetes mellitus
  Increased requirements for insulin or oral hypoglycemic agents in diabetics
Ophthalmic
  Posterior subcapsular cataracts
  Increased intraocular pressure
  Glaucoma
  Exophthalmos
Metabolic
  Negative nitrogen balance due to protein catabolism

Other
  Hypersensitivity
  Thromboembolism
  Weight gain
  Increased appetite
  Nausea
  Malaise

Dosage and Administration

DO NOT EXCEED THE RECOMMENDED DOSAGE.
The usual initial dosage of TURBINAIRE DECADRON Phosphate is:
  Adults—2 sprays in each nostril 2 or 3 times a day.
  Children (6 to 12 years of age)—1 or 2 sprays in each nostril 2 times a day depending on age.
See accompanying instructions on the proper use of TURBINAIRE.
When improvement occurs the dosage should be gradually reduced. Some patients will be symptom-free on one spray in each nostril 2 times a day. The maximum daily dosage for adults is 12 sprays, and for children, 8 sprays. Therapy should be discontinued as soon as feasible. It may be reinstituted if recurrence of symptoms occurs.

How Supplied

No. 7634—TURBINAIRE DECADRON Phosphate, aerosol for intranasal application, is supplied as follows: **NDC** 0006-7634-13 in a pressurized container and includes a plastic adapter. (6505-00-885-6302, 12.6 Grams, 170 Metered Doses)
No. 7642—Refill unit for TURBINAIRE DECADRON Phosphate aerosol for intranasal application is supplied as follows: **NDC** 0006-7642-13 in a pressurized container.
A.H.F.S. Category: 52:08
DC 6006419 Issued August 1981

DECADRON-LA® Suspension ℞
(dexamethasone acetate, MSD), U.S.P.
NOT FOR INTRAVENOUS USE

Description

Dexamethasone acetate, a synthetic adrenocortical steroid, is a white to practically white, odorless powder. It is a practically insoluble ester of dexamethasone.
Dexamethasone acetate is present in DECADRON-LA® (Dexamethasone Acetate, MSD) suspension as the monohydrate, with the empirical formula, $C_{24}H_{31}FO_6 \cdot H_2O$, and molecular weight, 452.52. Dexamethasone acetate is designated chemically as 21-(acetyloxy)-9-fluoro-11β,17-dihydroxy-16α-methylpregna-1,4-diene-3,20-dione.
DECADRON-LA suspension is a sterile white suspension (pH 5.0 to 7.5) that settles on standing, but is easily resuspended by mild shaking.
Each milliliter contains dexamethasone acetate equivalent to 8 mg dexamethasone. Inactive ingredients per ml: 6.67 mg sodium chloride; 5 mg creatinine; 0.5 mg disodium edetate; 5 mg sodium carboxymethylcellulose; 0.75 mg polysorbate 80; sodium hydroxide to adjust pH; and Water for Injection, q.s. 1 ml, with 9 mg benzyl alcohol, and 1 mg sodium bisulfite added as preservatives.

Actions

DECADRON-LA suspension is a long-acting, repository adrenocorticosteroid preparation with a prompt onset of action. It is suitable for intramuscular or local injection, but not when an immediate effect of short duration is desired.
Naturally occurring glucocorticoids (hydrocortisone and cortisone), which also have salt-retaining properties, are used as replacement therapy in adrenocortical deficiency states. Their synthetic analogs, including dexamethasone, are primarily used for their potent anti-inflammatory effects in disorders of many organ systems.
Glucocorticoids cause profound and varied metabolic effects. In addition, they modify the body's immune responses to diverse stimuli.

At equipotent anti-inflammatory doses, dexamethasone almost completely lacks the sodium-retaining property of hydrocortisone.

Indications

A. By intramuscular injection when oral therapy is not feasible:
  1. *Endocrine disorders*
Congenital adrenal hyperplasia
Nonsuppurative thyroiditis
Hypercalcemia associated with cancer
  2. *Rheumatic disorders*
As adjunctive therapy for short-term administration (to tide the patient over an acute episode or exacerbation) in:
Post-traumatic osteoarthritis
Synovitis of osteoarthritis
Rheumatoid arthritis, including juvenile rheumatoid arthritis (selected cases may require low-dose maintenance therapy)
Acute and subacute bursitis
Epicondylitis
Acute nonspecific tenosynovitis
Acute gouty arthritis
Psoriatic arthritis
Ankylosing spondylitis
  3. *Collagen diseases*
During an exacerbation or as maintenance therapy in selected cases of:
Systemic lupus erythematosus
Acute rheumatic carditis
  4. *Dermatologic diseases*
Pemphigus
Severe erythema multiforme (Stevens-Johnson syndrome)
Exfoliative dermatitis
Bullous dermatitis herpetiformis
Severe seborrheic dermatitis
Severe psoriasis
Mycosis fungoides
  5. *Allergic states*
Control of severe or incapacitating allergic conditions intractable to adequate trials of conventional treatment in:
Bronchial asthma
Contact dermatitis
Atopic dermatitis
Serum sickness
Seasonal or perennial allergic rhinitis
Drug hypersensitivity reactions
Urticarial transfusion reactions
  6. *Ophthalmic diseases*
Severe acute and chronic allergic and inflammatory processes involving the eye, such as:
Herpes zoster ophthalmicus
Iritis, Iridocyclitis
Chorioretinitis
Diffuse posterior uveitis and choroiditis
Optic neuritis
Sympathetic ophthalmia
Anterior segment inflammation
Allergic conjunctivitis
Keratitis
Allergic corneal marginal ulcers
  7. *Gastrointestinal diseases*
To tide the patient over a critical period of the disease in:
Ulcerative colitis (Systemic therapy)
Regional enteritis (Systemic therapy)
  8. *Respiratory diseases*
Symptomatic sarcoidosis
Berylliosis
Loeffler's syndrome not manageable by other means
Aspiration pneumonitis
  9. *Hematologic disorders*
Acquired (autoimmune) hemolytic anemia
Secondary thrombocytopenia in adults
Erythroblastopenia (RBC anemia)
Congenital (erythroid) hypoplastic anemia
  10. *Neoplastic diseases*
For palliative management of:
Leukemias and lymphomas in adults
Acute leukemia of childhood
  11. *Edematous states*
To induce diuresis or remission of proteinuria in the nephrotic syndrome, without uremia, of the

for possible revisions   Product Information   1293

Development of cushingoid state
Suppression of growth in children
Secondary adrenocortical and pituitary unresponsiveness, particularly in times of stress, as in trauma, surgery, or illness
Decreased carbohydrate tolerance
Manifestations of latent diabetes mellitus
Increased requirements for insulin or oral hypoglycemic agents in diabetics
Ophthalmic
Posterior subcapsular cataracts
Increased intraocular pressure
Glaucoma
Exophthalmos
Metabolic
Negative nitrogen balance due to protein catabolism
Other
Hypersensitivity
Thromboembolism
Weight gain
Increased appetite
Nausea
Malaise

Dosage and Administration

Recommended *initial dosage:*
  Adults   —3 inhalations 3 or 4 times per day.
  Children —2 inhalations 3 or 4 times per day.
Maximum dosage:
  Adults   —3 inhalations *per dose;* 12 inhalations *per day.*
  Children —2 inhalations *per dose;* 8 inhalations *per day.*

When a favorable response is attained, the dose may be gradually reduced. In patients on systemic corticosteroids, it is recommended that systemic therapy be reduced or eliminated before reduction of RESPIHALER dosage is begun. Gradual reduction of systemic corticosteroid therapy must be emphasized to avoid withdrawal symptoms.

How Supplied

No. 7626X—RESPIHALER DECADRON Phosphate, aerosol for oral inhalation, is supplied as follows: **NDC** 0006-7626-13 in a pressurized container, and includes a plastic adapter.
No. 7640—Refill Unit RESPIHALER DECADRON Phosphate is supplied as follows: **NDC** 0006-7640-13 in a pressurized container.
A.H.F.S. Category: 84:06
DC 6055714   Issued August 1981

DECADRON® Phosphate TURBINAIRE®   B
(dexamethasone sodium phosphate, MSD), U.S.P.

Description

TURBINAIRE® DECADRON® Phosphate (Dexamethasone Sodium Phosphate, MSD) is an aerosol for intranasal application. The inactive ingredients are fluorochlorohydrocarbons as propellants and alcohol 2%. One cartridge delivers an amount sufficient to ensure delivery of 170 metered sprays, each containing dexamethasone sodium phosphate equivalent to approximately 0.1 mg dexamethasone phosphate or to approximately 0.084 mg dexamethasone. Twelve sprays deliver a theoretical maximum of 1.0 mg dexamethasone. Dexamethasone sodium phosphate, a synthetic adrenocortical steroid, is a white or slightly yellow, crystalline powder. It is freely soluble in water and is exceedingly hygroscopic. The molecular weight is 516.41. It is designated chemically as 9-fluoro-11β, 17-dihydroxy-16α-methyl-21-(phosphonooxy) pregna-1, 4-diene-3, 20-dione disodium salt. The empirical formula is $C_{22}H_{28}FNa_2O_8P$.

Action

Inhibition of inflammatory response to inciting agents of mechanical, chemical or immunological nature.

Indications

Allergic or inflammatory nasal conditions, and nasal polyps (excluding polyps originating within the sinuses).

Contraindications

Systemic fungal infections.
Hypersensitivity to components.
Tuberculous, viral and fungal nasal conditions, ocular herpes simplex.

Warnings

In patients on therapy with TURBINAIRE DECADRON Phosphate subjected to unusual stress, increased dosage of rapidly acting corticosteroids before, during, and after the stressful situation is indicated.
Drug-induced secondary adrenocortical insufficiency may result from too rapid withdrawal of corticosteroids and may be minimized by gradual reduction of dosage. This type of relative insufficiency may persist for months after discontinuation of therapy; therefore, in any situation of stress occurring during that period, hormone therapy should be reinstituted. If the patient is receiving steroids already, dosage may have to be increased. Since mineralocorticoid secretion may be impaired, salt and/or a mineralocorticoid should be administered concurrently.
Dexamethasone may mask some signs of infection, and new infections may appear during its use. There may be decreased resistance and inability to localize infection when corticosteroids are used. Therefore, patients with bacterial infections should also be given appropriate antibiotic therapy if TURBINAIRE DECADRON Phosphate is used. Moreover, dexamethasone may affect the nitroblue-tetrazolium test for bacterial infection and produce false negative results.
Corticosteroids may activate latent amebiasis. Therefore, it is recommended that latent or active amebiasis be ruled out before initiating corticosteroid therapy in any patient who has spent time in the tropics or any patient with unexplained diarrhea.
Prolonged use of TURBINAIRE DECADRON Phosphate may produce posterior subcapsular cataracts, glaucoma with possible damage to the optic nerves, and may enhance the establishment of secondary ocular infections due to fungi or viruses.
Usage in pregnancy: Since adequate human reproduction studies have not been done with TURBINAIRE DECADRON Phosphate, use of this drug in pregnancy or in women of childbearing potential requires that the anticipated benefits be weighed against the possible hazards to the mother and embryo or fetus. Infants born of mothers who have received substantial doses of dexamethasone during pregnancy, should be carefully observed for signs of hypoadrenalism.
Dexamethasone appears in breast milk and could suppress growth, interfere with endogenous corticosteroid production, or cause other unwanted effects. Mothers taking pharmacologic doses of dexamethasone should be advised not to nurse.
Average and large doses of hydrocortisone or cortisone can cause elevation of blood pressure, salt and water retention, and increased excretion of potassium. These effects are less likely to occur with the synthetic derivatives and with TURBINAIRE DECADRON Phosphate, except when used in large doses. Dietary salt restriction and potassium supplementation may be necessary. All corticosteroids increase calcium excretion.
Administration of live virus vaccines, including smallpox, is contraindicated in individuals receiving immunosuppressive doses of corticosteroids. If inactivated viral or bacterial vaccines are administered to individuals receiving immunosuppressive doses of corticosteroids, the expected serum antibody response may not be obtained.
If TURBINAIRE DECADRON Phosphate is indicated in patients with latent tuberculosis or tuberculin reactivity, close observation is necessary as reactivation of the disease may occur. During prolonged therapy with TURBINAIRE DECADRON Phosphate, these patients should receive chemoprophylaxis.

Precautions

During local corticosteroid therapy, the possibility of pharyngeal candidiasis should be kept in mind. Although systemic absorption is low when TURBINAIRE DECADRON Phosphate is used in the recommended dosage, adrenal suppression may occur. In addition, other systemic effects of steroid administration must be considered as a possibility. Following prolonged therapy, withdrawal of corticosteroids may result in symptoms of the corticosteroid withdrawal syndrome including fever, myalgia, arthralgia, and malaise. This may occur in patients even without evidence of adrenal insufficiency. Replacement of systemic steroid with TURBINAIRE DECADRON Phosphate should be gradual and carefully monitored by the physician. There is an enhanced effect of dexamethasone in patients with hypothyroidism and in those with cirrhosis.
TURBINAIRE DECADRON Phosphate should be used cautiously in patients with ocular herpes simplex for fear of corneal perforation.
The lowest possible dose of TURBINAIRE DECADRON Phosphate should be used to control the condition under treatment, and when reduction in dosage is possible, the reduction must be gradual. If beneficial effect is not evident within 7 days after initiation of therapy, the patient should be re-evaluated.
Psychic derangements may appear when dexamethasone is used, ranging from euphoria, insomnia, mood swings, personality changes, and severe depression, to frank psychotic manifestations. Also, existing emotional instability or psychotic tendencies may be aggravated.
Aspirin should be used cautiously in conjunction with TURBINAIRE DECADRON Phosphate in hypoprothrombinemia.
TURBINAIRE DECADRON Phosphate should be used with caution in patients with nonspecific ulcerative colitis, if there is a probability of impending perforation, abscess or other pyogenic infection; also in diverticulitis; fresh intestinal anastomoses; active or latent peptic ulcer; renal insufficiency; hypertension; osteoporosis; and myasthenia gravis. Signs of peritoneal irritation following gastrointestinal perforation in patients receiving large doses of corticosteroids may be minimal or absent. Fat embolism has been reported as a possible complication of hypercortisonism.
Because clinical studies have not been done, the use of this product in children under the age of 6 years is not recommended. Growth and development of children 6 years of age or older on prolonged therapy with TURBINAIRE DECADRON Phosphate should be carefully followed.
Dexamethasone may increase or decrease motility and number of spermatozoa in some patients.
Phenytoin, phenobarbital, ephedrine and rifampin may enhance the metabolic clearance of dexamethasone, resulting in decreased blood levels and lessened physiologic activity, thus requiring adjustment in dexamethasone dosage.
The prothrombin time should be checked frequently in patients who are receiving TURBINAIRE DECADRON Phosphate and coumarin anticoagulants at the same time because of reports that corticosteroids have altered the response to these anticoagulants. Studies have shown that the usual effect produced by adding corticosteroids is inhibition of response to coumarins, although there have been some conflicting reports of potentiation, not substantiated by studies.
When TURBINAIRE DECADRON Phosphate is used concomitantly with potassium-depleting di-

Continued on next page

Information on the Merck Sharp & Dohme products listed on these pages is the full prescribing information from product circulars in use November 1, 1984.

tion. In contrast to aspirin, these effects of DOLOBID were reversible, because of the absence of the chemically labile and biologically reactive 0-acetyl group at the carbon 4 position. Bleeding time was not altered by a dose of 250 mg b.i.d., and was only slightly increased at 500 mg b.i.d. At 1000 mg b.i.d., a greater increase occurred, but was not statistically significantly different from the change in the placebo group.

Effect on Fecal Blood Loss
When DOLOBID was given to normal volunteers at the usual recommended dose of 500 mg twice daily, fecal blood loss was not significantly different from placebo. Aspirin at 1000 mg four times daily produced the expected increase in fecal blood loss. DOLOBID at 1000 mg twice daily (NOTE: exceeds the recommended dosage) caused a statistically significant increase in fecal blood loss, but this increase was only one-half as large as that associated with aspirin 1300 mg twice daily.

Effect on Blood Glucose
DOLOBID did not affect fasting blood sugar in diabetic patients who were receiving tolbutamide or placebo.

Indications and Usage

DOLOBID is indicated for acute or long-term use for symptomatic treatment of the following:
1. Mild to moderate pain
2. Osteoarthritis
3. Rheumatoid arthritis

Contraindications

Patients who are hypersensitive to this product. Patients in whom acute asthmatic attacks, urticaria, or rhinitis are precipitated by aspirin or other non-steroidal anti-inflammatory drugs.

Warnings

Peptic ulceration and gastrointestinal bleeding have been reported in patients receiving DOLOBID. In patients with active gastrointestinal bleeding or an active peptic ulcer, the physician must weigh the benefits of therapy with DOLOBID against possible hazards, institute an appropriate ulcer regimen, and carefully monitor the patient's progress. When DOLOBID is given to patients with a history of upper gastrointestinal tract disease, it should be given only after consulting the ADVERSE REACTIONS section and under close supervision.

Precautions

General
Although DOLOBID has less effect on platelet function and bleeding time than aspirin, at higher doses it is an inhibitor of platelet function; therefore, patients who may be adversely affected should be carefully observed when DOLOBID is administered (see CLINICAL PHARMACOLOGY).
Because of reports of adverse eye findings with agents of this class, it is recommended that patients who develop eye complaints during treatment with DOLOBID have ophthalmologic studies.
Since DOLOBID is eliminated primarily by the kidneys, patients with significantly impaired renal function should be closely monitored; a lower daily dosage should be anticipated to avoid excessive drug accumulation.
In studies in rats and dogs at high dosages, there was an occasional occurrence of mild renal toxicity as evidenced by papillary edema in some animals. Papillary necrosis occurred in mice in long-term studies.
Peripheral edema has been observed in some patients taking DOLOBID. Therefore, as with other drugs in this class, DOLOBID should be used with caution in patients with compromised cardiac function, hypertension, or other conditions predisposing to fluid retention.

Laboratory Tests
As with other non-steroidal anti-inflammatory drugs, borderline elevations of one or more liver tests may occur in up to 15% of patients. These abnormalities may progress, may remain essentially unchanged, or may be transient with continued therapy. The SGPT (ALT) test is probably the most sensitive indicator of liver dysfunction. Meaningful (3 times the upper limit of normal) elevations of SGPT or SGOT (AST) occurred in controlled clinical trials in less than 1% of patients. A patient with symptoms and/or signs suggesting liver dysfunction, or in whom an abnormal liver test has occurred, should be evaluated for evidence of the development of more severe hepatic reactions while on therapy with DOLOBID. Severe hepatic reactions, including jaundice, have been reported with DOLOBID as well as with other non-steroidal anti-inflammatory drugs. Although such reactions are rare, if abnormal liver tests persist or worsen, if clinical signs and symptoms consistent with liver disease develop, or if systemic manifestations occur (e.g. eosinophilia, rash, etc.), DOLOBID should be discontinued, since liver reactions can be fatal.

Drug Interactions
DOLOBID prolongs the prothrombin time in patients who are on oral anticoagulants. DOLOBID has not been shown to interact with tolbutamide. DOLOBID interacts with hydrochlorothiazide, furosemide, acetaminophen, aspirin, indomethacin, sulindac and naproxen (see below).

Oral Anticoagulants: In some normal volunteers, the concomitant administration of DOLOBID and warfarin, acenocoumarol, or phenprocoumon resulted in prolongation of prothrombin time. This may occur because diflunisal competitively displaces coumarins from protein binding sites. Accordingly, when DOLOBID is administered with oral anticoagulants, the prothrombin time should be closely monitored during and for several days after concomitant drug administration. Adjustment of dosage of oral anticoagulants may be required.

Tolbutamide: In diabetic patients receiving DOLOBID and tolbutamide, no significant effects were seen on tolbutamide plasma levels or fasting blood glucose.

Hydrochlorothiazide: In normal volunteers, concomitant administration of DOLOBID and hydrochlorothiazide resulted in significantly increased plasma levels of hydrochlorothiazide. DOLOBID decreased the hyperuricemic effect of hydrochlorothiazide.

Furosemide: In normal volunteers, the concomitant administration of DOLOBID and furosemide had no effect on the diuretic activity of furosemide. DOLOBID decreased the hyperuricemic effect of furosemide.

Antacids: Concomitant administration of antacids may reduce plasma levels of DOLOBID. This effect is small with occasional doses of antacids, but may be clinically significant when antacids are used on a continuous schedule.

Acetaminophen: In normal volunteers, concomitant administration of DOLOBID and acetaminophen resulted in an approximate 50% increase in plasma levels of acetaminophen. Acetaminophen had no effect on plasma levels of DOLOBID. Since acetaminophen in high doses has been associated with hepatotoxicity, concomitant administration of DOLOBID and acetaminophen should be used cautiously, with careful monitoring of patients. Concomitant administration of DOLOBID and acetaminophen in dogs, but not in rats, at approximately 2 times the recommended maximum human therapeutic dose of each (40-52 mg/kg/day of DOLOBID/acetaminophen), resulted in greater gastrointestinal toxicity than when either drug was administered alone. The clinical significance of these findings has not been established.

Drug Interactions: Non-steroidal Anti-inflammatory Drugs
The administration of diflunisal to normal volunteers receiving indomethacin decreased the renal clearance and significantly increased the plasma levels of indomethacin. In some patients the combined use of indomethacin and DOLOBID has been associated with fatal gastrointestinal hemorrhage. Therefore, indomethacin and DOLOBID should not be used concomitantly.

Since no further clinical data are available about the safety and effectiveness of DOLOBID when used in combination with other non-steroidal anti-inflammatory drugs, no recommendation for their concomitant use can be made. The following information was obtained from studies in normal volunteers.

Aspirin: In normal volunteers, a small decrease in diflunisal levels was observed when multiple doses of DOLOBID and aspirin were administered concomitantly.

Sulindac: The concomitant administration of DOLOBID and sulindac in normal volunteers resulted in lowering of the plasma levels of the active sulindac sulfide metabolite by approximately one-third.

Naproxen: The concomitant administration of DOLOBID and naproxen in normal volunteers had no effect on the plasma levels of naproxen, but significantly decreased the urinary excretion of naproxen and its glucuronide metabolite. Naproxen had no effect on plasma levels of DOLOBID.

Carcinogenesis, Mutagenesis, Impairment of Fertility
In a two-year study in the mouse, there was an apparent but not statistically significant increase in the incidence of pulmonary adenoma and hepatocellular adenoma. Since findings were inconclusive, the study is being repeated.
Diflunisal did not affect the type or incidence of neoplasia in a 105-week study in the rat.
Diflunisal passes the placental barrier to a minor degree in the rat. Diflunisal had no mutagenic activity after oral administration in the dominant lethal assay, in the Ames microbial mutagen test or in the V-79 Chinese hamster lung cell assay.
No evidence of impaired fertility was found in reproduction studies in rats at doses up to 50 mg/kg/day.

Pregnancy
Pregnancy Category C. A dose of 60 mg/kg/day of diflunisal (equivalent to two times the maximum human dose) was maternotoxic, embryotoxic, and teratogenic in rabbits. In three of six studies in rabbits, evidence of teratogenicity was observed at doses ranging from 40 to 50 mg/kg/day. Teratology studies in mice, at doses up to 45 mg/kg/day, and in rats at doses up to 100 mg/kg/day, revealed no harm to the fetus due to diflunisal. Aspirin and other salicylates have been shown to be teratogenic in a wide variety of species, including the rat and rabbit, at doses ranging from 50 to 400 mg/kg/day (approximately one to eight times the human dose). There are no adequate and well controlled studies with diflunisal in pregnant women. DOLOBID should be used during the first two trimesters of pregnancy only if the potential benefit justifies the potential risk to the fetus. Because of the known effect of drugs of this class on the human fetal cardiovascular system (closure of ductus arteriosus), use during the third trimester of pregnancy is not recommended.
In rats at a dose of one and one-half times the maximum human dose, there was an increase in the average length of gestation. Similar increases in the length of gestation have been observed with aspirin, indomethacin, and phenylbutazone, and may be related to inhibition of prostaglandin synthetase. Drugs of this class may cause dystocia and delayed parturition in pregnant animals.

Nursing Mothers
Diflunisal is excreted in human milk in concentrations of 2–7% of those in plasma. Because of the potential for serious adverse reactions in nursing infants from DOLOBID, a decision should be made whether to discontinue nursing or to discontinue the drug, taking into account the importance of the drug to the mother.

Continued on next page

Information on the Merck Sharp & Dohme products listed on these pages is the full prescribing information from product circulars in use November 1, 1984.

Merck Sharp & Dohme—Cont.

Pediatric Use
The adverse effects observed following diflunisal administration to neonatal animals appear to be species, age, and dose-dependent. At dose levels approximately 3 times the usual human therapeutic dose, both aspirin (200 to 400 mg/kg/day) and diflunisal (80 mg/kg/day) resulted in death, leukocytosis, weight loss, and bilateral cataracts in neonatal (4 to 5-day-old) beagle puppies after 2 to 10 doses. Administration of an 80 mg/kg/day dose of diflunisal to 25-day-old puppies resulted in lower mortality, and did not produce cataracts. In newborn rats, a 400 mg/kg/day dose of aspirin resulted in increased mortality and some cataracts, whereas the effects of diflunisal administration at doses up to 140 mg/kg/day were limited to a decrease in average body weight gain.
Safety and effectiveness in infants and children have not been established, and use of the drug in children below the age of 12 years is not recommended.

Adverse Reactions

The adverse reactions observed in controlled clinical trials encompass observations in 2,427 patients.
Listed below are the adverse reactions reported in the 1,314 of these patients who received treatment in studies of two weeks or longer. Five hundred thirteen patients were treated for at least 24 weeks, 255 patients were treated for at least 48 weeks, and 46 patients were treated for 96 weeks. In general, the adverse reactions listed below were 2 to 14 times less frequent in the 1,113 patients who received short-term treatment for mild to moderate pain.

Incidence Greater Than 1%
Gastrointestinal
The most frequent types of adverse reactions occurring with DOLOBID are gastrointestinal: these include nausea*, vomiting, dyspepsia*, gastrointestinal pain*, diarrhea*, constipation, and flatulence.
Psychiatric
Somnolence, insomnia.
Central Nervous System
Dizziness.
Special Senses
Tinnitus.
Dermatologic
Rash*.
Miscellaneous
Headache*, fatigue/tiredness.

Incidence Less Than 1 in 100
The following adverse reactions, occurring less frequently than 1 in 100, were reported in clinical trials or since the drug was marketed. The probability exists of a causal relationship between DOLOBID and these adverse reactions.
Dermatologic
Erythema multiforme, Stevens-Johnson syndrome, pruritus, sweating, dry mucous membranes, stomatitis.
Gastrointestinal
Peptic ulcer, gastrointestinal bleeding, anorexia, eructation, cholestatic jaundice, gastrointestinal perforation.
Hematologic
Thrombocytopenia.
Psychiatric
Nervousness.
Central Nervous System
Vertigo.
Miscellaneous
Asthenia, edema.

Causal Relationship Unknown
Other reactions have been reported in clinical trials or since the drug was marketed, but occurred under circumstances where a causal relationship could not be established. However, in these rarely reported events, that possibility cannot be excluded. Therefore, these observations are listed to serve as alerting information to physicians.
Respiratory
Dyspnea.
Cardiovascular
Palpitation, syncope.
Special Senses
Transient visual disturbances.
Nervous System
Paresthesias.
Musculoskeletal
Muscle cramps.
Psychiatric
Depression.
Genitourinary
Dysuria.
Miscellaneous
Chest pain, fever, malaise, hypersensitivity (including interstitial nephritis with renal failure), anaphylactic reaction with bronchospasm.

Potential Adverse Effects
In addition, a variety of adverse effects not observed with DOLOBID in clinical trials or in marketing experience, but reported with other non-steroidal analgesic/anti-inflammatory agents, should be considered potential adverse effects of DOLOBID.

Overdosage

Cases of overdosage have occurred and deaths have been reported. Most patients recovered without evidence of permanent sequelae. The most common signs and symptoms observed with overdosage were drowsiness, disorientation or stupor. A dose that is usually fatal has not yet been identified.
The oral LD$_{50}$ of the drug is 439 and 826 mg/kg in female mice and female rats, respectively.
In the event of overdosage, the stomach should be emptied by inducing vomiting or by gastric lavage, and the patient carefully observed and given symptomatic and supportive treatment. Because of the high degree of protein binding, hemodialysis may not be effective.

Dosage and Administration

Concentration-dependent pharmacokinetics prevail when DOLOBID is administered; a doubling of dosage produces a greater than doubling of drug accumulation. The effect becomes more apparent with repetitive doses.
For mild to moderate pain, an initial dose of 1000 mg followed by 500 mg every 12 hours is recommended for most patients. Following the initial dose, some patients may require 500 mg every 8 hours.
A lower dosage may be appropriate depending on such factors as pain severity, patient response, weight, or advanced age; for example, 500 mg initially, followed by 250 mg every 8–12 hours.
For osteoarthritis and rheumatoid arthritis, the suggested dosage range is 500 mg to 1000 mg daily in two divided doses. The dosage of DOLOBID may be increased or decreased according to patient response.
Maintenance doses higher than 1500 mg a day are not recommended.
DOLOBID may be administered with water, milk or meals. Tablets should be swallowed whole, not crushed or chewed.

How Supplied

Tablets DOLOBID are capsule-shaped, film-coated tablets supplied as follows:
No. 3390—250 mg peach colored, coded MSD 675
NDC 0006-0675-28 unit dose package of 100
NDC 0006-0675-61 unit of use bottles of 60.
Shown in Product Identification Section, page 421
No. 3392—500 mg orange colored, coded MSD 697
NDC 0006-0697-28 unit dose package of 100
NDC 0006-0697-61 unit of use bottles of 60.

*Incidence between 3% and 9%. Those reactions occurring in 1% to 3% are not marked with an asterisk.

Shown in Product Identification Section, page 421
A.H.F.S. Category: 28:08
DC 7170712 Issued August 1983
COPYRIGHT ©MERCK & CO., INC., 1983
All rights reserved

EDECRIN® Tablets ℞
(ethacrynic acid, MSD), U.S.P.
Intravenous
SODIUM EDECRIN® ℞
(ethacrynate sodium, MSD), U.S.P.

Warning

EDECRIN® (Ethacrynic Acid, MSD) is a potent diuretic which, if given in excessive amounts, may lead to profound diuresis with water and electrolyte depletion. Therefore, careful medical supervision is required, and dose and dose schedule must be adjusted to the individual patient's needs (see DOSAGE AND ADMINISTRATION).

Description

Ethacrynic acid is an unsaturated ketone derivative of an aryloxyacetic acid. Its chemical name is [2,3-dichloro-4-(2-methylenebutyryl) phenoxy]-acetic acid. It is a white, or practically white, crystalline powder, only very slightly soluble in water, but is soluble in most organic solvents such as alcohols, chloroform, and benzene. The sodium salt of ethacrynic acid is soluble in water at 25°C to the extent of about 7 percent. Solutions of the sodium salt are relatively stable at about pH 7 at room temperature for short periods, but as the pH or temperature increases the solutions are less stable.

Actions

EDECRIN acts on the ascending limb of the loop of Henle and on the proximal and distal tubules. Urinary output is usually dose dependent and related to the magnitude of fluid accumulation. Water and electrolyte excretion may be increased several times over that observed with thiazide diuretics, since EDECRIN inhibits reabsorption of a much greater proportion of filtered sodium than most other diuretic agents. Therefore, EDECRIN is effective in many patients who have significant degrees of renal insufficiency (see ADDITIONAL WARNINGS concerning deafness). EDECRIN has little or no effect on glomerular filtration or on renal blood flow, except following pronounced reductions in plasma volume when associated with rapid diuresis.
The electrolyte excretion pattern of ethacrynic acid varies from that of the thiazides and mercurial diuretics. Initial sodium and chloride excretion is usually substantial and chloride loss exceeds that of sodium. With prolonged administration, chloride excretion declines, and potassium and hydrogen ion excretion may increase. EDECRIN is effective whether or not there is clinical acidosis or alkalosis.
Although EDECRIN, in carefully controlled studies in animals and experimental subjects, produces a more favorable sodium/potassium excretion ratio than the thiazides, in patients with increased diuresis excessive amounts of potassium may be excreted.
Onset of action is rapid, usually within 30 minutes after an oral dose of EDECRIN or within 5 minutes after an intravenous injection of SODIUM EDECRIN® (Ethacrynate Sodium, MSD). Duration of action following oral administration is 6 to 8 hours, with peak activity occurring in about 2 hours.
The sulfhydryl binding propensity of ethacrynic acid differs somewhat from that of the organomercurials; its mode of action is not by carbonic anhydrase inhibition.

Indications

EDECRIN is especially useful in patients who require an agent with greater diuretic potential than those commonly employed.

1. Treatment of the edema associated with congestive heart failure, cirrhosis of the liver, and renal disease, including the nephrotic syndrome.
2. Short term management of ascites due to malignancy, idiopathic edema, and lymphedema.
3. Short term management of hospitalized pediatric patients with congenital heart disease or the nephrotic syndrome. Information in infants is insufficient to recommend therapy with EDECRIN.
4. Intravenous administration of SODIUM EDECRIN is indicated when a rapid onset of diuresis is desired, e.g., in acute pulmonary edema, or when gastrointestinal absorption is impaired or oral medication is not practicable.

Contraindications

All diuretics, including ethacrynic acid, are contraindicated in anuria. If increasing electrolyte imbalance, azotemia, and/or oliguria occur during treatment of severe, progressive renal disease, the diuretic should be discontinued.
In a few patients this diuretic has produced severe, watery diarrhea. If this occurs, it should be discontinued and not readministered.
Until further experience in infants is accumulated, therapy with oral and parenteral EDECRIN is contraindicated.
See also *Use in Pregnancy* under ADDITIONAL WARNINGS.
Hypersensitivity to any component of this product.

Additional Warnings

Frequent serum electrolyte, CO_2 and BUN determinations should be performed early in therapy and periodically thereafter during active diuresis. Any electrolyte abnormalities should be corrected or the drug temporarily withdrawn.
Initiation of diuretic therapy with EDECRIN in the cirrhotic patient with ascites is best carried out in the hospital. When maintenance therapy has been established, the individual can be satisfactorily followed as an outpatient.
EDECRIN should be given with caution to patients with advanced cirrhosis of the liver, particularly those with a history of previous episodes of electrolyte imbalance or hepatic encephalopathy. Like other diuretics it may precipitate hepatic coma and death.
Too vigorous a diuresis, as evidenced by rapid and excessive weight loss, may induce an acute hypotensive episode. In elderly cardiac patients, rapid contraction of plasma volume and the resultant hemoconcentration should be avoided to prevent the development of thromboembolic episodes, such as cerebral vascular thromboses and pulmonary emboli which may be fatal. Excessive loss of potassium in patients receiving digitalis glycosides may precipitate digitalis toxicity. Care should also be exercised in patients receiving potassium-depleting steroids.
The effects of EDECRIN on electrolytes are related to its renal pharmacologic activity and are dose dependent. The possibility of profound electrolyte and water loss may be avoided by weighing the patient throughout the treatment period, by careful adjustment of dosage, by initiating treatment with small doses, and by using the drug on an intermittent schedule when possible. When excessive diuresis occurs, the drug should be withdrawn until homeostasis is restored. When excessive electrolyte loss occurs, the dosage should be reduced or the drug temporarily withdrawn.
A number of possibly drug-related deaths have occurred in critically ill patients refractory to other diuretics. These generally have fallen into two categories: (1) patients with severe myocardial disease who have been receiving digitalis and presumably developed acute hypokalemia with fatal arrhythmia; (2) patients with severely decompensated hepatic cirrhosis with ascites, with or without accompanying encephalopathy, who were in electrolyte imbalance and died because of intensification of the electrolyte defect.
Deafness, tinnitus, and vertigo with a sense of fullness in the ears have occurred, most frequently in patients with severe impairment of renal function. These symptoms have been associated most often with intravenous administration and with doses in excess of those recommended. The deafness has usually been reversible and of short duration (one to 24 hours). However, in some patients the hearing loss has been permanent. A number of these patients were also receiving drugs known to be ototoxic.
Furthermore, EDECRIN may increase the ototoxic potential of other drugs such as aminoglycoside antibiotics. Their concurrent use should be avoided.
Lithium generally should not be given with diuretics because they reduce its renal clearance and add a high risk of lithium toxicity. Read circulars for lithium preparations before use of such concomitant therapy.
Nonspecific small bowel lesions consisting of stenosis with or without ulceration may occur in association with administration of enteric coated potassium tablets alone or in conjunction with diuretic therapy. Surgery was frequently required and deaths have occurred. Therefore, enteric coated potassium tablets should not be used when supplementary potassium administration is needed.

Use in Pregnancy

EDECRIN is not recommended for use in pregnant patients. Use of the drug in women of the childbearing age requires that its potential benefits be weighed against the possible hazards to the fetus. The safety and efficacy of the drug in toxemia of pregnancy have not been established. EDECRIN is contraindicated in nursing mothers. If use of the drug is deemed essential, the patient should stop nursing.

Precautions

Weakness, muscle cramps, paresthesias, thirst, anorexia, and signs of hyponatremia, hypokalemia, and/or hypochloremic alkalosis may occur following vigorous or excessive diuresis and these may be accentuated by rigid salt restriction. Rarely tetany has been reported following vigorous diuresis. *During therapy with ethacrynic acid, liberalization of salt intake and supplementary potassium chloride are often necessary.*
When a metabolic alkalosis may be anticipated, e.g., in cirrhosis with ascites, the use of potassium chloride with or without an aldosterone antagonist before and continuously during therapy with EDECRIN may mitigate or prevent the hypokalemia.
The safety and efficacy of ethacrynic acid in hypertension have not been established. However, the dosage of coadministered antihypertensive agents may require adjustment.
Orthostatic hypotension may occur in patients receiving other antihypertensive agents when given ethacrynic acid.
EDECRIN has little or no effect on glomerular filtration or on renal blood flow, except following pronounced reductions in plasma volume when associated with rapid diuresis. A transient increase in serum urea nitrogen may occur. Usually, this is readily reversible when the drug is discontinued.
As with other diuretics used in the treatment of renal edema, hypoproteinemia may reduce responsiveness to ethacrynic acid and the use of salt-poor albumin should be considered.
A number of drugs, including ethacrynic acid, have been shown to displace warfarin from plasma protein; a reduction in the usual anticoagulant dosage may be required in patients receiving both drugs.
EDECRIN may increase the risk of gastric hemorrhage associated with corticosteroid treatment.

Adverse Reactions

Gastrointestinal
Anorexia, malaise, abdominal discomfort or pain, dysphagia, nausea, vomiting, and diarrhea have occurred. These are more frequent with large doses or after one to three months of continuous therapy. A few patients have had sudden onset of watery, profuse diarrhea. Discontinue EDECRIN if diarrhea is severe and do not readminister it. Gastrointestinal bleeding has occurred in some patients.
Rarely, acute pancreatitis has been reported in patients receiving diuretics, including EDECRIN.

Renal
Reversible hyperuricemia and acute gout have been reported. Acute symptomatic hypoglycemia with convulsions occurred in two uremic patients who received doses above those recommended.

Carbohydrate Metabolism
Hyperglycemia has been reported in a few patients, most of whom had decompensated cirrhosis. However, patients who developed hyperglycemia on thiazide therapy have not done so when given EDECRIN.

Hemopoietic System
Agranulocytosis or severe neutropenia has been reported in a few critically ill patients also receiving agents known to produce this effect. Thrombocytopenia has been reported rarely. Rare instances of Henoch-Schönlein purpura have been reported in patients with rheumatic heart disease receiving many drugs, including EDECRIN.

Hepatic
Rarely, jaundice and abnormal liver function tests have been reported in seriously ill patients on multiple drug therapy that included EDECRIN.

Miscellaneous
Deafness, tinnitus, and vertigo, with a sense of fullness in the ears, have occurred (see ADDITIONAL WARNINGS). Infrequently, skin rash, headache, fever, chills, hematuria, blurred vision, fatigue, apprehension, and confusion have occurred.
SODIUM EDECRIN occasionally has caused local irritation and pain after intravenous use.

Dosage and Administration

Dosage must be regulated carefully to prevent a more rapid or substantial loss of fluid or electrolyte than is indicated or necessary. The magnitude of diuresis and natriuresis is largely dependent on the degree of fluid accumulation present in the patient. Similarly, the extent of potassium excretion is determined in large measure by the presence and magnitude of aldosteronism.

Oral Use
EDECRIN is available for oral use as 25 mg and 50 mg tablets.

Dosage: To Initiate Diuresis
The smallest dose required to produce gradual weight loss (about 1 to 2 pounds per day) is recommended. Onset of diuresis usually occurs at 50 to 100 mg for adults. After diuresis has been achieved, the minimally effective dose (usually from 50 to 200 mg daily) may be given on a continuous or intermittent dosage schedule. Dosage adjustments are usually in 25 to 50 mg increments to avoid derangement of water and electrolyte excretion.
The patient should be weighed under standard conditions before and during the institution of diuretic therapy with this compound. Small alterations in dose should effectively prevent a massive diuretic response. The following schedule may be helpful in determining the smallest effective dose.
  Day 1— 50 mg (single dose) after a meal
  Day 2— 50 mg twice daily after meals, if necessary

Continued on next page

Information on the Merck Sharp & Dohme products listed on these pages is the full prescribing information from product circulars in use November 1, 1984.

Merck Sharp & Dohme—Cont.

Day 3— 100 mg in the morning and 50 to 100 mg following the afternoon or evening meal, depending upon response to the morning dose

A few patients may require initial and maintenance doses as high as 200 mg twice daily. These higher doses, which should be achieved gradually, are most often required in patients with severe, refractory edema.

In children, the initial dose should be 25 mg. Careful stepwise increments in dosage of 25 mg should be made to achieve effective maintenance. A dosage for *infants* has not been established.

Maintenance Therapy

It is usually possible to reduce the dosage and frequency of administration once dry weight has been achieved.

EDECRIN (Ethacrynic Acid, MSD) may be given intermittently after an effective diuresis is obtained with the regimen outlined above. Dosage may be on an alternate daily schedule or more prolonged periods of diuretic therapy may be interspersed with rest periods. Such an intermittent dosage schedule allows time for correction of any electrolyte imbalance and may provide a more efficient diuretic response.

The chloruretic effect of this agent may give rise to retention of bicarbonate and a metabolic alkalosis. This may be corrected by giving chloride (ammonium chloride or arginine chloride). Ammonium chloride should not be given to cirrhotic patients. EDECRIN has additive effects when used with other diuretics. For example, a patient who is on maintenance dosage of an oral diuretic may require additional intermittent diuretic therapy, such as an organomercurial, for the maintenance of basal weight. The intermittent use of EDECRIN orally may eliminate the need for injections of organomercurials. Small doses of EDECRIN may be added to existing diuretic regimens to maintain basal weight. This drug may potentiate the action of carbonic anhydrase inhibitors, with augmentation of natriuresis and kaliuresis. Therefore, when adding EDECRIN the initial dose and changes of dose should be in 25 mg increments, to avoid electrolyte depletion. Rarely, patients who failed to respond to ethacrynic acid have responded to older established agents.

While many patients do not require supplemental potassium, the use of potassium chloride or aldosterone antagonists, or both, during treatment with EDECRIN is advisable, especially in cirrhotic or nephrotic patients and in patients receiving digitalis.

Salt liberalization usually prevents the development of hyponatremia and hypochloremia. During treatment with EDECRIN, salt may be liberalized to a greater extent than with other diuretics. Cirrhotic patients, however, usually require at least moderate salt restriction concomitant with diuretic therapy.

Intravenous Use

INTRAVENOUS SODIUM EDECRIN is for intravenous use when oral intake is impractical or in urgent conditions, such as acute pulmonary edema.

Each vial contains:
Ethacrynate sodium equivalent
  to ethacrynate acid.............................. 50 mg
Inactive ingredients:
Mannitol...62.5 mg
with 0.1 mg thimerosal added as preservative.
The usual intravenous dose for the average sized adult is 50 mg, or 0.5 to 1.0 mg per kg of body weight. Usually only one dose has been necessary; occasionally a second dose at a new injection site, to avoid possible thrombophlebitis, may be required. A single intravenous dose not exceeding 100 mg has been used in critical situations. Insufficient pediatric experience precludes recommendation for this age group.

To reconstitute the dry material, add 50 ml of 5 percent Dextrose Injection, or Sodium Chloride Injection to the vial. Occasionally, some 5 percent Dextrose Injection solutions may have a low pH (below 5). The resulting solution with such a diluent may be hazy or opalescent. Intravenous use of such a solution is not recommended.

The solution may be given slowly through the tubing of a running infusion or by direct intravenous injection over a period of several minutes. Do not mix this solution with whole blood or its derivatives. Discard unused reconstituted solution after 24 hours.

SODIUM EDECRIN should not be given subcutaneously or intramuscularly because of local pain and irritation.

How Supplied

No. 3321—Tablets EDECRIN, 25 mg, are white, capsule shaped, scored tablets, coded MSD 65. They are supplied as follows:
NDC 0006-0065-68 in bottles of 100
Shown in Product Identification Section, page 420
No. 3322—Tablets EDECRIN, 50 mg, are green, capsule shaped, scored tablets, coded MSD 90. They are supplied as follows:
NDC 0006-0090-68 in bottles of 100
(6505-00-834-0473 50 mg 100's)
Shown in Product Identification Section, page 420
No. 3330—INTRAVENOUS SODIUM EDECRIN is a dry white material either in a plug form or as a powder. It is supplied in vials containing ethacrynate sodium equivalent to 50 mg of ethacrynic acid, NDC 0006-3330-50.
(6505-00-875-7941 50 mg 50 ml vial)

A.H.F.S. Category: 40:28
DC 6073020 Issued September 1980

ELAVIL® Tablets ℞
(amitriptyline HCl, MSD), U.S.P.
ELAVIL® Injection ℞
(amitriptyline HCl, MSD), U.S.P.

Description

Amitriptyline HCl, a dibenzocycloheptadiene derivative, is a white or practically white, crystalline compound that is freely soluble in water.

It is designated chemically as 10,11-dihydro-N,N-dimethyl-5H-dibenzo $[a,d]$ cycloheptene-Δ^5,γ-propylamine hydrochloride. The molecular weight is 313.87. The empirical formula is $C_{20}H_{23}N\cdot HCl$.

ELAVIL® (Amitriptyline HCl, MSD) is supplied as 10 mg, 25 mg, 50 mg, 75 mg, 100 mg, and 150 mg tablets and as a sterile solution for intramuscular use. Each milliliter of the sterile solution contains:
Amitriptyline hydrochloride..........................10 mg
Dextrose..44 mg
Water for Injection, q.s.....................................1 ml
Added as preservatives:
Methylparaben..1.5 mg
Propylparaben...0.2 mg

Actions

ELAVIL is an antidepressant with sedative effects. Its mechanism of action in man is not known. It is not a monoamine oxidase inhibitor and it does not act primarily by stimulation of the central nervous system.

Amitriptyline inhibits the membrane pump mechanism responsible for uptake of norepinephrine and serotonin in adrenergic and serotonergic neurons. Pharmacologically this action may potentiate or prolong neuronal activity since reuptake of these biogenic amines is important physiologically in terminating transmitting activity. This interference with the reuptake of norepinephrine and /or serotonin is believed by some to underlie the antidepressant activity of amitriptyline.

Indications

For the relief of symptoms of depression. Endogenous depression is more likely to be alleviated than are other depressive states.

Contraindications

ELAVIL is contraindicated in patients who have shown prior hypersensitivity to it. It should not be given concomitantly with monoamine oxidase inhibitors. Hyperpyretic crises, severe convulsions, and deaths have occurred in patients receiving tricyclic antidepressant and monoamine oxidase inhibiting drugs simultaneously. When it is desired to replace a monoamine oxidase inhibitor with ELAVIL, a minimum of 14 days should be allowed to elapse after the former is discontinued. ELAVIL should then be initiated cautiously with gradual increase in dosage until optimum response is achieved.

This drug is not recommended for use during the acute recovery phase following myocardial infarction.

Warnings

ELAVIL may block the antihypertensive action of guanethidine or similarly acting compounds.

It should be used with caution in patients with a history of seizures and, because of its atropine-like action, in patients with a history of urinary retention, angle-closure glaucoma or increased intraocular pressure. In patients with angle-closure glaucoma, even average doses may precipitate an attack.

Patients with cardiovascular disorders should be watched closely. Tricyclic antidepressant drugs, including ELAVIL, particularly when given in high doses, have been reported to produce arrhythmias, sinus tachycardia, and prolongation of the conduction time. Myocardial infarction and stroke have been reported with drugs of this class. Close supervision is required when ELAVIL is given to hyperthyroid patients or those receiving thyroid medication.

This drug may impair mental and/or physical abilities required for performance of hazardous tasks, such as operating machinery or driving a motor vehicle.

ELAVIL may enhance the response to alcohol and the effects of barbiturates and other CNS depressants. In patients who may use alcohol excessively, it should be borne in mind that the potentiation may increase the danger inherent in any suicide attempt or overdosage. Delirium has been reported with concurrent administration of amitriptyline and disulfiram.

Usage in Pregnancy—Safe use of ELAVIL during pregnancy and lactation has not been established; therefore, in administering the drug to pregnant patients, nursing mothers, or women who may become pregnant, the possible benefits must be weighed against the possible hazards to mother and child.

Animal reproduction studies have been inconclusive and clinical experience has been limited.

Usage in Children—In view of the lack of experience with the use of this drug in children, it is not recommended at the present time for patients under 12 years of age.

Precautions

Schizophrenic patients may develop increased symptoms of psychosis; patients with paranoid symptomatology may have an exaggeration of such symptoms. Depressed patients, particularly those with known manic-depressive illness, may experience a shift to mania or hypomania. In these circumstances the dose of amitriptyline may be reduced or a major tranquilizer such as perphenazine may be administered concurrently.

When ELAVIL is given with anticholinergic agents or sympathomimetic drugs, including epinephrine combined with local anesthetics, close supervision and careful adjustment of dosages are required.

Paralytic ileus may occur in patients taking tricyclic antidepressants in combination with anticholinergic-type drugs.

Caution is advised if patients receive large doses of ethchlorvynol concurrently. Transient delirium has been reported in patients who were treated with one gram of ethchlorvynol and 75-150 mg of ELAVIL.

The possibility of suicide in depressed patients remains until significant remission occurs. Potentially suicidal patients should not have access to large quantities of this drug. Prescriptions should be written for the smallest amount feasible.

Concurrent administration of ELAVIL and electroshock therapy may increase the hazards associated with such therapy. Such treatment should be limited to patients for whom it is essential.

When possible, the drug should be discontinued several days before elective surgery.

Both elevation and lowering of blood sugar levels have been reported.

ELAVIL should be used with caution in patients with impaired liver function.

Adverse Reactions

Note: Included in the listing which follows are a few adverse reactions which have not been reported with this specific drug. However, pharmacological similarities among the tricyclic antidepressant drugs require that each of the reactions be considered when amitriptyline is administered.

Cardiovascular: Hypotension, particularly orthostatic hypotension; hypertension; tachycardia; palpitation; myocardial infarction; arrhythmias; heart block; stroke.

CNS and Neuromuscular: Confusional states; disturbed concentration; disorientation; delusions; hallucinations; excitement; anxiety; restlessness; insomnia; nightmares; numbness, tingling, and paresthesias of the extremities; peripheral neuropathy; incoordination; ataxia; tremors; seizures; alteration in EEG patterns; extrapyramidal symptoms; tinnitus; syndrome of inappropriate ADH (antidiuretic hormone) secretion.

Anticholinergic: Dry mouth, blurred vision, disturbance of accommodation, increased intraocular pressure, constipation, paralytic ileus, urinary retention, dilatation of urinary tract.

Allergic: Skin rash, urticaria, photosensitization, edema of face and tongue.

Hematologic: Bone marrow depression including agranulocytosis, leukopenia, eosinophilia, purpura, thrombocytopenia.

Gastrointestinal: Nausea, epigastric distress, vomiting, anorexia, stomatitis, peculiar taste, diarrhea, parotid swelling, black tongue. Rarely hepatitis (including altered liver function and jaundice).

Endocrine: Testicular swelling and gynecomastia in the male, breast enlargement and galactorrhea in the female, increased or decreased libido, elevation and lowering of blood sugar levels.

Other: Dizziness, weakness, fatigue, headache, weight gain or loss, edema, increased perspiration, urinary frequency, mydriasis, drowsiness, alopecia.

Withdrawal Symptoms: After prolonged administration, abrupt cessation of treatment may produce nausea, headache, and malaise. Gradual dosage reduction has been reported to produce, within two weeks, transient symptoms including irritability, restlessness, and dream and sleep disturbance. These symptoms are not indicative of addiction. Rare instances have been reported of mania or hypomania occurring within 2-7 days following cessation of chronic therapy with tricyclic antidepressants.

Dosage and Administration

Oral Dosage
Dosage should be initiated at a low level and increased gradually, noting carefully the clinical response and any evidence of intolerance.
Initial Dosage for Adults—For outpatients 75 mg of amitriptyline HCl a day in divided doses usually is satisfactory. If necessary, this may be increased to a total of 150 mg per day. Increases are made preferably in the late afternoon and/or bedtime doses. A sedative effect may be apparent before the antidepressant effect is noted, but an adequate therapeutic effect may take as long as 30 days to develop.

An alternate method of initiating therapy in outpatients is to begin with 50 to 100 mg amitriptyline HCl at bedtime. This may be increased by 25 or 50 mg as necessary in the bedtime dose to a total of 150 mg per day.

Hospitalized patients may require 100 mg a day initially. This can be increased gradually to 200 mg a day if necessary. A small number of hospitalized patients may need as much as 300 mg a day.

Adolescent and Elderly Patients—In general, lower dosages are recommended for these patients. Ten mg 3 times a day with 20 mg at bedtime may be satisfactory in adolescent and elderly patients who do not tolerate higher dosages.

Maintenance—The usual maintenance dosage of amitriptyline HCl is 50 to 100 mg per day. In some patients 40 mg per day is sufficient. For maintenance therapy the total daily dosage may be given in a single dose preferably at bedtime. When satisfactory improvement has been reached, dosage should be reduced to the lowest amount that will maintain relief of symptoms. It is appropriate to continue maintenance therapy 3 months or longer to lessen the possibility of relapse.

Intramuscular Dosage
Initially, 20 to 30 mg (2 to 3 ml) four times a day. When ELAVIL injection is administered intramuscularly, the effects may appear more rapidly than with oral administration.

When ELAVIL injection is used for initial therapy in patients unable or unwilling to take ELAVIL tablets, the tablets should replace the injection as soon as possible.

Usage in Children
In view of the lack of experience with the use of this drug in children, it is not recommended at the present time for patients under 12 years of age.

Plasma Levels
Because of the wide variation in the absorption and distribution of tricyclic antidepressants in body fluids, it is difficult to directly correlate plasma levels and therapeutic effect. However, determination of plasma levels may be useful in identifying patients who appear to have toxic effects and may have excessively high levels, or those in whom lack of absorption or noncompliance is suspected. Adjustments in dosage should be made according to the patient's clinical response and not on the basis of plasma levels.*

Overdosage

Manifestations—High doses may cause temporary confusion, disturbed concentration, or transient visual hallucinations. Overdosage may cause drowsiness; hypothermia; tachycardia and other arrhythmic abnormalities, such as bundle branch block; ECG evidence of impaired conduction; congestive heart failure; dilated pupils; disorders of ocular motility; convulsions; severe hypotension; stupor; and coma. Other symptoms may be agitation, hyperactive reflexes, muscle rigidity, vomiting, hyperpyrexia, or any of those listed under ADVERSE REACTIONS.

All patients suspected of having taken an overdosage should be admitted to a hospital as soon as possible. *Treatment* is symptomatic and supportive. Empty the stomach as quickly as possible by emesis followed by gastric lavage upon arrival at the hospital. Following gastric lavage, activated charcoal may be administered. Twenty to 30 g of activated charcoal may be given every four to six hours during the first 24 to 48 hours after ingestion. An ECG should be taken and close monitoring of cardiac function instituted if there is any sign of abnormality. Maintain an open airway and adequate fluid intake; regulate body temperature. The intravenous administration of 1-3 mg of physostigmine salicylate is reported to reverse the symptoms of tricyclic antidepressant poisoning. Because physostigmine is rapidly metabolized, the dosage of physostigmine should be repeated as required particularly if life threatening signs such as arrhythmias, convulsions, and deep coma recur or persist after the initial dosage of physostigmine. Because physostigmine itself may be toxic, it is not recommended for routine use.

---
*Hollister, L. E., *J. Amer. Med. Ass.* 241: 2530-2533, June 8, 1979.

Standard measures should be used to manage circulatory shock and metabolic acidosis. Cardiac arrhythmias may be treated with neostigmine, pyridostigmine, or propranolol. Should cardiac failure occur, the use of digitalis should be considered. Close monitoring of cardiac function for not less than five days is advisable.

Anticonvulsants may be given to control convulsions. Amitriptyline increases the CNS depressant action but not the anticonvulsant action of barbiturates; therefore, an inhalation anesthetic, diazepam, or paraldehyde is recommended for control of convulsions.

Dialysis is of no value because of low plasma concentrations of the drug.

Since overdosage is often deliberate, patients may attempt suicide by other means during the recovery phase.

Deaths by deliberate or accidental overdosage have occurred with this class of drugs.

How Supplied

No. 3287—Tablets ELAVIL, 10 mg, are blue, round, film coated tablets, coded MSD 23. They are supplied as follows:
NDC 0006-0023-68 bottles of 100
(6505-00-079-7453, 10 mg 100's)
NDC 0006-0023-28 single unit packages of 100
NDC 0006-0023-82 bottles of 1000
NDC 0006-0023-86 bottles of 5000.
Shown in Product Identification Section, page 420
No. 3288—Tablets ELAVIL, 25 mg, are yellow, round, film coated tablets, coded MSD 45. They are supplied as follows:
NDC 0006-0045-68 bottles of 100
(6505-00-082-2659, 25 mg 100's)
NDC 0006-0045-28 single unit packages of 100
(6505-00-118-2509, 25 mg individually sealed 100's)
NDC 0006-0045-82 bottles of 1000
(6505-00-724-6358, 25 mg 1000's)
NDC 0006-0045-86 bottles of 5000.
Shown in Product Identification Section, page 420
No. 3320—Tablets ELAVIL, 50 mg, are beige, round, film coated tablets, coded MSD 102. They are supplied as follows:
NDC 0006-0102-68 bottles of 100
NDC 0006-0102-28 single unit packages of 100
NDC 0006-0102-82 bottles of 1000.
Shown in Product Identification Section, page 420
No. 3348—Tablets ELAVIL, 75 mg, are orange, round, film coated tablets, coded MSD 430. They are supplied as follows:
NDC 0006-0430-68 bottles of 100
NDC 0006-0430-28 single unit packages of 100.
Shown in Product Identification Section, page 420
No. 3349—Tablets ELAVIL, 100 mg, are mauve, round, film coated tablets, coded MSD 435. They are supplied as follows:
NDC 0006-0435-68 bottles of 100
NDC 0006-0435-28 single unit packages of 100.
Shown in Product Identification Section, page 420
No. 3351—Tablets ELAVIL, 150 mg, are blue, capsule shaped, film coated tablets, coded MSD 673. They are supplied as follows:
NDC 0006-0673-30 bottles of 30
NDC 0006-0673-68 bottles of 100
NDC 0006-0673-28 single unit packages of 100.
Shown in Product Identification Section, page 420
No. 3286—Injection ELAVIL, 10 mg/ml, is a clear, colorless solution, and is supplied as follows:
NDC 0006-3286-10 in 10 ml vials.

Metabolism

Studies in man following oral administration of ^{14}C-labeled drug indicated that amitriptyline is rapidly absorbed and metabolized. Radioactivity of the plasma was practically negligible, although significant amounts of radioactivity appeared in

Continued on next page

Information on the Merck Sharp & Dohme products listed on these pages is the full prescribing information from product circulars in use November 1, 1984.

Merck Sharp & Dohme—Cont.

the urine by 4 to 6 hours and one-half to one-third of the drug was excreted within 24 hours. Amitriptyline is metabolized by N-demethylation and bridge hydroxylation in man, rabbit, and rat. Virtually the entire dose is excreted as glucuronide or sulfate conjugate of metabolites, with little unchanged drug appearing in the urine. Other metabolic pathways may be involved.

A.H.F.S. Category: 28:16:04
DC 6613123   Issued January 1983

ELSPAR® ℞
(asparaginase, MSD)

Warning

IT IS RECOMMENDED THAT ASPARAGINASE BE ADMINISTERED TO PATIENTS ONLY IN A HOSPITAL SETTING UNDER THE SUPERVISION OF A PHYSICIAN WHO IS QUALIFIED BY TRAINING AND EXPERIENCE TO ADMINISTER CANCER CHEMOTHERAPEUTIC AGENTS, BECAUSE OF THE POSSIBILITY OF SEVERE REACTIONS, INCLUDING ANAPHYLAXIS AND SUDDEN DEATH. THE PHYSICIAN MUST BE PREPARED TO TREAT ANAPHYLAXIS AT EACH ADMINISTRATION OF THE DRUG. IN THE TREATMENT OF EACH PATIENT THE PHYSICIAN MUST WEIGH CAREFULLY THE POSSIBILITY OF ACHIEVING THERAPEUTIC BENEFIT VERSUS THE RISK OF TOXICITY. THE FOLLOWING DATA SHOULD BE THOROUGHLY REVIEWED BEFORE ADMINISTERING THE COMPOUND.

Description

ELSPAR® (Asparaginase, MSD) contains the enzyme L-asparagine amidohydrolase, type EC-2, derived from *Escherichia coli*. It is a white crystalline powder that is freely soluble in water and practically insoluble in methanol, acetone and chloroform. Its activity is expressed in terms of International Units (I.U.) according to the recommendation of the International Union of Biochemistry. The specific activity of ELSPAR is at least 225 I.U. per milligram of protein and each vial contains 10,000 I.U. of asparaginase and 80 mg of mannitol, an inactive ingredient, as a sterile, white lyophilized plug or powder for intravenous or intramuscular injection after reconstitution.

Clinical Pharmacology

Action
In a significant number of patients with acute leukemia, particularly lymphocytic, the malignant cells are dependent on an exogenous source of asparagine for survival. Normal cells, however, are able to synthesize asparagine and thus are affected less by the rapid depletion produced by treatment with the enzyme asparaginase. This is a unique approach to therapy based on a metabolic defect in asparagine synthesis of some malignant cells. ELSPAR, derived from *Escherichia coli*, is effective in inducing remissions in some patients with acute lymphocytic leukemia.

Asparagine Dependence Test
An asparagine dependence test has been utilized during the investigational studies. In this test leukemic cells obtained from some marrow cultures could be shown to require asparagine in *vitro*, suggesting sensitivity to asparaginase therapy in *vivo*. However, present data indicate that the correlation between asparagine dependence in such tests and the final response to therapy is sufficiently poor that the test is not recommended as a basis for selection of patients for treatment.

Pharmacokinetics and Metabolism
In a study in patients with metastatic cancer and leukemia, initial plasma levels of L-asparaginase following intravenous administration were correlated to dose. Daily administration resulted in a cumulative increase in plasma levels. Plasma half-life varied from 8 to 30 hours; it did not appear to be influenced by dosage, either single or repetitive, and could not be correlated with age, sex, surface area, renal or hepatic function, diagnosis or extent of disease. Apparent volume of distribution was approximately 70–80% of estimated plasma volume. There was some slow movement of asparaginase from vascular to extravascular, extracellular space. L-asparaginase was detected in the lymph. Cerebrospinal fluid levels were less than 1% of concurrent plasma levels. Only trace amounts appeared in the urine.

In a study in which patients with leukemia and metastatic cancer received intramuscular L-asparaginase, peak plasma levels of asparaginase were reached 14 to 24 hours after dosing. Plasma half-life was 39 to 49 hours. No asparaginase was detected in the urine.

Indications and Usage

ELSPAR is indicated in the therapy of patients with acute lymphocytic leukemia. This agent is useful primarily in combination with other chemotherapeutic agents in the induction of remissions of the disease in children. ELSPAR should not be used as the sole induction agent unless combination therapy is deemed inappropriate. ELSPAR is not recommended for maintenance therapy.

Contraindications

ELSPAR is contraindicated in patients with pancreatitis or a history of pancreatitis. Acute hemorrhagic pancreatitis, in some instances fatal, has been reported following asparaginase administration. Asparaginase is also contraindicated in patients who have had previous anaphylactic reactions to it.

Warnings

Allergic reactions to asparaginase are frequent and may occur during the primary course of therapy. They are not completely predictable on the basis of the intradermal skin test. Anaphylaxis and death have occurred even in a hospital setting with experienced observers.

Once a patient has received ELSPAR as part of a treatment regimen, retreatment with this agent at a later time is associated with increased risk of hypersensitivity reactions. In patients found by skin testing to be hypersensitive to asparaginase, and in any patient who has received a previous course of therapy with asparaginase, therapy with this agent should be instituted or reinstituted only after successful desensitization, and then only if in the judgement of the physician the possible benefit is greater than the increased risk. Desensitization itself may be hazardous. (See DOSAGE AND ADMINISTRATION, *Intradermal Skin Test.*)

In view of the unpredictability of the adverse reactions to asparaginase, it is recommended that this product be used in a hospital setting. Asparaginase has an adverse effect on liver function in the majority of patients. Therapy with asparaginase may increase pre-existing liver impairment caused by prior therapy or the underlying disease. Because of this there is a possibility that asparaginase may increase the toxicity of other medications.

The administration of ELSPAR *intravenously concurrently with or immediately before* a course of vincristine and prednisone may be associated with increased toxicity. (See DOSAGE AND ADMINISTRATION, *Recommended Induction Regimens.*)

Precautions

General
This drug may be a contact irritant and both powder and solution must be handled and administered with care. Inhalation of dust or vapors and contact with skin or mucous membranes, especially those of the eyes, must be avoided. In case of contact, wash with copious amounts of water for at least 15 minutes.

Asparaginase has been reported to have immunosuppressive activity in animal experiments. Accordingly, the possibility that use of the drug in man may predispose to infection should be considered.

Asparaginase toxicity is reported to be greater in adults than in children.

Laboratory Tests
The fall in circulating lymphoblasts often is quite marked; normal or below normal leukocyte counts are noted frequently within the first several days after initiating therapy. This may be accompanied by a marked rise in serum uric acid. The possible development of uric acid nephropathy should be borne in mind. Appropriate preventive measures should be taken, e.g., allopurinol, increased fluid intake, alkalization of urine. As a guide to the effects of therapy, the patient's peripheral blood count and bone marrow should be monitored frequently.

Frequent serum amylase determinations should be obtained to detect early evidence of pancreatitis. If pancreatitis occurs, therapy should be stopped and not reinstituted.

Blood sugar should be monitored during therapy with ELSPAR because hyperglycemia may occur.

Drug Interactions
Tissue culture and animal studies indicate that ELSPAR can diminish or abolish the effect of methotrexate on malignant cells. This effect on methotrexate activity persists as long as plasma asparagine levels are suppressed. These results would seem to dictate against the clinical use of methotrexate with ELSPAR, or during the period following ELSPAR therapy when plasma asparagine levels are below normal.

Drug/Laboratory Test Interactions
L-asparaginase has been reported to interfere with the interpretation of thyroid function tests by producing a rapid and marked reduction in serum concentrations of thyroxine-binding globulin within two days after the first dose. Serum concentrations of thyroxine-binding globulin returned to pretreatment values within four weeks of the last dose of L-asparaginase.

Animal Toxicology
A one-month intravenous toxicity study of ELSPAR in dogs at doses of 250, 1000, and 2000 I.U./kg/day revealed reduced serum total protein and albumin with loss of body weight at the highest dose level and anorexia, emesis, and diarrhea at all dosage levels. A similar study in monkeys at doses of 100, 300, and 1000 I.U./kg/day also revealed reduction of serum total protein and albumin and body weight loss at all dosage levels. Bromsulfalein retention and fatty changes in the liver were noted in monkeys that were given 300 and 1000 I.U./kg/day. The rabbit was unusually sensitive to ELSPAR since a single intravenous dose of 1000 I.U./kg caused hypocalcemia associated with necrosis of the parathyroid cells, convulsions, and death in about one third of the animals. Some rabbits that died showed small thymic and lymph node hemorrhages and necrosis of the germinal centers in the lymph nodes and spleen. The intravenous administration of calcium gluconate alleviated or prevented the adverse effects.

Changes in the pancreatic islets (not pancreatitis) ranging from edema to necrosis were observed in the rabbits in the acute intravenous toxicity studies (doses of 12,500 to 50,000 I.U./kg) but not in rabbits that received 1000 I.U./kg. The anatomical changes and the hypocalcemia found in the rabbits were not observed in the subacute intravenous studies in the dogs and monkeys.

Carcinogenesis, Mutagenesis, Impairment of Fertility
The intraperitoneal injection of 2500 I.U./kg/ day for 4 days in newborn Swiss mice resulted in a small increase in pulmonary adenomas; lymphatic leukemia was not increased.

L-asparaginase at concentrations of 152-909 I.U./plate was not mutagenic in the Ames microbial mutagen test with or without metabolic activation.

There are no adequate studies on the effects of asparaginase on fertility.

Pregnancy

Pregnancy Category C. In mice and rats ELSPAR has been shown to retard the weight gain of mothers and fetuses when given in doses of more than 1000 I.U./kg (the recommended human dose). Resorptions, gross abnormalities and skeletal abnormalities were observed. The intravenous administration of 50 or 100 I.U./kg (one-twentieth or one-tenth of the human dose) to pregnant rabbits on Day 8 and 9 of gestation resulted in dose dependent embryotoxicity and gross abnormalities. There are no adequate and well-controlled studies in pregnant women. ELSPAR should be used during pregnancy only if the potential benefit justifies the potential risk to the fetus.

Nursing Mothers

It is not known whether this drug is secreted in human milk. Because many drugs are secreted in human milk and because of the potential for serious adverse reactions in nursing infants from ELSPAR, a decision should be made whether to discontinue nursing or to discontinue the drug, taking into account the importance of the drug to the mother.

Adverse Reactions

Allergic reactions, including skin rashes, urticaria, arthralgia, respiratory distress, and acute anaphylaxis have been reported. (See WARNINGS.) Acute reactions have occurred in the absence of a positive skin test and during continued maintenance of therapeutic serum levels of ELSPAR.

In children with advanced leukemia, a lower incidence of anaphylaxis has been reported with intramuscular administration, although there was a higher incidence of milder hypersensitivity reactions than with intravenous administration.

Fatal hyperthermia has been reported.

Pancreatitis, sometimes fulminant and fatal, has occurred during or following therapy with ELSPAR.

Hyperglycemia with glucosuria and polyuria has been reported in low incidence. Serum and urine acetone usually have been absent or negligible in these patients; this syndrome thus resembles hyperosmolar, nonketotic, hyperglycemia induced by a variety of other agents. This complication usually responds to discontinuance of ELSPAR, judicious use of intravenous fluid, and insulin, but may be fatal on occasion.

In addition to hypofibrinogenemia, depression of various other clotting factors has been reported. Most marked has been a decrease in plasma levels of factors V and VIII with a variable decrease in factors VII and IX. A decrease in circulating platelets has occurred in low incidence which, together with the increased levels of fibrin degradation products in the serum, may indicate development of a consumption coagulopathy. Bleeding has been a problem in only a minority of patients with demonstrable coagulopathy. However, intracranial hemorrhage and fatal bleeding associated with low fibrinogen levels have been reported. Increased fibrinolytic activity, apparently compensatory in nature, also has occurred.

Some patients have shown central nervous system effects consisting of depression, somnolence, fatigue, coma, confusion, agitation, and hallucinations varying from mild to severe. Rarely, a Parkinson-like syndrome has occurred, with tremor and a progressive increase in muscular tone. These side effects usually have reversed spontaneously after treatment was stopped. Therapy with ELSPAR is associated with an increase in blood ammonia during the conversion of asparagine to asparatic acid by the enzyme. No clear correlation exists between the degree of elevation of blood ammonia levels and the appearance of CNS changes. Chills, fever, nausea, vomiting, anorexia, abdominal cramps, weight loss, headache, and irritability may occur and usually are mild.

Azotemia, usually pre-renal, occurs frequently. Acute renal shut down and fatal renal insufficiency have been reported during treatment. Proteinuria has occurred infrequently.

A variety of liver function abnormalities have been reported, including elevations of SGOT, SGPT, alkaline phosphatase, bilirubin (direct and indirect), and depression of serum albumin, cholesterol (total and esters), and plasma fibrinogen. Increases and decreases of total lipids have occurred. Marked hypoalbuminemia associated with peripheral edema has been reported. However, these abnormalities usually are reversible on discontinuance of therapy and some reversal may occur during the course of therapy. Fatty changes in the liver have been documented by biopsy. Malabsorption syndrome has been reported.

Rarely, transient bone marrow depression has been observed, as evidenced by a delay in return of hemoglobin or hematocrit levels to normal in patients undergoing hematologic remission of leukemia. Marked leukopenia has been reported.

Overdosage

The acute intravenous LD_{50} of ELSPAR for mice was about 500,000 I.U./kg and for rabbits about 22,000 I.U./kg.

Dosage and Administration

As a component of selected multiple agent induction regimens, ELSPAR may be administered by either the intravenous or the intramuscular route. When administered intravenously this enzyme should be given over a period of not less than thirty minutes through the side arm of an already running infusion of Sodium Chloride Injection or Dextrose Injection 5% (D_5W). ELSPAR has little tendency to cause phlebitis when given intravenously. Anaphylactic reactions require the immediate use of epinephrine, oxygen, and intravenous steroids.

When administering ELSPAR intramuscularly, the volume at a single injection site should be limited to 2 ml. If a volume greater than 2 ml is to be administered two injection sites should be used.

Unfavorable interactions of ELSPAR with some antitumor agents have been demonstrated. It is recommended therefore, that ELSPAR be used in combination regimens only by physicians familiar with the benefits and risks of a given regimen. During the period of its inhibition of protein synthesis and cell replication ELSPAR may interfere with the action of drugs such as methotrexate which require cell replication for their lethal effect. ELSPAR may interfere with the enzymatic detoxification of other drugs, particularly in the liver.

Recommended Induction Regimens:

When using chemotherapeutic agents in combination for the induction of remissions in patients with acute lymphocytic leukemia, regimens are sought which provide maximum chance of success while avoiding excessive cumulative toxicity or negative drug interactions.

One of the following combination regimens incorporating ELSPAR is recommended for acute lymphocytic leukemia in children:

In the regimens below, Day 1 is considered to be the first day of therapy.

Regimen I

Prednisone 40 mg/square meter of body surface area per day orally in three divided doses for 15 days, followed by tapering of the dosage as follows: 20 mg/square meter for 2 days, 10 mg/square meter for 2 days, 5 mg/square meter for 2 days, 2.5 mg/square meter for 2 days and then discontinue.

Vincristine sulfate 2 mg/square meter of body surface area intravenously once weekly on Days 1, 8, and 15 of the treatment period. The maximum single dose should not exceed 2.0 mg.

Asparaginase 1,000 I.U./kg/day intravenously for ten successive days beginning on Day 22 of the treatment period.

Regimen II

Prednisone 40 mg/square meter of body surface area per day orally in three divided doses for 28 days (the total daily dose should be to the nearest 2.5 mg), following which the dosage of prednisone should be discontinued gradually over a 14 day period.

Vincristine sulfate 1.5 mg/square meter of body surface area intravenously weekly for four doses, on Days 1, 8, 15, and 22 of the treatment period. The maximum single dose should not exceed 2.0 mg.

Asparaginase 6,000 I.U./square meter of body surface area intramuscularly on Days 4, 7, 10, 13, 16, 19, 22, 25, and 28 of the treatment period. When a remission is obtained with either of the above regimens, appropriate maintenance therapy must be instituted. ELSPAR should not be used as part of a maintenance regimen. The above regimens do not preclude a need for special therapy directed toward the prevention of central nervous system leukemia.

It should be noted that ELSPAR has been used in combination regimens other than those recommended above. It is important to keep in mind that ELSPAR administered intravenously concurrently with or immediately before a course of vincristine and prednisone may be associated with increased toxicity. Physicians using a given regimen should be thoroughly familiar with its benefits and risks. Clinical data are insufficient for a recommendation concerning the use of combination regimens in adults. Asparaginase toxicity is reported to be greater in adults than in children. Use of ELSPAR as the sole induction agent should be undertaken only in an unusual situation when a combined regimen is inappropriate because of toxicity or other specific patient-related factors, or in cases refractory to other therapy. When ELSPAR is to be used as the sole induction agent for children or adults the recommended dosage regimen is 200 I.U./kg/ day intravenously for 28 days. When complete remissions were obtained with this regimen, they were of short duration, 1 to 3 months. ELSPAR has been used as the sole induction agent in other regimens. Physicians using a given regimen should be thoroughly familiar with its benefits and risks.

Patients undergoing induction therapy must be carefully monitored and the therapeutic regimen adjusted according to response and toxicity.

Such adjustments should always involve decreasing dosages of one or more agents or discontinuation depending on the degree of toxicity. Patients who have received a course of ELSPAR, if retreated, have an increased risk of hypersensitivity reactions. Therefore, retreatment should be undertaken only when the benefit of such therapy is weighed against the increased risk.

Intradermal Skin Test:

Because of the occurrence of allergic reactions, an intradermal skin test should be performed prior to the initial administration of ELSPAR and when ELSPAR is given after an interval of a week or more has elapsed between doses. The skin test solution may be prepared as follows: Reconstitute the contents of a 10,000 I.U. vial with 5.0 ml of diluent. From this solution (2,000 I.U./ml) withdraw 0.1 ml and inject it into another vial containing 9.9 ml of diluent, yielding a skin test solution of approximately 20.0 I.U./ml. Use 0.1 ml of this solution (about 2.0 I.U.) for the intradermal skin test. The skin test site should be observed for at least one hour for the appearance of a wheal or erythema either of which indicates a positive reaction. An allergic reaction even to the skin test dose in certain sensitized individuals may rarely occur. A negative skin test reaction does not preclude the possibility of the development of an allergic reaction.

Desensitization:
Desensitization should be performed before administering the first dose of ELSPAR on initiation of therapy in positive reactors, and

Continued on next page

Information on the Merck Sharp & Dohme products listed on these pages is the full prescribing information from product circulars in use November 1, 1984.

Merck Sharp & Dohme—Cont.

on retreatment of any patient in whom such therapy is deemed necessary after carefully weighing the increased risk of hypersensitivity reactions. Rapid desensitization of the patient may be attempted with progressively increasing amounts of intravenously administered ELSPAR provided adequate precautions are taken to treat an acute allergic reaction should it occur. One reported schedule begins with a total of 1 I.U. given intravenously and doubles the dose every 10 minutes, provided no reaction has occurred, until the accumulated total amount given equals the planned doses for that day.

For convenience the following table is included to calculate the number of doses necessary to reach the patient's total dose for that day:

Injection Number	ELSPAR Dose in I.U.	Accumulated Total Dose
1	1	1
2	2	3
3	4	7
4	8	15
5	16	31
6	32	63
7	64	127
8	128	255
9	256	511
10	512	1023
11	1024	2047
12	2048	4095
13	4096	8191
14	8192	16383
15	16384	32767
16	32768	65535
17	65536	131071
18	131072	262143

For example: A patient weighing 20 kg who is to receive 200 I.U./kg (total dose 4000 I.U.) would receive injections 1 through 12 during desensitization.

Directions for Reconstitution

Parenteral drug products should be inspected visually for particulate matter and discoloration prior to administration whenever solution and container permit. When reconstituted, ELSPAR should be a clear, colorless solution. If the solution becomes cloudy, discard.

For Intravenous Use
Reconstitute with Sterile Water for Injection or with Sodium Chloride Injection. The volume recommended for reconstitution is 5 ml for the 10,000 unit vials. Ordinary shaking during reconstitution does not inactivate the enzyme. This solution may be used for direct intravenous administration within an eight hour period following restoration. For administration by infusion, solutions should be diluted with the isotonic solutions, Sodium Chloride Injection or Dextrose Injection 5%. These solutions should be infused within eight hours and only if clear.

Occasionally, a very small number of gelatinous fiber-like particles may develop on standing. Filtration through a 5.0 micron filter during administration will remove the particles with no resultant loss in potency. Some loss of potency has been observed with the use of a 0.2 micron filter.

For Intramuscular Use
When ELSPAR is administered intramuscularly according to the schedule cited in the induction regimen, reconstitution is carried out by adding 2 ml Sodium Chloride Injection to the 10,000 unit vial. The resulting solution should be used within eight hours and only if clear.

How Supplied

No. 4612 — ELSPAR is a white lyophilized plug or powder supplied as follows:
NDC 0006-4612-00 in a sterile 10 ml vial containing 10,000 I.U. of asparaginase and 80 mg mannitol, an inactive ingredient.
Personnel preparing ELSPAR should avoid drug contact with skin, mucous membranes, or eyes and avoid inhaling the dust or vapor.
Store at 2–8°C (36–46°F). ELSPAR does not contain a preservative. Unused, reconstituted solution should be stored at 2 to 8°C (36 to 46°F) and discarded after eight hours, or sooner if it becomes cloudy.

A.H.F.S. Category: 44:00
DC 6680207 Issued September 1983
COPYRIGHT © MERCK & CO., INC., 1983
All rights reserved

FLEXERIL® Tablets ℞
(cyclobenzaprine HCl, MSD), U.S.P.

Description

Cyclobenzaprine hydrochloride is a white, crystalline tricyclic amine salt with the empirical formula $C_{20}H_{21}N \cdot HCl$ and a molecular weight of 311.9. It has a melting point of 217°C, and a pK_a of 8.47 at 25°C. It is freely soluble in water and alcohol, sparingly soluble in isopropanol, and insoluble in hydrocarbon solvents. If aqueous solutions are made alkaline, the free base separates. Cyclobenzaprine HCl is designated chemically as 3-(5H-dibenzo[a,d]cyclohepten-5-ylidene)-N, N-dimethyl-1-propanamine hydrochloride.
FLEXERIL® (Cyclobenzaprine HCl, MSD) is supplied as 10 mg tablets for oral administration.

Clinical Pharmacology

Cyclobenzaprine HCl relieves skeletal muscle spasm of local origin without interfering with muscle function. It is ineffective in muscle spasm due to central nervous system disease.
Cyclobenzaprine reduced or abolished skeletal muscle hyperactivity in several animal models. Animal studies indicate that cyclobenzaprine does not act at the neuromuscular junction or directly on skeletal muscle. Such studies show that cyclobenzaprine acts primarily within the central nervous system at brain stem as opposed to spinal cord levels, although its action on the latter may contribute to its overall skeletal muscle relaxant activity. Evidence suggests that the net effect of cyclobenzaprine is a reduction of tonic somatic motor activity, influencing both gamma (γ) and alpha (α) motor systems.
Pharmacological studies in animals showed a similarity between the effects of cyclobenzaprine and the structurally related tricyclic antidepressants, including reserpine antagonism, norepinephrine potentiation, potent peripheral and central anticholinergic effects, and sedation. Cyclobenzaprine caused slight to moderate increase in heart rate in animals.
Cyclobenzaprine is well absorbed after oral administration, but there is a large intersubject variation in plasma levels. Cyclobenzaprine is eliminated quite slowly with a half-life as long as one to three days. It is highly bound to plasma proteins, is extensively metabolized primarily to glucuronide-like conjugates, and is excreted primarily via the kidneys.
No significant effect on plasma levels or bioavailability of FLEXERIL or aspirin was noted when single or multiple doses of the two drugs were administered concomitantly. Concomitant administration of FLEXERIL and aspirin is usually well tolerated and no unexpected or serious clinical or laboratory adverse effects have been observed. No studies have been performed to indicate whether FLEXERIL enhances the clinical effect of aspirin or other analgesics, or whether analgesics enhance the clinical effect of FLEXERIL in acute musculoskeletal conditions.

Clinical Studies
Controlled clinical studies show that FLEXERIL significantly improves the signs and symptoms of skeletal muscle spasm as compared with placebo. The clinical responses include improvement in muscle spasm as determined by palpation, reduction in local pain and tenderness, increased range of motion, and less restriction in activities of daily living. When daily observations were made, clinical improvement was observed as early as the first day of therapy.
Eight double-blind controlled clinical studies were performed in 642 patients comparing FLEXERIL, diazepam*, and placebo. Muscle spasm, local pain and tenderness, limitation of motion, and restriction in activities of daily living were evaluated. In three of these studies there was a significantly greater improvement with FLEXERIL than with diazepam, while in the other studies the improvement following both treatments was comparable. Although the frequency and severity of adverse reactions observed in patients treated with FLEXERIL were comparable to those observed in patients treated with diazepam, dry mouth was observed more frequently in patients treated with FLEXERIL and dizziness more frequently in those treated with diazepam. The incidence of drowsiness, the most frequent adverse reaction, was similar with both drugs.
Analysis of the data from controlled studies shows that FLEXERIL produces clinical improvement whether or not sedation occurs.

Indications and Usage

FLEXERIL is indicated as an adjunct to rest and physical therapy for relief of muscle spasm associated with acute, painful musculoskeletal conditions.
Improvement is manifested by relief of muscle spasm and its associated signs and symptoms, namely, pain, tenderness, limitation of motion, and restriction in activities of daily living.
FLEXERIL (Cyclobenzaprine HCl, MSD) should be used only for short periods (up to two or three weeks) because adequate evidence of effectiveness for more prolonged use is not available and because muscle spasm associated with acute, painful musculoskeletal conditions is generally of short duration and specific therapy for longer periods is seldom warranted.
FLEXERIL has not been found effective in the treatment of spasticity associated with cerebral or spinal cord disease, or in children with cerebral palsy.

Contraindications

Hypersensitivity to the drug.
Concomitant use of monoamine oxidase inhibitors or within 14 days after their discontinuation.
Acute recovery phase of myocardial infarction, and patients with arrhythmias, heart block or conduction disturbances, or congestive heart failure.
Hyperthyroidism.

Warnings

Cyclobenzaprine is closely related to the tricyclic antidepressants, e.g., amitriptyline and imipramine. In short term studies for indications other than muscle spasm associated with acute musculoskeletal conditions, and usually at doses somewhat greater than those recommended for skeletal muscle spasm, some of the more serious central nervous system reactions noted with the tricyclic antidepressants have occurred (see WARNINGS, below, and ADVERSE REACTIONS).
FLEXERIL may interact with monoamine oxidase (MAO) inhibitors. Hyperpyretic crisis, severe convulsions, and deaths have occurred in patients

---
*VALIUM® (diazepam, Roche)

Surveillance Program
A post-marketing surveillance program was carried out in 7607 patients with acute musculoskeletal disorders, and included 297 patients treated for 30 days or longer. The overall effectiveness of FLEXERIL was similar to that observed in the double-blind controlled studies; the overall incidence of adverse effects was less (see ADVERSE REACTIONS).

receiving tricyclic antidepressants and MAO inhibitor drugs.
Tricyclic antidepressants have been reported to produce arrhythmias, sinus tachycardia, prolongation of the conduction time leading to myocardial infarction and stroke.
FLEXERIL may enhance the effects of alcohol, barbiturates, and other CNS depressants.

Precautions

General
Because of its atropine-like action, FLEXERIL should be used with caution in patients with a history of urinary retention, angle-closure glaucoma, increased intraocular pressure, and in patients taking anticholinergic medication.
Information for Patients
FLEXERIL may impair mental and/or physical abilities required for performance of hazardous tasks, such as operating machinery or driving a motor vehicle.
Drug Interactions
FLEXERIL may enhance the effects of alcohol, barbiturates, and other CNS depressants.
Tricyclic antidepressants may block the antihypertensive action of guanethidine and similarly acting compounds.
Carcinogenesis, Mutagenesis, Impairment of Fertility
In rats treated with FLEXERIL for up to 67 weeks at doses of approximately 5 to 40 times the maximum recommended human dose, pale, sometimes enlarged, livers were noted and there was a dose-related hepatocyte vacuolation with lipidosis. In the higher dose groups this microscopic change was seen after 26 weeks and even earlier in rats which died prior to 26 weeks; at lower doses, the change was not seen until after 26 weeks.
Cyclobenzaprine did not affect the onset, incidence or distribution of neoplasia in an 81-week study in the mouse or in a 105-week study in the rat.
At oral doses of up to 10 times the human dose, cyclobenzaprine did not adversely affect the reproductive performance or fertility of male or female rats. Cyclobenzaprine did not demonstrate mutagenic activity in the male mouse at dose levels of up to 20 times the human dose.
Pregnancy
Pregnancy Category B: Reproduction studies have been performed in rats, mice and rabbits at doses up to 20 times the human dose, and have revealed no evidence of impaired fertility or harm to the fetus due to FLEXERIL. There are, however, no adequate and well-controlled studies in pregnant women. Because animal reproduction studies are not always predictive of human response, this drug should be used during pregnancy only if clearly needed.
Nursing Mothers
It is not known whether this drug is excreted in human milk. Because cyclobenzaprine is closely related to the tricyclic antidepressants, some of which are known to be excreted in human milk, caution should be exercised when FLEXERIL is administered to a nursing woman.
Pediatric Use
Safety and effectiveness of FLEXERIL in children below the age of 15 have not been established.

Adverse Reactions

The following list of adverse reactions is based on the experience in 473 patients treated with FLEXERIL in controlled clinical studies, 7607 patients in the post-marketing surveillance program, and reports received since the drug was marketed. The overall incidence of adverse reactions among patients in the surveillance program was less than the incidence in the controlled clinical studies.
The adverse reactions reported most frequently with FLEXERIL were drowsiness, dry mouth and dizziness. The incidence of these common adverse reactions was lower in the surveillance program than in the controlled clinical studies:

	Clinical Studies	Surveillance Program
drowsiness	39%	16%
dry mouth	27%	7%
dizziness	11%	3%

Among the less frequent adverse reactions, there was no appreciable difference in incidence in controlled clinical studies or in the surveillance program. Adverse reactions which were reported in 1% to 3% of the patients were: fatigue/tiredness, asthenia, nausea, constipation, dyspepsia, unpleasant taste, blurred vision, headache, nervousness, and confusion.

Incidence Less Than 1 in 100
The following adverse reactions have been reported at an incidence of less than 1 in 100:
Body as a Whole: Syncope; facial edema; malaise.
Cardiovascular: Tachycardia; arrhythmia; vasodilatation; palpitation; hypotension.
Digestive: Vomiting; anorexia; diarrhea; gastrointestinal pain; gastritis; thirst; flatulence; edema of the tongue; abnormal liver function and rare reports of hepatitis, jaundice and cholestasis.
Musculoskeletal: Local weakness.
Nervous System and Psychiatric: Ataxia; vertigo; dysarthria; tremors; hypertonia; convulsions; muscle twitching; disorientation; insomnia; depressed mood; abnormal sensations; anxiety; agitation; abnormal thinking and dreaming; hallucinations; excitement; paresthesia.
Skin: Sweating; skin rash; urticaria.
Special Senses: Ageusia; tinnitus.
Urogenital: Urinary frequency and/or retention.

Causal Relationship Unknown
Other reactions, reported rarely for FLEXERIL under circumstances where a causal relationship could not be established or reported for other tricyclic drugs, are listed to serve as alerting information to physicians:
Body as a Whole: Chest pain; edema.
Cardiovascular: Hypertension; myocardial infarction; heart block; stroke.
Digestive: Paralytic ileus; tongue discoloration; stomatitis; parotid swelling.
Endocrine: Inappropriate ADH syndrome.
Hematic and Lymphatic: Purpura; bone marrow depression; leukopenia; eosinophilia; thrombocytopenia.
Metabolic, Nutritional and Immune: Elevation and lowering of blood sugar levels; weight gain or loss.
Musculoskeletal: Myalgia.
Nervous System and Psychiatric: Decreased or increased libido; abnormal gait; delusions; peripheral neuropathy; alteration in EEG patterns; extrapyramidal symptoms.
Respiratory: Dyspnea.
Skin: Pruritus; photosensitization; alopecia.
Urogenital: Impaired urination; dilatation of urinary tract; impotence; testicular swelling; gynecomastia; breast enlargement; galactorrhea.

Drug Abuse and Dependence

Pharmacologic similarities among the tricyclic drugs require that certain withdrawal symptoms be considered when FLEXERIL is administered, even though they have not been reported to occur with this drug. Abrupt cessation of treatment after prolonged administration may produce nausea, headache, and malaise. These are not indicative of addiction.

Overdosage

Manifestations: High doses may cause temporary confusion, disturbed concentration, transient visual hallucinations, agitation, hyperactive reflexes, muscle rigidity, vomiting, or hyperpyrexia, in addition to anything listed under ADVERSE REACTIONS. Based on the known pharmacologic actions of the drug, overdosage may cause drowsiness, hypothermia, tachycardia and other cardiac rhythm abnormalities such as bundle branch block, ECG evidence of impaired conduction, and congestive heart failure. Other manifestations may be dilated pupils, convulsions, severe hypotension, stupor, and coma.

The acute oral LD_{50} of FLEXERIL is approximately 338 and 425 mg/kg in mice and rats, respectively.
Treatment: Treatment is symptomatic and supportive. Empty the stomach as quickly as possible by emesis, followed by gastric lavage. After gastric lavage, activated charcoal may be administered. Twenty to 30 g of activated charcoal may be given every four to six hours during the first 24 to 48 hours after ingestion. An ECG should be taken and close monitoring of cardiac function must be instituted if there is any evidence of dysrhythmia. Maintenance of an open airway, adequate fluid intake, and regulation of body temperature are necessary.
The intravenous administration of 1-3 mg of physostigmine salicylate is reported to reverse symptoms of poisoning by atropine and other drugs with anticholinergic activity. Physostigmine may be helpful in the treatment of cyclobenzaprine overdose. Because physostigmine is rapidly metabolized, the dosage of physostigmine should be repeated as required, particularly if life-threatening signs such as arrhythmias, convulsions, and deep coma recur or persist after the initial dosage of physostigmine. Because physostigmine itself may be toxic, it is not recommended for routine use.
Standard medical measures should be used to manage circulatory shock and metabolic acidosis. Cardiac arrhythmias may be treated with neostigmine, pyridostigmine, or propranolol. When signs of cardiac failure occur, the use of a short-acting digitalis preparation should be considered. Close monitoring of cardiac function for not less than five days is advisable.
Anticonvulsants may be given to control seizures.
Dialysis is probably of no value because of low plasma concentrations of the drug.
Since overdosage is often deliberate, patients may attempt suicide by other means during the recovery phase. Deaths by deliberate or accidental overdosage have occurred with this class of drugs.

Dosage and Administration

The usual dosage of FLEXERIL is 10 mg three times a day, with a range of 20 to 40 mg a day in divided doses. Dosage should not exceed 60 mg a day. Use of FLEXERIL for periods longer than two or three weeks is not recommended. (See INDICATIONS AND USAGE.)

How Supplied

No. 3358—Tablets FLEXERIL, 10 mg, are butterscotch yellow, D-shaped, film coated tablets, coded MSD 931. They are supplied as follows:
NDC 0006-0931-68 in bottles of 100
NDC 0006-0931-28 unit dose packages of 100.
NDC 0006-0931-30 BACK-PACK® unit-of-use package of 30.
Shown in Product Identification Section, page 420
A.H.F.S. Category: 12:20
DC 6919207 Issued September 1983
COPYRIGHT © MERCK & CO., INC., 1977
All rights reserved

HEP-B-GAMMAGEE® ℞
(hepatitis B immune globulin [human], MSD), U.S.P.

Description

HEP-B-GAMMAGEE® [Hepatitis B Immune Globulin (Human), MSD] is a sterile solution of human immunoglobulin (10–18% protein) prepared by a patented process from the pooled plasma of a small group of well-monitored individuals who were hyperimmunized with hepatitis B vaccine to produce high levels of antibody to the

Continued on next page

Information on the Merck Sharp & Dohme products listed on these pages is the full prescribing information from product circulars in use November 1, 1984.

Merck Sharp & Dohme—Cont.

hepatitis B surface antigen (anti-HBs). HEP-B-GAMMAGEE is prepared from human plasma that was nonreactive when tested for hepatitis B surface antigen (HBsAg). The pooled plasma is processed by MSD and/or Armour Pharmaceutical Company using Cohn cold ethanol fractionation procedures. The product is dissolved in 0.3 molar glycine and contains thimerosal (mercury derivative) 1:10,000 added as a preservative. The solution has a pH of 6.8 ± 0.4 adjusted with hydrochloric acid or sodium hydroxide. Each vial of HEP-B-GAMMAGEE contains anti-HBs equivalent to or exceeding the potency of anti-HBs in a U.S. reference Hepatitis B Immune Globulin (Bureau of Biologics, FDA).

Clinical Pharmacology

Hepatitis B Immune Globulin (Human) provides passive immunization for individuals exposed to the hepatitis B virus (HBV) as evidenced by a reduction in the attack rate of hepatitis B following its use. The administration of the usual recommended dose of HEP-B-GAMMAGEE generally results in a detectable level of circulating antibody to hepatitis B surface antigen (anti-HBs) which persists for approximately 2 months or longer. The possibility of hepatitis B transmission is remote, as it is with other immune globulins prepared by the cold ethanol process.

Indications and Usage

HEP-B-GAMMAGEE is indicated for post-exposure prophylaxis following either parenteral exposure, direct mucous membrane contact, or oral ingestion involving HBsAg-positive materials such as blood, plasma or serum. Such exposures might occur by accidental "needle-stick", accidental splash, or a pipetting accident. HEP-B-GAMMAGEE is also indicated for post-exposure prophylaxis in infants born to hepatitis B-positive (HBsAg-positive) mothers.
Use of Hepatitis B Immune Globulin (Human) has been and continues to be evaluated in other situations which include nonparenteral exposure to hepatitis B, in dialysis patients and among hospital staffs. In addition, it has been tested as a prophylactic measure for susceptible individuals in close association with HBsAg-positive persons. These studies are still in progress and there are insufficient data at present on effectiveness, dosage and schedule for any of these uses to be included as definite indications.

Contraindications

None known.

Warnings

Persons with isolated immunoglobulin A deficiency have the potential for developing antibodies to immunoglobulin A and could have anaphylactic reactions to subsequent administration of blood products that contain immunoglobulin A. Therefore, as with any immune globulin preparation, Hepatitis B Immune Globulin (Human) should be given to such persons only if the expected benefits outweigh the potential risks.
In patients who have severe thrombocytopenia or any coagulation disorder that would contraindicate intramuscular injections, Hepatitis B Immune Globulin (Human) should be given only if the expected benefits outweigh the potential risks.

Precautions

General
HEP-B-GAMMAGEE should be given with caution to patients with a history of prior systemic allergic reactions following the administration of human immune globulin preparations. Hypersensitivity reactions to injections of immune serum globulin occur rarely. The incidence of these reactions may be increased in patients receiving large intramuscular doses or in patients receiving repeated injections of immune serum globulin.
HEP-B-GAMMAGEE *must not be administered intravenously* because of the potential for serious reactions. Injections should be made intramuscularly. Care should be taken to draw back on the plunger of the syringe before injection in order to be certain that the needle is not in a blood vessel. Epinephrine should be available for treatment of acute allergic symptoms.

Drug Interactions
Antibodies present in immune globulin preparations may interfere with the immune response to live virus vaccines such as measles, mumps, and rubella. Therefore, vaccination with live virus vaccines should be deferred until approximately three months after administration of Hepatitis B Immune Globulin. It may be necessary to revaccinate persons who received Hepatitis B Immune Globulin shortly after live virus vaccination.

Pregnancy
Pregnancy Category C. Animal reproduction studies have not been conducted with HEP-B-GAMMAGEE. Clinical experience with other immunoglobulin preparations administered during pregnancy suggests that there are no known adverse effects on the fetus from immune globulins per se. However, it is not known whether HEP-B-GAMMAGEE can cause fetal harm when administered to a pregnant woman or can affect reproduction capacity. HEP-B-GAMMAGEE should be given to a pregnant woman only if clearly needed.

Nursing Mothers
It is not known whether this drug is excreted in human milk. Because many drugs are excreted in human milk, caution should be exercised when HEP-B-GAMMAGEE is administered to a nursing woman.

Adverse Reactions

Local pain and tenderness at the injection site, urticaria and angioedema may occur. Anaphylactic reactions, although rare, have been reported following the injection of human immune globulin preparations. Anaphylaxis is more likely to occur if Hepatitis B Immune Globulin (Human) is given intravenously; therefore, Hepatitis B Immune Globulin (Human) must be administered *only* intramuscularly. In highly allergic individuals, repeated injections may lead to anaphylactic shock.

Overdosage

Although no data are available, clinical experience with other immunoglobulin preparations suggests that the only manifestations would be pain and tenderness at the injection site.

Dosage and Administration

Parenteral drug products should be inspected visually for particulate matter and discoloration prior to administration, whenever solution and container permit. HEP-B-GAMMAGEE is a clear, very slightly amber, moderately viscous liquid.
HEP-B-GAMMAGEE is administered *intramuscularly. It must not be injected intravenously.*
It is important to use a separate sterile syringe and needle for each individual patient to prevent transmission of hepatitis B and other infectious agents from one person to another.

Adults
The recommended dose is 0.06 ml per kilogram of body weight; the usual adult dose is 3 to 5 ml administered intramuscularly, preferably in the gluteal or deltoid region. The appropriate dose should be administered as soon after exposure as possible (preferably within 7 days) and repeated 28–30 days after exposure.

Newborns
The immunization regimen for infants born to hepatitis B-positive (HBsAg-positive) mothers consists of three doses. A dose of 0.5 ml should be administered intramuscularly in the anterolateral thigh as soon after birth as possible and repeated at 3 months and 6 months of age. Administration of the first dose later than 24 hours after birth results in a progressive loss of efficacy.

How Supplied

No. 4692—HEP-B-GAMMAGEE is supplied as follows:
NDC 0006-4692-00 in 5 ml vials.
Store at 2–8° C (35.6–46.4° F). Do not freeze. Do not use after expiration date.
A.H.F.S. Category: 80:04
DC 7062006 Issued November 1982
COPYRIGHT© MERCK & CO., INC., 1983
All rights reserved

HEPTAVAX-B®
(hepatitis B vaccine, MSD)

Description

HEPTAVAX-B® (Hepatitis B Vaccine, MSD) is a non-infectious formalin-inactivated subunit viral vaccine derived from surface antigen (HBsAg or Australia antigen) of hepatitis B virus. The antigen is harvested and purified from the plasma of human carriers of hepatitis B virus according to methods developed by Merck, Sharp and Dohme Research Laboratories.
The starting plasma from which the antigen is extracted is obtained from a small, closely monitored population of asymptomatic HBsAg-positive donors. Periodically each donor is required to undergo a health examination, and appropriate laboratory tests are performed prior to each plasmapheresis.
The vaccine production process uses purification and inactivation steps which are known to remove or inactivate not only infectious hepatitis B virus particles, but also representatives of all known groups of animal viruses. Such groups include rhabdo-, pox-, toga-, reo-, herpes-, corona-, myxo-, picorna-, parvo-, and retrovirus; delta agent, and slow viruses.
Initial purification is accomplished by double ultracentrifugation. This is followed by an inactivation process consisting of three sequential treatments using pepsin, 8 Molar urea, and formalin. Each of these treatments alone has been shown to inactivate 10^5 or more infectious doses of hepatitis B virus/ml, and one or more of the treatments also has been shown to inactivate many other virus groups, including those listed above. In addition, studies in chimpanzees and humans show that hepatitis B vaccine produced according to this process does not transmit the agent(s) of non-A/non-B hepatitis. Follow-up data from clinical trials of HEPTAVAX-B provide no evidence to suggest transmission of Acquired Immune Deficiency Syndrome (AIDS) by this vaccine.
Each lot of hepatitis B vaccine is tested for sterility and is inoculated into cell cultures and several species of animals including chimpanzees, to rule out the presence of adventitious viruses.
HEPTAVAX-B is a sterile suspension for intramuscular injection; however, it may be administered subcutaneously to persons at risk of hemorrhage following intramuscular injections (see DOSAGE AND ADMINISTRATION). Each 1.0 ml dose of vaccine contains 20 mcg of hepatitis B surface antigen formulated in an alum adjuvant, and thimerosal (mercury derivative) 1:20,000 added as a preservative. The vaccine is prepared without regard to subtype. HEPTAVAX-B is indicated for immunization of persons at risk of infection from hepatitis B virus including all known subtypes.

Clinical Pharmacology

Hepatitis B virus is one of at least three hepatitis viruses that cause a systemic infection, with a major pathology in the liver. The others are hepatitis A virus, and non-A, non-B hepatitis viruses.
Hepatitis B virus is an important cause of viral hepatitis. There is no specific treatment for this disease. The incubation period for type B hepatitis

is relatively long; six weeks to six months may elapse between exposure and the onset of clinical symptoms. The prognosis following infection with hepatitis B virus is variable and dependent on at least three factors: (1) Age—Infants and younger children usually experience milder initial disease than older persons; (2) Dose of Virus—The higher the dose, the more likely acute icteric hepatitis B will result; and, (3) Severity of Associated Underlying Disease—Underlying malignancy or pre-existing hepatic disease predisposes to increased mortality and morbidity.

Persistence of viral infection (the chronic hepatitis B virus carrier state) occurs in 5–10% of persons following acute hepatitis B, and occurs more frequently after initial anicteric hepatitis B than after initial icteric disease. Consequently, carriers of HBsAg frequently give no history of recognized acute hepatitis. It has been estimated that more than 170 million people in the world today are persistently infected with hepatitis B virus. The Centers for Disease Control (CDC) estimates that there are approximately 0.7 to 1.0 million chronic carriers of hepatitis B virus in the USA and that this pool of carriers grows by 2%–3% (8,000 to 16,000 individuals) annually. Chronic carriers represent the largest human reservoir of hepatitis B virus.

The serious complications and sequelae of hepatitis B virus infection include massive hepatic necrosis, cirrhosis of the liver, chronic active hepatitis, and hepatocellular carcinoma. Chronic carriers of HBsAg appear to be at increased risk of developing hepatocellular carcinoma, which accounts for 80 to 90 percent of primary liver carcinomas. Although a number of etiologic factors are associated with development of hepatocellular carcinoma, the single most important etiologic factor appears to be active infection with the hepatitis B virus. There is also evidence that several diseases other than hepatitis have been associated with hepatitis B virus infection through an immunologic mechanism involving antigen-antibody complexes. Such diseases include a syndrome with rash, urticaria, and arthralgia resembling serum sickness; polyarteritis nodosa; membranous glomerulonephritis; and infantile papular acrodermatitis.

Although the vehicles for transmission of the virus are predominantly blood and blood products, viral antigen has also been found in tears, saliva, breast milk, urine, semen and vaginal secretions. Hepatitis B virus is quite stable and capable of surviving for days on environmental surfaces. Infection may occur when hepatitis B virus, transmitted by infected body fluids, is implanted via mucous surfaces or percutaneously introduced through accidental or deliberate breaks in the skin.

Transmission of hepatitis B virus infection is often associated with close interpersonal contact with an infected individual and with crowded living conditions. In such circumstances, transmission by inoculation via routes other then overt parenteral ones may be quite common.

Hepatitis B is endemic throughout the world and is a serious medical problem in population groups at increased risk. (Refer to INDICATIONS AND USAGE)

Numerous epidemiological studies have shown that persons who develop anti-HBs following active infection with the hepatitis B virus are protected against the disease on re-exposure to the virus. Clinical studies have established that HEPTAVAX-B characteristically induces protective antibody (anti-HBs) in most individuals who receive the recommended 3-dose regimen. Responsiveness is age-dependent, with children showing a more vigorous response than adults. Immunocompromised and immunosuppressed persons respond less well than do healthy individuals.

The protective efficacy of HEPTAVAX-B has been demonstrated in human populations. In the three clinical studies described below, the vaccine was virtually 100% effective in preventing hepatitis B in those who developed anti-HBs.

In one study involving individuals with a high risk of contracting hepatitis B virus infection, HEPTAVAX-B was shown to reduce the incidence of infection by 92%. The vaccine protected against acute hepatitis B, asymptomatic infection, and chronic antigenemia. There was evidence of immunity in 87% of vaccinated subjects after administration of two doses of the 3-dose vaccine regimen. However, the third dose was necessary to attain both a higher percentage of responses to the vaccine (96%) and a long-term protective effect (i.e., vaccine-induced antibody persisting during the entire 24-month follow-up period). In a second study of similar design, administration of three doses of vaccine induced immunity in 85% of recipients.

In a third study, conducted in medical staff at hemodialysis units, protective antibody developed in 96% of vaccine recipients after administration of three doses of vaccine. Additionally, this study demonstrated the subtype cross-protection of HEPTAVAX-B. A lot of the vaccine selected to contain only the *ad* antigenic subtype induced protection against infection from the *ay* subtype hepatitis B virus. These results confirm that monovalent HBsAg/*ad* vaccine can provide protection in populations at high risk of infection with the *ay* subtype virus (e.g., patients and staff in hemodialysis units and users of illicit injectable drugs).

Although the duration of protective effect of HEPTAVAX-B is unknown at present, available data suggest that immunity will last for about 5 years in patients who have received all 3 doses, after which time a single booster dose of vaccine might be necessary to maintain immunity.

Further study is required to determine the effectiveness of HEPTAVAX-B in preventing hepatitis B when the vaccine regimen is begun after an exposure to the hepatitis B virus has already occurred (i.e., use for post-exposure prophylaxis). Until those studies are complete, Hepatitis B Immune Globulin remains the treatment of choice for post-exposure prophylaxis. However, it has been demonstrated that doses up to 3 ml of Hepatitis B Immune Globulin, when administered simultaneously with HEPTAVAX-B at separate body sites, do not interfere with the induction of protective antibodies against hepatitis B virus.

Indications and Usage

HEPTAVAX-B is indicated for immunization against infection caused by all known subtypes of hepatitis B virus.

HEPTAVAX-B will not prevent hepatitis caused by other agents, such as hepatitis A virus, non-A, non-B hepatitis viruses, or other viruses known to infect the liver.

Vaccination is recommended in persons of all ages, especially those who are or will be at increased risk of infection with hepatitis B virus, for example:

- *Health Care Personnel*
  Dentists and oral surgeons.
  Physicians and surgeons.
  Nurses.
  Paramedical personnel and custodial staff who may be exposed to the virus via blood or other patient specimens.
  Dental hygienists and dental nurses.
  Laboratory personnel handling blood, blood products and other patient specimens.
  Dental, medical and nursing students.
- *Selected Patients and Patient Contacts*
  Patients and staff in hemodialysis units and hematology/oncology units.
  Patients requiring frequent and/or large volume blood transfusions or clotting factor concentrates (e.g., persons with hemophilia, thalassemia).
  Clients (residents) and staff of institutions for the mentally handicapped.
  Classroom contacts of deinstitutionalized mentally handicapped persons who have persistent hepatitis B antigenemia and who show aggressive behavior.
  Household and other intimate contacts of persons with persistent hepatitis B antigenemia.
- *Populations with high incidence of the disease,* such as:
  Alaskan Eskimos.
  Indochinese refugees.
  Haitian refugees.
- *Military Personnel identified as being at increased risk*
- *Morticians and Embalmers*
- *Blood bank and plasma fractionation workers*
- *Persons at Increased Risk of the Disease Due to Their Sexual Practices,* such as:
  Persons who repeatedly contract sexually transmitted diseases.
  Homosexually active males.
  Female prostitutes.
- *Prisoners*
- *Users of illicit injectable drugs*

Revaccination
See CLINICAL PHARMACOLOGY

Contraindications

Hypersensitivity to any component of the vaccine.

Warnings

Persons with immuno-deficiency or those receiving immunosuppressive therapy require larger vaccine doses and respond less well than do healthy individuals. Refer to DOSAGE AND ADMINISTRATION for use in such individuals.

Because of the long incubation period for hepatitis B, it is possible for unrecognized infection to be present at the time HEPTAVAX-B is given. HEPTAVAX-B may not prevent hepatitis B in such patients.

Precautions

General
As with any parenteral vaccine, epinephrine should be available for immediate use should an anaphylactoid reaction occur.

Any serious active infection is reason for delaying use of HEPTAVAX-B, except when, in the opinion of the physician, withholding the vaccine entails a greater risk.

Caution and appropriate care should be exercised in administering HEPTAVAX-B to individuals with severely compromised cardiopulmonary status or to others in whom a febrile or systemic reaction could pose a significant risk.

Pregnancy
Pregnancy Category C. Animal reproduction studies have not been conducted with HEPTAVAX-B. It is also not known whether HEPTAVAX-B can cause fetal harm when administered to a pregnant woman or can affect reproductive capacity. HEPTAVAX-B should be given to a pregnant woman only if clearly needed.

Nursing Mothers
It is not known whether this drug is secreted in human milk. Because many drugs are secreted in human milk, caution should be exercised when HEPTAVAX-B is administered to a nursing woman.

Pediatric Use
HEPTAVAX-B has been shown to be well-tolerated and highly immunogenic in infants and children of all ages. Newborns also respond well; maternally transferred antibodies do not interfere with the active immune response to the vaccine. See DOSAGE AND ADMINISTRATION for recommended pediatric dosage.

Infants Born to HBsAg Positive Mothers
Hepatitis B Immune Globulin currently is the treatment of choice for infants born to HBsAg positive mothers. Ongoing clinical studies should show whether vaccine alone and/or vaccine plus Hepatitis B Immune Globulin are also effective in these infants.

Continued on next page

Information on the Merck Sharp & Dohme products listed on these pages is the full prescribing information from product circulars in use November 1, 1984.

Merck Sharp & Dohme—Cont.

Adverse Reactions

HEPTAVAX-B is generally well tolerated. No serious adverse reactions attributable to vaccination were reported during the course of clinical trials involving administration of HEPTAVAX-B to over 19,000 individuals. As with any vaccine, there is the possibility that broad use of the vaccine could reveal rare adverse reactions not observed in clinical trials.

In three double-blind placebo-controlled studies among 3,350 persons, the overall rates of adverse reactions reported by vaccine recipients (24.3%, 21.5% and 22.8%) did not differ significantly from those of placebo recipients (21.4%, 18.7% and 21.9%). Approximately half of all reported reactions were injection site soreness, which occurred somewhat more frequently among vaccine recipients.

Other less common local reactions have included erythema, swelling, warmth, or induration. These signs and symptoms of local inflammation are generally well tolerated and usually subside within 2 days of vaccination.

Low-grade fever (less than 101°F) occurs occasionally and is usually confined to the 48-hour period following vaccination. Although uncommon, fever over 102°F has been reported.

Systemic complaints including malaise, fatigue, headache, nausea, vomiting, dizziness, myalgia, and arthralgia are infrequent. Rash has been reported rarely.

Neurological disorders such as paresthesias and acute radiculoneuropathy including Guillain-Barré syndrome have been rarely reported in temporal association with administration of HEPTAVAX-B. No cause and effect relationship has been established.

Dosage and Administration

Do not inject intravenously or intradermally.
HEPTAVAX-B is for intramuscular injection. It may, however, be administered subcutaneously to persons at risk of hemorrhage following intramuscular injections. The immune responses and clinical reactions following intramuscular and subcutaneous administration of HEPTAVAX-B have been shown to be comparable. However, when other aluminum-absorbed vaccines have been administered subcutaneously, an increased incidence of local reactions including subcutaneous nodules has been observed. Therefore, subcutaneous administration should be used only in persons (e.g., hemophiliacs) at risk of hemorrhage following intramuscular injections.

Shake well before withdrawal and use. Thorough agitation at the time of administration is necessary to maintain suspension of the vaccine.
Parenteral drug products should be inspected visually for particulate matter and discoloration prior to administration. After thorough agitation, HEPTAVAX-B is a slightly opaque, white suspension. The immunization regimen consists of 3 doses of vaccine given according to the following schedule:

1st dose: at elected date
2nd dose: 1 month later
3rd dose: 6 months after the first dose
The volume of vaccine to be given on each occasion is as follows:
[See table below].
Revaccination (booster)—See CLINICAL PHARMACOLOGY.
Store unopened and opened vials at 2–8°C (35.6–46.4°F).
Do not freeze since freezing destroys potency. The vaccine is used as supplied; no dilution or reconstitution is necessary.
It is important to use a separate sterile syringe and needle for each individual patient to prevent transmission of hepatitis and other infectious agents from one person to another.
3.0 ml Vial
For Syringe Use Only: Withdraw the recommended dose from the vial using a sterile needle and syringe free of preservatives, antiseptics, and detergents.

How Supplied

No. 4720—HEPTAVAX-B is supplied as follows:
NDC 0006-4720-00 in a 3 ml vial.
A.H.F.S. Category: 80:12
DC 7207001 Issued March 1983
COPYRIGHT © MERCK & CO., INC., 1983
All rights reserved

**HYDELTRA–T.B.A.® Suspension   ℞
(prednisolone tebutate, MSD), U.S.P.**

For intra-articular, intralesional, and soft tissue injection only.

Description

Prednisolone tebutate, a synthetic adrenocortical steroid, is a white to slightly yellow powder sparingly soluble in alcohol, freely soluble in chloroform, and very slightly soluble in water. The molecular weight is 476.61 (monohydrate). It is designated chemically as 11β,17- dihydroxy - 21 - [(3,3-dimethyl-1-oxobutyl)oxy]   pregna-1,4-diene-3,20-dione. The empirical formula is $C_{27}H_{38}O_6$.
HYDELTRA-T.B.A.® (Prednisolone Tebutate, MSD) suspension is a white to slightly yellow suspension (pH 6.0 to 8.0) that settles upon standing. Each ml contains prednisolone tebutate, 20 mg. Inactive ingredients per ml: sodium citrate, 1 mg; polysorbate 80, 1 mg; sorbitol solution, 0.5 ml (equal to 450 mg d-sorbitol); Water for Injection, q.s., 1 ml. Benzyl alcohol, 9 mg, added as preservative.

Actions

HYDELTRA-T.B.A. has a slow onset but long duration of action when compared with more soluble preparations. Because of its slight solubility, it is suitable for intraarticular, intralesional, and soft tissue injection where its anti-inflammatory effects are confined mainly to the area in which it has been injected, although it is capable of producing systemic hormonal effects.
Naturally occurring glucocorticoids (hydrocortisone and cortisone), which also have salt-retaining properties, are used as replacement therapy in adrenocortical deficiency states. Their synthetic analogs, including prednisolone, are primarily used for their potent anti-inflammatory effects in disorders of many organ systems.
Glucocorticoids cause profound and varied metabolic effects. In addition, they modify the body's immune responses to diverse stimuli.

Indications

A. By intra-articular or soft tissue injection:
As adjunctive therapy for short-term administration (to tide the patient over an acute episode or exacerbation) in:
  Synovitis of osteoarthritis
  Rheumatoid arthritis
  Acute and subacute bursitis
  Acute gouty arthritis
  Epicondylitis
  Acute nonspecific tenosynovitis
  Post-traumatic osteoarthritis
B. By intralesional injection:
May be useful in cystic tumors of an aponeurosis or tendon (ganglia).

Contraindications

Systemic fungal infections
Hypersensitivity to any component of this product

Warnings

In patients on corticosteroid therapy subjected to any unusual stress, increased dosage of rapidly acting corticosteroids before, during, and after the stressful situation is indicated.
Drug-induced secondary adrenocortical insufficiency may result from too rapid withdrawal of corticosteroids and may be minimized by gradual reduction of dosage. This type of relative insufficiency may persist for months after discontinuation of therapy; therefore, in any situation of stress occurring during that period, hormone therapy should be reinstituted. If the patient is receiving steroids already, dosage may have to be increased. Since mineralocorticoid secretion may be impaired, salt and/or a mineralocorticoid should be administered concurrently.
Corticosteroids may mask some signs of infection, and new infections may appear during their use. There may be decreased resistance and inability to localize infection when corticosteroids are used. Moreover, corticosteroids may affect the nitro-blue-tetrazolium test for bacterial infection and produce false negative results.
In cerebral malaria, a double-blind trial has shown that the use of corticosteroids is associated with prolongation of coma and a higher incidence of pneumonia and gastrointestinal bleeding.
Corticosteroids may activate latent amebiasis. Therefore, it is recommended that latent or active amebiasis be ruled out before initiating corticosteroid therapy in any patient who has spent time in the tropics or any patient with unexplained diarrhea.
Prolonged use of corticosteroids may produce posterior subcapsular cataracts, glaucoma with possible damage to the optic nerves, and may enhance the establishment of secondary ocular infections due to fungi or viruses.
Usage in pregnancy. Since adequate human reproduction studies have not been done with corticosteroids, use of these drugs in pregnancy or in women of childbearing potential requires that the anticipated benefits be weighed against the possible hazards to the mother and embryo or fetus. Infants born of mothers who have received substantial doses of corticosteroids during pregnancy should be carefully observed for signs of hypoadrenalism.
Corticosteroids appear in breast milk and could suppress growth, interfere with endogenous corticosteroid production, or cause other unwanted effects. Mothers taking pharmacologic doses of corticosteroids should be advised not to nurse.
Average and large doses of cortisone or hydrocortisone can cause elevation of blood pressure, salt and water retention, and increased excretion of potas-

HEPTAVAX-B Group	Initial	1 month	6 months
Younger Children (Birth to 10 years of age)	0.5 ml	0.5 ml	0.5 ml
Adults and Older Children	1.0 ml	1.0 ml	1.0 ml
Dialysis Patients and Immunocompromised Patients	2.0 ml*	2.0 ml*	2.0 ml*

*Two 1.0 ml doses given at different sites.

sium. These effects are less likely to occur with the synthetic derivatives except when used in large doses. Dietary salt restriction and potassium supplementation may be necessary. All corticosteroids increase calcium excretion.

Administration of live virus vaccines, including smallpox, is contraindicated in individuals receiving immunosuppressive doses of corticosteroids. If inactivated viral or bacterial vaccines are administered to individuals receiving immunosuppressive doses of corticosteroids, the expected serum antibody response may not be obtained.

If corticosteroids are indicated in patients with latent tuberculosis or tuberculin reactivity, close observation is necessary as reactivation of the disease may occur. During prolonged corticosteroid therapy, these patients should receive chemoprophylaxis.

Because rare instances of anaphylactoid reactions have occurred in patients receiving parenteral corticosteroid therapy, appropriate precautionary measures should be taken prior to administration, especially when the patient has a history of allergy to any drug.

Precautions

This product, like many other steroid formulations, is sensitive to heat. Therefore, it should not be autoclaved when it is desirable to sterilize the exterior of the vial.

Following prolonged therapy, withdrawal of corticosteroids may result in symptoms of the corticosteroid withdrawal syndrome including fever, myalgia, arthralgia, and malaise. This may occur in patients even without evidence of adrenal insufficiency.

There is an enhanced effect of corticosteroids in patients with hypothyroidism and in those with cirrhosis.

Corticosteroids should be used cautiously in patients with ocular herpes simplex for fear of corneal perforation.

Psychic derangements may appear when corticosteroids are used, ranging from euphoria, insomnia, mood swings, personality changes, and severe depression to frank psychotic manifestations. Also, existing emotional instability or psychotic tendencies may be aggravated by corticosteroids.

Aspirin should be used cautiously in conjunction with corticosteroids in hypoprothrombinemia.

Steroids should be used with caution in nonspecific ulcerative colitis, if there is a probability of impending perforation, abscess, or other pyogenic infection, also in diverticulitis, fresh intestinal anastomoses, active or latent peptic ulcer, renal insufficiency, hypertension, osteoporosis, and myasthenia gravis. Signs of peritoneal irritation following gastrointestinal perforation in patients receiving large doses of corticosteroids may be minimal or absent. Fat embolism has been reported as a possible complication of hypercortisonism.

When large doses are given, some authorities advise that antacids be administered between meals to help to prevent peptic ulcer.

Growth and development of infants and children on prolonged corticosteroid therapy should be carefully followed.

Steroids may increase or decrease motility and number of spermatozoa in some patients.

Phenytoin, phenobarbital, ephedrine, and rifampin may enhance the metabolic clearance of corticosteroids, resulting in decreased blood levels and lessened physiologic activity, thus requiring adjustment in corticosteroid dosage.

The prothrombin time should be checked frequently in patients who are receiving corticosteroids and coumarin anticoagulants at the same time because of reports that corticosteroids have altered the response to these anticoagulants. Studies have shown that the usual effect produced by adding corticosteroids is inhibition of response to coumarins, although there have been some conflicting reports of potentiation not substantiated by studies.

When corticosteroids are administered concomitantly with potassium-depleting diuretics, patients should be observed closely for development of hypokalemia.

Intra-articular injection of a corticosteroid may produce systemic as well as local effects.

Appropriate examination of any joint fluid present is necessary to exclude a septic process.

A marked increase in pain accompanied by local swelling, further restriction of joint motion, fever, and malaise is suggestive of septic arthritis. If this complication occurs and the diagnosis of sepsis is confirmed, appropriate antimicrobial therapy should be instituted.

Injection of a steroid into an infected site is to be avoided.

Corticosteroids should not be injected into unstable joints.

Patients should be impressed strongly with the importance of not overusing joints in which symptomatic benefit has been obtained as long as the inflammatory process remains active.

Frequent intra-articular injection may result in damage to joint tissues.

Adverse Reactions

Fluid and electrolyte disturbances
  Sodium retention
  Fluid retention
  Congestive heart failure in susceptible patients
  Potassium loss
  Hypokalemic alkalosis
  Hypertension
Musculoskeletal
  Muscle weakness
  Steroid myopathy
  Loss of muscle mass
  Osteoporosis
  Vertebral compression fractures
  Aseptic necrosis of femoral and humeral heads
  Pathologic fracture of long bones
  Tendon rupture
Gastrointestinal
  Peptic ulcer with possible subsequent perforation and hemorrhage
  Perforation of the small and large bowel, particularly in patients with inflammatory bowel disease
  Pancreatitis
  Abdominal distention
  Ulcerative esophagitis
Dermatologic
  Impaired wound healing
  Thin fragile skin
  Petechiae and ecchymoses
  Erythema
  Increased sweating
  May suppress reactions to skin tests
  Other cutaneous reactions, such as allergic dermatitis, urticaria, angioneurotic edema
Neurologic
  Convulsions
  Increased intracranial pressure with papilledema (pseudotumor cerebri) usually after treatment
  Vertigo
  Headache
Endocrine
  Menstrual irregularities
  Development of cushingoid state
  Suppression of growth in children
  Secondary adrenocortical and pituitary unresponsiveness, particularly in times of stress, as in trauma, surgery, or illness
  Decreased carbohydrate tolerance
  Manifestations of latent diabetes mellitus
  Increased requirements for insulin or oral hypoglycemic agents in diabetics
  Hirsutism
Ophthalmic
  Posterior subcapsular cataracts
  Increased intraocular pressure
  Glaucoma
  Exophthalmos
Metabolic
  Negative nitrogen balance due to protein catabolism

Other
  Anaphylactoid or hypersensitivity reactions
  Thromboembolism
  Weight gain
  Increased appetite
  Nausea
  Malaise

Foreign body granulomatous reactions involving the synovium have been reported with repeated injections of HYDELTRA-T.B.A.

Localized pain and swelling, sometimes distal to the site of injection and persisting for several days, have been reported.

The following *additional* adverse reactions are related to injection of corticosteroids:
  Rare instances of blindness associated with intralesional therapy around the face and head
  Hyperpigmentation or hypopigmentation
  Subcutaneous and cutaneous atrophy
  Sterile abscess
  Postinjection flare (following intra-articular use)
  Charcot-like arthropathy

Dosage and Administration

For intra-articular, intralesional, and soft tissue injection only.

DOSAGE AND FREQUENCY OF INJECTION ARE VARIABLE AND MUST BE INDIVIDUALIZED ON THE BASIS OF THE DISEASE AND THE RESPONSE OF THE PATIENT.

The initial dose varies from 4 to 40 mg depending on the disease being treated and the size of the area to be injected. Frequency of injection depends on symptomatic response, and usually is once every two or three weeks. Severe conditions may require injection once a week. Frequent intra-articular injection may result in damage to joint tissues. If satisfactory clinical response does not occur after a reasonable period of time, discontinue HYDELTRA-T.B.A. suspension and transfer the patient to other therapy.

Patients should be observed closely for signs that might require dosage adjustment, including changes in clinical status resulting from remissions or exacerbations of the disease, and individual drug responsiveness.

For rapid onset of action, a soluble adrenocortical hormone preparation, such as DECADRON® phosphate (Dexamethasone Sodium Phosphate, MSD) injection or HYDELTRASOL® (Prednisolone Sodium Phosphate, MSD) injection, may be given with HYDELTRA-T.B.A.

If desired, a local anesthetic may be used, and may be injected before HYDELTRA-T.B.A., or mixed in a syringe with HYDELTRA-T.B.A. and given simultaneously.

If used prior to intra-articular injection of the steroid, inject most of the anesthetic into the soft tissues of the surrounding area and instill a small amount into the joint.

If given together, mixing should be done in the injection syringe by drawing the steroid in *first*, then the anesthetic. In this way, the anesthetic will not be introduced inadvertently into the vial of steroid. *The mixture must be used immediately and any unused portion discarded.*

Some of the usual single doses are:

Large Joints (e.g., Knee)	20 mg (1 ml), occasionally 30 mg (1.5 ml). Doses over 40 mg (2 ml) not recommended.

Continued on next page

Information on the Merck Sharp & Dohme products listed on these pages is the full prescribing information from product circulars in use November 1, 1984.

Merck Sharp & Dohme—Cont.

Small Joints (e.g., Interphalangeal, Temporomandibular)	8 to 10 mg (0.4 to 0.5 ml).
Bursae	20 to 30 mg (1 to 1.5 ml).
Tendon Sheaths	4 to 10 mg (0.2 to 0.5 ml).
Ganglia	10 to 20 mg (0.5 to 1 ml).

How Supplied

No. 7572—Suspenson HYDELTRA-T.B.A., 20 mg per ml, is a white, milky suspension, and is supplied as follows:
NDC 0006-7572-01 in 1 ml vials
(6505-00-225-7499 1 ml vial)
NDC 0006-7572-03 in 5 ml vials
(6505-00-890-1353 5 ml vial).
   A.H.F.S. Category: 68:04
   DC 6138622   Issued April 1983

HYDROCORTONE® Acetate ℞
Sterile Ophthalmic Ointment
(hydrocortisone acetate, MSD), U.S.P.
HYDROCORTONE® Acetate ℞
Sterile Ophthalmic Suspension
(hydrocortisone acetate, MSD), U.S.P.

Description

Sterile Ophthalmic Ointment HYDROCORTONE® Acetate (Hydrocortisone Acetate, MSD) 1.5% is a topical steroid preparation containing 15 mg of hydrocortisone acetate in a white petrolatum and mineral oil base in each gram.
Sterile Ophthalmic Suspension HYDROCORTONE® Acetate 2.5% contains 25 mg of hydrocortisone acetate in each milliliter. Inactive ingredients: sodium citrate, dibasic sodium phosphate, monobasic sodium phosphate, sodium chloride, polyethylene glycol 4000, polysorbate 80, and water for injection. Benzyl alcohol 0.5%, and benzalkonium chloride, 0.02%, are added as preservatives.

Action

Inhibition of inflammatory response to inciting agents of mechanical, chemical or immunological nature. No generally accepted explanation of this steroid property has been advanced.

Indications

For the treatment of the following conditions:
Ophthalmic:
Steroid responsive inflammatory conditions of the palpebral and bulbar conjunctiva, cornea, and anterior segment of the globe, such as allergic conjunctivitis, acne rosacea, superficial punctate keratitis, herpes zoster keratitis, iritis, cyclitis, selected infective conjunctivitis when the inherent hazard of steroid use is accepted to obtain an advisable diminution in edema and inflammation; corneal injury from chemical or thermal burns, or penetration of foreign bodies.
Otic:
Steroid responsive inflammatory conditions of the external auditory meatus, such as allergic otitis externa, selected purulent and nonpurulent infective otitis externa when the hazard of steroid use is accepted to obtain an advisable diminution in edema and inflammation.

Contraindications

Acute superficial herpes simplex keratitis. Fungal diseases of ocular or auricular structures.
Acute infectious stages of vaccinia, varicella and most other viral diseases of the cornea and conjunctiva.
Tuberculosis of the eye.
Hypersensitivity to a component of this medication.
Perforation of a drum membrane.

Warnings

Employment of steroid medication in the treatment of stromal herpes simplex requires great caution; frequent slit-lamp microscopy is mandatory.
Prolonged use may result in elevated intraocular pressure and/or glaucoma, damage to the optic nerve, defects in visual acuity and fields of vision, posterior subcapsular cataract formation, or may result in secondary ocular infections.
Viral, bacterial, and fungal infections of the cornea may be exacerbated by the application of steroids.
Acute purulent untreated infection of the eye or ear may be masked or activity enhanced by the presence of steroid medication.
In those diseases causing thinning of the cornea or sclera, perforation has been known to occur with the use of topical steroids.
Usage in Pregnancy
Safety of intensive or protracted use of topical steroids during pregnancy has not been substantiated.

Precautions

As fungal infections of the cornea are particularly prone to develop coincidentally with long-term local steroid applications, fungus invasion must be considered in any persistent corneal ulceration where a steroid has been used or is in use.
Intraocular pressure should be checked frequently.

Adverse Reactions

Glaucoma with optic nerve damage, visual acuity and field defects, posterior subcapsular cataract formation, secondary ocular infection from pathogens including herpes simplex, perforation of the globe.
Rarely, filtering blebs have been reported when topical steroids have been used following cataract surgery.
Rarely, stinging or burning may occur.

Dosage and Administration

The duration of treatment will vary with the type of lesion and may extend from a few days to several weeks, according to therapeutic response. Relapses, more common in chronic active lesions than in self-limited conditions, usually respond to retreatment.
Ophthalmic Suspension HYDROCORTONE Acetate (Hydrocortisone Acetate, MSD)
Eye—Instill one or two drops into the conjunctival sac every hour during the day and every two hours during the night as initial therapy. When a favorable response is observed, reduce dosage to one drop every four hours. Later, further reduction in dosage to one drop three or four times daily may suffice to control symptoms.
Ear—Clean the aural canal thoroughly and sponge dry. Instill ophthalmic suspension HYDROCORTONE acetate directly into the aural canal by use of the dropper. A suggested initial dosage is three or four drops two or three times a day. When a favorable response is obtained, reduce dosage gradually and eventually discontinue. If preferred, the aural canal may be packed with a gauze wick saturated with ophthalmic suspension HYDROCORTONE acetate. Keep the wick moist with the preparation and remove from the ear after 12 to 24 hours. Treatment may be repeated as often as necessary at the discretion of the physician.
Ophthalmic Ointment HYDROCORTONE Acetate (Hydrocortisone Acetate, MSD)
Eye—Apply a thin coating to the affected area three or four times a day. When a favorable response is observed, reduce the number of daily applications to two, and later to one a day as a maintenance dose if this proves sufficient to control symptoms.
Ophthalmic ointment HYDROCORTONE acetate is particularly convenient when an eye pad is used. It may also be the preparation of choice for patients in whom therapeutic benefit depends on prolonged contact of the active ingredients with ocular tissues.
Ear—Clean the aural canal thoroughly and sponge dry. With a cotton-tipped applicator, apply a thin coating of ophthalmic ointment HYDROCORTONE acetate to the affected canal area two or three times a day. When a favorable response is obtained, reduce the number of daily applications to one or two, and eventually discontinue.

Storage

Ophthalmic suspension HYDROCORTONE acetate should be protected from freezing to avoid the possibility of the formation of aggregates or larger crystals which may render the product unsuitable for use. It is supplied as a sterile preparation. Care should be exercised to avoid contamination.

How Supplied

No. 7504—1.5% Sterile Ophthalmic Ointment HYDROCORTONE Acetate, is a clear, unctuous ointment, supplied as follows:
NDC 0006-7504-04 in 3.5 g tubes, each gram containing 15 mg hydrocortisone acetate in a white petrolatum and mineral oil base.
No. 7506—2.5% Sterile Ophthalmic Suspension HYDROCORTONE Acetate, is a sterile, white suspension supplied as follows:
NDC 0006-7506-03 in 5 ml dropper bottles, each milliliter containing 25 mg hydrocortisone acetate.
   A.H.F.S. Category: 52:08
   DC 6007521   Issued May 1981

HydroDIURIL® Tablets ℞
(hydrochlorothiazide, MSD), U.S.P.

Description

HydroDIURIL® (Hydrochlorothiazide, MSD) is the 3,4-dihydro derivative of chlorothiazide. Its chemical name is 6-chloro-3,4-dihydro-2H-1,2,4-benzothiadiazine-7-sulfonamide 1,1-dioxide.
It is a white, or practically white, crystalline compound slightly soluble in water, but freely soluble in sodium hydroxide solution.

Actions

HydroDIURIL is a diuretic and antihypertensive. HydroDIURIL affects the renal tubular mechanism of electrolyte reabsorption. At maximal therapeutic dosage all thiazides are approximately equal in their diuretic efficacy.
HydroDIURIL increases excretion of sodium and chloride in approximately equivalent amounts. Natriuresis may be accompanied by some loss of potassium and bicarbonate.
After oral use diuresis begins within 2 hours, peaks in about 4 hours and lasts about 6 to 12 hours. HydroDIURIL is eliminated rapidly by the kidney.
The mechanism of the antihypertensive effect of thiazides is unknown. HydroDIURIL does not affect normal blood pressure.

Indications

HydroDIURIL is indicated as adjunctive therapy in edema associated with congestive heart failure, hepatic cirrhosis, and corticosteroid and estrogen therapy.
HydroDIURIL has also been found useful in edema due to various forms of renal dysfunction such as nephrotic syndrome, acute glomerulonephritis, and chronic renal failure.
HydroDIURIL is indicated in the management of hypertension either as the sole therapeutic agent or to enhance the effectiveness of other antihypertensive drugs in the more severe forms of hypertension.

Product Information

Use in Pregnancy. Routine use of diuretics during normal pregnancy is inappropriate and exposes mother and fetus to unnecessary hazard. Diuretics do not prevent development of toxemia of pregnancy and there is no satisfactory evidence that they are useful in the treatment of toxemia.

Edema during pregnancy may arise from pathologic causes or from the physiologic and mechanical consequences of pregnancy. Thiazides are indicated in pregnancy when edema is due to pathologic causes, just as they are in the absence of pregnancy (however, see WARNINGS). Dependent edema in pregnancy, resulting from restriction of venous return by the gravid uterus, is properly treated through elevation of the lower extremities and use of support stockings. Use of diuretics to lower intravascular volume in this instance is illogical and unnecessary. During normal pregnancy there is hypervolemia which is not harmful to the fetus or the mother in the absence of cardiovascular disease. However, it may be associated with edema, rarely generalized edema. If such edema causes discomfort, increased recumbency will often provide relief. Rarely this edema may cause extreme discomfort which is not relieved by rest. In these instances, a short course of diuretic therapy may provide relief and be appropriate.

Contraindications

Anuria.
Hypersensitivity to this product or to other sulfonamide-derived drugs.

Warnings

Use with caution in severe renal disease. In patients with renal disease, thiazides may precipitate azotemia. Cumulative effects of the drug may develop in patients with impaired renal function. Thiazides should be used with caution in patients with impaired hepatic function or progressive liver disease, since minor alterations of fluid and electrolyte balance may precipitate hepatic coma. Thiazides may add to or potentiate the action of other antihypertensive drugs.

Sensitivity reactions may occur in patients with or without a history of allergy or bronchial asthma. The possibility of exacerbation or activation of systemic lupus erythematosus has been reported. Lithium generally should not be given with diuretics because they reduce its renal clearance and add a high risk of lithium toxicity. Read circulars for lithium preparations before use of such concomitant therapy.

Use in Pregnancy. Thiazides cross the placental barrier and appear in cord blood. The use of thiazides in pregnancy requires that the anticipated benefit be weighed against possible hazards to the fetus. These hazards include fetal or neonatal jaundice, thrombocytopenia, and possibly other adverse reactions which have occurred in the adult.

Nursing Mothers. Thiazides appear in breast milk. If use of the drug is deemed essential, the patient should stop nursing.

Precautions

Periodic determination of serum electrolytes to detect possible electrolyte imbalance should be performed at appropriate intervals.
All patients receiving diuretic therapy should be observed for evidence of fluid or electrolyte imbalance: namely, hyponatremia, hypochloremic alkalosis, and hypokalemia. Serum and urine electrolyte determinations are particularly important when the patient is vomiting excessively or receiving parenteral fluids. Warning signs or symptoms of fluid and electrolyte imbalance include dryness of mouth, thirst, weakness, lethargy, drowsiness, restlessness, muscle pains or cramps, muscular fatigue, hypotension, oliguria, tachycardia, and gastrointestinal disturbances such as nausea and vomiting.

Hypokalemia may develop, especially with brisk diuresis, when severe cirrhosis is present, during concomitant use of corticosteroids or ACTH, or after prolonged therapy.

Interference with adequate oral electrolyte intake will also contribute to hypokalemia. Hypokalemia can sensitize or exaggerate the response of the heart to the toxic effects of digitalis (e.g., increased ventricular irritability). Hypokalemia may be avoided or treated by use of potassium supplements such as foods with a high potassium content.

Although any chloride deficit is generally mild and usually does not require specific treatment except under extraordinary circumstances (as in liver disease or renal disease), chloride replacement may be required in the treatment of metabolic alkalosis.

Dilutional hyponatremia may occur in edematous patients in hot weather; appropriate therapy is water restriction, rather than administration of salt, except in rare instances when the hyponatremia is life threatening. In actual salt depletion, appropriate replacement is the therapy of choice.

Hyperuricemia may occur or acute gout may be precipitated in certain patients receiving thiazides.

Insulin requirements in diabetic patients may be increased, decreased, or unchanged. Latent diabetes mellitus may become manifest during thiazide therapy.

Thiazides may increase the responsiveness to tubocurarine.

The antihypertensive effects of the drug may be enhanced in the postsympathectomy patient. Thiazides may decrease arterial responsiveness to norepinephrine. This diminution is not sufficient to preclude effectiveness of the pressor agent for therapeutic use.

If progressive renal impairment becomes evident, consider withholding or discontinuing diuretic therapy.

Thiazides may decrease serum PBI levels without signs of thyroid disturbance.

Thiazides may decrease urinary calcium excretion. Thiazides may cause intermittent and slight elevation of serum calcium in the absence of known disorders of calcium metabolism. Marked hypercalcemia may be evidence of hidden hyperparathyroidism. Thiazides should be discontinued before carrying out tests for parathyroid function.

Adverse Reactions

Body as a Whole: Weakness.
Cardiovascular: Orthostatic hypotension (may be aggravated by alcohol, barbiturates, or narcotics).
Digestive: Anorexia, gastric irritation, nausea, vomiting, cramping, diarrhea, constipation, jaundice (intrahepatic cholestatic jaundice), pancreatitis, sialadenitis.
Hematologic: Leukopenia, agranulocytosis, thrombocytopenia, aplastic anemia, hemolytic anemia.
Metabolic: Hyperglycemia, glycosuria, hyperuricemia, electrolyte imbalance (see PRECAUTIONS).
Musculoskeletal: Muscle spasm.
Nervous System/Psychiatric: Dizziness, vertigo, paresthesias, headache, restlessness.
Special Senses: Transient blurred vision, xanthopsia.
Hypersensitivity: Purpura, photosensitivity, rash, urticaria, necrotizing angiitis (vasculitis and cutaneous vasculitis), fever, respiratory distress including pneumonitis and pulmonary edema, anaphylactic reactions.
Whenever adverse reactions are moderate or severe, thiazide dosage should be reduced or therapy withdrawn.

Dosage and Administration

Therapy should be individualized according to patient response. Use the smallest dosage necessary to achieve the required response.

Adults
For Diuresis
The usual adult dosage is 50 to 100 mg once or twice a day. Many patients with edema respond to intermittent therapy, i.e., administration on alternate days or on three to five days each week. With an intermittent schedule, excessive response and the resulting undesirable electrolyte imbalance are less likely to occur.

For Control of Hypertension
The usual adult starting dosage is 50 or 100 mg a day as a single or divided dose. Dosage is increased or decreased according to blood pressure response. Rarely some patients may require up to 200 mg a day in divided doses.
When thiazides are used with other antihypertensives, the dose of the latter may need to be reduced to prevent excessive decrease in blood pressure.

Infants and Children
The usual pediatric dosage is based on 1.0 mg of HydroDIURIL per pound of body weight per day in two doses. Infants under 6 months of age may require up to 1.5 mg per pound per day in two doses. On this basis, infants up to 2 years of age may be given 12.5 to 37.5 mg daily in two doses. Children from 2 to 12 years of age may be given 37.5 to 100 mg daily in two doses. Dosage in both age groups should be based on body weight.

How Supplied

No. 3263—Tablets HydroDIURIL, 25 mg, are peach-colored, round, scored, compressed tablets, coded MSD 42. They are supplied as follows:
NDC 0006-0042-68 bottles of 100
NDC 0006-0042-28 unit dose packages of 100
NDC 0006-0042-82 bottles of 1000.
Shown in Product Identification Section, page 420
No. 3264—Tablets HydroDIURIL, 50 mg, are peach-colored, round, scored, compressed tablets, coded MSD 105. They are supplied as follows:
NDC 0006-0105-68 bottles of 100
NDC 0006-0105-28 unit dose packages of 100
NDC 0006-0105-82 bottles of 1000
NDC 0006-0105-86 bottles of 5000.
Shown in Product Identification Section, page 420
No. 3340—Tablets HydroDIURIL, 100 mg, are peach-colored, round, scored, compressed tablets, coded MSD 410. They are supplied as follows:
NDC 0006-0410-68 bottles of 100.
Shown in Product Identification Section, page 420
A.H.F.S. Category: 40:28
DC 6028533 Issued November 1983
COPYRIGHT © MERCK & CO., INC., 1983
All rights reserved

HYDROPRES® Tablets ℞
(reserpine-hydrochlorothiazide, MSD), U.S.P.

WARNING

This fixed combination drug is not indicated for initial therapy of hypertension. Hypertension requires therapy titrated to the individual patient. If the fixed combination represents the dosage so determined, its use may be more convenient in patient management. The treatment of hypertension is not static, but must be re-evaluated as conditions in each patient warrant.

Description

HYDROPRES® (Reserpine-Hydrochlorothiazide, MSD) combines two antihypertensive agents: HydroDIURIL® (Hydrochlorothiazide, MSD) and reserpine. The chemical name for hydrochlorothiazide is 6-chloro-3, 4-dihydro-2H-1,2,4-benzothiadiazine-7-sulfonamide 1,1-dioxide. Reserpine (11, 17α-dimethoxy -18β- [(3,4,5-trimethoxybenzoyl)oxy]-3β, 20α-yohimban-16β-carboxylic acid meth-

Continued on next page

Merck Sharp & Dohme—Cont.

yl ester) is a crystalline alkaloid derived from Rauwolfia serpentina.

Actions

Hydrochlorothiazide

Hydrochlorothiazide is a diuretic and antihypertensive. It affects the renal tubular mechanism of electrolyte reabsorption. At maximal therapeutic dosage all thiazides are approximately equal in their diuretic efficacy.

Hydrochlorothiazide increases excretion of sodium and chloride in approximately equivalent amounts. Natriuresis may be accompanied by some loss of potassium and bicarbonate.

The mechanism of the antihypertensive effect of thiazides is unknown. Hydrochlorothiazide does not affect normal blood pressure.

Hydrochlorothiazide is eliminated rapidly by the kidney.

Reserpine

Reserpine has antihypertensive, bradycardic, and tranquilizing properties. It lowers arterial blood pressure by depletion of catecholamines. Reserpine is beneficial in relieving anxiety, tension, and headache in the hypertensive patient. It acts at the hypothalamic level of the central nervous system to promote relaxation without hypnosis or analgesia. The sleep pattern shown by the electroencephalogram following barbiturates does not occur with this drug. In laboratory animals spontaneous activity and response to external stimuli are decreased, but confusion or difficulty of movement is not evident.

The bradycardic action of reserpine promotes relaxation and may eliminate sinus tachycardia. It is most pronounced in subjects with sinus tachycardia and usually is not prominent in persons with a normal pulse rate.

Miosis, relaxation of the nictitating membrane, ptosis, hypothermia, and increased gastrointestinal activity are noted in animals given reserpine, sometimes in subclinical doses. None of these effects, except increased gastrointestinal activity, has been found to be clinically significant in man with therapeutic doses.

Indication

Hypertension (see box warning).

Contraindications

Hydrochlorothiazide is contraindicated in anuria. HYDROPRES is contraindicated in hypersensitivity to hydrochlorothiazide or other sulfonamide-derived drugs or to reserpine.

Electroshock therapy should not be given to patients while on reserpine, as severe and even fatal reactions have been reported with minimal convulsive electroshock dosage. After discontinuing reserpine, allow at least seven days before starting electroshock therapy.

Active peptic ulcer, ulcerative colitis, and active mental depression, especially suicidal tendencies, are contraindications to reserpine therapy.

Warnings

Hydrochlorothiazide

Use with caution in severe renal disease. In patients with renal disease, thiazides may precipitate azotemia. Cumulative effects of the drug may develop in patients with impaired renal function.

Thiazides should be used with caution in patients with impaired hepatic function or progressive liver disease, since minor alterations of fluid and electrolyte balance may precipitate hepatic coma.

Thiazides may add to or potentiate the action of other antihypertensive drugs.

Sensitivity reactions may occur in patients with or without a history of allergy or bronchial asthma.

The possibility of exacerbation or activation of systemic lupus erythematosus has been reported.

Lithium generally should not be given with diuretics because they reduce its renal clearance and add a high risk of lithium toxicity. Read circulars for lithium preparations before use of such concomitant therapy.

Reserpine

The occurrence of mental depression due to reserpine in doses of 0.25 mg daily or less is unusual. In any event, HYDROPRES should be discontinued at the first sign of depression.

Use in Pregnancy

Reserpine has been demonstrated to cross the placental barrier in guinea pigs with depression of adrenal catecholamine stores in the newborn. There is some evidence that side effects such as nasal congestion, lethargy, depressed Moro reflex, and bradycardia may appear in infants born of reserpine-treated mothers.

Thiazides cross the placental barrier and appear in cord blood. The use of thiazides in pregnancy requires that the anticipated benefit be weighed against possible hazards to the fetus. These hazards include fetal or neonatal jaundice, thrombocytopenia, and possibly other adverse reactions which have occurred in the adult.

Nursing Mothers

Thiazides and reserpine appear in breast milk. If use of the drug is deemed essential, the patient should stop nursing.

Precautions

Hydrochlorothiazide

Periodic determination of serum electrolytes to detect possible electrolyte imbalance should be performed at appropriate intervals.

All patients receiving diuretic therapy should be observed for evidence of fluid or electrolyte imbalance: namely, hyponatremia, hypochloremic alkalosis, and hypokalemia. Serum and urine electrolyte determinations are particularly important when the patient is vomiting excessively or receiving parenteral fluids. Warning signs or symptoms of fluid and electrolyte imbalance include dryness of mouth, thirst, weakness, lethargy, drowsiness, restlessness, muscle pains or cramps, muscular fatigue, hypotension, oliguria, tachycardia, and gastrointestinal disturbances such as nausea and vomiting.

Hypokalemia may develop, especially with brisk diuresis, when severe cirrhosis is present, during concomitant use of corticosteroids or ACTH, or after prolonged therapy.

Interference with adequate oral electrolyte intake will contribute to hypokalemia. Hypokalemia can sensitize or exaggerate the response of the heart to the toxic effects of digitalis (e.g., increased ventricular irritability). Hypokalemia may be avoided or treated by use of potassium supplements such as foods with a high potassium content.

Although any chloride deficit is generally mild and usually does not require specific treatment except under extraordinary circumstances (as in liver disease or renal disease), chloride replacement may be required in the treatment of metabolic alkalosis.

Dilutional hyponatremia may occur in edematous patients in hot weather. Appropriate therapy is water restriction, rather than administration of salt, except in rare instances when the hyponatremia is life threatening. In actual salt depletion, appropriate replacement is the therapy of choice.

Hyperuricemia may occur or acute gout may be precipitated in certain patients receiving thiazides.

Insulin requirements in diabetic patients may be increased, decreased, or unchanged. Latent diabetes mellitus may become manifest during thiazide therapy.

Thiazides may increase the responsiveness to tubocurarine.

The antihypertensive effect of the drug may be enhanced in the postsympathectomy patient.

Thiazides may decrease arterial responsiveness to norepinephrine. This diminution is not sufficient to preclude effectiveness of the pressor agent for therapeutic use.

If progressive renal impairment becomes evident, consider withholding or discontinuing diuretic therapy.

Thiazides may decrease serum PBI levels without signs of thyroid disturbance.

Thiazides may decrease urinary calcium excretion. Thiazides may cause intermittent and slight elevation of serum calcium in the absence of known disorders of calcium metabolism. Marked hypercalcemia may be evidence of hidden hyperparathyroidism. Thiazides should be discontinued before carrying out tests for parathyroid function.

Reserpine

Since reserpine may increase gastric secretion and motility, it should be used cautiously in patients with a history of peptic ulcer, ulcerative colitis, or other gastrointestinal disorder. This compound may precipitate biliary colic in patients with gallstones, or bronchial asthma in susceptible persons. Reserpine may cause hypotension including orthostatic hypotension.

In hypertensive patients on reserpine therapy significant hypotension and bradycardia may develop during surgical anesthesia. The anesthesiologist should be aware that reserpine has been taken, since it may be necessary to give vagal blocking agents parenterally to prevent or reverse hypotension and/or bradycardia.

Anxiety or depression, as well as psychosis, may develop during reserpine therapy. If depression is present when therapy is begun, it may be aggravated. Mental depression is unusual with reserpine doses of 0.25 mg daily or less. In any case, HYDROPRES should be discontinued at the first sign of depression. Extreme caution should be used in treating patients with a history of mental depression, and the possibility of suicide should be kept in mind.

As with most antihypertensive therapy, caution should be exercised when treating hypertensive patients with renal insufficiency, since they adjust poorly to lowered blood pressure levels. Use reserpine cautiously with digitalis and quinidine; cardiac arrhythmias have occurred with reserpine preparations.

When two or more antihypertensives are given, the individual dosages may have to be reduced to prevent excessive drop in blood pressure. In hypertensive patients with coronary artery disease, it is important to avoid a precipitous drop in blood pressure.

Animal tumorigenicity: Rodent studies have shown that reserpine is an animal tumorigen, causing an increased incidence of mammary fibroadenomas in female mice, malignant tumors of the seminal vesicles in male mice, and malignant adrenal medullary tumors in male rats. These findings arose in 2 year studies in which the drug was administered in the feed at concentrations of 5 and 10 ppm-about 100 to 300 times the usual human dose. The breast neoplasms are thought to be related to reserpine's prolactin-elevating effect. Several other prolactin-elevating drugs have also been associated with an increased incidence of mammary neoplasia in rodents.

The extent to which these findings indicate a risk to humans is uncertain. Tissue culture experiments show that about one-third of human breast tumors are prolactin-dependent *in vitro*, a factor of considerable importance if the use of the drug is contemplated in a patient with previously detected breast cancer. The possibility of an increased risk of breast cancer in reserpine users has been studied extensively; however, no firm conclusion has emerged. Although a few epidemiologic studies have suggested a slightly increased risk (less than twofold in all studies except one) in women who have used reserpine, other studies of generally similar design have not confirmed this. Epidemiologic studies conducted using other drugs (neuroleptic agents) that, like reserpine, increase prolactin levels and therefore would be considered rodent mammary carcinogens, have not shown an association between chronic administration of the drug and human mammary tumorigenesis. While long-term clinical observation has not suggested such an association, the available evidence is considered too limited to be conclusive at this time. An association of reserpine intake with pheochromocytoma or tumors of the seminal vesicles has not been explored.

Adverse Reactions

Hydrochlorothiazide
Body as a Whole: Weakness.
Cardiovascular: Orthostatic hypotension (may be aggravated by alcohol, barbiturates, or narcotics).
Digestive: Anorexia, gastric irritation, nausea, vomiting, cramping, diarrhea, constipation, jaundice (intrahepatic cholestatic jaundice), pancreatitis, sialadenitis.
Hematologic: Leukopenia, agranulocytosis, thrombocytopenia, aplastic anemia, hemolytic anemia.
Metabolic: Hyperglycemia, glycosuria, hyperuricemia, electrolyte imbalance (see PRECAUTIONS).
Musculoskeletal: Muscle spasm.
Nervous System/Psychiatric: Dizziness, vertigo, paresthesias, headache, restlessness.
Special Senses: Transient blurred vision, xanthopsia.
Hypersensitivity: Purpura, photosensitivity, rash, urticaria, necrotizing angiitis (vasculitis and cutaneous vasculitis), fever, respiratory distress including pneumonitis and pulmonary edema, anaphylactic reactions.

Whenever adverse reactions are moderate or severe, thiazide dosage should be reduced or therapy withdrawn.

Reserpine
Cardiovascular: Bradycardia, angina pectoris, arrhythmia, premature ventricular contractions, and other direct cardiac effects (e.g., fluid retention, congestive failure).
Digestive: Hypersecretion and increased motility, nausea, vomiting, anorexia, diarrhea, dryness of mouth, increased salivation.
Hematologic: Excessive bleeding following prostatic surgery, thrombocytopenic purpura.
Metabolic: Weight gain.
Musculoskeletal: Muscular aches.
Nervous System/Psychiatric: Excessive sedation, mental depression, nightmares, headache, dizziness, syncope, nervousness, paradoxical anxiety, central nervous system sensitization (dull sensorium, deafness, glaucoma, uveitis, optic atrophy), parkinsonism (usually reversible with decreased dosage or discontinuance of therapy).
Respiratory: Nasal congestion, dyspnea, epistaxis, enhanced susceptibility to colds.
Hypersensitivity: Flushing of skin, pruritus, rash.
Urogenital: Dysuria, nonpuerperal lactation, impotence, decreased libido.

Dosage and Administration

The initial dosage of HYDROPRES should conform to the dosages of the individual components established during titration (see box warning). The usual adult dosage of HYDROPRES 25 is 1 or 2 tablets once or twice a day; that of HYDROPRES 50 is 1 tablet once or twice a day. Dosage may require adjustment according to the blood pressure response of the patient.
Careful observations for changes in blood pressure must be made when HYDROPRES is used with other antihypertensive drugs.

How Supplied

No. 3265—Tablets HYDROPRES 25 are green, round, scored, compressed tablets, coded MSD 53. Each tablet contains 25 mg of hydrochlorothiazide and 0.125 mg of reserpine. They are supplied as follows:
NDC 0006-0053-68 in bottles of 100
NDC 0006-0053-82 in bottles of 1000.
Shown in Product Identification Section, page 420
No. 3266—Tablets HYDROPRES 50 are green, round, scored, compressed tablets, coded MSD 127. Each tablet contains 50 mg of hydrochlorothiazide and 0.125 mg of reserpine. They are supplied as follows:

NDC 0006-0127-68 in bottles of 100
NDC 0006-0127-82 in bottles of 1000.
Shown in Product Identification Section, page 420
A.H.F.S. Category: 24:08
DC 6053230   Issued November 1983
COPYRIGHT © MERCK & CO., INC., 1983
All rights reserved

INDOCIN® Capsules and Suppositories ℞
(indomethacin, MSD)
INDOCIN® SR Capsules ℞
(indomethacin, MSD)

Description

INDOCIN® (Indomethacin, MSD) cannot be considered a simple analgesic and should not be used in conditions other than those recommended under INDICATIONS.
INDOCIN is supplied in three dosage forms. Capsules INDOCIN for oral administration contain either 25 mg or 50 mg of indomethacin, and Capsules INDOCIN SR for sustained release oral administration contain 75 mg of indomethacin. Suppositories INDOCIN for rectal use contain 50 mg of indomethacin and the following inactive ingredients: glycerin, polyethylene glycol 6000, polyethylene glycol 4000, sodium chloride, edetic acid, butylated hydroxyanisole and butylated hydroxytoluene. Indomethacin is a non-steroidal anti-inflammatory indole derivative designated chemically as 1-(4-chlorobenzoyl)-5-methoxy-2-methyl-1H-indole-3-acetic acid.

Clinical Pharmacology

INDOCIN is a non-steroidal drug with anti-inflammatory, antipyretic and analgesic properties. Its mode of action, like that of other anti-inflammatory drugs, is not known. However, its therapeutic action is not due to pituitary-adrenal stimulation. INDOCIN is a potent inhibitor of prostaglandin synthesis *in vitro*. Concentrations are reached during therapy which have been demonstrated to have an effect *in vivo* as well. Prostaglandins sensitize afferent nerves and potentiate the action of bradykinin in inducing pain in animal models. Moreover, prostaglandins are known to be among the mediators of inflammation. Since indomethacin is an inhibitor of prostaglandin synthesis, its mode of action may be due to a decrease of prostaglandins in peripheral tissues.
INDOCIN has been shown to be an effective anti-inflammatory agent, appropriate for long-term use in rheumatoid arthritis, ankylosing spondylitis, and osteoarthritis.
INDOCIN affords relief of symptoms; it does not alter the progressive course of the underlying disease.
INDOCIN suppresses inflammation in rheumatoid arthritis as demonstrated by relief of pain, and reduction of fever, swelling and tenderness. Improvement in patients treated with INDOCIN for rheumatoid arthritis has been demonstrated by a reduction in joint swelling, average number of joints involved, and morning stiffness; by increased mobility as demonstrated by a decrease in walking time; and by improved functional capability as demonstrated by an increase in grip strength.
Capsules INDOCIN have been found effective in relieving the pain, reducing the fever, swelling, redness, and tenderness of acute gouty arthritis. Capsules INDOCIN rather than Capsules INDOCIN SR are recommended for treatment of acute gouty arthritis—see INDICATIONS.
Following single oral doses of Capsules INDOCIN 25 mg or 50 mg, indomethacin is readily absorbed, attaining peak plasma concentrations of about 1 and 2 mcg/mL, respectively, at about 2 hours. Orally administered Capsules INDOCIN are virtually 100% bioavailable, with 90% of the dose absorbed within 4 hours.
Capsules INDOCIN SR 75 mg are designed to release 25 mg of the drug initially and the remaining 50 mg over approximately 12 hours (90% of dose absorbed by 12 hours). When measured over a 24-hour period, the cumulative amount and time-course of indomethacin absorption from a single Capsule INDOCIN SR are comparable to those of 3 doses of 25 mg Capsules INDOCIN given at 4–6 hour intervals.
Plasma concentrations of indomethacin fluctuate less and are more sustained following administration of Capsules INDOCIN SR than following administration of 25 mg Capsules INDOCIN given at 4–6 hour intervals. In multiple-dose comparisons, the mean daily steady-state plasma level of indomethacin attained with daily administration of Capsules INDOCIN SR 75 mg was indistinguishable from that following Capsules INDOCIN 25 mg given at 0, 6 and 12 hours daily. However, there was a significant difference in indomethacin plasma levels between the two dosage regimens especially after 12 hours.
Controlled clinical studies of safety and efficacy in patients with osteoarthritis have shown that one Capsule INDOCIN SR was clinically comparable to one 25 mg Capsule INDOCIN t.i.d.; and in controlled clinical studies in patients with rheumatoid arthritis, one Capsule INDOCIN SR taken in the morning and one in the evening were clinically indistinguishable from one 50 mg Capsule INDOCIN t.i.d.
Indomethacin is eliminated via renal excretion, metabolism, and biliary excretion. Indomethacin undergoes appreciable enterohepatic circulation. The mean half-life of indomethacin is estimated to be about 4.5 hours. With a typical therapeutic regimen of 25 or 50 mg t.i.d., the steady-state plasma concentrations of indomethacin are an average 1.4 times those following the first dose.
The rate of absorption is more rapid from the rectal suppository than from Capsules INDOCIN. Ordinarily, therefore, the total amount absorbed from the suppository would be expected to be at least equivalent to the capsule. In controlled clinical trials, however, the amount of indomethacin absorbed was found to be somewhat less (80–90%) than that absorbed from Capsules INDOCIN. This is probably because some subjects did not retain the material from the suppository for the one hour necessary to assure complete absorption. Since the suppository dissolves rather quickly rather than melting slowly, it is seldom recovered in recognizable form if the patient retains the suppository for more than a few minutes.
Indomethacin exists in the plasma as the parent drug and its desmethyl, desbenzoyl, and desmethyl-desbenzoyl metabolites, all in the unconjugated form. About 60 percent of an oral dosage is recovered in urine as drug and metabolites (26 percent as indomethacin and its glucuronide), and 33 percent is recovered in feces (1.5 percent as indomethacin).
About 90% of indomethacin is bound to protein in plasma over the expected range of therapeutic plasma concentrations.
In a gastroscopic study in 45 healthy subjects, the number of gastric mucosal abnormalities was significantly higher in the group receiving Capsules INDOCIN than in the group taking Suppositories INDOCIN or placebo.
In a double-blind comparative clinical study involving 175 patients with rheumatoid arthritis, however, the incidence of upper gastrointestinal adverse effects with Suppositories or Capsules INDOCIN was comparable. The incidence of lower gastrointestinal adverse effects was greater in the suppository group.

Indications

Because of its potential to cause adverse reactions, particularly at high dose levels, the use of INDOCIN in rheumatoid arthritis and osteoarthritis in adults should be carefully considered for active disease unresponsive to adequate trial with sali-

Continued on next page

Information on the Merck Sharp & Dohme products listed on these pages is the full prescribing information from product circulars in use November 1, 1984.

Merck Sharp & Dohme—Cont.

cylates and other measures of established value, such as appropriate rest.

In accord with this important concept indomethacin has been found effective in active stages of the following:

1. Moderate to severe rheumatoid arthritis including acute flares of chronic disease.
2. Moderate to severe ankylosing spondylitis.
3. Moderate to severe osteoarthritis.
4. Acute painful shoulder (bursitis and/or tendinitis).
5. Acute gouty arthritis.

Capsules INDOCIN SR are recommended for all of the indications for Capsules INDOCIN except acute gouty arthritis.

INDOCIN may enable the reduction of steroid dosage in patients receiving steroids for the more severe forms of rheumatoid arthritis. In such instances the steroid dosage should be reduced slowly and the patients followed very closely for any possible adverse effects.

The use of INDOCIN in conjunction with aspirin or other salicylates is not recommended. Controlled clinical studies have shown that the combined use of INDOCIN and aspirin does not produce any greater therapeutic effect than the use of INDOCIN alone. Furthermore, in one of these clinical studies, the incidence of gastrointestinal side effects was significantly increased with combined therapy (see DRUG INTERACTIONS).

Contraindications

INDOCIN is contraindicated in patients who are allergic to INDOCIN or who have nasal polyps associated with angioedema or a bronchospastic reaction to aspirin or other non-steroidal anti-inflammatory drugs.

Suppositories INDOCIN are contraindicated in patients with a history of proctitis or recent rectal bleeding.

Warnings

General:

Because of the variability of the potential of INDOCIN to cause adverse reactions in the individual patient, the following are strongly recommended:

1. The lowest possible effective dose for the individual patient should be prescribed. Increased dosage tends to increase adverse effects, particularly in doses over 150–200 mg/day, without corresponding increase in clinical benefits.
2. Careful instructions to, and observations of, the individual patient are essential to the prevention of serious adverse reactions. As advancing years appear to increase the possibility of adverse reactions, INDOCIN should be used with greater care in the aged.
3. Safe conditions for use in children have not been established; therefore, INDOCIN should not be prescribed for children 14 years of age and under except under circumstances where lack of efficacy or toxicity associated with other drugs warrants the risk. Such patients should be monitored closely.
4. If Capsules INDOCIN SR are used for initial therapy or during dosage adjustment, observe the patient closely (see DOSAGE AND ADMINISTRATION).

Gastrointestinal Effects:

Single or multiple ulcerations, including perforation and hemorrhage of the esophagus, stomach, duodenum or small intestine, have been reported to occur with INDOCIN. Fatalities have been reported in some instances. Rarely, intestinal ulceration has been associated with stenosis and obstruction.

Gastrointestinal bleeding without obvious ulcer formation and perforation of pre-existing sigmoid lesions (diverticulum, carcinoma, etc.) have occurred. Increased abdominal pain in ulcerative colitis patients or the development of ulcerative colitis and regional ileitis have been reported to occur rarely.

Because of the occurrence, and at times severity, of gastrointestinal reactions to INDOCIN, the prescribing physician must be continuously alert for any sign or symptom signaling a possible gastrointestinal reaction. The risks of continuing therapy with INDOCIN in the face of such symptoms must be weighed against the possible benefits to the individual patient.

INDOCIN should not be given to patients with active gastrointestinal lesions or with a history of recurrent gastrointestinal lesions except under circumstances which warrant the very high risk and where patients can be monitored very closely. The gastrointestinal effects may be reduced by giving Capsules INDOCIN or Capsules INDOCIN SR immediately after meals, with food, or with antacids.

Renal Effects:

Because adequate renal function can depend upon renal prostaglandin synthesis, INDOCIN can precipitate renal insufficiency, including acute renal failure. The risk is greater in patients with any of a number of underlying conditions, e.g., those with renal or hepatic dysfunction, complications associated with advanced age, extracellular volume depletion from any cause, congestive heart failure, sepsis, or concomitant use of any nephrotoxic drug. However, the drug should be given with caution and renal function should be monitored in any patient who may have reduced renal reserve. Most of the renal abnormalities have been reversible upon discontinuation of the drug.

Ocular Effects:

Corneal deposits and retinal disturbances, including those of the macula, have been observed in some patients who had received prolonged therapy with INDOCIN. The prescribing physician should be alert to the possible association between the changes noted and INDOCIN. It is advisable to discontinue therapy if such changes are observed. Blurred vision may be a significant symptom and warrants a thorough ophthalmological examination. Since these changes may be asymptomatic, ophthalmologic examination at periodic intervals is desirable in patients where therapy is prolonged.

Central Nervous System Effects:

INDOCIN may aggravate depression or other psychiatric disturbances, epilepsy, and parkinsonism, and should be used with considerable caution in patients with these conditions. If severe CNS adverse reactions develop, INDOCIN should be discontinued.

INDOCIN may cause drowsiness; therefore, patients should be cautioned about engaging in activities requiring mental alertness and motor coordination, such as driving a car. INDOCIN may also cause headache. Headache which persists despite dosage reduction requires cessation of therapy with INDOCIN.

Use in Pregnancy and the Neonatal Period

INDOCIN is not recommended for use in pregnant women, since safety for use has not been established, and because of the known effect of drugs of this class on the human fetal cardiovascular system (closure of the ductus arteriosus) during the third trimester of pregnancy.

Teratogenic studies were conducted in mice and rats at dosages of 0.5, 1.0, 2.0, and 4.0 mg/kg/day. Except for retarded fetal ossification at 4 mg/kg/day considered secondary to the decreased average fetal weights, no increase in fetal malformations was observed as compared with control groups. Other studies in mice reported in the literature using higher doses (5 to 15 mg/kg/day) have described maternal toxicity and death, increased fetal resorptions, and fetal malformations. Comparable studies in rodents using high doses of aspirin have shown similar maternal and fetal effects.

As with other non-steroidal anti-inflammatory agents which inhibit prostaglandin synthesis, indomethacin has been found to delay parturition in rats.

In rats and mice, 4.0 mg/kg/day given during the last three days of gestation caused a decrease in maternal weight gain and some maternal and fetal deaths. An increased incidence of neuronal necrosis in the diencephalon in the live-born fetuses was observed. At 2.0 mg/kg/day, no increase in neuronal necrosis was observed as compared with the control groups. Administration of 0.5 or 4.0 mg/kg/day during the first three days of life did not cause an increase in neuronal necrosis at either dose level.

Use in Nursing Mothers

INDOCIN is excreted in the milk of lactating mothers. INDOCIN is not recommended for use in nursing mothers.

Precautions

INDOCIN may mask the usual signs and symptoms of infection. Therefore, the physician must be continually on the alert for this and should use the drug with extra care in the presence of existing controlled infection.

INDOCIN, like other non-steroidal anti-inflammatory agents, can inhibit platelet aggregation. This effect is of shorter duration than that seen with aspirin and usually disappears within 24 hours after discontinuation of INDOCIN. INDOCIN has been shown to prolong bleeding time (but within the normal range) in normal subjects. Because this effect may be exaggerated in patients with underlying hemostatic defects, INDOCIN should be used with caution in persons with coagulation defects.

As with other non-steroidal anti-inflammatory drugs, borderline elevations of one or more liver tests may occur in up to 15% of patients. These abnormalities may progress, may remain essentially unchanged, or may be transient with continued therapy. The SGPT (ALT) test is probably the most sensitive indicator of liver dysfunction. Meaningful (3 times the upper limit of normal elevations of SGPT or SGOT (AST) occurred in controlled clinical trials in less than 1% of patients. A patient with symptoms and/or signs suggesting liver dysfunction, or in whom an abnormal liver test has occurred, should be evaluated for evidence of the development of more severe hepatic reaction while on therapy with INDOCIN. Severe hepatic reactions, including jaundice and cases of fatal hepatitis, have been reported with INDOCIN as with other non-steroidal anti-inflammatory drugs. Although such reactions are rare, if abnormal liver tests persist or worsen, if clinical signs and symptoms consistent with liver disease develop, or if systemic manifestations occur (e.g. eosinophilia, rash, etc.), INDOCIN should be discontinued.

Drug Interactions

In normal volunteers receiving indomethacin, the administration of diflunisal decreased the renal clearance and significantly increased the plasma levels of indomethacin. In some patients, combined use of INDOCIN and diflunisal has been associated with fatal gastrointestinal hemorrhage. Therefore, diflunisal and INDOCIN should not be used concomitantly.

In a study in normal volunteers, it was found that chronic concurrent administration of 3.6 g of aspirin per day decreases indomethacin blood levels approximately 20%.

Clinical studies have shown that INDOCIN does not influence the hypoprothrombinemia produced by anticoagulants. However, when any additional drug, including INDOCIN, is added to the treatment of patients on anticoagulant therapy, the patients should be observed for alterations of the prothrombin time.

When INDOCIN is given to patients receiving probenecid, the plasma levels of indomethacin are likely to be increased. Therefore, a lower total daily dosage of INDOCIN may produce a satisfactory therapeutic effect. When increases in the dose of INDOCIN are made, they should be made carefully and in small increments.

Capsules INDOCIN 50 mg t.i.d. produced a clinically relevant elevation of plasma lithium and reduction in renal lithium clearance in psychiatric patients and normal subjects with steady state plasma lithium concentrations. This effect has been attributed to inhibition of prostaglandin synthesis. As a consequence, when INDOCIN and lithium are given concomitantly, the patient should be carefully observed for signs of lithium toxicity. (Read circulars for lithium preparations before use of such concomitant therapy.) In addition, the frequency of monitoring serum lithium concentration should be increased at the outset of such combination drug treatment.

Clinical studies have shown that the administration of INDOCIN can reduce the natriuretic and anti-hypertensive effect of furosemide and thiazides in some patients. This response has been attributed to inhibition of renal prostaglandin synthesis by non-steroidal anti-inflammatory drugs. Therefore, when INDOCIN is added to the treatment of a patient receiving furosemide or thiazides, or furosemide or thiazides are added to the treatment of a patient receiving INDOCIN, the patient should be observed closely to determine if the desired effect of furosemide or thiazides is obtained.

INDOCIN blocks the furosemide-induced increase in plasma renin activity. This fact should be kept in mind when evaluating plasma renin activity in hypertensive patients.

There is a report of a clinical pharmacology study in which triamterene was added to a maintenance schedule of INDOCIN for four healthy volunteers. Two of the subjects developed azotemia and reduced creatinine clearance after several days of combined drug administration. This effect was reversible and may be mediated by prostaglandin inhibition. Nonetheless, INDOCIN and triamterene should not be used together.

Blunting of the antihypertensive effect of beta-adrenoceptor blocking agents by non-steroidal anti-inflammatory drugs including INDOCIN has been reported. Therefore, when using these blocking agents to treat hypertension, patients should be observed carefully in order to confirm that the desired therapeutic effect has been obtained. There are reports that INDOCIN can reduce the antihypertensive effect of captopril in some patients.

Adverse Reactions

The adverse reactions for Capsules INDOCIN listed in the following table have been arranged into two groups: (1) incidence greater than 1%; and (2) incidence less than 1%. The incidence for group (1) was obtained from 33 double-blind controlled clinical trials reported in the literature (1,092 patients). The incidence for group (2) was based on reports in clinical trials, in the literature, and on voluntary reports since marketing. The probability of a causal relationship exists between INDOCIN and these adverse reactions, some of which have been reported only rarely.

In controlled clinical trials, the incidence of adverse reactions to Capsules INDOCIN SR and equal 24-hour doses of Capsules INDOCIN were similar.

The adverse reactions reported with Capsules INDOCIN may occur with use of the suppositories. In addition, rectal irritation and tenesmus have been reported in patients who have received the suppositories.

[See table above].
[See table on next page].

Causal relationship unknown: Other reactions have been reported but occurred under circumstances where a causal relationship could not be established. However, in these rarely reported events, the possibility cannot be excluded. Therefore, these observations are being listed to serve as alerting information to physicians:

Hematologic: Although there have been several reports of leukemia, the supporting information is weak.

Genitourinary: Urinary frequency.

Dosage and Administration

INDOCIN is available as 25 and 50 mg Capsules INDOCIN and 75 mg Capsules INDOCIN SR for oral use, and 50 mg Suppositories INDOCIN for rectal use. Capsules INDOCIN SR 75 mg once a day can be substituted for Capsules INDOCIN 25 mg t.i.d. However, there will be significant differ-

Incidence greater than 1%	Incidence less than 1%	
GASTROINTESTINAL		
nausea* with or without vomiting	anorexia	gastrointestinal bleeding without obvious ulcer formation and perforation of pre-existing sigmoid lesions (diverticulum, carcinoma, etc.) development of ulcerative colitis and regional ileitis ulcerative stomatitis toxic hepatitis and jaundice (some fatal cases have been reported)
dyspepsia* (including indigestion, heartburn and epigastric pain)	bloating (includes distention) flatulence peptic ulcer gastro-enteritis rectal bleeding	
diarrhea	proctitis	
abdominal distress or pain	perforation and hemorrhage of the esophagus, stomach, duodenum or small intestines intestinal ulceration associated with stenosis and obstruction	
constipation		
CENTRAL NERVOUS SYSTEM		
headache**	anxiety (includes nervousness)	light-headedness
dizziness*	muscle weakness	syncope
vertigo	involuntary muscle movements	paresthesia
somnolence	insomnia	aggravation of epilepsy and parkinsonism
depression and fatigue (including malaise and listlessness)	muzziness psychic disturbances including psychotic episodes mental confusion drowsiness	depersonalization coma peripheral neuropathy convulsions
SPECIAL SENSES		
tinnitus	ocular—corneal deposits and retinal disturbances, including those of the macula, have been reported in some patients on prolonged therapy with INDOCIN	blurred vision hearing disturbances, deafness
CARDIOVASCULAR		
none	hypertension tachycardia chest pain	congestive heart failure arrhythmia; palpitations
METABOLIC		
none	edema weight gain fluid retention flushing or sweating	hyperglycemia glycosuria hyperkalemia
INTEGUMENTARY		
none	pruritus rash; urticaria petechiae or ecchymosis	exfoliative dermatitis erythema nodosum loss of hair Stevens-Johnson syndrome erythema multiforme toxic epidermal necrolysis
HEMATOLOGIC		
none	leukopenia bone marrow depression anemia secondary to obvious or occult gastrointestinal bleeding	aplastic anemia hemolytic anemia agranulocytosis thrombocytopenic purpura
HYPERSENSITIVITY		
none	acute respiratory distress rapid fall in blood pressure resembling a shock-like state angioedema	dyspnea asthma purpura angiitis pulmonary edema
GENITOURINARY		
none	hematuria vaginal bleeding	BUN elevation renal insufficiency, including renal failure

Continued on next page

Merck Sharp & Dohme—Cont.

MISCELLANEOUS
none   epistaxis
                        breast changes,
                          including
                          enlargement and
                          tenderness, or
                          gynecomastia

---

*Reactions occurring in 3% to 9% of patients treated with INDOCIN. (Those reactions occurring in less than 3% of the patients are unmarked.)
**Reactions occurring in over 10% of patients treated with INDOCIN.

ences between the two dosage regimens in indomethacin blood levels, especially after 12 hours (see CLINICAL PHARMACOLOGY). In addition, Capsules INDOCIN SR 75 mg b.i.d. can be substituted for Capsules INDOCIN 50 mg t.i.d. Capsules INDOCIN SR may be substituted for all the indications for Capsules INDOCIN except acute gouty arthritis.

Adverse reactions appear to correlate with the size of the dose of INDOCIN in most patients but not all. Therefore, every effort should be made to determine the smallest effective dosage for the individual patient.

Always give Capsules INDOCIN or Capsules INDOCIN SR with food, immediately after meals, or with antacids to reduce gastric irritation.

INDOCIN should not ordinarily be prescribed for children 14 years of age and under because safe conditions for use have not been established. (See WARNINGS.)

Dosage Recommendations for Active Stages of the Following:

1. Moderate to severe rheumatoid arthritis including acute flares of chronic disease; moderate to severe ankylosing spondylitis; and moderate to severe osteoarthritis.
   Suggested Dosage:
   Capsules INDOCIN 25 mg b.i.d. or t.i.d. If this is well tolerated, increase the daily dosage by 25 or by 50 mg, if required by continuing symptoms, at weekly intervals until a satisfactory response is obtained or until a total daily dose of 150–200 mg is reached. DOSES ABOVE THIS AMOUNT GENERALLY DO NOT INCREASE THE EFFECTIVENESS OF THE DRUG.
   In patients who have persistent night pain and/or morning stiffness, the giving of a large portion, up to a maximum of 100 mg, of the total daily dose at bedtime, either orally or by rectal suppositories, may be helpful in affording relief. The total daily dose should not exceed 200 mg. In acute flares of chronic rheumatoid arthritis, it may be necessary to increase the dosage by 25 mg or, if required, by 50 mg daily.
   If Capsules INDOCIN SR 75 mg are used for initiating indomethacin treatment, one capsule daily should be the usual starting dose in order to observe patient tolerance since 75 mg per day is the maximum recommended starting dose for indomethacin (see above). If Capsules INDOCIN SR are used to increase the daily dose, patients should be observed for possible signs and symptoms of intolerance since the daily increment will exceed the daily increment recommended for the other dosage forms. For patients who require 150 mg of INDOCIN per day and have demonstrated acceptable tolerance, INDOCIN SR may be prescribed as one capsule twice daily.
   If minor adverse effects develop as the dosage is increased, reduce the dosage rapidly to a tolerated dose and OBSERVE THE PATIENT CLOSELY.
   If severe adverse reactions occur, STOP THE DRUG. After the acute phase of the disease is under control, an attempt to reduce the daily dose should be made repeatedly until the patient is receiving the smallest effective dose or the drug is discontinued.
   Careful instructions to, and observations of, the individual patient are essential to the prevention of serious, irreversible, including fatal, adverse reactions.

As advancing years appear to increase the possibility of adverse reactions, INDOCIN should be used with greater care in the aged.

2. Acute painful shoulder (bursitis and/or tendinitis).
   Initial Dose:
   75–150 mg daily in 3 or 4 divided doses.
   The drug should be discontinued after the signs and symptoms of inflammation have been controlled for several days. The usual course of therapy is 7–14 days.

3. Acute gouty arthritis.
   Suggested Dosage:
   Capsules INDOCIN 50 mg t.i.d. until pain is tolerable. The dose should then be rapidly reduced to complete cessation of the drug. Definite relief of pain has been reported within 2 to 4 hours. Tenderness and heat usually subside in 24 to 36 hours, and swelling gradually disappears in 3 to 5 days.

How Supplied

No. 3316—Capsules INDOCIN, 25 mg are opaque blue and white capsules, coded MSD 25. They are supplied as follows:
  NDC 0006-0025-68 bottles of 100
  (6505-00-926-2154, 25 mg 100's)
  NDC 0006-0025-78 unit of use bottles of 100
  NDC 0006-0025-28 unit dose packages of 100
  (6505-00-118-2776, 25 mg individually sealed 100's)
  NDC 0006-0025-82 bottles of 1000
  (6505-00-931-0680, 25 mg 1000's).
Shown in Product Identification Section, page 420

No. 3317—Capsules INDOCIN, 50 mg are opaque blue and white capsules, coded MSD 50. They are supplied as follows:
  NDC 0006-0050-54 unit of use bottles of 60
  NDC 0006-0050-68 bottles of 100
  NDC 0006-0050-78 unit of use bottles of 100
  NDC 0006-0050-28 unit dose packages of 100.
Shown in Product Identification Section, page 420

No. 3370—Capsules INDOCIN SR, 75 mg each, are capsules with an opaque blue cap and clear body containing a mixture of blue and white pellets, coded MSD 693. They are supplied as follows:
  NDC 0006-0693-31 unit of use bottles of 30
  NDC 0006-0693-61 unit of use bottles of 60.
Shown in Product Identification Section, page 420
No. 3354—Suppositories INDOCIN, 50 mg each, are white, opaque, rectal suppositories and are supplied as follows:
  NDC 0006-0150-30, boxes of 30.
Shown in Product Identification Section, page 420

Suppositories INDOCIN are distributed by:
MERCK SHARP & DOHME, Division of Merck & Co., Inc.
West Point, Pa. 19486
Manufactured by:
MERCK SHARP & DOHME
(Italia) S.p.A.
27100—Pavia, Italy
Capsules INDOCIN® and INDOCIN® SR are distributed and manufactured by:

MERCK SHARP & DOHME, Division of Merck & Co., Inc.
West Point, Pa. 19486
  A.H.F.S. Category: 28:08
  DC 7286102   Issued June 1984
COPYRIGHT © MERCK & CO., INC., 1984
All rights reserved

LACRISERT® Sterile Ophthalmic Insert   R
(hydroxypropyl cellulose ophthalmic insert, MSD)

Description

LACRISERT® (Hydroxypropyl Cellulose Ophthalmic Insert, MSD) is a rod-shaped, water soluble, ophthalmic preparation made of hydroxypropyl cellulose, 5 mg. LACRISERT contains no preservatives or other ingredients. It is about 1.27 mm in diameter by about 3.5 mm long.
LACRISERT is supplied in packages of 60 units, together with illustrated instructions and a special applicator for removing LACRISERT from the unit dose blister and inserting it into the eye. A spare applicator is included in each package.

Actions

LACRISERT acts to stabilize and thicken the precorneal tear film and prolong the tear film breakup time which is usually accelerated in patients with dry eye states. LACRISERT also acts to lubricate and protect the eye. LACRISERT usually reduces the signs and symptoms resulting from moderate to severe dry eye syndromes.

Indications

LACRISERT is indicated in patients with moderate to severe dry eye syndromes, including keratoconjunctivitis sicca. LACRISERT is indicated especially in patients who remain symptomatic after an adequate trial of therapy with artificial tear solutions.
LACRISERT is also indicated for patients with:
  Exposure keratitis
  Decreased corneal sensitivity
  Recurrent corneal erosions
LACRISERT usually reduces the signs and symptoms resulting from moderate to severe dry eye syndromes, such as conjunctival hyperemia, corneal and conjunctival staining with rose bengal, exudation, itching, burning, foreign body sensation, smarting, photophobia, dryness and blurred or cloudy vision. Progressive visual deterioration which occurs in some patients may be retarded, halted, or sometimes reversed.
In a multicenter crossover study the 5 mg LACRISERT administered once a day during the waking hours was compared to artificial tears used four or more times daily. There was a significant prolongation of tear film breakup time and a significant decrease in foreign body sensation associated with dry eye syndrome in patients during treatment with inserts as compared to artificial tears. Improvement, as measured by amelioration of symptoms, by slit lamp examination and by rose bengal staining of the cornea and conjunctiva, was greater in most patients with moderate to severe symptoms during treatment with LACRISERT. Patient comfort was usually better with LACRISERT than with artificial tears solution, and most patients preferred LACRISERT.
In most patients treated with LACRISERT for over one year, improvement was observed as evidenced by amelioration of symptoms generally associated with keratoconjunctivitis sicca such as burning, tearing, foreign body sensation, itching, photophobia and blurred or cloudy vision.
During studies in healthy volunteers, a thickened precorneal tear film was usually observed through the slit lamp while LACRISERT was present in the conjunctival sac.

Contraindications

LACRISERT is contraindicated in patients who are hypersensitive to hydroxypropyl cellulose.

Warnings

Instructions for inserting and removing LACRISERT should be carefully followed.

Precautions

Because this product may produce transient blurring of vision, patients should be instructed to exercise caution when operating hazardous machinery or driving a motor vehicle.

Adverse Reactions

The following adverse reactions have been reported in patients treated with LACRISERT, but were in most instances mild and transient:
- Transient blurring of vision (See PRECAUTIONS)
- Ocular discomfort or irritation
- Matting or stickiness of eyelashes
- Photophobia
- Hypersensitivity
- Edema of the eyelids
- Hyperemia

Dosage and Administration

One LACRISERT ophthalmic insert in each eye once daily is usually sufficient to relieve the symptoms associated with moderate to severe dry eye syndromes. Individual patients may require more flexibility in the use of LACRISERT; some patients may require twice daily use for optimal results. Clinical experience with LACRISERT indicates that in some patients several weeks may be required before satisfactory improvement of symptoms is achieved.

LACRISERT is inserted into the inferior cul-de-sac of the eye beneath the base of the tarsus. Illustrated instructions are included in each package. While in the licensed practitioner's office, the patient should read the instructions, then practice insertion and removal of LACRISERT until proficiency is achieved.

NOTE: Occasionally LACRISERT is inadvertently expelled from the eye, especially in patients with shallow conjunctival fornices. The patient should be cautioned against rubbing the eye(s) containing LACRISERT, especially upon awakening, so as not to dislodge or expel the insert. If required, another LACRISERT ophthalmic insert may be inserted. If experience indicates that transient blurred vision develops in an individual patient, the patient may want to remove LACRISERT a few hours after insertion to avoid this. Another LACRISERT ophthalmic insert may be inserted if needed.

If LACRISERT causes worsening of symptoms, the patient should be instructed to inspect the conjunctival sac to make certain LACRISERT is in the proper location, deep in the inferior cul-de-sac of the eye beneath the base of the tarsus. If these symptoms persist, LACRISERT should be removed and the patient should contact the practitioner.

How Supplied

No. 3380—LACRISERT, a rod-shaped, water-soluble, ophthalmic preparation made of hydroxypropyl cellulose, 5 mg, is supplied as follows:
NDC 0006-3380-60 in packages containing 60 unit doses, two reusable applicators and a storage container.

Store below 30°C (86°F).
DC 7189404 Issued November 1981
Copyright © MERCK & CO., INC., 1979
All rights reserved

M-M-R® II
(measles, mumps and rubella virus vaccine, live, MSD), U.S.P.

Description

M-M-R® II (Measles, Mumps and Rubella Virus Vaccine, Live, MSD) is a live virus vaccine for immunization against measles (rubeola), mumps and rubella (German measles).

M-M-R II is a lyophilized preparation of (1) ATTENUVAX® (Measles Virus Vaccine, Live, Attenuated, MSD), a more attenuated line of measles virus, derived from Enders' attenuated Edmonston strain and grown in cell cultures of chick embryo; (2) MUMPSVAX® (Mumps Virus Vaccine, Live, MSD), the Jeryl Lynn (B level) mumps strain grown in cell cultures of chick embryo; and (3) MERUVAX® II (Rubella Virus Vaccine, Live, MSD), the Wistar RA 27/3 strain of live attenuated rubella virus grown in human diploid cell (WI-38) culture. The three viruses are mixed before being lyophilized. The product contains no preservative.

When reconstituted as directed, the dose for injection is 0.5 ml and contains not less than 1,000 $TCID_{50}$ (tissue culture infectious doses) of Measles Virus Vaccine, Live, Attenuated; 5,000 $TCID_{50}$ of Mumps Virus Vaccine, Live; and 1,000 $TCID_{50}$ of Rubella Virus Vaccine, Live, expressed in terms of the assigned titer of the FDA Reference Measles, Mumps and Rubella Viruses. Each dose contains approximately 25 mcg of neomycin.

Actions

Clinical studies of 279 triple seronegative children, 11 months to 7 years of age, demonstrated that M-M-R II is highly immunogenic and generally well tolerated. In these studies, a single injection of the vaccine induced measles hemagglutination-inhibition (HI) antibodies in 95 percent, mumps neutralizing antibodies in 96 percent, and rubella HI antibodies in 99 percent of susceptible persons.

The RA 27/3 rubella strain in M-M-R II elicits higher immediate postvaccination HI, complement-fixing and neutralizing antibody levels than other strains of rubella vaccine and has been shown to induce a broader profile of circulating antibodies including anti-theta and anti-iota precipitating antibodies. The RA 27/3 rubella strain immunologically simulates natural infection more closely than other rubella vaccine viruses. The increased levels and broader profile of antibodies produced by RA 27/3 strain rubella virus vaccine appear to correlate with greater resistance to subclinical reinfection with the wild virus, and provide greater confidence for lasting immunity.

Data relating to persistence of vaccine-induced antibodies are not available for M-M-R II at this time; however, it is expected that the antibodies against measles, mumps and rubella will be just as durable following administration of M-M-R II as after the single vaccines given separately. Antibody levels after immunization with ATTENUVAX (Measles Virus Vaccine, Live, Attenuated, MSD) have persisted for at least eight years without substantial decline; for ten years after MUMPSVAX (Mumps Virus Vaccine, Live, MSD); and for at least six years after administration of RA 27/3 strain rubella virus vaccine.

Indications

M-M-R II is indicated for simultaneous immunization against measles, mumps, and rubella in children 15 months of age or older, and adults.

Infants who are less than 15 months of age may fail to respond to one or all three components of the vaccine due to presence in the circulation of residual measles and/or mumps and/or rubella antibody of maternal origin; the younger the infant, the lower the likelihood of seroconversion. In geographically isolated or other relatively inaccessible populations for whom immunization programs are logistically difficult, and in population groups in which natural measles infection may occur in a significant proportion of infants before 15 months of age, it may be desirable to give the vaccine to infants at an earlier age. The advantage of early protection must be weighed against the chance for failure of response; infants vaccinated under these conditions should be revaccinated after reaching 15 months of age.

Previously unimmunized children of susceptible pregnant women should receive live attenuated rubella vaccine, because an immunized child will be less likely to acquire natural rubella and introduce the virus into the household.

Non-Pregnant Adolescent and Adult Females

Immunization of susceptible non-pregnant adolescent and adult females of child-bearing age with live attenuated rubella virus vaccine is indicated if certain precautions are observed (see below). Vaccinating susceptible postpubertal females confers individual protection against subsequently acquiring rubella infection during pregnancy, which in turn prevents infection of the fetus and consequent congenital rubella injury.

Pregnant females *must not* be given live attenuated rubella virus vaccine. It is not known to what extent infection of the fetus with attenuated virus might occur following vaccination, or whether damage to the fetus could result. Subjects should be considered for vaccination only if they agree that they will not become pregnant within three months following vaccination, and if they are informed of the reason for this precaution.* If a pregnant woman is inadvertently vaccinated or if she becomes pregnant within three months of vaccination, she should be counseled on the possible risks to the fetus.

It is recommended that rubella susceptibility be determined by serologic testing prior to immunization.** If immune, as evidenced by a specific rubella antibody titer of 1:8 or greater (hemagglutination inhibition test), vaccination is unnecessary. Congenital malformations do occur in up to seven percent of all live births. Their chance appearance after vaccination could lead to misinterpretation of the cause, particularly if the prior rubella-immune status of vaccinees is unknown.

Postpubertal females should be informed of the frequent occurrence of self-limited arthralgia and possible arthritis beginning 2 to 4 weeks after vaccination (See ADVERSE REACTIONS).

It has been found convenient in many instances to vaccinate rubella-susceptible women in the immediate post-partum period.

Revaccination: Based on available evidence, there is no reason to routinely revaccinate children originally vaccinated when 12 months of age or older; however, children vaccinated when younger than 12 months of age should be revaccinated. The decision to revaccinate should be based on evaluation of each individual case.

Use with Other Live Virus Vaccines

There are no data available concerning simultaneous use of M-M-R II, containing the RA 27/3 rubella strain, with monovalent or trivalent poliovirus vaccine, live, oral, or with killed poliovirus

---

* NOTE: The Immunization Practices Advisory Committee (ACIP) has recommended "In view of the importance of protecting this age group against rubella, asking females if they are pregnant, excluding those who say they are, and explaining the theoretical risks to the others are reasonable precautions in a rubella immunization program."

** NOTE: The Immunization Practices Advisory Committee (ACIP) has stated "When practical, and when reliable laboratory services are available, potential vaccinees of childbearing age can have serologic tests to determine susceptibility to rubella.... However, routinely performing serologic tests for all females of childbearing age to determine susceptibility so that vaccine is given only to proven susceptibles is expensive and has been ineffective in some areas. Accordingly, the ACIP believes that rubella vaccination of a woman who is not known to be pregnant and has no history of vaccination is justifiable without serologic testing."

Continued on next page

Information on the Merck Sharp & Dohme products listed on these pages is the full prescribing information from product circulars in use November 1, 1984.

Merck Sharp & Dohme—Cont.

vaccines. However, serologic evidence shows that when M-M-R, containing the HPV-77 rubella strain, is given simultaneously with trivalent poliovirus vaccine, live, oral, antibody responses can be expected to be comparable to those which follow administration of the vaccines at different times.

Contraindications

Do not give M-M-R$_{II}$ to pregnant females; the possible effects of the vaccine on fetal development are unknown at this time. If vaccination of postpubertal females is undertaken, pregnancy must be avoided for three months following vaccination. Hypersensitivity to neomycin (each dose of reconstituted vaccine contains approximately 25 mcg of neomycin).
Any febrile respiratory illness or other active febrile infection.
Active untreated tuberculosis.
Patients receiving therapy with ACTH, corticosteroids, irradiation, alkylating agents or antimetabolites. This contraindication does not apply to patients who are receiving corticosteroids as replacement therapy, e.g., for Addison's disease.
Individuals with blood dyscrasias, leukemia, lymphomas of any type, or other malignant neoplasms affecting the bone marrow or lymphatic systems. Primary immuno-deficiency states, including cellular immune deficiencies, hypogammaglobulinemic and dysgammaglobulinemic states.

Hypersensitivity to Eggs, Chicken, or Chicken Feathers

This vaccine is essentially devoid of potentially allergenic substances derived from host tissues (chick embryos).* However, because the attenuated measles and mumps viruses in this vaccine are propagated in cell cultures of chick embryo, there is a potential risk of hypersensitivity reactions in patients allergic to eggs, chicken or chicken feathers. Widespread use of the vaccine for more than a decade has resulted in only rare, isolated reports of minor allergic reactions attributed to allergens of this kind, possibly related to the vaccine. Significantly, when children with known allergies to eggs, chicken and chicken feathers were given a similarly prepared vaccine in a clinical study, none experienced reactions other than those reactions previously observed in non-allergic children.

Precautions

Administer M-M-R$_{II}$ subcutaneously; *do not give intravenously.*
Epinephrine should be available for immediate use in case an anaphylactoid reaction occurs. M-M-R$_{II}$ may be given simultaneously with monovalent or trivalent poliovirus vaccine, live, oral. M-M-R$_{II}$ should not be given less than one month before or after administration of other live virus vaccines. Due caution should be employed in administration of M-M-R$_{II}$ to children with a history of febrile convulsions, cerebral injury or any other condition in which stress due to fever should be avoided. The physician should be alert to the temperature elevation which may occur 5 to 12 days following vaccination.
Vaccination should be deferred for at least 3 months following blood or plasma transfusions, or administration of human immune serum globulin.
Excretion of small amounts of the live attenuated rubella virus from the nose or throat has occurred in the majority of susceptible individuals 7–28 days after vaccination. There is no confirmed evidence to indicate that such virus is transmitted to susceptible persons who are in contact with the vaccinated individuals. Consequently, transmission, while accepted as a theoretical possibility, is not regarded as a significant risk.**
There are no reports of transmission of live attenuated measles or mumps viruses from vaccinees to susceptible contacts.
It has been reported that live attenuated measles, mumps and rubella virus vaccines given individually may result in a temporary depression of tuberculin skin sensitivity. Therefore, if a tuberculin test is to be done, it should be administered either before or simultaneously with M-M-R$_{II}$.
As for any vaccine, vaccination with M-M-R$_{II}$ may not result in seroconversion in 100% of susceptible subjects given the vaccine.

Adverse Reactions

Because of the slightly acidic pH (6.2–6.6) of the vaccine, patients may complain of burning and/or stinging of short duration at the injection site.
The adverse clinical reactions associated with the use of M-M-R$_{II}$ are those expected to follow administration of the monovalent vaccines given separately. These may include malaise, sore throat, headache, fever, and rash; mild local reactions such as erythema, induration, tenderness and regional lymphadenopathy; parotitis; orchitis; thrombocytopenia and purpura; allergic reactions such as wheal and flare at the injection site or urticaria; and arthritis, arthralgia and polyneuritis.
Moderate fever [101–102.9°F (38.3–39.4°C)] occurs occasionally, and high fever [above 103°F (39.4°C)] occurs less commonly. On rare occasions, children developing fever may exhibit febrile convulsions. Rash occurs infrequently and is usually minimal, but rarely may be generalized.
Clinical experience with live attenuated measles, mumps and rubella virus vaccines given individually indicates that encephalitis and other nervous system reactions have occurred very rarely. These might occur also with M-M-R$_{II}$.
Experience from more than 80 million doses of all live measles vaccines given in the U.S. through 1975 indicates that significant central nervous system reactions such as encephalitis and encephalopathy, occurring within 30 days after vaccination, have been temporally associated with measles vaccine approximately once for every million doses. In no case has it been shown that reactions were actually caused by vaccine. The Center for Disease Control has pointed out that "a certain number of cases of encephalitis may be expected to occur in a large childhood population in a defined period of time even when no vaccines are administered". However, the data suggest the possibility that some of these cases may have been caused by measles vaccines. The risk of such serious neurological disorders following live measles virus vaccine administration remains far less than that for encephalitis and encephalopathy with natural measles (one per thousand reported cases).
There have been isolated reports of ocular palsies and Guillain-Barre syndrome occurring after immunization with vaccines containing live attenuated measles virus. The ocular palsies have occurred approximately 3–24 days following vaccination. No definite causal relationship has been established between either of these events and vaccination.
There have been reports of subacute sclerosing panencephalitis (SSPE) in children who did not have a history of natural measles but did receive measles vaccine. Some of these cases may have resulted from unrecognized measles in the first year of life or possibly from the measles vaccination. Based on estimated nationwide measles vaccine distribution, the association of SSPE cases to measles vaccination is about one case per million vaccine doses distributed. This is far less than the association with natural measles, 5–10 cases of SSPE per million cases of measles. The results of a retrospective case-controlled study conducted by the Center for Disease Control suggest that the overall effect of measles vaccine has been to protect against SSPE by preventing measles with its inherent higher risk of SSPE.
Local reactions characterized by marked swelling, redness and vesiculation at the injection site of attenuated live measles virus vaccines have occurred in children who received killed measles vaccine previously. M-M-R$_{II}$ was not given under this condition in clinical trials.
Transient arthritis, arthralgia and polyneuritis are features of natural rubella and vary in frequency and severity with age and sex, being greatest in adult females and least in prepubertal children. This type of involvement has also been reported following administration of MERUVAX$_{II}$ (Rubella Virus Vaccine, Live, MSD). In children, joint reactions are rare and of brief duration if they do occur. In women, incidence rates for arthritis and arthralgia are generally higher than those seen in children (children: 0–3%; women: 12–20%), and the reactions tend to be more marked and of longer duration. Rarely, symptoms may persist for a matter of months. In adolescent girls, the reactions appear to be intermediate in incidence between those seen in children and in adult women. Even in older women (35–45 years), these reactions are generally well tolerated and rarely interfere with normal activities.

Dosage and Administration

After suitably cleansing the immunization site, inject the total volume of reconstituted vaccine subcutaneously, preferably into the outer aspect of the upper arm. Do not inject M-M-R$_{II}$ intravenously. *Do not give immune serum globulin (ISG) concurrently with* M-M-R$_{II}$.

CAUTION: A sterile syringe free of preservatives, antiseptics, and detergents should be used for each injection of the vaccine because these substances may inactivate the live virus vaccine. A 25 gauge, $5/8''$ needle is recommended.

Shipment, Storage, and Reconstitution

During shipment, to insure that there is no loss of potency, the vaccine must be maintained at a temperature of 10°C (50°F) or less.
Before reconstitution, store M-M-R$_{II}$ at 2–8°C (35.6–46.4°F). *Protect from light.*
To reconstitute, use only the diluent supplied, since it is free of preservatives or other antiviral substances which might inactivate the vaccine. First withdraw the entire volume of diluent into the syringe to be used for reconstitution. Inject all the diluent in the syringe into the vial of lyophilized vaccine, and agitate to mix thoroughly. Withdraw the entire contents into a syringe and inject the total volume of restored vaccine subcutaneously.
It is important to use a separate sterile syringe and needle for each individual patient to prevent transmission of hepatitis B and other infectious agents from one person to another.
The color of the vaccine when reconstituted is yellow.
It is recommended that the vaccine be used as soon as possible after reconstitution. Protect vaccine from light at all times. Store reconstituted vaccine in a dark place at 2–8°C (35.6–46.4°F) and discard if not used within 8 hours.

How Supplied

No. 4749—M-M-R$_{II}$ is supplied as a single-dose vial of lyophilized vaccine, **NDC** 0006-4749-00, and a vial of diluent.
No. 4681/4309—M-M-R$_{II}$ is supplied as follows: (1) a box of 10 single-dose vials of lyophilized vaccine (package A), **NDC** 0006-4681-00; and (2) a box of 10 vials of diluent (package B). To conserve refrigerator space, the diluent may be stored separately at room temperature.
A.H.F.S. Category: 80:12
DC 7034405 Issued February 1983
Copyright © MERCK & CO., INC., 1983
All rights reserved

---

* Morbidity and Mortality Weekly Report 25(44): 350, Nov. 12, 1976.

** Recommendation of the Immunization Practices Advisory Committee (ACIP), Morbidity and Mortality Weekly Report 30(4): 37–42, 47, Feb. 6, 1981.

M-R-VAX®II
(measles and rubella virus vaccine, live, MSD), U.S.P.

Description

M-R-VAX®II (Measles and Rubella Virus Vaccine, Live, MSD) is a live virus vaccine for immunization against measles (rubeola) and rubella (German measles).

M-R-VAXII is a lyophilized preparation of (1) ATTENUVAX® (Measles Virus Vaccine, Live, Attenuated, MSD), a more attenuated line of measles virus, derived from Enders' attenuated Edmonston strain and grown in cell cultures of chick embryo; and (2) MERUVAX®II (Rubella Virus Vaccine, Live, MSD), the Wistar RA 27/3 strain of live attenuated rubella virus grown in human diploid cell (WI-38) culture. The two viruses are mixed before being lyophilized. The product contains no preservative.

When reconstituted as directed, the dose for injection is 0.5 ml and contains not less than 1,000 TCID$_{50}$ (tissue culture infectious doses) of Measles Virus Vaccine, Live, Attenuated; and 1,000 TCID$_{50}$ of Rubella Virus Vaccine, Live, expressed in terms of the assigned titer of the FDA Reference Measles and Rubella Viruses. Each dose contains approximately 25 mcg of neomycin.

Actions

Clinical studies of 237 double seronegative children, 10 months to 10 years of age, demonstrated that M-R-VAXII is highly immunogenic and generally well tolerated. In these studies, a single injection of the vaccine induced measles hemagglutination-inhibition (HI) antibodies in 95 percent and rubella HI antibodies in 99 percent of susceptible persons.

The RA 27/3 rubella strain in M-R-VAXII elicits higher immediate post-vaccination HI, complement-fixing and neutralizing antibody levels than other strains of rubella vaccine and has been shown to induce a broader profile of circulating antibodies including anti-theta and anti-iota precipitating antibodies. The RA 27/3 rubella strain immunologically simulates natural infection more closely than other rubella vaccine viruses. The increased levels and broader profile of antibodies produced by RA 27/3 strain rubella virus vaccine appear to correlate with greater resistance to subclinical reinfection with the wild virus, and provide greater confidence for lasting immunity.

Data relating to persistence of vaccine-induced antibodies are not available for M-R-VAXII at this time; however, it is expected that the antibodies against measles and rubella will be just as durable following administration of M-R-VAXII as after the single vaccines given separately. Antibody levels after immunization with ATTENUVAX (Measles Virus Vaccine, Live, Attenuated, MSD) have persisted for at least eight years without substantial decline; and for at least six years after administration of RA 27/3 strain rubella virus vaccine.

Indications

M-R-VAXII is indicated for simultaneous immunization against measles and rubella in children 15 months of age or older, and adults.

Infants who are less than 15 months of age may fail to respond to one or both components of the vaccine due to presence in the circulation of residual measles and/or rubella antibody of maternal origin; the younger the infant, the lower the likelihood of seroconversion. In geographically isolated or other relatively inaccessible populations for whom immunization programs are logistically difficult, and in population groups in which natural measles infection may occur in a significant proportion of infants before 15 months of age, it may be desirable to give the vaccine to infants at an earlier age. The advantage of early protection must be weighed against the chance for failure of response; infants vaccinated under these conditions should be revaccinated after reaching 15 months of age.

Previously unimmunized children of susceptible pregnant women should receive live attenuated rubella vaccine, because an immunized child will be less likely to acquire natural rubella and introduce the virus into the household.

Non-Pregnant Adolescent and Adult Females
Immunization of susceptible non-pregnant adolescent and adult females of childbearing age with live attenuated rubella virus vaccine is indicated if certain precautions are observed (see below). Vaccinating susceptible postpubertal females confers individual protection against subsequently acquiring rubella infection during pregnancy, which in turn prevents infection of the fetus and consequent congenital rubella injury.

Pregnant females *must not* be given live attenuated rubella virus vaccine. It is not known to what extent infection of the fetus with attenuated virus might occur following vaccination, or whether damage to the fetus could result. Subjects should be considered for vaccination only if they agree that they will not become pregnant within three months following vaccination, and if they are informed of the reason for this precaution.* If a pregnant woman is inadvertently vaccinated or if she becomes pregnant within three months of vaccination, she should be counseled on the possible risks to the fetus.

It is recommended that rubella susceptibility be determined by serologic testing prior to immunization.** If immune, as evidenced by a specific rubella antibody titer of 1:8 or greater (hemagglutination inhibition test), vaccination is unnecessary. Congenital malformations do occur in up to seven percent of all live births. Their chance appearance after vaccination could lead to misinterpretation of the cause, particularly if the prior rubella-immune status of vaccinees is unknown.

Postpubertal females should be informed of the frequent occurrence of self-limited arthralgia and possible arthritis beginning 2 to 4 weeks after vaccination (See ADVERSE REACTIONS).

It has been found convenient in many instances to vaccinate rubella-susceptible women in the immediate postpartum period.

Revaccination: Based on available evidence, there is no reason to routinely revaccinate children originally vaccinated when 12 months of age or older; however, children vaccinated when younger than 12 months of age should be revaccinated. The decision to revaccinate should be based on evaluation of each individual case.

Use with Other Live Virus Vaccines
There are no data available concerning simultaneous use of M-R-VAXII with monovalent or trivalent poliovirus vaccine, live, oral, or with killed poliovirus vaccines. However, serologic evidence shows that when M-M-R® (Measles, Mumps and Rubella Virus Vaccine, Live, MSD) containing the HPV-77 rubella strain, is given simultaneously with trivalent poliovirus vaccine, live, oral, antibody responses can be expected to be comparable to those which follow administration of the vaccines at different times. From this it follows that

* NOTE: The Immunization Practices Advisory Committee (ACIP) has recommended "In view of the importance of protecting this age group against rubella, asking females if they are pregnant, excluding those who say they are, and explaining the theoretical risks to the others are reasonable precautions in a rubella immunization program."
** NOTE: The Immunization Practices Advisory Committee (ACIP) has stated "When practical, and when reliable laboratory services are available, potential vaccinees of childbearing age can have serologic tests to determine susceptibility to rubella.... However, routinely performing serologic tests for all females of childbearing age to determine susceptibility so that vaccine is given only to proven susceptibles is expensive and has been ineffective in some areas. Accordingly, the ACIP believes that rubella vaccination of a woman who is not known to be pregnant and has no history of vaccination is justifiable without serologic testing."

when M-R-VAXII is given simultaneously with either monovalent or trivalent poliovirus vaccine, live, oral and/or MUMPSVAX® (Mumps Virus Vaccine, Live, MSD), antibody responses can be expected to be comparable to those which follow administration of the vaccines at different times.

Contraindications

Do not give M-R-VAXII to pregnant females; the possible effects of the vaccine on fetal development are unknown at this time. If vaccination of postpubertal females is undertaken, pregnancy must be avoided for three months following vaccination. Hypersensitivity to neomycin (each dose of reconstituted vaccine contains approximately 25 mcg of neomycin).

Any febrile respiratory illness or other active febrile infection.

Active untreated tuberculosis.

Patients receiving therapy with ACTH, corticosteroids, irradiation, alkylating agents or antimetabolites. This contraindication does not apply to patients who are receiving corticosteroids as replacement therapy, e.g., for Addison's disease. Individuals with blood dyscrasias, leukemia, lymphomas of any type, or other malignant neoplasms affecting the bone marrow or lymphatic systems. Primary immuno-deficiency states, including cellular immune deficiencies, hypogammaglobulinemic and dysgammaglobulinemic states.

Hypersensitivity to Eggs, Chicken, or Chicken Feathers

This vaccine is essentially devoid of potentially allergenic substances derived from host tissues (chick embryos).* However, because the attenuated measles virus in this vaccine is propagated in cell cultures of chick embryo, there is a potential risk of hypersensitivity reactions in patients allergic to eggs, chicken, or chicken feathers. Widespread use of the vaccine for more than a decade has resulted in only rare, isolated reports of minor allergic reactions attributed to allergens of this kind, possibly related to the vaccine. Significantly, when children with known allergies to eggs, chicken, and chicken feathers were given a similarly prepared vaccine in a clinical study, none experienced reactions other than those reactions previously observed in non-allergic children.

Precautions

Administer M-R-VAXII subcutaneously; *do not give intravenously.*
Epinephrine should be available for immediate use in case an anaphylactoid reaction occurs. M-R-VAXII may be given simultaneously with monovalent or trivalent poliovirus vaccine, live, oral and/or with MUMPSVAX (Mumps Virus Vaccine, Live, MSD). M-R-VAXII should not be given less than one month before or after administration of other live virus vaccines.

Due caution should be employed in administration of M-R-VAXII to children with a history of febrile convulsions, cerebral injury or any other condition in which stress due to fever should be avoided. The physician should be alert to the temperature elevation which may occur 5 to 12 days following vaccination.

Vaccination should be deferred for at least 3 months following blood or plasma transfusions, or administration of human immune serum globulin. Excretion of small amounts of the live attenuated

* Morbidity and Mortality Weekly Report 25(44): 350, Nov. 12, 1976.

Continued on next page

Information on the Merck Sharp & Dohme products listed on these pages is the full prescribing information from product circulars in use November 1, 1984.

Merck Sharp & Dohme—Cont.

rubella virus from the nose or throat has occurred in the majority of susceptible individuals 7–28 days after vaccination. There is no confirmed evidence to indicate that such virus is transmitted to susceptible persons who are in contact with the vaccinated individuals. Consequently, transmission, while accepted as a theoretical possibility, is not regarded as a significant risk.**

There are no reports of transmission of live attenuated measles virus from vaccinees to susceptible contacts.

It has been reported that live attenuated measles and rubella virus vaccines given individually may result in a temporary depression of tuberculin skin sensitivity. Therefore, if a tuberculin test is to be done, it should be administered either before or simultaneously with M-R-VAX$_{II}$.

As for any vaccine, vaccination with M-R-VAX$_{II}$ may not result in seroconversion in 100% of susceptible subjects given the vaccine.

Adverse Reactions

Because of the slightly acidic pH (6.2–6.6) of the vaccine, patients may complain of burning and/or stinging of short duration at the injection site.

The adverse clinical reactions associated with the use of M-R-VAX$_{II}$ are those expected to follow administration of the monovalent vaccines given separately. These may include malaise, sore throat, headache, fever and rash; mild local reactions such as erythema, induration, tenderness and regional lymphadenopathy; thrombocytopenia and purpura; allergic reactions such as wheal and flare at the injection site or urticaria; and arthritis, arthralgia and polyneuritis.

Moderate fever [101–102.9°F (38.3–39.4°C)] occurs occasionally, and high fever [above 103°F (39.4°C)] occurs less commonly. On rare occasions, children developing fever may exhibit febrile convulsions. Rash occurs infrequently and is usually minimal, but rarely may be generalized.

Clinical experience with live attenuated measles and rubella virus vaccines given individually indicates that encephalitis and other nervous system reactions have occurred very rarely. These might occur also with M-R-VAX$_{II}$.

Experience from more than 80 million doses of all live measles vaccines given in the U.S. through 1975 indicates that significant central nervous system reactions such as encephalitis and encephalopathy, occurring within 30 days after vaccination, have been temporally associated with measles vaccine approximately once for every million doses. In no case has it been shown that reactions were actually caused by vaccine. The Center for Disease Control has pointed out that "a certain number of cases of encephalitis may be expected to occur in a large childhood population in a defined period of time even when no vaccines are administered". However, the data suggest the possibility that some of these cases may have been caused by measles vaccines. The risk of such serious neurological disorders following live measles virus vaccine administration remains far less than that for encephalitis and encephalopathy with natural measles (one per thousand reported cases).

There have been isolated reports of ocular palsies and Guillain-Barre syndrome occurring after immunization with vaccines containing live attenuated measles virus. The ocular palsies have occurred approximately 3–24 days following vaccination. No definite causal relationship has been established between either of these events and vaccination.

There have been reports of subacute sclerosing panencephalitis (SSPE) in children who did not have a history of natural measles but did receive measles vaccine. Some of these cases may have resulted from unrecognized measles in the first year of life or possibly from the measles vaccination. Based on estimated nationwide measles vaccine distribution, the association of SSPE cases to measles vaccination is about one case per million vaccine doses distributed. This is far less than the association with natural measles, 5–10 cases of SSPE per million cases of measles. The results of a retrospective case-controlled study conducted by the Center for Disease Control suggest that the overall effect of measles vaccine has been to protect against SSPE by preventing measles with its inherent higher risk of SSPE.

Local reactions characterized by marked swelling, redness and vesiculation at the injection site of attenuated live measles virus vaccines have occurred in children who received killed measles vaccine previously. M-R-VAX$_{II}$ was not given under this condition in clinical trials.

Transient arthritis, arthralgia and polyneuritis are features of natural rubella and vary in frequency and severity with age and sex, being greatest in adult females and least in prepubertal children. This type of involvement has also been reported following administration of MERUVAX$_{II}$ (Rubella Virus Vaccine, Live, MSD). In children, joint reactions are rare and of brief duration if they do occur. In women, incidence rates for arthritis and arthralgia are generally higher than those seen in children (children: 0–3%; women: 12–20%), and the reactions tend to be more marked and of longer duration. Rarely, symptoms may persist for a matter of months. In adolescent girls, the reactions appear to be intermediate in incidence between those seen in children and in adult women. Even in older women (35–45 years), these reactions are generally well tolerated and rarely interfere with normal activities.

Dosage and Administration

After suitably cleansing the immunization site, inject the total volume of reconstituted vaccine subcutaneously, preferably into the outer aspect of the upper arm. Do not inject M-R-VAX$_{II}$ intravenously. *Do not give immune serum globulin (ISG) concurrently with* M-R-VAX$_{II}$.

CAUTION: A sterile syringe free of preservatives, antiseptics, and detergents should be used for each injection of the vaccine because these substances may inactivate the live virus vaccine. A 25 gauge, 5/8" needle is recommended.

Shipment, Storage, and Reconstitution

During shipment, to insure that there is no loss of potency, the vaccine must be maintained at a temperature of 10°C (50°F) or less.

Before reconstitution, store M-R-VAX$_{II}$ at 2–8°C (35.6–46.4°F). *Protect from light.*

To reconstitute, use only the diluent supplied, since it is free of preservatives or other antiviral substances which might inactivate the vaccine. First withdraw the entire volume of diluent into the syringe to be used for reconstitution. Inject all the diluent in the syringe into the vial of lyophilized vaccine, and agitate to mix thoroughly. Withdraw the entire contents into a syringe and inject the total volume of restored vaccine subcutaneously.

It is important to use a separate sterile syringe and needle for each individual patient to prevent transmission of hepatitis B and other infectious agents from one person to another.

The usual color of the vaccine when reconstituted is yellow.

It is recommended that the vaccine be used as soon as possible after reconstitution. Protect vaccine from light at all times. Store reconstituted vaccine in a dark place at 2–8°C (35.6– 46.4°F) and discard if not used within 8 hours.

How Supplied

No. 4751—M-R-VAX$_{II}$ is supplied as a single-dose vial of lyophilized vaccine, NDC 0006-4751-00, and a vial of diluent.

No. 4677/4309—M-R-VAX$_{II}$ is supplied as follows: (1) a box of 10 single-dose vials of lyophilized vaccine (package A), NDC 0006-4677-00; and (2) a box of 10 vials of diluent (package B). To conserve refrigerator space, the diluent may be stored separately at room temperature.

A.H.F.S. Category: 80:12
DC 7032906 Issued February 1983
Copyright © MERCK & CO., INC., 1983
All rights reserved

MEFOXIN® ℞
(cefoxitin sodium, MSD), U.S.P.

Description

MEFOXIN® (Sterile Cefoxitin Sodium, MSD) is a semi-synthetic, broad-spectrum cepha antibiotic for parenteral administration. It is derived from cephamycin C, which is produced by *Streptomyces lactamdurans*. It is the sodium salt of 3-(hydroxymethyl)-7α- methoxy-8-oxo -7- [2- (2-thienyl) acetamido]-5-thia-1-azabicyclo [4.2.0] oct-2-ene-2-carboxylate carbamate (ester). MEFOXIN contains approximately 53.8 mg (2.3 milliequivalents) of sodium per gram of cefoxitin activity. Solutions of MEFOXIN range from clear to light amber in color. The pH of freshly constituted solutions usually ranges from 4.2 to 7.0.

Actions

Clinical Pharmacology
After intramuscular administration of a 1 gram dose of MEFOXIN to normal volunteers, the mean peak serum concentration was 24 mcg/ml. The peak occurred at 20 to 30 minutes. Following an intravenous dose of 1 gram, serum concentrations were 110 mcg/ml at 5 minutes, declining to less than 1 mcg/ml at 4 hours. The half-life after an intravenous dose is 41 to 59 minutes; after intramuscular administration, the half-life is 64.8 minutes. Approximately 85 percent of cefoxitin is excreted unchanged by the kidneys over a 6-hour period, resulting in high urinary concentrations. Following an intramuscular dose of 1 gram, urinary concentrations greater than 3000 mcg/ml were observed. Probenecid slows tubular excretion and produces higher serum levels and increases the duration of measurable serum concentrations. Cefoxitin passes into pleural and joint fluids and is detectable in antibacterial concentrations in bile. Clinical experience has demonstrated that MEFOXIN can be administered to patients who are also receiving carbenicillin, kanamycin, gentamicin, tobramycin, or amikacin (see PRECAUTIONS and ADMINISTRATION).

Microbiology
The bactericidal action of cefoxitin results from inhibition of cell wall synthesis. Cefoxitin has *in vitro* activity against a wide range of gram-positive and gram-negative organisms. The methoxy group in the 7α position provides MEFOXIN with a high degree of stability in the presence of beta-lactamases, both penicillinases and cephalosporinases, of gram-negative bacteria. Cefoxitin is usually active against the following organisms *in vitro* and in clinical infections:

Gram-positive
  Staphylococcus aureus, including penicillinase and non-penicillinase producing strains.
  Staphylococcus epidermidis
  Beta-hemolytic and other streptococci (most strains of enterococci, e.g., *Streptococcus faecalis*, are resistant)
  Streptococcus pneumoniae (formerly *Diplococcus pneumoniae*)

Gram-negative
  Escherichia coli
  Klebsiella species (including *K. pneumoniae*)
  Hemophilus influenzae
  Neisseria gonorrhoeae, including penicillinase and non-penicillinase producing strains
  Proteus mirabilis
  Proteus rettgeri
  Proteus morganii
  Proteus vulgaris
  Providencia species

Anaerobic organisms
  Peptococcus species

** Recommendation of the Immunization Practices Advisory Committee (ACIP), Morbidity and Mortality Weekly Report *30*(4): 37–42, 47, Feb. 6, 1981.

Peptostreptococcus species
Clostridium species
Bacteroides species, including the *B. fragilis* group (includes *B. fragilis, B. distasonis, B. ovatus, B. thetaiotaomicron, B. vulgatus*)

MEFOXIN is inactive *in vitro* against most strains of *Pseudomonas aeruginosa* and enterococci and many strains of *Enterobacter cloacae*.

Methicillin-resistant staphylococci are almost uniformly resistant to MEFOXIN.

Susceptibility Tests

For fast-growing aerobic organisms, quantitative methods that require measurements of zone diameters give the most precise estimates of antibiotic susceptibility. One such procedure* has been recommended for use with discs to test susceptibility to cefoxitin. Interpretation involves correlation of the diameters obtained in the disc test with minimal inhibitory concentration (MIC) values for cefoxitin.

Reports from the laboratory giving results of the standardized single disc susceptibility test* using a 30 mcg cefoxitin disc should be interpreted according to the following criteria:

Organisms producing zones of 18 mm or greater are considered susceptible, indicating that the tested organism is likely to respond to therapy.

Organisms of intermediate susceptibility produce zones of 15 to 17 mm, indicating that the tested organism would be susceptible if high dosage is used or if the infection is confined to tissues and fluids (e.g., urine) in which high antibiotic levels are attained.

Resistant organisms produce zones of 14 mm or less, indicating that other therapy should be selected.

The cefoxitin disc should be used for testing cefoxitin susceptibility.

Cefoxitin has been shown by *in vitro* tests to have activity against certain strains of *Enterobacteriaceae* found resistant when tested with the cephalosporin class disc. For this reason, the cefoxitin disc should not be used for testing susceptibility to cephalosporins, and cephalosporin discs should not be used for testing susceptibility to cefoxitin.

Dilution methods, preferably the agar plate dilution procedure, are most accurate for susceptibility testing of obligate anaerobes.

A bacterial isolate may be considered susceptible if the MIC value for cefoxitin† is not more than 16 mcg/ml. Organisms are considered resistant if the MIC is greater than 32 mcg/ml.

Indications and Usage

Treatment

MEFOXIN is indicated for the treatment of serious infections caused by susceptible strains of the designated microorganisms in the diseases listed below.

(1) Lower respiratory tract infections, including pneumonia and lung abscess, caused by *Streptococcus pneumoniae* (formerly *Diplococcus pneumoniae*), other streptococci (excluding enterococci, e.g., *Streptococcus faecalis*), *Staphylococcus aureus* (penicillinase and non-penicillinase producing), *Escherichia coli, Klebsiella* species, *Hemophilus influenzae,* and *Bacteroides* species.

(2) Genitourinary infections. Urinary tract infections caused by *Escherichia coli, Klebsiella* species,

---

*Bauer, A. W.; Kirby, W. M. M.; Sherris, J. C.; Turck, M.: Antibiotic susceptibility testing by a standardized single disc method, Amer. J. Clin. Path. 45: 493-496, Apr. 1966. Standardized disc susceptibility test, Federal Register 37: 20527-20529, 1972. National Committee for Clinical Laboratory Standards: Approved Standard: ASM-2, Performance Standards for Antimicrobial Disc Susceptibility Tests, July 1975.

†Determined by the ICS agar dilution method (Ericsson and Sherris, Acta Path. Microbiol. Scand. (B) Suppl. No. 217, 1971) or any other method that has been shown to give equivalent results.

Proteus mirabilis, indole-positive Proteus (i.e., *Proteus morganii, rettgeri,* and *vulgaris*), and *Providencia* species. Uncomplicated gonorrhea due to *Neisseria gonorrhoeae* (penicillinase and non-penicillinase producing).

(3) Intra-abdominal infections, including peritonitis and intra-abdominal abscess, caused by *Escherichia coli, Klebsiella* species, *Bacteroides* species including the *Bacteroides fragilis* group**, and *Clostridium* species.

(4) Gynecological infections, including endometritis, pelvic cellulitis, and pelvic inflammatory disease caused by *Escherichia coli, Neisseria gonorrhoeae* (penicillinase and non-penicillinase producing), *Bacteroides* species including the *Bacteroides fragilis* group**, *Clostridium* species, *Peptococcus* species, *Peptostreptococcus* species, and Group B streptococci.

(5) Septicemia caused by *Streptococcus pneumoniae* (formerly *Diplococcus pneumoniae*), *Staphylococcus aureus* (penicillinase and non-penicillinase producing), *Escherichia coli, Klebsiella* species, and *Bacteroides* species including the *Bacteroides fragilis* group.**

(6) Bone and joint infections caused by *Staphylococcus aureus* (penicillinase and non-penicillinase producing).

(7) Skin and skin structure infections caused by *Staphylococcus aureus* (penicillinase and non-penicillinase producing), *Staphylococcus epidermidis,* streptococci (excluding enterococci, e.g., *Streptococcus faecalis*), *Escherichia coli, Proteus mirabilis, Klebsiella* species, *Bacteroides* species including the *Bacteroides fragilis* group**, *Clostridium* species, *Peptococcus* species, and *Peptostreptococcus* species.

Appropriate culture and susceptibility studies should be performed to determine the susceptibility of the causative organisms to MEFOXIN. Therapy may be started while awaiting the results of these studies.

In randomized comparative studies, MEFOXIN and cephalothin were comparably safe and effective in the management of infections caused by gram-positive cocci and gram-negative rods susceptible to the cephalosporins. MEFOXIN has a high degree of stability in the presence of bacterial beta-lactamases, both penicillinases and cephalosporinases.

Many infections caused by aerobic and anaerobic gram-negative bacteria resistant to some cephalosporins respond to MEFOXIN. Similarly, many infections caused by aerobic and anaerobic bacteria resistant to some penicillin antibiotics (ampicillin, carbenicillin, penicillin G) respond to treatment with MEFOXIN. Many infections caused by mixtures of susceptible aerobic and anaerobic bacteria respond to treatment with MEFOXIN.

Prevention

When compared to placebo in randomized controlled studies in patients undergoing gastrointestinal surgery, vaginal hysterectomy, abdominal hysterectomy and cesarean section, the prophylactic use of MEFOXIN resulted in a significant reduction in the number of postoperative infections. The prophylactic administration of MEFOXIN perioperatively (preoperatively, intraoperatively, and postoperatively) may reduce the incidence of certain postoperative infections in patients undergoing surgical procedures (e.g., hysterectomy, gastrointestinal surgery and transurethral prostatectomy) that are classified as contaminated or potentially contaminated.

The perioperative use of MEFOXIN may be effective in surgical patients in whom infection at the operative site would present a serious risk, e.g., prosthetic arthroplasty.

In patients undergoing cesarean section, intraoperative (after clamping the umbilical cord) and postoperative use of MEFOXIN may reduce the incidence of certain postoperative infections. Effective prophylactic use depends on the time of administration. MEFOXIN usually should be given one-half to one hour before the operation,

---

** *B. fragilis, B. distasonis, B. ovatus, B. thetaiotaomicron, B. vulgatus.*

which is sufficient time to achieve effective levels in the wound during the procedure. Prophylactic administration should usually be stopped within 24 hours since continuing administration of any antibiotic increases the possibility of adverse reactions but, in the majority of surgical procedures, does not reduce the incidence of subsequent infection. However, in patients undergoing prosthetic arthroplasty, it is recommended that MEFOXIN be continued for 72 hours after the surgical procedure.

If there are signs of infection, specimens for culture should be obtained for identification of the causative organism so that appropriate therapy may be instituted.

Contraindications

MEFOXIN is contraindicated in patients who have shown hypersensitivity to cefoxitin and the cephalosporin group of antibiotics.

Warnings

BEFORE THERAPY WITH MEFOXIN IS INSTITUTED, CAREFUL INQUIRY SHOULD BE MADE TO DETERMINE WHETHER THE PATIENT HAS HAD PREVIOUS HYPERSENSITIVITY REACTIONS TO CEFOXITIN, CEPHALOSPORINS, PENICILLINS, OR OTHER DRUGS. THIS PRODUCT SHOULD BE GIVEN WITH CAUTION TO PENICILLIN-SENSITIVE PATIENTS. ANTIBIOTICS SHOULD BE ADMINISTERED WITH CAUTION TO ANY PATIENT WHO HAS DEMONSTRATED SOME FORM OF ALLERGY, PARTICULARLY TO DRUGS. IF AN ALLERGIC REACTION TO MEFOXIN OCCURS, DISCONTINUE THE DRUG. SERIOUS HYPERSENSITIVITY REACTIONS MAY REQUIRE EPINEPHRINE AND OTHER EMERGENCY MEASURES.

Pseudomembranous colitis has been reported with virtually all antibiotics (including cephalosporins); therefore, it is important to consider its diagnosis in patients who develop diarrhea in association with antibiotic use. This colitis may range from mild to life threatening in severity.

Treatment with broad-spectrum antibiotics alters normal flora of the colon and may permit overgrowth of clostridia. Studies indicate a toxin produced by *Clostridium difficile* is one primary cause of antibiotic-associated colitis.

Mild cases of pseudomembranous colitis may respond to drug discontinuance alone. In more severe cases, management may include sigmoidoscopy, appropriate bacteriological studies, fluid, electrolyte and protein supplementation, and the use of a drug such as oral vancomycin as indicated. Isolation of the patient may be advisable. Other causes of colitis should also be considered.

Precautions

The total daily dose should be reduced when MEFOXIN is administered to patients with transient or persistent reduction of urinary output due to renal insufficiency (see DOSAGE), because high and prolonged serum antibiotic concentrations can occur in such individuals from usual doses.

Antibiotics (including cephalosporins) should be prescribed with caution in individuals with a history of gastrointestinal disease, particularly colitis.

As with other antibiotics, prolonged use of MEFOXIN may result in overgrowth of nonsusceptible organisms. Repeated evaluation of the patient's condition is essential. If superinfection occurs during therapy, appropriate measures should be taken.

Continued on next page

Information on the Merck Sharp & Dohme products listed on these pages is the full prescribing information from product circulars in use November 1, 1984.

Merck Sharp & Dohme—Cont.

Increased nephrotoxicity has been reported following concomitant administration of cephalosporins and aminoglycoside antibiotics.

Interference with Laboratory Tests
As with cephalothin, high concentrations of cefoxitin (>100 micrograms/ml) may interfere with measurement of serum and urine creatinine levels by the Jaffé reaction, and produce false increases of modest degree in the levels of creatinine reported. Serum samples from patients treated with cefoxitin should not be analyzed for creatinine if withdrawn within 2 hours of drug administration. High concentrations of cefoxitin in the urine may interfere with measurement of urinary 17-hydroxy-corticosteroids by the Porter-Silber reaction, and produce false increases of modest degree in the levels reported.

A false-positive reaction for glucose in the urine may occur. This has been observed with CLINITEST* reagent tablets.

Pregnancy
Reproduction and teratologic studies have been performed in mice and rats and have revealed no evidence of impaired fertility or harm to the fetus due to MEFOXIN. There are no well controlled studies with MEFOXIN in pregnant women. Use of the drug in women of childbearing potential requires that the anticipated benefit be weighed against the possible risks.

Nursing Mothers
MEFOXIN is excreted in human milk in low concentrations.

Infants and Children
Safety and efficacy in infants from birth to three months of age have not yet been established. In children three months of age and older, higher doses of MEFOXIN have been associated with an increased incidence of eosinophilia and elevated SGOT.

Adverse Reactions

MEFOXIN is generally well tolerated. The most common adverse reactions have been local reactions following intravenous or intramuscular injection. Other adverse reactions have been encountered infrequently.

Local Reactions
Thrombophlebitis has occurred with intravenous administration. Pain, induration, and tenderness after intramuscular injections have been reported.

Allergic Reactions
Rash (including exfoliative dermatitis), pruritus, eosinophilia, fever, and other allergic reactions have been noted.

Gastrointestinal
Symptoms of pseudomembranous colitis can appear during or after antibiotic treatment. Nausea and vomiting have been reported rarely.

---
*Registered trademark of Ames Company, Division of Miles Laboratories, Inc.

Blood
Transient eosinophilia, leukopenia, neutropenia, hemolytic anemia, and thrombocytopenia have been reported. A positive direct Coombs test may develop in some individuals, especially those with azotemia.

Liver Function
Transient elevations in SGOT, SGPT, serum LDH, and serum alkaline phosphatase have been reported.

Renal Function
Elevations in serum creatinine and/or blood urea nitrogen levels have been observed. As with the cephalosporins, acute renal failure has been reported rarely. The role of MEFOXIN in changes in renal function tests is difficult to assess, since factors predisposing to prerenal azotemia or to impaired renal function usually have been present.

Dosage

TREATMENT
Adults
The usual adult dosage range is 1 gram to 2 grams every six to eight hours. Dosage and route of administration should be determined by susceptibility of the causative organisms, severity of infection, and the condition of the patient (see Table 1 for dosage guidelines).
[See table below].
MEFOXIN may be used in patients with reduced renal function with the following dosage adjustments:
In adults with renal insufficiency, an initial loading dose of 1 gram to 2 grams may be given. After a loading dose, the recommendations for *maintenance dosage* (Table 2) may be used as a guide.
[See table above].
When only the serum creatinine level is available, the following formula (based on sex, weight, and age of the patient) may be used to convert this value into creatinine clearance. The serum creatinine should represent a steady state of renal function.

Males: $\dfrac{\text{Weight (kg)} \times (140 - \text{age})}{72 \times \text{serum creatinine (mg/100 ml)}}$

Females: $0.85 \times$ above value

In patients undergoing hemodialysis, the loading dose of 1 to 2 grams should be given after each hemodialysis, and the maintenance dose should be given as indicated in Table 2.
Antibiotic therapy for group A beta-hemolytic streptococcal infections should be maintained for at least 10 days to guard against the risk of rheumatic fever or glomerulonephritis. In staphylococcal and other infections involving a collection of pus, surgical drainage should be carried out where indicated.

The recommended dosage of MEFOXIN **for uncomplicated gonorrhea** is 2 grams intramuscularly, with 1 gram of BENEMID® (Probenecid, MSD) given by mouth at the same time or up to ½ hour before MEFOXIN.

Infants and Children
The recommended dosage in children three months of age and older is 80 to 160 mg/kg of body weight per day divided into four to six equal doses. The higher dosages should be used for more severe or serious infections. The total daily dosage should not exceed 12 grams.

At this time no recommendation is made for children from birth to three months of age (See PRECAUTIONS).

In children with renal insufficiency the dosage and frequency of dosage should be modified consistent with the recommendations for adults (see Table 2).

PREVENTION
For prophylactic use, the following doses are recommended:
Adults:
1) 2 grams administered intravenously or intramuscularly just prior to surgery (approximately one-half to one hour before the initial incision).
2) 2 grams every 6 hours after the first dose for no more than 24 hours (continued for 72 hours after prosthetic arthroplasty).

Children (3 months and older):
30 to 40 mg/kg doses may be given at the time designated above.

Cesarean section patients:
The first dose of 2.0 grams is administered intravenously as soon as the umbilical cord is clamped. The second and third doses should be given as 2.0 grams intravenously or intramuscularly 4 hours and 8 hours after the first dose. Subsequent doses may be given every 6 hours for no more than 24 hours.

Transurethral prostatectomy patients:
One gram administered just prior to surgery; 1 gram every 8 hours for up to five days.

Preparation of Solution

Table 3 is provided for convenience in constituting MEFOXIN for both intravenous and intramuscular administration.
[See table on next page].
For intravenous use, 1 gram should be constituted with at least 10 ml of Sterile Water for Injection, and 2 grams, with 10 or 20 ml. The 10 gram bulk package should be constituted with 50 or 100 ml of Sterile Water for Injection or any of the solutions listed under the *Intravenous* portion of the COMPATIBILITY AND STABILITY section. CAUTION: NOT FOR DIRECT INFUSION. One or 2 grams of MEFOXIN for infusion may be constituted with 50 or 100 ml of 0.9 percent Sodium Chloride Injection, 5 percent or 10 percent Dextrose Injection, or any of the solutions listed under the *Intravenous* portion of the COMPATIBILITY AND STABILITY section.

Benzyl alcohol as a preservative has been associated with toxicity in neonates. While toxicity has not been demonstrated in infants greater than three months of age, in whom use of MEFOXIN may be indicated, small infants in this age range may also be at risk for benzyl alcohol toxicity. Therefore, diluent containing benzyl alcohol should not be used when MEFOXIN is constituted for administration to infants.

Table 2—Maintenance Dosage of MEFOXIN in Adults with Reduced Renal Function

Renal Function	Creatinine Clearance (ml/min)	Dose (grams)	Frequency
Mild impairment	50–30	1–2	every 8–12 hours
Moderate impairment	29–10	1–2	every 12–24 hours
Severe impairment	9–5	0.5–1	every 12–24 hours
Essentially no function	<5	0.5–1	every 24–48 hours

Table 1—Guidelines for Dosage of MEFOXIN

Type of Infection	Daily Dosage	Frequency and Route
Uncomplicated forms* of infections such as pneumonia, urinary tract infection, cutaneous infection	3–4 grams	1 gram every 6–8 hours IV or IM
Moderately severe or severe infections	6–8 grams	1 gram every 4 hours *or* 2 grams every 6–8 hours IV
Infections commonly needing antibiotics in higher dosage (e.g., gas gangrene)	12 grams	2 grams every 4 hours *or* 3 grams every 6 hours IV

*Including patients in whom bacteremia is absent or unlikely

For intramuscular use, each gram of MEFOXIN may be constituted with 2 ml of Sterile Water for Injection, or
For intramuscular use ONLY: each gram of MEFOXIN may be constituted with 2 ml of 0.5 percent lidocaine hydrochloride solution* (without epinephrine) to minimize the discomfort of intramuscular injection.

Administration

MEFOXIN may be administered intravenously or intramuscularly after constitution.
Intravenous Administration
The intravenous route is preferable for patients with bacteremia, bacterial septicemia, or other severe or life-threatening infections, or for patients who may be poor risks because of lowered resistance resulting from such debilitating conditions as malnutrition, trauma, surgery, diabetes, heart failure, or malignancy, particularly if shock is present or impending.
For intermittent intravenous administration, a solution containing 1 gram or 2 grams in 10 ml of Sterile Water for Injection can be injected over a period of three to five minutes. Using an infusion system, it may also be given over a longer period of time through the tubing system by which the patient may be receiving other intravenous solutions. However, during infusion of the solution containing MEFOXIN, it is advisable to temporarily discontinue administration of any other solutions at the same site.
For the administration of higher doses by continuous intravenous infusion, a solution of MEFOXIN may be added to an intravenous bottle containing 5 percent Dextrose Injection, 0.9 percent Sodium Chloride Injection, 5 percent Dextrose and 0.9 percent Sodium Chloride Injection, or 5 percent Dextrose Injection with 0.02 percent sodium bicarbonate solution. BUTTERFLY** or scalp vein-type needles are preferred for this type of infusion. Solutions of MEFOXIN, like those of most beta-lactam antibiotics, should not be added to aminoglycoside solutions (e.g., gentamicin sulfate, tobramycin sulfate, amikacin sulfate) because of potential interaction. However, MEFOXIN and aminoglycosides may be administered separately to the same patient.

Intramuscular Administration
As with all intramuscular preparations, MEFOXIN should be injected well within the body of a relatively large muscle such as the upper outer quadrant of the buttock (i.e., gluteus maximus); aspiration is necessary to avoid inadvertent injection into a blood vessel.

Compatibility and Stability

Intravenous
MEFOXIN, as supplied in vials or the bulk package and constituted to 1 gram/10 ml with Sterile Water for Injection, Bacteriostatic Water for Injection (see PREPARATION OF SOLUTION), 0.9 percent Sodium Chloride Injection, or 5 percent Dextrose Injection, maintains satisfactory potency for 24 hours at room temperature, for one week under refrigeration (below 5°C), and for at least 30 weeks in the frozen state.
These primary solutions may be further diluted in 50 to 1000 ml of the following solutions and maintain potency for 24 hours at room temperature and at least 48 hours under refrigeration:
 Sterile Water for Injection‡
 0.9 percent Sodium Chloride Injection
 5 percent or 10 percent Dextrose Injection‡
 5 percent Dextrose and 0.9 percent Sodium Chloride Injection
 5 percent Dextrose Injection with 0.02 percent sodium bicarbonate solution

---

*See package circular of manufacturer for detailed information concerning contraindications, warnings, precautions, and adverse reactions.

** Registered trademark of Abbott Laboratories.

Table 3—Preparation of Solution
MEFOXIN

Strength	Amount of Diluent to be Added (ml)*	Approximate Withdrawable Volume (ml)	Approximate Average Concentration (mg/ml)
1 gram Vial	2 (Intramuscular)	2.5	400
2 gram Vial	4 (Intramuscular)	5	400
1 gram Vial	10 (IV)	10.5	95
2 gram Vial	10 or 20 (IV)	11.1 or 21.0	180 or 95
1 gram Infusion Bottle	50 or 100 (IV)	50 or 100	20 or 10
2 gram Infusion Bottle	50 or 100 (IV)	50 or 100	40 or 20
10 gram Bulk	50 or 100 (IV)	55 or 105	180 or 95

*Shake to dissolve and let stand until clear.

---

 5 percent Dextrose Injection with 0.2 percent or 0.45 percent saline solution
 Ringer's Injection
 Lactated Ringer's Injection‡
 5 percent dextrose in Lactated Ringer's Injection‡
 5 percent or 10 percent invert sugar in water
 10 percent invert sugar in saline solution
 5 percent Sodium Bicarbonate Injection
 Neut (sodium bicarbonate)*‡
 M/6 sodium lactate solution
 AMINOSOL* 5 percent Solution
 NORMOSOL-M in D5-W*‡
 IONOSOL B w/Dextrose 5 percent*‡
 POLYONIC M 56 in 5 percent Dextrose**
 Mannitol 5% and 2.5%
 Mannitol 10%‡
 ISOLYTE ***E
 ISOLYTE ***E with 5% dextrose
MEFOXIN, as supplied in infusion bottles and constituted with 50 to 100 ml of 0.9 percent Sodium Chloride Injection, or 5 percent or 10 percent Dextrose Injection, maintains satisfactory potency for 24 hours at room temperature or for 1 week under refrigeration (below 5°C).
Limited studies with solutions of MEFOXIN in 0.9 percent Sodium Chloride Injection, Lactated Ringer's Injection, and 5 percent Dextrose Injection in VIAFLEX† intravenous bags show stability for 24 hours at room temperature, 48 hours under refrigeration, 26 weeks in the frozen state, and 24 hours at room temperature thereafter. Also, solutions of MEFOXIN in 0.9 percent Sodium Chloride Injection show similar stability in plastic tubing, drip chambers, and volume control devices of common intravenous infusion sets.
After constitution with Sterile Water for Injection and subsequent storage in disposable plastic syringes, MEFOXIN is stable for 24 hours at room temperature and 48 hours under refrigeration.
After the periods mentioned above, any unused solutions or frozen material should be discarded. Do not refreeze.
Intramuscular
MEFOXIN, as constituted with Sterile Water for Injection, Bacteriostatic Water for Injection, or 0.5 percent or 1 percent lidocaine hydrochloride solution (without epinephrine), maintains satisfactory potency for 24 hours at room temperature, for one week under refrigeration (below 5°C), and for at least 30 weeks in the frozen state.
After the periods mentioned above, any unused solutions or frozen material should be discarded. Do not refreeze.
MEFOXIN has also been found compatible when admixed in intravenous infusions with the following:
 Heparin 0.1 units/ml at room temperature—8 hours

---

* Registered trademark of Abbott Laboratories.
** Registered trademark of Cutter Laboratories, Inc.
*** Registered trademark of American Hospital Supply Corporation.
† Travenol Laboratories, Inc.
‡ In these solutions, MEFOXIN has been found to be stable for a period of one week under refrigeration.

 Heparin 100 units/ml at room temperature—24 hours
 M.V.I.†† concentrate at room temperature 24 hours; under refrigeration 48 hours
 BEROCCA††† C-500 at room temperature 24 hours; under refrigeration 48 hours
 Insulin in Normal Saline at room temperature 24 hours; under refrigeration 48 hours
 Insulin in 10% invert sugar at room temperature 24 hours; under refrigeration 48 hours

How Supplied

Sterile MEFOXIN is a dry white to off-white powder supplied in vials and infusion bottles containing cefoxitin sodium as follows:
No. 3356—1 gram cefoxitin equivalent
NDC 0006-3356-71 in trays of 10 vials.
NDC 0006-3356-45 in trays of 25 vials.
No. 3368—1 gram cefoxitin equivalent
NDC 0006-3368-71 in trays of 10 infusion bottles.
No. 3357—2 gram cefoxitin equivalent
NDC 0006-3357-73 in trays of 10 vials.
NDC 0006-3357-53 in trays of 25 vials.
No. 3369—2 gram cefoxitin equivalent
NDC 0006-3369-73 in trays of 10 infusion bottles.
No. 3388—10 gram cefoxitin equivalent
NDC 0006-3388-10 in bulk bottles.
  A.H.F.S. Category: 8:12.28
  DC 7057117   Issued February 1983
COPYRIGHT© MERCK & CO., INC., 1983
All rights reserved

†† Registered trademark of USV Pharmaceutical Corp.
††† Registered trademark of Roche Laboratories.
Note: MEFOXIN in the dry state should be stored below 30°C. Avoid exposure to temperatures above 50°C. The dry material as well as solutions tend to darken, depending on storage conditions; product potency, however, is not adversely affected.

MERUVAX® II
(rubella virus vaccine, live, MSD), U.S.P.
(Wistar RA 27/3 Strain
Prepared in WI-38 Human Diploid Cells)

Description

MERUVAX® II (Rubella Virus Vaccine, Live, MSD) is a live virus vaccine for immunization against rubella (German measles).
MERUVAX II is a lyophilized preparation of the Wistar Institute RA 27/3 strain of live attenuated rubella virus. The virus was adapted to and propagated in human diploid cell (WI-38) culture.
When reconstituted as directed, the dose for injection is 0.5 ml and contains not less than the equivalent of 1,000 TCID$_{50}$ (tissue culture infective doses) of rubella virus vaccine expressed in terms of the assigned titer of the FDA Reference Rubella Virus. Each dose also contains approximately 25 mcg of neomycin.

Continued on next page

Information on the Merck Sharp & Dohme products listed on these pages is the full prescribing information from product circulars in use November 1, 1984.

Merck Sharp & Dohme—Cont.

Actions

Extensive clinical trials of rubella virus vaccines, prepared using RA 27/3 strain rubella virus, have been carried out in more than 28,000 human subjects (approximately 11,000 with MERUVAX II in the U.S.A. and more than 20 additional countries. Following subcutaneous inoculation, the vaccines have been shown to induce rubella hemagglutination-inhibiting (HI) antibodies in over 97% of susceptible subjects. The RA 27/3 rubella strain elicits higher immediate post-vaccination HI, complement-fixing and neutralizing antibody levels than other strains of rubella vaccine and has been shown to induce a broader profile of circulating antibodies including anti-theta and anti-iota precipitating antibodies. The RA 27/3 rubella strain immunologically simulates natural infection more closely than other rubella vaccine viruses. The increased levels and broader profile of antibodies produced by RA 27/3 strain rubella virus vaccine appear to correlate with greater resistance to subclinical reinfection with the wild virus, and provide greater confidence for lasting immunity.

Vaccine induced antibody levels have been shown to persist for at least six years without substantial decline. If the present pattern continues, it will provide a basis for the expectation that immunity following the vaccine will be permanent. However, continued surveillance will be required to demonstrate this point.

Indications†

1. *Children Between 12 Months of Age and Puberty*
MERUVAX II is indicated for immunization against rubella in boys and girls from 12 months of age to puberty. No booster is needed. It is not recommended for infants younger than 12 months because persons of that age may retain maternal rubella neutralizing antibodies that may interfere with the immune response. Children in kindergarten and the first grades of elementary school deserve priority for vaccination because often they are epidemiologically the major source of virus dissemination in the community. A history of rubella illness is usually not reliable enough to exclude children from immunization.

Previously unimmunized children of susceptible pregnant women should receive live attenuated rubella vaccine, because an immunized child will be less likely to acquire natural rubella and introduce the virus into the household.

2. *Adolescent and Adult Males*
Vaccination of adolescent or adult males may be a useful procedure in preventing or controlling outbreaks of rubella in circumscribed population groups (e.g., military bases and schools).

3. *Non-Pregnant Adolescent and Adult Females*
Immunization of susceptible non-pregnant adolescent and adult females of childbearing age with live attenuated rubella virus vaccine is indicated if certain precautions are observed (see below). Vaccinating susceptible postpubertal females confers individual protection against subsequently acquiring rubella infection during pregnancy, which in turn prevents infection of the fetus and consequent congenital rubella injury.

Pregnant females *must not* be given live attenuated rubella virus vaccine. It is not known to what extent infection of the fetus with attenuated virus might occur following vaccination, or whether damage to the fetus could result. Subjects should be considered for vaccination only if they agree that they will not become pregnant within three months following vaccination, and if they are informed of the reason for this precaution.* If a pregnant woman is inadvertently vaccinated or if she becomes pregnant within three months of vaccination, she should be counseled on the possible risks to the fetus.

It is recommended that rubella susceptibility be determined by serologic testing prior to immunization.** If immune, as evidenced by a specific rubella antibody titer of 1:8 or greater (hemagglutination inhibition test), vaccination is unnecessary. Congenital malformations do occur in up to seven percent of all live births. Their chance appearance after vaccination could lead to misinterpretation of the cause, particularly if the prior rubella-immune status of vaccinees is unknown.

Postpubertal females should be informed of the frequent occurrence of self-limited arthralgia and possible arthritis beginning 2 to 4 weeks after vaccination (See ADVERSE REACTIONS).

It has been found convenient in many instances to vaccinate rubella-susceptible women in the immediate postpartum period.

Revaccination
Based on available evidence, there is no reason to revaccinate children who were vaccinated originally when 12 months of age or older; however, children vaccinated when younger than 12 months of age should be revaccinated.

Use with Other Live Virus Vaccines
There are no data available concerning simultaneous use of MERUVAX II with monovalent or trivalent poliovirus vaccine, live, oral, or with killed poliovirus vaccines. However, serologic evidence shows that when M-M-R® (Measles, Mumps and Rubella Virus Vaccine, Live, MSD), containing the HPV-77 rubella strain, is given simultaneously with trivalent poliovirus vaccine, live, oral, antibody responses can be expected to be comparable to those which follow administration of the vaccines at different times. From this it follows that when MERUVAX II is given simultaneously with either monovalent or trivalent poliovirus vaccine, live, oral, ATTENUVAX® (Measles Virus Vaccine, Live, Attenuated, MSD) and/or MUMPSVAX® (Mumps Virus Vaccine, Live, MSD), antibody responses can be expected to be comparable to those which follow administration of the vaccines at different times.

Contraindications

Do not give MERUVAX II to pregnant females; the possible effects of the vaccine on fetal development are unknown at this time. When vaccination of post-pubertal females is undertaken, pregnancy must be avoided for three months following vaccination.

Hypersensitivity to neomycin (each dose of reconstituted vaccine contains approximately 25 mcg of neomycin).

Any febrile respiratory illness, or other active febrile infection.

Patients receiving therapy with ACTH, corticosteroids, irradiation, alkylating agents or antimetabolites. This contraindication does not apply to patients who are receiving corticosteroids as replacement therapy, e.g., for Addison's disease. Individuals with blood dyscrasias, leukemia, lymphomas of any type, or other malignant neoplasms affecting the bone marrow or lymphatic systems. Primary immuno-deficiency states, including cellular immune deficiencies, hypogammaglobulinemic and dysgammaglobulinemic states.

Precautions

The vaccine is to be given subcutaneously; *do not give intravenously.*

Epinephrine should be available for immediate use should an anaphylactoid reaction occur.

MERUVAX II may be given simultaneously with monovalent or trivalent poliovirus vaccine, live, oral, with ATTENUVAX (Measles Virus Vaccine, Live, Attenuated, MSD) and/or MUMPSVAX (Mumps Virus Vaccine, Live, MSD). MERUVAX II should not be given less than one month before or after administration of other live virus vaccines.

Excretion of small amounts of the live attenuated rubella virus from the nose or throat has occurred in the majority of susceptible individuals 7–28 days after vaccination. There is no confirmed evidence to indicate that such virus is transmitted to susceptible persons who are in contact with the vaccinated individuals. Consequently, transmission, while accepted as a theoretical possibility, is not regarded as a significant risk.*

There is no evidence that live rubella virus vaccine given after exposure to natural rubella virus will prevent illness. There is, however, no contraindication to vaccinating children already exposed to natural rubella.

Vaccination should be deferred for at least three months following blood or plasma transfusions, or administration of human immune serum globulin. However, susceptible postpartum patients who received blood products may receive MERUVAX II prior to discharge provided that a repeat HI titer is drawn 6–8 weeks after vaccination to insure seroconversion. Similarly, although studies with other live rubella virus vaccines suggest that MERUVAX II may be given in the immediate postpartum period to those non-immune women who have received anti-Rho (D) globulin (human) without interfering with vaccine effectiveness, a follow-up post-vaccination HI titer should also be determined.

It has been reported that attenuated rubella virus vaccine, live, may result in a temporary depression of tuberculin skin sensitivity. Therefore, if a tuberculin test is to be done, it should be administered either before or simultaneously with MERUVAX II.

As for any vaccine, vaccination with MERUVAX II may not result in seroconversion in 100% of susceptible subjects given the vaccine.

Adverse Reactions

Because of the slightly acidic pH (6.2–6.6) of the vaccine, patients may complain of burning and/or stinging of short duration at the injection site.

Adverse reactions are uncommon, but symptoms of the same kind as those seen following natural rubella may occur after vaccination. These include regional lymphadenopathy, urticaria, wheal and flare at the injection site, rash, malaise, sore throat, fever, headache, polyneuritis, and occasionally temporary arthralgia that is infrequently associated with signs of inflammation. Local pain, induration, and erythema may occur at the site of injection.

Moderate fever [101–102.9°F (38.3–39.4°C)] occurs occasionally, and high fever [above 103°F (39.4°C)] occurs less commonly.

Reactions are usually mild and transient.

In children, joint reactions are rare and of brief duration if they do occur. In women, incidence rates for arthritis and arthralgia are generally

---

† Based in part on the recommendation for rubella vaccine use of the Immunization Practices Advisory Committee (ACIP), Morbidity and Mortality Weekly Report *30*(4): 37–42, 47, Feb. 6, 1981.

* NOTE: The Immunization Practices Advisory Committee (ACIP) has recommended "In view of the importance of protecting this age group against rubella, asking females if they are pregnant, excluding those who say they are, and explaining the theoretical risks to the others are reasonable precautions in a rubella immunization program."

** NOTE: The Immunization Practices Advisory Committee (ACIP) has stated "When practical, and when reliable laboratory services are available, potential vaccinees of childbearing age can have serologic tests to determine susceptibility to rubella.... However, routinely performing serologic tests for all females of childbearing age to determine susceptibility so that vaccine is given only to proven susceptibles is expensive and has been ineffective in some areas. Accordingly, the ACIP believes that rubella vaccination of a woman who is not known to be pregnant and has no history of vaccination is justifiable without serologic testing."

* Recommendation of the Immunization Practices Advisory Committee (ACIP), Morbidity and Mortality Weekly Report *30*(4): 37–42, 47, Feb. 6, 1981.

higher than those seen in children (children: 0-3%; women: 12-20%) and the reactions tend to be more marked and of longer duration. Rarely, symptoms may persist for a matter of months. In adolescent girls, the reactions appear to be intermediate in incidence between those seen in children and in adult women. Even in older women (35-45 years), these reactions are generally well tolerated and rarely interfere with normal activities.

Clinical experience with live virus rubella vaccines thus far indicates that encephalitis and other nervous system reactions have occurred very rarely in subjects who were given the vaccines, but a cause and effect relationship has not been established.

In view of the decreases in platelet counts that have been reported, thrombocytopenic purpura is a theoretical hazard.

Dosage and Administration

Inject the total volume of reconstituted vaccine subcutaneously, preferably into the outer aspect of the upper arm, after suitable cleansing of the immunization site. MERUVAX II should not be injected intravenously, or administered intranasally. *Do not give immune serum globulin (ISG) concurrently with MERUVAX II.*

CAUTION: A sterile syringe free of preservatives, antiseptics, and detergents should be used for each injection of the vaccine because these substances may inactivate the live virus vaccine. A 25 gauge, 5/8" needle is recommended.

Shipment, Storage and Reconstitution

To insure that there is no loss of potency during shipment, the vaccine must be maintained at a temperature of 10°C (50°F) or less.
Before reconstitution, store MERUVAX II at 2-8°C (35.6-46.4°F). *Protect from light.*
To reconstitute, withdraw the entire volume of diluent into the syringe to be used for reconstitution. Inject all of the diluent in the syringe into the vial of lyophilized vaccine, and agitate to ensure thorough mixing. Withdraw the entire contents into a syringe and inject the total volume of restored vaccine subcutaneously.

It is important to use a separate sterile syringe and needle for each individual patient to prevent transmission of hepatitis B and other infectious agents from one person to another.

Each dose of reconstituted vaccine contains not less than 1000 $TCID_{50}$ (tissue culture infectious doses) of rubella virus vaccine expressed in terms of the assigned titer of the FDA Reference Rubella Virus.

The color of the vaccine when reconstituted is yellow.

Use only the diluent supplied to reconstitute the vaccine. It is recommended that the vaccine be used as soon as possible after reconstitution. Protect vaccine from light, at all times. Store reconstituted vaccine in a dark place at 2-8°C (35.6-46.4°F) and discard if not used within 8 hours.

How Supplied

No. 4747 MERUVAX II is supplied as a single-dose vial of lyophilized vaccine, **NDC** 0006-4747-00, and a vial of diluent.
No. 4673/4309 MERUVAX II is supplied as follows: (1) a box of 10 single-dose vials of lyophilized vaccine (package A), **NDC** 0006-4673-00; and (2) a box of 10 vials of diluent (package B). To conserve refrigerator space, the diluent may be stored separately at room temperature.

A.H.F.S. Category: 80:12
DC 7030807 Issued February 1983
COPYRIGHT © MERCK & CO., INC., 1983
All rights reserved

MIDAMOR® Tablets
(amiloride HCl, MSD), U.S.P.

Description

Amiloride HCl, an antikaliuretic-diuretic agent, is a pyrazinecarbonyl-guanidine that is unrelated chemically to other known antikaliuretic or diuretic agents. It is the salt of a moderately strong base (pKa 8.7). Its chemical name is 3,5-diamino-6-chloro-N-(diaminomethylene) pyrazinecarboxamide monohydrochloride. Its empirical formula is $C_6H_8ClN_7O \cdot HCl$.

MIDAMOR® (Amiloride HCl, MSD) is available for oral use as tablets containing 5 mg of amiloride HCl.

Clinical Pharmacology

MIDAMOR is a potassium-conserving (antikaliuretic) drug that possesses weak (compared with thiazide diuretics) natriuretic, diuretic, and antihypertensive activity. These effects have been partially additive to the effects of thiazide diuretics in some clinical studies. MIDAMOR has potassium-conserving activity in patients receiving kaliuretic-diuretic agents.

MIDAMOR is not an aldosterone antagonist and its effects are seen even in the absence of aldosterone.

MIDAMOR usually begins to act within 2 hours after an oral dose. Its effect on electrolyte excretion reaches a peak between 6 and 10 hours and lasts about 24 hours. Peak plasma levels are obtained in 3 to 4 hours and the plasma half-life varies from 6 to 9 hours. Effects on electrolytes increase with single doses of amiloride HCl up to approximately 15 mg.

Amiloride HCl is not metabolized by the liver but is excreted unchanged by the kidneys. About 50 percent of a 20 mg dose of MIDAMOR is excreted in the urine and 40 percent in the stool within 72 hours. MIDAMOR has little effect on glomerular filtration rate or renal blood flow. Because amiloride HCl is not metabolized by the liver, drug accumulation is not anticipated in patients with hepatic dysfunction, but accumulation can occur if the hepatorenal syndrome develops.

Indications and Usage

MIDAMOR is indicated as adjunctive treatment with thiazide diuretics or other kaliuretic-diuretic agents in congestive heart failure or hypertension to:

a. help restore normal serum potassium levels in patients who develop hypokalemia on the kaliuretic diuretic
b. prevent development of hypokalemia in patients who would be exposed to particular risk if hypokalemia were to develop, e.g., digitalized patients or patients with significant cardiac arrhythmias.

The use of potassium-conserving agents is often unnecessary in patients receiving diuretics for uncomplicated essential hypertension when such patients have a normal diet. MIDAMOR has little additive diuretic or antihypertensive effect when added to a thiazide diuretic.

MIDAMOR should rarely be used alone. It has weak (compared with thiazides) diuretic and antihypertensive effects. Used as single agents, potassium sparing diuretics, including MIDAMOR, result in an increased risk of hyperkalemia (approximately 10% with amiloride). MIDAMOR should be used alone only when persistent hypokalemia has been documented and only with careful titration of the dose and close monitoring of serum electrolytes.

Contraindications

Hyperkalemia
MIDAMOR should not be used in the presence of elevated serum potassium levels (greater than 5.5 mEq per liter).
Antikaliuretic Therapy or Potassium Supplementation
MIDAMOR should not be given to patients receiving other potassium-conserving agents, such as spironolactone or triamterene. Potassium supplementation in the form of medication or a potassium-rich diet should not be used with MIDAMOR except in severe and/or refractory cases of hypokalemia. Such concomitant therapy can be associated with rapid increases in serum potassium levels. If potassium supplementation is used, careful monitoring of the serum potassium level is necessary.

Impaired Renal Function
Anuria, acute or chronic renal insufficiency, and evidence of diabetic nephropathy are contraindications to the use of MIDAMOR. Patients with evidence of renal functional impairment (blood urea nitrogen [BUN] levels over 30 mg per 100 ml or serum creatinine levels over 1.5 mg per 100 ml) or diabetes mellitus should not receive the drug without careful, frequent and continuing monitoring of serum electrolytes, creatinine, and BUN levels. Potassium retention associated with the use of an antikaliuretic agent is accentuated in the presence of renal impairment and may result in the rapid development of hyperkalemia.
Hypersensitivity
MIDAMOR is contraindicated in patients who are hypersensitive to this product.

Warnings

Hyperkalemia

> Like other potassium-conserving agents, amiloride may cause hyperkalemia (serum potassium levels greater than 5.5 mEq per liter) which, if uncorrected, is potentially fatal. Hyperkalemia occurs commonly (about 10%) when amiloride is used without a kaliuretic diuretic. This incidence is greater in patients with renal impairment, diabetes mellitus (with or without recognized renal insufficiency), and in the elderly. When MIDAMOR is used concomitantly with a thiazide diuretic in patients without these complications, the risk of hyperkalemia is reduced to about 1-2%. It is thus essential to monitor serum potassium levels carefully in any patient receiving amiloride, particularly when it is first introduced, at the time of diuretic dosage adjustments, and during any illness that could affect renal function.

Warning signs or symptoms of hyperkalemia include paresthesias, muscular weakness, fatigue, flaccid paralysis of the extremities, bradycardia, shock, and ECG abnormalities. Monitoring of the serum potassium level is essential because mild hyperkalemia is not usually associated with an abnormal ECG.

When abnormal, the ECG in hyperkalemia is characterized primarily by tall, peaked T waves or elevations from previous tracings. There may also be lowering of the R wave and increased depth of the S wave, widening and even disappearance of the P wave, progressive widening of the QRS complex, prolongation of the PR interval, and ST depression.

Treatment of hyperkalemia: If hyperkalemia occurs in patients taking MIDAMOR, the drug should be discontinued immediately. If the serum potassium level exceeds 6.5 mEq per liter, active measures should be taken to reduce it. Such measures include the intravenous administration of sodium bicarbonate solution or oral or parenteral glucose with a rapid-acting insulin preparation. If needed, a cation exchange resin such as sodium polystyrene sulfonate may be given orally or by enema. Patients with persistent hyperkalemia may require dialysis.

Diabetes Mellitus
In diabetic patients, hyperkalemia has been reported with the use of all potassium-conserving diuretics, including MIDAMOR, even in patients without evidence of diabetic nephropathy. Therefore, MIDAMOR should be avoided, if possible, in diabetic patients and, if it is used, serum electro-

Continued on next page

Information on the Merck Sharp & Dohme products listed on these pages is the full prescribing information from product circulars in use November 1, 1984.

Merck Sharp & Dohme—Cont.

lytes and renal function must be monitored frequently.

MIDAMOR should be discontinued at least 3 days before glucose tolerance testing.

Metabolic or Respiratory Acidosis
Antikaliuretic therapy should be instituted only with caution in severely ill patients in whom respiratory or metabolic acidosis may occur, such as patients with cardiopulmonary disease or poorly controlled diabetes. If MIDAMOR is given to these patients, frequent monitoring of acid-base balance is necessary. Shifts in acid-base balance alter the ratio of extracellular/intracellular potassium, and the development of acidosis may be associated with rapid increases in serum potassium levels.

Precautions
General
Electrolyte Imbalance and BUN Increases
Hyponatremia and hypochloremia may occur when MIDAMOR is used with other diuretics and increases in BUN levels have been reported. These increases usually have accompanied vigorous fluid elimination, especially when diuretic therapy was used in seriously ill patients, such as those who had hepatic cirrhosis with ascites and metabolic alkalosis, or those with resistant edema. Therefore, when MIDAMOR is given with other diuretics to such patients, careful monitoring of serum electrolytes and BUN levels is important. In patients with pre-existing severe liver disease, hepatic encephalopathy, manifested by tremors, confusion, and coma, and increased jaundice, have been reported in association with diuretics, including amiloride HCl.

Drug Interactions
Lithium generally should not be given with diuretics because they reduce its renal clearance and add a high risk of lithium toxicity. Read circulars for lithium preparations before use of such concomitant therapy.

Carcinogenicity, Mutagenicity
There was no evidence of a tumorigenic effect when amiloride HCl was administered for 92 weeks to mice at doses up to 10 mg/kg/day (25 times the maximum daily human dose). Amiloride HCl has also been administered for 104 weeks to male and female rats at doses up to 6 and 8 mg/kg/day (15 and 20 times the maximum daily dose for humans, respectively) and showed no evidence of carcinogenicity.

Amiloride HCl was devoid of mutagenic activity in various strains of *Salmonella typhimurium* with or without a mammalian liver microsomal activation system (Ames test).

Pregnancy
Pregnancy Category B
Teratologic studies with amiloride HCl in rabbits and mice given 20 and 25 times the maximum human dose, respectively, revealed no evidence of harm to the fetus, although studies showed that the drug crossed the placenta in modest amounts. Reproduction studies in rats at 20 times the expected maximum daily dose for humans showed no evidence of impaired fertility. At approximately 5 or more times the expected maximum daily dose for humans, some toxicity was seen in adult rats and rabbits and a decrease in rat pup growth and survival occurred.

There are, however, no adequate and well-controlled studies in pregnant women. Because animal reproduction studies are not always predictive of human response, this drug should be used during pregnancy only if clearly needed.

Nursing Mothers
Studies in rats have shown that amiloride is excreted in milk in concentrations higher than that found in blood, but it is not known whether MIDAMOR is excreted in human milk. Because many drugs are excreted in human milk and because of the potential for serious adverse reactions in nursing infants from MIDAMOR, a decision should be made whether to discontinue nursing or to discontinue the drug, taking into account the importance of the drug to the mother.

Pediatric Use
Safety and effectiveness in children have not been established.

Adverse Reactions
MIDAMOR is usually well tolerated and, except for hyperkalemia (serum potassium levels greater than 5.5 mEq per liter—see WARNINGS), significant adverse effects have been reported infrequently. Minor adverse reactions were reported relatively frequently (about 20%) but the relationship of many of the reports to amiloride HCl is uncertain and the overall frequency was similar in hydrochlorothiazide treated groups. Nausea/anorexia, abdominal pain, flatulence, and mild skin rash have been reported and probably are related to amiloride. Other adverse experiences that have been reported with amiloride are generally those known to be associated with diuresis, or with the underlying disease being treated. The clinical adverse reactions listed in the following table have been arranged into two groups: 1) incidence greater than 1%; and 2) incidence equal to or less than 1%. The incidence was determined from clinical studies conducted in the United States (837 patients treated with MIDAMOR).

Incidence > 1%	Incidence ≤ 1%
Body as a Whole	
Headache*	Back pain
Weakness	Chest pain
Fatigability	Neck/shoulder ache
	Pain, extremities
Cardiovascular	
None	Angina pectoris
	Orthostatic hypotension
	Arrhythmia
	Palpitation
Digestive	
Nausea/anorexia*	Jaundice
Diarrhea*	GI bleeding
Vomiting*	Abdominal fullness
Abdominal pain	GI disturbance
Gas pain	Thirst
Appetite changes	Heartburn
Constipation	Flatulence
	Dyspepsia
Metabolic	
Elevated serum potassium levels (> 5.5 mEq per liter)†	None
Integumentary	
None	Skin rash
	Itching
	Dryness of mouth
	Pruritus
	Alopecia
Musculoskeletal	
Muscle cramps	Joint pain
	Leg ache
Nervous	
Dizziness	Paresthesia
Encephalopathy	Tremors
	Vertigo
Psychiatric	
None	Nervousness
	Mental confusion
	Insomnia
	Decreased libido
	Depression
	Somnolence
Respiratory	
Cough	Shortness of breath
Dyspnea	
Special Senses	
None	Visual disturbances
	Nasal congestion
	Tinnitus
	Increased intraocular pressure
Urogenital	
Impotence	Polyuria
	Dysuria
	Urinary frequency
	Bladder spasms

* Reactions occurring in 3% to 8% of patients treated with MIDAMOR. (Those reactions occurring in less than 3% of the patients are unmarked.)
† See WARNINGS.

Causal Relationship Unknown
Other reactions have been reported but occurred under circumstances where a causal relationship could not be established. However, in these rarely reported events, that possibility cannot be excluded. Therefore, these observations are listed to serve as alerting information to physicians.
  Activation of probable pre-existing peptic ulcer
  Aplastic anemia
  Neutropenia
  Abnormalities of liver function tests

Overdosage
No data are available in regard to overdosage in humans.
The oral LD_{50} of amiloride hydrochloride (calculated as the base) is 56 mg/kg in mice and 36 to 85 mg/kg in rats, depending on the strain.
It is not known whether the drug is dialyzable.
The most likely signs and symptoms to be expected with overdosage are dehydration and electrolyte imbalance. These can be treated by established procedures. Therapy with MIDAMOR should be discontinued and the patient observed closely. There is no specific antidote. Emesis should be induced or gastric lavage performed. Treatment is symptomatic and supportive. If hyperkalemia occurs, active measures should be taken to reduce the serum potassium levels.

Dosage and Administration
MIDAMOR should be administered with food.
MIDAMOR, one 5 mg tablet daily, should be added to the usual antihypertensive or diuretic dosage of a kaliuretic diuretic. The dosage may be increased to 10 mg per day, if necessary. More than two 5 mg tablets of MIDAMOR daily usually are not needed, and there is little controlled experience with such doses. If persistent hypokalemia is documented with 10 mg, the dose can be increased to 15 mg, then 20 mg, with careful monitoring of electrolytes.
In treating patients with congestive heart failure after an initial diuresis has been achieved, potassium loss may also decrease and the need for MIDAMOR should be reevaluated. Dosage adjustment may be necessary. Maintenance therapy may be on an intermittent basis.
If it is necessary to use MIDAMOR alone (see INDICATIONS), the starting dosage should be one 5 mg tablet daily. This dosage may be increased to 10 mg per day, if necessary. More than two 5 mg tablets usually are not needed, and there is little controlled experience with such doses. If persistent hypokalemia is documented with 10 mg, the dose can be increased to 15 mg, then 20 mg, with careful monitoring of electrolytes.

How Supplied
No. 3381—Tablets MIDAMOR, 5 mg, are yellow, diamond-shaped, compressed tablets, coded MSD 92. They are supplied as follows:
NDC 0006-0092-68 bottles of 100.
Shown in Product Identification Section, page 420
A.H.F.S. Category: 40:28
DC 7130004 Issued September 1981
COPYRIGHT© MERCK & CO., INC., 1978
All rights reserved

MINTEZOL® Chewable Tablets ℞
(thiabendazole, MSD)
MINTEZOL® Suspension ℞
(thiabendazole, MSD), U.S.P.

Description
MINTEZOL® (Thiabendazole, MSD) is an anthelmintic provided as 500 mg chewable tablets, and as a suspension, containing 500 mg thiabendazole per 5 ml. The suspension also contains sorbic

acid 0.1% added as a preservative. Thiabendazole is a white to off-white odorless powder with a molecular weight of 201.26, which is practically insoluble in water but readily soluble in dilute acid and alkali. Its chemical name is 2-(4-thiazolyl)-1H benzimidazole. The empirical formula is $C_{10}H_7N_3S$.

Clinical Pharmacology

In man, thiabendazole is rapidly absorbed and peak plasma concentration is reached within 1 to 2 hours after the oral administration of a suspension. It is metabolized almost completely to the 5-hydroxy form which appears in the urine as glucuronide or sulfate conjugates. In 48 hours, about 5% of the administered dose is recovered from the feces and about 90% from the urine. Most is excreted in the first 24 hours.

Mechanism of Action

The precise mode of action of thiabendazole on the parasite is unknown, but it may inhibit the helminth-specific enzyme fumarate reductase.

Thiabendazole is vermicidal and/or vermifugal against *Ascaris lumbricoides* ("common roundworm"), *Strongyloides stercoralis* (threadworm), *Necator americanus*, and *Ancylostoma duodenale* (hookworm), *Trichuris trichiura* (whipworm), *Ancylostoma braziliense* (dog and cat hookworm), *Toxocara canis* and *Toxocara cati* (ascarids), and *Enterobius vermicularis* (pinworm).

Its effect on larvae of *Trichinella spiralis* that have migrated to muscle is questionable.

Thiabendazole also suppresses egg and/or larval production and may inhibit the subsequent development of those eggs or larvae which are passed in the feces.

Indications and Usage

MINTEZOL is indicated for the treatment of:
Strongyloidiasis (threadworm)
Cutaneous larva migrans (creeping eruption)
Visceral larva migrans
Trichinosis: Relief of symptoms and fever and a reduction of eosinophilia have followed the use of MINTEZOL during the invasion stage of the disease.

Although not indicated as primary therapy, when enterobiasis (pinworm) occurs with any of the conditions listed above, additional therapy is not required for most patients. MINTEZOL should be used only in the following infestations when more specific therapy is not available or cannot be used or when further therapy with a second agent is desirable: Uncinariasis (hookworm: *Necator americanus* and *Ancylostoma duodenale*); Trichuriasis (whipworm); Ascariasis (large roundworm).

Contraindication

Hypersensitivity to this product.

Warnings

If hypersensitivity reactions occur, the drug should be discontinued immediately and not be resumed. Erythema multiforme has been associated with thiabendazole therapy; in severe cases (Stevens-Johnson syndrome), fatalities have occurred.

Because CNS side effects may occur quite frequently, activities requiring mental alertness should be avoided.

Precautions

General

MINTEZOL is not suitable for the treatment of mixed infections with ascaris because it may cause these worms to migrate.

Ideally, supportive therapy is indicated for anemic, dehydrated or malnourished patients prior to initiation of the anthelmintic therapy.

In the presence of hepatic or renal dysfunction, patients should be carefully monitored.

MINTEZOL should be used only in patients in whom susceptible worm infestation has been diagnosed and should not be used prophylactically.

Information for Patients

Because CNS side effects may occur quite frequently, activities requiring mental alertness should be avoided.

Laboratory Tests

Rarely, a transient rise in cephalin flocculation and SGOT has occurred in patients receiving MINTEZOL.

Drug Interactions

Thiabendazole may compete with other drugs, such as theophylline, for sites of metabolism in the liver, thus elevating the serum levels of such compounds to potentially toxic levels. Therefore, when concomitant use of thiabendazole and xanthine derivatives is anticipated, it may be necessary to monitor blood levels and/or reduce the dosage of such compounds. Such concomitant use should be administered under careful medical supervision.

Carcinogenesis, Mutagenesis, Impairment of Fertility

Thiabendazole has been used in numerous short- and long-term studies in animals at doses up to 15 times the usual human dose and was without carcinogenic effects. It did not adversely affect fertility in the mouse at 2½ times the usual human dose or in the rat at a dose equivalent to the usual human dose. Thiabendazole had no mutagenic activity in *in vitro* microbial mutagen test, the micronucleus test and the host mediated assay *in vivo*.

Pregnancy

Pregnancy Category C: Reproduction and teratogenic studies done in the rabbit at a dose up to 15 times the usual human dose, in the rat at a dose equivalent to the human dose, and in the mouse at a dose up to 2½ times the usual human dose, revealed no evidence of harm to the fetus. In an additional study in the mouse, no defects were observed when thiabendazole was given in an aqueous suspension, at a dose 10 times the usual human dose; however, cleft palate and axial skeletal defects were observed when thiabendazole was suspended in olive oil and given at the same dose. There are no adequate and well controlled studies in pregnant women. MINTEZOL should be used during pregnancy only if the potential benefit justifies the potential risk to the fetus.

Nursing Mothers

It is not known whether this drug is excreted in human milk. Because of the potential for serious adverse reactions in nursing infants from MINTEZOL, a decision should be made whether to discontinue nursing or to discontinue the drug, taking into account the importance of the drug to the mother.

Pediatric Use

The safety and effectiveness of thiabendazole for the treatment of Strongyloidiasis, Ascariasis, Uncinariasis, Trichuriasis and Trichinosis in children weighing less than 30 lbs has been limited.

Adverse Reactions

Gastrointestinal: anorexia, nausea, vomiting, diarrhea, epigastric distress, jaundice, cholestasis and parenchymal liver damage.

Central Nervous System: dizziness, weariness, drowsiness, giddiness, headache, numbness, hyperirritability, convulsions, collapse.

Special Senses: tinnitus, abnormal sensation in eyes, xanthopsia, blurring of vision.

Cardiovascular: hypotension.

Metabolic: hyperglycemia.

Hematologic: transient leukopenia.

Genitourinary: hematuria, enuresis, malodor of the urine, crystalluria.

Hypersensitivity: pruritus, fever, facial flush, chills, conjunctival injection, angioedema, anaphylaxis, skin rashes (including perianal), erythema multiforme (including Stevens-Johnson syndrome), and lymphadenopathy.

Miscellaneous: appearance of live Ascaris in the mouth and nose.

Overdosage

Overdosage may be associated with transient disturbances of vision and psychic alterations.

There is no specific antidote in the event of overdosage. Therefore, symptomatic and supportive measures should be employed. Emesis should be induced or gastric lavage performed carefully.

The oral LD_{50} of MINTEZOL is 3.6 g/kg, 3.1 g/kg and 3.8 g/kg in the mouse, rat, and rabbit respectively.

Dosage and Administration

The recommended maximum daily dose of MINTEZOL is 3 grams.

MINTEZOL should be given after meals if possible. Tablets MINTEZOL should be chewed before swallowing. Dietary restriction, complementary medications and cleansing enemas are not needed. The usual dosage schedule for all conditions is two doses per day. The dosage is determined by the patient's weight.

A weight-dose chart follows:

Weight	Each Dose	
	g	ml
30 lb	0.25	2.5
	(½ tablet)	(½ teaspoon)
50 lb	0.5	5.0
	(1 tablet)	(1 teaspoon)
75 lb	0.75	7.5
	(1½ tablets)	(1½ teaspoons)
100 lb	1.0	10.0
	(2 tablets)	(2 teaspoons)
125 lb	1.25	12.5
	(2½ tablets)	(2½ teaspoons)
150 lb & over	1.5	15.0
	(3 tablets)	(3 teaspoons)

The regimen for each indication follows:
[See table on next page].

How Supplied

No. 3331 — MINTEZOL Suspension, 500 mg per 5 ml, is white to off-white and is supplied as follows: NDC 0006-3331-60 in bottles of 120 ml (6505-00- 935-5835 0.5 g/5 ml 120 ml).

No. 3332 — MINTEZOL Chewable Tablets, 500 mg, are white to off-white, orange-flavored, round, scored, compressed tablets, coded MSD 907. They are supplied as follows:

NDC 0006-0907-36 in boxes of 36 strip packaged, individually foil-wrapped tablets.

Shown in Product Identification Section, page 420
A.H.F.S. Category: 8:08
DC 6857707 Issued August 1983
COPYRIGHT © MERCK & CO., INC., 1983
All rights reserved

MODURETIC® Tablets ℞
(amiloride HCl-hydrochlorothiazide, MSD), U.S.P.

Description

MODURETIC® (Amiloride HCl-Hydrochlorothiazide, MSD) combines the potassium-conserving action of amiloride HCl with the natriuretic action of hydrochlorothiazide. Each tablet contains 5 mg of amiloride HCl and 50 mg of hydrochlorothiazide.

Amiloride HCl is 3,5-diamino-6-chloro-N-(diaminomethylene) pyrazine-carboxamide monohydrochloride. Its empirical formula is $C_6H_8ClN_7O \cdot HCl$.

Hydrochlorothiazide is 6-chloro-3,4-dihydro-2H-1,2,4-benzothiadiazine-7-sulfonamide 1, 1-dioxide. Its empirical formula is $C_7H_8ClN_3O_4S_2$.

MODURETIC is available for oral use as tablets containing 5 mg of amiloride HCl and 50 mg of hydrochlorothiazide.

Continued on next page

Information on the Merck Sharp & Dohme products listed on these pages is the full prescribing information from product circulars in use November 1, 1984.

Merck Sharp & Dohme—Cont.

Clinical Pharmacology
MODURETIC provides diuretic and antihypertensive activity (principally due to the hydrochlorothiazide component), while acting through the amiloride component to prevent the excessive potassium loss that may occur in patients receiving a thiazide diuretic. The onset of the diuretic action of MODURETIC is within 1 to 2 hours and this action appears to be sustained for approximately 24 hours.

Amiloride HCl
Amiloride HCl is a potassium-conserving (antikaliuretic) drug that possesses weak (compared with thiazide diuretics) natriuretic, diuretic, and antihypertensive activity. These effects have been partially additive to the effects of thiazide diuretics in some clinical studies. Amiloride HCl has potassium-conserving activity in patients receiving kaliuretic-diuretic agents.

Amiloride HCl is not an aldosterone antagonist and its effects are seen even in the absence of aldosterone.

Amiloride HCl usually begins to act within 2 hours after an oral dose. Its effect on electrolyte excretion reaches a peak between 6 and 10 hours and lasts about 24 hours. Peak plasma levels are obtained in 3 to 4 hours and the plasma half-life varies from 6 to 9 hours. Effects on electrolytes increase with single doses of amiloride HCl up to approximately 15 mg.

Amiloride HCl is not metabolized by the liver but is excreted unchanged by the kidneys. About 50 percent of a 20 mg dose of amiloride HCl is excreted in the urine and 40 percent in the stool within 72 hours. Amiloride HCl has little effect on glomerular filtration rate or renal blood flow. Because amiloride HCl is not metabolized by the liver, drug accumulation is not anticipated in patients with hepatic dysfunction, but accumulation can occur if the hepatorenal syndrome develops.

Hydrochlorothiazide
Hydrochlorothiazide is a diuretic and antihypertensive agent. It affects the renal tubular mechanism of electrolyte reabsorption.

Hydrochlorothiazide increases excretion of sodium and chloride in approximately equivalent amounts. Natriuresis may be accompanied by some loss of potassium and bicarbonate.

The onset of the diuretic action of hydrochlorothiazide occurs in 2 hours and the peak action in about 4 hours. Diuretic activity lasts about 6 to 12 hours. Hydrochlorothiazide is eliminated rapidly by the kidney.

The mechanism of the antihypertensive effect of thiazides may be related to the excretion and redistribution of body sodium. Hydrochlorothiazide usually does not cause clinically important changes in normal blood pressure.

Indications and Usage
MODURETIC is indicated in those patients with hypertension or with congestive heart failure who develop hypokalemia when thiazides or other kaliuretic diuretics are used alone, or in whom maintenance of normal serum potassium levels is considered to be clinically important, e.g., digitalized patients, or patients with significant cardiac arrhythmias.

The use of potassium conserving agents is often unnecessary in patients receiving diuretics for uncomplicated essential hypertension when such patients have a normal diet.

MODURETIC may be used alone or as an adjunct to other antihypertensive drugs, such as methyldopa or beta blockers. Since MODURETIC enhances the action of these agents, dosage adjustments may be necessary to avoid an excessive fall in blood pressure and other unwanted side effects. **This fixed combination drug is not indicated for initial therapy of edema or hypertension. If the fixed combination represents the dose titrated to an individual patient's needs, it may be more convenient than the separate components.**

Contraindications
Hyperkalemia
MODURETIC should not be used in the presence of elevated serum potassium levels (greater than 5.5 mEq per liter).

Antikaliuretic Therapy or Potassium Supplementation
MODURETIC should not be given to patients receiving other potassium-conserving agents, such as spironolactone or triamterene. Potassium supplementation in the form of medication or a potassium-rich diet should not be used with MODURETIC except in severe and/or refractory cases of hypokalemia. Such concomitant therapy can be associated with rapid increases in serum potassium levels. If potassium supplementation is used, careful monitoring of the serum potassium level is necessary.

Impaired Renal Function
Anuria, acute or chronic renal insufficiency, and evidence of diabetic nephropathy are contraindications to the use of MODURETIC. Patients with evidence of renal functional impairment (blood urea nitrogen [BUN] levels over 30 mg per 100 mL or serum creatinine levels over 1.5 mg per 100 mL) or diabetes mellitus should not receive the drug without careful, frequent and continuing monitoring of serum electrolytes, creatinine, and BUN levels. Potassium retention associated with the use of an antikaliuretic agent is accentuated in the presence of renal impairment and may result in the rapid development of hyperkalemia.

Hypersensitivity
MODURETIC is contraindicated in patients who are hypersensitive to this product, or to other sulfonamide-derived drugs.

Warnings
Hyperkalemia

> Like other potassium-conserving diuretic combinations, MODURETIC may cause hyperkalemia (serum potassium levels greater than 5.5 mEq per liter). In patients without renal impairment or diabetes mellitus, the risk of hyperkalemia with MODURETIC is about 1-2%. This risk is higher in patients with renal impairment or diabetes mellitus (even without recognized diabetic nephropathy). Since hyperkalemia, if uncorrected, is potentially fatal, it is essential to monitor serum potassium levels carefully in any patient receiving MODURETIC, particularly when it is first introduced, at the time of dosage adjustments, and during any illness that could affect renal function.

Warning signs or symptoms of hyperkalemia include paresthesias, muscular weakness, fatigue, flaccid paralysis of the extremities, bradycardia, shock, and ECG abnormalities. Monitoring of the serum potassium level is essential because mild hyperkalemia is not usually associated with an abnormal ECG.

When abnormal, the ECG in hyperkalemia is characterized primarily by tall, peaked T waves or elevations from previous tracings. There may also be lowering of the R wave and increased depth of the S wave, widening and even disappearance of the P wave, progressive widening of the QRS complex, prolongation of the PR interval, and ST depression.

Treatment of hyperkalemia: If hyperkalemia occurs in patients taking MODURETIC, the drug should be discontinued immediately. If the serum potassium level exceeds 6.5 mEq per liter, active measures should be taken to reduce it. Such measures include the intravenous administration of sodium bicarbonate solution or oral or parenteral glucose with a rapid-acting insulin preparation. If needed, a cation exchange resin such as sodium polystyrene sulfonate may be given orally or by enema. Patients with persistent hyperkalemia may require dialysis.

Diabetes Mellitus
In diabetic patients, hyperkalemia has been reported with the use of all potassium-conserving diuretics, including amiloride HCl, even in patients without evidence of diabetic nephropathy. Therefore, MODURETIC should be avoided, if possible, in diabetic patients and, if it is used, serum electrolytes and renal function must be monitored frequently.

MODURETIC should be discontinued at least 3 days before glucose tolerance testing.

Metabolic or Respiratory Acidosis
Antikaliuretic therapy should be instituted only with caution in severely ill patients in whom respiratory or metabolic acidosis may occur, such as patients with cardiopulmonary disease or poorly controlled diabetes. If MODURETIC is given to these patients, frequent monitoring of acid-base

---

Therapeutic Regimens

Indication	Regimen	Comments
*STRONGYLOIDIASIS	2 doses per day for 2 successive days.	A single dose of 20 mg/lb or 50 mg/kg may be employed as an alternative schedule, but a higher incidence of side effects should be expected.
CUTANEOUS LARVA MIGRANS (Creeping Eruption)	2 doses per day for 2 successive days.	If active lesions are still present 2 days after completion of therapy, a second course is recommended.
VISCERAL LARVA MIGRANS	2 doses per day for 7 successive days.	Safety and efficacy data on the seven-day treatment course are limited.
*TRICHINOSIS	2 doses per day for 2–4 successive days according to the response of the patient.	The optimal dosage for the treatment of trichinosis has not been established.
Other Indications Intestinal roundworms (including Ascariasis, Uncinariasis and Trichuriasis)	2 doses per day for 2 successive days.	A single dose of 20 mg/lb or 50 mg/kg may be employed as an alternative schedule, but a higher incidence of side effects should be expected.

* Clinical experience with thiabendazole for treatment of each of these conditions in children weighing less than 30 lbs has been limited.

Product Information

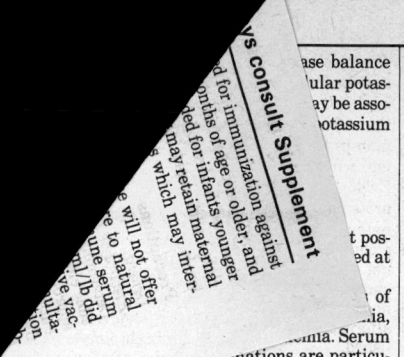

...ase balance
...ular potas-
...ay be asso-
...otassium

...of
...ia.
...mia. Serum
...inations are particu-
...en the patient is vomiting ex-
...or receiving parenteral fluids. Warning
signs or symptoms of fluid and electrolyte imbalance include dryness of mouth, thirst, weakness, lethargy, drowsiness, restlessness, muscle pains or cramps, muscular fatigue, hypotension, oliguria, tachycardia, and gastrointestinal disturbances such as nausea and vomiting.

Hyponatremia and hypochloremia may occur during the use of thiazides and other diuretics. Any chloride deficit during thiazide therapy is generally mild and may be lessened by the amiloride HCl component of MODURETIC. Hypochloremia usually does not require specific treatment except under extraordinary circumstances (as in liver disease or renal disease). Dilutional hyponatremia may occur in edematous patients in hot weather; appropriate therapy is water restriction, rather than administration of salt, except in rare instances when the hyponatremia is life threatening. In actual salt depletion, appropriate replacement is the therapy of choice.

Hypokalemia may develop during thiazide therapy, especially with brisk diuresis, when severe cirrhosis is present, during concomitant use of corticosteroids or ACTH, or after prolonged therapy. However, this usually is prevented by the amiloride HCl component of MODURETIC.

Interference with adequate oral electrolyte intake will also contribute to hypokalemia. Hypokalemia can sensitize or exaggerate the response of the heart to the toxic effects of digitalis (e.g., increased ventricular irritability).

Thiazides have been shown to increase the urinary excretion of magnesium; this may result in hypomagnesemia. Amiloride HCl, a component of MODURETIC, has been shown to decrease the enhanced urinary excretion of magnesium which occurs when a thiazide or loop diuretic is used alone.

Increases in BUN levels have been reported with amiloride HCl and with hydrochlorothiazide. These increases usually have accompanied vigorous fluid elimination, especially when diuretic therapy was used in seriously ill patients, such as those who had hepatic cirrhosis with ascites and metabolic alkalosis, or those with resistant edema. Therefore, when MODURETIC is given to such patients, careful monitoring of serum electrolyte and BUN levels is important. In patients with preexisting severe liver disease, hepatic encephalopathy, manifested by tremors, confusion, and coma, and increased jaundice, have been reported in association with diuretic therapy including amiloride HCl and hydrochlorothiazide.

In patients with renal disease, diuretics may precipitate azotemia. Cumulative effects of the components of MODURETIC may develop in patients with impaired renal function. If renal impairment becomes evident, MODURETIC should be discontinued (see CONTRAINDICATIONS and WARNINGS).

Drug Interactions

Thiazides may add to or potentiate the action of other antihypertensive drugs.

Thiazides may increase the responsiveness to tubocurarine.

Lithium generally should not be given with diuretics because they reduce its renal clearance and add a high risk of lithium toxicity. Read circulars for lithium preparations before use of such concomitant therapy.

Metabolic and Endocrine Effects

Thiazides may decrease serum PBI levels without signs of thyroid disturbance.

In diabetic patients, insulin requirements may be increased, decreased, or unchanged due to the hydrochlorothiazide component. Diabetes mellitus that has been latent may become manifest during administration of thiazide diuretics.

Because calcium excretion is decreased by thiazides, MODURETIC should be discontinued before carrying out tests for parathyroid function. Pathologic changes in the parathyroid glands, with hypercalcemia and hypophosphatemia have been observed in a few patients on prolonged thiazide therapy; however, the common complications of hyperparathyroidism such as renal lithiasis, bone resorption, and peptic ulceration have not been seen.

Hyperuricemia may occur or acute gout may be precipitated in certain patients receiving thiazide therapy.

Other Precautions

In patients receiving thiazides, sensitivity reactions may occur with or without a history of allergy or bronchial asthma. The possibility of exacerbation or activation of systemic lupus erythematosus has been reported with the use of thiazides.

Carcinogenicity, Mutagenicity

There was no evidence of a tumorigenic effect when amiloride HCl was administered for 92 weeks to mice at doses up to 10 mg/kg/day (25 times the maximum daily human dose). Amiloride HCl has also been administered for 104 weeks to male and female rats at doses up to 6 and 8 mg/kg/day (15 and 20 times the maximum daily dose for humans, respectively) and showed no evidence of carcinogenicity.

Amiloride HCl was devoid of mutagenic activity in various strains of *Salmonella typhimurium* with or without a mammalian liver microsomal activation system (Ames test).

Pregnancy

Pregnancy Category B: Teratogenicity studies have been performed with combinations of amiloride HCl and hydrochlorothiazide in rabbits and mice at doses up to 25 times the expected maximum daily dose for humans and have revealed no evidence of harm to the fetus. No evidence of impaired fertility in rats was apparent at dosage levels up to 25 times the expected maximum human daily dose. A perinatal and postnatal study in rats showed a reduction in maternal body weight gain during and after gestation at a daily dose of 25 times the expected maximum daily dose for humans. The body weights of alive pups at birth and at weaning were also reduced at this dose level. There are no adequate and well controlled studies in pregnant women. Because animal reproduction studies are not always predictive of human responses, and because of the data listed below with the individual components, this drug should be used during pregnancy only if clearly needed.

Amiloride HCl: Teratogenicity studies with amiloride HCl in rabbits and mice given 20 and 25 times the maximum human dose, respectively, revealed no evidence of harm to the fetus, although studies showed that the drug crossed the placenta in modest amounts. Reproduction studies in rats at 20 times the expected maximum daily dose for humans showed no evidence of impaired fertility. At approximately 5 or more times the expected maximum daily dose for humans, some toxicity was seen in adult rats and rabbits and a decrease in rat pup growth and survival occurred.

Hydrochlorothiazide: Thiazides cross the placental barrier and appear in cord blood. The possible hazards to the fetus include fetal or neonatal jaundice, thrombocytopenia, and possibly other adverse reactions which have occurred in the adult.

Nursing Mothers

Studies in rats have shown that amiloride is excreted in milk in concentrations higher than that found in blood, but it is not known whether amiloride HCl is excreted in human milk. However, thiazides appear in breast milk. Because of the potential for serious adverse reactions in nursing infants, a decision should be made whether to discontinue nursing or to discontinue the drug, taking into account the importance of the drug to the mother.

Pediatric Use

Safety and effectiveness in children have not been established.

Adverse Reactions

MODURETIC is usually well tolerated and significant clinical adverse effects have been reported infrequently. The risk of hyperkalemia (serum potassium levels greater than 5.5 mEq per liter) with MODURETIC is about 1-2% in patients without renal impairment or diabetes mellitus (see WARNINGS). Minor adverse reactions to amiloride HCl have been reported relatively frequently (about 20%) but the relationship of many of the reports to amiloride HCl is uncertain and the overall frequency was similar in hydrochlorothiazide treated groups. Nausea/anorexia, abdominal pain, flatulence, and mild skin rash have been reported and probably are related to amiloride. Other adverse experiences that have been reported with MODURETIC are generally those known to be associated with diuresis, thiazide therapy, or with the underlying disease being treated. Clinical trials have not demonstrated that combining amiloride and hydrochlorothiazide increases the risk of adverse reactions over those seen with the individual components. The clinical adverse reactions listed in the following table have been arranged into two groups: 1) incidence greater than 1%; and 2) incidence equal to or less than 1%. The incidence was obtained from clinical studies conducted in the United States (607 patients treated with MODURETIC).

Incidence > 1%	Incidence ≤ 1%
Body as a Whole	
Headache*	Malaise
Weakness*	Chest pain
Fatigue/tiredness	Back pain
Cardiovascular	
Arrhythmia	Tachycardia
	Digitalis toxicity
	Orthostatic hypotension
	Angina pectoris
Digestive	
Nausea/anorexia*	Constipation
Diarrhea	GI bleeding
Gastrointestinal pain	GI disturbance
	Appetite changes
Abdominal pain	Abdominal fullness
	Hiccups
	Thirst
	Vomiting
	Anorexia
	Flatulence
Metabolic	
Elevated serum potassium levels (> 5.5 mEq per liter)†	Gout
	Dehydration
Integumentary	
Rash*	Flushing
Pruritus	
Musculoskeletal	
Leg ache	Muscle cramps/spasm
	Joint pain
Nervous	
Dizziness*	Paresthesia/numbness
	Stupor
	Vertigo
Psychiatric	
None	Insomnia
	Nervousness
	Depression
	Sleepiness
	Mental confusion

Continued on next page

Information on the Merck Sharp & Dohme products listed on these pages is the full prescribing information from product circulars in use November 1.

Merck Sharp & Dohme—Cont.

Respiratory
Dyspnea — None

Special Senses
None — Bad taste
Visual disturbance
Nasal congestion

Urogenital
None — Impotence
Nocturia
Dysuria
Incontinence

* Reactions occurring in 3% to 8% of patients treated with MODURETIC. (Those reactions occurring in less than 3% of the patients are unmarked.)
† See WARNINGS.

Other adverse reactions that have been reported with the individual components are listed below:
Amiloride—Body as a Whole: Fatigability, neck/shoulder ache, painful extremities; *Cardiovascular:* Palpitation; *Digestive:* Abnormal liver function, jaundice, activation of probable pre-existing peptic ulcer, heartburn, dyspepsia; *Integumentary:* Itching, alopecia, dry mouth; *Nervous System/Psychiatric:* Encephalopathy, tremors, decreased libido; *Respiratory:* Cough, shortness of breath; *Special Senses:* Tinnitus, increased intraocular pressure; *Hematologic:* Aplastic anemia, neutropenia; *Urogenital:* Polyuria, urinary frequency, bladder spasms.

Hydrochlorothiazide—Digestive: Cramping, gastric irritation, jaundice (intrahepatic cholestatic jaundice), pancreatitis, sialadenitis; *Metabolic:* Glycosuria, hyperglycemia, hyperuricemia, electrolyte imbalance (see PRECAUTIONS); *Nervous System/Psychiatric:* Restlessness; *Special Senses:* Transient blurred vision, xanthopsia; *Hematologic:* Agranulocytosis, aplastic anemia, hemolytic anemia, leukopenia, thrombocytopenia; *Hypersensitivity:* Purpura, photosensitivity, urticaria, necrotizing angiitis (vasculitis, cutaneous vasculitis), fever, respiratory distress including pneumonitis and pulmonary edema, anaphylactic reactions.

Overdosage

No data are available in regard to overdosage in humans. The oral LD_{50} of the combination drug is 189 and 422 mg/kg for female mice and female rats, respectively.

It is not known whether the drug is dialyzable.

No specific information is available on the treatment of overdosage with MODURETIC, and no specific antidote is available. Treatment is symptomatic and supportive. Therapy with MODURETIC should be discontinued and the patient observed closely. Suggested measures include induction of emesis and/or gastric lavage.

Amiloride HCl: No data are available in regard to overdosage in humans.

The oral LD_{50} of amiloride HCl (calculated as the base) is 56 mg/kg in mice and 36 to 85 mg/kg in rats, depending on the strain.

The most common signs and symptoms to be expected with overdosage are dehydration and electrolyte imbalance. If hyperkalemia occurs, active measures should be taken to reduce the serum potassium levels.

Hydrochlorothiazide: The oral LD_{50} of hydrochlorothiazide is greater than 10.0 g/kg in both mice and rats.

The most common signs and symptoms observed are those caused by electrolyte depletion (hypokalemia, hypochloremia, hyponatremia) and dehydration resulting from excessive diuresis. If digitalis has also been administered, hypokalemia may accentuate cardiac arrhythmias.

Dosage and Administration

MODURETIC should be administered with food. The usual starting dosage is 1 tablet a day. The dosage may be increased to 2 tablets a day, if necessary. More than 2 tablets of MODURETIC daily usually are not needed and there is no controlled experience with such doses. The daily dose is usually given as a single dose but may be given in divided doses. Once an initial diuresis has been achieved, dosage adjustment may be necessary. Maintenance therapy may be on an intermittent basis.

How Supplied

No. 3385—Tablets MODURETIC are peach-colored, diamond-shaped, compressed tablets, coded MSD 917. Each tablet contains 5 mg of amiloride HCl and 50 mg of hydrochlorothiazide. They are supplied as follows:
NDC 0006-0917-68 in bottles of 100
NDC 0006-0917-28 unit dose packages of 100.
Shown in Product Identification Section, page 420
A.H.F.S. Category: 40:28
DC 7130507   Issued May 1984
COPYRIGHT © MERCK & CO., INC., 1984
All rights reserved

MUMPSVAX® R
(mumps virus vaccine, live, MSD), U.S.P.
Jeryl Lynn Strain

Usually, mumps is a mild disease. However, it may occasionally be severe and produce serious complications. For example, meningoencephalitis has been estimated to occur in about 10 percent of patients, and unilateral orchitis in about 20 to 30 percent of postpubertal males. Post-infectious encephalitis, oophoritis, pancreatitis, muscular weakness, myelitis, myocarditis, facial neuritis, arthritis, hepatitis, and deafness may also occur. The relationship of endocardial fibroelastosis in infants, and mumps in the mother during pregnancy, has not been conclusively established.

Studies in susceptible children and adults have assessed the safety and efficacy of MUMPSVAX® (Mumps Virus Vaccine, Live, MSD). A single dose induced an effective antibody response in approximately 97 percent of susceptible children and approximately 93 percent of susceptible adults. There were few reports of soreness at the site of injection during clinical studies. There was no significant difference in the incidence of fever in clinical trials when children vaccinated with mumps vaccine were compared with unvaccinated subjects studied concurrently. In studies which included more than 200 susceptible male adults inoculated with mumps vaccine, no significant clinical side effects were reported. (See ADVERSE REACTIONS.)

No reports have been received of transmission of mumps from vaccinees to susceptible contacts. Adequate antibody levels, with continuing protection of vaccinated children exposed to mumps, have persisted for ten years without substantial decline. The pattern of antibody closely resembles that observed for natural mumps although the antibody level is significantly lower than that following the natural infection. If this pattern continues it will provide a basis for expectation that immunity following the vaccine will be permanent. However, continued surveillance will be required to demonstrate this point.

Preparation

This vaccine is prepared from the Jeryl Lynn (B level) strain, named after the patient from whom the virus was initially recovered.

MUMPSVAX is grown in cell cultures of chick embryos, free of Avian leukosis, according to the general procedures used to prepare Enders' measles virus vaccine, live, attenuated. The vaccine is tested for safety and efficacy.

Indications

MUMPSVAX induces protective antibodies in essentially all non-immune recipients, provides protection against natural mumps in most cases, and has not been shown to cause significant systemic or local reactions. Evidence indicates that the mumps virus infection initiated by the vaccine is not contagious.

The vaccine is indicated [for prevention of] mumps in children 12 m[onths of age or older and] adults. It is not recommend[ed for children younger] than 12 months because they [may still possess] mumps neutralizing antibodie[s which could inter]fere with the immune response. [...]

Evidence indicates that the vaccin[e will afford some] protection when given after exposu[re to natural] mumps. It has been reported that imm[une serum] globulin (human) in a dosage of .01 to .02 [ml/lb does] not prevent the antibody response to the [mumps vac]cine when the two were administered sim[ulta]neously in opposite arms. However, protect[ion] afforded with this regimen has not been esta[b]lished.

Revaccination: Based on available evidence, there is no reason to routinely revaccinate children originally vaccinated when 12 months of age or older.

Use with Other Live Virus Vaccines

There are no data available concerning simultaneous use of MUMPSVAX with monovalent or trivalent poliovirus vaccine, live, oral, or with killed poliovirus vaccines. However, serologic evidence shows that when M-M-R® (Measles, Mumps and Rubella Virus Vaccine, Live, MSD), containing the HPV-77 rubella strain, is given simultaneously with trivalent oral poliovirus vaccine, live, oral, antibody responses can be expected to be comparable to those which follow administration of the vaccines at different times. From this it follows that when MUMPSVAX is given simultaneously with either monovalent or trivalent poliovirus vaccine, live, oral, ATTENUVAX® (Measles Virus Vaccine, Live, Attenuated, MSD) and/or MERUVAX®II (Rubella Virus Vaccine, Live, MSD), antibody responses can be expected to be comparable to those which follow administration of the vaccines at different times.

Contraindications

Hypersensitivity to neomycin (each dose of reconstituted vaccine contains approximately 25 micrograms of neomycin).

Individuals with blood dyscrasias, leukemia, lymphomas of any type, or other malignant neoplasms affecting the bone marrow or lymphatic systems. Patients receiving therapy with ACTH, corticosteroids, irradiation, alkylating agents or antimetabolites.

This contraindication does not apply to patients who are receiving corticosteroids as replacement therapy, e.g., for Addison's disease.

Primary immuno-deficiency states, including cellular immune deficiencies, hypogammaglobulinemic and dysgammaglobulinemic states. Any active infection is reason for delaying mumps vaccination.

Hypersensitivity to Eggs, Chicken, or Chicken Feathers

This vaccine is essentially devoid of potentially allergenic substances derived from host tissues (chick embryo)*. However, because the attenuated virus in this vaccine is propagated in cell cultures of chick embryo, there is a potential risk of hypersensitivity reactions in patients allergic to eggs, chicken, or chicken feathers. Widespread use of the vaccine for more than a decade has resulted in only rare, isolated reports of minor allergic reactions attributed to allergens of this kind, possibly related to the vaccine. Significantly, when children with known allergies to eggs, chicken, and chicken feathers were given a similarly prepared vaccine in a clinical study, none experienced reactions other than those reactions previously observed in non-allergic children.

Pregnancy

Do not give MUMPSVAX to pregnant females; the possible effects of the vaccine on fetal development are unknown at this time. When vaccination of

---

* Morbidity and Mortality Weekly Report 25(44): 350, Nov. 12, 1976.

post-pubertal females is undertaken, pregnancy at the time of vaccination must be ruled out and in addition, the possibility of pregnancy occurring in the three months following vaccination must be eliminated by medically acceptable methods.

Precautions

For subcutaneous use; *do not give intravenously.* MUMPSVAX may be given simultaneously with monovalent or trivalent poliovirus vaccine, live, oral, with ATTENUVAX (Measles Virus Vaccine, Live, Attenuated, MSD) and/or MERUVAX$_{II}$ (Rubella Virus Vaccine, Live, MSD). MUMPSVAX should not be given less than one month before or after administration of other live virus vaccines. Vaccination should be deferred for at least 3 months following blood or plasma transfusions, or administration of human immune serum globulin. It has been reported that mumps virus vaccine, live, may result in a temporary depression of tuberculin skin sensitivity. Therefore, if a tuberculin test is to be done, it should be administered either before or simultaneously with MUMPSVAX.
Epinephrine should be available for immediate use if needed.

Adverse Reactions

Because of the slightly acidic pH (6.2–6.6) of the vaccine, patients may complain of burning and/or stinging of short duration at the injection site. Mild fever occurs occasionally. Fever above 103°F (39.4°C) is uncommon.
Parotitis has been reported to occur in very low incidence, and orchitis rarely, in persons who were vaccinated. In most instances investigated, prior exposure to natural mumps was established. In other instances, whether or not this was due to vaccine or to prior natural mumps exposure or to other causes has not been established.
Reports of purpura and allergic reactions such as wheal and flare at the injection site or urticaria have been extremely rare.
Very rarely encephalitis and other nervous system reactions have occurred in vaccinees. A cause-effect relationship has not been established.

Shipment, Storage, and Reconstitution

During shipment, to insure that there is no loss of potency, the vaccine must be maintained at a temperature of 10°C (50°F) or less.
Prior to reconstitution, store the vaccine in a refrigerator at 2–8°C (35.6–46.4°F). *Protect from light.* To reconstitute, withdraw the entire volume of diluent into the syringe to be used for reconstitution. Inject all the diluent in the syringe into the vial of lyophilized vaccine, and agitate to ensure thorough mixing. Draw back entire contents into a syringe and inject total volume of restored vaccine subcutaneously. Each dose of reconstituted vaccine contains not less than 5,000 TCID$_{50}$ (tissue culture infectious doses) of mumps virus vaccine expressed in terms of the assigned titer of the FDA Reference Mumps Virus.
It is important to use a separate sterile syringe and needle for each individual patient to prevent transmission of hepatitis B virus and other infectious agents from one person to another.
Use only the diluent supplied and reconstitute the vaccine just before using. It is recommended that the vaccine be used as soon as possible after reconstitution. Protect the vaccine from light at all times. Store the reconstituted vaccine in a dark place at 2–8°C (35.6–46.4°F) and discard if not used within 8 hours.
Color: The color of the vaccine when reconstituted is yellow.

Dosage and Administration

After suitably cleansing the immunization site, inject total volume of reconstituted vaccine subcutaneously, preferably into the outer aspect of the upper arm. Do not inject intravenously.

The dosage of vaccine is the same for all patients. *Do not give immune serum globulin (ISG) concurrently with MUMPSVAX.*
CAUTION: A sterile syringe free of preservatives, antiseptics, and detergents should be used for each injection of the vaccine because these substances may inactivate the live virus vaccine. A 25 gauge, ⅝" needle is recommended.

How Supplied

No. 4753—MUMPSVAX—a single-dose vial of lyophilized vaccine, **NDC** 0006-4753-00, and a vial of diluent.
No. 4584X/4309—MUMPSVAX is supplied as follows: (1) a box of 10 single-dose vials of lyophilized vaccine (package A), **NDC** 0006-4584-00; and (2) a box of 10 vials of diluent (package B). To conserve refrigerator space, the diluent may be stored separately at room temperature.

A.H.F.S. Category: 80:12
DC 7075405 Issued February 1983
COPYRIGHT © MERCK & CO., INC. 1983
All rights reserved

MUSTARGEN®, Trituration of ℞
(mechlorethamine HCl for injection, MSD), U.S.P.

Description

MUSTARGEN® (Mechlorethamine HCl, MSD) a nitrogen mustard also known as HN2 hydrochloride, is a nitrogen analog of sulfur mustard. It is a white, crystalline, hygroscopic powder that is very soluble in water and also soluble in alcohol.
Mechlorethamine hydrochloride is designated chemically as 2-chloro- *N* -(2-chloroethyl)- *N* -methylethanamine hydrochloride. The molecular weight is 192.52 and the melting point is 108–111°C. The empirical formula is $C_5H_{11}Cl_2N \cdot HCl$, and the structural formula is: $CH_3N(CH_2CH_2Cl)_2 \cdot HCl$.
Trituration of MUSTARGEN is a white crystalline powder. Each vial of MUSTARGEN contains 10 mg of mechlorethamine hydrochloride triturated with sodium chloride q.s. 100 mg.

Actions

Mechlorethamine, a biologic alkylating agent, has a cytotoxic action which inhibits rapidly proliferating cells.

Indications

B re using MUSTARGEN see *Contraindications, Warnings, Precautions, Adverse Reactions, and Dosage and Administration.*
MUSTARGEN, administered intravenously, is indicated for the palliative treatment of Hodgkin's disease (Stages III and IV), lymphosarcoma, chronic myelocytic or chronic lymphocytic leukemia, polycythemia vera, mycosis fungoides, and bronchogenic carcinoma.
MUSTARGEN, administered intrapleurally, intraperitoneally, or intrapericardially, is indicated for the palliative treatment of metastatic carcinoma resulting in effusion.

Contraindications

Because of the toxicity of MUSTARGEN, and the unpleasant side effects following its use, the potential risk and discomfort from the use of this drug in patients with inoperable neoplasms or in the terminal stage of the disease must be balanced against the limited gain obtainable. These gains will vary with the nature and the status of the disease under treatment. The routine use of MUSTARGEN in all cases of widely disseminated neoplasms is to be discouraged.
The use of MUSTARGEN in patients with leukopenia, thrombocytopenia, and anemia, due to invasion of the bone marrow by tumor carries a greater risk. In such patients a good response to treatment with disappearance of the tumor from the bone marrow may be associated with improvement of bone marrow function. However, in the absence of

a good response or in patients who have been previously treated with chemotherapeutic agents, hematopoiesis may be further compromised, and leukopenia, thrombocytopenia and anemia may become more severe and lead to the demise of the patient.
Tumors of bone and nervous tissue have responded poorly to therapy. Its use is contraindicated in the presence of known infectious diseases. Results are unpredictable in disseminated and malignant tumors of different types.

Warnings

> Extravasation of the drug into subcutaneous tissues results in a painful inflammation. The area usually becomes indurated and sloughing may occur. If leakage of drug is obvious, prompt infiltration of the area with sterile isotonic sodium thiosulfate (⅙ molar) and application of an ice compress for 6 to 12 hours may minimize the local reaction. For a ⅙ molar solution of sodium thiosulfate, use 4.14 g of sodium thiosulfate per 100 ml of Sterile Water for Injection or 2.64 g of anhydrous sodium thiosulfate per 100 ml, or dilute 4 ml of Sodium Thiosulfate Injection U.S.P. (10%) with 6 ml of Sterile Water for Injection.

Before using MUSTARGEN, *an accurate histologic diagnosis of the disease, a knowledge of its natural course, and an adequate clinical history are important. The hematologic status of the patient must first be determined. It is essential to understand the hazards and therapeutic effects to be expected. Careful clinical judgment must be exercised in selecting patients. If the indication for its use is not clear, the drug should not be used.*
As nitrogen mustard therapy may contribute to extensive and rapid development of amyloidosis, it should be used only if foci of acute and chronic suppurative inflammation are absent.
Usage in Pregnancy
There is evidence that the nitrogen mustards have induced fetal abnormalities particularly when used early in pregnancy. The possible benefits of administration of MUSTARGEN in women of childbearing potential must be weighed against the considered risks; patients should be apprised of the risks involved. In pregnant patients requiring treatment for a life-threatening progressive tumor, use of MUSTARGEN should be avoided at least until the third trimester.
Nursing Mothers
Although breast milk studies have not been performed in animals or humans, breast feeding should be stopped before beginning treatment with MUSTARGEN.

Precautions

This drug is highly toxic and both powder and solution must be handled and administered with care. Since MUSTARGEN is a powerful vesicant, it is intended primarily for intravenous use, and in most instances is given by this route. Inhalation of dust or vapors and contact with skin or mucous membranes, especially those of the eyes, must be avoided. Should accidental eye contact occur, copious irrigation with water, normal saline or a balanced salt ophthalmic irrigating solution should be instituted immediately, followed by prompt ophthalmologic consultation. Should accidental skin contact occur, the affected part must be irrigated immediately with copious amounts of water, for at least 15 minutes, followed by 2 percent sodium thiosulfate solution. (See also box warning.) Do not use if the solution is discolored or if droplets of water are visible within the vial. Prepare fresh

Continued on next page

Information on the Merck Sharp & Dohme products listed on these pages is the full prescribing information from product circulars in use November 1, 1984.

Merck Sharp & Dohme—Cont.

solution for injection and dispose of the unused portion after neutralization. (See DOSAGE AND ADMINISTRATION.)

Precautions must be observed with the use of MUSTARGEN and x-ray therapy or other chemotherapy in alternating courses. Hematopoietic function is characteristically depressed by either form of therapy, and neither MUSTARGEN following x-ray therapy nor x-ray therapy subsequent to the drug should be given until bone marrow function has recovered. In particular, irradiation of such areas as sternum, ribs, and vertebrae shortly after a course of nitrogen mustard may lead to hematologic complications.

Therapy with alkylating agents such as MUSTARGEN may be associated with an increased incidence of a second malignant tumor, especially when such therapy is combined with other antineoplastic agents or radiation therapy.

Hyperuricemia may develop during therapy with MUSTARGEN. The problem of urate precipitation should be anticipated, particularly in the treatment of the lymphomas, and adequate methods for control of hyperuricemia should be instituted and careful attention directed toward adequate fluid intake before treatment.

Since drug toxicity, especially sensitivity to bone marrow failure, seems to be more common in chronic lymphatic leukemia than in other conditions, the drug should be given in this condition with great caution, if at all.

Adverse Reactions

Clinical use of MUSTARGEN usually is accompanied by toxic manifestations.

Local Toxicity
Thrombosis and thrombophlebitis may result from direct contact of the drug with the intima of the injected vein. Avoid high concentration and prolonged contact with the drug, especially in cases of elevated pressure in the antebrachial vein (e.g., in mediastinal tumor compression from severe vena cava syndrome).

Systemic Toxicity
Nausea, vomiting and depression of formed elements in the circulating blood are dose-limiting side effects and usually occur with the use of full doses of MUSTARGEN. Jaundice, alopecia, vertigo, tinnitus and diminished hearing may occur infrequently. Rarely, hemolytic anemia associated with such diseases as the lymphomas and chronic lymphocytic leukemia may be precipitated by treatment with alkylating agents including MUSTARGEN. Also, various chromosomal abnormalities have been reported in association with nitrogen mustard therapy.

MUSTARGEN is given preferably at night in case sedation for side effects is required. Nausea and vomiting usually occur 1 to 3 hours after use of the drug. Emesis may disappear in the first 8 hours, but nausea may persist for 24 hours. Nausea and vomiting may be so severe as to precipitate vascular accidents in patients with a hemorrhagic tendency. Premedication with antiemetics, in addition to sedatives, may help control severe nausea and vomiting. Anorexia, weakness and diarrhea may also occur.

The usual course of MUSTARGEN (total dose of 0.4 mg/kg either given as a single intravenous dose or divided into two or four daily doses of 0.2 or 0.1 mg/kg respectively) generally produces a lymphocytopenia within 24 hours after the first injection; significant granulocytopenia occurs within 6 to 8 days and lasts for 10 days to 3 weeks. Agranulocytosis appears to be relatively infrequent and recovery from leukopenia in most cases is complete within two weeks of the maximum reduction. Thrombocytopenia is variable but the time course of the appearance and recovery from reduced platelet counts generally parallels the sequence of granulocyte levels. In some cases severe thrombocytopenia may lead to bleeding from the gums and gastrointestinal tract, petechiae, and small subcutaneous hemorrhages; these symptoms appear to be transient and in most cases disappear with return to a normal platelet count. However, a severe and even uncontrollable depression of the hematopoietic system occasionally may follow the usual dose of MUSTARGEN, particularly in patients with widespread disease and debility and in patients previously treated with other antineoplastic agents or x-ray. Persistent pancytopenia has been reported. In rare instances, hemorrhagic complications may be due to hyperheparinemia. Erythrocyte and hemoglobin levels may decline during the first 2 weeks after therapy but rarely significantly. Depression of the hematopoietic system may be found up to 50 days or more after starting therapy. MUSTARGEN has been reported to have immunosuppressive activity. Therefore, it should be borne in mind that use of the drug may predispose the patient to bacterial, viral or fungal infection. This is more likely to occur when concomitant steroid therapy is employed.

Occasionally, a maculopapular skin eruption occurs, but this may be idiosyncratic and does not necessarily recur with subsequent courses of the drug. In one patient erythema multiforme has been observed. Herpes zoster, a common complicating infection in patients with lymphomas, may first appear after therapy is instituted and on occasion may be precipitated by treatment. Further treatment should be discontinued during the acute phase of this illness to avoid progression to generalized herpes zoster.

Since the gonads are susceptible to MUSTARGEN, treatment may be followed by delayed catamenia, oligomenorrhea, or temporary or permanent amenorrhea. Impaired spermatogenesis, azoospermia, and total germinal aplasia have been reported in male patients treated with alkylating agents, especially in combination with other drugs. In some instances spermatogenesis may return in patients in remission, but this may occur only several years after intensive chemotherapy has been discontinued. Patients should be warned of the potential risk to their reproductive capacity. With total doses exceeding 0.4 mg/kg of body weight for a single course, severe leukopenia, anemia, thrombocytopenia and a hemorrhagic diathesis with subsequent delayed bleeding may develop. Death may follow. The only treatment in instances of excessive dosage appears to be repeated blood product transfusions, antibiotic treatment of complicating infections and general supportive measures. *Extreme caution must be used in exceeding the average recommended dose.*

Dosage and Administration

Intravenous Administration
The dosage of MUSTARGEN varies with the clinical situation, the therapeutic response and the magnitude of hematologic depression. A total dose of 0.4 mg/kg of body weight for each course usually is given either as a single dose or in divided doses of 0.1 to 0.2 mg/kg per day. Dosage should be based on ideal dry body weight. The presence of edema or ascites must be considered so that dosage will be based on actual weight unaugmented by these conditions.

Within a few minutes after intravenous injection, MUSTARGEN undergoes chemical transformation, combines with reactive compounds, and is no longer present in its active form in the blood stream. Subsequent courses should not be given until the patient has recovered hematologically from the previous course; this is best determined by repeated studies of the peripheral blood elements awaiting their return to normal levels. It is often possible to give repeated courses of MUSTARGEN as early as three weeks after treatment. *The margin of safety in therapy with MUSTARGEN is narrow and considerable care must be exercised in the matter of dosage.* Repeated examinations of blood are *mandatory* as a guide to subsequent therapy.

Preparation of Solution and Intravenous Administration
Each vial of MUSTARGEN contains 10 mg of mechlorethamine hydrochloride triturated with sodium chloride q.s. 100 mg. In neutral or alkaline aqueous solution it undergoes rapid chemical transformation and is highly unstable. Although solutions prepared according to instructions are acidic and do not decompose as rapidly, they should be prepared immediately before each injection since they will decompose on standing.

Using a sterile 10 ml syringe, inject 10 ml of Sterile Water for Injection or 10 ml Sodium Chloride Injection into a vial of MUSTARGEN. With the needle still in the rubber stopper, shake the vial several times to dissolve the drug completely. The resultant solution contains 1 mg of mechlorethamine hydrochloride per ml.

Withdraw into the syringe the calculated volume of solution required for a single injection. *Dispose of any remaining solution after neutralization* (see below). Although the drug may be injected directly into any suitable vein, it is injected preferably into the rubber or plastic tubing of a flowing intravenous infusion set. This reduces the possibility of severe local reactions due to extravasation or high concentration of the drug. Injecting the drug into the tubing rather than adding it to the entire volume of the infusion fluid minimizes a chemical reaction between the drug and the solution. The rate of injection apparently is not critical provided it is completed within a few minutes.

Intracavitary Administration
Nitrogen mustard has been used by intracavitary administration with varying success in certain malignant conditions for the control of pleural, peritoneal, and pericardial effusions caused by malignant cells.

The technic and the dose used by any of these routes varies. Therefore, if MUSTARGEN is given by the intracavitary route, the published articles concerning such use should be consulted. *Because of the inherent risks involved, the physician should be experienced in the appropriate injection technics, and be thoroughly aware of the indications, dosages, hazards, and precautions as set forth in the published literature. When using MUSTARGEN by the intracavitary route, the general precautions concerning this agent should be borne in mind.*

As a general guide, reference is made especially to the technics of Weisberger et al. Intracavitary use is indicated in the presence of pleural, peritoneal, or pericardial effusion due to metastatic tumors. Local therapy with nitrogen mustard is used only when malignant cells are demonstrated in the effusion. Intracavitary injection is not recommended when the accumulated fluid is chylous in nature, since results are likely to be poor.

Paracentesis is first performed with most of the fluid being removed from the pleural or peritoneal cavity. The intracavitary use of MUSTARGEN may exert at least some of its effect through production of a chemical poudrage. Therefore, the removal of excess fluid allows the drug to more easily contact the peritoneal and pleural linings. For intrapleural or intrapericardial injection nitrogen mustard is introduced directly through the thoracentesis needle. For intraperitoneal injection it is given through a rubber catheter inserted into the trocar used for paracentesis or through a No. 18 gauge needle inserted at another site. This drug should be injected slowly, with frequent aspiration to ensure that a free flow of fluid is present. If fluid cannot be aspirated, pain and necrosis due to injection of solution outside the cavity may occur. Free flow of fluid also is necessary to prevent injection into a loculated pocket and to ensure adequate dissemination of nitrogen mustard.

The usual dose of nitrogen mustard for intracavitary injection is 0.4 mg/kg of body weight, though 0.2 mg/kg (or 10 to 20 mg) has been used by the intrapericardial route. The solution is prepared, as previously described for intravenous injection, by adding 10 ml of Sterile Water for Injection or 10 ml of Sodium Chloride Injection to the vial containing 10 mg of mechlorethamine hydrochloride. (Amounts of diluent of 50 to 100 ml of normal saline have also been used.) The position of the patient should be changed every 5 to 10 minutes for an hour after injection to obtain more uniform distribution of the drug throughout the serous cavity. The remaining fluid may be removed from the pleural or peritoneal cavity by paracentesis 24 to 36 hours later. The patient should be followed carefully by clinical and x-ray examination to detect reaccumulation of fluid.

Pain occurs rarely with intrapleural use; it is common with intraperitoneal injection and is often associated with nausea, vomiting, and diarrhea of 2 to 3 days duration. Transient cardiac irregularities may occur with intrapericardial injection. Death, possibly accelerated by nitrogen mustard, has been reported following the use of this agent by the intracavitary route. Although absorption of MUSTARGEN when given by the intracavitary route is probably not complete because of its rapid deactivation by body fluids, the systemic effect is unpredictable. The acute side effects such as nausea and vomiting are usually mild. Bone marrow depression is generally milder than when the drug is given intravenously. Care should be taken to avoid use by the intracavitary route when other agents which may suppress bone marrow function are being used systemically.

Neutralization of Equipment and Unused Solution

To clean rubber gloves, tubing, glassware, etc., after giving MUSTARGEN, soak them in an aqueous solution containing equal volumes of sodium thiosulfate (5%) and sodium bicarbonate (5%) for 45 minutes. Excess reagents and reaction products are washed away easily with water. Any unused injection solution should be neutralized by mixing with an equal volume of sodium thiosulfate/sodium bicarbonate solution. Allow the mixture to stand for 45 minutes. Vials that have contained MUSTARGEN should be treated in the same way with thiosulfate/bicarbonate solution before disposal.

How Supplied

No. 7753—Trituration of MUSTARGEN is a white crystalline powder, each vial containing 10 mg mechlorethamine hydrochloride with sodium chloride q.s. 100 mg, and is supplied as follows:
NDC 0006-7753-31 in treatment sets of 4 vials.

Special Handling

Due to the drug's toxic and mutagenic properties, appropriate precautions including the use of appropriate safety equipment are recommended for the preparation of MUSTARGEN for parenteral administration. The National Institutes of Health presently recommends that the preparation of injectable antineoplastic drugs should be performed in a Class II laminar flow biological safety cabinet and that personnel preparing drugs of this class should wear surgical gloves and a closed front surgical-type gown with knit cuffs.

A.H.F.S. Category: 10:00
DC 6382424 Issued September 1983
COPYRIGHT © MERCK & CO., INC., 1983
All rights reserved

MYOCHRYSINE® Injection R
(gold sodium thiomalate, MSD), U.S.P.

Physicians planning to use MYOCHRYSINE® (Gold Sodium Thiomalate, MSD) should thoroughly familiarize themselves with its toxicity and its benefits. The possibility of toxic reactions should always be explained to the patient before starting therapy. Patients should be warned to report promptly any symptoms suggesting toxicity. Before each injection of MYOCHRYSINE, the physician should review the results of laboratory work, and see the patient to determine the presence or absence of adverse reactions since some of these can be severe or even fatal.

Description

MYOCHRYSINE is a sterile aqueous solution of gold sodium thiomalate. It contains 0.5 percent benzyl alcohol added as a preservative. The pH of the product is 5.8–6.5.
Gold sodium thiomalate is a mixture of the mono- and di-sodium salts of gold thiomalic acid.

The molecular weight for $C_4H_3AuNa_2O_4S$ (the disodium salt) is 390.07 and for $C_4H_4AuNaO_4S$ (the monosodium salt) is 368.09.
MYOCHRYSINE is supplied as a solution for intramuscular injection containing 10 mg, 25 mg, 50 mg or 100 mg of gold sodium thiomalate per ml.

Clinical Pharmacology

The mode of action of gold sodium thiomalate is unknown. The predominant action appears to be a suppressive effect on the synovitis of active rheumatoid disease.

Indications and Usage

MYOCHRYSINE is indicated in the treatment of selected cases of active rheumatoid arthritis—both adult and juvenile type. The greatest benefit occurs in the early active stage. In late stages of the illness when cartilage and bone damage have occurred, gold can only check the progression of rheumatoid arthritis and prevent further structural damage to joints. It cannot repair damage caused by previously active disease.
MYOCHRYSINE should be used only as *one part* of a complete program of therapy; alone it is not a complete treatment.

Contraindications

Severe toxicity resulting from previous exposure to gold or other heavy metals.
Severe debilitation.
Systemic lupus erythematosus.

Warnings

Before treatment is started, the patient's hemoglobin, erythrocyte, white blood cell, differential and platelet counts should be determined, and urinalysis should be done to serve as basic reference. Urine should be analyzed for protein and sediment changes prior to each injection. Complete blood counts including platelet estimation should be made before every second injection throughout treatment. The occurrence of purpura or ecchymoses at any time always requires a platelet count. Danger signals of possible gold toxicity include: rapid reduction of hemoglobin, leukopenia below 4000 WBC/cu ml, eosinophilia above 5 percent, platelet decrease below 100,000/cu ml, albuminuria, hematuria, pruritus, skin eruption, stomatitis, or persistent diarrhea. No additional injections of MYOCHRYSINE should be given unless further studies show these abnormalities to be caused by conditions other than gold toxicity.

Precautions

General
Gold salts should not be used concomitantly with penicillamine.
The safety of coadministration with cytotoxic drugs has not been established.
Caution is indicated in the use of MYOCHRYSINE in patients with the following:
1. a history of blood dyscrasias such as granulocytopenia or anemia caused by drug sensitivity,
2. allergy or hypersensitivity to medications,
3. skin rash,
4. previous kidney or liver disease,
5. marked hypertension,
6. compromised cerebral or cardiovascular circulation.

Diabetes mellitus or congestive heart failure should be under control before gold therapy is instituted.

Carcinogenicity

Renal adenomas have been reported in long-term toxicity studies of rats receiving MYOCHRYSINE at high dose levels (2 mg/kg weekly for 45 weeks, followed by 6 mg/kg daily for 47 weeks), approximately 2 to 42 times the usual human dose. These adenomas are histologically similar to those produced in rats by chronic administration of experimental gold compounds and other heavy metals, such as lead. No reports have been received of renal adenomas in man in association with the use of MYOCHRYSINE.

Pregnancy
Pregnancy Category C.
MYOCHRYSINE has been shown to be teratogenic during the organogenetic period in rats and rabbits when given in doses, respectively, of 140 and 175 times the usual human dose. Hydrocephaly and microphthalmia were the malformations observed in rats when MYOCHRYSINE was administered subcutaneously at a dose of 25 mg/kg/day from day 6 through day 15 of gestation. In rabbits, limb malformations and gastroschisis were the malformations observed when MYOCHRYSINE was administered subcutaneously at doses of 20–45 mg/kg/day from day 6 through day 18 of gestation.
There are no adequate and well-controlled studies in pregnant women. MYOCHRYSINE should be used during pregnancy only if the potential benefit to the mother justifies the potential risk to the fetus.

Nursing Mothers
The presence of gold has been demonstrated in the milk of lactating mothers. In addition, gold has been found in the serum and red blood cells of a nursing infant. In view of the above findings and because of the potential for serious adverse reactions in nursing infants from MYOCHRYSINE, a decision should be made whether to discontinue nursing or to discontinue the drug, taking into account the importance of the drug to the mother. The slow excretion and persistence of gold in the mother, even after therapy is discontinued, must also be kept in mind.

Adverse Reactions

A variety of adverse reactions may develop during the initial phase (weekly injections) of therapy or during maintenance treatment. Adverse reactions are observed most frequently when the cumulative dose of MYOCHRYSINE administered is between 400 and 800 mg. Very uncommonly, complications occur days to months after cessation of treatment.
Cutaneous reactions: Dermatitis is the most common reaction. *Any eruption, especially if pruritic, that develops during treatment with MYOCHRYSINE should be considered a reaction to gold until proven otherwise.* Pruritus often exists before dermatitis becomes apparent, and therefore should be considered a warning signal of impending cutaneous reaction. The most serious form of cutaneous reaction is generalized exfoliative dermatitis which may lead to alopecia and shedding of nails. Gold dermatitis may be aggravated by exposure to sunlight or an actinic rash may develop.
Mucous membrane reactions: Stomatitis is the second most common adverse reaction. Shallow ulcers on the buccal membranes, on the borders of the tongue, and on the palate or in the pharynx may occur as the only adverse reaction, or along with dermatitis. Sometimes diffuse glossitis or gingivitis develops. A metallic taste may precede these oral mucous membrane reactions and should be considered a warning signal.
Conjunctivitis is a rare reaction.
Renal reactions: Gold may be toxic to the kidney and produce a nephrotic syndrome or glomerulitis with hematuria. These renal reactions are usually relatively mild and subside completely if recognized early and treatment is discontinued. They may become severe and chronic if treatment is continued after onset of the reaction. Therefore, it is important to perform a *urinalysis before every injection*, and to discontinue treatment promptly if proteinuria or hematuria develops.
Hematologic reactions: Blood dyscrasia due to gold toxicity is rare, but because of the potential serious consequences it must be constantly watched for and recognized early by frequent blood examinations done throughout treatment. Granulocytope-

Continued on next page

Information on the Merck Sharp & Dohme products listed on these pages is the full prescribing information from product circulars in use November 1, 1984.

Merck Sharp & Dohme—Cont.

nia; thrombocytopenia, with or without purpura; hypoplastic and aplastic anemia; and eosinophilia have all been reported. These hematologic disorders may occur separately or in combinations.

Nitritoid and allergic reactions: Reactions of the "nitritoid type" which may resemble anaphylactoid effects have been reported. Flushing, fainting, dizziness and sweating are most frequently reported. Other symptoms that may occur include: nausea, vomiting, malaise and weakness.

More severe, but less common effects include: anaphylactic shock, syncope, bradycardia, thickening of the tongue, difficulty in swallowing and breathing, and angioneurotic edema. These effects may occur almost immediately after injection or as late as 10 minutes following injection. They may occur at any time during the course of therapy and if observed, treatment with MYOCHRYSINE should be discontinued.

Miscellaneous reactions: Gastrointestinal reactions have been reported, including nausea, vomiting, anorexia, abdominal cramps and diarrhea. Ulcerative enterocolitis, which can be severe or even fatal, has been reported rarely.

There have been rare reports of reactions involving the eye such as iritis, corneal ulcers, and gold deposits in ocular tissues. There also have been rare reports of sensori-motor polyradiculoneuropathy (including Guillain-Barré syndrome).

Hepatitis with jaundice, gold bronchitis, pulmonary injury manifested by interstitial pneumonitis and fibrosis, partial or complete hair loss and fever have also been reported.

Sometimes arthralgia occurs for a day or two after an injection of MYOCHRYSINE; this reaction usually subsides after the first few injections.

Management of Adverse Reactions

Treatment with MYOCHRYSINE should be discontinued immediately when toxic reactions occur. Minor complications such as localized dermatitis, mild stomatitis, or slight proteinuria generally require no other therapy and resolve spontaneously with suspension of MYOCHRYSINE. Moderately severe skin and mucous membrane reactions often benefit from topical corticosteroids, oral antihistaminics, and soothing or anesthetic lotions.

If stomatitis or dermatitis becomes severe or more generalized, systemic corticosteroids (generally, prednisone 10 to 40 mg daily in divided doses) may provide symptomatic relief.

For serious renal, hematologic, pulmonary, and enterocolitic complications, high doses of systemic corticosteroids (prednisone 40 to 100 mg daily in divided doses) are recommended. The optimum duration of corticosteroid treatment varies with the response of the individual patient. Therapy may be required for many months when adverse effects are unusually severe or progressive.

In patients whose complications do not improve with high-dose corticosteroid treatment, or who develop significant steroid-related adverse reactions, a chelating agent may be given to enhance gold excretion. Dimercaprol (BAL) has been used successfully, but patients must be monitored carefully as numerous untoward reactions may attend its use. Corticosteroids and a chelating agent may be used concomitantly.

MYOCHRYSINE *should not be reinstituted after severe or idiosyncratic reactions.*

MYOCHRYSINE may be readministered following resolution of mild reactions, using a reduced dosage schedule. If an initial test dose of 5 mg MYOCHRYSINE is well-tolerated, progressively larger doses (5 to 10 mg increments) may be given at weekly to monthly intervals until a dose of 25 to 50 mg is reached.

Dosage and Administration

MYOCHRYSINE should be administered only by intramuscular injection, preferably intragluteally. It should be given with the patient lying down. He should remain recumbent for approximately 10 minutes after the injection.

Therapeutic effects from MYOCHRYSINE occur slowly. Early improvement, often limited to a reduction in morning stiffness, may begin after six to eight weeks of treatment, but beneficial effects may not be observed until after months of therapy. Parenteral drug products should be inspected visually for particulate matter and discoloration prior to administration. Do not use if material has darkened. Color should not exceed pale yellow.

For the adult of average size the following dosage schedule is suggested:

Weekly Injections

1st injection ....10 mg
2nd injection ....25 mg
3rd and subsequent injections ....25 to 50 mg

until there is toxicity or major clinical improvement, or, in the absence of either of these, the cumulative dose of MYOCHRYSINE reaches one gram.

MYOCHRYSINE is continued until the cumulative dose reaches one gram unless toxicity or major clinical improvement occurs. If significant clinical improvement occurs before a cumulative dose of one gram has been administered, the dose may be decreased or the interval between injections increased as with maintenance therapy. Maintenance doses of 25 to 50 mg every other week for two to 20 weeks are recommended. If the clinical course remains stable, injections of 25 to 50 mg may be given every third and subsequently every fourth week indefinitely. Some patients may require maintenance treatment at intervals of one to three weeks. Should the arthritis exacerbate during maintenance therapy, weekly injections may be resumed temporarily until disease activity is suppressed.

Should a patient fail to improve during initial therapy (cumulative dose of one gram), several options are available:

1—the patient may be considered to be unresponsive and MYOCHRYSINE is discontinued
2—the same dose (25 to 50 mg) of MYOCHRYSINE may be continued for approximately ten additional weeks
3—the dose of MYOCHRYSINE may be increased by increments of 10 mg every one to four weeks, not to exceed 100 mg in a single injection.

If significant clinical improvement occurs using option 2 or 3, the maintenance schedule described above should be initiated. If there is no significant improvement or if toxicity occurs, therapy with MYOCHRYSINE should be stopped. The higher the individual dose of MYOCHRYSINE, the greater the risk of gold toxicity. Selection of one of these options for chrysotherapy should be based upon a number of factors, including the physician's experience with gold salt therapy, the course of the patient's condition, the choice of alternative treatments, and the availability of the patient for the close supervision required.

Juvenile Rheumatoid Arthritis

The pediatric dose of MYOCHRYSINE is proportional to the adult dose on a weight basis. After the initial test dose of 10 mg, the recommended dose for children is one mg per kilogram body weight, not to exceed 50 mg for a single injection. Otherwise, the guidelines given above for administration to adults also apply to children.

Concomitant Drug Therapy—Gold salts should not be used concomitantly with penicillamine.

The safety of coadministration with cytotoxic drugs has not been established. Other measures, such as salicylates, other non-steroidal anti-inflammatory drugs, or systemic corticosteroids, may be continued when MYOCHRYSINE is initiated. After improvement commences, analgesic and anti-inflammatory drugs may be discontinued slowly as symptoms permit.

How Supplied

Injection MYOCHRYSINE is a clear colorless to light yellow solution, depending on potency, which must be protected from light. It is supplied as follows:

No. 7763—10 mg of gold sodium thiomalate per ml as
NDC 0006-7763-64 in boxes of 6 x 1 ml ampuls.
No. 7764—25 mg of gold sodium thiomalate per ml as
NDC 0006-7764-64 in boxes of 6 x 1 ml ampuls.
No. 7762—50 mg of gold sodium thiomalate per ml as
NDC 0006-7762-64 in boxes of 6 x 1 ml ampuls.
NDC 0006-7762-10 in 10 ml vials.
A.H.F.S. Category: 60:00
DC 6015523   Revised March 1984
COPYRIGHT © MERCK & CO., INC. 1982
All rights reserved

NEODECADRON® Sterile   R
Ophthalmic Ointment
Neomycin sulfate-dexamethasone
sodium phosphate ointment, U.S.P.

Description

Sterile ophthalmic ointment NEODECADRON® is a topical corticosteroid-antibiotic ointment for use in certain disorders of the anterior segment of the eye.

Ophthalmic ointment NEODECADRON contains in each gram: dexamethasone sodium phosphate equivalent to 0.5 mg (0.05%) dexamethasone phosphate and neomycin sulfate equivalent to 3.5 mg neomycin base. Inactive ingredients: white petrolatum and mineral oil.

Dexamethasone sodium phosphate is an inorganic ester of dexamethasone. Its empirical formula is $C_{22}H_{28}FNa_2O_8P$.

Neomycin sulfate is the sulfate salt of neomycin, an antibacterial substance produced by the growth of *Streptomyces fradiae* Waksman (Fam. Streptomycetaceae).

Clinical Pharmacology

Dexamethasone sodium phosphate, a corticosteroid, suppresses the inflammatory response to a variety of agents, and it probably delays or slows healing. Since corticosteroids may inhibit the body's defense mechanism against infection, a concomitant antimicrobial drug may be used when this inhibition is considered to be clinically significant in a particular case.

Neomycin sulfate, the anti-infective component in the combination, is included to provide action against specific organisms susceptible to it. Neomycin sulfate is considered active mainly against gram-negative organisms, except *Bacteroides* spp. and *Pseudomonas aeruginosa*, which are resistant. Gram-positive organisms except for *Staphylococcus aureus* are usually resistant.

When a decision to administer both a corticosteroid and an antimicrobial is made, the administration of such drugs in combination has the advantage of greater patient compliance and convenience, with the added assurance that the appropriate dosage of both drugs is administered, plus assured compatibility of ingredient when both types of drug are in the same formulation and, particularly, that the correct volume of drug is delivered and retained.

The relative potency of corticosteroids depends on the molecular structure, concentration, and release from the vehicle.

Indications and Usage

For steroid-responsive inflammatory ocular conditions for which a corticosteroid is indicated and where bacterial infection or a risk of bacterial ocular infection exists.

Ocular steroids are indicated in inflammatory conditions of the palpebral and bulbar conjunctiva, cornea, and anterior segment of the globe where the inherent risk of steroid use in certain infective conjunctivitides is accepted to obtain a diminution in edema and inflammation. They are also indicated in chronic anterior uveitis and corneal injury from chemical, radiation, or thermal burns, or penetration of foreign bodies.

The use of a combination drug with an anti-infective component is indicated where the risk of infection is high or where there is an expectation that potentially dangerous numbers of bacteria will be present in the eye.
The particular anti-infective drug in this product is active against the following common bacterial eye pathogens:

Staphylococcus aureus
Escherichia coli
Haemophilus influenzae
Klebsiella/Enterobacter species
Neisseria species

The product does not provide adequate coverage against:

Pseudomonas aeruginosa
Serratia marcescens
Streptococci, including *Streptococcus pneumoniae*

Contraindications

Epithelial herpes simplex keratitis (dendritic keratitis), acute infectious stages of vaccinia, varicella, and many other viral diseases of the cornea and conjunctiva. Mycobacterial infection of the eye. Fungal diseases of ocular structures. Hypersensitivity to a component of the medication (hypersensitivity to the antibiotic component occurs at a higher rate than for other components).
The use of these combinations is always contraindicated after uncomplicated removal of a corneal foreign body.

Warnings

Prolonged use may result in glaucoma, with damage to the optic nerve, defects in visual acuity and fields of vision, and posterior subcapsular cataract formation. Prolonged use may suppress the host response and thus increase the hazard of secondary ocular infections. In those diseases causing thinning of the cornea or sclera, perforations have been known to occur with the use of topical corticosteroids. In acute purulent conditions of the eye, corticosteroids may mask infection or enhance existing infection. If these products are used for 10 days or longer, intraocular pressure should be routinely monitored even though it may be difficult in children and uncooperative patients.
Employment of corticosteroid medication in the treatment of herpes simplex requires great caution: periodic slit-lamp microscopy is recommended.
Any substance (e.g. neomycin sulfate) may occasionally cause cutaneous sensitization. If any reaction indicating such sensitivity is observed, discontinue use.

Precautions

The initial prescriptions and renewal of the medication order beyond 8 grams should be made by a physician only after examination of the patient with the aid of magnification, such as slit lamp biomicroscopy and, where appropriate, fluorescein staining.
The possibility of persistent fungal infections of the cornea should be considered after prolonged corticosteroid dosing.
Usage in Pregnancy
Safety of intensive or protracted use of topical corticosteroids during pregnancy has not been substantiated.

Adverse Reactions

Adverse reactions have occurred with corticosteroid/anti-infective combination drugs which can be attributed to the corticosteroid component, the anti-infective component, or the combination. Exact incidence figures are not available since no denominator of treated patients is available.
Reactions occurring most often from the presence of the anti-infective ingredient are allergic sensitizations. The reactions due to the corticosteroid component in decreasing order of frequency are: elevation of intraocular pressure (IOP) with possible development of glaucoma, and infrequent optic nerve damage; posterior subcapsular cataract formation; and delayed wound healing.
Secondary Infection: The development of secondary infection has occurred after use of combinations containing corticosteroids and antimicrobials. Fungal infections of the cornea are particularly prone to develop coincidentally with long-term applications of corticosteroid. The possibility of fungal invasion must be considered in any persistent corneal ulceration where corticosteroid treatment has been used.
Secondary bacterial ocular infection following suppression of host responses also occurs.

Dosage and Administration

The duration of treatment will vary with the type of lesion and may extend from a few days to several weeks, according to therapeutic response. Relapses, more common in chronic active lesions than in self-limited conditions, usually respond to retreatment.
Apply a thin coating of ophthalmic ointment NEODECADRON three or four times a day. When a favorable response is observed, reduce the number of daily applications to two, and later to one a day as maintenance dose if this is sufficient to control symptoms.
Not more than 8 grams should be prescribed initially and the prescription should not be refilled without further evaluation as outlined in PRECAUTIONS above.
Ophthalmic ointment NEODECADRON is particularly convenient when an eye pad is used. It may also be the preparation of choice for patients in whom therapeutic benefit depends on prolonged contact of the active ingredients with ocular tissues.

How Supplied

No. 7617—Sterile Ophthalmic Ointment NEODECADRON is a clear, unctuous ointment, and is supplied as follows:
NDC 0006-7617-04 in 3.5 g tubes
(6505-00-823-7956 0.05% 3.5 g)
A.H.F.S. Category: 52:08
DC 6167721   Issued June 1982

NEODECADRON® Sterile   R
Ophthalmic Solution
(neomycin sulfate-dexamethasone sodium phosphate, MSD), U.S.P.

Description

Ophthalmic solution NEODECADRON® (Neomycin Sulfate-Dexamethasone Sodium Phosphate, MSD) is a topical corticosteroid-antibiotic solution for use in certain disorders of the anterior segment of the eye.
Each milliliter of buffered ophthalmic solution NEODECADRON in the OCUMETER® ophthalmic dispenser contains: dexamethasone sodium phosphate equivalent to 1 mg (0.1%) dexamethasone phosphate, and neomycin sulfate equivalent to 3.5 mg neomycin base. Inactive ingredients: creatinine, sodium citrate, sodium borate, polysorbate 80, disodium edetate, hydrochloric acid to adjust pH to 6.6–7.8, and water for injection. Benzalkonium chloride 0.02% and sodium bisulfite 0.1% added as preservatives.
Dexamethasone sodium phosphate is a water soluble, inorganic ester of dexamethasone. Its empirical formula is $C_{22}H_{28}FNa_2O_8P$. It is approximately three thousand times more soluble in water at 25°C than hydrocortisone.
Neomycin sulfate is the sulfate salt of neomycin, an antibacterial substance produced by the growth of *Streptomyces fradiae* Waksman (Fam. Streptomycetaceae).

Clinical Pharmacology

Dexamethasone sodium phosphate, a corticosteroid, suppresses the inflammatory response to a variety of agents, and it probably delays or slows healing. Since corticosteroids may inhibit the body's defense mechanism against infection, a concomitant antimicrobial drug may be used when this inhibition is considered to be clinically significant in a particular case. Neomycin sulfate, the anti-infective component in the combination, is included to provide action against specific organisms susceptible to it. Neomycin sulfate is considered active mainly against gram-negative organisms, except *Bacteroides* spp. and *Pseudomonas aeruginosa*, which are resistant. Gram-positive organisms except for *Staphylococcus aureus* are usually resistant.
When a decision to administer both a corticosteroid and an antimicrobial is made, the administration of such drugs in combination has the advantage of greater patient compliance and convenience, with the added assurance that the appropriate dosage of both drugs is administered, plus assured compatibility of ingredients when both types of drug are in the same formulation and, particularly, that the correct volume of drug is delivered and retained.
The relative potency of corticosteroids depends on the molecular structure, concentration, and release from the vehicle.

Indications and Usage

For steroid-responsive inflammatory ocular conditions for which a corticosteroid is indicated and where bacterial infection or a risk of bacterial ocular infection exists.
Ocular steroids are indicated in inflammatory conditions of the palpebral and bulbar conjunctiva, cornea, and anterior segment of the globe where the inherent risk of steroid use in certain infective conjunctivitides is accepted to obtain a diminution in edema and inflammation. They are also indicated in chronic anterior uveitis and corneal injury from chemical, radiation, or thermal burns, or penetration of foreign bodies.
The use of a combination drug with an anti-infective component is indicated where the risk of infection is high or where there is an expectation that potentially dangerous numbers of bacteria will be present in the eye.
The particular anti-infective drug in this product is active against the following common bacterial eye pathogens:

Staphylococcus aureus
Escherichia coli
Haemophilus influenzae
Klebsiella/Enterobacter species
Neisseria species

The product does not provide adequate coverage against:

Pseudomonas aeruginosa
Serratia marcescens
Streptococci, including *Streptococcus pneumoniae*

Contraindications

Epithelial herpes simplex keratitis (dendritic keratitis), acute infectious stages of vaccinia, varicella, and many other viral diseases of the cornea and conjunctiva. Mycobacterial infection of the eye. Fungal diseases of ocular structures. Hypersensitivity to a component of the medication (hypersensitivity to the antibiotic component occurs at a higher rate than for other components).
The use of these combinations is always contraindicated after uncomplicated removal of a corneal foreign body.

Warnings

Prolonged use may result in glaucoma, with damage to the optic nerve, defects in visual acuity and fields of vision, and posterior subcapsular cataract formation. Prolonged use may suppress the host response and thus increase the hazard of secon-

Continued on next page

Information on the Merck Sharp & Dohme products listed on these pages is the full prescribing information from product circulars in use November 1, 1984.

Merck Sharp & Dohme—Cont.

dary ocular infections. In those diseases causing thinning of the cornea or sclera, perforations have been known to occur with the use of topical corticosteroids. In acute purulent conditions of the eye, corticosteroids may mask infection or enhance existing infection. If these products are used for 10 days or longer, intraocular pressure should be routinely monitored even though it may be difficult in children and uncooperative patients.
Employment of corticosteroid medication in the treatment of herpes simplex requires great caution: periodic slit-lamp microscopy is recommended.
Any substance (e.g. neomycin sulfate) may occasionally cause cutaneous sensitization. If any reaction indicating such sensitivity is observed, discontinue use.

Precautions

The initial prescription and renewal of the medication order beyond 20 milliliters should be made by a physician only after examination of the patient with the aid of magnification, such as slit-lamp biomicroscopy and, where appropriate, fluorescein staining.
The possibility of persistent fungal infections of the cornea should be considered after prolonged corticosteroid dosing.
Usage in Pregnancy
Safety of intensive or protracted use of topical corticosteroids during pregnancy has not been substantiated.

Adverse Reactions

Adverse reactions have occurred with corticosteroid/anti-infective combination drugs which can be attributed to the corticosteroid component, the anti-infective component, or the combination. Exact incidence figures are not available since no denominator of treated patients is available.
Reactions occurring most often from the presence of the anti-infective ingredient are allergic sensitizations. The reactions due to the corticosteroid component in decreasing order of frequency are: elevation of intraocular pressure (IOP) with possible development of glaucoma, and infrequent optic nerve damage; posterior subcapsular cataract formation; and delayed wound healing.
Secondary Infection: The development of secondary infection has occurred after use of combinations containing corticosteroids and antimicrobials. Fungal infections of the cornea are particularly prone to develop coincidentally with long-term applications of corticosteroid. The possibility of fungal invasion must be considered in any persistent corneal ulceration where corticosteroid treatment has been used. Secondary bacterial ocular infection following suppression of host responses also occurs.

Dosage and Administration

The duration of treatment will vary with the type of lesion and may extend from a few days to several weeks, according to therapeutic response. Relapses, more common in chronic active lesions than in self-limited conditions, usually respond to retreatment.
Instill one or two drops of ophthalmic solution NEODECADRON into the conjunctival sac every hour during the day and every two hours during the night as initial therapy. When a favorable response is observed, reduce dosage to one drop every four hours. Later, further reduction in dosage to one drop three or four times daily may suffice to control symptoms. Not more than 20 milliliters should be prescribed initially and the prescription should not be refilled without further evaluation as outlined in PRECAUTIONS above.

How Supplied

Sterile ophthalmic solution NEODECADRON is a clear, colorless to pale yellow solution.

No. 7639—Ophthalmic solution NEODECADRON is supplied as follows:
NDC 0006-7639-03 in 5 mL white opaque, plastic OCUMETER ophthalmic dispenser with a controlled drop tip.
(6505-01-039-4325 0.1% 5 mL).
A.H.F.S. Category: 52:08
DC 6361414 Issued June 1982

PERIACTIN® Tablets ℞
(cyproheptadine HCl, MSD), U.S.P.
PERIACTIN® Syrup ℞
(cyproheptadine HCl, MSD), U.S.P.

Description

PERIACTIN® (Cyproheptadine HCl, MSD) is an antihistaminic and antiserotonergic agent.
Cyproheptadine hydrochloride is a white to slightly yellowish, crystalline solid, with a molecular weight of 350.89, which is soluble in water, freely soluble in methanol, sparingly soluble in ethanol, soluble in chloroform, and practically insoluble in ether. It is the sesquihydrate of 4-(5H-dibenzo $[a,d]$ cyclohepten-5-ylidene)-1-methylpiperidine hydrochloride. The empirical formula of the anhydrous salt is $C_{21}H_{21}N \cdot HCl$.
PERIACTIN is available in tablets, containing 4 mg of cyproheptadine hydrochloride, and as a syrup in which 5 ml contains 2 mg of cyproheptadine hydrochloride.

Clinical Pharmacology

PERIACTIN is a serotonin and histamine antagonist with anticholinergic and sedative effects. Antiserotonin and antihistamine drugs appear to compete with serotonin and histamine, respectively, for receptor sites.
Pharmacokinetics and Metabolism
After a single 4 mg oral dose of ^{14}C-labelled cyproheptadine HCl in normal subjects, given as tablets or syrup, 2-20% of the radioactivity was excreted in the stools. Only about 34% of the stool radioactivity was unchanged drug, corresponding to less than 5.7% of the dose. At least 40% of the administered radioactivity was excreted in the urine. No significant difference in the mean urinary excretion exists between the tablet and syrup formulations. No detectable amounts of unchanged drug were present in the urine of patients on chronic 12-20 mg daily doses of PERIACTIN Syrup. The principle metabolite found in human urine has been identified as a quaternary ammonium glucuronide conjugate of cyproheptadine. Elimination is diminished in renal insufficiency.

Indications and Usage

Perennial and seasonal allergic rhinitis
Vasomotor rhinitis
Allergic conjunctivitis due to inhalant allergens and foods
Mild, uncomplicated allergic skin manifestations of urticaria and angioedema
Amelioration of allergic reactions to blood or plasma
Cold urticaria
Dermatographism
As therapy for anaphylactic reactions *adjunctive* to epinephrine and other standard measures after the acute manifestations have been controlled

Contraindications

Newborn or Premature Infants
This drug should *not* be used in newborn or premature infants.
Nursing Mothers
Because of the higher risk of antihistamines for infants generally and for newborns and prematures in particular, antihistamine therapy is contraindicated in nursing mothers.
Lower Respiratory Disease
Antihistamines should not be used to treat lower respiratory tract symptoms including asthma.
Other Conditions
Hypersensitivity to cyproheptadine and other drugs of similar chemical structure:

Monoamine oxidase inhibitor therapy (see DRUG INTERACTIONS)
Angle-closure glaucoma
Stenosing peptic ulcer
Symptomatic prostatic hypertrophy
Bladder neck obstruction
Pyloroduodenal obstruction
Elderly, debilitated patients

Warnings

Children
Overdosage of antihistamines, particularly in infants and children, may produce hallucinations, central nervous system depression, convulsions, and death.
Antihistamines may diminish mental alertness; conversely, particularly, in the young child, they may occasionally produce excitation.
CNS Depressants
Antihistamines may have additive effects with alcohol and other CNS depressants, e.g., hypnotics, sedatives, tranquilizers, antianxiety agents.
Activities Requiring Mental Alertness
Patients should be warned about engaging in activities requiring mental alertness and motor coordination, such as driving a car or operating machinery.
Antihistamines are more likely to cause dizziness, sedation, and hypotension in elderly patients.

Precautions

General
Cyproheptadine has an atropine-like action and, therefore, should be used with caution in patients with:
   History of bronchial asthma
   Increased intraocular pressure
   Hyperthyroidism
   Cardiovascular disease
   Hypertension
Information for Patients
Antihistamines may diminish mental alertness; conversely, particularly, in the young child, they may occasionally produce excitation.
Patients should be warned about engaging in activities requiring mental alertness and motor coordination, such as driving a car or operating machinery.
Drug Interactions
MAO Inhibitors prolong and intensify the anticholinergic effects of antihistamines.
Antihistamines may have additive effects with alcohol and other CNS depressants, e.g., hypnotics, sedatives, tranquilizers, antianxiety agents.
Carcinogenesis, Mutagenesis, Impairment of Fertility
Long-term carcinogenic studies have not been done with cyproheptadine.
Cyproheptadine had no effect on fertility in a two-litter study in rats or a two generation study in mice at about 10 times the human dose.
Cyproheptadine did not produce chromosome damage in human lymphocytes or fibroblasts *in vitro;* high doses (10^{-4} M) were cytotoxic. Cyproheptadine did not have any mutagenic effect in the Ames microbial mutagen test; concentrations of above 500 mcg/plate inhibited bacterial growth.
Pregnancy
Pregnancy Category B: Reproduction studies have been performed in rabbits, mice, and rats at doses up to 32 times the human dose and have revealed no evidence of impaired fertility or harm to the fetus due to cyproheptadine. There are, however, no adequate and well-controlled studies in pregnant women. Because animal reproduction studies are not always predictive of human response, this drug should be used during pregnancy only if clearly needed.
Nursing Mothers
It is not known whether this drug is excreted in human milk. Because many drugs are excreted in human milk, and because of the potential for serious adverse reactions in nursing infants from PERIACTIN, a decision should be made whether to discontinue nursing or to discontinue the drug,

taking into account the importance of the drug to the mother (see CONTRAINDICATIONS).
Pediatric Use
Safety and effectiveness in children below the age of two have not been established. See CONTRAINDICATIONS, *Newborn Premature Infants,* and WARNINGS, *Children.*

Adverse Reactions

Adverse reactions which have been reported with the use of antihistamines are as follows:
Central Nervous System: Sedation and sleepiness (often transient), dizziness, disturbed coordination, confusion, restlessness, excitation, nervousness, tremor, irritability, insomnia, paresthesias, neuritis, convulsions, euphoria, hallucinations, hysteria, faintness.
Integumentary: Allergic manifestation of rash and edema, excessive perspiration, urticaria, photosensitivity.
Special Senses: Acute labyrinthitis, blurred vision, diplopia, vertigo, tinnitus.
Cardiovascular: Hypotension, palpitation, tachycardia, extrasystoles, anaphylactic shock.
Hematologic: Hemolytic anemia, leukopenia, agranulocytosis, thrombocytopenia.
Digestive System: Dryness of mouth, epigastric distress, anorexia, nausea, vomiting, diarrhea, constipation.
Genitourinary: Urinary frequency, difficult urination, urinary retention, early menses.
Respiratory: Dryness of nose and throat, thickening of bronchial secretions, tightness of chest and wheezing, nasal stuffiness.
Miscellaneous: Fatigue, chills, headache.

Overdosage

Antihistamine overdosage reactions may vary from central nervous system depression to stimulation especially in children. Also, atropine-like signs and symptoms (dry mouth; fixed, dilated pupils; flushing, etc.) as well as gastrointestinal symptoms may occur.
If vomiting has not occurred spontaneously the patient should be induced to vomit. This is best done by having him drink a glass of water after which he should be made to gag. Precautions against aspiration must be taken especially in infants and children.
If patient is unable to vomit, gastric lavage is indicated. Isotonic or ½ isotonic saline is the lavage of choice.
Saline cathartics, as milk of magnesia, by osmosis draw water into the bowel and, therefore, are valuable for their action in rapid dilution of bowel content.
Stimulants should *not* be used.
Vasopressors may be used to treat hypotension.
The oral LD$_{50}$ of cyproheptadine is 123 mg/kg, and 295 mg/kg in the mouse and rat, respectively.

Dosage and Administration

DOSAGE SHOULD BE INDIVIDUALIZED ACCORDING TO THE NEEDS AND THE RESPONSE OF THE PATIENT.
Each PERIACTIN tablet contains 4 mg of cyproheptadine hydrochloride. Each 5 ml of PERIACTIN syrup contains 2 mg of cyproheptadine hydrochloride.
Although intended primarily for administration to children, the syrup is also useful for administration to adults who cannot swallow tablets.
Children
The total daily dosage for children may be calculated on the basis of body weight or body area using approximately 0.25 mg/kg/day (0.11 mg/lb/day) or 8 mg per square meter of body surface (8 mg/M^2). In small children for whom the calculation of dosage based upon body size is most important, it may be necessary to use PERIACTIN syrup to permit accurate dosage.
Age 2 to 6 years
The usual dose is 2 mg (½ tablet or 1 teaspoon) two or three times a day, adjusted as necessary to the size and response of the patient. The dose is not to exceed 12 mg a day.

Age 7 to 14 years
The usual dose is 4 mg (1 tablet or 2 teaspoons) two or three times a day, adjusted as necessary to the size and response of the patient. The dose is not to exceed 16 mg a day.
Adults
The total daily dose for adults should not exceed 0.5 mg/kg/day (0.23 mg/lb/day).
The therapeutic range is 4 to 20 mg a day, with the majority of patients requiring 12 to 16 mg a day. An occasional patient may require as much as 32 mg a day for adequate relief. It is suggested that dosage be initiated with 4 mg (1 tablet or 2 teaspoons) three times a day and adjusted according to the size and response of the patient.

How Supplied

No. 3276—Tablets PERIACTIN, containing 4 mg of cyproheptadine hydrochloride each, are white, round, scored compressed tablets, coded MSD 62. They are supplied as follows:
NDC 0006-0062-68 bottles of 100.
(6505-00-890-1884 4 mg 100's)
Shown in Product Identification Section, page 420
No. 3289X—Syrup PERIACTIN, 2 mg per 5 ml is a clear, yellow, syrupy liquid. Contains alcohol 5%, with sorbic acid 0.1% added as preservative and is supplied as follows:
NDC 0006-3289-74 bottles of 473 ml.
A.H.F.S. Category: 4:00
DC 6589614 Issued April 1983
COPYRIGHT © MERCK & CO., INC., 1983
All rights reserved

PNEUMOVAX® 23
(pneumococcal vaccine, polyvalent, MSD)

Description

PNEUMOVAX® 23 (Pneumococcal Vaccine, Polyvalent, MSD), is a sterile, liquid vaccine for intramuscular or subcutaneous injection. It consists of a mixture of highly purified capsular polysaccharides from the 23 most prevalent or invasive pneumococcal types accounting for at least 90% of pneumococcal blood isolates and at least 85% of all pneumococcal isolates from sites which are generally sterile as determined by ongoing surveillance of U.S. data.
PNEUMOVAX 23 is manufactured according to methods developed by the MERCK SHARP & DOHME Research Laboratories. Each 0.5 ml dose of vaccine contains 25 µg of each polysaccharide type dissolved in isotonic saline solution containing 0.25% phenol as preservative.
Type 6B pneumococcal polysaccharide exhibits somewhat greater stability in purified form than does Type 6A. A high degree of cross-reactivity between the two types has been demonstrated in adult volunteers. Therefore, Type 6B has replaced Type 6A, which had been used in the 14-valent vaccine. Although contained in the 14-valent vaccine, Type 25 is not included in PNEUMOVAX 23 because it has recently become a rare isolate in many parts of the world including the United States, Canada and Europe.
[See table above].

Clinical Pharmacology

Pneumococcal infection is a leading cause of death throughout the world and a major cause of pneumonia, meningitis, and otitis media. The emergence of strains of pneumococci with increased resistance to one or more of the common antibiotics and recent isolations of pneumococci with multiple antibiotic resistance emphasize the importance of vaccine prophylaxis against pneumococcal disease. Based on projection from limited observations in the United States, it has been esti-

23 Pneumococcal Capsular Types Included in PNEUMOVAX 23

Nomenclature	Pneumococcal Types
Danish	1 2 3 4 5 6B 7F 8 9N 9V 10A 11A 12F 14 15B 17F 18C 19F 19A 20 22F 23F 33F
U.S.	1 2 3 4 5 26 51 8 9 68 34 43 12 14 54 17 56 19 57 20 22 23 70

mated that 400,000 to 500,000 cases of pneumococcal pneumonia may occur annually. The overall case fatality rate ranges from 5–10%. Populations at high risk are the elderly; individuals with immune deficiencies; patients with asplenia or splenic deficiencies, including sickle cell anemia and other severe hemoglobinopathies; alcoholics; and patients with the following diseases: Hodgkin's disease, multiple myeloma and nephrotic syndrome. About 25% of all persons with pneumococcal pneumonia develop bacteremia. Death occurs in about 28% of these bacteremic patients over 50 years of age. Of all patients with pneumococcal bacteremia who died despite treatment with penicillin or tetracycline, as many as 60% died within five days of onset of the illness.
The annual incidence of pneumococcal meningitis is approximately 1.5 to 2.5 per 100,000 population. One-half of the cases occur in children, in whom the fatality rate is about 40%. Children with sickle cell disease have been estimated to have a risk of pneumococcal meningitis nearly 600 times greater than normal children. Within the first two years of life, about 15 to 20% of all children develop otitis media caused by pneumococci, and 50% of all children develop such illness within the first 10 years of life (see under INDICATIONS AND USAGE). Other illnesses caused by pneumococci include acute exacerbations of chronic bronchitis, sinusitis, arthritis and conjunctivitis.
Invasive pneumococcal disease causes high morbidity and mortality in spite of effective antimicrobial control by antibiotics. These effects of pneumococcal disease appear due to irreversible physiologic damage caused by the bacteria during the first 5 days following onset of illness, and occur irrespective of antimicrobial therapy. Vaccination offers an effective means of further reducing the mortality and morbidity of this disease.
Pneumococci can be isolated from 38–55% of all cases of acute otitis media and from two-thirds of those in which pathogenic bacteria are cultured from the middle-ear fluid (MEF). The demonstration of soluble pneumococcal antigens in many MEF samples that are negative by bacteriological culture methods points to an even greater role of pneumococci in otitis media.
At present, there are 83 known pneumococcal capsular types. However, the preponderance of pneumococcal diseases is caused by only some capsular types. For example, a 10-year (1952–1962) surveillance at a New York medical center, showed that 56% of all deaths due to pneumococcal pneumonia were caused by 6 capsular types and that approximately 78% of all pneumococcal pneumonias were caused by 12 capsular types. Such unequal distribution of pneumococcal capsular types causing disease has been shown throughout the world. It is on the basis of this information that the pneumococcal vaccine is composed of 23 capsular types, designed to provide coverage of approximately 90% of the most frequently reported types.
It has been established that the purified pneumococcal capsular polysaccharides induce antibody production and that such antibody is effective in preventing pneumococcal disease. Studies in humans have demonstrated the immunogenicity (antibody-stimulating capability) of each of the 23 capsular types when tested in polyvalent vaccines. Adults of all ages responded immunologically to the vaccines. Earlier studies with 12- and 14-valent pneumococcal vaccines in children two years

Continued on next page

Information on the Merck Sharp & Dohme products listed on these pages is the full prescribing information from product circulars in use November 1, 1984.

Merck Sharp & Dohme—Cont.

of age and older and in adults showed immunogenic responses. Protective capsular type-specific antibody levels develop by the third week following vaccination.

The protective efficacy of pneumococcal vaccines containing 6 and 12 capsular polysaccharides was investigated in controlled studies of gold miners in South Africa, in whom there is a high attack rate for pneumococcal pneumonia. Capsular type-specific attack rates for pneumococcal pneumonia were observed for the period from 2 weeks through about 1 year after vaccination. The rates for pneumonia caused by the same capsular types represented in the vaccines are given in the table. Protective efficacy was 76% and 92%, respectively, in the two studies for the capsular types represented. [See table below].

In similar studies carried out by Dr. R. Austrian and associates using similar pneumococcal vaccines prepared for the National Institute of Allergy and Infectious Diseases, the reduction in pneumonias caused by the capsular types contained in the vaccines was 79%. Reduction in type-specific pneumococcal bacteremia was 82%. A preliminary report suggests that in patients with sickle cell anemia and/or anatomical or functional asplenia, the vaccine was highly effective in persons over two years of age in preventing severe pneumococcal disease and bacteremia.

In a controlled study conducted in Finland among 455 children 2 to 6 years of age with one or more prior episodes of acute otitis media, PNEUMOVAX (Pneumococcal Vaccine, Polyvalent, MSD) (14-valent) was found to effect a significant reduction in the number of clinical cases of pneumococcal otitis media during a six-month postvaccination period of analysis. There was an overall 73% reduction in the frequency of cases caused by serotypes in the vaccine other than type 6. No protection was found for type 6.

Another trial conducted in Sweden among children attending day-care nurseries showed a 30% reduction in visits for acute otitis media of all causes in children over 2 years of age. This reduction was noted over a one-year follow-up and was seen both in children with a history of otitis prior to vaccination and in those children with no such history.

The duration of protective effect of PNEUMOVAX 23 is presently unknown, but it has been shown in previous studies with other pneumococcal vaccines that antibody induced by the vaccine may persist for as long as 5 years. Type-specific antibody levels induced by PNEUMOVAX (Pneumococcal Vaccine, Polyvalent, MSD) (14-valent) have been observed to decline over a 42-month period of observation, but remain significantly above pre-vaccination levels in almost all recipients who manifest an initial response.

Indications and Usage

PNEUMOVAX 23 is indicated for immunization against pneumococcal disease caused by those pneumococcal types included in the vaccine. Effectiveness of the vaccine in the prevention of pneumococcal pneumonia and pneumococcal bacteremia has been demonstrated in controlled trials. PNEUMOVAX 23 *will not immunize against capsular types of pneumococcus other than those contained in the vaccine.*

PNEUMOVAX 23

Number of Capsular Types in Pneumococcal Vaccine	Rate/1000 for Pneumonia Caused by Homologous Capsular Types		Protective Efficacy
	Vaccinated Group	Control Group	
6	9.2	38.3	76%
12	1.8	22.0	92%

Use in selected individuals over 2 years of age as follows: (1) patients who have anatomical asplenia or who have splenic dysfunction due to sickle cell disease or other causes; (2) persons with chronic illnesses in which there is an increased risk of pneumococcal disease, such as functional impairment of cardiorespiratory, hepatic and renal systems; (3) persons 50 years of age or older; (4) patients with other chronic illnesses who may be at greater risk of developing pneumococcal infection or experiencing more severe pneumococcal illness as a result of alcohol abuse or coexisting diseases including diabetes mellitus, chronic cerebrospinal fluid leakage, or conditions associated with immunosuppression; (5) patients with Hodgkin's disease if immunization can be given at least 10 days prior to treatment. For maximal antibody response immunization should be given at least 14 days prior to the start of treatment with radiation or chemotherapy. Immunization of patients less than 10 days prior to or during treatment is not recommended. (see CONTRAINDICATIONS.)

Use in communities. Persons over 2 years of age as follows: (1) closed groups such as those in residential schools, nursing homes and other institutions. (To decrease the likelihood of acute outbreaks of pneumococcal disease in closed institutional populations where there is increased risk that the disease may be severe, vaccination of the entire closed population should be considered where there are no other contraindications.); (2) groups epidemiologically at risk in the community when there is a generalized outbreak in the population due to a single pneumococcal type included in the vaccine; (3) patients at high risk of influenza complications, particularly pneumonia.

Use in preventing pneumococcal otitis media. Children 2 years of age or older who, in the judgment of the physician, are at risk for developing middle ear infections. See CLINICAL PHARMACOLOGY for results of clinical studies.

PNEUMOVAX 23 may not be effective in preventing infection resulting from basilar skull fracture or from external communication with cerebrospinal fluid.

Simultaneous administration of pneumococcal polysaccharide vaccine and whole-virus influenza vaccine gives satisfactory antibody response without increasing the occurrence of adverse reactions. Simultaneous administration of the pneumococcal vaccine and split-virus influenza vaccine may also be expected to yield satisfactory results.

Revaccination
Revaccination of adults is not recommended. Adults previously immunized with any polyvalent pneumococcal vaccine should not receive PNEUMOVAX 23 or PNEUMOVAX (Pneumococcal Vaccine, Polyvalent, MSD) (14-valent) since an increased incidence and severity of adverse reactions among healthy adults receiving such reinjections have been noted, most likely due to sustained high antibody levels.

Certain groups of children at very high risk for pneumococcal disease (e.g., children with sickle cell disease or nephrotic syndrome) may have lower peak levels of antibody response and/or more rapid rates of decline in antibody levels than do healthy adults. However, insufficient data are available at this time to permit formulation of guidelines for reimmunization of high-risk children.

Contraindications

Hypersensitivity to any component of the vaccine. Epinephrine injection (1:1000) must be immediately available should an acute anaphylactoid reaction occur due to any component of the vaccine.

Revaccination of adults is contraindicated. Adults previously immunized with any polyvalent pneumococcal vaccine should not receive PNEUMOVAX 23 or PNEUMOVAX (Pneumococcal Vaccine, Polyvalent, MSD) (14-valent) since an increased incidence and severity of adverse reactions among healthy adults receiving such reinjections have been noted, most likely due to sustained high antibody levels.

Patients with Hodgkin's disease immunized less than 7 to 10 days prior to immunosuppressive therapy have in some instances been found to have post-immunization antibody levels below their pre-immunization levels. Because of these results, immunization less than 10 days prior to or during treatment is contraindicated.

Patients with Hodgkin's disease who have received extensive chemotherapy and/or nodal irradiation have been shown to have an impaired antibody response to a 12-valent pneumococcal vaccine. Because, in some intensively treated patients, administration of that vaccine depressed pre-existing levels of antibody to some pneumococcal types, PNEUMOVAX 23 is not recommended at this time for patients who have received these forms of therapy for Hodgkin's disease.

Warnings

If the vaccine is used in persons receiving immunosuppressive therapy, the expected serum antibody response may not be obtained.

Intradermal administration may cause severe local reactions.

Precautions

General
Caution and appropriate care should be exercised in administering PNEUMOVAX 23 to individuals with severely compromised cardiac and/or pulmonary function in whom a systemic reaction would pose a significant risk.

Any febrile respiratory illness or other active infection is reason for delaying use of PNEUMOVAX 23, except when, in the opinion of the physician, withholding the agent entails even greater risk.

In patients who require penicillin (or other antibiotic) prophylaxis against pneumococcal infection, such prophylaxis should not be discontinued after vaccination with PNEUMOVAX 23.

Pregnancy
Pregnancy Category C: Animal reproduction studies have not been conducted with PNEUMOVAX 23. It is also not known whether PNEUMOVAX 23 can cause fetal harm when administered to a pregnant woman or can affect reproduction capacity. PNEUMOVAX 23 should be given to a pregnant woman only if clearly needed.

Nursing Mothers
It is not known whether this drug is excreted in human milk. Because many drugs are excreted in human milk, caution should be exercised when PNEUMOVAX 23 is administered to a nursing woman.

Pediatric Use
Children less than 2 years of age do not respond satisfactorily to the capsular types of PNEUMOVAX 23 that are most often the cause of pneumococcal disease in this age group. Safety and effectiveness in children below the age of 2 years have not been established. Accordingly, PNEUMOVAX 23 is not recommended in this age group.

Adverse Reactions

Local erythema and soreness at the injection site, usually of less than 48 hours duration, occurs commonly; local induration occurs less commonly. In a study of PNEUMOVAX 22 (containing 22 capsular types) in 29 adults, 21 (71%) showed local reaction characterized principally by local soreness

and/or induration at the injection site within 2 days after vaccination.
Rash and arthralgia have been reported rarely. Low grade fever (less than 100.9°F) occurs occasionally and is usually confined to the 24-hour period following vaccination. Although rare, fever over 102°F has been reported.
Patients with otherwise stabilized idiopathic thrombocytopenic purpura have, on rare occasions, experienced a relapse in their thrombocytopenia, occurring 2 to 14 days after vaccination, and lasting up to 2 weeks.
Reactions of greater severity, duration, or extent are unusual. Neurological disorders such as paresthesias and acute radiculoneuropathy including Guillain-Barré syndrome have been rarely reported in temporal association with administration of pneumococcal vaccine. No cause and effect relationship has been established. Rarely, anaphylactoid reactions have been reported.

Dosage and Administration

Do not inject intravenously. Intradermal administration should be avoided.
Parenteral drug products should be inspected visually for particulate matter and discoloration prior to administration, whenever solution and container permit. PNEUMOVAX 23 is a clear, colorless solution.
Administer a single 0.5 ml dose of PNEUMOVAX 23 subcutaneously or intramuscularly (preferably in the deltoid muscle or lateral mid-thigh), with appropriate precautions to avoid intravascular administration.

Single-Dose and 5-Dose Vials
For Syringe Use Only: Withdraw 0.5 ml from the vial using a sterile needle and syringe free of preservatives, antiseptics and detergents.
It is important to use a separate sterile syringe and needle for each individual patient to prevent transmission of hepatitis B and other infectious agents from one person to another.
Store unopened and opened vials at 2–8°C (35.6–46.4°F). The vaccine is used directly as supplied. No dilution or reconstitution is necessary. Phenol 0.25% added as preservative. All vaccine must be discarded after the expiration date.

How Supplied

No. 4739—PNEUMOVAX 23 contains one 5-dose vial of liquid vaccine, **NDC** 0006-4739-00. For use with syringe only.
No. 4741—PNEUMOVAX 23 is supplied as follows: **NDC** 0006-4741-00. A box of 5 individual cartons, each containing a single-dose vial of vaccine.
A.H.F.S. Category: 80:12
DC 7267001 Issued May 1983
COPYRIGHT © MERCK & CO., INC., 1983
All rights reserved

SINEMET® Tablets ℞
(carbidopa-levodopa, MSD), U.S.P.

Description

When SINEMET® (Carbidopa-Levodopa, MSD) is to be given to patients who are being treated with levodopa, levodopa must be discontinued at least eight hours before therapy with SINEMET is started. In order to reduce adverse reactions, it is necessary to individualize therapy. See the WARNINGS and DOSAGE AND ADMINISTRATION sections before initiating therapy.
Carbidopa, an inhibitor of aromatic amino acid decarboxylation, is a white, crystalline compound, slightly soluble in water, with a molecular weight of 244.3. It is designated chemically as (—)-L-α-hydrazino-α-methyl-β-(3,4-dihydroxybenzene) propanoic acid monohydrate.
Tablet content is expressed in terms of anhydrous carbidopa which has a molecular weight of 226.3.
Levodopa, an aromatic amino acid, is a white, crystalline compound, slightly soluble in water, with a molecular weight of 197.2. It is designated chemically as (—)-L-α-amino-β-(3,4-dihydroxybenzene) propanoic acid.

SINEMET is supplied as tablets in three strengths:
SINEMET 10/100, containing 10 mg of carbidopa and 100 mg of levodopa
SINEMET 25/100, containing 25 mg of carbidopa and 100 mg of levodopa
SINEMET 25/250, containing 25 mg of carbidopa and 250 mg of levodopa

Actions

Current evidence indicates that symptoms of Parkinson's disease are related to depletion of dopamine in the corpus striatum. Administration of dopamine is ineffective in the treatment of Parkinson's disease apparently because it does not cross the blood-brain barrier. However, levodopa, the metabolic precursor of dopamine, does cross the blood-brain barrier, and presumably is converted to dopamine in the basal ganglia. This is thought to be the mechanism whereby levodopa relieves symptoms of Parkinson's disease.
When levodopa is administered orally it is rapidly converted to dopamine in extracerebral tissues so that only a small portion of a given dose is transported unchanged to the central nervous system. For this reason, large doses of levodopa are required for adequate therapeutic effect and these may often be attended by nausea and other adverse reactions, some of which are attributable to dopamine formed in extracerebral tissues.
Carbidopa inhibits decarboxylation of peripheral levodopa. It does not cross the blood-brain barrier and does not affect the metabolism of levodopa within the central nervous system.
Since its decarboxylase inhibiting activity is limited to extracerebral tissues, administration of carbidopa with levodopa makes more levodopa available for transport to the brain. In dogs, reduced formation of dopamine in extracerebral tissues, such as the heart, provides protection against the development of dopamine-induced cardiac arrhythmias. Clinical studies tend to support the hypothesis of a similar protective effect in humans although controlled data are too limited at the present time to draw firm conclusions.
Carbidopa reduces the amount of levodopa required by about 75 percent and, when administered with levodopa, increases both plasma levels and the plasma half-life of levodopa, and decreases plasma and urinary dopamine and homovanillic acid.
In clinical pharmacologic studies, simultaneous administration of carbidopa and levodopa produced greater urinary excretion of levodopa in proportion to the excretion of dopamine than administration of the two drugs at separate times.
Pyridoxine hydrochloride (vitamin B_6), in oral doses of 10 mg to 25 mg, may reverse the effects of levodopa by increasing the rate of aromatic amino acid decarboxylation. Carbidopa inhibits this action of pyridoxine.

Indications

SINEMET is indicated in the treatment of the symptoms of idiopathic Parkinson's disease (paralysis agitans), postencephalitic parkinsonism, and symptomatic parkinsonism which may follow injury to the nervous system by carbon monoxide intoxication and manganese intoxication. SINEMET is indicated in these conditions to permit the administration of lower doses of levodopa with reduced nausea and vomiting, with more rapid dosage titration, with a somewhat smoother response, and with supplemental pyridoxine (vitamin B_6).
The incidence of levodopa-induced nausea and vomiting is less with SINEMET than with levodopa. In many patients this reduction in nausea and vomiting will permit more rapid dosage titration.
In some patients a somewhat smoother antiparkinsonian effect results from therapy with SINEMET than with levodopa. However, patients with markedly irregular ("on-off") responses to levodopa have not been shown to benefit from SINEMET.

Since carbidopa prevents the reversal of levodopa effects caused by pyridoxine, SINEMET can be given to patients receiving supplemental pyridoxine (vitamin B_6).
Although the administration of carbidopa permits control of parkinsonism and Parkinson's disease with much lower doses of levodopa, there is no conclusive evidence at present that this is beneficial other than in reducing nausea and vomiting, permitting more rapid titration, and providing a somewhat smoother response to levodopa. *Carbidopa does not decrease adverse reactions due to central effects of levodopa. By permitting more levodopa to reach the brain, particularly when nausea and vomiting is not a dose-limiting factor, certain adverse CNS effects, e.g., dyskinesias, may occur at lower dosages and sooner during therapy with SINEMET than with levodopa.*
Certain patients who responded poorly to levodopa have improved when SINEMET was substituted. This is most likely due to decreased peripheral decarboxylation of levodopa which results from administration of carbidopa rather than to a primary effect of carbidopa on the nervous system. Carbidopa has not been shown to enhance the intrinsic efficacy of levodopa in parkinsonian syndromes.
In considering whether to give SINEMET to patients already on levodopa who have nausea and/or vomiting, the practitioner should be aware that, while many patients may be expected to improve, some do not. Since one cannot predict which patients are likely to improve, this can only be determined by a trial of therapy. It should be further noted that in controlled trials comparing SINEMET with levodopa, about half of the patients with nausea and/or vomiting on levodopa improved spontaneously despite being retained on the same dose of levodopa during the controlled portion of the trial.

Contraindications

Monoamine oxidase inhibitors and SINEMET should not be given concomitantly. These inhibitors must be discontinued at least two weeks prior to initiating therapy with SINEMET.
SINEMET is contraindicated in patients with known hypersensitivity to this drug, and in narrow angle glaucoma.
Because levodopa may activate a malignant melanoma, it should not be used in patients with suspicious, undiagnosed skin lesions or a history of melanoma.

Warnings

When patients are receiving levodopa, it must be discontinued at least eight hours before SINEMET is started. SINEMET should be substituted at a dosage that will provide approximately 25 percent of the previous levodopa dosage (see DOSAGE AND ADMINISTRATION). Patients who are taking SINEMET should be instructed not to take additional levodopa unless it is prescribed by the physician.
As with levodopa, SINEMET may cause involuntary movements and mental disturbances. These reactions are thought to be due to increased brain dopamine following administration of levodopa. All patients should be observed carefully for the development of depression with concomitant suicidal tendencies. Patients with past or current psychoses should be treated with caution. *Because carbidopa permits more levodopa to reach the brain and, thus, more dopamine to be formed, dyskinesias may occur at lower dosages and sooner with SINEMET than with levodopa.* The occurrence of dyskinesias may require dosage reduction.

Continued on next page

Information on the Merck Sharp & Dohme products listed on these pages is the full prescribing information from product circulars in use November 1, 1984.

Merck Sharp & Dohme—Cont.

SINEMET should be administered cautiously to patients with severe cardiovascular or pulmonary disease, bronchial asthma, renal, hepatic or endocrine disease.
Care should be exercised in administering SINEMET, as with levodopa, to patients with a history of myocardial infarction who have residual atrial, nodal, or ventricular arrhythmias. In such patients, cardiac function should be monitored with particular care during the period of initial dosage adjustment, in a facility with provisions for intensive cardiac care.
As with levodopa there is a possibility of upper gastrointestinal hemorrhage in patients with a history of peptic ulcer.
Usage in Pregnancy and Lactation: Although the effects of SINEMET on human pregnancy and lactation are unknown, both levodopa and combinations of carbidopa and levodopa have caused visceral and skeletal malformations in rabbits. Use of SINEMET in women of childbearing potential requires that the anticipated benefits of the drug be weighed against possible hazards to mother and child. SINEMET should not be given to nursing mothers.
Usage in Children: The safety of SINEMET in patients under 18 years of age has not been established.

Precautions

As with levodopa, periodic evaluations of hepatic, hematopoietic, cardiovascular, and renal function are recommended during extended therapy.
Patients with chronic wide angle glaucoma may be treated cautiously with SINEMET provided the intraocular pressure is well controlled and the patient is monitored carefully for changes in intraocular pressure during therapy.
Laboratory Tests
Abnormalities in laboratory tests may include elevations of blood urea nitrogen, SGOT, SGPT, lactic dehydrogenase, bilirubin, alkaline phosphatase, protein-bound iodine and positive Coombs test. More commonly, levels of blood urea nitrogen, creatinine, and uric acid are lower during administration of SINEMET than with levodopa.
SINEMET may cause a false-positive reaction for urinary ketone bodies when a test tape is used for determination of ketonuria. This reaction will not be altered by boiling the urine specimen. False-negative tests may result with the use of glucose-oxidase methods of testing for glucosuria.
Drug Interactions
Caution should be exercised when the following drugs are administered concomitantly with SINEMET:
Symptomatic postural hypotension can occur when SINEMET is added to the treatment of a patient receiving antihypertensive drugs. Therefore, when therapy with SINEMET is started, dosage adjustment of the antihypertensive drug may be required. For patients receiving monoamine oxidase inhibitors, see CONTRAINDICATIONS.
There have been rare reports of adverse reactions, including hypertension and dyskinesia, resulting from the concomitant use of tricyclic antidepressants and SINEMET.
Phenothiazines and butyrophenones may reduce the therapeutic effects of levodopa. In addition, the beneficial effects of levodopa in Parkinson's disease have been reported to be reversed by phenytoin and papaverine. Patients taking these drugs with SINEMET should be carefully observed for loss of therapeutic response.

Adverse Reactions

The most common serious adverse reactions occurring with SINEMET are choreiform, dystonic, and other involuntary movements. Other serious adverse reactions are mental changes including paranoid ideation and psychotic episodes, depression with or without development of suicidal tendencies, and dementia. Convulsions also have occurred; however, a causal relationship with SINEMET has not been established.
A common but less serious effect is nausea.
Less frequent adverse reactions are cardiac irregularities and/or palpitations, orthostatic hypotensive episodes, bradykinetic episodes (the "on-off" phenomenon), anorexia, vomiting, and dizziness. Rarely, gastrointestinal bleeding, development of duodenal ulcer, hypertension, phlebitis, hemolytic anemia, leukopenia, and agranulocytosis have occurred.
Other adverse reactions that have been reported with levodopa include dry mouth, dysphagia, sialorrhea, abdominal pain and distress, ataxia, increased hand tremor, headache, numbness, weakness and faintness, bruxism, confusion, insomnia and nightmares, hallucinations and delusions, agitation and anxiety, malaise, fatigue, euphoria, muscle twitching, and blepharospasm (which may be taken as an early sign of excess dosage; consideration of dosage reduction may be made at this time), trismus, burning sensation of tongue, bitter taste, diarrhea, constipation, flatulence, flushing, skin rash, increased sweating, bizarre breathing patterns, urinary retention, urinary incontinence, diplopia, blurred vision, dilated pupils, hot flashes, weight gain or loss, dark sweat and/or urine, oculogyric crises, sense of stimulation, hiccups, edema, loss of hair, hoarseness, priapism, and activation of latent Horner's syndrome.

Dosage and Administration

The optimum daily dosage of SINEMET must be determined by careful titration in each patient. SINEMET tablets are available in a 1:4 ratio of carbidopa to levodopa (SINEMET 25/100) as well as a 1:10 ratio (SINEMET 25/250 and SINEMET 10/100). Tablets of the two ratios may be given separately or combined as needed to provide the optimum dosage.
Studies show that peripheral dopa decarboxylase is saturated by carbidopa at approximately 70 to 100 mg a day. Patients receiving less than this amount of carbidopa are more likely to experience nausea and vomiting.
Usual Initial Dosage
Dosage is best initiated with one tablet of SINEMET 25/100 three times a day. This dosage schedule provides 75 mg of carbidopa per day. Dosage may be increased by one tablet every day or every other day, as necessary, until a dosage of six tablets of SINEMET 25/100 a day is reached. If SINEMET 10/100 is used, dosage may be initiated with one tablet three or four times a day and increased by one tablet every day or every other day until a total of eight tablets (2 tablets q.i.d.) is reached.
How to Transfer Patients from Levodopa
Levodopa must be discontinued at least eight hours before starting SINEMET (Carbidopa-Levodopa, MSD). A daily dosage of SINEMET should be chosen that will provide approximately 25 percent of the previous levodopa dosage. Patients who are taking less than 1500 mg of levodopa a day should be started on one tablet of SINEMET 25/100 three or four times a day. The suggested starting dosage for most patients taking more than 1500 mg of levodopa is one tablet of SINEMET 25/250 three or four times a day.
Maintenance
Therapy should be individualized and adjusted according to the desired therapeutic response. When a greater proportion of carbidopa is required, one tablet of SINEMET 25/100 may be substituted for each tablet of SINEMET 10/100. When more levodopa is required, SINEMET 25/250 should be substituted at a dosage of one tablet three or four times a day. If necessary, the dosage may be increased by one-half or one tablet every day or every other day to a maximum of eight tablets a day. Experience with total daily dosages of carbidopa greater than 200 mg is limited.
Because both therapeutic and adverse responses occur more rapidly with SINEMET than with levodopa alone, patients should be monitored closely during the dose adjustment period. Specifically, involuntary movements will occur more rapidly with SINEMET than with levodopa. The occurrence of involuntary movements may require dosage reduction. Blepharospasm may be a useful early sign of excess dosage in some patients.
Current evidence indicates that other standard drugs for Parkinson's disease (except levodopa) may be continued while SINEMET is being administered, although their dosage may have to be adjusted.
If general anesthesia is required, SINEMET may be continued as long as the patient is permitted to take fluids and medication by mouth. If therapy is interrupted temporarily, the usual daily dosage may be administered as soon as the patient is able to take oral medication.

Overdosage

Management of acute overdosage with SINEMET is basically the same as management of acute overdosage with levodopa; however, pyridoxine is not effective in reversing the actions of SINEMET. General supportive measures should be employed, along with immediate gastric lavage. Intravenous fluids should be administered judiciously and an adequate airway maintained. Electrocardiographic monitoring should be instituted and the patient carefully observed for the development of arrhythmias; if required, appropriate antiarrhythmic therapy should be given. The possibility that the patient may have taken other drugs as well as SINEMET should be taken into consideration. To date, no experience has been reported with dialysis; hence, its value in overdosage is not known.

How Supplied

No. 3346—Tablets SINEMET 10/100 are dark dapple-blue, oval, scored, uncoated tablets, coded MSD 647. They are supplied as follows:
NDC 0006-0647-68 bottles of 100
(6505-01-020-8280 100's)
NDC 0006-0647-28 single unit packages of 100
NDC 0006-0647-78 unit of use bottles of 100.
Shown in Product Identification Section, page 420
No. 3365—Tablets SINEMET 25/100 are yellow, oval, scored tablets, coded MSD 650. They are supplied as follows:
NDC 0006-0650-68 bottles of 100
NDC 0006-0650-28 single unit packages of 100
NDC 0006-0650-78 unit of use bottles of 100.
Shown in Product Identification Section, page 420
No. 3347—Tablets SINEMET 25/250 are light dapple-blue, oval, scored, uncoated tablets, coded MSD 654. They are supplied as follows:
NDC 0006-0654-68 bottles of 100
(6505-01-020-8279 100's)
NDC 0006-0654-28 single unit packages of 100
NDC 0006-0654-78 unit of use bottles of 100.
Shown in Product Identification Section, page 420
A.H.F.S. Category: 92:00
DC6834812 Issued April 1983
COPYRIGHT © MERCK & CO., INC., 1983
All rights reserved

TIMOLIDE® Tablets R
(timolol maleate-hydrochlorothiazide, MSD)

Description

TIMOLIDE® (Timolol Maleate-Hydrochlorothiazide, MSD) is for the treatment of hypertension. It combines the antihypertensive activity of two agents: a non-selective beta-adrenergic receptor blocking agent (timolol maleate) and a diuretic (hydrochlorothiazide). Each tablet of TIMOLIDE contains 10 mg of timolol maleate and 25 mg of hydrochlorothiazide.
Timolol maleate is (S)-1-[(1, 1-dimethylethyl) amino]-3-[[4-(4-morpholinyl)-1, 2, 5-thiadiazol-3-yl] oxy]-2-propanol, (Z)-butenedioate (1:1) salt. Its empirical formula is $C_{13}H_{24}N_4O_3S \cdot C_4H_4O_4$.
Hydrochlorothiazide is 6-chloro-3,4-dihydro-2H-1,2,4-benzothiadiazine-7-sulfonamide 1, 1- dioxide. Its empirical formula is $C_7H_8ClN_3O_4S_2$.
TIMOLIDE is supplied as tablets containing 10 mg of timolol maleate and 25 mg of hydrochlorothiazide for oral administration.

Clinical Pharmacology

TIMOLIDE

Timolol maleate and hydrochlorothiazide have been used singly and concomitantly for the treatment of hypertension. The antihypertensive effects of these agents are additive. The two components of TIMOLIDE have similar dosage schedules, and studies have shown that there is no interference with bioavailability when these agents are given together in the single combination tablet. Therefore, this combination provides a convenient formulation for the concomitant administration of these two entities.

In controlled clinical trials with TIMOLIDE in selected patients with mild to moderate essential hypertension, about 90 percent had a good to excellent response. In patients with more severe hypertension, TIMOLIDE may be administered with other antihypertensives such as ALDOMET® (Methyldopa, MSD) or a vasodilator.

Although the mechanisms of action of timolol maleate and hydrochlorothiazide in the treatment of hypertension have not been established, they are thought to be different; for example, hydrochlorothiazide increases plasma renin activity while timolol maleate reduces plasma renin activity.

Timolol Maleate

Timolol maleate is a beta$_1$ and beta$_2$ (non-selective) adrenergic receptor blocking agent that does not have significant intrinsic sympathomimetic, direct myocardial depressant, or local anesthetic activity.

Pharmacodynamics

Clinical pharmacology studies have confirmed the beta-adrenergic blocking activity as shown by (1) changes in resting heart rate and response of heart rate to changes in posture; (2) inhibition of isoproterenol-induced tachycardia; (3) alteration of the response to the Valsalva maneuver and amyl nitrite administration; and (4) reduction of heart rate and blood pressure changes on exercise.

Timolol maleate decreases the positive chronotropic, positive inotropic, bronchodilator, and vasodilator responses caused by beta-adrenergic receptor agonists. The magnitude of this decreased response is proportional to the existing sympathetic tone and the concentration of timolol maleate at receptor sites.

In normal volunteers, the reduction in heart rate response to a standard exercise was dose dependent over the test range of 0.5 to 20 mg, with a peak reduction at 2 hours of approximately 30% at higher doses.

Beta-adrenergic receptor blockade reduces cardiac output in both healthy subjects and patients with heart disease. In patients with severe impairment of myocardial function beta-adrenergic receptor blockade may inhibit the stimulatory effect of the sympathetic nervous system necessary to maintain adequate cardiac function.

Beta-adrenergic receptor blockade in the bronchi and bronchioles results in increased airway resistance from unopposed parasympathetic activity. Such an effect in patients with asthma or other bronchospastic conditions is potentially dangerous.

Clinical studies indicate that timolol maleate at a dosage of 20-60 mg/day reduces blood pressure without causing postural hypotension in most patients with essential hypertension. Administration of timolol maleate to patients with hypertension results initially in a decrease in cardiac output, little immediate change in blood pressure, and an increase in calculated peripheral resistance. With continued administration of timolol maleate blood pressure decreases within a few days, cardiac output usually remains reduced, and peripheral resistance falls toward pretreatment levels. Plasma volume may decrease or remain unchanged during therapy with timolol maleate. In the majority of patients with hypertension timolol maleate also decreases plasma renin activity. Dosage adjustment to achieve optimal antihypertensive effect may require a few weeks. When therapy with timolol maleate is discontinued, the blood pressure tends to return to pretreatment levels gradually. In most patients the antihypertensive activity of timolol maleate is maintained with long-term therapy and is well tolerated.

The mechanism of the antihypertensive effects of beta-adrenergic receptor blocking agents is not established at this time. Possible mechanisms of action include reduction in cardiac output, reduction in plasma renin activity, and a central nervous system sympatholytic action.

Pharmacokinetics and Metabolism

Timolol maleate is rapidly and nearly completely absorbed (about 90%) following oral ingestion. Detectable plasma levels of timolol occur within one-half hour and peak plasma levels occur in about one to two hours. The drug half-life in plasma is approximately 4 hours and this is essentially unchanged in patients with moderate renal insufficiency. Timolol is partially metabolized by the liver and timolol and its metabolites are excreted by the kidney. Timolol is not extensively bound to plasma proteins; i.e., <10% by equilibrium dialysis and approximately 60% by ultrafiltration. An *in vitro* hemodialysis study, using ^{14}C timolol added to human plasma or whole blood, showed that timolol was readily dialyzed from these fluids; however, a study of patients with renal failure showed that timolol did not dialyze readily. Plasma levels following oral administration are about half those following intravenous administration indicating approximately 50% first pass metabolism. The level of beta sympathetic activity varies widely among individuals, and no simple correlation exists between the dose or plasma level of timolol maleate and its therapeutic activity. Therefore, objective clinical measurements such as reduction of heart rate and/or blood pressure should be used as guides in determining the optimal dosage for each patient.

Hydrochlorothiazide

Hydrochlorothiazide is a diuretic and antihypertensive agent. It affects the renal tubular mechanism of electrolyte reabsorption. Hydrochlorothiazide increases excretion of sodium and chloride in approximately equivalent amounts. Natriuresis may be accompanied by some loss of potassium and bicarbonate. The mechanism of the antihypertensive effect of thiazides may be related to the excretion and redistribution of body sodium. Hydrochlorothiazide usually does not cause clinically important changes in normal blood pressure.

Indications and Usage

TIMOLIDE is indicated for the treatment of hypertension.

This fixed combination drug is not indicated for initial therapy of hypertension. If the fixed combination represents the dose titrated to an individual patient's needs, it may be more convenient than the separate components.

Contraindications

TIMOLIDE is contraindicated in patients with bronchial asthma or with a history of bronchial asthma, or severe chronic obstructive pulmonary disease (see WARNINGS); sinus bradycardia; second and third degree atrioventricular block; overt cardiac failure (see WARNINGS); cardiogenic shock; anuria; hypersensitivity to this product or to sulfonamide-derived drugs.

Warnings

Cardiac Failure

Sympathetic stimulation may be essential for support of the circulation in individuals with diminished myocardial contractility, and its inhibition by beta-adrenergic receptor blockade may precipitate more severe failure. Although beta-blockers should be avoided in overt congestive heart failure, they can be used, if necessary, with caution in patients with a history of failure who are well-compensated, usually with digitalis and diuretics. Both digitalis and timolol maleate slow AV conduction. If cardiac failure persists, therapy with TIMOLIDE should be withdrawn.

In Patients Without a History of Cardiac Failure continued depression of the myocardium with beta-blocking agents over a period of time can, in some cases, lead to cardiac failure. At the first sign or symptom of cardiac failure, patients receiving TIMOLIDE should be digitalized and/or be given additional diuretic therapy. Observe the patient closely. If cardiac failure continues, despite adequate digitalization and diuretic therapy, TIMOLIDE should be withdrawn.

Renal and Hepatic Disease and Electrolyte Disturbances

Since timolol maleate is partially metabolized in the liver and excreted mainly by the kidneys, dosage reductions may be necessary when hepatic and/or renal insufficiency is present.

Although the pharmacokinetics of timolol maleate are not greatly altered by renal impairment, marked hypotensive responses have been seen in patients with marked renal impairment undergoing dialysis after 20 mg doses. Dosing in such patients should therefore be especially cautious.

In patients with renal disease, thiazides may precipitate azotemia, and cumulative effects may develop in the presence of impaired renal function. If progressive renal impairment becomes evident, TIMOLIDE should be discontinued.

In patients with impaired hepatic function or progressive liver disease, even minor alterations in fluid and electrolyte balance may precipitate hepatic coma. Hepatic encephalopathy, manifested by tremors, confusion, and coma, has been reported in association with diuretic therapy including hydrochlorothiazide.

Exacerbation of Ischemic Heart Disease Following Abrupt Withdrawal—Hypersensitivity to catecholamines has been observed in patients withdrawn from beta blocker therapy; exacerbation of angina and, in some cases, myocardial infarction have occurred after *abrupt* discontinuation of such therapy. When discontinuing chronically administered timolol maleate, particularly in patients with ischemic heart disease, the dosage should be gradually reduced over a period of one to two weeks and the patient should be carefully monitored. If angina markedly worsens or acute coronary insufficiency develops, timolol maleate administration should be reinstituted promptly, at least temporarily, and other measures appropriate for the management of unstable angina should be taken. Patients should be warned against interruption or discontinuation of therapy without the physician's advice. Because coronary artery disease is common and may be unrecognized, it may be prudent not to discontinue timolol maleate therapy abruptly even in patients treated only for hypertension.

Non-Allergic Bronchospasm

In patients with non-allergic bronchospasm or with a history of non-allergic bronchospasm (e.g., chronic bronchitis, emphysema), TIMOLIDE should be administered with caution since it may block bronchodilation produced by endogenous and exogenous catecholamine stimulation of beta$_2$ receptors.

Major Surgery

The necessity or desirability of withdrawal of beta-blocking therapy prior to major surgery is controversial. Beta-adrenergic receptor blockade impairs the ability of the heart to respond to beta-adrenergically mediated reflex stimuli. This may augment the risk of general anesthesia in surgical procedures. Some patients receiving beta-adrenergic receptor blocking agents have been subject to protracted severe hypotension during anesthesia. Difficulty in restarting and maintaining the heartbeat has also been reported. For these reasons, in patients undergoing elective surgery, some au-

Continued on next page

Information on the Merck Sharp & Dohme products listed on these pages is the full prescribing information from product circulars in use November 1, 1984.

Merck Sharp & Dohme—Cont.

thorities recommend gradual withdrawal of beta-adrenergic receptor blocking agents.

If necessary during surgery, the effects of beta-adrenergic blocking agents may be reversed by sufficient doses of such agonists as isoproterenol, dopamine, dobutamine or levarterenol (see OVERDOSAGE).

Metabolic and Endocrine Effects

Beta-adrenergic blockade may mask certain clinical signs (e.g., tachycardia) of hyperthyroidism. Patients suspected of developing thyrotoxicosis should be managed carefully to avoid abrupt withdrawal of beta blockade which might precipitate a thyroid storm. Thiazides may decrease serum PBI levels without signs of thyroid disturbance.

Beta-adrenergic receptor blocking agents may mask the signs and symptoms of acute hypoglycemia. Therefore, TIMOLIDE should be administered with caution to patients subject to spontaneous hypoglycemia, or to diabetic patients (especially those with labile diabetes) who are receiving insulin or oral hypoglycemic agents. Insulin requirements in diabetic patients may be increased, decreased, or unchanged by thiazides. Diabetes mellitus which has been latent may become manifest during administration of thiazide diuretics.

Because calcium excretion is decreased by thiazides, TIMOLIDE should be discontinued before carrying out tests for parathyroid function. Pathologic changes in the parathyroid glands, with hypercalcemia and hypophosphatemia, have been observed in a few patients on prolonged thiazide therapy; however, the common complications of hyperparathyroidism such as renal lithiasis, bone resorption, and peptic ulceration have not been seen.

Hyperuricemia may occur or acute gout may be precipitated in certain patients receiving thiazide therapy.

Precautions

General

Electrolyte and Fluid Balance Status: Periodic determination of serum electrolytes to detect possible electrolyte imbalance should be performed at appropriate intervals.

Patients should be observed for clinical signs of fluid or electrolyte imbalance, i.e., hyponatremia, hypochloremic alkalosis, and hypokalemia. Serum and urine electrolyte determinations are particularly important when the patient is vomiting excessively or receiving parenteral fluids. Warning signs or symptoms of fluid and electrolyte imbalance include dryness of the mouth, thirst, weakness, lethargy, drowsiness, restlessness, muscle pains or cramps, muscular fatigue, hypotension, oliguria, tachycardia, and gastrointestinal disturbances such as nausea and vomiting.

Hypokalemia may develop, especially with brisk diuresis, when severe cirrhosis is present, or during concomitant use of corticosteroids or ACTH. Interference with adequate oral electrolyte intake will also contribute to hypokalemia. Hypokalemia can sensitize or exaggerate the response of the heart to the toxic effects of digitalis (e.g., increased ventricular irritability). Hypokalemia may be avoided or treated by use of potassium supplements or foods with a high potassium content.

Any chloride deficit during thiazide therapy is generally mild and usually does not require specific treatment except under extraordinary circumstances (as in liver disease or renal disease). Dilutional hyponatremia may occur in edematous patients in hot weather; appropriate therapy is water restriction rather than administration of salt except in rare instances when the hyponatremia is life threatening. In actual salt depletion, appropriate replacement is the therapy of choice.

Muscle Weakness: Beta-adrenergic blockade has been reported to potentiate muscle weakness consistent with certain myasthenic symptoms (e.g., diplopia, ptosis, and generalized weakness). Timolol has been reported rarely to increase muscle weakness in some patients with myasthenic symptoms.

Drug Interactions

TIMOLIDE may potentiate the action of other antihypertensive agents used concomitantly. Close observation of the patient is recommended when TIMOLIDE is administered to patients receiving catecholamine-depleting drugs such as reserpine, because of possible additive effects and the production of hypotension and/or marked bradycardia, which may produce vertigo, syncope, or postural hypotension.

Blunting of the antihypertensive effect of beta-adrenoceptor blocking agents by non-steroidal anti-inflammatory drugs has been reported. When using these agents concomitantly, patients should be observed carefully to confirm that the desired therapeutic effect has been obtained.

Thiazides may decrease arterial responsiveness to norepinephrine. This diminution is not sufficient to preclude the therapeutic effectiveness of norepinephrine. Thiazides may increase the responsiveness to tubocurarine.

Lithium generally should not be given with diuretics because they reduce its renal clearance and add a high risk of lithium toxicity. Read circulars for lithium preparations before use of such preparations with TIMOLIDE.

Other Precautions

In patients receiving thiazides, sensitivity reactions may occur with or without a history of allergy or bronchial asthma. The possible exacerbation or activation of systemic lupus erythematosus has been reported. The antihypertensive effects of thiazides may be enhanced in the post-sympathectomy patient.

Carcinogenesis, Mutagenesis, Impairment of Fertility

In two-year study of timolol maleate in rats, there was a statistically significant (P ≤ 0.05) increase in the incidence of adrenal pheochromocytomas in male rats administered 300 times the maximum recommended human dose (1 mg/kg/day). Similar differences were not observed in rats administered doses equivalent to 25 or 100 times the maximum recommended human dose. In a lifetime study in mice, there were statistically significant (P ≤ 0.05) increases in the incidence of benign and malignant pulmonary tumors and benign uterine polyps in female mice at doses 500 mg/kg/day, but not at 5 or 50 mg/kg/day. There was also a significant increase in mammary adenocarcinomas at the 500 mg/kg/day dose. This was associated with elevations in serum prolactin which occurred in female mice administered timolol at 500 mg/kg, but not at doses of 5 or 50 mg/kg/day. An increased incidence of mammary adenocarcinomas in rodents has been associated with administration of several other therapeutic agents which elevate serum prolactin, but no correlation between serum prolactin levels and mammary tumors has been established in man. Furthermore, in adult human female subjects who received oral dosages of up to 60 mg of timolol maleate, the maximum recommended human oral dosage, there were no clinically meaningful changes in serum prolactin.

There was a statistically significant increase (P ≤ 0.05) in the overall incidence of neoplasms in female mice at the 500 mg/kg/day dosage level. Timolol maleate was devoid of mutagenic potential when evaluated *in vivo* (mouse) in the micronucleus test and cytogenetic assay (doses up to 800 mg/kg) and *in vitro* in a neoplastic cell transformation assay (up to 100 μg/ml). In Ames tests the highest concentrations of timolol employed, 5000 or 10,000 μg/plate, were associated with statistically significant elevations (P ≤ 0.05) of revertants observed with tester strain TA100 (in seven replicate assays), but not in the remaining three strains. In the assays with tester strain TA100, no consistent dose response relationship was observed, nor did the ratio of test to control revertants reach 2. A ratio of 2 is usually considered the criterion for a positive Ames test.

Reproduction and fertility studies in rats showed no adverse effect on male or female fertility at doses up to 150 times the maximum recommended human dose.

Pregnancy

Pregnancy Category C. Combinations of timolol maleate and hydrochlorothiazide were studied for teratogenic potential in the mouse and rabbit. The timolol maleate/hydrochlorothiazide combinations were administered orally to pregnant mice and pregnant rabbits at dosage levels of 1/2.5, 4/10, or 8/10 mg/kg/day. No teratogenic, embryotoxic, fetotoxic, or maternotoxic effects attributable to treatment were observed in either species. There are no adequate and well-controlled studies in pregnant women with TIMOLIDE. Because of the data listed below with the individual components, TIMOLIDE should be used during pregnancy only if the potential benefit justifies the potential risk to the fetus.

Timolol Maleate: Teratogenic studies with timolol maleate in mice and rabbits at doses up to 50 mg/kg/day (50 times the maximum recommended human dose) showed no evidence of fetal malformations. Although delayed fetal ossification was observed at this dose in rats, there were no adverse effects on postnatal development of offspring. Doses of 1000 mg/kg/day (1,000 times the maximum recommended human dose) were maternotoxic in mice and resulted in an increased number of fetal resorptions. Increased fetal resorptions were also seen in rabbits at doses of 100 times the maximum recommended human dose, in this case without apparent maternotoxicity.

Hydrochlorothiazide: TIMOLIDE contains hydrochlorothiazide. Thiazides cross the placental barrier and appear in cord blood. The possible hazards to the fetus include fetal or neonatal jaundice, thrombocytopenia, and possibly other adverse reactions which have occurred in the adult.

Nursing Mothers

Because of the potential for serious adverse reactions from timolol and hydrochlorothiazide in nursing infants, a decision should be made whether to discontinue nursing or to discontinue the drug, taking into account the importance of the drug to the mother.

Pediatric Use

Safety and effectiveness in children have not been established.

Adverse Reactions

TIMOLIDE is usually well tolerated in properly selected patients. Most adverse effects have been mild and transient.

The adverse reactions listed in the following table were spontaneously reported and have been arranged into two groups: (1) incidence greater than 1%; and (2) incidence less than 1%. The incidence was obtained from clinical studies conducted in the United States (257 patients treated with TIMOLIDE).

Incidence Greater Than 1%	Incidence Less Than 1%
BODY AS A WHOLE	
fatigue/tiredness (1.9%)	chest pain
asthenia (1.9%)	headache
CARDIOVASCULAR	
hypotension (1.6%)	arrhythmia
bradycardia (1.2%)	syncope
	cardiac failure
DIGESTIVE SYSTEM	
none	diarrhea
	dyspepsia
	nausea
	gastrointestinal pain
	constipation
INTEGUMENTARY	
none	rash
	increased pigmentation
	dry mucous membranes
MUSCULOSKELETAL	
none	myalgia
NERVOUS SYSTEM	
dizziness (1.2%)	none
PSYCHIATRIC	
none	insomnia

decreased libido
nervousness
confusion
trouble concentrating
somnolence

RESPIRATORY
bronchial spasm (1.6%)
dyspnea (1.2%)
rales

UROGENITAL
none
renal colic

The following additional adverse effects have been reported in clinical experience with the drug: cerebral ischemia, cerebral vascular accident, gout, muscle cramps, oculogyric crisis, worsening of chronic obstructive pulmonary disease, earache, and impotence.

Other adverse reactions that have been reported with the individual components are listed below:
Timolol Maleate—*Body as a Whole:* extremity pain, decreased exercise tolerance, weight loss; *Cardiovascular:* cerebral vascular accident, worsening of angina pectoris, sinoatrial block, AV block, worsening of arterial insufficiency, Raynaud's phenomenon, claudication, palpitations, vasodilitation, cold hands and feet, edema; *Digestive:* hepatomegaly, vomiting; *Hematologic:* non-thrombocytopenic purpura; *Endocrine:* hyperglycemia, hypoglycemia; *Skin:* skin irritation, pruritus, sweating; *Musculoskeletal:* arthralgia; *Nervous System:* local weakness, vertigo, paresthesia; *Psychiatric:* depression, nightmares, hallucinations; *Respiratory:* cough; *Special Senses:* visual disturbances, diplopia, ptosis, eye irritation, dry eyes, tinnitus; *Urogenital:* urination difficulties.
There have been reports of retroperitoneal fibrosis in patients receiving timolol maleate and in patients receiving other beta-adrenergic blocking agents. A causal relationship between this condition and therapy with beta-adrenergic blocking agents has not been established.
Hydrochlorothiazide—*Body as a Whole:* weakness; *Digestive:* anorexia, gastric irritation, vomiting, cramping, jaundice (intrahepatic cholestatic jaundice), pancreatitis, sialadenitis; *Nervous System/Psychiatric:* vertigo, paresthesias, restlessness; *Hematologic:* Leukopenia, agranulocytosis, thrombocytopenia, aplastic anemia, hemolytic anemia; *Cardiovascular:* orthostatic hypotension (may be aggravated by alcohol, barbiturates, or narcotics); *Hypersensitivity:* purpura, photosensitivity, urticaria, necrotizing angiitis (vasculitis, cutaneous vasculitis), fever, respiratory distress including pneumonitis and pulmonary edema, anaphylactic reactions; *Metabolic:* hyperglycemia, glycosuria, hyperuricemia, electrolyte imbalance (see PRECAUTIONS); *Musculoskeletal:* muscle spasm; *Special Senses:* transient blurred vision, xanthopsia.
Potential Adverse Effects: In addition, a variety of adverse effects not observed in clinical trials with timolol maleate, but reported with other beta-adrenergic blocking agents, should be considered potential adverse effects of timolol maleate: *Nervous System:* Reversible mental depression progressing to catatonia; an acute reversible syndrome characterized by disorientation for time and place, short-term memory loss, emotional lability, slightly clouded sensorium, and decreased performance on neuropsychometrics; *Cardiovascular:* Intensification of AV block (see CONTRAINDICATIONS); *Digestive:* Mesenteric arterial thrombosis, ischemic colitis; *Hematologic:* Agranulocytosis, thrombocytopenic purpura; *Allergic:* Erythematous rash, fever combined with aching and sore throat, laryngospasm and respiratory distress; *Miscellaneous:* Reversible alopecia, Peyronie's disease.
There have been reports of a syndrome comprising psoriasiform skin rash, conjunctivitis sicca, otitis, and sclerosing serositis attributed to the beta-adrenergic receptor blocking agent, practolol. This syndrome has not been reported with TIMOLIDE or BLOCADREN® (Timolol Maleate, MSD).
Clinical Laboratory Test Findings: Clinically important changes in standard laboratory parameters were rarely associated with the administration of TIMOLIDE. The changes in laboratory parameters were not progressive and usually were not associated with clinical manifestations. The most common changes were increases in serum triglycerides and uric acid and decreases in serum potassium and chloride.

Overdosage

No data are available in regard to overdosage in humans. Pretreatment of mice with hydrochlorothiazide (5 mg/kg) did not alter the LD$_{50}$ of timolol (1320 mg/kg compared to 1300 mg/kg without pretreatment).
No specific information is available on the treatment of overdosage with TIMOLIDE, and no specific antidote is available. Treatment is symptomatic and supportive. Therapy with TIMOLIDE should be discontinued and the patient observed closely. Suggested measures include induction of emesis and/or gastric lavage, and correction of dehydration, electrolyte imbalance, and hypotension by established procedures.

Timolol Maleate
No data are available in regard to overdosage in humans.
The oral LD$_{50}$ of the drug is 1190 and 900 mg/kg in female mice and female rats, respectively.
An *in vitro* hemodialysis study, using ^{14}C timolol added to human plasma or whole blood, showed that timolol was readily dialyzed from these fluids; however, a study of patients with renal failure showed that timolol did not dialyze readily.
The most common signs and symptoms to be expected with overdosage with a beta-adrenergic receptor blocking agent are symptomatic bradycardia, hypotension, bronchospasm, and acute cardiac failure. If overdosage occurs the following therapeutic measures should be considered:
(1) *Gastric lavage.*
(2) *Symptomatic bradycardia:* Use atropine sulfate intravenously in a dosage of 0.25 mg to 2 mg to induce vagal blockade. If bradycardia persists, intravenous isoproterenol hydrochloride should be administered cautiously. In refractory cases the use of a transvenous cardiac pacemaker may be considered.
(3) *Hypotension:* Use sympathomimetic pressor drug therapy, such as dopamine, dobutamine or levarterenol. In refractory cases the use of glucagon hydrochloride has been reported to be useful.
(4) *Bronchospasm:* Use isoproterenol hydrochloride. Additional therapy with aminophylline may be considered.
(5) *Acute cardiac failure:* Conventional therapy with digitalis, diuretics, and oxygen should be instituted immediately. In refractory cases the use of intravenous aminophylline is suggested. This may be followed, if necessary, by glucagon hydrochloride which has been reported to be useful.
(6) *Heart block (second or third degree):* Use isoproterenol hydrochloride or a transvenous cardiac pacemaker.

Hydrochlorothiazide
The most common signs and symptoms observed with hydrochlorothiazide overdosage are those caused by electrolyte depletion (hypokalemia, hypochloremia, hyponatremia) and dehydration resulting from excessive diuresis. If digitalis has also been administered, hypokalemia may accentuate cardiac arrhythmias.

Dosage and Administration

The recommended starting and maintenance dosage is 1 tablet twice a day. If the antihypertensive response is not satisfactory, another antihypertensive agent may be added.

How Supplied

No. 3373—Tablets TIMOLIDE 10-25 are light blue, flat, hexagonal-shaped, compressed tablets, with MSD 67 code on one side and TIMOLIDE on the other. Each tablet contains 10 mg of timolol maleate and 25 mg of hydrochlorothiazide. They are supplied as follows:

NDC 0006-0067-68 bottles of 100
NDC 0006-0067-28 unit dose packages of 100.
Shown in Product Identification Section, page 420
A.H.F.S. Category: 24:08
DC 7119518   Issued November 1983
COPYRIGHT © MERCK & CO., INC., 1983
All rights reserved

TIMOPTIC® Sterile
Ophthalmic Solution
(timolol maleate, MSD), U.S.P.

Description

TIMOPTIC® (Timolol Maleate, MSD) Ophthalmic Solution is a non-selective beta-adrenergic receptor blocking agent. Its chemical name is (S)-1-[(1,1-dimethylethyl)amino]-3-[[4-(4-morpholinyl)-1,2,5-thiadiazol-3-yl]oxy]-2-propanol, (Z)-butenedioate (1:1) salt. Timolol maleate possesses an asymmetric carbon atom in its structure and is provided as the levo isomer. The nominal optical rotation of timolol maleate is

$$[\alpha]^{25°}_{405\,nm} \text{ in } 0.1\text{ N HCl } (C = 5\%) = -12.2°.$$

Its empirical formula is $C_{13}H_{24}N_4O_3S \cdot C_4H_4O_4$.
TIMOPTIC Ophthalmic Solution is supplied as a sterile, isotonic, buffered, aqueous solution of timolol maleate in two dosage strengths: Each ml of TIMOPTIC 0.25% contains 2.5 mg of timolol (3.4 mg of timolol maleate). Each ml of TIMOPTIC 0.5% contains 5.0 mg of timolol (6.8 mg of timolol maleate). Inactive ingredients: monobasic and dibasic sodium phosphate, sodium hydroxide to adjust pH, and water for injection. Benzalkonium chloride 0.01% is added as preservative.
Timolol maleate has a molecular weight of 432.49. It is a white, odorless, crystalline powder which is soluble in water, methanol, and alcohol. TIMOPTIC is stable at room temperature.

Clinical Pharmacology

Timolol maleate is a beta$_1$ and beta$_2$ (non-selective) adrenergic receptor blocking agent that does not have significant intrinsic sympathomimetic, direct myocardial depressant, or local anesthetic (membrane-stabilizing) activity.
Beta-adrenergic receptor blockade reduces cardiac output in both healthy subjects and patients with heart disease. In patients with severe impairment of myocardial function beta-adrenergic receptor blockade may inhibit the stimulatory effect of the sympathetic nervous system necessary to maintain adequate cardiac function.
Beta-adrenergic receptor blockade in the bronchi and bronchioles results in increased airway resistance from unopposed para-sympathetic activity. Such an effect in patients with asthma or other bronchospastic conditions is potentially dangerous.
TIMOPTIC Ophthalmic Solution, when applied topically in the eye, has the action of reducing elevated as well as normal intraocular pressure, whether or not accompanied by glaucoma. Elevated intraocular pressure is a major risk factor in the pathogenesis of glaucomatous visual field loss. The higher the level of intraocular pressure, the greater the likelihood of glaucomatous visual field loss and optic nerve damage.
The onset of reduction in intraocular pressure following administration of TIMOPTIC can usually be detected within one-half hour after a single dose. The maximum effect usually occurs in one to two hours and significant lowering of intraocular pressure can be maintained for periods as long as 24 hours with a single dose. Repeated observations over a period of one year indicate that the intraocular pressure-lowering effect of TIMOPTIC is well maintained.

Continued on next page

Information on the Merck Sharp & Dohme products listed on these pages is the full prescribing information from product circulars in use November 1, 1984.

Merck Sharp & Dohme—Cont.

The precise mechanism of the ocular hypotensive action of TIMOPTIC is not clearly established at this time. Tonography and fluorophotometry studies in man suggest that its predominant action may be related to reduced aqueous formation. However, in some studies a slight increase in outflow facility was also observed. Unlike miotics, TIMOPTIC reduces intraocular pressure with little or no effect on accommodation or pupil size. Thus, changes in visual acuity due to increased accommodation are uncommon, and dim or blurred vision and night blindness produced by miotics are not evident. In addition, in patients with cataracts the inability to see around lenticular opacities when the pupil is constricted is avoided.

In the clinical studies which are reported below, ocular pressure reductions to less than 22 mmHg were used as a reasonable reference point to allow comparisons between treatments. Reduction of ocular pressure to just below 22 mmHg may not be optimal for all patients; therapy should be individualized.

In controlled multiclinic studies in patients with untreated intraocular pressures of 22 mmHg or greater, TIMOPTIC 0.25 percent or 0.5 percent administered twice a day produced a greater reduction in intraocular pressure than 1, 2, 3, or 4 percent pilocarpine solution administered four times a day or 0.5, 1, or 2 percent epinephrine hydrochloride solution administered twice a day.

In the multiclinic studies comparing TIMOPTIC with pilocarpine, 61 percent of patients treated with TIMOPTIC had intraocular pressure reduced to less than 22 mmHg compared to 32 percent of patients treated with pilocarpine. For patients completing these studies, the mean reduction in pressure at the end of the study from pretreatment was 30.7 percent for patients treated with TIMOPTIC and 21.7 percent for patients treated with pilocarpine.

In the multiclinic studies comparing TIMOPTIC with epinephrine, 69 percent of patients treated with TIMOPTIC had intraocular pressure reduced to less than 22 mmHg compared to 42 percent of patients treated with epinephrine. For patients completing these studies, the mean reduction in pressure at the end of the study from pretreatment was 33.2 percent for patients treated with TIMOPTIC and 28.1 percent for patients treated with epinephrine.

In these studies, TIMOPTIC was generally well tolerated and produced fewer and less severe side effects than either pilocarpine or epinephrine. A slight reduction of resting heart rate in some patients receiving TIMOPTIC (mean reduction 2.9 beats/minute standard deviation 10.2) was observed.

TIMOPTIC has also been used in patients with glaucoma wearing conventional (PMMA) hard contact lenses, and has generally been well tolerated. TIMOPTIC has not been studied in patients wearing lenses made with materials other than PMMA.

Indications and Usage

TIMOPTIC Ophthalmic Solution has been shown to be effective in lowering intraocular pressure and may be used in:
Patients with chronic open-angle glaucoma
Patients with aphakic glaucoma
Some patients with secondary glaucoma
Other patients with elevated intraocular pressure who are at sufficient risk to require lowering of the ocular pressure.

Clinical trials have also shown that in patients who respond inadequately to multiple antiglaucoma drug therapy the addition of TIMOPTIC may produce a further reduction of intraocular pressure.

Contraindications

TIMOPTIC is contraindicated in patients with bronchial asthma or with a history of bronchial asthma, or severe chronic obstructive pulmonary disease (see WARNINGS); sinus bradycardia; second and third degree atrioventricular block; overt cardiac failure (see WARNINGS); cardiogenic shock; hypersensitivity to any component of this product.

Warnings

As with other topically applied ophthalmic drugs, this drug may be absorbed systemically.
The same adverse reactions found with systemic administration of beta-adrenergic blocking agents may occur with topical administration. For example, severe respiratory reactions and cardiac reactions, including death due to bronchospasm in patients with asthma, and rarely death in association with cardiac failure, have been reported following administration of TIMOPTIC (see CONTRAINDICATIONS).

Cardiac Failure
Sympathetic stimulation may be essential for support of the circulation in individuals with diminished myocardial contractility, and its inhibition by beta-adrenergic receptor blockade may precipitate more severe failure.

In Patients Without a History of Cardiac Failure continued depression of the myocardium with beta-blocking agents over a period of time can, in some cases, lead to cardiac failure. At the first sign or symptom of cardiac failure TIMOPTIC should be discontinued.

Non-Allergic Bronchospasm
In patients with non-allergic bronchospasm or with a history of non-allergic bronchospasm (e.g., chronic bronchitis, emphysema), TIMOPTIC should be administered with caution since it may block bronchodilation produced by endogenous and exogenous catecholamine stimulation of beta$_2$ receptors.

Major Surgery
The necessity or desirability of withdrawal of beta-adrenergic blocking agents prior to major surgery is controversial. Beta-adrenergic receptor blockade impairs the ability of the heart to respond to beta-adrenergically mediated reflex stimuli. This may augment the risk of general anesthesia in surgical procedures. Some patients receiving beta-adrenergic receptor blocking agents have been subject to protracted severe hypotension during anesthesia. Difficulty in restarting and maintaining the heartbeat has also been reported. For these reasons, in patients undergoing elective surgery, some authorities recommend gradual withdrawal of beta-adrenergic receptor blocking agents.

If necessary during surgery, the effects of beta-adrenergic blocking agents may be reversed by sufficient doses of such agonists as isoproterenol, dopamine, dobutamine or levarterenol (see OVERDOSAGE).

Diabetes Mellitus
Beta-adrenergic blocking agents should be administered with caution in patients subject to spontaneous hypoglycemia or to diabetic patients (especially those with labile diabetes) who are receiving insulin or oral hypoglycemic agents. Beta-adrenergic receptor blocking agents may mask the signs and symptoms of acute hypoglycemia.

Thyrotoxicosis
Beta-adrenergic blocking agents may mask certain clinical signs (e.g., tachycardia) of hyperthyroidism. Patients suspected of developing thyrotoxicosis should be managed carefully to avoid abrupt withdrawal of beta-adrenergic blocking agents which might precipitate a thyroid storm.

Precautions

Patients who are receiving a beta-adrenergic blocking agent orally and TIMOPTIC should be observed for a potential additive effect either on the intraocular pressure or on the known systemic effects of beta blockade.

Muscle Weakness: Beta-adrenergic blockade has been reported to potentiate muscle weakness consistent with certain myasthenic symptoms (e.g., diplopia, ptosis, and generalized weakness). Timolol has been reported rarely to increase muscle weakness in some patients with myasthenic symptoms.

In patients with angle-closure glaucoma, the immediate objective of treatment is to reopen the angle. This requires constricting the pupil with a miotic. TIMOPTIC has little or no effect on the pupil. When TIMOPTIC is used to reduce elevated intraocular pressure in angle-closure glaucoma, it should be used with a miotic and not alone.

As with the use of other antiglaucoma drugs, diminished responsiveness to TIMOPTIC after prolonged therapy has been reported in some patients. However, in one long-term study in which 96 patients have been followed for at least 3 years, no significant difference in mean intraocular pressure has been observed after initial stabilization.

Drug Interactions
Although TIMOPTIC used alone has little or no effect on pupil size, mydriasis resulting from concomitant therapy with TIMOPTIC and epinephrine has been reported occasionally.

Close observation of the patient is recommended when a beta blocker is administered to patients receiving catecholamine-depleting drugs such as reserpine, because of possible additive effects and the production of hypotension and/or marked bradycardia, which may produce vertigo, syncope, or postural hypotension.

Animal Studies
No adverse ocular effects were observed in rabbits and dogs administered TIMOPTIC topically in studies lasting one and two years respectively.

Carcinogenesis, Mutagenesis, Impairment of Fertility
In a two-year oral study of timolol maleate in rats, there was a statistically significant ($P \le 0.05$) increase in the incidence of adrenal pheochromocytomas in male rats administered 300 times the maximum recommended human oral dose* (1 mg/kg/day). Similar differences were not observed in rats administered oral doses equivalent to 25 or 100 times the maximum recommended human oral dose. In a lifetime oral study in mice, there were statistically significant ($P \le 0.05$) increases in the incidence of benign and malignant pulmonary tumors and benign uterine polyps in female mice at 500 mg/kg/day, but not at 5 or 50 mg/kg/day. There was also a significant increase in mammary adenocarcinomas at the 500 mg/kg/day dose. This was associated with elevations in serum prolactin which occurred in female mice administered timolol at 500 mg/kg, but not at doses of 5 or 50 mg/kg/day. An increased incidence of mammary adenocarcinomas in rodents has been associated with administration of several other therapeutic agents which elevate serum prolactin, but no correlation between serum prolactin levels and mammary tumors has been established in man. Furthermore, in adult human female subjects who received oral dosages of up to 60 mg of timolol maleate, the maximum recommended human oral dosage, there were no clinically meaningful changes in serum prolactin.

There was a statistically significant increase ($P \le 0.05$) in the overall incidence of neoplasms in female mice at the 500 mg/kg/day dosage level. Timolol maleate was devoid of mutagenic potential when evaluated *in vivo* (mouse) in the micronucleus test and cytogenetic assay (doses up to 800 mg/kg) and *in vitro* in a neoplastic cell transformation assay (up to 100 μg/ml). In Ames tests the highest concentrations of timolol employed, 5000 or 10,000 μg/plate, were associated with statistically significant elevations ($P \le 0.05$) of revertants observed with tester strain TA100 (in seven replicate assays), but not in the remaining three strains. In the assays with tester strain TA100, no consistent dose response relationship was observed, nor did the ratio of test to control revertants reach 2. A ratio of 2 is usually considered the criterion for a positive Ames test.

---
*The maximum recommended single oral dose is 30 mg of timolol. One drop of TIMOPTIC 0.5% contains about 1/150 of this dose which is about 0.2 mg.

Reproduction and fertility studies in rats showed no adverse effect on male or female fertility at doses up to 150 times the maximum recommended human oral dose.

Pregnancy

Pregnancy Category C. Teratogenic studies with timolol in mice and rabbits at doses up to 50 mg/kg/day (50 times the maximum recommended human oral dose) showed no evidence of fetal malformations. Although delayed fetal ossification was observed at this dose in rats, there were no adverse effects on postnatal development of offspring. Doses of 1000 mg/kg/day (1,000 times the maximum recommended human oral dose) were maternotoxic in mice and resulted in an increased number of fetal resorptions. Increased fetal resorptions were also seen in rabbits at doses of 100 times the maximum recommended human oral dose, in this case without apparent maternotoxicity. There are no adequate and well-controlled studies in pregnant women. TIMOPTIC should be used during pregnancy only if the potential benefit justifies the potential risk to the fetus.

Nursing Mothers

Because of the potential for serious adverse reactions from timolol in nursing infants, a decision should be made whether to discontinue nursing or to discontinue the drug, taking into account the importance of the drug to the mother.

Pediatric Use

Safety and effectiveness in children have not been established by adequate and well-controlled studies.

Adverse Reactions

TIMOPTIC Ophthalmic Solution is usually well tolerated. The following adverse reactions have been reported either in clinical trials of up to 3 years duration prior to release in 1978 or since the drug has been marketed.

BODY AS A WHOLE
 Headache.
CARDIOVASCULAR
 Bradycardia, arrhythmia, hypotension, syncope, heart block, cerebral vascular accident, cerebral ischemia, congestive heart failure, palpitation.
DIGESTIVE
 Nausea.
NERVOUS SYSTEM
 Dizziness.
PSYCHIATRIC
 Depression.
SKIN
 Hypersensitivity, including localized and generalized rash; urticaria.
RESPIRATORY
 Bronchospasm (predominantly in patients with pre-existing bronchospastic disease), respiratory failure.
ENDOCRINE
 Masked symptoms of hypoglycemia in insulin-dependent diabetics (See WARNINGS).
SPECIAL SENSES
 Signs and symptoms of ocular irritation, including conjunctivitis, blepharitis, keratitis, blepharoptosis, decreased corneal sensitivity, visual disturbances including refractive changes (due to withdrawal of miotic therapy in some cases), diplopia, ptosis.

Casual Relationship Unknown: The following adverse effects have been reported rarely, and a casual relationship to therapy with TIMOPTIC has not been established: *Body as a Whole:* Fatigue; *Cardiovascular:* Hypertension; *Digestive:* Dyspepsia, anorexia, dry mouth; *Nervous System:* Confusion; *Psychiatric:* Somnolence, anxiety; *Special Senses:* Aphakic cystoid macular edema; *Urogenital:* Retroperitoneal fibrosis.

The following additional adverse effects have been reported in clinical experience with oral timolol maleate, and may be considered potential effects of ophthalmic timolol maleate: *Body as a Whole:* Chest pain, asthenia, extremity pain, decreased exercise tolerance, weight loss; *Cardiovascular:* Edema, pulmonary edema (non-fatal), cardiac failure, heart rate < 40 beats/minute, worsening of angina pectoris, worsening of arterial insufficiency, AV block, sinoatrial block, Raynaud's phenomenon, vasodilatation; *Digestive:* Gastrointestinal pain, hepatomegaly, vomiting, diarrhea; *Hematologic:* Nonthrombocytopenic purpura; *Endocrine:* Hyperglycemia, hypoglycemia; *Skin:* Pruritus, skin irritation, increased pigmentation, sweating, cold hands and feet; *Musculoskeletal:* Arthralgia, claudication; *Nervous System:* Vertigo, paresthesia, local weakness; *Psychiatric:* Decreased libido, nightmares, insomnia, nervousness, diminished concentration, hallucinations; *Respiratory:* Dyspnea, rales, cough, bronchial obstruction; *Special Senses:* Tinnitus, dry eyes; *Urogenital:* Impotence, urination difficulties.

Potential Adverse Effects: In addition, a variety of adverse effects have been reported with other beta-adrenergic blocking agents and may be considered potential effects of ophthalmic timolol maleate: *Digestive:* Mesenteric arterial thrombosis, ischemic colitis; *Hematologic:* Agranulocytosis, thrombocytopenic purpura; *Nervous System:* Reversible mental depression progressing to catatonia; an acute reversible syndrome characterized by disorientation for time and place, short-term memory loss, emotional lability, slightly clouded sensorium, and decreased performance on neuropsychometrics; *Allergic:* Erythematous rash, fever combined with aching and sore throat, laryngospasm and respiratory distress; *Miscellaneous:* Reversible alopecia, Peyronie's disease.

There have been reports of a syndrome comprising psoriasiform skin rash, conjunctivitis sicca, otitis and sclerosing serositis attributed to the beta-adrenergic receptor blocking agent, practolol. This syndrome has not been reported with timolol maleate.

Overdosage

No data are available in regard to overdosage in humans.

The oral LD$_{50}$ of the drug is 1190 and 900 mg/kg in female mice and female rats, respectively.

An *in vitro* hemodialysis study, using ^{14}C timolol added to human plasma or whole blood, showed that timolol was readily dialyzed from these fluids; however, a study of patients with renal failure showed that timolol did not dialyze readily.

The most common signs and symptoms to be expected with overdosage with administration of a systemic beta-adrenergic receptor blocking agent are symptomatic bradycardia, hypotension, bronchospasm, and acute cardiac failure. The following additional therapeutic measures should be considered:

(1) *Gastric lavage:* If ingested.
(2) *Symptomatic bradycardia:* Use atropine sulfate intravenously in a dosage of 0.25 mg to 2 mg to induce vagal blockade. If bradycardia persists, intravenous isoproterenol hydrochloride should be administered cautiously. In refractory cases the use of a transvenous cardiac pacemaker may be considered.
(3) *Hypotension:* Use sympathomimetic pressor drug therapy, such as dopamine, dobutamine or levarterenol. In refractory cases the use of glucagon hydrochloride has been reported to be useful.
(4) *Bronchospasm:* Use isoproterenol hydrochloride. Additional therapy with aminophylline may be considered.
(5) *Acute cardiac failure:* Conventional therapy with digitalis, diuretics, and oxygen should be instituted immediately. In refractory cases the use of intravenous aminophylline is suggested. This may be followed if necessary by glucagon hydrochloride which has been reported to be useful.
(6) *Heart block (second or third degree):* Use isoproterenol hydrochloride or a transvenous cardiac pacemaker.

Dosage and Administration

TIMOPTIC Ophthalmic Solution is available in concentrations of 0.25 and 0.5 percent. The usual starting dose is one drop of 0.25 percent TIMOPTIC in the affected eye(s) twice a day. If the clinical response is not adequate, the dosage may be changed to one drop of 0.5 percent solution in the affected eye(s) twice a day.

Since in some patients the pressure-lowering response to TIMOPTIC may require a few weeks to stabilize, evaluation should include a determination of intraocular pressure after approximately 4 weeks of treatment with TIMOPTIC.

If the intraocular pressure is maintained at satisfactory levels, the dosage schedule may be changed to one drop once a day in the affected eye(s). Because of diurnal variations in intraocular pressure, satisfactory response to the once-a-day dose is best determined by measuring the intraocular pressure at different times during the day.

Dosages above one drop of 0.5 percent TIMOPTIC twice a day generally have not been shown to produce further reduction in intraocular pressure. If the patient's intraocular pressure is still not at a satisfactory level on this regimen, concomitant therapy with pilocarpine and other miotics, and/or epinephrine, and/or systemically administered carbonic anhydrase inhibitors, such as acetazolamide, can be instituted.

When a patient is transferred from a single antiglaucoma agent, continue the agent already being used and add one drop of 0.25 percent TIMOPTIC in the affected eye(s) twice a day. On the following day, discontinue the previously used antiglaucoma agent completely and continue with TIMOPTIC. If a higher dosage of TIMOPTIC is required, substitute one drop of 0.5 percent solution in the affected eye(s) twice a day.

When a patient is transferred from several concomitantly administered antiglaucoma agents, individualization is required. Adjustments should involve one agent at a time and usually should be made at intervals of not less than one week. A recommended approach is to continue the agents being used and to add one drop of 0.25 percent TIMOPTIC in the affected eye(s) twice a day. On the following day, discontinue one of the other antiglaucoma agents. The remaining antiglaucoma agents may be decreased or discontinued according to the patient's response to treatment. If a higher dosage of TIMOPTIC is required, substitute one drop of 0.5 percent solution in the affected eye(s) twice a day. The physician may be able to discontinue some or all of the other antiglaucoma agents.

How Supplied

Sterile Ophthalmic Solution TIMOPTIC is a clear, colorless to light yellow solution.

No. 3366—TIMOPTIC Ophthalmic Solution, 0.25% timolol equivalent, is supplied in a white, opaque, plastic OCUMETER® ophthalmic dispenser with a controlled drop tip as follows:
NDC 0006-3366-03, 5 ml
NDC 0006-3366-10, 10 ml
NDC 0006-3366-12, 15 ml.

No. 3367—TIMOPTIC Ophthalmic Solution, 0.5% timolol equivalent, is supplied in a white, opaque, plastic OCUMETER ophthalmic dispenser with a controlled drop tip as follows:
NDC 0006-3367-03, 5 ml
NDC 0006-3367-10, 10 ml
NDC 0006-3367-12, 15 ml.

A.H.F.S. Category: 52:36
DC 7046019 Issued June 1983
COPYRIGHT © MERCK & CO., INC., 1983
All rights reserved

TONOCARD® Tablets   R
(tocainide HCl, MSD)

Description: TONOCARD* (Tocainide HCl, MSD) is a primary amine analog of lidocaine with

Continued on next page

Information on the Merck Sharp & Dohme products listed on these pages is the full prescribing information from product circulars in use November 1, 1984.

Merck Sharp & Dohme—Cont.

antiarrhythmic properties useful in the treatment of ventricular arrhythmias. The chemical name for tocainide hydrochloride is 2-amino-N-(2,6-dimethylphenyl) propanamide hydrochloride. Its empirical formula is $C_{11}H_{16}N_2O \cdot HCl$, with a molecular weight of 228.72. The structural formula is:

Tocainide hydrochloride is a white crystalline powder with a bitter taste and is freely soluble in water. It is supplied as 400 mg and 600 mg tablets for oral administration.

Clinical Pharmacology
Action
Tocainide, like lidocaine, produces dose dependent decreases in sodium and potassium conductance, thereby decreasing the excitability of myocardial cells. In experimental animal models, the dose-related depression of sodium current is more pronounced in ischemic tissue than in normal tissue.
Electrophysiology
Tocainide is a Class I antiarrhythmic compound with electrophysiologic properties in man similar to those of lidocaine, but dissimilar from quinidine, procainamide, and disopyramide.
In studies of ioslated dog Purkinje fibers, tocainide in concentrations of 1–50 mcg/mL had no significant effect on resting membrane potential, but reduced the amplitude and rate of depolarization (dv/dt) of the action potential. Tocainide decreased the effective refractory period (ERP) to a lesser extent than the action potential duration (APD) resulting in an increase in the ERP/APD ratio.
In patients with cardiac disease, TONOCARD produced no clinically significant changes in sinus nodal function, effective refractory periods, or intracardiac conduction times when studied under electrophysiologic testing procedures.
Tocainide, like lidocaine, characteristically does not prolong ventricular depolarization (QRS duration) or repolarization (QT intervals) as measured by electrocardiography. Theoretically, therefore, TONOCARD may be useful in the treatment of ventricular arrhythmias associated with a prolonged QT interval.
Patients who respond to lidocaine also respond to TONOCARD in a majority of cases. Failure to respond to lidocaine usually predicts failure to respond to TONOCARD, but there are exceptions to this.
Pharmacokinetics
Following oral administration of tocainide, peak plasma concentrations occur within 0.5 to 2 hours. The average plasma half-life in patients is approximately 15 hours. Although the effective plasma concentration may vary from patient to patient, the usual therapeutic plasma range (as defined by 50–80 percent PVC suppression) is 4–10 mcg/mL (18–45 micromole/L), expressed as tocainide hydrochloride. Tocainide is approximately 10 percent bound to plasma protein.
In contrast to lidocaine, tocainide undergoes negligible first pass hepatic degradation. Following oral administration, the bioavailability of TONOCARD approaches 100 percent. The extent of its bioavailability is unaffected by food. Tocainide has no cardioactive metabolites. Approximately 40 percent of the administered dose of tocainide is excreted unchanged in the urine. Acidification of the urine has not been shown to significantly alter tocainide excretion in the urine, but alkalinization of the urine results in a significant decrease in the percent of tocainide excreted unchanged in the urine. Animal data indicate that tocainide crosses the blood-brain barrier; however, it has less lipid solubility than lidocaine.

Hemodynamics
Cardiac catheterization studies in man utilizing intravenous tocainide infusions (0.5–0.75 mg/kg/min over 15 min) have shown that tocainide usually produces a small degree of depression of parameters of left ventricular function, such as left ventricular dP/dt, and left ventricular end diastolic pressure. There were usually no changes in cardiac output or clinical evidence of increasing congestive heart failure in the well-compensated patients studied. Small but statistically significant increases in aortic and pulmonary arterial pressures have been consistently observed and are probably related to small increases in vascular resistance. When used concomitantly with a beta-blocking drug, tocainide further reduced cardiac index and left ventricular dP/dt and further increased pulmonary wedge pressure.
No clinically significant changes in heart rate, blood pressure, or signs of myocardial depression were observed in a study of 72 post-myocardial infarction patients receiving long-term therapy with oral TONOCARD at usual doses (400 mg q8h). When tocainide was administered orally at a dose of 120 mg/kg to anesthetized dogs (14 times the initial maximum dose recommended for humans), a negative inotropic effect was observed: the rate of change of left ventricular pressure decreased by up to 29 percent of control at 3 hours after administration. This effect was not observed at lower doses (60 mg/kg). Tocainide has been used safely in patients with acute myocardial infarction and various degrees of congestive heart failure. It has, however, a small negative inotropic effect and can increase peripheral resistance slightly. It therefore should be used cautiously in patients with known heart failure, particularly if a beta blocker is given as well. (See PRECAUTIONS.)

Indications and Usage
TONOCARD is indicated for the suppression of symptomatic ventricular arrhythmias, including frequent premature ventricular contractions, unifocal or multifocal, couplets, and ventricular tachycardia.
In a controlled comparison with quinidine, 600 mg b.i.d. of TONOCARD produced a mean reduction of 42 percent in PVC count, compared to a 54 percent reduction by quinidine 300 mg every 6 hours. Among all patients entered into the study, about one-fifth of tocainide recipients and one-third of quinidine recipients had 75 percent or greater reductions in PVC count or had elimination of ventricular tachycardia.
Like other antiarrhythmics, tocainide has not been shown to prevent sudden death in patients with serious ventricular ectopic activity, and also, like other antiarrhythmics, it has potentially serious adverse effects, including the ability to worsen arrhythmias. It is therefore essential that each patient given tocainide be evaluated electrocardiographically and clinically prior to, and during, tocainide therapy to determine whether the response to tocainide supports continued treatment.

Contraindications
Patients who are hypersensitive to this product or to local anesthetics of the amide type.
Patients with second or third degree atrioventricular block in the absence of an artificial ventricular pacemaker.

Warnings
Blood Dyscrasias: Leukopenia, agranulocytosis, hypoplastic anemia, and thrombocytopenia, possibly drug related, have been reported in patients receiving TONOCARD. Many of these events occurred in patients who were seriously ill and who were receiving concomitant drugs. Patients should be instructed to promptly report the development of bruising or bleeding and any signs of infection such as fever, sore throat, or chills. Periodic blood counts are recommended, particularly during the first six months of therapy. If any of these hematologic disorders is identified, TONOCARD should be discontinued and appropriate treatment should be instituted if necessary. Blood counts usually return to normal within one month of discontinuation. (See ADVERSE REACTIONS).
Acceleration of Ventricular Rate: Acceleration of ventricular rate occurs infrequently when antiarrhythmics are administered to patients with atrial flutter or fibrillation (see ADVERSE REACTIONS).

Precautions
General
Pulmonary Fibrosis: Pulmonary fibrosis, pneumonitis, alveolitis, pulmonary edema, and pneumonia, possibly drug related, have been reported in patients receiving TONOCARD. Many of these events occurred in patients who were seriously ill. The experiences are usually characterized by bilateral infiltrates on x-ray and are frequently associated with dyspnea and cough. Fever may or may not be present. Patients should be instructed to promptly report the development of any pulmonary symptoms such as exertional dyspnea, cough or wheezing. Chest x-rays are advisable at that time. If these pulmonary disorders develop, TONOCARD should be discontinued. (See ADVERSE REACTIONS).
In patients with known heart failure or minimal cardiac reserve, TONOCARD should be used with caution because of the potential for aggravating the degree of heart failure.
Caution should be used in the institution or continuation of antiarrhythmic therapy in the presence of signs of increasing depression of cardiac conductivity.
In patients with severe liver or kidney disease, the rate of drug elimination may be significantly decreased (see DOSAGE AND ADMINISTRATION).
Since antiarrhythmic drugs may be ineffective in patients with hypokalemia, the possibility of a potassium deficit should be explored and, if present, the deficit should be corrected.
Like all other oral antiarrhythmics, TONOCARD has been reported to increase arrhythmias in some patients (see ADVERSE REACTIONS).
Drug Interactions
Specific interaction studies with digoxin and metoprolol have been conducted, no clinically significant interaction was seen with digoxin, but tocainide and metoprolol had additive effects on wedge pressure and cardiac index. TONOCARD has also been used in open studies with digitalis, beta-blocking agents, other antiarrhythmic agents, anticoagulants, and diuretics, without evidence of clinically significant interactions. Nevertheless, caution should be exercised in the use of multiple drug therapy.
TONOCARD is equally effective in digitalized and non-digitalized patients. In 17 patients with refractory ventricular arrhythmias on concomitant therapy, serum digoxin levels $(1.1 \pm 0.4$ ng/mL) remained in the expected normal range (0.5–2.5 ng/mL) during tocainide administration.
Carcinogenesis, Mutagenesis, Impairment of Fertility
The carcinogenic potential of tocainide was studied in mice using oral doses up to 300 mg/kg/day (about 6 times the maximum recommended human dose) for up to 94 weeks in males and 102 weeks in females and in rats at doses up to 200 mg/kg/day for 24 months. Tocainide did not affect the type or incidence of neoplasia in the two studies.
Tocainide did not show any mutagenic potential when evaluated *in vivo* in the micronucleus test using mice at oral doses up to 187.5 mg/kg/day (about 7 times the usual human dose). Also, no mutagenic activity was seen *in vitro* in the Ames microbial mutagen test or in the mouse lymphoma forward mutation assay.
Reproduction and fertility studies in rats showed no adverse effects on male or female fertility at oral doses up to 200 mg/kg/day (about 8 times the usual human dose).
Pregnancy
Pregnancy Category C. In a teratogenicity study in rabbits, tocainide was administered orally at doses of 25, 50, and 100 mg/kg/day (about 1 to 4 times the usual human dose). No evidence of a

---
*Registered trademark of Astra Pharmaceutical Products, Inc.

drug-related teratogenic effect was noted; however, these doses were maternotoxic and produced a dose-related increase in abortions and stillbirths. In a teratogenicity study in rats, an oral dose of 300 mg/kg/day (about 12 times the usual human dose) showed no evidence of treatment-related fetal malformations, but maternotoxicity and an increase in fetal resorptions were noted. An oral dose of 30 mg/kg/day (about twice the usual human dose) did not produce any adverse effects.

In reproduction studies in rats at maternotoxic oral doses of 200 and 300 mg/kg/day (about 8 and 12 times the usual human dose, respectively), dystocia, and delayed parturition occurred which was accompanied by an increase in stillbirths and decreased survival in offspring during the first week postpartum. Growth and viability of surviving offspring were not affected for the remainder of the lactation period.

There are no adequate and well-controlled studies in pregnant women. TONOCARD should be used during pregnancy only if the potential benefit justifies the potential risk to the fetus.

Nursing Mothers

It is not known whether tocainide is secreted in human milk. Because many drugs are secreted in human milk and because of the potential for serious adverse reactions in nursing infants from TONOCARD, a decision should be made whether to discontinue nursing or to discontinue the drug, taking into account the importance of the drug to the mother.

Pediatric Use

Safety and effectiveness in children have not been established.

Adverse Reactions

TONOCARD commonly produces minor, transient, nervous system and gastrointestinal adverse reactions, but is otherwise generally well tolerated. TONOCARD has been evaluated in both short-term (n = 1,358) and long-term (n = 262) controlled studies as well as a compassionate use program. Dosages were lower in most of the controlled studies (1200 mg/day) and higher in the compassionate use program (1800 mg and more). In long-term (2–6 months) controlled studies, the most frequent adverse reactions were lightheadedness/dizziness (15.3 percent), nausea (14.5 percent), paresthesia/numbness (9.2 percent), and tremor (8.4 percent). These reactions were generally mild, transient, dose-related and reversible with a reduction in dosage, by taking the drug with food, or by therapy discontinuation. Tremor, when present, may be useful as a clinical indicator that the maximum dose is being approached. Adverse reactions leading to therapy discontinuation occurred in 21 percent of patients in long-term controlled trials and were usually related to the nervous system or gastrointestinal system.

Adverse reactions occurring in greater than one percent of patients from the short-term and long-term controlled studies appear in the following table:

	Percent of Patients Controlled Studies	
	Short-Term (n = 1,358)	Long-Term (n = 262)
NERVOUS SYSTEM		
Lightheadedness/dizziness/vertigo/giddiness	8.0	15.3
Paresthesia/numbness	3.5	9.2
Tremor/quivering/tremulousness	2.9	8.4
Confusion/disorientation/hallucinations	2.1	2.7
Altered mood/awareness	1.5	3.4
Restlessness/shakiness/nervousness	1.5	0.4
Blurred vision/visual disturbances	1.3	1.5
Discoordination/unsteadiness/walking disturbances	1.2	0.0
Anxiety	1.1	1.5
Tinnitus/hearing loss	0.4	1.5
Ataxia	0.2	3.0
Nystagmus	0.0	1.1
GASTROINTESTINAL SYSTEM		
Nausea	15.2	14.5
Vomiting	8.3	4.6
Anorexia	1.2	1.9
Diarrhea/loose stools	0.0	3.8
CARDIOVASCULAR SYSTEM		
Hypotension	3.4	2.7
Bradycardia	1.8	0.4
Palpitations	1.8	0.4
Chest pain	1.6	0.4
Conduction disturbances	1.5	0.0
Left ventricular failure	1.4	0.0
OTHER		
Sweating/cold sweat/night sweats/clammy	5.1	2.3
Headache	2.1	4.6
Tiredness/drowsiness/fatigue/lethargy/lassitude/sleepiness	1.6	0.8
Hot/cold feelings	0.5	1.5
Rash/skin lesion	0.4	8.4

An additional group of about 2,000 patients has been treated in a program allowing for the use of TONOCARD under compassionate use circumstances. These patients were seriously ill with the large majority on multiple drug therapy, and comparatively high doses of TONOCARD were used. Fifty-four percent of the patients continued in the program for one year or longer, and 12 percent were treated for longer than three years, with the longest duration of therapy being nine years. Adverse reactions leading to therapy discontinuation occurred in 12 percent of patients (usually central nervous system effects or rash). A tabulation of adverse reactions occurring in one percent or more of patients follows:

	Percent of Patients Compassionate Use (n = 1,927)
NERVOUS SYSTEM	
Lightheadedness/dizziness/vertigo/giddiness	25.3
Tremor/quivering/tremulousness	21.6
Restlessness/shakiness/nervousness	11.5
Confusion/disorientation/hallucinations	11.2
Altered mood/awareness	11.0
Ataxia	10.8
Blurred vision/visual disturbances	10.0
Paresthesia/numbness	9.2
Nystagmus	1.1
GASTROINTESTINAL SYSTEM	
Nausea	24.6
Anorexia	11.3
Vomiting	9.0
Diarrhea/loose stools	6.8
CARDIOVASCULAR SYSTEM	
Increased ventricular arrhythmias/PVCs	10.9
CHF/progression of CHF	4.0
Tachycardia	3.2
Hypotension	1.8
Conduction disturbances	1.3
Bradycardia	1.0
OTHER	
Rash/skin lesion	12.2
Sweating/cold sweat/night sweats/clammy	8.3
Arthritis/arthralgia	4.7
Myalgia	1.7
Lupus	1.6

Adverse reactions occurring in less than one percent of patients in either the controlled studies or the compassionate use program are as follows:

Nervous System: Coma, convulsions/seizures, depression, psychosis, mental change, agitation, altered taste/smell, difficulty concentrating, diplopia, dysarthria, impaired memory, increased stuttering/slurred speech, insomnia/sleeping disturbance, local anesthesia, nightmares, thirst, weakness, myasthenia gravis.

Gastrointestinal System: Abdominal pain/discomfort, constipation, dysphagia, gastrointestinal symptoms (including dyspepsia).

Cardiovascular System: Ventricular fibrillation, extension of acute myocardial infarction, cardiogenic shock, angina, AV block, hypertension, increased QRS duration, pleurisy/pericarditis, prolonged QT interval, right bundle branch block, syncope, vasovagal episodes, cardiomegaly, sinus arrest.

Pulmonary System: Respiratory arrest, pulmonary edema, pulmonary embolism, pulmonary fibrosis, alveolitis, pneumonia, pneumonitis, dyspnea.

Other: Hematologic disorder (agranulocytosis, hypoplastic anemia, anemia, leukopenia, thrombocytopenia), increased ANA, urinary retention, polyuria/increased diuresis, alopecia, cinchonism, claudication, cold extremities, dry mouth, earache, edema, fever, hiccups, itching, leg cramps, malaise, metallic/menthol taste, muscle twitching/spasm, neck pain, pain radiating from neck, pallor/flushed face, pressure on shoulder, yawning.

Leukopenia, agranulocytosis, hypoplastic anemia, and thrombocytopenia, possibly drug related, have been reported (0.10 percent) in patients receiving TONOCARD in controlled trials and the compassionate use program. These hematologic disorders usually occurred after 2–12 weeks of therapy and two patients died. These events usually occurred in seriously ill patients who were receiving concomitant drugs known to be associated with hematologic disorders. (See WARNINGS.)

Pulmonary fibrosis, pneumonitis, alveolitis, pulmonary edema, and pneumonia, possibly drug related, have been reported in patients receiving TONOCARD. The incidence of pulmonary fibrosis was 0.03 percent in controlled trials and the compassionate use program. These events usually occurred in seriously ill patients. Symptoms of these pulmonary disorders and/or x-ray changes usually occurred following 3–18 weeks of therapy and two patients died. (See PRECAUTIONS).

Drug Abuse and Dependence

Drug withdrawal after chronic treatment has not shown any indication of psychological or physical dependence.

Overdosage

The initial and most important signs and symptoms of overdosage would be expected to be related to the central nervous system. Other adverse reactions, such as gastrointestinal disturbances, may follow. (See ADVERSE REACTIONS).

Should convulsions or respiratory depression or arrest develop, the patency of the airway and adequacy of ventilation must be assured immediately. Should convulsions persist despite ventilatory therapy with oxygen, small increments of anticonvulsive agents may be given intravenously. Examples of such agents include a benzodiazepine (e.g., diazepam), an ultrashort-acting barbiturate (e.g., thiopental or thiamylal), or a short-acting barbiturate (e.g., pentobarbital or secobarbital).

Continued on next page

Information on the Merck Sharp & Dohme products listed on these pages is the full prescribing information from product circulars in use November 1, 1984.

Merck Sharp & Dohme—Cont.

The oral LD_{50} of tocainide was calculated to be about 800 mg/kg in mice, 1000 mg/kg in rats, and 230 mg/kg in guinea pigs; deaths were usually preceded by convulsions.
Studies in normal individuals to date indicate that tocainide has a hemodialysis clearance approximately equivalent to its renal clearance.

Dosage and Administration

The dosage of TONOCARD must be individualized on the basis of antiarrhythmic response and tolerance, both of which are dose-related. Clinical and electrocardiographic evaluation (including Holter monitoring if necessary for evaluation) are needed to determine whether the desired antiarrhythmic response has been obtained and to guide titration and dose adjustment. Adverse effects appearing shortly after dosing, for example, suggest a need for dividing the dose further with a shorter dose-interval. Loss of arrhythmia control prior to the next dose suggests use of a shorter dose interval and/or a dose increase. Absence of a clear response suggests reconsideration of therapy.
The recommended initial dosage is 400 mg every 8 hours. The usual adult dosage is between 1200 and 1800 mg/day in a three dose daily divided regimen. Doses beyond 2400 mg per day have been administered infrequently. Patients who tolerate the t.i.d. regimen may be tried on a twice daily regimen with careful monitoring.
Some patients, particularly those with renal or hepatic impairment, may be adequately treated with less than 1200 mg/day.

How Supplied

No. 3409—Tablets TONOCARD, 400 mg, are oval, yellow, film-coated tablets, coded MSD 707. They are supplied as follows:
NDC 0006-0707-68 bottles of 100
NDC 0006-0707-28 unit dose packages of 100.
Shown in Product Identification Section, page 421
No. 3410—Tablets TONOCARD, 600 mg, are oval, yellow, film-coated tablets, coded MSD 709. They are supplied as follows:
NDC 0006-0709-68 bottles of 100
NDC 0006-0709-28 unit dose packages of 100.
Shown in Product Identification Section, page 421
Manufactured for:
MERCK SHARP & DOHME
DIV. OF MERCK & CO., INC.
WEST POINT, PA 19486
by:
AB ASTRA
SÖDERTÄLJE, SWEDEN
A.H.F.S. Category:24:04
DC 7299002   Issued November 1984
COPYRIGHT © MERCK & CO., INC., 1984
All rights reserved

TRIAVIL® Tablets   R
Tranquilizer-antidepressant

Description

TRIAVIL®, a broad-spectrum psychotherapeutic agent for the management of outpatients and hospitalized patients with psychoses or neuroses characterized by mixtures of anxiety or agitation with symptoms of depression, is a combination of perphenazine and ELAVIL® (Amitriptyline HCl, MSD). Since such mixed syndromes can occur in patients with various degrees of intensity of mental illness, TRIAVIL tablets are provided in multiple combinations to afford dosage flexibility for optimum management.

Actions

Perphenazine—In common with all members of the piperazine group of phenothiazine derivatives, perphenazine has greater behavioral potency than phenothiazine derivatives of other groups without a corresponding increase in autonomic, hematologic, or hepatic side effects.
Extrapyramidal effects, however, may occur more frequently. These effects are interpreted as neuropharmacologic. They usually regress after discontinuation of the drug.
Perphenazine is a potent tranquilizer and also a potent antiemetic. Orally, its milligram potency is about five or six times that of chlorpromazine with respect to behavioral effects. It is capable of alleviating symptoms of anxiety, tension, psychomotor excitement, and other manifestations of emotional stress without apparent dulling of mental acuity.
ELAVIL (Amitriptyline HCl, MSD) is an antidepressant with sedative effects. Its mechanism of action in man is not known. It is not a monoamine oxidase inhibitor and it does not act primarily by stimulation of the central nervous system.

Indications

TRIAVIL is recommended for treatment of (1) patients with *moderate to severe anxiety and/or agitation and depressed mood*, (2) patients with *depression in whom anxiety and/or agitation are severe*, and (3) patients with *depression and anxiety in association with chronic physical disease*. In many of these patients, anxiety masks the depressive state so that, although therapy with a tranquilizer appears to be indicated, the administration of a tranquilizer alone will not be adequate.
Schizophrenic patients who have associated depressive symptoms should be considered for therapy with TRIAVIL.
Many patients presenting symptoms such as agitation, anxiety, insomnia, psychomotor retardation, functional somatic complaints, a feeling of tiredness, loss of interest, and anorexia have responded well to therapy with TRIAVIL.

Contraindications

TRIAVIL is contraindicated in depression of the central nervous system from drugs (barbiturates, alcohol, narcotics, analgesics, antihistamines); in the presence of evidence of bone marrow depression; and in patients known to be hypersensitive to phenothiazines or amitriptyline.
It should not be given concomitantly with monoamine oxidase inhibitors. Hyperpyretic crises, severe convulsions, and deaths have occurred in patients receiving tricyclic antidepressants and monoamine oxidase inhibitors simultaneously. When it is desired to replace a monoamine oxidase inhibitor with TRIAVIL, a minimum of 14 days should be allowed to elapse after the former is discontinued. TRIAVIL should then be initiated cautiously with gradual increase in dosage until optimum response is achieved.
Amitriptyline HCl is not recommended for use during the acute recovery phase following myocardial infarction.

Warnings

TRIAVIL should not be given concomitantly with guanethidine or similarly acting compounds, since amitriptyline, like other tricyclic antidepressants, may block the antihypertensive effect of these compounds.
Because of the atropine-like activity of amitriptyline, TRIAVIL should be used with caution in patients with a history of urinary retention, or with angle-closure glaucoma or increased intraocular pressure. In patients with angle-closure glaucoma, even average doses may precipitate an attack.
It should be used with caution also in patients with convulsive disorders. Dosage of anticonvulsive agents may have to be increased.
Patients with cardiovascular disorders should be watched closely. Tricyclic antidepressants, including amitriptyline HCl, particularly when given in high doses, have been reported to produce arrhythmias, sinus tachycardia, and prolongation of the conduction time. Myocardial infarction and stroke have been reported with drugs of this class. Close supervision is required when amitriptyline HCl is given to hyperthyroid patients or those receiving thyroid medication.
This drug may impair mental and/or physical abilities required for performance of hazardous tasks, such as operating machinery or driving a motor vehicle.
TRIAVIL may enhance the response to alcohol and the effects of barbiturates and other CNS depressants. In patients who may use alcohol excessively, it should be borne in mind that the potentiation may increase the danger inherent in any suicide attempt or overdosage. Delirium has been reported with concurrent administration of amitriptyline and disulfiram.
Usage in Pregnancy—TRIAVIL is not recommended for use in pregnant patients or in nursing mothers at this time. Reproduction studies in rats have shown no fetal abnormalities; however, clinical experience and follow-up in pregnancy have been limited, and the possibility of adverse effects on fetal development must be considered.
Usage in Children—Since dosage for children has not been established, TRIAVIL is not recommended for use in children.

Precautions

The possibility of suicide in depressed patients remains during treatment and until significant remission occurs. Such patients should not have access to large quantities of this drug.

Perphenazine
As with all phenothiazine compounds, perphenazine should not be used indiscriminately. Caution should be observed in giving it to patients who have previously exhibited severe adverse reactions to other phenothiazines.
Some of the untoward actions of perphenazine tend to appear more frequently when high doses are used. However, as with other phenothiazine compounds, patients receiving perphenazine in any dosage should be kept under close supervision. The antiemetic effect of perphenazine may obscure signs of toxicity due to overdosage of other drugs, or render more difficult the diagnosis of disorders such as brain tumors or intestinal obstruction.
A significant, not otherwise explained, rise in body temperature may suggest individual intolerance to perphenazine, in which case TRIAVIL should be discontinued.
If hypotension develops, epinephrine should not be employed, as its action is blocked and partially reversed by perphenazine.
Phenothiazines may potentiate the action of central nervous system depressants (opiates, analgesics, antihistamines, barbiturates, alcohol) and atropine. In concurrent therapy with any of these, TRIAVIL should be given in reduced dosage. Phenothiazines also may potentiate the action of heat and phosphorous insecticides.
Neuroleptic drugs elevate prolactin levels; the elevation persists during chronic administration. Tissue culture experiments indicate that approximately one-third of human breast cancers are prolactin dependent *in vitro*, a factor of potential importance if the prescription of these drugs is contemplated in a patient with a previously detected breast cancer. Although disturbances such as galactorrhea, amenorrhea, gynecomastia, and impotence have been reported, the clinical significance of elevated serum prolactin levels is unknown for most patients. An increase in mammary neoplasms has been found in rodents after chronic administration of neuroleptic drugs. Neither clinical studies nor epidemiologic studies conducted to date, however, have shown an association between chronic administration of these drugs and mammary tumorigenesis; the available evidence is considered too limited to be conclusive at this time.

ELAVIL (Amitriptyline HCl, MSD)
Depressed patients, particularly those with known manic depressive illness, may experience a shift to mania or hypomania. Patients with paranoid symptomatology may have an exaggeration of such symptoms. The tranquilizing effect of TRIAVIL seems to reduce the likelihood of these effects.
When ELAVIL (Amitriptyline HCl, MSD) is given with anticholinergic agents or sympathomimetic drugs, including epinephrine combined with local anesthetics, close supervision and careful adjustment of dosages are required.

Paralytic ileus may occur in patients taking tricyclic antidepressants in combination with anticholinergic-type drugs.

Caution is advised if patients receive large doses of ethchlorvynol concurrently. Transient delirium has been reported in patients who were treated with 1 g of ethchlorvynol and 75-150 mg of ELAVIL (Amitriptyline HCl, MSD).

Concurrent administration of amitriptyline HCl and electroshock therapy may increase the hazards associated with such therapy. Such treatment should be limited to patients for whom it is essential.

Discontinue the drug several days before elective surgery if possible.

Both elevation and lowering of blood sugar levels have been reported.

ELAVIL (Amitriptyline HCl, MSD) should be used with caution in patients with impaired liver function.

Adverse Reactions

To date, clinical evaluation of TRIAVIL has not revealed any adverse reactions peculiar to the combination. The adverse reactions that occurred were limited to those that have been reported previously for perphenazine and amitriptyline.

Perphenazine

Extrapyramidal symptoms (opisthotonus, oculogyric crisis, hyper-reflexia, dystonia, akathisia, acute dyskinesia, ataxia, parkinsonism) have been reported. Their incidence and severity usually increase with an increase in dosage, but there is considerable individual variation in the tendency to develop such symptoms. Extrapyramidal symptoms can usually be controlled by the concomitant use of effective antiparkinsonian drugs, such as benztropine mesylate, and/or by reduction in dosage. In some instances, they may persist after discontinuation of the drug.

Tardive dyskinesia may appear in some patients on long-term therapy or may occur after drug therapy with phenothiazines and related agents has been discontinued. The risk appears to be greater in elderly patients on high-dose therapy, especially females. The symptoms are persistent and in some patients appear to be irreversible. The syndrome is characterized by rhythmical involuntary movements of the tongue, face, mouth or jaw (e.g., protrusion of tongue, puffing of cheeks, puckering of mouth, chewing movements). Involuntary movements of the extremities sometimes occur. There is no known treatment for tardive dyskinesia; antiparkinsonism agents usually do not alleviate the symptoms. It is advised that all antipsychotic agents be discontinued if the above symptoms appear. If treatment is reinstituted, or dosage of the particular drug increased, or another drug substituted, the syndrome may be masked. It has been suggested that fine vermicular movements of the tongue may be an early sign of the syndrome, and that the full-blown syndrome may not develop if medication is stopped when lingual vermiculation appears.

Skin disorders have occurred with phenothiazine compounds (photosensitivity, itching, erythema, urticaria, eczema, up to exfoliative dermatitis); as well as other allergic reactions (asthma, laryngeal edema, angioneurotic edema, anaphylactoid reactions); peripheral edema; reversed epinephrine effect; hyperglycemia; endocrine disturbances (lactation, galactorrhea, gynecomastia, disturbances in the menstrual cycle); altered cerebrospinal fluid proteins; paradoxical excitement; hypertension, hypotension, tachycardia, and EKG abnormalities (quinidine-like effect). Reactivation of psychotic processes and the production of catatonic-like states have been described.

Autonomic reactions, such as dry mouth or salivation, headache, anorexia, nausea, vomiting, constipation, obstipation, urinary frequency or incontinence, blurred vision, nasal congestion, and a change in the pulse rate occasionally may occur. Other adverse reactions reported with various phenothiazine compounds, but not with perphenazine, include grand mal convulsions, cerebral edema, polyphagia, photophobia, skin pigmentation, and failure of ejaculation.

The phenothiazine compounds have produced blood dyscrasias (pancytopenia, thrombocytopenic purpura, leukopenia, agranulocytosis, eosinophilia); and liver damage (jaundice, biliary stasis).

Pigmentary retinopathy has been reported to occur after administration of some phenothiazines with a piperidylethyl side chain, but not with perphenazine which has a piperazine side chain.

Pigmentation of the cornea and lens has been reported to occur after long-term administration of some phenothiazines. Although it has not been reported in patients receiving TRIAVIL, the possibility that it might occur should be considered.

Hypnotic effects appear to be minimal, particularly in patients who are permitted to remain active.

A few patients have reported lassitude, muscle weakness, and mild insomnia.

False positive pregnancy tests, including immunologic, have been reported with phenothiazines.

ELAVIL (Amitriptyline HCl, MSD)

Note: Included in the listing which follows are a few adverse reactions which have not been reported with this specific drug. However, pharmacological similarities among the tricyclic antidepressant drugs require that each of the reactions be considered when amitriptyline is administered.

Cardiovascular: Hypotension, particularly orthostatic hypotension; hypertension; tachycardia; palpitation; myocardial infarction; arrhythmias; heart block; stroke.

CNS and Neuromuscular: Confusional states; disturbed concentration; disorientation; delusions; hallucinations; excitement; anxiety; restlessness; insomnia; nightmares; numbness, tingling, and paresthesias of the extremities; peripheral neuropathy; incoordination; ataxia; tremors; seizures; alteration in EEG patterns; extrapyramidal symptoms; tinnitus; syndrome of inappropriate ADH (antidiuretic hormone) secretion.

Anticholinergic: Dry mouth, blurred vision, disturbance of accommodation, increased intraocular pressure, constipation, paralytic ileus, urinary retention, dilatation of urinary tract.

Allergic: Skin rash, urticaria, photosensitization, edema of face and tongue.

Hematologic: Bone marrow depression including agranulocytosis, leukopenia, eosinophilia, purpura, thrombocytopenia.

Gastrointestinal: Nausea, epigastric distress, vomiting, anorexia, stomatitis, peculiar taste, diarrhea, parotid swelling, black tongue. Rarely hepatitis (including altered liver function and jaundice).

Endocrine: Testicular swelling and gynecomastia in the male, breast enlargement and galactorrhea in the female, increased or decreased libido, elevation and lowering of blood sugar levels.

Other: Dizziness, weakness, fatigue, headache, weight gain or loss, edema, increased perspiration, urinary frequency, mydriasis, drowsiness, alopecia.

Withdrawal Symptoms: After prolonged administration, abrupt cessation of treatment may produce nausea, headache, and malaise. Gradual dosage reduction has been reported to produce, within two weeks, transient symptoms including irritability, restlessness, and dream and sleep disturbance. These symptoms are not indicative of addiction. Rare instances have been reported of mania or hypomania occurring within 2-7 days following cessation of chronic therapy wih tricyclic antidepressants.

Dosage and Administration

TRIAVIL tablets are provided as:
TRIAVIL 2-25, containing 2 mg of perphenazine and 25 mg of amitriptyline HCl.
TRIAVIL 4-25, containing 4 mg of perphenazine and 25 mg of amitriptyline HCl.
TRIAVIL 4-50, containing 4 mg of perphenazine and 50 mg of amitriptyline HCl.
TRIAVIL 2-10, containing 2 mg of perphenazine and 10 mg of amitriptyline HCl.
TRIAVIL 4-10, containing 4 mg of perphenazine and 10 mg of amitriptyline HCl.

Since dosage for children has not been established, TRIAVIL is not recommended for use in children. The total daily dose of TRIAVIL should not exceed four tablets of the 4-50 or eight tablets of any other dosage strength.

Initial Dosage

In psychoneurotic patients when anxiety and depression are of such a degree as to warrant combined therapy, one tablet of TRIAVIL 2-25 or TRIAVIL 4-25 three or four times a day or one tablet of TRIAVIL 4-50 twice a day is recommended.

In more severely ill patients with schizophrenia, TRIAVIL 4-25 is recommended in an initial dose of two tablets three times a day. If necessary, a fourth dose may be given at bedtime.

In elderly patients and adolescents, and some other patients in whom anxiety tends to predominate, TRIAVIL 4-10 may be administered three or four times a day initially, then adjusted as required for subsequent adequate therapy.

Maintenance Dosage

Depending on the condition being treated, therapeutic response may take from a few days to a few weeks or even longer. After a satisfactory response is noted, dosage should be reduced to the smallest amount necessary to obtain relief from the symptoms for which TRIAVIL is being administered. A useful maintenance dosage is one tablet of TRIAVIL 2-25 or 4-25 two to four times a day or one tablet of TRIAVIL 4-50 twice a day. TRIAVIL 2-10 and 4-10 can be used to increase flexibility in adjusting maintenance dosage to the lowest amount consistent with relief of symptoms. In some patients, maintenance dosage is required for many months.

Overdosage

Manifestations—High doses may cause temporary confusion, disturbed concentration, or transient visual hallucinations. Overdosage may cause drowsiness; hypothermia; tachycardia and other arrhythmic abnormalities, such as bundle branch block; ECG evidence of impaired conduction; congestive heart failure; dilated pupils; disorders of ocular motility; convulsions; severe hypotension; stupor; and coma. Other symptoms may be agitation, hyperactive reflexes, muscle rigidity, vomiting, hyperpyrexia, or any of the adverse reactions listed for perphenazine or amitriptyline.

Levarterenol (norepinephrine) may be used to treat hypotension, but not epinephrine.

All patients suspected of having taken an overdosage should be admitted to a hospital as soon as possible. *Treatment* is symptomatic and supportive. Empty the stomach as quickly as possible by emesis followed by gastric lavage upon arrival at the hospital. Saline emetics should not be used as the antiemetic effect of perphenazine may cause retention of the saline load and subsequent hypernatremia. Following gastric lavage, activated charcoal may be administered. Twenty to 30 g of activated charcoal may be given every four to six hours during the first 24 to 48 hours after ingestion. An ECG should be taken and close monitoring of cardiac function instituted if there is any sign of abnormality. Maintain an open airway and adequate fluid intake; regulate body temperature. The intravenous administration of 1–3 mg of physostigmine salicylate is reported to reverse the symptoms of tricyclic antidepressant poisoning. Because physostigmine is rapidly metabolized, the dosage of physostigmine should be repeated as required particularly if life threatening signs such as arrhythmias, convulsions, and deep coma recur

Continued on next page

Information on the Merck Sharp & Dohme products listed on these pages is the full prescribing information from product circulars in use November 1, 1984.

Merck Sharp & Dohme—Cont.

or persist after the initial dosage of physostigmine. On this basis, in severe overdosage with perphenazine-amitriptyline combinations, symptomatic treatment of central anticholinergic effects with physostigmine salicylate should be considered. Because physostigmine itself may be toxic, it is not recommended for routine use.

Standard measures should be used to manage circulatory shock and metabolic acidosis. Cardiac arrhythmias may be treated with neostigmine, pyridostigmine, or propranolol. Should cardiac failure occur, the use of digitalis should be considered. Close monitoring of cardiac function for not less than five days is advisable.

Anticonvulsants may be given to control convulsions. Amitriptyline and perphenazine increase the CNS depressant action but not the anticonvulsant action of barbiturates; therefore, an inhalation anesthetic, diazepam, or paraldehyde is recommended for control of convulsions. The management of acute symptoms of parkinsonism resulting from perphenazine intoxication may be treated with appropriate doses of COGENTIN® (Benztropine Mesylate, MSD) or diphenhydramine hydrochloride.*

Dialysis is of no value because of low plasma concentrations of the drug.

Since overdosage is often deliberate, patients may attempt suicide by other means during the recovery phase.

Deaths by deliberate or accidental overdosage have occurred with this class of drugs.

How Supplied

No. 3328—Tablets TRIAVIL 2-10 are blue, triangular, film coated tablets, coded MSD 914. They are supplied as follows:
NDC 0006-0914-68 bottles of 100
NDC 0006-0914-28 single unit package of 100
NDC 0006-0914-74 bottles of 500.
Shown in Product Identification Section, page 420
No. 3311—Tablets TRIAVIL 2-25 are orange, triangular, film coated tablets, coded MSD 921. They are supplied as follows:
NDC 0006-0921-68 bottles of 100
NDC 0006-0921-28 single unit package of 100
NDC 0006-0921-74 bottles of 500.
(6505-00-931-4303 500's)
Shown in Product Identification Section, page 420
No. 3310—Tablets TRIAVIL 4-10 are salmon, triangular, film coated tablets, coded MSD 934. They are supplied as follows:
NDC 0006-0934-68 bottles of 100
NDC 0006-0934-28 single unit package of 100
NDC 0006-0934-74 bottles of 500.
Shown in Product Identification Section, page 420
No. 3312—Tablets TRIAVIL 4-25 are yellow, triangular, film coated tablets, coded MSD 946. They are supplied as follows:
NDC 0006-0946-68 bottles of 100
(6505-01-012-7558 100's)
NDC 0006-0946-28 single unit package of 100
NDC 0006-0946-74 bottles of 500.
Shown in Product Identification Section, page 420
No. 3364—Tablets TRIAVIL 4-50 are orange, diamond shaped, film coated tablets, coded MSD 517. They are supplied as follows:
NDC 0006-0517-60 bottles of 60
NDC 0006-0517-68 bottles of 100
NDC 0006-0517-28 single unit package of 100.
Shown in Product Identification Section, page 420
A.H.F.S. Categories: 28:16:04, 28:16:08
DC 6613122   Issued January 1983

---

*BENADRYL® (Diphenhydramine Hydrochloride), Parke, Davis & Co.

**TURBINAIRE®—see under
DECADRON® Phosphate, TURBINAIRE®
(dexamethasone sodium phosphate, MSD)**

URECHOLINE® Tablets   ℞
(bethanechol chloride, MSD), U.S.P.
URECHOLINE® Injection   ℞
(bethanechol chloride, MSD), U.S.P.

Description

Bethanechol chloride is an ester of a choline-like compound.
It is designated chemically as 2-[(aminocarbonyl) oxy] -N, N, N-trimethyl-1-propanaminium chloride.
It is a white, hygroscopic crystalline compound having a slight amine-like odor and is freely soluble in water.
URECHOLINE® (Bethanechol Chloride, MSD) is available as 5 mg, 10 mg, 25 mg, and 50 mg tablets for oral use, and as a sterile solution for subcutaneous use only.
The sterile solution is essentially neutral. Each milliliter contains bethanechol chloride, 5 mg, and Water for Injection, q.s., 1 ml. It may be autoclaved at 120° C for 20 minutes without discoloration or loss of potency.

Actions

Bethanechol chloride acts principally by producing the effects of stimulation of the parasympathetic nervous system. It increases the tone of the detrusor urinae muscle, usually producing a contraction sufficiently strong to initiate micturition and empty the bladder. It stimulates gastric motility, increases gastric tone, and often restores impaired rhythmic peristalsis.

Stimulation of the parasympathetic nervous system releases acetylcholine at the nerve endings. When spontaneous stimulation is reduced and therapeutic intervention is required, acetylcholine can be given, but it is rapidly hydrolyzed by cholinesterase, and its effects are transient. Bethanechol chloride is not destroyed by cholinesterase and its effects are more prolonged than those of acetylcholine.

It has predominant muscarinic action and only feeble nicotinic action. Doses that stimulate micturition and defecation and increase peristalsis do not ordinarily stimulate ganglia or voluntary muscles. Therapeutic test doses in normal human subjects have little effect on heart rate, blood pressure, or peripheral circulation.

A clinical study* was conducted on the relative effectiveness of oral and subcutaneous doses of bethanechol chloride on the stretch response of bladder muscle in patients with urinary retention. Results showed that 5 mg of the drug given subcutaneously stimulated a response that was more rapid in onset and of larger magnitude than an oral dose of 50 mg, 100 mg, or 200 mg. All the oral doses, however, had a longer duration of effect than the subcutaneous dose. Although the 50 mg oral dose caused little change in intravesical pressure in this study, this dose has been found in other studies to be clinically effective in the rehabilitation of patients with decompensated bladders.

Indications

For the treatment of acute postoperative and postpartum nonobstructive (functional) urinary retention and for neurogenic atony of the urinary bladder with retention.

Contraindications

Hypersensitivity to URECHOLINE tablets or to any component of URECHOLINE injection, hyperthyroidism, pregnancy, peptic ulcer, latent or active bronchial asthma, pronounced bradycardia or hypotension, vasomotor instability, coronary artery disease, epilepsy, and parkinsonism.
URECHOLINE should not be employed when the strength or integrity of the gastrointestinal or bladder wall is in question, in the presence of mechanical obstruction; when increased muscular activity of the gastrointestinal tract or urinary

---

*Diokno, A. C.; Lapides, J., Urol. 10: 23-24, July 1977.

---

bladder might prove harmful, as following recent urinary bladder surgery, gastrointestinal resection and anastomosis, or when there is possible gastrointestinal obstruction; in bladder neck obstruction, spastic gastrointestinal disturbances, acute inflammatory lesions of the gastrointestinal tract, or peritonitis; or in marked vagotonia.

Warning

The sterile solution is for subcutaneous use only. It should never be given intramuscularly or intravenously. Violent symptoms of cholinergic over-stimulation, such as circulatory collapse, fall in blood pressure, abdominal cramps, bloody diarrhea, shock, or sudden cardiac arrest are likely to occur if the drug is given by either of these routes. Although rare, these same symptoms have occurred after subcutaneous injection, and may occur in cases of hypersensitivity or overdosage.

Precautions

Special care is required if this drug is given to patients receiving ganglion blocking compounds because a critical fall in blood pressure may occur. Usually, severe abdominal symptoms appear before there is such a fall in the blood pressure.
In urinary retention, if the sphincter fails to relax as URECHOLINE contracts the bladder, urine may be forced up the ureter into the kidney pelvis. If there is bacteriuria, this may cause reflux infection.

Adverse Reactions

Abdominal discomfort, salivation, flushing of the skin ("hot feeling"), sweating.
Large doses more commonly result in effects of parasympathetic stimulation, such as malaise, headache, sensation of heat about the face, flushing, colicky pain, diarrhea, nausea and belching, abdominal cramps, borborygmi, asthmatic attacks, and fall in blood pressure.
Atropine is a specific antidote. The recommended dose for adults is 0.6 mg (1/100 grain). The recommended dosage in infants and children up to 12 years of age is 0.01 mg/kg repeated every two hours as needed until the desired effect is obtained, or adverse effects of atropine preclude further usage. The maximum single dose should not exceed 0.4 mg. Subcutaneous injection of atropine is preferred except in emergencies when the intravenous route may be employed.
When URECHOLINE is administered subcutaneously, a syringe containing a dose of atropine sulfate should always be available to treat symptoms of toxicity.

Dosage and Administration

Dosage and route of administration must be individualized, depending on the type and severity of the condition to be treated.
Preferably give the drug when the stomach is empty. If taken soon after eating, nausea and vomiting may occur.
Oral—The usual adult dosage is 10 to 50 mg three or four times a day. The minimum effective dose is determined by giving 5 or 10 mg initially and repeating the same amount at hourly intervals until satisfactory response occurs or until a maximum of 50 mg has been given. The effects of the drug sometimes appear within 30 minutes and usually within 60 to 90 minutes. They persist for about an hour.
Subcutaneous—The usual dose is 1 ml (5 mg), although some patients respond satisfactorily to as little as 0.5 ml (2.5 mg). The minimum effective dose is determined by injecting 0.5 ml (2.5 mg) initially and repeating the same amount at 15 to 30 minute intervals to a maximum of four doses until satisfactory response is obtained, unless disturbing reactions appear. The minimum effective dose may be repeated thereafter three or four times a day as required.
Rarely, single doses up to 2 ml (10 mg) may be required. Such large doses may cause severe reactions and should be used only after adequate trial

of single doses of 0.5 to 1 ml (2.5 to 5 mg) has established that smaller doses are not sufficient.
URECHOLINE is usually effective in 5 to 15 minutes after subcutaneous injection.
If necessary, the effects of the drug can be abolished promptly by atropine (see ADVERSE REACTIONS).

How Supplied

Tablets URECHOLINE are round, compressed tablets, scored on one side. They are supplied as follows:
No. 7785—5 mg, white in color, coded MSD 403.
NDC 0006-0403-68 in bottles of 100.
NDC 0006-0403-28 unit dose packages of 100.
Shown in Product Identification Section, page 421
No. 7787—10 mg, pink in color, coded MSD 412.
NDC 0006-0412-68 in bottles of 100.
(6505-00-616-7856 10 mg 100's)
NDC 0006-0412-28 unit dose packages of 100.
Shown in Product Identification Section, page 421
No. 7788—25 mg, yellow in color, coded MSD 457.
NDC 0006-0457-68 in bottles of 100.
NDC 0006-0457-28 unit dose packages of 100.
Shown in Product Identification Section, page 421
No. 7790—50 mg, yellow in color, coded MSD 460.
NDC 0006-0460-68 in bottles of 100.
NDC 0006-0460-28 in unit dose packages of 100.
Shown in Product Identification Section, page 421
No. 7786—Injection URECHOLINE, 5 mg per ml, is a clear, colorless solution, and is supplied as follows:
NDC 0006-7786-29 in box of 6 × 1 ml vials.
(6505-00-616-8947 in box of 6 × 1 ml vials.)
A.H.F.S. Category: 12:04
DC 6208427   Issued May 1980

VIVACTIL® Tablets ℞
(protriptyline HCl, MSD), U.S.P.

Description

Protriptyline HCl, a dibenzocycloheptene derivative, is a white to yellowish powder freely soluble in water.
It is designated chemically as N-methyl-5H-dibenzo[a,d]cycloheptene-5-propylamine hydrochloride. The molecular weight is 299.8. The empirical formula is $C_{19}H_{21}N \cdot HCl$.
VIVACTIL® (Protriptyline HCl, MSD) is supplied as 5 mg and 10 mg film coated tablets.

Actions

VIVACTIL is an antidepressant agent. The mechanism of its antidepressant action in man is not known. It is not a monoamine oxidase inhibitor, and it does not act primarily by stimulation of the central nervous system.
VIVACTIL has been found in some studies to have a more rapid onset of action than imipramine or amitriptyline. The initial clinical effect may occur within one week. Sedative and tranquilizing properties are lacking. The rate of excretion is slow.

Indications

VIVACTIL is indicated for the treatment of symptoms of mental depression in patients who are under close medical supervision. Its activating properties make it particularly suitable for withdrawn and anergic patients.

Contraindications

VIVACTIL is contraindicated in patients who have shown prior hypersensitivity to it.
It should not be given concomitantly with a monoamine oxidase inhibiting compound. Hyperpyretic crises, severe convulsions, and deaths have occurred in patients receiving tricyclic antidepressant and monoamine oxidase inhibiting drugs simultaneously. When it is desired to substitute VIVACTIL for a monoamine oxidase inhibitor, a minimum of 14 days should be allowed to elapse after the latter is discontinued. VIVACTIL should then be initiated cautiously with gradual increase in dosage until optimum response is achieved.

This drug should not be used during the acute recovery phase following myocardial infarction.

Warnings

VIVACTIL may block the antihypertensive effect of guanethidine or similarly acting compounds.
It may impair mental and/or physical abilities required for the performance of hazardous tasks, such as operating machinery or driving a motor vehicle.
VIVACTIL should be used with caution in patients with a history of seizures, and, because of its autonomic activity, in patients with a tendency to urinary retention, or increased intraocular tension.
Tachycardia and postural hypotension may occur more frequently with VIVACTIL than with other antidepressant drugs. VIVACTIL should be used with caution in elderly patients and patients with cardiovascular disorders; such patients should be observed closely because of the tendency of the drug to produce tachycardia, hypotension, arrhythmias, and prolongation of the conduction time. Myocardial infarction and stroke have occurred with drugs of this class.
On rare occasions, hyperthyroid patients or those receiving thyroid medication may develop arrhythmias when this drug is given.
In patients who may use alcohol excessively, it should be borne in mind that the potentiation may increase the danger inherent in any suicide attempt or overdosage.

Usage in Children
This drug is not recommended for use in children because safety and effectiveness in the pediatric age group have not been established.

Usage in Pregnancy
Safe use in pregnancy and lactation has not been established; therefore, use in pregnant women, nursing mothers or women who may become pregnant requires that possible benefits be weighed against possible hazards to mother and child.
In mice, rats, and rabbits, doses about ten times greater than the recommended human doses had no apparent adverse effects on reproduction.

Precautions

When protriptyline HCl is used to treat the depressive component of schizophrenia, psychotic symptoms may be aggravated. Likewise, in manic-depressive psychosis, depressed patients may experience a shift toward the manic phase if they are treated with an antidepressant drug. Paranoid delusions, with or without associated hostility, may be exaggerated. In any of these circumstances, it may be advisable to reduce the dose of VIVACTIL or to use a major tranquilizing drug concurrently.
Symptoms, such as anxiety or agitation, may be aggravated in overactive or agitated patients.
When VIVACTIL is given with anticholinergic agents or sympathomimetic drugs, including epinephrine combined with local anesthetics, close supervision and careful adjustment of dosages are required.
It may enhance the response to alcohol and the effects of barbiturates and other CNS depressants.
The possibility of suicide in depressed patients remains during treatment and until significant remission occurs. This type of patient should not have access to large quantities of the drug.
Concurrent administration of VIVACTIL and electroshock therapy may increase the hazards of therapy. Such treatment should be limited to patients for whom it is essential.
Discontinue the drug several days before elective surgery, if possible.
Both elevation and lowering of blood sugar levels have been reported.

Adverse Reactions

Note: Included in the listing which follows are a few adverse reactions which have not been reported with this specific drug. However, the pharmacological similarities among the tricyclic antidepressant drugs require that each of the reactions be considered when protriptyline is administered. VIVACTIL is more likely to aggravate agitation and anxiety and produce cardiovascular reactions such as tachycardia and hypotension.
Cardiovascular: hypotension, particularly orthostatic hypotension; hypertension; tachycardia; palpitation; myocardial infarction; arrhythmias; heart block; stroke.
Psychiatric: confusional states (especially in the elderly) with hallucinations, disorientation, delusions, anxiety, restlessness, agitation; insomnia, panic, and nightmares; hypomania; exacerbation of psychosis.
Neurological: numbness, tingling, and paresthesias of extremities; incoordination, ataxia, tremors, peripheral neuropathy; extrapyramidal symptoms; seizures; alteration in EEG patterns, tinnitus; syndrome of inappropriate ADH (antidiuretic hormone) secretion.
Anticholinergic: dry mouth and rarely associated sublingual adenitis; blurred vision, disturbance of accommodation, increased intraocular pressure, mydriasis; constipation, paralytic ileus; urinary retention, delayed micturition, dilatation of the urinary tract.
Allergic: skin rash, petechiae, urticaria, itching, photosensitization (avoid excessive exposure to sunlight), edema (general, or of face and tongue), drug fever.
Hematologic: bone marrow depression; agranulocytosis; leukopenia; eosinophilia; purpura; thrombocytopenia.
Gastrointestinal: nausea and vomiting, anorexia, epigastric distress, diarrhea, peculiar taste, stomatitis, abdominal cramps, black tongue.
Endocrine: gynecomastia in the male; breast enlargement and galactorrhea in the female; increased or decreased libido, impotence; testicular swelling; elevation or depression of blood sugar levels.
Other: jaundice (simulating obstructive); altered liver function; weight gain or loss; perspiration; flushing; urinary frequency, nocturia; drowsiness, dizziness, weakness and fatigue; headache; parotid swelling; alopecia.
Withdrawal Symptoms: Though not indicative of addiction, abrupt cessation of treatment after prolonged therapy may produce nausea, headache, and malaise.

Dosage and Administration

Dosage should be initiated at a low level and increased gradually, noting carefully the clinical response and any evidence of intolerance.
Usual Adult Dosage—Fifteen to 40 mg a day divided into 3 or 4 doses. If necessary, dosage may be increased to 60 mg a day. Dosages above this amount are not recommended. Increases should be made in the morning dose.
Adolescent and Elderly Patients—In general, lower dosages are recommended for these patients. Five mg 3 times a day may be given initially, and increased gradually if necessary. In elderly patients, the cardiovascular system must be monitored closely if the daily dose exceeds 20 mg.
When satisfactory improvement has been reached, dosage should be reduced to the smallest amount that will maintain relief of symptoms.
Minor adverse reactions require reduction in dosage. Major adverse reactions or evidence of hypersensitivity require prompt discontinuation of the drug.
Usage in Children—This drug is not recommended for use in children because safety and effectiveness in the pediatric age group have not been established.

Overdosage

Manifestations—High doses may cause temporary

Continued on next page

Information on the Merck Sharp & Dohme products listed on these pages is the full prescribing information from product circulars in use November 1, 1984.

Merck Sharp & Dohme—Cont.

confusion, disturbed concentration, or transient visual hallucinations. Overdosage may cause drowsiness; hypothermia; tachycardia and other arrhythmic abnormalities, for example, bundle branch block; ECG evidence of impaired conduction; congestive heart failure; dilated pupils; convulsions; severe hypotension; stupor; and coma. Other symptoms may be agitation, hyperactive reflexes, muscle rigidity, vomiting, hyperpyrexia, or any of those listed under ADVERSE REACTIONS.

Experience in the management of overdosage with protriptyline is limited. The following recommendations are based on the management of overdosage with other tricyclic antidepressants.

All patients suspected of having taken an overdosage should be admitted to a hospital as soon as possible. *Treatment* is symptomatic and supportive. Empty the stomach as quickly as possible by emesis followed by gastric lavage upon arrival at the hospital. Following gastric lavage, activated charcoal may be administered. Twenty to 30 g of activated charcoal may be given every four to six hours during the first 24 to 48 hours after ingestion. An ECG should be taken and close monitoring of cardiac function instituted if there is any sign of abnormality. Maintain an open airway and adequate fluid intake; regulate body temperature. The intravenous administration of 1-3 mg of physostigmine salicylate is reported to reverse the symptoms of other tricyclic antidepressant poisoning in humans. Because physostigmine is rapidly metabolized, the dosage of physostigmine should be repeated as required particularly if life threatening signs such as arrhythmias, convulsions, and deep coma recur or persist after the initial dosage of physostigmine. Because physostigmine itself may be toxic, it is not recommended for routine use.

Standard measures should be used to manage circulatory shock and metabolic acidosis. Cardiac arrhythmias may be treated with neostigmine, pyridostigmine, or propranolol. Should cardiac failure occur, the use of digitalis should be considered. Close monitoring of cardiac function for not less than five days is advisable.

Anticonvulsants may be given to control convulsions.

Dialysis is of no value because of low plasma concentrations of the drug.

Since overdosage is often deliberate, patients may attempt suicide by other means during the recovery phase.

Deaths by deliberate or accidental overdosage have occurred with this class of drugs.

How Supplied

No. 3313—Tablets VIVACTIL, 5 mg, are orange, oval, film coated tablets, coded MSD 26. They are supplied as follows:
NDC 0006-0026-68 bottles of 100
NDC 0006-0026-82 bottles of 1000.
Shown in Product Identification Section, page 421
No. 3314—Tablets VIVACTIL, 10 mg, are yellow, oval, film coated tablets, coded MSD 47. They are supplied as follows:
NDC 0006-0047-68 bottles of 100
NDC 0006-0047-28 unit dose packages of 100
NDC 0006-0047-82 bottles of 1000.
Shown in Product Identification Section, page 421

Metabolism

Metabolic studies indicate that protriptyline is well absorbed from the gastrointestinal tract and is rapidly sequestered in tissues. Relatively low plasma levels are found after administration, and only a small amount of unchanged drug is excreted in the urine of dogs and rabbits. Preliminary studies indicate that demethylation of the secondary amine moiety occurs to a significant extent, and that metabolic transformation probably takes place in the liver. It penetrates the brain rapidly in mice and rats, and moreover that which is present in the brain is almost all unchanged drug.

Studies on the disposition of radioactive protriptyline in human test subjects showed significant plasma levels within 2 hours, peaking at 8 to 12 hours, then declining gradually.

Urinary excretion studies in the same subjects showed significant amounts of radioactivity in 2 hours. The rate of excretion was slow. Cumulative urinary excretion during 16 days accounted for approximately 50% of the drug. The fecal route of excretion did not seem to be important.

A.H.F.S. Category: 28:16:04
DC 6380615 Issued April 1984

Information on the Merck Sharp & Dohme products listed on these pages is the full prescribing information from product circulars in use November 1, 1984.

Mericon Industries, Inc.
8819 N. PIONEER ROAD
PEORIA, IL 61615

ORAZINC CAPSULES OTC
(zinc sulfate USP)

(See PDR For Nonprescription Drugs)

Merieux Institute, Inc.
P. O. BOX 52-3980
MIAMI, FL 33152

IMOGAM® RABIES ℞
[ĭm′o-găm]
(Rabies Immune Globulin-Human)

NDC 50361-180200 2ml (300IU) pediatric vial
NDC 50361-181000 10ml (1500IU) adult vial
Supplied in tamper proof plastic box.

IMOVAX® RABIES ℞
[ĭm′o-vak]
(Rabies Vaccine Human Diploid Cell)

NDC 50361-250100 1ml IM pre-exposure/post-exposure single dose vial
Supplied in tamper proof unit dose plastic box containing disposable syringe with 1 ml of Sterile Water for Injection U.S.P. for reconstitution and sterile disposable needles for reconstitution and administration, and 1 ml vial of lyophilized vaccine.

MONO-VACC® TEST (O.T.) ℞
[mon′ō-vak]
TUBERCULIN, MONO-VACC®TEST (O.T.)
(old tuberculin)
Multiple Puncture Device

NDC 50361-772425 25 test per box
Supplied in plastic tamper proof box of 25 test/box also available test reading cards in English or Spanish.

MULTITEST® CMI™ ℞
[mul′tĭ-test]
(Skin Test Antigens for Cellular Hypersensitivity)

NDC 50361-780001
Description: Skin Test Antigens for Cellular Hypersensitivity, MULTITEST® CMI™ is a disposable, plastic applicator consisting of eight sterile test heads preloaded with the following seven delayed hypersensitivity skin test antigens and glycerin negative control for precutaneous administration: Tetanus Toxoid Antigen, Diphtheria Toxoid Antigen, Streptococcus Antigen, Old Tuberculin, Candida Antigen, Trichophyton Antigen, and Proteus Antigen.
MULTITEST® CMI™ provides a quick, convenient and uniform procedure for delayed cutaneous hypersensitivity testing.

Supplied in box of 10 individual cartons containing one preloaded MULTITEST® CMI™ per carton.

EDUCATIONAL MATERIAL

BOOKLETS
"Rabies a Preventable Disease", Merieux Institute, Inc., Editor. Written for lay public on ways to prevent rabies exposure and what to do in case of exposure. 10 each, free to Physicians; 10 each, free to Pharmacists For additional quantities and prices, please write or call.
"Rabies Concepts for the Medical Professional", William G. Winkler, Editor. Chapters dealing with rabies in humans, animals, diagnosis, pre and post-exposure prophylaxis, etiology, glossary and bibliography. 1 each, free to Physicians; 1 each, free to Pharmacists. For additional quantities and prices, please write or call.
NEWSLETTER
"Rabies Update", Merieux Institute, Inc., Editor. Quarterly newsletter on recently published articles on rabies, coverage of rabies conferences and rabies enzootic and epizootic updates.
Free to Physicians by subscription only (no charge)
Free to Pharmacists by subscription only (no charge)
VIDEO CASSETTE
"Play it Safe", Merieux Institute, Inc., Editor. A 30 second Public Service Announcement available for Professional Organization, ie. State or County Medical Societies for commercial. T.V. Broadcast warning about rabies danger and prophylaxis available in $3/4''$ V.H.S. Suitable for duplication for T.V. broadcast and with space available to identify Medical or Pharmaceutical Society available on a No Charge loan basis for duplication. Call or write for additional information.
FILM
"Rabies/La Rage", Institut Merieux, Editor. A 30 minute 16 mm. color film on rabies and its treatment in humans. Available free of charge for showing at group functions, society meetings, etc. Allow 8 weeks (minimum) prior to desired date. Call or write for additional information.
CHARTS
"Rabies—What to do in an Emergency", Merieux Institute, Inc. Editor. Wall chart and pocket chart with ACIP/CDC recommendations on what to do in rabies exposure.
Free to Physicians
Free to Pharmacists
REPRINTS
Latest articles on rabies, prophylaxis, product information, etc.
Free to Physicians
Free to Pharmacists

Merrell Dow Pharmaceuticals Inc.

Subsidiary of The Dow Chemical Company
CINCINNATI, OH 45242-9553

AVC™ Cream/Suppositories ℞
AVAILABLE ONLY ON PRESCRIPTION

Description:
AVC Cream
Each tube contains:
Sulfanilamide 15.0%
Aminacrine hydrochloride 0.2%
Allantoin 2.0%
with lactose, in a water-miscible base made from propylene glycol, stearic acid, diglycol stearate, and trolamine; buffered with lactic acid to an acid pH.
AVC Suppositories
Each suppository contains:
Sulfanilamide ....1.05 g

Aminacrine hydrochloride ....0.014 g
Allantoin ....0.14 g
with lactose, in a base made from polyethylene glycol 400, polysorbate 80, polyethylene glycol 4000, and glycerin; buffered with lactic acid to an acid pH. AVC Suppositories have an inert covering, which dissolves promptly in the vagina. The covering is composed of gelatin, glycerin, water, methylparaben, and propylparaben. Contains color additives including FD&C Yellow No. 5 (tartrazine).

Actions: AVC is a vaginal preparation combining aminacrine hydrochloride and sulfanilamide. Sulfanilamide is believed to block certain metabolic processes essential for the growth of susceptible bacteria. Aminacrine hydrochloride, a highly ionized acridine derivative, is thought to act by interfering or competing with certain hydrogen ions in microbial enzyme systems.

These ingredients are combined in a specially compounded base buffered to the pH of the normal vagina to encourage the presence of the normally occurring Döderlein's bacilli of the vagina.

Indications
Based on a review of AVC by the National Academy of Sciences—National Research Council and/or other information, FDA has classified the indications as follows:

"Probably" effective: For the relief of symptoms of vulvovaginitis where isolation of the specific organism responsible (usually *Trichomonas vaginalis*, *Candida albicans*, or *Hemophilus vaginalis*) is not possible. NOTE: When the offending organism is known, treatment with a specific agent known to be active against that microorganism is preferred.

"Possibly" effective: For the treatment of trichomoniasis, vulvovaginal candidiasis, and vaginitis due to *Hemophilus vaginalis* or other susceptible bacteria.

Final classification of the less-than-effective indications requires further investigation.

Contraindications: AVC should not be used in patients known to be sensitive to the sulfonamides.
Precautions: As with all sulfonamides, the usual precautions apply. Patients should be observed for manifestations such as skin rash or other evidence of systemic toxicity, and if these develop, the medication should be discontinued.

AVC Suppositories contain FD&C Yellow No. 5 (tartrazine), which may cause allergic-type reactions (including bronchial asthma) in certain susceptible individuals. Although the overall incidence of FD&C Yellow No. 5 (tartrazine) sensitivity in the general population is low, it is frequently seen in patients who also have aspirin hypersensitivity.

Adverse Reactions: Although some absorption of sulfanilamide may occur through the vaginal mucosa, systemic manifestations attributable to this drug are infrequent. Local sensitivity reactions such as increased discomfort or a burning sensation have occasionally been reported following the use of topical sulfonamides. Treatment should be discontinued if either local or systemic manifestations of sulfonamide toxicity or sensitivity occur.

Dosage and Administration: 1 applicatorful (about 6 g) or 1 suppository intravaginally once or twice daily. Improvements in symptoms should occur within a few days, but treatment should be continued through one complete menstrual cycle unless a definite diagnosis is made and specific therapy initiated.

If there is no response within a few days or if symptoms recur, AVC should be discontinued and another attempt made by appropriate laboratory methods to isolate the organism responsible (*Trichomonas vaginalis*, *Candida albicans*, *Hemophilus vaginalis*) and institute specific therapy.

Douching with a suitable solution before insertion may be recommended for hygienic purposes. A pad may be used to prevent staining of clothing.

How Supplied:
AVC Cream
0068-0110-13: 4 oz. tube with applicator
AVC Suppositories
0068-0111-16: Box of 16 suppositories with inserter

Product Information as of August, 1979
Suppositories are
Manufactured by
R. P. Scherer, North America
Clearwater, Florida 33518 for
MERRELL DOW PHARMACEUTICALS INC.
Subsidiary of The Dow Chemical Company
Cincinnati, Ohio 45242-9553, U.S.A.

ACCURBRON® ℞
[ăk′ĕr-brŏn]
(theophylline)

Description: Each ml of ACCURBRON (theophylline) elixir for oral use contains anhydrous theophylline 10 mg (50 mg per 5 ml teaspoonful) and alcohol 7.5% in a pleasant-tasting vehicle. Theophylline is a bronchodilator. Chemically theophylline is 1,3-dimethylxanthine.

Clinical Pharmacology: Theophylline is rapidly absorbed when given as an elixir. It acts by inhibiting the enzyme phosphodiesterase which degrades cyclic AMP. Its plasma half-life ($T\frac{1}{2}$) varies widely because of differences in the rate of metabolism. The approximate average half-life of theophylline is 4 hours with a range for children of 2 to 10 hours, and up to 16 hours for adults. Steady state levels are reached in approximately three days. Theophylline relaxes the smooth muscle of the respiratory tract and relieves bronchospasm. Its bronchodilator effect is minimal in the absence of bronchospasm.

Other actions of theophylline include dilation of pulmonary, coronary and renal arteries, increased cardiac output and CNS stimulation. Usual doses increase blood pressure only slightly. Theophylline also has a mild diuretic action.

Indications and Usage: For the relief of bronchial asthma and reversible bronchospasm associated with obstructive pulmonary diseases such as chronic bronchitis and emphysema. Epinephrine is the drug of choice in severe acute asthma attacks.

Theophylline relieves the shortness of breath, wheezing and dyspnea associated with asthma and improves pulmonary function (increases flow rates and vital capacity). In doses sufficient to produce therapeutic serum concentrations (10–20 $\mu g/ml$), theophylline may also prevent the symptoms of chronic asthma and suppress exercise-induced asthma. It is especially useful for long-term treatment of bronchospasm because tolerance to the bronchodilator effect of theophylline rarely occurs.

Corticosteroids may be given in conjunction with theophylline, if needed.

Contraindications: Patients with peptic ulcers, active gastritis, and hypersensitivity or idiosyncrasy to theophylline and other methylxanthines.

Warnings: Should not be given concomitantly with other xanthine-containing drugs because of the potential for serious toxicity from elevated xanthine serum levels. Patients who exhibit idiosyncratic reactions to other xanthines (coffee, tea, colas, cocoas, chocolates, etc.) may also have similar reactions to theophylline and ACCURBRON should be used with caution for these patients.

Precautions: *General:* Use with caution in patients with cardiovascular disease, young children and the elderly, and patients with liver, kidney and heart disease.

Laboratory Tests: Serum theophylline levels may be helpful in following the patient's response to therapy with ACCURBRON.

Drug Interactions: Theophylline increases the excretion of lithium carbonate and may enhance the sensitivity and toxicity of digitalis derivatives and sympathomimetic amines. Doses higher than usual may increase the effect of oral anticoagulants. Concomitant use with erythromycin, clindamycin, lincomycin and troleandomycin may increase theophylline serum levels.

Drug/Laboratory Test Interactions: Colorimetric methods for serum uric acid are affected by theophylline. Spectrophotometric methods for theophylline in serum are affected by furosemide, sulfathiazole, phenylbutazone, probenecid and theobromine.

Pregnancy Category C: Animal reproduction studies have not been conducted with ACCURBRON. It is also not known whether ACCURBRON can cause fetal harm when administered to a pregnant women or can affect reproduction capacity. ACCURBRON may be given to a pregnant woman only if clearly needed.

Nursing Mothers: Theophylline is excreted in the milk. Use during lactation and in women of childbearing potential requires that benefits be weighed against possible hazards to fetus or child.

Adverse Reactions: *Gastrointestinal:* loss of appetite, nausea, vomiting, gastric irritation.
CNS: irritability, especially in children, insomnia, headache, dizziness and convulsions. These side effects are usually associated with high theophylline serum levels (exceeding 20 $\mu g/ml$).
Cardiovascular: palpitations, sinus tachycardia and increased pulse rate, usually mild and transient.

Other side-effects may include increased irritation with dehydration, muscle twitching and increased SGOT levels.

Overdosage: Theophylline has a narrow therapeutic index and toxicity is likely to occur when serum levels exceed 20 $\mu g/ml$. Usual signs of overdosage are anorexia, nausea, vomiting, irritability, headache. Gross overdosage, especially in children, may lead to seizures and death without preceding symptoms of toxicity. Treatment is symptomatic (prompt induction of emesis and gastric lavage, supportive therapy, hemodialysis, etc.).

Dosage and Administration: Dosage must be individualized. Accepted therapeutic serum levels of theophylline are 10–20 $\mu g/ml$. Its metabolism may vary greatly with age, among individuals and in patients with liver, kidney and heart disease. Metabolism may be stable within the same individual. Careful monitoring for manifestations of toxicity and periodic determinations of theophylline serum levels are necessary, especially for prolonged therapy and with high doses.

Children: The following table may be used with the graduated measuring spoon for ACCURBRON:
[See table on next page].

Adults: Recommended starting dose is 100 to 200 mg (10 to 20 ml) every 6 hours. The adequacy of the dose should be determined by clinical response and periodic monitoring of theophylline serum levels. May be given after meals with water to minimize possible G.I. irritation.

Caution: Federal law prohibits dispensing without prescription.

How Supplied: As a dye-free liquid in pint bottles (NDC 0068-5002-16) with a graduated measuring spoon for ACCURBRON.

BENTYL® ℞
[bĕn′til]
(dicyclomine hydrochloride USP)
Tablets, Capsules, Syrup, Injection

Caution: Federal law prohibits dispensing without prescription.
Description:
1. Bentyl 10 mg capsules
   10 mg dicyclomine hydrochloride USP in each blue capsule.
2. Bentyl 20 mg tablets
   20 mg dicyclomine hydrochloride USP in each blue tablet.
3. Bentyl syrup
   10 mg dicyclomine hydrochloride USP in each 5 ml (1 teaspoonful) pink syrup.

Continued on next page

Information on Merrell Dow products is based on labeling in effect in August, 1984.

Merrell Dow—Cont.

4. Bentyl Injection
Ampul—2 ml—Each ml contains 10 mg dicyclomine hydrochloride USP, in water for injection, made isotonic with sodium chloride.
Vial—10 ml—Each ml contains 10 mg dicyclomine hydrochloride USP, in water for injection, made isotonic with sodium chloride. 0.5% chlorobutanol hydrous (chloral derivative) added as a preservative.
Prefilled Syringe—2 ml—Each ml contains 10 mg dicyclomine hydrochloride USP, in water for injection, made isotonic with sodium chloride.

Indications: For the treatment of Functional Bowel/Irritable Bowel Syndrome (irritable colon, spastic colon, and mucous colitis).

Clinical Pharmacology: Bentyl relieves smooth muscle spasm of the gastrointestinal tract. In two controlled clinical trials, 82 percent of the patients treated with initial doses of 160 mg daily demonstrated a favorable clinical response. In these trials, however, 61 percent of the patients on the drug experienced one or more of the following typical anticholinergic side effects: (See "Adverse Reactions" for full information).

Side effect	Dicyclomine hydrochloride (40 mg q.i.d.) %	Placebo %
Dry Mouth	33	5
Dizziness	29	2
Blurred Vision	27	2
Nausea	14	6
Light-headedness	11	3
Drowsiness	9	1
Weakness	7	1
Nervousness	6	2

In these trials, approximately 9 percent of the dicyclomine (and 2 percent of the placebo) patients discontinued therapy because of one or more of these side effects. For the most part, however, these side effects were neither severe nor intolerable, and generally did not interfere with successful treatment of the patient. In 25 percent of the patients who had these side effects, the side effects disappeared or were tolerated with no dose reduction. A total of 28 percent of the patients in these trials had their dose reduced (to an average dose of 90 mg daily) because of side effects. These patients generally continued to experience a favorable clinical response and their side effects either disappeared or were tolerated.

Contraindications: Obstructive uropathy (for example, bladder neck obstruction due to prostatic hypertrophy); obstructive disease of the gastrointestinal tract (as in achalasia, pyloroduodenal stenosis); paralytic ileus, intestinal atony of the elderly or debilitated patient; unstable cardiovascular status in acute hemorrhage; severe ulcerative colitis; toxic megacolon complicating ulcerative colitis; myasthenia gravis, and glaucoma.
Infants less than 6 months of age. (See PRECAUTIONS and WARNINGS.)

Warnings: In the presence of a high environmental temperature, heat prostration can occur with drug use (fever and heat stroke due to decreased sweating).
Diarrhea may be an early symptom of incomplete intestinal obstruction, especially in patients with ileostomy or colostomy. In this instance, treatment with this drug would be inappropriate and possibly harmful.
Bentyl may produce drowsiness or blurred vision. In this event, the patient should be warned not to engage in activities requiring mental alertness such as operating a motor vehicle or other machinery or perform hazardous work while taking this drug.
Anticholinergic psychosis has been reported in sensitive individuals given anticholinergic drugs. CNS signs and symptoms include confusion, disorientation, short-term memory loss, hallucinations, dysarthria, ataxia, coma, euphoria, decreased anxiety, fatigue, insomnia, agitation and mannerisms, and inappropriate effect. These CNS signs and symptoms usually resolve within 12 to 24 hours after discontinuation of the drug.
There are reports of infants who, in their first 3 months of life, were given dicyclomine hydrochloride syrup and evidenced respiratory symptoms (breathing difficulty, shortness of breath, breathlessness, respiratory collapse, apnea), as well as seizures, syncope, asphyxia, pulse rate fluctuations, muscular hypotonia, and coma. In some instances, these symptoms occurred within minutes of ingestion and lasted up to 20 to 30 minutes. The symptoms were reported in association with dicyclomine hydrochloride syrup therapy but the cause and effect relationship has neither been disproved nor proved. The timing and nature of the reactions suggest that they may have been a consequence of local irritation, aspiration and/or sensitization.
Worldwide, a few deaths have been reported in infants three months of age or less who had been given dicyclomine hydrochloride syrup. Two of these were reported to have been associated with excessively high dicyclomine blood levels.
Although no causal relationship between these effects, observed in infants, and dicyclomine administration has been established, Bentyl is contraindicated in infants less than 6 months of age. (See CONTRAINDICATIONS.)

Precautions: Although studies have failed to demonstrate adverse effects of dicyclomine hydrochloride in patients with prostatic hypertrophy, it should be prescribed with caution in patients known to have or suspected of having prostatic hypertrophy.
Use with caution in patients with:
- Autonomic neuropathy.
- Hepatic or renal disease.
- Ulcerative colitis. Large doses may suppress intestinal motility to the point of producing a paralytic ileus and the use of this drug may precipitate or aggravate the serious complication of toxic megacolon.
- Hyperthyroidism, coronary heart disease, congestive heart failure, cardiac arrhythmias, and hypertension.
- Hiatal hernia associated with reflux esophagitis since anticholinergic drugs may aggravate this condition.

Do not rely on the use of the drug in the presence of complication of biliary tract disease.
Investigate any tachycardia before giving anticholinergic (atropine-like) drugs since they may increase the heart rate.
With overdosage, a curare-like action may occur.
Pediatric Use (See CONTRAINDICATIONS and WARNINGS.)
Safety and effectiveness in children have not been adequately established.

Adverse Reactions: Anticholinergics/antispasmodics produce certain effects which may be physiologic or toxic depending upon the individual patient's response. The physician must delineate these.
Adverse reactions may include xerostomia; urinary hesitancy and retention; blurred vision and tachycardia; palpitations; mydriasis; cycloplegia; increased ocular tension; loss of taste; headache; nervousness; drowsiness; weakness; dizziness; insomnia; nausea; vomiting; impotence; suppression of lactation; constipation; bloated feeling; severe allergic reaction or drug idiosyncrasies including anaphylaxis; urticaria and other dermal manifestations; some degree of mental confusion and/or excitement, especially in elderly persons; and decreased sweating.
With the injectable form there may be a temporary sensation of light-headedness and occasionally local irritation.

Dosage and Administration: DOSAGE MUST BE ADJUSTED TO INDIVIDUAL PATIENT NEEDS. (See CLINICAL PHARMACOLOGY.)
Adults—oral
The only oral dose clearly shown to be effective is 160 mg per day (in four equally divided doses). Since this dose is associated with a significant incidence of side effects, it is prudent to begin with 80 mg per day (in four equally divided doses). Depending upon the patient's response, during the first week of therapy the dose should be increased to 160 mg per day unless side effects limit dosage escalation.
If efficacy is not achieved within two weeks or side effects require doses below 80 mg per day, the drug should be discontinued. Documented safety data are not available for doses of 80 to 160 mg daily for periods longer than two weeks.
Adults—intramuscular injection
The intramuscular dosage form is to be used temporarily when the patient cannot take oral medication. Intramuscular injection is about twice as bioavailable as oral dosage forms; consequently the recommended intramuscular dose is 80 mg daily (in four divided doses). Oral dicyclomine should be started as soon as possible and the intramuscular form should not be used for periods longer than one or two days.

NOT FOR INTRAVENOUS USE.

Management of Overdose: The signs and symptoms of overdose are headache, nausea, vomiting, blurred vision, dilated pupils, hot, dry skin, dizziness, dryness of the mouth, difficulty in swallowing, CNS stimulation.
Treatment should consist of gastric lavage, emetics, and activated charcoal. Barbiturates may be used either orally or intramuscularly for sedation but they should not be used if Bentyl with Phenobarbital has been ingested. If indicated, parenteral cholinergic agents such as Urecholine® (bethanecol chloride USP) should be used.

How Supplied:
20 mg Tablets debossed MERRELL 123
 Bottles of 100, 500, and 1,000 and unit dose dispenser of 100
Syrup
 16-ounce bottles
10 mg Capsules imprinted MERRELL 120/BENTYL®
 Bottles of 100, 500, and unit dose dispenser of 100
Injection
 10 ml multiple dose vials
 Boxes of five 2 ml ampuls
 Cartons of five 2 ml prefilled syringes
Product Information as of November, 1984
Injectable dosage forms manufactured by

ACCURBRON® (theophylline) - PEDIATRIC DOSAGE CALCULATION TABLE

Starting dosage: 4 mg/kg body wt every 6 hours
(All ages for first 3 days) not to exceed 100 mg (10 ml Accurbron)

Age	Body Weight lbs	kgs	3 mg/kg	4 mg/kg	5 mg/kg	6 mg/kg	7 mg/kg
Under 9 years* average dose 4–6 mg/kg/6 hrs.	10	4.5	1 ml	2 ml	2 ml	3 ml	3 ml
	20	9	3 ml	4 ml	5 ml	5 ml	6 ml
	30	14	4 ml	6 ml	7 ml	8 ml	10 ml
	40	18	5 ml	7 ml	9 ml	11 ml	13 ml
	50	23	7 ml	9 ml	12 ml	14 ml	16 ml
	60	27	8 ml	11 ml	14 ml	16 ml	19 ml
	70	32	10 ml	13 ml	16 ml	19 ml	22 ml
9—12 years* average dose 4–5 mg/kg/6 hrs.	80	36	11 ml	14 ml	18 ml	22 ml	25 ml
	90	41	12 ml	16 ml	20 ml	25 ml	29 ml
	100	45	14 ml	18 ml	22 ml	27 ml	32 ml

ACCURBRON contains 10 mg theophylline (anhydrous) per ml.
*Do not exceed this dosage without careful clinical monitoring or checking theophylline serum level because of the increased risk of side effects when serum levels exceed 20 µg/ml.

CONNAUGHT LABORATORIES, INC.
Swiftwater, Pennsylvania 18370 or
TAYLOR PHARMACAL COMPANY
Decatur, Illinois 62525 for
MERRELL DOW PHARMACEUTICALS INC.
Subsidiary of The Dow Chemical Company
Cincinnati, Ohio 45242-9553, U.S.A.
Shown in Product Identification Section, page 421

BRICANYL® ℞
[brĭk'ă-nĭl]
(terbutaline sulfate)
Injection

Name of Drug: Bricanyl® (terbutaline sulfate) Subcutaneous Injection
Description: Terbutaline sulfate, a synthetic sympathomimetic amine, may be chemically described as α-[(tert-butylamine) methyl]-3,5-dihydroxybenzyl alcohol sulfate. The structural formula is as follows:

$$\left[\text{HO-} \bigcirc \text{-CHCH}_2\text{NHC(CH}_3)_3 \right]_2 \cdot \text{H}_2\text{SO}_4$$
$$\text{OH}$$

Terbutaline sulfate is a water soluble, colorless, crystalline solid. Solutions are sensitive to excessive heat and light. Ampules should therefore be stored at controlled room temperature with protection from light by storage in their original carton until dispensed. Solutions should not be used if discolored.
Each milliliter of sterile isotonic solution contains 1.0 mg of terbutaline sulfate (equivalent to 0.82 mg of the free base), 8.9 mg of sodium chloride, and hydrochloric acid to adjust the pH to 3.0–5.0.
Actions: Bricanyl, brand of terbutaline sulfate, is a β-adrenergic receptor agonist which has been shown by *in vitro* and *in vivo* pharmacological studies in animals to exert a preferential effect on β_2 adrenergic receptors such as those located in bronchial smooth muscle. Controlled clinical studies in patients who were administered the drug orally have revealed proportionally greater changes in pulmonary function parameters than in heart rate or blood pressure. While this suggests a relative preference for the β_2 receptor in man, the usual cardiovascular effects commonly associated with sympathomimetic agents were also observed with terbutaline sulfate.
Bricanyl (terbutaline sulfate) Subcutaneous Injection has been shown in controlled clinical studies to relieve acute bronchospasm in acute and chronic obstructive pulmonary disease, resulting in a clinically significant increase in pulmonary flow rates, e.g., an increase of 15% or greater in FEV_1. Following administration of 0.25 mg by subcutaneous injection, a measurable change in flow rate is usually observed within five minutes, and a clinically significant increase in FEV_1 occurs by 15 minutes following the injection. The maximum effect usually occurs within 30–60 minutes and clinically significant bronchodilator activity has been observed to persist for 90 minutes to four hours. The duration of clinically significant improvement is comparable to that found with equimilligram doses of epinephrine.
Indications: Bricanyl (terbutaline sulfate) Subcutaneous Injection is indicated as a bronchodilator for bronchial asthma and for reversible bronchospasm which may occur in association with bronchitis and emphysema.
Contraindications: Bricanyl (terbutaline sulfate) Subcutaneous Injection is contraindicated when there is known hypersensitivity to sympathomimetic amines.
Warnings:
Usage in Pregnancy: Animal reproductive studies have been negative with respect to adverse effects on fetal development. The safe use of terbutaline sulfate has not, however, been established in human pregnancy. As with any medication, the use of the drug in pregnancy, lactation, or women of childbearing potential requires that the expected therapeutic benefit of the drug be weighed against its possible hazards to the mother or child.
Usage in Pediatrics: Bricanyl (terbutaline sulfate) Subcutaneous Injection is not presently recommended for children below the age of twelve years due to insufficient clinical data in this pediatric group.
Usage in Labor and Delivery: Serious adverse reactions have been reported following administration of terbutaline sulfate to women in labor. These reports have included transient hypokalemia, pulmonary edema and hypoglycemia in the mother and hypoglycemia in the neonatal children of women treated with terbutaline parenterally.
Precautions: Bricanyl (terbutaline sulfate) Subcutaneous Injection should be used with caution in patients with diabetes, hypertension, hyperthyroidism, and history of seizures.
As with other sympathomimetic bronchodilator agents, Bricanyl (terbutaline sulfate) Subcutaneous Injection should be administered cautiously to cardiac patients, especially those with associated arrhythmias.
The concomitant use of Bricanyl (terbutaline sulfate) Subcutaneous Injection with other sympathomimetic agents is not recommended, since their combined effect on the cardiovascular system may be deleterious to the patient.
Preparation of Other Dosage Forms: Use of the subcutaneous injection for preparation of other dosage forms, i.e., IV infusion, is inappropriate. Sterility and accurate dosing cannot be assured if the ampules are not used in accordance with *Dosage and Administration.*
Adverse Reactions: Commonly observed side effects include increases in heart rate, nervousness, tremor, palpitations and dizziness. These occur more frequently at doses in excess of 0.25 mg. Other reported reactions include headache, nausea, vomiting, anxiety, and muscle cramps. These reactions are transient in nature and usually do not require treatment. In general, all side effects are characteristic of those commonly seen with sympathomimetic amines such as epinephrine.
Dosage and Administration: The usual subcutaneous dose of Bricanyl, brand of terbutaline sulfate, is 0.25 mg injected into the lateral deltoid area. If significant clinical improvement does not occur by 15–30 minutes, a second dose of 0.25 mg may be administered. A total dose of 0.5 mg should not be exceeded within a four hour period. If a patient fails to respond to a second 0.25 mg dose within 15–30 minutes, other therapeutic measures should be considered.
Overdosage: Overdosage experience is limited. Excessive β-adrenergic receptor stimulation may augment the signs or symptoms listed under Adverse Reactions and they may be accompanied by other adrenergic effects. In the case of terbutaline overdosage, the patient should be treated symptomatically for the sympathomimetic overdosage with careful consideration to the appropriateness of any chosen therapy and possible effect on the patient's underlying disease state.
How Supplied: Bricanyl (terbutaline sulfate) Subcutaneous Injection is supplied in packages of ten 2 ml size ampules each containing one ml of solution [1.0 mg of Bricanyl (terbutaline sulfate)]. Thus, 0.25 ml of solution will provide the usual clinical dose of 0.25 mg. Ampules are expiration dated.

Product Information as of June, 1982
Manufactured by
Astra Pharmaceutical Products, Inc.
Worcester, Mass. 01606, U.S.A. for
MERRELL DOW PHARMACEUTICALS INC.
Subsidiary of The Dow Chemical Company
Cincinnati, Ohio 45242-9553, U.S.A.
U.S. Patent No. 3,937,838
Shown in Product Identification Section, page 421

BRICANYL® ℞
[brĭk'ă-nĭl]
(terbutaline sulfate)
Tablets

Name of Drug: Bricanyl® (terbutaline sulfate) tablets
Description: Terbutaline sulfate, a synthetic sympathomimetic amine, may be chemically described as α-[(tert-butylamino) methyl]-3,5-dihydroxybenzyl alcohol sulfate. The structural formula is as follows:

$$\left[\text{HO-} \bigcirc \text{-CHCH}_2\text{NHC(CH}_3)_3 \right]_2 \cdot \text{H}_2\text{SO}_4$$
$$\text{OH}$$

Terbutaline sulfate is a water soluble, colorless, crystalline solid. Tablets containing Bricanyl (terbutaline sulfate) should be stored at controlled room temperature.
Tablets containing 2.5 mg (equivalent to 2.05 mg of free base) and 5 mg (equivalent to 4.1 mg of free base) of terbutaline sulfate are white in color, and carry an inscription which represents the last 3 digits of the NDC product code (i.e., 725 for 2.5 mg tablets, and 750 for 5 mg tablets).
Actions: Bricanyl brand of terbutaline sulfate is a β-adrenergic receptor agonist which has been shown by *in vitro* and *in vivo* pharmacological studies in animals to exert a preferential effect on adrenergic receptors such as those located in bronchial smooth muscle. Controlled clinical studies in patients who were administered the drug orally have revealed proportionally greater changes in pulmonary function parameters than in heart rate or blood pressure. While this suggests a relative preference for the β_2 receptor in man, the usual cardiovascular effects commonly associated with sympathomimetic agents were also observed with terbutaline sulfate.
Bricanyl (terbutaline sulfate) tablets have been shown in controlled clinical studies to relieve bronchospasm in chronic obstructive pulmonary disease. This action is manifested by a clinically significant increase in pulmonary function as demonstrated by an increase of 15% or more in FEV_1 and $FEF_{25-75}\%$. Following administration of Bricanyl tablets, a measurable change in pulmonary function occurs at 60–120 minutes. The maximum effect usually occurs within 120–180 minutes. There is a clinically significant decrease in airway and pulmonary resistance which persists for at least 4 hours or longer. Significant bronchodilator action, as measured by various pulmonary function determinations (airway resistance, MMEFR, PEFR) has been demonstrated in studies for periods up to 8 hours.
Clinical studies were conducted in which the effectiveness of Bricanyl brand of terbutaline sulfate was evaluated in comparison with ephedrine over periods up to 3 months. Both drugs continued to produce significant improvement in pulmonary function throughout this period of treatment.
Indications: Bricanyl, brand of terbutaline sulfate, is indicated as a bronchodilator for bronchial asthma and for reversible bronchospasm which may occur in association with bronchitis and emphysema.
Contraindications: Bricanyl (terbutaline sulfate) tablets are contraindicated when there is known hypersensitivity to sympathomimetic amines.
Warnings:
Usage in Pregnancy: Animal reproductive studies have been negative with respect to adverse effects on hypertension, development. The safe use of terbutaline sulfate has not, however, been established in human pregnancy. As with any medication, the use of the drug in pregnancy, lactation, or women of childbearing potential requires that the expected therapeutic benefit of the drug be weighed against its possible hazards to the mother or child.
Usage in Pediatrics: Bricanyl (terbutaline sulfate) tablets are not presently recommended for children below the age of twelve years due to insufficient clinical data in this pediatric group.
Precautions: Bricanyl (terbutaline sulfate) tablets should be used with caution in patients with diabetes, hypertension, hyperthyroidism, and a history of seizures.
As with other sympathomimetic bronchodilator agents, Bricanyl (terbutaline sulfate) tablets should be administered cautiously to cardiac patients, especially those with associated arrhythmias.

Continued on next page

Merrell Dow—Cont.

The concomitant use of terbutaline sulfate with other sympathomimetic agents is not recommended, since their combined effect on the cardiovascular system may be deleterious to the patient. However, this does not preclude the use of an aerosol bronchodilator of the adrenergic stimulant type for the relief of an acute bronchospasm in patients receiving chronic oral terbutaline sulfate therapy.

Adverse Reactions: Commonly observed side effects include nervousness and tremor. The frequency of these side effects appears to diminish with continued therapy. Other reported reactions include headache, increased heart rate, palpitations, drowsiness, nausea, vomiting, sweating, and muscle cramps. These reactions are generally transient in nature and usually do not require treatment. In general, all the side effects observed are characteristic of those commonly seen with sympathomimetic amines.

Dosage and Administration: The usual oral dose of Bricanyl (terbutaline sulfate) tablets for adults is 5 mg administered at approximately six-hour intervals three times daily, during the hours the patient is usually awake. If side effects are particularly disturbing, the dose may be reduced to 2.5 mg three times daily and still provide a clinically significant improvement in pulmonary function. A dose of 2.5 mg three times daily also is recommended for children in the 12-15 year group. Bricanyl is not recommended at present for use in children below the age of twelve years. In adults, a total dose of 15 mg should not be exceeded in a 24-hour period.

Overdosage: Overdosage experience is limited. Excessive β-adrenergic receptor stimulation may augment the signs or symptoms listed under Adverse Reactions and they may be accompanied by other adrenergic effects. Treat the alert patient who has taken excessive oral medication by emptying the stomach by means of induced emesis, followed by gastric lavage. In the unconscious patient, secure the airway with a cuffed endotracheal tube before beginning lavage (do not induce emesis). Instillation of activated charcoal slurry may help reduce absorption of terbutaline sulfate. Maintain adequate respiratory exchange. Provide cardiac and respiratory support as needed. Continue observation until symptom-free.

How Supplied: Both 2.5 mg and 5 mg Bricanyl® (terbutaline sulfate) tablets are supplied in bottles of 100 and 1,000 and in hospital (unit dose) packs of 100 individually packaged tablets.

Product Information as of June, 1982
Manufactured by
Astra Pharmaceutical Products, Inc.
Worcester, Mass. 01606, U.S.A. for
MERRELL DOW PHARMACEUTICALS INC.
Subsidiary of The Dow Chemical Company
Cincinnati, Ohio 45242-9553, U.S.A.
U.S. Patent No. 3,937,838
Shown in Product Identification Section, page 421

CANTIL® ℞
[kăn'tĭl]
(mepenzolate bromide USP)
Tablets

Caution: Federal law prohibits dispensing without prescription.

Description: Cantil (mepenzolate bromide USP) chemically is 3-[(hydroxydiphenylacetyl) oxy]-1,1-dimethylpiperidinium bromide.
Mepenzolate bromide occurs as a white or light cream-colored powder, which is freely soluble in methanol, slightly soluble in water and chloroform, and practically insoluble in ether.
Each yellow tablet contains 25 mg mepenzolate bromide USP.

Clinical Pharmacology: Cantil diminishes gastric acid and pepsin secretion. Cantil also suppresses spontaneous contractions of the colon. Pharmacologically, it is a post-ganglionic parasympathetic inhibitor.

Radiotracer studies in which Cantil-^{14}C was used in animals and humans indicate that absorption following oral administration, as with other quaternary ammonium compounds, is low. Between 3 and 22% of an orally administered dose is excreted in the urine over a 5-day period, with the majority of the radioactivity appearing on Day 1. The remainder appears in the next 5 days in the feces and presumably has not been absorbed.

Indication: Cantil is indicated for use as adjunctive therapy in the treatment of peptic ulcer. Cantil has not been shown to be effective in contributing to the healing of peptic ulcer, decreasing the rate of recurrence or preventing complications.

Contraindications: Glaucoma, obstructive uropathy (for example, bladder neck obstruction due to prostatic hypertrophy), obstructive disease of the gastrointestinal tract (for example, pyloroduodenal stenosis, achalasia), paralytic ileus, intestinal atony of the elderly or debilitated patient, unstable cardiovascular status in acute hemorrhage, severe ulcerative colitis, toxic megacolon complicating ulcerative colitis, myasthenia gravis, allergic or idiosyncratic reactions to Cantil or related compounds.

Warnings: In the presence of high environmental temperature, heat prostration (fever and heat stroke due to decreased sweating) can occur with use of Cantil.
Cantil may produce drowsiness or blurred vision. The patient should be cautioned regarding activities requiring mental alertness such as operating a motor vehicle or other machinery or performing hazardous work while taking this drug.
With overdosage, a curare-like action may occur, i.e., neuromuscular blockade leading to muscular weakness and possible paralysis.
It should be noted that the use of anticholinergic drugs in the treatment of gastric ulcer may produce a delay in gastric emptying time and may complicate such therapy (antral stasis).

Pregnancy
Reproduction studies in rats and rabbits have shown no evidence of impaired fertility or harm to the animal fetus. Information on possible adverse effects in the pregnant female is limited to uncontrolled data derived from marketing experience. Such experience has revealed no reports of the effect of Cantil on human pregnancies. No controlled studies to establish the safety of the drug in pregnancy have been performed.

Pediatric Use
Since there is no adequate experience in children who have received this drug, safety and efficacy in children have not been established. Newborn animal studies have been undertaken that show that younger animals are more sensitive to the toxic effects of mepenzolate bromide than are older animals.

Precautions: Use Cantil with caution in the elderly and in all patients with:
Autonomic neuropathy
Hepatic or renal disease
Ulcerative colitis. Large doses may suppress intestinal motility to the point of producing a paralytic ileus and for this reason precipitate or aggravate "toxic megacolon," a serious complication of the disease.
Hyperthyroidism, coronary heart disease, congestive heart failure, "cardiac tachyarrhythmias," tachycardia, hypertension, and prostatic hypertrophy.
Hiatal hernia associated with reflux esophagitis, since anticholinergic drugs may aggravate this condition.
This product contains FD&C Yellow No. 5 (tartrazine), which may cause allergic-type reactions (including bronchial asthma) in certain susceptible individuals. Although the overall incidence of FD&C Yellow No. 5 (tartrazine) sensitivity in the general population is low, it is frequently seen in patients who also have aspirin hypersensitivity.

Nursing Mothers
It is not known whether this drug is secreted in human milk. As a general rule, nursing should not be undertaken while a patient is on a drug since many drugs are excreted in human milk.

Adverse Reactions: Xerostomia, decreased sweating, urinary hesitancy and retention, blurred vision, tachycardia, palpitations, dilatation of the pupil, cycloplegia, increased ocular tension, loss of taste, headaches, nervousness, mental confusion, drowsiness, weakness, dizziness, insomnia, nausea, vomiting, constipation, bloated feeling, impotence, suppression of lactation, severe allergic reaction or drug idiosyncrasies including anaphylaxis, urticaria and other dermal manifestations.

Overdosage: The symptoms of overdosage with Cantil progress from an intensification of the usual adverse effects to CNS disturbances (from restlessness and excitement to psychotic behavior), circulatory changes (flushing, fall in blood pressure, circulatory failure), respiratory failure, paralysis, and coma.
Measures to be taken are (1) immediate lavage of the stomach and (2) injection of physostigmine 0.5 to 2 mg intravenously, repeated as necessary up to a total of 5 mg. Fever may be treated symptomatically (alcohol sponging, ice packs). Excitement of a degree that demands attention may be managed with sodium thiopental 2% solution given slowly intravenously or chloral hydrate (100-200 ml of a 2% solution) by rectal infusion. In the event of progression of the curare-like effect to paralysis of the respiratory muscles, artificial respiration should be instituted and maintained until effective respiratory action returns.

Dosage and Administration: Usual Adult Dose: 1 or 2 tablets three times a day preferably with meals and 1 or 2 tablets at bedtime. Begin with the lower dosage when possible and adjust subsequently according to the patient's response. Since there is no adequate experience in children who have received this drug, safety and efficacy in children have not been established.

Drug Interactions: Concomitant administration of anticholinergic drugs and any other drugs which would increase the anticholinergic effects of Cantil is to be avoided.

How Supplied: Tablets (25 mg) debossed MERRELL 037: bottles of 100 and 1000
Product Information as of July, 1979
Shown in Product Identification Section, page 421

CEPACOL® Mouthwash/Gargle
[sēp'ă-cŏl]
(See PDR For Nonprescription Drugs)

CEPACOL® Throat Lozenges
[sēp'ă-cŏl]
(See PDR For Nonprescription Drugs)

CEPACOL® Anesthetic Lozenges (Troches)
[sēp'ă-cŏl]
(See PDR For Nonprescription Drugs)

CEPASTAT® Lozenges
[sēp'ă-stăt]
(See PDR For Nonprescription Drugs)

Cherry Flavor
CEPASTAT® Sore Throat Lozenges
[sēp'ă-stăt]
(See PDR For Nonprescription Drugs)

CEPHULAC® (lactulose) Syrup ℞
[sĕf'ū-lăk]
FOR ORAL OR RECTAL ADMINISTRATION
AVAILABLE ONLY ON PRESCRIPTION

Description: Lactulose is 4-O-β-D-galactopyranosyl-D-fructofuranose. The structural formula is: (See next page)
The molecular formula is $C_{12}H_{22}O_{11}$ and the molecular weight is 342.30. Each 15 ml of Cephulac contains: 10 g lactulose (and less than 2.2 g galactose, less than 1.2 g lactose, and 1.2 g or less of other sugars), water, flavoring, and coloring. Sodium hydroxide used to adjust pH.

Clinical Pharmacology: Lactulose causes a

decrease in blood ammonia concentration and reduces the degree of portal-systemic encephalopathy. These actions are considered to be results of the following:

Bacterial degradation of lactulose in the colon acidifies the colonic contents.

This acidification of colonic contents results in the retention of ammonia in the colon as the ammonium ion. Since the colonic contents are then more acid than the blood, ammonia can be expected to migrate from the blood into the colon to form the ammonium ion.

The acid colonic contents convert NH_3 to the ammonium ion $[NH_4]^+$, trapping it and preventing its absorption.

The laxative action of the metabolites of lactulose then expels the trapped ammonium ion from the colon.

Experimental data indicate that lactulose is poorly absorbed. Lactulose given orally to man and experimental animals resulted in only small amounts reaching the blood. Urinary excretion has been determined to be 3% or less and is essentially complete within 24 hours.

When incubated with extracts of human small intestinal mucosa, lactulose was not hydrolyzed during a 24-hour period and did not inhibit the activity of these extracts on lactose. Lactulose reaches the colon essentially unchanged. There it is metabolized by bacteria with the formation of low molecular weight acids that acidify the colonic contents.

Indications: For the prevention and treatment of portal-systemic encephalopathy, including the stages of hepatic pre-coma and coma.

Controlled studies have shown that lactulose syrup therapy reduces the blood ammonia levels by 25–50%; this is generally paralleled by an improvement in the patients' mental state and by an improvement in EEG patterns. The clinical response has been observed in about 75% of patients, which is at least as satisfactory as that resulting from neomycin therapy. An increase in patients' protein tolerance is also frequently observed with lactulose therapy. In the treatment of chronic portal-systemic encephalopathy, Cephulac has been given for over 2 years in controlled studies.

Contraindications: Since Cephulac contains galactose (less than 2.2 g/15 ml), it is contraindicated in patients who require a low galactose diet.

Warnings:

A theoretical hazard may exist for patients being treated with lactulose syrup who may be required to undergo electrocautery procedures during proctoscopy or colonoscopy. Accumulation of H_2 gas in significant concentration in the presence of an electrical spark may result in an explosive reaction. Although this complication has not been reported with lactulose, patients on lactulose therapy undergoing such procedures should have a thorough bowel cleansing with a non-fermentable solution. Insufflation of CO_2 as an additional safeguard may be pursued but is considered to be a redundant measure.

Use in Pregnancy

Studies in laboratory animals have not revealed a teratogenic potential of lactulose. The safety of lactulose syrup during pregnancy and its effect on the mother or the fetus have not been evaluated in humans. The physician and patient should understand that the possibility that lactulose syrup might cause damage to the human fetus cannot be excluded. Lactulose syrup should not be given during pregnancy unless, in the opinion of the physician, the possible benefits outweigh the possible risks.

Precautions: Lactulose syrup contains galactose (less than 2.2 g/15 ml) and lactose (less than 1.2 g/15 ml) and it should be used with caution in diabetics.

There have been conflicting reports about the concomitant use of neomycin and lactulose syrup. Theoretically, the elimination of certain colonic bacteria by neomycin and possibly other anti-infective agents may intefere with the desired degradation of lactulose and thus prevent the acidification of colonic contents. Thus the status of the lactulose-treated patient should be closely monitored in the event of concomitant oral anti-infective therapy.

Other laxatives should not be used especially during the initial phase of therapy for portal-systemic encephalopathy because the loose stools resulting from their use may falsely suggest that adequate Cephulac dosage has been achieved.

In the overall management of portal-systemic encephalopathy it should be recognized that there is serious underlying liver disease with complications such as electrolyte disturbance (e.g., hypokalemia) for which other specific therapy may be required.

Adverse Reactions: Cephulac may produce gaseous distention with flatulence or belching and abdominal discomfort such as cramping in about 20% of patients. Excessive dosage can lead to diarrhea. Nausea and vomiting have been reported infrequently.

Overdosage: There have been no reports of accidental overdosage. In the event of overdosage it is expected that diarrhea and abdominal cramps would be the major symptoms.

Dosage and Administration:

Oral

Adult: The usual adult, oral dosage is 2 to 3 tablespoonfuls (30 to 45 ml, containing 20 g to 30 g of lactulose) three or four times daily. The dosage may be adjusted every day or two to produce 2 or 3 soft stools daily.

Hourly doses of 30 to 45 ml of Cephulac may be used to induce the rapid laxation indicated in the initial phase of the therapy of portal-systemic encephalopathy. When the laxative effect has been achieved, the dose of Cephulac may then be reduced to the recommended daily dose. Improvement in the patient's condition may occur within 24 hours but may not begin before 48 hours or even later.

Continuous long-term therapy is indicated to lessen the severity and prevent the recurrence of portal-systemic encephalopathy. The dose of Cephulac for this purpose is the same as the recommended daily dose.

Pediatric: Very little information on the use of lactulose in young children and adolescents has been recorded. As with adults, the subjective goal in proper treatment is to produce 2 or 3 soft stools daily. On the basis of information available, the recommended initial daily oral dose in infants is 2.5 to 10 ml in divided doses. For older children and adolescents the total daily dose is 40 to 90 ml. If the initial dose causes diarrhea, the dose should be reduced immediately. If diarrhea persists, lactulose should be discontinued.

Rectal

When the adult patient is in the impending coma or coma stage of portal-systemic encephalopathy and the danger of aspiration exists, or when the necessary endoscopic or intubation procedures physically interfere with the administration of the recommended oral doses, Cephulac may be given as a retention enema via a rectal balloon catheter. Cleansing enemas containing soap suds or other alkaline agents should not be used.

Three hundred ml of Cephulac should be mixed with 700 ml of water or physiologic saline and retained for 30 to 60 minutes. Cephulac enema may be repeated every 4 to 6 hours. If the enema is inadvertently evacuated too promptly, it may be repeated immediately.

The goal of treatment is reversal of the coma stage in order that the patient may be able to take oral medication. Reversal of coma may take place within 2 hours of the first enema in some patients. Cephulac given orally in the recommended doses should be started before Cephulac by enema is stopped entirely.

How Supplied:

1 pint (473 ml containing 315 g of lactulose)
2 quarts (1.89 liters containing 1260 g or 1.26 kg of lactulose)
30 ml (containing 20 g of lactulose) unit dose containers

Product Information as of April, 1981

Store at room temperature, below 86°F (30°C). Do not freeze.

Under recommended storage conditions, a normal darkening of color may occur. Such darkening is characteristic of sugar solutions and does not affect therapeutic action. Prolonged exposure to temperatures above 86°F (30°C) or to direct light may cause extreme darkening and turbidity which may be pharmaceutically objectionable. If this condition develops do not use.

Prolonged exposure to freezing temperatures may cause change to a semisolid, too viscous to pour. Viscosity will return to normal upon warming to room temperature.

Shown in Product Identification Section, page 421

CHRONULAC®

[krŏn´ ū-lăk]
(lactulose)
Syrup

Caution: Federal law prohibits dispensing without a prescription.

Description: Chronulac is 4-O-β-D-galactopyranosyl-D-fructofuranose.

The molecular formula is $C_{12}H_{22}O_{11}$ and the molecular weight is 342.30. Each 15 ml of Chronulac contains: 10 g lactulose (and less than 2.2 g galactose, less than 1.2 g lactose, and 1.2 g or less of other sugars).

Clinical Pharmacology: Chronulac is poorly absorbed from the gastrointestinal tract and no enzyme capable of hydrolysis of this disaccharide is present in human gastrointestinal tissue. As a result, oral doses of Chronulac reach the colon virtually unchanged. In the colon, Chronulac is broken down primarily to lactic acid, and also to small amounts of formic and acetic acids, by the action of colonic bacteria, which results in an increase in osmotic pressure and slight acidification of the colonic contents. This in turn causes an increase in stool water content and softens the stool. Since Chronulac does not exert its effect until it reaches the colon, and since transit time through the colon may be slow, 24 to 48 hours may be required to produce a normal bowel movement. Chronulac given orally to man and experimental animals resulted in only small amounts reaching the blood. Urinary excretion has been determined to be 3% or less and is essentially complete within 24 hours.

Indication: For the treatment of constipation. In patients with a history of chronic constipation, lactulose syrup (Chronulac) therapy increases the number of bowel movements per day and the number of days on which bowel movements occur.

Contraindications: Since Chronulac contains galactose (less than 2.2 g/15 ml), it is contraindicated in patients who require a low galactose diet.

Warnings:

A theoretical hazard may exist for patients being treated with lactulose syrup who may be required to undergo electrocautery procedures during proctoscopy or colonoscopy. Accumulation of H_2 gas in

Continued on next page

Information on Merrell Dow products is based on labeling in effect in August, 1984.

Merrell Dow—Cont.

significant concentration in the presence of an electrical spark may result in an explosive reaction. Although this complication has not been reported with lactulose, patients on lactulose therapy undergoing such procedures should have a thorough bowel cleansing with a non-fermentable solution. Insufflation of CO_2 as an additional safeguard may be pursued but is considered to be a redundant measure.

Use in Pregnancy
Studies in laboratory animals (mice, rats, rabbits) have not revealed a teratogenic potential of Chronulac. The safety of Chronulac syrup during pregnancy and its effect on the mother or the fetus have not been evaluated in humans.
The physician and patient should understand that the possibility that Chronulac might cause damage to the human fetus cannot be excluded. Chronulac should not be given during pregnancy unless, in the opinion of the physician, the possible benefits outweigh the possible risks.

Use in Nursing Mothers
There are no data on secretion of Chronulac in human milk or effect on the nursing infant.

Use in Children
There is insufficient experience to recommend a dose of Chronulac that is safe and effective for treatment of constipation in children.

Precautions: Elderly, debilitated patients who receive Chronulac for more than six months should have serum electrolytes (potassium, chloride, carbon dioxide) measured periodically. Also, since Chronulac contains galactose (less than 2.2 g/15 ml) and lactose (less than 1.2 g/15 ml), it should be used with caution in diabetics.

Adverse Reactions: Initial dosing may produce flatulence and intestinal cramps, which are usually transient. Excessive dosage can lead to diarrhea. Nausea has been reported.

Overdosage: There have been no reports of accidental overdosage. In the event of overdosage it is expected that diarrhea and abdominal cramps would be the major symptoms. Medication should be terminated.

Dosage and Administration: The usual dose is 1 to 2 tablespoonfuls (15 to 30 ml, containing 10 g to 20 g of lactulose) daily. The dose may be increased to 60 ml daily if necessary. Twenty-four to 48 hours may be required to produce a normal bowel movement.

Note: Some patients have found that Chronulac may be more acceptable when mixed with fruit juice, water, or milk.

How Supplied:
8 fl. oz. bottles (237 ml)
30 ml unit dose cups (containing 20 g of lactulose) in trays of 10 cups
1 quart bottles (946 ml)

Product Information as of April, 1981
Store at room temperature, below 86°F (30°C). Do not freeze.
Under recommended storage conditions, a normal darkening of color may occur. Such darkening is characteristic of sugar solutions and does not affect therapeutic action. Prolonged exposure to temperatures above 86°F (30°C) or to direct light may cause extreme darkening and turbidity which may be pharmaceutically objectionable. If this condition develops do not use.
Prolonged exposure to freezing temperatures may cause change to a semisolid, too viscous to pour. Viscosity will return to normal upon warming to room temperature.
Shown in Product Identification Section, page 421

CLOMID®
[klăhm'ĭd]
(clomiphene citrate)

For prescribing information, write to:
Professional Relations Manager
MERRELL DOW PHARMACEUTICALS INC.
Subsidiary of The Dow Chemical Company
Cincinnati, Ohio 45242-9553, U.S.A.

DV® (dienestrol USP)
Cream
AVAILABLE ONLY ON PRESCRIPTION
Warnings:

1. ESTROGENS HAVE BEEN REPORTED TO INCREASE THE RISK RATIO FOR ENDOMETRIAL CARCINOMA.
Three independent case control studies have reported an increased risk ratio of endometrial cancer in postmenopausal women exposed to exogenous estrogens for prolonged periods.[1-3] This reported risk was independent of the other risk factors studied. Additionally, the incidence rates of endometrial cancer have increased since 1969 in 8 different areas of the United States with population-based cancer reporting systems, an increase that may [or may not] be related to the expanded use of estrogens during the last decade.[4]
The 3 case control studies reported that the estimated risk ratio for endometrial cancer in estrogen users was about 4.5 to 13.9 times greater than in nonusers. The risk appeared to depend on both duration of treatment[1] and on estrogen dose.[3] In view of these reports, when estrogens are used for the treatment of menopausal symptoms, the lowest dose that will control symptoms should be utilized and medication should be discontinued as soon as possible. When prolonged treatment is medically indicated, the patient should be reassessed on at least a semiannual basis to determine the need for continued therapy. Although the evidence must be considered preliminary, one study suggests that cyclic administration of low doses of estrogen may carry less risk than continuous administration;[3] it therefore appears prudent to utilize such a regimen.
Close clinical surveillance of all women taking estrogens is important. In all cases of undiagnosed persistent or recurring abnormal vaginal bleeding, adequate diagnostic measures should be undertaken to rule out malignancy.
There is no evidence at present that "natural" estrogens are more or less hazardous than "synthetic" estrogens at equiestrogenic doses.

2. ESTROGENS SHOULD NOT BE USED DURING PREGNANCY.
The use of exogenous estrogens and progestagens during early pregnancy has been reported to damage the offspring. An association has been reported between *in utero* exposure of the female fetus to diethylstilbestrol, a non-steroidal estrogen, and an increased risk of the post-pubertal development of an ordinarily rare form of vaginal or cervical cancer.[5,6] This risk for diethylstilbestrol was recently estimated to be in the range of 0.14 to 1.4 per 1000 exposures,[7] consistent with a previous risk estimate of not greater than 4 per 1000 exposures.[8] Furthermore, a high percentage of such females exposed *in utero* (30 to over 90%) has been reported to have vaginal adenosis, epithelial changes of the vagina and cervix.[9-12] Although these changes are histologically benign, it is not known whether they are precursors of adenocarcinoma. Although similar data are not available with the use of other estrogens, it cannot be presumed they would not induce similar changes.
Several reports suggest a possible association between fetal exposure to exogenous estrogens and progestagens and congenital anomalies, including congenital heart defects and limb reduction defects.[13-16] One case control study[16] estimated a 4.7 fold increased risk of limb reduction defects in infants exposed *in utero* to exogenous steroids (oral contraceptives, hormone withdrawal tests for pregnancy, or attempted treatment for threatened abortion). Some of these exposures were very short and involved only a few days of treatment. The data suggest that the risk of limb reduction defects in exposed fetuses is somewhat less than 1 per 1000.
This product is not for use in therapy of threatened or habitual abortion.
If DV (dienestrol USP) Cream is used during pregnancy, or if the patient becomes pregnant while using this drug, she should be apprised of the potential risks to the fetus, and the advisability of pregnancy continuation.

Description: DV (dienestrol USP) is a synthetic estrogen in cream form suitable for vaginal administration.
DV Cream (dienestrol cream USP)—Each tube contains:
Dienestrol USP 0.01%
with lactose, in a water-miscible base made from propylene glycol, stearic acid, diglycol stearate, trolamine, benzoic acid, butylated hydroxytoluene and disodium edetate; buffered with lactic acid to an acid pH.

Chemistry
Generic name: Dienestrol USP
Chemical name: Phenol,4,4'-(1,2-diethylidene-1,2-ethanediyl)bis,(E,E)- 4,4 -(Diethylidene-ethylene)diphenol.
Dienestrol occurs as colorless, white, or practically white needlelike crystals or as a white or practically white crystalline powder. It is odorless. It is practically insoluble in water, is slightly soluble in chloroform and fatty oils, and is soluble in alcohol, acetone, ether, and propylene glycol.

Indications: For the treatment of atrophic vaginitis and kraurosis vulvae.
DV (dienestrol USP) CREAM HAS NOT BEEN SHOWN TO BE EFFECTIVE FOR ANY PURPOSE DURING PREGNANCY AND THE USE MAY HAVE POTENTIAL RISKS TO THE FETUS. (SEE BOXED WARNING.)

Contraindications: DV (dienestrol USP) should not be used in patients with any of the following conditions:
1. Known or suspected cancer of the breast except in appropriately selected patients being treated for metastatic disease.
2. Known or suspected estrogen-dependent neoplasia.
3. Known or suspected pregnancy. (See Boxed Warning.)
4. Undiagnosed abnormal genital bleeding.
5. Active thrombophlebitis or thromboembolic disorders.
6. A past history of thrombophlebitis, thrombosis, or thromboembolic disorders.
7. Hypersensitivity to the ingredients of the cream or suppositories.

Warnings:
1. *Induction of malignant neoplasms.* Long-term continuous administration of natural and synthetic estrogens in certain animal species increases the frequency of carcinomas of the breast, cervix, vagina, and liver. There are now reports that estrogens increase the risk of carcinoma of the endometrium in humans. (See Boxed Warning.)
At the present time there is no satisfactory evidence that estrogens given to postmenopausal women increase the risk of cancer of the breast,[17] although a recent long-term followup of a single physician's practice has raised this possibility.[18] Because of the animal data, there is a need for caution in prescribing estrogens for women with a strong family history of breast cancer or who have breast nodules, fibrocystic disease, or abnormal mammograms.
2. *Gallbladder disease.* A recent study has reported a two to threefold increase in the risk of surgically confirmed gallbladder disease in women receiving postmenopausal estrogens,[17] similar to the twofold increase previously noted in users of oral contraceptives.[19] In the case of oral contraceptives the increased risk appeared after a period of use.[19]

3. *Effects similar to those caused by estrogen-progestagen oral contraceptives.* There are several adverse effects reported in association with oral contraceptives, most of which have not been documented as consequences of postmenopausal estrogen therapy, although it has been reported that there is an increased risk of thrombosis in men receiving high doses of estrogens for prostatic cancer and in women receiving estrogens for postpartum breast engorgement.[20-23] The possibility that the adverse effects reported in association with oral contraceptives may be associated with larger doses of estrogen cannot be excluded.

a. *Thromboembolic disease.* Studies have now shown that users of oral contraceptives have an increased risk of various thromboembolic, thrombotic, and vascular diseases, such as thrombophlebitis, pulmonary embolism, stroke, and myocardial infarction.[24-31] Cases of retinal thrombosis, mesenteric thrombosis, and optic neuritis have been reported in oral contraceptive users. There is evidence that the risk of several of these adverse reactions is related to the dose of the drug.[32,33] An increased risk of post-surgery thromboembolic complications has also been reported in users of oral contraceptives.[34,35] If feasible, estrogen should be discontinued at least 4 weeks before surgery of the type associated with an increased risk of thromboembolism, or during periods of prolonged immobilization.

While an increased rate of thromboembolic and thrombotic disease in postmenopausal users of estrogens has not been found,[17,36] this does not rule out the possibility that such an increase may be present, or that subgroups of women who have underlying risk factors, or who are receiving relatively large doses of estrogens may have an increased risk. Therefore, estrogens should not be used in persons with active thrombophlebitis or thromboembolic disorders, and they should not be used (except in treatment of malignancy) in persons with a history of such disorders. They should be used with caution in patients with cerebral vascular or coronary artery disease and only for those in whom estrogens are needed.

Doses of estrogen (5 mg. conjugated estrogens per day), comparable to those used to treat cancer of the prostate and breast, have been reported in a large prospective clinical trial in men[37] to increase the risk of nonfatal myocardial infarction, pulmonary embolism, and thrombophlebitis. When estrogen doses of this size are used, any of the thromboembolic and thrombotic adverse effects associated with oral contraceptive use should be considered as a risk.

b. *Hepatic adenoma.* Benign hepatic adenomas have been reported to be associated with the use of oral contraceptives.[38-40] Although benign and rare, these may rupture and may cause death through intra-abdominal hemorrhage. Such lesions have not yet been reported in association with other estrogen or progestagen preparations but should be considered in estrogen users having abdominal pain and tenderness, abdominal mass, or hypovolemic shock. Hepatocellular carcinoma has also been reported in women taking estrogen-containing oral contraceptives.[39] The relationship of this malignancy to these drugs is not known at this time.

c. *Elevated blood pressure.* Increased blood pressure is not uncommon in women using oral contraceptives and there is now a report that this may occur with use of estrogens in the menopause[41] and blood pressure should be monitored with estrogen use, especially if high doses are used.

d. *Glucose tolerance.* A worsening of glucose tolerance has been observed in a significant percentage of patients on estrogen-containing oral contraceptives. For this reason diabetic patients should be carefully observed while receiving estrogen.

4. *Hypercalcemia.* Administration of estrogens may lead to hypercalcemia in patients with breast cancer and bone metastases. If this occurs, the drug should be stopped and appropriate measures taken to reduce the serum calcium level.

Precautions:
A. General Precautions
1. A complete medical and family history should be taken prior to the initiation of any estrogen therapy. The pretreatment and periodic physical examinations should include special reference to blood pressure, breasts, abdomen, and pelvic organs, and should include a Papanicolaou smear. As a general rule, estrogen should not be prescribed for longer than 1 year without another physical examination being performed.
2. For conditions due to infection with known organisms, specific treatment should be given for the organism responsible.
3. Fluid retention—Because estrogens may cause some degree of fluid retention, conditions that might be influenced by this factor such as epilepsy, migraine, and cardiac or renal dysfunction require careful observation.
4. Certain patients may develop undesirable manifestations of excessive estrogenic stimulation, such as abnormal or excessive uterine bleeding, mastodynia, etc. In order to avoid this, the dosage should be reduced or the estrogens should be administered intermittently in the menopausal or hypogonadal patient.
5. The age of the patient constitutes no absolute limiting factor, although treatment with estrogens may mask the onset of the climacteric.
6. Oral contraceptives have been reported to be associated with an increased incidence of mental depression. Although it is not clear whether this is possibly due to the estrogenic or progestagenic component of the contraceptive, patients with a history of depression should be carefully observed.
7. Patients having pre-existing uterine leiomyomata should be observed for increased growth of myomata during estrogen therapy.
8. The pathologist should be advised of estrogen therapy when relevant specimens are submitted.
9. Patients with a past history of jaundice during pregnancy have an increased risk of recurrence of jaundice while receiving estrogen-containing oral contraceptive therapy. If jaundice develops in any patient receiving estrogen, the medication should be discontinued while the cause is investigated.
10. Estrogens may be poorly metabolized in patients with impaired liver function and they should be administered with caution in such patients.
11. Because estrogens influence the metabolism of calcium and phosphorus, they should be used with caution in patients with metabolic bone diseases that are associated with hypercalcemia or in patients with renal insufficiency.
12. Because of the effects of estrogens on epiphyseal closure, they should be used judiciously in young patients in whom bone growth is not complete.
13. Judicious assessment of the following changes in certain endocrine and liver function tests is necessary for patients receiving large doses of estrogen:
 a. Increased sulfobromophthalein retention.
 b. Increased prothrombin and factors VII, VIII, IX, and X; decreased antithrombin 3; increased norepinephrine-induced platelet aggregability.
 c. Increased thyroid binding globulin (TBG) leading to increased circulating total thyroid hormone, as measured by PBI, T4 by column, or T4 by radioimmunoassay. Free T3 resin uptake is decreased, reflecting the elevated TBG; free T4 concentration is unaltered.
 d. Impaired glucose tolerance.
 e. Decreased pregnanediol excretion.
 f. Reduced response to metyrapone test.
 g. Reduced serum folate concentration.
 h. Increased serum triglyceride, phospholipid, or cholesterol.
B. Information For The Patient
A patient package insert accompanies this drug product. This insert is available from pharmacists who carry this product and from the company upon request.

C. Pregnancy Category X
See Contraindications and Boxed Warning.
D. Nursing Mothers
As a general principle, the administration of any drug to nursing mothers should be done only when clearly necessary since many drugs are excreted in human milk.

Adverse Reactions: (See Warnings regarding reports of induction of neoplasia, adverse effects on the fetus, increased incidence of gallbladder disease, and adverse effects similar to those of oral contraceptives, including thromboembolism.)

Since there is a possibility of dienestrol absorption through the vaginal mucosa, uterine bleeding might be provoked by excessive administration of dienestrol in menopausal women. Cytologic study or D & C may be required to differentiate this uterine bleeding from carcinoma. Tenderness of the breasts and vaginal discharge due to mucus hypersecretion may result from excessive estrogenic stimulation; endometrial withdrawal bleeding may occur if use of dienestrol is suddenly discontinued. Such reactions indicate overdosage.
Menstrual irregularity may be made worse by dienestrol if a sufficient amount is absorbed. Dienestrol may cause serious bleeding in a woman sterilized because of endometriosis and in whom remaining foci of endometrium could be activated.
The following additional adverse reactions have been reported with estrogenic therapy including oral contraceptives:
1. *Genitourinary system*
Breakthrough bleeding, spotting, change in menstrual flow and cycle.
Dysmenorrhea.
Premenstrual-like syndrome.
Amenorrhea during and after treatment.
Increase in size of uterine fibromyomata.
Vaginal candidiasis.
Change in cervical eversion and in degree of cervical secretion.
Cystitis-like syndrome.
2. *Breasts*
Tenderness, enlargement, secretion.
3. *Gastrointestinal*
Nausea, vomiting.
Abdominal cramps, bloating.
Cholestatic jaundice.
4. *Skin*
Chloasma or melasma which may persist when drug is discontinued.
Erythema multiforme.
Erythema nodosum.
Hemorrhagic eruption.
Loss of scalp hair.
Hirsutism.
Urticaria.
5. *Eyes*
Steepening of corneal curvature.
Intolerance to contact lenses.
6. *CNS*
Headache, migraine, dizziness.
Mental depression.
Chorea.
7. *Miscellaneous*
Increase or decrease in weight.
Reduced carbohydrate tolerance.
Aggravation of porphyria.
Edema.
Changes in libido and/or potency.
Acute Overdosage: Numerous reports of ingestion of large doses of estrogen-containing oral contraceptives by young children indicate that serious ill effects usually do not occur. Overdosage of estrogen may cause nausea, and withdrawal bleeding may occur in females.
Dosage and Administration: 1 or 2 applicatorfuls of cream intravaginally per day for 1 or 2 weeks, then reduced to either one-half initial dosage or 1 applicatorful (about 6 g) every other day for a similar period.

Continued on next page

Information on Merrell Dow products is based on labeling in effect in August, 1984.

Merrell Dow—Cont.

Maintenance Dose
1 applicatorful of cream one to three times a week may be used after restoration of the vaginal mucosa has been effected.

How Supplied:
DV Cream
NDC 0068-0293-13: 3 oz. tube with applicator

References:
1. Ziel, H.K. and Finkel, W.D.: Increased risk of endometrial carcinoma among users of conjugated estrogens. New Eng. J. Med. 293:1167-1170, 1975.
2. Smith, D.C., Prentice, R., Thompson, D.J., and Hermann, W.L.: Association of exogenous estrogen and endometrial carcinoma. New Eng. J. Med. 293:1164-1167, 1975.
3. Mack, T.M., Pike, M.C., Henderson, B.E., Pfeffer, R.I., Gerkins, V.R., Arthur, M., and Brown, S.E.: Estrogens and endometrial cancer in a retirement community. New Eng. J. Med. 294:1262-1267, 1976.
4. Weiss, N.S., Szekely, D.R., and Austin, D.F.: Increasing incidence of endometrial cancer in the United States. New Eng. J. Med. 294:1259-1262, 1976.
5. Herbst, A.L., Ulfelder, H., and Poskanzer, D.C.: Adenocarcinoma of the vagina. New Eng. J. Med. 284:878-881, 1971.
6. Greenwald, P., Barlow, J.J., Nasca, P.C., and Burnett, W.S.: Vaginal cancer after maternal treatment with synthetic estrogens. New Eng. J. Med. 285:390-392, 1971.
7. Herbst, A.L., Cole, P., Colton, T., Robboy, S.J., and Scully, R.E.: Age-incidence and risk of diethylstilbestrol-related clear cell adenocarcinoma of the vagina and cervix. Amer. J. Obstet. Gynec. 128:43-50, 1977.
8. Lanier, A.P., Noller, K.L., Decker, D.G., Elveback, L.R., and Kurland, L.T.: Cancer and stilbestrol. A follow-up of 1719 persons exposed to estrogens in utero and born 1943-1959. Mayo Clin. Proc. 48:793-799, 1973.
9. Herbst, A.L., Kurman, R.J., and Scully, R.E.: Vaginal and cervical abnormalities after exposure to stilbestrol in utero. Obstet. Gynec. 40:287-298, 1972.
10. Herbst, A.L., Poskanzer, D.C., Robboy, S.J., Friedlander, L., and Scully, R.E.: Prenatal exposure to stilbestrol. A prospective comparison of exposed female offspring with unexposed controls. New Eng. J. Med. 292:334-339, 1975.
11. Stafl, A., Mattingly, R.F., Foley, D.V., and Fetherston, W.C.: Clinical diagnosis of vaginal adenosis. Obstet. Gynec. 43:118-128, 1974.
12. Sherman, A.I., Goldrath, M., Berlin, A., Vakhariya, V., Banooni, F., Michaels, W., Goodman, P., and Brown, S.: Cervical-vaginal adenosis after *in utero* exposure to synthetic estrogens. Obstet. Gynec. 44:531-545, 1974.
13. Gal, I., Kirman, B., and Stern, J.: Hormone pregnancy tests and congenital malformation. Nature 216:83, 1967.
14. Levy, E.P., Cohen, A., and Fraser, F.C.: Hormone treatment during pregnancy and congenital heart defects. Lancet 1:611, 1973.
15. Nora, J.J. and Nora, A.H.: Birth defects and oral contraceptives. Lancet 1:941-942, 1973.
16. Janerich, D.T., Piper, J.M., and Glebatis, D.M.: Oral contraceptives and congenital limb-reduction defects. New Eng. J. Med. 291:697-700, 1974.
17. Boston Collaborative Drug Surveillance Program: Surgically confirmed gall bladder disease, venous thromboembolism, and breast tumors in relation to post menopausal estrogen therapy. New Eng. J. Med. 290:15-19, 1974.
18. Hoover, R., Gray, L.A., Sr., Cole, P., and MacMahon, B.: Menopausal estrogens and breast cancer. New Eng. J. Med. 295:401-405, 1976.
19. Boston Collaborative Drug Surveillance Program: Oral contraceptives and venous thromboembolic disease, surgically confirmed gall-bladder disease, and breast tumors. Lancet 1:1399-1404, 1973.
20. Daniel, D.G., Campbell, H., and Turnbull, A.C.: Puerperal thromboembolism and suppression of lactation. Lancet 2:287-289, 1967.
21. Bailar, J.C., III: Thromboembolism and oestrogen therapy. Lancet 2:560, 1967.
22. The Veterans Administration Cooperative Urological Research Group: Carcinoma of the prostate: Treatment comparisons. J. Urol. 98:516-522, 1967.
23. Blackard, C.E., Doe, R.P., Mellinger, G.T., and Byar, D.P.: Incidence of cardiovascular disease and death in patients receiving diethylstilbestrol for carcinoma of the prostate. Cancer 26:249-256, 1970.
24. Royal College of General Practitioners: Oral contraception and thromboembolic disease. J. Roy. Coll. Gen. Pract. 13:267-269, 1967.
25. Inman, W.H.W. and Vessey, M.P.: Investigation of deaths from pulmonary, coronary, and cerebral thrombosis and embolism in women of child-bearing age. Brit. Med. J. 2:193-199, 1968.
26. Vessey, M.P. and Doll, R.: Investigation of relation between use of oral contraceptives and thromboembolic disease. A further report. Brit. Med. J. 2:651-657, 1969.
27. Sartwell, P.E., Masi, A.T., Arthes, F.G., Greene, G.R., and Smith, H.E.: Thromboembolism and oral contraceptives: An epidemiological case-control study. Amer. J. Epidem. 90:365-380, 1969.
28. Collaborative Group for the Study of Stroke in Young Women: Oral contraception and increased risk of cerebral ischemia or thrombosis. New Eng. J. Med. 288:871-878, 1973.
29. Collaborative Group for the Study of Stroke in Young Women: Oral contraceptives and stroke in young women: Associated risk factors. J.A.M.A. 231:718-722, 1975.
30. Mann, J.I. and Inman, W.H.W.: Oral contraceptives and death from myocardial infarction. Brit. Med. J. 2:245-248, 1975.
31. Mann, J.I., Vessey, M.P., Thorogood, M., and Doll, R.: Myocardial infarction in young women with special reference in oral contraceptive practice. Brit. Med. J. 2:241-245, 1975.
32. Inman, W.H.W., Vessey, M.P., Westerholm, B., and Engelund, A.: Thromboembolic disease and the steroidal content of oral contraceptives. A report to the Committee on Safety of Drugs. Brit. Med. J. 2:203-209, 1970.
33. Stolley, P.D., Tonascia, J.A., Tockman, M.S., Sartwell, P.E., Rutledge, A.H., and Jacobs, M.P.: Thrombosis with low-estrogen oral contraceptives. Amer. J. Epidem. 102:197-208, 1975.
34. Vessey, M.P., Doll, R., Fairbairn, A.S., and Glober, G.: Post-operative thromboembolism and the use of the oral contraceptives. Brit. Med. J. 3:123-126, 1970.
35. Greene, G.R. and Sartwell, P.E.: Oral contraceptive use in patients with thromboembolism following surgery, trauma, or infection. Amer. J. Public Health 62:680-685, 1972.
36. Rosenberg, L., Armstrong, B., Phil, D., and Jick, H.: Myocardial infarction and estrogen therapy in post-menopausal women. New Eng. J. Med. 294:1256-1259, 1976.
37. Coronary Drug Project Research Group: The coronary drug project: Initial findings leading to modifications of its research protocol. J.A.M.A. 214:1303-1313, 1970.
38. Baum, J., Holtz, F., Bookstein, J.J., and Klein, E.W.: Possible association between benign hepatomas and oral contraceptives. Lancet 2:926-928, 1973.
39. Mays, E.T., Christopherson, W.M., Mahr, M.M., and Williams, H.C.: Hepatic changes in young women ingesting contraceptive steroids. Hepatic hemorrhage and primary hepatic tumors. J.A.M.A. 235:730-732, 1976.
40. Edmondson, H., Henderson, A.B., and Benton, B.: Liver-cell adenomas associated with the use of oral contraceptives. New Eng. J. Med. 294:470-472, 1976.
41. Pfeffer, R.I. and Van Den Noort, S.: Estrogen use and stroke risk in postmenopausal women. Amer. J. Epidem. 103:445-456, 1976.

Product Information as of August, 1979
DV Suppositories are manufactured by R. P. Scherer, North America

Clearwater, Florida 33518 for
MERRELL DOW PHARMACEUTICALS INC.
Subsidiary of The Dow Chemical Company
Cincinnati, Ohio 45242-9553, U.S.A.

HIPREX® ℞
[hĭp′rĕx]
(methenamine hippurate)

AVAILABLE ONLY ON PRESCRIPTION

Description: Hiprex (methenamine hippurate) is the hippuric acid salt of methenamine (hexamethylenetetramine).

Actions: Microbiology: Hiprex (methenamine hippurate) has antibacterial activity because the methenamine component is hydrolyzed to formaldehyde in acid urine. Hippuric acid, the other component, has some antibacterial activity and also acts to keep the urine acid. The drug is generally active against *E. coli*, enterococci and staphylococci. *Enterobacter aerogenes* is generally resistant. The urine must be kept sufficiently acid for urea-splitting organisms such as *Proteus* and *Pseudomonas* to be inhibited.

Human Pharmacology: Within $\frac{1}{2}$ hour after ingestion of a single 1-gram dose of Hiprex, antibacterial activity is demonstrable in the urine. Urine has continuous antibacterial activity when Hiprex is administered at the recommended dosage schedule of 1 gram twice daily. Over 90% of methenamine moiety is excreted in the urine within 24 hours after administration of a single 1-gram dose. Similarly, the hippurate moiety is rapidly absorbed and excreted, and it reaches the urine by both tubular secretion and glomerular filtration. This action may be important in older patients or in those with some degree of renal impairment.

Indications: Hiprex is indicated for prophylactic or suppressive treatment of frequently recurring urinary tract infections when long-term therapy is considered necessary. This drug should only be used after eradication of the infection by other appropriate antimicrobial agents.

Contraindications: Hiprex (methenamine hippurate) is contraindicated in patients with renal insufficiency, severe hepatic insufficiency, or severe dehydration. Methenamine preparations should not be given to patients taking sulfonamides because some sulfonamides may form an insoluble precipitate with formaldehyde in the urine.

Warnings: Large doses of methenamine (8 grams daily for 3 to 4 weeks) have caused bladder irritation, painful and frequent micturition, albuminuria, and gross hematuria.

Precautions:
1. Care should be taken to maintain an acid pH of the urine, especially when treating infections due to urea-splitting organisms such as *Proteus* and strains of *Pseudomonas*.
2. In a few instances in one study, the serum transaminase levels were slightly elevated during treatment but returned to normal while the patients were still taking Hiprex. Because of this report, it is recommended that liver function studies be performed periodically on patients taking the drug, especially those with liver dysfunction.
3. *Use in pregnancy:* In early pregnancy the safe use of Hiprex is not established. In the last trimester, safety is suggested, but not definitely proved. No adverse effects on the fetus were seen in studies in pregnant rats and rabbits.

Hiprex taken during pregnancy can interfere with laboratory tests of urine estriol (resulting in unmeasurably low values) when acid hydrolysis is used in the laboratory procedure. This interference is due to the presence in the urine of methenamine and/or formaldehyde. Enzymatic hydrolysis, in place of acid hydrolysis, will circumvent this problem.

4. This product contains FD&C Yellow No. 5 (tartrazine), which may cause allergic-type reactions (including bronchial asthma) in certain susceptible individuals. Although the overall incidence of FD&C Yellow No. 5 (tartrazine) sensitivity in the

general population is low, it is frequently seen in patients who also have aspirin hypersensitivity.
Adverse Reactions: Minor adverse reactions have been reported in less than 3.5% of patients treated. These reactions have included nausea, upset stomach, dysuria, and rash.
Dosage and Administration:
1 tablet (1.0 g) twice daily (morning and night) for adults and children over 12 years of age.
½ to 1 tablet (0.5 to 1.0 g) twice daily (morning and night) for children 6 to 12 years of age.
Since the antibacterial activity of Hiprex is greater in acid urine, restriction of alkalinizing foods and medications is desirable. If necessary, as indicated by urinary pH and clinical response, supplemental acidification of the urine should be instituted. The efficacy of therapy should be monitored by repeated urine cultures.
How Supplied: 1-gram scored, capsule-shaped yellow tablets debossed MERRELL 277 in bottles of 100

Product Information as of August, 1979
Shown in Product Identification Section, page 421

IMFERON®
[ĭm'fĕr-ŏn]
(iron dextran injection USP)
AVAILABLE ONLY ON PRESCRIPTION
Warning:

> THE PARENTERAL USE OF COMPLEXES OF IRON AND CARBOHYDRATES HAS RESULTED IN FATAL ANAPHYLACTIC-TYPE REACTIONS. DEATHS ASSOCIATED WITH SUCH ADMINISTRATION HAVE BEEN REPORTED. THEREFORE, IMFERON SHOULD BE USED ONLY IN THOSE PATIENTS IN WHOM THE INDICATIONS HAVE BEEN CLEARLY ESTABLISHED AND LABORATORY INVESTIGATIONS CONFIRM AN IRON DEFICIENT STATE NOT AMENABLE TO ORAL IRON THERAPY.

Description: Imferon is a dark brown, slightly viscous liquid complex of ferric hydroxide and dextran in a 0.9% sodium chloride solution for injection. It contains the equivalent of 50 mg elemental iron (as an iron dextran complex) per ml. Multiple dose vial also contains 0.5% phenol.
Action: The iron dextran complex is dissociated by the reticuloendothelial system, and the ferric iron is transported by transferrin and incorporated into hemoglobin.
Indications: Intravenous or intramuscular injections of iron dextran USP are advisable solely for use in those patients in whom an iron deficiency state is present, its cause has been determined, and, if possible, corrected, and in whom oral administration of iron is unsatisfactory or impossible.
Contraindications: Hypersensitivity to the product. All anemias other than iron deficiency anemia.
Warnings: Two ml of undiluted iron dextran is the maximum recommended daily dose. (See DOSAGE AND ADMINISTRATION.)
Large intravenous doses, such as those used in Total Dose Infusions, may be associated with an increased incidence of adverse effects, particularly, delayed reactions typified by arthralgia, myalgia, and fever.
The following pattern of signs/symptoms has been reported as a delayed (1-2 days) reaction at recommended doses: modest-high fever, chills, backache, headache, myalgia, malaise, nausea, vomiting, and dizziness. These reactions have been reported in an unexpectedly high incidence with certain batches. Therefore, in estimating the benefit/risk of treatment for an individual patient, it must be assumed that there is a real possibility that such a delayed reaction may occur.
This preparation should be used with extreme care in patients with serious impairment of liver function.

A risk of carcinogenesis may attend the intramuscular injection of iron-carbohydrate complexes. Such complexes have been found under experimental conditions to produce sarcomas when large doses are injected in rats, mice, and rabbits, and possibly in hamsters. The number of tumors produced was relatively small. Such tumors have not been produced in guinea pigs.
The long latent period between the injection of a potential carcinogen and the appearance of a tumor makes it impossible to measure the risk in man accurately. There have, however, been several reports in the literature describing tumors at the injection site in humans who had previously received intramuscular injections of iron-carbohydrate complexes.
Use in Pregnancy
Animal studies have shown that administration of iron dextran injection USP during pregnancy caused an increase in the number of stillbirths and fetal anomalies, and a decrease in neonatal survival. Thus, iron dextran injection USP should not be used in pregnancy, or in women of childbearing potential unless, in the judgment of the physician, the potential benefits outweigh the possible hazards.
Precautions: Unwarranted therapy with parenteral iron will cause excess storage of iron with the consequent possibility of exogenous hemosiderosis. Such iron overload is particularly apt to occur in patients with hemoglobinopathies and other refractory anemias that might be erroneously diagnosed as iron deficiency anemias.
Imferon should be used with caution in individuals with histories of significant allergies and/or asthma.
Epinephrine should be immediately available in the event of acute hypersensitivity reactions. (Usual adult dose: 0.5 ml of a 1:1000 solution, by subcutaneous or intramuscular injection.)
Patients with both iron deficiency anemia and rheumatoid arthritis may have an acute exacerbation of joint pain and swelling following the intravenous administration of Imferon.
Reports in the literature from countries outside the United States (in particular, New Zealand) have suggested that the use of intramuscular iron dextran in neonates has been associated with an increased incidence of gram-negative sepsis, primarily due to *E. coli*. This effect from the use of Imferon in the United States has not been reported.
Drug/Laboratory Test Interactions
Interactions described below have been reported with intravenous doses of Imferon larger than the maximum dose (2 ml) in the currently approved labeling. (See WARNINGS.)
A. Serum iron: Caution should be used in interpreting results of serum iron values when blood samples are obtained within 1 or 2 weeks following administration of large doses of Imferon.
B. Serum discoloration: An intravenous injection of 5 ml of Imferon has been reported to impart a brownish color to serum from a blood sample drawn 4 hours after Imferon administration.
Interference with Laboratory Tests
Bone scans involving Tc-99 m diphosphonate have been reported to show dense, crescentic areas of activity following the contour of the iliac crest, visualized 1 to 6 days after intramuscular injections of Imferon.
Adverse Reactions: Anaphylactic reactions including fatal anaphylaxis; other hypersensitivity reactions including dyspnea, urticaria, other rashes and itching, arthralgia, myalgia, febrile episodes, and sweating; variable degree of soreness and inflammation at or near injection site, including sterile abscesses (I.M. injection); brown skin discoloration at injection site (I.M. injection); lymphadenopathy; local phlebitis at injection site (I.V. injection); peripheral vascular flushing with overly rapid I.V. administration; hypotensive reaction; convulsions; possible arthritic reactivation in patients with quiescent rheumatoid arthritis; leucocytosis, frequently with fever; headache, backache, dizziness, malaise, transitory paresthesias, nausea, vomiting, and shivering.

Dosage and Administration:
Oral iron should be discontinued prior to administration of Imferon.
Dosage
Serum ferritin assays have been shown to correlate satisfactorily with iron stores. It is recommended that periodic serum ferritin testing be done in patients who are administered Imferon over prolonged periods.
Iron Deficiency Anemia
Periodic hematologic determinations should be used as a guide in therapy. It should be recognized that iron storage may lag behind the appearance of normal blood morphology. Although there are significant variations in body build and weight distribution among males and females, the accompanying table and formula represent a simple and convenient means for estimating the total iron required. This total iron requirement reflects the amount of iron needed to restore hemoglobin to normal or near normal levels plus an additional 50% allowance to provide adequate replenishment of iron stores in most individuals with moderately or severely reduced levels of hemoglobin. Factors contributing to the formula are shown below.
[See table above].

$$\frac{\text{mg blood iron}}{\text{lb body weight}} = \frac{\text{ml blood}}{\text{lb body weight}} \times \frac{\text{g hemoglobin}}{\text{ml blood}} \times \frac{\text{mg iron}}{\text{g hemoglobin}}$$

a) Blood volume	8.5% body weight
b) Normal hemoglobin (males and females)	
over 30 pounds	14.8 g/dl
(30 pounds or less	12.0 g/dl)
c) Iron content of hemoglobin	0.34%
d) Hemoglobin deficit	
e) Weight	

Based on the above factors, individuals with normal hemoglobin levels will have approximately 20 mg of blood iron per pound of body weight.
The formula should not be used for patients weighing 30 pounds or less. (Adjustments have been made in the table values to account for the lower normal hemoglobins for those weighing 30 pounds or less.)
Note: The table and accompanying formula are applicable for dosage determinations only in patients with *iron deficiency anemia;* they are not to be used for dosage determinations in patients requiring *iron replacement for blood loss.*
[See table on next page].
Iron Replacement for Blood Loss
Some individuals sustain blood losses on an intermittent or repetitive basis. Such blood losses may occur periodically in patients with hemorrhagic diatheses (familial telangiectasia; hemophilia; gastrointestinal bleeding) and on a repetitive basis from procedures such as renal hemodialysis.
Iron therapy in these patients should be directed toward replacement of the equivalent amount of iron represented in the blood loss. The table and formula described under iron deficiency anemia are *not* applicable for simple iron replacement values.
Quantitative estimates of the individual's periodic blood loss and hematocrit during the bleeding episode provide a convenient method for the calculation of the required iron dose.

Continued on next page

Information on Merrell Dow products is based on labeling in effect in August, 1984.

Merrell Dow—Cont.

The formula shown below is based on the approximation that 1 ml of normocytic, normochromic red cells contains 1 mg of elemental iron:

Replacement iron (in mg) = Blood loss (in ml) × hematocrit

Example: Blood loss of 500 ml with 20% hematocrit

Replacement iron = 500 × 0.20 = 100 mg

Imferon dose = $\frac{100 \text{ mg}}{50}$ = 2 ml

Administration
The total amount of Imferon required for the treatment of *iron deficiency anemia* or *iron replacement for blood loss* is determined from the table or appropriate formula. (See Dosage.)

Intravenous Injection
Test dose: Prior to receiving their first Imferon therapeutic dose, all patients should be given an intravenous test dose of 0.5 ml. Although anaphylactic reactions known to occur following Imferon administration are usually evident within a few minutes, or sooner, it is recommended that a period of an hour or longer elapse before the remainder of the initial therapeutic dose is given.

Individual doses of 2 ml or less may be given on a daily basis until the calculated total amount required has been reached.

Imferon is given undiluted and *slowly* (1 ml or less per minute).

Intramuscular Injection
Test dose: Prior to receiving their first Imferon therapeutic dose, all patients should be given an intramuscular test dose of 0.5 ml, administered in the same recommended test site and by the same technique as described in the last paragraph of this section. Although anaphylactic reactions known to occur following Imferon administration are usually evident within a few minutes or sooner, it is recommended that a period of an hour or longer elapse before the remainder of the initial therapeutic dose is given.

If no adverse reactions are observed, Imferon can be given according to the following schedule until the calculated total amount required has been reached. Each day's dose should ordinarily not exceed 0.5 ml (25 mg of iron) for infants under 10 lb; 1.0 ml (50 mg of iron) for children under 20 lb; 2.0 ml (100 mg of iron) for other patients.

Imferon should be injected only into the muscle mass of the upper outer quadrant of the buttock —never into the arm or other exposed areas—and should be injected deeply, with a 2-inch or 3-inch 19 or 20 gauge needle. If the patient is standing, he should be bearing his weight on the leg opposite the injection site, or if in bed, he should be in the lateral position with injection site uppermost. To avoid injection or leakage into the subcutaneous tissue, a Z-track technique (displacement of the skin laterally prior to injection) is recommended.

How Supplied:
For intramuscular or intravenous use
2 ml ampuls
NDC 0068-0050-09: boxes of 10
For intramuscular use ONLY
10 ml multiple dose vial containing 0.5% phenol as a preservative
NDC 0068-0052-22: boxes of 2

Imferon is distributed under license from Fisons Pharmaceuticals, Ltd.

Product Information as of August, 1983
Manufactured by
Fisons plc
Pharmaceutical Division
Loughborough, England for
MERRELL DOW PHARMACEUTICALS INC.
Subsidiary of The Dow Chemical Company
Cincinnati, Ohio 45242-9553, U.S.A.

LORELCO® Tablets ℞
[lō-rĕl'cō]
(probucol tablets)

Caution: Federal law prohibits dispensing without prescription.

Description: Lorelco (probucol) film-coated tablets for oral administration contain 250 mg of probucol per tablet. Lorelco is an agent for the reduction of elevated serum cholesterol. The chemical name is 4,4'-(isopropylidenedithio) bis (2,6-di-t-butylphenol). Its chemical structure does not resemble that of any other available cholesterol-lowering agent. It is lipophilic.

(See next column)

Clinical Pharmacology: Lorelco (probucol) lowers serum cholesterol and has relatively little effect on serum triglycerides. Patients responding to probucol exhibit a decrease in low density lipoprotein cholesterol. Cholesterol is reduced not only in the low density lipoprotein fraction, but also in some high density lipoprotein fractions with proportionately greater effect on the high density portion in some patients. Epidemiological studies have shown that both low HDL-cholesterol and high LDL-cholesterol are independent risk factors for coronary heart disease. The risk of lowering HDL-cholesterol while lowering LDL-cholesterol remains unknown. There is little or no effect reported on very low density lipoprotein.

Studies on the mode of action of Lorelco indicate that it increases the fractional rate of catabolism of low density lipoproteins. This effect may be linked to the observed increased excretion of fecal bile acids, a final metabolic pathway for the elimination of cholesterol from the body. Lorelco also exhibits inhibition of early stages of cholesterol synthesis and slight inhibition of absorption of dietary cholesterol. There is no increase in the cyclic precursors of cholesterol, namely desmosterol and 7-dehydrocholesterol. On this basis, it is concluded that Lorelco does not affect the later stages of cholesterol biosynthesis.

Absorption of Lorelco from the gastrointestinal tract is limited and variable. When it is administered with food, peak blood levels are higher and less variable. With continuous administration in a dosage of 500 mg b.i.d., the blood levels of an individual gradually increase over the first three to four months and thereafter remain fairly constant. In 116 patients treated with Lorelco for periods of three months to one year, the mean blood level was 23.6 ± 17.2 mcg/ml (± S.D.) ranging to 78.3 mcg/ml. Levels observed after seven years of treatment in 40 patients yielded an average value of 21.5 ± 16.5 mcg/ml (± S.D.) ranging to 62.0 mcg/ml.

At the end of 12 months of treatment in eight patients blood levels averaged 19.0 mcg/ml. Six weeks after cessation of therapy, the average had fallen by 60 percent. After six months the average had fallen by 80 percent.

Indications and Usage: Serious animal toxicity has been encountered with probucol. See WARNINGS and ANIMAL PHARMACOLOGY AND TOXICOLOGY sections. Probucol is not an innocuous drug and strict attention should be paid to the INDICATIONS and WARNINGS.

Drug therapy should not be used for the routine treatment of elevated blood lipids for the prevention of coronary heart disease. Dietary therapy specific for the type of hyperlipidemia is the initial treatment of choice. Excess body weight may be an important factor and should be addressed prior to any drug therapy. Physical exercise can be an important ancillary measure. Contributory disease such as hypothyroidism or diabetes mellitus should be looked for and adequately treated. The use of drugs should be considered only when reasonable attempts have been made to obtain satisfactory results with non-drug methods. If the decision ultimately is to use drugs, the patient should be instructed that this does not reduce the importance of adhering to diet.

The selection of patients for cholesterol-lowering drug therapy should take into account other important coronary risk factors such as smoking, hypertension, and diabetes mellitus. Consideration should be given to the efficacy, safety, and compliance factors for each of the cholesterol-lowering drugs prior to selecting the one most appropriate for an individual patient.

Lorelco may be indicated for the reduction of elevated serum cholesterol in patients with primary hypercholesterolemia (elevated low density lipoproteins) who have not responded adequately to diet, weight reduction and control of diabetes mellitus. Lorelco may be useful to lower elevated cho-

Total Amount of Imferon Required (to the nearest ml) for Restoration of Hemoglobin and Replacement of Depleted Iron Stores, Based on Observed Hemoglobin and Body Weight

Patient Weight		Milliliter Requirement Based on Observed Hemoglobin of			
lb	kg	4.0 (g/dl)	6.0 (g/dl)	8.0 (g/dl)	10.0 (g/dl)
10	4.5	3 ml	3 ml	2 ml	2 ml
20	9.1	7	6	4	3
30	13.6	10	8	7	5
40	18.1	18	14	11	8
50	22.7	22	18	14	10
60	27.2	26	21	17	12
70	31.8	31	25	19	14
80	36.3	35	28	22	16
90	40.8	39	32	25	18
100	45.4	44	35	28	20
110	49.9	48	39	30	21
120	54.4	53	42	33	23
130	59.0	57	46	36	25
140	63.5	61	50	39	27
150	68.1	66	53	41	29
160	72.6	70	57	44	31
170	77.1	74	60	47	33
180	81.7	79	64	50	35

The total amount of iron (in mg) required to restore hemoglobin to normal levels and to replenish iron stores may be approximated from the formula:

$$0.3 \times \text{Body Weight in Pounds} \times \left(100 - \frac{\text{hemoglobin in g/dl} \times 100}{14.8}\right)$$

(To calculate dose in ml of Imferon, divide this result by 50.)

lesterol that occurs in patients with combined hypercholesterolemia and hypertriglyceridemia, but it is not indicated where hypertriglyceridemia is the abnormality of most concern.

It is not always possible to predict from the lipoprotein type or other factors which patients will exhibit favorable results. Lipid levels should be periodically assessed. Small or transient changes in high density lipoprotein cholesterol may be due to inaccuracies in the method of determination. Substantial changes are sometimes seen with diet. The effect of drug-induced reduction of serum cholesterol or triglyceride levels or alteration of HDL-cholesterol levels on morbidity or mortality due to coronary heart disease has not been established. Several years may be required before ongoing long-term investigations will resolve this question.

Contraindications: (See also PRECAUTIONS.) Lorelco is contraindicated in patients who are known to have a hypersensitivity to it.

Warnings: SERIOUS ANIMAL TOXICITY HAS BEEN ENCOUNTERED WITH PROBUCOL IN RHESUS MONKEYS FED AN ATHEROGENIC DIET AND IN BEAGLE DOGS. (SEE ANIMAL PHARMACOLOGY AND TOXICOLOGY SECTION.)

Although QT prolongation can occur in patients on probucol, the arrhythmias observed in monkeys fed large doses of probucol added to an atherogenic diet have not been reported in man; nevertheless, the following precautions are deemed prudent:

1. At the start of treatment with Lorelco and throughout the treatment period, patients should be advised to adhere to a low cholesterol, low fat diet.
2. As part of an overall evaluation, a baseline, six month, and one year repeat ECG tracing should be considered. If marked prolongation of the QT interval (after correction for rate) occurs, the possible benefits and risks should be carefully considered before making the decision to continue the probucol administration.

Lorelco should not be used in patients with evidence of recent or progressive myocardial damage or findings suggestive of ventricular arrhythmias. No instances of increase in ectopy attributed to Lorelco have been reported. However, patients with unexplained syncope while on Lorelco should have ECG surveillance.

Precautions:

General: Because Lorelco is intended for long-term administration, adequate baseline studies should be performed to determine that the patient has elevated serum cholesterol levels. Serum lipid levels should be determined before treatment and repeated during the first few months of treatment and periodically thereafter. A favorable trend in cholesterol reduction should be evident during the first three to four months of administration of Lorelco. In evaluating response, the effect of probucol on LDL-cholesterol and HDL-cholesterol should be considered. (See CLINICAL PHARMACOLOGY.) If satisfactory lipid alteration is not achieved, the drug should be discontinued.

Information for Patients: The patient should be instructed to adhere to a prudent diet. Females should be cautioned against becoming pregnant for at least six months after discontinuing Lorelco and should not breast feed their infants during therapy with Lorelco.

Laboratory Tests: The physician should schedule periodic blood lipid determinations and should consider periodic electrocardiograms. (See WARNINGS.)

Elevations of the serum transaminases (glutamic-oxalacetic and glutamic-pyruvic), bilirubin, alkaline phosphatase, creatine phosphokinase, uric acid, blood urea nitrogen and blood glucose above the normal range were observed on one or more occasions in various patients treated with Lorelco. Most often these were transient and/or could have been related to the patient's clinical state or other modes of therapy. Although the basis for the relationship between probucol and these abnormalities is not firm, the possibility that some of these are drug-related cannot be excluded. In the controlled trials, the incidence of abnormal laboratory values was no higher in the patients treated with probucol than in the patients who received placebo. If abnormal laboratory tests persist or worsen, if clinical signs consistent with the abnormal laboratory tests develop, or if systemic manifestations occur, probucol should be discontinued.

Drug Interactions: The addition of clofibrate to probucol is not recommended since the lowering effect on mean serum levels of either LDL or total cholesterol is generally not significantly additive and, in some patients, there may be a pronounced lowering of HDL-cholesterol. Neither oral hypoglycemic agents nor oral anticoagulants alter the effect of Lorelco on serum cholesterol. The dosage of these agents is not usually modified when given with Lorelco. Monkeys fed a high fat, high cholesterol diet admixed with probucol exhibited serious toxicity. The toxicity observed in monkeys has not been reported in man. (See WARNINGS and ANIMAL PHARMACOLOGY AND TOXICOLOGY sections.)

Carcinogenesis, Mutagenesis, Impairment of Fertility: In chronic studies of two years' duration in rats, no toxicity or carcinogenicity was observed. These results are consistent with the lack of any adverse effect on fertility and the negative findings in tests for mutagenic activity in rats.

Pregnancy:

Teratogenic Effects

Pregnancy—Category B: Reproduction studies have been performed in rats and rabbits at doses up to 50 times the human dose, and have revealed no evidence of impaired fertility or harm to the fetus due to Lorelco. There are, however, no adequate and well-controlled studies in pregnant women. Because animal reproduction studies are not always predictive of human response, this drug should be used during pregnancy only if clearly needed. Furthermore, if a patient wishes to become pregnant it is recommended that the drug be withdrawn and birth control procedures be used for at least six months because of persistence of the drug in the body for prolonged periods. (See CLINICAL PHARMACOLOGY.)

Labor and Delivery: The effect of Lorelco on human labor and delivery is unknown.

Nursing Mothers: It is not known whether this drug is secreted in human milk, but it is likely to be since such excretion has been shown in animals. It is recommended that nursing not be undertaken while a patient is on Lorelco.

Pediatric Use: Safety and effectiveness in children have not been established.

Adverse Reactions:

Gastrointestinal: diarrhea or loose stools, flatulence, abdominal pain, nausea and vomiting, indigestion, gastrointestinal bleeding

Cardiovascular: prolongation of the QT interval on ECG

Neurologic: headache, dizziness, paresthesias, insomnia, tinnitus, peripheral neuritis

Hematologic: eosinophilia, low hemoglobin and/or hematocrit, thrombocytopenia

Dermatologic: rash, pruritus, ecchymosis, petechiae, hyperhidrosis, fetid sweat

Genitourinary: impotency, nocturia

Ophthalmic: conjunctivitis, tearing, blurred vision

Endocrine: enlargement of multinodular goiter

Idiosyncrasies: An idiosyncratic reaction observed with initiation of therapy and characterized by dizziness, palpitations, syncope, nausea, vomiting and chest pain has been observed.

Other: diminished sense of taste and smell, anorexia, angioneurotic edema

Drug Abuse and Dependence: No evidence of abuse potential has been associated with Lorelco, nor is there evidence of psychological or physical dependence in humans.

Overdosage: There is a single report of a 15 kg, three-year-old male child who ingested 5 gm of probucol. Emesis was induced by ipecac. The child remained well, apart from a brief episode of loose stools and flatulence. No specific information is available on the treatment of overdosage with Lorelco and no specific antidote is available. Probucol is not dialyzable. Treatment is symptomatic and supportive. Probucol has shown no identifiable acute toxicity in mice and rats. In these animals the LD_{50} (oral) is in excess of 5 gm/kg of body weight.

Dosage and Administration: For adult use only. The recommended and maximal dose is 500 mg (two tablets of 250 mg each) twice daily with the morning and evening meals.

How Supplied: Each white film-coated tablet contains 250 mg probucol and is imprinted with the DOW diamond trademark over the code number 51.

Bottles of 120 tablets, a 30-day supply for one patient (NDC 0068-0051-52)

Keep well closed. Store in a dry place. Avoid excessive heat. Dispense in well closed light-resistant container with child-resistant closure.

Animal Pharmacology and Toxicology: In rhesus monkeys administration of probucol in diets containing unusually high amounts of cholesterol and saturated fat resulted in the death of four of eight animals after several weeks. Premonitory syncope was frequently observed and was associated with a pronounced prolongation of the QT intervals (30 to 50 percent longer than that observed in untreated monkeys). Serum levels of probucol greater than 20 mcg/ml were generally associated with some prolongation in the QT interval in the cholesterol-fed monkey. A 75 msec or greater increase in QT interval from control values was usually seen at 40 mcg/ml and above. Blood levels in humans receiving probucol average approximately 20 mcg/ml and not uncommonly reach levels of 40 mcg/ml and higher. Rhesus monkeys fed normal (low fat) chow and receiving probucol three to thirty times the human dose equivalent achieved blood levels only one-third those of many human subjects. No adverse effects were detected in these monkeys over an eight-year period of continuous drug administration. In another study in rhesus monkeys, an atherogenic diet was fed for two years and daily treatment with probucol, separated in time from the atherogenic meal, was carried out during the second year. Serum probucol levels ranged 20 to 50 mcg/ml in five of ten monkeys and less in the remaining animals. Marked prolongation of the QT_c interval in the electrocardiogram or syncopal behavior was never observed over the entire one-year treatment period. Regression of gross aortic lesions comparable to that observed in a parallel group of monkeys receiving cholestyramine was seen in animals receiving probucol. It should be emphasized that both HDL-cholesterol and LDL-cholesterol were markedly reduced in this regression study. During the performance of a two-year chronic study involving 32 probucol-treated dogs (beagles) there were 12 fatalities. Subsequent experiments have indicated that probucol sensitizes the canine myocardium to epinephrine, resulting in ventricular fibrillation in many dogs. Among the animal species in which probucol has been studied, the dog is peculiar with respect to the phenomenon of sudden death due to the sensitization of the myocardium to epinephrine. In contrast to findings in the dog, injections of epinephrine to probucol-treated monkeys did not induce ventricular fibrillation. In other studies, monkeys were given probucol either before and after, or only after myocardial infarction induced by coronary artery ligation. In these studies there was no difference between probucol- and placebo-treated groups with respect to either survival or detailed blind quantitation of myocardial changes (gross and histopathologic). Probucol has shown no identifiable toxicity in mice and rats. In these animals the LD_{50} (oral) is in excess of five gm/kg of body weight. In chronic studies of two-year duration in rats, no toxicity or carcinogenicity was observed.

From studies in rats, dogs and monkeys, it is known that probucol accumulates slowly in adipose tissue. Approximately 90 percent of probucol administered orally is unabsorbed. For that which is absorbed, the biliary tract is the major pathway for clearance from the body and very little is excreted by way of the kidneys.

Information on Merrell Dow products is based on labeling in effect in August, 1984.

Continued on next page

Merrell Dow—Cont.

Myocardial injury was produced in various groups of rats by one of the following procedures: aortic coarctation, coronary ligation, or cobalt or isoproterenol injection. After probucol administration no deleterious effects related to treatment occurred as measured by survival and microscopic examination of myocardial damage.

Probucol was administered to minipigs beginning ten days before ligation of coronary artery and continued for 60 days post surgery. Challenge wth epinephrine at the end of 60 days failed to induce ventricular fibrillation in any of the coronary-ligated, probucol-treated minipigs.

Product Information as of October, 1984
MERRELL DOW PHARMACEUTICALS INC.
Subsidiary of The Dow Chemical Company
Cincinnati, Ohio 45242-9553, U.S.A.
Shown in Product Identification Section, page 421

METAHYDRIN®
[mĕt″ăh-hī′drĭn]
(trichlormethiazide USP)

AVAILABLE ONLY ON PRESCRIPTION

Description: Metahydrin is an oral diuretic and antihypertensive of the thiazide class. Differing from other thiazides by the inclusion of a dichloromethyl radical at the 3 position on the benzothiadiazine structure.

Action: The mechanism of action results in an interference with the renal tubular mechanism of electrolyte reabsorption. At maximal therapeutic dosage all thiazides are approximately equal in their diuretic potency. The mechanism whereby thiazides function in the control of hypertension is unknown.

Indications: Metahydrin is indicated as adjunctive therapy in edema associated with congestive heart failure, hepatic cirrhosis, and corticosteroid and estrogen therapy.

Metahydrin has also been found useful in edema due to various forms of renal dysfunction as:
  Nephrotic syndrome;
  Acute glomerulonephritis; and
  Chronic renal failure.

Metahydrin is indicated in the management of hypertension either as the sole therapeutic agent or to enhance the effectiveness of other antihypertensive drugs in the more severe forms of hypertension.

Usage in Pregnancy. The routine use of diuretics in an otherwise healthy woman is inappropriate and exposes mother and fetus to unnecessary hazard. Diuretics do not prevent development of toxemia of pregnancy, and there is no satisfactory evidence that they are useful in the treatment of developed toxemia.

Edema during pregnancy may arise from pathologic causes or from the physiologic and mechanical consequences of pregnancy. Thiazides are indicated in pregnancy when edema is due to pathologic causes, just as they are in the absence of pregnancy. (However, see Warnings, below.) Dependent edema in pregnancy, resulting from restriction of venous return by the expanded uterus, is properly treated through elevation of the lower extremities and use of support hose; use of diuretics to lower intravascular volume in this case is illogical and unnecessary. There is hypervolemia during normal pregnancy, which is harmful to neither the fetus nor the mother (in the absence of cardiovascular disease), but which is associated with edema, including generalized edema, in the majority of pregnant women. If this edema produces discomfort, increased recumbency will often provide relief. In rare instances, this edema may cause extreme discomfort which is not relieved by rest. In these cases, a short course of diuretics may provide relief and may be appropriate.

Contraindications:
Anuria.
Hypersensitivity to this or other sulfonamide-derived drugs.

Warnings: Thiazides should be used with caution in severe renal disease. In patients with renal disease, thiazides may precipitate azotemia. Cumulative effects of the drug may develop in patients with impaired renal function.

Thiazides should be used with caution in patients with impaired hepatic function or progressive liver disease, since minor alterations of fluid and electrolyte balance may precipitate hepatic coma. Thiazides may add to or potentiate the action of other antihypertensive drugs. Potentiation occurs with ganglionic or peripheral adrenergic blocking drugs.

Sensitivity reactions may occur in patients with a history of allergy or bronchial asthma.

The possibility of exacerbation or activation of systemic lupus erythematosus has been reported.

Usage in Pregnancy. Thiazides cross the placental barrier and appear in cord blood. The use of thiazides in pregnant women requires that the anticipated benefit be weighed against possible hazards to the fetus. These hazards include fetal or neonatal jaundice, thrombocytopenia, and possibly other adverse reactions which have occurred in the adult.

Nursing Mothers. Thiazides appear in the breast milk. If use of the drug is deemed essential, the patient should stop nursing.

Precautions: Periodic determination of serum electrolytes to detect possible electrolyte imbalance should be performed at appropriate intervals. All patients receiving thiazide therapy should be observed for clinical signs of fluid or electrolyte imbalance; namely, hyponatremia, hypochloremic alkalosis, and hypokalemia. Serum and urine electrolyte determinations are particularly important when the patient is vomiting excessively or receiving parenteral fluids. Medication such as digitalis may also influence serum electrolytes. Warning signs, irrespective of cause, are: dryness of mouth, thirst, weakness, lethargy, drowsiness, restlessness, muscle pains or cramps, muscular fatigue, hypotension, oliguria, tachycardia, and gastrointestinal disturbances such as nausea and vomiting.

Hypokalemia may develop with thiazides as with any other potent diuretic, especially with brisk diuresis, when severe cirrhosis is present, or during concomitant use of corticosteroids or ACTH. Interference with adequate oral electrolyte intake will also contribute to hypokalemia. Digitalis therapy may exaggerate metabolic effects of hypokalemia especially with reference to myocardial activity.

Any chloride deficit is generally mild and usually does not require specific treatment except under extraordinary circumstances (as in liver disease or renal disease). Dilutional hyponatremia may occur in edematous patients in hot weather; appropriate therapy is water restriction, rather than administration of salt except in rare instances when the hyponatremia is life threatening. In actual salt depletion, appropriate replacement is the therapy of choice.

Hyperuricemia may occur or frank gout may be precipitated in certain patients receiving thiazide therapy.

Insulin requirements in diabetic patients may be increased, decreased, or unchanged. Latent diabetes mellitus may become manifest during thiazide administration.

Thiazide drugs may increase the responsiveness to tubocurarine.

The antihypertensive effects of the drug may be enhanced in the postsympathectomy patient.

Thiazides may decrease arterial responsiveness to norepinephrine. This diminution is not sufficient to preclude effectiveness of the pressor agent for therapeutic use.

If progressive renal impairment becomes evident, as indicated by a rising nonprotein nitrogen or blood urea nitrogen, a careful reappraisal of therapy is necessary with consideration given to withholding or discontinuing diuretic therapy.

Thiazides may decrease serum PBI levels without signs of thyroid disturbance.

This product contains FD&C Yellow No. 5 (tartrazine), which may cause allergic-type reactions (including bronchial asthma) in certain susceptible individuals. Although the overall incidence of FD&C Yellow No. 5 (tartrazine) sensitivity in the general population is low, it is frequently seen in patients who also have aspirin hypersensitivity.

Adverse Reactions:
1. Gastrointestinal System Reactions: anorexia, gastric irritation, nausea, diarrhea, constipation, jaundice (intrahepatic cholestatic jaundice), vomiting, cramping, pancreatitis.
2. Central Nervous System Reactions: dizziness, vertigo, parasthesias, headache, xanthopsia.
3. Hematologic Reactions: leukopenia, agranulocytosis, thrombocytopenia, aplastic anemia.
4. Dermatologic-Hypersensitivity Reactions: purpura, photosensitivity, rash, urticaria, necrotizing angiitis (vasculitis) (cutaneous vasculitis).
5. Cardiovascular Reaction: orthostatic hypotension may occur and may be aggravated by alcohol, barbiturates, or narcotics.
6. Other: hyperglycemia, glycosuria, hyperuricemia, muscle spasm, weakness, restlessness.

Whenever adverse reactions are moderate or severe, Metahydrin dosage should be reduced or therapy withdrawn.

Dosage and Administration: Therapy should be individualized according to patient response. This therapy should be titrated to gain maximal therapeutic response as well as the minimal dose possible to maintain that therapeutic response.

The usual daily doses of Metahydrin for antihypertensive and diuretic effect are as follows:
  The usual dose is one 2 mg or 4 mg tablet once daily.
  In initiating therapy, these doses may be given twice daily.

How Supplied:
2 mg pink tablets debossed MERRELL 62: bottles of 100
4 mg aqua blue tablets debossed MERRELL 63: bottles of 100 and 1000

Product Information as of August, 1979
Shown in Product Identification Section, page 421

METATENSIN®
[mĕt″ăh-tĕn′sĭn]
(trichlormethiazide USP and reserpine)

AVAILABLE ONLY ON PRESCRIPTION

> **Warning**
> This fixed combination drug is not indicated for initial therapy of hypertension. Hypertension requires therapy titrated to the individual patient. If the fixed combination represents the dosage so determined, its use may be more convenient in patient management. The treatment of hypertension is not static, but must be re-evaluated as conditions in each patient warrant.

Description: Each tablet contains Metahydrin® (trichlormethiazide USP) 2 mg or 4 mg and reserpine 0.1 mg.

Metahydrin (trichlormethiazide USP) is an orally effective diuretic and antihypertensive of the thiazide class, differing from other thiazides by the inclusion of a dichloromethyl radical at the 3 position on the benzothiadiazine structure.

Reserpine is a pure crystalline alkaloid derived from the root of Rauwolfia serpentina.

Action:

Trichlormethiazide
The mechanism of action results in an interference with the renal tubular mechanism of electrolyte reabsorption. At maximal therapeutic dosage all thiazides are approximately equal in their diuretic potency. The mechanism whereby thiazides function in the control of hypertension is unknown.

Reserpine
Reserpine probably produces its antihypertensive effects through depletion of tissue stores of epinephrine and norepinephrine from peripheral sites. By contrast, its sedative and tranquilizing properties are thought to be related to depletion of 5-hydroxytryptamine from the brain.

Reserpine is characterized by slow onset of action and sustained effect. Both its cardiovascular and central nervous system effects may persist following withdrawal of the drug.

Indications: Hypertension (See box Warning.)
Usage in Pregnancy. The routine use of diuretics in an otherwise healthy woman is inappropriate and exposes mother and fetus to unnecessary hazard. Diuretics do not prevent development of toxemia of pregnancy, and there is no satisfactory evidence that they are useful in the treatment of developed toxemia.

Edema during pregnancy may arise from pathologic causes or from the physiologic and mechanical consequences of pregnancy. Thiazides are indicated in pregnancy when edema is due to pathologic causes, just as they are in the absence of pregnancy. (However, see Warnings, below.) Dependent edema in pregnancy, resulting from restriction of venous return by the expanded uterus, is properly treated through elevation of the lower extremities and use of support hose; use of diuretics to lower intravascular volume in this case is illogical and unnecessary. There is hypervolemia during normal pregnancy, which is harmful to neither the fetus nor the mother (in the absence of cardiovascular disease), but which is associated with edema, including generalized edema, in the majority of pregnant women. If this edema produces discomfort, increased recumbency will often provide relief. In rare instances, this edema may cause extreme discomfort which is not relieved by rest. In these cases, a short course of diuretics may provide relief and may be appropriate.

Contraindications:
Trichlormethiazide
Trichlormethiazide is contraindicated in patients with anuria and in patients known to be hypersensitive to this or other sulfonamide derived drugs.
Reserpine
Hypersensitivity, mental depression especially with suicidal tendencies, active peptic ulcer and ulcerative colitis.
Warnings:
Trichlormethiazide
Use with caution in severe renal disease. In patients with renal disease, thiazides may precipitate azotemia. Cumulative effects of the drug may develop in patients with impaired renal function. Thiazides should be used with caution in patients with impaired hepatic function or progressive liver disease, since minor alterations of fluid and electrolyte balance may precipitate hepatic coma. Thiazides may add to or potentiate the action of other antihypertensive drugs. Potentiation occurs with ganglionic or peripheral adrenergic blocking drugs. Sensitivity reactions may occur in patients with a history of allergy or bronchial asthma. Exacerbation or activation of systemic lupus erythematosis has been reported.
Reserpine
As suicide is always a possible result of mental depression, discontinue treatment if mood depression develops.
Reserpine may induce peptic ulceration; discontinue use if peptic ulcer develops.
Electroshock therapy should not be given to patients taking reserpine, since severe and even fatal reactions have been reported. The drug should be discontinued for two weeks before giving electroshock therapy.
MAO inhibitors should be avoided or used with extreme caution.
Usage in Pregnancy. Trichlormethiazide: Thiazides cross the placental barrier and appear in cord blood. The use of thiazides in pregnant women requires that the anticipated benefit be weighed against possible hazards to the fetus. These hazards include fetal or neonatal jaundice, thrombocytopenia, and possibly other adverse reactions which have occurred in the adult.
Reserpine: The safety of reserpine for use during pregnancy or lactation has not been established; therefore, the drug should be used in pregnant patients or in women of childbearing potential only when, in the judgment of the physician, it is essential to the welfare of the patient.
Increased respiratory secretions, nasal congestion, cyanosis, and anorexia may occur in infants born to reserpine-treated mothers, since reserpine crosses the placental barrier and appears in maternal breast milk.

Nursing Mothers. Thiazides and reserpine appear in breast milk. If use of Metatensin is deemed essential, the patient should stop nursing.

Precautions: The #2 tablet contains FD&C Yellow No. 5 (tartrazine), which may cause allergic-type reactions (including bronchial asthma) in certain susceptible individuals. Although the overall incidence of FD&C Yellow No. 5 (tartrazine) sensitivity in the general population is low, it is frequently seen in patients who also have aspirin hypersensitivity.

Trichlormethiazide
Periodic determinations of serum electrolytes to detect possible electrolyte imbalance should be performed at appropriate intervals.
All patients receiving thiazide therapy should be observed for clinical signs of fluid or electrolyte imbalance; namely, hyponatremia, hypochloremic alkalosis, and hypokalemia. Serum and urine electrolyte determinations are particularly important when the patient is vomiting excessively or receiving parenteral fluids.
Medication such as digitalis may also influence serum electrolytes. Warning signs, irrespective of cause, are: dryness of mouth, thirst, weakness, lethargy, drowsiness, restlessness, muscle pains or cramps, muscular fatigue, hypotension, oliguria, tachycardia, and gastrointestinal disturbances such as nausea and vomiting.
Hypokalemia may develop with thiazides as with any other potent diuretic, especially with brisk diuresis, when severe cirrhosis is present, or during concomitant use of corticosteroids or ACTH. Interference with adequate oral electrolyte intake will also contribute to hypokalemia. Digitalis therapy may exaggerate metabolic effects of hypokalemia especially with reference to myocardial activity.
Any chloride deficit is generally mild and usually does not require specific treatment except under extraordinary circumstances (as in liver disease or renal disease). Dilutional hyponatremia may occur in edematous patients in hot weather; appropriate therapy is water restriction, rather than administration of salt except in rare instances when the hyponatremia is life threatening. In actual salt depletion, appropriate replacement is the therapy of choice.
Hyperuricemia may occur or frank gout may be precipitated in certain patients receiving thiazide therapy.
Insulin requirements in diabetic patients may be increased, decreased, or unchanged. Latent diabetes mellitus may become manifest during thiazide administration.
Thiazide drugs may increase the responsiveness to tubocurarine.
The antihypertensive effects of the drug may be enhanced in the postsympathectomy patient.
Thiazides may decrease arterial responsiveness to norepinephrine. This diminution is not sufficient to preclude effectiveness of the pressor agent for therapeutic use.
If progressive renal impairment becomes evident, as indicated by a rising non-protein nitrogen or blood urea nitrogen, a careful reappraisal of therapy is necessary with consideration given to withholding or discontinuing diuretic therapy.
Thiazides may decrease serum PBI levels without signs of thyroid disturbance.

Reserpine
Caution should be used in treating hypertensive patients with renal insufficiency.
Cardiac arrhythmias have occurred in patients receiving digitalis and quinidine with reserpine.
Reserpine potentiates many anesthetic agents; hypotension and bradycardia have been noted during anesthesia. In addition, a relative sensitivity to norepinephrine or other pressor agents may exist due to the previous action of reserpine; thus usual doses of the pressor agent may be excessive.
Use with caution in patients with a previous history of depression, peptic ulcer or other gastrointestinal disorders and in hypertensive patients with functionally severe coronary artery disease.

Animal tumorigenicity. Rodent studies have shown that reserpine is an animal tumorigen, causing an increased incidence of mammary fibroadenomas in female mice, malignant tumors of the seminal vesicles in male mice, and malignant adrenal medullary tumors in male rats. These findings arose in 2-year studies in which the drug was administered in the feed at concentrations of 5 and 10 ppm—about 100 to 300 times the usual human dose. The breast neoplasms are thought to be related to reserpine's prolactin-elevating effect. Several other prolactin-elevating drugs have also been associated with an increased incidence of mammary neoplasia in rodents.
The extent to which these findings indicate a risk to humans is uncertain. Tissue culture experiments show that about one-third of human breast tumors are prolactin-dependent in vitro, a factor of considerable importance if the use of the drug is contemplated in a patient with previously detected breast cancer. The possibility of an increased risk of breast cancer in reserpine users has been studied extensively; however, no firm conclusion has emerged. Although a few epidemiologic studies have suggested a slightly increased risk (less than twofold in all studies except one) in women who have used reserpine, other studies of generally similar design have not confirmed this. Epidemiologic studies conducted using other drugs (neuroleptic agents) that, like reserpine, increase prolactin levels and therefore would be considered rodent mammary carcinogens, have not shown an association between chronic administration of the drug and human mammary tumorigenesis. While long-term clinical observation has not suggested such an association, the available evidence is considered too limited to be conclusive at this time. An association of reserpine intake with pheochromocytoma or tumors of the seminal vesicles has not been explored.

Adverse Reactions:
Trichlormethiazide
1. Gastrointestinal System Reactions: anorexia, gastric irritation, nausea, diarrhea, constipation, jaundice (intrahepatic cholestatic jaundice), vomiting, cramping, pancreatitis.
2. Central Nervous System Reactions: dizziness, vertigo, paresthesias, headache, xanthopsia.
3. Hematologic Reactions: leukopenia, agranulocytosis, thrombocytopenia, aplastic anemia.
4. Dermatologic-Hypersensitivity Reactions: purpura, photosensitivity, rash, urticaria, necrotizing angiitis (vasculitis) (cutaneous vasculitis).
5. Cardiovascular Reaction: orthostatic hypotension may occur and may be aggravated by alcohol, barbiturates, or narcotics.
6. Other: hyperglycemia, glycosuria, hyperuricemia, muscle spasm, weakness, restlessness.

Reserpine
Gastric hypersecretion; vomiting; nervousness; paradoxical anxiety, CNS sensitization manifested by deafness, glaucoma, uveitis, and optic atrophy; purpura; nasal stuffiness; loose stools; reversible parkinsonism; muscular fatigue and weakness; and nightmares. Mental depression, particularly when doses of reserpine of over 1.0 mg daily are used, has been reported. Other side effects of reserpine reported include anorexia, nausea, dizziness, headaches, impotence, flushing of the skin, dryness of the mouth, biliary colic, blurring of vision, muscular aches and pruritus. Hypotension, including the orthostatic variety, may occur in some patients. Angina pectoris, arrhythmias and congestive heart failure have also been reported but are uncommon.
After the onset of therapy with reserpine, a turbulent phase of short duration may occur. Very rare additional adverse effects that have been observed in association with reserpine therapy include epistaxis, skin eruptions and edema due to sodium retention. Bradycardia may occur as an exagger-

Continued on next page

Information on Merrell Dow products is based on labeling in effect in August, 1984.

Merrell Dow—Cont.

ated response related to the pharmacodynamic effect of reserpine.

Dosage: As determined by individual titration. (See box Warning.)

In the stabilized hypertensive patient, administration may be continued on a once-daily basis administered in the morning. The maximum single effective dose of Metatensin is 8 mg (in some patients 4 mg). Doses in excess of 8 mg normally will not produce any increase in sodium and water excretion and in refractory patients may increase excretion of potassium.

How Supplied:
Metatensin #2
(trichlormethiazide 2.0 mg and reserpine 0.1 mg)
Bottles of 100 and 1000 yellow tablets debossed MERRELL 64
Metatensin #4
(trichlormethiazide 4.0 mg and reserpine 0.1 mg)
Bottles of 100 and 1000 lavender tablets debossed MERRELL 65

Product Information as of April, 1983
Shown in Product Identification Section, page 421

NEO-POLYCIN®
[nē″ō-pŏl′ĭ-sĭn]
neomycin sulfate, polymyxin B sulfate and bacitracin zinc ointment
Topical Antibiotic

Description: Each gram of Neo-Polycin topical antibiotic ointment contains: neomycin sulfate equivalent to 3.5 mg neomycin; polymyxin B sulfate, 5000 units; bacitracin zinc, 400 units in a unique Fuzene® ointment base. Inert ingredients are polyethylene glycol dilaurate, polyethylene glycol distearate, light liquid petrolatum, white petrolatum and synthetic glyceride wax.

Actions: All three antibiotics in Neo-Polycin meet most criteria for ideal topical agents. They are rarely used systemically and there is apparently minimal risk of systemic toxicity from their topical use because they are not absorbed to an appreciable extent from denuded skin or mucous membranes. They are essentially non-irritating to the tissues. They are active in the presence of blood or pus, and they diffuse readily into tissue exudates.

Neomycin acts against most of the bacteria that cause topical infection and is especially active against species of *Proteus* and *Staphylococcus*. Bacitracin is primarily effective against gram-positive bacteria, and is especially effective against hemolytic streptococci. Polymyxin is primarily effective against gram-negative bacteria, particularly *Pseudomonas aeruginosa*. This combination of antibiotics makes Neo-Polycin effective against practically all pyogenic bacteria that cause topical infections. Because the Fuzene base is miscible with both tissue exudate and the oils and waxes of the skin, Neo-Polycin can be used in weeping exudative lesions.

Indications: Neo-Polycin may be used in the treatment of bacterial infections of the skin and mucous membrane caused by susceptible bacteria. These include such pyogenic conditions as impetigo, folliculitis, paronychia, and sycosis barbae. It is also effective in controlling secondary bacterial infections in skin carcinoma, burns, eczemas, contact dermatitis, fungal infections, acne, psoriasis, varicose ulcers and neurodermatitis. Its broad antibacterial spectrum and special base make Neo-Polycin especially useful for treating chronic lesions, where mixed infections with relatively resistant bacteria may be present and difficult to identify for definitive therapy.

Neo-Polycin is also indicated as a non-irritating, non-staining dressing for the prevention of bacterial infection of traumatic lesions and surgical incisions.

Contraindications: Hypersensitivity to product ingredients. Not for use in the eyes. Do not use in external ear canal if the eardrum is perforated.

Warning: Because of the potential hazard of nephrotoxicity and ototoxicity due to neomycin, care should be exercised when using Neo-Polycin in treating extensive burns, trophic ulceration and other extensive conditions where absorption of neomycin is possible. Not more than one application a day is recommended where widespread body surfaces are affected, especially if the patient has impaired renal function or is receiving other aminoglycoside antibiotics concurrently.

Precautions: As with any antibacterial preparation, prolonged use may result in overgrowth of nonsusceptible organisms, including fungi. If this occurs, treatment should be discontinued and appropriate therapy instituted.

Adverse Reactions: Sensitivity, especially to the neomycin ingredient, may develop after continuous, chronic therapy. If itching, burning or inflammation follows application, usage should be discontinued. Articles in the current medical literature indicate an increase in the prevalence of persons sensitive to neomycin.

Administration: Spread Neo-Polycin thinly, with or without a dressing. Reapplication 2 or 3 times daily may be desirable. Avoid using excessive amounts of ointment since it is unnecessary and tends to result in the deposition of undesirable residue.

How Supplied: In $\frac{1}{2}$ ounce tubes (NDC 0068-2010-93).

NICORETTE®
[nĭk′ō-rĕt″]
(nicotine polacrilex)

Caution: Federal law prohibits dispensing without prescription.

Description: Nicorette (nicotine polacrilex) contains nicotine bound to an ion exchange resin in a sugar-free flavored chewing gum base. Nicotine is absorbed through the buccal mucosa when Nicorette is chewed. Each piece of Nicorette contains nicotine polacrilex equivalent to 2 mg nicotine to be used as an adjunct to smoking cessation programs. The chemical name for nicotine is (S)-3-(1-methyl-2-pyrrolidinyl)pyridine.

Clinical Pharmacology: Nicotine is an agonist at nicotinic receptors in the peripheral and central nervous systems. In man, as in animals, nicotine has been shown to produce both behavioral stimulation and depression.

Nicotine's effects are generally dose-dependent, and extremely high doses (achievable through parenteral, rectal, and perhaps percutaneous routes), can produce toxic symptoms, i.e., delirium. These effects can occur in nicotine-tolerant individuals. In nonsmokers, CNS mediated symptoms of hiccups, nausea, and emesis are commonly associated with the use of even small doses of inhaled smoke or chewed Nicorette gum. However, in smokers, these symptoms occur only with much larger doses.

Nicotine has actions at the sympathetic ganglia and on the chemoreceptors of the aorta and carotid bodies. Nicotine also affects the adrenal medulla, with the attendant release of catecholamines. The overall effect on the cardiovascular system leads to acceleration of the heart, peripheral vasoconstriction, and elevation of blood pressure with an attendant increase in the work of the heart. Nicotine may induce vasospasm and cardiac arrhythmias. Tolerance does not develop to the catecholamine-releasing effects of nicotine.

Results of cardiovascular studies comparing Nicorette with cigarettes document that each source of nicotine produces similar dose-dependent effects on cardiovascular performance (see *Biopharmaceutics and Pharmacokinetics* section). However, if Nicorette gum (2 mg/piece) is used by smokers at a rate not exceeding one piece per hour, the cardiovascular effects produced do not differ from those seen with placebo.

Reinforcement of cigarette smoking behavior is considered to have both psychological (or learned) and pharmacological components. Buffered nicotine-containing gum is designed to provide an alternative source of nicotine for nicotine-dependent individuals acutely withdrawing from tobacco smoking.

Biopharmaceutics and Pharmacokinetics
The nicotine in Nicorette is bound to an ion exchange resin and is released only during chewing; nicotine will not be released in significant amounts if the gum is swallowed. The blood level of nicotine obtained with Nicorette will depend upon the vigor and duration of chewing.

In studies comparing the nicotine blood level achieved with Nicorette to that achieved with smoking, it was found that the trough level of nicotine obtained by smoking one cigarette per hour is approximately twice that of chewing one 2 mg Nicorette.

The pronounced early peak in nicotine blood levels seen with the inhalation of cigarette smoke is not observed with the chewing of Nicorette. Swallowing Nicorette does not produce clinically significant blood levels of nicotine. Nicotine is metabolized mainly by the liver, but may also be metabolized to a lesser extent by the kidney and the lung. The principal metabolites are cotinine and nicotine-1′-N-oxide. Both nicotine and its metabolites are excreted through the kidneys with about 10 to 20% of absorbed nicotine excreted unchanged in the urine. Excretion of nicotine is increased in acid urine and by high urine output. The metabolism of nicotine absorbed buccally from Nicorette is qualitatively similar to the metabolism observed when nicotine is absorbed through inhalation of cigarette smoke.

Indication and Usage: Nicorette is indicated as a temporary aid to the cigarette smoker seeking to give up his or her smoking habit while participating in a behavioral modification program under medical supervision.

The efficacy of Nicorette as an aid to smoking cessation was demonstrated in clinical studies which showed that Nicorette gum, in comparison to control chewing gums, increased the likelihood of smoking cessation among participants in behavior modification programs. As used in the context of this labeling, behavioral modification refers to supervised programs of education, counselling and psychological support. The efficacy of Nicorette use without concomitant participation in a behavioral modification program has not been established.

In general, smokers who have a high 'physical' type of nicotine dependence are most likely to benefit from the use of Nicorette. The following subject characteristics are correlated with a 'physical' type of nicotine dependence: (1) smoke more than 15 cigarettes per day, (2) prefer brands of cigarettes with nicotine levels of greater than 0.9 mg, (3) usually inhale the smoke, (4) smoke the first cigarette within 30 minutes of arising, (5) find the first cigarette in the morning the hardest to give up, (6) smoke more frequently during the morning than the rest of the day, (7) find it difficult to refrain from smoking in places where it is forbidden, or (8) smoke even when they are so ill they are confined to bed most of the day.

The benefits of Nicorette use beyond three months has not been demonstrated.

Contraindications: Nicorette is contraindicated in non-smokers.

Nicorette is contraindicated in patients during the immediate post-myocardial infarction period, patients with life-threatening arrhythmias, and patients with severe or worsening angina pectoris (see WARNINGS). Also, Nicorette is contraindicated in patients with active temporomandibular joint disease.

Current medical opinion indicates that nicotine in any form may be harmful to an unborn child. Nicorette and cigarettes both contain nicotine.

Nicorette may cause fetal harm when administered to a pregnant woman.

Use of cigarettes or Nicorette during the last trimester has been associated with a decrease in fetal breathing movements. These effects may be the result of decreased placental perfusion caused by nicotine. One miscarriage during Nicorette therapy has been reported, and the relation to drug therapy as a contributing factor cannot be excluded. Studies in pregnant rhesus monkeys have shown that maternal nicotine administration produced acidosis, hypoxia and hypercarbia in the fetus.

Nicotine has been shown to be teratogenic in mice treated subcutaneously with 25 mg/kg, which is approximately 300 times the human buccal dose. Studies in rats and monkeys have not demonstrated a teratogenic effect of nicotine in doses which would occur during cigarette smoking.

Nicorette is therefore contraindicated in women who are or may become pregnant, and female patients should be advised to take adequate precautions to avoid becoming pregnant. The physician may wish to consider a pregnancy test before instituting therapy with Nicorette. If this drug is used during pregnancy, or if the patient becomes pregnant while taking this drug, the patient should be apprised of the potential hazard to the fetus.

Warnings: The risks of nicotine in patients with certain cardiovascular and endocrine diseases should be carefully weighed against the benefits of including Nicorette in a smoking cessation program in these patients. Specifically, patients with coronary heart disease (history of myocardial infarction and/or angina pectoris), serious cardiac arrhythmias, or vasospastic diseases (Buerger's disease, Prinzmetal variant angina) should be carefully screened and evaluated before Nicorette is prescribed.

As the action of nicotine on the adrenal medulla (release of catecholamines) does not appear to be affected by tolerance, Nicorette should be used with caution in patients with hyperthyroidism, pheochromocytoma or insulin-dependent diabetes. Cigarette smoking is felt to play a perpetuating role in hypertension and peptic ulcer disease. Therefore, Nicorette should be used in patients with systemic hypertension or inactive peptic ulcer only when the benefits of including Nicorette in a smoking cessation program outweigh the risks.

Precautions: Nicorette should be used with caution in patients with oral or pharyngeal inflammation and in patients with a history of esophagitis or peptic ulcer.

The dosage form of Nicorette dictates that it be used with caution in patients whose dental problems might be exacerbated by chewing gum.

Nicorette is sugar-free and has been formulated to minimize stickiness. As with other gums, however, the degree to which Nicorette may stick to dentures, dental caps or partial bridges may depend on the materials from which they are made and other factors such as amount of saliva produced, possible interaction with denture adhesives, denture cleaning compounds, dryness of mouth due to other causes and salivary constituents. Should an excessive degree of stickiness to dental work occur, there is the possibility that as with other gums, Nicorette may damage dental work; if this should occur, the patient should discontinue its use and consult a physician or dentist.

The sustained use of Nicorette by ex-smokers is not to be encouraged because the chronic consumption of nicotine is toxic and addicting. The physician must, however, weigh the relative risks of a possible return to smoking and continued, long-term use of the gum.

Information for Patients: The patient instruction sheet is attached at the end of the professional labeling text. It is intended for detachment by the pharmacist and inclusion in the package of Nicorette dispensed to the patient. It contains important selected information on patient selection, risks, adverse effects and instructions on how to use Nicorette properly.

Drug Interactions: Smoking cessation, with or without nicotine substitutes, may alter response to concomitant medication in ex-smokers. Smoking is considered to increase metabolism and thus lower blood levels of drugs such as phenacetin, caffeine, theophylline, imipramine and pentazocine, through enzyme induction. Cessation of smoking may result in increased levels of these drugs. Absorption of glutethimide may be decreased, and the "first pass" metabolism of propoxyphene decreased by smoking cessation. Other reported effects of smoking, which do not involve enzyme induction, include reduced diuretic effects of furosemide and decreased cardiac output, and increased blood pressure with propranolol, which may also relate to the hormonal effects of nicotine. Smoking cessation may reverse these actions.

Both smoking and nicotine can increase circulating cortisol and catecholamines. Therapy with adrenergic agonists or with adrenergic blockers may need to be adjusted according to changes in nicotine therapy or smoking status.

Carcinogenesis, Mutagenesis, Impairment of Fertility

Nicotine was not mutagenic in the Ames *Salmonella* test.

Literature reports indicate that nicotine is neither an initiator nor a tumor-promoter in mice. There is inconclusive evidence to suggest that cotinine, an oxidized metabolite of nicotine, may be carcinogenic in rats. Cotinine was not mutagenic in the Ames *Salmonella* test.

Studies have shown a decrease of litter size in rats treated with nicotine during the time of fertilization.

Pregnancy: Pregnancy Category X. See "Contraindications" section.

Nursing Mothers: Nicotine passes freely into the breast milk. Because of the potential for serious adverse reactions in nursing infants from nicotine, a decision should be made whether to discontinue nursing or to discontinue the drug, taking into account the importance of the drug to the mother.

Pediatric Use: Safety and effectiveness in children and adolescents who smoke has not been evaluated.

Adverse Reactions: Adverse reactions reported in association with the use of Nicorette include both local effects and systemic effects representing the pharmacologic action of nicotine.

Local side effects: Mechanical effects of gum chewing include traumatic injury to oral mucosa or teeth, jaw ache, and eructation secondary to air swallowing. These side effects may be minimized by modifying chewing technique.

Systemic side effects: Although the systemic effects seen in trials were generally similar, the reported frequency of adverse drug effects was highly variable, as illustrated by the variation observed in adverse event incidence estimated from the results of two well-controlled studies (one performed in the United States, and the other in England) designed to evaluate the safety and efficacy of Nicorette. (See table, below.) Given this variability, the table can be used only as an indication of the relative frequency of adverse events reported in representative clinical trials. It can not predict expected incidences of these effects during the course of usual medical practice. [See table above].

In addition to the more frequently reported effects listed in the table above, the following events were reported at a rate of less than one percent in clinical trials with Nicorette: systemic nicotine intoxication (see below), laxative effect, constipation, vomiting, hoarseness, dry mouth, flushing, sneezing, cough, euphoria, insomnia and gas pains. One miscarriage during Nicorette therapy has been reported, and a relation to drug therapy as a contributing factor cannot be excluded.

The only potentially serious systemic adverse effect observed among the 152 patients evaluated in the controlled clinical trials used to support the efficacy of Nicorette was cardiac irritability; a patient displayed what may have been nicotine-induced, but reversible, atrial fibrillation. Cardiac irritability is a well known consequence of cigarette smoking.

Adverse reactions reported in settings other than controlled clinical trials are similar to those reported in the trials. A 46-year-old male patient participating in a clinical trial of Nicorette was reported to have developed nicotine intoxication requiring hospitalization. After 4 days, he was discharged, fully recovered. He died suddenly one month later. Nicorette was not used during this one-month interval. The relationship of the patient's death to his prior treatment is undetermined.

Drug Abuse and Dependence: While nicotine dependence from the use of substances other than tobacco products has not been reported, the possibility of transference of nicotine dependence to Nicorette exists. The use of the Nicorette gum beyond three months has not been demonstrated to increase the smoking cessation rate. To minimize the risk of dependence, patients should be encouraged to gradually withdraw or stop gum usage altogether at 3 months. Usage beyond three months should be discouraged. In patients who have used the gum for longer periods, gradual withdrawal should be instituted.

Overdosage: Overdosage could occur if many pieces were chewed simultaneously or in rapid succession. Risk of poisoning by swallowing the gum is small because absorption in the absence of chewing is slow and incomplete. The consequences of overdose will most likely be minimized by the early nausea and vomiting known to occur with

Treatment Emergent Symptom Incidence for the 2 mg Gum

	U.S. Drug	U.S. Placebo	British Drug	British Placebo
Number of Subjects Reporting	94	95	58	58
Percent of Subjects Reporting				
Autonomic				
Excess Salivation	2.1	0.0		
CNS				
Insomnia	1.1	1.1		
Dizziness/Light-headedness	2.1	2.1	19.0	13.8
Irritable/Fussy	1.1	1.1		
Headache	1.1	5.3	24.1	29.3
Gastrointestinal				
Nonspecific GI Distress	9.6	6.3		
Eructation	6.4	1.1		
Indigestion			41.4	20.7
Nausea/Vomiting	18.1	4.2	31.0	15.5
Reactions Referable to Mouth, Throat, Jaw, or Teeth				
Mouth or Throat Soreness	37.2	31.6	56.9	53.4
Jaw Muscle Ache	18.1	9.5	44.8	44.8
Others				
Anorexia	1.1	1.1		
Hiccups	14.9	0.0	22.4	3.4

Continued on next page

Information on Merrell Dow products is based on labeling in effect in August, 1984.

Merrell Dow—Cont.

excessive nicotine intake. However, toxic systemic effects may occur. Should an overdose occur, the symptoms would be those of acute nicotine poisoning. Symptoms and signs include nausea, salivation, abdominal pain, vomiting, diarrhea, cold sweat, headache, dizziness, disturbed hearing and vision, mental confusion and marked weakness. Faintness and prostration will likely ensue and hypotension may occur; breathing is difficult; the pulse may be rapid, weak and irregular; collapse may follow by terminal convulsions. Death may result within a few minutes from respiratory failure caused by paralysis of the muscles of respiration.

The oral LD_{50} for nicotine in rodents varies with species but is in excess of 24 mg/kg. Death in rodents was due to respiratory paralysis. The oral minimum lethal dose of nicotine in dogs is greater than 5 mg/kg. The oral minimum lethal dose for nicotine in human adults is 40–60 mg.

Treatment of Overdosage: In view of the lack of actual experience in the treatment of Nicorette overdose, the procedures recommended are those that have been suggested for the treatment of acute nicotine poisoning.

If emesis has not occurred, it should be induced with ipecac syrup in conscious patients. A saline cathartic will speed gastrointestinal passage of the gum. In unconscious patients with a secure airway, gastric lavage with a wide-bore tube followed by suspension of activated charcoal will aid in nicotine removal. Mechanical ventilation for respiratory paralysis may be necessary in severe nicotine poisoning. Hypotension and/or cardiovascular collapse may occur and should be treated vigorously.

Dosage and Administration: Nicorette is an adjunct to smoking cessation programs (see *Indication and Usage* section), and dosage should be individualized. A patient who is a candidate for Nicorette therapy must desire to stop smoking and should be instructed to *stop smoking immediately*. The patient should be given an instruction sheet on Nicorette gum chewing, and be allowed to read the instruction sheet and ask any questions. The patient should arrange for followup visits at intervals not greater than one month. At followup visits the patient's progress in smoking cessation should be evaluated and the continued usage of Nicorette reassessed. It is recommended that patients be evaluated at not greater than monthly intervals and that those successful abstainers at three months should stop using gum or gradually withdraw from gum usage. Patients who chew gum beyond a three-month period should be considered as possibly using Nicorette as a substitute source of nicotine for their nicotine dependence. (See *Drug Abuse and Dependence* section.)

At the initial office or group visit, patients should be instructed to chew one piece of gum whenever they have the urge to smoke. Each piece should be chewed slowly and intermittently for about 30 minutes. The aim of this chewing is to promote even, slow, buccal absorption of the nicotine released from the buffered gum. Chewing quickly can release the nicotine too rapidly, leading to effects similar to oversmoking, e.g., nausea, hiccups or irritation of the throat.

As the nature of adverse effects experienced by an individual patient will be primarily related to the balance between the degree of nicotine tolerance and the rate and degree of absorption of nicotine from the gum, it is important for the patient to learn to chew the gum slowly and to self-titrate the nicotine dose, in order to minimize side effects. (SEE PATIENT INSTRUCTION SHEET AT END OF PRODUCT LABELING.)

Most patients require approximately 10 pieces of gum per day during the first month of treatment. Patients should be instructed not to exceed 30 pieces of the Nicorette per day.

Patients should be assessed after one month of treatment to determine smoking status, and the use of Nicorette as an adjunct should be reevaluated.

Most patients who have returned to smoking in Nicorette assisted programs did so within six months of treatment. Therefore, a gradual withdrawal from Nicorette should be instituted if gum consumption has not been spontaneously reduced by the patient by six months. The use of Nicorette beyond six months is not recommended.

How Supplied: Nicorette is available in 2 mg (beige) square chewing pieces, packaged in child-resistant blister strips of 12 chewing pieces per strip with 8 strips per box.

Boxes of 96 chewing pieces, 2 mg (NDC 0068-0045-55). Store at room temperature, below 86°F (30°C). Protect from light.

Product Information as of August, 1984
Manufactured by AB LEO, Helsingborg, Sweden
for
MERRELL DOW PHARMACEUTICALS INC.
Subsidiary of The Dow Chemical Company
Cincinnati, Ohio 45242-9553, U.S.A.

NICORETTE®
(nicotine polacrilex)

Instructions for Use

You must read these instructions carefully before using Nicorette. While this pamphlet contains important information about Nicorette, it does not contain all information about the drug. If you have questions on the use of Nicorette, you should consult your physician.

WARNING TO FEMALE PATIENTS: NICORETTE CONTAINS NICOTINE WHICH MAY CAUSE FETAL HARM WHEN ADMINISTERED TO A PREGNANT WOMAN. DO NOT TAKE NICORETTE IF YOU ARE PREGNANT OR NURSING. TAKE PRECAUTIONS TO AVOID PREGNANCY WHILE USING NICORETTE, BUT IF YOU SUSPECT YOU ARE PREGNANT, STOP MEDICATION AND TELL YOUR DOCTOR AT ONCE.

THIS DRUG HAS BEEN PRESCRIBED FOR YOU BY YOUR PHYSICIAN. DO NOT LET ANYONE ELSE USE IT. KEEP THIS AND ALL OTHER DRUGS OUT OF THE REACH OF CHILDREN.

1. Starting now you must give up smoking completely. Gradually cutting down your tobacco consumption will not work.
2. Your physician has prescribed Nicorette as part of a program to help you stop smoking.
3. Whenever you feel that you want to smoke, put *one* piece of gum into your mouth.
4. When you chew the gum, nicotine is slowly released and is absorbed through the lining of your mouth.
5. Chew the gum *very slowly* until you taste it or feel a slight tingling in your mouth. (This is *usually* after about 15 chews—the number of chews is not the same for all people.) Because of its nicotine content, the gum does not taste like ordinary chewing gum.
6. As soon as you get the taste of the gum, stop chewing.
7. After the taste or tingling is almost gone (about one minute), chew *slowly* again until you taste the gum. Then stop chewing again.
8. The gum should be chewed slowly and intermittently for about 30 minutes to release most of the nicotine.
9. Most people find that 10 to 12 pieces per day of 2 mg Nicorette are enough to control their urge to smoke. Depending on your needs, you can adjust the rate of chewing and the time between pieces.
10. WARNING: If you chew the gum too fast, you may get effects like people get when they inhale a cigarette for the first time, or when they smoke too fast. These effects include lightheadedness, nausea and vomiting, throat and mouth irritation, hiccups, and stomach upset. Most of these side effects are controlled by chewing more slowly. See instructions above. Some other effects sometimes seen—particularly during the first few days of using the gum—include mouth ulcers, jaw muscle ache, headaches, heart palpitations, and more than the usual amount of saliva in the mouth. In addition, the mechanical effects of gum chewing (any gum) include traumatic injury to oral mucosa or teeth, jaw ache and belching from swallowing air. These side effects may be minimized by proper chewing technique (see steps 5 through 8 above). *There are other side effects which have been infrequently reported with the use of Nicorette. Your physician can answer any questions you may have as to possible side effects. Report any disturbing symptoms to your doctor.*
11. *Not more than 30 pieces of 2 mg gum should be chewed in any one day.*
12. If you accidentally swallow a piece of gum, you should not experience adverse effects. If you do experience adverse effects, call your doctor. Overdosage could occur if many pieces are chewed simultaneously or in rapid succession. IN CASE OF ACCIDENTAL OVERDOSE OR IF A CHILD CHEWS OR SWALLOWS ONE OR MORE PIECES OF THE GUM, YOU SHOULD CONTACT YOUR PHYSICIAN OR LOCAL POISON CONTROL CENTER IMMEDIATELY.
13. As your urge to smoke fades, gradually reduce the number of pieces of gum you chew each day. This may be possible within two to three months. Unless your physician tells you otherwise, do not attempt to stop using the gum until your craving is satisfied with one or two pieces a day, but do not use the gum for more than 6 months.
14. Remember to carry the gum with you at all times in case you feel the sudden urge to smoke again. DO NOT FORGET THAT ONE CIGARETTE IS ENOUGH TO START YOU ON THE SMOKING HABIT AGAIN.

PLEASE NOTE: Nicorette is sugar-free and has been formulated to minimize stickiness. As with other gums, however, the degree to which Nicorette may stick to your dentures, dental caps or partial bridges may depend on the materials from which they are made and other factors. Should an excessive degree of stickiness to your dental work occur, there is the possibility that as with other gums, Nicorette may damage dental work, and you should discontinue its use and consult your physician or dentist.

To remove the gum, tear off single unit.

Peel off backing starting at corner with loose edge.

Push gum through foil.

Shown in Product Identification Section, page 421

NORPRAMIN® ℞
[nŏr′prăm-ĭn]
(desipramine hydrochloride tablets USP)

AVAILABLE ONLY ON PRESCRIPTION

Description: Norpramin (desipramine hydrochloride USP) is an antidepressant drug of the tricyclic type, and is chemically: 5H-Dibenz[b,f]azepine-5-propanamine, 10, 11-dihydro-N-methyl-, monohydrochloride.

Clinical Pharmacology:
Mechanism of Action

Available evidence suggests that many depressions have a biochemical basis in the form of a relative deficiency of neurotransmitters such as norepinephrine and serotonin. Norepinephrine deficiency may be associated with relatively low urinary 3-methoxy-4-hydroxyphenyl glycol (MHPG) levels, while serotonin deficiencies may be associated with low spinal fluid levels of 5-hydroxyindolacetic acid.

While the precise mechanism of action of the tricyclic antidepressants is unknown, a leading theory suggests that they restore normal levels of neurotransmitters by blocking the re-uptake of these substances from the synapse in the central nervous system. Evidence indicates that the secondary amine tricyclic antidepressants, including Norpramin, may have greater activity in blocking the re-uptake of norepinephrine. Tertiary amine tricyclic antidepressants, such as amitriptyline, may have greater effect on serotonin re-uptake. Norpramin (desipramine hydrochloride) is not a monoamine oxidase (MAO) inhibitor and does not act primarily as a central nervous system stimulant. It has been found in some studies to have a more rapid onset of action than imipramine. Earliest therapeutic effects may occasionally be seen in 2 to 5 days, but full treatment benefit usually requires 2 to 3 weeks to obtain.

Metabolism
Tricyclic antidepressants, such as desipramine hydrochloride, are rapidly absorbed from the gastrointestinal tract. Tricyclic antidepressants or their metabolites are to some extent excreted through the gastric mucosa and re-absorbed from the gastrointestinal tract. Desipramine is metabolized in the liver and approximately 70% is excreted in the urine.

The rate of metabolism of tricyclic antidepressants varies widely from individual to individual, chiefly on a genetically determined basis. Up to a thirty-sixfold difference in plasma level may be noted among individuals taking the same oral dose of desipramine. In general, the elderly metabolize tricyclic antidepressants more slowly than do younger adults.

Certain drugs, particularly the psychostimulants and the phenothiazines, increase plasma levels of concomitantly administered tricyclic antidepressants through competition for the same metabolic enzyme systems. Other substances, particularly barbiturates and alcohol, induce liver enzyme activity and thereby reduce tricyclic antidepressant plasma levels. Similar effects have been reported with tobacco smoke.

Research on the relationship of plasma level to therapeutic response with the tricyclic antidepressants has produced conflicting results. While some studies report no correlation, many studies cite therapeutic levels for most tricyclics in the range of 50 to 300 nanograms per milliliter. The therapeutic range is different for each tricyclic antidepressant. For desipramine, an optimal range of therapeutic plasma levels has not been established.

Indications: Norpramin (desipramine hydrochloride) is indicated for relief of symptoms in various depressive syndromes, especially endogenous depression.

Contraindications: Desipramine hydrochloride should not be given in conjunction with, or within 2 weeks of, treatment with an MAO inhibitor drug; hyperpyretic crises, severe convulsions, and death have occurred in patients taking MAO inhibitors and tricyclic antidepressants. When Norpramin (desipramine hydrochloride) is substituted for an MAO inhibitor, at least 2 weeks should elapse between treatments. Norpramin should then be started cautiously and should be increased gradually.

The drug is contraindicated in the acute recovery period following myocardial infarction. It should not be used in those who have shown prior hypersensitivity to the drug. Cross sensitivity between this and other dibenzazepines is a possibility.

Warnings:
1. Extreme caution should be used when this drug is given in the following situations:
   a. In patients with cardiovascular disease, because of the possibility of conduction defects, arrhythmias, tachycardias, strokes, and acute myocardial infarction.
   b. In patients with a history of urinary retention or glaucoma, because of the anticholinergic properties of the drug.
   c. In patients with thyroid disease or those taking thyroid medication, because of the possibility of cardiovascular toxicity, including arrhythmias.
   d. In patients with a history of seizure disorder, because this drug has been shown to lower the seizure threshold.

2. This drug is capable of blocking the antihypertensive effect of guanethidine and similarly acting compounds.

3. USE IN PREGNANCY
Safe use of desipramine hydrochloride during pregnancy and lactation has not been established; therefore, if it is to be given to pregnant patients, nursing mothers, or women of childbearing potential, the possible benefits must be weighed against the possible hazards to mother and child. Animal reproductive studies have been inconclusive.

4. USE IN CHILDREN
Norpramin (desipramine hydrochloride) is not recommended for use in children since safety and effectiveness in the pediatric age group have not been established.

5. The patient should be cautioned that this drug may impair the mental and/or physical abilities required for the performance of potentially hazardous tasks such as driving a car or operating machinery.

6. In patients who may use alcohol excessively, it should be borne in mind that the potentiation may increase the danger inherent in any suicide attempt or overdosage.

Precautions:
1. It is important that this drug be dispensed in the least possible quantities to depressed outpatients, since suicide has been accomplished with this class of drug. Ordinary prudence requires that children not have access to this drug or to potent drugs of any kind; if possible this drug should be dispensed in containers with child-resistant safety closures. Storage of this drug in the home must be supervised responsibly.

2. If serious adverse effects occur, dosage should be reduced or treatment should be altered.

3. Norpramin (desipramine hydrochloride) therapy in patients with manic-depressive illness may induce a hypomanic state after the depressive phase terminates.

4. The drug may cause exacerbation of psychosis in schizophrenic patients.

5. Close supervision and careful adjustment of dosage are required when this drug is given concomitantly with anticholinergic or sympathomimetic drugs.

6. Patients should be warned that while taking this drug their reponse to alcoholic beverages may be exaggerated.

7. Clinical experience in the concurrent administration of ECT and antidepressant drugs is limited. Thus, if such treatment is essential, the possibility of increased risk relative to benefits should be considered.

8. If Norpramin (desipramine hydrochloride) is to be combined with other psychotropic agents such as tranquilizers or sedative/hypnotics, careful consideration should be given to the pharmacology of the agents employed since the sedative effects of Norpramin and benzodiazepines (e.g., chlordiazepoxide or diazepam) are additive. Both the sedative and anticholinergic effects of the major tranquilizers are also additive to those of Norpramin.

9. This drug should be discontinued as soon as possible prior to elective surgery because of the possible cardiovascular effects. Hypertensive episodes have been observed during surgery in patients taking desipramine hydrochloride.

10. Both elevation and lowering of blood sugar levels have been reported.

11. Leukocyte and differential counts should be performed in any patient who develops fever and sore throat during therapy; the drug should be discontinued if there is evidence of pathologic neutrophil depression.

12. Norpramin 25, 50, 75, and 100 mg tablets contain FD&C Yellow No. 5 (tartrazine), which may cause allergic-type reactions (including bronchial asthma) in certain susceptible individuals. Although the overall incidence of FD&C Yellow No. 5 (tartrazine) sensitivity in the general population is low, it is frequently seen in patients who also have aspirin hypersensitivity.

Adverse Reactions:
Note: Included in the following listing are a few adverse reactions that have not been reported with this specific drug. However, the pharmacologic similarities among the tricyclic antidepressant drugs require that each of the reactions be considered when Norpramin (desipramine hydrochloride) is given.

Cardiovascular: hypotension, hypertension, tachycardia, palpitation, arrhythmias, heart block, myocardial infarction, stroke.

Psychiatric: confusional states (especially in the elderly) with hallucinations, disorientation, delusions; anxiety, restlessness, agitation; insomnia and nightmares; hypomania; exacerbation of psychosis.

Neurologic: numbness, tingling, paresthesias of extremities; incoordination, ataxia, tremors; peripheral neuropathy; extrapyramidal symptoms; seizures; alteration in EEG patterns; tinnitus.

Anticholinergic: dry mouth, and rarely associated sublingual adenitis; blurred vision, disturbance of accommodation, mydriasis, increased intraocular pressure; constipation, paralytic ileus; urinary retention, delayed micturition, dilatation of urinary tract.

Allergic: skin rash, petechiae, urticaria, itching, photosensitization (avoid excessive exposure to sunlight), edema (of face and tongue or general), drug fever, cross sensitivity with other tricyclic drugs.

Hematologic: Bone marrow depressions including agranulocytosis, eosinophilia, purpura, thrombocytopenia.

Gastrointestinal: anorexia, nausea and vomiting, epigastric distress, peculiar taste, abdominal cramps, diarrhea, stomatitis, black tongue.

Endocrine: gynecomastia in the male, breast enlargement and galactorrhea in the female; increased or decreased libido, impotence, testicular swelling; elevation or depression of blood sugar levels.

Other: jaundice (simulating obstructive), altered liver function; weight gain or loss; perspiration, flushing; urinary frequency, nocturia; parotid swelling; drowsiness, dizziness, weakness and fatigue, headache; alopecia.

Withdrawal Symptoms: Though not indicative of addiction, abrupt cessation of treatment after prolonged therapy may produce nausea, headache, and malaise.

Dosage and Administration: Not recommended for use in children.

Lower dosages are recommended for elderly patients and adolescents. Lower dosages are also recommended for outpatients compared to hospitalized patients, who are closely supervised. Dosage should be initiated at a low level and increased according to clinical response and any evidence of intolerance. Following remission, maintenance medication may be required for a period of time and should be at the lowest dose that will maintain remission.

Usual Adult Dose:
The usual adult dose is 100 to 200 mg per day. In more severely ill patients, dosage may be further increased gradually to 300 mg/day if necessary. Dosages above 300 mg/day are not recommended. Dosage should be initiated at a lower level and increased according to tolerance and clinical response.

Treatment of patients requiring as much as 300 mg should generally be initiated in hospitals, where regular visits by the physician, skilled nursing care, and frequent electrocardiograms (ECG's) are available.

The best available evidence of impending toxicity from very high doses of Norpramin is prolongation of the QRS or QT intervals on the ECG. Prolongation of the PR interval is also significant, but less closely correlated with plasma levels. Clinical symptoms of intolerance, especially drowsiness, dizziness, and postural hypotension, should also alert the physician to the need for reduction in

Continued on next page

Information on Merrell Dow products is based on labeling in effect in August, 1984.

Merrell Dow—Cont.

dosage. Plasma desipramine measurement would constitute the optimal guide to dosage monitoring. Initial therapy may be administered in divided doses or a single daily dose.

Maintenance therapy may be given on a once-daily schedule for patient convenience and compliance.

Adolescent and Geriatric Dose:

The usual adolescent and geriatric dose is 25 to 100 mg daily.

Dosage should be initiated at a lower level and increased according to tolerance and clinical response to a usual maximum of 100 mg daily. In more severely ill patients, dosage may be further increased to 150 mg/day. Doses above 150 mg/day are not recommended in these age groups.

Initial therapy may be administered in divided doses or a single daily dose.

Maintenance therapy may be given on a once-daily schedule for patient convenience and compliance.

Overdosage: There is no specific antidote for desipramine, nor are there specific phenomena of diagnostic value characterizing poisoning by the drug.

Within an hour of ingestion the patient may become agitated or stuporous and then comatose. Hypotension, shock, and renal shutdown may ensue. Grand mal seizures, both early and late after ingestion, have been reported. Hyperactive reflexes, hyperpyrexia, muscle rigidity, vomiting, and ECG evidence of impaired conduction may occur. Serious disturbances of cardiac rate, rhythm, and output can occur. The precepts of early evacuation of the ingested material and subsequent support of respiration (airway and movement), circulation, and renal output apply.

The principles of management of coma and shock by means of the mechanical respirator, cardiac pacemaker, monitoring of central venous pressure, and regulation of fluid and acid-base balance are well known in most medical centers and are not further discussed here.

Because CNS involvement, respiratory depression, and cardiac arrhythmia can occur suddenly, hospitalization and close observation are generally advisable, even when the amount ingested is thought to be small or the initial degree of intoxication appears slight or moderate. Most patients with ECG abnormalities should have continuous cardiac monitoring for at least 72 hours and be closely observed until well after cardiac status has returned to normal; relapses may occur after apparent recovery.

The slow intravenous administration of physostigmine salicylate has been reported to reverse most of the anticholinergic cardiovascular and CNS effects of overdose with tricyclic antidepressants. In adults, 1 to 3 mg has been reported to be effective. In children, the dose should be started with 0.5 mg and repeated at 5-minute intervals to determine the minimum effective dose; no more than 2 mg. should be given. Because of the short duration of action of physostigmine, the effective dose should be repeated at 30-minute to 60-minute intervals, as necessary. Rapid injection should be avoided to reduce the possibility of physostigmine-induced convulsions.

Other possible therapeutic considerations include:

(a) Dialysis: Desipramine is found in low concentration in the serum, even after a massive oral dose. In vitro experiments in which blood bank blood was used indicate that it is very poorly dialyzed. Because of indications that the drug is secreted in gastric juice, constant gastric lavage has been suggested.

(b) Pharmacologic treatment of shock: Since desipramine potentiates the action of such vasopressor agents as levarterenol and metaraminol, they should be used only with caution.

(c) Pharmacologic control of seizures: Intravenous barbiturates are the treatment of choice for the control of grand mal seizures. One may, alternately, consider the parenteral use of diphenylhydantoin, which has less central depressant effect but also has an effect on heart rhythm that has not yet been fully defined.

(d) Pharmacologic control of cardiac function: Severe disturbances of cardiac rate, rhythm, and output are probably the initiating events in shock. Intravascular volume must be maintained by i.v. fluids. Digitalization should be carried out early in view of the fact that a positive inotropic effect can be achieved without increase in cardiac work. Many of the cardiodynamic effects of digital- is are the exact opposite of those of massive doses of desipramine (animal studies).

How Supplied:

10 mg blue coated tablets imprinted 68-7
Bottles of 100
25 mg yellow coated tablets imprinted MERRELL 11
Bottles of 100 and 1000 and unit dose dispenser of 100
50 mg green coated tablets imprinted MERRELL 15
Bottles of 100 and 1000 and unit dose dispenser of 100
75 mg orange coated tablets imprinted MERRELL 19
Bottles of 100
100 mg peach coated tablets imprinted MERRELL 20
Bottles of 100
150 mg white coated tablets imprinted MERRELL 21
Bottles of 50

U.S. Patent Numbers 3,454,554
3,454,698

Product Information as of May, 1980
(10 mg tablet added July, 1982)
Shown in Product Identification Section, page 421

NOVAFED® Capsules
[nō'vă-fĕd]
pseudoephedrine hydrochloride
Controlled-Release Decongestant

Description: Each Novafed capsule contains 120 mg of pseudoephedrine hydrochloride in specially formulated pellets designed to provide continuous therapeutic effect for 12 hours. About one-half of the active ingredient is released soon after administration and the rest slowly over the remaining time period.

Actions: Pseudoephedrine (a sympathomimetic) is an orally effective nasal decongestant with peripheral effects similar to epinephrine and central effects similar to, but less intense than, amphetamines. It has the potential for excitatory side effects. At the recommended oral dosage, it has little or no pressor effect in normotensive adults. Patients have not been reported to experience the rebound congestion sometimes experienced with frequent, repeated use of topical decongestants.

Indications: Relief of nasal congestion or eustachian tube congestion. May be given concomitantly with analgesics, antihistamines, expectorants and antibiotics.

Contraindications: Patients with severe hypertension, severe coronary artery disease, and patients on MAO inhibitor therapy. Also contraindicated in patients with hypersensitivity or idiosyncrasy to sympathomimetic amines which may be manifested by insomnia, dizziness, weakness, tremor or arrhythmias.

Children under 12: Should not be used by children under 12 years.

Nursing Mothers: Contraindicated because of the higher than usual risk for infants from sympathomimetic amines.

Warnings: Use judiciously and sparingly in patients with hypertension, diabetes mellitus, ischemic heart disease, increased intraocular pressure, hyperthyroidism or prostatic hypertrophy. See, however, Contraindications. Sympathomimetics may produce central nervous stimulation with convulsions or cardiovascular collapse with accompanying hypotension.

Do not exceed recommended dosage.

Use in Pregnancy: Safety in pregnancy has not been established.

Use in Elderly: The elderly (60 years and older) are more likely to have adverse reactions to sympathomimetics. Overdosage of sympathomimetics in this age group may cause hallucinations, convulsions, CNS depression, and death. Safe use of a short-acting sympathomimetic should be demonstrated in the individual elderly patient before considering the use of a sustained-action formulation.

Precautions: Patients with diabetes, hypertension, cardiovascular disease and hyper-reactivity to ephedrine.

Adverse Reactions: Hyper-reactive individuals may display ephedrine-like reactions such as tachycardia, palpitations, headache, dizziness or nausea. Sympathomimetics have been associated with certain untoward reactions including fear, anxiety, tenseness, restlessness, tremor, weakness, pallor, respiratory difficulty, dysuria, insomnia, hallucinations, convulsions, CNS depression, arrhythmias, and cardiovascular collapse with hypotension.

Drug Interactions: MAO inhibitors and beta adrenergic blockers increase the effects of pseudoephedrine. Sympathomimetics may reduce the antihypertensive effects of methyldopa, mecamylamine, reserpine and veratrum alkaloids.

Dosage and Administration: One capsule every 12 hours. Do not give to children under 12 years of age.

Caution: Federal law prohibits dispensing without prescription.

How Supplied: Brown and orange colored hard gelatin capsules, monographed with the Dow diamond followed by the number 104. Bottle of 100 capsules (NDC 0068-0104-61).

Manufactured by KV Pharmaceutical Company, St. Louis, MO 63144

Shown in Product Identification Section, page 421

NOVAFED® Liquid
[nō'vă-fĕd]
pseudoephedrine hydrochloride
Decongestant

Description: Each 5 ml teaspoonful of Novafed liquid contains 30 mg of pseudoephedrine hydrochloride, the salt of a pharmacologically active stereoisomer of ephedrine (1-phenyl-2-methylamino propanol). The formulation also contains 7.5% alcohol.

Actions: Pseudoephedrine hydrochloride is an orally effective nasal decongestant. Pseudoephedrine is a sympathomimetic amine with peripheral effects similar to epinephrine and central effects similar to, but less intense than, amphetamines. Therefore, it has the potential for excitatory side effects. At the recommended oral dosage, pseudoephedrine has little or no pressor effect in normotensive adults. Patients taking pseudoephedrine orally have not been reported to experience the rebound congestion sometimes experienced with frequent, repeated use of topical decongestants. Pseudoephedrine is not known to produce drowsiness.

Indications: Novafed liquid is indicated for the relief of nasal congestion associated, for example, with the common cold, acute upper respiratory infections, sinusitis, and hay fever or upper respiratory allergies. Decongestants have been used for many years to relieve eustachian tube congestion associated with acute eustachian salpingitis, aerotitis media, acute otitis media and serous otitis media. Novafed liquid may be given concurrently, when indicated, with analgesics, antihistamines, expectorants and antibiotics.

Contraindications: Patients with severe hypertension, severe coronary artery disease and patients on MAO inhibitor therapy. Also contraindicated in patients with hypersensitivity or idiosyncrasy to sympathomimetic amines which may be manifested by insomnia, dizziness, weakness, tremor or arrhythmias.

Nursing Mothers: Contraindicated because of the higher than usual risk for infants from sympathomimetic amines.

Warnings: Use judiciously and sparingly in patients with hypertension, diabetes mellitus, ischemic heart disease, increased intraocular pressure, hyperthyroidism, or prostatic hypertrophy. See, however, Contraindications. Sympathomimetics may produce central nervous stimulation with convulsions or cardiovascular collapse with accompanying hypotension.

Do not exceed recommended dosage.

Use in Pregnancy: Safety has not been established.

Use in Elderly: The elderly (60 years and older) are more likely to have adverse reactions to sympathomimetics. Overdosage of sympathomimetics in this age group may cause hallucinations, convulsions, CNS depression, and death.

Precautions: Patients with diabetes, hypertension, cardiovascular disease and hyperreactivity to ephedrine.

Adverse Reactions: Hyperreactive individuals may display ephedrine-like reactions such as tachycardia, palpitations, headache, dizziness, or nausea. Sympathomimetics have been associated with certain untoward reactions including fear, anxiety, tenseness, restlessness, tremor, weakness, pallor, respiratory difficulty, dysuria, insomnia, hallucinations, convulsions, CNS depression, arrhythmias, and cardiovascular collapse with hypotension.

Drug Interactions: MAO inhibitors and beta adrenergic blockers increase the effects of pseudoephedrine. Sympathomimetics may reduce the antihypertensive effects of methyldopa, mecamylamine, reserpine and veratrum alkaloids.

Dosage and Administration: Adults, and children over 12 years of age, 2 teaspoonfuls; children 6 to 12 years, 1 teaspoonful; and children under 6 years, $\frac{1}{2}$ teaspoonful, every 4 to 6 hours, not to exceed 4 doses in a 24-hour period. However, this dosage may be modified at the discretion of the physician.

Note: Novafed liquid does not require a prescription. The package label has dosage instructions as follows: Adults, and children over 12 years of age, 2 teaspoonfuls, every 4 to 6 hours. Children 6 to 12 years, 1 teaspoonful, every 4 to 6 hours. Children 2 to 5 years, $\frac{1}{2}$ teaspoonful, every 4 to 6 hours. Do not exceed four doses in a 24-hour period. For children younger than 2 years, consult a physician.

How Supplied: As a lime green liquid in 4 fluid ounce bottles (NDC 0068-1011-04).

NOVAFED® A CAPSULES   ℞
[nō′ vă-fĕd]
Controlled-Release
Decongestant plus Antihistamine

Description: Each NOVAFED A capsule for oral use contains 120 mg pseudoephedrine hydrochloride, and 8 mg of chlorpheniramine maleate. The specially formulated pellets in each capsule are designed to provide continuous therapeutic effect for about 12 hours. Nearly one-half of the active ingredients is released soon after administration and the remainder is released slowly over the remaining time period.

Pseudoephedrine hydrochloride is a nasal decongestant. Chemically it is α-[1-(methyl-amino)ethyl]-benzenemethanol hydrochloride.

Chlorpheniramine maleate is an antihistamine. Chemically it is α-(4-chlorophenyl)-N,N-dimethyl-2-pyridinepropanamine.

Clinical Pharmacology: Pseudoephedrine is an orally active sympathomimetic amine and exerts a decongestant action on the nasal mucosa. Pseudoephedrine produces peripheral effects similar to those of ephedrine and central effects similar to, but less intense than amphetamines. It has the potential for excitatory side effects. At the recommended oral dosages it has little or no pressor effect in normotensive adults. The serum half-life (T-$\frac{1}{2}$) of pseudoephedrine is approximately 4 to 6 hours. T-$\frac{1}{2}$ is decreased with increased excretion of drug at urine pH lower than 6 and may be increased with decreased excretion at urine pH higher than 8.

Chlorpheniramine is an antihistaminic that possesses anticholinergic and sedative effects. It is considered one of the most effective and least toxic of the histamine antagonists. Chlorpheniramine is an H_1 receptor antagonist. It antagonizes many of the pharmacologic actions of histamine. It prevents released histamine from dilating capillaries and causing edema of the respiratory mucosa. Chlorpheniramine has a duration of action of 4 to 6 hours in clinical studies. Its half-life in serum, however, is 12 to 16 hours.

Indications and Usage: Relief of nasal congestion and eustachian tube congestion associated with the common cold, sinusitis and acute upper respiratory infections. It is also indicated for symptomatic relief of perennial and seasonal allergic rhinitis, vasomotor rhinitis, allergic conjunctivitis due to inhalant allergens and foods and mild, uncomplicated allergic skin manifestations of urticaria and angioedema. Decongestants in combination with antihistamines have been used for many years to relieve eustachian tube congestion associated with acute eustachian salpingitis, aerotitis media, acute otitis media and serous otitis media. May be given concomitantly with analgesics and antibiotics.

Contraindications: Patients with severe hypertension, severe coronary artery disease, and in patients on MAO inhibitor therapy. Antihistamines are contraindicated in patients with narrow-angle glaucoma, urinary retention, peptic ulcer, during an asthmatic attack, and in patients receiving MAO inhibitors.

Hypersensitivity: Contraindicated in patients with hypersensitivity or idiosyncrasy to sympathomimetic amines or phenanthrene derivatives.

Nursing Mothers: Contraindicated because of the higher than usual risk for infants from sympathomimetic amines.

Warnings: Sympathomimetic amines should be used judiciously and sparingly in patients with hypertension, diabetes mellitus, ischemic heart disease, increased intraocular pressure, hyperthyroidism or prostatic hypertrophy (see CONTRAINDICATIONS). Sympathomimetics may produce CNS stimulation with convulsions or cardiovascular collapse with accompanying hypotension.

Chlorpheniramine maleate has an atropine-like action and should be used with caution in patients with increased intraocular pressure, cardiovascular disease, hypertension or in patients with a history of bronchial asthma (see CONTRAINDICATIONS). Do not exceed recommended dose.

Use in Elderly: The elderly (60 years and older) are more likely to have adverse reactions to sympathomimetics. Overdosage of sympathomimetics in this age group may cause hallucinations, convulsions, CNS depression and death.

Precautions: *General:* Should be used with caution in patients with diabetes, hypertension, cardiovascular disease and hyperreactivity to ephedrine. The antihistaminic may cause drowsiness and ambulatory patients who operate machinery or motor vehicles should be cautioned accordingly.

Information for Patients: Antihistamines may impair mental and physical abilities required for the performance of potentially hazardous tasks, such as driving a vehicle or operating machinery, and mental alertness in children.

Drug Interactions: MAO inhibitors and beta adrenergic blockers increase the effect of sympathomimetics. Sympathomimetics may reduce the antihypertensive effects of methyldopa, mecamylamine, reserpine and veratrum alkaloids. Concomitant use of antihistamines with alcohol, tricyclic antidepressants, barbiturates and other CNS depressants may have an additive effect.

Pregnancy Category C: Animal reproduction studies have not been conducted with NOVAFED A capsules. It is also not known whether NOVAFED A capsules can cause fetal harm when administered to a pregnant woman or can affect reproduction capacity. NOVAFED A capsules may be given to a pregnant woman only if clearly needed.

Nursing Mothers: Pseudoephedrine is contraindicated in nursing mothers because of the higher than usual risk for infants from sympathomimetic amines.

Adverse Reactions: Hyperreactive individuals may display ephedrine-like reactions such as tachycardia, palpitations, headache, dizziness, or nausea. Patients sensitive to antihistamines may experience mild sedation. Sympathomimetic drugs have been associated with certain untoward reactions including fear, anxiety, tenseness, restlessness, tremor, weakness, pallor, respiratory difficulty, dysuria, insomnia, hallucinations, convulsions, CNS depression, arrhythmias, and cardiovascular collapse with hypotension.

Possible side effects of antihistamines are drowsiness, restlessness, dizziness, weakness, dry mouth, anorexia, nausea, headache, nervousness, blurring of vision, heartburn, dysuria and very rarely dermatitis. Patient idiosyncrasy to adrenergic agents may be manifested by insomnia, dizziness, weakness, tremor, or arrhythmias.

Overdosage: Acute overdosage with NOVAFED A capsules may produce clinical signs of CNS stimulation and variable cardiovascular effects. Pressor amines should be used with great caution in the presence of pseudoephedrine. Patients with signs of stimulation should be treated conservatively.

Dosage and Administration: One capsule every 12 hours. Do not give to children under 12 years of age.

Caution: Federal law prohibits dispensing without prescription.

How Supplied: NOVAFED A is supplied in red and orange colored hard gelatin capsules monogrammed with the Dow diamond followed by the number 106, in bottles of 100 capsules (NDC 0068-0106-61).

Manufactured by KV Pharmaceutical Company, St. Louis, MO 63144

Shown in Product Identification Section, page 421

NOVAFED® A
[nō′ vă-fĕd]
Decongestant Plus Antihistamine
Liquid

Description: Each 5 ml teaspoonful of Novafed A liquid contains: pseudoephedrine hydrochloride, 30 mg, and chlorpheniramine maleate, 2 mg. Pseudoephedrine hydrochloride is the salt of a pharmacologically active stereoisomer of ephedrine (1-phenyl-2-methylamino propanol). Chlorpheniramine is an antihistamine drug of the alkylamine type. Other ingredients include alcohol, 5%.

Actions: Combines the actions of an orally effective nasal decongestant, pseudoephedrine, and an antihistamine, chlorpheniramine. The antihistamine also possesses anticholinergic and sedative effects.

Indications: Novafed A liquid is indicated for the relief of nasal congestion associated, for example, with the common cold, acute upper respiratory infections, sinusitis, and hay fever or upper respiratory allergies. Decongestants in combination with antihistamines have been used for many years to relieve eustachian tube congestion associated with acute eustachian salpingitis, aerotitis media, acute otitis media and serous otitis media. Novafed A liquid may be given concurrently, when indicated, with analgesics and antibiotics.

Contraindications: Patients with severe hypertension, severe coronary artery disease; patients on MAO inhibitor therapy; patients with narrow-angle glaucoma, urinary retention, peptic ulcer and during an asthmatic attack. Also contraindicated in patients with hypersensitivity or idiosyncrasy to sympathomimetic amines or antihistamines which may be manifested by insomnia, dizziness, weakness, tremor or arrhythmias, dry mouth, drowsiness and vomiting.

Continued on next page

Information on Merrell Dow products is based on labeling in effect in August, 1984.

Merrell Dow—Cont.

Nursing Mothers: Contraindicated because of the higher than usual risk for infants from sympathomimetic amines.

Warnings: Sympathomimetic amines should be used judiciously and sparingly in patients with hypertension, diabetes mellitus, ischemic heart disease, increased intraocular pressure, hyperthyroidism or prostatic hypertrophy. See, however, Contraindications. Sympathomimetics may produce central nervous system stimulation with convulsions or cardiovascular collapse with accompanying hypotension.

Antihistamines may impair mental and physical abilities required for the performance of potentially hazardous tasks, such as driving a vehicle or operating machinery, and may impair mental alertness in children. Chlorpheniramine has an atropine-like action and should be used with caution in patients with increased intraocular pressure, cardiovascular disease, hypertension or in patients with a history of bronchial asthma. See, however, Contraindications.

Do not exceed recommended dosage.

Use in Pregnancy: Safety of pseudoephedrine has not been established.

Use in Elderly: The elderly (60 years and older) are more likely to have adverse reactions to sympathomimetics. Overdosage of sympathomimetics in this age group may cause hallucinations, convulsions, CNS depression, and death.

Precautions: Patients with diabetes, hypertension, cardiovascular disease and hyperreactivity to ephedrine. The antihistamine may cause drowsiness and ambulatory patients who operate machinery or motor vehicles should be cautioned accordingly.

Adverse Reactions: Hyperreactive individuals may display ephedrine-like reactions such as tachycardia, palpitations, headache, dizziness or nausea. Patients sensitive to antihistamines may experience mild sedation.

Sympathomimetics have been associated with certain untoward reactions including fear, anxiety, tenseness, restlessness, tremor, weakness, pallor, respiratory difficulty, dysuria, insomnia, hallucinations, convulsions, CNS depression, arrhythmias, and cardiovascular collapse with hypotension.

Possible side effects of antihistamines are drowsiness, dry mouth, anorexia, nausea, vomiting, headache and nervousness, blurring of vision, polyuria, heartburn, dysuria and very rarely, dermatitis.

Drug Interactions: MAO inhibitors and beta adrenergic blockers increase the effects of sympathomimetics. Sympathomimetics may reduce the antihypertensive effects of methyldopa, mecamylamine, reserpine and veratrum alkaloids. Concomitant use of antihistamines with alcohol, tricyclic antidepressants, barbiturates and other CNS depressants may have an additive effect.

Dosage and Administration: Adults, and children over 12 years of age, 2 teaspoonfuls; children 6 to 12 years, 1 teaspoonful; and children under 6 years, ½ teaspoonful, every 4 to 6 hours, not to exceed 4 doses in a 24-hour period. However, this dosage may be modified at the discretion of the physician.

Note: Novafed A liquid does not require a prescription. The package label has dosage instructions as follows: Adults, and children over 12 years of age, 2 teaspoonfuls every 4 to 6 hours. Children 6 to 12 years, 1 teaspoonful, every 4 to 6 hours. For children under 6 years of age, consult a physician. Do not exceed 4 doses in a 24-hour period.

How Supplied: As a green liquid in 4 fluid ounce bottles (NDC 0068-1010-04).

NOVAHISTINE® COUGH FORMULA
[nō″ vă-hĭs′ tēn]
(See PDR For Nonprescription Drugs)

NOVAHISTINE® COUGH & COLD FORMULA
[nō″ vă-hĭs′ tēn]
(See PDR For Nonprescription Drugs)

NOVAHISTINE® DH
[nō″ vă-hĭs′ tēn]
Antitussive-Decongestant-Antihistamine Modified Formula

Description: Each 5 ml teaspoonful contains codeine phosphate, 10 mg (Warning: may be habit forming), pseudoephedrine hydrochloride, 30 mg, chlorpheniramine maleate, 2 mg, and alcohol, 5%.

Actions: Antitussive, decongestant and antihistaminic actions. Codeine, at the recommended dose, causes suppression of the cough reflex by a direct effect on the cough center in the medulla of the brain. Codeine has antitussive, mild analgesic and sedative effects.

Pseudoephedrine hydrochloride, an orally effective nasal decongestant, is a sympathomimetic amine with peripheral effects similar to epinephrine and central effects similar to, but less intense than, amphetamines. Therefore, it has the potential for excitatory side effects. Pseudoephedrine at the recommended oral dosage has little or no pressor effect in normotensive adults. Patients taking pseudoephedrine orally have not been reported to experience the rebound congestion sometimes experienced with frequent, repeated use of topical decongestants. Pseudoephedrine is not known to produce drowsiness.

Chlorpheniramine possesses antihistaminic, mild anticholinergic and sedative effects. It antagonizes many of the pharmacologic actions of histamine. It prevents released histamine from dilating capillaries and causing edema of the respiratory mucosa.

Indications: For the temporary relief of cough associated with minor throat and bronchial irritation or nasal congestion due to the common cold, sinusitis, and hay fever (allergic rhinitis).

A minimum dosage of codeine is provided for the symptomatic relief of nonproductive cough. Decongestants have been used to relieve eustachian salpingitis, aerotitis, otitis, and serous otitis media. Chlorpheniramine maleate provides temporary relief from runny nose, sneezing, itching of nose or throat, and itchy and watery eyes as may occur in hay fever (allergic rhinitis).

May be used as supportive therapy for acute otitis media and relief of mild otalgia.

May be given concomitantly, when indicated, with analgesics and antibiotics.

Contraindications: Patients with severe hypertension, severe coronary artery disease, and in patients on MAO inhibitor therapy.

Nursing Mothers: Pseudoephedrine is contraindicated in nursing mothers because of the higher than usual risk for infants from sympathomimetic amines.

Hypersensitivity: This drug is contraindicated in patients with hypersensitivity or idiosyncrasy to its ingredients. Patient idiosyncrasy to adrenergic agents may be manifested by insomnia, dizziness, weakness, tremor or arrhythmias.

Warnings: Codeine should be prescribed and administered with the same degree of caution as all oral medications containing a narcotic analgesic. Codeine appears in the milk of nursing mothers.

If sympathomimetic amines are used in patients with hypertension, diabetes mellitus, ischemic heart disease, hyperthyroidism, increased intraocular pressure or prostatic hypertrophy, judicious caution should be exercised. See, however, Contraindications. Sympathomimetics may produce CNS stimulation with convulsions or cardiovascular collapse with accompanying hypotension. Do not exceed recommended dosage.

The elderly (60 years and older) are more likely to have adverse reactions to sympathomimetics. Safety for use during pregnancy has not been established.

Antihistamines may cause excitability, especially in children.

Precautions: If cough persists for more than one week, tends to recur or is accompanied by fever, rash or headache, discontinue treatment. Other medications containing a narcotic analgesic, phenothiazines, tranquilizers, sedatives, hypnotics and other CNS depressants, including alcohol, may have an additive CNS depressant effect when used concomitantly. The dose should be reduced when such combined therapy is contemplated.

Caution should be exercised if used in patients with high blood pressure, heart disease, asthma, emphysema, diabetes, thyroid disease and hyperreactivity to ephedrine.

The antihistamine may cause drowsiness, and ambulatory patients who operate machinery or motor vehicles should be cautioned accordingly.

Adverse Reactions: Nausea, vomiting, constipation, dizziness, sedation, palpitations or pruritus may occur. More frequent or higher than recommended dosage may cause respiratory depression, especially in patients with respiratory disease associated with carbon dioxide retention.

Drugs containing sympathomimetic amines have been associated with certain untoward reactions including fear, anxiety, tenseness, restlessness, tremor, weakness, pallor, respiratory difficulty, dysuria, insomnia, hallucinations, convulsions, CNS depression, arrhythmias and cardiovascular collapse with hypotension.

Patients sensitive to antihistamine drugs may experience mild sedation. Other side effects from antihistamines may include dry mouth, dizziness, weakness, anorexia, nausea, vomiting, headache, nervousness, polyuria, heartburn, diplopia, dysuria, and very rarely, dermatitis.

Drug Interactions: Codeine may potentiate the effects of other narcotics, general anesthetics, tranquilizers, sedatives and hypnotics, tricyclic antidepressants, MAO inhibitors, alcohol and other CNS depressants.

Beta adrenergic blockers and MAO inhibitors potentiate the sympathomimetic effects of pseudoephedrine. Sympathomimetics may reduce the antihypertensive effects of methyldopa, mecamylamine, reserpine and veratrum alkaloids.

Antihistamines have been shown to enhance one or more of the effects of alcohol, tricyclic antidepressants, barbiturates and other CNS depressants.

Dosage: Adults, 2 teaspoonfuls; children 50–90 lbs, ½ to 1 teaspoonful; 25–50 lbs, ¼ to ½ teaspoonful. Repeat every 4 to 6 hours. May be given to children under 2 at the discretion of the physician. *Do not exceed 4 doses in a 24-hour period.*

Product label dosage is as follows: Adults, 2 teaspoonfuls; children 6 to 12 years, 1 teaspoonful. May be given every 4 to 6 hours, *but do not exceed 4 doses in 24 hours.* For children under 6 years, consult a physician.

How Supplied: In 4 fluid ounce bottles (NDC 0068-1027-04), and pints (NDC 0068-1027-16).

Shown in Product Identification Section, page 421

NOVAHISTINE® DMX
[nō″ vă-hĭs′ tēn]
Antitussive-Decongestant Liquid
(See PDR For Nonprescription Drugs)

NOVAHISTINE® ELIXIR
[nō″ vă-hĭs′ tēn]
Decongestant—Antihistaminic
(See PDR For Nonprescription Drugs)

NOVAHISTINE® EXPECTORANT
[nō″ vă-hĭs′ tēn]
Antitussive-Decongestant-Expectorant Modified Formula

Description: Each 5 ml teaspoonful contains codeine phosphate, 10 mg (Warning: may be habit forming), pseudoephedrine hydrochloride, 30 mg, guaifenesin (glyceryl guaiacolate), 100 mg, and alcohol, 7.5%.

Actions: Expectorant, antitussive and decongestant actions. Codeine, at the recommended dose, causes suppression of the cough reflex by a direct effect on the cough center in the medulla of the brain. Codeine has antitussive and mild analgesic and sedative effects.

Pseudoephedrine hydrochloride, an orally effective nasal decongestant, is a sympathomimetic amine with peripheral effects similar to epinephrine and central effects similar to, but less intense than, amphetamines. Therefore, it has the potential for excitatory side effects. Pseudoephedrine at the recommended oral dosage has little or no pressor effect in normotensive adults. Patients taking pseudoephedrine orally have not been reported to experience the rebound congestion sometimes experienced with frequent, repeated use of topical decongestants. Pseudoephedrine is not known to produce drowsiness.

Guaifenesin helps drainage of bronchial tubes by thinning the mucus, and facilitates expectoration by loosening phlegm and bronchial secretions.

Indications: For loosening tenacious pulmonary secretions associated with cough and respiratory congestion.

A minimum dosage of codeine phosphate is provided for the symptomatic relief of nonproductive cough. Decongestants have been used to relieve eustachian tube congestion associated with acute eustachian salpingitis, aerotitis, otitis and serous otitis media. Guaifenesin helps loosen phlegm (sputum) and bronchial secretions.

May be used as supportive therapy for acute otitis media and relief of mild otalgia.

May be given concomitantly, when indicated, with analgesics and antibiotics.

Contraindications: Patients with severe hypertension, severe coronary artery disease, and in patients on MAO inhibitor therapy.

Nursing Mothers: Pseudoephedrine is contraindicated in nursing mothers because of the higher than usual risk for infants from sympathomimetic amines.

Hypersensitivity: This drug is contraindicated in patients with hypersensitivity or idiosyncrasy to its ingredients. Patient idiosyncrasy to adrenergic agents may be manifested by insomnia, dizziness, weakness, tremor or arrhythmias.

Warnings: Codeine should be prescribed and administered with the same degree of caution as all oral medications containing a narcotic analgesic. Codeine appears in the milk of nursing mothers.

If sympathomimetic amines are used in patients with hypertension, diabetes mellitus, ischemic heart disease, hyperthyroidism, increased intraocular pressure and prostatic hypertrophy, judicious caution should be exercised. See, however, Contraindications. Sympathomimetics may produce CNS stimulation with convulsions or cardiovascular collapse with accompanying hypotension. Do not exceed recommended dosage.

The elderly (60 years and older) are more likely to have adverse reactions to sympathomimetics. Safety for use during pregnancy has not been established.

Precautions: If cough persists for more than one week, tends to recur or is accompanied by fever, rash or headache, discontinue treatment. Other medications containing a narcotic analgesic, phenothiazines, tranquilizers, sedatives, hypnotics, and other CNS depressants, including alcohol, may have an additive CNS depressant effect when used concomitantly. The dose should be reduced when such combined therapy is contemplated.

Caution should be exercised if used in patients with high blood pressure, heart disease, asthma, emphysema, diabetes, thyroid disease and hyperreactivity to ephedrine.

Adverse Reactions: Nausea, vomiting, constipation, dizziness, sedation, palpitations, or pruritus may occur. More frequent or higher than recommended dosage may cause respiratory depression, especially in patients with respiratory disease associated with carbon dioxide retention. Drugs containing sympathomimetic amines have been associated with certain untoward reactions including fear, anxiety, tenseness, restlessness, tremor, weakness, pallor, respiratory difficulty, dysuria, insomnia, hallucinations, convulsions, CNS depression, arrhythmias and cardiovascular collapse with hypotension.

Note: Guaifenesin interferes with the colorimetric determination of 5-hydroxyindoleacetic acid (5-HIAA) and vanillylmandelic acid (VMA).

Drug Interactions: Codeine may potentiate the effects of other narcotics, general anesthetics, tranquilizers, sedatives and hypnotics, tricyclic antidepressants, MAO inhibitors, alcohol and other CNS depressants.

Beta adrenergic blockers and MAO inhibitors potentiate the sympathomimetic effects of pseudoephedrine. Sympathomimetics may reduce the antihypertensive effects of methyldopa, mecamylamine, reserpine and veratrum alkaloids.

Dosage: Adults, 2 teaspoonfuls; children 50–90 lbs, ½ to 1 teaspoonful; 25–50 lbs, ¼ to ½ teaspoonful. Repeat every 4 to 6 hours. May be given to children under 2 at the discretion of the physician. *Do not exceed 4 doses in a 24-hour period.*

Product label dosage is as follows: Adults, 2 teaspoonfuls; children 6 to 12 years, 1 teaspoonful; children 2 to 5 years, ½ teaspoonful. May be given every 4 to 6 hours but *do not exceed 4 doses in 24 hours.* For children under 2 years, consult a physician.

How Supplied: As a liquid in 4 fluid ounce bottles (NDC 0068-1028-04) and pints (NDC 0068-1028-16).

Shown in Product Identification Section, page 421

ORENZYME®
[ŏr-ĕn'zīm]
(Oral enteric coated enzyme tablet)
ORENZYME® BITABS™
(Double strength oral enteric coated enzyme tablet)

AVAILABLE ONLY ON PRESCRIPTION

Description:
Orenzyme
Each red, enteric coated tablet of Orenzyme contains:
trypsin ....50,000 USP Units
chymotrypsin ....4,000 USP Units
equivalent in tryptic activity to 20 mg of USP trypsin.

Orenzyme Bitabs
Each yellow, enteric coated tablet of Orenzyme Bitabs contains:
trypsin ....100,000 USP Units
chymotrypsin ....8,000 USP Units
equivalent in tryptic activity to 40 mg of USP trypsin.

The tablets have a special enteric coating designed to permit intact passage through the stomach, followed by disintegration in the intestinal tract.

Action: The mode of action of Orenzyme has not been established.

Indications:
Based on a review of this drug by the National Academy of Sciences—National Research Council and/or other information, FDA has classified the indications as follows:
"Possibly" effective: Relief of symptomatology related to episiotomy.
Lack of substantial evidence of effectiveness: Adjunctive therapy for the resolution of inflammation and edema resulting from serious accidental trauma or surgical trauma.
Final classification of the less-than-effective indications requires further investigation.

Contraindications: Orenzyme should not be given to patients with a known sensitivity to trypsin or chymotrypsin.

Precautions: Orenzyme should be used with caution in patients with abnormality of the blood clotting mechanism such as hemophilia or with severe hepatic or renal disease. Safe use in pregnancy has not been established.

This product contains FD&C Yellow No. 5 (tartrazine), which may cause allergic-type reactions (including bronchial asthma) in certain susceptible individuals. Although the overall incidence of FD&C Yellow No. 5 (tartrazine) sensitivity in the general population is low, it is frequently seen in patients who also have aspirin hypersensitivity.

Adverse Reactions: Adverse reactions with Orenzyme have been reported infrequently. Reports include allergic manifestations (rash, urticaria, itching), gastrointestinal upset, and increased speed of dissolution of animal-origin surgical sutures. There have been isolated reports of anaphylactic shock, albuminuria, and hematuria. Increased tendency to bleed has also been reported, but in controlled studies it has been seen with equal incidence in placebo-treated groups. (See Precautions.)

It is recommended that if side effects occur, medication be discontinued.

Dosage and Administration:
Orenzyme: 1 or 2 tablets q.i.d.
Orenzyme Bitabs: 1 tablet q.i.d.

How Supplied:
Orenzyme Tablets imprinted MERRELL 441
NDC 0068-0441-13: bottles of 48
Orenzyme Bitabs imprinted MERRELL 442
NDC 0068-0442-15: bottles of 100

Product Information as of August, 1979

QUIDE®
[kwīd]
piperacetazine

Description: Quide (piperacetazine) is a piperidine derivative of phenothiazine having the following chemical designation: 10-{3-[4-(2-Hydroxyethyl)-piperidino] propyl}phenothiazin-2-yl methyl ketone.

Actions: The exact mode of action of the phenothiazines is unclear, but drugs of this class produce changes at all levels of the central nervous system, as well as on multiple organ systems.

Indications: Quide is indicated for use in the management of the manifestations of psychotic disorders.

Quide has not been shown effective in the management of behavioral complications in patients with mental retardation.

Contraindications: Quide is contraindicated in patients who are comatose or markedly depressed from any cause and in the presence of preexisting thrombocytopenia and other blood dyscrasias, bone marrow depression and in patients with significant liver disease. Quide is contraindicated in women who are or may become pregnant since animal reproductive studies adequate to establish safety during pregnancy have not been carried out. Quide is contraindicated in patients who have shown hypersensitivity to the drug. Cross sensitivity between phenothiazine derivatives may occur.

Warnings: Like other phenothiazines, Quide may impair the mental and/or physical abilities required for the performance of potentially hazardous tasks such as driving a car or operating machinery, especially during the first few days of therapy. Therefore, patients should be cautioned accordingly. Concomitant use with alcohol should be avoided due to the potential additive effect. Patients with known suicidal tendencies should not be given Quide except under strict medical supervision.

Use in Children: The use of Quide (piperacetazine) in children under 12 years of age is not recommended because safe conditions for its use have not been established.

Precautions: Use with caution in persons who:
1. are receiving barbiturates or narcotics, because of additive effects on central nervous system depression. The dosage of the narcotic or barbiturate should be reduced when given concomitantly with Quide.

Continued on next page

Information on Merrell Dow products is based on labeling in effect in August, 1984.

Merrell Dow—Cont.

2. are receiving atropine or related drugs, because of additive anticholinergic effects.
3. have a history of epilepsy, because this drug may lower the convulsive threshold. Adequate anticonvulsant therapy must be maintained concomitantly.
4. are exposed to extreme heat or phosphorus insecticides.
5. have cardiovascular disease.
6. have respiratory impairment due to acute pulmonary infections or chronic respiratory disorders such as severe asthma or emphysema.

Keep in mind that the antiemetic effect may mask the toxicity of other drugs or obscure the diagnosis of such conditions as intestinal obstruction or brain tumor.

Any sign of blood dyscrasias requires immediate discontinuance of the drug and the institution of appropriate therapy.

The possibility of liver damage, pigmentary retinopathy, lenticular or corneal deposits, and development of irreversible dyskinesias should be kept in mind when patients are on prolonged therapy. Neuroleptic drugs elevate prolactin levels; the elevation persists during chronic administration. Tissue culture experiments indicate that approximately one-third of human breast cancers are prolactin dependent in vitro, a factor of potential importance if the prescription of these drugs is contemplated in a patient with a previously detected breast cancer. Although disturbances such as galactorrhea, amenorrhea, gynecomastia, and impotence have been reported, the clinical significance of elevated serum prolactin levels is unknown for most patients. An increase in mammary neoplasms has been found in rodents after chronic administration of neuroleptic drugs. Neither clinical studies nor epidemiologic studies conducted to date, however, have shown an association between chronic administration of these drugs and mammary tumorigenesis; the available evidence is considered too limited to be conclusive at this time.

Abrupt Withdrawal: In general, phenothiazines do not produce psychic dependence, but gastritis, nausea and vomiting, dizziness and tremulousness have been reported following abrupt cessation of high-dose therapy. Reports suggest that these symptoms can be reduced if concomitant antiparkinson agents are continued for several weeks after the phenothiazine is withdrawn.

Both QUIDE 10 mg and QUIDE 25 mg tablets contain FD&C Yellow No. 5 (tartrazine) which may cause allergic-type reactions (including bronchial asthma) in certain susceptible individuals. Although the overall incidence of FD&C Yellow No. 5 (tartrazine) sensitivity in the general population is low, it is frequently seen in patients who also have aspirin hypersensitivity.

Adverse Reactions: Not all of the following adverse reactions have been reported with Quide (piperacetazine) but pharmacological similarities among various phenothiazine derivatives require that each be considered.

Note: Sudden Death has occasionally been reported in patients who have received phenothiazines. In some cases death was apparently due to cardiac arrest, in others the cause appeared to be asphyxia due to failure of the cough reflex. In some patients the cause could not be determined, nor could it be established that death was due to the phenothiazine.

Drowsiness: May occur particularly during the first or second week, after which it generally disappears. If troublesome, lower the dosage.

Jaundice: Incidence is low. When it occurs (usually between the second and fourth weeks of therapy) it is generally regarded as a sensitivity reaction. The clinical picture resembles infectious hepatitis with laboratory features of obstructive jaundice It is usually reversible although chronic jaundice has been reported with phenothiazine therapy.

Hematological Disorders: Agranulocytosis, eosinophilia, leukopenia, hemolytic anemia, thrombocytopenic purpura, aplastic anemia and pancytopenia.

Agranulocytosis: Most cases have occurred between the fourth and tenth weeks of therapy. Patients should be watched closely during that period for the sudden appearance of sore throat or other signs of infection. If white blood count and differential show significant cellular depression, discontinue the drug and start appropriate therapy. A slightly lowered white count, however, is not in itself an indication to discontinue the drug.

Cardiovascular: Postural hypotension, tachycardia (especially following rapid increase in dosage), bradycardia, cardiac arrest, faintness and dizziness. Occasionally the hypotensive effect may produce a shock-like condition. In the event a vasoconstrictor is required, levarterenol and phenylephrine are the most suitable. Other pressor agents, including epinephrine, should not be used because a paradoxical further lowering of the blood pressure may ensue.

EKG changes, nonspecific, usually reversible, have been observed in some patients receiving phenothiazine tranquilizers. Their relationship to myocardial damage has not been confirmed.

CNS Effects: Neuromuscular (extrapyramidal) Reactions: These are usually dose related and take three forms: (1) pseudoparkinsonism; (2) akathisia; and (3) dystonias (dystonias include spasms of the neck muscles, extensor rigidity of back muscles, carpopedal spasm, eyes rolled back, convulsions, trismus and swallowing difficulties). These resemble serious neurological disorders but usually subside within 48 hours. Management of the extrapyramidal symptoms, depending upon the type and severity, includes sedation, injectable diphenhydramine, and the use of antiparkinsonism agents. Hyperreflexia has been reported in the newborn when a phenothiazine was used during pregnancy.

Persistent Tardive Dyskinesia: As with all antipsychotic agents, tardive dyskinesia may appear in some patients on long-term therapy or may appear after drug therapy has been discontinued. The risk appears to be greater in elderly patients on high-dose therapy, especially females. The symptoms are persistent and in some patients appear to be irreversible. The syndrome is characterized by rhythmical involuntary movements of the tongue, face, mouth or jaw (e.g., protrusion of tongue, puffing of cheeks, puckering of the mouth, chewing movements). Sometimes these may be accompanied by involuntary movements of extremities.

There is no known effective treatment for tardive dyskinesia; anti-parkinsonism agents usually do not alleviate the symptoms of this syndrome. It is suggested that all antipsychotic agents be discontinued if these symptoms appear. Should it be necessary to reinstitute treatment, or increase the dosage of the agent, or switch to a different antipsychotic agent, the syndrome may be masked. It has been reported that fine vermicular movements of the tongue may be an early sign of the syndrome and if the medication is stopped at that time the syndrome may not develop.

Other CNS Effects: Cerebral edema. Abnormality of cerebral spinal fluid proteins. Convulsive seizures, particularly in patients with EEG abnormalities or a history of such disorders. Hyperpyrexia.

Adverse Behavioral Effects: Paradoxical exacerbation of psychotic symptoms.

Allergic Reactions: Urticaria, itching, erythema, photosensitivity (avoid undue exposure to the sun), eczema. Severe reactions include: exfoliative dermatitis (rare); contact dermatitis in nursing personnel administering the drug; asthma; laryngeal edema; angioneurotic edema; and anaphylactoid reactions.

Endocrine Disorders: Lactation and moderate breast engorgement in females and gynecomastia in males on large doses; changes in libido; false-positive pregnancy tests; amenorrhea; hyperglycemia, hypoglycemia, glycosuria.

Autonomic Reactions: Dry mouth, nasal congestion, constipation, adynamic ileus, myosis, mydriasis, urinary retention.

Special Considerations in Long-term Therapy: After prolonged administration of phenothiazines, pigmentation of the skin has occurred chiefly in the exposed areas, especially in females on large doses. Ocular changes consisting of deposition of fine particulate matter in the cornea and lens, progressing in more severe cases to star-shaped lenticular opacities; epithelial keratopathies; pigmentary retinopathy.

Other Adverse Reactions: Increases in appetite and weight; peripheral edema; systemic lupus erythematosus-like syndrome.

Dosage and Administration: Dosage should be individualized, not only initially but during the course of therapy, and the minimal effective dose should always be employed.

A starting dosage of 10 mg two to four times daily is recommended for adults. The dose may be increased up to 160 mg daily within a three to five day period. Should side effects occur, dosage should be reduced or discontinued as indicated. For maintenance therapy, up to 160 mg daily in divided doses may be given.

Overdosage with Phenothiazines:
Manifestations: One of three clinical pictures may be seen.

1. Extreme somnolence; patient can usually be roused with prodding, but if permitted, will fall asleep. General condition is usually satisfactory. The skin, though pale, is warm and dry. Slight blood pressure, respiratory and pulse changes may occur but are not problems.
2. Mild to moderate drop in blood pressure (patient may be conscious or unconscious). Skin is markedly gray, but warm and dry. Nail beds are pink. Respiration is slow and regular. Pulse is strong but rate slightly increased.
3. Severe hypotension, possibly accompanied by weakness, cyanosis, perspiration, rapid, thready pulse and respiratory depression.

TREATMENT: Is essentially symptomatic and supportive. Early gastric lavage and intestinal purges may help. Centrally acting emetics may not help because of the possible antiemetic effect of Quide. Give hot tea or coffee. Severe hypotension usually responds to measures described under hypotensive effects (see ADVERSE REACTIONS: Cardiovascular). Additional measures include pressure bandages to lower limbs, oxygen and I.V. fluids.

Avoid stimulants that may cause convulsions (e.g., picrotoxin and pentylenetetrazol).

Limited experience with dialysis indicates that it is not helpful.

Caution: Federal law prohibits dispensing without prescription.

How Supplied:
Quide (piperacetazine) Tablets-10 mg (orange)-bottles of 100 (NDC 0183-0052-02). Quide (piperacetazine) Tablets-25 mg (yellow)-bottles of 100 (NDC 0183-0053-02).

Note: Dispense only in light-resistant containers; the coatings on the tablets contain light-sensitive colors.

QUINAMM™ ℞
[kwĭ′ năm]
(quinine sulfate tablets)

Caution: Federal law prohibits dispensing without prescription.

Description:
Each white, beveled, compressed tablet for oral administration contains 260 mg quinine sulfate.
Neuromuscular Agent
Quinine sulfate has the following structural formula:

Quinine sulfate occurs as a white, crystalline powder, which darkens on exposure to light. It is odorless and has a persistent, very bitter taste. It is slightly soluble in water, alcohol, chloroform, and ether.

Clinical Pharmacology: Quinine, a cinchona alkaloid, acts on skeletal muscle by three mechanisms: it increases the refractory period by direct action on the muscle fiber, it decreases the excitability of the motor end-plate, an action similar to that of curare, and it affects the distribution of calcium within the muscle fiber.

Quinine is readily absorbed when given orally. Absorption occurs mainly from the upper part of the small intestine, and is almost complete even in patients with marked diarrhea.

The cinchona alkaloids in large measure are metabolically degraded in the body, especially in the liver; less than 5% of an administered dose is excreted unaltered in the urine. It is reported that there is no accumulation of the drugs in the body upon continued administration. The metabolic degradation products are excreted in the urine, where many of them have been identified as hydroxy derivatives, but small amounts also appear in the feces, gastric juice, bile, and saliva. Renal excretion of quinine is twice as rapid when the urine is acidic as when it is alkaline, due to the greater tubular reabsorption of the alkaloidal base that occurs in an alkaline media. Excretion is also limited by the binding of a large fraction of cinchona alkaloids to plasma proteins.

Peak plasma concentrations of cinchona alkaloids occur within 1 to 3 hours after a single oral dose. The half-life is 4 to 5 hours. After chronic administration of total daily doses of 1 g of drug, the average plasma quinine concentration is approximately 7 μg/ml. After termination of quinine therapy, the plasma level falls rapidly and only a negligible concentration is detectable after 24 hours.

A large fraction (approximately 70%) of the plasma quinine is bound to proteins. This explains in part why the concentration of the alkaloid in cerebrospinal fluid is only 2 to 5% of that in the plasma. However, it can traverse the placental membrane and readily reach fetal tissues.

Tinnitus and impairment of hearing rarely should occur at plasma quinine concentrations of less than 10 μg/ml. While this level would not be anticipated from use of 1 or 2 tablets of Quinamm daily, an occasional patient may have some evidence of cinchonism on this dosage, such as tinnitus. (See WARNINGS section.)

Indications and Usage: For the prevention and treatment of nocturnal recumbency leg muscle cramps.

Contraindications: Quinamm may cause fetal harm when administered to a pregnant woman. Congenital malformations in the human have been reported with the use of quinine, primarily with large doses (up to 30 g) for attempted abortion. In about half of these reports, the malformation was deafness related to auditory nerve hypoplasia. Among the other abnormalities reported were limb anomalies, visceral defects, and visual changes. In animal tests, teratogenic effects were found in rabbits and guinea pigs and were absent in mice, rats, dogs, and monkeys. Quinamm is contraindicated in women who are or may become pregnant. If this drug is used during pregnancy, or if the patient becomes pregnant while taking this drug, the patient should be apprised of the potential hazard to the fetus.

Because of the quinine content, Quinamm is contraindicated in patients with known quinine hypersensitivity and in patients with glucose-6-phosphate dehydrogenase (G-6-PD) deficiency.

Since thrombocytopenic purpura may follow the administration of quinine in highly sensitive patients, a history of this occurrence associated with previous quinine ingestion contraindicates its further use. Recovery usually occurs following withdrawal of the medication and appropriate therapy.

This drug should not be used in patients with tinnitus or optic neuritis or in patients with a history of blackwater fever.

Warnings: Repeated doses or overdosage of quinine in some individuals may precipitate a cluster of symptoms referred to as cinchonism. Such symptoms, in the mildest form, include ringing in the ears, headache, nausea, and slightly disturbed vision; however, when medication is continued or after large single doses, symptoms also involve the gastrointestinal tract, the nervous and cardiovascular systems, and the skin.

Hemolysis (with the potential for hemolytic anemia) has been associated with a G-6-PD deficiency in patients taking quinine. Quinamm should be stopped immediately if evidence of hemolysis appears.

If symptoms occur, drug should be discontinued and supportive measures instituted. In case of overdosage, see OVERDOSAGE section of prescribing information.

Precautions:
General
Quinamm should be discontinued if there is any evidence of hypersensitivity. (See CONTRAINDICATIONS.) Cutaneous flushing, pruritus, skin rashes, fever, gastric distress, dyspnea, ringing in the ears, and visual impairment are the usual expressions of hypersensitivity, particularly if only small doses of quinine have been taken. Extreme flushing of the skin accompanied by intense, generalized pruritus is the most common form. Hemoglobinuria and asthma from quinine are rare types of idiosyncrasy.

In patients with atrial fibrillation, the administration of quinine requires the same precautions as those for quinidine. (See *Drug Interactions*.)

Drug Interactions
Increased plasma levels of digoxin and digitoxin have been demonstrated in individuals after concomitant quinidine administration. Because of possible similar effects from use of quinine, it is recommended that plasma levels for digoxin and digitoxin be determined for those individuals taking these drugs and Quinamm concomitantly.

Concurrent use of aluminum-containing antacids may delay or decrease absorption of quinine.

Cinchona alkaloids, including quinine, have the potential to depress the hepatic enzyme system that synthesizes the vitamin K-dependent factors. The resulting hypoprothrombinemic effect may enhance the action of warfarin and other oral anticoagulants.

The effects of neuromuscular blocking agents (particularly pancuronium, succinylcholine, and tubocurarine) may be potentiated with quinine and result in respiratory difficulties.

Urinary alkalizers (such as acetazolamide and sodium bicarbonate) may increase quinine blood levels with potential for toxicity.

Drug/Laboratory Interactions
Quinine may produce an elevated value for urinary 17-ketogenic steroids when the Zimmerman method is used.

Carcinogenesis, Mutagenesis, Impairment of Fertility
A study of quinine sulfate administered in drinking water (0.1%) to rats for periods up to 20 months showed no evidence of neoplastic changes. Mutation studies of quinine (dihydrochloride) in male and female mice gave negative results by the micronucleus test. Intraperitoneal injections (0.5 mM/kg) were given twice, 24 hours apart. Direct *Salmonella typhimurium* tests were negative; when mammalian liver homogenate was added, positive results were found.

Mutation studies of quinine hydrochloride, 100 mg/kg, p.o. in Chinese hamsters showed no genotoxic activity in the sister chromatid exchange (SCE) test, micronucleus test, or chromosome aberration test. In mice given quinine hydrochloride, 100 mg/kg, p.o., the micronucleus test and chromosome aberration test were negative; the SCE test exhibited an increase of SCEs/cell. Tests were repeated in two inbred strains of mice using 55, 75, and 110 mg/kg, p.o. The effect was more pronounced in these mice and the increase in SCEs/cell demonstrated a linear dose relationship. One of the inbred strains had positive micronucleus test findings. The chromosome aberration test also revealed an increase of chromatid breaks. The Ames test system results were negative for point mutation.

No information relating to the effect of quinine upon fertility in animal or in man has been found.

Pregnancy
Category X. See CONTRAINDICATIONS.

Nonteratogenic Effects
Because quinine crosses the placenta in humans, the potential for fetal effects is present. Stillbirths in mothers taking quinine have been reported in which no obvious cause for the fetal deaths was shown. Quinine in toxic amounts has been associated with abortion. Whether this action is always due to direct effect on the uterus is questionable.

Nursing Mothers
Caution should be exercised when Quinamm is given to nursing women because quinine is excreted in breast milk (in small amounts).

Adverse Reactions: The following adverse reactions have been reported with Quinamm in therapeutic or excessive dosage. (Individual or multiple symptoms may represent cinchonism or hypersensitivity.)

Hematologic: acute hemolysis, thrombocytopenic purpura, agranulocytosis, hypoprothrombinemia
CNS: visual disturbances, including blurred vision with scotomata, photophobia, diplopia, diminished visual fields, and disturbed color vision; tinnitus, deafness, and vertigo; headache, nausea, vomiting, fever, apprehension, restlessness, confusion, and syncope
Dermatologic/Allergic: cutaneous rashes (urticarial, the most frequent type of allergic reaction, papular, or scarlatinal), pruritus, flushing of the skin, sweating, occasional edema of the face
Respiratory: asthmatic symptoms
Cardiovascular: anginal symptoms
Gastrointestinal: nausea and vomiting (may be CNS-related), epigastric pain, hepatitis

Drug Abuse and Dependence: Tolerance, abuse, or dependence with Quinamm has not been reported.

Overdosage: The more common signs and symptoms of overdosage are tinnitus, dizziness, skin rash, and gastrointestinal disturbance (intestinal cramping). With higher doses, cardiovascular and CNS effects may occur, including headache, fever, vomiting, apprehension, confusion, and convulsions. Other effects are listed in the ADVERSE REACTIONS section.

A fatal oral dose of quinine in adults has been reported as 8 grams. In a report of overdosage with a tablet containing quinine sulfate 260 mg and aminophylline 195 mg, a 43-year-old male ingested perhaps as many as 100 tablets, but gastric lavage was performed within 5 to 6 hours. The clinical picture was described as normal, but a massive elevation of the serum CPK was noted. Cardiac arrhythmias did not occur and the patient denied any symptoms of cinchonism. The CPK value was stated to have returned to normal in 4 days. Tinnitus and impaired hearing may occur at plasma quinine concentrations over 10 μg/ml. This level would not be normally attained with the use of 1 or 2 Quinamm tablets daily, but in a hypersensitive patient, as little as 0.3 g of quinine may produce tinnitus.

Treatment
Treatment for overdosage should include initially efforts to remove any residual Quinamm from the stomach by gastric lavage or by emesis induced with syrup of ipecac. The blood pressure should be supported and measures used to maintain renal function. Artificial respiration may be needed. Sedatives, oxygen, and other supportive measures should be used as necessary.

Fluid and electrolyte balance with intravenous fluids should be maintained. Acidification of the

Continued on next page

Information on Merrell Dow products is based on labeling in effect in August, 1984.

Merrell Dow—Cont.

urine will promote renal excretion of quinine. In the presence of hemoglobinuria, however, acidification of the urine may augment renal blockade. Quinine should be readily dialyzable by hemodialysis and/or hemoperfusion procedures.

Evidence of angioedema or asthma may require the use of epinephrine, corticosteroids, and antihistamines. In the acute phase of toxic amaurosis caused by quinine, vasodilators administered intravenously may have a salutary effect. Stellate block has also been used effectively for quinine-associated blindness. Residual visual impairment occasionally yields to vasodilators.

Dosage and Administration: 1 tablet upon retiring. If needed, 2 tablets may be taken nightly—1 following the evening meal and 1 upon retiring.

After several consecutive nights in which recumbency leg cramps do not occur, Quinamm may be discontinued in order to determine whether continued therapy is needed.

How Supplied: White tablets debossed W one side, Merrell 547 other side
NDC 0068-0547-15: bottles of 100 white tablets
NDC 0068-0547-16: bottles of 500 white tablets

Product Information as of September, 1983
MERRELL DOW PHARMACEUTICALS INC.
Subsidiary of The Dow Chemical Company
Cincinnati, Ohio 45242-9553, U.S.A.

Shown in Product Identification Section, p. 421

RIFADIN® ℞
[rif'ă-dĭn]
rifampin

Description: Rifadin (rifampin) is a semi-synthetic antibiotic derivative of rifamycin B. Specifically, Rifadin is the hydrazone, 3-(4-methyl-piperazinyliminomethyl) rifamycin SV.

Actions: Rifadin inhibits DNA-dependent RNA polymerase activity in susceptible cells. Specifically, it interacts with bacterial RNA polymerase, but does not inhibit the mammalian enzyme. This is the mechanism of action by which rifampin exerts its therapeutic effect. Cross resistance to Rifadin has only been shown with other rifamycins. Peak blood levels in normal adults vary widely from individual to individual. Peak levels occur between 2 and 4 hours following the oral administration of a 600 mg dose. The average peak value is 7 mcg/ml; however, the peak level may vary from 4 to 32 mcg/ml.

In normal subjects the $T\frac{1}{2}$ (biological half-life) of Rifadin in blood is approximately three hours. Elimination occurs mainly through the bile and, to a much lesser extent, the urine.

Indications: Pulmonary tuberculosis. In the initial treatment and in retreatment of patients with pulmonary tuberculosis Rifadin must be used in conjunction with at least one other antituberculosis drug. Frequently used regimens have been the following:
 isoniazid and Rifadin
 ethambutol and Rifadin
 isoniazid, ethambutol and Rifadin

Neisseria meningitidis carriers: Rifadin is indicated for the treatment of asymptomatic carriers of *N. meningitidis* to eliminate meningococci from the nasopharynx.
Rifadin is not indicated for the treatment of meningococcal infection.

To avoid the indiscriminate use of Rifadin, diagnostic laboratory procedures, including serotyping and susceptibility testing, should be performed to establish the carrier state and the correct treatment. In order to preserve the usefulness of Rifadin in the treatment of asymptomatic meningococcal carriers, it is recommended that the drug be reserved for situations in which the risk of meningococcal meningitis is high.

Both in the treatment of tuberculosis and in the treatment of meningococcal carriers, small numbers of resistant cells, present within large populations of susceptible cells, can rapidly become the predominating type. Since rapid emergence of resistance can occur, culture and susceptibility tests should be performed in the event of persistent positive cultures.

Contraindications: A history of previous hypersensitivity reaction to any of the rifamycins.

Warnings: Rifampin has been shown to produce liver dysfunction. There have been fatalities associated with jaundice in patients with liver disease or receiving rifampin concomitantly with other hepatoxic agents. Since an increased risk may exist for individuals with liver disease, benefits must be weighed carefully against the risk of further liver damage. Periodic liver function monitoring is mandatory.

The possibility of rapid emergence of resistant meningococci restricts the use of Rifadin to short-term treatment of the asymptomatic carrier state. Rifadin is not to be used for the treatment of meningococcal disease.

Several studies of tumorigenicity potential have been done in rodents. In one strain of mice known to be particularly susceptible to the spontaneous development of hepatomas, rifampin given at a level 2–10 times the maximum dosage used clinically, resulted in a significant increase in the occurrence of hepatomas in female mice of this strain after one year of administration. There was no evidence of tumorigenicity in the males of this strain, in males or females of another mouse strain or in rats.

Usage in Pregnancy: Although rifampin has been reported to cross the placental barrier and appear in cord blood, the effect of Rifadin, alone or in combination with other antituberculosis drugs, on the human fetus is not known. An increase in congenital malformations, primarily spina bifida and cleft palate, has been reported in the offspring of rodents given oral doses of 150–250 mg/kg/day of rifampin during pregnancy.

The possible teratogenic potential in women capable of bearing children should be carefully weighed against the benefits of therapy.

Precautions: Rifadin is not recommended for intermittent therapy; the patient should be cautioned against intentional or accidental interruption of the daily dosage regimen since rare renal hypersensitivity reactions have been reported when therapy was resumed in such cases.

Rifampin has been observed to increase the requirement for anticoagulant drugs of the coumarin type. The cause of this phenomenon is unknown. In patients receiving anticoagulants and rifampin concurrently, it is recommended that the prothrombin time be performed daily or as frequently as necessary to establish and maintain the required dose of anticoagulant.

Urine, feces, saliva, sputum, sweat and tears may be colored red-orange by rifampin and its metabolites. Soft contact lenses may be permanently stained. Individuals to be treated should be made aware of these possibilities.

It has been reported that the reliability of oral contraceptives may be affected in some patients being treated for tuberculosis with rifampin in combination with at least one other antituberculosis drug. In such cases, alternative contraceptive measures may need to be considered.

It has also been reported that rifampin given in combination with other antituberculosis drugs may decrease the pharmacologic activity of methadone, oral hypoglycemics, digitoxin, quinidine, disopyramide, dapsone and corticosteroids. In these cases, dosage adjustment of the interacting drugs is recommended.

Therapeutic levels of rifampin have been shown to inhibit standard microbiological assays for serum folate and vitamin B_{12}. Alternative methods must be considered when determining folate and vitamin B_{12} concentrations in the presence of rifampin.

Since rifampin has been reported to cross the placental barrier and appear in cord blood, neonates of rifampin-treated mothers should be carefully observed for any evidence of adverse effects.

Adverse Reactions: Gastrointestinal disturbances such as heartburn, epigastric distress, anorexia, nausea, vomiting, gas, cramps, and diarrhea have been noted in some patients. Headache, drowsiness, fatigue, menstrual disturbances, ataxia, dizziness, inability to concentrate, mental confusion, visual distur- bances, muscular weakness, fever, pains in the extremities and generalized numbness have also been noted.

Hypersensitivity reactions have been reported. Encountered occasionally have been pruritus, urticaria, rash, pemphigoid reaction, eosinophilia, sore mouth, sore tongue and exudative conjunctivitis. Rarely, hepatitis or a shock-like syndrome with hepatic involvement and abnormal liver function tests have been reported. Transient abnormalities in liver function tests (e.g., elevations in serum bilirubin, BSP, alkaline phosphatase, serum transaminases) have also been observed.

Thrombocytopenia, transient leukopenia, hemolytic anemia and decreased hemoglobin have been observed. Thrombocytopenia has occurred when Rifadin and ethambutol were administered concomitantly according to an intermittent dose schedule twice weekly, and in high doses.

Elevations in BUN and serum uric acid have occurred. Rarely, hemolysis, hemoglobinuria, hematuria, renal insufficiency or acute renal failure have been reported and are generally considered to be hypersensitivity reactions. These have usually occurred during intermittent therapy or when treatment was resumed following intentional or accidental interruption of a daily dosage regimen and were reversible when rifampin was discontinued and appropriate therapy instituted.

Although rifampin has been reported to have an immunosuppressive effect in some animal experiments, available human data indicate that this has no clinical significance.

Dosage and Administration: It is recommended that Rifadin be administered once daily, either one hour before, or two hours after a meal. Data are not available for determination of dosage for children under 5.

Pulmonary tuberculosis:
 Adults: 600 mg (two 300 mg or four 150 mg capsules) in a single daily administration.
 Children: 10–20 mg/kg not to exceed 600 mg/day.

In the treatment of pulmonary tuberculosis, Rifadin must be used in conjunction with at least one other antituberculous agent. In general, therapy should be continued until bacterial conversion and maximal improvement have occurred.

Meningococcal carriers:
It is recommended that Rifadin be administered once daily for four consecutive days in the following doses:
 Adults: 600 mg (two 300 mg or four 150 mg capsules) in a single daily administration.
 Children: 10–20 mg/kg not to exceed 600 mg/day.

Preparation of Extemporaneous Oral Suspension:
For pediatric and adult patients, in whom capsule swallowing is difficult or where lower doses are needed, a liquid suspension may be prepared as follows.

Rifadin 1% w/v suspension (10 mg/ml) can be compounded using one of five syrups—Simple Syrup (Syrup NF), Simple Syrup (Humco Laboratories), Simple Syrup (Whiteworth Inc.), Wild Cherry Syrup (Eli Lilly and Company) and Syrpalta® Syrup (Emerson Laboratories).

1. Empty contents of four Rifadin 300 mg capsules or eight Rifadin 150 mg capsules onto a piece of weighing paper.
2. If necessary, gently crush the capsule contents with a spatula to produce a fine powder.
3. Transfer rifampin powder blend to a four-ounce amber glass prescription bottle.
4. Rinse the paper and spatula with 20 ml of one of the above recommended syrups and add the rinse to the bottle. Shake vigorously.

5. Add 100 ml of syrup to the bottle and shake vigorously.

This compounding procedure results in a 1% w/v suspension containing 10 mg rifampin/ml. Stability studies indicate that the suspension is stable for four weeks when stored at room temperature (25 ± 3°C) or in a refrigerator (2–8°C).

This extemporaneously prepared suspension must be shaken well prior to administration.

Susceptibility testing: Pulmonary tuberculosis. Rifampin susceptibility powders are available for both direct and indirect methods of determining the susceptibility of strains of mycobacteria. The MIC's of susceptible clinical isolates when determined in 7H10 or other non-egg-containing media have ranged from 0.1 to 2 mcg/ml.

Meningococcal carriers: Susceptibility discs containing 5 mcg of rifampin are available for susceptibility testing of *N. meningitidis.*

Quantitative methods that require measurement of zone diameters give the most precise estimates of antibiotic susceptibility. One such procedure* has been recommended for use with discs for testing susceptibility to rifampin. Interpretations correlate zone diameters from the disc test with MIC (minimal inhibitory concentration) values for rifampin. A range of MIC's from 0.1 to 1 mcg/ml has been found *in vitro* for susceptible strains of *N. meningitidis.* With this procedure, a report from the laboratory of "resistant" indicates that the organism is not likely to be eradicated from the nasopharynx of asymptomatic carriers.

Overdosage:

Signs and Symptoms:

Nausea, vomiting, and increasing lethargy will probably occur within a short time after ingestion; actual unconsciousness may occur with severe hepatic involvement. Brownish-red or orange discoloration of the skin, urine, sweat, saliva, tears, and feces is proportional to amount ingested.

Liver enlargement, possibly with tenderness, can develop within a few hours after severe overdosage and jaundice may develop rapidly. Hepatic involvement may be more marked in patients with prior impairment of hepatic function. Other physical findings remain essentially normal.

Direct and total bilirubin levels may increase rapidly with severe overdosage; hepatic enzyme levels may be affected, especially with prior impairment of hepatic function. A direct effect upon the hematopoietic system, electrolyte levels, or acid-base balance is unlikely.

Treatment:

Since nausea and vomiting are likely to be present, gastric lavage is probably preferable to induction of emesis. Activated charcoal slurry instilled into the stomach following evacuation of gastric contents can help absorb any remaining drug in the G.I. tract. Antiemetic medication may be required to control severe nausea/vomiting.

Active diuresis (with measured intake and output) will help promote excretion of the drug. Bile drainage may be indicated in presence of serious impairment of hepatic function lasting more than 24–48 hours; under these circumstances, extracorporeal hemodialysis may be required.

In patients with previously adequate hepatic function, reversal of liver enlargement and impaired hepatic excretory function probably will be noted within 72 hours, with rapid return toward normal thereafter.

Caution: Federal law prohibits dispensing without prescription.

How Supplied:

150 mg maroon and scarlet capsules imprinted with the Dow diamond trademark over the code number 510.

Bottles of 30 (NDC 0068-0510-30)

300 mg maroon and scarlet capsules imprinted with the Dow diamond trademark and the code number 508.

Bottles of 30 (NDC 0068-0508-30)
Bottles of 60 (NDC 0068-0508-60)
Bottles of 100 (NDC 0068-0508-61)

*Bauer, A.W., Kirby, W.M., Sherris, J.C., and Turck, M. Antibiotic susceptibility testing by a standardized single disk method. Am. J. Clin. Path. 45:493-496, 1966.

Revised: April, 1984

Rifadin 150 mg capsules are manufactured by
DOW PHARMACEUTICALS
Dow Chemical of Canada, Limited
Richmond Hill, Ontario, L4C 5H2
Canada for
MERRELL DOW PHARMACEUTICALS INC.
Subsidiary of The Dow Chemical Company
Cincinnati, Ohio 45242-9553, U.S.A.

Shown in Product Identification Section, page 421

RIFAMATE® B
[*rif' ăh-māt*]
rifampin-isoniazid
Capsules

WARNING

Severe and sometimes fatal hepatitis associated with isoniazid therapy may occur and may develop even after many months of treatment. The risk of developing hepatitis is age related. Approximate case rates by age are: 0 per 1,000 for persons under 20 years of age, 3 per 1,000 for persons in the 20–34 year age group, 12 per 1,000 for persons in the 35–49 year age group, 23 per 1,000 for persons in the 50–64 year age group, and 8 per 1,000 for persons over 65 years of age. The risk of hepatitis is increased with daily consumption of alcohol. Precise data to provide a fatality rate for isoniazid-related hepatitis are not available; however, in a U.S. Public Health Service Surveillance Study of 13,838 persons taking isoniazid, there were 8 deaths among 174 cases of hepatitis.

Therefore, patients given isoniazid should be carefully monitored and interviewed at monthly intervals. Serum transaminase concentration becomes elevated in about 10–20 percent of patients, usually during the first few months of therapy, but it can occur at any time. Usually enzyme levels return to normal despite continuance of drug, but in some cases progressive liver dysfunction occurs. Patients should be instructed to report immediately any of the prodromal symptoms of hepatitis, such as fatigue, weakness, malaise, anorexia, nausea, or vomiting. If these symptoms appear or if signs suggestive of hepatic damage are detected, isoniazid should be discontinued promptly, since continued use of the drug in these cases has been reported to cause a more severe form of liver damage.

Patients with tuberculosis should be given appropriate treatment with alternative drugs. If isoniazid must be reinstituted, it should be reinstituted only after symptoms and laboratory abnormalities have cleared. The drug should be restarted in very small and gradually increasing doses and should be withdrawn immediately if there is any indication of recurrent liver involvement.

Treatment should be deferred in persons with acute hepatic diseases.

Description: Rifamate is a combination capsule contaning 300 mg rifampin and 150 mg isoniazid. Rifampin is a semisynthetic antibiotic derivative of rifamycin B. Specifically, rifampin is the hydrazone, 3-(4-methylpiperazinylimino- methyl) rifamycin SV.

Isoniazid is the hydrazide of isonicotinic acid. It exists as colorless or white crystals or as a white, crystalline powder that is water soluble, ordorless, and slowly affected by exposure to air and light.

Actions:

Rifampin

Rifampin inhibits DNA-dependent RNA polymerase activity in susceptible cells. Specifically, it interacts with bacterial RNA polymerase but does not inhibit the mammalian enzyme. This is the mechanism of action by which rifampin exerts its therapeutic effect. Rifampin cross resistance has only been shown with other rifamycins.

In a study of 14 normal human adult males, peak blood levels of rifampin occured 1½ to 3 hours following oral administration of two Rifamate capsules. The peaks ranged from 6.9 to 14 mcg/ml with an average of 10 mcg/ml.

In normal subjects the $T_{1/2}$ (biological half-life) of rifampin in blood is approximately 3 hours. Elimination occurs mainly through the bile and, to a much lesser extent the urine.

Isoniazid

Isoniazid acts against actively growing tubercle bacilli.

After oral administration isoniazid produces peak blood levels within 1 to 2 hours which decline to 50% or less within 6 hours. It diffuses readily into all body fluids (cerebrospinal, pleural, and ascitic fluids), tissues, organs and excreta (saliva, sputum, and feces). The drug also passes through the placental barrier and into milk in concentrations comparable to those in the plasma. From 50 to 70% of a dose of isoniazid is excreted in the urine in 24 hours.

Isoniazid is metabolized primarily by acetylation and dehydrazination. The rate of acetylation is genetically determined. Approximately 50% of Blacks and Caucasians are "slow inactivators"; the majority of Eskimos and Orientals are "rapid inactivators."

The rate of acetylation does not significantly alter the effectiveness of isoniazid. However, slow acetylation may lead to higher blood levels of the drug, and thus an increase in toxic reactions.

Pyridoxine deficiency (B_6) is sometimes observed in adults with high doses of isoniazid and is considered probably due to its competition with pyridoxal phosphate for the enzyme apotryptophanase.

Indications: For pulmonary tuberculosis in which organisms are susceptible, and when the patient has been titrated on the individual components and it has therefore been established that this fixed dosage is therapeutically effective.

This fixed-dosage combination drug is not recommended for initial therapy of tuberculosis or for preventive therapy.

In the treatment of tuberculosis, small numbers of resistant cells, present within large populations of susceptible cells, can rapidly become the predominating type. Since rapid emergence of resistance can occur, culture and susceptibility tests should be performed in the event of persistent positive cultures.

This drug is *not* indicated for the treatment of meningococcal infections or asymptomatic carriers of *N. meningitidis* to eliminate meningococci from the nasopharynx.

Contraindications: Previous isoniazid-associated hepatic injury; severe adverse reactions to isoniazid, such as drug fever, chills, and arthritis; acute liver disease of any etiology.

A history of previous hypersensitivity reaction to any of the rifamycins or to isoniazid, including drug-induced hepatitis.

Warnings: Rifamate (rifampin-isoniazid) is a combination of two drugs, each of which has been associated with liver dysfunction. Liver function tests should be performed prior to therapy with Rifamate and periodically during treatment.

Rifampin

Rifampin has been shown to produce liver dysfunction. There have been fatalities associated with jaundice in patients with liver disease or receiving rifampin concomitantly with other hepatoxic agents. Since an increased risk may exist for individuals with liver disease, benefits must be weighed carefully against the risk of further liver damage.

Several studies of tumorigenicity potential have been done in rodents. In one strain of mice known to be particularly susceptible to the spontaneous development of hepatomas, rifampin given at a

Continued on next page

Information on Merrell Dow products is based on labeling in effect in August, 1984.

Merrell Dow—Cont.

level 2-10 times the maximum dosage used clinically, resulted in a significant increase in the occurrence of hepatomas in female mice of this strain after one year of administration. There was no evidence of tumorigenicity in the males of this strain, in males or females of another mouse strain, or in rats.

Isoniazid
See the boxed warning.

Precautions:
Rifampin
Rifampin is not recommended for intermittent therapy; the patient should be cautioned against intentional or accidental interruption of the daily dosage regimen since rare renal hypersensitivity reactions have been reported when therapy was resumed in such cases.

Rifampin has been observed to increase the requirements for anticoagulant drugs of the coumarin type. The cause of the phenomenon is unknown. In patients receiving anticoagulants and rifampin concurrently, it is recommended that the prothrombin time be performed daily or as frequently as necessary to establish and maintain the required dose of anticoagulant.

Urine, feces, saliva, sputum, sweat and tears may be colored red-orange by rifamin and its metabolites. Soft contact lenses may be permanently stained. Individuals to be treated should be made aware of these possibilities.

It has been reported that the reliability of oral contraceptives may be affected in some patients being treated for tuberculosis with rifampin in combination with at least one other antituberculosis drug. In such cases, alternative contraceptive measures may need to be considered.

It has also been reported that rifampin given in combination with other antituberculosis drugs may affect the blood concentration of methadone, oral hypoglycemics, digitalis derivatives, dapsone and corticosteroids. In these cases, dosage adjustment of the interacting drugs is recommended.

Therapeutic levels of rifampin have been shown to inhibit standard assays for serum folate and vitamin B_{12}. Alternative methods must be considered when determining folate and vitamin B_{12} concentrations in the presence of rifampin.

Since rifampin has been reported to cross the placental barrier and appear in cord blood and in maternal milk, neonates and newborns of rifampin-treated mothers should be carefully observed for any evidence of untoward effects.

Isoniazid
All drugs should be stopped and an evaluation of the patient should be made at the first sign of a hypersensitivity reaction.

Use of isoniazid should be carefully monitored in the following:
1. Patients who are receiving phenytoin (diphenylhydantoin) concurrently. Isoniazid may decrease the excretion of phenytoin or may enhance its effects. To avoid phenytoin intoxication, appropriate adjustment of the anticonvulsant dose should be made.
2. Daily users of alcohol. Daily ingestion of alcohol may be associated with a higher incidence of isoniazid hepatitis.
3. Patients with current chronic liver disease or severe renal dysfunction.

Periodic ophthalmoscopic examination during isoniazid therapy is recommended when visual symptoms occur.

Usage in Pregnancy and Lactation
Rifampin
Although rifampin has been reported to cross the placental barrier and appear in cord blood, the effect of rifampin, alone or in combination with other antituberculosis drugs, on the human fetus is not known. An increase in congenital malformations, primarily spina bifida and cleft palate, has been reported in the offspring of rodents given oral doses of 150-250 mg/kg/day of rifampin during pregnancy.

The possible teratogenic potential in women capable of bearing children should be carefully weighed against the benefits of therapy.

Isoniazid
It has been reported that in both rats and rabbits, isoniazid may exert an embryocidal effect when administered orally during pregnancy, although no isoniazid-related congenital anomalies have been found in reproduction studies in mammalian species (mice, rats, and rabbits). Isoniazid should be prescribed during pregnancy only when therapeutically necessary. The benefit of preventive therapy should be weighed against a possible risk to the fetus. Preventive treatment generally should be started after delivery because of the increased risk of tuberculosis for new mothers.

Since isoniazid is known to cross the placental barrier and to pass into maternal breast milk, neonates and breast-fed infants of isoniazid treated mothers should be carefully observed for any evidence of adverse effects.

Carcinogenesis:
Isoniazid has been reported to induce pulmonary tumors in a number of strains of mice.

Adverse Reactions:
Rifampin
Nervous system reactions: headache, drowsiness, fatigue, ataxia, dizziness, inability to concentrate, mental confusion, visual disturbances, muscular weakness, pain in extremities and generalized numbness.

Gastrointestinal disturbances: in some patients heartburn, epigastric distress, anorexia, nausea, vomiting, gas, cramps, and diarrhea.

Hepatic reactions: transient abnormalities in liver function tests (e.g. elevations in serum bilirubin, BSP, alkaline phosphatase, serum transaminases) have been observed. Rarely, hepatitis or a shocklike syndrome with hepatic involvement and abnormal liver function tests.

Hematologic reactions: thrombocytopenia, transient leukopenia, hemolytic anemia, eosinophilia and decreased hemoglobin have been observed. Thrombocytopenia has occurred when rifampin and ethambutol were administered concomitantly according to an intermittent dose schedule twice weekly and in high doses.

Allergic and immunological reactions: occasionally pruritus, urticaria, rash, pemphigus, acneiform lesions, eosinophilia, sore mouth, sore tongue and exudative conjunctivitis. Rarely, hemolysis, hemoglobinuria, hematuria, renal insufficiency or acute renal failure have been reported which are generally considered to be hypersensitivity reactions. These have usually occurred during intermittent therapy or when treatment was resumed following intentional or accidental interruption of a daily dosage regimen and were reversible when rifampin was discontinued and appropriate therapy instituted.

Although rifampin has been reported to have an immunosuppressive effect in some animal experiments, available human data indicate that this has no clinical significance.

Metabolic reactions: elevations in BUN and serum uric acid have occurred.

Miscellaneous reactions: fever and menstrual distrubances have been noted.

Isoniazid
The most frequent reactions are those affecting the nervous system and the liver.

Nervous system reactions: Peripheral neuropathy is the most common toxic effect. It is dose-related, occurs most often in the malnourished and in those predisposed to neuritis (e.g., alcoholics and diabetics), and is usually preceded by paresthesias of the feet and hands. The incidence is higher in "slow inactivators".

Other neurotoxic effects, which are uncommon with conventional doses, are convulsions, toxic encephalopathy, optic neuritis and atrophy, memory impairment, and toxic psychosis.

Gastrointestinal reactions: Nausea, vomiting, and epigastric distress.

Hepatic reactions: Elevated serum transaminases (SGOT; SGPT), bilirubinemia, bilirubinuria, jaundice, and occasionally severe and sometimes fatal hepatitis. The common prodromal symptoms are anorexia, nausea, vomiting, fatigue, malaise, and weakness. Mild and transient elevation of serum transaminase levels occurs in 10 to 20 percent of persons taking isoniazid. The abnormality usually occurs in the first 4 to 6 months of treatment but can occur at any time during therapy. In most instances, enzyme levels return to normal with no necessity to discontinue medication. In occasional instances, progressive liver damage occurs, with accompanying symptoms. In these cases, the drug should be discontinued immediately. The frequency of progressive liver damage increases with age. It is rare in persons under 20, but occurs in up to 2.3 percent of those over 50 years of age.

Hematologic reactions: agranulocytosis, hemolytic sideroblastic or aplastic anemia, thrombocytopenia and eosinophilia.

Hypersensitivity reactions: fever, skin eruptions (morbilliform, maculopapular, purpuric, or exfoliative), lymphadenopathy and vasculitis.

Metabolic and endocrine reactions: pyridoxine deficiency, pellagra, hyperglycemia, metabolic acidosis, and gynecomastia.

Miscellaneous reactions: rheumatic syndrome and systemic lupus erythematosus-like syndrome.

Overdosage:
Rifampin
Signs and Symptoms
Nausea, vomiting, and increasing lethargy will probably occur within a short time after ingestion; actual unconsciousness may occur with severe hepatic involvement. Brownish-red or orange discoloration of the skin, urine, sweat, saliva, tears, and feces is proportional to amount ingested.

Liver enlargement, possibly with tenderness, can develop within a few hours after severe overdosage and jaundice may develop rapidly. Hepatic involvement may be more marked in patients with prior impairment of hepatic function. Other physical findings remain essentially normal.

Direct and total bilirubin levels may increase rapidly with severe overdosage; hepatic enzyme levels may be affected, especially with prior impairment of hepatic function. A direct effect upon hemopoietic system, electrolyte levels or acid-base balance is unlikely.

Isoniazid
Signs and Symptoms
Isoniazid overdosage produces signs and symptoms within 30 minutes to 3 hours. Nausea, vomiting, dizziness, slurring of speech, blurring of vision, visual hallucinations (including bright colors and strange designs), are among the early manifestations. With marked overdosage, respiratory distress and CNS depression, progessing rapidly from stupor to profound coma, are to be expected, along with severe, intractable seizures. Severe metabolic acidosis, acetonuria, and hyperglycemia are typical laboratory findings.

Rifamate (rifampin-isoniazid)
Treatment
The airway should be secured and adequate respiratory exchange established. Only then should gastric emptying (lavage-aspiration) be attempted; this may be difficult because of seizures. Since nausea and vomiting are likely to be present, gastric lavage is probably preferable to induction of emesis.

Activated charcoal slurry instilled into the stomach following evacuation of gastric contents can help absorb any remaining drug in the GI tract. Antiemetic medication may be required to control severe nausea and vomiting.

Blood samples should be obtained for immediate determination of gases, electrolytes, BUN, glucose, etc. Blood should be typed and crossmatched in preparation for possible hemodialysis.

Rapid control of metabolic acidosis is fundamental to management. Intravenous sodium bicarbonate should be given at once and repeated as needed, adjusting subsequent dosage on the basis of laboratory findings (i.e. serum sodium, pH, etc.). At the same time, anticonvulsants should be given intravenously (i.e. barbiturates, diphenylhydantoin, diazepam) as required, and large doses of intravenous pyridoxine.

Forced osmotic diuresis must be started early and should be continued for some hours after clinical improvement to hasten renal clearance of drug and help prevent relapse. Fluid intake and output should be monitored.

Bile drainage may be indicated in presence of serious impairment of hepatic function lasting more than 24–48 hours. Under these circumstances, and for severe cases extra-corporeal hemodialysis may be required; if this is not available, peritoneal dialysis can be used along with forced diuresis.

Along with measures based on initial and repeated determination of blood gases and other laboratory tests as needed, meticulous respiratory and other intensive care should be utilized to protect against hypoxia, hypotension, aspiration, pneumonitis, etc.

In patients with previously adequate hepatic function, reversal of liver enlargement and impaired hepatic excretory function probably will be noted within 72 hours, with rapid return toward normal thereafter.

Untreated or inadequately treated cases of gross isoniazid overdosage can terminate fatally, but good response has been reported in most patients brought under adequate treatment within the first few hours after drug ingestion.

Dosage and Administration: In general, therapy should be continued until bacterial conversion and maximal improvement have occured.

Adults: Two Rifamate (rifampin-isoniazid) capsules (600 mg rifampin, 300 mg isoniazid) once daily, administered one hour before or two hours after a meal.

Concomitant administration of pyridoxine (B_6) is recommended in the malnourished, in those predisposed to neuropathy (e.g. diabetics) and in adolescents.

Susceptibility Testing
Rifampin
Rifampin susceptibility powders are available for both direct and indirect methods of determining the susceptibility of strains of mycobacteria. The MIC's of susceptible clinical isolates when determined in 7H10 or other non-egg-containing media have ranged from 0.1 to 2 mcg/ml.

Quantitative methods that require measurement of zone diameters give the most precise estimates of antibiotic susceptibility. One such procedure has been recommended for use with discs for testing susceptibility to rifampin, Interpretations correlate zone diameters from the disc test with MIC (minimal inhibitory concentration) values for rifampin.

Caution: Federal law prohibits dispensing without prescription.

How Supplied: Capsules (opaque red), containing 300 mg rifampin and 150 mg isoniazid; bottles of 60 (NDC 0068-0509-60).

Shown in Product Identification Section, page 421

SINGLET® ℞
[sĭn'glĕt]
Long-Acting Tablets
Decongestant-Antihistamine-Analgesic

Description: Each SINGLET long-acting tablet for oral use contains phenylephrine hydrochloride 40 mg, chlorpheniramine maleate 8 mg, and acetaminophen 500 mg.

Phenylephrine hydrochloride is a nasal decongestant. Chemically it is: (R)-3-Hydroxy-α-[(methylamino)methyl] benzenemethanol hydrochloride.
Chlorpheniramine maleate is an antihistamine. Chemically it is: α-(4-Chlorophenyl)-N,N-dimethyl-2-pyridinepropanamine.
Acetaminophen is an analgesic-antipyretic. Chemically it is: (N-acetyl-p-aminophenol).

Clinical Pharmacology: Phenylephrine is a nasal decongestant. Its effects are similar to epinephrine, but it is less potent on a weight basis, and has a longer duration of action. Phenylephrine produces peripheral effects similar to epinephrine, but has little or no central nervous system stimulation. After oral administration, nasal decongestion may occur within 15 to 20 minutes and persist for 2 to 4 hours.

Chlorpheniramine is an antihistaminic drug that possesses anticholinergic and sedative effects. It is considered one of the most effective and least toxic of the histamine antagonists. Chlorpheniramine is an H_1 receptor antagonist. It antagonizes many of the pharmacologic actions of histamine. It prevents released histamine from dilating capillaries and causing edema of the respiratory mucosa. Chlorpheniramine has a duration of action of 4 to 6 hours. Its half-life in serum, however, is 12 to 16 hours.

Acetaminophen is an analgesic and antipyretic. Its actions are similar to salicylates, but it has a weak anti-inflammatory effect. Acetaminophen has a half-life of 1 to 3 hours.

Indications and Usage: For the relief of multiple symptoms of nasal and eustachian tube congestion, sneezing, runny nose, watery eyes, myalgia, headache and fever associated with colds and other viral infections, sinusitis, influenza, and seasonal and perennial nasal allergies.

May be given concomitantly, when indicated, with antibiotics.

Contraindications: Patients with severe hypertension, severe coronary artery disease, on MAO inhibitor therapy, narrow angle glaucoma, urinary retention, peptic ulcer, during an asthmatic attack, and seriously impaired liver and kidney function. Contraindicated in children under 12 years.

Hypersensitivity: Contraindicated in patients with hypersensitivity or idiosyncrasy to sympathomimetic amines, phenanthrene derivatives, or to any other formula ingredients.

Nursing Mothers: Contraindicated because of the higher than usual risk for infants from sympathomimetic amines.

Warning: If sympathomimetic amines are used in patients with hypertension, diabetes mellitus, ischemic heart disease, hyperthyroid- ism, increased intraocular pressure, and prostatic hypertrophy, judicious caution should be exercised (see **Contraindications**).

Use in Elderly: The elderly (60 years and older) are more likely to have adverse reactions to sympathomimetics. Overdosage of sympathomimetics in this age group may cause hallucinations, convulsions, CNS depression, and death.

Precautions: *General:* Caution should be exercised if used in patients with diabetes, hypertension, cardiovascular disease, hyperreactivity to ephedrine or decreased respiratory drive (see **Contraindications**).

Information for Patient: Antihistamines may impair mental and physical abilities required for the performance of potentially hazardous tasks, such as driving a vehicle or operating machinery, and mental alertness in children.

Do not exceed the prescribed dosage.

Drug Interactions: MAO inhibitors and beta adrenergic blockers increase the effect of sympathomimetics and the anticholinergic (drying) effects of antihistamines. Sympathomimetics may reduce the antihypertensive effects of methyldopa, mecamylamine, reserpine and veratrum alkaloids. Concomitant use of antihistamines with alcohol, tricyclic antidepressants, barbiturates and other CNS depressants may have an additive effect.

Pregnancy Category C: Animal reproduction studies have not been conducted with SINGLET. It is also not known whether SINGLET can cause fetal harm when administered to a pregnant woman or can affect reproduction capacity. SINGLET may be given to a pregnant woman only if clearly needed.

Nursing Mothers: Because of the potential for serious adverse reactions in nursing infants from sympathomimetic amines, phenylephrine is contraindicated in nursing mothers.

Adverse Reactions: Individuals hyperreactive to phenylephrine may display ephedrine-like reactions such as tachycardia, palpitation, headache, dizziness, or nausea. Sympathomimetic drugs have been associated with certain untoward reactions including fear, anxiety, tenseness, restlessness, tremor, weakness, pallor, respiratory difficulty, dysuria, insomnia, hallucinations, convulsions, CNS depression, arrhythmias, and cardio-

vascular collapse with hypotension. Possible side effects of antihistamines are drowsiness, restlessness, dizziness, weakness, dry mouth, anorexia, nausea, headache, nervousness, blurring of vision, heartburn, dysuria and very rarely dermatitis. Patient idiosyncrasy to adrenergic agents may be manifested by insomnia, dizziness, weakness, tremor or arrhythmias.

Overdosage: Pressor amines should be used with great caution in the presence of phenylephrine. Patients with signs of stimulation should be treated conservatively. Acetaminophen in massive overdosage has caused liver damage and fatal hepatic necrosis.

Recent studies have indicated that n-acetylcysteine may prevent hepatic damage if given within 24 hours of acetaminophen ingestion. Since n-acetylcysteine has not yet been approved for use as an antidote, except as an investigational drug, consult the Rocky Mountain Poison Center (toll-free number (800) 526-6115).[1]

Dosage and Administration: Adults: one table three times daily. In severe cases, a fourth dose may be indicated. The interval between doses should not be less than six hours. (NOTE: This product is specifically formulated to provide therapeutic effect for up to eight hours. Do not break or crush the tablets.)

Caution: Federal law prohibits dispensing without prescription.

How Supplied: The long-acting, pink, capsule-shaped tablet is monogrammed with the Dow diamond and 103 for positive identification. In bottles of 100 tablets (NDC 0068-0103-61).

[1] Peterson R G and Rumack BH: Toxicity of acetaminophen overdose. *JACEP* 7:5, 202, 1978.
  Glynn JP and Kendall SE: *Lancet*, 1147-48, May 17, 1975.

Shown in Product Identification Section, page 421

TACE® ℞
[tās]
(CHLOROTRIANISENE USP)
12 mg and 25 mg
Capsules

AVAILABLE ONLY ON PRESCRIPTION

Warnings:

1. ESTROGENS HAVE BEEN REPORTED TO INCREASE THE RISK RATIO FOR ENDOMETRIAL CARCINOMA.
Three independent case control studies have reported an increased risk ratio of endometrial cancer in postmenopausal women exposed to exogenous estrogens for prolonged periods.[1-3] This reported risk was independent of the other risk factors studied. Additionally, the incidence rates of endometrial cancer have increased since 1969 in 8 different areas of the United States with population-based cancer reporting systems, an increase that may [or may not] be related to the expanded use of estrogens during the last decade.[2]
The 3 case control studies reported that the estimated risk ratio for endometrial cancer in estrogen users was about 4.5 to 13.9 times greater than in nonusers. The risk appeared to depend on both duration of treatment[1] and on estrogen dose.[3] In view of these reports, when estrogens are used for the treatment of menopausal symptoms, the lowest dose that will control symptoms should be utilized and medication should be discontinued as soon as possible. When prolonged treatment is medically indicated, the patient should be reassessed on at least a semiannual basis to determine the need for continued therapy. Al-

Continued on next page

Information on Merrell Dow products is based on labeling in effect in August, 1984.

Merrell Dow—Cont.

though the evidence must be considered preliminary, one study suggests that cyclic administration of low doses of estrogen may carry less risk than continuous administration;[3] it therefore appears prudent to utilize such a regimen.

Close clinical surveillance of all women taking estrogens is important. In all cases of undiagnosed persistent or recurring abnormal vaginal bleeding, adequate diagnostic measures should be undertaken to rule out malignancy.

There is no evidence at present that "natural" estrogens are more or less hazardous than "synthetic" estrogens at equiestrogenic doses.

2. ESTROGENS SHOULD NOT BE USED DURING PREGNANCY.

The use of exogenous estrogens and progestagens during early pregnancy has been reported to damage the offspring. An association has been reported between *in utero* exposure of the female fetus to diethylstilbestrol, a nonsteroidal estrogen, and an increased risk of the post-pubertal development of an ordinarily rare form of vaginal or cervical cancer.[5,6] This risk for diethylstilbestrol was recently estimated to be in the range of 0.14 to 1.4 per 1000 exposures,[7] consistent with a previous risk estimate of not greater than 4 per 1000 exposures.[8] Furthermore, a high percentage of such females exposed *in utero* (30 to over 90%) has been reported to have vaginal adenosis, epithelial changes of the vagina and cervix.[9-12] Although these changes are histologically benign, it is not known whether they are precursors of adenocarcinoma. Although similar data are not available with the use of other estrogens, it cannot be presumed they would not induce similar changes.

Several reports suggest a possible association between fetal exposure to exogenous estrogens and progestagens and congenital anomalies, including congenital heart defects and limb reduction defects.[13-16] One case control study[16] estimated a 4.7 fold increased risk of limb reduction defects in infants exposed *in utero* to exogenous steroids (oral contraceptives, hormone withdrawal tests for pregnancy, or attempted treatment for threatened abortion). Some of these exposures were very short and involved only a few days of treatment. The data suggest that the risk of limb reduction defects in exposed fetuses is somewhat less than 1 per 1000.

This product is not for use in therapy of threatened or habitual abortion.

If TACE (CHLOROTRIANISENE USP) is used during pregnancy, or if the patient becomes pregnant while taking this drug, she should be apprised of the potential risks to the fetus, and the advisability of pregnancy continuation.

Description: TACE (CHLOROTRIANISENE USP) is a long-acting, synthetic estrogen in capsule form suitable for oral administration.

Each green, soft gelatin capsule contains 12 mg of chlorotrianisene in corn oil. Each two-tone green, hard gelatin capsule contains 25 mg of chlorotrianisene in tristearin.

Chemistry

Generic name: Chlorotrianisene USP

Chemical name: Benzene, 1, 1′, 1″-(1-chloro- 1 - ethenyl - 2 - ylidene) tris [4 - methoxy]-. Chlorotris (*p*-methoxyphenyl) ethylene.

Chlorotrianisene occurs as small, white crystals or as a crystalline powder. It is odorless. It is slightly soluble in alcohol and very slightly soluble in water.

Indications:

1. Postpartum breast engorgement—Although estrogens have been widely used for the prevention of postpartum breast engorgement, controlled studies have demonstrated that the incidence of significant painful engorgement in patients not receiving such hormonal therapy is low and usually responsive to appropriate analgesic or other supportive therapy. Consequently, the benefit to be derived from estrogen therapy for this indication must be carefully weighed against the potential risk of puerperal thromboembolism associated with the use of estrogens.[17]

2. Prostatic carcinoma—palliative therapy of advanced disease.

3. Moderate to severe *vasomotor* symptoms associated with the menopause. (There is no well-documented evidence that estrogens are effective for nervous symptoms or depression which might occur during menopause and they should not be used to treat these conditions.)

4. Atrophic vaginitis.

5. Kraurosis vulvae.

6. Female hypogonadism.

TACE (CHLOROTRIANISENE USP) HAS NOT BEEN SHOWN TO BE EFFECTIVE FOR ANY PURPOSE DURING PREGNANCY, AND ITS USE MAY HAVE POTENTIAL RISKS TO THE FETUS. (SEE BOXED WARNING.)

Contraindications: TACE (CHLOROTRIANISENE USP) should not be used in women or men with any of the following conditions:

1. Known or suspected cancer of the breast except in appropriately selected patients being treated for metastatic disease.

2. Known or suspected estrogen-dependent neoplasia.

3. Known or suspected pregnancy (See Boxed Warning.)

4. Undiagnosed abnormal genital bleeding.

5. Active thrombophlebitis or thromboembolic disorders.

6. A past history of thrombophlebitis, thrombosis, or thromboembolic disorders (except when used in treatment of prostatic malignancy).

Warnings:

1. *Induction of malignant neoplasms*. Long-term continuous administration of natural and synthetic estrogens in certain animal species increases the frequency of carcinomas of the breast, cervix, vagina, and liver. There are now reports that estrogens increase the risk of carcinoma of the endometrium in humans. (See Boxed Warning.)

At the present time there is no satisfactory evidence that estrogens given to postmenopausal women increase the risk of cancer of the breast,[18] although a recent long-term followup of a single physician's practice has raised this possibility.[19] Because of the animal data, there is a need for caution in prescribing estrogens for women with a strong family history of breast cancer or who have breast nodules, fibrocystic disease, or abnormal mammograms.

2. *Gallbladder disease*. A recent study has reported a two to threefold increase in the risk of surgically confirmed gallbladder disease in women receiving postmenopausal estrogens,[18] similar to the twofold increase previously noted in users of oral contraceptives.[20] In the case of oral contraceptives the increased risk appeared after a period of use.[20]

3. *Effects similar to those caused by estrogen-progestagen oral contraceptives*. There are several adverse effects reported in association with oral contraceptives, most of which have not been documented as consequences of postmenopausal estrogen therapy, although it has been reported that there is an increased risk of thrombosis in men receiving high doses of estrogens for prostatic cancer and in women receiving estrogens for postpartum breast engorgement.[17,21-23] The possibility that the adverse effects reported in association with oral contraceptives may be associated with larger doses of estrogen cannot be excluded.

a. *Thromboembolic disease*. Studies have now shown that users of oral contraceptives have an increased risk of various thromboembolic, thrombotic, and vascular diseases, such as thrombophlebitis, pulmonary embolism, stroke, and myocardial infarction.[24-31] Cases of retinal thrombosis, mesenteric thrombosis, and optic neuritis have been reported in oral contraceptive users. There is evidence that the risk of several of these adverse reactions is related to the dose of the drug.[32,33] An increased risk of post-surgery thromboembolic complications has also been reported in users of oral contraceptives.[34,35] If feasible, estrogen should be discontinued at least 4 weeks before surgery of the type associated with an increased risk of thromboembolism, or during periods of prolonged immobilization.

While an increased rate of thromboembolic and thrombotic disease in postmenopausal users of estrogens has not been found,[18,36] this does not rule out the possibility that such an increase may be present, or that subgroups of women who have underlying risk factors, or who are receiving relatively large doses of estrogens may have an increased risk. Therefore, estrogens should not be used in persons with active thrombophlebitis or thromboembolic disorders, and they should not be used (except in treatment of malignancy) in persons with a history of such disorders. They should be used with caution in patients with cerebral vascular or coronary artery disease and only for those in whom estrogens are needed.

Doses of estrogen (5 mg conjugated estrogens per day), comparable to those used to treat cancer of the prostate and breast, have been reported in a large prospective clinical trial in men[37] to increase the risk of nonfatal myocardial infarction, pulmonary embolism, and thrombophlebitis. When estrogen doses of this size are used, any of the thromboembolic and thrombotic adverse effects associated with oral contraceptive use should be considered as a risk.

b. *Hepatic adenoma*. Benign hepatic adenomas have been reported to be associated with the use of oral contraceptives.[38-40] Although benign and rare, these may rupture and may cause death through intra-abdominal hemorrhage. Such lesions have not yet been reported in association with other estrogen or progestagen preparations but should be considered in estrogen users having abdominal pain and tenderness, abdominal mass, or hypovolemic shock. Hepatocellular carcinoma has also been reported in women taking estrogen-containing oral contraceptives.[39] The relationship of this malignancy to these drugs is not known at this time.

c. *Elevated blood pressure*. Increased blood pressure is not uncommon in women using oral contraceptives and there is now a report that this may occur with use of estrogens in the menopause[41] and blood pressure should be monitored with estrogen use, especially if high doses are used.

d. *Glucose tolerance*. A worsening of glucose tolerance has been observed in a significant percentage of patients on estrogen-containing oral contraceptives. For this reason diabetic patients should be carefully observed while receiving estrogen.

4. *Hypercalcemia*. Administration of estrogens may lead to hypercalcemia in patients with breast cancer and bone metastases. If this occurs, the drug should be stopped and appropriate measures taken to reduce the serum calcium level.

Precautions:

A. General Precautions

1. A complete medical and family history should be taken prior to the initiation of any estrogen therapy. The pretreatment and periodic physical examinations should include special reference to blood pressure, breasts, abdomen, and pelvic organs, and should include a Papanicolaou smear. As a general rule, estrogen should not be prescribed for longer than 1 year without another physical examination being performed.

2. Fluid retention—Because estrogens may cause some degree of fluid retention, conditions that might be influenced by this factor such as epilepsy, migraine, and cardiac or renal dysfunction require careful observation.

3. Certain patients may develop undesirable manifestations of excessive estrogenic stimulation, such as abnormal or excessive uterine bleeding, mastodynia, etc.

4. Oral contraceptives have been reported to be associated with an increased incidence of mental depression. Although it is not clear whether this is possibly due to the estrogenic or progestagenic component of the contraceptive, patients with a history of depression should be carefully observed.
5. Patients having pre-existing uterine leiomyomata should be observed for increased growth of myomata during estrogen therapy.
6. The pathologist should be advised of estrogen therapy when relevant specimens are submitted.
7. Patients with a past history of jaundice during pregnancy have an increased risk of recurrence of jaundice while receiving estrogen-containing oral contraceptive therapy. If jaundice develops in any patient receiving estrogen, the medication should be discontinued while the cause is investigated.
8. Estrogens may be poorly metabolized in patients with impaired liver function and they should be administered with caution in such patients.
9. Because estrogens influence the metabolism of calcium and phosphorus, they should be used with caution in patients with metabolic bone diseases that are associated with hypercalcemia or in patients with renal insufficiency.
10. Because of the effects of estrogens on epiphyseal closure, they should be used judiciously in young patients in whom bone growth is not complete.
11. Judicious assessment of the following changes in certain endocrine and liver function tests is necessary for patients receiving large doses of estrogen:
 a. Increased sulfobromophthalein retention.
 b. Increased prothrombin and factors VII, VIII, IX, and X; decreased antithrombin 3; increased norepinephrine-induced platelet aggregability.
 c. Increased thyroid binding globulin (TBG) leading to increased circulating total thyroid hormone, as measured by PBI, T4 by column, or T4 by radioimmunoassay. Free T3 resin uptake is decreased, reflecting the elevated TBG; free T4 concentration is unaltered.
 d. Impaired glucose tolerance.
 e. Decreased pregnanediol excretion.
 f. Reduced response to metyrapone test.
 g. Reduced serum folate concentration.
 h. Increased serum triglyceride, phospholipid, or cholesterol.
12. This product contains FD&C Yellow No. 5 (tartrazine), which may cause allergic-type reactions (including bronchial asthma) in certain susceptible individuals. Although the overall incidence of FD&C Yellow No. 5 (tartrazine) sensitivity in the general population is low, it is frequently seen in patients who also have aspirin hypersensitivity.

B. Information For The Patient
A patient package insert accompanies this drug product. This insert is available from pharmacists who carry this product and from the company upon request.
C. Pregnancy Category X
See Contraindications and Boxed Warning.
D. Nursing Mothers
As a general principle, the administration of any drug to nursing mothers should be done only when clearly necessary since many drugs are excreted in human milk.

Adverse Reactions: (See Warnings regarding reports of induction of neoplasia, adverse effects on the fetus, increased incidence of gallbladder disease, and adverse effects similar to those of oral contraceptives, including thromboembolism.) The following additional adverse reactions have been reported with estrogenic therapy including oral contraceptives:
1. *Genitourinary system*
Breakthrough bleeding, spotting, change in menstrual flow and cycle.
Dysmenorrhea.
Premenstrual-like syndrome.
Amenorrhea during and after treatment.
Increase in size of uterine fibromyomata.
Vaginal candidiasis.
Change in cervical eversion and in degree of cervical secretion.
Cystitis-like syndrome.
2. *Breasts*
Tenderness, enlargement, secretion.
3. *Gastrointestinal*
Nausea, vomiting.
Abdominal cramps, bloating.
Cholestatic jaundice.
4. *Skin*
Chloasma or melasma, which may persist when drug is discontinued.
Erythema multiforme.
Erythema nodosum.
Hemorrhagic eruption.
Loss of scalp hair.
Hirsutism.
Urticaria.
5. *Eyes*
Steepening of corneal curvature.
Intolerance to contact lenses.
6. *CNS*
Headache, migraine, dizziness.
Mental depression.
Chorea.
7. *Miscellaneous*
Increase or decrease in weight.
Reduced carbohydrate tolerance.
Aggravation of porphyria.
Edema.
Changes in libido and/or potency.

Acute Overdosage: Numerous reports of ingestion of large doses of estrogen-containing oral contraceptives by young children indicate that serious ill effects usually do not occur. Overdosage of estrogen may cause nausea, and withdrawal bleeding may occur in females.

Dosage and Administration:
Given for a few days
Prevention of postpartum breast engorgement.
 The usual dosage is one 12 mg capsule four times daily for 7 days, or two 25 mg capsules every six hours for 6 doses. For immediate postpartum use, the first dose should be given within 8 hours after delivery.
Given chronically
Inoperable progressing prostatic cancer.
 The usual dosage is 12 to 25 mg daily (one or two 12 mg capsules or one 25 mg capsule).
Given cyclically for short-term use only
For treatment of moderate to severe *vasomotor* symptoms, atrophic vaginitis, or kraurosis vulvae associated with the menopause.
The lowest dose that will control symptoms should be chosen and medication should be discontinued as promptly as possible.
Administration should be cyclic (*e.g.,* 3 weeks on and 1 week off).
Attempts to discontinue or taper medication should be made at 3-month to 6-month intervals.
 The usual dosage range for vasomotor symptoms associated with the menopause is 12 to 25 mg daily (one or two 12 mg capsules or one 25 mg capsule) for 30 days; one or more courses may be prescribed.
 The usual dosage range for atrophic vaginitis or kraurosis vulvae is 12 to 25 mg daily (one or two 12 mg capsules or one 25 mg capsule) for 30 to 60 days.
Given cyclically
For female hypogonadism.
 The usual dosage is 12 to 25 mg daily (one or two 12 mg capsules or one 25 mg capsule) for 21 days. This course may, if desired, be followed immediately by the intramuscular injection of 100 mg of progesterone; alternatively, an oral progestogen such as medroxyprogesterone may be given during the last 5 days of TACE (CHLOROTRIANISENE USP) therapy. The next course may begin on the 5th day of the induced uterine bleeding.
Treated patients with an intact uterus should be monitored closely for signs of endometrial cancer, and appropriate diagnostic measures should be taken to rule out malignancy in the event of persistent or recurrent abnormal vaginal bleeding.

How Supplied:
TACE 12 mg (CHLOROTRIANISENE CAPSULES USP) green capsules imprinted MERRELL 690
NDC 0068-0690-61: bottles of 100
TACE 25 mg (CHLOROTRIANISENE CAPSULES USP) two-tone green capsules imprinted MERRELL 691
NDC 0068-0691-60: bottles of 60

References:
1. Ziel, H.K. and Finkel, W.D.: Increased risk of endometrial carcinoma among users of conjugated estrogens. New Eng. J. Med. 293:1167–1170, 1975.
2. Smith, D.C., Prentice, R., Thompson, D.J., and Hermann, W.L.: Association of exogenous estrogen and endometrial carcinoma. New Eng. J. Med. 293:1164–1167, 1975.
3. Mack, T.M., Pike, M.C., Henderson, B.E., Pfeffer, R. I., Gerkins, V.R., Arthur, M., and Brown, S.E.: Estrogens and endometrial cancer in a retirement community. New Eng. J. Med. 294:1262–1267, 1976.
4. Weiss, N.S., Szekely, D.R., and Austin, D.F.: Increasing incidence of endometrial cancer in the United States. New Eng. J. Med. 294:1259–1262, 1976.
5. Herbst, A.L., Ulfelder, H., and Poskanzer, D.C.: Adenocarcinoma of the vagina. New Eng. J. Med. 284:878–881, 1971.
6. Greenwald, P., Barlow, J.J., Nasca, P.C., and Burnett, W.S.: Vaginal cancer after maternal treatment with synthetic estrogens. New Eng. J. Med. 285: 390–392, 1971.
7. Herbst, A.L., Cole, P., Colton, T., Robboy, S.J., and Scully, R.E.: Age-incidence and risk of diethylstilbestrol-related clear cell adenocarcinoma of the vagina and cervix. Amer. J. Obstet. Gynec. 128:43–50, 1977.
8. Lanier, A.P., Noller, K.L., Decker, D.G., Elveback, L.R., and Kurland, L.T.: Cancer and Stilbestrol. A follow-up of 1719 persons exposed to estrogens in utero and born 1943–1959. Mayo Clin. Proc. 48:793–799, 1973.
9. Herbst, A.L., Kurman, R.J., and Scully, R.E.: Vaginal and cervical abnormalities after exposure to stilbestrol in utero. Obstet. Gynec. 40:287-298, 1972.
10. Herbst, A.L., Poskanzer, D.C., Robboy, S.J., Friedlander, L. and Scully, R.E.: Prenatal exposure to stilbestrol. A prospective comparison of exposed female offspring with unexposed controls. New Eng. J. Med. 292:334–339, 1975.
11. Stafl, A., Mattingly, R.F., Foley, D.V., and Fetherston, W.C.: Clinical diagnosis of vaginal adenosis. Obstet. Gynec. 43:118–128, 1974.
12. Sherman, A.I., Goldrath, M., Berlin A., Vakhariya, V., Banooni, F., Michaels, W., Goodman, P., and Brown, S.: Cervical-vaginal adenosis after *in utero* exposure to synthetic estrogens. Obstet. Gynec. 44:531–545, 1974.
13. Gal, I., Kirman, B., Stern, J.: Hormone pregnancy tests and congenital malformation. Nature 216:83, 1967.
14. Levy, E.P., Cohen, A., and Fraser, F.C.: Hormone treatment during pregnancy and congenital heart defects. Lancet 1:611, 1973.
15. Nora, J.J. and Nora, A.H.: Birth defects and oral contraceptives. Lancet 1:941–942, 1973.
16. Janerich, D.T., Piper, J.M., and Glebatis, D.M.: Oral contraceptives and congenital limb-reduction defects. New Eng. J. Med. 291:697–700, 1974.
17. Daniel, D.G., Campbell, H., and Turnbull, A.C.: Puerperal thromboembolism and suppression of lactation. Lancet 2:287–289, 1967.
18. Boston Collaborative Drug Surveillance Program: Surgically confirmed gall bladder disease, venous thromboembolism, and breast tumors in relation to post menopausal estrogen therapy. New Eng. J. Med. 290:15–19, 1974.

Continued on next page

Information on Merrell Dow products is based on labeling in effect in August, 1984.

Merrell Dow—Cont.

19. Hoover, R., Gray, L.A., Sr., Cole, P., and MacMahon, B.: Menopausal estrogens and breast cancer. New Eng. J. Med. 295:401–405, 1976.
20. Boston Collaborative Drug Surveillance Program: Oral contraceptives and venous thromboembolic disease, surgically confirmed gall-bladder disease, and breast tumors. Lancet 1:1399–1404, 1973.
21. Bailar, J.C., III: thromboembolism and oestrogen therapy. Lancet 2:560, 1967.
22. The Veterans Administration Cooperative Urological Research Group: Carcinoma of the prostate: Treatment comparisons. J. Urol. 98:516–522, 1967.
23. Blackard, C.E., Doe, R.P., Mellinger, G.T., and Byar, D.P.: Incidence of cardiovascular disease and death in patients receiving diethylstilbestrol for carcinoma of the prostate. Cancer 26:249–256, 1970.
24. Royal College of General Practitioners: Oral contraception and thromboembolic disease. J. Roy. Coll. Gen. Pract. 13:267–269, 1967.
25. Inman, W.H.W. and Vessey, M.P.: Investigation of deaths from pulmonary, coronary, and cerebral thrombosis and embolism in women of childbearing age. Brit. Med. J. 2:193–199, 1968.
26. Vessey, M.P. and Doll, R.: Investigation of relation between use of oral contraceptives and thromboembolic disease. A further report. Brit. Med. J. 2:651–657, 1969.
27. Sartwell, P.E., Masi, A.T., Arthes, F.G., Greene, G.R. and Smith, H.E.: Thromboembolism and oral contraceptives: An epidemiological case-control study. Amer. J. Epidem. 90:365-380, 1969.
28. Collaborative Group for the Study of Stroke in Young Women: Oral contraception and increased risk of cerebral ischemia or thrombosis. New Eng. J. Med. 288:871–878, 1973.
29. Collaborative Group for the Study of Stroke in Young Women: Oral contraceptives and stroke in young women: Associated risk factors. J.A.M.A. 231:718–722, 1975.
30. Mann, J.I. and Inman, W.H.W.: Oral contraceptives and death from myocardial infarction. Brit. Med. J. 2:245–248, 1975.
31. Mann, J.I., Vessey, M.P., Thorogood, M., and Doll, R.: Myocardial infarction in young women with special reference in oral contraceptive practice. Brit. Med. J. 2:241–245, 1975.
32. Inman, W.H.W., Vessey, M.P., Westerholm, B., and Engelund, A.: Thromboembolic disease and the steroidal content of oral contraceptives. A report to the Committee on Safety of Drugs. Brit. Med. J. 2:203–209, 1970.
33. Stolley, P.D., Tonascia, J.A., Tockman, M.S., Sartwell, P.E., Rutledge, A.H., and Jacobs, M.P.: Thrombosis with low-estrogen oral contraceptives. Amer. J. Epidem. 102:197–208, 1975.
34. Vessey, M.P., Doll, R., Fairbairn, A.S., and Glober, G.: Post-operative thromboembolism and the use of the oral contraceptives. Brit. Med. J. 3:123–126, 1970.
35. Greene, G.R. and Sartwell, P.E.: Oral contraceptive use in patients with thromboembolism following surgery, trauma, or infection. Amer. J. Public Health 62:680–685, 1972.
36. Rosenberg, L., Armstrong, B., Phil. D., and Jick H.: Myocardial infarction and estrogen therapy in post-menopausal women. New Eng. J. Med. 294:1256–1259, 1976.
37. Coronary Drug Project Research Group: The coronary drug project: initial findings leading to modifications of its research protocol. J.A.M.A. 214:1303–1313, 1970.
38. Baum, J., Holtz, F., Bookstein, J.J., and Klein, E.W.: Possible association between benign hepatomas and oral contraceptives. Lancet 2:926–928, 1973.
39. Mays, E.T., Christopherson, W.M., Mahr, M.M., and Williams, H.C.: Hepatic changes in young women ingesting contraceptive steroids. Hepatic hemorrhage and primary hepatic tumors. J.A.M.A. 235:730–732, 1976.
40. Edmondson, H., Henderson, A.B., and Benton, B.: Liver-cell adenomas associated with the use of oral contraceptives. New Eng. J. Med. 294:470–472, 1976.
41. Pfeffer, R.I. and Van Den Noort, S.: Estrogen use and stroke risk in postmenopausal women. Amer. J. Epidem. 103:445–456, 1976.

*Product Information as of August, 1979
(Package information amended February, 1983)*
TACE 12 mg Capsules
Manufactured by
R. P. Scherer, North America
Clearwater, Florida 33518 for
MERRELL DOW PHARMACEUTICALS INC.
Subsidiary of The Dow Chemical Company
Cincinnati, Ohio 45242-9553, U.S.A.

TACE®   R
(CHLOROTRIANISENE)
12 mg and 25 mg
Capsules
Information for Patients

> TACE (CHLOROTRIANISENE) is a synthetic estrogen supplied in 12 mg, 25 mg, and 72 mg capsules.

What You Should Know About Estrogens: Estrogens are female hormones produced by the ovaries. The ovaries make several different kinds of estrogens. In addition, scientists have been able to make a variety of synthetic estrogens. As far as we know, all these estrogens have many similar properties and therefore much the same usefulness, side effects, and risks. This leaflet is intended to help you understand what estrogens are sometimes used for, the risk involved in their use, and how to use them as safely as possible.

This leaflet includes important information about estrogens, but not all the information. If you want to know more, you can ask your doctor or pharmacist to let you read the package insert for this product prepared for the doctor.

Uses of Estrogen: Estrogens are prescribed by doctors for a number of purposes, including:
1. To provide estrogen during a period of adjustment when a woman's ovaries produce it in decreased amounts in order to prevent certain uncomfortable symptoms of estrogen deficiency. (All women normally produce less estrogen, generally between the ages of 45 and 55; this is called the menopause.)
2. To prevent symptoms of estrogen deficiency when a woman's ovaries have been removed surgically before the natural menopause.
3. To prevent pregnancy. (Estrogens are given along with a progestagen, another female hormone; these combinations are called oral contraceptives or birth control pills. Patient labeling is available to women taking oral contraceptives and they will not be discussed in this leaflet.) *This product is not intended to prevent pregnancy.*
4. To treat certain cancers in women and men. *This product is not intended to treat cancers in women.*
5. To prevent painful swelling of the breasts after pregnancy in women who choose not to nurse their babies.

THERE IS NO PROPER USE OF TACE IN A PREGNANT WOMAN.

Estrogens in the Menopause: In the natural course of their lives, all women eventually experience a decrease in estrogen production. This usually occurs between ages 45 and 55 but may occur earlier or later. Sometimes the ovaries may need to be removed before or during natural menopause by an operation, producing a "surgical menopause."

When the amount of estrogen in the blood begins to decrease, many women may develop typical symptoms: feelings of warmth in the face, neck, and chest or sudden intense episodes of heat and sweating throughout the body (called "hot flashes" or "hot flushes"). These symptoms are sometimes very uncomfortable. A few women eventually develop changes in the vagina (called "atrophic vaginitis") which cause discomfort, especially during and after intercourse.

Estrogens can be prescribed to treat these symptoms of the menopause. It is estimated that considerably more than half of all women undergoing the menopause have only mild symptoms or no symptoms at all and therefore do not need estrogens. Other women may need estrogens for a few months, while their bodies adjust to lower estrogen levels. Sometimes the need will be for periods longer than six months. In an attempt to avoid overstimulation of the uterus (womb), estrogens are usually given cyclically during each month of use, that is, three weeks of pills followed by one week without pills.

Sometimes women experience nervous symptoms or depression during menopause. There is no well-documented evidence that estrogens are effective for such symptoms and they should not be used to treat them, although other treatment may be needed.

You may have heard that taking estrogens for long periods (years) after the menopause will keep your skin soft and supple and keep you feeling young. There is no evidence that this is so, however, and such long-term treatment carries important risks.

Estrogens To Prevent Swelling of the Breasts After Pregnancy: If you do not breast feed your baby after delivery, your breasts may fill up with milk and become engorged and painful. This usually begins about 3 to 4 days after delivery and may last for a few days to up to a week or more. Sometimes the discomfort is severe, but usually it is not and can be controlled by pain relieving drugs such as aspirin and by binding the breasts up tightly. Estrogens can be used to try to prevent the breasts from filling up.

While this treatment is usually successful in reducing amount of filling, in many cases the breasts fill up to some degree in spite of treatment. The daily dose of estrogens needed to prevent pain and swelling of the breasts is larger than the dose needed to treat symptoms of the menopause and this may increase your chances of developing blood clots in the legs or lungs. (See below.) Therefore, it is important that you discuss the benefits and the risks of estrogen use with your doctor if you have decided not to breast feed your baby.

The Dangers of Estrogens:
1. *Cancer of the uterus.* Several independent studies have reported an increased risk ratio of endometrial cancer (cancer of the lining of the uterus) if estrogens are used in the post-menopausal period for more than a year. Women taking estrogens are reported to have roughly 5 to 10 times as great a chance of getting this cancer as women who take no estrogens. To put this another way, while a postmenopausal woman not taking estrogens has 1 chance in 1,000 each year of getting cancer of the uterus, a woman taking estrogens has 5 to 10 chances in 1,000 each year. For this reason *it is important to take estrogens only when you really need them.*

The risk of this cancer is reported to be greater the longer estrogens are used and also seems to be greater when larger doses are taken. For this reason *it is important to take the lowest dose of estrogen that will control symptoms and to take it only as long as it is needed.* If estrogens are needed for longer periods of time, your doctor will want to reevaluate your need for estrogens at least every six months.

Women using estrogens should report any irregular vaginal bleeding to their doctors; such bleeding may be of no importance, but it can be an early warning of cancer of the uterus. If you have undiagnosed vaginal bleeding, you should not use estrogens until a diagnosis is made that there is no cancer of the uterus.

If you have had your uterus completely removed (total hysterectomy), there is no danger of developing cancer of the uterus.

2. *Other possible cancers.* Long-term continuous

administration of estrogens in certain animal species increases the frequency of cancers of the breast, cervix, vagina, and liver. At present there is no satisfactory evidence that women using estrogen in the menopause have an increased risk of such tumors, but there is no way yet to be sure they do not; and one study raises the possibility that use of estrogens in the menopause may increase the risk of breast cancer many years later. This is a further reason to use estrogens only when clearly needed. While you are taking estrogens, it is important that you go to your doctor at least every six months for an examination. Also, if members of your family have had breast cancer or if you have breast nodules or abnormal mammograms (breast x-rays), your doctor may wish to carry out more frequent examinations of your breasts.

3. *Gall bladder disease.* Women who use estrogens after menopause are reported to be more likely to develop gall bladder disease needing surgery than women who do not use estrogens. Birth control pills have a similar effect.

4. *Abnormal blood clotting.* Oral contraceptives increase the risk of blood clotting in various parts of the body. This can result in a stroke (if the clot is in the brain), a heart attack (clot in a blood vessel of the heart), or a pulmonary embolus (a clot which forms in the legs or pelvis, then breaks off and travels to the lungs). Any of these can be fatal.
At this time use of estrogens in the menopause is not known to cause such blood clotting, but the possibility that such clotting in association with oral contraceptives may be associated with larger doses of estrogen cannot be excluded. It is recommended that if you have had clotting in the legs or lungs or a heart attack or stroke while you were using estrogens or birth control pills, you should not use estrogens (unless they are being used to treat cancer of the breast or prostate). If you have had a stroke or heart attack or if you have angina pectoris, estrogens should be used with caution and only if clearly needed (for example, if you have severe symptoms of the menopause).
The large doses of estrogen used to prevent swelling of the breasts after pregnancy have been reported to increase the risk of clotting in the legs and lungs.

Special Warning About Pregnancy: You should not receive estrogen if you are pregnant. It has been reported that there is a greater than usual chance that the developing child will be born with a birth defect, although the possibility remains fairly small. It is also reported that a female child may have an increased risk of developing cancer of the vagina or cervix later in life (in the teens or twenties). Every possible effort should be made to avoid exposure to TACE during pregnancy. If exposure occurs, see your doctor.

Other Effects of Estrogens: In addition to the serious reported risks of estrogens described above, estrogens have the following side effects and potential risks:

1. *Nausea and vomiting.* The most common side effect of estrogen therapy is nausea. Vomiting is less common.

2. *Effects on breasts.* Estrogens may cause breast tenderness or enlargement and may cause the breasts to secrete a liquid. These effects are not dangerous.

3. *Effects on the uterus.* Estrogens may cause benign fibroid tumors of the uterus to get larger. Some women will have menstrual bleeding when estrogens are stopped. But if the bleeding occurs on days you are still taking estrogens you should report this to your doctor.

4. *Effects on liver.* Women taking oral contraceptives develop on rare occasions a tumor of the liver which can rupture and bleed into the abdomen. So far, these tumors have not been reported in women using estrogens in the menopause, but you should report any swelling or unusual pain or tenderness in the abdomen to your doctor immediately.
Women with a past history of jaundice (yellowing of the skin and white parts of the eyes) may get jaundice again during estrogen use. If this occurs, stop taking estrogens and see your doctor.

5. *Other effects.* Estrogens may cause excess fluid to be retained in the body. This may make some conditions worse, such as epilepsy, migraine, heart disease, or kidney disease.

Summary: Estrogens have important uses, but they have reported risks of potentially serious conditions developing as well. You must decide, with your doctor, whether the risks are acceptable to you in view of the benefits of treatment. Except where your doctor has prescribed TACE for use in special cases of cancer of the prostate, you should not use TACE if you have cancer of the breast or uterus, are pregnant, have undiagnosed abnormal vaginal bleeding, clotting in the legs or lungs, or have had a stroke, heart attack or angina, or clotting in the legs or lungs in the past while you were taking estrogens.
You can use TACE as safely as possible by understanding that your doctor will require regular physical examinations while you are taking it and will try to discontinue the drug as soon as possible and use the smallest dose possible. Be alert for signs of trouble including:
1. Abnormal bleeding from the vagina.
2. Pains in the calves or chest or sudden shortness of breath, or coughing blood (indicating possible clots in the legs, heart, or lungs).
3. Severe headache, dizziness, faintness, or changes in vision (indicating possible developing clots in the brain or eye).
4. Breast lumps. (You should ask your doctor how to examine your own breasts.)
5. Jaundice (yellowing of the skin).
6. Mental depression.
Based on his or her assessment of your medical needs, your doctor has prescribed this drug for you. Do not give this drug to anyone else.

How Supplied: TACE (CHLOROTRIANISENE) is a long-acting synthetic estrogen in capsule form. The capsule is suitable for taking by mouth.
Each green, soft gelatin capsule imprinted MERRELL 690 contains 12 mg of chlorotrianisene in corn oil.
Each two-tone green, hard gelatin capsule imprinted MERRELL 691 contains 25 mg of chlorotrianisene in tristearin.
This product contains color additives including FD&C Yellow No. 5 (tartrazine).

Patient Information as of August, 1979
Shown in Product Identification Section, page 421

TACE® ℞
[tās]
(CHLOROTRIANISENE USP)
72 mg Capsules
AVAILABLE ONLY ON PRESCRIPTION
Warnings

1. ESTROGENS HAVE BEEN REPORTED TO INCREASE THE RISK RATIO FOR ENDOMETRIAL CARCINOMA.
Three independent case control studies have reported an increased risk ratio of endometrial cancer in postmenopausal women exposed to exogenous estrogens for prolonged periods.[1-3] This reported risk was independent of the other risk factors studied. Additionally, the incidence rates of endometrial cancer have increased since 1969 in 8 different areas of the United States with population-based cancer reporting systems, an increase that may [or may not] be related to the expanded use of estrogens during the last decade.[4]
The 3 case control studies reported that the estimated risk ratio for endometrial cancer in estrogen users was about 4.5 to 13.9 times greater than in nonusers. The risk appeared to depend on both duration of treatment[1] and on estrogen dose.[3] In view of these reports, when estrogens are used for the treatment of menopausal symptoms, the lowest dose that will control symptoms should be utilized and medication should be discontinued as soon as possible. When prolonged treatment is medically indicated, the patient should be reassessed on at least a semiannual basis to determine the need for continued therapy. Although the evidence must be considered preliminary, one study suggests that cyclic administration of low doses of estrogen may carry less risk than continuous administration;[3] it therefore appears prudent to utilize such a regimen.
Close clinical surveillance of all women taking estrogens is important. In all cases of undiagnosed persistent or recurring abnormal vaginal bleeding, adequate diagnostic measures should be undertaken to rule out malignancy.
There is no evidence at present that "natural" estrogens are more or less hazardous than "synthetic" estrogens at equiestrogenic doses.

2. ESTROGENS SHOULD NOT BE USED DURING PREGNANCY.
The use of exogenous estrogens and progestagens during early pregnancy has been reported to damage the offspring. An association has been reported between *in utero* exposure of the female fetus to diethylstilbestrol, a non-steroidal estrogen, and an increased risk of the postpubertal development of an ordinarily rare form of vaginal or cervical cancer.[5,6] This risk for diethylstilbestrol was recently estimated to be in the range of 0.14 to 1.4 per 1000 exposures,[7] consistent with a previous risk estimate of not greater than 4 per 1000 exposures.[8] Furthermore, a high percentage of such females exposed *in utero* (30 to over 90%) has been reported to have vaginal adenosis, epithelial changes of the vagina and cervix.[9-12] Although these changes are histologically benign, it is not known whether they are precursors of adenocarcinoma. Although similar data are not available with the use of other estrogens, it cannot be presumed they would not induce similar changes.
Several reports suggest a possible association between fetal exposure to exogenous estrogens and progestagens and congenital anomalies, including congenital heart defects and limb reduction defects.[13-16] One case control study[16] estimated a 4.7 fold increased risk of limb reduction defects in infants exposed *in utero* to exogenous steriods (oral contraceptives, hormone withdrawal tests for pregnancy, or attempted treatment for threatened abortion). Some of these exposures were very short and involved only a few days of treatment. The data suggest that the risk of limb reduction defects in exposed fetuses is somewhat less than 1 per 1000.
This product is not for use in therapy of threatened or habitual abortion.
If TACE (CHLOROTRIANISENE USP) is used during pregnancy, or if the patient becomes pregnant while taking this drug, she should be apprised of the potential risks to the fetus, and the advisability of pregnancy continuation.

Description:
TACE (CHLOROTRIANISENE USP) is a long-acting, synthetic estrogen in capsule form suitable for oral administration.
Each two-tone green and yellow soft gelatin capsule contains 72 mg of TACE (CHLOROTRIANISENE) in Dispex®, an emulsifiable vehicle containing corn oil, sorbitan trioleate, polysorbate 80, and benzyl benzoate.

Continued on next page

Information on Merrell Dow products is based on labeling in effect in August, 1984.

Merrell Dow—Cont.

Chemistry
Generic name: Chlorotrianisene USP
Chemical name: Benzene, 1, 1', 1''-(1-chloro- 1 - ethenyl - 2 - ylidene) tris [4 - methoxy]-. Chlorotris (*p*-methoxyphenyl) ethylene.
Chlorotrianisene occurs as small, white crystals or as a crystalline powder. It is odorless. It is slightly soluble in alcohol and very slightly soluble in water.

Indications: Postpartum breast engorgement—Although estrogens have been widely used for the prevention of postpartum breast engorgement, controlled studies have demonstrated that the incidence of significant painful engorgement in patients not receiving such hormonal therapy is low and usually responsive to appropriate analgesic or other supportive therapy. Consequently, the benefit to be derived from estrogen therapy for this indication must be carefully weighed against the potential risk of puerperal thromboembolism associated with the use of estrogens.[17]
TACE (CHLOROTRIANISENE USP) HAS NOT BEEN SHOWN TO BE EFFECTIVE FOR ANY PURPOSE DURING PREGNANCY, AND ITS USE MAY HAVE POTENTIAL RISKS TO THE FETUS. (SEE BOXED WARNING.)

Contraindications: TACE (CHLOROTRIANISENE USP) should not be used in women or men with any of the following conditions:
1. Known or suspected cancer of the breast except in appropriately selected patients being treated for metastatic disease.
2. Known or suspected estrogen-dependent neoplasia.
3. Known or suspected pregnancy. (See Boxed Warning.)
4. Undiagnosed abnormal genital bleeding.
5. Active thrombophlebitis or thromboembolic disorders.
6. A past history of thrombophlebitis, thrombosis, or thromboembolic disorders (except when used in treatment of prostatic malignancy).

Warnings:
1. *Induction of malignant neoplasms.* Long-term continuous administration of natural and synthetic estrogens in certain animal species increases the frequency of carcinomas of the breast, cervix, vagina, and liver. There are now reports that estrogens increase the risk of carcinoma of the endometrium in humans. (See Boxed Warning.)
At the present time there is no satisfactory evidence that estrogens given to postmenopausal women increase the risk of cancer of the breast,[18] although a recent long-term followup of a single physician's practice has raised this possibility.[19] Because of the animal data, there is a need for caution in prescribing estrogens for women with a strong family history of breast cancer or who have breast nodules, fibrocystic disease, or abnormal mammograms.
2. *Gallbladder disease.* A recent study has reported a two to threefold increase in the risk of surgically confirmed gallbladder disease in women receiving postmenopausal estrogens,[18] similar to the twofold increase previously noted in users of oral contraceptives.[20] In the case of oral contraceptives the increased risk appeared after a period of use.[20]
3. *Effects similar to those caused by estrogen-progestagen oral contraceptives.* There are several adverse effects reported in association with oral contraceptives, most of which have not been documented as consequences of postmenopausal estrogen therapy, although it has been reported that there is an increased risk of thrombosis in men receiving high doses of estrogens for prostatic cancer and in women receiving estrogens for postpartum breast engorgement.[17,21-23] The possibility that the adverse effects reported in association with oral contraceptives may be associated with larger doses of estrogen cannot be excluded.
   a. *Thromboembolic disease.* Studies have now shown that users of oral contraceptives have an increased risk of various thromboembolic, thrombotic, and vascular diseases, such as thrombophlebitis, pulmonary embolism, stroke, and myocardial infarction.[24-31] Cases of retinal thrombosis, mesenteric thrombosis, and optic neuritis have been reported in oral contraceptive users. There is evidence that the risk of several of these adverse reactions is related to the dose of the drug.[32, 33] An increased risk of post-surgery thromboembolic complications has also been reported in users of oral contraceptives.[34,35] If feasible, estrogen should be discontinued at least 4 weeks before surgery of the type associated with an increased risk of thromboembolism, or during periods of prolonged immobilization.
While an increased rate of thromboembolic and thrombotic disease in postmenopausal users of estrogens has not been found,[18, 36] this does not rule out the possibility that such an increase may be present, or that subgroups of women who have underlying risk factors, or who are receiving relatively large doses of estrogens may have an increased risk. Therefore, estrogens should not be used in persons with active thrombophlebitis or thromboembolic disorders, and they should not be used (except in treatment of malignancy) in persons with a history of such disorders. They should be used with caution in patients with cerebral vascular or coronary artery disease and only for those in whom estrogens are needed.
Doses of estrogen (5 mg conjungated estrogens per day), comparable to those used to treat cancer of the prostate and breast, have been reported in a large prospective clinical trial in men[37] to increase the risk of nonfatal myocardial infarction, pulmonary embolism, and thrombophlebitis. When estrogen doses of this size are used, any of the thromboembolic and thrombotic adverse effects associated with oral contraceptive use should be considered as a risk.
   b. *Hepatic adenoma.* Benign hepatic adenomas have been reported to be associated with the use of oral contraceptives.[38-40] Although benign and rare, these may rupture and may cause death through intra-abdominal hemorrhage. Such lesions have not yet been reported in association with other estrogen or progestagen preparations but should be considered in estrogen users having abdominal pain and tenderness, abdominal mass, or hypovolemic shock. Hepatocellular carcinoma has also been reported in women taking estrogen-containing oral contraceptives.[39] The relationship of this malignancy to these drugs is not known at this time.
   c. *Elevated blood pressure.* Increased blood pressure is not uncommon in women using oral contraceptives and there is now a report that this may occur with use of estrogens in the menopause[41] and blood pressure should be monitored with estrogen use, especially if high doses are used.
   d. *Glucose tolerance.* A worsening of glucose tolerance has been observed in a significant percentage of patients on estrogen-containing oral contraceptives. For this reason diabetic patients should be carefully observed while receiving estrogen.
4. *Hypercalcemia.* Administration of estrogens may lead to hypercalcemia in patients with breast cancer and bone metastases. If this occurs, the drug should be stopped and appropriate measures taken to reduce the serum calcium level.

Precautions:
A. General Precautions
1. A complete medical and family history should be taken prior to the initiation of any estrogen therapy. The pretreatment and periodic physical examinations should include special reference to blood pressure, breasts, abdomen, and pelvic organs, and should include a Papanicolaou smear. As a general rule, estrogen should not be prescribed for longer than 1 year without another physical examination being performed.
2. Fluid retention—Because estrogens may cause some degree of fluid retention, conditions that might be influenced by this factor such as epilepsy, migraine, and cardiac or renal dysfunction require careful observation.
3. Certain patients may develop undersirable manifestations of excessive estrogenic stimulation, such as abnormal or excessive uterine bleeding, mastodynia, etc.
4. Oral contraceptives have been reported to be associated with an increased incidence of mental depression. Although it is not clear whether this is possibly due to the estrogenic or progestagenic component of the contraceptive, patients with a history of depression should be carefully observed.
5. Patients having pre-existing uterine leiomyomata should be observed for increased growth of myomata during estrogen therapy.
6. The pathologist should be advised of estrogen therapy when relevant specimens are submitted.
7. Patients with a past history of jaundice during pregnancy have an increased risk of recurrence of jaundice while receiving estrogen-containing oral contraceptive therapy. If jaundice develops in any patient receiving estrogen, the medication should be discontinued while the cause is investigated.
8. Estrogens may be poorly metabolized in patients with impaired liver function and they should be administered with caution in such patients.
9. Because estrogens influence the metabolism of calcium and phosphorus, they should be used with caution in patients with metabolic bone diseases that are associated with hypercalcemia or in patients with renal insufficiency.
10. Because of the effects of estrogens on epiphyseal closure, they should be used judiciously in young patients in whom bone growth is not complete.
11. Judicious assessment of the following changes in certain endocrine and liver function tests is necessary for patients receiving large doses of estrogen:
   a. Increased sulfobromophthalein retention.
   b. Increased prothrombin and factors VII, VIII, IX and X; decreased antithrombin 3; increased norepinephrine-induced platelet aggregability.
   c. Increased thyroid binding globulin (TBG) leading to increased circulating total thyroid hormone, as measured by PBI, T4 by column, or T4 by radioimmunoassay. Free T3 resin uptake is decreased, reflecting the elevated TBG; free T4 concentration is unaltered.
   d. Impaired glucose tolerance.
   e. Decreased pregnanediol excretion.
   f. Reduced response to metyrapone test.
   g. Reduced serum folate concentration.
   h. Increased serum triglyceride, phospholipid, or cholesterol.
12. This product contains FD&C Yellow No. 5 (tartrazine), which may cause allergic-type reactions (including bronchial asthma) in certain susceptible individuals. Although the overall incidence of FD&C Yellow No. 5 (tartrazine) sensitivity in the general population is low, it is frequently seen in patients who also have aspirin hypersensitivity.
B. Information For The Patient
A patient package insert accompanies this drug product. This insert is available from pharmacists who carry this product and from the company upon request.
C. Pregnancy Category X
See Contraindications and Boxed Warning.
D. Nursing Mothers
As a general principle, the administration of any drug to nursing mothers should be done only when clearly necessary since many drugs are excreted in human milk.

Adverse Reactions: (See Warnings regarding reports of induction of neoplasia, adverse effects on the fetus, increased incidence of gallbladder disease, and adverse effects similar to those of oral contraceptives, including thromboembolism.) The following additional adverse reactions have been reported with estrogenic therapy including oral contraceptives:
1. *Genitourinary system*
Breakthrough bleeding, spotting, change in menstrual flow and cycle.

Dysmenorrhea.
Premenstrual-like syndrome.
Amenorrhea during and after treatment.
Increase in size of uterine fibromyomata.
Vaginal candidiasis.
Change in cervical eversion and in degree of cervical secretion.
Cystitis-like syndrome.
2. *Breasts*
Tenderness, enlargement, secretion.
3. *Gastrointestinal*
Nausea, vomiting.
Abdominal cramps, bloating.
Cholestatic jaundice.
4. *Skin*
Chloasma or melasma, which may persist when drug is discontinued.
Erythema multiforme.
Erythema nodosum.
Hemorrhagic eruption.
Loss of scalp hair.
Hirsutism.
Urticaria.
5. *Eyes*
Steepening of corneal curvature.
Intolerance to contact lenses.
6. *CNS*
Headache, migraine, dizziness.
Mental depression.
Chorea.
7. *Miscellaneous*
Increase or decrease in weight.
Reduced carbohydrate tolerance.
Aggravation of porphyria.
Edema.
Changes in libido and/or potency.
Acute Overdosage: Numerous reports of ingestion of large doses of estrogen-containing oral contraceptives by young children indicate that serious ill effects usually do not occur. Overdosage of estrogen may cause nausea, and withdrawal bleeding may occur in females.
Dosage and Administration:
Given for a few days
Prevention of postpartum breast engorgement.
The usual dosage is 1 TACE 72 mg capsule twice daily for 2 days. The first dose should be given as soon as possible after delivery but within 8 hours.
How Supplied:
TACE 72 mg (CHLOROTRIANISENE CAPSULES USP) green and yellow capsules imprinted MERRELL 692
NDC 0068-0692-48: packages of 48 capsules.
References:
1. Ziel, H. K. and Finkel, W. D.: Increased risk of endometrial carcinoma among users of conjugated estrogens. New Eng. J. Med. 293: 1167–1170, 1975.
2. Smith, D.C., Prentice, R., Thompson, D.J., and Hermann, W.L.: Association of exogenous estrogen and endometrial carcinoma. New Eng. J. Med. 293:1164–1167, 1975.
3. Mack, T.M., Pike, M.C., Henderson, B.E., Pfeffer, R.I., Gerkins, V.R., Arthur, M., and Brown, S.E.: Estrogens and endometrial cancer in a retirement community. New Eng. J. Med. 294:1262–1267, 1976.
4. Weiss, N.S., Szekely, D.R., and Austin, D.F.: Increasing incidence of endometrial cancer in the United States. New Eng. J. Med. 294:1259–1262, 1976.
5. Herbst, A.L., Ulfelder, H., and Poskanzer, D.C.: Adenocarcinoma of the vagina. New Eng. J. Med. 284:878–881, 1971.
6. Greenwald, P., Barlow, J.J., Nasca, P.C., and Burnett, W.S.: Vaginal cancer after maternal treatment with synthetic estrogens. New Eng. J. Med. 285:390–392, 1971.
7. Herbst, A.L., Cole, P., Colton, T., Robboy, S.J., and Scully, R.E.: Age-incidence and risk of diethylstilbestrol-related clear cell adenocarcinoma of the vagina and cervix. Amer. J. Obstet. Gynec. 128:43-50, 1977.
8. Lanier, A.P., Noller, K.L., Decker, D.G., Elveback, L.R., and Kurland, L.T.: Cancer and stilbestrol. A follow-up of 1719 persons exposed to estrogens in utero and born 1943-1959. Mayo Clin. Proc. 48:793–799, 1973.

9. Herbst, A.L., Kurman, R.J., and Scully, R.E.: Vaginal and cervical abnormalities after exposure to stilbestrol in utero. Obstet. Gynec. 40:287–298, 1972.
10. Herbst, A.L., Poskanzer, D.C., Robboy, S.J., Friedlander, L., and Scully, R.E.: Prenatal exposure to stilbestrol. A prospective comparison of exposed female offspring with unexposed controls. New Eng. J. Med. 292:334–339, 1975.
11. Stafl, A., Mattingly, R.F., Foley, D.V., and Fetherston, W.C.: Clincial diagnosis of vaginal adenosis. Obstet. Gynec. 43:118–128, 1974.
12. Sherman, A.I., Goldrath, M., Berlin, A., Vakhariya, V., Banooni, F., Michaels, W., Goodman, P., and Brown, S.: Cervical-vaginal adenosis after *in utero* exposure to synthetic estrogens. Obstet. Gynec. 44:531–545, 1974.
13. Gal, I., Kirman, B., and Stern. J.: Hormone pregnancy tests and congenital malformation. Nature 216:83, 1967.
14. Levy, E.P., Cohen, A., and Fraser, F.C.: Hormone treatment during pregnancy and congenital heart defects. Lancet 1:611, 1973.
15. Nora, J.J. and Nora, A.H.: Birth defects and oral contraceptives. Lancet 1:941–942, 1973.
16. Janerich, D.T., Piper, J.M., and Glebatis, D.M.: Oral contraceptives and congenital limb-reduction defects. New Eng. J. Med. 291:697–700, 1974.
17. Daniel, D.G., Campbell, H., and Turnbull, A.C.: Puerperal thromboembolism and suppression of lactation. Lancet 2:287–289, 1967.
18. Boston Collaborative Drug Surveillance Program: Surgically confirmed gall bladder disease, venous thromboembolism, and breast tumors in relation to post menopausal estrogen therapy. New Eng. J. Med. 290:15–19, 1974.
19. Hoover, R., Gray, L.A., Sr., Cole, P., and MacMahon, B.: Menopausal estrogens and breast cancer. New Eng. J. Med. 295:401–405, 1976.
20. Boston Collaborative Drug Surveillance Program: Oral contraceptives and venous thromboembolic disease, surgically confirmed gall-bladder disease, and breast tumors. Lancet 1:1399–1404, 1973.
21. Bailar, J.C., III: Thromboembolism and oestrogen therapy. Lancet 2:560, 1967.
22. The Veterans Administration Cooperative Urological Research Group: Carcinoma of the prostate: Treatment comparisons. J. Urol. 98:516–522, 1967.
23. Blackard, C.E., Doe, R.P., Mellinger, G.T., and Byar, D.P.: Incidence of cardiovascular disease and death in patients receiving diethylstilbestrol for carcinoma of the prostate. Cancer 26:249–256, 1970.
24. Royal College of General Practitioners: Oral contraception and thromboembolic disease. J. Roy. Coll. Gen. Pract. 13:267–269, 1967.
25. Inman, W.H.W. and Vessey, M.P.: Investigation of deaths from pulmonary, coronary, and cerebral thrombosis and embolism in women of childbearing age. Brit. Med. J. 2:193–199, 1968.
26. Vessey, M.P. and Doll, R.: Investigation of relation between use of oral contraceptives and thromboembolic disease. A further report. Brit. Med. J. 2:651–657, 1969.
27. Sartwell, P.E., Masi, A.T., Arthes, F.G., Greene, G.R., and Smith, H.E.: Thromboembolism and oral contraceptives: An epidemiological case-control study. Amer. J. Epidem. 90:365–380, 1969.
28. Collaborative Group for the Study of Stroke in Young Women: Oral contraception and increased risk of cerebral ischemia or thrombosis. New Eng. J. Med. 288:871–878, 1973.
29. Collaborative Group for the Study of Stroke in Young Women: Oral contraceptives and stroke in young women: Associated risk factors. J.A.M.A. 231:718–722, 1975.
30. Mann, J.I. and Inman, W.H.W.: Oral contraceptives and death from myocardial infarction. Brit. Med. J. 2:245–248, 1975.
31. Mann, J.I., Vessey, M.P., Thorogood, M., and Doll, R.: Myocardial infarction in young women with special reference in oral contraceptive practice. Brit. Med. J. 2:241–245, 1975.
32. Inman, W.H.W., Vessey, M.P., Westerholm, B., and Engeland, A.: Thromboembolic disease and the steroidal content of oral contraceptives. A re-

port to the Committee on Safety of Drugs. Brit. Med. J. 2:203–209, 1970.
33. Stolley, P.D., Tonascia, J.A., Tockman, M.S., Sartwell, P.E., Rutledge, A.H., and Jacobs, M.P.: Thrombosis with low-estrogen oral contraceptives. Amer. J. Epidem. 102:197–208, 1975.
34. Vessey, M.P., Doll, R., Fairbairn, A.S., and Glober, G.: Post-operative thromboembolism and the use of the oral contraceptives. Brit. Med. J. 3:123-126, 1970.
35. Greene, G.R. and Sartwell, P.E.: Oral contraceptive use in patients with thromboembolism following surgery, trauma, or infection. Amer. J. Public Health 62:680–685, 1972.
36. Rosenberg, L., Armstrong, B., Phil, D., and Jick, H.: Myocardial infarction and estrogen therapy in post-menopausal women. New Eng. J. Med. 294:1256–1259, 1976.
37. Coronary Drug Project Research Group: The coronary drug project: Initial findings leading to modifications of its research protocol. J.A.M.A. 214:1303–1313, 1970.
38. Baum, J., Holtz, F., Bookstein, J.J., and Klein, E.W.: Possible association between benign hepatomas and oral contraceptives. Lancet 2:926–928, 1973.
39. Mays, E.T., Christopherson, W.M., Mahr, M.M., and Williams, H.C.: Hepatic changes in young women ingesting contraceptive steroids. Hepatic hemorrhage and primary hepatic tumors. J.A.M.A. 235:730–732, 1976.
40. Edmondson, H., Henderson, A.B., and Benton, B.: Liver-cell adenomas associated with the use of oral contraceptives. New Eng. J. Med. 294:470–472, 1976.
41. Pfeffer, R.I. and Van Den Noort, S.: Estrogen use and stroke risk in postmenopausal women. Amer. J. Epidem. 103:445–456, 1976.

Product Information as of August, 1979
Manufactured by
R. P. Scherer, North America
Clearwater, Florida 33518 for
MERRELL DOW PHARMACEUTICALS INC.
Subsidiary of The Dow Chemical Company
Cincinnati, Ohio 45242-9553, U.S.A.

TACE® B
(CHLOROTRIANISENE)
72 mg Capsules
Information for Patients

TACE (CHLOROTRIANISENE) is a synthetic estrogen supplied in 12 mg, 25 mg, and 72 mg capsules.

What You Should Know About Estrogens: Estrogens are female hormones produced by the ovaries. The ovaries make several different kinds of estrogens. In addition, scientists have been able to make a variety of synthetic estrogens. As far as we know, all these estrogens have many similar properties and therefore much the same usefulness, side effects, and risks. This leaflet is intended to help you understand what estrogens are sometimes used for, the risks involved in their use, and how to use them as safely as possible.
This leaflet includes important information about estrogens, but not all the information. If you want to know more, you can ask your doctor or pharmacist to let you read the package insert for this product prepared for the doctor.
Uses of Estrogen: Estrogens are prescribed by doctors for a number of purposes, including:
1. To provide estrogen during a period of adjustment when a woman's ovaries produce it in decreased amounts in order to prevent certain uncomfortable symptoms of estrogen deficiency. (All women normally produce less estrogen, generally

Continued on next page

Information on Merrell Dow products is based on labeling in effect in August, 1984.

Merrell Dow—Cont.

between the ages of 45 and 55; this is called the menopause.)
2. To prevent symptoms of estrogen deficiency when a woman's ovaries have been removed surgically before the natural menopause.
3. To prevent pregnancy. (Estrogens are given along with a progestagen, another female hormone; these combinations are called oral contraceptives or birth control pills. Patient labeling is available to women taking oral contraceptives and they will not be discussed in this leaflet.) *This product is not intended to prevent pregnancy.*
4. To treat certain cancers in women and men. *This product is not intended to treat cancers in women.*
5. To prevent painful swelling of the breasts after pregnancy in women who choose not to nurse their babies.
THERE IS NO PROPER USE OF TACE IN A PREGNANT WOMAN.
Estrogens in the Menopause: In the natural course of their lives, all women eventually experience a decrease in estrogen production. This usually occurs between ages 45 and 55 but may occur earlier or later. Sometimes the ovaries may need to be removed before or during natural menopause by an operation, producing a "surgical menopause."
When the amount of estrogen in the blood begins to decrease, many women will develop typical symptoms: feelings of warmth in the face, neck, and chest or sudden intense episodes of heat and sweating throughout the body called "hot flashes" or "hot flushes"). These symptoms are sometimes very uncomfortable. A few women eventually develop changes in the vagina (called "atrophic vaginitis") which cause discomfort, especially during and after intercourse.
Estrogens can be prescribed to treat these symptoms of the menopause. It is estimated that considerably more than half of all women undergoing the menopause have only mild symptoms or no symptoms at all and therefore do not need estrogens. Other women may need estrogens for a few months, while their bodies adjust to lower estrogen levels. Sometimes the need will be for periods longer than six months. In an attempt to avoid overstimulation of the uterus (womb), estrogens are usually given cyclically during each month of use, that is, three weeks of pills followed by one week without pills.
Sometimes women experience nervous symptoms or depression during menopause. There is no well-documented evidence that estrogens are effective for such symptoms and they should not be used to treat them, although other treatment may be needed.
You may have heard that taking estrogens for long periods (years) after the menopause will keep your skin soft and supple and keep you feeling young. There is no evidence that this is so, however, and such long-term treatment carries important risks.
Estrogens To Prevent Swelling of the Breasts After Pregnancy: If you do not breast feed your baby after delivery, your breasts may fill up with milk and become engorged and painful. This usually begins about 3 to 4 days after delivery and may last for a few days to up to a week or more. Sometimes the discomfort is severe, but usually it is not and can be controlled by pain relieving drugs such as aspirin and by binding the breasts up tightly. Estrogens can be used to try to prevent the breasts from filling up.
While this treatment is usually successful in reducing amount of filling, in many cases the breasts fill up to some degree in spite of treatment. The daily dose of estrogens needed to prevent pain and swelling of the breasts is larger than the dose needed to treat symptoms of the menopause and this may increase your chances of developing blood clots in the legs or lungs. (See below.) Therefore, it is important that you discuss the benefits and the risks of estrogen use with your doctor if you have decided not to breast feed your baby.

The Dangers of Estrogens:
1. *Cancer of the uterus.* Several independent studies have reported an increased risk ratio of endometrial cancer (cancer of the lining of the uterus) if estrogens are used in the post-menopausal period for more than a year. Women taking estrogens are reported to have roughly 5 to 10 times as great a chance of getting this cancer as women who take no estrogens. To put this another way, while a postmenopausal woman not taking estrogens has 1 chance in 1,000 each year of getting cancer of the uterus, a woman taking estrogens has 5 to 10 chances in 1,000 each year. For this reason *it is important to take estrogens only when you really need them.*
The risk of this cancer is reported to be greater the longer estrogens are used and also seems to be greater when larger doses are taken. For this reason *it is important to take the lowest dose of estrogen that will control symptoms and to take it only as long as it is needed.* If estrogens are needed for longer periods of time, your doctor will want to reevaluate your need for estrogens at least every six months.
Women using estrogens should report any irregular vaginal bleeding to their doctors; such bleeding may be of no importance, but it can be an early warning of cancer of the uterus. If you have undiagnosed vaginal bleeding, you should not use estrogens until a diagnosis is made that there is no cancer of the uterus.
If you have had your uterus completely removed (total hysterectomy), there is no danger of developing cancer of the uterus.

2. *Other possible cancers.* Long-term continuous administration of estrogens in certain animal species increases the frequency of cancers of the breast, cervix, vagina, and liver. At present there is no satisfactory evidence that women using estrogen in the menopause have an increased risk of such tumors, but there is no way yet to be sure they do not; and one study raises the possibility that use of estrogens in the menopause may increase the risk of breast cancer many years later. This is a further reason to use estrogens only when clearly needed. While you are taking estrogens, it is important that you go to your doctor at least every six months for an examination. Also, if members of your family have had breast cancer or if you have breast nodules or abnormal mammograms (breast x-rays), your doctor may wish to carry out more frequent examinations of your breasts.

3. *Gall bladder disease.* Women who use estrogens after menopause are reported to be more likely to develop gall bladder disease needing surgery than women who do not use estrogens. Birth control pills have a similar effect.

4. *Abnormal blood clotting.* Oral contraceptives increase the risk of blood clotting in various parts of the body. This can result in a stroke (if the clot is in the brain), a heart attack (clot in a blood vessel of the heart), or a pulmonary embolus (a clot which forms in the legs or pelvis, then breaks off and travels to the lungs). Any of these can be fatal.
At this time use of estrogens in the menopause is not known to cause such blood clotting, but the possibility that such clotting in association with oral contraceptives may be associated with larger doses of estrogen cannot be excluded. It is recommended that if you have had clotting in the legs or lungs or a heart attack or stroke while you were using estrogens or birth control pills, you should not use estrogens (unless they are being used to treat cancer of the breast or prostate). If you have had a stroke or heart attack or if you have angina pectoris, estrogens should be used with caution and only if clearly needed (for example, if you have severe symptoms of the menopause).
The larger doses of estrogen used to prevent swelling of the breasts after pregnancy have been reported to increase the risk of clotting in the legs and lungs.

Special Warning About Pregnancy: You should not receive estrogen if you are pregnant. It has been reported that there is a greater than usual chance that the developing child will be born with a birth defect, although the possibility remains fairly small. It is also reported that a female child may have an increased risk of developing cancer of the vagina or cervix later in life (in the teens or twenties). Every possible effort should be made to avoid exposure to TACE during pregnancy. If exposure occurs, see your doctor.

Other Effects of Estrogens: In addition to the serious reported risks of estrogens described above, estrogens have the following side effects and potential risks:
1. *Nausea and vomiting.* The most common side effect of estrogen therapy is nausea. Vomiting is less common.
2. *Effects on breasts.* Estrogens may cause breast tenderness or enlargement and may cause the breasts to secrete a liquid. These effects are not dangerous.
3. *Effects on the uterus.* Estrogens may cause benign fibroid tumors of the uterus to get larger. Some women will have menstrual bleeding when estrogens are stopped. But if the bleeding occurs on days you are still taking estrogens you should report this to your doctor.
4. *Effects on liver.* Women taking oral contraceptives develop on rare occasions a tumor of the liver which can rupture and bleed into the abdomen. So far, these tumors have not been reported in women using estrogens in the menopause, but you should report any swelling or unusual pain or tenderness in the abdomen to your doctor immediately.
Women with a past history of jaundice (yellowing of the skin and white parts of the eyes) may get jaundice again during estrogen use. If this occurs, stop taking estrogens and see your doctor.
5. *Other effects.* Estrogens may cause excess fluid to be retained in the body. This may make some conditions worse, such as epilepsy, migraine, heart disease, or kidney disease.

Summary: Estrogens have important uses, but they have reported risks of potentially serious conditions developing as well. You must decide, with your doctor, whether the risks are acceptable to you in view of the benefits of treatment. Except where your doctor has prescribed TACE for use in special cases of cancer of the prostate, you should not use TACE if you have cancer of the breast or uterus, are pregnant, have undiagnosed abnormal vaginal bleeding, clotting in the legs or lungs, have had a stroke, heart attack or angina, or clotting in the legs or lungs in the past while you were taking estrogens.
You can use TACE as safely as possible by understanding that your doctor will require regular physical examinations while you are taking it and will try to discontinue the drug as soon as possible and use the smallest dose possible. Be alert for signs of trouble including:
1. Abnormal bleeding from the vagina.
2. Pains in the calves or chest or sudden shortness of breath, or coughing blood (indicating possible clots in the legs, heart, or lungs).
3. Severe headache, dizziness, faintness, or changes in vision (indicating possible developing clots in the brain or eye).
4. Breast lumps. (You should ask your doctor how to examine your own breasts.)
5. Jaundice (yellowing of the skin).
6. Mental depression.
Based on his or her assessment of your medical needs, your doctor has prescribed this drug for you. Do not give this drug to anyone else.

How Supplied: TACE (CHLOROTRIANISENE) is a long-acting synthetic estrogen in capsule form. The capsule is suitable for taking by mouth.
Each two-tone green and yellow, soft gelatin capsule imprinted MERRELL 692 contains 72 mg of chlorotrianisene in Dispex®, an emulsifiable vehicle containing corn oil, sorbitan trioleate, polysorbate 80, and benzyl benzoate.
This product contains color additives including FD&C Yellow No. 5 (tartrazine).
Patient Information as of August, 1979
Shown in Product Identification Section, page 421

TENUATE®
[těn' ū-āt] © ℞
(diethylpropion hydrochloride USP)
TENUATE DOSPAN®
(diethylpropion hydrochloride USP)
controlled-release tablets

AVAILABLE ONLY ON PRESCRIPTION

Description: Diethylpropion hydrochloride, a sympathomimetic agent, is 1-phenyl-2-diethylamino-1-propanone hydrochloride.

In Tenuate Dospan tablets, diethylpropion hydrochloride is dispersed in a hydrophilic matrix. On exposure to water the diethylpropion hydrochloride is released at a relatively uniform rate as a result of slow hydration of the matrix. The result is controlled release of the anorexic agent.

Actions: Tenuate is a sympathomimetic amine with some pharmacologic activity similar to that of the prototype drugs of this class used in obesity, the amphetamines. Actions include some central nervous system stimulation and elevation of blood pressure. Tolerance has been demonstrated with all drugs of this class in which these phenomena have been looked for.

Drugs of this class used in obesity are commonly known as "anorectics" or "anorexigenics." It has not been established, however, that the action of such drugs in treating obesity is primarily one of appetite suppression. Other central nervous system actions, or metabolic effects may be involved, for example.

Adult obese subjects instructed in dietary management and treated with "anorectic" drugs lose more weight on the average than those treated with placebo and diet, as determined in relatively short-term clinical trials.

The magnitude of increased weight loss of drug-treated patients over placebo-treated patients is some fraction of a pound a week. However, some patients lose more weight than this and some lose less. The rate of weight loss is greatest in the first weeks of therapy for both drug and placebo subjects and tends to decrease in succeeding weeks. The possible origins of the increased weight loss due to the various drug effects are not established. The amount of weight loss associated with the use of an "anorectic" drug varies from trial to trial, and the increased weight loss appears to be related in part to variables other than the drug prescribed, such as the physician-investigator, the population treated, and the diet prescribed. Studies do not permit conclusions as to the relative importance of the drug and non-drug factors on weight loss.

The natural history of obesity is measured in years, whereas most studies cited are restricted to a few weeks duration; thus, the total impact of drug-induced weight loss over that of diet alone must be considered clinically limited.

The controlled-release characteristics of Tenuate Dospan have been demonstrated by studies in humans in which plasma levels of diethylpropion-related material were measured by phosphorescence analysis. Plasma levels obtained with the 75 mg Dospan formulation administered once daily indicated a more gradual release than the standard formulation. The formulation has not been shown superior in effectiveness to the same dosage of the standard, noncontrolled-release formulation.

Indication: Tenuate and Tenuate Dospan are indicated in the management of exogenous obesity as a short-term adjunct (a few weeks) in a regimen of weight reduction based on caloric restriction. The limited usefulness of agents of this class (see ACTIONS) should be measured against possible risk factors inherent in their use such as those described below.

Contraindications: Advanced arteriosclerosis, hyperthyroidism, known hypersensitivity, or idiosyncrasy to the sympathomimetic amines, glaucoma.
Agitated states.
Patients with a history of drug abuse.
During or within 14 days following the administration of monoamine oxidase inhibitors, (hypertensive crises may result).

Warnings: If tolerance develops, the recommended dose should not be exceeded in an attempt to increase the effect; rather, the drug should be discontinued. Tenuate may impair the ability of the patient to engage in potentially hazardous activities such as operating machinery or driving a motor vehicle; the patient should therefore be cautioned accordingly.
When central nervous system active agents are used, consideration must always be given to the possibility of adverse interactions with alcohol.

Drug Dependence
Tenuate has some chemical and pharmacologic similarities to the amphetamines and other related stimulant drugs that have been extensively abused. There have been reports of subjects becoming psychologically dependent on diethylpropion. The possibility of abuse should be kept in mind when evaluating the desirability of including a drug as part of a weight reduction program. Abuse of amphetamines and related drugs may be associated with varying degrees of psychologic dependence and social dysfunction which, in the case of certain drugs, may be severe. There are reports of patients who have increased the dosage to many times that recommended. Abrupt cessation following prolonged high dosage administration results in extreme fatigue and mental depression; changes are also noted on the sleep EEG. Manifestations of chronic intoxication with anorectic drugs include severe dermatoses, marked insomnia, irritability, hyperactivity, and personality changes. The most severe manifestation of chronic intoxications is psychosis, often clinically indistinguishable from schizophrenia.

Use in Pregnancy
Although rat and human reproductive studies have not indicated adverse effects, the use of Tenuate by women who are pregnant or may become pregnant requires that the potential benefits be weighed against the potential risks.

Use in Children
Tenuate is not recommended for use in children under 12 years of age.

Precautions: Caution is to be exercised in prescribing Tenuate for patients with hypertension or with symptomatic cardiovascular disease, including arrhythmias. Tenuate should not be administered to patients with severe hypertension.
Insulin requirements in diabetes mellitus may be altered in association with the use of Tenuate and the concomitant dietary regimen.
Tenuate may decrease the hypotensive effect of guanethidine.
The least amount feasible should be prescribed or dispensed at one time in order to minimize the possibiltiy of overdosage.
Reports suggest that Tenuate may increase convulsions in some epileptics. Therefore, epileptics receiving Tenuate should be carefully monitored. Titration of dose or discontinuance of Tenuate may be necessary.

Adverse Reactions:
Cardiovascular: Palpitation, tachycardia, elevation of blood pressure, precordial pain, arrhythmia. One published report described T-wave changes in the ECG of a healthy young male after ingestion of diethylpropion hydrochloride.
Central Nervous System: Overstimulation, nervousness, restlessness, dizziness, jitteriness, insomnia, anxiety, euphoria, depression, dysphoria, tremor, dyskinesia, mydriasis, drowsiness, malaise, headache; rarely psychotic episodes at recommended doses. In a few epileptics an increase in convulsive episodes has been reported.
Gastrointestinal: Dryness of the mouth, unpleasant taste, nausea, vomiting, abdominal discomfort, diarrhea, constipation, other gastrointestinal disturbances.
Allergic: Urticaria, rash, ecchymosis, erythema.
Endocrine: Impotence, changes in libido, gynecomastia, menstrual upset.
Hematopoietic System: Bone marrow depression, agranulocytosis, leukopenia.
Miscellaneous: A variety of miscellaneous adverse reactions has been reported by physicians. These include complaints such as dyspnea, hair loss, muscle pain, dysuria, increased sweating, and polyuria.

Dosage and Administration:
Tenuate (diethylpropion hydrochloride):
  One 25 mg tablet three times daily, one hour before meals, and in midevening if desired to overcome night hunger.
Tenuate Dospan (diethylpropion hydrochloride) controlled-release:
  One 75 mg tablet daily, swallowed whole, in midmorning.
Tenuate is not recommended for use in children under 12 years of age.

Overdosage: Manifestations of acute overdosage include restlessness, tremor, hyperreflexia, rapid respiration, confusion, assaultiveness, hallucinations, panic states.
Fatigue and depression usually follow the central stimulation.
Cardiovascular effects include arrhythmias, hypertension or hypotension and circulatory collapse. Gastrointestinal symptoms include nausea, vomiting, diarrhea, and abdominal cramps. Overdose of pharmacologically similar compounds has resulted in fatal poisoning, usually terminating in convulsions and coma.
Management of acute Tenuate intoxication is largely symptomatic and includes lavage and sedation with a barbiturate. Experience with hemodialysis or peritoneal dialysis is inadequate to permit recommendation in this regard. Intravenous phentolamine (Regitine®) has been suggested on pharmacologic grounds for possible acute, severe hypertension, if this complicates Tenuate overdosage.

How Supplied: White 25 mg Tenuate tablets debossed MERRELL 697: bottles of 100
White capsule-shaped 75 mg Tenuate Dospan tablets debossed MERRELL 698: bottles of 100 and 250
Product Information as of June, 1980
MERRELL DOW PHARMACEUTICALS INC.
Subsidiary of The Dow Chemcial Company
Cincinnati, Ohio 45242-9553, U.S.A.

Shown in Product Identification Section, page 421

TUSSEND®
[tŭs' ĕnd] © ℞
Antitussive-Decongestant
Liquid and Tablets

Description: Each 5 ml teaspoonful or tablet of TUSSEND for oral use contains hydrocodone bitartrate, 5 mg (Warning: may be habit forming) and pseudoephedrine hydrochloride 60 mg. The liquid also contains alcohol 5%.
Hydrocodone bitartrate is an antitussive. Chemically it is 4,5α-epoxy-3-methoxy-17-methylmorphinan-6-one tartrate (1:1) hydrate (2:5).
Pseudoephedrine hydrochloride is a nasal decongestant. Chemically it is α-[1-(methyl-amino) ethyl] - benzenemethanol hydrochloride.

Clinical Pharmacology: Hydrocodone is a narcotic-analgesic chemically and pharmacologically related to codeine. Hydrocodone suppresses the cough reflex by depressing the medullary cough center. The duration of antitussive action of hydrocodone in man after oral administration is 4 to 8 hours. Hydrocodone is approximately three times more potent than codeine on a weight basis.

Continued on next page

Information on Merrell Dow products is based on labeling in effect in August, 1984.

Merrell Dow—Cont.

Pseudoephedrine is an orally active sympathomimetic amine and exerts a decongestant action on the nasal mucosa. Pseudoephedrine produces peripheral effects similar to those of ephedrine and central effects similar to, but less intense than amphetamines. It has the potential for excitatory side effects. At the recommended oral dosages it has little or no pressor effect in normotensive adults. The serum half-life ($T\frac{1}{2}$) of pseudoephedrine is approximately 4 to 6 hours. $T\frac{1}{2}$ is decreased with increased excretion of drug at a urine pH lower than 6 and may be increased with decreased excretion at urine pH higher than 8.

Indications and Usage: For exhausting cough spasms accompanying upper respiratory tract congestion associated with the common cold, influenza, bronchitis and sinusitis.

Contraindications: Patients with severe hypertension, severe coronary artery disease, and in patients on MAO inhibitor therapy.

Hypersensitivity: Contraindicated in patients with hypersensitivity or idiosyncrasy to sympathomimetic amines, phenanthrene derivatives, or to any other formula ingredients.

Nursing Mothers: Contraindicated because of the higher than usual risk for infants from sympathomimetic amines.

Warnings: Hydrocodone should be prescribed and administered with the same degree of caution as all oral medications containing a narcotic-analgesic. Extreme caution should be exercised in the use of hydrocodone in patients with severe respiratory impairment or patients with impaired respiratory drive.

If sympathomimetic amines are used in patients with hypertension, diabetes mellitus, ischemic heart disease, hyperthyroidism, increased intraocular pressure or prostatic hypertrophy, judicious caution should be exercised (see CONTRAINDICATIONS).

Use in elderly: The elderly (60 years and older) are more likely to have adverse reactions to sympathomimetics. Overdosage of sympathomimetics in this age group may cause hallucinations, convulsions, CNS depression and death.

Precautions: *General:* Caution should be exercised if used in patients with diabetes, hypertension, cardiovascular disease, hyperreactivity to ephedrine, or decreased respiratory drive (see CONTRAINDICATIONS).

Information for Patients: Hydrocodone may produce drowsiness. Persons who perform hazardous tasks requiring mental alertness or physical coordination should be cautioned accordingly. Concomitant use of hydrocodone with tranquilizers, alcohol or other depressants may produce additive depressant effects. Do not exceed the prescribed dosage.

Drug Interactions: Hydrocodone may potentiate the effects of other narcotics, general anesthetics, tranquilizers, sedatives and hypnotics, tricyclic antidepressants, MAO inhibitors, alcohol, and other CNS depressants. Beta adrenergic blockers and MAO inhibitors potentiate the sympathomimetic effects of pseudoephedrine. Sympathomimetics may reduce the antihypertensive effects of methyldopa, mecamylamine, reserpine and veratrum alkaloids.

Pregnancy Category C: Animal reproduction studies have not been conducted with pseudoephedrine or hydrocodone. It is also not known whether pseudoephedrine or hydrocodone can cause fetal harm when administered to a pregnant woman or can affect reproduction capacity. Pseudoephedrine or hydrocodone may be given to a pregnant woman only if clearly needed.

Nursing Mothers: Because of the potential for serious adverse reactions in nursing infants from sympathomimetic amines, pseudoephedrine is contraindicated in nursing mothers.

Adverse Reactions: Gastrointestinal upset, nausea, drowsiness and constipation. A slight elevation in serum transaminase levels has been noted.

Individuals hyperreactive to pseudoephedrine may display ephedrine-like reactions such as tachycardia, palpitations, headache, dizziness or nausea. Sympathomimetic drugs have been associated with certain untoward reactions including fear, anxiety, tenseness, restlessness, tremor, weakness, pallor, respiratory difficulty, dysuria, insomnia, hallucinations, convulsions, CNS depression, arrhythmias, and cardiovascular collapse with hypotension.

Patient idiosyncrasy to adrenergic agents may be manifested by insomina, dizziness, weakness, tremor or arrhythmias.

Drug Abuse and Dependence:

Controlled Substance: Hydrocodone in TUSSEND mixture is controlled by the Drug Enforcement Administration. TUSSEND is a Schedule III controlled substance.

Abuse: Human experience indicates that abuse of TUSSEND is uncommon. However, hydrocodone is a narcotic drug related to codeine with roughly three times the abuse potential of codeine on a weight basis.

Dependence: Hydrocodone can produce drug dependence of the morphine type. Psychic dependence, physical dependence and tolerance may develop if dosage recommendations are greatly exceeded over a prolonged period of time.

Overdosage: Acute overdosage with TUSSEND may produce variable clinical signs as hydrocodone produces CNS depression and cardiovascular depression while pseudoephedrine produces CNS stimulation and variable cardiovascular effects. Hydrocodone is likely to be responsible for most of the severe reactions from overdosage. Pressor amines should be used with great caution when taking pseudoephedrine. Patients with signs of stimulation should be treated conservatively and depressant medications should be avoided if possible because of potential drug interaction with hydrocodone.

Dosage and Administration: Adults and children over 90 lbs, 1 tablet or one teaspoonful; children 50 to 90 lbs, $\frac{1}{2}$ teaspoonful; children 25 to 50 lbs, $\frac{1}{4}$ teaspoonful. May be given four times a day as needed. May be taken with meals.

Caution: Federal law prohibits dispensing without prescription.

How Supplied: Tussend liquid is supplied in pints (NDC 0068-1018-16). Tussend tablets are supplied in bottles of 100 (NDC 0068-0042-61).

Shown in Product Identification Section, page 421

TUSSEND® EXPECTORANT   ℞ ©
[tŭs'ĕnd]
Antitussive-Decongestant
Liquid

Description: Each 5 ml teaspoonful of TUSSEND Expectorant liquid for oral use contains hydrocodone bitartrate, 5 mg (Warning: May be habit forming), pseudoephedrine hydrochloride 60 mg, guaifenesin (glyceryl guaiacolate) 200 mg, and alcohol 12.5%.

Hydrocodone bitartrate is an antitussive. Chemically it is 4,5α-epoxy-3-methoxy-17-methylmorphinan-6-one tartrate (1:1) hydrate (2:5).

Pseudoephedrine hydrochloride is a nasal decongestant. Chemically it is α-[1-(methylamino)ethyl]-benzenemethanol hydrochloride.

Guaifenesin is an expectorant. Chemically it is 3-(O-methoxyphenoxy)-1,2 propanediol.

Clinical Pharmacology: Hydrocodone is a narcotic-analgesic chemically and pharmacologically related to codeine. Hydrocodone suppresses the cough reflex by depressing the medullary cough center. The duration of antitussive action of hydrocodone in man after oral administration is 4 to 8 hours. Hydrocodone is approximately three times more potent than codeine on a weight basis.

Pseudoephedrine is an orally active sympathomimetic amine and exerts a decongestant action on the nasal mucosa. Pseudoephedrine produces peripheral effects similar to those of ephedrine and central effects similar to, but less intense than amphetamines. It has the potential for excitatory side effects. At the recommended oral dosages it has little or no pressor effect in normotensive adults. The serum half-life ($T-\frac{1}{2}$) of pseudoephedrine is approximately 4 to 6 hours. $T-\frac{1}{2}$ is decreased with increased excretion of drug at a urine pH lower than 6 and may be increased with decreased excretion at urine pH higher than 8.

Guaifenesin is used as an expectorant. On the basis of studies in animals, guaifenesin is thought to increase mucus flow in the lung by stimulation of gastric mucosal reflexes. Objective human data are lacking.

Indications and Usage: For exhausting, nonproductive cough accompanying respiratory tract congestion associated with the common cold, influenza, sinusitis and bronchitis.

Contraindications: Patients with severe hypertension, severe coronary artery disease, and in patients on MAO inhibitor therapy.

Hypersensitivity: Contraindicated in patients with hypersensitivity or idiosyncrasy to sympathomimetic amines, phenanthrene derivatives, or to any other formula ingredients.

Nursing Mothers: Contraindicated because of the higher than usual risk for infants for sympathomimetic amines.

Warnings: Hydrocodone should be prescribed and administered with the same degree of caution as all oral medications containing a narcotic analgesic. Extreme caution should be exercised in the use of hydrocodone in patients with severe respiratory impairment or patients with impaired respiratory drive.

If sympathomimetic amines are used in patients with hypertension, diabetes mellitus, ischemic heart disease, hyperthyroidism, increased intraocular pressure or prostatic hypertrophy, judicious caution should be exercised (see CONTRAINDICATIONS).

Use in Elderly: The elderly (60 years and older) are more likely to have adverse reactions to sympathomimetics. Overdosage of sympathomimetics in this age group may cause hallucinations, convulsions, CNS depression and death.

Precautions: *General:* Caution should be exercised if used in patients with diabetes, hypertension, cardiovascular diseases, hyperreactivity to ephedrine, or decreased respiratory drive (see CONTRAINDICATIONS).

Information for Patients: Hydrocodone may produce drowsiness. Persons who perform hazardous tasks requiring mental alertness or physical coordination should be cautioned accordingly. Concomitant use of hydrocodone with tranquilizers, alcohol or other depressants may produce additive depressant effects. Do not exceed the prescribed dosage.

Drug Interactions: Hydrocodone may potentiate the effects of other narcotics, general anesthetics, tranquilizers, sedatives and hypnotics, tricyclic antidepressants, MAO inhibitors, alcohol, and other CNS depressants. Beta adrenergic blockers and MAO inhibitors potentiate the sympathomimetic effects of pseudoephedrine. Sympathomimetics may reduce the antihypertensive effects of methyldopa, mecamylamine, reserpine and veratrum alkaloids.

Laboratory Test Interactions: Guaifenesin interferes with the colorimetric determination of 5-hydroxyindoleacetic acid (5-HIAA) and vanilmandelic acid (VMA).

Pregnancy Category C: Animal reproduction studies have not been conducted with pseudoephedrine, guaifenesin, or hydrocodone. It is also not known whether pseudoephedrine, guaifenesin or hydrocodone can cause fetal harm when administered to a pregnant woman or can affect reproduction capacity. Pseudoephedrine or hydrocodone may be given to a pregnant woman only if clearly needed.

Nursing Mothers: Because of the potential for serious adverse reactions in nursing infants from sympathomimetic amines, pseudoephedrine is contraindicated in nursing mothers.

Adverse Reactions: Gastrointestinal upset, nausea, drowsiness and constipation. A slight elevation in serum transaminase levels has been noted.

Individuals hyperreactive to pseudoephedrine may display ephedrine-like reactions such as tachycardia, palpitations, headache, dizziness or nausea. Sympathomimetic drugs have been associated with certain untoward reactions including fear, anxiety, tenseness, restlessness, tremor, weakness, pallor, respiratory difficulty, dysuria, insomnia, hallucinations, convulsions, CNS depression, arrhythmias, and cardiovascular collapse with hypotension.

Patient idiosyncrasy to adrenergic agents may be manifested by insomnia, dizziness, weakness, tremor or arrhythmias.

Drug Abuse and Dependence:
Controlled Substance: Hydrocodone in TUSSEND Expectorant mixture is controlled by the Drug Enforcement Administration. TUSSEND Expectorant is a Schedule III controlled substance.
Abuse: Human experience indicates that abuse of TUSSEND Expectorant is uncommon. However, hydrocodone is a narcotic drug related to codeine with roughly three times the abuse potential of codeine on a weight basis.
Dependence: Hydrocodone can produce drug dependence of the morphine type. Psychic dependence, physical dependence and tolerance may develop if dosage recommendations are greatly exceeded over a prolonged period of time.
Overdosage: Acute overdosage with TUSSEND Expectorant may produce variable clinical signs as hydrocodone produces CNS depression and cardiovascular depression while pseudoephedrine produces CNS stimulation and variable cardiovascular effects. Hydrocodone is likely to be responsible for most of the severe reactions from overdosage. Pressor amines should be used with great caution when taking pseudoephedrine. Patients with signs of stimulation should be treated conservatively and depressant medications should be avoided if possible because of potential drug interaction with hydrocodone.
Dosage and Administration: Adults and children over 90 lbs, 1 teaspoonful; children 50 to 90 lbs, $1/2$ teaspoonful; children 25 to 50 lbs, $1/4$ teaspoonful. May be given four times a day as needed. May be taken with meals.
Caution: Federal law prohibits dispensing without prescription.
How Supplied: TUSSEND Expectorant is supplied in pints (NDC 0068-1016-16).
Shown in Product Identification Section, page 421

Information on Merrell Dow products is based on labeling in effect in August, 1984.

Miles Laboratories, Inc.
P. O. BOX 340
ELKHART, IN 46515

ALKA-SELTZER® Effervescent Pain Reliever & Antacid With Specially Buffered Aspirin
[al-kuh-selt-sir]

Active Ingredients: Each tablet contains: aspirin 324 mg., heat treated sodium bicarbonate 1916 mg., citric acid 1000 mg. ALKA-SELTZER® in water contains principally the antacid sodium citrate and the analgesic sodium acetylsalicylate. Buffered pH is between 6 and 7.
Indications: ALKA-SELTZER® Effervescent Pain Reliever & Antacid is an analgesic and an antacid and is indicated for relief of sour stomach, acid indigestion or heartburn with headache or body aches and pains. Also for fast relief of upset stomach with headache from overindulgence in food and drink—especially recommended for taking before bed and again on arising. Effective for pain relief alone: headache or body and muscular aches and pains.
Actions: When the ALKA-SELTZER® Effervescent Pain Reliever & Antacid tablet is dissolved in water, the acetylsalicylate ion differs from acetylsalicylic acid chemically, physically and pharmacologically. Being fat insoluble, it is not absorbed by the gastric mucosal cells. Studies and observations in animals and man including radiochrome determinations of fecal blood loss, measurement of ion fluxes and direct visualization with gastrocamera, have shown that, as contrasted with acetylsalicylic acid, the acetylsalicylate ion delivered in the solution does not alter gastric mucosal permeability to permit back-diffusion of hydrogen ion, and gastric damage and acute gastric mucosal lesions are therefore not seen after administration of the product.

ALKA-SELTZER® Effervescent Pain Reliever & Antacid has the capacity to neutralize gastric hydrochloric acid quickly and effectively. In-vitro, 154 ml. of 0.1 N hydrochloric acid are required to decrease the pH of one tablet of ALKA-SELTZER® Effervescent Pain Reliever & Antacid in solution to 4.0. Measured against the in vitro standard established by the Food and Drug Administration one tablet neutralizes 17.2 mEq of acid. In vivo, the antacid activity of two ALKA-SELTZER® Effervescent Pain Reliever & Antacid tablets is comparable to that of 10 ml. of milk of magnesia. ALKA-SELTZER® Effervescent Pain Reliever & Antacid is able to resist pH changes caused by the continuing secretion of acid in the normal individual and to maintain an elevated pH until emptying occurs.

ALKA-SELTZER® Effervescent Pain Reliever & Antacid provides highly water soluble acetylsalicylate ions which are fat soluble. Acetylsalicylate ions are not absorbed from the stomach. They empty from the stomach and thereby become available for absorption from the duodenum. Thus, fast drug absorption and high plasma acetylsalicylate levels are achieved. Plasma levels of salicylate following the administration of ALKA-SELTZER® Effervescent Pain Reliever & Antacid solution (acetylsalicylate equivalent to 648 mg. acetylsalicylic acid) can reach 29 mg./liter in 10 minutes and rise to peak levels as high as 55 mg./liter within 30 minutes.

Warnings: Except under the advice and supervision of a physician, do not take more than, Adults: 8 tablets in a 24 hour period. (60 years of age or older: 4 tablets in a 24 hour period), Children (6–12), 4 tablets in a 24 hour period, (3–5) 2 tablets in a 24 hour period, or use the maximum dosage for more than 10 days (5 days for children). Do not use if you are allergic to aspirin or have asthma, if you have a coagulation (bleeding) disease, or if you are on a sodium restricted diet. Each tablet contains 554 mg. of sodium. As with any drug, if you are pregnant or nursing a baby, seek the advice of a health professional before using this product. Keep this and all drugs out of the reach of children.
Dosage and Administration:
ALKA-SELTZER® Effervescent Pain Reliever & Antacid is taken in solution, approximately three ounces of water per tablet is sufficient.
Adults: 2 tablets every 4 hours. Children: (6–12) 1 tablet, (3–5) $1/2$ tablet, every 4–6 hours; children under 3, as directed by a physician. CAUTION: If symptoms persist or recur frequently, or if you are under treatment for ulcer, consult your physician.
How Supplied: Tablets: in bottles of 8 and 26; foil sealed; box of 12; dispenser boxes of 36 tablets in 18 foil twin packs; 100 tablets in 50 foil twin packs; carton of 72 tablets in 36 foil twin packs. Product Identification Mark: "Alka-Seltzer" embossed on each tablet.

ALKA-SELTZER® Effervescent Antacid
[al-kuh-selt-sir]

Active Ingredients: Each tablet contains heat treated sodium bicarbonate 958 mg., citric acid 832 mg., potassium bicarbonate 312 mg. ALKA-SELTZER® Effervescent Antacid in water contains principally the antacids sodium citrate and potassium citrate.
Indications: ALKA-SELTZER® Effervescent Antacid is indicated for relief of acid indigestion, sour stomach or heartburn.
Actions: The ALKA-SELTZER® Effervescent Antacid solution provides quick and effective neutralization of gastric acid. Measured by the in vitro standard established by the Food and Drug Administration one tablet will neutralize 10.6 mEq of acid.
Warnings: Except under the advice and supervision of a physician, do not take more than: Adults: 8 tablets in a 24 hour period (60 years of age or older: 7 tablets in a 24 hour period), Children 4 tablets in a 24 hour period; or use the maximum dosage of this product for more than 2 weeks.
Do not use this product if you are on a sodium restricted diet. Each tablet contains 296 mg. of sodium.
Keep this and all drugs out of the reach of children. As with any drug, if you are pregnant or nursing a baby, seek the advice of a health professional before using this product.
Dosage and Administration:
ALKA-SELTZER® Effervescent Antacid is taken in solution; approximately 3 oz. of water per tablet is sufficient. Adults: one or two tablets every 4 hours as needed. Children: $1/2$ the adult dosage.
How Supplied: Tablets: foil sealed, box of 12; dispenser boxes of 20 tablets in 10 foil twin packs; 36 tablets in 18 foil twin packs.

ALKA-SELTZER PLUS® Cold Medicine
[al-kuh-selt-sir]

Active Ingredients:
Each dry ALKA-SELTZER PLUS® Cold Tablet contains the following active ingredients: Phenylpropanolamine bitartrate 24 mg., chlorpheniramine maleate 2 mg., aspirin 324 mg. The product is dissolved in water prior to ingestion and the aspirin is converted into its soluble ionic form, sodium acetylsalicylate.
Indications: For relief of the symptoms of head colds, common flu, sinus congestion and hay fever.
Actions: Each tablet contains: A decongestant which helps restore free breathing, shrink swollen nasal tissue and relieve sinus congestion due to head colds or hay fever. An antihistamine which helps relieve the runny nose, sneezing, sniffles, itchy watering eyes that accompany colds or hay fever. Specially buffered aspirin which relieves headache, scratchy sore throat, general body aches and the feverish feeling of a cold and common flu.
Warnings: Do not use if you are allergic to aspirin or have asthma, or if you have a coagulation (bleeding) disease. If symptoms do not improve in 7 days or are accompanied by high fever or if fever persists for more than 3 days consult a physician before continuing use. Do not take this product if you have glaucoma or difficulty in urination due to enlargement of the prostate gland except under the advice and supervision of a physician. Avoid alcoholic beverages while taking this product.
Caution: Individuals with high blood pressure, diabetes, heart or thyroid disease or on a sodium restricted diet should use only as directed by a physician. Each tablet contains 515 mg. of sodium. Product may cause drowsiness: use caution if operating heavy machinery or driving a vehicle. Keep this and all drugs out of the reach of children. As with any drug, if you are pregnant or nursing a baby, seek the advice of a health professional before using this product.
Dosage and Administration:
ALKA-SELTZER PLUS® is taken in solution; approximately 3 ounces of water per tablet is sufficient. Adults: two tablets every 4 hours up to 8 tablets in 24 hours. Children (6–12): Half of adult dosage. Children under 6 years: Consult your physician.
How Supplied: Tablets: carton of 20 tablets in 10 foil twin packs; carton of 36 tablets in 18 foil twin packs.
Product Identification Mark:
"Alka-Seltzer Plus" embossed on each tablet.

BACTINE® Antiseptic·Anesthetic First Aid Spray
[bak-tēn]

(See PDR for Nonprescription Drugs)

Continued on next page

Miles Labs.—Cont.

BACTINE® Hydrocortisone (0.5%) Skin Care Cream
[bak-tēn]

(See PDR for Non-prescription drugs)

BIOCAL™ 250 mg Chewable Tablets
[bī'ō-căl]
Calcium Supplement

Each Tablet Contains: 625 mg of calcium carbonate, U.S.P. which provides: 250 mg Elemental calcium.
Indication: Calcium supplementation
Description: BIOCAL™ 250 mg Tablets are round, white, pleasant-tasting mint flavored chewable tablets containing pure calcium carbonate. No sugar, salt, preservatives, or artificial colors added.
Directions: Four chewable tablets daily provide:

Elemental Calcium	For Adults and Children Over 4 % U.S. RDA	For Pregnant or Lactating Women
1000 mg	100%	77%

Chew 2 to 4 tablets daily or as recommended by a physician. Keep out of reach of children.
How Supplied: Bottles of 60 tablets in tamper-resistant package.

BIOCAL™ 500 mg Tablets
[bī'ō-căl]
Calcium Supplement

Each Tablet Contains: 1250 mg of calcium carbonate, U.S.P. which provides: 500 mg

Indications: Calcium supplementation.
Description: BIOCAL™ 500 mg Tablets are white, capsule-shaped tablets containing pure calcium carbonate. No sugar, salt, preservatives, artificial colors or flavors added.
Directions: Two tablets daily provide:

Elemental Calcium	For Adults % U.S. RDA	For Pregnant or Lactating Women % U.S. RDA
1000 mg	100%	77%

Take one or two tablets daily or as recommended by a physician.
Keep out of reach of children.
How Supplied: Bottles of 60 tablets in tamper-resistant package.

BUGS BUNNY® Children's Chewable Vitamins (Sugar Free)
(Multivitamin Supplement)
BUGS BUNNY® Children's Chewable Vitamins Plus Iron (Sugar Free)
(Multivitamin Supplement with Iron)
BUGS BUNNY® Vitamins Plus Minerals (Sugar Free)

FLINTSTONES® Children's Chewable Vitamins Plus Iron
(Multivitamin Supplement with Iron)
FLINTSTONES® Children's Chewable Vitamins
(Multivitamin Supplement)
FLINTSTONES® COMPLETE
With Iron, Calcium & Minerals
Children's Chewable Vitamins

(See PDR For Nonprescription Drugs)

BUGS BUNNY® With Extra C (Sugar Free)
Multivitamin Supplement

(See PDR For Nonprescription Drugs)

FLINTSTONES® With Extra C
Multivitamin Supplement

(See PDR For Nonprescription Drugs)

MILES® NERVINE
NIGHTTIME SLEEP-AID

(See PDR For Nonprescription Drugs)

ONE-A-DAY® Essential
(Multivitamin Supplement)
ONE-A-DAY® Within
(Multivitamin Plus Iron and Calcium)

(See PDR For Nonprescription Drugs)

ONE-A-DAY® Maximum Formula
(Multivitamin/Multimineral Supplement for adults and teens)

(See PDR For Nonprescription Drugs)

ONE-A-DAY® Plus Extra C
High Potency 500 mg Vitamin C Plus 10 Essential Vitamins
(For Adults and Teens)

(See PDR For Nonprescription Drugs)

ONE-A-DAY® STRESSGARD™
Vitamins
(B Complex Plus C Stress Formula)
High Potency
Multivitamin/Multimineral Supplement For Adults

(See PDR For Nonprescription Drugs)

Important Notice

Before prescribing or administering any product described in PHYSICIANS' DESK REFERENCE always consult the PDR Supplement for possible new or revised information.

Miles Pharmaceuticals
Division of Miles Laboratories, Inc.
400 MORGAN LANE
WEST HAVEN, CT 06516

PRODUCT IDENTIFICATION CODES

To provide an accurate identification of Miles Pharmaceuticals products, each solid dosage form is coded with the name Miles and a 3 digit product identification number.

PRODUCT ORAL DOSAGE FORMS	PRODUCT IDENTIFICATION CODE NUMBER
Decholin® Tablets 250 mg (dehydrocholic acid)	121
Lithane® Tablets 300 mg (lithium carbonate)	951
Mycelex® Troche 10 mg (clotrimazole)	095
Niclocide® Chewable Tablets 500 mg (niclosamide)	721
Stilphostrol® Tablets 50 mg (diethylstilbestrol diphosphate)	132

NON-ORAL DOSAGE FORMS

Domeboro® Tablets (aluminum sulfate, calcium acetate)	411
Mycelex®-G Vaginal Tablets 100 mg (clotrimazole)	093

AZLIN® ℞
Sterile azlocillin sodium
for intravenous use.

Description: AZLIN® (sterile azlocillin sodium) is a semisynthetic broad spectrum penicillin antibiotic for parenteral administration. It is the monosodium salt of 6-D-2 (2-OXO-imidazolidine-1-carboxamido)-2- phenyl- acetamido -penicillanic acid.
Structural Formula:

Empirical Formula: $C_{20}H_{22}N_5O_6S$ Na
AZLIN® has a molecular weight of 483.5 and contains 49.8 mg (2.17 mEq) of sodium per one gram of azlocillin activity. The dosage form is supplied as a sterile white to pale yellow powder, which is freely soluble in water. When reconstituted, aqueous solutions of AZLIN® are clear and range from colorless to pale yellow with a pH of 6.0 to 8.0.
Clinical Pharmacology: Intravenous Administration. In healthy adult volunteers, means serum levels of azlocillin 30 minutes after a 5–10 minute intravenous injection of 1g, 2g, or 5g are 35, 106 and 256 mcg/ml, respectively. Serum levels, as noted below, lack dose proportionality:
[See table below].
After an intravenous infusion (30 min) of 2g or 3 g azlocillin, mean serum levels 5 minutes after dos-

---

AZLIN®
AZLOCILLIN SERUM LEVELS IN ADULTS (mcg/ml) 5-10 MIN IV INJECTION

DOSE	5 min	15 min	30 min	1 hr	2 hr	3 hr	4 hr	6 hr	8 hr
1g			35 (29–41)	22 (18–26)	9.4 (7.2–14)	4.3 (2.6–6.8)	2.2 (1.2–4.0)		
2g	239 (142–363)	139 (85–188)	106 (83–134)	47 (30–60)	19 (16–26)	12 (8.7–13)	7.4 (5.7–11)	2.1 (1.8–2.9)	0.5 (0–0.7)
5g	527 (470–604)	353 (258–440)	256 (184–287)	174 (116–231)	85 (43–121)	55 (26–91) 91	33 (15–58)	7.7 (1.6–19)	4.1 (1.4–7.8)

AZLIN®

AZLOCILLIN SERUM LEVELS IN ADULTS (mcg/ml) 30 MIN IV INFUSION

DOSE	0	5 min	15 min	30 min	45 min	1 hr	1.5 hr	2 hr	3 hr	4 hr	6 hr	8 hr
2g		165 (55–278)	130 (73–189)	104 (62–175)	85 (42–121)	62 (23–85)	49 (27–82)	36 (19–57)	26 (13–48)	13 (5–25)	6 (2–11)	2 (1–4)	1 (1–4)
3g		214 (155–273)	180 (133–235)	139 (119–186)	104 (61–159)	82 (58–121)	68 (38–94)	58 (35–74)	39 (17–53)	24 (9–36)	10 (3–14)	3 (1–5)	1 (1–4)

ing are 130 mcg/ml (73–189) and 180 mcg/ml (133–235), respectively.
[See table above].

Following intravenous infusion (30 min) of a 3g dose of azlocillin every 6 hours for 5 days, mean peak serum concentrations were higher than 150 mcg/ml; trough levels were between 4–12 mcg/ml. From the first to the last day of dosing, the serum half-life increased from 61 minutes to approximately 77 minutes.

General: As with other penicillins, azlocillin is excreted primarily by the kidney through glomerular filtration and tubular secretion. The rate of elimination is dose dependent and also related to the status of renal function. In patients with normal renal function, 50 to 70% of the administered dose is recovered from the urine within 24 hours after dosing. Two hours after an intravenous injection of 2g, concentrations of active drug in urine generally exceed 4000 mcg/ml. By 4–8 hours after injection, concentrations are still above 500 mcg/ml. The serum elimination half-life of azlocillin is dose dependent and ranges from approximately 55 minutes after an intravenous dose of 2g to about 70 minutes after intravenous dose of 5g. Probenecid interferes with the renal tubular secretion of azlocillin, thereby increasing serum concentrations and prolonging serum half-life of the antibiotic.

In patients with reduced renal function, the serum half-life of azlocillin is prolonged, depending on degree of renal impairment. Dosage adjustments are usually not necessary except in patients with moderate to severe renal impairment. (See Dosage and Administration). As with other penicillins, azlocillin is metabolized only slightly; less than 10% of the administered dose is found in the urine in the form of the penicilloate or penilloate. The drug is readily removed from the serum by hemodialysis.

Following an intravenous dose of 2g azlocillin, peak concentrations of active drug in bile generally exceed 1000 mcg/ml. The bile levels are approximately 15 times higher than the corresponding serum levels. Biliary excretion is reduced in patients with common bile duct obstruction.

Following parenteral administration, the apparent volume of distribution is approximately 20% of body weight. The drug is present in active form in the serum, urine, bile, bronchial and wound secretions, bone and other tissues. As with other penicillins, penetration into the cerebrospinal fluid (CSF) is generally poor, however, higher CSF concentrations are obtained in the presence of meningeal inflammation.

The serum level of uric acid has been noted to be depressed in some patients receiving azlocillin; this effect appears to be transient.

Protein binding studies indicate that the degree of azlocillin binding is low (25–45%) and depends upon testing methods and concentrations of drug studied.

Microbiology
Azlocillin is a bactericidal antibiotic which acts by interfering with synthesis of cell wall components. It is active against *Pseudomonas aeruginosa* and other species of Pseudomonas, many of which are resistant to other broad spectrum antibiotics. Azlocillin is also active *in vitro* against many strains of the following organisms, however, clinical efficacy for infections other than those included in the indication section has not been documented:

Gram-negative bacteria
Escherichia coli
Proteus Mirabilis
Proteus vulgaris
Morganella morganii (formerly *P. morganii*)
Providencia rettgeri (formerly *P. rettgeri*)
Providencia stuartii
Enterobacter species
Shigella species
Haemophilus influenzae
Haemophilus parainfluenzae
Neisseria species
Citrobacter species
Some strains of *Klebsiella, Serratia, Salmonella,* and *Acinetobacter* are also susceptible.

Gram-positive bacteria
Staphylococcus aureus (non-penicillinase producing strains)
Beta-hemolytic streptococci (Groups A and B)
Streptococcus pneumoniae (formerly *Diplococcus pneumoniae*)
Streptococcus faecalis (enterococcus)
Listeria monocytogenes

Anaerobic Organisms
Peptococcus species
Peptostreptococcus species
Clostridium species
Bacteroides species (including *B. fragilis* group)
Fusobacterium species
Veillonella species
Eubacterium species

Azlocillin is inactive against penicillinase-producing strains of *Staphylococcus aureus* and is susceptible to inactivation by beta-lactamases produced by the Enterobacteriaceae.

In vitro studies have shown that azlocillin combined with an aminoglycoside (e.g., gentamicin, tobramycin, amikacin, sisomicin) acts synergistically against many strains of *Pseudomonas aeruginosa*.

Azlocillin is slightly more active when tested at alkaline pH and, as with other penicillins, has reduced activity when tested *in vitro* with increasing inoculum. The minimal bactericidal concentration (MBC) may exceed the minimal inhibitory concentration (MIC) by four-fold or more depending on medium used. Resistance to azlocillin *in vitro* develops slowly (multiple step mutation). Some strains of *Pseudomonas aeruginosa* have developed resistance fairly rapidly.

Susceptibility Tests
Quantitative methods that require measurement of zone diameters give good estimates of bacterial susceptibility. One such procedure* has been recommended for use with discs to test susceptibility to antimicrobials. When the causative organism is tested by the Kirby-Bauer disc diffusion method, a 75 mcg azlocillin disc should give a zone of 18 mm or greater to indicate susceptibility. Zone sizes of 14 mm or less indicate resistance. Zone sizes of 15 to 17 mm indicate intermediate susceptibility. With this procedure, a report from the laboratory of "Susceptible" indicates that the infecting organism is likely to respond to therapy. A report of "Resistant" indicates that the infecting organism is not likely to respond to therapy; other therapy should be selected. A report of "Intermediate Susceptibility" suggests that the organism may be susceptible if the infection is confined to tissues and fluids (e.g., urine), in which high antibiotic levels are attained. The azlocillin disc should be used for testing susceptibility to azlocillin. Standardized procedure requires use of control organisms. The 75 mcg azlocillin disc should give zone diameters between 24 and 30 mm for *P. aeruginosa* ATCC 27853. For *E. coli* ATCC 25922 the zone diameters should be between 21 and 24 mm.

* Bauer, A.W., Kirby, W.M., Sherris, J.C., and Turck, M.: Antibiotic Testing by a Standardized Single Disc Method, Am. J. Clin. Pathol., 45:493, 1966; Standardized Disc Susceptibility Test, FEDERAL REGISTER, 39: 19182–19184, 1974.

In certain conditions, it may be desirable to do additional susceptibility testing by broth or agar dilution techniques. Dilution methods, preferably the agar plate dilution procedure, are most accurate for susceptibility testing of obligate anaerobes. *Pseudomonas* species and the *Enterobacteriaceae* are considered susceptible if the MIC of azlocillin is no greater than 64 mcg/ml and are considered resistant if the MIC is greater than 128 mcg/ml. The MIC values of azlocillin for the control strains are the following:

P. aeruginosa ATCC 27853, 4–8 mcg/ml and
E. coli ATCC 25922, 8–16 mcg/ml.

Azlocillin standard is available for broth or agar dilution studies.

Indications and Usage: AZLIN® is indicated primarily for the treatment of serious infections caused by susceptible strains of *Pseudomonas aeruginosa* in the conditions listed below:

LOWER RESPIRATORY TRACT INFECTIONS including pneumonia and lung abscess.

URINARY TRACT INFECTIONS both complicated and uncomplicated of the lower and upper urinary tract.

SKIN AND SKIN STRUCTURE INFECTIONS including ulcers, abscesses, burns and severe external otitis.

BONE AND JOINT INFECTIONS including osteomyelitis.

BACTERIAL SEPTICEMIA

Azlocillin has also been shown to be effective for the treatment of Lower Respiratory Tract Infections caused by *Escherichia coli* and *Haemophilus influenzae;* Urinary Tract Infections and Skin Structure Infections caused by *Escherichia coli, Proteus mirabilis* or *Streptococcus faecalis;* and Septicemia caused by *Escherichia coli.*

Appropriate culture and susceptibility tests should be performed before treatment in order to isolate and identify organisms causing infections and to determine their susceptibility to azlocillin. Therapy with AZLIN® may be initiated before results of these tests are known; once results become available, appropriate therapy should be continued.

In certain severe infections, when the causative organisms are unknown and *Pseudomonas aeruginosa* is suspected, AZLIN® may be administered in conjunction with an aminoglycoside or a cephalosporin antibiotic as initial therapy. As soon as results of culture and susceptibility tests become available, antimicrobial therapy should be adjusted as indicated. Culture and susceptibility testing, performed periodically during therapy, will provide information on the therapeutic effect of the antimicrobial and will monitor for the possible emergence of bacterial resistance.

AZLIN® has been used effectively in combination with an aminoglycoside antibiotic for the treatment of life-threatening infections caused by *Pseudomonas aeruginosa* including acute pulmonary exacerbation in patients with cystic fibrosis. For the treatment of febrile episodes in immunosuppressed patients with granulocytopenia, AZLIN® should be combined with an aminoglycoside or a cephalosporin antibiotic.

Contraindications: AZLIN® is contraindicated in patients with a history of hypersensitivity reactions to any of the penicillins.

Warnings: Serious and occasionally fatal hypersensitivity (anaphylactic) reactions have occurred in patients receiving a penicillin. These reactions are more apt to occur in individuals with a history

Continued on next page

Miles Pharm.—Cont.

of sensitivity to multiple allergens. There have been reports of individuals with a history of penicillin hypersensitivity reactions who have experienced severe hypersensitivity reactions when treated with a cephalosporin. Before therapy with azlocillin is instituted, careful inquiry should be made to determine whether the patient has had previous hypersensitivity reactions to penicillins, cephalosporins or other drugs. Antibiotics should be used with caution in any patient who has demonstrated some form of allergy, particularly to drugs.

If an allergic reaction occurs during therapy with azlocillin, the drug should be discontinued. SERIOUS ANAPHYLACTOID REACTIONS REQUIRE IMMEDIATE EMERGENCY TREATMENT WITH EPINEPHRINE. OXYGEN, INTRAVENOUS STEROIDS, AND AIRWAY MANAGEMENT, INCLUDING INTUBATION, SHOULD ALSO BE PROVIDED AS INDICATED.

Precautions: Although AZLIN® shares with other penicillins the low potential for toxicity, as with any potent drug, periodic assessment of organ system functions, including renal, hepatic and hematopoietic, is advisable during prolonged therapy.

Bleeding manifestations have occurred in some patients receiving beta-lactam antibiotics. These reactions have been associated with abnormalities of coagulation tests, such as clotting time, platelet aggregation and prothrombin time and are more likely to occur in patients with renal impairment. Although AZLIN® has rarely been associated with any bleeding abnormalities, the possibility of this occurring should be kept in mind, particularly in patients with severe renal impairment receiving maximum doses of the drug.

AZLIN® has only rarely been reported to cause hypokalemia; however, the possibility of this occurring should also be kept in mind, particularly when treating patients with fluid and electrolyte imbalance. Periodic monitoring of serum potassium may be advisable in patients receiving prolonged therapy.

AZLIN® is a monosodium salt containing only 49.8 mg (2.17 mEq) of sodium per gram of azlocillin. This should be considered when treating patients requiring restricted salt intake.

As with any penicillin, an allergic reaction, including anaphylaxis, may occur during AZLIN® administration, particularly in a hypersensitive individual.

The rapid intravenous administration of AZLIN® has been associated with transient chest discomfort. Therefore, the drug should not be infused over a period of less than five minutes.

As with other antibiotics, prolonged use of AZLIN® may result in overgrowth of non-susceptible organisms. If this occurs, appropriate measures should be taken.

Interactions with Drugs and Laboratory Tests
As with other penicillins, the mixing of azlocillin with an aminoglycoside in solutions for parenteral administration can result in substantial inactivation of the aminoglycoside.

Probenecid interferes with the renal tubular secretion of azlocillin, thereby increasing serum concentrations and prolonging serum half-life of the antibiotic.

The serum level of uric acid has been noted to be depressed in some patients receiving azlocillin; this effect appears to be transient.

High urine concentrations of azlocillin may produce false positive protein reactions (pseudoproteinuria) with the following methods: sulfosalicylic acid and boiling test, acetic acid test, biuret reaction, and nitric acid test. The bromphenol blue (Multi-stix®) reagent strip test has been reported to be reliable.

Pregnancy Category B
Reproduction studies have been performed in rats and mice at doses up to 2 times the human dose, and have revealed no evidence of impaired fertility or harm to the fetus, due to AZLIN®. There are however no adequate and well controlled studies in pregnant women. Because animal reproductive studies are not always predictive of human response, this drug should be used during pregnancy only if clearly needed. Azlocillin crosses the placenta and is found in cord blood and amniotic fluid.

Nursing Mothers
Azlocillin is detected in low concentrations in the milk of nursing mothers, therefore caution should be exercised when AZLIN® is administered to a nursing woman.

Drug Abuse and Dependence
Neither AZLIN® abuse nor AZLIN® dependence has been reported.

Adverse Reactions: As with other penicillins, the following adverse reactions may occur:
Hypersensitivity reactions: skin rash, pruritus, urticaria, arthralgia, myalgia, drug fever, chills, chest discomfort, and anaphylactic reactions.
Central nervous system: headache, giddiness, neuromuscular hyperirritability or convulsive seizures.
Gastro-intestinal disturbances: disturbances of taste and smell, stomatitis, flatulence, nausea, vomiting and diarrhea, epigastric pain.
Hemic and Lymphatic Systems: thrombocytopenia, leukopenia, neutropenia, eosinophilia and reduction of hemoglobin or hematocrit. Prolongation of prothrombin time and bleeding time.
Abnormalities of hepatic and renal function tests: elevation of serum aspartate aminotransferase (SGOT), serum alanine aminotransferase (SGPT), serum alkaline phosphatase, serum LDH, serum bilirubin. Elevation of serum creatinine and/or BUN, hypernatremia. Reduction in serum potassium and uric acid.
Local reactions: pain and thrombophlebitis with intravenous administration.

Overdosage: As with other penicillins, AZLIN® in overdosage has the potential to cause neuromuscular hyperirritability or convulsive seizures. Hemodialysis, if necessary, will aid in removal of the drug from the blood.

Dosage and Administration: AZLIN® (sterile azlocillin sodium) may be administered by slow intravenous injection (5 min or longer) or by intravenous infusion (30 min).

The recommended adult dosage for serious infections is 200–300 mg/kg per day given in 4 to 6 divided doses. The usual dose is 3g given every 4 hours (18g/day). For life-threatening infections, up to 350 mg/kg per day may be administered, but the total daily dosage should ordinarily not exceed 24g.

[See table below].

For patients with life-threatening infections, 4g may be administered every 4 hours (24g/day).

Dosage for any individual patient must take into consideration the site and severity of infection, the susceptibility of the organisms causing infection, and the status of the patient's host defense mechanisms.

The duration of therapy depends upon the severity of infection. Generally, AZLIN® should be continued for at least 2 days after the signs and symptoms of infection have disappeared. The usual duration is 10 to 14 days; however, in difficult and complicated infections, more prolonged therapy may be required (e.g., osteomyelitis).

In certain deep-seated infections, involving abscess formation, appropriate surgical drainage should be performed in conjunction with antimicrobial therapy.

Patients with Impaired Renal Function
The rate of elimination of azlocillin is dose dependent and related to the degree of renal function impairment. After an intravenous dose of 5g, the serum half-life is approximately 1 hour in patients with creatinine clearances above 80 ml/min, 2.0 hr in those with clearances of 30–79 ml/min, 4.0 hr in those with clearances of 10–29 ml/min and approximately 5.9 hr in patients with clearances of less than 10 ml/min. Dosage adjustments of AZLIN® are not required in patients with mild impairment of renal function. For patients with a creatinine clearance of ≤ 30 ml/min (serum creatinine of approximately 3.0 mg% or greater), the following dosage guide may be used.

[See table above].

For patients undergoing hemodialysis for renal failure, 3g may be administered after each dialysis and then every 12 hours

For patients with renal failure, particularly those with concomitant hepatic insufficiency, measurement of serum levels of azlocillin will provide additional guidance for adjusting dosage.

Intravenous Administration
AZLIN® may be administered intravenously by intermittent infusion or by direct slow intravenous injection.

Infusion. Each gram of azlocillin should be reconstituted by vigorous shaking with at least 10 ml of Sterile Water for Injection, 5% Dextrose Injection or 0.9% Sodium Chloride Injection. The dissolved drug should be further diluted to desired volume (50-100 ml) with an appropriate intravenous solution. (See Compatibility and Stability section). The solution of reconstituted drug may then be administered over a period of 30 minutes by direct infusion or through a Y-type intravenous infusion set which may already be in place. If this method or

AZLIN® DOSAGE GUIDE FOR PATIENTS WITH IMPAIRED RENAL FUNCTION

Creatinine Clearance ml/min	Urinary Tract Infection (Uncomplicated)	Urinary Tract Infection (Complicated)	Serious Systemic Infection
> 30	Usual Recommended Dosage		
10–30	1.5 g every 12 hours	1.5g every 8 hours	2g every 8 hours
< 10	1.5 g every 12 hours	2g every 12 hours	3g every 12 hours

AZLIN® DOSAGE GUIDE (ADULTS)

Condition	Daily Dosage Range	Usual Daily Dosage	Frequency and Route of Administration
Urinary tract infection (uncomplicated)	100–125 mg/kg	8g	2g every 6 hours IV
Urinary tract infection (complicated)	150–200 mg/kg	12g	3g every 6 hours IV
Lower respiratory tract infection			
Skin & skin structure infection			3g every 4 hours or 4g every 6 hours
Bone & joint infection Septicemia	225–300 mg/kg	16–18g	IV

the "piggyback" method of administration is used, it is advisable to discontinue temporarily the administration of any other solutions during the infusion of AZLIN®.

Injection. The reconstituted solution of AZLIN® may also be injected directly into a vein or into intravenous tubing; when administered in this way, the injection should be given slowly over a period of 5 minutes or longer. To minimize venous irritation, the concentration of drug should not exceed 10%.

When AZLIN® is given in combination with another antimicrobial, such as an aminoglycoside, each drug should be given separately in accordance with the recommended dosage and routes of administration for each drug.

After reconstitution and prior to administration, AZLIN® as with other parenteral drugs, should be inspected visually for particulate matter and discoloration.

Pediatric Use

Only limited data are available on the safety and effectiveness of AZLIN® in the treatment of infants with documented serious infection. Until further experience is gained, the drug should not be used in the newborn period.

In children with acute pulmonary exacerbation of cystic fibrosis, azlocillin may be administered at a dose of 75 mg/kg every 4 hours (450 mg/kg/day). The total daily dosage should not exceed 24g. The drug may be infused intravenously over a period of about 30 minutes.

Compatibility and Stability: AZLIN® at concentrations of 10 mg/ml and 50 mg/ml is stable (loss of potency less than 10%) when stored at room temperature in the following intravenous solutions for the time periods stated. When stored under refrigeration (below 8°C), AZLIN® at concentrations up to 100 mg/ml is stable for the time periods stated:

INTRAVENOUS SOLUTION	STABILITY
Sterile Water for Injection, U.S.P.	24 hours
0.9% Sodium Chloride Injection, U.S.P.	24 hours
5% Dextrose Injection, U.S.P.	24 hours
5% Dextrose in 0.225% Sodium Chloride Injection, U.S.P.	24 hours
Lactated Ringer's Injection, U.S.P.	24 hours
5% Dextrose in 0.45% Sodium Chloride Injection, U.S.P.	24 hours

Unused portion must be discarded after the time period stated

How Supplied: AZLIN® (sterile azlocillin sodium) is a white to pale yellow powder supplied in vials and infusion bottles. Each vial contains azlocillin sodium equivalent to 2g, 3g or 4g azlocillin. Each infusion bottle contains azlocillin sodium equivalent to 2g, 3g or 4g azlocillin.

AZLIN® vials and infusion bottles should be stored at or below 30°C (86°F). The powder as well as the reconstituted solution of drug may darken slightly, depending upon storage conditions, but potency is not affected.

Issued: June, 1982   PD 100565 18958

BILTRICIDE®
(praziquantel)   ℞

Description: BILTRICIDE (praziquantel) is a trematodicide provided in tablet form for the oral treatment of schistosome infections.

BILTRICIDE (praziquantel) is 2-(cyclohexylcarbonyl)-1,2,3,6,7,11b-hexahydro4H-pyrazino [2,1-a] isoquinolin-4-one with the molecular formula: $C_{19}H_{24}N_2O_2$.

The structural formula is as follows:

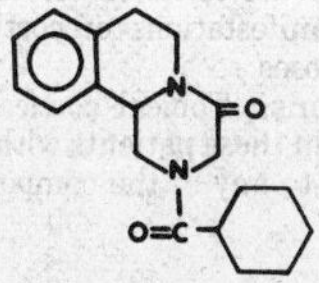

Praziquantel is a colorless crystalline powder of bitter taste. The compound is stable under normal conditions and melts at 136–140°C with decomposition. The active substance is hygroscopic. Praziquantel is easily soluble in chloroform and dimethylsulfoxide, soluble in ethanol and very slightly soluble in water.

BILTRICIDE lacquered tablets contain 600 mg of praziquantel.

Clinical Pharmacology: BILTRICIDE induces a rapid contraction of schistosomes by a specific effect on the permeability of the cell membrane. The drug further causes vacuolization and disintegration of the schistosome tegument.

After oral administration BILTRICIDE is rapidly absorbed (80%), subjected to a first pass effect, metabolized and eliminated by the kidneys. Maximal serum concentration is achieved 1–3 hours after dosing. The half-life of praziquantel in serum is 0.8–1.5 hours.

Indications and Usage: BILTRICIDE® is indicated for the treatment of infections due to: *Schistosoma mekongi, Schistosoma japonicum, Schistosoma mansoni* and *Schistosoma hematobium*.

Contraindications: BILTRICIDE should not be given to patients who previously have shown hypersensitivity to the drug. Since parasite destruction within the eye may cause irreparable lesions, ocular cysticercosis should not be treated with this compound.

Precautions: Information for the patient: Patients should be warned not to drive a car and not to operate machinery on the day of BILTRICIDE treatment and the following day. Minimal increases in liver enzymes have been reported in some patients.

When schistosomiasis or fluke infection is found to be associated with cerebral cysticercosis it is advised to hospitalize the patient for the duration of treatment.

Drug Interactions: No data are available regarding interaction of BILTRICIDE with other drugs.

Mutagenesis, Carcinogenesis: Mutagenic effects in Salmonella tests found by one laboratory have not been confirmed in the same tested strain by other laboratories. Long term carcinogenicity studies in rats and golden hamsters did not reveal any carcinogenic effect.

Pregnancy Category B: Reproduction studies have been performed in rats and rabbits at doses up to 40 times the human dose and have revealed no evidence of impaired fertility or harm to the fetus due to BILTRICIDE. There are, however, no adequate and well-controlled studies in pregnant women. An increase of the abortion rate was found in rats at three times the single human therapeutic dose. While animal reproduction studies are not always predictive of human response this drug should be used during pregnancy only if clearly needed.

Nursing mothers: BILTRICIDE® appeared in the milk of nursing women at a concentration of about $\frac{1}{4}$ that of maternal serum. Women should not nurse on the day of BILTRICIDE treatment and during the subsequent 72 hours.

Pediatric use: Safety in children under 4 years of age has not been established.

Adverse Effects: In general BILTRICIDE is very well tolerated. Side effects are usually mild and transient and do not require treatment. The following side effects were observed generally in order of severity: malaise, headache, dizziness, abdominal discomfort with or without nausea, rise in temperature and, rarely, urticaria. Such symptoms can, however, also result from the infection itself. Such side effects may be more frequent and/or serious in patients with a heavy worm burden. In patients with liver impairment caused by the infection, no adverse effects of BILTRICIDE have occurred which would necessitate restriction in use.

Overdosage: In rats and mice the acute LD_{50} was about 2,500 mg/kg. No data are available in humans. In the event of overdose a fast-acting laxative should be given.

Dosage and Administration: The dosage recommended for the treatment of schistosomiasis is: 3 × 20 mg/kg bodyweight as a one day treatment. The tablets should be washed down unchewed with some liquid during meals. Keeping the tablets or segments thereof in the mouth can reveal a bitter taste which can promote gagging or vomiting. The interval between the individual doses should not be less than 4 and not more than 6 hours.

How Supplied: BILTRICIDE is supplied as a 600 mg white, film-coated, oblong tablet with three scores. When broken each of the four segments contains 150 mg of active ingredient so that the dosage can be easily adjusted to the patient's bodyweight. Segments are broken off by pressing the score (notch) with thumbnails. If $\frac{1}{4}$ of a tablet is required, this is best achieved by breaking the segment from the outer end.

BILTRICIDE® is available in bottles of 6.

Storage Conditions: Store below 86°F (30°C).
PD100576   19253   April 1983
Shown in Product Identification Section, page 421

CORT-DOME®   ℞
1%, ½%, ¼% and ⅛%
(hydrocortisone) creme   acid pH

Description: Cort-Dome® Creme contains microdispersed hydrocortisone (the active ingredient) in a compatible vehicle buffered to the acid pH range of normal skin. Each gram of Cort-Dome® Creme contains 10.0mg/g (1%), 5.0mg/g (½%), 2.5mg/g (¼%) or 1.25 mg/g (⅛%) of hydrocortisone. Cort-Dome® Creme is applied topically. Hydrocortisone is a corticosteroid. Chemically, hydrocortisone is Pregn-4-ene-3, 20-dione,11,17,21-trihydroxy-,(11β)-. with the following structural formula:

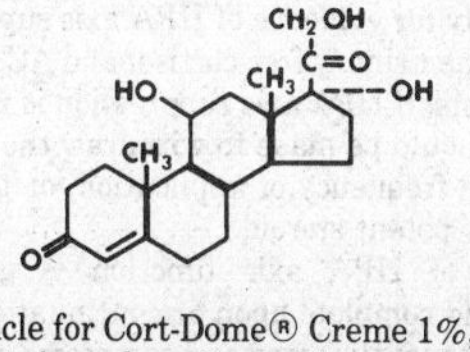

The vehicle for Cort-Dome® Creme 1%, ½%, and ¼% contains glycerin, calcium acetate, cetylstearyl alcohol-sodium lauryl sulfate, aluminum sulfate, purified water, synthetic beeswax (B-wax), white petrolatum, dextrin, and light mineral oil, preserved with methylparaben. The emollient vehicle for Cort-Dome® Creme ⅛% is composed of isopropyl myristate, cholesterol, white petrolatum, synthetic beeswax (B-wax), stearic acid, polyoxyethylene sorbitan monostearate, sorbitan monostearate, aluminum sulfate, propylene glycol, calcium acetate, dextrin, perfume, and purified water, preserved with methyl and propyl parabens.

EMPIRICAL FORMULA	MOLECULAR WEIGHT	CAS REGISTRY NUMBER
$C_{21}H_{30}O_5$	362.47	50-23-7

Clinical Pharmacology: Topical corticosteroids share anti-inflammatory, anti-pruritic and vasoconstrictive actions.

The mechanism of anti-inflammatory activity of the topical corticosteroids is unclear. Various laboratory methods, including vasoconstrictor assays, are used to compare and predict potencies and/or clinical efficacies of the topical corticosteroids. There is some evidence to suggest that a recognizable correlation exists between vasoconstrictor potency and therapeutic efficacy in man.

Pharmacokinetics

The extent of percutaneous absorption of topical corticosteroids is determined by many factors including the vehicle, the integrity of the epidermal barrier, and the use of occlusive dressings.

Topical corticosteroids can be absorbed from normal intact skin. Inflammation and/or other disease processes in the skin increase percutaneous absorption. Occlusive dressings substantially increase the percutaneous absorption of topical corticosteroids. Thus, occlusive dressings may be a valuable therapeutic adjunct for treatment of resistant dermatoses. (See DOSAGE AND ADMINISTRATION).

Once absorbed through the skin, topical corticosteroids are handled through pharmacokinetic

Continued on next page

Miles Pharm.—Cont.

pathways similar to systemically administered corticosteroids. Corticosteroids are bound to plasma proteins in varying degrees. Corticosteroids are metabolized primarily in the liver and are then excreted by the kidneys. Some of the topical corticosteroids and their metabolites are also excreted into the bile.

Indications and Usage: Topical corticosteroids are indicated for the relief of the inflammatory and pruritic manifestations of corticosteroid-responsive dermatoses.

Contraindications: Topical corticosteroids are contraindicated in those patients with a history of hypersensitivity to any of the components of the preparation.

Precautions:
General
Systemic absorption of topical corticosteroids has produced reversible hypothalamic-pituitary-adrenal (HPA) axis suppression, manifestations of Cushing's syndrome, hyperglycemia, and glucosuria in some patients.

Conditions which augment systemic absorption include the application of the more potent steroids, use over large surface areas, prolonged use, and the addition of occlusive dressings.

Therefore, patients receiving a large dose of a potent topical steroid applied to a large surface area or under an occlusive dressing should be evaluated periodically for evidence of HPA axis suppression by using the urinary free cortisol and ACTH stimulation tests. If HPA suppression is noted, an attempt should be made to withdraw the drug, to reduce the frequency of application, or to substitute a less potent steroid.

Recovery of HPA axis function is generally prompt and complete upon discontinuation of the drug. Infrequently, signs and symptoms of steroid withdrawal may occur, requiring supplemental systemic corticosteroids.

Children may absorb proportionally larger amounts of topical corticosteroids and thus be more susceptible to systemic toxicity. (See PRECAUTIONS—Pediatric Use.)

If irritation develops, topical corticosteroids should be discontinued and appropriate therapy instituted.

In the presence of dermatological infections, the use of an appropriate antifungal or antibacterial agent should be instituted. If a favorable response does not occur promptly, the corticosteroid should be discontinued until the infection has been adequately controlled.

Information for the Patient
Patients using topical corticosteroids should receive the following information and instructions:
1. This medication is to be used as directed by the physician. It is for external use only. Avoid contact with the eyes.
2. Patients should be advised not to use this medication for any disorder other than for which it was prescribed.
3. The treated skin area should not be bandaged or otherwise covered or wrapped as to be occlusive unless directed by the physician.
4. Patients should report any signs of local adverse reactions especially under occlusive dressing.
5. Parents of pediatric patients should be advised not to use tight-fitting diapers or plastic pants on a child being treated in the diaper area, as these garments may constitute occlusive dressings.

Laboratory Tests
The following tests may be helpful in evaluating the HPA axis suppression:
Urinary free cortisol test
ACTH stimulation test

Carcinogenesis, Mutagenesis, and Impairment of Fertility
Long-term animal studies have not been performed to evaluate the carcinogenic potential or the effect on fertility of topical corticosteroids.

Studies to determine mutagenicity with prednisolone and hydrocortisone have revealed negative results.

Pregnancy Category C
Corticosteroids are generally teratogenic in laboratory animals when administered systemically at relatively low-dosage levels. The more potent corticosteroids have been shown to be teratogenic after dermal application in laboratory animals. There are no adequate and well-controlled studies in pregnant women on teratogenic effects from topically applied corticosteroids. Therefore, topical corticosteroids should be used during pregnancy only if the potential benefit justifies the potential risk to the fetus. Drugs of this class should not be used extensively on pregnant patients, in large amounts, or for prolonged periods of time.

Nursing Mothers
It is not known whether topical administration of corticosteroids could result in sufficient systemic absorption to produce detectable quantities in breast milk. Systemically administered corticosteroids are secreted into breast milk in quantities *not* likely to have a deleterious effect on the infant. Nevertheless, caution should be exercised when topical corticosteroids are administered to a nursing woman.

Pediatric Use
Pediatric patients may demonstrate greater susceptibility to topical corticosteroid-induced HPA axis suppression and Cushing's syndrome than mature patients because of a larger skin surface area to body weight ratio.

Hypothalamic-pituitary-adrenal (HPA) axis suppression, Cushing's syndrome, and intracranial hypertension have been reported in children receiving topical corticosteroids. Manifestations of adrenal suppression in children include linear growth retardation, delayed weight gain, low plasma cortisol levels, and absence of response to ACTH stimulation. Manifestations of intracranial hypertension include bulging fontanelles, headaches, and bilateral papilledema.

Administration of topical corticosteroids to children should be limited to the least amount compatible with an effective therapeutic regimen. Chronic corticosteroid therapy may interfere with the growth and development of children.

Adverse Reactions: The following local adverse reactions are reported infrequently with topical corticosteroids, but may occur more frequently with the use of occlusive dressings. These reactions are listed in an approximate decreasing order of occurrence:
Burning
Itching
Irritation
Dryness
Folliculitis
Hypertrichosis
Acneiform eruptions
Hypopigmentation
Perioral dermatitis
Allergic contact dermatitis
Maceration of the skin
Secondary infection
Skin atrophy
Striae
Miliaria

Overdosage: Topically applied corticosteroids can be absorbed in sufficient amounts to produce systemic effects. (See PRECAUTIONS).

Dosage and Administration: Topical corticosteroids are generally applied to the affected area as a thin film from two to four times daily depending on the severity of the condition.

Occlusive dressings may be used for the management of psoriasis or recalcitrant conditions.

If an infection develops, the use of occlusive dressings should be discontinued and appropriate antimicrobial therapy instituted.

How Supplied: Cort-Dome® (hydrocortisone) Creme 1/8%-1 oz. tube. Cort-Dome® Creme 1/4%-1 oz. tube and 4 oz. dispensajar. Cort-Dome® Creme 1/2%-1/2 oz. tube, 1 oz tube and 4 oz. Cort-Dome® Creme 1%-1/2 oz. tube, 1 oz. tube.

Cort-Dome® Creme is a white semi-solid.
Store below 86°F (30°C), avoid freezing.
Caution: Federal (USA) law prohibits dispensing without a prescription.
July, 1982   PD100569   18876

CORT-DOME®   ℞
1%, 1/2%, 1/4% and 1/8%
(hydrocortisone)
lotion   acid pH

Description: Cort-Dome® Lotion contains microdispersed hydrocortisone (the active ingredient) in a compatible vehicle buffered to the acid pH range of normal skin. Each ml of Cort-Dome® Lotion contains 10.0mg/ml (1%). 5.0mg/ml(1/2%), 2.5mg/ml (1/4%) or 1.25mg/ml (1/8%) of hydrocortisone. Cort-Dome® Lotion is applied topically. Hydrocortisone is a corticosteroid. Chemically, hydrocortisone is Pregn-4-ene-3,20-dione,11,17,21-trihydroxy-(11β)-. with the following structural formula:

The vehicle for Cort-Dome® Lotion 1%, 1/2%, 1/4% and 1/8% is composed of glyceryl monostearyl, cetyl-stearyl alcohol-sodium lauryl sulfate, butyl stearate, aluminum sulfate, calcium acetate, dextrin, isopropyl myristate, polyoxyethylene sorbitan monolaurate, glycerin, and purified water preserved with methyl and propyl parabens.

EMPIRICAL FORMULA	MOLECULAR WEIGHT	CAS REGISTRY NUMBER
$C_{21}H_{30}O_5$	362.47	50-23-7

Clinical Pharmacology: Topical corticosteroids share anti-inflammatory, anti-pruritic and vasoconstrictive actions.

The mechanism of anti-inflammatory activity of the topical corticosteroids is unclear. Various laboratory methods, including vasoconstrictor assays, are used to compare and predict potencies and/or clinical efficacies of the topical corticosteroids. There is some evidence to suggest that a recognizable correlation exists between vasoconstrictor potency and therapeutic efficacy in man.

Pharmacokinetics
The extent of percutaneous absorption of topical corticosteroids is determined by many factors including the vehicle, the integrity of the epidermal barrier, and the use of occlusive dressings.

Topical corticosteroids can be absorbed from normal intact skin. Inflammation and/or other disease processes in the skin increase percutaneous absorption. Occlusive dressings substantially increase the percutaneous absorption of topical corticosteroids. Thus, occlusive dressings may be a valuable therapeutic adjunct for treatment of resistant dermatoses. (See DOSAGE AND ADMINISTRATION).

Once absorbed through the skin, topical corticosteroids are handled through pharmacokinetic pathways similar to systemically administered corticosteroids. Corticosteroids are bound to plasma proteins in varying degrees. Corticosteroids are metabolized primarily in the liver and are then excreted by the kidneys. Some of the topical corticosteroids and their metabolites are also excreted into the bile.

Indications and Usage: Topical corticosteroids are indicated for the relief of the inflammatory and pruritic manifestations of corticosteroid-responsive dermatoses.

Contraindications: Topical corticosteroids are contraindicated in those patients with a history of hypersensitivity to any of the components of the preparation.

Precautions:
General
Systemic absorption of topical corticosteroids has produced reversible hypothalamic-pituitary-adrenal (HPA) axis suppression, manifestations of

Cushing's syndrome, hyperglycemia, and glucosuria in some patients.
Conditions which augment systemic absorption include the application of the more potent steroids, use over large surface areas, prolonged use, and the addition of occlusive dressings.
Therefore, patients receiving a large dose of a potent topical steroid applied to a large surface area or under an occlusive dressing should be evaluated periodically for evidence of HPA axis suppression by using the urinary free cortisol and ACTH stimulation tests. If HPA axis suppression is noted, an attempt should be made to withdraw the drug, to reduce the frequency of application, or to substitute a less potent steroid.
Recovery of HPA axis function is generally prompt and complete upon discontinuation of the drug. Infrequently, signs and symptoms of steroid withdrawal may occur, requiring supplemental systemic corticosteroids.
Children may absorb proportionally larger amounts of topical corticosteroids and thus be more susceptible to systemic toxicity. (See PRECAUTIONS—Pediatric Use).
If irritation develops, topical corticosteroids should be discontinued and appropriate therapy instituted.
In the presence of dermatological infections, the use of an appropriate antifungal or antibacterial agent should be instituted. If a favorable response does not occur promptly, the corticosteroid should be discontinued until the infection has been adequately controlled.

Information for the Patient
Patients using topical corticosteroids should receive the following information and instructions:
1. This medication is to be used as directed by the physician. It is for external use only. Avoid contact with the eyes.
2. Patients should be advised not to use this medication for any disorder other than for which it was prescribed.
3. The treated skin area should not be bandaged or otherwise covered or wrapped as to be occlusive unless directed by the physician.
4. Patients should report any signs of local adverse reactions especially under occlusive dressing.
5. Parents of pediatric patients should be advised not to use tightfitting diapers or plastic pants on a child being treated in the diaper area, as these garments may constitute occlusive dressings.

Laboratory Tests
The following tests may be helpful in evaluating the HPA axis suppression:
Urinary free cortisol test
ACTH stimulation test

Carcinogenesis, Mutagenesis, and Impairment of Fertility
Long-term animal studies have not been performed to evaluate the carcinogenic potential or the effect on fertility of topical corticosteroids.
Studies to determine mutagenicity with prednisolone and hydrocortisone have revealed negative results.

Pregnancy Category C
Corticosteroids are generally teratogenic in laboratory animals when administered systemically at relatively low dosage levels. The more potent corticosteroids have been shown to be teratogenic after dermal application in laboratory animals. There are no adequate and well-controlled studies in pregnant women on teratogenic effects from topically applied corticosteroids. Therefore, topical corticosteroids should be used during pregnancy only if the potential benefit justifies the potential risk to the fetus. Drugs of this class should not be used extensively on pregnant patients, in large amounts, or for prolonged periods of time.

Nursing Mothers
It is not known whether topical administration of corticosteroids could result in sufficient systemic absorption to produce detectable quantities in breast milk. Systemically administered corticosteroids are secreted into breast milk in quantities *not* likely to have a deleterious effect on the infant. Nevertheless, caution should be exercised when topical corticosteroids are administered to a nursing woman.

Pediatric Use
Pediatric patients may demonstrate greater susceptibility to topical corticosteroid-induced HPA axis suppression and Cushing's syndrome than mature patients because of a larger skin surface area to body weight ratio.
Hypothalamic-pituitary-adrenal (HPA) axis suppression, Cushing's syndrome, and intracranial hypertension have been reported in children receiving topical corticosteroids. Manifestations of adrenal suppression in children include linear growth retardation, delayed weight gain, low plasma cortisol levels, and absence of response to ACTH stimulation. Manifestations of intracranial hypertension include bulging fontaneiles, headaches, and bilateral papilledema.
Administration of topical corticosteroids to children should be limited to the least amount compatible with an effective therapeutic regimen. Chronic corticosteroid therapy may interfere with the growth and development of children.

Adverse Reactions: The following local adverse reactions are reported infrequently with topical corticosteroids, but may occur more frequently with the use of occlusive dressings. These reactions are listed in an approximate decreasing order of occurrence:
Burning
Itching
Irritation
Dryness
Folliculitis
Hypertrichosis
Acneiform eruptions
Hypopigmentation
Perioral dermatitis
Allergic contact dermatitis
Maceration of the skin
Secondary infection
Skin atrophy
Striae
Miliaria

Overdosage: Topically applied corticosteroids can be absorbed in sufficient amounts to produce systemic effects. (See PRECAUTIONS).

Dosage and Administration: Topical corticosteroids are generally applied to the affected area as a thin film from two to four times daily depending on the severity of the condition.
Occlusive dressings may be used for the management of psoriasis or recalcitrant conditions.
In an infection develops, the use of occlusive dressings should be discontinued and appropriate antimicrobial therapy instituted.

How Supplied: Cort-Dome® (hydrocortisone) Lotion 1/8%-6 fl. oz. bottle, Cort-Dome® Lotion 1/4%-4 fl. oz. bottles. Cort-Dome® Lotion 1/2%-4 fl. oz. bottles. Cort-Dome® Lotion 1%-1 fl. oz. bottles.
Cort-Dome® Lotion is a white semi-fluid liquid.
Store below 86°F (30°C), avoid freezing.

Caution: Federal (USA) law prohibits dispensing without a prescription.

July, 1982   PD100570   18872

CORT-DOME® ℞
(hydrocortisone acetate)
regular potency suppositories

Description: Each Cort-Dome Regular Potency Suppository contains 15 mg hydrocortisone acetate in a monoglyceride base. Hydrocortisone acetate is a corticosteroid. Chemically, hydrocortisone acetate is pregn-4-ene-3, 20-dione, 21-(acetyloxy)-11, 17-dihydroxy-(11β)- with the following structural formula:

Clinical Pharmacology: In normal subjects, about 26 percent of hydrocortisone acetate is absorbed when the hydrocortisone acetate suppository is applied to the rectum. Absorption of hydrocortisone acetate may vary across abraded or inflamed surfaces.
Topical steroids are primarily effective because of their anti-inflammatory, anti-pruritic and vasoconstrictive action.

Indications and Usage: For use in inflamed hemorrhoids, post irradiation (factitial) proctitis, as an adjunct in the treatment of chronic ulcerative colitis, cryptitis, other inflammatory conditions of the anorectum, and pruritus ani.

Contraindications: Cort-Dome suppositories are contraindicated in those patients with a history of hypersensitivity to any of its components.

Precautions: Do not use unless adequate proctologic examination is made.
If irritation develops, the product should be discontinued and appropriate therapy instituted.
In the presence of an infection the use of an appropriate antifungal or antibacterial agent should be instituted. If a favorable response does not occur promptly, the corticosteroid should be discontinued until the infection has been adequately controlled.
No long term studies in animals have been performed to evaluate the carcinogenic potential of corticosteroid suppositories.
Pregnancy Category C. In laboratory animals, topical steroids have been associated with an increase in the incidence of fetal abnormalities when gestating females have been exposed to rather low dosage levels. There are no adequate and well controlled studies in pregnant women. Cort-Dome Regular Potency Suppositories should only be used during pregnancy if the potential benefit justifies the risk to the fetus. Drugs of this class should not be used extensively on pregnant patients, in large amounts, or for prolonged periods of time.
It is not known whether this drug is excreted in human milk. Because many drugs are excreted in human milk and because of the potential for serious adverse reactions in nursing infants from Cort-Dome Regular Potency Suppositories, a decision should be made whether to discontinue nursing or to discontinue the drug, taking into account the importance of the drug to the mother.

Adverse Reactions: The following local adverse reactions have been reported with corticosteroid suppositories:
1. Burning
2. Itching
3. Irritation
4. Dryness
5. Folliculitis
6. Hypopigmentation
7. Allergic Contact Dermatitis
8. Secondary infection

Drug Abuse and Dependence: Drug abuse and dependence has not been reported in patients treated with Cort-Dome Suppositories.

Overdosage: If signs and symptoms of systemic overdosage occur discontinue use.

Dosage and Administration: Usual dosage: One suppository in the rectum morning and night for two weeks, in non-specific proctitis. In more severe cases, one suppository three times daily; or two suppositories twice daily. In factitial proctitis, recommended therapy is six to eight weeks or less, according to response.

How Supplied: Cort-Dome Regular Potency Suppository is yellowish-white, waxy, smooth surfaced rod shaped with one rounded end, approximately 38 mm. long by 9.5 mm. in diameter. Package of 12 suppositories.
Store below 86°F (30°C), avoid freezing.

CORT-DOME® ℞
(hydrocortisone acetate)
high potency suppositories

Description: Each Cort-Dome High Potency Suppository contains 25 mg hydrocortisone ace-

Continued on next page

Miles Pharm.—Cont.

tate in a monoglyceride base. Hydrocortisone acetate is a corticosteroid. Chemically, hydrocortisone acetate is pregn-4-ene-3, 20-dione, 21-(acetyloxy)-11, 17-dihydroxy-(11β)- with the following structural formula:

Clinical Pharmacology: In normal subjects, about 26 percent of hydrocortisone acetate is absorbed when the hydrocortisone acetate suppository is applied to the rectum. Absorption of hydrocortisone acetate may vary across abraded or inflamed surfaces.
Topical steroids are primarily effective because of their anti-inflammatory, anti-pruritic and vasoconstrictive action.
Indications and Usage: For use in inflamed hemorrhoids, post-irradiation (factitial) proctitis, as an adjunct in the treatment of chronic ulcerative colitis, cryptitis, other inflammatory conditions of the anorectum, and pruritis ani.
Contraindication: Cort-Dome suppositories are contraindicated in those patients with a history of hypersensitivity to any of the components.
Precautions: Do not use unless adequate proctologic examination is made.
If irritation develops, the product should be discontinued and appropriate therapy instituted.
In the presence of an infection, the use of an appropriate antifungal or antibacterial agent should be instituted. If a favorable response does not occur promptly, the corticosteroids should be discontinued until the infection has been adequately controlled.
No long term studies in animals have been performed to evaluate the carcinogenic potential of corticosteroid suppositories.
Pregnancy Category C. In laboratory animals, topical steroids have been associated with an increase in the incidence of fetal abnormalities when gestating females have been exposed to rather low dosage levels. There are no adequate and well controlled studies in pregnant women. Cort-Dome High Potency Suppositories should only be used during pregnancy if the potential benefit justifies the risk to the fetus. Drugs of this class should not be used extensively on pregnant patients, in large amounts, or for prolonged periods of time.
It is not known whether this drug is excreted in human milk and because many drugs are excreted in human milk and because of the potential for serious adverse reactions in nursing infants from Cort-Dome High Potency Suppositories, a decision should be made whether to discontinue nursing or to discontinue the drug, taking into account the importance of the drug to the mother.
Adverse Reactions: The following local adverse reactions have been reported with corticosteroid suppositories.
1. Burning
2. Itching
3. Irritation
4. Dryness
5. Folliculitis
6. Hypopigmentation
7. Allergic Contact Dermatitis
8. Secondary infection

Drug Abuse and Dependence: Drug abuse and dependence has not been reported in patients treated with Cort-Dome Suppositories.
Overdosage: If signs and symptoms of systemic overdosage occur discontinue use.
Dosage and Administration: Usual dosage: One suppository in the rectum morning and night for two weeks, in non-specific proctitis. In more severe cases, one suppository three times daily; or two suppositories twice daily. In factitial proctitis, recommended therapy is six to eight weeks or less, according to response.
How Supplied: Cort-Dome High Potency Suppository is yellowish-white, waxy, smooth surfaced rod shaped with one rounded end, approximately 33 mm. long by 9.5 mm. in diamter. Package of 12 suppositories.
Store below 86°F (30°C), avoid freezing.

DECHOLIN® Tablets
(dehydrocholic acid)

Composition: Dehydrocholic acid 250 mg. contained in each tablet.
Indications: For the temporary relief of constipation.
Average Adult Dose: One or two tablets, three times daily or as directed by physician.
Warning: Do not use when abdominal pain, nausea or vomiting are present. Frequent use of this preparation may result in dependence on laxatives.
Store at controlled room temperature (59°–86°F.).
KEEP THIS AND ALL MEDICATIONS OUT OF THE REACH OF CHILDREN.
How Supplied: White tablets coded with number 121-Miles in bottles of 100 and 500.
Shown in Product Identification Section, page 421

DOMEBORO® Powder Packets, Effervescent Tablets (acid pH) Astringent Wet Dressing

One packet or tablet dissolved in a pint of water makes a modified Burow's Solution approximately equivalent to a 1:40 dilution, two packets or tablets a 1:20 dilution, and four packets or tablets a 1:10 dilution.
Buffered to an acid pH.
Contains: Aluminum sulfate and calcium acetate.
Indications: A soothing wet dressing for relief of inflammatory conditions of the skin such as insect bites, poison ivy, swellings and bruises or athlete's foot.
Directions: Dissolve one or two packets or tablets in a pint (large glass) of water and stir. When the powder disperses, shake resulting mixture. Do not strain or filter. Bandage the site of application loosely. Pour mixture on bandage every 15 to 30 minutes to keep dressing moist. Continue for 4 to 8 hours unless otherwise directed by physician. Do not use plastic or other impervious material to prevent evaporation without consulting your physician.
Caution: Keep away from eyes. For external use only. Store below 86°F. (30°C.), avoid freezing. Material in diluted form may be stored for 7 days at room temperature.
How Supplied:
Powder Packets: Boxes of 12 and 100. Each packet contains 2.2 gm. Individually foil-wrapped *Tablets:* Boxes of 12, 100 and 1000.
White tablets coded with number 411-Miles.
Shown in Product Identification Section, page 422

DOME-PASTE® Bandage
3″ and 4″ Bandages
(Medicated Bandage for Leg or Arm, Improved Unna's boot)

Composition: Each medicated bandage is impregnated with zinc oxide, calamine and gelatin. No heating or painting necessary.
Indications: For those conditions of the extremities (e.g. varicose veins and associated ulcers, stasis edema, thrombophlebitis, lymphangitis).
Caution: If skin sensitivity or irritation develops discontinue use and consult a physician.
Administration and Dosage: Detailed instructions for application are supplied on each carton.
How Supplied: 3″ and 4″ cotton bandage by 360″ (10 yd.). Each carton contains one medicated bandage in polyethylene bag.

DOMOL® Bath and Shower Oil
(diisopropyl sebacate, isopropyl myristate)

Composition: Contains sebacate*, a special skin moisturizing agent, refined mineral oil and skin softener.
*Diisopropyl sebacate.
Action and Uses: Effective, pleasant way to lubricate skin and relieve itchy discomfort. It lubricates skin and restores the protective action of skin oils washed away by soaps and detergents. DOMOL helps maintain skin's normal condition by retarding evaporation of skin's moisture.
Directions for Use:
Bath—Add 1 or 2 capfuls to bathtub or water. Soak for 10-20 minutes.
Shower—Pour 1 capful on wet sponge or washcloth. Rub gently over body, rinse under shower.
Infant's Bath—Add 1 capful to basin or bathinette of water.
Sponge Bath—Add 1 or 2 capfuls to about a pint of water. Sponge body gently with washcloth or cellulose sponge. After bathing the skin should be patted dry rather than rubbed.
How Supplied: 8 fl. oz. unbreakable plastic bottle.

DTIC–Dome®
(dacarbazine)
Sterile

℞

> **Warning:** It is recommended that DTIC-Dome (dacarbazine) be administered under the supervision of a qualified physician experienced in the use of cancer chemotherapeutic agents.
> 1. Hemopoietic depression is the most common toxicity with DTIC-Dome (See Warnings).
> 2. Hepatic necrosis has been reported (See Warnings).
> 3. Studies have demonstrated this agent to have a carcinogenic and teratogenic effect when used in animals.
> 4. In treatment of each patient, the physician must weigh carefully the possibility of achieving therapeutic benefit against the risk of toxicity.

Description: DTIC-Dome Sterile (dacarbazine) is a colorless to an ivory colored solid which is light sensitive. Each vial contains 100mg of dacarbazine, or 200mg of dacarbazine (the active ingredient), anhydrous citric acid and mannitol. DTIC-Dome is reconstituted and administered intravenously (pH 3-4) DTIC-Dome is an anticancer agent. Chemically, DTIC-Dome is 5-(3, 3-dimethyl-l-triazeno)-imidazole-4-carboxamide (DTIC).
Clinical Pharmacology: After intravenous administration of DTIC-Dome, the volume of distribution exceeds total body water content suggesting localization in some body tissue, probably the liver. Its disappearance from the plasma is biphasic with initial half-life of 19 minutes and a terminal half-life of 5 hours. In a patient with renal and hepatic dysfunctions, the half-lives were lengthened to 55 minutes and 7.2 hours. The average cumulative excretion of unchanged DTIC in the urine is 40% of the injected dose in 6 hours. DTIC is subject to renal tubular secretion rather than glomerular filtration. At therapeutic concentrations DTIC is not appreciably bound to human plasma protein.
In man, DTIC is extensively degraded. Besides unchanged DTIC, 5-aminoimidazole -4 carboxamide (AIC) is a major metabolite of DTIC excreted in the urine. AIC is not derived endogenously but from the injected DTIC, because the administration of radioactive DTIC labeled with ^{14}C in the imidazole portion of the molecule (DTIC-2-^{14}C) gives rise to AIC-2-^{14}C.
Although the exact mechanism of action of DTIC-Dome is not known, three hypotheses have been offered:
1. inhibition of DNA synthesis by acting as a purine analog

2. action as an alkylating agent
3. interaction with SH groups

Indications and Usage: DTIC-Dome is indicated in the treatment of metastatic malignant melanoma. In addition, DTIC-Dome is also indicated for Hodgkin's disease as a second-line therapy when used in combination with other effective agents.

Contraindications: DTIC-Dome is contraindicated in patients who have demonstrated a hypersensitivity to it in the past.

Warnings: Hemopoietic depression is the most common toxicity with DTIC-Dome and involves primarily the leukocytes and platelets, although, anemia may sometimes occur. Leukopenia and thrombocytopenia may be severe enough to cause death. The possible bone marrow depression requires careful monitoring of white blood cells, red blood cells, and platelet levels. Hemopoietic toxicity may warrant temporary suspension or cessation of therapy with DTIC-Dome.

Hepatic toxicity accompanied by hepatic vein thrombosis and hepatocellular necrosis resulting in death, has been reported. The incidence of such reactions has been low; approximately 0.01% of patients treated. This toxicity has been observed mostly when DTIC-Dome has been administered concomitantly with other anti-neoplastic drugs; however, it has also been reported in some patients treated with DTIC-Dome alone.

Anaphylaxis can occur following the administration of DTIC-Dome.

Precautions: Hospitalization is not always necessary but adequate laboratory study capability must be available. Extravasation of the drug subcutaneously during intravenous administration may result in tissue damage and severe pain. Local pain, burning sensation, and irritation at the site of injection may be relieved by locally applied hot packs.

Carcinogenicity of DTIC was studied in rats and mice. Proliferative endocardial lesions, including fibrosarcomas and sarcomas were induced by DTIC in rats. In mice, administration of DTIC resulted in the induction of angiosarcomas of the spleen.

Pregnancy Category C—DTIC-Dome has been shown to be teratogenic in rats when given in doses 20 times the human daily dose on day 12 of gestation. DTIC when administered in 10 times the human daily dose to male rats (twice weekly for 9 weeks) did not affect the male libido, although female rats mated to male rats had higher incidence of resorptions than controls. In rabbits, DTIC daily dose 7 times the human daily dose given on Days 6–15 of gestation resulted in fetal skeletal anomalies. There are no adequate and well controlled studies in pregnant women. DTIC-Dome should be used during pregnancy only if the potential benefit justifies the potential risk to the fetus.

It is not known whether this drug is excreted in human milk. Because many drugs are excreted in human milk and because of the potential for tumorigenicity shown for DTIC-Dome in animal studies, a decision should be made whether to discontinue nursing or to discontinue the drug, taking into account the importance of the drug to the mother.

Adverse Reactions: Symptoms of anorexia, nausea, and vomiting are the most frequently noted of all toxic reactions. Over 90% of patients are affected with the initial few doses. The vomiting lasts 1–12 hours and is incompletely and unpredictably palliated with phenobarbital and/or prochlorperazine. Rarely, intractable nausea and vomiting have necessitated discontinuance of therapy with DTIC-Dome. Rarely, DTIC-Dome has caused diarrhea. Some helpful suggestions include restricting the patient's oral intake of food for 4–6 hours prior to treatment. The rapid toleration of these symptoms suggests that a central nervous system mechanism may be involved, and usually these symptoms subside after the first 1 or 2 days. There are a number of minor toxicities that are infrequently noted. Patients have experienced an influenza-like syndrome of fever to 39°C, myalgias and malaise. These symptoms occur usually after large single doses, may last for several days, and they may occur with successive treatments.

Alopecia has been noted as has facial flushing and facial paresthesia. There have been few reports of significant liver or renal function test abnormalities in man. However, these abnormalities have been observed more frequently in animal studies. Erythematous and urticarial rashes have been observed infrequently after administration of DTIC-Dome. Rarely, photosensitivity reactions may occur.

Overdosage: Give supportive treatment and monitor blood cell counts.

Dosage and Administration: MALIGNANT MELANOMA—The recommended dosage is 2 to 4.5mg/kg/day for 10 days. Treatment may be repeated at 4 week intervals.

An alternate recommended dosage is 250mg/square meter body surface/day I.V. for 5 days. Treatment may be repeated every 3 weeks.
HODGKIN'S DISEASE: The recommended dosage of DTIC-Dome in the treatment of Hodgkin's Disease is 150mg/square meter body surface/day for 5 days, in combination with other effective drugs. Treatment may be repeated every 4 weeks. An alternative recommended dosage is 375mg/square meter body surface on day 1, in combination with other effective drugs, to be repeated every 15 days.
DTIC-Dome (dacarbazine) 100mg/vial and 200mg/vial are reconstituted with 9.9 ml and 19.7 ml, respectively, of Sterile Water for Injection, U.S.P. The resulting solution contains 10mg/ml of dacarbazine having a pH of 3.0 to 4.0. The calculated dose of the resulting solution is drawn into a syringe and administered *only* intravenously.

The reconstituted solution may be further diluted with 5% dextrose injection, U.S.P. or sodium chloride injection, U.S.P. and administered as an intravenous infusion.

After reconstitution and prior to use, the solution in the vial may be stored at 4°C for up to 72 hours or at normal room conditions (temperature and light) for up to 8 hours. If the reconstituted solution is further diluted in 5% dextrose, injection, U.S.P. or sodium chloride injection, U.S.P., the resulting solution may be stored at 4°C for up to 24 hours or at normal room conditions for up to 8 hours.

How Supplied: 10 ml vials containing 100mg or 20 ml vials containing 200 mg of DTIC-Dome as sterile dacarbazine in boxes of 12.

Manufactured by:
Ben Venue Laboratories
Bedford, Ohio 44146
Distributed by:
Miles Pharmaceuticals
Division of Miles Laboratories, Inc.
West Haven, Connecticut 06516 USA
PD100546   October 1981   18265

LITHANE® R
(lithium carbonate)
TABLETS
For Control of Manic Episodes in Manic-Depressive Psychosis

Warning

Lithium toxicity is closely related to serum lithium levels, and can occur at doses close to therapeutic levels. Facilities for prompt and accurate serum lithium determinations should be available before initiating therapy.

Description: Lithium carbonate is a white, light, alkaline powder with molecular formula Li_2CO_3 and molecular weight 73.89. Lithium is an element of the alkali-metal group with atomic number 3, atomic weight 6.94, and an emission line at 671 nm on the flame photometer.

Actions: Preclinical studies have shown that lithium alters sodium transport in nerve and muscle cells and effects a shift toward intraneuronal metabolism of catecholamines, but the specific biochemical mechanism of lithium action in mania is unknown.

Indications: Lithium carbonate is indicated in the treatment of manic episodes of manic-depressive illness. Maintenance therapy prevents or diminishes the intensity of subsequent episodes in those manic-depressive patients with a history of mania.

Typical symptoms of mania include pressure of speech, motor hyperactivity, reduced need for sleep, flight of ideas, grandiosity, elation, poor judgment, aggressiveness, and possibly hostility. When given to a patient experiencing a manic episode, lithium may produce a normalization of symptomatology within 1 to 3 weeks.

Warnings: Lithium should generally not be given to patients with significant renal or cardiovascular disease, severe debilitation or dehydration, or sodium depletion, and to patients receiving diuretics, since the risk of lithium toxicity is very high in such patients. If the psychiatric indication is life-threatening, and if such a patient fails to respond to other measures, lithium treatment may be undertaken with extreme caution, including daily serum lithium determinations and adjustment to the usually low doses ordinarily tolerated by these individuals. In such instances, hospitalization is a necessity.

Lithium therapy has been reported in some cases to be associated with morphologic changes in the kidneys. The relationship between such changes and renal function has not been established.

An encephalopathic syndrome (characterized by weakness, lethargy, fever, tremulousness and confusion, extrapyramidal symptoms, leukocytosis, elevated serum enzymes, BUN and FBS) followed by irreversible brain damage has occurred in a few patients treated with lithium plus haloperidol. A causal relationship between these events and the concomitant administration of lithium and haloperidol has not been established; however, patients receiving such combined therapy should be monitored closely for early evidence of neurologic toxicity and treatment discontinued promptly if such signs appear. The possibility of similar adverse interactions with other antipsychotic medication exists.

Lithium toxicity is closely related to serum lithium levels, and can occur at doses close to therapeutic levels (see DOSAGE AND ADMINISTRATION).

Outpatients and their families should be warned that the patient must discontinue lithium carbonate therapy and contact his physician if such clinical signs of lithium toxicity as diarrhea, vomiting, tremor, mild ataxia, drowsiness, or muscular weakness occur.

Lithium carbonate may impair mental and/or physical abilities. Caution patients about activities requiring alertness (e.g., operating vehicles or machinery).

Lithium may prolong the effects of neuromuscular blocking agents. Therefore, neuromuscular blocking agents should be given with caution to patients receiving lithium.

Usage in Pregnancy: Adverse effects on nidation in rats, embryo viability in mice, and metabolism *in vitro* of rat testis and human spermatozoa have been attributed to lithium, as have teratogenicity in submammalian species and cleft palates in mice. Studies in rats, rabbits, and monkeys have shown no evidence of lithium-induced teratology. There are lithium birth registries in the United States and elsewhere; however there is at the present time insufficient data to determine the effects of lithium carbonate on human fetuses. Therefore, at this point, lithium should not be used in pregnancy, especially the first trimester, unless in the opinion of the physician, the potential benefits outweigh the possible hazards.

Usage in Nursing Mothers: Lithium is excreted in human milk. Nursing should not be undertaken during lithium therapy except in rare and unusual circumstances where, in the view of the physician, the potential benefits to the mother outweigh possible hazards to the child.

Continued on next page

Miles Pharm.—Cont.

Usage in Children: Since information regarding the safety and effectiveness of lithium carbonate in children under 12 years of age is not available, its use in such patients is not recommended at this time.

Precautions: The ability to tolerate lithium is greater during the acute manic phase and decreases when manic symptoms subside (see DOSAGE AND ADMINISTRATION).

The distribution space of lithium approximates that of total body water. Lithium is primarily excreted in urine with insignificant excretion in feces. Renal excretion of lithium is proportional to its plasma concentration. The half-life of elimination of lithium is approximately 24 hours. Lithium decreases sodium reabsorption by the renal tubules which could lead to sodium depletion. Therefore, it is essential for the patient to maintain a normal diet, including salt, and an adequate fluid intake (2500–3000 ml) at least during the initial stabilization period. Decreased tolerance to lithium has been reported to ensue from protracted sweating or diarrhea and, if such occur, supplemental fluid and salt should be administered.

In addition to sweating and diarrhea, concomitant infection with elevated temperatures may also necessitate a temporary reduction or cessation of medication.

Previously existing underlying thyroid disorders do not necessarily constitute a contraindication to lithium treatment; where hypothyroidism exists, careful monitoring of thyroid function during lithium stabilization and maintenance allows for correction of changing thyroid parameters, if any; where hypothroidism occurs during lithium stabilization and maintenance, supplemental thyroid treatment may be used.

This product contains FD&C Yellow No. 5 (tartrazine) which may cause allergic-type reactions (including bronchial asthma) in certain susceptible individuals. Although the over-all incidence of FD&C Yellow No. 5 (tartrazine) sensitivity in the general population is low, it is frequently seen in patients who also have aspirin hypersensitivity. Indomethacin (50 mg t.i.d.) has been reported to increase steady state plasma lithium levels from 30 to 59 percent. There is also evidence that other nonsteroidal, anti-inflammatory may have a similar effect. When such combinations are used, increased plasma lithium level monitoring is recommended.

Adverse Reactions: Adverse reactions are seldom encountered at serum lithium levels below 1.5 mEq./l., except in the occasional patient sensitive to lithium. Mild to moderate toxic reactions may occur at levels from 1.5–2.5 mEq./l., and moderate to severe reactions may be seen at levels from 2.0–2.5 mEq./l., depending upon individual response to the drug.

Fine hand tremor, polyuria, and mild thirst may occur during initial therapy for the acute manic phase, and may persist throughout treatment. Transient and mild nausea and general discomfort may also appear during the first few days of lithium administration.

These side effects are an inconvenience rather than a disabling condition, and usually subside with continued treatment or a temporary reduction or cessation of dosage. If persistent, a cessation of dosage is indicated.

Diarrhea, vomiting, drowsiness, muscular weakness, and lack of coordination may be early signs of lithium intoxication, and can occur at lithium levels below 2.0 mEq./l. At higher levels, giddiness, ataxia, blurred vision, tinnitus, and a large output of dilute urine may be seen. Serum lithium levels above 3.0 mEq./l. may produce a complex clinical picture involving multiple organs and organ systems. Serum lithium levels should not be permitted to exceed 2.0 mEq./l, during the acute treatment phase.

The following reactions have been reported and appear to be related to serum lithium levels, including levels within the therapeutic range:

Neuromuscular: tremor, muscle hyperirritability (fasciculations, twitching, clonic movements of whole limbs), ataxia, choreo-athetotic movements, hyperactive deep tendon reflexes.

Central Nervous System: blackout spells, epileptiform seizures, slurred speech, dizziness, vertigo, incontinence of urine or feces, somnolence, psychomotor retardation, restlessness, confusion stupor, coma.

Cardiovascular: cardiac arrhythmia, hypotension, peripheral circulatory collapse.

Gastrointestinal: anorexia, nausea, vomiting, diarrhea.

Genitourinary: albuminuria, oliguria, polyuria, glycosuria.

Dermatologic: drying and thinning of hair, anesthesia of skin, chronic folliculitis, xerosis cutis, alopecia, and exacerbation of psoriasis.

Autonomic Nervous System: blurred vision, dry mouth.

Thyroid Abnormalities: Euthyroid goiter and/or hypothyroidism (including myxedema) accompanied by lower T_3 and T_4. I^{131} iodine uptake may be elevated. (See **Precautions**.) Paradoxically, rare cases of hyperthroidism have been reported.

EEG. Changes: diffuse slowing, widening of frequency spectrum, potentiation and disorganization of background rhythm.

EKG. Changes: reversible flattening, isoelectricity or inversion of T-waves.

Miscellaneous: fatigue, lethargy, tendency to sleep, dehydration, weight loss, transient scotomata.

Miscellaneous reactions unrelated to dosage are: transient electroencephalographic and electrocardiographic changes, leucocytosis, headache, diffuse non-toxic goiter with or without hypothyroidism, transient hyperglycemia, generalized pruritus with or without rash, cutaneous ulcers, albuminuria, worsening of organic brain syndromes, excessive weight gain, edematous swelling of ankles or wrists, and thirst or polyuria, sometimes resembling diabetes insipidus, and metallic taste. A single report has been received of the development of painful discoloration of fingers and toes and coldness of the extremities within one day of the starting of treatment of lithium. The mechanism through which these symptoms (resembling Raynaud's Syndrome) developed is not known. Recovery followed discontinuance.

Dosage and Administration:

Acute Mania: Optimal patient response to lithium carbonate usually can be established and maintained with 600 mg t.i.d. Such doses will normally produce an effective serum lithium level ranging between 1.0 and 1.5 mEq./l. Dosage must be individualized according to serum levels and clinical response. Regular monitoring of the patient's clinical state and of serum lithium levels is necessary. Serum levels should be determined twice per week during the acute phase, and until the serum level and clinical condition of the patient have been stabilized.

Long term Control: The desirable lithium levels are 0.6 to 1.2 mEq./l. Dosage will vary from one individual to another, but usually 300 mg t.i.d. or q.i.d. will maintain this level. Serum lithium levels in uncomplicated cases receiving maintenance therapy during remission should be monitored at least every two months.

Patients abnormally sensitive to lithium may exhibit toxic signs at serum levels of 1.0 to 1.5 mEq./l. Elderly patients often respond to reduced dosage, and may exhibit signs of toxicity at serum levels ordinarily tolerated by other patients.

N.B.: Blood samples for serum lithium determinations should be drawn immediately prior to the next dose when lithium concentrations are relatively stable (i.e., 8–12 hours after the previous dose). Total reliance must not be placed on serum levels alone. Accurate patient evaluation requires both clinical and laboratory analysis.

Overdosage: The toxic levels for lithium are close to the therapeutic levels. It is therefore important that patients and their families be cautioned to watch for early toxic symptoms and to discontinue the drug and inform the physician should they occur. Toxic symptoms are listed in detail under ADVERSE REACTIONS.

Treatment: No specific antidote for lithium poisoning is known. Early symptoms of lithium toxicity can usually be treated by reduction or cessation of dosage of the drug and resumption of the treatment at a lower dose after 24 to 48 hours. In severe cases of lithium poisoning, the first and foremost goal of treatment consists of elimination of this ion from the organism.

Treatment is essentially the same as that used in barbiturate poisoning: 1) lavage, 2) correction of fluid and electrolyte imbalance, and 3) regulation of kidney functioning. Urea, mannitol, and aminophylline all produce significant increases in lithium excretion. Hemodialysis is an effective and rapid means of removing the ion from the severely toxic patient. Infection prophylaxis, regular chest X-rays, and preservation of adequate respiration are essential.

How Supplied: Lithane (lithium carbonate) is available as round, green, scored tablets containing 300 mg of lithium carbonate coded with the word Miles and the three digit code 951 in bottles of 100.

PD100591 Revised July 1983
Manufactured for
Miles Pharmaceuticals
Division of Miles Laboratories, Inc.
West Haven, Connecticut 06516 USA
by Pfizer, Inc., New York, N.Y. 10017
©1980, Miles Laboratories, Inc.
Shown in Product Identification Section, page 422

MEZLIN® ℞
(sterile mezlocillin sodium)
for intravenous or intramuscular use.

Description: MEZLIN® (sterile mezlocillin sodium) is a semisynthetic broad spectrum penicillin antibiotic for parenteral administration. It is the monohydrate sodium salt of 6-{D-2 [3-(methylsulfonyl) -2- OXO-imidazolidine-1-carboxamido]-2-phenyl-acetamido} penicillanic acid.

Structural Formula:

Empirical Formula: $C_{21}H_{24}N_5O_8S_2Na \cdot H_2O$

MEZLIN® has a molecular weight of 579.6 and contains 42.6 mg (1.85 mEq) of sodium per one gram of mezlocillin activity. The dosage form is supplied as a sterile white to pale yellow crystalline powder, which is freely soluble in water. When reconstituted, solutions of MEZLIN® are clear and range from colorless to pale yellow with a pH of 4.5 to 8.0.

Clinical Pharmacology: **Intravenous Administration.** In healthy adult volunteers, mean serum levels of mezlocillin 5 minutes after a 5-minute intravenous injection of 1g, 2g, or 5g are 100, 253 or 411 mcg/ml, respectively. Serum levels, as

MEZLIN®
MEZLOCILLIN SERUM LEVELS IN ADULTS (mcg/ml) 2–5 MIN IV INJECTION

DOSE	0	15 min	30 min	45 min	1 hr	2 hr	3 hr	4 hr	6 hr
4g	—	254 (155–400)	163 (99–260)	122 (78–215)	93 (67–133)	47 (22–96)	20 (8–45)	9.1 (6–13)	8.4 (5–17)

MEZLIN® — Product Information

MEZLOCILLIN SERUM LEVELS IN ADULTS (mcg/ml) 5 MIN IV INJECTION

DOSE	0	5 min	10 min	20 min	30 min	1 hr	2 hr	3 hr	4 hr	6 hr	8 hr
1g	149 (132–185)	100 (64–143)	66 (47–87)	50 (31–87)	40 (22–83)	18 (8–31)	5.3 (3.3–7.7)	2.5 (1.7–3.7)	1.7 (0.7–2.8)	0.5 (0–1.2)	0.1 (0–0.2)
2g	314 (207–362)	253 (161–364)	161 (113–214)	117 (76–174)	82 (55–112)	56 (23–88)	20 (7.5–32)	11 (3.8–16)	4.4 (1.6–8.7)	1.5 (0.5–2.6)	0.6 (0.1–1.4)
5g	547 (268–854)	411 (199–597)	357 (246–456)	250 (203–353)	226 (190–333)	131 (104–193)	76 (59–104)	31 (20–40)	13 (6.4–17)	4.6 (2.1–9.4)	1.9 (1.1–3.6)

noted below, lack dose proportionality. [See table above].

Fifteen minutes after a 4g intravenous injection (2–5 min), the concentration in serum is 254 mcg/ml; 1 hour and 4 hours later levels are 93 mcg/ml and 9.1 mcg/ml, respectively: (See table on preceding page)

After an intravenous infusion (15 min) of 3g, mean levels 15 minutes after dosing are 269 mcg/ml (170–280).

A 30-minute intravenous infusion of 3g produces mean peak concentrations of 263 mcg/ml; 1 hour and 4 hours later the concentrations are 57 mcg/ml and 4.4 mcg/ml, respectively: (See table below)

Following intravenous infusion (2 hr) of a 3g dose of mezlocillin every 4 hours for 7 days, mean peak serum concentrations are higher than 100 mcg/ml, and levels above 50 mcg/ml are maintained throughout dosing.

Intramuscular Administration. MEZLIN® is rapidly absorbed after intramuscular injection. In healthy volunteers, the mean peak serum concentration occurs approximately 45 minutes after a single dose of 1g and is about 15 mcg/ml. The oral administration of 1g probenecid before injection produces an increase in mezlocillin serum levels of about 50%. After repetitive intramuscular doses of 1g mezlocillin every 6 hours, peak levels in the serum generally range between 35 and 45 mcg/ml. The relationship between the pharmacokinetics of intramuscular and intravenous dosing has not yet been clearly established.

General. As with other penicillins, mezlocillin is excreted primarily by glomerular filtration and tubular secretion. The rate of elimination is dose dependent and related to the degree of renal functional impairment. In patients with normal renal function, approximately 55% of the administered dose is recovered from the urine within the first 6 hours after dosing. Two hours after an intravenous injection of 2g, concentrations of active drug in urine generally exceed 4000 mcg/ml. By 4–6 hours after injection, concentrations usually decline to a range of about 50 to 200 mcg/ml. The serum elimination half-life of mezlocillin after intravenous dosing is approximately 55 minutes.

In patients with reduced renal function, the half-life is only slightly prolonged. Dosage adjustments are usually not necessary except in patients with severe renal impairment. (See Dosage and Administration). As with other penicillins, mezlocillin is metabolized only slightly; less than 10% of the drug excreted in the urine is in the form of the penicilloate or penilloate. The drug is readily removed from the serum by hemodialysis and, to a lesser extent, by peritoneal dialysis.

Up to 26% of a dose of mezlocillin is recovered from the bile of patients with normal liver function. Following intravenous doses of 2 to 5g, concentrations of active drug in bile generally range from 500 to 2500 mcg/ml. The biliary excretion of mezlocillin is reduced in patients with common bile duct obstruction.

Mezlocillin is not appreciably absorbed when given orally. Following parenteral administration, the apparent volume of distribution is approximately equal to the extracellular fluid volume.

The drug is present in active form in the serum, urine, bile, peritoneal fluid, pleural fluid, bronchial and wound secretions, bone and other tissues. As with other penicillins, penetration into the cerebrospinal fluid (CSF) is generally poor, however higher CSF concentrations are obtained in the presence of meningeal inflammation.

Protein binding studies indicate that the degree of mezlocillin binding is low (16–42%) and depends upon testing methods and concentrations of drug studied.

Microbiology

Mezlocillin is a bactericidal antibiotic which acts by interfering with synthesis of cell wall components. It is active against a variety of gram-negative and gram-positive bacteria, including aerobic and anaerobic strains. Mezlocillin is usually active *in vitro* against most strains of the following organisms:

Gram-negative bacteria

Escherichia coli
Klebsiella species (including *K. pneumoniae*)
Proteus mirabilis
Proteus vulgaris
Morganella morganii (formerly *P. morganii*)
Providencia rettgeri (formerly *Proteus rettgeri*)
Providencia stuartii
Citrobacter species*
Enterobacter species
Shigella species*
Pseudomonas aeruginosa (and other species)
Haemophilus influenzae
Haemophilus parainfluenzae
Neisseria species

Many strains of *Serratia, Salmonella**, and *Acinetobacter** are also susceptible.

Gram-positive bacteria

Staphylococcus aureus (non-penicillinase producing strains)
Beta-hemolytic *streptococci* (Groups A and B)
Streptococcus pneumoniae (formerly *Diplococcus pneumoniae*)
Streptococcus faecalis (enterococcus)

Anaerobic Organisms

Peptococcus species
Peptostreptococcus species
Clostridium species*
Bacteroides species (including *B. fragilis* group)
Fusobacterium species*
Veillonella species*
Eubacterium species*

*Mezlocillin has been shown to be active *in vitro* against these organisms, however clinical efficacy has not yet been established.

Noteworthy is mezlocillin's broadened spectrum of *in vitro* activity against important pathogenic aerobic gram-negative bacteria, including strains of *Pseudomonas, Klebsiella, Enterobacter, Serratia, Proteus, Escherichia* and *Haemophilus*, as well as *Bacteroides* and other anaerobes; and its excellent inhibitory effect against gram-positive organisms including *Streptococcus faecalis* (enterococcus). It is inactive against penicillinase-producing strains of *Staphylococcus aureus*.

In vitro studies have shown that mezlocillin combined with an aminoglycoside (e.g., gentamicin, tobramycin, amikacin, sisomicin) acts synergistically against strains of *Streptococcus faecalis* and *Pseudomonas aeruginosa*. In some instances, this combination also acts synergistically *in vitro* against other gram-negative bacteria such as *Serratia, Klebsiella* and *Acinetobacter* species.

Mezlocillin is slightly more active when tested at alkaline pH and, as with other penicillins, has reduced activity when tested *in vitro* with increasing inoculum. The minimum bactericidal concentration (MBC) generally exceeds the minimum inhibitory concentration (MIC) by a factor of 2 or 3. Resistance to mezlocillin *in vitro* develops slowly (multiple step mutation). Some strains of *Pseudomonas aeruginosa* have developed resistance fairly rapidly. Mezlocillin is not stable in the presence of penicillinase and strains of *Staphylococcus aureus* resistant to penicillin are also resistant to mezlocillin.

Susceptibility Tests

Quantitative methods that require measurement of zone diameters give good estimates of bacterial susceptibility. One such procedure* has been recommended for use with discs to test susceptibility to antimicrobials. When the causative organism is tested by the Kirby-Bauer method of disc susceptibility, a 75 mcg mezlocillin disc should give a zone of 18 mm or greater to indicate susceptibility. Zone sizes of 14 mm or less indicate resistance. Zone sizes of 15 to 17 mm indicate intermediate susceptibility. Susceptible strains of *Haemophilus* and *Neisseria* species give zones of ≥ 29 mm resistant strains ≤ 28 mm. With this procedure, a report from the laboratory of "Susceptible" indicates that the infecting organism is likely to respond to therapy. A report of "Resistant" indicates that the infecting organism is not likely to respond to therapy; other therapy should be selected. A report of "Intermediate Susceptibility" suggests that the organism may be susceptible if the infection is confined to tissues and fluids (e.g., urine), in which high antibiotic levels are attained. The mezlocillin disc should be used for testing susceptibility to mezlocillin. In certain conditions, it may be desirable to do additional susceptibility testing by broth or agar dilution techniques. Dilution methods, preferably the agar plate dilution procedure, are most accurate for susceptibility testing of obligate anaerobes. *Enterobacteriaceae Pseudomonas* species and *Acinetobacter* species are considered susceptible if the MIC of mezlocillin is no greater than 64 mcg/ml and are considered resistant if the MIC is greater than 128 mcg/ml. *Haemophilus* species and *Neisseria* species considered susceptible if the MIC of mezlocillin is less than or equal to 1 mcg/ml. Mezlocillin standard is available for broth or agar dilution studies.

*Bauer, A.W., Kirby, W.M., Sherris, J.C. and Turck, M.: Antibiotic Testing by a Standardized Single Disc Method, Am. J. Clin. Pathol., 45:493, 1966. Standardized Disc Susceptibility Test, FEDERAL REGISTER 39: 19182-19184, 1974.

Indications and Usage: MEZLIN® is indicated for the treatment of serious infections caused by susceptible strains of the designated microorganisms in the conditions listed below:

LOWER RESPIRATORY TRACT INFECTIONS including pneumonia and lung abscess caused by *Haemophilus influenzae, Klebsiella* species including *K. pneumoniae, Proteus mirabilis, Pseudomonas* species including *P. aeruginosa, E. Coli,* and *Baceroides* species including *B. fragilis*.

INTRA-ABDOMINAL INFECTIONS including acute cholecystitis, cholangitis, peritonitis, he-

MEZLOCILLIN SERUM LEVELS IN ADULTS (mcg/ml) 30 MIN IV INFUSION

DOSE	0	5 min	15 min	30 min	45 min	1 hr	2 hr	3 hr	4 hr	6 hr	8 hr
3g	263 (87–489)	170 (63–371)	141 (75–301)	109 (56–288)	79 (41–135)	57 (28–100)	26 (14–55)	12 (5.8–26)	4.4 (2.2–6.5)	1.6 (1.0–3.4)	<1

Miles Pharm.—Cont.

patic abscess and intra-abdominal abscess caused by susceptible *E. coli, Proteus mirabilis, Klebsiella* species, *Pseudomonas* species, *S. faecalis (enterococcus), Bacteroides* species, *Peptococcus* species, and *Peptostreptococcus* species.

URINARY TRACT INFECTIONS caused by susceptible *E. coli, Proteus mirabilis,* the indole positive *Proteus* species, *Morganella morganii; Klebsiella* species, *Enterobacter* species, *Serratia* species, *Pseudomonas* species *S. faecalis* (enterococcus).
Uncomplicated gonorrhea due to susceptible *Neisseria gonorrhoeae.*

GYNECOLOGICAL INFECTIONS including endometritis, pelvic cellulitis, and pelvic inflammatory disease associated with susceptible *Neisseria gonorrhoeae, Peptococcus* species, *Peptostreptococcus* species, *Bacteroides* species, *E. coli, Proteus mirabilis, Klebsiella* species, and *Enterobacter* species.

SKIN AND SKIN STRUCTURE INFECTIONS caused by susceptible *S. faecalis* (enterococcus), *E. coli, Proteus mirabilis,* the indole positive *Proteus* species, *Proteus vulgaris,* and *Providencia rettgeri; Klebsiella* species, *Enterobacter* species, *Pseudomonas* species, *Peptococcus* species, and *Bacteroides* species.

SEPTICEMIA including bacteremia caused by susceptible *E. coli, Klebsiella* species, *Enterobacter* species, *Pseudomonas* species, *Bacteroides* species, and *Peptoccocus* species.

Mezlocillin has also been shown to be effective for the treatment of infections caused by *Streptococcus* species including Group A Beta-hemolytic *Streptococcus* and *Streptococcus pneumoniae* (formerly *Diplococcus pneumoniae*) however, infections caused by these organisms are ordinarily treated with more narrow spectrum penicillins.

Appropriate culture and susceptibility tests should be performed before treatment in order to isolate and identify organisms causing infection and to determine their susceptibility to mezlocillin Therapy with MEZLIN® may be initiated before results of these tests are known, once results become available, appropriate therapy should be continued.

Mezlocillin's broad spectrum of activity makes it particularly useful for treating mixed infections caused by susceptible strains of both gram-negative and gram-positive aerobic or anaerobic bacteria. It is not effective, however, against infections caused by penicillinase-producing *Staphylococcus-aureus.*

In certain severe infections, when the causative organisms are unknown, MEZLIN® may be administered in conjunction with an aminoglycoside or a cephalosporin antibiotic as initial therapy. As soon as results of culture and susceptibility tests become available, antimicrobial therapy should be adjusted if indicated. Culture and sensitivity testing, performed periodically during therapy, will provide information on the therapeutic effect of the antimicrobal and will monitor for the possible emergence of bacterial resistance.

MEZLIN® has been used effectively in combination with an aminoglycoside antibiotic for the treatment of life-threatening infections caused by *Pseudomonas aeruginosa.* For the treatment of febrile episodes in immunosuppressed patients with granulocytopenia. MEZLIN® should be combined with an aminoglycoside or a cephalosporin antibiotic.

Contraindications: MEZLIN® is contraindicated in patients with a history of hypersensitivity reactions to any of the penicillins.

Warnings: Serious and occasionally fatal hypersensitivity (anaphylactic) reactions have occurred in patients receiving a penicillin. These reactions are more apt to occur in individuals with a history of sensitivity to multiple allergens. There have been reports of individuals with a history of penicillin hypersensitivity reactions who have experienced severe hypersensitivity reactions when treated with a cephalosporin. Before therapy with mezlocillin is instituted, careful inquiry should be made to determine whether the patient has had previous hypersensitivity reactions to penicillins, cephalosporins or other drugs. Antibiotics should be used with caution in any patient who has demonstrated some form of allergy, particularly to drugs.

If an allergic reaction occurs during therapy with mezlocillin, the drug should be discontinued. SERIOUS ANAPHYLACTOID REACTIONS REQUIRE IMMEDIATE EMERGENCY TREATMENT WITH EPINEPHRINE, OXYGEN, INTRAVENOUS STERIODS, AND AIRWAY MANAGEMENT, INCLUDING INTUBATION, SHOULD ALSO BE PROVIDED AS INDICATED.

Precautions: Although MEZLIN™ shares with other pencillins the low potential for toxicity as with any potent drug, periodic assessment of organ system functions, including renal hepatic and hematopoietic, is advisable during prolonged therapy.

Bleeding manifestations have occurred in some patients receiving beta-lactam antibiotics. These reactions have been associated with abnormalities of coagulation tests such as clotting time, platelet aggregation and prothrombin time and are more likely to occur in patients with renal impairment. Although MEZLIN® has rarely been associated with any bleeding abnormalities, the possibility of this occurring should be kept in mind, particularly in patients with severe renal impairment receiving maximum doses of the drug.

MEZLIN® has only rarely been reported to cause hypokalemia, however, the possibility of this occurring should also be kept in mind particularly when treating patients with fluid and electrolyte imbalance. Periodic monitoring of serum potassium may be advisable in patients receiving prolonged therapy.

MEZLIN® is a monosodium salt containing only 42.6 mg (1.85 mEq) of sodium per gram of mezlocillin. This should be considered when treating patients requiring restricted salt intake.

As with any penicillin, an allergic reaction, including anaphylaxis, may occur during MEZLIN® administration, particularly in a hypersensitive individual.

As with other antibiotics prolonged use of MEZLIN® may result in overgrowth of non-susceptible organisms. If this occurs, appropriate measures should be taken.

Antimicrobials used in high doses for short periods to treat gonorrhea may mask or delay the symptoms of incubating syphilis. Therefore, prior to treatment, patients with gonorrhea should also be evaluated for syphillis. Specimens for dark field examination should be obtained from any suspected primary lesion and serologic tests should be performed. Patients treated with MEZLIN® should undergo follow-up serologic tests three months after therapy.

Interactions with Drugs and Laboratory Tests
As with other penicillins, the mixing of mezlocillins with a aminoglycoside in solutions for parenteral administration can result in substantial inactivation of the aminoglycoside.

Probenecid interferes with the renal tubular secretion of mezlocillin, therby increasing serum concentrations and prolonging serum half-life of the antibiotic.

High urine concentrations of mezlocillin may produce false positive protein reactions (pseudoproteinuria) with the following methods sulfosalicyclic acid and boiling test, acetic acid test, biuret reaction, and nitric acid test. The bromphenol blue (Multi-stix®) reagent strip test has been reported to be reliable.

Pregnancy Category B
Reproduction studies have been performed in rats and mice at doses up to 2 times the human dose, and have revealed no evidence of impaired fertility or harm to the fetus, due to MEZLIN®. There are however no adequate and well controlled studies in pregnant women. Because animal reproductive studies are not always predictive of human response, this drug should be used during pregnancy only if clearly needed. Mezlocillin crosses the placenta and is found in low concentrations in cord blood and amniotic fluid.

Nursing Mothers
Mezlocillin is detected in low concentrations in the milk of nursing mothers, therefore caution should be exercised when MEZLIN® is administered to a nursing woman.

Adverse Reactions: As with other penicillins, the following adverse reactions may occur.
Hypersensitivity reactions: skin rash, pruritus, urticaria, drug fever, and anaphylactic reactions.
Gastro-intestinal distrubances: abnormal taste sensation, nausea, vomiting and diarrhea.
Hemic and Lymphatic Systems: thrombocytopenia, leukopenia, neutropenia, eosinophilia and reduction of hemoglobin or hematocrit.
Abnormalities of hepatic and renal function tests: elevation of serum aspartate aminotransferase (SGOT), serum alanine aminotransferase (SGPT), serum alkaline phosphatase, serum bilirubin. Elevation of serum creatinine and/or BUN. Reduction in serum potassium.
Central nervous system: convulsive seizures or neuromuscular hyperirritability
Local reactions: thrombophlebitis with intravenous administration, pain with intramsucular injection.

Overdosage: As with other penicillins, MEZLIN® in overdosage has the potential to cause neuromusuclar hyperirritability or convulsive seizures. Hemodialysis, if necessary, will aid in removal of the drug from the blood.

Dosage and Administration: MEZLIN® (sterile mezlocillin sodium) may be administered intravenously or intramuscularly. For serious infections, the intravenous route of administration should be used. Intramuscular doses should not exceed 2g per injection.

The recommended adult dosage for serious infections is 200-300 mg/kg per day given in 4 to 6 divided doses. The usual dose is 3g given every 4 hours (18g/day) or 4g given every 6 hours (16g/day). For life-threatening infections, up to 350 mg/kg per day may be administered, but the total daily dosage should ordinarily not exceed 24g.

[See table below].

For patients with life-threatening infections, 4g may be administered every 4 hours (24g/day).
Dosage for any individual patient must take into consideration the site and severity of infection, the susceptibility of the organisms causing infection, and the status of the patient's host defense mechanism.

The duration of therapy depends upon the severity

MEZLIN® DOSAGE GUIDE (ADULTS)

Condition	Daily Dosage Range	Usual Daily Dosage	Frequency and Route of Administration
Urinary tract infection (uncomplicated)	100–125 mg/kg	6-8g	1.5–2g every 6 hours IV or IM
Urinary tract infection (complicated)	150–200 mg/kg	12g	3g every 6 hours IV
Lower respiratory tract infection			
Intra-abdominal infection			4g every 6 hours or
Gynecological infection	225–300 mg/kg	16–18g	3g every 4 hours
Skin & skin structure infection			IV
Septicemia			

MEZLIN® DOSAGE GUIDE FOR PATIENTS WITH IMPAIRED RENAL FUNCTION

Creatinine Clearance ml/min	Urinary Tract Infection (Uncomplicated)	Urinary Tract Infection (Complicated)	Serious Systemic Infection
> 30	Usual Recommended Dosage		
10–30	1.5g every 8 hours	1.5g every 6 hours	3g every 8 hours
< 10	1.5g every 8 hours	1.5g every 8 hours	2g every 8 hours

of infection. Generally, MEZLIN® should be continued for at least 2 days after the signs and symptoms of infection have disappeared. The usual duration is 7 to 10 days; however, in difficult and complicated infections, more prolonged therapy may be required. Antibiotic therapy for Group A beta-hemolytic streptococcal infections should be maintained for at least 10 days to reduce the risk of rheumatic fever or glomerulonephritis.

In certain deep-seated infections, involving abscess formation, appropriate surgical drainage should be performed in conjunction with antimicrobial therapy.

For acute, uncomplicated gonococcal urethritis, the usual dose is 1–2g given once intravenously or by intramuscular injection. Probenecid 1g may be given orally at the time of dosing or up to ½-hour before. (For full prescribing information, refer to probenecid package insert.)

Patients with Impaired Renal Function
The rate of elimination of mezlocillin is dose dependent and related to the degree of renal function impairment. After an intravenous dose of 3g. the serum half-life is approximately 1 hour in patients with creatinine clearances above 60 ml/min, 1.3 hr in those with clearances of 30–59 ml/min, 1.6 hr in those with clearances of 10–29 ml/min and approximately 3.6 hr in patients with clearances of less than 10 ml/min. Dosage adjustments of MEZLIN® are not required in patients with mild impairment of renal function. For patients with a creatinine clearance of ≤ 30 ml/min (serum creatinine of approximately 3.0 mg% or greater), the following dosage guide may be used. (See above)

For life-threatening infections, 3g may be given every 6 hours to patients with creatinine clearances between 10–30 ml/min and 2g every 6 hours to those with clearances less than 10 ml/min.

For patients with serious systemic infection undergoing hemodialysis for renal failure, 3-4g may be administered after each dialysis and then every 12 hours. Patients undergoing peritoneal dialysis may receive 3g every 12 hours.

For patients with renal failure and hepatic insufficiency, measurement of serum levels of mezlocillin will provide additional guidance for adjusting dosage.

Intravenous Administration
MEZLIN® may be administered intravenously by intermittent infusion or by direct intravenous injection.

Infusion. Each gram of mezlocillin should be reconstituted by vigorous shaking with at least 10 ml of Sterile Water for Injection, 5% Dextrose Injection or 0.9% Sodium Chloride Injection. The dissolved drug should be further diluted to desired volume (50-100 ml) with an appropriate intravenous solution (See Compatibility and Stability section). The solution of reconstituted drug may then be administered over a period of 30 minutes by direct infusion or through a Y-type intravenous infusion set which may already be in place. If this method or the "piggyback" method of administration is used, it is advisable to discontinue temporarily the administration of any other solutions during the infusion of MEZLIN®.

Injection. The reconstituted solution of MEZLIN® may also be injected directly into a vein or into intravenous tubing, when administered this way, the injection should be given slowly over a period of 3–5 minutes. To minimize venous irritation, the concentration of drug should not exceed 10%.

When MEZLIN® is given in combination with another antimicrobial, such as an aminoglycoside, each drug should be given separately in accordance with the recommended dosage and routes of administration for each drug.

Intramuscular Administration
Each gram of mezlocillin may be reconstituted by vigorous shaking with 3-4 ml of sterile water for injection or with 3-4 ml of 0.5 or 1.0% lidocaine hydrochloride solution (without epinephrine). (For Full prescribing information, refer to lidocaine package insert). Intramuscular doses of MEZLIN® should not exceed 2g per injection.

As with all intramuscular preparations, MEZLIN® should be injected well within the body of a relatively large muscle, such as the upper outer quadrant of the buttock (i.e., gluteus maximus), aspiration will help avoid unintentional injection into a blood vesel. Slow injection (12-15 sec) will minimize the discomfort associated with intramuscular administration.

Infants and Children
Only limited data are available on the safety and effectiveness of MEZLIN® in the treatment of infants and children with documented serious infection. In the event a child has an infection for which MEZLIN® may be judged particularly appropriate, the following dosage guide may be used:

[See table below].

For infants beyond one month of age and children up to the age of 12 years, 50 mg/kg may be administered every 4 hours (300 mg/kg/day).

The drug may be infused intravenously over 30-minutes or be given by intramuscular injection.

Compatibility and Stability: MEZLIN® at concentrations of 10 mg/ml and 100 mg/ml is stable (loss of potency less than 10%) in the following intravenous solutions for the time periods stated. [See table on next page].

If precipitation should occur under refrigeration, the product should be warmed to 37°C for 20 minutes in a water bath and shaken well.

*This solution is stable from 10 mg/ml to 50 mg/ml under refrigeration.

MEZLIN® at concentrations up to 250 mg/ml is stable for 24 hours at room temperature in the following diluents
  Sterile Water for Injection, USP
  0.9% Sodium Chloride Injection, USP
  0.5% and 1.0% Lidocaine Hydrochloride solution (without epinephrine)

MEZLIN® is stable for up to 28 days when frozen at - 12 C at concentrations up to 100 mg/ml in the following diluents.
  Sterile Water for Injection, USP
  0.9% Sodium Chloride Injection, USP or 5% Dextrose Injection, USP

How Supplied: MEZLIN® (sterile mezolin sodium) is a white to pale yellow crystalline powder supplied in vials and infusion bottles.

Each vial contains mezlocillin sodium equivalent to 1g, 2g, 3g or 4g mezlocillin. Each infusion bottle contains mezlocillin sodium equivalent to 2g, 3g or 4g mezlocillin.

MEZLIN® vials and infusion bottles should be stored at or below 30°C (86°F). The powder as well as the reconstituted solution of drug may darken slightly, depending upon storage conditions, but potency is not affected.

Miles Pharmaceuticals
Division of Miles Laboratories, Inc.
West Haven, Connecticut 06516 USA

MITHRACIN®
(plicamycin)
FOR INTRAVENOUS USE

Warning: IT IS RECOMMENDED THAT MITHRACIN (plicamycin) BE ADMINISTERED ONLY TO HOSPITALIZED PATIENTS BY OR UNDER THE SUPERVISION OF A QUALIFIED PHYSICIAN WHO IS EXPERIENCED IN THE USE OF CANCER CHEMOTHERAPEUTIC AGENTS, BECAUSE OF THE POSSIBILITY OF SEVERE REACTIONS. FACILITIES FOR THE DETERMINATION OF NECESSARY LABORATORY STUDIES MUST BE AVAILABLE.

SEVERE THROMBOCYTOPENIA, A HEMORRHAGIC TENDENCY AND EVEN DEATH MAY RESULT FROM THE USE OF MITHRACIN. ALTHOUGH SEVERE TOXICITY IS MORE APT TO OCCUR IN PATIENTS WHO HAVE FAR-ADVANCED DISEASE OR ARE OTHERWISE CONSIDERED POOR RISKS FOR THERAPY, SERIOUS TOXICITY MAY ALSO OCCASIONALLY OCCUR EVEN IN PATIENTS WHO ARE IN RELATIVELY GOOD CONDITION.

IN THE TREATMENT OF EACH PATIENT, THE PHYSICIAN MUST WEIGH CAREFULLY THE POSSIBILITY OF ACHIEVING THERAPEUTIC BENEFIT VERSUS THE RISK OF TOXICITY WHICH MAY OCCUR WITH MITHRACIN THERAPY. THE FOLLOWING DATA CONCERNING THE USE OF MITHRACIN IN THE TREATMENT OF TESTICULAR TUMORS, HYPERCALCEMIC AND/OR HYPERCALCIURIC CONDITIONS ASSOCIATED WITH VARIOUS ADVANCED MALIGNANCIES, SHOULD BE THOROUGHLY REVIEWED BEFORE ADMINISTERING THIS COMPOUND.

Description: Mithracin is a yellow crystalline compound which is produced by a microorganism, *Streptomyces plicatus*. It has an empirical formula of $C_{52}H_{75}O_{24}$.

Actions: Although the exact mechanism by which Mithracin causes tumor inhibition is not yet known, studies have indicated that this compound forms a complex with deoxyribonucleic acid (DNA) and inhibits cellular ribonucleic acid (RNA) and enzymic RNA synthesis. The binding of Mithracin to DNA in the presence of Mg^{11} (or other divalent cations) is responsible for the inhibition of DNA-dependent or DNA-directed RNA synthesis. This action presumably accounts for the biological properties of Mithracin.

MEZLIN® DOSAGE GUIDE (NEWBORNS)

BODY WEIGHT (gm)	AGE ≤7 DAYS	AGE >7 DAYS
≤ 2000	75 mg/kg every 12 hours (150 mg/kg/day)	75 mg/kg every 8 hours (225 mg/kg/day)
> 2000	75 mg/kg every 12 hours (150 mg/kg/day)	75 mg/kg every 6 hours (300 mg/kg/day)

Continued on next page

Miles Pharm.—Cont.

Mithracin shows potent cytotoxicity against malignant cells of human origin (Hela cells) growing in tissue culture. Mithracin is lethal to Hela cells in 48 hours at concentrations as low as 0.5 micrograms per milliliter of tissue culture medium. Mithracin has shown significant anti-tumor activity against experimental leukemia in mice when administered intraperitoneally.

Indications: Mithracin is a potent antineoplastic agent which has been shown to be useful in the treatment of carefully selected hospitalized patients with malignant tumors of the testis in whom successful treatment by surgery and/or radiation is impossible. Also, on the basis of limited clinical experience to date, it may be considered in the treatment of certain symptomatic patients with hypercalcemia and hypercalciuria associated with a variety of advanced neoplasms.

The use of Mithracin in other types of neoplastic disease is not recommended at the present time.

Contraindications: Mithracin (plicamycin) is contraindicated in patients with thrombocytopenia, thrombocytopathy, coagulation disorder or an increased susceptibility to bleeding due to other causes. Mithracin should not be administered to any patient with impairment of bone marrow function.

Mithracin should not be used in the treatment of patients who are not hospitalized and who cannot be observed carefully and frequently during and after therapy, or whenever appropriate laboratory facilities are unavailable.

Precautions: Mithracin should be administered only to patients who are hospitalized and who can be observed carefully and frequently during and after therapy.

Severe thrombocytopenia, a hemorrhagic tendency and even death may result from the use of Mithracin. Although severe toxicity is more apt to occur in patients who have far-advanced disease or are otherwise considered poor risks for therapy, serious toxicity may also occasionally occur even in patients who are in relatively good condition. Electrolyte imbalance, especially hypocalcemia, hypokalemia, and hypophosphatemia, should be corrected with appropriate electrolyte therapy prior to treatment with Mithracin.

Mithracin should be used with extreme caution in patients with significant impairment of renal or hepatic function.

In the treatment of each patient, the physician must weigh carefully the possiblity of achieving therapeutic benefit versus the risk of toxicity which may occur with Mithracin therapy. The following laboratory studies should be obtained frequently during therapy and for several days following the last dose: platelet count, prothrombin time, bleeding time. The occurrence of thrombocytopenia or a significant prolongation of prothrombin time or bleeding time is an indication for the termination of therapy.

Adverse Reactions: THE MOST IMPORTANT FORM OF TOXICITY ASSOCIATED WITH THE USE OF MITHRACIN CONSISTS OF A BLEEDING SYNDROME WHICH USUALLY BEGINS WITH AN EPISODE OF EPISTAXIS. This bleeding tendency may only consist of a single or several episodes of epistaxis and progress no further. However, in some cases, this hemorrhagic syndrome can start with an episode of hematemesis which may progress to more wide-spread hemorrhage in the gastrointestinal tract or to a more generalized bleeding tendency. This hemorrhagic diathesis is most likely due to abnormalities in multiple clotting factors.

A detailed analysis of the clinical data in 1,160 patients treated with Mithracin indicates that the hemorrhagic syndrome is dose related. With doses of 30 mcg/kg/day or less for 10 or fewer doses, the incidence of bleeding episodes has been 5.4% with an associated drug-related mortality rate of 1.6%. With doses greater than 30 mcg/kg/day and/or for more than 10 doses, a significantly larger number of bleeding episodes occurred (11.9%) and the associated drug-related mortality rate was also significantly higher (5.7%).

The most common side effects reported with the use of Mithracin consist of gastrointestinal symptoms: anorexia, nausea, vomiting, diarrhea, and stomatitis. Other less frequently reported side effects include fever, drowsiness, weakness, lethargy, malaise, headache, depression, phlebitis, facial flushing, and skin rash.

The following laboratory abnormalities have been reported during therapy with Mithracin (plicamycin) and in most instances were reversible following cessation of treatment:

Hematologic Abnormalities: Depression of platelet count, white count, hemoglobin and prothrombin content; elevation of clotting time and bleeding time; abnormal clot retraction.

Thrombocytopenia may be rapid in onset and may occur at any time during therapy or within several days following the last dose. With the occurrence of severe thrombocytopenia, the infusion of platelet concentrates or platelet-rich plasma may be helpful in elevating the platelet count.

The occurrence of leukopenia with the use of Mithracin is relatively uncommon, occurring only in approximately 6% of patients.

It has been uncommon for abnormalities in clotting time or clot retraction to be demonstrated prior to the onset of an overt bleeding episode noted in some patients treated with Mithracin. Nevertheless, the performance of these tests periodically is recommended because in a few instances, an abnormality in one of these studies may have served as a warning to terminate therapy because of impeding serious toxicity.

Abnormal Liver Function Tests: Increased levels of serum glutamic oxalacetic transaminase, serum glutamic pyruvic transaminase, lactic dehydrogenase, alkaline phosphatase, serum bilirubin, ornithine carbamyl transferase, isocitric dehydrogenase, and increased retention of bromsulphalein.

Abnormal Renal Function Tests: Increased blood urea nitrogen and serum creatinine; proteinuria.

Abnormalities in Electrolyte Concentrations: Depression of serum calcium, phosphorus, and potassium.

Dosage: The daily dose of Mithracin is based on the patient's body weight. If a patient has abnormal fluid retention such as edema, hydrothorax or ascites, the patient's ideal weight rather than actual body weight should be used to calculate the dose.

Treatment of Testicular Tumors: In the treatment of patients with testicular tumors the recommended daily dose of Mithracin (plicamycin) is 25 to 30 micrograms per kilogram of body weight. Therapy should be continued for a period of 8 to 10 days unless significant side effects or toxicity occur during therapy. A course of therapy consisting of more than 10 daily doses is not recommended. Individual daily doses should not exceed 30 micrograms per kilogram of body weight.

In those patients with responsive tumors, some degree of tumor regression is usually evident within 3 or 4 weeks following the initial course of therapy. If tumor masses remain unchanged following an initial course of therapy, additional courses of therapy at monthly intervals are warranted.

When a significant tumor regression is obtained, it is suggested that additional courses of therapy be given at monthly intervals until a complete regression of tumor masses is achieved or until definite tumor progression or new tumor masses occur in spite of continued courses of therapy.

Treatment of Hypercalcemia and Hypercalciuria: Reversal of hypercalcemia and hypercalciuria can usually be achieved with Mithracin at doses considerably lower than those recommended for use in the treatment of testicular tumors.

In hypercalcemia and hypercalciuria associated with advanced malignancy the recommended course of treatment with Mithracin is 25 micrograms per kilogram of body weight per day for 3 or 4 days.

If the desired degree of reversal of hypercalcemia or hypercalciuria is not achieved with the initial course of therapy, additional courses of therapy may then be administered at intervals of one week or more to achieve the desired result or to maintain serum calcium and urinary calcium excretion at normal levels. It may be possible to maintain normal calcium balance with single, weekly doses or with a schedule of 2 or 3 doses per week.

NOTE: BECAUSE OF THE DRUG'S TOXICITY AND THE LIMITED CLINICAL EXPERIENCE TO DATE IN THESE INDICATIONS, THE FOLLOWING RECOMMENDATIONS SHOULD BE KEPT IN MIND BY THE PHYSICIAN.

1. **CONSIDER CASES OF HYPERCALCEMIA AND HYPERCALCIURIA NOT RESPONSIVE TO CONVENTIONAL TREATMENT.**
2. **APPLY SAME CONTRAINDICATIONS AND PRECAUTIONARY MEASURES AS IN ANTITUMOR TREATMENT.**
3. **RENAL FUNCTION SHOULD BE CAREFULLY MONITORED BEFORE, DURING, AND AFTER TREATMENT.**
4. **BENEFITS OF USE DURING PREGNANCY OR IN WOMEN OF CHILDBEARING AGE SHOULD BE WEIGHED AGAINST POTENTIAL TOXICITY TO EMBRYO OR FETUS.**

Administration: By IV administration only. The appropriate daily dose of Mithracin should be diluted in one liter of 5% Dextrose Injection, USP or Sodium Chloride Injection, USP and administered by slow intravenous infusion over a period of 4 to 6 hours. Rapid direct intravenous injection of Mithracin should be avoided as it may be associated with a higher incidence and greater severity of gastrointestinal side effects. Extravasation of solutions of Mithracin may cause local irritation and cellulitis at injection sites. Should thrombophlebitis or perivascular cellulitis occur, the infusion should be terminated and reinstituted at another site. The application of moderate heat to the site of extravasation may help to disperse the compound and minimize discomfort and local tissue irritation. The use of antiemetic compounds prior to and during treatment with Mithracin may be helpful in relieving nausea and vomiting.

How Supplied: Mithracin is available in vials as a freeze-dried preparation for intravenous administration. Each vial contains 2500 mcg of Mithracin with 100 mg of mannitol and sufficient disodium phosphate to adjust to pH 7. These vials should be stored at refrigerator temperatures between 2°C. to 8°C. (36°F. to 46°F.).

MEZLIN

STABILITY

INTRAVENOUS SOLUTION	Controlled Room Temperature	Refrigeration
Sterile Water for Injection, USP	48 hours	7 days
0.9% Sodium Chloride Injection, USP	48 hours	7 days
5% Dextrose Injection, USP	48 hours	7 days
5% Dextrose in 0.225% Sodium Chloride Injection, USP	72 hours	7 days
Lactated Ringer's Injection, USP	72 hours	7 days
5% Dextrose in Electrolyte #75 Injection	72 hours	7 days
5% Dextrose in 0.45% Sodium Chloride Injection, USP	48 hours	48 hours
Ringers Injection	24 hours	24 hours
10% Dextrose Injection	24 hours	24 hours
5% Fructose Injection	24 hours	24 hours

MITHRACIN

RESULTS IN 305 TESTICULAR TUMOR CASES BY TUMOR TYPE

TYPE OF TESTICULAR TUMOR	TOTAL	COMPLETE RESPONSE	PARTIAL RESPONSE	NO RESPONSE
EMBRYONAL CELL	173	26	42	105
TERATOMA	5	0	1	4
TERATOCARCINOMA	23	0	5	18
SEMINOMA	18	0	7	11
CHORIOCARCINOMA	13	1	6	6
MIXED TUMOR	73	6	19	48
TOTALS	305	33	80	192

To reconstitute, add aseptically 4.9 ml of Sterile Water for Injection to the contents of the vial and shake to dissolve. Each ml of the resulting solution will then contain 500 mcg of Mithracin. AFTER REMOVAL OF THE APPROPRIATE DOSE, THE REMAINING UNUSED SOLUTION MUST BE DISCARDED, FRESH SOLUTIONS MUST BE PREPARED IN THE ABOVE MANNER EACH DAY OF THERAPY.

Pharmacology and Toxicology: In mice the average intravenous LD_{50} of Mithracin is 2,000 mcg/kg of body weight. When administered orally, it is not toxic to mice even at doses 100 times greater than the intravenous LD_{50}. In rats the average intravenous LD_{50} of Mithracin is 1,700 mcg/kg of body weight. It is not toxic to rats when administered orally at doses 17 times greater than the intravenous LD_{50}. In dogs and monkeys Mithracin is essentially non-toxic when administered intravenously for 24 days at daily doses as high as 50 and 24 mcg/kg of body weight, respectively. However, at higher doses of 100 mcg/kg/day intravenously it is lethal to dogs and monkeys. Signs of toxicity in dogs and monkeys included anorexia, vomiting, listlessness, melena, anemia, lymphopenia, elevated alkaline phosphatase, serum glutamic oxalacetic transaminase, serum glutamic pyruvic transaminase values, hypochloremia, and azotemia. Dogs also showed marked thrombocytopenia, hyponatremia, hypokalemia, hypocalcemia, and decreased prothrombin consumption. Necropsy findings consisted of necrosis of lymphoid tissue and multiple generalized hemorrhages. Mithracin (plicamycin) was only mildly irritating when injected intramuscularly in rabbits and subcutaneously in guinea pigs. Histologic evidence of inhibition of spermatogenesis was observed in a substantial number of male rats receiving doses of 0.6 mg/kg/day and above. This preclinical finding of selective drug effect constituted the scientific rationale for clinical trials in testicular tumors.

Clinical Reports:

Treatment of Patients with Inoperable Testicular Tumors: In a combined series of 305 patients with inoperable testicular tumors treated with Mithracin, 33 patients (10.8%) showed a complete disappearance of tumor masses and an additional 80 patients (26.2%) responded with significant partial regression of tumor masses. The longest duration of a continuing complete response is now over 8½ years. The therapeutic responses in this series of patients have been summarized by type of testicular tumor in the accompanying table. [See table above].

Mithracin may be useful in the treatment of patients with testicular tumors which are resistant to other chemotherapeutic agents. Prior radiation therapy or prior chemotherapy did not alter the response rate with Mithracin. This suggests that there is no significant cross resistance between Mithracin (plicamycin) and other chemotherapeutic agents.

Treatment of Patients with Hypercalcemia and Hypercalciuria: A limited number of patients with hypercalcemia (range: 12.0–25.8 mg%) and patients with hypercalciuria (range 215–492 mg/day) associated with malignant disease were treated with Mithracin. Hypercalcemia and hypercalciuria were promptly reversed in all patients. In some patients, the primary malignancy was of non-testicular origin.

Manufactured for
Miles Pharmaceuticals
Division of Miles Laboratories, Inc.
West Haven, Connecticut 06516 USA
by Pfizer Laboratories, New York, N.Y. 10017

MYCELEX® 1% ℞
(clotrimazole) cream
For dermatologic use only

Description: Mycelex is clotrimazole [1-(o-Chloro-α, α-diphenylbenzyl) imidazole], a synthetic anti-fungal agent having the chemical formula, $C_{22}H_{17}ClN_2$.

Each gram of Mycelex contains 10 mg clotrimazole in a vanishing cream base of sorbitan monostearate, polysorbate 60, cetyl esters wax, cetostearyl alcohol, 2-octyldodecanol, purified water and, as preservative, benzyl alcohol (1%).

Actions: Clotrimazole is a broad-spectrum, antifungal agent that inhibits the growth of pathogenic dermatophytes, yeasts, and *Malassezia furfur*. Clotrimazole exhibits fungicidal activity in vitro against isolates of *Trichophyton rubrum*, *Trichophyton mentagrophytes*, *Epidermophyton floccosum*, *Microsporum canis*, and *Candida albicans*.

No single-step or multiple-step resistance to clotrimazole has developed during successive passages of *Candida albicans* and *trichophyton mentagrophytes*.

Indications: Mycelex Cream is indicated for the topical treatment of the following dermal infections: tinea pedis, tinea cruris, and tinea corporis due to *Trichophyton rubrum*, *Trichophyton mentagrophytes*, *Epidermophyton folccosum*, and *Microsporum canis*; candidiasis due to *Candida albicans*; and tinea versicolor due to *Malassezia furfur*.

Contraindications: Mycelex Cream is contraindicated in individuals who have shown hypersensitivity to any of its components.

Warnings: Mycelex Cream is not for ophthalmic use.

Precautions: In the first trimester of pregnancy, Mycelex Cream should be used only when considered essential to the welfare of the patient. If irritation or sensitivity develops with the use of Mycelex, treatment should be discontinued and appropriate therapy instituted.

Adverse Reactions: The following adverse reactions have been reported in connection with the use of this product: erythema, stinging, blistering, peeling, edema, pruritus, urticaria, and general irritation of the skin.

Dosage and Administration: Gently massage sufficient Mycelex Cream into the affected and surrounding skin areas twice a day, in the morning and evening.

Clinical improvement, with relief of pruritus, usually occurs within the first week of treatment. If a patient shows no clinical improvement after four weeks of treatment with Mycelex the diagnosis should be reviewed.

How Supplied: Mycelex Cream 1% is supplied in 15, 30 and 2 x 45 gram tubes.
DPSC Stocked:
15 gram—NSN 6505-01-023-5011
30 gram—NSN 6505-01-05-1405
VA Stocked: 15 gram—SN 6505-01-023-5011
30 gram—SN 6505-01-015-1405
Store between 35° and 86° F.
U.S. Patents No. 3,660,577 and 3,705,172.
April, 1981   PD 100504
Copyright © 1980, Miles Pharmaceuticals, Division Miles Laboratories, Inc.

MYCELEX® 1% ℞
(clotrimazole) Solution
For dermatologic use only

Description: Mycelex is clotrimazole [1-(o-Chloro-α, α-diphenylbenzyl) imidazole], a synthetic antifungal agent having the chemical formula $C_{22}H_{17}ClN_2$.

Each ml. of Mycelex Solution contains 10 mg. clotrimazole in a nonaqueous vehicle of polyethylene glycol 400.

Actions: Clotrimazole is a broad-spectrum, antifungal agent that inhibits the growth of pathogenic dermatophytes, yeasts and *Malassezia furfur*. Clotrimazole exhibits fungicidal activity *in vitro* against isolates of *Trichophyton rubrum*, *Trichophyton mentagrophytes*, *Epidermophyton floccosum*, *Microsporum canis*, and *Candida albicans*.

No single-step or multiple-step resistance to clotrimazole has developed during successive passages of *Candida albicans* and *Trichophyton mentagrophytes*.

Indications: Mycelex Solution is indicated for the topical treatment of the following dermal infections: tinea pedis, tinea cruris, and tinea corporis due to *Trichophyton rubum*, *Trichophyton mentagrophytes*, *Epidermophyton floccosum*, and *Microsporum canis*; candidiasis due to *Candida albicans*; and tinea versicolor due to *Malassezia furfur*.

Contraindications: Mycelex Solution is contraindicated in individuals who have shown hypersensitivity to any of its components.

Warnings: Mycelex Solution is not for ophthalmic use.

Precautions: In the first trimester of pregnancy, Mycelex Solution should be used only when considered essential to the welfare of the patient. If irritation or sensitivity develops with the use of Mycelex, treatment should be discontinued and appropriate therapy instituted.

Adverse Reactions: The following adverse reactions have been reported in connection with the use of this product: erythema, stinging, blistering, peeling, edema, pruritus, urticaria, and general irritation of the skin.

Dosage and Administration: Gently massage sufficient Mycelex Solution into the affected and surrounding skin areas twice a day, in the morning and evening.

Clinical improvement, with relief of pruritus, usually occurs within the first week of treatment. If a patient shows no clinical improvement after four weeks of treatment with Mycelex the diagnosis should be reviewed.

How Supplied: Mycelex Solution 1% is supplied in 10 ml. and 30 ml. plastic bottles.
DPSC Stocked: 10 ml—NSN 6505-01-015-1406
VA Stocked: 10 ml—SN 6505-01-015-1406
30 ml—SN 6505-01-016-5675
Store between 35° and 86°F.
U.S. Patents No. 3,660,577 and 3,705,172.
PD100510   November, 1980   17370
Copyright© 1980, Miles Pharmaceuticals, Division of Miles Laboratories, Inc.

MYCELEX® ℞
(clotrimazole)
Troche

Description: Each Mycelex® Troche contains 10 mg clotrimazole [1(o-chloro-α, α-diphenylbenzyl) imidazole], a synthetic antifungal agent, for topical use in the mouth.

Continued on next page

Miles Pharm.—Cont.

Structural Formula:

Chemical Formula:
$C_{22}H_{17}ClN_2$

The troche dosage form is a large, slow-dissolving tablet (lozenge) containing 10 mg of clotrimazole dispersed in dextrose, microcrystalline cellulose, povidone, and magnesium stearate.

Clinical Pharmacology: Clotrimazole is a broad-spectrum antifungal agent that inhibits the growth of pathogenic yeasts by altering the permeability of cell membranes. It exhibits fungicidal activity *in vitro* against *Candida albicans* and other species of the genus *Candida*. No single-step or multiple-step resistance to clotrimazole has developed during successive passages of *Candida albicans* in the laboratory.

After oral administration of a 10 mg clotrimazole troche to healthy volunteers concentrations sufficient to inhibit most species of *Candida* persist in saliva for up to three hours following the approximately 30 minutes needed for a troche to dissolve. The long term effective concentration of drug in saliva appears to be related to the slow release of clotrimazole from the oral mucosa to which the drug is apparently bound. Repetitive dosing at three hour intervals maintains effective salivary levels above the minimum inhibitory concentration of most strains of *Candida*. The amount of drug absorbed has not been measured.

Indications and Usage: Mycelex Troches are indicated for the local treatment of oropharyngeal candidiasis. The diagnosis should be confirmed by a KOH smear and/or culture prior to treatment.

Contraindications: Mycelex Troches are contraindicated in patients who are hypersensitive to any of its components.

Warning: Mycelex Troches are not indicated for the treatment of systemic mycoses.

Precautions: Abnormal liver function tests have been reported in patients treated with clotrimazole troches; elevated SGOT levels were reported in about 15% of patients in the clinical trials. In most cases the elevations were minimal and it was often impossible to distinguish effects of clotrimazole from those of other therapy and the underlying disease (malignancy in most cases). Periodic assessment of hepatic function is advisable particularly in patients with pre-existing hepatic impairment.

Since patients must be instructed to allow each troche to dissolve slowly in the mouth in order to achieve maximum effect of the medication, they must be of such an age and physical and/or mental condition to comprehend such instructions.

Carcinogenesis: An 18 month dosing study with clotrimazole in rats has not revealed any carcinogenic effect.

Usage in Pregnancy: Pregnancy Category C: Clotrimazole has been shown to be embryotoxic in rats and mice when given in doses 100 times the adult human dose (in mg/kg), possibly secondary to maternal toxicity. The drug was not teratogenic in mice, rabbits, and rats when given in doses up to 200, 180, and 100 times the human dose.

Clotrimazole given orally to mice from nine weeks before mating through weaning at a dose 120 times the human dose was associated with impairment of mating, decreased number of viable young, and decreased survival to weaning. No effects were observed at 60 times the human dose. When the drug was given to rats during a similar time period at 50 times the human dose, there was a slight decrease in the number of pups per litter and decreased pup viability.

There are no adequate and well controlled studies in pregnant women. Clotrimazole troches should be used during pregnancy only if the potential benefit justifies the potential risk to the fetus.

Pediatric Use: Safety and effectiveness of clotrimazole in children below the age of 3 years have not been established; therefore, its use in such patients is not recommended.

Adverse Reactions: Abnormal liver function tests have been reported in patients treated with clotrimazole troches; elevated SGOT levels were reported in about 15% of patients in the clinical trials (see **Precautions** section).

Nausea and vomiting was reported in about one in twenty patients.

Overdose: No data available.

Drug Abuse and Dependence: No data available.

Dosage and Administration: Mycelex® Troches are administered only as a lozenge that must be dissolved slowly in the mouth. The recommended dose is one troche five times a day for fourteen consecutive days. Only limited data are available on the safety and effectiveness of the clotrimazole troche after prolonged administration; therefore, therapy should be limited to short term use, if possible.

How Supplied: Mycelex® Troches, white discoid, uncoated tablets are supplied in bottles of 70 and 140. Each tablet will be identified with the following: Miles 095.

Store below 86°F (30°C), avoid freezing.

PD100552   19329   June, 1983

Shown in Product Identification Section, page 422

MYCELEX®-G 1% ℞
(clotrimazole) Vaginal Cream

Description: Mycelex-G is clotrimazole [1-(o-Chloro-α,α-diphenylbenzyl) imidazole], a synthetic antifungal agent having the chemical formula, $C_{22}H_{17}ClN_2$, and following chemical structure:

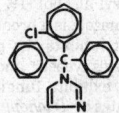

Each applicatorful of Mycelex-G Vaginal Cream contains approximately 50 mg. clotrimazole dispersed in sorbitan monostearate, polysorbate 60, cetyl esters wax, cetostearyl alcohol, 2-octyldodecanol, purified water, and as a preservative, benzyl alcohol (1%).

Actions: Clotrimazole is a broad spectrum antifungal agent that inhibits the growth of pathogenic yeasts. Clotrimazole exhibits fungicidal activity *in vitro* against *Candida albicans* and other species of the genus *Candida*.

No single-step or multiple-step resistance to clotrimazole has developed during successive passages of *Candida albicans*.

Indications: Mycelex-G Vaginal Cream is indicated for the local treatment of patients with vulvovaginal candidiasis (moniliasis). As Mycelex-G Vaginal Cream has been shown to be effective only for candidal vulvovaginitis, the diagnosis should be confirmed by KOH smears and/or cultures. Other pathogens commonly associated with vulvovaginitis (*Trichomonas* and *Hemophilus vaginalis*) should be ruled out by appropriate laboratory methods.

Studies have shown that women taking oral contraceptives had a cure rate similar to those not taking oral contraceptives.

Contraindications: Mycelex-G Vaginal Cream is contraindicated in women who have shown hypersensitivity to any of the components of the preparation.

Precautions: Laboratory Tests: If there is a lack of response to Mycelex-G Vaginal Cream, appropriate microbiological studies should be repeated to confirm the diagnosis and rule out other pathogens before instituting another course of antimycotic therapy.

Usage in Pregnancy: While Mycelex-G Vaginal Cream has not been studied in the first trimester of pregnancy, use in the second and third trimesters has not been associated with ill effects. Application of ^{14}C labeled clotrimazole has shown negligible absorption (peak serum level of 0.01 mcg/ml 24 hours after insertion of vaginal cream containing 50 mg. of active drug) from both normal and inflamed human vaginal mucosa.

Adverse Reactions: Three (0.5%) of the 653 patients treated with Mycelex-G Vaginal Cream reported complaints during therapy that were possibly drug related. Vaginal burning occurred in one patient; erythema, irritation and burning in another; intercurrent cystitis was reported in the third.

Dosage and Administration: Mycelex-G Vaginal Cream has been found to be effective when used from seven to fourteen days; studies have shown that patients treated for fourteen days had a significantly higher cure rate. The recommended dose is one applicatorful a day for seven to fourteen consecutive days; using the applicator supplied, insert one applicatorful of cream (approximately 5 grams) intravaginally preferably at bedtime.

How Supplied: Mycelex-G Vaginal Cream 1% is supplied in 45 and 90 gram tubes with a measured-dose applicator; for seven-day and for fourteen-day treatments.

Store between 35° and 86° F (2° and 30° C).

February, 1981   PD 100526

Copyright © 1980, Miles Pharmaceuticals, Division of Miles Laboratories, Inc.

MYCELEX®-G 100 mg ℞
(clotrimazole) Vaginal Tablets

Description: Mycelex-G is clotrimazole [1-(o-Chloro-α, α-diphenylbenzyl) imidazole], a synthetic antifungal agent having the chemical formula, $C_{22}H_{17}ClN_2$.

Each Mycelex-G Vaginal Tablet contains 100 mg clotrimazole dispersed in lactose, povidone, corn starch and magnesium stearate.

Actions: Clotrimazole is a broad-spectrum antifungal agent that inhibits the growth of pathogenic yeasts. Clotrimazole exhibits fungicidal activity *in vitro* against *Candida albicans* and other species of the genus *Candida*.

No single-step or multiple-step resistance to clotrimazole has developed during successive passages of *Candida albicans*.

Indications: Mycelex-G Vaginal Tablets are indicated for the local treatment of vulvovaginal candidiasis. The diagnosis should be confirmed by KOH smears and/or cultures. Other pathogens commonly associated with vulvovaginitis (*Trichomonas* and *Hemophilus vaginalis*) should be ruled out by appropriate laboratory methods.

Contraindications: Mycelex-G Vaginal Tablets are contraindicated in women who have shown hypersensitivity to any components of the preparation.

Precautions: Laboratory Tests: If there is a lack of response to Mycelex-G Vaginal Tablets, appropriate microbiological studies should be repeated to confirm the diagnosis and rule out other pathogens before instituting another course of antimycotic therapy.

Application of ^{14}C-labeled clotrimazole has shown negligible absorption (peak of 0.03 mcg/ml of serum 24 hours after insertion of a 100 mg tablet) from both normal and inflammed human vaginal mucosa.

Usage in Pregnancy: While Mycelex-G Vaginal Tablets have not been studied in the first trimester of pregnancy, use in the second and third trimesters has not been associated with ill effects. Follow-up reports now available on 71 neonates of 117 pregnant patients reveal no adverse effects or complications attributable to Mycelex-G therapy.

Adverse Reactions: Eighteen (1.6%) of the 1116 patients treated with Mycelex-G in double-blind studies reported complaints during therapy that were possibly drug-related. Mild burning occured in six patients while other complaints, such as skin rash, itching, vulval irritation, lower abdominal cramps and bloating, slight cramping, slight urinary frequency, and burning or irritation in the sexual partner, occurred rarely.

Dosage and Administration: The recommended dose is one tablet a day for seven consecutive days. Recent studies indicate that an alternative regimen of two tablets a day for three consecutive days is similarly effective in non-pregnant patients; however, in pregnant patients the three-day treatment course did not prove to be effective and is therefore not recommended. They should receive the seven-day treatment. Using the applicator supplied, insert one or two tablets intravaginally preferably at bedtime.

In the event of treatment failure, other pathogens commonly responsible for vaginitis should be ruled out before instituting another course of antimycotic therapy. There are no studies to show whether a second course of clotrimazole would be effective in patients who fail to respond to the initial course.

How Supplied: Mycelex-G Vaginal Tablets 100 mg, white, tear-drop-shaped, uncoated tablets coded with number 093-Miles, supplied in a strip of seven tablets with plastic applicator and patient leaflet of instructions.

DPSC Stocked: NSN 6505-01-090-6795
Do not store above 35°C [95°F].
U.S. Patent No. 3,660,577 and 3,705,172
PD100513   November, 1980   17372
Shown in Product Identification Section, page 422

NICLOCIDE®   ℞
(niclosamide)
Chewable Tablets

Description: NICLOCIDE (niclosamide) is an anthelmintic provided in chewable tablet form at a strength of 500 mg per tablet. Niclosamide is 2′,5-Dichloro-4′-nitrosalicylanilide. The empirical formula is $C_{13}H_8Cl_2N_2O_4$ with the following structural formula.

Clinical Pharmacology: NICLOCIDE inhibits oxidative phosphorylation in the mitochondria of cestodes. Both *in vitro* and *in vivo*, the scolex and proximal segments are killed on contact with the drug. The scolex of the tapeworm, loosened from the gut wall, may be digested in the intestine, and thus may not be identified in the feces even after extensive purging.

The use of NICLOCIDE has not been associated with the development of anemia, leukopenia or thrombocytopenia nor have there been any effects on normal renal and hepatic functions.

Indications and Usage: NICLOCIDE (niclosamide) is indicated for the treatment of tapeworm infections by *Taenia saginata* (beef tapeworm), *Diphyllobothrium latum* (fish tapeworm) and *Hymenolepis nana* (dwarf tapeworm).

Contraindications: NICLOCIDE™ Tablets are contraindicated in individuals who have shown hypersensitivity to any of its components.

Precautions: NICLOCIDE affects the cestodes of the intestine only. It is without effect in cysticercosis.

Drug Interactions: No data are available regarding interaction of niclosamide with other drugs.

Carcinogenesis, mutagenesis, impairment of fertility:

Carcinogenetic Potential: Although carcinogenicity studies on niclosamide *per se* have not been done, long-term feeding studies on its ethanolamine salt in rats and mice did not show carcinogenicity. Mutagenicity tests have not been performed.

Pregnancy: Pregnancy Category B: Reproduction studies in rabbits and rats at doses of 25 times the human therapeutic dose and in mice at 12 times the human therapeutic dose, have revealed no evidence of impaired fertility or harm to the fetus due to niclosamide. There are, however, no adequate and well-controlled studies in pregnant women. Because animal studies are not always predictive of human response, the drug should be used during pregnancy only if clearly needed.

Nursing Mothers: No studies are available.

Pediatric Use: In children under 2 years of age, the safety of the drug has not been established.

Adverse Reactions: The incidence of side effects has been reported as follows: nausea/vomiting 4.1%, abdominal discomfort including loss of appetite 3.4%, diarrhea 1.6%, drowsiness, dizziness, and or headache 1.4%, and skin rash including pruritus ani 0.3%. Other side effects listed in decreasing order of frequency were: oral irritation, fever, rectal bleeding, weakness, bad taste in mouth, sweating, palpitations, constipation, alopecia, edema of an arm, backache and irritability. There was also one instance of a transient rise in SGOT in an i.v. narcotic addict. Two cases of urticaria reported may be related to the breakdown products of the tapeworm. All side effects were mild or moderate and transitory and did not necessitate discontinuation of the treatment.

Overdosage: Insufficient data are available. In the event of overdose a fast-acting laxative and enema should be given. Vomiting should not be induced.

Dosage and Administration:
1. *Taenia saginata* and *Diphyllobothrium latum*
   a. Adults: 4 tablets (2.0 g) chewed thoroughly in a single dose.
   b. Children weighing more than 34 kg (75 lbs): 3 tablets (1.5 g) chewed thoroughly in a single dose.
   c. Children weighing between 11 and 34 kg (25 to 75 lbs): 2 tablets (1.0 g) chewed thoroughly in a single dose.
2. *Hymenolepis nana*
   a. Adults: 4 tablets (2.0 g) chewed thoroughly as a single daily dose for 7 days.
   b. Children weighing more than 34 kg (75 lbs): 3 tablets (1.5g) chewed thoroughly on the first day, then 2 tablets (1.0 g) daily for next 6 days.
   c. Children weighing between 11 and 34 kg (25 to 75 lbs): 2 tablets (1.0 g) to be chewed thoroughly on the first day, then one tablet (0.5 g) daily for next 6 days.

   T. saginata and *D. latum* infections are usually due to a single adult worm and require an intermediate host in their life cycle. With *Hymenolepis nana* multiple infections are the rule. No intermediate host is required; both larval and adult stages of the worm may be found in the human intestine where the complete life cycle occurs. Since the drug is more effective against the mature than the larval stage, therapy must be extended over several days to cover all stages of maturation. Patients with *H. nana* must be instructed to observe strict personal and environmental hygiene to avoid autoinfection with this parasite.
3. NICLOCIDE™ must be thoroughly chewed and then swallowed with a little water. No special dietary restrictions are necessary before or after treatment. The best time to take the drug is after a light meal (e.g., breakfast). A mild laxative may be desirable in constipated patients to achieve a normal bowel movement.

   Young children should have the tablets crushed to a fine powder and mixed with a small amount of water to form a paste.
   NICLOCIDE has a vanilla taste which is not unpleasant to most persons.
   NICLOCIDE is suitable for administration on an ambulatory or outpatient basis.
4. Follow-up:
   As the vermicidal action of NICLOCIDE renders the tapeworm, especially the scolex and proximal segments, vulnerable to destruction during their passage through the gut, it is not always possible to identify the scolex in stools. The sooner the tapeworm is passed and examined after treatment, the better the chance of identification of the scolex. Segments and/or ova of beef or fish tapeworm may be present in the stool for up to 3 days after therapy. Persistent *T. saginata* or *D. latum* segments and/or ova on the seventh day post therapy indicate failure. A second identical course of treatment may be given at that time.

   No patient should be considered cured unless the stool has been negative for a minimum of three months.

How Supplied: NICLOCIDE is available as round, light yellow chewable tablets, scored on one side, coded with the word Miles and number 721, each containing 500 mg of niclosamide, and is supplied in boxes of 4 tablets.

Storage Conditions: Store below 86°F (30°C), avoid freezing.

Manufactured: by
Bayvet Division Cutter Laboratories, Inc.
Shawnee, Kansas 66201

Distributed by:
Miles Pharmaceuticals
Division of Miles Laboratories, Inc.
West Haven, Connecticut 06516

April, 1982
Shown in Product Identification Section, page 422

NYSTAFORM® Ointment   ℞
(nystatin-iodochlorhydroxyquin ointment)

Description: NYSTAFORM Ointment contains nystatin U.S.P. 100,000 units/Gm and iodochlorhydroxyquin 1% in a water-dispersible, white petrolatum base containing octylphenoxyethanol and paraffin wax.

Actions: Nystatin acts against Candida species (Monilia). Iodochlorhydroxyquin has antibacterial action against bacteria sensitive to this chemotherapeutic agent.

Indications: NYSTAFORM Ointment is indicated for the treatment of cutaneous or mucocutaneous mycotic infections caused by Candida species (Monilia) complicated by iodochlorhydroxyquin-sensitive bacteria.

Contraindications: Lesions caused by pathogens not susceptible to nystatin and iodochlorhydroxyquin and hypersensitivity to any of the components.

Precautions: If irritation or sensitivity occurs and/or infection persists, discontinue use. If new infections appear, appropriate therapy should be instituted. Trace amounts of iodochlorhydroxyquin present in the diaper or urine can yield a false positive test for phenylketonuria (PKU). Percutaneous absorption of iodochlorhydroxyquin may interfere with thyroid function tests. Therapy should be discontinued for one month before these tests are conducted.

Caution: Federal (U.S.A.) law prohibits dispensing without prescription. For external use only. Not for ophthalmic use. Store below 30°C (86°F), avoid freezing. May stain clothing and hair.

Dosage and Administration: Apply two or three times daily. Continue use for one week after clinical cure.

How Supplied: NYSTAFORM Ointment ½ oz. tube

Otic DOMEBORO® Solution (acid pH)   ℞
(acetic acid 2%)

Composition: Acetic acid 2% in aluminum acetate (modified Burow's) solution.

Indications: For the treatment of superficial infections of the external auditory canal caused by organisms susceptible to the action of the antimicrobial.

Precautions: If undue irritation or sensitivity develops, discontinue treatment.

Caution: Federal (U.S.A.) law prohibits dispensing without prescription.
For external use only. Not for ophthalmic use. Store below 86°F (30°C), avoid freezing.

Administration and Dosage: 4 to 6 drops every 2 to 3 hours.

How Supplied: 2 fl. oz. (60 cc.) plastic squeeze bottle with otic tip.

Continued on next page

Miles Pharm.—Cont.

STILPHOSTROL®
(diethylstilbestrol diphosphate)

Actions: Although the mode of action is not known, diethylstilbestrol diphosphate acts in a similar fashion as estrogens and synthetic estrogens in the treatment of prostatic carcinoma.

Important Notes: An increased risk of thromboembolic disease associated with the use of estrogens has now been conclusively established. Retrospective studies have shown a statistically significant association between thrombophlebitis, pulmonary embolism, and cerebral thrombosis and embolism and the use of these drugs. There have been three principal studies in Great Britain[1-3] and one in the United States[4] leading to this conclusion. As a result of these studies, it has been estimated that users of estrogens are 4 to 7 times more likely than nonusers to develop thromboembolic disease without evident cause. The American study also indicated that the increased risk did not persist after discontinuance nor was it enhanced by long-continued administration.

In a more recent analysis of data derived from several national adverse reaction reporting system(s), British investigators concluded that the risk of thromboembolism, including coronary thrombosis, is directly related to the dose of estrogen. Their analysis did suggest, however, that the quantity of estrogen may not be the sole factor involved. Nevertheless, in view of this study, as well as others that have demonstrated a positive relationship between estrogens and thromboembolism, it would seem prudent and in keeping with basic therapeutic principles, to utilize, whenever feasible, the smallest effective dose of estrogen in treating patients.

Risks associated with certain other known adverse reactions, such as elevated blood pressure, liver dysfunction, and reduced tolerance to carbohydrate, have not as yet been quantitated.

Long-term administration of both natural and synthetic estrogens in subprimate animal species in multiples of the human dose increases the frequency for some animal carcinomas. These data cannot be transposed directly to man. The possible carcinogenicity due to the estrogens can neither be confirmed nor refuted at this time. Close clinical surveillance of all persons taking estrogens must be continued.

Indications: STILPHOSTROL (diethylstilbestrol diphosphate) is indicated for the treatment of inoperable progressing prostatic cancer (for palliation only when castration is not feasible or when castration failures or delayed escape following a response to castration have occurred).

Contraindications: 1. Patients with markedly impaired liver function.
2. Patients with thrombophlebitis, thromboembolic disorders, cerebral apoplexy or with a past history of these conditions.

Warning: 1. The physician should be alert to the earliest manifestations of thrombotic disorders (thrombophlebitis, cerebrovascular disorders, pulmonary embolism and retinal thrombosis). If these occur or are suspected, the drugs should be discontinued immediately.
2. Discontinue medication pending examination if there is sudden onset of proptosis, diplopia or migraine. If examination reveals papilledema or retinal vascular lesions, medication should be withdrawn.

Precautions: 1. Because of estrogen-induced salt and water retention, these drugs should be used with caution in patients with epilepsy, migraine, asthma, cardiac or renal disease.
2. Patients with a history of psychic depression should be carefully observed and the drug discontinued if the depression recurs to a serious degree.
3. Because of a possible decrease in glucose tolerance, diabetic patients should be followed closely.
4. Because estrogens influence the metabolism of calcium and phosphorus, they should be used with caution in patients with certain metabolic bone diseases that are associated with hypercalcemia or in patients with renal insufficiency.
5. The pathologist should be advised of estrogen therapy when relevant specimens are submitted.
6. Certain endocrine and liver function tests may be affected by treatment with estrogens. If such tests are abnormal in a patient taking these drugs it is recommended that they be repeated after the drug has been withdrawn for two months.

Adverse Reactions: A statistically significant association has been demonstrated between use of estrogen-containing drugs and the following serious reactions: thrombophlebitis, pulmonary embolism and cerebral thrombosis.

Although available evidence is suggestive of an association, such a relationship has been neither confirmed nor refuted for the following serious reactions: coronary thrombosis and neuro-ocular lesions (e.g., retinal thrombosis and optic neuritis). The following adverse reactions are known to occur in patients receiving estrogens: nausea, vomiting, anorexia, gastrointestinal symptoms (such as abdominal cramps or bloating), edema, breast tenderness and enlargement, change in body weight (increase or decrease), headache, allergic rash, loss of libido and gynecomastia in the male, sterile abscess (injectable forms only), pain at the site of injection (injectable forms only), post-injection flare (injectable forms only), aggravation of migraine headaches, hepatic cutaneous porphyria becoming manifest, cholestatic jaundice, rise in blood pressure in susceptible individuals, mental depression, cystitis-like syndrome, loss of scalp hair, erythema nodosum, hemorrhagic eruption, changes in libido, changes in appetite, nervousness, dizziness, fatigue, backache, erythema multiforme, itching, irritability, malaise.

Dosage and Administration: TABLETS 50 mg: Start with one tablet t.i.d. and increase this dose level to four or more tablets t.i.d. depending on the tolerance of the patient. Alternatively, if relief is not obtained with high oral dosages, STILPHOSTROL (diethylstilbestrol diphosphate) may be administered intravenously. STILPHOSTROL (diethylstilbestrol diphosphate) solution must be diluted before intravenous infusion.

AMPULS 0.25 g: It is recommended that 0.5 g (2 ampuls) dissolved in 300 ml of saline or 5% dextrose be given intravenously the first day, and that each day thereafter 1 g (4 ampuls) be similarly administered in 300 ml of saline or dextrose. The infusion should be administered slowly (20-30 drops per minute) during the first 10-15 minutes and then the rate of flow adjusted so that the entire amount is given in a period of one hour. This procedure should be followed for five days or more depending on the response of the patient. Following the first intensive course of therapy, 0.25-0.5 g (1 or 2 ampuls) may be administered in a similar manner once or twice weekly or maintenance obtained with STILPHOSTROL (diethylstilbestrol diphosphate) Tablets.

How Supplied: STILPHOSTROL Tablets—Bottles of 50 tablets. Each mottled gray/white tablet contains diethylstilbestrol diphosphate 50 mg and is coded with number 132-Miles. Store at controlled room temperature (59°-86°F).
STILPHOSTROL Ampuls—Boxes of 20 ampuls. Each 5 ml ampul contains diethylstilbestrol diphosphate 0.25 g as a solution of its sodium salts. Store at controlled room temperature (59°-86°F). Ampules manufactured by Taylor Pharmacal Co., Decatur, Illinois 62525
Distributed by Miles Pharmaceuticals, West Haven, Conn. 06516

References: 1. Royal College of General Practitioners: Oral contraception and thromboembolic disease. *J Coll Gen Pract* 13:267-279, 1967. 2. Inman WHW, Vessey MP: Investigation of deaths from pulmonary, coronary and cerebral thrombosis and embolism in women in childbearing age. *Brit Med J* 2:193-199, 1968. 3. Vessey MP, Doll R: Investigation of relation between use of oral contraceptives and thromboembolic disease. A further report. *Brit Med J* 2:651-657, 1969. 4. Sartwell PE, et al: Thromboembolism and oral contraceptives: An epidemiological case-control study. *Am J Epidemiol* 90:365-380, 1969. 5. Inman, WHW, et al: Thromboembolic disease and the steroidal content of oral contraceptives. *Brit Med J* 2:203-209, 1970. 6. Herbst AL, Ulfelder H, Poskanzer DR: Adenocarcinoma of the vagina. *N Engl J Med* 284:878-881, 1971.

Shown in Product Identification Section, page 422

TRIDESILON® 0.05%
(desonide)
creme

Description: Tridesilon® Creme contains microdispersed desonide (the active ingredient) in a compatible vehicle buffered to the pH range of normal skin. Each gram of Tridesilon® Creme contains 0.5 milligrams of desonide. Tridesilon® Creme is applied topically.

Tridesilon® (desonide) is a non-fluorinated corticosteroid. Chemically, desonide is Pregna-1,4-diene-3,20-dione,11,21-dihydroxy-16,17-[(1-methylethylidene)bis(oxy)]-,(11β,16α)- with the following structural formula:

The vehicle for Tridesilon® Creme 0.05% contains glycerin, sodium lauryl sulfate, aluminum sulfate, calcium acetate, dextrin, purified water, cetyl stearyl alcohol, synthetic beeswax, (B-wax), white petrolatum, and light mineral oil. Preserved with methylparaben.

EMPIRICAL FORMULA	MOLECULAR WEIGHT	CAS REGISTRY NUMBER
$C_{24}H_{32}O_6$	416.51	638-94-8

Clinical Pharmacology: Topical corticosteroids share anti-inflammatory, anti-pruritic and vasoconstrictive actions.

The mechanism of anti-inflammatory activity of the topical corticosteroids is unclear. Various laboratory methods, including vasoconstrictor assays, are used to compare and predict potencies and/or clinical efficacies of the topical corticosteroids. There is some evidence to suggest that a recognizable correlation exists between vasoconstrictor potency and therapeutic efficacy in man.

Pharmacokinetics

The extent of percutaneous absorption of topical corticosteroids is determined by many factors including the vehicle, the integrity of the epidermal barrier, and the use of occlusive dressings.

Topical corticosteroids can be absorbed from normal intact skin. Inflammation and/or other disease processes in the skin increase percutaneous absorption. Occlusive dressings substantially increase the percutaneous absorption of topical corticosteroids. Thus, occlusive dressings may be a valuable therapeutic adjunct for treatment of resistant dermatoses. (See DOSAGE AND ADMINISTRATION).

Once absorbed through the skin, topical corticosteroids are handled through pharmacokinetic pathways similar to systemically administered corticosteroids. Corticosteroids are bound to plasma proteins in varying degrees. Corticosteroids are metabolized primarily in the liver and are then excreted by the kidneys. Some of the topical corticosteroids and their metabolites are also excreted into the bile.

Indications and Usage: Topical corticosteroids are indicated for the relief of the inflammatory and pruritic manifestations of corticosteroid-responsive dermatoses.

Contraindications: Topical corticosteroids are contraindicated in those patients with a history of hypersensitivity to any of the components of the preparation.

Precautions:
General

Systemic absorption of topical corticosteroids has produced reversible hypothalmic-pituitary-adrenal (HPA) axis suppression, manifestations of Cushing's syndrome, hyperglycemia, and glucose in some patients.

Conditions which augment systemic absorption include the application of the more potent steroids, use over large surface areas, prolonged use, and the addition of occlusive dressings.

Therefore, patients, receiving a large dose of a potent topical steroid applied to a large surface area or under an occlusive dressing should be evaluated periodically for evidence of HPA axis suppression by using the urinary free cortisol and ACTH stimulation tests. If HPA axis suppression is noted, an attempt should be made to withdraw the drug, to reduce the frequency of application, or to substitute a less potent steroid.

Recovery of HPA axis function is generally prompt and complete upon discontinuation of the drug. Infrequently, signs and symptoms of steroid withdrawal may occur, requiring supplemental systemic corticosteroids.

Children may absorb proportionally larger amounts of topical corticosteroids and thus be more susceptible to systemic toxicity. (See PRECAUTIONS—Pediatric Use).

If irritation develops, topical corticosteroids should be discontinued and appropriate therapy instituted.

In the presence of dermatological infections, the use of an appropriate antifungal or antibacterial agent should be instituted. If a favorable response does not occur promptly, the corticosteroid should be discontinued until the infection has been adequately controlled.

Information for the Patient
Patients using topical corticosteroids should receive the following information and instructions:
1. This medication is to be used as directed by the physician. It is for external use only. Avoid contact with eyes.
2. Patients should be advised not to use this medication for any disorder other than for which it was prescribed.
3. The treated skin area should not be bandaged or otherwise covered or wrapped as to be occlusive unless directed by the physician.
4. Patients should report any signs of local adverse reactions especially under occlusive dressing.
5. Parents of pediatric patients should be advised not to use tightfitting diapers or plastic pants on a child being treated in the diaper area, as these garments may constitute occlusive dressings.

Laboratory Tests
The following tests may be helpful in evaluating the HPA axis suppression:
Urinary free cortisol test
ACTH stimulation test

Carcinogenesis, Mutagenesis, and Impairment of Fertility
Long-term animal studies have not been performed to evaluate the carcinogenic potential or the effect on fertility of topical corticosteroids. Studies to determine mutagenicity with prednisolone and hydrocortisone have revealed negative results.

Pregnancy Category C
Corticosteroids are generally teratogenic in laboratory animals when administered systemically at relatively low dosage levels. The more potent corticosteroids have been shown to be teratogenic after dermal application in laboratory animals. There are no adequate and well-controlled studies in pregnant women on teratogenic effects from topically applied corticosteroids. Therefore, topical corticosteroids should be used during pregnancy only if the potential benefit justifies the potential risk to the fetus. Drugs of this class should not be used extensively on pregnant patients, in large amounts, or for prolonged periods of time.

Nursing Mothers
It is not known whether topical administration of corticosteroids could result in sufficient systemic absorption to produce detectable quantities in breast milk. Systemically administered corticosteroids are secreted into breast milk in quantities *not* likely to have a deleterious effect on the infant. Nevertheless, caution should be exercised when topical corticosteroids are administered to a nursing woman.

Pediatric Use
Pediatric patients demonstrate greater susceptibility to topical corticosteroid-induced HPA axis suppression and Cushing's syndrome than mature patients because of a larger skin surface area to body weight ratio.

Hypothalamic-pituitary-adrenal (HPA) axis suppression. Cushing's syndrome, and intracranial hypertension have been reported in children receiving topical corticosteroids. Manifestations of adrenal supression in children include linear growth retardation, delayed weight gain, low plasma cortisol levels, and absence of response to ACTH stimulation. Manifestations of intracranial hypertension include bulging fontanelles, headaches, and bilateral papilledema.

Administration of topical corticosteroids to children should be limited to the least amount compatible with an effective therapeutic regimen. Chronic corticosteroid therapy may interfere with the growth and development of children.

Adverse Reactions: The following local adverse reactions are reported infrequently with topical corticosteroids, but may occur more frequently with the use of occlusive dressings. These reactions are listed in an approximate decreasing order of occurrence:
Burning
Itching
Irritation
Dryness
Folliculitis
Hypertrichosis
Acneiform eruptions
Hypopigmentation
Perioral dermatitis
Allergic contact dermatitis
Maceration of the skin
Secondary infection
Skin atrophy
Striae
Miliaria

Overdosage: Topically applied corticosteroids can be absorbed in sufficient amounts to produce systemic effects. (See PRECAUTIONS).

Dosage and Administration: Topical Corticosteroids are generally applied to the affected area as a thin film from two to four times daily depending on the severity of the condition.

Occlusive dressings may be used for management of psoriasis or recalcitrant conditions.

If an infection develops, the use of occlusive dressings should be discontinued and appropriate antimicrobial therapy instituted.

How Supplied: Tridesilon® (desonide) Creme 0.05% is supplied in 15 and 60 gram tubes and in 5 pound jars. It is a white semi-solid.
DPSC Stocked:
  15 gram—NSN 6505-00-148-6969
  60 gram—NSN 6505-001-148-6968
  5 pound—NSN 6505-01-004-9217
VA Stocked: 60 gram—SN 6505-01-027-6866A
Store below 86°F (30°C), avoid freezing.
Caution: Federal (USA) law prohibits dispensing without a prescription.
July, 1982   PD100573   18873

TRIDESILON® 0.05%   R
(desonide)
ointment

Description: Tridesilon® Ointment contains microdispersed desonide (the active ingredient) in a compatible vehicle buffered to the pH range of normal skin. Each gram of Tridesilon® Ointment contains 0.5 miligrams of desonide. Tridesilon® Ointment is applied topically.

Tridesilon® (desonide) is a non-fluorinated corticosteroid. Chemically, desonide is Pregna-1,4-diene-3,20-dione,11,21-dihydroxy-16,17-[(1-methylethylidene)bis(oxy)]-,11β,16α)- with the following structural formula:

The vehicle for Tridesilon® Ointment is white petrolatum.

EMPIRICAL FORMULA	MOLECULAR WEIGHT	CAS REGISTRY NUMBER
$C_{24}H_{32}O_6$	416.51	638-94-8

Clinical Pharmacology: Topical corticosteroids share anti-inflammatory, anti-puritic and vasoconstrictive actions.

The mechanism of anti-inflammatory activity of the topical corticosteroids is unclear. Various laboratory methods, including vasoconstrictor assays, are used to compare and predict potencies and/or clinical efficacies of the topical corticosteroids. There is some evidence to suggest that a recognizable correlation exists between vasoconstrictor potency and therapeutic efficacy in man.

Pharmacokinetics
The extent of percutaneous absorption of topical corticosteroids is determined by many factors including the vehicle, the integrity of the epidermal barrier, and the use of occlusive dressings.

Topical corticosteroids can be absorbed from normal intact skin. Inflammation and/or other disease processes in the skin increase percutaneous absorption. Occlusive dressings substantially increase the percutaneous absorption of topical corticosteroids. Thus, occlusive dressings may be a valuable therapeutic adjunct for treatment of resistant dermatoses. (See DOSAGE AND ADMINISTRATION).

Once absorbed through the skin, topical corticosteroids are handled through pharmacokinetic pathways similar to systemically administered corticosteroids. Corticosteroids are bound to plasma proteins in varying degrees. Corticosteroids are metabolized primarily in the liver and are then excreted by the kidneys. Some of the topical corticosteroids and their metabolites are also excreted into the bile.

Indications and Usage: Topical corticosteroids are indicated for the relief of the inflammatory and pruritic manifestations of corticosteroid-responsive dermatoses.

Contraindications: Topical corticosteroids are contraindicated in those patients with a history of hypersensitivity to any of the components of the preparation.

Precautions:
General
Systemic absorption of topical corticosteroids has produced reversible hypothalamic-pituitary-adrenal (HPA) axis suppression, manifestations of Cushing's syndrome, hyperglycemia, and glucosuria in some patients.

Conditions which augment systemic absorption include the application of the more potent steroids, use over large surface areas, prolonged use, and the addition of occlusive dressings.

Therefore, patients receiving a large dose of a potent topical steroid applied to a large surface area or under an occlusive dressing should be evaluated periodically for evidence of HPA axis suppression by using the urinary free cortisol and ACTH stimulation tests. If HPA axis suppression is noted, an attempt should be made to withdraw the drug, to reduce the frequency of application, or to substitute a less potent steroid.

Recovery of HPA axis functions is generally prompt and complete upon discontinuation of the drug. Infrequently, signs and symptoms of steroid withdrawal may occur, requiring supplemental systemic corticosteroids.

Children may absorb proportionally larger amounts of topical corticosteroids and thus be more susceptible to systemic toxicity. (See PRECAUTIONS—Pediatric Use).

If irritation develops, topical corticosteroids should be discontinued and appropriate therapy instituted.

In the presence of dermatological infections, the use of an appropriate antifungal or antibacterial agent should be instituted. If a favorable response does not occur promptly, the corticosteroid should

Continued on next page

Miles Pharm.—Cont.

be discontinued until the infection has been adequately controlled.

Information for the Patient
Patients using topical corticosteroids should receive the following information and instructions:
1. This medication is to be used as directed by the physician. It is for external use only. Avoid contact with the eyes.
2. Patients should be advised not to use this medication for any disorder other than for which it was prescribed.
3. The treated skin area should not be bandaged or otherwise covered or wrapped as to be occlusive unless directed by the physician.
4. Patients should report any signs of local adverse reactions especially under occlusive dressing.
5. Parents of pediatric patients should be advised not to use tight-fitting diapers or plastic pants on a child being treated in the diaper area, as these garments may constitute occlusive dressings.

Laboratory Tests
The following tests may be helpful in evaluating the HPA axis suppression.
Urinary free cortisol test
ACTH stimulation test

Carcinogenesis, Mutagenesis, and Impairment of Fertility
Long-term animal studies have not been performed to evaluate the carcinogenic potential or the effect on fertility of topical corticosteroids.
Studies to determine mutagenicity with prednisolone and hydrocortisone have revealed negative results.

Pregnancy Category C
Corticosteroids are generally teratogenic in laboratory animals when administered systemically at relatively low dosage levels. The more potent corticosteroids have been shown to be teratogenic after dermal application in laboratory animals. There are no adequate and well-controlled studies in pregnant women on teratogenic effects from topically applied corticosteroids. Therefore, topical corticosteroids should be used during pregnancy only if the potential benefit justifies the potential risk to the fetus. Drugs of this class should not be used extensively on pregnant patients, in large amounts, or for prolonged periods of time.

Nursing Mothers
It is not known whether topical administration of corticosteroids could result in sufficient systemic absorption to produce detectable quantities in breast milk. Systemically administered corticosteroids are secreted into breast milk in quantities *not* likely to have a deleterious effect on the infant. Nevertheless, caution should be exercised when topical corticosteroids are administered to a nursing woman.

Pediatric Use
Pediatric patients may demonstrate greater susceptibility to topical corticosteroid-induced HPA axis and Cushing's syndrome than mature patients because of a larger skin surface area to body weight ratio.
Hypothalmic-pituitary-adrenal (HPA) axis suppression, Cushing's syndrome, and intracranial hypertension have been reported in children receiving topical corticosteroids. Manifestations of adrenal suppression in children include linear growth retardation, delayed weight gain, low plasma cortisol levels, and absence of response to ACTH stimulation. Manifestations of intracranial hypertension include bulging fontanelles, headaches, and bilateral papilledema.
Administration of topical costicosteroids to children should be limited to the least amount compatible with an effective therapeutic regimen. Chronic corticosteroid therapy may interfere with the growth and development of children.

Adverse Reactions.
The following local adverse reactions are reported infrequently with topical corticosteroids, but may occur more frequently with the use of occlusive dressings. These reactions are listed in an approximate decreasing order of occurrence:
Burning
Itching
Irritation
Dryness
Folliculitis
Hypertrichosis
Acneiform eruptions
Hypopigmentation
Perioral dermatitis
Allergic contact dermatitis
Maceration of the skin
Secondary infection
Skin atrophy
Striae
Miliaria

Overdosage: Topically applied corticosteroids can be absorbed in sufficient amounts to produce systemic effects. (See PRECAUTIONS).

Dosage and Administration: Topical corticosteroids are generally applied to the affected area as a thin film from two to four times daily depending on the severity of the condition.
Occlusive dressings may be used for the management of psoriasis or recalcitrant conditions.
In an infection develops, the use of occlusive dressings should be discontinued and appropriate antimicrobial therapy instituted.

How Supplied: Tridesilon® (desonide) Ointment 0.05% is supplied in 15 and 60 gram tubes. It is white or faintly yellowish, transparent semi-solid.

DPSC Stocked:
15 gram—NSN 6505-00-148-6969
60 gram—NSN 6505-00-148-6968
VA Stocked: 60 gram—SN 6505-01-027-6866A
Store below 86°F (30°C), avoid freezing.

Caution: Federal (USA) law prohibits dispensing without a prescription.

July, 1982   PD100574   18871

TRIDESILON® 0.05% R
Otic
(desonide 0.05%-acetic acid 2%)
solution

Description: Otic Tridesilon® Solution contains desonide 0.05% and acetic acid 2% (the active ingredients) in a compatible vehicle buffered to the pH range of the normal ear. Otic Tridesilon® Solution is instilled into the external auditory canal.
Tridesilon® (desonide) is a non-fluorinated corticosteroid. Chemically, desonide is Pregna-1,4-diene-3,20-dione,11,21-dihydroxy-16,17-[(1-methylethylidene)bis(oxy)]-,(11β,16α)- with the following structural formula:

EMPIRICAL FORMULA	MOLECULAR WEIGHT	CAS REGISTRY NUMBER
$C_{24}H_{32}O_6$	416.51	638-94-8

Acetic acid is an astringent and antimicrobial agent. Chemically, it is $C_2H_4O_2$ with the following structural formula:

The base is composed of purified water, propylene glycol, sodium acetate, and citric acid.

Clinical Pharmacology: Topical corticosteroids share anti-inflammatory, anti-pruritic and vasoconstrictive actions.
The mechanism of anti-inflammatory activity of the topical corticosteroids is unclear. Various laboratory methods, including vasoconstrictor assays, are used to compare and predict potencies and/or clinical efficacies of the topical corticosteroids. There is some evidence to suggest that a recognizable correlation exists between vasoconstrictor potency and therapeutic efficacy in man.

Pharmacokinetics
The extent of percutaneous absorption of topical corticosteroids is determined by many factors including the vehicle, the integrity of the epidermal barrier, and the use of occlusive dressings.
Topical corticosteroids can be absorbed from normal intact skin. Inflammation and/or other disease processes in the skin increase percutaneous absorption. Occlusive dressings substantially increase the percutaneous absorption of topical corticosteroids.
Once absorbed through the skin, topical corticosteroids are handled through pharmacokinetic pathways similar to systemically administered corticosteroids. Corticosteroids are bound to plasma proteins in varying degrees. Corticosteroids are metabolized primarily in the liver and are then excreted by the kidneys. Some of the topical corticosteroids and their metabolites are also excreted into the bile.

Indications and Usage: Otic Tridesilon Solution is indicated for the treatment of superficial infections of the external auditory canal caused by organisms susceptible to the action of the antimicrobial and accompanied by inflammation.

Contraindications: Otic Tridesilon Solution (desonide 0.05%-acetic acid 2%) is contraindicated in those patients who have shown hypersensitivity to any of the components of the preparation. Perforated tympanic membranes are frequently considered a contraindication to the use of external ear canal medication.

Precautions:
General
Systemic absorption of topical corticosteroids has produced reversible hypothalamic-pituitary-adrenal (HPA) axis suppression, manifestations of Cushing's syndrome, hyperglycemia, and glucosuria in some patients.
Conditions which augment systemic absorption include the application of the more potent steroids, use over large surface areas, prolonged use, and the addition of occlusive dressings.
Children may absorb proportionally larger amounts of topical corticosteroids and thus be more susceptible to systemic toxicity. (See PRECAUTIONS—Pediatric Use).
If irritation develops, the product should be discontinued and appropriate therapy instituted.
If infection persists or new infection appears, appropriate therapy should be instituted. If a favorable response does not occur promptly, the corticosteroid should be discontinued until the infection has been adequately controlled.

Information for the Patient
Patients using topical corticosteroids should receive the following information and instructions:
1. This medication is to be used as directed by the physician. It is for external use only. Avoid contact with the eyes.
2. Patients should be advised not to use this medication for any disorder other than for which it was prescribed.

Laboratory Tests
The following tests may be helpful in evaluating the HPA axis suppression:
Urinary free cortisol test
ACTH stimulation test

Carcinogenesis, Mutagenesis, and Impairment of Fertility
Long-term animal studies have not been preformed to evaluate the carcinogenic potential or the effect on fertility of topical corticosteroids.
Studies to determine mutagenicity with prednisolone and hydrocortisone have revealed negative results.

Pregnancy Category C
Corticosteroids are generally teratogenic in laboratory animals when administered systemically at relatively low dosage levels. The more potent corticosteroids have been shown to be teratogenic after dermal application in laboratory animals. There

are no adequate and well-controlled studies in pregnant women on teratogenic effects from topically applied corticosteroids. Therefore, topical corticosteroids should be used during pregnancy only if the potential benefit justifies the potential risk to the fetus. Drugs of this class should not be used extensively on pregnant patients, in large amounts, or for prolonged periods of time.

Nursing Mothers
It is not known whether topical administration of corticosteroids could result in sufficient systemic absorption to produce detectable quantities in breast milk. Systemically administered corticosteroids are secreted into breast milk in quantities *not* likely to have a deleterious effect on the infant. Nevertheless, caution should be exercised when topical corticosteroids are administered to a nursing woman.

Pediatric Use
Pediatric patients may demonstrate greater susceptibility to topical corticosteroid-induced HPA axis suppression and Cushing's syndrome than mature patients because of a larger skin surface area to body weight ratio.
Hypothalamic-pituitary-adrenal (HPA) axis suppression, Cushing's syndrome, and intracranial hypertension have been reported in children receiving topical corticosteroids. Manifestations of adrenal suppression in children include linear growth retardation, delayed weight gain, low plasma cortisol levels, and absence of response to ACTH stimulation. Manifestations of intracranial hypertension include bulging fontanelles, headaches, and bilateral papilledema.
Administration of topical corticosteroids to children should be limited to the least amount compatible with an effective therapeutic regimen.
Chronic corticosteroid therapy may interfere with the growth and development of children.

Adverse Reactions: The following local adverse reactions may occur infrequently with otic use of topical corticosteroids. These reactions are listed in an approximate decreasing order of occurrence.

Burning   Hypopigmentation
Itching   Allergic contact dermatitis
Irritation   Maceration of the skin
Dryness   Secondary infection
Folliculitis   Skin atrophy
Hypertrichosis

Overdosage: Topically applied corticosteroids can be absorbed in sufficient amounts to produce systemic effects. (See PRECAUTIONS.)

Dosage and Administration: All ceruminous material and debris should be carefully removed to permit Otic Tridesilon® Solution (desonide 0.05%–acetic acid 2%) to contact the infected surfaces. Instill 3 to 4 drops into the ear 3 to 4 times daily. If preferred, a gauze or cotton wick saturated with the solution may be inserted in the ear canal and allowed to remain in situ. It should be kept moist by further addition of the solution, as required.

How Supplied: Otic Tridesilon® Solution (desonide 0.05%–acetic acid 2%) is supplied in 10cc bottles with dropper.
Otic Tridesilon® is a clear colorless solution.
Store below 86°F (30°C), avoid freezing.

Caution: Federal (USA) law prohibits dispensing without a prescription. For external use only.
Aug., 1983   PD100572   19386

Products are cross-indexed by generic and chemical names in the
YELLOW SECTION

Milex Products, Inc.
5915 NORTHWEST HIGHWAY
CHICAGO, IL 60631

AMINO-CERV™ R
[ah-me'no-serv]
pH 5.5 Cervical Creme

Active Ingredients: Urea 8.34%, Sodium Propionate 0.50%, Methionine 0.83%, Cystine 0.35%, Inositol 0.83%, Benzalkonium Chloride 0.000004%. Buffered to pH of 5.5 in a water-miscible creme base.

Description: An AMINO-ACID and UREA creme specifically formulated for cervical treatment: Cervicitis (mild), postpartum cervicitis, postpartum cervical tears, post cauterization, post cryosurgery and post conization.

Advantages: METHIONINE and CYSTINE are amino-acids necessary for wound healing and forming of epithelial tissue. INOSITOL acts as an essential growth factor and promotes epithelialization.
UREA aids in debridement, dissolves the coagulum and promotes epithelialization. Its solvent action on fibroblasts prevents the formation of excessive tissue—thus preventing stenosis when used as directed.
BENZALKONIUM CHLORIDE serves to lower surface tension and thus aids in spreading the medication. Along with SODIUM PROPIONATE it also exerts a bacteriostatic effect.
AMINO-CERV is geared to the higher pH of the healthy cervix in contrast with pH 4 vaginal preparations. With its pH factor of 5.5 Amino-Cerv promotes faster healing of the cervix, yet will not adversely affect a healthy vagina.

Directions: When immediate postpartum bleeding has subsided (usually from 24 to 48 hours after delivery), one Milex-Jector full of AMINO-CERV creme should be applied nightly for four weeks. In mild CERVICITIS (not requiring cautery or cryosurgery) one applicatorful of AMINO-CERV should be injected in the vagina nightly upon retiring for 2 weeks.
A small amount of AMINO-CERV should be applied immediately after HOT CAUTERIZATION, HOT CONIZATION and CRYOSURGERY. One applicatorful should be injected nightly upon retiring for 2 to 4 weeks (the duration of treatment depends on extent of cauterization or hot conization or cryosurgery). During the weekly office visit for (2 to 4 visits) the physician should again apply a small amount of AMINO-CERV with a probe or applicator. The canal is to be completely probed on the last visit.
After COLD CONING, one applicatorful should be injected upon retiring about 24 hours after surgery and nightly thereafter for four weeks. During the four weekly office visits following cold coning, a small amount of AMINO-CERV should be applied with a probe or applicator into the canal by the physician. The canal is to be completely probed on the last visit.

Reasons For Variation of Directions:
(1) After hot conization, cauterization and cryosurgery immediate use of AMINO-CERV is indicated to aid in dissolving dead or burned tissue.
(2) After cold coning, there is no dead tissue to slough off. Therefore, a wait of 24 hours or longer is desirable for normal healing to take place and for some fibroblasts to be laid down before applying the AMINO-CERV (which has a solvent action on both the fibroblasts and the absorbable sutures). When NONABSORBABLE sutures are used, AMINO-CERV can be used immediately.

Contraindications: Deleterious side effects have not been a problem at the doses recommended. The usual precautions against allergic reactions should be observed.

Storage: Store at room temperature.

Packaging: 2¾ oz. tube with Milex-Jector (2 weeks supply, 14 applications).
Available only on hospital direct orders: 5½ oz. tube with MILEX-JECTOR (4 weeks supply, 28 applications).

PRO–CEPTION
[pro-sep'shun]

Description: PRO-CEPTION is a precoital douche to help promote conception. It provides in a convenient form supplementary nutrient immediately available to the sperm for metabolism and movement. Also effective for removal of a thick tenacious mucous plug of the cervix.

Directions: The screw cap is used as a measuring device and filled level with the powder which is then dissolved in eight ounces of lukewarm water. The woman is told to douche while in a recumbent position and to retain the solution (10 to 15 minutes). Following coitus the patient should remain recumbent for two hours or more. May be used as a companion with Milex Oligospermia Cups. Frequently used in connection with PRO-CEPTION Basal Thermometers.

Contraindications: None.

Packaging: Available in 12 douche container.

Mission Pharmacal Company
1325 E. DURANGO ST.
SAN ANTONIO, TX 78210

CALCET®
[kăl'cet]
Calcium Supplement
NDC-0178-0251-01

Composition: Each tablet contains:

	% US RDA*	
Calcium Lactate		240 mg.
Calcium Gluconate		240 mg.
Calcium Carbonate		240 mg.
(Calcium	15	152.8 mg.)
Vitamin D2	25	100. Units

* Percent of U.S. Recommended Daily Allowance for adults and children 4 or more years of age.

Indications: CALCET® tablets are indicated as a daily supplement to provide a dietary source of calcium. CALCET® tablets are of particular value in people who have milk allergies, in people who have low calcium leg cramps or calcium deficiencies due to low dietary calcium.

Dosage: TWO CALCET® TABLETS AT BEDTIME as a general or prenatal supplement. In calcium deficiency states or in nocturnal leg cramping, dosage should be increased to TWO CALCET® TABLETS AT BEDTIME plus one tablet mid-morning and one tablet mid-afternoon.

How Supplied: CALCET® tablets are supplied as yellow, oval shaped, coated tablets in bottles of 100 tablets.

Literature Available: Yes.

CALCET PLUS™
[kăl'cet]
Calcium-Iron-Zinc-Multivitamin
NDC 0178-0252-60

Composition: Each tablet contains:

	%USRDA*	
Vitamin C	800	500 mg.
(Calcium Ascorbate, Ascorbic Acid)		
Vitamin B$_1$	150	2.25 mg.
(Thiamine Mononitrate)		
Vitamin B$_2$	150	2.55 mg.
(Riboflavin)		
Vitamin B$_3$	150	30.0 mg.
(Niacinamide)		
Vitamin B$_5$	150	15.0 mg.
(d-Calcium Pantothenate)		
Vitamin B$_6$	150	3.0 mg.
(Pyridoxine Hydrochloride)		

Continued on next page

Mission—Cont.

Vitamin B_{12} (Crystalline on Resin)	150	9 mcg.
Folic Acid	200	0.8 mg.
Vitamin A (Vitamin A Acetate)	100	5000 USPU
Vitamin D	100	400 USPU
Vitamin E (d-Alpha Tocopheryl Acid Succinate)	100	30 USPU
Calcium (Calcium Ascorbate, Calcium Carbonate)	15	152.8 mg.
Iron (Ferrous Fumarate)	100	18.0 mg.
Zinc (Zinc Sulfate, dried)	100	15.0 mg.

*USRDA: U.S. recommended daily allowance for adults and children 4 or more years of age.
Indications: CALCET PLUS tablets are indicated as adjunctive therapy in osteoporosis, pre- and post-operative patients, low calcium leg cramping, for patients with milk allergies and nursing mothers.
Dosage: Two CALCET PLUS tablets at bedtime.
How Supplied: CALCET PLUS tablets are supplied as white, oval shaped, coated tablets in bottles of 60's.
Literature Available: Yes.

COMPETE®
[kŏm'pēt]
Multivitamins with Iron and Zinc
NDC-0178-0221-01

Description: COMPETE® is a multivitamin with iron and zinc formulated to provide an especially well tolerated group of nutritional components for the active, stressful lifestyle of the 1980's. COMPETE® provides 150% of the U.S.R.D.A. of all components except vitamins A and D, which have been maintained at a 100% level, and vitamin B_6 which is provided in a level of 1250% U.S.R.D.A. for the particular needs of today's active woman using birth control tablets.
Composition: Each tablet contains:

	Quantity/Tablet	%USRDA
Vitamin A	5000 I.U.	100%
Vitamin D	400 I.U.	100%
Vitamin E	45 I.U.	150%
Vitamin C	90 mg	150%
Folic Acid	0.4 mg	150%
Thiamine Mononitrate	2.25 mg	150%
Riboflavin	2.6 mg	150%
Niacinamide	30 mg	150%
Pyridoxine HCl	25.0 mg	1250%
Vitamin B_{12}	9 mcg	150%
Iron (As Ferrous Gluconate 233 mg)	27 mg	150%
Zinc (As Zinc Sulfate)	22.5 mg	150%

Dosage: One tablet at bedtime as directed by your physician.
Warning: KEEP THIS AND ALL MEDICATIONS OUT OF THE REACH OF CHILDREN. In case of accidental overdose, seek professional assistance or contact a poison control center immediately.
Precaution: Folic Acid, especially in doses above 0.1 mg. daily, may obscure pernicious anemia in that hematologic remission may occur while neurological manifestations remain progressive.
How Supplied: COMPETE® is supplied as orange, football-shaped, sugar coated tablets in bottles of 100.

FERRALET®
[fer″alét]
Ferrous Gluconate
NDC-0178-0082-01

Composition: Each tablet contains:

		% US RDA*
Ferrous Gluconate	320 mg	
(Iron	37.0 mg.)	206.0

*Percent of U.S. recommended daily allowance for adults and children 4 or more years of age.
Description: The FERRALET® tablet contains only one active ingredient, iron, as ferrous gluconate. FERRALET® is particularly well tolerated in most patients because ferrous gluconate is non-astringent, non-irritating, and will not precipitate protein from aqueous media. FERRALET® provides a more efficient source of ferrous ion because of the low ionization constant of ferrous gluconate, coupled with high solubility and stability over the entire pH range of the gastrointestinal tract. FERRALET® provides utilizable iron throughout the entire length of the intestinal absorption bed. With FERRALET®, heavy iron loading is not necessary due to the superior efficiency of the iron component. The result of moderate ferrous ion dosage is usually improved patient acceptance and excellent dosage continuity. FERRALET® is manufactured in a unique, easy to swallow shape, to further enhance patient acceptance of the product. FERRALET® has a tailored disintegration rate to minimize gastric intoleration with a rapid dissolution rate to assure rapid availability for absorption.
Indications: Anemias amenable to iron therapy.
Dosage: One to three tablets a day depending upon the severity of the anemia and the particular toleration of the patient.
How Supplied: FERRALET® is packaged in bottles of 100 tablets.
Literature Available: Yes.

FOSFREE®
[fos'frē]
Calcium—Vitamins—Iron
NDC-0178-0031-01

Composition: Each tablet contains:

	One Tablet	% US RDA
Calcium Lactate	250.0 mg.	
Calcium Gluconate	250.0 mg.	
Calcium Carbonate	300.0 mg.	
(Calcium	175.7 mg.)	17
Ferrous Gluconate	125.0 mg.	
(Iron	14.5 mg.)	80
Vitamin D_2	150.0 USP U. optional	
Vitamin A Acetate	1500.0 USP U.	30
Ascorbic Acid (C)	50.0 mg.	83
Pyridoxine HCl (B_6)	3.0 mg.	150
Thiamine Mononitrate (B_1)	5.0 mg.	333
Riboflavin (B_2)	2.0 mg.	117
Niacinamide (B_3)	10.0 mg.	50
d-Calcium Pantothenate (B_5)	1.0 mg.	10
Vitamin B_{12} (Crystalline on resin)	2.0 mcg.	33

Action and Uses: FOSFREE® tablets are primarily indicated as a prenatal, postpartum or geriatric supplement particularly when soluble calcium salt supplementation is desired. FOSFREE® is a specific for hypocalcemic tetany (nocturnal leg cramping).
Administration and Dosage: One or two FOSFREE® tablets at bedtime as a general or prenatal supplement. In calcium deficiency states or in nocturnal leg cramping, dosage should be increased to two FOSFREE® tablets at bedtime plus one tablet mid-morning and one tablet mid-afternoon.
How Supplied: FOSFREE® is supplied as yellow capsule shaped coated tablets in bottles of 100 tablets.
Literature Available: Yes.

IROMIN-G®
[i'rō-min]
Hematinic Supplement
NDC-0178-0081-01

Composition: Each tablet contains:

	% US RDA	
Ferrous Gluconate		333.3 mg.
(Iron	214	38.6 mg.)
Ascorbic Acid (C)	166	100.0 mg.
Thiamine Mononitrate (B_1)	333	5.0 mg.
Pyridoxine HCl (B_6)	1250	25.0 mg.
Riboflavin (B_2)	117	2.0 mg.
Niacinamide	50	10.0 mg.
Folic Acid	200	0.8 mg.
d-Calcium Pantothenate	10	1.0 mg.
Vitamin B_{12} (Crystalline on resin)	33	2.0 mcg.
Vitamin A Acetate	80	4000.0 USP U.
Vitamin D_2	Optional	400.0 USP U.
Calcium Carbonate		70.0 mg.
Calcium Gluconate		100.0 mg.
Calcium Lactate		100.0 mg.
(Calcium	5	50.0 mg.)

Action and Uses: Secondary anemias, and as a supplement for the prenatal, teenage and geriatric diet.
Administration and Dosage: One to three tablets daily after meals or as directed by a physician.
Precaution: Folic Acid, especially in doses above 0.1 mg. daily, may obscure pernicious anemia in that hematologic remission may occur while neurological manifestations remain progressive.
Side Effects: IROMIN-G® is virtually free of side effects when given in the recommended dosage. The rare constipation, diarrhea, or gastric upset can usually be controlled by dosage adjustment.
How Supplied: IROMIN-G® is supplied as red football shaped coated tablets in bottles of 100 tablets.
Literature Available: Yes.

MISSION PHARMACAL UROLOGICALS

CALCIBIND™ ℞
[kal'sē-bīnd]
Cellulose Sodium Phosphate (CSP)

Description: Cellulose Sodium Phosphate (CSP), the active ingredient in CALCIBIND™, is a synthetic compound made by phosphorylation of cellulose and has the following structural formula:

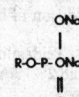

It has an inorganic phosphate content of approximately 34% and sodium content of approximately 11%. It is insoluble in water and non-absorbable. It has excellent ion exchange properties, the sodium ion exchanging for calcium. When taken orally, CSP binds calcium, the complex of calcium and cellulose phosphate being excreted in feces. The dosage of CALCIBIND™ is powder for oral administration.
Clinical Pharmacology: CSP alters urinary composition of calcium, magnesium, phosphate and oxalate by affecting their absorption in the intestinal tract. When it is given orally with meals, CSP binds dietary and secreted calcium, and reduces urinary calcium by approximately 50 mg/5 grams of CSP. It also binds dietary Mg and lowers urinary Mg. Oral magnesium supplementation given separately from CSP partly overcomes this effect.
CSP administration increases urinary phosphorus (P) and oxalate. The usual rise in urinary P of 150–250 mg/15 grams CSP largely reflects the

CALCIBIND™
Diagnostic Criteria

Criteria	Absorptive Hypercalciuria Type I	Absorptive Hypercalciuria Type II	Renal Hypercalciuria	Primary Hyperparathyroidism	Control Subjects
Serum calcium (mg/dl)	normal	normal	normal	high	normal
Phosphorus (mg/dl)	> 2.5	> 2.5	> 2.5	normal or low	> 2.5
PTH	normal	normal	high	high	normal
Urinary calcium					
Restricted diet (mg/day)	> 200	< 200	> 200	> 200	< 200
Fasting (mg/100 ml glomerular filtrate)	< 0.11	< 0.11	> 0.11	> 0.11	< 0.11
After calcium load (mg/mg creatinine)	> 0.2	> 0.2	> 0.2	> 0.2	< 0.2

Restricted diet, representing 400 mg calcium and 100 meq sodium/day, may be imposed in an outpatient setting. The fasting sample is obtained in a 2-hour specimen collected after an overnight fast, and after calcium load sample is obtained in a 4-hour specimen following an oral calcium load (1 gram).

hydrolysis of 7–30% in CSP in the intestinal tract and absorption of released P. An increase in urinary oxalate occurs. Since CSP binds divalent cations, the cations are not available to complex oxalate and thereby limit its absorption. The rise in urinary oxalate may be largely prevented by moderate dietary oxalate restriction and the use of a modest dose of CSP (10–15 grams/day).

The marked reduction in urinary calcium with only slightly increased urinary phosphorus and oxalate leads to a reduction in urinary saturation and propensity for spontaneous nucleation of calcium oxalate and calcium phosphate (brushite). CSP does not apparently alter the metabolism of trace metals, since it does not significantly change the serum concentration of copper, zinc or iron.

Indications and Usage: CSP is indicated only for absorptive hypercalciuria Type I with recurrent calcium oxalate or calcium phosphate nephrolithiasis. Appropriate use (see Dosage and Administration) of CSP substantially reduces the incidence of new stone formation in these patients. Causes of hypercalciuria other than hyperabsorption cannot be expected to respond to CSP 1 Treatment with CSP is not needed for absorptive hypercalciuria Type II because dietary calcium restriction provides adequate treatment. In patients without hyperabsorption of calcium, CSP would be expected to cause excessive parathyroid hormone secretion and possible hyperparathyroid bone disease.

Absorptive hypercalciuna Type I is characterized by (a) recurrent passage or formation of calcium oxalate and/or calcium phosphate renal stones, (b) no evidence of bone disease, (c) normal serum calcium and phosphorus, (d) increased intestinal calcium absorption, (e) hypercalciuria, (f) normal urinary calcium during fasting, (g) normal parathyroid function, and (h) lack of renal "leak" or excessive skeletal mobilization of calcium. Absorptive hypercalciuria Type II is identical except that hypercalciuria can be eliminated by a low calcium diet. The enclosed tabulation of diagnostic criteria for different causes of hypercalciuria is intended as a guide for patient selection. **Minimal diagnostic tests include serum calcium and phosphorus, parathyroid hormone (PTH) level obtained before breakfast, 24-hour urinary calcium on a diet restricted in calcium and sodium, and a fasting urinary excretion of calcium.**

The diagnosis of absorptive hypercalciuria Type I can be made if there is: a) recurrent calcium nephrolithiasis without clinical evidence of bone disease, b) normal serum calcium and phosphorus (borderline values should be repeated), c) 24-hour urinary calcium greater than 200 mg/day on a diet of 400 mg calcium and 100 mEq sodium/day, d) normal serum immunoreactive PTH, and e) normal fasting urinary calcium. A definitive diagnosis requires, in addition, evidence of high intestinal calcium absorption (e.g. urinary calcium > 0.2 mg/mg creatinine after oral load of 1 gram calcium.)

Contraindications: CSP is contraindicated in (a) primary or secondary hyperparathyroidism, including renal hypercalciuria (renal calcium leak), (b) hypomagnesemic states (serum magnesium < 1.5 mg/dl), (c) bone disease (osteoporosis, osteomalacia, osteitis), (d) hypocalcemic states (e.g. hypoparathyroidism, intestinal malabsorption), (e) normal or low intestinal absorption and renal excretion of calcium, and (f) enteric hyperoxaluria. It should not be used in patients with high fasting urinary calcium or hypophosphatemia, unless a high skeletal mobilization of calcium can be excluded.

Warnings: In patients with congestive heart failure or ascites, sodium contained in CSP (35–48 mEq exchangeable sodium/15 grams CSP) may represent a hazard.

Precautions: By inhibiting intestinal calcium absorption, CSP may stimulate parathyroid function leading to hyperparathyroid bone disease. It is therefore essential to monitor parathyroid hormone levels. CSP treatment has been shown to maintain parathyroid function within normal limits, if it is used only in patients with absorptive hypercalciuria Type I (increased intestinal calcium absorption and high urinary calcium even on calcium absorption and high urinary calcium even on calcium restricted diet), at a dosage just sufficient to restore normal calcium absorption but not sufficient to cause subnormal absorption.

The following additional complications may potentially develop during long-term use of CSP: a) hyperoxaluria and hypomagnesiuria, which would negate the beneficial effect of hypocalciuria on new stone formation, b) magnesium depletion, and c) depletion of trace metals (copper, zinc, iron). All of these effects may be minimized by restricting the use of CSP to absorptive hypercalciuria Type I only (see Indications for diagnostic criteria), and by taking precautionary measures (see Administration and Dosage) and by monitoring serum calcium, magnesium, copper, zinc, iron, parathyroid hormone, and complete blood count every 3 to 6 mouths. Borderline values for parathyroid hormone and calcium should be repeated promptly. Serum PTH should be obtained at least once between the first 2 weeks to 3 months of treatment and the treatment should be adjusted or stopped if a rise in serum PTH above normal appears. If there is an inadequate hypocalciuric response to CSP treatment (a reduction in urinary calcium of less than 30 mg/5 grams of CSP), while patients are maintained on moderate calcium and sodium restriction, the treatment may be considered ineffective and should be stopped. Cessation of treatment should be considered if urinary oxalate exceeds 55 mg/day on moderate dietary oxalate restriction.

Carcinogenesis, mutagenesis, impairment of fertility: No long-term studies were conducted to determine the carcinogenic potential of CSP.

Pregnancy: Pregnancy category C: Animal reproduction studies have not been conducted with CSP. It is also not known whether CSP can cause fetal harm when administered to a pregnant woman or can affect reproduction capacity. However, because of the increased requirement of dietary calcium in pregnant women, CSP should be given to pregnant women only if clearly needed.

Pediatric use: Because of the increased requirement for dietary calcium in growing children, the use of CSP in children less than 16 years of age is not recommended.

Adverse Reactions: Some patients may have gastrointestinal complaints, manifested by poor taste of the drug, loose bowel movements, diarrhea or dyspepsia.

Dosage and Administration: The amount of dietary calcium bound depends upon actual mixing of CSP with a meal. Consequently, CSP should be taken with a meal; the amount of dietary calcium bound by CSP is considerably reduced when CSP is administered more than 1 hour after a meal. Both the initial and maintenance doses of CSP are based on measurements of 24-hour urinary calcium excretion. The recommended initial dose of CSP is 15 grams/day (5 grams with each meal) in patients with urinary calcium greater than 300 mg/day (on moderate calcium—restricted diet, i.e., avoidance of dairy products). When urinary calcium declines to less than 150 mg/day, the dosage of CSP should be reduced to 10 grams/day (5 grams with supper, 2.5 grams each with remaining meal). Patients with controlled urinary calcium on moderate calcium—restricted diet of less than 300 mg/day (but greater than 200 mg/day) should begin on CSP 10 grams/day.

The following general measures should be imposed during CSP therapy. A moderate calcium intake is recommended, by avoidance of dairy products. A moderate dietary oxalate restriction should be imposed by discouraging ingestion of spinach (and similar dark greens), rhubarb, chocolate and brewed tea. Vitamin C supplementation should be denied because of its potential metabolism to oxalate. A high sodium intake should be discouraged by advising avoidance of "salty" foods and salt shakers, in an attempt to achieve an intake of less than 150 mEq/day. Fluid intake should be encouraged, to achieve a minimum urine output of 2 liters/day.

The dose of oral magnesium supplements, given as magnesium gluconate, depends upon the dose of CSP. Those receiving 15 grams of CSP/day should take 1.5 grams of magnesium gluconate before breakfast and again at bedtime (separately from CSP). Those taking 10 grams of CSP/day should take 1 gram of magnesium gluconate twice a day. To avoid binding of magnesium by CSP, supplemental magnesium should be given at least 1 hour before or after a dose of CSP.

It is recommended that each dose of CSP (in the powder form) be suspended in a glass of water, soft drink or fruit juice, and ingested within ½ hour of the meal. It should not be given with magnesium gluconate.

[See table above].

How Supplied: CALCIBIND™ NDC 0178-0255-90, is available for oral administration in boxes of 90 packets containing 2.5 grams of CSP powder each. CALCIBIND™ NDC 0178-0255-30 is available for oral administration in bottles of 300 grams of CSP bulk powder.

Continued on next page

Mission—Cont.

LITHOSTAT™ ℞
[lith'o-stat]
Acetohydroxamic Acid (AHA)

Description: Acetohydroxamic acid (AHA) is a stable, synthetic compound derived from hydroxylamine and ethyl acetate. Its molecular structure is similar to urea:

ACETOHYDROXAMIC ACID (AHA)

AHA is weakly acidic, highly soluble in water, and chelates metals - notably iron. The molecular weight is 75.068. AHA has a PKA of 9.32 and a melting point of 89–91°C. Available as 250 mg tablets.

Clinical Pharmacology: AHA reversibly inhibits the bacterial enzyme urease, thereby inhibiting the hydrolysis of urea and production of ammonia in urine infected with urea-splitting organisms. The reduced ammonia levels and decreased pH enhance the effectiveness of antimicrobial agents and allow an increased cure rate of these infections.

AHA is well absorbed from the gastrointestinal tract after oral administration; peak blood levels occur from 0.25 to 1 hour after dosing. The compound is distributed throughout body water, and there is no known binding to any tissue. AHA chelates with dietary iron within the gut. This reaction may interfere with absorption of AHA and with iron. Concomitant hypochromic anemia should be treated with intramuscular iron.

In rodents, the metabolic fate of AHA is well known; 55% is excreted unchanged in urine, 25% is excreted as acetamide or acetate and 7% is excreted by the lungs as carbon dioxide. Less than 1% is excreted in the feces. Approximately 5% of the administered dose is unaccounted for. In rodents, AHA shows a dose-related change in pharmacokinetics; with increasing dose, there is an increase in the half-life and an increase in the percent of the administered dose recovered in urine as unchanged AHA.

Pharmacokinetics in man are generally similar to rodents including the dose-related increase in half-life, but they are not as well characterized as in the rodent. Thirty-six to sixty-five percent (36–65%) of the oral dosage is excreted unchanged in the urine. It is unaltered AHA in urine that provides the therapeutic effect, but the precise concentration of AHA in urine that is necessary to inhibit urease is incompletely delineated. Therapeutic benefit may be obtained from concentrations as low as 8 mcg/ml; higher concentrations (i.e., 30 mcg/ml) are expected to provide more complete inhibition of urease. The plasma half-life of AHA is approximately 5–10 hours in subjects with normal renal function and is prolonged in patients with reduced renal function.

Acetohydroxamic acid has been evaluated clinically in patients with urea-splitting urinary infections, often accompanied by struvite stone disease, that were recalcitrant to other forms of medical and surgical management. In these clinical trials, AHA reduced the pathologically elevated urinary ammonia and pH levels that result from the hydrolysis of urea by the enzyme, urease.

AHA does not acidify urine directly nor does it have a direct anti-bacterial effect. The usefulness of reducing ammonia levels and decreasing urinary pH is suggested by single (not yet replicated) clinical trials in which urease inhibition 1) allowed successful antibiotic treatment of urea-splitting Proteus infections after surgical removal of struvite stones in patients not cured by 3 months of antibacterial treatment alone, and 2) reduced the rate of stone growth in patients who were not candidates for surgical removal of stones.

Indications and Usage: Acetohydroxamic acid (AHA) is indicated as adjunctive therapy in patients with chronic urea-splitting urinary infection. AHA is intended to decrease urinary ammonia and alkalinity, but it should not be used in lieu of curative surgical treatment (for patients with stones) or antimicrobial treatment. Long-term treatment with AHA may be warranted to maintain urease inhibition as long as urea-splitting infection is present. Experience with AHA does not go beyond 7 years. A patient package insert should be distributed to each patient who receives AHA.

Contraindications: Acetohydroxamic acid (AHA) should not be used in:
a. patients whose physical state and disease are amenable to definitive surgery and appropriate antimicrobial agents
b. patients whose urine is infected by non-urease producing organisms
c. patients whose urinary infections can be controlled by culture-specific oral antimicrobial agents
d. patients whose renal function is poor (i.e., serum creatinine more than 2.5 mg/dl and/or creatinine clearance less than 20 ml/min)
e. female patients who do not evidence a satisfactory methods of contraception
f. patients who are pregnant

Acetohydroxamic acid (AHA) may cause fetal harm when administered to a pregnant woman. AHA was teratogenic (retarded and/or clubbed rear leg at 750 mg/kg and above and exencephaly and encephalocele at 1,500 mg/kg) when given intraperitoneally to rats. AHA is contraindicated in women who are or may become pregnant. If this drug is used during pregnancy, or if the patient becomes pregnant while taking this drug, the patient should be informed of the potential hazard to the fetus.

Warnings: A Coombs negative hemolytic anemia has occurred in patients receiving AHA. Gastrointestinal upset characterized by nausea, vomiting, anorexia and generalized malaise have accompanied the most severe forms of hemolytic anemia. Approximately 15% of patients receiving AHA have had only laboratory findings of an anemia. However, most patients developed a mild reticulocytosis. The untoward reactions have reverted to normal following cessation of treatment. A complete blood count, including a reticulocyte count, is recommended after two weeks of treatment. If the reticulocyte count exceeds 6%, a reduced dosage should be entertained. A CBC and reticulocyte count are recommended at 3-month intervals for the duration of treatment.

Precautions:
General:
Hematologic Effects:
Bone marrow depression (leukopenia, anemia, and thrombocytopenia) has occurred in experimental animals receiving large doses of AHA, but has not been seen in man to date. AHA is a known inhibitor of DNA synthesis and also chelates metals notably iron. Its bone marrow suppressant effect is probably related to its ability to inhibit DNA synthesis, but anemia could also be related to depletion of iron stores. To date, the only clinical effect noted has been hemolysis, with a decrease in the circulating red blood cells, hemoglobin and hematocrit. Abnormalities in platelet or white blood cell count have not been noted. However, clinical monitoring of the platelet and white cell count is recommended.

Monitoring Liver Function:
Abnormalities of liver function have not been reported to date. However, a chloro-benzene derivative of acetohydroxamic acid caused significant liver dysfunction in an unrelated study. Therefore, close monitoring of liver function is recommended. (See Carcinogenesis for discussion of possible hepatic carcinogenesis.)

Use In Patients With Renal Impairment:
Since AHA is eliminated primarily by the kidneys, patients with significantly impaired renal function should be closely monitored, and a reduction of daily dose may be needed to avoid excessive drug accumulation. (See Dosage and Administration.)

Drug Interactions: AHA has been used concomitantly with insulin, oral and parenteral antibiotics, and progestational agents. No clinically significant interactions have been noted, but until wider clinical experience is obtained, AHA should be used with caution in patients receiving other therapeutic agents.

AHA taken in association with alcoholic beverages has resulted in a rash. (See Adverse Reactions.)
AHA chelates heavy metals - notably iron. The absorption of iron and AHA from the intestinal lumen may be reduced when both drugs are taken concomitantly. When iron administration is indicated, intramuscular iron is probably the product of choice.

Carcinogenesis, Mutagenesis, Impairment of Fertility:
Well controlled, long-term animal studies that identify the carcinogenic potential of AHA treatment have not been conducted. Acetamide, a metabolite of AHA, has been shown to cause hepatocellular carcinoma in rats at oral doses 1,500 times the human dose. AHA is cytotoxic and was positive for mutagenicity in the Ames test.

Pregnancy:
Pregnancy Category X. (See Contraindications.)

Nursing Mothers:
It is not known whether AHA is secreted in human milk. Because many drugs are excreted in human milk, and because of the potential for serious adverse reactions in nursing infants from AHA, a decision should be made to discontinue nursing or the drug, taking into account the significance of the drug to the mother's well being.

Pediatric Use:
Children with chronic, recalcitrant, urea-splitting urinary infection may benefit from treatment with AHA. However, detailed studies involving dosage and dose intervals in children have not been established. Children have tolerated a dose of 10 mg/kg/day, taken in two or three divided doses, satisfactorily for periods up to one year. Close monitoring of such patients is mandatory.

Adverse Reactions: Experience with AHA is limited. About 150 patients have been treated, most for periods of more than a year.
Adverse reactions have occurred in up to thirty percent (30%) of the patients receiving AHA. In some instances the reactions were symptomatic; in others only changes in laboratory parameters were noted. Adverse reactions seem to be more prevalent in patients with preexisting thrombophlebitis or phlebothrombosis and/or in patients with advanced degrees of renal insufficiency. The risk of adverse reactions is highest during the first year of treatment. Chronic treatment does not seem to increase the risk nor the severity of adverse reactions.

The following reactions have been reported:
Neurological:
Mild headaches are commonly reported (about 30%) during the first 48 hours of treatment. These headaches are mild, responsive to oral salicylate-type analgesics, and usually disappear spontaneously. The headaches have not been associated with vertigo, tinnitus, or visual or auditory abnormalities. Tremulousness and nervousness have also been reported.

Gastrointestinal:
Gastrointestinal symptoms, nausea, vomiting, anorexia, and malaise have occurred in 20–5% of patients. In most patients the symptoms were mild, transitory, and did not result in interruption of treatment. Approximately 3% of patients developed a hemolytic anemia of sufficient magnitude to warrant interruption in treatment; several of these patients also had symptoms of gastrointestinal upset.

Hematological:
Approximately 15% of patients have had laboratory findings characteristic of a hemolytic anemia. A mild reticulocytosis (5–%) without anemia, is even more prevalent. The laboratory findings are occasionally accompanied by systemic symptoms such as malaise, lethargy and fatigue, and gastrointestinal symptoms. Symptoms and laboratory findings have invariably improved following cessation of treatment with AHA. The hematological abnormalities are more prevalent in patients with advanced renal failure.

Product Information

Dermatological:
A nonpruritic, macular skin rash has occurred in the upper extremities and on the face of several patients taking AHA on a long-term basis, usually when AHA has been taken concomitantly with alcoholic beverages, but in a few patients in the absence of alcohol consumption. The rash commonly appears 30–45 minutes after ingestion of alcoholic beverages; it characteristically disappears spontaneously in 30–60 minutes. The rash may be associated with a general sensation of warmth. In some patients the rash is sufficiently severe to warrant discontinuation of treatment, but most patients have continued treatment, avoiding alcohol or using smaller quantities of it. Alopecia has also been reported in patients taking AHA.

Cardiovascular:
Superficial phlebitis involving the lower extremities has occurred in several patients on AHA during the early (Phase II) clinical trials. Several of the affected patients had had phlebitic episodes prior to treatment. One patient developed deep vein thrombosis of the lower extremities. The patient with phlebothrombosis had an associated traumatic injury to the groin. It is unclear whether the phlebitis was related to or exacerbated by treatment with AHA. No patient in the three (3) year controlled (Phase III) clinical trial developed phlebitis. In all instances these vascular abnormalities returned to normal following appropriate medical therapy. Embolic phenomena have been reported in three patients taking AHA in the Phase II trial. The phlebitis and emboli resolved following discontinuation of AHA and implementation of appropriate medical therapy. Several patients have resumed treatment with AHA without ill effect. Palpitations have also been reported in patients taking AHA.

Respiratory:
No symptoms have been reported. Radiographic evidence of small pulmonary emboli has been seen in three patients with phlebitis in their lower legs.

Psychiatric:
Depression, anxiety, nervousness, and tremulousness have been observed in approximately 20% of patients taking AHA. In most patients the symptoms were mild and transitory, but in about 6% of patients the symptoms were sufficiently distressing to warrant interruption or discontinuation of treatment.

Overdosage: Acute deliberate overdosage in man has not occurred, but would be expected to induce the following symptoms: anorexia, malaise, lethargy, diminished sense of well being, tremulousness, anxiety, nausea and vomiting. Laboratory findings are likely to include an elevated reticulocyte count and a severe hemolytic reaction requiring hospitalization, symptomatic treatment, and possibly blood transfusions. Concomitant reduction in platelets and/or white blood cells should be anticipated.

Milder overdosages resulting in hemolysis have occurred in an occasional patient with reduced renal function after several weeks or months of continuous treatment.

The acute LD 50 of AHA in animals (rats) is 4.8 gm/kg.

Recommended treatment for an overdosage reaction consists of (1) cessation of treatment, (2) close monitoring of hematologic status, (3) symptomatic treatment, and (4) blood transfusions as required by the clinical circumstances. The drug is probably dialyzable, but this property has not been tested clinically.

Dosage and Administration: AHA should be administered orally, one tablet 3–4 times a day in a total daily dose of 10–15 mg/kg/day. The recommended starting dose is 12 mg/kg/day, administered at 6–8 hour intervals at a time when the stomach is empty. The maximum daily dose should be no more than 1.5 grams, regardless of body weight.

The dosage should be reduced in patients with reduced renal function. Patients whose serum creatinine is greater than 1.8 mg/dl should take no more than 1.0 gm/day; such patients should be dosed at q-12-h intervals. Further reductions in dosage to prevent the accumulation of toxic concentrations in the blood may also be desirable. Insufficient data exists to accurately characterize the optimum dose and/or dose interval in patients with moderate degrees of renal insufficiency.

Patients with advanced renal insufficiency (i.e., serum creatinine more than 2.5 mg/dl) should not be treated with AHA. The risk of accumulation of toxic blood levels of AHA seems to be greater than the chances for a beneficial effect in such patients.

In children an initial dose of 10 mg/kg/day is recommended. Close monitoring of the patient's clinical condition and hematologic status is recommended. Titration of the dose to higher or lower levels may be required to obtain an optimum therapeutic effect and/or to reduce the risk of side effects.

How Supplied: LITHOSTAT™, NDC 0178-0500-12, is available for oral administration as 250 mg scored tablets, in unit of use packages of 120 tablets.

MISSION PRENATAL SERIES

MISSION PRENATAL®
Vitamins—Iron—Calcium—.4 mg. Folic Acid
NDC 0178-132-01

MISSION PRENATAL® F.A.
Vitamins—Iron—Calcium—.8 mg. Folic Acid and Zinc
NDC 0178-0153-01

MISSION PRENATAL® H.P.
Vitamins—Iron—Calcium—0.8 mg. Folic Acid
NDC 0178-0161-01

Composition: Each tablet contains:

		%U.S.R.D.A.
Ferrous Gluconate		333.3 mg.
(Iron	214	38.6 mg.)
Ascorbic Acid (C)	167	100.0 mg.
Thiamine Mononitrate (B$_1$)	270	5.0 mg.
*† Pyridoxine HCl (B$_6$)	99	3.0 mg.
Riboflavin (B$_2$)	100	2.0 mg.
Niacinamide	50	10.0 mg.
d-Calcium Pantothenate	9	1.0 mg.
Vitamin B$_{12}$ (Crystalline on Resin)	25	2.0 mcg.
*† Folic Acid	50	0.4 mg.
Vitamin A Acetate	50	4000.0 USPU
Vitamin D$_2$	100	400.0 USPU
Calcium Carbonate		70.0 mg.
Calcium Gluconate		100.0 mg.
Calcium Lactate		100.0 mg.
(Calcium	4	50.0 mg.)
Zinc (as Zinc Sulfate)		15.0 mg.

*Pyridoxine HCL—Mission® Prenatal F.A. =10mg., 329%U.S.R.D.A.
*Folic Acid—Mission® Prenatal F.A. =.8mg., 100%U.S.R.D.A.
†Pyridoxine HCL—Mission®Prenatal H.P. =25 mg., 1250%U.S.R.D.A.
†Folic Acid—Mission® Prenatal H.P. =1.0 mg., 125%U.S.R.D.A.
Zinc—only in Mission® Prenatal F.A.

Indications: ALL MISSION® PRENATALS are prenatal and postpartum supplements.

Dosage: Take one tablet at bedtime or as directed by your physician. Keep this and all medications out of the reach of children.

Precaution: Folic Acid, especially in doses above 0.1 mg. daily, may obscure pernicious anemia in that hematologic remission may occur while neurological manifestations remain progressive.

How Supplied: MISSION® PRENATAL is supplied as pink, football-shaped, sugar-coated tablets in bottles of 100.
MISSION® PRENATAL F.A. is supplied as blue, football-shaped, sugar coated tablets in bottles of 100.
MISSION® PRENATAL H.P. is supplied as green, football-shaped, sugar-coated tablets in bottles of 100.

MISSION PRENATAL™ RX ℞

Prenatal Supplement with Vitamins and Minerals
NDC 0178-0007-01

COMPOSITION: Each Tablet Contains:

		%USRDA*
Vitamin A	8000 I.U.	100
(as Vitamin A Acetate)		
Vitamin D	400 I.U.	100
Vitamin C	240 mg.	400
(as Ascorbic Acid, Calcium Ascorbate)		
Vitamin B$_1$	4 mg.	235
(as Thiamine Mononitrate)		
Vitamin B$_2$	2 mg.	100
(as Riboflavin)		
Vitamin B$_3$	20 mg.	100
(as Niacinamide)		
Vitamin B$_5$	10 mg.	100
(as Calcium Pantothenate)		
Vitamin B$_6$	20 mg.	800
(as Pyridoxine Hydrochloride)		
Vitamin B$_{12}$	8 mcg.	100
(as Cyanocobalamine on resin)		
Folic Acid	1 mg.	125
Iron	60 mg.	333
(as Ferrous Fumarate)		
Calcium	175 mg.	13.5
(as Calcium Carbonate and Calcium Ascorbate)		
Iodine	0.3 mg.	200
(as Potassium Iodide)		
Zinc	15 mg.	100
(as Zinc Sulfate, dried)		
Copper	2 mg.	100
(as Cupric Oxide)		

*USRDA: U.S. recommended daily allowance for pregnant or lactating women.

Indications: MISSION PRENATAL Rx is a prenatal and postpartum supplement.

Dosage: Take one tablet at bedtime or as directed by your physician.

Caution: Federal law prohibits dispensing without a prescription.

How Supplied: MISSION PRENATAL Rx is supplied as pink, football shape, film-coated tablets in bottles of 100.

Literature Available: Yes.

MISSION® PRE-SURGICAL

A dietary supplement for pre-surgical and post-surgical patients. NDC 0178-0168-01

Composition: Each tablet contains:

		%USRDA*
Ascorbic Acid (C)	500.0 mg	833
Thiamine Mononitrate (B$_1$)	2.5 mg	150
Riboflavin(B$_2$)	2.6 mg	150
Niacinamide (B$_3$)	30.0 mg	150
Calcium Pantothenate (B$_5$)	16.3 mg	150
Pyridoxine Hydrochloride (B$_6$)	3.6 mg	150
Vitamin B$_{12}$	9.0 mcg	150
Vitamin A Acetate	5000 USPU	100
Vitamin D$_2$	400 USPU	100
Vitamin E Succinate	45 IU	150
Iron (as Ferrous Gluconate)	27.0 mg	150
Zinc (as Zinc Sulfate)	22.5 mg	150

*USRDA: U.S. Receommended Daily Allowance for adults and children 4 or more years of age.

Action and Uses: A dietary supplement specifically designed to provide the vitamin and mineral nutritional assistance needed by the pre- and post-surgical patient for optimal recovery from the stress of surgery.

Administration and Dosage: One tablet at bedtime or as directed by physician.

Warning: KEEP THIS AND ALL MEDICATIONS OUT OF THE REACH OF CHILDREN. In case of accidental overdose, seek professional assis-

Continued on next page

Mission—Cont.

tance or contact a poison control center immediately.
How Supplied: MISSION® PRE-SURGICAL is supplied as a light green, bolus-shaped, sugar coated tablet in bottles of 100.
Literature available: Yes.

PRULET®
[prū-let']
White Phenolphthalein tablets N.F.
NDC 0178-0090-01

Composition: Each tablet contains:
White phenolphthalein N.F. ...... 60 mg.
Action and Uses: PRULET® is a mild and gentle, effective laxative for patients with atonic or hypotonic bowel syndrome.
PRULET® is a chewable tablet in lemon—lime flavor.
Administration and Dosage: Take one to three tablets administered at bedtime; then adjust to need.
Contraindications: Not to be taken in the presence of nausea, vomiting, abdominal pains, or other symptoms of appendicitis.
Precautions: Phenolphthalein is known to produce skin eruptions in sensitized individuals. If a skin rash or eruption appears, do not take this or any other preparation containing phenolphthalein. PRULET® may cause pink to red urine coloration in patients with an alkaline urine.
How Supplied: PRULET® is supplied in green scored tablets in film strip packages of 12 and 40 tablets.
Literature Available: Yes.

SUPAC®
[sū'pac]
Analgesic Compound
NDC-0178-0100-01

Composition: Each tablet contains:
Acetaminophen .... 160 mg.
Aspirin .... 230 mg.
Caffeine .... 33 mg.
Calcium Gluconate .... 60 mg.
Action and Uses: For temporary relief of pain accompanying simple head colds, temporary relief of pain accompanying menstruation, sinus and tension headache, minor traumatic pain, tooth extractions, arthritic and rheumatic pain syndromes.
Administration and Dosage: Adults—One or two tablets. This dose may be repeated in 4 hours. Do not exceed 4 tablets at a single dose or 16 tablets in a 24 hour period. Children—6 to 12 years of age, ½ of the maximum adult dose or dosage; 3 to 6 years of age, ⅓ of the maximum adult dose or dosage.
Precautions: If pain persists for more than 10 days, or redness is present, or in conditions affecting children under 12 years of age, physicians should be alert to other possible complications.
How Supplied: SUPAC® is supplied as white scored tablets in bottles of 100 and 1000 tablets.
Literature Available: Yes.

THERABID®
[thēr'a-bid]
Therapeutic Multivitamin
NDC 0178-0171-01

Composition: Each Tablet Contains:
		% US RDA
Ascorbic Acid (Vitamin C)	500 mg.	833
Thiamine Mononitrate (Vitamin B$_1$)	15 mg.	1000
Riboflavin (Vitamin B$_2$)	10 mg.	588
Niacinamide (Vitamin B$_3$)	100 mg.	500
Calcium Pantothenate (Vitamin B$_5$)	20 mg.	200
Pyridoxine Hydrochloride (Vitamin B$_6$)	10 mg.	500
Vitamin B$_{12}$	5 mcg.	83
Vitamin A Acetate	5,000 U.	100
Vitamin D$_2$	200 U.	optional
Vitamin E (as a-tocopheryl acetate)	30 IU	100

Action and Uses: THERABID® is a therapeutic multivitamin preparation.
Administration and Dosage: One to two tablets per day or at the discretion of the physician.
Precautions: Do not exceed a dosage of four tablets per day.
How Supplied: THERABID® is supplied as green capsule shaped sugar coated tablets in bottles of 100 tablets.
Literature Available: Yes.

THERA–GESIC®
[ther'a-jē-zik]
Analgesic Creme Balm
Methyl Salicylate and Menthol

Description: THERA-GESIC® contains Methyl Salicylate and Menthol in a rapidly absorbed greaseless base.
Actions: Topical analgesic, counter irritant.
Indications: For the temporary relief of pain associated with musculo-skeletal soreness and discomfort; additionally, as a topical adjunct in arthritis, rheumatism, and bursitis.
Contraindications: Do not use in patients with Aspirin or Salicylate idiosyncrasy.
Warnings: Use only as directed. Keep away from children to avoid accidental poisoning. Keep away from eyes, mucous membranes, broken or irritated skin. If skin irritation develops, or if pain lasts 10 days or more, or if redness is present, discontinue use and consult a physician. DO NOT SWALLOW. If swallowed, induce vomiting, call a physician.
Precautions: Do not use excessive amounts of THERA-GESIC® or occlude a fresh application of THERA-GESIC®. Do not heat pack THERA-GESIC® covered skin. For use by adults only.
Adverse Reactions: Adverse reactions related to the Salicylate and Menthol components are possible. These include excessive irritation, tinnitus, nausea or vomiting if excessive or extreme dosage is employed.
Dosage and Administration: Gently massage THERA-GESIC® in thin applications into the sore or painful area as well as into the area immediately surrounding the painful area. The number of thin applications applied controls the intensity of the action of THERA-GESIC®. One application provides a mild effect, two provide a strong effect and three applications provide a very strong effect. Once THERA-GESIC® has penetrated the skin, the area may be washed, leaving the area dry, clean and free from the typical wintergreen odor without decreasing the effectiveness of the product. If you intend to bandage or wrap the area, the area should be washed first to avoid excessive irritation.
How Supplied:
NDC-0178-0320-03   Tubes-3 oz.
NDC-0178-0320-05   Tubes-5 oz.

Important Notice
Before prescribing or administering any product described in PHYSICIANS' DESK REFERENCE always consult the PDR Supplement for possible new or revised information

---

Muro Pharmaceutical, Inc.
890 EAST STREET
TEWKSBURY, MA 01876-9987

BROMFED® CAPSULES ℞
[brŏm'fĕd]

A green and clear capsule containing white beads.
Each capsule contains:
Brompheniramine maleate .... 12 mg.
Pseudoephedrine hydrochloride .... 120 mg.
in a specially prepared base to provide prolonged action.

BROMFED-PD® CAPSULES ℞

A blue—green and clear capsule containing white beads.
Each capsule contains:
Brompheniramine maleate .... 6 mg.
Pseudoephedrine hydrochloride .... 60 mg.
in a specially prepared base to provide prolonged action.

BROMFED® TABLETS ℞

A white scored tablet.
Each tablet contains:
Brompheniramine maleate .... 4 mg.
Pseudoephedrine hydrochloride .... 60 mg.
BROMFED contains ingredients of the following therapeutic classes: antihistamine and decongestant.
Clinical Pharmacology: Brompheniramine maleate is an alkylamine type antihistamine. This group of antihistamines are among the most active histamine antagonists and are generally effective in relatively low doses. The drugs are not so prone to produce drowsiness and are among the most suitable agents for day time use; but again, a significant proportion of patients do experience this effect. Pseudoephedrine hydrochloride is a sympathomimetic which acts predominently on alpha receptors and has little action on beta receptors. It therefore functions as an oral nasal decongestant with minimal CNS stimulation.
Indications: For the temporary relief of symptoms of the common cold, allergic rhinitis (hay fever) and sinusitis.
Contraindications: Hypersensitivity to any of the ingredients. Also contraindicated in patients with severe hypertension, severe coronary artery disease, patients on MAO inhibitor therapy, patients with narrow-angle glaucoma, urinary retention, peptic ulcer and during an asthmatic attack.
Warnings: Considerable caution should be exercised in patients with hypertension, diabetes mellitus, ischemic heart disease, hyperthyroidism, increased intraocular pressure and prostatic hypertrophy. The elderly (60 years or older) are more likely to exhibit adverse reactions.
Antihistamines may cause excitability, especially in children. At dosages higher than the recommended dose, nervousness, dizziness or sleeplessness may occur.
Precautions: General: Caution should be exercised in patients with high blood pressure, heart disease, diabetes or thyroid disease. The antihistamine in this product may exhibit additive effects with other CNS depressants, including alcohol.
Information for Patients: Antihistamine may cause drowsiness and ambulatory patients who operate machinery or motor vehicles should be cautioned accordingly.
Drug Interactions: MAO inhibitors and beta adrenergic blockers increase the effects of sympathomimetics. Sympathomimetics may reduce the antihypertensive effects of methyldopa, mecamylamine, reserpine and veratrum alkaloids. Concomitant use of antihistamines with alcohol and other CNS depressants may have an additive effect.
Pregnancy: The safety of use of this product in pregnancy has not been established.
Adverse Reactions: Adverse reactions include drowsiness, lassitude, nausea, giddiness, dryness of mouth, blurred vision, cardiac palpitations, flushing, increased irritability or excitement (especially in children).

Dosage and Administration:
BROMFED® CAPSULES Adults and children over 12 years of age —1 capsule orally every 12 hours.
BROMFED-PD® CAPSULES Children 6 to 12 years of age —1 capsule orally every 12 hours. Adults —2 capsules every 12 hours.
BROMFED® TABLETS Adults and children 12 and over: One tablet every 4 hours not to exceed 6 doses in 24 hours. Children 6 to 12 years: One-half tablet every 4 hours not to exceed 6 doses in 24 hours. Do not give to children under 6 years except under the advice and supervision of a physician.
How Supplied: Bottles of 100 and 500.
Dispense in tight containers as defined in USP. Store between 15°–30°C (59°–86°F).

GUAIFED® Capsules ℞
[gwi'ah-fĕd]

Description: Each capsule contains:
Pseudoephedrine hydrochloride ....120 mg.
in a specially prepared base to provide prolonged action.
Guaifenesin...250 mg.
designed for immediate release to provide rapid action.
This product contains ingredients of the following therapeutic classes: decongestant and expectorant.
Clinical Pharmacology: Pseudoephedrine hydrochloride is a sympathomimetic which acts predominently on alpha receptors and has little action on beta receptors. It therefore functions as an oral nasal decongestant with minimal CNS stimulation. This product is designed to release the pseudoephedrine hydrochloride gradually over a period of 5 to 7 hours resulting in activity up to 10 to 12 hours. Guaifenesin is an expectorant which thins the mucous in the bronchial tract due to reflex action on the stomach. The guaifenesin, therefore, is not in a sustained release form. It is available immediately to trigger the reflex action.
Indications: For temporary relief of nasal congestion and dry non-productive cough associated with the common cold and other respiratory allergies.
Contraindications: This product is contraindicated in patients with a known hypersensitivity to any of its ingredients. Also contraindicated in patients with severe hypertension, severe coronary artery disease and patients on MAO inhibitor therapy. Should not be used in children under 12 years or in nursing mothers.
Warnings: Considerable caution should be exercised in patients with hypertension, diabetes mellitus, ischemic heart disease, hyperthroidism and prostatic hypertrophy. The elderly (60 years or older) are more likely to exhibit adverse reactions. At doses higher than the recommended dose, nervousness, dizziness or sleeplessness may occur.
Precautions:
General: Caution should be exercised in patients with high blood pressure, heart disease, diabetes or thyroid disease.
Drug Interactions: MAO inhibitors and beta adrenergic blockers increase the effects of sympathomimetics. Sympathomimetics may reduce the antihypertensive effect of methyldopa, mecamylamine, reserpine and veratrum alkaloids.
Pregnancy: The safety of use of this product in pregnancy has not been established.
Adverse Reactions: Adverse reactions include nausea, cardiac, palpitations, increased irritability or excitement, headache, dizziness and tachycardia.
Dosage and Administration: Adults and children over 12 years of age: 1 capsule orally every 12 hours.
How Supplied: Bottle of 100
STORE AND DISPENSE IN TIGHT CONTAINERS AS DEFINED IN THE USP/NF. STORE BETWEEN 15°–30°C (59°–86°F).

LIQUID PRED® Syrup ℞
Each teaspoonful contains:
Prednisone 5mg/5ml
How Supplied:
NDC-0451-1201-04–4 fl. oz. (120 ml)
NDC-0451-1201-08–8 fl. oz. (240 ml)

MURO TEARS®
[mū'rō terz]
Artificial Tears
(See PDR For Nonprescription Drugs)

SALINEX Nasal Mist and Drops
[sal'i-nĕx]
(Buffered isotonic sodium chloride solution)
(See PDR for Nonprescription Drugs)

National Dermaceutical Products, Inc.
8749 SURREY PLACE
MAINEVILLE, OH 45039

STIMUZYME PLUS® ℞
Composition: Each 0.82 cc. of medication delivered to the wound site contains Trypsin crystallized 0.1 mg., Balsam Peru 72.5 mg., Castor Oil 650.0 mg., and an emulsifier.
Action: Trypsin is intended for debridement of eschar and other necrotic tissue. Balsam Peru is an effective capillary bed stimulant used to increase circulation in the wound site area. Also, Balsam Peru has a mildly bactericidal action. Castor Oil is used to improve epithelialization by reducing premature epithelial desiccation and cornification. Also, it can act as a protective covering and aids in the reduction of pain.
Indications: For the treatment of decubitus ulcers, varicose ulcers, debridement of eschar, dehiscent wounds and sunburn.
Uses: Stimuzyme Plus is in aerosol form which can be important to healing. It must be remembered, healing starts with a thin sheath of epithelium no more than a cell or two thick. Any rough movement or trauma can quickly destroy the healing tissue. Aerosols have the advantage of eliminating all extraneous physical contact with the wound. Stimuzyme Plus is easy to apply and quickly reduces odor frequently accompanying a decubitus ulcer. The wound may be left open or a wet bandage may be applied.
Warning: Do not spray on fresh arterial clots. Avoid spraying in eyes or nostrils. Flammable, do not use near fire or open flame. Contents under pressure. Do not puncture or incinerate. Do not store at temperatures above 120°F. Keep out of reach of children. Use only as directed. Intentional misuse by deliberately concentrating and inhaling the contents can be harmful or fatal.
Dosage: Apply three times daily or as often as necessary. Shake well, press the aerosol valve and coat the wound rapidly but not excessively.
How Supplied:
2 oz. Aerosol NDC 51268-075-02
4 oz. Aerosol NDC 51268-075-04

IDENTIFICATION PROBLEM?
Consult PDR's
Product Identification Section
where you'll find over 1200
products pictured actual size
and in full color.

Neutrogena Dermatologics
Division of
Neutrogena Corporation
5755 W. 96TH STREET
P.O. BOX 45036
LOS ANGELES, CA 90045

MELANEX® ℞
[mel'an-ex]
(3% hydroquinone) Topical Solution

Composition: Melanex (3% hydroquinone) Topical Solution contains 30 mg hydroquinone per ml in a vehicle of 47.3% alcohol, purified water, laureth-4, isopropyl alcohol 4%, propylene glycol and ascorbic acid.
Pharmacological class: Depigmenting agent.
Clinical Pharmacology: It has been suggested that the primary action of hydroquinone is directed at tyrosinase. The selective inhibition of the enzyme affects melanogenesis in the melanocytes resulting in cessation of melanin formation and subsequent reduction in pigmentation. Additional studies indicate that hydroquinone acts on the essential subcellular metabolic processes of melanocytes with resultant cytolysis, i.e., nonenzyme-medicated depigmentation.
Indications and Usage: Melanex is indicated in the temporary bleaching of hyperpigmented skin conditions such as chloasma, melasma, freckles, senile lentigines, and other forms of melanin hyperpigmentation.
Dosage and Administration: Apply to affected areas twice daily, in the morning and before bedtime. During the day, an effective broad spectrum sunscreen should be used and unnecessary solar exposure avoided, or protective clothing should be worn to cover bleached skin in order to prevent repigmentation from occurring.
Contraindications: Melanex is contraindicated in persons who have shown hypersensitivity to hydroquinone or any of the other ingredients. The safety of topical treatment with hydroquinone during pregnancy has not been established.
Precautions: Concurrent use of Melanex with benzoyl peroxide may result in transient dark staining of skin areas so treated. This is due to the oxidation of hydroquinone by the benzoyl peroxide. This transient staining can be removed by discontinuing concurrent usage and normal soap cleansing.
For external use only. Hydroquinone preparations may produce skin irritation in susceptible individuals and have a slight potential to produce an allergic response. Therefore, the physician should use appropriate caution. If rash or irritation develops, discontinue use and consult physician. Do not use on children under 12. If no improvement is seen after three months of treatment, use of product should be discontinued. Avoid contact with eyes. In case of accidental contact, patient should rinse eyes thoroughly with water and contact physician. A bitter taste and anesthetic effect may occur if applied to lips. Keep out of the reach of children. Use of Melanex in paranasal and infraorbital areas increases the chance of irritation (see Adverse Reactions). A Patient Instruction Sheet for using Melanex is provided (to the physician) to be given to the patient at the discretion of the physician.
Adverse Reactions: The following have been reported: dryness and fissuring of paranasal and infraorbital areas, erythema and stinging. Hydroquinone has been known to produce irritation and sensitization in susceptible individuals.
How Supplied: 1.0 fl oz (30 ml) bottle with Appliderm™ Applicator Unit.
Note: Slight darkening of the Melanex solution is normal and will not affect potency. See expiration date on bottle.
For additional information, call Neutrogena Corporation, Technical Department, (800) 421-6857. In California, call (213) 642-1150, collect.
NDC #10812-9300-1

Continued on next page

Neutrogena—Cont.

VEHICLE/N®
VEHICLE/N® MILD

Composition: Vehicle/N and Vehicle/N MILD are both versatile liquid vehicles for extemporaneous compounding of topical drugs. Both formulations solubilize selected dermatologic agents and provide astringent and drying actions.
The Appliderm™ Applicator Unit automatically filters the compounded drug and provides a convenient, spill-proof, self-contained unit for topical application.

Vehicle/N contains:
Alcohol	47.5%
Purified Water	
Laureth-4	
Isopropyl Alcohol	4.0%
Propylene Glycol	

Vehicle/N MILD contains:
Alcohol	41.5%
Purified Water	
Isopropyl Alcohol	6.0%
Laureth-4	

Precautions: Do not use near fire or flame due to alcohol content. Both Neutrogena Vehicle/N and Vehicle/N MILD preparations contain substantial alcohol and are not suitable for use in acute dermatoses. Stinging may be noted if used on irritated or abraded skin. Avoid contact with eyes or eyelids. If the product accidentally comes in contact with eyes, rinse thoroughly with water and contact physician. For external use only. Keep out of reach of children.
Contraindications: Vehicle/N and Vehicle/N MILD are contraindicated in persons who have shown hypersensitivity to any of their listed ingredients.
Availability: 50 ml in plastic bottle with applicator top. (Bottle filled to ¾ capacity to ensure proper mixing.)
Note: Laboratory and clinical evaluations necessary to determine the safety and efficacy of the preparations resulting from the addition of any drugs to Neutrogena Vehicle/N and Vehicle/N MILD have not been conducted. Neutrogena Corporation makes no claims regarding the safety or efficacy of extemporaneously prepared products.
For additional information, call Neutrogena Corporation, Technical Department, (800) 421-6857. In California, call (213) 642-1150 collect.
Vehicle/N: NDC #10812-9100-1
Vehicle/N MILD: NDC #10812-9400-1
Patent Pending

Norcliff Thayer Inc.
303 SOUTH BROADWAY
TARRYTOWN, NY 10591

A-200 Pyrinate® Pediculicide Shampoo
Liquid, Gel

A-200 Pyrinate® Liquid
Description: Active ingredients: pyrethrins 0.17%, piperonyl butoxide technical 2% (equivalent to 1.6% (butylcarbityl) (6-propylpiperonyl) ether and 0.4% related compounds. Inert ingredients: petroleum distillate 5%, other inert ingredients 92.83%.

A-200 Pyrinate® Gel
Description: Active ingredients: pyrethrins 0.33%, piperonyl butoxide technical 4% (equivalent to 3.2% (butylcarbityl) (6-propylpiperonyl) ether and 0.8% related compounds. Inert ingredients: petroleum distillate 5.33%, other inert ingredients 90.34%.
Actions: A-200 Pyrinate is an effective pediculicide for control of head lice (Pediculus humanus capitis), pubic lice (Phthirus pubis) and body lice (Pediculus humanus corporis), and their nits.
Indications: A-200 Pyrinate Liquid and Gel are indicated for the treatment of human pediculosis—head lice, body lice and pubic lice, and their eggs. A-200 Pyrinate Gel is specially formulated for pubic lice and head lice in children, where control of application is desirable.
Contraindications: A-200 Pyrinate is contraindicated in individuals hypersensitive to any of its ingredients or allergic to ragweed.
Precautions: A-200 Pyrinate is for external use only. It is harmful if swallowed or inhaled. It may be irritating to the eyes and mucous membranes. In case of accidental contact with eyes, they should be immediately flushed with water. In order to prevent reinfestation with lice, all clothing and bedding must be sterilized or treated concurrent with the application of this preparation. If skin irritation or signs of infection are present, a physician should be consulted.
Administration and Dosage: Apply sufficient A-200 Pyrinate to completely "wet" the hair and scalp or skin of any infested area. Allow applicaton to remain no longer than 10 minutes. Wash and rinse with plenty of warm water. Remove dead lice and eggs from hair with fine comb. To restore body and luster to hair following scalp applications, follow with a good shampoo. If necessary, this treatment may be repeated, but should not exceed two applications within 24 hours.
How Supplied: A-200 Pyrinate Liquid in 2 and 4 fl. oz. bottles with special comb. A-200 Pyrinate Gel in 1 oz. tubes.
Literature Available: Patient literature available upon request.
Shown in Product Identification Section, page 422

ESOTÉRICA® MEDICATED FADE CREAM
Regular
Facial
Fortified with Sunscreen Scented
Fortified with Sunscreen Unscented
(See PDR For Nonprescription Drugs)

LIQUIPRIN®
(acetaminophen)
(See PDR For Nonprescription Drugs)

NATURE'S REMEDY® Laxative
(See PDR For Nonprescription Drugs)

NoSalt™
Salt Alternative
Regular and Seasoned
(See PDR For Nonprescription Drugs)

OXY CLEAN™ Lathering Facial Scrub
(See PDR For Nonprescription Drugs)

OXY CLEAN™ MEDICATED
Cleanser
Pads
Soap
(See PDR Nonprescription Drugs)

OXY-5® Lotion with Sorboxyl
OXY-10® Lotion and Cover with Sorboxyl
Benzoyl Peroxide Lotion 5% and 10%
(See PDR For Nonprescription Drugs)

OXY-10® WASH Antibacterial Skin Wash
(See PDR For Nonprescription Drugs)

TUMS® Antacid Tablets, Regular and Extra Strength
(See PDR For Nonprescription Drugs)

Products are cross-indexed by generic and chemical names in the **YELLOW SECTION**

Nordisk-USA
6500 ROCK SPRING DRIVE
SUITE 304
BETHESDA, MD 20817

PURIFIED PORK INSULIN PRODUCTS

INSULATARD™ NPH
[in′sŭl-ă″tard]
U-100 Pork, Isophane purified pork insulin suspension.

WARNING: ANY CHANGE OF INSULIN SHOULD BE MADE CAUTIOUSLY ONLY UNDER MEDICAL SUPERVISION. WHEN CHANGING TO PURIFIED PORK INSULIN FROM ANY OTHER INSULIN A DOSAGE ADJUSTMENT, IF ANY, IS LIKELY TO BE A REDUCTION TO AVOID HYPOGLYCEMIA. CHANGES IN PURITY, STRENGTH (U-40, U-80, U-100), BRAND (MANUFACTURER), TYPE (LENTE, NPH, REGULAR, ETC.) AND/OR SPECIES SOURCE (BEEF, PORK, BEEF/PORK) MAY RESULT IN THE NEED FOR A CHANGE IN DOSAGE. IT IS NOT POSSIBLE TO IDENTIFY WHICH PATIENTS WILL REQUIRE A REDUCTION IN DOSAGE TO AVOID HYPOGLYCEMIA WHEN USING THIS INSULIN. ADJUSTMENT MAY BE NEEDED WITH THE FIRST DOSE OR OVER A PERIOD OF SEVERAL WEEKS. (SEE DOSAGE ADJUSTMENT SECTION). BE AWARE OF THE POSSIBILITY OF SYMPTOMS OF EITHER HYPOGLYCEMIA OR HYPERGLYCEMIA. SEE SECTIONS ENTITLED INSULIN REACTION AND HYPERGLYCEMIA.
Description: INSULATARD NPH is a suspension of protamine insulin crystals. It has a slower speed of action than VELOSULIN (Regular) and a shorter duration than Protamine Zinc Insulin. The effect on the blood sugar begins approximately 1½ hours after the injection and lasts up to approximately 24 hours, having its maximum effect between the 4th and 12th hour.
Directions: Shake vial carefully to obtain a uniformly cloudy suspension of the crystals. Avoid heavy foaming. Do not use a vial if the insulin remains clear after it has been shaken. Also do not use it if you see lumps that float or stick to the sides.
INSULATARD NPH can be mixed with any other Nordisk insulin preparation. In the mixture the different insulins will keep their original effect (stable mixtures).
Keep INSULATARD NPH in a cold place (refrigerator) at 2 degrees to 10 degrees C (35–50 degrees F), but do not let it freeze or be exposed to direct sunlight. Do not use the insulin after the expiration date stamped on the label.
Dosage Adjustment: Reductions in dosage resulting from the switchover to this purified pork insulin from any other insulin have been observed to be in the neighborhood of 10–20% initially to maintain control.
Adjustment may be needed either with the first dose or over a period of several weeks, and it is therefore recommended that the patient be monitored closely by a physician during the changeover and that dosage be adjusted downwards as necessary.
It is not possible to identify which patients will require a reduction in dose to avoid hypoglycemia when using purified pork insulins.
Be aware of the possibility of symptoms indicating the need for adjustment. See sections on Insulin Reaction or Hyperglycemia.
Use the Correct Syringe: INSULATARD NPH is available in the U-100 strength (100 units per ml). The patient must understand the markings on the syringe and use only a syringe marked for U-100. Avoid contamination and possible infection by following these instructions:
Reusable syringes and needles must be sterile when used. The best method of sterilization is to boil the syringe, plunger and needle in water for 5 minutes. If this is not possible, as when travelling, the parts may be sterilized by immersion for at least 5 minutes in a sterilizing liquid like ethyl

alcohol, 70%. Do not use bathing, rubbing or medicated alcohol for sterilization. Remove all liquid from the syringe by pushing the plunger in and out several times and leave it to dry if alcohol has been used for sterilization. To prepare the dose, clean the rubber cap with cotton dipped in alcohol such as ethyl alcohol, 70%. The rubber cap must never be removed. Air is drawn into the syringe corresponding in amount to the prescribed amount of insulin. The needle is plunged through the cap in a downward position and the vial and syringe then inverted so that the air may be pushed out of the syringe into the vial. The prescribed amount of insulin is drawn into the syringe, and this is best done by drawing up slightly more insulin than required and then pushing the piston back to the desired mark. In this way any air bubbles are forced out of the syringe. Withdraw the needle from the vial without changing the position of the plunger in the syringe and lay aside the syringe so that it will not come in contact with any object. Disinfect the skin with a cotton swab dipped in a suitable antiseptic, such as ethyl alcohol, 70%. Pinch up the skin that has been disinfected and push the needle at a right angle quickly into the tissue under the skin. Do not inject deeper into a muscle or a vein. Give each injection in a different place from the previous one. If you instruct the patient to mix two types of insulin in the syringe, air should be injected into each vial first.

Warning: Patients who have been directed to mix two types of insulin should be aware that insulin hypodermic syringes may vary in amount of space between the bottom line and the needle. Because of this, the patient should not change:
1. The order of mixture prescribed, or
2. The model and brand of the syringe or needle.

Failure to heed this warning can result in a dosage error.

Insulin injections, a balanced diet, and regular exercise are required to secure proper control of diabetes. Urine should be tested regularly for sugar. Consistent presence of sugar in the urine indicates that diabetes is not properly controlled. As with any drug, if you are pregnant or nursing a baby, seek professional advice before using this product.

Adverse Reactions: Insulin allergy occurs very rarely, but when it does, it may cause a serious reaction including a general skin rash over the body, shortness of breath, fast pulse, sweating, and a drop in blood pressure.

In a very few diabetics, the skin where insulin has been injected may become red, swollen and itchy. This local reaction may occur if the injection is not properly made, if the skin is sensitive to the cleansing solution or if the patient is allergic to insulin. Patients with severe systemic reactions to insulin (i.e. generalized urticaria, angioedema, anaphylaxis) should be skin tested with each new preparation to be used prior to initiation of therapy with that preparation.

Insulin Reaction: Insulin reaction (hypoglycemia) can occur if the patient takes too much insulin, misses a meal or exercises or works harder than normal. The symptoms, which usually come on suddenly, are hunger, dizziness, and sweating. Eating sugar or a sugar-sweetened product will normally correct the condition.

Hyperglycemia: Hyperglycemia can occur if the patient takes too little insulin, eats significantly more than usual, or develops a cold or other infection. The symptoms are thirst, frequent passing of urine, and in severe cases nausea and abdominal pain. These symptoms generally come on gradually.

How Supplied: 10 ml vials
100 units per ml.
NDC # 50445-200-01

MIXTARD®
[mix′tard]
U-100 Pork, Isophane purified pork insulin suspension and purified pork insulin injection

WARNING: ANY CHANGE OF INSULIN SHOULD BE MADE CAUTIOUSLY ONLY UNDER MEDICAL SUPERVISION. WHEN CHANGING TO PURIFIED PORK INSULIN FROM ANY OTHER INSULIN A DOSAGE ADJUSTMENT, IF ANY, IS LIKELY TO BE A REDUCTION TO AVOID HYPOGLYCEMIA. CHANGES IN PURITY, STRENGTH (U-40, U-80, U-100), BRAND (MANUFACTURER), TYPE (LENTE, NPH, REGULAR, ETC.) AND/OR SPECIES SOURCE (BEEF, PORK, BEEF/PORK) MAY RESULT IN THE NEED FOR A CHANGE IN DOSAGE. IT IS NOT POSSIBLE TO IDENTIFY WHICH PATIENTS WILL REQUIRE A REDUCTION IN DOSAGE TO AVOID HYPOGLYCEMIA WHEN USING THIS INSULIN. ADJUSTMENT MAY BE NEEDED WITH THE FIRST DOSE OR OVER A PERIOD OF SEVERAL WEEKS. (SEE DOSAGE ADJUSTMENT SECTION). BE AWARE OF THE POSSIBILITY OF SYMPTOMS OF EITHER HYPOGLYCEMIA OR HYPERGLYCEMIA. SEE SECTIONS ENTITLED INSULIN REACTION AND HYPERGLYCEMIA.

Description: MIXTARD is a standard mixture of 30% VELOSULIN (corresponding to Regular insulin) and 70% INSULATARD NPH. The content of VELOSULIN gives the preparation a rapid onset of effect on the blood sugar, approximately ½ hour after the injection. The content of INSULATARD NPH gives it a duration of up to 24 hours, depending on the size of the dose. The maximal effect lies between the 4th and the 8th hour after injection.

Directions: Shake vial carefully to obtain a uniformly cloudy suspension of the crystals. Avoid heavy foaming. Do not use a vial if the insulin remains clear after it has been shaken. Also do not use it if you see lumps that float or stick to the sides.

MIXTARD can be mixed with any other Nordisk insulin preparation. In the mixture the different insulins will keep their original effect (stable mixtures).

Keep MIXTARD in a cold place (refrigerator) at 2 degrees to 10 degrees C (35–50 degrees F), but do not let it freeze or be exposed to direct sunlight. Do not use the insulin after the expiration date stamped on the label.

Dosage Adjustment: Reductions in dosage resulting from the switchover to this purified pork insulin from any other insulin have been observed to be in the neighborhood of 10–20% initially to maintain control. Adjustment may be needed either with the first dose or over a period of several weeks, and it is therefore recommended that the patient be monitored closely by a physician during the changeover and that dosage be adjusted downwards as necessary.

It is not possible to identify which patients will require a reduction in dose to avoid hypoglycemia when using purified pork insulins.

Be aware of the possibility of symptoms indicating the need for adjustment. See sections on Insulin Reaction or Hyperglycemia.

Use the Correct Syringe: MIXTARD is available in the U-100 strength (100 units per ml). The patient must understand the markings on the syringe and use only a syringe marked for U-100.

Avoid contamination and possible infection by following these instructions:

Reusable syringes and needles must be sterile when used. The best method of sterilization is to boil the syringe, plunger and needle in water for 5 minutes. If this is not possible, as when travelling, the parts may be sterilized by immersion for at least 5 minutes in a sterilizing liquid like ethyl alcohol, 70%. Do not use bathing, rubbing or medicated alcohol for sterilization. Remove all liquid from the syringe by pushing the plunger in and out several times and leave it to dry if alcohol has been used for sterilization. To prepare the dose, clean the rubber cap with cotton dipped in alcohol such as ethyl alcohol, 70%. The rubber cap must never be removed. Air is drawn into the syringe corresponding in amount to the prescribed amount of insulin. The needle is plunged through the cap in a downward position and the vial and syringe then inverted so that the air may be pushed out of the syringe into the vial. The prescribed amount of insulin is drawn into the syringe, and this is best done by drawing up slightly more insulin than required and then pushing the piston back to the desired mark. In this way any air bubbles are forced out of the syringe. Withdraw the needle from the vial without changing the position of the plunger in the syringe and lay aside the syringe so that it will not come in contact with any object. Disinfect the skin with a cotton swab dipped in a suitable antiseptic, such as ethyl alcohol, 70%. Pinch up the skin that has been disinfected and push the needle at a right angle quickly into the tissue under the skin. Do not inject deeper into a muscle or a vein. Give each injection in a different place from the previous one. If you instruct the patient to mix two types of insulin in the syringe, air should be injected into each vial first.

Warning: Insulin injections, a balanced diet, and regular exercise are required to secure proper control of diabetes. Urine should be tested regularly for sugar. Consistent presence of sugar in the urine indicates that diabetes is not properly controlled.

As with any drug, if you are pregnant or nursing a baby, seek professional advice before using this product.

Adverse Reactions: Insulin allergy occurs very rarely, but when it does, it may cause a serious reaction including a general skin rash over the body, shortness of breath, fast pulse, sweating, and a drop in blood pressure.

In a very few diabetics, the skin where insulin has been injected may become red, swollen and itchy. This local reaction may occur if the injection is not properly made, if the skin is sensitive to the cleansing solution or if the patient is allergic to insulin. Patients with severe systemic reactions to insulin (i.e. generalized urticaria, angioedema, anaphylaxis) should be skin tested with each new preparation to be used prior to initiation of therapy with that preparation.

Insulin Reaction: Insulin reaction (hypoglycemia) can occur if the patient takes too much insulin, misses a meal or exercises or works harder than normal. The symptoms, which usually come on suddenly, are hunger, dizziness, and sweating. Eating sugar or a sugar-sweetened product will normally correct the condition.

Hyperglycemia: Hyperglycemia can occur if the patient takes too little insulin, eats significantly more than usual, or develops a cold or other infection. The symptoms are thirst, frequent passing of urine, and in severe cases nausea and abdominal pain. These symptoms generally come on gradually.

How Supplied: 10 ml vials
100 units per ml.
NDC #50445-300-01

VELOSULIN™
[vĕl″ ŏ′sul″ in]
U-100 Pork, Purified pork insulin injection

WARNING: ANY CHANGE OF INSULIN SHOULD BE MADE CAUTIOUSLY ONLY UNDER MEDICAL SUPERVISION. WHEN CHANGING TO PURIFIED PORK INSULIN FROM ANY OTHER INSULIN A DOSAGE ADJUSTMENT, IF ANY, IS LIKELY TO BE A REDUCTION TO AVOID HYPOGLYCEMIA. CHANGES IN PURITY, STRENGTH (U-40, U-80, U-100), BRAND (MANUFACTURER), TYPE (LENTE, NPH, REGULAR, ETC.) AND/OR SPECIES SOURCE (BEEF, PORK, BEEF/PORK) MAY RESULT IN THE NEED FOR A CHANGE IN DOSAGE. IT IS NOT POSSIBLE TO IDENTIFY WHICH PATIENTS WILL REQUIRE A REDUCTION IN DOSAGE TO AVOID HYPOGLYCEMIA WHEN USING THIS INSULIN. ADJUSTMENT MAY BE NEEDED WITH THE FIRST DOSE OR OVER A PERIOD OF SEVERAL WEEKS. (SEE DOSAGE ADJUSTMENT SECTION). BE AWARE OF THE POSSIBILITY OF SYMPTOMS OF EITHER HYPOGLYCEMIA OR HYPERGLYCEMIA. SEE SECTIONS ENTITLED INSULIN REACTION AND HYPERGLYCEMIA.

Description: VELOSULIN is a clear solution of insulin obtained from pork pancreas. It has a rapid onset of effect on the blood sugar, approximately ½ hour after the injection. The effect lasts up to

Continued on next page

Nordisk-USA—Cont.

approximately 8 hours with a maximal effect between the 1st and 3rd hour.

Directions: Do not use the preparation if the color has become other than water clear or if the liquid has become viscous. VELOSULIN can be mixed with any other Nordisk insulin preparation. In the mixture the different insulins will keep their original effect (stable mixtures).

Keep VELOSULIN in a cold place (refrigerator) at 2 degrees to 10 degrees C (35–50 degrees F), but do not let it freeze or be exposed to direct sunlight. Do not use the insulin after the expiration date stamped on the label.

Dosage Adjustment: Reductions in dosage resulting from the switchover to this purified pork insulin from any other insulin have been observed to be in the neighborhood of 10–20% initially to maintain control.

Adjustment may be needed either with the first dose or over a period of several weeks, and it is therefore recommended that the patient be monitored closely by a physician during the changeover and that dosage be adjusted downwards as necessary.

It is not possible to identify which patients will require a reduction in dose to avoid hypoglycemia when using purified pork insulins.

Be aware of the possibility of symptoms indicating the need for adjustment. See sections on Insulin Reaction or Hyperglycemia.

Use the Correct Syringe: VELOSULIN is available in the U-100 strength (100 units per ml). The patient must understand the markings on the syringe and use only a syringe marked for U-100.

Avoid contamination and possible infection by following these instructions:

Reusable syringes and needles must be sterile when used. The best method of sterilization is to boil the syringe, plunger and needle in water for 5 minutes. If this is not possible, as when travelling, the parts may be sterilized by immersion for at least 5 minutes in a sterilizing liquid like ethyl alcohol, 70%. Do not use bathing, rubbing or medicated alcohol for sterilization. Remove all liquid from the syringe by pushing the plunger in and out several times and leave it to dry if alcohol has been used for sterilization. To prepare the dose, clean the rubber cap with cotton dipped in alcohol such as ethyl alcohol, 70%. The rubber cap must never be removed. Air is drawn into the syringe corresponding in amount to the prescribed amount of insulin. The needle is plunged through the cap in a downward position and the vial and syringe then inverted so that the air may be pushed out of the syringe into the vial. The prescribed amount of insulin is drawn into the syringe, and this is best done by drawing up slightly more insulin than required and then pushing the piston back to the desired mark. In this way any air bubbles are forced out of the syringe. Withdraw the needle from the vial without changing the position of the plunger in the syringe and lay aside the syringe so that it will not come in contact with any object. Disinfect the skin with a cotton swab dipped in a suitable antiseptic, such as ethyl alcohol, 70%. Pinch up the skin that has been disinfected and push the needle at a right angle quickly into the tissue under the skin. Do not inject deeper into a muscle or vein. Give each injection in a different place from the previous one. If you instruct the patient to mix two types of insulin in the syringe, air should be injected into each vial first.

Warning: Patients who have been directed to mix two types of insulin should be aware that insulin hypodermic syringes may vary in amount of space between the bottom line and the needle. Because of this, the patient should not change:
1. The order of mixture prescribed, or
2. The model and brand of the syringe or needle.

Failure to heed this warning can result in a dosage error.

Insulin injections, a balanced diet, and regular exercise are required to secure proper control of diabetes. Urine should be tested regularly for sugar. Consistent presence of sugar in the urine indicates that diabetes is not properly controlled. As with any drug, if you are pregnant or nursing a baby, seek professional advice before using this product.

Adverse Reactions: Insulin allergy occurs very rarely, but when it does, it may cause a serious reaction including a general skin rash over the body, shortness of breath, fast pulse, sweating, and a drop in blood pressure.

In a very few diabetics, the skin where insulin has been injected may become red, swollen and itchy. This local reaction may occur if the injection is not properly made, if the skin is sensitive to the cleansing solution or if the patient is allergic to insulin. Patients with severe systemic reactions to insulin (i.e. generalized urticaria, angioedema, anaphylaxis) should be skin tested with each new preparation to be used prior to initiation of therapy with that preparation.

Insulin Reaction: Insulin reaction (hypoglycemia) can occur if the patient takes too much insulin, misses a meal or exercises or works harder than normal. The symptoms, which usually come on suddenly, are hunger, dizziness, and sweating. Eating sugar or a sugar-sweetened product will normally correct the condition.

Hyperglycemia: Hyperglycemia can occur if the patient takes too little insulin, eats significantly more than usual, or develops a cold or other infection. The symptoms are thirst, frequent passing of urine, and in severe cases nausea and abdominal pain. These symptoms generally come on gradually.

How Supplied: 10 ml vials
100 units per ml.
NDC # 50445-100-01

Norgine Laboratories, Inc.
2 OVERHILL ROAD
SCARSDALE, NY 10583

ENZYPAN® Tablets
[en'zĭ-pan]

Composition: Each tablet contains pancreatin sufficient to digest in 2 hours time: 19 g. of protein, 43 g. of starch and 10 g. of fat; in addition it provides Ox Bile (des.), 0.056 g. and peptic potency equivalent to Pepsin 1-3,000, 9 mg.

Action and Uses: Releases the principal digestive enzymes consecutively from two specially constructed tablet sections. Valuable in digestive enzyme deficiencies leading to fat, protein or starch intolerance and such enzyme-deficiency-linked symptoms as fermentative or putrefactive dyspepsia, postprandial distress, epigastric fullness, flatulence, regurgitation.

Administration and Dosage: *Adults*—2 to 3 tablets during or after each meal. To be taken whole, with water.

How Supplied: Containers of 120, 500.

MOVICOL® Granules
[mo'vic-all]

Composition: Gum Karaya and cortex rhamni frangulae in a pleasantly sweetened mixture.

Action and Uses: Treatment of constipation with natural mucilage (for bulk formation) and small amounts of well-aged frangula (for initial peristalsis). Especially in cardiovascular, hernial, rectal cases; diverticulosis; invalid, surgical, convalescent cases; geriatric patients; dieters; patients with sedentary habits. In bulk-producing capacity, 1 teaspoonful of Movicol equals 2 lbs. of consumed vegetables.

Administration and Dosage: *Adults*—1 or 2 heaped teaspoonfuls once or twice daily after the main meals, or on retiring. Dry granules are placed on the tongue in small amounts and, without chewing or crushing, swallowed with plenty of water. As bowel tone and rhythm are gradually restored, dosage may be reduced and ultimately discontinued.

Warning: Not to be used if abdominal pain, nausea or vomiting are present. Frequent or prolonged use may result in dependence on laxatives.

Contraindications: Intestinal obstruction, fecal impaction.

How Supplied: Containers of 200 and 500 grams.

MURIPSIN® Tablets
[mu-rip'sin]

Composition: Each tablet contains: glutamic acid hydrochloride 500 mg.; pepsin 35 mg.; in a special base.*

Action and Uses: Gastric hydrochloric acid therapy in a solid tablet. Muripsin avoids corrosive unpleasantness and uncontrolled acid release; formulated with glutamic acid hydrochloride, it not only substitutes hydrochloric acid but also stimulates secretagogue action. Each tablet provides the equivalent of 15 minims of dilute hydrochloric acid. Useful in hydrochloric acid deficiencies, primary or secondary.

Administration and Dosage: For adults one to two tablets with each meal to be swallowed whole with water.

Contraindications: Hyperacidity or if peptic ulcers are present.

How Supplied: Containers of 100 and 500. *U.S. Patent 2,958,627

Norwich Eaton Pharmaceuticals, Inc.
A Proctor & Gamble Company
(formerly Eaton Laboratories, Professional Products Group, Norwich Products or Consumer Products Group)
NORWICH, NY 13815
(See also Procter & Gamble)

Literature on Norwich Eaton products sent to physicians on request.

ALPHADERM® ℞
[al'fa-derm]
(1% hydrocortisone)
CREAM

The following text is based on official labeling in effect August 1, 1984.

Description: Alphaderm Cream contains hydrocortisone 1% in a powder-in-cream base with urea 10% incorporated as a hypermolar solution, purified water, sorbitol, polyoxyethylene fatty glyceride, starch, white petrolatum, triglycerides of saturated fatty acids, isopropyl myristate, and sorbitan monolaurate. The near neutral pH of the formulation is made possible by the stabilized delivery system in which urea is absorbed by a polysaccharide powder matrix. Alphaderm (1% hydrocortisone) Cream is hypoallergenic and contains no parabens or lanolin.

HYDROCORTISONE
Molecular Weight: 362.47
Molecular Formula: $C_{21}H_{30}O_5$
CAS: 50-23-7

Pregn-4-ene-3,20-dione,11,17,21-trihydroxy-,(11β)-

Clinical Pharmacology: Topical corticosteroids are effective primarily because of their anti-inflammatory, antipruritic and vasoconstrictive actions.

The mechanism of anti-inflammatory activity of the topical corticosteroids is unclear. Various laboratory methods, including vasoconstrictor assays, are used to compare and predict potencies and/or clinical efficacies of the topical corticosteroids. There is some evidence to suggest that a recognizable correlation exists between vasoconstrictor potency and therapeutic efficacy in man.

Pharmacokinetics: The extent of percutaneous absorption of topical corticosteroids is determined by many factors including the use of occlusive dressings, the integrity of the epidermal barrier and the vehicle itself. The Alphaderm Cream base contains 10% urea which has been shown to increase the penetration of the active ingredient, hydrocortisone 1%, into the epidermis.

Topical corticosteroids can be absorbed from normal intact skin. Inflammation and/or other disease processes in the skin increase percutaneous absorption. Occlusive dressings substantially increase the percutaneous absorption of topical corticosteroids. Thus, occlusive dressings may be a valuable therapeutic adjunct for treatment of resistant dermatoses. (See DOSAGE AND ADMINISTRATION.)

Once absorbed through the skin, topical corticosteroids are handled through pharmacokinetic pathways similar to systemically administered corticosteroids. Corticosteroids are bound to plasma proteins in varying degrees. Corticosteroids are metabolized primarily in the liver and are then excreted by the kidneys. Some of the topical corticosteroids and their metabolites are also excreted into the bile.

Indications and Usage: Alphaderm (1% hydrocortisone) Cream is indicated for the relief of the inflammatory and pruritic manifestations of corticosteroid-responsive dermatoses.

Contraindications: Topical steroids are contraindicated in those patients with a history of hypersensitivity to any of the components of the preparation.

Precautions: General: Systemic absorption of topical corticosteroids has produced reversible hypothalamic-pituitary-adrenal (HPA) axis suppression, manifestations of Cushing's syndrome, hyperglycemia, and glucosuria in some patients. Conditions which augment systemic absorption include the application of the more potent steroids, use over large surface areas, prolonged use, and the addition of occlusive dressings.

Patients receiving a large dose of a potent topical steroid applied to a large surface area or under an occlusive dressing should be evaluated periodically for evidence of HPA axis suppression by using the urinary free cortisol and ACTH stimulation tests. If HPA axis suppression is noted, an attempt should be made to withdraw the drug, to reduce the frequency of application, or to substitute a less potent steroid.

Recovery of HPA axis function is generally prompt and complete upon discontinuation of the drug. Infrequently, signs and symptoms of steroid withdrawal may occur, requiring supplemental systemic corticosteroids.

Children may absorb proportionally larger amounts of topical corticosteroids and thus be more susceptible to systemic toxicity. (See Pediatric Use.) However, serious side effects secondary to topical 1% hydrocortisone are rare.

If irritation develops, topical corticosteroids should be discontinued and appropriate therapy instituted.

In the presence of dermatological infections, the use of an appropriate antifungal or antibacterial agent should be instituted. If a favorable response does not occur promptly, the corticosteroid should be discontinued until the infection has been adequately controlled.

Information for the Patient: Patients using topical corticosteroids should receive the following information and instructions:

1. This medication is to be used as directed by the physician. It is for external use only. Avoid contact with the eyes.
2. Patients should be advised not to use this medication for any disorder other than for which it was prescribed.
3. The treated skin area should not be bandaged or otherwise covered or wrapped as to be occlusive unless directed by the physician.
4. Patients should report any signs of local adverse reactions especially under occlusive dressing.
5. Parents of pediatric patients should be advised not to use tight-fitting diapers or plastic pants on a child being treated in the diaper area, as these garments may constitute occlusive dressings.

Laboratory Tests: The following tests may be helpful in evaluating the HPA axis suppression:
Urinary free cortisol test
ACTH stimulation test

Carcinogenesis, Mutagenesis, Impairment of Fertility: Long-term animal studies have not been performed to evaluate the carcinogenic potential or the effect on fertility of topical corticosteroids. Studies to determine mutagenicity with prednisolone and hydrocortisone have revealed negative results.

Pregnancy: Pregnancy Category C: Corticosteroids are generally teratogenic in laboratory animals when administered systemically at relatively low dosage levels. The more potent corticosteroids have been shown to be teratogenic after dermal application in laboratory animals. There are no adequate and well-controlled studies in pregnant women on teratogenic effects from topically applied corticosteroids. Therefore, topical corticosteroids should be used during pregnancy only if the potential benefit justifies the potential risk to the fetus. Drugs of this class should not be used extensively on pregnant patients, in large amounts, or for prolonged periods of time.

Nursing Mothers: It is not known whether topical administration of corticosteroids could result in sufficient systemic absorption to produce detectable quantities in breast milk. Systemically administered corticosteroids are secreted into breast milk in quantities *not* likely to have a deleterious effect on the infant. Nevertheless, caution should be exercised when topical corticosteroids are administered to a nursing woman.

Pediatric Use: *Pediatric patients may demonstrate greater susceptibility to topical corticosteroid-induced HPA axis suppression and Cushing's syndrome than mature patients because of a larger skin surface area to body weight ratio.*

Hypothalamic-pituitary-adrenal (HPA) axis suppression, Cushing's syndrome, and intracranial hypertension have been reported in children receiving topical corticosteroids. Manifestations of adrenal suppression in children include linear growth retardation, delayed weight gain, low plasma cortisol levels, and absence of response to ACTH stimulation. Manifestations of intracranial hypertension include bulging fontanelles, headaches, and bilateral papilledema.

Administration of topical corticosteroids to children should be limited to the least amount compatible with an effective therapeutic regimen. Chronic corticosteroid therapy may interfere with the growth and development of children.

Adverse Reactions: The following local adverse reactions are reported infrequently with topical corticosteroids, but may occur more frequently with the use of occlusive dressings. These reactions are listed in an approximate decreasing order of occurrence:

1. Burning
2. Itching
3. Irritation
4. Dryness
5. Folliculitis
6. Hypertrichosis
7. Acneiform eruptions
8. Hypopigmentation
9. Perioral dermatitis
10. Allergic contact dermatitis
11. Maceration of the skin
12. Secondary infection
13. Skin atrophy
14. Striae
15. Miliaria

Overdosage: Topically applied corticosteroids can be absorbed in sufficient amounts to produce systemic effects (see PRECAUTIONS).

Dosage and Administration: Apply a thin film of Alphaderm (1% hydrocortisone) Cream to affected areas two to four times a day, and rub in well.

Occlusive dressings may be used for the management of recalcitrant conditions. If an infection develops, the use of occlusive dressings should be discontinued and appropriate antimicrobial therapy instituted.

How Supplied: Alphaderm (1% hydrocortisone) Cream is available in:
NDC 0149-0705-12   tubes of 30 grams
NDC 0149-0705-51   tubes of 100 grams
Store below 59°F (15°C). Do not freeze.

Caution: Federal law prohibits dispensing without a prescription.

ALPHA-P6

COMHIST® LA   ℞
[kŏm'hist]

The following text is based on official labeling in effect August 1, 1984.

Description: Each COMHIST LA yellow and clear capsule for oral administration contains:
chlorpheniramine maleate .... 4 mg
phenyltoloxamine citrate ....50 mg
phenylephrine hydrochloride ....20 mg
in a special base to provide a prolonged therapeutic effect.

This product contains ingredients of the following therapeutic classes: antihistamine and decongestant.

Chlorpheniramine maleate is an antihistamine having the chemical name γ-(4-chlorophenyl)-N,N-dimethyl-2-pyridinepropanamine,(Z)-2-butenedioate(1:1) with the following structure:

Phenyltoloxamine citrate is an antihistamine having the chemical name N,N-dimethyl-2-(α-phenyl-o-tolyloxy) ethylamine dihydrogen citrate with the following structure:

Phenylephrine hydrochloride is a decongestant having the chemical name 3-hydroxy-α[methylamino)methyl] benzenemethanol hydrochloride with the following structure:

Clinical Pharmacology: Chlorpheniramine maleate is an alkylamine-type antihistamine while phenyltoloxamine citrate belongs to the ethanolamine chemical class. The antihistamines in COMHIST LA act by competing with histamine for H_1 histamine receptor sites, thereby preventing the action of histamine on the cell. Clinically, chlorpheniramine and phenyltoloxamine suppress the histamine-mediated symptoms of allergic rhinitis, relieving sneezing, rhinorrhea, and itching of the eyes, nose, and throat.

Phenylephrine hydrochloride is an α-adrenergic receptor agonist (sympathomimetic) which produces vasoconstriction by stimulating α-receptors within the mucosa of the respiratory tract. Clinically, phenylephrine shrinks swollen mucous membranes, reduces tissue hyperemia, edema, and nasal congestion, and increases nasal airway patency.

Indications and Usage: COMHIST LA is indicated for the relief of rhinorrhea and congestion associated with seasonal and/or perennial allergic rhinitis and vasomotor rhinitis.

Contraindications: COMHIST LA is contraindicated in persons hypersensitive to any of its components. It should not be administered to children under 12 years of age, patients with severe hypertension, narrow angle glaucoma, or asthmatic

Continued on next page

Norwich Eaton—Cont.

symptoms, or patients taking monoamine oxidase inhibitors.

Warnings: Chlorpheniramine maleate and phenyltoloxamine citrate should be used with extreme caution in patients with stenosing peptic ulcer, pyloroduodenal obstruction, prostatic hypertrophy, or bladder neck obstruction. These compounds have an atropine-like action and therefore should be used with caution in patients with a history of bronchial asthma, increased intraocular pressure, cardiovascular disease, or hypertension. Sympathomimetic amines should be used with caution in patients with hypertension, diabetes mellitus, heart disease, increased intraocular pressure, hyperthyroidism, or prostatic hypertrophy.

Precautions:
Information for Patients: This product may cause sedation. Patients should be cautioned against engaging in activities requiring mental alertness, such as driving a car or operating machinery.
Drug Interactions: The sedative effects of chlorpheniramine maleate and phenyltoloxamine citrate are additive to the CNS depressant effects of alcohol, hypnotics, sedatives, and tranquilizers. COMHIST LA should not be used in patients taking monoamine oxidase inhibitors.
Pregnancy: Pregnancy Category C. Animal reproduction studies have not been conducted with COMHIST LA. It is also not known whether COMHIST LA can cause fetal harm when administered to a pregnant woman or can affect reproduction capacity. COMHIST LA should be given to a pregnant woman only if clearly needed.
Nursing Mothers: It is not known whether the drugs in COMHIST LA are excreted in human milk. Because many drugs are excreted in human milk and because of the potential for serious adverse reactions in nursing infants, a decision should be made whether to discontinue nursing or to discontinue the product, taking into account the importance of the drug to the mother.
Pediatric Use: Safety and effectiveness of COMHIST LA in children below the age of 12 have not been established.
Adverse Reactions: General: Urticaria, drug rash, dryness of mouth, nose, and throat.
Cardiovascular System: Hypotension, headache, palpitations.
Hematologic System: Thrombocytopenia, agranulocytosis, leukopenia.
Nervous System: Sedation, dizziness, excitation (especially in children), nervousness, insomnia, blurred vision, convulsions.
Gastrointestinal System: Epigastric distress, anorexia, nausea, vomiting, diarrhea, constipation.
Genitourinary System: Urinary frequency, urinary retention.
Respiratory System: Thickening of bronchial secretions, tightness of chest and wheezing, nasal stuffiness.
Overdosage: The treatment of overdosage should provide symptomatic and supportive care. If the amount ingested is considered dangerous or excessive, induce vomiting with ipecac syrup unless the patient is convulsing, comatose, or has lost the gag reflex, in which case perform gastric lavage using a large-bore tube. If indicated, follow with activated charcoal and a saline cathartic. Since the effects of COMHIST LA may last up to 12 hours, treatment should be continued for at least that length of time.
Dosage and Administration: Adults and children 12 years of age and older—1 capsule every 8 to 12 hours; not recommended for children under 12 years of age.
How Supplied: COMHIST LA is available as a yellow and clear capsule imprinted "COMHIST LA" and "01490446".
NDC 0149-0446-01 Bottle of 100
Caution: Federal law prohibits dispensing without prescription.

Manufactured for
Norwich Eaton Pharmaceuticals, Inc.
Norwich, New York 13815
A Procter & Gamble Company
by KV Pharmaceutical Company
St. Louis, Missouri 63144
REVISED MARCH 1984
COMLA-X5
Shown in Product Identification Section, page 422

COMHIST® ℞
[kom′hist]
The following text is based on official labeling in effect August 1, 1984.
Description: Each COMHIST yellow, scored tablet for oral administration contains:
Chlorpheniramine maleate ....2 mg
Phenyltoloxamine citrate ....25 mg
Phenylephrine hydrochloride ....10 mg
This product contains ingredients of the following therapeutic classes: antihistamine and decongestant.
Chlorpheniramine maleate is an antihistamine having the chemical name γ-(4-chlorophenyl)-N,N-dimethyl-2-pyridinepropanamine,(Z)-2-butenedioate(1:1) with the following structure:

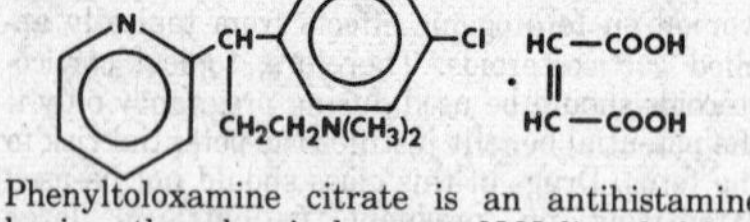

Phenyltoloxamine citrate is an antihistamine having the chemical name N,N-dimethyl-2-(α-phenyl-o-tolyloxy) ethylamine dihydrogen citrate with the following structure:

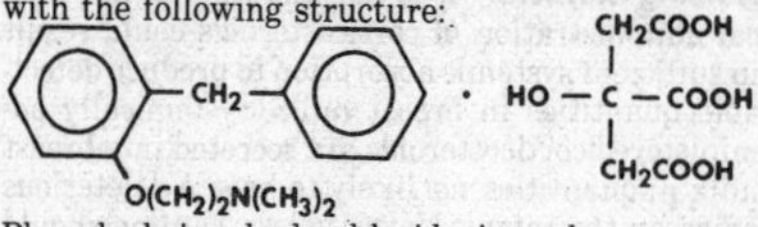

Phenylephrine hydrochloride is a decongestant having the chemical name 3-hydroxy-α[(methylamino)methyl]benzenemethanol hydrochloride with the following structure:

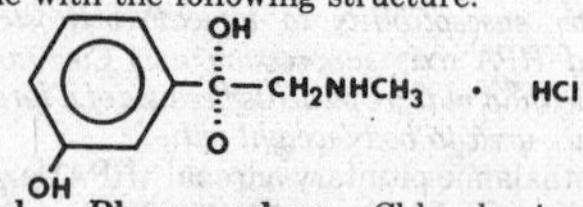

Clinical Pharmacology: Chlorpheniramine maleate is an alkylamine-type antihistamine while phenyltoloxamine citrate belongs to the ethanolamine chemical class. The antihistamines in COMHIST act by competing with histamine for H_1 histamine receptor sites, thereby preventing the action of histamine on the cell. Clinically, chlorpheniramine and phenyltoloxamine suppress the histamine-mediated symptoms of allergic rhinitis, relieving sneezing, rhinorrhea, and itching of the eyes, nose, and throat.
Phenylephrine hydrochloride is an α-adrenergic receptor agonist (sympathomimetic) which produces vasoconstriction by stimulating α-receptors within the mucosa of the respiratory tract. Clinically, phenylephrine shrinks swollen mucous membranes, reduces tissue hyperemia, edema, and nasal congestion, and increases nasal airway patency.
Indications and Usage: COMHIST is indicated for the relief of rhinorrhea and congestion associated with seasonal and/or perennial allergic rhinitis and vasomotor rhinitis.
Contraindications: COMHIST is contraindicated in persons hypersensitive to any of its components. It should not be administered to children under 6 years of age, patients with severe hypertension, narrow angle glaucoma, or asthmatic symptoms, or patients taking monoamine oxidase inhibitors.
Warnings: Chlorpheniramine maleate and phenyltoloxamine citrate should be used with extreme caution in patients with stenosing peptic ulcer, pyloroduodenal obstruction, prostatic hypertrophy, or bladder neck obstruction. These compounds have an atropine-like action and therefore should be used with caution in patients with a history of bronchial asthma, increased intraocular pressure, cardiovascular disease, or hypertension. Sympathomimetic amines should be used with caution in patients with hypertension, diabetes mellitus, heart disease, increased intraocular pressure, hyperthyroidism, or prostatic hypertrophy.

Precautions:
Information for Patients: This product may cause sedation. Patients should be cautioned against engaging in activities requiring mental alertness, such as driving a car or operating machinery.
Drug Interactions: The sedative effects of chlorpheniramine maleate and phenyltoloxamine citrate are additive to the CNS depressant effects of alcohol, hypnotics, sedatives, and tranquilizers. COMHIST should not be used in patients taking monoamine oxidase inhibitors.
Pregnancy: Pregnancy Category C. Animal reproduction studies have not been conducted with COMHIST. It is also not known whether COMHIST can cause fetal harm when administered to a pregnant woman or can affect reproduction capacity. COMHIST should be given to a pregnant woman only if clearly needed.
Nursing Mothers: It is not known whether the drugs in COMHIST are excreted in human milk. Because many drugs are excreted in human milk and because of the potential for serious adverse reactions in nursing infants, a decision should be made whether to discontinue nursing or to discontinue the product, taking into account the importance of the drug to the mother.
Pediatric Use: Safety and effectiveness of COMHIST in children below the age of 6 have not been established.
Adverse Reactions:
General: Urticaria, drug rash, dryness of mouth, nose, and throat.
Cardiovascular System: Hypotension, headache, palpitations.
Hematologic System: Thrombocytopenia, agranulocytosis, leukopenia.
Nervous System: Sedation, dizziness, excitation (especially in children), nervousness, insomnia, blurred vision, convulsions.
Gastrointestinal System: Epigastric distress, anorexia, nausea, vomiting, diarrhea, constipation.
Genitourinary System: Urinary frequency, urinary retention.
Respiratory System: Thickening of bronchial secretions, tightness of chest and wheezing, nasal stuffiness.
Overdosage: The treatment of overdosage should provide symptomatic and supportive care. If the amount ingested is considered dangerous or excessive, induce vomiting with ipecac syrup unless the patient is convulsing, comatose, or has lost the gag reflex, in which case perform gastric lavage using a large-bore tube. If indicated, follow with activated charcoal and a saline cathartic.
Dosage and Administration: Adults and children 12 years of age and older—1 or 2 tablets three times daily (every 8 hours); children 6 to under 12 years of age—1 tablet three times daily (every 8 hours); not recommended for children under 6 years of age.
How Supplied: COMHIST is available as a round, yellow, scored tablet imprinted "COMHIST" on the smooth side and "0149-0444" on the scored side.
NDC 0149-0444-01 Bottle of 100
Caution: Federal law prohibits dispensing without prescription.
COMTB-P6

DANTRIUM® ℞
[dan′trē-um]
(dantrolene sodium)
CAPSULES
The following text is based on official labeling in effect August 1, 1984.

> Dantrium (dantrolene sodium) has a potential for hepatotoxicity, and should not be used in conditions other than those recommended. Symptomatic hepatitis (fatal and non-fatal) has been reported at various dose levels of the drug. The incidence reported in patients taking up to 400 mg/day is much lower than in those taking doses of 800 mg or more per day. Even sporadic short courses of these higher

dose levels within a treatment regimen markedly increased the risk of serious hepatic injury. Liver dysfunction as evidenced by blood chemical abnormalities alone (liver enzyme elevations) have been observed in patients exposed to Dantrium for varying periods of time. Overt hepatitis has occurred at varying intervals after initiation of therapy, but has been most frequently observed between the third and twelfth month of therapy. The risk of hepatic injury appears to be greater in females, in patients over 35 years of age, and in patients taking other medication(s) in addition to Dantrium (dantrolene sodium). Dantrium should be used only in conjunction with appropriate monitoring of hepatic function including frequent determination of SGOT or SGPT. If no observable benefit is derived from the administration of Dantrium after a total of 45 days, therapy should be discontinued. The lowest possible effective dose for the individual patient should be prescribed.

Description: The chemical formula of Dantrium (dantrolene sodium) is hydrated 1-[[[5-(4-nitrophenyl)-2-furanyl]methylene]amino]-2, 4-imidazolidinedione sodium salt. It is an orange powder, slightly soluble in water, but due to its slightly acidic nature the solubility increases somewhat in alkaline solution. The anhydrous salt has a molecular weight of 336. The hydrated salt contains approximately 15% water (3½ moles) and has a molecular weight of 399. The structural formula for the hydrated salt is:

Dantrium is supplied in capsules of 25-mg, 50-mg, and 100-mg.

Clinical Pharmacology: In isolated nerve-muscle preparation, Dantrium has been shown to produce relaxation by affecting the contractile response of the skeletal muscle at a site beyond the myoneural junction, directly on the muscle itself. In skeletal muscle, Dantrium dissociates the excitation-contraction coupling, probably by interfering with the release of Ca^{++} from the sarcoplasmic reticulum. This effect appears to be more pronounced in fast muscle fibers as compared to slow ones, but generally affects both. A central nervous system effect occurs, with drowsiness, dizziness and generalized weakness occasionally present. Although Dantrium does not appear to directly affect the CNS, the extent of its indirect effect is unknown. The absorption of Dantrium after oral administration in humans is incomplete and slow but consistent, and dose-related blood levels are obtained. The duration and intensity of skeletal muscle relaxation is related to the dosage and blood levels. The mean biologic half-life of Dantrium in adults is 8.7 hours after a 100-mg dose. Specific metabolic pathways in the degradation and elimination of Dantrium in human subjects have been established. Metabolic patterns are similar in adults and children. In addition to the parent compound, dantrolene, which is found in measurable amounts in blood and urine, the major metabolites noted in body fluids are the 5-hydroxy analog and the acetamido analog. Since Dantrium is probably metabolized by hepatic microsomal enzymes, enhancement of its metabolism by other drugs is possible. However, neither phenobarbital nor diazepam appears to affect Dantrium metabolism.

Clinical experience in the management of fulminant human malignant hyperthermia, as well as experiments conducted in malignant hyperthermia susceptible swine, have revealed that the administration of intravenous dantrolene, combined with indicated supportive measures, is effective in reversing the hypermetabolic process of malignant hyperthermia. Known differences between human and swine malignant hyperthermia are minor. The prophylactic administration of oral or intravenous dantrolene to malignant hyperthermia susceptible swine will attenuate or prevent the development of signs of malignant hyperthermia in a manner dependent upon the dosage of dantrolene administered and the intensity of the malignant hyperthermia triggering stimulus. Limited clinical experience with the administration of oral dantrolene to patients judged malignant hyperthermia susceptible, when combined with clinical experience in the use of intravenous dantrolene for the treatment of malignant hyperthermia and data derived from the above cited animal model experiments, suggest that oral dantrolene will also attenuate or prevent the development of signs of human malignant hyperthermia, provided that currently accepted practices in the management of such patients are adhered to (see INDICATIONS AND USAGE); intravenous dantrolene should also be available for use should the signs of malignant hyperthermia appear.

Indications and Usage:
In Chronic Spasticity:
Dantrium is indicated in controlling the manifestations of clinical spasticity resulting from upper motor neuron disorders (e.g. spinal cord injury, stroke, cerebral palsy, or multiple sclerosis). It is of particular benefit to the patient whose functional rehabilitation has been retarded by the sequelae of spasticity. Such patients must have presumably reversible spasticity where relief of spasticity will aid in restoring residual function. Dantrium is not indicated in the treatment of skeletal muscle spasm resulting from rheumatic disorders.

If improvement occurs, it will ordinarily occur within the dosage titration (see DOSAGE AND ADMINISTRATION), and will be manifested by a decrease in the severity of spasticity and the ability to resume a daily function not quite attainable without Dantrium.

Occasionally, subtle but meaningful improvement in spasticity may occur with Dantrium therapy. In such instances information regarding improvement should be solicited from the patient and those who are in constant daily contact and attendance with him. Brief withdrawal of Dantrium for a period of 2 to 4 days will frequently demonstrate exacerbation of the manifestations of spasticity and may serve to confirm a clinical impression.

A decision to continue the administration of Dantrium on a long-term basis is justified if introduction of the drug into the patient's regimen:
  produces a significant reduction in painful and/or disabling spasticity such as clonus, or
  permits a significant reduction in the intensity and/or degree of nursing care required, or
  rids the patient of any annoying manifestation of spasticity considered important by the patient himself.

In Malignant Hyperthermia:
Oral Dantrium is also indicated preoperatively to prevent or attenuate the development of signs of malignant hyperthermia in known, or strongly suspect, malignant hyperthermia susceptible patients who require anesthesia and/or surgery. Currently accepted clinical practices in the management of such patients must still be adhered to (careful monitoring for early signs of malignant hyperthermia, minimizing exposure to triggering mechanisms and prompt use of intravenous dantrolene sodium and indicated supportive measures should signs of malignant hyperthermia appear); see also the package insert for Dantrium (dantrolene sodium) Intravenous.

Oral Dantrium should be administered following a malignant hyperthermic crisis to prevent recurrence of the signs of malignant hyperthermia.

Contraindications: Active hepatic disease, such as hepatitis and cirrhosis, is a contraindication for use of Dantrium. Dantrium is contraindicated where spasticity is utilized to sustain upright posture and balance in locomotion or whenever spasticity is utilized to obtain or maintain increased function.

Warnings: It is important to recognize that fatal and non-fatal liver disorders of an idiosyncratic or hypersensitivity type may occur with Dantrium therapy.

At the start of Dantrium therapy, it is desirable to do liver function studies (SGOT, SGPT, alkaline phosphatase, total bilirubin) for a baseline or to establish whether there is pre-existing liver disease. If baseline liver abnormalities exist and are confirmed, there is a clear possibility that the potential for Dantrium hepatotoxicity could be enhanced, although such a possibility has not yet been established.

Liver function studies (e.g. SGOT or SGPT) should be performed at appropriate intervals during Dantrium therapy. If such studies reveal abnormal values, therapy should generally be discontinued. Only where benefits of the drug have been of major importance to the patient, should reinitiation or continuation of therapy be considered. Some patients have revealed a return to normal laboratory values in the face of continued therapy while others have not.

If symptoms compatible with hepatitis, accompanied by abnormalities in liver functions tests or jaundice appear, Dantrium should be discontinued. If caused by Dantrium and detected early, the abnormalities in liver function characteristically have reverted to normal when the drug was discontinued.

Dantrium therapy has been reinstituted in a few patients who have developed clinical and/or laboratory evidence of hepatocellular injury. If such reinstitution of therapy is done, it should be attempted only in patients who clearly need Dantrium and only after previous symptoms and laboratory abnormalities have cleared. The patient should be hospitalized and the drug should be restarted in very small and gradually increasing doses. Laboratory monitoring should be frequent and the drug should be withdrawn immediately if there is any indication of recurrent liver involvement. Some patients have reacted with unmistakable signs of liver abnormality upon administration of a challenge dose, while others have not. Dantrium should be used with particular caution in females and in patients over 35 years of age in view of apparent greater likelihood of drug-induced, potentially fatal, hepatocellular disease in these groups.

Long-term safety of Dantrium in humans has not been established. Chronic studies in rats, dogs and monkeys at dosages greater than 30 mg/kg/day showed growth or weight depression and signs of hepatopathy and possible occlusion nephropathy, all of which were reversible upon cessation of treatment. Sprague-Dawley female rats fed dantrolene sodium for 18 months at dosage levels of 15, 30 and 60 mg/kg/day showed an increased incidence of benign and malignant mammary tumors compared with concurrent controls and, at the highest dosage, an increase in the incidence of hepatic lymphangiomas and hepatic angiosarcomas. These effects were not seen in 2½-year studies in Sprague-Dawley or Fischer 344 rats or in 2-year studies in mice of the HaM/ICR strain. Carcinogenicity in humans cannot be fully excluded, so that this possible risk of chronic administration must be weighed against the benefits of the drug (i.e., after a brief trial) for the individual patient.

Usage in Pregnancy: The safety of Dantrium for use in women who are or who may become pregnant has not been established. Dantrium should not be used in nursing mothers.

Usage in Children: The long-term safety of Dantrium in children under the age of 5 years has not been established. Because of the possibility that adverse effects of the drug could become apparent only after many years, a benefit-risk consideration of the long-term use of Dantrium is particularly important in pediatric patients.

Drug Interactions: While a definite drug interaction with estrogen therapy has not yet been established, caution should be observed if the two drugs are to be given concomitantly. Hepatotoxicity has occurred more often in women over 35 years of age receiving concomitant estrogen therapy.

Continued on next page

Norwich Eaton—Cont.

Precautions: Dantrium should be used with caution in patients with impaired pulmonary function, particularly those with obstructive pulmonary disease, and in patients with severely impaired cardiac function due to myocardial disease. It should be used with caution in patients with a history of previous liver disease or dysfunction (See WARNINGS).

Patients should be cautioned against driving a motor vehicle or participating in hazardous occupations while taking Dantrium. Caution should be exercised in the concomitant administration of tranquilizing agents.

Dantrium might possibly evoke a photosensitivity reaction; patients should be cautioned about exposure to sunlight while taking it.

Adverse Reactions: The most frequently occurring side effects of Dantrium have been drowsiness, dizziness, weakness, general malaise, fatigue, and diarrhea. These are generally transient, occurring early in treatment, and can often be obviated by beginning with a low dose and increasing dosage gradually until an optimal regimen is established. Diarrhea may be severe and may necessitate temporary withdrawal of Dantrium therapy. If diarrhea recurs upon readministration of Dantrium, therapy should probably be withdrawn permanently.

Other less frequent side effects, listed according to system are:

Gastrointestinal: Constipation, GI bleeding, anorexia, swallowing difficulty, gastric irritation, abdominal cramps.
Hepatobiliary: Hepatitis (See WARNINGS).
Neurologic: Speech disturbance, seizure, headache, light-headedness, visual disturbance, diplopia, alteration of taste, insomnia.
Cardiovascular: Tachycardia, erratic blood pressure, phlebitis.
Psychiatric: Mental depression, mental confusion, increased nervousness.
Urogenital: Increased urinary frequency, crystalluria, hematuria, difficult erection, urinary incontinence and/or nocturia, difficult urination and/or urinary retention.
Integumentary: Abnormal hair growth, acnelike rash, pruritus, urticaria, eczematoid eruption, sweating.
Musculoskeletal: Myalgia, backache.
Respiratory: Feeling of suffocation.
Special Senses: Excessive tearing.
Hypersensitivity: Pleural effusion with pericarditis.
Other: Chills and fever.

Dosage and Administration:
For Use in Chronic Spasticity:
Prior to the administration of Dantrium, consideration should be given to the potential response to treatment. A decrease in spasticity sufficient to allow a daily function not otherwise attainable should be the therapeutic goal of treatment with Dantrium. Refer to INDICATIONS AND USAGE section for description of response to be anticipated.

It is important to establish a therapeutic goal (regain and maintain a specific function such as therapeutic exercise program, utilization of braces, transfer maneuvers, etc.) before beginning Dantrium therapy. Dosage should be increased until the maximum performance compatible with the dysfunction due to underlying disease is achieved. No further increase in dosage is then indicated.

Usual Dosage: It is important that the dosage be titrated and individualized for maximum effect. The lowest dose compatible with optimal response is recommended.

In view of the potential for liver damage in long-term Dantrium use, therapy should be stopped if benefits are not evident within 45 days.

Adults: Begin therapy with 25 mg once daily; increase to 25 mg two, three, or four times daily and then by increments of 25 mg up to as high as 100 mg two, three, or four times daily if necessary. As most patients will respond to a dose of 400 mg/day or less, rarely should doses higher than 400 mg/day be used (see Box Warning.)

Each dosage level should be maintained for four to seven days to determine the patient's response. The dose should not be increased beyond, and may even have to be reduced to, the amount at which the patient received maximal benefit without adverse effects.

Children: A similar approach should be utilized starting with 0.5 mg/kg of body weight twice daily; this is increased to 0.5 mg/kg three or four times daily and then by increments of 0.5 mg/kg up to as high as 3.0 mg/kg two, three, or four times daily, if necessary. Doses higher than 100 mg four times daily should not be used in children.

For Malignant Hyperthermia:
Preoperatively: Administer 4 to 8 mg/kg/day of oral Dantrium in 3 or 4 divided doses for one or two days prior to surgery, with the last dose being given approximately 3 to 4 hours before scheduled surgery with a minimum of water.

This dosage will usually be associated with skeletal muscle weakness and sedation (sleepiness or drowsiness); adjustment can usually be made within the recommended dosage range to avoid incapacitation or excessive gastrointestinal irritation (including nausea and/or vomiting).

Post Crisis Follow-up:
Oral Dantrium should also be administered following a malignant hyperthermia crisis, in doses of 4 to 8 mg/kg per day in four divided doses, for a one to three day period to prevent recurrence of the manifestations of malignant hyperthermia.

Overdosage: For acute overdosage, general supportive measures should be employed along with immediate gastric lavage.

Intravenous fluids should be administered in fairly large quantities to avert the possibility of crystalluria. An adequate airway should be maintained and artificial resuscitation equipment should be at hand. Electrocardiographic monitoring should be instituted, and the patient carefully observed. To date, no experience has been reported with dialysis and its value in Dantrium overdosage is not known.

How Supplied: Dantrium (dantrolene sodium) is available in:

25 mg opaque, orange and light brown capsules:
NDC 0149-0030-05 bottle of 100
NDC 0149-0030-66 bottle of 500
NDC 0149-0030-77 hospital unit-dose strips in boxes of 100.
50-mg opaque, orange and dark brown capsules:
NDC 0149-0031-05 bottle of 100.
100-mg opaque, orange and light brown capsules:
NDC 0149-0033-05 bottle of 100
NDC 0149-0033-77 hospital unit-dose strips in boxes of 100.

Address medical inquiries to Norwich Eaton Pharmaceuticals, Medical Department, Norwich, NY 13815.
Manufactured by
Eaton Laboratories, Inc.
Manati, Puerto Rico 00701
Distributed by
Norwich Eaton Pharmaceuticals, Inc.
Norwich, New York 13815
A Procter & Gamble Company

DANCP-P6

DANTRIUM®   ℞
[*dan' trē-um*]
(dantrolene sodium)
INTRAVENOUS

Description: Dantrium Intravenous is a sterile, lyophilized formulation of dantrolene sodium, and in this form provides a preparation for intravenous use. Each 70 ml vial contains 20 mg dantrolene sodium, 3000 mg mannitol, and sufficient sodium hydroxide to yield a pH of approximately 9.5 when reconstituted with 60 ml sterile water for injection U.S.P. (without a bacteriostatic agent). Dantrolene sodium is classified as a direct-acting skeletal muscle relaxant. Chemically, dantrolene sodium is hydrated 1-[[[5-(4-nitrophenyl)-2-furanyl]methylene]amino]-2,4-imidazolidinedione sodium salt. The structural formula for the hydrated salt is:

$$O_2N\text{—}\bigcirc\text{—}CH=NN\diagdown\begin{array}{c}C=O\\C=O\end{array}\diagup NNa \cdot 3\tfrac{1}{2}H_2O$$
$$\phantom{O_2N\text{—}\bigcirc\text{—}}CH_2$$

The hydrated salt contains approximately 15% water (3½ moles) and has a molecular weight of 399. The anhydrous salt (dantrolene) has a molecular weight of 336.

Actions: Dantrolene sodium is a muscle relaxant acting specifically on skeletal muscle. It does not affect neuromuscular transmission nor does it have measurable effects on the electrically excitable surface membrane. Studies have shown that in the presence of dantrolene sodium, the responses of the muscle to caffeine are decreased or delayed.

In isolated muscle preparations, dantrolene sodium uncouples the excitation and contraction of skeletal muscle, probably by interfering with the release of calcium from the sarcoplasmic reticulum.

In the anesthetic-induced malignant hyperthermia syndrome, evidence points to an intrinsic abnormality of muscle tissue. In affected humans and swine, it has been postulated that "triggering agents" induce a sudden rise in myoplasmic calcium either by preventing the sarcoplasmic reticulum from accumulating calcium adequately, or by accelerating its release. This rise in myoplasmic calcium activates acute catabolic processes common to the malignant hyperthermia crisis.

Dantrolene sodium may prevent the increase in myoplasmic calcium and the acute catabolism within the muscle cell by interfering with the release of calcium from the sarcoplasmic reticulum to the myoplasm. Thus, the physiologic, metabolic, and biochemical changes associated with the crisis may be reversed or attenuated.

Specific metabolic pathways in the degradation and elimination of dantrolene sodium in humans have been established. Dantrolene is found in measurable amounts in blood and urine. In addition, its major metabolites in body fluids are the 5-hydroxy analog and the acetamido analog. Another metabolite with an unknown structure appears related to acetylaminodantrolene. Dantrolene sodium may also undergo hydrolysis and subsequent oxidation forming nitrophenylfuroic acid. Since dantrolene sodium is metabolized by the liver, enhancement of its metabolism by other drugs is possible. However, neither phenobarbital nor diazepam appears to affect dantrolene sodium metabolism.

The mean biologic half-life of dantrolene sodium after intravenous administration is about 5 hours. Based on assays of whole blood and plasma, slightly greater amounts of dantrolene are associated with red blood cells than with the plasma fraction of blood. Significant amounts of dantrolene are bound to plasma proteins, mostly albumin, and this binding is readily reversible. Binding to plasma protein is not significantly altered by diazepam, diphenylhydantoin, or phenylbutazone. Binding to plasma proteins is reduced by warfarin and clofibrate and increased by tolbutamide.

In animals, dantrolene sodium given intravenously has no appreciable effect on the cardiovascular system or on respiratory function. A transient inconsistent effect on smooth muscles has been observed at high doses.

Because of the low drug concentration requiring the administration of large volumes of fluid, acute toxicity of a dantrolene sodium intravenous formulation could not be assessed. In 14-day (subacute) studies, the intravenous formulation of dantrolene sodium was relatively non-toxic to rats at doses of 10 mg/kg/day and 20 mg/kg/day. While 10 mg/kg/day in dogs for 14 days evoked little toxicity, 20 mg/kg/day for 14 days caused hepatic changes of questionable biologic significance.

Indications: Dantrium Intravenous is indicated, along with appropriate supportive measures, for the management of the fulminant hypermetabolism of skeletal muscle characteristic of malignant hyperthermia crisis. It should be administered by intravenous injection as soon as the malignant hyperthermia reaction is recognized (i.e. tachycardia, tachypnea, central venous desaturation, hypercarbia, metabolic acidosis, skeletal muscle rigidity, increased utilization of anesthesia circuit carbon dioxide absorber, cyanosis and mottling of the skin, and, in many cases, fever).

Contraindications: None.
Warnings: *The use of Dantrium Intravenous in the management of malignant hyperthermia crisis is not a substitute for previously known supportive measures. These measures must be individualized, but it will usually be necessary to discontinue the suspect triggering agents, attend to increased oxygen requirements, manage the metabolic acidosis, institute cooling when necessary, attend to urinary output and monitor for electrolyte imbalance.*

Precautions:
a) Because of the high pH of the intravenous formulation of Dantrium, care must be taken to prevent extravasation of the intravenous solution into the surrounding tissues.
b) Pregnancy: The safety of Dantrium Intravenous in women who are or who may become pregnant has not been established; it should be given only when the potential benefits have been weighed against the possible risk to mother and child.
c) Drug Intractions: The combination of therapeutic doses of intravenous dantrolene sodium and verapamil in halothane/α-chloralose anesthetized swine has resulted in ventricular fibrillation and cardiovascular collapse in association with marked hyperkalemia. It is recommended that the combination of intravenous dantrolene sodium and calcium channel blockers, such as verapamil, not be used during reversal of a malignant hyperthermia crisis until the relevance of these findings to humans is established.

Adverse Reactions: The serious reactions reported with chronic oral Dantrium use have been hepatitis, seizures, and pleural effusion with pericarditis. Hypersensitivity with attendant skin reactions has been infrequently noted. None of the reactions reported in patients taking oral Dantrium have been reported in patients treated with short-term Dantrium Intravenous therapy for malignant hyperthermia.

Dosage and Administration: As soon as the malignant hyperthermia reaction is recognized, all anesthetic agents should be discontinued. Dantrium Intravenous should be administered by continuous rapid intravenous push beginning at a minimum dose of 1 mg/kg, and continuing until symptoms subside or the maximum cumulative dose of 10 mg/kg has been reached. If the physiologic and metabolic abnormalities reappear, the regimen may be repeated. It is important to note that administration of Dantrium Intravenous should be continuous until symptoms subside. The effective dose to reverse the crisis is directly dependent upon the individual's degree of susceptibility to malignant hyperthermia, the amount and time of exposure to the triggering agent, and the time elapsed between onset of the crisis and initiation of treatment.

Children's Dose: Experience to date indicates that the dose for children is the same as for adults.
Preoperatively: Dantrium (dantrolene sodium) Capsules are indicated preoperatively as possible protection against the development of a malignant hyperthermia crisis in individuals thought to be susceptible.
Oral administration of Dantrium Capsules: Administer 4 to 8 mg/kg/day of oral dantrolene in 3 or 4 divided doses for one or two days prior to surgery, with the last dose being given approximately 3 to 4 hours before scheduled surgery with a minimum of water.
This dosage usually will be associated with skeletal muscle weakness and sedation (sleepiness or drowsiness); adjustment can usually be made within the recommended dosage range to avoid incapacitation or excessive gastrointestinal irritation (including nausea and/or vomiting). See also the package insert for oral dantrolene sodium (Dantrium Capsules).

Post Crisis Follow-up: Dantrium (dantrolene sodium) Capsules should also be administered following a malignant hyperthermia crisis in doses of 4 to 8 mg/kg per day in four divided doses, for a one to three day period to prevent recurrence of the manifestations of malignant hyperthermia.

Preparation: Each vial of Dantrium Intravenous should be reconstituted by adding 60 ml of sterile water for injection U.S.P. (without a bacteriostatic agent), and the vial shaken until the solution is clear. The contents of the vial must be *protected from direct light* and *used within 6 hours* after reconstitution. Store reconstituted solutions at controlled room temperature (59°F to 86°F or 15°C to 30°C).

How Supplied: Dantrium Intravenous (NDC 0149-0734-02) is available in vials containing a sterile lyophilized mixture of 20 mg dantrolene sodium, 3000 mg mannitol, and sufficient sodium hydroxide to yield a pH of approximately 9.5 when reconstituted with 60 ml sterile water for injection U.S.P. (without a bacteriostatic agent).
Store unreconstituted product below 86°F (30°C) and avoid prolonged exposure to light.
Address medical inquiries to Norwich Eaton Pharmaceuticals Inc., Medical Department, Norwich, NY 13815.
Manufactured by
Eaton Laboratories, Inc.
Manati, Puerto Rico 00701
Distributed by
Norwich Eaton Pharmaceuticals, Inc.
Norwich, New York 13815
A Procter & Gamble Company
REVISED DECEMBER 1983   DANIV-P6

DIDRONEL® ℞
[dī'drō-nel]
(etidronate disodium)

The following text is based on official labeling in effect August 15, 1984.
Description: DIDRONEL tablets contain 200 mg of etidronate disodium, the disodium salt of (1-hydroxyethylidene) diphosphonic acid, for oral administration. This compound, also known as EHDP, regulates bone metabolism. It is a white powder, highly soluble in water, with a molecular weight of 250 and the following structural formula:

$$HO-\underset{\underset{O}{|}}{\overset{\overset{ONa}{|}}{P}}-\underset{\underset{CH_3}{|}}{\overset{\overset{OH}{|}}{C}}-\underset{\underset{O}{|}}{\overset{\overset{ONa}{|}}{P}}-OH$$

Clinical Pharmacology: DIDRONEL acts primarily on bone. It can inhibit the formation, growth and dissolution of hydroxyapatite crystals and their amorphous precursors by chemisorption to calcium phosphate surfaces. Inhibition of crystal resorption occurs at lower doses than are required to inhibit crystal growth. Both effects increase as the dose increases.
DIDRONEL is not metabolized. Absorption averages about 1% of an oral dose of 5 mg/kg body weight/day. This increases to about 2.5% at 10 mg/kg/day and 6% at 20 mg/kg/day. Most of the absorbed drug is cleared from the blood within 6 hours. Within 24 hours about half of the absorbed dose is excreted in the urine. The remainder is chemically adsorbed to bone, especially to areas of elevated osteogenesis, and is slowly eliminated. Unabsorbed drug is excreted intact in the feces. DIDRONEL therapy does not adversely affect serum levels of parathyroid hormone or calcium. Hyperphosphatemia has been observed in DIDRONEL patients, usually in association with doses of 10–20 mg/kg/day. No adverse effects have been traced to this, and it is not a contraindication for therapy. It is apparently due to drug-related increased tubular reabsorption of phosphate by the kidney. Serum phosphate levels generally return to normal 2–4 weeks post-therapy.

PAGET'S DISEASE
Paget's disease of bone (osteitis deformans) is an idiopathic, progressive disease characterized by abnormal and accelerated bone metabolism in one or more bones. Signs and symptoms may include bone pain and/or deformity, neurologic disorders, elevated cardiac output and other vascular disorders, and increased serum alkaline phosphatase and/or urinary hydroxyproline levels. Bone fractures are common in patients with Paget's disease. DIDRONEL slows accelerated bone turnover (resorption and accretion) in pagetic lesions and, to a lesser extent, in normal bone. This has been demonstrated histologically, scintigraphically, biochemically, and through calcium kinetic and balance studies. Reduced bone turnover is often accompanied by symptomatic improvement, including reduced bone pain. Also, the incidence of pagetic fractures may be reduced, and elevated cardiac output and other vascular disorders may be improved by DIDRONEL therapy.

HETEROTOPIC OSSIFICATION
Heterotopic ossification, also referred to as myositis ossificans (circumscripta, progressiva or traumatica), ectopic calcification, periarticular ossification, or paraosteoarthropathy, is characterized by metaplastic osteogenesis. It usually presents with signs of localized inflammation or pain, elevated skin temperature, and redness. When tissues near joints are involved, functional loss may also be present. Heterotopic ossification may occur for no known reason as in myositis ossificans progressiva or may follow a wide variety of surgical, occupational, and sports trauma (e.g., hip arthroplasty, spinal cord injury, head injury, burns and severe thigh bruises). Heterotopic ossification has also been observed in non-traumatic conditions (e.g., infections of the central nervous system, peripheral neuropathy, tetanus, biliary cirrhosis, Peyronie's disease, as well as in association with a variety of benign and malignant neoplasms). Clinical trials have demonstrated the efficacy of Didronel in heterotopic ossification following total hip replacement, or due to spinal cord injury.

— *Heterotopic ossification complicating total hip replacement* typically develops radiographically 3–8 weeks post-operatively in the pericapsular area of the affected hip joint. The overall incidence is about 50%; about one-third of these cases are clinically significant.

— *Heterotopic ossification due to spinal cord injury* typically develops radiographically 1–4 months after injury. It occurs below the level of injury, usually at major joints. The overall incidence is about 40%; about one-half of these cases are clinically significant.

DIDRONEL chemisorbs to calcium hydroxyapatite crystals and their amorphous precursors, blocking the aggregation, growth and mineralization of these crystals. This is thought to be the mechanism by which DIDRONEL presents or retards heterotopic ossification. There is no evidence DIDRONEL affects mature heterotopic bone.

Indications and Usage:
PAGET'S DISEASE
DIDRONEL is indicated for the treatment of symptomatic Paget's disease of bone.
DIDRONEL therapy usually arrests or significantly impedes the disease process as evidenced by:
—Symptomatic relief, including decreased pain and/or increased mobility (experienced by 3 out of 5 patients).
—Reductions in serum alkaline phosphatase and urinary hydroxyproline levels (30% or more in 4 out of 5 patients).
—Histomorphometry showing reduced numbers of osteoclasts and osteoblasts, and more lamellar bone formation.
—Bone scans showing reduced radionuclide uptake at pagetic lesions.
In addition, reductions in pagetically elevated cardiac output and skin temperature have been observed in some patients. Also, the incidence of pagetic fractures may be reduced when DIDRONEL is administered intermittently over a period of years.

Continued on next page

Norwich Eaton—Cont.

In many patients, the disease process will be suppressed for a period of at least one year following cessation of therapy. The upper limit of this period has not been determined.

DIDRONEL's effects have not been studied in patients with asymptomatic Paget's disease. However, DIDRONEL treatment of such patients may be warranted if extensive involvement threatens irreversible neurologic damage, major joints, or major weight-bearing bones.

HETEROTOPIC OSSIFICATION

DIDRONEL is indicated in the prevention and treatment of heterotopic ossification following total hip replacement or due to spinal cord injury. DIDRONEL reduces the incidence of clinically important heterotopic bone by about two-thirds. Among those patients who form heterotopic bone, DIDRONEL retards the progression of immature lesions and reduces the severity by at least half. Follow-up data (at least nine months post-therapy) suggest these benefits persist.

In total hip replacement patients, DIDRONEL does not promote loosening of the prosthesis or impede trochanteric reattachment.

In spinal cord injury patients, DIDRONEL does not inhibit fracture healing or stabilization of the spine.

Contraindications: None known.

Warnings: *In Paget's patients* the response to therapy may be of slow onset and continue for months after DIDRONEL therapy is discontinued. Dosage should not be increased prematurely. A 90-day drug-free interval should be provided between courses of therapy.

Heterotopic ossification: No specific warnings.

Precautions:

General. Patients should maintain an adequate nutritional status, particularly an adequate intake of calcium and vitamin D.

Therapy has been withheld from some patients with enterocolitis since diarrhea may be experienced, particularly at higher doses.

DIDRONEL is not metabolized and is excreted intact via the kidney. There is no experience to specifically guide treatment in patients with impaired renal function. DIDRONEL dosage should be reduced when reductions in glomerular filtration rates are present. Patients with renal impairment should be closely monitored. DIDRONEL suppresses bone turnover, and may retard mineralization of osteoid laid down during the bone accretion process. These effects are dose and time dependent. Osteoid, which may accumulate noticeably at doses of 10–20 mg/kg/day, mineralizes normally post-therapy. In patients with fractures, especially of long bones, it may be advisable to delay or interrupt treatment until callus is evident.

Carcinogenesis. Long-term studies in rats have indicated that DIDRONEL is not carcinogenic.

Pregnancy: Teratogenic Effects. Pregnancy Category B.

Reproduction/teratology studies performed in rats and rabbits at doses up to five times the maximum human dose by the intended route of administration have revealed no evidence of impaired fertility or harm to the fetus due to DIDRONEL. At doses of twenty-two times the maximum human dose, a decrease in live fetuses were observed in rats. The only incidence of malformations occurred in rats at exaggerated doses following parenteral administration and were skeletal in nature. These malformations were deemed the result of the pharmacological action of the drug. There are no adequate, well-controlled studies in pregnant women. Because animal reproduction studies are not always predictive of human response, this drug should be used during pregnancy only if clearly needed.

Nursing Mothers. It is not known whether this drug is excreted in human milk. Because many drugs are excreted in human milk, caution should be exercised when DIDRONEL is administered to a nursing woman.

Pediatric Use. Safety and effectiveness in children have not been established.

Adverse Reactions: The incidence of gastrointestinal complaints (diarrhea, nausea) is the same for DIDRONEL at 5 mg/kg/day as for placebo, about 1 patient in 15. At 10–20 mg/kg/day the incidence may increase to 2 or 3 in 10. These complaints are often alleviated by dividing the total daily dose.

In Paget's patients increased or recurrent bone pain at pagetic sites, and/or the onset of pain at previously asymptomatic sites has been reported. At 5 mg/kg/day about 1 patient in 10 (verus 1 in 15 in the placebo group) report these phenomena. At higher doses the incidence rises to about 2 in 10. When therapy continues, pain resolves in some patients but persists in others.

Heterotopic ossification: No specific adverse reactions.

Overdosage: While there is no experience with acute overdosage, it is theoretically possible that enough DIDRONEL could be taken to result in hypocalcemia.

Dosage and Administration: DIDRONEL should be taken as a single, oral dose. However, should gastrointestinal discomfort occur, the dose may be divided. To maximize absorption, patients should avoid taking the following items within two hours of dosing:

—Food, especially those high in calcium, such as milk or milk products.
—Vitamins with mineral supplements or antacids which are high in metals such as calcium, iron, magnesium or aluminum.

PAGET'S DISEASE

Initial Treatment Regimens:

5–10 mg/kg/day, not to exceed 6 months, or
11–20 mg/kg/day, not to exceed 3 months.

The recommended initial dose is 5 mg/kg/day for a period not to exceed six months. Doses above 10 mg/kg/day should be reserved for when 1) lower doses are ineffective or 2) there is an overriding need to suppress rapid bone turnover (especially when irreversible neurologic damage is possible) or reduce elevated cardiac output. Doses in excess of 20 mg/kg/day are not recommended.

Retreatment Guidelines. Retreatment should be initiated only after: 1) a DIDRONEL-free period of at least 90 days and 2) there is biochemical, symptomatic or other evidence of active disease process. It is advisable to monitor patients every 3–6 months although some patients may go drug free for extended periods. Retreatment regimens are the same as for initial treatment. For most patients the original dose will be adequate for retreatment. If not, consideration should be given to increasing the dose within the recommended guidelines.

HETEROTOPIC OSSIFICATION

The following treatment regimens have been shown to be effective:

—*Total Hip Replacement Patients: 20 mg/kg/day for 1 month before and 3 months after surgery (4 months total).*
—*Spinal Cord Injured Patients: 20 mg/kg/day for 2 weeks followed by 10 mg/kg/day for 10 weeks (12 weeks total). DIDRONEL therapy should begin as soon as medically feasible following the injury, preferably prior to evidence of heterotopic ossification.*

Retreatment has not been studied.

How Supplied: Didronel is available as 200-mg, white, rectangular tablets with "P&G" on one face and "402" on the other.

NDC 0149-0405-60 bottle of 60

400-mg, white, scored, capsule-shaped tablets with "N E" on one face and "406" on the other.

NDC 0149-0406-60 bottle of 60

Caution: Federal law prohibits dispensing without prescription.

Shown in Product Identification Section, page 422

DID-P3

DUVOID®
[dū′void]
(bethanechol chloride—oral)

The following text is based on official labeling in effect August 1, 1984.

Description: Duvoid (bethanechol chloride), an ester of a choline-like compound, is 2-[(aminocarbonyl)oxy]-N,N,N-trimethyl-1-propanaminium chloride. Bethanechol chloride is a white, hygroscopic, crystalline powder having a slight amine-like odor and is freely soluble in water.

$$\left[\begin{array}{c} CH_3CH-CH_2N+(CH_3)_3 \\ O-CO-NH_2 \end{array} \right] Cl-$$

Molecular weight: 196.68
Molecular formula: $C_7H_{17}ClN_2O_2$

Duvoid, a cholinergic agent, is available as 10-mg, 25-mg, and 50-mg tablets intended for oral administration.

Clinical Pharmacology: Duvoid acts principally by producing the effects of stimulation of the parasympathetic nervous system. It increases the tone of the detrusor urinae muscle, usually producing a contraction sufficiently strong to initiate micturition and empty the bladder. It stimulates gastric motility, increases gastric tone, and often restores impaired rhythmic peristalsis.

Stimulation of the parasympathetic nervous system releases acetylcholine at the nerve endings. When spontaneous stimulation is reduced and therapeutic intervention is required, acetylcholine can be given, but is rapidly hydrolyzed by cholinesterase, and its effects are transient. Bethanechol chloride is not destroyed by cholinesterase and its effects are more prolonged than those of acetylcholine.

It has predominant muscarinic action and only feeble nicotinic action. Doses that stimulate micturition and defecation and increase peristalsis do not ordinarily stimulate ganglia or voluntary muscles. Therapeutic test doses in normal human subjects have little effect on heart rate, blood pressure, or peripheral circulation.

Indications and Usage: Duvoid is indicated for the treatment of acute postoperative and postpartum nonobstructive (functional) urinary retention, and neurogenic atony of the urinary bladder with retention.

Contraindications: Duvoid is contraindicated in the presence of mechanical obstruction of the gastrointestinal or urinary tracts, or in conditions where the integrity of the gastrointestinal or bladder wall is questionable. Also, it is contraindicated in spastic gastrointestinal disturbances, peptic ulcer, acute inflammatory conditions of the gastrointestinal tract, or peritonitis, or in marked vagotonia.

Duvoid is also contraindicated in latent or active asthma, hyperthyroidism, coronary occlusion, bradycardia, vasomotor instability, hypotension, coronary artery disease, epilepsy, and parkinsonism.

Warnings: Asthmatic attacks may be precipitated, especially in susceptible individuals. Substernal pressure or pain may occur; however, it is uncertain whether this is due to bronchoconstriction, or spasm of the esophagus. Myocardial hypoxia must be considered if a marked fall in blood pressure occurs.

Transient syncope with cardiac arrest, transient complete heart block, dyspnea, and orthostatic hypotension may be associated with large doses. Patients with hypertension may react to the drug with a precipitous fall in blood pressure. Short periods of atrial fibrillation have been observed in hyperthyroid individuals following the administration of cholinergic drugs. Involuntary defecation and urinary urgency may occur after large doses.

Precautions:

General: In urinary retention, if the sphincter fails to relax as Duvoid contracts the bladder, urine may be forced up the ureter into the kidney

pelvis. If there is bacteriuria, this may cause a reflux infection.
Drug Interactions: Special care and consideration are required when Duvoid is administered to patients concomitantly being treated with other drugs with which pharmacologic interactions may occur. Examples of drugs with potential for such interactions are: quinidine and procainamide, which may antagonize cholinergic effects; cholinergic drugs, particularly cholinesterase inhibitors, where additive effects may occur. When administered to patients receiving ganglionic blocking compounds a critical fall in blood pressure may occur, usually preceded by severe abdominal symptoms.
Pregnancy: Pregnancy Category C. Animal reproduction studies have not been conducted with Duvoid. It is also not known whether Duvoid can cause fetal harm when administered to a pregnant woman or can affect reproduction capacity. Duvoid should be given to a pregnant woman only if clearly needed.
Nursing Mothers: It is not known whether this drug is excreted in human milk. Because many drugs are excreted in human milk, caution should be exercised when Duvoid is administered to a nursing woman.
Pediatric Use: Safety and effectiveness in children below the age of 8 years have not been established.
Adverse Reactions: Adverse reactions are infrequent with Duvoid. The following may occur:
Cardiovascular: Fall in blood pressure. (See **Warnings**.)
Gastrointestinal: Involuntary defecation, vomiting, colicky pain, abdominal cramps, diarrhea, nausea and belching, salivation, and borborygmi.
Respiratory: Asthmatic attacks and dyspnea.
Neurologic: Headache, facial flushing.
Urogenital: Urinary urgency.
Miscellaneous: Substernal pressure or pain (see **Warnings**), malaise.
Overdosage: Maintain artificial respiration until antidote can be given. Atropine sulfate is a specific antidote and may be given in doses of 0.6 mg–1.2 mg intravenously (slowly), intramuscularly, or subcutaneously to counteract severe toxic cardiovascular or bronchoconstrictor responses to bethanechol chloride.
Dosage and Administration: Dosage must be individualized, depending on type and severity of the condition to be treated.
Preferably give the drug on an empty stomach to minimize the possibility of nausea and vomiting. The usual adult oral dose ranges from 10 to 50 mg three or four times a day. The minimum effective dose is determined by giving 5 or 10 mg initially, and repeating the same amount at hourly intervals until satisfactory response occurs, or until a maximum of 50 mg has been given. The effects of the drug sometimes appear within 30 minutes, and are usually maximal within 90 minutes. The drug's effects persist for about one hour.
How Supplied: Duvoid is available as follows:
10 mg: pale orange, scored tablets coded "Eaton 045"
NDC 0149-0045-05 bottle of 100
NDC 0149-0045-77 hospital unit-dose strips in box of 100.
25 mg: white, scored tablets coded "Eaton 046"
NDC 0149-0046-05 bottle of 100
NDC 0149-0046-77 hospital unit-dose strips in box of 100.
50 mg: tan, scored tablets coded "Eaton 047"
NDC 0149-0047-05 bottle of 100
NDC 0149-0047-77 hospital unit-dose strips in box of 100.
Keep container tightly closed. Avoid excessive heat (over 104°F or 40°C).
Caution: Federal law prohibits dispensing without prescription.   DUV-P6

ENTEX®   ℞
[n'tex]

The following text is based on official labeling in effect August 1, 1984.
Description: Each ENTEX orange and white capsule for oral administration contains:
phenylephrine hydrochloride .... 5 mg
phenylpropanolamine hydrochloride .... 45 mg
guaifenesin .... 200 mg
This product contains ingredients of the following therapeutic classes: decongestant and expectorant.
Phenylephrine hydrochloride is a decongestant having the chemical name, 3-hydroxy-α-[(methylamino)methyl]benzenemethanol hydrochloride, with the following structure:

Phenylpropanolamine hydrochloride is a decongestant having the chemical name, benzenemethanol, α-(1-aminoethyl)-, hydrochloride (R*, S*), (±), with the following structure:

Guaifenesin is an expectorant having the chemical name, 1,2-propanediol,3-(2-methoxyphenoxy)-, with the following structure:

Clinical Pharmacology: Phenylephrine hydrochloride and phenylpropanolamine hydrochloride are α-adrenergic receptor agonists (sympathomimetics) which produce vasoconstriction by stimulating α-receptors within the mucosa of the respiratory tract. Clinically, phenylephrine and phenylpropanolamine shrink swollen mucous membranes, reduce tissue hyperemia, edema, and nasal congestion, and increase nasal airway patency. Guaifenesin promotes lower respiratory tract drainage by thinning bronchial secretions, lubricates irritated respiratory tract membranes through increased mucus flow, and facilitates removal of viscous, inspissated mucus. As a result, sinus and bronchial drainage is improved, and dry, nonproductive coughs become more productive and less frequent.
Indications and Usage: ENTEX is indicated for the symptomatic relief of sinusitis, bronchitis, pharyngitis, and coryza when these conditions are associated with nasal congestion and viscous mucus in the lower respiratory tract.
Contraindications: ENTEX is contraindicated in individuals with known hypersensitivity to sympathomimetics, severe hypertension, or in patients receiving monoamine oxidase inhibitors.
Warnings: Sympathomimetic amines should be used with caution in patients with hypertension, diabetes mellitus, heart disease, peripheral vascular disease, increased intraocular pressure, hyperthyroidism, or prostatic hypertrophy.
Precautions:
Drug Interactions: ENTEX should not be used in patients taking monoamine oxidase inhibitors or other sympathomimetics.
Drug/Laboratory Test Interactions: Guaifenesin has been reported to interfere with clinical laboratory determinations of urinary 5-hydroxyindoleacetic acid (5-H1AA) and urinary vanilmandelic acid (VMA).
Pregnancy: Pregnancy Category C. Animal reproduction studies have not been conducted with ENTEX. It is also not known whether ENTEX can cause fetal harm when administered to a pregnant woman or can affect reproduction capacity. ENTEX should be given to a pregnant woman only if clearly needed.
Nursing Mothers: It is not known whether the drugs in ENTEX are excreted in human milk. Because many drugs are excreted in human milk and because of the potential for serious adverse reactions in nursing infants, a decision should be made whether to discontinue nursing or to discontinue the product, taking into account the importance of the drug to the mother.
Pediatric Use: Safety and effectiveness of EN-
TEX capsules in children below the age of 12 have not been established.
Adverse Reactions: Possible adverse reactions include nervousness, insomnia, restlessness, headache, nausea, or gastric irritation. These reactions seldom, if ever, require discontinuation of therapy. Urinary retention may occur in patients with prostatic hypertrophy.
Overdosage: The treatment of overdosage should provide symptomatic and supportive care. If the amount ingested is considered dangerous or excessive, induce vomiting with ipecac syrup unless the patient is convulsing, comatose, or has lost the gag reflex, in which case perform gastric lavage using a large-bore tube. If indicated, follow with activated charcoal and a saline cathartic.
Dosage and Administration: Adults and children 12 years of age and older—one capsule four times daily (every 6 hours) with food or fluid. ENTEX is not recommended for children under 12 years of age.
How Supplied: ENTEX orange and white capsules are imprinted with "ENTEX" and "0149 0412".
NDC 0149-0412-01 Bottle of 100
NDC 0149-0412-05 Bottle of 500
Caution: Federal law prohibits dispensing without prescription.
                                                                    ENXCP-P4

ENTEX® LIQUID   ℞
[n'tex]

The following text is based on official labeling in effect August 1, 1984.
Description: Each 5 ml (one teaspoonful) for oral administration contains:
phenylephrine hydrochloride .... 5 mg
phenylpropanolamine hydrochloride .... 20 mg
guaifenesin .... 100 mg
alcohol 5%
This product contains ingredients of the following therapeutic classes: decongestant and expectorant.
Phenylephrine hydrochloride is a decongestant having the chemical name, 3-hydroxy-α-[(methylamino)methyl]benzenemethanol hydrochloride, with the following structure:

Phenylpropanolamine hydrochloride is a decongestant having the chemical name, benzenemethanol, α-(1-aminoethyl)-, hydrochloride (R*, S*), (±), with the following structure:

Guaifenesin is an expectorant having the chemical name, 1,2-propanediol, 3-(2-methoxyphenoxy)-, with the following structure:

Clinical Pharmacology: Phenylephrine hydrochloride and phenylpropanolamine hydrochloride are α-adrenergic receptor agonists (sympathomimetics) which produce vasoconstriction by stimulating α-receptors within the mucosa of the respiratory tract. Clinically, phenylephrine and phenylpropanolamine shrink swollen mucous membranes, reduce tissue hyperemia, edema, and nasal congestion, and increase nasal airway patency. Guaifenesin promotes lower respiratory tract drainage by thinning bronchial secretions, lubricates irritated respiratory tract membranes through increased mucus flow, and facilitates removal of viscous, inspissated mucus. As a result, sinus and bronchial drainage is improved, and dry, nonproductive coughs become more productive and less frequent.

Continued on next page

Norwich Eaton—Cont.

Indications and Usage: ENTEX LIQUID is indicated for the symptomatic relief of sinusitis, bronchitis, pharyngitis, and coryza when these conditions are associated with nasal congestion and inspissated mucus in the lower respiratory tract.

Contraindications: ENTEX LIQUID is contraindicated in individuals with hypersensitivity to sympathomimetics, severe hypertension, or in patients receiving monoamine oxidase inhibitors.

Warnings: Sympathomimetic amines should be used with caution in patients with hypertension, diabetes mellitus, heart disease, peripheral vascular disease, increased intraocular pressure, hyperthyroidism, or prostatic hypertrophy.

Precautions:
Drug Interactions: ENTEX LIQUID should not be used in patients taking monoamine oxidase inhibitors or other sympathomimetics.
Drug/Laboratory Test Interactions: Guaifenesin has been reported to interfere with clinical laboratory determinations of urinary 5-hydroxyindoleacetic acid (5-HIAA) and urinary vanilmandelic acid (VMA).
Pregnancy: Pregnancy Category C. Animal reproduction studies have not been conducted with ENTEX LIQUID. It is also not known whether ENTEX LIQUID can cause fetal harm when administered to a pregnant woman or can affect reproduction capacity. ENTEX LIQUID should be given to a pregnant woman only if clearly needed.
Nursing Mothers: It is not known whether the drugs in EXTEX LIQUID are excreted in human milk. Because many drugs are excreted in human milk and because of the potential for serious adverse reactions in nursing infants, a decision should be made whether to discontinue nursing or to discontinue the product, taking into account the importance of the drug to the mother.
Pediatric Use: Safety and effectiveness of ENTEX LIQUID in children below the age of 2 have not been established.
Adverse Reactions: Possible adverse reactions include nervousness, insomnia, restlessness, headache, nausea, or gastric irritation. These reactions seldom, if ever, require discontinuation of therapy. Urinary retention may occur in patients with prostatic hypertrophy.
Overdosage: The treatment of overdosage should provide symptomatic and supportive care. If the amount ingested is considered dangerous or excessive, induce vomiting with ipecac syrup unless the patient is convulsing, comatose, or has lost the gag reflex, in which case perform gastric lavage using a large-bore tube. If indicated, follow with activated charcoal and a saline cathartic.
Dosage and Administration: All dosage should be administered four times daily (every 6 hours). Children:
2 to under 4 years .... ½ teaspoonful (2.5 ml)
4 to under 6 years .... 1 teaspoonful (5.0 ml)
6 to under 12 years .... 1½ teaspoonfuls (7.5 ml)
Adults and children 12 years
of age and older .... 2 teaspoonfuls (10.0 ml)
How Supplied: ENTEX LIQUID is available as an orange-colored, pleasant-tasting liquid.
NDC 0149-0414-16 16 FL. OZ. (1 Pint) bottle
Caution: Federal law prohibits dispensing without prescription.
ENXLQ-P3

ENTEX® LA
[n'tex]

The following text is based on official labeling in effect August 1, 1984.
Description: Each ENTEX LA blue, scored, long-acting tablet for oral administration contains:
phenylpropanolamine hydrochloride .... 75 mg
guaifenesin .... 400 mg
in a special base to provide a prolonged therapeutic effect.
This product contains ingredients of the following therapeutic classes: decongestant and expectorant.
Phenylpropanolamine hydrochloride is a decongestant having the chemical name, benzenemethanol, α-(1-aminoethyl)-, hydrochloride (R*, S*), (±), with the following structure:

Guaifenesin is an expectorant having the chemical name, 1,2-propanediol, 3-(2-methoxyphenoxy)-, with the following structure:

Clinical Pharmacology: Phenylpropanolamine hydrochloride is an α-adrenergic receptor agonist (sympathomimetic) which produces vasoconstriction by stimulating α-receptors within the mucosa of the respiratory tract. Clinically, phenylpropanolamine shrinks swollen mucous membranes, reduces tissue hyperemia, edema, and nasal congestion, and increases nasal airway patency. Guaifenesin promotes lower respiratory tract drainage by thinning bronchial secretions, lubricates irritated respiratory tract membranes through increased mucus flow, and facilitates removal of viscous, inspissated mucus. As a result, sinus and bronchial drainage is improved, and dry, nonproductive coughs become more productive and less frequent.
Indications and Usage: ENTEX LA is indicated for the symptomatic relief of sinusitis, bronchitis, pharyngitis, and coryza when these conditions are associated with nasal congestion and viscous mucus in the lower respiratory tract.
Contraindications: ENTEX LA is contraindicated in individuals with known hypersensitivity to sympathomimetics, severe hypertension, or in patients receiving monoamine oxidase inhibitors.
Warnings: Sympathomimetic amines should be used with caution in patients with hypertension, diabetes mellitus, heart disease, peripheral vascular disease, increased intraocular pressure, hyperthyroidism, or prostatic hypertrophy.
Precautions:
Information for Patients: Do not crush or chew ENTEX LA tablets prior to swallowing.
Drug Interactions: ENTEX LA should not be used in patients taking monoamine oxidase inhibitors or other sympathomimetics.
Drug/Laboratory Test Interactions: Guaifenesin has been reported to interfere with clinical laboratory determinations of urinary 5-hydroxyindoleacetic acid (5-HIAA) and urinary vanilmandelic acid (VMA).
Pregnancy: Pregnancy Category C. Animal reproduction studies have not been conducted with ENTEX LA. It is also not known whether ENTEX LA can cause fetal harm when administered to a pregnant woman or can affect reproduction capacity. ENTEX LA should be given to a pregnant woman only if clearly needed.
Nursing Mothers: It is not known whether the drugs in ENTEX LA are excreted in human milk. Because many drugs are excreted in human milk and because of the potential for serious adverse reactions in nursing infants, a decision should be made whether to discontinue nursing or to discontinue the product, taking into account the importance of the drug to the mother.
Pediatric Use: Safety and effectiveness of ENTEX LA tablets in children below the age of 6 have not been established.
Adverse Reactions: Possible adverse reactions include nervousness, insomnia, restlessness, headache, nausea, or gastric irritation. These reactions seldom, if ever, require discontinuation of therapy. Urinary retention may occur in patients with prostatic hypertrophy.
Overdosage: The treatment of overdosage should provide symptomatic and supportive care. If the amount ingested is considered dangerous or excessive, induce vomiting with ipecac syrup unless the patient is convulsing, comatose, or has lost the gag reflex, in which case perform gastric lavage using a large-bore tube. If indicated, follow with activated charcoal and a saline cathartic. Since the effects of ENTEX LA may last up to 12 hours, treatment should be continued for at least that length of time.
Dosage and Administration: Adults and children 12 years of age and older—one tablet twice daily (every 12 hours); children 6 to under 12 years—one-half (½) tablet twice daily (every 12 hours). ENTEX LA is not recommended for children under 6 years of age. Tablets may be broken in half for ease of administration without affecting release of medication but should not be crushed or chewed prior to swallowing.
How Supplied: ENTEX LA is available as a blue, scored tablet imprinted with "ENTEX LA" on the smooth side and "0149 0436" on the scored side.
NDC 0149-0436-01 bottle of 100
Caution: Federal law prohibits dispensing without prescription.
Shown in Product Identification Section, page 422
ENXLATB-P5

FURADANTIN®
[fewr-a-dan'tin]
(nitrofurantoin)

The following text is based on official labeling in effect August 1, 1984.
Description: Furadantin is 1-[[(5-nitro-2-furanyl)methylene]amino]-2, 4-imidazolidinedione, a synthetic antimicrobial agent. It is a yellow, stable crystalline compound:

Actions: Clinical Pharmacology: Orally administered Furadantin is readily absorbed and rapidly excreted in urine. Blood concentrations at therapeutic dosage are usually low. It is highly soluble in urine, to which it may impart a brown color. Following a therapeutic dose regimen (100 mg q.i.d. for 7 days) average urinary drug recoveries (0–24 hours) on day 1 and day 7 were 42.7% and 43.6%, respectively, for Furadantin.
Microbiology: Furadantin, *in vitro*, is bacteriostatic in low concentrations (10 mcg/ml to 5 mcg/ml) and is considered to be bactericidal in higher concentrations. Its presumed mode of action is based upon its interference with several bacterial enzyme systems. Bacteria develop only a limited resistance to furan derivatives clinically. Furadantin is usually active against the following organisms *in vitro: Escherichia coli*, enterococci (e.g. *Streptococcus faecalis*) *Staphylococcus aureus*.
Note: Some strains of *Enterobacter* species and *Klebsiella* species are resistant to Furadantin. It is not active against most strains of *Proteus* species, and *Serratia* species. It has no activity against *Pseudomonas* species.
Susceptibility Tests—Quantitative methods that require measurement of zone diameters give the most precise estimates of antimicrobial susceptibility. One recommended procedure, (NCCLS, ASM-2)*, uses a disc containing 300 micrograms for testing susceptibility; interpretations correlate zone diameters of this disc test with MIC values for nitrofurantoin. Reports from the laboratory should be interpreted according to the following criteria:
Susceptible organisms produce zones of 17 mm or greater, indicating that the tested organism is likely to respond to therapy.
Organisms of intermediate susceptibility produce zones of 15 to 16 mm, indicating that the tested organism would be suceptible if high dosage is used.
Resistant organisms produce zones of 14 mm or less, indicating that other therapy should be selected.
A bacterial isolate may be considered susceptible if the MIC value for nitrofurantoin is not more than 25 micrograms per ml. Organisms are considered

resistant if the MIC is not less than 100 micrograms per ml.

Indications: Furadantin is indicated for the treatment of urinary tract infections when due to susceptible strains of *E. coli*, enterococci, *S. aureus* (it is not indicated for the treatment of associated renal cortical or perinephric abscesses), and certain susceptible strains of *Klebsiella* species, *Enterobacter* species, and *Proteus* species.

Note: Specimens for culture and susceptibility testing should be obtained prior to and during drug administration.

Contraindications: Anuria, oliguria, or significant impairment of renal function (creatinine clearance under 40 ml per minute) are contraindications to therapy with this drug. Treatment of this type of patient carries an increased risk of toxicity because of impaired excretion of the drug. For the same reason, this drug is much less effective under these circumstances.

The drug is contraindicated in pregnant patients at term as well as in infants under one month of age because of the possibility of hemolytic anemia due to immature enzyme systems (glutathione instability).

The drug is also contraindicated in those patients with known hypersensitivity to Furadantin, Macrodantin® (nitrofurantoin macrocrystals), and other nitrofurantoin preparations.

Warnings: Acute, subacute and chronic pulmonary reactions have been observed in patients treated with nitrofurantoin products. If these reactions occur, the drug should be withdrawn and appropriate measures should be taken.

An insidious onset of pulmonary reactions (diffuse interstitial pneumonitis or pulmonary fibrosis, or both) in patients on long-term therapy warrants close monitoring of these patients.

There have been isolated reports giving pulmonary reactions as a contributing cause of death. (See Hypersensitivity reactions.)

Cases of hemolytic anemia of the primaquine sensitivity type have been induced by Furadantin. The hemolysis appears to be linked to a glucose-6-phosphate dehydrogenase deficiency in the red blood cells of the affected patients. This deficiency is found in 10 percent of Negroes and a small percentage of ethnic groups of Mediterranean and Near-Eastern origin. Any sign of hemolysis is an indication to discontinue the drug. Hemolysis ceases when the drug is withdrawn.

Hepatitis, including chronic active hepatitis, occurs rarely. Fatalities have been reported. The onset of chronic active hepatitis may be insidious, and patients receiving long-term therapy should be monitored periodically for changes in liver function. If hepatitis occurs, the drug should be withdrawn immediately and appropriate measures should be taken.

Precautions: Peripheral neuropathy may occur with Furadantin therapy; this may become severe or irreversible. Fatalities have been reported. Predisposing conditions such as renal impairment (creatinine clearance under 40 ml per minute), anemia, diabetes, electrolyte imbalance, vitamin B deficiency, and debilitating disease may enhance such occurrence.

Usage in Pregnancy: The safety of Furadantin during pregnancy and lactation has not been established. Use of this drug in women of childbearing potential requires that the anticipated benefit be weighed against the possible risks.

Adverse Reactions: Gastrointestinal reactions: Anorexia, nausea and emesis are the most frequent reactions; abdominal pain and diarrhea occur less frequently. These dose-related toxicity reactions can be minimized by reduction of dosage, especially in the female patient. Hepatitis, including chronic active hepatitis, has been observed rarely. The mechanism appears to be of an idiosyncratic hypersensitive type.

Hypersensitivity reactions: Pulmonary sensitivity reactions may occur, which can be acute, subacute, or chronic.

Acute reactions are commonly manifested by fever, chills, cough, chest pain, dyspnea, pulmonary infiltration with consolidation or pleural effusion on x-ray, and eosinophilia. The acute reactions usually occur within the first week of treatment and are reversible with cessation of therapy. Resolution may be dramatic.

In subacute reactions, fever and eosinophilia are observed less often. Recovery is somewhat slower, perhaps as long as several months. If the symptoms are not recognized as being drug related and nitrofurantoin is not withdrawn, symptoms may become more severe.

Chronic pulmonary reactions are more likely to occur in patients who have been on continuous nitrofurantoin therapy for six months or longer. The insidious onset of malaise, dyspnea on exertion, cough, and altered pulmonary function are common manifestations. Roentgenographic and histologic findings of diffuse interstitial pneumonitis or fibrosis, or both, are also common manifestations. Fever is rarely prominent.

The severity of these chronic pulmonary reactions and the degree of their resolution appear to be related to the duration of therapy after the first clinical signs appear. Pulmonary function may be permanently impaired even after cessation of nitrofurantoin therapy. This risk is greater when pulmonary reactions are not recognized early.

Dermatologic reactions: Exfoliative dermatitis and erythema multiforme (including Stevens-Johnson Syndrome) have been reported rarely. Maculopapular, erythematous or eczematous eruption, pruritus, urticaria, and angioedema.

Other hypersensitivity reactions: Anaphylaxis, asthmatic attack in patients with history of asthma, cholestatic jaundice, hepatitis, drug fever, and arthralgia.

Hematologic reactions: Hemolytic anemia, granulocytopenia, agranulocytosis, leukopenia, thrombocytopenia, eosinophilia, and megaloblastic anemia. Return of the blood picture to normal has followed cessation of therapy. Aplastic anemia has been reported rarely.

Neurological reactions: Peripheral neuropathy, headache, dizziness, nystagmus, and drowsiness.

Miscellaneous reactions: Transient alopecia. As with other antimicrobial agents, superinfections by resistant organisms, e.g., *Pseudomonas*, may occur. With Furadantin, however, these are limited to the genitourinary tract because suppression of normal bacterial flora elsewhere in the body does not occur.

Dosage and Administration: Furadantin should be given with food to improve drug absorption and, in some patients, tolerance.

Adults: 50-100 mg four times a day—the lower dosage level is recommended for uncomplicated urinary tract infections.

Children: 5-7 mg/kg of body weight per 24 hours, to be given in four divided doses (contraindicated under one month of age). The following table can be used to calculate an average dose of Furadantin Oral Suspension (5 mg/ml) for children (one 5 ml teaspoon of Furadantin Oral Suspension contains 25 mg of Furadantin):

Body Weight		No. Teaspoonfuls
Pounds	Kilograms	4 Times Daily
15 to 26	7 to 11	½ (2.5 ml)
27 to 46	12 to 21	1 (5 ml)
47 to 68	22 to 30	1½ (7.5 ml)
69 to 91	31 to 41	2 (10 ml)

Therapy should be continued for at least one week and for at least 3 days after sterility of the urine is obtained. Continued infection indicates the need for reevaluation.

For long-term suppressive therapy in adults, a reduction of dosage to 50-100 mg at bedtime may be adequate. See WARNINGS section regarding risks associated with long-term therapy. For long-term suppressive therapy in children, doses as low as 1 mg/kg per 24 hours, given in a single or in two divided doses, may be adequate.

How Supplied: Furadantin is available in: 50-mg scored, yellow tablets coded "Eaton 036"
NDC 0149-0036-05   bottle of 100
NDC 0149-0036-66   bottle of 500
NDC 0149-0036-06   hospital unit-dose strips in box of 100
100-mg scored, yellow tablets coded "Eaton 037"
NDC 0149-0037-05   bottle of 100
NDC 0149-0037-66   bottle of 500
NDC 0149-0037-07   hospital unit-dose strips in box of 100

It should be dispensed in amber bottles.
Furadantin (nitrofurantoin) Oral Suspension is available in:
NDC 0149-0735-15   amber bottle of 60 ml
NDC 0149-0735-61   amber bottle of 470 ml

Avoid exposure to strong light which may darken the drug. It is stable in storage. It should be dispensed in amber bottles.

Furadantin 300 mcg Sensi-Discs for the laboratory determination of bacterial sensitivity are available from BBL, division of BioQuest. For information on simple Furadantin assays in blood, serum, and urine, write or call the Medical Department. Literature sent to physicians on request.

Address medical inquiries to Norwich Eaton Pharmaceuticals, Inc., Medical Department, Norwich, NY 13815.

* National Committee for Clinical Laboratory Standards. Approved Standard: ASM-2, Performance Standards for Antimicrobial Disc Susceptibility Tests, July, 1975.

Manufactured by
Eaton Laboratories, Inc.
Manati, Puerto Rico 00701
Distributed by
Norwich Eaton Pharmaceuticals, Inc.
Norwich, New York 13815
A Procter & Gamble Company

FDN-P5

FURACIN®   ℞
[*fewr′ a-sin*]
(nitrofurazone) SOLUBLE DRESSING

The following text is based on official labeling in effect August 1, 1984.

Description: Chemically, Furacin is nitrofurazone, 2-[(5-nitro-2-furanyl)methylene]hydrazinecarboxamide, with the following structure:

$$O_2N - \bigcirc - CH = NNHCONH_2$$

Furacin Soluble Dressing is a preparation containing 0.2% nitrofurazone in Solubase® (a water-soluble base of polyethylene glycols 3350, 900, and 300).

Furacin Soluble Dressing is an antibacterial agent for topical use.

Clinical Pharmacology: Furacin Soluble Dressing (nitrofurazone) is a nitrofuran that is bactericidal for most pathogens commonly causing surface infections, including *Staphylococcus aureus*, *Streptococcus*, *Escherichia coli*, *Clostridium perfringens*, *Aerobacter aerogenes*, and *Proteus*. Furacin Soluble Dressing inhibits a number of bacterial enzymes, especially those involved in the aerobic and anaerobic degradation of glucose and pyruvate. The activity appears to involve the pyruvate dehydrogenase system as well as citrate synthetase, malate dehydrogenase, glutathione reductase, and pyruvate decarboxylase. Glutathione reductase inhibition may be caused by control of pentose phosphate metabolism. Although Furacin Soluble Dressing inhibits a variety of enzymes, it is not considered to be a general enzyme inactivator since many enzymes are not inhibited by this compound.

Indications and Usage: Furacin Soluble Dressing is a topical antibacterial agent indicated for adjunctive therapy of patients with second- and third-degree burns when bacterial resistance to other agents is a real or potential problem.

It is also indicated in skin grafting where bacterial contamination may cause graft rejection and/or donor site infection particularly in hospitals with historical resistant-bacteria epidemics.

Continued on next page

Norwich Eaton—Cont.

There is no known evidence of effectiveness of this product in the treatment of minor burns or surface bacterial infections involving wounds, cutaneous ulcers, or the various pyodermas.

Contraindications: Known sensitization to any of the components of this preparation is a contraindication for use.

Warnings: Nitrofurazone has been shown to produce mammary tumors when fed at high doses to female Sprague-Dawley rats. The relevance of this to topical use in humans is unknown.

Furacin Soluble Dressing should be used with caution in patients with known or suspected renal impairment. The polyethylene glycols in the base can be absorbed through denuded skin and may not be excreted normally by the compromised kidney. This may lead to symptoms of progressive renal impairment such as increased BUN, anion gap, and metabolic acidosis. (NOTE: Furacin (nitrofurazone) Topical Cream does not contain polyethylene glycols.)

Precautions:
General: Use of topical antimicrobials occasionally allows overgrowth of nonsusceptible organisms including fungi. If this occurs, or if irritation, sensitization or superinfection develops, treatment with Furacin Soluble Dressing should be discontinued and appropriate therapy instituted.

Carcinogenesis, mutagenesis, and impairment of fertility: Nitrofurazone has been shown to produce mammary tumors when fed at high doses to female Sprague-Dawley rats. The relevance of this to topical use in humans is unknown. Dietary dosage levels of 60 and 30 mg/kg/day shortened the onset time of the typical mammary gland tumors associated with older female rats. These tumors exhibited the same histological characteristics seen in the spontaneously occurring tumors, and were seen only in the female animals. No mammary tumors were seen in rats treated with nitrofurazone orally in the diet for 1 year at levels of approximately 11 mg/kg/day. Spermatogenic arrest was noted in the male rats in dietary dosage levels of 30 mg/kg/day and above, after one year on test.

Usage in Pregnancy: Pregnancy Category C: Nitrofurazone has been shown to have an embryocidal effect in rabbits when given in oral doses thirty times the human dose. There are no adequate and well controlled studies in pregnant women.

Furacin Soluble Dressing should be used during pregnancy only if the potential benefit justifies the potential risk to the fetus.

Nursing mothers: It is not known whether this drug is excreted in human milk. Because many drugs are excreted in human milk and because of the potential for tumorigenicity shown for nitrofurazone in animal studies, a decision should be made whether to discontinue nursing or to discontinue the drug, taking into account the importance of the drug to the mother.

Pediatric use: Safety and effectiveness in children have not been established.

Adverse Reactions: In quantitative studies published during the period 1945-70, 206 instances of clinical skin reaction were reported out of 18,249 patients (an incidence of 1.1%) treated with Furacin formulations. Symptoms appeared as varying degrees of contact dermatitides such as rash, pruritus, and local edema.

Allergic reactions to Furacin Soluble Dressing should be treated symptomatically.

Dosage and Administration:
Burns: Apply directly to the lesion with a spatula, or first place on gauze. Impregnated gauze may be used. Reapply depending on the preferred dressing technique. Flushing the dressing with sterile saline facilitates its removal.

Preparation of Impregnated Gauze: Sterile gauze strips are placed in a tray and covered with Furacin Soluble Dressing. Repeat the procedure, adding several layers of gauze for each layer of Furacin Soluble Dressing. Sprinkling a little sterile water on each layer of dressing will minimize any color change from autoclaving. Cover the tray very loosely and autoclave at 121°C for 30 minutes at 15 to 20 pounds pressure.

To impregnate bandage rolls, place some Furacin Soluble Dressing in the bottom of a glass jar. Stand rolls on end. Place more Furacin Soluble Dressing on top. Cover top of jar with aluminum foil. Autoclave at 121°C for 45 minutes at 15 to 20 pounds pressure. Do not store impregnated bandage rolls for more than 24 hours.

Autoclaving more than once is not recommended.

How Supplied: Furacin Soluble Dressing is available in:
NDC 0149-0704-12 tube of 28 grams
NDC 0149-0704-11 tube of 56 grams
NDC 0149-0704-51 jar of 135 grams
NDC 0149-0704-61 jar of 454 grams

Animal Toxicology: The oral administration of nitrofurazone for 7 days to rats at extremely high dosage levels of 240 mg/kg/day produced severe hepatorenal lesions whereas only renal changes were seen when the dosage level was reduced to 60 mg/kg/day for 60 days.

Dogs treated orally with nitrofurazone for 400 days at levels of 11 mg/kg/day showed no toxic effects related to drug treatment. The single intravenous administration in dogs of 20, 35, or 75 mg/kg nitrofurazone produced clinical signs of lacrimation, salivation, emesis, diarrhea, excitation, weakness, ataxia, and weight loss, whereas 100 mg/kg produced convulsions and death.

There was no evidence of toxicosis in rhesus monkeys treated with doses of nitrofurazone as high as 58 mg/kg/day for 10 weeks and 23 mg/kg/day for 63 weeks.

The peroral LD_{50} of nitrofurazone in mice and rats is 747 and 590 mg/kg respectively.

For bacterial sensitivity tests: Furacin Sensi-Discs are available from BBL, Division of Bio-Quest.

FSD-P9

FURACIN® TOPICAL CREAM ℞
[fewr′a-sin]
(nitrofurazone)

The following text is based on official labeling in effect August 1, 1984.

Description: Chemically, Furacin is nitrofurazone, 2-[(5-nitro-2-furanyl)methylene]hydrazinecarboxamide, with the following structure:

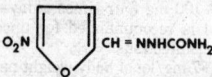

Furacin Topical Cream is a preparation containing 0.2% Furacin in a water-miscible base consisting of glycerin, cetyl alcohol, mineral oil, an ethoxylated fatty alcohol, methylparaben, propylparaben, and purified water.

Furacin Topical Cream is an antibacterial agent for topical use.

Clinical Pharmacology: Furacin Topical Cream is a nitrofuran that is bactericidal for most pathogens commonly causing surface infections, including *Staphylococcus aureus, Streptococcus, Escherichia coli, Clostridium perfringens, Aerobacter aerogenes,* and *Proteus.*

Furacin Topical Cream inhibits a number of bacterial enzymes, especially those involved in the aerobic and anaerobic degradation of glucose and pyruvate. The activity appears to involve the pyruvate dehydrogenase system as well as citrate synthetase, malate dehydrogenase, glutathione reductase, and pyruvate decarboxylase. Glutathione reductase inhibition may be caused by control of pentose phosphate metabolism. Although Furacin Topical Cream inhibits a variety of enzymes, it is not considered to be a general enzyme inactivator since many enzymes are not inhibited by this compound.

Indications and Usage: Furacin Topical Cream is a topical antibacterial agent indicated for adjunctive therapy of patients with second- and third-degree burns when bacterial resistance to other agents is a real or potential problem.

It is also indicated in skin grafting where bacterial contamination may cause graft rejection and/or donor site infection particularly in hospitals with historical resistant-bacteria epidemics.

There is no known evidence of effectiveness of this product in the treatment of minor burns or surface bacterial infections involving wounds, cutaneous ulcers or the various pyodermas.

Contraindications: Known sensitization to any of the components of this preparation is a contraindication for use.

Warnings: None.

Precautions:
General: Use of Furacin Topical Cream occasionally allows overgrowth of nonsusceptible organisms including fungi and *Pseudomonas*. If this occurs, or if irritation, sensitization or superinfection develops, treatment with Furacin Topical Cream should be discontinued and appropriate therapy instituted.

Information for Patients: Patients should be told to use Furacin Topical Cream only as directed by a physician. Patients should be advised to discontinue the drug and contact a physician should rash or irritation occur.

Carcinogenesis, Mutagenesis, and Impairment of Fertility: Nitrofurazone has been shown to produce mammary tumors when fed at high doses to female Sprague-Dawley rats. The relevance of this to topical use in humans is unknown.

Dietary dosage levels of 60 and 30 mg/kg/day shortened the onset time of the typical mammary gland tumors associated with older female rats. These tumors exhibited the same histological characteristics seen in the spontaneously occurring tumors, and were seen only in the female animals. No mammary tumors were seen in rats treated with nitrofurazone orally in the diet for 1 year at levels approximately 11 mg/kg/day. Spermatogenic arrest was noted in the male rats in dietary dosage levels of 30 mg/kg/day and above, after one year on test.

Usage in Pregnancy: Pregnancy Category C: Nitrofurazone, when administered orally to pregnant rabbits, caused a slight increase in the frequency of stillbirths when given in doses thirty times the human dose. There are no adequate and well controlled studies in pregnant women. Furacin Topical Cream should be used during pregnancy only if the potential benefit justifies the potential risk to the fetus.

Nursing Mothers: It is not known whether this drug is excreted in human milk. Because many drugs are excreted in human milk and because of the potential for tumorigenicity shown for nitrofurazone in animal studies, a decision should be made whether to discontinue nursing or to discontinue the drug, taking into account the importance of the drug to the mother.

Adverse Reactions: In quantitative studies published during the period 1945–70, 206 instances of clinical skin reaction were reported out of 18,249 patients (an incidence of 1.1%) treated with Furacin formulations. Symptoms appeared as varying degrees of contact dermatitides such as rash, pruritus, and local edema.

Allergic reactions to Furacin Topical Cream should be treated symptomatically.

Dosage and Administration: Apply Furacin Topical Cream directly to the lesion, or first place on gauze. Reapply once daily or every few days, depending on the usual dressing technique.

How Supplied: Furacin Topical Cream is available in:
NDC 0149-0777-15 tube of 14 grams
NDC 0149-0777-12 tube of 28 grams
NDC 0149-0777-61 jar of 368 grams

Storage: Avoid exposure to direct sunlight, strong fluorescent lighting, alkaline materials, and excessive heat (over 104°F or 40°C).

Animal Toxicology: The oral administration of nitrofurazone for 7 days to rats at extremely high dosage levels of 240 mg/kg/day produced severe hepatorenal lesions whereas only renal changes were seen when the dosage level was reduced to 60 mg/kg/day for 60 days.

Dogs treated orally with nitrofurazone for 400 days at levels of 11 mg/kg/day showed no toxic effects related to drug treatment.

There was no evidence of toxicosis in rhesus monkeys treated with doses of nitrofurazone as high as 58 mg/kg/day for 10 weeks and 23 mg/kg/day for 63 weeks.

The peroral LD_{50} of nitrofurazone in mice and rats is 747 and 590 mg/kg respectively.

For bacterial sensitivity tests: Furacin Sensi-Discs are available from BBL, Division of BioQuest.

Caution: Federal law prohibits dispensing without prescription.

FTOPCR-P4

FUROXONE® R
[fewr-ox'ōne]
(Brand of Furazolidone Eaton)
Available both in Tablet Form
and as a Liquid Suspension

The following text is based on official labeling in effect August 1, 1984.

Description: Furoxone (furazolidone) is one of the synthetic antimicrobial nitrofurans. It is a stable, yellow, crystalline compound with the following structure:

3-(5-nitrofurfurylideneamino)-2-oxazolidinone

Action: Furoxone (furazolidone) has a broad antibacterial spectrum covering the majority of gastrointestinal tract pathogens including E. coli, staphylococci, Salmonella, Shigella, Proteus, Aerobacter aerogenes, Vibrio cholerae[9,10,11] and Giardia lamblia.[5,6] Its bactericidal activity is based upon its interference with several bacterial enzyme systems; this antimicrobial action minimizes the development of resistant organisms. It neither significantly alters the normal bowel flora nor results in fungal overgrowth. The brown color found in the urine with adequate dosage is of no clinical significance.

Indications: Indicated in the specific and symptomatic treatment of bacterial or protozoal diarrhea and enteritis caused by susceptible organisms. Furoxone (furazolidone) products are well tolerated, have a very low incidence of adverse reactions.

Contraindications:
1. To obviate an Antabuse® (disulfiram-)like reaction which may occur in some patients the ingestion of alcohol should be avoided during or within four days after Furoxone (furazolidone) therapy. (See Adverse Reactions.)
2. IN GENERAL, MAOI DRUGS, TYRAMINE CONTAINING FOODS AND INDIRECTLY ACTING SYMPATHOMIMETIC AMINES ARE CONTRAINDICATED OR SHOULD BE USED WITH CAUTION IN PATIENTS RECEIVING FUROXONE (FURAZOLIDONE). (SEE PRECAUTIONS.)
3. INFANTS UNDER 1 MONTH SHOULD NOT RECEIVE FUROXONE (FURAZOLIDONE) (SEE ADVERSE REACTIONS AND DOSAGE FOR CHILDREN).[4] THE FUROXONE (FURAZOLIDONE) CONCENTRATION IN THE BREAST MILK OF LACTATING WOMEN HAS NOT BEEN DETERMINED, THEREFORE THE SAFETY IN THIS CIRCUMSTANCE HAS NOT BEEN ESTABLISHED.
4. Prior sensitivity to Furoxone (furazolidone) is a contraindication.

Warnings: (See Contraindications listed above.)

Use in Pregnancy: The safety of Furoxone (furazolidone) during the childbearing age has not been established; as with any potent antibacterial, Furoxone (furazolidone) must be administered with caution during the childbearing age. However, animal breeding studies have revealed no evidence of teratogenicity following the administration of Furoxone (furazolidone) for long periods of time and at doses far in excess of those recommended for the human. There have been no clinical reports regarding this possible adverse effect on the fetus or the newborn infant.

Precautions: Monoamine Oxidase Inhibition:[7] Effective inhibition of monoamine oxidase by furazolidone has been demonstrated experimentally in man by the enhancement of tyramine and amphetamine sensitivity and by the directly measured monamine oxidase inhibition.

A period of five days of furazolidone administration in the recommended doses in these patients was required to give an enhancement of the tyramine and amphetamine sensitivities by two to threefold. Administration of furazolidone in the recommended dose of 400 mg/day for a period of five days should not subject the adult patient to an undue hazard of hypertensive crisis due to monoamine oxidase inhibition. Hypertensive crises have never been reported even after the peroral administration of larger doses and/or for longer periods of time. Controlled studies reveal no signs or symptoms of hypertensive crisis even after the peroral administration of Furoxone (furazolidone) in doses of 400 mg/day in excess of 48 consecutive months.[8]

If administered in doses larger than recommended or in excess of five days the indications must be weighed against the possible hazards of hypertensive crisis related to the accumulation of monoamine oxidase inhibition. If indications are sufficient, the patients should be informed of drugs and foods which predispose to hypertensive crises:

(A) Other known MAOI drugs; however, when indicated they should be prescribed with caution and at a reduced dosage.
(B) Tyramine containing foods such as broad beans, yeast extracts, strong unpasteurized cheeses, beer, wine, pickled herring, chicken livers and fermented products are contraindicated.
(C) Indirectly acting sympathomimetic amines such as those found in nasal decongestants (phenylephrine, ephedrine) and anorectics (amphetamines) are contraindicated.
(D) Likewise, sedatives, antihistamines, tranquilizers and narcotics should be used in reduced dosages and with caution.

Orthostatic hypotension and hypoglycemia may occur.

Adverse Reactions: A few hypersensitivity reactions to Furoxone (furazolidone) have been reported including a fall in blood pressure, urticaria, fever, arthralgia and a vesicular morbilliform rash. These reactions subsided following withdrawal of the drug.

Nausea, emesis, headache or malaise occur occasionally and may be minimized or eliminated by reduction in dosage or withdrawal of the drug.

Rarely, individuals receiving Furoxone (furazolidone) have exhibited an Antabuse® (disulfiram)-like reaction to alcohol characterized by flushing, slight temperature elevation, dyspnea, and in some instances a sense of constriction within the chest. All symptomatology disappeared within 24 hours with no lasting ill effects. During nine years of clinical use and approximately 3.5 million courses of therapy (in the U.S.A. alone) in the published literature and documented case reports 43 cases have been reported—of which 14 were produced under experimental conditions with planned doses of the compound in excess of those recommended. Three of these experienced a fall in blood pressure necessitating active therapy. Indications are that levarterenol (Levophed®) may be used to combat such hypotensive episodes since human studies show that this drug is not potentiated in patients treated with Furoxone (furazolidone). (Indirectly acting pressor agents should be avoided.) The ingestion of alcohol in any form should be avoided during Furoxone (furazolidone) therapy and for four days thereafter to prevent this reaction.

Furoxone (furazolidone) may cause mild reversible intravascular hemolysis in certain ethnic groups of Mediterranean and Near-Eastern origin, and Negroes.[1,3] This is due to an intrinsic defect of red blood cell metabolism in a small percentage of these ethnic groups, making them unusually susceptible to hemolysis by numerous compounds.[2] It is necessary to observe such patients closely while receiving Furoxone (furazolidone) and to discontinue its use if there is any indication of hemolysis. Should not be administered to infants under 1 month of age because of the possibility of producing a hemolytic anemia due to immature enzyme systems (glutathione instability) in the early neonatal period.[4]

Colitis, proctitis, anal pruritus, staphylococcic enteritis, renal or hepatic toxicity have not been a significant problem with Furoxone (furazolidone).

Dosage and Administration:

FUROXONE (furazolidone) TABLETS, 100 mg each, are brown and scored to facilitate adjustment of dosage.

Average Adult Dosage: One 100 mg tablet four times daily.

Average Dosage for Children: Those 5 years of age or older should receive 25 to 50 mg (¼ to ½ tablet) four times daily. The tablet dosage may be crushed and given in a spoonful of corn syrup.

FUROXONE (furazolidone) LIQUID composition: each 15 ml tablespoonful contains Furoxone (furazolidone) 50 mg per 15 ml (3.33 mg per ml) in a light-yellow aqueous vehicle. Suitable flavoring, suspending and preservative agents complete the formulation. It is stable in storage. Prior to administering Furoxone (furazolidone) Liquid shake the bottle vigorously. It should be dispensed in amber bottles.

Average Adult Dosage: Two tablespoonfuls four times daily.

Average Dosage for Children:
5 years or older—½ to 1 tablespoonful four times daily (7.5–15.0 ml)
1 to 4 years old—1 to 1½ teaspoonfuls four times daily (5.0–7.5 ml)
1 month to 1 year—½ to 1 teaspoonful four times daily (2.5–5.0 ml)

This dosage is based on an average dose of 5 mg of Furoxone (furazolidone) per Kg (2.3 mg per lb) of body weight given in four equally divided doses during 24 hours. The maximal dose of 8.8 mg of Furoxone (furazolidone) per Kg (4 mg per lb) of body weight per 24 hours should probably not be exceeded because of the possibility of producing nausea or emesis. If these are severe, the dosage should be reduced.

The average case of diarrhea treated with Furoxone (furazolidone) will respond within 2 to 5 days of therapy. Occasional patients may require a longer term of therapy. If satisfactory clinical response is not obtained within 7 days it indicates that the pathogen is refractory to Furoxone (furazolidone) and the drug should be discontinued. Adjunctive therapy with other antibacterial agents or bismuth salts is not contraindicated. (N.B. Refer to Warnings.)

In order to administer furazolidone in doses larger than recommended or in excess of five days the indications must be weighed against the possible hazards of hypertensive crisis related to the accumulation of monoamine oxidase inhibition. If indications are sufficient, the patient should be informed of drugs and foods which predispose to hypertensive crisis. (See Precautions.)

How Supplied: Furoxone (furazolidone) Tablets, 100 mg each, coded "Eaton 072", are supplied in amber bottles containing 20 and 100 tablets. (Should be dispensed in amber bottles.)

Furoxone (furazolidone) Liquid is supplied in amber bottles containing 60 ml and 473 ml. (Should be dispensed in amber bottles.)

References:
(1) Kellermeyer, R.S.; Tarlov, A.R.; Schrier, S.L., and Alving, A.S.: J. Lab. Clin. Med. 52:827–828 (Nov.) 1958.

Continued on next page

Norwich Eaton—Cont.

(2) Tarlov et al.: Arch. Int. Med. 109:209–234, 1962.
(3) Kellermeyer et al.: J.A.M.A. 180: No. 5, 388–394, 1962.
(4) Zinkham, Pediatrics, 23:18–32, 1959; Gross & Hurwitz, Pediatrics 22:453, 1958.
(5) Fallas Vargas, M. Un Nuevo Tratamiento para la Giardiasis (A New Treatment for Giardiasis). Rev. Med. Costa Rica 19:269–284 (July 1962).
(6) Webster, B.H. Furazolidone in the Treatment of Giardiasis. Amer. J. Dig. Diseases 5:618–622 (July) 1960.
(7) Oates, J.A.; Pettinger, W.A. Inhibition of Monoamine Oxidase by Furazolidone in Man. Data on file: Office of the Medical Director, Norwich-Eaton Pharmaceuticals. Available upon request.
(8) Kirsner, Joseph B., M.D., Ph.D. Data on file: Office of the Medical Director, Norwich-Eaton Pharmaceuticals. Available upon request.
(9) Neogy, K.N., et al. Furazolidone in Cholera. Journ. Indian Med. Assoc. 48:137, 1967.
(10) Chaudhuri, R.N. et al. Furazolidone in Cholera. Lancet 2:909 (Oct. 30) 1965.
(11) Curlin, G. Comparison of Antibiotic Regimens in Cholera. Abstracts of papers, Epidemiological Intelligence Service Conference, Atlanta, Ga., April 11–14, 1967, p. 11.

FUROXONE (FURAZOLIDONE) SENSI-DISCS for laboratory determination of bacterial sensitivity are available from BBL, division of BioQuest.

Caution: Federal law prohibits dispensing without prescription.

Literature available to physicians on request.

FUROX-P3

LABID™ 250 mg
[lā'bid]
(anhydrous theophylline)

The following text is based on official labeling in effect August 1, 1984.

Description: LāBID contains 250 mg anhydrous theophylline in a scored, long-acting, dye-free tablet. Theophylline is a white, odorless, crystalline powder, having a bitter taste, and is chemically related to theobromine and caffeine. LāBID has been specially formulated to provide therapeutic serum levels when administered every 12 hours, and minimizes the peaks and valleys of serum levels commonly found with shorter-acting theophylline products.

Clinical Pharmacology: The pharmacologic actions of theophylline include stimulation of respiration, augmentation of cardiac inotropy and chronotropy, relaxation of smooth muscles, including those in the bronchi and blood vessels (other than cerebral vessels) and diuresis. The main use of theophylline has been in the treatment of reversible airway obstruction. Theophylline is considered a potent medication for the control of chronic asthma. No development of tolerance occurs with chronic use of theophylline. The half-life is shortened with cigarette smoking and prolonged in alcoholism, reduced hepatic or renal function, congestive heart failure, and in patients receiving antibiotics such as lincomycin, clindamycin, troleandomycin, or erythromycin. High fever for prolonged periods and certain viral illnesses may decrease theophylline elimination. Newborn infants have extremely slow clearances and half-lives exceeding 24 hours.

Older adults with chronic obstructive pulmonary disease, any patients with cor pulmonale or other causes of heart failure, and patients with liver pathology may have much lower clearances with half-lives that exceed 24 hours.

In comparative cross-over steady-state studies with immediate-release theophylline dosed at an average of 2.1 mg/K every 6 hours, LāBID 250 produced identical areas under curve when dosed at an average of 4.5 mg/K every 12 hours and adjusted for dosage difference. This confirms that LāBID 250 bioavailability dosed q12h is identical to liquid theophylline preparations dosed q6h. Data from the study also confirms a uniform and constant rate of absorption of theophylline from LāBID 250 in each subject. At steady-state, LāBID 250 provides adequate therapeutic theophylline levels. In single dose studies, LāBID 250 produces mean peak theophylline serum levels of 13.3 ± 4.6 mcg/ml at 4.9 ± 2.3 hours when dosed at an average of 7.9 mg/K.

Indications: For relief and/or prevention of symptoms from asthma and reversible bronchospasm associated with chronic bronchitis and emphysema.

Contraindications: LāBID is contraindicated in individuals who have shown hypersensitivity to any of its components or to xanthine derivatives.

Warnings: Status asthmaticus is a medical emergency. Optimal therapy frequently requires additional medication including corticosteroids when the patient is not rapidly responsive to bronchodilators. LāBID, as a long-acting theophylline, should not be used in status asthmaticus.

Since excessive theophylline doses may be associated with toxicity, periodic measurement of serum theophylline levels is recommended to assure maximal benefit without excessive risk. Incidence of toxicity increases at serum levels greater than 20 mcg/ml. Although early signs of theophylline toxicity, such as nausea and restlessness, are often seen, in some cases ventricular arrhythmias or seizures may be the first signs of toxicity.

Many patients who have excessive theophylline serum levels exhibit a tachycardia.

Theophylline preparations may worsen pre-existing arrhythmias.

Usage in Pregnancy: Safe use in pregnancy has not been established relative to possible adverse effects on fetal development, but neither have adverse effects on fetal development been established. This is, unfortunately, true for most antiasthmatic medications. Therefore, use of theophylline in pregnant women should be balanced against the risk of uncontrolled asthma.

Precautions: DO NOT CRUSH OR CHEW LāBID 250 TABLETS BEFORE INGESTION. Mean half-life in smokers is shorter than non-smokers. Therefore, smokers may require larger doses of theophylline.

Theophylline should not be administered concurrently with other xanthine preparations. Use with caution in patients with severe cardiac disease, severe hypoxemia, hypertension, hyperthyroidism, acute myocardial injury, cor pulmonale, congestive heart failure, liver disease, in the elderly (especially males), and in neonates. Great caution should be used in giving theophylline to patients with congestive heart failure. Such patients have shown markedly prolonged theophylline blood levels with theophylline persisting in serum for long periods following discontinuation of the drug.

Use theophylline cautiously in patients with a history of peptic ulcer.

Theophylline may occasionally act as a local gastrointestinal irritant, although G.I. symptoms are more commonly centrally mediated and associated with high serum concentration.

Adverse Reactions: The most consistent adverse reactions are due usually to overdose, and are:

Gastrointestinal: anorexia, nausea, vomiting, epigastric pain, hematemesis, diarrhea.
Central nervous system: headaches, irritability, restlessness, insomnia, reflex hyperexcitability, muscle twitching, clonic and tonic generalized convulsions.
Cardiovascular: palpitation, tachycardia, extrasystoles, flushing, hypotension, circulatory failure, ventricular arrhythmias.
Respiratory: tachypnea, respiratory arrest.
Renal: albuminuria, increased excretion of renal tubular cells and red blood cells; potentiation of diuresis.
Others: hyperglycemia, inappropriate ADH syndrome, fever, dehydration.

Drug Interactions:

Drug	Effect
Aminophylline with lithium carbonate	Increased excretion of lithium carbonate
Aminophylline with propranolol	Antagonism of propranolol effect
Theophylline with furosemide	Increased diuresis
Theophylline with hexamethonium	Decreased chronotropic effect
Theophylline with reserpine	Tachycardia
Theophylline with clindamycin, lincomycin, troleandomycin, or erythromycin	Increased theophylline blood levels
Theophylline with chlordiazepoxide	Chlordiazepoxide-induced fatty acid metabolism

Dosage and Administration: THE AVERAGE INITIAL ADULT DOSE IS ONE TO TWO LāBID 250 mg TABLETS EVERY 12 HOURS.

The recommended starting dose of LāBID for adolescents and adults is 6 mg per kg body weight every 12 hours based upon ideal body weight. If the desired relief is not achieved with this dose, and there are no systemic side effects (see Adverse Reactions), the dose may be increased by 1 mg per kg body weight every 2 days. With doses above 8 mg per kg every 12 hours, serum theophylline levels should be monitored.

Doses should be increased until therapeutic responses or side effects occur (higher doses may be necessary and well tolerated).

Occasional patients may require every 8 hours dosing.

THE AVERAGE INITIAL CHILDREN'S DOSE IS ONE-HALF TO ONE LāBID 250 mg TABLET EVERY 12 HOURS.

The recommended starting dose for children is 6 mg per kg body weight every 12 hours, and this dose can be increased by 1 mg per kg body weight every two days. With doses above 8 mg/kg every 12 hours, serum theophylline levels should be monitored.

Overdosage: Management
A. If potential overdose is established and seizure has not occurred:
  1) Induce vomiting.
  2) Administer activated charcoal.
  3) Administer a cathartic (this is particularly important if sustained release preparations have been taken).
B. If patient is having seizure:
  1) Establish an airway.
  2) Administer oxygen.
  3) Treat the seizure with intravenous diazepam 0.1 to 0.3 mg/kg up to 10 mg.
  4) Monitor vital signs, maintain blood pressure and provide adequate hydration.
C. Post-Seizure Coma:
  1) Maintain airway and oxygenation.
  2) Follow above recommendations to prevent absorption of drug, but intubation and lavage will have to be performed instead of inducing emesis, and the cathartic and charcoal will need to be introduced via a large-bore gastric lavage tube.
  3) Continue to provide full supportive care and adequate hydration while waiting for drug to be metabolized. In general, the drug is metabolized sufficiently rapidly so as to not warrant consideration of dialysis.

How Supplied: LāBID 250 mg tablets are supplied in bottles of 100
NDC 0149-0402-01.

LBD-P2

MACRODANTIN®
[mak″rō-dan′tin]
(nitrofurantoin macrocrystals)
CAPSULES

The following text is based on official labeling in effect August 1, 1984.

Description: Macrodantin is a synthetic chemical of controlled crystal size. It is a stable, yellow crystalline compound. It is supplied in capsules containing 25 mg, 50 mg, and 100 mg.

1-[[(5-nitro-2-furanyl)methylene]
amino]-2, 4-imidazolidinedione

Actions: Clinical Pharmacology: Macrodantin is a larger crystal form of Furadantin® (nitrofurantoin). The absorption of Macrodantin is slower and its excretion somewhat less when compared to Furadantin. Blood concentrations at therapeutic dosage are usually low. A number of patients who cannot tolerate Furadantin (nitrofurantoin) Tablets are able to take Macrodantin Capsules without nausea. It is highly soluble in urine, to which it may impart a brown color. Following a therapeutic dose regimen (100 mg q.i.d. for 7 days) average urinary drug recoveries (0-24 hours) on day 1 and 7 were 37.9% and 35.0%, respectively, for Macrodantin.

Microbiology: Macrodantin, in vitro, is bacteriostatic in low concentrations (10 mcg/ml to 5 mcg/ml) and is considered to be bactericidal in higher concentrations. Its presumed mode of action is based upon its interference with several bacterial enzyme systems. Bacteria develop only a limited resistance to furan derivatives clinically. Macrodantin is usually active against the following organisms in vitro: Escherichia coli, enterococci (e.g. Streptococcus faecalis), Staphylococcus aureus.

Note: Some strains of Enterobacter species and Klebsiella species are resistant to Macrodantin. It is not active against most strains of Proteus species, and Serratia species. It has no activity against Pseudomonas species.

Susceptibility Tests—Quantitative methods that require measurement of zone diameters give the most precise estimates of antimicrobial susceptibility. One recommended procedure, (NCCLS, ASM-2)*, uses a disc containing 300 micrograms for testing susceptibility; interpretations correlate zone diameters of this disc test with MIC values for nitrofurantoin.

Reports from the laboratory should be interpreted according to the following criteria:
Susceptible organisms produce zones of 17 mm or greater, indicating that the tested organism is likely to respond to therapy.
Organisms of intermediate susceptibility produce zones of 15 to 16 mm, indicating that the tested organism would be susceptible if high dosage is used.
Resistant organisms produce zones of 14 mm or less, indicating that other therapy should be selected.
A bacterial isolate may be considered susceptible if the MIC value for nitrofurantoin is not more than 25 micrograms per ml. Organisms are considered resistant if the MIC is not less than 100 micrograms per ml.

Indications: Macrodantin is indicated for the treatment of urinary tract infections when due to susceptible strains of E. coli, enterococci, S. aureus (it is not indicated for the treatment of associated renal cortical or perinephric abscesses), and certain susceptible strains of Klebsiella species, Enterobacter species and Proteus species.

Note: Specimens for culture and susceptibility testing should be obtained prior to and during drug administration.

Contraindications: Anuria, oliguria, or significant impairment of renal function (creatinine clearance under 40 ml per minute) are contraindications to therapy with this drug. Treatment of this type of patient carries an increased risk of toxicity because of impaired excretion of the drug. For the same reason, this drug is much less effective under these circumstances.
The drug is contraindicated in pregnant patients at term as well as in infants under one month of age because of the possibility of hemolytic anemia due to immature enzyme systems (glutathione instability).
The drug is also contraindicated in those patients with known hypersensitivity to Macrodantin, Furadantin (nitrofurantoin), and other nitrofurantoin preparations.

Warnings: Acute, subacute and chronic pulmonary reactions have been observed in patients treated with nitrofurantoin products. If these reactions occur, the drug should be withdrawn and appropriate measures should be taken.
An insidious onset of pulmonary reactions (diffuse interstitial pneumonitis or pulmonary fibrosis, or both) in patients on long-term therapy warrants close monitoring of these patients.
There have been isolated reports giving pulmonary reactions as a contributing cause of death. (See Hypersensitivity reactions.)
Cases of hemolytic anemia of the primaquine sensitivity type have been induced by Macrodantin. The hemolysis appears to be linked to a glucose-6-phosphate dehydrogenase deficiency in the red blood cells of the affected patients. This deficiency is found in 10 percent of Negroes and a small percentage of ethnic groups of Mediterranean and Near-Eastern origin. Any sign of hemolysis is an indication to discontinue the drug. Hemolysis ceases when the drug is withdrawn.
Hepatitis, including chronic active hepatitis, occurs rarely. Fatalities have been reported. The onset of chronic active hepatitis may be insidious, and patients receiving long-term therapy should be monitored periodically for changes in liver function. If hepatitis occurs, the drug should be withdrawn immediately and appropriate measures should be taken.

Precautions: Peripheral neuropathy may occur with Macrodantin therapy; this may become severe or irreversible. Fatalities have been reported. Predisposing conditions such as renal impairment (creatinine clearance under 40 ml per minute), anemia, diabetes, electrolyte imbalance, vitamin B deficiency, and debilitating disease may enhance such occurrence.

Usage in Pregnancy: The safety of Macrodantin during pregnancy and lactation has not been established. Use of this drug in women of childbearing potential requires that the anticipated benefit be weighed against the possible risks.

Adverse Reactions: Gastrointestinal reactions: Anorexia, nausea and emesis are the most frequent reactions; abdominal pain and diarrhea occur less frequently. These dose-related toxicity reactions can be minimized by reduction of dosage, especially in the female patient.
Hepatitis, including chronic active hepatitis, has been observed rarely. The mechanism appears to be of an idiosyncratic hypersensitive type.
Hypersensitivity reactions: Pulmonary sensitivity reactions may occur, which can be acute, subacute, or chronic.
Acute reactions are commonly manifested by fever, chills, cough, chest pain, dyspnea, pulmonary infiltration with consolidation or pleural effusion on x-ray, and eosinophilia. The acute reactions usually occur within the first week of treatment and are reversible with cessation of therapy. Resolution may be dramatic.
In subacute reactions, fever and eosinophilia are observed less often. Recovery is somewhat slower, perhaps as long as several months. If the symptoms are not recognized as being drug related and nitrofurantoin is not withdrawn, symptoms may become more severe.
Chronic pulmonary reactions are more likely to occur in patients who have been on continuous nitrofurantoin therapy for six months or longer. The insidious onset of malaise, dyspnea on exertion, cough, and altered pulmonary function are common manifestations. Roentgenographic and histologic findings of diffuse interstitial pneumonitis or fibrosis, or both, are also common manifestations. Fever is rarely prominent. The severity of these chronic pulmonary reactions and the degree of their resolution appear to be related to the duration of therapy after the first clinical signs appear. Pulmonary function may be permanently impaired even after cessation of nitrofurantoin therapy. This risk is greater when pulmonary reactions are not recognized early.
Dermatologic reactions: Exfoliative dermatitis and erythema multiforme (including Stevens-Johnson Syndrome) has been reported rarely. Maculopapular, erythematous, or eczematous eruption, pruritus, urticaria and angioedema.
Other hypersensitivity reactions: Anaphylaxis, asthmatic attack in patients with history of asthma, cholestatic jaundice, hepatitis, drug fever, and arthralgia.
Hematologic reactions: Hemolytic anemia, granulocytopenia, agranulocytosis, leukopenia, thrombocytopenia, eosinophilia, and megaloblastic anemia. Return of the blood picture to normal has followed cessation of therapy. Aplastic anemia has been reported rarely.
Neurological reactions: Peripheral neuropathy, headache, dizziness, nystagmus, and drowsiness.
Miscellaneous reactions: Transient alopecia. As with other antimicrobial agents, superinfections by resistant organisms, e.g., Pseudomonas, may occur. With Macrodantin, however, these are limited to the genitourinary tract because suppression of normal bacterial flora elsewhere in the body does not occur.

Dosage and Administration: Macrodantin should be given with food to improve drug absorption and, in some patients tolerance.
Adults: 50–100 mg four times a day—the lower dosage level is recommended for uncomplicated urinary tract infections.
Children: 5-7 mg/kg of body weight per 24 hours given in four divided doses (contraindicated under one month of age).
Therapy should be continued for at least one week and for at least 3 days after sterility of the urine is obtained. Continued infection indicates the need for reevaluation.
For long-term suppressive therapy in adults, a reduction of dosage to 50–100 mg at bedtime may be adequate. See WARNINGS section regarding risks associated with long-term therapy. For long-term suppressive therapy in children, doses as low as 1 mg/kg per 24 hours, given in a single or in two divided doses, may be adequate.

How Supplied: Macrodantin is available as follows:
100 mg: opaque, yellow capsule imprinted with three black lines encircling the capsule and coded "Macrodantin 100 mg" and "0149 0009".*
NDC 0149-0009-05 bottle of 100
NDC 0149-0009-66 bottle of 500
NDC 0149-0009-67 bottle of 1000
NDC 0149-0009-77 hospital unit-dose strips in box of 100
50 mg: opaque, yellow and white capsule imprinted with two black lines encircling the capsule and coded "Macrodantin 50 mg" and "0149 0008".*
NDC 0149-0008-05 bottle of 100
NDC 0149-0008-66 bottle of 500
NDC 0149-0008-67 bottle of 1000
NDC 0149-0008-77 hospital unit-dose strips in box of 100
25 mg: opaque, white capsule imprinted with one black line encircling the capsule and coded "Macrodantin 25 mg" and "0149 0007".
NDC 0149-0007-05 bottle of 100
*capsule design, registered trademark of Eaton Laboratories, Inc.
Furadantin (nitrofurantoin)/Macrodantin Sensi-Discs for the laboratory determination of bacterial sensitivity are available from BBL, Division of BioQuest. For information on simple nitrofurantoin assays in blood, serum, and urine, write or call the Medical Department. Literature sent to physicians on request.
Address medical inquires to Norwich Eaton Pharmaceuticals, Inc. Medical Department, Norwich, NY 13815.
Manufactured by
Eaton Laboratories, Inc.
Manati, Puerto Rico 00701
Distributed by
Norwich Eaton Pharmaceuticals, Inc.
Norwich, New York 13815
A Procter & Gamble Company
Shown in Product Identification Section, page 422
MACRO-P6

Norwich Eaton—Cont.

TOPICYCLINE® ℞
[top'i-sī-klēn"]
(tetracycline hydrochloride for topical solution)

The following text is based on official labeling in effect August 1, 1984.

Description: TOPICYCLINE is a topical antibiotic preparation containing 2.2 mg of tetracycline hydrochloride per ml as the active ingredient, as well as 4-epitetracycline hydrochloride and sodium bisulfite in an aqueous base of 40% ethanol, citric acid and n-decyl methyl sulfoxide.

Tetracycline is 4-(dimethylamino)-1,4,4a,5,5a, 6, 11, 12a-octahydro-3, 6, 10, 12, 12a-pentahydroxy-6-methyl-1, 11-dioxo-2-naphthacenecarboxamide, the structural formula of which is:

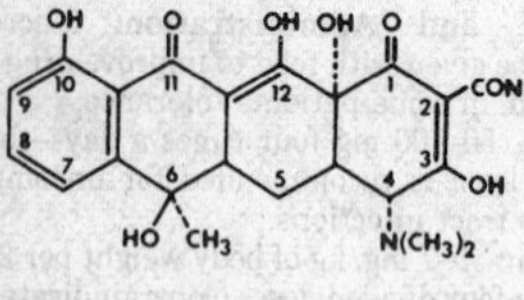

Clinical Pharmacology: TOPICYCLINE delivers tetracycline to the pilosebaceous apparatus and the adjacent tissues. TOPICYCLINE reduces inflammatory acne lesions, but its mode of action is not fully understood.

In clinical studies, use of TOPICYCLINE on the face and neck twice daily delivered to the skin an average dose of 2.9 mg of tetracycline hydrochloride per day. Patients who used the medication twice daily on other acne-involved areas in addition to the face and neck applied an average dose of 4.8 mg of tetracycline hydrochloride per day. TOPICYCLINE has been formulated such that the recrystallization properties of the tetracyclines on the skin greatly reduce or eliminate the yellow color often associated with topical tetracycline.

Indications and Usage: TOPICYCLINE is indicated in the treatment of acne vulgaris.

Contraindications: TOPICYCLINE is contraindicated in persons who have shown hypersensitivity to any of its ingredients or to any of the other tetracyclines.

Precautions: This drug is for external use only and care should be taken to keep it out of the eyes, nose, and mouth.

A two-year dermal study in mice has been performed with TOPICYCLINE and indicates there is no carcinogenic potential with this drug.

Pregnancy Category B. Reproduction studies have been performed in rats and rabbits at doses of up to 246 times the human dose (assuming the human dose to be 1.3 ml/40kg/day) and have revealed no evidence of impaired fertility or harm to the fetus from TOPICYCLINE. There are, however, no adequate and well-controlled studies in pregnant women. Because animal reproduction studies are not always predictive of human response, this drug should be used during pregnancy only if clearly needed.

It is not known whether tetracycline or any other component of TOPICYCLINE administered in this topical form, is excreted in human milk. Because many drugs are excreted in human milk, caution should be exercised when TOPICYCLINE is administered to a nursing woman.

Safety and effectiveness in children below the age of eleven have not been established.

Adverse Reactions: Among the 838 patients treated with TOPICYCLINE under normal usage conditions during clinical evaluation, there was one instance of severe dermatitis requiring systemic steroid therapy.

About one-third of patients are likely to experience a stinging or burning sensation upon application of TOPICYCLINE. The sensation ordinarily lasts no more than a few minutes, and does not occur at every application. There has been no indication that patients experience sufficient discomfort to reduce the frequency of use or to discontinue use of the product.

The kinds of side effects often associated with oral or parenteral administration of tetracyclines (e.g., various gastrointestinal complaints, vaginitis, hematologic abnormalities, manifestations of systemic hypersensitivity reactions, and dental and skeletal disorders) have not been observed with TOPICYCLINE. Because of TOPICYCLINE's topical form of administration, it is highly unlikely that such side effects will occur from its use.

Dosage and Administration: It is recommended that TOPICYCLINE be applied generously twice-daily to the entire affected area (not just to individual lesions) until the skin is thoroughly wet. Instructions to the patients for proper application are provided on the TOPICYCLINE bottle label. Patients may continue their normal use of cosmetics.

Concomitant use with benzoyl peroxide or oral tetracycline has been reported without observed problems.

How Supplied: TOPICYCLINE is supplied in a single carton containing a powder and a liquid which must be combined prior to using. Complete instructions for mixing are provided on the carton. Once combined, the TOPICYCLINE bottle contains 70 ml of medication. This constitutes about an eight-week supply for treating the face and neck, or about a four-week supply for treating the face, neck and additional acne-involved areas. Differences in individual usage habits will result in variation from these averages.

TOPICYCLINE should be kept at controlled room temperature or below.

Caution: Federal law prohibits dispensing without prescription.

NDC 37000-401-03

Made in U.S.A. by Taylor Pharmacal, Decatur, Illinois 62525 for Norwich Eaton Pharmaceuticals, Inc., Norwich, New York 13815, a Procter & Gamble Company.

TOPI-P3

STANDARD VIVONEX®
[vī'vō-nex"]

The following text is based on official labeling in effect August 1, 1984.

NUTRITIONAL INFORMATION AND USE INSTRUCTIONS

Standard Vivonex® is a patented, nutritionally complete elemental diet formulated for the nutritional management of patients with impaired digestion and/or malabsorption.

Composition: Standard Vivonex is a chemically defined diet composed of all essential nutrients in simple, readily absorbable form: free amino acids, predigested carbohydrates, safflower oil, vitamins, minerals, electrolytes and trace elements. One 80-gram packet provides 300 Calories and 0.98 grams of available nitrogen with a caloric density of 1 Calorie per ml when diluted with 255 ml water to a total standard dilution volume of 300 ml: [See table left].

Six 80-g packets of Standard Vivonex supply 5.88 grams of available nitrogen, 2.61 grams fat, 407 grams carbohydrate, and the following vitamins, minerals, electrolytes and amino acid profile: [See table above].

Vitamins, Minerals and Trace Elements	Per 1000 ml (Standard dilution)		Per 6 Packets (480 Grams)		% U.S. RDA Per 6 Packets
Vitamin A	2778	IU	5000	IU	100
Vitamin D₃	222	IU	400	IU	100
Vitamin E	16.7	IU	30	IU	100
Vitamin C	33.3	mg	60	mg	100
Folic Acid	0.22	mg	0.4	mg	100
Thiamine	0.83	mg	1.5	mg	100
Riboflavin	0.94	mg	1.7	mg	100
Niacin	11.1	mg	20	mg	100
Vitamin B₆	1.11	mg	2	mg	100
Vitamin B₁₂	3.33	mcg	6	mcg	100
Biotin	0.17	mg	0.3	mg	100
Pantothenic Acid	5.55	mg	10	mg	100
Vitamin K₁	37.2	mcg	67	mcg	*
Choline	40.9	mg	73.7	mg	*
Calcium	0.55	g	1	g	100
Phosphorus	0.55	g	1	g	100
Iodine	83.3	mcg	150	mcg	100
Iron	10	mg	18	mg	100
Magnesium	222	mg	400	mg	100
Copper	1.11	mg	2	mg	100
Zinc	8.33	mg	15	mg	100
Manganese	1.56	mg	2.81	mg	*
Selenium+	83.3	mcg	150	mcg	*
Molybdenum+	83.3	mcg	150	mcg	*
Chromium+	27.8	mg	50	mcg	*

* No U.S. RDA established
+ Represents amounts of these elements added.

	Amount per 80 g	Amount per 1000 ml (Standard dilution)		Energy Distribution
Total energy (Calories)	300	1000		
Amino acids (free base equivalent)	6.18 g	20.6 g		8.2%
Carbohydrate (dry basis)	67.9 g	226.3 g		90.5%
Fat	0.435 g	1.45		1.3%
Linoleic acid	0.348 g	1.16 g		1.0%

Electrolytes	mEq per 1000 ml (Standard dilution)	Wt per 1000 ml (Standard dilution)
CATIONS		
Sodium	20.4	468 mg
Potassium	30.0	1172 mg
Calcium	27.7	556 mg
Magnesium	18.3	222 mg
Manganese	0.057	1.56 mg
Iron	0.358	10 mg

Copper	0.035	1.11 mg		
Zinc	0.255	8.33 mg		
Selenium+	0.002*	83.3 mcg		
Molybdenum+	0.002**	83.3 mcg		
Chromium+	0.002	27.8 mcg		
ANIONS				
Chloride	20.4	722 mg		
Phosphorous	54.0‡	556 mg		
Acetate	18.7	1106 mg		
Iodide	0.0007	83.3 mcg		

+ Represents amounts of these elements added.
* Calculated as Selenite SeO_3^{-2}
** Calculated as Molybdate MoO_4^{-2}
‡ Calculated as Phosphate PO_4

Amino Acid Profile	% Total Amino Acids
ESSENTIALS	
L-Isoleucine	4.55
L-Leucine	7.20
L-Valine	5.02
L-Lysine	5.41
L-Methionine	4.66
L-Phenylalanine	5.18
L-Threonine	4.55
L-Tryptophan	1.41
Total essential amino acids	37.98
NON-ESSENTIAL	
L-Alanine	4.85
L-Arginine	8.87
L-Aspartic Acid	10.35
L-Glutamine	17.07
Glycine	7.91
L-Histidine	2.21
L-Proline	6.48
L-Serine	3.34
L-Tyrosine	0.94
Total non-essential amino acids	62.02

In the standard solution of 1 Calorie/ml, Standard Vivonex has a pH of approximately 5.5 and an average osmolality of 550 mOsm/kg.

Actions and Uses: Standard Vivonex is a nutritionally complete, elemental diet that is rapidly utilized, since digestion is virtually obviated, and absorption can take place without the aid of peptidases. Standard Vivonex is absorbed within the first 100 cm of functional small intestine. It is essentially a non-residue diet. There is minimal stimulation of biliary, pancreatic, and intestinal secretions, because of its free L-amino acid nitrogen (protein) source, glucose oligosaccharide primary energy source, and low fat content. The low fat content also permits rapid gastric emptying and eliminates gastric residuals, thus minimizing the possibility of aspiration.

The balanced amino acid profile of Standard Vivonex insures optimum utilization and retention of its readily absorbed, elemental nitrogen source.

Standard Vivonex is useful in the dietary management of patients with impaired digestion and absorption which are secondary to a variety of diseases and disorders such as gastrointestinal disease, e.g. inflammatory bowel disease, cancer, intestinal atresia; conditions leading to partial function of the gastrointestinal tract, e.g. pancreatitis, fistula, partial obstruction, short-gut syndrome. Standard Vivonex is also useful in the dietary management of neonates and infants suffering from intractable diarrhea, as an aid in preparing the bowel for diagnostic and surgical procedures, and as a transition diet between parenteral and normal oral feeding. It is synthetically derived and contains no whole foodstuffs and therefore is hypoallergenic and well tolerated by patients with known food sensitivites. Standard Vivonex has been proven useful as an elimination diet for patients undergoing diagnosis of specific food allergens.

One packet diluted with 255 ml (8½ oz.) of water makes a single serving. Six packets of Standard Vivonex mixed thoroughly with 1530 ml of water provide a full day's supply for the average adult with 1800 Calories, 5.88 grams available nitrogen, 2.61 grams fat, and 415 grams carbohydrate. Standard Vivonex is a perishable liquid food when in solution. A full day's supply may be prepared at one time and stored in the refrigerator for up to 24 hours; shake the liquid briefly before serving. Do not leave at room temperature for more than 8 hours.

For oral use, Standard Vivonex must be flavored and served chilled over ice. Vivonex Flavor Packets were specifically developed for this purpose, although other flavoring agents may be used if their contribution to the elemental and nutritional qualities of the diet are kept in mind. Standard Vivonex should be sipped slowly, preferably with a straw, when served as a beverage. Initiate oral feeding with dilute solution, e.g. one packet diluted with 555 ml (18½ oz.), and gradually increase volume and concentration.

Oral feedings of elemental diets are sometimes met by poor patient acceptance because of taste and the lack of the usual appetite cues of normal meals. Varying the available flavors, serving chilled over ice and sipping through a straw, and educating and motivating the patient as to the therapeutic importance of this form of diet, are reportedly effective in improving patient acceptability.

Standard Vivonex may also be administered via feeding tube placed nasogastrically or into an esophagostomy, gastrostomy, or jejunostomy. Because of its homogeneity and low viscosity, as small as a 16 gauge catheter or #5 French feeding tube may be used to optimize patient tolerance. It is suggested that the diet be given at room temperature by continuous drip technique using the Vivonex® Acutrol® Enteral Feeding System, the Vivonex® Delivery System, or a suitable infusion pump. At the 1 Calorie per ml dilution, Standard Vivonex supplies most of the daily fluid requirements. Additional fluids should be given when necessary to maintain adequate urine output.

During the first two days of use, Standard Vivonex may need to be over-diluted for the osmotically sensitive patient, gradually titrating up to full strength. The following administration schedule will facilitate GI adaptation, in most patients, within three days:
[See table above].

If diarrhea is encountered, revert one step to a more dilute solution, maintaining the patient at the last tolerated rate until free of symptoms for 8 hours. Then continue with progressive schedule until desired caloric/nitrogen intake is achieved.

Precautions: DO NOT ADMINISTER STANDARD VIVONEX PARENTERALLY.

Day	Strength	Approx. Rate (ml/hour)	Standard Vivonex (No. of Packets)	+	Total Water (ml)	=	Volume (ml)	Calories (Cal.)	Nitrogen (g)
1	½	75	3	+	1,665	=	1,800	900	3
2	⅔	75	4	+	1,620	=	1,800	1,200	4
3	Full	75	6	+	1,530	=	1,800	1,800	6

For use only under medical supervision.

Nausea, vomiting, abdominal cramps and distention, and diarrhea have been reported. Nausea is usually due to feeding rate, while diarrhea may also be caused by the diet concentration. If encountered, revert one step in the above administration schedule, and then continue slowly with a progressive schedule until desired caloric/nitrogen intake is achieved. Local water conditions have also been implicated in instances of diarrhea. Using deionized or distilled water in diet preparation, until patient tolerance with full strength diet is achieved, has been reported to be effective in this circumstance.

Aspiration is an uncommon complication with Standard Vivonex because of its low fat content. However, in patients suspected at risk, radiologically confirm the anatomic position of the feeding tube, elevate the head of the bed 30° while the patient is receiving diet intragastrically, and control the administration to 150 ml/hour or less, depending upon patient tolerance. Jejunal administration should also be considered.

Additional professional and technical information on all Vivonex products is available through your local Norwich Eaton Pharmaceuticals representative.

Supply Information: Standard Vivonex (NDC 0149-0052-01) is available in cartons of six 80-g sealed packets for individual servings. Each packet provides 300 Calories in a total volume of 300 ml when mixed with 255 ml water.

Vivonex Flavor Packets are available in Vanilla (NDC 0149-0054-02), Strawberry (NDC 0149-0056-02), Orange-Pineapple (NDC 0149-0058-02), and Lemon-Lime (NDC 0149-0057-02) flavors.

The Vivonex Acutrol Enteral Feeding System (NDC 0149-0065-06) is a one-liter, universal, gravity feeding system offering a unique rapid-fill funnel cap, easy-to-read fluid level graduations, macro-drip sight chamber, precise control roller clamp, universal luer adapter, and a built-in burette. The Vivonex Delivery System (NDC 0149-0050-10) is a disposable, gravity-drip tube feeding system with one liter capacity, complete with micro-drop cannula and connecting tubing.

Patent No. 3,697,287   STDVIV-P6

HIGH NITROGEN VIVONEX®
[hī nī-trō-jen vī' vō-nex]
(80-gram packet)
The following text is based on official labeling in effect August 1, 1984.

NUTRITIONAL INFORMATION AND USE INSTRUCTIONS

High Nitrogen Vivonex® is a patented, nutritionally complete, high nitrogen elemental diet formulated for the nutritional management of patients at risk for, or who are suffering from, protein/calorie malnutrition, or for patients with impaired digestion and/or malabsorption.

Composition: High Nitrogen Vivonex is a chemically defined diet composed of all essential nutrients in simple, readily absorbable form: free amino acids, predigested carbohydrates, safflower oil, vitamins, minerals, electrolytes and trace elements. One 80-gram packet provides 300 Calories and 2 grams of available nitrogen with a caloric density of 1 Calorie per ml when diluted with 225 ml water to a total standard dilution volume of 300 ml:
[See table left].

Ten 80-g packets of High Nitrogen Vivonex meet or exceed the quantity of nutrients and energy

	Amount per 80 g	Amount per 1000 ml (Standard dilution)	Energy Distribution
Total energy (Calories)	300	1000	
Amino acids (free base equivalent)	13.3 g	44.3 g	17.7%
Carbohydrate (dry basis)	61.1 g	203.7 g	81.5%
Fat	0.261 g	0.87 g	0.8%
Linoleic acid	0.209 g	0.70 g	0.6%

Continued on next page

Norwich Eaton—Cont.

required daily by the average catabolic adult: 20.0 grams of available nitrogen, 133 grams amino acids, 2.61 grams fat, 611 grams carbohydrate, and the following vitamins, minerals, electrolytes and amino acid profile:
[See table right].

Electrolytes	mEq per 1000 ml (Standard dilution)	Wt per 1000 ml (Standard dilution)
CATIONS		
Sodium	23	529 mg
Potassium	30	1173 mg
Calcium	16.6	333 mg
Magnesium	11	133 mg
Manganese	0 0.34	937 mcg
Iron	0.215	6 mg
Copper	0.021	670 mcg
Zinc	0.153	5 mg
Selenium+	0.001*	50 mcg
Molybdenum+	0.001**	50 mcg
Chromium+	0.001	17 mcg
ANIONS		
Chloride	23.1	815 mg
Phosphorous	31.6‡	333 mg
Acetate	26.0	1533 mg
Iodide	0.0004	50 mcg

+ Represents amounts of these elements added.
* Calculated as Selenite SeO_3^{-2}
** Calculated as Molybdate MoO_4^{-2}
‡ Calculated as Phosphate PO_4

Amino Acid Profile	% Total Amino Acids
ESSENTIAL	
L-Isoleucine	4.15
L-Leucine	6.57
L-Valine	4.58
L-Lysine	4.94
L-Methionine	4.58
L-Phenylalanine	7.10
L-Threonine	4.16
L-Tryptophan	1.28
Total essential amino acids	37.36
NON-ESSENTIAL	
L-Alanine	5.18
L-Arginine	4.07
L-Aspartic Acid	11.06
L-Glutamine	18.22
Glycine	9.84
L-Histidine	2.36
L-Proline	6.92
L-Serine	4.15
L-Tyrosine	0.84
Total non-essential amino acids	62.64

In the standard dilution of 1 Calorie/ml, High Nitrogen Vivonex has a pH of approximately 5.0 and an average osmolality of 810 mOsm/kg.

Actions and Uses: High Nitrogen Vivonex is a nutritionally complete, high nitrogen elemental diet that is rapidly utilized, since digestion is virtually obviated, and absorption can take place without the aid of peptidases. High Nitrogen Vivonex is absorbed within the first 100 cm of functional small intestine. It is essentially a no-residue diet. There is minimal stimulation of biliary, pancreatic, and intestinal secretions, because of its free L-amino acid nitrogen (protein) source, glucose oligosaccharide primary energy source, and low fat content. The low fat content also permits rapid gastric emptying and eliminates gastric residuals, therefore minimizing the possibility of aspiration. High Nitrogen Vivonex, by virtue of its balanced amino acid profile and nitrogen to Calorie ratio of 1:150, spares nitrogen for anabolic purposes and promotes efficient protein synthesis.

High Nitrogen Vivonex is useful in the dietary management of patients with impaired digestion and absorption which are secondary to a variety of diseases and disorders such as gastrointestinal disease, e.g. inflammatory bowel disease, cancer, intestinal atresia; conditions leading to partial function of the gastrointestinal tract, e.g. pancreatitis, fistula, partial obstruction, short-gut syndrome; conditions causing increased metabolic needs, e.g. head and neck cancer, multiple trauma, severe burns; and in the nutritional management of malnourished and cachectic patients. High Nitrogen Vivonex is also useful in the dietary management of neonates and infants suffering from intractable diarrhea, as an aid in preparing the bowel for diagnostic and surgical procedures, and as a transition diet between parenteral and normal oral feeding. High Nitrogen Vivonex has also been shown to be useful in obtaining positive protein balance and an earlier return to normal nutrition following major abdominal surgery by its administration during the immediate postoperative period. It is synthetically derived and contains no whole foodstuffs and therefore is hypoallergenic and well tolerated by patients with known food sensitivities.

One packet diluted with 255 ml (8½ oz.) of water makes a single serving. Ten packets of High Nitrogen Vivonex mixed thoroughly with 2550 ml of water provide the quantity of nutrients and energy required daily by the average catabolic adult. High Nitrogen Vivonex is a perishable liquid food when in solution. A full day's supply may be prepared at one time and stored in the refrigerator for up to 24 hours; shake the liquid briefly before serving. Do not leave at room temperature for more than 8 hours.

Oral Administration: For oral use, High Nitrogen Vivonex must be flavored and served chilled over ice. Vivonex Flavor Packets were specifically developed for this purpose, although other flavoring agents may be used if their contribution to the elemental and nutritional qualities of the diet are kept in mind. High Nitrogen Vivonex should be sipped slowly, preferably with a straw, when served as a beverage. Initiate oral feeding with dilute solution, e.g. one packet diluted with 555 ml (18½ oz.), and gradually increase volume and concentration.

Oral feedings of elemental diets are sometimes met by poor patient acceptance because of taste and the lack of the usual appetite cues of normal meals. Varying the available flavors, serving chilled over ice and sipping through a straw, and educating and motivating the patient as to the therapeutic importance of this form of diet, are reportedly effective in improving patient acceptability.

Feeding Tube Administration: High Nitrogen Vivonex may also be administered via feeding tube placed nasogastrically, or into an esophagostomy, gastrostomy, or jejunostomy. Because of its homogeneity and low viscosity, as small as a 16 gauge catheter or #5 French feeding tube may be used to optimize patient tolerance. It is suggested that the

Vitamins, Minerals and Trace Elements	Per 1000 ml (Standard dilution)	Per 10 Packets 800 Grams	% U.S. RDA Per 10 Packets
Vitamin A	1667 IU	5000 IU	100
Vitamin D_3	133 IU	400 IU	100
Vitamin E	10 IU	30 IU	100
Vitamin C	20 mg	60 mg	100
Folic Acid	0.13 mg	0.4 mg	100
Thiamine	0.5 mg	1.5 mg	100
Riboflavin	0.57 mg	1.7 mg	100
Niacin	6.7 mg	20 mg	100
Vitamin B_6	0.67 mg	2 mg	100
Vitamin B_{12}	2 mcg	6 mcg	100
Biotin	0.1 mg	0.3 mg	100
Pantothenic Acid	3.3 mg	10 mg	100
Vitamin K_1	22.3 mcg	67 mcg	*
Choline	24.6 mg	73.7 mg	*
Calcium	0.33 g	1 g	100
Phosphorus	0.33 g	1 g	100
Iodine	50 mcg	150 mcg	100
Iron	6 mg	18 mg	100
Magnesium	133 mg	400 mg	100
Copper	0.67 mg	2 mg	100
Zinc	5 mg	15 mg	100
Manganese	0.94 mg	2.81 mg	*
Selenium†	50 mcg	150 mcg	*
Molybdenum†	50 mcg	150 mcg	*
Chromium†	17 mcg	50 mcg	*

* No U.S. RDA established
† Represents amounts of these elements added.

diet be given at room temperature by continuous drip technique, using the Vivonex® Acutrol® Enteral Feeding System, The Vivonex® Delivery System, or a suitable infusion pump. At the 1 Calorie per ml dilution, High Nitrogen Vivonex supplies most of the daily fluid requirements. Additional fluids should be given when necessary to maintain adequate urine output.

During the first few days of use, High Nitrogen Vivonex should be overdiluted, gradually titrating up to full strength. The following administration schedules are offered as guidelines and will facilitate adaptation in most patients:
[See table on next page].

In patients with severely compromised GI function, several days may be required to allow for adaptation to full strength diet. If diarrhea is encountered, revert one step to a more dilute solution, maintaining the patient at the last tolerated rate until free of symptoms for eight hours. Then continue with progressive schedule until desired caloric/nitrogen intake is achieved.

Precautions: DO NOT ADMINISTER HIGH NITROGEN VIVONEX PARENTERALLY.

For use only under medical supervision.

Nausea, vomiting, abdominal cramps and distention, and diarrhea have been reported. Nausea is usually due to feeding rate, while diarrhea may also be caused by the diet concentration. If encountered, revert one step in the administration schedule, and then continue slowly with a progressive schedule until desired caloric/nitrogen intake is achieved. Local water conditions have also been implicated in instances of diarrhea. Using deionized or distilled water in diet preparation, until patient tolerance with full strength diet is achieved, has been reported effective in this circumstance.

Aspiration is an uncommon complication with High Nitrogen Vivonex because of its low fat content. However, in patients suspected at risk, radiologically confirm the anatomic position of the feeding tube, elevate the head of the bed 30° while the patient is receiving diet intragastrically, and control the administration to 150 ml/hour or less, depending upon patient tolerance. Jejunal administration should also be considered.

Additional professional and technical information on all Vivonex products is available through your local Norwich Eaton Pharmaceuticals representative.

Supply Information: High Nitrogen Vivonex (NDC 0149-0051-01) is supplied in cartons of ten 80-g sealed packets, each providing 300 Calories in a total volume of 300 ml when mixed with 255 ml water. Vivonex Flavor Packets are available in Vanilla (NDC 0149-0054-02), Strawberry (NDC

0149-0056-02), Orange-Pineapple (NDC 0149-0058-02), and Lemon-Lime (NDC 0149-0057-02) flavors. The Vivonex Acutrol Enteral Feeding System (NDC 0149-0065-06) is a one-liter, universal, gravity feeding system offering a unique rapid-fill funnel cap, easy-to-read fluid level graduations, macro-drip sight chamber, precise control roller clamp, universal luer adapter, and a built-in burette. The Vivonex Delivery System is a disposable, gravity-drip tube feeding system with one liter capacity, complete with micro-drop cannula and connecting tubing.
Patent No. 3,697,287   HNVIV-P6

VIVONEX®
[vī'vō-nex"]
FLAVOR PACKETS
NONNUTRITIVE
Exclusively for use with High Nitrogen Vivonex or Standard Vivonex.

The following text is based on official labeling in effect August 1, 1984.
Mixing Instructions: For normal dilution, place 8½ ounces (255 ml) of water in a blender. Add contents of one 80-gram packet of **High Nitrogen Vivonex** or **Standard Vivonex** and one flavor packet. Blend at high speed until in solution. Flavor packets are readily dispersible and may also be added by stirring into the prepared unflavored diet solution. Serve well chilled.
See package insert enclosed in diet package for complete nutritional information and use instructions.
Storage: Store Vivonex Flavor Packets away from excessive heat. In normal dilution, **Vivonex** diets are perishable liquid foods, and refrigeration is necessary.
Nutritional Information: In addition to the nutritional values of **Vivonex T.E.N., High Nitrogen Vivonex,** and **Standard Vivonex,** each flavor packet contains the following:

Artificial Lemon-Lime Flavor
Calories 6
Protein .... 0 gram
Carbohydrate .... 0.77 gram
Fat .... 0 gram
Saccharin .... 20 mg
Citric Acid .... 1.2 gram
(providing 2.5 Cals/gm)
Osmolality: One flavor packet in 300 ml full-strength diet increases the osmolality by approximately 45 mOsm/kg, giving the following values: Vivonex T.E.N.: approximately 675 mOsm/kg. High Nitrogen Vivonex: approximately 855 mOsm/kg. Standard Vivonex: approximately 595 mOsm/kg.

Artificial Orange-Pineapple Flavor
Calories 6
Protein .... 0 gram
Carbohydrate .... 0.93 gram
Fat .... 0 gram
Saccharin .... 20 mg
Citric Acid .... 1.0 gram
(providing 2.5 Cals/gm)
Osmolality: One flavor packet in 300 ml full-strength diet increases the osmolality by approximately 45 mOsm/kg, giving the following values: Vivonex T.E.N.: approximately 675 mOsm/kg. High Nitrogen Vivonex: approximately 855 mOsm/kg. Standard Vivonex: approximately 595 mOsm/kg.

Artificial Strawberry Flavor
Calories 8
Protein .... 0 gram
Carbohydrate .... 1.71 gram

Gastric Administration Schedule

Day	Strength	Approx. Rate (ml/hour)	High Nitrogen Vivonex (No. of Packets) +	Water (ml) =	Total Volume (ml)	Calories (Cal.)	Nitrogen (g)
1	½	50	2 +	1,110 =	1,200	600	4
2	½	100	4 +	2,220 =	2,400	1,200	8
3	¾	100	6 +	2,130 =	2,400	1,800	12
4	Full	100	8 +	2,040 =	2,400	2,400	16
5	Full	125	10 +	2,550 =	3,000	3,000	20

Intestinal Administration Schedule

Day	Strength	Approx. Rate (ml/hour)	High Nitrogen Vivonex (No. of Packets) +	Water (ml) =	Total Volume (ml)	Calories (Cal.)	Nitrogen (g)
1	¼	50	1 +	1,155 =	1,200	300	2
2	¼	100	2 +	2,310 =	2,400	600	4
3	½	100	4 +	2,220 =	2,400	1,200	8
4	¾	100	6 +	2,130 =	2,400	1,800	12
5	Full	100	8 +	2,040 =	2,400	2,400	16
6	Full	125	10 +	2,550 =	3,000	3,000	20

Fat .... 0 gram
Saccharin .... 20 mg
Citric Acid .... 0.3 gram
(providing 2.5 Cals/gm)
Osmolality: One flavor packet in 300 ml full-strength diet increases the osmolality by approximately 45 mOsm/kg, giving the following values: Vivonex T.E.N.: approximately 675 mOsm/kg. High Nitrogen Vivonex: approximately 855 mOsm/kg. Standard Vivonex: approximately 595 mOsm/kg.

Artificial Vanilla Flavor
Calories 9
Protein .... 0 gram
Carbohydrate .... 2.2 gram
Fat .... 0 gram
Saccharin .... 20 mg
Osmolality: One flavor packet in 300 ml full-strength diet increases the osmolality by approximately 45 mOsm/kg, giving the following values: Vivonex T.E.N.: approximately 675 mOsm/kg. High Nitrogen Vivonex: approximately 855 mOsm/kg. Standard Vivonex: approximately 595 mOsm/kg.
How Supplied: SIXTY 0.088 OZ. (2.5 GRAM) PACKETS—NET WT. 5.28 OZ. (150.0 GRAMS).
VIVFLAV-C2,3,3,4

VIVONEX® ACUTROL® ℞
[vī'vō-nex" ak'ū-trawl]
Enteral Feeding System

VIVONEX® Delivery System
[vī'vō-nex"]
Tube Feeding System

VIVONEX® JEJUNOSTOMY KIT
[vī'vō-nex" jā-jū-nos'tō-me]
Needle catheter jejunostomy kit

VIVONEX® MOSS TUBE
[vī'vō-nex"]
Naso-esophago-gastric decompression tube with duodenal feeding tube.

	Amount per 80.4 g	Amount per 1000 ml (standard dilution)	Energy Distribution
Total energy (Calories)	300	1000	
Amino acids (free base equivalent)	11.46 g	38.20 g	15.3%
Carbohydrate (dry basis)	61.67 g	205.57 g	82.2%
Fat	0.83 g	2.77 g	2.5%
Linoleic acid	0.65 g	2.17 g	2.0%

VIVONEX® T.E.N.
[vī'vō-nex]
Elemental Diet For TOTAL ENTERAL NUTRITION

The following text is based on official labeling in effect August 1, 1984.
Vivonex® T.E.N. is a high nitrogen, elemental diet for total enteral nutrition. Its high essential-to-non-essential amino acid ration (52:48), enhanced branched-chain amino acid content (33% of total amino acids), and optimal quantity of protein-sparing carbohydrate in a 175:1 Calorie to nitrogen ration, make it especially useful in stressed, catabolic patients. Vivonex T.E.N. will further benefit those patients requiring a low residue feeding that permits maximal absorption with minimal digestion. Vivonex T.E.N. is an enteral equivalent to T.P.N. (total parenteral nutrition).
Indications: Vivonex T.E.N. is recommended in the dietary management of the following conditions:
- Stress
  - multiple trauma
  - burns
  - immediate postoperative malnutrition
  - sepsis
- Impaired digestion and absorption
  - inflammatory bowel disease
  - cancer
  - intestinal atresia
  - pancreatitis
  - fistula
  - partial obstruction
  - short-gut syndrome
- Malnutrition and cachexia
- Bowel preparation prior to diagnostic and surgical procedures
- Transition diet between parenteral and normal oral feeding
- Food sensitivities

Composition: Vivonex T.E.N. is a chemically defined diet composed of all essential nutrients in simple, readily absorbable form: free amino acids, predigested carbohydrates, safflower oil, vitamins, minerals, electrolytes, and trace elements. One 80.4-gram packet provides 300 Calories and 1.71 grams of available nitrogen with a caloric density of 1 Calorie per ml when diluted with 250 ml water to a total standard dilution volume of 300 ml: [See table left].
Ten 80.4-gram packets of Vivonex T.E.N. meet or exceed the quantity of nutrients and energy required by the average catabolic adult: 17.1 grams of available nitrogen, 115 grams amino acids, 8.33 grams fat, 617 grams carbohydrate, and the follow-

Continued on next page

Norwich Eaton—Cont.

ing vitamins, minerals, electrolytes, and amino acid profile:
[See table below].

Electrolytes	mEq per 1000 ml (standard dilution)	Wt. Per 1000 ml (standard dilution)
Cations		
Sodium	20	460 mg
Potassium	20	782 mg
Calcium	25	500 mg
Magnesium	16.5	200 mg
Manganese	0.034	937 mcg
Iron	0.322	9 mg
Copper	0.032	1 mg
Zinc	0.306	10 mg
Selenium†	0.001*	50 mcg
Molybdenum†	0.001**	50 mcg
Chromium†	0.001	17 mcg
Anions		
Chloride	23.1	819 mg
Phosphorus	48.5‡	500 mg
Acetate	31.0	1830 mg
Iodide	0.0006	75 mcg

† Represents amounts of these elements added
* Calculated as Selenite, SeO_3^{-2}
** Calculated as Molybdate, MoO_4^{-2}
‡ Calculated as Phosphate, PO_4^{-3}

Amino Acid Profile	% Total Amino Acids
Essential	
L-Isoleucine	8.27
L-Leucine	16.56
L-Valine	8.27
L-Lysine	5.10
L-Methionine	3.66
L-Phenylalanine	5.16
L-Threonine	4.00
L-Tryptophan	1.28
Total essential amino acids	52.30
Non-essential	
L-Alanine	5.18
L-Arginine	7.64
L-Aspartic Acid	7.01
L-Glutamine	12.85
Glycine	4.01
L-Histidine	2.36
L-Proline	4.88
L-Serine	2.93
L-Tryosine	0.84
Total non-essential amino acids	47.70

Vitamins, Minerals and Trace Elements	Per 1000 ml (standard dilution)	Per 10 Packets (804 Grams)	% U.S. RDA Per 10 Packets
Vitamin A	2500 IU	7500 IU	150
Vitamin D_3	200 IU	600 IU	150
Vitamin E	15 IU	45 IU	150
Vitamin C	60 mg	180 mg	300
Folic Acid	0.4 mg	1.2 mg	300
Thiamine	1.5 mg	4.5 mg	300
Riboflavin	1.7 mg	5.1 mg	300
Niacin	20 mg	60 mg	300
Vitamin B_6	2 mg	6 mg	300
Vitamin B_{12}	6 mcg	18 mcg	300
Biotin	0.3 mg	0.9 mg	300
Pantothenic Acid	10 mg	30 mg	300
Vitamin K_1	22.3 mcg	67 mcg	*
Choline	73.7 mg	221 mg	*
Calcium	0.5 g	1.5 g	150
Phosphorus	0.5 g	1.5 g	150
Iodine	75 mcg	225 mcg	150
Iron	9 mg	27 mg	150
Magnesium	200 mg	600 mg	150
Copper	1 mg	3 mg	150
Zinc	10 mg	30 mg	200
Manganese	0.94 mg	2.81 mg	*
Selenium†	50 mcg	150 mcg	*
Molybdenum†	50 mcg	150 mcg	*
Chromium†	16.67 mcg	50 mcg	*

* No U.S. RDA established.
† Represents amounts of these elements added.

Gastric Administration Schedule

Day	Strength	Approx. Rate (ml/hour)	Vivonex T.E.N. (no. of packets)	+	Water (ml)	=	Total Volume (ml)	Calories (Cal.)	Nitrogen (g)
1	½	50	2	+	1100	=	1200	600	3.42
2	Full	50	4	+	1000	=	1200	1200	6.84
3	Full	100	8	+	2000	=	2400	2400	13.68
4	Full	125	10	+	2500	=	3000	3000	17.10

Intestinal Administration Schedule

Day	Strength	Approx. Rate (ml/hour)	Vivonex T.E.N. (no. of packets)	+	Water (ml)	=	Total Volume (ml)	Calories (Cal.)	Nitrogen (g)
1	½	50	2	+	1100	=	1200	600	3.42
2	½	100	4	+	2200	=	2400	1200	6.84
3	¾	100	6	+	2100	=	2400	1800	10.26
4	Full	100	8	+	2000	=	2400	2400	13.68
5	Full	125	10	+	2500	=	3000	3000	17.10

Branched-chain amino acids
(Isoleucine, Leucine, Valine)   33.10
Aromatic amino acids   6.00
(Phenylalanine, Tyrosine)
Branched-chain: Aromatic amino acid   7.4 : 1 molar ratio

In the standard dilution of 1 Calorie/ml, Vivonex T.E.N. has a pH of approximately 5.0 and an average osmolality of 630 mOsm/kg.

Mixing and Storage: Each packet should be blended with 250 ml (8-1/3 oz.) water to make a 300 ml serving of standard dilution diet.
1. Measure the total water needed into the blender.
2. Start blender at slow speed.
3. Slowly add contents of the Vivonex T.E.N. packet(s).
4. Blend at high speed until in solution, 30-60 seconds. Add flavoring, e.g., Vivonex® Flavor Packet(s), for oral use.
5. Pour formula into container and label.

Vivonex T.E.N. is a perishable liquid food when in solution. A full day's supply may be prepared at one time and stored in the refrigerator for up to 48 hours; shake the liquid briefly before serving. Do not leave at room temperature for more than 8 hours.

Feeding Tube Administration: VIVONEX T.E.N. may be administered via a nasogastric, nasointestinal, esophagostomy, gastrostomy, or jejunostomy feeding tube. Because of its homogeneity and low viscosity, small bore feeding tubes (16 gauge catheter or #5 French tube) may be used to optimize patient tolerance. The diet should be given at room temperature by continuous drip technique, using the Vivonex® Acutrol® Enteral Feeding System, the Vivonex® Delivery System, or a suitable infusion pump. At the 1 Calorie per ml dilution, Vivonex T.E.N. supplies most of the daily fluid requirements. Additional fluids should be given when necessary to maintain hydration and adequate urine output.

During the first few days of use, Vivonex T.E.N. should be diluted. Concentration should be gradually increased up to full strength (1 Calorie/ml). The following administration schedules are offered as guidelines and will facilitate adaptation in most patients:
[See table above].

If diarrhea is encountered, revert one step to a more dilute solution, maintaining the patient at the last tolerated rate until free of symptoms for eight hours. Then continue with progressive schedule until desired caloric/nitrogen intake is achieved.

Oral Administration: For oral use, Vivonex T.E.N. should be flavored and served chilled over ice. Vivonex Flavor Packets were specifically developed for this purpose, although other flavoring agents may be used if their contribution to the elemental and nutritional qualities of the diet are kept in mind. Vivonex T.E.N. should be sipped slowly, preferably through a straw, when served as a beverage. Initiate oral feeding with dilute solution, e.g., one packet diluted with 550 ml (18-1/3 oz.), and gradually increase volume and concentration.

Oral feedings of elemental diets are sometimes met with poor patient acceptance because of taste and the lack of the usual appetite cues of normal meals. Varying the available flavors, serving chilled over ice and sipping through a straw, and educating and motivating the patient as to the therapeutic importance of this form of diet, are reportedly effective in improving patient acceptability.

Precautions: DO NOT ADMINISTER Vivonex T.E.N. PARENTERALLY. For use only under medical supervision. Nausea, vomiting, abdominal cramps, distention, and diarrhea are possible. Nausea and diarrhea are usually due to feeding rate or diet concentration. If encountered, revert one step in the administration schedule, and then continue slowly with a progressive schedule until desired caloric/nitrogen intake is achieved. Local water conditions may be implicated in instances of diarrhea. Preparing diet with deionized or distilled water may be effective in this circumstance. Aspiration is an uncommon complication with Vivonex T.E.N. because of its low fat content. However, radiologically confirm the anatomic position of the feeding tube, elevate the head of the bed 30° while the patient is receiving diet intragastrically, and control the administration to 150 ml/hour or less, depending upon patient tolerance. Jejunal administration should also be considered. Diabetics and patients with renal insufficiency receiving this diet should be closely monitored. Use in children may require adjusting the daily

consumption to meet the Recommended Daily Allowance for the age group involved.
Supply Information: Vivonex T.E.N. (NDC 0149-0067-01) is available in cartons of ten 80.4-gram sealed packets, each providing 300 Calories. Vivonex Flavor Packets are available in Vanilla (NDC 0149-0054-02), Strawberry (NDC 0149-0056-02), Orange-Pineapple (NDC 0149-0058-02), and Lemon-Lime (NDC 0149-0057-02) flavors.
The Vivonex Acutrol Enteral Feeding System (NDC 0149-0065-06) is a one-liter, universal, gravity feeding system offering a unique rapid-fill funnel cap, easy-to-read fluid level graduations, macro-drip sight chamber, precise control roller clamp, universal luer adapter, and a built-in burette. The Vivonex Delivery System (NDC 0149-0050-10) is a disposable, gravity-drip tube feeding system with one liter capacity, complete with micro-drop cannula and connecting tubing.
Additional professional and technical information on all Vivonex products is available through local Norwich Eaton Pharmaceuticals representatives.

VIVTEN-P2

EDUCATIONAL MATERIAL

Norwich Eaton offers a wide range of Professional Services to the medical profession free of charge. Please write to the Director of Professional Services, Norwich Eaton Pharmaceuticals, Inc., Norwich, NY 13815, for further information.
- *The Norwich Eaton Audio-Visual Library*—over 225 film, slide and videotape programs are available on free-loan (Directory available upon request)
- *Professional Speaker Bureaus* (Urology, Nutrition, Respiratory Diseases, and Clinical Disorders of Bone)
- *Calendars of CME Events* (Ob/Gyn, Urology, Allergy)
- *Patient Education Brochures and Films* (Urology)
- *ACOG Physician Placement Service*
- *AUA Physician Placement Service*

NTRON International Sales Co.
3833 REDWOOD HWY.
P.O. BOX 7000
SAN RAFAEL, CA 94912

NTRON TTS-2500 ℞
[ĕn′trŏn]
Transcutaneous Electrical Nerve Stimulator

Description: The NTRON TTS-2500 TENS is a portable, battery-powered electrical generator. It produces small amounts of pulsatile alternating current which is transported through the patient's skin by non-invasive surface electrodes. The effects are comfortable for most patients.
Actions: The physiological means by which TENS produces analgesia is as yet incompletely understood. Current theory suggests that electrical stimulation of the large, faster-conducting nonnociceptive A-beta nerve fibers may block impulses from the smaller, slower-conducting nociceptive A-delta and C fibers at the substantia gelatinosa. It is also suggested that TENS may increase the body's production of endogenous opiates.
Indications: TENS may be indicated for the treatment of chronic intractable pain as a conservative alternative to pharmaceutical or surgical analgesic treatments. It has been shown to be effective in reducing or eliminating pain associated with a wide variety of syndromes, including low back pain, sciatica, causalgia, phantom limb, osteoarthritis, post herpetic neuralgias, bursitis, and tension and migraine headaches.
TENS therapy may also be effective in relieving acute pain due to trauma, and to relieve incisional pain following surgery, while reducing ileus and atelectasis.
Contraindications: There are no known short or long term complications. The possibility that TENS may effect the nervous system in some presently unknown way should not be overlooked.
Warnings: The stimulation of the NTRON TTS-2500 TENS is not enough to effect the function of the heart in normal individuals. Adequate precautions should be taken with suspected heart patients. Electrical stimulation may interfere with the proper functioning of demand-type pacemakers. Care should be exercised in avoiding stimulation in paths that include the pacemaker and pacemaker cables. Electrodes should not be placed directly over the eye, in the mouth, or over the carotid sinus. Power should be increased slowly so as not to startle the patient or cause a secondary accident. The conductive gel under the electrodes should not be allowed to dry, as this may result in skin burn or irritation.
Precautions: Though no adverse effects have been reported, the safety of TENS during pregnancy, labor and delivery has not been established. As with all analgesics, TENS should be used only to relieve pain and not replace proper medical procedure for a correctable condition.
Adverse Reactions: Cases of skin irritation under the electrodes may be avoided by periodic relocation of the electrodes after extended wear or by selection of a compatible electrode gel, adhesive and/or use of a skin barrier preparation.
Dosage and Administration: The efficacy of TENS therapy is quite patient-specific. The most effective electrode placements, number of electrodes, device settings, and length of treatment time for optimum results may vary from patient to patient. One or more clinical training sessions will be necessary to establish the most effective regimen and to train the patient in the proper use of the instrument. After clinical training, unsupervised self-administration by the patient can be considered. Treatment time should be determined by patient comfort and clinical effect. Treatments may vary from a few minutes up to 24 hours per day. Once a trial period of self-administered patient use has been evaluated, TENS may be considered for long term use.
Overdosage: Within the strictures of the aforementioned warnings and precautions, treatment with the TTS-2500 TENS has been used indefinitely with no reported ill effects. It is a non-addictive and completely reversible form of analgesia with no known combinatory disadvantages.
How Supplied: NTRON TTS-2500 Transcutaneous Electrical Nerve Stimulator. The device is housed in an attractive 3 × 2 × 1″ grey plastic case. Electrodes and cables, 9 Volt alkaline battery, electrode gel, adhesives, and Patient Instruction Booklet are supplied. Accessories are available for special requirements. Clinical training materials are available.
Caution: Federal law prohibits dispensing without prescription.

IDENTIFICATION PROBLEM?
Consult PDR's
Product Identification Section
where you'll find over 1200
products pictured actual size
and in full color.

O'Neal, Jones & Feldman Pharmaceuticals
2510 METRO BLVD.
MARYLAND HEIGHTS MO 63043

A.C.T.H. "40" INJECTABLE ℞
Each ml. contains:
Adrenocorticotropic hormone ....40 unit
How Supplied: 5 ml. multiple dose vials.

A.C.T.H. "80" INJECTABLE ℞
Each ml. contains:
Adrenocorticotropic hormone ....80 unit
How Supplied: 5 ml. multiple dose vials.

ANTILIRIUM ℞
(physostigmine salicylate)

Description: ANTILIRIUM (Physostigmine Salicylate) is a derivative of the Calabar bean, and its active moiety, physostigmine, is also known as eserine.
It is soluble in water and a 0.5% aqueous solution has a pH of 5.8.
ANTILIRIUM Injection is available in 2 ml ampuls, each ml containing 1 mg of Physostigmine Salicylate in a vehicle composed of sodium bisulfite 0.1%, benzyl alcohol 2.0% as a preservative in water for injection.
Clinical Pharmacology: ANTILIRIUM is a reversible anticholinesterase which effectively increases the concentration of acetylcholine at the sites of cholinergic transmission. The action of acetylcholine is normally very transient because of its hydrolysis by the enzyme, acetylcholinesterase. ANTILIRIUM inhibits the destructive action of acetylcholinesterase and thereby prolongs and exaggerates the effect of the acetylcholine.
ANTILIRIUM contains a tertiary amine and easily penetrates the blood brain barrier, while an anticholinesterase, such as neostigmine, which has a quaternary ammonium ion is not capable of crossing the barrier. ANTILIRIUM can reverse both central and peripheral anticholinergia. The anticholinergic syndrome has both central and peripheral signs and symptoms. Central toxic effects include anxiety, delirium, disorientation, hallucinations, hyper-activity and seizures. Severe poisoning may produce coma, medullary paralysis and death. Peripheral toxicity is characterized by tachycardia, hyperpyrexia, mydriasis, vasodilatation, urinary retention, diminution of gastrointestinal motility, decrease of secretion in salivary and sweat glands, and loss of secretions in the pharynx, bronchi, and nasal passages.
Dramatic reversal of the effects of anticholinergic symptoms can be expected in minutes after the intravenous administration of ANTILIRIUM, if the diagnosis is correct and the patient has not suffered anoxia or other insult. The duration of action of ANTILIRIUM is relatively short, approx. 45 to 60 minutes.
Numerous drugs and some plants produce the anticholinergic syndrome either directly or as a side effect; this undesirable or potentially dangerous phenomenon may be brought about by either therapeutic doses or overdoses of the drugs. Such drugs include among others, atropine, other derivatives of the belladonna alkaloids, tricyclic antidepressants, phenothiazines, and antihistamines.
Indications and Usages: To reverse the effect upon the central nervous system, caused by clinical or toxic dosages of drugs capable of producing the anticholinergic syndrome.
Contraindications: ANTILIRIUM should not be used in the presence of asthma, gangrene, diabetes, cardiovascular disease, mechanical obstruction of the intestine or urogenital tract or any vagotonic state, and in patients receiving choline esters or depolarizing neuromuscular blocking agents (decamethonium succinylcholine).

Continued on next page

O'Neal, Jones & Feldman—Cont.

For post-anesthesia, the concomitant use of atropine with the physostigmine salicylate is not recommended, since the atropine antagonizes the action of physostigmine.

Warnings: If excessive symptoms of salivation, emesis, urination and defecation occur, the use of ANTILIRIUM should be terminated. If excessive sweating or nausea occur, the dosage should be reduced.

Intravenous administration should be a slow, controlled rate, no more than 1 mg per minute (see dosage). Rapid administration can cause bradycardia, hypersalivation leading to respiratory difficulties and possible convulsions.

An overdosage of ANTILIRIUM can cause a cholinergic crisis.

Precautions: Because of the possibility of hypersensitivity in an occasional patient, atropine sulfate injection should always be at hand since it is an antagonist and antidote for physostigmine.

Usage in Pregnancy: Safe use in pregnancy and lactation has not been established; therefore, use in pregnant women, nursing mothers or women who may become pregnant requires that possible benefits be weighed against possible hazards to mother and child.

Adverse Reactions: Nausea, vomiting and salivation; can be offset by reducing dosage. Bradycardia and convulsions, if intravenous administration is too rapid. See DOSAGE AND ADMINISTRATION.

Overdosage: Can cause a cholinergic crisis. Appropriate antidote is atropine sulfate.

Dosage and Administration: Post Anesthesia Care: 0.5 to 1.0 mg intramuscularly or intravenously. INTRAVENOUS ADMINISTRATION SHOULD BE AT A SLOW CONTROLLED RATE OF NO MORE THAN 1 MG PER MINUTE. Dosage may be repeated at intervals of 10 to 30 minutes if desired patient response is not obtained.

Overdosages of Drugs That Cause Anticholinergia: 2.0 mg intramuscularly or INTRAVENOUSLY AT SLOW CONTROLLED RATE (SEE ABOVE). Dosage may be repeated if life threatening signs, such as arrhythmia, convulsions or coma occurs.

Pediatric Dosage: Recommended dosage is .02 mg/kg, intramuscularly or by slow intravenous injection, no more than 0.5 mg per minute. If the toxic effects persist, and there is no sign of cholinergic effects, the dosage may be repeated at 5 to 10 minute intervals until a therapeutic effect is obtained or a maximum dose of 2 mg is attained. IN ALL CASES OF POISONING, THE USUAL SUPPORTIVE MEASURES SHOULD BE UNDERTAKEN.

How Supplied: Ampuls, 2 ml packed 12 per box, 1 mg per ml.

Caution: Federal law prohibits dispensing without prescription.

BANALG® HOSPITAL STRENGTH ARTHRITIC PAIN RELIEVER
BANALG® LINIMENT

(See PDR For Nonprescription Drugs)

BANCAP CAPSULES   ℞
BANCAP c̄ CODEINE CAPSULES   ℞

BANCAP CAPSULES
Each capsule contains:
Acetaminophen ....325 mg
Butalbital ....50 mg
(Warning: May be habit forming)

BANCAP c̄ CODEINE CAPSULES
Each capsule contains:
Acetaminophen ....325 mg
Butalbital ....50 mg
(Warning: May be habit forming)
Codeine phosphate ....30 mg
(Warning: May be habit forming)

How Supplied: Bottles of 100 and 500.

BANCAP HC CAPSULES   ℞

Description:
Each hard gelatin capsule contains:
Hydrocodone Bitartrate ....5 mg
(WARNING: May be habit forming)
Acetaminophen ....500 mg

Acetaminophen is a nonopiate, non-salicylate analgesic and antipyretic which occurs as a white, odorless crystalline powder possessing a slightly bitter taste. Hydrocodone bitartrate is an opioid analgesic and antitussive and occurs as fine, white crystals or as a crystalline powder. It is affected by light.

Clinical Pharmacology: Hydrocodone is a semisynthetic narcotic analgesic and antitussive with multiple actions qualitatively similar to those of codeine. Most of these involve the central nervous system and smooth muscle. The precise mechanism of action of hydrocodone and other opiates is not known, although it is believed to relate to the existence of opiate receptors in the central nervous system. In addition to analgesia, narcotics may produce drowsiness, changes in mood and mental clouding.

Radioimmunoassay techniques have recently been developed for the analysis of hydrocodone in human plasma. After a 10 mg oral dose of hydrocodone bitartrate, a mean peak serum drug level of 23.6 ng/ml and an elimination half-life of 3.8 hours were found.

The analgesic action of acetaminophen involves peripheral and central influences, but the specific mechanism is as yet undetermined. Antipyretic activity is mediated through hypothalmic heat regulating centers. Acetaminophen inhibits prostaglandin synthetase. Therapeutic doses of acetaminophen have neglible effects on the cardiovascular or respiratory systems; however, toxic doses, may cause circulatory failure and rapid, shallow breathing. Acetaminophen is rapidly and almost completely absorbed from the gastrointestinal tract, producing maximum serum concentrations within 30 minutes to one hour. The plasma half-life in adults and children ranges from 0.90 hours to 3.25 hours with an average of approximately 2 hours. The drug distributes uniformly in most body fluids and is approximately 25% protein bound. Acetaminophen is conjugated in the liver, with less than 3% of the dose excreted unchanged in 24 hours. The primary metabolic pathway is conjugation to sulfate and glucuronide by-products. A minor oxidative pathway forms cysteine and mercapturic acid. These compounds are subsequently excreted by the kidneys into the urine.

Indications and Usage: For the relief of moderate to moderately severe pain.

Contraindications: Hypersensitivity to acetaminophen or hydrocodone.

Warnings: Respiratory Depression: At high doses or in sensitive patients, hydrocodone may produce dose-related respiratory depression by acting directly on brain stem respiratory centers. Hydrocodone also affects centers that control respiratory rhythm, and may produce irregular and periodic breathing.

Head Injury and Increased Intracranial Pressure: The respiratory depressant effects of narcotics and their capacity to elevate cerebrospinal fluid pressure may be markedly exaggerated in the presence of head injury, other intracranial lesions or a preexisting increase in intracranial pressure. Furthermore, narcotics produce adverse reactions which may obscure the clinical course of patients with head injuries.

Acute Abdominal Conditions: The administration of narcotics may obscure the diagnosis or clinical course of patients with acute abdominal conditions.

Precautions: Special Risk Patients: As with any narcotic analgesic agent, BANCAP HC Capsules should be used with caution in elderly or debilitated patients and those with severe impairment of hepatic or renal function, hypothyroidism, Addison's disease, prostatic hypertrophy or urethral stricture. The usual precautions should be observed and the possibility of respiratory depression should be kept in mind.

Information for Patients: BANCAP HC Capsules like all narcotics, may impair the mental and/or physical abilities required for the performance of potentially hazardous tasks such as driving a car or operating machinery; patients should be cautioned accordingly.

Cough Reflex: Hydrocodone suppresses the cough reflex; as with all narcotics, caution should be exercised when BANCAP HC Capsules are used postoperatively and in patients with pulmonary disease.

Drug Interactions: Patients receiving other narcotic analgesic, antipsychotics, antianxiety agents, or other CNS depressants (including alcohol) concommitantly with BANCAP HC Capsules may exhibit an additive CNS depression. When combined therapy is contemplated, the dose of one or both agents should be reduced.

The use of MAO inhibitors or tricyclic antidepressants with hydrocodone preparations may increase the effect of either the antidepressant or hydrocodone.

The concurrent use of anticholinergics with hydrocodone may produce paralytic ileus.

Usage in Pregnancy: Pregnancy Category C. Hydrocodone has been shown to be teratogenic in hamsters when given in doses 700 times the human dose. There are no adequate and well-controlled studies in pregnant women. BANCAP HC Capsules should be used during pregnancy only if the potential benefit justifies the potential risk to the fetus.

Nonteratogenic Effects: Babies born to mothers who have been taking opioids regularly prior to delivery will be physically dependent. The withdrawal signs include irritability and excessive crying, tremors, hyperactive reflexes, increased respiratory rate, increased stools, sneezing, yawning, vomiting, and fever. The intensity of the syndrome does not always correlate with the duration of maternal opiod use or dose. There is no consensus on the best method of managing withdrawal. Chlorpromazine 0.7 to 1.0 mg/kg q6h, and paregoric 2 to 4 drops/kg q4h, have been used to treat withdrawal symptoms in infants. The duration of therapy is 4 to 28 days, with the dosage decreased as tolerated.

Labor and Delivery: As with all narcotics, administration of BANCAP HC Capsules to the mother shortly before delivery may result in some degree of respiratory depression in the newborn, especially if higher doses are used.

Nursing Mothers: It is not known whether this drug is excreted in human milk. Because many drugs are excreted in human milk and because of the potential for serious adverse reactions in nursing infants from BANCAP HC Capsules, a decision should be made whether to discontinue nursing or to discontinue the drug, taking into account the importance of the drug to the mother.

Pediatric Use: Safety and effectiveness in children have not been established.

Adverse Reactions: Central Nervous System: Sedation, drowsiness, mental clouding, lethargy, impairment of mental and physical performance, anxiety, fear, dysphoria, dizziness, psychic dependence, mood changes.

Gastrointestinal System: Nausea and vomiting may occur; they are more frequent in ambulatory than in recumbent patients. The antiemetic phenothiazines are useful in suppressing these effects; however, some phenothiazine derivatives seem to be antianalgesic and to increase the amount of narcotic required to produce pain relief, while other phenothiazines reduce the amount of narcotic required to produce a given level of analgesia. Prolonged administration of BANCAP HC Capsules may produce constipation.

Genitourinary System: Ureteral spasm, spasm of vesical sphincters and urinary retention have been reported.

Respiratory Depression: BANCAP HC Capsules may produce dose-related respiratory depression by acting directly on brain stem respiratory centers. Hydrocodone also affects centers that control respiratory rhythm, and may produce irregular and periodic breathing. If significant respiratory depression occurs, it may be antagonized by the use of naloxone hydrochloride. Apply other supportive measures when indicated.

Drug-Abuse and Dependence: BANCAP HC Capsules are subject to the Federal Controlled Substance Act (Schedule III). Psychic dependence, physical dependence, and tolerance may develop upon repeated administration of narcotics; therefore, BANCAP HC Capsules should be prescribed and administered with caution. However, psychic dependence is unlikely to develop when BANCAP HC Capsules are used for a short time for the treatment of pain.

Physical dependence, the condition in which continued administration of the drug is required to prevent the appearance of a withdrawal syndrome, assumes clinically significant proportions only after several weeks of continued narcotic use, although some mild degree of physical dependence may develop after a few days of narcotic therapy. Tolerance, in which increasingly large doses are required in order to produce the same degree of analgesia, is manifested initially by a shortened duration of analgesic effect, and subsequently by decreases in the intensity of analgesia. The rate of development of tolerance varies among patients.

Overdosage: Acetaminophen: Signs and Symptoms: Acetaminophen in massive overdosage may cause hepatic toxicity in some patients. In all cases of suspected overdose, immediately call your regional poison center or the Rocky Mountain Poison Center's toll-free number (800-525-5115) for assistance in diagnosis and for directions in the use of N-acetylcysteine as an antidote, a use currently restricted to investigational status.

In adults, hepatic toxicity has rarely been reported with acute overdoses of less than 10 grams and fatalities with less than 15 grams. Importantly, young children seem to be more resistant than adults to the hepatotoxic effect of an acetaminophen overdose. Despite this, the measures outlined below should be initiated in any adult or child suspected of having ingested an acetaminophen overdose.

Early symtoms following a potentially hepatotoxic overdose may include: nausea, vomiting, diaphoresis and general malaise. Clinical and laboratory evidence of hepatic toxicity may not be apparent until 48 to 72 hours post-ingestion.

Treatment: The stomach should be emptied promptly by lavage or by induction of emesis with syrup of ipecac. Patients' estimates of the quantity of a drug ingested are notoriously unreliable. Therefore, if an acetaminophen overdose is suspected, a serum acetaminophen assay should be obtained as early as possible, but no sooner than four hours following ingestion. Liver function studies should be obtained initially and repeated at 24-hour intervals.

The antidote, N-acetylcysteine, should be administered as early as possible, and within 16 hours of the overdose ingestion for optimal results. Following recovery, there are no residual, structural or functional hepatic abnormalities.

Hydrocodone: Signs and Symptoms: Serious overdose with hydrocodone is characterized by respiratory depression (a decrease in respiratory rate and Cortidial volume, Cheyne-Stokes respiration, cyanosis), extreme somnolence progressing to stupor or coma, skeletal muscle flaccidity, cold and clammy skin, and sometimes bradycardia and hypotension. In severe overdosage, apnea, circulatory collapse, cardiac arrest and death may occur.

Treatment: Primary attention should be given to the reestablishment of adequate respiratory exchange through provision of a patent airway and the institution of assisted or controlled ventilation. The narcotic antagonist, naloxone is a specific antidote against respiratory depression which may result from overdosage or unusual sensitivity to narcotics, including hydrocodone. Therefore, an appropriate dose of naloxone should be administered, preferably by the intravenous route, and simultaneously with efforts at respiratory resuscitation. Since the duration of action of hydrocodone may exceed that of the antagonist, the patient should be kept under continued surveillance and repeated doses of the antagonist should be administered as needed to maintain adequate respiration.

An antagonist should not be administered in the absence of clinically significant respiratory or cardiovascular depression. Oxygen, intravenous fluids, vasopressors and other supportive measures should be employed as indicated. Gastric emptying may be useful in removing unabsorbed drug.

Dosage and Administration: Dosage should be adjusted according to the severity of the pain and the response of the patient. However, it should be kept in mind that tolerance to hydrocodone can develop with continued use and that the incidence of untoward effects is dose related.

The usual dose is one capsule every six hours as needed for pain. If necessary, this dose may be repeated at four hour intervals. In cases of more severe pain, two capsules every six hours (up to 8 capsules in 24 hours) may be required.

How Supplied: Black and red capsules imprinted OJF 610.
Bottles of 100—NDC 0456-0610-01
Bottles of 500—NDC 0456-0610-02
Caution: Federal law prohibits dispensing without prescription.
Revised: MARCH 7, 1982
Shown in Product Identification Section, page 422

CONEX OTC
CONEX with CODEINE

Composition: CONEX: Each 5 ml contains:
Guaifenesin ....100 mg
Phenylpropanolamine HC1 ....12.5 mg
CONEX WITH CODEINE: Each 5 ml contains:
Phenylpropanolamine HCl ....12.5 mg
Guaifenesin ....100 mg
Codeine Phosphate ....10 mg
(Warning: May be habit forming)
How Supplied: Bottles of 4 ounces.

DALALONE INJECTION

Each ml. contains:
Dexamethasone Sodium Phosphate equivalent to
Dexamethasone Phosphate ....4 mg.
How Supplied: 5 ml multiple dose vial.

DALALONE D.P. INJECTION

Each ml. contains:
Dexamethasone Acetate, equivalent
to Dexamethasone ....16 mg.
How Supplied: 5 ml. multiple dose vial.
1 ml. unit dose vial, Box of 5.

DALALONE L.A. INJECTION

Each ml. contains:
Dexamethasone Acetate
equivalent to Dexamethasone..........................8 mg
How Supplied: 5 ml multiple dose vial.

DALCAINE INJECTION

Each ml. contains:
Lidocaine HCl 2% without preservative
How Supplied: 5 ml. unit dose vial (box of 6).

DEHIST

Composition: Each **Capsule** contains:
Phenylpropanolamine HCl ....75 mg
Chlorpheniramine Maleate ....12 mg
in a special base, providing timed release for the Chlorpheniramine Maleate and Phenypropanolamine HCl.
How Supplied: Capsules, bottles of 100 and 1000.

depMEDALONE "40" INJECTABLE

Each ml. contains:
Methylprednisolone Acetate
in aqueous suspension ....40 mg.
How Supplied: 5 ml. multiple dose vials.

depMEDALONE "80" INJECTABLE

Each ml. contains:
Methylprednisolone Acetate
in aqueous suspension ....80 mg.
How Supplied: 5 ml. multiple dose vials.

DURADYNE DHC TABLET

Description: Each green, scored tablet contains:
Hydrocodone Bitartrate ....5 mg.
(WARNING: May be habit forming.)
Acetaminophen ....500 mg.
How Supplied: Bottles of 100 and 1000.

FEOSTAT Tablets OTC
FEOSTAT Suspension
FEOSTAT Drops
(Ferrous Fumarate)

FEOSTAT Tablets
Each chocolate-flavored chewable tablet contains:
Ferrous fumarate ....100 mg.
(Elemental iron ....33 mg.)
FEOSTAT Suspension
Each 5 cc. (teaspoonful) contains:
Ferrous fumarate ....100 mg.
(Elemental iron ....33 mg.)
FEOSTAT Drops
Each 12 drops (0.6 cc.) contains:
Ferrous fumarate ....45 mg.
(Elemental iron ....15 mg.)
How Supplied:
Tablets: Bottles of 100 and 1000.
Suspension: 8 ounce bottle.
Drops: 2 ounce bottle.

HEPARIN SODIUM
without preservatives

Each ml. contains:
Heparin Sodium (w/o pres.) ....1000 units
How Supplied: 5 ml. ampuls, Box 25

IODO-NIACIN® TABLETS

Description: Each controlled action tablet contains:
Potassium Iodide ....135 mg
Niacinamide Hydroiodide ....25 mg
How Supplied: Bottles of 100 and 500.

MAGNESIUM SULFATE INJECTION

Each ml. contains:
Magnesium Sulfate ....500 mg.
How Supplied: 30 ml. vial.

OXYMYCIN INJECTION

Each ml. contains:
Oxytetracycline ....50 mg.
How Supplied: 10 ml. multiple dose vial.

PEDAMETH® CAPSULE
PEDAMETH® LIQUID
(racemethionine)

Composition:
CAPSULES—200 mg. racemethionine.
LIQUID—75 mg. racemethionine per 5 cc. (teaspoon) in a fruit flavored base.
Indications:
Control of urine odor, dermatitis and ulcerations caused by ammoniacal urine in the incontinent adult patient.
Diaper rash caused by ammoniacal urine.
Contraindication: Do not administer to patients with history of liver disease as large doses of methionine may exaggerate the toxemia of the disease.
Precautions: It has been pointed out by Goldstein and in animal studies that excessive dosage of methionine, added alone to the diet over extended periods, may result in a weight gain below normal when protein intake is insufficient. Thus, it is essential that adequate protein intake be main-

Continued on next page

O'Neal, Jones & Feldman—Cont.

tained during therapy and that recommended dosage not be exceeded. Methionine should not be administered on an empty stomach.
Dosage and Administration:
Capsules—Adults: one capsule three or four times a day after meals.
Liquid—Infants: 2 months to 6 months—one teaspoon (5 cc.) three times per day for 3-5 days. May be added to formula, milk or juice; 6 months to 14 months—one teaspoon (5 cc.) four times per day for 3-5 days. In severe cases it may be necessary to double the dosage the first two days of treatment.
How Supplied:
CAPSULES: Bottles of 50 and 500.
LIQUID: Pint Bottle.
Shown in Product Identification Section, page 422

ROGENIC INJECTION ℞

Each ml. contains:
Cyanocobalamin .... 500 mcg
Peptonized Iron .... 20 mg
Liver (equiv. to Vit. B-12) .... 10 mcg
How Supplied: 10 ml multiple dose vial.

Organon Pharmaceuticals
A Division of Organon Inc.
375 MT. PLEASANT AVE.
WEST ORANGE, NJ 07052

Below are listed the currently available products. For a complete catalog and price list direct inquiries to Customer Service. For specific product information, direct inquiries to the Professional Services Department.

BILOGEN®
How Supplied: Tablets—bottle of 100.

CORTROPHIN®—Zinc ℞
ACTH
How Supplied: Vials, 5 ml (40 USP Units/ml).

CORTROSYN® ℞
Cosyntropin is α 1-24 corticotropin, a synthetic subunit of ACTH.
How Supplied: Available as a lyophilized powder in vials containing 0.25 mg of Cortrosyn and 10 mg of mannitol, (Boxes of 10 × 1 ml vials of powder and 10 × 1 ml amps diluent).

COTAZYM® ℞
[kōt′a zīm]
(Pancrelipase Capsules, USP)
Description: Cotazym (Pancrelipase, USP) is a powder containing enzymes obtained from the pancreas of the hog. These include amylase and protease but principally lipase. Each capsule (regular or cherrry flavored) contains:
Lipase—8,000 USP Units
Protease—30,000 USP Units
Amylase—30,000 USP Units
Precipitated calcium carbonate 25 mg.
Indications and Usage: It is indicated in conditions where pancreatic enzymes are either absent or deficient with resultant inadequate fat digestion. Such conditions include but are not limited to chronic pancreatitis, pancreatectomy, cystic fibrosis and steatorrhea of diverse etiologies.
Contraindications: Known hypersensitivity to pork protein.
Precautions: In the event that capsules are opened for any reason care should be taken so that powder is not inhaled or spilled on hands since it may prove irritating to the skin or mucous membranes.
Adverse Reactions: No adverse reactions have been reported. It should be noted, however, that extremely high doses of exogenous pancreatic enzymes have been associated with hyperuricosuria and hyperuricemia.
Dosage and Administration: One to three capsules just prior to each meal or snack or as directed by physician. Severe cases may require higher dosage and dietary adjustment.
Storage: Not to exceed 25°C (77°F). Dry place when opened.
Dispense: In tight container as defined in the USP.
Supplied: Cotazym capsules (regular) bottles of 100 and 500. NDC # 0052-0381-91, NDC # 0052-0381-95.
Cotazym capsules (cherry flavored) bottles of 100.
NDC # 0052-0386-91.
Shown in Product Identification Section, page 422

COTAZYM-S™ ℞
[kōt′a zīm-s]
Enteric coated spheres
(Pancrelipase USP)
Description: Cotazym-S contains enteric coated spheres of pancrelipase, a substance containing enzymes, principally lipase, with amylase and protease, obtained from the pancreas of the hog.
Each capsule contains:
Lipase—5,000 USP Units
Protease—20,000 USP Units
Amylase—20,000 USP Units
COTAZYM-S™
Clinical Pharmacology: Cotazym-S is protected against inactivation by gastric acidity, and active enzymes are released in the duodenum. The enzymes promote hydrolysis of fats into glycerol and fatty acids, protein into proteases and derived substances, and starch into dextrans and sugars.
Indications and Usage: Cotazym-S is indicated in conditions where pancreatic enzymes are either absent or deficient with resultant inadequate fat digestion. Such conditions include but are not limited to chronic pancreatitis, pancreatectomy, cystic fibrosis and steatorrhea of diverse etiologies.
Contraindications: Known hypersensitivity to pork protein.
Precautions: To maintain enteric coating integrity, do not chew or crush spheres.
Adverse Reactions: No adverse reactions have been reported. It should be noted, however, that extremely high doses of exogenous pancreatic enzymes have been associated with hyperuricosuria and hyperuricemia.
Dosage and Administration: One to two capsules with each meal or snack as directed by physician. Severe cases may require higher dosage and dietary adjustment. Cotazym-S capsules are usually easy to swallow, but in case of any difficulty, capsules may be opened and the spheres taken with liquids or soft foods which do not require chewing.
Storage: Not to exceed 25°C (77°F). Dry place when opened.
Dispense: In tight container as defined in the USP.
Supplied: Cotazym-S bottles of 100. NDC #0052-0388-91. Bottles of 500. NDC #0052-0388-95.
Shown in Product Identification Section, page 422

DECA–DURABOLIN® ℞
(Nandrolone Decanoate Injection, USP)
How Supplied:
50 mg/ml—1 ml ampuls, 2 ml vials, 1 ml prefilled syringe.
100 mg/ml—2 ml vials, 1 ml prefilled syringe.
200 mg/ml—1 ml vials, 1 ml prefilled syringe.

DOCA® ACETATE ℞
(Desoxycorticosterone Acetate Injection, USP)
How Supplied: Vials, 10 ml (5 mg/ml).

DURABOLIN® ℞
(Nandrolone Phenpropionate Injection, USP)
How Supplied:
25 mg/ml—1 ml ampuls, 5 ml vials.
50 mg/ml—2 ml vials.

HEPARIN SODIUM ℞
Injection, USP
(From Beef Lung)
How Supplied:
1,000 USP Units/ml (aqueous) Vials, 10 ml and 30 ml
5,000 USP Units/ml (aqueous) Vials, 1 ml and 10 ml
10,000 USP Units/ml (aqueous) Vials, 1 ml and 4 ml

HEXADROL® Elixir
(Dexamethasone Elixir, USP)
Each 5 ml contains: 0.5 mg dexamethasone with 5% alcohol.
How Supplied: Elixir (0.5 mg/5 ml)—Bottle of 120 ml

HEXADROL® ℞
(Dexamethasone Tablets, USP)
How Supplied:
Tablets (0.5 mg yellow, scored)—bottle of 100 & 500.
Tablets (0.75 mg white, scored)—bottle of 100 & 500
Tablets (1.5 mg peach, scored)—bottle of 100
Tablets (4 mg green, scored)—bottle of 100
Shown in Product Identification Section, page 422

HEXADROL® STRIP PACKS ℞
(Dexamethasone Tablets, USP)
How Supplied:
Tablets (0.5 mg yellow, scored)
  Box of 100 (10 strips—10 per strip)
Tablets (0.75 mg white, scored)
  Box of 100 (10 strips—10 per strip)
Tablets (1.5 mg peach, scored)
  Box of 100 (10 strips—10 per strip)
Tablets (4 mg green, scored)
  Box of 100 (10 strips—10 per strip)
Shown in Product Identification Section, page 422

HEXADROL® ℞
Therapeutic Pack
(Dexamethasone, Tablets, USP)
How Supplied: Each pack contains: 6 × 1.5 mg tablets, (peach scored); 8 × 0.75 mg tablets, (white, scored).
Shown in Product Identification Section, page 422

HEXADROL®
Phosphate Injection
(Dexamethasone Sodium Phosphate Injection, USP)
Aqueous Solutions
How Supplied: Available in three potencies:
4 mg/ml—1 ml vials, 5 ml vials, 1 ml prefilled syringe.
10 mg/ml—10 ml vials, 1 ml prefilled syringe.
20 mg/ml—5 ml vial, 5 ml prefilled syringe.

HYDROCORTISONE, USP ℞
Micronized Powder
Non-Sterile: For Prescription Compounding Only
How Supplied: Available in 10, 25 and 100 gram containers.

LIQUAEMIN® Sodium ℞
Heparin Sodium Injection, USP
(from porcine intestinal mucosa)
How Supplied:
1,000 USP Units/ml (aqueous) Vials, 10 ml & 30 ml
5,000 USP Units ml (aqueous) Ampuls, 1 ml Vials, 1 ml & 10 ml
10,000 USP Units/ml (aqueous) Ampuls, 1 ml Vials, 1 ml & 4 ml
20,000 USP Units/ml (aqueous) Vials, 1 ml, 2 ml & 5 ml
40,000 USP Units/ml (aqueous) Vials, 1 ml

LIQUAMAR®
(Phenprocoumon Tablets, USP) ℞

How Supplied: Tablets, 3 mg—bottle of 100.

MAXIBOLIN®
(ethylestrenol) ℞

How Supplied:
Tablets, 2 mg—bottle of 100.
Elixir, 2 mg/5 ml—120 ml bottle.
Shown in Product Identification Section, page 422

METHYLPREDNISOLONE
Sodium Succinate
for Injection, USP ℞

How Supplied:
500 mg vials of Lyophilized Powder with vial of Diluent
1000 mg vials of Lyophilized Powder with vial of Diluent

NORCURON® (NC–45)
(vecuronium bromide for injection) ℞

> THIS DRUG SHOULD BE ADMINISTERED BY ADEQUATELY TRAINED INDIVIDUALS FAMILIAR WITH ITS ACTIONS, CHARACTERISTICS, AND HAZARDS.

Description: NORCURON® (vecuronium bromide for injection) is a nondepolarizing neuromuscular blocking agent of intermediate duration, chemically designated as piperidinium, 1-[(2β,3α,5α,16β,17)-3, 17-bis(acetyloxy)-2-(1-piperidinyl)androstan-16-yl]-1-methyl-, bromide. The structural formula is:

Norcuron® is supplied as a sterile freeze-dried buffered cake of very fine microscopic crystalline particles for intravenous injection only. Following reconstitution with solvent (water for injection) the resultant solution is isotonic and has a pH of 4. Each 5 ml vial contains 10 mg vecuronium bromide. Each vial also contains citric acid, dibasic sodium phosphate, sodium hydroxide, and/or phosphoric acid to buffer and adjust pH and mannitol to make isotonic.

Clinical Pharmacology: Norcuron® (vecuronium bromide for injection) is a nondepolarizing neuromuscular blocking agent possessing all of the characteristic pharmacological actions of this class of drugs (curariform). It acts by competing for cholinergic receptors at the motor endplate. The antagonism to acetylcholine is inhibited and neuromuscular block is reversed by acetylcholinesterase inhibitors such as neostigmine, edrophonium, and pyridostigmine. Norcuron® is about ⅓ more potent than pancuronium; the duration of neuromuscular blockade produced by Norcuron® is shorter than that of pancuronium at initially equipotent doses. The time to onset of paralysis decreases and the duration of maximum effect increases with increasing Norcuron® doses. The use of a peripheral nerve stimulator is of benefit in assessing the degree of muscular relaxation. The ED_{90} (dose required to produce 90% suppression of the muscle twitch response with balanced anesthesia) has averaged 0.057 mg/kg (0.049 to 0.062 mg/kg in various studies). An initial Norcuron® dose of 0.08 to 10 mg/kg generally produces first depression of twitch in approximately 1 minute, good or excellent intubation conditions within 2.5 to 3.0 minutes, and maximum neuromuscular blockade within 3 to 5 minutes of injection in most patients. Under balanced anesthesia, the time to recovery to 25% of control (clinical duration) is approximately 25 to 40 minutes after injection and recovery is usually 95% complete approximately 45–65 minutes after injection of intubating dose. The neuromuscular blocking action of Norcuron® is slightly enhanced in the presence of potent inhalation anesthetics. If Norcuron® is first administered more than 5 minutes after the start of the inhalation of enflurane, isoflurane, or halothane, or when steady state has been achieved, the intubating dose of Norcuron® may be decreased by approximately 15% (see DOSAGE AND ADMINISTRATION section). Prior administration of succinylcholine may enhance the neuromuscular blocking effect of Norcuron® and its duration of action. With succinylcholine as the intubating agent, initial doses of 0.04–0.06 mg/kg of Norcuron® will produce complete neuromuscular block with clinical duration of action of 25–30 minutes. If succinylcholine is used prior to Norcuron®, the administration of Norcuron® should be delayed until the patient starts recovering from succinylcholine-induced neuromuscular blockade. The effect of prior use of other nondepolarizing neuromuscular blocking agents on the activity of Norcuron® has not been studied (see Drug Interactions).

Repeated administration of maintenance doses of Norcuron® has little or no cumulative effect on the duration of neuromuscular blockade. Therefore, repeat doses can be administered at relatively regular intervals with predictable results. After an initial dose of 0.08 to 0.1 mg/kg under balanced anesthesia, the first maintenance dose (suggested maintenance dose is 0.01 to 0.015 mg/kg) is generally required within 25 to 40 minutes; subsequent maintenance doses, if required, may be administered at approximately 12 to 15 minute intervals. Halothane anesthesia increases the clinical duration of the maintenance dose only slightly. Under enflurane a maintenance dose of 0.01 mg/kg is approximately equal to 0.015 mg/kg dose under balanced anesthesia.

The recovery index (time from 25% to 75% recovery) is approximately 15–25 minutes under balanced or halothane anesthesia. When recovery from Norcuron® neuromuscular blocking effect begins, it proceeds more rapidly than recovery from pancuronium. Once spontaneous recovery has started, the neuromuscular block produced by Norcuron® is readily reversed with various anticholinesterase agents, e.g. pyridostigmine, neostigmine, or edrophonium in conjunction with an anticholinergic agent such as atropine or glycopyrrolate. There have been no reports of recurarization following satisfactory reversal of Norcuron® induced neuromuscular blockade; rapid recovery is a finding consistent with its short elimination half-life.

Pharmacokinetics: At clinical doses of 0.04–0.1 mg/kg, 60–80% of Norcuron® is usually bound to plasma protein. The distribution half-life following a single intravenous dose (range 0.025–0.28 mg/kg) is approximately 4 minutes. Elimination half-life over this same dosage range is approximately 65–75 minutes in healthy surgical patients and in renal failure patients undergoing transplant surgery. In late pregnancy, elimination half-life may be shortened to approximately 35–40 minutes. The volume of distribution at steady state is approximately 300–400 ml/kg; systemic rate of clearance is approximately 3–4.5 ml/minute/kg. In man, urine recovery of Norcuron® varies from 3–35% within 24 hours. Data derived from patients requiring insertion of a T-tube in the common bile duct suggests that 25–50% of a total intravenous dose of vecuronium may be excreted in bile within 42 hours. Only unchanged Norcuron® (vecuronium bromide for injection) has been detected in human plasma following clinical use. One metabolite, 3-deacetyl vecuronium, has been recovered in the urine of some patients in quantities that account for up to 10% of injected dose; 3-deacetyl vecuronium has also been recovered by T-tube in some patients accounting for up to 25% of the injected dose.

This metabolite has been judged by animal screening (dogs and cats) to have 50% or more of the potency of Norcuron®; equipotent doses are of approximately the same duration as Norcuron® in dogs and cats. Biliary excretion accounts for about half the dose of Norcuron® within 7 hours in the anesthetized rat. Circulatory bypass of the liver (cat preparation) prolongs recovery from Norcuron®. Limited data derived from patients with cirrhosis or cholestasis suggests that some measurements of recovery may be doubled in such patients. In patients with renal failure, measurements of recovery do not differ significantly from similar measurements in healthy patients.

Studies involving routine hemodynamic monitoring in good risk surgical patients reveal that the administration of Norcuron® in doses up to three times that needed to produce clinical relaxation (0.15 mg/kg) did not produce clinically significant changes in systolic, diastolic or mean arterial pressure. The heart rate, under similar monitoring, remained unchanged in some studies and was lowered by a mean of up to 8% in other studies. A large dose of 0.28 mg/kg administered during a period of no stimulation, while patients were being prepared for coronary artery bypass grafting, was not associated with alterations in rate-pressure-product or pulmonary capillary wedge pressure. Systemic vascular resistance was lowered slightly and cardiac output was increased insignificantly. (The drug has not been studied in patients with hemodynamic dysfunction secondary to cardiac valvular disease). Limited clinical experience (3 patients) with use of Norcuron® during surgery for pheochromocytoma has shown that administration of this drug is not associated with changes in blood pressure or heart rate.

Unlike other nondepolarizing skeletal muscle relaxants, Norcuron® has no clinically significant effects on hemodynamic parameters and will not counteract those hemodynamic changes or known side effects produced by or associated with anesthetic agents.

Preliminary data on histamine assay in 16 patients and available clinical experience in more than 600 patients indicate that hypersensitivity reactions such as bronchospasm, flushing, redness, hypotension, tachycardia, and other reactions commonly associated with histamine release are unlikely to occur.

Indications and Usage: Norcuron® is indicated as an adjunct to general anesthesia, to facilitate endotracheal intubation and to provide skeletal muscle relaxation during surgery or mechanical ventilation.

Contraindications: None known.

Warning: NORCURON® SHOULD BE ADMINISTERED IN CAREFULLY ADJUSTED DOSAGE BY OR UNDER THE SUPERVISION OF EXPERIENCED CLINICIANS WHO ARE FAMILIAR WITH ITS ACTIONS AND THE POSSIBLE COMPLICATIONS THAT MIGHT OCCUR FOLLOWING ITS USE. THE DRUG SHOULD NOT BE ADMINISTERED UNLESS FACILITIES FOR INTUBATION, ARTIFICAL RESPIRATION, OXYGEN THERAPY, AND REVERSAL AGENTS ARE IMMEDIATELY AVAILABLE. THE CLINICIAN MUST BE PREPARED TO ASSIST OR CONTROL RESPIRATION. In patients who are known to have myasthenia gravis or the myasthenic (Eaton-Lambert) syndrome, small doses of Norcuron® may have profound effects. In such patients, a peripheral nerve stimulator and use of a small test dose may be of value in monitoring the response to administration of muscle relaxants.

Precautions: *Renal Failure:* Norcuron® is well-tolerated without clinically significant prolongation of neuromuscular blocking effect in patients with renal failure who have been optimally prepared for surgery by dialysis. Under emergency conditions in anephric patients some prolongation of neuromuscular blockade may occur; therefore, if anephric patients cannot be prepared

Continued on next page

Organon—Cont.

for non-elective surgery, a lower initial dose of Norcuron® should be considered.

Altered Circulation Time: Conditions associated with slower circulation time in cardiovascular disease, old age, edematous states resulting in increased volume of distribution may contribute to a delay in onset time; therefore dosage should not be increased.

Hepatic Disease: Limited experience in patients with cirrhosis or cholestasis has revealed prolonged recovery time in keeping with the role the liver plays in recovery from Norcuron® metabolism and excretion (see Pharmacokinetics). Data currently available do not permit dosage recommendations in patients with impaired liver function.

UNDER THE ABOVE CONDITIONS, USE OF A PERIPHERAL NERVE STIMULATOR FOR ADEQUATE MONITORING OF NEUROMUSCULAR BLOCKING EFFECT WILL PRECLUDE INADVERTANT EXCESS DOSING.

Severe Obesity or Neuromuscular Disease: Patients with severe obesity or neuromuscular disease may pose airway and/or ventilatory problems requiring special care before, during and after the use of neuromuscular blocking agents such as Norcuron®.

Malignant Hyperthermia: Many drugs used in anesthetic practice are suspected of being capable of triggering a potentially fatal hypermetabolism of skeletal muscle known as malignant hyperthermia. There are insufficient data derived from screening in susceptible animals (swine) to establish whether or not Norcuron® is capable of triggering malignant hyperthermia.

Norcuron® has no known effect on consciousness, the pain threshold or cerebration. Administration must be accompanied by adequate anesthesia.

Drug Interactions: Prior administraion of succinylcholine may enhance the neuromuscular blocking effect of Norcuron® (vecuronium bromide for injection) and its duration of action. If succinylcholine is used before Norcuron®, the administration of Norcuron® should be delayed until the succinylcholine effect shows signs of wearing off. With succinylcholine as the intubating agent, initial doses of 0.04–0.06 mg/kg of Norcuron® may be administered to produce complete neuromuscular block with clinical duration of action of 25–30 minutes (see CLINICAL PHARMACOLOGY). The use of Norcuron® before succinylcholine, in order to attenuate some of the side effects of succinylcholine, has not been sufficiently studied.

Other nondepolarizing neuromuscular blocking agents (pancuronium, d-tubocurarine, metocurine, and gallamine) act in the same fashion as does Norcuron®, therefore these drugs and Norcuron® may manifest an additive effect when used together. There are insufficient data to support concomitant use of Norcuron® and other competitive muscle relaxants in the same patient.

Inhalational Anesthetics: Use of volatile inhalational anesthetics such as enflurane, isoflurane, and halothane with Norcuron® will enhance neuromuscular blockade. Potentiation is most prominent with use of enflurane and isoflurane. With the above agents the initial dose of Norcuron® may be the same as with balanced anesthesia unless the inhalational anesthetic has been administered for a sufficient time at a sufficient dose to have reached clinical equilibrium (see CLINICAL PHARMACOLOGY).

Antibiotics: Parenteral/intraperitoneal administration of high doses of certain antibiotics may intensify or produce neuromuscular block on their own. The following antibiotics have been associated with various degrees of paralysis; aminoglycosides (such as neomycin, streptomycin, kanamycin, gentamicin, and dihydrostreptomycin); tetracyclines; bacitracin; polymyxin B; colistin; and sodium colistimethate. If these or other newly introduced antibiotics are used in conjunction with Norcuron® during surgery, unexpected prolongation of neuromuscular block should be considered a possibility.

Other: Experience concerning injection of quinidine during recovery from use of other muscle relaxants suggests that recurrent paralysis may occur. This possiblity must also be considered for Norcuron®. Norcuron® induced neuromuscular blockade has been counteracted by alkalosis and enhanced by acidosis in experimental animals (cat). Electrolyte imbalance and diseases which lead to electrolyte imbalance, such as adrenal cortical insufficiency, have been shown to alter neuromuscular blockade. Depending on the nature of the imbalance, either enhancement or inhibition may be expected. Magnesium salts, administered for the management of toxemia of pregnancy, may enhance the neuromuscular blockade.

Drug/laboratory test interactions: None known.

Carcinogenesis, Mutagenesis, Impairment of Fertility: Long-term studies in animals have not been performed to evaluate carcinogenic or mutagenic potential or impairment of fertility.

Pregnancy: Pregnancy Category C: Animal reproduction studies have not been conducted with Norcuron®. It is also not known whether Norcuron® can cause fetal harm when administered to a pregnant woman or can affect reproduction capacity. Norcuron® should be given to a pregnant woman only if clearly needed.

Pediatric Use: Infants under 1 year of age but older than 7 weeks, also tested under halothane anesthesia, are moderately more sensitive to Norcuron® on a mg/kg basis than adults and take about 1½ times as long to recover. Information presently available does not permit recommendations for usage in neonates.

Adverse Reactions: Norcuron® was well-tolerated and produced no adverse reactions during extensive clinical trials. The most frequent adverse reaction to nondepolarizing blocking agents as a class consists of an extension of the drug's pharmacological action beyond the time period needed for surgery and anesthesia. This may vary from skeletal muscle weakness to profound and prolonged skeletal muscle paralysis resulting in respiratory insufficiency or apnea.

Inadequate reversal of the neuromuscular blockade, although not yet reported, is possible with Norcuron® as with all curariform drugs. These adverse reactions are managed by manual or mechanical ventilation until recovery is judged adequate. Little or no increase in intensity of blockade or duration of action of Norcuron® is noted from the use of thiobarbiturates, narcotic analgesics, nitrous oxide, or droperidol. See OVERDOSAGE for discussion of other drugs used in anesthetic practice which also cause respiratory depression.

Overdosage: There has been no experience with Norcuron® overdosage. The possibility of iatrogenic overdosage can be minimized by carefully monitoring muscle twitch response to peripheral nerve stimulation.

Excessive doses of Norcuron® can be expected to produce enhanced pharmacological effects. Residual neuromuscular blockade beyond the time period needed for surgery and anesthesia may occur with Norcuron® as with other neuromuscular blockers. This may be manifested by skeletal muscle weakness, decreased respiratory reserve, low tidal volume, or apnea. A peripheral nerve stimulator may be used to assess the degree of residual neuromuscular blockade and help to differentiate residual neuromuscular blockade from other causes of decreased respiratory reserve.

Respiratory depression may be due either wholly or in part to other drugs used during the conduct of general anesthesia such as narcotics, thiobarbiturates and other central nervous system depressants. Under such circumstances the primary treatment is maintenance of a patent airway and manual or mechanical ventilation until complete recovery of normal respiration is assured. Regonol® (pyridostigmine bromide injection), neostigmine, or edrophonium, in conjunction with atropine or glycopyrrolate will usually antagonize the skeletal muscle relaxant action of Norcuron®. Satisfactory reversal can be judged by adequacy of skeletal muscle tone and by adequacy of respiration. A peripheral nerve stimulator may also be used to monitor restoration of twitch height. Failure to prompt reversal (within 30 minutes) may occur in the presence of extreme debilitation, carcinomatosis, and with concomitant use of certain broad spectrum antibiotics, or anesthetic agents and other drugs which enhance neuromuscular blockade or cause respiratory depression of their own. Under such circumstances the management is the same as that of prolonged neuromuscular blockade. Ventilation must be supported by artificial means until the patient has resumed control of his respiration. Prior to the use of reversal agents, reference should be made to the specific package insert of the reversal agent.

Dosage and Administration: Norcuron® (vecuronium bromide for injection) is for intravenous use only. This drug should be administered by or under the supervision of experienced clinicians familiar with the use of neuromuscular blocking agents. Dosage must be individualized in each case. The dosage information which follows is derived from studies based upon units of drug per unit of body weight and is intended to serve as a guide only, especially regarding enhancement of neuromuscular blockade of Norcuron® by volatile anesthetics and by prior use of succinylcholine (see PRECAUTIONS/Drug Interactions). Parenteral drug products should be inspected visually for particulate matter and discoloration prior to administration, whenever solution and container permit.

To obtain maximum clinical benefits of Norcuron® and to minimize the possibility of overdosage, the monitoring of muscle twitch response to peripheral nerve stimulation is advised.

The recommended initial dose of Norcuron® is 0.08 to 0.1 mg/kg (1.4 to 1.75 times the ED_{90}) given as intravenous bolus injection. This dose can be expected to produce good or excellent non-emergency intubation conditions in 2.5 to 3 minutes after injection. Under balanced anesthesia, clinically required neuromuscular blockade lasts approximately 25–30 minutes, with recovery to 25% of control achieved approximately 25 to 40 minutes after injection and recovery to 95% of control achieved approximately 45–65 minutes after injection. In the presence of potent inhalation anesthetics, the neuromuscular blocking effect of Norcuron® is enhanced. If Norcuron® is first administered more than 5 minutes after the start of inhalation agent or when steady state has been achieved, the initial Norcuron® dose may be reduced by approximately 15%, i.e., 0.06 to 0.085 mg/kg.

Prior administration of succinylcholine may enhance the neuromuscular blocking effect and duration of action of Norcuron®. If intubation is performed using succinylcholine, a reduction of initial dose of Norcuron® to 0.04–0.06 mg/kg with inhalation anesthesia and 0.05–0.06 mg/kg with balanced anesthesia may be required.

During prolonged surgical procedures, maintenance doses of 0.01 to 0.015 mg/kg of Norcuron® are recommended; after the initial Norcuron® injection, the first maintenance dose will generally be required within 25 to 40 minutes. However, clinical criteria should be used to determine the need for maintenance doses. Since Norcuron® lacks clinically important cumulative effects, subsequent maintenance doses, if required, may be administered at relatively regular intervals for each patient, ranging approximately from 12 to 15 minutes under balanced anesthesia, slightly longer under inhalation agents. (If less frequent administration is desired, higher maintenance doses may be administered.)

Should there be reason for the selection of larger doses in individual patients, initial doses ranging from 0.15 mg/kg up to 0.28 mg/kg have been administered during surgery under halothane anesthesia without ill effects to the cardiovascular system being noted as long as ventilation is properly maintained (see CLINICAL PHARMACOLOGY).

Dosage in Children: Older children (10 to 17 years of age) have approximately the same dosage requirements (mg/kg) as adults and may be managed the same way. Younger children (1 to 10 years of age) may require a slightly higher initial dose and may also require supplementation slightly more often than adults. Infants under one year of age but older than 7 weeks are moderately more sensitive to Norcuron® on a mg/kg basis than adults and take about $1\frac{1}{2}$ times as long to recover. See also subsection of PRECAUTIONS titled Pediatric Use. Information presently available does not permit recommendation on usage in neonates (see PRECAUTIONS).

Compatibility: Norcuron® is compatible in solution with:
0.9% NaCl solution   5% glucose in saline
5% glucose in water   Lactated Ringers
How Supplied: 5 ml vials (contains 10 mg of active ingredient) and 5 ml ampul of preservative-free sterile water for injection as the diluent. Boxes of 12. NDC #0052-0442-10
Storage: PROTECT FROM LIGHT Store at 15°–30°C (59°–86°F)
After Reconstitution: Solution may be stored in refrigerator or kept at room temperature not to exceed 30°C (86°F) DISCARD SOLUTION AFTER 24 HOURS.
DISCARD UNUSED PORTION.
SINGLE USE VIALS
Manufactured for ORGANON INC.
By BEN VENUE LABORATORIES, INC.
Bedford, Ohio 44146

ORGATRAX® R
(Hydroxyzine Hydrochloride Injection, USP)

How Supplied:
Vials 10 ml (50 mg/ml)
Vials 25 × 2 ml (50 gm/ml)

PAVULON® R
[păv-u-lon]
(pancuronium bromide injection)

THIS DRUG SHOULD ONLY BE ADMINISTERED BY ADEQUATELY TRAINED INDIVIDUALS FAMILIAR WITH ITS ACTIONS, CHARACTERISTICS, AND HAZARDS.

Description: Pavulon (pancuronium bromide injection) is the aminosteroid 2 beta, 16 beta-dipiperidine-5 alpha-androstane-3 alpha, 17-beta-diol diacetate dimethobromide. It has the following structural formula:

Actions: Pavulon is a non-depolarizing neuromuscular blocking agent possessing all of the characteristic pharmacological actions of this class of drugs (curariform) on the myoneural junction. Pavulon is approximately 5 times as potent as d-tubocurarine chloride.
The onset and duration of action of Pavulon is dose dependent. With the administration of 0.04 mg. per kg. the onset of action, as measured by a peripheral nerve stimulator, is usually within 45 seconds, and its peak effect is usually within $4\frac{1}{2}$ minutes; recovery to 90% of control twitch height usually takes place in less than one hour. Larger doses, more suitable for endotracheal intubation, such as 0.08 mg. per kg. of Pavulon have an onset of action of about 30 seconds, and a peak effect within 3 minutes. Supplemental incremental doses of Pavulon, following the initial dose, slightly increase the magnitude of blockade, and significantly increase the duration of the blockade. Pavulon has little effect upon the circulatory system. The most frequently reported observation is a slight rise in pulse rate.
Human histamine assays, and clinical observations, as well as in *vivo* guinea pig testing, and in *vitro* mast cell testing, indicate that histamine release rarely, if ever, occurs.
Pavulon (pancuronium bromide injection) is antagonized by acetylcholine, anticholinesterases, and potassium ion. Its action is increased by inhalational anesthetics such as halothane, diethyl ether, enflurane and methoxyflurane, as well as by quinine, magnesium salts, hypokalemia, some carcinomas, and certain antibiotics such as neomycin, streptomycin, kanamycin, gentamicin and bacitracin. The action of Pavulon may be altered by dehydration, electrolyte imbalance, acid-base imbalance, renal disease, and concomitant administration of other neuromuscular agents.
Pavulon has no known effect on consciousness, the pain threshold, or cerebration.
Indications: Pavulon is indicated as an adjunct to anesthesia to induce skeletal muscle relaxation. It may also be employed to facilitate the management of patients undergoing mechanical ventilation.
Contraindications: Pavulon is contraindicated in patients known to be hypersensitive to the drug or to the bromide ion.
Warnings: PAVULON SHOULD BE ADMINISTERED IN CAREFULLY ADJUSTED DOSAGE BY OR UNDER THE SUPERVISION OF EXPERIENCED CLINICIANS, WHO ARE FAMILIAR WITH ITS ACTIONS AND THE POSSIBLE COMPLICATIONS THAT MIGHT OCCUR FOLLOWING ITS USE. THE DRUG SHOULD NOT BE ADMINISTERED UNLESS FACILITIES FOR INTUBATION, ARTIFICIAL RESPIRATION, OXYGEN THERAPY, AND REVERSAL AGENTS ARE IMMEDIATELY AVAILABLE. THE CLINICIAN MUST BE PREPARED TO ASSIST OR CONTROL RESPIRATION.
In patients who are known to have myasthenia gravis small doses of Pavulon may have profound effects. A peripheral nerve stimulator is especially valuable in assessing the effects of Pavulon in such patients.
Usage in Pregnancy: The safe use of pancuronium bromide has not been established with respect to the possible adverse effects upon fetal development. Therefore, it should not be used in women of childbearing potential and particularly during early pregnancy unless in the judgment of the physician the potential benefits outweigh the unknown hazards.
Pavulon may be used in operative obstetrics (Cesarean section), but reversal of pancuronium may be unsatisfactory in patients receiving magnesium sulfate for toxemia of pregnancy, because magnesium salts enhance neuromuscular blockade. Dosage should usually be reduced, as indicated, in such cases.
Precautions: Although Pavulon has been used successfully in many patients with pre-existing pulmonary, hepatic, or renal disease, caution should be exercised in these situations. This is particularly true of renal disease since a major portion of administered Pavulon is excreted unchanged in the urine.
Adverse Reactions: Neuromuscular: the most frequently noted adverse reactions consist primarily of an extension of the drug's pharmacological actions beyond the time period needed for surgery and anesthesia. This may vary from skeletal muscle weakness to profound and prolonged skeletal muscle relaxation resulting in respiratory insufficiency or apnea. Inadequate reversal of the neuromuscular blockade by anticholinesterase agents has also been observed with Pavulon (pancuronium bromide injection) as with all curariform drugs. These adverse reactions are managed by manual or mechanical ventilation until recovery is judged adequate.
Cardiovascular: A slight increase in pulse rate is frequently noted.
Gastrointestinal: Salivation is sometimes noted during very light anesthesia, especially if no anticholinergic premedication is used.
Skin: An occasional transient rash is noted accompanying the use of Pavulon.
Respiratory: One case of wheezing, responding to deepening of the inhalational anesthetic, has been reported.
Drug Interaction: The intensity of blockade and duration of action of Pavulon is increased in patients receiving potent volatile inhalational anesthetics such as halothane, diethyl ether, enflurane and methoxyflurane. No increase in intensity of blockade or duration of action of Pavulon is noted from the use of thiobarbiturates, narcotic analgesics, nitrous oxide, or droperidol.
Prior administration of succinylcholine, such as that used for endotracheal intubation, enhances the relaxant effect of Pavulon and the duration of action. If succinylcholine is used before Pavulon, the administration of Pavulon should be delayed until the succinylcholine shows signs of wearing off.
Dosage and Administration: Pavulon should be administered only by or under the supervision of experienced clinicians. DOSAGE MUST BE INDIVIDUALIZED IN EACH CASE. The dosage information which follows has been derived from dose-response studies based on body weight and is intended to serve as a guide only. Since potent inhalational agents or prior administration of succinylcholine enhance the intensity of blockade and duration of Pavulon (see DRUG INTERACTION), these factors should be taken into consideration in selection of initial and incremental dosage.
In adults the initial intravenous dosage range is 0.04 to 0.1 mg. per kg. Later incremental doses starting at 0.01 mg. per kg. may be used. These increments slightly increase the magnitude of the blockade, and significantly increase the duration of blockade, because a significant number of myoneural junctions are still blocked when there is clinical need for more drug.
If Pavulon is used to provide skeletal muscle relaxation for endotracheal intubation, doses of 0.06 to 0.1 mg. per kg. are recommended. Conditions satisfactory for intubation are usually present within 2 to 3 minutes. The ability of the anesthetist to intubate with Pavulon (pancuronium bromide injection) improves with experience.
Dosage in Children: Dose response studies in children indicate that, with the exception of neonates, dosage requirements are the same as for adults. Neonates are especially sensitive to non-depolarizing neuromuscular blocking agents, such as Pavulon, (pancuronium bromide injection) during the first month of life. It is recommended that a test dose of 0.02 mg. per kg. be given first in this group to measure responsiveness.
Cesarean Section: The dosage to provide relaxation for intubation and operation is the same as for general surgical procedures. The dosage to provide relaxation, following usage of succinylcholine for intubation (see DRUG INTERACTION), is the same as for general surgical procedures.
Management of Prolonged Neuromuscular Blockade: Residual neuromuscular blockade beyond the time period needed for surgery and anesthesia may occur with Pavulon as with other neuromuscular blockers. This may be manifested by skeletal muscle weakness, decreased respiratory reserve, low tidal volume or apnea. A peripheral nerve stimulator may be used to assess the degree of residual neuromuscular blockade. Under such circumstances the primary treatment is manual or mechanical ventilation and maintenance of a patent airway until complete recovery of normal respiration is assured. Regonol (pyridostigmine bromide injection) or neostigmine, in conjunction with atropine, will usually antagonize the skeletal muscle relaxant action of Pavulon. These should be accompanied by or preceded by injection of atropine sulfate to minimize the incidence of cholinergic side effects, notably excessive secretions and bradycardia. Satisfactory reversal can be judged by adequacy of skeletal muscle tone, and by adequacy of respiration. A peripheral nerve stimula-

Continued on next page

Organon—Cont.

tor may also be used to monitor restoration of twitch height. Failure of prompt reversal (within 30 minutes) may occur in the presence of extreme debilitation, carcinomatosis, and with concomitant use of certain broad spectrum antibiotics, or anesthetic agents and adjuncts which enhance neuromuscular blockade or cause respiratory depression of their own. Under such circumstances the management is the same as that of prolonged neuromuscular blockade; ventilation must be supported by artificial means until the patient has resumed control of his respiration. Prior to the use of reversal agents, reference to the specific package insert of the reversal agents should be made.

How Supplied:
2 ml. ampuls—2 mg./ml.—boxes of 25 NDC 0052-0444-26
5 ml. ampuls—2 mg./ml.—boxes of 25 NDC 0052-0444-25
10 ml. vials—1 mg./ml.—boxes of 25 NDC 0052-0443-25

PREGNYL®
(Chorionic Gonadotropin For Injection U.S.P.)

Description: Human chorionic gonadotropin (HCG), a polypeptide hormone produced by the human placenta, is composed of an alpha and a beta sub-unit. The alpha sub-unit is essentially identical to the alpha sub-units of the human pituitary gonadotropins, luteinizing hormone (LH) and follicle-stimulating hormone (FSH), as well as to the alpha sub-unit of human thyroid-stimulating hormone (TSH). The beta sub-units of these hormones differ in amino acid sequence. Chorionic Gonadotropin is derived from the urine of pregnant women. It is standardized by a biological assay procedure.

Clinical Pharmacology: The action of HCG is virtually identical to that of pituitary LH although HCG appears to have a small degree of FSH activity as well. It stimulates production of gonadal steroid hormones by stimulating the interstitial cells (Leydig cells) of the testis to produce androgens and the corpus luteum of the ovary to produce progesterone. Androgen stimulations in the male leads to the development of secondary sex characteristics and may stimulate testicular descent when no anatomical impediment to descent is present. This descent is usually reversible when HCG is discontinued. During the normal menstrual cycle, LH participates with FSH in the development and maturation of the normal ovarian follicle and the mid-cyclew LH surge triggers ovulation. HCG can substitute for LH in this function. During a normal pregnancy, HCG is secreted by the placenta maintains the corpus luteum after LH secretion decreases, supporting continued secretion of estrogen and progesterone and preventing menstruation. HCG HAS NO KNOWN EFFECT ON FAT MOBILIZATION, APPETITE OR SENSE OF HUNGER, OR BODY FAT DISTRIBUTION.

Indications: HCG HAS NOT BEEN DEMONSTRATED TO BE EFFECTIVE ADJUNCTIVE THERAPY IN THE TREATMENT OF OBESITY THERE IS NO SUBSTANTIAL EVIDENCE THAT IT INCREASES WEIGHT LOSS BEYOND THAT RESULTING FROM CALORIC RESTRICTION THAT IT CAUSES A MORE ATTRACTIVE OR "NORMAL" DISTRIBUTION OF FAT, OR THAT IT DECREASES THE HUNGER AND DISCOMFORT ASSOCIATED WITH CALORIE-RESTRICTED DIETS.

1. Prepubertal cryptorchidism not due to anatomical obstruction in general, HCG is thought to induce testicular descent in situations when descent would have occurred at puberty. HCG thus may help predict whether or not orchiopexy will be needed in the future. Although in some cases, descent following HCG administration is permanent in most cases, the response is temporary. Therapy is usually instituted between the ages 4 and 9.

2. Selected cases of hypogonadotropic hypogonadism (hypogonadism secondary to a pituitary deficiency) in males.
3. Induction of ovulation and pregnancy in the anovulatory, infertile woman in whom the cause of anovulation is secondary and not due to primary ovarian failure and who has been appropiately pretreated with human menotropins.

Contraindications: Precocious puberty, prostatic carcinoma or other androgen-dependent neoplasm, prior allergic reaction to HCG.

Warnings: HCG should be used in conjunction with human menopausal gonadotropins only by physicians experienced with infertility problems who are familiar with the criteria for patient selection, contraindication,, warning, precautions and adverse reactions described in the package insert for menotropins. The principal serious adverse reactions during this use are (1) Ovarian hyperstimulation a syndrome of sudden ovarian enlargement ascites with or without pain, and/or pleural effusion. (2) Rupture of ovarian cysts with resultant hemoperitoneum. (3) Multiple births, and (4) Arterial thromboembolism.

Precautions: Induction of androgen secretion by HCG may induce precocious puberty in patients treated for cryptorchidism. Therapy should be discontinued if signs of precocious puberty occur. Since androgens may cause fluid retention, HCG should be used with caution in patients with cardiac or renal disease, epilepsy, migrane, or asthma.

Adverse Reactions: Headache, irritability, restlessness, despression, fatigue, edema, precocious puberty, gynecomastia, pain at the site of injection.

Dosage and Administration: (Intramuscular Use Only): The dosage regimen employed in any particular case will depend upon the indication for use, the age and weight of the patient, and the physicians preference. The following regimens have been advocated by various authorities.

Prepubertal crylorchidism not due to anatomical obstruction.
1 4,000 U.S.P. Units three times, weekly for three weeks
2 5,000 U.S.P. Units every second day for four injections
3 15 injections of 500 to 1,000 U.S.P. Units over a period of six weeks
4 500 U.S.P. Units three times weekly for four to six weeks. If this course of treatment is not successful, another is begun one month later giving 1,000 U.S.P. Units per injection.

Selected cases of hypogonadotropic hypogonadism in males
1 500 to 1,000 U.S.P. Units three times a week for three weeks, followed by the same dose twice a week for three weeks.
2 4,000 U.S.P. Units three times weekly for six to nine months, following which the dosage my be reduced to 2,000 U.S.P. Units three times weekly for an additional three months.

Induction ov ovulation and pregnancy in the anovulatory infertile woman in whom the cause of anovulation is secondary and not due to primary ovarian failure and who has been approximately pre-treated with human menotropins. (See prescribing information for menotropins for dosage and administration for that drug product. 5,000 to 10,000 U.S.P. Units one day following the last dose of menotropins. (A dosage of 10,000 U.S.P. Units is recommended in the labeling for menotropins).

IMPORTANT USE COMPLETELY WITHIN 60 DAYS AFTER RECONSTITUTION REFRIGERATE AFTER RECONSTITUTION

How Supplied: The freeze-dried stabilized active principle is supplied in a two vial package including Bacterostatic Water for Injection as diluent

When reconstituted, each vial contains in U.S.P. Units:

VIAL SIZE	10 ml
Chorionic Gonadotropin	10,000 U.
Mannitol, U.S.P.	100 mg.
Benzyl Alcohol, N F	0.9%

with Sodium Phosphate Dibasic and Sodium Phosphate Monobasic to adjust pH.

The product is assayed in accord with the U.S.P. method and potencies refer to U.S.P. Units (International Units) defined in terms of the U.S.P. Chorionic Gonadotropin Reference Standard

Caution: Federal (USA) law prohibits dispensing without prescription.

Directions For Reconstitution: TWO-VIAL PACKAGE: withdraw sterile air from lyophilized vial and inject into diluent vial. Remove 10 ml from diluent and add to lyophilized vial, agitate gently until solution is complete.

Refrigerate after reconstitution and use within 60 days.

REGONOL®
[re-gō-nol]
(pyridostigmine bromide injection USP)

Description: Regonol (pyridostigmine bromide injection, USP) is an active cholinesterase inhibitor. Chemically, pyridostigmine bromide is 3-hydroxy-1-methylpyridinium bromide dimethylcarbamate. Its structural formula is:

Each ml. contains 5 mg. of pyridostigmine bromide compounded with 1% benzyl alcohol as the preservative. The pH is buffered with sodium citrate and citric acid and adjusted with sodium hydroxide if necessary.

Actions: Pyridostigmine bromide facilitates the transmission of impulses across the myoneural junction by inhibiting the destruction of acetylcholine by cholinesterase. Pyridostigmine is an analog of neostigmine but differs from it clinically by having fewer side effects. Currently available data indicate that pyridostigmine may have a significantly lower degree and incidence of bradycardia, salivation and gastrointestinal stimulation. Animal studies using the injectable form of pyridostigmine and human studies using the oral preparation have indicated that pyridostigmine has a longer duration of action than does neostigmine measured under similar circumstances.

Indications: Pyridostigmine bromide is useful as a reversal agent or antagonist to nondepolarizing muscle relaxants.

Contraindications: Known hypersensitivity to anticholinesterase agents; intestinal and urinary obstructions of mechanical type.

Warnings: Pyridostigmine bromide should be used with particular caution in patients with bronchial asthma or cardiac dysrhythmias. Transient bradycardia may occur and be relieved by atropine sulfate. Atropine should also be used with caution in patients with cardiac dysrhythmias. When large doses of pyridostigmine bromide are administered, as during reversal of muscle relaxants, prior or simultaneous injection of atropine sulfate is advisable. Because of the possibility of hypersensitivity in an occasional patient, atropine and antishock medication should always be readily available.

When used as an antagonist to nondepolarizing muscle relaxants, adequate recovery of voluntary respiration and neuromuscular transmission must be obtained prior to discontinuation of respiratory assistance and there should be continuous patient observation. Satisfactory recovery may be defined by a combination of clinical judgement, respiratory measurements and observation of the effects of peripheral nerve stimulation. If there is any doubt concerning the adequacy of recovery from the effects of the nondepolarizing muscle relaxant, artificial ventilation should be continued until all doubt has been removed.

Use in Pregnancy—The safety of pyridostigmine bromide during pregnancy or lactation in humans has not been established. Therefore its use in women who are pregnant requires weighing the drug's potential benefits against its possible hazards to mother and child.

Adverse Reactions: The side effects of pyridostigmine bromide are most commonly related to overdosage and generally are of two varieties, muscarinic and nicotinic. Among those in the former group are nausea, vomiting, diarrhea, abdominal cramps, increased peristalsis, increased salivation, increased bronchial secretions, miosis and diaphoresis. Nicotinic side effects are comprised chiefly of muscle cramps, fasciculation and weakness. Muscarinic side effects can usually be counteracted by atropine. As with any compound containing the bromide radical, a skin rash may be seen in an occasional patient. Such reactions usually subside promptly upon discontinuance of the medication. Thrombophlebitis has been reported subsequent to intravenous administration.

Dosage and Administration: When pyridostigmine bromide is given intravenously to reverse the action of muscle relaxant drugs, it is recommended that atropine sulfate (0.6 to 1.2 mg.) or glycopyrrolate in equipotent doses be given intravenously immediately prior to or simultaneous with its administration. Side effects, notably excessive secretions and bradycardia are thereby minimized. Reversal dosages range from 0.1 - 0.25 mg/kg. Usually 10 to 20 mg. of pyridostigmine bromide will be sufficient for antagonism of the effects of the nondepolarizing muscle relaxants. Although full recovery may occur within 15 minutes in most patients, others may require a half hour or more. Satisfactory reversal can be evident by adequate voluntary respiration, respiratory measurements and use of a peripheral nerve stimulator device. It is recommended that the patient be well ventilated and a patent airway maintained until complete recovery of normal respiration is assured. Once satisfactory reversal has been attained, recurarization has not been reported.

Failure of pyridostigmine bromide to provide prompt (within 30 minutes) reversal may occur, e.g. in the presence of extreme debilitation, carcinomatosis, or with concomitant use of certain broad spectrum antibiotics or anesthetic agents, notably ether. Under these circumstances ventilation must be supported by artificial means until the patient has resumed control of his respiration.

How Supplied: Regonol is available in:
5 mg./ml.: 2 ml. ampuls—boxes of 25—NDC-0052-0460-02
5mg/ml, 5 ml. vials—boxes of 25—NDC-0052-0460-05
Protect from light.

WIGRAINE® Tablets and Suppositories ℞
WIGRAINE®-PB Suppositories ℞

Description: Wigraine Tablet: Each tablet contains the following:
Ergotamine tartrate, USP ....1 mg
Caffeine, USP...100 mg
Wigraine tablets are uncoated and prepared to insure rapid disintegration (by an exclusive manufacturing process) and facilitate quick absorption. Rapid onset of effect is important for the satisfactory treatment of acute attacks of vascular headaches.
Wigraine Suppository: Each suppository contains the following:
Ergotamine tartrate, USP ....2 mg
Caffeine, USP...100 mg
Tartaric Acid..21.5 mg
Wigraine suppositories contain the active ingredients in a synthetic cocoa butter base which melts rapidly at room temperature.
Wigraine-PB Suppositories: Each suppository contains the following:
Ergotamine Tartrate, USP.............................2 mg
Caffeine, USP...100 mg
Belladonna Alkaloids (Levorotatory).........0.25 mg
Pentobarbital, USP.......................................60 mg
(Warning: May be habit forming)
Wigraine-PB Suppositories are sealed in foil to afford protection from cocoa butter leakage. If exposure to heat softens the suppository, it should be chilled in ice-cold water to re-solidify it before removing the foil.

Clinical Pharmacology: Ergotamine is an alpha adrenergic blocking agent with a direct stimulating effect on the smooth muscle of peripheral and cranial blood vessels and produces depression of central vasomotor centers. The compound also has the properties of serotonin antagonism. In comparison to hydrogenated ergotamine, the adrenergic blocking actions are less pronounced and vasoconstrictive actions are greater.

Caffeine, also a cranial vasoconstrictor, is added to further enhance the vasoconstrictive effect without the necessity of increasing ergotamine dosage. For individuals experiencing excessive nausea and vomiting during migraine attacks the further addition of the anticholinergic and antiemetic alkaloids of belladonna and pentobarbital for reduction of nervous tension has been provided.

Many migraine patients experience excessive nausea and vomiting during attacks, making it impossible for them to retain any oral medication. In such cases, therefore, the only practical means of medication is through the rectal route, where medication may reach the cranial vessels directly, evading the splanchnic vasculature and the liver.

Indications:
Wigraine—Indicated as therapy to abort or prevent vascular headaches such as migraine, migraine variants, or so-called histamine cephalalgia.
Wigraine-PB—Indicated as therapy to abort or prevent vascular headache complicated by tension and gastrointestinal disturbances.

Contraindications: Wigraine can cause fetal harm when administered to a pregnant women. It can produce prolonged uterine contractions which can result in abortion. Wigraine is contraindicated in women who are or may become pregnant. If this drug is used during pregnancy or if the patient becomes pregnant while taking this drug, the patient should be advised of the potential hazard to the fetus.

Peripheral vascular disease, coronary heart disease, hypertension, impaired hepatic or renal function, sepsis, and hypersensitivity to any of the components.

Precautions: Although signs and symptoms of ergotism rarely develop even after long term intermittent use of the orally or rectally administered drugs, care should be exercised to remain within the limits of recommended dosage.

Pregnancy Category X. See Contraindications section.

Nursing Mothers. It is not known whether the ergotamine tartrate in Wigraine is excreted in human milk. Because some ergot alkoids have been found in the milk of nursing mothers resulting in symptoms of ergotism in their children, a decision should be made whether to discontinue nursing or to discontinue the drug, taking into account the importance of the drug to the mother.

Pediatric Usage. Safety and effectiveness in children have not been established.

Adverse Reactions: Vasoconstrictive complications, at times of a serious nature, may occur. These include pulselessness, weakness, muscle pains and paresthesias of the extremities and precordial distress and pain. Although these effects occur most commonly with long term therapy at relatively high doses, they have also been reported with short term or normal doses. Other adverse effects include transient tachycardia or bradycardia, nausea, vomiting, localized edema and itching. Drowsiness may occur with Wigraine-PB.

Dosage and Administration: Best results are obtained if the tablets and suppositories are administered at the first sign of an attack.
Wigraine Tablet: The average oral adult dose is 2 tablets at the start of a vascular headache (migraine) attack; followed by one additional tablet every half hour if needed, up to 6 tablets per attack. Total weekly dosage should not exceed 10 tablets.
Wigraine and Wigraine-PB Suppositories: Rectally—1 suppository at start of attack; second suppository after 1 hour, if needed for full relief (maximum two suppositories per attack, 5 per week).
Maximum Adult Dosage: Orally: Total dose for any one attack should not exceed six tablets. Rectally: Two suppositories is the maximum dose for an individual attack. Total weekly dosage should not exceed ten (10) tablets or five (5) suppositories. In carefully selected patients, with due consideration of maximum dosage recommendations, administration of the drug at bedtime may be an appropriate short-term preventative measure.

Overdosage: The toxic effects of an acute overdosage of Wigraine and Wigraine-PB are due primarily to the ergotamine component. The amount of caffeine is such that its toxic effects will be overshadowed by those of ergotamine. Symptoms include vomiting, numbness, tingling, pain and cyanosis of the extremities associated with diminished or absent peripheral pulses, hypertension or hypotension: drowsiness, stupor, coma, convulsions, and shock. A case has been reported of reversible bilateral papillitis with ring scotomata in a patient who received five times the recommended daily adult dose over a period of 14 days. Treatment consists of removal of the offending drug by induction of emesis, gastric lavage, and catharsis. Maintenance of adequate pulmonary ventilation, correction of hypotension and control of convulsions are important considerations. Treatment of peripheral vasospasm should consist of warmth, but not heat and protection of the ischemic limbs. Vasodilators may be used with benefit but caution must be exercised to avoid aggravating an already existent hypotension.

The LD_{50} limits of the various components as outlined in NIOSH 1978 Registry of Toxic Effects of Chemical Substances, published by U.S. Department of Health, Education, and Welfare are as follows: Ergotamine Tartrate IV LD_{50} in rats = 80mg/kg, Caffeine IV LD_{50} in rats = 105mg/kg.

How Supplied: Wigraine tablets are individually foil stripped and packaged in boxes of 20 NDC #0052-0542-20 and 100's NDC #0052-0542-91. Wigraine suppositories are individually foil wrapped and packaged in boxes of 12. NDC #0052-0548-12 Wigraine tablets should be stored at a maximum of 30°C (86°F) and the suppositories should be refrigerated at 2°-8°C (36°-46°F).

Wigraine-PB Suppositories are sealed in aluminum foil and packaged in boxes of 12, NDC #0052-0549-12. Store Below 77°F.

Wigraine tablets are manufactured by ORGANON INC., WEST ORANGE, NEW JERSEY 07052

Wigraine Suppositories and Wigraine-PB Suppositories are manufactured by G&W Laboratories, Inc., South Plainfield, New Jersey 07080 and distributed by ORGANON INC., WEST ORANGE, NEW JERSEY 07052

WIGRETTES® ℞
[wĭ-grets']
(ergotamine tartrate sublingual tablets)

Description: Each sublingual tablet contains 2 mg ergotamine tartrate.
Pharmacological Category: Vasoconstrictor, uterine stimulant, alpha adrenoreceptor antagonist.
Therapeutic Class: Anti-migraine.
Chemical Name: Ergotaman-3', 6', 18-trione, 12'-hydroxy - 2' - methyl - 5' - (phenyl-methyl)-, (5 α)-, [R-(R*, R*)]- 2,3 - dihydroxybutanedioate (2:1) tartrate.
Structural Formula:

Clinical Pharmacology: The pharmacological properties of ergotamine are extremely complex, some of its actions are unrelated to each other, and

Continued on next page

Organon—Cont.

even mutually antagonistic. The drug has partial agonist and/or antagonist activity against tryptaminergic, dopaminergic and alpha adrenergic receptors depending upon their site, and it is a highly active uterine stimulant. It causes constriction of peripheral and cranial blood vessels and produces depression of central vasomotor centers. The pain of a migraine attack is believed to be due to greatly increased amplitude of pulsations in the cranial arteries, especially the meningeal branches of the external carotid artery. Ergotamine reduces extracranial bloodflow, causes a decline in the amplitude of pulsation in the cranial arteries, and decreases hyperperfusion of the territory of the basilar artery. It does not reduce cerebral hemispheric blood flow. Long term usage has established the fact that ergotamine tartrate is effective in controlling up to 70% of acute migraine attacks, so that it is now considered specific for the treatment of this headache syndrome. Ergotamine produces constriction of both arteries and veins. In doses used in the treatment of vascular headaches, ergotamine usually produces only small increases in blood pressure, but it does increase peripheral resistance and decrease blood flow in various organs. Small doses of the drug increase the force and frequency of uterine contraction, larger doses increase the resting tone of the uterus also. The gravid uterus is particularly sensitive to these effects of ergotamine. Although specific teratogenic effects attributable to ergotamine have not been found, the fetus suffers if ergotamine is given to the mother. Retarded fetal growth and an increase in intrauterine death and resorption have been seen in animals. These are thought to result from ergotamine induced increases in uterine motility and vasoconstriction in the placental vascular bed.

The bioavailability of sublingually administered ergotamine has not been determined.

Ergotamine is metabolized by the liver by largely undefined pathways, and 90% of the metabolites are excreted in the bile. The unmetabolized drug is erratically secreted in the saliva, and only traces of unmetabolized drug appear in the urine and feces. Ergotamine is secreted into breast milk. The elimination half-life of ergotamine from plasma is about 2 hours, but the drug may be stored in some tissues, which would account for its long lasting therapeutic and toxic actions.

Indications and Usage: Ergotamine tartrate is indicated as therapy to abort or prevent vascular headache, e.g., migraine, migraine variants, or so called "histaminic cephalalgia."

Contraindications: Ergotamine is contraindicated in peripheral vascular disease, (thromboangiitis obliterans, luetic arteritis, severe arteriosclerosis, thrombophlebitis, Raynaud's disease), coronary heart disease, hypertension, impaired hepatic or renal function, severe pruritis, and sepsis. It is also contraindicated in patients who are hypersensitive to any of its components. Ergotamine may cause fetal harm when administered to a pregnant woman by virtue of its powerful uterine stimulant actions. It is contraindicated in women who are, or may become, pregnant.

Precautions:
General: Although signs and symptoms of ergotism rarely develop even after long term intermittent use of ergotamine, care should be exercised to remain within the limits of recommended dosage.

Drug Interactions: The effects of ergotamine tartrate may be potentiated by triacetyloleandomycin which inhibits the metabolism of ergotamine. The pressor effects of ergotamine and other vasoconstrictor drugs can combine to cause dangerous hypertension.

Carcinogenesis: No studies have been performed to investigate ergotamine tartrate for carcinogenic effects.

Pregnancy: Pregnancy Category X—See 'Contraindications' section.

Nursing Mothers: Ergotamine is secreted into human milk. It can reach the breast-fed infant by this route and exert pharmacologic effects in it. Caution should be exercised when ergotamine is administered to a nursing woman. Excessive dosing or prolonged administration of ergotamine may inhibit lactation.

Adverse Reactions: Nausea and vomiting occur in up to 10% of patients after ingestion of therapeutic doses or ergotamine. Weakness of the legs and pain in limb muscles are also frequently complaints. Numbness and tingling of the fingers and toes, precordial pain, transient changes in heart rate and localized edema and itching may also occur, particularly in patients who are sensitive to the drug.

Drug Abuse and Dependence: Patients who take ergotamine for extended periods of time may become dependent upon it and require progressively increasing doses for relief of vascular headaches, and for prevention of dysphoric effects which follow withdrawal of the drug.

Overdosage: Overdosage with ergotamine causes nausea, vomiting, weakness of the legs, pain in limb muscles, numbness and tingling of the fingers and toes, precordial pain, tachycardia or bradycardia, hypertension or hypotension and localized edema and itching together with signs and symptoms of ischemia due to vasoconstriction of peripheral arteries and arterioles. The feet and hands become cold, pale and numb. Muscle pain occurs while walking and later at rest also. Gangrene may ensue. Confusion, depression, drowsiness, and convulsions are occasional signs of ergotamine toxicity. Overdosage is particularly likely to occur in patients with sepsis or impaired renal or hepatic function. Patients with peripheral vascular disease are specially at risk of developing peripheral ischemia following treatment with ergotamine. Some cases of ergotamine poisoning have been reported in patients who have taken less than 5 mg of the drug. Usually however, toxicity is seen at doses of ergotamine tartrate in excess of about 15 mg in 24 hours or 40 mg in a few days.

Treatment of ergotamine overdosage consists of the withdrawal of the drug followed by symptomatic measures including attempts to maintain an adequate circulation in the affected parts. Anticoagulant drugs, low molecular weight dextran and potent vasodilator drugs may all be beneficial. Intravenous infusion of sodium nitroprusside has also been reported to be successful. Vasodilators must be used with special care in the presence of hypotension.

Nausea and vomiting may be relieved by atropine or antiemetic compounds of the phenothiazine group. Ergotamine is dialyzable.

Dosage and Administration: All efforts should be made to initiate therapy as soon as possible after the first symptoms of the attack are noted; since success is proportional to rapidity of treatment, lower dosages will be effective. At the first sign of an attack or to relieve symptoms after onset of an attack, one 2 mg tablet is placed under the tongue. Another tablet should be taken at half-hourly intervals thereafter, if necessary, but dosage must not exceed three tablets in any 24 hour period. Dosage should be limited to not more than five tablets (10 mg) in any one week.

How Supplied: Each Wigrettes® sublingual tablet (white) contains 2 mg of ergotamine tartrate. Wigrettes® are individually foiled, stripped and packaged in boxes of 24. NDC #0052-0547-24. Store at maximum of 30°C (86°F).

Shown in Product Identification Section, page 422

Products are cross-indexed by
generic and chemical names
in the
YELLOW SECTION

Ortho Diagnostic Systems Inc.
ROUTE 202
RARITAN, NEW JERSEY 08869

MICRhoGAM™ ℞
[mike'ro-gam]
Rh₀(D) Immune Globulin (Human) Micro-Dose
For Intramuscular Use Only

Micro-Dose for use *only* after spontaneous or induced abortion or termination of ectopic pregnancy up to and including 12 weeks gestation.

Description: MICRhoGAM Rh₀(D) Immune Globulin (Human) Micro-Dose is a sterile concentrated solution of specific immunoglobulin (lgG) containing anti-Rh₀(D) for intramuscular injection, prepared from fractionated human plasma (cold alcohol method). It may include immunoglobulin derived from a plasma fraction which does not contain anti-Rh₀(D) prepared by other licensed manufacturers. All plasma used in the manufacture of this product was tested for hepatitis B surface antigen by a licensed third generation test and found to be nonreactive.

Active Ingredient
Anti-Rh₀(D) in 15% ± 1.5% serum globulin
Inactive Ingredients
15 mg/ml glycine—approximately
2.9 mg/ml sodium chloride—approximately
Preservative: 0.01% thimerosal (mercury derivative)

Clinical Pharmacology: MICRhoGAM acts by suppressing the specific immune response of Rh negative individuals to Rh positive red blood cells. Exposure to Rh positive red blood cells can occur as a consequence of spontaneous or induced abortion or termination of ectopic pregnancy. The injection of Rh₀(D) antibody to an Rh negative mother suppresses the antibody response and the formation of anti-Rh₀(D). Prevention of isoimmunization by Rh positive red cells in susceptible females prevents hemolytic disease of the newborn in the subsequent pregnancy. The mechanism of action of MICRhoGAM is not fully understood; however, an immunostat hypothesis has been proposed.

The risk of isoimmunization is directly related to the number of Rh positive red cells to which the Rh negative individual is exposed. The risk was found to be three percent when 0.1 ml of fetal red blood cells are present in the mother and 65 percent when 5 ml are present. In the first 12 weeks of gestation the total volume of red cells in the fetus is estimated at less than 2.5 ml.

Clinical studies demonstrated that administration of MICRhoGAM within three (3) hours following abortion reduced the incidence of Rh isoimmunization from 12–13% to 1–2%. Additional studies in male volunteers showed MICRhoGAM to be effective when given as long as 72 hours after the infusion of Rh positive red cells. A lesser degree of protection is afforded if the antibody is administered beyond this time period.

Indications and Usage: MICRhoGAM is indicated for the prevention of isoimmunization in Rh negative women following spontaneous or induced abortion or termination of ectopic pregnancy up to and including 12 weeks gestation, unless the father is conclusively shown to be Rh negative.

Contraindications: MICRhoGAM should not be administered after 12 weeks gestation because it does not contain sufficient antibody to provide protection against the larger volume of fetal red cells that may be present in the second and third trimesters of pregnancy.

Warnings: None
Precautions: None
Adverse Reactions: Reactions of Rh negative individuals given Rh immune globulin are infrequent, of a mild nature and mostly confined to the area of injection.

Immune Serum Globulin (Human) prepared from plasma negative for HBsAg by third generation tests has not been reported to transmit hepatitis.

Dosage and Administration: One vial of MICRhoGAM will completely suppress the im-

mune response to 2.5 ml of Rh positive red blood cells (packed cells, not whole blood).
Administer one vial of MICRhoGAM intramuscularly as soon as possible after termination of a pregnancy up to and including 12 weeks gestation. At or beyond 13 weeks gestation it is recommended that one vial of RhoGAM™ Rh$_o$(D) Immune Globulin (Human) be given instead of MICRhoGAM.

How Supplied: MICRhoGAM is supplied in a package containing:
- one single-dose vial of MICRhoGAM
- package insert
- control form
- patient identification card

MICRhoGAM is also supplied in a package containing:
- 50 single-dose vials of MICRhoGAM
- package insert
- 50 control forms
- 50 patient identification cards

Storage: Store at 2° to 8°C. DO NOT FREEZE.

RhoGAM™
[ro'gam]
Rh$_o$ (D) Immune Globulin (Human)
For Intramuscular Use Only

Description: RhoGAM Rh$_o$(D) Immune Globulin (Human) is a sterile concentrated solution of specific immunoglobulin (IgG) containing anti-Rh$_o$(D) for intramuscular injection, prepared from fractionated human plasma (cold alcohol method). It may include immunoglobulin derived from a plasma fraction which does not contain anti-Rh$_o$(D) prepared by other licensed manufacturers. All plasma used in the manufacture of this product was tested for hepatitis B surface antigen by a licensed third generation test and found to be nonreactive.

Active Ingredient
Anti-Rh$_o$(D) in 15% ± 1.5% serum globulin

Inactive Ingredients—
15 mg/ml glycine—approximately
2.9 mg/ml sodium chloride—approximately
Preservative: 0.01% thimerosal (mercury derivative)

Clinical Pharmacology: RhoGAM acts by suppressing the specific immune response of Rh negative individuals to Rh positive red blood cells. Exposure to Rh positive red blood cells can occur as a consequence of pregnancy, abortion or delivery or transfusion of an Rh negative recipient with Rh positive red blood cells. Prevention of isoimmunization by Rh positive red cells in susceptible females who may have Rh positive babies prevents hemolytic disease of the newborn. The injection of Rh$_o$(D) antibody to an Rh negative mother or to the Rh negative recipient of Rh positive red cells suppresses the antibody response and the formation of anti-Rh$_o$(D). The mechanism of action of RhoGAM is not fully understood; however, an immunostat hypothesis has been proposed.

The risk of isoimmunization is directly related to the number of Rh positive red cells to which the Rh negative individual is exposed. The risk was found to be three percent when 0.1 ml of fetal red blood cells are present in the mother and 65 percent when 5 ml are present.

Immunization of Rh negative women not previously exposed to Rh positive red cells occurs most frequently during the third stage of labor when fetal red cells enter the maternal circulation. However fetal-maternal hemorrhage has been noted as early as the second trimester of pregnancy and increases in size and frequency as gestation proceeds.

Clinical studies proved that administration of RhoGAM within 72 hours of delivery of a full-term infant reduced the incidence of Rh isoimmunization as a result of pregnancy from 12–13% to 1–2%. A lesser degree of protection is afforded if Rh antibody is administered beyond this time period. Data from Canada, Sweden and England indicate 1.5 to 1.8% of Rh negative women carrying Rh positive fetuses who are given Rh immune globulin postpartum may be immunized to Rh during the latter part of their pregnancies or following delivery. Bowman has reported that the incidence of immunization can be further reduced from approximately 1.6% to less than 0.1% by administering Rh immune globulin in two doses, one antepartum at 28 weeks gestation and another following delivery.

Abortion, either spontaneous or induced, and amniocentesis may cause fetal-maternal hemorrhage. The number of Rh negative women immunized to Rh has been reduced by administering Rh immune globulin following these procedures. Similarly, immunization resulting in the production of anti-Rh$_o$(D) following transfusion of Rh positive red cells to an Rh negative recipient may be prevented by administering Rh immune globulin.

Indications and Usage: RhoGAM is indicated for the prevention of isoimmunization in Rh negative individuals exposed to Rh positive red cells.

Pregnancy
1. RhoGAM is unequivocally indicated postpartum for an unsensitized Rh negative woman delivering an Rh$_o$(D) positive or D^u positive baby. If the Rh type of the baby cannot be determined, it should be presumed to be Rh positive. If RhoGAM is administered antepartum, it is essential that the mother receive another dose of RhoGAM after delivering an Rh$_o$(D) positive or D^u positive infant.
2. RhoGAM is indicated for an Rh negative woman after abortion or ectopic pregnancy unless the products of conception or the father are conclusively shown to be Rh negative.
3. Amniocentesis and other abdominal trauma resulting in fetal cells entering the maternal circulation are indications for RhoGAM.

Transfusion
RhoGAM may be indicated following transfusion of an Rh negative, premenopausal female with Rh positive red cells or whole blood, or components such as platelets or granulocytes prepared from Rh positive blood.

Contraindications: None known.

Warnings: Babies born of women given Rh immune globulin antepartum may have a weakly positive direct Coombs test at birth. Passively acquired anti-Rh$_o$(D) may be detected in maternal serum if antibody screening tests are performed subsequent to antepartum or postpartum administration of Rh immune globulin.

Precautions: The presence of fetal cells in a maternal blood sample or passive antibody given to the mother antepartum can affect the interpretation of laboratory tests to identify and monitor the candidate for RhoGAM. In case of doubt as to the patient's Rh type or immune status, RhoGAM should be administered.

Adverse Reactions: Reactions of Rh negative individuals given Rh immune globulin are infrequent, of a mild nature and mostly confined to the area of injection. An occasional patient may react more strongly both locally and generally. A slight elevation of temperature has been noted in a small number of postpartum women. There is no evidence that the safety of the fetus is jeopardized by the administration of RhoGAM antepartum.

Following mismatched transfusions and injection of several vials of RhoGAM, approximately five out of 22 subjects noted fever, myalgia and lethargy. Bilirubin levels of 0.4–6.8 mg% were observed in some of the treated subjects and one had splenomegaly. Systemic reactions are rare and sensitization due to repeated injection of immune globulins is unusual. Immune Serum Globulin (Human) prepared from plasma negative for HBsAg by third generation tests has not been reported to transmit hepatitis.

Dosage and Administration: One vial of RhoGAM will completely suppress the immune response to 15 ml of Rh positive red blood cells (packed cells, not whole blood).

Pregnancy
1. For postpartum prophylaxis, administer one vial of RhoGAM intramuscularly, preferably within three days of delivery. If an unusually large fetal-maternal hemorrhage is suspected, an approved laboratory procedure such as the Kleihauer-Betke technique should be used to estimate the volume of Rh positive red cells in the maternal circulation. The number of vials of RhoGAM to be given can be determined by dividing the volume of Rh positive red cells by 15.
2. For antepartum prophylaxis, one vial of RhoGAM is administered intramuscularly at approximately 28 weeks. This *must* be followed by another full dose (one vial) preferably within three days following delivery, if the infant is Rh positive.
3. Following amniocentesis, miscarriage, abortion, or ectopic pregnancy at or beyond the thirteenth week of gestation, it is recommended that one vial of RhoGAM be given. (If the products of conception are passed or removed prior to the thirteenth week of gestation, one vial of MICRhoGAM™ Rh$_o$(D) Immune Globulin (Human) Micro-Dose may be used instead of RhoGAM.)

Transfusion
Rh Positive Red Cells to an Rh Negative Recipient. RhoGAM may be administered intramuscularly to prevent isoimmunization in eligible Rh negative premenopausal females who receive Rh positive red cells by transfusion, whether inadvertently or in association with leukocyte or platelet therapy. One vial protects against each 15 ml of transfused red cells.

How Supplied: RhoGAM is supplied in packages containing:
- one single-dose vial of RhoGAM
- package insert
- control form
- patient identification card
  and
- 25 single-dose vials of RhoGAM
- package insert
- 25 control forms
- 25 patient identification cards
  and
- 72 single-dose vials of RhoGAM
- package insert
- 75 control forms
- 75 patient identification cards
  and
- six vials each containing a single dose of RhoGAM
- package insert
- suggested office protocol
- six injection records
- six patient information booklets
- six patient identification cards
- six labels for patient's chart

Storage: Store at 2° to 8° C. DO NOT FREEZE.

Ortho Pharmaceutical Corporation
RARITAN, NJ 08869

ACI–JEL® Therapeutic Vaginal Jelly

Description: ACI-JEL Vaginal Jelly is a bland, non-irritating, water-dispersible, buffered acid jelly for intravaginal use. ACI-JEL is classified as a Vaginal Therapeutic Jelly. ACI-JEL contains 0.921% glacial acetic acid ($C_2H_4O_2$), 0.025% oxyquinoline sulfate ($C_{18}H_{16}N_2O_6S$), 0.7% ricinoleic acid ($C_{18}H_{34}O_3$), and 5% glycerin ($C_3H_8O_3$) compounded with tragacanth, acacia, propylparaben, potassium hydroxide, stannous chloride, egg albumen, potassium bitartrate, perfume and purified water. ACI-JEL is formulated to pH 3.9–4.1.

Clinical Pharmacology: ACI-JEL acts to restore and maintain normal vaginal acidity through its buffer action.

Indications and Usage: ACI-JEL is indicated as adjunctive therapy in those cases where restoration and maintenance of vaginal acidity are desirable.

Contraindications: None known.

Warnings: No serious adverse reactions or potential safety hazards have been reported with the use of ACI-JEL.

Continued on next page

Ortho Pharm.—Cont.

Precautions: *General:* No special care is required for the safe and effective use of ACI-JEL. *Drug Interactions:* No incidence of drug interactions have been reported with concomitant use of ACI-JEL and any other medications. *Laboratory Tests:* The monitoring of vaginal acidity (pH) may be helpful in following the patient's response. (The normal vaginal pH has been shown to be in the range of 4.0 to 5.0.) *Carcinogenesis:* No long-term studies in animals have been performed to evaluate carcinogenic potential. *Pregnancy:* Pregnancy Category C. Animal reproduction studies have not been conducted with ACI-JEL. It is also not known whether ACI-JEL can cause fetal harm when administered to a pregnant woman or can affect reproduction capacity. ACI-JEL should be given to a pregnant woman only if clearly needed. *Nursing Mothers:* It is not known whether this drug is excreted in human milk. Because many drugs are excreted in human milk, caution should be exercised when ACI-JEL is administered to a nursing woman.

Adverse Reactions: Occasional cases of local stinging and burning have been reported.

Dosage and Administration: The usual dose is one applicatorful, administered intravaginally, morning and evening. Duration of treatment may be determined by the patient's response to therapy.

How Supplied: 85g Tube with ORTHO® Measured-Dose Applicator.
NDC 0062-5421-01

CONCEPTROL® Birth Control Cream
(See PDR For Nonprescription Drugs)

CONCEPTROL® Contraceptive Gel Disposable
(See PDR For Nonprescription Drugs)

DELFEN® Contraceptive Foam
(See PDR For Nonprescription Drugs)

DIENESTROL Cream   R
(See ORTHO® Dienestrol Cream)

GYNOL II® Contraceptive Jelly
(See PDR For Nonprescription Drugs)

LIPPES LOOP®   R
Intrauterine Device

Description: The LIPPES LOOP is made of polyethylene in the shape of a double S. Four different sizes are manufactured to allow for the variability in the size of the uterus. (See below.) A fine, double thread or "tail" made of polyethylene suture (monofilament) is attached to the lower end to facilitate removal. In addition, palpation of the tail through the cervix by the patient, or visualization by the physician, can assist in determining whether or not an undetected expulsion has occurred. A LIPPES LOOP comes prepackaged and sterilized with an introducer, together with an insertion tube in a polyethylene pouch. The insertion tube is equipped with a flange to aid in gauging the depth to which the insertion tube should be inserted through the cervical canal and into the uterine cavity. The four available sizes are as follows:

Loop A—22.5 mm. Blue thread. For nulliparous females.
Loop B—27.5 mm. WITH REDUCED RADII. Black thread. Suggested for women who have had premature pregnancy losses and multiparous females whose uteri sound out less than 6 cm.
Loop C—30 mm. WITH REDUCED RADII. Yellow thread. Suggested for use when Loop D is removed for bleeding or pain. The physician is advised to wait two to four weeks between removing a loop for bleeding and reinserting a second loop.
Loop D—30 mm. White thread. Suggested for use in women with one or more children.

Mode of Action or Principles of IUD Design: The exact mechanism of action of the LIPPES LOOP is not known. However, it is believed to interfere in some manner with nidation in the endometrium, probably through foreign body reaction in the uterus.

Indications and Usage: LIPPES LOOP is indicated for contraception.

Contraindications: IUD's should not be inserted when the following conditions exist:
1. Pregnancy or suspicion of pregnancy.
2. Abnormalities of the uterus resulting in distortion of the uterine cavity.
3. Pelvic inflammatory disease or a history of repeated pelvic inflammatory disease.
4. Postpartum endometritis or infected abortion in the past three months.
5. Known or suspected uterine or cervical malignancy including unresolved, abnormal "Pap" smear.
6. Genital bleeding of unknown etiology.
7. Cervicitis until infection is controlled.

Warnings:
1. Pregnancy. a. Long-term effects. Long-term effects on the offspring when pregnancy occurs with LIPPES LOOP in place are unknown.
b. Septic abortion. Reports have indicated an increased incidence of septic abortion associated in some instances with septicemia, septic shock, and death in patients becoming pregnant with an IUD in place. Most of these reports have been associated with the mid-trimester of pregnancy. In some cases, the initial symptoms have been insidious and not easily recognized. If pregnancy should occur with an IUD in place, the IUD should be removed if the string is visible or, if removal proves to be or would be difficult, termination of the pregnancy should be considered and offered the patient as an option, bearing in mind that the risks associated with an elective abortion increase with gestational age.
c. Continuation of pregnancy. If the patient chooses to continue the pregnancy, she must be warned of the increased risk of spontaneous abortion and of the increased risk of sepsis, including death, if the pregnancy continues with the IUD in place. The patient must be closely observed and she must be advised to report all abnormal symptoms, such as flu-like syndrome, fever, abdominal cramping and pain, bleeding, or vaginal discharge, immediately because generalized symptoms of septicemia may be insidious.
2. Ectopic pregnancy. a. A pregnancy that occurs with an IUD in place is more likely to be ectopic than a pregnancy occuring without an IUD in place. Accordingly, patients who become pregnant while using the IUD should be carefully evaluated for the possibility of an ectopic pregnancy.
b. Special attention should be directed to patients with delayed menses, slight metrorrhagia and/or unilateral pelvic pain, and to those patients who wish to terminate a pregnancy because of IUD failure, to determine whether ectopic pregnancy has occurred.
3. Pelvic Infection. An increased risk of pelvic infection has been reported with the IUD in place. Although the etiology of this risk is not understood, it has been suggested that the tail may act as a mechanism for the passage of vaginal bacteria into the uterus. This, at times, may result in the development of bilateral or unilateral tubo-ovarian abscesses or general peritonitis which may lead to hospitalization or surgery and infertility. Appropriate aerobic and anaerobic bacteriological studies should be done and antibiotic therapy initiated. The IUD should be removed and the continuing treatment reassessed based upon the results of culture and sensitivity tests.
Because of the increased risk of pelvic infection, the physician may wish each woman who has an IUD in place to have a periodic cervical vaginal "Pap" smear and pelvic exam. All "Pap" smears should include specific evaluation for actinomycosis.
4. Embedment. Partial penetration or lodging of the IUD in the endometrium can result in difficult removals.
5. Perforation. Partial or total perforation of the uterine wall or cervix may occur with the use of IUDs. The possibility of perforation must be kept in mind during insertion and at the time of any subsequent examination. If perforation occurs, the IUD should be removed. Adhesions, foreign body reactions, and intestinal obstruction may result if an IUD is left in the peritoneal cavity. There are a few reports that there has been migration after insertion apparently in the absence of perforation at insertion. In any event, it is possible for the IUD to perforate outside the uterus.

Precautions:
1. Patient counseling. Prior to insertion, the physician, nurse, or other trained health professional must provide the patient with the Patient Brochure. The patient should be given the opportunity to read the brochure and discuss fully any questions she may have concerning the IUD as well as other methods of contraception.
2. Patient evaluation and clinical considerations. a. A complete medical history should be obtained to determine conditions that might influence the selection of an IUD. Physical examination should include a pelvic examination, "Pap" smear, gonorrhea culture and, if indicated, appropriate tests for other forms of venereal disease. Papanicolaou smears should include specific evaluation for actinomycosis.
b. The uterus should be carefully sounded prior to insertion to determine the degree of patency of the endocervical canal and the internal os, and the direction and depth of the uterine cavity. In occasional cases, severe cervical stenosis may be encountered. Do not use excessive force to overcome this resistance.
c. The uterus should sound to a depth of 6 to 8 centimeters (cm). Insertion of an IUD into a uterine cavity measuring less than 6.5 cm by sounding may increase the incidence of expulsion, bleeding, pain and perforation.
d. The possibility of insertion in the presence of an existing undetermined pregnancy is reduced if insertion is performed during or shortly following a menstrual period. The IUD should not be inserted postpartum or postabortion until involution of the uterus is completed. The incidence of perforation and expulsion is greater if involution is not completed.
e. IUD's should be used with caution in those patients who have anemia or a history of menorrhagia or hypermenorrhea. Patients experiencing menorrhagia and/or metrorrhagia following IUD insertion may be at risk for the development of hypochromic microcytic anemia. Also, IUD's should be used with caution in patients receiving anticoagulants or having a coagulopathy.
f. Syncope, bradycardia, or other neurovascular episodes may occur during insertion or removal of IUD's, especially in patients with a previous disposition to these conditions.
g. Patients with valvular or congenital heart disease are more prone to develop subacute bacterial endocarditis than patients who do not have valvular or congenital heart disease. Use of an IUD in these patients may represent a potential source of septic emboli.
h. Use of an IUD in those patients with cervicitis should be postponed until treatment has cured the infection (see CONTRAINDICATIONS Section).
i. Since an IUD may be expelled or displaced, patients should be reexamined and evaluated shortly after the first postinsertion menses, but definitely within three months after insertion. Thereafter, annual examination with appropriate medical and laboratory examination should be carried out.
j. The patient should be told that some bleeding and cramps may occur during the first few weeks after insertion, but if these symptoms continue or are severe, she should report them to her physician. The patient should be instructed on how to check to make certain that the thread still pro-

trudes from the cervix, and she should be cautioned that there is no contraceptive protection if the IUD is expelled. She should be instructed to check the tail as often as possible, but at least after each menstrual period. The patient should be cautioned not to pull on the thread and displace the IUD. If partial expulsion occurs, removal is indicated and a new IUD may be inserted.

k. The use of medical diathermy (shortwave and microwave) in patients with metal-containing IUD's may cause heat injury to the surrounding tissue. Therefore, medical diathermy to the abdominal and sacral areas should not be used. [LIPPES LOOP contains no metals. This section does not apply to LIPPES LOOP].

Adverse Reactions: These adverse reactions are not listed in any order of frequency or severity. Reported adverse reactions include: endometritis, spontaneous abortion, septic abortion, septicemia, perforation of the uterus and cervix, embedment, migration resulting in partial or complete perforation, fragmentation of the IUD, pelvic infection (pelvic inflammatory disease), vaginitis, leukorrhea, cervical erosion, pregnancy, ectopic pregnancy, difficult removal, complete or partial expulsion of the IUD, intermenstrual spotting, prolongation of menstrual flow, anemia, pain and cramping, dysmenorrhea, backaches, dyspareunia, neurovascular episodes, including bradycardia and syncope secondary to insertion. Perforation into the abdomen has been followed by abdominal adhesions, intestinal penetration, intestinal obstruction, and cystic masses in the pelvis.

Directions For Use:
Preinsertion

1. It is imperative that sterile technique be maintained throughout the insertion procedure.
2. Perform a thorough pelvic examination to determine freedom from overt disease and to determine position and shape of the uterus. RULE OUT PREGNANCY AND OTHER CONTRAINDICATIONS.
3. With a speculum in place, gently insert a sterile sound to determine the depth and direction of the uterine canal. Be sure to determine the position of the uterus before insertion.

Occasionally a tenaculum is required if the uterine canal needs to be straightened. If a stenotic cervix must be dilated, use a sterile Hank's dilator rather than a Hegar's; dilation to a Hank's 16 to 18 should be sufficient.

Insertion
Caution: It is generally felt that perforations are caused at the time of insertion, although the perforation may not be detected until some time later. The position of the uterus should be determined during the preinsertion examination. Great care must be exercised during the preinsertion sounding and subsequent insertion. No attempt should be made to force the insertion. There are a few reports, however, that there has been migration after insertion apparently in the absence of perforation at insertion. In any event, it is possible for the IUD to perforate outside the uterus.

1. How to prepare the LIPPES LOOP Intrauterine Double-S inserter.

Using sterile gloves, hold tube in one hand and with the other draw LOOP into inserter by pulling the push rod. As the LOOP is drawn into the inserter you will encounter some resistance. It is important to use a slow steady pulling action until all but the bulbous tip of the LOOP is entirely within the inserter. At this point, insure that both the flat surface of the bulbous tip and the inserter flange are in a horizontal plane.

Do this not more than one minute before insertion.

2. How to insert LIPPES LOOP Intrauterine Double-S.

Insert the loaded inserter gently through the endocervical canal, with the flange in a horizontal plane. DO NOT FORCE THE INSERTION. If resistance is encountered, do not proceed; perforation of the uterus may occur. If the flange makes contact with the cervix WITHOUT the inserter touching the fundal wall, withdraw 1/4 inch before pressing the push rod to release the device in utero. Should the inserter touch the fundal wall BEFORE the flange makes contact, withdraw 1/2 inch prior to pressing the push rod to release the device in utero. With the inserter now in place, proceed, and WITHOUT UNDUE PRESSURE, push the rod slowly as far as it will go. LIPPES LOOP Intrauterine Double-S should now be in place. Withdraw the inserter tube and push rod from the cervical os until the tail is visible. Cut the tail leaving it as long as possible.

Time of Insertion
LIPPES LOOP Intrauterine Double-S should be inserted preferably the last one or two days of a normal menstrual period or the two days following the last day.

The expulsion and perforation rate may be increased when insertions are made before normal uterine involution occurs (usually four to six weeks postpartum or postabortion).

To Remove
To remove LIPPES LOOP Intrauterine Double-S, pull gently on the exposed tail. On those rare occasions that the tail is not available, the device should be carefully removed.

Clinical Studies: Different event rates have been recorded with the use of different IUD's. Inasmuch as these rates are usually derived from separate studies conducted by different investigators in several population groups, they cannot be compared with precision. Furthermore, event rates tend to be lower as clinical experience is expanded, possibly due to retention in the cinical study of those patients who accept the treatment regimen and do not discontinue due to adverse reactions or pregnancy. In clinical trials conducted by The Population Council with the LIPPES LOOP, use effectiveness was determined as follows for women, as tabulated by the life table method. (Rates are expressed as events per 100 women through 12 and 24 months of use.) This experience is based on 198,257 woman/months of use, including 121,489 woman/months of use in first year after insertion, and 76,768 woman/months of use in second year after insertion. LIPPES LOOP Intrauterine Double-S devices are manufactured in four different sizes, and the figures given above represent the totals for the four sizes. The following table presents these figures individually for each size LOOP:

[See table above].

Tables II–V below give the pregnancy expulsion, medical removal and continuation rates for each individual size LOOP.

TABLE I

LIPPES LOOP Size	Number Woman/Months	Woman/Months of Use 1st Year After Insertion	Woman/Months of Use 2nd year After Insertion
A	13,453	8,751	4,702
B	12,463	9,660	2,803
C	50,775	31,032	19,743
D	121,566	72,046	49,520

TABLE II
LOOP A
(Annual Rates Per 100 Users)

	12 Months	24 Months (cumulative)
Pregnancy	5.3	9.7
Expulsion	23.9	27.7
Medical Removal	12.2	20.0
Continuation Rate	75.2	63.6

TABLE III
LOOP B
(Annual Rates Per 100 Users)

	12 Months	24 Months (cumulative)
Pregnancy	3.4	6.3
Expulsion	18.9	24.9
Medical Removal	15.1	23.8
Continuation Rate	74.6	59.2

TABLE IV
LOOP C
(Annual Rates Per 100 Users)

	12 Months	24 Months (cumulative)
Pregnancy	3.0	4.8
Expulsion	19.1	24.6
Medical Removal	14.3	22.1
Continuation Rate	76.5	62.8

TABLE V
LOOP D
(Annual Rates Per 100 Users)

	12 Months	24 Months (cumulative)
Pregnancy	2.7	4.2
Expulsion	12.7	16.0
Medical Removal	15.2	23.3
Continuation Rate	77.4	65.6

MASSE'® Breast Cream

(See PDR For Nonprescription Drugs)

MONISTAT® 7 Vaginal Cream ℞
(miconazole nitrate 2%)

Description: MONISTAT 7 Vaginal Cream (miconazole nitrate 2%) is a water-miscible, white cream containing as the active ingredient, 2% miconazole nitrate, 1-[2,4-dichloro-β-(2,4-dichlorobenzyloxy) phenethyl] imidazole nitrate.

Actions: MONISTAT 7 Vaginal Cream exhibits fungicidal activity *in vitro* against species of the genus *Candida*. The pharmacologic mode of action is unknown.

Indications: MONISTAT 7 Vaginal Cream is indicated for the local treatment of vulvovaginal candidiasis (moniliasis). As MONISTAT 7 Vaginal Cream is effective only for candidal vulvovaginitis, the diagnosis should be confirmed by KOH smears and/or cultures. Other pathogens commonly associated with vulvovaginitis (*Trichomonas* and *Haemophilus vaginalis* [*Gardnerella*]) should be ruled out by appropriate laboratory methods.

MONISTAT 7 is effective in both pregnant and non-pregnant women, as well as in women taking oral contraceptives. (See PRECAUTIONS.)

Contraindications: Patients known to be hypersensitive to this drug.

Precautions:
General: Discontinue drug if sensitization or irritation is reported during use. Laboratory Tests: If there is a lack of response to MONISTAT 7, appropriate microbiological studies should be repeated to confirm the diagnosis and rule out other pathogens.

Pregnancy: Since MONISTAT is absorbed in small amounts from the human vagina, it should be used in the first trimester of pregnancy only when the physician considers it essential to the welfare of the patient.

Clinical studies, during which MONISTAT was used for 14 days, included 209 pregnant patients. Follow-up reports now available in 174 of these patients reveal no adverse effects or complications attributable to MONISTAT therapy in infants born to these women.

Adverse Reactions: During clinical studies with MONISTAT for a 14-day regimen, 39 of the 528 patients (7.4%) treated with MONISTAT reported complaints during therapy that were possibly drug-related. Most complaints were reported during the first week of therapy.

Continued on next page

Ortho Pharm.—Cont.

Vulvovaginal burning, itching or irritation occurred in 6.6%, while other complaints such as vaginal burning, pelvic cramps, hives, skin rash and headache occurred rarely (each less than 0.2% patient incidence). The therapy-related dropout rate was 0.9%.
Clinical: Statistical analysis of randomized clinical trials, conducted to determine the shortest effective course of therapy with MONISTAT, demonstrates that a regimen of seven or more days has a cure rate equivalent to the 14-day regimen. The graphic representation of this conclusion plots days of therapy versus cure rates. The solid line represents the mean therapeutic cure rate and the shaded area represents the 95% confidence interval.

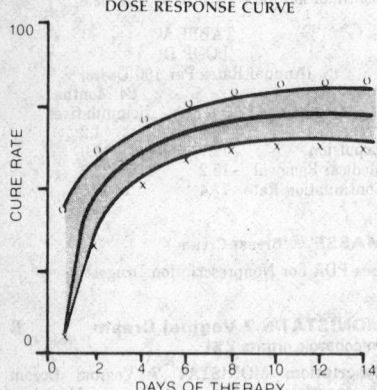

Dosage and Administration: One applicatorful is administered intravaginally once daily at bedtime for seven days. Course of therapy may be repeated after other pathogens have been ruled out by appropriate smears and cultures.
Supplied: MONISTAT 7 Vaginal Cream is available in 1.59 oz. (45 g) tubes with ORTHO® Measured-Dose Applicator.
Shown in Product Identification Section, page 423

MONISTAT® 3   ℞
(miconazole nitrate, 200 mg)
Vaginal Suppositories

Description: MONISTAT 3 Vaginal Suppositories are water-miscible, white to off-white suppositories, each containing the antifungal agent, miconazole nitrate, 1-[2,4-dichloro-β(2,4-dichlorobenzyloxy) phenethyl] imidazole nitrate, 200 mg, in a hydrogenated vegetable oil base. Miconazole nitrate for vaginal use is also available as MONISTAT 7 Vaginal Cream and MONISTAT 7 Vaginal Suppositories.

MICONAZOLE NITRATE

Clinical Pharmacology: Miconazole nitrate exhibits fungicidal activity *in vitro* against species of the genus *Candida*. The pharmacologic mode of action is unknown. Following intravaginal administration of miconazole nitrate, small amounts are absorbed. Administration of a single dose of miconazole nitrate suppositories (100mg) to healthy subjects resulted in a total recovery from the urine and feces of 0.85% (±0.43%) of the administered dose.
Animal studies indicate that the drug crossed the placenta and doses above those used in humans result in embryo and feto-toxicity (80 mg/kg, orally), although this has not been reported in human subjects (See PRECAUTIONS).
In multi-center clinical trials in 440 women with vulvovaginal candidiasis, the efficacy of treatment with the MONISTAT 3 Vaginal Suppository for 3 days was compared with treatment for 7 days with MONISTAT 7 Vaginal Cream. The clinical cure rates (free of microbiological evidence and clinical signs and symptoms of candidiasis at 8–10 days and 30–35 days post-therapy) were numerically lower, although not statistically different, with the 3-Day Suppository when compared with the 7-Day Cream.
Indications and Usage: MONISTAT 3 Vaginal Suppositories are indicated for the local treatment of vulvovaginal candidiasis (moniliasis). Effectiveness in pregnancy and in diabetic patients has not been established. As MONISTAT is effective only for candidal vulvovaginitis, the diagnosis should be confirmed by KOH smear and/or cultures. Other pathogens commonly associated with vulvovaginitis (*Trichomonas* and *Haemophilus vaginalis* [*Gardnerella*]) should be ruled out by appropriate laboratory methods.
Contraindications: Patients known to be hypersensitive to this drug.
Precautions: General: Discontinue drug if sensitization or irritation is reported during use. The base contained in the suppository formulation may interact with certain latex products, such as that used in vaginal contraceptive diaphragms. Concurrent use is not recommended. MONISTAT 7 Vaginal Cream may be considered for use under these conditions.
Laboratory Tests: If there is a lack of response to MONISTAT 3 Vaginal Suppositories, appropriate microbiological studies (standard KOH smear and/or cultures) should be repeated to confirm the diagnosis and rule out other pathogens.
Carcinogenesis, Mutagenesis, Impairment of Fertility: Long-term animal studies to determine carcinogenic potential have not been performed.
Fertility (Reproduction): Oral administration of miconazole nitrate in rats has been reported to produce prolonged gestation. However, this effect was not observed in oral rabbit studies. In addition, signs of fetal and embryo toxicity were reported in rat and rabbit studies, and dystocia was reported in rat studies after oral doses at and above 80 mg per kg. Intravaginal administration did not produce these effects in rats.
Pregnancy: Since imidazoles are absorbed in small amounts from the human vagina, they should not be used in the first trimester of pregnancy unless the physician considers it essential to the welfare of the patient.
Clinical studies, during which miconazole nitrate vaginal cream and suppositories were used for up to 14 days, were reported to include 514 pregnant patients. Follow-up reports available in 471 of these patients reveal no adverse effects or complications attributable to miconazole nitrate therapy in infants born to these women.
Nursing Mothers: It is not known whether miconazole nitrate is excreted in human milk. Because many drugs are excreted in human milk, caution should be exercised when miconazole nitrate is administered to a nursing woman.
Adverse Reactions: During clinical studies with the MONISTAT 3 Vaginal Suppository (miconazole nitrate, 200 mg) 301 patients were treated. The incidence of vulvovaginal burning, itching or irritation was 2%. Complaints of cramping (2%) and headaches (1.3%) were also reported. Other complaints (hives, skin rash) occurred with less than a 0.5% incidence. The therapy-related dropout rate was 0.3%.
Overdose: Overdose of miconazole nitrate in humans has not been reported to date. In mice, rats, guinea pigs and dogs, the oral LD 50 values were found to be 578.1, >640, 275.9 and >160 mg/kg, respectively.
Dosage and Administration: MONISTAT 3 Vaginal Suppositories: One suppository (miconazole nitrate, 200 mg) is inserted intravaginally once daily at bedtime for three consecutive days. Before prescribing another course of therapy, the diagnosis should be reconfirmed by smears and/or cultures to rule out other pathogens.
How Supplied: MONISTAT 3 Suppositories (miconazole nitrate, 200 mg) are available as 2.5 gm, elliptically shaped white to off-white suppositories in packages of three (NDC 0062-5437-01) with a vaginal applicator. Store at 59°–86° F (13–30° C).

MONISTAT® 7 Vaginal Suppositories   ℞
(100 mg miconazole nitrate)

Description: MONISTAT 7 Vaginal Suppositories are water-miscible, white to off-white suppositories, each containing the antifungal agent, miconazole nitrate, 1-[2,4-dichloro-β-(2,4-dichlorobenzyloxy) phenethyl] imidazole nitrate, 100 mg, in a hydrogenated vegetable oil base. Miconazole nitrate for vaginal use is also available as MONISTAT 7 Vaginal Cream.
Clinical Pharmacology: Miconazole nitrate exhibits fungicidal activity *in vitro* against species of the genus *Candida*. The pharmacologic mode of action is unknown. Following intravaginal administration of MONISTAT 7 Vaginal Suppositories or MONISTAT 7 Vaginal Cream, small amounts are absorbed. Administration of a single dose of MONISTAT 7 Vaginal Suppositories to healthy subjects resulted in a total recovery from the urine and feces of 0.85% (±0.43%) of the administered dose. For MONISTAT 7 Vaginal Cream the corresponding figure was 1.03% (±0.51%) of the administered dose.
Animal studies indicate that the drug crossed the placenta and doses above those used in humans result in embryo and feto-toxicity (80 mg/kg-orally) although this has not been reported in human subjects (see Precautions).
Indications and Usage: MONISTAT 7 Vaginal Suppositories are indicated for the local treatment of vulvovaginal candidiasis (moniliasis). Effectiveness in pregnancy has not been established. As MONISTAT 7 is effective only for candidal vulvovaginitis, the diagnosis should be confirmed by KOH smear and/or cultures. Other pathogens commonly associated with vulvovaginitis (*Trichomonas* and *Haemophilus vaginalis* [*Gardnerella*]) should be ruled out by appropriate laboratory methods.
Clinical: Statistical analyses of randomized clinical trials, conducted to determine the shortest effective course of therapy with miconazole nitrate vaginal cream and suppositories, demonstrate that a regimen of seven or more days had a cure rate equivalent to a 14-day regimen.
The graphic representation of this conclusion plots Days of Therapy versus Cure Rate for miconazole nitrate vaginal cream. (Results were similar with suppositories.) The solid line represents the mean therapeutic cure rate and the shaded area represents the 95% confidence interval.

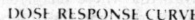
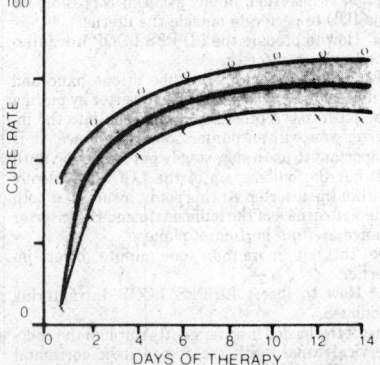

Contraindications: Patients known to be hypersensitive to this drug.
Precautions: General: Discontinue drug if sensitization or irritation is reported during use. The base contained in the suppository formulation

may interact with certain latex products, such as that used in vaginal contraceptive diaphragms. Concurrent use is not recommended. MONISTAT 7 Vaginal Cream may be considered for use under these conditions.

Laboratory Tests: If there is a lack of response to MONISTAT 7, appropriate microbiological studies (standard KOH smear and/or cultures) should be repeated to confirm the diagnosis and rule out other pathogens.

Carcinogenesis, Mutagenesis, Impairment of Fertility: Long-term animal studies to determine carcinogenic potential have not been performed.

Fertility (reproduction): Oral administration of miconazole nitrate in rats has been reported to produce prolonged gestation. However, this effect was not observed in oral rabbit studies. In addition, signs of fetal and embryotoxicity were reported in rat and rabbit studies and dystocia in rat studies after oral doses at and above 80 mg/kg. Intravaginal administration did not produce these effects in rats.

Pregnancy: Since imidazoles are absorbed in small amounts from the human vagina, they should not be used in the first trimester of pregnancy unless the physician considers it essential to the welfare of the patient.

Clinical studies, during which miconazole nitrate vaginal cream and suppositories were used for up to 14 days, were reported to include 487 pregnant patients. Follow-up reports available on 446 of these patients reveal no adverse effects or complications attributable to miconazole nitrate therapy in infants born to these women.

Nursing Mothers: It is not known whether miconazole nitrate is excreted in human milk. Because many drugs are excreted in human milk, caution should be exercised when miconazole nitrate is administered to a nursing woman.

Adverse Reactions: During clinical studies with miconazole nitrate cream for a 14-day regimen, 39 of the 528 patients (7.4%) treated with miconazole nitrate cream reported complaints during therapy that were possibly drug-related. Most complaints were reported during the first week of therapy. Vulvovaginal burning, itching or irritation occurred in 6.6%, while other complaints such as vaginal burning, pelvic cramps, hives, skin rash and headache occurred rarely (each less than 0.2% patient incidence). The therapy-related dropout rate was 0.9%.

During clinical studies with regimens which varied from 1 to 14 days, 1,057 patients were treated with miconazole nitrate suppositories. The incidence of vulvovaginal burning, itching or irritation was 0.5%, while complaints of skin rash occurred at only a 0.2% incidence.

Overdose: Overdosage of miconazole nitrate in humans has not been reported to date. In mice, rats, guinea pigs and dogs, the oral LD_{50} values were found to be 578.1, >640, 275.9 and >160 mg/kg, respectively.

Dosage and Administration: MONISTAT 7 Vaginal Suppositories: One suppository (100 mg miconazole nitrate) is inserted intravaginally once daily at bedtime for seven days. Before prescribing another course of therapy, the diagnosis should be reconfirmed by smears and/or cultures to rule out other pathogens.

How Supplied: MONISTAT 7 Vaginal Suppositories are available as 2.5g (100 mg miconazole nitrate) elliptically shaped white to off-white suppositories in packages of seven with a vaginal applicator. Store at 59°–86°F (13°–30°C).

Shown in Product Identification Section, page 423

ORTHO-CREME® Contraceptive Cream

(See PDR For Nonprescription Drugs)

ORTHO™ DIAPHRAGM KITS

Description: ORTHO Diaphragm Kits include three different types in a variety of sizes.

1. The ALL-FLEX* Arcing Spring Diaphragm is a molded, buff-colored, latex vaginal diaphragm containing a distortion-free, dual spring-within-a-spring which provides unique arcing action no matter where the rim is compressed. It is ideal not only where ordinary diaphragms are indicated, but also in patients with mild cystocele, rectocele or retroversion.
2. The ORTHO* Coil Spring Diaphragm is a molded latex vaginal diaphragm. The rim encases a tension-adjusted, cadmium-plated coil spring.
3. The ORTHO-WHITE* Flat Spring Diaphragm is a molded, pure white, latex vaginal diaphragm containing a flat, watch-type spring which allows compressibility in one plane only, thus facilitating insertion.

ORTHO Diaphragms are used in conjunction with spermicides, e.g., GYNOL II* Contraceptive Jelly, ORTHO-GYNOL* Contraceptive Jelly or ORTHO-CREME* Contraceptive Cream in conception control.

Action: These diaphragms when properly fitted serve two purposes:
a. To stop the sperm from entering the cervical canal;
b. To hold the spermicide.

Indications: ORTHO Diaphragms, in conjunction with an appropriate spermicide, are indicated for the prevention of pregnancy in women who elect to use diaphragms as a method of contraception.

Precautions: Although an association has not been established between diaphragm use and toxic shock syndrome (TSS), symptoms of this condition have been reported in a few women using diaphragms. In most of these cases, the women wore a diaphragm continuously for more than 24 hours. Therefore, continuous wearing of the diaphragm for more than 24 hours is not recommended.

Primary symptoms of TSS are sudden high fever (usually 102°F or more) and vomiting, diarrhea, fainting or near fainting when standing up, dizziness or a rash that looks like a sunburn. There may also be other signs of TSS, such as aching of muscles and joints, redness of the eyes, sore throat and weakness. The patient should be instructed that if she has sudden high fever and one or more of the other symptoms, she should remove her diaphragm and consult her physician immediately.

Instructions:
1. Proper placement of the diaphragm is vital for effectiveness.
2. To be fully effective the diaphragm should never be used without contraceptive cream or jelly. This contraceptive cream or jelly must be spread around the inner surface of the diaphragm as well as around the rim.
3. The diaphragm may be inserted up to six hours before intercourse. If more than six hours has elapsed between insertion of the diaphragm and intercourse, additional contraceptive jelly or cream must be applied. The diaphragm should not be removed to apply this additional cream or jelly.
4. The diaphragm should not be removed nor should the patient douche for six to eight hours after intercourse. The diaphragm should not remain in position for more than 24 hours.

How Supplied: All ORTHO Diaphragm Kits are available individually and contain a sample tube of GYNOL II Contraceptive Jelly. Each diaphragm is contained in an attractive plastic compact.

1. The ALL-FLEX Arcing Spring Diaphragm is available in sizes 55mm through 95mm in 5mm increments.
2. The ORTHO Coil Spring Diaphragm is available in sizes 50mm through 105mm in 5mm increments.
3. The ORTHO-WHITE Flat Spring Diaphragm is available in sizes 55mm through 95mm in 5mm increments.

*Trademark

ORTHO® Dienestrol Cream ℞

1. ESTROGENS HAVE BEEN REPORTED TO INCREASE THE RISK OF ENDOMETRIAL CARCINOMA.

Three independent case control studies have shown an increased risk of endometrial cancer in postmenopausal women exposed to exogenous estrogens for prolonged periods.[1–3] This risk was independent of the other known risk factors for endometrial cancer. These studies are further supported by the finding that incidence rates of endometrial cancer have increased sharply since 1969 in eight different areas of the United States with population-based cancer reporting systems, an increase which may be related to the rapidly expanding use of estrogens during the last decade.[4]

The three case control studies reported that the risk of endometrial cancer in estrogen users was about 4.5 to 13.9 times greater than in nonusers. The risk appears to depend on both duration of treatment[1] and on estrogen dose.[3] In view of these findings, when estrogens are used for the treatment of menopausal symptoms, the lowest dose that will control symptoms should be utilized and medication should be discontinued as soon as possible. When prolonged treatment is medically indicated, the patient should be reassessed on at least a semiannual basis to determine the need for continued therapy. Although the evidence must be considered preliminary, one study suggests that cyclic administration of low doses of estrogen may carry less risk than continuous administration;[3] it therefore appears prudent to utilize such a regimen.

Close clinical surveillance of all women taking estrogens is important. In all cases of undiagnosed persistent or recurring abnormal vaginal bleeding, adequate diagnostic measures should be undertaken to rule out malignancy.

There is no evidence at present that "natural" estrogens are more or less hazardous than "synthetic" estrogens at equiestrogenic doses.

2. ESTROGENS SHOULD NOT BE USED DURING PREGNANCY

The use of female sex hormones, both estrogens and progestogens, during early pregnancy may seriously damage the offspring. It has been shown that females exposed *in utero* to diethylstilbestrol, a non-steroidal estrogen, have an increased risk of developing in later life a form of vaginal or cervical cancer that ordinarily is extremely rare.[5,6] This risk has been estimated as not greater than 4 per 1000 exposures.[7] Furthermore, a high percentage of such exposed women (from 30 to 90 percent) have been found to have vaginal adenosis,[8,13] epithelial changes of the vagina and cervix. Although these changes are histologically benign, it is not known whether they are precursors of malignancy. Although similar data are not available with the use of other estrogens, it cannot be presumed they would not induce similar changes.

Several reports suggest an association between intrauterine exposure to female sex hormones and congenital anomalies, including congenital heart defects and limb reduction defects.[13–16] One case control study[16] estimated a 4.7 fold increased risk of limb reduction defects in infants exposed in utero to sex hormones (oral contraceptives, hormone withdrawal tests for pregnancy, or attempted treatment for threatened abortion). Some of these exposures were very short and involved only a few days of treatment. The data suggest that the risk of limb reduction defects in exposed fetuses is somewhat less than 1 per 1000.

Continued on next page

Ortho Pharm.—Cont.

In the past, female sex hormones have been used during pregnancy in an attempt to treat threatened or habitual abortion. There is considerable evidence that estrogens are ineffective for these indications, and there is no evidence from well controlled studies that progestogens are effective for these uses.

If ORTHO Dienestrol Cream is used during pregnancy, or if the patient becomes pregnant while using this drug, she should be apprised of the potential risks to the fetus, and the advisability of pregnancy continuation.

Description:
ORTHO Dienestrol Cream
Cream for Intravaginal use only
Active ingredient: Dienestrol 0.01%.
Dienestrol is a synthetic, non-steroidal estrogen. It is compounded in a cream base suitable for intravaginal use only. The cream base is composed of glyceryl monostearate, peanut oil, glycerin, benzoic acid, glutamic acid, butylated hydroxyanisole, citric acid, sodium hydroxide and water. The pH is approximately 4.3.

Clinical Pharmacology: Systemic absorption and mode of action are undetermined.

Indications: ORTHO Dienestrol Cream is indicated in the treatment of atrophic vaginitis and kraurosis vulvae.

ORTHO DIENESTROL CREAM HAS NOT BEEN SHOWN TO BE EFFECTIVE FOR ANY PURPOSE DURING PREGNANCY AND ITS USE MAY CAUSE SEVERE HARM TO THE FETUS (*SEE* BOXED WARNING).

Contraindications: Estrogens may cause fetal harm when administered to a pregnant woman (see Boxed Warning). Estrogens are contraindicated in women who are or may become pregnant. If this drug is used during pregnancy, or if the patient becomes pregnant while using this drug, the patient should be apprised of the potential hazard to the fetus.

Estrogens should also not be used in women with any of the following conditions:
1. Known or suspected cancer of the breast.
2. Known or suspected estrogen-dependent neoplasia.
3. Undiagnosed abnormal genital bleeding.
4. Active thrombophlebitis or thromboembolic disorders.
5. A past history of thrombophlebitis, thrombosis, or thromboembolic disorders associated with previous estrogen use.

Warnings:
1. *Induction of malignant neoplasms.* Long-term continuous administration of natural and synthetic estrogens in certain animal species increases the frequency of carcinomas of the breast, cervix, vagina, and liver. There is now evidence that estrogens increase the risk of carcinoma of the endometrium in humans. (*See* Boxed Warning.)

At the present time there is no satisfactory evidence that estrogens given to postmenopausal women increase the risk of cancer of the breast,[18] although a recent long-term followup of a single physician's practice has raised this possibility.[18a] Because of the animal data, there is a need for caution in prescribing estrogens for women with a strong family history of breast cancer or who have breast nodules, fibrocystic disease, or abnormal mammograms.

2. *Gall bladder disease.* A recent study has reported a 2 to 3-fold increase in the risk of surgically confirmed gall bladder disease in women receiving postmenopausal estrogens,[18] similar to the 2-fold increase previously noted in users of oral contraceptives.[19,24] In the case of oral contraceptives the increased risk appeared after two years of use.[24]

3. *Effects similar to those caused by estrogen-progestogen oral contraceptives.* There are several serious adverse effects of oral contraceptives, most of which have not, up to now, been documented as consequences of postmenopausal estrogen therapy. This may reflect the comparatively low doses of estrogen used in postmenopausal women. It would be expected that the larger doses of estrogen used to treat prostatic or breast cancer or postpartum breast engorgement are more likely to result in these adverse effects, and, in fact, it has been shown that there is an increased risk of thrombosis in men receiving estrogens for prostatic cancer and women for postpartum breast engorgement.[20-23]

a. *Thromboembolic disease.* It is now well established that users of oral contraceptives have an increased risk of various thromboembolic and thrombotic vascular diseases, such as thrombophlebitis, pulmonary embolism, stroke, and myocardial infarction.[24-31] Cases of retinal thrombosis, mesenteric thrombosis, and optic neuritis have been reported in oral contraceptive users. There is evidence that the risk of several of these adverse reactions is related to the dose of the drug.[32,33] An increased risk of postsurgery thromboembolic complications has also been reported in users of oral contraceptives.[34,35] If feasible, estrogen should be discontinued at least 4 weeks before surgery of the type associated with an increased risk of thromboembolism, or during periods of prolonged immobilization.

While an increased risk of thromboembolic and thrombotic disease in postmenopausal users of estrogens has not been found,[18,36] this does not rule out the possibility that such an increase may be present or that subgroups of women who have underlying risk factors or who are receiving relatively large doses of estrogens may have increased risk. Therefore estrogens should not be used in persons with active thrombophlebitis or thromboembolic disorders, and they should not be used (except in treatment of malignancy) in persons with a history of such disorders in association with estrogen use. They should be used with caution in patients with cerebral vascular or coronary artery disease and only for those in whom estrogens are clearly needed.

Large doses of estrogen (5 mg conjugated estrogens per day), comparable to those used to treat cancer of the prostate and breast, have been shown in a large prospective clinical trial in men to increase the risk of nonfatal myocardial infarction, pulmonary embolism and thrombophlebitis. When estrogen doses of this size are used, any of the thromboembolic and thrombotic adverse effects associated with oral contraceptive use should be considered a clear risk.

b. *Hepatic adenoma.* Benign hepatic adenomas appear to be associated with the use of oral contraceptives.[38-40] Although benign, and rare, these may rupture and may cause death through intraabdominal hemorrhage. Such lesions have not yet been reported in association with other estrogen or progestogen preparations but should be considered in estrogen users having abdominal pain and tenderness, abdominal mass, or hypovolemic shock. Hepatocellular carcinoma has also been reported in women taking estrogen-containing oral contraceptives.[39] The relationship of this malignancy to these drugs is not known at this time.

c. *Elevated blood pressure.* Increased blood pressure is not uncommon in women using oral contraceptives. There is now a report that this may occur with use of estrogens during menopause.[41] Blood pressure should be monitored with estrogen use, especially if high doses are used.

d. *Glucose tolerance.* A worsening of glucose tolerance has been observed in a significant percentage of patients on estrogen-containing oral contraceptives. For this reason, diabetic patients should be carefully observed while receiving estrogen.

4. *Hypercalcemia.* Administration of estrogens may lead to severe hypercalcemia in patients with breast cancer and bone metastases. If this occurs, the drug should be stopped and appropriate measures taken to reduce the serum calcium level.

Precautions:
A. General
1. A complete medical and family history should be taken prior to the initiation of any estrogen therapy. The pretreatment and periodic physical examinations should include special reference to blood pressure, breasts, abdomen, and pelvic organs, and should include a Papanicolaou smear. As a general rule, estrogen should not be prescribed for longer than one year without another physical examination being performed.

2. Fluid retention—Because estrogens may cause some degree of fluid retention, conditions which might be influenced by this factor such as epilepsy, migraine, and cardiac or renal dysfunction, require careful observation.

3. Certain patients may develop undesirable manifestations of excessive estrogenic stimulation, such as abnormal or excessive uterine bleeding, mastodynia, etc.

4. Oral contraceptives appear to be associated with an increased incidence of mental depression.[24] Although it is not clear whether this is due to the estrogenic or progestogenic component of the contraceptive, patients with a history of depression should be carefully observed.

5. Preexisting uterine leiomyomata may increase in size during estrogen use.

6. The pathologist should be advised of estrogen therapy when relevant specimens are submitted.

7. Patients with a past history of jaundice during pregnancy have an increased risk of recurrence of jaundice while receiving estrogen-containing oral contraceptive therapy. If jaundice develops in any patient receiving estrogen, the medication should be discontinued while the cause is investigated.

8. Estrogens may be poorly metabolized in patients with impaired liver function and they should be administered with caution in such patients.

9. Because estrogens influence the metabolism of calcium and phosphorus, they should be used with caution in patients with metabolic bone diseases that are associated with hypercalcemia or in patients with renal insufficiency.

10. Because of the effects of estrogens on epiphyseal closure, they should be used judiciously in young patients in whom bone growth is not complete.

B. Information for Patients: See text of Patient Package Information which is reproduced below.

C. Drug/Laboratory Test Interactions
Certain endocrine and liver function tests may be affected by estrogen-containing oral contraceptives. The following similar changes may be expected with larger doses of estrogen:
1. Increased sulfobromophthalein retention.
2. Increased prothrombin and factors VII, VIII, IX and X; decreased antithrombin 3; increased norepinephrine-induced platelet aggregability.
3. Increased thyroid-binding globulin (TBG) leading to increased circulating total thyroid hormone, as measured by PBI, T4 by column, or T4 by radioimmunoassay. Free T3 resin uptake is decreased, reflecting the elevated TBG; free T4 concentration is unaltered.
4. Impaired glucose tolerance.
5. Decreased pregnanediol excretion.
6. Reduced response to metyrapone test.
7. Reduced serum folate concentration.
8. Increased serum triglyceride and phospholipid concentration.

D. Carcinogenesis, Mutagenesis, Impairment of Fertility: See "Warnings" section for information on carcinogenesis, mutagenesis and impairment of fertility.

E. Pregnancy:
Teratogenic Effects.
Pregnancy Category X.
See "Contraindications" section.

F. Nursing Mothers: It is not known whether this drug is excreted in human milk. Because many drugs are excreted in human milk, caution should be exercised when estrogens are administered to a nursing woman.

Adverse Reactions: (*See* Warnings regarding induction of neoplasia, adverse effects on the fetus, increased incidence of gall bladder disease, and adverse effects similar to those of oral contraceptives, including thromboembolism.) The following additional adverse reactions have been reported

with estrogenic therapy, including oral contraceptives:
1. *Genitourinary system.*
Increase in size of uterine fibromyomata.
Vaginal candidiasis.
Breakthrough bleeding, spotting, change in menstrual flow.
Dysmenorrhea.
Premenstrual-like syndrome.
Amenorrhea during and after treatment.
Change in cervical eversion and in degree of cervical secretion.
Cystitis-like syndrome.
2. *Breasts.*
Tenderness, enlargement, secretion.
3. *Gastrointestinal.*
Cholestatic jaundice.
Nausea, vomiting.
Abdominal cramps, bloating.
4. *Skin.*
Erythema multiforme.
Erythema nodosum.
Hemorrhagic eruption.
Loss of scalp hair.
Hirsutism.
Chloasma or melasma which may persist when drug is discontinued.
5. *Eyes.*
Steepening of corneal curvature.
Intolerance to contact lenses.
6. *CNS.*
Mental depression.
Headache, migraine, dizziness.
Chorea.
7. *Miscellaneous.*
Reduced carbohydrate tolerance.
Aggravation of porphyria.
Edema.
Changes in libido.
Increase or decrease in weight.

Overdosage: Numerous reports of ingestion of large doses of estrogen-containing oral contraceptives by young children indicate that serious ill effects do not occur. Overdosage of estrogen may cause nausea, and withdrawal bleeding may occur in females.

Dosage and Administration: *Given cyclically for short term use only:*
For treatment of atrophic vaginitis, or kraurosis vulvae associated with the menopause.
The lowest dose that will control symptoms should be chosen and medication should be discontinued as promptly as possible.
Attempts to discontinue or taper medication should be made at 3 to 6 month intervals.
The usual dosage range is one or two applicatorsful per day for one or two weeks, then gradually reduced to one half initial dosage for a similar period. A maintenance dosage of one applicatorful, one to three times a week, may be used after restoration of the vaginal mucosa has been achieved.
Treated patients with an intact uterus should be monitored closely for signs of endometrial cancer and appropriate diagnostic measures should be taken to rule out malignancy in the event of persistent or recurring abnormal vaginal bleeding.

Supplied: Available in 2.75 oz. (78g) tubes with or without ORTHO® Measured-Dose Applicator.
With applicator: NDC 0062-5450-77
Without applicator: NDC 0062-5450-00
Store at controlled room temperature.

1. Ziel, H.K. and W.D. Finkle, "Increased Risk of Endometrial Carcinoma Among Users of Conjugated Estrogens," *New England Journal of Medicine,* 293:1167–1170, 1975.
2. Smith, D.C., R. Prentic, D.J. Thompson, and W.L. Hermann, "Association of Exogenous Estrogen and Endometrial Carcinoma," *New England Journal of Medicine,* 293:1164–1167, 1975.
3. Mack, T.M., M.C. Pike, B.E. Henderson, R.I. Pfeffer, V.R. Gerkins, M. Arthur, and S.E. Brown, "Estrogens and Endometrial Cancer in a Retirement Community," *New England Journal of Medicine,* 294:1267–1287, 1976.
4. Weiss, N.S., D.R. Szekely and D.F. Austin, "Increasing Incidence of Endometrial Cancer in the United States," *New England Journal of Medicine,* 294:1259–1262, 1976.
5. Herbst, A.L., H. Ulfelder and D.C. Poskanzer, "Adenocarcinoma of Vagina," *New England Journal of Medicine,* 284:878–881, 1971.
6. Greenwald, P., J. Barlow, P. Nasca, and W. Burnett, "Vaginal Cancer after Maternal Treatment with Synthetic Estrogens," *New England Journal of Medicine,* 285:390–392, 1971.
7. Lanier, A., K. Noller, D. Decker, L. Elveback, and L. Kurland, "Cancer and Stilbestrol. A Follow-up of 1719 Persons Exposed to Estrogens in Utero and Born 1943–1959," *Mayo Clinic Proceedings,* 48:793–799, 1973.
8. Herbst, A., R. Kurman, and R. Scully, "Vaginal and Cervical Abnormalities After Exposure to Stilbestrol In Utero," *Obstetrics and Gynecology,* 40:287–298, 1972.
9. Herbst, A., S. Robboy, G. Macdonald, and R. Scully, "The Effects of Local Progesterone on Stilbestrol-Associated Vaginal Adenosis," *American Journal of Obstetrics and Gynecology* 118:607–615, 1974.
10. Herbst, A., D. Poskanzer, S. Robboy, L. Friedlander, and R. Scully, "Prenatal Exposure to Stilbestrol, A Prospective Comparison of Exposed Female Offspring with Unexposed Controls," *New England Journal of Medicine,* 292:334–339, 1975.
11. Staffi, A., R. Mattingly, D. Foley, and W. Fetherston, "Clinical Diagnosis of Vaginal Adenosis," *Obstetrics and Gynecology,* 43:118–128, 1974.
12. Sherman, A.I., M. Goldrath, A. Berlin, V. Vakhariya, F. Banooni, W. Michaels, P. Goodman, S. Brown, "Cervical-Vaginal Adenosis After *In Utero* Exposure to Synthetic Estrogens," *Obstetrics and Gynecology,* 44:531–545, 1974.
13. Gal, I., B. Kirman, and J. Stern, "Hormone Pregnancy Tests and Congenital Malformation," *Nature,* 216:83, 1967.
14. Levy, E.P., A. Cohen, and F.C. Fraser, "Hormone Treatment During Pregnancy and Congenital Heart Defects," *Lancet,* 1:611, 1973.
15. Nora, J. and A. Nora, "Birth Defects and Oral Contraceptives," *Lancet,* 1:941–942, 1973.
16. Janerich, D.T., J.M. Piper, and D.M. Glebatis, "Oral Contraceptives and Congenital Limb-Reduction Defects," *New England Journal of Medicine,* 291:697–700, 1974.
17. "Estrogens for Oral or Parenteral Use," *Federal Register,* 40:8212, 1975.
18. Boston Collaborative Drug Surveillance Program, "Surgically Confirmed Gall Bladder Disease, Venous Thromboembolism and Breast Tumors in Relation to Post-Menopausal Estrogen Therapy," *New England Journal of Medicine,* 290:15–19, 1974.
18a. Hoover, R., L.A. Gray, Sr., P. Cole, and B. MacMahon, "Menopausal Estrogens and Breast Cancer," *New England Journal of Medicine,* 295:401–405, 1976.
19. Boston Collaborative Drug Surveillance Program, "Oral Contraceptives and Venous Thromboembolic Disease, Surgically Confirmed Gall Bladder Disease, and Breast Tumors," *Lancet* 1:1399–1404, 1973.
20. Daniel, D.G., H. Campbell, and A.C. Turnbull, "Puerperal Thromboembolism and Suppression of Lactation," *Lancet,* 2:287–289, 1967.
21. The Veterans Administration Cooperative Urological Research Group, "Carcinoma of the Prostate: Treatment Comparisons," *Journal of Urology,* 98:516–522, 1967.
22. Bailer, J.C., "Thromboembolism and Oestrogen Therapy," *Lancet,* 2:560, 1967.
23. Blackard, C., R. Doe, G. Mellinger, and D. Byar, "Incidence of Cardiovascular Disease and Death In Patients Receiving Diethylstilbestrol for Carcinoma of the Prostate," *Cancer,* 26:249–256, 1970.
24. Royal College of General Practitioners, "Oral Contraception and Thromboembolic Disease," *Journal of the Royal College of General Practitioners,* 13:267–279, 1967.
25. Inman, W.H.W. and M.P. Vessey, "Investigation of Deaths from Pulmonary, Coronary, and Cerebral Thrombosis and Embolism in Women of Child-Bearing Age," *British Medical Journal,* 2:193–199, 1968.
26. Vessey, M.P. and R. Doll, "Investigation of Relation Between Use of Oral Contraceptives and Thromboembolic Disease, A Further Report," *British Medical Journal,* 2:651–657, 1969.
27. Sartwell, P.E., A.T. Masi, F.G. Arthes, G.R. Greene, and H.E. Smith, "Thromboembolism and Oral Contraceptives: An Epidemiological Case Control Study," *American Journal of Epidemiology,* 90:365–380, 1969.
28. Collaborative Group for the Study of Stroke In Young Women, "Oral Contraception and Increased Risk of Cerebral Ischemia or Thrombosis," *New England Journal of Medicine,* 288:871–878, 1973.
29. Collaborative Group for the Study of Stroke in Young Women, "Oral Contraceptives and Stroke in Young Women: Associated Risk Factors," *Journal of the American Medical Association,* 231:718–722, 1975.
30. Mann, J.I. and W.H.W. Inman, "Oral Contraceptives and Death from Myocardial Infarction," *British Medical Journal,* 2:245–248, 1975.
31. Mann, J.I., M.P. Vessey, M. Thorogood, and R. Doll., "Myocardial Infarction in Young Women with Special Reference to Oral Contraceptive Practice," *British Medical Journal,* 2:241–245, 1975.
32. Inman, W.H.W., V.P. Vessey, B. Westerholm, and A. Engelund, "Thromboembolic Disease and the Steroidal Content of Oral Contraceptives," *British Medical Journal,* 2:203–209, 1970.
33. Stolley, P.D., J.A. Tonascia, M.S. Tockman, P.E. Sartwell, A.H. Rutledge, and M.P. Jacobs, "Thrombosis with Low-Estrogen Oral Contraceptives," *American Journal of Epidemiology,* 102:197–208, 1975.
34. Vessey, M.P., R. Doll, A.S. Fairbairn, and G. Glober, "Post-Operative Thromboembolism and the Use of the Oral Contraceptives," *British Medical Journal,* 3:123–126, 1970.
35. Greene, G.R. and P.E. Sartwell, "Oral Contraceptive Use in Patients with Thromboembolism Following Surgery, Trauma or Infection," *American Journal of Public Health,* 62:680–685, 1972.
36. Rosenberg, L., M.B. Armstrong and H. Jick, "Myocardial Infarction and Estrogen Therapy in Postmenopausal Women," *New England Journal of Medicine,* 294:1256–1259, 1976.
37. Coronary Drug Project Research Group, "The Coronary Drug Project: Initial Findings Leading to Modifications of Its Research Protocol," *Journal of the American Medical Association,* 214:1303–1313, 1970.
38. Baum, J., F. Holtz, J.J. Bookstein, and E.W. Klein, "Possible Association between Benign Hepatomas and Oral Contraceptives," *Lancet,* 2:926–928, 1973.
39. Mays, E.T., W.M. Christopherson, M.M. Mahr, and H.C. Williams, "Hepatic Changes in Young Women Ingesting Contraceptive Steroids, Hepatic Hemorrhage and Primary Hepatic Tumors." *Journal of the American Medical Association,* 235:730–782, 1976.
40. Edmondson, H.A., B. Henderson, and B. Benton, "Liver Cell Adenomas Associated with the Use of Oral Contraceptives," *New England Journal of Medicine,* 294:470–472, 1976.
41. Pfeffer, R.I. and S. Van Den Noore, "Estrogen Use and Stroke Risk in Postmenopausal Women," *American Journal of Epidemiology,* 103:445–456, 1976.

PATIENT INFORMATION ABOUT ESTROGENS

Estrogens are female hormones produced by the ovaries. The ovaries make several different kinds of estrogens. In addition, scientists have been able to make a variety of synthetic estrogens. As far as we know, all these synthetic estrogens have similar properties and therefore much the same usefulness, side effects, and risks. This leaflet is intended to help you understand what estrogens are used for, some of the risks involved in their use, and to help minimize these risks.
This leaflet includes important information about estrogens, but not all the information. If you want

Continued on next page

Ortho Pharm.—Cont.

to know more, you can ask your doctor or pharmacist to let you read the package insert prepared for the doctor.

Uses of Estrogen: THERE IS NO PROPER USE OF ESTROGENS IN A PREGNANT WOMAN
Estrogens are prescribed by doctors for a number of purposes, including:
1. To provide estrogen during a period of adjustment when a woman's ovaries no longer produce it, in order to prevent certain uncomfortable symptoms of estrogen deficiency. (All women normally decrease the production of estrogens, generally between the ages of 45 and 55; this is called the menopause.)
2. To prevent symptoms of estrogen deficiency when a woman's ovaries have been removed surgically before the natural menopause.
3. To prevent pregnancy. (Estrogens are given along with a progestogen, another female hormone; these combinations are called oral contraceptives or birth control pills. Patient labeling is available to women taking oral contraceptives and they will not be discussed in this leaflet.)
4. To treat certain cancers in women and men.
5. To prevent painful swelling of the breasts after pregnancy in women who choose not to nurse their babies.

Estrogens in the Menopause: In the natural course of their lives, all women eventually experience a decrease in estrogen production. This usually occurs between ages 45 and 55 but may occur earlier or later. Sometimes the ovaries may need to be removed by an operation before natural menopause, producing a "surgical menopause."
When the amount of estrogen in the blood begins to decrease, many women may develop typical symptoms: Feelings of warmth in the face, neck, and chest or sudden intense episodes of heat and sweating throughout the body (called "hot flashes" or "hot flushes"). These symptoms are sometimes very uncomfortable. A few women eventually develop changes in the vagina (called "atrophic vaginitis") which cause discomfort, especially during and after intercourse.
Estrogens can be prescribed to treat these symptoms of the menopause. It is estimated that considerably more than half of all women undergoing the menopause have only mild symptoms or no symptoms at all and therefore do not need estrogens. Other women may need estrogens for a few months, while their bodies adjust to lower estrogen levels. Sometimes the need will be for periods longer than six months. In an attempt to avoid over-stimulation of the uterus (womb), estrogens are usually given cyclically during each month of use, that is three weeks of pills followed by one week without pills.
Sometimes women experience nervous symptoms or depression during menopause. There is no evidence that estrogens are effective for such symptoms and they should not be used to treat them, although other treatment may be needed.
You may have heard that taking estrogens for long periods (years) after the menopause will keep your skin soft and supple and keep you feeling young. There is no evidence that this is so, however, and such long-term treatment carries important risks.

Estrogens to Prevent Swelling of the Breasts After Pregnancy: If you do not breast-feed your baby after delivery, your breasts may fill up with milk and become painful and engorged. This usually begins about three to four days after delivery and may last for a few days to up to a week or more. Sometimes the discomfort is severe, but usually it is not and can be controlled by pain-relieving drugs such as aspirin and by binding the breasts up tightly. Estrogens can be used to try to prevent the breasts from filling up. While this treatment is sometimes successful, in many cases the breasts fill up to some degree in spite of treatment. The dose of estrogens needed to prevent pain and swelling of the breasts is much larger than the dose needed to treat symptoms of the menopause and this may increase your chances of developing blood clots in the legs or lungs (see below). Therefore, it is important that you discuss the benefits and the risks of estrogen use with your doctor if you have decided not to breast-feed your baby.

Some of the Dangers of Estrogen:
1. *Cancer of the uterus.* If estrogens are used in the postmenopausal period for more than a year, there is an increased risk of *endometrial cancer* (cancer of the uterus). Women taking estrogens have roughly five to ten times as great a chance of getting this cancer as women who take no estrogens. To put this another way, while a postmenopausal woman not taking estrogens has one chance in 1,000 each year of getting cancer of the uterus, a woman taking estrogens has five to ten chances in 1,000 each year. For this reason *it is important to take estrogens only when you really need them.*
The risk of this cancer is greater the longer estrogens are used and also seems to be greater when larger doses are taken. For this reason *it is important to take the lowest dose of estrogen that will control symptoms and to take it only as long as it is needed.* If estrogens are needed for longer periods of time, your doctor will want to reevaluate your need for estrogens at least every six months.
Women using estrogens should report any irregular vaginal bleeding to their doctors; such bleeding may be of no importance, but it can be an early warning of cancer of the uterus. If you have undiagnosed vaginal bleeding, you should not use estrogens until a diagnosis is made and you are certain there is no cancer of the uterus.
If you have had your uterus completely removed (total hysterectomy), there is no danger of developing cancer of the uterus.
2. *Other possible cancers.* Estrogens can cause development of other tumors in animals, such as tumors of the breast, cervix, vagina, or liver, when given for a long time. At present there is no good evidence that women using estrogen in the menopause have an increased risk of such tumors, but there is no way yet to be sure they do not; and one study raises the possibility that use of estrogens in the menopause may increase the risk of breast cancer many years later. This is a further reason to use estrogens only when clearly needed. While you are taking estrogens, it is important that you go to your doctor at least once a year for a physical examination. Also, if members of your family have had breast cancer or if you have breast nodules or abnormal mammograms (breast x-rays), your doctor may wish to carry out more frequent examinations of your breasts.
3. *Gall bladder disease.* Women who use estrogens after menopause are more likely to develop gall bladder disease needing surgery than women who do not use estrogens. Birth control pills have a similar effect.
4. *Abnormal blood clotting.* Oral contraceptives, some of which contain estrogens, increase the risk of blood clotting in various parts of the body. This can result in a stroke (if the clot is in the brain), a heart attack (clot in a blood vessel of the heart), or a pulmonary embolus (a clot which forms in the legs or pelvis, then breaks off and travels to the lungs). Any of these can be fatal. Blood clots may result in the loss of a limb, paralysis or loss of sight, depending on where the blood clot is formed or lodges if it breaks loose.
The larger doses of estrogen used to prevent swelling of the breasts after pregnancy have been reported to cause clotting in the legs and lungs.
It is recommended that if you have had any blood clotting disorders including clotting in the legs or lungs, or a heart attack or stroke, you should not use estrogens.

Special Warning About Pregnancy: You should not receive estrogen if you are pregnant. If this should occur, there is a greater than usual chance that the developing child will be born with a birth defect, although the possibility remains fairly small. A female child may have an increased risk of developing cancer of the vagina or cervix later in life (in the teens or twenties). Every possible effort should be made to avoid exposure to estrogens during pregnancy. If exposure occurs, see your doctor.

Some Other Effects of Estrogens: In addition to the serious known risks of estrogens described above, estrogens have the following side effects and potential risks:
1. *Nausea and vomiting.* The most common side effect of estrogen therapy is nausea. Vomiting is less common.
2. *Effects on breasts.* Estrogens may cause breast tenderness or enlargement and may cause the breasts to secrete a liquid.
3. *Effects on the uterus.* Estrogens may cause benign fibroid tumors of the uterus to get larger. Some women will have menstrual bleeding when estrogens are stopped. But if the bleeding occurs on days you are still taking estrogens you should report this to your doctor.
4. *Effects on liver.* Women taking estrogens develop on rare occasions a tumor of the liver which can rupture and bleed into the abdomen. You should report any swelling or unusual pain or tenderness in the abdomen to your doctor immediately.
Women with a past history of jaundice (yellowing of the skin and white parts of the eyes) may get jaundice again during estrogen use.
5. *Other effects.* Estrogens may cause excess fluid to be retained in the body. This may make some conditions worse, such as epilepsy, migraine, heart disease, or kidney disease.
If any of the above occur, stop taking estrogens and call your doctor.

Summary: Estrogens have important uses, but they have serious risks as well. You must decide, with your doctor, whether the risks are acceptable to you in view of the benefits of treatment. Except where your doctor has prescribed estrogens for use in special cases of cancer of the breast or prostate, you should not use estrogens if you have cancer of the breast or uterus, are pregnant, have undiagnosed abnormal vaginal bleeding, blood clotting disorders including clotting in the legs or lungs, or have had a stroke, heart attack or angina.
You must understand that your doctor will require regular physical examinations while you are taking them and will try to discontinue the drug as soon as possible and use the smallest dose possible. You can help minimize the risk by being alert for signs of trouble including:
1. Abnormal bleeding from the vagina.
2. Pains in the calves or chest or sudden shortness of breath, or coughing blood (indicating possible clots in the legs, heart or lungs).
3. Severe headache, dizziness, faintness, or changes in vision (indicating possible developing clots in the brain or eye).
4. Breast lumps (you should ask your doctor how to examine your own breasts).
5. Jaundice (yellowing of the skin).
6. Mental depression.
7. *Any* other unusual condition or problem.
Based on his or her assessment of your medical needs, your doctor has prescribed this drug for you. Do not give the drug to anyone else.

How Supplied: Available in 2.75 oz. (78g) tubes with or without ORTHO® Measured-Dose Applicator.
With applicator: NDC 0062-5450-77
Without applicator: NDC 0062-5450-00
Store at controlled room temperature.

ORTHO® Disposable Applicator

(See PDR For Nonprescription Drugs)

ORTHO® Personal Lubricant

(See PDR For Nonprescription Drugs)

ORTHO-GYNOL® Contraceptive Jelly

(See PDR For Nonprescription Drugs)

Product Information

ORTHO–NOVUM® Tablets ℞
(norethindrone/mestranol) or
(norethindrone/ethinyl estradiol)
and

MODICON® Tablets ℞
(norethindrone/ethinyl estradiol)
and

MICRONOR® Tablets ℞
(norethindrone)

Description:
ORTHO-NOVUM 7/7/7□21 Tablets are a combination oral contraceptive. Each white ORTHO-NOVUM 7/7/7□21 Tablet contains 0.5 mg of the progestational compound, norethindrone (17-hydroxy-19-nor-17α-pregn-4-en-20-yn-one), together with 0.035 mg of the estrogenic compound ethinyl estradiol (19-nor-17α-pregna-1,3,5(10)-trien-20-yne-3,17-diol). Each light peach ORTHO-NOVUM 7/7/7□21 Tablet contains 0.75 mg of the progestational compound, norethindrone (17-hydroxy-19-nor-17α-pregn-4-en-20-yn-3-one), together with 0.035 mg of the estrogenic compound, ethinyl estradiol (19-nor-17α-pregna-1,3,5(10)-trien-20-yne-3,17-diol). Each peach ORTHO-NOVUM 7/7/7□21 Tablet contains 1 mg of the progestational compound, norethindrone (17-hydroxy-19-nor-17α-pregn-4-en-20-yn-3-one), together with 0.035 mg of the estrogenic compound, ethinyl estradiol (19-nor-17α-pregna-1,3,5(10)-trien-20-yne-3,17-diol).

ORTHO-NOVUM 7/7/7□28 Tablets are a combination oral contraceptive. Each white ORTHO-NOVUM 7/7/7□28 Tablet contains 0.5 mg of the progestational compound, norethindrone (17-hydroxy-19-nor-17α-pregn-4-en-20-yn-3-one), together with 0.035 mg of the estrogenic compound, ethinyl estradiol (19-nor-17α-pregna-1,3,5(10)-trien-20-yne-3,17-diol). Each light peach ORTHO-NOVUM 7/7/7□28 Tablet contains 0.75 mg of the progestational compound, norethindrone (17-hydroxy-19-nor-17α-pregn-4-en-20-yn-3-one), together with 0.035 mg of the estrogenic compound, ethinyl estradiol (19-nor-17α-pregna-1,3,5(10)-trien-20-yne-3,17-diol). Each peach ORTHO-NOVUM 7/7/7□28 Tablet contains 1 mg of the progestational compound norethindrone (17-hydroxy-19-nor-17α-pregn-4-en-20-yn-3-one), together with 0.035 mg of the estrogenic compound, ethinyl estradiol (19-nor-17α-pregna-1,3,5(10)-trien-20-yne-3,17-diol). Each green tablet contains inert ingredients.

ORTHO-NOVUM 10/11□21 Tablets are a combination oral contraceptive. Each white ORTHO-NOVUM 10/11□21 Tablet contains 0.5 mg of the progestational compound, norethindrone (17-hydroxy-19-nor-17α-pregn-4-en-20-yn-3-one), together with 0.035 mg of the estrogenic compound, ethinyl estradiol (19-nor-17α-pregna-1,3,5(10)-trien-20-yne-3,17-diol). Each peach ORTHO-NOVUM 10/11□21 Tablet contains 1 mg of the progestational compound, norethindrone (17-hydroxy-19-nor-17α-pregn-4-en-20-yn-3-one), together with 0.035 mg of the estrogenic compound, ethinyl estradiol (19-nor-17α-pregna-1,3,5(10)-trien-20-yne-3,17-diol).

ORTHO-NOVUM 10/11□28 Tablets are a combination oral contraceptive. Each white ORTHO-NOVUM 10/11□28 Tablet contains 0.5 mg of the progestational compound, norethindrone (17-hydroxy-19-nor-17α-pregn-4-en-20-yn-3-one), together with 0.035 mg of the estrogenic compound, ethinyl estradiol (19-nor-17α-pregna-1,3,5(10)-trien-20-yne-3,17-diol). Each peach ORTHO-NOVUM 10/11□28 Tablet contains 1 mg of the progestational compound, norethindrone (17-hydroxy-19-nor-17α-pregn-4-en-20-yn-3-one), together with 0.035 mg of the estrogenic compound, ethinyl estradiol (19-nor-17α-pregna-1,3,5(10)-trien-20-yne-3,17-diol). Each green tablet contains inert ingredients.

ORTHO-NOVUM 1/35□21 Tablets are a combination oral contraceptive. Each ORTHO-NOVUM 1/35□21 Tablet contains 1 mg of the progestational compound, norethindrone (17- hydroxy-19-nor-17α -pregn- 4 -en- 20-yn-3- one), together with 0.035 mg of the estrogenic compound, ethinyl estradiol (19-nor-17α-pregna-1,3,5(10)-trien-20-yne-3,17-diol).

ORTHO-NOVUM 1/35□28 Tablets are a combination oral contraceptive. Each peach ORTHO-NOVUM 1/35□28 Tablet contains 1 mg of the progestational compound, norethindrone (17-hydroxy-19-nor-17α-pregn-4-en-20-yn-3-one), together with 0.035 mg of the estrogenic compound ethinyl estradiol (19-nor-17α-pregna-1,3,5(10)-trien-20-yne-3, 17-diol). Each green tablet contains inert ingredients.

MODICON 21 Tablets are a combination oral contraceptive. Each MODICON 21 Tablet contains 0.5 mg of the progestational compound, norethindrone (17-hydroxy-19-nor-17α-pregn-4-en-20-yn-3-one), together with 0.035 mg of the estrogenic compound, ethinyl estradiol (19-nor-17α-pregna-1,3,5(10)-trien-20-yne-3,17-diol).

MODICON 28 Tablets are a combination oral contraceptive. Each white MODICON 28 Tablet contains 0.5 mg of the progestational compound, norethindrone (17-hydroxy-19-nor-17α-pregn-4-en-20-yn-3-one), together with 0.035 mg of the estrogenic compound, ethinyl estradiol (19-nor-17α-pregna-1,3,5(10)-trien-20-yne-3,17-diol). Each green tablet contains inert ingredients.

ORTHO-NOVUM 1/50□21 Tablets are a combination oral contraceptive. Each ORTHO-NOVUM 1/50□21 Tablet contains 1 mg of the progestational compound, norethindrone (17-hydroxy-19-nor- 17α -pregn-4-en-20-yn-3-one), together with 0.05 mg of the estrogenic compound, mestranol (3-methoxy-19-nor-17α-pregna-1,3,5(10)-trien-20-yn-17-ol).

ORTHO-NOVUM 1/50□28 Tablets are a combination oral contraceptive. Each yellow ORTHO-NOVUM 1/50□28 Tablet contains 1 mg of the progestational compound, norethindrone (17-hydroxy-19-nor-17α-pregn-4-en-20-yn-3-one), together with 0.05 mg of the estrogenic compound, mestranol (3-methoxy-19-nor-17α-pregna-1,3,5(10)-trien-20-yn-17-ol). Each green tablet contains inert ingredients.

ORTHO-NOVUM 1/80□21 Tablets are a combination oral contraceptive. Each ORTHO-NOVUM 1/80□21 Tablet contains 1 mg of the progestational compound, norethindrone (17-hydroxy-19-nor- 17α -pregn-4-en-20-yn-3-one), together with 0.08 mg of the estrogenic compound, mestranol (3-methoxy-19-nor-17α-pregna-1,3,5(10)-trien-20-yn-17-ol).

ORTHO-NOVUM 1/80□28 Tablets are a combination oral contraceptive. Each white ORTHO-NOVUM 1/80□28 Tablet contains 1 mg of the progestational compound, norethindrone (17-hydroxy-19-nor-17α-pregn-4-en-20-yn-3-one), together with 0.08 mg of the estrogenic compound, mestranol (3-methoxy-19-nor-17α-pregna-1,3,5(10)-trien-20-yn-17-ol). Each green tablet contains inert ingredients.

ORTHO-NOVUM 2 mg□21 Tablets are a combination oral contraceptive. Each ORTHO-NOVUM 2 mg□21 Tablet contains 2 mg of the progestational compound, norethindrone (17- hydroxy-19-nor-17α -pregn- 4 -en- 20-yn-3- one), together with 0.10 mg of the estrogenic compound, mestranol (3-methoxy-19-nor-17α-pregna-1,3,5(10)-trien-20-yn-17-ol).

MICRONOR Tablets are a progestogen-only oral contraceptive. Each MICRONOR Tablet contains 0.35 mg of the progestational compound, norethindrone (17-hydroxy-19-nor-17α-pregn-4-en-20-yn-3-one), a synthetic progestogen.

Clinical Pharmacology Combination Oral Contraceptives Only: Combination oral contraceptives act primarily through the mechanism of gonadotropin suppression due to the estrogenic and progestational activity of the ingredients. Although the primary mechanism of action is inhibition of ovulation, alterations in the genital tract including changes in the cervical mucus (which increase the difficulty of sperm penetration) and the endometrium (which reduce the likelihood of implantation) may also contribute to contraceptive effectiveness.

Clinical Pharmacology Progestogen Oral Contraceptives: The primary mechanism through which MICRONOR prevents conception is not known, but progestogen-only contraceptives are known to alter the cervical mucus, exert a progestational effect on the endometrium, interfering with implantation, and, in some patients, suppress ovulation.

Indications and Usage: ORTHO-NOVUM 7/7/7□21, ORTHO-NOVUM 7/7/7□28, ORTHO-NOVUM 10/11□21, ORTHO-NOVUM 10/11□28, ORTHO-NOVUM 1/35□21, ORTHO-NOVUM 1/35□28, MODICON 21, MODICON 28, ORTHO-NOVUM 1/50□21, ORTHO-NOVUM 1/50□28, ORTHO-NOVUM 1/80□21, ORTHO-NOVUM 1/80□28, and MICRONOR are indicated for the prevention of pregnancy in women who elect to use oral contraceptives as a method of contraception.

ORTHO-NOVUM 2 mg□21 is indicated for the treatment of hypermenorrhea. ORTHO-NOVUM 2 mg□21 is indicated for the prevention of pregnancy in women who elect to use oral contraceptives as a method of contraception. (See first paragraph immediately following the opening WARNINGS statement.)

Oral contraceptives are highly effective. The pregnancy rate in women using conventional combination oral contraceptives (containing 35 mcg or more of ethinyl estradiol or 50 mcg or more of mestranol) is generally reported as less than one pregnancy per 100 woman-years of use. Slightly higher rates (somewhat more than one pregnancy per 100 woman-years of use) are reported for some combination products containing 35 mcg or less of ethinyl estradiol, and rates on the order of three pregnancies per 100 woman-years are reported for the progestogen-only oral contraceptives.

These rates are derived from separate studies conducted by different investigators in several population groups and cannot be compared precisely. Furthermore, pregnancy rates tend to be lower as clinical studies are continued, possibly due to selective retention in the longer studies of those patients who accept the treatment regimen and do not discontinue as a result of adverse reactions, pregnancy or other reasons.

The ORTHO-NOVUM 7/7/7□21 Tablet regimen consists of 7 white tablets containing 0.5 mg norethindrone together with 0.035 mg ethinyl estradiol, followed by 7 light peach tablets containing 0.75 mg norethindrone together with 0.035 mg ethinyl estradiol, followed by 7 peach tablets containing 1 mg norethindrone together with 0.035 mg ethinyl estradiol.

The ORTHO-NOVUM 7/7/7□28 Tablet regimen consists of 7 white tablets containing 0.5 mg norethindrone together with 0.035 mg ethinyl estradiol, followed by 7 light peach tablets containing 0.75 mg norethindrone together with 0.035 mg ethinyl estradiol, followed by 7 peach tablets containing 1 mg norethindrone together with 0.035 mg ethinyl estradiol and 7 green placebo tablets.

7 WHITE TABLETS
In clinical trials with a formulation containing 0.5 mg of norethindrone and 0.035 mg of ethinyl estradiol, 1,168 patients completed 16,345 cycles of use and a total of 3 pregnancies was reported. This represents a pregnancy rate of 0.22 per 100 woman-years.

7 PEACH TABLETS
In clinical trials with a formulation containing 1 mg of norethindrone and 0.035 mg of ethinyl estradiol, 940 subjects completed 14,366 cycles of use. Two pregnancies were reported for a pregnancy rate of 0.17 per 100 woman-years.

Table 1 gives ranges of pregnancy rates reported in the literature for other means of contraception. The efficacy of these means of contraception (except the IUD) depends upon the degree of adherence to the method.

The ORTHO-NOVUM 10/11□21 Tablet regimen consists of 10 white tablets followed by 11 peach tablets.

The ORTHO-NOVUM 10/11□28 Tablet regimen consists of 10 white tablets followed by 11 peach tablets and 7 green placebo tablets.

Continued on next page

Ortho Pharm.—Cont.

10 WHITE TABLETS
In clinical trials with a formulation containing 0.5 mg of norethindrone and 0.035 mg of ethinyl estradiol, 1,168 patients completed 16,345 cycles of use and a total of three pregnancies was reported. This represents a pregnancy rate of 0.22 per 100 woman-years.

11 PEACH TABLETS
In clinical trials with a formulation containing 1 mg norethindrone and 0.035 mg of ethinyl estradiol, 940 subjects completed 14,366 cycles of use. Two pregnancies were reported for a pregnancy rate of 0.17 per 100 woman-years.

The dropout rate for medical reasons, as observed in the clinical trials conducted with ORTHO-NOVUM 1/35 and MODICON, appears to be somewhat higher than observed with higher dose combination products. The dropout rate due to menstrual disorders and irregularities was also somewhat higher, dropouts being equally split between menstrual disorders and irregularities and other medical reasons attributable to the drug.

In clinical trials with ORTHO-NOVUM 1/35□21 and ORTHO-NOVUM 1/35□28, 940 subjects completed 14,366 cycles of use. Two pregnancies were reported for a pregnancy rate of 0.17 per 100 woman-years.

In clinical trials with MODICON and MODICON 28, 1,168 patients completed 16,345 cycles of use, and a total of three pregnancies was reported. This represents a pregnancy rate of 0.22 per 100 woman-years.

In clinical trials with ORTHO-NOVUM 1/50□21, 3,852 patients completed 45,937 cycles, and a total of 10 pregnancies was reported. This represents a pregnancy rate of 0.26 per 100 woman-years.

In clinical trials with ORTHO-NOVUM 1/50□28, 1,590 patients completed 7,330 cycles, and a total of three pregnancies was reported. This represents a pregnancy rate of 0.5 per 100 woman-years.

In clinical trials with ORTHO-NOVUM 1/80□21, and ORTHO-NOVUM 1/80□28, 3,464 patients completed 34,068 cycles, and a total of five pregnancies was reported. This represents a pregnancy rate of 0.18 per 100 woman-years.

In clinical trials with ORTHO-NOVUM 2 mg□20, 6,097 patients completed 121,233 cycles, and a total of 13 pregnancies was reported. This represents a pregnancy rate of 0.13 per 100 woman-years. In clinical trials with ORTHO-NOVUM 2 mg□21, 965 patients completed 3,743 cycles, and no pregnancies were reported. This represents a pregnancy rate of 0.0 per 100 woman-years.

In clinical trials with MICRONOR, 2,963 patients completed 25,901 cycles of therapy, and a total of 55 pregnancies was reported. This represents an average pregnancy rate of 2.54 per 100 woman-years.

A higher pregnancy rate of 3.72 was recorded in "fresh" patients (those who had never taken oral contraceptives prior to starting MICRONOR therapy) to a large extent because of incorrect tablet intake. This compares to the lower pregnancy rate of 1.95 recorded in "changeover" patients (those switched from other oral contraceptives).

This difference was found to be statistically significant. Furthermore, an even greater statistically significant difference in pregnancy rates between these two groups was found during the first six months of MICRONOR therapy. Therefore, it is especially important for "fresh" patients to strictly adhere to the regimen.

Table 1 gives ranges of pregnancy rates reported in the literature[1] for other means of contraception. The efficacy of these means of contraception (except the IUD) depends upon the degree of adherence to the method.

Table 1
Pregnancies Per 100 Woman-Years
IUD, less than 1–6;
Diaphragm with spermicidal product (creams or jellies), 2–20; Condom, 3–36; Aerosol foams, 2–29; Jellies and creams, 4–36; Periodic abstinence (rhythm) all types, less than 1–47;
1. Calendar method, 14–47;
2. Temperature method, 1–20;
3. Temperature method—intercourse only in postovulatory phase, less than 1–7;
4. Mucus method, 1–25;
No contraception, 60–80.

Dose-Related Risk of Thromboembolism From Oral Contraceptives: Two studies have shown a positive association between the dose of estrogens in oral contraceptives and the risk of thromboembolism.[2,3] For this reason, it is prudent and in keeping with good principles of therapeutics to minimize exposure to estrogen. The oral contraceptive product prescribed for any given patient should be that product which contains the least amount of estrogen that is compatible with an acceptable pregnancy rate and patient acceptance. It is recommended that new acceptors of oral contraceptives be started on preparations containing .05 mg or less of estrogen.

Contraindications: Oral contraceptives should not be used in women with any of the following conditions:
1. Thrombophlebitis or thromboembolic disorders.
2. A past history of deep vein thrombophlebitis or thromboembolic disorders.
3. Cerebral vascular or coronary artery disease.
4. Known or suspected carcinoma of the breast.
5. Known or suspected estrogen-dependent neoplasia.
6. Undiagnosed, abnormal genital bleeding.
7. Oral contraceptive tablets may cause fetal harm when administered to a pregnant woman. Oral contraceptive tablets are contraindicated in women who are pregnant. If the patient becomes pregnant while taking this drug, the patient should be apprised of the potential hazard to the fetus (see WARNINGS, No. 5).
8. Benign or malignant liver tumor which developed during the use of oral contraceptives or other estrogen-containing products.

WARNINGS

> Cigarette smoking increases the risk of serious cardiovascular side effects from oral contraceptive use. This risk increases with age and with heavy smoking (15 or more cigarettes per day) and is quite marked in women over 35 years of age. Women who use oral contraceptives should be strongly advised not to smoke.
>
> The use of oral contraceptives is associated with increased risk of several serious conditions including thromboembolism, stroke, myocardial infarction, hepatic adenoma, gallbladder disease, hypertension. Practitioners prescribing oral contraceptives should be familiar with the following information relating to these risks.

ORTHO-NOVUM 2 mg□21 should only be used for contraception when lower dose formulations prove unacceptable.

1. THROMBOEMBOLIC DISORDERS AND OTHER VASCULAR PROBLEMS. An increased risk of thromboembolic and thrombotic disease associated with the use of oral contraceptives is well-established. Four principal studies in Great Britain[4,5,6,26] and three in the United States[7-10] have demonstrated an increased risk of fatal and nonfatal venous thromboembolism and stroke, both hemorrhagic and thrombotic. These studies estimate that users of oral contraceptives are 4 to 11 times more likely than nonusers to develop these diseases without evident cause (Tables 2,4). Overall excess mortality due to pulmonary embolism or stroke is on the order of 1.0 to 3.5 deaths annually per 100,000 users and increases with age (Table 3).

Table 2
Hospitalization Rates Due to Venous Thromboembolic Disease[6]
Admissions annually per 100,000 women, age 20–44
Users of oral contraceptives 45
Nonusers 5

Table 3
Death Rates Due to Pulmonary Embolism or Cerebral Thrombosis[5]—Deaths Annually Per 100,000 Nonpregnant Women

	Age 20 to 34	Age 35 to 44
Users of oral contraceptives	1.5	3.9
Nonusers	.2	.5

Cerebrovascular Disorders: In a collaborative American study,[9,10] of cerebrovascular disorders in women with and without predisposing causes, it was estimated that the risk of hemorrhagic stroke was 2.0 times greater in users than in nonusers and the risk of thrombotic stroke was 4.0 to 9.5 times greater in users than in nonusers (Table 4).

Table 4
Summary of Relative Risk of Thromboembolic Disorders and Other Vascular Problems in Oral Contraceptive Users Compared to Nonusers

Relative risk, times greater
Idiopathic thromboembolic disease 4–11
Post surgery thromboembolic
complications 4–6
Thrombotic stroke 4–9.5
Hemorrhagic stroke 2
Myocardial infarction 2–12

A prospective study conducted in Great Britain[57] estimated that former users have a risk for all cerebrovascular disease 2.6 times greater than that of non-users. This risk remained elevated for at least six years after last oral contraceptive use. A prospective study conducted in the United States[55] found that past use of oral contraceptives was associated with increased risk of subarachnoid hemorrhage, the relative risk being 5.3. There was also some evidence from this study that the degree of risk may be related to duration of oral contraceptive use.

Myocardial Infarction: An increased risk of myocardial infarction associated with the use of oral contraceptives has been reported[11,12,13] confirming a previously suspected association (Tables 5 & 6). These studies, conducted in the United Kingdom, found, as expected, that the greater the number of underlying risk factors for coronary artery disease (cigarette smoking, hypertension, hypercholesterolemia, obesity, diabetes, history of preeclamptic toxemia), the higher the risk of developing myocardial infarction, regardless of whether the patient was an oral contraceptive user or not. Oral contraceptives, however, were found to be a clear additional risk factor.

The annual excess case rate (increased risk) of myocardial infarction (fatal and nonfatal) in oral contraceptive users was estimated to be approximately 7 cases per 100,000 women users in the 30–39 age group and 67 cases per 100,000 women users in the 40–44 age group.

In terms of relative risk, it has been estimated[52] that oral contraceptive users who do not smoke (smoking is considered a major predisposing condition to myocardial infarction) are about twice as likely to have a fatal myocardial infarction as nonusers who do not smoke. Oral contraceptive users who are also smokers have about a 5-fold increased risk of fatal infarction compared to users who do not smoke, but about a 10- to 12-fold increased risk compared to nonusers who do not smoke. Furthermore, the amount of smoking is also an important factor. In determining the importance of these relative risks, however, the baseline rates for various age groups, as shown in Table 5, must be given serious consideration. The importance of other predisposing conditions mentioned above in determining relative and absolute risks have not as yet been quantified; it is quite likely that the same synergistic action exists, but perhaps to a lesser extent.

A study[56] suggests that some increased risk of myocardial infarction in oral contraceptive users persists following discontinuation of oral contraceptives and that the degree of the residual risk is related to the duration of past use.

Table 6
Myocardial Infarction Rates in Users And Nonusers Of Oral Contraceptives in Britain[11,12,13]—Cases Annually Per 100,000 Women

	Nonfatal		Fatal	
	Age 30 to 39	Age 40 to 44	Age 30 to 39	Age 40 to 44
Users of oral contraceptives	5.6	56.9	5.4	32.0
Nonusers of oral contraceptives	2.1	9.9	1.9	12.0
Relative risk	2.7	5.7	2.8	2.8

Table 5
Estimated Annual Mortality Rate Per 100,000 Women From Myocardial Infarction By Use Of Oral Contraceptives, Smoking Habits, And Age (in years)

	Myocardial Infarction	
	Women aged 30–39	Women aged 40–44
Smoking habits	Users / Nonusers	Users / Nonusers
All smokers	10.2 / 2.6	62.0 / 15.9
Heavy[1]	13.0 / 5.1	78.7 / 31.3
Light	4.7 / .9	28.6 / 5.7
Nonsmokers	1.8 / 1.2	10.7 / 7.4
Smokers and nonsmokers	5.4 / 1.9	32.8 / 11.7

[1]Heavy smoker: 15 or more cigarettes per day. From Jain, A.K., Studies in Family Planning. 8:50, 1977.
[See table above].

Risk of dose: In an analysis of data derived from several national adverse reaction reporting systems,[2] British investigators concluded that the risk of thromboembolism including coronary thrombosis is directly related to the dose of estrogen used in oral contraceptives. Preparations containing 100 mcg or more of estrogen were associated with a higher risk of thromboembolism than those containing 50–80 mcg of estrogen. Their analysis did suggest, however, that the quantity of estrogen may not be the sole factor involved. This finding has been confirmed in the United States.[3] Careful epidemiological studies to determine the degree of thromboembolic risk associated with progestogen-only oral contraceptives have not been performed. Cases of thromboembolic disease have been reported in women using these products, and they should not be presumed to be free of excess risk.

The risk of thromboembolic and thrombotic disorders, in both users and nonusers of oral contraceptives, increases with age. Oral contraceptives are, however, an independent risk factor for these events.

Estimate of Excess Mortality From Circulatory Diseases: A large prospective study[53] carried out in the United Kingdom estimated the mortality rate per 100,000 women per year from diseases of the circulatory system for users and nonusers of oral contraceptives according to age, smoking habits, and duration of use. The overall excess death rate annually from circulatory diseases for oral contraceptive users was estimated to be 20 per 100,000 (ages 15–34—5/100,000; ages 35–44—33/100,000; ages 45–49—140/100,000), the risk being concentrated in older women, in those with a long duration of use and in cigarette smokers. It was not possible, however, to examine the interrelationships of age, smoking, and duration of use, nor to compare the effects of continuous versus intermittent use. Although the study showed a 10-fold increase in death due to circulatory diseases in users for five or more years, all of these deaths occurred in women 35 or older. Until larger numbers of women under 35 with continuous use for five or more years are available, it is not possible to assess the magnitude of the relative risk for this younger age group.

This study reports that the increased risk of circulatory disease mortatilty[57] may persist after the pill is discontinued.

Another study published at the same time confirms a previously reported increase of mortality in pill users from cardiovascular disease.[54]

The available data from a variety of sources have been analyzed[14] to estimate the rate of death associated with various methods of contraception. The estimates of risk of death for each method include the combined risk of the contraceptive method (e.g., thromboembolic and thrombotic disease in the case of oral contraceptives) plus the risk attributable to pregnancy or abortion in the event of method failure. This latter risk varies with the effectiveness of the contraceptive method. The findings of this analysis are shown in Figure 1 below.[14] The study concluded that the mortality associated with all methods of birth control is low and below that associated with childbirth, with the exception of oral contraceptives in women over 40 who smoke. (The rates given for pill only/smokers for each age group are for smokers as a class. For "heavy" smokers [more than 15 cigarettes a day], the rates given would be about double; for "light" smokers [less than 15 cigarettes a day], about 50 percent.)

The mortality associated with oral contraceptive use in nonsmokers over 40 is higher than with any other method of contraception in that age group.

The lowest mortality is associated with the condom or diaphragm backed up by early abortion.

The risk of thromboembolic and thrombotic disease associated with oral contraceptives increases with age after approximately age 30 and, for myocardial infarction, is further increased by hypertension, hypercholesterolemia, obesity, diabetes, or history of preeclamptic toxemia and especially by cigarette smoking. The risk of myocardial infarction in oral contraceptive users is substantially increased in women age 40 and over, especially those with other risk factors.

Based on the data currently available, the following chart gives a gross estimate of the risk of death from circulatory disorders associated with the use of oral contraceptives:

Smoking Habits and Other Predisposing Conditions—Risk Associated With Use Of Oral Contraceptives

Age	Below 30	30–39	40+
Heavy smokers	C	B	A
Light smokers	D	C	B
Nonsmokers (no predisposing conditions)	D	C,D	C
Nonsmokers (other predisposing conditions)	C	C,B	B,A

A—Use associated with very high risk.
B—Use associated with high risk.
C—Use associated with moderate risk.
D—Use associated with low risk.

The physician and the patient should be alert to the earliest manifestations of thromboembolic and thrombotic disorders (e.g., thrombophlebitis, pulmonary embolism, cerebrovascular insufficiency, coronary occlusion, retinal thrombosis, and mesenteric thrombosis). Should any of these occur or be suspected, the drug should be discontinued immediately.

A four- to six-fold increased risk of post surgery thromboembolic complications has been reported in oral contraceptives users.[15,16] If feasible, oral contraceptives should be discontinued at least four weeks before surgery of a type associated with an increased risk of thromboembolism or prolonged immobilization.

2. OCULAR LESIONS. There have been reports of neuro-ocular lesions such as optic neuritis or retinal thrombosis associated with the use of oral contraceptives. Discontinue oral contraceptive medication if there is unexplained, sudden or gradual, partial or complete loss of vision; onset of proptosis or diplopia; papilledema; or retinal vascular lesions and institute appropriate diagnostic and therapeutic measures.

3. CARCINOMA. Long-term continuous administration of either natural or synthetic estrogen in certain animal species increases the frequency of carcinoma of the breast, cervix, vagina, and liver. Certain synthetic progestogens, none currently contained in oral contraceptives, have been noted to increase the incidence of mammary nodules, benign and malignant, in dogs.

In humans, three case control studies have reported an increased risk of endometrial carcinoma associated with the prolonged use of exogenous estrogen in postmenopausal women.[17,18,19] One publication[20] reported on the first 21 cases submitted by physicians to a registry of cases of adenocarcinoma of the endometrium in women under 40 on oral contraceptives. Of the cases found in women without predisposing risk factors for adenocarcinoma of the endometrium (e.g., irregular bleeding at the time oral contraceptives were first given, polycystic ovaries), nearly all occurred in women who had used a sequential oral contraceptive. These products are no longer marketed. No evidence has been reported suggesting an increased risk of endometrial cancer in users of conventional combination or progestogen-only oral contraceptives.

Several studies[8,21-24] have found no increases in breast cancer in women taking oral contraceptives or estrogens. One study[25] however, while also noting no overall increased risk of breast cancer in women treated with oral contraceptives, found an excess risk in the subgroups of oral contraceptive users with documented benign breast disease. A reduced occurrence of benign breast tumors in users of oral contraceptives has been well-documented.[8,21,25,26,27]

In summary, there is at present no confirmed evidence from human studies of an increased risk of cancer associated with oral contraceptives. Close

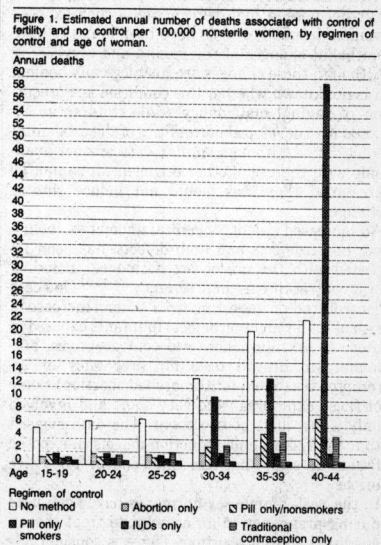

Figure 1. Estimated annual number of deaths associated with control of fertility and no control per 100,000 nonsterile women, by regimen of control and age of woman.

Continued on next page

Ortho Pharm.—Cont.

clinical surveillance of all women taking oral contraceptives is, nevertheless, essential. In all cases of undiagnosed persistent or recurrent abnormal vaginal bleeding, appropriate diagnostic measures should be taken to rule out malignancy. Women with a strong family history of breast cancer or who have breast nodules, fibrocystic disease or abnormal mammograms should be monitored with particular care if they elect to use oral contraceptives instead of other methods of contraception.

4. HEPATIC TUMORS. Benign hepatic adenomas have been found to be associated with the use of oral contraceptives.[28,29,30,46] One study[46] showed that oral contraceptive formulations with high hormonal potency were associated with a higher risk than lower potency formulations and use of oral contraceptives with high hormonal potency and age over 30 years may further increase the woman's risk of hepatocellular adenoma. Although benign, hepatic adenomas may rupture and may cause death through intra-abdominal hemorrhage. This has been reported in short-term as well as long-term users of oral contraceptives. Two studies relate risk with duration of use of the contraceptive, the risk being much greater after four or more years of oral contraceptive use.[30,46] While hepatic adenoma is a rare lesion, it should be considered in women presenting abdominal pain and tenderness, abdominal mass or shock.

A few cases of hepatocellular carcinoma have been reported in women taking oral contraceptives. The relationship of these drugs to this type of malignancy is not known at this time.

5. USE IN OR IMMEDIATELY PRECEDING PREGNANCY, BIRTH DEFECTS IN OFFSPRING, AND MALIGNANCY IN FEMALE OFFSPRING. The use of female sex hormones—both estrogenic and progestational agents—during early pregnancy may seriously damage the offspring. It has been shown that females exposed in utero to diethylstilbestrol, a nonsteroidal estrogen, have an increased risk of developing in later life a form of vaginal or cervical cancer that is ordinarily extremely rare.[31,32] This risk has been estimated to be of the order of 1 to 4 in 1000 exposures.[33,47] Although there is no evidence at the present time that oral contraceptives further enhance the risk of developing this type of malignancy, such patients should be monitored with particular care if they elect to use oral contraceptives instead of other methods of contraception. Furthermore, a high percentage of such exposed women (from 30 to 90%) have been found to have epithelial changes of the vagina and cervix.[34-38] Although these changes are histologically benign, it is not known whether this condition is a precursor of vaginal malignancy. Male children so exposed may develop abnormalities of the urogenital tract.[48,49,50] Although similar data are not available with the use of other estrogens, it cannot be presumed that they would not induce similar changes.

An increased risk of congenital anomalies, including heart defects and limb defects, has been reported with the use of sex hormones, including oral contraceptives, in pregnancy.[39-42,51] One case control study[42] has estimated a 4.7-fold increase in risk of limb-reduction defects in infants exposed in utero to sex hormones (oral contraceptives, hormonal withdrawal tests for pregnancy or attempted treatment for threatened abortion). Some of these exposures were very short and involved only a few days of treatment. The data suggest that the risk of limb-reduction defects in exposed fetuses is somewhat less than one in 1,000 live births.

In the past, female sex hormones have been used during pregnancy in an attempt to treat threatened or habitual abortion. There is considerable evidence that estrogens are ineffective for these indications, and there is no evidence from well-controlled studies that progestogens are effective for these uses.

There is some evidence that triploidy and possibly other types of polyploidy are increased among abortuses from women who become pregnant soon after ceasing oral contraceptives.[43] Embryos with these anomalies are virtually always aborted spontaneously. Whether there is an overall increase in spontaneous abortion of pregnancies conceived soon after stopping oral contraceptives is unknown. It is recommended that for any patient who has missed two consecutive periods, pregnancy should be ruled out before continuing the contraceptive regimen. If the patient has not adhered to the prescribed schedule, the possibility of pregnancy should be considered at the time of the first missed period (or after 45 days from the last menstrual period if the progestogen-only oral contraceptives are used), and further use of oral contraceptives should be withheld until pregnancy has been ruled out. If pregnancy is confirmed, the patient should be apprised of the potential risks to the fetus and the advisability of continuation of the pregnancy should be discussed in the light of these risks.

It is also recommended that women who discontinue oral contraceptives with the intent of becoming pregnant use an alternate form of contraception for a period of time before attempting to conceive. Many clinicians recommend three months although no precise information is available on which to base this recommendation.

The administration of progestogen-only or progestogen-estrogen combinations to induce withdrawal bleeding should not be used as a test of pregnancy.

6. GALLBLADDER DISEASE. Studies[8,23,26] report an increased risk of surgically confirmed gallbladder disease in users of oral contraceptives and estrogens. In one study, an increased risk appeared after two years of use and doubled after four or five years of use. In one of the other studies, an increased risk was apparent between six and twelve months of use.

7. CARBOHYDRATE AND LIPID METABOLIC EFFECTS. A decrease in glucose tolerance has been observed in a significant percentage of patients on oral contraceptives. For this reason, prediabetic and diabetic patients should be carefully observed while receiving oral contraceptives.

An increase in triglycerides and total phospholipids has been observed in patients receiving oral contraceptives.[44] The clinical significance of this finding remains to be defined.

8. ELEVATED BLOOD PRESSURE. An increase in blood pressure has been reported in patients receiving oral contraceptives.[26] In some women hypertension may occur within a few months of beginning oral contraceptive use. In the first year of use, the prevalence of women with hypertension is low in users and may be no higher than that of a comparable group of nonusers. The prevalence in users increases, however, with longer exposure, and in the fifth year of use is two and a half to three times the reported prevalence in the first year. Age is also strongly correlated with the development of hypertension in oral contraceptive users. Women who previously have had hypertension during pregnancy may be more likely to develop elevation of blood pressure when given oral contraceptives. Hypertension that develops as a result of taking oral contraceptives usually returns to normal after discontinuing the drug.

9. HEADACHE. The onset or exacerbation of migraine or development of headache of a new pattern which is recurrent, persistent, or severe, requires discontinuation of oral contraceptives and evaluation of the cause.

10. BLEEDING IRREGULARITIES. Breakthrough bleeding, spotting, and amenorrhea are frequent reasons for patients discontinuing oral contraceptives. In breakthrough bleeding, as in all cases of irregular bleeding from the vagina, nonfunctional causes should be borne in mind. In undiagnosed persistent or recurrent abnormal bleeding from the vagina, adequate diagnostic measures are indicated to rule out pregnancy or malignancy. If pathology has been excluded, time or a change to another formulation may solve the problem. Changing to an oral contraceptive with a higher estrogen content, while potentially useful in minimizing menstrual irregularity, should be done only if necessary since this may increase the risk of thromboembolic disease.

An alteration in menstrual patterns is likely to occur in women using progestogen-only oral contraceptives. The amount and duration of flow, cycle length, breakthrough bleeding, spotting and amenorrhea will probably be quite variable. Bleeding irregularities occur more frequently with the use of progestogen-only oral contraceptives than with the combinations and the dropout rate due to such conditions is higher.

Women with a past history of oligomenorrhea or secondary amenorrhea or young women without regular cycles may have a tendency to remain anovulatory or to become amenorrheic after discontinuation of oral contraceptives. Women with these preexisting problems should be advised of this possibility and encouraged to use other contraceptive methods. Postuse anovulation, possibly prolonged, may also occur in women without previous irregularities.

11. ECTOPIC PREGNANCY. Ectopic as well as intrauterine pregnancy may occur in contraceptive failures. However, in progestogen-only oral contraceptive failures, the ratio of ectopic to intrauterine pregnancies is higher than in women who are not receiving oral contraceptives, since the drugs are more effective in preventing intrauterine than ectopic pregnancies.

12. BREAST FEEDING. Oral contraceptives given in the postpartum period may interfere with lactation. There may be a decrease in the quantity and quality of the breast milk. Furthermore, a small fraction of the hormonal agents in oral contraceptives has been identified in the milk of mothers receiving these drugs.[45] The effects, if any, on the breast-fed child have not been determined. If feasible, the use of oral contraceptives should be deferred until the infant has been weaned.

Precautions:

General

1. A complete medical and family history should be taken prior to the initiation of oral contraceptives. The pretreatment and periodic physical examinations should include special reference to blood pressure, breasts, abdomen and pelvic organs, including Papanicolaou smear and relevant laboratory tests. As a general rule, oral contraceptives should not be prescribed for longer than one year without another physical examination being performed.

2. Under the influence of estrogen-progestogen preparations, preexisting uterine leiomyomata may increase in size.

3. Patients with a history of psychic depression should be carefully observed and the drug discontinued if depression recurs to a serious degree. Patients becoming significantly depressed while taking oral contraceptives should stop the medication and use an alternate method of contraception in an attempt to determine whether the symptom is drug-related.

4. Oral contraceptives may cause some degree of fluid retention. They should be prescribed with caution, and only with careful monitoring, in patients with conditions which might be aggravated by fluid retention, such as convulsive disorders, migraine syndrome, asthma, or cardiac or renal insufficiency.

5. Patients with a past history of jaundice during pregnancy have an increased risk of recurrence of jaundice while receiving oral contraceptive therapy. If jaundice develops in any patient receiving such drugs, the medication should be discontinued.

6. Steroid hormones may be poorly metabolized in patients with impaired liver function and should be administered with caution in such patients.

7. Oral contraceptive users may have disturbances in normal tryptophan metabolism which may result in a relative pyridoxine deficiency. The clinical significance of this is yet to be determined.

8. Serum folate levels may be depressed by oral contraceptive therapy. Since the pregnant woman

1975. 4. Royal College of General Practitioners, "Oral contraception and thromboembolic disease," J Coll Gen Pract 13:267-279, 1967. 5. Inman, W.H.W. and M.P. Vessey, "Investigation of deaths from pulmonary, coronary, and cerebral thrombosis and embolism in women of childbearing age," Brit Med J 2:193-199, 1968. 6. Vessey, M.P. and R. Doll, "Investigation of relation between use of oral contraceptives and thromboembolic disease. A further report," Brit Med J 2:651-657, 1969. 7. Sartwell, P.E., A.T. Masi, F.G. Arthes, G.R. Greene and H.E. Smith, "Thromboembolism and oral contraceptives: an epidemiological case control study," Am J Epidemiol 90:365-380, 1969. 8. Boston Collaborative Drug Surveillance Program, "Oral contraceptives and venous thromboembolic disease, surgically confirmed gall bladder disease and breast tumors," Lancet 1:1399-1404, 1973. 9. Collaborative Group for the Study of Stroke in Young Women, "Oral contraception and increased risk of cerebral ischemia or thrombosis," N Engl J Med 288:871-878, 1973. 10. Collaborative Group for the Study of Stroke in Young Women, "Oral contraceptives and strokes in young women: associated risk factors," JAMA 231:718-722, 1975. 11. Mann, J.I. and W.H.W. Inman, "Oral contraceptives and death from myocardial infarction," Brit Med J 2:245-248, 1975. 12. Mann, J.I., W.H.W. Inman, and M. Thorogood, "Oral contraceptive use in older women and fatal myocardial infarction," Brit Med J 2:445-447, 1976. 13. Mann. J.I., M.P. Vessey, M. Thorogood, and R. Doll, "Myocardial infarction in young women with special reference to oral contraceptive practice," Brit Med J 2:241-245, 1975. 14. Tietze, C., "New Estimate of Mortality Associated with Fertility Control," Family Planning Perspectives Vol. 9, No. 2, 74-76, 1977. 15. Vessey, M.P., R. Doll, A.S. Fairbairn, and G. Glober, "Post-operative thromboembolism and the use of oral contraceptives," Brit Med J 3:123-126, 1970. 16. Greene, G.R., and P.E. Sartwell, "Oral contraceptive use in patients with thromboembolism following surgery, trauma, or infection," Am J Pub Health 62:680-685, 1972. 17. Smith, D.C., R. Prentice, D.J. Thompson, and W.L. Herrmann, "Association of exogenous estrogen and endometrial carcinoma," N Engl J Med 293:1164-1167, 1975. 18. Ziel, H.K. and W.D. Finkle, "Increased risk of endometrial carcinoma among users of conjugated estrogens," N Engl J Med 293:1167-1170, 1975. 19. Mack, T.N., M.C. Pike, B.E. Henderson, R.I. Pfeffer, V.R. Gerkins, M. Arthur, and S.E. Brown, "Estrogens and endometrial cancer in a retirement community," N Engl J Med 294:1262-1267, 1976. 20. Silverberg, S.G., and E.L. Makowski, "Endometrial carcinoma in young women taking oral contraceptive agents," Obstet Gynecol 46:503-506, 1975. 21. Vessey, M.P., R. Doll, and P.M. Sutton, "Oral contraceptives and breast neoplasia: a retrospective study," Brit Med J 3:719-724, 1972. 22. Vessey, M.P., R. Doll, and K. Jones, "Oral contraceptives and breast cancer. Progress report of an epidemiological study," Lancet 1:941-943, 1975. 23. Boston Collaborative Drug Surveillance Program, "Surgically confirmed gall bladder disease, venous thromboembolism and breast tumors in relation to postmenopausal estrogen therapy," N Engl J Med 290:15-19, 1974. 24. Arthes, F.G., P.E. Sartwell, and E.F. Lewison, "The Pill, estrogens, and the breast. Epidemiological aspects," Cancer 28:1391-1394, 1971. 25. Fasal, E., and R.S. Paffenbarger, "Oral contraceptives as related to cancer and benign lesions of the breast," J Natl Cancer Inst 55:767-773, 1975. 26. Royal College of General Practitioners, "Oral Contraceptives and Health," London, Pitman, 1974. 27. Ory, H., P. Cole, B. MacMahon and R. Hoover, "Oral contraceptives and reduced risk of benign breast diseases," N Engl J Med 294:419-422, 1976. 28. Baum, J., F. Holtz, J.J. Bookstein, and E.W. Klein, "Possible association between benign hepatomas and oral contraceptives," Lancet 2:926-928, 1973. 29. Mays, E.T., W.M. Christopherson, M.M. Mahr, and H.C. Williams, "Hepatic changes in young women ingesting contraceptive steroids. Hepatic hemorrhage and primary hepatic tumors," JAMA 235:730-732, 1976. 30. Edmonsen, H.A., B. Henderson, and B. Benton, "Liver-cell adenomas associated with the use of oral contraceptives," N Engl J Med 294:470-472, 1976. 31. Herbst, A.L., H. Ulfedler, and D.C. Poskanzer, "Adenocarcinoma of the vagina," N Engl J Med 284:878-881, 1971. 32. Greenwald, P., J.J. Barlow, P.C. Nasca, and W. Burnett, "Vaginal cancer after maternal treatment with synthetic estrogens," N Engl J Med 285:390-392, 1971. 33. Lanier, A.P., K.L. Noller, D.G. Decker, L. Elveback, and L.T. Kurland, "Cancer and stilbestrol. A follow-up of 1719 persons exposed to estrogen in utero and born 1943-1959," Mayo Clinic Pro 48:793-799, 1973. 34. Herbst, A.L., R.J. Kurman, and R.E. Scully, "Vaginal and cervical abnormalities after exposure to stilbestrol in utero," Obstet Gynecol 40:287-298, 1972. 35. Herbst, A.L., S.J. Robboy, G.J. Macdonald, and R.E. Scully, "The effects of local progesterone on stilbestrol-associated vaginal adenosis," Am J Obstet Gynecol 118:607-615, 1974. 36. Herbst, A.L., D.C. Poskanzer, S.J. Robboy, L. Friedlander, and R.E. Scully, "Prenatal exposure to stilbestrol: a prospective comparison of exposed female offspring with unexposed controls," N Engl J Med 292:334-339, 1975. 37. Stafl, A., R.F. Mattingly, D.V. Foley, W. Fetherston, "Clinical diagnosis of vaginal adenosis," Obstet Gynecol 43:118-128, 1974. 38. Sherman, A.I., M. Goldrath, A. Berlin, V. Vakhariya, F. Banooni, W. Michaels, P. Goodman, and S. Brown, "Cervical-vaginal adenosis after in utero exposure to synthetic estrogens," Obstet Gynecol 44:531-545, 1974. 39. Gal, I., B. Kirman, and J. Stern, "Hormone pregnancy tests and congenital malformation," Nature 216:83, 1967. 40. Levy, E.P., A. Cohen, and F.C. Fraser, "Hormone treatment during pregnancy and congenital heart defects," Lancet 1:611, 1973. 41. Nora, J.J. and A.H. Nora, "Birth defects and oral contraceptives," Lancet 1:941-942, 1973. 42. Janerich, D.T., J.M. Piper, and D.M. Glebatis, "Oral contraceptives and congenital limb-reduction defects," N Engl J Med 291:697-700, 1974. 43. Carr, D.H., "Chromosome studies in selected spontaneous abortions: I. Conception after oral contraceptives," Canad Med Assoc J 103:343-348, 1970. 44. Wynn, V., J.W.H. Doar, and G.L. Mills, "Some effects of oral contraceptives on serum-lipid and lipoprotein levels," Lancet 2:720-723, 1966. 45. Laumas, K.R., P.K. Malkani, S. Bhatnagar, and V. Laumas, "Radioactivity in the breast milk of lactating women after oral administration of 3 H-norethynodrel," Amer J Obstet Gynecol 98:411-413, 1967. 46. Rooks, et al., "Epidemiology of Hepatocellular Ademona, the Role of Oral Contraceptive Use," JAMA 242:644, 1979. 47. Herbst, A.L., P. Cole, T. Colton, S.J. Robboy, R. E. Scully, "Age-incidence and Risk of Diethylstilbestrol-related Clear Cell Adenocarcinoma of the Vagina and Cervix," Am J Obstet Gynecol, 128:43-50, 1977. 48. Bibbo, M., M. Al-Naqeeb, I. Baccarini, W. Gill, M. Newton, K.M. Sleeper, M. Sonek, G.L. Wied, "Follow-up Study of Male and Female Offspring of DES-treated Mothers. A Preliminary Report," Jour of Repro Med, 15:29-32, 1975. 49. Gill, W.B., G.F.B. Schumacher, M. Bibbo, "Structural and Functional Abnormalities in the Sex Organs of Male Offspring of Mothers Treated with Diethylstilbestrol (DES)," Jour of Repro Med, 16:147-153, 1976. 50. Henderson, B.E., B.Senton, M. Cosgrove, J. Baptista, J. Aldrich, D. Townsend, W. Hart, T. Mack, "Urogenital Tract Abnormalities in Sons of Women Treated with Diethylstilbestrol," Pediatrics, 58:505-507, 1976. 51. Heinonen, O.P., D. Slone, R.R. Nonson, E.B. Hook, S. Shapiro, "Cardiovascular Birth Defects and Antenatal Exposure to Female Sex Hormones," N Engl J Med, 296:67-70, 1977. 52. Jain, A.K., "Mortality Risk Associated with the Use of Oral Contraceptives," Studies in Family Planning, 8:50-54, 1977. 53. Beral, V., "Mortality Among Oral Contraceptive Users," Lancet, 2:727-731, 1977. 54. Vessey, M.P., McPherson, K., and Johnson, B., "Mortality Among Women Participating in the Oxford/Family Planning Association Contraceptive Study," Lancet 2:731-733, 1977. 55. Petitti, D.B., Wingerd, J., "Use of Oral Contraceptives, Cigarette Smoking, and Risk of Subarachnoid Haemorrhage," Lancet, 2:234-6, 1978. 56. Slone, D., et al, "Risk of Myocardial Infarction in Relation of Current and Discontinued Use of Oral Contraceptives," N Engl J Med, 305:420-424, 1981. 57. Royal College of General Practitioners, "Incidence of Arterial Disease Among Oral Contraceptive Users." J Coll Gen Pract 33:75-82, 1983.

Brief Summary Patient Package Insert

> Cigarette smoking increases the risk of serious adverse effects on the heart and blood vessels from oral contraceptive use. This risk increases with age and with heavy smoking (15 or more cigarettes per day) and is quite marked in women over 35 years of age. Women who use oral contraceptives should not smoke.

Oral contraceptives taken as directed are about 99% effective in preventing pregnancy. (The mini-pill, however, is somewhat less effective.) Forgetting to take your pills increases the chance of pregnancy. Various drugs, such as antibiotics, may also decrease the effectiveness of oral contraceptives. Women who have or have had clotting disorders, cancer of the breast or sex organs, unexplained vaginal bleeding, a stroke, heart attack, angina pectoris, or who suspect they may be pregnant should not use oral contraceptives.

Most side effects of the pill are not serious. The most common side effects are nausea, vomiting, bleeding between menstrual periods, weight gain, and breast tenderness. However, proper use of oral contraceptives requires that they be taken under your doctor's continuous supervision, because they can be associated with serious side effects which may be fatal. Fortunately, these occur very infrequently. The serious side effects are:

1. Blood clots in the legs, lungs, brain, heart or other organs and hemorrhage into the brain due to bursting of a blood vessel.
2. Liver tumors, which may rupture and cause severe bleeding.
3. Birth defects if the pill is taken while you are pregnant.
4. High blood pressure.
5. Gallbladder disease.

Some of the symptoms associated with these serious side effects are discussed in the detailed leaflet given you with your supply of pills. Notify your doctor if you notice any unusual physical disturbance while taking the pill.

The estrogen in oral contraceptives has been found to cause breast cancer and other cancers in certain animals. These findings suggest that oral contraceptives may also cause cancer in humans. However, studies to date in women taking currently marketed oral contraceptives have not confirmed that oral contraceptives cause cancer in humans.

The detailed leaflet describes more completely the benefits and risks of oral contraceptives. It also provides information on other forms of contraception. Read it carefully. If you have any questions, consult your doctor.

Caution: Oral contraceptives are of no value in the prevention or treatment of venereal disease.

Detailed Patient Labeling

What You Should Know About Oral Contraceptives: Oral contraceptives ("the pill") are the most effective way (except for sterilization) to prevent pregnancy. They are also convenient and, for most women, free of serious or unpleasant side effects. Oral contraceptives must always be taken under the continuous supervision of a physician. The information in this leaflet under the headings "Who Should Not Use Oral Contraceptives," "The Dangers of Oral Contraceptives," and "How to Use Oral Contraceptives As Effectively As Possible, Once You Have Decided to Use Them" is also applicable when these drugs are used for other indications.

ORTHO-NOVUM 2 mg☐21 may be prescribed for the treatment of hypermenorrhea.

Continued on next page

Ortho Pharm.—Cont.

It is important that any woman who considers using an oral contraceptive understand the risks involved. Although the oral contraceptives have important advantages over other methods of contraception, they have certain risks that no other method has. Only you can decide whether the advantages are worth these risks. This leaflet will tell you about the most important risks. It will explain how you can help your doctor prescribe the pill as safely as possible by telling him about yourself and being alert for the earliest signs of trouble. And it will tell you how to use the pill properly, so that it will be as effective as possible. There is more detailed information available in the leaflet prepared for doctors. Your pharmacist can show you a copy; you may need your doctor's help in understanding parts of it.

Who Should Not Use Oral Contraceptives:

A. If you have now, or have had in the past, any of the following conditions you should not use the pill:
1. Heart attack or stroke.
2. Clots in the legs or lungs.
3. Angina pectoris.
4. Known or suspected cancer of the breast or sex organs.
5. Unusual vaginal bleeding that has not yet been diagnosed.

B. If you are pregnant or suspect that you are pregnant, do not use the pill.

C. Cigarette smoking increases the risk of serious adverse effects on the heart and blood vessels from oral contraceptive use. This risk increases with age and with heavy smoking (15 or more cigarettes per day) and is quite marked in women over 35 years of age. Women who use oral contraceptives should not smoke.

D. If you have scanty or irregular periods or are a young woman without a regular cycle, you should use another method of contraception because, if you use the pill, you may have difficulty becoming pregnant or may fail to have menstrual periods after discontinuing the pill.

Deciding To Use Oral Contraceptives: If you do not have any of the conditions listed above and are thinking about using oral contraceptives, to help you decide, you need information about the advantages and risks of oral contraceptives and of other contraceptive methods as well. This leaflet describes the advantages and risks of oral contraceptives. Except for sterilization, the IUD and abortion, which have their own exclusive risks, the only risks of other methods of contraception are those due to pregnancy should the method fail. Your doctor can answer questions you may have with respect to other methods of contraception. He can also answer any questions you may have after reading this leaflet on oral contraceptives.

1. What Oral Contraceptives Are and How They Work. Oral contraceptives are of two types. The most common, often simply called "the pill," is a combination of an estrogen and a progestogen, the two kinds of female hormones. The amount of estrogen and progestogen can vary, but the amount of estrogen is most important because both the effectiveness and some of the dangers of oral contraceptives are related to the amount of estrogen. This kind of oral contraceptive works principally by preventing release of an egg from the ovary. When the amount of estrogen is 50 micrograms or more, and the pill is taken as directed, oral contraceptives are more than 99% effective (i.e., there would be less than one pregnancy if 100 women used the pill for one year). Pills that contain 20 to 35 micrograms of estrogen vary slightly in effectiveness, ranging from 98% to more than 99% effective.

The second type of oral contraceptive, often called the "mini-pill," contains only a progestogen. It works in part by preventing release of an egg from the ovary but also by keeping sperm from reaching the egg and by making the uterus (womb) less receptive to any fertilized egg that reaches it. The mini-pill is less effective than the combination oral contraceptive, about 97% effective. In addition, the progestogen-only pill has a tendency to cause irregular bleeding which may be quite inconvenient, or cessation of bleeding entirely. The progestogen-only pill is used despite its lower effectiveness in the hope that it will prove not to have some of the serious side effects of the estrogen-containing pill (see below) but it is not yet certain that the mini-pill does in fact have fewer serious side effects. The discussion below, while based mainly on information about the combination pills, should be considered to apply as well to the mini-pill.

2. Other Nonsurgical Ways to Prevent Pregnancy. As this leaflet will explain, oral contraceptives have several serious risks. Other methods of contraception have lesser risks or none at all. They are also less effective than oral contraceptives, but, used properly, may be effective enough for many women. The following table gives reported pregnancy rates (the number of women out of 100 who would become pregnant in one year) for these methods:

Pregnancies Per 100 Women Per Year
Intrauterine device (IUD), less than 1–6;
Diaphragm with spermicidal products (creams or jellies), 2–20;
Condom (rubber), 3–36; Aerosol foams, 2–29;
Jellies and creams, 4–36;
Periodic abstinence (rhythm) all types, less than 1–47;
  1. Calendar method, 14–47;
  2. Temperature method, 1–20;
  3. Temperature method—intercourse only in postovulatory phase, less than 1–7;
  4. Mucus method, 1–25;
No contraception, 60–80.

The figures (except for the IUD) vary widely because people differ in how well they use each method. Very faithful users of the various methods obtain very good results, except for users of the calendar method of periodic abstinence (rhythm). Except for the IUD, effective use of these methods requires somewhat more effort than simply taking a single pill every morning, but it is an effort that many couples undertake successfully. Your doctor can tell you a great deal more about these methods of contraception.

3. The Dangers of Oral Contraceptives.
a. *Circulatory disorders (abnormal blood clotting, heart attack, and stroke due to hemorrhage).* Blood clots (in various blood vessels of the body) are the most common of the serious side effects of oral contraceptives. A clot can result in a stroke (if the clot is in the brain), a heart attack (if the clot is in a blood vessel of the heart), or a pulmonary embolus (a clot which forms in the legs or pelvis, then breaks off and travels to the lungs). Any of these can be fatal. Clots also occur rarely in the blood vessels of the eye, resulting in blindness or impairment of vision in that eye. There is evidence that the risk of clotting increases with higher estrogen doses. It is therefore important to keep the dose of estrogen as low as possible, so long as the oral contraceptive used has an acceptable pregnancy rate and doesn't cause unacceptable changes in the menstrual pattern. Furthermore, cigarette smoking by oral contraceptive users increases the risk of serious adverse effects on the heart and blood vessels. This risk increases with age and with heavy smoking (15 or more cigarettes per day) and begins to become quite marked in women over 35 years of age. For this reason, women who use oral contraceptives should not smoke.

The risk of abnormal blood clotting increases with age in both users and nonusers of oral contraceptives, but the increased risk from the oral contraceptive appears to be present at all ages. For women aged 20 to 44 it is estimated that about 1 in 2,000 using oral contraceptives will be hospitalized each year because of abnormal clotting. Among nonusers in the same age group, about 1 in 20,000 would be hospitalized each year. For oral contraceptive users in general, it has been estimated that in women between the ages of 15 and 34 the risk of death due to a circulatory disorder is about 1 in 12,000 per year, whereas for nonusers the rate is about 1 in 50,000 per year. In the age group 35 to 44, the risk is estimated to be about 1 in 2,500 per year for oral contraceptive users and about 1 in 10,000 per year for nonusers.

Even without the pill the risk of having a heart attack increases with age and is also increased by such heart attack risk factors as high blood pressure, high cholesterol, obesity, diabetes, and cigarette smoking. Without any risk factors present, the use of oral contraceptives alone may double the risk of heart attack. However, the combination of cigarette smoking, especially heavy smoking, and oral contraceptive use greatly increases the risk of heart attack. Oral contraceptive users who smoke are about five times more likely to have a heart attack than users who do not smoke and about ten times more likely to have a heart attack than nonusers who do not smoke. It has been estimated that users between the ages of 30 and 39 who smoke have about a 1-in-10,000 chance each year of having a fatal heart attack compared to about a 1-in-50,000 chance in users who do not smoke, and about a 1-in-100,000 chance in nonusers who do not smoke. In the age group 40 to 44, the risk is about 1 in 1,700 per year for users who smoke compared to about 1 in 10,000 for users who do not smoke and to about one in 14,000 per year for nonusers who do not smoke. Heavy smoking (about 15 cigarettes or more a day) further increases the risk. If you do not smoke and have none of the other heart attack risk factors described above, you will have a smaller risk than listed. If you have several heart attack risk factors, the risk may be considerably greater than listed.

In addition to blood clotting disorders, it has been estimated that women taking oral contraceptives are twice as likely as nonusers to have a stroke due to rupture of a blood vessel in the brain.

One report suggests that the risk of circulatory diseases appears to increase the longer you are on the pill.

Several reports suggest that an increased risk of heart attack, stroke and other blood clotting disorders may continue for a number of years after stopping oral contraceptives. There is also some evidence that the size of this continuing risk may be greater with longer duration of oral contraceptive use.

b. *Formation of tumors.* Studies have found that when certain animals are given the female sex hormone estrogen, which is an ingredient of oral contraceptives, continuously for long periods, cancers may develop in the breast, cervix, vagina, and liver.

These findings suggest that oral contraceptives may cause cancer in humans. However, studies to date in women taking currently marketed oral contraceptives have not confirmed that oral contraceptives cause cancer in humans. Several studies have found no increase in breast cancer in users, although one study suggested oral contraceptives might cause an increase in breast cancer in women who already have benign breast disease (e.g., cysts).

Women with a strong family history of breast cancer or who have breast nodules, fibrocystic disease, or abnormal mammograms or who were exposed to DES (diethylstilbestrol), an estrogen, during their mother's pregnancy must be followed very closely by their doctors if they choose to use oral contraceptives instead of another method of contraception. Many studies have shown that women taking oral contraceptives have less risk of getting benign breast disease than those who have not used oral contraceptives. Recently, strong evidence has emerged that estrogens (one component of oral contraceptives), when given for periods of more than one year to women after the menopause, increase the risk of cancer of the uterus (womb). There is also some evidence that a kind of oral contraceptive which is no longer marketed, the sequential oral contraceptive, may increase the risk of cancer of the uterus. There remains no evidence, however, that the oral contraceptives now available increase the risk of this cancer.

Oral contraceptives do cause, although rarely, a benign (non-malignant) tumor of the liver. These tumors do not spread, but they may rupture and cause internal bleeding, which may be fatal. A few cases of cancer of the liver have been reported in women using oral contraceptives, but it is not yet known whether the drug caused them.

c. *Dangers to a developing child if oral contraceptives are used in or immediately preceding pregnancy.* Oral contraceptives should not be taken by pregnant women because they may damage the developing child. An increased risk of birth defects, including heart defects and limb defects, has been associated with the use of sex hormones, including oral contraceptives, in pregnancy. In addition, the developing female child whose mother has received DES (diethylstilbestrol), an estrogen, during pregnancy has a risk of getting cancer of the vagina or cervix in her teens or young adulthood. This risk is estimated to be about 1 to 4 in 1000 exposures. Abnormalities of the urinary and sex organs have been reported in male offspring so exposed. It is possible that other estrogens, such as the estrogens in oral contraceptives, could have the same effect in the child if the mother takes them during pregnancy.

If you stop taking oral contraceptives to become pregnant, your doctor may recommend that you use another method of contraception for a short while, for example three months. The reason for this is that there is evidence from studies in women who have had "miscarriages" soon after stopping the pill, that the lost fetuses are more likely to be abnormal. Whether there is an overall increase in "miscarriage" in women who become pregnant soon after stopping the pill as compared with women who do not use the pill is not known, but it is possible that there may be. If, however, you do become pregnant soon after stopping oral contraceptives, and do not have a miscarriage, there does not appear to be evidence that the baby has an increased risk of being abnormal.

d. *Gallbladder disease.* Women who use oral contraceptives have a greater risk than nonusers of having gallbladder disease requiring surgery. The increased risk may first appear within one year of use and may double after four or five years of use.

e. *Other side effects of oral contraceptives.* Some women using oral contraceptives experience unpleasant side effects. Some of these may be temporary. Your breasts may feel tender, nausea and vomiting may occur, you may gain or lose weight, and your ankles may swell. A spotty darkening of the skin, particularly of the face, is possible and may persist. You may notice unexpected vaginal bleeding or changes in your menstrual period. Irregular bleeding is frequently seen when using the mini-pill or combination oral contraceptives containing less than 50 micrograms of estrogen. More serious side effects include worsening of migraine, asthma, epilepsy, and kidney or heart disease because of a tendency for water to be retained in the body when oral contraceptives are used. Other side effects are growth of preexisting fibroid tumors of the uterus; mental depression; and liver problems with jaundice (yellowing of the skin). Your doctor may find that levels of sugar and fatty substances in your blood are elevated; the long-term effects of these changes are not known. Some women develop high blood pressure while taking oral contraceptives, which ordinarily returns to the original levels when the oral contraceptive is stopped.

Other reactions, although not proved to be caused by oral contraceptives, are occasionally reported. These include more frequent urination and some discomfort when urinating, kidney disease including blood cell breakdown with kidney failure, nervousness, dizziness, some loss of scalp hair, an increase in body hair, an increase or decrease in sex drive, appetite changes, cataracts, and a need for a change in contact lens prescription or inability to use contact lenses.

After you stop using oral contraceptives there may be a delay before you are able to become pregnant or before you resume having menstrual periods. This is especially true of women who had irregular menstrual cycles prior to the use of oral contraceptives. As discussed previously, your doctor may recommend that you wait a short while after stopping the pill before you try to become pregnant. During this time, use another form of contraception. You should consult your physician before resuming use of oral contraceptives after childbirth, especially if you plan to nurse your baby. Drugs in oral contraceptives are known to appear in the milk, and the long-range effect on infants is not known at this time. Furthermore, oral contraceptives may cause a decrease in your milk supply as well as in the quality of the milk.

4. Comparison of the Risks of Oral Contraceptives and Other Contraceptive Methods. The many studies on the risks and effectiveness of oral contraceptives and other methods of contraception have been analyzed to estimate the risk of death associated with various methods of contraception. This risk has two parts: (a) the risk of the method itself (e.g., the risk that oral contraceptives will cause death due to abnormal clotting), and (b) the risk of death due to pregnancy or abortion in the event the method fails. The results of this analysis are shown in the bar graph (Figure 1). The height of the bars is the number of deaths per 100,000 women each year. There are six sets of bars, each set referring to a specific age group of women. Within each set of bars there is a single bar for each of the different contraceptive methods. For oral contraceptives, there are two bars—one for smokers and the other for nonsmokers. The analysis is based on present knowledge and new information could, of course, alter it. The analysis shows that the risk of death from all methods of birth control is low and below that associated with childbirth, except for oral contraceptives in women over 40 who smoke. It shows that the lowest risk of death is associated with the condom or diaphragm (traditional contraception) backed up by early abortion in case of failure of the condom or diaphragm to prevent pregnancy. Also, at any age the risk of death (due to unexpected pregnancy) from the use of traditional contraception, even without a backup of abortion, is generally the same as or less than that from use of oral contraceptives.

How To Use Oral Contraceptives As Effectively As Possible, Once You Have Decided To Use Them:

1. What to Tell your Doctor.

You can make use of the pill as effectively as possible by telling your doctor if you have any of the following:

a. Conditions that mean you should not use oral contraceptives:
Clots in the legs or lungs.
Clots in the legs or lungs in the past.
A stroke, heart attack, or angina pectoris.
Known or suspected cancer of the breast or sex organs.
Unusual vaginal bleeding that has not been diagnosed.
Known or suspected pregnancy.

b. Conditions that your doctor will want to watch closely or which might cause him to suggest another method of contraception:
A family history of breast cancer.
Breast nodules, fibrocystic disease of the breast, or an abnormal mammogram.

Diabetes.	Heart or kidney disease.
High blood pressure.	Epilepsy.
High cholesterol.	Mental depression.
Cigarette smoking.	Fibroid tumors of the uterus.
Migraine headaches.	Gallbladder disease.

c. Once you are using oral contraceptives, you should be alert for signs of a serious adverse effect and call your doctor if they occur:
Sharp pain in the chest, coughing blood, or sudden shortness of breath (indicating possible clots in the lungs).
Pain in the calf (possible clot in the leg).
Crushing chest pain or heaviness (indicating possible heart attack).
Sudden severe headache or vomiting, dizziness or fainting, disturbance of vision or speech or weakness or numbness in an arm or leg (indicating a possible stroke).
Sudden partial or complete loss of vision (indicating a possible clot in the eye).
Breast lumps (you should ask your doctor to show you how to examine your own breasts).
Severe pain in the abdomen (indicating a possible ruptured tumor of the liver).
Severe depression.
Yellowing of the skin (jaundice).

2. How to Take the Pill So That it is Most Effective. Reduced effectiveness and an increased incidence of breakthrough bleeding have been associated with the use of oral contraceptives with antibiotics such as rifampicin, ampicillin, griseofulvin, and tetracycline or with certain other drugs, such as barbiturates, phenylbutazone or phenytoin sodium. You should use an additional means of contraception during any cycle in which any of these drugs are taken.

To achieve maximum contraceptive effectiveness, ORTHO-NOVUM, MODICON, and MICRONOR must be taken exactly as directed and at intervals not exceeding 24 hours.

ORTHO-NOVUM 7/7/7 Sunday-Start Package:
21-Day Regimen: The first white tablet should be taken on the first Sunday after the menstrual period begins. If period begins on Sunday, the first white tablet is taken on that day. Take one white tablet at the same time each day for 7 consecutive days, take one light peach tablet daily for 7 days, then take one peach tablet daily for 7 days. During the FIRST cycle, it is important that you use another method of birth control until you have taken a white tablet daily for seven consecutive days. After taking your last peach tablet, wait for seven days during which time a menstrual period usually occurs. After the seven-day waiting period, on Sunday, start taking a white tablet each day for the next 7 days; a light peach tablet for the next 7 days; then a peach tablet for the next 7 days, thus using a three-week-on, one-week-off regimen.

28-Day Regimen: The first white tablet should be taken on the first Sunday after the menstrual period begins. If period begins on Sunday, begin taking tablets that day. Take one white tablet at the same time each day for 7 consecutive days; take one light peach tablet daily for 7 days; take one peach tablet daily for 7 days, then take one green tablet daily for 7 days, during which time your period usually occurs. During the FIRST cycle, it is important that you use another method of birth control until you have taken a white tablet daily for seven consecutive days. After 28 tablets have been taken, (last green tablet will always be taken on Saturday) take the first tablet (white) from your next package the following day (Sunday) whether or not you are still menstruating. With the 28-day regimen, tablets are taken every day of the year.

ORTHO-NOVUM 10/11 — Sunday-Start Package
21-Day Regimen: The first white tablet should be taken on the first Sunday after the menstrual period begins. If period begins on Sunday, begin taking tablets that day. Take one white tablet at the same time each day for 10 consecutive days, then take one peach tablet daily for 11 days. During the FIRST cycle, it is important that you use another method of birth control until you have taken a white tablet daily for seven consecutive days. After taking your last peach tablet, wait for seven days during which time a menstrual period usually occurs. After the seven-day waiting period, on Sunday, start taking a white tablet each day for the next 10 days, then a peach tablet for the next 11 days, thus using a three-week-on, one-week-off regimen.

28-Day Regimen: The first white tablet should be taken on the first Sunday after the menstrual period begins. If period begins on Sunday, begin taking tablets that day. Take one white tablet at the same time each day for 10 consecutive days, take one peach tablet daily for 11 days, then

Continued on next page

Ortho Pharm.—Cont.

take one green tablet daily for 7 days, during which time your period usually occurs. During the FIRST cycle, it is important that you use another method of birth control until you have taken a white tablet daily for seven consecutive days. After 28 tablets have been taken, (last green tablet will always be taken on a Saturday) take the first tablet (white) from your next package the following day (Sunday) whether or not you are still menstruating. With the 28-day regimen, pills are taken every day of the year.

ORTHO-NOVUM 1/35, MODICON, ORTHO-NOVUM 1/50, ORTHO-NOVUM 1/80 and ORTHO-NOVUM 2 mg

21-day Regimen: Counting the first day of menstrual flow as "Day 1," take one tablet daily from the 5th through the 25th day of the menstrual cycle. If the first tablet is taken later than the 5th day of the menstrual cycle or postpartum, contraceptive reliance should not be placed on ORTHO-NOVUM or MODICON until after the first seven consecutive days of administration. Take a tablet the same time each day, preferably at bedtime, for 21 days, then wait for 7 days during which time a menstrual period usually occurs. Following this 7-day waiting period, start taking a tablet each day for the next 21 days, thus using a three-weeks-on, one-week-off dosage regimen.

When ORTHO-NOVUM 2 mg☐21 Tablets are used for the treatment of hypermenorrhea, your physician will discuss the regimen with you.

ORTHO-NOVUM 1/35, MODICON, ORTHO-NOVUM 1/50 and ORTHO-NOVUM 1/80.

28-Day Regimen: The first white, yellow or peach tablet should be taken on the first Sunday after the menstrual period begins. If period begins on Sunday, begin taking tablets that day. Take one white, yellow or peach tablet at the same time each day for 21 consecutive days, then take one green tablet daily for 7 days during which time your menstrual period usually occurs. During the FIRST cycle, it is important that you use another method of birth control until you have taken a white, yellow or peach tablet daily for seven consecutive days. After 28 tablets have been taken, (last green tablet will always be taken on a Saturday) take the first tablet (white, yellow or peach) from your next package the following day (Sunday) whether or not you are still menstruating. With the 28-day regimen, pills are taken every day of the year.

Continuous Regimen (MICRONOR): The first MICRONOR Tablet should be taken on the first day of the menstrual period.

Take one tablet at the same time each day without interruption for as long as contraceptive protection is desired.

The effectiveness of progestogen-only oral contraceptives, such as MICRONOR, is lower than that of the combination oral contraceptives containing both estrogen and progestogen. If 100 women utilized an estrogen-containing oral contraceptive for a period of one year, generally less than one pregnancy would be expected to occur; however, if MICRONOR had been utilized, approximately three pregnancies might occur.

Women who participated in the clinical studies with MICRONOR and who had not taken other oral contraceptives before starting MICRONOR had a higher pregnancy rate (four women out of 100), particularly during the first six months of therapy, and to a large extent because they did not take their tablets correctly.

Of course, if you don't take your tablets as directed, or forget to take them every day, the chance you may become pregnant is naturally greater.

MICRONOR (norethindrone) will probably cause some changes in your menstrual pattern. Your cycle, that is the time between menstrual periods, will vary. For example, you might have a 28-day cycle, followed by a 17-day cycle, followed by a 35-day cycle, etc. This is common with MICRONOR.

While using MICRONOR, your period may be longer or shorter than before. If bleeding lasts more than eight days, be sure to let your doctor know.

At times there may be no menstrual period after a cycle of pills. Therefore, if you miss one menstrual period but have taken the pills *exactly as you were supposed to*, continue as usual into the next cycle. If you have not taken them correctly and miss a menstrual period, or if you are taking mini-pills and it is 45 days or more from the start of your last menstrual period, you may be pregnant and should stop taking oral contraceptives until your doctor determines whether or not you are pregnant. Until you can get to your doctor, use another form of contraception. If two consecutive menstrual periods are missed, you should stop taking pills until it is determined whether you are pregnant. If you do become pregnant while using oral contraceptives, you should discuss the risks to the developing child with your doctor.

3. Periodic Examination.

Your doctor will take a complete medical and family history before prescribing oral contraceptives. At that time and about once a year thereafter, he will generally examine your blood pressure, breasts, abdomen, and pelvic organs (including a Papanicolaou smear, i.e., test for cancer).

Summary: Oral contraceptives are the most effective method, except sterilization, for preventing pregnancy. Other methods, when used conscientiously, are also very effective and have fewer risks.

Women who use oral contraceptives should not smoke.

In addition, if you have certain conditions or have had these conditions in the past, you should not use oral contraceptives because the risk is too great. These conditions are listed in the booklet. If you do not have these conditions and decide to use the "pill," please read the booklet carefully so that you can use the "pill."

Based on his or her assessment of your medical needs, your doctor has prescribed this drug for you. Do not give the drug to anyone else.

Revised December 1984
Shown in Product Identification Section, pages 422, 423

PROTOSTAT® ℞
(metronidazole) Tablets

> **Warning:** Metronidazole has been shown to be carcinogenic in mice and rats. *(See Warnings.)* Unnecessary use of this drug should be avoided. Its use should be reserved for the conditions described in the *Indications And Usage* section below.

Description: PROTOSTAT (metronidazole) is a 1-(β-hydroxyethyl)-2-methyl-5-nitroimidazole.
Metronidazole is classified therapeutically as an antiprotozoal *(Trichomonas)*, and antibacterial (antianaerobic) agent. It occurs as pale yellow crystals that are slightly soluble in water and alcohol. Metronidazole has the following structural formula:

Clinical Pharmacology: Metronidazole is usually well absorbed after oral administration, with peak plasma concentrations occurring between one and two hours. An average elimination half-life is 8 hours in healthy humans. Plasma concentrations of metronidazole are proportional to the administered dose. Oral administration of 250 mg., 500 mg., or 2,000 mg. produced peak plasma concentrations of 6 mcg/ml, 12 mcg/ml, and 40 mcg/ml, respectively. Studies reveal no significant bioavailability differences between males and females; however, because of weight differences, the resulting plasma levels in males are generally lower.

Metronidazole is the major component appearing in the plasma, with lesser quantities of the 2-hydroxymethyl metabolite also being present. Less than 20% of the circulating metronidazole is bound to plasma proteins. Both the parent compound and the metabolite possess *in vitro* trichomonacidal activity and *in vitro* bactericidal activity against most strains of anaerobic bacteria.

The major route of elimination of metronidazole and its metabolites is via the urine (60-80% of the dose), with fecal excretion accounting for 6-15% of the dose. The metabolites that appear in the urine result primarily from side-chain oxidation [1-(β-hydroxyethyl)-2-hydroxymethyl-5-nitroimidazole and 2-methyl-5-nitroimidazole-1-yl-acetic acid] and glucuronide conjugation, with unchanged metronidazole accounting for approximately 20% of the total. Renal clearance of metronidazole is approximately 10 ml/min/1.73m^2.

Decreased renal function does not alter the single-dose pharmacokinetics of metronidazole. However, plasma clearance of metronidazole is decreased in patients with decreased liver function.

Metronidazole appears in cerebrospinal fluid, saliva, and breast milk in concentrations similar to those found in plasma. Bactericidal concentrations of metronidazole have also been detected in pus from hepatic abscesses.

Microbiology: Metronidazole possesses direct trichomonacidal and amoebicidal activity against *Trichomonas Vaginalis* and *Entamoeba histolytica*. The *in vitro* minimal inhibitory concentration (MIC) for most strains of these organisms is 1 mcg/ml or less. Metronidazole's mechanism of antiprotozoal action is unknown.

Anaerobic Bacteria: Metronidazole is active *in vitro* against obligate anaerobes, but does not appear to possess any clinically relevant activity against facultative anaerobes or obligate aerobes. Against susceptible organisms, metronidazole is generally bactericidal at concentrations equal to or slightly higher than the minimal inhibitory concentrations (MIC). Metronidazole has been shown to have *in vitro* and clinical activity against the following organisms:

Anaerobic gram-negative bacilli, including:
Bacteroides species, including the *Bacteroides fragilis* group (*B. fragilis*, *B. distasonis*, *B. ovatus*, *B. thetaiotaomicron*, *B. vulgatus*)
Fusobacterium species
Anaerobic gram-positive bacilli, including:
Clostridium species and susceptible strains of *Eubacterium*
Anaerobic gram-positive cocci, including:
Peptococcus species
Peptostreptococcus species

Susceptibility tests: Bacteriologic studies should be performed to determine the causative organisms and their susceptibility to metronidazole; however, the rapid, routine susceptibility testing of individual isolates of anaerobic bacteria is not always practical, and therapy may be started while awaiting these results.

Quantitative methods give the most precise estimates of susceptibility to antibacterial drugs. A standardized agar dilution method and a broth microdilution method are recommended.[1]

Control strains are recommended for standardized susceptibility testing. Each time the test is performed, one or more of the following strains should be included: *Clostridium perfringens* ATCC 13124, *Bacteroides fragilis* ATCC 25285, and *Bacteroides thetaiotaomicron* ATCC 29741. The mode metronidazole MIC's for those three strains are reported to be 0.25, 0.25, and 0.5 mcg/ml, respectively.

A clinical laboratory is considered under acceptable control if the results of the control strains are within one doubling dilution of the mode MIC's reported for metronidazole.

A bacterial isolate may be considered susceptible if the MIC value for metronidazole is not more than 16 mcg/ml. An organism is considered resistant if the MIC is greater than 16 mcg/ml. A report of "resistant" from the laboratory indicates that the infecting organism is not likely to respond to therapy.

Indications and Usage: *Symptomatic Trichomoniasis:* PROTOSTAT is indicated for the treatment of symptomatic trichomoniasis in females and males when the presence of trichomonad has been confirmed by appropriate laboratory procedures (wet smears and/or cultures).

Asymptomatic Trichomoniasis: PROTOSTAT is indicated in the treatment of asymptomatic females when the organism is associated with endocervicitis, cervicitis, or cervical erosion. Since there is evidence that presence of the trichomonad can interfere with accurate assessment of abnormal cytological smears, additional smears should be performed after eradication of the parasite.

Treatment of Asymptomatic Consorts: T. vaginalis infection is a venereal disease. Therefore, asymptomatic sexual partners of treated patients should be treated simultaneously if the organism has been found to be present in order to prevent reinfection of the partner. The decision as to whether to treat an asymptomatic male partner with a negative culture or one in whom no culture has been attempted is an individual one. In making this decision, it should be noted that there is evidence that women may become reinfected if the consort is not treated. Also, since there can be considerable difficulty in isolating the organism from the asymptomatic male carrier, negative smears and cultures cannot be relied upon in this regard. In any event, the consort should be treated with PROTOSTAT in cases of reinfection.

Amoebiasis: PROTOSTAT is indicated in the treatment of acute intestinal amoebiasis (amoebic dysentery) and amoebic liver abscess.

In amoebic liver abscess, PROTOSTAT therapy does not obviate the need for aspiration or drainage of pus.

Anaerobic Bacterial Infections: PROTOSTAT is indicated in the treatment of serious infections caused by susceptible anaerobic bacteria. Indicated surgical procedures should be performed in conjunction with PROTOSTAT therapy. In a mixed aerobic and anaerobic infection, antibiotics appropriate for the treatment of aerobic infection should be used in addition to PROTOSTAT. In the treatment of most serious anaerobic infections the intravenous form of metronidazole is usually administered initially. This may be followed by oral therapy with PROTOSTAT at the discretion of the physician.

INTRA-ABDOMINAL INFECTION, including peritonitis, intra-abdominal abscess, and liver abscess, caused by *Bacteroides* species including the *B. fragilis* group (*B. fragilis, B. distasonis, B. ovatus, B. thetaiotaomicron, B. vulgatus), Clostridium* species, *Eubacterium* species, *Peptococcus* species, and *Peptostreptococcus* species.

SKIN AND SKIN STRUCTURE INFECTIONS caused by *Bacteroides* species including the *B. fragilis* group, *Clostridium* species, *Peptococcus* species, *Peptostreptococcus* species, and *Fusobacterium* species.

GYNECOLOGIC INFECTIONS, including endometritis, endyometritis, tubo-ovarian abscess, and post-surgical vaginal cuff infection, caused by *Bacteroides* species including the *B. fragilis* group, *Clostridium* species, *Peptococcus* species, and *Peptostreptococcus* species.

BACTERIAL SEPTICEMIA caused by *Bacteroides* species including the *B. fragilis* group, and *Clostridium* species.

BONE AND JOINT INFECTIONS, as adjunctive therapy, caused by *Bacteroides* species including the *B. fragilis* group.

CENTRAL NERVOUS SYSTEM (CNS) INFECTIONS, including meningitis and brain abscess, caused by *Bacteroides* species including the *B. fragilis* group.

LOWER RESPIRATORY TRACT INFECTIONS, including pneumonia, empyema, and lung abscess, caused by *Bacteroides* species including the *B. fragilis* group.

ENDOCARDITIS caused by *Bacteroides* species including the *B. fragilis* group.

Contraindications: PROTOSTAT is contraindicated in patients with a prior history of hypersensitivity to metronidazole or other nitroimidazole derivatives. In patients with trichomoniasis, PROTOSTAT is contraindicated during the first trimester of pregnancy. *(See Warnings.)*

Warnings: *Convulsive Seizures and Peripheral Neuropathy:* Convulsive seizures and peripheral neuropathy, the latter characterized mainly by numbness or paresthesia of an extremity, have been reported in patients treated with metronidazole. The appearance of abnormal neurologic signs demands the prompt discontinuation of PROTOSTAT therapy. PROTOSTAT should be administered with caution to patients with central nervous system diseases.

Tumorigenicity Studies in Rodents: Metronidazole has shown evidence of carcinogenic activity in a number of studies involving chronic, oral administration in mice and rats.

Prominent among the effects in the mouse was the promotion of pulmonary tumorigenesis. This has been observed in all six reported studies in that species, including one study in which the animals were dosed on an intermittent schedule (administration during every fourth week only). At very high dose levels (approx. 500mg/kg/day) there was a statistically significant increase in the incidence of malignant liver tumors in males. Also, the published results of one of the mouse studies indicated an increase in the incidence of malignant lymphomas as well as pulmonary neoplasms associated with lifetime feeding of the drug. All these effects are statistically significant.

Several long-term oral dosing studies in the rats have been completed. There was a statistically significant increase in the incidence of various neoplasms, particularly in mammary and hepatic tumors, among female rats administered metronidazole over those noted in the concurrent female control groups.

Two lifetime tumorigenicity studies in hamsters have been performed and reported to be negative.

Mutagenicity Studies: Although metronidazole has shown mutagenic activity in a number of *in vitro* assay systems, studies in mammals (*in vivo*) have failed to demonstrate a potential for genetic damage.

Precautions: *General:* Patients with severe hepatic disease metabolize metronidazole slowly, with resultant accumulation of metronidazole and its metabolites in the plasma. Accordingly, for such patients, doses below those usually recommended should be administered cautiously.

Known or previously unrecognized candidiasis may present more prominent symptoms during therapy with PROTOSTAT and requires treatment with a candicidal agent.

Laboratory Tests: PROTOSTAT (metronidazole) is a nitroimidazole and should be used with care in patients with evidence of, or history of, blood dyscrasia. A mild leukopenia has been observed during its administration; however, no persistent hematologic abnormalities attributable to metronidazole have been observed in clinical studies. Total and differential leukocyte counts are recommended before and after therapy for trichomoniasis and amoebiasis, especially if a second course of therapy is necessary, and before and after therapy for anaerobic infection.

Drug Interactions: Metronidazole has been reported to potentiate the anticoagulant effect of coumarin and warfarin resulting in a prolongation of prothrombin time. This possible drug interaction should be considered when PROTOSTAT is prescribed for patients on this type of anti-coagulant therapy.

Alcoholic beverages should not be consumed during PROTOSTAT therapy because abdominal cramps, nausea, vomiting, headache, and flushing may occur.

The simultaneous administration of drugs that induce microsomal liver enzymes, such as phenytoin or phenobarbital, may accelerate the elimination of metronidazole, resulting in reduced plasma levels.

Drug/Laboratory Test Interactions: Metronidazole may interfere with certain chemical analyses for serum glutamic oxalacetic transaminase, resulting in decreased values. Values of zero may be observed.

Carcinogenesis: (See Warnings.)

Pregnancy: Teratogenic Effects—Pregnancy Category B: Metronidazole crosses the placental barrier and enters the fetal circulation rapidly. Reproduction studies have been performed in rabbits and rats at doses up to five times the human dose and have revealed no evidence of impaired fertility or harm to the fetus due to metronidazole. There are, however, no adequate and well-controlled studies in pregnant women. Because animal reproduction studies are not always predictive of human response, and because metronidazole is a carcinogen in rodents, this drug should be used during pregnancy only if clearly needed. *(See Contraindications.)*

Use of PROTOSTAT for trichomoniasis in the second and third trimesters should be restricted to those in whom local palliative treatment has been inadequate to control symptoms.

Nursing Mothers: Because of the potential for tumorigenicity shown for metronidazole in mouse and rat studies, a decision should be made whether to discontinue nursing or to discontinue the drug, taking into account the importance of the drug to the mother. Metronidazole is secreted in breast milk in concentrations similar to those found in plasma.

Pediatric Use: Safety and effectiveness in children have not been established, except for the treatment of amoebiasis.

Adverse Reactions: The two most serious adverse reactions reported in patients treated with PROTOSTAT (metronidazole) have been convulsive seizures and peripheral neuropathy, the latter characterized mainly by numbness or paresthesia of an extremity. Since persistent peripheral neuropathy has been reported in some patients receiving prolonged administration of PROTOSTAT, patients should be specifically warned about these reactions and should be told to stop the drug and report immediately to their physicians if any neurologic symptoms occur.

The most common adverse reactions reported have been referable to the gastrointestinal tract, particularly nausea, sometimes accompanied by headache, anorexia, and occasionally vomiting; diarrhea; epigastric distress; and abdominal cramping. Constipation has also been reported.

The following reactions have also been reported during treatment with PROTOSTAT (metronidazole):

Mouth: A sharp, unpleasant metallic taste is not unusual. Furry tongue, glossitis, and stomatitis have occurred; these may be associated with a sudden overgrowth of *Candida* which may occur during effective therapy.

Hematopoietic: Reversible neutropenia (leukopenia).

Cardiovascular: Flattening of the T-wave may be seen in electrocardiographic tracings.

Central Nervous System: Convulsive seizures, peripheral neuropathy, dizziness, vertigo, incoordination, ataxia, confusion, irritability, depression, weakness, and insomnia.

Hypersensitivity: Urticaria, erythematous rash, flushing, nasal congestion, dryness of mouth (or vagina or vulva), and fever.

Renal: Dysuria, cystitis, polyuria, incontinence, and a sense of pelvic pressure. Instances of darkened urine have been reported, and this manifestation has been the subject of a special investigation. Although the pigment which is probably responsible for this phenomenon has not been positively identified, it is almost certainly a metabolite of metronidazole and seems to have no clinical significance.

Other: Proliferation of *Candida* in the vagina, dyspareunia, decrease of libido, proctitis, and fleeting joint pains sometimes resembling "serum sickness." If patients receiving PROTOSTAT drink alcoholic beverages, they may experience abdominal distress, nausea,

Continued on next page

Ortho Pharm.—Cont.

vomiting, flushing, or headache. A modification of the taste of alcoholic beverages has also been reported.

Overdosage: Single oral doses of metronidazole, up to 15 g, have been reported in suicide attempts and accidental overdoses. Symptoms reported include nausea, vomiting, and ataxia. Oral metronidazole has been studied as a radiation sensitizer in the treating of malignant tumors. Neurotoxic effects, including seizures and peripheral neuropathy, have been reported after 5 to 7 days of doses of 6 to 10.4 g every other day.

Treatment: There is no specific antidote for PROTOSTAT overdose; therefore, management of the patient should consist of symptomatic and supportive therapy.

Dosage and Administration:
Trichomoniasis:
In The Female: One-day treatment—two grams of PROTOSTAT given either as a single dose or in two divided doses of one gram each given in the same day.

Seven-day course of treatment—250 mg three times daily for seven consecutive days. There is some indication from controlled comparative studies that cure rates as determined by vaginal smears, signs and symptoms, may be higher after a seven-day course of treatment than after a one-day treatment regimen.

The dosage regimen should be individualized. Single-dose treatment can assure compliance, especially if administered under supervision, in those patients who cannot be relied on to continue the seven-day regimen.

A seven-day course of treatment may minimize reinfection of the female long enough to treat sexual contacts. Further, some patients may tolerate one course of therapy better than the other.

Pregnant patients should not be treated during the first trimester with either regimen. If treated during the second or third trimester, the one-day course of therapy should not be used, as it results in higher serum levels which reach the fetal circulation. *(See Contraindications and Precautions.)*

When repeated courses of the drug are required, it is recommended that an interval of four to six weeks elapse between courses and that the presence of the trichomonad be reconfirmed by appropriate laboratory measures. Total and differential leukocyte counts should be made before and after treatment.

In The Male: Treatment should be individualized as for the female.

Amoebiasis: Adults: For Acute Intestinal Amoebiasis (Acute Amoebic Dysentery):
750 mg. orally 3 times daily for 5 to 10 days.
For Amoebic Liver Abscess: 500 mg or 750 mg orally 3 times daily for 5 to 10 days.
Children: 35 to 50 mg/kg of body weight/24 hours divided into 3 doses, orally for 10 days.

Anaerobic Bacterial Infections: In the treatment of most serious anaerobic infections the intravenous form of metronidazole is usually administered initially.

Following intravenous therapy, oral metronidazole may be used when conditions warrant based upon the severity of the disease and the response of the patient to intravenous treatment. The usual adult *oral* dosage is 7.5 mg/kg every six hours (approximately 500 mg for a 70 kg adult). A maximum of 4.0 g should not be exceeded during a 24-hour period.

The usual duration of therapy is 7 to 10 days; however, infections of the bone and joint, lower respiratory tract, and endocardium may require longer treatment.

Patients with severe hepatic disease metabolize metronidazole slowly, with resultant accumulation of metronidazole and its metabolites in the plasma. Accordingly, for such patients, doses below those usually recommended should be administered cautiously. Close monitoring of plasma metronidazole levels[2] and toxicity is recommended.

The dose of PROTOSTAT should not be specifically reduced in anuric patients since accumulated metabolites may be rapidly removed by dialysis.

How Supplied: Available in tablets containing 250 mg. and 500 mg. of metronidazole, USP. PROTOSTAT 250 mg. is a white to off-white capsule-shaped, convex tablet. Each 250 mg. PROTOSTAT Tablet is scored on one side and imprinted with ORTHO 1570 on the other side, packaged in a bottle of 100 tablets (NDC 0062-1570-01). PROTOSTAT 500 mg. is a white to off-white capsule-shaped, convex tablet. Each 500 mg. PROTOSTAT tablet is scored on one side and imprinted with ORTHO 1571 on the other side, packaged in a bottle of 50 tablets (NDC 0062-1571-01). Dispense in well-closed, light-resistant containers as defined in the USP.

Store below 86°F (30°C).

1. Proposed standard: PSM-11—Proposed Reference Dilution Procedure for Antimicrobic Susceptibility Testing of Anaerobic Bacteria, National Committee for Clinical Laboratory Standards, and Sutter, et al: Collaborative Evaluation of a Proposed Reference Dilution Method of Susceptibility Testing of Anaerobic Bacteria, Antimicrob. Agents Chemother. *16*:495-502 (Oct.) 1979; and Talley, et al: *In Vitro* Activity of Thienamycin Antimicrob. Agents Chemother. *14*:436–438 (Sept.) 1978.

2. Ralph, E.D., and Kirby, W.M.M.: Bioassay of Metronidazole With Either Anaerobic or Aerobic Incubation, J. Infect. Dis. *132*:587–591 (Nov.) 1975; or Gulaid, et al: Determination of Metronidazole and Its Major Metabolites in Biological Fluids by High Pressure Liquid Chromatography, Br. J. Clin. Pharmacol. *6*:430–432, 1978.

Shown in Product Identification Section, page 423

SULTRIN® Triple Sulfa Cream and Vaginal Tablets ℞

Composition: SULTRIN Cream contains sulfathiazole 3.42%, sulfacetamide 2.86%, sulfabenzamide 3.7% and urea 0.64%, compounded with glyceryl monostearate, cetyl alcohol, stearic acid, cholesterol, lanolin, lecithin, peanut oil, propylparaben, propylene glycol, diethylaminoethyl stearamide, phosphoric acid, methylparaben and purified water.

Composition: Each SULTRIN Tablet contains sulfathiazole 172.5 mg, sulfacetamide 143.75 mg, and sulfabenzamide 184.0 mg, compounded with urea, lactose, guar gum, starch and magnesium stearate.

Indications: SULTRIN Cream and SULTRIN Tablets are indicated for treatment of *Haemophilus vaginalis* (*Gardnerella*) vaginitis.

Contraindications: Sulfonamide sensitivity and kidney disease.

Dosage: SULTRIN Cream. One applicatorful intravaginally twice daily for 4 to 6 days. The dosage may then be reduced one-half to one-quarter.
SULTRIN Vaginal Tablets. 1 tablet intravaginally before retiring and again in the morning for 10 days. This course may be repeated if necessary.

Packaging: Cream—78 g tubes with the ORTHO® Measured-Dose Applicator.
Vaginal Tablets—Package of 20 foil-wrapped tablets with vaginal applicator.

EDUCATIONAL MATERIAL

THE ORTHO FILM LIBRARY
Ortho Pharmaceutical Corporation can provide a number of educational films on a free-loan basis to hospitals, medical schools and health care professionals for use in training and educational programs.

These films, which are available directly from the distributor, KAROL MEDIA, 22 Riverview Drive, Wayne, New Jersey 07470, or by calling (201) 628-9111 are:

Modern Obstetrics: Cesarean Section
Modern Obstetrics: Fetal Evaluation
Modern Obstetrics: Normal Labor and Delivery
Modern Obstetrics: Postpartum Hemorrhage
Modern Obstetrics: Pre-Eclampsia—Eclampsia

Printed narrations of these Modern Obstetrics films are available upon written request from: Professional Affairs Department, Ortho Pharmaceutical Corporation, U.S. Route 202, Raritan, New Jersey 08869.

Ortho Pharmaceutical Corporation
DERMATOLOGICAL DIVISION
ROUTE 202
RARITAN, NJ 08869

CLODERM® ℞
(clocortolone pivalate)
Cream 0.1%
For Topical Use Only

Description: CLODERM Cream 0.1% contains the medium potency topical corticosteroid, clocortolone pivalate, in a specially formulated water-washable emollient cream base consisting of purified water, white petrolatum, mineral oil, stearyl alcohol, polyoxyl 40 stearate, carbomer 934P, edetate disodium, sodium hydroxide, with methylparaben and propylparaben as preservatives.

Chemically, clocortolone pivalate is 9-chloro-6α-fluoro-11β, 21- dihydroxy -16α-methylpregna-1,4-diene-3,20-dione 21-pivalate.

Clinical Pharmacology: Topical corticosteroids share anti-inflammatory, anti-pruritic and vasoconstrictive actions.

The mechanism of anti-inflammatory activity of the topical corticosteroids is unclear. Various laboratory methods, including vasoconstrictor assays, are used to compare and predict potencies and/or clinical efficacies of the topical corticosteroids. There is some evidence to suggest that a recognizable correlation exists between vasoconstrictor potency and therapeutic efficacy in man.

Pharmacokinetics: The extent of percutaneous absorption of topical corticosteroids is determined by many factors including the vehicle, the integrity of the epidermal barrier, and the use of occlusive dressings.

Topical corticosteroids can be absorbed from normal intact skin. Inflammation and/or other disease processes in the skin increase percutaneous absorption. Occlusive dressings substantially increase the percutaneous absorption of topical corticosteroids. Thus, occlusive dressings may be a valuable therapeutic adjunct for treatment of resistant dermatoses. (See *DOSAGE AND ADMINISTRATION*).

Once absorbed through the skin, topical corticosteroids are handled through pharmacokinetic pathways similar to systemically administered corticosteroids. Corticosteroids are bound to plasma proteins in varying degrees. Corticosteroids are metabolized primarily in the liver and are then excreted by the kidneys. Some of the topical corticosteroids and their metabolites are also excreted into the bile.

Indications and Usage: Topical corticosteroids are indicated for the relief of the inflammatory and pruritic manifestations of corticosteroid-responsive dermatoses.

Contraindications: Topical corticosteroids are contraindicated in those patients with a history of hypersensitivity to any of the components of the preparation.

Precautions
General: Systemic absorption of topical corticosteroids has produced reversible hypothalamic-pituitary-adrenal (HPA) axis suppression, manifestations of Cushing's syndrome, hyperglycemia, and glucosuria in some patients.

Conditions which augment systemic absorption include the application of the more potent steroids, use over large surface areas, prolonged use, and the addition of occlusive dressings.

Therefore, patients receiving a large dose of a potent topical steroid applied to a large surface area or under an occlusive dressing should be evaluated periodically for evidence of HPA axis suppression by using the urinary free cortisol and ACTH stimulation tests. If HPA axis suppression is noted, an attempt should be made to withdraw the drug, to reduce the frequency of application, or to substitute a less potent steroid.

Recovery of HPA axis function is generally prompt and complete upon discontinuation of the drug. Infrequently, signs and symptoms of steroid withdrawal may occur, requiring supplemental systemic corticosteroids.

Children may absorb proportionally larger amounts of topical corticosteroids and thus be more susceptible to systemic toxicity (See *PRECAUTIONS—Pediatric Use*).

If irritation develops, topical corticosteroids should be discontinued and appropriate therapy instituted.

In the presence of dermatological infections, the use of an appropriate antifungal or antibacterial agent should be instituted. If a favorable response does not occur promptly, the corticosteroid should be discontinued until the infection has been adequately controlled.

Information for the Patient: Patients using topical corticosteroids should receive the following information and instructions:
1. This medication is to be used as directed by the physician. It is for external use only. Avoid contact with the eyes.
2. Patients should be advised not to use this medication for any disorder other than for which it was prescribed.
3. The treated skin area should not be bandaged or otherwise covered or wrapped as to be occlusive unless directed by the physician.
4. Patients should report any signs of local adverse reactions especially under occlusive dressing.
5. Parents of pediatric patients should be advised not to use tight-fitting diapers or plastic pants on a child being treated in the diaper area, as these garments may constitute occlusive dressings.

Laboratory Tests: The following tests may be helpful in evaluating the HPA axis suppression:
  Urinary free cortisol test
  ACTH stimulation test

Carcinogenesis, Mutagenesis, and Impairment of Fertility: Long-term animal studies have not been performed to evaluate the carcinogenic potential or the effect on fertility of topical corticosteroids.

Studies to determine mutagenicity with prednisolone and hydrocortisone have revealed negative results.

Pregnancy Category C: Corticosteroids are generally teratogenic in laboratory animals when administered systemically at relatively low dosage levels. The more potent corticosteroids have been shown to be teratogenic after dermal application in laboratory animals. There are no adequate and well-controlled studies in pregnant women on teratogenic effects from topically applied corticosteroids. Therefore, topical corticosteroids should be used during pregnancy only if the potential benefit justifies the potential risk to the fetus. Drugs of this class should not be used extensively on pregnant patients, in large amounts, or for prolonged periods of time.

Nursing Mothers: It is not known whether topical administration of corticosteroids could result in sufficient systemic absorption to produce detectable quantities in breast milk. Systemically administered corticosteroids are secreted into breast milk in quantities *not* likely to have a deleterious effect on the infant. Nevertheless, caution should be exercised when topical corticosteroids are administered to a nursing woman.

Pediatric Use: Pediatric patients may demonstrate greater susceptibility to topical cortico- steroid-induced HPA axis suppression and Cushing's syndrome than mature patients because of a larger skin surface area to body weight ratio.

Hypothalamic-pituitary-adrenal (HPA) axis suppression, Cushing's syndrome, and intracranial hypertension have been reported in children receiving topical corticosteroids. Manifestations of adrenal suppression in children include linear growth retardation, delayed weight gain, low plasma cortisol levels, and absence of response to ACTH stimulation. Manifestations of intracranial hypertension include bulging fontanelles, headaches, and bilateral papilledema.

Administration of topical corticosteroids to children should be limited to the least amount compatible with an effective therapeutic regimen. Chronic corticosteroid therapy may interfere with the growth and development of children.

Adverse Reactions: The following local adverse reactions are reported infrequently with topical corticosteroids, but may occur more frequently with the use of occlusive dressings. These reactions are listed in an approximate decreasing order of occurrence:
  Burning
  Itching
  Irritation
  Dryness
  Folliculitis
  Hypertrichosis
  Acneiform eruptions
  Hypopigmentation
  Perioral dermatitis
  Allergic contact dermatitis
  Maceration of the skin
  Secondary infection
  Skin atrophy
  Striae
  Miliaria

Overdosage: Topically applied corticosteroids can be absorbed in sufficient amounts to produce systemic effects (see *PRECAUTIONS*).

Dosage and Administration: Apply CLODERM (clocortolone pivalate) Cream 0.1% sparingly to the affected areas three times a day and rub in gently.

Occlusive dressings may be used for the management of psoriasis or recalcitrant conditions.

If an infection develops, the use of occlusive dressings should be discontinued and appropriate antimicrobial therapy instituted.

How Supplied: CLODERM (clocortolone pivalate) Cream 0.1% is supplied in tubes containing 15 grams and 45 grams.

Store CLODERM Cream between 59° and 86°F. Avoid freezing.

GRIFULVIN V®
(griseofulvin microsize)
Tablets/Suspension

Description: Griseofulvin microsize is an antibiotic derived from a species of *Penicillium*.

Clinical Pharmacology: GRIFULVIN V (griseofulvin microsize) acts systemically to inhibit the growth of Trichophyton, Microsporum and Epidermophyton genera of fungi. Fungistatic amounts are deposited in the keratin, which is gradually exfoliated and replaced by noninfected tissue. Griseofulvin absorption from the gastrointestinal tract varies considerably among individuals, mainly because of insolubility of the drug in aqueous media of the upper G.I. tract. The peak serum level found in fasting adults given 0.5 gm. occurs at about four hours and ranges between 0.5 and 2.0 mcg./ml.

It should be noted that some individuals are consistently "poor absorbers" and tend to attain lower blood levels at all times. This may explain unsatisfactory therapeutic results in some patients. Better blood levels can probably be attained in most patients if the tablets are administered after a meal with a high fat content.

Indications and Usage: Major indications for GRIFULVIN V griseofulvin microsize are:
  Tinea capitis (ringworm of the scalp)
  Tinea corporis (ringworm of the body)
  Tinea pedis (athlete's foot)
  Tinea unguium (onychomycosis; ringworm of the nails)
  Tinea cruris (ringworm of the thigh)
  Tinea barbae (barber's itch)

GRIFULVIN V (griseofulvin microsize) inhibits the growth of those genera of fungi that commonly cause ringworm infections of the hair, skin, and nails, such as:
  Trichophyton rubrum
  Trichophyton tonsurans
  Trichophyton mentagrophytes
  Trichophyton interdigitalis
  Trichophyton verrucosum
  Trichophyton sulphureum
  Trichophyton schoenleini
  Microsporum audouini
  Microsporum canis
  Microsporum gypseum
  Epidermophyton floccosum
  Trichophyton megnini
  Trichophyton gallinae
  Trichophyton crateriform

Note: Prior to therapy, the type of fungi responsible for the infection should be indentified. The use of the drug is not justified in minor or trivial infections which will respond to topical antifungal agents alone.

It is *not* effective in:
  Bacterial infections
  Candidiasis (Moniliasis)
  Histoplasmosis
  Actinomycosis
  Sporotrichosis
  Chromoblastomycosis
  Coccidioidomycosis
  North American Blastomycosis
  Cryptococcosis (Torulosis)
  Tinea versicolor
  Nocardiosis

Contraindications: This drug is contraindicated in patients with porphyria, hepatocellular failure, and in individuals with a history of hypersensitivity to griseofulvin.

Warnings:

Usage in Pregnancy: Safe use of GRIFULVIN V (griseofulvin microsize) in pregnancy has not been established.

Prophylactic Usage: Safety and efficacy of prophylactic use of this drug has not been established.

Chronic feeding of griseofulvin, at levels ranging from 0.5-2.5% of the diet, resulted in the development of liver tumors in several strains of mice, particularly in males. Smaller particle sizes result in an enhanced effect. Lower oral dosage levels have not been tested. Subcutaneous administration of relatively small doses of griseofulvin once a week during the first three weeks of life has also been reported to induce hepatomata in mice. Although studies in other animal species have not yielded evidence of tumorigenicity, these studies were not of adequate design to form a basis for conclusions in this regard.

In subacute toxicity studies, orally administered griseofulvin produced hepatocellular necrosis in mice, but this has not been seen in other species. Disturbances in porphyrin metabolism have been reported in griseofulvin-treated laboratory animals. Griseofulvin has been reported to have a colchicine-like effect on mitosis and cocarcinogenicity with methylcholanthrene in cutaneous tumor induction in laboratory animals.

Reports of animal studies in the Soviet literature state that a griseofulvin preparation was found to be embryotoxic and teratogenic on oral administration to pregnant Wistar rats. Rat reproduction studies done thus far in the United States and Great Britain have been inconclusive in this regard, and additional animal reproduction studies are underway. Pups with abnormalities have been reported in the litters of a few bitches treated with griseofulvin.

Suppression of spermatogenesis has been reported to occur in rats but investigation in man failed to confirm this.

Precautions: Patients on prolonged therapy with any potent medication should be under close

Continued on next page

Ortho Derm.—Cont.

observation. Periodic monitoring of organ system function, including renal, hepatic and hemopoietic, should be done.

Since griseofulvin is derived from species of penicillin, the possibility of cross sensitivity with penicillin exists; however, known penicillin-sensitive patients have been treated without difficulty.

Since a photosensitivity reaction is occasionally associated with griseofulvin therapy, patients should be warned to avoid exposure to intense natural or artificial sunlight. Should a photosensitivity reaction occur, lupus erythematosus may be aggravated.

Patients on warfarin-type anticoagulant therapy may require dosage adjustment of the anticoagulant during and after griseofulvin therapy. Concomitant use of barbiturates usually depresses griseofulvin activity and may necessitate raising the dosage.

Adverse Reactions: When adverse reactions occur, they are most commonly of the hypersensitivity type such as skin rashes, urticaria and rarely, angioneurotic edema, and may necessitate withdrawal of therapy and appropriate countermeasures. Paresthesias of the hands and feet have been reported rarely after extended therapy. Other side effects reported occasionally are oral thrush, nausea, vomiting, epigastric distress, diarrhea; headache, fatigue, dizziness, insomnia, mental confusion and impairment of performance of routine activities.

Proteinuria and leukopenia have been reported rarely. Administration of the drug should be discontinued if granulocytopenia occurs.

When rare, serious reactions occur with griseofulvin, they are usually associated with high dosages, long periods of therapy, or both.

Dosage and Administration: Accurate diagnosis of the infecting organism is essential. Identification should be made either by direct microscopic examination of a mounting of infected tissue in a solution of potassium hydroxide or by culture on an appropriate medium.

Medication must be continued until the infecting organism is completely eradicated as indicated by appropriate clinical or laboratory examination. Representative treatment periods are tinea capitis, 4 to 6 weeks; tinea corporis, 2 to 4 weeks; tinea pedis, 4 to 8 weeks; tinea unguium—depending on rate of growth —fingernails, at least 4 months; toenails, at least 6 months.

General measures in regard to hygiene should be observed to control sources of infection or reinfection. Concomitant use of appropriate topical agents is usually required, particularly in treatment of tinea pedis since in some forms of athlete's foot, yeasts and bacteria may be involved. Griseofulvin will not eradicate the bacterial or monilial infection.

Adults: A daily dose of 500 mg. will give a satisfactory response in most patients with tinea corporis, tinea cruris, and tinea capitis.

For those fungus infections more difficult to eradicate such as tinea pedis and tinea unguium, a daily dose of 1.0 gram is recommended.

Children: Approximately 5 mg. per pound of body weight per day is an effective dose for most children. On this basis the following dosage schedule for children is suggested:
  Children weighing 30 to 50 pounds—125 mg. to 250 mg. daily.
  Children weighing over 50 pounds—250 mg. to 500 mg. daily.

How Supplied: GRIFULVIN V (griseofulvin microsize) 250 mg. Tablets in bottles of 100 (NDC 0062-0211-60) (white, scored, imprinted "ORTHO 211").

GRIFULVIN V (griseofulvin microsize) 500 mg. Tablets in bottles of 100 (NDC 0062-0214-60) and 500 (NDC 0062-0214-70) (white, scored, imprinted "ORTHO 214").

Dispense GRIFULVIN V tablets in well-closed container as defined in the official compendia.

GRIFULVIN V (griseofulvin microsize) Suspension 125 mg. per 5 cc. in bottles of 4 fl. oz. (NDC 0062-0206-04).

Dispense GRIFULVIN V suspension in tight, light-resistant container as defined in the official compendia.

STORE AT ROOM TEMPERATURE

MECLAN® ℞
(meclocycline sulfosalicylate)
Cream 1%

Description: MECLAN (meclocycline sulfosalicylate) Cream 1% is a homogeneous smooth yellow cream, each gram of which contains meclocycline sulfosalicylate equivalent to 10 mg. of meclocycline activity in an aqueous cream vehicle consisting of glyceryl stearate, propylene glycol stearate, caprylic/capric triglyceride, paraffin, trihydroxystearin, polysorbate 40, sorbitol solution, propyl gallate, sorbic acid, sodium formaldehyde sulfoxylate, perfume, and water. The vehicle is pharmaceutically compatible with both oil- and water-based systems.

Chemically meclocycline sulfosalicylate is [4S-(4α, 4aα, 5α, 5aα, 12aα)]-7-chloro-4-(dimethyl- amino) 1, 4,4a,5,5a,6,11,12a-octahydro-3,5,10, 12,12a-pentahydroxy-6-methylene-1, 11- dioxo- 2-napthacenecarboxamide 5-sulfosalicylate.

Actions (Clinical Pharmacology): The mode of action of MECLAN Cream in the treatment of acne is not fully understood. However, it appears that meclocycline possesses a localized effect, since it is not absorbed through the skin in sufficient quantities to be detected systemically. In subtotal body inunction studies, up to 40 times the average treatment dose was applied to 20 human subjects daily for 28 days. No measurable amounts of meclocycline appeared in the blood (0.1 microgram/ml. level of detectability) or urine (0.02 microgram/ml. level of detectability).

Indication: MECLAN Cream (meclocycline sulfosalicylate) is indicated for topical application in the treatment of acne vulgaris.

Contraindications: MECLAN is contraindicated in persons who have shown hypersensitivity to any of its ingredients or to any of the other tetracyclines.

Warnings: Although no absorption has been demonstrated by 28-day inunction studies in humans, the possibility exists that significant percutaneous absorption may result from prolonged use. Therefore, caution is advised in administering MECLAN (meclocycline sulfosalicylate) to persons with hepatic or renal dysfunction.

Precautions: This drug is for external use only and should be kept out of the eyes, nose, and mouth. It should be used with caution by patients who are sensitive to formaldehyde.

Pregnancy: Pregnancy Category B. Reproduction studies have been performed in rats and rabbits at oral doses up to 1000 times the human dose (assuming the human dose to be one gram of cream per day) and have revealed no evidence of impaired fertility or harm to the fetus due to meclocycline sulfosalicylate. There was, however, a slight delay in ossification in rabbits when meclocycline was applied topically. There are no adequate and well-controlled studies in pregnant women. Because animal reproduction studies are not always predictive of human response, this drug should be used during pregnancy only if clearly needed.

Nursing Mothers: It is not known whether this drug is excreted in human milk. Because many drugs are excreted in human milk, caution should be exercised when meclocycline sulfosalicylate is administered to a nursing woman.

Adverse Reactions: MECLAN is well tolerated by the skin. In the clinical trials there was one report of acute contact dermatitis. There were isolated reports of skin irritation. Temporary follicular staining may occur with excessive application. Patch testing has demonstrated no photosensitivity or contact allergy potential.

Dosage and Administration: It is recommended that MECLAN be applied to the affected area twice daily, morning and evening. Less frequent application may be used depending on patient response. Excessive use of MECLAN Cream may cause staining of some fabrics.

How Supplied: MECLAN (meclocycline sulfosalicylate) Cream 1% is supplied in 20 gram and 45 gram sealed tubes.

MONISTAT-DERM™ ℞
(miconazole nitrate 2%)
Cream and Lotion
For Topical Use Only

Description: MONISTAT-DERM (miconazole nitrate 2%) Cream and Lotion each contain miconazole nitrate* 2%, formulated into a water-miscible base consisting of pegoxol 7 stearate, peglicol 5 oleate, mineral oil, benzoic acid, and butylated hydroxyanisole and purified water.

*Chemical name: 1-[2,4-dichloro-β-{(2,4-di- chlorobenzyl)oxy} phenethyl] imidazole mononitrate.

Actions: Miconazole nitrate is a synthetic antifungal agent which inhibits the growth of the common dermatophytes, *Trichophyton rubrum, Trichophyton mentagrophytes,* and *Epidermophyton floccosum,* the yeast-like fungus. *Candida albicans,* and the organism responsible for tinea versicolor *(Malassezia furfur).*

Indications: For topical application in the treatment of tinea pedis (athlete's foot), tinea cruris, and tinea corporis caused by *Trichophyton rubrum, Trichophyton mentagrophytes,* and *Epidermophyton floccosum,* in the treatment of cutaneous candidiasis (moniliasis), and in the treatment of tinea versicolor.

Contraindications: MONISTAT-DERM (miconazole nitrate 2%) Cream and Lotion have no known contraindications.

Precautions: If a reaction suggesting sensitivity or chemical irritation should occur, use of the medication should be discontinued.

For external use only. Avoid introduction of MONISTAT-DERM Cream and Lotion into the eyes.

Adverse Reactions: There have been isolated reports of irritation, burning, and maceration, and allergic contact dermatitis associated with application of MONISTAT-DERM.

Dosage and Administration: Sufficient MONISTAT-DERM Cream should be applied to cover affected areas twice daily (morning and evening) in patients with tinea pedis, tinea cruris, tinea corporis, and cutaneous candidiasis, and once daily in patients with tinea versicolor. It is preferable to use MONISTAT-DERM Lotion in intertriginous areas; if the cream is used, it should be applied sparingly and smoothed in well to avoid maceration effects.

Early relief of symptoms (2 to 3 days) is experienced by the majority of patients and clinical improvement may be seen fairly soon after treatment is begun; however, *Candida* infections and tinea cruris and corporis should be treated for two weeks and tinea pedis for one month in order to reduce the possibility of recurrence. If a patient shows no clinical improvement after a month of treatment, the diagnosis should be redetermined. Patients with tinea versicolor usually exhibit clinical and mycological clearing after two weeks of treatment.

How Supplied: MONISTAT-DERM (miconazole nitrate 2%) Cream containing miconazole nitrate at 2% strength is supplied in 15 g., 1 oz. and 3 oz. tubes. MONISTAT-DERM (miconazole nitrate 2%) Lotion containing miconazole nitrate at 2% w/w strength is supplied in polyethylene squeeze bottles in quantities of 30 ml. and 60 ml.

PERSA-GEL® 5% & 10% ℞
(benzoyl peroxide)
acetone-base gel
PERSA-GEL W 5% & 10%
(benzoyl peroxide)
water-base gel

Description: PERSA-GEL and PERSA-GEL W 5% and 10% (benzoyl peroxide 5% and 10%) are topical gel preparations for use in the treatment of acne vulgaris. Benzoyl peroxide is an oxidizing agent which possesses antibacterial properties and is classified as a keratolytic.

PERSA-GEL contains benzoyl peroxide 5% or 10% as the active ingredient in a gel base containing acetone, carbomer 940, trolamine, sodium lauryl sulfate, propylene glycol and purified water.

PERSA-GEL W contains benzoyl peroxide 5% or 10% as the active ingredient containing purified water, carbomer, sodium hydroxide, hydroxypropyl methylcellulose 2906, and laureth 4.

Clinical Pharmacology: The mechanism of action of benzoyl peroxide has not been determined but may be related to its antibacterial activity against **Propionibacterium acnes** and its ability to cause drying and peeling. Benzoyl peroxide reduces the concentration of free fatty acids in the sebum. Little is known about the percutaneous penetration, metabolism, and excretion of benzoyl peroxide, although it is likely that benzoic acid is a major metabolite. There is no evidence of systemic toxicity caused by benzoyl peroxide in humans.

Indications and Usage: These products are indicated for the topical treatment of acne vulgaris.

Contraindications: These products are contraindicated in patients with a history of hypersensitivity to any of the components of the preparations.

Precautions: General: For external use only. If severe irritation develops, discontinue use and institute appropriate therapy. After the reaction clears, treatment may often be resumed with less frequent application. This preparation should not be used in or near the eyes or on mucous membranes.

Information for Patients: Avoid contact with eyes, eyelids, lips and mucous membranes. If accidental contact occurs, rinse with water. May bleach hair and colored fabrics. If excessive irritation develops, discontinue use and consult your physician.

Carcinogenesis, Mutagenesis, Impairment of Fertility: There is no evidence in the published literature that benzoyl peroxide is carcinogenic, mutagenic or that it impairs fertility.

Pregnancy: Pregnancy Category C: Animal reproduction studies have not been conducted with benzoyl peroxide. It is also not known whether benzoyl peroxide can cause fetal harm when administered to a pregnant woman or can affect reproduction capacity. Benzoyl per- oxide should be used by a pregnant woman only if clearly needed. There are no data available on the effect of benzoyl peroxide on the growth, development and functional maturation of the unborn child.

Nursing Mothers: It is not known whether this drug is excreted in human milk. Because many drugs are excreted in human milk, caution should be exercised when benzoyl peroxide is administered to a nursing woman.

Pediatric Use: Safety and effectiveness in children have not been established.

Adverse Reactions: Allergic contact dermatitis has been reported with topical benzoyl peroxide therapy.

Dosage and Administration: PERSA-GEL or PERSA-GEL W 5% or 10% should be applied once or twice daily to affected areas after washing with a mild cleanser and water. The degree of drying and peeling can be adjusted by modification of the dosage schedule.

How Supplied:
PERSA-GEL 5%, 1.5 oz. tubes
(NDC 0062-8610-31)
PERSA-GEL 5%, 3 oz. tubes
(NDC 0062-8610-03)
PERSA-GEL 10%, 1.5 oz. tubes
(NDC 0062-8600-31)
PERSA-GEL 10%, 3 oz. tubes
(NDC 0062-8600-03)
PERSA-GEL W 5% 1.5 oz. tubes
(NDC 0062-8630-31)
PERSA-GEL W 5% 3.0 oz. tubes
(NDC 0062-8630-03)
PERSA-GEL W 10% 1.5 oz. tubes
(NDC 0062-8620-31)
PERSA-GEL W 10% 3.0 oz. tubes

(NDC 0062-8620-03)
Store at controlled room temperature (59°-86°F).

PURPOSE® Dry Skin Cream
(See PDR For Nonprescription Drugs)

PURPOSE® Shampoo
(See PDR For Nonprescription Drugs)

PURPOSE® Soap
(See PDR For Nonprescription Drugs)

RETIN-A™
(tretinoin)
Cream•Gel•Liquid
For Topical Use Only

Description: RETIN-A Gel, Cream and Liquid, containing tretinoin, are used for the topical treatment of acne vulgaris. RETIN-A Gel contains tretinoin (retinoic acid; vitamin A acid) in either of two strengths, 0.025% of 0.01% by weight, in a gel vehicle of butylated hydroxytoluene, hydroxypropyl cellulose, and alcohol 90% w/w. RETIN-A (tretinoin) Cream contains tretinoin in either of two strengths, 0.1% or 0.05% by weight, in a hydrophilic cream vehicle of stearic acid, isopropyl myristate, polyoxyl 40 stearate, stearyl alcohol, xanthan gum, sorbic acid, butylated hydroxytoluene, and purified water. RETIN-A Liquid contains tretinoin 0.05% by weight, polyethylene glycol 400, butylated hydroxytoluene, and alcohol 55%.

Clinical Pharmacology: Although the exact mode of action of tretinoin is unknown, current evidence suggests that topical tretinoin decreases cohesiveness of follicular epithelial cells with decreased microcomedo formation. Additionally, tretinoin stimulates mitotic activity and increased turnover of follicular epithelial cells, causing extrusion of the comedones.

Indications and Usage: RETIN-A is indicated for topical application in the treatment of acne vulgaris.

Contraindications: Use of the product should be discontinued if hypersensitivity to any of the ingredients is noted.

Precautions: General: If a reaction suggesting sensitivity or chemical irritation occurs, use of the medication should be discontinued. Exposure to sunlight, including sunlamps, should be minimized during the use of RETIN-A, and patients with sunburn should be advised not to use the product until fully recovered because of heightened susceptibility to sunlight as a result of the use of tretinoin. Patients who may be required to have considerable sun exposure due to occupation and those with inherent sensitivity to the sun should exercise particular caution. Use of sunscreen products and protective clothing over treated areas may be prudent when exposure cannot be avoided. Weather extremes, such as wind or cold, also may be irritating to patients under treatment with tretinoin.

RETIN-A (tretinoin) acne treatment should be kept away from the eyes, the mouth, angles of the nose, and mucous membranes. Topical use may induce severe local erythema and peeling at the site of application. If the degree of local irritation warrants, patients should be directed to use the medication less frequently, discontinue use temporarily, or discontinue use altogether. Tretinoin has been reported to cause severe irritation on eczematous skin and should be used with utmost caution in patients with this condition.

Drug Interactions: Concomitant topical medication, medicated or abrasive soaps and cleansers, soaps and cosmetics that have a strong drying effect, and products with high concentrations of alcohol, astringents, spices or lime should be used with caution because of possible interaction with tretinoin. Particular caution should be exercised in using preparations containing sulfur, resorcinol, or salicylic acid with RETIN-A. It is also advisable to "rest" a patient's skin until the effects of such preparations subside before use of RETIN-A is begun.

Carcinogenesis: Long-term animal studies to determine the carcinogenic potential of tretinoin have not been performed. Studies in hairless albino mice suggest that tretinoin may accelerate the tumorigenic potential of ultraviolet radiation. Although the significance to man is not clear, patients should avoid or minimize exposure to sun.

Pregnancy: Pregnancy Category B. Reproduction studies performed in rats and rabbits at dermal doses up to 50 times the human dose (assuming the human dose to be 500 mg of gel per day) have revealed no evidence of impaired fertility or harm to the fetus due to tretinoin (retinoic acid). There was, however, a slightly higher incidence of irregularly contoured or partially ossified skull bones in some rat and rabbit fetuses. There are no adequate and well-controlled studies in pregnant women. Because animal reproduction studies are not always predictive of human response, this drug should be used during pregnancy only if clearly needed.

Nursing Mothers: It is not known whether this drug is excreted in human milk. Because many drugs are excreted in human milk, caution should be exercised when tretinoin is administered to a nursing woman.

Adverse Reactions: The skin of certain sensitive individuals may become excessively red, edematous, blistered, or crusted. If these effects occur, the medication should either be discontinued until the integrity of the skin is restored, or the medication should be adjusted to a level the patient can tolerate. True contact allergy to topical tretinoin is rarely encountered. Temporary hyper- or hypopigmentation has been reported with repeated application of RETIN-A. Some individuals have been reported to have heightened susceptibility to sunlight while under treatment with RETIN-A. To date, all adverse effects of RETIN-A have been reversible upon discontinuation of therapy (see Dosage and Administration Section).

Overdosage: If medication is applied excessively, no more rapid or better results will be obtained or marked redness, peeling, or discomfort may occur.

Oral LD_{50} values for the various dosage forms of RETIN-A were found to be:

	0.05% Solution	0.1% Cream	0.05% Gel*
Mice	19.0 ml/Kg	Sublethal	11.83 ml/Kg
Rats	20.9 ml/Kg	Sublethal	20.21 ml/Kg

The intravenous LD_{50} values of the 0.05% solution in mice and rats were found to be 5.2 ml/Kg and 8.7 ml/Kg respectively.

Dosage and Administration: RETIN-A Gel, Cream or Liquid should be applied once a day, before retiring, to the skin where acne lesions appear, using enough to cover the entire affected area lightly. Liquid: The liquid may be applied using a fingertip, gauze pad, or cotton swab. If gauze or cotten is employed, care should be taken not to oversaturate it to the extent that the liquid would run into areas where treatment is not intended. Gel: Excessive application results in "pilling" of the gel, which minimizes the likelihood of overapplication by the patient.

Application may cause a transitory feeling of warmth or slight stinging. In cases where it has been necessary to temporarily discontinue therapy or to reduce the frequency of application, therapy may be resumed or frequency of application increased when the patients become able to tolerate the treatment.

It should be noted that just as some patients require less frequent applications or other dosage forms, others may respond better to more frequent application of tretinoin. Alterations of vehicle, drug concentration, or dose frequency should be closely monitored by careful observation of the clinical therapeutic response and skin tolerance. During the early weeks of therapy, an *apparent* exacerbation of inflammatory lesions may occur. This is due to the action of the medication on deep,

Continued on next page

Ortho Derm.—Cont.

previously unseen lesions and should not be considered a reason to discontinue therapy.

Therapeutic results should be noticed after two to three weeks but more than six weeks of therapy may be required before definite beneficial effects are seen.

Once the acne lesions have responded satisfactorily, it may be possible to maintain the improvement with less frequent applications or other dosage forms.

Patients treated with RETIN-A (tretinoin) acne treatment may use cosmetics, but the areas to be treated should be cleansed thoroughly before the medication is applied.

How Supplied: RETIN-A (tretinoin) is supplied as:

1. A 0.025% Gel in tubes of 15 grams (NDC 0062-0475-42) and 45 grams (NDC 0062-0475-45) and a 0.01% Gel in tubes of 15 grams (NDC 0062-0575-44) and 45 grams (NDC 0062-0575-46).
2. A 0.1% Cream in tubes of 20 grams (NDC 0062-0275-23) and a 0.05% Cream in tubes of 20 grams (NDC 0062-0175-12) and 45 grams (NDC 0062-0175-13).
3. A 0.05% Liquid in amber bottles containing 28 ml (NDC 0062-0075-07).

Storage Conditions: RETIN-A Liquid 0.05%, and RETIN-A Gel 0.025% and 0.01%; store below 86°F. RETIN-A Cream 0.1% and 0.05% store below 80°F.
The 0.05% Gel was never marketed.

SPECTAZOLE™   ℞
(econazole nitrate 1%)
Cream
For Topical Use Only

Description: SPECTAZOLE Cream contains the antifungal agent, econazole nitrate 1%, in a water-miscible base consisting of pegoxol 7 stearate, peglicol 5 oleate, mineral oil, benzoic acid, butylated hydroxyanisole, and purified water. The white to off-white soft cream is for topical use only. Chemically, econazole nitrate is 1-[2-[(4-chlorophenyl)methoxy]-2-(2,4-dichlorophenyl)ethyl]-1H-imidazole mononitrate. Its structure is as follows:

Clinical Pharmacology: After topical application to the skin of normal subjects, systemic absorption of econazole nitrate is extremely low. Although most of the applied drug remains on the skin surface, drug concentrations were found in the stratum corneum which, by far, exceeded the minimum inhibitory concentration for dermatophytes. Inhibitory concentrations were achieved in the epidermis and as deep as the middle region of the dermis. Less than 1% of the applied dose was recovered in the urine and feces.

Microbiology: In *in-vitro* studies, econazole nitrate exhibits broad-spectrum antifungal activity against the dermatophytes, *Trichophyton rubrum*, *Trichophyton mentagrophytes*, *Trichophyton tonsurans*, *Microsporum canis*, *Microsporum audouini*, *Microsporum gypseum*, and *Epidermophyton floccosum*, the yeasts, *Candida albicans* and *Pityrosporum orbiculare* (the organism responsible for tinea versicolor), and certain gram positive bacteria.

Indications and Usage: SPECTAZOLE Cream is indicated for topical application in the treatment of tinea pedis, tinea cruris, and tinea corporis caused by *Trichophyton rubrum*, *Trichophyton mentagrophytes*, *Trichophyton tonsurans*, *Microsporum canis*, *Microsporum audouini*, *Microsporum gypseum*, and *Epidermophyton floccosum*, in the treatment of cutaneous candidiasis, and in the treatment of tinea versicolor.

Contraindications: SPECTAZOLE Cream is contraindicated in individuals who have shown hypersensitivity to any of its ingredients.

Warnings: SPECTAZOLE is not for ophthalmic use.

Although not observed in clinical studies using SPECTAZOLE, several cases of hepatocellular dysfunction have been reported during systemic treatment with another imidazole.

Precautions:

General: If a reaction suggesting sensitivity or chemical irritation should occur, use of the medication should be discontinued.

For external use only. Avoid introduction of SPECTAZOLE Cream into the eyes.

Carcinogenicity Studies: Long-term animal studies to determine carcinogenic potential have not been performed.

Fertility (Reproduction): Oral administration of econazole nitrate in rats has been reported to produce prolonged gestation. Intravaginal administration in humans has not shown prolonged gestation or other adverse reproductive effects attributable to econazole nitrate therapy.

Pregnancy: Pregnancy Category C. Econazole nitrate has not been shown to be teratogenic when administered orally to mice, rabbits or rats. Fetotoxic or embryotoxic effects were observed in Segment I oral studies with rats receiving 10 to 40 times the human dermal dose. Similar effects were observed in Segment II or Segment III studies with mice, rabbits and/or rats receiving oral doses 80 or 40 times the human dermal dose.

Econazole should be used in the first trimester of pregnancy only when the physician considers it essential to the welfare of the patient. The drug should be used during the second and third trimesters of pregnancy only if clearly needed.

Nursing Mothers: It is not known whether econazole nitrate is excreted in human milk. Following oral administration of econazole nitrate to lactating rats, econazole and/or metabolites were excreted in milk and were found in nursing pups. Also, in lactating rats receiving large oral doses (40 or 80 times the human dermal dose), there was a reduction in post partum viability of pups and survival to weaning; however, at these high doses, maternal toxicity was present and may have been a contributing factor. Caution should be exercised when econazole nitrate is administered to a nursing woman.

Adverse Reactions: During clinical trials, 12 (3.3%) of 366 patients treated with econazole nitrate 1% cream reported side effects, consisting mainly of burning, itching, stinging and erythema.

Overdose: Overdosage of econazole nitrate in humans has not been reported to date. In mice, rats, guinea pigs and dogs, the oral LD 50 values were found to be 462, 668, 272, and > 160 mg/kg, respectively.

Dosage and Administration: Sufficient SPECTAZOLE Cream should be applied to cover affected areas twice daily (morning and evening) in patients with tinea pedis, tinea cruris, tinea corporis, and cutaneous candidiasis, and once daily in patients with tinea versicolor.

Early relief of symptoms is experienced by the majority of patients and clinical improvement may be seen fairly soon after treatment is begun; however, candidal infections and tinea cruris and corporis should be treated for two weeks and tinea pedis for one month in order to reduce the possibility of recurrence. If a patient shows no clinical improvement after the treatment period, the diagnosis should be redetermined. Patients with tinea versicolor usually exhibit clinical and mycological clearing after two weeks of treatment.

How Supplied: SPECTAZOLE (econazole nitrate 1%) Cream is supplied in tubes of 15 grams (NDC 0062-5460-02), 30 grams (NDC 0062-5460-01), and 85 grams (NDC 0062-5460-03).

Store SPECTAZOLE Cream below 86°F.

Palisades Pharmaceuticals, Inc.
219 COUNTY ROAD
TENAFLY, NEW JERSEY 07670

YOCON®   ℞
(brand of yohimbine hydrochloride)

Description: Yohimbine is a $3\alpha\text{-}15\alpha\text{-}20\beta\text{-}17\alpha$-hydroxy Yohimbine-16α-carboxylic acid methyl ester. The alkaloid is found in Rubaceae and related trees. Also in Rauwolfia Serpentina (L) Benth.

Yohimbine is an indolalkylamine alkaloid with chemical similarity to reserpine. It is a crystalline powder, odorless. Each compressed tablet contains (1/12 gr.) 5.4 mg of Yohimbine Hydrochloride.

Action: Yohimbine blocks presynaptic alpha-2 adrenergic receptors. Its action on peripheral blood vessels resembles that of reserpine, though it is weaker and of short duration. Yohimbine's peripheral autonomic nervous system effect is to increase parasympathetic (cholinergic) and decrease sympathetic (adrenergic) activity. It is to be noted that in male sexual performance, erection is linked to cholinergic activity and to alpha-2 adrenergic blockade which may theoretically result in increased penile inflow, decreased penile outflow or both.

Yohimbine exerts a stimulating action on the mood and may increase anxiety. Such actions have not been adequately studied or related to dosage although they appear to require high doses of the drug. Yohimbine has a mild anti-diuretic action, probably via stimulation of hypothalmic centers and release of posterior pituitary hormone.

Reportedly, Yohimbine exerts no significant influence on cardiac stimulation and other effects mediated by β-adrenergic receptors, its effect on blood pressure, if any, would be to lower it; however, no adequate studies are at hand to quantitate this effect in terms of Yohimbine dosage.

Indications: YOCON® is indicated as a sympathicolytic and mydriatic. It may have activity as an aphrodisiac.

Contraindications: Renal diseases, and patient's sensitive to the drug. In view of the limited and inadequate information at hand, no precise tabulation can be offered of additional contraindications.

Warning: Generally, this drug is not proposed for use in females and certainly must not be used during pregnancy. Neither is this drug proposed for use in pediatric, geriatric or cardio-renal patients with gastric or duodenal ulcer history. Nor should it be used in conjunction with mood-modifying drugs such as antidepressants, or in psychiatric patients in general.

Adverse Reactions: Yohimbine readily penetrates the (CNS) and produces a complex pattern of responses in lower doses than required to produce peripheral α-adrenergic blockade. These include, anti-diuresis, a general picture of central excitation including elevation of blood pressure and heart rate increased motor activity, irritability and tremor. Sweating, nausea and vomiting are common after parenteral administration of the drug.[1,2] Also dizziness, headache, skin flushing reported when used orally[1,3].

Dosage and Administration: Experimental dosage reported in treatment of erectile impotence:[1,3,4] 1 tablet (5.4 mg) 3 times a day, to adult males taken orally. Occasional side effects reported with this dosage are nausea, dizziness or nervousness. In the event of side effects dosage is to be reduced to $\frac{1}{2}$ tablet 3 times a day, followed by gradual increases to 1 tablet 3 times a day. Reported therapy not more than 10 weeks[9].

How Supplied: Oral tablets of Yocon® 1/12 gr 5.4 mg in bottles of 100's **NDC** 53159-001-01 and 1000's **NDC** 53159-001-10.

References:

1. A. Morales et al., New England Journal of Medicine: 1221. November 12, 1981.
2. Goodman, Gilman —The Pharmacological basis of Therapeutics 6th ed., p. 176-188, McMillan

3. Weekly Urological Clinical letter, 27:2, July 4, 1983.
4. A. Morales et al., The Journal of Urology 128: 45-47, 1982.

Rev. December 24, 1984

Parke-Davis
Division of Warner-Lambert Company
201 TABOR ROAD
MORRIS PLAINS, NEW JERSEY
07950

PARCODE®
(Parke-Davis Accurate Recognition Code)

Code Number	Product Name
001	**Peritrate® Tablets**
	Each tablet contains 20 mg pentaerythritol tetranitrate.
002- 003	*Unassigned*
004	**Peritrate® SA Sustained Action Tablets**
	Each tablet contains 80 mg pentaerythritol tetranitrate (20 mg in the immediate release layer and 60 mg in the sustained release base).
005- 006	*Unassigned*
007	**Dilantin® Infatabs®**
	Each tablet contains 50 mg phenytoin sodium, USP.
008	**Peritrate® Tablets**
	Each tablet contains 40 mg pentaerythritol tetranitrate.
009	*Unassigned*
010	**Chlorpromazine Hydrochloride Tablets, USP (Promapar®)**
	Each tablet contains 10 mg chlorpromazine hydrochloride, USP.
011- 012	*Unassigned*
013	**Peritrate® Tablets**
	Each tablet contains 10 mg pentaerythritol tetranitrate.
014- 024	*Unassigned*
025	**Chlorpromazine Hydrochloride Tablets, USP (Promapar®)**
	Each tablet contains 25 mg chlorpromazine hydrochloride, USP.
026- 033	*Unassigned*
034	**Gelusil® Tablets**
	Each tablet contains 200 mg aluminum hydroxide, 200 mg magnesium hydroxide, and 25 mg simethicone.
035- 036	*Unassigned*
037	**Ferrous Sulfate Filmseals®, USP (325 mg)**
038- 042	*Unassigned*
043	**Gelusil-II® Tablets**
	Each tablet contains 400 mg aluminum hydroxide, 400 mg magnesium hydroxide, and 30 mg simethicone.
044	*Unassigned*
045	**Gelusil-M® Tablets**
	Each tablet contains 300 mg aluminum hydroxide, 200 mg magnesium hydroxide, and 25 mg simethicone.
046- 049	*Unassigned*
050	**Chlorpromazine Hydrochloride Tablets, USP (Promapar®)**
	Each tablet contains 50 mg chlorpromazine hydrochloride, USP.
051- 099	*Unassigned*
100	**Chlorpromazine Hydrochloride Tablets, USP (Promapar®)**
	Each tablet contains 100 mg chlorpromazine hydrochloride, USP.
101- 110	*Unassigned*
111	**Ergostat® Sublingual Tablets**
	Each tablet contains 2 mg ergotamine tartrate.
112- 116	*Unassigned*
117	**Diphenoxylate Hydrochloride and Atropine Sulfate Tablets, USP**
	Each tablet contains 2.5 mg diphenoxylate hydrochloride and 0.025 mg atropine sulfate, USP.
118- 120	*Unassigned*
121	**Chlorthalidone Tablets, USP**
	Each tablet contains 50 mg chlorthalidone, USP.
122	*Unassigned*
123	**Chlorthalidone Tablets, USP**
	Each tablet contains 25 mg chlorthalidone, USP.
124- 165	*Unassigned*
166	**Mandelamine® Tablets**
	Each tablet contains 0.5 gram methenamine mandelate, USP.
167	**Mandelamine® Tablets**
	Each tablet contains 1.0 gram methenamine mandelate, USP.
168- 176	*Unassigned*
177	**Sinubid® Tablets**
	Each tablet contains 300 mg acetaminophen, 100 mg phenylpropanolamine hydrochloride, and 66 mg phenyltoloxamine citrate.
180	**Pyridium® Tablets**
	Each tablet contains 100 mg phenazopyridine hydrochloride, USP.
181	**Pyridium® Tablets**
	Each tablet contains 200 mg phenazopyridine hydrochloride, USP.
182	**Pyridium® Plus Tablets**
	Each tablet contains 150 mg phenazopyridine hydrochloride (Pyridium®), 0.3 mg hyoscyamine hydrobromide, and 15 mg butabarbital.
183- 199	*Unassigned*
200	**Brondecon® Tablets**
	Each tablet contains 200 mg oxtriphylline and 100 mg guaifenesin.
201	**Chlorpromazine Hydrochloride Tablets, USP (Promapar®)**
	Each tablet contains 200 mg chlorpromazine hydrochloride, USP.
202	**Procan® SR Tablets, 250 mg**
	Each sustained-release tablet contains 250 mg procainamide hydrochloride.
203	*Unassigned*
204	**Procan® SR Tablets, 500 mg**
	Each sustained-release tablet contains 500 mg procainamide hydrochloride.
205	**Procan® SR Tablets, 750 mg**
	Each sustained-release tablet contains 750 mg procainamide hydrochloride.
206- 209	*Unassigned*
210	**Choledyl® Tablets**
	Each tablet contains 100 mg oxtriphylline, USP.
211	**Choledyl® Tablets**
	Each tablet contains 200 mg oxtriphylline, USP.
212- 213	*Unassigned*
214	**Choledyl® SA Tablets**
	Each sustained-action tablet contains 400 mg oxtriphylline, USP.
215- 220	*Unassigned*
221	**Choledyl® SA Tablets**
	Each sustained-action tablet contains 600 mg oxtriphylline, USP.
222- 229	*Unassigned*
230	**Tedral® Tablets**
	Each tablet contains 130 mg theophylline, 24 mg ephedrine hydrochloride, and 8 mg phenobarbital.
231	**Tedral® SA Tablets**
	Each sustained-action tablet contains 180 mg anhydrous theophylline (90 mg in the immediate release layer and 90 mg in the sustained-release layer); 48 mg ephedrine hydrochloride (16 mg in the immediate release layer and 32 mg in the sustained-release layer); 25 mg phenobarbital in the immediate release layer.
232- 236	*Unassigned*
237	**Zarontin® Capsules**
	Each capsule contains 250 mg ethosuximide, USP.
238	**Tedral-25® Tablets**
	Each tablet contains 130 mg theophylline, 24 mg ephedrine hydrochloride, and 25 mg butabarbital.
239- 246	*Unassigned*
247	**D-S-S Capsules**
	Each capsule contains 100 mg docusate sodium.
248	**D-S-S Plus Capsules**
	Each capsule contains 100 mg docusate sodium and 30 mg casanthranol.
249- 250	*Unassigned*
251	**Proloid® Tablets**
	Each tablet contains ½ grain thyroglobulin, USP.
252	**Proloid® Tablets**
	Each tablet contains 1 grain thyroglobulin, USP.
253	**Proloid® Tablets**
	Each tablet contains 1½ grains thyroglobulin, USP.
254	**Proloid® Tablets**
	Each tablet contains 3 grains thyroglobulin, USP.
255- 256	*Unassigned*
257	**Proloid® Tablets**
	Each tablet contains 2 grains thyroglobulin, USP.
258- 259	*Unassigned*
260	**Euthroid®-½ Tablets**
	Each tablet contains 30 mcg levothyroxine sodium (T_4), 7.5 mcg liothyronine sodium (T_3).
261	**Euthroid®-1 Tablets**
	Each tablet contains 60 mcg levothyroxine sodium (T_4), 15 mcg liothyronine sodium (T_3).
262	**Euthroid®-2 Tablets**
	Each tablet contains 120 mcg levothyroxine sodium (T_4), 30 mcg liothyronine sodium (T_3).
263	**Euthroid®-3 Tablets**
	Each tablet contains 180 mcg levothyroxine sodium (T_4), 45 mcg liothyronine sodium (T_3).
264- 267	*Unassigned*
268	**Meclomen® Capsules**
	Each capsule contains 50 mg meclofenamate sodium.
269	**Meclomen® Capsules**
	Each capsule contains 100 mg meclofenamate sodium.

Continued on next page

This product information was prepared in August, 1984. On these and other Parke-Davis Products, information may be obtained by addressing PARKE-DAVIS, Division of Warner-Lambert Company, Morris Plains, New Jersey 07950.

Parke-Davis—Cont.

270 Nardil® Tablets
Each tablet contains 15 mg phenelzine sulfate, USP.

271 Amitriptyline Hydrochloride Tablets
Each tablet contains 100 mg amitriptyline hydrochloride, USP.

272 Amitriptyline Hydrochloride Tablets
Each tablet contains 10 mg amitriptyline hydrochloride, USP.

273 Amitriptyline Hydrochloride Tablets
Each tablet contains 25 mg amitriptyline hydrochloride, USP.

274 Amitriptyline Hydrochloride Tablets
Each tablet contains 50 mg amitriptyline hydrochloride, USP.

275 Amitriptyline Hydrochloride Tablets
Each tablet contains 75 mg amitriptyline hydrochloride, USP.

276 Centrax® Tablets
Each tablet contains 10 mg prazepam.

277 Unassigned

278 Amitriptyline Hydrochloride Tablets
Each tablet contains 150 mg amitriptyline hydrochloride, USP.

279-281 Unassigned

282 Natafort® Filmseal®
Each tablet represents vitamin A (acetate), 6,000 IU; vitamin D 400 IU; folic acid, 1 mg; vitamin B_1 (thiamine mononitrate), 3 mg; vitamin B_2 (riboflavin), 2 mg; vitamin B_6 (pyridoxine hydrochloride), 15 mg; vitamin B_{12} (cyanocobalamin), crystalline, 6 mcg; vitamin C (ascorbic acid), 120 mg; nicotinamide (niacinamide), 20 mg; vitamin E (dl-alpha tocopheryl acetate), 30 IU; calcium (as calcium carbonate), 350 mg; magnesium (as magnesium oxide), 100 mg; iodine (as potassium iodide), 0.15 mg; iron (as ferrous fumarate), 65 mg; zinc (as zinc oxide), 25 mg.

283-319 Unassigned

320 Parsidol® Tablets
Each tablet contains 10 mg ethopropazine hydrochloride, USP.

321 Parsidol® Tablets
Each tablet contains 50 mg ethopropazine hydrochloride, USP.

322-336 Unassigned

337 Eldec® Kapseals®
Each capsule represents vitamin A (acetate), (0.5 mg) 1,667 IU; vitamin C (ascorbic acid), 66.7 mg; vitamin B_1 (thiamine mononitrate), 10 mg; vitamin B_2 (riboflavin), 0.87 mg; vitamin B_6 (pyridoxine hydrochloride), 0.67 mg; nicotinamide (niacinamide), 16.7 mg; dl-panthenol, 10 mg; ferrous sulfate, dried, 16.7 mg; iodine (as potassium iodide), 0.05 mg; calcium carbonate, 66.7 mg; vitamin E (dl-alpha tocopheryl acetate), (10 mg) 10 IU; vitamin B_{12} (cyanocobalamin), 2 mcg; folic acid, 0.33 mg. The Kapseal is a Dark Blue No. 1 capsule with Light Blue opaque band.

338-361 Unassigned

362 Dilantin® Kapseals®
Each Kapseal contains 100 mg extended phenytoin sodium, USP. The Kapseal is a No. 3 capsule with Orange band. (The Orange band on White capsule is a trademark registered in the US Patent Office.)

363-364 Unassigned

365 Dilantin® Kapseals®
Each Kapseal contains 30 mg extended phenytoin sodium, USP. The Kapseal is a No. 4 capsule with Pink opaque band.

366-372 Unassigned

373 Benadryl® Kapseals®
Each Kapseal contains 50 mg diphenhydramine hydrochloride. The Kapseal is a Pink No. 4 capsule with White opaque band. (The White band on Pink capsule is a trademark registered in the US Patent Office.)

374 Unassigned

375 Dilantin® with Phenobarbital ($\frac{1}{4}$ grain) Kapseals®
Each Kapseal contains Dilantin (phenytoin sodium), 100 mg; phenobarbital, 16 mg ($\frac{1}{4}$ grain). The Kapseal is a No. 3 capsule with Garnet band.

376-378 Unassigned

379 Chloromycetin® Kapseals®
Each Kapseal contains 250 mg chloramphenicol. The Kapseal is a White opaque No. 2 capsule with Gray opaque band. (The Gray band on White capsule is a trademark registered in the US Patent Office.)

380-389 Unassigned

390 Natabec® Kapseals®
Each Kapseal represents vitamin A (acetate), (1.2 mg), 4,000 IU*; vitamin D, 400 IU; vitamin C (ascorbic acid), 50 mg; vitamin B_1 (thiamine mononitrate), 3 mg; vitamin B_2 (riboflavin), 2 mg; nicotinamide +, 10 mg; vitamin B_6 (pyridoxine HCl), 3 mg; vitamin B_{12} crystalline (cyanocobalamin), 5 mcg; precipitated calcium carbonate, 600 mg; iron (as dried ferrous sulfate), 30 mg.

---
*IU = International Units
+Supplied as niacinamide

391-392 Unassigned

393 Milontin® Kapseals®
Each Kapseal contains 500 mg phensuximide, USP. The Kapseal is a Light Orange No. 0 capsule with Orange band.

394-401 Unassigned

402 Amcill® Capsules, 250 mg
Each capsule contains ampicillin trihydrate equivalent to 250 mg ampicillin.

403 Unassigned

404 Amcill® Capsules, 500 mg
Each capsule contains ampicillin trihydrate equivalent to 500 mg ampicillin.

405-406 Unassigned

407 Tetracycline Hydrochloride Capsules, USP, 250 mg (Cyclopar®)
Each capsule contains 250 mg tetracycline hydrochloride, USP.

408-419 Unassigned

420 Quinine Sulfate Capsules, USP
Each capsule contains 0.325 g (5 grains) quinine sulfate.

421-436 Unassigned

437 Estrovis® Tablets
Each tablet contains 100 mcg quinestrol.

438-439 Unassigned

440 Furosemide Tablets, USP, 20 mg
Each tablet contains 20 mg furosemide, USP.

441 Furosemide Tablets, USP, 40 mg
Each tablet contains 40 mg furosemide, USP.

442-470 Unassigned

471 Benadryl® Capsules
Each capsule contains 25 mg diphenhydramine hydrochloride.

472-489 Unassigned

490 Easprin® Enteric Coated Tablets
Each tablet contains 15 grains (975 mg) aspirin, USP.

491-524 Unassigned

525 Celontin® Kapseals®
Each Kapseal contains 300 mg methsuximide, USP. The Kapseal is a Yellow Tint No. 2 capsule with Orange band.

526-528 Unassigned

529 Humatin® Capsules
Each capsule contains paromomycin sulfate, USP, equivalent to 250 mg paromomycin.

530 Unassigned

531 Dilantin® with Phenobarbital ($\frac{1}{2}$ grain) Kapseals®
Each Kapseal contains Dilantin (phenytoin sodium), 100 mg; phenobarbital, 32 mg ($\frac{1}{2}$ grain). The Kapseal is a No. 3 capsule with Black band.

532 Unassigned

533 Calcium Lactate Tablets, USP
Each tablet contains 325 mg calcium lactate.

534 Natabec® with Fluoride Kapseals®
Each Kapseal represents vitamin A (acetate) (1.2 mg), 4,000 IU*; vitamin D (ergocalciferol) (10 mcg), 400 IU; vitamin C (ascorbic acid), 50 mg; thiamine mononitrate (vitamin B_1), 3 mg; riboflavin (vitamin B_2), 2.0 mg; nicotinamide (niacinamide), 20 mg; vitamin B_6 (pyridoxine hydrochloride), 3 mg; vitamin B_{12}, crystalline (cyanocobalamin), 5 mcg; ferrous sulfate, 150 mg; calcium carbonate, 600 mg; sodium fluoride, 2.2 mg.

---
*International Units
The Kapseal is a Pastel Pink No. 0 capsule with Ruby Red opaque band.

535-536 Unassigned

537 Celontin® (Half Strength) Kapseals®
Each Kapseal contains 150 mg methsuximide, USP. The Kapseal is a Yellow Tint No. 4 capsule with Brown opaque band.

538-539 Unassigned

540 Ponstel® Kapseals®
Each Kapseal contains 250 mg mefenamic acid. The Kapseal is an Ivory opaque No. 1 capsule with Light Blue opaque band. The blue band on ivory capsule combination is a Parke-Davis trademark.

541 Natabec-FA® Kapseals®
Each Kapseal represents vitamin A (acetate), (1.2 mg) 4,000 IU; ergocalciferol (10 mcg), 400 IU; ascorbic acid, 50 mg; thiamine mononitrate, 3 mg; riboflavin, 2 mg; pyridoxine hydrochloride, 3 mg; cyanocobalamin, 5 mcg; folic acid, 0.1 mg; niacinamide, 20 mg; calcium carbonate, 600 mg; ferrous sulfate,* 150 mg.

*Supplied as dried ferrous sulfate equivalent to the labeled amount of ferrous sulfate.
The Kapseal is a Pink Tint opaque No. 0 capsule with White opaque band.

542-543 Unassigned

544 Geriplex-FS® Kapseals®
Each capsule represents vitamin A (acetate) (1.5 mg), 5,000 IU; ascorbic acid,* 50 mg; thiamine mononitrate, 5 mg; riboflavin, 5 mg; cyanocobalamin, 2 mcg; choline dihydrogen citrate, 20 mg; niacinamide, 15 mg; dl-alpha tocopheryl acetate (5 mg), 5 IU; iron,† 6 mg; copper sulfate, 4 mg; manganese sulfate (monohydrate), 4 mg; zinc sulfate, 2 mg; calcium phosphate, dibasic (anhydrous), 200 mg; Taka-Diastase® (aspergillus oryzae enzymes); $2\frac{1}{2}$ gr; docusate sodium, 100 mg.

*Supplied as sodium ascorbate.
†Supplied as dried ferrous sulfate.
The Kapseal is a Blue No. 0 capsule with White opaque band.

545-
546 *Unassigned*
547 **Natabec R® Kapseals®**
Each Kapseal represents vitamin A (acetate) (1.2 mg), 4,000 IU; Vitamin D (10 mcg) 400 IU; ascorbic acid, 50 mg; thiamine mononitrate, 3 mg; riboflavin, 2 mg; pyridoxine hydrochloride, 3 mg; cyanocobalamin, 5 mcg; niacinamide, 10 mg; folic acid, 1 mg; calcium carbonate, precipitated, 600 mg; iron* 30 mg.

*Supplied as dried ferrous sulfate.
The Kapseal is a Blue opaque No. 0 capsule with Pink opaque band. The banded capsule is a Warner-Lambert trademark registered in the US Patent Office.

548-
549 *Unassigned*
550 **Thera-Combex H-P® Kapseals®**
Each Kapseal contains: ascorbic acid, 500 mg; thiamine mononitrate, 25 mg; riboflavin, 15 mg; pyridoxine hydrochloride, 10 mg; cyanocobalamin, 5 mcg; niacinamide, 100 mg; *dl*-panthenol, 20 mg.
The Kapseal is a Brown No. 0 capsule with Green opaque band.
551 *Unassigned*
552 **©Centrax® Capsules**
Each capsule contains 5 mg prazepam.
553 **©Centrax® Capsules**
Each capsule contains 10 mg prazepam.
554 **©Centrax® Capsules**
Each capsule contains 20 mg prazepam.
555-
603 *Unassigned*
604 **Calcium Lactate Tablets, USP**
Each tablet contains 650 mg (10 grains) calcium lactate.
605 *Unassigned*
606 **Aspirin Tablets, USP (White)**
Each tablet contains 325 mg (5 grains) aspirin.
607 **©Phenobarbital Tablets, USP**
Each tablet contains 60 mg (1 grain) phenobarbital.
608-
617 *Unassigned*
618 **Placebo tablet in Norlestrin 28 1/50.**
619-
621 *Unassigned*
622 **Ferrous Fumarate Tablets**
Each tablet contains 75 mg ferrous fumarate, USP.
623-
633 *Unassigned*
634 **©Acetaminophen with Codeine Phosphate Tablets, No. 2**
Each tablet contains 300 mg acetaminophen and 15 mg (¼ grain) codeine phosphate.
635 **©Acetaminophen with Codeine Phosphate Tablets, No. 3**
Each tablet contains 300 mg acetaminophen and 30 mg (½ grain) codeine phosphate.
636 *Unassigned*
637 **©Acetaminophen with Codeine Phosphate Tablets, No. 4**
Each tablet contains 300 mg acetaminophen and 60 mg (1 grain) codeine phosphate.
638 **Tabron® Filmseal®**
Each tablet represents ferrous fumarate, 304.2 mg (represents 100 mg of elemental iron); vitamin C (ascorbic acid), 500 mg; vitamin B₁ (thiamine mononitrate), 6 mg; vitamin B₂ (riboflavin), 6 mg; vitamin B₆ (pyridoxine hydrochloride), 5 mg; vitamin B₁₂ (cyanocobalamin), crystalline, 25 mcg; folic acid, 1 mg; nicotinamide (niacinamide), 30 mg; calcium pantothenate, 10 mg; vitamin E (*dl*-alpha tocopheryl acetate), (30 mg), 30 IU; docusate sodium, 50 mg.

639
640 **Acetaminophen Tablets, USP (Tapar®)**
Each tablet contains 325 mg (5 grains) acetaminophen, USP.
641-
646 *Unassigned*
647 **©Meprobamate Tablets, USP**
Each tablet contains 400 mg meprobamate, USP.
648 **Penicillin V Potassium Tablets, USP, 250 mg (Penapar VK®)**
Each tablet contains penicillin V potassium equivalent to 250 mg (400,000 units) penicillin V.
649-
668 *Unassigned*
669 **Lopid® Capsules**
Each capsule contains 300 mg gemfibrozil.
670-
671 *Unassigned*
672 **Erythromycin Stearate Filmseals (Erypar®)**
Each Filmseal® contains 250 mg erythromycin as erythromycin stearate.
673 **Penicillin V Potassium Tablets, USP, 500 mg (Penapar VK®)**
Each tablet contains penicillin V potassium equivalent to 500 mg (800,000 units) penicillin V.
674-
691 *Unassigned*
692 **©Propoxyphene Hydrochloride Capsules, USP**
Each capsule contains 65 mg propoxyphene hydrochloride.
693-
695 *Unassigned*
696 **ERYC® Capsules**
Each capsule contains 250 mg erythromycin, USP.
697 **Tetracycline Hydrochloride Capsules, USP, 500 mg (Cyclopar® 500)**
Each capsule contains 500 mg tetracycline hydrochloride, USP.
698 **©Phenobarbital Tablets, USP**
Each tablet contains 100 mg (1½ grains) phenobarbital.
699 **©Phenobarbital Tablets, USP**
Each tablet contains 15 mg (¼ grain) phenobarbital.
700 **©Phenobarbital Tablets, USP**
Each tablet contains 30 mg (½ grain) phenobarbital.
701 *Unassigned*
702 **Hydrochlorothiazide Tablets, USP (Thiuretic®)**
Each tablet contains 25 mg hydrochlorothiazide.
703-
709 *Unassigned*
710 **Hydrochlorothiazide Tablets, USP (Thiuretic®)**
Each tablet contains 50 mg hydrochlorothiazide.
711-
712 **Spironolactone with Hydrochlorothiazide Tablets**
Each tablet contains 25 mg spironolactone and 25 mg hydrochlorothiazide.
713 **Spironolactone Tablets, USP**
Each tablet contains 25 mg spironolactone, USP.
714-
724 *Unassigned*
725 **©Aspirin with Codeine Phosphate Tablets, No. 2**
Each tablet contains codeine phosphate, ¼ grain; aspirin, 325 mg.
726 **©Aspirin with Codeine Phosphate Tablets, No. 3**
Each tablet contains codeine phosphate, ½ grain; aspirin, 325 mg.

727 **©Aspirin with Codeine Phosphate Tablets, No. 4**
Each tablet contains codeine phosphate, 1 grain; aspirin, 325 mg.
728-
729 *Unassigned*
730 **Amoxicillin Capsules (Utimox®), USP, 250 mg**
Each capsule contains 250 mg amoxicillin.
731 **Amoxicillin Capsules (Utimox®), USP, 500 mg**
Each capsule contains 500 mg amoxicillin.
732-
746 *Unassigned*
747 **Povan® Filmseal®**
Each film-coated tablet contains pyrvinium pamoate equivalent to 50 mg pyrvinium.
748-
799 *Unassigned*
800 **©Chlordiazepoxide Hydrochloride Capsules, USP**
Each capsule contains 5 mg chlordiazepoxide hydrochloride.
801 **©Chlordiazepoxide Hydrochloride Capsules, USP**
Each capsule contains 10 mg chlordiazepoxide hydrochloride.
802 **©Chlordiazepoxide Hydrochloride Capsules, USP**
Each capsule contains 25 mg chlordiazepoxide hydrochloride.
803-
848 *Unassigned*
849 **Quinidine Sulfate Tablets, USP**
Each tablet contains 3 grains (200 mg) quinidine sulfate.
850 **Duraquin® (quinidine gluconate) Tablets, 330 mg**
Each scored, white, sustained-release tablet contains 330 mg quinidine gluconate.
851-
881 *Unassigned*
882 **Norlutin® Tablets**
Each tablet contains 5 mg norethindrone, USP.
883 **Nitrostat SR Capsules, 2.5 mg**
Each capsule contains 2.5 mg nitroglycerin in a special base for prolonged therapeutic effect.
884 **Nitrostat SR Capsules, 6.5 mg**
Each capsule contains 6.5 mg nitroglycerin in a special base for prolonged therapeutic effect.
885 **Nitrostat SR Capsules, 9.0 mg**
Each capsule contains 9.0 mg nitroglycerin in a special base for prolonged therapeutic effect.
886-
900 *Unassigned*
901 **Norlestrin® 2.5/50 Tablets**
Each tablet contains norethindrone acetate, 2.5 mg; ethinyl estradiol, 50 mcg.
902-
903 *Unassigned*
904 **Norlestrin® 1/50 Tablets**
Each tablet contains norethindrone acetate, 1 mg; ethinyl estradiol, 50 mcg.
905-
914 *Unassigned*
915 **Loestrin® 1/20 Tablets**
Each tablet contains norethindrone acetate, 1 mg; ethinyl estradiol, 20 mcg.
916 **Loestrin® 1.5/30 Tablets**
Each tablet contains norethindrone acetate, 1.5 mg; ethinyl estradiol, 30 mcg.

This product information was prepared in August, 1984. On these and other Parke-Davis Products, information may be obtained by addressing PARKE-DAVIS, Division of Warner-Lambert Company, Morris Plains, New Jersey 07950.

Continued on next page

Parke-Davis—Cont.

917 *Unassigned*
918 **Norlutate® Tablets**
Each tablet contains 5 mg norethindrone acetate.
919 **Erythromycin Stearate Filmseals (Erypar®)**
Each Filmseal® contains 500 mg erythromycin as erythromycin stearate.
920–
999 *Unassigned*

ADRENALIN® CHLORIDE SOLUTION ℞
[ă-drĕn'ă-lĭn" chlō'rīde]
(Epinephrine Injection, USP), 1:1000

Description: A sterile solution intended for subcutaneous or intramuscular injection. When diluted, it may also be administered intracardially or intravenously. Each milliliter contains 1 mg Adrenalin (epinephrine) as the hydrochloride dissolved in Water for Injection, USP, with sodium chloride added for isotonicity. The ampoules contain not more than 0.1% sodium bisulfite as an antioxidant, and the air in the ampoule has been displaced by nitrogen. The Steri-Vials® contain 0.5% Chloretone® (chlorobutanol) (chloroform derivative) as a preservative and not more than 0.15% sodium bisulfite as an antioxidant. Epinephrine is the active principle of the adrenal medulla, chemically described as (−)-3,4-Dihydroxy-α-[(methylamino) methyl] benzyl alcohol.

Clinical Pharmacology: Adrenalin (epinephrine) is a sympathomimetic drug. It activates an adrenergic receptive mechanism on effector cells and imitates all actions of the sympathetic nervous system except those on the arteries of the face and sweat glands. Epinephrine acts on both alpha and beta receptors and is the most potent alpha receptor activator.

Indications and Usage: In general, the most common uses of epinephrine are to relieve respiratory distress due to bronchospasm, to provide rapid relief of hypersensitivity re- actions to drugs and other allergens, and to prolong the action of infiltration anesthetics. Its cardiac effects may be of use in restoring cardiac rhythm in cardiac arrest due to various causes, but it is not used in cardiac failure or in hemorrhagic, traumatic, or cardiogenic shock.

Epinephrine is used as a hemostatic agent. It is also used in treating mucosal congestion of hay fever, rhinitis, and acute sinusitis; to relieve bronchial asthmatic paroxysms; in syncope due to complete heart block or carotid sinus hypersensitivity; for symptomatic relief of serum sickness, urticaria, angioneurotic edema; for resuscitation in cardiac arrest following anesthetic accidents; in simple (open angle) glaucoma; for relaxation of uterine musculature and to inhibit uterine contractions. Epinephrine Injection can be utilized to prolong the action of intraspinal and local anesthetics (see Contraindications).

Contraindications: Epinephrine is contraindicated in narrow angle (congestive) glaucoma, shock, during general anesthesia with halogenated hydrocarbons or cyclopropane and in individuals with organic brain damage. Epinephrine is also contraindicated with local anesthesia of certain areas, eg, fingers, toes, because of the danger of vasoconstriction producing sloughing of tissue; in labor because it may delay the second stage; in cardiac dilatation and coronary insufficiency.

Warnings: Administer with caution to elderly people; to those with cardiovascular disease, hypertension, diabetes or hyperthyroidism; in psychoneurotic individuals, and in pregnancy.

Patients with long-standing bronchial asthma and emphysema who have developed degenerative heart disease should be administered the drug with extreme caution.

Overdosage or inadvertent intravenous injection of epinephrine may cause cerebrovascular hemorrhage resulting from the sharp rise in blood pressure. Fatalities may also result from pulmonary edema because of the peripheral constriction and cardiac stimulation produced. Rapidly acting vasodilators such as nitrites, or alpha blocking agents may counteract the marked pressor effects of epinephrine.

Precautions:
General: Adrenalin (epinephrine injection) should be protected from exposure to light. Do not remove ampoules or syringes from carton until ready to use. The solution should not be used if it is brown in color or contains a precipitate.

Epinephrine is readily destroyed by alkalies and oxidizing agents. In the latter category are oxygen, chlorine, bromine, iodine, permanganates, chromates, nitrites and salts of easily reducible metals, especially iron.

Drug Interactions: Use of epinephrine with excessive doses of digitalis, mercurial diuretics, or other drugs that sensitize the heart to arrhythmias is not recommended. Anginal pain may be induced when coronary insufficiency is present. The effects of epinephrine may be potentiated by tricyclic antidepressants; certain antihistamines, eg, diphenhydramine, tripelennamine, d-chlorpheniramine; and sodium l-thyroxine.

Usage in Pregnancy: Pregnancy Category C. Adrenalin (epinephrine) has been shown to be teratogenic in rats when given in doses about 25 times the human dose. There are no adequate and well controlled studies in pregnant women. Adrenalin should be used during pregnancy only if the potential benefit justifies the potential risk to the fetus.

Adverse Reactions: Transient and minor side effects of anxiety, headache, fear and palpitations often occur with therapeutic doses, especially in hyperthyroid individuals. Repeated local injections can result in necrosis at sites of injection from vascular constriction. "Epinephrine-fastness" can occur with prolonged use.

Dosage and Administration: Subcutaneously or intramuscularly—0.2 to 1 ml (mg). Start with a small dose and increase if required.

Note: The subcutaneous is the preferred route of administration. If given intramuscularly, injection into the buttocks should be avoided.

For bronchial asthma and certain allergic manifestations, eg, angioedema, urticaria, serum sickness, anaphylactic shock, use epinephrine subcutaneously. For bronchial asthma in pediatric patients, administer 0.01 mg/kg or 0.3 mg/m² to a maximum of 0.5 mg subcutaneously, repeated every four hours if required.

For cardiac resuscitation—A dose of 0.5 ml (0.5 mg) diluted to 10 ml with sodium chloride injection can be administered intravenously or intracardially to restore myocardial contractility. External cardiac massage should follow intracardial administration to permit the drug to enter coronary circulation. The drug should be used secondarily to unsuccessful attempts with physical or electromechanical methods.

Ophthalmologic use (for producing conjunctival decongestion, to control hemorrhage, produce mydriasis and reduce intraocular pres- sure)—use a concentration of 1:10,000 (0.1 mg/ml) to 1:1,000 (1 mg/ml).

Intraspinal use (Amp 88)—Usual dose is 0.2 to 0.4 ml (0.2 to 0.4 mg) added to anesthetic spinal fluid mixture (may prolong anesthetic action by limiting absorption). For use with local anesthetic—Epinephrine 1:100,000 (0.01 mg /ml) to 1:20,000 (0.05 mg/ml) is the usual concentration employed with local anesthetics.

How Supplied:
N 0071-4188-03 (Amp 88) Sterile solution containing 1 mg Adrenalin (epinephrine) as the hydrochloride in each 1-ml ampoule (1:1000). For intramuscular or subcutaneous use. When diluted, it may also be administered intracardially, intravenously, or intraspinally. Supplied in packages of ten.

N 0071-4011-13 (S.V. 11) Sterile solution containing 1 mg Adrenalin (epinephrine) as the hydrochloride (1:1000). For intramuscular or subcutaneous use. When diluted, it may also be administered intracardially or intravenously. Supplied in a 30 ml Steri-Vial® (rubber-diaphragm-capped vial.)

4188G040

AGORAL® PLAIN
[ă'gō-răl"]
AGORAL® RASPBERRY
AGORAL® MARSHMALLOW

Description: Each tablespoonful (15 ml) of Agoral Plain (white) contains 4.2 grams mineral oil in a thoroughly homogenized emulsion with agar, tragacanth, acacia, egg albumin, glycerin and water.

Each tablespoonful (15 ml) of Agoral Raspberry (pink) or of Agoral Marshmallow (white) contains 4.2 grams mineral oil and 0.2 gram phenolphthalein in a thoroughly homogenized emulsion with agar, tragacanth, acacia, egg albumin, glycerin and water.

Actions: Agoral, containing mineral oil, facilitates defecation by lubricating the fecal mass and softening the stool. More effective than nonemulsified oil in penetrating the feces, Agoral thereby greatly reduces the possibility of oil leakage at the anal sphincter. Phenolphthalein gently stimulates motor activity of the lower intestinal tract. Agoral's combined lubricating-softening and peristaltic actions can help to restore a normal pattern of evacuation.

Indications: Relief of constipation. Agoral may be especially required when straining at stool is a hazard, as in hernia, cardiac, or hypertensive patients; during convalescence from surgery; before and after surgery for hemorrhoids or other painful anorectal disorders; for obstetrical patients; for patients confined to bed.

The management of chronic constipation should also include attention to fluid intake, diet and bowel habits.

Contraindications: Sensitivity to phenolphthalein.

Dosage and Management:
(Taken at bedtime, laxation may be expected the next morning.)

	Adults	Children over 6 years
Agoral Plain (without phenolphthalein)	1 to 2 tablespoonfuls	2 to 4 teaspoonfuls
Agoral Raspberry	½ to 1 tablespoonful	1 to 2 teaspoonfuls
Agoral Marshmallow	½ to 1 tablespoonful	1 to 2 teaspoonfuls

Take at bedtime only, unless other time is advised by physician.

Agoral may be taken alone or in milk, water, fruit juice, or any miscible food.

Expectant or nursing mothers, bedridden or aged patients, young children or infants should use only on advice of physician.

Supplied: Agoral Plain (without phenolphthalein), plastic bottles of 16 fl oz (N 0071-2071-23). Agoral (raspberry flavor), plastic bottles of 16 fl oz (N 0071-2072-23). Agoral (marshmallow flavor), plastic bottles of 8 fl oz (N 0071-2070-20) and 16 fl oz (N 0071-2070-23).

AMCILL® ℞
[ăm'cĭll"]
(ampicillin, USP) as the trihydrate
Ampicillin Capsules, USP—250 mg and 500 mg
Ampicillin for Oral Suspension, USP 125 mg/5 ml and 250 mg/5 ml

Description: Ampicillin is a semisynthetic penicillin derived from the basic penicillin nucleus, 6-aminopenicillanic acid.

Actions: Microbiology: *In vitro* studies have shown sensitivity of the following microorganisms to ampicillin:

Gram Positive: Alpha- and beta-hemolytic streptococci, *Diplococcus pneumoniae*, staphylococci (non-penicillinase-producing), *Bacillus anthracis*,

Clostridia spp, *Corynebacterium xerose*, and most strains of enterococci.

The drug does not resist destruction by penicillinase, hence is not effective against penicillin G-resistant staphylococci.

Gram Negative: *Haemophilus influenzae, Neisseria gonorrhoeae, N meningitidis, Proteus mirabilis,* and many strains of *Salmonella* (including *S typhosa), Shigella* spp, and *Escherichia coli*.

Testing for Susceptibility: The invading organism should be cultured and its sensitivity demonstrated as a guide to therapy. If the Kirby-Bauer method of disc sensitivity is used, a 10-mcg ampicillin disc should be used to determine the relative *in vitro* susceptibility.

Human Pharmacology: Ampicillin is stable in the presence of gastric acid and is well-absorbed from the gastrointestinal tract. It diffuses readily into most body tissues and fluids. However, penetration into the cerebrospinal fluid and brain occurs only with meningeal inflammation. Ampicillin is excreted largely unchanged in the urine. Its excretion can be delayed by concurrent administration of probenecid. Ampicillin is the least serum bound of all the penicillins, averaging 20% compared to 60% to 90% for other penicillins. Average peak blood serum levels of approximately 3 mcg/ml are attained in approximately two hours following a 500-mg dose of ampicillin in the capsule form. A dose of 250 mg ampicillin, as the oral suspension, produces average blood serum levels of approximately 2 mcg/ml within one and one-half hours.

Indications: Ampicillin is indicated primarily in the treatment of infections caused by susceptible strains of the following microorganisms: *Shigella, Salmonella* (including *S typhosa), E coli, H influenzae, P mirabilis,* and *N gonorrhoeae*. Ampicillin may also be indicated in certain infections caused by susceptible gram positive organisms: penicillin G-sensitive staphylococci, streptococci, pneumococci, and enterococci.

Bacteriology studies to determine the causative organisms and their sensitivity to ampicillin should be performed. Therapy may be instituted prior to the results of sensitivity testing.

Contraindication: Ampicillin is contraindicated in patients with a history of a hypersensitivity reaction to the penicillins.

Warning: Serious and occasionally fatal hypersensitivity (anaphylactic) reactions have been reported in patients on penicillin therapy. Although anaphylaxis is more frequent following parenteral therapy, it has occurred in patients on oral penicillins. These reactions are more apt to occur in individuals with a history of sensitivity to multiple allergens.

There have been reports of individuals with a history of penicillin hypersensitivity who experienced severe reactions when treated with cephalosporins. Before therapy with any penicillin, careful inquiry should be made concerning previous hypersensitivity reactions to penicillins, cephalosporins, or other allergens. Serious anaphylactoid reactions require immediate emergency treatment with epinephrine. Oxygen, intravenous steroids, and airway management, including intubation, should also be administered as indicated.

Usage in Pregnancy: Safety for use in pregnancy has not been established.

Precautions: As with any potent drug, periodic assessment of renal, hepatic, and hematopoietic functions should be made during prolonged therapy.

The possibility of superinfections with mycotic or bacterial pathogens should be kept in mind during therapy. If superinfections occur, appropriate therapy should be instituted.

Adverse Reactions: As with other penicillins, it may be expected that untoward reactions will be essentially related to sensitivity phenomena. They are more likely to occur in individuals who have previously demonstrated hypersensitivity to penicillins and in those with a history of allergy, asthma, hay fever, or urticaria.

The following adverse reactions have been reported as associated with the use of ampicillin.

Gastrointestinal—Glossitis, stomatitis, black "hairy" tongue, nausea, vomiting, enterocolitis, pseudomembranous colitis, and diarrhea have been reported. (These reactions are usually associated with oral dosage forms.)

Hypersensitivity Reactions—Erythematous maculopapular rashes have been reported fairly frequently. Urticaria, erythema multiforme, and an occasional case of exfoliative dermatitis have been reported. Anaphylaxis is the most serious reaction experienced and has usually been associated with the parenteral dosage form.

NOTE: Urticaria, other skin rashes, and serum sickness-like reactions may be controlled with antihistamines and, if necessary, systemic corticosteroids. Whenever such reactions occur, ampicillin should be discontinued unless, in the opinion of the physician, the condition being treated is life-threatening and amenable only to ampicillin therapy. Serious anaphylactic reactions require the immediate use of epinephrine, oxygen, and intravenous steroids.

Liver—A moderate rise in serum glutamic oxaloacetic transaminase (SGOT) has been noted, particularly in infants, but the significance of this finding is unknown.

Hemic and Lymphatic Systems—Anemia, thrombocytopenia, thrombocytopenic purpura, eosinophilia, leukopenia, and agranulocytosis have been reported during therapy with the penicillins. These reactions are usually reversible on discontinuation of therapy and are believed to be hypersensitivity phenomena.

Other—Since infectious mononucleosis is viral in origin, ampicillin should not be used in the treatment. A high percentage of patients with mononucleosis who received ampicillin developed a skin rash.

Dosage and Administration:

Infections of the respiratory tract and soft tissues

Patients weighing 20 kg (44 lb) or more: 250 mg every six hours

Patients weighing less than 20 kg (44 lb): 50 mg/kg/day in equally divided doses at 6- or 8-hour intervals

Infections of the gastrointestinal and genitourinary tracts

Patients weighing 20 kg (44 lb) or more: 500 mg every six hours

Patients weighing less than 20 kg (44 lb): 100 mg/kg/day in equally divided doses at 6- or 8-hour intervals

In the treatment of chronic urinary tract and intestinal infections, frequent bacteriologic and clinical appraisal is necessary. Smaller doses than those recommended above should not be used. Higher doses should be used for stubborn or severe infections. In stubborn infections, therapy may be required for several weeks. It may be necessary to continue clinical and/or bacteriologic follow-up for several months after cessation of therapy.

Urethritis in males or females due to *N gonorrhoeae*:

3.5 grams with 1 gram probenecid, administered simultaneously.

In the treatment of complications of gonorrheal urethritis, such as prostatitis and epididymitis, prolonged and intensive therapy is recommended. Cases of gonorrhea with a suspected primary lesion of syphilis should have darkfield examinations before receiving treatment. In all other cases where concomitant syphilis is suspected, monthly serologic tests should be made for a minimum of four months.

Treatment of all infections should be continued for a minimum of 48 to 72 hours beyond the time that the patient becomes asymptomatic or evidence of bacterial eradication has been obtained. A minimum of ten days treatment is recommended for any infection caused by Group A beta-hemolytic streptococci to help prevent the occurrence of acute rheumatic fever or acute glomerulonephritis.

Directions For Dispensing Oral Suspensions

Prepare suspension at time of dispensing. For ease in preparation, add water to the bottle in two portions, and shake well after each addition.

125 MG/5 ML

Add a total of 88 ml to the 100-ml package and 173 ml to the 200-ml package. This will provide 100 and 200 ml of suspension. Each 5 ml (teaspoonful) will contain ampicillin trihydrate equivalent to 125 mg ampicillin. The reconstituted suspension is stable for 14 days under refrigeration.

250 MG/5 ML

Add a total of 70 ml to the 100-ml package and 140 ml to the 200-ml package. This will provide 100 and 200 ml of suspension. Each 5 ml (teaspoonful) will contain ampicillin trihydrate equivalent to 250 mg ampicillin. The reconstituted suspension is stable for 14 days under refrigeration.

How Supplied:

N 0071-0402 (Capsule 402)—Amcill Capsules, 250 mg. Each capsule contains ampicillin trihydrate equivalent to 250 mg ampicillin. Bottles of 100 and 500, and unit-dose packages of 100 (10 strips of 10 capsules each).

N 0071-0404 (Capsule 404)—Amcill Capsules, 500 mg. Each capsule contains ampicillin trihydrate equivalent to 500 mg ampicillin. Bottles of 100 and 500, and unit-dose packages of 100 (10 strips of 10 capsules each).

Shown in Product Identification Section, page 423

N 0071-2301—Amcill for Oral Suspension 125 mg/5 ml. Each 5 ml of reconstituted suspension contains ampicillin trihydrate equivalent to 125 mg ampicillin. Available in 100-ml and 200-ml individual bottles and packs of six.

N 0071-2302—Amcill for Oral Suspension 250 mg/5 ml. Each 5 ml of reconstituted suspension contains ampicillin trihydrate equivalent to 250 mg ampicillin. Available in 100-ml and 200-ml individual bottles and packs of six.

AHFS 8:12.16   7000G092

Amcill products are manufactured by John D. Copanos Inc., Baltimore, MD 21225 and distributed by Parke-Davis, Morris Plains, NJ 07950.

AMITRIPTYLINE HYDROCHLORIDE   ℞

[ă"mĭ-trĭp'ty-līne]

Tablets USP

(Amitril®)

Description: Amitriptyline HCl, a dibenzocycloheptadiene derivative, is a white, crystalline compound that is readily soluble in water.

It is designated chemically as 5-(3-dimethylaminopropylidene)-dibenzo [a,d] [1,4] cycloheptadiene hydrochloride. The molecular weight is 313.87. The empirical formula is $C_{20}H_{23}N \cdot HCl$.

Clinical Pharmacology: Amitriptyline HCl is an antidepressant with sedative effects. Its mechanism of action in man is not known. It is not a monoamine oxidase inhibitor and it does not act primarily by stimulation of the central nervous system.

Amitriptyline inhibits the membrane pump mechanism responsible for reuptake of norepinephrine and serotonin into adrenergic and serotonergic neurons. Pharmacologically this action may potentiate or prolong neuronal activity since reuptake of these biogenic amines is important physiologically in terminating its transmitting activity. This interference with reuptake of norepinephrine and/or serotonin is believed by some to underlie the antidepressant activity of amitriptyline.

Indications and Usage: For the relief of symptoms of depression. Endogenous depression is more likely to be alleviated than are other depressive states.

Contraindications: Amitriptyline HCl is contraindicated in patients who have shown prior hypersensitivity to it. It should not be given concomitantly with a monoamine oxidase inhibitor. Hyperpyretic crises, severe convulsions, and deaths have occurred in patients receiving tricyclic antidepressant and monoamine oxidase inhibiting drugs simultaneously. When it is desired to replace a monoamine oxidase inhibitor with ami-

Continued on next page

This product information was prepared in August, 1984. On these and other Parke-Davis Products, information may be obtained by addressing PARKE-DAVIS, Division of Warner-Lambert Company, Morris Plains, New Jersey 07950.

Parke-Davis—Cont.

triptyline, a minimum of 14 days should be allowed to elapse after the former is discontinued. Amitriptyline HCl should then be initiated cautiously with gradual increase in dosage until optimum response is achieved.

This drug is not recommended for use during the acute recovery phase following myocardial infarction.

Warnings: Amitriptyline HCl may block the antihypertensive action of guanethidine or similarly acting compounds.

It should be used with caution in patients with a history of seizures and because of its atropine-like action, in patients with a history of urinary retention, angle-closure glaucoma, or increased intraocular pressure. In patients with angle-closure glaucoma, even average doses may precipitate an attack.

Patients with cardiovascular disorders should be watched closely. Tricyclic antidepressant drugs, including amitriptyline, particularly when given in high doses, have been reported to produce arrhythmias, sinus tachycardia, and prolongation of the conduction time. Myocardial infarction and stroke have been reported with drugs of this class. Close supervision is required when amitriptyline is given to hyperthyroid patients or those receiving thyroid medication.

This drug may impair mental and/or physical abilities required for performance of hazardous tasks, such as operating machinery or driving a motor vehicle.

Amitriptyline may enhance the response to alcohol and the effects of barbiturates and other CNS depressants. In patients who may use alcohol excessively, it should be borne in mind that the potentiation may increase the danger inherent in any suicide attempt or overdosage.

Usage in Pregnancy—Safe use of amitriptyline during pregnancy and lactation has not been established; therefore, in administering the drug to pregnant patients, nursing mothers, or women who may become pregnant, the possible benefits must be weighed against the possible hazards to mother and child.

Animal reproduction studies have been inconclusive and clinical experience has been limited.

Usage in Children—In view of the lack of experience in children, the drug is not recommended at the present time for patients under 12 years of age.

Precautions: Schizophrenic patients may develop increased symptoms of psychosis; patients with paranoid symptomatology may have an exaggeration of such symptoms; manic depressive patients may experience a shift to the manic phase. In these circumstances the dose of amitriptyline may be reduced or a major tranquilizer such as perphenazine may be administered concurrently. When this drug is given with anticholinergic agents or sympathomimetic drugs, including epinephrine combined with local anesthetics, close supervision and careful adjustment of dosages are required.

Paralytic ileus may occur in patients taking tricyclic antidepressants in combination with anticholinergic-type drugs.

Caution is advised if patients receive large doses of ethclorvynol concurrently. Transient delirium has been reported in patients who were treated with one gram of ethchlorvynol and 75 to 150 mg of amitriptyline.

The possibility of suicide in depressed patients remains until significant remission occurs. Potentially suicidal patients should not have access to large quantities of this drug. Prescriptions should be written for the smallest amount feasible.

Concurrent administration of amitriptyline and electroshock therapy may increase the hazards associated with such therapy. Such treatment should be limited to patients for whom it is essential.

Discontinue the drug several days before elective surgery if possible.

Both elevation and lowering of blood sugar levels have been reported.

Amitriptyline should be used with caution in patients with impaired liver function.

Adverse Reactions:

Note: Included in the listing which follows are a few adverse reactions which have not been reported with this specific drug. However, pharmacological similarities among the tricyclic antidepressant drugs require that each of the reactions be considered when amitriptyline is administered.

Cardiovascular: Hypotension, hypertension, tachycardia, palpitation, myocardial infarction, arrhythmias, heart block, stroke.

CNS and Neuromuscular: Confusional states, disturbed concentration; disorientation; delusions; hallucinations; excitement; anxiety; restlessness; insomnia; nightmares; numbness, tingling, and paresthesias of the extremities; peripheral neuropathy; incoordination; ataxia; tremors; seizures; alteration in EEG patterns; extrapyramidal symptoms; tinnitus; syndrome of inappropriate ADH (antidiuretic hormone) secretion.

Anticholinergic: Dry mouth, blurred vision, disturbance of accommodation, constipation, paralytic ileus, urinary retention, dilatation of urinary tract.

Allergic: Skin rash, urticaria, photosensitization, edema of face and tongue.

Hematologic: Bone marrow depression including agranulocytosis, leukopenia, eosinophilia, purpura, thrombocytopenia.

Gastrointestinal: Nausea, epigastric distress, vomiting, anorexia, stomatitis, peculiar taste, diarrhea, parotid swelling, black tongue. Rarely hepatitis (including altered liver function and jaundice).

Endocrine: Testicular swelling and gynecomastia in the male, breast enlargement and galactorrhea in the female, increased or decreased libido, elevation and lowering of blood sugar levels.

Other: Dizziness, weakness, fatigue, headache, weight gain or loss, increased perspiration, urinary frequency, mydriasis, drowsiness, alopecia.

Withdrawal Symptoms: Abrupt cessation of treatment after prolonged administration may produce nausea, headache, and malaise. These are not indicative of addiction.

Overdosage:

Manifestations—High doses may cause temporary confusion, disturbed concentration, or transient visual hallucinations. Overdosage may cause drowsiness; hypothermia; tachycardia and other arrhythmic abnormalities, such as bundle branch block; ECG evidence of impaired conduction; congestive heart failure; dilated pupils; convulsions; severe hypotension; stupor; and coma. Other symptoms may be agitation, hyperactive reflexes, muscle rigidity, vomiting, hyperpyrexia, or any of those listed under ADVERSE REACTIONS.

All patients suspected of having taken an overdosage should be admitted to a hospital as soon as possible.

Treatment is symptomatic and supportive. Empty the stomach as quickly as possible by emesis followed by gastric lavage upon arrival at the hospital. Following gastric lavage, activated charcoal may be administered. Twenty to 30 g of activated charcoal may be given every four to six hours during the first 24 to 48 hours after ingestion. An ECG should be taken and close monitoring of cardiac function instituted if there is any sign of abnormality. Maintain an open airway and adequate fluid intake; regulate body temperature.

The intravenous administration of 1–3 mg of physostigmine salicylate has been reported to reverse the symptoms of tricyclic antidepressant poisoning. Because physostigmine is rapidly metabolized, the dosage of physostigmine should be repeated as required particularly if life threatening signs such as arrhythmias, convulsions, and deep coma recur or persist after the initial dosage of physostigmine. Because physostigmine itself may be toxic, it is not recommended for routine use.

Standard measures should be used to manage circulatory shock and metabolic acidosis. Cardiac arrhythmias may be treated with neostigmine, pyridostigmine, or propranolol. Should cardiac failure occur, the use of digitalis should be considered. Close monitoring of cardiac function for not less than five days is advisable.

Anticonvulsants may be given to control convulsions. Amitriptyline increases the CNS depressant action, but not the anticonvulsant action of barbiturates; therefore, an inhalation anesthetic, diazepam, or paraldehyde is recommended for control of convulsions.

Dialysis is of no value because of low plasma concentrations of the drug.

Since overdosage is often deliberate, patients may attempt suicide by other means during the recovery phase.

Deaths by deliberate or accidental overdosage have occurred with this class of drugs.

Dosage and Administration:

Oral Dosage—Dosage should be initiated at a low level and increased gradually, noting carefully the clinical response and any evidence of intolerance.

Initial Dosage for Adults—Twenty-five mg three times a day usually is satisfactory for outpatients. If necessary this may be increased to a total of 150 mg a day. Increases are made preferably in the late afternoon and/or bedtime doses. A sedative effect may be apparent before the antidepressant effect is noted, but an adequate therapeutic effect may take as long as 30 days to develop.

An alternative method of initiating therapy in outpatients is to begin with 50 to 100 mg amitriptyline HCl at bedtime. This may be increased by 25 to 50 mg as necessary in the bedtime dose to a total of 150 mg per day.

Hospitalized patients may require 100 mg a day initially. This can be increased gradually to 200 mg a day if necessary. A small number of hospitalized patients may need as much as 300 mg a day.

Adolescent and Elderly Patients—In general, lower dosages are recommended for these patients. Ten mg three times a day with 20 mg at bedtime may be satisfactory in adolescent and elderly patients who do not tolerate higher dosages.

Maintenance—The usual maintenance dose is 25 mg two to four times a day. In some patients 10 mg four times a day is sufficient. When satisfactory improvement has been reached, dosage should be reduced to the lowest amount that will maintain relief of symptoms. It is appropriate to continue maintenance therapy three months or longer to lessen the possibility of relapse.

Usage in Children—In view of the lack of experience in children, this drug is not recommended at the present time for patients under 12 years of age.

How Supplied: Amitriptyline HCl tablets are supplied as film-coated tablets as follows:

N 0071-0272   10 mg (tan, P-D 272), in bottles of 100 and unit-dose packages of 100 (10 strips of 10 tablets each).

N 0071-0273   25 mg (coral, P-D 273), in bottles of 100 and 1000 and unit-dose packages of 100 (10 strips of 10 tablets each).

N 0071-0274   50 mg (blue/purple, P-D 274), in bottles of 100 and 1000 and unit-dose packages of 100 (10 strips of 10 tablets each).

N 0071-0275   75 mg (green, P-D 275), in bottles of 100.

N 0071-0271   100 mg (brown/mustard, P-D 271), in bottles of 100 and unit-dose packages of 100 (10 strips of 10 tablets each).

N 0071-0278   150 mg (orange, P-D 278), in bottles of 100.

Store at controlled room temperature between 15°–30°C (59°–86°F).

6000G033

Shown in Product Identification Section, p. 423

AMOXICILLIN   R
[ă-mŏx'ă-cĭll″ĭn]
(Utimox®)
Amoxicillin Capsules, USP—250 and 500 mg
Amoxicillin for Oral Suspension, USP—125 mg/5 ml and 250 mg/5 ml

Description: Amoxicillin is a semisynthetic penicillin, an analogue of ampicillin, with a broad spectrum of bactericidal activity against many gram-positive and gram-negative microorganisms.

for possible revisions   **Product Information**

Chemically, it is D-(-)-α-amino-*p*-hydroxybenzyl penicillin trihydrate.

Actions:
Pharmacology
Amoxicillin is stable in the presence of gastric acid and may be given with no regard for food. It is rapidly absorbed after oral administration. It diffuses readily into most body tissues and fluids, with the exception of brain and spinal fluid, except when meninges are inflamed. The half-life of amoxicillin is 1 hour. Most of the amoxicillin is excreted unchanged in the urine; its excretion can be delayed by concurrent administration of probenecid. Amoxicillin is not highly protein-bound. In blood serum, amoxicillin is approximately 20% protein-bound as compared to 60% for penicillin G.

Orally administered doses of 250 mg and 500 mg amoxicillin capsules result in average peak blood levels, one to two hours after administration, in the range of 3.5 mcg/ml to 5.0 mcg/ml, and 5.5 mcg/ml to 7.5 mcg/ml, respectively.

Orally administered doses of amoxicillin suspension 125 mg/5 ml and 250 mg/5 ml result in average peak blood levels, one to two hours after administration, in the range of 1.5 mcg/ml to 3.0 mcg/ml, and 3.5 mcg/ml to 5.0 mcg/ml, respectively.

Detectable serum levels are observed up to 8 hours after an orally administered dose of amoxicillin. Approximately 60% of an orally administered dose of amoxicillin is excreted in the urine within six to eight hours.

Microbiology
Amoxicillin is similar to ampicillin in its bactericidal action against susceptible organisms during the stage of active multiplication. It acts through the inhibition of biosynthesis of cell wall mucopeptide. *In vitro* studies have demonstrated the susceptibility of most strains of the following gram-positive bacteria: alpha- and beta-hemolytic streptococci, *Diplococcus pneumoniae*, nonpenicillinase-producing staphylococci, and *Streptococcus faecalis*. Amoxicillin is active *in vitro* against many strains of *Haemophilus influenzae*, *Neisseria gonorrhoeae*, *Escherichia coli*, and *Proteus mirabilis*. Because it does not resist destruction by penicillinase, the drug is not effective against penicillinase-producing bacteria, particularly resistant staphylococci. All strains of *Pseudomonas* and most strains of *Klebsiella* and *Enterobacter* are resistant.

Disc Susceptibility Tests
Quantitative methods that require measurement of zone diameters give the most precise estimates of antibiotic susceptibility. One such procedure* has been recommended for use with discs for testing susceptibility to ampicillin class antibiotics. Interpretations correlate diameters of the disc test with MIC values for amoxicillin. With this procedure, a report from the laboratory of "susceptible" indicates that the infecting organism is likely to respond to therapy. A report of "resistant" indicates that the infecting organism is not likely to respond to therapy. A report of "intermediate susceptibility" suggests that the organism would be susceptible if high dosage is used, or if the infection is confined to tissues and fluids (eg, urine), in which high antibiotic levels are attained.

Indications: Amoxicillin is indicated in the treatment of infections due to susceptible strains of the following.

Gram-negative organisms—*H influenzae, E coli, P mirabilis,* and *N gonorrhoeae*

Gram-positive organisms—Streptococci (including *Str faecalis*), *D pneumoniae*, and nonpenicillinase-producing staphylococci

Therapy may be instituted prior to obtaining results from bacteriological and susceptibility studies to determine the causative organisms and their susceptibility to amoxicillin.

Indicated surgical procedures should be performed.

Contraindication: The use of this drug is contraindicated in individuals with a history of an allergic reaction to the penicillins.

Warnings: SERIOUS AND OCCASIONALLY FATAL HYPERSENSITIVITY (ANAPHYLACTOID) REACTIONS HAVE BEEN REPORTED IN PATIENTS ON PENICILLIN THERAPY. ALTHOUGH ANAPHYLAXIS IS MORE FREQUENT FOLLOWING PARENTERAL THERAPY, IT HAS OCCURRED IN PATIENTS ON ORAL PENICILLINS. THESE REACTIONS ARE MORE APT TO OCCUR IN INDIVIDUALS WITH A HISTORY OF SENSITIVITY TO MULTIPLE ALLERGENS.

THERE HAVE BEEN REPORTS OF INDIVIDUALS WITH A HISTORY OF PENICILLIN HYPERSENSITIVITY WHO HAVE EXPERIENCED SEVERE REACTIONS WHEN TREATED WITH CEPHALOSPORINS. BEFORE THERAPY WITH ANY PENICILLIN, CAREFUL INQUIRY SHOULD BE MADE CONCERNING PREVIOUS HYPERSENSITIVITY REACTIONS TO PENICILLINS, CEPHALOSPORINS, AND OTHER ALLERGENS. IF AN ALLERGIC REACTION OCCURS, APPROPRIATE THERAPY SHOULD BE INSTITUTED AND DISCONTINUANCE OF AMOXICILLIN THERAPY CONSIDERED. SERIOUS ANAPHYLACTOID REACTIONS REQUIRE IMMEDIATE EMERGENCY TREATMENT WITH EPINEPHRINE. OXYGEN, INTRAVENOUS STEROIDS, AND AIRWAY MANAGEMENT, INCLUDING INTUBATION, SHOULD ALSO BE ADMINISTERED AS INDICATED.

Usage in Pregnancy—Safety for use in pregnancy has not been established.

Precautions: As with any potent drug, periodic assessment of renal, hepatic, and hematopoietic functions should be made during prolonged therapy.

The possibility of superinfections with mycotic or bacterial pathogens should be kept in mind during therapy. If superinfections occur (usually involving *Enterobacter, Pseudomonas,* or *Candida)*, the drug should be discontinued and/or appropriate therapy instituted.

Adverse Reactions: As with other penicillins, it may be expected that untoward reactions will be essentially limited to sensitivity phenomena. They are more likely to occur in individuals who have previously demonstrated hypersensitivity to penicillins and in those with a history of allergy, asthma, hay fever, or urticaria.

The following adverse reactions have been reported as associated with the use of penicillins.

Gastrointestinal—Nausea, vomiting, and diarrhea

Hypersensitivity Reactions—Erythematous maculopapular rashes and urticaria have been reported.

Note—Urticaria, other skin rashes, and serum sickness-like reactions may be controlled with antihistamines and, if necessary, systemic corticosteroids. Whenever such reactions occur, amoxicillin should be discontinued unless, in the opinion of the physician, the condition being treated is life-threatening and amenable only to amoxicillin therapy.

Liver—A moderate rise in serum glutamic oxaloacetic transaminase (SGOT) has been noted, but the significance of this finding is unknown.

Hemic and Lymphatic Systems—Anemia, thrombocytopenia, thrombocytopenic purpura, eosinophilia, leukopenia, and agranulocytosis have been reported during therapy with the penicillins. These reactions are usually reversible on discontinuation of therapy and are believed to be hypersensitivity phenomena.

Dosage and Administration: Infections of the ear, nose, and throat due to streptococci, pneumococci, nonpenicillinase-producing staphylococci, and *H influenzae*:

Infections of the genitourinary tract due to *E coli, P mirabilis,* and *Str faecalis:*

Infections of the skin and soft tissues due to streptococci, susceptible staphylococci, and *E coli:*

Usual Dosage:
Adults: 250 mg every 8 hours
Children: 20 mg/kg/day in divided doses every 8 hours.

Children weighing 20 kg or more should be dosed according to the adult recommendations.

In severe infections or those caused by less susceptible organisms: 500 mg every 8 hours for adults, and 40 mg/kg/day in divided doses every 8 hours for children may be needed.

Infections of the lower respiratory tract due to streptococci, pneumococci, nonpenicillinase-producing staphylococci, and *H influenzae*:

Usual Dosage:
Adults: 500 mg every 8 hours
Children: 40/kg/day in divided doses every 8 hours

Children weighing 20 kg or more should be dosed according to the adult recommendations.

Gonorrhea, acute, uncomplicated anogenital and urethral infections due to *N gonorrhoeae:* (males and females) 3 grams as a single dose.

Cases of gonorrhea with a suspected lesion of syphilis should have darkfield examinations before receiving amoxicillin and monthly serological tests for a minimum of four months.

Larger doses may be required for stubborn or severe infections.

The children's dosage is intended for individuals whose weight will not cause a dosage to be calculated greater than that recommended for adults. It should be recognized that in the treatment of chronic urinary tract infections, frequent bacteriological and clinical appraisals are necessary. Smaller doses than those recommended above should not be used. Even higher doses may be needed at times. In stubborn infections, therapy may be required for several weeks. It may be necessary to continue clinical and/or bacteriological follow-up for several months after cessation of therapy. Except for gonorrhea, treatment should be continued for a minimum of 48 to 72 hours beyond the time that the patient becomes asymptomatic or evidence of bacterial eradication has been obtained.

It is recommended that there be at least 10 days' treatment for any infection caused by hemolytic streptococci to prevent the occurrence of acute rheumatic fever or glomerulonephritis.

After reconstitution, the required amount of suspension should be placed directly on the child's tongue for swallowing. Alternate means of administration are to add the required amount of suspension to formula, milk, fruit juice, water, ginger ale, or cold drinks. These preparations should then be taken immediately. To be certain the child is receiving full dosage, such preparations should be consumed in entirety.

Directions for Preparing Oral Suspension: Prepare suspension at the time of dispensing. Shake bottle to loosen powder or break up the cake that may have formed. For ease of preparation, add water to the bottle in two portions and shake well after each addition. Each teaspoonful (5 ml) will contain 125 mg or 250 mg amoxicillin.

Product	Bottle Size	Amount of Water Required for Reconstitution
125 mg/5 ml	80 ml	70 ml
	100 ml	87 ml
	150 ml	130 ml
	200 ml	170 ml
250 mg/5 ml	80 ml	56 ml
	100 ml	70 ml
	150 ml	105 ml
	200 ml	140 ml

NOTE: SHAKE THE ORAL SUSPENSION WELL BEFORE USING.

Keep bottle tightly closed. The reconstituted suspension is stable for 14 days. Refrigeration is preferable but not required.

How Supplied:
Amoxicillin Capsules are supplied as:
N 0071-0730-24   250 mg—Bottles of 100
N 0071-0730-30   250 mg—Bottles of 500
N 0071-0730-40   250 mg—Unit dose packages of 100 (10 strips of 10)

Continued on next page

This product information was prepared in August, 1984. On these and other Parke-Davis Products, information may be obtained by addressing PARKE-DAVIS, Division of Warner-Lambert Company, Morris Plains, New Jersey 07950.

Parke-Davis—Cont.

Each capsule contains amoxicillin trihydrate equivalent to 250 mg amoxicillin.
N 0071-0731-24 500 mg—Bottles of 100
N 0071-0731-40 500 mg—Unit dose packages of 100 (10 strips of 10)
Each capsule contains amoxicillin trihydrate equivalent to 500 mg amoxicillin.
Shown in Product Identification Section, page 423
Amoxicillin for Oral Suspension is supplied as:
N 0071-2500-16 125 mg/5 ml—80 ml individual bottles and packs of six.
N 0071-2500-17 125 mg/5 ml—100 ml individual bottles and packs of six.
N 0071-2500-18 125 mg/5 ml—150 ml individual bottles and packs of six.
N 0071-2500-20 125 mg/5 ml—200 ml individual bottles and packs of six.
When reconstituted according to directions, each 5 ml of reconstituted suspension contains amoxicillin trihydrate equivalent to 125 mg amoxicillin.
N 0071-2501-16 250 mg/5 ml—80 ml individual bottles and packs of six.
N 0071-2501-17 250 mg/5 ml—100 ml individual bottles and packs of six.
N 0071-2501-18 250 mg/5 ml—150 ml individual bottles and packs of six.
N 0071-2501-20 250 mg/5 ml—200 ml individual bottles and packs of six.
When reconstituted according to directions, each 5 ml of reconstituted suspension contains amoxicillin trihydrate equivalent to 250 mg amoxicillin.

* Bauer, A.W., Kirby, W.M.M., Sherris, J.C., and Turck, M.: Antibiotic Testing by a Standardized Single Disc Method, *Am. J. Clin. Pathol.*, 45:493, 1966; Standardized Disc Susceptibility Test, *FEDERAL REGISTER* 37:20527-29, 1972.
Manufactured by John D. Copanos Inc., Baltimore, MD 21225 and distributed by Parke-Davis, Morris Plains, NJ 07950.
AHFS: 8:12.16   7000G084

ANUSOL® Suppositories/Ointment
[ăn′ ū-sōl″]
Description:

	Anusol Suppositories each contains	Anusol Ointment each gram
Bismuth subgallate	2.25%	—
Bismuth Resorcin Compound	1.75%	—
Benzyl Benzoate	1.2 %	12 mg
Peruvian Balsam	1.8 %	18 mg
Zinc Oxide	11.0 %	110 mg
Analgine® (pramoxine hydrochloride)	—	10 mg

Also contains the following inactive ingredients: dibasic calcium phosphate and certified coloring in a hydrogenated vegetable oil base.

Also contains the following inactive ingredients: dibasic calcium phosphate and kaolin in a liquid petrolatum-cocoa butter-polyethylene wax base containing glyceryl monooleate and glyceryl stearate.

Actions: Anusol Suppositories and Anusol Ointment help to relieve pain, itching and discomfort arising from irritated anorectal tissues. They have a soothing, lubricant action on mucous membranes.
Analgine (pramoxine hydrochloride) in Anusol Ointment is a rapidly acting local anesthetic for the skin and mucous membranes of the anus and rectum. Analgine is also chemically distinct from procaine, cocaine, and dibucaine and can often be used in the patient previously sensitized to other surface anesthetics. Surface analgesia lasts for several hours.

Indications: Anusol Suppositories and Anusol Ointment are adjunctive therapy for the symptomatic relief of pain and discomfort in: external and internal hemorrhoids, proctitis, papillitis, cryptitis, anal fissures, incomplete fistulas, and relief of local pain and discomfort following anorectal surgery.
Anusol Ointment is also indicated for pruritus ani.

Contraindications: Anusol Suppositories and Anusol Ointment are contraindicated in those patients with a history of hypersensitivity to any of the components of the preparations.

Precautions: Symptomatic relief should not delay definitive diagnoses or treatment.
If irritation develops, these preparations should be discontinued. These preparations are not for ophthalmic use.

Adverse Reactions: Upon application of Anusol Ointment which contains Analgine, a patient may occasionally experience burning, especially if the anoderm is not intact. Sensitivity reactions have been rare; discontinue medication if suspected.

Dosage and Administration: Anusol Suppositories—Adults: Remove foil wrapper and insert suppository into the anus. Insert one suppository in the morning and one at bedtime, and one immediately following each evacuation.
Anusol Ointment—Adults: After gentle bathing and drying of the anal area, remove tube cap and apply freely to the exterior surface and gently rub in. Ointment should be applied every 3 or 4 hours, or, when necessary, every 2 hours.

NOTE: If staining from either of the above products occurs, the stain may be removed from fabric by hand or machine washing with household detergent.

How Supplied: Anusol Suppositories—boxes of 12 (N 0071-1088-07), 24 (N 0071-1088-13) and 48 (N 0071-1088-18) in silver foil strips.
Shown in Product Identification Section, page 423
Anusol Ointment—one-ounce (N 0071-3075-13) and two-ounce (N 0071-3075-15) tubes with plastic applicator.
Store between 15°–30° C (59°–86° F).

ANUSOL-HC® SUPPOSITORIES ℞
[ăn′ ū-sōl″]
Hemorrhoidal Suppositories

ANUSOL-HC® CREAM ℞
Rectal Cream
with Hydrocortisone Acetate

Description:

	Anusol-HC Suppositories each contains	Anusol-HC Cream each gram
Hydrocortisone Acetate	10.0 mg	5.0 mg
Bismuth Sub-gallate	2.25%	22.5 mg
Bismuth Resorcin Compound	1.75%	17.5 mg
Benzyl Benzoate	1.2 %	12.0 mg
Peruvian Balsam	1.8 %	18.0 mg
Zinc Oxide	11.0 %	110.0 mg

Also contains the following inactive ingredients: dibasic calcium phosphate and certified coloring in a hydrogenated vegetable oil base.

Also contains the following inactive ingredients: propylene glycol, propylparaben, methylparaben, polysorbate 60 and sorbitan monostearate in a water-miscible base of mineral oil, glyceryl monostearate and water.

Actions: Anusol-HC Suppositories and Anusol-HC Cream help to relieve pain, itching and discomfort arising from irritated anorectal tissues. These preparations have a soothing, lubricant action on mucous membranes, and the antiinflammatory action of hydrocortisone acetate in Anusol-HC helps to reduce hyperemia and swelling. The hydrocortisone acetate in Anusol-HC is primarily effective because of its antiinflammatory, antipruritic and vasoconstrictive actions.

Indications: Anusol-HC Suppositories and Anusol-HC Cream are adjunctive therapy for the symptomatic relief of pain and discomfort in: external and internal hemorrhoids, proctitis, papillitis, cryptitis, anal fissures, incomplete fistulas and relief of local pain and discomfort following anorectal surgery.
Anusol-HC Cream is also indicated for pruritus ani.
Anusol-HC is especially indicated when inflammation is present. After acute symptoms subside, most patients can be maintained on regular Anusol® Suppositories or Ointment.

Contraindications: Anusol-HC Suppositories and Anusol-HC Cream are contraindicated in those patients with a history of hypersensitivity to any of the components of the preparations.

Warnings: The safe use of topical steroids during pregnancy has not been fully established. Therefore, during pregnancy, they should not be used unnecessarily on extensive areas, in large amounts, or for prolonged periods of time.

Precautions: Symptomatic relief should not delay definitive diagnoses or treatment.
If irritation develops, Anusol-HC Suppositories and Anusol-HC Cream should be discontinued and appropriate therapy instituted.
In the presence of an infection the use of an appropriate antifungal or antibacterial agent should be instituted. If a favorable response does not occur promptly, the corticosteroid should be discontinued until the infection has been adequately controlled.
Care should be taken when using the corticosteroid hydrocortisone acetate in children and infants. Anusol-HC is not for ophthalmic use.

Dosage and Administration: Anusol-HC Suppositories—Adults: Remove foil wrapper and insert suppository into the anus. Insert one suppository in the morning and one at bedtime, for 3 to 6 days or until inflammation subsides. Then maintain patient comfort with regular Anusol Suppositories.
Anusol-HC Cream—Adults: After gentle bathing and drying of the anal area, remove tube cap and apply to the exterior surface and gently rub in. For internal use, attach the plastic applicator and insert into the anus by applying gentle continuous pressure. Then squeeze the tube to deliver medication. Cream should be applied 3 or 4 times a day for 3 to 6 days until inflammation subsides. Then maintain patient comfort with regular Anusol Ointment.

NOTE: If staining from either of the above products occurs, the stain may be removed from fabric by hand or machine washing with household detergent.

How Supplied: Anusol-HC Suppositories—boxes of 12 (N 0071-1089-07) and boxes of 24 (N 0071-1089-13); in silver foil strips.
Shown in Product Identification Section, page 423
Anusol-HC Cream—one-ounce tube (N 0071-3090-13); with plastic applicator.
Store between 15°–30° C (59°–86° F).
Shown in Product Identification Section, page 423
1089 G 010

APLISOL® ℞
[ă′ plĭ-sōl″]
(tuberculin purified protein derivative, diluted
[Stabilized Solution])

For complete product information, consult Diagnostic Products Information Section.

APLITEST® ℞
[ă′ plĭ-tĕst″]
(tuberculin purified protein derivative)
Multiple-Puncture Device

For complete product information, consult Diagnostic Products Information Section.

for possible revisions

BENADRYL®
[bĕ' nă-dryl"]
(diphenhydramine hydrochloride, USP)
Kapseals®
Capsules
Elixir
Parenteral

Description: Benadryl (diphenhydramine hydrochloride) is 2-(diphenylmethoxy)-N, N-dimethylethylamine hydrochloride, and occurs as a white, crystalline powder, and is freely soluble in water and alcohol.

Actions: Diphenhydramine hydrochloride is an antihistamine with anticholinergic (drying) and sedative side effects. Antihistamines appear to compete with histamine for cell receptor sites on effector cells.

Indications: *Oral:* Benadryl in the oral form is effective for the following indications.

Antihistaminic: For perennial and seasonal (hay fever) allergic rhinitis; vasomotor rhinitis, allergic conjunctivitis due to inhalant allergens and foods; mild, uncomplicated allergic skin manifestations of urticaria and angioedema; amelioration of allergic reactions to blood or plasma, dermatographism; as therapy for anaphylactic reactions *adjunctive* to epinephrine and other standard measures after the acute manifestations have been controlled

Motion sickness: For active and prophylactic treatment of motion sickness

Antiparkinsonism: For parkinsonism (including drug-induced extrapyramidal reactions) in the elderly unable to tolerate more potent agents; mild cases of parkinsonism (including drug-induced) in other age groups; in other cases of parkinsonism (including drug-induced) in combination with centrally acting anticholinergic agents

Parenteral: Benadryl in the injectable form is effective for the following conditions when Benadryl in the oral form is impractical.

Antihistaminic: For amelioration of allergic reactions to blood or plasma; in anaphylaxis as an adjunct to epinephrine and other standard measures after the acute symptoms have been controlled; and for other uncomplicated allergic conditions of the immediate type when oral therapy is impossible or contraindicated.

Motion Sickness: For active treatment of motion sickness

Antiparkinsonism: For use in parkinsonism when oral therapy is impossible or contraindicated, as follows: parkinsonism in the elderly who are unable to tolerate more potent agents, mild cases of parkinsonism in other age groups, and in other cases of parkinsonism in combination with centrally acting anticholinergic agents.

Contraindications: *Oral and Parenteral:*

Use in Newborn or Premature Infants: This drug should *not* be used in newborn or premature infants.

Use in Nursing Mothers: Because of the higher risk of antihistamines for infants generally and for newborns and prematures in particular, antihistamine therapy is contraindicated in nursing mothers.

Use in Lower Respiratory Disease: Antihistamines *should NOT* be used to treat lower respiratory tract symptoms, including asthma.

Antihistamines are also contraindicated in the following conditions.
  Hypersensitivity to diphenhydramine hydrochloride and other antihistamines of similar chemical structure
  Monoamine oxidase inhibitor therapy (See Drug Interactions section.)

Warnings: *Oral and Parenteral:* Antihistamines should be used with considerable caution in patients with narrow-angle glaucoma, stenosing peptic ulcer, pyloroduodenal obstruction, symptomatic prostatic hypertrophy, or bladder-neck obstruction.

Use in Children: In infants and children, especially, antihistamines in *overdosage* may cause hallucinations, convulsions, or death.

Product Information

As in adults, antihistamines may diminish mental alertness in children. In the young child, particularly, they may produce excitation.

Use in Pregnancy: Experience with this drug in pregnant women is inadequate to determine whether there exists a potential for harm to the developing fetus.

Use With CNS Depressants: Diphenhydramine hydrochloride has additive effects with alcohol and other CNS depressants (hypnotics, sedatives, tranquilizers, etc).

Use in Activities Requiring Mental Alertness: Patients should be warned about engaging in activities requiring mental alertness, such as driving a car or operating appliances, machinery, etc.

Use in the Elderly (approximately 60 years or older): Antihistamines are more likely to cause dizziness, sedation, and hypotension in elderly patients.

Precautions: *Oral and Parenteral:* Diphenhydramine hydrochloride has an atropine-like action and, therefore, should be used with caution in patients with a history of bronchial asthma, increased intraocular pressure, hyperthyroidism, cardiovascular disease, or hypertension.

Drug Interactions: *Oral and Parenteral:* MAO inhibitors prolong and intensify the anticholinergic (drying) effects of antihistamines.

Adverse Reactions: *Oral and Parenteral:* The most frequent adverse reactions are underscored.
1. *General:* Urticaria, drug rash, anaphylactic shock, photosensitivity, excessive perspiration, chills, dryness of mouth, nose, and throat
2. *Cardiovascular System:* Hypotension, headache, palpitations, tachycardia, extrasystoles
3. *Hematologic System:* Hemolytic anemia, thrombocytopenia, agranulocytosis
4. *Nervous System:* Sedation, sleepiness, dizziness, disturbed coordination, fatigue, confusion, restlessness, excitation, nervousness, tremor, irritability, insomnia, euphoria, paresthesia, blurred vision, diplopia, vertigo, tinnitus, acute labyrinthitis, hysteria, neuritis, convulsions
5. *GI System:* Epigastric distress, anorexia, nausea, vomiting, diarrhea, constipation
6. *GU System:* Urinary frequency, difficult urination, urinary retention, early menses
7. *Respiratory System:* Thickening of bronchial secretions, tightness of chest and wheezing, nasal stuffiness

Overdosage: *Oral and Parenteral:* Antihistamine overdosage reactions may vary from central nervous system depression to stimulation. Stimulation is particularly likely in children. Atropine-like signs and symptoms—dry mouth; fixed, dilated pupils; flushing—and gastrointestinal symptoms may also occur.

If vomiting has not occurred spontaneously, the patient should be induced to vomit. This is best done by having the patient drink a glass of water or milk, after which the patient should be made to gag. Precautions against aspiration must be taken, especially in infants and children.

If vomiting is unsuccessful, gastric lavage is indicated within 3 hours after ingestion and even later if large amounts of milk or cream were given beforehand. Isotonic or ½ isotonic saline is the lavage solution of choice.

Saline cathartics, as milk of magnesia, by osmosis draw water into the bowel and therefore are valuable for their action in rapid dilution of bowel content.

Stimulants should *not* be used.

Vasopressors may be used to treat hypotension.

Dosage and Administration: *Oral and Parenteral:*
DOSAGE SHOULD BE INDIVIDUALIZED ACCORDING TO THE NEEDS AND THE RESPONSE OF THE PATIENT.

Oral:
A single oral dose of diphenhydramine hydrochloride is quickly absorbed, with maximum activity occurring in approximately one hour. The duration of activity following an average dose of Benadryl (diphenhydramine hydrochloride) is from four to six hours.

ADULTS: 25 to 50 mg three or four times daily
CHILDREN (over 20 lb): 12.5 to 25 mg three to four times daily. Maximum daily dosage not to exceed 300 mg. For physicians who wish to calculate the dose on the basis of body weight or surface area, the recommended dosage is 5 mg/kg/24 hours or 150 mg/m^2/24 hours.

The basis for determining the most effective dosage regimen will be the response of the patient to medication and the condition under treatment.

In motion sickness, full dosage is recommended for prophylactic use, the first dose to be given 30 minutes before exposure to motion and similar doses before meals and upon retiring for the duration of exposure.

Parenteral: Benadryl in the injectable form is indicated when the oral form is impractical.
CHILDREN: 5 mg/kg/24 hours or 150 mg/m^2/24 hours. Maximum daily dosage is 300 mg. Divide into four doses, administered intravenously or deeply intramuscularly.
ADULTS: 10 to 50 mg intravenously or deeply intramuscularly; 100 mg if required; maximum daily dosage is 400 mg.

How Supplied:
Benadryl is supplied in the oral form as:
N 0071-0373-24—Bottle of 100
N 0071-0373-32—Bottle of 1000
N 0071-0373-40—Unit dose (10/10's)
Each capsule contains 50 mg diphenhydramine hydrochloride.
N 0071-0471-24—Bottle of 100
N 0071-0471-32—Bottle of 1000
N 0071-0471-40—Unit dose (10/10's)
Each capsule contains 25 mg diphenhydramine hydrochloride.   0373G011
Shown in Product Identification Section, page 423
Benadryl is also supplied in the following oral dosage form:
Elixir
N 0071-2220-17—4-oz bottle
N 0071-2220-23—Pint bottle
N 0071-2220-32—Gallon bottle
N 0071-2220-40—Unit-dose (5 ml × 100)
Each 5 ml of elixir contains 12.5 mg diphenhydramine hydrochloride with 14% alcohol.
                                        2220G301
Benadryl in parenteral form is supplied as:
N 0071-4015-10 (10-ml vial)
N 0071-4015-13 (30-ml vial)
Sterile solution for parenteral use containing 10 mg diphenhydramine hydrochloride in each milliliter of solution with 0.1 mg/ml benzethonium chloride as a germicidal agent. Supplied in multiple-dose vials (Steri-Vials®).
N 0071-4402-10 (10-ml vial)
Sterile solution for parenteral use containing 50 mg diphenhydramine hydrochloride in each milliliter of solution with 0.1 mg/ml benzethonium chloride as a germicidal agent. Supplied in multiple-dose vials.
N 0071-4259-03 1-ml ampoule
Sterile solution for parenteral use containing 50 mg diphenhydramine hydrochloride. Supplied in packages of 10.
N 0071-4259-40 (individual cartons)
N 0071-4259-41 (2 trays of 5 syringes each)
Sterile solution for parenteral use containing 50 mg diphenhydramine hydrochloride in a 1-ml disposable syringe. (Steri-Dose®). Supplied in packages of ten.
The pH of the solutions for parenteral use have been adjusted with either sodium hydroxide or hydrochloric acid.   4259G010

Continued on next page

This product information was prepared in August, 1984. On these and other Parke-Davis Products, information may be obtained by addressing PARKE-DAVIS, Division of Warner-Lambert Company, Morris Plains, New Jersey 07950.

Parke-Davis—Cont.

BENYLIN®   OTC
[bĕ″ ny-lĭn″]
Cough Syrup

Description: Each teaspoonful (5 ml) contains Benadryl® (diphenhydramine hydrochloride), 12.5 mg. Alcohol, 5%.

Indications: For the temporary relief of cough due to minor throat and bronchial irritation as may occur with the common cold or with inhaled irritants.

Warnings: May cause marked drowsiness. Keep this and all drugs out of the reach of children. In case of accidental overdosage, seek professional assistance or contact a poison control center immediately. Do not give to children under 6 years of age except under the advice and supervision of a physician. May cause excitability, especially in children. Do not take this product for persistent or chronic cough such as occurs with smoking, asthma, emphysema, or when cough is accompanied by excessive secretions, or if you have epilepsy, glaucoma, or difficulty in urination due to enlargement of the prostate gland except under the advice and supervision of a physician. As with any drug, if you are pregnant or nursing a baby, seek the advice of a health professional before using this product.

Caution: Avoid driving a motor vehicle or operating heavy machinery, or drinking alcoholic beverages. A persistent cough may be a sign of a serious condition. If cough persists for more than one week, tends to recur, or is accompanied by high fever, rash, or persistent headache, consult a physician.

Directions: Adults—two teaspoonfuls every four hours, not to exceed twelve teaspoonfuls in twenty-four hours; Children (6 to under 12 years), one teaspoonful every four hours not to exceed six teaspoonfuls in twenty-four hours; or as directed by a physician. Your physician should be contacted for the recommended dosage for children 2 to under 6 years. Do not give to children under 2 years except under the advice and supervision of a physician.

How Supplied: N 0071-2195-Benylin Cough Syrup is supplied in 4-oz, 8-oz, 1-pt, 1-gal bottles, and unit-dose bottles of 5 ml and 10 ml.
Store below 30°C (86°F).
Protect from freezing.

BENYLIN DM® Cough Syrup
[bĕ″ ny-lĭn″]
(See PDR For Nonprescription Drugs)

BRONDECON®   ℞
[brŏn′ dĕ-cŏn″]
oxtriphylline and guaifenesin

Description: Each tablet contains 200 mg oxtriphylline and 100 mg guaifenesin. Each 5 ml teaspoonful of elixir contains 100 mg oxtriphylline and 50 mg guaifenesin; alcohol 20%.
NOTE: 100 mg oxtriphylline is equivalent to 64 mg anhydrous theophylline.

Actions: Brondecon, a bronchodilator and expectorant, helps to relieve symptoms of bronchospasm as well as obstruction caused by viscid mucus in the bronchioles.
Oxtriphylline, the choline salt of theophylline, is a xanthine bronchodilating agent. Compared to aminophylline, oxtriphylline is less irritating to the gastric mucosa, better absorbed from the gastrointestinal tract, more stable and more soluble.
The expectorant component of Brondecon is guaifenesin, which tends to increase the secretion and decrease the viscosity of fluids of the respiratory tract. These physiologic fluids help to lubricate the inflamed mucous membranes of the bronchi and also help the patient to expel viscid mucus thus making cough more productive.

Indications: Brondecon is an adjunct in the management of bronchitis, bronchial asthma, asthmatic bronchitis, pulmonary emphysema, and similar chronic obstructive lung disease. It is indicated when both relaxation of bronchospasm and expectorant action are desirable.

Precautions: Concurrent use of other xanthine preparations may lead to adverse reactions, particularly CNS stimulation in children.

Adverse Reactions: Gastric distress and, occasionally, palpitation and CNS stimulation have been reported.

Dosage: Tablets—over 12 years of age: one tablet, 4 times a day.
Elixir—over 12 years of age: two teaspoonfuls, 4 times a day; from 2 to 12 years: one teaspoonful per 60 lb body weight, 4 times a day.
Above recommendations are averages. Dosage should be individualized.

Supplied: Salmon-pink tablets in bottles of 100 (N 0071-0200-24). Elixir, dark red, cherry-flavored in 237 ml (8 fl oz) (N 0071-2201-20) and 474 ml (16 fl oz) (N 0071-2201-23) bottles.
Store between 15° and 30°C (59° and 86°F).
Shown in Product Identification Section, page 423
0200 G 010

CALADRYL® Cream
[că′ lă-dryl″]
CALADRYL® Lotion

Description: *Caladryl Lotion*—A drying, antihistaminic, calamine-Benadryl® lotion containing calamine; 1% Benadryl (diphenhydramine hydrochloride); camphor; and 2% alcohol
Caladryl Cream—a drying, antihistaminic, calamine-Benadryl cream containing 1% Benadryl (diphenhydramine hydrochloride) and camphor

Indications: For relief of itching due to mild poison ivy or oak, insect bites, or other minor skin irritations, and soothing relief of mild sunburn.

Warnings: Should not be applied to blistered, raw, or oozing areas of the skin. Discontinue use if burning sensation or rash develops or condition persists. Remove by washing with soap and water. Use on extensive areas of the skin or for longer than seven days only as directed by a physician.

Caution: Keep away from eyes or other mucous membranes.
FOR EXTERNAL USE ONLY
Keep this and all drugs out of the reach of children. In case of accidental ingestion, seek professional assistance or contact a Poison Control Center immediately.

Directions: Caladryl Cream—Apply topically three or four times daily. Cleanse skin with soap and water and dry area before each application.
Caladryl Lotion—SHAKE WELL. Apply topically three or four times daily. Cleanse skin with soap and water and dry area before each application.

How Supplied: N 0071-3226-14: Caladryl Cream; 1½-oz tubes
N 0071-3181: Caladryl Lotion—2½-oz (75 ml) squeeze bottles and 6-oz bottles.

CELONTIN® KAPSEALS®   ℞
[cĕ″ lŏn′ tĭn]
(methsuximide capsules, USP)

Description: Celontin (methsuximide) is an anticonvulsant succinimide, chemically designated as N,2-Dimethyl-2-phenylsuccinimide.

Action: Methsuximide suppresses the paroxysmal three-cycle-per-second spike and wave activity associated with lapses of consciousness which is common in absence (petit mal) seizures. The frequency of epileptiform attacks is reduced, apparently by depression of the motor cortex and elevation of the threshold of the central nervous system to convulsive stimuli.

Indication: Celontin is indicated for the control of absence (petit mal) seizures that are refractory to other drugs.

Contraindication: Methsuximide should not be used in patients with a history of hypersensitivity to succinimides.

Warnings: Blood dyscrasias, including some with fatal outcome, have been reported to be associated with the use of succinimides; therefore, periodic blood counts should be performed.
It has been reported that succinimides have produced morphological and functional changes in animal liver. For this reason, methsuximide should be administered with extreme caution to patients with known liver or renal disease. Periodic urinalysis and liver function studies are advised for all patients receiving the drug.
Cases of systemic lupus erythematosus have been reported with the use of succinimides. The physician should be alert to this possibility.

Usage in Pregnancy: The effects of Celontin in human pregnancy and nursing infants are unknown.
Recent reports suggest an association between the use of anticonvulsant drugs by women with epilepsy and an elevated incidence of birth defects in children born to these women. Data are more extensive with respect to phenytoin and phenobarbital, but these are also the most commonly prescribed anticonvulsants; less systematic or anecdotal reports suggest a possible similar association with the use of all known anticonvulsant drugs. The reports suggesting an elevated incidence of birth defects in children of drug-treated epileptic women cannot be regarded as adequate to prove a definite cause-and-effect relationship. There are intrinsic methodologic problems in obtaining adequate data on drug teratogenicity in humans; the possibility also exists that other factors, eg, genetic factors or the epileptic condition itself, may be more important than drug therapy in leading to birth defects. The great majority of mothers on anticonvulsant medication deliver normal infants. It is important to note that anticonvulsant drugs should not be discontinued in patients in whom the drug is administered to prevent major seizures because of the strong possibility of precipitating status epilepticus with attendant hypoxia and threat to life. In individual cases where the severity and frequency of the seizure disorder are such that the removal of medication does not pose a serious threat to the patient, discontinuation of the drug may be considered prior to and during pregnancy, although it cannot be said with any confidence that even minor seizures do not pose some hazard to the developing embryo or fetus.
The prescribing physician will wish to weigh these considerations in treating or counseling epileptic women of childbearing potential.

Hazardous Activities: Methsuximide may impair the mental and/or physical abilities required for the performance of potentially hazardous tasks, such as driving a motor vehicle or other such activity requiring alertness; therefore, the patient should be cautioned accordingly.

Precautions: It is recommended that the physician withdraw the drug slowly on the appearance of unusual depression, aggressiveness, or other behavioral alterations.
As with other anticonvulsants, it is important to proceed slowly when increasing or decreasing dosage, as well as when adding or eliminating other medication. Abrupt withdrawal of anticonvulsant medication may precipitate absence (petit mal) status.
Methsuximide, when used alone in mixed types of epilepsy, may increase the frequency of grand mal seizures in some patients.
ADVICE TO THE PHARMACIST AND PATIENT: Since methsuximide has a relatively low melting temperature (124°F), storage conditions which may promote high temperatures (closed cars, delivery vans, or storage near steam pipes) should be avoided. Do not dispense or use capsules that are not full or in which contents have melted. Effectiveness may be reduced. Protect from excessive heat (104°F).

Adverse Reactions: Gastrointestinal System: Gastrointestinal symptoms occur frequently and have included nausea or vomiting, anorexia, diarrhea, weight loss, epigastric and abdominal pain, and constipation.

Hemopoietic System: Hemopoietic complications associated with the administration of methsuximide have included eosinophilia, leukopenia, monocytosis, and pancytopenia.

Nervous System: Neurologic and sensory reactions reported during therapy with methsuximide have included drowsiness, ataxia or dizziness, irritability and nervousness, headache, blurred vi-

sion, photophobia, hiccups, and insomnia. Drowsiness, ataxia, and dizziness have been the most frequent side effects noted. Psychologic abnormalities have included confusion, instability, mental slowness, depression, hypochondriacal behavior, and aggressiveness. There have been rare reports of psychosis, suicidal behavior, and auditory hallucinations.
Integumentary System: Dermatologic manifestations which have occurred with the administration of methsuximide have included urticaria, Stevens-Johnson syndrome, and pruritic erythematous rashes.
Other: Miscellaneous reactions reported include periorbital edema and hyperemia.
Dosage and Administration: Optimum dosage of Celontin must be determined by trial. A suggested dosage schedule is 300 mg per day for the first week. If required, dosage may be increased thereafter at weekly intervals by 300 mg per day for the three weeks following to a daily dosage of 1.2 g. Because therapeutic effect and tolerance vary among patients, therapy with Celontin must be individualized according to the response of each patient. Optimal dosage is that amount of Celontin which is barely sufficient to control seizures so that side effects may be kept to a minimum. The smaller capsule (150 mg) facilitates administration to small children.
Celontin may be administered in combination with other anticonvulsants when other forms of epilepsy coexist with absence (petit mal.)
How Supplied:
N 0071-0525-24 (P-D 525)—Celontin Kapseals, each containing 300 mg methsuximide; bottles of 100.
N 0071-0537-24 (P-D 537)—Celontin Kapseals, Half Strength, each containing 150 mg methsuximide, bottles of 100.
Store at controlled room temperature 15°–30°C (59°–86°F).
Protect from light and moisture.

0537G011

Shown in Product Identification Section, page 423

CENTRAX®
[cĕn'trăx]
(prazepam)

Description: Centrax (prazepam) is a benzodiazepine derivative. Chemically, prazepam is 7-chloro-1-(cyclopropylmethyl)-1, 3-dihydro-5-phenyl-2H-1,4-benzodiazepin-2-one, and has a molecular weight of 324.8.
Clinical Pharmacology: Studies in normal subjects have shown that Centrax (prazepam) has depressant effects on the central nervous system. Oral administration of single doses as high as 60 mg and of divided doses up to 100 mg three times a day (300 mg total daily dosage) were without toxic effects.
Single, oral doses of Centrax (prazepam) in normal subjects produced average peak blood levels of the major metabolite norprazepam at 6 hours postadministration, with significant amounts still present after 48 hours. Prazepam was slowly absorbed over a prolonged period; rather constant blood levels were maintained on multiple-dose schedules; and excretion was prolonged. The mean half-life of norprazepam measured in subjects given 10 mg prazepam three times a day for one week was 63 ($\pm$ 15 SD) hours before and 70 ($\pm$ 10 SD) hours after multiple dosing—a nonsignificant difference. Human metabolism studies showed that prior to elimination from the body, prazepam is metabolized in large part to 3-hydroxyprazepam and oxazepam.
Indications: Centrax is indicated for the management of anxiety disorders or for the short-term relief of the symptoms of anxiety. Anxiety or tension associated with the stress of everyday life usually does not require treatment with an anxiolytic.
The effectiveness of Centrax in long-term use, that is, more than 4 months, has not been assessed by systematic clinical studies. The physician should periodically reassess the usefulness of the drug for the individual patient.

Contraindications: Centrax (prazepam) is contraindicated in patients with a known hypersensitivity to the drug and in those with acute narrow-angle glaucoma.
Warnings: Centrax (prazepam) is not recommended in psychotic states and in those psychiatric disorders in which anxiety is not a prominent feature.
Patients taking Centrax should be cautioned against engaging in hazardous occupations requiring mental alertness, such as operating dangerous machinery including motor vehicles.
Because Centrax has a central nervous system depressant effect, patients should be advised against the simultaneous use of other CNS-depressant drugs, including phenothiazines, narcotics, barbiturates, MAO inhibitors, and other antidepressants. The effects of alcohol may also be increased with prazepam.
Physical and Psychological Dependence: Withdrawal symptoms similar in character to those noted with barbiturates and alcohol have occurred following abrupt discontinuance of benzodiazepine drugs. These symptoms include convulsions, tremor, abdominal and muscle cramps, vomiting and sweating. Addiction-prone individuals, such as drug addicts and alcoholics, should be under careful surveillance when receiving benzodiazepines because of the predisposition of such patients to habituation and dependence.
Withdrawal symptoms have also been reported following abrupt discontinuance of benzodiazepines taken continuously at therapeutic levels for several months.
Precautions: *Usage in Pregnancy and Lactation:* An increased risk of congenital malformations associated with the use of minor tranquilizers (chlordiazepoxide, diazepam, and meprobamate) during the first trimester of pregnancy has been suggested in several studies. Prazepam, a benzodiazepine derivative, has not been studied adequately to determine whether it, too, may be associated with an increased risk of fetal abnormality. Because use of these drugs is rarely a matter of urgency, their use during this period should almost always be avoided. The possibility that a woman of childbearing potential may be pregnant at the time of institution of therapy should be considered. Patients should be advised that if they become pregnant during therapy or intend to become pregnant, they should communicate with their physicians about the desirability of discontinuing the drug. In view of their molecular size, prazepam and its metabolites are probably excreted in human milk. Therefore, this drug should not be given to nursing mothers.
In those patients in whom a degree of depression accompanies the anxiety, suicidal tendencies may be present and protective measures may be required. The least amount of drug that is feasible should be available to the patient at any one time.
Patients taking Centrax (prazepam) for prolonged periods should have blood counts and liver function tests periodically. The usual precautions in treating patients with impaired renal or hepatic functions should also be observed. Hepatomegaly and cholestasis were observed in chronic toxicity studies in rats and dogs.
In elderly or debilitated patients, the initial dose should be small, and increments should be made gradually, in accordance with the response of the patient, to preclude ataxia or excessive sedation.
Pediatric Use: Safety and effectiveness in patients below the age of 18 have not been established.
Adverse Reactions: The side effects most frequently reported during double-blind, placebo-controlled trials employing a typical 30-mg divided total daily dosage and the percent incidence in the prazepam group were fatigue (11.6%), dizziness (8.7%), weakness (7.7%), drowsiness (6.8%), light-headedness (6.8%), and ataxia (5.0%). Less frequently reported were headache, confusion, tremor, vivid dreams, slurred speech, palpitation, stimulation, dry mouth, diaphoresis, and various gastrointestinal complaints. Other side effects included pruritus, transient skin rashes, swelling of feet, joint pains, various genitourinary com-

plaints, blurred vision, and syncope. Single, nightly dose, controlled trials of variable dosages showed a dose-related incidence of these same side effects. Transient and reversible aberrations of liver function tests have been reported, as have been slight decreases in blood pressure and increases in body weight.
These findings are characteristic of benzodiazepine drugs.
Overdosage: As in the management of overdosage with any drug, it should be borne in mind that multiple agents may have been taken.
Vomiting should be induced if it has not occurred spontaneously. Immediate gastric lavage is also recommended. General supportive care, including frequent monitoring of vital signs and close observation of the patient, is indicated. Hypotension, though unlikely, may be controlled with Levophed® (levarterenol bitartrate), or Aramine® (metaraminol bitartrate).
Dosage and Administration: Centrax (prazepam) is administered orally in divided doses. The usual daily dose is 30 mg. The dose should be adjusted gradually within the range of 20 mg to 60 mg daily in accordance with the response of the patient. In elderly or debilitated patients it is advisable to initiate treatment at a divided daily dose of 10 mg to 15 mg (see Precautions).
Centrax may also be administered as a single, daily dose at bedtime. The recommended starting nightly dose is 20 mg. The response of the patient to several days' treatment will permit the physician to adjust the dose upwards or, occasionally, downwards to maximize antianxiety effect with a minimum of daytime drowsiness. The optimum dosage will usually range from 20 mg to 40 mg.
Drug Interactions: If Centrax (prazepam) is to be combined with other drugs acting on the central nervous system, careful consideration should be given to the pharmacology of the agents to be employed. The actions of the benzodiazepines may be potentiated by barbiturates, narcotics, phenothiazines, monoamine oxidase inhibitors, or other antidepressants.
If Centrax (prazepam) is used to treat anxiety associated with somatic disease states, careful attention must be paid to possible drug interaction with concomitant medication.
How Supplied:
Centrax 5 mg—Each capsule contains 5 mg prazepam. Available in bottles of 100 (N 0710-0552-24), and 500 (N 0710-0552-30). Centrax 10 mg—Each capsule contains 10 mg prazepam. Available in bottles of 100 (N 0710-0553-24), and 500 (N 0710-0553-30). Centrax 20 mg—Each capsule contains 20 mg prazepam. Available in bottles of 100 (N 0710-0554-24).
Also supplied as Centrax Tablets (prazepam tablets, USP) 10 mg light blue, scored tablets in bottles of 100 (N 0710-0276-24) and unit dose (N 0710-0276-40).
Direct Medical Inquiries to:
Parke-Davis, Div Warner-Lambert Inc
c/o Warner-Lambert Co
201 Tabor Road, Morris Plains, NJ 07950.
Attn: Medical Affairs Dept

0552G120

Shown in Product Identification Section, page 423

CHLOROMYCETIN® CREAM, 1%
[chlō″ rō-my-cē' tin]
(chloramphenicol cream, USP) 1%

Description: Each gram of Chloromycetin Cream, 1%, contains 10 mg chloramphenicol with 0.1% propylparaben in a water-miscible ointment base of liquid petrolatum, cetyl alcohol, sodium lauryl sulfate, sodium phosphate buffer, and water.

Continued on next page

This product information was prepared in August, 1984. On these and other Parke-Davis Products, information may be obtained by addressing PARKE-DAVIS, Division of Warner-Lambert Company, Morris Plains, New Jersey 07950.

Parke-Davis—Cont.

Clinical Pharmacology: Chloramphenicol is a broad-spectrum antibiotic originally isolated from *Streptomyces venezuelae*. It is primarily bacteriostatic and acts by inhibition of protein synthesis by interfering with the transfer of activated amino acids from soluble RNA to ribosomes. Development of resistance to chloramphenicol can be regarded as minimal for staphylococci and many other species of bacteria.

Indications and Usage: Chloromycetin (chloramphenicol) Cream, 1%, is indicated for the treatment of surface skin infections caused by bacteria susceptible to chloramphenicol. Deeper cutaneous infections should be treated with appropriate systemic antibiotics.

Contraindication: This product is contraindicated in persons sensitive to any of its components.

Warnings: Bone marrow hypoplasia, including aplastic anemia and death, has been reported following the local application of chloramphenicol.

Precautions: The prolonged use of antibiotics may occasionally result in overgrowth of nonsusceptible organisms, including fungi. If new infections appear during medication, the drug should be discontinued and appropriate measures should be taken.

In all except very superficial infections, the topical use of chloramphenicol should be supplemented by appropriate systemic medication.

Adverse Reactions: Signs of local irritation with subjective symptoms of itching or burning, angioneurotic edema, urticaria, vesicular and maculopapular dermatitis have been reported in patients sensitive to chloramphenicol and are causes for discontinuing the medication. Similar sensitivity reactions to other materials in topical preparations may also occur. Blood dyscrasias have been reported in association with the use of chloramphenicol (See WARNINGS).

Dosage and Administration: Apply to the infected area three or four times daily after cleansing.

How Supplied:
N 0071-3166-13 (Ointment 66)
Chloromycetin Cream (chloramphenicol cream), 1%, is supplied in 1-oz tubes.
AHFS 84:04.04   3166G012

CHLOROMYCETIN® ℞
[*chlō″rō-my-cē′tĭn*]
HYDROCORTISONE OPHTHALMIC
(Chloramphenicol and Hydrocortisone Acetate for Suspension, USP)

> **Warning**
> Bone marrow hypoplasia including aplastic anemia and death has been reported following local application of chloramphenicol. Chloramphenicol should not be used when less potentially dangerous agents would be expected to provide effective treatment.

Description: Chloromycetin® Hydrocortisone Ophthalmic (Chloramphenicol and Hydrocortisone Acetate for Suspension, USP) is a sterile, buffered antibiotic/antiinflammatory dry mixture for suspension for ophthalmic administration. Each vial of Chloromycetin Hydrocortisone Ophthalmic contains 12.5 mg chloramphenicol and 25 mg hydrocortisone acetate with boric acid-sodium borate buffer, cholesterol, methylcellulose, sodium chloride, and Phemerol® (benzethonium chloride), 0.1 mg per ml, in the suspension when prepared as directed.

The chemical names for chloramphenicol are:
(1) Acetamide,2,2-dichloro-N-[2-hydroxy-1-(hydroxymethyl)-2-(4-nitrophenyl) ethyl]-, and
(2) D-*threo*-(-)-2,2-Dichloro-N-[β-hydroxy-α-(hydroxymethyl)-*p*-nitrophenethyl] acetamide

The chemical names for hydrocortisone acetate are:
(1) Pregn-4-ene-3,20-dione,21-(acetyloxy)-11,17-dihydroxy-,(11β)-, and
(2) 17-Hydroxycorticosterone 21-acetate

Clinical Pharmacology: Corticoids suppress the inflammatory response to a variety of agents and they probably delay or slow healing. Since corticoids may inhibit the body's defense mechanism against infection, a concomitant antimicrobial drug may be used when this inhibition is considered to be clinically significant in a particular case.

The antiinfective component in this combination is included to provide action against specific organisms susceptible to it. Chloramphenicol is considered active against a wide spectrum of gram-negative and gram-positive organisms such as *Escherichia coli*, *Hemophilus influenzae*, *Staphylococcus aureus*, *Streptococcus hemolyticus*, and *Moraxella lacunata* (Morax-Axenfeld bacillus). Development of resistance to chloramphenicol can be regarded as minimal for staphylococci and many other species of bacteria. Chloramphenicol is primarily bacteriostatic and acts by inhibition of protein synthesis by interfering with the transfer of activated amino acids from soluble RNA to ribosomes. It has been noted that chloramphenicol is found in measurable amounts in the aqueous humor following local application to the eye.

When a decision to administer both a corticoid and an antimicrobial is made, the administration of such drugs in combination has the advantage of greater patient compliance and convenience, with the added assurance that the appropriate dosage of both drugs is administered, plus assured compatibility of ingredients when both types of drug are in the same formulation and, particularly, that the correct volume of drug is delivered and retained.

The relative potency of corticosteroids depends on the molecular structure, concentration, and release from the vehicle.

Indications and Usage: Chloramphenicol should be used only in those serious infections for which less potentially dangerous drugs are ineffective or contraindicated. Bacteriological studies should be performed to determine the causative organisms and their sensitivity to chloramphenicol (See Box Warning).

For steroid-responsive inflammatory ocular conditions for which a corticosteroid is indicated and where bacterial infection or a risk of bacterial ocular infection exists.

Ocular steroids are indicated in inflammatory conditions of the palpebral and bulbar conjunctiva, cornea, and anterior segment of the globe where the inherent risk of steroid use in certain infective conjunctivitides is accepted to obtain a diminution in edema and inflammation. They are also indicated in chronic anterior uveitis and corneal injury from chemical radiation, thermal burns, or penetration of foreign bodies.

The use of a combination drug with an antiinfective component is indicated where the risk of infection is high or where there is an expectation that potentially dangerous numbers of bacteria will be present in the eye.

The particular antiinfective drug in this product is active against the following common bacterial eye pathogens:
Staphylococcus aureus
Streptococci, including *Streptococcus pneumoniae*
Escherichia coli
Hemophilus influenzae
Klebsiella/Enterobacter species
Moraxella lacunata (Morax-Axenfeld bacillus)
Neisseria species
The product does not provide adequate coverage against:
Pseudomonas aeruginosa
Serratia marcescens

Contraindications: Epithelial herpes simplex keratitis (dendritic keratitis), vaccinia, varicella, and many other viral diseases of the cornea and conjunctiva. Mycobacterial infection of the eye. Fungal diseases of ocular structures. Hypersensitivity to a component of the medication. (Hypersensitivity to the antibiotic component occurs at a higher rate than for other components).

The use of these combinations is always contraindicated after uncomplicated removal of a corneal foreign body.

Warnings: SEE BOX WARNING
Prolonged use of steroids may result in glaucoma, with damage to the optic nerve, defects in visual acuity and fields of vision, and posterior subcapsular cataract formation. Prolonged use may suppress the host response and thus increase the hazard of secondary ocular infections. In those diseases causing thinning of the cornea or sclera, perforations have been known to occur with the use of topical steroids. In acute purulent conditions of the eye, steroids may mask infection or enhance existing infection. If these products are used for 10 days or longer, intraocular pressure should be routinely monitored even though it may be difficult in children and uncooperative patients. Employment of steroid medication in the treatment of herpes simplex requires great caution.

Precautions: The initial prescription and renewal of the medication order beyond 20 milliliters should be made by a physician only after examination of the patient with the aid of magnification, such as slit lamp biomicroscopy and, where appropriate, fluorescein staining.

The possibility of persistent fungal infections of the cornea should be considered after prolonged steroid dosing.

The prolonged use of antibiotics may occasionally result in overgrowth of nonsusceptible organisms, including fungi. If new infections appear during medication, the drug should be discontinued and appropriate measures should be taken.

In all serious infections the topical use of chloramphenicol should be supplemented by appropriate systemic medication.

Adverse Reactions: Blood dyscrasias have been reported in association with the use of chloramphenicol. (See **Warnings**).

Adverse reactions have occurred with steroid/antiinfective combination drugs which can be attributed to the steroid component, the antiinfective component, or the combination. Exact incidence figures are not available since no denominator of treated patients is available.

Reactions occurring most often from the presence of the antiinfective ingredient are allergic sensitizations. The reactions due to the steroid component in decreasing order of frequency are: elevation of intraocular pressure (IOP) with possible development of glaucoma, and infrequent optic nerve damage; posterior subcapsular cataract formation; and delayed wound healing.

Secondary Infection: The development of secondary infection has occurred after use of combinations containing steroids and antimicrobials. Fungal infections of the cornea are particularly prone to develop coincidentally with long-term applications of steroid. The possibility of fungal invasion must be considered in any persistent corneal ulceration where steroid treatment has been used. Secondary bacterial ocular infection following suppression of host responses also occurs.

Dosage and Administration: Two drops applied to the affected eye every three hours, or more frequently if deemed advisable by the prescribing physician. Administration should be continued day and night for the first 48 hours, after which the interval between applications may be increased. Treatment should be continued for at least 48 hours after the eye appears normal.

Directions for dispensing—Add 5 ml sterile distilled water to contents of vial under aseptic conditions. Shake to make uniform suspension. Place sterile dropper in vial. Each ml of suspension prepared as directed contains 2.5 mg Chloromycetin (chloramphenicol) and 5 mg Hydrocortisone Acetate.

Not more than 20 milliliters should be prescribed initially and the prescription should not be refilled without further evaluation as outlined in Precautions above.

How Supplied: N 0071-3228-35 Chloromycetin Hydrocortisone Ophthalmic (Chloramphenicol and Hydrocortisone Acetate for Suspension, USP) is supplied in a package containing dry ingredients in a 5 ml vial for preparation of the ophthalmic suspension. After dispensing, the product may be stored at room temperature for a period of not more than 10 days. A sterilized dropper-cap assembly for use with the vial is included in the package. Chloromycetin, brand of chloramphenicol, Reg US Pat Off.

3228G013

KAPSEALS®/CAPSULES CHLOROMYCETIN® ℞
[chlō″ rō-my-cē′ tin]
(chloramphenicol capsules, USP)

WARNING
Serious and fatal blood dyscrasias (aplastic anemia, hypoplastic anemia, thrombocytopenia, and granulocytopenia) are known to occur after the administration of chloramphenicol. In addition, there have been reports of aplastic anemia attributed to chloramphenicol which later terminated in leukemia. Blood dyscrasias have occurred after both short-term and prolonged therapy with this drug. Chloramphenicol must not be used when less potentially dangerous agents will be effective, as described in the Indications section. *It must not be used in the treatment of trivial infections or where it is not indicated, as in colds, influenza, infections of the throat; or as a prophylactic agent to prevent bacterial infections.*

Precautions: It is essential that adequate blood studies be made during treatment with the drug. While blood studies may detect early peripheral blood changes, such as leukopenia, reticulocytopenia, or granulocytopenia, before they become irreversible, such studies cannot be relied on to detect bone marrow depression prior to development of aplastic anemia. To facilitate appropriate studies and observation during therapy, it is desirable that patients be hospitalized.

Description: Chloramphenicol is an antibiotic that is clinically useful for, *and should be reserved for,* serious infections caused by organisms susceptible to its antimicrobial effects when less potentially hazardous therapeutic agents are ineffective or contraindicated. Sensitivity testing is essential to determine its indicated use, but may be performed concurrently with therapy initiated on clinical impression that one of the indicated conditions exists (see Indications section).

Actions and Pharmacology: *In vitro* chloramphenicol exerts mainly a bacteriostatic effect on a wide range of gram-negative and gram-positive bacteria and is active *in vitro* against rickettsiae, the lymphogranuloma psittacosis group, and *Vibrio cholerae.* It is particularly active against *Salmonella typhi* and *Hemophilus influenzae.* The mode of action is through interference or inhibition of protein synthesis in intact cells and in cell-free systems.

Chloramphenicol administered orally is absorbed rapidly from the intestinal tract. In controlled studies in adult volunteers using the recommended dosage of 50 mg/kg/day, a dosage of 1 g every 6 hours for 8 doses was given. Using the microbiological assay method, the average peak serum level was 11.2 mcg/ml one hour after the first dose. A cumulative effect gave a peak rise to 18.4 mcg/ml after the fifth dose of 1 g. Mean serum levels ranged from 8 to 14 mcg/ml over the 48-hour period. Total urinary excretion of chloramphenicol in these studies ranged from a low of 68% to a high of 99% over a three-day period. From 8 to 12% of the antibiotic excreted is in the form of free chloramphenicol; the remainder consists of microbiologically inactive metabolites, principally the conjugate with glucuronic acid. Since the glucuronide is excreted rapidly, most chloramphenicol detected in the blood is in the microbiologically active free form. Despite the small proportion of unchanged drug excreted in the urine, the concentration of free chloramphenicol is relatively high, amounting to several hundred mcg/ml in patients receiving divided doses of 50 mg/kg/day. Small amounts of active drug are found in bile and feces. Chloramphenicol diffuses rapidly, but its distribution is not uniform. Highest concentrations are found in liver and kidney, and lowest concentrations are found in brain and cerebrospinal fluid. Chloramphenicol enters cerebrospinal fluid even in the absence of meningeal inflammation, appearing in concentrations about half of those found in the blood. Measurable levels are also detected in pleural and in ascitic fluids, saliva, milk, and in the aqueous and vitreous humors. Transport across the placental barrier occurs with somewhat lower concentration in cord blood of newborn infants than in maternal blood.

Indications: In accord with the concepts in the warning box and this indications section, chloramphenicol must be used only in those serious infections for which less potentially dangerous drugs are ineffective or contraindicated. However, chloramphenicol may be chosen to initiate antibiotic therapy on the clinical impression that one of the conditions below is believed to be present; *in vitro* sensitivity tests should be performed concurrently so that the drug may be discontinued as soon as possible if less potentially dangerous agents are indicated by such tests. The decision to continue use of chloramphenicol rather than another antibiotic when both are suggested by *in vitro* studies to be effective against a specific pathogen should be based upon severity of the infection, susceptibility of the pathogen to the various antimicrobial drugs, efficacy of the various drugs in the infection, and the important additional concepts contained in the Warning Box above:

1. Acute infections caused by *Salmonella typhi*
Chloramphenicol is a drug of choice.* It is not recommended for the routine treatment of the typhoid carrier state.
2. Serious infections caused by susceptible strains in accordance with the concepts expressed above:
   a. *Salmonella* species
   b. *H influenzae,* specifically meningeal infections
   c. Rickettsia
   d. Lymphogranuloma-psittacosis group
   e. Various gram-negative bacteria causing bacteremia, meningitis, or other serious gram-negative infections
   f. Other susceptible organisms which have been demonstrated to be resistant to all other appropriate antimicrobial agents.
3. Cystic fibrosis regimens

Contraindications: Chloramphenicol is contraindicated in individuals with a history of previous hypersensitivity and/or toxic reaction to it. *It must not be used in the treatment of trivial infections or where it is not indicated, as in colds, influenza, infections of the throat; or as a prophylactic agent to prevent bacterial infections.*

---

* In the treatment of typhoid fever, some authorities recommend that chloramphenicol be administered at therapeutic levels for 8 to 10 days after the patient has become afebrile to lessen the possibility of relapse.

Precautions: 1. Baseline blood studies should be followed by periodic blood studies approximately every two days during therapy. The drug should be discontinued upon appearance of reticulocytopenia, leukopenia, thrombocytopenia, anemia, or any other blood study findings attributable to chloramphenicol. However, it should be noted that such studies do not exclude the possible later appearance of the irreversible type of bone marrow depression.
2. Repeated courses of the drug should be avoided if at all possible. Treatment should not be continued longer than required to produce a cure with little or no risk of relapse of the disease.
3. Concurrent therapy with other drugs that may cause bone marrow depression should be avoided.
4. Excessive blood levels may result from administration of the recommended dose to patients with impaired liver or kidney function, including that due to immature metabolic processes in the infant. The dosage should be adjusted accordingly or, preferably, the blood concentration should be determined at appropriate intervals.
5. There are no studies to establish the safety of this drug in pregnancy.
6. Since chloramphenicol readily crosses the placental barrier, caution in use of the drug is particularly important during pregnancy at term or during labor because of potential toxic effects on the fetus ("gray syndrome").
7. Precaution should be used in therapy of premature and full-term infants to avoid "gray syndrome" toxicity. (See Adverse Reactions.) Serum drug levels should be carefully followed during therapy of the newborn infant.
8. Precaution should be used in therapy during lactation because of the possibility of toxic effects on the nursing infant.
9. The use of this antibiotic, as with other antibiotics, may result in an overgrowth of nonsusceptible organisms, including fungi. If infections caused by nonsusceptible organisms appear during therapy, appropriate measures should be taken.

Adverse Reactions:
1. Blood Dyscrasias
The most serious adverse effect of chloramphenicol is bone marrow depression. Serious and fatal blood dyscrasias (aplastic anemia, hypoplastic anemia, thrombocytopenia, and granulocytopenia) are known to occur after the administration of chloramphenicol. An irreversible type of marrow depression leading to aplastic anemia with a high rate of mortality is characterized by the appearance weeks or months after therapy of bone marrow aplasia or hypoplasia. Peripherally, pancytopenia is most often observed, but in a small number of cases only one or two of the three major cell types (erythrocytes, leukocytes, platelets) may be depressed.

A reversible type of bone marrow depression, which is dose-related, may occur. This type of marrow depression is characterized by vacuolization of the erythroid cells, reduction of reticulocytes, and leukopenia, and responds promptly to the withdrawal of chloramphenicol.

An exact determination of the risk of serious and fatal blood dyscrasias is not possible because of lack of accurate information regarding (1) the size of the population at risk, (2) the total number of drug-associated dyscrasias, and (3) the total number of nondrug-associated dyscrasias.
In a report to the California State Assembly by the California Medical Association and the State Department of Public Health in January 1967, the risk of fatal aplastic anemia was estimated at 1:24,200 to 1:40,500 based on two dosage levels. There have been reports of aplastic anemia attributed to chloramphenicol which later terminated in leukemia.

Paroxysmal nocturnal hemoglobinuria has also been reported.
2. Gastrointestinal Reactions
Nausea, vomiting, glossitis and stomatitis, diarrhea, and enterocolitis may occur in low incidence.
3. Neurotoxic Reactions
Headache, mild depression, mental confusion, and delirium have been described in patients receiving chloramphenicol. Optic and peripheral neuritis have been reported, usually following long-term therapy. If this occurs, the drug should be promptly withdrawn.
4. Hypersensitivity Reactions
Fever, macular and vesicular rashes, angioedema, urticaria, and anaphylaxis may occur. Herxheimer reactions have occurred during therapy for typhoid fever.

Continued on next page

This product information was prepared in August, 1984. On these and other Parke-Davis Products, information may be obtained by addressing PARKE-DAVIS, Division of Warner-Lambert Company, Morris Plains, New Jersey 07950.

Parke-Davis—Cont.

5. "Gray Syndrome"
Toxic reactions including fatalities have occurred in the premature and newborn; the signs and symptoms associated with these reactions have been referred to as the "gray syndrome". One case of "gray syndrome" has been reported in an infant born to a mother having received chloramphenicol during labor. One case has been reported in a 3-month-old infant. The following summarizes the clinical and laboratory studies that have been made on these patients:
(a) In most cases, therapy with chloramphenicol had been instituted within the first 48 hours of life.
(b) Symptoms first appeared after 3 to 4 days of continued treatment with high doses of chloramphenicol.
(c) The symptoms appeared in the following order:
 (1) abdominal distention with or without emesis;
 (2) progressive pallid cyanosis;
 (3) vasomotor collapse, frequently accompanied by irregular respiration;
 (4) death within a few hours of onset of these symptoms.
(d) The progression of symptoms from onset to exitus was accelerated with higher dose schedules.
(e) Preliminary blood serum level studies revealed unusually high concentrations of chloramphenicol (over 90 mcg/ml after repeated doses).
(f) Termination of therapy upon early evidence of the associated symptomatology frequently reversed the process with complete recovery.

Dosage and Administration:
Dosage Recommendations For Oral Chloramphenicol Preparations
The majority of microorganisms susceptible to chloramphenicol will respond to a concentration between 5 and 20 mcg/ml. The desired concentration of active drug in blood should fall within this range over most of the treatment period. Dosage of 50 mg/kg/day divided into 4 doses at intervals of 6 hours will usually achieve and sustain levels of this magnitude.
Except in certain circumstances (eg, premature and newborn infants and individuals with impairment of hepatic or renal function), lower doses may not achieve these concentrations. Chloramphenicol, like other potent drugs, should be prescribed at recommended doses known to have therapeutic activity. Close observation of the patient should be maintained and in the event of any adverse reactions, dosage should be reduced or the drug discontinued, if other factors in the clinical situation permit.

Adults
Adults should receive 50 mg/kg/day (approximately one 250-mg capsule per each 10 lbs body weight) in divided doses at 6-hour intervals. In exceptional cases, patients with infections due to moderately resistant organisms may require increased dosage up to 100 mg/kg/day to achieve blood levels inhibiting the pathogen, but these high doses should be decreased as soon as possible. Adults with impairment of hepatic or renal function or both may have reduced ability to metabolize and excrete the drug. In instances of impaired metabolic processes, dosages should be adjusted accordingly. (See discussion under Newborn Infants.) Precise control of concentration of the drug in the blood should be carefully followed in patients with impaired metabolic processes by the available microtechniques (information available on request).

Children
Dosage of 50 mg/kg/day divided into 4 doses at 6-hour intervals yields blood levels in the range effective against most susceptible organisms. Severe infections (eg, bacteremia or meningitis), especially when adequate cerebrospinal fluid concentrations are desired, may require dosage up to 100 mg/kg/day; however, it is recommended that dosage be reduced to 50 mg/kg/day as soon as possible. Children with impaired liver or kidney function may retain excessive amounts of the drug.

Newborn Infants
(See section titled "Gray Syndrome" under Adverse Reactions.)
A total of 25 mg/kg/day in 4 equal doses at 6-hour intervals usually produces and maintains concentrations in blood and tissues adequate to control most infections for which the drug is indicated. Increased dosage in these individuals, demanded by severe infections, should be given only to maintain the blood concentration within a therapeutically effective range. After the first two weeks of life, full-term infants ordinarily may receive up to a total of 50 mg/kg/day equally divided into 4 doses at 6-hour intervals. **These dosage recommendations are extremely important because blood concentration in all premature infants and full-term infants under two weeks of age differs from that of other infants.** This difference is due to variations in the maturity of the metabolic functions of the liver and the kidneys.
When these functions are immature (or seriously impaired in adults), high concentrations of the drug are found which tend to increase with succeeding doses.

Infants and Children with Immature Metabolic Processes
In young infants and other children in whom immature metabolic functions are suspected, a dose of 25 mg/kg/day will usually produce therapeutic concentrations of the drug in the blood. In this group particularly, the concentration of the drug in the blood should be carefully following by microtechniques. (Information available on request.)

How Supplied:
Kapseals No. 379, Chloromycetin (Chloramphenicol Capsules), each contain 250 mg chloramphenicol.
N 0071-0379-09 Bottles of 16.
N 0071-0379-24 Bottles of 100.
N 0071-0379-40 Unit dose packages of 100 (10/10's).
Shown in Product Identification Section, page 423
AHFS 8:12.08   0379G100

Chloromycetin, brand of chloramphenicol.
Reg. US Pat Off
Storage: Store at a room temperature below 86°F(30°C). Protect from moisture and excessive heat.

CHLOROMYCETIN® OPHTHALMIC ℞
[chlō″ rō-my-cē′ tin]
(Chloramphenical for Ophthalmic Solution, USP)

Warning
Bone marrow hypoplasia including aplastic anemia and death has been reported following local application of chloramphenicol. Chloramphenicol should not be used when less potentially dangerous agents would be expected to provide effective treatment.

Description: Each vial of Chloromycetin Ophthalmic contains 25 mg of Chloromycetin (chloramphenicol) with boric acid-sodium borate buffer. Sodium hydroxide may have been added for adjustment of pH. A 15 ml bottle of Sterile Distilled Water is included in each package for use as a diluent in the preparation of a solution of Chloromycetin suitable for ophthalmic use. By varying the quantity of diluent used solutions ranging in strength from 0.16% to 0.5% may be prepared. Both the powder for solution and the diluent contain no preservatives. Sterile powder.
The chemical names for chloramphenicol are:
(1) Acetamide,2,2-dichloro-N-[2-hydroxy-1-(hydroxymethyl)-2-(4-nitrophenyl) ethyl]-, and
(2) D-threo-(-)-2,2-Dichloro-N-[β-hydroxy-α-(hydroxymethyl)-p-nitrophenethyl] acetamide
Clinical Pharmacology: Chloramphenicol is a broad-spectrum antibiotic originally isolated from Streptomyces venezuelae. It is primarily bacteriostatic and acts by inhibition of protein synthesis by interfering with the transfer of activated amino acids from soluble RNA to ribosomes. It has been noted that chloramphenicol is found in measurable amounts in the aqueous humor following local application to the eye. Development of resistance to chloramphenicol can be regarded as minimal for staphylococci and many other species of bacteria.
Indications and Usage: Chloramphenicol should be used only in those serious infections for which less potentially dangerous drugs are ineffective or contraindicated. Bacteriological studies should be performed to determine the causative organisms and their sensitivity to chloramphenicol (See Box Warning).
Chloromycetin (chloramphenicol) Ophthalmic is indicated for the treatment of surface ocular infections involving the conjunctiva and/or cornea caused by chloramphenicol-susceptible organisms. The particular antiinfective drug in this product is active against the following common bacterial eye pathogens:
Staphylococcus aureus
Streptococci, including *Streptococcus pneumoniae*
Escherichia coli
Haemophilus influenzae
Klebsiella/Enterobacter species
Moraxella lacunata (Morax-Axenfeld bacillus)
Neisseria species
The product does not provide adequate coverage against:
Pseudomonas aeruginosa
Serratia marcescens
Contraindications: This product is contraindicated in persons sensitive to any of its components.
Warnings: SEE BOX WARNING
Precautions: The prolonged use of antibiotics may occasionally result in overgrowth of nonsusceptible organisms, including fungi. If new infections appear during medication, the drug should be discontinued and appropriate measures should be taken.
In all serious infections the topical use of chloramphenicol should be supplemented by appropriate systemic medication.
Adverse Reactions: Blood dyscrasias have been reported in association with the use of chloramphenicol (See WARNINGS).
Dosage and Administration: Two drops applied to the affected eye every three hours, or more frequently if deemed advisable by the prescribing physician. Administration should be continued day and night for the first 48 hours, after which the interval between applications may be increased. Treatment should be continued for at least 48 hours after the eye appears normal.
Directions for dispensing—Prepare solution by adding sterile distilled water to the vial as follows:

Strength of solution desired	Add sterile distilled water
0.5%	5 ml
0.25%	10 ml
0.16%	15 ml

Solutions remain stable at room temperature for ten days.
How Supplied: N 0071-3213-35 Chloromycetin (chloramphenicol) Ophthalmic is supplied in a package containing dry ingredients in a 15 ml vial and also a vial containing 15 ml of Sterile Distilled Water for use as a diluent in preparing the solution for ophthalmic use. A sterilized dropper-cap assembly for use on the vial of solution is included in the package.
Store below 30°C (86°F).
Chloromycetin, brand of chloramphenicol. Reg US Pat Off

3213G011

CHLOROMYCETIN®
[chlō″rō-my-cē′tĭn]
OPHTHALMIC OINTMENT, 1%
(chloramphenicol ophthalmic ointment, USP)

> **WARNING**
> Bone marrow hypoplasia including aplastic anemia and death has been reported following local application of chloramphenicol. Chloramphenicol should not be used when less potentially dangerous agents would be expected to provide effective treatment.

Description: Each gram of Chloromycetin Ophthalmic Ointment, 1% contains 10 mg chloramphenicol in a special base of liquid petrolatum and polyethylene. It contains no preservatives. Sterile ointment.
The chemical names for chloramphenicol are:
(1) Acetamide,2,2-dichloro-N-[2-hydroxy-1-(hydroxymethyl)-2-(4-nitrophenyl) ethyl]-, and
(2) D-$threo$-(–)-2,2-Dichloro-N-[β-hydroxy-α-(hydroxymethyl)-p-nitrophenethyl] acetamide

Clinical Pharmacology: Chloramphenicol is a broad-spectrum antibiotic originally isolated from *Streptomyces venezuelae*. It is primarily bacteriostatic and acts by inhibition of protein synthesis by interfering with the transfer of activated amino acids from soluble RNA to ribosomes. It has been noted that chloramphenicol is found in measurable amounts in the aqueous humor following local application to the eye. Development of resistance to chloramphenicol can be regarded as minimal for staphylococci and many other species of bacteria.

Indications and Usage: Chloramphenicol should be used only in those serious infections for which less potentially dangerous drugs are ineffective or contraindicated. Bacteriological studies should be performed to determine the causative organisms and their sensitivity to chloramphenicol (See Box Warning).
Chloromycetin (chloramphenicol) Ophthalmic Ointment, 1% is indicated for the treatment of surface ocular infections involving the conjunctiva and/or cornea caused by chloramphenicol-susceptible organisms.
The particular antiinfective drug in this product is active against the following common bacterial eye pathogens:
Staphylococcus aureus
Streptococci, including *Streptococcus pneumoniae*
Escherichia coli
Haemophilus influenzae
Klebsiella/Enterobacter species
Moraxella lacunata (Morax-Axenfeld bacillus)
Neisseria species
The product does not provide adequate coverage against:
Pseudomonas aeruginosa
Serratia marcescens

Contraindications: This product is contraindicated in persons sensitive to any of its components.
Warnings: SEE BOX WARNING
Ophthalmic ointments may retard corneal wound healing.
Precautions: The prolonged use of antibiotics may occasionally result in overgrowth of nonsusceptible organisms, including fungi. If new infections appear during medication, the drug should be discontinued and appropriate measures should be taken.
In all serious infections the topical use of chloramphenicol should be supplemented by appropriate systemic medication.
Adverse Reactions: Blood dyscrasias have been reported in association with the use of chloramphenicol (See WARNINGS).
Dosage and Administration: A small amount of ointment placed in the lower conjunctival sac every three hours, or more frequently if deemed advisable by the prescribing physician. Administration should be continued day and night for the first 48 hours, after which the interval between applications may be increased. Treatment should be continued for at least 48 hours after the eye appears normal.
How Supplied:
N 0071-3070-07
Chloromycetin Ophthalmic Ointment, 1% (Chloramphenicol Ophthalmic Ointment, USP) is supplied, sterile, in ophthalmic ointment tubes of 3.5 grams.
Chloromycetin, brand of chloramphenicol. Reg US Pat Off
AHFS Category 52:04.04   3070G021

CHLOROMYCETIN® OTIC
[chlō″rō-my-cē′tĭn ō′-tĭc]
(chloramphenicol otic)

Description: Each milliliter of Chloromycetin Otic contains 5 mg (0.5%) chloramphenicol in propylene glycol. Sterile.
Clinical Pharmacology: Chloramphenicol is a broad-spectrum antibiotic originally isolated from *Streptomyces venezuelae*. It is primarily bacteriostatic and acts by inhibition of protein synthesis by interfering with the transfer of activated amino acids from soluble RNA to ribosomes. Development of resistance to chloramphenicol can be regarded as minimal for staphylococci and many other species of bacteria.
Indications and Usage: Chloromycetin (chloramphenicol) Otic is indicated for the treatment of superficial infections of the external auditory canal caused by susceptible strains of various gram-positive and gram-negative organisms including:
Staphylococcus aureus, Escherichia coli, Hemophilus influenzae, Pseudomonas aeruginosa, Aerobacter aerogenes, Klebsiella pneumoniae, and *Proteus* species.
Deeper infections should be treated with appropriate systemic antibiotics.
Contraindication: This product is contraindicated in persons sensitive to any of its components.
Warnings: Bone marrow hypoplasia, including aplastic anemia and death, has been reported following the local application of chloramphenicol.
Precautions: The prolonged use of antibiotics may occasionally result in overgrowth of nonsusceptible organisms, including fungi. If new infections appear during medication, the drug should be discontinued and appropriate measures should be taken.
In all except very superficial infections, the topical use of chloramphenicol should be supplemented by appropriate systemic medication.
Adverse Reactions: Signs of local irritation, with subjective symptoms of itching or burning, angioneurotic edema, urticaria, vesicular and maculopapular dermatitis, have been reported in patients sensitive to chloramphenicol and are causes for discontinuing the medication. Similar sensitivity reactions to other materials in topical preparations may also occur. Blood dyscrasias have been reported in association with the use of chloramphenicol (See WARNINGS).
Dosage and Administration: Instill 2 or 3 drops into the ear three times daily.
How Supplied: N 0071-3313-35—Chlor-omycetin (chloramphenicol) Otic is supplied in 15-ml vials with droppers.
AHFS 52:04.04   3313G021
                       121 870600/21

ORAL SUSPENSION
CHLOROMYCETIN® PALMITATE
[chlō″rō-my-ce′tĭn păl′mĭ-tāte″]
(chloramphenicol palmitate oral suspension)

> **WARNING**
> Serious and fatal blood dyscrasias (aplastic anemia, hypoplastic anemia, thrombocytopenia, and granulocytopenia) are known to occur after the administration of chloramphenicol. In addition, there have been reports of aplastic anemia attributed to chloramphenicol which later terminated in leukemia. Blood dyscrasias have occurred after both short-term and prolonged therapy with this drug. Chloramphenicol must not be used when less potentially dangerous agents will be effective, as described in the Indications section. *It must not be used in the treatment of trivial infections or where it is not indicated, as in colds, influenza, infections of the throat; or as a prophylactic agent to prevent bacterial infections.*
> **Precautions:** It is essential that adequate blood studies be made during treatment with the drug. While blood studies may detect early peripheral blood changes, such as leukopenia, reticulocytopenia, or granulocytopenia, before they become irreversible, such studies cannot be relied on to detect bone marrow depression prior to development of aplastic anemia. To facilitate appropriate studies and observation during therapy, it is desirable that patients be hospitalized.

Description: Chloramphenicol is an antibiotic that is clinically useful for, *and should be reserved for,* serious infections caused by organisms susceptible to its antimicrobial effects when less potentially hazardous therapeutic agents are ineffective or contraindicated. Sensitivity testing is essential to determine its indicated use, but may be performed concurrently with therapy initiated on clinical impression that one of the indicated conditions exists (see Indications section).
Actions and Pharmacology: *In vitro* chloramphenicol exerts mainly a bacteriostatic effect on a wide range of gram-negative and gram-positive bacteria and is active *in vitro* against rickettsiae, the lymphogranuloma-psittacosis group and *Vibrio cholerae*. It is particularly active against *Salmonella typhi* and *Hemophilus influenzae*. The mode of action is through interference or inhibition of protein synthesis in intact cells and in cell-free systems.
Chloramphenicol administered orally is absorbed rapidly from the intestinal tract. In controlled studies in adult volunteers using the recommended dosage of 50 mg/kg/day, a dosage of 1 g every 6 hours for 8 doses was given. Using the microbiological assay method, the average peak serum level was 11.2 mcg/ml one hour after the first dose.
A cumulative effect gave a peak rise to 18.4 mcg/ml after the fifth dose of 1 g. Mean serum levels ranged from 8 to 14 mcg/ml over the 48-hour period. Total urinary excretion of chloramphenicol in these studies ranged from a low of 68% to a high of 99% over a three-day period. From 8% to 12% of the antibiotic excreted is in the form of free chloramphenicol; the remainder consists of microbiologically inactive metabolites, principally the conjugate with glucuronic acid. Since the glucuronide is excreted rapidly, most chloramphenicol detected in the blood is in the microbiologically active free form. Despite the small proportion of unchanged drug excreted in the urine, the concentration of free chloramphenicol is relatively high, amounting to several hundred mcg/ml in patients receiving divided doses of 50 mg/kg/day. Small amounts of active drug are found in bile and feces. Chloramphenicol diffuses rapidly, but its distribution is not uniform. Highest concentrations are found in liver and kidney, and lowest concentrations are found in brain and cerebrospinal fluid. Chloramphenicol enters cerebrospinal fluid even in the absence of meningeal inflammation, appearing in concentrations about half of those found in the blood. Measurable levels are also detected in pleural and in ascitic fluids, saliva, milk and in the aqueous and vitreous humors. Transport across the placental barrier occurs with some-

Continued on next page

This product information was prepared in August, 1984. On these and other Parke-Davis Products, information may be obtained by addressing PARKE-DAVIS, Division of Warner-Lambert Company, Morris Plains, New Jersey 07950.

Parke-Davis—Cont.

what lower concentration in cord blood of newborn infants than in maternal blood.

Indications: In accord with the concepts in the Warning Box and this Indications section, chloramphenicol must be used only in those serious infections for which less potentially dangerous drugs are ineffective or contraindicated. However, chloramphenicol may be chosen to initiate antibiotic therapy on the clinical impression that one of the conditions below is believed to be present; *in vitro* sensitivity tests should be performed concurrently so that the drug may be discontinued as soon as possible if less potentially dangerous agents are indicated by such tests. The decision to continue use of chloramphenicol rather than another antibiotic when both are suggested by *in vitro* studies to be effective against a specific pathogen should be based upon severity of the infection, susceptibility of the pathogen to the various antimicrobial drugs, efficacy of the various drugs in the infection, and the important additional concepts contained in the Warning Box above.

1. **Acute infections caused by *Salmonella typhi***
Chloramphenicol is a drug of choice.* It is not recommended for the routine treatment of the typhoid carrier state.
2. **Serious infections caused by susceptible strains in accordance with the concepts expressed above:**
   a. Salmonella species
   b. *H influenzae,* specifically meningeal infections
   c. Rickettsia
   d. Lymphogranuloma-psittacosis group
   e. Various gram-negative bacteria causing bacteremia, meningitis or other serious gram-negative infections
   f. Other susceptible organisms which have been demonstrated to be resistant to all other appropriate antimicrobial agents.
3. **Cystic fibrosis regimens**

* In the treatment of typhoid fever some authorities recommend that chloramphenicol be administered at therapeutic levels for 8 to 10 days after the patient has become afebrile to lessen the possibility of relapse.

Contraindications: Chloramphenicol is contraindicated in individuals with a history of previous hypersensitivity and/or toxic reaction to it. *It must not be used in the treatment of trivial infections or where it is not indicated, as in colds, influenza, infections of the throat; or as a prophylactic agent to prevent bacterial infections.*

Precautions:
1. Baseline blood studies should be followed by periodic blood studies approximately every two days during therapy. The drug should be discontinued upon appearance of reticulocytopenia, leukopenia, thrombocytopenia, anemia, or any other blood study findings attributable to chloramphenicol. However, it should be noted that such studies do not exclude the possible later appearance of the irreversible type of bone marrow depression.
2. Repeated courses of the drug should be avoided if at all possible. Treatment should not be continued longer than required to produce a cure with little or no risk of relapse of the disease.
3. Concurrent therapy with other drugs that may cause bone marrow depression should be avoided.
4. Excessive blood levels may result from administration of the recommended dose to patients with impaired liver or kidney function, including that due to immature metabolic processes in the infant. The dosage should be adjusted accordingly or, preferably, the blood concentration should be determined at appropriate intervals.
5. There are no studies to establish the safety of this drug in pregnancy.
6. Since chloramphenicol readily crosses the placental barrier, caution in use of the drug is particularly important during pregnancy at term or during labor because of potential toxic effects on the fetus (gray syndrome).
7. Precaution should be used in therapy of premature and full-term infants to avoid "gray syndrome" toxicity. (See "Adverse Reactions.") Serum drug levels should be carefully followed during therapy of the newborn infant.
8. Precaution should be used in therapy during lactation because of the possibility of toxic effects on the nursing infant.
9. The use of this antibiotic, as with other antibiotics, may result in an overgrowth of nonsusceptible organisms, including fungi. If infections caused by nonsusceptible organisms appear during therapy, appropriate measures should be taken.

Adverse Reactions:
1. **Blood Dyscrasias**
The most serious adverse effect of chloramphenicol is bone marrow depression. Serious and fatal blood dyscrasias (aplastic anemia, hypoplastic anemia, thrombocytopenia, and granulocytopenia) are known to occur after the administration of chloramphenicol. An irreversible type of marrow depression leading to aplastic anemia with a high rate of mortality is characterized by the appearance weeks or months after therapy of bone marrow aplasia or hypoplasia. Peripherally, pancytopenia is most often observed, but in a small number of cases only one or two of the three major cell types (erythrocytes, leukocytes, platelets) may be depressed.

A reversible type of bone marrow depression, which is dose related, may occur. This type of marrow depression is characterized by vacuolization of the erythroid cells, reduction of reticulocytes and leukopenia, and responds promptly to the withdrawal of chloramphenicol.

An exact determination of the risk of serious and fatal blood dyscrasias is not possible because of lack of accurate information regarding 1) the size of the population at risk, 2) the total number of drug-associated dyscrasias, and 3) the total number of nondrug associated dyscrasias.

In a report to the California State Assembly by the California Medical Association and the State Department of Public Health in January 1967, the risk of fatal aplastic anemia was estimated at 1:24,200 to 1:40,500 based on two dosage levels. There have been reports of aplastic anemia attributed to chloramphenicol which later terminated in leukemia.

Paroxysmal nocturnal hemoglobinuria has also been reported.

2. **Gastrointestinal Reactions**
Nausea, vomiting, glossitis and stomatitis, diarrhea and enterocolitis may occur in low incidence.

3. **Neurotoxic Reactions**
Headache, mild depression, mental confusion and delirium have been described in patients receiving chloramphenicol. Optic and peripheral neuritis have been reported, usually following long-term therapy. If this occurs, the drug should be promptly withdrawn.

4. **Hypersensitivity Reactions**
Fever, macular and vesicular rashes, angioedema, urticaria and anaphylaxis may occur. Herxheimer reactions have occurred during therapy for typhoid fever.

5. **"Gray Syndrome"**
Toxic reactions including fatalities have occurred in the premature and newborn, the signs and symptoms associated with these reactions have been referred to as the gray syndrome. One case of gray syndrome has been reported in an infant born to a mother having received chloramphenicol during labor. One case has been reported in a 3-month-old infant. The following summarizes the clinical and laboratory studies that have been made on these patients.
(a) In most cases therapy with chloramphenicol had been instituted within the first 48 hours of life.
(b) Symptoms first appeared after 3 to 4 days of continued treatment with high doses of chloramphenicol
(c) The symptoms appeared in the following order:
   1) abdominal distention with or without emesis;
   2) progressive pallid cyanosis;
   3) vasomotor collapse, frequently accompanied by irregular respiration;
   4) death within a few hours of onset of these symptoms.
(d) The progression of symptoms from onset to exitus was accelerated with higher dose schedules.
(e) Preliminary blood serum level studies revealed unusually high concentrations of chloramphenicol (over 90 mcg/ml after repeated doses).
(f) Termination of therapy upon early evidence of the associated symptomatology frequently reversed the process with complete recovery.

Dosage and Administration:

Dosage Recommendations
The majority of microorganisms susceptible to chloramphenicol will respond to a concentration between 5 and 20 mcg/ml. The desired concentration of active drug in blood should fall within this range over most of the treatment period. Dosage of 50 mg/kg/day divided into 4 doses at intervals of 6 hours will usually achieve and sustain levels of this magnitude.

Except in certain circumstances (eg. premature and newborn infants and individuals with impairment of hepatic or renal function) lower doses may not achieve these concentrations. Chloramphenicol, like other potent drugs, should be prescribed at recommended doses known to have therapeutic activity. Close observation of the patient should be maintained and in the event of any adverse reactions, dosage should be reduced or the drug discontinued, if other factors in the clinical situation permit.

Adults
Adults should receive 50 mg/kg/day in divided doses at 6-hour intervals. In exceptional cases patients with infections due to moderately resistant organisms may require increased dosage up to 100 mg/kg/day to achieve blood levels inhibiting the pathogen, but these high doses should be decreased as soon as possible. Adults with impairment of hepatic or renal function or both may have reduced ability to metabolize and excrete the drug. In instances of impaired metabolic processes, dosages should be adjusted accordingly. (See discussion under Newborn Infants.) Precise control of concentration of the drug in the blood should be carefully followed in patients with impaired metabolic processes by the available microtechniques (information available on request).

Children
Dosage of 50 mg/kg/day divided into 4 doses at 6-hour intervals yields blood levels in the range effective against most susceptible organisms. Severe infections (eg. bacteremia or meningitis), especially when adequate cerebrospinal fluid concentrations are desired, may require dosage up to 100 mg/kg/day; however, it is recommended that dosage be reduced to 50 mg/kg/day as soon as possible. Children with impaired liver or kidney function may retain excessive amounts of the drug.

Newborn Infants
(See section titled "Gray Syndrome" under Adverse Reactions.)
A total of 25 mg/kg/day in 4 equal doses at 6-hour intervals usually produces and maintains concentrations in blood and tissues adequate to control most infections for which the drug is indicated. Increased dosage in these individuals, demanded by severe infections, should be given only to maintain the blood concentration within a therapeutically effective range. After the first two weeks of life, full-term infants ordinarily may receive up to a total of 50 mg/kg/day equally divided into 4 doses at 6-hour intervals. *These dosage recommendations are extremely important because blood concentration in all premature infants and full-term infants under two weeks of age differs from that of other infants.* This difference is due to variations in the maturity of the metabolic functions of the liver and the kidneys.

When these functions are immature (or seriously impaired in adults), high concentrations of the drug are found which tend to increase with succeeding doses.

Infants and Children with Immature Metabolic Processes
In young infants and other children in whom immature metabolic functions are suspected, a dose of 25 mg/kg/day will usually produce therapeutic

concentrations of the drug in the blood. In this group particularly, the concentration of the drug in the blood should be carefully followed by microtechniques. (Information available on request.)

How Supplied:
N 0071-2310-15
Oral Suspension Chloromycetin (chloramphenicol) Palmitate, each 5 ml contains chloramphenicol palmitate equivalent to 150 mg chloramphenicol with 0.5% sodium benzoate as preservative, in bottles of 60 ml.

Chloramphenicol Palmitate is hydrolyzed to chloramphenicol before absorption. Resulting blood concentration is similar to that produced by the oral administration of chloramphenicol.

Chloromycetin, brand of chloramphenicol. Reg. US Pat Off

2310G040

CHLOROMYCETIN® ℞
[chlō″rō-my-cē′tin sŭc′cĭ-nāte″]
SODIUM SUCCINATE
(sterile chloramphenicol sodium succinate, USP)
FOR INTRAVENOUS ADMINISTRATION

WARNING
Serious and fatal blood dyscrasias (aplastic anemia, hypoplastic anemia, thrombocytopenia, and granulocytopenia) are known to occur after the administration of chloramphenicol. In addition, there have been reports of aplastic anemia attributed to chloramphenicol which later terminated in leukemia. Blood dyscrasias have occurred after both short-term and prolonged therapy with this drug. Chloramphenicol must not be used when less potentially dangerous agents will be effective, as described in the Indications section. *It must not be used in the treatment of trivial infections or where it is not indicated, as in colds, influenza, infections of the throat; or as a prophylactic agent to prevent bacterial infections.*
Precautions: It is essential that adequate blood studies be made during treatment with the drug. While blood studies may detect early peripheral blood changes, such as leukopenia, reticulocytopenia, or granulocytopenia, before they become irreversible, such studies cannot be relied on to detect bone marrow depression prior to development of aplastic anemia. To facilitate appropriate studies and observation during therapy, it is desirable that patients be hospitalized.

IMPORTANT CONSIDERATIONS IN PRESCRIBING INJECTABLE CHLORAMPHENICOL SODIUM SUCCINATE
CHLORAMPHENICOL SODIUM SUCCINATE IS INTENDED FOR INTRAVENOUS USE ONLY. IT HAS BEEN DEMONSTRATED TO BE INEFFECTIVE WHEN GIVEN INTRAMUSCULARLY.
1. Chloramphenicol sodium succinate must be hydrolyzed to its microbiologically active form and there is a lag in achieving adequate blood levels compared with the base given intravenously.
2. The oral form of chloramphenicol is readily absorbed and adequate blood levels are achieved and maintained on the recommended dosage.
3. Patients started on intravenous chloramphenicol sodium succinate should be changed to the oral form as soon as practicable.
Description: Chloramphenicol is an antibiotic that is clinically useful for, *and should be reserved for,* serious infections caused by organisms susceptible to its antimicrobial effects when less potentially hazardous therapeutic agents are ineffective or contraindicated. Sensitivity testing is essential to determine its indicated use, but may be performed concurrently with therapy initiated on clinical impression that one of the indicated conditions exists (see Indications section).

Each gram (10 ml of a 10% solution) of chloramphenicol sodium succinate contains approximately 52 mg (2.25 mEq) of sodium.
Actions and Pharmacology: *In vitro* chloramphenicol exerts mainly a bacteriostatic effect on a wide range of gram-negative and gram-positive bacteria and is active *in vitro* against rickettsiae, the lymphogranuloma-psittacosis group, and *Vibrio cholerae.* It is particularly active against *Salmonella typhi* and *Hemophilus influenzae.* The mode of action is through interference or inhibition of protein synthesis in intact cells and in cell-free systems.

Chloramphenicol administered orally is absorbed rapidly from the intestinal tract. In controlled studies in adult volunteers using the recommended dosage of 50 mg/kg/day, a dosage of 1 g every 6 hours for 8 doses was given. Using the microbiological assay method, the average peak serum level was 11.2 mcg/ml one hour after the first dose. A cumulative effect gave a peak rise to 18.4 mcg/ml after the fifth dose of 1 g. Mean serum levels ranged from 8 to 14 mcg/ml over the 48-hour period. Total urinary excretion of chloramphenicol in these studies ranged from a low of 68% to a high of 99% over a three-day period. From 8 to 12% of the antibiotic excreted is in the form of free chloramphenicol; the remainder consists of microbiologically inactive metabolites, principally the conjugate with glucuronic acid. Since the glucuronide is excreted rapidly, most chloramphenicol detected in the blood is in the microbiologically active free form. Despite the small proportion of unchanged drug excreted in the urine, the concentration of free chloramphenicol is relatively high, amounting to several hundred mcg/ml in patients receiving divided doses of 50 mg/kg/day. Small amounts of active drug are found in bile and feces. Chloramphenicol diffuses rapidly, but its distribution is not uniform. Highest concentrations are found in liver and kidney, and lowest concentrations are found in brain and cerebrospinal fluid. Chloramphenicol enters cerebrospinal fluid even in the absence of meningeal inflammation, appearing in concentrations about half of those found in the blood. Measurable levels are also detected in pleural and in ascitic fluids, saliva, milk, and in the aqueous and vitreous humors. Transport across the placental barrier occurs with somewhat lower concentration in cord blood of newborn infants than in maternal blood.

Indications: In accord with the concepts in the warning box and this Indications section, chloramphenicol must be used only in those serious infections for which less potentially dangerous drugs are ineffective or contraindicated. However, chloramphenicol may be chosen to initiate antibiotic therapy on the clinical impression that one of the conditions below is believed to be present; *in vitro* sensitivity tests should be performed concurrently so that the drug may be discontinued as soon as possible if less potentially dangerous agents are indicated by such tests. The decision to continue use of chloramphenicol rather than another antibiotic when both are suggested by *in vitro* studies to be effective against a specific pathogen should be based upon severity of the infection, susceptibility of the pathogen to the various antimicrobial drugs, efficacy of the various drugs in the infection, and the important additional concepts contained in the Warning Box above:
1. Acute infections caused by *S typhi**
It is not recommended for the routine treatment of the typhoid carrier state.
2. Serious infections caused by susceptible strains in accordance with the concepts expressed above:
 a. *Salmonella* species
 b. *H influenzae,* specifically meningeal infections
 c. Rickettsia
 d. Lymphogranuloma-psittacosis group
 e. Various gram-negative bacteria causing bacteremia, meningitis, or other serious gram-negative infections
 f. Other susceptible organisms which have been demonstrated to be resistant to all other appropriate antimicrobial agents.

3. Cystic fibrosis regimens

*In the treatment of typhoid fever, some authorities recommend that chloramphenicol be administered at therapeutic levels for 8 to 10 days after the patient has become afebrile to lessen the possibility of relapse.
Contraindications: Chloramphenicol is contraindicated in individuals with a history of previous hypersensitivity and/or toxic reaction to it. *It must not be used in the treatment of trivial infections or where it is not indicated, as in colds, influenza, infections of the throat; or as a prophylactic agent to prevent bacterial infection.*
Precautions:
1. Baseline blood studies should be followed by periodic blood studies approximately every two days during therapy. The drug should be discontinued upon appearance of reticulocytopenia, leukopenia, thrombocytopenia, anemia, or any other blood study findings attributable to chloramphenicol. However, it should be noted that such studies do not exclude the possible later appearance of the irreversible type of bone marrow depression.
2. Repeated courses of the drug should be avoided if at all possible. Treatment should not be continued longer than required to produce a cure with little or no risk of relapse of the disease.
3. Concurrent therapy with other drugs that may cause bone marrow depression should be avoided.
4. Excessive blood levels may result from administration of the recommended dosage to patients with impaired liver or kidney function, including that due to immature metabolic processes in the infant. The dosage should be adjusted accordingly or, preferably, the blood concentration should be determined at appropriate intervals.
5. There are no studies to establish the safety of this drug in pregnancy.
6. Since chloramphenicol readily crosses the placental barrier, caution in use of the drug is particularly important during pregnancy at term or during labor because of potential toxic effects on the fetus (gray syndrome).
7. Precaution should be used in therapy of premature and full-term infants to avoid gray syndrome toxicity (see Adverse Reactions). Serum drug levels should be carefully followed during therapy of the newborn infant.
8. Precaution should be used in therapy during lactation because of the possibility of toxic effects on the nursing infant.
9. The use of this antibiotic, as with other antibiotics, may result in an overgrowth of nonsusceptible organisms, including fungi. If infections caused by nonsusceptible organisms appear during therapy, appropriate measures should be taken.
Adverse Reactions:
1. Blood Dyscrasias
The most serious adverse effect of chloramphenicol is bone marrow depression. Serious and fatal blood dyscrasias (aplastic anemia, hypoplastic anemia, thrombocytopenia, and granulocytopenia) are known to occur after the administration of chloramphenicol. An irreversible type of marrow depression leading to aplastic anemia with a high rate of mortality is characterized by the appearance weeks or months after therapy of bone marrow aplasia or hypoplasia. Peripherally, pancytopenia is most often observed, but in a small number of cases only one or two of the three major cell types (erythrocytes, leukocytes, platelets) may be depressed.

A reversible type of bone marrow depression, which is dose-related, may occur. This type of marrow depression is characterized by vacuolization of the erythroid cells, reduction of reticulocytes, and

Continued on next page

This product information was prepared in August, 1984. On these and other Parke-Davis Products, information may be obtained by addressing PARKE-DAVIS, Division of Warner-Lambert Company, Morris Plains, New Jersey 07950.

Parke-Davis—Cont.

leukopenia, and responds promptly to the withdrawal of chloramphenicol.

An exact determination of the risk of serious and fatal blood dyscrasias is not possible because of lack of accurate information regarding (1) the size of the population at risk, (2) the total number of drug-associated dyscrasias, and (3) the total number of nondrug-associated dyscrasias.

In a report to the California State Assembly by the California Medical Association and the State Department of Public Health in January 1967, the risk of fatal aplastic anemia was estimated at 1:24,200 to 1:40,500 based on two dosage levels. There have been reports of aplastic anemia attributed to chloramphenicol which later terminated in leukemia.

Paroxysmal nocturnal hemoglobinuria has also been reported.

2. Gastrointestinal Reactions
Nausea, vomiting, glossitis and stomatitis, diarrhea, and enterocolitis may occur in low incidence.

3. Neurotoxic Reactions
Headache, mild depression, mental confusion, and delirium have been described in patients receiving chloramphenicol. Optic and peripheral neuritis have been reported, usually following long-term therapy. If this occurs, the drug should be promptly withdrawn.

4. Hypersensitivity Reactions
Fever, macular and vesicular rashes, angioedema, urticaria, and anaphylaxis may occur. Herxheimer reactions have occurred during therapy for typhoid fever.

5. "Gray Syndrome"
Toxic reactions including fatalities have occurred in the premature and newborn; the signs and symptoms associated with these reactions have been referred to as the gray syndrome. One case of gray syndrome has been reported in an infant born to a mother having received chloramphenicol during labor. One case has been reported in a 3-month-old infant. The following summarizes the clinical and laboratory studies that have been made on these patients:

a) In most cases, therapy with chloramphenicol had been instituted within the first 48 hours of life.
b) Symptoms first appeared after 3 to 4 days of continued treatment with high doses of chloramphenicol.
c) The symptoms appeared in the following order:
  (1) abdominal distention with or without emesis;
  (2) progressive pallid cyanosis;
  (3) vasomotor collapse, frequently accompanied by irregular respiration;
  (4) death within a few hours of onset of these symptoms.
d) The progression of symptoms from onset to exitus was accelerated with higher dose schedules.
e) Preliminary blood serum level studies revealed unusually high concentrations of chloramphenicol (over 90 mcg/ml after repeated doses).
f) Termination of therapy upon early evidence of the associated symptomatology frequently reversed the process with complete recovery.

Administration: Chloramphenicol, like other potent drugs, should be prescribed at recommended doses known to have therapeutic activity. Administration of 50 mg/kg/day in divided doses will produce blood levels of the magnitude to which the majority of susceptible microorganisms will respond.

As soon as feasible, an oral dosage form of chloramphenicol should be substituted for the intravenous form because adequate blood levels are achieved with chloramphenicol by mouth.

The following method of administration is recommended:

Intravenously as a 10% (100 mg/ml) solution to be injected over at least a one-minute interval. This is prepared by the addition of 10 ml of an aqueous diluent, such as water for injection or 5% dextrose injection.

Dosage:
Adults
Adults should receive 50 mg/kg/day in divided doses at 6-hour intervals. In exceptional cases, patients with infections due to moderately resistant organisms may require increased dosage up to 100 mg/kg/day to achieve blood levels inhibiting the pathogen, but these high doses should be decreased as soon as possible. Adults with impairment of hepatic or renal function or both may have reduced ability to metabolize and excrete the drug. In instances of impaired metabolic processes, dosages should be adjusted accordingly. (See discussion under Newborn Infants.) Precise control of concentration of the drug in the blood should be carefully followed in patients with impaired metabolic processes by the available microtechniques (information available on request).

Children
Dosage of 50 mg/kg/day divided into 4 doses at 6-hour intervals yields blood levels in the range effective against most susceptible organisms. Severe infections (eg, bacteremia or meningitis), especially when adequate cerebrospinal fluid concentrations are desired, may require dosage up to 100 mg/kg/day; however, it is recommended that dosage be reduced to 50 mg/kg/day as soon as possible. Children with impaired liver or kidney function may retain excessive amounts of the drug.

Newborn Infants
(See section titled Gray Syndrome under Adverse Reactions.)
A total of 25 mg/kg/day in 4 equal doses at 6-hour intervals usually produces and maintains concentrations in blood and tissues adequate to control most infections for which the drug is indicated. Increased dosage in these individuals, demanded by severe infections, should be given only to maintain the blood concentration within a therapeutically effective range. After the first two weeks of life, full-term infants ordinarily may receive up to a total of 50 mg/kg/day equally divided into 4 doses at 6-hour intervals. *These dosage recommendations are extremely important because blood concentration in all premature infants and full-term infants under two weeks of age differs from that of other infants.* This difference is due to variations in the maturity of the metabolic functions of the liver and the kidneys.

When these functions are immature (or seriously impaired in adults), high concentrations of the drug are found which tend to increase with succeeding doses.

Infants and Children with Immature Metabolic Processes
In young infants and other children in whom immature metabolic functions are suspected, a dose of 25 mg/kg/day will usually produce therapeutic concentrations of the drug in the blood. In this group particularly, the concentration of the drug in the blood should be carefully followed by microtechniques. (Information available on request.)

How Supplied: N 0071-4057-03—(Steri-Vial® No. 57) Chloromycetin Sodium Succinate (Chloramphenicol Sodium Succinate for Injection, USP) is freeze-dried in the vial and supplied in Steri-Vials (rubber diaphragm-capped vials). When reconstituted as directed, each vial contains a sterile solution equivalent to 100 mg of chloramphenicol per milliliter (1 g/10 ml). Available in packages of 10 vials.

Chloromycetin, brand of chloramphenicol, Reg US Pat Off

AHFS 8:12.08   4057G020

CHLORTHALIDONE ℞
[*chlōr-thăl' lǐ-dōne"*]
Tablets, USP

Description: Chlorthalidone is a monosulfamyl diuretic that differs chemically from thiazide diuretics in that a double-ring system is incorporated in its structure. Chemically it is designated 2-chloro-5-(1-hydroxy-3-oxo-1-isoindo-linyl) benzenesulfonamide. Its empirical formula is $C_{14}H_{11}ClN_2O_4S$.

Chlorthalidone Tablets, USP are available in strengths of 25 mg and 50 mg for oral administration.

Clinical Pharmacology: Chlorthalidone is an oral diuretic with prolonged action (48 to 72 hours) and low toxicity. The diuretic effect of the drug occurs within two hours of an oral dose and continues for up to 72 hours. It produces copious diuresis with greatly increased excretion of sodium and chloride. At maximal therapeutic dosage, chlorthalidone is approximately equal in its diuretic effect to comparable maximal therapeutic doses of benzothiadiazine diuretics. The site of action appears to be the cortical diluting segment of the ascending limb of Henle's loop of the nephron.

Indications and Usage: Diuretics such as chlorthalidone are indicated in the management of hypertension either as the sole therapeutic agent or to enhance the effect of other antihypertensive drugs in the more severe forms of hypertension. Chlorthalidone is indicated as adjunctive therapy in edema associated with congestive heart failure, hepatic cirrhosis, and corticosteroid and estrogen therapy.

Chlorthalidone has also been found useful in edema due to various forms of renal dysfunction such as nephrotic syndrome, acute glomerulonephritis, and chronic renal failure.

Usage in Pregnancy: The routine use of diuretics in an otherwise healthy woman is inappropriate and exposes mother and fetus to unnecessary hazard. Diuretics do not prevent development of toxemia of pregnancy, and there is no satisfactory evidence that they are useful in the treatment of developed toxemia.

Edema during pregnancy may arise from pathological causes or from the physiologic and mechanical consequences of pregnancy. Chlorthalidone is indicated in pregnancy when edema is due to pathologic causes, just as it is in the absence of pregnancy (however, see PRECAUTIONS, below). Dependent edema in pregnancy, resulting from restriction of venous return by the expanded uterus, is properly treated through elevation of the lower extremities and use of support hose; use of diuretics to lower intravascular volume in this case is illogical and unnecessary. There is hypervolemia during normal pregnancy which is harmful to neither the fetus nor the mother (in the absence of cardiovascular disease), but which is associated with edema, including generalized edema, in the majority of pregnant women. If this edema produces discomfort, increased recumbency will often provide relief. In rare instances, this edema may cause extreme discomfort that is not relieved by rest. In these cases, a short course of diuretics may provide relief and may be appropriate.

Contraindications: Anuria.
Hypersensitivity to chlorthalidone or other sulfonamide-derived drugs.

Warnings: Should be used with caution in severe renal disease. In patients with renal disease, chlorthalidone or related drugs may precipitate azotemia. Cumulative effects of the drug may develop in patients with impaired renal function.
Chlorthalidone should be used with caution in patients with impaired hepatic function or progressive liver disease, since minor alterations of fluid and electrolyte balance may precipitate hepatic coma.
Chlorthalidone may add to or potentiate the action of the other antihypertensive drugs. Potentiation occurs with ganglionic or peripheral adrenergic blocking drugs.
Sensitivity reactions may occur in patients with a history of allergy or bronchial asthma.
The possibility of exacerbation or activation of systemic lupus erythematosus has been reported with thiazide diuretics, which are structurally related to chlorthalidone. However, systemic lupus erythematosus has not been reported following chlorthalidone administration.

Precautions: Periodic determination of serum electrolytes to detect possible electrolyte imbalance should be performed at appropriate intervals. All patients receiving chlorthalidone should be observed for clinical signs of fluid or electrolyte imbalance; namely, hyponatremia, hypochloremic alkalosis, and hypokalemia. Serum and urine electrolyte determinations are particularly important when the patient is vomiting excessively or receiving parenteral fluids. Medication such as digitalis may also influence serum electrolytes. Warning signs, irrespective of cause are: dryness of mouth, thirst, weakness, lethargy, drowsiness, restlessness, muscle pains or cramps, muscular fatigue, hypotension, oliguria, tachycardia, and gastrointestinal disturbances such as nausea and vomiting.

Hypokalemia may develop with chlorthalidone as with any other potent diuretic, especially with brisk diuresis, when severe cirrhosis is present, or during concomitant use of corticosteroids or ACTH.

Interference with adequate oral electrolyte intake will also contribute to hypokalemia. Digitalis therapy may exaggerate metabolic effects of hypokalemia especially with reference to myocardial activity.

Any chloride deficit is generally mild and usually does not require specific treatment except under extraordinary circumstances (as in liver disease or renal disease). Dilutional hyponatremia may occur in edematous patients in hot weather; appropriate therapy is water restriction rather than administration of salt except in rare instances when the hyponatremia is life-threatening. In actual salt depletion, appropriate replacement is the therapy of choice.

Hyperuricemia may occur or frank gout may be precipitated in certain patients receiving chlorthalidone.

Insulin requirements in diabetic patients may be increased, decreased, or unchanged. Latent diabetes mellitus may become manifest during chlorthalidone administration.

Chlorthalidone and related drugs may increase the responsiveness to tubocurarine.

The antihypertensive effects of the drug may be enhanced in the postsympathectomy patient.

Chlorthalidone and related drugs may decrease arterial responsiveness to norepinephrine. This diminution is not sufficient to preclude effectiveness of the pressor agent for therapeutic use.

If progressive renal impairment becomes evident, as indicated by a rising nonprotein nitrogen or blood urea nitrogen, a careful reappraisal of therapy is necessary with consideration given to withholding or discontinuing diuretic therapy.

Chlorthalidone and related drugs may decrease serum PBI levels without signs of thyroid disturbance.

Usage in Pregnancy: Reproduction studies in various animal species at multiples of the human dose showed no significant level of teratogenicity; no fetal or congenital abnormalities were observed. Animal data should not be extrapolated for clinical application.

Thiazides cross the placental barrier and appear in cord blood. The use of chlorthalidone and related drugs in pregnant women requires that the anticipated benefits of the drug be weighed against possible hazards to the fetus. These hazards include fetal or neonatal jaundice, thrombocytopenia, and possibly other adverse reactions which have occurred in the adult.

Nursing Mothers: Thiazides cross the placental barrier and appear in breast milk. If use of the drug is deemed essential, the patient should stop nursing.

Adverse Reactions:
Gastrointestinal System Reactions:
anorexia
gastric irritation
nausea
vomiting
cramping
diarrhea
constipation
jaundice (intrahepatic cholestatic jaundice)
pancreatitis
Central Nervous System Reactions:
dizziness
vertigo
paresthesias
headache
xanthopsia
Hematologic Reactions:
leukopenia
agranulocytosis
thrombocytopenia
aplastic anemia
Dermatologic-Hypersensitivity Reactions:
purpura
photosensitivity
rash
urticaria
necrotizing angiitis (vasculitis) (cutaneous vasculitis)
Lyell's syndrome (toxic epidermal necrolysis)
Cardiovascular Reaction: Orthostatic hypotension may occur and may be aggravated by alcohol, barbiturates or narcotics.
Other Adverse Reactions:
hyperglycemia
glycosuria
hyperuricemia
muscle spasm
weakness
restlessness
impotence

Whenever adverse reactions are moderate or severe, chlorthalidone dosage should be reduced or therapy withdrawn.

Overdosage: Symptoms of overdosage include nausea, weakness, dizziness and disturbances of electrolyte balance. There is no specific antidote, but gastric lavage is recommended, followed by supportive treatment. Where necessary, this may include intravenous dextrose-saline with potassium, administered with caution.

Dosage and Administration: Therapy should be individualized according to patient response. This therapy should be titrated to gain maximal therapeutic response as well as the minimal dose possible to maintain that therapeutic response. A single dose given in the morning with food is recommended; divided doses are unnecessary.

Hypertension. Initiation: Therapy should be initiated with a dose of 25 mg or 50 mg as a single daily dose. In some patients a 100-mg dose may lower the blood pressure further, but dosage above this level usually does not increase effectiveness. Increases in serum uric acid and decreases in serum potassium are dose-related over the 25–100 mg/day range.

Maintenance: Maintenance doses may often be lower than initial doses and should be adjusted according to the individual patient. Effectiveness is well sustained during continued use.

Edema. Initiation: Adults, initially 50 to 100 mg daily, or 100 mg on alternate days. Some patients may require 150 to 200 mg at these intervals, or up to 200 mg daily. Dosages above this level, however, do not usually produce a greater response.

Maintenance: Maintenance doses may often be lower than initial doses and should be adjusted according to the individual patient. Effectiveness is well sustained during continued use.

How Supplied: Chlorthalidone Tablets, USP 25 mg (orange, P-D 123) are supplied as:
N 0071-0123-24 Bottle of 100
N 0071-0123-32 Bottle of 1000
N 0071-0123-40 Unit-Dose packages of 100 (10 strips of 10 tablets each).
Chlorthalidone Tablets, USP 50 mg (light blue, P-D 121) are supplied as:
N 0071-0121-24 Bottle of 100
N 0071-0121-32 Bottle of 1000
N 0071-0121-40 Unit-Dose packages of 100 (10 strips of 10 tablets each).

Animal Pharmacology: Biochemical studies in animals have suggested reasons for the prolonged effect of chlorthalidone. Absorption from the gastrointestinal tract is slow because of low solubility. After passage to the liver, some of the drug enters the general circulation, while some is excreted in the bile to be reabsorbed later. In the general circulation, it is distributed widely to the tissues, but is taken up in highest concentrations by the kidneys, where amounts have been found 72 hours after ingestion, long after it has disappeared from other tissues. The drug is excreted unchanged in the urine.

0123G010

CHOLEDYL® ℞
[clō'lĕ-dyl"]
Tablets/Elixir
(oxtriphylline, USP)

Description: Each partially enteric coated tablet contains 200 mg or 100 mg oxtriphylline. Each 5 ml teaspoonful of the elixir contains 100 mg oxtriphylline; alcohol 20%.

NOTE: 100 mg oxtriphylline is equivalent to 64 mg anhydrous theophylline.

Actions: Choledyl (oxtriphylline) is a xanthine bronchodilator—the choline salt of theophylline. Choledyl, compared to aminophylline, is less irritating to the gastric mucosa, more readily absorbed from the gastrointestinal tract, more stable and more soluble.

Like other xanthines, oxtriphylline is known to increase vital capacity which has been impaired by bronchospasm and air-trapping. Development of tolerance has been reported infrequently, and therefore Choledyl is useful for long-term therapy of bronchospasm.

Indications: Choledyl (oxtriphylline) is indicated for relief of acute bronchial asthma and for reversible bronchospasm associated with chronic bronchitis and emphysema.

Warning: Use in pregnancy—animal studies revealed no evidence of teratogenic potential. Safety in human pregnancy has not been established; use during lactation or in patients who are or who may become pregnant requires that the potential benefits of the drug be weighed against its possible hazards to the mother and child.

Precautions: Concurrent use of other xanthine-containing preparations may lead to adverse reactions, particularly CNS stimulation in children.

Adverse Reactions: Gastric distress and, occasionally, palpitation and CNS stimulation have been reported.

Dosage:
Tablets—Adults: 200 mg, 4 times a day.
Elixir—Adults: 200 mg (two teaspoonfuls or 10 ml), 4 times a day; Children (2 to 12): 100 mg (one teaspoonful or 5 ml) per 60 lb body weight, 4 times a day.

Above recommendations are averages. Dosage should be individualized.

Supplied: N 0071-0211—Choledyl 200 mg, yellow, partially enteric coated tablets in bottles of 100, 1000, and unit dose packages (10 x 10 strips);
N 0071-0210-24 Choledyl 100 mg, red partially enteric coated tablets in bottles of 100;
N 0071-2215-23 Choledyl elixir, sherry-flavored in bottles of 16 fl oz (1 pint) 474 ml.
Store between 59° and 86°F (15° and 30°C).

Toxicity:
Oxtriphylline, aminophylline and caffeine appear to be more toxic to newborn than to adult rats. No teratogenic effects have been seen.

Shown in Product Identification Section, page 423
0210 G 010

CHOLEDYL® PEDIATRIC SYRUP ℞
[chō'lĕ-dyl"]
(oxtriphylline)

Description: Choledyl (oxtriphylline) is a xanthine bronchodilator—the choline salt of theophylline.

Each 5 ml of Choledyl Pediatric Syrup contains 50 mg oxtriphylline (equivalent to 32 mg of anhydrous theophylline).

Clinical Pharmacology: Theophylline directly relaxes the smooth muscle of the bronchial air-

Continued on next page

This product information was prepared in August, 1984. On these and other Parke-Davis Products, information may be obtained by addressing PARKE-DAVIS, Division of Warner-Lambert Company, Morris Plains, New Jersey 07950.

Parke-Davis—Cont.

ways and pulmonary blood vessels, thus acting mainly as a bronchodilator, pulmonary vasodilator and smooth muscle relaxant. The drug also possesses other actions typical of the xanthine derivatives: coronary vasodilator, diuretic, cardiac stimulant, cerebral stimulant and skeletal muscle stimulant. The actions of theophylline may be mediated through inhibition of phosphodiesterase and a resultant increase in intracellular cyclic AMP which could mediate smooth muscle relaxation. At concentrations higher than attained *in vivo*, theophylline also inhibits the release of histamine by mast cells.

Theophylline has been shown to react additively with beta agonists that increase intracellular cyclic AMP through the stimulation of adenyl cyclase (isoproterenol).

Apparently, the development of tolerance does not occur with chronic use of theophylline.

The half-life is shortened with cigarette smoking. The half-life is prolonged in alcoholism, reduced hepatic or renal function, congestive heart failure, and in patients receiving antibiotics such as TAO (troleandomycin), erythromycin and clindamycin. High fever for prolonged periods may decrease theophylline elimination.

Theophylline Elimination Characteristics

	Theophylline Clearance Rates (mean ± S.D.)	Half-life Average (mean ± S.D.)
Children (over 6 months of age)	1.45 ± .58 ml/kg/min	3.7 ± 1.1 hours
Adult non-smokers with uncomplicated asthma	.65 ± .19 ml/kg/min	8.7 ± 2.2 hours

Newborn infants have extremely slow clearances and half-lives exceeding 24 hours, which approach those seen for older children after about 3–6 months.

The half-life of theophylline is prolonged in patients with congestive heart failure, in those with reduced hepatic or renal function, and in alcoholism. The half-life of theophylline may also be prolonged by concurrent use of various drugs such as phenobarbital, and certain antibiotics, including troleandomycin, erythromycin, and lincomycin. Theophylline half-life is shortened in cigarette smokers (1 to 2 packs/day) as compared to non-smokers. The increase in theophylline clearance caused by smoking is probably the result of induction of drug metabolizing enzymes that do not readily normalize after cessation of smoking. It appears that between 3 months and 2 years may be necessary for normalization of the effect of smoking on theophylline pharmacokinetics.

Actions: Choledyl (oxtriphylline), the choline salt of theophylline, effects significant improvement in pulmonary function parameters which have been impaired by bronchospasm. It is more soluble than either aminophylline or theophylline.

Indications: Choledyl (oxtriphylline) is indicated for relief of acute and chronic bronchial asthma and for reversible bronchospasm associated with chronic bronchitis and emphysema.

Contraindications: Choledyl is contraindicated in individuals who have shown hypersensitivity to theophylline or to Choledyl (oxtriphylline) or any of its components.

Warnings: Status asthmaticus is a medical emergency. Optimal therapy frequently requires additional medication including corticosteroids when the patient is not rapidly responsive to bronchodilators.

Excessive theophylline doses may be associated with toxicity, and serum theophylline levels are recommended to assure maximal benefit without excessive risk; incidence of toxicity increases at levels greater than 20 mcg theophylline/ml. Morphine, curare, and stilbamidine should be used with caution in patients with airflow obstruction since they stimulate histamine release and can induce asthmatic attacks. These drugs may also suppress respiration leading to respiratory failure. Alternative drugs should be chosen whenever possible.

There is excellent correlation between high blood levels of theophylline resulting from conventional doses and associated clinical manifestations of toxicity in patients with liver dysfunction or chronic obstructive lung disease.

There is excellent correlation between high serum levels of theophylline (over 20 mcg/ml) and the clinical manifestations of toxicity. Careful reduction of dosage and monitoring of serum levels are especially important in patients manifesting a decrease in total body theophylline clearance rate, including those with generalized debility, acute hypoxia, cardiac decompensation, hepatic dysfunction, or renal failure. Dosage reduction may also be necessary in patients who are older than 55 years of age, particularly males.

Serious toxic effects may occur suddenly and are not invariably preceded by minor adverse effects such as nausea, vomiting, and restlessness. Convulsions, tachycardia, or ventricular arrhythmias may be the first sign of toxicity.

Children have a marked sensitivity to the CNS stimulant action of theophylline. Serious toxic effects, including fatalities have been reported in children as well as adults.

Theophylline products may worsen pre-existing arrhythmias.

Precautions: General: Mean half-life in smokers is shorter than nonsmokers. Therefore, smokers may require larger doses of theophylline. Theophylline should not be administered concurrently with other xanthine medications or with xanthine-containing beverages or foods. Use with caution in patients with severe cardiac disease, severe hypoxemia, hypertension, hyperthyroidism, acute myocardial injury, cor pulmonale, congestive heart failure, or liver disease, and in the elderly (especially males) and in neonates. Great caution should especially be used in giving theophylline to patients in congestive heart failure. Such patients have shown markedly prolonged theophylline blood level curves with theophylline persisting in serum for long periods following discontinuation of the drug.

Use theophylline cautiously in patients with a history of peptic ulcer. Theophylline may occasionally act as a local irritant to the G.I. tract although gastrointestinal symptoms are more commonly central and associated with serum theophylline concentrations over 20 mcg/ml.

Drug Interactions: Theophylline-containing preparations have exhibited interaction with the following drugs:

Drug	Effect
Lithium carbonate	Increased excretion of lithium carbonate.
Propranolol	Antagonism of propranolol effect.
Furosemide	Increased furosemide diuresis.
Hexamethonium	Decreased hexamethonium-induced chronotropic effect.
Reserpine	Reserpine-induced tachycardia.
Chlordiazepoxide	Chlordiazepoxide-induced fatty acid mobilization.
Troleandomycin erythromycin or lincomycin	Increased theophylline plasma levels.

Usage in Pregnancy: Safe use of Choledyl (oxtriphylline) in pregnancy and lactation has not been established relative to possible adverse effects on fetal or neonatal development. Therefore Choledyl (oxtriphylline) should not be used in patients who are pregnant or who may become pregnant, or during lactation unless, in the judgment of the physician, the potential benefits outweigh the possible hazards.

Adverse Reactions: The most consistent adverse reactions are usually due to overdose and are:

1. Gastrointestinal: nausea, vomiting, epigastric pain, hematemesis, diarrhea.
2. Central nervous system: headaches, irritability, restlessness, insomnia, reflex hyperexcitability, muscle twitching, clonic and tonic generalized convulsions.
3. Cardiovascular: palpitation, tachycardia, extrasystoles, flushing, hypotension, circulatory failure, life-threatening ventricular arrhythmias.
4. Respiratory: tachypnea.
5. Renal: albuminuria, increased excretion of renal tubular cells and red blood cells, diuresis.
6. Others: hyperglycemia and inappropriate antidiuretic hormone (ADH) syndrome.

Dosage and Administration: Therapeutic serum levels associated with optimal likelihood of benefit and minimal risk of toxicity are considered to be between 10 mcg/ml and 20 mcg/ml. Levels above 20 mcg/ml may produce toxic effects. There is great variation from patient to patient in dosage needed in order to achieve a therapeutic blood level because of variable rates of elimination. Because of this wide variation from patient to patient and the relatively narrow therapeutic blood level range, dosage must be individualized; monitoring of theophylline serum levels is highly recommended.

Dosage should be calculated on the basis of lean (ideal) body weight—mg/kg. Theophylline does not distribute into fatty tissue.

Giving theophylline with food may prevent the rare case of stomach irritation, and although absorption may be slower, it is still complete.

When rapidly absorbed products such as solutions are used, dosing to maintain "around the clock" blood levels generally requires administration every 6 hours to obtain the greatest efficacy for use in children; dosing intervals up to 8 hours may be satisfactory for adults because of their slower elimination. Children and adults requiring higher than average doses may benefit from products with slower absorption. This may allow longer dosing intervals and/or less fluctuation in serum concentration over a dosing interval during chronic therapy. In patients receiving concurrent bronchodilator therapy, eg, beta agonists, downward adjustment of Choledyl (oxtriphylline) dosage is necessary.

[See table on top next page].

II. *Those currently receiving theophylline products:* Determine where possible, the time, amount, route of administration and form of the patient's last dose.

The loading dose for theophylline will be based on the principle that each 0.8 mg/kg of Choledyl (oxtriphylline) (0.5 mg/kg of theophylline) administered as a loading dose will result in a 1 mcg/ml increase in serum theophylline concentration. Ideally, then, the loading dose should be deferred if a serum theophylline concentration can be rapidly obtained. If this is not possible, the clinician must exercise his judgment in selecting a dose based on the potential for benefit and risk. When there is sufficient respiratory distress to warrant a small risk, 4 mg/kg Choledyl (oxtriphylline) (2.5 mg/kg of theophylline) is likely to increase the serum concentration when administered as a loading dose in rapidly absorbed form by only about 5 mcg/ml. If the patient is not already experiencing theophylline toxicity, this is unlikely to result in dangerous adverse effects.

Following the decision regarding loading dose in this group of patients, the subsequent maintenance dosage recommendations are the same as those described above.

To achieve optimal therapeutic theophylline dosage, monitoring of serum theophylline concentrations is recommended. However, it is not always possible or practical to obtain a serum theophylline level.

Patients should be closely monitored for signs of toxicity. The present data suggest that the above dosage recommendations will achieve therapeutic serum concentrations with minimal risk of toxicity for most patients. However, some risk of toxic serum concentration is still present.

Adverse reactions to theophylline often occur when serum theophylline levels exceed 20 mcg/ml.

Chronic Asthma

Theophyllinization is a treatment of first choice for the management of chronic asthma (to prevent symptoms and maintain patent airways). Slow clinical titration is generally preferred to assure acceptance and safety of the medication.

Choledyl (oxtriphylline)

Initial dose: 25 mg*/kg/day or 625 mg/day (whichever is lower) in 3 to 4 divided doses at 6–8 hour intervals.

Increased dose: The above dosage may be increased in approximately 25 percent increments at 2 to 3 day intervals so long as no intolerance is observed until the maximum, indicated below, is reached.

*25 mg Choledyl = 16 mg anhydrous theophylline

Maximum dose of Choledyl Pediatric Syrup without measurement of serum theophylline concentration:

Not to exceed the following: (WARNING: DO NOT ATTEMPT TO MAINTAIN ANY DOSE THAT IS NOT TOLERATED)

Age < 9 years —37.5 mg/kg/day
 **(24 mg/kg/day)
Age 9–12 years —31 mg/kg/day
 **(20 mg/kg/day)
Age 12–16 years —28 mg/kg/day
 **(18 mg/kg/day)
Age > 16 years —20 mg/kg/day
 or 1400 mg/day
 (WHICHEVER IS LESS)
 **(13 mg/kg/day
 or 900 mg/day)
 (WHICHEVER IS LESS)

NOTE: Use ideal body weight for obese patients.
**anhydrous theophylline indicated in ( )

To assist in determining dosage of Choledyl Pediatric Syrup in chronic asthma the above information has been summarized in the Approximate Choledyl Pediatric Syrup Dosage table. [See table below].

Measurement of serum theophylline concentration during chronic therapy

If the above maximum dosages are to be maintained or exceeded, serum theophylline measurement is recommended. This should be obtained at the approximate time of peak absorption (1 to 1½ hours after dosing) during chronic therapy. It is important that the patient will have missed *no* doses during the previous 48 hours and that dosing intervals will have been reasonably typical, with no added doses during that period of time.

DOSAGE ADJUSTMENT BASED ON SERUM THEOPHYLLINE MEASUREMENTS IF THE ABOVE INSTRUCTIONS HAVE NOT BEEN FOLLOWED MAY RESULT IN RISK OF TOXICITY TO THE PATIENT.

Caution should be exercised for younger children who cannot complain of minor side effects. Older adults, those with cor pulmonale, congestive heart failure, and/or liver disease, may have unusually low dosage requirements and thus may experience toxicity at the maximal dosage recommended above.

It is important that no patient be maintained on any dosage that he is not tolerating. In instructing patients to increase dosage according to the schedule above, they should be instructed to not take a subsequent dose if apparent side effects occur and to resume therapy at a lower dose once adverse effects have disappeared.

Overdosage: Serious toxic effects due to overdosage may occur suddenly and are not invariably preceded by minor adverse effects. Therefore, careful observation of the patient and prompt institution of appropriate therapeutic measures are essential in all cases of overdosage. All patients suspected of overdosage should be hospitalized.

Signs and symptoms of overdosage are related primarily to the cardiovascular, gastrointestinal, and central nervous systems.

Cardiovascular symptoms include precordial pain, tachycardia, ventricular and other arrhythmias; also varying degrees of hypotension including in extreme cases, severe shock, cardiovascular collapse and death.

Gastrointestinal symptoms include abdominal pain, nausea, persistent vomiting, and hematemesis.

Central nervous system symptoms include headache, dizziness, restlessness, irritability, tremors, hyperactivity, and agitation followed, in severe cases, by convulsions, drowsiness, coma and death. Treatment of overdosage should be directed toward minimizing absorption and supporting vital functions.

In the alert patient emesis should be induced, followed by appropriate additional measures, as listed below. In the obtunded patient, the airway should be secured immediately by means of an endotracheal tube with cuff inflated. After the airway has been secured, lavage should be carried out, and activated charcoal slurry and a cathartic should be administered.

CNS stimulation may be controlled with diazepam, 0.1–0.3 mg/kg intravenously in children, and 10 mg intravenously in adults. Respiration should be supported by appropriate means. Hypotension and shock should be treated with appropriate fluid replacement, avoiding the use of vasopressors, if possible. Additional supportive measures should be carried out as required.

Serial serum theophylline levels are of value in following the patient's course and in guiding further management.

Forced diuresis is of no value because of the small amount of theophylline excreted unchanged by the kidney. There has been a single report of survival with the use of an activated charcoal column (hemoperfusion) in massive theophylline overdosage.

How Supplied:

N 0071-2217-23—Choledyl Pediatric Syrup, 50 mg oxtriphylline/5 ml (equivalent to 32 mg anhydrous theophylline), is supplied as a vanilla-mint flavored syrup in bottles of 16 fl oz (474 ml).

2217G051

CHOLEDYL® SA ℞
[*chō' lĕ-dyl"*]
(Oxtriphylline)
Sustained Action

Description: Choledyl (oxtriphylline) is a xanthine bronchodilator—the choline salt of theophylline.

Each film-coated Choledyl SA tablet contains 400 mg or 600 mg oxtriphylline (equivalent to 256 mg or 384 mg anhydrous theophylline, respectively). Each tablet of Choledyl SA contains oxtriphylline in a tablet matrix specially designed for the prolonged release of the drug in the gastrointestinal tract. Following release of the drug, the expended wax tablet matrix, which is not absorbed, may be detected in the stool.

Clinical Pharmacology: Choledyl (oxtriphylline), the choline salt of theophylline, effects significant improvement in pulmonary function parameters which have been impaired by bronchospasm. It is more soluble than either aminophylline or theophylline. Film-coated Choledyl SA tablets are less irritating to the gastric mucosa than aminophylline.

Choledyl SA tablets have been formulated to provide therapeutic serum levels when administered

Continued on next page

This product information was prepared in August, 1984. On these and other Parke-Davis Products, information may be obtained by addressing PARKE-DAVIS, Division of Warner-Lambert Company, Morris Plains, New Jersey 07950.

CHOLEDYL (OXTRIPHYLLINE) DOSAGE FOR PATIENT POPULATION

Acute Symptoms of Asthma Requiring Rapid Theophyllinization:

I. *Not currently receiving theophylline products:*

GROUP	ORAL LOADING DOSE CHOLEDYL	MAINTENANCE DOSE FOR NEXT 12 HOURS CHOLEDYL	MAINTENANCE DOSE BEYOND 12 HOURS CHOLEDYL
1. Children 6 months to 9 years	9.4 mg/kg *(6 mg/kg)	6.2 mg/kg q4 hrs *(4 mg/kg q4 hrs)	6.2 mg/kg q6 hrs *(4 mg/kg q6 hrs)
2. Children age 9–16 and young adult smokers	9.4 mg/kg *(6 mg/kg)	4.7 mg/kg q4 hrs *(3 mg/kg q4 hrs)	4.7 mg/kg q6 hrs *(3 mg/kg q6 hrs)
3. Otherwise healthy nonsmoking adults	9.4 mg/kg *(6 mg/kg)	4.7 mg/kg q6 hrs *(3 mg/kg q6 hrs)	4.7 mg/kg q8 hrs *(3 mg/kg q8 hrs)
4. Older patients and patients with cor pulmonale	9.4 mg/kg *(6 mg/kg)	3.1 mg/kg q6 hrs *(2 mg/kg q6 hrs)	3.1 mg/kg q8 hrs *(2 mg/kg q8 hrs)
5. Patients with congestive heart failure, liver failure	9.4 mg/kg *(6 mg/kg)	3.1 mg/kg q8 hrs *(2 mg/kg q8 hrs)	1.6–3.1 mg/kg q12 hrs *(1–2 mg/kg q12 hrs)

*Anhydrous theophylline indicated in ( )

Approximate Choledyl Pediatric Syrup Dosage
(administered every 6 hours)

		< 9 years		9–12 years		12–16 years		> 16 years	
Body Weight		Initial Dose	Max. Dose	Initial Dose	Max. Dose	Initial Dose	Max. Dose	Initial Dose	Max. Dose
lbs.	Kg.	6.2 mg/kg	9.4 mg/kg	6.2 mg/kg	7.8 mg/kg	6.2 mg/kg	7 mg/kg	6.2 mg/kg	5
18	8	1 tsp	1½ tsp	—	—	—	—	—	—
36	16	2 tsp	3 tsp	2 tsp	2½ tsp	—	—	—	—
54	24	3 tsp*	4½ tsp	3 tsp*	3½ tsp	3 tsp*	3½ tsp	—	—
72	32	3 tsp*	6 tsp	3 tsp*	5 tsp	3 tsp*	4½ tsp	3 tsp*	3 tsp
90	40	3 tsp*	7 tsp**	3 tsp*	6 tsp	3 tsp*	5½ tsp	3 tsp*	4 tsp
108	48	3 tsp*	7 tsp**	3 tsp*	7 tsp**	3 tsp*	6½ tsp	3 tsp*	5 tsp

NOTE: The initial dosage may be increased in approximately 25 percent increments at 2 to 3 day intervals as clinically indicated and tolerated until the maximum dosage is reached.

1 mg Choledyl (oxtriphylline) = 0.64 mg anhydrous theophylline

*Initial Dosage should not exceed 625 mg/day Choledyl (400 mg/day theophylline)
**Maximum Dosage should not exceed 1400 mg/day Choledyl (900 mg/day theophylline)

Parke-Davis—Cont.

every 12 hours and minimize the peaks and valleys of serum levels commonly found with shorter acting theophylline products.

The sustained action characteristic of Choledyl SA tablets has been demonstrated in studies in human subjects. Single and multiple dose studies have shown equivalent steady-state theophylline plasma levels of Choledyl SA tablets given every 12 hours when compared with an equal total daily dose of (the nonsustained action) Choledyl Elixir given every six hours.

Theophylline directly relaxes the smooth muscle of the bronchial airways and pulmonary blood vessels, thus acting mainly as a bronchodilator, pulmonary vasodilator and smooth muscle relaxant. The drug also possesses other actions typical of the xanthine derivatives: coronary vasodilator, diuretic, cardiac stimulant, cerebral stimulant and skeletal muscle stimulant. The actions of theophylline may be mediated through inhibition of phosphodiesterase and a resultant increase in intracellular cyclic AMP which could mediate smooth muscle relaxation. At concentrations higher than attained *in vivo*, theophylline also inhibits the release of histamine by mast cells.

Theophylline has been shown to react synergistically with beta agonists that increase intracellular cyclic AMP through the stimulation of adenyl cyclase (isoproterenol).

Apparently, the development of tolerance does not occur with chronic use of theophylline.

The half-life is shortened with cigarette smoking. The half-life is prolonged in alcoholism, reduced hepatic or renal function, congestive heart failure, and in patients receiving antibiotics such as TAO (troleandomycin), erythromycin and clindamycin. High fever for prolonged periods may decrease theophylline elimination.

Theophylline Elimination Characteristics

	Theophylline Clearance Rates (mean ± S.D.)	Half-Life Average (mean ± S.D.)
Children (over 6 months of age)	1.45 ± .58 ml/kg/min	3.7 ± 1.1 hours
Adult non-smokers with uncomplicated asthma	.65 ± .19 ml/kg/min	8.7 ± 2.2 hours

Newborn infants have extremely slow clearance and half-lives exceeding 24 hours, which approach those seen for older children after about 3–6 months.

Older adults with chronic obstructive pulmonary disease, and patients with cor pulmonale or other causes of heart failure, and patients with liver pathology may have much lower clearances with half-lives that may exceed 24 hours.

The half-life of theophylline is prolonged in patients with congestive heart failure, in those with reduced hepatic or renal function, and in alcoholism. The half-life of theophylline may also be prolonged by concurrent use of various drugs such as phenobarbital, and certain antibiotics, including troleandomycin, erythromycin, and lincomycin.

Theophylline half-life is shortened in cigarette smokers (1 to 2 packs/day) as compared to nonsmokers. The increase in theophylline clearance caused by smoking is probably the result of induction of drug metabolizing enzymes that do not readily normalize after cessation of smoking. It appears that between 3 months and 2 years may be necessary for normalization of the effect of smoking on theophylline pharmacokinetics.

Indications: Choledyl (oxtriphylline) is indicated for relief of acute and chronic bronchial asthma and for reversible bronchospasm associated with chronic bronchitis and emphysema.

Contraindications: Choledyl is contraindicated in individuals who have shown hypersensitivity to theophylline or to Choledyl (oxtriphylline) or any of its components.

Warnings: Status asthmaticus is a medical emergency. Optimal therapy frequently requires additional medication including corticosteroids when the patient is not rapidly responsive to bronchodilators.

Excessive theophylline doses may be associated with toxicity, and serum theophylline levels are recommended to assure maximal benefit without excessive risk; incidence of toxicity increases at levels greater than 20 mcg theophylline/ml. Morphine, curare, and stilbamidine should be used with caution in patients with airflow obstruction since they stimulate histamine release and can induce asthmatic attacks. These drugs may also suppress respiration leading to respiratory failure. Alternative drugs should be chosen whenever possible.

There is an excellent correlation between high blood levels of theophylline resulting from conventional doses and associated clinical manifestations of toxicity in patients with liver dysfunction or chronic obstructive lung disease.

There is excellent correlation between high serum levels of theophylline (over 20 mcg/ml) and the clinical manifestations of toxicity. Careful reduction of dosage and monitoring of serum levels is especially important in patients manifesting a decrease in total body theophylline clearance rate, including those with generalized debility, acute hypoxia, cardiac decompensation, hepatic dysfunction, or renal failure. Dosage reduction may also be necessary in patients who are older than 55 years of age, particularly males.

Serious toxic effects may occur suddenly and are not invariably preceded by minor adverse effects such as nausea, vomiting, and restlessness. Convulsions, tachycardia, or ventricular arrhythmias may be the first sign of toxicity.

Children have a marked sensitivity to the CNS stimulant action of theophylline. Serious toxic effects, including fatalities have been reported in children as well as adults.

Theophylline products may worsen pre-existing arrhythmias.

Usage in Pregnancy: Safe use of Choledyl (oxtriphylline) in pregnancy and lactation has not been established relative to possible adverse effects on fetal or neonatal development. Therefore Choledyl (oxtriphylline) should not be used in patients who are pregnant or who may become pregnant, or during lactation unless, in the judgment of the physician, the potential benefits outweigh the possible hazards.

Precautions: Mean half-life in smokers is shorter than nonsmokers, therefore, smokers may require larger doses of theophylline. Theophylline should not be administered concurrently with other xanthine medications or with xanthine-containing beverages or foods. Use with caution in patients with severe cardiac disease, severe hypoxemia, hypertension, hyperthyroidism, acute myocardial injury, cor pulmonale, congestive heart failure, or liver disease, and in the elderly (especially males) and in neonates. Great caution should especially be used in giving theophylline to patients in congestive heart failure. Such patients have shown markedly prolonged theophylline blood level curves with theophylline persisting in serum for long periods following discontinuation of the drug.

Use theophylline cautiously in patients with a history of peptic ulcer. Theophylline may occasionally act as a local irritant to the GI tract although gastrointestinal symptoms are more commonly central and associated with serum theophylline concentrations over 20 mcg/ml.

Adverse Reactions: The most consistent adverse reactions are usually due to overdose and are:
1. Gastrointestinal: nausea, vomiting, epigastric pain, hematemesis, diarrhea.
2. Central nervous system: headaches, irritability, restlessness, insomnia, reflex hyperexcitability, muscle twitching, clonic and tonic generalized convulsions.
3. Cardiovascular: palpitation, tachycardia, extrasystoles, flushing, hypotension, circulatory failure, life-threatening ventricular arrhythmias.
4. Respiratory: tachypnea.
5. Renal: albuminuria, increased excretion of renal tubular cells and red blood cells, diuresis.
6. Others: hyperglycemia, and inappropriate antidiuretic hormone (ADH) syndrome.

Drug Interactions: Theophylline-containing preparations have exhibited interaction with the following drugs:

Drug	Effect
Lithium carbonate	Increased excretion of lithium carbonate.
Propranolol	Antagonism of propranolol effect.
Furosemide	Increased furosemide diuresis.
Hexamethonium	Decreased hexamethonium-induced chronotropic effect
Reserpine	Reserpine-induced tachycardia.
Chlordiazepoxide	Chlordiazepoxide-induced fatty acid mobilization.
Troleandomycin, erythromycin or lincomycin	Increased theophylline plasma levels.

Dosage and Administration: Therapy should be initiated and daily dosage requirements established utilizing a nonsustained-action form of Choledyl (oxtriphylline) (eg, Choledyl Tablets, Elixir).

If the total daily maintenance dosage requirement of the Choledyl (oxtriphylline) nonsustained preparation is established at approximately 1200 mg, Choledyl SA 600 mg Sustained Action Tablets, one every 12 hours, may be substituted to provide smoother steady-state theophylline levels and the convenience of bid dosage. Similarly, if the total daily maintenance dosage is established at approximately 800 mg, Choledyl SA 400 mg Sustained Action Tablets, one every 12 hours, may be substituted.

Therapeutic serum levels associated with optimal likelihood of benefit and minimal risk of toxicity are considered to be between 10 mcg/ml and 20 mcg/ml. Levels above 20 mcg/ml may produce toxic effects.

There is great variation from patient to patient in dosage needed in order to achieve a therapeutic blood level because of variable rates of elimination. Because of this wide variation from patient to patient and the relatively narrow therapeutic blood level range, dosage must be individualized; monitoring of theophylline serum levels is highly recommended.

Dosage should be calculated on the basis of lean (ideal) body weight—mg/kg. Theophylline does not distribute into fatty tissue.

Giving Choledyl (oxtriphylline) with food may prevent the rare case of stomach irritation, and although absorption may be slower, it is still complete.

When rapidly absorbed products such as solutions are used, dosing to maintain "around the clock" blood levels generally requires administration every 6 hours to obtain the greatest efficacy for use in children, dosing intervals up to 8 hours may be satisfactory for adults because of their slower elimination. Children and adults requiring higher than average doses may benefit from products with slower absorption. This may allow longer dosing intervals and/or less fluctuation in serum concentration over a dosing interval during chronic therapy. In patients receiving concurrent bronchodilator therapy, eg, beta agonists, downward adjustment of Choledyl (oxtriphylline) dosage is necessary.

The following dosage information relates to initiation and titration of daily dosage requirements

Product Information

utilizing a nonsustained action form of Choledyl (eg Choledyl Tabs, Elixir).
[See table at right].

II. *Those currently receiving theophylline products:*

Determine where possible, the time, amount, route of administration and form of the patient's last dose.

The loading dose for theophylline will be based on the principle that each 0.8 mg/kg of Choledyl (oxtriphylline) (0.5 mg/kg of theophylline) administered as a loading dose will result in a 1 mcg/ml increase in serum theophylline concentration. Ideally, then, the loading dose should be deferred if a serum theophylline concentration can be rapidly obtained. If this is not possible, the clinician must exercise his judgment in selecting a dose based on the potential for benefit and risk. When there is sufficient respiratory distress to warrant a small risk, 4 mg/kg Choledyl (oxtriphylline) (2.5 mg/kg of theophylline) is likely to increase the serum concentration when administered as a loading dose in rapidly absorbed form by only about 5 mcg/ml. If the patient is not already experiencing theophylline toxicity, this is unlikely to result in dangerous adverse effect.

Following the decision regarding loading dose in this group of patients, the subsequent maintenance dosage recommendations are the same as those described above.

To achieve optimal therapeutic theophylline dosage, monitoring of serum theophylline concentrations is recommended. However, it is not always possible or practical to obtain a serum theophylline level.

Patients should be closely monitored for signs of toxicity. The present data suggests that the above dosage recommendations will achieve therapeutic serum concentrations with minimal risk of toxicity for most patients. However, some risk of toxic serum concentrations is still present.

Adverse reactions to theophylline often occur when serum theophylline levels exceed 20 mcg/ml.

Chronic Asthma

Theophyllinization is a treatment of first choice for the management of chronic asthma (to prevent symptoms and maintain patent airways). Slow clinical titration is generally preferred to assure acceptance and safety of the medication.
[See table below].

Maximum dose of Choledyl (oxtriphylline) without measurement of serum theophylline concentration:

Not to exceed the following: (WARNING: DO NOT ATTEMPT TO MAINTAIN ANY DOSE THAT IS NOT TOLERATED)

Age <9 years	—37.5 mg/kg/day **(24 mg/kg/day)
Age 9–12 years	—31 mg/kg/day **(20 mg/kg/day)
Age 12–16 years	—28 mg/kg/day **(18 mg/kg/day)
Age >16 years	—20 mg/kg/day or 1400 mg/day (WHICHEVER IS LESS) **(13 mg/kg/day or 900 mg/day) (WHICHEVER IS LESS)

Note: Use ideal body weight for obese patients.
**anhydrous theophylline indicated in ( )

If the total daily maintenance dosage requirement of the Choledyl (oxtriphylline) nonsustained preparation is established at approximately 1200 mg, Choledyl SA 600 mg Sustained Action Tablets, one every 12 hours, may be substituted to provide smoother steady-state theophylline levels and the convenience of bid dosage. Similarly, if the total daily maintenance dosage is established at approximately 800 mg, Choledyl SA 400 mg Sustained Action Tablets, one every 12 hours, may be substituted.

Measurement of serum theophylline concentration during chronic therapy

If the above maximum dosages are to be maintained or exceeded, serum theophylline measurement is recommended. This should be obtained at the approximate time of peak absorption (1 to 2 hours after dosing) during chronic therapy. It is important that the patient will have missed *no* doses during the previous 48 hours and that dosing intervals will have been reasonably typical, with no added doses during that period of time.

DOSAGE ADJUSTMENT BASED ON SERUM THEOPHYLLINE MEASUREMENTS IF THE ABOVE INSTRUCTIONS HAVE NOT BEEN FOLLOWED MAY RESULT IN RISK OF TOXICITY TO THE PATIENT.

Caution should be exercised for younger children who cannot complain of minor side effects. Older adults, those with cor pulmonale, congestive heart failure, and/or liver disease, may have unusually low dosage requirements and thus may experience toxicity at the maximal dosage recommended above.

It is important that no patient be maintained on any dosage that he is not tolerating. In instructing patients to increase dosage according to the schedule above, they should be instructed to not take a subsequent dose if apparent side effects occur and to resume therapy at a lower dose once adverse effects have disappeared.

Overdosage: Serious toxic effects due to overdosage may occur suddenly and are not invariably preceded by minor adverse effects. Therefore, careful observation of the patient and prompt institution of appropriate therapeutic measures are essential in all cases of overdosage. All patients suspected of overdosage should be hospitalized.

Signs and symptoms of overdosage are related primarily to the cardiovascular, gastrointestinal, and central nervous systems.

Cardiovascular symptoms include precordial pain, tachycardia, ventricular and other arrhythmias; also varying degrees of hypotension including, in extreme cases, severe shock, cardiovascular collapse and death.

Gastrointestinal symptoms include abdominal pain, nausea, persistent vomiting, and hematemesis.

Central nervous system symptoms include headache, dizziness, restlessness, irritability, tremors, hyperactivity, and agitation followed, in severe cases, by convulsions, drowsiness, coma and death.

Treatment of overdosage should be directed toward minimizing absorption and supporting vital functions.

In the alert patient emesis should be induced, followed by appropriate additional measures, as listed below.

In the obtunded patient, the airway should be secured immediately by means of an endotracheal tube with cuff inflated. After the airway has been secured, lavage should be carried out, and activated charcoal slurry and a cathartic should be administered.

CNS stimulation may be controlled with diazepam, 0.1–0.3 mg/kg intravenously in children, and 10 mg intravenously in adults. Respiration should be supported by appropriate means. Hypotension and shock should be treated with appropriate fluid replacement, avoiding the use of vasopressors, if possible. Additional supportive measures should be carried out as required.

Serial serum theophylline levels are of value in following the patient's course and in guiding further management.

Forced diuresis is of no value because of the small amount of theophylline excreted unchanged by the kidney. There has been a single report of survival with the use of an activated charcoal column (hemoperfusion) in massive theophylline overdosage.

How Supplied:

Choledyl SA 400 mg—each sustained action tablet contains 400 mg oxtriphylline. Available as pink film-coated tablets in bottles of 100 (N 0071-0214-24), and unit-dose 100's (N 0071-0214-40).

Choledyl SA 600 mg—each sustained action tablet contains 600 mg oxtriphylline. Available as tan film-coated tablets in bottles of 100 (N 0071-0221-24), and unit-dose 100's (N 0071-0221-40).

0214G090

Shown in Product Identification Section, page 423

Continued on next page

CHOLEDYL (OXTRIPHYLLINE) DOSAGE FOR PATIENT POPULATION

Acute Symptoms of Asthma Requiring Rapid Theophyllinization:

1. *Not currently receiving theophylline products:*

GROUP	ORAL LOADING DOSE CHOLEDYL	MAINTENANCE DOSE FOR NEXT 12 HOURS CHOLEDYL	MAINTENANCE DOSE BEYOND 12 HOURS CHOLEDYL
1. Children 6 months to 9 years	9.4 mg/kg *(6 mg/kg)	6.2 mg/kg q4 hrs *(4 mg/kg q4 hrs)	6.2 mg/kg q6 hrs *(4 mg/kg q6 hrs)
2. Children age 9–16 and young adult smokers	9.4 mg/kg *(6 mg/kg)	4.7 mg/kg q4 hrs *(3 mg/kg q4 hrs)	4.7 mg/kg q6 hrs *(3 mg/kg q6 hrs)
3. Otherwise healthy nonsmoking adults	9.4 mg/kg *(6 mg/kg)	4.7 mg/kg q6 hrs *(3 mg/kg q6 hrs)	4.7 mg/kg q8 hrs *3 mg/kg q8 hrs)
4. Older patients and patients with cor pulmonale	9.4 mg/kg *(6 mg/kg)	3.1 mg/kg q6 hrs *(2 mg/kg q6 hrs)	3.1 mg/kg q8 hrs *(2 mg/kg q8 hrs)
5. Patients with congestive heart failure, liver failure	9.4 mg/kg *(6 mg/kg)	3.1 mg/kg q8 hrs *(2 mg/kg q8 hrs)	1.6–3.1 mg/kg q12 hrs *(1–2 mg/kg q12 hrs)

*Anhydrous theophylline indicated in ( )

Choledyl (oxtriphylline)

Initial dose:	25 mg*/kg/day or 625 mg/day (whichever is lower) in 3 to 4 divided doses at 6–8 hour intervals.
Increased dose:	The above dosage may be increased in approximately 25 percent increments at 2 to 3 day intervals so long as no intolerance is observed until the maximum indicated below is reached.

*25 mg Choledyl = 16 mg anhydrous theophylline

This product information was prepared in August, 1984. On these and other Parke-Davis Products, information may be obtained by addressing PARKE-DAVIS, Division of Warner-Lambert Company, Morris Plains, New Jersey 07950.

Parke-Davis—Cont.

COLY-MYCIN® M PARENTERAL ℞
[cō″ ly-my′ cĭn pă″ rĕn′ tĕr-ăl]
(sterile colistimethate sodium, USP)
for intramuscular and intravenous use

Description: Coly-Mycin M Parenteral (sterile colistimethate sodium) contains the sodium salt of colistimethate. Colistimethate sodium is a polypeptide antibiotic with an approximate molecular weight of 1750; the empirical formula is $C_{58}H_{105}N_{16}Na_5O_{28}S_5$.

Clinical Pharmacology:
Microbiology
Coly-Mycin M Parenteral has bactericidal activity against the following gram-negative bacilli: *Enterobacter aerogenes, Escherichia coli, Klebsiella pneumoniae,* and *Pseudomonas aeruginosa.*

Human Pharmacology
Typical serum and urine levels following a single 150 mg dose of Coly-Mycin M Parenteral IM or IV in normal adult subjects are shown in Figure 1.

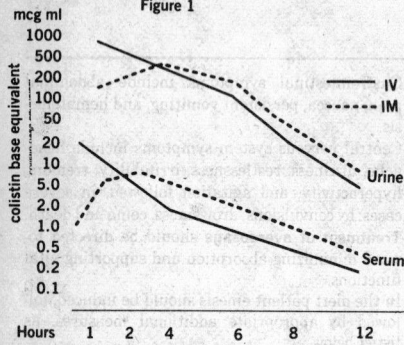

Figure 1. Urine and serum values in adults following parenteral (IM or IV) administration of Coly-Mycin M Parenteral

Higher serum levels were obtained at 10 minutes following IV administration. Serum concentration declined with a half-life of 2-3 hours following either intravenous or intramuscular administration in adults and children, including premature infants.

Colistimethate sodium is transferred across the placental barrier, and blood levels of about 1 mcg/ml are obtained in the fetus following intravenous administration to the mother.

Average urine levels ranged from about 270 mcg/ml at 2 hours to about 15 mcg/ml at 8 hours after intravenous administration and from about 200 to about 25 mcg/ml during a similar period following intramuscular administration.

Indications and Usage: Coly-Mycin M Parenteral (sterile colistimethate sodium) is indicated for the treatment of acute or chronic infections due to sensitive strains of certain gram-negative bacilli. It is particularly indicated when the infection is caused by sensitive strains of *Pseudomonas aeruginosa.* This antibiotic is not indicated for infections due to *Proteus* or *Neisseria.* Coly-Mycin M Parenteral has proven clinically effective in treatment of infections due to the following gram-negative organisms:
Enterobacter aerogenes, Escherichia coli, Klebsiella pneumoniae, and *Pseudomonas aeruginosa.*
Pending results of appropriate bacteriologic cultures and sensitivity tests, Coly-Mycin M Parenteral may be used to initiate therapy in serious infections that are suspected to be due to gram-negative organisms.

Contraindications: The use of Coly-Mycin M Parenteral is contraindicated for patients with a history of sensitivity to the drug.

Warning: Maximum daily dose should not exceed 5 mg/kg/day (2.3 mg/lb) with normal renal function.
Transient neurological disturbances may occur. These include circumoral paresthesias or numbness, tingling or formication of the extremities, generalized pruritus, vertigo, dizziness, and slurring of speech. For these reasons, patients should be warned not to drive vehicles or use hazardous machinery while on therapy. Reduction of dosage may alleviate symptoms. Therapy need not be discontinued, but such patients should be observed with particular care. Overdosage can result in renal insufficiency, muscle weakness and apnea. See PRECAUTIONS for use concomitantly with curariform drugs, and DOSAGE and ADMINISTRATION Section for use in renal impairment.

Precautions: Since Coly-Mycin M Parenteral (sterile colistimethate sodium) is eliminated mainly by renal excretion, it should be used with caution when the possibility of impaired renal function exists. The decline in renal function with advanced age should be considered.

When actual renal impairment is present, Coly-Mycin M Parenteral may be used, but the greatest caution should be exercised and the dosage should be reduced in proportion to the extent of the impairment. Administration of amounts of Coly-Mycin M Parenteral in excess of renal excretory capacity will lead to high serum levels and can result in further impairment of renal function, initiating a cycle which, if not recognized, can lead to acute renal insufficiency, renal shutdown and further concentration of the antibiotic to toxic levels in the body. At this point, interference of nerve transmission at neuromuscular junctions may occur and result in muscle weakness and apnea.

Easily recognized signs indicating the development of impaired renal function are diminishing urine output, rising BUN and serum creatinine. If present, therapy with Coly-Mycin M Parenteral (sterile colistimethate sodium) should be discontinued immediately.

If a life-threatening situation exists, therapy may be reinstated at a lower dosage after blood levels have fallen.

Certain other antibiotics (kanamycin, streptomycin, dihydrostreptomycin, polymyxin, neomycin) have also been reported to interfere with the nerve transmission at the neuromuscular junction. Based on this reported activity, they should not be given concomitantly with Coly-Mycin M Parenteral except with the greatest caution. The antibiotics with a gram-positive antimicrobial spectrum, e.g., penicillin, tetracycline, sodium cephalothin, have not been reported to interfere with nerve transmission and, accordingly, would not be expected to potentiate this activity of Coly-Mycin M Parenteral.

Other drugs, including curariform muscle relaxants (ether, tubocurarine, succinylcholine, gallamine, decamethonium and sodium citrate), potentiate the neuromuscular blocking effect and should be used with extreme caution in patients being treated with Coly-Mycin M Parenteral.

If apnea occurs, it may be treated with assisted respiration, oxygen, and calcium chloride injections.

Use in Pregnancy: The safety of colistimethate sodium during human pregnancy has not been established.

Adverse Reactions: Respiratory arrest has been reported following intramuscular administration of colistimethate sodium. Impaired renal function increases the possibility of apnea and neuromuscular blockade following administration of colistimethate sodium. This has been generally due to failure to follow recommended guidelines, usually overdosage, failure to reduce dose commensurate with degree of renal impairment, and/or concomitant use of other antibiotics or drugs with neuromuscular blocking potential.

A decrease in urine output or increase in blood urea nitrogen or serum creatinine can be interpreted as signs of nephrotoxicity, which is probably a dose-dependent effect of colistimethate sodium. These manifestations of nephrotoxicity are reversible following discontinuation of the antibiotic.

Increases of blood urea nitrogen have been reported for patients receiving Coly-Mycin M Parenteral (sterile colistimethate sodium) at dose levels of 1.6-5 mg/kg per day. The BUN values returned to normal following cessation of Coly-Mycin M Parenteral administration.

Paresthesia, tingling of the extremities or tingling of the tongue and generalized itching or urticaria have been reported by patients who received Coly-Mycin M Parenteral by intravenous or intramuscular injection. In addition, the following adverse reactions have been reported for colistimethate sodium: drug fever and gastrointestinal upset, vertigo, and slurring of speech. The subjective symptoms reported by the adult may not be manifest in infants or young children, thus requiring close attention to renal function.

Dosage and Administration:
Important: Coly-Mycin M Parenteral (sterile colistimethate sodium) is supplied in vials containing colistimethate sodium equivalent to 150 mg colistin base activity per vial.

Reconstitution: The *150-mg* vial should be reconstituted with *2.0 ml* Sterile Water for Injection USP. The reconstituted solution provides colistimethate sodium at a concentration of 75 mg/ml. During reconstitution swirl *gently* to avoid frothing.

Dosage: *Adults and children—intravenous or intramuscular administration*—Coly-Mycin M Parenteral should be given in 2 to 4 divided doses at dose levels of 2.5 to 5 mg/kg per day for patients with normal renal function, depending on the severity of the infection.

The daily dose should be reduced in the presence of any renal impairment, which can often be anticipated from the history.

Modifications of dosage in the presence of renal impairment are presented in Table 1.
[See table on next page].

INTRAVENOUS ADMINISTRATION
1. Direct Intermittent Administration — slowly inject one-half of the total daily dose over a period of 3 to 5 minutes every 12 hours.
2. Continuous Infusion — slowly inject one-half the total daily dose over 3 to 5 minutes. Add the remaining half of the total daily dose of Coly-Mycin M Parenteral to one of the following: 0.9% NaCl; 5% dextrose in 0.9% NaCl; 5% dextrose in water; 5% dextrose in 0.45% NaCl; 5% dextrose in 0.225% NaCl; lactated Ringer's solution, or 10% invert sugar solution. There are not sufficient data to recommend usage of Coly-Mycin M Parenteral with other drugs or with other than the above listed infusion solutions. Administer by slow intravenous infusion starting 1 to 2 hours after the initial dose at a rate of 5-6 mg/hr in the presence of normal renal function. In the presence of impaired renal function, reduce the infusion rate depending on the degree of renal impairment. The choice of intravenous solution and the volume to be employed are dictated by the requirements of fluid and electrolyte management.

Any infusion solution containing colistimethate sodium should be freshly prepared and used for no longer than 24 hours.

How Supplied: Coly-Mycin M Parenteral (sterile colistimethate sodium) is supplied in vials containing colistimethate sodium (150 mg colistin base equivalent per vial) as a white to slightly yellow lyophilized cake and is available as one vial per carton (N 0071-4145-01) or as 50 vials per carton (N 0071-4145-47).

STORE AT CONTROLLED ROOM TEMPERATURE (15° to 30°C) (59° to 86°F).
STORE RECONSTITUTED SOLUTION IN REFRIGERATOR (2° to 8°C) (36° to 46°F) OR AT CONTROLLED ROOM TEMPERATURE (15° to 30°C) (59° to 86°F), and use within 7 days.

Toxicology and Animal Pharmacology:
Acute Toxicity: The intravenous LD_{50} was 41.5 mg/kg in the dog and 739 mg/kg in the mouse;

intramuscular toxicity was 42 mg/kg in the dog and 267 mg/kg in the mouse.

Subacute Toxicity: In albino rabbits and beagle dogs, IV doses of 5, 10 and 20 mg/kg/day for 28 days resulted in elevated blood urea nitrogen in the dog (10 mg/kg/day dose group) and in both 20 mg/kg dose groups.

Clinical Studies: Clinically, Coly-Mycin M Parenteral (sterile colistimethate sodium) has been of particular therapeutic value in acute and chronic urinary tract infections caused by sensitive strains of *Pseudomonas aeruginosa*. Colistimethate sodium is clinically effective in the treatment of infections due to other sensitive gram-negative pathogenic bacilli that have become resistant to broad-spectrum antibiotics.

Colistimethate sodium has been used to treat bacteriuria and overt urinary infections in pregnant women during the third trimester. However, in view of the evidence of possible embryotoxic and teratogenic effects of colistimethate sodium in pregnant rabbits, caution should be exercised in use of this drug in women of childbearing potential.

4145G013

Table 1
SUGGESTED MODIFICATION OF DOSAGE SCHEDULES OF COLY-MYCIN M PARENTERAL (STERILE COLISTIMETHATE SODIUM) FOR ADULTS WITH IMPAIRED RENAL FUNCTION

RENAL FUNCTION	Normal	Mild	Moderate	Considerable
Plasma creatinine, (mg/100 ml)	0.7–1.2	1.3–1.5	1.6–2.5	2.6–4.0
Urea clearance, % of normal	80–100	40–70	25–40	10–25
DOSAGE				
Unit dose of Coly-Mycin M, mg	100–150	75–115	66–150	100–150
Frequency, times/day	4 to 2	2	2 or 1	every 36 hr
Total daily dose, mg	300	150–230	133–150	100
Approximate daily dose, mg/kg/day	5.0	2.5–3.8	2.5	1.5

Note: The suggested unit dose is 2.5–5 mg/kg; however, the time INTERVAL between injections should be increased in the presence of impaired renal function.

COLY-MYCIN® S FOR ORAL SUSPENSION ℞
[cō″ly-my′cĭn]
(colistin sulfate for oral suspension, USP)
FOR ORAL USE ONLY

Description: Coly-Mycin S For Oral Suspension (colistin sulfate for oral suspension) contains the sulfate salt of colistin, a polypeptide antibiotic with a molecular weight of approximately 1170. The empirical formula of colistin is $C_{53}H_{100}N_{16}O_{13}$.

Clinical Pharmacology: Colistin sulfate has *in vitro* bactericidal activity against most gram-negative enteric pathogens, especially enteropathogenic E. coli and *Shigella* (but not *Proteus*). In infants and children, it has effectively controlled acute infections of the intestinal tract due to these pathogens. Susceptible strains of *E. coli* and *Shigella in vitro* or *in vivo* rarely develop resistance to colistin sulfate. Cross resistance to polymyxin B sulfate does exist, but cross resistance to broad spectrum antibiotics has not been encountered.

Indications and Usage: Diarrhea in infants and children, caused by susceptible strains of enteropathogenic *E. coli*.

Gastroenteritis due to *Shigella* organisms. Clinical response may vary due to the absence of tissue levels in the bowel wall.

Contraindications: Known hypersensitivity to the drug.

Warnings: Although colistin sulfate is not absorbed systemically in measurable amounts, it is assumed that slight absorption may occur. Therefore, in the presence of azotemia or, if dosages above the recommended range are used, a potential for possible renal toxicity exists.

With prolonged usage, suppression of intestinal bacterial flora may occur. There may be a resultant overgrowth of organisms (such as *Proteus*); appropriate therapy should be initiated immediately.

Precautions: Renal function should be assessed prior to initiation of therapy.

Adverse Reactions: Within the recommended dosage range, none reported.

Dosage and Administration: The usual dosage of colistin base (supplied as the sulfate) is 5–15 mg/kg/day (2.3–6.8 mg/pound/day) given in three divided doses. Higher doses may be necessary. Each 5 ml of suspension contains the equivalent of 25 mg colistin base. A 10-pound infant would require a total daily dose of 23–68 mg colistin base, given in divided doses (approximately ⅓ to 1 teaspoonful three times a day). A 50-pound patient would require a total daily dose of 115–340 mg colistin base, given in divided doses (approximately 1½–4½ teaspoonfuls three times a day).

Preparation: Coly-Mycin S For Oral Suspension (colistin sulfate for oral suspension) is a dry powder which is reconstituted with 37 ml of distilled water. To reconstitute, slowly add one half of the diluent, replace the cap and shake well. Add the remaining diluent and repeat shaking. Volume after reconstitution is 60 ml. When reconstituted, Coly-Mycin S Oral Suspension is a chocolate-flavored mixture, each 5 ml teaspoonful containing the equivalent of 25 mg of colistin base. Reconstituted Coly-Mycin S Oral Suspension is stable for two weeks when kept below 15°C (59°F).

Supplied: Bottles containing colistin sulfate equivalent to 300 mg colistin base (N 0071-2142-15).

Before reconstitution store between 15° and 30°C.

2142G011

COLY-MYCIN® S OTIC ℞
[cō″ly-my′cĭn s ō′tĭc]
with Neomycin and Hydrocortisone
(colistin sulfate—neomycin sulfate—thonzonium bromide—hydrocortisone acetate otic suspension)

Description: Coly-Mycin S Otic with Neomycin and Hydrocortisone (colistin sulfate-neomycin sulfate-thonzonium bromide-hydrocortisone acetate otic suspension) is a sterile aqueous suspension containing in each ml: Colistin base activity, 3 mg (as the sulfate); Neomycin base activity, 3.3 mg (as the sulfate); Hydrocortisone acetate, 10 mg (1%); Thonzonium bromide, 0.5 mg (0.05%); Polysorbate 80, acetic acid, and sodium acetate in a buffered aqueous vehicle. Thimerosal (mercury derivative), 0.002%, added as a preservative. It is a nonviscous liquid, buffered at pH 5, for instillation into the canal of the external ear or direct application to the affected aural skin.

Clinical Pharmacology:
1. Colistin sulfate—an antibiotic with bactericidal action against most gram-negative organisms, notably *Pseudomonas aeruginosa, E. coli.*, and *Klebsiella-Aerobacter*.
2. Neomycin sulfate—a broad-spectrum antibiotic, bactericidal to many pathogens, notably *Staph aureus* and *Proteus* sp.
3. Hydrocortisone acetate—a corticosteroid that controls inflammation, edema, pruritus and other dermal reactions.
4. Thonzonium bromide—a surface-active agent that promotes tissue contact by dispersion and penetration of the cellular debris and exudate.

Indications and Usage: For the treatment of superficial bacterial infections of the external auditory canal, caused by organisms susceptible to the action of the antibiotics; and for the treatment of infections of mastoidectomy and fenestration cavities, caused by organisms susceptible to the antibiotics.

Contraindications: This product is contraindicated in those individuals who have shown hypersensitivity to any of its components, and in herpes simplex, vaccinia and varicella.

Warnings: As with other antibiotic preparations, prolonged treatment may result in overgrowth of nonsusceptible organisms and fungi.

If the infection is not improved after one week, cultures and susceptibility tests should be repeated to verify the identity of the organism and to determine whether therapy should be changed. Patients who prefer to warm the medication before using should be cautioned against heating the solution above body temperature, in order to avoid loss of potency.

Precautions: General: If sensitization or irritation occurs, medication should be discontinued promptly.

This drug should be used with care in cases of perforated eardrum and in longstanding cases of chronic otitis media because of the possibility of ototoxicity caused by neomycin.

Treatment should not be continued for longer than ten days.

Allergic cross-reactions may occur which could prevent the use of any or all of the following antibiotics for the treatment of future infections: kanamycin, paromomycin, streptomycin, and possibly gentamicin.

Adverse Reactions: Neomycin is a not uncommon cutaneous sensitizer. There are articles in the current literature that indicate an increase in the prevalence of persons sensitive to neomycin.

Dosage and Administration: The external auditory canal should be thoroughly cleansed and dried with a sterile cotton applicator.

For adults, 4 drops of the suspension should be instilled into the affected ear 3 or 4 times daily. For infants and children, 3 drops are suggested because of the smaller capacity of the ear canal. The patient should lie with the affected ear upward and then the drops should be instilled. This position should be maintained for 5 min- utes to facilitate penetration of the drops into the ear canal. Repeat, if necessary, for the opposite ear.

If preferred, a cotton wick may be inserted into the canal and then the cotton may be saturated with the solution. This wick should be kept moist by adding further solution every 4 hours. The wick should be replaced at least once every 24 hours.

Continued on next page

This product information was prepared in August, 1984. On these and other Parke-Davis Products, information may be obtained by addressing PARKE-DAVIS, Division of Warner-Lambert Company, Morris Plains, New Jersey 07950.

Parke-Davis—Cont.

How Supplied:
Coly-Mycin S Otic is supplied as:
N 0071-3141-08—5 ml bottle
N 0071-3141-10—10 ml bottle
Each ml contains: Colistin sulfate equivalent to 3 mg of colistin base, Neomycin sulfate equivalent to 3.3 mg neomycin base, Hydrocortisone acetate 10 mg (1%), Thonzonium bromide 0.5 mg (0.05%), and Polysorbate 80 in an aqueous vehicle buffered with acetic acid and sodium acetate. Thimerosal (mercury derivative) 0.002% added as a preservative.
Shake well before using.
Store at controlled room temperature 15°–30°C (59°–86°F). Stable for 18 months at room temperature; prolonged exposure to higher temperatures should be avoided.

3141G032
121 888150/32

KAPSEALS®
DILANTIN® ℞
[dī-lăn'tĭn"]
(Extended Phenytoin Sodium Capsules, USP)

Description: Phenytoin Sodium is an antiepileptic drug. Phenytoin sodium is related to the barbiturates in chemical structure, but has a five-membered ring. The chemical name is sodium 5,5-diphenyl-2,4-imidazolidinedione.
Each Dilantin—*Extended Phenytoin Sodium Capsule* USP contains 30 mg or 100 mg phenytoin sodium. Product *in vivo* performance is characterized by a slow and extended rate of absorption with peak blood concentrations expected in 4 to 12 hours as contrasted to *Prompt Phenytoin Sodium Capsules* USP with a rapid rate of absorption with peak blood concentration expected in 1½ to 3 hours.
Clinical Pharmacology: Phenytoin is an antiepileptic drug which can be useful in the treatment of epilepsy. The primary site of action appears to be *the motor cortex* where spread of seizure activity is inhibited. Possibly by promoting sodium efflux from neurons, phenytoin tends to *stabilize* the threshold against hyperexcitability caused by excessive stimulation or environmental changes capable of reducing membrane sodium gradient. This includes the reduction of posttetanic potentiation at synapses. Loss of posttetanic potentiation prevents cortical seizure foci from detonating adjacent cortical areas. Phenytoin reduces the maximal activity of brain stem centers responsible for the tonic phase of tonic-clonic (grand mal) seizures. The plasma half-life in man after oral administration of phenytoin averages 22 hours, with a range of 7 to 42 hours. Steady-state therapeutic levels are achieved 7 to 10 days after initiation of therapy with recommended doses of 300 mg/day.
Optimum control without clinical signs of toxicity occurs more often with serum levels between 10 and 20 mcg/ml, although some mild cases of tonic-clonic (grand mal) epilepsy may be controlled with lower-serum levels of phenytoin.
In most patients maintained at a steady dosage, stable phenytoin serum levels are achieved. There may be wide interpatient variability in phenytoin serum levels with equivalent dosages. Patients with unusually low levels may be noncompliant or hypermetabolizers of phenytoin. Unusually high levels result from liver disease, congenital enzyme deficiency or drug interactions which result in metabolic interference. The patient with large variations in phenytoin plasma levels, despite standard doses, presents a difficult clinical problem. Serum level determinations in such patients may be particularly helpful.
Most of the drug is excreted in the bile as inactive metabolites which are then reabsorbed from the intestinal tract and excreted in the urine. Urinary excretion of phenytoin and its metabolites occurs partly through glomerular filtration but more importantly, by tubular secretion. Because phenytoin is hydroxylated in the liver by an enzyme system which is saturable, small incremental doses may produce very substantial increases in serum levels, when these are in the upper range. The steady-state level may be double or triple from an increase in dosage of 10% or more, resulting in toxicity.
Indications and Usage: Dilantin is indicated for the control of tonic-clonic and psychomotor (grand mal and temporal lobe) seizures and prevention and treatment of seizures occurring during or following neurosurgery.
Phenytoin serum level determinations may be necessary for optimal dosage adjustments (see Dosage and Administration).
Contraindications: Phenytoin is contraindicated in those patients who are hypersensitive to phenytoin or other hydantoins.
Warnings: Abrupt withdrawal of phenytoin in epileptic patients may precipitate status epilepticus. When, in the judgment of the clinician, the need for dosage reduction, discontinuation, or substitution of alternative antiepileptic medication arises, this should be done gradually. However, in the event of an allergic or hypersensitivity reaction, rapid substitution of alternative therapy may be necessary. In this case, alternative therapy should be an antiepileptic drug not belonging to the hydantoin chemical class.
There have been a number of reports suggesting a relationship between phenytoin and the development of lymphadenopathy (local or generalized) including benign lymph node hyperplasia, pseudolymphoma, lymphoma, and Hodgkin's Disease. Although a cause and effect relationship has not been established, the occurrence of lymphadenopathy indicates the need to differentiate such a condition from other types of lymph node pathology. Lymph node involvement may occur with or without symptoms and signs resembling serum sickness eg, fever, rash and liver involvement.
In all cases of lymphadenopathy, follow-up observation for an extended period is indicated and every effort should be made to achieve seizure control using alternative antiepileptic drugs.
Acute alcoholic intake may increase phenytoin serum levels while chronic alcoholic use may decrease serum levels.
Usage in Pregnancy:
A number of reports suggests an association between the use of antiepileptic drugs by women with epilepsy and a higher incidence of birth defects in children born to these women. Data are more extensive with respect to phenytoin and phenobarbital, but these are also the most commonly prescribed antiepileptic drugs; less systematic or anecdotal reports suggest a possible similar association with the use of all known antiepileptic drugs. The reports suggesting a higher incidence of birth defects in children of drug-treated epileptic women cannot be regarded as adequate to prove a definite cause and effect relationship. There are intrinsic methodologic problems in obtaining adequate data on drug teratogenicity in humans; genetic factors or the epileptic condition itself may be more important than drug therapy in leading to birth defects. The great majority of the mothers on antiepileptic medication deliver normal infants. It is important to note that antiepileptic drugs should not be discontinued in patients in whom the drug is administered to prevent major seizures, because of the strong possibility of precipitating status epilepticus with attendant hypoxia and threat to life. In individual cases where the severity and frequency of the seizure disorder are such that the removal of medication does not pose a serious threat to the patient, discontinuation of the drug may be considered prior to and during pregnancy, although it cannot be said with any confidence that even minor seizures do not pose some hazards to the developing embryo or fetus. The prescribing physician will wish to weigh these considerations in treating and counseling epileptic women of childbearing potential.
In addition to the reports of increased incidence of congenital malformation, such as cleft lip/palate and heart malformations in children of women receiving phenytoin and other antiepileptic drugs, there have more recently been reports of a fetal hydantoin syndrome. This consists of prenatal growth deficiency, microcephaly and mental deficiency in children born to mothers who have received phenytoin, barbiturates, alcohol, or trimethadione. However, these features are all interrelated and are frequently associated with intrauterine growth retardation from other causes.
There have been isolated reports of malignancies, including neuroblastoma, in children whose mothers received phenytoin during pregnancy.
An increase in seizure frequency during pregnancy occurs in a high proportion of patients, because of altered phenytoin absorption or metabolism. Periodic measurement of serum phenytoin levels is particularly valuable in the management of a pregnant epileptic patient as a guide to an appropriate adjustment of dosage. However, postpartum restoration of the original dosage will probably be indicated.
Neonatal coagulation defects have been reported within the first 24 hours in babies born to epileptic mothers receiving phenobarbital and/or phenytoin. Vitamin K_1 has been shown to prevent or correct this defect and has been recommended to be given to the mother before delivery and the neonate after birth.
Precautions:
General:
The liver is the chief site of biotransformation of phenytoin; patients with impaired liver function, elderly patients, or those who are gravely ill may show early signs of toxicity.
A small percentage of individuals who have been treated with phenytoin have been shown to metabolize the drug slowly. Slow metabolism may be due to limited enzyme availability and lack of induction; it appears to be genetically determined.
Phenytoin should be discontinued if a skin rash appears (see "Warnings" section regarding drug discontinuation). If the rash is exfoliative, purpuric, or bullous or if lupus erythematosus or Stevens-Johnson syndrome is suspected, use of the drug should not be resumed. (See Adverse Reactions.) If the rash is of a milder type (measles-like or scarlatiniform), therapy may be resumed after the rash has completely disappeared. If the rash recurs upon reinstitution of therapy, further phenytoin medication is contraindicated.
Hyperglycemia, resulting from the drug's inhibitory effects on insulin release, has been reported. Phenytoin may also raise the serum glucose level in diabetic patients.
Osteomalacia has been associated with phenytoin therapy and is considered to be due to phenytoin's interference with Vitamin D metabolism.
Phenytoin is not indicated for seizures due to hypoglycemic or other causes. Appropriate diagnostic procedures should be performed as indicated.
Phenytoin is not effective for absence (petit mal) seizures. If tonic-clonic (grand-mal) and absence (petit mal) seizures are present, combined drug therapy is needed.
Information for Patients:
Patients taking phenytoin should be advised of the importance of adhering strictly to the prescribed dosage regimen, and of informing the physician of any clinical condition in which it is not possible to take the drug orally as prescribed, eg, surgery, etc. Patients should also be cautioned on the use of other drugs or alcoholic beverages without first seeking the physician's advice.
The importance of good dental hygiene should be stressed in order to minimize the development of gingival hyperplasia and its complications.
Laboratory Tests:
Phenytoin serum level determinations may be necessary to achieve optimal dosage adjustments.
Drug Interactions:
1. Drugs which may *increase* phenytoin serum levels include: tolbutamide, chloramphenicol, dicumarol, disulfiram, isoniazid, chlordane, phenylbutazone, acute alcohol intake, aminosalicylic acid, chlordiazepoxide HCl, chlorpromazine, diazepam, estrogens, ethosuximide, halothane, methylphenidate, prochlorperazine, sulfaphenazole.
2. Drugs which may *decrease* phenytoin serum levels include: carbamazepine, chronic alcohol abuse, reserpine. Molindon Hydrochloride contains calcium ions which interfere with the absorption of phenytoin.

3. Drugs which may either increase or decrease phenytoin serum levels include: phenobarbital, valproic acid, and sodium valproate. Similarly, the effect of phenytoin on phenobarbital, valproic acid and sodium valproate serum levels is unpredictable.

4. Although not a true drug interaction, tricyclic antidepressants may precipitate seizures in susceptible patients and phenytoin dosage may need to be adjusted.

5. Drugs whose efficacy is impaired by phenytoin include: corticosteroids, coumarin anticoagulants, oral contraceptives, quinidine, and vitamin D. Serum level determinations are especially helpful when possible drug interactions are suspected.

Drug/Laboratory Test Interactions:
Phenytoin may cause decreased serum levels of protein-bound iodine (PBI). It may also produce lower than normal values for dexamethasone or metyrapone tests. Phenytoin may cause raised serum levels of glucose, alkaline phosphatase, and gamma glutamyl transpeptidase (GGT).

Carcinogenesis:
See 'Warnings' section for information on carcinogenesis.

Pregnancy:
See Warnings

Nursing Mothers:
Infant breast feeding is not recommended for women taking this drug because phenytoin appears to be secreted in low concentrations in human milk.

Adverse Reactions:
Central Nervous System: The most common manifestations encountered with phenytoin therapy are referable to this system and are usually dose-related. These include nystagmus, ataxia, slurred speech, and mental confusion. Dizziness, insomnia, transient nervousness, motor twitchings, and headaches have also been observed. There have also been rare reports of phenytoin induced dyskinesias, including chorea, dystonia, tremor and asterixis, similar to those induced by phenothiazine and other neuroleptic drugs.
Gastrointestinal System: Nausea, vomiting and constipation.
Integumentary System: Dermatological manifestations sometimes accompanied by fever have included scarlatiniform or morbilliform rashes. A morbilliform rash (measles-like) is the most common; other types of dermatitis are seen more rarely. Other more serious forms which may be fatal have included bullous, exfoliative or purpuric dermatitis, lupus erythematosus, and Stevens-Johnson syndrome (see Precautions).
Hemopoietic System: Hemopoietic complications, some fatal, have occasionally been reported in association with administration of phenytoin. These have included thrombocytopenia, leukopenia, granulocytopenia, agranulocytosis, and pancytopenia. While macrocytosis and megaloblastic anemia have occurred, these conditions usually respond to folic acid therapy. Lymphadenopathy including benign lymph node hyperplasia, pseudolymphoma, lymphoma, and Hodgkin's Disease have been reported (see Warnings).
Connective Tissue System: Coarsening of the facial features, enlargement of the lips, gingival hyperplasia, hirsutism, and Peyronie's Disease.
Other: Systemic lupus erythematosus, periarteritis nodosa, toxic hepatitis, liver damage, and immunoglobulin abnormalities may occur.

Overdosage: The lethal dose in children is not known. The lethal dose in adults is estimated to be 2 to 5 grams. The initial symptoms are nystagmus, ataxia, and dysarthria. Other signs are tremor, hyperflexia, lethargy, slurred speech, nausea, vomiting. The patient may become comatose and hypertensive. Death is due to respiratory and circulatory depression.
There are marked variations among individuals with respect to phenytoin plasma levels where toxicity may occur. Nystagmus, on lateral gaze, usually appears at 20 mcg/ml, ataxia at 30 mcg/ml, dysarthria and lethargy appear when the plasma concentration is over 40 mcg/ml, but as high a concentration as 50 mcg/ml has been reported without evidence of toxicity. As much as 25 times the therapeutic dose has been taken to result in a serum concentration over 100 mcg/ml with complete recovery.

Treatment:
Treatment is nonspecific since there is no known antidote.
The adequacy of the respiratory and circulatory systems should be carefully observed and appropriate supportive measures employed. Hemodialysis can be considered since phenytoin is not completely bound to plasma proteins. Total exchange transfusion has been used in the treatment of severe intoxication in children.
In acute overdosage the possibility of other CNS depressants, including alcohol, should be borne in mind.

Dosage and Administration:
*Serum concentrations should be monitored in changing from Extended Phenytoin Sodium Capsules USP (Dilantin) to Prompt Phenytoin Sodium Capsules USP.
General:
Dosage should be individualized to provide maximum benefit. In some cases serum blood level determinations may be necessary for optimal dosage adjustments—the clinically effective serum level is usually 10-20 mcg/ml. With recommended dosage, a period of seven to ten days may be required to achieve steady-state blood levels with phenytoin and changes in dosage (increase or decrease) should not be carried out at intervals shorter than seven to ten days.
Adult Dosage:
Divided Daily Dosage
Patients who have received no previous treatment may be started on one 100 mg Dilantin (Extended Phenytoin Sodium Capsule) three times daily and the dosage then adjusted to suit individual requirements. For most adults, the satisfactory maintenance dosage will be one capsule three to four times a day. An increase up to two capsules three times a day may be made, if necessary.
Once-a-Day Dosage:
In adults, if seizure control is established with divided doses of three 100 mg Dilantin capsules daily, once-a-day dosage with 300 mg of extended phenytoin sodium capsules may be considered. Studies comparing divided doses of 300 mg with a single daily dose of this quantity indicated absorption, peak plasma levels, biologic half-life, difference between peak and minimum values, and urinary recovery were equivalent. Once-a-day dosage offers a convenience to the individual patient or to nursing personnel for institutionalized patients and is intended to be used only for patients requiring this amount of drug daily. A major problem in motivating noncompliant patients may also be lessened when the patient can take this drug once a day. However, patients should be cautioned not to miss a dose, inadvertently.
Only extended phenytoin sodium capsules are recommended for once-a-day dosing. Inherent differences in dissolution characteristics and resultant absorption rates of phenytoin due to different manufacturing procedures and/or dosage forms preclude such recommendation for other phenytoin products. When a change in the dosage form or brand is prescribed, careful monitoring of phenytoin serum levels should be carried out.
Loading Dose:
Some authorities have advocated use of an oral loading dose of phenytoin in adults who require rapid steady-state serum levels and where intravenous administration is not desirable. This dosing regimen should be reserved for patients in a clinic or hospital setting where phenytoin serum levels can be closely monitored. Patients with a history of renal or liver disease should not receive the oral loading regimen.
Initially, one gram of phenytoin capsules is divided into 3 doses (400 mg, 300 mg, 300 mg) and administered at two-hourly intervals. Normal maintenance dosage is then instituted 24 hours after the loading dose, with frequent serum level determinations.
Pediatric Dosage:
Initially, 5 mg/kg/day in two or three equally divided doses, with subsequent dosage individualized to a maximum of 300 mg daily. A recommended daily maintenance dosage is usually 4 to 8 mg/kg. Children over 6 years old may require the minimum adult dose (300 mg/day).

How Supplied:
N 0071-0362 (Kapseal 362)—Dilantin 100 mg; in 100's, 1,000's, and unit dose 100's and in a Memo Pack containing 84 unit dose capsules (28 days dosage regimen).
N 0071-0365 (Kapseal 365)—Dilantin 30 mg; in 100's, 1,000's and unit dose 100's.
Shown in Product Identification Section, page 423
Also available as:
N 0071-2214—Dilantin-125® Suspension 125 mg phenytoin/5 ml with a maximum alcohol content not greater than 0.6 percent, available in 8-oz bottles and individual unit dose foil pouches which deliver 5 ml (125 mg phenytoin). The minimum sales unit is 100 pouches.
N 0071-2315—Dilantin-30® Pediatric Suspension 30 mg phenytoin/5 ml with a maximum alcohol content not greater than 0.6 percent; available in 8-oz bottles and individual unit dose foil pouches which deliver 5 ml (30 mg phenytoin). The minimum sales unit is 100 pouches.
N 0071-0375 (Kapseal 375)—Dilantin with Phenobarbital each contain 100 mg phenytoin sodium with 16 mg (¼ gr) phenobarbital; in 100's and 1,000's.
N 0071-0531 (Kapseal 531)—Dilantin with Phenobarbital each contain 100 mg phenytoin sodium with 32 mg (½ gr) phenobarbital; in 100's, 1,000's and unit dose 100's.
N 0071-0007 (Tablet 7)—Dilantin Infatabs® each contain 50 mg phenytoin, 100's and unit dose 100's.
For Parenteral Use:
N 0071-4488-05 (Ampoule 1488)—Dilantin ready-mixed solution containing 50 mg phenytoin sodium per milliliter is supplied in 2-ml ampoules. Packages of ten.
N 0071-4488-41 (Steri-Dose® 4488)—Dilantin ready-mixed solution containing 50 mg phenytoin sodium per milliliter is supplied in a 2-ml sterile disposable syringe (22 gauge × 1¼ inch needle). Packages of ten individually cartoned syringes.
N 0071-4475-35 (Ampoule 1475)—Dilantin ready-mixed solution containing 50 mg phenytoin sodium per milliliter is supplied in 5-ml ampoules with one 6-ml sterile disposable syringe (22 gauge × 1¼ inch needle). Packages of ten.
N 0071-4475-08 (Ampoule 1475)—Dilantin ready-mixed solution containing 50 mg phenytoin sodium per milliliter is supplied in packages of ten 5-ml ampoules without syringes.
Store below 30°C (86°F). Protect from light and moisture.

0362G021

INFATABS®
DILANTIN® ℞
[dī-lăn'tĭn" ĭn'fă-tăbs"]
(Phenytoin Tablets, USP)

NOT FOR ONCE A DAY DOSING
Description: Dilantin is an antiepileptic drug. Dilantin (phenytoin) is related to the barbiturates in chemical structure, but has a five-membered ring. The chemical name is 5,5-diphenyl-2,4-imidazolidinedione.
Each Dilantin Infatab, for oral administration, contains 50 mg phenytoin.
Clinical Pharmacology: Phenytoin is an antiepileptic drug which can be useful in the treatment of epilepsy. The primary site of action appears to be the motor cortex where spread of seizure activity is inhibited. Possibly by promoting sodium efflux from neurons, phenytoin tends to stabilize the threshold against hyperexcitability

Continued on next page

This product information was prepared in August, 1984. On these and other Parke-Davis Products, information may be obtained by addressing PARKE-DAVIS, Division of Warner-Lambert Company, Morris Plains, New Jersey 07950.

Parke-Davis—Cont.

caused by excessive stimulation or environmental changes capable of reducing membrane sodium gradient. This includes the reduction of posttetanic potentiation at synapses. Loss of posttetanic potentiation prevents cortical seizure foci from detonating adjacent cortical areas. Phenytoin reduces the maximal activity of brain stem centers responsible for the tonic phase of tonic-clonic (grand mal) seizures.

Clinical studies using Dilantin Infatabs have shown an average plasma half-life of 14 hours with a range of 7 to 29 hours. Steady-state therapeutic levels are achieved 7 to 10 days after initiation of therapy with recommended doses of 300 mg/day. Optimum control without clinical signs of toxicity occurs more often with serum levels between 10 and 20 mcg/ml, although some mild cases of tonic-clonic (grand mal) epilepsy may be controlled with lower-serum levels of phenytoin.

In most patients maintained at a steady dosage, stable phenytoin serum levels are achieved. There may be wide interpatient variability in phenytoin serum levels with equivalent dosages. Patients with unusually low levels may be noncompliant or hypermetabolizers of phenytoin. Unusually high levels result from liver disease, congenital enzyme deficiency or drug interactions which result in metabolic interference. The patient with large variations in phenytoin plasma levels, despite standard doses, presents a difficult clinical problem. Serum level determinations in such patients may be particularly helpful.

Most of the drug is excreted in the bile as inactive metabolites which are then reabsorbed from the intestinal tract and excreted in the urine. Urinary excretion of phenytoin and its metabolites occurs partly with glomerular filtration but more importantly, by tubular secretion. Because phenytoin is hydroxylated in the liver by an enzyme system which is saturable, small incremental doses may produce very substantial increases in serum levels, when these are in the upper range. The steady-state level may be double or triple from an increase in dosage of 10% or more, resulting in toxicity.

Clinical studies show that chewed and unchewed Dilantin Infatabs are bioequivalent, yield approximately equivalent plasma levels, and are more rapidly absorbed than 100-mg Dilantin Kapseals.®

Indications and Usage: Dilantin Infatabs (Phenytoin Tablets, USP) are indicated for the control of tonic-clonic and psychomotor (grand mal and temporal lobe) seizures and prevention and treatment of seizures occurring during or following neurosurgery. Phenytoin serum level determinations may be necessary for optimal dosage adjustments (see Dosage and Administration).

Contraindications: Phenytoin is contraindicated in those patients who are hypersensitive to phenytoin or other hydantoins.

Warnings: Abrupt withdrawal of phenytoin in epileptic patients may precipitate status epilepticus. When, in the judgment of the clinician, the need for dosage reduction, discontinuation, or substitution of alternative antiepileptic medication arises, this should be done gradually. However, in the event of an allergic or hypersensitivity reaction, rapid substitution of alternative therapy may be necessary. In this case, alternative therapy should be an antiepileptic drug not belonging to the hydantoin chemical class.

There have been a number of reports suggesting a relationship between phenytoin and the development of lymphadenopathy (local or generalized) including benign lymph node hyperplasia, pseudolymphoma, lymphoma, and Hodgkin's Disease. Although a cause and effect relationship has not been established, the occurrence of lymphadenopathy indicates the need to differentiate such a condition from other types of lymph node pathology. Lymph node involvement may occur with or without symptoms and signs resembling serum sickness eg, fever, rash and liver involvement. In all cases of lymphadenopathy, follow-up observation for an extended period is indicated and every effort should be made to achieve seizure control using alternative antiepileptic drugs.

Acute alcoholic intake may increase phenytoin serum levels while chronic alcoholic use may decrease serum levels.

Usage in Pregnancy

A number of reports suggest an association between the use of antiepileptic drugs by women with epilepsy and a higher incidence of birth defects in children born to these women. Data are more extensive with respect to phenytoin and phenobarbital, but these are also the most commonly prescribed antiepileptic drugs; less systematic or anecdotal reports suggest a possible similar association with the use of all known antiepileptic drugs. The reports suggesting a higher incidence of birth defects in children of drug-treated epileptic women cannot be regarded as adequate to prove a definite cause and effect relationship. There are intrinsic methodologic problems in obtaining adequate data on drug teratogenicity in humans: genetic factors or the epileptic condition itself, may be more important than drug therapy in leading to birth defects. The great majority of mothers on antiepileptic medication deliver normal infants. It is important to note that antiepileptic drugs should not be discontinued in patients in whom the drug is administered to prevent major seizures, because of the strong possibility of precipitating status epilepticus with attendant hypoxia and threat to life. In individual cases where the severity and frequency of the seizure disorder are such that the removal of medication does not pose a serious threat to the patient, discontinuation of the drug may be considered prior to and during pregnancy, although it cannot be said with any confidence that even minor seizures do not pose some hazard to the developing embryo or fetus. The prescribing physician will wish to weigh these considerations in treating or counseling epileptic women of childbearing potential.

In addition to the reports of increased incidence of congenital malformations, such as cleft lip/palate and heart malformations in children of women receiving phenytoin and other antiepileptic drugs, there have more recently been reports of a fetal hydantoin syndrome. This consists of prenatal growth deficiency, microcephaly and mental deficiency in children born to mothers who have received phenytoin, barbiturates, alcohol, or trimethadione. However, these features are all interrelated and are frequently associated with intrauterine growth retardation from other causes.

There have been isolated reports of malignancies, including neuroblastoma, in children whose mothers received phenytoin during pregnancy.

An increase in seizure frequency during pregnancy occurs in a high proportion of patients, because of altered phenytoin absorption or metabolism. Periodic measurement of serum phenytoin levels is particularly valuable in the management of a pregnant epileptic patient as a guide to an appropriate adjustment of dosage. However, postpartum restoration of the original dosage will probably be indicated.

Neonatal coagulation defects have been reported within the first 24 hours in babies born to epileptic mothers receiving phenobarbital and/or phenytoin. Vitamin K has been shown to prevent or correct this defect and has been recommended to be given to the mother before delivery and to the neonate after birth.

Precautions:
General

The liver is the chief site of biotransformation of phenytoin; patients with impaired liver function, elderly patients, or those who are gravely ill may show early signs of toxicity.

A small percentage of individuals who have been treated with phenytoin have been shown to metabolize the drug slowly. Slow metabolism may be due to limited enzyme availability and lack of induction; it appears to be genetically determined.

Phenytoin should be discontinued if a skin rash appears (see "Warnings" section regarding drug discontinuation). If the rash is exfoliative, purpuric, or bullous or if lupus erythematosus or Stevens-Johnson syndrome is suspected, use of the drug should not be resumed, (see Adverse Reactions). If the rash is of a milder type (measles-like or scarlatiniform), therapy may be resumed after the rash has completely disappeared. If the rash recurs upon reinstitution of therapy, further phenytoin medication is contraindicated.

Hyperglycemia, resulting from the drug's inhibitory effects on insulin release, has been reported. Phenytoin may also raise the serum glucose level in diabetic patients.

Osteomalacia has been associated with phenytoin therapy and is considered to be due to phenytoin's interference with Vitamin D metabolism.

Phenytoin is not indicated for seizures due to hypoglycemic or other causes. Appropriate diagnostic procedures should be performed as indicated.

Phenytoin is not effective for absence (petit mal) seizures. If tonic-clonic (grand-mal) and absence (petit mal) seizures are present, combined drug therapy is needed.

Information for Patients

Patients taking phenytoin should be advised of the importance of adhering strictly to the prescribed dosage regimen, and of informing the physician of any clinical condition in which it is not possible to take the drug orally as prescribed, eg, surgery, etc. Patients should also be cautioned on the use of other drugs or alcoholic beverages without first seeking the physician's advice.

The importance of good dental hygiene should be stressed in order to minimize the development of gingival hyperplasia and its complications.

Laboratory Tests

Phenytoin serum level determinations may be necessary to achieve optimal dosage adjustments.

Drug Interactions

1. Drugs which may <u>increase</u> phenytoin serum levels include: tolbutamide, chloramphenicol, dicumarol, disulfiram, isoniazid, chlordane, phenylbutazone, acute alcohol intake, aminosalicylic acid, chlordiazepoxide HCl, chlorpromazine, diazepam, estrogens, ethosuximide, halothane, methylphenidate, prochlorperazine, sulfaphenazole.

2. Drugs which may <u>decrease</u> phenytoin serum levels include: carbamazepine, chronic alcohol abuse, reserpine. Molindon Hydrochloride contains calcium ions which interfere with the absorption of phenytoin.

3. Drugs which may either increase or decrease phenytoin serum levels include: Phenobarbital, valproic acid, and sodium valproate. Similarly, the effect of phenytoin on phenobarbital, valproic acid and sodium valproate serum levels is unpredictable.

4. Although not a true drug interaction, tricyclic antidepressants may precipitate seizures in susceptible patients and phenytoin dosage may need to be adjusted.

5. Drugs whose efficacy is impaired by phenytoin include: corticosteroids, coumarin anticoagulants, oral contraceptives, quinidine, and vitamin D.

Serum level determinations are especially helpful when possible drug interactions are suspected.

Drug/Laboratory Test Interactions

Phenytoin may cause decreased serum levels of protein-bound iodine (PBI). It may also produce lower than normal values for dexamethasone or metyrapone tests. Phenytoin may cause raised serum levels of glucose, alkaline phosphatase, and gamma glutamyl transpeptidase (GGT).

Carcinogenesis

See 'Warnings' section for information on carcinogenesis.

Pregnancy

See Warnings

Nursing Mothers

Infant breast-feeding is not recommended for women taking this drug because phenytoin appears to be secreted in low concentrations in human milk.

Adverse Reactions:

Central Nervous System: The most common manifestations encountered with phenytoin therapy are referable to this system and are usually dose-related. These include nystagmus, ataxia, slurred speech, and mental confusion. Dizziness,

insomnia, transient nervousness, motor twitchings, and headache have also been observed.
There have also been rare reports of phenytoin induced dyskinesias, including chorea, dystonia, tremor and asterixis, similar to those induced by phenothiazine and other neuroleptic drugs.

Gastrointestinal System: Nausea, vomiting, and constipation.

Integumentary System: Dermatological manifestations sometimes accompanied by fever have included scarlatiniform or morbilliform rashes. A morbilliform rash (measles-like) is the most common; other types of dermatitis are seen more rarely. Other more serious forms which may be fatal have included bullous, exfoliative or purpuric dermatitis, lupus erythematosus, and Stevens-Johnson syndrome (see Precautions).

Hemopoietic System: Hemopoietic complications, some fatal, have occasionally been reported in association with administration of phenytoin. These have included thrombocytopenia, leukopenia, granulocytopenia, agranulocytosis, and pancytopenia. While macrocytosis and megaloblastic anemia have occurred, these conditions usually respond to folic acid therapy. Lymphadenopathy including benign lymph node hyperplasia, pseudolymphoma, lymphoma, and Hodgkin's Disease have been reported (see Warnings).

Connective Tissue System: Coarsening of the facial features, enlargement of the lips, gingival hyperplasia, hirsutism, and Peyronie's Disease.

Other: Systemic lupus erythematosus, periarteritis nodosa, toxic hepatitis, liver damage, and immunoglobulin abnormalities may occur.

Overdosage: The lethal dose in children is not known. The lethal dose in adults is estimated to be 2 to 5 grams. The initial symptoms are nystagmus, ataxia, and dysarthria. Other signs are tremor, hyperflexia, lethargy, slurred speech, nausea, vomiting. The patient may become comatose and hypertensive. Death is due to respiratory and circulatory depression.

There are marked variations among individuals with respect to phenytoin plasma levels where toxicity may occur. Nystagmus on lateral gaze usually appears at 20 mcg/ml, ataxia at 30 mcg/ml, dysarthria and lethargy appear when the plasma concentration is over 40 mcg/ml, but as high a concentration as 50 mcg/ml has been reported without evidence of toxicity. As much as 25 times the therapeutic dose has been taken to result in a serum concentration over 100 mcg/ml with complete recovery.

Treatment
Treatment is nonspecific since there is no known antidote.
The adequacy of the respiratory and circulatory systems should be carefully observed and appropriate supportive measures employed. Hemodialysis can be considered since phenytoin is not completely bound to plasma proteins. Total exchange transfusion has been used in the treatment of severe intoxication in children.
In acute overdosage the possibility of other CNS depressants, including alcohol, should be borne in mind.

Dosage and Administration: When given in equal doses, Dilantin Infatabs yield higher plasma levels than Dilantin Kapseals.® For this reason, care should be taken when switching a patient from one dosage form to the other.

General
Not for once a day dosing.
Dosage should be individualized to provide maximum benefit. In some cases, serum blood level determinations may be necessary for optimal dosage adjustments—the clinically effective serum level is usually 10–20 mcg/ml. With recommended dosage, a period of seven to ten days may be required to achieve steady-state blood levels with phenytoin and changes in dosage (increase or decrease) should not be carried out at intervals shorter than seven to ten days.
Dilantin Infatabs can be either chewed thoroughly before being swallowed or swallowed whole.

Adult Dosage
Patients who have received no previous treatment may be started on two Infatabs three times daily, and the dose is then adjusted to suit individual requirements. For most adults, the satisfactory maintenance dosage will be six to eight Infatabs daily; an increase to twelve Infatabs daily may be made, if necessary.

Pediatric Dosage
Initially, 5 mg/kg/day in two or three equally divided doses, with subsequent dosage individualized to a maximum of 300 mg daily. A recommended daily maintenance dosage is usually 4 to 8 mg/kg. Children over 6 years old may require the minimum adult dose (300 mg/day). If the daily dosage cannot be divided equally, the larger dose should be given before retiring.

How Supplied:
Dilantin Infatabs are supplied as:
N 0071-0007-24—Bottle of 100.
N 0071-0007-40—Unit dose (10/10's).
Each tablet contains 50 mg phenytoin.
Shown in Product Identification Section, page 423
Store at controlled room temperature (59°–86°F).
Protect from moisture.
Dilantin is also supplied in the following forms:
N 0071-0362-24—Bottle of 100.
N 0071-0362-32—Bottle of 1000.
N 0071-0362-40—Unit dose (10/10's).
Each capsule contains 100 mg phenytoin sodium.
N 0071-0365-24—Bottle of 100.
N 0071-0365-32—Bottle of 1000.
N 0071-0365-40—Unit dose (10/10's).
Each capsule contains 30 mg phenytoin sodium.
N 0071-2214-20—8 oz bottle.
N 0071-2214-40—Unit dose pouches (5 ml × 100).
Each 5 ml of suspension contains 125 mg phenytoin with a maximum alcohol content not greater than 0.6 percent.
N 0071-2315-20—8 oz bottle.
N 0071-2315-40—Unit dose pouches (5 ml × 100).
Each 5 ml of suspension contains 30 mg phenytoin with a maximum alcohol content not greater than 0.6 percent.
N 0071-0375-24—Bottle of 100.
N 0071-0375-32—Bottle of 1000.
Each capsule contains phenytoin sodium 100 mg and phenobarbital 16 mg (¼ gr).
N 0071-0531-24—Bottle of 100.
N 0071-0531-32—Bottle of 1000.
N 0071-0531-40—Unit dose (10/10's).
Each capsule contains phenytoin sodium 100 mg and phenobarbital 32 mg (½ gr).
N 0071-4488-05—2-ml ampoules.
A sterile solution for parenteral use containing 50 mg phenytoin sodium per ml. Supplied in packages of ten.
N 0071-4488-41—2-ml prefilled syringes.
A sterile solution for parenteral use containing 50 mg phenytoin sodium per ml in an individually cartoned disposable syringe (22 gauge × 1 ¼ inch needle). Supplied in packages of ten.
N 0071-4475-35—5-ml ampoules with syringes.
A sterile solution for parenteral use containing 50 mg phenytoin sodium per ml. One 6-ml sterile disposable syringe (22 gauge × 1 ¼ inch needle). Supplied in packages of ten.
N 0071-4475-08—5-ml ampoules.
A sterile solution for parenteral use containing 50 mg phenytoin sodium per ml. Supplied in packages of ten.

0007G041

Parenteral
DILANTIN®
[dī-lăn' tĭn"]
(Phenytoin Sodium Injection, USP)

IMPORTANT NOTE
This drug must be administered slowly. Do not exceed 50 mg per minute intravenously.

Description: Dilantin (phenytoin sodium injection, USP) is a ready-mixed solution of phenytoin sodium in a vehicle containing 40% propylene glycol and 10% alcohol in water for injection, adjusted to pH 12 with sodium hydroxide. Phenytoin sodium is related to the barbiturates in chemical structure, but has a five-membered ring. The chemical name is sodium 5,5-diphenyl-2,4-imidazolidinedione.

Clinical Pharmacology: Phenytoin is an anticonvulsant which may be useful in the treatment of status epilepticus of the grand mal type. The primary site of action appears to be the motor cortex where spread of seizure activity is inhibited. Possibly by promoting sodium efflux from neurons, phenytoin tends to stabilize the threshold against hyperexcitability caused by excessive stimulation or environmental changes capable of reducing membrane sodium gradient. This includes the reduction of posttetanic potentiation at synapses. Loss of posttetanic potentiation prevents cortical seizure foci from detonating adjacent cortical areas. Phenytoin reduces the maximal activity of brain stem centers responsible for the tonic phase of grand mal seizures.

A fall in plasma levels may occur when patients are changed from oral to intramuscular administration. The drop is caused by slower absorption, as compared to oral administration, due to the poor water solubility of phenytoin. Intravenous administration is the preferred route for producing rapid therapeutic serum levels.

There are occasions when intramuscular administration may be required, ie, postoperatively, in comatose patients, for GI upsets. During these periods, a sufficient dose must be administered intramuscularly to maintain the plasma level within the therapeutic range. Where oral dosage is resumed following intramuscular usage, the oral dose should be properly adjusted to compensate for the slow, continuing IM absorption to avoid toxic symptoms.

Patients stabilized on a daily oral regimen of Dilantin experience a drop in peak blood levels to 50–60 percent of stable levels if crossed over to an equal dose administered intramuscularly. However, the intramuscular depot of poorly soluble material is eventually absorbed, as determined by urinary excretion of 5-(p-hydroxyphenyl)-5-phenylhydantoin (HPPH), the principal metabolite, as well as the total amount of drug eventually appearing in the blood.

A short-term (one week) study indicates that patients do not experience the expected drop in blood levels when crossed over to the intramuscular route, if the Dilantin IM dose is increased by 50 percent over the previously established oral dose. To avoid drug cumulation due to absorption from the muscle depots, it is recommended that for the first week back on oral Dilantin, the dose be reduced to half of the original oral dose (one-third of the IM dose). Experience for periods greater than one week is lacking and blood level monitoring is recommended. For administration of Dilantin in patients who cannot take oral medication for periods greater than a week gastric intubation may be considered.

Indications: Parenteral Dilantin is indicated for the control of status epilepticus of the grand mal type, and prevention and treatment of seizures occurring during neurosurgery.

Contraindications: Phenytoin is contraindicated in patients with a history of hypersensitivity to hydantoin products.
Because of its effect on ventricular automaticity, phenytoin is contraindicated in sinus bradycardia, sino-atrial block, second and third degree A-V block, and patients with Adams-Stokes syndrome.

Warnings:
Intravenous administration should not exceed 50 mg per minute.
Phenytoin sodium injection is not indicated in seizures due to hypoglycemia or other causes which may be immediately identified and corrected.

Continued on next page

This product information was prepared in August, 1984. On these and other Parke-Davis Products, information may be obtained by addressing PARKE-DAVIS, Division of Warner-Lambert Company, Morris Plains, New Jersey 07950.

Parke-Davis—Cont.

Appropriate diagnostic procedures should be performed as indicated.

Phenytoin metabolism may be significantly altered by the concomitant use of other drugs, such as:

a. Barbiturates may enhance the rate of metabolism of phenytoin. This effect, however, is variable and unpredictable. It has been reported that in some patients the concomitant administration of carbamazepine resulted in an increased rate of phenytoin metabolism.

b. Coumarin anticoagulants, disulfiram, phenylbutazone, and sulfaphenazole may inhibit the metabolism of phenytoin, resulting in signs of phenytoin toxicity. The effect of dicumarol in inhibiting the metabolism of phenytoin in the liver has been well documented.

c. Isoniazid inhibits the metabolism of phenytoin so that with combined therapy patients who are slow acetylators may suffer from phenytoin intoxication.

d. Tricyclic antidepressants in high doses may precipitate seizures and the dosage of phenytoin may have to be adjusted.

The results of certain clinical laboratory tests, eg, metyrapone, 1-mg dexamethasone, and protein-bound iodine, may be altered if the patient has been receiving phenytoin.

Phenytoin should be used with caution in patients with hypotension and severe myocardial insufficiency.

The intramuscular route is not recommended for the treatment of status epilepticus since blood levels of phenytoin in the therapeutic range cannot be readily achieved with doses and methods of administration ordinarily employed.

Usage in Pregnancy: The effects of Dilantin in human pregnancy and nursing infants are unknown.

Recent reports suggest an association between the use of anticonvulsant drugs by women with epilepsy and an elevated incidence of birth defects in children born to these women. Data are more extensive with respect to phenytoin and phenobarbital, but these are also the most commonly prescribed anticonvulsants; less systematic or anecdotal reports suggest a possible similar association with the use of all known anticonvulsant drugs.

The reports suggesting an elevated incidence of birth defects in children of drug-treated epileptic women cannot be regarded as adequate to prove a definite cause and effect relationship. There are intrinsic methodologic problems in obtaining adequate data on drug teratogenicity in humans; the possibility also exists that other factors, eg, genetic factors or the epileptic condition itself, may be more important than drug therapy in leading to birth defects. The great majority of mothers on anticonvulsant medication deliver normal infants. It is important to note that anticonvulsant drugs should not be discontinued in patients in whom the drug is administered to prevent major seizures because of the strong possibility of precipitating status epilepticus with attendant hypoxia and threat to life. In individual cases where the severity and frequency of the seizure disorder are such that the removal of medication does not pose a serious threat to the patient, discontinuation of the drug may be considered prior to and during pregnancy, although it cannot be said with any confidence that even minor seizures do not pose some hazard to the developing embryo or fetus. The prescribing physician will wish to weigh these considerations in treating or counseling epileptic women of child-bearing potential.

Precautions: The addition of Dilantin solution to intravenous infusion is not recommended due to lack of solubility and resultant precipitation.

The liver is the site of biotransformation. Patients with impaired liver function, elderly patients, or those who are gravely ill may show early toxicity.

A small percentage of individuals who have been treated with phenytoin have been shown to metabolize the drug slowly. Slow metabolism may be due to limited enzyme availability and lack of induction; it appears to be genetically determined.

Drugs that control grand mal are not effective against petit mal seizures. Therefore, if both conditions are present, combined drug therapy is needed.

Each injection of intravenous Dilantin should be followed by an injection of sterile saline through the same needle or intravenous catheter to avoid local venous irritation due to the alkalinity of the solution. Continuous infusion should be avoided.

Hyperglycemia, resulting from the drug's inhibitory effect on insulin release, has been reported. Phenytoin may also raise the blood sugar level in persons already suffering from hyperglycemia.

Adverse Reactions: The most notable signs of toxicity associated with the intravenous use of this drug are cardiovascular collapse and/or central nervous system depression. Hypotension does occur when the drug is administered rapidly by the intravenous route. The *rate* of administration is very important; it should not exceed 50 mg per minute. At this rate, toxicity should be minimized. Severe cardiotoxic reactions and fatalities have been reported with atrial and ventricular conduction depression and ventricular fibrillation. Severe complications are most commonly encountered in elderly or gravely ill patients.

Parenteral Dilantin sometimes causes drowsiness, nystagmus, circumoral tingling, vertigo, nausea and rarely vomiting. When these effects are observed, the plasma concentration is usually above 20 mcg/ml which is just above the usual therapeutic plasma concentration.

Administration of this drug has produced an elevation in plasma glucose concentration.

Dosage and Administration: The addition of Dilantin solution to intravenous infusion is not recommended due to lack of solubility and resultant precipitation.

Not to exceed 50 mg per minute, intravenously.

There is a relatively small margin between full therapeutic effect and minimally toxic doses of this drug.

The solution is suitable for use as long as it remains free of haziness and precipitate. Upon refrigeration or freezing a precipitate might form; this will dissolve again after the solution is allowed to stand at room temperature. The product is still suitable for use. Only a clear solution should be used. A faint yellow coloration may develop, however, this has no effect on the potency of the solution.

In the treatment of status epilepticus, the intravenous route is preferred because of the delay in absorption of phenytoin when administered intramuscularly.

Status Epilepticus:

Intravenously: 150 to 250 mg administered slowly, then 100 to 150 mg 30 minutes later if necessary. Higher doses may be required to control seizures. Dosage for children is usually determined according to weight in proportion to the dosage for a 150-pound adult. Pediatric dosage may also be calculated on the basis of 250 mg per square meter of body surface.

If the state of the patient is such that immobilization of an extremity is impossible due to convulsions, or veins are inaccessible, medication can be given intramuscularly during the attack.

If administration of phenytoin does not terminate the seizure, the clinician may consider the use of other anticonvulsants, intravenous barbiturates, general anesthesia, or other measures.

Neurosurgery: Prophylactic dosage—100 to 200 mg (2 to 4 ml) intramuscularly at approximately 4-hour intervals during surgery and continued during the postoperative period.

When intramuscular administration is required for a patient previously stabilized orally, compensating dosage adjustments are necessary to maintain therapeutic plasma levels. An intramuscular dose 50% greater than the oral dose is necessary to maintain these levels. When returned to oral administration, the dose should be reduced by 50% of the original oral dose for one week to prevent excessive plasma levels due to sustained release from intramuscular tissue sites.

If the patient requires more than a week of IM Dilantin, alternative routes should be explored, such as gastric intubation. For time periods less than one week, the patient shifted back from IM administration should receive one half the original oral dose for the same period of time the patient received IM Dilantin. Monitoring plasma levels would help prevent a fall into the subtherapeutic range. Serum blood level determinations are especially helpful when possible drug interactions are suspected.

Overdosage: The mean lethal dose in adults is estimated to be 2 to 5 grams. The cardinal initial symptoms are nystagmus, ataxia and dysarthria. The patient then becomes comatose, pupils unresponsive and hypotension occurs. Death is due to respiratory depression and apnea. Treatment is nonspecific since there is no known antidote. If the gag reflex is absent, the airway should be supported. Oxygen, vasopressors and assisted ventilation may be necessary for central nervous system, respiratory and cardiovascular depression.

Finally, hemodialysis can be considered since phenytoin is not completely bound to plasma proteins. Total exchange transfusion has been utilized in the treatment of severe intoxication in children.

How Supplied:

N 0071-4488-05 (Ampoule 1488) Dilantin ready-mixed solution containing 50 mg phenytoin sodium per milliliter is supplied in 2-ml ampoules. Packages of ten.

N 0071-4488-41 (Steri-Dose® 4488) Dilantin ready-mixed solution containing 50 mg phenytoin sodium per milliliter is supplied in a 2-ml sterile disposable syringe (22 gauge x 1¼ inch needle). Packages of ten individually cartoned syringes.

N 0071-4475-35 (Ampoule 1475) Dilantin ready-mixed solution containing 50 mg phenytoin sodium per milliliter is supplied in 5-ml ampoules with one 6-ml sterile disposable syringe (22 gauge x 1¼ inch needle). Packages of ten.

N 0071-4475-08 (Ampoule 1475) Dilantin ready-mixed solution containing 50 mg phenytoin sodium per milliliter is supplied in packages of ten 5-ml ampoules without syringes.

AHFS Category 28:12   4475G022

DILANTIN-30® PEDIATRIC/ DILANTIN-125® ℞
[dī-lăn' tĭn]
(Phenytoin Oral Suspension, USP)

Description: Dilantin (phenytoin) is related to the barbiturates in chemical structure, but has a five-membered ring. The chemical name is 5,5-diphenyl-2,4 imidazolidinedione.

Action: Phenytoin is an anticonvulsant drug which can be useful in the treatment of epilepsy. The primary site of action appears to be the motor cortex where spread of seizure activity is inhibited. Possibly by promoting sodium efflux from neurons, phenytoin tends to stabilize the threshold against hyperexcitability caused by excessive stimulation or environmental changes capable of reducing membrane sodium gradient. This includes the reduction of posttetanic potentiation at synapses. Loss of posttetanic potentiation prevents cortical seizure foci from detonating adjacent cortical areas. Phenytoin reduces the maximal activity of brain stem centers responsible for the tonic phase of grand mal seizures.

Indications: Dilantin (phenytoin) is indicated for the control of grand mal and psychomotor seizures.

Contraindication: Dilantin is contraindicated in those patients with a history of hypersensitivity to hydantoin products.

Warnings: Abrupt withdrawal of phenytoin in epileptic patients may precipitate status epilepticus. When in the judgment of the clinician the need for dosage reduction, discontinuation, or substitution of alternative anticonvulsant medication arises, this should be done gradually. In the event of an allergic or hypersensitivity reaction, more rapid substitution of alternative therapy may be necessary. In this case, alternative therapy should be an anticonvulsant not belonging to the hydantoin chemical class. Phenytoin is not indicated in seizures due to hypoglycemia or other causes which may be immediately identified and corrected. Appropriate diagnostic procedures should be performed as indicated.

Phenytoin metabolism may be significantly altered by the concomitant use of other drugs such as:

a. Barbiturates may enhance the rate of metabolism of phenytoin. This effect, however, is variable and unpredictable. It has been reported that in some patients the concomitant administration of carbamazepine resulted in an increased rate of phenytoin metabolism.

b. Coumarin anticoagulants, disulfiram, phenylbutazone, and sulfaphenazole may inhibit the metabolism of phenytoin, resulting in increased serum levels of the drug. This may lead to an increased incidence of nystagmus, ataxia, or other toxic signs. The effect of dicumarol in inhibiting the metabolism of phenytoin in the liver has been well documented.

c. Isoniazid inhibits the metabolism of phenytoin so that with combined therapy, patients who are slow acetylators may suffer from phenytoin intoxication.

d. Tricyclic antidepressants in high doses may precipitate seizures, and the dosage of phenytoin may have to be adjusted accordingly.

Phenytoin may interfere with the metyrapone and the 1-mg dexamethasone tests. It may also suppress the protein-bound iodine. However, this has not been associated with any clinical signs of hypothyroidism, the T-3 is normal.

Usage in Pregnancy: The effects of Dilantin (phenytoin) in human pregnancy and nursing infants are unknown.

Recent reports suggest an association between the use of anticonvulsant drugs by women with epilepsy and an elevated incidence of birth defects in children born to these women. Data are more extensive with respect to phenytoin and phenobarbital, but these are also the most commonly prescribed anticonvulsants; less systematic or anecdotal reports suggest a possible similar association with the use of all known anticonvulsant drugs. The reports suggesting an elevated incidence of birth defects in children of drug-treated epileptic women cannot be regarded as adequate to prove a definite cause and effect relationship. There are intrinsic methodologic problems in obtaining adequate data on drug teratogenicity in humans; the possibility also exists that other factors, eg, genetic factors or the epileptic condition itself, may be more important than drug therapy in leading to birth defects. The great majority of mothers on anticonvulsant medication deliver normal infants. It is important to note that anticonvulsant drugs should not be discontinued in patients in whom the drug is administered to prevent major seizures because of the strong possibility of precipitating status epilepticus with attendant hypoxia and threat to life. In individual cases where the severity and frequency of the seizure disorder are such that the removal of medication does not pose a serious threat to the patient, discontinuation of the drug may be considered prior to and during pregnancy, although it cannot be said with any confidence that even minor seizures do not pose some hazard to the developing embryo or fetus. The prescribing physician will wish to weigh these considerations in treating or counseling epileptic women of childbearing potential.

Precautions: The liver is the chief site of biotransformation of phenytoin; patients with impaired liver function may show early signs of toxicity. Elderly patients or those who are gravely ill may show early signs of toxicity.

A small percentage of individuals who have been treated with phenytoin have been shown to metabolize the drug slowly. Slow metabolism may be due to limited enzyme availability and lack of induction; it appears to be genetically determined.

Phenytoin has been associated with reversible lymph node hyperplasia. If lymph node enlargement occurs in patients on phenytoin, every effort should be made to substitute another anticonvulsant drug or drug combination.

Drugs that control grand mal are not effective for petit mal seizures. Therefore, if both conditions are present, combined drug therapy is needed.

The phenytoin should be discontinued if a skin rash appears (see Warnings section regarding drug discontinuation). If the rash is exfoliative, purpuric, or bullous, use of the drug should not be resumed. If the rash is a milder type (measles-like or scarlatiniform), therapy may be resumed after the rash has completely disappeared. If the rash recurs upon reinstitution of therapy, further phenytoin medication is contraindicated.

Osteomalacia has been associated with anticonvulsant therapy, including phenytoin.

Hyperglycemia, resulting from the drug's inhibitory effect on insulin release, has been reported. Phenytoin may also raise the blood sugar level in persons already suffering from hyperglycemia.

Adverse Reactions:

Central Nervous System: The most common manifestations encountered with phenytoin therapy are referable to this system. These include nystagmus, ataxia, slurred speech, and mental confusion. Dizziness, insomnia, transient nervousness, motor twitchings, and headache have also been observed. These side effects may disappear with continuing therapy at a reduced dosage level.

Gastrointestinal System: Phenytoin may cause nausea, vomiting, and constipation. Administration of the drug with or immediately after meals may help prevent gastrointestinal discomfort.

Integumentary System: Dermatological manifestations sometimes accompanied by fever have included scarlatiniform or morbilliform rashes. A morbilliform rash (measles-like) is the most common; other types of dermatitis are seen more rarely. Rashes are more frequent in children and young adults. Other more serious forms which may be fatal have included bullous, exfoliative, or purpuric dermatitis, lupus erythematosus, and Stevens-Johnson syndrome.

Hemopoietic System: Hemopoietic complications, some fatal, have occasionally been reported in association with administration of phenytoin. These have included thrombocytopenia, leukopenia, granulocytopenia, agranulocytosis, and pancytopenia. While macrocytosis and megaloblastic anemia have occurred, these conditions usually respond to folic acid therapy. The occasional occurrence of lymphadenopathy indicates the need to differentiate such a condition from other lymph gland pathology.

Other: Gingival hyperplasia occurs frequently; this incidence may be reduced by good oral hygiene including gum massage, frequent brushing and appropriate dental care. Polyarthropathy and hirsutism occur occasionally. Hyperglycemia has been reported. Toxic hepatitis, liver damage, and periarteritis nodosa may occur and can be fatal.

Dosage and Administration: Dosage should be individualized to provide maximum benefit. In some cases, serum blood level determinations may be necessary for optimal dosage adjustments—the clinically effective serum level is usually 10–20 mcg/ml. Serum blood level determinations are especially helpful when possible drug interactions are suspected. With recommended dosage, a period of seven to ten days may be required to achieve therapeutic blood levels with Dilantin (phenytoin).

Adult Dose: Patients who have received no previous treatment may be started on one teaspoonful of Dilantin-125 Suspension three times daily, and the dose then adjusted to suit individual requirements. An increase to five teaspoonfuls daily may be made, if necessary.

Pediatric Dose: Initially, 5 mg/kg/day in two or three equally divided doses, with subsequent dosage individualized to a maximum of 300 mg daily. A recommended daily maintenance dosage is usually 4 to 8 mg/kg. Children over 6 years may require the minimum adult dose (300 mg/day).

Management of Overdosage: The mean lethal dose in adults is estimated to be 2 to 5 grams. The cardinal initial symptoms are nystagmus, ataxia, and dysarthria. The patient then becomes comatose, the pupils are unresponsive and hypotension occurs. Death is due to respiratory depression and apnea.

Treatment is nonspecific since there is no known antidote. First, the stomach should be emptied. If the gag reflex is absent, the airway should be supported. Oxygen, vasopressors, and assisted ventilation may be necessary for central nervous system, respiratory, and cardiovascular depression. Finally, hemodialysis can be considered since phenytoin is not completely bound to plasma proteins. Total exchange transfusion has been utilized in the treatment of severe intoxication in children.

How Supplied:

N 0071-2214—Dilantin-125® Suspension (phenytoin oral suspension, USP), 125 mg phenytoin/5 ml with a maximum alcohol content not greater than 0.6 percent; available in 8-oz bottles and individual unit dose foil pouches which deliver 5 ml (125 mg phenytoin). The minimum sales unit is 100 pouches.

N 0071-2315—Dilantin-30® Pediatric Suspension (phenytoin oral suspension, USP), 30 mg phenytoin/5 ml with a maximum alcohol content not greater than 0.6 percent, available in 8-oz bottles and individual unit dose foil pouches which deliver 5 ml (30 mg phenytoin). The minimum sales unit is 100 pouches.

Also available as:

N 0071-0362 (Kapseal® 362)—Dilantin (extended phenytoin sodium capsules, USP) 100 mg; in 100's, 1000's and unit dose 100's.

N 0071-0365 (Kapseal 365)—Dilantin (extended phenytoin sodium capsules, USP) 30 mg. in 100's, 1000's and unit dose 100's.

N 0071-0375 (Kapseal 375)—Dilantin with Phenobarbital each contain 100 mg phenytoin sodium with 16 mg (¼ gr) phenobarbital; in 100's and 1000's.

N 0071-0531 (Kapseal 531)—Dilantin with Phenobarbital each contain 100 mg phenytoin sodium with 32 mg (½ gr) phenobarbital; in 100's, 1000's and unit dose 100's.

N 0071-0007 (Tablet 7)—Dilantin Infatabs® (phenytoin tablets, USP) each contain 50 mg phenytoin; 100's and unit dose 100's.

For Parenteral Use:

N 0071-4488-05 (Ampoule 1488)—Dilantin readymixed solution containing 50 mg phenytoin sodium per milliliter is supplied in 2-ml ampoules. Packages of ten.

N 0071-4475-35 (Ampoule 1475)—Dilantin (phenytoin sodium injection) ready-mixed solution containing 50 mg phenytoin sodium per milliliter is supplied in 5-ml ampoules with one 6-ml sterile disposable syringe (22 gauge x 1¼ inch needle). Packages of ten.

N 0071-4475-08 (Ampoule 1475)—Dilantin readymixed solution containing 50 mg phenytoin sodium per milliliter is supplied in packages of ten 5-ml ampoules without syringes.

N 0071-4488-41 (Steri-Dose® 4488)—Dilantin ready-mixed solution containing 50 mg phenytoin sodium per milliliter is supplied in a 2-ml sterile disposable syringe (22 gauge x 1¼ inch needle). Packages of ten individually cartoned syringes.

2214G102

KAPSEALS®
DILANTIN® ℞
[di-lău'tin]
(Phenytoin Sodium) with Phenobarbital

Each Dilantin® with ¼ gr Phenobarbital Kapseal® contains:
Dilantin (phenytoin sodium) ....100 mg
Phenobarbital ....16 mg (¼ gr)
(Warning—May be habit forming)
Each Dilantin with ½ gr Phenobarbital Kapseal contains:

Continued on next page

This product information was prepared in August, 1984. On these and other Parke-Davis Products, information may be obtained by addressing PARKE-DAVIS, Division of Warner-Lambert Company, Morris Plains, New Jersey 07950.

Parke-Davis—Cont.

Dilantin (phenytoin sodium) ....100 mg
Phenobarbital ....32 mg (½ gr)
(Warning—May be habit forming)

Description: Dilantin (phenytoin sodium) is related to the barbiturates in chemical structure, but has a five-membered ring. The chemical name is sodium 5,5-diphenyl-2,4- imidazolidinedione.
Phenobarbital is a derivative of barbituric acid and is chemically described as 5-ethyl-5-phenylbarbituric acid.

Clinical Pharmacology:
Phenytoin
Phenytoin is an anticonvulsant drug which can be useful in the treatment of epilepsy. The primary site of action appears to be the motor cortex where spread of seizure activity is inhibited. Possibly by promoting sodium efflux from neurons, phenytoin tends to stabilize the threshold against hyperexcitability caused by excessive stimulation or environmental changes capable of reducing membrane sodium gradient. This includes the reduction of posttetanic potentiation at synapses. Loss of posttetanic potentiation prevents cortical seizure foci from detonating adjacent cortical areas. Phenytoin reduces the maximal activity of brain stem centers responsible for the tonic phase of grand mal seizures.

The plasma half-life in man after oral administration of phenytoin averages 22 hours, with a range of 7 to 42 hours. Steady-state therapeutic levels are achieved 7 to 10 days after initiation of therapy with recommended doses of 300 mg/day. The clinically effective serum level is usually 10 to 20 mcg/ml.

The majority of phenytoin is excreted in the bile as inactive metabolites, which are then reabsorbed from the intestinal tract and excreted in the urine. Urinary excretion of phenytoin and its metabolites occurs partly with glomerular filtration, but more importantly, by tubular secretion.

In most patients maintained at a steady dosage, a stable phenytoin blood level is achieved. Some patients manifest a large variation in plasma levels despite equivalent doses. Patients with unusually low levels may not be absorbing phenytoin, may be noncompliant, or are hypermetabolizers of phenytoin. Unusually high levels result from liver disease, congenital enzyme deficiency, or drug interactions which result in metabolic interference. The patient with large variations in phenytoin plasma levels, despite standard doses, presents a difficult clinical problem and may benefit from serum level determinations.

Phenobarbital
Phenobarbital produces its anticonvulsant effect by depressing the motor cortex and raising the seizure threshold.
Phenobarbital is absorbed completely, although slowly, following oral administration and undergoes partial biotransformation in the liver by hydroxylation. Phenobarbital is excreted via the kidneys, 10 to 25% as free drug and the remainder primarily as the inactive para-hydroxyphenyl metabolite. The plasma half-life is long, approximately two to six days in adults, and shorter and more variable in children.

In adults, the oral anticonvulsant dose of 1 to 3 mg/kg will produce therapeutic concentrations of 10 to 30 mcg/ml in the serum, the levels usually necessary for seizure control. At this dose, approximately three weeks may be required for the serum levels to achieve steady-state.
High serum levels occur when liver disease, diminished urinary flow, acidosis, or obesity is present. Low serum levels in adults may be due to poor patient compliance.

When used as an anticonvulsant, the clinical phenomenon of breakthrough seizures has been seen. Whether this is a case of true pharmacologic tolerance or some form of spontaneous variation is not known. Physical dependence does develop and may produce accentuation of seizures in epileptics when the drug is abruptly withdrawn.

Indications and Usage: Dilantin with Phenobarbital is indicated for the control of grand mal and psychomotor seizures, only in those patients who require both drugs for seizure control and who previously have had their daily anticonvulsant requirements determined by the administration of the two drugs separately. Combinations should not be used to initiate anticonvulsant therapy and are provided as a convenience for epileptic patients.

Contraindications: Phenytoin is contraindicated in those patients with a history of hypersensitivity to hydantoin products.
Phenobarbital is contraindicated in the following conditions: latent or manifest porphyria or familial history of intermittent porphyria, history of confusion or restlessness from hypnotics, history of abnormal reaction or known hypersensitivity to barbital and its derivatives, including phenobarbital, or a known previous addiction to sedative-hypnotics. Other contraindications include renal and hepatic impairment and severe pulmonary insufficiency.

Warnings:
Warning—Phenobarbital may be habit forming.
Abrupt withdrawal of phenytoin in epileptic patients may precipitate status epilepticus. When, in the judgment of the clinician, the need for dosage reduction, discontinuation, or substitution of alternative anticonvulsant medication arises, this should be done gradually. In the event of an allergic or hypersensitivity reaction, more rapid substitution of alternative therapy may be necessary. In this case, alternative therapy should be an anticonvulsant not belonging to the hydantoin chemical class. Phenytoin is not indicated in seizures due to hypoglycemia or other causes which may be immediately identified and corrected. Appropriate diagnostic procedures should be performed as indicated.

Usage in Pregnancy: The effects of phenytoin and phenobarbital in human pregnancy and nursing infants are unknown.
Recent reports suggest an association between the use of anticonvulsant drugs by women with epilepsy and an elevated incidence of birth defects in children born to these women. Data are more extensive with respect to phenytoin and phenobarbital, but these are also the most commonly prescribed anticonvulsants; less systematic or anecdotal reports suggest a possible similar association with the use of all known anticonvulsant drugs.
The reports suggesting an elevated incidence of birth defects in children of drug-treated epileptic women cannot be regarded as adequate to prove a definite cause and effect relationship. There are intrinsic methodologic problems in obtaining adequate data on drug teratogenicity in humans; the possibility also exists that other factors, e.g., genetic factors or the epileptic condition itself, may be more important than drug therapy in leading to birth defects. The great majority of mothers on anticonvulsant medication deliver normal infants. It is important to note that anticonvulsant drugs should not be discontinued in patients in whom the drug is administered to prevent major seizures because of the strong possibility of precipitating status epilepticus with attendant hypoxia and threat to life. In individual cases where the severity and frequency of the seizure disorder are such that the removal of medication does not pose a serious threat to the patient, discontinuation of the drug may be considered prior to and during pregnancy, although it cannot be said with any confidence that even minor seizures do not pose some hazard to the developing embryo or fetus. The prescribing physician will wish to weigh these considerations in treating or counseling epileptic women of childbearing potential.

Precautions:
Phenytoin
The liver is the chief site of biotransformation of phenytoin; patients with impaired liver function may show early signs of toxicity. Elderly patients or those who are gravely ill may show early signs of toxicity.
A small percentage of individuals who have been treated with phenytoin have been shown to metabolize the drug slowly. Slow metabolism may be due to limited enzyme availability and lack of induction; it appears to be genetically determined.
Phenytoin has been associated with reversible lymph node hyperplasia. If lymph node enlargement occurs in patients on phenytoin, every effort should be made to substitute another anticonvulsant drug or drug combination.
Drugs that control grand mal are not effective for absence (petit mal) seizures. Therefore, if both conditions are present, combined therapy with an anticonvulsant effective against absence (petit mal) epilepsy is necessary.
The phenytoin should be discontinued if a skin rash appears (see Warnings section regarding drug discontinuation). If the rash is exfoliative, purpuric, or bullous, use of the drug should not be resumed. If the rash is a milder type (measles-like or scarlatiniform), therapy may be resumed after the rash has completely disappeared. If the rash occurs upon reinstitution of therapy, further phenytoin medication is contraindicated.
Hyperglycemia, resulting from the drug's inhibitory effect on insulin release, has been reported. Phenytoin may also raise the blood sugar level in persons already suffering from hyperglycemia.
Osteomalacia has been associated with anticonvulsant therapy including phenytoin and/or phenobarbital.

Clinically Significant Drug Interactions
Phenytoin metabolism may be significantly altered by the concomitant use of other drugs such as:
a. Barbiturates may enhance the rate of metabolism of phenytoin. This effect, however, is variable and unpredictable. It has been reported that in some patients the concomitant administration of carbamazepine resulted in an increased rate of phenytoin metabolism.
b. Coumarin anticoagulants, disulfiram, phenylbutazone, and sulfaphenazole may inhibit the metabolism of phenytoin, resulting in increased serum levels of the drug. This may lead to increased incidence of nystagmus, ataxia, or other toxic signs. The effect of dicumarol in inhibiting the metabolism of phenytoin in the liver has been well documented.
c. Isoniazid inhibits the metabolism of phenytoin so that with combined therapy, patients who are slow acetylators may suffer from phenytoin intoxication.
d. Tricyclic antidepressants in high doses may precipitate seizures, and the dosage of phenytoin may have to be adjusted accordingly.
Phenytoin may interfere with the metyrapone and the 1-mg dexamethasone tests. It may also suppress the protein-bound iodine. However, this has not been associated with any clinical signs of hypothyroidism, the T-3 is normal.

Pregnancy
See WARNINGS.

Nursing Mothers
Evidence that phenytoin is secreted in human milk is inadequate. The drug appears to be secreted in low concentrations which are unlikely to affect the infant. If the mother is receiving large doses of phenytoin, however, the drug concentration in milk might increase. For this reason, artificial feeding of the infant is recommended for women taking this drug.

Phenobarbital
Withdrawal symptoms, including convulsions and delirium, may occur upon discontinuance of phenobarbital in patients with chronic intoxication. Analgesics, if used with phenobarbital, should be prescribed with caution because of possible additive effects. Caution should be exercised in prescribing this drug to patients with suicidal tendencies or with a predilection to abusive use of barbiturates.
Phenobarbital should be used with caution in debilitating and pulmonary diseases.
Phenobarbital should be used with caution in patients with severely impaired liver function, severe anemia, congestive heart failure, fever, neuroses, hyperthyroidism, diabetes mellitus, and any conditions in which respiratory depression may be characteristic. Marked excitement rather than depression may occur in aged or debilitated pa-

tients, particularly those with cerebral arteriosclerosis.

Confusion or euphoria may result from use of this drug. Symptoms in mentally ill, phobic, and emotionally disturbed patients may be accentuated. Prolonged usage may produce psychological habituation. Sudden discontinuation or radical reduction of dosage may precipitate withdrawal symptoms in patients who have taken the drug for prolonged periods; dosage should be gradually reduced to the point of complete discontinuation.

Barbiturates should be prescribed with extreme caution for persons known or suspected of routinely or periodically consuming large quantities of alcoholic beverages. Potentiation of effect, even to the extent of causing death, may result from consumption of barbiturates by patients with a high serum alcohol level.

Information for the Patient
Phenobarbital may impair the mental and/or physical abilities required for the performance of potentially hazardous tasks, such as driving a motor vehicle or other such activity requiring alertness; therefore, the patient should be cautioned accordingly.

Clinically Significant Drug Interactions
The effects of phenobarbital may be increased by many drugs, including antihistamines, tranquilizers, corticosteroids, monoamine oxidase inhibitors, narcotic analgesics, amitriptyline, imipramine, and rauwolfia alkaloids.

Pregnancy
See WARNINGS.

Nursing Mothers
Evidence that phenobarbital is secreted in human milk is inadequate. The drug appears to be secreted in low concentrations which are unlikely to affect the infant. If the mother is receiving large doses of phenobarbital, however, the drug concentration in milk might increase. For this reason, artificial feeding of the infant is recommended for women taking this drug.

Labor and Delivery
Barbiturates readily cross the placental barrier and, if administered during labor, may have a depressant effect on the fetus; infants born of mothers receiving barbiturates may have difficulty breathing spontaneously.

Adverse Reactions:
Phenytoin
Central Nervous System: The most common manifestations encountered with phenytoin therapy are referable to this system. These include nystagmus, ataxia, slurred speech, and mental confusion. Dizziness, insomnia, transient nervousness, motor twitchings, and headache have also been observed. These side effects may disappear with continuing therapy at a reduced dosage level.
Gastrointestinal System: Phenytoin may cause nausea, vomiting, and constipation. Administration of the drug with or immediately after meals may help prevent gastrointestinal discomfort.
Integumentary System: Dermatological manifestations sometimes accompanied by fever have included scarlatiniform or morbilliform rashes. A morbilliform rash (measles-like) is the most common; other types of dermatitis are seen more rarely. Rashes are more frequent in children and young adults. Other, more serious forms which may be fatal have included bullous, exfoliative, or purpuric dermatitis, lupus erythematosus, and Stevens-Johnson syndrome.
Hemopoietic System: Hemopoietic complications, some fatal, have occasionally been reported in association with administration of phenytoin. These have included thrombocytopenia, leukopenia, granulocytopenia, agranulocytosis, and pancytopenia. While macrocytosis and megaloblastic anemia have occurred; these conditions usually respond to folic acid therapy. The occasional occurrence of lymphadenopathy indicates the need to differentiate such a condition from other lymph gland pathology.
Other: Gingival hyperplasia occurs frequently; this incidence may be reduced by good oral hygiene including gum massage, frequent brushing, and appropriate dental care. Hyperglycemia has been reported. Polyarthropathy and hirsutism occur occasionally. Toxic hepatitis, liver damage, and periarteritis nodosa may occur and can be fatal.

Phenobarbital
Central Nervous System: With larger doses, the most common manifestations relate to this system. These include drowsiness, vertigo, ataxia, hebetude, headache, delirium, and stupor.
Gastrointestinal System: Phenobarbital may cause gastrointestinal discomfort and nausea.
Integumentary System: Hypersensitivity reactions are rare. Cutaneous eruptions are principally due to idiosyncrasy. Fatalities from exfoliative dermatitis and cutaneous eruptions have been reported. There are two syndromes associated with phenobarbital administration: Stevens-Johnson and a phenobarbital sensitivity syndrome. The phenobarbital sensitivity syndrome, which has resulted in fatalities, is characterized by an erythematous rash, high fever, jaundice, mental confusion, and toxic damage of "parenchymatous organs."
Hemopoietic System: Megaloblastic anemia has been reported; this condition usually responds to folic acid therapy.

OVERDOSAGE
The therapeutic ranges for phenytoin and phenobarbital in adults are 10 to 20 mcg/ml and 10 to 30 mcg/ml, respectively. Following acute overdosage of this combination, the patient at steady-state may experience evidence of phenytoin toxicity ahead of phenobarbital toxicity because phenytoin plasma levels rise more rapidly than phenobarbital levels. Phenytoin also has a narrower margin between therapeutic and toxic levels than does phenobarbital.

Phenytoin
The mean lethal dose of Dilantin in adults is estimated to be 2 to 5 grams. The cardinal initial symptoms are nystagmus, ataxia, and dysarthria. The patient then becomes comatose, the pupils unresponsive and hypotension occurs. Death is due to respiratory depression and apnea.

There are marked variations among individuals with respect to phenytoin plasma levels where toxicity may occur. Nystagmus, on lateral gaze, usually appears at 20 mcg/ml, ataxia at 30 mcg/ml, dysarthria and lethargy appear when the plasma concentration is over 40 mcg/ml, but as high a concentration as 50 mcg/ml has been reported without evidence of toxicity.[1] As much as 25 times the therapeutic dose has been taken to give a serum concentration over 100 mcg/ml with complete recovery.[2]

Treatment is nonspecific because there is no known antidote. First, the stomach should be emptied. If the gag reflex is absent, the airway should be supported. Oxygen, vasopressors, and assisted ventilation may be necessary for central nervous system, respiratory, and cardiovascular depression. Finally, hemodialysis can be considered because phenytoin is not completely bound to plasma proteins. Total exchange transfusion has been utilized in the treatment of severe intoxication in children.

Phenobarbital
The lethal dose of phenobarbital is believed to be 5 grams. The highest known blood level from which a patient recovered was 580 mcg/ml. An overdose of phenobarbital will induce the classical picture of progressive central nervous system depression. In its severest form, this syndrome leads to respiratory arrest as a result of general reflex paralysis. The milder forms of this syndrome may mimic any stage of clinical anesthesia. Except for a rapid (and weak) pulse, vital signs are characteristically reduced. In addition to direct inhibition of the cardiac contractile mechanism with consequent hypotension, circulatory insufficiency may be aggravated by hypoxia from inadequate pulmonary ventilation. Early deaths are usually due to respiratory arrest, but delayed fatalities may arise from one or any combination of the following complications; hypostatic pneumonia, bronchopneumonia, lung abscess, pulmonary edema, cerebral edema, circulatory collapse, and irreversible renal shutdown.

The treatment of barbiturate poisoning consists in removing any unabsorbed drug from the stomach, supporting the respiration and circulation, and expediting elimination of the drug which has been absorbed.

Dosage and Administration:
The combination of Dilantin with Phenobarbital Kapseals is provided as a convenience for epileptic patients who require both drugs for seizure control. Anticonvulsant therapy should be initiated with either phenytoin or phenobarbital and, if indicated, the other drug can then be added. If the total daily doses of the two drugs used separately are within those given below, the combination of Dilantin with Phenobarbital Kapseals can then be substituted in equivalent amounts. When plasma level determinations are necessary for optimal dosage adjustments, the clinically effective level of Dilantin is usually 10 to 20 mcg/ml and for phenobarbital 10 to 30 mcg/ml in adults. Serum blood level determinations are especially helpful when possible drug interactions are suspected.

If either the phenytoin or phenobarbital dosage requires adjustment, this should be done by switching the patient to separate phenytoin and phenobarbital dosage forms in order to enable subsequent dosage adjustment of either or both drugs.

The recommended starting phenobarbital dose for children is 2 to 3 mg/kg/day in two or three equally divided doses.

The recommended starting Dilantin dose for children is 5 mg/kg/day in two or three equally divided doses.

Adult Dosage: For maintenance (see above) —usually three or four capsules daily. An increase to six capsules daily may be made, if necessary.

Pediatric Dosage: For maintenance (see above) —individualized to a maximum of 300 mg Dilantin daily.

How Supplied: N 0071-0375 (Kapseal 375)—Dilantin with Phenobarbital each contain 100 mg phenytoin sodium with 16 mg ($\frac{1}{4}$ gr) phenobarbital; in 100's, and 1000's.
N 0071-0531 (Kapseal 531)—Dilantin with Phenobarbital each contain 100 mg phenytoin sodium with 32 mg ($\frac{1}{2}$ gr) phenobarbital in 100's, 1000's and unit dose 100's.
Store at room temperature below 86° F (30° C). Protect from moisture and light.

Also Available As:
N 0071-0362 (Kapseal 362)—Dilantin (phenytoin sodium) 100 mg; in 100's, 1000's and unit dose 100's.
N 0071-0365 (Kapseal 365)—Dilantin (phenytoin sodium) 30 mg; in 100's, 1000's and unit dose 100's.
N 0071-0007 (Tablet 7)—Dilantin Infatabs® each contain 50 mg phenytoin; 100's, and unit dose 100's
N 0071-2214—Dilantin-125® Suspension (phenytoin oral suspension USP) 125 mg phenytoin/5 ml with a maximum alcohol content not greater than 0.6 percent; available in 8-oz bottles and individual dose foil pouches which deliver 5 ml (125 mg phenytoin). The minimum sales unit is 100 pouches.
N 0071-2315—Dilantin-30® Pediatric Suspension (phenytoin oral suspension, USP) 30 mg phenytoin/5 ml with a maximum alcohol content not greater than 0.6 percent; available in 8-oz bottles and individual unit dose foil pouches which deliver 5 ml (30 mg phenytoin). The minimum sales unit is 100 pouches.

For Parenteral Use:
N 0071-4488-05 (Ampoule 1488)—Dilantin ready-mixed solution containing 50 mg phenytoin sodium per milliliter is supplied in 2-ml ampoules. Packages of ten. N 0071-4488-41 (Steri-Dose® 4488)—Dilantin ready-mixed solution containing

Continued on next page

This product information was prepared in August, 1984. On these and other Parke-Davis Products, information may be obtained by addressing PARKE-DAVIS, Division of Warner-Lambert Company, Morris Plains, New Jersey 07950.

Parke-Davis—Cont.

50 mg phenytoin sodium per milliliter is supplied in a 2-ml sterile disposable syringe (22 gauge × 1¼ inch needle). Packages of ten individually cartoned syringes. N 0071-4475-35 (Ampoule 1475)—Dilantin ready-mixed solution containing 50 mg phenytoin sodium per milliliter is supplied in 5-ml ampoules with one 6-ml sterile disposable syringe (22 gauge × 1¼ inch needle). Packages of ten. N 0071-4475-08 (Ampoule 1475)—Dilantin ready-mixed solution containing 50 mg phenytoin sodium per milliliter is supplied in packages of ten 5-ml ampoules without syringes.

References:
1. Woodbury, DM and Fingl, E. "Drugs Effective in the Therapy of the Epilepsies," in Goodman, LS and Gilman, A (eds): The Pharmacological Basis of Therapeutics ed 5. New York, Macmillan Publishing Co, Inc, 1975, pp 201–226.
2. Henn, K. "Diphenylhydantoin: Relation of Plasma Levels to Clinical Control," in Woodbury, DM, Penry, JK, and Schmidt, RP, (eds): Antiepileptic Drugs, New York, Raven Press, Publishers, 1972, pp 211–218.

Shown in Product Identification Section, page 423
0375G010

DOPASTAT™ ℞
[dō'pă-stăt"]
Brand of
(Dopamine Hydrochloride)

Description: Dopamine hydrochloride is 3,4 dihydroxyphenethylamine hydrochloride, a naturally-occurring biochemical catecholamine precursor of norepinephrine.
Dopamine hydrochloride is a white, odorless crystalline powder, freely soluble in water and soluble in alcohol. It is sensitive to light, alkalis, iron salts and oxidizing agents.
Each milliliter of the clear, practically colorless, sterile, pyrogen-free dopamine hydrochloride injection contains 40 mg of dopamine hydrochloride (equivalent to 32.31 mg of dopamine base) in Water for Injection, USP, containing 1% sodium bisulfite as a preservative.

Actions: Dopamine hydrochloride exerts an inotropic effect on the myocardium resulting in an increased cardiac output. Dopamine hydrochloride produces less increase in myocardial oxygen consumption than isoproterenol and its use is usually not associated with a tachyarrhythmia. Clinical studies indicate that dopamine hydrochloride usually increases systolic and pulse pressure with either no effect or a slight increase in diastolic pressure. Total peripheral resistance at low and intermediate therapeutic doses is usually unchanged. Blood flow to peripheral vascular beds may decrease while mesenteric flow increases. Dopamine hydrochloride has also been reported to dilate the renal vasculature presumptively by activation of a "dopaminergic" receptor. This action is accompanied by increases in glomerular filtration rate, renal blood flow, and sodium excretion. An increase in urinary output produced by dopamine is usually not associated with a decrease in osmolality of the urine.

Indications: Dopamine hydrochloride is indicated for the correction of hemodynamic imbalances present in the shock syndrome due to myocardial infarctions, trauma, endotoxic septicemia, open heart surgery, renal failure, and chronic cardiac decompensation as in congestive failure.
Where appropriate, restoration of blood volume with a suitable plasma expander or whole blood should be instituted or completed prior to administration of dopamine hydrochloride.
Patients most likely to respond adequately to dopamine hydrochloride are those in whom physiological parameters, such as urine flow, myocardial function, and blood pressure, have not undergone profound deterioration. Multiclinic trials indicate that the shorter the time interval between onset of signs and symptoms and initiation of therapy with volume correction and dopamine hydrochloride, the better the prognosis.

Poor Perfusion of Vital Organs—Urine flow appears to be one of the better diagnostic signs by which adequacy of vital organ perfusion can be monitored. Nevertheless, the physician should also observe the patient for signs of reversal of confusion or comatose condition. Loss of pallor, increase in toe temperature, and/or adequacy of nail bed capillary filling may also be used as indices of adequate dosage. Clinical studies have shown that when dopamine hydrochloride is administered before urine flow has diminished to levels approximately 0.3 ml/minute, prognosis is more favorable. Nevertheless, in a number of oliguric or anuric patients, administration of dopamine hydrochloride has resulted in an increase in urine flow which in some cases reached normal levels. Dopamine hydrochloride may also increase urine flow in patients whose output is within normal limits and thus may be of value in reducing the effect of pre-existing fluid accumulation. It should be noted that at doses above those optimal for the individual patient, urine flow may decrease, necessitating reduction of dosage. Concurrent administration of dopamine hydrochloride and diuretic agents may produce an additive or potentiating effect.

Low Cardiac Output—Increased cardiac output is related to dopamine hydrochloride's direct inotropic effect on the myocardium. Increased cardiac output at low or moderate doses appears to be related to a favorable prognosis. Increase in cardiac output has been associated with either static or decreased systemic vascular resistance (SVR). Static or decreased SVR associated with low or moderate movements in cardiac output is believed to be a reflection of differential effects on specific vascular beds with increased resistance in peripheral beds (eg, femoral) and concomitant decreases in mesenteric and renal vascular beds.
Redistribution of blood flow parellels these changes so that an increase in cardiac output is accompanied by an increase in mesenteric and renal blood flow. In many instances the renal fraction of the total cardiac output has been found to increase. Increase in cardiac output produced by dopamine hydrochloride is not associated with substantial decreases in systemic vascular resistance as may occur with isoproterenol.

Hypotension—Hypotension due to inadequate cardiac output can be managed by administration of low to moderate doses of dopamine hydrochloride, which have little effect on SVR. At high therapeutic doses, dopamine hydrochloride's alpha adrenergic activity becomes more prominent and thus may correct hypotension due to diminished SVR. As in the case of other circulatory decompensation states, prognosis is better in patients whose blood pressure and urine flow have not undergone profound deterioration. Therefore, it is suggested that the physician administer dopamine hydrochloride as soon as a definite trend toward decreased systolic and diastolic pressure becomes evident.

Contraindications: Dopamine hydrochloride should not be used in patients with pheochromocytoma.

Warnings: Dopamine hydrochloride should not be administered in the presence of uncorrected tachyarrhythmias or ventricular fibrillation.
Do NOT add dopamine hydrochloride to any alkaline solution, since the drug is inactivated in alkaline solution.
Patients who have been treated with monoamine oxidase (MAO) inhibitors prior to the administration of dopamine hydrochloride will require substantially reduced dosage. Dopamine is metabolized by MAO, and inhibition of this enzyme prolongs and potentiates the effect of dopamine hydrochloride. The starting dose in such patients should be reduced to at least one-tenth (1/10) of the usual dose.

Usage in Pregnancy—Animal studies have revealed no evidence of teratogenic effects from dopamine hydrochloride. In one study, administration of dopamine hydrochloride to pregnant rats resulted in a decreased survival rate of the newborn and a potential for cataract formation in the survivors. The drug may be used in pregnant women when, in the judgment of the physician, the expected benefits outweigh the potential risk to the fetus.

Usage in Children—The safety and efficacy of this drug in children has not been established. Dopamine hydrochloride has been used in a limited number of pediatric patients but such use has been inadequate to fully define proper dosage and limitations for use. Further studies are in progress.

Precautions:
Avoid Hypovolemia—Prior to treatment with dopamine hydrochloride, hypovolemia should be fully corrected, if possible, with either whole blood or plasma as indicated.

Decreased Pulse Pressure—If a disproportionate rise in the diastolic pressure (ie, a marked decrease in the pulse pressure) is observed in patients receiving dopamine hydrochloride, the infusion rate should be decreased and the patient observed carefully for further evidence of predominant vasoconstrictor activity, unless such an effect is desired.

Extravasation—Dopamine hydrochloride should be infused into a large vein whenever possible to prevent the possibility of extravasation into tissue adjacent to the infusion site. Extravasation may cause necrosis and sloughing of surrounding tissue. Large veins of the antecubital fossa are preferred to veins in the dorsum of the hand or ankle. Less suitable infusion sites should be used only if the patient's condition requires immediate attention. The physician should switch to more suitable sites as rapidly as possible. The infusion site should be continuously monitored for free flow.

Occlusive Vascular Disease—Patients with a history of occlusive vascular disease (for example, atherosclerosis, arterial embolism, Raynaud's disease, cold injury, diabetic endarteritis, and Buerger's disease) should be closely monitored for any changes in color or temperature of the skin in the extremities. If a change in skin color or temperature occurs and is thought to be the result of compromised circulation to the extremities, the benefits of continued dopamine hydrochloride infusion should be weighed against the risk of possible necrosis. This condition may be reversed by either decreasing or discontinuing the rate of infusion.

IMPORTANT
Antidote for Peripheral Ischemia: To prevent sloughing and necrosis in ischemic areas, the area should be infiltrated as soon as possible with 10 to 15 ml of Saline solution containing from 5 to 10 mg of Regitine® (brand of phentolamine), an adrenergic blocking agent. A syringe with a fine hypodermic needle should be used, and the solution liberally infiltrated throughout the ischemic area. Sympathetic blockade with phentolamine causes immediate and conspicuous local hyperemic changes if the area is infiltrated within 12 hours. Therefore, *phentolamine should be given as soon as possible* after the extravasation is noted.

Avoid Cyclopropane or Halogenated Hydrocarbon Anesthetics—Cyclopropane or halogenated hydrocarbon anesthetics increase cardiac autonomic irritability and therefore may sensitize the myocardium to the action of certain intravenously administered catecholamines. This interaction appears to be related both to pressor activity and to beta adrenergic stimulating properties of these catecholamines. Therefore, as with certain other catecholamines, and because of the theoretical arrhythmogenic potential, dopamine hydrochloride should be used with EXTREME CAUTION in patients inhaling cyclopropane or halogenated hydrocarbon anesthetics.

Careful Monitoring Required—Close monitoring of the following indices—urine flow, cardiac output and blood pressure—during dopamine hydrochloride infusion is necessary as in the case of any adrenergic agent.

Adverse Reactions: The most frequent adverse reactions observed in clinical evaluation of dopamine hydrochloride included ectopic beats, nausea, vomiting, tachycardia, anginal pain, palpitation, dyspnea, headache, hypotension, and vasoconstriction. Other adverse reactions which have been reported infrequently were aberrant conduction, bradycardia, piloerection, widened QRS complex, azotemia, and elevated blood pressure.

Dosage and Administration:
WARNING: This is a potent drug. It must be diluted before administration to patient.
Suggested Dilution—Transfer contents of one ampoule (5 ml containing 200 mg dopamine hydrochloride) by aseptic technique to either a 250 ml or 500 ml bottle of one of the following sterile intravenous solutions:
1. Sodium Chloride Injection, USP
2. Dextrose 5% Injection, USP
3. Dextrose (5%) and Sodium Chloride (0.9%) Injection, USP
4. 5% Dextrose in 0.45% Sodium Chloride Solution
5. Dextrose (5%) in Lactated Ringer's Solution
6. Sodium Lactate (1/6 Molar) Injection, USP
7. Lactated Ringer's Injection, USP

Dopamine hydrochloride has been found to be stable for a minimum of 24 hours after dilution in the sterile intravenous solutions listed above. However, as with all intravenous admixtures, dilution should be made just prior to administration.
Do NOT add dopamine hydrochloride injection to 5% Sodium Bicarbonate or other alkaline intravenous solutions, since the drug is inactivated in alkaline solution.
Rate of Administration—Dopamine hydrochloride, after dilution, is administered intravenously through a suitable intravenous catheter or needle. An IV drip chamber or other suitable metering device is essential for controlling the rate of flow in drops/minute. Each patient must be individually titrated to the desired hemodynamic and/or renal response with dopamine hydrochloride. In titrating to the desired increase in systolic blood pressure, the optimum dosage rate for renal response may be exceeded, thus necessitating a reduction in rate after the hemodynamic condition is stabilized. Administration at rates greater than 50 mcg/kg/minute have safely been used in advanced circulatory decompensation states. If unnecessary fluid expansion is of concern, adjustment of drug concentration may be preferred over increasing the flow rate of a less concentrated dilution.
Suggested Regimen:
1. When appropriate, increase blood volume with whole blood or plasma until central venous pressure is 10 to 15 cm. H$_2$O or pulmonary wedge pressure is 14-18 mm Hg.
2. Begin administration of diluted solution at doses of 2-5 mcg/kg/minute dopamine hydrochloride in patients who are likely to respond to modest increments of heart force and renal perfusion. In more seriously ill patients, begin administration of diluted solution at doses of 5 mcg/kg/minute dopamine hydrochloride and increase gradually using 5-10 mcg/kg/minute increments up to 20-50 mcg/kg/minute as needed. If doses of dopamine hydrochloride in excess of 50 mcg/kg/minute are required, it is suggested that urine output be checked frequently. Should urine flow begin to decrease in the absence of hypotension, reduction of dopamine hydrochloride dosage should be considered. Multiclinic trials have shown that more than 50% of the patients were satisfactorily maintained on doses of dopamine hydrochloride less than 20 mcg/kg/minute. In patients who do not respond to these doses with adequate arterial pressures or urine flow, additional increments of dopamine hydrochloride may be employed in an effort to produce an appropriate arterial pressure and central perfusion.
3. Treatment of all patients requires constant evaluation of therapy in terms of the blood volume, augmentation of myocardial contractility, and distribution of peripheral perfusion. Dosage of dopamine hydrochloride should be adjusted according to the patient's response, with particular attention to diminution of established urine flow rate, increasing tachycardia or development of new dysrhythmias as indices for decreasing or temporarily suspending the dosage.
4. As with all potent intravenously administered drugs, care should be taken to control the rate of administration so as to avoid inadvertent administration of a bolus of drug.

Overdosage: In case of accidental overdosage, as evidenced by excessive blood pressure elevation, reduce rate of administration or temporarily discontinue dopamine hydrochloride until patient's condition stabilizes. Since dopamine hydrochloride's duration of action is quite short, no additional remedial measures are usually necessary. If these measures fail to stabilize the patient's condition, use of the short acting alpha adrenergic blocking agent phentolamine should be considered.

How Supplied:
Dopamine hydrochloride is supplied as:
N 0071-4210-08—5-ml ampoules. Each ml contains 40 mg dopamine hydrochloride (equivalent to 32.31 mg dopamine base). Supplied as packages of ten individually cartoned 5-ml ampoules.

4210G041

DURAQUIN® ℞
[dū'rǎ-quĭn]
(quinidine gluconate tablets)
SUSTAINED RELEASE

Description: Quinidine gluconate is the gluconate of an alkaloid which may be obtained from various species of Cinchona and their hybrids, from *Remijia pedunculata* Fluckiger (Fam. Rubiaceae), or prepared from quinine. Quinidine gluconate contains, on the dry basis, not less than 99% of $C_{20}H_{24}N_2O_2 \cdot C_6H_{12}O_7$ (520.58). Quinidine is chemically described as 6-methoxy-alpha-(5-vinyl-2 quinuclidinyl)-4 quinolinemethanol and is the dextrorotatory isomer of quinine. Each 330-mg sustained-release tablet, representing 206 mg of quinidine base, is equivalent to 248 mg of quinidine sulfate.

Actions: The antiarrhythmic activity consists of two actions: (a) prolongation of effective refractory period of the atrial or ventricular muscle which leads to termination of arrhythmia; (b) decrease in excitability of ectopic foci of the heart. In addition, quinidine blocks vagal innervation and facilitates conduction in the atrial-ventricular junction.

Clinical Pharmacology: In clinical studies, single doses of Duraquin produced a mean maximum plasma level at 2 hours which was maintained for 12 hours. This broad plateau indicates slow, continuous absorption from the gastrointestinal tract.
In multiple-dose studies, administration of Duraquin tablets, 660 mg every 12 hours, produced steady state (equilibrium) plasma levels shortly after 24 hours. The average quinidine plasma levels (Cramer and Isaksson assay[1]) were 0.81 mcg/ml and the mean peak levels were 1.16 mcg/ml in a group of normal male subjects weighing 75 kg. Following the last dose at steady state, quinidine plasma levels decreased at an approximate rate of 50% in 10 hours. This compares to the expected plasma half-life of 6.3 hours for quinidine sulfate tablets, USP.
Therapeutic and toxic effects coordinate better with plasma levels than with dosage. While therapeutic levels of 3 to 6 mcg/ml with a range of 1.5 to 9 mcg/ml have been reported, these values are based on peak plasma levels determined by the less specific Edgar and Sokolow assay.[2] This procedure yields quinidine levels averaging 22% higher than the Cramer and Isaksson assay. Plasma levels vary considerably in patients receiving identical doses. Therefore, it is advisable to adjust the dosage by monitoring plasma quinidine levels.

Indications: Duraquin tablets are indicated for the prevention of premature atrial, nodal, or ventricular contractions. They are also indicated for the maintenance of normal sinus rhythm following spontaneous reversion or electrical conversion of atrial, nodal, or ventricular tachycardia, atrial flutter and fibrillation (either paroxysmal or chronic).

Contraindications:
1. History of hypersensitivity to quinidine manifested by thrombocytopenia, skin eruption, febrile reactions, etc.
2. Complete A-V block
3. Complete bundle branch block or other severe intraventricular conduction defects exhibiting marked QRS widening or bizarre complexes
4. Myasthenia gravis
5. Arrhythmias associated with digitalis toxicity

Warnings:
1. (a) In the treatment of atrial fibrillation with rapid ventricular response, ventricular rate should be controlled with digitalis glycosides *prior* to administration of quinidine.
   (b) In the treatment of atrial flutter with quinidine, reversion to sinus rhythm may be preceded by progressive reduction in the degree of A-V block to a 1:1 ratio resulting in an extremely high ventricular rate. This potential hazard may be reduced by digitalization prior to administration of quinidine.

Recent reports have described increased, potentially toxic, digoxin plasma levels when quinidine is administered concurrently. When concurrent use is necessary, digoxin dosage should be reduced and plasma concentration should be monitored and patients observed closely for digitalis intoxication.

2. Quinidine cardiotoxicity may be manifested by increased PR and QT intervals, 50% widening of QRS, and/or ventricular ectopic beats or tachycardia. Appearance of these toxic signs during quinidine administration mandates immediate discontinuation of the drug, and/or close clinical and electrocardiographic monitoring. Note: Quinidine effect is enhanced by potassium and reduced in the presence of hypokalemia.
3. "Quinidine Syncope" may occur as a complication of long-term therapy. It is manifested by sudden loss of consciousness and ventricular arrhythmias with bizarre QRS complexes. This syndrome does not appear to be related to dose or plasma levels but occurs more often with prolonged QT intervals.
4. Because quinidine antagonizes the effect of vagal excitation upon the atrium and the A-V node, the administration of parasympathomimetic drugs (choline esters) or the use of any other procedure to enhance vagal activity may fail to terminate paroxysmal supraventricular tachycardia in patients receiving quinidine.
5. Quinidine should be used with extreme caution in: a) the presence of incomplete A-V block, since a complete block and asystole may result. Quinidine may cause unpredictable abnormalities of rhythm in digitalized hearts. Therefore, it should be used with caution in the presence of digitalis intoxication. (See 1.(b) above).
   b) Partial bundle branch block.
   c) Severe congestive heart failure and hypotensive states due to the depressant effects of quinidine on myocardial contractility and arterial pressure.
   d) Poor renal function, especially renal tubular acidosis, because of the potential accumulation of quinidine in plasma leading to toxic concentrations.

Precautions:
1. Test Dose
A preliminary test dose of a single tablet of quinidine *sulfate* should be administered prior to the initiation of the sustained release gluconate to determine whether the patient has an idiosyncrasy to the quinidine molecule.

Continued on next page

This product information was prepared in August, 1984. On these and other Parke-Davis Products, information may be obtained by addressing PARKE-DAVIS, Division of Warner-Lambert Company, Morris Plains, New Jersey 07950.

Parke-Davis—Cont.

2. Hypersensitivity
During the first weeks of therapy; hypersensitivity to quinidine, although rare, should be considered (eg, angioedema, purpura, acute asthmatic episode, vascular collapse).

3. Long-Term Therapy
Periodic blood counts and liver and kidney function tests should be performed during long-term therapy and the drug should be discontinued if blood dyscrasias or signs of hepatic or renal disorders occur.

4. Large Doses
ECG monitoring and determination of plasma quinidine levels are recommended when doses greater than 2.5 g/day are administered.

5. Usage in Pregnancy
The use of quinidine, in pregnancy, should be reserved only for those cases where the benefits outweigh the possible hazards to the patient and fetus.

6. Nursing Mothers
The drug should be used with extreme caution in nursing mothers because the drug is excreted in breast milk.

7. General
In patients exhibiting asthma, muscle weakness, and infection with fever *prior* to quinidine administration, hypersensitivity reactions to the drug may be masked.

Drug Interactions:
1. Caution should be used when quinidine and its analogs are administered concurrently with coumarin anticoagulants. This combination may reduce prothrombin levels and cause bleeding.
2. Quinidine, a weak base, may have its half-life prolonged in patients who are concurrently taking drugs that can alkalize the urine, such as thiazide diuretics, sodium bicarbonate, and carbonic anhydrase inhibitors. Quinidine and drugs which alkalize the urine should be used together cautiously.
3. Quinidine exhibits a distinct anticholinergic activity in the myocardial tissues. An additive vagolytic effect may be seen when quinidine and drugs having anticholinergic blocking activity are used together. Drugs having cholinergic activity may be antagonized by quinidine.
4. Quinidine and other antiarrhythmic agents may produce additive cardiac depressant effects when administered together.
5. Quinidine interaction with cardiac glycosides (digoxin); See Warnings.
6. Antacids may delay absorption of quinidine but appear unlikely to cause incomplete absorption.
7. Phenobarbital and phenytoin may reduce plasma half-life of quinidine by 50%.
8. Quinidine may potentiate the neuromuscular blocking effect in ventilatory depression of patients receiving decamethonium, tubocurare, or succinylcholine.

Adverse Reactions: Symptoms of cinchonism (ringing in the ears, headache, disturbed vision) may appear in sensitive patients after a single dose of the drug.
Gastrointestinal: The most common side effects encountered with quinidine are referable to this system. Diarrhea frequently occurs, but it rarely necessitates withdrawal of the drug. Nausea, vomiting, and abdominal pain also occur. Some of these effects may be minimized by administering the drug with meals.
Cardiovascular: Widening of QRS complex, cardiac asystole, ventricular ectopic beats, idioventricular rhythms including ventricular tachycardias and fibrillation; paradoxical tachycardia, arterial embolism and hypotension.
Hematologic: acute hemolytic anemia, hypoprothrombinemia, thrombocytopenic purpura, agranulocytosis.
CNS: headache, fever, vertigo, apprehension, excitement, confusion, delirium and syncope, disturbed hearing (tinnitus, decreased auditory acuity), disturbed vision (mydriasis, blurred vision, disturbed color perception, photophobia, diplopia, night blindness, scotomata); optic neuritis.
Dermatologic: cutaneous flushing with intense pruritus.
Hypersensitivity reactions: angioedema, acute asthmatic episode, vascular collapse, respiratory arrest.

Dosage and Administration: Dosage should be titrated to give the desired clinical effect, e.g., elimination of paroxysmal rhythm or reduction in premature contractions (See Clinical Pharmacology). This will often require prolonged ambulatory ECG monitoring, as hour-to-hour variability renders brief ECG recordings unreliable. When doses larger than 2.5g/day are used, quinidine blood levels should be monitored, if possible, and serial ECGs should be followed (See Warnings and Precautions).
For prevention of premature contractions and maintenance of normal sinus rhythm following spontaneous reversion or electrical conversion, the usual dosage is from 330 mg to 660 mg every eight hours, most patients requiring the higher dosage.
In elderly patients, and in patients in the lower end of the normal weight range, plasma quinidine determinations should be considered. Dosage adjustments may be required.
Overdosage: Cardiotoxic effects of quinidine may be reversed in part by molar sodium lactate; the hypotension may be reversed by vasoconstrictors and by catecholamines (since the vasodilation is partly due to alpha-adrenergic blockade).
How Supplied: N 0071-0850 (P-D 850) Duraquin (quinidine gluconate tablets) 330-mg tablets are supplied in bottles of 100 and in unit-dose packages of 100 (10 strips of 10 tablets each).

0850G010

[1] Cramer, G. and Isaksson, B. Quantitative Determination of Quinidine in Plasma, Scandinavian J. Clin. & Lab Investigation 15, 553, 1963.
[2] Edgar, A.L. and Sokolow, M. Experiences with the Photofluorometric Determination of Quinidine in Blood J. Lab Clin. Med. 36, 478, 1950.

Shown in Product Identification Section, page 423

EASPRIN®
[ēas'prin"]
(Aspirin Tablets, USP)
Enteric Coated Tablets

Caution—Federal law prohibits dispensing without prescription.
Description: Easprin (Aspirin Tablets, USP) enteric coated tablets contain 15 grains (975 mg) aspirin for oral administration. The enteric coating is designed to prevent the release of aspirin in the stomach and thereby reduce gastric irritation and total occult blood loss. The pharmacologic effects of aspirin include analgesia, antipyresis, antiinflammatory activity, and antirheumatic activity.
Clinical Pharmacology: Aspirin is a salicylate that has demonstrated antiinflammatory, analgesic, antipyretic, and antirheumatic activity.
Aspirin's mode of action as an antiinflammatory and antirheumatic agent may be due to inhibition of synthesis and release of prostaglandins.
Aspirin appears to produce analgesia by virtue of both a peripheral and CNS effect. Peripherally, aspirin acts by inhibiting the synthesis and release of prostaglandins. Acting centrally, it would appear to produce analgesia at a hypothalamic site in the brain, although the mode of action is not known.
Aspirin also acts on the hypothalamus to produce antipyresis; heat dissipation is increased as a result of vasodilation and increased peripheral blood flow. Aspirin's antipyretic activity may also be related to inhibition of synthesis and release of prostaglandins.
In a crossover study, Easprin at a dose of one tablet (15 grains) three times a day produced an average fecal blood loss of 1.54 ml per day. Uncoated aspirin at a dosage of three 5 grain tablets given three times a day caused an average fecal blood loss of 4.33 ml per day.
Easprin Tablets are enteric coated. This coating acts to prevent the release of aspirin in the stomach but permits the tablet to dissolve with resultant absorption in the upper portion of the small intestine. This reduces any gastric irritation that may occur with uncoated aspirin but does delay the onset of action. Aspirin is rapidly hydrolyzed primarily in the liver to salicylic acid, which is conjugated with glycine (forming salicyluric acid) and glucuronic acid and excreted largely in the urine. As a result of the rapid hydrolysis, plasma concentrations of aspirin are always low and rarely exceed 20 mcg/ml at ordinary therapeutic doses. The peak salicylate level for uncoated aspirin occurs in about 2 hours; however with enteric coated aspirin tablets this is delayed. A direct correlation between salicylate plasma levels and clinical analgesic effectiveness has not been definitely established, but effective analgesia is usually achieved at plasma levels of 15 to 30 mg per 100 ml. Effective antiinflammatory activity is usually achieved at salicylate plasma levels of 20 to 30 mg per 100 ml. There is also poor correlation between toxic symptoms and plasma salicylate concentrations, but most patients exhibit symptoms of salicylism at plasma salicylate levels of 35 mg per 100 ml. The plasma half-life for aspirin is approximately 15 minutes; that for salicylate lengthens as the dose increases: Doses of 300 to 650 mg have a half-life of 3.1 to 3.2 hours; with doses of 1 gram, the half-life is increased to 5 hours and with 2 grams it is increased to about 9 hours.
Salicylates are excreted mainly by the kidney. Studies in man indicate that salicylate is excreted in the urine as free salicylic acid (10%), salicyluric acid (75%), salicylic phenolic (10%), and acyl (5%) glucuronides and gentisic acid.
Indications and Usage: Easprin is indicated in patients who need the higher 15 grain dose of aspirin in the long-term palliative treatment of mild to moderate pain and inflammation of arthritic and other inflammatory conditions.
Contraindications: Easprin should not be used in patients who have previously exhibited hypersensitivity to aspirin and/or nonsteroidal antiinflammatory agents.
Easprin should not be given to patients with a recent history of gastrointestinal bleeding or in patients with bleeding disorders (eg, hemophilia).
Warnings: Easprin Tablets should be used with caution when anticoagulants are prescribed concurrently, for aspirin may depress the concentration of prothrombin in plasma and thereby increase bleeding time. Large doses of salicylates have a hypoglycemic action and may enhance the effect of the oral hypoglycemics. Consequently, they should not be given concomitantly; if however, this is necessary, the dosage of the hypoglycemic agent must be reduced while the salicylate is given. This hypoglycemic action may also affect the insulin requirements of diabetics.
Although salicylates in large doses are uricosuric agents, smaller amounts may decrease the uricosuric effects of probenecid, sulfinpyrazone, and phenylbutazone.
Precautions:
General: Easprin Tablets should be administered with caution to patients with asthma, nasal polyps, or nasal allergies.
In patients receiving large doses of aspirin and/or prolonged therapy, mild salicylate intoxication (salicylism) may develop that may be reversed by reduction in dosage.
Although the fecal blood loss with Easprin is less than that with uncoated aspirin tablets, Easprin Tablets should be administered with caution to patients with a history of gastric distress, ulcer, or bleeding problems. Occult gastrointestinal bleeding occurs in many patients but is not correlated with gastric distress. The amount of blood lost is usually insignificant clinically, but with prolonged administration, it may result in iron deficiency anemia.
Sodium excretion produced by spironolactone may be decreased in the presence of salicylates.

Salicylates can produce changes in thyroid function tests.

Salicylates should be used with caution in patients with severe hepatic damage, preexisting hypoprothrombinemia, or Vitamin K deficiency, and in those undergoing surgery.

Drug Interactions:
Anticoagulants: See Warnings.
Hypoglycemic Agents: See Warnings.
Uricosuric Agents: Aspirin may decrease the effects of probenecid, sulfinpyrazone, and phenylbutazone.
Spironolactone: See general precautions above.
Alcohol: Has a synergistic effect with aspirin in causing gastrointestinal bleeding.
Corticosteroids: Concomitant administration with aspirin may increase the risk of gastrointestinal ulceration.
Pyrazolone Derivatives (phenylbutazone, oxyphenbutazone, and possibly dipyrone): Concomitant administration with aspirin may increase the risk of gastrointestinal ulceration.
Nonsteroidal Antiinflammatory Agents: Aspirin is contraindicated in patients who are hypersensitive to nonsteroidal antiinflammatory agents.
Urinary Alkalinizers: Decrease aspirin effectiveness by increasing the rate of salicylate renal excretion.
Phenobarbital: Decreases aspirin effectiveness by enzyme induction.
Propranolol: May decrease aspirin's antiinflammatory action by competing for the same receptors.
Antacids: Easprin should not be given concurrently with antacids, since an increase in the pH of the stomach may affect the enteric coating of the tablets.

Usage in Pregnancy: Aspirin does not appear to have any teratogenic effects. However, it has been reported that adverse effects were increased in the mother and fetus following chronic ingestion of aspirin. Prolonged pregnancy and labor with increased bleeding before and after delivery, as well as decreased birth weight and increased rate of stillbirth were correlated with high blood salicylate levels. Because of possible adverse effects on the neonate and the potential for increased maternal blood loss, aspirin should be avoided during the last three months of pregnancy.

Adverse Reactions:
Gastrointestinal: Dyspepsia, nausea, vomiting, diarrhea, gastrointestinal bleeding, and/or ulceration.
Ear: Tinnitus, vertigo, reversible hearing loss.
Hematologic: Prolongation of bleeding time, leukopenia, thrombocytopenia, purpura, decreased plasma iron concentration and shortened erythrocyte survival time.
Dermatologic and Hypersensitivity: Urticaria, angioedema, pruritus, various skin eruptions, asthma, and anaphylaxis.
Miscellaneous: Acute reversible hepatotoxicity, mental confusion, drowsiness, sweating, dizziness, headache, fever, thirst, and dimness of vision.

Overdosage:
Overdosage of 200 to 500 mg/kg is in the fatal range. Early symptoms are CNS stimulation with vomiting, hyperpnea, hyperactivity, and possibly convulsions. This progresses quickly to depression, coma, respiratory failure, and collapse. These symptoms are accompanied by severe electrolyte disturbances.

In the treatment of salicylate overdosage, intensive supportive therapy should be instituted immediately. Plasma salicylate levels should be measured in order to determine the severity of the poisoning and to provide a guide for therapy. Emptying of the stomach should be accomplished as soon as possible with ipecac syrup unless the patient is depressed. In depressed patients use airway protected gastric lavage. Delay absorption with activated charcoal and give a saline cathartic. Proceed according to Standard Reference Procedures for Salicylate Intoxication.

Dosage and Administration:
Usual Adult Dosage: One tablet 3 to 4 times daily.

Patients who have displayed no significant adverse effects on a long term qid regimen and who receive a total daily dosage of aspirin no greater than 3.9 grams may be considered for a bid regimen (2 tablets of Easprin twice daily). Patients on the bid Easprin regimen should be closely monitored for serum salicylate levels, increased incidence of CNS-related adverse effects, increased fecal blood loss, or any other signs or symptoms suggestive of significant blood loss.

If necessary, dosage may be increased until relief is obtained, but dosage should be maintained slightly below that which produces tinnitus. Plasma salicylate levels may also be helpful in determining proper dosage (see Clinical Pharmacology section).

How Supplied: Easprin enteric coated tablets each containing 15 grains (975 mg) aspirin are available:
N 0071-0490-24—Bottles of 100
Storage: Store at controlled room temperature 15° to 30°C (59° to 86°F).
AHFS Category 28:08   0490G013
Shown in Product Identification Section, page 424

ELASE® ℞
[ē′ lāse″]
(fibrinolysin and desoxyribonuclease, combined [bovine])
ELASE OINTMENT ℞
(fibrinolysin and desoxyribonuclease, combined [bovine], ointment)
ELASE–CHLOROMYCETIN® ℞
OINTMENT
(fibrinolysin and desoxyribonuclease, combined [bovine], with chloramphenicol ointment)

Description: Elase is a combination of two lytic enzymes, fibrinolysin and desoxyribonuclease, supplied as a lyophilized powder and in an ointment base of liquid petrolatum and polyethylene. The fibrinolysin component is derived from bovine plasma and the desoxyribonuclease is isolated in a purified form from bovine pancreas. The fibrinolysin used in the combination is activated by chloroform.

Elase-Chloromycetin Ointment: Elase-Chloromycetin Ointment contains two lytic enzymes, fibrinolysin and desoxyribonuclease, combined with chloramphenicol in an ointment base.

Chloramphenicol is a broad-spectrum antibiotic originally isolated from *Streptomyces venezuelae*. It is therapeutically active against a wide variety of susceptible organisms, both gram-positive and gram-negative. Chemically, chloramphenicol may be identified as D(-)- threo-1-p-nitrophenyl -2 - dichloroacetamido- 1, 3-propanediol.

Action: Combination of these two enzymes is based on the observation that purulent exudates consist largely of fibrinous material and nucleoprotein. Desoxyribonuclease attacks the desoxyribonucleic acid (DNA) and fibrinolysin attacks principally fibrin of blood clots and fibrinous exudates.

The activity of desoxyribonuclease is limited principally to the production of large polynucleotides, which are less likely to be absorbed than the more diffusible protein fractions liberated by certain enzyme preparations obtained from bacteria. The fibrinolytic action of Elase and of the enzymes in Elase Ointment and Elase-Chloromycetin Ointment is directed mainly against denatured proteins, such as those found in devitalized tissue, while protein elements of living cells remain relatively unaffected.

Elase, Elase Ointment, and Elase-Chloromycetin Ointment are combinations of active enzymes. This is an important consideration in treating patients suffering from lesions resulting from impaired circulation.

The enzymatic action of Elase helps to produce clean surfaces and thus supports healing in a variety of exudative lesions.

Elase-Chloromycetin Ointment:
Chloramphenicol is a broad-spectrum antibiotic that is primarily bacteriostatic and acts by inhibition of protein synthesis by interfering with the transfer of activated amino acids from soluble RNA to ribosomes. Development of resistance to chloramphenicol can be regarded as minimal for staphylococci and many other species of bacteria. The action of Elase-Chloromycetin helps to produce clean surfaces and thus supports healing in a variety of exudative lesions.

Indications: Elase and Elase Ointment are indicated for topical use as debriding agents in a variety of inflammatory and infected lesions. These include: (1) general surgical wounds; (2) ulcerative lesions—trophic, decubitus, stasis, arteriosclerotic; (3) second- and third-degree burns; (4) circumcision and episiotomy. Elase and Elase Ointment are used intravaginally in: (1) cervicitis—benign, postpartum, and postconization, and (2) vaginitis. Elase is used as an irrigating agent in the following conditions: (1) infected wounds—abscesses, fistulae, and sinus tracts; (2) otorhinolaryngologic wounds; (3) superficial hematomas (except when the hematoma is adjacent to or within adipose tissue).

Elase-Chloromycetin Ointment:
Elase-Chloromycetin Ointment is indicated for use in the treatment of infected lesions, such as burns, ulcers, and wounds where the actions of both a debriding agent and a topical antibiotic are desired. This dual-purpose approach is especially useful in the treatment of infections caused by organisms that utilize a process of fibrin deposition as protective device (ie, coagulase and the staphylococcus). Appropriate measures should be taken to determine the susceptibility of the pathogen to chloramphenicol.

Contraindications: These products (Elase, Elase Ointment, Elase-Chloromycetin Ointment) are contraindicated in individuals with a history of hypersensitivity reactions to any of their components. Elase is not recommended for parenteral use because the bovine fibrinolysin may be antigenic.

Warnings: *Elase-Chloromycetin Ointment:*
Bone marrow hypoplasia, including aplastic anemia and death, has been reported following the local application of chloramphenicol.

Precautions: *Elase-Chloromycetin Ointment:* The prolonged use of antibiotics may occasionally result in overgrowth of nonsusceptible organisms, including fungi. If new infections appear during medication, the drug should be discontinued and appropriate measures should be taken.

In all except very superficial infections, the topical use of chloramphenicol should be supplemented by appropriate systemic medication.

Elase, Elase Ointment, Elase-Chloromycetin Ointment: The usual precautions against allergic reactions should be observed, particularly in persons with a history of sensitivity to materials of bovine origin or to mercury compounds.

Elase: To be maximally effective, Elase solutions must be freshly prepared before use. The loss in activity is reduced by refrigeration; however, even when stored in a refrigerator, the solution should not be used 24 hours or more after reconstitution.

Adverse Reactions: Side effects attributable to the enzymes have not been a problem at the dose and for the indications recommended herein. With higher concentrations, side effects have been minimal, consisting of local hyperemia.

Chills and fever attributable to antigenic action of profibrinolysin activators of bacterial origin are not a problem with Elase, Elase Ointment, or Elase-Chloromycetin Ointment.

Elase-Chloromycetin Ointment: Signs of local irritation, with subjective symptoms of itching or burning, angioneurotic edema, urticaria, vesicular and maculopapular dermatitis have been reported in patients sensitive to chloramphenicol and are

Continued on next page

This product information was prepared in August, 1984. On these and other Parke-Davis Products, information may be obtained by addressing **PARKE-DAVIS**, *Division of Warner-Lambert Company, Morris Plains, New Jersey 07950.*

Parke-Davis—Cont.

causes for discontinuing the medication. Similar sensitivity reactions to other materials in topical preparations may also occur. Blood dyscrasias have been associated with the use of chloramphenicol.

Preparation of Elase Solution: The contents of each vial may be reconstituted with 10 ml of isotonic sodium chloride solution. Higher or lower concentrations can be prepared if desired by varying the amount of the diluent.

Dosage and Administration: Since the conditions for which Elase and Elase Ointment and Elase-Chloromycetin Ointment are helpful vary considerably in severity, dosage must be adjusted to the individual case; however, the following general recommendations can be made.

Successful use of enzymatic debridement depends on several factors: (1) dense, dry eschar, if present, should be removed surgically before enzymatic debridement is attempted; (2) the enzyme must be in constant contact with the substrate; (3) accumulated necrotic debris must be periodically removed; (4) the enzyme must be replenished at least once daily; and (5) secondary closure or skin grafting must be employed as soon as possible after optimal debridement has been attained. It is further essential that wound-dressing techniques be performed carefully under aseptic conditions and that appropriate systemically acting antibiotics be administered concomitantly if, in the opinion of the physician, they are indicated.

General Topical Uses: *Elase Ointment:* Local application should be repeated at intervals for as long as enzyme action is desired. After application Elase Ointment becomes rapidly and progressively less active and is probably exhausted for practical purposes at the end of 24 hours. A recommended procedure for application of Elase Ointment follows.
1. Clean the wound with water, peroxide, or normal saline and dry area gently. If there is a dense, dry eschar present, it should be removed surgically before applying Elase.
2. Apply a *thin* layer of Elase Ointment.
3. Cover with petrolatum gauze or another type of nonadhering dressing.
4. Change the dressing at least ONCE a day, preferably two or three times daily. Frequency of application is more important than the amount of Elase used. Flush away the necrotic debris and fibrinous exudates with saline, peroxide, or warm water so that newly applied ointment can be in direct contact with the substrate.

Elase: Local application should be repeated at intervals for as long as enzyme action is desired. Elase solution may be applied topically as a liquid, spray, or wet dressing. Application of a gentle spray of the solution can be accomplished by using a conventional atomizer. After application, Elase, especially in solution, becomes rapidly and progressively less active and is probably exhausted for practical purposes at the end of 24 hours. The dry material for solution is stable at room temperature through the expiration date printed on the package. A recommended procedure for application of a solution of Elase using a Wet-to-Dry method follows.
1. Mix one vial of Elase powder with 10 to 50 ml of saline and saturate strips of fine-mesh gauze or an unfolded sterile gauze sponge with the Elase solution.
2. Pack ulcerated area with the Elase-saturated gauze, making sure the gauze remains in contact with the necrotic substrate (if the lesion is covered with a heavy eschar, it must be removed surgically before wet-to-dry debridement is begun).
3. ALLOW GAUZE TO DRY IN CONTACT WITH THE ULCERATED LESION (approximately six to eight hours). As the gauze dries, the necrotic tissues slough and become enmeshed in the gauze.
4. Remove dried gauze. This mechanically debrides the area. Repeat wet-to-dry procedure three or four times daily, since frequent dressing changes greatly enhance results. After two, three, or four days, the area becomes clean and starts to fill in with granulation tissue.

Intravaginal use: *Elase Ointment:* In mild to moderate vaginitis and cervicitis, 5 ml of Elase Ointment should be deposited deep in the vagina once nightly at bedtime for approximately five applications, or until the entire contents of one 30-g tube has been used. The patient should be checked by her physician to determine possible need for further therapy. In more severe cervicitis and vaginitis, some physicians prefer to initiate therapy with an application of Elase (fibrinolysin and desoxyribonuclease, combined, [bovine]) in solution. See Elase package insert.

Elase: In severe cervicitis and vaginitis, the physician may instill 10 ml of the solution intravaginally, wait one or two minutes for the enzyme to disperse and then insert a cotton tampon in the vaginal canal. The tampon should be removed the next day. Continuing therapy should then be instituted with Elase Ointment (fibrinolysin and desoxyribonuclease, combined [bovine] ointment). See Elase Ointment package insert.

Abscesses, empyema cavities, fistulae, sinus tracts or subcutaneous hematomas: Despite the contraindication against parenteral use, Elase has been used in irrigating these specific conditions. The Elase solution should be drained and replaced at intervals of six to ten hours to reduce the amount of by-product accumulation and minimize loss of enzyme activity. Traces of blood in the discharge usually indicate active filling in of the cavity.

How Supplied:
ELASE (fibrinolysin and desoxyribonuclease, combined [bovine])
N 0071-4256-01 Elase—lyophilized powder for solution
Elase is supplied in rubber diaphragm-capped vials of 30-ml capacity containing 25 units (Loomis) of fibrinolysin and 15,000 units (modified Christensen method) of desoxyribonuclease with 0.1 mg thimerosal (mercury derivative).
This product also contains sodium chloride and sucrose as incidental ingredients.
Shown in Product Identification Section, page 424
121 876350/ZF

ELASE OINTMENT (fibrinolysin and desoxyribonuclease, combined [bovine], ointment)
N 0071-4279-10 Elase Ointment, 10 g.
The 10-g tube contains 10 units of fibrinolysin and 6,666 units of desoxyribonuclease with 0.04 mg thimerosal (mercury derivative) in a special ointment base of liquid petrolatum and polyethylene.
N 0071-4279-13 Elase Ointment, 30 g.
The 30-g tube contains 30 units of fibrinolysin and 20,000 units of desoxyribonuclease with 0.12 mg thimerosal (mercury derivative) in a special ointment base of liquid petrolatum and polyethylene.
For gynecologic use, six disposable vaginal applicators (V-Applicator*) as a separate package are available for this tube when required to facilitate administration of the proper dose.
These products also contain sodium chloride and sucrose as incidental ingredients.
Shown in Product Identification Section, page 424
4279G020
121 855100/ZF

ELASE-CHLOROMYCETIN OINTMENT (fibrinolysin and desoxyribonuclease, combined [bovine], with chloramphenicol ointment)
Elase-Chloromycetin (fibrinolysin-desoxyribonuclease-chloramphenicol) is supplied in 30-g and 10-g ointment tubes. The 10-g tubes have an elongated nozzle to facilitate the application to surface lesions.
The 30-g tubes contain 30 units (Loomis) of fibrinolysin (bovine) and 20,000 units** of desoxyribonuclease with 0.12 mg thimerosal (mercury derivative) (as a preservative) and 0.3 g† chloramphenicol in a special ointment base of liquid petrolatum and polyethylene.
The 10-g tubes contain 10 units (Loomis) of fibrinolysin (bovine) and 6,666 units** of desoxyribonuclease with 0.04 mg thimerosal (mercury derivative) (as a preservative) and 0.1 g† chloramphenicol in a special ointment base of liquid petrolatum and polyethylene.
The ointment contains sodium chloride and sucrose used in its manufacture.
*Trademark
**Modified Christensen method.
†10 mg chloramphenicol per gram, or 1%.
Shown in Product Identification Section, page 424
4281G020
121 863300/ZD

ELDEC® KAPSEALS® ℞
[ĕl′dĕc″]

Composition: Each capsule contains vitamin A (acetate), 1,667 IU; vitamin C (ascorbic acid), 66.7 mg; vitamin B_1 (thiamine mononitrate), 10 mg; vitamin B_2 (riboflavin), 0.87 mg; vitamin B_6 (pyridoxine hydrochloride), 0.67 mg; nicotinamide (niacinamide), 16.7 mg; dl-panthenol, 10 mg; ferrous sulfate, dried, 16.7 mg; iodine (as potassium iodide), 0.05 mg; calcium carbonate, precipitated, 66.7 mg; vitamin E (dl-alpha tocopheryl acetate), (10 mg) 10 IU; vitamin B_{12} (cyanocobalamin), 2 mcg; folic acid, 0.33 mg.

Action and Uses: For certain vitamin and mineral deficiencies.

Caution—Folic acid in doses above 0.1 mg daily may obscure pernicious anemia in that hematologic remission can occur while neurological manifestations remain progressive.

Dosage: The usual dosage of Eldec is one capsule three times a day.

How Supplied: N 0071-0337-24 Eldec (Kapseal 398), bottles of 100. Parcode® No. 337; new ID code imprint, formerly 398—no formula change.
Shown in Product Identification Section, page 424

ERGOSTAT® ℞
(Ergotamine Tartrate Tablets) sublingual

Description: Each sublingual tablet contains 2 mg ergotamine tartrate.

Pharmacological Category: Vasoconstrictor, uterine stimulant, alpha adrenoreceptor antagonist.

Therapeutic Class: Antimigraine.

Chemical Name: Ergotaman-3′,6′,18-trione,12′-hydroxy-2′-methyl-5′-(phenylmethyl)-,(5′α)-,[R-(R*, R*)]-2,3-dihydroxybutanedioate (2:1) salt.

Clinical Pharmacology: The pharmacological properties of ergotamine are extremely complex; some of its actions are unrelated to each other, and even mutually antagonistic. The drug has partial agonist and/or antagonist activity against tryptaminergic, dopaminergic and alpha adrenergic receptors depending upon their site, and it is a highly active uterine stimulant. It causes constriction of peripheral and cranial blood vessels and produces depression of central vasomotor centers. The pain of a migraine attack is believed to be due to greatly increased amplitude of pulsations in the cranial arteries, especially the meningeal branches of the external carotid artery. Ergotamine reduces extracranial blood flow, causes a decline in the amplitude of pulsation in the cranial arteries, and decreases hyperperfusion of the territory of the basilar artery. It does not reduce cerebral hemispheric blood flow. Long-term usage has established the fact that ergotamine tartrate is effective in controlling up to 70% of acute migraine attacks, so that it is now considered specific for the treatment of this headache syndrome. Ergotamine produces constriction of both arteries and veins. In doses used in the treatment of vascular headaches, ergotamine usually produces only small increases in blood pressure, but it does increase peripheral resistance and decrease blood flow in various organs. Small doses of the drug increase the force and frequency of uterine contraction; larger doses increase the resting tone of the uterus also. The gravid uterus is particularly sensitive to these effects of ergotamine. Although specific teratogenic effects attributable to ergotamine have not been found, the fetus suffers if ergotamine is given to the mother. Retarded fetal growth and an increase in intrauterine death and resorption have been seen in animals. These are thought to result from ergotamine-induced increases in uterine motility and vasoconstriction in the placental vascular bed.

The bioavailability of sublingually administered ergotamine has not been determined.

Ergotamine is metabolized in the liver by largely undefined pathways, and 90% of the metabolites are excreted in the bile. The unmetabolized drug is erratically secreted in the saliva, and only traces of unmetabolized drug appear in the urine and feces. Ergotamine is secreted into breast milk. The elimination half-life of ergotamine from plasma is about 2 hours, but the drug may be stored in some tissues, which would account for its long-lasting therapeutic and toxic actions.

Indications and Usage: Ergotamine tartrate is indicated as therapy to abort or prevent vascular headache, e.g., migraine, migraine variants, or so called "histaminic cephalalgia".

Contraindications: Ergotamine is contraindicated in peripheral vascular disease (thromboangiitis obliterans, luetic arteritis, severe arteriosclerosis, thrombophlebitis, Raynaud's disease), coronary heart disease, hypertension, impaired hepatic or renal function, severe pruritus, and sepsis. It is also contraindicated in patients who are hypersensitive to any of its components. Ergotamine may cause fetal harm when administered to a pregnant woman by virtue of its powerful uterine stimulant actions. It is contraindicated in women who are, or may become, pregnant.

Precautions:
General: Although signs and symptoms of ergotism rarely develop even after long-term intermittent use of ergotamine, care should be exercised to remain within the limits of recommended dosage.

Drug Interactions: The effects of ergotamine tartrate may be potentiated by triacetyloleandomycin which inhibits the metabolism of ergotamine. The pressor effects of ergotamine and other vasoconstrictor drugs can combine to cause dangerous hypertension.

Carcinogenesis: No studies have been performed to investigate ergotamine tartrate for carcinogenic effects.

Pregnancy: Pregnancy Category X—See CONTRAINDICATIONS.

Nursing Mothers: Ergotamine is secreted into human milk. It can reach the breast-fed infant by this route and exert pharmacologic effects in it. Caution should be exercised when ergotamine is administered to a nursing woman. Excessive dosing or prolonged administration of ergotamine may inhibit lactation.

Adverse Reactions: Nausea and vomiting occur in up to 10% of patients after ingestion of therapeutic doses of ergotamine. Weakness of the legs and pain in limb muscles are also frequent complaints. Numbness and tingling of the fingers and toes, precordial pain, transient changes in heart rate and localized edema and itching may also occur, particularly in patients who are sensitive to the drug.

Drug Abuse and Dependence: Patients who take ergotamine for extended periods of time may become dependent upon it and require progressively increasing doses for relief of vascular headaches, and for prevention of dysphoric effects which follow withdrawal of the drug.

Overdosage: Overdosage with ergotamine causes nausea, vomiting, weakness of the legs, pain in limb muscles, numbness and tingling of the fingers and toes, precordial pain, tachycardia or bradycardia, hypertension or hypotension and localized edema and itching together with signs and symptoms of ischemia due to vasoconstriction of peripheral arteries and arterioles. The feet and hands become cold, pale and numb. Muscle pain occurs while walking and later at rest also. Gangrene may ensue. Confusion, depression, drowsiness, and convulsions are occasional signs of ergotamine toxicity. Overdosage is particularly likely to occur in patients with sepsis or impaired renal or hepatic function. Patients with peripheral vascular disease are especially at risk of developing peripheral ischemia following treatment with ergotamine. Some cases of ergotamine poisoning have been reported in patients who have taken less than 5 mg of the drug. Usually, however, toxicity is seen at doses of ergotamine tartrate in excess of about 15 mg in 24 hours or 40 mg in a few days.

Treatment of ergotamine overdosage consists of the withdrawal of the drug followed by symptomatic measures including attempts to maintain an adequate circulation in the affected parts. Anticoagulant drugs, low molecular weight dextran and potent vasodilator drugs may all be beneficial. Intravenous infusion of sodium nitroprusside has also been reported to be successful. Vasodilators must be used with special care in the presence of hypotension.

Nausea and vomiting may be relieved by atropine or antiemetic compounds of the phenothiazine group. Ergotamine is dialyzable.

Dosage and Administration: All efforts should be made to initiate therapy as soon as possible after the first symptoms of the attack are noted, because success is proportional to rapidity of treatment, and lower dosages will be effective. At the first sign of an attack or to relieve the symptoms of the full-blown attack, one sublingual tablet (2 mg) is placed under the tongue. Another sublingual tablet (2 mg) should be placed under the tongue at half-hourly intervals thereafter, if necessary, for a total of three tablets (6 mg). Dosage must not exceed three tablets (6 mg) in any 24-hour period. Limit dosage to not more than five tablets (10 mg) in any one week.

How Supplied: Ergostat (Ergotamine Tartrate Tablets) sublingual, 2 mg (round, orange, coded P-D 111), is supplied as follows:

N 0071-0111-13 Vial containing 24 individually packaged tablets.

Store at controlled room temperature 15°–30°C (59°–86°F).

AHFS Category 12:16   0111G012

Shown in Product Identification Section, page 424

ERYC®   R
[ē'ryc]
(Erythromycin Capsules, USP)

Description: ERYC Capsules contain enteric-coated pellets of erythromycin base for oral administration. Erythromycin is produced by a strain of *Streptomyces erythraeus* and belongs to the macrolide group of antibiotics. It is basic and readily forms salts with acids, but it is the base which is microbiologically active. Each ERYC Capsule contains 250 milligrams of erythromycin base. Erythromycin base is 14-Ethyl-7, 12, 13-trihydroxy-3, 5, 7, 9, 11, 13-hexamethyl-2, 10-dioxo-6-[(3, 4, 6-trideoxy-3-(dimethylamino) -β- D*xylo*-hexapyranosyl) oxy] oxacyclotetradec-4-yl 2, 6-dideoxy-3-C-methyl-3-O-methyl -α L-*ribo*-hexopyranoside.

Clinical Pharmacology: Orally administered erythromycin base and its salts are readily absorbed in the microbiologically active form. Interindividual variations in the absorption of erythromycin are, however, observed, and some patients do not achieve acceptable serum levels. Erythromycin is largely bound to plasma proteins, and the freely dissociating bound fraction after administration of erythromycin base represents 90% of the total erythromycin absorbed. After absorption erythromycin diffuses readily into most body fluids. In the absence of meningeal inflammation, low concentrations are normally achieved in the spinal fluid but the passage of the drug across the blood-brain barrier increases in meningitis. Erythromycin is excreted in breast milk. The drug crosses the placental barrier but fetal plasma levels are low.

In the presence of normal hepatic function erythromycin is concentrated in the liver and is excreted in the bile; the effect of hepatic dysfunction on biliary excretion of erythromycin is not known. After oral administration less than 5% of the administered dose can be recovered in the active form in the urine.

The enteric coating of pellets in ERYC Capsules protects the erythromycin base from inactivation by gastric acidity. Because of their small size and enteric coating, the pellets readily pass intact from the stomach to the small intestine and dissolve efficiently to allow absorption of erythromycin in a uniform manner. After administration of a single dose of a 250 mg ERYC capsule, peak serum levels in the range of 1.13 to 1.68 mcg/ml are attained in approximately 3 hours and decline to 0.30-0.42 mcg/ml in 6 hours. Optimal conditions for stability in the presence of gastric secretion and for complete absorption are attained when ERYC is taken on an empty stomach.

Microbiology Erythromycin acts by inhibition of protein synthesis by binding 50 S ribosomal subunits of susceptible organisms. It does not affect nucleic acid synthesis. Antagonism has been demonstrated between clindamycin and erythromycin. Resistance to erythromycin by some strains of *Haemophilus influenzae* and staphylococci has been demonstrated. Specimens should be obtained for culture and susceptibility testing.

Erythromycin is usually active against the following organisms in *vitro* and in clinical infections:

Streptococcus pyogenes
Alpha hemolytic streptococci (viridans group)
Staphylococcus aureus (Resistant organisms may emerge during treatment.)
Streptococcus pneumoniae
Mycoplasma pneumoniae (Eaton's Agent)
Haemophilus influenzae (Many strains are resistant to erythromycin alone, but are susceptible to erythromycin and sulfonamides together.)
Treponema pallidum
Corynebacterium diphtheriae
Corynebacterium minutissimum
Entamoeba histolytica
Listeria monocytogenes
Neisseria gonorrhoeae
Bordetella pertussis
Legionella pneumophila (agent of Legionnaires' Disease)

Susceptibility Testing Quantitative methods that require measurement of zone diameters give the most precise estimates of antibiotic susceptibility. One such standardized single disc procedure has been recommended for use with discs to test susceptibility to erythromycin.[1] Interpretation involves correlation of the zone diameters obtained in the disc test with minimum inhibitory concentration (MIC) values for erythromycin.

Reports from the laboratory giving results of the standardized single-disc susceptibility test using a 15 mcg erythromycin disc should be interpreted according to the following criteria:

Susceptible organisms produce zones of 18 mm or greater indicating that the tested organism is likely to respond to therapy.

Resistant organisms produce zones of 13 mm or less, indicating that other therapy should be selected.

Organisms of intermediate susceptibility produce zones of 14 to 17 mm. The "intermediate" category provides a "buffer zone" which should prevent small uncontrolled technical factors from causing major discrepancies in interpretations, thus when a zone diameter falls within the "intermediate" range, the results may be considered equivocal. If alternate drugs are not available, confirmation by dilution tests may be indicated.

A bacterial isolate may be considered susceptible if the MIC value[2] (minimal inhibitory concentration) for erythromycin is not more than 2 mcg/ml. Organisms are considered resistant if the MIC is 8 mcg/ml or higher.

Indications and Usage:
ERYC is indicated in children and adults for the treatment of the following conditions:

Upper respiratory tract infections of mild to moderate degree caused by *Streptococcus pyogenes* (group A beta hemolytic streptococci);

Continued on next page

This product information was prepared in August, 1984. On these and other Parke-Davis Products, information may be obtained by addressing PARKE-DAVIS, Division of Warner-Lambert Company, Morris Plains, New Jersey 07950.

Parke-Davis—Cont.

Streptococcus pneumoniae (Diplococcus pneumoniae); Haemophilus influenzae (when used concomitantly with adequate doses of sulfonamides, since not all strains of *H influenzae* are susceptible at the erythromycin concentrations ordinarily achieved). (See appropriate sulfonamide labeling for prescribing information.)

Lower respiratory tract infections of mild to moderate severity caused by *Streptococcus pyogenes* (group A beta hemolytic streptococci): *Streptococcus pneumoniae (Diplococcus pneumoniae).*

Respiratory tract infections due to *Mycoplasma pneumoniae (Eaton's agent).*

Pertussis (whooping cough) caused by *Bordetella pertussis.* Erythromycin is effective in eliminating the organism from the nasopharynx of infected individuals, rendering them noninfectious. Some clinical studies suggest that erythromycin may be helpful in the prophylaxis of pertussis in exposed susceptible individuals.

Diphtheria—As an adjunct to antitoxin in infections due to *Corynebacterium diphtheriae*, to prevent establishment of carriers and to eradicate the organism in carriers.

Erythrasma—In the treatment of infections due to *Corynebacterium minutissimum.*

Intestinal amebiasis caused by *Entamoeba histolytica* (oral erythromycins only). Extraenteric amebiasis requires treatment with other agents.

Infections due to *Listeria monocytogenes.*

Skin and soft tissue infections of mild to moderate severity caused by *Streptococcus pyogenes* and *Staphylococcus aureus* (Resistant staphylococci may emerge during treatment.)

Primary syphilis caused by *Treponema pallidum.* Erythromycin (oral forms only) is an alternate choice of treatment for primary syphilis in patients allergic to the penicillins. In treatment of primary syphilis, spinal fluid should be examined before treatment and as part of the follow-up after therapy. The use of erythromycin for the treatment of *in utero* syphilis is not recommended (See CLINICAL PHARMACOLOGY).

Erythromycins are indicated for treatment of the following infections caused by *Chlamydia trachomatis:* conjunctivitis of the newborn, pneumonia of infancy, urogenital infections during pregnancy. When tetracyclines are contraindicated or not tolerated, erythromycin is indicated for the treatment of uncomplicated urethral, endocervical, or rectal infections in adults due to *Chlamydia trachomatis*[4].

Legionnaires' disease caused by *Legionella pneumophila.*

Although no controlled clinical efficacy studies have been conducted, *in vitro* and limited preliminary clinical data suggest that erythromycin may be effective in treating Legionnaires' disease.

Therapy with erythromycin should be monitored by bacteriological studies and by clinical response (See CLINICAL PHARMACOLOGY—Microbiology).

Injectable benzathine penicillin G is considered by the American Heart Association to be the drug of choice in the treatment and prevention of streptococcal pharyngitis and in long-term prophylaxis of rheumatic fever. When oral medication is preferred for treatment of the above conditions, penicillin G, V, or erythromycin are alternate drugs of choice.

Although no controlled clinical efficacy trials have been conducted, erythromycin has been suggested by the American Heart Association and the American Dental Association for use in a regimen for prophylaxis against bacterial endocarditis in patients allergic to penicillin who have congenital and/or rheumatic or other acquired valvular heart disease when they undergo dental procedures and surgical procedures of the upper respiratory tract.[3] (Erythromycin is not suitable prior to genitourinary surgery where the organisms likely to lead to bacteremia are gram-negative bacilli or the enterococcal group of streptococci).

NOTE: When selecting antibiotics for the prevention of bacterial endocarditis the physician or dentist should read the full joint 1977 statement of the American Heart Association and the American Dental Association.[3]

Contraindication: ERYC is contraindicated in patients with known hypersensitivity to this antibiotic.

Warning: There have been a few reports of hepatic dysfunction, with or without jaundice, occurring in patients receiving erythromycin ethylsuccinate, base, and stearate products.

Precautions: Caution should be exercised when erythromycin is administered to patients with impaired hepatic function (see CLINICAL PHARMACOLOGY and WARNING).

Erythromycin use in patients who are receiving high doses of theophylline may be associated with an increase in serum theophylline levels and potential theophylline toxicity. In case of theophylline toxicity and/or elevated serum theophylline levels, the dose of theophylline should be reduced while the patient is receiving concomitant erythromycin therapy.

Erythromycin interferes with the fluorometric determination of urinary catecholamines.

Prolonged or repeated use of erythromycin may result in an overgrowth of nonsusceptible bacteria or fungi. If superinfection occurs, erythromycin should be discontinued and appropriate therapy instituted.

When indicated, incision and drainage or other surgical procedures should be performed in conjunction with antibiotic therapy.

Pregnancy Category B—Reproduction studies have been performed in rats, mice and rabbits using erythromycin and its various salts and esters, at doses which were several times multiples of the usual human dose. No evidence of impaired fertility or harm to the fetus that appeared related to erythromycin was reported in these studies. There are, however, no adequate and well-controlled studies in pregnant women. Because animal reproduction studies are not always predictive of human response, this drug should be used during pregnancy only if clearly needed.

Labor and Delivery—The effect of ERYC on labor and delivery is unknown.

Nursing Mothers—Erythromycin is excreted in milk (see CLINICAL PHARMACOLOGY).

Pediatric Use—See INDICATIONS AND USAGE and DOSAGE AND ADMINISTRATION.

Adverse Reactions: The most frequent side effects of oral erythromycin preparations are gastrointestinal and are dose-related. They include nausea, vomiting, abdominal pain, diarrhea and anorexia. Symptoms of hepatic dysfunction and/or abnormal liver function test results may occur (see WARNING).

Mild allergic reactions such as rashes with or without pruritus, urticaria, bullous fixed eruptions, and eczema have been reported with erythromycin. Serious allergic reactions, including anaphylaxis have been reported.

A few cases of transient deafness have been reported with high doses of erythromycin.

Dosage and Administration: Administration of a dose of ERYC in the presence of food lowers the blood levels of systemically available erythromycin. Although the blood levels obtained upon administration of enteric-coated erythromycin products in the presence of food are still above minimum inhibitory concentrations (MICs) of most organisms for which erythromycin is indicated, optimum blood levels are obtained on a fasting stomach (administration of at least ½ hour and preferably two hours before or after a meal).

ADULTS: The usual dose is 250 mg every 6 hours taken one hour before meals. If twice-a-day dosage is desired, the recommended dose is 500 mg every 12 hours. Dosage may be increased up to 4 grams per day, according to the severity of infection. Twice-a-day dosing is not recommended when doses larger than 1 gram daily are administered.

CHILDREN: Age, weight, and severity of the infection are important factors in determining the proper dosage. The usual dosage is 30 to 50 mg/kg/day in divided doses. For the treatment of more severe infections, this dose may be doubled.

Streptococcal infections: A therapeutic dosage of oral erythromycin should be administered for at least 10 days. For continuous prophylaxis against recurrences of streptococcal infections in persons with a history of rheumatic heart disease, the dose is 250 mg twice a day.

For the prevention of bacterial endocarditis in penicillin-allergic patients with valvular heart disease who are to undergo dental procedures or surgical procedures of the upper respiratory tract, the adult dose is 1.0 grams orally (20 mg/kg for children) one and one-half to 2 hours prior to the procedure and then 500 mg (10 mg/kg for children) orally every 6 hours for 8 doses.[3] (See INDICATIONS AND USAGE).

Primary syphilis: 30-40 grams given in divided doses over a period of 10-15 days.

Intestinal amebiasis: 250 mg four times daily for 10 to 14 days for adults; 30 to 50 mg/kg/day in divided doses for 10 to 14 days for children.

Legionnaires' Disease: Although optimal doses have not been established, doses utilized in reported clinical data were those recommended above (1 to 4 grams daily in divided doses).

Urogenital infections during pregnancy due to *Chlamydia trachomatis:* Although the optimal dose and duration of therapy have not been established, the suggested treatment is erythromycin 500 mg, by mouth, 4 times a day on an empty stomach for at least 7 days. For women who cannot tolerate this regimen, a decreased dose of 250 mg, by mouth, 4 times a day should be used for at least 14 days[4].

For adults with uncomplicated urethral, endocervical, or rectal infections caused by *Chlamydia trachomatis* in whom tetracyclines are contraindicated or not tolerated: 500 mg. by mouth, 4 times a day for at least 7 days[4].

Pertussis: Although optimum dosage and duration of therapy have not been established, doses of erythromycin utilized in reported clinical studies were 40-50 mg/kg/day, given in divided doses for 5 to 14 days.

How Supplied:

ERYC (Capsule 696), clear and orange opaque capsules, each containing 250 mg erythromycin as enteric coated pellets, are available as follows:
N 0071-0696-24 Bottles of 100
N 0071-0696-30 Bottles of 500
N 0071-0696-40 Unit dose package of 100 (10 strips of 10 capsules each).

Storage Conditions: Store at a room temperature below 30°C (86°F). Protect from moisture and light.

References:

1. Approved Standard ASM-2 "Performance Standards for Anti-microbial Disc Susceptibility Test." National Committee for Clinical Laboratory Standards. 771 East Lancaster Avenue, Villanova. PA 19085.
2. Ericson, H.M. and Sherris, J.C.: "Antibiotic Sensitivity Testing Report of an International Collaborative Study." *Acta Pathologica et Microbiologica Scandinavica.* Section B. Supp. 217, 1971, pp. 1-90.
3. Am. Heart Assoc. and Am. Dental Assoc. "Prevention of Bacterial Endocarditis." *Circulation.* Vol. 56, No. 1, July, 1977. 139A-143A.
4. CDC Sexually Transmitted Diseases Treatment Guidelines 1982.

Shown in Product Identification Section, page 424

0696G012

ERYTHROMYCIN STEARATE R
[ĕ-ry'thrō-my"cĭn stēa'rāte"]
TABLETS, USP
(Erypar®)

Description: Erythromycin is produced by a strain of *Streptomyces erythraeus* and belongs to the macrolide group of antibiotics. It is basic and readily forms salts with acids. The base, the stea-

rate salt, and the esters are poorly soluble in water, and are suitable for oral administration.
The film-coated tablets contain 250 mg or 500 mg of erythromycin as erythromycin stearate, USP. Each tablet is buffered with sodium citrate.

Clinical Pharmacology: The mode of action of erythromycin is by inhibition of protein synthesis without affecting nucleic acid synthesis. Resistance to erythromycin of some strains of *Hemophilus influenzae* and staphylococci has been demonstrated. Culture and susceptibility testing should be done. If the Kirby-Bauer method of disc susceptibility is used, a 15-mcg erythromycin disc should give a zone diameter of at least 18 mm when tested against an erythromycin-susceptible organism.

Orally administered erythromycin is readily absorbed by most patients, especially on an empty stomach, but patient variation is observed.

After absorption, erythromycin diffuses readily into most body fluids. In the absence of meningeal inflammation, low concentrations are normally achieved in the spinal fluid, but passage of the drug across the blood-brain barrier increases in meningitis. In the presence of normal hepatic function, erythromycin is concentrated in the liver and excreted in the bile; the effect of hepatic dysfunction on excretion of erythromycin by the liver into the bile is not known. After oral administration, less than 5 percent of the activity of the administered dose can be recovered in the urine.

Erythromycin crosses the placental barrier but fetal plasma levels are generally low.

Indications and Usage: *Streptococcus pyogenes* (Group A beta-hemolytic *Streptococcus*): Upper and lower respiratory tract, skin, and soft-tissue infections of mild to moderate severity

Injectable benzathine penicillin G is considered by the American Heart Association to be the drug of choice in the treatment and prevention of streptococcal pharyngitis and in the long-term prophylaxis of rheumatic fever.

When oral medication is preferred for treatment of streptococcal pharyngitis, penicillin G, V, or erythromycin are alternate drugs of choice.

When oral medication is given, the importance of strict adherence by the patient to the prescribed dosage regimen must be stressed. A therapeutic dose should be administered for at least 10 days.

Although no controlled clinical efficacy trials have been conducted, oral erythromycin has been suggested by the American Heart Association and American Dental Association for use in a regimen for prophylaxis against bacterial endocarditis in patients hypersensitive to penicillin who have congenital heart disease or rheumatic or other acquired valvular heart disease when they undergo dental procedures and surgical procedures of the upper respiratory tract.[1] Erythromycin is not suitable prior to genitourinary or gastrointestinal tract surgery.

Note: When selecting antibiotics for the prevention of bacterial endocarditis, the physician or dentist should read the full joint statement of the American Heart Association and the American Dental Association.[1]

Staphylococcus aureus: Acute infections of skin and soft tissue of mild to moderate severity. Resistant organisms may emerge during treatment.

Diplococcus pneumoniae: Upper respiratory tract infections (eg, otitis media, pharyngitis) and lower respiratory tract infections (eg, pneumonia) of mild to moderate degree

Mycoplasma pneumoniae (Eaton agent, PPLO): In the treatment of primary atypical pneumonia, when due to this organism

Treponema pallidum: Erythromycin is an alternate choice of treatment for primary syphilis in patients allergic to the penicillins. In treatment of primary syphilis, spinal fluid examinations should be done before treatment and as part of follow-up after therapy.

Erythromycins are indicated for treatment of the following infections caused by *Chlamydia trachomatis:* conjunctivitis of the newborn, pneumonia of infancy, urogenital infections during pregnancy. When tetracyclines are contraindicated or not tolerated, erythromycin is indicated for the treatment of uncomplicated urethral, endocervical, or rectal infections in adults due to *Chlamydia trachomatis.*[2]

Corynebacterium diphtheriae and *C minutissimum:* As an adjunct to antitoxin, to prevent establishment of carriers, and to eradicate the organism in carriers

In the treatment of erythrasma

Entamoeba histolytica: In the treatment of intestinal amebiasis only. Extra-enteric amebiasis requires treatment with other agents.

Listeria monocytogenes: Infections due to this organism

Legionnaires' Disease: Although no controlled clinical efficacy studies have been conducted, *in vitro* and limited preliminary clinical data suggest that erythromycin may be effective in treating Legionnaires' Disease.

Contraindication: Erythromycin is contraindicated in patients with known hypersensitivity to this antibiotic.

Precautions: Erythromycin is principally excreted by the liver. Caution should be exercised in administering the antibiotic to patients with impaired hepatic function. There have been reports of hepatic dysfunction, with or without jaundice, occurring in patients receiving oral erythromycin products.

Recent data from studies of erythromycin reveal that its use in patients who are receiving high doses of theophylline may be associated with an increase of serum theophylline levels and potential theophylline toxicity. In case of theophylline toxicity and/or elevated serum theophylline levels, the dose of theophylline should be reduced while the patient is receiving concomitant erythromycin therapy.

Surgical procedures should be performed when indicated.

Usage during pregnancy and lactation: The safety of erythromycin for use during pregnancy has not been established.

Erythromycin crosses the placental barrier. Erythromycin also appears in breast milk.

Adverse Reactions: The most frequent side effects of oral erythromycin preparations are gastrointestinal, such as abdominal cramping and discomfort, and are dose-related. Nausea, vomiting, and diarrhea occur infrequently with usual oral doses.

During prolonged or repeated therapy, there is a possibility of overgrowth of nonsusceptible bacteria or fungi. If such infections occur, the drug should be discontinued and appropriate therapy instituted.

Mild allergic reactions, such as urticaria and other skin rashes, have occurred. Serious allergic reactions, including anaphylaxis, have been reported.

Dosage and Administration: Optimum blood levels are obtained when doses are given on an empty stomach.

Adults: 250 mg every six hours is the usual dose; or 500 mg every 12 hours, one hour before meals. Dosage may be increased up to 4 grams per day according to the severity of the infection.

Children: Age, weight, and severity of the infection are important factors in determining the proper dosage: 30 to 50 mg/kg/day, in divided doses, is the usual dose. For more severe infections, this dosage may be doubled.

If dosage is desired on a twice-a-day schedule in either adults or children, one half of the total daily dose may be given every 12 hours, one hour before meals.

In the treatment of streptococcal infections, a therapeutic dosage of erythromycin should be administered for at least 10 days. In continuous *prophylaxis* of streptococcal infections in persons with a history of rheumatic heart disease, the dose is 250 mg twice a day.

For prophylaxis against bacterial endocarditis[1] in patients with congenital heart disease or rheumatic or other acquired valvular heart disease when undergoing dental procedures or surgical procedures of the upper respiratory tract, give 1.0 gm (20 mg/kg for children) orally 1½-2 hours before the procedure, and then 500 mg (10 mg/kg for children) orally every 6 hours for 8 doses.

For treatment of primary syphilis: 30 to 40 grams given in divided doses over a period of 10 to 15 days.

For dysenteric amebiasis: Adults: 250 mg four times daily for 10 to 14 days. Children: 30 to 50 mg/kg/day in divided doses for 10 to 14 days.

For treatment of Legionnaires' Disease: Although optimal doses have not been established, doses utilized in reported clinical data were those recommended above (1 to 4 grams erythromycin stearate daily in divided doses).

How Supplied:
Erythromycin Stearate Tablets, USP are supplied as:
N 0071-0672-24—bottle of 100
N 0071-0672-30—bottle of 500
N 0071-0672-40—unit dose (10/10's)
Each film-coated tablet contains 250 mg erythromycin as erythromycin stearate.
N 0071-0919-24—bottle of 100
Each film-coated tablet contains 500 mg erythromycin as erythromycin stearate.
AHFS 8:12.12   0672G011
Shown in Product Identification Section, page 424
Reference:
1. American Heart Association. Prevention of bacterial endocarditis. *Circulation.* 56:139A-143A 1977.

ESTROVIS® ℞
[ĕs-trō' vĭs]
(Quinestrol tablets, USP)*

*Product of Warner-Lambert Inc

Warning:
1. Estrogens Have Been Reported to Increase the Risk of Endometrial Carcinoma.
Three independent case control studies have shown an increased risk of endometrial cancer in postmenopausal women exposed to exogenous estrogens for prolonged periods.[1-3] This risk was independent of the other known risk factors for endometrial cancer. These studies are further supported by the finding that incidence rates of endometrial cancer have increased sharply since 1969 in eight different areas of the United States with population-based cancer reporting systems, an increase which may be related to the rapidly expanding use of estrogens during the last decade.[4]

The three case control studies reported that the risk of endometrial cancer in estrogen users was about 4.5 to 13.9 times greater than in nonusers. The risk appears to depend on both duration of treatment[1] and on estrogen dose.[3] In view of these findings, when estrogens are used for the treatment of menopausal symptoms, the lowest dose that will control symptoms should be utilized and medication should be discontinued as soon as possible. When prolonged treatment is medically indicated, the patient should be reassessed on at least a semiannual basis to determine the need for continued therapy. Although the evidence must be considered preliminary, one study suggests that cyclic administration of low doses of estrogen may carry less risk than continuous administration.[3] Therefore, while it appears prudent to utilize such a regimen with other orally administered estrogens, Estrovis may be administered, following a seven-day priming schedule, on a once weekly maintenance dosage beginning two weeks after the start of treatment.

Close clinical surveillance of all women taking estrogens is important. In all cases of un-

Continued on next page

This product information was prepared in August, 1984. On these and other Parke-Davis Products, information may be obtained by addressing PARKE-DAVIS, Division of Warner-Lambert Company, Morris Plains, New Jersey 07950.

Parke-Davis—Cont.

diagnosed persistent or recurring abnormal vaginal bleeding, adequate diagnostic measures should be undertaken to rule out malignancy.

There is no evidence at present that "natural" estrogens are more or less hazardous than "synthetic" estrogens at equiestrogenic doses.

2. Estrogens Should not be Used During Pregnancy.

The use of female sex hormones, both estrogens and progestogens, during early pregnancy may seriously damage the offspring. It has been shown that females exposed *in utero* to diethylstilbestrol, a nonsteroidal estrogen, have an increased risk of developing in later life a form of vaginal or cervical cancer that is ordinarily extremely rare.[5-6] This risk has been estimated as not greater than 4 per 1,000 exposures.[7] Furthermore, a high percentage of such exposed women (from 30 to 90%) have been found to have vaginal adenosis,[8-12] epithelial changes of the vagina and cervix. Although these changes are histologically benign, it is not known whether they are precursors of malignancy. Although similar data are not available with the use of other estrogens, it cannot be presumed they would not induce similar changes.

Several reports suggest an association between intrauterine exposure to female sex hormones and congenital anomalies, including congenital heart defects and limb- reduction defects.[13-16] One case control study[16] estimated a 4.7-fold increased risk of limb-reduction defects in infants exposed *in utero* to sex hormones (oral contraceptives, hormone withdrawal tests for pregnancy, or attempted treatment for threatened abortion). Some of these exposures were very short and involved only a few days of treatment. The data suggest that the risk of limb-reduction defects in exposed fetuses is somewhat less than 1 per 1,000.

In the past, female sex hormones have been used during pregnancy in an attempt to treat threatened or habitual abortion. There is considerable evidence that estrogens are ineffective for these indications, and there is no evidence from well-controlled studies that progestogens are effective for these uses.

If Estrovis (quinestrol) is used during pregnancy, or if the patient becomes pregnant while taking this drug, she should be apprised of the potential risks to the fetus and the advisability of pregnancy continuation.

Description: Estrovis (quinestrol) is available as a 100-mcg oral tablet. It is an estrogen.

Estrovis (quinestrol) is the 3-cyclopentylether of ethinyl estradiol. The chemical name is 3-cyclopentyloxy-17α-ethynylestra-1, 3, 5 (10) - trien-17β-ol.

It is a white, essentially odorless powder, insoluble in water and soluble in alcohol, chloroform, and ether.

Clinical Pharmacology: Estrovis (quinestrol) is an orally effective estrogen as judged by conventional assay procedures employing vagina and uterine end-points in mice, rats and rabbits.

The estrogenic effects of Estrovis have been demonstrated in clinical studies by its effects on the endometrium, maturation of the vaginal epithelium, thinning of cervical mucus, suppression of pituitary gonadotropin, inhibition of ovulation, and prevention of postpartum breast discomfort.

Indications: Estrovis (quinestrol) is indicated in the treatment of:

1. Moderate to severe vasomotor symptoms associated with the menopause. (There is no evidence that estrogens are effective for nervous symptoms or depression which might occur during menopause, and they should not be used to treat these conditions.)
2. Atrophic vaginitis
3. Kraurosis vulvae
4. Female hypogonadism
5. Female castration
6. Primary ovarian failure

Estrovis (Quinestrol) Has Not Been Shown to be Effective for any Purpose during Pregnancy and Its Use May Cause Severe Harm to the Fetus (See Boxed Warning).

Contraindications: Estrogens should not be used in women (or men) with any of the following conditions:

1. Known or suspected cancer of the breast except in appropriately selected patients being treated for metastatic disease
2. Known or suspected estrogen-dependent neoplasia
3. Known or suspected pregnancy (See Boxed Warning)
4. Undiagnosed abnormal genital bleeding
5. Active thrombophlebitis or thromboembolic disorders
6. A past history of thrombophlebitis, thrombosis, or thromboembolic disorders associated with previous estrogen use (except when used in treatment of breast or prostatic malignancy)

Warnings:

1. *Induction of malignant neoplasms.* Long-term continuous administration of natural and synthetic estrogens in certain animal species increases the frequency of carcinomas of the breast, cervix, vagina, and liver. There is now evidence that estrogens increase the risk of carcinoma of the endometrium in humans. (See Boxed Warning.)

At the present time, there is no satisfactory evidence that estrogens given to postmenopausal women increase the risk of cancer of the breast,[18] although a recent long-term follow up of a single physician's practice has raised this possibility.[18a] Because of the animal data, there is a need for caution in prescribing estrogens for women with a strong family history of breast cancer or who have breast nodules, fibrocystic disease, or abnormal mammograms.

2. *Gallbladder disease.* A recent study has reported a 2- to 3-fold increase in the risk of surgically confirmed gallbladder disease in women receiving postmenopausal estrogens,[18] similar to the 2-fold increase previously noted in users of oral contraceptives.[19-24] In the case of oral contraceptives, the increased risk appeared after two years of use.[24]

3. *Effects similar to those caused by estrogen-progestogen oral contraceptives.* There are several serious adverse effects of oral contraceptives, most of which have not, up to now, been documented as consequences of postmenopausal estrogen therapy. This may reflect the comparatively low doses of estrogen used in postmenopausal women. It would be expected that the larger doses of estrogen used to treat prostatic or breast cancer or postpartum breast engorgement are more likely to result in these adverse effects, and, in fact, it has been shown that there is an increased risk of thrombosis in men receiving estrogens for prostatic cancer and women for postpartum breast engorgement.[20-23]

a. *Thromboembolic disease.* It is now well established that users of oral contraceptives have an increased risk of various thromboembolic and thrombotic vascular diseases, such as thrombophlebitis, pulmonary embolism, stroke, and myocardial infarction.[24-31] Cases of retinal thrombosis, mesenteric thrombosis, and optic neuritis have been reported in oral contraceptive users. There is evidence that the risk of several of these adverse reactions is related to the dose of the drug.[32,33] An increased risk of postsurgery thromboembolic complications has also been reported in users of oral contraceptives.[34,35] If feasible, estrogen should be discontinued at least 4 weeks before surgery of the type associated with an increased risk of thromboembolism, or during periods of prolonged immobilization.

While an increased rate of thromboembolic and thrombotic disease in postmenopausal users of estrogens has not been found,[18,36] this does not rule out the possibility that such an increase may be present or that subgroups of women who have underlying risk factors or who are receiving relatively large doses of estrogens may have increased risk. Therefore, estrogens should not be used in persons with active thrombophlebitis or thromboembolic disorders, and they should not be used (except in treatment of malignancy) in persons with a history of such disorders in association with estrogen use. They should be used with caution in patients with cerebral vascular or coronary artery disease and only for those in whom estrogens are clearly needed.

Large doses of estrogen (5 mg conjugated estrogens per day), comparable to those used to treat cancer of the prostate and breast, have been shown in a large prospective clinical trial in men[37] to increase the risk of nonfatal myocardial infarction, pulmonary embolism, and thrombophlebitis. When estrogen doses of this size are used, any of the thromboembolic and thrombotic adverse effects associated with oral contraceptive use should be considered a clear risk.

b. *Hepatic adenoma.* Benign hepatic adenomas appear to be associated with the use of oral contraceptives.[38-40] Although benign, and rare, these may rupture and may cause death through intra-abdominal hemorrhage. Such lesions have not yet been reported in association with other estrogen or progestogen preparations but should be considered in estrogen users having abdominal pain and tenderness, abdominal mass, or hypovolemic shock. Hepatocellular carcinoma has also been reported in women taking estrogen-containing oral contraceptives.[39] The relationship of this malignancy to these drugs is not known at this time.

c. *Elevated blood pressure.* Increased blood pressure is not uncommon in women using oral contraceptives. There is now a report that this may occur with use of estrogens in the menopause[11] and blood pressure should be monitored with estrogen use, especially if high doses are used.

d. *Glucose tolerance.* A worsening of glucose tolerance has been observed in a significant percentage of patients on estrogen-containing oral contraceptives. For this reason, diabetic patients should be carefully observed while receiving estrogen.

4. *Hypercalcemia.* Administration of estrogens may lead to severe hypercalcemia in patients with breast cancer and bone metastases. If this occurs, the drug should be stopped and appropriate measures taken to reduce the serum calcium level.

Precautions:

A. General Precautions

1. A complete medical and family history should be taken prior to the initiation of any estrogen therapy. The pretreatment and periodic physical examinations should include special reference to blood pressure, abdomen, and pelvic organs, and should include a Papanicolaou smear. As a general rule, estrogen should not be prescribed for longer than one year without another physical examination being performed.
2. Fluid retention—Because estrogens may cause some degree of fluid retention, conditions which might be influenced by this factor, such as epilepsy, migraine, and cardiac or renal dysfunction, require careful observation.
3. Certain patients may develop undesirable manifestations of excessive estrogenic stimulation, such as abnormal or excessive uterine bleeding, mastodynia, etc.
4. Oral contraceptives appear to be associated with an increased incidence of mental depression.[24] Although it is not clear whether this is due to the estrogenic or progestogenic component of the contraceptive, patients with a history of depression should be carefully observed.
5. Preexisting uterine leiomyomata may increase in size during estrogen use.
6. The pathologist should be advised of estrogen therapy when relevant specimens are submitted.
7. Patients with a past history of jaundice during pregnancy have an increased risk of recurrence of jaundice while receiving estrogen-containing oral contraceptive therapy. If jaundice develops in any patient receiving estrogen, the medication should be discontinued while the cause is investigated.

8. Estrogens may be poorly metabolized in patients with impaired liver function and they should be administered with caution in such patients.
9. Because estrogens influence the metabolism of calcium and phosphorus, they should be used with caution in patients with metabolic bone diseases that are associated with hypercalcemia or in patients with renal insufficiency.
10. Because of the effects of estrogens on epiphyseal closure, they should be used judiciously in young patients in whom bone growth is not complete.
11. Certain endocrine and liver function tests may be affected by estrogen-containing oral contraceptives. The following similar changes may be expected with larger doses of estrogen:
a. Increased sulfobromophthalein retention.
b. Increased prothrombin and factors VII, VIII, IX, and X; decreased antithrombin 3; increased norepinephrine-induced platelet aggregability.
c. Increased thyroid binding globulin (TBG) leading to increased circulating total thyroid hormone, as measured by PHI, T4 by column, or T4 by radioimmunoassay. Free T3 resin uptake is decreased, reflecting the elevated TBG; free T4 concentration is unaltered.
d. Impaired glucose tolerance.
e. Decreased pregnanediol excretion.
f. Reduced response to metyrapone test.
g. Reduced serum folate concentration.
h. Increased serum triglyceride and phospholipid concentration.
B. Information for the patient. See text of Patient Package Insert.
C. Pregnancy. See Contraindications and Boxed Warning.
D. Nursing Mothers. As a general principle, the administration of any drug to nursing mothers should be done only when clearly necessary because many drugs are excreted in human milk.

Adverse Reactions: (See Warnings regarding induction of neoplasia, adverse effects on the fetus, increased incidence of gallbladder disease, and adverse effects similar to those of oral contraceptives, including thromboembolism.) The following additional adverse reactions have been reported with estrogenic therapy, including oral contraceptives:
1. *Genitourinary system.*
Breakthrough bleeding, spotting, change in menstrual flow
Dysmenorrhea
Premenstrual-like syndrome
Amenorrhea during and after treatment
Increase in size of uterine fibromyomata
Vaginal candidiasis
Change in cervical eversion and in degree of cervical secretion
Cystitis-like syndrome
2. *Breasts.*
Tenderness, enlargement, secretion
3. *Gastrointestinal.*
Nausea, vomiting
Abdominal cramps, bloating
Cholestatic jaundice
4. *Skin.*
Chloasma or melasma which may persist when drug is discontinued
Erythema multiforme
Erythema nodosum
Hemorrhagic eruption
Loss of scalp hair
Hirsutism
5. *Eyes.*
Steepening of corneal curvature
Intolerance to contact lenses
6. *CNS.*
Headache, migraine, dizziness
Mental depression
Chorea
7. *Miscellaneous.*
Increase or decrease in weight
Reduced carbohydrate tolerance
Aggravation of porphyria
Edema
Changes in libido

Acute Overdosage: Numerous reports of ingestion of large doses of estrogen-containing oral contraceptives by young children indicate that serious ill effects do not occur. Overdosage of estrogen may cause nausea, and withdrawal bleeding may occur in females.

Dosage and Administration: For treatment of moderate to severe vasomotor symptoms associated with the menopause, and for atrophic vaginitis, kraurosis vulvae, female hypogonadism, female castration, and primary ovarian failure.
One Estrovis (quinestrol) 100-mcg tablet once daily for seven days, followed by one 100-mcg tablet weekly as a maintenance schedule, commencing two weeks after inception of treatment. The dosage may be increased to 200 mcg weekly if the therapeutic response is not that which may be desirable or considered optimal.
The lowest maintenance dose that will control symptoms should be chosen and medication should be discontinued as promptly as possible.
Attempts to discontinue or taper medication should be made at three- to six-month intervals.
Treated patients with an intact uterus should be monitored closely for signs of endometrial cancer and appropriate diagnostic measures should be taken to rule out malignancy in the event of persistent or recurring abnormal vaginal bleeding.

How Supplied: N 0071-0437-24 (P-D 437) Estrovis (quinestrol) 100-mcg tablets are supplied in bottles of 100.

0437G023

Physician References:
1. Ziel, H.K. and W.D. Finkle, "Increased Risk of Endometrial Carcinoma Among Users of Conjugated Estrogens." *New England Journal of Medicine*, 293:1167–1170, 1975.
2. Smith, D.C., R. Prentic, D.J. Thompson, and W.L. Hermann, "Association of Exogenous Estrogen and Endometrial Carcinoma." *New England Journal of Medicine*, 293:1164–1167, 1975.
3. Mack, T.M., M.C. Pike, B.E. Henderson, R.I. Pfeffer, V.R. Gerkins, M. Arthur, and S.E. Brown, "Estrogens and Endometrial Cancer in a Retirement Community." *New England Journal of Medicine*, 294:1262–1267, 1976.
4. Weiss, N.D., D.R. Szekely and D.F. Austin, "Increasing Incidence of Endometrial Cancer in the United States." *New England Journal of Medicine*, 294:1259–1262, 1976.
5. Herbst, A.L., H. Ulfelder and D.C. Poskanzer, "Adenocarcinoma of Vagina." *New England Journal of Medicine*, 284:878–881, 1971.
6. Greenwald, P., J. Barlow, P. Nasca, and W. Burnett, "Vaginal Cancer after Maternal Treatment with Synthetic Estrogens." *New England Journal of Medicine*, 285:390–392, 1971.
7. Lanier, A., K. Noller, D. Decker, L. Elveback, and L. Kurland, "Cancer and Stilbestrol, A Follow-Up of 1719 Persons Exposed to Estrogens in *Utero* and Born 1943–1959." *Mayo Clinic Proceedings*, 48:793–799, 1973.
8. Herbst, A., R. Kurman, and R. Scully, "Vaginal and Cervical Abnormalities After Exposure to Stilbestrol in Utero." *Obstetrics and Gynecology*, 40:287–298, 1972.
9. Herbst, A., S. Robboy, G. Macdonald, and R. Scully, "The Effects of Local Progesterone on Stilbestrol-Associated Vaginal Adenosis." *American Journal of Obstetrics and Gynecology*, 118:607–615, 1974.
10. Herbst, A., D. Poskanzer, S. Robboy, L. Friedlander, and R. Scully, "Prenatal Exposure to Stilbestrol, A Prospective Comparison of Exposed Female Offspring with Unexpected Controls." *New England Journal of Medicine*, 292:334–339, 1975.
11. Stafl, A., R. Mattingly, D. Foley, and W. Fetherston, "Clinical Diagnosis of Vaginal Adenosis." *Obstetrics and Gynecology*, 43:118–128, 1974.
12. Sherman, A.I., M. Goldrath, A. Berlin, V. Vakhariya, F. Banooni, W. Michaels, P. Goodman, S. Brown, "Cervical-Vaginal Adenosis After *In Utero* Exposure to Synthetic Estrogens," *Obstetrics and Gynecology*, 44:531–545, 1974.
13. Gal, I., B. Kirman, and J. Stern, "Hormone Pregnancy Tests and Congenital Malformation," *Nature*, 216:83, 1967.
14. Levy, E.P., A. Cohen, and F.C. Fraser, "Hormone Treatment During Pregnancy and Congenital Heart Defects," *Lancet*, 1:611, 1973.
15. Nora, J. and A. Nora, "Birth Defects and Oral Contraceptives," *Lancet*, 1:941–942, 1973.
16. Janerich, D.T., J.M. Piper, and D.M. Glebatis, "Oral Contraceptives and Congenital Limb-Reduction Defects," *New England Journal of Medicine*, 291:697–700, 1974.
17. "Estrogens for Oral or Parenteral Use," *Federal Register*, 40:8212, 1975.
18. Boston Collaborative Drug Surveillance Program "Surgically Confirmed Gallbladder Disease, Venous Thromboembolism and Breast Tumors in Relation to Post-Menopausal Estrogen Therapy," *New England Journal of Medicine*, 210:15–19, 1974.
18a. Hoover, R., L.A. Gray, Sr., P. Cole, and B. MacMahon, "Menopausal Estrogens and Breast Cancer." *New England Journal of Medicine*, 295:401–405, 1976.
19. Boston Collaborative Drug Surveillance Program, "Oral Contraceptives and Venous Thromboembolic Disease, Surgically Confirmed Gallbladder Disease, and Breast Tumors," *Lancet*, 1:1399–1404, 1973.
20. Daniel, D.G., H. Campbell, and A.C. Turnbull, "Puerperal Thromboembolism and Suppression of Lactation." *Lancet*, 2:287–289, 1967.
21. The Veterans Administration Cooperative Urological Research Group, "Carcinoma of the Prostate: Treatment Comparisons," *Journal of Urology*, 98:516–522, 1967.
22. Ballar, J.C., "Thromboembolism and Oestrogen Therapy," *Lancet*, 2, 560. 1967.
23. Blackard, C., R. Doe, G. Mellinger, and D. Byar, "Incidence of Cardiovascular Disease and Death in Patients Receiving Diethylstilbestrol for Carcinoma of the Prostate," *Cancer*, 26:249–256, 1970.
24. Royal College of General Practitioners, "Oral Contraception and Thromboembolic Disease," *Journal of the Royal College of General Practitioners*, 13, 267–279, 1967.
25. Inman, W.H.W. and M.P. Vessey, "Investigation of Deaths from Pulmonary, Coronary, and Cerebral Thrombosis and Embolism in Women of Child-Bearing Age." *British Medical Journal*, 2:193–199, 1968.
26. Vessey, M.P. and R. Doll, "Investigation of Relation Between Use of Oral Contraceptives and Thromboembolic Disease, A Further Report," *British Medical Journal*, 2:651–657, 1969.
27. Sartwell, P.E., A.T. Masi, F.G. Arthes, G.R. Greene and H.E. Smith, "Thromboembolism and Oral Contraceptives: An Epidemiological Case Control Study." *American Journal of Epidemiology*, 90:365–380, 1969.
28. Collaborative Group for the Study of Stroke in Young Women, "Oral Contraception and Increased Risk of Cerebral Ischemia or Thrombosis," *New England Journal of Medicine*, 288:871–878, 1973.
29. Collaborative Group for the Study of Stroke in Young Women: "Oral Contraceptives and Stroke in Young Women: Associated Risk Factors," 231:718–722, 1975. *Journal of the American Medical Assoc.* 231:718–722, 1975.
30. Mann, J.I. and W.H.W. Inman, "Oral Contraceptives and Death from Myocardial Infarction," *British Medical Journal*, 2:245–248, 1975.
31. Mann, J.I., M.P. Vessey, M. Thorogood, and R. Doll, "Myocardial Infarction in Young Women with Special Reference to Oral Contraceptive

Continued on next page

This product information was prepared in August, 1984. On these and other Parke-Davis Products, information may be obtained by addressing PARKE-DAVIS, Division of Warner-Lambert Company, Morris Plains, New Jersey 07950.

Parke-Davis—Cont.

Practice," *British Medical Journal,* 2:241–245, 1975.
32. Inman, W.H.W., M.P. Vessey, B. Westerholm, and A. Engelund. "Thromboembolic Disease and the Steroidal Content of Oral Contraceptives," *British Medical Journal,* 2:203–209, 1970.
33. Stolley, P.D., J.A. Tonascia, M.S. Tockman, P.E. Sartwell, A.H. Rutledge, and M.P. Jacobs, "Thrombosis with Low-Estrogen Oral Contraceptives," *American Journal of Epidemiology,* 102:197–208, 1975.
34. Vessey, M.P., R. Doll, A.S. Fairbairn, and G. Glober, "Post-Operative Thromboembolism and the use of the Oral Contraceptives," *British Medical Journal,* 3:123–126, 1970.
35. Greene, G.R. and P.E. Sartwell, "Oral Contraceptive Use in Patients with Thromboembolism Following Surgery, Trauma or Infection," *American Journal of Public Health,* 62:680–685, 1972.
36. Rosenberg, L., M.B. Armstrong and H. Jick "Myocardial Infarction and Estrogen Therapy in Post-menopausal Women," *New England Journal of Medicine,* 294:1256–1259, 1976.
37. Coronary Drug Project Research Group, "The Coronary Drug Project: Initial Findings Leading to Modifications of Its Research Protocol," *Journal of the American Medical Association,* 214:1303–1313, 1970.
38. Baum, J., F. Holtz, J.J. Bookstein, and E.W. Klein, "Possible Association between Benign Hepatomas and Oral Contraceptives," *Lancet,* 2:926–928, 1973.
39. Mays, E.T., W.M. Christopherson, M.M. Mahr, and H.C. Williams, "Hepatic Changes in Young Women Ingesting Contraceptive Steroids, Hepatic Hemorrhage and Primary Hepatic Tumors," *Journal of the American Medical Association,* 235:780–782, 1976.
40. Edmondson, H.A., B. Henderson, and B. Benton, "Liver Cell Adenomas Association with the Use of Oral Contraceptives," *New England Journal of Medicine,* 294:470–472, 1976.
41. Pfeffer, A.I. and S. Van Den Noore, "Estrogen use and Stroke Risk in Post-menopausal Women," *American Journal of Epidemiology,* 103:545–546, 1976.

Shown in Product Identification Section, page 424

EUTHROID® ℞
[*ūth'roid*]
(Liotrix Tablets, USP)

Description: Thyroid hormone drugs are natural or synthetic preparations containing tetraiodothyronine (T_4, levothyroxine) sodium or triiodothyronine (T_3, liothyronine) sodium or both. T_4 and T_3 are produced in the human thyroid gland by the iodination and coupling of the amino acid tyrosine. T_4 contains four iodine atoms and is formed by the coupling of two molecules of diiodotyrosine (DIT). T_3 contains three atoms of iodine and is formed by the coupling of one molecule of DIT with one molecule of monoiodotyrosine (MIT). Both hormones are stored in the thyroid colloid as thyroglobulin.

Thyroid hormone preparations belong to two categories: (1) natural hormonal preparations derived from animal thyroid, and (2) synthetic preparations. Natural preparations include desiccated thyroid and thyroglobulin. Desiccated thyroid is derived from domesticated animals that are used for food by man (either beef or hog thyroid), and thyroglobulin is derived from thyroid glands of the hog. The United States Pharmacopeia (USP) has standardized the total iodine content of natural preparations. Thyroid USP contains not less than (NLT) 0.17 percent and not more than (NMT) 0.23 percent iodine, and thyroglobulin contains not less than 0.7 percent of organically bound iodine. Iodine content is only an indirect indicator of true hormonal biologic activity.

There are five (5) preparations in the USP. They are: (1) Thyroid Tablets, (2) Thyroglobulin Tablets, (3) Levothyroxine Sodium Tablets, (4) Liothyronine Sodium Tablets, and (5) Liotrix Tablets (a ratio, by weight, of 4 to 1, of the sodium salts of T_4 and T_3, respectively).

Clinical Pharmacology: The steps in the synthesis of the thyroid hormones are controlled by thyrotropin (Thyroid Stimulating Hormone, TSH) secreted by the anterior pituitary. This hormone's secretion is in turn controlled by a feedback mechanism effected by the thyroid hormones themselves and by thyrotropin releasing hormone (TRH), a tripeptide of hypothalamic origin. Endogenous thyroid hormone secretion is suppressed when exogenous thyroid hormones are administered by euthyroid individuals in excess of the normal gland's secretion.

The mechanisms by which thyroid hormones exert their physiologic action are not well understood. These hormones enhance oxygen consumption by most tissues of the body, increase the basal metabolic rate, and the metabolism of carbohydrates, lipids and proteins. Thus, they exert a profound influence on every organ system in the body and are of particular importance in the development of the central nervous system.

The normal thyroid gland contains approximately 200 mcg of levothyroxine (T_4) per gram of gland, and 15 mcg of triiodothyronine (T_3) per gram. The ratio of these two hormones in the circulation does not represent the ratio in the thyroid gland, since about 80 percent of peripheral triiodothyronine comes from the monodeiodination of levothyroxine. Peripheral monodeiodination of levothyroxine at the 5 position (inner ring) also results in the formation of reverse triiodothyronine (r T_3), which is calorigenically inactive. These facts would seem to advocate levothyroxine as the treatment of choice for the hypothyroid patient and to militate against the administration of hormone combinations, which while normalizing thyroxine levels may produce triiodothyronine levels in the thyrotoxic range.

Triiodothyronine (T_3) level is low in the fetus and newborn, in old age, in chronic caloric deprivation, hepatic cirrhosis, renal failure, surgical stress, and chronic illnesses representing what has been called the "low triiodothyronine syndrome."

Pharmacokinetics: Animal studies have shown that T_4 is only partially absorbed from the gastrointestinal tract. The degree of absorption is dependent on the vehicle used for its administration and by the character of the intestinal contents, the intestinal flora, including plasma protein, soluble dietary factors, all of which bind thyroid and thereby make it unavailable for diffusion. Only 41 percent is absorbed when given in a gelatin capsule as opposed to a 74 percent absorption when given with an albumin carrier.

Depending on other factors, absorption has varied from 48 to 79 percent of the administered dose. Fasting increases absorption. Malabsorption syndromes, as well as dietary factors (children's soybean formula, concomitant use of anionic exchange resins such as cholestyramine), causes excessive fecal loss. T_3 is almost totally absorbed, 95 percent in 4 hours. The hormones contained in the natural preparations are absorbed in a manner similar to the synthetic hormones.

More than 99 percent of circulating hormones are bound to serum proteins, including thyroid-binding globulin (TBg), thyroid-binding prealbumin (TBPA), and albumin (TBa), whose capacities and affinities vary for the hormones. The higher affinity of levothyroxine (T_4) for both TBg and TBPA as compared to triiodothyronine (T_3) partially explains the higher serum levels and longer half-life of the former hormone. Both protein-bound hormones exist in reverse equilibrium with minute amounts of free hormone, the latter accounting for the metabolic activity.

Deiodination of levothyroxine (T_4) occurs at a number of sites, including liver, kidney, and other tissues. The conjugated hormone, in the form of glucuronide or sulfate, is found in the bile and gut where it may complete an enterohepatic circulation. Eighty-five percent of levothyroxine (T_4) metabolized daily is deiodinated.

Indications and Usage: Thyroid hormone drugs are indicated:

1. As replacement or supplemental therapy in patients with hypothyroidism of any etiology, except transient hypothyroidism during the recovery phase of subacute thyroiditis. This category includes cretinism, myxedema, and ordinary hypothyroidism in patients of any age (children, adults, the elderly), or state (including pregnancy), primary hypothyroidism resulting from functional deficiency, primary atrophy, partial or total absence of thyroid gland, or the effects of surgery, radiation, or drugs, with or without the presence of goiter, and secondary (pituitary) or tertiary (hypothalamic) hypothyroidism (see WARNINGS).
2. As pituitary TSH suppressants, in the treatment or prevention of various types of euthyroid goiters, including thyroid nodules, subacute or chronic lymphocytic thyroiditis (Hashimoto's), multinodular goiter, and in the management of thyroid cancer.
3. As diagnostic agents in suppression tests to differentiate suspected mild hyperthyroidism or thyroid gland autonomy.

Contraindications: Thyroid hormone preparations are generally contraindicated in patients with diagnosed but as yet uncorrected adrenal cortical insufficiency, untreated thyrotoxicosis, and apparent hypersensitivity to any of their active or extraneous constituents. There is no well documented evidence from the literature, however, of true allergic or idiosyncratic reactions to thyroid hormone.

Warnings:

> Drugs with thyroid hormone activity, alone or together with other therapeutic agents, have been used for the treatment of obesity. In euthyroid patients, doses within the range of daily hormonal requirements are ineffective for weight reduction. Larger doses may produce serious or even life-threatening manifestations of toxicity, particularly when given in association with sympathomimetic amines such as those used for their anorectic effects.

The use of thyroid hormones in the therapy of obesity, alone or combined with other drugs, is unjustified and has been shown to be ineffective. Neither is their use justified for the treatment of male or female infertility unless this condition is accompanied by hypothyroidism.

Precautions:

General: Thyroid hormones should be used with great caution in a number of circumstances where the integrity of the cardiovascular system, particularly the coronary arteries, is suspect. These include patients with angina pectoris or the elderly, in whom there is a greater likelihood of occult cardiac disease. In these patients, therapy should be initiated with low doses, ie, 25–50 mcg levothyroxine (T_4) or its isocaloric equivalents. When, in such patients, a euthyroid state can only be reached at the expense of an aggravation of the cardiovascular disease, thyroid hormone dosage should be reduced.

Thyroid hormone therapy in patients with concomitant diabetes mellitus or insipidus or adrenal cortical insufficiency aggravates the intensity of their symptoms. Appropriate adjustments of the various therapeutic measures directed at these concomitant endocrine diseases are required. The therapy of myxedema coma requires simultaneous administration of glucocorticoids (See DOSAGE AND ADMINISTRATION).

Hypothyroidism decreases and hyperthyroidism increases the sensitivity to oral anticoagulants. Prothrombin time should be closely monitored in thyroid-treated patients on oral anticoagulants and dosage of the latter agents adjusted on the basis of frequent prothrombin time determination. In infants, excessive doses of thyroid hormone preparations may produce craniosynostosis.

Information for the Patient: Patients on thyroid hormone preparations and parents of children on thyroid therapy should be informed that:

1. Replacement therapy is to be taken essentially for life, with the exception of cases of transient

hypothyroidism, usually associated with thyroiditis, and in those patients receiving a therapeutic trial of the drug.
2. They should immediately report during the course of therapy any signs or symptoms of thyroid hormone toxicity, eg, chest pain, increased pulse rate, palpitations, excessive sweating, heat intolerance, nervousness, or any other unusual event.
3. In case of concomitant diabetes mellitus, the daily dosage of antidiabetic medication may need readjustment as thyroid hormone replacement is achieved. If thyroid medication is stopped, a downward readjustment of the dosage of insulin or oral hypoglycemic agent may be necessary to avoid hypoglycemia. At all times, close monitoring of urinary glucose levels is mandatory in such patients.
4. In case of concomitant oral anticoagulant therapy, the prothrombin time should be measured frequently to determine if the dosage of oral anticoagulants is to be readjusted.
5. Partial loss of hair may be experienced by children in the first few months of thyroid therapy, but this is usually a transient phenomenon and later recovery is usually the rule.

Laboratory Tests: Treatment of patients with thyroid hormones requires the periodic assessment of thyroid status by means of appropriate laboratory tests besides the full clinical evaluation. The TSH suppression test can be used to test the effectiveness of any thyroid preparation, bearing in mind the relative insensitivity of the infant pituitary to the negative feedback effect of thyroid hormones. Serum T_4 levels can be used to test the effectiveness of all thyroid medications except T_3. When the total serum T_4 is low but TSH is normal, a test specific to assess unbound (free) T_4 levels is warranted. Specific measurements of T_4 and T_3 by competitive protein binding or radioimmunoassay are not influenced by blood levels of organic or inorganic iodine and have essentially replaced older tests of thyroid hormone measurements, ie, PBI, BEI, and T_4 by column.

Drug Interactions: Oral Anticoagulants—Thyroid hormones appear to increase catabolism of vitamin K-dependent clotting factors. If oral anticoagulants are also being given, compensatory increases in clotting factor synthesis are impaired. Patients stabilized on oral anticoagulants who are found to require thyroid replacement therapy should be watched very closely when thyroid is started. If a patient is truly hypothyroid, it is likely that a reduction in anticoagulant dosage will be required. No special precautions appear to be necessary when oral anticoagulant therapy is begun in a patient already stabilized on maintenance thyroid replacement therapy.

Insulin or Oral Hypoglycemics—Initiating thyroid replacement therapy may cause increases in insulin or oral hypoglycemic requirements. The effects seen are poorly understood and depend upon a variety of factors such as dosage and type of thyroid preparations and endocrine status of the patient. Patients receiving insulin or oral hypoglycemics should be closely watched during initiation of thyroid replacement therapy.

Cholestyramine—Cholestyramine binds both T_4 and T_3 in the intestine, thus impairing absorption of these thyroid hormones. *In vitro* studies indicate that the binding is not easily removed. Therefore, four to five hours should elapse between administration of cholestyramine and thyroid hormones.

Estrogen, Oral Contraceptives—Estrogens tend to increase serum thyroxine-binding globulin (TBg). In a patient with a nonfunctioning thyroid gland who is receiving thyroid replacement therapy, free levothyroxine may be decreased when estrogens are started thus increasing thyroid requirements. However, if the patient's thyroid gland has sufficient function, the decreased free thyroxine will result in a compensatory increase in thyroxine output by the thyroid. Therefore, patients without a functioning thyroid gland who are on thyroid replacement therapy may need to increase their thyroid dose if estrogens or estrogen-containing oral contraceptives are given.

Drug/Laboratory Test Interactions: The following drugs or moieties are known to interfere with laboratory tests performed in patients on thyroid hormone therapy: androgens, corticosteroids, estrogens, oral contraceptives containing estrogens, iodine-containing preparations, and the numerous preparations containing salicylates.
1. Changes in TBg concentration should be taken into consideration in the interpretation of T_4 and T_3 values. In such cases, the unbound (free) hormone should be measured. Pregnancy, estrogens, and estrogen-containing oral contraceptives increase TBg concentrations. TBg may also be increased during infectious hepatitis. Decreases in TBg concentrations are observed in nephrosis, acromegaly, and after androgen or corticosteroid therapy. Familial hyper- or hypothyroxine-binding-globulinemias have been described. The incidence of TBg deficiency approximates 1 in 9000. The binding of thyroxine by TBPA is inhibited by salicylates.
2. Medicinal or dietary iodine interferes with all *in vivo* tests of radioiodine uptake, producing low uptakes which may not be reflective of a true decrease in hormone synthesis.
3. The persistence of clinical and laboratory evidence of hypothyroidism in spite of adequate dosage replacement indicates poor patient compliance, poor absorption, excessive fecal loss, or inactivity of the preparation. Intracellular resistance to thyroid hormone is quite rare.

Carcinogenesis, Mutagenesis, and Impairment of Fertility: A reportedly apparent association between prolonged thyroid therapy and breast cancer has not been confirmed and patients on thyroid for established indications should not discontinue therapy. No confirmatory long-term studies in animals have been performed to evaluate carcinogenic potential, mutagenicity, or impairment of fertility in either males or females.

Pregnancy—Category A: Thyroid hormones do not readily cross the placental barrier. The clinical experience to date does not indicate any adverse effect on fetuses when thyroid hormones are administered to pregnant women. On the basis of current knowledge, thyroid replacement therapy to hypothyroid women should not be discontinued during pregnancy.

Nursing Mothers: Minimal amounts of thyroid hormones are excreted in human milk. Thyroid is not associated with serious adverse reactions and does not have a known tumorigenic potential. However, caution should be exercised when thyroid is administered to a nursing woman.

Pediatric Use: Pregnant mothers provide little or no thyroid hormone to the fetus. The incidence of congenital hypothyroidism is relatively high (1:4,000) and the hypothyroid fetus would not derive any benefit from the small amounts of hormone crossing the placental barrier. Routine determinations of serum T_4 and/or TSH are strongly advised in neonates in view of the deleterious effects of thyroid deficiency on growth and development.
Treatment should be initiated immediately upon diagnosis and maintained for life, unless transient hypothyroidism is suspected; in which case, therapy may be interrupted for 2 to 8 weeks after the age of 3 years to reassess the condition. Cessation of therapy is justified in patients who have maintained a normal TSH during those 2 to 8 weeks.

Adverse Reactions: Adverse reactions other than those indicative of hyperthyroidism because of therapeutic overdosage, either initially or during the maintenance period, are rare (See OVERDOSAGE).

Overdosage:
Signs and Symptoms: Excessive doses of thyroid result in a hypermetabolic state resembling in every respect the condition of endogenous origin. The condition may be self-induced.
Treatment of Overdosage: Dosage should be reduced or therapy temporarily discontinued if signs and symptoms of overdosage appear. Treatment may be reinstituted at a lower dosage. In normal individuals, normal hypothalamic-pituitary-thyroid axis function is restored in 6 to 8 weeks after thyroid suppression.

Treatment of acute massive thyroid hormone overdosage is aimed at reducing gastrointestinal absorption of the drugs and counteracting central and peripheral effects, mainly those of increased sympathetic activity. Vomiting may be induced initially if further gastrointestinal absorption can reasonably be prevented and barring contraindications such as coma, convulsions, or loss of the gagging reflex. Treatment is symptomatic and supportive. Oxygen may be administered and ventilation maintained. Cardiac glycosides may be indicated if congestive heart failure develops. Measures to control fever, hypoglycemia, or fluid loss should be instituted if needed. Antiadrenergic agents, particularly propranolol, have been used advantageously in the treatment of increased sympathetic activity. Propranolol may be administered intravenously at a dosage of 1 to 3 mg over a 10 minute period or orally, 80 to 160 mg/day, especially when no contraindications exist for its use.

Dosage and Administration: The dosage of thyroid hormones is determined by the indication and must in every case be individualized according to patient response and laboratory findings.
Thyroid hormones are given orally. In acute, emergency conditions, injectable sodium levothyroxine may be given intravenously when oral administration is not feasible or desirable, as in the treatment of myxedema coma, or during total parenteral nutrition. Injectable sodium liothyronine is also available upon request from the manufacturer, under investigational status, for the treatment of myxedema coma. Intramuscular administration of these two preparations is not advisable because of reported poor absorption.

Hypothyroidism: Therapy is usually instituted using low doses, with increments which depend on the cardiovascular status of the patient. The usual starting dose is 50 mcg of levothyroxine (T_4) or its isocaloric equivalent, with increments of 25 mcg every 2 to 3 weeks. A lower starting dosage, 25 mcg/day, is recommended in patients with longstanding myxedema, particularly if cardiovascular impairment is suspected, in which case extreme caution is recommended. The appearance of angina is an indication for a reduction in dosage. The 200 to 400 mcg levothyroxine (T_4) recommended in the early trials are now considered excessive and most patients require 100 to 200 mcg/day or the caloric equivalent. Failure to respond to doses of 300 mcg suggests lack of compliance or malabsorption. Maintenance dosages of 100–200 mcg/day usually result in normal serum levothyroxine (T_4) and triiodothyronine (T_3) levels. Adequate therapy usually results in normal TSH and T_4 levels after 2 to 3 weeks of therapy.
Readjustment of thyroid hormone dosage should be made within the first four weeks of therapy, after proper clinical and laboratory evaluations, including serum levels of T_4, bound and free, and TSH.
The rapid onset and dissipation of action of sodium liothyronine (T_3), as compared with sodium levothyroxine (T_4), has led some clinicians to prefer its use in patients who might be more susceptible to the untoward effects of thyroid medication. However, the wide swings in serum T_3 levels that follow its administration and the possibility of more pronounced cardiovascular side effects tend to counterbalance the stated advantages. Many physicians continue to use thyroid tablets, USP, a T_3/T_4 combination, or a newer synthetic combination.
T_3 may be used in preference to levothyroxine (T_4) during radioisotope scanning procedures, since induction of hypothyroidism in those cases is more abrupt and can be of shorter duration. It may also

Continued on next page

This product information was prepared in August, 1984. On these and other Parke-Davis Products, information may be obtained by addressing PARKE-DAVIS, Division of Warner-Lambert Company, Morris Plains, New Jersey 07950.

Parke-Davis—Cont.

be preferred when impairment of peripheral conversion of T_4 and T_3 is suspected.

Myxedema Coma: Myxedema coma is usually precipitated in the hypothyroid patient of long standing by intercurrent illness or drugs such as sedatives and anesthetics and should be considered a medical emergency. Therapy should be directed at the correction of electrolyte disturbances and possible infection besides the administration of thyroid hormones. Corticosteroids should be administered routinely. T_4 and T_3 may be administered via a nasogastric tube, but the preferred route of administration of both hormones is intravenous. Sodium levothyroxine (T_4) is given at a starting dose of 400 mcg (100 mcg/ml) given rapidly and is usually well tolerated, even in the elderly. This initial dose is followed by daily supplements of 100 to 200 mcg given IV. Normal T_4 levels are achieved in 24 hours followed in 3 days by threefold elevation of T_3. Triiodothyronine (T_3) (which is obtained only by special request from the manufacturer) is given at doses of 200 mcg IV followed by 25 mcg supplements at 8-hour intervals. Oral therapy with either hormone would be resumed as soon as the clinical situation has been stabilized and the patient is able to take oral medication.

Thyroid Cancer: Exogenous thyroid hormone may produce regression of metastases from follicular and papillary carcinoma of the thyroid and is used as ancillary therapy of these conditions with radioactive iodine. TSH should be suppressed to low or undetectable levels. Therefore, larger amounts of thyroid hormone than those used for replacement therapy are required. Medullary carcinoma of the thyroid is usually unresponsive to this therapy.

Thyroid Suppression Therapy: Administration of thyroid hormone in doses higher than those produced physiologically by the gland results in suppression of the production of endogenous hormone. This is the basis for the thyroid suppression test and is used as an aid in the diagnosis of patients with signs of mild hyperthyroidism in whom baseline laboratory tests appear normal or to demonstrate thyroid gland autonomy in patients with Graves' ophthalmopathy. [131]I uptake is determined before and after the administration of the exogenous hormone. A fifty percent or greater suppression of uptake indicates a normal thyroid-pituitary axis and thus rules out thyroid gland autonomy.

For adults, the usual suppressive dose of levothyroxine (T_4) is 2.6 mcg/kg of body weight per day given for 7 to 10 days. These doses usually yield normal serum T_4 and T_3 levels and lack of response to TSH.

T_3 is given in doses of 75–100 mcg/day for 7 days and radioactive iodine uptake is determined before and after administration of the hormone. If thyroid function is under normal control, the radioiodine uptake will drop significantly after treatment with either hormone.

Either hormone or combination therapy should be administered cautiously to patients in whom there is a strong suspicion of thyroid gland autonomy, in view of the fact that the exogenous hormone effects will be additive to the endogenous source.

Pediatric Dosage: Pediatric dosage should follow the recommendations summarized in Table 1. In infants with congenital hypothyroidism, therapy with full doses should be instituted as soon as the diagnosis has been made.
[See table below].

How Supplied: Square monogrammed tablets of four potencies, each identified by a different color (see Table 2).
Euthroid-½ is supplied as:
N 0710-0260-24—Bottles of 100.
Euthroid-1 is supplied as:
N 0710-0261-24—Bottles of 100.
N 0710-0261-32—Bottles of 1000.
Euthroid-2 is supplied as:
N 0710-0262-24—Bottles of 100.
Euthroid-3 is supplied as:
N 0710-0263-24—Bottles of 100.
Store between 15°–30°C (59°–86°F).
Licensed under U.S. Patent 2,823,164

0260G022
Shown in Product Identification Section, page 424

FLUOGEN®
[flū'ō-jĕn"]
(influenza virus vaccine)

The formulation of influenza virus vaccine for use during each season is established by the Bureau of Biologics, Food and Drug Administration, Public Health Service. For information regarding the current formulation, please refer to the product package insert, contact your Parke-Davis representative, or call (201) 540-2000.

FUROSEMIDE INJECTION, USP
[fū-rō'sĕ-mīde"]
(10 mg/ml)

Warning: Furosemide is a potent diuretic which, if given in excessive amounts, can lead to a profound diuresis with water and electrolyte depletion. Therefore, careful medical supervision is required and dose and dose schedule have to be adjusted to the individual patient's needs. (See under "DOSAGE AND ADMINISTRATION.")

Description: Furosemide is an anthranilic acid derivative. It is a white to slightly yellow, odorless, crystalline powder. It is practically insoluble in water; freely soluble in acetone, in dimethylformamide, and in solutions of alkali hydroxides; soluble in methanol; sparingly soluble in alcohol; slightly soluble in ether; very slightly soluble in chloroform. Chemically it is 4-chloro-N-furfuryl-5-sulfamoyl-anthranilic acid.

Actions: Investigations into the mode of action of furosemide have utilized micropuncture studies in rats, stop flow experiments in dogs and various clearance studies in both humans and experimental animals. It has been demonstrated that furosemide inhibits primarily the reabsorption of sodium and chloride not only in the proximal and distal tubules but also in the loop of Henle. The high degree of efficacy is largely due to this unique site of action. The action of the distal tubule is independent of any inhibitory effect on carbonic anhydrase and aldosterone.

The onset of diuresis following intravenous administration is within 5 minutes and somewhat later after intramuscular administration. The peak effect occurs within the first half hour. The duration of diuretic effect is approximately 2 hours.

Indications: Parenteral therapy should be reserved for patients unable to take oral medication or for patients in emergency clinical situations.

Furosemide is indicated for the treatment of edema associated with congestive heart failure, cirrhosis of the liver, and renal disease, including the nephrotic syndrome. Furosemide is particularly useful when an agent with greater diuretic potential than that of those commonly employed is desired.

Furosemide is indicated as adjunctive therapy in acute pulmonary edema. The intravenous administration of furosemide is indicated when a rapid onset of diuresis is desired, eg, in acute pulmonary edema.

If gastrointestinal absorption is impaired or oral medication is not practical for any reason, furosemide is indicated by the intravenous or intramuscular route. Parenteral use should be replaced with oral furosemide as soon as practical.

Contraindications: Furosemide is contraindicated in anuria. It is contraindicated in patients with a history of hypersensitivity to this compound.

Warnings: Excessive diuresis may result in dehydration and reduction in blood volume with circulatory collapse and with the possibility of vascular thrombosis and embolism, particularly in elderly patients. Excessive loss of potassium in patients receiving digitalis glycosides may precipitate digitalis toxicity. Care should also be exercised in patients receiving potassium-depleting steroids.

Frequent serum electrolyte, CO_2 and BUN determinations should be performed during the first few months of therapy and periodically thereafter, and abnormalities corrected or the drug temporarily withdrawn.

In patients with hepatic cirrhosis and ascites, initiation of therapy with furosemide is best carried out in the hospital. In hepatic coma and in states of electrolyte depletion, therapy should not be instituted until the basic condition is improved. Sudden alterations of fluid and electrolyte balance in patients with cirrhosis may precipitate hepatic coma; therefore, strict observation is necessary during the period of diuresis. Supplemental potassium chloride and, if required, an aldosterone antagonist are helpful in preventing hypokalemia and metabolic alkalosis.

If increasing azotemia and oliguria occur during treatment of severe progressive renal disease, the drug should be discontinued.

As with many other drugs, patients should be observed regularly for the possible occurrence of blood dyscrasias, liver damage, or other idiosyncratic reactions.

Patients with known sulfonamide sensitivity may show allergic reactions to furosemide.

Furosemide may add to or potentiate the therapeutic effect of other antihypertensive drugs. Potentiation occurs with ganglionic or peripheral adrenergic blocking drugs.

The possibility exists of exacerbation or activation of systemic lupus erythematosus.

Table 1 Recommended Pediatric Dosage for Congenital Hypothyroidism

	Tetraiodothyronine (T_4, levothyroxine) sodium	
Age	Dose per day	Daily dose per kg of body weight
0–6 mos	25–50 mcg	8–10 mcg
6–12 mos	50–75 mcg	6–8 mcg
1–5 yrs	75–100 mcg	5–6 mcg
6–12 yrs	100–150 mcg	4–5 mcg
over 12 yrs	over 150 mcg	2–3 mcg

Table 2 Approximate Equivalent of Euthroid

Euthroid (liotrix tablets, USP)			Natural	Synthetic	
Tablet	T_4*/T_3** mcg	Color	Thyroid USP	T_4*	T_3**
Euthroid-½	(30/75)	pale orange	½ grain	0.05 mg	12.5 mcg
Euthroid-1	(60/15)	light brown	1 grain	0.1 mg	25.0 mcg
Euthroid-2	(120/30)	violet	2 grains	0.2 mg	50.0 mcg
Euthroid-3	(180/45)	gray	3 grains	0.3 mg	75.0 mcg

*T_4 = levothyroxine sodium (l-thyroxine)   **T_3 = liothyronine sodium (l-triiodothyronine)

for possible revisions

Furosemide appears in breast milk. If use of the drug is deemed essential, the patient should stop nursing.

Parenterally administered furosemide may increase the ototoxic potential of aminoglycoside antibiotics. Especially in the presence of impaired renal function, the use of parenterally administered furosemide in patients to whom aminoglycoside antibiotics are also being given should be avoided, except in life-threatening situations.

Cases of tinnitus and reversible hearing impairments have been reported. There have also been some reports of cases in which irreversible hearing impairment occurred. Usually, ototoxicity has been reported when furosemide was injected rapidly in patients with severe impairment of renal function at doses exceeding several times the usual recommended dose and in whom other drugs known to be ototoxic were given. If the physician elects to use high dose parenteral therapy in patients with severely impaired renal function, controlled intravenous infusion is advisable [for adults, an infusion rate not exceeding 4 mg furosemide per minute has been used].

Precautions: As with any effective diuretic, electrolyte depletion may occur during therapy with furosemide, especially in patients receiving higher doses and a restricted salt intake. Periodic determinations of serum electrolytes to detect possible imbalance should be performed at appropriate intervals.

All patients receiving furosemide therapy should be observed for signs of fluid or electrolyte imbalance: namely, hyponatremia, hypochloremic alkalosis and hypokalemia. Serum and urine electrolyte determinations are particularly important when the patient is vomiting excessively or receiving parenteral fluids. Medication such as digitalis may also influence serum electrolytes. Warning signs, irrespective of cause, are dryness of mouth, thirst, weakness, lethargy, drowsiness, restlessness, muscle pains or cramps, muscular fatigue, hypotension, oliguria, tachycardia, arrhythmia and gastrointestinal disturbances such as nausea and vomiting.

Hypokalemia may develop with furosemide as with any other potent diuretic, especially with brisk diuresis, when cirrhosis is present, or during concomitant use of corticosteroids or ACTH.

Interference with adequate oral electrolyte intake will also contribute to hypokalemia. Digitalis therapy may exaggerate metabolic effects of hypokalemia, especially with reference to myocardial activity.

Asymptomatic hyperuricemia can occur and gout may rarely be precipitated.

Periodic checks on urine and blood glucose should be made in diabetics and even those suspected of latent diabetes when receiving furosemide. Increases in blood glucose and alterations in glucose tolerance tests with abnormalities of the fasting and 2-hour postprandial sugar have been observed, and rare cases of precipitation of diabetes mellitus have been reported.

Furosemide may lower serum calcium levels, and rare cases of tetany have been reported. Accordingly, periodic serum calcium levels should be obtained.

Reversible elevations of BUN may be seen. These have been observed in association with dehydration, which should be avoided, particularly in patients with renal insufficiency.

Patients receiving high doses of salicylates, as in rheumatic disease, in conjunction with furosemide may experience salicylate toxicity at lower doses because of competitive renal excretory sites.

Furosemide has a tendency to antagonize the skeletal muscle relaxing effect of tubocurarine and may potentiate the action of succinylcholine.

Lithium generally should not be given with diuretics because they reduce its renal clearance and add a high risk of lithium toxicity.

It has been reported in the literature that diuretics such as furosemide may enhance the nephrotoxicity of cephaloridine. Therefore, furosemide and cephaloridine should not be administered simultaneously.

Product Information

Furosemide may decrease arterial responsiveness to norepinephrine. This diminution is not sufficient to preclude effectiveness of the pressor agent for therapeutic use.

Pregnancy:

Pregnancy Category C. Furosemide has been shown to cause unexplained maternal deaths and abortions in rabbits at 2, 4 and 8 times the human dose. There are no adequate and well-controlled studies in pregnant women. Furosemide should be used during pregnancy only if the potential benefit justifies the potential risk to the fetus.

The effects of furosemide on embryonic and fetal development and on pregnant dams were studied in mice, rats and rabbits.

Furosemide caused unexplained maternal deaths and abortions in the rabbit when 50 mg/kg (4 times the maximal recommended human dose of 600 mg per day) was administered between days 12 and 17 of gestation. In a previous study the lowest dose of only 25 mg/kg (2 times the maximal recommended human dose of 600 mg per day) caused maternal deaths and abortions. In a third study, none of the pregnant rabbits survived a dose of 100 mg/kg. Data from the above studies indicate fetal lethality that can precede maternal deaths.

The results of the mouse study and one of the three rabbit studies also showed an increased incidence of hydronephrosis (distention of the renal pelvis and, in some cases, of the ureters) in fetuses derived from treated dams as compared to the incidence in fetuses from the control group.

Adverse Reactions:
Gastrointestinal System Reactions
1. anorexia
2. oral and gastric irritation
3. nausea
4. vomiting
5. cramping
6. diarrhea
7. constipation
8. jaundice (intrahepatic cholestatic jaundice)
9. pancreatitis

Central Nervous System Reactions
1. dizziness
2. vertigo
3. paresthesias
4. headache
5. xanthopsia
6. blurred vision
7. tinnitus and hearing loss

Hematologic Reactions
1. anemia
2. leukopenia
3. agranulocytosis (rare)
4. thrombocytopenia
5. aplastic anemia (rare)

Dermatologic-Hypersensitivity Reactions
1. purpura
2. photosensitivity
3. rash
4. uticaria
5. necrotizing angiitis (vasculitis, cutaneous vasculitis)
6. exfoliative dermatitis
7. erythema multiforme
8. pruritus

Cardiovascular Reactions
Orthostatic hypotension may occur and be aggravated by alcohol, barbiturates or narcotics.

Other
1. hyperglycemia
2. glycosuria
3. hyperuricemia
4. muscle spasm
5. weakness
6. restlessness
7. urinary bladder spasm
8. thrombophlebitis
9. transient pain at the injection site following intramuscular injection

Whenever adverse reactions are moderate or severe, furosemide dosage should be reduced or therapy withdrawn.

Dosage and Administration:
Adults—Parenteral therapy should be reserved for patients for whom oral medication is not practical or in emergency situations where prompt

1523

diuresis is desired. Parenteral therapy should be replaced by oral therapy as soon as this is practical for continued mobilization of edema.

Edema The usual initial dose of furosemide is 20 to 40 mg given as a single dose, injected intramuscularly or intravenously. The intravenous injection should be given slowly (1 to 2 minutes). Ordinarily, a prompt diuresis ensues. Depending on the patient's response, a second dose can be administered 2 hours after the first dose or later.

If the diuretic response with a single dose of 20 to 40 mg is not satisfactory, increase this dose by increments of 20 mg not sooner than 2 hours after the previous dose until the desired diuretic effect has been obtained. This individually determined single dose should then be given once or twice daily.

If the physician elects to use high dose parenteral therapy it should be administered as a controlled infusion at a rate not exceeding 4 mg/min. Furosemide Injection, USP is a mildly buffered alkaline solution which should not be mixed with acidic solutions of pH below 5.5. To prepare infusion solutions, isotonic saline and lactated Ringer's injection and 5% dextrose injection have been used after pH has been adjusted when necessary.

Therapy should be individualized according to patient response. This therapy should be titrated to gain maximal therapeutic response as well as the minimal dose possible to maintain that therapeutic response. Close medical supervision is necessary.

Acute Pulmonary Edema The usual initial dose of furosemide is 40 mg injected intravenously. The injection should be given slowly (1 to 2 minutes). If 40 mg furosemide does not produce a satisfactory response within 1 hour, the dose may be increased to 80 mg given intravenously (over 1 to 2 minutes). If deemed necessary, additional therapy (eg, digitalis, oxygen) can be administered concomitantly.

Infants and Children—Parenteral therapy should be reserved for patients for whom oral medication is not practical or in emergency situations where prompt diuresis is desired. Parenteral therapy should be replaced by oral therapy as soon as this is practical for continued mobilization of edema. The usual initial dose of furosemide, injected intravenously or intramuscularly, in infants and children is 1 mg/kg body weight and should be given slowly under close medical supervision. If the diuretic response after the initial dose is not satisfactory, dosage may be increased by 1 mg/kg not sooner than 2 hours after the previous dose, until the desired diuretic effect has been obtained. Doses greater than 6 mg/kg body weight are not recommended.

How Supplied: Furosemide Injection, USP is supplied as a sterile solution for parenteral use as follows:

N 0071-4143-05 2 ml amber ampoule, carton of 10 ampoules
N 0071-4143-08 4 ml amber ampoule, carton of 10 ampoules
N 0071-4143-10 10 ml amber ampoule, carton of 10 ampoules

Each milliliter of solution contains 10 mg furosemide, with sodium chloride for isotonicity and sodium hydroxide to make the solution slightly alkaline.

Store at controlled room temperature, 15°-30°C (59°-86°F). Do not use if solution is discolored.

4143G010

Continued on next page

This product information was prepared in August, 1984. On these and other Parke-Davis Products, information may be obtained by addressing PARKE-DAVIS, Division of Warner-Lambert Company, Morris Plains, New Jersey 07950.

Parke-Davis—Cont.

FUROSEMIDE Tablets, USP ℞
[fū″rō′sĕ-mīde]

Warning:
Furosemide is a potent diuretic which, if given in excessive amounts, can lead to a profound diuresis with water and electrolyte depletion. Therefore, careful medical supervision is required and dose and dose schedule have to be adjusted to the individual patient's needs. (See under "DOSAGE AND ADMINISTRATION.")

Description: Furosemide is an anthranilic acid derivative. It is a white to slightly yellow, odorless, crystalline powder. It is practically insoluble in water; freely soluble in acetone, in dimethylformamide, and in solutions of alkali hydroxides; soluble in methanol; sparingly soluble in alcohol; slightly soluble in ether; very slightly soluble in chloroform. Chemically it is 4-chloro-N-furfuryl-5-sulfamoyl-anthranilic acid.
Furosemide Tablets, USP are available in strengths of 20 mg and 40 mg for oral administration.

Clinical Pharmacology: Investigations into the mode of action of furosemide have utilized micropuncture studies in rats, stop flow experiments in dogs and various clearance studies in both humans and experimental animals. It has been demonstrated that furosemide inhibits primarily the reabsorption of sodium and chloride not only in the proximal and distal tubules but also in the loop of Henle. The high degree of efficacy is largely due to this unique site of action. The action on the distal tubule is independent of any inhibitory effect on carbonic anhydrase and aldosterone.
The onset of diuresis following oral administration is within 1 hour. The peak effect occurs within the first or second hour. The duration of diuretic effect is 6 to 8 hours.

Indications:
Edema: Furosemide is indicated for the treatment of edema associated with congestive heart failure, cirrhosis of the liver, and renal disease, including the nephrotic syndrome. Furosemide is particularly useful when an agent with greater diuretic potential than that of those commonly employed is desired.
If gastrointestinal absorption is impaired or oral medication is not practical for any reason, furosemide is indicated by the intravenous or intramuscular route. Parenteral use should be replaced with oral furosemide as soon as practical.
Hypertension: Furosemide may be used for the treatment of hypertension alone or in combination with other antihypertensive agents. Hypertensive patients who cannot be adequately controlled with thiazides will probably also not be adequately controlled with furosemide alone.

Contraindications: Furosemide is contraindicated in anuria. It is contraindicated in patients with a history of hypersensitivity to this compound.

Warnings: Excessive diuresis may result in dehydration and reduction in blood volume with circulatory collapse and with the possibility of vascular thrombosis and embolism, particularly in elderly patients. Excessive loss of potassium in patients receiving digitalis glycosides may precipitate digitalis toxicity. Care should also be exercised in patients receiving potassium-depleting steroids.
Frequent serum electrolyte, CO_2 and BUN determinations should be performed during the first few months of therapy and periodically thereafter, and abnormalities corrected or the drug temporarily withdrawn.
In patients with hepatic cirrhosis and ascites, initiation of therapy with furosemide is best carried out in the hospital. In hepatic coma and in states of electrolyte depletion, therapy should not be instituted until the basic condition is improved. Sudden alterations of fluid and electrolyte balance in patients with cirrhosis may precipitate hepatic coma; therefore, strict observation is necessary during the period of diuresis. Supplemental potassium chloride and, if required, an aldosterone antagonist are helpful in preventing hypokalemia and metabolic alkalosis.
If increasing azotemia and oliguria occur during treatment of severe progressive renal disease, the drug should be discontinued.
As with many other drugs, patients should be observed regularly for the possible occurrence of blood dyscrasias, liver damage, or other idiosyncratic reactions.
Patients with known sulfonamide sensitivity may show allergic reactions to furosemide.
Furosemide may add to or potentiate the therapeutic effect of other antihypertensive drugs. Potentiation occurs with ganglionic or peripheral adrenergic blocking drugs.
The possibility exists of exacerbation or activation of systemic lupus erythematosus.
Furosemide appears in breast milk. If use of the drug is deemed essential, the patient should stop nursing.
When parenteral use of furosemide precedes its oral use, it should be kept in mind that cases of tinnitus and reversible hearing impairments have been reported. There have also been some reports of cases in which irreversible hearing impairment occurred. Usually ototoxicity has been reported when furosemide was injected rapidly in patients with severe impairment of renal function at doses exceeding several times the usual recommended dose and in whom other drugs known to be ototoxic were given. If the physician elects to use high dose parenteral therapy in patients with severely impaired renal function, controlled intravenous infusion is advisable [for adults, an infusion rate not exceeding 4 mg furosemide per minute has been used].

Precautions: As with any effective diuretic, electrolyte depletion may occur during therapy with furosemide, especially in patients receiving higher doses and a restricted salt intake. Periodic determinations of serum electrolytes to detect possible imbalance should be performed at appropriate intervals.
All patients receiving furosemide therapy should be observed for signs of fluid or electrolyte imbalance: namely, hyponatremia, hypochloremic alkalosis and hypokalemia. Serum and urine electrolyte determinations are particularly important when the patient is vomiting excessively or receiving parenteral fluids. Medication such as digitalis may also influence serum electrolytes. Warning signs, irrespective of cause are dryness of mouth, thirst, weakness, lethargy, drowsiness, restlessness, muscle pains or cramps, muscular fatigue, hypotension, oliguria, tachycardia, arrhythmia and gastrointestinal disturbances such as nausea and vomiting.
Hypokalemia may develop with furosemide as with any other potent diuretic, especially with brisk diuresis, when cirrhosis is present, or during concomitant use of corticosteroids or ACTH.
Interference with adequate oral electrolyte intake will also contribute to hypokalemia. Digitalis therapy may exaggerate metabolic effects of hypokalemia, especially with reference to myocardial activity.
Asymptomatic hyperuricemia can occur and gout may rarely be precipitated.
Periodic checks on urine and blood glucose should be made in diabetics and even those suspected of latent diabetes when receiving furosemide. Increases in blood glucose and alterations in glucose tolerance tests with abnormalities of the fasting and 2-hour postprandial sugar have been observed, and rare cases of precipitation of diabetes mellitus have been reported.
Furosemide may lower serum calcium levels, and rare cases of tetany have been reported. Accordingly, periodic serum calcium levels should be obtained.
Reversible elevations of BUN may be seen. These have been observed in association with dehydration, which should be avoided, particularly in patients with renal insufficiency.
Patients receiving high doses of salicylates, as in rheumatic disease, in conjunction with furosemide may experience salicylate toxicity at lower doses because of competitive renal excretory sites.
Furosemide has a tendency to antagonize the skeletal muscle relaxing effect of tubocurarine and may potentiate the action of succinylcholine.
Lithium generally should not be given with diuretics because they reduce its renal clearance and add a high risk of lithium toxicity.
It has been reported in the literature that diuretics such as furosemide may enhance the nephrotoxicity of cephaloridine. Therefore, furosemide and cephaloridine should not be administered simultaneously.
Furosemide may decrease arterial responsiveness to norepinephrine. This diminution is not sufficient to preclude effectiveness of the pressor agent for therapeutic use.
It has been reported in the literature that coadministration of indomethacin may reduce the natriuretic and antihypertensive effects of furosemide in some patients. This effect has been attributed to inhibition of prostaglandin synthesis by indomethacin. Indomethacin may also affect plasma renin levels and aldosterone excretion; this should be borne in mind when a renin profile is evaluated in hypertensive patients. Patients receiving both indomethacin and furosemide should be observed closely to determine if the desired diuretic and/or antihypertensive effect of furosemide is achieved.

Pregnancy:
Pregnancy Category C. Furosemide has been shown to cause unexplained maternal deaths and abortions in rabbits at 2, 4 and 8 times the human dose. There are no adequate and well-controlled studies in pregnant women. Furosemide should be used during pregnancy only if the potential benefit justifies the potential risk to the fetus.
The effects of furosemide on embryonic and fetal development and on pregnant dams were studied in mice, rats and rabbits.
Furosemide caused unexplained maternal deaths and abortions in the rabbit when 50 mg/kg (4 times the maximal recommended human dose of 600 mg per day) was administered between days 12 and 17 of gestation. In a previous study the lowest dose of only 25 mg/kg (2 times the maximal recommended human dose of 600 mg per day) caused maternal deaths and abortions. In a third study, none of the pregnant rabbits survived a dose of 100 mg/kg. Data from the above studies indicate fetal lethality that can precede maternal deaths.
The results of the mouse study and one of the three rabbit studies also showed an increased incidence of hydronephrosis (distention of the renal pelvis and, in some cases, of the ureters) in fetuses derived from treated dams as compared to the incidence in fetuses from the control group.

Adverse Reactions:
Gastrointestinal System Reactions
1. anorexia
2. oral and gastric irritation
3. nausea
4. vomiting
5. cramping
6. diarrhea
7. constipation
8. jaundice (intrahepatic cholestatic jaundice)
9. pancreatitis

Central Nervous System Reactions
1. dizziness
2. vertigo
3. paresthesias
4. headache
5. xanthopsia
6. blurred vision
7. tinnitus and hearing loss

Hematologic Reactions
1. anemia
2. leukopenia
3. agranulocytosis (rare)
4. thrombocytopenia
5. aplastic anemia (rare)

Dermatologic-Hypersensitivity Reactions
1. purpura
2. photosensitivity
3. rash
4. urticaria
5. necrotizing angiitis (vasculitis, cutaneous vasculitis)
6. exfoliative dermatitis
7. erythema multiforme
8. pruritus

Product Information

Cardiovascular Reactions
Orthostatic hypotension may occur and be aggravated by alcohol, barbiturates or narcotics.

Other
1. hyperglycemia
2. glycosuria
3. hyperuricemia
4. muscle spasm
5. weakness
6. restlessness
7. urinary bladder spasm
8. thrombophlebitis

Whenever adverse reactions are moderate or severe, furosemide dosage should be reduced or therapy withdrawn.

Dosage and Administration:
Edema

Therapy should be individualized according to patient response. This therapy should be titrated to gain maximal therapeutic response as well as the minimal dose possible to maintain that therapeutic response.

Parenteral therapy should be reserved for patients unable to take oral medication or in emergency situations.

Adults: The usual daily dose of furosemide is 20 to 80 mg given as a single dose. Ordinarily a prompt diuresis ensues. Depending on the patient's response, a second dose can be administered 6 to 8 hours later.

If the diuretic response to a single dose of 20 to 80 mg is not satisfactory, increase this dose by increments of 20 or 40 mg not sooner than 6 to 8 hours after the previous dose until the desired diuretic effect has been obtained. This individually determined single dose should then be given once or twice daily (eg, at 8:00 a.m. and 2:00 p.m.). The dose of furosemide may be carefully titrated up to 600 mg/day in those patients with severe clinical edematous states.

The mobilization of edema may be most efficiently and safely accomplished by utilizing an intermittent dosage schedule in which the diuretic is given for 2 to 4 consecutive days each week.

When doses exceeding 80 mg/day are given for prolonged periods, careful clinical and laboratory observations are particularly advisable.

Infants and Children: The usual initial dose of furosemide in infants and children is 2 mg/kg body weight, given as a single dose. If the diuretic response is not satisfactory after the initial dose, dose may be increased by 1 or 2 mg/kg no sooner than 6 to 8 hours after the previous dose. Doses greater than 6 mg/kg body weight are not recommended.

For maintenance therapy in infants and children, the dose should be adjusted to the minimum effective level.

Hypertension

Therapy should be individualized according to patient response. This therapy should be titrated to gain maximal therapeutic response as well as the minimal dose possible to maintain that therapeutic response.

Adults: The usual initial daily dose of furosemide for antihypertensive therapy is 80 mg, usually divided into 40 mg twice a day. Dosage should then be adjusted according to response. If the patient does not respond, add other antihypertensive agents.

Careful observations for changes in blood pressure must be made when this compound is used with other antihypertensive drugs, especially during initial therapy. The dosage of other agents must be reduced by at least 50 percent as soon as furosemide is added to the regimen, to prevent excessive drop in blood pressure. As the blood pressure falls under the potentiating effect of furosemide, a further reduction in dosage or even discontinuation of other antihypertensive drugs may be necessary.

How Supplied:
Furosemide Tablets, USP, 20 mg are supplied as white, oval tablets (P-D 440).
N 0071-0440-24 Bottles of 100
Furosemide Tablets, USP, 40 mg are supplied as white, round scored tablets (P-D 441).

N 0071-0441-24 Bottles of 100
N 0071-0441-30 Bottles of 500
N 0071-0441-40 Unit-dose packages of 100 (10 strips of 10 tablets each)

Note: Dispense in well-closed, light resistant containers. Discolored tablets should not be dispensed.

Store bottles at room temperature below 30°C (86°F) and unit-dose packages at controlled room temperature 15°-30°C (59°-86°F).

Protect from light and moisture.

0440G012

GELUSIL®
[jĕl'ū-sĭl"]
Antacid-Anti-gas
Liquid/Tablets

Each teaspoonful (5 ml) or tablet contains:
200 mg aluminum hydroxide
200 mg magnesium hydroxide
25 mg simethicone

Advantages:
- High acid-neutralizing capacity
- Low sodium content
- Simethicone for antiflatulent activity
- Good taste for better patient compliance
- Fast dissolution of chewed tablets for prompt relief

Indications: Gelusil, a carefully balanced combination of two widely used antacids and the antiflatulent simethicone, is effective for the relief of symptoms associated with heartburn, sour stomach and acid indigestion with gas. Gelusil provides symptomatic relief of hyperacidity associated with the diagnosis of peptic ulcer, gastritis, peptic esophagitis, gastric hyperacidity and hiatal hernia, and it alleviates or relieves the symptoms of gas and postoperative gas pain.

Actions and Uses: The proven neutralizing power of aluminum hydroxide and of magnesium hydroxide combine to give Gelusil dependable antacid action without the acid rebound sometimes associated with calcium carbonate.

The pleasant peppermint-flavored taste of Gelusil Liquid and Tablets encourages patient acceptance of, and compliance with, recommended antacid-anti-gas regimens.

Gelusil Tablets are easy to chew and are specifically formulated to dissolve readily, providing prompt onset of action and reliable relief of symptoms.

Gelusil is appropriate whenever there is a need for well-accepted, effective antacid-anti-gas therapy.

Dosage and Administration: Two or more teaspoonfuls or tablets one hour after meals and at bedtime, or as directed by a physician. Tablets should be chewed.

The following information is provided to facilitate treatment:

Gelusil	LIQUID	TABLETS
Acid-neutralizing capacity	24 mEq/ 10 ml	22 mEq/ 2 tabs
Sodium	0.7 mg/ 5 ml	0.8 mg/ tab
Lactose	0	0

Warnings: Do not take more than 12 tablets or teaspoonfuls in a 24-hour period, or use this maximum dosage for more than 2 weeks, or use this product if you have kidney disease, except under the advice and supervision of a physician.

Keep this and all drugs out of the reach of children.

Drug Interaction Precaution: Do not take this product if you are presently taking a prescription antibiotic drug containing any form of tetracycline.

All aluminum-containing antacids, including Gelusil, may prevent proper absorption of tetracycline.

How Supplied:
N 0071-2036—**Liquid**—In plastic bottles of 6 fl oz and 12 fl oz.

N 0071-0034—**Tablets**—White, embossed Gelusil P-D 034—individual strips of 10 in boxes of 50, 100 and 1000; 165 tablets loose-packed in plastic bottles.

Shown in Product Identification Section, page 424

GELUSIL-M®
[jĕl'ū-sĭl"]
Antacid-Anti-gas
Liquid/Tablets

Each teaspoonful (5 ml) or tablet contains:
300 mg aluminum hydroxide
200 mg magnesium hydroxide
25 mg simethicone

Advantages:
- High acid-neutralizing capacity
- Low sodium content
- Simethicone for antiflatulent activity
- Good taste for better patient compliance
- Fast dissolution of chewed tablets for prompt relief

Indications: Gelusil-M, a carefully balanced combination of two widely used antacids and the antiflatulent simethicone, is effective for the relief of symptoms associated with heartburn, sour stomach, and acid indigestion with gas. Gelusil-M provides symptomatic relief of hyperacidity associated with the diagnosis of peptic ulcer, gastritis, peptic esophagitis, gastric hyperacidity and hiatal hernia, and it alleviates or relieves the symptoms of gas and postoperative gas pain.

Actions and Uses: The proven neutralizing power of aluminum hydroxide and magnesium hydroxide combine to give Gelusil-M dependable antacid action without the acid rebound sometimes associated with calcium carbonate.

The pleasant spearmint-flavored taste of Gelusil-M Liquid and Tablets encourages patient acceptance of, and compliance with, recommended antacid-anti-gas regimens.

Gelusil-M Tablets are easy to chew and are specifically formulated to dissolve readily providing prompt onset of action and reliable relief of symptoms.

Gelusil-M is appropriate whenever there is a need for well-accepted, effective antacid-anti-gas therapy.

Dosage and Administration: Two or more teaspoonfuls or tablets one hour after meals and at bedtime, or as directed by a physician. Tablets should be chewed.

The following information is provided to facilitate treatment:

Gelusil-M	LIQUID	TABLETS
Acid-neutralizing capacity	30 mEq/ 10 ml	25 mEq/ 2 tabs
Sodium	1.2 mg/ 5 ml	1.3 mg/ tab
Lactose	0	0

Warnings: Do not take more than 10 teaspoonfuls or tablets in a 24-hour period, or use this maximum dosage for more than 2 weeks, or use this product if you have kidney disease, except under the advice and supervision of a physician.

Keep this and all drugs out of the reach of children.

Drug Interaction Precaution: Do not take this product if you are presently taking a prescription antibiotic drug containing any form of tetracycline.

All aluminum-containing antacids, including Gelusil-M, may prevent proper absorption of tetracycline.

Continued on next page

This product information was prepared in August, 1984. On these and other Parke-Davis Products, information may be obtained by addressing **PARKE-DAVIS**, Division of Warner-Lambert Company, Morris Plains, New Jersey 07950.

Parke-Davis—Cont.

How Supplied:
N 0071-2043- **Liquid**—In plastic bottles of 12 fl oz.
N 0071-0045-**Tablets**—White, embossed P-D 045—individual strips of 10 in boxes of 100.

GELUSIL–II®
[jĕl'ū-sil"]
Antacid-Anti-gas
Liquid/Tablets
High Potency

Each teaspoonful (5 ml) or tablet contains:
400 mg aluminum hydroxide
400 mg magnesium hydroxide
30 mg simethicone

Advantages:
- High acid-neutralizing capacity
- Low sodium content
- Simethicone for antiflatulent activity
- Good taste for better patient compliance
- Fast dissolution of chewed tablets for prompt relief
- Double strength antacid

Indications: Gelusil-II, a carefully balanced, high-potency combination of two widely used antacids and the antiflatulent simethicone, is effective for the relief of symptoms associated with heartburn, sour stomach and acid indigestion with gas. Gelusil-II provides symptomatic relief of hyperacidity associated with the diagnosis of peptic ulcer, gastritis, peptic esophagitis, gastric hyperacidity and hiatal hernia, and it alleviates or relieves the symptoms of gas and postoperative gas pain.

Actions and Uses: The proven neutralizing power of aluminum hydroxide and magnesium hydroxide combine to give Gelusil-II dependable antacid action without the acid rebound sometimes associated with calcium carbonate. The higher potency of Gelusil-II is achieved by greater concentration of antacid ingredients per dosage unit.

The pleasant taste of Gelusil-II Liquid (citrus-flavored) and Tablets (orange-flavored) encourages patient acceptance of, and compliance with, recommended antacid-anti-gas regimens.

Gelusil-II Tablets are easy to chew and are specifically formulated to dissolve readily, providing prompt onset of action and reliable relief of symptoms.

Gelusil-II is appropriate whenever there is a need for well-accepted, effective antacid-anti-gas therapy.

Dosage and Administration: Two or more teaspoonfuls or tablets one hour after meals and at bedtime, or as directed by a physician. Tablets should be chewed.

The following information is provided to facilitate treatment:

Gelusil-II	LIQUID	TABLETS
Acid-neutralizing capacity	48 mEq/ 10 ml	42 mEq/ 2 tabs
Sodium	1.3 mg/ 5 ml	2.1 mg/ tab
Lactose	0	0

Warnings: Do not take more than 8 tablets or teaspoonfuls in a 24-hour period, or use this maximum dosage for more than 2 weeks, or use this product if you have kidney disease, except under the advice and supervision of a physician.
Keep this and all drugs out of the reach of children.

Drug Interaction Precaution: Do not take this product if you are presently taking a prescription antibiotic containing any form of tetracycline.
All aluminum-containing antacids, including Gelusil-II, may prevent proper absorption of tetracycline.

How Supplied:
N 0071-0042-**Liquid**—In plastic bottles of 12 fl oz.
N 0071-0043-**Tablets**—Double-layered white/ orange, embossed W/C 043 or P-D 043 - individual strips of 10 in boxes of 80.
Shown in Product Identification Section, page 424

GENERICS
The following is a list of the generic names of all Parke-Davis solid-oral product forms which are marketed under the generic name or a trade name.

Code	Product
0634-	℞ Acetaminophen with Codeine Phosphate Tablets, No. 2
0635-	℞ Acetaminophen with Codeine Phosphate Tablets, No. 3
0637-	℞ Acetaminophen with Codeine Phosphate Tablets, No. 4
0640-	Acetaminophen Tablets, USP (Tapar®), 325 mg
0272-	Amitriptyline Hydrochloride Tablets, USP (Amitril®), 10 mg
0273-	Amitriptyline Hydrochloride Tablets, USP (Amitril®), 25 mg
0274-	Amitriptyline Hydrochloride Tablets, USP (Amitril®), 50 mg
0275-	Amitriptyline Hydrochloride Tablets, USP (Amitril®), 75 mg
0271-	Amitriptyline Hydrochloride Tablets, USP (Amitril®), 100 mg
0278-	Amitriptyline Hydrochloride Tablets, USP (Amitril®), 150 mg
0730-	Amoxicillin (Utimox®) Capsules, 250 mg
0731-	Amoxicillin (Utimox®) Capsules, 500 mg
0402-	Ampicillin Capsules, USP (Amcill® Capsules), 250 mg
0404-	Ampicillin Capsules, USP (Amcill® Capsules), 500 mg
0606-	Aspirin Tablets, USP, 325 mg
0533-	Calcium Lactate Tablets, USP, 325 mg
0604-	Calcium Lactate Tablets, USP, 650 mg
0379-	Chloramphenicol Capsules, USP (Chloromycetin® Kapseals), 250 mg
0800-	℞ Chlordiazepoxide Hydrochloride Capsules, USP, 5 mg
0801-	℞ Chlordiazepoxide Hydrochloride Capsules, USP, 10 mg
0802-	℞ Chlordiazepoxide Hydrochloride Capsules, USP, 25 mg
0010-	Chlorpromazine Hydrochloride Tablets, USP (Promapar®), 10 mg
0025-	Chlorpromazine Hydrochloride Tablets, USP, 25 mg
0050-	Chlorpromazine Hydrochloride Tablets, USP, 50 mg
0100-	Chlorpromazine Hydrochloride Tablets, USP, 100 mg
0201-	Chlorpromazine Hydrochloride Tablets, USP, 200 mg
0123-	Chlorthalidone Tablets, USP, 25 mg
0121-	Chlorthalidone Tablets, USP, 50 mg
0471-	Diphenhydramine Hydrochloride Capsules, USP (Benadryl®), 25 mg
0373-	Diphenhydramine Hydrochloride Capsules, USP (Benadryl® Kapseals), 50 mg
0247-	Docusate Sodium Capsules, USP (DSS Capsules), 100 mg
0248-	Docusate Sodium with Casanthranol Capsules (DSS Plus Capsules)
0111-	Ergotamine Tartrate Tablets (Ergostat® Sublingual Tablets), 2 mg
0672-	Erythromycin Stearate Tablets, USP (Erypar® Filmseal), 250 mg
0919-	Erythromycin Stearate Tablets, USP (Erypar® Filmseal), 500 mg
0237-	Ethosuximide Capsules, USP (Zarontin® Capsules), 250 mg
0037-	Ferrous Sulfate Filmseal, 325 mg
0440-	Furosemide Tablets, USP, 20 mg
0441-	Furosemide Tablets, USP, 40 mg
0702-	Hydrochlorothiazide Tablets, USP (Thiuretic®), 25 mg
0710-	Hydrochlorothiazide Tablets, USP (Thiuretic®), 50 mg
0268-	Meclofenamate Sodium (Meclomen®) Capsules, 50 mg
0269-	Meclofenamate Sodium (Meclomen) Capsules, 100 mg
0540-	Mefenamic Acid (Ponstel® Kapseals), 250 mg
0932-	℞ Meprobamate Tablets, USP, 200 mg
0647-	℞ Meprobamate Tablets, USP, 400 mg
0525-	Methsuximide Capsules, USP (Celontin® Kapseals), 300 mg
0537-	Methsuximide Capsules, USP (Celontin® Kapseals), 150 mg
1460-	Nitroglycerin Tablets, USP (Nitrostat® Sublingual Tablets), 0.15 mg
1469-	Nitroglycerin Tablets, USP (Nitrostat® Sublingual Tablets), 0.3 mg
1470-	Nitroglycerin Tablets, USP (Nitrostat® Sublingual Tablets), 0.4 mg
1471-	Nitroglycerin Tablets, USP (Nitrostat® Sublingual Tablets), 0.6 mg
0882-	Norethindrone Tablets, USP (Norlutin® Tablets), 5 mg
0918-	Norethindrone Acetate Tablets, USP (Norlutate® Tablets), 5 mg
0210-	Oxtriphylline (Choledyl®) Tablets, USP, 100 mg
0211-	Oxtriphylline (Choledyl®) Tablets, USP, 200 mg
0529-	Paromomycin Sulfate Capsules, USP (Humatin® Capsules), 250 mg
0648-	Penicillin V Potassium Tablets, USP (Penapar VK®), 250 mg
0673-	Penicillin V Potassium Tablets, USP (Penapar VK®), 500 mg
0699-	℞ Phenobarbital Tablets, USP, 15 mg
0700-	℞ Phenobarbital Tablets, USP, 30 mg
0607-	℞ Phenobarbital Tablets, USP, 60 mg
0698-	℞ Phenobarbital Tablets, USP, 100 mg
0393-	Phensuximide Capsules, USP (Milontin® Kapseals), 500 mg
0007-	Phenytoin Tablets, USP (Dilantin® Infatabs®), 50 mg
0362-	Phenytoin Sodium, Extended, Capsules, USP (Dilantin® Kapseals), 100 mg
0365-	Phenytoin Sodium, Extended, Capsules, USP (Dilantin® Kapseals), 30 mg
0552-	℞ Prazepam (Centrax®) Capsules, 5 mg
0553-	℞ Prazepam (Centrax®) Capsules, 10 mg
0554-	℞ Prazepam (Centrax®) Capsules, 20 mg
0276-	℞ Prazepam (Centrax®) Tablets, 10 mg
0202-	Procainamide Hydrochloride Tablets, Sustained Release (Procan® SR), 250 mg
0204-	Procainamide Hydrochloride Tablets, Sustained Release (Procan® SR), 500 mg
0205-	Procainamide Hydrochloride Tablets, Sustained Release (Procan® SR), 750 mg
0692-	℞ Propoxyphene Hydrochloride Capsules, USP, 65 mg
0747-	Pyrvinium Pamoate Tablets, USP (Povan® Filmseal), 50 mg
0437-	Quinestrol Tablets (Estrovis® Tablets), 100 mcg

0850-	Quinidine Gluconate Tablets, Sustained Release, (Duraquin® Tablets), 330 mg
0849-	Quinidine Sulfate Tablets, USP, 200 mg
0420-	Quinine Sulfate Capsules, USP, 325 mg
0713-	Spironolactone Tablets, USP
0712-	Spironolactone with Hydrochlorothiazide Tablets
0407-	Tetracycline Hydrochloride Capsules, USP (Cyclopar®), 250 mg
0697-	Tetracycline Hydrochloride Capsules, USP (Cyclopar® 500), 500 mg
0251-	Thyroglobulin Tablets (Proloid®), ½ grain
0252-	Thyroglobulin Tablets (Proloid®), 1 grain
0253-	Thyroglobulin Tablets (Proloid®), 1½ grains
0257-	Thyroglobulin Tablets (Proloid®), 2 grains
0254-	Thyroglobulin Tablets (Proloid®), 3 grains

GERIPLEX-FS® KAPSEALS®
[jĕ'-rĭ-plĕx"]

Composition: Each capsule represents:
Vitamin A ....(1.5 mg) 5,000 IU*
  (acetate)
Vitamin C .... 50 mg
  (ascorbic acid)†
Vitamin B$_1$ .... 5 mg
  (thiamine mononitrate)
Vitamin B$_2$ .... 5 mg
  (riboflavin)
Vitamin B$_{12}$, crystalline
  (cyanocobalamin) .... 2 mcg
Choline dihydrogen
  citrate... 20 mg
Nicotinamide .... 15 mg
  (niacinamide)
Vitamin E (dl-alpha tocopheryl acetate, 5 mg) ....5 IU*
Iron‡.. 6 mg
Copper sulfate .... 4 mg
Manganese sulfate
  (monohydrate)... 4 mg
Zinc sulfate .... 2 mg
Calcium phosphate, dibasic
  (anhydrous)... 200 mg
Taka-Diastase® (aspergillus
  oryzae enzymes).. 2½ gr
Docusate sodium .... 100 mg

* International Units
†Supplied as sodium ascorbate
‡Supplied as dried ferrous sulfate

Action and Uses: A preparation containing vitamins, minerals, and a fecal softener for middle-aged and older individuals. The fecal softening agent, docusate sodium, acts to soften stools and make bowel movements easier.
Administration and Dosage: USUAL DOSAGE—One capsule daily, with or immediately after a meal.
How Supplied: N 0071-0544-24—Bottles of 100. Parcode® No. 544.
Shown in Product Identification Section, page 424

GERIPLEX-FS®
[jĕ'-rĭ-plĕx"]
LIQUID
Geriatric Vitamin Formula with Iron and a Fecal Softener

Composition: Each 30 ml represents vitamin B$_1$ (thiamine hydrochloride), 1.2 mg; vitamin B$_2$ (as riboflavin-5'-phosphate sodium), 1.7 mg; vitamin B$_6$ (pyridoxine hydrochloride), 1 mg; vitamin B$_{12}$ (cyanocobalamin) crystalline, 5 mcg; niacinamide, 15 mg; iron (as ferric ammonium citrate, green), 15 mg; Pluronic® F-68,* 200 mg; alcohol, 18%.
Administration and Dosage: USUAL ADULT DOSAGE—Two tablespoonfuls (30 ml) daily or as recommended by the physician.

How Supplied: N 0071-2454-23—16-oz bottles.

*Pluronic is a registered trademark of BASF Wyandotte Corporation for polymers of ethylene oxide and propylene oxide.

HUMATIN®
[hu'mah-tin]
(Paromomycin Sulfate, USP)

Description: Humatin is a broad spectrum antibiotic produced by *Streptomyces rimosus* var. *paromomycinus*. It is a white, amorphous, stable, water-soluble product supplied as capsules containing the equivalent of 250 mg paromomycin.
Action: The *in vitro* and *in vivo* antibacterial action of paromomycin closely parallels that of neomycin. It is poorly absorbed after oral administration, with almost 100% of the drug recoverable in the stool.
Indications: Humatin is indicated for intestinal amebiasis—acute and chronic (NOTE—It is not effective in extra-intestinal amebiasis); management of hepatic coma—as adjunctive therapy.
Contraindications: Paromomycin sulfate is contraindicated in individuals with a history of previous hypersensitivity reactions to it. It is also contraindicated in intestinal obstruction.
Precautions: The use of this antibiotic, as with other antibiotics, may result in an overgrowth of nonsusceptible organisms, including fungi. Constant observation of the patient is essential. If new infections caused by nonsusceptible organisms appear during therapy, appropriate measures should be taken.
The drug should be used with caution in individuals with ulcerative lesions of the bowel to avoid renal toxicity through inadvertent absorption.
Adverse Reactions: Nausea, abdominal cramps, and diarrhea have been reported in patients on doses over 3 g daily.
Dosage and Administration: *Intestinal amebiasis:* Adults and Children: Usual dose—25 to 35 mg/kg body weight daily, administered in three doses with meals, for five to ten days.
Management of hepatic coma: Adults: Usual dose—4 g daily in divided doses, given at regular intervals for five to six days.
How Supplied: N0071-0529-09 Humatin Capsules, each containing paromomycin sulfate equivalent to 250 mg paromomycin, are supplied in bottles of 16.
Shown in Product Identification Section, page 424
0529G030

HYDROCHLOROTHIAZIDE TABLETS,
[hy"drō-chlō"rō-thī'ă-zīde]
USP
(Thiuretic®)

Description: Hydrochlorothiazide is a member of the benzothiadiazine (thiazide) family of drugs, closely related to chlorothiazide. Its chemical name is 6-chloro-3,4-dihydro-2H-1,2, 4-benzothiadiazine-7-sulfonamide 1,1-dioxide.
Hydrochlorothiazide is a white, or practically white, crystalline compound which is slightly soluble in water and soluble in alcohol.
Clinically, hydrochlorothiazide is a diuretic-antihypertensive agent, available in 25 mg and 50 mg strength tablets for oral administration.
Clinical Pharmacology: The diuretic and saluretic effects of hydrochlorothiazide result from a drug-induced inhibition of the renal tubular reabsorption of electrolytes. The excretion of sodium and chloride is greatly enhanced. Potassium excretion is also enhanced to a variable degree, as it is with the other thiazides. Although urinary excretion of bicarbonate is increased slightly, there is usually no significant change in urinary pH. Hydrochlorothiazide has a per mg natriuretic activity approximately 10 times that of the prototype thiazide, chlorothiazide. At maximal therapeutic dosages, all thiazides are approximately equal in their diuretic/natriuretic effects.
There is significant natriuresis and diuresis within two hours after administration of a single oral dose of hydrochlorothiazide. These effects reach a peak in about six hours and persist for about 12 hours following oral administration of a single dose.
Like other benzothiadiazines, hydrochlorothiazide also has antihypertensive properties, and may be used for this purpose either alone or to enhance the antihypertensive action of other drugs. The mechanism by which the benzothiadiazines, including hydrochlorothiazide, produce a reduction of elevated blood pressure is not known. However, sodium depletion appears to be involved.
Hydrochlorothiazide is readily absorbed from the gastrointestinal tract and is excreted unchanged by the kidneys. Excretion of the drug is essentially complete within 24 hours.
Indications and Usage: Hydrochlorothiazide is indicated in the management of hypertension either as the sole therapeutic agent or to enhance the effectiveness of other antihypertensive drugs in the more severe forms of hypertension.
Hydrochlorothiazide is indicated as adjunctive therapy in edema associated with congestive heart failure, hepatic cirrhosis, and corticosteroid and estrogen therapy.
Hydrochlorothiazide has also been found useful in edema due to various forms of renal dysfunction such as the nephrotic syndrome, acute glomerulonephritis, and chronic renal failure.
Usage in Pregnancy: The routine use of diuretics in an otherwise healthy pregnant woman is inappropriate and exposes mother and fetus to unnecessary hazard. Diuretics do not prevent development of toxemia of pregnancy, and there is no satisfactory evidence that they are useful in the treatment of developed toxemia.
Edema during pregnancy may arise from pathological causes or from the physiological and mechanical consequences of pregnancy. Thiazides are indicated in pregnancy when edema is due to pathological causes, just as they are in the absence of pregnancy (however, see PRECAUTIONS below). Dependent edema in pregnancy, resulting from restriction of venous return by the expanded uterus, is properly treated through elevation of the lower extremities and use of support hose; use of diuretics to lower intravascular volume in this case is illogical and unnecessary. There is hypervolemia during normal pregnancy which is harmful to neither the fetus nor the mother (in the absence of cardiovascular disease), but which is associated with edema, including generalized edema, in the majority of pregnant women. If this edema produces discomfort, increased recumbency will often provide relief. In rare instances, this edema may cause extreme discomfort which is not relieved by rest. In these cases, a short course of diuretics may provide relief and may be appropriate.
Contraindications: Anuria.
Hypersensitivity to this or other sulfonamide-derived drugs.
Warnings: Thiazides should be used with caution in patients with renal disease or significant impairment of renal function. In patients with renal disease, thiazides may precipitate azotemia. Cumulative effects of the drug may develop in patients with impaired renal function.
Thiazides should be used with caution in patients with impaired hepatic function or progressive liver disease, since minor alterations of fluid and electrolyte balance may precipitate hepatic coma. Thiazides may add to or potentiate the action of other antihypertensive drugs. Potentiation occurs with ganglionic or peripheral adrenergic blocking drugs.
Sensitivity reactions may occur in patients with a history of allergy or bronchial asthma.
The possibility of exacerbation or activation of systemic lupus erythematosus has been reported.

Continued on next page

This product information was prepared in August, 1984. On these and other Parke-Davis Products, information may be obtained by addressing PARKE-DAVIS, Division of Warner-Lambert Company, Morris Plains, New Jersey 07950.

Parke-Davis—Cont.

Precautions: Periodic determinations of serum electrolytes should be performed at appropriate intervals for the purpose of detecting possible electrolyte imbalances. All patients receiving thiazide therapy should be observed for clinical signs of fluid or electrolyte imbalance, namely, hyponatremia, hypochloremic alkalosis, and hypokalemia. Serum and urine electrolyte determinations are particularly important when a patient is vomiting excessively or receiving parenteral fluids. Warning signs of electrolyte imbalance include dryness of mouth, thirst, weakness, lethargy, drowsiness, restlessness, muscle pains or cramps, muscular fatigue, hypotension, oliguria, tachycardia, and gastrointestinal disturbances such as nausea and vomiting.

Hypokalemia may develop with thiazides as with any other potent diuretic, especially when brisk diuresis occurs, severe cirrhosis is present, or when corticosteroids or ACTH are given concomitantly. Interference with the adequate oral intake of electrolytes will also contribute to the possible development of hypokalemia. Potassium depletion, even of a mild degree, resulting from thiazide use may sensitize a patient to the effects of cardiac glycosides such as digitalis.

Any chloride deficit is generally mild and usually does not require specific treatment except under extraordinary circumstances (as in liver disease or renal disease). Dilutional hyponatremia may occur in edematous patients in hot weather; appropriate therapy is water restriction rather than administration of salt except in rare instances where the hyponatremia is life threatening.

In actual salt depletion, appropriate replacement is the therapy of choice.

Hyperuricemia may occur or frank gout may be precipitated in certain patients receiving thiazide therapy.

Insulin requirements in diabetic patients may be increased, decreased or unchanged. Latent diabetes mellitus may become manifest during thiazide administration.

Thiazide drugs may increase the responsiveness to tubocurarine.

The antihypertensive effects of the drug may be enhanced in the postsympathectomy patient.

Thiazides may decrease arterial responsiveness to norepinephrine. This diminution is not sufficient to preclude effectiveness of the pressor agent for therapeutic use.

If progressive renal impairment becomes evident as indicated by a rising nonprotein nitrogen or blood urea nitrogen, a careful reappraisal of therapy is necessary with consideration given to withholding or discontinuing diuretic therapy.

Thiazides may decrease serum PBI levels without signs of thyroid disturbance.

Thiazides have been reported, on rare occasions, to have elevated serum calcium to hypercalcemic levels. The serum calcium levels have returned to normal when the medication has been stopped. This phenomenon may be related to the ability of the thiazide diuretics to lower the amount of calcium excreted in the urine.

Usage in Pregnancy: Thiazides cross the placental barrier and appear in cord blood. The use of thiazides in pregnant women requires that the anticipated benefit be weighed against possible hazards to the fetus. These hazards include fetal or neonatal jaundice, thrombocytopenia, and possible other adverse reactions that have occurred in the adults. (Also see INDICATIONS AND USAGE, above.)

Nursing Mothers: Thiazides appear in breast milk. If use of the drug is deemed essential, the patient should stop nursing.

Adverse Reactions:
A. *Gastrointestinal System*
 1. anorexia
 2. gastric irritation
 3. nausea
 4. vomiting
 5. cramping
 6. diarrhea
 7. constipation
 8. jaundice (intrahepatic cholestatic jaundice)
 9. pancreatitis
B. *Central Nervous System*
 1. dizziness
 2. vertigo
 3. paresthesias
 4. headache
 5. xanthopsia
C. *Hematologic*
 1. leukopenia
 2. agranulocytosis
 3. thrombocytopenia
 4. aplastic anemia
D. *Dermatologic-Hypersensitivity*
 1. purpura
 2. photosensitivity
 3. rash
 4. urticaria
 5. necrotizing angiitis
  (vasculitis)
  (cutaneous vasculitis)
E. *Cardiovascular*
 Orthostatic hypotension may occur and may be aggravated by alcohol, barbiturates, or narcotics.
F. *Other*
 1. hyperglycemia
 2. glycosuria
 3. hypercalcemia
 4. hyperuricemia
 5. muscle spasm
 6. weakness
 7. restlessness
 8. severe fluid and electrolyte derangements (rarely)
Whenever adverse reactions are moderate or severe, thiazide dosage should be reduced or therapy withdrawn.

Overdosage: Symptoms of overdosage include electrolyte imbalance and signs of potassium deficiency such as confusion, dizziness, muscular weakness and gastrointestinal disturbances. General supportive measures including replacement of fluids and electrolytes may be indicated in treatment of overdosage.

Dosage and Administration: Hydrochlorothiazide is administered orally. Therapy should be individualized according to the patient's requirements and response. The response of the patient depends on factors such as the nature and degree of the disease, state of hydration, cardiac output, physical activity, diet, and concurrent administration of other drugs. Therapy should be titrated to attain the maximum therapeutic effect at minimum dosage.

Adult Dose: For the management of edema, the usual initial adult dosage is 25 to 200 mg daily given in 1 to 3 doses. When nonedematous weight is attained, a maintenance dosage of 25 to 100 mg daily or intermittently may be instituted. Occasionally, up to 200 mg daily is required in refractory patients.

For the management of hypertension, the usual initial adult dosage is 50 to 100 mg daily, given in 2 divided doses. The dosage may be increased if necessary to a maximum of 200 mg daily, given in 2 divided doses. Maintenance dosage is determined by the patient's blood pressure and usually ranges from 25 to 100 mg daily in a single dose.

When therapy is prolonged or large doses are used, particular attention should be given to the patient's electrolyte status. Supplemental potassium may be required.

In the treatment of hypertension, hydrochlorothiazide may be employed either alone or concurrently with other antihypertensive drugs. Combined therapy may provide adequate control of hypertension with lower dosage of the component drugs and fewer or less severe side effects.

For treatment of moderate to severe hypertension, supplemental use of other more potent antihypertensive agents may be indicated.

When other antihypertensive agents are to be added to the regimen, this should be accomplished gradually. Additional potent antihypertensive agents should be given at only half the usual dose since their effect is potentiated by pretreatment with hydrochlorothiazide.

Pediatric Dose: The usual pediatric dosage is 1 mg hydrochlorothiazide per pound of body weight per day, given in 2 divided doses. Infants younger than 6 months of age may require up to 1.5 mg per pound per day in 2 divided doses.

How Supplied: Hydrochlorothiazide Tablets, USP, 25 mg (white, round, scored, coded P-D 702) are available in bottles of 100 (N 0071-0702-24). Hydrochlorothiazide Tablets, USP, 50 mg (white, round, scored, coded P-D 710) are available in bottles of 100 (N 0071-0710-24), bottles of 1000 (N 0071-0710-32), and unit dose packages of 100 (N 0071-0710-40).

0702G011

KETALAR® ℞
[ke' tă-lär"]
(Ketamine Hydrochloride Injection, USP)

SPECIAL NOTE

EMERGENCE REACTIONS HAVE OCCURRED IN APPROXIMATELY 12 PERCENT OF PATIENTS.

THE PSYCHOLOGICAL MANIFESTATIONS VARY IN SEVERITY BETWEEN PLEASANT DREAM-LIKE STATES, VIVID IMAGERY, HALLUCINATIONS, AND EMERGENCE DELIRIUM. IN SOME CASES THESE STATES HAVE BEEN ACCOMPANIED BY CONFUSION, EXCITEMENT, AND IRRATIONAL BEHAVIOR WHICH A FEW PATIENTS RECALL AS AN UNPLEASANT EXPERIENCE. THE DURATION ORDINARILY IS NO MORE THAN A FEW HOURS; IN A FEW CASES, HOWEVER, RECURRENCES HAVE TAKEN PLACE UP TO 24 HOURS POSTOPERATIVELY. NO RESIDUAL PSYCHOLOGICAL EFFECTS ARE KNOWN TO HAVE RESULTED FROM USE OF KETALAR.

THE INCIDENCE OF THESE EMERGENCE PHENOMENA IS LEAST IN THE YOUNG (15 YEARS OF AGE OR LESS) AND ELDERLY (OVER 65 YEARS OF AGE) PATIENT. ALSO, THEY ARE LESS FREQUENT WHEN THE DRUG IS GIVEN INTRAMUSCULARLY AND THE INCIDENCE IS REDUCED AS EXPERIENCE WITH THE DRUG IS GAINED.

THE INCIDENCE OF PSYCHOLOGICAL MANIFESTATIONS DURING EMERGENCE, PARTICULARLY DREAM-LIKE OBSERVATIONS AND EMERGENCE DELIRIUM, MAY BE REDUCED BY USING LOWER RECOMMENDED DOSAGES OF KETALAR IN CONJUNCTION WITH INTRAVENOUS DIAZEPAM DURING INDUCTION AND MAINTENANCE OF ANESTHESIA. (See Dosage and Administration.) ALSO, THESE REACTIONS MAY BE REDUCED IF VERBAL, TACTILE AND VISUAL STIMULATION OF THE PATIENT IS MINIMIZED DURING THE RECOVERY PERIOD. THIS DOES NOT PRECLUDE THE MONITORING OF VITAL SIGNS. IN ORDER TO TERMINATE A SEVERE EMERGENCE REACTION THE USE OF A SMALL HYPNOTIC DOSE OF A SHORT-ACTING OR ULTRASHORT-ACTING BARBITURATE MAY BE REQUIRED.

WHEN KETALAR IS USED ON AN OUTPATIENT BASIS, THE PATIENT SHOULD NOT BE RELEASED UNTIL RECOVERY FROM ANESTHESIA IS COMPLETE AND THEN SHOULD BE ACCOMPANIED BY A RESPONSIBLE ADULT.

Description: Ketalar is a nonbarbiturate anesthetic, chemically designated *dl* 2-(o-chlorophenyl)-2-(methylamino) cyclohexanone hy- drochloride. It is formulated as a slightly acid (pH 3.5-5.5) sterile solution for intravenous or intramuscular injection in concentrations containing the equivalent of either 10, 50 or 100 mg ketamine base per milliliter and contains not more than 0.1 mg/ml Phemerol® (benzethonium chloride) added as a preservative. The 10 mg/ml solution has been made isotonic with sodium chloride.

Clinical Pharmacology: Ketalar is a rapid-acting general anesthetic producing an anesthetic state characterized by profound analgesia, normal pharyngeal-laryngeal reflexes, normal or slightly enhanced skeletal muscle tone, cardiovascular and respiratory stimulation, and occasionally a transient and minimal respiratory depression.

A patent airway is maintained partly by virtue of unimpaired pharyngeal and laryngeal reflexes. (See Warnings and Precautions.)

The biotransformation of Ketalar includes N-dealkylation (metabolite I), hydroxylation of the cyclohexone ring (metabolites III and IV), conjugation with glucuronic acid and dehydration of the hydroxylated metabolites to form the cyclohexene derivative (metabolite II).

Following intravenous administration, the ketamine concentration has an initial slope (alpha phase) lasting about 45 minutes with a half-life of 10 to 15 minutes. This first phase corresponds clinically to the anesthetic effect of the drug. The anesthetic action is terminated by a combination of redistribution from the CNS to slower equilibrating peripheral tissues and by hepatic biotransformation to metabolite I. This metabolite is about $1/3$ as active as ketamine in reducing halothane requirements (MAC) of the rat. The later half-life of ketamine (beta phase) is 2.5 hours.

The anesthetic state produced by Ketalar has been termed "dissociative anesthesia" in that it appears to selectively interrupt association pathways of the brain before producing somesthetic sensory blockade. It may selectively depress the thalamoneocortical system before significantly obtunding the more ancient cerebral centers and pathways (reticular-activating and limbic systems).

Elevation of blood pressure begins shortly after injection, reaches a maximum within a few minutes and usually returns to preanesthetic values within 15 minutes after injection. In the majority of cases, the systolic and diastolic blood pressure peaks from 10% to 50% above preanesthetic levels shortly after induction of anesthesia, but the elevation can be higher or longer in individual cases (see Contraindications.)

Ketamine has a wide margin of safety; several instances of unintentional administration of overdoses of Ketalar (up to ten times that usually required) have been followed by prolonged but complete recovery.

Ketalar has been studied in over 12,000 operative and diagnostic procedures, involving over 10,000 patients from 105 separate studies. During the course of these studies Ketalar was administered as the sole agent, as induction for other general agents, or to supplement low-potency agents. Specific areas of application have included the following:

1. debridement, painful dressings, and skin grafting in burn patients, as well as other superficial surgical procedures.
2. neurodiagnostic procedures such as pneumoencephalograms, ventriculograms, myelograms, and lumbar punctures. See also Precaution concerning increased intracranial pressure.
3. diagnostic and operative procedures of the eye, ear, nose, and mouth, including dental extractions.
4. diagnostic and operative procedures of the pharynx, larynx, or bronchial tree. NOTE: Muscle relaxants, with proper attention to respiration, may be required (see Precautions).
5. sigmoidoscopy and minor surgery of the anus and rectum, and circumcision.
6. extraperitoneal procedures used in gynecology such as dilatation and curettage.
7. orthopedic procedures such as closed reductions, manipulations, femoral pinning, amputations, and biopsies.
8. as an anesthetic in poor-risk patients with depression of vital functions.
9. in procedures where the intramuscular route of administration is preferred.
10. in cardiac catheterization procedures.

In these studies, the anesthesia was rated either "excellent" or "good" by the anesthesiologist and the surgeon at 90% and 93%, respectively; rated "fair" at 6% and 4%, respectively; and rated "poor" at 4% and 3%, respectively. In a second method of evaluation, the anesthesia was rated "adequate" in at least 90%, and "inadequate" in 10% or less of the procedures.

Indications and Usage: Ketalar is indicated as the sole anesthetic agent for diagnostic and surgical procedures that do not require skeletal muscle relaxation. Ketalar is best suited for short procedures but it can be used, with additional doses, for longer procedures.

Ketalar is indicated for the induction of anesthesia prior to the administration of other general anesthetic agents.

Ketalar is indicated to supplement low-potency agents, such as nitrous oxide.

Specific areas of application are described in the Clinical Pharmacology section.

Contraindications: Ketamine hydrochloride is contraindicated in those in whom a significant elevation of blood pressure would constitute a serious hazard and in those who have shown hypersensitivity to the drug.

Warnings: Cardiac function should be continually monitored during the procedure in patients found to have hypertension or cardiac decompensation.

Postoperative confusional states may occur during the recovery period. (See Special Note.)

Respiratory depression may occur with overdosage or too rapid a rate of administration of Ketalar, in which case supportive ventilation should be employed. Mechanical support of respiration is preferred to administration of analeptics.

Precautions:
General
Ketalar should be used by or under the direction of physicians experienced in administering general anesthetics and in maintenance of an airway and in the control of respiration.

Because pharyngeal and laryngeal reflexes are usually active, Ketalar should not be used alone in surgery or diagnostic procedures of the pharynx, larynx, or bronchial tree. Mechanical stimulation of the pharynx should be avoided, whenever possible, if Ketalar is used alone. Muscle relaxants, with proper attention to respiration, may be required in both of these instances.

Resuscitative equipment should be ready for use.

The incidence of emergence reactions may be reduced if verbal and tactile stimulation of the patient is minimized during the recovery period. This does not preclude the monitoring of vital signs (see Special Note).

The intravenous dose should be administered over a period of 60 seconds. More rapid administration may result in respiratory depression or apnea and enhanced pressor response.

In surgical procedures involving visceral pain pathways, Ketalar should be supplemented with an agent which obtunds visceral pain.

Use with caution in the chronic alcoholic and the acutely alcohol-intoxicated patient.

An increase in cerebrospinal fluid pressure has been reported following administration of ketamine hydrochloride. Use with extreme caution in patients with preanesthetic elevated cerebrospinal fluid pressure.

Information for Patients
As appropriate, especially in cases where early discharge is possible, the duration of Ketalar and other drugs employed during the conduct of anesthesia should be considered. The patients should be cautioned that driving an automobile, operating hazardous machinery or engaging in hazardous activities should not be undertaken for 24 hours or more (depending upon the dosage of Ketalar and consideration of other drugs employed) after anesthesia.

Drug Interactions
Prolonged recovery time may occur if barbiturates and/or narcotics are used concurrently with Ketalar.

Ketalar is clinically compatible with the commonly used general and local anesthetic agents when an adequate respiratory exchange is maintained.

Usage in Pregnancy
Since the safe use in pregnancy, including obstetrics (either vaginal or abdominal delivery), has not been established, such use is not recommended (see Animal Reproduction).

Adverse Reactions:
Cardiovascular: Blood pressure and pulse rate are frequently elevated following administration of Ketalar alone. However, hypotension and bradycardia have been observed. Arrhythmia has also occurred.

Respiration: Although respiration is frequently stimulated, severe depression of respiration or apnea may occur following rapid intravenous administration of high doses of Ketalar. Laryngospasms and other forms of airway obstruction have occurred during Ketalar anesthesia.

Eye: Diplopia and nystagmus have been noted following Ketalar administration.

It also may cause a slight elevation in intraocular pressure measurement.

Psychological: (See Special Note).

Neurological: In some patients, enhanced skeletal muscle tone may be manifested by tonic and clonic movements sometimes resembling seizures (see Dosage and Administration).

Gastrointestinal: Anorexia, nausea and vomiting have been observed; however this is not usually severe and allows the great majority of patients to take liquids by mouth shortly after regaining consciousness (see Dosage and Administration).

General: Local pain and exanthema at the injection site have infrequently been reported. Transient erythema and/or morbilliform rash have also been reported.

Overdosage: Respiratory depression may occur with overdosage or too rapid a rate of administration of Ketalar, in which case supportive ventilation should be employed. Mechanical support of respiration is preferred to administration of analeptics.

Dosage and Administration:
Note: Barbiturates and Ketalar, being chemically incompatible because of precipitate formation, *should not* be injected from the same syringe. If the Ketalar dose is augmented with diazepam, the two drugs must be given separately. Do not mix Ketalar and diazepam in syringe or infusion flask. For additional information on the use of diazepam, refer to the Warnings and Dosage and Administration Sections of the diazepam insert.

Preoperative Preparations:
1. While vomiting has been reported following Ketalar administration, some airway protection may be afforded because of active laryngeal-pharyngeal reflexes. However, since aspiration may occur with Ketalar and since protective reflexes may also be diminished by supplementary anesthetics and muscle relaxants, the possibility of aspiration must be considered. Ketalar is recommended for use in the patient whose stomach is not empty when, in the judgment of the practitioner, the benefits of the drug outweigh the possible risks.

2. Atropine, scopolamine, or another drying agent should be given at an appropriate interval prior to induction.

Onset and Duration:
Because of rapid induction following the initial intravenous injection, the patient should be in a supported position during administration.

The onset of action of Ketalar is rapid; an intravenous dose of 2 mg/kg (1 mg/lb) of body weight usually produces surgical anesthesia within 30 seconds after injection, with the anesthetic effect usually lasting five to ten minutes. If a longer effect is desired, additional increments can be administered intravenously or intramuscularly to maintain anesthesia without producing significant cumulative effects.

Continued on next page

This product information was prepared in August, 1984. On these and other Parke-Davis Products, information may be obtained by addressing PARKE-DAVIS, Division of Warner-Lambert Company, Morris Plains, New Jersey 07950.

Parke-Davis—Cont.

Intramuscular doses, from experience primarily in children, in a range of 9 to 13 mg/kg (4 to 6 mg/lb) usually produce surgical anesthesia within 3 to 4 minutes following injection, with the anesthetic effect usually lasting 12 to 25 minutes.

Dosage:

As with other general anesthetic agents, the individual response to Ketalar is somewhat varied depending on the dose, route of administration, and age of patient, so that dosage recommendation cannot be absolutely fixed. The drug should be titrated against the patient's requirements.

Induction:

Intravenous Route: The initial dose of Ketalar administered intravenously may range from 1 mg/kg to 4.5 mg/kg (0.5 to 2 mg/lb). The average amount required to produce five to ten minutes of surgical anesthesia has been 2 mg/kg (1 mg/lb). Alternatively, in adult patients an induction dose of 1.0 mg to 2.0 mg/kg intravenous ketamine at a rate of 0.5 mg/kg/min may be used for induction of anesthesia. In addition, diazepam in 2 mg to 5 mg doses, administered in a separate syringe over 60 seconds, may be used. In most cases, 15.0 mg of intravenous diazepam *or less* will suffice. The incidence of psychological manifestations during emergence, particularly dream-like observations and emergence delirium, may be reduced by this induction dosage program.

Note: The 100 mg/ml concentration of Ketalar *should not* be injected intravenously without proper dilution. It is recommended the drug be diluted with an equal volume of either Sterile Water for Injection, USP, Normal Saline, or 5% Dextrose in Water.

Rate of Administration: It is recommended that Ketalar be administered slowly (over a period of 60 seconds). More rapid administration may result in respiratory depression and enhanced pressor response.

Intramuscular Route: The initial dose of Ketalar administered intramuscularly may range from 6.5 to 13 mg/kg (3 to 6 mg/lb). A dose of 10 mg/kg (5 mg/lb) will usually produce 12 to 25 minutes of surgical anesthesia.

Maintenance of Anesthesia:

The maintenance dose should be adjusted according to the patient's anesthetic needs and whether an additional anesthetic agent is employed.

Increments of one-half to the full induction dose may be repeated as needed for maintenance of anesthesia. However, it should be noted that purposeless and tonic-clonic movements of extremities may occur during the course of anesthesia. These movements do not imply a light plane and are not indicative of the need for additional doses of the anesthetic.

It should be recognized that the larger the total dose of Ketalar administered, the longer will be the time to complete recovery.

Adult patients induced with Ketalar augmented with intravenous diazepam may be maintained on Ketalar given by slow microdrip infusion technique at a dose of 0.1 to 0.5 mg/minute, augmented with diazepam 2 to 5 mg administered intravenously as needed. In many cases 20 mg *or less* of intravenous diazepam total for combined induction and maintenance will suffice. However, slightly more diazepam may be required depending on the nature and duration of the operation, physical status of the patient, and other factors. The incidence of psychological manifestations during emergence, particularly dream-like observations and emergence delirium, may be reduced by this maintenance dosage program.

Dilution: To prepare a dilute solution containing 1 mg of ketamine per ml, aseptically transfer 10 ml (50 mg per ml Steri-Vial) or 5 ml (100 mg per ml Steri-Vial) to 500 ml of 5% Dextrose Injection, USP or Sodium Chloride (0.9%) Injection, USP (Normal Saline) and mix well. The resultant solution will contain 1 mg of ketamine per ml.

The fluid requirements of the patient and duration of anesthesia must be considered when selecting the appropriate dilution of Ketalar. If fluid restriction is required, Ketalar can be added to a 250 ml infusion as described above to provide a Ketalar concentration of 2 mg/ml.

Ketalar Steri-Vials, 10 mg/ml are not recommended for dilution.

Supplementary Agents:

Ketalar is clinically compatible with the commonly used general and local anesthetic agents when an adequate respiratory exchange is maintained.

The regimen of a reduced dose of Ketalar supplemented with diazepam can be used to produce balanced anesthesia by combination with other agents such as nitrous oxide and oxygen.

How Supplied:
Ketalar is supplied as the hydrochloride in concentrations equivalent to ketamine base.

N 0071-4581-15—Each 50-ml vial contains 10 mg/ml. Supplied in cartons of 10.
N 0071-4581-13—Each 25-ml vial contains 10 mg/ml. Supplied in cartons of 10.
N 0071-4581-12—Each 20-ml vial contains 10 mg/ml. Supplied in cartons of 10.
N 0071-4582-10—Each 10-ml vial contains 50 mg/ml. Supplied in cartons of 10.
N 0071-4585-08—Each 5-ml vial contains 100 mg/ml. Supplied in cartons of 10.

Animal Pharmacology and Toxicology:

Toxicity: The acute toxicity of Ketalar has been studied in several species. In mature mice and rats, the intraperitoneal LD_{50} values are approximately 100 times the average human intravenous dose and approximately 20 times the average human intramuscular dose. A slightly higher acute toxicity observed in neonatal rats was not sufficiently elevated to suggest an increased hazard when used in children. Daily intravenous injections in rats of five times the average human intravenous dose and intramuscular injections in dogs at four times the average human intramuscular dose demonstrated excellent tolerance for as long as 6 weeks. Similarly, twice weekly anesthetic sessions of one, three, or six hours' duration in monkeys over a four-to six-week period were well tolerated.

Interaction With Other Drugs Commonly Used For Preanesthetic Medication: Large doses (three or more times the equivalent effective human dose) of morphine, meperidine, and atropine increased the depth and prolonged the duration of anesthesia produced by a standard anesthetizing dose of Ketalar in Rhesus monkeys. The prolonged duration was not of sufficient magnitude to contraindicate the use of these drugs for preanesthetic medication in human clinical trials.

Blood Pressure: Blood pressure responses to Ketalar vary with the laboratory species and experimental conditions. Blood pressure is increased in normotensive and renal hypertensive rats with and without adrenalectomy and under pentobarbital anesthesia.

Intravenous Ketalar produces a fall in arterial blood pressure in the Rhesus monkey and a rise in arterial blood pressure in the dog. In this respect the dog mimics the cardiovascular effect observed in man. The pressor response to Ketalar injected into intact, unanesthetized dogs is accompanied by a tachycardia, rise in cardiac output and a fall in total peripheral resistance. It causes a fall in perfusion pressure following a large dose injected into an artificially perfused vascular bed (dog hindquarters), and it has little or no potentiating effect upon vasoconstriction responses of epinephrine or norepinephrine. The pressor response to Ketalar is reduced or blocked by chlorpromazine (central depressant and peripheral α-adrenergic blockade), by β-adrenergic blockade, and by ganglionic blockade. The tachycardia and increase in myocardial contractile force seen in intact animals does not appear in isolated hearts (Langendorff) at a concentration of 0.1 mg of Ketalar nor in Starling dog heart-lung preparations at a Ketalar concentration of 50 mg/kg of HLP. These observations support the hypothesis that the hypertension produced by Ketalar is due to selective activation of central cardiac stimulating mechanisms leading to an increase in cardiac output. The dog myocardium is not sensitized to epinephrine and Ketalar appears to have a weak antiarrhythmic activity.

Metabolic Disposition: Ketalar is rapidly absorbed following parenteral administration. Animal experiments indicated that Ketalar was rapidly distributed into body tissues, with relatively high concentrations appearing in body fat, liver, lung, and brain; lower concentrations were found in the heart, skeletal muscle, and blood plasma. Placental transfer of the drug was found to occur in pregnant dogs and monkeys. No significant degree of binding to serum albumin was found with Ketalar.

Balance studies in rats, dogs, and monkeys resulted in the recovery of 85% to 95% of the dose in the urine, mainly in the form of degradation products. Small amounts of drug were also excreted in the bile and feces. Balance studies with tritium-labeled Ketalar in human subjects (1 mg/lb given intravenously) resulted in the mean recovery of 91% of the dose in the urine and 3% in the feces. Peak plasma levels averaged about 0.75 $\mu g/ml$, and CSF levels were about 0.2 $\mu g/ml$, 1 hour after dosing.

Ketalar undergoes N-demethylation and hydroxylation of the cyclohexanone ring, with the formation of water-soluble conjugates which are excreted in the urine. Further oxidation also occurs with the formation of a cyclohexanone derivative. The unconjugated N-demethylated metabolite was found to be less than one-sixth as potent as Ketalar. The unconjugated demethyl cyclohexanone derivative was found to be less than one-tenth as potent as Ketalar. Repeated doses of Ketalar administered to animals did not produce any detectable increase in microsomal enzyme activity.

Reproduction: Male and female rats, when given five times the average human intravenous dose of Ketalar for three consecutive days about one week before mating, had a reproductive performance equivalent to that of saline-injected controls. When given to pregnant rats and rabbits intramuscularly at twice the average human intramuscular dose during the respective periods of organogenesis, the litter characteristics were equivalent to those of saline-injected controls. A small group of rabbits was given a single large dose (six times the average human dose) of Ketalar on Day 6 of pregnancy to simulate the effect of an excessive clinical dose around the period of nidation. The outcome of pregnancy was equivalent in control and treated groups.

To determine the effect of Ketalar on the perinatal and postnatal period, pregnant rats were given twice the average human intramuscular dose during Days 18 to 21 of pregnancy. Litter characteristics at birth and through the weaning period were equivalent to those of the control animals. There was a slight increase in incidence of delayed parturition by one day in treated dams of this group. Three groups each of mated beagle bitches were given 2.5 times the average human intramuscular dose twice weekly for the three weeks of the first, second, and third trimesters of pregnancy, respectively, without the development of adverse effects in the pups.

4581G030

LOESTRIN® 21 1/20 ℞
[lō"ĕs'trĭn]
(Each white tablet contains 1 mg norethindrone acetate and 20 mcg ethinyl estradiol.)

LOESTRIN® 21 1.5/30 ℞
(Each green tablet contains 1.5 mg norethindrone acetate and 30 mcg ethinyl estradiol.)

LOESTRIN® Fe 1/20 ℞
(Each white tablet contains 1 mg norethindrone acetate and 20 mcg ethinyl estradiol. Each brown tablet contains 75 mg ferrous fumarate, USP.)

LOESTRIN® Fe 1.5/30 ℞
(Each green tablet contains 1.5 mg norethindrone acetate and 30 mcg ethinyl estradiol. Each brown tablet contains 75 mg ferrous fumarate, USP)

Each white tablet contains: norethindrone acetate (17 alpha-ethinyl-19-nortestosterone acetate), 1 mg; ethinyl estradiol (17 alpha-ethinyl-1,3,5(10)-estratriene-3,17 beta-diol), 20 mcg.

Each green tablet contains: norethindrone acetate (17 alpha-ethinyl-19-nortestosterone acetate). 1.5 mg; ethinyl estradiol (17 alpha-ethinyl-1,3,5(10)-estratriene-3, 17 beta-diol), 30 mcg.

Each brown tablet contains 75 mg ferrous fumarate, USP.

Description: Loestrin is a progestogen-estrogen combination.

Loestrin Fe 1/20 and 1.5/30 provides a continuous dosage regimen consisting of 21 oral contraceptive tablets and seven ferrous fumarate tablets. The ferrous fumarate tablets are present to facilitate ease of drug administration via a 28-day regimen and are not intended to serve any therapeutic purpose.

Clinical Pharmacology: Combination oral contraceptives act primarily through the mechanism of gonadotropin suppression due to the estrogenic and progestational activity of the ingredients. Although the primary mechanism of action is inhibition of ovulation, alterations in the genital tract, including changes in the cervical mucus (which increase the difficulty of sperm penetration) and the endometrium (which reduce the likelihood of implantation) may also contribute to contraceptive effectiveness.

Indications and Usage: Loestrin is indicated for the prevention of pregnancy in women who elect to use oral contraceptives as a method of contraception.

Oral contraceptives are highly effective. The pregnancy rate in women using conventional combination oral contraceptives (containing 35 mcg or more of ethinyl estradiol or 50 mcg or more of mestranol) is generally reported as less than one pregnancy per 100 women-years of use. Slightly higher rates (somewhat more than one pregnancy per 100 woman-years of use) are reported for some combination products containing 35 mcg or less of ethinyl estradiol, and rates on the order of three pregnancies per 100 woman-years are reported for the progestogen-only oral contraceptives.

These rates are derived from separate studies conducted by different investigators in several population groups and cannot be compared precisely. Furthermore, pregnancy rates tend to be lower as clinical studies are continued, possibly due to selective retention in the longer studies of those patients who accept the treatment regimen and do not discontinue as a result of adverse reactions, pregnancy, or other reasons.

In clinical trials with Loestrin 1/20, 1,431 patients completed 15,899 cycles and a total of 10 pregnancies were reported. This represents a pregnancy rate of 0.75 per 100 woman-years based upon data that include the cases where patients failed to comply with the dosage regimen. The pregnancy rate in patients who adhered to the dosage regimen was 0.30 per 100 woman-years (four pregnancies in these trials).

In clinical trials with Loestrin 1.5/30, 1,289 patients completed 17,139 cycles and a total of 7 pregnancies were reported. This represents a pregnancy rate of 0.49 per 100 woman-years based upon data that include the cases where patients failed to comply with the dosage regimen. The pregnancy rate in patients who adhered to the dosage regimen was 0.07 per 100 woman-years (one pregnancy in these trials).

Table 1 gives ranges of pregnancy rates reported in the literature[1] for other means of contraception. The efficacy of these means of contraception (except the IUD) depends upon the degree of adherence to the method.

Table 1 Pregnancies per 100 Woman-Years
IUD, less than 1–6; Diaphragm with spermicidal products (creams or jellies), 2–20; Condom, 3–36; Aerosol foams, 2–29; Jellies and creams, 4–36; Periodic abstinence (rhythm) all types less than 1–47; 1. Calendar method, 14–47; 2. Temperature method, 1–20; 3. Temperature method—intercourse only in post-ovulatory phase, less than 1–7; 4. Mucus method, 1–25; No contraception, 60–80.

Dose-Related Risk of Thromboembolism from Oral Contraceptives
Two studies have shown a positive association between the dose of estrogens in oral contraceptives and the risk of thromboembolism.[2,3] For this reason, it is prudent and in keeping with good principles of therapeutics to minimize exposure to estrogen. The oral contraceptive product prescribed for any given patient should be that product which contains the least amount of estrogen that is compatible with an acceptable pregnancy rate and patient acceptance. It is recommended that new acceptors of oral contraceptives be started on preparations containing 0.05 mg or less of estrogen.

Contraindications: Oral contraceptives should not be used in women with any of the following conditions.
1. Thrombophlebitis or thromboembolic disorders
2. A past history of deep vein thrombophlebitis or thromboembolic disorders.
3. Cerebral vascular or coronary artery disease
4. Known or suspected carcinoma of the breast
5. Known or suspected estrogen-dependent neoplasia
6. Undiagnosed abnormal genital bleeding
7. Known or suspected pregnancy (see Warning No. 5)
8. Benign or malignant liver tumor which developed during the use of oral contraceptives or other estrogen-containing products.

Warnings:

Cigarette smoking increases the risk of serious cardiovascular side effects from oral contraceptive use. This risk increases with age and with heavy smoking (15 or more cigarettes per day) and is quite marked in women over 35 years of age. Women who use oral contraceptives should be strongly advised not to smoke.

The use of oral contraceptives is associated with increased risk of several serious conditions including thromboembolism, stroke, myocardial infarction, hepatic adenoma, gallbladder disease, and hypertension. Practitioners prescribing oral contraceptives should be familiar with the following information relating to these risks.

1. *Thromboembolic Disorders and Other Vascular Problems.* An increased risk of thromboembolic and thrombotic disease associated with the use of oral contraceptives is well established. Three principal studies in Great Britain[4–6] and three in the United States[7–10] have demonstrated an increased risk of fatal and nonfatal venous thromboembolism and stroke, both hemorrhagic and thrombotic. These studies estimate that users of oral contraceptives are 4 to 11 times more likely than nonusers to develop these diseases without evident cause (Table 2).

Cerebrovascular Disorders
In a collaborative American study[9,10] of cerebrovascular disorders in women with and without predisposing causes, it was estimated that the risk of hemorrhagic stroke was 2.0 times greater in users than nonusers and the risk of thrombotic stroke was 4 to 9.5 times greater in users than in nonusers (Table 2).

Table 2
Summary of relative risk of thromboembolic disorders and other vascular problems in oral contraceptive users compared to nonusers

	Relative risk, times greater
Idiopathic thromboembolic disease	4–11
Postsurgery thromboembolic complications	4–6
Thrombotic stroke	4–9.5
Hemorrhagic stroke	2
Myocardial infarction	2–12

Myocardial Infarction
An increased risk of myocardial infarction associated with the use of oral contraceptives has been reported[11–13] confirming a previously suspected association. These studies, conducted in the United Kingdom, found, as expected, that the greater the number of underlying risk factors for coronary artery disease (cigarette smoking, hypertension, hypercholesterolemia, obesity, diabetes, history of preeclamptic toxemia) the higher the risk of developing myocardial infarction, regardless of whether the patient was an oral contraceptive user or not. Oral contraceptives, however, were found to be a clear additional risk factor.

In terms of relative risk, it has been estimated[52] that oral contraceptive users who do not smoke (smoking is considered a major predisposing condition to myocardial infarction) are about twice as likely to have a fatal myocardial infarction as nonusers who do not smoke. Oral contraceptive users who are also smokers have about a 5-fold increased risk of fatal infarction compared to users who do not smoke, but about a 10- to 12-fold increased risk compared to nonusers who do not smoke. Furthermore, the amount of smoking is also an important factor. In determining the importance of these relative risks, however, the baseline rates for various age groups, as shown in Table 3, must be given serious consideration. The importance of other predisposing conditions mentioned above in determining relative and absolute risks has not as yet been quantified; it is quite likely that the same synergistic action exists, but perhaps to a lesser extent.

Table 3
Estimated annual mortality rate per 100,000 women from myocardial infarction by use of oral contraceptives, smoking habits, and age (in years) [See table on next page].

Risk of Dose
In an analysis of data derived from several national adverse reaction reporting systems,[2] British investigators concluded that the risk of thromboembolism, including coronary thrombosis, is directly related to the dose of estrogen used in oral contraceptives. Preparations containing 100 mcg or more of estrogen were associated with a higher risk of thromboembolism than those containing 50 to 80 mcg of estrogen. Their analysis did suggest, however, that the quantity of estrogen may not be the sole factor involved. This finding has been confirmed in the United States. Careful epidemiological studies to determine the degree of thromboembolic risk associated with progestogen-only oral contraceptives have not been performed. Cases of thromboembolic disease have been reported in women using these products, and they should not be presumed to be free of excess risk.

Estimate of Excess Mortality from Circulatory Diseases
A large prospective study[53] carried out in the U.K. estimated the mortality rate per 100,000 women per year from diseases of the circulatory system

Continued on next page

This product information was prepared in August, 1984. On these and other Parke-Davis Products, information may be obtained by addressing PARKE-DAVIS, Division of Warner-Lambert Company, Morris Plains, New Jersey 07950.

Parke-Davis—Cont.

for users and nonusers of oral contraceptives according to age, smoking habits, and duration of use. The overall excess death rate annually from circulatory diseases for oral contraceptive users was estimated to be 20 per 100,000 (ages 15 to 34—5/100,000; ages 35 to 44— 33/100,000; ages 45 to 49—140/100,000), the risk being concentrated in older women, in those with a long duration of use, and in cigarette smokers. It was not possible, however, to examine the interrelationships of age, smoking, and duration of use, nor to compare the effects of continuous versus intermittent use. Although the study showed a 10-fold increase in death due to circulatory diseases in users for 5 or more years, all of these deaths occurred in women 35 or older. Until larger numbers of women under 35 with continuous use for 5 or more years are available, it is not possible to assess the magnitude of the relative risk for this younger age group.

The available data from a variety of sources have been analyzed[14] to estimate the risk of death associated with various methods of contraception. The estimates of risk of death for each method include the combined risk of the contraceptive method (eg, thromboembolic and thrombotic disease in the case of oral contraceptives) plus the risk attributable to pregnancy or abortion in the event of method failure. This latter risk varies with the effectiveness of the contraceptive method. The findings of this analysis are shown in Figure 1 which follows.[14] The study concluded that the mortality associated with all methods of birth control is low and below that associated with childbirth, with the exception of oral contraceptives in women over 40 who smoke. (The rates given for pill only/smokers for each age group are for smokers as a class. For "heavy" smokers [more than 15 cigarettes a day] the rates given would be about double, for "light" smokers [less than 15 cigarettes a day] about 50 percent.) The lowest mortality is associated with the condom or diaphragm backed up by early abortion.
[See table above].

The risk of thromboembolic and thrombotic disease associated with oral contraceptives increases with age after approximately age 30 and, for myocardial infarction, is further increased by hypertension, hypercholesterolemia, obesity, diabetes, or history of preeclamptic toxemia and especially by cigarette smoking.

Based on the data currently available, the following chart gives a gross estimate of the risk of death from circulatory disorders associated with the use of oral contraceptives.

Smoking Habits and Other Predisposing Conditions—Risk Associated with Use of Oral Contraceptives

Age	Below 30	30–39	40+
Heavy smokers	C	B	A
Light smokers	D	C	B
Nonsmokers (no predisposing conditions)	D	C,D	C
Nonsmokers (other predisposing conditions)	C	C,B	B,A

A—Use associated with very high risk
B—Use associated with high risk
C—Use associated with moderate risk
D—Use associated with low risk

The physician and the patient should be alert to the earliest manifestations of thromboembolic and thrombotic disorders (eg, thrombophlebitis, pulmonary embolism, cerebrovascular insufficiency, coronary occlusion, retinal thrombosis, and mesenteric thrombosis). Should any of these occur or be suspected, the drug should be discontinued immediately.

A four- to six-fold increased risk of postsurgery thromboembolic complications has been reported in oral contraceptive users.[15,16] If feasible, oral contraceptives should be discontinued at least 4 weeks before surgery of a type associated with an increased risk of thromboembolism or prolonged immobilization.

2. *Ocular Lesions.* There have been reports of neuro-ocular lesions, such as optic neuritis or retinal thrombosis, associated with the use of oral contraceptives. Discontinue oral contraceptive medication if there is unexplained, sudden or gradual, partial or complete loss of vision; onset of proptosis or diplopia; papilledema; or retinal vascular lesions and institute appropriate diagnostic and therapeutic measures.

3. *Carcinoma.* Long-term continuous administration of either natural or synthetic estrogen in certain animal species increases the frequency of carcinoma of the breast, cervix, vagina, and liver. Certain synthetic progestogens, none currently contained in oral contraceptives, have been noted to increase the incidence of mammary nodules, benign and malignant, in dogs.

In humans, three case control studies have reported an increased risk of endometrial carcinoma associated with the prolonged use of exogenous estrogen in post-menopausal women.[17-19] One publication[20] reported on the first 21 cases submitted by physicians to a registry of cases of adenocarcinoma of the endometrium in women under 40 on oral contraceptives. Of the cases found in women without predisposing risk factors for adenocarcinoma of the endometrium (eg, irregular bleeding at the time oral contraceptives were first given, polycystic ovaries), nearly all occurred in women who had used a sequential oral contraceptive. These products are no longer marketed. No evidence has been reported suggesting an increased risk of endometrial cancer in users of convention-

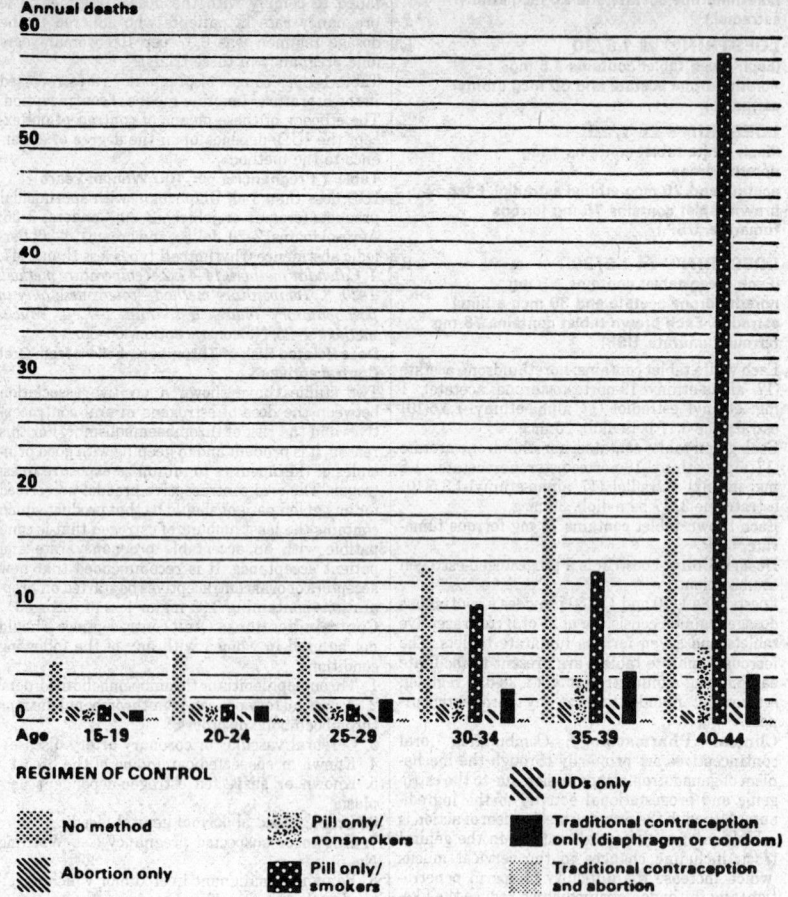

Figure 1. Estimated annual number of deaths associated with control of fertility and no control per 100,000 nonsterile women, by regimen of control and age of woman.

Loestrin

	Myocardial infarction			
	Women aged 30–39		Women aged 40–44	
Smoking habits	Users	Nonusers	Users	Nonusers
All smokers	10.2	2.6	62.0	15.9
Heavy*	13.0	5.1	78.7	31.3
Light	4.7	0.9	28.6	5.7
Nonsmokers	1.8	1.2	10.7	7.4
Smokers and nonsmokers	5.4	1.9	32.8	11.7

*Heavy smoker: 15 or more cigarettes per day. From Jain, A.K., Studies in Family Planning 8:50, 1977.

al-combination or progestogen-only oral contraceptives.
Several studies[8,21–24] have found no increase in breast cancer in women taking oral contraceptives or estrogens. One study,[25] however, while also noting no overall increased risk of breast cancer in women treated with oral contraceptives, found an excess risk in the subgroups of oral contraceptive users with documented benign breast disease. A reduced occurrence of benign breast tumors in users of oral contraceptives has been well-documented.[8,21,25–27]
In summary, there is at present no confirmed evidence from human studies of an increased risk of cancer associated with oral contraceptives. Close clinical surveillance of all women taking oral contraceptives is, nevertheless, essential. In all cases of undiagnosed persistent or recurrent abnormal vaginal bleeding, appropriate diagnostic measures should be taken to rule out malignancy. Women with a strong family history of breast cancer or who have breast nodules, fibrocystic disease, or abnormal mammograms, should be monitored with particular care if they elect to use oral contraceptives instead of other methods of contraception.
4. *Hepatic Tumors.* Benign hepatic adenomas have been found to be associated with the use of oral contraceptives.[28–30,46] One study[46] showed that oral contraceptive formulations with high hormonal potency were associated with a higher risk than lower potency formulations. Although benign, hepatic adenomas may rupture and may cause death through intra-abdominal hemorrhage. This has been reported in short-term as well as long-term users of oral contraceptives. Two studies relate risk with duration of use of the contraceptive, the risk being much greater after 4 or more years of oral contraceptive use.[30,46] While hepatic adenoma is a rare lesion, it should be considered in women presenting abdominal pain and tenderness, abdominal mass or shock.
A few cases of hepatocellular carcinoma have been reported in women taking oral contraceptives. The relationship of these drugs to this type of malignancy is not known at this time.
5. *Use in or Immediately Preceding Pregnancy, Birth Defects in Offspring, and Malignancy in Female Offspring.* The use of female sex hormones—both estrogenic and progestational agents—during early pregnancy may seriously damage the offspring. It has been shown that females exposed *in utero* to diethylstilbestrol, a nonsteroidal estrogen, have an increased risk of developing in later life a form of vaginal or cervical cancer that is ordinarily extremely rare.[31,32] This risk has been estimated to be of the order of 1 in 1,000 exposures or less.[33,47] Although there is no evidence at the present time that oral contraceptives further enhance the risk of developing this type of malignancy, such patients should be monitored with particular care if they elect to use oral contraceptives instead of other methods of contraception. Furthermore, a high percentage of such exposed women (from 30% to 90%) have been found to have epithelial changes of the vagina and cervix.[34–38] Although these changes are histologically benign, it is not known whether this condition is a precursor of vaginal malignancy. Male children so exposed may develop abnormalities of the urogenital tract.[48–50] Although similar data are not available with the use of other estrogens, it cannot be presumed that they would not induce similar changes.
An increased risk of congenital anomalies, including heart defects and limb defects, has been reported with the use of sex hormones, including oral contraceptives, in pregnancy.[39–42,51] One case control study[42] has estimated a 4.7-fold increase in risk of limb-reduction defectes in infants exposed *in utero* to sex hormones (oral contraceptives, hormonal withdrawal tests for pregnancy or attempted treatment for threatened abortion). Some of these exposures were very short and involved only a few days of treatment. The data suggest that the risk of limb-reduction defects in exposed fetuses is somewhat less than 1 in 1,000 live births.
In the past, female sex hormones have been used during pregnancy in an attempt to treat threatened or habitual abortion. There is considerable evidence that estrogens are ineffective for these indications, and there is no evidence from well-controlled studies that progestogens are effective for these uses.
There is some evidence that triploidy and possibly other types of polyploidy are increased among abortuses from women who become pregnant soon after ceasing oral contraceptives.[43] Embryos with these anomalies are virtually always aborted spontaneously. Whether there is an overall increase in spontaneous abortion of pregnancies conceived soon after stopping oral contraceptives is unknown.
It is recommended that for any patient who has missed two consecutive periods, pregnancy should be ruled out before continuing the contraceptive regimen. If the patient has not adhered to the prescribed schedule, the possibility of pregnancy should be considered at the time of the first missed period, and further use of oral contraceptives should be withheld until pregnancy has been ruled out. If pregnancy is confirmed, the patient should be apprised of the potential risks to the fetus and the advisability of continuation of the pregnancy should be discussed in the light of these risks.
It is also recommended that women who discontinue oral contraceptives with the intent of becoming pregnant use an alternate form of contraception for a period of time before attempting to conceive. Many clinicians recommend 3 months although no precise information is available on which to base this recommendation.
The administration of progestogen-only or progestogen-estrogen combinations to induce withdrawal bleeding should not be used as a test of pregnancy.
6. *Gallbladder Disease.* Studies[8,23,26] report an increased risk of surgically confirmed gallbladder disease in users of oral contraceptives and estrogens. In one study, an increased risk appeared after 2 years of use and doubled after 4 or 5 years of use. In one of the other studies, an increased risk was apparent between 6 and 12 months of use.
7. *Carbohydrate and Lipid Metabolic Effects.* A decrease in glucose tolerance has been observed in a significant percentage of patients on oral contraceptives. For this reason, prediabetic and diabetic patients should be carefully observed while receiving oral contraceptives.
An increase in triglycerides and total phospholipids has been observed in patients receiving oral contraceptives.[44] The clinical significance of this finding remains to be defined.
8. *Elevated Blood Pressure.* An increase in blood pressure has been reported in patients receiving oral contraceptives.[26] In some women, hypertension may occur within a few months of beginning oral contraceptive use. In the first year of use, the prevalence of women with hypertension is low in users and may be no higher than that of a comparable group of nonusers. The prevalance in users increases, however, with longer exposure, and in the fifth year of use is two and a half to three times the reported prevalence in the first year. Age is also strongly correlated with the development of hypertension in oral contraceptive users. Women who previously have had hypertension during pregnancy may be more likely to develop elevation of blood pressure when given oral contraceptives. Hypertension that develops as a result of taking oral contraceptives usually returns to normal after discontinuing the drug.
9. *Headache.* The onset or exacerbation of migraine or development of headache of a new pattern which is recurrent, persistent, or severe, requires discontinuation of oral contraceptives and evaluation of the cause.
10. *Bleeding Irregularities.* Breakthrough bleeding, spotting and amenorrhea are frequent reasons for patients discontinuing oral contraceptives. In breakthrough bleeding, as in all cases of irregular bleeding from the vagina, nonfunctional causes should be borne in mind. In undiagnosed persistent or recurrent abnormal bleeding from the vagina, adequate diagnostic measures are indicated to rule out pregnancy or malignancy. If pathology has been excluded, time or a change to another formulation may solve the problem. Changing to an oral contraceptive with a higher estrogen content, while potentially useful in minimizing menstrual irregularity, should be done only if necessary since this may increase the risk of thromboembolic disease.
Women with a past history of oligomenorrhea or secondary amenorrhea or young women without regular cycles may have a tendency to remain anovulatory or to become amenorrheic after discontinuation of oral contraceptives. Women with these preexisting problems should be advised of this possibility and encouraged to use other contraceptive methods. Post-use anovulation, possibly prolonged, may also occur in women without previous irregularities.
11. *Ectopic Pregnancy.* Ectopic as well as intrauterine pregnancy may occur in contraceptive failures. However, in progestogen-only oral contraceptive failures, the ratio of ectopic to intrauterine pregnancies is higher than in women who are not receiving oral contraceptives, since the drugs are more effective in preventing intrauterine than ectopic pregnancies.
12. *Breast-Feeding.* Oral contraceptives given in the postpartum period may interfere with lactation. There may be a decrease in the quantity and quality of the breast milk. Furthermore, a small fraction of the hormonal agents in oral contraceptives has been identified in the milk of mothers receiving these drugs.[45] The effects, if any, on the breast-fed child have not been determined. If feasible, the use of oral contraceptives should be deferred until the infant has been weaned.

Precautions:

General

1. A complete medical and family history should be taken prior to the initiation of oral contraceptives. The pretreatment and periodic physical examinations should include special reference to blood pressure, breasts, abdomen and pelvic organs, including Papanicolaou smear and relevant laboratory tests. As a general rule, oral contraceptives should not be prescribed for longer than 1 year without another physical examination being performed.
2. Under the influence of estrogen-progestogen preparations preexisting uterine leiomyomata may increase in size.
3. Patients with a history of psychic depression should be carefully observed and the drug discontinued if depression recurs to a serious degree. Patients becoming significantly depressed while taking oral contraceptives should stop the medication and use an alternate method of contraception in an attempt to determine whether the symptom is drug related.
4. Oral contraceptives may cause some degree of fluid retention. They should be prescribed with caution, and only with careful monitoring, in patients with conditions which might be aggravated by fluid retention, such as convulsive disorders, migraine syndrome, asthma, or cardiac or renal insufficiency.
5. Patients with a past history of jaundice during pregnancy have an increased risk of recurrence of jaundice while receiving oral contraceptive therapy. If jaundice develops in any patient receiving such drugs, the medication should be discontinued.
6. Steroid hormones may be poorly metabolized in patients with impaired liver function and should be administered with caution in such patients.
7. Oral contraceptive users may have disturbances in normal tryptophan metabolism which may result in a relative pyridoxine deficiency. The clinical significance of this is yet to be determined.
8. Serum folate levels may be depressed by oral contraceptive therapy. Since the pregnant woman

Continued on next page

This product information was prepared in August, 1984. On these and other Parke-Davis Products, information may be obtained by addressing PARKE-DAVIS, Division of Warner-Lambert Company, Morris Plains, New Jersey 07950.

Parke-Davis—Cont.

is predisposed to the development of folate deficiency and the incidence of folate deficiency increases with increasing gestation, it is possible that if a woman becomes pregnant shortly after stopping oral contraceptives, she may have a greater chance of developing folate deficiency and complications attributed to this deficiency.
9. The pathologist should be advised of oral contraceptive therapy when relevant specimens are submitted.
10. Certain endocrine and liver function tests and blood components may be affected by estrogen-containing oral contraceptives:
a. Increased sulfobromophthalein retention
b. Increased prothrombin and factors VII, VIII, IX, and X; decreased antithrombin 3; increased norepinephrine-induced platelet aggregability
c. Increased thyroid binding globulin (TBG) leading to increased circulating total thyroid hormone, as measured by protein-bound iodine (PBI), T4 by column, or T4 by radioimmunoassay. Free T3 resin uptake is decreased, reflecting the elevated TBG, free T4 concentration is unaltered
d. Decreased pregnanediol excretion
e. Reduced response to metyrapone test
Information For The Patient: See Patient Labeling printed following the reference section.
Drug Interactions: Reduced efficacy and increased incidence of breakthrough bleeding have been associated with concomitant use of rifampin. A similar association has been suggested with barbiturates, phenylbutazone, phenytoin sodium, tetracycline, and ampicillin.
Carcinogenesis: See Warnings section for information on the carcinogenic potential of oral contraceptives.
Pregnancy: Pregnancy category X. See Contraindications and Warnings.
Nursing Mothers: See Warnings.
Adverse Reactions: An increased risk of the following serious adverse reactions has been associated with the use of oral contraceptives (see Warnings):
   Thrombophlebitis
   Pulmonary embolism
   Coronary thrombosis
   Cerebral thrombosis
   Cerebral hemorrhage
   Hypertension
   Gallbladder disease
   Benign hepatomas
   Congenital anomalies
There is evidence of an association between the following conditions and the use of oral contraceptives, although additional confirmatory studies are needed:
   Mesenteric thrombosis
   Neuro-ocular lesions, eg, retinal thrombosis and optic neuritis
The following adverse reactions have been reported in patients receivng oral contraceptives and are believed to be drug related:
Nausea and/or vomiting, usually the most common adverse reactions, occur in approximately 10 percent or less of patients during the first cycle. Other reactions, as a general rule, are seen much less frequently or only occasionally:
   Gastrointestinal symptoms (such as abdominal cramps and bloating)
   Breakthrough bleeding
   Spotting
   Change in menstrual flow
   Dysmenorrhea
   Amenorrhea during and after treatment
   Temporary infertility after discontinuance of treatment
   Edema
   Chloasma or melasma which may persist
   Breast changes: tenderness, enlargement and secretion
   Change in weight (increase or decrease)
   Change in cervical erosion and cervical secretion
   Possible diminution in lactation when given immediately postpartum
   Cholestatic jaundice
   Migraine
   Increase in size of uterine leiomyomata
   Rash (allergic)
   Mental depression
   Reduced tolerance to carbohydrates
   Vaginal candidiasis
   Change in corneal curvature (steepening)
   Intolerance to contact lenses
The following adverse reactions have been reported in users of oral contraceptives, and the association has been neither confirmed nor refuted:
   Premenstrual-like syndrome
   Cataracts
   Changes in libido
   Chorea
   Changes in appetite
   Cystitis-like syndrome
   Headache
   Nervousness
   Dizziness
   Hirsutism
   Loss of scalp hair
   Erythema multiforme
   Erythema nodosum
   Hemorrhagic eruption
   Vaginitis
   Porphyria
Acute Overdose: Serious ill effects have not been reported following acute ingestion of large doses of oral contraceptives by young children. Overdosage may cause nausea, and withdrawal bleeding may occur in females.
Dosage and Administration For 21-Day Dosage Regimen: To achieve maximum contraceptive effectiveness, Loestrin must be taken exactly as directed and at intervals not exceeding 24 hours. Loestrin 21 provides the patient with a convenient tablet schedule of "3 weeks on—1 week off."
The first day of menstrual flow is considered Day 1. Initially, the patient begins taking tablets on Day 5 and takes one tablet daily for 21 days. She then takes no tablets for seven days.
After the seven days during which no tablets are taken, the patient begins a new course of one tablet daily for 21 days. Each course of tablets will begin on the same day of the week as the first course. Likewise, the interval of no tablets will always start on the same day of the week.
Tablets should be taken regularly with a meal or at bedtime. It should be stressed that efficacy of medication depends on strict adherence to the dosage schedule.
Special Notes on Administration
Menstruation usually begins two or three days, but may begin as late as the fourth or fifth day after discontinuing medication. Because of the relatively low estrogenic content, Loestrin is not a good cyclic regulator. There are patients whose inherent hormone balance will require larger amounts of estrogen to achieve cyclic regularity than that contained in Loestrin. These patients experience altered bleeding patterns, which do not conform to treatment schedules, while taking Loestrin tablets. However, it is important that patients adhere to the dosage schedule regardless of when bleeding occurs.
The occurrence of altered bleeding is highest in Cycle 1. The majority of patients will have seven days or less of total bleeding during the 28-day cycle (including both withdrawal bleeding and breakthrough bleeding and spotting). Should irregular bleeding occur, patients should be reassured and instructed to continue taking the tablets as directed. If by the third cycle the irregular patterns are unacceptable, consideration should be given to changing the medication to a product with a higher estrogen content (Norlestrin® *1/50 or Norlestrin 2.5/50). The physician should be alert to the fact that the irregular bleeding patterns could mask bleeding from organic causes, and appropriate diagnostic measures should be taken if the bleeding persists or continues after changing to a higher estrogen-content product.
If a patient forgets to take one or more tablets, the following is suggested. If one tablet is missed, take it as soon as remembered, or take two tablets the next day. If two consecutive tablets are missed, take two tablets daily for the next two days, then resume the regular schedule. While there is little likelihood of pregnancy occurring if the patient misses only one or two tablets, the possibility of pregnancy increases with each successive day that tablets are missed. *However if the patient is taking* Loestrin **21** 1/20, *in addition to taking two white tablets a day for two days the patient should use an additional means of contraception for seven consecutive days.* If three consecutive tablets are missed, begin a new compact of tablets starting seven days after the last tablet was taken. The patient should use an alternate means of contraception, other than oral tablets, until the start of the next menstrual period.
The possibility of ovulation occurring increases with each successive day that scheduled tablets are missed. While there is little likelihood of ovulation occurring if only one tablet is missed, the possibility of spotting or bleeding is increased. This is particularly likely to occur if two or more consecutive tablets are missed.

---
*Norlestrin (Norethindrone Acetate and Ethinyl Estradiol Tablets, USP)
Dosage and Administration For 28-Day Dosage Regimen: To achieve maximum contraceptive effectiveness, Loestrin must be taken exactly as directed and at intervals not exceeding 24 hours. Loestrin Fe provides a continuous administration regimen consisting of 21 *light-colored* tablets of Loestrin and 7 brown tablets of ferrous fumarate. There is no need for the patient to count days between cycles because there are no "off-tablet days."
The dosage schedule is one *light-colored* tablet daily for 21 days, starting initially on Day 5 of the menstrual cycle, followed without interruption by one brown tablet daily for 7 days. The first day of menstrual flow is considered Day 1. Upon completion of this first course of tablets, a second course of tablets is started without interruption. All subsequent courses also are taken without interruption.
Tablets should be taken regularly with a meal or at bedtime. It should be stressed that efficacy of medication depends on strict adherence to the dosage schedule.
Special Notes on Administration
Menstruation usually begins two or three days, but may begin as late as the fourth or fifth day, after the brown tablets have been started. Because of the relatively low estrogenic content, Loestrin is not a good cyclic regulator. There are patients whose inherent hormone balance will require larger amounts of estrogen to achieve cyclic regularity than that contained in Loestrin. These patients experience altered bleeding patterns, which do not conform to treatment schedules, while taking the *light-colored* Loestrin tablets. However, it is important that patients adhere to the dosage schedule regardless of when bleeding occurs.
The occurrence of altered bleeding is highest in Cycle 1. The majority of patients will have seven days or less of total bleeding during the 28-day cycle (including both withdrawal bleeding and breakthrough bleeding and spotting). Should irregular bleeding occur, patients should be reassured and instructed to continue taking the tablets as directed. If by the third cycle the irregular patterns are unacceptable, consideration should be given to changing the medication to a product with a higher estrogen content (Norlestrin *1/50 or Norlestrin 2.5/50). The physician should be alert to the fact that the irregular bleeding patterns could mask bleeding from organic causes, and appropriate diagnostic measures should be taken if the bleeding persists or continues after changing to a higher estrogen-content product.
If a patient forgets to take one or more *light-colored* tablets, the following is suggested. If one *light-colored* tablet is missed, take it as soon as remembered, or take two *light-colored* tablets the next day. If two consecutive *light-colored* tablets are missed, take two *light-colored* tablets daily for the next two days, then resume the regular sched-

ule. While there is little likelihood of pregnancy occurring if the patient misses only one or two *light-colored* tablets, the possibility of pregnancy increases with each successive day that *light-colored* tablets are missed. However, *if the patient is taking* Loestrin Fe 1/20, *in addition to taking two white tablets a day for two days, the patient should use an additional means of contraception for seven consecutive days.* If three consecutive *light-colored* tablets are missed, begin a new compact of tablets, starting seven days after the last *light-colored* tablet was taken. The patient should use an alternate means of contraception, other than oral tablets, until the start of the next menstrual period.

The possibility of ovulation occurring increases with each successive day that scheduled *light-colored* tablets are missed. While there is little likelihood of ovulation occurring if only one *light-colored* tablet is missed, the possibility of spotting or bleeding is increased. This is particularly likely to occur if two or more consecutive *light-colored* tablets are missed.

If one or more brown tablets are missed, the *light-colored* tablets should be started no later than the eighth day after the last *light-colored* tablet was taken. The possibility of conception occurring is not increased if brown tablets are missed.

*Norlestrin (Norethindrone Acetate and Ethinyl Estradiol Tablets, USP)

Use of oral contraceptives in the event of a missed menstrual period:

1. If the patient has not adhered to the prescribed dosage regimen, the possibility of pregnancy should be considered after the first missed period and oral contraceptives should be withheld until pregnancy has been ruled out.

2. If the patient has adhered to the prescribed regimen and misses two consecutive periods, pregnancy should be ruled out before continuing the contraceptive regimen.

After several months on treatment, bleeding may be reduced to a point of virtual absence. This reduced flow may occur as a result of medication, in which event it is not indicative of pregnancy.

How Supplied:

Loestrin 21 1/20 is available in compacts each containing 21 tablets. Each tablet contains 1 mg of norethindrone acetate and 20 mcg of ethinyl estradiol. Available in packages of five compacts and packages of five refills.

Loestrin Fe 1/20 is available in compacts each containing 21 white tablets and 7 brown tablets. Each white tablet contains 1 mg of norethindrone acetate and 20 mcg of ethinyl estradiol. Each brown tablet contains 75 mg ferrous fumarate, USP. Available in packages of five compacts and packages of five refills.

Loestrin 21 1.5/30 is available in compacts each containing 21 tablets. Each tablet contains 1.5 mg of norethindrone acetate and 30 mcg of ethinyl estradiol. Available in packages of five compacts and packages of five refills.

Loestrin Fe 1.5/30 is available in compacts each containing 21 green tablets and 7 brown tablets. Each green tablet contains 1.5 mg of norethindrone acetate and 30 mcg of ethinyl estradiol. Each brown tablet contains 75 mg ferrous fumarate, USP. Available in packages of five compacts and packages of five refills.

References:

1. "*Population Reports,*" Series H, Number 2, May 1974; Series 1, Number 1, June 1974; Series B, Number 2, January 1975; Series H, Number 3, 1975; Series H, Number 4, January 1976 (published by the Population Information Program, The George Washington University Medical Center, 2001 S. St. NW., Washington, D.C.)
2. Inman, W. H. W., M. P. Vessey, B. Westerholm, and A. Engelund. "Thromboembolic disease and the steroidal content of oral contraceptives. A report to the Committee on Safety of Drugs," *Brit Med J* 2:203–209, 1970.
3. Stolley, P.D., J. A. Tonascia, M. S. Tockman, P. E. Sartwell, A. H. Rutledge, and M. P. Jacobs, "Thrombosis with low-estrogen oral contraceptives," *Am J Epidemiol* 102: 197–208, 1975.
4. Royal College of General Practitioners, "Oral contraception and thromboembolic disease," *J Coll Gen Pract* 13:267–279, 1967.
5. Inman, W. H. W. and M. P. Vessey, "Investigation of deaths from pulmonary, coronary and cerebral thrombosis and embolism in women of childbearing age," *Brit Med. J* 2-193–199, 1968.
6. Vessey, M. P. and R. Doll, "Investigation of relation between use of oral contraceptives and thromboembolic disease. A further report," *Brit Med J* 2:651–657, 1969.
7. Sartwell, P. E., A. T. Masi, F. G. Arthes, G. R. Greene, and H. E. Smith, "Thromboembolism and oral contraceptives an epidemiological case control study," *Am J Epidemiol* 90:365–380, 1969.
8. Boston Collaborative Drug Surveillance Program. "Oral contraceptives and venous thromboembolic disease, surgically confirmed gallbladder disease and breast tumors," *Lancet* 1:1399–1404, 1973.
9. Collaborative Group for the Study of Stroke in Young Women, "Oral contraception and increased risk of cerebral ischemia or thrombosis," *N Engl J Med* 288:871–878, 1973.
10. Collaborative Group for the Study of Stroke in Young Women, "Oral contraceptives and stroke in young women: associated risk factors," *JAMA* 231:718–722, 1975.
11. Mann, J. I., and W. H. W. Inman, "Oral contraceptives and death from myocardial infarction," *Brit Med J* 2:245–248, 1975.
12. Mann, J. I., W. H. W. Inman, and M. Thorogood, "Oral contraceptive use in older women and fatal myocardial infarction," *Brit Med J* 2:445–447, 1976.
13. Mann, J. I., M. P. Vessey, M. Thorogood and R. Doll, "Myocardial infarction in young women with special reference to oral contraceptive practice," *Brit Med J* 2:241–245, 1975.
14. Tietze, C., "New Estimates of Mortality Associated with Fertility Control," *Family Planning Perspectives,* 9:74–76, 1977.
15. Vessey, M. P., R. Doll, A. S. Fairbairn, and G. Glober, "Post-operative thromboembolism and the use of oral contraceptives," *Brit Med J* 3:123–126, 1970.
16. Greene, G. R., P. E. Sartwell, "Oral contraceptive use in patients with thromboembolism following surgery, trauma or infection," *Am J Pub Health* 62:680–685, 1972.
17. Smith, D. C., R. Prentice, D. J. Thompson and W. L. Herrmann, "Association of exogenous estrogen and endometrial carcinoma," *N Engl J Med* 293:1164–1167, 1975.
18. Ziel, H. K., and W. D. Finkle, "Increased risk of endometrial carcinoma among users of conjugated estrogens," *N Engl J Med* 293: 1167–1170, 1975.
19. Mack, T. N., M. C. Pike, B. E. Henderson, R. I. Pfeffer, V. R. Gerkins, M. Arthur and S. E. Brown, "Estrogens and endometrial cancer in a retirement community," *N Engl J Med* 294: 1262–1267, 1976.
20. Silverberg, S. G., and E. L. Makowski, "Endometrial carcinoma in young women taking oral contraceptive agents," *Obstet Gynecol* 46:503–506, 1975.
21. Vessey, M. P., R. Doll, and P. M. Sutton, "Oral contraceptives and breast neoplasia: a retrospective study," *Brit Med J* 3:719–724, 1972.
22. Vessey, M. P., R. Doll, and K. Jones, "Oral contraceptives and breast cancer. Progress report of an epidemiological study," *Lancet* 1:941–943, 1975.
23. Boston Collaborative Drug Surveillance Program, "Surgically confirmed gallbladder disease, venous thromboembolism and breast tumors in relation to postmenopausal estrogen therapy," *N Engl J Med* 290:14–19, 1974.
24. Arthes, F. G., P. E. Sartwell, and E. F. Lewison, "The pill, estrogens, and the breast, Epidemiologic aspects," *Cancer* 28:1391–1394, 1971.
25. Fasal, E., and R. S. Paffenbarger, "Oral contraceptives as related to cancer and benign lesions of the breast." *J Natl Cancer Inst* 55:767–773, 1975.
26. Royal College of General Practitioners, "Oral Contraceptives and Health," London, Pitman, 1974.
27. Ory, H., P. Cole, B. MacMahon, and R. Hoover, "Oral contraceptives and reduced risk of benign breast diseases," *N Engl J Med* 294:419–422, 1976.
28. Baum, J., F. Holtz, J. J. Bookstein, and E. W. Klein, "Possible association between benign hepatomas and oral contraceptives," *Lancet* 2:926–928, 1973.
29. Mays, E. T., W. M. Christopherson, M. M. Mahr, and H. C. Williams, "Hepatic changes in young women ingesting contraceptive steroids. Hepatic hemorrhage and primary hepatic tumors," *JAMA* 235:730–732, 1976.
30. Edmondson, H. A., B. Henderson, and B. Benton, "Liver-cell adenomas associated with use of oral contraceptives," *N Engl J Med* 294:470–472, 1976.
31. Herbst, A. L., H. Ulfelder, and D. C. Poskanzer, "Adenocarcinoma of the vagina," *N Engl J Med* 284:878–881, 1971.
32. Greenwald, P., J. J. Barlow, P. C. Nasca and W. Burnett, "Vaginal cancer after maternal treatment with synthetic estrogens," *N Engl J Med* 285:390–392, 1971.
33. Lanier, A. P., K. L. Noller, D. G. Decker, L. Elveback, and L. T. Kurland, "Cancer and stilbestrol. A follow-up of 1719 persons exposed to estrogens in utero and born 1943–1959," *Mayo Clin Pro* 48:793–799, 1973.
34. Herbst, A. L., R. J. Kurman, and R. E. Scully, "Vaginal and cervical abnormalities after exposure to stilbestrol in utero," *Obstet Gynecol* 40:287–298, 1972.
35. Herbst, A. L., S. J. Robboy, G. J. Macdonald, and R. E. Scully, "The effects of local progesterone on stilbestrol-associated vaginal adenosis," *Am J. Obstet Gynecol* 118:607–615, 1974.
36. Herbst, A. L., D. C. Poskanzer, S. J. Robboy, L. Friedlander, and R. E. Scully, "Prenatal exposure to stilbestrol: a prospective comparison of exposed female offspring with unexposed controls," *N Engl J Med* 292:334–339, 1975.
37. Stafl, A., R. F. Mattingly, D. V. Foley, W. Fetherston, "Clinical diagnosis of vaginal adenosis," *Obstet Gynecol* 43:118–128, 1974.
38. Sherman, A. I., M. Goldrath, A. Berlin, V. Vakhariya, F. Banooni, W. Michaels, P. Goodman, and S. Brown, "Cervical-vaginal adenosis after in utero exposure to synthetic estrogens," *Obstet Gynecol* 44:531–545, 1974.
39. Gal, I., B. Kirman, and J. Stern, "Hormone pregnancy tests and congenital malformation," *Nature* 216:83, 1967.
40. Levy, E. P., A. Cohen, and F. C. Fraser, "Hormone treatment during pregnancy and congenital heart defects," *Lancet* 1:611, 1973.
41. Nora, J. J., and A. H. Nora, "Birth defects and oral contraceptives," *Lancet* 1:941–942, 1973.
42. Janerich, D. T., J. M. Piper, and M. D. Glebatis, "Oral contraceptives and congenital limb-reduction defects," *N Engl J Med* 291:697–700, 1974.
43. Carr, D. H., "Chromosome studies in selected spontaneous abortions: I. Conception after oral contraceptives," *Canad Med Assoc J* 103:343–348, 1970.
44. Wynn, V., J. W. H. Doar, and G. L. Mills, "Some effects of oral contraceptives on serum-lipid and lipoprotein levels," *Lancet* 2:720–723, 1966.
45. Laumas, K. R., P. K. Malkani, S. Bhatnagar, and V. Laumas, "Radioactivity in the breast milk of lactating women after oral administration of 3 H-norethynodrel," *Amer J Obstet Gynecol* 98:411–413, 1967.
46. Center for Disease Control, "Increased Risk of Hepatocellular Adenoma in Women with Long-term use of Oral Contraceptives," *Morbidity and Mortality Weekly Report* 26:293–294, 1977.
47. Herbst, A. L., P. Cole, T. Colton, S. J. Robboy, R. E. Scully, "Age-incidence and Risk of Diethylstil-

Continued on next page

This product information was prepared in August, 1984. On these and other Parke-Davis Products, information may be obtained by addressing PARKE-DAVIS, Division of Warner-Lambert Company, Morris Plains, New Jersey 07950.

Parke-Davis—Cont.

bestrol-related Clear Cell Adenocarcinoma of the Vagina and Cervix," *Am J. Obstet Gynecol* 128:43–50, 1977.
48. Bibbo, M., M. Al-Naqeeb, I. Baccarini, W. Gill, M. Newton, K. M. Sleeper, M. Sonek, G. L. Wied, "Follow-Up Study of Male and Female Offspring of DES-treated Mothers. A Preliminary Report," *Jour of Repro Med* 15:29–32, 1975.
49. Gill, W. B., G. F. B. Schumacher, M. Bibbo, "Structural and Functional Abnormalities in the Sex Organs of Male Offspring of Mothers Treated with Diethylstilbestrol (DES)," *Jour of Repro Med* 16:147–153, 1976.
50. Henderson, B. E., B. Benton, M. Cosgrove, J. Baptista, J. Aldrich, D. Townsend, W. Hart, T. Mack, "Urogenital Tract Abnormalities in Sons of Women Treated with Diethylstilbestrol," *Pediatrics* 58:505–507, 1976.
51. Heinonen, O. P., D. Slone, R. R. Nonson, E. B. Hook, S. Shapiro, "Cardiovascular Birth Defects and Antenatal Exposure to Female Sex Hormones," *N Engl J Med* 296:67–70, 1977.
52. Jain, A. K., "Mortality Risk Associated with the Use of Oral Contraceptives," *Studies in Family Planning* 8:50–54, 1977.
53. Beral, V., "Mortality Among Oral Contraceptive Users," *Lancet* 2:727–731, 1977.
The patient labeling for oral contraceptive drug products is set forth below:

Brief Summary Patient Package Insert

> Cigarette smoking increases the risk of serious adverse effects on the heart and blood vessels from oral contraceptive use. This risk increases with age and with heavy smoking (15 or more cigarettes per day) and is quite marked in women over 35 years of age. Women who use oral contraceptives should not smoke.

Oral contraceptives taken as directed are about 99% effective in preventing pregnancy. (The mini-pill, however is somewhat less effective.) Forgetting to take your pills increases the chance of pregnancy. Various drugs, such as antibiotics, may also decrease the effectiveness of oral contraceptives.
Women who have or have had clotting disorders, cancer of the breast or sex organs, unexplained vaginal bleeding, a stroke, heart attack, angina pectoris, or who suspect they may be pregnant should not use oral contraceptives.
Most side effects of the pill are not serious. The most common side effects are nausea, vomiting, bleeding between menstrual periods, weight gain, and breast tenderness. However, proper use of oral contraceptives requires that they be taken under your doctor's continuous supervision, because they can be associated with serious side effects which may be fatal. Fortunately, these occur very infrequently.
The serious side effects are:
1. Blood clots in the legs, lungs, brain, heart or other organs and hemorrhage into the brain due to bursting of a blood vessel
2. Liver tumors, which may rupture and cause severe bleeding
3. Birth defects if the pill is taken while you are pregnant
4. High blood pressure
5. Gallbladder disease
The symptoms associated with these serious side effects are discussed in the detailed leaflet given you with your supply of pills. Notify your doctor if you notice any unusual physical disturbance while taking the pill.
The estrogen in oral contraceptives has been found to cause breast cancer and other cancers in certain animals. These findings suggest that oral contraceptives may also cause cancer in humans. However, studies to date in women taking currently marketed oral contraceptives have not confirmed that oral contraceptives cause cancer in humans.

The detailed leaflet describes more completely the benefits and risks of oral contraceptives. It also provides information on other forms of contraception. Read it carefully. If you have any questions, consult your doctor.
Caution: Oral contraceptives are of no value in the prevention or treatment of venereal disease.

Detailed Patient Labeling
What You Should Know About Oral Contraceptives
Oral contraceptives ("the pill") are the most effective way (except for sterilization) to prevent pregnancy. They are also convenient and, for most women, free of serious or unpleasant side effects. Oral contraceptives must always be taken under the continuous supervision of a physician.
It is important that any woman who considers using an oral contraceptive understand the risks involved. Although the oral contraceptives have important advantages over other methods of contraception, they have certain risks that no other method has. Only you can decide whether the advantages are worth these risks. This leaflet will tell you about the most important risks. It will explain how you can help your doctor prescribe the pill as safely as possible by telling him about yourself and being alert for the earliest signs of trouble. And it will tell you how to use the pill properly, so that it will be as effective as possible. There is more detailed information available in the leaflet prepared for doctors. Your pharmacist can show you a copy; you may need your doctor's help in understanding parts of it.

Who Should Not Use Oral Contraceptives
A. If you have any of the following conditions you should not use the pill:
1. Clots in the legs or lungs
2. Angina pectoris
3. Known or suspected cancer of the breast or sex organs
4. Unusual vaginal bleeding that has not yet been diagnosed
5. Known or suspected pregnancy
B. If you have had any of the following conditions you should not use the pill:
1. Heart attack or stroke
2. Clots in the legs or lungs

> C. Cigarette smoking increases the risk of serious adverse effects on the heart and blood vessels from oral contraceptive use. This risk increases with age and with heavy smoking (15 or more cigarettes per day) and is quite marked in women over 35 years of age. Women who use oral contraceptives should not smoke.

D. If you have scanty or irregular periods or are a young woman without a regular cycle, you should use another method of contraception because, if you use the pill, you may have difficulty becoming pregnant or may fail to have menstrual periods after discontinuing the pill.

Deciding To Use Oral Contraceptives
If you do not have any of the conditions listed above and are thinking about using oral contraceptives, to help you decide, you need information about the advantages and risks of oral contraceptives and of other contraceptive methods as well. This leaflet describes the advantages and risks of oral contraceptives. Except for sterilization, the IUD and abortion, which have their own exclusive risks, the only risks of other methods of contraception are those due to pregnancy should the method fail. Your doctor can answer questions you may have with respect to other methods of contraception. He can also answer any questions you may have after reading this leaflet on oral contraceptives.
1. What Oral Contraceptives Are and How They Work. Oral contraceptives are of two types. The most common, often simply called "the pill," is a combination of an estrogen and a progestogen, the two kinds of female hormones. The amount of estrogen and progestogen can vary, but the amount of estrogen is most important because both the effectiveness and some of the dangers of oral contraceptives are related to the amount of estrogen. This kind of oral contraceptive works principally by preventing release of an egg from the ovary. When the amount of estrogen is 50 micrograms or more, and the pill is taken as directed, oral contraceptives are more than 99% effective (ie, there would be less than one pregnancy if 100 women used the pill for 1 year). Pills that contain 20 to 35 micrograms of estrogen vary slightly in effectiveness, ranging from 98% to more than 99% effective. Norlestrin was shown in clinical trials to be more than 99% effective.
The second type of oral contraceptive, often called the "mini-pill," contains only a progestogen. It works in part by preventing release of an egg from the ovary but also by keeping sperm from reaching the egg and by making the uterus (womb) less receptive to any fertilized egg that reaches it. The mini-pill is less effective than the combination oral contraceptive, about 97% effective.
In addition, the progestogen-only pill has a tendency to cause irregular bleeding which may be quite inconvenient, or cessation of bleeding entirely. The progestogen-only pill is used despite its lower effectiveness in the hope that it will prove not to have some of the serious side effects of the estrogen-containing pill (which follows) but it is not yet certain that the mini-pills does in fact have fewer serious side effects. The discussion which follows, while based mainly on information about the combination pills, should be considered to apply, as well, to the mini-pill.
2. Other Nonsurgical Ways to Prevent Pregnancy. As this leaflet will explain, oral contraceptives have several serious risks. Other methods of contraception have lesser risks or none at all. They are also less effective than oral contraceptives but, used properly, may be effective enough for many women. The following gives reported pregnancy rates (the number of women out of 100 who would become pregnant in 1 year) for these methods:
Pregnancies Per 100 Women Per Year
Intrauterine device (IUD), less than 1-6; Diaphragm with spermicidal products (creams or jellies), 2-20; Condom (rubber), 3-36; Aerosol foams, 2-29; Jellies and creams, 4-36; Periodic abstinence (rhythm) all types, less than 1-47; *1. Calendar method, 14-47; 2. Temperature method, 1-20; 3. Temperature method—intercourse only in postovulatory phase, less than 1-7; 4. Mucus method, 1-25;* No contraception, 60-80.
The figures (except for the IUD) vary considerably because people differ in how well they use each method. Very faithful users of the various methods obtain very good results except for users of the calendar method of periodic abstinence (rhythm). Except for the IUD, effective use of these methods requires somewhat more effort than simply taking a single pill every morning, but it is an effort that many couples undertake successfully. Your doctor can tell you a great deal more about these methods of contraception.
3. The Dangers of Oral Contraceptives.
a. *Circulatory disorders (abnormal blood clotting and stroke due to hemorrhage).* Blood clots (in various blood vessels of the body) are the most common of the serious side effects of oral contraceptives. A clot can result in a stroke (if the clot is in the brain), a heart attack (if the clot is in a blood vessel of the heart), or a pulmonary embolus (a clot which forms in the legs or pelvis, then breaks off and travels to the lungs). Any of these can be fatal. Clots also occur rarely in the blood vessels of the eye, resulting in blindness or impairment of vision in that eye. There is evidence that the risk of clotting increases with higher estrogen doses. It is, therefore, important to keep the dose of estrogen as low as possible, so long as the oral contraceptive used has an acceptable pregnancy rate and doesn't cause unacceptable changes in the menstrual pattern. Furthermore, cigarette smoking by oral contraceptive users increases the risk of serious adverse effects on the heart and blood vessels. This risk increases with age and with heavy smoking (15 or more cigarettes per day) and begins to become quite marked in women over 35 years of age. For this reason, women who use oral contraceptives should not smoke.

The risk of abnormal clotting increases with age in both users and nonusers of oral contraceptives, but the increased risk from the contraceptives appears to be present at all ages. For oral contraceptive users in general, it has been estimated that in women between the ages of 15 and 34 the risk of death due to a circulatory disorder is about 1 in 12,000 per year, whereas for nonusers the rate is about 1 in 50,000 per year. In the age group 35 to 44, the risk is estimated to be about 1 in 2,500 per year for oral contraceptive users and about 1 in 10,000 per year for nonusers.

Even without the pill the risk of having a heart attack increases with age and is also increased by such heart attack risk factors as high blood pressure, high cholesterol, obesity, diabetes, and cigarette smoking. Without any risk factors present, the use of oral contraceptives alone may double the risk of heart attack. However, the combination of cigarette smoking, especially heavy smoking, and oral contraceptive use greatly increases the risk of heart attack. Oral contraceptive users who smoke are about 5 times more likely to have a heart attack than users who do not smoke and about 10 times more likely to have a heart attack than nonusers who do not smoke. It has been estimated that users between the ages of 30 and 39 who smoke have about a 1 in 10,000 chance each year of having a fatal heart attack compared to about a 1 in 50,000 chance in users who do not smoke, and about a 1 in 100,000 chance in nonusers who do not smoke. In the age group 40 to 44, the risk is about 1 in 1,700 per year for users who smoke compared to about 1 in 10,000 for users who do not smoke and to about 1 in 14,000 per year for nonusers who do not smoke. Heavy smoking (about 15 cigarettes or more a day) further increases the risk. If you do not smoke and have none of the other heart attack risk factors described above, you will have a smaller risk than listed. If you have several heart attack risk factors, the risk may be considerably greater than listed.

In addition to blood-clotting disorders, it has been estimated that women taking oral contraceptives are twice as likely as nonusers to have a stroke due to rupture of a blood vessel in the brain.

b. *Formation of tumors.* Studies have found that when certain animals are given the female sex hormone estrogen, which is an ingredient of oral contraceptives, continuously for long periods, cancers may develop in the breast, cervix, vagina, and liver.

These findings suggest that oral contraceptives may cause cancer in humans. However, studies to date in women taking currently marketed oral contraceptives have not confirmed that oral contraceptives cause cancer in humans. Several studies have found no increase in breast cancer in users, although one study suggested oral contraceptives might cause an increase in breast cancer in women who already have benign breast disease (eg, cysts).

Women with a strong family history of breast cancer or who have breast nodules, fibrocystic disease, or abnormal mammograms or who were exposed to DES (diethylstilbestrol), an estrogen, during their mother's pregnancy must be followed very closely by their doctors if they choose to use oral contraceptives instead of another method of contraception. Many studies have shown that women taking oral contraceptives have less risk of getting benign breast disease than those who have not used oral contraceptives. Recently, strong evidence has emerged that estrogens (one component of oral contraceptives), when given for periods of more than one year to women after the menopause, increase the risk of cancer of the uterus (womb). There is also some evidence that a kind of oral contraceptive which is no longer marketed, the sequential oral contraceptive, may increase the risk of cancer of the uterus. There remains no evidence, however, that the oral contraceptives now available increase the risk of this cancer.

Oral contraceptives do cause, although rarely, a benign (nonmalignant) tumor of the liver. These tumors do not spread, but they may rupture and cause internal bleeding, which may be fatal. A few cases of cancer of the liver have been reported in women using oral contraceptives, but it is not yet known whether the drug caused them.

c. *Dangers to a developing child if oral contraceptives are used in or immediately preceding pregnancy.* Oral contraceptives should not be taken by pregnant women because they may damage the developing child. An increased risk of birth defects, including heart defects and limb defects, has been associated with the use of sex hormones, including oral contraceptives, in pregnancy. In addition, the developing female child whose mother has received DES (diethylstilbestrol), an estrogen, during pregnancy has a risk of getting cancer of the vagina or cervix in her teens or young adulthood. This risk is estimated to be about 1 in 1,000 exposures or less. Abnormalities of the urinary and sex organs have been reported in male offspring so exposed. It is possible that other estrogens, such as the estrogens in oral contraceptives, could have the same effect in the child if the mother takes them during pregnancy.

If you stop taking oral contraceptives to become pregnant, your doctor may recommend that you use another method of contraception for a short while. The reason for this is that there is evidence from studies in women who have had "miscarriages" soon after stopping the pill, that the lost fetuses are more likely to be abnormal. Whether there is an overall increase in "miscarriage" in women who become pregnant soon after stopping the pill, as compared with women who do not use the pill, is not known, but it is possible that there may be. If, however, you do become pregnant soon after stopping oral contraceptives, and do not have a miscarriage, there is no evidence that the baby has an increased risk of being abnormal.

d. *Gallbladder disease.* Women who use oral contraceptives have a greater risk than nonusers of having gallbladder disease requiring surgery. The increased risk may first appear within 1 year of use and may double after 4 or 5 years of use.

e. *Other side effects of oral contraceptives.* Some women using oral contraceptives experience unpleasant side effects that are not dangerous and are not likely to damage their health. Some of these may be temporary. Your breasts may feel tender, nausea and vomiting may occur, you may gain or lose weight, and your ankles may swell. A spotty darkening of the skin, particularly of the face, is possible and may persist. You may notice unexpected vaginal bleeding or changes in your menstrual period. Irregular bleeding is frequently seen when using the mini-pill or combination oral contraceptives containing less than 50 micrograms of estrogen.

More serious side effects include worsening of migraine, asthma, epilepsy, and kidney or heart disease because of a tendency for water to be retained in the body when oral contraceptives are used. Other side effects are growth of preexisting fibroid tumors of the uterus, mental depression, and liver problems with jaundice (yellowing of the skin). Your doctor may find that levels of sugar and fatty substances in your blood are elevated; the long-term effects of these changes are not known. Some women develop high blood pressure while taking oral contraceptives, which ordinarily returns to the original levels when the oral contraceptive is stopped.

Other reactions, although not proved to be caused by oral contraceptives, are occasionally reported. These include more frequent urination and some discomfort when urinating, nervousness, dizziness, some loss of scalp hair, an increase in body hair, an increase or decrease in sex drive, appetite changes, cataracts, and a need for a change in contact lens prescription or inability to use contact lenses.

After you stop using oral contraceptives there may be a delay before you are able to become pregnant or before you resume having menstrual periods. This is especially true of women who had irregular menstrual cycles prior to the use of oral contraceptives. As discussed previously, your doctor may recommend that you wait a short while after stopping the pill before you try to become pregnant. During this time, use another form of contraception. You should consult your physician before resuming use of oral contraceptives after childbirth, especially if you plan to nurse your baby. Drugs in oral contraceptives are known to appear in the milk, and the long-range effect on infants is not known at this time. Furthermore, oral contraceptives may cause a decrease in your milk supply as well as in the quality of the milk.

4. Comparison of the Risks of Oral Contraceptives and Other Contraceptive Methods. The many studies on the risks and effectiveness of oral contraceptives and other methods of contraception have been analyzed to estimate the risk of death associated with various methods of contraception. This risk has two parts: (a) the risk of the method itself (eg, the risk that oral contraceptives will cause death due to abnormal clotting); and (b) the risk of death due to pregnancy or abortion in the event the method fails. The results of this analysis are shown in the following bar graph. The height of the bars is the number of deaths per 100,000 women each year. There are six sets of bars, each set referring to a specific age group of women. Within each set of bars, there is a single bar for each of the different contraceptive methods. For oral contraceptives, there are two bars—one for smokers and the other for nonsmokers. The analysis is based on present knowledge and new information could, of course, alter it. The analysis shows that the risk of death from all methods of birth control is low and below that associated with childbirth, except for oral contraceptives in women over 40 who smoke. It shows that the lowest risk of death is associated with the condom or diaphragm (traditional contraception) backed up by early abortion in case of failure of the condom or diaphragm to prevent pregnancy. Also, at any age the risk of death (due to unexpected pregnancy) from the use of traditional contraception, even without a backup of abortion, is generally the same as or less than that from use of oral contraceptives.

[See table on next page].

How to Use Oral Contraceptives As Safely and Effectively As Possible, Once You Have Decided to Use Them

1. What to Tell your Doctor.

You can make use of the pill as safely as possible, by telling your doctor if you have any of the following:

a. Conditions that mean you should not use oral contraceptives:

Clots in the legs or lungs
Clots in the legs or lungs in the past
A stroke, heart attack, or angina pectoris
Known or suspected cancer of the breast or sex organs
Unusual vaginal bleeding that has not yet been diagnosed
Known or suspected pregnancy

b. Conditions that your doctor will want to watch closely or which might cause him to suggest another method of contraception:

A family history of breast cancer
Breast nodules, fibrocystic disease of the breast, or an abnormal mammogram
Diabetes
High blood pressure
High cholesterol
Cigarette smoking
Migraine headaches
Heart or kidney disease
Epilepsy
Mental depression
Fibroid tumors of the uterus
Gallbladder disease

c. Once you are using oral contraceptives, you should be alert for signs of a serious adverse effect and call your doctor if they occur:

Continued on next page

This product information was prepared in August, 1984. On these and other Parke-Davis Products, information may be obtained by addressing PARKE-DAVIS, Division of Warner-Lambert Company, Morris Plains, New Jersey 07950.

Parke-Davis—Cont.

Sharp pain in the chest, coughing blood, or sudden shortness of breath (indicating possible clots in the lungs)
Pain in the calf (possible clot in the leg)
Crushing chest pain or heaviness (indicating possible heart attack)
Sudden severe headache or vomiting, dizziness or fainting, disturbance of vision or speech, or weakness or numbness in an arm or leg (indicating a possible stroke)
Sudden partial or complete loss of vision (indicating a possible clot in the eye)
Breast lumps (you should ask your doctor to show you how to examine your own breasts)
Severe pain in the abdomen (indicating a possible ruptured tumor of the liver)
Severe depression
Yellowing of the skin (jaundice)
2. How to Take the Pill So That It Is Most Effective.
Reduced effectiveness and an increased incidence of breakthrough bleeding have been associated with the use of oral contraceptives with antibiotics such as rifampin, ampicillin, and tetracycline or with certain other drugs, such as barbiturates, phenylbutazone or phenytoin sodium. You should use an additional means of contraception during any cycle in which any of these drugs are taken.

Directions For 21-Day Dosage Regimen

a. The first day of your period is Day 1. On the fifth day (Day 5), start taking one tablet daily, beginning with the tablet in the upper left corner of the Petipac. In the space provided, write the day you start. To remove a tablet, press down on it with your thumb or finger. The tablet will drop through a hole in the bottom of the Petipac. Do not press on the tablet with your thumbnail or fingernail, or any other sharp object.

If your period begins on:	Start taking tablets on:
Sunday	Thursday
Monday	Friday
Tuesday	Saturday
Wednesday	Sunday
Thursday	Monday
Friday	Tuesday
Saturday	Wednesday

b. Continue to take one tablet daily until all the tablets have been taken.
c. After you have taken all 21 tablets, stop and don't take any tablets for the next seven days. You should have a menstrual period one to three days after you stop taking tablets; sometimes, it may take a day or so longer.
d. After seven days, during which you take no tablets, put a new refill in your Petipac and begin a new course of tablets, taking one tablet daily for 21 days. You will always start each new course of 21 tablets on the same day of the week. Likewise, the interval of no tablets will always start on the same day of the week.
e. If spotting should occur at an unexpected time, continue to take your tablets as directed. Spotting is usually temporary and without significance. However, if bleeding should occur at an unexpected time, consult your physician. Call your physician regarding any problem or change in your general health that may concern you.
f. If you forget to take a tablet, take it as soon as you remember, even if it is the next day. Then take the next scheduled tablet at the usual time. If you miss two consecutive tablets, take two tablets daily for the next two days. Then resume the regular schedule. While there is little likelihood of pregnancy occurring if you miss only one or two tablets, the possibility of pregnancy increases with each successive day that tablets are missed. *However, if you are taking* Loestrin 21 1/20, *in addition to taking two white tablets a day for two days, you should use an additional means of contraception for seven consecutive days.* If you miss three consecutive tablets, discard any tablets remaining and begin a new course of tablets, starting seven days after the last tablet was taken, even if you are still menstruating. You should use an alternate means of contraception, other than oral tablets, until the start of your next menstrual period.
Remembering to take tablets according to schedule is stressed because of its importance in providing you the greatest degree of protection.

Directions For 28-Day Dosage Regimen

a. The first day of your period is Day 1. On the fifth day (Day 5), start taking one *light-colored* tablet daily, beginning with the tablet in the upper left corner of the Petipac. In the space provided, write the day you start. Take all the tablets in the top row first, followed by the second row, and so on. To remove a tablet, press down on it with your thumb or finger. The tablet will drop through a hole in the bottom of the Petipac. Do not press on the tablet with your thumbnail or fingernail, or any other sharp object.

If your period begins on:	Start taking tablets on:
Sunday	Thursday
Monday	Friday
Tuesday	Saturday
Wednesday	Sunday
Thursday	Monday
Friday	Tuesday
Saturday	Wednesday

b. On the day after taking the last *light-colored* tablet, begin taking one *brown* tablet daily until all the tablets have been taken.
c. When the last tablet has been taken, put a new refill in your Petipac and, without interruption, begin a new course of tablets by taking the *light-colored* tablets first, followed by the *brown* tablets. There should never be a day when you are not taking a tablet.
d. Continue taking *light-colored* tablets without interruption whether or not your period has occurred or is still in progress. Your period will usually occur during the time you are taking *brown* tablets.
e. If spotting should occur at an unexpected time, continue to take your tablets as directed. Spotting is usually temporary and without significance. However, if bleeding should occur at an unexpected time, consult your physician. Call your physician regarding any problem or change in your general health that may concern you.
f. If you forget to take a *light-colored* tablet, take it as soon as you remember, even if it is the next day. Then take the next scheduled *light-colored* tablet at the usual time. If you miss two consecutive *light-colored* tablets, take two *light-colored*

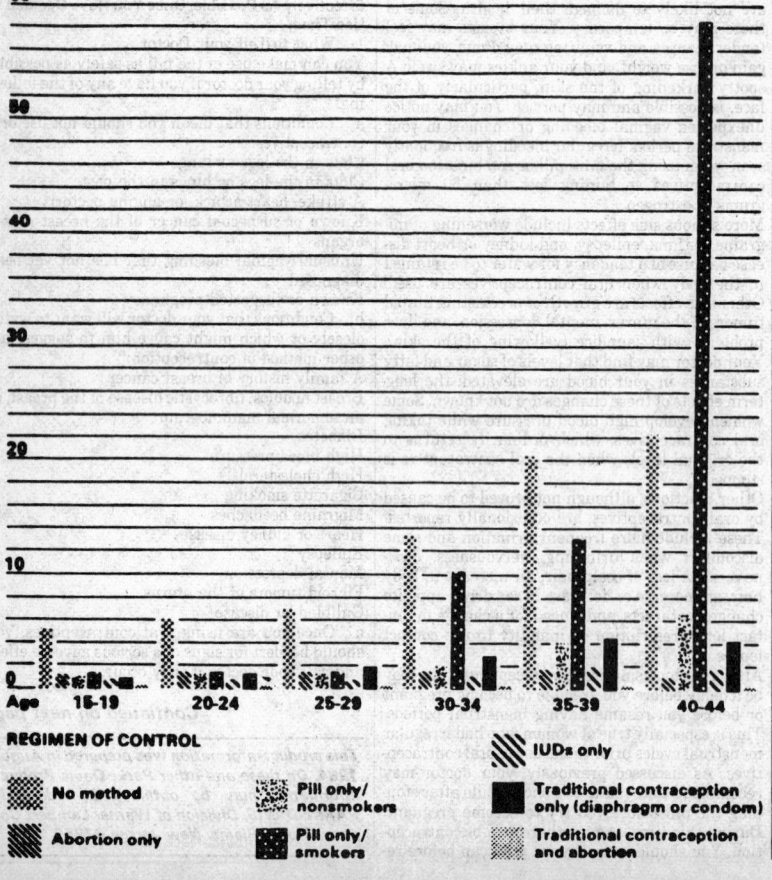

Figure 1. Estimated annual number of deaths associated with control of fertility and no control per 100,000 nonsterile women, by regimen of control and age of woman.

tablets daily for the next two days. Then resume the regular schedule. While there is little likelihood of pregnancy occurring if you miss only one or two tablets, the possibility of pregnancy increases with each successive day that tablets are missed. *However, if you are taking* Loestrin Fe 1/20, *in addition to taking two white tablets a day for two days, you should use an additional means of contraception for seven consecutive days.* If you miss three consecutive *light-colored* tablets discard any tablets remaining and begin a new course of tablets, starting seven days after the last *light-colored* tablet was taken, even if you are still menstruating. You should use an alternate means of contraception, other than oral tablets, until the start of your next menstrual period.

g. If you miss one or more *brown* tablets discard the remainder and begin a new course of tablets no later than the eighth day after you took the last *light-colored* tablet. Under no circumstances should you substitute a *brown* tablet for a *light-colored* one, or take any *brown* tablet before you have taken all the *light-colored* tablets, unless your physician advises you to do so. Remembering to take tablets according to schedule is stressed because of its importance in providing you the greatest degree of protection.

Missed Menstrual Periods For Both Dosage Regimens: At times there may be no menstrual period after a cycle of pills. Therefore, if you miss one menstrual period but have taken the pills *exactly as your were supposed to,* continue as usual into the next cycle. If you have not taken the pills correctly and miss a menstrual period, *you may be pregnant* and should stop taking oral contraceptives until your doctor determines whether or not you are pregnant. Until you can get to your doctor, use another form of contraception. If two consecutive menstrual periods are missed, you should stop taking pills until it is determined whether you are pregnant. If you do become pregnant while using oral contraceptives, you should discuss the risks to the developing child with your doctor.

Periodic Examination
Your doctor will take a complete medical and family history before prescribing oral contraceptives. At that time and about once a year thereafter, he will generally examine your blood pressure, breasts, abdomen, and pelvic organs (including a Papanicolaou smear, ie, test for cancer).

Summary: Oral contraceptives are the most effective method, except sterilization, for preventing pregnancy. Other methods, when used conscientiously, are also very effective and have fewer risks. The serious risks of oral contraceptives are uncommon and the "pill" is a very convenient method of preventing pregnancy.

If you have certain conditions or have had these conditions in the past, you should not use oral contraceptives because the risk is too great. These conditions are listed in this leaflet. If you do not have these conditions, and decide to use the "pill," please read this leaflet carefully so that you can use the "pill" most safely and effectively.

Based on his or her assessment of your medical needs, your doctor has prescribed this drug for you. Do not give this drug to anyone else.

0913G150
Shown in Product Identification Section, page 424

LOPID®
[lō′ pĭd]
(gemfibrozil capsules, USP)

Description: LOPID (gemfibrozil) is a lipid regulating agent. It is available as capsules for oral administration. Each capsule contains 300 mg gemfibrozil. The chemical name is 5-(2,5-dimethylphenoxy)-2,2-dimethylpentanoic acid.

The empirical formula is $C_{15}H_{22}O_3$ and the molecular weight is 250.35; the solubility in water and acid is 0.0019% and in dilute base it is greater than 1%. The melting point is 58°-61°C. Gemfibrozil is a white solid which is stable under ordinary conditions.

Clinical Pharmacology: LOPID is a lipid regulating agent which lowers elevated serum lipids primarily by decreasing serum triglyceride with a variable reduction in total serum cholesterol. These decreases occur primarily in the very low density lipoprotein (VLDL) fraction and less frequently in the low density lipoprotein (LDL) fraction. In addition, LOPID may increase the high density lipoprotein (HDL) cholesterol fraction, an action considered of possible benefit to inhibition of the atherosclerotic process. The mechanism of action has not been definitively established. In man, LOPID has been shown to inhibit peripheral lipolysis and to decrease the hepatic extraction of free fatty acids, thus reducing hepatic triglyceride production. LOPID also inhibits synthesis of VLDL carrier apoprotein, leading to a decrease in VLDL production.

Animal studies suggest that LOPID may, in addition to elevating HDL cholesterol, reduce incorporation of long-chain fatty acids into newly formed triglycerides, accelerate turnover and removal of cholesterol from the liver, and increase excretion of cholesterol in the feces.

LOPID is well absorbed from the gastrointestinal tract after oral administration. Peak plasma levels occur in one to two hours with a plasma half-life of 1.5 hours following single doses and 1.3 hours following multiple doses. Plasma levels appear proportional to dose and do not demonstrate accumulation across time following multiple doses.

LOPID mainly undergoes oxidation of a ring methyl group to successively form a hydroxymethyl and a carboxyl metabolite. Approximately seventy percent of the administered human dose is excreted in the urine, primarily as unchanged gemfibrozil. Six percent of the dose is accounted for in the feces. In a large, controlled multicenter trial of 427 patients, lipid and lipoprotein changes from average baseline (%) by hyperlipoproteinemic (HLP) type are summarized below for those patients receiving gemfibrozil, 1200 mg/day, at the end of 12 weeks.
[See table above].

Lopid HLP Type	TRIGLYCERIDE	CHOLESTEROL Total	VLDL	LDL	HDL	RATIO: HDL Cholesterol / Total Cholesterol
IIa	−44%	−4.2%	−44.3%	−5.8%	+24.6%	+33%
IIb	−45%	−8.6%	−45.0%	−6.4%	+19.5%	+34%
IV	−40%	−1.8%	−40.8%	+14.6%	+17.4%	+23%

Indications and Usage: Drug therapy should not be used for the routine treatment of elevated blood lipids for the prevention of coronary heart disease. Dietary therapy specific for the type of hyperlipidemia is the initial treatment of choice. Excess body weight and excess alcoholic intake may be important factors in hypertriglyceridemia and should be addressed prior to any drug therapy. Physical exercise can be an important ancillary measure.

Contributory diseases such as hypothyroidism or diabetes mellitus should be looked for and adequately treated. The use of drugs should be considered only when reasonable attempts have been made to obtain satisfactory results with nondrug methods. If the decision is to use drugs, the patient should be instructed that this does not reduce the importance of adhering to diet.

Because of chemical, pharmacological, and clinical similarities between gemfibrozil and clofibrate, and the adverse findings with clofibrate in two large clinical studies (see Warnings), use of gemfibrozil should be restricted to the following indications. LOPID may be considered for the treatment of adult patients with very high serum triglyceride levels (type IV hyperlipidemia) who present a risk of abdominal pain and pancreatitis and who do not respond adequately to a determined dietary effort to control them. Patients with triglyceride levels in excess of 750 mg per deciliter are likely to present such risk. LOPID (gemfibrozil) has little effect on elevated cholesterol levels in most subjects. A minority of subjects show a more pronounced response. However, it must be understood that there is no evidence that use of any lipid-altering drug will be beneficial in preventing death from coronary heart disease (See WARNINGS). Therefore, the physician should be very selective and confine gemfibrozil treatment to patients with clearly defined risk due to severe hypercholesterolemia (eg, individuals with familial hypercholesterolemia starting in childhood) who inadequately respond to appropriate diet and more effective cholesterol-lowering drugs.

LOPID is not useful for the hypertriglyceridemia of Type I hyperlipidemia.

The biochemical response to gemfibrozil is variable, and it is not always possible to predict from the lipoprotein type or other factors which patients will obtain favorable results. It is essential that lipid levels be assessed and that the drug be discontinued after three months in any patient in whom lipids do not show significant improvement. The effect of drug-induced reduction of serum cholesterol or triglyceride levels or elevation of HDL cholesterol levels on morbidity or mortality due to coronary heart disease has not been established. Several years may be required before ongoing long-term investigations will resolve this question.

Contraindications:
1. Hepatic or severe renal dysfunction, including primary biliary cirrhosis.
2. Preexisting gallbladder disease. (See Warnings).
3. Hypersensitivity to gemfibrozil.

Warnings:
1. Because of chemical, pharmacological, and clinical similarities between gemfibrozil and clofibrate, the adverse findings with clofibrate in two large clinical studies may also apply to gemfibrozil. In the first of those studies, the Coronary Drug Project, 1000 subjects with previous myocardial infarction were treated for five years with clofibrate. There was no difference in mortality between the clofibrate-treated subjects and 3000 placebo-treated subjects, but twice as many clofibrate-treated subjects developed cholelithiasis and cholecystitis requiring surgery. In the other study, conducted by the World Health Organization, 5000 subjects without known coronary heart disease were treated with clofibrate for five years and followed one year beyond. There was a statistically significant 36% higher total mortality in the clofibrate-treated than in a comparable placebo-treated control group. The excess mortality was due to noncardiovascular causes, including malignancy, postcholecystectomy complications, and pancreatitis. The higher risk of clofibrate-treated subjects for gallbladder disease was confirmed.

2. Long-Term Toxicity and Animal Tumorigenicity Studies: Long-term studies have been conducted in rats and mice at one and ten times the human dose. The incidence of benign liver nodules and liver carcinomas was significantly increased in high dose male rats. The incidence of liver carcinomas increased also in low dose males, but this increase was not statistically significant (p greater than 0.05). There were no statistically significant differences from controls in the incidence of liver tumors in female rats, and in male and female mice.

Continued on next page

This product information was prepared in August, 1984. On these and other Parke-Davis Products, information may be obtained by addressing PARKE-DAVIS, Division of Warner-Lambert Company, Morris Plains, New Jersey 07950.

Parke-Davis—Cont.

Electron microscopy studies have demonstrated a florid hepatic peroxisome proliferation following LOPID administration to the male rat. Similar changes have not been found in the human liver. Male rats had a dose-related increase of benign Leydig cell tumors. Subcapsular bilateral cataracts occurred in 10%, and unilateral in 6.3% of the high dose males.

3. Since a reduction of mortality from coronary artery disease has not been demonstrated and liver and interstitial cell testicular tumors were increased in male rats, LOPID should be administered only to those patients described in the Indications and Usage Section. If a significant serum lipid response is not obtained, LOPID should be discontinued.

4. Cholelithiasis—LOPID may increase cholesterol excretion into the bile leading to cholelithiasis. If cholelithiasis is suspected gallbladder studies are indicated. LOPID therapy should be discontinued if gallstones are found.

5. Concomitant Anticoagulants—Caution should be exercised when anticoagulants are given in conjunction with LOPID. The dosage of the anticoagulant should be reduced to maintain the prothrombin time at the desired level to prevent bleeding complications. Frequent prothrombin determinations are advisable until it has been definitely determined that the prothrombin level has stabilized.

Precautions:
1. **Initial Therapy**—Before instituting LOPID (gemfibrozil) therapy, every attempt should be made to control serum lipids with appropriate diet, exercise, weight loss in obese patients, and other medical problems such as diabetes mellitus and hypothyroidism.
2. **Continued Therapy**—Pretreatment laboratory studies should be performed to ensure that patients have abnormal levels of serum lipids. Periodic determinations of serum lipids should be obtained during LOPID administration. The drug should be withdrawn after three months if the lipid response is inadequate.
3. **Seasonal Variation of Lipid Levels**—LOPID is not expected to alter seasonal variations of higher serum lipid values in midwinter and late summer or the lower values in fall and spring.
4. **Impairment of Fertility**—Administration of approximately three and ten times the human dose to male rats for 10 weeks resulted in a dose-related decrease of fertility. Subsequent studies demonstrated that this effect was reversed after a drug-free period of about eight weeks, and it was not transmitted to their offspring.
5. **Pregnancy Category B**—Reproduction studies have been performed in the rat at doses 3 and 9 times the human dose, and in the rabbit at 2 and 6.7 times the human dose. These studies have revealed no evidence of impaired fertility in females or harm to the fetus due to LOPID. Minor fetotoxicity was manifested by reduced birth rates observed at the high dose levels. No significant malformations were found among almost 400 offspring from 36 litters of rats and 100 fetuses from 22 litters of rabbits.
There are no studies in pregnant women. In view of the fact that LOPID is tumorigenic in male rats, the use of LOPID in pregnancy should be reserved for those patients where the benefit clearly outweighs the possible risk to the patient or fetus.
6. **Nursing Mothers**—Because of the potential for tumorigenicity shown for gemfibrozil in male rats, a decision should be made whether to discontinue nursing or discontinue the drug, taking into account the importance of the drug to the mother.
7. **Hematologic Changes**—Mild hemoglobin, hematocrit and white blood cell decreases have been observed in occasional patients following initiation of LOPID therapy. However, these levels stabilize during long-term administration. Therefore, periodic blood counts are recommended during the first 12 months of LOPID administration.

8. **Liver Function**—Abnormal liver function tests have been observed occasionally during LOPID administration, including elevations of SGOT, SGPT, LDH, and alkaline phosphatase. These are usually reversible when LOPID is discontinued. Therefore periodic liver function studies are recommended and LOPID therapy should be terminated if abnormalities persist.
9. **Cardiac Arrhythmias**—Although no clinically significant abnormalities occurred that could be attributed to LOPID, the possibility exists that such abnormalities may occur.
10. **Use in Children**—Safety and efficacy in children have not been established.

Adverse Reactions: In controlled clinical trials of 805 patients, including 245 who received LOPID for at least one year, the most frequently reported adverse reactions associated with LOPID involved the gastrointestinal system. In decreasing order of frequency, these were abdominal pain (6.0%), epigastric pain (4.9%), diarrhea (4.8%), nausea (4.0%), vomiting (1.6%), and flatulence (1.1%). Other adverse reactions where the probability of a causal relationship to LOPID therapy exists are listed by system.

Integumentary: rash, dermatitis, pruritus, urticaria
Central Nervous System: headache, dizziness, blurred vision
Musculoskeletal: painful extremities
Hematopoietic: anemia, eosinophilia, leukopenia
Other reactions have been reported under conditions where a causal relationship is difficult to establish, thus the physician should be alert to these occurrences. Reports of viral and bacterial infections (common cold, cough, and urinary tract infections) were more common in gemfibrozil than in placebo-treated patients.

Other reactions were:
Gastrointestinal: dry mouth, constipation, anorexia, gas pain, dyspepsia
Musculoskeletal: back pain, arthralgia, muscle cramps, myalgia, swollen joints
Central Nervous System: vertigo, insomnia, paresthesia, tinnitus
Clinical Laboratory: hypokalemia, liver function abnormalities (increased SGOT, SGPT, LDH, CPK, alkaline phosphatase)
Miscellaneous: fatigue, malaise, syncope

Dosage and Administration: The recommended dose for adults is 1200 mg administered in two divided doses 30 minutes before the morning and evening meal. Some patients will experience therapeutic effects on 900 mg/day; a few may require 1500 mg/day for satisfactory results.

Drug Interactions: CAUTION SHOULD BE EXERCISED WHEN ANTICOAGULANTS ARE GIVEN IN CONJUNCTION WITH LOPID (GEMFIBROZIL). THE DOSAGE OF THE ANTICOAGULANT SHOULD BE REDUCED TO MAINTAIN THE PROTHROMBIN TIME AT THE DESIRED LEVEL TO PREVENT BLEEDING COMPLICATIONS. FREQUENT PROTHROMBIN DETERMINATIONS ARE ADVISABLE UNTIL IT HAS BEEN DEFINITELY DETERMINED THAT THE PROTHROMBIN LEVEL HAS STABILIZED.

Management of Overdosage: While there has been no reported case of overdosage, symptomatic supportive measures should be taken should it occur.

How Supplied:
N 0071-0669-24 (Capsule 669) LOPID Capsules, each containing 300 mg gemfibrozil, are available in 100's.
Parcode® No. 669.
Storage: Store below 30°C (86°F).

0669G013
Shown in Product Identification Section, page 424

MANDELAMINE® TABLETS ℞
[măn″dĕ′ lă-mĭne]
(methenamine mandelate tablets, USP)

MANDELAMINE SUSPENSION FORTE, ℞
500 mg/5ml
MANDELAMINE SUSPENSION, ℞
250 mg/5ml
(methenamine mandelate oral suspension, USP)

MANDELAMINE GRANULES ℞
(methenamine mandelate)

Description: Mandelamine (methenamine mandelate, USP), a urinary antibacterial agent, is the chemical combination of mandelic acid with methenamine. Mandelamine is available for oral use as film-coated tablets, suspension, and granules.

Clinical Pharmacology: Mandelamine is readily absorbed but remains essentially inactive until it is excreted by the kidney and concentrated in the urine. An acid urine is essential for antibacterial action, with maximum efficacy occurring at pH 5.5 or less. In an acid urine, mandelic acid exerts its antibacterial action and also contributes to the acidification of the urine. Mandelic acid is excreted by both glomerular filtration and tubular excretion. The methenamine component, in an acid urine, is hydrolyzed to ammonia and to the bactericidal agent formaldehyde. There is equally effective antibacterial activity against both gram-positive and gram-negative organisms, since the antibacterial action of mandelic acid and formaldehyde is nonspecific. There are reports that Mandelamine is ineffective in some infections with *Proteus vulgaris* and urea-splitting strains of *Pseudomonas aeruginosa* and *A aerogenes*. Since urea-splitting strains may raise the pH of the urine, particular attention to supplementary acidification is required. However, results in any single case will depend to a large extent on the underlying pathology and the overall management.

Indications and Usage: Mandelamine is indicated for the suppression or elimination of bacteriuria associated with pyelonephritis, cystitis, and other chronic urinary tract infections; also for infected residual urine sometimes accompanying neurologic diseases. When used as recommended, Mandelamine is particularly suitable for long-term therapy because of its safety and because resistance to the nonspecific bactericidal action of formaldehyde does not develop. Pathogens resistant to other antibacterial agents may respond to Mandelamine because of the non-specific effect of formaldehyde formed in an acid urine.

Prophylactic use rationale: Urine is a good culture medium for many urinary pathogens. Inoculation by a few organisms (relapse or reinfection) may lead to bacteriuria in susceptible individuals. Thus, the rationale of management in recurring urinary tract infection (bacteriuria) is to change the urine from a growth-supporting to a growth-inhibiting medium. There is a growing body of evidence that long-term administration of Mandelamine can prevent the recurrence of bacteriuria in patients with chronic pyelonephritis.

Therapeutic use rationale: Mandelamine helps to sterilize the urine, and in some situations in which underlying pathologic conditions prevent sterilization by any means, it can help to suppress the bacteriuria. Mandelamine should not be used alone for acute infections with parenchymal involvement causing systemic symptoms such as chills and fever. A thorough diagnostic investigation as a part of the overall management of the urinary tract infection should accompany the use of Mandelamine.

Contraindications: Contraindicated in renal insufficiency.
Mandelamine should not be used in patients who have previously exhibited hypersensitivity to it.

Precautions:
General: Dysuria may occur (usually at higher than recommended dosage). This can be controlled by reducing the dosage and the acidification. When urine acidification is contraindicated or unattainable (as with some urea-splitting bacteria), the drug is not recommended.

To avoid inducing lipid pneumonia, administer Mandelamine Suspension Forte and Mandelamine Suspension with care to elderly, debilitated or otherwise susceptible patients.

Drug Interactions: Formaldehyde and sulfamethizole form an insoluble precipitate in acid urine; therefore, Mandelamine should not be administered concurrently with sulfamethizole.

Drug/Laboratory Test Interactions: Formaldehyde interferes with fluorometric procedures for determination of urinary catecholamines and vanilmandelic acid (VMA) causing erroneously high results. Formaldehyde also causes falsely decreased urine estriol levels by reacting with estriol when acid hydrolysis techniques are used; estriol determinations which use enzymatic hydrolysis are unaffected by formaldehyde. Formaldehyde causes falsely elevated 17-hydroxy-corticosteroid levels when the Porter-Silber method is used and falsely decreased 5-hydroxy-indoleacetic acid (5HIAA) levels by inhibiting color development when nitrosonaphthol methods are used.

Pregnancy Category C. Animal reproduction studies have not been conducted with Mandelamine. It is also not known whether Mandelamine can cause fetal harm when administered to a pregnant woman or can affect reproduction capacity. Mandelamine should be given to a pregnant woman only if clearly needed.

Since introduction, published reports on the use of Mandelamine in pregnant women have not shown an increased risk of fetal abnormalities from use during pregnancy.

Adverse Reactions: An occasional patient may experience gastrointestinal disturbance or a generalized skin rash. Microscopic and rarely gross hematuria have been described.

Dosage and Administration: Directions for using Granules: dissolve contents of packet in 2-4 oz of water immediately before using. Solution formed may remain turbid.

Suspensions: Shake well before using.

The average adult dosage is 4 grams daily given as 1.0 gram after each meal and at bedtime. Children 6 to 12 should receive half the adult dose and children under 6 years of age should receive 250 mg per 30 lb body weight, four times daily. (See chart.) Since an acid urine is essential for antibacterial activity, with maximum efficacy occurring at pH 5.5 or below, restriction of alkalinizing foods and medication is thus desirable. If testing of urine pH reveals the need, supplemental acidification should be given.

DOSAGES

Dosage	Adults	Children
Tablets and Granules		
1.0 gram	1 tablet qid	—
	1 packet qid	—
0.5 gram	2 tablets qid	(Ages 6–12) 1 tablet qid
	—	(Ages 6–12) 1 packet qid
Suspension Forte		
500 mg/5 ml teasp.	2 teaspoonfuls (10 ml) qid	(Ages 6–12) 1 teaspoonful (5 ml) qid
Suspension		
250 mg/5 ml teasp.	—	(Age under 6) 1 teaspoonful (5 ml) per 30 lb body weight qid

How Supplied:
Mandelamine Tablets are supplied as:
N 0071-0166-24 0.5 g—Bottles of 100
N 0071-0166-32 0.5 g—Bottles of 1000
N 0071-0166-40 0.5 g—Unit dose packages of 100 (10 × 10 strips)
Each tablet is film coated, brown, and bears the P-D 166 monogram.
N 0071-0167-24 1.0 g—Bottles of 100
N 0071-0167-30 1.0 g—Bottles of 500
N 0071-0167-40 1.0 g—Unit dose packages of 100 (10 × 10 strips)
Each tablet is film coated, and bears the P-D 167 monogram.

Mandelamine Granules are supplied as:
N 0071-2177-02 0.5 g—Cartons of 56 individual packets.
N 0071-2176-03 1.0 g—Cartons of 56 individual packets.
Granules are orange flavored.

Mandelamine Suspension is supplied as:
N 0071-2173-23 250 mg/5 ml—Bottles of 16 fl oz
Suspension is cream colored, coconut flavored, and in vegetable oil.

Mandelamine Suspension Forte is supplied as:
N 0071-2174-20 500 mg/5 ml—Bottles of 8 fl oz
N 0071-2174-23 500 mg/5 ml—Bottles of 16 fl oz
Suspension is rosy pink, cherry flavored, and in vegetable oil.

Store between 15°–30°C (59°–86°F).

0166G034
Shown in Product Identification Section, page 424

MECLOMEN®   ℞
[mĕ'clō" mĕn]
(Meclofenamate Sodium Capsules, USP)

Description: Meclomen (meclofenamate sodium) is N-(2, 6-dichloro-m-tolyl) anthranilic acid, sodium salt, monohydrate. It is an antiinflammatory drug for oral administration. Meclomen capsules contain 50 mg or 100 mg meclofenamic acid as the sodium salt.

It is a white powder with melting point 287° to 291°C, molecular weight 336.15, and water solubility greater than 250 mg/ml.

Clinical Pharmacology: Meclomen is a nonsteroidal agent which has demonstrated antiinflammatory, analgesic, and antipyretic activity in laboratory animals. The mode of action, like that of other nonsteroidal antiinflammatory agents, is not known. Therapeutic action does not result from pituitary-adrenal stimulation. In animal studies, Meclomen was found to inhibit prostaglandin synthesis and to compete for binding at the prostaglandin receptor site. These properties may be responsible for the antiinflammatory action of Meclomen. There is no evidence that Meclomen alters the course of the underlying disease. Following a single oral dose to normal human volunteers, peak plasma levels occurred in 0.5 to 1 hr, with a half-life of 2 hr (3.3 hr following multiple doses). Plasma levels are proportional to dose. There is no evidence of accumulation of drug. Urinary and fecal excretion of tritium-labeled Meclomen account for 80% to 102% of the total dose, with about two thirds appearing in urine and one third in feces. Most of the urinary excretion occurs as the glucuronide conjugates of the metabolites, with only small amounts of free drug recovered.

In several human isotope studies, Meclomen, at a dosage of 300 mg/day, produced a fecal blood loss of 1 to 2 ml per day, and 2 to 3 ml per day at 400 mg/day. Aspirin, at a dosage of 3.6 g/day, caused a fecal blood loss of 6 ml per day.

In a multiple-dose, one-week study in normal human volunteers, Meclomen had little or no effect on collagen-induced platelet aggregation, platelet count, or bleeding time. In comparison, aspirin suppressed collagen-induced platelet aggregation and increased bleeding time. The concomitant administration of antacids (aluminum and magnesium hydroxides) does not interfere with absorption of Meclomen.

Controlled clinical trials comparing Meclomen with aspirin demonstrated comparable efficacy in rheumatoid arthritis. The Meclomen-treated patients had fewer reactions involving the special senses, specifically tinnitus, but more gastrointestinal reactions, specifically diarrhea.

The incidence of patients who discontinued therapy due to adverse reactions was similar for both the Meclomen and aspirin-treated groups.

The improvement with Meclomen reported by patients and the reduction of the disease activity as evaluated by both physicians and patients with rheumatoid arthritis are associated with a significant reduction in number of tender joints, severity of tenderness, and duration of morning stiffness.

The improvement reported by patients and as evaluated by physicians in patients treated with Meclomen for osteoarthritis is associated with a significant reduction in night pain, pain on walking, degree of starting pain, and pain on passive motion. The function of knee joints also improved significantly.

Meclomen has been used in combination with gold salts or corticosteroids in patients with rheumatoid arthritis. Studies have demonstrated that Meclomen contributes to the improvement of patients' conditions while maintained on gold salts or corticosteroids. Data are inadequate to demonstrate that Meclomen in combination with salicylates produces greater improvement than that achieved with Meclomen alone.

Indications and Usage: Meclomen is indicated for relief of the signs and symptoms of acute and chronic rheumatoid arthritis and osteoarthritis. Meclomen is not recommended as the initial drug for treatment because of gastrointestinal side effects, including diarrhea which is sometimes severe. Selection of Meclomen requires a careful assessment of the benefit/risk ratio. (See Precautions, Warnings, and Adverse Reactions sections.) The safety and effectiveness of Meclomen have not been established in those patients with rheumatoid arthritis who are designated by the American Rheumatism Association as Functional Class IV (incapacitated, largely or wholly bedridden, or confined to a wheelchair, little or no self-care).

Meclomen is not recommended in children because adequate studies to demonstrate safety and efficacy have not been carried out.

Contraindications: Meclomen should not be used in patients who have previously exhibited hypersensitivity to it.

Because the potential exists for cross sensitivity to aspirin or other nonsteroidal antiinflammatory drugs, Meclomen should not be given to patients in whom these drugs induce symptoms of bronchospasm, allergic rhinitis, or urticaria.

Warnings: In patients with a history of upper gastrointestinal tract disease, Meclomen should be given under close supervision and only after consulting the Adverse Reactions section. Peptic ulceration and gastrointestinal bleeding, sometimes severe, including one fatality, have been reported in patients receiving Meclomen.

Diarrhea, gastrointestinal irritation, and abdominal pain may be associated with Meclomen therapy. Dosage reduction or temporarily stopping the drug have generally controlled these symptoms. (See Adverse Reactions and Dosage and Administration sections.)

Precautions:
General: Patients receiving nonsteroidal antiinflammatory agents, such as Meclomen, should be evaluated periodically to insure that the drug is still necessary and well tolerated. (See other Precautions, Warnings, and Adverse Reactions.)

Decreases in hemoglobin and/or hematocrit levels have occurred in approximately 1 of 6 patients, but rarely required discontinuation of Meclomen therapy. The clinical data revealed no evidence of in-

Continued on next page

This product information was prepared in August, 1984. On these and other Parke-Davis Products, information may be obtained by addressing PARKE-DAVIS, Division of Warner-Lambert Company, Morris Plains, New Jersey 07950.

Parke-Davis—Cont.

creased chronic blood loss, bone-marrow suppression, or hemolysis to account for the decreases in hemoglobin or hematocrit levels. Patients who are receiving long-term Meclomen therapy should have hemoglobin and hematocrit values determined if anemia is suspected on clinical grounds. If a patient develops visual symptoms (see Adverse Reactions) during Meclomen therapy, the drug should be discontinued and the patient should have a complete ophthalmologic examination.

When Meclomen is used in combination with steroid therapy, any reduction in steroid dosage should be gradual to avoid the possible complications of sudden steroid withdrawal.

Adverse effects are seen more commonly in the elderly, therefore a lower starting dose and careful follow-up are advised.

As with other nonsteroidal antiinflammatory drugs, borderline evaluations of one or more liver tests may occur in some patients. These abnormalities may progress, may remain essentially unchanged, or may be transient with continued therapy. The SGPT (ALT) test is probably the most sensitive indicator of liver dysfunction. Meaningful (3 times the upper limit of normal) elevations of SGPT or SGOT (AST) occurred in controlled clinical trials in less than 1% of patients. A patient with symptoms and/or signs suggesting liver dysfunction, or in whom an abnormal liver test has occurred, should be evaluated for evidence of the development of more severe hepatic reaction while on therapy with Meclomen. Severe hepatic reactions, including jaundice and cases of fatal hepatitis, have been reported with other nonsteroidal antiinflammatory drugs. Although such reactions are rare, if abnormal liver tests persist or worsen, if clinical signs and symptoms consistent with liver disease develop, or if systemic manifestations occur (eg, eosinophilia, rash), Meclomen should be discontinued.

Information for Patients: Patients should be advised that nausea, vomiting, diarrhea, and abdominal pain have been associated with the use of Meclomen. The patient should be made aware of a possible drug connection and accordingly should consider discontinuing the drug and contacting his or her physician if any of these conditions are severe.

Meclomen may be taken with meals or milk to control gastrointestinal complaints. Concomitant administration of an antacid (specifically, aluminum and magnesium hydroxides) does not interfere with the absorption of the drug.

Laboratory Tests: Patients receiving long-term Meclomen therapy should have hemoglobin and hematocrit values determined if signs or symptoms of anemia occur.

Low white blood cell counts were rarely observed in clinical trials. These low counts were transient and usually returned to normal while the patient continued on Meclomen therapy. Persistent leukopenia, granulocytopenia, or thrombocytopenia warrant further clinical evaluation and may require discontinuation of the drug.

When abnormal blood chemistry values are obtained, follow-up studies are indicated.

Elevations of serum transaminase levels and of alkaline phosphatase levels occurred in approximately 4% of patients. An occasional patient had elevations of serum creatinine or BUN levels.

Drug Interactions:
1. **Warfarin:** Meclomen enhances the effect of warfarin. Therefore, when Meclomen is given to a patient receiving warfarin, the dosage of warfarin should be reduced to prevent excessive prolongation of the prothrombin time.
2. **Aspirin:** Concurrent administration of aspirin may lower Meclomen plasma levels, possibly by competing for protein-binding sites. The urinary excretion of Meclomen is unaffected by aspirin, indicating no change in Meclomen absorption. Meclomen does not affect serum salicylate levels. Greater fecal blood loss results from concomitant administration of both drugs than from either drug alone.
3. **Propoxyphene:** The concurrent administration of propoxyphene hydrochloride does not affect the bioavailability of Meclomen.
4. **Antacids:** Concomitant administration of aluminum and magnesium hydroxides does not interfere with absorption of Meclomen.

Carcinogenesis: An 18-month study in rats revealed no evidence of carcinogenicity.

Usage in Pregnancy: Meclomen like aspirin and other nonsteroidal antiinflammatory drugs causes fetotoxicity, minor skeletal malformations, eg, supernumerary ribs, and delayed ossification in rodent reproduction trials, but no major teratogenicity. Similarly, it prolongs gestation and interferes with parturition and with normal development of young before weaning. Meclomen is not recommended for use during pregnancy, particularly in the 1st and 3rd trimesters based on these animal findings. There are, however, no adequate and well-controlled studies in pregnant women.

Usage in Nursing Mothers: It is not known whether Meclomen is excreted in human milk. Because of the effects on suckling rodents and the fact that many drugs are excreted in human milk, Meclomen is not recommended for nursing women.

Pediatric Use: Safety and effectiveness in children below the age of 14 have not been established.

Adverse Reactions:
Incidence Greater than 1%
The following adverse reactions were observed in clinical trials and included observations from more than 2,700 patients, 594 of whom were treated for one year and 248 for at least two years.
Gastrointestinal: The most frequently reported adverse reactions associated with Meclomen involve the gastrointestinal system. In controlled studies of up to six months duration, these disturbances occurred in the following decreasing order of frequency with the approximate incidences in parentheses: diarrhea (10–33%), nausea with or without vomiting (11%), other gastrointestinal disorders (10%), and abdominal pain.* In long-term uncontrolled studies of up to four years duration, one third of the patients had at least one episode of diarrhea some time during Meclomen therapy.

In approximately 4% of the patients in controlled studies, diarrhea was severe enough to require discontinuation of Meclomen. The occurrence of diarrhea is dose related, generally subsides with dose reduction, and clears with termination of therapy. The incidence of diarrhea in patients with osteoarthritis is generally lower than that reported in patients with rheumatoid arthritis.

Other reactions less frequently reported were pyrosis,* flatulence,* anorexia, constipation, stomatitis, and peptic ulcer. The majority of the patients with peptic ulcer had either a history of ulcer disease or were receiving concomitant antiinflammatory drugs, including corticosteroids which are known to produce peptic ulceration.
Cardiovascular: edema
Dermatologic: rash,* urticaria, pruritus
Central Nervous System: headache,* dizziness*
Special Senses: tinnitus
*Incidence between 3% and 9%. Those reactions occurring in 1% to 3% of patients are not marked with an asterisk.

Incidence Less than 1%.
Probably Causally Related
The following adverse reactions were reported less frequently than 1% during controlled clinical trials and through voluntary reports since marketing. The probability of a causal relationship exists between the drug and these adverse reactions.
Gastrointestinal: Bleeding and/or perforation with or without obvious ulcer formation
Renal: Renal failure.
Hematologic: Neutropenia, thrombocytopenic purpura, leukopenia, agranulocytosis, hemolytic anemia, eosinophilia, decrease in hemoglobin and/or hematocrit
Dermatologic: Erythema multiforme, Stevens-Johnson syndrome, exfoliative dermatitis
Hepatic: Alteration of liver function tests
Allergic: Lupus and serum sickness-like symptoms
Incidence Less than 1%
Causal Relationship Unknown
Other reactions have been reported but under conditions where a causal relationship could not be established. However, in these rarely reported events, that possibility cannot be excluded. Therefore, these observations are listed to alert physicians.
Cardiovascular: palpitations
Central Nervous System: malaise, fatigue, paresthesia, insomnia, depression
Special Senses: blurred vision, taste disturbances, decreased visual acuity, temporary loss of vision, reversible loss of color vision, retinal changes including macular fibrosis, macular and perimacular edema, conjunctivitis, iritis
Renal: nocturia
Gastrointestinal: paralytic ileus
Dermatologic: erythema nodosum, hair loss
Overdosage: The following is based on the little information available concerning overdosage with Meclomen and related compounds. After a massive overdose, CNS stimulation may be manifested by irrational behavior, marked agitation and generalized seizures. Following this phase, renal toxicity (falling urine output, rising creatinine, abnormal urinary cellular elements) may be noted with possible oliguria or anuria and azotemia. One patient was anuric for about a week before diuresis and recovery occurred.

Management consists of emptying the stomach by emesis or lavage and instilling an ample dose of activated charcoal into the stomach. There is some evidence that charcoal will actively absorb Meclomen, but dialysis or hemoperfusion may be less effective because of plasma protein binding. The seizures should be controlled by an appropriate anticonvulsant regimen. Attention should be directed throughout, by careful monitoring, to the preservation of vital functions and fluid-electrolyte balance. Dialysis may be required to correct serious azotemia or electrolyte imbalance.

Dosage and Administration:
Usual Dosage: For rheumatoid arthritis and osteoarthritis, including acute exacerbations of chronic disease, the dosage is 200 to 400 mg per day, administered in three or four equal doses.

Therapy should be initiated at the lower dosage, then increased as necessary to improve clinical response. The dosage should be individually adjusted for each patient depending on the severity of the symptoms and the clinical response. The daily dosage should not exceed 400 mg per day. The smallest dosage of Meclomen that yields clinical control should be employed.

Although improvement may be seen in some patients in a few days, two to three weeks of treatment may be required to obtain the optimum therapeutic benefit.

After a satisfactory response has been achieved, the dosage should be adjusted as required. A lower dosage may suffice for long-term administration. If gastrointestinal complaints occur, see Warnings and Precautions. Meclomen may be administered with meals or with milk. If intolerance occurs, the dosage may need to be reduced. Therapy should be terminated if any severe adverse reactions occur.

How Supplied: (Capsule 268) Meclomen Capsules, each containing meclofenamate sodium monohydrate equivalent to 50 mg meclofenamic acid, are available:
N 0710-0268-24—bottles of 100
N 0710-0268-40—Uni/Use® 100's (10 × 10)
(Capsule 269) Meclomen Capsules, each containing meclofenamate sodium monohydrate equivalent to 100 mg meclofenamic acid, are available:
N 0710-0269-24—bottles of 100
N 0710-0269-30—bottles of 500
N 0710-0269-40—Uni/Use 100's (10 × 10)
Storage: Store at room temperature below 30°C (86°F). Protect from moisture and light.

0268G130

Shown in Product Identification Section, page 424

MILONTIN® ℞
[mĭl″ lŏn′ tĭn]
(phensuximide, USP)

Description: Milontin (phensuximide) is an anticonvulsant succinimide, chemically designated as N-methyl-2-phenylsuccinimide.

Action: Phensuximide suppresses the paroxysmal three-cycle-per-second spike and wave activity associated with lapses of consciousness which is common in absence (petit mal) seizures. The frequency of epileptiform attacks is reduced, apparently by depression of the motor cortex and elevation of the threshold of the central nervous system to convulsive stimuli.

Indication: Milontin is indicated for the control of absence (petit mal) seizures.

Contraindication: Phensuximide should not be used in patients with a history of hypersensitivity to succinimides.

Warnings: Blood dyscrasias, including some with fatal outcome, have been reported to be associated with the use of succinimides; therefore, periodic blood counts should be performed.

It has been reported that succinimides have produced morphological and functional changes in animal liver. For this reason, phensuximide should be administered with extreme caution to patients with known liver or renal diseases. Periodic urinalysis and liver function studies are advised for all patients receiving the drug.

Cases of systemic lupus erythematosus have been reported with the use of succinimides. The physician should be alert to this possibility.

Usage in pregnancy: The effects of Milontin in human pregnancy and nursing infants are unknown.

Recent reports suggest an association between the use of anticonvulsant drugs by women with epilepsy and an elevated incidence of birth defects in children born to these women. Data is more extensive with respect to phenytoin and phenobarbital, but these are also the most commonly prescribed anticonvulsants; less systematic or anecdotal reports suggest a possible similar association with the use of all known anticonvulsant drugs.

The reports suggesting an elevated incidence of birth defects in children of drug-treated epileptic women cannot be regarded as adequate to prove a definite cause-and-effect relationship. There are intrinsic methodologic problems in obtaining adequate data on drug teratogenicity in humans; the possibility also exists that other factors, eg, genetic factors or the epileptic condition itself, may be more important than drug therapy in leading to birth defects. The great majority of mothers on anticonvulsant medication deliver normal infants. It is important to note that anticonvulsant drugs should not be discontinued in patients in whom the drug is administered to prevent major seizures because of the strong possibility of precipitating status epilepticus with attendant hypoxia and threat to life. In individual cases where the severity and frequency of the seizure disorder are such that the removal of medication does not pose a serious threat to the patient, discontinuation of the drug may be considered prior to and during pregnancy, although it cannot be said with any confidence that even minor seizures do not pose some hazard to the developing embryo or fetus. The prescribing physician will wish to weigh these considerations in treating or counseling epileptic women of childbearing potential.

Hazardous activities: Phensuximide may impair the mental and/or physical abilities required for the performance of potentially hazardous tasks, such as driving a motor vehicle or other such activity requiring alertness; therefore, the patient should be cautioned accordingly.

Precautions: Phensuximide, when used alone in mixed types of epilepsy, may increase the frequency of grand mal seizures in some patients. As with other anticonvulsants, it is important to proceed slowly when increasing or decreasing dosage, as well as when adding or eliminating other medication. Abrupt withdrawal of anticonvulsant medication may precipitate absence (petit mal) status.

Adverse Reactions:
Gastrointestinal System: Gastrointestinal symptoms, such as nausea, vomiting, and anorexia, occur frequently, but may be the result of overdosage.
Nervous System: Neurologic and sensory reactions reported during therapy with phensuximide have included drowsiness, dizziness, ataxia, headache, dreamlike state, and lethargy. Side effects, such as drowsiness and dizziness, may be relieved by a reduction in total dosage.
Integumentary System: Dermatologic manifestations reported to be associated with the administration of phensuximide have included pruritus, skin eruptions, erythema multiforme, and erythematous rashes.
Genitourinary System: Genitourinary complications which have been reported include urinary frequency, renal damage, and hematuria.
Hemopoietic System: Hemopoietic complications associated with the administration of phensuximide include granulocytopenia, transient leukopenia, and pancytopenia.
Other: Miscellaneous reactions reported have been alopecia and muscular weakness.

Dosage and Administration: Milontin (phensuximide capsules, USP) is administered by the oral route in doses of 500 mg to 1 g two or three times daily. As with other anticonvulsant medication, the dosage should be adjusted to suit individual requirements. The total dosage, irrespective of age, may, therefore, vary between 1 and 3 g per day, the average being 1.5 g.

Milontin may be administered in combination with other anticonvulsants when other forms of epilepsy coexist with absence (petit mal).

How Supplied:
N 0071-0393-24 (Kapseal® 393)—Milontin Kapseals, each containing 0.5 g phensuximide; bottles of 100.

0393G0011
Shown in Product Identification Section, page 424

MYADEC®
[my′ă-dĕc″]

Each tablet represents:		% of US Recommended Daily Allowances (US RDA)
Vitamins	
Vitamin A	10,000 IU*	200%
Vitamin D	400 IU	100%
Vitamin E	30 IU	100%
Vitamin C (ascorbic acid)	250 mg	417%
Folic Acid	0.4 mg	100%
Thiamine (vitamin B₁)	10 mg	667%
Riboflavin (vitamin B₂)	10 mg	588%
Niacin†	100 mg	500%
Vitamin B₆	5 mg	250%
Vitamin B₁₂	6 mcg	100%
Pantothenic Acid	20 mg	200%
Minerals	
Iodine	150 mcg	100%
Iron	20 mg	111%
Magnesium	100 mg	25%
Copper	2 mg	100%
Zinc	20 mg	133%
Manganese	1.25 mg	‡

Ingredients: Sodium ascorbate, magnesium oxide, niacinamide, microcrystalline cellulose, ferrous fumarate, zinc sulfate monohydrate, ascorbic acid, gelatin, hydroxypropyl methylcellulose, vitamin E acetate, povidone, calcium pantothenate, FD and C yellow no 6 lake, silicon dioxide, riboflavin, thiamine mononitrate, polyethylene glycol 3350, magnesium stearate, pyridoxine hydrochloride, cupric sulfate anhydrous, sugar, vitamin A, manganese sulfate monohydrate, titanium dioxide, FD and C blue no 2 lake, FD and C red no 3 lake, ethylcellulose, methylparaben, candelilla wax, citric acid anhydrous, hydroxypropyl cellulose, polysorbate 80, folic acid, vanillin, potassium iodide, propylparaben, vitamin D, vitamin B₁₂.

* International Units
† Supplied as niacinamide
‡ No US Recommended Daily Allowance (US RDA) has been established for this nutrient.

Actions and Uses: High-potency vitamin supplement with minerals for adults.
Dosage: One tablet daily with a full meal.
How Supplied: N 0071-0335. In bottles of 130 and 250 and unit-dose packages of 100 (10 strips of 10 tablets).

NARDIL® ℞
[năr′dĭl″]
(Phenelzine Sulfate Tablets, USP)

Description: Nardil (phenelzine sulfate) is a potent inhibitor of monoamine oxidase (MAO). Chemically, it is a hydrazine derivative.

Actions: Monoamine oxidase is a complex enzyme system, widely distributed throughout the body. Drugs that inhibit monoamine oxidase in the laboratory are associated with a number of clinical effects. Thus, it is unknown whether MAO inhibition *per se*, other pharmacologic actions, or an interaction of both is responsible for the clinical effects observed. Therefore, the physician should become familiar with all the effects produced by drugs of this class.

Indications: Nardil has been found to be effective in depressed patients clinically characterized as "atypical," "nonendogenous," or "neurotic." These patients often have mixed anxiety and depression and phobic or hypochondriacal features. There is less conclusive evidence of its usefulness with severely depressed patients with endogenous features.

Nardil should rarely be the first antidepressant drug used. Rather, it is more suitable for use with patients who have failed to respond to the drugs more commonly used for these conditions. Nardil has had considerable use in combination with certain dibenzazepine derivatives in treatment-resistant patients without a significant incidence of serious side effects.

Contraindications: Nardil is contraindicated in patients with known sensitivity to the drug, pheochromocytoma, congestive heart failure, a history of liver disease, or abnormal liver function tests. The potentiation of sympathomimetic substances and related compounds by MAO inhibitors may result in hypertensive crises (See WARNINGS). Therefore, patients being treated with Nardil should not take sympathomimetic drugs (including amphetamines, cocaine, methylphenidate, dopamine, epinephrine and norepinephrine) or related compounds (including methyldopa, L-dopa, L-tryptophan, L-tyrosine, and phenylalanine). Hypertensive crises during Nardil therapy may also be caused by the ingestion of foods with a high concentration of tyramine or dopamine. Therefore, patients being treated with Nardil should avoid high protein food that has undergone protein breakdown by aging, fermentation, pickling, smoking, or bacterial contamination; patients should also avoid cheeses (especially aged varieties), pickled herring, beer, wine, liver, yeast extract (including brewer's yeast in large quantities), dry sausage (including Genoa salami, hard salami, pepperoni, and Lebanon bologna), pods of broad beans (Fava beans), and yogurt. Excessive amounts of caffeine and chocolate may also cause hypertensive reactions.

Nardil should not be used in combination with CNS depressants such as alcohol and certain narcotics. Excitation, seizures, delirium, hyperpy-

Continued on next page

This product information was prepared in August, 1984. On these and other Parke-Davis Products, information may be obtained by addressing PARKE-DAVIS, Division of Warner-Lambert Company, Morris Plains, New Jersey 07950.

Parke-Davis—Cont.

rexia, circulatory collapse, coma, and death have been reported in patients receiving MAOI therapy who have been given a single dose of meperidine. Nardil should not be administered together with or in rapid succession to other MAO inhibitors because HYPERTENSIVE CRISES and convulsive seizures, fever, marked sweating, excitation, delirium, tremor, coma, and circulatory collapse may occur.

List of MAO Inhibitors

Generic Name	Trademark
pargyline hydrochloride	Eutonyl® (Abbott Laboratories)
pargyline hydrochloride and methylclothiazide	Eutron® (Abbott Laboratories)
furazolidone	Furoxone® (Eaton Laboratories)
isocarboxazid	Marplan® (Roche)
procarbazine	Matulane® (Roche)
tranylcypromine	Parnate® (Smith Kline & French Laboratories)

Patients taking Nardil should not undergo elective surgery requiring general anesthesia. Also, they should not be given cocaine or local anesthesia containing sympathomimetic vasoconstrictors. The possible combined hypotensive effects of Nardil and spinal anesthesia should be kept in mind. Nardil should be discontinued at least 10 days prior to elective surgery.

Important:
Warnings: The most serious reactions to Nardil involve changes in blood pressure.
Hypertensive Crises: The most important reaction associated with Nardil administration is the occurrence of hypertensive crises, which have sometimes been fatal.
These crises are characterized by some or all of the following symptoms: occipital headache which may radiate frontally, palpitation, neck stiffness or soreness, nausea, vomiting, sweating (sometimes with fever and sometimes with cold, clammy skin), dilated pupils, and photophobia. Either tachycardia or bradycardia may be present and can be associated with constricting chest pain.
NOTE: Intracranial bleeding has been reported in association with the increase in blood pressure.
Blood pressure should be observed frequently to detect evidence of any pressor response in all patients receiving Nardil. Therapy should be discontinued immediately upon the occurrence of palpitation or frequent headaches during therapy.
Recommended treatment in hypertensive crisis: If a hypertensive crisis occurs, Nardil should be discontinued immediately and therapy to lower blood pressure should be instituted immediately. On the basis of present evidence, phentolamine is recommended. (The dosage reported for phentolamine is 5 mg intravenously.) Care should be taken to administer this drug slowly in order to avoid producing an excessive hypotensive effect. Fever should be managed by means of external cooling.
Warning to the patient: All patients should be warned that the following foods, beverages and medications must be avoided while taking Nardil, and for two weeks after discontinuing use.
Foods and Beverages To Avoid
Meat and Fish
Pickled herring
Liver
Dry sausage (including Genoa salami, hard salami, pepperoni, and Lebanon bologna)
Vegetables
Broad bean pods (fava bean pods)
Dairy Products
Cheese (cottage cheese and cream cheese are allowed)
Yogurt
Beverages
Beer and wine
Miscellaneous
Yeast extract (including brewer's yeast in large quantities)
Excessive amounts of chocolate and caffeine
Also, any spoiled or improperly refrigerated, handled or stored protein-rich foods such as meats, fish, and dairy products, including foods that may have undergone protein changes by aging, pickling, fermentation, or smoking to improve flavor should be avoided.
OTC Medications To Avoid
Cold tablets or liquids
Nasal decongestants (tablets, drops or spray)
Hay-fever medications
Sinus medications
Asthma inhalant medications
Antiappetite medicines
Weight-reducing preparations
"Pep" pills
Also, certain prescription drugs should be avoided. Therefore, patients under the care of another physician or dentist, should inform him/her they are taking Nardil.
Patients should be warned that the use of the above foods, beverages or medications may cause a reaction characterized by headache and other serious symptoms due to a rise in blood pressure.
Patients should be instructed to report promptly the occurrence of headache or other unusual symptoms.
Concomitant Use with Dibenzazepine Derivative Drugs
If the decision is made to administer Nardil concurrently with other antidepressant drugs, or within less than 10 days after discontinuation of antidepressant therapy, the patient should be cautioned by the physician regarding the possibility of adverse drug interaction.

List of Dibenzazepine Derivative Drugs

Generic Name	Trademark
nortriptyline hydrochloride	Aventyl® (Eli Lilly & Co.)
amitriptyline hydrochloride	Amitril® (Parke-Davis)
amitriptyline hydrochloride	Elavil® (Merck Sharp & Dohme)
amitriptyline hydrochloride	Endep® (Roche)
perphenazine and amitriptyline hydrochloride	Etrafon® (Schering Corporation)
perphenazine and amitriptyline hydrochloride	Triavil® (Merck Sharp & Dohme)
desipramine hydrochloride	Norpramin® (Merrell-National)
desipramine hydrochloride	Pertofrane® (USV)
imipramine hydrochloride	Tofranil® (Geigy)
doxepin	Adapin® (Pennwalt)
doxepin	Sinequan® (Pfizer)
carbamazepine	Tegretol® (Geigy)
cyclobenzaprine HCl	Flexeril® (Merck Sharp & Dohme)
amoxapine	Asendin® (Lederle)
maprotiline HCl	Ludiomil® (CIBA)
trimipramine maleate	Surmontil® (Ives)

Nardil should be used with caution in combination with antihypertensive drugs, including thiazide diuretics and β-blockers, since exaggerated hypotensive effects may result. MAO inhibitors including Nardil are contraindicated in patients receiving guanethidine.
Use in Pregnancy: The safe use of Nardil during pregnancy or lactation has not been established. The potential benefit of this drug, if used during pregnancy, lactation, or in women of childbearing age, should be weighed against the possible hazard to the mother or fetus.
Doses of Nardil in pregnant mice well exceeding the maximum recommended human dose have caused a significant decrease in the number of viable offspring per mouse. In addition, the growth of young dogs and rats has been retarded by doses exceeding the maximum human dose.

Use in Children: Nardil is not recommended for patients under 16 years of age since there are no controlled studies of safety in this age group.
Nardil, as with other hydrazine derivatives, has been reported to induce pulmonary and vascular tumors in an uncontrolled lifetime study in mice.
Precautions: In depressed patients, the possibility of suicide should always be considered and adequate precautions taken. It is recommended that careful observations of patients undergoing Nardil treatment be maintained until control of depression is achieved. If necessary, additional measures (ECT, hospitalization, etc.) should be instituted.
All patients undergoing treatment with Nardil should be closely followed for symptoms of postural hypotension. Hypotensive side effects have occurred in hypertensive as well as normal and hypotensive patients. Blood pressure usually returns to pretreatment levels rapidly when the drug is discontinued or the dosage is reduced.
Because the effect of Nardil on the convulsive threshold may be variable, adequate precautions should be taken when treating epileptic patients.
Of the more severe side effects that have been reported with any consistency, hypomania has been the most common. This reaction has been largely limited to patients in whom disorders characterized by hyperkinetic symptoms coexist with, but are obscured by, depressive affect; hypomania usually appeared as depression improved. If agitation is present, it may be increased with Nardil. Hypomania and agitation have also been reported at higher than recommended doses, or following long-term therapy.
Nardil may cause excessive stimulation in schizophrenic patients; in manic-depressive states it may result in a swing from a depressive to a manic phase.
MAO inhibitors, including Nardil potentiate hexobarbital hypnosis in animals. Therefore, barbiturates should be given at a reduced dose with Nardil.
MAO inhibitors inhibit the destruction of serotonin and norepinephrine, which are believed to be released from tissue stores by rauwolfia alkaloids. Accordingly, caution should be exercised when rauwolfia is used concomitantly with an MAO inhibitor, including Nardil.
There is conflicting evidence as to whether or not MAO inhibitors affect glucose metabolism or potentiate hypoglycemic agents. This should be kept in mind if Nardil is administered to diabetics.
Adverse Reactions: Nardil is a potent inhibitor of monoamine oxidase. Because this enzyme is widely distributed throughout the body, diverse pharmacologic effects can be expected to occur. When they occur, such effects tend to be mild or moderate in severity (see below), often subside as treatment continues, and can be minimized by adjusting dosage; rarely is it necessary to institute counteracting measures or to discontinue Nardil. Common side effects include dizziness, constipation, dry mouth, postural hypotension, drowsiness, weakness and fatigue, edema, gastrointestinal disturbances, tremors, twitching, and hyperreflexia.
Less common mild to moderate side effects, some of which have been reported in a single patient or by a single physician, include blurred vision, glaucoma, sweating, skin rash, jitteriness, palilalia, urinary retention, weight gain, euphoria, nystagmus, sexual disturbances and hypernatremia.
Although reported less frequently, and sometimes only once, additional severe side effects have included ataxia, shock-like coma, edema of the glottis, transient respiratory and cardiovascular depression following ECT, leukopenia, toxic delirium, reversible jaundice, manic reaction, convulsions, acute anxiety reaction and precipitation of schizophrenia. To date, fatal progressive necrotizing hepatocellular damage has been reported in a very few patients.
Dosage and Administration:
Initial dose: the usual starting dose of Nardil is one tablet (15 mg) three times a day.
Early phase treatment: dosage should be increased to at least 60 mg per day at a fairly rapid pace consistent with patient tolerance. It may be

necessary to increase dosage up to 90 mg per day to obtain sufficient MAO inhibition. Many patients do not show a clinical response until treatment at 60 mg has been continued for at least 4 weeks.
Maintenance dose: after maximum benefit from Nardil is achieved, dosage should be reduced slowly over several weeks. Maintenance dose may be as low as 1 tablet, 15 mg, a day or every other day, and should be continued for as long as is required.

Overdosage:
Note—For management of *hypertensive crises* see Warnings.
Accidental or intentional overdosage may be more common in patients who are depressed. It should be remembered that multiple drugs and/or alcohol may have been ingested.
Depending on the amount of overdosage with Nardil, a varying and mixed clinical picture may develop, involving signs and symptoms of central nervous system and cardiovascular stimulation and/or depression. Signs and symptoms may be absent or minimal during the initial 12-hour period following ingestion and may develop slowly thereafter, reaching a maximum in 24–48 hours. Death has been reported following overdosage. Therefore, immediate hospitalization, with continuous patient observation and monitoring throughout this period, is essential.
Signs and symptoms of overdosage may include, alone or in combination, any of the following: drowsiness, dizziness, faintness, irritability, hyperactivity, agitation, severe headache, hallucinations, trismus, opisthotonus, convulsions and coma; rapid and irregular pulse, hypertension, hypotension and vascular collapse; precordial pain, respiratory depression and failure, hyperpyrexia, diaphoresis, and cool, clammy skin.
Intensive symptomatic and supportive treatment may be required. Induction of emesis or gastric lavage with instillation of charcoal slurry may be helpful in early poisoning, provided the airway has been protected against aspiration. Signs and symptoms of central nervous system stimulation, including convulsions, should be treated with diazepam, given slowly intravenously. Phenothiazine derivatives and central nervous system stimulants should be avoided. Hypotension and vascular collapse should be treated with intravenous fluids and, if necessary, blood pressure titration with an intravenous infusion of dilute pressor agent. It should be noted that adrenergic agents may produce a markedly increased pressor response.
Respiration should be supported by appropriate measures, including management of the airway, use of supplemental oxygen, and mechanical ventilatory assistance, as required.
Body temperature should be monitored closely. Intensive management of hyperpyrexia may be required. Maintenance of fluid and electrolyte balance is essential.
There are no data on the lethal dose in man. The pathophysiologic effects of massive overdosage may persist for several days, since the drug acts by inhibiting physiologic enzyme systems. With symptomatic and supportive measures, recovery from *mild* overdosage may be expected within 3 to 4 days.
Hemodialysis, peritoneal dialysis, and charcoal hemoperfusion may be of value in massive overdosage, but sufficient data are not available to recommend their routine use in these cases.
Toxic blood levels of phenelzine have not been established, and assay methods are not practical for clinical or toxicological use.
How Supplied: Tablets—each orange-coated tablet bears the P-D 270 monogram and contains phenelzine sulfate equivalent to 15 mg of phenelzine base; bottles of 100 (N 0071-0270-24). Store between 15°–30°C (59°–86°F).
US Patent 3,314,855
Shown in Product Identification Section, page 424
0270G022

NATABEC® KAPSEALS®
[nā′ tă-bĕc]

Each capsule represents:

Vitamins
Vitamin A (acetate) .... (1.2 mg) 4,000 IU*
Vitamin D .... 400 IU
Vitamin C (ascorbic acid) .... 50 mg
Vitamin B₁ (thiamine
    mononitrate) .... 3 mg
Vitamin B₂ (riboflavin) .... 2.0 mg
Nicotinamide + ... 10 mg
Vitamin B₆ (pyridoxine HCl) .... 3 mg
Vitamin B₁₂ crystalline
    (cyanocobalamin) .... 5 mcg
Minerals
Precipitated Calcium Carbonate .... 600 mg
Iron (as dried ferrous sulfate) .... 30 mg

*IU = International Units
+Supplied as niacinamide
Action and Uses: A multivitamin and mineral supplement for use during pregnancy and lactation
Dosage: One capsule daily, or as directed by physician
How Supplied: N 0071-0390-24. In bottles of 100, Parcode® 390
The color combination of the banded capsule is a Warner-Lambert trademark.
Shown in Product Identification Section, page 424

NATABEC Rx® KAPSEALS® ℞
[nā′ tă-bĕc″]
Vitamin and Mineral Formula Containing Folic Acid

Each Kapseal Represents:
Vitamin A (acetate) .... 4,000 units
Vitamin D .... 400 units
Vitamin C (ascorbic acid) .... 50 mg
Vitamin B₁ (thiamine mononitrate) .... 3 mg
Vitamin B₂ (riboflavin) .... 2 mg
Vitamin B₆ (pyridoxine
    hydrochloride) .... 3 mg
Vitamin B₁₂ (cyanocobalamin)
    crystalline .... 5 mcg
Nicotinamide (niacinamide) .... 10 mg
Folic acid .... 1 mg
Calcium carbonate,
    precipitated .... 600 mg
Iron* .... 30 mg

* Supplied as dried ferrous sulfate.
Action and Uses: Vitamin and mineral formula containing 1 mg folic acid for use during pregnancy and lactation
Caution—Folic acid in doses above 0.1 mg daily may obscure pernicious anemia in that hematologic remission can occur while neurological manifestations remain progressive.
Dosage: One capsule daily or as directed by the physician.
How Supplied: N 0071-0547-24—bottles of 100. The pink band on blue capsule is a Warner-Lambert trademark registered in the US Patent Office.
Shown in Product Identification Section, page 424

NATAFORT® FILMSEAL® ℞
[nā′ tă-fōrt″]

Each tablet represents:
Vitamin A (acetate) .... 6,000 IU*
Vitamin D .... 400 IU
Vitamin C (ascorbic acid) .... 120 mg
Thiamine (vitamin B₁) (thiamine
    mononitrate) .... 3 mg
Riboflavin (vitamin B₂)(riboflavin) .... 2 mg
Vitamin B₆ (pyridoxine HCl) .... 15 mg
Vitamin B₁₂ (cyanocobalamin
    crystalline .... 6 mcg
Folic acid .... 1 mg
Nicotinamide (niacinamide) .... 20 mg
Vitamin E (dl alpha tocopheryl
    acetate) .... 30 IU
Calcium† .... 350 mg
Iodine† .... 0.15 mg
Iron† .... 65 mg

Magnesium† .... 100 mg
Zinc† .... 25 mg

* IU = International Units
† The minerals are supplied as calcium carbonate, magnesium oxide, potassium iodide, ferrous fumarate, and zinc oxide.
Indications: Comprehensive prenatal vitamin and mineral formula including 1 mg of folic acid to prevent megaloblastic anemia of pregnancy.
Caution—Folic acid in doses above 0.1 mg daily may obscure pernicious anemia in that hematologic remission can occur while neurological manifestations remain progressive.
Usual Dosage: One tablet daily.
How Supplied: N 0071-0282-24 bottles of 100.
Shown in Product Identification Section, page 424

NITROSTAT® Ointment 2% ℞
[nĭ′ trō″ stăt]
(Nitroglycerin)

Description: Nitrostat® ointment contains 2% nitroglycerin in an ointment base composed of lanolin, lactose, and white petrolatum, formulated to provide a controlled release of the active ingredient. Each inch, as squeezed from the tube, contains 15 mg nitroglycerin.
Actions: When the ointment is spread on the skin, nitroglycerin is absorbed continuously into the systemic circulation. Nitrostat ointment reduces the work load of the heart by virtue of its smooth muscle relaxation. This results predominantly in peripheral venous dilatation, which reduces preload, but also to a lesser degree in peripheral arteriolar dilatation, which reduces afterload. These hemodynamic effects have been advanced as explanations for the beneficial actions of nitroglycerin ointment in angina pectoris.
Computerized digital plethysmographic studies have shown the duration of action of nitroglycerin ointment (2 inches applied to the chest) to be eight hours in comparison to placebo; the onset of action occurred within thirty minutes of administration. Controlled clinical studies have demonstrated that nitroglycerin ointment increased measured exercise tolerance in patients with angina pectoris up to three hours after application (the maximal time interval studied).

Indications:
This drug product has been conditionally approved by the FDA for the prevention and treatment of angina pectoris due to coronary artery disease. The conditional approval reflects a determination that the drug may be marketed while further investigation of its effectiveness is undertaken. A final evaluation of the effectiveness of the product will be announced by the FDA.

Contraindications: In patients known to be intolerant of the organic nitrate drugs.
Warnings: In acute myocardial infarction or congestive heart failure, Nitrostat ointment should be used under careful clinical and/or hemodynamic monitoring.
Precautions: Nitrostat ointment should not be used for treatment of acute anginal attacks. Symptoms of hypotension, particularly during sudden arising from the recumbent position, are signs of overdosage. When they occur, the dosage should be reduced.
Adverse Reactions: Transient headaches are the most common side effect, especially at higher dosages. Headaches should be treated with mild analgesics, and nitroglycerin ointment continued.

Continued on next page

This product information was prepared in August, 1984. On these and other Parke-Davis Products, information may be obtained by addressing PARKE-DAVIS, Division of Warner-Lambert Company, Morris Plains, New Jersey 07950.

Parke-Davis—Cont.

Only with untreatable headaches should the dosage be reduced. Although uncommon, hypotension, an increase in heart rate, faintness, flushing, dizziness, and nausea may occur. These are all attributable to the pharmacologic effects of nitroglycerin on the cardiovascular system but are symptoms of overdosage. When they occur and persist, the dosage should be reduced.

Dosage and Administration: When applying the ointment, place the specially designed dose-measuring applicator supplied with the package on a flat surface with the printed side down and squeeze the necessary amount of ointment from the tube onto the applicator. Then place the applicator with the ointment side down onto the desired area of skin, usually the chest (although other areas can be used).

Using the applicator, spread the ointment in a thin, uniform layer over an area approximately the size of the applicator or larger. Cover the area, including the applicator, with plastic wrap, which can be held in place by adhesive tape. The applicator allows the patient to measure the necessary amount of ointment and to spread it without its being absorbed through the fingers during application to the skin surface.

The usual therapeutic dose is 2 inches (50 mm) applied every eight hours, although some patients may require as much as 4 to 5 inches (100 to 125 mm) and/or application every four hours.

Start at ½ inch (12.5 mm) every eight hours and increase the dose by ½ inch (12.5 mm) with each successive application to achieve the desired clinical effects. The optimal dosage should be selected based upon the clinical response, side effects, and the effects of therapy upon blood pressure. The greatest attainable decrease in resting blood pressure that is not associated with clinical symptoms of hypotension, especially during orthostasis, indicates the optimal dosage. To decrease adverse reactions, the dose and frequency of application should be tailored to the individual patient's needs.

Keep the tube tightly closed and store at controlled room temperature 15° to 30°C (59° to 86°F). Avoid excessive heat.

Patient Instructions For Application: Information furnished with dose-measuring applicators.

How Supplied: Nitrostat ointment 2% is supplied as:
N 0071-3001-13—30-gram tube
N 0071-3001-15—60-gram tube
Each gram of ointment contains 20 mg of nitroglycerin.

3001G032
Shown in Product Identification Section, page 425

NITROSTAT®
[nīʹ trō″stăt]
(nitroglycerin tablets, USP)

Description: Nitrostat is a stabilized sublingual nitroglycerin tablet manufactured by a patented process* which prevents the migration of nitroglycerin by adding the nonvolatile fixing agent polyethylene glycol 3350. This stabilized formulation has been shown to be more stable and more uniform than conventional molded tablets. Nitrostat tablets contain 0.15 mg (1/400 grain), 0.3 mg (1/200 grain), 0.4 mg (1/150 grain) and 0.6 mg (1/100 grain) nitroglycerin.

Nitroglycerin, an organic nitrate, is a vasodilating agent. The chemical name for nitroglycerin is 1,2,3 propanetriol trinitrate.

Clinical Pharmacology: Relaxation of vascular smooth muscle is the principal pharmacologic action of nitroglycerin. The mechanism by which nitroglycerin produces relaxation of smooth muscle is unknown. Although venous effects predominate, nitroglycerin produces, in a dose-related manner, dilation of both arterial and venous beds. Dilation of the postcapillary vessels, including large veins, promotes peripheral pooling of blood and decreases venous return to the heart, reducing left ventricular end-diastolic pressure (preload).

Arteriolar relaxation reduces systemic vascular resistance and arterial pressure (afterload). Myocardial oxygen consumption or demand (as measured by the pressure-rate product, tension-time index and stroke-work index) is decreased by both the arterial and venous effects of nitroglycerin, and a more favorable supply-demand ratio can be achieved.

Therapeutic doses of nitroglycerin may reduce systolic, diastolic and mean arterial blood pressure. Effective coronary perfusion pressure is usually maintained, but can be compromised if blood pressure falls excessively or increased heart rate decreases diastolic filling time.

Elevated central venous and pulmonary capillary wedge pressures, pulmonary vascular resistance and systemic vascular resistance are also reduced by nitroglycerin therapy. Heart rate is usually slightly increased, presumably a reflex response to the fall in blood pressure. Cardiac index may be increased, decreased, or unchanged. Patients with elevated left ventricular filling pressure and systemic vascular resistance values in conjunction with a depressed cardiac index are likely to experience an improvement in cardiac index. On the other hand, when filling pressures and cardiac index are normal, cardiac index may be slightly reduced by intravenous nitroglycerin.

Nitroglycerin is rapidly absorbed following sublingual administration. Its onset of action is approximately one to three minutes. Significant pharmacologic effects are present for 30 to 60 minutes following administration by the above route.

Nitroglycerin is rapidly metabolized to dinitrates and mononitrates, with a short half-life, estimated at 1 to 4 minutes. At plasma concentrations of between 50 and 500 ng/ml, the binding of nitroglycerin to plasma proteins is approximately 60%, while that of 1,2 dinitroglycerin and 1,3 dinitroglycerin is 60% and 30% respectively. The activity and half-life of 1,2 dinitroglycerin and 1,3 dinitroglycerin are not well characterized. The mononitrate is not active.

Indications and Usage: Nitroglycerin is indicated for the prophylaxis, treatment and management of patients with angina pectoris.

Contraindications: Sublingual nitroglycerin therapy is contraindicated in patients with early myocardial infarction, severe anemia, increased intracranial pressure, and those with a known hypersensitivity to nitroglycerin.

Precautions:
General: Only the smallest dose required for effective relief of the acute anginal attack should be used. Excessive use may lead to the development of tolerance. Nitrostat tablets are intended for sublingual or buccal administration and should not be swallowed. The drug should be discontinued if blurring of vision or drying of the mouth occurs. Excessive dosage of nitroglycerin may produce severe headaches.

Information for Patients: If possible, patients should sit down when taking Nitrostat tablets. This eliminates the possibility of falling due to lightheadedness or dizziness.

Drug Interactions: Concomitant use of nitrates and alcohol may cause hypotension. Patients receiving antihypertensive drugs, beta-adrenergic blockers, or phenothiazines and nitrates should be observed for possible additive hypotensive effects.

Drug/Laboratory Test Interactions: Nitrates may interfere with the Zlatkis-Zak color reaction causing a false report of decreased serum cholesterol.

Carcinogenesis, Mutagenesis, Impairment of Fertility: No long-term studies in animals were performed to evaluate the carcinogenic potential of nitroglycerin.

Pregnancy Category C: Animal reproduction studies have not been conducted with nitroglycerin. It is also not known whether nitroglycerin can cause fetal harm when administered to a pregnant woman or can affect reproduction capacity. Nitroglycerin should be given to a pregnant woman only if clearly needed.

Nursing Mother: It is not known whether nitroglycerin is excreted in human milk. Because many drugs are excreted in human milk, caution should be exercised when intravenous nitroglycerin is administered to a nursing woman.

Pediatric Use: The safety and effectiveness of nitroglycerin in children have not been established.

Adverse Reactions: Transient headache may occur immediately after use. Vertigo, weakness, palpitation, and other manifestations of postural hypotension may develop occasionally, particularly in erect, immobile patients. Syncope due to nitrate vasodilation has been reported.

Dosage and Administration: One tablet should be dissolved under the tongue or in the buccal pouch at the first sign of an acute anginal attack. The dose may be repeated approximately every five minutes until relief is obtained. If the pain persists after a total of 3 tablets in a 15-minute period, the physician should be notified. Nitrostat may be used prophylactically five to ten minutes prior to engaging in activities which might precipitate an acute attack.

How Supplied: Nitrostat is supplied in four strengths in bottles containing 100 tablets each, with color-coded labels, and in color-coded Patient Convenience Packages of four bottles of 25 tablets each.

0.15 mg (1/400 grain):
N 0071-0568-24—Bottle of 100 tablets
N 0071-0568-13—Convenience Package
0.3 mg (1/200 grain):
N 0071-0569-24—Bottle of 100 tablets
N 0071-0569-13—Convenience Package
0.4 mg (1/150 grain):
N 0071-0570-24—Bottle of 100 tablets
N 0071-0570-13—Convenience Package
0.6 mg (1/100 grain):
N 0071-0571-24—Bottle of 100 tablets
N 0071-0571-13—Convenience Package

Store at controlled room temperature 15°-30°C (59°-86°F).
Protect from moisture.
*US Patent No. 3,789,119

0568G062
Shown in Product Identification Section, page 424

NITROSTAT® IV
[nīʹ trō″stăt]
(Nitroglycerin for Infusion)
FOR INTRAVENOUS USE ONLY

NOT FOR DIRECT INTRAVENOUS INJECTION. NITROSTAT IV IS A CONCENTRATED, POTENT DRUG WHICH MUST BE DILUTED IN DEXTROSE (5%) INJECTION, USP OR SODIUM CHLORIDE (0.9%) INJECTION, USP PRIOR TO ITS INFUSION. THE CONTAINER AND ADMINISTRATION SET USED FOR INFUSION MAY AFFECT THE AMOUNT OF INTRAVENOUS NITROGLYCERIN DELIVERED TO THE PATIENT. (SEE WARNINGS AND DOSAGE AND ADMINISTRATION SECTIONS.)

CAUTION: SEVERAL PREPARATIONS OF NITROGLYCERIN FOR INJECTION ARE AVAILABLE. THEY DIFFER IN CONCENTRATION AND/OR VOLUME PER VIAL. WHEN SWITCHING FROM ONE PRODUCT TO ANOTHER, ATTENTION MUST BE PAID TO THE DILUTION AND DOSAGE AND ADMINISTRATION INSTRUCTIONS.

Description: Nitrostat IV is a clear, practically colorless additive solution for intravenous infusion after dilution. Each milliliter contains 0.8 mg nitroglycerin, with citric acid and sodium citrate as buffers, and 5% alcohol in Water for Injection, USP.

The solution is sterile, nonpyrogenic, and nonexplosive. Intravenous nitroglycerin, an organic nitrate, is a vasodilator. The chemical name for nitroglycerin is 1,2,3 propanetriol trinitrate and its chemical structure is:

$$H_2C-O-NO_2$$
$$|$$
$$HC-O-NO_2$$
$$|$$
$$H_2C-O-NO_2$$

Clinical Pharmacology: Relaxation of vascular smooth muscle is the principal pharmacologic action of intravenous nitroglycerin. Although venous effects predominate, nitroglycerin produces, in a dose-related manner, dilation of both arterial and venous beds. Dilation of the postcapillary vessels, including large veins, promotes peripheral pooling of blood and decreases venous return to the heart, reducing left ventricular end-diastolic pressure (preload). Arteriolar relaxation reduces systemic vascular resistance and arterial pressure (afterload). Myocardial oxygen consumption or demand (as measured by the pressure-rate product, tension-time index and stroke-work index) is decreased by both the arterial and venous effects of nitroglycerin, and a more favorable supply-demand ratio can be achieved.

Therapeutic doses of intravenous nitroglycerin reduce systolic, diastolic and mean arterial blood pressure. Effective coronary perfusion pressure is usually maintained, but can be compromised if blood pressure falls excessively or increased heart rate decreases diastolic filling time.

Elevated central venous and pulmonary capillary wedge pressures, pulmonary vascular resistance and systemic vascular resistance are also reduced by nitroglycerin therapy. Heart rate is usually slightly increased, presumably a reflex response to the fall in blood pressure. Cardiac index may be increased, decreased, or unchanged. Patients with elevated left ventricular filling pressure and systemic vascular resistance values in conjunction with a depressed cardiac index are likely to experience an improvement in cardiac index. On the other hand, when filling pressures and cardiac index are normal, cardiac index may be slightly reduced by intravenous nitroglycerin.

Nitroglycerin is widely distributed in the body with an apparent volume of distribution of approximately 200 liters in adult male subjects, and is rapidly metabolized to dinitrates and mononitrates, with a short half-life, estimated at 1 to 4 minutes. This results in a low plasma concentration after intravenous infusion. At plasma concentrations of between 50 and 500 ng/ml, the binding of nitroglycerin to plasma proteins is approximately 60%, while that of 1,2 dinitroglycerin and 1,3 dinitroglycerin is 60% and 30% respectively. The activity and half-life of 1,2 dinitroglycerin and 1,3 dinitroglycerin are not well characterized. The mononitrate is not active.

Indications and Usage:
Nitrostat IV is indicated for:
1. *Control of blood pressure in perioperative hypertension*, ie, hypertension associated with surgical procedures, especially cardiovascular procedures, such as the hypertension seen during intratracheal intubation, anesthesia, skin incision, sternotomy, cardiac bypass, and in the immediate postsurgical period.
2. *Congestive Heart Failure Associated with Acute Myocardial Infarction.*
3. *Treatment of Angina Pectoris* in patients who have not responded to recommended doses of organic nitrates and/or a beta blocker.
4. *Production of controlled hypotension during surgical procedures.*

Contraindications:
Nitrostat IV should not be administered to individuals with:
1. A known hypersensitivity to nitroglycerin or a known idiosyncratic reaction to organic nitrates.
2. Hypotension or uncorrected hypovolemia, as the use of Nitrostat IV in such states could produce severe hypotension or shock.
3. Increased intracranial pressure (eg, head trauma or cerebral hemorrhage).
4. Constrictive pericarditis and pericardial tamponade.

Warnings:
1. Nitroglycerin readily migrates into many plastics. To avoid absorption of nitroglycerin into plastic parenteral solution containers, the dilution and storage of nitroglycerin for intravenous infusion should be made only in glass parenteral solution bottles.
2. Some filters also absorb nitroglycerin; they should be avoided if possible.
3. Forty to 80% of the total amount of nitroglycerin in the final diluted solution for infusion is absorbed by the polyvinyl chloride (PVC) tubing of the intravenous administration sets currently in general use. The higher rates of absorption occur when flow rates are low, nitroglycerin concentrations are high, and tubing is long. Although the rate of loss is highest during the early phase of administration (when flow rates are lowest), the loss is neither constant nor self-limiting; consequently no simple calculation or correction can be performed to convert the theoretical infusion rate (based on the concentration of the infusion solution) to the actual delivery rate.

Because of this problem, Parke-Davis, Division of Warner-Lambert Company has developed a nonabsorbing infusion set, Nitrostat IV intravenous infusion set, in which the loss of nitroglycerin is minimal (less than 5%). The Nitrostat IV intravenous infusion set or a similar infusion set is recommended for infusions of intravenous nitroglycerin.

Dosage instructions must be followed with care. It should be noted that when these infusion sets are used, the calculated dose will be delivered to the patient because the loss of nitroglycerin due to absorption in standard PVC tubing will be kept to a minimum. Note that the dosages commonly used in published studies utilized general-use PVC infusion sets and recommended doses based on this experience are too high if the new infusion sets are used.

Precautions: Nitrostat IV should be used with caution in patients who have severe hepatic or renal disease.

Excessive hypotension, especially for prolonged periods of time, must be avoided because of possible deleterious effects on the brain, heart, liver, and kidney from poor perfusion and the attendant risk of ischemia, thrombosis, and altered function of these organs. Paradoxical bradycardia and increased angina pectoris may accompany nitroglycerin-induced hypotension. Patients with normal or low pulmonary capillary wedge pressure are especially sensitive to the hypotensive effects of intravenous nitroglycerin. If pulmonary capillary wedge pressure is being monitored, it will be noted that a fall in wedge pressure precedes the onset of arterial hypotension, and the pulmonary capillary wedge pressure is thus a useful guide to safe titration of the drug.

NITROSTAT IV CONTAINS ALCOHOL. SAFETY FOR INTRACORONARY INJECTION HAS NOT BEEN SHOWN.

Carcinogenesis, Mutagenesis, Impairment of Fertility:
No long-term studies in animals were performed to evaluate the carcinogenic potential of nitroglycerin.

Pregnancy:
Category C: Animal reproduction studies have not been conducted with nitroglycerin. It is also not known whether nitroglycerin can cause fetal harm when administered to a pregnant woman or can affect reproduction capacity. Nitroglycerin should be given to a pregnant woman only if clearly needed.

Nursing Mother:
It is not known whether nitroglycerin is excreted in human milk. Because many drugs are excreted in human milk, caution should be exercised when intravenous nitroglycerin is administered to a nursing woman.

Pediatric Use:
The safety and effectiveness of nitroglycerin in children have not been established.

Adverse Reactions: The most frequent adverse reaction in patients treated with nitroglycerin is headache, which occurs in approximately 2% of patients. Other adverse reactions occurring in less than 1% of patients are the following: tachycardia, nausea, vomiting, apprehension, restlessness, muscle twitching, retrosternal discomfort, palpitations, dizziness and abdominal pain.

The following additional adverse reactions have been reported with the oral and/or topical use of nitroglycerin: cutaneous flushing, weakness, and occasionally drug rash or exfoliative dermatitis.

Overdosage: Accidental overdosage of nitroglycerin may result in severe hypotension and reflex tachycardia which can be treated by elevating the legs and decreasing or temporarily terminating the infusion until the patient's condition stabilizes. Since the duration of the hemodynamic effects following nitroglycerin administration is quite short, additional corrective measures are usually not required. However, if further therapy is indicated, administration of an intravenous alpha adrenergic agonist (eg, methoxamine or phenylephrine) should be considered.

Dosage and Administration:
NOT FOR DIRECT INTRAVENOUS INJECTION
NITROSTAT IV IS A CONCENTRATED, POTENT DRUG WHICH MUST BE DILUTED IN DEXTROSE (5%) INJECTION, USP OR SODIUM CHLORIDE (0.9%) INJECTION, USP PRIOR TO ITS INFUSION.
NITROSTAT IV SHOULD NOT BE ADMIXED WITH OTHER DRUGS.

Dilution: It is important to consider the fluid requirements of the patient as well as the expected duration of infusion in selecting the appropriate dilution of nitroglycerin.

Solution Preparation for an Infusion Pump (60 microdrops = 1 ml)
Aseptically transfer 10 ml (8 mg nitroglycerin) of Nitrostat IV into a *glass* IV bottle containing 250 ml of 5% Dextrose Injection, USP or 0.9% Sodium Chloride Injection, USP and mix well. The resultant solution will contain approximately 30 mcg/ml of nitroglycerin and is stable for at least 96 hours at controlled room temperature (15° to 30° C) or under refrigeration.

RATE OF ADMINISTRATION
(microdrops per minute or milliliters per hour)

10 ml in 250 ml = 30 mcg/ml (approx)

Desired Dose (mcg/min)	Microdrops Per Minute	ml/hour
5	10	10
10	20	20
15	30	30
20	40	40
30	60	60
40	80	80
50	100	100

The tables below contain dosage information if a higher concentration of nitroglycerin or a longer duration of infusion is desired. Aseptically transfer the required volume from the ampoules to 250 ml of either 5% Dextrose Injection, USP or 0.9% Sodium Chloride Injection, USP.

If the concentration is adjusted, it is imperative to flush or replace the Nitrostat IV infusion set before a new concentration is utilized. The dead space of the set is approximately 15 ml and, depending on the flow rate, it could take from 9 minutes to 3 hours for the new concentration to reach the patient if the set were not flushed or replaced.

RATE OF ADMINISTRATION
(microdrops per minute or milliliters per hour)

20 ml in 250 ml = 60 mcg/ml (approx)

Desired Dose (mcg/min)	Microdrops Per Minute	ml/hour
5	5	5
10	10	10

This product information was prepared in August, 1984. On these and other Parke-Davis Products, information may be obtained by addressing PARKE-DAVIS, Division of Warner-Lambert Company, Morris Plains, New Jersey 07950.

Continued on next page

Parke-Davis—Cont.

15	15	15
20	20	20
30	30	30
40	40	40
50	50	50
60	60	60
80	80	80
100	100	100

30 ml in 250 ml = 85 mcg/ml (approx)

Desired Dose (mcg/min)	Microdrops Per Minute	ml/hour
5	3	3.529
10	7	7.058
15	10	10.588
20	14	14.117
30	21	21.176
40	28	28.235
50	35	35.294
60	42	42.352
80	56	56.47
100	70	70.588

Dosage: *IMPORTANT NOTICE:* Dosage is affected by the type of container used as well as the type of infusion set used (See Warnings). Although the usual starting adult dose range reported in clinical studies was 25 mcg/min or more, those studies used *PVC TUBING. The use of nonabsorbing tubing will result in the need to use reduced doses.*

The recommended dosage when using the nonabsorbing Nitrostat IV Intravenous Infusion Set should initially be 5 mcg/min delivered through an infusion pump capable of exact and constant delivery of the drug. Subsequent titration must be adjusted to the clinical situation, with dose increments becoming more cautious as partial response is seen. Initial titration should be 5 mcg/min increments, with increases every 3 to 5 minutes until some response is noted. If no response is seen at 20 mcg/min, increments of 10 and later 20 mcg/min can be used. Once a partial blood pressure response is observed, the dose increase should be reduced and the interval between increments should be lengthened. Patients with normal or low left ventricular filling pressure or pulmonary capillary wedge pressure (eg, angina patients without other complications) may be hypersensitive to the effects of nitroglycerin and may respond fully to doses as small as 5 mcg/min. These patients require especially careful titration and monitoring. There is no fixed optimum dose of nitroglycerin. Due to variations in the responsiveness of individual patients to the drug, each patient must be titrated to the desired level of hemodynamic function. Therefore, continuous monitoring of physiologic parameters (blood pressure and heart rate in all patients, other measurements such as pulmonary capillary wedge pressure, as appropriate) MUST BE PERFORMED to achieve the correct dose. Adequate systemic blood pressure and coronary perfusion pressure must be maintained.

Directions For Preparing Nitrostat IV Infusion Set:

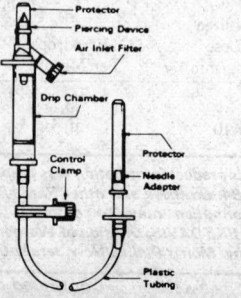

Caution—The fluid path and areas under the protectors of the intravenous infusion set are sterile. Do not use if damaged or if end protectors are not in place.
1. Position control clamp 6 to 8 inches from the needle adapter end of set, then close clamp. (To close clamp, rotate screw stem clockwise.)
2. With IV solution bottle in the upright position,
   a) remove plastic protector from the piercing device,
   b) THRUST the piercing device STRAIGHT DOWN through the CENTER of the target area in the rubber stopper (push straight down, do not twist).
   c) squeeze drip chamber and hold.
3. Invert the bottle and suspend from suitable stand.
4. Release pressure from drip chamber.
5. Remove needle adapter protector by pulling straight off (do not twist off).
If required, place needle on needle adapter. Hold this end of the tubing above the level of the nitroglycerin solution in the bottle. Loosen the control clamp and allow the solution to run into and to fill the tubing and needle. Displace the air in the entire injection set by raising or lowering the intravenous needle end of tubing until all the air bubbles are expelled.
(NOTE: Drip chamber should not be completely filled.)
6. Attach the infusion set to a suitable mechanical infusion control device.
7. Tighten control clamp and proceed with venipuncture or connect to needle.
8. Adjust infusion control device for precise measurement of flow rate.

How Supplied:
N 0071-4572-35 Nitrostat IV Infusion Kit containing one 10-ml ampoule of Nitrostat IV, 8 mg (0.8 mg/ml) and one disposable intravenous infusion set.
N 0071-4572-10 Carton of 10 × 10-ml ampoules of Nitrostat IV.
Store at controlled room temperature 15°–30° C (59°–86° F).

4572G022

Shown in Product Identification Section, page 424

NORLESTRIN® 21 1/50   ℞
[nōr″ lĕs′ trĭn]
(Each tablet contains 1 mg norethindrone acetate and 50 mcg ethinyl estradiol.)

NORLESTRIN® 21 2.5/50   ℞
(Each tablet contains 2.5 mg norethindrone acetate and 50 mcg ethinyl estradiol.)

NORLESTRIN® Fe 1/50   ℞
(Each yellow tablet contains 1 mg norethindrone acetate and 50 mcg ethinyl estradiol. Each brown tablet contains 75 mg ferrous fumarate, USP.)

NORLESTRIN® Fe 2.5/50   ℞
(Each pink tablet contains 2.5 mg norethindrone acetate and 50 mcg ethinyl estradiol. Each brown tablet contains 75 mg ferrous fumarate, USP.)

NORLESTRIN® 28 1/50   ℞
(Each yellow tablet contains 1 mg norethindrone acetate and 50 mcg ethinyl estradiol. Each white tablet is inert.)

Each yellow tablet contains: norethindrone acetate (17 alpha-ethinyl-19-nortestosterone acetate), 1 mg; ethinyl estradiol (17 alpha-ethinyl-1,3,5(10)-estratriene-3, 17 beta-diol), 50 mcg.
Each pink tablet contains: norethindrone acetate (17 alpha-ethinyl-19-nortestosterone acetate), 2.5 mg; ethinyl estradiol (17 alpha-ethinyl-1,3,5(10)-estratriene-3, 17 beta-diol), 50 mcg.
Each brown tablet contains 75 mg ferrous fumarate, USP.
Each white tablet is inert.
Description: Norlestrin is a progestogen-estrogen combination.
Norlestrin Fe 1/50 and 2.5/50 provides a continuous dosage regimen consisting of 21 oral contraceptive tablets and seven ferrous fumarate tablets. The ferrous fumarate tablets are present to facilitate ease of drug administration via a 28-day regimen and are not intended to serve any therapeutic purpose.
Norlestrin 28 1/50 provides a continuous dosage regimen consisting of 21 oral contraceptive tablets and 7 inert tablets.
Clinical Pharmacology: Combination oral contraceptives act primarily through the mechanism of gonadotropin suppression due to the estrogenic and progestational activity of the ingredients. Although the primary mechanism of action is inhibition of ovulation, alterations in the genital tract, including changes in the cervical mucus (which increase the difficulty of sperm penetration) and the endometrium (which reduce the likelihood of implantation) may also contribute to contraceptive effectiveness.
Indications and Usage: Norlestrin is indicated for the prevention of pregnancy in women who elect to use oral contraceptives as a method of contraception.
Oral contraceptives are highly effective. The pregnancy rate in women using conventional combination oral contraceptives (containing 35 mcg or more of ethinyl estradiol or 50 mcg or more of mestranol) is generally reported as less than one pregnancy per 100 woman-years of use. Slightly higher rates (somewhat more than 1 pregnancy per 100 woman-years of use) are reported for some combination products containing 35 mcg or less of ethinyl estradiol, and rates on the order of 3 pregnancies per 100 woman-years are reported for the progestogen-only oral contraceptives.
These rates are derived from separate studies conducted by different investigators in several population groups and cannot be compared precisely. Furthermore, pregnancy rates tend to be lower as clinical studies are continued, possibly due to selective retention in the longer studies of those patients who accept the treatment regimen and do not discontinue as a result of adverse reactions, pregnancy, or other reasons.
In clinical trials with Norlestrin 1/50, 1,156 patients completed 25,983 cycles and a total of one pregnancy was reported. This represents a pregnancy rate of 0.05 per 100 woman-years.
In clinical trials with Norlestrin 2.5/50, 3,829 patients completed 96,388 cycles and a total of 18 pregnancies were reported. This represents a pregnancy rate of 0.22 per 100 woman-years based upon data that include the cases where patients failed to comply with the dosage regimen. The pregnancy rate in patients who adhered to the dosage regimen was 0.02 per 100 woman-years (two pregnancies in these trials).
Table 1 gives ranges of pregnancy rates reported in the literature[1] for other means of contraception. The efficacy of these means of contraception (except the IUD) depends upon the degree of adherence to the method.

Table 1 Pregnancies per 100 Woman-Years
IUD, less than 1–6; Diaphragm with spermicidal products (creams or jellies), 2–20; Condom, 3–36; Aerosol foams, 2–29; Jellies and creams, 4–36; Periodic abstinence (rhythm) all types, less than 1–47; *1. Calendar method, 14–47; 2. Temperature method, 1–20; 3. Temperature method—intercourse only in post-ovulatory phase, less than 1–7; 4. Mucus method, 1–25;* No contraception, 60–80.

Dose-Related Risk of Thromboembolism from Oral Contraceptives
Two studies have shown a positive association between the dose of estrogens in oral contraceptives and the risk of thromboembolism.[2,3] For this reason, it is prudent and in keeping with good principles of therapeutics to minimize exposure to estrogen. The oral contraceptive product prescribed for any given patient should be that product which contains the least amount of estrogen that is compatible with an acceptable pregnancy rate and patient acceptance. It is recommended that new acceptors of oral contraceptives be started on preparations containing 0.05 mg or less of estrogen.
Contraindications: Oral contraceptives should not be used in women with any of the following conditions.

for possible revisions — Product Information

1. Thrombophlebitis or thromboembolic disorders
2. A past history of deep vein thrombophlebitis or thromboembolic disorders
3. Cerebral vascular or coronary artery disease
4. Known or suspected carcinoma of the breast
5. Known or suspected estrogen-dependent neoplasia
6. Undiagnosed abnormal genital bleeding
7. Known or suspected pregnancy (see Warning No. 5)
8. Benign or malignant liver tumor which developed during the use of oral contraceptives or other estrogen-containing products.

Warnings:

> Cigarette smoking increases the risk of serious cardiovascular side effects from oral contraceptive use. This risk increases with age and with heavy smoking (15 or more cigarettes per day) and is quite marked in women over 35 years of age. Women who use oral contraceptives should be strongly advised not to smoke.
>
> The use of oral contraceptives is associated with increased risk of several serious conditions including thromboembolism, stroke, myocardial infarction, hepatic adenoma, gallbladder disease, and hypertension. Practitioners prescribing oral contraceptives should be familiar with the following information relating to these risks.

1. *Thromboembolic Disorders and Other Vascular Problems.* An increased risk of thromboembolic and thrombotic disease associated with the use of oral contraceptives is well established. Three principal studies in Great Britain[4-6] and three in the United States[7-10] have demonstrated an increased risk of fatal and nonfatal venous thromboembolism and stroke, both hemorrhagic and thrombotic. These studies estimate that users of oral contraceptives are 4 to 11 times more likely than nonusers to develop these diseases without evident cause (Table 2).

Cerebrovascular Disorders

In a collaborative American study[9,10] of cerebrovascular disorders in women with and without predisposing causes, it was estimated that the risk of hemorrhagic stroke was 2.0 times greater in users than nonusers and the risk of thrombotic stroke was 4 to 9.5 times greater in users than in nonusers (Table 2).

Table 2

Summary of relative risk of thromboembolic disorders and other vascular problems in oral contraceptive users compared to nonusers

	Relative risk, times greater
Idiopathic thromboembolic disease	4–11
Postsurgery thromboembolic complications	4–6
Thrombotic stroke	4–9.5
Hemorrhagic stroke	2
Myocardial infarction	2–12

Myocardial Infarction

An increased risk of myocardial infarction associated with the use of oral contraceptives has been reported[11-13] confirming a previously suspected association. These studies, conducted in the United Kingdom, found, as expected, that the greater the number of underlying risk factors for coronary artery disease (cigarette smoking, hypertension, hypercholesterolemia, obesity, diabetes, history of preeclamptic toxemia) the higher the risk of developing myocardial infarction, regardless of whether the patient was an oral contraceptive user or not. Oral contraceptives, however, were found to be a clear additional risk factor.

In terms of relative risk, it has been estimated[52] that oral contraceptive users who do not smoke (smoking is considered a major predisposing condition to myocardial infarction) are about twice as likely to have a fatal myocardial infarction as nonusers who do not smoke. Oral contraceptive users who are also smokers have about a 5-fold increased risk of fatal infarction compared to users who do not smoke, but about a 10- to 12-fold increased risk compared to nonusers who do not smoke. Furthermore, the amount of smoking is also an important factor. In determining the importance of these relative risks, however, the baseline rates for various age groups, as shown in Table 3, must be given serious consideration. The importance of other predisposing conditions mentioned above in determining relative and absolute risks has not yet been quantified; it is quite likely that the same synergistic action exists, but perhaps to a lesser extent.

Table 3

Estimated annual mortality rate per 100,000 women from myocardial infarction by use of oral contraceptives, smoking habits, and age (in years) [See table above].

Risk of Dose

In an analysis of data derived from several national adverse reaction reporting systems,[2] British investigators concluded that the risk of thromboembolism, including coronary thrombosis, is directly related to the dose of estrogen used in oral contraceptives. Preparations containing 100 mcg or more of estrogen were associated with a higher risk of thromboembolism than those containing 50 to 80 mcg of estrogen. Their analysis did suggest, however, that the quantity of estrogen may not be the sole factor involved. This finding has been confirmed in the United States. Careful epidemiological studies to determine the degree of thromboembolic risk associated with progestogen-only oral contraceptives have not been performed. Cases of thromboembolic disease have been reported in women using these products, and they should not be presumed to be free of excess risk.

Estimate of Excess Mortality from Circulatory Diseases

A large prospective study[53] carried out in the U.K. estimated the mortality rate per 100,000 women per year from diseases of the circulatory system for users and nonusers of oral contraceptives according to age, smoking habits, and duration of use. The overall excess death rate annually from circulatory diseases for oral contraceptive users was estimated to be 20 per 100,000 (ages 15 to 34—5/100,000; ages 35 to 44—33/100,000; ages 45 to 49—140/100,000), the risk being concentrated in older women, in those with a long duration of use, and in cigarette smokers. It was not possible, however, to examine the interrelationships of age, smoking, and duration of use, nor to compare the effects of continuous versus intermittent use. Although the study showed a 10-fold increase in death due to circulatory diseases in users for 5 or more years, all of these deaths occurred in women 35 or older. Until larger numbers of women under 35 with continuous use for 5 or more years are available, it is not possible to assess the magnitude of the relative risk for this younger age group.

The available data from a variety of sources have been analyzed[14] to estimate the risk of death associated with various methods of contraception. The estimates of risk of death for each method include the combined risk of the contraceptive method (eg, thromboembolic and thrombotic disease in the case of oral contraceptives) plus the risk attributable to pregnancy or abortion in the event of method failure. This latter risk varies with the effectiveness of the contraceptive method. The findings of this analysis are shown in Figure 1 which follows.[14] The study concluded that the mortality associated with all methods of birth control is low and below that associated with childbirth, with the exception of oral contraceptives in women over 40 who smoke. (The rates given for pill only/smokers for each age group are for smokers as a class. For "heavy" smokers [more than 15 cigarettes a day] the rates given would be about double, for "light" smokers [less than 15 cigarettes a day] about 50 percent.) The lowest mortality is associated with the condom or diaphragm backed up by early abortion.

[See table on next page].

The risk of thromboembolic and thrombotic disease associated with oral contraceptives increases with age after approximately age 30 and, for myocardial infarction, is further increased by hypertension, hypercholesterolemia, obesity, diabetes, or history of preeclamptic toxemia and especially by cigarette smoking.

Based on the data currently available, the following chart gives a gross estimate of the risk of death from circulatory disorders associated with the use of oral contraceptives.

Smoking Habits and Other Predisposing Conditions—Risk Associated with Use of Oral Contraceptives

Age:	Below 30	30–39	40+
Heavy smokers	C	B	A
Light smokers	D	C	B
Nonsmokers (no predisposing conditions)	D	C,D	C
Nonsmokers (other predisposing conditions)	C	C,B	B,A

A—Use associated with very high risk
B—Use associated with high risk
C—Use associated with moderate risk
D—Use associated with low risk

The physician and the patient should be alert to the earliest manifestations of thromboembolic and thrombotic disorders (eg, thrombophlebitis, pulmonary embolism, cerebrovascular insufficiency, coronary occlusion, retinal thrombosis, and mesenteric thrombosis). Should any of these occur or be suspected, the drug should be discontinued immediately.

A four- to six-fold increased risk of postsurgery thromboembolic complications has been reported in oral contraceptive users.[15,16] If feasible, oral contraceptives should be discontinued at least 4 weeks before surgery of a type associated with an increased risk of thromboembolism or prolonged immobilization.

2. *Ocular Lesions.* There have been reports of neuro-ocular lesions, such as optic neuritis or retinal thrombosis, associated with the use of oral contraceptives. Discontinue oral contraceptive medication if there is unexplained, sudden or gradual, partial or complete loss of vision; onset of proptosis or diplopia; papilledema; or retinal vascular

Continued on next page

Norlestrin

Myocardial infarction

Smoking habits	Women aged 30–39 Users	Women aged 30–39 Nonusers	Women aged 40–44 Users	Women aged 40–44 Nonusers
All smokers	10.2	2.6	62.0	15.9
Heavy*	13.0	5.1	78.7	31.3
Light	4.7	0.9	28.6	5.7
Nonsmokers	1.8	1.2	10.7	7.4
Smokers and nonsmokers	5.4	1.9	32.8	11.7

*Heavy smoker: 15 or more cigarettes per day. From Jain, A.K., Studies in Family Planning 8:50, 1977.

This product information was prepared in August, 1984. On these and other Parke-Davis Products, information may be obtained by addressing PARKE-DAVIS, Division of Warner-Lambert Company, Morris Plains, New Jersey 07950.

Parke-Davis—Cont.

lesions and institute appropriate diagnostic and therapeutic measures.

3. *Carcinoma.* Long-term continuous administration of either natural or synthetic estrogen in certain animal species increases the frequency of carcinoma of the breast, cervix, vagina, and liver. Certain synthetic progestogens, none currently contained in oral contraceptives, have been noted to increase the incidence of mammary nodules, benign and malignant, in dogs.

In humans, three case control studies have reported an increased risk of endometrial carcinoma associated with the prolonged use of exogenous estrogen in post-menopausal women.[17-19] One publication[20] reported on the first 21 cases submitted by physicians to a registry of cases of adenocarcinoma of the endometrium in women under 40 on oral contraceptives. Of the cases found in women without predisposing risk factors for adenocarcinoma of the endometrium (eg, irregular bleeding at the time oral contraceptives were first given, polycystic ovaries), nearly all occurred in women who had used a sequential oral contraceptive. These products are no longer marketed. No evidence has been reported suggesting an increased risk of endometrial cancer in users of conventional-combination or progestogen-only oral contraceptives.

Several studies[8,21-24] have found no increase in breast cancer in women taking oral contraceptives or estrogens. One study,[25] however, while also noting no overall increased risk of breast cancer in women treated with oral contraceptives, found an excess risk in the subgroups of oral contraceptive users with documented benign breast disease. A reduced occurrence of benign breast tumors in users of oral contraceptives has been well-documented.[8,21,25-27]

In summary, there is at present no confirmed evidence from human studies of an increased risk of cancer associated with oral contraceptives. Close clinical surveillance of all women taking oral contraceptives is, nevertheless, essential. In all cases of undiagnosed persistent or recurrent abnormal vaginal bleeding, appropriate diagnostic measures should be taken to rule out malignancy. Women with a strong family history of breast cancer or who have breast nodules, fibrocystic disease, or abnormal mammograms, should be monitored with particular care if they elect to use oral contraceptives instead of other methods of contraception.

4. *Hepatic Tumors.* Benign hepatic adenomas have been found to be associated with the use of oral contraceptives.[28-30,46] One study[46] showed that oral contraceptive formulations with high hormonal potency were associated with a higher risk than lower potency formulations. Although benign, hepatic adenomas may rupture and may cause death through intra-abdominal hemorrhage. This has been reported in short-term as well as long-term users of oral contraceptives. Two studies relate risk with duration of use of the contraceptive, the risk being much greater after 4 or more years of oral contraceptive use.[30,46] While hepatic adenoma is a rare lesion, it should be considered in women presenting abdominal pain and tenderness, abdominal mass or shock.

A few cases of hepatocellular carcinoma have been reported in women taking oral contraceptives. The relationship of these drugs to this type of malignancy is not known at this time.

5. *Use in or Immediately Preceding Pregnancy, Birth Defects in Offspring, and Malignancy in Female Offspring.* The use of female sex hormones—both estrogenic and progestational agents—during early pregnancy may seriously damage the offspring. It has been shown that females exposed *in utero* to diethylstilbestrol, a nonsteroidal estrogen, have an increased risk of developing in later life a form of vaginal or cervical cancer that is ordinarily extremely rare.[31,32] This risk has been estimated to be of the order of 1 in 1,000 exposures or less.[33,47] Although there is no evidence at the present time that oral contraceptives further enhance the risk of developing this type of malignancy, such patients should be monitored with particular care if they elect to use oral contraceptives instead of other methods of contraception. Furthermore, a high percentage of such exposed women (from 30% to 90%) have been found to have epithelial changes of the vagina and cervix.[34-38] Although these changes are histologically benign, it is not known whether this condition is a precursor of vaginal malignancy. Male children so exposed may develop abnormalities of the urogenital tract.[48-50] Although similar data are not available with the use of other estrogens, it cannot be presumed that they would not induce similar changes. An increased risk of congenital anomalies, including heart defects and limb defects, has been reported with the use of sex hormones, including oral contraceptives, in pregnancy.[39-42,51] One case control study[42] has estimated a 4.7-fold increase in risk of limb-reduction defects in infants exposed *in utero* to sex hormones (oral contraceptives, hormonal withdrawal tests for pregnancy or attempted treatment for threatened abortion). Some of these exposures were very short and involved only a few days of treatment. The data suggest that the risk of limb-reduction defects in exposed fetuses is somewhat less than 1 in 1,000 live births. In the past, female sex hormones have been used during pregnancy in an attempt to treat threatened or habitual abortion. There is considerable evidence that estrogens are ineffective for these indications, and there is no evidence from well-controlled studies that progestogens are effective for these uses.

There is some evidence that triploidy and possibly other types of polyploidy are increased among abortuses from women who become pregnant soon after ceasing oral contraceptives.[43] Embryos with these anomalies are virtually always aborted spontaneously. Whether there is an overall increase in spontaneous abortion of pregnancies conceived soon after stopping oral contraceptives is unknown.

It is recommended that for any patient who has missed two consecutive periods, pregnancy should be ruled out before continuing the contraceptive regimen. If the patient has not adhered to the prescribed schedule, the possibility of pregnancy should be considered at the time of the first missed period, and further use of oral contraceptives should be withheld until pregnancy has been ruled out. If pregnancy is confirmed, the patient should be apprised of the potential risks to the fetus and the advisability of continuation of the pregnancy should be discussed in the light of these risks.

It is also recommended that women who discontinue oral contraceptives with the intent of becoming pregnant use an alternate form of contraception for a period of time before attempting to conceive. Many clinicians recommend 3 months although no precise information is available on which to base this recommendation.

The administration of progestogen-only or progestogen-estrogen combinations to induce withdrawal bleeding should not be used as a test of pregnancy.

6. *Gallbladder Disease.* Studies[8,23,26] report an increased risk of surgically confirmed gallbladder disease in users of oral contraceptives and estrogens. In one study, an increased risk appeared after 2 years of use and doubled after 4 or 5 years

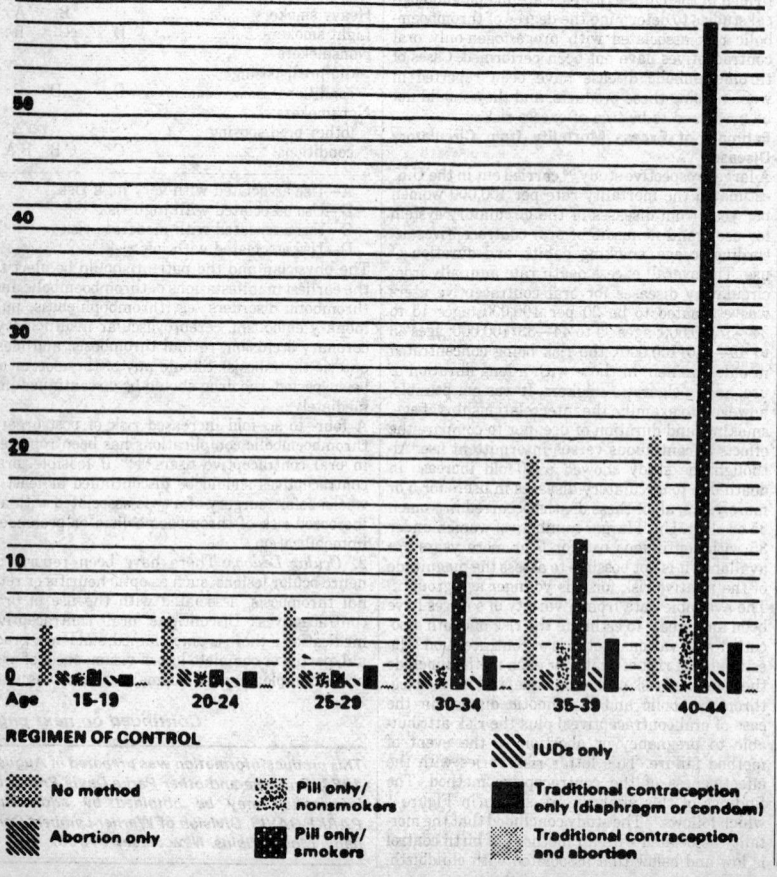

Figure 1. Estimated annual number of deaths associated with control of fertility and no control per 100,000 nonsterile women, by regimen of control and age of woman.

of use. In one of the other studies, an increased risk was apparent between 6 and 12 months of use.

7. *Carbohydrate and Lipid Metabolic Effects.* A decrease in glucose tolerance has been observed in a significant percentage of patients on oral contraceptives. For this reason, prediabetic and diabetic patients should be carefully observed while receiving oral contraceptives.

An increase in triglycerides and total phospholipids has been observed in patients receiving oral contraceptives.[44] The clinical significance of this finding remains to be defined.

8. *Elevated Blood Pressure.* An increase in blood pressure has been reported in patients receiving oral contraceptives.[26] In some women, hypertension may occur within a few months of beginning oral contraceptive use. In the first year of use, the prevalence of women with hypertension is low in users and may be no higher than that of a comparable group of nonusers. The prevalence in users increases, however, with longer exposure, and in the fifth year of use is two and a half to three times the reported prevalence in the first year. Age is also strongly correlated with the development of hypertension in oral contraceptive users. Women who previously have had hypertension during pregnancy may be more likely to develop elevation of blood pressure when given oral contraceptives. Hypertension that develops as a result of taking oral contraceptives usually returns to normal after discontinuing the drug.

9. *Headache.* The onset or exacerbation of migraine or development of headache of a new pattern which is recurrent, persistent, or severe, requires discontinuation of oral contraceptives and evaluation of the cause.

10. *Bleeding Irregularities.* Breakthrough bleeding, spotting and amenorrhea are frequent reasons for patients discontinuing oral contraceptives. In breakthrough bleeding, as in all cases of irregular bleeding from the vagina, nonfunctional causes should be borne in mind. In undiagnosed persistent or recurrent abnormal bleeding from the vagina, adequate diagnostic measures are indicated to rule out pregnancy or malignancy. If pathology has been excluded, time or a change to another formulation may solve the problem. Changing to an oral contraceptive with a higher estrogen content, while potentially useful in minimizing menstrual irregularity, should be done only if necessary since this may increase the risk of thromboembolic disease.

Women with a past history of oligomenorrhea or secondary amenorrhea or young women without regular cycles may have a tendency to remain anovulatory or to become amenorrheic after discontinuation of oral contraceptives. Women with these preexisting problems should be advised of this possibility and encouraged to use other contraceptive methods. Post-use anovulation, possibly prolonged, may also occur in women without previous irregularities.

11. *Ectopic Pregnancy.* Ectopic as well as intrauterine pregnancy may occur in contraceptive failures. However, in progestogen-only oral contraceptive failures, the ratio of ectopic to intrauterine pregnancies is higher than in women who are not receiving oral contraceptives, since the drugs are more effective in preventing intrauterine than ectopic pregnancies.

12. *Breast-Feeding.* Oral contraceptives given in the postpartum period may interfere with lactation. There may be a decrease in the quantity and quality of the breast milk. Furthermore, a small fraction of the hormonal agents in oral contraceptives has been identified in the milk of mothers receiving these drugs.[45] The effects, if any, on the breast-fed child have not been determined. If feasible, the use of oral contraceptives should be deferred until the infant has been weaned.

Precautions:
General
1. A complete medical and family history should be taken prior to the initiation of oral contraceptives. The pretreatment and periodic physical examinations should include special reference to blood pressure, breasts, abdomen and pelvic organs, including Papanicolaou smear and relevant laboratory tests. As a general rule, oral contraceptives should not be prescribed for longer than 1 year without another physical examination being performed.

2. Under the influence of estrogen-progestogen preparations preexisting uterine leiomyomata may increase in size.

3. Patients with a history of psychic depression should be carefully observed and the drug discontinued if depression recurs to a serious degree. Patients becoming significantly depressed while taking oral contraceptives should stop the medication and use an alternate method of contraception in an attempt to determine whether the symptom is drug related.

4. Oral contraceptives may cause some degree of fluid retention. They should be prescribed with caution, and only with careful monitoring, in patients with conditions which might be aggravated by fluid retention, such as convulsive disorders, migraine syndrome, asthma, or cardiac or renal insufficiency.

5. Patients with a past history of jaundice during pregnancy have an increased risk of recurrence of jaundice while receiving oral contraceptive therapy. If jaundice develops in any patient receiving such drugs, the medication should be discontinued.

6. Steroid hormones may be poorly metabolized in patients with impaired liver function and should be administered with caution in such patients.

7. Oral contraceptive users may have disturbances in normal tryptophan metabolism which may result in a relative pyridoxine deficiency. The clinical significance of this is yet to be determined.

8. Serum folate levels may be depressed by oral contraceptive therapy. Since the pregnant woman is predisposed to the development of folate deficiency and the incidence of folate deficiency increases with increasing gestation, it is possible that if a woman becomes pregnant shortly after stopping oral contraceptives, she may have a greater chance of developing folate deficiency and complications attributed to this deficiency.

9. The pathologist should be advised of oral contraceptive therapy when relevant specimens are submitted.

10. Certain endocrine and liver function tests and blood components may be affected by estrogen-containing oral contraceptives:
 a. Increased sulfobromophthalein retention
 b. Increased prothrombin and factors VII, VIII, IX, and X; decreased antithrombin 3; increased norepinephrine-induced platelet aggregability
 c. Increased thyroid binding globulin (TBG) leading to increased circulating total thyroid hormone, as measured by protein-bound iodine (PBI), T4 by column, or T4 by radioimmunoassay. Free T3 resin uptake is decreased, reflecting the elevated TBG, free T4 concentration is unaltered
 d. Decreased pregnanediol excretion
 e. Reduced response to metyrapone test

Information For The Patient: See Patient Labeling printed following the reference section.

Drug Interactions: Reduced efficacy and increased incidence of breakthrough bleeding have been associated with concomitant use of rifampin. A similar association has been suggested with barbiturates, phenylbutazone, phenytoin sodium, tetracycline, and ampicillin.

Carcinogenesis: See Warnings section for information on the carcinogenic potential of oral contraceptives.

Pregnancy: Pregnancy category X. See Contraindications and Warnings.

Nursing Mothers: See Warnings.

Adverse Reactions: An increased risk of the following serious adverse reactions has been associated with the use of oral contraceptives (see Warnings):
 Thrombophlebitis
 Pulmonary embolism
 Coronary thrombosis
 Cerebral thrombosis
 Cerebral hemorrhage
 Hypertension
 Gallbladder disease
 Benign hepatomas
 Congenital anomalies

There is evidence of an association between the following conditions and the use of oral contraceptives, although additional confirmatory studies are needed:
 Mesenteric thrombosis
 Neuro-ocular lesions, eg, retinal thrombosis and optic neuritis

The following adverse reactions have been reported in patients receiving oral contraceptives and are believed to be drug related:

Nausea and/or vomiting, usually the most common adverse reactions, occur in approximately 10 percent or less of patients during the first cycle. Other reactions, as a general rule, are seen much less frequently or only occasionally.
 Gastrointestinal symptoms (such as abdominal cramps and bloating)
 Breakthrough bleeding
 Spotting
 Change in menstrual flow
 Dysmenorrhea
 Amenorrhea during and after treatment
 Temporary infertility after discontinuance of treatment
 Edema
 Chloasma or melasma which may persist
 Breast changes: tenderness, enlargement and secretion
 Change in weight (increase or decrease)
 Change in cervical erosion and cervical secretion
 Possible diminution in lactation when given immediately postpartum
 Cholestatic jaundice
 Migraine
 Increase in size of uterine leiomyomata
 Rash (allergic)
 Mental depression
 Reduced tolerance to carbohydrates
 Vaginal candidiasis
 Change in corneal curvature (steepening)
 Intolerance to contact lenses

The following adverse reactions have been reported in users of oral contraceptives, and the association has been neither confirmed nor refuted:
 Premenstrual-like syndrome
 Cataracts
 Changes in libido
 Chorea
 Changes in appetite
 Cystitis-like syndrome
 Headache
 Nervousness
 Dizziness
 Hirsutism
 Loss of scalp hair
 Erythema multiforme
 Erythema nodosum
 Hemorrhagic eruption
 Vaginitis
 Porphyria

Acute Overdose: Serious ill effects have not been reported following acute ingestion of large doses of oral contraceptives by young children. Overdosage may cause nausea, and withdrawal bleeding may occur in females.

Dosage and Administration For 21-Day Dosage Regimen: To achieve maximum contraceptive effectiveness, Norlestrin must be taken exactly as directed and at intervals not exceeding 24 hours. Norlestrin 21 provides the patient with a convenient tablet schedule of "3 weeks on—1 week off." The first day of menstrual flow is considered Day 1. Initially, the patient begins taking tablets on Day 5 and takes one tablet daily for 21 days. She then takes no tablets for seven days.

Continued on next page

This product information was prepared in August, 1984. On these and other Parke-Davis Products, information may be obtained by addressing PARKE-DAVIS, Division of Warner-Lambert Company, Morris Plains, New Jersey 07950.

Parke-Davis—Cont.

After the seven days during which no tablets are taken, the patient begins a new course of one tablet daily for 21 days. Each course of tablets will begin on the same day of the week as the first course. Likewise, the interval of no tablets will always start on the same day of the week.

Tablets should be taken regularly with a meal or at bedtime. It should be stressed that efficacy of medication depends on strict adherence to the dosage schedule.

Special Notes on Administration

Menstruation usually begins two or three days, but may begin as late as the fourth or fifth day, after discontinuing medication.

If spotting occurs while on the usual regimen of one tablet daily, the patient should continue medication without interruption.

If a patient forgets to take one or more tablets, the following is suggested: If one tablet is missed, take it as soon as remembered, or take two tablets the next day. If two consecutive tablets are missed, take two tablets daily for the next two days, then resume the regular schedule. If three consecutive tablets are missed, begin a new compact of tablets, starting seven days after the last tablet was taken. The possibility of ovulation occurring increases with each successive day that scheduled tablets are missed. When three consecutive tablets are missed the patient should use an alternate means of contraception, other than oral tablets, until the start of the next menstrual period.

While there is little likelihood of ovulation occurring if only one tablet is missed, the possibility of spotting or bleeding is increased. This is particularly likely to occur if two or more consecutive tablets are missed.

In the rare case of bleeding which resembles menstruation, the patient should be advised to discontinue medication and then begin taking tablets from a new compact on the fifth day (Day 5). Persistent bleeding which is not controlled by this method indicates the need for re-examination of the patient at which time nonfunctional causes should be borne in mind.

Dosage and Administration For 28-Day Dosage Regimen:

To achieve maximum contraceptive effectiveness, Norlestrin must be taken exactly as directed and at intervals not exceeding 24 hours. Norlestrin Fe and 28 provides a continuous administration regimen consisting of 21 *light-colored* tablets of Norlestrin and 7 brown tablets of ferrous fumarate or 7 white inert tablets. There is no need for the patient to count days between cycles because there are no "off-tablet days."

The dosage schedule is one *light-colored* tablet daily for 21 days, starting initially on Day 5 of the menstrual cycle, followed without interruption by one brown or white tablet daily for 7 days. The first day of menstrual flow is considered Day 1. Upon completion of this first course of tablets, a second course of tablets is started without interruption. All subsequent courses also are taken without interruption.

Tablets should be taken regularly with a meal or at bedtime. It should be stressed that efficacy of medication depends on strict adherence to the dosage schedule.

Special Notes on Administration

Menstruation usually begins two or three days, but may begin as late as the fourth or fifth day, after the brown or white tablets have been started. In any event, the next course of tablets should be started without interruption. There should never be a day when the patient is not taking a tablet.

If spotting occurs while the patient is taking *light-colored* tablets, continue medication without interruption.

If a patient forgets to take one or more *light-colored* tablets, the following is suggested: If one *light-colored* tablet is missed, take it as soon as remembered, or take two *light-colored* tablets the next day. If two consecutive *light-colored* tablets are missed, take two *light-colored* tablets daily for the next two days, then resume the regular sched-

ule. If three consecutive *light-colored* tablets are missed, begin a new compact of tablets, starting seven days after the last *light-colored* tablet was taken.

The possibility of ovulation occurring increases with each successive day that scheduled *light-colored* tablets are missed. When three consecutive *light-colored* tablets are missed, the patient should use an alternate means of contraception, other than oral tablets, until the start of the next menstrual period.

While there is little likelihood of ovulation occurring if only one *light-colored* tablet is missed, the possibility of spotting or bleeding is increased. This is particularly likely to occur if two or more consecutive *light-colored* tablets are missed.

If one or more brown or white tablets are missed, the *light-colored* tablets should be started no later than the eighth day after the last *light-colored* tablet was taken. The possibility of conception occurring is not increased if brown or white tablets are missed.

In the rare case of bleeding which resembles menstruation, the patient should be advised to discontinue medication and then begin taking tablets from a new compact on the fifth day (Day 5). Persistent bleeding which is not controlled by this method indicates the need for re-examination of the patient, at which time nonfunctional causes should be borne in mind.

Use of oral contraceptives in the event of a missed menstrual period:

1. If the patient has not adhered to the prescribed dosage regimen, the possibility of pregnancy should be considered after the first missed period and oral contraceptives should be withheld until pregnancy has been ruled out.

2. If the patient has adhered to the prescribed regimen and misses two consecutive periods, pregnancy should be ruled out before continuing the contraceptive regimen.

After several months on treatment, bleeding may be reduced to a point of virtual absence. This reduced flow may occur as a result of medication, in which event it is not indicative of pregnancy.

How Supplied:

Norlestrin 21 1/50 is available in compacts each containing 21 tablets. Each tablet contains 1 mg of norethindrone acetate and 50 mcg of ethinyl estradiol. Available in packages of five compacts and packages of five refills.

Norlestrin 21 2.5/50 is available in compacts each containing 21 tablets. Each tablet contains 2.5 mg of norethindrone acetate and 50 mcg of ethinyl estradiol. Available in packages of five compacts and packages of five refills.

Norlestrin Fe 1/50 is available in compacts each containing 21 yellow tablets and 7 brown tablets. Each yellow tablet contains 1 mg of norethindrone acetate and 50 mcg of ethinyl estradiol. Each brown tablet contains 75 mg ferrous fumarate, USP. Available in packages of five compacts and packages of five refills.

Norlestrin Fe 2.5/50 is available in compacts each containing 21 pink tablets and 7 brown tablets. Each pink tablet contains 2.5 mg of norethindrone acetate and 50 mcg of ethinyl estradiol. Each brown tablet contains 75 mg ferrous fumarate, USP. Available in packages of five compacts and packages of five refills.

Norlestrin 28 1/50 is available in compacts each containing 21 yellow tablets and 7 white inert tablets. Each yellow tablet contains 1 mg of norethindrone acetate and 50 mcg of ethinyl estradiol. Available in packages of five compacts and packages of five refills.

References:

1. "*Population Reports*," Series H, Number 2, May 1974; Series 1, Number 1, June 1974; Series B, Number 2, January 1975; Series H, Number 3, 1975; Series H, Number 4, January 1976 (published by the Population Information Program, The George Washington University Medical Center, 2001 S. St. NW., Washington, D.C.)
2. Inman, W. H. W., M. P. Vessey, B. Westerholm, and A. Engelund. "Thromboembolic disease and the steroidal content of oral contraceptives. A report to the Committee on Safety of Drugs," *Brit Med J* 2:203–209, 1970.
3. Stolley, P.D., J. A. Tonascia, M. S. Tockman, P. E. Sartwell, A. H. Rutledge, and M. P. Jacobs, "Thrombosis with low-estrogen oral contraceptives," *Am J Epidemiol* 102: 197–208, 1975.
4. Royal College of General Practitioners, "Oral contraception and thromboembolic disease," *J Coll Gen Pract* 13:267–279, 1967.
5. Inman, W. H. W. and M. P. Vessey, "Investigation of deaths from pulmonary, coronary and cerebral thrombosis and embolism in women of childbearing age," *Brit Med. J* 2-193–199, 1968.
6. Vessey, M. P. and R. Doll, "Investigation of relation between use of oral contraceptives and thromboembolic disease. A further report," *Brit Med J* 2:651–657, 1969.
7. Sartwell, P. E., A. T. Masi, F. G. Arthes, G. R. Greene, and H. E. Smith, "Thromboembolism and oral contraceptives an epidemiological case control study," *Am J Epidemiol* 90:365–380, 1969.
8. Boston Collaborative Drug Surveillance Program. "Oral contraceptives and venous thromboembolic disease, surgically confirmed gallbladder disease and breast tumors," *Lancet* 1:1399–1404, 1973.
9. Collaborative Group for the Study of Stroke in Young Women, "Oral contraception and increased risk of cerebral ischemia or thrombosis," *N Engl J Med* 288:871–878, 1973.
10. Collaborative Group for the Study of Stroke in Young Women, "Oral contraceptives and stroke in young women: associated risk factors," *JAMA* 231:718–722, 1975.
11. Mann, J. I., and W. H. W. Inman, "Oral contraceptives and death from myocardial infarction," *Brit Med J* 2:245–248, 1975.
12. Mann, J. I., W. H. W. Inman, and M. Thorogood, "Oral contraceptive use in older women and fatal myocardial infarction," *Brit Med J* 2:445–447, 1976.
13. Mann, J. I., M. P. Vessey, M. Thorogood and R. Doll, "Myocardial infarction in young women with special reference to oral contraceptive practice," *Brit Med J* 2:241–245, 1975.
14. Tietze, C., "New Estimates of Mortality Associated with Fertility Control," *Family Planning Perspectives*, 9:74–76, 1977.
15. Vessey, M. P., R. Doll, A. S. Fairbairn, and G. Glober, "Post-operative thromboembolism and the use of oral contraceptives," *Brit Med J* 3:123–126, 1970.
16. Greene, G. R., P. E. Sartwell, "Oral contraceptive use in patients with thromboembolism following surgery, trauma or infection," *Am J Pub Health* 62:680–685, 1972.
17. Smith, D. C., R. Prentice, D. J. Thompson and W. L. Herrmann, "Association of exogenous estrogen and endometrial carcinoma," *N Engl J Med* 293:1164–1167, 1975.
18. Ziel, H. K., and W. D. Finkle, "Increased risk of endometrial carcinoma among users of conjugated estrogens," *N Engl J Med* 293: 1167–1170, 1975.
19. Mack, T. N., M. C. Pike, B. E. Henderson, R. I. Pfeffer, V. R. Gerkins, M. Arthur and S. E. Brown, "Estrogens and endometrial cancer in a retirement community," *N Engl J Med* 294: 1262–1267, 1976.
20. Silverberg, S. G., and E. L. Makowski, "Endometrial carcinoma in young women taking oral contraceptive agents," *Obstet Gynecol* 46:503–506, 1975.
21. Vessey, M. P., R. Doll, and P. M. Sutton, "Oral contraceptives and breast neoplasia: a retrospective study," *Brit Med J* 3:719–724, 1972.
22. Vessey, M. P., R. Doll, and K. Jones, "Oral contraceptives and breast cancer. Progress report of an epidemiological study," *Lancet* 1:941–943, 1975.
23. Boston Collaborative Drug Surveillance Program, "Surgically confirmed gallbladder disease, venous thromboembolism and breast tumors in relation to postmenopausal estrogen therapy," *N Engl J Med* 290:14–19, 1974.
24. Arthes, F. G., P. E. Sartwell, and E. F. Lewison, "The pill, estrogens, and the breast, Epidemiologic aspects," *Cancer* 28:1391–1394, 1971.
25. Fasal, E., and R. S. Paffenbarger, "Oral contraceptives as related to cancer and benign lesions

of the breast." *J Natl Cancer Inst* 55:767–773, 1975.
26. Royal College of General Practitioners, "Oral Contraceptives and Health," London, Pitman, 1974.
27. Ory, H., P. Cole, B. MacMahon, and R. Hoover, "Oral contraceptives and reduced risk of benign breast diseases," *N Engl J Med* 294:419–422, 1976.
28. Baum, J., F. Holtz, J. J. Bookstein, and E. W. Klein, "Possible association between benign hepatomas and oral contraceptives," *Lancet* 2:926–928, 1973.
29. Mays, E. T., W. M. Christophersen, M. M. Mahr, and H. C. Williams, "Hepatic changes in young women ingesting contraceptive steroids. Hepatic hemorrhage and primary hepatic tumors," *JAMA* 235:730–732, 1976.
30. Edmondson, H. A., B. Henderson, and B. Benton, "Liver-cell adenomas associated with use of oral contraceptives," *N Engl J Med* 294:470–472, 1976.
31. Herbst, A. L., H. Ulfelder, and D. C. Poskanzer, "Adenocarcinoma of the vagina," *N Engl J Med* 284:878–881, 1971.
32. Greenwald, P., J. J. Barlow, P. C. Nasca and W. Burnett, "Vaginal cancer after maternal treatment with synthetic estrogens," *N Engl J Med* 285:390–392, 1971.
33. Lanier, A. P., K. L. Noller, D. G. Decker, L. Elveback, and L. T. Kurland, "Cancer and stilbestrol. A follow-up of 1719 persons exposed to estrogens in utero and born 1943–1959," *Mayo Clin Pro* 48:793–799, 1973.
34. Herbst, A. L., R. J. Kurman, and R. E. Scully, "Vaginal and cervical abnormalities after exposure to stilbestrol in utero," *Obstet Gynecol* 40:287–298, 1972.
35. Herbst, A. L., S. J. Robboy, G. J. Macdonald, and R. E. Scully, "The effects of local progesterone on stilbestrol-associated vaginal adenosis," *Am J Obstet Gynecol* 118:607–615, 1974.
36. Herbst, A. L., D. C. Poskanzer, S. J. Robboy, L. Friedlander, and R. E. Scully, "Prenatal exposure to stilbestrol: a prospective comparison of exposed female offspring with unexposed controls," *N Engl J Med* 292:334–339, 1975.
37. Stafl, A., R. F. Mattingly, D. V. Foley, W. Fetherston, "Clinical diagnosis of vaginal adenosis," *Obstet Gynecol* 43:118–128, 1974.
38. Sherman, A. I., M. Goldrath, A. Berlin, V. Vakhariya, F. Banooni, W. Michaels, P. Goodman, and S. Brown, "Cervical-vaginal adenosis after in utero exposure to synthetic estrogens," *Obstet Gynecol* 44:531–545, 1974.
39. Gal, I., B. Kirman, and J. Stern, "Hormone pregnancy tests and congenital malformation," *Nature* 216:83, 1967.
40. Levy, E. P., A. Cohen, and F. C. Fraser, "Hormone treatment during pregnancy and congenital heart defects," *Lancet* 1:611, 1973.
41. Nora, J. J., and A. H. Nora, "Birth defects and oral contraceptives," *Lancet* 1:941–942, 1973.
42. Janerich, D. T., J. M. Piper, and D. M. Glebatis, "Oral contraceptives and congenital limb-reduction defects," *N Engl J Med* 291:697–700, 1974.
43. Carr, D. H., "Chromosome studies in selected spontaneous abortions: I. Conception after oral contraceptives," *Canad Med Assoc J* 103:343–348, 1970.
44. Wynn, V., J. W. H. Doar, and G. L. Mills, "Some effects of oral contraceptives on serum-lipid and lipoprotein levels," *Lancet* 2:720–723, 1966.
45. Laumas, K. R., P. K. Malkani, S. Bhatnagar, and V. Laumas, "Radioactivity in the breast milk of lactating women after oral administration of 3 H-norethynodrel," *Amer J Obstet Gynecol* 98:411–413, 1967.
46. Center for Disease Control, "Increased Risk of Hepatocellular Adenoma in Women with Long-term use of Oral Contraceptives," *Morbidity and Mortality Weekly Report* 26:293–294, 1977.
47. Herbst, A. L., P. Cole, T. Colton, S. J. Robboy, R. E. Scully, "Age-incidence and Risk of Diethylstilbestrol-related Clear Cell Adenocarcinoma of the Vagina and Cervix," *Am J Obstet Gynecol* 128:43–50, 1977.
48. Bibbo, M., M. Al-Naqeeb, I. Baccarini, W. Gill, M. Newton, K. M. Sleeper, M. Sonek, G. L. Wied, "Follow-Up Study of Male and Female Offspring of DES-treated Mothers. A Preliminary Report," *Jour of Repro Med* 15:29–32, 1975.
49. Gill, W. B., G. F. B. Schumacher, M. Bibbo, "Structural and Functional Abnormalities in the Sex Organs of Male Offspring of Mothers Treated with Diethylstilbestrol (DES)," *Jour of Repro Med* 16:147–153, 1976.
50. Henderson, B. E., B. Benton, M. Cosgrove, J. Baptista, J. Aldrich, D. Townsend, W. Hart, T. Mack, "Urogenital Tract Abnormalities in Sons of Women Treated with Diethylstilbestrol," *Pediatrics* 58:505–507, 1976.
51. Heinonen, O. P., D. Slone, R. R. Nonson, E. B. Hook, S. Shapiro, "Cardiovascular Birth Defects and Antenatal Exposure to Female Sex Hormones," *N Engl J Med* 296:67–70, 1977.
52. Jain, A. K., "Mortality Risk Associated with the Use of Oral Contraceptives," *Studies in Family Planning* 8:50–54, 1977.
53. Beral, V., "Mortality Among Oral Contraceptive Users," *Lancet* 2:727–731, 1977.

The patient labeling for oral contraceptive drug products is set forth below:

Brief Summary Patient Package Insert

> Cigarette smoking increases the risk of serious adverse effects on the heart and blood vessels from oral contraceptive use. This risk increases with age and with heavy smoking (15 or more cigarettes per day) and is quite marked in women over 35 years of age. Women who use oral contraceptives should not smoke.

Oral contraceptives taken as directed are about 99% effective in preventing pregnancy. (The mini-pill, however is somewhat less effective.) Forgetting to take your pills increases the chance of pregnancy. Various drugs, such as antibiotics, may also decrease the effectiveness of oral contraceptives. Women who have or have had clotting disorders, cancer of the breast or sex organs, unexplained vaginal bleeding, a stroke, heart attack, angina pectoris, or who suspect they may be pregnant should not use oral contraceptives.

Most side effects of the pill are not serious. The most common side effects are nausea, vomiting, bleeding between menstrual periods, weight gain, and breast tenderness. However, proper use of oral contraceptives requires that they be taken under your doctor's continuous supervision, because they can be associated with serious side effects which may be fatal. Fortunately, these occur very infrequently.

The serious side effects are:
1. Blood clots in the legs, lungs, brain, heart or other organs and hemorrhage into the brain due to bursting of a blood vessel
2. Liver tumors, which may rupture and cause severe bleeding
3. Birth defects if the pill is taken while you are pregnant
4. High blood pressure
5. Gallbladder disease

The symptoms associated with these serious side effects are discussed in the detailed leaflet given you with your supply of pills. Notify your doctor if you notice any unusual physical disturbance while taking the pill.

The estrogen in oral contraceptives has been found to cause breast cancer and other cancers in certain animals. These findings suggest that oral contraceptives may also cause cancer in humans. However, studies to date in women taking currently marketed oral contraceptives have not confirmed that oral contraceptives cause cancer in humans.

The detailed leaflet describes more completely the benefits and risks of oral contraceptives. It also provides information on other forms of contraception. Read it carefully. If you have any questions, consult your doctor.

Caution: Oral contraceptives are of no value in the prevention or treatment of venereal disease.

Detailed Patient Labeling
What You Should Know About Oral Contraceptives

Oral contraceptives ("the pill") are the most effective way (except for sterilization) to prevent pregnancy. They are also convenient and, for most women, free of serious or unpleasant side effects. Oral contraceptives must always be taken under the continuous supervision of a physician.

It is important that any woman who considers using an oral contraceptive understand the risks involved. Although the oral contraceptives have important advantages over other methods of contraception, they have certain risks that no other method has. Only you can decide whether the advantages are worth these risks. This leaflet will tell you about the most important risks. It will explain how you can help your doctor prescribe the pill as safely as possible by telling him about yourself and being alert for the earliest signs of trouble. And it will tell you how to use the pill properly, so that it will be as effective as possible. There is more detailed information available in the leaflet prepared for doctors. Your pharmacist can show you a copy; you may need your doctor's help in understanding parts of it.

Who Should Not Use Oral Contraceptives
A. If you have any of the following conditions you should not use the pill:
1. Clots in the legs or lungs
2. Angina pectoris
3. Known or suspected cancer of the breast or sex organs
4. Unusual vaginal bleeding that has not yet been diagnosed
5. Known or suspected pregnancy
B. If you have had any of the following conditions you should not use the pill:
1. Heart attack or stroke
2. Clots in the legs or lungs

> C. Cigarette smoking increases the risk of serious adverse effects on the heart and blood vessels from oral contraceptive use. This risk increases with age and with heavy smoking (15 or more cigarettes per day) and is quite marked in women over 35 years of age. Women who use oral contraceptives should not smoke.

D. If you have scanty or irregular periods or are a young woman without a regular cycle, you should use another method of contraception because, if you use the pill, you may have difficulty becoming pregnant or may fail to have menstrual periods after discontinuing the pill.

Deciding To Use Oral Contraceptives
If you do not have any of the conditions listed above and are thinking about using oral contraceptives, to help you decide, you need information about the advantages and risks of oral contraceptives and of other contraceptive methods as well. This leaflet describes the advantages and risks of oral contraceptives. Except for sterilization, the IUD and abortion, which have their own exclusive risks, the only risks of other methods of contraception are those due to pregnancy should the method fail. Your doctor can answer questions you may have with respect to other methods of contraception. He can also answer any questions you may have after reading this leaflet on oral contraceptives.

1. What Oral Contraceptives Are and How They Work. Oral contraceptives are of two types. The most common, often simply called "the pill," is a combination of an estrogen and a progestogen, the two kinds of female hormones. The amount of estrogen and progestogen can vary, but the amount

Continued on next page

This product information was prepared in August, 1984. On these and other Parke-Davis Products, information may be obtained by addressing PARKE-DAVIS, Division of Warner-Lambert Company, Morris Plains, New Jersey 07950.

Parke-Davis—Cont.

of estrogen is most important because both the effectiveness and some of the dangers of oral contraceptives are related to the amount of estrogen. This kind of oral contraceptive works principally by preventing release of an egg from the ovary. When the amount of estrogen is 50 micrograms or more, and the pill is taken as directed, oral contraceptives are more than 99% effective (ie, there would be less than one pregnancy if 100 women used the pill for 1 year). Pills that contain 20 to 35 micrograms of estrogen vary slightly in effectiveness, ranging from 98% to more than 99% effective. Norlestrin was shown in clinical trials to be more than 99% effective.

The second type of oral contraceptive, often called the "mini-pill," contains only a progestogen. It works in part by preventing release of an egg from the ovary but also by keeping sperm from reaching the egg and by making the uterus (womb) less receptive to any fertilized egg that reaches it. The mini-pill is less effective than the combination oral contraceptive, about 97% effective.

In addition, the progestogen-only pill has a tendency to cause irregular bleeding which may be quite inconvenient, or cessation of bleeding entirely. The progestogen-only pill is used despite its lower effectiveness in the hope that it will prove not to have some of the serious side effects of the estrogen-containing pill (which follows) but it is not yet certain that the mini-pill does in fact have fewer serious side effects. The discussion which follows, while based mainly on information about the combination pills, should be considered to apply, as well, to the mini-pill.

2. Other Nonsurgical Ways to Prevent Pregnancy. As this leaflet will explain, oral contraceptives have several serious risks. Other methods of contraception have lesser risks or none at all. They are also less effective than oral contraceptives but, used properly, may be effective enough for many women. The following gives reported pregnancy rates (the number of women out of 100 who would become pregnant in 1 year) for these methods:

Pregnancies Per 100 Women Per Year
Intrauterine device (IUD), less than 1-6; Diaphragm with spermicidal products (creams or jellies), 2-20; Condom (rubber), 3-36; Aerosol foams, 2-29; Jellies and creams, 4-36; Periodic abstinence (rhythm) all types, less than 1-47; 1. Calendar method, 14-47; 2. Temperature method, 1-20; 3. Temperature method—intercourse only in postovulatory phase, less than 1-7; 4. Mucus method, 1-25; No contraception, 60-80.

The figures (except for the IUD) vary widely because people differ in how well they use each method. Very faithful users of the various methods obtain very good results except for users of the calendar method of periodic abstinence (rhythm). Except for the IUD, effective use of these methods requires somewhat more effort than simply taking a single pill every morning, but it is an effort that many couples undertake successfully. Your doctor can tell you a great deal more about these methods of contraception.

3. The Dangers of Oral Contraceptives.
a. *Circulatory disorders (abnormal blood clotting and stroke due to hemorrhage).* Blood clots (in various blood vessels of the body) are the most common of the serious side effects of oral contraceptives. A clot can result in a stroke (if the clot is in the brain), a heart attack (if the clot is in a blood vessel of the heart), or a pulmonary embolus (a clot which forms in the legs or pelvis, then breaks off and travels to the lungs). Any of these can be fatal. Clots also occur rarely in the blood vessels of the eye, resulting in blindness or impairment of vision in that eye. There is evidence that the risk of clotting increases with higher estrogen doses. It is, therefore, important to keep the dose of estrogen as low as possible, so long as the oral contraceptive used has an acceptable pregnancy rate and doesn't cause unacceptable changes in the menstrual pattern. Furthermore, cigarette smoking by oral contraceptive users increases the risk of serious adverse effects on the heart and blood vessels. This risk increases with age and with heavy smoking (15 or more cigarettes per day) and begins to become quite marked in women over 35 years of age. For this reason, women who use oral contraceptives should not smoke.

The risk of abnormal clotting increases with age in both users and nonusers of oral contraceptives, but the increased risk from the contraceptives appears to be present at all ages. For oral contraceptive users in general, it has been estimated that in women between the ages of 15 and 34 the risk of death due to a circulatory disorder is about 1 in 12,000 per year, whereas for nonusers the rate is about 1 in 50,000 per year. In the age group 35 to 44, the risk is estimated to be about 1 in 2,500 per year for oral contraceptive users and about 1 in 10,000 per year for nonusers.

Even without the pill the risk of having a heart attack increases with age and is also increased by such heart attack risk factors as high blood pressure, high cholesterol, obesity, diabetes, and cigarette smoking. Without any risk factors present, the use of oral contraceptives alone may double the risk of heart attack. However, the combination of cigarette smoking, especially heavy smoking, and oral contraceptive use greatly increases the risk of heart attack. Oral contraceptive users who smoke are about 5 times more likely to have a heart attack than users who do not smoke and about 10 times more likely to have a heart attack than nonusers who do not smoke. It has been estimated that users between the ages of 30 and 39 who smoke have about a 1 in 10,000 chance each year of having a fatal heart attack compared to about a 1 in 50,000 chance in users who do not smoke, and about a 1 in 100,000 chance in nonusers who do not smoke. In the age group 40 to 44, the risk is about 1 in 1,700 per year for users who smoke compared to about 1 in 10,000 for users who do not smoke and to about 1 in 14,000 per year for nonusers who do not smoke. Heavy smoking (about 15 cigarettes or more a day) further increases the risk. If you do not smoke and have none of the other heart attack risk factors described above, you will have a smaller risk than listed. If you have several heart attack risk factors, the risk may be considerably greater than listed.

In addition to blood-clotting disorders, it has been estimated that women taking oral contraceptives are twice as likely as nonusers to have a stroke due to rupture of a blood vessel in the brain.

b. *Formation of tumors.* Studies have found that when certain animals are given the female sex hormone estrogen, which is an ingredient of oral contraceptives, continuously for long periods, cancers may develop in the breast, cervix, vagina, and liver.

These findings suggest that oral contraceptives may cause cancer in humans. However, studies to date in women taking currently marketed oral contraceptives have not confirmed that oral contraceptives cause cancer in humans. Several studies have found no increase in breast cancer in users, although one study suggested oral contraceptives might cause an increase in breast cancer in women who already have benign breast disease (eg, cysts).

Women with a strong family history of breast cancer or who have breast nodules, fibrocystic disease, or abnormal mammograms or who were exposed to DES (diethylstilbestrol), an estrogen, during their mother's pregnancy must be followed very closely by their doctors if they choose to use oral contraceptives instead of another method of contraception. Many studies have shown that women taking oral contraceptives have less risk of getting benign breast disease than those who have not used oral contraceptives. Recently, strong evidence has emerged that estrogens (one component of oral contraceptives), when given for periods of more than one year to women after the menopause, increase the risk of cancer of the uterus (womb). There is also some evidence that a kind of oral contraceptive which is no longer marketed, the sequential oral contraceptive, may increase the risk of cancer of the uterus. There remains no evidence, however, that the oral contraceptives now available increase the risk of this cancer.

Oral contraceptives do cause, although rarely, a benign (nonmalignant) tumor of the liver. These tumors do not spread, but they may rupture and cause internal bleeding, which may be fatal. A few cases of cancer of the liver have been reported in women using oral contraceptives, but it is not yet known whether the drug caused them.

c. *Dangers to a developing child if oral contraceptives are used in or immediately preceding pregnancy.* Oral contraceptives should not be taken by pregnant women because they may damage the developing child. An increased risk of birth defects, including heart defects and limb defects, has been associated with the use of sex hormones, including oral contraceptives, in pregnancy. In addition, the developing female child whose mother has received DES (diethylstilbestrol), an estrogen, during pregnancy has a risk of getting cancer of the vagina or cervix in her teens or young adulthood. This risk is estimated to be about 1 in 1,000 exposures or less. Abnormalities of the urinary and sex organs have been reported in male offspring so exposed. It is possible that other estrogens, such as the estrogens in oral contraceptives, could have the same effect in the child if the mother takes them during pregnancy.

If you stop taking oral contraceptives to become pregnant, your doctor may recommend that you use another method of contraception for a short while. The reason for this is that there is evidence from studies in women who have had "miscarriages" soon after stopping the pill, that the lost fetuses are more likely to be abnormal. Whether there is an overall increase in "miscarriage" in women who become pregnant soon after stopping the pill, as compared with women who do not use the pill, is not known, but it is possible that there may be. If, however, you do become pregnant soon after stopping oral contraceptives, and do not have a miscarriage, there is no evidence that the baby has an increased risk of being abnormal.

d. *Gallbladder disease.* Women who use oral contraceptives have a greater risk than nonusers of having gallbladder disease requiring surgery. The increased risk may first appear within 1 year of use and may double after 4 or 5 years of use.

e. *Other side effects of oral contraceptives.* Some women using oral contraceptives experience unpleasant side effects that are not dangerous and are not likely to damage their health. Some of these may be temporary. Your breasts may feel tender, nausea and vomiting may occur, you may gain or lose weight, and your ankles may swell. A spotty darkening of the skin, particularly of the face, is possible and may persist. You may notice unexpected vaginal bleeding or changes in your menstrual period. Irregular bleeding is frequently seen when using the mini-pill or combination oral contraceptives containing less than 50 micrograms of estrogen.

More serious side effects include worsening of migraine, asthma, epilepsy, and kidney or heart disease because of a tendency for water to be retained in the body when oral contraceptives are used. Other side effects are growth of preexisting fibroid tumors of the uterus, mental depression, and liver problems with jaundice (yellowing of the skin). Your doctor may find that levels of sugar and fatty substances in your blood are elevated; the long-term effects of these changes are not known. Some women develop high blood pressure while taking oral contraceptives, which ordinarily returns to the original levels when the oral contraceptive is stopped.

Other reactions, although not proved to be caused by oral contraceptives, are occasionally reported. These include more frequent urination and some discomfort when urinating, nervousness, dizziness, some loss of scalp hair, an increase in body hair, an increase or decrease in sex drive, appetite changes, cataracts, and a need for a change in contact lens prescription or inability to use contact lenses.

After you stop using oral contraceptives there may be a delay before you are able to become pregnant or before you resume having menstrual periods.

This is especially true of women who had irregular menstrual cycles prior to the use of oral contraceptives. As discussed previously, your doctor may recommend that you wait a short while after stopping the pill before you try to become pregnant. During this time, use another form of contraception. You should consult your physician before resuming use of oral contraceptives after childbirth, especially if you plan to nurse your baby. Drugs in oral contraceptives are known to appear in the milk, and the long-range effect on infants is not known at this time. Furthermore, oral contraceptives may cause a decrease in your milk supply as well as in the quality of the milk.

4. Comparison of the Risks of Oral Contraceptives and Other Contraceptive Methods. The many studies on the risks and effectiveness of oral contraceptives and other methods of contraception have been analyzed to estimate the risk of death associated with various methods of contraception. This risk has two parts: (a) the risk of the method itself (eg, the risk that oral contraceptives will cause death due to abnormal clotting); and (b) the risk of death due to pregnancy or abortion in the event the method fails. The results of this analysis are shown in the following bar graph. The height of the bars is the number of deaths per 100,000 women each year. There are six sets of bars, each set referring to a specific age group of women. Within each set of bars, there is a single bar for each of the different contraceptive methods. For oral contraceptives, there are two bars—one for smokers and the other for nonsmokers. The analysis is based on present knowledge and new information could, of course, alter it. The analysis shows that the risk of death from all methods of birth control is low and below that associated with childbirth, except for oral contraceptives in women over 40 who smoke. It shows that the lowest risk of death is associated with the condom or diaphragm (traditional contraception) backed up by early abortion in case of failure of the condom or diaphragm to prevent pregnancy. Also, at any age the risk of death (due to unexpected pregnancy) from the use of traditional contraception, even without a backup of abortion, is generally the same as or less than that from use of oral contraceptives.
[See table above].

How to Use Oral Contraceptives As Safely and Effectively As Possible, Once You Have Decided to Use Them

1. What to Tell your Doctor.
You can make use of the pill as safely as possible, by telling your doctor if you have any of the following:
a. Conditions that mean you should not use oral contraceptives:
Clots in the legs or lungs
Clots in the legs or lungs in the past
A stroke, heart attack, or angina pectoris
Known or suspected cancer of the breast or sex organs
Unusual vaginal bleeding that has not yet been diagnosed
Known or suspected pregnancy
b. Conditions that your doctor will want to watch closely or which might cause him to suggest another method of contraception:
A family history of breast cancer
Breast nodules, fibrocystic disease of the breast, or an abnormal mammogram
Diabetes
High blood pressure
High cholesterol
Cigarette smoking
Migraine headaches
Heart or kidney disease
Epilepsy
Mental depression
Fibroid tumors of the uterus
Gallbladder disease
c. Once you are using oral contraceptives, you should be alert for signs of a serious adverse effect and call your doctor if they occur:
Sharp pain in the chest, coughing blood, or sudden shortness of breath (indicating possible clots in the lungs)
Pain in the calf (possible clot in the leg)
Crushing chest pain or heaviness (indicating possible heart attack)
Sudden severe headache or vomiting, dizziness or fainting, disturbance of vision or speech, or weakness or numbness in an arm or leg (indicating a possible stroke)
Sudden partial or complete loss of vision (indicating a possible clot in the eye)
Breast lumps (you should ask your doctor to show you how to examine your own breasts)
Severe pain in the abdomen (indicating a possible ruptured tumor of the liver)
Severe depression
Yellowing of the skin (jaundice)

2. How to Take the Pill So That It Is Most Effective.
Reduced effectiveness and an increased incidence of breakthrough bleeding have been associated with the use of oral contraceptives with antibiotics such as rifampin, ampicillin, and tetracycline or with certain other drugs, such as barbiturates, phenylbutazone or phenytoin sodium. You should use an additional means of contraception during any cycle in which any of these drugs are taken.

Directions For 21-Day Dosage Regimen
a. The first day of your period is Day 1. On the fifth day (Day 5), start taking a tablet daily, beginning with the tablet in the upper left corner of the Petipac. In the space provided, write the day you start. To remove a tablet, press down on it with your thumb or finger. The tablet will drop through a hole in the bottom of the Petipac. Do not press on the tablet with your thumbnail or fingernail, or any other sharp object.

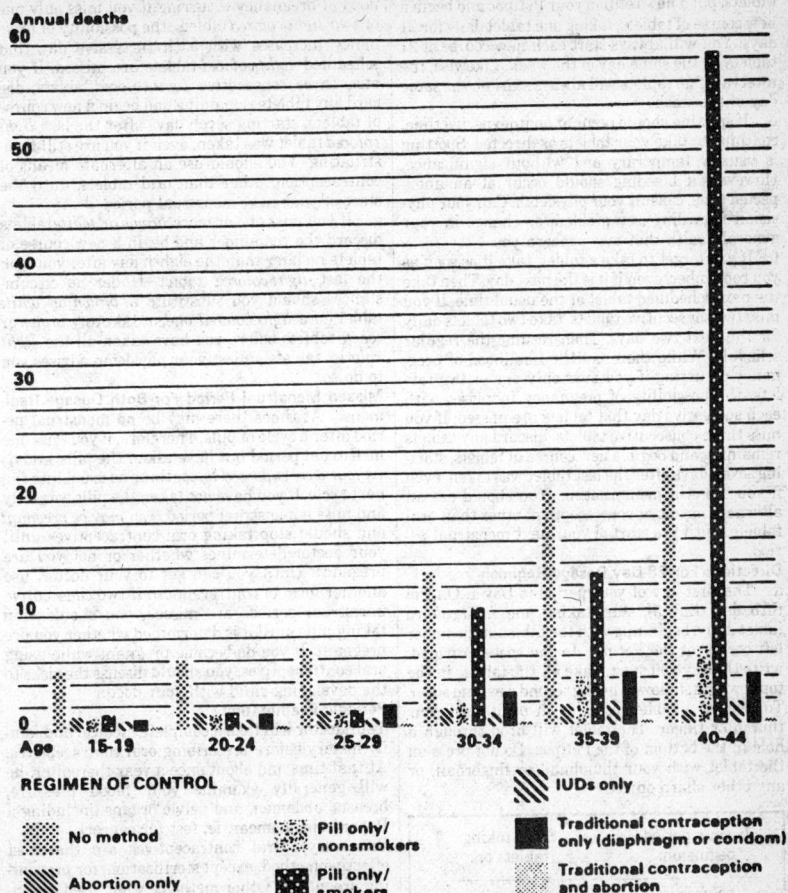

Figure 1. Estimated annual number of deaths associated with control of fertility and no control per 100,000 nonsterile women, by regimen of control and age of woman.

If your period begins on:	Start taking tablets on:
Sunday	Thursday
Monday	Friday
Tuesday	Saturday
Wednesday	Sunday
Thursday	Monday
Friday	Tuesday
Saturday	Wednesday

b. Continue to take one tablet daily until all the tablets have been taken.
c. After you have taken all 21 tablets, stop and don't take any tablets for the next seven days. You should have a menstrual period one to three days after you stop taking tablets; sometimes, it may take a day or so longer.

Continued on next page

This product information was prepared in August, 1984. On these and other Parke-Davis Products, information may be obtained by addressing PARKE-DAVIS, Division of Warner-Lambert Company, Morris Plains, New Jersey 07950.

Parke-Davis—Cont.

d. After seven days, during which you take no tablets, put a new refill in your Petipac and begin a new course of tablets, taking one tablet daily for 21 days. You will always start each new course of 21 tablets on the same day of the week. Likewise, the interval of no tablets will always start on the same day of the week.

e. If spotting should occur at an unexpected time, continue to take your tablets as directed. Spotting is usually temporary and without significance. However, if bleeding should occur at an unexpected time, consult your physician. Call your physician regarding any problem or change in your general health that may concern you.

f. If you forget to take a tablet, take it as soon as you remember, even if it is the next day. Then take the next scheduled tablet at the usual time. If you miss two consecutive tablets, take two tablets daily for the next two days. Then resume the regular schedule. While there is little likelihood of pregnancy occurring if you miss only one or two tablets, the possibility of pregnancy increases with each successive day that tablets are missed. If you miss three consecutive tablets, discard any tablets remaining and begin a new course of tablets, starting seven days after the last tablet was taken, even if you are still menstruating. You should use an alternate means of contraception, other than oral tablets, until the start of your next menstrual period.

Directions For 28-Day Dosage Regimen

a. The first day of your period is Day 1. On the fifth day (Day 5), start taking one *light-colored* tablet daily, beginning with the tablet in the upper left corner of the Petipac. In the space provided, write the day you start. Take all the tablets in the top row first, followed by the second row, and so on. To remove a tablet, press down on it with your thumb or finger. The tablet will drop through a hole in the bottom of the Petipac. Do not press on the tablet with your thumbnail or fingernail, or any other sharp object.

If your period begins on:	Start taking tablets on:
Sunday	Thursday
Monday	Friday
Tuesday	Saturday
Wednesday	Sunday
Thursday	Monday
Friday	Tuesday
Saturday	Wednesday

b. On the day after taking the last *light-colored* tablet, begin taking one *brown* or *white* tablet daily until all the tablets have been taken.

c. When the last tablet has been taken, put a new refill in your Petipac and, without interruption, begin a new course of tablets by taking the *light-colored* tablets first, followed by the *brown* or *white* tablets. There should never be a day when you are not taking a tablet.

d. Continue taking *light-colored* tablets without interruption whether or not your period has occurred or is still in progress. Your period will usually occur during the time you are taking *brown* or *white* tablets.

e. If spotting should occur at an unexpected time, continue to take your tablets as directed. Spotting is usually temporary and without significance. However, if bleeding should occur at an unexpected time, consult your physician. Call your physician regarding any problem or change in your general health that may concern you.

f. If you forget to take a *light-colored* tablet, take it as soon as you remember, even if it is the next day. Then take the next scheduled *light-colored* tablet at the usual time. If you miss two consecutive *light-colored* tablets, take two *light-colored* tablets daily for the next two days. Then resume the regular schedule. While there is little likelihood of pregnancy occurring if you miss only one or two *light-colored* tablets, the possibility of pregnancy increases with each successive day that scheduled *light-colored* tablets are missed. If you miss three consecutive *light-colored* tablets, discard any tablets remaining and begin a new course of tablets, starting seven days after the last *light-colored* tablet was taken, even if you are still menstruating. You should use an alternate means of contraception, other than oral tablets, until the start of your next menstrual period.

g. If you miss one or more *brown* or *white* tablets discard the remainder and begin a new course of tablets no later than the eighth day after you took the last *light-colored* tablet. Under no circumstances should you substitute a *brown* or *white* tablet for a *light-colored* one, or take any *brown* or *white* tablets before you have taken all the *light-colored* tablets, unless your physician advises you to do so.

Missed Menstrual Period For Both Dosage Regimens:

At times there may be no menstrual period after a cycle of pills. Therefore, if you miss one menstrual period but have taken the pills *exactly as your were supposed to*, continue as usual into the next cycle. If you have not taken the pills correctly and miss a menstrual period, *you may be pregnant* and should stop taking oral contraceptives until your doctor determines whether or not you are pregnant. Until you can get to your doctor, use another form of contraception. If two consecutive menstrual periods are missed, you should stop taking pills until it is determined whether you are pregnant. If you do become pregnant while using oral contraceptives, you should discuss the risks to the developing child with your doctor.

Periodic Examination

Your doctor will take a complete medical and family history before prescribing oral contraceptives. At that time and about once a year thereafter, he will generally examine your blood pressure, breasts, abdomen, and pelvic organs (including a Papanicolaou smear, ie, test for cancer).

Summary: Oral contraceptives are the most effective method, except sterilization, for preventing pregnancy. Other methods, when used conscientiously, are also very effective and have fewer risks. The serious risks of oral contraceptives are uncommon and the "pill" is a very convenient method of preventing pregnancy.

If you have certain conditions or have had these conditions in the past, you should not use oral contraceptives because the risk is too great. These conditions are listed in this leaflet. If you do not have these conditions, and decide to use the "pill," please read this leaflet carefully so that you can use the "pill" most safely and effectively.

Based on his or her assessment of your medical needs, your doctor has prescribed this drug for you. Do not give this drug to anyone else.

0907G130

Shown in Product Identification Section, page 425

NORLUTIN® ℞
[nōr″ lū′ tin]
(norethindrone tablets, USP)*

NORLUTATE® ℞
[nōr″ lū′ tāte]
(norethindrone acetate tablets, USP)*

*Product of Warner-Lambert Inc

WARNING
THE USE OF PROGESTATIONAL AGENTS DURING THE FIRST FOUR MONTHS OF PREGNANCY IS NOT RECOMMENDED.
Progestational agents have been used beginning with the first trimester of pregnancy in an attempt to prevent habitual abortion or to treat threatened abortion. There is no adequate evidence that such use is effective and there is evidence of potential harm to the fetus when such drugs are given during the first four months of pregnancy. Furthermore, in the vast majority of women, the cause of abortion is a defective ovum, which progestational agents could not be expected to influence. In addition, the use of progestational agents, with their uterine-relaxant properties, in patients with fertilized defective ova may cause a delay in spontaneous abortion. Therefore, the use of such drugs during the first four months of pregnancy is not recommended.

Several reports suggest an association between intrauterine exposure to female sex hormones and congenital anomalies, including congenital heart defects and limb reduction defects.[1-5] One study[4] estimated a 4.7 fold increased risk of limb reduction defects in infants exposed *in utero* to sex hormones (oral contraceptives, hormone withdrawal test for pregnancy, or attempted treatment for threatened abortion). Some of these exposures were very short and involved only a few days of treatment. The data suggest that the risk of limb reduction defects in exposed fetuses is somewhat less than 1 in 1,000.

If the patient is exposed to Norlutin or Norlutate during the first four months of pregnancy or if she becomes pregnant while taking either of these drugs, she should be apprised of the potential risk to the fetus.

Description: Norlutin is the 17 alpha-ethinyl derivative of 19-nortestosterone. It is a purified crystalline compound that provides orally potent progestational action. The use of norethindrone is indicated in those clinical conditions associated with a deficiency in the secretion of progesterone. Norlutate is the acetic acid ester of norethindrone, which is the 17 alpha-ethinyl derivative of 19-nortestosterone. The use of norethindrone acetate is indicated in those clinical conditions associated with a deficiency in the secretion of progesterone. Norethindrone acetate differs from norethindrone only in potency; the acetate is approximately twice as potent.

Actions: Transforms proliferative endometrium into secretory endometrium

Inhibits (at the usual dosage range) the secretion of pituitary gonadotropins, which in turn prevents follicular maturation and ovulation.

May also demonstrate some estrogenic, anabolic, or androgenic activity but should not be relied upon.

Indications: Norlutin and Norlutate are indicated in amenorrhea; in abnormal uterine bleeding due to hormonal imbalance in the absence of organic pathology, such as submucous fibroids or uterine cancer; and in endometriosis.

Contraindications:
1. Thrombophlebitis, thromboembolic disorders, cerebral apoplexy, or patients with a past history of these conditions
2. Known or suspected carcinoma of the breast
3. Undiagnosed vaginal bleeding
4. Missed abortion
5. As a diagnostic test for pregnancy

Warnings:
1. Discontinue medication pending examination if there is a sudden partial or complete loss of vision, or if there is sudden onset of proptosis, diplopia, or migraine. If examination reveals papilledema or retinal vascular lesions, medication should be withdrawn.
2. Detectable amounts of progestogens have been identified in the milk of mothers receiving them. The effect of this on the nursing infant has not been determined.
3. Because of the occasional occurrence of thrombophlebitis and pulmonary embolism in patients taking progestogens, the physician should be alert to the earliest manifestations of the disease.
4. Masculinization of the female fetus has occurred when progestogens have been used in pregnant women.
5. Some beagle dogs treated with medroxyprogesterone acetate developed mammary nodules.

Although nodules occasionally appeared in control animals, they were intermittent in nature, whereas nodules in treated animals were larger and more numerous, and persisted. There is no general agreement as to whether the nodules are benign or malignant. Their significance with respect to humans has not been established.

Precautions:
1. The pretreatment physical examination should include special reference to breasts and pelvic organs, as well as a Papanicolaou smear.
2. Because this drug may cause some degree of fluid retention, conditions which might be influenced by this factor, such as epilepsy, migraine, asthma, cardiac or renal dysfunction, require careful observation.
3. In cases of breakthrough bleeding, as in all cases of irregular bleeding per vaginum, nonfunctional causes should be borne in mind. In cases of undiagnosed vaginal bleeding, adequate diagnostic measures are indicated.
4. Patients who have a history of psychic depression should be carefully observed and the drug discontinued if the depression recurs to a serious degree.
5. Any possible influence of prolonged progestogen therapy on pituitary, ovarian, adrenal, hepatic, or uterine functions awaits further study.
6. A decrease in glucose tolerance has been observed in a small percentage of patients on estrogen-progestogen combination drugs. The mechanism of this decrease is obscure. For this reason, diabetic patients should be carefully observed while receiving progestogen therapy.
7. The age of the patient constitutes no absolute limiting factor, although treatment with progestogens may mask the onset of the climacteric.
8. The pathologist should be advised of progestogen therapy when relevant specimens are submitted.
9. Steroid hormones are metabolized by the liver, therefore, these drugs should be administered with caution in patients with impaired liver function.
10. Information for the Patient. See text of Patient Package Insert which is printed following references.

Adverse Reactions: The following adverse reactions have been observed in women taking progestogens.
1. Breakthrough bleeding
2. Spotting
3. Change in menstrual flow
4. Amenorrhea
5. Edema
6. Changes in weight (increase or decrease)
7. Changes in cervical erosion and cervical secretions
8. Cholestatic jaundice
9. Rash (allergic) with and without pruritus
10. Melasma or chloasma
11. Mental depression

The following laboratory result may be altered by the use of progestogens:
Pregnanediol determination.
In addition, the following laboratory results may be altered by the concomitant use of estrogens with progestogens.
1. Hepatic function
2. Coagulation tests: increase in prothrombin, factors VII, VIII, IX, and X
3. Increase in PBI, BEI, and a decrease in T3 uptake
4. Metyrapone test

A statistically significant association has been demonstrated between use of estrogen-progestogen combination drugs and the following serious adverse reactions: thrombophlebitis; pulmonary embolism, and cerebral thrombosis and embolism. For this reason, patients on progestogen therapy should be carefully observed.

Although available evidence is suggestive of an association, such a relationship has been neither confirmed nor refuted for the following serious adverse reactions:

Neuro-ocular lesions, eg, retinal thrombosis and optic neuritis.
The following adverse reactions have been observed in patients receiving estrogen-progestogen combination drugs.
1. Rise in blood pressure in susceptible individuals
2. Premenstrual-like syndrome
3. Changes in libido
4. Changes in appetite
5. Cystitis-like syndrome
6. Headache
7. Nervousness
8. Dizziness
9. Fatigue
10. Backache
11. Hirsutism
12. Loss of scalp hair
13. Erythema multiforme
14. Erythema nodosum
15. Hemorrhagic eruption
16. Itching

In view of these observations, patients on progestogen therapy should be carefully observed for their occurrence.

Dosage and Administration: Norlutin (norethindrone tablets, USP): *Therapy with Norlutin must be adapted to the specific indications and therapeutic response of the individual patient.*
This dosage schedule assumes the interval between menses to be 28 days.
Amenorrhea, abnormal uterine bleeding due to hormonal imbalance in the absence of organic pathology: 5 to 20 mg Norlutin starting with the fifth day of the menstrual cycle and ending on the 25th day.
Endometriosis: Initial daily dosage of 10 mg Norlutin for two weeks with increments of 5 mg per day of Norlutin every two weeks until 30 mg per day of Norlutin is reached. Therapy may be held at this level for from six to nine months or until annoying breakthrough bleeding demands temporary termination.

Norlutate (norethindrone acetate tablets, USP): *Therapy with Norlutate must be adapted to the specific indications and therapeutic response of the individual patient.*
This dosage schedule assumes the interval between menses to be 28 days.
Amenorrhea, abnormal uterine bleeding due to hormonal imbalance in the absence of organic pathology: 2.5 to 10 mg Norlutate starting with the fifth day of the menstrual cycle and ending on the 25th day.
Endometriosis: Initial daily dosage of 5 mg Norlutate for two weeks, with increments of 2.5 mg per day of Norlutate every two weeks until 15 mg per day of Norlutate is reached. Therapy may be held at this level for from six to nine months or until annoying breakthrough bleeding demands temporary termination.

How Supplied: N 0710-0882-19 (Tablet 882)—Norlutin is supplied as 5-mg scored tablets in bottles of 50. 0882G010
Shown in Product Identification Section, page 425
N 0710-0918-50 (Tablet 918)—Norlutate is supplied as 5-mg scored tablets in bottles of 50.
AHFS 68:32   0918 G 040
Shown in Product Identification Section, page 425

PATIENT LABELING FOR PROGESTOGENS
WARNING FOR WOMEN
There is an increased risk of birth defects in children whose mothers take these drugs during the first four months of pregnancy.
Norlutin and Norlutate are similar to the progesterone hormones naturally produced by the body. Progesterone and progesterone-like drugs are used to treat menstrual disorders, to test if the body is producing certain hormones, and to treat some forms of cancer in women.
These drugs have been used as a test for pregnancy but such use is no longer considered safe because of possible damage to a developing baby. Also, more rapid methods for testing for pregnancy are now available.
These drugs have also been used to prevent miscarriage in the first few months of pregnancy. No adequate evidence is available to show that they are effective for this purpose and there is evidence of an increased risk of birth defects, such as heart or limb defects, if these drugs are taken during the first four months of pregnancy. Furthermore, most cases of early miscarriage are due to causes which could not be helped by these drugs.
The exact risk of taking these drugs early in pregnancy and having a baby with a birth defect is not known. However, one study found that babies born to women who had taken sex hormones (such as progesterone-like drugs) during the first three months of pregnancy were 4 to 5 times more likely to have abnormalities of the arms or legs than if their mothers had not taken such drugs. Some of these women had taken these drugs for only a few days. The chance that an infant whose mother had taken this drug will have this type of defect is about 1 in 1,000.
If you take Norlutin or Norlutate and later find you were pregnant when you took it, be sure to discuss this with your doctor as soon as possible.

OPHTHOCHLOR®   ℞
[ŏph'thō"chlōr]
(chloramphenicol ophthalmic solution)
0.5%

> **Warning**
> Bone marrow hypoplasia including aplastic anemia and death has been reported following local application of chloramphenicol. Chloramphenicol should not be used when less potentially dangerous agents would be expected to provide effective treatment.

Description: Ophthochlor (Chloramphenicol Ophthalmic Solution, USP), 0.5%, is a sterile, buffered solution containing 0.5% (5 mg/ml) of chloramphenicol. It contains no preservatives.
The chemical names for chloramphenicol are:
(1) Acetamide,2,2-dichloro-N-[2-hydroxy-1-(hydroxymethyl)-2-(4-nitrophenyl) ethyl]-, and
(2) D-*threo*-(-)-2,2-Dichloro-N-[β-hydroxy-α-(hydroxymethyl)-p-nitrophenethyl] acetamide

Clinical Pharmacology: Chloramphenicol is a broad-spectrum antibiotic originally isolated from *Streptomyces venezuelae*. It is primarily bacteriostatic and acts by inhibition of protein synthesis by interfering with the transfer of activated amino acids from soluble RNA to ribosomes. It has been noted that chloramphenicol is found in measurable amounts in the aqueous humor following local application to the eye. Development of resistance to chloramphenicol can be regarded as minimal for staphylococci and many other species of bacteria.

Indications and Usage: Chloramphenicol should be used only in those serious infections for which less potentially dangerous drugs are ineffective or contraindicated. Bacteriological studies should be performed to determine the causative organisms and their sensitivity to chloramphenicol (See Box Warning).
Ophthochlor (chloramphenicol ophthalmic solution) 0.5% is indicated for the treatment of surface ocular infections involving the conjunctiva and/or cornea caused by chloramphenicol-susceptible organisms.
The particular antiinfective drug in this product is active against the following common bacterial eye pathogens:
Staphylococcus aureus
Streptococci, including *Streptococcus pneumoniae*
Escherichia coli
Haemophilus influenzae

Continued on next page

This product information was prepared in August, 1984. On these and other Parke-Davis Products, information may be obtained by addressing PARKE-DAVIS, Division of Warner-Lambert Company, Morris Plains, New Jersey 07950.

Parke-Davis—Cont.

Klebsiella/Enterobacter species
Moraxella lacunata (Morax-Axenfeld bacillus)
Neisseria species
The product does not provide adequate coverage against:
Pseudomonas aeruginosa
Serratia marcescens
Contraindications: This product is contraindicated in persons sensitive to any of its components.
Warnings: SEE BOX WARNING
Precautions: The prolonged use of antibiotics may occasionally result in overgrowth of nonsusceptible organisms, including fungi. If new infections appear during medication, the drug should be discontinued and appropriate measures should be taken. In all serious infections the topical use of chloramphenicol should be supplemented by appropriate systemic medication.
Adverse Reactions: Blood dyscrasias have been reported in association with the use of chloramphenicol (See WARNINGS).
Dosage and Administration: Two drops applied to the affected eye every three hours or more frequently if deemed advisable by the prescribing physician. Administration should be continued day and night for the first 48 hours, after which the interval between applications may be increased. Treatment should be continued for at least 48 hours after the eye appears normal.
How Supplied: N 0071-3395-11 15 ml bottle.
Ophthochlor (Chloramphenicol Ophthalmic Solution, USP), 0.5% is supplied in plastic dropper bottles and contains no preservatives. Each ml contains 5 mg chloramphenicol in a boric acid-sodium borate buffer solution. Sodium hydroxide may have been added for adjustment of pH. To protect it from light, the solution should be dispensed in the carton. This product should be stored in a refrigerator until dispensed. Discard solution within 21 days from date dispensed.
AHFS Category 52:04.04   3395G011
Shown in Product Identification Section, p. 425

OPHTHOCORT®
[ŏph'thō"cŏrt]
(Chloramphenicol, Polymyxin B Sulfate, and Hydrocortisone Acetate Ophthalmic Ointment, USP)

WARNING
Bone marrow hypoplasia including aplastic anemia and death has been reported following local application of chloramphenicol. Chloramphenicol should not be used when less potentially dangerous agents would be expected to provide effective treatment.

Description: Ophthocort® (Chloramphenicol, Polymyxin B Sulfate, and Hydrocortisone Acetate Ophthalmic Ointment, USP) is a sterile antibiotic-/antiinflammatory ointment for ophthalmic administration. Each gram of Ophthocort contains 10 mg chloramphenicol, 10,000 units polymyxin B (as the sulfate), and 5 mg hydrocortisone acetate in a special base of liquid petrolatum and polyethylene. It contains no preservatives.
Clinical Pharmacology: Corticoids suppress the inflammatory response to a variety of agents and they probably delay or slow healing. Since corticoids may inhibit the body's defense mechanism against infection, a concomitant antimicrobial drug may be used when this inhibition is considered to be clinically significant in a particular case.
The antiinfective components in this combination are included to provide action against specific organisms susceptible to them. Chloramphenicol is considered active against a wide spectrum of gram-negative and gram-positive organisms such as *Escherichia coli, Hemophilus influenzae, Staphylococcus aureus, Streptococcus hemolyticus,* and *Moraxella lacunata* (Morax-Axenfeld bacillus). Development of resistance to chloramphenicol can be regarded as minimal for staphylococci and many other species of bacteria. Chloramphenicol is primarily bacteriostatic and acts by inhibition of protein synthesis by interfering with the transfer of activated amino acids from soluble RNA to ribosomes. It has been noted that chloramphenicol is found in measurable amounts in the aqueous humor following local application to the eye.
Polymyxin B sulfate has a bactericidal action against almost all gram-negative bacilli except the *Proteus* group. All gram-positive bacteria, fungi, and the gram-negative cocci, *Neisseria gonorrhoeae* and *N meningitidis,* are resistant.
When a decision to administer both a corticoid and an antimicrobial is made, the administration of such drugs in combination has the advantage of greater patient compliance and convenience, with the added assurance that the appropriate dosage of both drugs is administered, plus assured compatibility of ingredients when both types of drug are in the same formulation and, particularly, that the correct volume of drug is delivered and retained.
The relative potency of corticosteroids depends on the molecular structure, concentration, and release from the vehicle.
Indications and Usage: Chloramphenicol should be used only in those serious infections for which less potentially dangerous drugs are ineffective or contraindicated. Bacteriological studies should be performed to determine the causative organisms and their sensitivity to chloramphenicol (See Box Warning).
For steroid-responsive inflammatory ocular conditions for which a corticosteroid is indicated and where bacterial infection or a risk of bacterial ocular infection exists.
Ocular steroids are indicated in inflammatory conditions of the palpebral and bulbar conjunctiva, cornea, and anterior segment of the globe where the inherent risk of steroid use in certain infective conjunctivitides is accepted to obtain a diminution in edema and inflammation. They are also indicated in chronic anterior uveitis and corneal injury from chemical radiation, thermal burns, or penetration of foreign bodies.
The use of a combination drug with an antiinfective component is indicated where the risk of infection is high or where there is an expectation that potentially dangerous numbers of bacteria will be present in the eye.
The particular antiinfective drugs in this product are active against the following common bacterial eye pathogens.
Staphylococcus aureus
Streptococci, including *Streptococcus pneumoniae*
Escherichia coli
Hemophilus influenzae
Klebsiella/Enterobacter species
Neisseria species
Moraxella lacunata (Morax-Axenfeld bacillus)
Pseudomonas aeruginosa
The product does not provide adequate coverage against:
Serratia marcescens
Contraindications: Epithelial herpes simplex keratitis (dendritic keratitis), vaccinia, varicella, and many other viral diseases of the cornea and conjunctiva. Mycobacterial infection of the eye. Fungal diseases of ocular structures. Hypersensitivity to a component of the medication. (Hypersensitivity to the antibiotic component occurs at a higher rate than for other components.)
The use of these combinations is always contraindicated after uncomplicated removal of a corneal foreign body.
Warnings: SEE BOX WARNING
Prolonged use of steroids may result in glaucoma, with damage to the optic nerve, defects in visual acuity and fields of vision, and posterior subcapsular cataract formation. Prolonged use may suppress the host response and thus increase the hazard of secondary ocular infections. In those diseases causing thinning of the cornea or sclera, perforations have been known to occur with the use of topical steroids. In acute purulent conditions of the eye, steroids may mask infection or enhance existing infection. If these products are used for 10 days or longer, intraocular pressure should be routinely monitored even though it may be difficult in children and uncooperative patients. Employment of steroid medication in the treatment of herpes simplex requires great caution. Ophthalmic ointments may retard corneal wound healing.
Precautions: The initial prescription and renewal of the medication order beyond 8 grams should be made by a physician only after examination of the patient with the aid of magnification, such as slit lamp biomicroscopy and, where appropriate, fluorescein staining.
The possibility of persistent fungal infections of the cornea should be considered after prolonged steroid dosing.
The prolonged use of antibiotics may occasionally result in overgrowth of nonsusceptible organisms, including fungi. If new infections appear during medication, the drug should be discontinued and appropriate measures should be taken.
In all serious infections the topical use of chloramphenicol should be supplemented by appropriate systemic medication.
Adverse Reactions: There have been reports of punctate staining of the cornea following intensive treatment (every one to two hours during the waking day) of corneal ulcers with Ophthocort. In each reported case, the staining has disappeared after discontinuation of the medication.
Blood dyscrasias have been reported in association with the use of chloramphenicol (See WARNINGS).
Adverse reactions have occurred with steroid/antiinfective combination drugs which can be attributed to the steroid component, the antiinfective component, or the combination. Exact incidence figures are not available since no denominator of treated patients is available.
Reactions occurring most often from the presence of the antiinfective ingredient are allergic sensitizations. The reactions due to the steroid component in decreasing order of frequency are: elevation of intraocular pressure (IOP) with possible development of glaucoma, and infrequent optic nerve damage; posterior subcapsular cataract formation; and delayed wound healing.
Secondary Infection: The development of secondary infection has occurred after use of combinations containing steroids and antimicrobials. Fungal infections of the cornea are particularly prone to develop coincidentally with long-term applications of steroid. The possibility of fungal invasion must be considered in any persistent corneal ulceration where steroid treatment has been used.
Secondary bacterial ocular infection following suppression of host responses also occurs.
Dosage and Administration: Application of a small amount of ointment, placed in the lower conjunctival sac, is made to the affected eye every three hours, or more frequently if deemed advisable by the prescribing physician. Administration should be continued day and night for the first 48 hours, after which the interval between applications may be increased. Treatment should be continued for at least 48 hours after the eye appears normal.
Not more than 8 grams should be prescribed initially and the prescription should not be refilled without further evaluation as outlined in Precautions above.
How Supplied: N 0071-3079-07 Ophthocort (Chloramphenicol, Polymyxin B Sulfate, and Hydrocortisone Acetate Ophthalmic Ointment, USP); Each gram of ointment contains 10 mg chloramphenicol, 10,000 units polymyxin B (as the sulfate), and 5 mg hydrocortisone acetate in a special base of liquid petrolatum and polyethylene. Supplied in 3.5 g tubes.
AHFS Category 52:04.04   3079G011

PAPASE®
[păp'āse"]
(proteolytic enzymes extracted from *Carica papaya*)
Description: Each tablet of Papase contains proteolytic enzymes extracted from *Carica papaya*;

the tablet is standardized to 10,000 Warner-Lambert Units of enzyme activity. Tablets may be administered orally or buccally.
Actions: Papase is an anti-inflammatory agent standardized to provide optimal therapeutic activity.

Indications
Based on a review of this drug by the National Academy of Sciences—National Research Council and/or other information, FDA has classified the indications as follows:
"Possibly" effective for relieving symptomatology related to episiotomy.
Final classification of the less-than-effective indications requires further investigation.

Contraindications: Concomitant use with anticoagulants is the only known contraindication. However, it is not recommended in generalized or systemic infections, or in severe disorders of blood clotting, or in patients with a prior allergic reaction to Papase or papain.
Warning—Use in Pregnancy: Safe use of this drug in pregnancy has not been established.
Precautions: This drug should be used with caution in patients with severe renal or hepatic disease.
Adverse Reactions: The incidence of side effects is low. The following reactions have been described: nausea, vomiting, diarrhea, dizziness, pruritus, rash, and urticaria. To date, buccal ulceration has not been observed in patients, even those receiving Papase (proteolytic enzymes extracted from *Carica papaya*) for prolonged periods. An occasional patient, however, has experienced a mild, local tingling at the site of buccal absorption; this sensation usually subsided when the tablet was moved.
Dosage and Administration: Usual Prophylactic Dosage—Two tablets, 1 or 2 hours before episiotomy.
Usual Therapeutic Dosage—Two tablets 4 times a day for at least five days.
Tablets may be administered buccally or orally, swallowed with water, or chewed.
Supplied: Green peppermint-flavored tablets (with desiccant) in bottles of 100 (N 0071-0301-24) and 1000 (N 0071-0301-32).
Standardization — Since anti-inflammatory action is related to proteolytic enzyme activity, Papase has been specially prepared and carefully standardized on this basis. The method used is a milk-clotting assay,[1] the results of which are expressed in Warner-Lambert Units. One Warner-Lambert Unit is that quantity of proteolytic enzymes extracted from *Carica papaya* which, under the conditions specified in the method of assay, will clot 2.64 microliters of milk substrate in 2 minutes at 40° C.
Store between 15° and 30°C (59° and 86°F).
Reference: 1. Hinkle ET Jr, Alford, AC: *Ann. New York Acad. Sc.* 54(2):208, 1951.
Shown in Product Identification Section, page 425
0301 G 010

PARSIDOL® ℞
[păr′sĭ-dōl″]
(Ethopropazine Hydrochloride Tablets, USP)

Description: Parsidol, an orally effective antiparkinsonism drug, is a phenothiazine derivative. The chemical name is: 10H-Phenothiazine-10-ethanamine, N,N-diethyl-α-methyl-,monohydrochloride.
Actions: Among a wide variety of pharmacologic effects, Parsidol exerts significant anticholinergic (para-sympatholytic) actions. Although its specific mode of action in parkinsonism is unknown, it exerts a marked influence upon the neuromuscular symptoms of the disease. Most of the symptoms of parkinsonism—rigidity, spasms, tremors, sialorrhea, oculogyric crises, and festination—will respond to therapy with this drug. Parsidol is one of the drugs effective against tremor; in certain instances, however, rigidity may respond better to treatment than tremor. It is highly effective given alone or in combination with other drugs such as atropine, stramonium, dextroamphetamine, and antihistamines. Combination therapy with appropriate agents increases its efficacy in the control of specific symptoms in extreme cases, e.g., atropine plus Parsidol in refractory oculogyric crises. Unlike other phenothiazine derivatives, Parsidol does not potentiate central nervous system depressants nor does it have an antiemetic action.
Indications: Parsidol is effective as an adjunct in the therapy of all forms of parkinsonism (postencephalitic, idiopathic, and arteriosclerotic). Although chemically a phenothiazine derivative, Parsidol is distinct from other drugs of its class and is useful in the control of extrapyramidal disorders due to central nervous system drugs such as reserpine and phenothiazines.
Contraindications: Glaucoma or prostatic hypertrophy. Hypersensitivity.
Warning: Safety of use during pregnancy and lactation has not been established. This drug should not be used in pregnant patients unless the expected benefits outweigh the potential risk. Patients receiving this drug should be cautioned against hazardous activities requiring complete mental alertness, such as operating machinery or driving a motor vehicle.
Precautions: Use with caution in patients for whom anticholinergic action would be undesirable. Because chronic use may predispose elderly persons toward glaucoma, older patients should be checked periodically for glaucoma.
Antiparkinsonism agents, when used to treat extrapyramidal reactions resulting from phenothiazines or reserpine in patients with mental disorders, may exacerbate mental symptoms and precipitate a toxic psychosis.
Permanent extrapyramidal symptoms have been described with prolonged phenothiazine therapy. The possibility that ethopropazine might mask the development of these symptoms has not been investigated.
Adverse Reactions: The most common side effects reported to occur with Parsidol are drowsiness and cerebral reaction (this latter effect has been described as fogginess, inability to think, lassitude, forgetfulness and confusion). Additional side effects (dryness of mouth, nausea, vomiting, blurring of vision and diplopia, constipation, and urinary retention—signs of the drug's anticholinergic effects) are rarely severe and either disappear as the drug is continued, or diminish when the dose is reduced.
Less commonly observed side effects include epigastric discomfort, muscular cramping, paresthesia, a sensation of heaviness of the limbs, skin rash and, following high dosages, mild, transient hypotension. Although Parsidol is different from other drugs of the phenothiazine class, the following side effects are theoretically possible with its use: EEG slowing, seizures, ECG abnormalities (e.g., tachycardia), rare hematologic reactions (agranulocytosis, pancytopenia, purpura), certain endocrinologic disturbances, jaundice, pigmentation of the cornea, lens, retina, or skin, and visual hallucinations.
Dosage: Initial dosage is usually 50 mg once or twice a day, increase gradually if necessary. Patients with mild-to-moderate symptoms are frequently controlled with 100 to 400 mg daily. Severe cases may require further gradual increase to 500 to 600 mg or more daily.
How Supplied:
Parsidol Tablets are supplied as:
N 0071-0320-24 10 mg (white) bottles of 100
N 0071-0321-24 50 mg (white, scored) bottles of 100
0320G010
Shown in Product Identification Section, page 425

PENICILLIN V POTASSIUM, USP ℞
[pĕ″nĭ-cĭ″llĭn v pō″tă′ssĭ-ŭm]
(Penapar VK®)
[pĕ″nă-pär″]
Description: Penicillin V is the phenoxymethyl analog of penicillin G.

Action and Pharmacology: Penicillin V exerts a bactericidal action against penicillin-sensitive microorganisms during the stage of active multiplication. It acts through the inhibition of biosynthesis of cell wall mucopeptide. It is not active against the penicillinase-producing bacteria, which include many strains of staphylococci. The drug exerts high *in vitro* activity against staphylococci (except penicillinase-producing strains), streptococci (groups A, C, G, H, L, and M), and pneumococci. Other organisms sensitive *in vitro* to penicillin V are *Corynebacterium diphtheriae, Bacillus anthracis,* Clostridia, *Actinomyces bovis, Streptobacillus moniliformis, Listeria monocytogenes,* Leptospira, and *N gonorrhoeae. Treponema pallidum* is extremely sensitive.
Penicillin V has the distinct advantage over penicillin G in resistance to inactivation by gastric acid. It may be given with meals; however, blood levels are slightly higher when the drug is given on an empty stomach. Average blood levels are two to five times higher than the levels following the same dose of oral penicillin G and also show much less individual variation.
Once absorbed, penicillin V is about 80% bound to serum protein. Tissue levels are highest in the kidneys, with lesser amounts in the liver, skin, and intestines. Small amounts are found in all other body tissues and the cerebrospinal fluid. The drug is excreted as rapidly as it is absorbed in individuals with normal kidney function; however, recovery of the drug from the urine indicates that only about 25% of the dose given is absorbed. In neonates, young infants, and individuals with impaired kidney function, excretion is considerably delayed.
Indications: Penicillin V is indicated in the treatment of mild to moderately severe infections due to penicillin G-sensitive microorganisms that are sensitive to the low serum levels common to this particular dosage form. Therapy should be guided by bacteriologic studies (including sensitivity tests) and by clinical response.
NOTE: Severe pneumonia, empyema, bacteremia, pericarditis, meningitis, and arthritis should not be treated with penicillin V during the acute stage.
Indicated surgical procedures should be performed.
The following infections will usually respond to adequate dosage of penicillin V:
Streptococcal infections (without bacteremia); mild to moderate infections of the upper respiratory tract, scarlet fever, and mild erysipelas
NOTE: Streptococci in groups A, C, G, H, L, and M are very sensitive to penicillin. Other groups, including group D (enterococcus), are resistant.
Pneumococcal infections. Mild to moderately severe infections of the respiratory tract
Staphylococcal infections—penicillin G-sensitive; mild infections of the skin and soft tissues.
NOTE: Reports indicate an increasing number of strains of staphylococci resistant to penicillin G, emphasizing the need for culture and sensitivity studies in treating suspected staphylococcal infections.
Fusospirochetosis (Vincent's gingivitis and pharyngitis); mild to moderately severe infections of the oropharynx usually respond to therapy with oral penicillin.
NOTE: Necessary dental care should be accomplished in infections involving the gum tissue.
Medical conditions in which oral penicillin therapy is indicated as prophylaxis:
For the prevention of recurrence following rheumatic fever and/or chorea: prophylaxis with oral penicillin on a continuing basis has proved effective in preventing recurrence of these conditions.

Continued on next page

This product information was prepared in August, 1984. On these and other Parke-Davis Products, information may be obtained by addressing PARKE-DAVIS, Division of Warner-Lambert Company, Morris Plains, New Jersey 07950.

Parke-Davis—Cont.

Although no controlled clinical efficacy studies have been conducted, penicillin V has been suggested by the American Heart Association and the American Dental Association for use as part of a parenteral-oral regimen and as an alternative oral regimen for prophylaxis against bacterial endocarditis in patients with congenital heart disease or rheumatic or other acquired valvular heart disease when they undergo dental procedures and surgical procedures of the respiratory tract.[1] Since it may happen that *alpha* hemolytic streptococci relatively resistant to penicillin may be found when patients are receiving continuous oral penicillin for secondary prevention of rheumatic fever, prophylactic agents other than penicillin may be chosen for these patients and prescribed in addition to their continuous rheumatic fever prophylactic regimen. Oral penicillin should not be used as adjunctive prophylaxis for genitourinary instrumentation or surgery, lower intestinal tract surgery, sigmoidoscopy, and childbirth.

NOTE: When selecting antibiotics for the prevention of bacterial endocarditis, the physician or dentist should read the full joint statement of the American Heart Association and the American Dental Association.[1]

Contraindications: A previous hypersensitivity reaction to any penicillin is a contraindication.

Warning: Serious and occasionally fatal hypersensitivity (anaphylactoid) reactions have been reported in patients on penicillin therapy. Although anaphylaxis is more frequent following parenteral therapy, it has occurred in patients on oral penicillins. These reactions are more apt to occur in individuals with a history of sensitivity to multiple allergens.

There have been well-documented reports of individuals with a history of penicillin hypersensitivity reactions who have experienced severe hypersensitivity reactions when treated with a cephalosporin. Before therapy with a penicillin, careful inquiry should be made concerning previous hypersensitivity reactions to penicillins, cephalosporins, and other allergens. If an allergic reaction occurs, the drug should be discontinued and the patient treated with the usual agents, eg, pressor amines, antihistamines, and corticosteroids.

Precautions: Penicillin should be used with caution in individuals with histories of significant allergies and/or asthma.

The oral route of administration should not be relied upon in patients with severe illness, or with nausea, vomiting, gastric dilatation, cardiospasm, or intestinal hypermotility.

Occasional patients will not absorb therapeutic amounts of orally administered penicillin.

In streptococcal infections, therapy must be sufficient to eliminate the organism (ten days minimum); otherwise, the sequelae of streptococcal disease may occur. Cultures should be taken following completion of treatment to determine whether streptococci have been eradicated.

Prolonged use of antibiotics may promote the overgrowth of nonsusceptible organisms, including fungi. Should superinfection occur, appropriate measures should be taken.

Adverse Reactions: Although the incidence of reactions to oral penicillins has been reported with much less frequency than following parenteral therapy, it should be remembered that all degrees of hypersensitivity, including fatal anaphylaxis, have been reported with oral penicillin.

The most common reactions to oral penicillin are nausea, vomiting, epigastric distress, diarrhea, and black hairy tongue. The hypersensitivity reactions reported are skin eruptions (maculopapular to exfoliative dermatitis), urticaria and other serum sickness reactions, laryngeal edema, and anaphylaxis. Fever and eosinophilia may frequently be the only reaction observed. Hemolytic anemia, leukopenia, thrombocytopenia, neuropathy, and nephropathy are infrequent reactions and usually associated with high doses of parenteral penicillin.

Dosage and Administration: The dosage of penicillin V should be determined according to the sensitivity of the causative microorganisms and the severity of the infection, and adjusted to the clinical response of the patient.

The usual dosage recommendations for adults and children 12 years and over are as follows.

Streptococcal infections—mild to moderately severe—of the upper respiratory tract and including scarlet fever and erysipelas: 125 to 250 mg (200,000 to 400,000 units) every six to eight hours for ten days

Pneumococcal infections—mild to moderately severe—of the respiratory tract, including otitis media: 250 mg (400,000 units) every six hours until the patient has been afebrile for at least two days

Staphylococcal infections—mild infections of skin and soft tissue (culture and sensitivity tests should be performed): 250 mg (400,000 units) every six to eight hours

Fusospirochetosis (Vincent's infection) of the oropharynx—mild to moderately severe infections: 250 mg (400,000 units) every six to eight hours

For the prevention of recurrence following rheumatic fever and/or chorea: 125 mg (200,000 units) twice daily on a continuing basis.

NOTE: Therapy for children under 12 years of age is calculated on the basis of body weight. For infants and small children, the suggested dosage is 15 to 56 mg (25,000 to 90,000 units) per kg per day in three to six divided doses.

For prophylaxis against bacterial endocarditis[1] in patients with congenital heart disease or rheumatic or other acquired valvular heart disease when undergoing dental procedures or surgical procedures of the upper respiratory tract, one of two regimens may be selected:

(1) For the oral regimen, give 2.0 gm of penicillin V (1.0 gm for children under 60 lbs) ½ to 1 hour before the procedure, and then, 500 mg (250 mg for children under 60 lbs) every 6 hours for 8 doses; or

(2) For the combined parenteral-oral regimen give one million units of aqueous crystalline penicillin G (30,000 units/kg in children) intramuscularly mixed with 600,000 units procaine penicillin G (600,000 units for children) ½ to 1 hour before the procedure, and then oral penicillin V, 500 mg for adults or 250 mg for children under 60 lbs, every 6 hours for 8 doses. Doses for children should not exceed recommendations for adults for a single dose or for a 24 hour period.

How Supplied:

Penicillin V Tablets are supplied as:

N 0071-0648-24 250 mg—Bottle of 100.
N 0071-0648-32 250 mg—Bottle of 1000.
N 0071-0648-40 250 mg—Unit dose Package of 100 (10 strips of 10).

Each tablet contains penicillin V potassium equivalent to 250 mg (400,000 units) penicillin V.

N 0071-0673-24 500 mg—Bottle of 100.
N 0071-0673-30 500 mg—Bottle of 500.

Each tablet contains penicillin V potassium equivalent to 500 mg (800,000 units) penicillin V.

Shown in Product Identification Section, page 425

Penicillin V For Oral Solution is supplied as:

N 0071-2449-17 125 mg/5 ml—100 ml individual bottles and packs of six.
N 0071-2449-20 125 mg/5 ml—200 ml individual bottles and packs of six.

When reconstituted according to directions, each 5 ml contains penicillin V potassium equivalent to 125 mg (200,000 units) penicillin V.

N 0071-2506-17 250 mg/5 ml—100 ml individual bottles and packs of six.
N 0071-2506-20 250 mg/5 ml—200 ml individual bottles and packs of six.

When reconstituted according to directions, each 5 ml contains penicillin V potassium equivalent to 250 mg (400,000 units) penicillin V.

Reference:
1. American Heart Association: Prevention of bacterial endocarditis. *Circulation* 56: 139A-143A, 1977.

Manufactured by John D. Copanos Inc., Baltimore, MD 21225 and distributed by Parke-Davis, Warner-Lambert Co, Morris Plains, NJ 07950

AHFS 8:12.16   7000 G 103

PERITRATE® SA
[pĕ'rĭ-trāte]
(pentaerythritol tetranitrate tablets)
Sustained Action*

PERITRATE®
(pentaerythritol tetranitrate tablets, USP)

Description: Peritrate SA Sustained Action 80 mg: each tablet contains pentaerythritol tetranitrate 80 mg (20 mg in the immediate release layer and 60 mg in sustained release base).

Peritrate 40 mg: each tablet contains pentaerythritol tetranitrate 40 mg.

Peritrate 20 mg: each tablet contains pentaerythritol tetranitrate 20 mg.

Peritrate 10 mg: each tablet contains pentaerythritol tetranitrate 10 mg.

Pentaerythritol tetranitrate is a nitric acid ester of a tetrahydric alcohol (pentaerythritol).

Actions: The exact cause of angina pectoris (that is, the pain associated with coronary artery disease) remains obscure, despite the numerous and often conflicting hypotheses concerning its pathophysiology. Therapy at the present time, therefore, remains essentially empirical. Customarily, clinical improvement has been measured by: reduction in (1) number, intensity and duration of angina pectoris attacks and (2) necessity for glyceryl trinitrate intake for prevention or relief of anginal attacks. Peritrate SA (pentaerythritol tetranitrate) Sustained Action and Peritrate (pentaerythritol tetranitrate) have been reported in clinical usage to reduce in number and severity the incidence of angina pectoris attacks, with concomitant reduction in glyceryl trinitrate intake. In the evaluation of Peritrate and Peritrate SA in angina pectoris, clinical improvement has been customarily measured subjectively by: reduction in number and severity of attacks and necessity for glyceryl trinitrate intake for prevention or abortion of anginal attacks. Individual patterns of angina pectoris differ widely as does the symptomatic response to antianginal agents such as pentaerythritol tetranitrate. The published literature contains both favorable and unfavorable clinical reports. In conjunction with total management of the patient with angina pectoris, Peritrate and Peritrate SA have been accepted as safe for prolonged administration and widely regarded as useful.

Indications

Based on a review of this drug by the National Academy of Sciences—National Research Council and/or other information, FDA has classified the indications as follows:

"Possibly" effective: Peritrate is indicated for the relief of angina pectoris (pain associated with coronary artery disease). It is not intended to abort the acute anginal episode but is widely regarded as useful in the prophylactic treatment of angina pectoris.

Final classification of the less-than-effective indications requires further investigation.

Contraindications: Peritrate SA and Peritrate are contraindicated in patients who have a history of sensitivity to the drug.

Warnings: Data supporting the use of Peritrate or Peritrate SA during the early days of the acute phase of myocardial infarction (the period during which clinical and laboratory findings are unstable) are insufficient to establish safety.

This drug can act as a physiological antagonist to norepinephrine, acetylcholine, histamine, and many other agents.

Precautions: Should be used with caution in patients who have glaucoma. Tolerance to this drug and cross-tolerance to other nitrites and nitrates may occur.

Adverse Reactions: Side effects reported to date have been predominantly related to rash (which requires discontinuation of medication) and headache and gastrointestinal distress, which are usually mild and transient with continuation of medication. In some cases severe persistent headaches may occur. In addition, the following adverse reac-

tions to nitrates such as pentaerythritol tetranitrate have been reported in the literature:
(a) Cutaneous vasodilatation with flushing.
(b) Transient episodes of dizziness and weakness, as well as other signs of cerebral ischemia associated with postural hypotension, may occasionally develop.
(c) An occasional individual exhibits marked sensitivity to the hypotensive effects of nitrite and severe responses (nausea, vomiting, weakness, restlessness, pallor, perspiration and collapse) can occur, even with the usual therapeutic doses. Alcohol may enhance this effect.

Dosage: Peritrate may be administered in individualized doses up to 160 mg a day. Dosage can be initiated at one 10 mg or 20 mg tablet q.i.d. and titrated upward to 40 mg (two 20 mg tablets or one 40 mg tablet) q.i.d. one-half hour before or one hour after meals and at bedtime. Tablets can be chewed or swallowed whole. Alternatively, Peritrate SA can be administered on a convenient b.i.d. (on an empty stomach) dosage schedule. One tablet immediately on arising and 1 tablet 12 hours later. Tablets should not be chewed.

Supplied:
Peritrate SA Sustained Action 80 mg—double layer, biconvex, dark green/light green tablets in bottles of 100 (N 0710-0004-24) and 1000 (N 0710-0004-32).

Shown in Product Identification Section, page 425
Also in unit dose package of 10 × 10 strips (N 0710-0004-40).
Peritrate 40 mg—coral scored tablets in bottles of 100 (N 0710-0008-24).

Shown in Product Identification Section, page 425
Peritrate 20 mg—light green, scored tablets in bottles of 100 (N 0710-0001-24) and 1000 (N 0710-0001-32).

Shown in Product Identification Section, page 425
Also in unit dose package of 10 × 10 strips (N 0710-0001-40).
Peritrate 10 mg—light green, unscored tablets in bottles of 100 (N 0710-0013-24) and 1000 (N 0710-0013-32).

Shown in Product Identification Section, page 425

Animal Pharmacology: In a series of carefully designed studies in pigs, Peritrate was administered for 48 hours before an artificially induced occlusion of a major coronary artery and for seven days thereafter. The pigs were sacrificed at various intervals for periods up to six weeks. The result showed a significantly larger number of survivors in the drug-treated group. Damage to myocardial tissue in the drug-treated survivors was less extensive than in the untreated group. Studies in dogs subjected to oligemic shock through progressive bleeding have demonstrated that Peritrate is vasoactive at the postarteriolar level, producing increased blood flow and better tissue perfusion. These animal experiments cannot be translated to the drug's actions in humans.

0001G020/0001G010

PITOCIN® ℞
[pĭ″tō′cĭn]
(oxytocin injection, USP) synthetic

IMPORTANT NOTICE
Pitocin is not indicated for the elective induction of labor because available data and information are inadequate to define the benefits-to-risks considerations in the use of the drug product. Elective induction of labor is defined as the initiation of labor in an individual with a term pregnancy who is free of medical indications for the initiation of labor.

Description: Pitocin (oxytocin injection, USP) is a sterile, aqueous solution of synthetic oxytocic hormone standardized to contain 10 units/ml and containing 0.5% Chloretone® (chlorobutanol) (chloroform derivative) as a preservative, with the acidity adjusted with acetic acid. The drug is prepared synthetically to avoid possible contamination with vasopressin (ADH) and its antidiuretic and cardiovascular effects. However, the physician should be cognizant of the fact that even highly purified synthetic oxytocin contains inherent pressor-antidiuretic properties which may become manifest following administration of large doses (see Precautions).

Action: Uterine motility is controlled by a variety of biochemical and regulatory processes. Oxytocin appears to act primarily on uterine myofibril activity by increasing the permeability of the cell membranes to sodium ions, thus augmenting the number of contracting myofibrils, and thereby enabling the uterus to produce the necessary number of contractions. The effect depends on the uterine threshold of excitability. The sensitivity of the uterus to oxytocin increases gradually during gestation; then increases sharply before parturition.

Indications: Antepartum: Pitocin is indicated for the initiation or improvement of uterine contractions, where this is desirable and considered suitable, for the following purposes: induction of labor in patients with a medical indication for the initiation of labor, such as mild preeclampsia at or near term, when delivery is in the best interest of mother and fetus or when membranes are prematurely ruptured and delivery is indicated; stimulation or reinforcement of labor, as in selected cases of uterine inertia; as adjunctive therapy in the management of incomplete or inevitable abortion. In the first trimester, curettage is generally considered primary therapy. In second trimester abortion, oxytocin infusion will often be successful in emptying the uterus. Other means of therapy, however, may be required in such cases.

Postpartum: Pitocin is indicated to produce uterine contractions during the third stage of labor and to control postpartum bleeding or hemorrhage.

Contraindications: Pitocin is contraindicated in any of the following conditions: significant cephalopelvic disproportion; unfavorable fetal positions or presentations which are undeliverable without conversion prior to delivery (as, for example, transverse lies); in obstetrical emergencies where the benefit-to-risk ratio for either the fetus or the mother favors surgical intervention; in cases of fetal distress where delivery is not imminent; prolonged use in uterine inertia or severe toxemia; hypertonic uterine patterns; patients with hypersensitivity to the drug; induction or augmentation of labor in those cases where vaginal delivery is contraindicated, such as invasive cervical carcinoma, cord presentation or prolapse, total placenta previa, and vasa previa.

Warnings: Pitocin, when given for induction or stimulation of labor, must be administered only by the intravenous route and with adequate medical supervision in a hospital.

Precautions:
1. All patients receiving intravenous oxytocin must be under continuous observation by trained personnel with a thorough knowledge of the drug and qualified to identify complications. A physician qualified to manage any complications should be immediately available.
2. When properly administered, oxytocin should stimulate uterine contractions comparable to those seen in normal labor. Overstimulation of the uterus by improper administration can be hazardous to both mother and fetus. Even with proper administration and adequate supervision, hypertonic contractions can occur in patients whose uteri are hypersensitive to oxytocin. This fact must be considered by the physician in exercising judgment regarding patient selection.
3. Except in unusual circumstances, oxytocin should not be administered in the following conditions: fetal distress, partial placenta previa, prematurity, borderline cephalopelvic disproportion, and in any conditions where there is a predisposition for uterine rupture, such as previous major surgery on the cervix or uterus including cesarean section, overdistention of the uterus, grand multiparity, or past history of uterine sepsis or of traumatic delivery. Because of the variability of the combinations of factors which may be present in the conditions listed above, the definition of "unusual circumstances" must be left to the judgment of the physician. The decision can only be made by carefully weighing the potential benefits which oxytocin can provide in a given case against rare but definite potential for the drug to produce hypertonicity or tetanic spasm.
4. Maternal deaths due to hypertensive episodes, subarachnoid hemorrhage, rupture of the uterus, and fetal deaths due to various causes have been reported associated with the use of parenteral oxytocic drugs for induction of labor or for augmentation in the first and second stages of labor.
5. Oxytocin has been shown to have an intrinsic antidiuretic effect, acting to increase water reabsorption from the glomerular filtrate. Consideration should, therefore, be given to the possibility of water intoxication, particularly when oxytocin is administered continuously by infusion and the patient is receiving fluids by mouth.
6. When oxytocin is used for induction or reinforcement of already existent labor, patients should be carefully selected. Pelvic adequacy must be considered and maternal and fetal conditions evaluated before use of the drug.

Adverse Reactions: Fetal bradycardia, anaphylactic reaction, postpartum hemorrhage, cardiac arrhythmia, and pelvic hematoma have been reported.

Excessive dosage or hypersensitivity to the drug may result in uterine hypertonicity, spasm, tetanic contraction, or rupture.

Side effects that may also occur during spontaneous labor, such as nausea, vomiting, and premature ventricular contractions, have been noted occasionally with oxytocin.

A fatality due to afibrinogenemia has been reported, naming oxytocin injection as a possible cause. The possibility of increased blood loss and afibrinogenemia should be kept in mind when administering the drug.

Severe water intoxication with convulsions and coma has occurred, associated with a slow oxytocin infusion over a 24-hour period. Maternal death due to oxytocin-induced water intoxication has been reported.

Dosage and Administration: Dosage of oxytocin is determined by uterine response. The following dosage information is based upon the various regimens and indications in general use.

A. Induction or Stimulation of Labor
Intravenous infusion (drip method) is the only acceptable method of parenteral administration for the induction or stimulation of labor. Accurate control of the rate of infusion flow is essential. An infusion pump or other such device and at least external electronic monitoring are necessary for the safe administration of oxytocin for the induction or stimulation of labor. If uterine contractions become too powerful, the infusion can be abruptly stopped, and oxytocic stimulation of the uterine musculature will soon wane.
1. An intravenous infusion of non-oxytocin containing solution should be started. (Physiologic electrolyte solution should be used.)
2. To prepare the standard solution for infusion, the contents of one 1-ml ampoule is combined aseptically with 1,000 ml of 0.9% aqueous sodium chloride solution or other nonhydrating diluent. The combined solution (1 ml = 10 milliunits) is rotated in the infusion bottle to insure thorough mixing. Add the container with dilute oxytocic solution to the system through use of a constant infusion pump.
3. The initial dose should be 1 to 2 mU/min- ute. At 15 to 30 minute intervals, the dose should be gradually increased in increments of 1 to 2 mU/minute until the desired contraction pattern has been established, which should be comparable to that seen in normal labor.

Continued on next page

This product information was prepared in August, 1984. On these and other Parke-Davis Products, information may be obtained by addressing PARKE-DAVIS, Division of Warner-Lambert Company, Morris Plains, New Jersey 07950.

Parke-Davis—Cont.

4. The fetal heart rate, resting uterine tone, and the frequency, duration, and force of contractions should be monitored.
5. The oxytocin infusion should be discontinued immediately in the event of uterine hyperactivity or fetal distress. Oxygen should be administered to the mother. The mother and the fetus must be evaluated by the responsible physician.

B. Control of Postpartum Uterine Bleeding
1. Intravenous Infusion (Drip Method)
To control postpartum bleeding, 10 to 40 units of oxytocin may be added to 1,000 ml of 5% dextrose injection and run at a rate necessary to control uterine atony.

Intramuscular Administration
1 ml (10 units) of oxytocin can be given after delivery of the placenta.

C. Treatment of Incomplete or Inevitable Abortion:
Intravenous infusion with physiologic saline solution, 500 ml, or 5% dextrose in physiologic saline solution to which 10 units of Pitocin have been added should be infused at a rate of 10 to 20 milliunits (20 to 40 drops) per minute.

How Supplied: N 0071-4160-02 (Ampoule 163) Contains 5 units in a 0.5-ml ampoule, packages of ten
N 0071-4160-03 (Ampoule 160)
Contains 10 units in a 1-ml ampoule, packages of ten
N 0071-4160-40 (Steri-Dose® syringe 1489)
Contains 10 units in a 1-ml sterile disposable syringe, packages of ten
N 0071-4160-10 (Steri-Vial® 1541)
Contains 10 units per milliliter in a 10-ml Steri-Vial (multiple dose vial)
AHFS 76:00
121 858950/60
4160 G060

PITRESSIN® ℞
[pĭ'' trĕ' sĭn]
(vasopressin injection, USP)
synthetic

Description: Pitressin (vasopressin injection) is a sterile, aqueous solution of synthetic vasopressin (8-arginine vasopressin) of the posterior pituitary gland. It is substantially free from the oxytocic principle and is standardized to contain 20 pressor units/ml. The solution contains 0.5% Chloretone® (chlorobutanol) (chloroform derivative) as a preservative. The acidity of the solution is adjusted with acetic acid.
Action: The antidiuretic action of vasopressin is ascribed to increasing reabsorption of water by the renal tubules.
Vasopressin can cause contraction of smooth muscle of the gastrointestinal tract and of all parts of the vascular bed, especially the capillaries, small arterioles and venules, with less effect on the smooth musculature of the large veins. The direct effect on the contractile elements is neither antagonized by adrenergic blocking agents nor prevented by vascular denervation.
Contraindication: Anaphylaxis or hypersensitivity to the drug or its components.
Indications: Pitressin is indicated for prevention and treatment of postoperative abdominal distention, in abdominal roentgenography to dispel interfering gas shadows, and in diabetes insipidus.
Warnings: This drug should not be used in patients with vascular disease, especially disease of the coronary arteries, except with extreme caution. In such patients, even small doses may precipitate anginal pain, and with larger doses, the possibility of myocardial infarction should be considered.
Vasopressin may produce water intoxication. The early signs of drowsiness, listlessness, and headaches should be recognized to prevent terminal coma and convulsions.
Precautions: Vasopressin should be used cautiously in the presence of epilepsy, migraine, asthma, heart failure, or any state in which a rapid addition to extracellular water may produce hazard for an already overburdened system. Chronic nephritis with nitrogen retention contraindicates the use of vasopressin until reasonable nitrogen blood levels have been attained.
Adverse Reactions: Local or systemic allergic reactions may occur in hypersensitive individuals. The following side effects have been reported following the administration of vasopressin: tremor, sweating, vertigo, circumoral pallor, "pounding" in head, abdominal cramps, passage of gas, nausea, vomiting, urticaria, bronchial constriction. Anaphylaxis (cardiac arrest and/or shock) has been observed shortly after injection of vasopressin.
Dosage and Administration: Pitressin may be administered subcutaneously or intramuscularly. Ten units of Pitressin (0.5 ml) will usually elicit full physiologic response in adult patients; 5 units will be adequate in many cases. Pitressin should be given intramuscularly at three- or four-hour intervals as needed. The dosage should be proportionately reduced for children. (For an additional discussion of dosage, consult the sections below).
When determining the dose of Pitressin for a given case, the following should be kept in mind.
It is particularly desirable to give a dose not much larger than is just sufficient to elicit the desired physiologic response. Excessive doses may cause undesirable side actions—blanching of the skin, abdominal cramps, nausea— which, though not serious, may be alarming to the patient. Spontaneous recovery from such side actions occurs in a few minutes. It has been found that one or two glasses of water given at the time Pitressin is administered reduces such symptoms.
Abdominal Distention: In the average post- operative adult patient, give 5 units (0.25 ml) initially; increase to 10 units (0.5 ml) at subsequent injections if necessary. It is recommended that Pitressin be given intramuscularly and that injections be repeated at three- or four-hour intervals as required. Dosage to be reduced proportionately for children.
Pitressin used in this manner will frequently prevent, or relieve, postoperative distention. These recommendations apply also to distention complicating pneumonia or other acute toxemias.
Abdominal Roentgenography: For the average case, two injections of 10 units each (0.5 ml) are suggested. These should be given two hours and one half hour, respectively, before films are exposed. Many roentgenologists advise giving an enema prior to the first dose of Pitressin.
Diabetes Insipidus: Pitressin may be given by injection or administered intranasally on cotton pledgets, by nasal spray, or by dropper. The dose by injection is 5 to 10 units (0.25 to 0.5 ml) repeated two or three times daily as needed. When Pitressin is administered intranasally by spray or on pledgets, the dosage and interval between treatments must be determined for each patient.
How Supplied: Pitressin (vasopressin injection, USP) synthetic is supplied in ampoules as follows.
N 0071-4200-02
0.5 ml (10 pressor units). Packages of 10
N 0071-4200-03
1 ml (20 pressor units). Packages of 10
Note: When ordering Pitressin Ampoules, Synthetic, be sure to state whether the 10- or 20-unit is desired.
4200G041

PITRESSIN® TANNATE IN OIL ℞
[pĭ'' trĕ' sĭn tă' nāte]
(vasopressin tannate)
FOR INTRAMUSCULAR USE ONLY

Description: Pitressin Tannate (vasopressin tannate) is a water-insoluble chemical compound of vasopressin, the pressor fraction of the posterior lobe of the pituitary gland, and tannic acid.
Action: The antidiuretic action of vasopressin tannate is ascribed to increasing reabsorption of water by the renal tubules.
Vasopressin can cause contraction of smooth muscle of the gastrointestinal tract and of all parts of the vascular bed, especially the capillaries, small arterioles, and venules, with less effect on the smooth musculature of the large veins. These effects are ordinarily not seen to a significant degree with recommended antidiuretic doses of vasopressin tannate. The direct effect on the contractile elements is neither antagonized by adrenergic blocking agents nor prevented by vascular denervation.
Indications: Pitressin Tannate in Oil is indicated for the control or prevention of the symptoms and complications of diabetes insipidus due to a deficiency of endogenous posterior pituitary antidiuretic hormone.
Contraindication: Anaphylaxis or hypersensitivity to the drug or its components.
Warnings:
This preparation should never be administered intravenously.
This drug should not be used in patients with vascular disease, especially disease of the coronary arteries, except with extreme caution. In such patients, even small doses may precipitate anginal pain.
Vasopressin may produce water intoxication. The early signs of drowsiness, listlessness, and headaches should be recognized to prevent terminal coma and convulsions.
Precautions: Vasopressin should be used cautiously in the presence of epilepsy, migraine, asthma, heart failure, or any state in which a rapid addition to extracellular water may produce hazard for an already overburdened system. Chronic nephritis with nitrogen retention contraindicates the use of vasopressin until reasonable nitrogen blood levels have been attained.
Adverse Reactions: Local or systemic allergic reactions may occur in hypersensitive individuals. The following side effects have been reported following the administration of vasopressin: tremor, sweating, vertigo, circumoral pallor, "pounding" in head, abdominal cramps, passage of gas, nausea, vomiting, urticaria, bronchial constriction, anaphylaxis, cardiac arrest.
Dosage and Administration: Intramuscular—0.3 to 1 ml repeated as required. The duration of action varies with the patient and his condition, and may be as prolonged as 48 to 96 hours.
How Supplied:
N 0071-4302-03 (Ampoule 302)
Pitressin Tannate in Oil is supplied as a suspension containing 5 pressor units per ml in peanut oil, in 1-ml ampoules, packages of 10.
AHFS 68:28
4302G040

PONSTEL® ℞
[pŏn' stĕl'']
(mefenamic acid)

Description: Ponstel (mefenamic acid) is N-(2,3-xylyl)-anthranilic acid. It is an analgesic agent for oral administration. Ponstel is available in capsules containing 250 mg of mefenamic acid.
It is a white powder with a melting point of 230-231° C, molecular weight 241.28, and water solubility of 0.004% at pH 7.1.
Clinical Pharmacology: Ponstel is a nonsteroidal agent with demonstrated antiinflammatory, analgesic, and antipyretic activity in laboratory animals.[1,2] The mode of action is not known. In animal studies, Ponstel was found to inhibit prostaglandin synthesis and to compete for binding at the prostaglandin receptor site.[3]
Pharmacologic studies show Ponstel did not relieve morphine abstinence signs in abstinent, morphine-habituated monkeys.[1]
Following a single 1-gram oral dose, peak plasma levels of 10 µg/ml occurred in 2 to 4 hours with a half-life of 2 hours. Following multiple doses, plasma levels are proportional to dose with no evidence of drug accumulation. One gram of Ponstel given four times daily produces peak blood levels of 20 µg/ml by the second day of administration.[4]
Following a single dose, sixty-seven percent of the total dose is excreted in the urine as unchanged drug or as one of two metabolites. Twenty to twenty-five percent of the dose is excreted in the feces during the first three days.[4]
In controlled, double-blind, clinical trials, Ponstel was evaluated for the treatment of primary spas-

modic dysmenorrhea. The parameters used in determining efficacy included pain assessment by both patient and investigator; the need for concurrent analgesic medication; and evaluation of change in frequency and severity of symptoms characteristic of spasmodic dysmenorrhea. Patients received either Ponstel, 500 mg (2 capsules) as an initial dose and 250 mg every 6 hours, or placebo at onset of bleeding or of pain, whichever began first. After three menstrual cycles, patients were crossed over to the alternate treatment for an additional three cycles. Ponstel was significantly superior to placebo in all parameters, and both treatments (drug and placebo) were equally tolerated.

Indications and Usage: Ponstel is indicated for the relief of moderate pain[5] when therapy will not exceed one week. Ponstel is also indicated for the treatment of primary dysmenorrhea.[5,6]
Studies in children under 14 years of age have been inadequate to evaluate the safety and effectiveness of Ponstel.

Contraindications: Ponstel should not be used in patients who have previously exhibited hypersensitivity to it.
Because the potential exists for cross-sensitivity to aspirin or other nonsteroidal antiinflammatory drugs, Ponstel should not be given to patients in whom these drugs induce symptoms of bronchospasm, allergic rhinitis, or urticaria.
Ponstel is contraindicated in patients with active ulceration or chronic inflammation of either the upper or lower gastrointestinal tract.
Ponstel should be avoided in patients with preexisting renal disease.

Warnings: In patients with a history of ulceration or chronic inflammation of the upper or lower gastrointestinal tract, Ponstel should be given under close supervision and only after consulting the Adverse Reactions Section.
If diarrhea occurs, the dosage should be reduced or temporarily suspended (see Adverse Reactions and Dosage and Administration). Certain patients who develop diarrhea may be unable to tolerate the drug because of recurrence of the symptoms on subsequent exposure.

Precautions: If rash occurs, administration of the drug should be stopped.
A false-positive reaction for urinary bile, using the diazo tablet test, may result after mefenamic acid administration. If biliuria is suspected, other diagnostic procedures, such as the Harrison spot test, should be performed.
In chronic animal toxicity studies of Ponstel at doses 7 to 28 times the recommended human dose, rats had minor microscopic renal papillary necrosis, dogs had edema and blunting of the renal papilla, and monkeys had renal papillary edema.[5]
Normal human volunteers had mild BUN elevations with prolonged administration at greater than therapeutic doses.[5] The significance of these findings is unknown. However, since Ponstel is eliminated primarily through the kidneys,[4] the drug should not be administered to patients with significantly impaired renal function.
As with other nonsteroidal antiinflammatory drugs, borderline elevations of one or more liver tests may occur in some patients. These abnormalities may progress, may remain essentially unchanged, or may be transient with continued therapy. The SGPT (ALT) test is probably the most sensitive indicator of liver dysfunction. Meaningful (3 times the upper limit of normal) elevations of SGPT or SGOT (AST) occurred in controlled clinical trials in less than 1% of patients. A patient with symptoms and/or signs suggesting liver dysfunction, or in whom an abnormal liver test has occurred, should be evaluated for evidence of the development of more severe hepatic reaction while on therapy with Ponstel. Severe hepatic reactions, including jaundice and cases of fatal hepatitis, have been reported with other nonsteroidal antiinflammatory drugs. Although such reactions are rare, if abnormal liver tests persist or worsen, if clinical signs and symptoms consistent with liver disease develop, or if systemic manifestations occur (eg eosinophilia, rash, etc), Ponstel should be discontinued.

Information for Patients: Patients should be advised that if rash, diarrhea or other digestive problems arise, they should stop the drug and consult their physician.
Patients in whom aspirin or other nonsteroidal antiinflammatory drugs induce symptoms of bronchospasm, allergic rhinitis, or urticaria should be made aware that the potential exists for cross-sensitivity to Ponstel.
The long-term effects, if any, of intermittent Ponstel therapy for dysmenorrhea are not known. Women on such therapy should consult their physician if they should decide to become pregnant.

Drug Interactions: Ponstel may prolong prothrombin time.[5] Therefore, when the drug is administered to patients receiving oral anticoagulant drugs, frequent monitoring of prothrombin time is necessary.

Use in Pregnancy: Pregnancy Category C. Reproduction studies have been performed in rats, rabbits and dogs. Rats given up to 10 times the human dose showed decreased fertility, delay in parturition, and a decreased rate of survival to weaning. Rabbits at 2.5 times the human dose showed an increase in the number of resorptions. There were no fetal anomalies observed in these studies nor in dogs at up to 10 times the human dose.[5]
There are no adequate and well-controlled studies in pregnant women. Because animal reproduction studies are not always predictive of human response, this drug should be used only if clearly needed.
The use of Ponstel in late pregnancy is not recommended because of the effects on the fetal cardiovascular system of drugs of this class.

Nursing Mothers: Trace amounts of Ponstel may be present in breast milk and transmitted to the nursing infant[7]; thus Ponstel should not be taken by the nursing mother because of the effects on the infant cardiovascular system of drugs of this class.

Use in Children: Safety and effectiveness in children below the age of 14 have not been established.

Adverse Reactions:

Gastrointestinal: The most frequently reported adverse reactions associated with the use of Ponstel involve the gastrointestinal tract. In controlled studies for up to eight months, the following disturbances were reported in decreasing order of frequency: diarrhea (approximately 5% of patients), nausea with or without vomiting, other gastrointestinal symptoms, and abdominal pain.
In certain patients, the diarrhea was of sufficient severity to require discontinuation of medication. The occurrence of the diarrhea is usually dose related, generally subsides on reduction of dosage, and rapidly disappears on termination of therapy. Other gastrointestinal reactions less frequently reported were anorexia, pyrosis, flatulence, and constipation.
Gastrointestinal ulceration with and without hemorrhage has been reported.

Hematopoietic: Cases of autoimmune hemolytic anemia have been associated with the continuous administration of Ponstel for 12 months or longer. In such cases the Coombs test results are positive with evidence of both accelerated RBC production and RBC destruction. The process is reversible upon termination of Ponstel administration.
Decreases in hematocrit have been noted in 2-5% of patients and primarily in those who have received prolonged therapy. Leukopenia, eosinophilia, thrombocytopenic purpura, agranulocytosis, pancytopenia, and bone marrow hypoplasia have also been reported on occasion.

Nervous System: Drowsiness, dizziness, nervousness, headache, blurred vision, and insomnia have occurred.

Integumentary: Urticaria, rash, and facial edema have been reported.

Renal: As with other nonsteroidal antiinflammatory agents, renal failure, including papillary necrosis, has been reported. In elderly patients renal failure has occurred after taking Ponstel for 2-6 weeks. The renal damage may not be completely reversible. Hematuria and dysuria have also been reported with Ponstel.

Other: Eye irritation, ear pain, perspiration, mild hepatic toxicity, and increased need for insulin in a diabetic have been reported. There have been rare reports of palpitation, dyspnea, and reversible loss of color vision.

Overdosage: Although doses up to 6000 mg/day have been given, no specific information is available on the management of acute massive overdosage.
Should accidental overdosage occur, the stomach should be emptied by inducing emesis or by careful gastric lavage followed by the administration of activated charcoal.[8] Laboratory studies indicate that Ponstel should be adsorbed from the gastrointestinal tract by activated charcoal.[4] Vital functions should be monitored and supported. Because mefenamic acid and its metabolites are firmly bound to plasma proteins, hemodialysis and peritoneal dialysis may be of little value.[4]

Dosage and Administration: Administration is by the oral route, preferably with food.
The recommended regimen in acute pain for adults and children over 14 years of age is 500 mg as an initial dose followed by 250 mg every six hours as needed, usually not to exceed one week.[5] For the treatment of primary dysmenorrhea, the recommended dosage is 500 mg as an initial dose followed by 250 mg every 6 hours, starting with the onset of bleeding and associated symptoms. Clinical studies indicate that effective treatment can be initiated with the start of menses and should not be necessary for more than 2 to 3 days.[6]

How Supplied: N 0710-0540-24 (P-D 540) Ponstel (mefenamic acid) is available as 250 mg capsules in bottles of 100.

Shown in Product Identification Section, page 425

References:
1. Winder CV, et al: Antiinflammatory, antipyretic and antinociceptive properties of N-(2,3-xylyl) anthranilic acid (mefenamic acid). *J Pharmacol Exp Ther* 138: 405-413, 1962.
2. Wax J, et al: Comparative activities, tolerances and safety of nonsteroidal antiinflammatory agents in rats. *J Pharmacol Exp Ther* 192: 172-178, 1975.
3. Ferreira SH, Vane JR: Aspirin and prostaglandins, in *The Prostaglandins,* Ramwell PW Ed, Plenum Press, NY, vol. 2, 1974, pp 1-47.
4. Glazko AJ: Experimental observations of flufenamic, mefenamic, and meclofenamic acids. Part III. Metabolic disposition, in *Fenamates in Medicine.* A Symposium, London 1966; *Annals of Physical Medicine,* supplement, pp 23-36, 1967.
5. Data on file, Medical Affairs Dept, Parke-Davis.
6. Budoff PW: Use of mefenamic acid in the treatment of primary dysmenorrhea. *JAMA* 241: 2713-2716, 1979.
7. Buchanan RA, et al: The breast milk excretion of mefenamic acid. *Curr Ther Res* 10:592, 1968.
8. Corby DG, Decker WJ: Management of acute poisoning with activated charcoal. *Pediatrics* 54:324, 1974.

Direct Medical Inquiries to: Parke-Davis
Div of Warner-Lambert Inc, 201 Tabor Road
Morris Plains, NJ 07950
Att: Medical Affairs Department

0540G013

POVAN® FILMSEAL® ℞
[pō'văn"]
(pyrvinium pamoate tablets, USP)*

*Product of Warner-Lambert Inc

Description: Pyrvinium pamoate, a cyanine dye, is 6-dimethylamino-2-(2-[2,5-dimethyl-1-phenyl-3-pyrrolyl]-vinyl)-1-methylquinolinium as the pamoate. It is a deep red crystalline powder which is stable to heat, light, and air, and is practically insoluble in water.

Continued on next page

This product information was prepared in August, 1984. On these and other Parke-Davis Products, information may be obtained by addressing PARKE-DAVIS, Division of Warner-Lambert Company, Morris Plains, New Jersey 07950.

Parke-Davis—Cont.

Actions: Pyrvinium pamoate appears to exert its anthelmintic effect by preventing the parasite from using exogenous carbohydrates. The parasite's endogenous reserves are depleted, and it dies. Povan is not appreciably absorbed from the gastrointestinal tract.

Indication: Povan is indicated for the treatment of enterobiasis.

Warnings: No animal or human reproduction studies have been performed. Therefore, the use of this drug during pregnancy requires that the potential benefits be weighed against its possible hazards to the mother and fetus.

Precautions: To forestall undue concern and help avoid accidental staining, patients and parents should be advised of the staining properties of Povan. Tablets should be swallowed whole to avoid staining of teeth. Parents and patients should be informed that pyrvinium pamoate will color the stool a bright red. This is not harmful to the patient. If emesis occurs, the vomitus will probably be colored red and will stain most materials.

Adverse Reactions: Nausea, vomiting, cramping, diarrhea, and hypersensitivity reactions (photosensitization and other allergic reactions) have been reported. The gastrointestinal reactions occur more often in older children and adults who have received large doses.

Emesis is more frequently seen with Povan Suspension than with Povan Filmseals.

Dosage and Administration: For control of pinworm infections in children and adults, Povan is administered orally in a single dose of 5 mg pyrvinium per kilogram body weight. If necessary, the dose may be repeated in two or three weeks.

Pinworm infection can pass easily from person to person by transfer of eggs through direct contact, handling contaminated objects, and breathing airborne eggs in dust. Therefore, if an infection is detected in any member of a family or institution group, treatment of all members should be considered for complete parasite eradication.

Dosage may be conveniently determined by referring to the Table.

Povan (pyrvinium pamoate): Dosage Table

BODY WEIGHT		DOSAGE
lb	kg	(Number of Tablets)
154*	70	7
143	65	7
132	60	6
121	55	6
110	50	5
99	45	5
88	40	4
77	35	4
66	30	3
55	25	3
44	20	2
33	15	2

*Because the gastrointestinal tract of adults does not appreciably increase in size with increased weight gain, the dosage for adults need not exceed that recommended for a patient weighing 154 lb. A single dose of seven tablets should be adequate for patients who weigh more than 154 lb.

How Supplied:
N 0710-0747-19 (Tablet 747)—Each Povan Filmseal contains pyrvinium pamoate equivalent to 50 mg pyrvinium. Supplied in bottles of 50.

Shown in Product Identification Section, page 425
NSN: 6505-00-890-1093
AHFS 8:08   0747 G 050

PROCAN® SR
[prō'căn″]
(procainamide hydrochloride tablets)
SUSTAINED RELEASE

> The prolonged administration of procainamide often leads to the development of a positive antinuclear antibody (ANA) test with or without symptoms of lupus erythematosus-like syndrome. If a positive ANA titer develops, the benefit/risk ratio related to continued procainamide therapy should be assessed. This may necessitate consideration of alternative antiarrhythmic therapy.

Description: Procan SR is an antiarrhythmic drug. Each tablet of Procan SR contains procainamide hydrochloride in a tablet matrix specially designed for the prolonged release of the drug in the gastrointestinal tract. Following release of the drug, the expended wax tablet matrix, which is not absorbed, may be detected in the stool. Procan SR is available for oral administration as green, film-coated tablets containing 250 mg procainamide hydrochloride; as yellow, scored, film-coated tablets containing 500 mg procainamide hydrochloride; and as orange scored film-coated tablets containing 750 mg procainamide hydrochloride.

Procainamide hydrochloride is the amide analogue of procaine hydrochloride. The chemical name is 4-amino-N-[2-(diethylamino)ethyl]benzamide monohydrochloride.

Clinical Pharmacology: Procainamide depresses the excitability of cardiac muscle to electrical stimulation, and slows conduction in the atrium, the bundle of His, and the ventricle. The refractory period of the atrium is considerably more prolonged than that of the ventricle. Contractility of the heart is usually not affected nor is cardiac output decreased to any extent unless myocardial damage exists. In the absence of any arrhythmia, the heart rate may occasionally be accelerated by conventional doses, suggesting that the drug possesses anticholinergic properties. Larger doses can induce atrioventricular block and ventricular extrasystoles which may proceed to ventricular fibrillation. These effects on the myocardium are reflected in the electrocardiogram; a widening of the QRS complex occurs most consistently; less regularly, the P-R and Q-T intervals are prolonged; and the QRS and T waves show some decrease in voltage.

The sustained-release characteristic of Procan SR tablets has been demonstrated in studies in human subjects. A multiple-dose study has shown equivalent steady-state plasma levels of Procan SR tablets given every six hours when compared with an equal total daily dose of Pronestyl® (procainamide hydrochloride capsules, E.R. Squibb and Sons) given every three hours.

Procainamide is less readily hydrolyzed than procaine, and plasma levels decline slowly—about 10% to 20% per hour for standard dosage forms of procainamide. The drug is excreted primarily in the urine, about 10% as free and conjugated p-aminobenzoic acid and about 60% in the unchanged form. The fate of the remainder is unknown.

Indications and Usage: Oral procainamide is indicated in the treatment of premature ventricular contractions and ventricular tachycardia, atrial fibrillation, and paroxysmal atrial tachycardia.

Contraindications: It has been suggested that procainamide be contraindicated in patients with myasthenia gravis. Hypersensitivity to the drug is an absolute contraindication; in this connection, cross-sensitivity to procaine and related drugs must be borne in mind. Procainamide should not be administered to patients with complete atrioventricular heart block. Procainamide is also contraindicated in cases of second degree and third degree A-V block unless an electrical pacemaker is operative.

Precautions:
General—During administration of the drug, evidence of untoward myocardial responses should be carefully watched for in all patients. In the presence of an abnormal myocardium, procainamide may at times produce untoward responses. In atrial fibrillation or flutter, the ventricular rate may increase suddenly as the atrial rate is slowed. Adequate digitalization reduces, but does not abolish, this danger. If myocardial damage exists, ventricular tachysystole is particularly hazardous. Correction of atrial fibrillation, with resultant forceful contractions of the atrium, may cause a dislodgement of mural thrombi and produce an embolic episode. However, it has been suggested that in a patient who is already discharging emboli, procainamide is more likely to stop than to aggravate the process.

Attempts to adjust the heart rate in a patient who has developed ventricular tachycardia during an occlusive coronary episode should be carried out with extreme caution. Caution is also required in marked disturbances of atrioventricular conduction such as A-V block, bundle branch block, or severe digitalis intoxication, where the use of procainamide may result in additional depression of conduction and ventricular asystole or fibrillation. Because patients with severe organic heart disease and ventricular tachycardia may also have complete heart block, which is difficult to diagnose under these circumstances, this complication should always be kept in mind when treating ventricular arrhythmias with procainamide. If the ventricular rate is significantly slowed by procainamide without attainment of regular atrioventricular conduction, the drug should be stopped and the patient reevaluated since asystole may result under these circumstances.

In patients receiving normal dosage, but who have both liver and kidney disease, symptoms of overdosage (principally ventricular tachycardia and severe hypotension) may occur due to drug accumulation.

Instances of a syndrome resembling lupus erythematosus have been reported in connection with maintenance procainamide therapy. The mechanism of this syndrome is uncertain. Polyarthralgia, arthritis, and pleuritic pain are common symptoms; to a lesser extent fever, myalgia, skin lesions, pleural effusion, and pericarditis may occur. Rare cases of thrombocytopenia or Coombs-positive hemolytic anemia have been reported which may be related to this syndrome.

Laboratory Tests—Patients receiving procainamide for extended periods of time, or in whom symptoms suggestive of a lupus-like reaction appear, should have antinuclear antibody titers measured at regular intervals.

The drug should be discontinued if there is a rising titer (antinuclear antibody) or clinical symptoms of LE appear. The LE syndrome may be reversible upon discontinuation of the drug. If discontinuation of the drug does not cause remission of the symptoms, steroid therapy may be effective. If the syndrome develops in a patient with recurrent life-threatening arrhythmias not controllable by other antiarrhythmic agents, steroid suppressive therapy may be used concomitantly with procainamide. It is recommended that tests for lupus erythematosus be carried out at regular intervals in patients receiving maintenance procainamide therapy.

Routine blood counts are advisable during maintenance procainamide therapy.

Adverse Reactions: Agranulocytosis has occasionally followed the repeated use of the drug, and deaths have occurred. Therefore, routine blood counts are advisable during maintenance procainamide therapy. The patient should be instructed to report any soreness of the mouth, throat or gums, unexplained fever, or any symptoms of upper respiratory tract infection. If any of these should occur, and leucocyte counts indicate cellular depression, procainamide therapy should be discontinued and appropriate treatment should be instituted immediately.

Hypersensitivity reactions, such as angioneurotic edema and maculopapular rash have also occurred.

A syndrome resembling lupus erythematosus has been reported (see PRECAUTIONS).

Hypotension following oral administration is rare. Large oral doses of procainamide may sometimes produce anorexia, nausea, urticaria, and/or pruritus.

Reactions consisting of fever and chills have also been reported, including a case with fever and chills plus nausea, vomiting, abdominal pain, acute hepatomegaly, and a rise in serum glutamic oxaloacetic transaminase following single doses of the drug. Bitter taste, diarrhea, weakness, mental depression, giddiness, and psychosis with hallucinations have been reported. The possibility of such untoward effects should be borne in mind.

Dosage and Administration: Procan SR tablets are a sustained-release product form. The duration of action of procainamide hydrochloride supplied in this sustained-release product form allows dosing at intervals of every six hours instead of the more frequent every-three-hour dosing interval required for standard preparations of oral procainamide hydrochloride. The convenient six-hour dosing schedule may encourage patient compliance.

Ventricular tachycardia—Treatment with standard procainamide hydrochloride is recommended until the tachycardia is interrupted or the limit of tolerance is reached. Maintenance may then be continued with Procan SR.

The suggested dosage is as follows. An initial dose of 1 g of standard procainamide hydrochloride followed thereafter by a total daily dose of 50 mg/kg of body weight given at three-hour intervals. The suggested oral dosage for premature ventricular contractions is 50 mg/kg of body weight daily given in divided doses at three-hour intervals.

The suggested maintenance dosage of Procan SR is 50 mg/kg of body weight daily given in divided doses at six-hour intervals.

Although the dosage for each patient must be determined on an individual basis, the following may be used as a guide for providing the total daily dosage: patients weighing less than 55 kg (120 lb), 0.5 g every six hours; patients weighing between 55 and 91 kg (120 and 200 lb) 0.75 g every six hours; and patients weighing over 91 kg (200 lb), 1 g every six hours.

Atrial fibrillation and paroxysmal atrial tachycardia.

Treatment with standard procainamide hydrochloride is recommended until the arrhythmia is interrupted or the limit of tolerance is reached. Maintenance may then be continued with Procan SR.

The suggested dosage is as follows. An initial dose of 1.25 g of standard procainamide hydrochloride may be followed in one hour by 0.75 g if there have been no electrocardiographic changes. Standard procainamide hydrochloride may then be given at a dose of 0.5 g to 1 g every two hours until interruption of the arrhythmia or the tolerance limit is reached.

The suggested maintenance dosage for Procan SR is 1 g every six hours.

If procainamide therapy is continued for appreciable periods, electrocardiograms should be made occasionally to determine the need for the drug.

How Supplied:
Procan SR 250 mg (green, film-coated, coded PD 202) is a sustained-release tablet that contains 250 mg of procainamide hydrochloride. It is supplied as follows:

N 0071-0202-24	Bottles of 100
N 0071-0202-30	Bottles of 500
N 0071-0202-40	Unit-dose packages of 100 (10 strips of 10 tablets each)

Procan SR 500 mg (yellow, scored, film-coated, coded PD 204) is a sustained-release tablet that contains 500 mg of procainamide hydrochloride. It is supplied as follows:

N 0071-0204-24	Bottles of 100
N 0071-0204-30	Bottles of 500
N 0071-0204-40	Unit-dose packages of 100 (10 strips of 10 tablets each)

Procan SR 750 mg (orange, scored, film-coated, coded PD 205) is a sustained-release tablet that contains 750 mg of procainamide hydrochloride. It is supplied as follows:

N 0071-0205-24	Bottles of 100
N 0071-0205-40	Unit-dose packages of 100 (10 strips of 10 tablets each)

Storage Conditions
Protect from moisture.
Store bottles below 30°C (86°F).
Store unit-dose packages at contolled room temperature, 15°–30°C (59°–86°F).

0202G012
Shown in Product Identification Section, page 425

PROLOID® ℞
[prō′ loid]
(Thyroglobulin Tablets, USP)

Description: Thyroid hormone drugs are natural or synthetic preparations containing tetraiodothyronine (T_4, levothyroxine) sodium or triiodothyronine (T_3, liothyronine) sodium or both. T_4 and T_3 are produced in the human thyroid gland by the iodination and coupling of the amino acid tyrosine. T_4 contains four iodine atoms and is formed by the coupling of two molecules of diiodotyrosine (DIT). T_3 contains three atoms of iodine and is formed by the coupling of one molecule of DIT with one molecule of monoiodotyrosine (MIT). Both hormones are stored in the thyroid colloid as thyroglobulin.

Thyroid hormone preparations belong to two categories: (1) natural hormonal preparations derived from animal thyroid, and (2) synthetic preparations. Natural preparations include desiccated thyroid and thyroglobulin. Desiccated thyroid is derived from domesticated animals that are used for food by man (either beef or hog thyroid), and thyroglobulin is derived from thyroid glands of the hog. The United States Pharmacopeia (USP) has standardized the total iodine content of natural preparations. Thyroid USP contains not less than (NLT) 0.17 percent and not more than (NMT) 0.23 percent iodine, and thyroglobulin contains not less than (NLT) 0.7 percent of organically bound iodine. Iodine content is only an indirect indicator of true hormonal biologic activity.

There are five (5) preparations in the USP. They are: (1) Thyroid Tablets, (2) Thyroglobulin Tablets, (3) Levothyroxine Sodium Tablets, (4) Liothyronine Sodium Tablets, and (5) Liotrix Tablets (a ratio, by weight, of 4 to 1, of the sodium salts of T_4 and T_3, respectively).

Clinical Pharmacology: The steps in the synthesis of the thyroid hormones are controlled by thyrotropin (Thyroid Stimulating Hormone, TSH) secreted by the anterior pituitary. This hormone's secretion is in turn controlled by a feedback mechanism effected by the thyroid hormones themselves and by thyrotropin releasing hormone (TRH), a tripeptide of hypothalamic origin. Endogenous thyroid hormone secretion is suppressed when exogenous thyroid hormones are administered to euthyroid individuals in excess of the normal gland's secretion.

The mechanisms by which thyroid hormones exert their physiologic action are not well understood. These hormones enhance oxygen consumption by most tissues of the body, increase the basal metabolic rate, and the metabolism of carbohydrates, lipids, and proteins. Thus, they exert a profound influence on every organ system in the body and are of particular importance in the development of the central nervous system.

The normal thyroid gland contains approximately 200 mcg of levothyroxine (T_4) per gram of gland, and 15 mcg of triiodothyronine (T_3) per gram. The ratio of these two hormones in the circulation does not represent the ratio in the thyroid gland, since about 80 percent of peripheral triiodothyronine comes from monodeiodination of levothyroxine. Peripheral monodeiodination of levothyroxine at the 5 position (inner ring) also results in the formation of reverse triiodothyronine (r T_3), which is calorigenically inactive. These facts would seem to advocate levothyroxine as the treatment of choice for the hypothyroid patient and to militate against the administration of hormone combinations, which while normalizing thyroxine levels may produce triiodothyronine levels in the thyrotoxic range.

Triiodothyronine (T_3) level is low in the fetus and newborn, in old age, in chronic caloric deprivation, hepatic cirrhosis, renal failure, surgical stress, and chronic illnesses representing what has been called the "low triiodothyronine syndrome."

Pharmacokinetics: Animal studies have shown that T_4 is only partially absorbed from the gastrointestinal tract. The degree of absorption is dependent on the vehicle used for its administration and by the character of the intestinal contents, the intestinal flora, including plasma protein, soluble dietary factors, all of which bind thyroid and thereby make it unavailable for diffusion. Only 41 percent is absorbed when given in a gelatin capsule as opposed to a 74 percent absorption when given with an albumin carrier.

Depending on other factors, absorption has varied from 48 to 79 percent of the administered dose. Fasting increases absorption. Malabsorption syndromes, as well as dietary factors (children's soybean formula, concomitant use of anionic exchange resins such as cholestyramine), cause excessive fecal loss. T_3 is almost totally absorbed, 95 percent in 4 hours. The hormones contained in the natural preparations are absorbed in a manner similar to the synthetic hormones.

More than 99 percent of circulating hormones are bound to serum proteins, including thyroid-binding globulin (TBg), thyroid-binding prealbumin (TBPA), and albumin (TBa), whose capacities and affinities vary for the hormones. The higher affinity of levothyroxine (T_4) for both TBg and TBPA as compared to triiodothyronine (T_3) partially explains the higher serum levels and longer half-life of the former hormone. Both protein-bound hormones exist in reverse equilibrium with minute amounts of free hormone, the latter accounting for the metabolic activity.

Deiodination of levothyroxine (T_4) occurs at a number of sites, including liver, kidney, and other tissues. The conjugated hormone, in the form of glucuronide or sulfate, is found in the bile and gut where it may complete an enterohepatic circulation. Eighty-five percent of levothyroxine (T_4) metabolized daily is deiodinated.

Indications and Usage: Thyroid hormone drugs are indicated:

1. As replacement or supplemental therapy in patients with hypothyroidism of any etiology, except transient hypothyroidism during the recovery phase of subacute thyroiditis. This category includes cretinism, myxedema, and ordinary hypothyroidism in patients of any age (children, adults, the elderly), or state (including pregnancy); primary hypothyroidism resulting from functional deficiency, primary atrophy, partial or total absence of thyroid gland, or the effects of surgery, radiation, or drugs, with or without the presence of goiter; and secondary (pituitary) or tertiary (hypothalamic) hypothyroidism (See WARNINGS).

2. As pituitary TSH suppressants, in the treatment or prevention of various types of euthyroid goiters, including thyroid nodules, subacute or chronic lymphocytic thyroiditis (Hashimoto's),

Continued on next page

This product information was prepared in August, 1984. On these and other Parke-Davis Products, information may be obtained by addressing PARKE-DAVIS, Division of Warner-Lambert Company, Morris Plains, New Jersey 07950.

Parke-Davis—Cont.

multinodular goiter, and in the management of thyroid cancer.
3. As diagnostic agents in suppression tests to differentiate suspected mild hyperthyroidism or thyroid gland autonomy.

Contraindications: Thyroid hormone preparations are generally contraindicated in patients with diagnosed but as yet uncorrected adrenal cortical insufficiency, untreated thyrotoxicosis, and apparent hypersensitivity to any of their active or extraneous constituents. There is no well documented evidence from the literature, however, of true allergic or idiosyncratic reactions to thyroid hormone.

Warnings:

> Drugs with thyroid hormone activity, alone or together with other therapeutic agents, have been used for the treatment of obesity. In euthyroid patients, doses within the range of daily hormonal requirements are ineffective for weight reduction. Larger doses may produce serious or even life-threatening manifestations of toxicity, particularly when given in association with sympathomimetic amines such as those used for their anorectic effects.

The use of thyroid hormones in the therapy of obesity, alone or combined with other drugs, is unjustified and has been shown to be ineffective. Neither is their use justified for the treatment of male or female infertility unless this condition is accompanied by hypothyroidism.

Precautions:

General: Thyroid hormones should be used with great caution in a number of circumstances where the integrity of the cardiovascular system, particularly the coronary arteries, is suspect. These include patients with angina pectoris or the elderly, in whom there is a greater likelihood of occult cardiac disease. In these patients, therapy should be initiated with low doses, ie, 25–50 mcg levothyroxine (T_4) or its isocaloric equivalents. When, in such patients, a euthyroid state can only be reached at the expense of an aggravation of the cardiovascular disease, thyroid hormone dosage should be reduced.

Thyroid hormone therapy in patients with concomitant diabetes mellitus or insipidus or adrenal cortical insufficiency aggravates the intensity of their symptoms. Appropriate adjustments of the various therapeutic measures directed at these concomitant endocrine diseases are required. The therapy of myxedema coma requires simultaneous administration of glucocorticoids (See DOSAGE AND ADMINISTRATION).

Hypothyroidism decreases and hyperthyroidism increases the sensitivity to oral anticoagulants. Prothrombin time should be closely monitored in thyroid-treated patients on oral anticoagulants and dosage of the latter agents adjusted on the basis of frequent prothrombin time determination. In infants, excessive doses of thyroid hormone preparations may produce craniosynostosis.

Information for the Patient: Patients on thyroid hormone preparations and parents of children on thyroid therapy should be informed that:
1. Replacement therapy is to be taken essentially for life, with the exception of cases of transient hypothyroidism, usually associated with thyroiditis, and in those patients receiving a therapeutic trial of the drug.
2. They should immediately report during the course of therapy any signs or symptoms of thyroid hormone toxicity, eg, chest pain, increased pulse rate, palpitations, excessive sweating, heat intolerance, nervousness, or any other unusual event.
3. In case of concomitant diabetes mellitus, the daily dosage of antidiabetic medication may need readjustment as thyroid hormone replacement is achieved. If thyroid medication is stopped, a downward readjustment of the dosage of insulin or oral hypoglycemic agent may be necessary to avoid hypoglycemia. At all times, close monitoring of urinary glucose levels is mandatory in such patients.
4. In case of concomitant oral anticoagulant therapy, the prothrombin time should be measured frequently to determine if the dosage of oral anticoagulants is to be readjusted.
5. Partial loss of hair may be experienced by children in the first few months of thyroid therapy, but this is usually a transient phenomenon and later recovery is usually the rule.

Laboratory Tests: Treatment of patients with thyroid hormones requires the periodic assessment of thyroid status by means of appropriate laboratory tests besides the full clinical evaluation. The TSH suppression test can be used to test the effectiveness of any thyroid preparation, bearing in mind the relative insensitivity of the infant pituitary to the negative feedback effect of thyroid hormones. Serum T_4 levels can be used to test the effectiveness of all thyroid medications except T_3. When the total serum T_4 is low but TSH is normal, a test specific to assess unbound (free) T_4 levels is warranted. Specific measurements of T_4 and T_3 by competitive protein binding or radioimmunoassay are not influenced by blood levels of organic or inorganic iodine and have essentially replaced older tests of thyroid hormone measurements, ie, PBI, BEI, and T_4 by column.

Drug Interactions: Oral Anticoagulants—Thyroid hormones appear to increase catabolism of vitamin K-dependent clotting factors. If oral anticoagulants are also being given, compensatory increases in clotting factor synthesis are impaired. Patients stabilized on oral anticoagulants who are found to require thyroid replacement therapy should be watched very closely when thyroid is started. If a patient is truly hypothyroid, it is likely that a reduction in anticoagulant dosage will be required. No special precautions appear to be necessary when oral anticoagulant therapy is begun in a patient already stabilized on maintenance thyroid replacement therapy.

Insulin or Oral Hypoglycemics—Initiating thyroid replacement therapy may cause increases in insulin or oral hypoglycemic requirements. The effects seen are poorly understood and depend upon a variety of factors such as dosage and type of thyroid preparations and endocrine status of the patient. Patients receiving insulin or oral hypoglycemics should be closely watched during initiation of thyroid replacement therapy.

Cholestyramine—Cholestyramine binds both T_4 and T_3 in the intestine, thus impairing absorption of these thyroid hormones. *In vitro* studies indicate that the binding is not easily removed. Therefore, four to five hours should elapse between administration of cholestyramine and thyroid hormones.

Estrogen, Oral Contraceptives—Estrogens tend to increase serum thyroxine-binding globulin (TBg). In a patient with a nonfunctioning thyroid gland who is receiving thyroid replacement therapy, free levothyroxine may be decreased when estrogens are started thus increasing thyroid requirements. However, if the patient's thyroid gland has sufficient function, the decreased free thyroxine will result in a compensatory increase in thyroxine output by the thyroid. Therefore, patients without a functioning thyroid gland who are on thyroid replacement therapy may need to increase their thyroid dose if estrogens or estrogen-containing oral contraceptives are given.

Drug/Laboratory Test Interactions: The following drugs or moieties are known to interfere with laboratory tests performed in patients on thyroid hormone therapy: androgens, corticosteroids, estrogens, oral contraceptives containing estrogens, iodine-containing preparations, and the numerous preparations containing salicylates.
1. Changes in TBg concentration should be taken into consideration in the interpretation of T_4 and T_3 values. In such cases, the unbound (free) hormone should be measured. Pregnancy, estrogens, and estrogen-containing oral contraceptives increase TBg concentrations. TBg may also be increased during infectious hepatitis. Decreases in TBg concentrations are observed in nephrosis, acromegaly, and after androgen or corticosteroid therapy. Familial hyper- or hypothyroxine-binding-globulinemias have been described. The incidence of TBg deficiency approximates 1 in 9000. The binding of thyroxine by TBPA is inhibited by salicylates.
2. Medicinal or dietary iodine interferes with all *in vivo* tests of radioiodine uptake, producing low uptakes which may not be reflective of a true decrease in hormone synthesis.
3. The persistence of clinical and laboratory evidence of hypothyroidism in spite of adequate dosage replacement indicates poor patient compliance, poor absorption, excessive fecal loss, or inactivity of the preparation. Intracellular resistance to thyroid hormone is quite rare.

Carcinogenesis, Mutagenesis, and Impairment of Fertility: A reportedly apparent association between prolonged thyroid therapy and breast cancer has not been confirmed and patients on thyroid for established indications should not discontinue therapy. No confirmatory long-term studies in animals have been performed to evaluate carcinogenic potential, mutagenicity, or impairment of fertility in either males or females.

Pregnancy-Category A: Thyroid hormones do not readily cross the placental barrier. The clinical experience to date does not indicate any adverse effect on fetuses when thyroid hormones are administered to pregnant women. On the basis of current knowledge, thyroid replacement therapy to hypothyroid women should not be discontinued during pregnancy.

Nursing Mothers: Minimal amounts of thyroid hormones are excreted in human milk. Thyroid is not associated with serious adverse reactions and does not have a known tumorigenic potential. However, caution should be exercised when thyroid is administered to a nursing woman.

Pediatric Use: Pregnant mothers provide little or no thyroid hormone to the fetus. The incidence of congenital hypothyroidism is relatively high (14,000) and the hypothyroid fetus would not derive any benefit from the small amounts of hormone crossing the placental barrier. Routine determinations of serum (T_4) and/or TSH are strongly advised in neonates in view of the deleterious effects of thyroid deficiency on growth and development.

Treatment should be initiated immediately upon diagnosis and maintained for life, unless transient hypothyroidism is suspected; in which case, therapy may be interrupted for 2 to 8 weeks after the age of 3 years to reassess the condition. Cessation of therapy is justified in patients who have maintained a normal TSH during those 2 to 8 weeks.

Adverse Reactions: Adverse reactions other than those indicative of hyperthyroidism because of therapeutic overdosage, either initially or during the maintenance period, are rare (See **Overdosage**).

Overdosage:

Signs and Symptoms: Excessive doses of thyroid result in a hypermetabolic state resembling in every respect the condition of endogenous origin. The condition may be self-induced.

Treatment of Overdosage: Dosage should be reduced or therapy temporarily discontinued if signs and symptoms of overdosage appear. Treatment may be reinstituted at a lower dosage. In normal individuals, normal hypothalamic-pituitary-thyroid axis function is restored in 6 to 8 weeks after thyroid suppression.

Treatment of acute massive thyroid hormone overdosage is aimed at reducing gastrointestinal absorption of the drugs and counteracting central and peripheral effects, mainly those of increased sympathetic activity. Vomiting may be induced initially if further gastrointestinal absorption can reasonably be prevented and barring contraindications such as coma, convulsions, or loss of the gagging reflex. Treatment is symptomatic and supportive. Oxygen may be administered and ventilation maintained. Cardiac glycosides may be indicated if congestive heart failure develops. Measures to control fever, hypoglycemia, or fluid loss should be instituted if needed. Antiadrenergic agents, particularly propranolol, have been used advantageously in the treatment of increased sympathetic activity. Propranolol may be administered intravenously at a dosage of 1 to 3 mg over a 10 minute period or orally, 80 to 160 mg/day, especially when no contraindications exist for its use.

Dosage and Administration: The dosage of thyroid hormones is determined by the indication and must in every case be individualized according to patient response and laboratory findings.

Thyroid hormones are given orally. In acute, emergency conditions, injectable sodium levothyroxine may be given intravenously when oral administration is not feasible or desirable, as in the treatment of myxedema coma, or during total parenteral nutrition. Injectable sodium liothyronine is also available upon request from the manufacturer, under investigational status, for the treatment of myxedema coma. Intramuscular administration of these two preparations is not advisable because of reported poor absorption.

Hypothyroidism: Therapy is usually instituted using low doses, with increments which depend on the cardiovascular status of the patient. The usual starting dose is 50 mcg of levothyroxine (T_4) or its isocaloric equivalent, with increments of 25 mcg every 2 to 3 weeks. A lower starting dosage, 25 mcg/day, is recommended in patients with long-standing myxedema, particularly if cardiovascular impairment is suspected, in which case extreme caution is recommended. The appearance of angina is an indication for a reduction in dosage. The 200 to 400 mcg levothyroxine (T_4) recommended in the early trials are now considered excessive and most patients require 100 to 200 mcg/day or the caloric equivalent. Failure to respond to doses of 300 mcg suggests lack of compliance or malabsorption. Maintenance dosages of 100–200 mcg/day usually result in normal serum levothyroxine (T_4) and triiodothyronine (T_3) levels. Adequate therapy usually results in normal TSH and T_4 levels after 2 to 3 weeks of therapy.

Readjustment of thyroid hormone dosage should be made within the first four weeks of therapy, after proper clinical and laboratory evaluations, including serum levels of T_4, bound and free, and TSH.

The rapid onset and dissipation of action of sodium liothyronine (T_3), as compared with sodium levothyroxine (T_4), has led some clinicians to prefer its use in patients who might be more susceptible to the untoward effects of thyroid medication. However, the wide swings in serum T_3 levels that follow its administration and the possibility of more pronounced cardiovascular side effects tend to counterbalance the stated advantages. Many physicians continue to use thyroid tablets, USP, a T_3/T_4 combination, or a newer synthetic combination.

T_3 may be used in preference to levothyroxine (T_4) during radioisotope scanning procedures, since induction of hypothyroidism in those cases is more abrupt and can be of shorter duration. It may also be preferred when impairment of peripheral conversion of T_4 and T_3 is suspected.

Myxedema Coma: Myxedema coma is usually precipitated in the hypothyroid patient of long-standing by intercurrent illness or drugs such as sedatives and anesthetics and should be considered a medical emergency. Therapy should be directed at the correction of electrolyte disturbances and possible infection besides the administration of thyroid hormones. Corticosteroids should be administered routinely. T_4 and T_3 may be administered via a nasogastric tube, but the preferred route of administration of both hormones is intravenous. Sodium levothyroxine (T_4) is given at a starting dose of 400 mcg (100 mcg/ml) given rapidly and is usually well tolerated, even in the elderly. This initial dose is followed by daily supplements of 100 to 200 mcg given IV. Normal T_4 levels are achieved in 24 hours followed in 3 days by threefold elevation of T_3. Triiodothyronine (T_3) (which is obtained only by special request from the manufacturer) is given at doses of 200 mcg IV followed by 25 mcg supplements at 8-hour intervals. Oral therapy with either hormone would be resumed as soon as the clinical situation has been stabilized and the patient is able to take oral medication.

Thyroid Cancer: Exogenous thyroid hormone may produce regression of metastases from follicular and papillary carcinoma of the thyroid and is used as ancillary therapy of these conditions with radioactive iodine: TSH should be suppressed to low or undetectable levels. Therefore, larger amounts of thyroid hormone than those used for replacement therapy are required. Medullary carcinoma of the thyroid is usually unresponsive to this therapy.

Thyroid Suppression Therapy: Administration of thyroid hormone in doses higher than those produced physiologically by the gland results in suppression of the production of endogenous hormone. This is the basis for the thyroid suppression test and is used as an aid in the diagnosis of patients with signs of mild hyperthyroidism in whom baseline laboratory tests appear normal or to demonstrate thyroid gland autonomy in patients with Graves' ophthalmopathy. $_{131}$I uptake is determined before and after the administration of the exogenous hormone. A fifty percent or greater suppression of uptake indicates a normal thyroid-pituitary axis and thus rules out thyroid gland autonomy.

For adults, the usual suppressive dose of levothyroxine (T_4) is 2.6 mcg/kg of body weight per day given for 7 to 10 days. These doses usually yield normal serum T_4 and T_3 levels and lack of response to TSH.

T_3 is given in doses of 75–100 mcg/day for 7 days and radioactive iodine uptake is determined before and after administration of the hormone. If thyroid function is under normal control, the radioiodine uptake will drop significantly after treatment with either hormone.

Either hormone or combination therapy should be administered cautiously to patients in whom there is a strong suspicion of thyroid gland autonomy, in view of the fact that the exogenous hormone effects will be additive to the endogenous source.

Pediatric Dosage: Pediatric dosage should follow the recommendations summarized in Table 1. In infants with congenital hypothyroidism, therapy with full doses should be instituted as soon as the diagnosis has been made.

Table 1 Recommended Pediatric Dosage for Congenital Hypothyroidism

Age	Tetraiodothyronine (T_4, levothyroxine) sodium Dose per day	Daily dose per kg of body weight
0–6 mos	25–50 mcg	8–10 mcg
6–12 mos	50–75 mcg	6–8 mcg
1–5 yrs	75–100 mcg	5–6 mcg
6–12 yrs	100–150 mcg	4–5 mcg
over 12 yrs	over 150 mcg	2–3 mcg

N 0710-0251-24	½ grain (32 mg)	Bottles of 100
N 0710-0251-32	½ grain (32 mg)	Bottles of 1000
N 0710-0252-24	1 grain (65 mg) Scored	Bottles of 100
N 0710-0252-32	1 grain (65 mg) Scored	Bottles of 1000
N 0710-0253-24	1½ grain (100 mg)	Bottles of 100
N 0710-0253-32	1½ grain (100 mg)	Bottles of 1000
N 0710-0257-24	2 grain (130 mg) Scored	Bottles of 100
N 0710-0254-24	3 grain (200 mg)	Bottles of 100
N 0710-0254-32	3 grain (200 mg)	Bottles of 1000

How Supplied: Proloid tablets are supplied: [See table above].
Tablets are gray and uncoated.
Store at controlled room temperature 15°–30°C (59°–86°F).

0250G012

Shown in Product Identification Section, page 425

PYRIDIUM®   ℞
[pў″ rĭ″ dĭ-ŭm]
(Phenazopyridine Hydrochloride Tablets, USP)

Description: Pyridium (phenazopyridine hydrochloride) is chemically designated 2,6-Pyridinediamine, 3-(phenylazo), monohydrochloride. It is a urinary tract analgesic agent for oral administration. Pyridium tablets contain 100 mg or 200 mg phenazopyridine hydrochloride.

Clinical Pharmacology: Pyridium is excreted in the urine where it exerts a topical analgesic effect on the mucosa of the urinary tract. This action helps to relieve pain, burning, urgency and frequency. The precise mechanism of action is not known.

The pharmacokinetic properties of Pyridium have not been determined. Phenazopyridine is rapidly excreted by the kidneys, with as much as 65% of an oral dose being excreted unchanged in the urine.

Indications and Usage: Pyridium is indicated for the symptomatic relief of pain, burning, urgency, frequency, and other discomforts arising from irritation of the lower urinary tract mucosa caused by infection, trauma, surgery, endoscopic procedures, or the passage of sounds or catheters. The use of Pyridium for relief of symptoms should not delay definitive diagnosis and treatment of causative conditions. Because it provides only symptomatic relief, prompt appropriate treatment of the cause of pain must be instituted and Pyridium should be discontinued when symptoms are controlled.

The analgesic action may reduce or eliminate the need for systemic analgesics or narcotics. It is, however, compatible with antibacterial therapy and can help to relieve pain and discomfort during the interval before antibacterial therapy controls the infection. Treatment of a urinary tract infection with Pyridium should not exceed 2 days because there is a lack of evidence that the combined administration of Pyridium and an antibacterial provides greater benefit than administration of the antibacterial alone after 2 days. (See Dosage and Administration Section.)

Contraindications: Pyridium should not be used in patients who have previously exhibited hypersensitivity to it. The use of Pyridium is contraindicated in patients with renal insufficiency.

Continued on next page

This product information was prepared in August, 1984. On these and other Parke-Davis Products, information may be obtained by addressing PARKE-DAVIS, Division of Warner-Lambert Company, Morris Plains, New Jersey 07950.

Parke-Davis—Cont.

Precautions:
General: A yellowish tinge of the skin or sclera may indicate accumulation due to impaired renal excretion and the need to discontinue therapy. The decline in renal function associated with advanced age should be kept in mind.
Information for Patients: Pyridium produces an orange to red color in the urine and may stain fabric.
Laboratory Test Interactions: Due to its properties as an azo dye, Pyridium may interfere with urinalysis based on spectrometry or color reactions.
Carcinogenesis, Mutagenesis, Impairment of Fertility: Long-term administration of phenazopyridine hydrochloride has induced neoplasia in rats (large intestine) and mice (liver). Although no association between phenazopyridine hydrochloride and human neoplasia has been reported, adequate epidemiological studies along these lines have not been conducted.
Pregnancy Category B: Reproduction studies have been performed in rats at doses up to 50 mg/kg/day and have revealed no evidence of impaired fertility or harm to the fetus due to Pyridium. There are, however, no adequate and well controlled studies in pregnant women. Because animal reproduction studies are not always predictive of human response, this drug should be used during pregnancy only if clearly needed.
Nursing Mothers: No information is available on the appearance of Pyridium or its metabolites in human milk.
Adverse Reactions: Headache, rash and occasional gastrointestinal disturbance. Methemoglobinemia, hemolytic anemia, renal and hepatic toxicity have been described, usually at overdose levels (see Overdosage section).
Overdosage: Exceeding the recommended dose in patients with good renal function or administering the usual dose to patients with impaired renal function (common in elderly patients), may lead to increased serum levels and toxic reactions. Methemoglobinemia generally follows a massive, acute overdose. Methylene blue, 1 to 2 mg/kg body weight intravenously, or ascorbic acid 100 to 200 mg given orally should cause prompt reduction of the methemoglobinemia and disappearance of the cyanosis which is an aid in diagnosis. Oxidative Heinz body hemolytic anemia may also occur, and "bite cells" (degmacytes) may be present in a chronic overdosage situation. Red blood cell G-6-PD deficiency may predispose to hemolysis. Renal and hepatic impairment and occasional failure, usually due to hypersensitivity, may also occur.
Dosage and Administration: 100 mg tablets: Adult dosage is two tablets 3 times a day after meals. 200 mg tablets: Adult dosage is one tablet 3 times a day after meals.
When used concomitantly with an antibacterial agent for the treatment of a urinary tract infection, the administration of Pyridium should not exceed 2 days.
How Supplied:
N 0710-0180-24 100 mg tablets
  Bottles of 100
N 0710-0180-32 100 mg tablets
  Bottles of 1000
N 0710-0180-40 100 mg tablets Unit dose packages of 100 (10 strips of 10)
Tablets are dark maroon and coated.
N 0710-0181-24 200 mg tablets
  Bottles of 100
N 0710-0181-32 200 mg tablets
  Bottles of 1000
N 0710-0181-40 200 mg tablets Unit dose packages of 100 (10 strips of 10)
Tablets are dark maroon and coated.
Store at controlled room temperature 15° to 30° C (59° to 86° F).
Direct Medical Inquiries to Parke-Davis, Div Warner-Lambert Company, 201 Tabor Road, Morris Plains, NJ 07950, Attn: Medical Affairs Department
AHFS Category 84:08   0180G011
Shown in Product Identification Section, p. 425

PYRIDIUM® PLUS Tablets   ℞
[pў″ rĭ′ dĭ-ŭm]

Description: Each Pyridium Plus tablet contains:
150 mg phenazopyridine hydrochloride (Pyridium®)
0.3 mg hyoscyamine hydrobromide
15 mg butabarbital

Clinical Pharmacology: Pyridium Plus relieves lower urinary symptoms of pain, frequency, urgency, burning and dysuria arising from inflammation of the urothelium, the mucosal lining of the lower urinary tract.
Lower urinary tract pain can cause reflex spasm of the detrusor. Pain and spasm are often aggravated by apprehension to promote a pain-spasm-apprehension cycle. Each of the three pharmacologic components of Pyridium Plus acts against a phase of this cycle.
Phenazopyridine hydrochloride (Pyridium), excreted in the urine, is a topical analgesic to relieve pain and discomfort.
Hyoscyamine hydrobromide, a parasympatholytic, acts to relieve detrusor muscle spasm. Butabarbital, a short-to-intermediate-acting sedative, helps to allay associated anxiety and apprehension.

Indications and Usage: Pyridium Plus is indicated for the symptomatic relief of pain, burning, frequency, urgency, and dysuria, particularly when accompanied by detrusor muscle spasm and apprehension.
These symptoms may arise from infection, trauma, surgery, endoscopic procedures, or passage of sounds or catheters.
Therapy with Pyridium Plus does not interfere with antibacterial therapy and can help to relieve symptoms of pain and discomfort before definitive treatment is effective. The use of Pyridium Plus for symptomatic relief should not delay definitive diagnosis and treatment. Treatment of a urinary tract infection with Pyridium Plus should not exceed 2 days because there is a lack of evidence that the combined administration of phenazopyridine hydrochloride and an antibacterial provides greater benefit than administration of the antibacterial alone after 2 days. (See Dosage and Administration Section.)
In the absence of infection, Pyridium Plus may be the only medication required.

Contraindications: Pyridium Plus should not be used in patients who have previously exhibited hypersensitivity to any component. The use of Pyridium Plus is contraindicated in patients with renal or hepatic insufficiency, glaucoma, bladder neck obstruction, porphyria.

Warning: BUTABARBITAL MAY BE HABIT-FORMING. Drowsiness or dizziness may occur. Patients should be instructed to use caution in driving or operating machinery.

Precautions:
General: A yellowish tinge of the skin or sclera may indicate accumulation due to impaired renal excretion of phenazopyridine (Pyridium) and the need to discontinue therapy.
The decline in renal function asssociated with advanced age should be kept in mind.
Information for Patients: Phenazopyridine hydrochloride produces an orange to red color in the urine and may stain fabric. Butabarbital may cause drowsiness or dizziness, patients should be instructed to use caution in driving or operating machinery.
Laboratory Test Interactions: Due to its properties as an azo dye, phenazopyridine hydrochloride may interfere with urinalysis based on spectrometry or color reactions.
Carcinogenesis, Mutagenesis, Impairment of Fertility: Pyridium Plus has not undergone adequate studies relating to carcinogenesis, mutagenesis, or impairment of fertility; however, the component phenazopyridine hydrochloride has induced neoplasia in rats (large intestine) and mice (liver). Although no association between phenazopyridine hydrochloride and human neoplasia has been reported, adequate epidemiological studies along these lines have not been conducted.

Pregnancy Category C: Animal reproduction studies have not been conducted with Pyridium Plus. It is also not known whether Pyridium Plus can cause fetal harm when administered to a pregnant woman or can affect reproduction capacity. Pyridium Plus should be given to a pregnant woman only if clearly needed.
Nursing Mothers: No information is available on the appearance of the components of Pyridium Plus in human milk.
Adverse Reactions: Methemoglobinemia, hemolytic anemia, and renal and hepatic toxicity have been described for phenazopyridine, usually at overdosage levels (see Overdosage Section).
Hyoscyamine hydrobromide is an atropinic drug that may produce adverse effects characteristic of this class of drugs. Dry mouth, drowsiness, or dizziness is noted in more than one third of patients (and may occur in half of the patients of older age groups). Other atropine-like effects, such as blurred vision, may occur. There may be occasional gastrointestinal disturbances.
Butabarbital is a short- to intermediate-acting barbiturate which has the potential for adverse reactions attributable to barbiturates.
Overdosage: Pyridium Plus is a combination of three active drugs, and overdosage can be expected to show the effects related to each ingredient. Management includes the usual measures to empty the stomach by emesis or lavage, administration of a charcoal slurry, and supportive measures as needed.
Toxicity and management suggestions relating to the individual ingredients are as follows:
Phenazopyridine Hydrochloride (Pyridium): Exceeding the recommended dose in patients with good renal function or administering the usual dose to patients with impaired renal function (common in elderly patients), may lead to increased serum levels and toxic reactions. Methemoglobinemia generally follows a massive, acute overdose. Methylene blue, 1 to 2 mg/kg body weight intravenously or ascorbic acid 100 to 200 mg given orally should cause prompt reduction of the methemoglobinemia and disappearance of cyanosis which is an aid in diagnosis. Oxidative Heinz body hemolytic anemia may also occur, and "bite cells" (degmacytes) may be present in a chronic overdosage situation. Red blood cell G-6-PD deficiency may predispose to hemolysis. Renal and hepatic impairment and occasional failure, usually due to hypersensitivity, may also occur.
Hyoscyamine Hydrobromide: Overdosage of hyoscyamine, a form of atropine, will cause dilated pupils, blurred vision, rapid pulse, increased intraocular tension, hot, dry, red skin, dry mouth, disorientation, delirium, fever, convulsions, and coma. As an antidote, physostigmine salicylate may be given IV slowly. Dilute 1 mg in 5 ml of saline and use 1 ml of this dilution in children. Repeat every five minutes as needed up to a total of 2 mg in children, or 6 mg in adults every 30 minutes.
Butabarbital: This drug may produce sedation and respiratory depression progressing to coma, depending on the amount ingested. General and supportive measures should be instituted.
Dosage and Administration:
Adult Dosage: One tablet four times a day (after meals and at bedtime).
When used concomitantly with an antibacterial agent for the treatment of a urinary tract infection, the administration of Pyridium Plus should not exceed 2 days.
How Supplied:
N 0710-0182-24 Bottles of 100. Tablets are dark maroon and square.
Store at controlled room temperature 15° to 30°C (59° to 86°F).
Direct Medical Inquiries to: Parke-Davis, Div Warner-Lambert Inc, c/o Warner-Lambert Company, 201 Tabor Road, Morris Plains, NJ 07950. Attn: Medical Affairs Department
AHFS Category 8:12.24   0182G062
Shown in Product Identification Section, p. 425

SINUBID®
[sīn'ū-bĭd"]

Description: Each Sinubid tablet contains:
600 mg acetaminophen
100 mg phenylpropanolamine hydrochloride
66 mg phenyltoloxamine citrate

Clinical Pharmacology: Sinubid is designed to provide symptomatic relief of coryza and nasal congestion when given twice a day (every 12 hours). Sinubid can provide symptomatic relief of headache, fever, and other symptoms associated with mucosal congestion (nasopharyngeal), general malaise, and irritability associated with the common cold, allergic and vasomotor disorders, sinusitis, and rhinitis.

Sinubid contains an analgesic-antipyretic (acetaminophen) to relieve the pain of sinus headache and nasal congestion. This analgesic-antipyretic is rapidly absorbed and as effective as aspirin in raising the pain threshold, but has the advantage of causing little or no gastric irritation. Sinubid, because it contains no salicylates, can be used by patients who are allergic to aspirin.

Decongestion of the nasopharyngeal mucosa is provided by phenylpropanolamine hydrochloride, a sympathomimetic amine which provides symptomatic relief. Because its vasoconstrictor activity is similar to that of ephedrine, but less likely to cause CNS stimulation, Sinubid may eliminate the need for topical decongestants.

Phenyltoloxamine citrate is a mild antihistamine which may provide symptomatic relief of seasonal and perennial allergic rhinitis, vasomotor rhinitis, nasal and sinus symptoms of sinusitis, and adjunctive therapy for bacterial sinusitis in uncomplicated upper respiratory infections.

Indications and Usage: Sinubid is indicated for the rapid, prolonged, symptomatic relief of nasal congestion in sinus or other frontal headache; allergic and vasomotor manifestations of upper respiratory disorders such as sinusitis, allergic rhinitis, vasomotor rhinitis, coryza; facial pain and "pressure" of acute and chronic sinusitis; and for the relief of accompanying fever. Sinubid is indicated only for intermittent treatment of the above noted acute symptoms.

Contraindications: This compound should not be used in patients whose oversensitivity to small doses of sympathomimetic amines produces sleeplessness, dizziness, lightheadedness, weakness, tremulousness, or cardiac arrhythmias. The drug is contraindicated in any patient hypersensitive to any of the ingredients of the formulation.

Warnings: Instruct patients not to drive or operate machinery if drowsiness occurs. Individuals should not ingest alcoholic beverages, monoamine oxidase inhibitors, or barbiturates while taking this medication.

Precautions

General: Individuals with high blood pressure, heart disease, diabetes mellitus, chronic renal disease, or thyroid disease should use only as directed by a physician.

Drug Interactions: See Warnings

Pregnancy: Pregnancy Category C. Animal reproduction studies have not been conducted with Sinubid. It is also not known whether Sinubid can cause fetal harm when administered to a pregnant woman or can affect reproduction capacity. Sinubid should be given to a pregnant woman only if clearly needed.

Nursing mothers: This drug should not be used in nursing mothers.

Adverse Reactions: The following adverse reactions have been reported for each of the individual or combinations of ingredients: Acetaminophen—urticaria, epigastric distress, dizziness, and palpitation. Phenylpropanolamine HCl—anxiety, restlessness, tension, insomnia, tremor, weakness, headache, vertigo, sweating, arrhythmia, nausea, and vomiting. Phenyltoloxamine Citrate—urticaria, drowsiness, disturbed coordination, inability to concentrate, dizziness, insomnia, tremors, nervousness, palpitation, convulsions, muscular weakness, gastric distress, diarrhea, intestinal cramps, blurred vision, hypotension, urinary retention, dryness of mouth, throat and nose.

Dosage and Administration:
Adults: One tablet twice daily (every 12 hours).
Children (6-12 years of age): One-half tablet twice daily (every 12 hours).
Tablets should not be chewed.

How Supplied: Sinubid (P-D 177) is an ellipsoid, bi-layered (light pink/pink), scored tablet, supplied in bottles of 100 (N 0071-0177-24).

Store between 15°-30°C (59°-86°F).

0177G020

Shown in Product Identification Section, page 425

SPIRONOLACTONE
[spī-rō" nō-lăc' tōne]
Tablets, USP

Warning
Spironolactone has been shown to be a tumorigen in chronic toxicity studies in rats. This drug should be used only in those conditions described under INDICATIONS. Unnecessary use of this drug should be avoided.

Description: Spironolactone is a potassium-sparing, diuretic-antihypertensive agent, available in 25 mg strength tablets for oral administration.

Spironolactone is a synthetic steroidal aldosterone antagonist, occurring as a light cream-colored to light tan, crystalline powder which is practically insoluble in water and soluble in alcohol. Its chemical name is 17-hydroxy-7α-mercapto-3-oxo-17α-pregn-4-ene-21-carboxylic acid γ-lactone acetate; its empirical formula is $C_{24}H_{32}O_4S$.

Clinical Pharmacology: Spironolactone specifically inhibits the physiologic effects of the adrenocortical hormone aldosterone through competitive binding of receptors at the aldosterone-dependent sodium potassium exchange site in the distal convoluted renal tubule, thereby producing increased excretion of sodium, chloride, and water while potassium is retained.

Spironolactone is rapidly and extensively metabolized, primarily to the pharmacologically active derivative canrenone. Peak plasma levels of canrenone occur two to four hours after administration of a single oral dose of spironolactone. After multiple doses, the half-life of canrenone is between 13 and 24 hours. Both spironolactone and canrenone are more than 90% bound to plasma proteins. Spironolactone metabolites are excreted primarily in urine, but also in bile. After withdrawal of spironolactone, diuresis persists for two to three days.

Spironolactone has diuretic activity only in the presence of aldosterone, with the most pronounced effect in patients with aldosteronism. Through its action in antagonizing the effect of aldosterone, it inhibits the exchange of sodium for potassium in the distal renal tubule and helps to prevent potassium loss.

Spironolactone is also effective in significantly lowering the systolic and diastolic blood pressure in many patients with essential hypertension, even when aldosterone secretion is within normal limits.

Indications and Usage: Spironolactone is indicated in the management of:
1. Primary hyperaldosteronism for:
   a. Establishing the diagnosis of primary hyperaldosteronism by therapeutic trial.
   b. Short-term preoperative treatment for patients with primary hyperaldosteronism.
   c. Long-term maintenance therapy for patients with discrete aldosterone-producing adrenal adenomas who are judged to be poor operative risks, or who decline surgery.
   d. Long-term maintenance therapy for patients with bilateral micro- or macro-nodular adrenal hyperplasia (idiopathic hyperaldosteronism).
2. **Edematous conditions** for patients with:
   a. **Congestive heart failure:** For the management of edema and sodium retention when the patient is only partially responsive to, or is intolerant of, other therapeutic measures.

Spironolactone is also indicated for patients with congestive heart failure taking digitalis, when other therapies are considered inappropriate.

b. **Cirrhosis of the liver accompanied by edema and/or ascites:** Aldosterone levels may be exceptionally high in this condition. Spironolactone is indicated for maintenance therapy together with bed rest and restriction of fluid and sodium.

c. **The nephrotic syndrome:** For nephrotic patients when treatment of the underlying disease, restriction of fluid and sodium intake, and the use of other diuretics do not provide an adequate response.

3. **Essential hypertension:** Usually in combination with other drugs, spironolactone is indicated for patients who cannot be treated adequately with other agents or for whom other agents are considered inappropriate.

4. **Hypokalemia:** For the treatment of patients with hypokalemia when other measures are considered inappropriate or inadequate. Spironolactone is also indicated for the prophylaxis of hypokalemia in patients taking digitalis when other measures are considered inadequate or inappropriate.

Usage in Pregnancy: The routine use of diuretics in an otherwise healthy woman is inappropriate and exposes mother and fetus to unnecessary hazard. Diuretics do not prevent development of toxemia of pregnancy, and there is no satisfactory evidence that they are useful in the treatment of developed toxemia.

Edema during pregnancy may arise from pathological causes or from the physiological and mechanical consequences of pregnancy. Spironolactone is indicated in pregnancy when edema is due to pathological causes just as it is in the absence of pregnancy (however, see PRECAUTIONS below). Dependent edema in pregnancy, resulting from restriction of venous return by the expanded uterus, is properly treated through elevation of the lower extremities and use of support hose; use of diuretics to lower intravascular volume in this case is unsupported and unnecessary. There is hypervolemia during normal pregnancy which is harmful to neither the fetus nor the mother (in the absence of cardiovascular disease), but which is associated with edema, including generalized edema, in the majority of pregnant women. If this edema produces discomfort, increased recumbency will often provide relief. In rare instances, this edema may cause extreme discomfort that is not relieved by rest. In these cases, a short course of diuretics may provide relief and may be appropriate.

Contraindications: Anuria, acute renal insufficiency, significant impairment of renal function, hyperkalemia.

Warnings: Excessive potassium intake may cause hyperkalemia in patients receiving spironolactone (see PRECAUTIONS). Potassium supplementation, either in the form of medication or as a diet rich in potassium, should not ordinarily be given in association with spironolactone.

Spironolactone should not be administered concurrently with other potassium-sparing diuretics.

Spironolactone has been shown to be a tumorigen in chronic toxicity studies performed in rats, with its proliferative effects being manifested on endocrine organs and the liver.

Precautions

General: Periodic determinations of serum electrolytes should be performed at appropriate intervals for the purpose of detecting possible fluid and electrolyte imbalance. Serum and urine electrolyte determinations are particularly important

Continued on next page

This product information was prepared in August, 1984. On these and other Parke-Davis Products, information may be obtained by addressing PARKE-DAVIS, Division of Warner-Lambert Company, Morris Plains, New Jersey 07950.

Parke-Davis—Cont.

when a patient is vomiting excessively or receiving parenteral fluids.

Hyperkalemia may occur in patients with impaired renal function or excessive potassium intake and can cause cardiac irregularities that may be fatal. Consequently, no potassium supplement should ordinarily be given with spironolactone. Hyperkalemia can be treated promptly by the rapid intravenous administration of glucose (20% to 50%) and regular insulin, using 0.25 to 0.5 units of insulin per gram of glucose. This is a temporary measure to be repeated as required. Spironolactone should be discontinued and potassium intake (including dietary potassium) restricted.

Reversible hyperchloremic metabolic acidosis, usually in association with hyperkalemia,, has been reported to occur in some patients with decompensated hepatic cirrhosis, even in the presence of normal renal function.

Spironolactone may cause a transient elevation of BUN. This appears to represent a concentration phenomenon rather than renal toxicity since the BUN returns to normal after the drug is discontinued. Progressive elevation of BUN is suggestive of the presence of preexisting renal impairment. Spironolactone may cause mild acidosis.

Hyponatremia, manifested by dryness of the mouth, thirst, lethargy and drowsiness and confirmed by a low serum level, may be induced or aggravated, especially when spironolactone is administered in combination with other diuretics.

Gynecomastia may develop in association with the use of spironolactone, and physicians should be alert to its possible onset. The development of gynecomastia appears to be related to both dosage levels and duration of therapy and is normally reversible when spironolactone therapy is discontinued. In rare instances some breast enlargement may persist.

Drug Interactions: Excessive potassium intake or concurrent administration of other potassium-sparing diuretics may cause hyperkalemia in patients receiving spironolactone.

Spironolactone reduces vascular responsiveness to norepinephrine. Therefore, caution should be used in the management of patients subjected to regional or general anesthesia while they are being treated with spironolactone.

When used in combination with other diuretics or antihypertensive agents, spironolactone potentiates their effects. Therefore, the dosage of such drugs, particularly the ganglionic blocking agents, should be reduced by at least fifty percent when spironolactone is added to the regimen.

Usage in Pregnancy: Spironolactone or its metabolites may cross the placental barrier. Therefore, the use of this drug in pregnant women requires that the anticipated benefit be weighed against possible hazards to the fetus. These hazards include fetal or neonatal jaundice, thrombocytopenia, and other possible adverse reactions that have been reported in the adult. Also see INDICATIONS AND USAGE above.

Nursing Mothers: Canrenone, a metabolite of spironolactone, appears in breast milk. If use of spironolactone is deemed essential, an alternative method of infant feeding should be instituted.

Adverse Reactions: Adverse reactions are usually reversible upon discontinuation of spironolactone.

A. **Gastrointestinal System**
  1. cramping
  2. diarrhea
B. **Central Nervous System**
  1. drowsiness
  2. lethargy
  3. headache
  4. mental confusion
  5. ataxia
C. **Endocrine System**
  1. gynecomastia
  2. inability to achieve or maintain erection
  3. irregular menses or amenorrhea
  4. postmenopausal bleeding
  5. hirsutism
  6. deepening of the voice
  7. hypochloremic acidosis in cirrhosis
D. **Other**
  1. maculopapular or erythematous cutaneous eruptions
  2. urticaria
  3. drug fever
  4. carcinoma of the breast has been reported in patients taking spironolactone, but a cause-and-effect relationship has not been established.

Dosage and Administration: Spironolactone is administered orally. Therapy should be individualized according to the patient's requirements and response. The response of the patient depends on factors such as the nature and degree of the disease, state of hydration, cardiac output, physical activity, diet, and concurrent administration of other drugs.

Primary hyperaldosteronism. Spironolactone may be employed as an initial diagnostic measure to provide presumptive evidence of primary hyperaldosteronism while patients are on normal diets.

Long test: Administer a daily dosage of 400 mg for three to four weeks. Correction of hypokalemia and hypertension provides presumptive evidence for the diagnosis of primary hyperaldosteronism.

Short test: Administer a daily dosage of 400 mg for four days. If serum potassium increases during spironolactone administration but drops when spironolactone is discontinued, a presumptive diagnosis of primary hyperaldosteronism should be considered.

After establishing the diagnosis of hyperaldosteronism by more definitive testing procedures, administer spironolactone in doses of 100 to 400 mg daily in preparation for surgery. For patients who are considered unsuitable for surgery, spironolactone may be employed for long-term maintenance therapy at the lowest effective dosage determined for the individual patient.

Edema in adults (congestive heart failure, hepatic cirrhosis or nephrotic syndrome). An initial daily dosage of 100 mg spironolactone administered in either single or divided doses is recommended, but may range from one to eight tablets (25 to 200 mg) daily. When given as the sole agent for diuresis, spironolactone should be continued for at least five days at the initial dosage level, after which it may be adjusted to the optimal therapeutic or maintenance level administered in either single or divided daily doses. If after five days an adequate diuretic response to spironolactone has not occurred, a second diuretic that acts more proximally in the renal tubule may be added to the regimen. Because of the additive effect of spironolactone when administered concurrently with such diuretics, an enhanced diuresis usually begins on the first day of combined treatment; combined therapy is indicated when more rapid diuresis is desired. The dosage of spironolactone should remain unchanged when other diuretic therapy is added.

Edema in children: The initial daily dosage should provide approximately 1.5 mg of spironolactone per pound of body weight (3.3 mg/kg) administered in either single or divided doses. For small children, spironolactone tablets may be pulverized and administered as a suspension in Cherry Syrup, NF. When refrigerated, such a suspension is stable for one month.

Essential hypertension: For adults, an initial daily dosage of 50 to 100 mg of spironolactone administered in either single or divided doses is recommended. Spironolactone may also be given with diuretics that act more proximally in the renal tubule or with other antihypertensive agents. Treatment with spironolactone should be continued for at least two weeks, since the maximum response may not occur before this time. Subsequently, dosage should be adjusted according to the response of the patient.

Hypokalemia: Spironolactone in a dosage ranging from 25 to 100 mg daily is useful in treating a diuretic-induced hypokalemia, when oral potassium supplements or other potassium-sparing regimens are considered inappropriate.

How Supplied: Spironolactone Tablets, USP, 25 mg (round, white, scored tablets coded P-D 713) are supplied as follows:
N 0071-0713-24 Bottles of 100
N 0071-0713-32 Bottles of 1000
N 0071-0713-40 Unit-dose packages of 100 individually sealed tablets
Store at room temperature below 30°C (86°F).
Protect from moisture and light.

0713G010

SPIRONOLACTONE WITH HYDROCHLOROTHIAZIDE ℞
[spī-rō" nō-lăc' tōne with hy" drō-chlō" rō-thī' ă-zīde]
Tablets

> **Warning**
> Spironolactone has been shown to be a tumorigen in chronic toxicity studies in rats (see WARNINGS). Spironolactone with Hydrochlorothiazide Tablets should be used only in those conditions described under INDICATIONS. Unnecessary use of this drug should be avoided.
> Fixed-dose combination drugs are not indicated for initial therapy of edema or hypertension. Edema or hypertension requires therapy titrated to the individual patient. If the fixed combination represents the dosage so determined, its use may be more convenient in patient management. The treatment of hypertension and edema is not static, but must be reevaluated as conditions in each patient warrant.

Description: Spironolactone with Hydrochlorothiazide is a combination of two diuretic agents with different but complementary mechanisms and sites of action, thereby providing additive diuretic and antihypertensive effects. In addition, spironolactone helps to decrease the potassium excretion characteristically induced by hydrochlorothiazide.

Spironolactone with Hydrochlorothiazide is available as tablets for oral administration, with each tablet containing:
Spironolactone ....25 mg
Hydrochlorothiazide ....25 mg
Spironolactone is a synthetic steroid aldosterone antagonist, occurring as a light cream-colored to light tan, crystalline powder that is practically insoluble in water and soluble in alcohol. Its chemical name is 17-hydroxy-7α-mercapto-3-oxo-17α-pregn-4-ene-21-carboxylic acid γ-lactone acetate; its empirical formula is $C_{24}H_{32}O_4S$.

Hydrochlorothiazide is a member of the benzothiadiazine (thiazide) family of drugs, closely related to chlorothiazide. It occurs as a white, or practically white, crystalline compound that is slightly soluble in water and soluble in alcohol. Its chemical name is 6-chloro-3,4-dihydro-2H-1,2,4-benzothiadiazine-7-sulfonamide 1,1-dioxide; its empirical formula is $C_7H_8ClN_3O_4S_2$.

Clinical Pharmacology: Spironolactone inhibits the physiologic effects of the adrenocortical hormone aldosterone through competitive binding of receptors at the aldosterone-dependent sodium-potassium exchange site in the distal convoluted renal tubule, thereby producing increased excretion of sodium, chloride, and water while potassium is retained. Spironolactone has diuretic activity only in the presence of aldosterone, with the most pronounced effect in patients with aldosteronism.

Spironolactone is rapidly and extensively metabolized, primarily to the pharmacologically active derivative canrenone. Peak plasma levels of canrenone occur two to four hours after administration of a single oral dose of spironolactone. After multiple doses, the half-life of canrenone is between 13 and 24 hours. Both spironolactone and canrenone are more than 90% bound to plasma proteins. Spironolactone metabolites are excreted primarily in urine, but also in bile. After withdrawal of spironolactone, diuresis persists for two to three days.

The diuretic and saluretic effects of hydrochlorothiazide result from a drug-induced inhibition of the renal tubular reabsorption of electrolytes. The excretion is enhanced to a variable degree.

Hydrochlorothiazide is readily absorbed from the gastrointestinal tract. There is significant natriuresis and diuresis within two hours after administration of a single oral dose. These effects reach a peak in about six hours and persist for about twelve hours. Hydrochlorothiazide is excreted unchanged by the kidneys, and excretion is essentially complete within 24 hours.

Spironolactone with Hydrochlorothiazide is effective in significantly lowering the systolic and diastolic blood pressure in many patients with essential hypertension, even when aldosterone secretion is within normal limits.

Both spironolactone and hydrochlorothiazide reduce exchangeable sodium, plasma volume, body weight, and blood pressure. The diuretic and antihypertensive effects of the individual components are potentiated when spironolactone and hydrochlorothiazide are given concurrently.

Indications and Usage: Spironolactone has been shown to be a tumorigen in chronic toxicity studies in rats. Spironolactone with Hydrochlorothiazide Tablets should be used only in those conditions described below. Unnecessary use of this drug should be avoided.

Edematous conditions associated with:

Congestive heart failure: Management of edema and sodium retention when the patient is only partially responsive to or is intolerant of other therapeutic measures. Treatment of diuretic-induced hypokalemia in patients with congestive heart failure when other measures are considered inappropriate. For patients with congestive heart failure who are taking digitalis, when other therapies are considered inadequate or inappropriate.

Cirrhosis of the liver accompanied by edema and /or ascites:

Maintenance therapy together with bed rest and restriction of fluid and sodium. Aldosterone levels may be exceptionally high in this condition.

The nephrotic syndrome: For nephrotic patients when treatment of the underlying disease, restriction of fluid and sodium intake, and the use of other diuretics do not provide an adequate response.

Essential hypertension

For patients with essential hypertension in whom other measures are considered inadequate or inappropriate.

For hypertensive patients for the treatment of a diuretic-induced hypokalemia when other measures are considered inappropriate.

Usage in Pregnancy: The routine use of diuretics in an otherwise healthy pregnant woman is inappropriate and exposes mother and fetus to unnecessary hazard. Diuretics do not prevent development of toxemia of pregnancy, and there is no satisfactory evidence that they are useful in the treatment of developed toxemia.

Edema during pregnancy may arise from pathological causes or from physiological and mechanical consequences of pregnancy. This drug is indicated in pregnancy when edema is due to pathological causes, just as it is in the absence of pregnancy (however, see PRECAUTIONS below). Dependent edema in pregnancy, resulting from restriction of venous return by the expanded uterus, is properly treated through elevation of the lower extremities and use of support hose; use of diuretics to lower intravascular volume in this case is illogical and unnecessary. There is hypervolemia during normal pregnancy which is harmful to neither the fetus nor the mother (in the absence of cardiovascular disease), but which is associated with edema, including generalized edema, in the majority of pregnant women. If this edema produces discomfort, increased recumbency will often provide relief. In rare instances, this edema may cause extreme discomfort that is not relieved by rest. In these cases, a short course of diuretics may provide relief and may be appropriate.

Contraindications: Anuria, acute renal insufficiency, significant impairment of renal function, hyperkalemia, allergy to thiazide diuretics or to other sulfonamide-derived drugs. This drug may also be contraindicated in acute or severe hepatic failure.

Warnings: Excessive potassium intake may cause hyperkalemia in patients receiving Spironolactone with Hydrochlorothiazide Tablets (see PRECAUTIONS). Potassium supplementation, either in the form of medication or as a diet rich in potassium, should not ordinarily be given in association with this drug. Spironolactone with Hydrochlorothiazide should not be administered concurrently with other potassium-sparing diuretics.

The possibility of exacerbation or activation of systemic lupus erythematosus has been reported with sulfonamide derivatives, including thiazides. Spironolactone has been shown to be a tumorigen in chronic toxicity studies performed in rats, with its proliferative effects manifested on endocrine organs and the liver.

Precautions

General: Periodic determinations of serum electrolytes should be performed at appropriate intervals for the purpose of detecting possible fluid and electrolyte imbalance. Patients receiving Spironolactone with Hydrochlorothiazide Tablets should be observed for clinical signs of fluid or electrolyte imbalance, namely hyponatremia, hypochloremic alkalosis, hypokalemia and hyperkalemia. Serum and urine electrolyte determinations are particularly important when a patient is vomiting excessively or receiving parenteral fluids. Warning signs of fluid and electrolyte imbalance include dryness of mouth, thirst, weakness, lethargy, drowsiness, restlessness, muscle pains or cramps, muscular fatigue, hypotension, oliguria, tachycardia, and gastrointestinal disturbances such as nausea and vomiting.

Hyperkalemia may occur in patients with impaired renal function or excessive potassium intake and can cause cardiac irregularities that may be fatal. Consequently, no potassium supplement should ordinarily be given with this drug. Hyperkalemia can be treated promptly by the rapid intravenous administration of glucose (20% to 50%) and regular insulin, using 0.25 to 0.5 units of insulin per gram of glucose. This is a temporary measure to be repeated as required. Spironolactone with Hydrochlorothiazide should be discontinued and potassium intake (including dietary potassium) restricted.

Reversible hyperchloremic metabolic acidosis, usually in association with hyperkalemia, has been reported to occur in some patients with decompensated hepatic cirrhosis, even in the presence of normal renal function.

Spironolactone with Hydrochlorothiazide may cause a transient elevation of BUN. This appears to represent a concentration phenomenon rather than renal toxicity since the BUN returns to normal after the drug is discontinued. Progressive elevation of BUN is suggestive of the presence of preexisting renal impairment.

Dilutional hyponatremia, manifested by dryness of the mouth, thirst, lethargy and drowsiness and confirmed by a low serum sodium level, may be induced, especially when Spironolactone with Hydrochlorothiazide is administered in combination with other diuretics. A true low-salt syndrome may rarely develop with Spironolactone with Hydrochlorothiazide therapy and may be manifested by increasing mental confusion similar to that observed with hepatic coma. This syndrome is differentiated from dilutional hyponatremia in that it does not occur with obvious fluid retention. Its treatment requires that diuretic therapy be discontinued and sodium administered.

Gynecomastia may develop in association with the use of spironolactone, and physicians should be alert to its possible onset. The development of gynecomastia appears to be related to both dosage level and duration of therapy and is normally reversible when Spironolactone with Hydrochlorothiazide is discontinued. In rare instances some breast enlargement may persist.

Thiazides have been shown to alter the metabolism of uric acid and carbohydrates, with possible development of hyperuricemia, gout, and decreased glucose tolerance. Thiazides may temporarily exaggerate abnormalities of glucose metabolism in diabetic patients or cause latent diabetes mellitus to become manifest.

The antihypertensive effects of hydrochlorothiazide may be enhanced in patients who have undergone sympathectomy.

Pathologic changes in the parathyroid gland with hypercalcemia and hypophosphatemia have been observed in patients on prolonged thiazide therapy. Thiazides may decrease serum PBI levels without evidence of thyroid disturbance.

Drug Interactions: Excessive potassium intake or concurrent administration of other potassium-sparing diuretics may cause hyperkalemia in patients receiving Spironolactone with Hydrochlorothiazide Tablets.

Hypokalemia may develop as a result of brisk diuresis, particularly when loop diuretics, glucocorticoids, or ACTH are given concomitantly with Spironolactone with Hydrochlorothiazide. Hypokalemia may exaggerate the effects of digitalis therapy. Potassium depletion may induce signs of digitalis intoxication at previously tolerated levels.

Both spironolactone and hydrochlorothiazide reduce vascular responsiveness to norepinephrine. Therefore, caution should be used in the management of patients subjected to regional or general anesthesia while they are being treated with Spironolactone with Hydrochlorothiazide.

Thiazides may increase the responsiveness to tubocurarine.

Usage in Pregnancy: Spironolactone or its metabolites may, and hydrochlorothiazide does, cross the placental barrier. Therefore, the use of this combination drug in pregnant women requires that the anticipated benefit be weighed against possible hazards to the fetus. These hazards include fetal or neonatal jaundice, thrombocytopenia and other possible adverse reactions that have been reported in the adult. Also see INDICATIONS AND USAGE above.

Nursing Mothers: Canrenone, a metabolite of spironolactone, and hydrochlorothiazide appear in breast milk. If use of Spironolactone with Hydrochlorothiazide is deemed essential, an alternative method of infant feeding should be instituted.

Adverse Reactions: Adverse reactions are usually reversible upon discontinuation of Spironolactone with Hydrochlorothiazide.

The following adverse reactions have been reported in association with the use of spironolactone:

A. Gastrointestinal System
1. cramping
2. diarrhea

B. Central Nervous System
1. drowsiness
2. lethargy
3. headache
4. mental confusion
5. ataxia

C. Endocrine System
1. gynecomastia
2. inability to achieve or maintain erection
3. irregular menses or amenorrhea
4. postmenopausal bleeding
5. hirsutism
6. deepening of the voice
7. hypochloremic acidosis in cirrhosis

D. Other
1. maculopapular or erythematous cutaneous eruptions

Continued on next page

This product information was prepared in August, 1984. On these and other Parke-Davis Products, information may be obtained by addressing PARKE-DAVIS, Division of Warner-Lambert Company, Morris Plains, New Jersey 07950.

Parke-Davis—Cont.

2. urticaria
3. drug fever
4. Carcinoma of the breast has been reported in patients taking spironolactone, but a cause-and-effect relationship has not been established.

The following adverse reactions have been reported in association with the use of hydrochlorothiazide:

A. Gastrointestinal System
1. anorexia
2. gastric irritation
3. nausea
4. vomiting
5. cramping
6. diarrhea
7. constipation
8. jaundice (intrahepatic cholestatic jaundice)
9. pancreatitis

B. Central Nervous System
1. dizziness
2. vertigo
3. paresthesias
4. headache
5. xanthopsia

C. Hematologic
1. leukopenia
2. agranulocytosis
3. thrombocytopenia
4. aplastic anemia

D. Dermatologic-Hypersensitivity
1. purpura
2. photosensitivity
3. rash
4. urticaria
5. necrotizing angiitis (vasculitis, cutaneous vasculitis)

E. Cardiovascular
Orthostatic hypotension may occur and may be aggravated by alcohol, barbiturates, or narcotics.

F. Other
1. hyperglycemia
2. glycosuria
3. hyperuricemia
4. muscle spasm
5. weakness
6. restlessness
7. hypercalcemia
8. severe fluid and electrolyte derangements (rare)

Dosage and Administration: Spironolactone with Hydrochlorothiazide is administered orally. Therapy should be individualized according to the patient's requirements and response. The response of the patient depends on factors such as the nature and degree of the disease, state of hydration, cardiac output, physical activity, diet, and concurrent administration of other drugs. Optimal dosage should be established by individual titration of the components (see Box Warning).
Edema in adults (congestive heart failure, hepatic cirrhosis or nephrotic syndrome). The usual maintenance dose is four tablets daily, administered in either single or divided doses, but it may range from one to eight tablets daily, depending on the response to the initial titration. In some instances it may be desirable to administer, in addition to Spironolactone with Hydrochlorothiazide Tablets, separate tablets of either spironolactone or hydrochlorothiazide in order to provide optimal individual therapy.
The onset of diuresis occurs promptly and, due to prolonged effect of the spironolactone component, persists for two to three days after discontinuance of the drug.
Edema in children. The usual daily maintenance dose should be that which provides 0.75 to 1.5 mg of spironolactone per pound of body weight (1.65 to 3.3 mg/kg), administered in either single or divided doses.
Essential hypertension. Although the dosage will vary depending on the results of titration of the individual ingredients, many patients will be found to have an optimal response to the amount of hydrochlorothiazide and spironolactone contained in two to four tablets of Spironolactone with Hydrochlorothiazide Tablets per day, administered in single or divided doses.
Concurrent potassium supplementation is not recommended when this drug is used in the long-term management of hypertension or in the treatment of most edematous conditions, since the spironolactone content is usually sufficient to minimize loss induced by the hydrochlorothiazide component.
How Supplied: Spironolactone with Hydrochlorothiazide Tablets (round, white, scored tablets coded P-D 712) are supplied as follows::
N 0071-0712-24 Bottles of 100
N 0071-0712-32 Bottles of 1000
N 0071-0712-40 Unit-dose packages of 100 individually sealed tablets
Store at room temperature below 30°C (86°F).
Protect from moisture and light.

0712G010

SURITAL®
[sū'rĭ-tăl"]
(thiamylal sodium for injection, USP)

Description: Surital (thiamylal sodium for injection, USP) is sodium-5-allyl-5-(1-methylbutyl)-2-thiobarbiturate.
Actions: Thiamylal sodium is a rapid, ultra-short-acting barbiturate, intravenous, anesthetic agent.
Indications: Surital is indicated for induction of anesthesia, for supplementing other anesthetic agents, as intravenous anesthesia for short surgical procedures with minimal painful stimuli, or as an agent for inducing a hypnotic state.
Contraindications: Thiamylal sodium is contraindicated when general anesthesia is contraindicated, in patients with latent or manifest porphyria, or in patients with a known hypersensitivity to barbiturates.
Warnings: RESUSCITATIVE EQUIPMENT AND DRUGS SHOULD BE IMMEDIATELY AVAILABLE. This drug should be administered by persons qualified in the use of intravenous anesthetics.
Repeated and continuous infusion may cause cumulative effects resulting in prolonged somnolence, and respiratory and circulatory depression.
Usage in pregnancy: Safe use of thiamylal sodium has not been established with respect to adverse effects upon fetal development. Therefore, thiamylal sodium should not be used in women of childbearing potential, and particularly during early pregnancy, unless, in the judgment of the physician, the expected benefits outweigh the potential hazards.
Precautions: Respiratory depression, apnea, or hypotension may occur due to variations in tolerance from individual to individual or to physical status of patient. Caution should be exercised in debilitated patients, or those with impaired function of respiratory, circulatory, renal, hepatic, and endocrine systems.
Thiamylal sodium should be used with extreme caution in patients in status asthmaticus.
Extravascular injection may cause pain, swelling, ulceration, and necrosis. Intra-arterial injection is dangerous and may produce gangrene of an extremity.
Adverse Reactions: The following adverse reactions have been reported: circulatory depression, thrombophlebitis, pain at injection site, and respiratory depression, including apnea, laryngospasm, bronchospasm, salivation, hiccups, emergence delirium, headache, injury to nerves adjacent to injection site, skin rashes, urticaria, nausea, and emesis.
Dosage and Administration: The dosage is individualized according to the patient's response.
A 2.5% solution is recommended for induction of anesthesia as well as for maintenance by intermittent intravenous injection. A dilute solution (0.3%) may be used by continuous drip for maintenance. The rate of injection during induction should be approximately 1 ml of 2.5% solution every five seconds; an initial injection of 3 to 6 ml of 2.5% solution is generally sufficient to produce short periods of surgical anesthesia.
Sterile Water for Injection is the preferred solvent for preparing Surital (thiamylal sodium for injection, USP) solutions. Initially, Surital solutions are clear, but they may become cloudy on aging. Thiamylal sodium cannot be reconstituted with Ringer's Solution or solutions containing bacteriostatic or buffer agents, because they may tend to cause precipitation. In preparing dilute solutions for continuous drip maintenance, either 5% dextrose or isotonic sodium chloride should be used instead of sterile water for injection to avoid extreme hypotonicity. Dextrose solutions are occasionally sufficiently acid, however, to cause precipitation. Injection of air into the solution should be avoided because this may hasten the development of cloudiness.
Solutions of atropine sulfate, d-tubocurarine, or succinylcholine may be given concurrently with Surital, but they should not be mixed prior to administration.
Thiamylal sodium solutions should be prepared under aseptic conditions. Solutions cannot be heated for sterilization. The solutions should be stored in a refrigerator and used within six days. If kept at room temperature, the solution should be used within 24 hours. Only clear solutions should be used; discard if cloudiness or precipitate form. Refrigeration of the reconstituted Surital contributes to the maintenance of a clear solution.
[See table below].

How Supplied: Surital is supplied as follows:
N 0071-4064-03 (35-64-25)
1 g, in packages of 25 (Steri-Vial® 64)
N 0071-4122-08 (35-122-10)
5 g, in packages of 10 (Steri-Vial 122)
N 0071-4123-10 (35-123-10)
10 g, in packages of 10 (Steri-Vial 123)
AHFS 28:24   4064G020

TABRON® FILMSEAL®
[tăb'rŏn"]

Each tablet represents:
Ferrous fumarate .... 304.2 mg
(represents 100 mg of elemental iron)
Vitamin C (ascorbic acid) .... 500 mg
Vitamin B₁ (thiamine
 mononitrate) .... 6 mg
Vitamin B₂ (riboflavin) .... 6 mg
Vitamin B₆ (pyridoxine
 hydrochloride) .... 5 mg
Vitamin B₁₂ (cyanocobalamin),
 crystalline .... 25 mcg
Folic acid .... 1 mg
Nicotinamide (niacinamide) .... 30 mg
Calcium pantothenate .... 10 mg
Vitamin E (dl-alpha
 tocopheryl acetate) .... (30 mg) 30 IU
Docusate sodium .... 50 mg
Caution—Folic acid in doses above 0.1 mg daily may obscure pernicious anemia in that hematologic remission can occur while neurological manifestations remain progressive.

PREPARING SURITAL SOLUTIONS

Surital (g)	Amount of solvent required (in ml) for percentage solutions shown								
	0.2%	0.3%	0.4%	2%	2.5%	3%	4%	5%	10%
1	500	333	250	50	40	33.3	25	20	10
5	2,500	1,670	1,250	250	200	167	125	100	50
10	5,000	3,333	2,500	500	400	333	250	200	100

Indications: Tabron is a hematinic for the treatment of iron-deficiency anemia and folate deficiency.
Dosage: Usual adult dose: One tablet per day.
How Supplied: N 0071-0638—Bottles of 100 and unit-dose packages of 100 (ten 10s). Parcode® No. 638
Shown in Product Identification Section, page 425

TEDRAL®   ℞
[tĕd′ral]
TEDRAL® SUSPENSION
TEDRAL ELIXIR
Description:
Tedral Suspension: Each 5 ml teaspoonful of suspension contains 65 mg theophylline (59.1 mg anhydrous), 12 mg ephedrine hydrochloride, and 4 mg phenobarbital.
Tedral Elixir: Each 5 ml teaspoonful contains 32.5 mg theophylline (29.5 mg anhydrous), 6 mg ephedrine hydrochloride, and 2 mg phenobarbital; the alcohol content is 15%.
Actions: Tedral combines theophylline and ephedrine—widely accepted oral bronchodilators, with differing modes of action—with the sedative phenobarbital.
From experimental evidence,[1] it appears that a combination of a sympathomimetic and methylxanthine is more effective than either drug alone in inhibiting the release of bronchoconstricting mediators (histamine and slow-reacting substance of anaphylaxis) produced by antigen-antibody (IgE) interaction on sensitive cells. The β-adrenergic stimulation by the sympathomimetics produces cyclic 3′5′-adenosine monophosphate (cAMP), and the degradation of cAMP by the specific enzyme, phosphodiesterase, is inhibited by methylxanthines. Thus, at present, the principal action of the Tedral formulations in the relief or prevention of bronchoconstriction appears to be involved with the cAMP system.
Phenobarbital is incorporated to counteract possible stimulation by ephedrine and to provide a mild, long-acting sedative for the apprehensive asthmatic patient.
Tedral Suspension and Tedral Elixir are convenient formulations for children and other persons who may have difficulty in swallowing tablets.
Indications: Tedral Suspension and Tedral Elixir are indicated for the symptomatic relief of bronchial asthma, asthmatic bronchitis, and other bronchospastic disorders. They may also be used prophylactically to abort or minimize asthmatic attacks and are of value in managing occasional, seasonal or perennial asthma.
Tedral Suspension and Tedral Elixir are convenient for persons who may have difficulty in swallowing tablets.
These Tedral formulations are adjuncts in the total management of the asthmatic patient. Acute or severe asthmatic attacks may necessitate supplemental therapy with others drugs by inhalation or other parenteral routes.
Contraindications: Sensitivity to any of the ingredients; porphyria.
Warnings: Drowsiness may occur. Phenobarbital may be habit-forming.
Precautions: Use with caution in the presence of cardiovascular disease, severe hypertension, hyperthyroidism, prostatic hypertrophy, or glaucoma.
Adverse Reactions: Mild epigastric distress, palpitation, tremulousness, insomnia, difficulty of micturition, and CNS stimulation have been reported.
Dosage and Administration:
Tedral Suspension
Adults—two to four teaspoonfuls every 4 hours.
Children—one teaspoonful per 60 lb body weight, every 4-6 hours. Should be given to children under 2 years of age only with extreme caution.
SHAKE BOTTLE WELL.
Tedral Elixir
Children—one teaspoonful per 30 lb body weight, every 4-6 hours. Should be given to children under 2 years of age only with extreme caution.
Adults—one to two tablespoonfuls every four hours.
How Supplied:
Tedral Suspension is supplied as a yellow, licorice-flavored suspension in bottles of 8 fl oz (237 ml) (N 0071-2237-20) and in bottles of 16 fl oz (474 ml) (N 0071-2237-23).
Tedral Elixir is supplied as a dark red, cherry-flavored elixir in bottles of 16 fl oz (474 ml) (N 0071-2242-23).
Store between 15°-30°C (59°-86°F).
Reference: 1. Koopman WJ, Orange RP, Austen KF: *J. Immunol* 105:1096, November 1970.

0230G012

TEDRAL®SA   ℞
[tĕd′ral]
Description: Tedral SA: Each tablet contains 180 mg anhydrous theophylline (90 mg in the immediate release layer and 90 mg in the sustained release layer); 48 mg ephedrine hydrochloride (16 mg in the immediate release layer and 32 mg in the sustained release layer); 25 mg phenobarbital in the immediate release layer.
Actions: Tedral SA combines theophylline and ephedrine—widely accepted oral bronchodilators with differing modes of action.
From experimental evidence,[1] it appears that a combination of a sympathomimetic and methylxanthine is more effective than either drug alone in inhibiting the release of bronchoconstricting mediators (histamine and slow-reacting substance of anaphylaxis) produced by antigen-antibody (IgE) interaction on sensitive cells. Th β-adrenergic stimulation by the sympathomimetics produces cyclic 3′5′-adenosine monophosphate (cAMP), and the degradation of cAMP by the specific enzyme, phosphodiesterase, is inhibited by methylxanthines. Thus, at present, the principal action of Tedral SA in the relief or prevention of bronchoconstriction appears to be involved with the cAMP system.
Phenobarbital is incorporated into Tedral SA to counteract possible stimulation by ephedrine and to provide a mild, long-acting sedative for the apprehensive asthmatic patient.
Tedral SA provides sustained as well as immediate bronchodilatation for the asthmatic patient, with the convenience of bid dosage.
Indications: Tedral SA is indicated for the symptomatic relief of bronchial asthma, asthmatic bronchitis, and other bronchospastic disorders. It may also be used prophylactically to abort or minimize asthmatic attacks and is of value in managing occasional, seasonal, or perennial asthma.
Tedral SA (Sustained Action) offers the convenience of bid dosage.
This Tedral formulation is an adjunct in the total management of the asthmatic patient. Acute or severe asthmatic attacks may necessitate supplemental therapy with other drugs by inhalation or other parenteral routes.
Contraindications: Sensitivity to any of the ingredients; porphyria.
Warnings: Drowsiness may occur. Phenobarbital may be habit forming.
Precautions: Use with caution in the presence of cardiovascular disease, severe hypertension, hyperthyroidism, prostatic hypertrophy, or glaucoma.
Adverse Reactions: Mild epigastric distress, palpitation, tremulousness, insomnia, difficulty of micturition, and CNS stimulation have been reported.
Dosage and Administration: Adults—one tablet on arising and one tablet 12 hours later. Tablets should not be chewed.
Children—not established for children under 12.
How Supplied: Tedral SA is supplied as double-layered, uncoated, coral/mottled white tablets in bottles of 100 (N 0710-0231-24). 1000 (N 0710-0231-32) and unit dose (10/10) (N 0710-0231-40).
Store between 15°-30°C (59°-86°F).
Reference: 1. Koopman WJ, Orange RP, Austen KF. *J Immunol* 105:1096, November 1970.

Shown in Product Identification Section, page 425

0231G011

TETRACYCLINE HCl CAPSULES, USP   ℞
[tĕ″ trȧ-cy′clīne]
Cyclopar®/Cyclopar® 500
Description: Tetracycline hydrochloride capsules, USP, contain the broad-spectrum antibiotic, tetracycline hydrochloride. Tetracycline hydrochloride is a yellow, odorless, crystalline powder with the chemical formula $C_{22}H_{24}N_2O_8 \cdot HCl$.
Actions: The tetracyclines are primarily bacteriostatic and are thought to exert their antimicrobial effect by the inhibition of protein synthesis. Tetracyclines are active against a wide range of gram-negative and gram-positive organisms.
The drugs in the tetracycline class have closely similar antimicrobial spectra, and cross-resistance among them is common. Microorganisms may be considered susceptible if the MIC (minimum inhibitory concentration) is not more than 4.0 mcg/ml, and intermediate if the MIC is 4.0 to 12.5 mcg/ml.
Susceptibility plate testing: A tetracycline disc may be used to determine microbial susceptibility to drugs in the tetracycline class. If the Kirby-Bauer method of disc susceptibility testing is used, a 30-mcg tetracycline disc should give a zone of at least 19 mm when tested against a tetracycline-susceptible bacterial strain.
Tetracyclines are readily absorbed and are bound to plasma proteins in varying degrees. They are concentrated by the liver in the bile and excreted in the urine and feces at high concentrations and in a biologically active form.
Indications: Tetracycline is indicated in infections caused by the following microorganisms.
  Rickettsiae (Rocky Mountain spotted fever, typhus fever and the typhus group, Q fever, rickettsialpox, and tick fevers)
  Mycoplasma pneumoniae (PPLO, Eaton agent)
  Agents of psittacosis and ornithosis
  Agents of lymphogranuloma venereum and granuloma inguinale
  The spirochetal agent of relapsing fever (*Borrelia recurrentis*)
  The following gram-negative microorganisms:
  Haemophilus ducreyi (chancroid)
  Pasteurella pestis and *Pasteurella tularensis*
  Bartonella bacilliformis
  Bacteroides species
  Vibrio comma and *Vibrio fetus*
  Brucella species (in conjunction with streptomycin)
Because many strains of the following groups of microorganisms have been shown to be resistant to tetracyclines, culture and susceptibility testing is recommended.
Tetracycline is indicated for treatment of infections caused by the following gram-negative microorganisms when bacteriologic testing indicates appropriate susceptibility to the drug.
  Escherichia coli
  Enterobacter aerogenes (formerly *Aerobacter aerogenes*)
  Shigella species
  Mima species and *Herellea* species
  Haemophilus influenzae (respiratory infections)
  Klebsiella species (respiratory and urinary infections)
Tetracycline is indicated for treatment of infections caused by the following gram-positive microorganisms when bacteriologic testing indicates appropriate susceptibility to the drug.
  Streptococcus species:
    Up to 44 percent of strains of *Streptococcus pyogenes* and 74 percent of *Streptococcus faecalis* have been found to be resistant to tetracycline drugs. Therefore, tetracyclines should not be

Continued on next page

This product information was prepared in August, 1984. On these and other Parke-Davis Products, information may be obtained by addressing PARKE-DAVIS, Division of Warner-Lambert Company, Morris Plains, New Jersey 07950.

Parke-Davis—Cont.

used for streptococcal disease unless the organism has been demonstrated to be sensitive.

For upper respiratory infections due to group A beta-hemolytic streptococci, penicillin is the usual drug of choice, including prophylaxis of rheumatic fever.

Diplococcus pneumoniae
Staphylococcus aureus
 Skin and soft-tissue infections. Tetracyclines are not the drugs of choice in the treatment of any type of staphylococcal infection.

When penicillin is contraindicated, tetracyclines are alternative drugs in the treatment of infections due to:

Neisseria gonorrhoeae,
Treponema pallidum and *Treponema pertenue* (syphilis and yaws),
Listeria monocytogenes,
Clostridium species,
Bacillus anthracis,
Fusobacterium fusiforme (Vincent's infection),
Actinomyces species.

Tetracycline hydrochloride is indicated for the treatment of uncomplicated urethral, endocervical or rectal infections in adults caused by *Chlamydia trachomatis*.[1]

In acute intestinal amebiasis, the tetracyclines may be a useful adjunct to amebicides.

In severe acne, the tetracyclines may be useful adjunctive therapy.

Tetracyclines are indicated in the treatment of trachoma, although the infectious agent is not always eliminated, as judged by immunofluorescence.

Inclusion conjunctivitis may be treated with oral tetracyclines or with a combination of oral and topical agents.

Contraindication: This drug is contraindicated in persons who have shown hypersensitivity to any of the tetracyclines.

Warnings: THE USE OF DRUGS OF THE TETRACYCLINE CLASS DURING TOOTH DEVELOPMENT (LAST HALF OF PREGNANCY, INFANCY, AND CHILDHOOD TO THE AGE OF 8 YEARS) MAY CAUSE PERMANENT DISCOLORATION OF THE TEETH (YELLOW-GRAY-BROWN). This adverse reaction is more common during long-term use of the drugs but has been observed following repeated short-term courses. Enamel hypoplasia has also been reported. TETRACYCLINE DRUGS, THEREFORE, SHOULD NOT BE USED IN THIS AGE GROUP UNLESS OTHER DRUGS ARE NOT LIKELY TO BE EFFECTIVE OR ARE CONTRAINDICATED.

If renal impairment exists, even usual oral or parenteral doses may lead to excessive systemic accumulation of the drug and possible liver toxicity. Under such conditions, lower than usual total doses are indicated and, if therapy is prolonged, serum level determinations of the drug may be advisable.

Photosensitivity manifested by an exaggerated sunburn reaction has been observed in some individuals taking tetracyclines. Patients apt to be exposed to direct sunlight or ultraviolet light should be advised that this reaction can occur with tetracycline drugs, and treatment should be discontinued at the first evidence of skin erythema.

The antianabolic action of the tetracyclines may cause an increase in BUN. While this is not a problem in those with normal renal function, in patients with significantly impaired function, higher serum levels of tetracycline may lead to azotemia, hyperphosphatemia, and acidosis.

Usage in pregnancy. (See above Warnings about use during tooth development).

Results of animal studies indicate that tetracyclines cross the placenta, are found in fetal tissues, and can have toxic effects on the developing fetus (often related to retardation of skeletal development.) Evidence of embryotoxicity has also been noted in animals treated early in pregnancy.

Usage in newborns, infants, and children. (See above Warnings about use during tooth development.)

All tetracyclines form a stable calcium complex in any bone-forming tissue. A decrease in the fibula growth rate has been observed in prematures given oral tetracycline in doses of 25 mg/kg every 6 hours. This reaction was shown to be reversible when the drug was discontinued.

Tetracyclines are present in the milk of lactating women who are taking a drug in this class.

Precautions: As with other antibiotic preparations, use of this drug may result in overgrowth of nonsusceptible organisms, including fungi. If superinfection occurs, the antibiotic should be discontinued and appropriate therapy instituted.

In venereal diseases when coexistent syphilis is suspected, darkfield examination should be done before treatment is started and the blood serology repeated monthly for at least four months.

Because tetracyclines have been shown to depress plasma prothrombin activity, patients who are on anticoagulant therapy may require downward adjustment of their anticoagulant dosage.

In long-term therapy, periodic laboratory evaluation of organ systems, including hematopoietic, renal, and hepatic studies, should be performed.

All infections due to Group A beta-hemolytic streptococci should be treated for at least 10 days. Since bacteriostatic drugs may interfere with the bactericidal action of penicillin, it is advisable to avoid giving tetracycline in conjunction with penicillin.

Adverse Reactions: Gastrointestinal: anorexia, nausea, vomiting, diarrhea, glossitis, dysphagia, enterocolitis, and inflammatory lesions (with monilial overgrowth) in the anogenital region. These reactions have been caused by both the oral and parenteral administration of tetracyclines.

Skin: maculopapular and erythematous rashes. Exfoliative dermatitis has been reported but is uncommon. Photosensitivity is discussed above. (See Warnings.)

Renal toxicity: rise in BUN has been reported and is apparently dose-related. (See Warnings.)

Hypersensitivity reactions: urticaria, angioneurotic edema, anaphylaxis, anaphylactoid purpura, pericarditis, and exacerbation of systemic lupus erythematosus

Bulging fontanels have been reported in young infants following full therapeutic dosage. This sign disappeared rapidly when the drug was discontinued.

Blood: hemolytic anemia, thrombocytopenia, neutropenia, and eosinophilia have been reported.

When given over prolonged periods, tetracyclines have been reported to produce brown-black microscopic discoloration of thyroid glands. No abnormalities of thyroid function studies are known to occur.

Dosage and Administration: Therapy should be continued for at least 24 to 48 hours after symptoms and fever have subsided.

Concomitant therapy: Antacids containing aluminum, calcium, or magnesium impair absorption and should not be given to patients taking oral tetracycline.

Food and some dairy products also interfere with absorption. Oral forms of tetracycline should be given 1 hour before or 2 hours after meals. Pediatric oral dosage forms should not be given with milk formulas and should be given at least 1 hour prior to feeding.

In patients with renal impairment (See Warnings.): Total dosage should be decreased by reduction of recommended individual doses and/or by extending time intervals between doses.

In the treatment of streptococcal infections, a therapeutic dose of tetracycline should be administered for at least 10 days.

Adults: Usual daily dosage, 1 to 2 grams divided in two or four equal doses, depending on the severity of the infection.

For children above eight years of age: Usual daily dosage, 10 to 20 mg (25 to 50 mg/kg) per pound of body weight divided in four equal doses.

For treatment of brucellosis, 500 mg tetracycline four times daily for three weeks should be accompanied by streptomycin, 1 gram, intramuscularly twice daily the first week and once daily the second week.

For treatment of syphilis, a total of 30 to 40 grams in equally divided doses over a period of 10 to 15 days should be given. Close follow-up, including laboratory tests, is recommended.

For the treatment of acute gonococcal urethritis, a single, initial dose of 1.5 grams followed by 0.5 grams every 4 to 6 hours for 4 to 6 days should be given. Female patients may require more prolonged therapy.

Uncomplicated urethral, endocervical, or rectal infection in adults caused by *Chlamydia trachomatis;* 500 mg, by mouth, 4 times a day for at least 7 days.[1]

How Supplied:
Tetracycline hydrochloride capsules, USP (Cyclopar)
N 0071-0407-24 250 mg Bottles of 100.
N 0071-0407-32 250 mg Bottles of 1000.
Each capsule contains 250 mg tetracycline hydrochloride.
Tetracycline hydrochloride capsules, USP (Cyclopar 500)
N 0071-0697-24 500 mg Bottles of 100.
Each capsule contains 500 mg tetracycline hydrochloride.

Reference: 1. CDC Sexually Transmitted Diseases Treatment Guidelines 1982.
AHFS 8:12.24   0407G101
Shown in Product Identification Section, page 425

THERA-COMBEX H-P®
[thĕ″ rā″ cŏm′ bĕx″]
High-Potency Vitamin B Complex with 500 mg Vitamin C

Composition: Each Kapseal contains:
Ascorbic acid (vitamin C) .... 500 mg
Thiamine (vitamin B$_1$)
 mononitrate .... 25 mg
Riboflavin (vitamin B$_2$) .... 15 mg
Pyridoxine hydrochloride
 (vitamin B$_6$) .... 10 mg
Vitamin B$_{12}$ (cyanocobalamin) .... 5 mcg
Niacinamide .... 100 mg
dl-Panthenol .... 20 mg

Uses: For the prevention or treatment of vitamin B complex and vitamin C deficiencies.
Dosage: One or two capsules daily
How Supplied: N 0071-0550-24—Bottles of 100.
Parcode® No. 550
Shown in Product Identification Section, page 425

THROMBOSTAT™ ℞
(Thrombin, USP) Bovine Origin

Thrombostat must not be injected! Apply on the surface of bleeding tissue as a solution or powder.

Description: Thrombostat (Thrombin, USP) is a protein substance produced through a conversion reaction in which prothrombin of bovine origin is activated by tissue thromboplastin in the presence of calcium chloride. It is supplied as a sterile powder that has been freeze-dried in the final container. Also contained in this preparation are calcium chloride, sodium chloride, aminoacetic acid (glycine) and Phemerol® (benzethonium chloride). Glycine is included to make the dried product friable and more readily soluble, and benzethonium chloride as a preservative as follows: 0.4 mg per 1000 unit vial, 0.1 mg per 5000 unit vial, 0.2 mg per 10,000 unit vial, and 0.4 mg per 20,000 unit vial.

A 5 ml, 10 ml, or 20 ml vial of Isotonic Saline is enclosed to be used as a diluent with the 5 ml, 5000 unit; 10 ml, 10,000 unit; or 20 ml, 20,000 unit vial, respectively, of Thrombostat.

Isotonic Saline is a sterile, isotonic solution of sodium chloride in Water For Injection, USP. It contains Phemerol® (benzethonium chloride) 0.02 mg per ml as a preservative. (See Dosage and Administration for additional information on diluents which may be used.)

This product is prepared under rigid assay control. A unit is defined as the amount required to clot 1 ml of standardized fibrinogen solution in 15 sec-

onds. Approximately 2 units are required to clot 1 ml of oxalated human plasma in the same period of time.
Clinical Pharmacology: Thrombostat requires no intermediate physiological agent for its action. It clots the fibrinogen of the blood directly. **Failure to clot blood occurs in the rare case where the primary clotting defect is the absence of fibrinogen itself.** The speed with which thrombin clots blood is dependent upon its concentration. For example, the contents of a 5000 unit vial of Thrombostat dissolved in 5 ml of saline diluent is capable of clotting an equal volume of blood in less than a second, or 1000 ml in less than a minute.
Indications and Usage: Thrombostat (Thrombin, USP) is indicated as an aid in hemostasis wherever oozing blood from capillaries and small venules is accessible.
In various types of surgery solutions of Thrombostat may be used in conjunction with Absorbable Gelatin Sponge, USP for hemostasis.
Contraindication: Thrombostat is contraindicated in persons known to be sensitive to any of its components and/or to material of bovine origin.
Warning: Because of its action in the clotting mechanism, Thrombostat must not be injected or otherwise allowed to enter large blood vessels. Extensive intravascular clotting and even death may result. Thrombostat is an antigenic substance and has caused sensitivity and allergic reactions when injected into animals.
Precautions:
General:
Consult the absorbable gelatin sponge product labeling for complete information for use prior to utilizing the thrombin-saturated sponge procedure.
Pregnancy—
Teratogenic effects: Pregnancy Category C. Animal reproduction studies have not been conducted with Thrombin, Topical (Bovine). It is also not known whether Thrombin, Topical (Bovine) can cause fetal harm when administered to a pregnant woman or can affect reproduction capacity. Thrombin, Topical (Bovine) should be given to a pregnant woman only if clearly indicated.
Pediatric Use:
Safety and effectiveness in children have not been established.
Adverse Reactions: An allergic type reaction following the use of Thrombostat for treatment of epistaxis has been reported. Febrile reactions have also been observed following the use of Thrombostat in certain surgical procedures but no cause-effect relationship has been established.
Dosage and Administration:
General: Solutions of Thrombostat may be prepared in sterile distilled water or isotonic saline. The intended use determines the strength of the solution to prepare. For general use in plastic surgery, dental extractions, skin grafting, neurosurgery, etc., solutions containing approximately 100 units per ml are frequently used. For this, 10 ml of diluent added to the 1000 unit package is suitable. Where bleeding is profuse, as from cut surfaces of liver and spleen, concentrations as high as 1000 to 2000 units per ml may be required. For this the 5000 unit vial dissolved in 5 ml or 2.5 ml respectively of the diluent supplied in the package is convenient. Intermediate strengths to suit the needs of the case may be prepared by selecting the proper strength package and dissolving the contents in an appropriate volume of diluent. In many situations, it may be advantageous to use Thrombostat in dry form on oozing surfaces.
Caution: Solutions should be used the day they are prepared. The solution may be used for up to 6 hours when stored at room temperature, up to 24 hours when stored under refrigeration, and, if necessary, up to 48 hours when stored frozen.
The following techniques are suggested for the topical application of Thrombostat.
1. The recipient surface should be sponged (not wiped) free of blood before Thrombostat is applied.
2. A spray may be used or the surface may be flooded using a sterile syringe and small gauge needle. The most effective hemostasis results when the Thrombostat mixes freely with the blood as soon as it reaches the surface.
3. In instances where Thrombostat in dry form is needed, the vial is opened by removing the metal ring by flipping up the plastic cap and tearing counterclockwise. The rubber-diaphragm cap may be easily removed and the dried Thrombostat is then broken up into a powder by means of a sterile glass rod or other suitable sterile instrument.
4. Sponging of treated surfaces should be avoided in order that the clot remain securely in place.
Thrombostat may be used in conjunction with Absorbable Gelatin Sponge, USP as follows:
1. Prepare Thrombostat solution of the desired strength.
2. Immerse sponge strips of the desired size in the Thrombostat solution. Knead the sponge strips vigorously with moistened gloved fingers to remove trapped air, thereby facilitating saturation of the sponge.
3. Apply saturated sponge to bleeding area. Hold in place for 10 to 15 seconds with a pledget of cotton or a small gauze sponge.
Thrombostat Kit
Thrombostat Kit contains one sterile 20,000 unit vial of Thrombostat, one sterile vial of Isotonic Saline Diluent, and one sterile pump sprayer cap. The Kit may be used as folllows:
1. Remove the Tyvek blister lid by pulling up at the indicated corner. The sterile inner tray can be lifted out or introduced into the operating field.
2. The cover to the sterile inner tray is removed by pulling up on the finger tab, exposing the sterile contents.
3. Thrombostat solution of the desired strength is prepared and the pump sprayer cap inserted and seated on the Thrombostat solution vial. Note: Several strokes of the pump sprayer will be required before the Thrombostat solution is expelled.
4. Alternatively, when Thrombostat in dry form is needed, the vial is opened as described above and the dried Thrombostat broken up into a powder by means of a sterile glass rod or other suitable sterile instrument.
How Supplied: Thrombostat is supplied as:
N 0071-4173-35—Package contains one 5000 unit vial of Thrombostat and one 5 ml vial of Isotonic Saline Diluent with Phemerol, 0.02 mg per ml, as a preservative.
N 0071-4176-35—Package contains one 10,000 unit vial of Thrombostat and one 10 ml vial of Isotonic Saline Diluent with Phemerol, 0.02 mg per ml, as a preservative.
N 0071-4177-01—Package contains one 1000 unit vial of Thrombostat.
N 0071-4180-35—Package contains one 20,000 unit vial of Thrombostat and one 20 ml vial of Isotonic Saline Diluent with Phemerol, 0.02 mg per ml, as a preservative.
N 0071-4180-36—Kit contains one sterile 20,000 unit vial of Thrombostat, one sterile 20 ml vial of Isotonic Saline Diluent with Phemerol, 0.02 mg per ml, as a preservative, and one sterile pump sprayer cap in a sterile tray with a Tyvek lid.
Storage: This product should be stored at 2° to 8°C (36° to 46°F).
AHFS Category 20:12.16   4173G014

TUCKS®
[tŭcks]
Pre-Moistened Hemorrhoidal/Vaginal Pads

Indications: Temporarily relieve external discomfort of simple hemorrhoids.
—Soothe, cool, and comfort itching, burning, and irritation of sensitive rectal and outer vaginal areas.
—As a compress, to help relieve discomfort from rectal/vaginal surgical stitches.
—Effective hygienic wipe to cleanse rectal area of irritation-causing residue.
—Solution buffered to help prevent further irritation.
Directions: For external use only. Use as a wipe following bowel movement, during menstruation, or after napkin or tampon change. Or, as a compress, apply to affected area 10 to 15 minutes as needed. Change compresses every 5 minutes.
Warning: In case of rectal bleeding, consult physician promptly. In case of continued irritation, discontinue use and consult a physician. Keep this and all medication out of the reach of children. In case of accidental ingestion seek professional assistance or contact a Poison Control Center immediately.
Contains: Soft pads pre-moistened with a solution containing 50% Witch Hazel, 10% Glycerin USP, Purified Water USP deionized q.s., Methylparaben USP 0.1% and Benzalkonium Chloride USP 0.003% as preservatives. Buffered to acid pH.
Store between 59° and 86°F.
How Supplied: Jars of 40 and 100. Also available as Tucks Take-Alongs®, individual, foil-wrapped, nonwoven wipes, 12 packets per box
Tucks—N 0071-1703.
Tucks Take-Alongs—N 0071-1704-01

TUCKS® OINTMENT, CREAM
[tŭcks]

Composition: Tucks Ointment and Cream contain a specially formulated aqueous phase of 50% witch hazel (hamamelis water).
Both nonstaining Tucks Ointment and Tucks Cream exert a temporary soothing, cooling, mildly astringent effect on such superficial irritations as simple hemorrhoids, vaginal and rectal area itch, postepisiotomy discomfort and anorectal surgical wounds. Neither the Ointment nor the Cream contains steroids or skin sensitizing "caine" type topical anesthetics.
Warning: If itching or irritation continues, discontinue use and consult physician. In case of rectal bleeding, consult physician promptly. Keep this and all drugs out of the reach of children. In case of accidental ingestion seek professional assistance or contact a poison control center immediately.
Dosage and Administration: Apply locally three or four times daily. Applicator provided for rectal instillation.
How Supplied: Tucks Ointment and Tucks Cream (water-washable) in 1.4-oz tubes with rectal applicators
Tucks Ointment—N 0071-3021-14
Tucks Cream—N 0071-3022-14   7000G071

UITICORT®   ℞
[ū'tĭ-cŏrt"]
(betamethasone benzoate)
Cream, 0.025%
Gel, 0.025%
Lotion, 0.025%
Ointment, 0.025%

For external use only
Caution: Federal law prohibits dispensing without prescription.
Description: Uticort Gel/Cream/Ointment/Lotion contain the active fluorinated corticosteroid compound betamethasone benzoate, the 17-benzoate ester of betamethasone, having the chemical formula of 9-fluoro-11β, 17, 21-trihydroxy-16β-methylpregna-1, 4-diene-3, 20-dione 17-benzoate.
Each gram of 0.025% Gel contains 0.25 mg of betamethasone benzoate in a specially formulated gel base consisting of 13.8% (w/w) alcohol, carboxyvinyl polymer, propylene glycol, disodium edetate, diisopropanolamine and purified water. The gel is self-liquefying, clear, greaseless and non-staining. The active ingredient is completely solubilized and remains in the clear film without crys-

Continued on next page

This product information was prepared in August, 1984. On these and other Parke-Davis Products, information may be obtained by addressing PARKE-DAVIS, Division of Warner-Lambert Company, Morris Plains, New Jersey 07950.

Parke-Davis—Cont.

tallization after evaporation of volatile substances.

Each gram of 0.025% Cream contains 0.25 mg of betamethasone benzoate in a water-washable emollient cream base consisting of cetyl alcohol, glyceryl stearate, light mineral oil, propylene glycol, disodium monooleamidosulfosuccinate, citric acid and purified water.

Each gram of 0.025% Ointment contains 0.25 mg of betamethasone benzoate in an emollient ointment base of light mineral oil, glyceryl stearate, food starch-modified and polyethylene.

In this formulation the active ingredient is micronized to provide uniform distribution and optimal activity.

Each gram of 0.025% Lotion contains 0.25 mg of betamethasone benzoate in a water miscible, oil- and fat-free vehicle consisting of cetyl alcohol, stearyl alcohol, propylene glycol, sodium lauryl sulfate, purified water, and propyl-, butyl-, and methylparabens as preservatives.

Clinical Pharmacology: Topical corticosteroids share antiinflammatory, antipruritic and vasoconstrictive actions.

The mechanism of antiinflammatory activity of the topical corticosteroids is unclear. Various laboratory methods, including vasoconstrictor assays, are used to compare and predict potencies and/or clinical efficacies of the topical corticosteroids. There is some evidence to suggest that a recognizable correlation exists between vasoconstrictor potency and therapeutic efficacy in man.

Pharmacokinetics

The extent of percutaneous absorption of topical corticosteroids is determined by many factors including the vehicle, the integrity of the epidermal barrier, and the use of occlusive dressings.

Topical corticosteroids can be absorbed from normal intact skin. Inflammation and/or other disease processes in the skin increase percutaneous absorption.

Occlusive dressings substantially increase the percutaneous absorption of topical corticosteroids. Thus, occlusive dressings may be a valuable therapeutic adjunct for treatment of resistant dermatoses (See *DOSAGE AND ADMINISTRATION*)

Once absorbed through the skin, topical corticosteroids are handled through pharmacokinetic pathways similar to systemically administered corticosteroids. Corticosteroids are bound to plasma proteins in varying degrees. Corticosteroids are metabolized primarily in the liver and are then excreted by the kidneys. Some of the topical corticosteroids and their metabolites are also excreted into the bile.

Indications and Usage: Topical corticosteroids are indicated for the relief of the inflammatory and pruritic manifestations of corticosteroid-responsive dermatoses.

Contraindications: Topical corticosteroids are contraindicated in those patients with a history of hypersensitivity to any of the components of the preparation.

Precautions:
General
Systemic absorption of topical corticosteroids has produced reversible hypothalamic-pituitary-adrenal (HPA) axis suppression, manifestations of Cushing's syndrome, hyperglycemia and glucosuria in some patients.

Conditions which augment systemic absorption include the application of the more potent steroids, use over large surface areas, prolonged use, and the addition of occlusive dressings.

Therefore, patients receiving a large dose of a potent topical steroid applied to a large surface area or under an occlusive dressing should be evaluated periodically for evidence of HPA axis suppression by using the urinary free cortisol and ACTH stimulation tests. If HPA axis suppression is noted, an attempt should be made to withdraw the drug, to reduce the frequency of application, or to substitute a less potent steroid.

Recovery of HPA axis function is generally prompt and complete upon discontinuation of the drug. Infrequently, signs and symptoms of steroid withdrawal may occur, requiring supplemental systemic corticosteroids.

Children may absorb proportionally larger amounts of topical corticosteroids and thus be more susceptible to systemic toxicity (See *PRECAUTIONS—Pediatric Use*).

If irritation develops, topical corticosteroids should be discontinued and appropriate therapy instituted.

In the presence of dermatological infections, the use of an appropriate antifungal or antibacterial agent should be instituted. If a favorable response does not occur promptly, the corticosteroid should be discontinued until the infection has been adequately controlled.

Information for the Patient

Patients using topical corticosteroids should receive the following information and instructions:
1. This medication is to be used as directed by the physician. It is for external use only. Avoid contact with the eyes.
2. Patients should be advised not to use this medication for any disorder other than for which it was prescribed.
3. The treated skin area should not be bandaged or otherwise covered or wrapped as to be occlusive unless directed by the physician.
4. Patients should report any signs of local adverse reactions especially under occlusive dressing.
5. Parents of pediatric patients should be advised not to use tight-fitting diapers or plastic pants on a child being treated in the diaper area, as these garments may constitute occlusive dressings.

Laboratory Tests

The following tests may be helpful in evaluating the HPA axis suppression:
Urinary free cortisol test
ACTH stimulation test

Carcinogenesis, Mutagenesis, and Impairment of Fertility

Long-term animal studies have not been performed to evaluate the carcinogenic potential or the effect on fertility of topical corticosteroids.

Studies to determine mutagenicity with prednisolone and hydrocortisone have revealed negative results.

Pregnancy Category C

Corticosteroids are generally teratogenic in laboratory animals when administered systemically at relatively low dosage levels. The more potent corticosteroids have been shown to be teratogenic after dermal application in laboratory animals. There are no adequate and well-controlled studies in pregnant women on teratogenic effects from topically applied corticosteroids. Therefore, topical corticosteroids should be used during pregnancy only if the potential benefit justifies the potential risk to the fetus. Drugs of this class should not be used extensively on pregnant patients, in large amounts, or for prolonged periods of time.

Nursing Mothers

It is not known whether topical administration of corticosteroids could result in sufficient systemic absorption to produce detectable quantities in breast milk. Systemically administered corticosteroids are secreted into breast milk in quantities *not* likely to have a deleterious effect on the infant. Nevertheless, caution should be exercised when topical corticosteroids are administered to a nursing woman.

Pediatric Use

Pediatric patients may demonstrate greater susceptibility to topical corticosteroid-induced HPA axis suppression and Cushing's syndrome than mature patients because of a larger skin surface area to body weight ratio.

Hypothalamic-pituitary-adrenal (HPA) axis suppression, Cushing's syndrome, and intracranial hypertension have been reported in children receiving topical corticosteroids. Manifestations of adrenal suppression in children include linear growth retardation, delayed weight gain, low plasma cortisol levels, and absence of response to ACTH stimulation. Manifestations of intracranial hypertension include bulging fontanelles, headaches, and bilateral papilledema.

Administration of topical corticosteroids to children should be limited to the least amount compatible with an effective therapeutic regimen. Chronic corticosteroid therapy may interfere with the growth and development of children.

Uticort (Betamethasone Benzoate) Gel/Cream/Ointment/Lotion are not for ophthalmic use.

Adverse Reactions: The following local adverse reactions are reported infrequently with topical corticosteroids, but may occur more frequently with the use of occlusive dressings. These reactions are listed in an approximate decreasing order of occurrence.

Burning
Itching
Irritation
Dryness
Folliculitis
Hypertrichosis
Acneiform eruptions
Hypopigmentation
Perioral dermatitis
Allergic contact dermatitis
Maceration of the skin
Secondary infection
Skin atrophy
Striae
Miliaria

Overdosage: Topically applied corticosteroids can be absorbed in sufficient amounts to produce systemic effects (See *PRECAUTIONS*).

Dosage and Administration: Topical corticosteroids are generally applied to the affected area as a thin film from two to four times daily depending on the severity of the condition.

Occlusive dressings may be used for the management of psoriasis or recalcitrant conditions.

If an infection develops, the use of occlusive dressings should be discontinued and appropriate antimicrobial therapy instituted.

How Supplied:

Uticort Gel 0.025% is supplied as:
N 0071-3025-11—15 gram tube
N 0071-3025-15—60 gram tube
Each gram of Uticort Gel contains 0.25 mg of betamethasone benzoate

Uticort Cream 0.025% is supplied as:
N 0071-3027-11—15 gram tube
N 0071-3027-15—60 gram tube
Each gram of Uticort Cream contains 0.25 mg of betamethasone benzoate

Uticort Ointment 0.025% is supplied as:
N 0071-3026-11—15 gram tube
N 0071-3026-15—60 gram tube
Each gram of Uticort Ointment contains 0.25 mg of betamethasone benzoate

Uticort Lotion 0.025% is supplied as:
N 0071-3029-11—15 ml plastic bottle
N 0071-3029-15—60 ml plastic bottle
US Patent Nos. 3,529,060 and 3,749,773

Store between 59°-86° F.

3026G010

Shown in Product Identification Section, page 426

VIRA-A®   ℞
[vī″ ră ā′]
(vidarabine concentrate for infusion, USP)

Description: Vira-A is the trade name for vidarabine (also known as adenine arabinoside and Ara-A), an antiviral drug. Vira-A is a purine nucleoside obtained from fermentation cultures of *Streptomyces antibioticus*. Each milliliter of sterile suspension contains 200 milligrams of vidarabine monohydrate equivalent to 187.4 milligrams of vidarabine. Each milliliter contains 0.1 milligrams Phemerol® (benzethonium chloride) as a preservative; sodium phosphate, USP, 1.8 milligrams, and sodium biphosphate, USP, 4.8 milligrams, as buffering agents. Hydrochloric acid may have been added to adjust pH. Vira-A is a white, crystalline solid with this empirical formula: $C_{10}H_{13}N_5O_4 \cdot H_2O$. The molecular weight is 285.2; the solubility is 0.45 mg/ml at 25 C; and the melting point ranges from 260 to 270 C. The chemical

for possible revisions

name is 9-β-D-arabinofuranosyladenine monohydrate.

Clinical Pharmacology: Following intravenous administration, Vira-A is rapidly deaminated into arabinosylhypoxanthine (Ara-Hx), the principal metabolite, which is promptly distributed into the tissues. Peak Ara-Hx and Ara-A plasma levels ranging from 3 to 6 μg/ml and 0.2 to 0.4 μg/ml, respectively, are attained after slow intravenous infusion of Vira-A doses of 10 mg/kg of body weight. These levels reflect the rate of infusion and show no accumulation across time. The mean half-life of Ara-Hx is 3.3 hours. Ara-Hx penetrates into the cerebrospinal fluid (CSF) to give a CSF/plasma ratio of approximately 1:3.

Excretion of Vira-A is principally via the kidneys. Urinary excretion is constant over 24 hours. Forty-one to 53% of the daily dose is recovered in the urine as Ara-Hx with 1 to 3% appearing as the parent compound. There is no evidence of fecal excretion of drug or metabolites. In patients with impaired renal function Ara-Hx may accumulate in the plasma and reach levels several-fold higher than those described above.

Vira-A possesses *in vitro* and *in vivo* antiviral activity against Herpes simplex virus types 1 and 2, and *in vitro* activity against varicella-zoster virus. The antiviral mechanism of action has not yet been established. The drug is converted into nucleotides which appear to be involved with the inhibition of viral replication. In KB cells infected with Herpes simplex virus type 1, Vira-A inhibits viral DNA synthesis. Vira-A is rapidly deaminated to Ara-Hx, the principal metabolite, in cell cultures, laboratory animals, and humans.

Ara-Hx also possesses *in vitro* antiviral activity but this activity is significantly less than the activity of Vira-A.

Indications and Usage: Herpes Simplex Virus Encephalitis—Vira-A is indicated in the treatment of Herpes simplex virus encephalitis. Controlled studies indicated that Vira-A therapy will reduce the mortality caused by Herpes simplex virus encephalitis from 70 to 28% 30 days following onset. In a larger uncontrolled study of 75 patients with biopsy-proven herpes simplex encephalitis, the mortality 6 months from onset was 39%, similar to 44% in the initial controlled study at 6 months. Morbidity from both studies one year after onset was: normal 53%, moderately debilitated 29%, and severely damaged 18%. Vira-A does not appear to alter morbidity and resulting serious neurological sequelae in the comatose patient. Therefore early diagnosis and treatment are essential. Herpes simplex virus encephalitis should be suspected in patients with a history of an acute febrile encephalopathy associated with disordered mentation, altered level of consciousness and focal cerebral signs.

Studies which may support the suspected diagnosis include examination of cerebrospinal fluid and localization of an intra-cerebral lesion by brain scan, electroencephalography or computerized axial tomography (CAT).

Brain biopsy is required in order to confirm the etiological diagnosis by means of viral isolation in cell cultures.

Detection of Herpes simplex virus in the biopsied brain tissue can also be reliably done by specific fluorescent antibody techniques. Detection of Herpes virus-like particles by electron microscopy or detection of intranuclear inclusions by histopathologic techniques only provides a presumptive diagnosis.

Herpes zoster—Vira-A is indicated in the treatment of herpes zoster (shingles) due to reactivated varicella-zoster virus infections in immunosuppressed patients. Placebo-controlled studies have shown that Vira-A significantly reduced the severity of acute pain, new vesicle formation, time to pustulation and scabbing, cutaneous dissemination inside and outside the primary dermatome(s), and the overall frequency of visceral complications (uveitis or keratitis, hepatitis, encephalitis and peripheral neuropathy). To be effective, Vira-A therapy should be initiated as early as possible, within 72 hours after the appearance of vesicular lesions.

Herpes zoster is recognized by the formation of clear skin vesicles progressing to pustules and scabs along a sensory nerve distribution. The appearance of vesicles may be preceded by fever, local pain and erythema. Varicella-zoster virus can be isolated from vesicular lesions or detected by fluorescent antibody techniques.

Contraindications: Vira-A is contraindicated in patients who develop hypersensitivity reactions to it.

Warnings: Vira-A should not be administered by the intramuscular or subcutaneous route because of its low solubility and poor absorption.

There are no reports available to indicate that Vira-A for infusion is effective in the management of encephalitis due to varicella-zoster or vaccinia viruses. Vira-A is not effective against infections caused by adenovirus or RNA viruses. It is also not effective against bacterial or fungal infections. There are no data to support efficacy of Vira-A against cytomegalovirus, vaccinia virus, or smallpox virus.

Precautions:

General—Treatment should be discontinued in the patient with a brain biopsy negative for Herpes simplex virus in cell culture.

Special care should be exercised when administering Vira-A to patients susceptible to fluid overloading or cerebral edema. Examples are patients with CNS infections and impaired renal function. Patients with impaired renal function, such as post-operative renal transplant recipients, may have a slower rate of renal excretion of Ara-Hx. Therefore, the dose of Vira-A may need to be adjusted according to the severity of impairment. These patients should be carefully monitored.

Patients with impaired liver function should also be observed for possible adverse effects.

Although clear evidence of adverse experience in humans from simultaneous Vira-A and allopurinol administration has not been reported, laboratory studies indicate that allopurinol may interfere with Vira-A metabolism. Therefore, caution is recommended when administering Vira-A to patients receiving allopurinol.

Laboratory Tests—Appropriate hematologic tests are recommended during Vira-A administration since hemoglobin, hematocrit, white blood cells, and platelets may be depressed during therapy. Some degree of immunocompetence must be present in order for Vira-A to achieve clinical response.

Carcinogenesis—Chronic parenteral (IM) studies of vidarabine have been conducted in mice and rats.

In the mouse study, there was a statistically significant increase in liver tumor incidence among the vidarabine-treated females. In the same study, some vidarabine-treated male mice developed kidney neoplasia. No renal tumors were found in the vehicle-treated control mice or the vidarabine-treated female mice.

In the rat study, intestinal, testicular, and thyroid neoplasia occurred with greater frequency among the vidarabine-treated animals than in the vehicle-treated controls. The increases in thyroid adenoma incidence in the high-dose (50 mg/kg) males and the low-dose (30 mg/kg) females were statistically significant.

Hepatic megalocytosis, associated with vidarabine treatment, has been found in short- and long-term rodent (rat and mouse) studies. It is not clear whether or not this represents a preneoplastic change.

In the Balb/3T3 *in vitro* neoplastic transformation assay, used to provide preliminary assessment of potential oncogenicity, vidarabine induced a significant and dose-related increase in transformed foci over the concentration range of 0.5–3.0 μg/ml.

Mutagenesis—Results of *in vitro* experiments indicate that vidarabine can be incorporated into mammalian DNA and can induce mutation in mammalian cells (mouse L5178Y cell line). Thus far, *in vivo* studies have not been as conclusive, but there is some evidence (dominant lethal assay in mice) that vidarabine may be capable of producing mutagenic effects in male germ cells.

It has also been reported that vidarabine causes chromosome breaks and gaps when added to human leukocytes *in vitro*. While the significance of these effects in terms of mutagenicity is not fully understood, there is a well-known correlation between the ability of various agents to produce such effects and their ability to produce heritable genetic damage.

Pregnancy Category C—Vira-A given parenterally is teratogenic in rats and rabbits. Doses of 5 mg/kg or higher given intramuscularly to pregnant rabbits during organogenesis induced fetal abnormalities. Doses of 3 mg/kg or less did not induce teratogenic changes in pregnant rabbits. Vira-A doses ranging from 30 to 250 mg/kg were given intramuscularly to pregnant rats during organogenesis; signs of maternal toxicity were induced at doses of 100 mg/kg or higher and frank fetal anomalies were found at doses of 150 to 250 mg/kg.

A safe dose for the human embryo or fetus has not been established.

There are no adequate and well controlled studies in pregnant women. Vira-A should be used during pregnancy only if the potential benefit justifies the potential risk to the fetus.

Nursing Mothers—It is not known whether Vira-A is excreted in human milk. Because many drugs are excreted in human milk and because of the potential tumorigenicity shown for Vira-A in animal studies, a decision should be made whether to discontinue nursing or to discontinue the drug, taking into account the importance of the drug to the mother.

Adverse Reactions: The principal adverse reactions involve the gastrointestinal tract and are anorexia, nausea, vomiting, and diarrhea. These reactions are mild to moderate, and seldom require termination of Vira-A therapy.

CNS disturbances have been reported at therapeutic doses. These are tremor, dizziness, hallucinations, confusion, psychosis, ataxia, headache and encephalopathy.

Hematologic clinical laboratory changes noted in controlled and uncontrolled studies were a decrease in hemoglobin or hematocrit, white blood cell count, and platelet count. SGOT elevations were also observed. Other changes occasionally observed were decreases in reticulocyte count and elevated total bilirubin.

Other symptoms which have been reported are weight loss, malaise, pruritus, rash, hematemesis, and pain at the injection site.

Overdosage: Acute massive overdose of the intravenous form has been reported without any serious evidence of adverse effect. Because of the low solubility of Vira-A, acute water overloading would pose a greater threat to the patient than Vira-A. Doses of Vira-A over 20 mg/kg/day can produce bone marrow depression with concomitant thrombocytopenia and leukopenia. If a massive overdose of the intravenous form occurs, hematologic, liver, and renal functions should be carefully monitored.

Dosage and Administration: CAUTION—THE CONTENTS OF THE VIAL MUST BE DILUTED IN AN APPROPRIATE INTRAVENOUS SOLUTION PRIOR TO ADMINISTRATION. RAPID OR BOLUS INJECTION MUST BE AVOIDED.

Dosage— Herpes simplex virus encephalitis—15 mg/kg/day for 10 days.

Herpes zoster—10 mg/kg/day for 5 days.

Method of Preparation—Each 5-ml vial contains 1 gram of Vira-A (200 mg per ml of suspension). The solubility of Vira-A in intravenous infusion fluids is limited. Each one mg of Vira-A requires 2.22 ml

Continued on next page

This product information was prepared in August, 1984. On these and other Parke-Davis Products, information may be obtained by addressing PARKE-DAVIS, Division of Warner-Lambert Company, Morris Plains, New Jersey 07950.

Parke-Davis—Cont.

of intravenous infusion fluid for complete solubilization. Therefore, each one liter of intravenous infusion fluid will solubilize a maximum of 450 mg of Vira-A.

Any appropriate intravenous solution is suitable for use as a diluent *EXCEPT* biologic or colloidal fluids (e.g., blood products, protein solutions, etc.). Shake the Vira-A vial well to obtain a homogeneous suspension before measuring and transferring. Prepare the Vira-A solution for intravenous administration by aseptically transferring the proper dose of Vira-A into an appropriate intravenous infusion fluid. The intravenous infusion fluid used to prepare the Vira-A solution should be prewarmed to 35° to 40°C (95° to 100°F) to facilitate solution of the drug following its transference. Depending on the dose to be given, more than one liter of intravenous infusion fluid may be required. Thoroughly agitate the prepared admixture until *completely* clear. Complete solubilization of the drug, as indicated by a completely clear solution, is ascertained by careful visual inspection. Final filtration with an in-line membrane filter (0.45 μ pore size or smaller) is necessary.

Dilution should be made just prior to administration and used at least within 48 hours. Subsequent agitation, shaking, or inversion of the bottle is unnecessary once the drug is completely in solution. DO NOT REFRIGERATE THE DILUTION.

Administration—Using aseptic technique, slowly infuse the total daily dose by intravenous infusion (prepared as discussed above) at a constant rate over a 12- to 24-hour period.

How Supplied:
N 0071-4150-08 (Steri-Vial® 4150) Vira-A (Vidarabine Concentrate for Infusion, USP), a sterile suspension containing 200 mg/ml, is supplied in 5 ml Steri-Vials; packages of 10.

Animal Pharmacology and Toxicity:
Acute Toxicity: The intraperitoneal LD₅₀ for Vira-A ranged from 3,890 to 4,500 mg/kg in mice, and from 2,239 to 2,512 mg/kg in rats, suggesting a low order of toxicity to a single parenteral dose. Hepatic megalocytosis was observed in rats after single, intraperitoneal injections at doses near and exceeding the LD₅₀ value. The hepatic megalocytosis appeared to regress completely over several months. Acute intravenous LD₅₀ values could not be obtained because of the limited solubility of Vira-A.

Subacute Toxicity: Rats, dogs, and monkeys have been given daily intramuscular injections of Vira-A as a 20% suspension for 28 days. These animal species showed dose related decreases in hemoglobin, hematocrit, and lymphocytes. Bone marrow depression was also observed in monkeys. Except for localized, injection-site injury and weight gain inhibition or loss, rats tolerated daily doses up to 150 mg/kg, and dogs tolerated daily doses up to 50 mg/kg. Megalocytosis was not seen in the rats dosed by the intramuscular route for 28 days. Rhesus monkeys were particularly sensitive to Vira-A. Daily intramuscular doses of 15 mg/kg were tolerable, but doses of 25 mg/kg or higher induced progressively severe clinical signs of CNS toxicity. Three monkeys given slow intravenous infusions of Vira-A in solution at a dose of 15 mg/kg daily for 28 days had no significant adverse reactions.

4150G021

VIRA-A®   R
[vī″ră ā′]
(vidarabine ophthalmic ointment, USP), 3%

Description: VIRA-A is the trade name for vidarabine (also known as adenine arabinoside and Ara-A), an antiviral drug for the topical treatment of epithelial keratitis caused by Herpes simplex virus. The chemical name is 9-β-D-arabinofuranosyladenine. Each gram of the ophthalmic ointment contains 30 mg of vidarabine monohydrate equivalent to 28.11 mg of vidarabine in a sterile, inert, petrolatum base.

Clinical Pharmacology: Vira-A is a purine nucleoside obtained from fermentation cultures of *Streptomyces antibioticus*. Vira-A possesses *in vitro* and *in vivo* antiviral activity against Herpes simplex types 1 and 2, Varicella-Zoster, and Vaccinia viruses. Except for Rhabdovirus and Oncornavirus, Vira-A does not display *in vitro* antiviral activity against other RNA or DNA viruses, including Adenovirus.

The antiviral mechanism of action has not been established. Vira-A appears to interfere with the early steps of viral DNA synthesis. Vira-A is rapidly deaminated to arabinosyl-hypoxanthine (Ara-Hx), the principal metabolite. Ara-Hx also possesses *in vitro* antiviral activity but this activity is less than that of Vira-A. Because of the low solubility of Vira-A, trace amounts of both Vira-A and Ara-Hx can be detected in the aqueous humor only if there is an epithelial defect in the cornea. If the cornea is normal, only trace amounts of Ara-Hx can be recovered from the aqueous humor.

Systemic absorption of Vira-A should not be expected to occur following ocular administration and swallowing lacrimal secretions. In laboratory animals, Vira-A is rapidly deaminated in the gastrointestinal tract to Ara-Hx.

In contrast to topical idoxuridine, Vira-A demonstrated less cellular toxicity in the regenerating corneal epithelium in the rabbit.

Indications and Usage: Vira-A Ophthalmic Ointment, 3%, is indicated for the treatment of acute keratoconjunctivitis and recurrent epithelial keratitis due to Herpes simplex virus types 1 and 2. It is also effective in superficial keratitis caused by Herpes simplex virus which has not responded to topical idoxuridine or when toxic or hypersensitivity reactions to idoxuridine have occurred. The effectiveness of Vira-A Ophthalmic Ointment, 3%, against stromal keratitis and uveitis due to Herpes simplex virus has not been established.

The clinical diagnosis of keratitis caused by Herpes simplex virus is usually established by the presence of typical dendritic or geographic lesions on slit-lamp examination.

In controlled and uncontrolled clinical trials, an average of seven and nine days of continuous Vira-A Ophthalmic Ointment, 3%, therapy was required to achieve corneal re-epithelialization. In the controlled trials, 70 of 81 subjects (86%) re-epithelialized at the end of three weeks of therapy. In the uncontrolled trials, 101 of 142 subjects (71%) re-epithelialized at the end of three weeks. Seventy-five percent of the subjects in these uncontrolled trials had either not healed previously or had developed hypersensitivity to topical idoxuridine therapy.

The following topical antibiotics: gentamicin, erythromycin, and chloramphenicol; or topical steroids: prednisolone or dexamethasone, have been administered concurrently with Vira-A Ophthalmic Ointment, 3%, without an increase in adverse reactions.

Contraindication: Vira-A Ophthalmic Ointment, 3%, is contraindicated in patients who develop hypersensitivity reactions to it.

Warnings: Normally, corticosteroids alone are contraindicated in Herpes simplex virus infections of the eye. If Vira-A Ophthalmic Ointment, 3%, is administered concurrently with topical corticosteroid therapy, corticosteroid-induced ocular side effects must be considered. These include corticosteroid-induced glaucoma or cataract formation and progression of a bacterial or viral infection. Vira-A is not effective against RNA virus or adenoviral ocular infections. It is also not effective against bacterial, fungal, or chlamydial infections of the cornea or nonviral trophic ulcers.

Although viral resistance to VIRA-A has not been observed, this possibility may exist.

Precautions:
General—The diagnosis of keratoconjunctivitis due to Herpes simples virus should be established clinically prior to prescribing VIRA-A Ophthalmic Ointment, 3%.

Patients should be forewarned that VIRA-A Ophthalmic Ointment, 3%, like any ophthalmic ointment, may produce a temporary visual haze.

Carcinogenesis—Chronic parenteral (IM) studies of vidarabine have been conducted in mice and rats.

In the mouse study, there was a statistically significant increase in liver tumor incidence among the vidarabine-treated females. In the same study some vidarabine-treated male mice developed kidney neoplasia. No renal tumors were found in the vehicle-treated control mice or the vidarabine-treated female mice.

In the rat study, intestinal, testicular, and thyroid neoplasia occurred with greater frequency among the vidarabine-treated animals than in the vehicle-treated controls. The increases in thyroid adenoma incidence in the high dose (50 mg/kg) males and the low dose (30 mg/kg) females were statistically significant.

Hepatic megalocytosis, associated with vidarabine treatment, has been found in short- and long-term rodent (rat and mouse) studies. It is not clear whether or not this represents a preneoplastic change.

The recommended frequency and duration of administration should not be exceeded (See Dosage and Administration).

Mutagenesis—Results of *in vitro* experiments indicate that vidarabine can be incorporated into mammalian DNA and can induce mutation in mammalian cells (mouse L5178Y cell line). Thus far, *in vivo* studies have not been as conclusive, but there is some evidence (dominant lethal assay in mice) that vidarabine may be capable of producing mutagenic effects in male germ cells.

It has also been reported that vidarabine causes chromosome breaks and gaps when added to human leukocytes *in vitro*. While the significance of these effects in terms of mutagenicity is not fully understood, there is a well-known correlation between the ability of various agents to produce such effects and their ability to produce heritable genetic damage.

Pregnancy Category C—VIRA-A parenterally is teratogenic in rats and rabbits. Ten percent VIRA-A ointment applied to 10% of the body surface during organogenesis induced fetal abnormalities in rabbits. When 10% VIRA-A ointment was applied to 2% to 3% of the body surface of rabbits, no fetal abnormalities were found. This dose greatly exceeds the total recommended ophthalmic dose in humans. The possibility of embryonic or fetal damage in pregnant women receiving VIRA-A Ophthalmic Ointment, 3%, is remote. The topical ophthalmic dose is small, and the drug relatively insoluble. Its ocular penetration is very low. However, a safe dose for a human embryo or fetus has not been established. There are no adequate and well controlled studies in pregnant women. VIRA-A should be used during pregnancy only if the potential benefit justifies the potential risk to the fetus.

Nursing Mothers—It is not known whether VIRA-A is secreted in human milk. Because many drugs are excreted in human milk and because of the potential for tumorigenicity shown for VIRA-A in animal studies, a decision should be made whether to discontinue nursing or to discontinue the drug, taking into account the importance of the drug to the mother. However, breast milk excretion is unlikely because VIRA-A is rapidly deaminated in the gastrointestinal tract.

Adverse Reactions: Lacrimation, foreign body sensation, conjunctival injection, burning, irritation, superficial punctate keratitis, pain, photophobia, punctal occlusion, and sensitivity have been reported with VIRA-A Ophthalmic Ointment, 3%. The following have also been reported but appear disease-related: uveitis, stromal edema, secondary glaucoma, trophic defects, corneal vascularization, and hyphema.

Overdosage: Acute massive overdosage by oral ingestion of the ophthalmic ointment has not occurred. However, the rapid deamination to arabinosylhypoxanthine should preclude any difficulty. The oral LD₅₀ for vidarabine is greater than 5020 mg/kg in mice and rats. No untoward effects should result from ingestion of the entire contents of a tube.

Overdosage by ocular instillation is unlikely because any excess should be quickly expelled from the conjunctival sac. Too frequent administration should be avoided.

Dosage and Administration: Administer approximately one half inch of VIRA-A Ophthalmic Ointment, 3%, into the lower conjunctival sac five times daily at three-hour intervals.

If there are no signs of improvement after 7 days, or complete re-epithelialization has not occurred by 21 days, other forms of therapy should be considered. Some severe cases may require longer treatment.

After re-epithelialization has occurred, treatment for an additional seven days at a reduced dosage (such as twice daily) is recommended in order to prevent recurrence.

How Supplied: N 0071-3677-07 (Stock 18-1677-139)

VIRA-A Ophthalmic Ointment, 3%, is supplied sterile in ophthalmic ointment tubes of 3.5 g. The base is a 60:40 mixture of solid and liquid petrolatum.

3677G020
121 880400/20
Shown in Product Identification Section, page 426

ZARONTIN®
[ză″ rŏn′ tĭn]
(ethosuximide, USP)
Capsules

Description: Zarontin (ethosuximide) is an anticonvulsant succinimide, chemically designated as alpha-ethyl-alpha-methyl-succinimide.

Action: Ethosuximide suppresses the paroxysmal three-cycle-per-second spike and wave activity associated with lapses of consciousness which is common in absence (petit mal) seizures. The frequency of epileptiform attacks is reduced, apparently by depression of the motor cortex and elevation of the threshold of the central nervous system to convulsive stimuli.

Indication: Zarontin is indicated for the control of absence (petit mal) epilepsy.

Contraindication: Ethosuximide should not be used in patients with a history of hypersensitivity to succinimides.

Warnings: Blood dyscrasias, including some with fatal outcome, have been reported to be associated with the use of ethosuximide; therefore, periodic blood counts should be performed.

Ethosuximide is capable of producing morphological and functional changes in the animal liver. In humans, abnormal liver and renal function studies have been reported.

Ethosuximide should be administered with extreme caution to patients with known liver or renal diseases. Periodic urinalysis and liver function studies are advised for all patients receiving the drug.

Cases of systemic lupus erythematosus have been reported with the use of ethosuximide. The physician should be alert to this possibility.

Usage in Pregnancy: The effects of Zarontin in human pregnancy and nursing infants are unknown.

Recent reports suggest an association between the use of anticonvulsant drugs by women with epilepsy and an elevated incidence of birth defects in children born to these women. Data are more extensive with respect to phenytoin and phenobarbital, but these are also the most commonly prescribed anticonvulsants. Less systematic or anecdotal reports suggest a possible similar association with the use of all known anticonvulsant drugs. The reports suggesting an elevated incidence of birth defects in children of drug-treated epileptic women cannot be regarded as adequate to prove a definite cause-and-effect relationship. There are intrinsic methodologic problems in obtaining adequate data on drug teratogenicity in humans. The possibility also exists that other factors, eg, genetic factors or the epileptic condition itself, may be more important than drug therapy in leading to birth defects. The great majority of mothers on anticonvulsant medication deliver normal infants. It is important to note that anticonvulsant drugs should not be discontinued in patients in whom the drug is administered to prevent major seizures because of the strong possibility of precipitating status epilepticus with attendant hypoxia and threat to life. In individual cases where the severity and frequency of the seizure disorder are such that the removal of medication does not pose a serious threat to the patient, discontinuation of the drug may be considered prior to and during pregnancy, although it cannot be said with any confidence that even minor seizures do not pose some hazard to the developing embryo or fetus.

The prescribing physician will wish to weigh these considerations in treating or counseling epileptic women of childbearing potential.

Hazardous Activities: Ethosuximide may impair the mental and/or physical abilities required for the performance of potentially hazardous tasks, such as driving a motor vehicle or other such activity requiring alertness; therefore, the patient should be cautioned accordingly.

Precautions: Ethosuximide, when used alone in mixed types of epilepsy, may increase the frequency of grand mal seizures in some patients.

As with other anticonvulsants, it is important to proceed slowly when increasing or decreasing dosage, as well as when adding or eliminating other medication. Abrupt withdrawal of anticonvulsant medication may precipitate absence (petit mal) status.

Adverse Reactions:

Gastrointestinal System: Gastrointestinal symptoms occur frequently and include anorexia, vague gastric upset, nausea and vomiting, cramps, epigastric and abdominal pain, weight loss, and diarrhea.

Hemopoietic System: Hemopoietic complications associated with the administration of ethosuximide have included leukopenia, agranulocytosis, pancytopenia, aplastic anemia, and eosinophilia.

Nervous System: Neurologic and sensory reactions reported during therapy with ethosuximide have included drowsiness, headache, dizziness, euphoria, hiccups, irritability, hyperactivity, lethargy, fatigue, and ataxia. Psychiatric or psychological aberrations associated with ethosuximide administration have included disturbances of sleep, night terrors, inability to concentrate, and aggressiveness. These effects may be noted particularly in patients who have previously exhibited psychological abnormalities. There have been rare reports of paranoid psychosis, increased libido, and increased state of depression with overt suicidal intentions.

Integumentary System: Dermatologic manifestations which have occurred with the administration of ethosuximide have included urticaria, Stevens-Johnson syndrome, systemic lupus erythematosus, and pruritic erythematous rashes.

Miscellaneous: Other reactions reported have included myopia, vaginal bleeding, swelling of the tongue, gum hypertrophy, and hirsutism.

Dosage and Administration:

Zarontin Capsules (ethosuximide capsules, USP): Zarontin is administered by the oral route. The initial dose for patients 3 to 6 years of age is one capsule (250 mg) per day; for patients 6 years of age and older, 2 capsules (500 mg) per day. The dose thereafter must be individualized according to the patient's response. Dosage should be increased by small increments. One useful method is to increase the daily dose by 250 mg every four to seven days until control is achieved with minimal side effects. Dosages exceeding 1.5 g daily, in divided doses, should be administered only under the strictest supervision of the physician. The *optimal* dose for most children is 20 mg/kg/day. This dose has given average plasma levels within the accepted therapeutic range of 40 to 100 mcg/ml. Subsequent dose schedules can be based on effectiveness and plasma level determinations.

Zarontin may be administered in combination with other anticonvulsants when other forms of epilepsy coexist with absence (petit mal). The *optimal* dosage for most children is 20 mg/kg/day.

How Supplied:

N 0071-0237-24 Bottle of 100. Each capsule contains 250 mg ethosuximide.

0237G021
Shown in Product Identification Section, page 426

ZARONTIN®
[ză″ rŏn′ tĭn]
(ethosuximide)
Syrup

Description: Zarontin (ethosuximide) is an anticonvulsant succinimide, chemically designated as alpha-ethyl-alpha-methyl-succinimide.

Each teaspoonful (5 ml), for oral administration, contains 250 mg ethosuximide in a raspberry flavored base.

Clinical Pharmacology: Ethosuximide suppresses the paroxysmal three cycle per second spike and wave activity associated with lapses of consciousness which is common in absence (petit mal) seizures. The frequency of epileptiform attacks is reduced, apparently by depression of the motor cortex and elevation of the threshold of the central nervous system to convulsive stimuli.

Indication and Usage: Zarontin is indicated for the control of absence (petit mal) epilepsy.

Contraindication: Ethosuximide should not be used in patients with a history of hypersensitivity to succinimides.

Warnings: Blood dyscrasias, including some with fatal outcome, have been reported to be associated with the use of ethosuximide; therefore, periodic blood counts should be performed. Ethosuximide is capable of producing morphological and functional changes in the animal liver. In humans, abnormal liver and renal function studies have been reported.

Ethosuximide should be administered with extreme caution to patients with known liver or renal disease. Periodic urinalysis and liver function studies are advised for all patients receiving the drug.

Cases of systemic lupus erythematosus have been reported with the use of ethosuximide. The physician should be alert to this possibility.

Hazardous Activities: Ethosuximide may impair the mental and/or physical abilities required for the performance of potentially hazardous tasks, such as driving a motor vehicle or other such activity requiring alertness; therefore, the patient should be cautioned accordingly.

Usage in Pregnancy: The effects of Zarontin in human pregnancy and nursing infants are unknown.

Recent reports suggest an association between the use of anticonvulsant drugs by women with epilepsy and an elevated incidence of birth defects in children born to these women. Data are more extensive with respect to phenytoin and phenobarbital, but these are also the most commonly prescribed anticonvulsants; less systematic or anecdotal reports suggest a possible similar association with the use of all known anticonvulsant drugs. The reports suggesting an elevated incidence of birth defects in children of drug-treated epileptic women cannot be regarded as adequate to prove a definite cause and effect relationship. There are intrinsic methodologic problems in obtaining adequate data on drug teratogenicity in humans; the possibility also exists that other factors, eg. genetic factors or the epileptic condition itself, may be more important than drug therapy in leading to birth defects. The great majority of mothers on anticonvulsant medication deliver normal infants. It is important to note that anticonvulsant drugs should not be discontinued in patients in whom the drug is administered to prevent major seizures because of the strong possibility of precipitating status epilepticus with attendant hypoxia and threat to life. In individual cases where the severity and frequency of the seizure disorder are such

Continued on next page

This product information was prepared in August, 1984. On these and other Parke-Davis Products, information may be obtained by addressing PARKE-DAVIS, Division of Warner-Lambert Company, Morris Plains, New Jersey 07950.

Parke-Davis—Cont.

that the removal of medication does not pose a serious threat to the patient, discontinuation of the drug may be considered prior to and during pregnancy, although it cannot be said with any confidence that even minor seizures do not pose some hazard to the developing embryo or fetus. The prescribing physician will wish to weigh these considerations in treating or counseling epileptic women of childbearing potential.

Precautions:
General: Ethosuximide, when used alone in mixed types of epilepsy, may increase the frequency of grand mal seizures in some patients.
As with other anticonvulsants, it is important to proceed slowly when increasing or decreasing dosage, as well as when adding or eliminating other medication. Abrupt withdrawal of anticonvulsant medication may precipitate absence (petit mal) status.
Information for Patient: Ethosuximide may impair the mental and/or physical abilities required for the performance of potentially hazardous tasks such as driving a motor vehicle or other such activity requiring alertness; therefore, the patient should be cautioned accordingly.
Pregnancy: See WARNINGS

Adverse Reactions:
Gastrointestinal System: Gastrointestinal symptoms occur frequently and include anorexia, vague gastric upset, nausea and vomiting, cramps, epigastric and abdominal pain, weight loss, and diarrhea.
Hemopoietic System: Hemopoietic complications associated with the administration of ethosuximide have included leukopenia, agranulocytosis, pancytopenia, aplastic anemia, and eosinophilia.
Nervous System: Neurologic and sensory reactions reported during therapy with ethosuximide have included drowsiness, headache, dizziness, euphoria, hiccups, irritability, hyperactivity, lethargy, fatigue, and ataxia.
Psychiatric or psychological aberrations associated with ethosuximide administration have included disturbances of sleep, night terrors, inability to concentrate, and aggressiveness. These effects may be noted particularly in patients who have previously exhibited psychological abnormalities. There have been rare reports of paranoid psychosis, increased libido, and increased state of depression with overt suicidal intentions.
Integumentary System: Dermatologic manifestations which have occurred with the administration of ethosuximide have included urticaria, Stevens-Johnson syndrome, systemic lupus erythematosus, and pruritic erythematous rashes.
Miscellaneous: Other reactions reported have included myopia, vaginal bleeding, swelling of the tongue, gum hypertrophy, and hirsutism.
Dosage and Administration: Zarontin is administered by the oral route. The *initial* dose for patients 3 to 6 years of age is one teaspoonful (250 mg) per day; for patients 6 years of age and older, 2 teaspoonfuls (500 mg) per day. The dose thereafter must be individualized according to the patient's response. Dosage should be increased by small increments. One useful method is to increase the daily dose by 250 mg every four to seven days until control is achieved with minimal side effects. Dosages exceeding 1.5 g daily, in divided doses, should be administered only under the strictest supervision of the physician. The *optimal* dose for most children is 20 mg/kg/day. This dose has given average plasma levels within the accepted therapeutic range of 40 to 100 mcg/ml. Subsequent dose schedules can be based on effectiveness and plasma level determinations.
Zarontin may be administered in combination with other anticonvulsants when other forms of epilepsy coexist with absence (petit mal). The optimal dose for most children is 20 mg/kg/day.
How Supplied:
Zarontin is supplied as:
N0071-2418-23–1 pint bottles. Each 5 ml of syrup contains 250 mg ethosuximide in a raspberry flavored base. Store below 30°C (86°F). Protect from freezing and light.
Zarontin is also supplied in the following form:
N0071-0237-24–Bottle of 100. Each capsule contains 250 mg ethosuximide. Store below 30°C (86°F).

2418G021

ZIRADRYL® Lotion
[zī′ră-dryl″]

Description: A zinc oxide-Benadryl lotion of 2% Benadryl® (diphenhydramine hydrochloride) and 2% zinc oxide; contains 2% alcohol.
Indications: For relief of itching in ivy or oak poisoning.
Warning: Should not be applied to extensive, or raw, oozing areas, or for a prolonged time, except as directed by a physician. Hypersensitivity to any of the components may occur.
Caution: Do not use in the eyes. If the condition for which this preparation is used persists or if a rash or irritation develops, discontinue use and consult a physician. *FOR EXTERNAL USE ONLY*
Directions: *SHAKE WELL*
For relief of itching, cleanse affected area and apply generously three or four times daily. Temporary stinging sensation may follow application. Discontinue use if stinging persists. Easily removed with water.
How Supplied: N 0071-3224-19—6-oz bottles

Pedinol Pharmacal Inc.
110 BELL STREET
W. BABYLON, NY 11704

BREEZEE MIST FOOT POWDER   OTC
Composition: Aluminum Chlorhydrate, Menthol, Undecylenic Acid.
Indications: Topical treatment for hyperhidrosis, bromidrosis and tinea pedis (athlete's foot).
How Supplied: 4 oz. aerosol can.

CASTELLANI PAINT   ℞
Composition: Basic Fuchsin, Phenol, Resorcinol, Acetone, Alcohol.
Indications: Topical antifungal agent for macerations and ulcerations.
Precautions: If irritation or sensitivity develops, discontinue treatment and consult podiatrist or physician.
Administration: Apply to affected areas once or twice a day.
How Supplied: 1 oz. and 1 pt. plastic bottle. Colorless (without basic fuchsin), 1 oz. and 1 pt. plastic bottle.

FUNGOID CREME and SOLUTION   ℞
Composition: Cetyl Pyridinium Chloride, Triacetin, Chloroxylenol, Vanishing Creme Base and Oil Base Solution.
Indications: Topical treatment for fungus, yeast and bacterial infections of the skin.
Precautions: If irritation or sensitivity develops, discontinue treatment and consult podiatrist or physician.
Administration: Apply to affected areas three times a day.
How Supplied: 1 oz. plastic tube; 15cc plastic bottle with controlled dropper.

FUNGOID TINCTURE   ℞
Composition: Cetyl Pyridinium Chloride, Triacetin, Chloroxylenol.
Indications: Topical treatment for ringworm infections of the nails, tinea unguium (onychomycosis).
Precautions: If irritation or sensitivity develops, discontinue treatment and consult podiatrist or physician.
Administration: Apply to affected nails twice a day.
How Supplied: 1 oz. bottle with brush applicator, 1 pt. bottle.

G-MYTICIN CREME and OINTMENT 0.1%   ℞
(gentamicin sulfate 0.1%)

Composition: Creme and ointment—each gram contains gentamicin sulfate equivalent to 1 mg. of gentamicin base.
Indications: Topical wide-spectrum antibiotic provides highly effective treatment in primary and secondary bacterial infections of the skin.
NOTE: G-myticin Creme/Ointment is not effective against viruses or fungi skin infections.
Adverse Reactions: In patients with dermatoses treated with G-myticin erythema and pruritis that did not usually require discontinuance of treatment has been reported in a small percentage of cases.
Contraindications: G-myticin creme/ointment, is contraindicated in those patients with a history of hypersensitivity to any of the components of this preparation.
Precautions: The overgrowth of nonsusceptible organisms, including fungi, occasionally occurs with the use of topical antibiotics. If this occurs, or if irritation, sensitization, or superinfection develops, treatment with G-myticin should be discontinued and consult Podiatrist or Physician.
Administration: Apply 3 to 4 times daily.
How Supplied: G-myticin Creme/Ointment—15 grm tubes.

HYDRISALIC GEL   ℞
Composition: Salicyclic Acid 6%, Isopropanol, Propylene Glycol, Hydroxypropyl Cellulose.
Indications: Topical treatment for hyperkeratotic skin.
Precautions: Use should be limited to children under 12 years of age. If irritation or sensitivity develops, discontinue treatment and consult podiatrist or physician.
Administration: Apply to affected area in the evening. Wash hands thoroughly following application. The medication is washed off the following morning.
How Supplied: 1 oz. plastic tubes.

HYDRISEA LOTION   OTC
Composition: Dead Sea Salts Concentrate 8%, Coloring Agent.
Indications: Topical treatment for scaly, dry skin.
Precautions: If irritation or sensitivity develops, discontinue treatment and consult podiatrist or physician.
Administration: Apply twice daily.
How Supplied: 4 oz. plastic bottle.

HYDRISINOL CREME AND LOTION   OTC
Composition: Sulfonated Hydrogenated Castor Oil, N.F. IX, Hydrogenated Vegetable Oil.
Indications: Topical emollient to soften dry, cracked, calloused skin.
Administration: Apply as needed.
How Supplied: 4 oz. and 1 lb. jars; 8 oz. plastic bottle.

OSTI–DERM LOTION   OTC
Composition: Liquified Phenol, Glycerin, Zinc Oxide, Magnesium Carbonate, Aluminum Acetate Solution (Burow's Solution), Camphor Water, in a Hydrated Aluminum Silicate Gel.
Indications: Topical treatment for bromidrosis, hyperhidrosis, decubitus ulcers, blisters, itching, poison ivy and dermatitis.
Precautions: Check skin sensitivity to phenol. If irritation or sensitivity develops, discontinue treatment and consult podiatrist or physician.
Administration: Apply 2–3 times a day.
How Supplied: 45cc plastic tube.

PEDI-BATH SALTS — OTC
Composition: Colloidal Sulphur, Sodium, Magnesium Sulphate, Potassium Iodide, Sodium Chloride, Sodium Bicarb., Pine Needle Oil.
Indications: Topical foot bath; soak for tired aching feet.
Dosage and Administration: Two capsful in a foot bath.
How Supplied: 6 oz. plastic bottle.

PEDI-BORO SOAKS PAKS — OTC
Composition: Aluminum Sulfate, Calcium Acetate, Coloring Agent.
Actions: A soothing astringent wet dressing of a modified Burow's Solution, buffered.
Dosage and Administration: Dissolve 1 or 2 paks in a pint of water. Prepare fresh daily.
How Supplied: Box of 12 and Box of 100.

PEDI-CORT V CREME — ℞
Composition: Hydrocortisone 1%, Iodochlorhydroxyquin 3%.
Indications: Topical anti-inflammatory antifungal, antibacterial, antipruritic creme for the skin.
Contraindications: Hypersensitivity to any of the ingredients. Not for use in the presence of tuberculosis, vaccinia, varicella or other viral skin conditions.
Precautions: Observe all precautions for using a steroid preparation. If irritation or sensitivity develops, discontinue treatment and consult podiatrist or physician.
Administration: Apply 1-3 times a day.
How Supplied: 20 gm. tubes.

PEDI-DRI FOOT POWDER — ℞
Composition: Aluminum Chlorhydroxide, Menthol, Zinc Undecylenate, Formaldehyde.
Indications: Topical treatment for hyperhidrosis, bromidrosis and tinea pedis (athlete's foot).
Precautions: External use only. Check for skin sensitivity to formaldehyde. If irritation or sensitivity develops, discontinue treatment and consult podiatrist or physician.
Administration: Apply twice a day.
How Supplied: 2 oz. plastic bottle.

PEDI-PRO FOOT POWDER — OTC
Composition: Aluminum Chlorhydroxide, Chloroxylenol, Zinc Undecylenate, Menthol, Micro-Kaolin, Starch.
Indications: Athlete's Foot: Aids in temporary relief of burning, itching and cracking skin in athlete's foot.
Caution: External use only. Do not use near eyes or mucous membranes. Keep out of reach of children. Persons with impaired circulation, including diabetes, should consult a Podiatrist before using medication. If symptoms persist consult your Podiatrist or Physician.
Contraindications: Do not use in patients known to be sensitive to any ingredients in Pedi-Pro Foot Powder.
Administration: Apply twice a day.
How Supplied: 2 oz. plastic bottle.

PEDI-VIT A CREME — OTC
Composition: Vitamin A.
Indications: Topical treatment for irritated, dry, sensitive skin.
Administration: Apply daily as needed.
How Supplied: 2 oz. jar and 1 lb. jar.

SALACTIC FILM — ℞
Composition: Salicyclic Acid 16.7% U.S.P., Lactic Acid 16.7% U.S.P., Flexible Collodion U.S.P., Coloring Agent.
Indications: Topical treatment as a keratolytic agent for removal of verrucae.
Contraindications: Diabetics or patients with impaired blood circulation. Do not use on moles, birthmarks or warts with hair growing from them.
Precautions: Highly flammable. Keep bottle tightly capped when not in use. If irritation or sensitivity develops, discontinue treatment and consult podiatrist or physician.
Administration: Apply once daily as directed.
How Supplied: ½ oz. bottle with brush applicator.

UREACIN-10 Lotion — OTC
UREACIN-20 Creme — OTC
UREACIN-40 Creme — ℞
Composition: Urea 10%, Urea 20% and 40%, Vegetable Oil Base.
Indications: Ureacin-10 Lotion, Ureacin-20 Creme is a topical treatment for rough, dry, cracked, calloused skin. Ureacin-40 Creme is indicated for the treatment of nail destruction and dissolution.
Precautions: If irritation or sensitivity develops, discontinue treatment and consult podiatrist or physician.
Administration: Rub in gently two or three times a day to affected area. Ureacin-40 Creme to be applied to diseased nail surface by podiatrist or physician only.
How Supplied: 8 oz. plastic bottle, 2½ oz. plastic jar, 1 oz. plastic jar.

For further product information please contact Pedinol Pharmacal Inc.

Pennwalt Corp.
Prescription Division
ROCHESTER, NY 14623

ADAPIN® — ℞
[ad′uh-pin″]
(doxepin HCl)

Description: Adapin (doxepin HCl) is an isomeric mixture of 1-Propanamine,3-dibenz[b,e]oxepin-11 (6H) ylidene -N, N- dimethyl-,hydrochloride.
Actions: Adapin has a variety of pharmacological actions with its predominant action on the central nervous system. While its mechanism of action is not known, studies have demonstrated that it is neither a monoamine oxidase inhibitor nor a primary stimulant of the central nervous system.
In a large series of patients systematically observed for withdrawal symptoms, none were reported—a finding which is consistent with the virtual absence of euphoria as a side effect and the lack of addictive potential characteristic of this type of chemical compound.
Indications: In controlled clinical evaluations, Adapin has shown marked antianxiety and significant antidepressant effects. Adapin has been found to be well tolerated even in elderly patients. Adapin is indicated for the treatment of patients with:
1. Psychoneurotic anxiety and/or depressive reactions.
2. Mixed symptoms of anxiety and depression.
3. Anxiety and/or depression associated with alcoholism.
4. Anxiety associated with organic disease.
5. Psychotic depressive disorders including involutional depression and manic-depressive reactions.

Target symptoms of psychoneurosis that respond particularly well to Adapin include: anxiety, tension, depression, somatic symptoms and concerns, insomnia, guilt, lack of energy, fear, apprehension and worry.
Because Adapin provides antidepressant as well as antianxiety effects, it is of particular value in patients in whom anxiety masks depression. Patients who have not responded to other antianxiety or antidepressant drugs may benefit from Adapin.
Contraindications: Because Adapin has an anticholinergic effect, it is contraindicated in patients with glaucoma or a tendency toward urinary retention.

Use of Adapin is contraindicated in patients who have been found hypersensitive to it.
Warnings: *Usage in Pregnancy:* Adapin has not been evaluated in pregnant patients. Therefore, it should not be used during pregnancy unless, in the judgment of the physician, it is essential to the welfare of the patient.
In animal reproduction studies of Adapin, gross and microscopic examination of the offspring gave no evidence of drug-related teratogenic effect. Following doses of up to 25 mg./kg./day for 8 to 9 months, no changes were observed in the number of live births, litter size, or lactation. A decreased rate of conception was observed when male rats were given 25 mg./kg./day for prolonged periods—an effect which has occurred with other psychotropic drugs and has been attributed to drug effect on the central and/or autonomic nervous systems.
Usage in Children: The use of Adapin in children under 12 years of age is not recommended, because safe conditions for its use have not been established.
MAO Inhibitors: Serious side effects and even death have been reported following the concomitant use of certain drugs with MAO inhibitors. Therefore, MAO inhibitors should be discontinued at least two weeks prior to the cautious initiation of therapy with Adapin (doxepin HCl). The exact length of time may vary and is dependent upon the particular MAO inhibitor being used, the length of time it has been administered, and the dosage involved.
Alcohol: In patients who may use alcohol excessively, it should be borne in mind that the potentiation may increase the danger inherent in any suicide attempt or overdosage.
Precautions: Drowsiness may occur with Adapin (doxepin HCl); therefore, patients should be warned of its possible occurrence and cautioned against driving a motor vehicle or operating hazardous machinery while taking the drug.
Patients should also be cautioned that the effects of alcoholic beverages may be increased.
Since suicide is an inherent risk in depressed patients and remains a risk through the initial phases of improvement, depressed patients should be closely supervised.
Although Adapin has shown effective tranquilizing activity, the possibility of activating or unmasking latent psychotic symptoms should be kept in mind.
Compounds structurally related to Adapin can block the effects of guanethidine and similarly acting compounds. However, at the usual clinical dosages, 75 mg. to 150 mg. per day, Adapin has been given concomitantly with guanethidine without blocking its antihypertensive effect. But at dosages of 300 mg. per day or higher, Adapin has exerted a significant blocking effect.
Adapin, like other structurally related psychotropic drugs, potentiates norepinephrine response in animals. But this effect has not been observed with Adapin in humans, which is in accord with the low incidence of tachycardia reported clinically.
Adverse Reactions: *Anticholinergic Effects:* Dry mouth, blurred vision and constipation have been reported. These are usually mild, and often subside as therapy is continued or dosage reduced.
Central Nervous System Effects: Drowsiness has been observed. It usually occurs early in the course of therapy and tends to subside as therapy continues.
Cardiovascular Effects: Tachycardia and hypotension have been reported infrequently.
Other infrequently reported adverse effects with tricyclic antidepressants include extrapyramidal symptoms, syndrome of inappropriate ADH (antidiuretic hormone) secretion, gastrointestinal reactions, secretory effects such as increased sweating, weakness, dizziness, fatigue, weight gain, edema, paresthesias, flushing, chills, tinnitus, photophobia, decreased libido, rash, and pruritus.
Withdrawal Symptoms: Abrupt cessation of treatment after prolonged administration may

Continued on next page

Pennwalt—Cont.

produce nausea, headache and malaise. These are not indicative of addiction.

Dosage and Administration: *In most patients with mild to moderate anxiety and/or depression:* A starting dose of 25 mg. t.i.d. is recommended. Decrease or increase the dosage at appropriate intervals according to individual response. Usual optimum dosage is 75 mg. to 150 mg. per day. As an alternate regimen the total daily dosage, up to 150 mg., may be given at bedtime without loss of effectiveness.

In some patients with mild symptomatology or emotional symptoms accompanying organic disease, dosage as low as 25 mg. to 50 mg. per day has provided effective control.

In more severe anxiety and/or depression: 50 mg. t.i.d. may be required to start—if necessary, gradually increase to 300 mg. per day. Additional effectiveness is rarely obtained by exceeding 300 mg. per day.

Although optimal antidepressant response may not be evident for two to three weeks, antianxiety activity is rapidly apparent.

Overdosage: Symptoms—An increase of any of the reported adverse reactions, primarily excessive sedation and anticholinergic effects such as blurred vision and dry mouth. Other effects may be: pronounced tachycardia, hypotension and extrapyramidal symptoms. Treatment—Essentially symptomatic; supportive therapy in the case of hypotension and excessive sedation.

How Supplied: Each capsule contains doxepin, as the hydrochloride, 10 mg. (NDC 0018-0356), 25 mg. (NDC 0018-0357), 50 mg. (NDC 0018-0358), 75 mg. (NDC 0018-0361) and 100 mg (NDC 0018-0359) capsules in bottles of 100, and 1000.

Rev 10/83

Shown in Product Identification Section, page 426

CORSYM™ OTC
[kŏr'sim]
(phenylpropanolamine polistirex and chlorpheniramine polistirex)

Description: Provides 12-hour relief of nasal congestion. Each teaspoonful (5 ml) contains phenylpropanolamine polistirex equivalent to 37.5 mg phenylpropanolamine HCl, plus chlorpheniramine polistirex equivalent to 4 mg chlorpheniramine maleate.

Indications: For temporary relief of nasal congestion due to the common cold. For temporary relief of nasal congestion associated with sinusitis. For temporary relief of running nose, sneezing, itching of the nose or throat and itchy and watery eyes as may occur in allergic rhinitis (such as hay fever).

Warnings: Do not exceed recommended dosage because at higher doses nervousness, dizziness, or sleeplessness may occur. May cause excitability, especially in children. Do not take this product if you have asthma, glaucoma, high blood pressure, heart disease, diabetes, thyroid disease, or difficulty in urination due to enlargement of the prostate gland, except under the advice and supervision of a physician. Do not give this product to children under 6, except under the advice and supervision of a physician. If symptoms do not improve within 7 days or are accompanied by high fever, consult a physician before continuing use. May cause drowsiness. As with any drug, if you are pregnant or nursing a baby, seek the advice of a health professional before using this product. Keep this and all drugs out of the reach of children. In case of accidental overdose, seek professional assistance or contact a Poison Control Center immediately.

Caution: Avoid driving a motor vehicle or operating heavy machinery. Avoid alcoholic beverages while taking this product.

Drug Interaction Precaution: Do not take this product if you are presently taking a prescription antihypertensive or antidepressant drug containing a monoamine oxidase inhibitor except under the advice and supervision of a physician.

Directions: Shake well before using. Adults: 2 teaspoonsful every 12 hours; do not exceed 4 teaspoonsful in 24 hours. Children 6–12: 1 teaspoonful every 12 hours; do not exceed 2 teaspoonsful in 24 hours. Children 2–5 (use under the supervision of a physician): ½ teaspoonful every 12 hours; do not exceed 1 teaspoonful in 24 hours.

How Supplied: 3 fl. oz. bottles (NDC 0018-0842-61) and 1 pint bottles (NDC 0018-0842-67).

DELSYM®
[del'sim]
(dextromethorphan polistirex)

Description: Provides 12-hour relief of cough due to minor throat and bronchial irritation. Each teaspoonful (5 ml) contains dextromethorphan polistirex equivalent to 30 mg dextromethorphan hydrobromide.

Indications: For temporary relief of cough due to minor throat and bronchial irritation as may occur with the common cold or with inhaled irritants.

Warnings: Do not give this product to children under 2 years except under the advice and supervision of a physician. Do not take this product for persistent or chronic cough such as occurs with smoking, asthma, or emphysema, or where cough is accompanied by excessive phlegm (mucus) unless directed by a physician.

As with any drug, if you are pregnant or nursing a baby, seek the advice of a health professional before using this product.

Caution: A persistent cough may be a sign of a serious condition. If cough persists for more than 1 week, tends to recur or is accompanied by high fever, rash or persistent headache, consult a physician. Keep this and all drugs out of reach of children. In case of accidental overdose, seek professional assistance or contact a Poison Control Center immediately.

Directions: Shake well before using. Adults: 2 teaspoonsful every 12 hours; do not exceed 4 teaspoonsful in 24 hours. Children 6–12: 1 teaspoonful every 12 hours; do not exceed 2 teaspoonsful in 24 hours. Children 2–5: ½ teaspoonful every 12 hours; do not exceed 1 teaspoonful in 24 hours. Children under 2: Use only under the advice and supervision of a physician.

How Supplied: 3 fl. oz. bottles (NDC 0018-0842-61)

HYLOREL® Tablets ℞
[hi'lō-rel"]
(guanadrel sulfate)
10 and 25 mg

Description: HYLOREL Tablets for oral administration contain guanadrel sulfate, an antihypertensive agent belonging to the class of adrenergic neuron blocking drugs. The tablets are available in two strengths: 10 mg and 25 mg. Guanadrel sulfate is (1,4-dioxaspiro[4.5]decan-2-ylmethyl) guanidine sulfate with a molecular weight of 524.63. It is a white to off-white crystalline powder, which melts with decomposition at about 235°C. It is soluble in water to the extent of 76 mg/ml.

Clinical Pharmacology: Guanadrel sulfate is an orally effective antihypertensive agent that lowers both systolic and diastolic arterial blood pressures. Guanadrel sulfate inhibits sympathetic vasoconstriction by inhibiting norepinephrine release from neuronal storage sites in response to stimulation of the nerve and also causes depletion of norepinephrine from the nerve ending. This results in relaxation of vascular smooth muscle which decreases total peripheral resistance, and decreases venous return, both of which reduce the ability to maintain blood pressure in the upright position. The result is a hypotensive effect that is greater in the standing than in the supine position by about 10 mmHg systolic and 3.5 mmHg diastolic, on the average. Heart rate is also decreased usually by about 5 beats/minute. Fluid retention occurs during treatment with guanadrel, particularly when it is not accompanied by a diuretic. The drug does not inhibit parasympathetic nerve function nor does it enter the central nervous system.

Guanadrel sulfate is rapidly absorbed after oral administration. Plasma concentrations generally peak 1½ to 2 hours after ingestion. The half life is about 10 hours, but individual variability is great. Approximately 85% of the drug is eliminated in the urine. Urinary excretion is approximately 85% complete within 24 hours after administration; about 40% of a dose is excreted as unchanged drug. There is no information available regarding pharmacokinetics in patients with impaired renal function.

Guanadrel sulfate begins to decrease blood pressure within 2 hours and produces maximal decreases in 4 to 6 hours. No significant change in cardiac output accompanies the blood pressure decline in normal individuals.

Because drugs of the adrenergic neuron blocking class are transported into the neuron by the "norepinephrine pump," drugs that compete for the pump may block their effects. The ability of tricyclic antidepressants to reverse the blood pressure effect of guanethidine and bethanidine is well documented and a similar effect with guandarel should be presumed. Chlorpromazine seems to have a similar effect on guanethidine and may affect guanadrel as well. Indirectly acting adrenergic amines are transported into the neuron by the "norepinephrine pump" and may interfere with uptake or may displace blocking agents. Ephedrine rapidly reverses the effects of guanadrel but other agents have not been studied.

[See table on next page].

Agents of the guanethidine class cause increased sensitivity to circulating norepinephrine, probably by preventing uptake of norepinephrine by adrenergic neurons, the usual mechanism for terminating norepinephrine effects. Agents of this class are thus dangerous in the presence of excess norepinephrine, eg, in the presence of a pheochromocytoma.

In controlled clinical studies comparing guanadrel to guanethidine and methyldopa, involving about 2000 patients exposed to guanadrel, patients with supine blood pressures averaging 160-170/105-110 mmHg had decreases in blood pressure of 20-25/15-20 mmHg in the standing position. The decreases in supine blood pressure were less than the decreases in standing blood pressure by 6-10/2-7 mmHg in different studies. Guanethidine and guanadrel were very similar in effectiveness while methyldopa had a larger effect on supine systolic pressure. Side effects of guanadrel and guanethidine were generally similar in type (see **Adverse Reactions**) while methyldopa had more central nervous system effects (depression, drowsiness) but fewer orthostatic effects and less diarrhea.

Indications and Usage: HYLOREL Tablets are indicated for the treatment of hypertension in patients not responding adequately to a thiazide type diuretic. HYLOREL is Step-2 therapy and should be added to a diuretic regimen for optimum blood pressure control.

Contraindications: HYLOREL Tablets are contraindicated in known or suspected pheochromocytoma.

HYLOREL should not be used concurrently with, or within one week of, monoamine oxidase inhibitors.

HYLOREL should not be used in patients hypersensitive to the drug.

HYLOREL should not be used in patients with frank congestive heart failure.

Warnings:

a. Orthostatic Hypotension: Orthostatic hypotension and its consequences (dizziness and weakness) are frequent in people treated with HYLOREL Tablets. Rarely, fainting upon standing or exercise is seen. Careful instructions to the patient can minimize these symptoms, as can recognition by the physician that the supine blood pressure does not constitute an adequate assessment of the effects of this drug. Patients with known regional vascular disease (cerebral, coronary) are at particular risk from marked orthostatic hypotension and HYLOREL should be avoided in them unless drugs with lesser degrees of orthostatic hypotension are ineffective or unacceptable. In such patients hypotensive episodes should be avoided,

FREQUENCY OF SIDE EFFECTS
Percent of Clinic Visits in Which Side Effect was Reported

	Guanadrel			Methyldopa			Guanethidine		
Week	Pre-Drug 0	1-8	9-52	Pre-Drug 0	1-8	9-52	Pre-Drug 0	1-8	9-52
Number of clinic visits analyzed	470	3003	4260	266	1610	2216	215	1421	2009
Side Effect									
Morning orthostatic faintness	6.6	9.4	6.8	6.8	8.1	7.4	4.6	10.7	7.9
Orthostatic faintness during the day	7.5	10.8	8.5	7.5	8.0	7.8	5.6	8.9	6.3
Other faintness	7.8	4.8	4.5	6.2	3.7	3.8	5.9	2.7	2.0
Increased bowel movements	4.9	7.9	6.1	4.9	5.9	3.8	3.7	7.9	9.4
Drowsiness	15.3	14.4	8.7	13.2	21.2	18.6	10.2	10.3	6.4
Fatigue	25.7	26.6	23.7	32.9	22.6	27.6	21.4	20.5	17.5
Ejaculation disturbance	7.0	17.5	12.0	10.3	13.4	11.5	6.9	16.6	18.2

The frequency of side effects over time may be reduced by the discontinuation of patients due to intolerable side effects. Reasons for discontinuation of therapy with guanadrel are shown in the following table.

PERCENT OF PATIENTS WHO DISCONTINUED

	Guanadrel	Methyldopa	Guanethidine
Orthostatic faintness	0.6	0.7	6.0
Syncope	0.4	0.3	2.0
Other faintness	1.2	0.0	0.0
Increased bowel movements	0.8	0.7	1.4
Drowsiness	0.0	1.9	0.0
Fatigue	0.2	2.6	0.0
Ejaculation disturbances	0.4	0.0	0.0

even if this requires accepting a poorer degree of blood pressure control.

Instructions to patients: Patients should be advised about the risk of orthostatic hypotension and told to sit or lie down immediately at the onset of dizziness or weakness so that they can prevent loss of consciousness. They should be told that postural hypotension is worst in the morning and upon arising and may be exaggerated by alcohol, fever, hot weather, prolonged standing, or exercise.

Surgery: To reduce the possibility of vascular collapse during anesthesia, guanadrel should be discontinued 48-72 hours before elective surgery. If emergency surgery is required, the anesthesiologist should be made aware that the patient has been taking HYLOREL and that preanesthetic and anesthetic agents should be administered cautiously in reduced dosage. If vasopressors are needed they must be used cautiously, as guanadrel can enhance the pressor response to such agents and increase their arrhythmogenicity.

b. Drug Interactions: As discussed above (**Clinical Pharmacology**), tricyclic antidepressants and indirect-acting sympathomimetics such as ephedrine or phenylpropanolamine, and possibly phenothiazines, can reverse the effects of neuronal blocking agents. IN VIEW OF THE PRESENCE OF SYMPATHOMIMETIC AMINES IN MANY NON-PRESCRIPTION DRUGS FOR THE TREATMENT OF COLDS, ALLERGY, OR ASTHMA, PATIENTS GIVEN GUANADREL SHOULD BE SPECIFICALLY WARNED NOT TO USE SUCH PREPARATIONS WITHOUT THEIR PHYSICIAN'S ADVICE.

Guanadrel enhances the activity of direct-acting sympathomimetics, like norepinephrine, by blocking neuronal uptake.

Drugs that affect the adrenergic response by the same or other mechanisms would be expected to potentiate the effects of guanadrel, causing excessive postural hypotension and bradycardia. These include alpha- or beta-adrenergic blocking agents and reserpine. There is no clinical experience with such combinations.

c. Asthmatic patients: Special care is needed in patients with bronchial asthma, as their condition may be aggravated by catecholamine depletion and sympathomimetic amines may interfere with the hypotensive effect of guanadrel.

Precautions:
General: Salt and water retention may occur with the use of HYLOREL Tablets. In clinical studies major problems did not arise because of concomitant diuretic use. Patients with heart failure have not been studied on HYLOREL, but guanadrel could interfere with the adrenergic mechanisms that maintain compensation.

In patients with a history of peptic ulcer, which could be aggravated by a relative increase in parasympathetic tone, HYLOREL should be used cautiously.

HYLOREL has not been studied in patients with renal failure.

Information for patients: See **Warnings** section.
Drug interactions: See **Warnings** section.

Carcinogenesis, mutagenesis, impairment of fertility: No evidence of carcinogenic potential appeared in a 2-year mouse study of guanadrel sulfate. In a 22-month rat study, endometrial fibromatous polyps were observed at a dosage of 100 mg/kg per day. The polyps are common, spontaneous lesions of aged rats, and their relationship to drug therapy is unknown. Salmonella testing (Ames test) showed no evidence of mutagenic activity.

Pregnancy Category B: Teratogenic effects: Reproduction studies have been performed in rats and rabbits at doses up to 12 times the maximum recommended human dose and have revealed no evidence of impaired fertility or harm to the fetus due to guanadrel sulfate. There are, however, no adequate and well-controlled studies in pregnant women. Because animal reproduction studies are not always predictive, HYLOREL should be used in pregnant women only when the potential benefit outweighs the potential risk to mother and infant.

Nursing mothers: Whether guanadrel sulfate is excreted in human milk is not known, but because many drugs are excreted in human milk and because of the potential for serious adverse reactions in nursing infants from guanadrel, a decision should be made whether to discontinue nursing or discontinue the drug, taking into account the importance of the drug to the mother.

Pediatric Use: Safety and effectiveness in children have not been established.

Adverse Reactions: The adverse reaction data for guanadrel are derived principally from comparative long-term (6 months to 3 years) studies with guanethidine and methyldopa in which side effects were assessed through use of periodic questionnaires, a method that tends to give high adverse reaction rates. In the tables that follow, some of the adverse effects reported may not be drug-related, but in the absence of a placebo-treated group, these cannot be readily distinguished. Comparative results with two well-known drugs, guanethidine and methyldopa, should aid in interpretation of these adverse reaction rates.

The following table displays the frequency of side effects which are believed to be related to sympathetic blocking agents: orthostatic faintness, increased bowel movements and ejaculation disturbances for peripherally acting drugs such as guanadrel and drowsiness for centrally acting drugs such as methyldopa. The frequencies observed were generally higher during the first 8 weeks of therapy. Week 0 frequencies, which were recorded just prior to administration of the antihypertensive drugs while the patients were receiving diuretics, serve as a reference point. Frequency while on therapy is shown for the first 8 weeks and for weeks 9 to 52.

The following paragraph shows the incidence of reactions often associated with adrenergic neuron blockers as the percent of patients who reported the event at least once over the treatment periods of 6 months to 3 years. For such long-term studies these incidence rates of side effects, which are found often in untreated patients, tend to be high and accumulate with time. The incidence rates for two well-known comparison drugs, guanethidine and methyldopa, should aid in interpreting the high rates. It can be seen that the serious consequences of the orthostatic effect of guanadrel, such as syncope, were very uncommon.

1544 guanadrel, 330 guanethidine and 743 methyldopa patients were evaluated in comparison studies. The observed incidence rates of major drug related side effects for guanadrel, guanethidine and methyldopa, respectively, are as follows: orthostatic faintness: 49%, 48% 41%; other faintness: 47%, 45% 46%; increased bowel movements: 31%, 36%, 28%; ejaculation disturbances: 18%, 22%, 21%; impotence: 5.1% 7.2%, 12.2%; syncope: 0.4%, 2%, 0.3%; urine retention: 0.2%, 0%, 0%. Apart from these adverse effects, many others were reported. Relationship to therapy is less clear, although some (such as peripheral edema with all three drugs, depression with methyldopa) are in part drug related. All adverse effects reported in at least 1% of guanadrel patients are listed in the following table:
[See table on bottom next page].

Overdosage: Overdosage usually produces marked dizziness and blurred vision related to postural hypotension and may progress to syncope on standing. The patient should lie down until these symptoms subside.

If excessive hypotension occurs and persists despite conservative treatment, intensive therapy may be needed to support vital functions. A vasoconstrictor such as phenylephrine will ameliorate the effect of HYLOREL Tablets (guanadrel sulfate), but great care must be used because patients may be hypersensitive to such agents.

Dosage and Administration: As with other sympathetic suppressant drugs, the dose response to HYLOREL Tablets varies widely and must be adjusted for each patient until the therapeutic goal is achieved. With long-term therapy, some tolerance may occur and the dosage may have to be increased.

Because HYLOREL has a substantial orthostatic effect, monitoring both supine and standing pres-

Continued on next page

Pennwalt—Cont.

sures is essential, especially while dosage is being adjusted.

HYLOREL should be administered in divided doses. The usual starting dosage for treating hypertension is 10 mg per day, which can be given as 5 mg b.i.d. by breaking the 10 mg tablet. Because the half-life is approximately ten hours, the dosages should be adjusted weekly or monthly until blood pressure is controlled. Most patients will require daily dosage of the range of 20 to 75 mg usually in twice daily doses. For larger doses 3 or 4 times daily dosing may be needed.

Combination Therapy: HYLOREL Tablets have not been studied in combination with antihypertensive drugs other than thiazide diuretics.

How Supplied: HYLOREL Tablets are available as follows:

10 mg. scored elliptical tablets (light orange)
  Bottles of 100—NDC 0018-0787-71
25 mg. scored elliptical tablets (white)
  Bottles of 100—NDC 0018-0788-71

Caution: Federal law prohibits dispensing without a prescription.
Rev 4/21/83
Mkt by
PENNWALT CORP.
PRESCRIPTION DIVISION
Rochester, NY 14623
Shown in Product Identification Section, page 426

INFALYTE™
[in'fa-lit"]
Oral Electrolyte Replenisher Powder

The remarkable success of the diarrheal-disease program of the World Health Organization (WHO) has demonstrated that, even in the presence of vomiting which often accompanies diarrhea, oral rehydration therapy with a standard glucose-electrolyte solution is the most simple and effective way to:

1. restore water and electrolyte losses in patients of all ages, including newborns, with mild to moderate dehydration caused by acute diarrhea—and—
2. compensate for the losses during continuing diarrhea.

The sodium content of the oral rehydration solution recommended by WHO is designed to replace the large sodium losses seen in cholera. Physicians in developed countries where cholera rarely occurs have been hesitant to use the WHO formula feeling it might cause hypernatremia in patients with milder types of diarrhea. Infalyte contains 45% less sodium chloride than the WHO formula. Therefore, the sodium content of Infalyte in solution (50 mEq/L) is more in keeping with the fecal sodium losses which occur in mild to moderate diarrhea thereby reducing the possibility of inducing hypernatremia while retaining the effectiveness of the WHO formulation.[1]

In addition to its safety, simplicity and effectiveness, oral rehydration and maintenance with Infalyte in solution is less expensive and more comfortable for the patient than intravenous therapy. Since intravenous therapy usually requires hospitalization, oral rehydration could eliminate this additional expense and inconvenience in many cases.

In cases of severe dehydration requiring intravenous therapy, once the patient's blood pressure and pulse rate have stabilized and the estimated dehydration reduced to 5 to 8%, the patient may be switched from intravenous to oral replacement therapy for the completion of rehydration.

[1]Santosham M, Daum RS, Dillman L, et al: Oral rehydration therapy of infantile diarrhea. N Engl J Med 306: 1070-6, 1982.

Indications: When diluted as directed, Infalyte provides a solution suitable for oral administration to restore water and electrolytes lost in patients of all ages, including newborns, with mild to moderate dehydration due to acute diarrhea of mild to moderate severity. It is also indicated to maintain hydration and electrolyte balance as long as diarrhea continues.

Ingredients: D-glucose, sodium bicarbonate, potassium chloride and sodium chloride.

Infalyte

Body Weight		(A) Replacement to Correct Dehydration	(B) Maintenance to Prevent Dehydration
lb	kg	Approximate fl. oz.	Approximate fl. oz.
5	2.3	14	8
10	4.5	22	14
15	6.8	30	19
20	9.1	37	23
25	11.4	44	27
30	13.6	50	31
35	15.9	56	35
40	18.2	61	38

Composition of the Solution Made with Infalyte™

Ingredient	mEq/liter	mmol/liter
Sodium	50	50
Potassium	20	20
Chloride	40	40
Bicarbonate	30	30
Glucose		111

Osmolarity (mOsm/liter) 251
Each liter provides 77 calories

Preparation of Solution: Dissolve contents of 24 g. packet in 1 quart (32 fl. oz. or 960 ml) of drinking water. Dissolve contents of 6 g. packet in 8 fl. oz. of drinking water. Prepared solution should be covered, refrigerated and used within 24 hours.

Therapy:
Dosage Information for Infants and Young Children
(NOTE: Breast feeding may be continued during rehydration and maintenance therapy with Infalyte in solution even in the presence of vomiting.)

See appropriate column of the following table for the approximate volume of Infalyte in solution to be given. Lesser amounts would be needed by those also receiving breast milk.

Recommended Total Daily Intake of Infalyte in Solution for Infants and Young Children to:
(A) Replace fluid and electrolyte deficit in mild to moderate dehydration due to diarrhea of mild to moderate severity.
(B) Maintain fluid and electrolyte balance during continuing diarrhea:
[See table above].

1. It is recommended that no food or other liquids (except for breast feeding as noted above) be given during the first eight hours of rehydration therapy with Infalyte in solution. Infalyte in solution should be offered at frequent intervals.
2. After eight hours of Infalyte therapy, food may be offered even if diarrhea has not stopped. For those not being breast fed, cow's milk or commercial lactose-containing products prepared from cow's milk should not be given. Instead, a soy-based, lactose-free formula diluted 1 to 1 with water may be given.

Drug	Guanadrel	Methyldopa	Guanethidine
No. patients treated	1544	743	330
Event	%	%	%
Cardiovascular-Respiratory			
Chest Pain	27.9%	37.4%	27.3%
Coughing	26.9%	36.2%	21.5%
Palpitations	29.5%	35.0%	24.5%
Shortness of breath at rest	18.3%	22.3%	17.0%
Shortness of breath on exertion	45.9%	53.2%	48.8%
Central Nervous System-Special Senses			
Confusion	14.8%	22.6%	10.9%
Depression	1.9%	3.9%	1.8%
Drowsiness	44.6%	64.1%	28.5%
Headache	58.1%	69.0%	49.7%
Paresthesias	25.1%	35.1%	16.4%
Psychological problems	3.8%	4.8%	3.9%
Sleep disorders	2.1%	2.3%	2.7%
Visual disturbances	29.2%	35.3%	26.1%
Gastrointestinal			
Abdominal distress or pain	1.7%	1.9%	1.5%
Anorexia	18.7%	23.0%	17.6%
Constipation	21.0%	29.1%	20.3%
Dry mouth, dry throat	1.7%	4.0%	0.6%
Gas pain	32.0%	39.7%	29.4%
Glossitis	8.4%	10.8%	4.8%
Indigestion	23.7%	30.8%	18.5%
Nausea and/or vomiting	3.9%	4.8%	3.6%
Genitourinary			
Hematuria	2.3%	4.2%	2.1%
Nocturia	48.4%	52.4%	41.5%
Peripheral edema	28.6%	37.4%	22.7%
Urination urgency or frequency	33.6%	39.8%	27.6%
Miscellaneous			
Excessive weight gain	44.3%	53.7%	42.4%
Excessive weight loss	42.2%	51.1%	41.5%
Fatigue	63.6%	76.2%	57.0%
Musculoskeletal			
Aching limbs	42.9%	51.7%	33.9%
Backache or neckache	1.5%	1.1%	1.8%
Joint pain or inflammation	1.7%	2.0%	2.4%
Leg cramps during the day	21.1%	26.0%	20.0%
Leg cramps during the night	25.6%	32.6%	21.2%

Those capable of eating should be offered such things as rice cereal mixed with water, pureed fruit such as applesauce or bananas mixed with water, etc.
3. When diarrhea stops, discontinue Infalyte therapy. Avoid cow's milk and other lactose-containing liquids for the next 24 hours at which time the normal diet may be resumed.

Dosage Information for Older Children and Adults
See appropriate column of table below for approximate volume of Infalyte™ in solution to be given.
Recommended Total Daily Intake of Infalyte in solution for Older Children and Adults to:
(A) Replace fluid and electrolyte deficit in mild to moderate dehydration due to diarrhea of mild to moderate severity.
(B) Maintain fluid and electrolyte balance during continuing diarrhea.
[See table above].

1. It is recommended that no food or other liquids be given during the first eight hours of rehydration therapy with Infalyte in solution. Infalyte in solution should be taken at frequent intervals.
2. After eight hours of Infalyte therapy, age-appropriate food may be offered even if the diarrhea has not stopped. Cow's milk should be avoided until the diarrhea has stopped for 24 hours.
3. When diarrhea stops discontinue Infalyte therapy and resume normal diet. 8/82

Infalyte	(A) Replacement to Correct Dehydration	(B) Maintenance to Prevent Dehydration
Children 4 to 12 years old	Approximate amount 2 to 3 quarts	Approximate amount 1 to 2 quarts
Older children and adults	3 to 4 quarts	2 to 3 quarts

IONAMIN®
[i″on'uh-min]
(phentermine resin)

Description: Ionamin '15' and Ionamin '30' contain 15 mg. and 30 mg. respectively of phentermine as the cationic exchange resin complex. Phentermine is α, α-dimethyl phenylethylamine (phenyl-tertiary-butylamine).
Actions: Ionamin is a sympathomimetic amine with pharmacologic activity similar to the prototype drug of this class used in obesity, amphetamine (d- and dl-amphetamine). Actions include central nervous system stimulation and elevation of blood pressure. Tachyphylaxis and tolerance have been demonstrated with all drugs of this class in which this phenomena have been looked for.
Drugs of this class used in obesity are commonly known as "anorectics" or "anorexigenics." It has not been established, however, that the action of such drugs in treating obesity is primarily one of appetite suppression. Other central nervous system actions, or metabolic effects may be involved.
Adult obese subjects instructed in dietary management and treated with "anorectic" drugs, lose more weight on the average than those treated with placebo and diet, as determined in relatively short-term clinical trials.
The magnitude of increased weight loss of drug-treated patients over placebo-treated patients is only a fraction of a pound a week. The rate of weight loss is greatest in the first weeks of therapy for both drug and placebo subjects and tends to decrease in succeeding weeks. The possible origins of the increased weight loss due to the various drug effects are not established. The amount of weight loss associated with the use of an "anorectic" drug varies from trial to trial, and the increased weight loss appears to be related in part to variables other than the drugs prescribed, such as the physician-investigator, the population treated, and the diet prescribed. Studies do not permit conclusions as to the relative importance of the drug and non-drug factors on weight loss.
The natural history of obesity is measured in years, whereas the studies cited are restricted to a few weeks or months duration; thus, the total impact of drug-induced weight loss over that of diet alone must be considered clinically limited.
The bioavailability of Ionamin has been studied in humans in which blood levels of phentermine were measured by a gas-chromatography method. Blood levels obtained with the 15 mg. and 30 mg. resin complex formulations indicated slower absorption with a reduced but prolonged peak concentration and without a significant difference in prolongation of blood levels when compared with the same doses of phentermine hydrochloride. The clinical significance of these differences is not known. In clinical trials establishing the efficacy of Ionamin, a single daily dose produced an effect comparable to that produced by other regimens of "anorectic" drug therapy.
Indication: Ionamin is indicated in the management of exogenous obesity as a short-term (a few weeks) adjunct in a regimen of weight reduction based on caloric restriction. The limited usefulness of agents of this class (see ACTIONS) should be measured against possible risk factors inherent in their use such as those described below.
Contraindications: Advanced arteriosclerosis, symptomatic cardiovascular disease, moderate to severe hypertension, hyperthyroidism, known hypersensitivity, or idiosyncrasy to the sympathomimetic amines, glaucoma.
Agitated states.
Patients with a history of drug abuse.
During or within 14 days following the administration of monoamine oxidase inhibitors (hypertensive crises may result).
Warnings: If tolerance to the "anorectic" effect develops, the recommended dose should not be exceeded in an attempt to increase the effect: rather, the drug should be discontinued.
Ionamin may impair the ability of the patient to engage in potentially hazardous activities such as operating machinery or driving a motor vehicle; the patient should therefore be cautioned accordingly.
When using CNS active agents, consideration must always be given to the possibility of adverse interactions with alcohol.
Drug Dependence: Ionamin is related chemically and pharmacologically to amphetamine (d- and dl- amphetamine) and other stimulant drugs that have been extensively abused. The possibility of abuse of Ionamin should be kept in mind when evaluating the desirability of including a drug as part of a weight reduction program. Abuse of amphetamine (d- and dl- amphetamine) and related drugs may be associated with intense psychological dependence and severe social dysfunction. There are reports of patients who have increased the dosage of some of these drugs to many times that recommended. Abrupt cessation following prolonged high dosage administration results in extreme fatigue and mental depression; changes are also noted on the sleep EEG. Manifestations of chronic intoxication with anorectic drugs include severe dermatoses, marked insomnia, irritability, hyperactivity, and personality changes. The most severe manifestation of chronic intoxications is psychosis, often clinically indistinguishable from schizophrenia.
Usage in Pregnancy: Safe use in pregnancy has not been established. Use of Ionamin by women who are or may become pregnant requires that the potential benefit be weighed against the possible hazard to mother and infant.
Usage in Children: Ionamin is not recommended for use in children under 12 years of age.
Precautions: Caution is to be exercised in prescribing Ionamin for patients with even mild hypertension. Insulin requirements in diabetes mellitus may be altered in association with the use of Ionamin and the concomitant dietary regimen. Ionamin may decrease the hypotensive effect of adrenergic neuron blocking drugs.
The least amount feasible should be prescribed or dispensed at one time in order to minimize the possibility of overdosage.
Adverse Reactions:
Cardiovascular: Palpitation, tachycardia, elevation of blood pressure.
Central Nervous System: Overstimulation, restlessness, dizziness, insomnia, euphoria, dysphoria, tremor, headache; rarely psychotic episodes at recommended doses with some drugs in this class.
Gastrointestinal: Dryness of the mouth, unpleasant taste, diarrhea, constipation, other gastrointestinal disturbances.
Allergic: Urticaria.
Endocrine: Impotence, changes in libido.
Dosage and Administration: One capsule daily, before breakfast or 10–14 hours before retiring. For individuals exhibiting greater drug responsiveness, Ionamin '15' will usually suffice. Ionamin '30' is recommended for less responsive patients. Ionamin is not recommended for use in children under 12 years of age.
Overdosage: Manifestations of acute overdosage may include restlessness, tremor, hyperreflexia, rapid respiration, confusion, assaultiveness, hallucinations, panic states.
Fatigue and depression usually follow the central stimulation.
Cardiovascular effects include arrhythmias, hypertension, or hypotension and circulatory collapse. Gastrointestinal symptoms include nausea, vomiting, diarrhea, and abdominal cramps. Overdosage of pharmacologically similar compounds has resulted in fatal poisoning, usually terminating in convulsions and coma.
Management of acute Ionamin intoxication is largely symptomatic and includes lavage and sedation with a barbiturate. Experience with hemodialysis or peritoneal dialysis is inadequate to permit recommendation in this regard. Intravenous phentolamine (Regitine) has been suggested on pharmacologic grounds for possible acute, severe hypertension, if this complicates overdosage.
How Supplied: Two strengths: Ionamin (phentermine resin) 15 mg. (NDC 0018-0903) yellow and gray capsules; Ionamin (phentermine resin) 30 mg. (NDC 0018-0904) yellow capsules. Available on prescription only. Stock bottles of 100 and 400.
Rev 7/83
Shown in Product Identification Section, page 426

Antitussive
TUSSIONEX®
[tus'e-uh-nex]
(Resin Complexes of Hydrocodone and Phenyltoloxamine)

TUSSIONEX® Capsules, Suspension and Tablets
Composition: Each capsule, teaspoonful (5 ml.) or tablet contains 5 mg. hydrocodone (*Warning:* may be habit-forming), and 10 mg. phenyltoloxamine as cationic resin complexes.
Effects: An effective antitussive which acts for approximately 12 hours.
Dosage: *Adults:* 1 teaspoonful (5 ml.), capsule or tablet every 8-12 hours. May be adjusted to individual requirements. *Children:* Under 1 year: ¼ teaspoonful every 12 hours. From 1-5 years: ½ teaspoonful every 12 hours. Over 5 years: 1 teaspoonful every 12 hours.
Side Effects: Negligible, but when encountered may include mild constipation, nausea, facial pruritus, drowsiness, which disappear with adjustment of dose or discontinuance of treatment.
Precaution: In young children the respiratory center is especially susceptible to the depressant action of narcotic cough suppressants. Benefit to risk ratio should be carefully considered especially in children with respiratory embarrassment. Estimation of dosage relative to the age and weight of the child is of great importance.

Continued on next page

Pennwalt—Cont.

Overdosage: Immediately evacuate the stomach. Respiratory depression, if any, can be counteracted by respiratory stimulants. Convulsions, sometimes seen in children, can be controlled by intravenous administration of short-acting barbiturates. Hypothermia can be controlled by the usual supportive methods.

How Supplied: Tussionex Suspension, neutral in taste, golden color; 16 oz. and 900 ml. bottles. Tussionex Tablets, light brown, scored; bottles of 100. Tussionex Capsules, green and white; bottles of 50. A prescription for 2 oz. of the Suspension, or 12 Capsules or Tablets, constitutes a 6 day supply in the average case.

Rev 11/79

Diuretic, Antihypertensive
ZAROXOLYN® ℞
[zar″ox′uh-lin]
(Metolazone)

Each ZAROXOLYN Tablet contains 2½, 5, or 10 mg of metolazone.

Description: ZAROXOLYN (metolazone) has the molecular formula $C_{16}H_{16}ClN_3O_3S$ and a molecular weight of 365.84 and its chemical name is 7-chloro-1,2,3,4-tetrahydro-2-methyl-4-oxo-3-o-tolyl-6-quinazolinesulfonamide. Metolazone is only sparingly soluble in water, but more soluble in plasma, blood, alkali, and organic solvents.

Actions: ZAROXOLYN (metolazone) is a diuretic/saluretic/antihypertensive drug. The action of ZAROXOLYN results in an interference with the renal tubular mechanism of electrolyte reabsorption. The mechanism of this action is unknown. ZAROXOLYN acts primarily to inhibit sodium reabsorption at the cortical diluting site and in the proximal convoluted tubule. Sodium and chloride ions are excreted in approximately equivalent amounts. The increased delivery of sodium to the distal-tubular exchange site may result in increased potassium excretion.

DRUG INTERACTION STUDIES: In animals pretreated with ZAROXOLYN, the drug did not alter the characteristic effect of heparin on clotting time nor protamine antagonism; dicumarol on prothrombin time nor Vitamin K antagonism; the response of guanethidine, reserpine and hydralazine to cardiovascular parameters nor the pressor response of the subsequent dose of norepinephrine.

ZAROXOLYN and furosemide, administered concurrently have produced marked diuresis in some patients where edema or ascites was refractory to treatment with maximum recommended doses of these or other diuretics administered alone. The mechanism of this interaction is not known.

In clinical usage, ZAROXOLYN does not inhibit carbonic anhydrase. Its proximal action has been evidenced in humans by increased excretion of phosphate and magnesium ions, by markedly increased fractional excretion of sodium in patients with severely compromised glomerular filtration, and in animals by the results of micropuncture studies. Decrease in calcium ion excretion has not been noted.

At maximum therapeutic dosage ZAROXOLYN is approximately equal to thiazide diuretics in its diuretic potency. However, ZAROXOLYN may produce diuresis in patients with glomerular filtration rates below 20 ml/min.

When ZAROXOLYN is given, diuresis and saluresis usually begin within one hour and persist for 12 to 24 hours depending on dosage. Maximum effect occurs about two hours after administration. At the higher recommended dosages, effect may be prolonged beyond 24 hours. *A single daily dose is recommended.* For most patients the duration of effect can be varied by adjusting the daily dose. The prolonged duration of action of ZAROXOLYN is attributed to protein-binding and enterohepatic recycling. A small amount of ZAROXOLYN is metabolized and the fraction so changed is nontoxic. The primary route of excretion is renal.

The mechanism whereby diuretics function in the control of hypertension is unknown; both renal and extra-renal actions may be involved. An antihypertensive effect may be seen as early as three to four days after ZAROXOLYN has been started. Administration for three to four weeks, however, is usually required for optimum antihypertensive effect.

Indications: ZAROXOLYN (metolazone) is indicated in the management of hypertension either as the sole therapeutic agent or to enhance the effectiveness of other antihypertensive drugs in the more severe forms of hypertension.

ZAROXOLYN (metolazone) is indicated for the treatment of salt and water retention including
—edema accompanying congestive heart failure
—edema accompanying renal diseases, including the nephrotic syndrome, and states of diminished renal function

Usage in Pregnancy

The routine use of diuretics in an otherwise healthy woman is inappropriate and exposes mother and fetus to unnecessary hazard. Diuretics do not prevent development of toxemia of pregnancy, and there is no satisfactory evidence that they are useful in the treatment of developed toxemia.

Edema during pregnancy may arise from pathological causes or from the physiologic and mechanical consequences of pregnancy. ZAROXOLYN is indicated in pregnancy when edema is due to pathologic causes, just as it is in the absence of pregnancy (however, see Warnings, below). Dependent edema in pregnancy, resulting from restriction of venous return by the expanded uterus, is properly treated through elevation of the lower extremities and use of support hose; use of diuretics to lower intravascular volume in this case is illogical and unnecessary. There is hypervolemia during normal pregnancy which is harmful to neither the fetus nor the mother (in the absence of cardiovascular disease), but which is associated with edema, including generalized edema, in the majority of pregnant women. If this edema produces discomfort, increased recumbency will often provide relief. In rare instances, this edema may cause extreme discomfort which is not relieved by rest. In these cases, a short course of diuretics may provide relief and may be appropriate.

Contraindications: Anuria.

Hepatic coma or pre-coma; known allergy or hypersensitivity to ZAROXOLYN (metolazone).

Warnings: While not reported to date, cross-allergy theoretically may occur when ZAROXOLYN (metolazone) is given to patients known to be allergic to sulfonamide-derived drugs, thiazides, or quinethazone.

Hypokalemia may occur, with consequent weakness, cramps, and cardiac dysrhythmias. Hypokalemia is a particular hazard in digitalized patients; dangerous or fatal arrhythmias may be precipitated.

Azotemia and hyperuricemia may be noted or precipitated during the administration of ZAROXOLYN. (Infrequently, gouty attacks have been reported in persons with history of gout.)

If azotemia and oliguria worsen during treatment of patients with severe renal disease, ZAROXOLYN should be discontinued.

Until additional data have been obtained, ZAROXOLYN is not recommended for patients in the pediatric age group.

Unusually large or prolonged effects on volume and electrolytes may result when ZAROXOLYN and furosemide are administered concurrently. It is recommended that concurrent administration of these diuretics for treatment of resistant edema be started under hospital conditions in order to provide for adequate monitoring.

When ZAROXOLYN is used with other antihypertensive drugs, particular care must be taken, especially during initial therapy. Dosage of other antihypertensive agents, especially the ganglionic blockers, should be reduced.

ZAROXOLYN may be given with a potassium-sparing diuretic when indicated. In this circumstance, diuresis may be potentiated and dosages should be reduced. Potassium retention and hyperkalemia may result; the serum potassium should be determined frequently. Potassium supplementation is contraindicated when a potassium-sparing diuretic is given.

Usage in Pregnancy

ZAROXOLYN crosses the placental barrier and appears in cord blood. The use of ZAROXOLYN in pregnant women requires that the anticipated benefit be weighed against possible hazards to the fetus. These hazards include fetal or neonatal jaundice, thrombocytopenia, and possibly other adverse reactions which have occurred in the adult.

Nursing Mothers

ZAROXOLYN appears in breast milk. If use of the drug is deemed essential, the patient should stop nursing.

Precautions: Periodic determination of serum electrolytes to detect possible electrolyte imbalance should be performed at appropriate intervals. Blood urea nitrogen, uric acid, and glucose levels should be assessed at intervals during diuretic therapy.

All patients receiving ZAROXOLYN (metolazone) therapy should be observed for clinical signs of fluid and/or electrolyte imbalance; namely, hyponatremia, hypochloremic alkalosis, and hypokalemia. Serum and urine electrolyte determinations are particularly important when the patient is vomiting excessively or receiving parenteral fluids. Medication such as digitalis may also influence serum electrolytes. Warning signs, irrespective of cause, are: dryness of mouth, thirst, weakness, lethargy, drowsiness, restlessness, muscle pains or cramps, muscular fatigue, hypotension, oliguria, tachycardia, and gastrointestinal disturbances such as nausea and vomiting.

The serum potassium should be determined at regular intervals, and potassium supplementation instituted whenever indicated. Hypokalemia will be more common in association with intensive or prolonged diuretic therapy, with concomitant steroid or ACTH therapy, and with inadequate electrolyte intake.

While not reported to date for ZAROXOLYN, related diuretics have increased responsiveness to tubocurarine and decreased arterial responsiveness to norepinephrine. Accordingly, it may be advisable to discontinue ZAROXOLYN three days before elective surgery.

Caution should be observed when administering ZAROXOLYN to hyperuricemic or gouty patients. ZAROXOLYN exerts minimal effects on glucose metabolism; insulin requirements may be affected in diabetics, and hyperglycemia and glycosuria may occur in patients with latent diabetes.

Chloride deficit and hypochloremic alkalosis may occur. In patients with severe edema accompanying cardiac failure or renal disease, a low-salt syndrome may be produced; hot weather and a low-salt diet will contribute.

Caution should be observed when administering ZAROXOLYN to patients with severely impaired renal function. As most of the drug is excreted by the renal route, cumulative effects may be seen in this circumstance.

Orthostatic hypotension may occur, this may be potentiated by alcohol, barbiturates, narcotics, or concurrent therapy with other antihypertensive drugs.

While not reported for ZAROXOLYN, use of other diuretics has been associated on rare occasions with pathological changes in the parathyroid glands and with hypercalcemia. This possibility should be kept in mind with clinical use of ZAROXOLYN.

Adverse Reactions: Adverse reactions encountered during therapy with potent medications should be considered in two groups: those that represent extensions of the expected pharmacologic actions of the drug, and those which are pharmacologically unexpected, idiosyncratic, specially toxic, due to allergy or hypersensitivity, or due to unexplained causes.

For ZAROXOLYN (metolazone), adverse reactions constituting extensions of the expected pharmacologic actions of this potent diuretic/saluretic/antihypertensive drug may include:

Gastrointestinal reactions: constipation.
Central nervous system reactions: syncope, dizziness, drowsiness.
Cardiovascular reactions: orthostatic hypotension, excessive volume depletion, hemoconcentration, venous thrombosis.
Other reactions: dryness of the mouth, symptomatic and asymptomatic hypokalemia, hyponatremia, hypochloremia; hypochloremic alkalosis, hypophosphatemia, hyperuricemia, hyperglycemia, glycosuria, increase in BUN or creatinine, fatigue, muscle cramps or spasm, weakness, restlessness sometimes resulting in insomnia.
In the second classification, adverse reactions to ZAROXOLYN may include:
Gastrointestinal reactions: nausea, vomiting, anorexia, diarrhea, abdominal bloating, epigastric distress, intrahepatic cholestatic jaundice, hepatitis.
Central nervous system reactions: vertigo, headache, paresthesias.
Hematologic reactions: leukopenia, aplastic anemia.
Dermatologic-hypersensitivity reactions: urticaria and other skin rashes, purpura, necrotizing angiitis (cutaneous vasculitis).
Cardiovascular reactions: palpitation, chest pain.
Other reactions: chills, acute gouty attacks, transient blurred vision.
Adverse reactions which have occurred with other diuretics, but which have not been reported to date for ZAROXOLYN (metolazone), include: pancreatitis, xanthopsia, agranulocytosis, thrombocytopenia, and photosensitivity. These reactions should be considered as possible occurrences with clinical usage of ZAROXOLYN.
Whenever adverse reactions are moderate or severe, ZAROXOLYN dosage should be reduced or therapy withdrawn.
Dosage and Administration: Therapy should be individualized according to patient response. Programs of therapy with ZAROXOLYN (metolazone) shbuld be titrated to gain a maximal initial therapeutic response, and to determine the minimal dose possible to maintain that therapeutic response.
ZAROXOLYN is a potent drug with a prolonged, 12-to-24-hour duration of action. When an initially-desired therapeutic effect has been obtained, it is ordinarily advisable to reduce the dosage of ZAROXOLYN to a lower maintenance level. The time interval required for the initial higher-dosage regimen may vary from days in edematous states to three or four weeks in the treatment of elevated blood pressure.
The daily dosage depends on the severity of each patient's condition, his sodium intake, and his responsiveness. Therefore, dosage adjustment is usually necessary during the course of therapy. A decision to reduce the daily dosage of ZAROXOLYN from a higher induction level to a lower maintenance level should be based on the results of thorough clinical and laboratory evaluations. If antihypertensive drugs or diuretics are given concurrently with ZAROXOLYN, careful dosage adjustment may be necessary.
Usual single daily dosage schedules
Suitable initial dosages will usually fall in the ranges given:
Mild to moderate essential hypertension: ZAROXOLYN 2½–5 mg. once daily
Edema of cardiac failure: ZAROXOLYN 5–10 mg. once daily
Edema of renal disease: ZAROXOLYN 5–20 mg. once daily
For patients with congestive cardiac failure who tend to experience paroxysmal nocturnal dyspnea, it is usually advisable to employ a dosage near the upper end of the range, to ensure prolongation of diuresis and saluresis for a full 24-hour period.
How Supplied: ZAROXOLYN (metolazone) is provided as: pink 2½ mg tablets, blue 5 mg tablets, and yellow 10 mg tablets; in package sizes of 100, 500, 1000 and unit-dose strip packages of 100 (10 × 10's).

Rev 8/83
Shown in Product Identification Section, page 426

Persōn & Covey, Inc.
616 ALLEN AVENUE
GLENDALE, CA 91201

A.C.N®   OTC
Water-miscible Vitamin A, C, and Niacinamide Tablets
Description:
Each tablet contains: % of U.S. RDA*
Vitamin A .... 25,000 I.U.   500
Ascorbic Acid .... 250 mg   417
Niacinamide .... 25 mg   125
*Percentage of U.S. Recommended Daily Allowance.
Indication: For use as a dietary supplement.
Dosage: One tablet daily as a dietary supplement. For adults and children 4 or more years of age.
Warnings: Keep all medication out of the reach of children. Keep in tight, light-resistant container.
How Supplied: In bottles of 100 tablets.
NDC 0096-0014-11

DHS™ Conditioning Rinse   OTC
DHS Conditioning Rinse is specially formulated for dermatological hair care.
DHS Conditioning Rinse helps control static electricity, eliminate tangles, mend split ends and improve elasticity.
DHS Conditioning Rinse helps make hair easier to comb and manage while adding lustre and body.
Directions: Shampoo and rinse well. (We suggest DHS™ Shampoo.) Then apply a generous amount of DHS Conditioning Rinse and work evenly through the hair to the ends for 60 seconds. Rinse with warm water for 30 seconds.
Caution: For external use only. Keep out of the reach of children. Avoid contact with the eyes.
Contains: Purified Water, Glyceryl Stearate, Quaternium-31, Panthenol, Cetearyl Alcohol, Dimethicone Copolyol, Fragrance, FD&C Yellow #6.
How Supplied: 8 fluid ounce plastic bottles with easy to use dispenser.
NDC #0096-0726-08

DHS™ Shampoo   OTC
Dermatological Hair and Scalp Shampoo
DHS™ contains a unique blend of special cleansing agents that provide a luxurious lather which cleans the hair and scalp.
DHS™ conditioners reduce the need for after rinses and leave the hair lustrously clean.
DHS™ is especially formulated for pH balance. DHS may be used daily.
Directions: (1) Wet hair thoroughly; apply DHS, lather and rinse. Reapply DHS, later and rinse again. Repeat as necessary or as directed by your physician.
Caution: For external use only. Keep out of the reach of children. Avoid contact with the eyes.
Contents: purified water, TEA-lauryl sulfate, sodium-chloride, PEG-8 distearate, cocamide DEA, cocamide MEA, fragrance and FD&C yellow #6.
How Supplied: 8 fluid and 16 fluid ounce plastic bottles with easy to use dispenser.
NDC 0096-0727-08
NDC 0096-0727-16

DHS™ Tar Shampoo   OTC
Dermatological Hair and Scalp Shampoo
DHS™ Tar Shampoo aids in the control of the scaling of seborrhea (dandruff) and psoriasis of the scalp.
Directions: (1) Wet hair thoroughly; apply a liberal quantity of DHS™ Tar Shampoo and massage into a lather. (2) Rinse thoroughly and repeat application. (3) Allow lather to remain on scalp for about 5 minutes. (4) Use DHS Tar Shampoo once or twice weekly or as directed by your physician.
Caution: Avoid contact with eyes. In case of contact wash out with water. If irritation occurs, discontinue use and consult physician.
Warning: Keep out of the reach of children. For external use only.
DHS™ Tar Shampoo contains: Tar, equivalent to 0.5% Coal Tar U.S.P., TEA-lauryl sulfate, purified water, sodium chloride, PEG-8 disterate, cocamide DEA, cocamide MEA.
How Supplied: 4 and 8 fluid ounce plastic bottles with easy to use dispenser.
NDC 0096-0728-04
NDC 0096-0728-08

DHS™ Zinc Dandruff Shampoo   OTC
2% Zinc Pyrithione
DHS™ Zinc Shampoo aids in the control of dandruff/seborrheic dermatitis of the scalp.
Directions: Shake well before using. (1) Wet hair thoroughly; apply a liberal quantity of DHS™ Zinc and massage into a lather. (2) Rinse thoroughly and repeat application. (3) Allow lather to remain on scalp for about 5 minutes. (4) Use DHS Zinc at least twice weekly for the first two weeks, then regularly thereafter, or as directed by physician.
Caution: Avoid contact with eyes. In case of contact, wash out with water. If irritation occurs, discontinue use and consult physician.
Warning: Keep out of the reach of children. For external use only.
DHS™ Zinc contains: 2% zinc pyrithione, purified water, TEA-lauryl sulfate, PEG-8 distearate, sodium chloride, cocamide DEA, cocamide MEA, magnesium aluminum silicate, hydroxypropyl methylcellulose, fragrance, and FD&C yellow #6.
How Supplied: 6 and 12 fluid ounce plastic bottles.
NDC 0096-0729-06
NDC 0096-0729-12

DRYSOL™   ℞
A Solution of:
Aluminum Chloride (Hexahydrate) 20% w/v in Anhydrous Ethyl Alcohol (S.D. Alcohol 40) 93% v/v.
Indication: An aid in the management of hyperhidrosis.
Directions: Apply Drysol™ to the affected area once a day, only at bedtime. To help prevent irritation, the area should be completely dry prior to application. Do not apply Drysol to broken, irritated or recently shaved skin.
For Maximum Effect: Your doctor may instruct you to cover the treated area with saran wrap held in place by a snug fitting "T" or body shirt, mitten or sock. (Never hold saran in place with tape.) Wash the treated area the following morning. Excessive sweating may be stopped after two or more treatments. Thereafter, apply Drysol™ once or twice weekly or as needed.
Notice: Drysol™ will probably produce a burning or prickling sensation. Keep cap tightly closed when not in use to prevent evaporation.
Warning: For external use only. Keep out of the reach of children. Avoid contact with the eyes. If irritation or sensitization occurs, discontinue use or consult with a physician. Drysol™ may be harmful to certain fabrics. Keep away from open flame.
Package: 37.5 cc polyethylene bottle. NDC 0096-0707-37.
35 cc bottle with convenient Dab-O-Matic™ applicator head. NDC 0096-0707-35.
Assembly Instructions: (For 35cc Dab-O-Matic™ bottle only.) Remove and discard original cap. Push special Dab-O-Matic applicator into bottle opening using the white cap as a holder. Screw cap down to seat applicator.
Patient instruction sheets are available upon request.

Continued on next page

Person & Covey—Cont.

ENISYL™ 500 Tablets   OTC
ENISYL™ 334 Tablets
Lysine Hydrochloride
(L-Lysine Monohydrochloride)

Composition: Each tablet contains Lysine 334 mg and 500 mg respectively (from the hydrochloride).
Indication: For use as a dietary supplement.
Dosage: Adults: one to three tablets daily as a dietary supplement.
Actions: Improves utilization of vegetable proteins such as rice, wheat, corn, etc.
Warnings: Keep out of the reach of children. Keep in tight, light-resistant container.
How Supplied: In bottles of 100 and 250 tablets. 334 and 500 mg.

| NDC 0096-0777-11 | NDC 0096-0777-52 |
| NDC 0096-0778-11 | NDC 0096-0778-52 |

SOLBAR® PF (PABA FREE)   OTC
SPF 10

PABA FREE SOLBAR PF is specially formulated for extra protection from the sun's burning rays. Oxybenzone and Dioxybenzone give superior protection from long wave ultraviolet (UVA) which is particularly important to the photosensitive or photoallergic person.
Fragrance free-alcohol free
Liberal and regular use of this product over the years may help reduce the chance of premature aging of the skin and skin cancer.
Directions: Apply liberally to all exposed areas before sun exposure. To insure the greater benefit reapply after swimming or excessive sweating.
Caution: For external use only, not to be swallowed. If irritation or sensitization occurs, discontinue use and consult a physician. Avoid contact with the eyes. Keep this and all drugs out of the reach of children.
Contains: Oxybenzone USP 5%, Dioxybenzone USP 2%, Purified Water, Isopropyl Myristate, PPG-20 Lanolin Ether, PPG-2 Lanolin Ether, Glyceryl Stearate, PEG-100 Stearate, Carbomer 934, PEG-15 Cocamine, Sodium Hydroxide, Methylparaben Propylparaben.
How Supplied: Packaged in 2½ oz. plastic tube. NDC 0096-0682-75

SOLBAR® PLUS 15   OTC
Sun Protectant Cream

Solbar® Plus 15: Specially formulated to provide ultra protection from the sun's burning and tanning rays. Provides a high degree of sunburn protection for sun sensitive skin and fair skinned persons, blondes, brunettes and redheads.
Fragrant-free formula ... contains no drying alcohol.
Directions: Smooth evenly on all exposed skin. To ensure maximum protection reapply after swimming or exercise.
Caution: For external use only. If irritation or sensitization occurs discontinue use and consult a physician. Avoid contact with the eyes. Keep this and all drugs out of the reach of children. Solbar® Plus 15 contains: Oxybenzone USP 6%, Oxtyl Dimethyl PABA 6%, Purified Water, Isopropyl Palmitate, PPG-20 Lanolin Ether, PPG-2 Lanolin Ether, Glyceryl Stearate, PEG-100 Stearate, Carbomer 934, PEG-15 Cocamine, Sodium Hydroxide, Methylparaben, Propylparaben.
How Supplied: 4 ounce plastic tube.
NDC 0096-0681-04

XERAC®   OTC
(alcohol gel)

Composition:
Isopropyl Alcohol..................................44%
Microcrystalline Sulfur..........................4%
Effects: A medicated antiseptic gel to promote drying and peeling of the skin. An aid in the management of acne. Invisible when applied to the skin.
Directions: Apply a thin film to affected areas one to three times daily, or as directed by physician.
Precautions: Avoid overuse. If undue skin irritation develops or becomes excessive, discontinue use and consult physician. Avoid contact with eyes. Keep this and all medication out of the reach of children. For eternal use only.
How Supplied: 45 g (1-½ oz.) plastic tube.
NDC 0096-0787-45

XERAC AC™   ℞
Aluminum Chloride Hexahydrate in Anhydrous Ethanol

CAUTION: FEDERAL LAW PROHIBITS DISPENSING WITHOUT PRESCRIPTION.
Description: A solution of Aluminum Chloride (Hexahydrate) 6.25% (w/v) in Anhydrous Ethyl Alcohol (S.D. Alcohol 40) 96% (v/v).
Indication: For topical application as an antiperspirant (anhidrotic).
Directions: Apply Xerac AC* to the axillae at bedtime or as directed by physician. Application of Xerac AC is facilitated by the special swab applicator head of the Xerac AC dispenser. To help prevent irritation, the area should be completely dry prior to application. Do not apply Xerac AC to broken or irritated skin. Keep container tightly closed.
Adverse Reactions: Transient stinging or itching may occur. It is not evidence of contact sensitivity and may be prevented or reduced by applying Xerac AC* only to skin which is completely dry or by removing the solution with soap and water.
Warning: For External Use Only. Some users of this product will experience skin irritation. If this occurs, discontinue use. Avoid contact with the eyes. This product may be harmful to certain fabrics. Keep the container tightly closed when not in use to prevent evaporation. Keep this and all medication out of the reach of children.
Assembly Instructions: Remove and discard original cap. Push special Dab-O-Matic™ applicator into bottle opening using the white cap as a holder. Screw cap down to seat applicator.
How Supplied: Xerac AC*—35 and 60 cc bottle with special swab applicator head.
NDC 0096-0709-35.
NDC 0096-0709-60

XERAC BP5™   OTC
XERAC BP10™   OTC
(benzoyl peroxide water gel)

Composition: Xerac BP5™ contains 5% Benzoyl Peroxide, Laureth-4, Carbomer-934, Triethanolamine, Disodium EDTA and Purified Water.
Xerac BP10™ contains 10% Benzoyl Peroxide, Laureth-4, Carbomer-934, Triethanolamine, Disodium EDTA and Purified Water.
Indication: For the treatment of acne.
Xerac BP10™ helps dry and clear acne blemishes, reduce blackheads and prevent the development of new acne lesions.
Directions: Cleanse the skin thoroughly before applying medication. Cover the entire affected area with a thin layer one to three times daily. Because excessive drying of the skin may occur start with one application daily, then gradually increase to two or three times daily or as directed by a physician.
Caution: Persons with very sensitive skin or known allergy to benzoyl peroxide should not use this medication. If uncomfortable irritation or excessive dryness and/or peeling occurs, reduce frequency of use or dosage. If excessive itching, redness, burning, or swelling occurs, discontinue use. If these symptoms persist, consult a doctor promptly. Keep away from eyes, lips and other mucous membranes. May bleach hair or dyed fabrics.
Warning: For external use only. Keep this and all drugs out of the reach of children. Other topical acne medications should not be used at the same time as this medication.
How Supplied: 45 g (1.5 oz.) and 90 g (3 oz.) plastic tubes.
45 g tubes
Xerac BP5™ - NDC 0096-0790-45
Xerac BP10™ - NDC 0096-0791-45
90 g tubes
Xerac BP5™ - NDC 0096-0790-90
Xerac BP10™ - NDC 0096-0791-90

Personal Care Products Division
RICHARDSON-VICKS INC.
TEN WESTPORT ROAD
WILTON, CT 06897

CLEARASIL® Adult Care™
(Sulfur/Resorcinol)
(See PDR For Nonprescription Drugs)

CLEARASIL® Super Strength Acne Treatment Cream
(10% Benzoyl Peroxide)
Vanishing and Tinted
(See PDR For Nonprescription Drugs)

CLEARASIL® 5% Benzoyl Peroxide Lotion Acne Treatment
(See PDR For Nonprescription Drugs)

CLEARASIL® Pore Deep Cleanser
(Salicylic Acid 0.5%)
(See PDR For Nonprescription Drugs)

DENQUEL® Sensitive Teeth Toothpaste
Desensitizing Dentifrice
(See PDR For Nonprescription Drugs)

TOPEX® 10% Benzoyl Peroxide Lotion Buffered* Acne Medication
*With special emollients to help prevent the overdrying effects of benzoyl peroxide
(See PDR For Nonprescription Drugs)

Pfipharmecs Division
PFIZER INC.
235 EAST 42ND STREET
NEW YORK, NY 10017

Pfipharmecs is a division of Pfizer Inc. which provides economical distribution of a line of time honored products and certain over-the-counter products to community and hospital pharmacists. These products include those listed here. Full color identification photographs of selected products can be found in the Product Identification Section.

PRODUCT IDENTIFICATION CODES
To provide quick and positive identification of Pfipharmecs Division products, we have imprinted the product identification number of the National Drug Code on tablets and capsules.
In order that you may quickly identify a product by its code number, we have compiled below a numerical list of code numbers of prescription products with their corresponding product names.

Product Identification Code	NUMERICAL PRODUCT INDEX Product
010	Bacitracin Sterile Powder 50,000 units/vial
050	Polymyxin B Sulfate Sterile 500,000 units/vial
051	Pfizerpen for Injection (penicillin G potassium) 1,000,000 units/vial

052	Pfizerpen for Injection (penicillin G potassium) 5,000,000 units/vial
053	Pfizerpen for Injection (penicillin G potassium) 20,000,000 units/vial
054	Pfizerpen-AS Aqueous Suspension (pencillin G procaine) 3,000,000 units/vial
062	Streptomycin Sulfate 1 gm/vial
063	Streptomycin Sulfate 5 gm/vial
067	Terra-Cortril Ophthalmic Suspension (oxytetracycline HCl and hydrocortisone acetate) 5 ml/vial
073	Terramycin (oxytetracycline HCl) capsules 250 mg.
075	Terramycin Intramuscular Injection (oxytetracycline) 50 mg/ml, 10 ml
080	Terramycin Ophthalmic Ointment with Polymyxin B Sulfate (oxytetracycline HCl with polymyxin B sulfate)
085	Terramycin Topical Ointment (oxytetracycline HCl with polymyxin B sulfate)
545	Vistaril Intramuscular Solution (hydroxyzine HCl) 25 mg/ml
546	Vistaril Intramuscular Solution (hydroxyzine HCl) 50 mg/ml
546	Vistaril Intramuscular Solution Unit-Dose Vials (hydroxyzine HCl) 50 mg/ml, 100 mg/2 ml
640	Antiminth (pyrantel pamoate) 60 ml oral suspension (50 mg of pyrantel base/ml)
1643	Isoject Permapen Aqueous Suspension (penicillin G benzathine) 1,200,000 units/2 ml

ANTIMINTH®
(pyrantel pamoate) ℞
ORAL SUSPENSION

Actions: Antiminth has demonstrated anthelmintic activity against *Enterobius vermicularis* (pinworm) and *Ascaris Lumbricoides* (common roundworm). The anthelmintic action is probably due to the neuromuscular blocking property of the drug.
Antiminth is partially absorbed after an oral dose. Plasma levels of unchanged drug are low. Peak levels (0.05–0.13 µg.ml.) are reached in 1–3 hours. Quantities greater than 50% of administered drug are excreted in feces as the unchanged form, whereas only 7% or less of the dose is found in urine as the unchanged form of the drug and its metabolites.
Indications: For the treatment of ascariasis (common roundworm infection) and enterobiasis (pinworm infection).
Warnings:
Usage in Pregnancy
Reproduction studies have been performed in animals and there was no evidence of propensity for harm to the fetus. The relevance to the human is not known.
There is no experience in pregnant women who have received this drug.
This drug has not been extensively studied in children under two years; therefore, in the treatment of children under the age of two years, the relative benefit/risk should be considered.
Precautions: Minor transient elevations of SGOT have occurred in a small percentage of patients. Therefore, this drug should be used with caution in patients with pre-existing liver dysfunction.
Adverse Reactions: The most frequently encountered adverse reactions are related to the gastrointestinal system.
Gastrointestinal and hepatic reactions: anorexia, nausea, vomiting, gastralgia, abdominal cramps, diarrhea and tenesmus, transient elevation of SGOT.
CNS reactions: headache, dizziness, drowsiness, and insomnia.
Skin reactions: rashes.
Dosage and Administration:
Children and Adults
Antiminth Oral Suspension (50 mg. of pyrantel base/ml.) should be administered in a single dose of 11 mg. of pyrantel base per kg. of body weight (or 5 mg./lb.); maximum total dose 1 gram. This corresponds to a simplified dosage regimen of 1 ml. of Antiminth per 10 lb. of body weight. (One teaspoonful = 5 ml.)
Antiminth (pyrantel pamoate) Oral Suspension may be administered without regard to ingestion of food or time of day, and purging is not necessary prior to, during, or after therapy. It may be taken with milk or fruit juices.
How Supplied: Antiminth Oral Suspension is available as a pleasant tasting caramel flavored suspension which contains the equivalent of 50 mg. pyrantel base per ml., supplied in 60 ml. bottles.
Shown in Product Identification Section, page 426

BONINE®
(meclizine hydrochloride)
Chewable Tablets

Actions: BONINE is an antihistamine which shows marked protective activity against nebulized histamine and lethal doses of intravenously injected histamine in guinea pigs. It has a marked effect in blocking the vasodepressor response to histamine, but only a slight blocking action against acetylcholine. Its activity is relatively weak in inhibiting the spasmogenic action of histamine on isolated guinea pig ileum.
Indications: BONINE is effective in the management of nausea, vomiting and dizziness associated with motion sickness.
Contraindications: Meclizine HCl is contraindicated in individuals who have shown a previous hypersensitivity to it.
Warnings: Since drowsiness may, on occasion, occur with the use of this drug, patients should be warned of this possibility and cautioned against driving a car or operating dangerous machinery. Patients should avoid alcoholic beverages while taking this drug. Due to its potential anticholinergic action, this drug should be used with caution in patients with asthma, glaucoma, or enlargement of the prostate gland.
Usage in Children:
Clinical studies establishing safety and effectiveness in children have not been done; therefore, usage is not recommended in children under 12 years of age.
Usage in Pregnancy:
As with any drug, if you are pregnant or nursing a baby, seek advice of a health care professional before taking this product.
Adverse Reactions: Drowsiness, dry mouth, and on rare occasions, blurred vision have been reported.
Dosage and Administration: For motion sickness 1 or 2 tablets of BONINE should be taken one hour prior to embarkation against motion sickness. Therefore, the dose may be repeated every 24 hours for the duration of the journey.
How Supplied: BONINE (meclizine HCl) is available in convenient packets of 8 chewable tablets of 25 mg. meclizine HCl.
Shown in Product Identification Section, page 426

CORTRIL®
(hydrocortisone) ℞
Topical Ointment

How Supplied: Topical Ointment 1.0%: ½ oz. (14.2 Gm.) tube containing 10 mg./Gm. of hydrocortisone.

CORYBAN®–D CAPSULES
Decongestant Cold Capsules

Composition: Each capsule contains:
Caffeine U.S.P. .... 30 mg.
Chlorpheniramine maleate U.S.P. .... 2 mg.
Phenylpropanolamine HCl .... 25 mg.
How Supplied: In bottles of 24, light and dark blue capsules.

CORYBAN®–D COUGH SYRUP
With Decongestant
(Sugar and Saccharin Free Formula)

Composition: Each 5 ml (1 teaspoonful) contains:
Dextromethorphan HBr U.S.P. .... 7.5 mg.
Guaifenesin .... 50 mg.
Phenylephrine HCl .... 5 mg.
Acetaminophen .... 120 mg.
Alcohol* 7.5%
* Small loss unavoidable
How Supplied: Coryban-D Cough Syrup is available in 4-ounce dripless spout bottles. Sorbitol, which is contained in this product, is a nutritive, carbohydrate sweetening agent which is metabolized more slowly than sugar.

LI-BAN™ Spray
Lice Control Spray

THIS PRODUCT IS NOT FOR USE ON HUMANS OR ANIMALS

Active Ingredient:
(5-Benzyl-3-Furyl) methyl 2, 2-dimethyl-3-(2-methylpropenyl) cyclopropanecarboxylate
                                                    0.500%
Related Compounds   0.068%
Aromatic petroleum
  hydrocarbons   0.664%
Inert Ingredients   98.768%
                                                 100.000%
Actions: A highly active synthetic pyrethroid for the control of lice and louse eggs on garments, bedding, furniture and other inanimate objects.
Warnings: Avoid contamination of feed and foodstuffs. Cover or remove fishbowls. HARMFUL IF SWALLOWED. This product is not for use on humans or animals. If lice infestations should occur on humans, consult either your physician or pharmacist for a product for use on humans.
Physical and Chemical Hazards: Contents under pressure. Do not use or store near heat or open flame. Do not puncture or incinerate container. Exposure to temperatures above 130° F may cause bursting.
Direction For Use: It is a violation of Federal law to use this product in a manner inconsistent with its labeling.
Shake well before each use. Remove protective cap. Aim spray opening away from person. Push button to spray. CAUTION! Avoid spraying in eyes. Avoid breathing spray mist. Use only in well ventilated areas. Avoid contact with skin. In case of contact wash immediately with soap and water. Vacate room after treatment and ventilate before reoccupying.
To kill lice and louse eggs: Spray in an inconspicuous area to test for possible staining or discoloration. Inspect again after drying, then proceed to spray entire area to be treated.
Hold container upright with nozzle away from you. Depress valve and spray from a distance of 8 to 10 inches.
Spray each square foot for 3 seconds. Spray only those garments, parts of bedding, including mattresses and furniture that cannot be either laundered or dry cleaned.
Allow all sprayed articles to dry thoroughly before use. Repeat treatment as necessary.
Buyer assumes all risks of use, storage or handling of this material not in strict accordance with direction given herewith.

Continued on next page

Pfipharmecs—Cont.

DISPOSAL OF CONTAINER
Wrap container and dispose of in trash. Do not incinerate.
How Supplied: 5 ounce aerosol can.

PERMAPEN® Isoject® ℞
(penicillin G benzathine)
in Aqueous Suspension
1,200,000 units
For Intramuscular Use Only

STORE BETWEEN 2°-8°C. (36°-46°F.)
SHAKE WELL BEFORE USING

Description: Permapen (penicillin G benzathine) is a repository penicillin compound which provides blood levels for long periods following its intramuscular injection. This property is the result of its extremely low solubility in water. Chemically, this compound is dibenzylethylenediamine dipenicillin G.

Actions and Pharmacology: Penicillin G exerts a bactericidal action against penicillin-sensitive microorganisms during the stage of active multiplication. It acts through the inhibition of biosynthesis of cell wall mucopeptide. It is not active against the penicillinase-producing bacteria, which includes many strains of staphylococci. Penicillin G exerts high in vitro activity against staphylococci (except penicillinase-producing strains), streptococci (groups A, C, G, H, L and M), and pneumococci. Other organisms sensitive to penicillin G are: *Corynebacterium diphtheriae, Bacillus anthracts,* Clostridia, *Actinomyces bovis, Streptobacillus moniliformis, Listeria monocytogenes,* and Leptospira. *Treponema pallidum* is extremely sensitive to the bactericidal action of penicillin G.
Intramuscular penicillin G benzathine is absorbed very slowly into the blood stream from the intramuscular site and converted by hydrolysis to penicillin G. This combination of hydrolysis and slow absorption results in blood serum levels much lower than other parenteral penicillins.
Approximately 60% of penicillin G is bound to serum protein. The drug is distributed throughout the body tissues in widely varying amounts. Highest levels are found in the kidneys with lesser amounts in the liver, skin and intestines. Penicillin G penetrates into all other tissues and the spinal fluid to a lesser degree. With normal kidney function the drug is excreted rapidly by tubular excretion. In neonates and young infants and in individuals with impaired kidney function, excretion is considerably delayed.

Indications: Intramuscular penicillin G benzathine is indicated in the treatment of infections due to penicillin G-sensitive microorganisms that are susceptible to the low and very prolonged serum levels common to this particular dosage form. Therapy should be guided by bacteriological studies (including sensitivity tests) and by clinical response.
The following infections will usually respond to adequate dosage of intramuscular penicillin G benzathine.
Streptococcal infections (Group A—without bacteremia). Mild to moderate infections of the upper respiratory tract (pharyngitis).
Venereal infections—Syphilis, yaws, bejel and pinta.
Medical Conditions in Which Penicillin G Benzathine Therapy Is Indicated as Prophylaxis:
Rheumatic fever and/or chorea—Prophylaxis with penicillin G benzathine has proven effective in preventing recurrence of these conditions. It has also been used as followup prophylactic therapy for rheumatic heart disease and acute glomerulonephritis.

Contraindications: A history of a previous hypersensitivity reaction to any of the penicillins is a contraindication.

Warning: Serious and occasionally fatal hypersensitivity (anaphylactoid) reactions have been reported in patients on penicillin therapy. Although anaphylaxis is more frequent following parenteral therapy it has occurred in patients on oral penicillins. These reactions are more apt to occur in individuals with a history of sensitivity to multiple allergens.
There have been well documented reports of individuals with a history of penicillin hypersensitivity reactions who have experienced severe hypersensitivity reactions when treated with a cephalosporin. Before therapy with a penicillin, careful inquiry should be made concerning previous hypersensitivity reactions to penicillins, cephalosporins, and other allergens. If an allergic reaction occurs, the drug should be discontinued and the patient treated with the usual agents, e.g., pressor amines, antihistamines and corticosteroids.

Precautions: Penicillin should be used with caution in individuals with histories of significant allergies and/or asthma.
In intramuscular therapy, care should be taken to avoid accidental intravenous administration.
As with all intramuscular preparations, penicillin G benzathine should be injected well within the body of a relatively large muscle. ADULTS: The preferred sites are the upper outer quadrant of the buttock, (i.e., gluteus maximus), and the mid-lateral thigh. CHILDREN: It is recommended that intramuscular injections be given preferably in the mid-lateral muscles of the thigh. In infants and small children the periphery of the upper outer quadrant of the gluteal region should only be used when necessary, such as in burn patients, in order to minimize the possibility of damage to the sciatic nerve.
The deltoid area should be used only if well developed such as in certain adults and older children, and then only with caution to avoid radial nerve injury. Intramuscular injections should not be made into the lower and mid-third of the upper arm. As with all intramuscular injections, aspiration is necessary to help avoid inadvertent injection into a blood vessel.
Irritation at the site of injection may occur. In addition, subcutaneous and fat-layer injections should be avoided since they may cause pain and induration. If these occur, they may be relieved by the application of an ice pack.
In streptococcal infections, therapy must be sufficient to eliminate the organism; otherwise the sequelae of streptococcal disease may occur. Cultures should be taken following completion of treatment to determine whether streptococci have been eradicated.
Prolonged use of antibiotics may promote the overgrowth of nonsusceptible organisms, including fungi. Should superinfection occur, appropriate measures should be taken.

Adverse Reactions: The hypersensitivity reactions reported are skin eruptions (maculopapular to exfoliative dermatitis), urticaria and other serum sickness reactions, laryngeal edema and anaphylaxis. Fever and eosinophilia may frequently be the only reaction observed. Hemolytic anemia, leucopenia, thrombocytopenia, neuropathy and nephropathy are infrequent reactions and usually associated with high doses of parenteral penicillin.

Administration and Dosage:
Pediatric Dosage Schedules: In children under 12 years of age, dosage should be adjusted in accordance with the age and weight of the child and the severity of the infection.
Under 2 years of age, the dose may be divided between the two buttocks if necessary.
Streptococcal infections (group A) pharyngitis—A single injection of—900,000 units for older children; 1,200,000 units for adults.
Venereal infections—
Syphilis—Primary, secondary and latent—2.4 million units (1 dose).
Late Syphilis (tertiary and neurosyphilis)—3 million units at 7 day intervals for a total of 6-9 million units.
Congenital Syphilis—under 2 years of age—50,000 units/kg body weight; age 2-12 years—adjust dosage based on adult dosage schedule.
Yaws, Bejel and Pinta—1.2 million units (1 injection).

Prophylaxis—for rheumatic fever and glomerulonephritis.
Following an acute attack, penicillin G benzathine (parenteral) may be given in doses of 1,200,000 units once a month or 600,000 units every 2 weeks.
How Supplied: Permapen (penicillin G benzathine) Aqueous Suspension is supplied in ISOJECT syringe filled with 2 ml. ISOJECT is a pre-filled disposable syringe unit with a 20-gauge, 1¼ inch needle. Each ml contains: 600,000 units penicillin G benzathine; 0.006 g sodium citrate; 0.003 g polyvinylpyrrolidone; 0.010 g lecithin, and 0.003 g sodium carboxymethylcellulose. Preservatives: methylparaben 0.09%; propylparaben 0.01%.

Buffered PFIZERPEN® ℞
(penicillin G potassium)
for Injection

Description: Buffered Pfizerpen (penicillin G potassium) for Injection is a sterile, pyrogen-free powder which is stable for 36 months when stored at room temperature.
Each million units contains approximately 6.8 milligrams of sodium (0.3 mEq.) and 65.6 milligrams of potassium (1.68 mEq.).

Actions and Pharmacology: Penicillin G exerts a bactericidal action against penicillin-sensitive microorganisms during the stage of active multiplication. It acts through the inhibition of biosynthesis of cell wall mucopeptide. It is not active against the penicillinase-producing bacteria, which include many strains of staphylococci. Penicillin G exerts high *in vitro* activity against staphylococci (except penicillinase-producing strains), streptococci (groups A, C, G, H, L, and M) and pneumococci. Other organisms sensitive to penicillin G are *N. gonorrhoeae, Corynebacterium diphtheriae, Bacillus anthracis,* Clostridia, *Actinomyces bovis, Streptobacillus moniliformis, Listeria monocytogenes* and Leptospira. *Treponema pallidum* is extremely sensitive to the bactericidal action of penicillin G. Some species of gram-negative bacilli are sensitive to moderate to high concentrations of the drug obtained with intravenous administration. These include most strains of *Escherichia coli,* all strains of *Proteus mirabilis,* Salmonella and Shigella and some strains of *Aerobacter aerogenes* and *Alcaligenes fecalis.*
Sensitivity Plate Testing: If the Kirby-Bauer method of disc sensitivity is used, a 10 unit penicillin disc should give a zone greater than 28 mm when tested against a penicillin-sensitive bacterial strain.
Aqueous penicillin G is rapidly absorbed following both intramuscular and subcutaneous injection. Approximately 60 percent of the total dose of 300,000 units is excreted in the urine within this 5-hour period. For this reason high and frequent doses are required to maintain the elevated serum levels desirable in treating certain severe infections in individuals with normal kidney function. In neonates and young infants and in individuals with impaired kidney function, excretion is considerably delayed.

Indications: Aqueous penicillin G (parenteral) is indicated in the therapy of severe infections caused by penicillin G-sensitive microorganisms when rapid and high penicillinemia is required. Therapy should be guided by bacteriological studies (including sensitivity tests) and by clinical response.
The following infections will usually respond to adequate dosage of aqueous penicillin G (parenteral):
Streptococcal infections.
NOTE: Streptococci in groups A, C, H, G, L, and M are very sensitive to penicillin G. Some group D organisms are sensitive to the high serum levels obtained with aqueous penicillin G.
Aqueous penicillin (parenteral) is the penicillin dosage form of choice for bacteremia, empyema, severe pneumonia, pericarditis, endocarditis, meningitis and other severe infections caused by sensitive strains of the gram-positive species listed above.

Product Information

Pneumococcal infections.
Staphylococcal infections—penicillin G sensitive.
Other infections:
Anthrax.
Actinomycosis.
Clostridial infections (including tetanus).
Diphtheria (to prevent carrier state).
Erysipeloid (*Erysipelothrix insidiosa*) endocarditis.
Fusospirochetal infections—severe infections of the oropharynx (Vincent's), lower respiratory tract and genital area due to *Fusobacterium fusiformisans* spirochetes.
Gram-negative bacillary infections (bateremias)—(*E. coli, A. aero genes, A. faecalis,* Salmonella, Shigella and *P. mirabilis*).
Listeria infections (*Listeria monocytogenes*).
Meningitis and endocarditis.
Pasteurella infections (*Pasteurella multocida*).
Bacteremia and meningitis.
Rat-bite fever (*Spirillum minus* or *Streptobacillus moniliformis*).
Gonorrheal endocarditis and arthritis (*N. gonorrhoeae*).
Syphilis (*T. pallidum*) including congenital syphilis.
Meningococcic meningitis.

Although no controlled clinical efficacy studies have been conducted, aqueous crystalline penicillin G for injection and penicillin G procaine suspension have been suggested by the American Heart Association and the American Dental Association for use as part of a combined parenteral-oral regimen for prophylaxis against bacterial endocarditis in patients with congenital heart disease or rheumatic, or other acquired valvular heart disease when they undergo dental procedures and surgical procedures of the upper respiratory tract.[1] Since it may happen that *alpha* hemolytic streptococci relatively resistant to penicillin may be found when patients are receiving continuous oral penicillin for secondary prevention of rheumatic fever, prophylactic agents other than penicillin may be chosen for these patients and prescribed in addition to their continuous rheumatic fever prophylactic regimen.

NOTE: When selecting antibiotics for the prevention of bacterial endocarditis the physician or dentist should read the full joint statement of the American Heart Association and the American Dental Association.[1]

Contraindications: A history of a previous hypersensitivity reaction to any of the penicillins is a contraindication.

Warnings: Serious and occasionally fatal hypersensitivity (anaphylactoid) reactions have been reported in patients on penicillin therapy. Although anaphylaxis is more frequent following parenteral therapy it has occurred in patients on oral penicillins. These reactions are more apt to occur in individuals with a history of sensitivity to multiple allergens.

There have been well documented reports of individuals with a history of penicillin hypersensitivity reactions who have experienced severe hypersensitivity reactions when treated with a cephalosporin. Before therapy with a penicillin, careful inquiry should be made concerning previous hypersensitivity reactions to penicillins, cephalosporins, and other allergens. If an allergic reaction occurs, the drug should be discontinued and the patient treated with the usual agents, e.g., pressor amines, antihistamines, and corticosteroids.

Precautions: Penicillin should be used with caution in individuals with histories of significant allergies and/or asthma.

In streptococcal infections, therapy must be sufficient to eliminate the organism (10 days minimum) otherwise the sequelae of streptococcal disease may occur. Cultures should be taken following the completion of treatment to determine whether streptococci have been eradicated.

Aqueous penicillin G by the intravenous route in high doses (above 10 million units), should be administered slowly because of the adverse effects of electrolyte imbalance from either the potassium or sodium content of the penicillin. The patient's renal, cardiac and vascular status should be evaluated and if impairment of function is suspected or known to exist a reduction in the total dosage should be considered. Frequent evaluation of electrolyte balance, renal and hematopoietic function is recommended during therapy when high doses of intravenous aqueous penicillin G are used.

Prolonged use of antibiotics may promote overgrowth of non-susceptible organisms, including fungi. Should superinfection occur, appropriate measures should be taken. Indwelling intravenous catheters encourage superinfections and should be avoided whenever possible.

Therapy of susceptible infections should be accompanied by any indicated surgical procedures.

Adverse Reactions: Penicillin is a substance of low toxicity but does have a significant index of sensitization. The following hypersensitivity reactions have been reported: skin rashes ranging from maculopapular eruptions to exfoliative dermatitis: urticaria and reactions resembling serum sickness, including chills, fever, edema, arthralgia and prostration. Severe and occasionally fatal anaphylaxis has occurred (see "Warnings").

Hemolytic anemia, leucopenia, thrombocytopenia, nephropathy, and neuropathy are rarely observed adverse reactions and are usually associated with high intravenous dosage. Patients given continuous intravenous therapy with penicillin G potassium in high dosage (10 million to 100 million units daily) may suffer severe or even fatal potassium poisoning, particularly if renal insufficiency is present. Hyperreflexia, convulsions and coma may be indicative of this syndrome.

Cardiac arrhythmias and cardiac arrest may also occur. (High dosage of penicillin G sodium may result in congestive heart failure due to high sodium intake.)

The Jarisch-Herxheimer reaction has been reported in patients treated for syphilis.

Administration and Dosage: *Severe infections due to Susceptible Strains of Streptococci, Pneumococci and Staphylococci*—bacteremia, pneumonia, endocarditis, pericarditis, empyema, meningitis and other severe infections—a minimum of 5 million units daily.

Syphilis—Aqueous penicillin G may be used in the treatment of acquired and congenital syphilis, but because of the necessity of frequent dosage, hospitalization is recommended. Dosage and duration of therapy will be determined by age of patient and stage of the disease.

Gonorrheal endocarditis—a minimum of 5 million units daily.

Meningococcic meningitis—1-2 million units intramuscularly every 2 hours, or continuous I.V. drip of 20–30 million units/day.

Actinomycosis—1-6 million units/day for cervico-facial cases; 10–20 million units/day for thoracic and abdominal disease.

Clostridial infections—20 million units/day; penicillin is adjunctive therapy to antitoxin.

Fusospirochetal infections—severe infections of oropharynx, lower respiratory tract and genital area—5–10 million units/day.

Rat-bite fever (*Spirillum minus* or *Streptobacillus moniliformis*)—12-15 million units/day for 3-4 weeks.

Listeria infections (*Listeria monocytogenes*).
Neonates—500,000 to 1 million units/day.
Adults with meningitis—15–20 million units/day for 2 weeks.
Adults with endocarditis—15–20 million units/day for 4 weeks.

Pasteurella infections (*Pasteurella multocida*).
Bacteremia and meningitis—4–6 million units/day for 2 weeks.

Erysipeloid (*Erysipelothrix insidiosa*).
Endocarditis—2–20 million units/day for 4-6 weeks.

Gram-negative bacillary infections (*E. coli, A. aerogenes, A. faecalis,* Salmonella, Shigella and *Proteus mirabilis*).
Bacteremia—20–80 million units/day.

Diphtheria (carrier state)—300,000–400,000 units of penicillin/day in divided doses for 10–12 days.

Anthrax—a minimum of 5 million units of penicillin/day in divided doses until cure is effected.

For prophylaxis against bacterial endocarditis[1] in patients with congenital heart disease or rheumatic, or other acquired valvular heart disease when undergoing dental procedures or surgical procedures of the upper respiratory tract, use a combined parenteral-oral regimen. One million units of aqueous crystalline penicillin G (30,000 units/kg in children) intramuscularly mixed with 600,000 units procaine penicillin G (600,000 units for children) should be given one-half to one hour before the procedure. Oral penicillin V (phenoxymethyl penicillin), 500 mg for adults or 250 mg for children less than 60 lb, should be given every 6 hours for 8 doses. Doses for children should not exceed recommendations for adults for a single dose or for a 24 hour period.

The following table shows the amount of solvent required for solution of various concentrations. [See table above].

When the required volume of solvent is greater than the capacity of the vial, the penicillin can be dissolved by first injecting only a portion of the solvent into the vial, then withdrawing the resultant solution and combining it with the remainder of the solvent in a larger sterile container.

Buffered Pfizerpen (penicillin G potassium) for Injection is highly water soluble. It may be dissolved in small amounts of Water for Injection, or Sterile Isotonic Sodium Chloride Solution for Parenteral Use. All solutions should be stored in a refrigerator. When refrigerated, penicillin solutions may be stored for seven days without significant loss of potency.

Buffered Pfizerpen (penicillin G potassium) for Injection may be given intramuscularly or by continuous intravenous drip for dosages of 500,000, 1,000,000, or 5,000,000 units. It is also suitable for intrapleural, intraarticular, and other local instillations.

THE 20,000,000 UNIT DOSAGE MAY BE ADMINISTERED BY INTRAVENOUS INFUSION ONLY.

(1) Intramuscular Injection: Keep total volume of injection small. The intramuscular route is the preferred route of administration. Solutions containing up to 100,000 units of penicillin per ml of diluent may be used with a minimum of discomfort. Greater concentration of penicillin G per ml is physically possible and may be employed where therapy demands. When large dosages are required, it may be advisable to administer aqueous solutions of penicillin by means of continuous intravenous drip.

(2) Continuous Intravenous Drip: Determine the volume of fluid and rate of its administration required by the patient in a 24-hour period in the usual manner for fluid therapy, and add the appropriate daily dosage of penicillin to this fluid. For example, if an adult patient requires 2 liters of

Continued on next page

Pfizerpen

Desired Concentration (units/ml)	Approx. Volume (ml) 1,000,000 units	Solvent for Vial of 5,000,000 units	Infusion Only 20,000,000 units
50,000	19.6	...	...
100,000	9.6	...	...
250,000	3.6	18.2	74.2
500,000	1.6	8.2	32.4
750,000	...	4.8	...
1,000,000	...	3.2	11.5

Pfipharmecs—Cont.

fluid in 24 hours and a daily dosage of 10 million units of penicillin, add 5 million units to 1 liter and adjust the rate of flow so that the liter will be infused in 12 hours.

(3) Intrapleural or Other Local Infusion: If fluid is aspirated, give infusion in a volume equal to ¼ or ½ the amount of fluid aspirated, otherwise, prepare as for intramuscular injection.

(4) Intrathecal Use: The intrathecal use of penicillin in meningitis must be highly individualized. It should be employed only with full consideration of the possible irritating effects of penicillin when used by this route. The preferred route of therapy in bacterial meningitides is intravenous, supplemental by intramuscular injection.

How Supplied: Buffered Pfizerpen (penicillin G potassium) for Injection is available in vials containing respectively 1,000,000 units × 10's (NDC 0995-0510-83), 1,000,000 units × 100's (NDC 0995-0510-95), 5,000,000 units × 10's (NDC 0995-0520-83), 5,000,000 units × 100's (NDC 0995-0520-95), 20,000,000 units × 1's (NDC 0995-0530-28) and 20,000,000 units × 10 's (NDC 0995-0530-83) of dry powder for reconstitution; buffered with sodium citrate and citric acid to an optimum pH.

Each million units contains approximately 6.8 milligrams of sodium (0.3 mEq.) and 65.6 milligrams of potassium (1.68 mEq.).

Reference:
1. American Heart Association. 1977. Prevention of bacterial endocarditis. Circulation. **56**:139A-143A.

PFIZERPEN®-AS   R
(penicillin G procaine)
in Aqueous Suspension
For Intramuscular Use Only

Description: Pfizerpen-AS (penicillin G procaine) is a highly potent antibacterial agent effective against a wide variety of pathogenic organisms. It is an equimolecular compound of procaine and penicillin G in aqueous suspension for intramuscular administration.

Actions and Pharmacology: Penicillin G exerts a bactericidal action against penicillin-sensivitive micoorganisms during the stage of active multiplication. It acts through the inhibition of biosynthesis of cell wall mucopeptide. It is not active against the penicillinase-producing bacteria, which include many strains of staphylococci. Penicillin G exerts high in vitro activity against staphylococci (except penicillinase-producing strains), streptococci (groups A.C.G.H.L. and M.) and pneumococci. Other organisms sensitive to penicillin G are *N. gonorrhoeae, Corvnebacterium diphtheriae, Bacillus anthracis,* Clostrida, *Actinomyces bovis, Streptobacillus moniliformis, Listera monocytogenes* and Leptospira. *Treponema pallidum* is extremely sensitive to the bactericidal action of penicillin G.

Sensitivity plate testing: If the Kirby-Bauer method of disc sensitivity is used, a 10-unit penicillin disc should give a zone greater than 28 mm when tested against a penicillin-sensitive bacterial strain.

Penicillin G procaine is an equimolecular compound of procaine and penicillin G administered intramuscularly as a suspension. It dissolves slowly at the site of injection, giving a plateau type of blood level at about 4 hours which falls slowly over a period of the next 15-20 hours.

Approximately 60% of penicillin G is bound to serum protein. The drug is distributed throughout the body tissues in widely varying amounts. Highest levels are found in the kidneys with lesser amounts in the liver, skin and intestines. Penicillin G penetrates into all other tissues to a lesser degree with a very small level found in the cerebrospinal fluid. With normal kidney function the drug is excreted rapidly by tubular excretion. In neonates and young infants and in individuals with impaired kidney functions, excretion is considerably delayed. Approximately 60-90% of a dose of parenteral penicillin G is excreted in the urine within 24-36 hours.

Indications: Penicillin G procaine is indicated in the treatment of moderately severe infections due to penicillin G-sensitive microorganisms that are sensitive to the low and persistent serum levels common to this paritcular dosage form. Therapy should be guided by bacteriological studies (including sensitivity tests) and by clinical response.

NOTE: When high sustained serum levels are required, aqueous penicillin G either IM or IV should be used.

The following infections will usually respond to adequate dosages of intramuscular penicillin G procaine.

Streptococcal infections: Group A (without bacteremia). Moderately severe to severe infections of the upper respiratory tract (including middle ear infections—otitis media), skin and soft tissue infections, scarlet fever, and erysipelas.

NOTE: Streptococci in groups A.C.H.G.L. and M are very sensitive to penicillin G. Other groups, including group D (enterococcus) are resistant. Aqueous penicillin is recommended for streptococcal infections with bacteremia.

Pneumococcal infections: Moderately severe infections of the respiratory tract (including middled ear infections—otitis media).

NOTE: Severe pneumonia, empyema, bacteremia, pericarditis, meningitis, peritonitis, and purulent or septic arthritis of pneumococcal etiology are better treated with aqueous penicillin G during the acute stage.

Staphylococcal infections: penicillin G-sensitive. Moderately severe infections of the skin and soft tissues.

NOTE: Reports indicate an increasing number of strains of staphylococci resistant to penicillin G emphasizing the need for culture and sensitivity studies in treating suspected staphylococcal infections.

Indicated surgical procedures should be performed.

Fusospirochetosis (Vincent's gingivitis and pharyngitis). Moderately severe infections of the oropharynx respond to therapy with penicillin G procaine.

NOTE: Necessary dental care should be accomplished in infections involving the gum tissue.

Treponema pallidum (syphilis): all stages.

N. gonorrhoeae; acute and chronic (without bacteremia).

Yaws, Bejel, Pinta.

C. diphtheriae—penicillin G procaine as an adjunct to antitoxin for prevention of the carrier stage.

Anthrax.

Streptobacillus monoliformis and *Spirillum minus* infections (rat bite fever).

Erysipeloid.

Subacute bacterial endocarditis (group A streptococcus) only in extremely sensitive infections.

Prophylaxis Against Bacterial Endocarditis— Penicillin G procaine may be given to patients with congenital and/or rheumatic heart lesions who are to undergo dental or upper respiratory tract surgery or instrumentation. Prophylaxis should be instituted the day of the procedure and continued for 2 or more days following.

NOTE: Since patients who have a past history of rheumatic fever and are receiving continuous prophylaxis may harbor increased numbers of penicillin-resistant organisms, use of another prophylactic anti-infective agent should be considered. If penicillin is to be used in these patients at surgery, the regular rheumatic fever program should be interrupted 1 week prior to the contemplated surgery. At the time of surgery, penicillin may be reinstituted as a prophylactic measure against the hazards of surgically induced bacteremia.

Contraindications: A previous hypersensitivity reaction to any penicillin or procaine is a contraindication.

Warnings: Serious and occasionally fatal hypersensitivity (anaphylactoid) reactions have been reported in patients on penicillin therapy. Although anaphylaxis is more frequent following parenteral therapy it has occurred in patients on oral penicillins. These reactions are more apt to occur in individuals with a history of sensitivity to multiple allergens.

There have been well documented reports of individuals with a history of penicillin hypersensitivity reactions who have experienced severe hypersensitivity reactions when treated with a cephalosporin. Before therapy with a penicillin, careful inquiry should be made concerning previous hypersensitivity reactions to penicillins, cephalosporins, and other allergens. If an allergic reaction occurs, the drug should be discontinued and the patient treated with the usual agents *e.g.*, pressor amines, antihistamines and corticosteroids.

Immediate toxic reactions to procaine may occur in some individuals, particularly when a large single dose is administered in the treatment of gonorrhea (4.8 million units). These reactions may be manifested by mental disturbances including anxiety, confusion, agitation, depression, weakness, seizures, hallucinations, combativeness, and expressed "fear of impending death". The reactions noted in carefully controlled studies occurred in approximately one in 500 patients treated for gonorrhea. Reactions are transient, lasting from 15-30 minutes.

Precautions: Penicillin should be used with caution in individuals with histories of significant allergies and/or asthma.

In intramuscular therapy, care should be taken to avoid accidental intravenous administration.

As with all intramuscular preparations, Pfizerpen-AS (penicillin G procaine) should be injected well within the body of a relatively large muscle. ADULTS: The preferred site is the upper outer quadrant of the buttock, (i.e., gluteus maximus), or the mid-lateral thigh. CHILDREN: It is recommended that intramuscular injections be given preferably in the mid-lateral muscles of the thigh. In infants and small children the periphery of the upper outer quadrant of the gluteal region should only be used when necessary, such as in burn patients, in order to minimize the possibility of damage to the sciatic nerve.

The deltoid area should be used only if well developed such as in certain adults and older children, and then only with caution to avoid radial nerve injury. Intramuscular injections should not be made into the lower and mid-third of the upper arm. As with all intramuscualr injections, aspiration is necessary to help avoid inadvertent injection into a blood vessel.

In suspected staphylococcal infections, proper laboratory studies, including sensitivity tests, should be performed.

A small percentage of patients are sensitive to procaine. If there is a history of sensitivity make the usual test: Inject intradermally 0.1 ml of a 1 to 2 percent procaine solution. Development of an erythema, wheal, flare or eruption indicates procaine sensitivity. Sensitivity should be treated by the usual methods, including barbiturates, and penicillin G procaine preparations should not be used. Antihistamines appear beneficial in treatment of procaine reactions.

The use of antibiotics may result in overgrowth of nonsusceptible organisms. Constant observation of the patient is essential. If new infections due to bacteria or fungi appear during therapy, the drug should be discontinued and appropriate measures taken. Whenever allergic reactions occur, penicillin should be withdrawn unless, in the opinion of the physician, the condition being treated is life threatening and amenable only to penicillin therapy.

In prolonged therapy with penicillin, and particularly with high dosage schedules, periodic evaluation of the renal and hematopoietic systems are recommended.

When treating gonococcal infections in which primary or secondary syphilis may be suspected, proper diagnostic procedures, including dark field examinations should be done. In all cases in which concomitant syphilis is suspected, monthly serological tests should be made for at least four months.

Adverse Reactions: Penicillin is a substance of low toxicity, but does possess a significant index of sensitization. The following hypersensitivity reactions associated with use of penicillin have been reported: skin rashes, ranging from maculopapular eruptions to exfoliative dermatitis; urticaria; serum sickness-like reactions, including chills, fever, edema, arthralgia and prostration. Severe and often fatal anaphylaxis has been reported (see "Warnings"). As with other treatments for syphilis, the Jarisch-Herxheimer reaction has been reported.

Procaine toxicity manifestations have been reported (see Warnings). Procaine hypersensitivity reactions have not been reported with this drug.

Administration and Dosage:
Pediatric Dosage Schedules: In children under 3 months of age, the absorption of aqueous penicillin G produces such high and sustained levels that penicillin G procaine dosage forms offer no advantages and are usually unnecessary.

In children under 12 years of age, dosage should be adjusted in accordance with the age and weight of the child and the severity of the infection.

Under 2 years of age, the dose may be divided between the two buttocks if necessary.

Penicillin G procaine (aqueous) is for intramuscular injection only.

Recommended dosage for penicillin G procaine aqueous:

Pneumonia (pneumococcal), moderately severe (uncomplicated): 600,000-1,000,000 units daily.
Streptococcal infections (group A), moderately severe to severe tonsillitis, erysipelas, scarlet fever, upper respiratory tract, skin and soft tissue: 600,000-1,000,000 units daily for 10 day minimum.
Staphylococcal infections, moderately severe to severe: 600,000-1,000,000 units daily.
Bacterial endocarditis (group A streptococci) only in extremely sensitive infections: 600,000-1,000,000 units daily.
To prevent bacterial endocarditis in patients with rheumatic or congenital heart lesions who are to undergo dental or upper respiratory tract surgery or instrumentation:
  600,000 units penicillin G procaine aqueous the day of the procedure.
  600,000 units aqueous penicillin G 1-2 hours before surgery.
  600,000 units penicillin G procaine aqueous daily for 2 days following surgery.
Syphilis
Primary, secondary and latent with a negative spinal fluid in adults and children over 12 years of age: 600,000 units daily for 8 days—total 4,800,000 units.
Late (tertiary, neurosyphilis and latent syphilis with positive spinal fluid examination or no spinal fluid examination): 600,000 units daily for 10-15 days—total 6-9 million units.
Congenital syphilis (early and late) under 70 lb. body weight 50,000 units/kg/day for 10 days.
Yaws, Bejel, and Pinta—Treatment as syphilis in corresponding stage of disease.
Gonorrheal infections (uncomplicated): Men or women—4.8 million units intramuscularly divided into at least two doses and injected at different sites at one visit, together with 1 gram of oral probenecid, preferably given at least 30 minutes prior to the injection.
  NOTE: gonorrheal endocarditis should be treated intensively with aqueous penicillin G.
  Diphtheria-adjunctive therapy with antitoxin: 300,000-600,000 units daily.
  Diphtheria carrier state—300,000 units daily for 10 days.
  Anthrax-cutaneous: 600,000-1,000,000 units/day.
  Vincent's infection (fusopirochetosis): 600,000-1,000,000 units/day.
  Erysipeloid: 600,000-1,000,000 units/day.
Streptobacillus moniliformis and spirillum minus (rat bite fever): 600,000-1,000,000 units/day.

How Supplied: Pfizerpen-AS (penicillin G procaine) in Aqueous Suspension is supplied in 10 ml vials (3,000,000 units). Each ml contains 300,000 units penicillin G procaine; and as w/v: 0.8% Sodium citrate; 0.15% sodium carboxymethylcellulose; 25% of sorbitol solution U.S.P.; 0.06% polyvinylpyrrolidone, and 0.6% lecithin.

Preservatives: 0.103% methylparaben; 0.011% propylparaben.

RID™
Liquid Pediculicide

Description: Rid is a liquid pediculicide whose active ingredients are: pyrethrins 0.3%, piperonyl butoxide, technical 3.00%, equivalent to 2.4% (butylcarbityl) (6-propylpiperonyl) ether and to 0.6% related compounds, petroleum distillate 1.20% and benzyl alcohol 2.4%. Inert ingredients 93.1%.

Actions: RID kills head lice (*Pediculus humanus capitis*), body lice (*Pediculus humanus humanus*), and pubic or crab lice (*Phthirus pubis*), and their eggs on contact.

The pyrethrins act as a contact poison and affect the parasite's nervous system, resulting in paralysis and death. The efficacy of the pyrethrins is enhanced by the synergist, piperonyl butoxide.

Indications: RID is indicated for the treatment of infestations of head lice, body lice and pubic (crab) lice and their eggs.

Warning: RID should be used with caution by ragweed sensitized persons.

Precautions: This product is for external use only. It is harmful if swallowed. It should not be inhaled. It should be kept out of the eyes and contact with mucous membranes should be avoided. If accidental contact with eyes occurs, flush immediately with water. In case of infection or skin irritation, discontinue use and consult a physician. Consult a physician if infestation of eyebrows or eyelashes occurs. Avoid contamination of feed or foodstuffs. Do not reuse container. Rinse thoroughly and wrap container in several layers of newspaper and discard in trash.

Do not transport or store below 32°F (0°C).

Dosage and Administration: (1) Apply RID undiluted to hair and scalp or to any other infested area until entirely wet. Do not use on eyelashes or eyebrows. (2) Allow RID to remain on area for 10 minutes but no longer. (3) Wash thoroughly with warm water and soap or shampoo. (4) Dead lice and eggs may require removal with fine-toothed comb provided. A second application should be made in 7 to 10 days to kill any newly hatched lice. Do not exceed two consecutive applications within 24 hours.

Since lice infestations are spread by contact, each family member should be examined carefully. If infested, he or she should be treated promptly to avoid spread or reinfestation of previously treated individuals. Contaminated clothing and other articles, such as hats, etc. should be dry cleaned, boiled or otherwise treated until decontaminated to prevent reinfestation or spread.

How Supplied: In 2 and 4 fl. oz. bottles and one gallon plastic containers. Special fine-tooth comb that removes all the nits and patient instruction booklet are included in each package of RID.

Shown in Product Identification Section, page 426

STREPTOMYCIN SULFATE ℞
Dry Powder: Vials of 1 g and 5 g
Injection (400 mg/ml): Vials of 1 g (2.5 ml) and 5 g (12.5 ml)

WARNING

THE RISK OF SEVERE NEUROTOXIC REACTIONS IS SHARPLY INCREASED IN PATIENTS WITH IMPAIRED KIDNEY FUNCTION OR PRERENAL AZOTEMIA. THESE INCLUDE DISTURBANCES OF THE AUDITORY NERVE, OPTIC NERVE, PERIPHERAL NEURITIS, ARACHNOIDITIS, AND ENCEPHALOPATHY. RENAL FUNCTION SHOULD BE CAREFULLY DETERMINED AND PATIENTS WITH RENAL DAMAGE AND NITROGEN RETENTION SHOULD HAVE REDUCED DOSAGE. THE PEAK SERUM CONCENTRATION IN INDIVIDUALS WITH KIDNEY DAMAGE SHOULD NOT EXCEED 20 TO 25 MCG PER MILLILITER.

THE CONCURRENT OR SEQUENTIAL USE OF OTHER NEUROTOXIC AND/OR NEPHROTOXIC DRUGS WITH STREPTOMYCIN SULFATE, PARTICULARLY NEOMYCIN, KANAMYCIN, GENTAMICIN, CEPHALORIDINE, PAROMOMYCIN, VIOMYCIN, POLYMYXIN B, COLISTIN, AND TOBRAMYCIN SHOULD BE AVOIDED.
THE NEUROTOXICITY OF STREPTOMYCIN CAN RESULT IN RESPIRATORY PARALYSIS FROM NEUROMUSCULAR BLOCKADE, ESPECIALLY WHEN THE DRUG IS GIVEN SOON AFTER ANESTHESIA AND THE USE OF MUSCLE RELAXANTS.
THE ADMINISTRATION OF STREPTOMYCIN IN PARENTERAL FORM SHOULD BE RESERVED FOR PATIENTS WHERE ADEQUATE LABORATORY FACILITIES ARE AVAILABLE AND CONSTANT SUPERVISION OF THE PATIENT IS POSSIBLE.

Description: Streptomycin is a water-soluble aminoglycoside derived from *Streptomyces griseus*. It is marketed as the sulfate salt of streptomycin.

Actions: Streptomycin sulfate is a bactericidal antibiotic in therapeutic dosage. The mode of action is the interference with normal protein synthesis and production of "faulty proteins."

Following intramuscular injection of 1 g of the drug, a peak serum level of 25 to 50 mcg per milliliter is reached within 1 hour, diminishing slowly to about 50 percent after 5 to 6 hours. Appreciable concentrations are found in all organ tissues except the brain. Significant amounts have been found in pleural fluid and tuberculous cavities. Streptomycin passes through the placenta with serum levels in the cord blood similar to maternal levels. Small amounts are excreted in milk, saliva, and sweat.

Streptomycin is excreted rapidly in the urine by glomerular filtration. In patients with normal kidney function, between 29 and 89 percent of a single 0.6 g dose is excreted within 24 hours. Any reduction of glomerular activity results in decreased excretion of the drug and concurrent rise in serum and tissue levels.

Sensitivity plate testing: If the Kirby-Bauer method of disc sensitivity is used, a 10 mcg streptomycin disc should give a zone of over 15 millimeters when tested against a streptomycin-sensitive bacterial strain.

Indications:
1. Mycobacterium tuberculosis: Streptomycin may be indicated for all forms of this infection when the infecting organisms are susceptible. It should be used only in combination with other antituberculosis drugs. The common combined drug therapy is streptomycin, PAS, and isoniazid; this combination is effective only where the organisms are susceptible to the drugs being used in combination.
2. Nontuberculosis infections: Streptomycin should be used only in those serious nontuberculosis infections caused by organisms shown by *in vitro* sensitivity studies to be susceptible to it and when less potentially hazardous therapeutic agents are ineffective or contraindicated.
  a. *Pasteurella pestis* (plague).
  b. *Pasteurella tularensis* (tularemia).
  c. *Brucella.*
  d. *Donovanosis* (granuloma inguinale).
  e. *H. ducreyi* (chancroid).
  f. *H. influenzae* (in respiratory, endocardial, and meningeal infections—concomitantly with another antibacterial agent).
  g. *K. pneumoniae* pneumonia (concomitantly with another antibacterial agent).
  h. *E. coli, Proteus, A. aerogenes, K. pneumoniae,* and *Streptococcus faecalis* in urinary tract infections.
  i. *Strep. viridans, Strep. faecalis* (in endocardial infections—concomitantly with penicillin).
  j. Gram-negative bacillary bacteremia (concomitantly with another antibacterial agent).

Note: The use of streptomycin should be limited to the treatment of infections caused by bacteria

Continued on next page

Pfipharmecs—Cont.

which have been shown to be susceptible to the antibacterial effects of streptomycin and which are not amenable to therapy with less potentially toxic agents.

Contraindications: Streptomycin is contraindicated in those individuals who have shown previous toxic or hypersensitivity reaction to it.

Warnings: Ototoxicity: Streptomycin may frequently affect the vestibular branch of the auditory nerve causing severe nausea, vomiting, and vertigo. The incidence is directly proportional to duration and amount of the drug administered. Advanced age and renal impairment predispose to ototoxicity. Symptoms subside and recovery is usually complete following discontinuance of the drug.

Loss of hearing has been reported following long term therapy; however, ototoxic effect on the auditory branch of the eighth nerve is infrequent and usually is preceded by vestibular symptoms. Hearing loss, when extensive, is usually permanent.

USAGE IN PREGNANCY: Since streptomycin readily crosses the placental barrier, caution in use of the drug is important to prevent ototoxicity in the fetus.

Precautions: Baseline and periodic caloric stimulation tests and audiometric tests are advisable with extended streptomycin therapy. Tinnitus, roaring noises, or a sense of fullness in the ears indicates need for audiometric examination or termination of streptomycin therapy or both.

Care should be taken by individuals handling or preparing streptomycin for injection to avoid skin sensitivity reactions.

As with all intramuscular preparations, Streptomycin Sulfate Injection should be injected well within the body of a relatively large muscle. ADULTS: The preferred site is the upper outer quadrant of the buttock, (i.e., gluteus maximus), or the mid-lateral thigh. CHILDREN: It is recommended that intramuscular injections be given preferably in the mid-lateral muscles of the thigh. In infants and small children the periphery of the upper outer quadrant of the gluteal region should be used only when necessary, such as in burn patients, in order to minimize the possibility of damage to the sciatic nerve.

The deltoid area should be used only if well developed such as in certain adults and older children, and then only with caution to avoid radial nerve injury. Intramuscular injections should not be made into the lower and mid-third of the upper arm. As with all intramuscular injections, aspiration is necessary to help avoid inadvertent injection into a blood vessel.

Injection sites should be alternated, and solutions of concentration greater than 500 mg/ml are not recommended.

As higher doses or more prolonged therapy with streptomycin may be indicated for more severe or fulminating infections (endocarditis, meningitis, etc.), the physician should always take adequate measures to be immediately aware of any toxic signs or symptoms occurring in the patient as a result of streptomycin therapy.

While disturbances in renal function due to streptomycin have been reported in the past, purification of the drug has minimized this side effect. In the presence of pre-existing renal insufficiency, however, extreme caution must be exercised in the administration of streptomycin. Since in severely uremic patients a single dose may produce reasonably high blood levels for several days, the cumulative effect may produce ototoxic sequelae. When streptomycin must be given for prolonged periods of time, alkalinization of the urine may minimize or prevent renal irritation.

A syndrome of apparent central nervous system depression, characterized by stupor and flaccidity, at times to the extent of coma and deep respiratory depression, has been reported in very young infants in whom streptomycin dosage had materially exceeded the recommended limits. Thus, infants should not receive streptomycin in excess of the recommended dosage.

In the treatment of venereal infections such as granuloma inguinale, and chancroid, if concomitant syphilis is suspected, suitable laboratory procedures such as a dark field examination should be performed before the start of treatment, and monthly serologic tests should be done for at least four months.

As with other antibiotics, use of this drug may result in overgrowth of nonsusceptible organisms, including fungi. If superinfection occurs, appropriate therapy should be instituted.

Adverse Reactions: The following reactions are common: ototoxicity—nausea, vomiting, and vertigo; paresthesia of face; rash; fever; urticaria; angioneurotic edema; and eosinophilia.

The following reactions are less frequent: deafness, exfoliative dermatitis, anaphylaxis, azotemia, leucopenia, thrombocytopenia, pancytopenia, hemolytic anemia, muscular weakness, and amblyopia.

Vestibular dysfunction resulting from the parenteral administration of streptomycin is cumulatively related to the total daily dose. When 1.8 to 2.0 g/day are given, symptoms are likely to develop in the large percentage of patients—especially in the elderly or patients with impaired renal function—within four weeks. Therefore, it is recommended that caloric and audiometric tests be done prior to, during, and following intensive therapy with streptomycin in order to facilitate detection of any vestibular dysfunction and/or impairment of hearing which may occur.

Vestibular symptoms generally appear early and usually are reversible with early detection and cessation of administration of the drug. After two to three months, gross vesibular symptoms usually disappear, except for the relative inability to walk in total darkness or on very rough terrain.

Clinical judgment as to termination of therapy must be exercised when side effects occur.

Dosage and Administration:
Intramuscular Route Only

1. Tuberculosis: All forms when organisms are known or believed to be drug susceptible.

Adult, combined therapy: Streptomycin—1 g daily with PAS 5 g t.i.d. and isoniazid 200 to 300 mg daily. Elderly patients should have a smaller daily dose of streptomycin, based on age, renal function, and eighth nerve function. Ultimately the streptomycin should be discontinued or reduced in dosage to 1 g 2 to 3 times weekly. Therapy with streptomycin may be terminated when toxic symptoms have appeared, when impending toxicity is feared, when organisms become resistant, or when full treatment effect has been obtained. The total period of drug treatment of tuberculosis is a minimum of 1 year; however, indications for terminating therapy with streptomycin may occur at any time as noted above.

2. Tularemia: One to 2 g daily in divided doses for 7 to 10 days until the patient is afebrile for 5 to 7 days.

3. Plague: Two to 4 g daily in divided doses until the patient is afebrile for at least 3 days.

4a. Bacterial endocarditis: In penicillin-sensitive alpha and nonhemolytic streptococcal endocarditis (penicillin sensitive to 0.1 mcg per milliliter or less), streptomycin may be used for 2-week treatment concomitantly with penicillin. Streptomycin dosage is 1 g b.i.d. for 1 week, and 0.5 g b.i.d. for the 2d week. If the patient is over 60 years of age, the dosage should be 0.5 g b.i.d. for the entire 2-week period.

b. Enterococcal endocarditis: Streptomycin in doses of 1 g b.i.d. for 2 weeks and 0.5 g b.i.d. for 4 weeks is given in combination with penicillin. Ototoxicity may require termination of the streptomycin prior to completion of the 6-week course of treatment.

5. For use concomitantly with other agents to which the infecting organism is also sensitive. Streptomycin in these conditions is considered as a drug of secondary choice: gram-negative bacillary bacteremia, meningitis, and pneumonia; brucellosis; granuloma inguinale; chancroid, and urinary tract infection.

For adults:
a. Severe fulminating infection: 2 to 4 g daily, administered intramuscularly in divided doses every 6 to 12 hours.
b. With less severe infections and with highly susceptible organisms: 1 to 2 g daily.
For children: 20 to 40 mg per kg of body weight daily (8 to 20 mg per pound) in divided doses every 6 to 12 hours. (Particular care should be taken to avoid excessive dosage in children.)

The dry powder is dissolved by adding Water for Injection, U.S.P. or Isotonic Sodium Chloride Solution, U.S.P. in an amount to yield the desired concentration as indicated in the following table:

Approx. Conc. (mg/ml)	Volume (ml) of Solvent 1 g Vial	5 g Vial
200	4.2	—
250	3.2	—
400	1.8	9.0

Sterile reconstituted solutions may be stored at room temperature for four weeks without significant loss of potency.

Supply: Streptomycin Sulfate is supplied as a sterile powder in packages of 100 vials, each vial containing streptomycin sulfate equivalent to 1.0 g and 5.0 g of streptomycin base.

Streptomycin Sulfate Injection is supplied in 2.5 ml vials, packages of 100 (streptomycin sulfate equivalent to 1.0 g of streptomycin base) and 12.5 ml vials, packages of 100 (streptomycin sulfate equivalent to 5.0 g of streptomycin base). Each 2.5 ml of injection also contains 0.03 g sodium citrate; 0.005 g sodium bisulfite; with phenol 0.25% w/v as preservative.

Also available as ISOJECT SYRINGES, packages of 10. Each contains (2.0 ml) streptomycin sulfate equivalent to 1.0 g of streptomycin base; 0.026 g sodium citrate; 0.004 g sodium bisulfite, with phenol 0.25 w/v as preservative.

TERRA–CORTRIL® ℞
Terramycin® (oxytetracycline HCl)
—Cortril® (hydrocortisone acetate)
OPHTHALMIC SUSPENSION

Description: Terra-Cortril suspension combines the antibiotic, oxytetracycline HCl ($C_{22}H_{24}N_2O_9 \cdot HCl$) and the adrenocorticoid, hydrocortisone acetate ($C_{23}H_{32}O_6$). Each ml of Terra-Cortril contains Terramycin (oxytetracycline HCl) equivalent to 5 mg of oxytetracycline, and 15 mg of Cortril (hydrocortisone acetate) incorporated in mineral oil with aluminum tristearate.

For Ophthalmic Use Only.

Clinical Pharmacology: Corticosteroids suppress the inflammatory response to a variety of agents and they probably delay or slow healing. Since corticoids may inhibit the body's defense mechanism against infection, a concomitant antimicrobial drug may be used when this inhibition is considered to be clinically significant in a particular case.

The anti-infective component in the combination is included to provide action against specific organisms suspectible to it.

Terramycin is considered active against the following microorganisms:

Rickettsiae (Rocky Mountain spotted fever, typhus fever and the typhus group, Q fever, rickettsialpox and tick fevers),
Mycoplasma pneumoniae (PPLO, Eaton Agent),
Agents of psittacosis and ornithosis,
Agents of lymphogranuloma venereum and granuloma inguinale,
The spirochetal agent of relapsing fever (*Borrelia recurrentis*).
The following gram-negative microorganisms:
Haemophilus ducreyi (chancroid),
Pasteurella pestis and *Pasteurella tularensis*,
Bartonella bascilloformis,
Bacteroides species,
Vibrio comma and *Vibrio fetus*,
Brucella species (in conjunction with streptomycin).
Because many strains of the following groups of microorganisms have been shown to be resistant to

tetracyclines, culture and susceptibility testing are recommended.
Oxytetracycline is indicated for treatment of infections caused by the following gram-negative microorganisms, when bacteriologic testing indicates appropriate susceptibility to the drug:
Escherichia coli,
Enterobacter aerogenes (formerly *Aerobacter aerogenes*),
Shigella species,
Mima species and *Herellea* species,
Haemophilus influenzae (respiratory infections),
Klebsiella species (respiratory and urinary infections).
Oxytetracycline is indicated for treatment of infections caused by the following gram-positive microorganisms when bacteriologic testing indicates appropriate suspectibility to the drug:
Streptococcus species:
Up to 44 percent of strains of *Streptococcus pyogenes* and 74 percent of *Streptococcus faecalis* have been found to be resistant to tetracycline drugs. Therefore, tetracyclines should not be used for streptococcal disease unless the organism has been demonstrated to be sensitive.
For upper respiratory infections due to Group A beta-hemolytic streptococci, pencillin is the usual drug of choice, including prophylaxis of rheumatic fever.
Diplococcus pneumoniae,
Staphylococcus aureus, skin and soft tissue infections. Oxytetracycline is not the drug of choice in the treatment of any type of staphylococcus infections.
When penicillin is contraindicated, tetracyclines are alternative drugs in the treatment of infections due to:
Neisseria gonorrhoeae,
Treponema pallidum and *Treponema pertenue* (syphilis and yaws),
Listeria monocytogenes,
Clostridium species,
Bacillus anthracis,
Fusobacterium fusiforme (Vincent's infection),
Actinomyces species.
Tetracyclines are indicated in the treatment of trachoma, although the infectious agent is not always eliminated, as judged by immunofluorescence.
Inclusion conjunctivitis may be treated with oral tetracyclines or with a combination of oral and topical agents.
When a decision to administer both a corticoid and an antimicrobial is made, the administration of such drugs in combination has the advantage of greater patient compliance and convenience, with the added assurance that the appropriate dosage of both drugs is administered, plus assured compatibility of ingredients when both types of drug are in the same formulation and, particularly, that the correct volume of drug is delivered and retained.
The relative potency of corticosteroids depends on the molecular structure, concentration, and release from the vehicle.
Indications and Usage: A steroid/anti-infective combination is indicated in ocular inflammation when concurrent use of an antimicrobial is judged necessary.
Contraindications: Epithelial herpes simplex keratitis (dendritic keratitis), vaccinia, varicella, and many other viral diseases of the cornea and conjunctiva. Mycobacterial infection of the eye. Fungal diseases of ocular structures. Hypersensitivity to a component of the medication. (Hypersensitivity to the antibiotic component occurs at a higher rate than for other components.)
The use of these combinations is always contraindicated after uncomplicated removal of a corneal foreign body.
Warnings: Prolonged use may result in glaucoma, with damage to the optic nerve, defects in visual acuity and fields of vision, and posterior subcapsular cataract formation. Prolonged use may suppress the host response and thus increase the hazard of secondary ocular infections. In those diseases causing thinning of the cornea or sclera, perforations have been known to occur with the use of topical steroids. In acute purulent conditions of the eye, steroids may mask infection or enhance existing infection. If these products are used for 10 days or longer, intraocular pressure should be routinely monitored even though it may be difficult in children and uncooperative patients. Employment of steroid medication in the treatment of herpes simplex requires great caution.
Precautions: The initial prescription and renewal of the medication order beyond 20 milliliters should be made by a physician only after examination of the patient with the aid of magnification, such as slit lamp biomicroscopy and, where appropriate, fluorescein staining.
The possibility of persistent fungal infections of the cornea should be considered after prolonged steroid dosing.
Adverse Reactions: Adverse reactions have occurred with steroid/anti-infective combination drugs which can be attributed to the steroid component, the anti-infective component, or the combination. Exact incidence figures are not available since no denominator of treated patients is available.
Reactions occurring most often from the presence of the anti-infective ingredient are allergic sensitizations. The reactions due to the steroid component in decreasing order of frequency are: elevation of intraocular pressure (IOP) with possible development of glaucoma, and infrequent optic nerve damage; posterior subcapsular cataract formation; and delayed wound healing.
Secondary Infection: The development of secondary infection has occurred after use of combinations containing steroids and antimicrobials. Fungal infections of the cornea are particularly prone to develop coincidentally with long-term applications of steroid. The possibility of fungal invasion must be considered in any persistent corneal ulceration where steroid treatment has been used.
Secondary bacterial ocular infection following suppression of host responses also occurs.
Dosage and Administration: Instill 1 or 2 drops of Terra-Cortril Ophthalmic Suspension into the affected eye three times daily.
Not more than 20 milliliters should be prescribed initially and the prescription should not be refilled without further evaluation as outlined in "Precautions" above.
How Supplied: Terra-Cortril Ophthalmic Suspension is supplied in 5 ml vials with separate sterile dropper.

TERRAMYCIN® ℞
Capsules
(oxytetracycline HCl)
Film–coated Tablets
(oxytetracycline)

Description: Oxytetracycline is a product of the metabolism of *Streptomyces rimosus* and is one of the family of tetracycline antibiotics.
Oxytetracycline diffuses readily through the placenta into the fetal circulation, into the pleural fluid and, under some circumstances, into the cerebrospinal fluid. It appears to be concentrated in the hepatic system and excreted in the bile, so that it appears in the feces, as well as in the urine, in a biologically active form.
Actions: Oxytetracycline is primarily bacteriostatic and is thought to exert its antimicrobial effect by the inhibition of protein synthesis. Oxytetracycline is active against a wide range of gram-negative and gram-positive organisms. The drugs in the tetracycline class have closely similar antimicrobial spectra, and cross-resistance among them is common. Microorganisms may be considered susceptible if the M.I.C. (minimum inhibitory concentration) is not more than 4.0 mcg/ml and intermediate if the M.I.C. is 4.0 to 12.5 mcg/ml.
Susceptibility plate testing: A tetracycline disc may be used to determine microbial susceptiblity to drugs in the tetracycline class. If the Kirby-Bauer method of disc susceptibility testing is used, a 30 mcg tetracycline disc should give a zone of at least 19 mm when tested against a tetracycline-susceptible bacterial strain.

Tetracyclines are readily absorbed and are bound to plasma proteins in varying degree. They are concentrated by the liver in the bile and excreted in the urine and feces at high concentrations and in a biologically active form.
Indications: Oxytetracycline is indicated in infections caused by the following microorganisms:
Rickettsiae (Rocky Mountain spotted fever, typhus fever and the typhus group, Q fever, rickettsialpox and tick fevers),
Mycoplasma pneumoniae(PPLO, Eaton Agent), Agents of psittacosis and ornithosis,
Agents of lymphogranuloma venereum and granuloma inguinale,
The spirochetal agent of relapsing fever *(Borrelia recurrentis).*
The following gram-negative microorganisms:
Haemophilus ducreyi (chancroid),
Pasteurella pestis and *Pasteurella tularensis,*
Bartonella bacilliformis,
Bacteroides species,
Vibrio comma and *Vibrio fetus,*
Brucella species (in conjunction with streptomycin).
Because many strains of the following groups of microorganisms have been shown to be resistant to tetracyclines, culture and susceptibility testing are recommended.
Oxytetracycline is indicated for treatment of infections caused by the following gram- negative microorganisms, when bacteriologic testing indicates appropriate susceptibility to the drug:
Escherichia coli,
Enterobacter aerogenes (formerly *Aerobacter aerogenes*),
Shigella species,
Mima species and *Herellea* species,
Haemophilus influenzae (respiratory infections),
Klebsiella species (respiratory and urinary infections).
Oxytetracycline is indicated for treatment of infections caused by the following gram-positive microorganisms when bacteriologic testing indicates appropriate susceptibility to the drug:
Streptococcus species:
Up to 44 percent of strains of *Streptococcus pyogenes* and 74 percent of *Streptococcus faecalis* have been found to be resistant to tetracycline drugs. Therefore, tetracyclines should not be used for streptococcal disease unless the organism has been demonstrated to be sensitive.
For upper respiratory infections due to Group A beta-hemolytic streptococci, penicillin is the usual drug of choice, including prophylaxis of rheumatic fever.
Diplococcus pneumoniae,
Staphylococcus aureus, skin and soft tissue infections. Oxytetracycline is not the drug of choice in the treatment of any type of staphylococcal infections.
When penicillin is contraindicated, tetracyclines are alternative drugs in the treatment of infections due to:
Neisseria gonorrhoeae
In acute intestinal amebiasis, the tetracyclines may be a useful adjunct to amebicides.
In severe acne, the tetracyclines may be useful adjunctive therapy. (This indication is for the oral use only, not for I.M. or I.V.)
Tetracyclines are indicated in the treatment of trachoma, although the infectious agent is not always eliminated, as judged by immunofluorescence.
Inclusion conjunctivitis may be treated with oral tetracyclines or with a combination of oral and topical agents.
Contraindications: This drug is contraindicated in persons who have shown hypersensitivity to any of the tetracyclines.
Warnings: THE USE OF DRUGS OF THE TETRACYCLINE CLASS DURING TOOTH DEVELOPMENT (LAST HALF OF PREGNANCY, INFANCY, AND CHILDHOOD TO THE AGE OF 8 YEARS) MAY CAUSE PERMANENT DISCOL-

Continued on next page

Pfipharmecs—Cont.

ORATION OF THE TEETH (YELLOW-GRAY-BROWN). This adverse reaction is more common during long term use of the drugs but has been observed following repeated short term courses. Enamel hypoplasia has also been reported. *TETRACYCLINE DRUGS, THEREFORE, SHOULD NOT BE USED IN THIS AGE GROUP UNLESS OTHER DRUGS ARE NOT LIKELY TO BE EFFECTIVE OR ARE CONTRAINDICATED.*

When the need for intensive treatment outweighs its potential dangers (mostly during pregnancy or in individuals with known or suspected renal or liver impairment), it is advisable to perform renal and liver function tests before and during therapy. Also, tetracycline serum concentrations should be followed. If renal impairment exists, even usual oral or parenteral doses may lead to excessive systemic accumulation of the drug and possible liver toxicity. Under such conditions, lower than usual total doses are indicated, and if therapy is prolonged, serum level determinations of the drug may be advisable. This hazard is of particular importance in the parenteral administration of tetracyclines to pregnant or postpartum patients with pyelonephritis.

When used under these circumstances, the blood level should not exceed 15 mcg/ml and liver function tests should be made at frequent intervals. Other potentially hepatotoxic drugs should not be prescribed concomitantly.

Photosensitivity manifested by an exaggerated sunburn reaction has been observed in some individuals taking tetracyclines. Patients apt to be exposed to direct sunlight or ultraviolet light should be advised that this reaction can occur with tetracycline drugs, and treatment should be discontinued at the first evidence of skin erythema. The antianabolic action of the tetracyclines may cause an increase in BUN. While this is not a problem in those with normal renal function, in patients with significantly impaired function, higher serum levels of tetracycline may lead to azotemia, hyperphosphatemia, and acidosis.

Usage in pregnancy. (See above "Warnings" about use during tooth development.)

Results of animal studies indicate that tetracyclines cross the placenta, are found in fetal tissues and can have toxic effects on the developing fetus (often related to retardation of skeletal development). Evidence of embryotoxicity has also been noted in animals treated early in pregnancy.

Usage in newborns, infants, and children. (See above "Warnings" about use during tooth development.)

All tetracyclines form a stable calcium complex in any bone forming tissue. A decrease in the fibula growth rate has been observed in prematures given oral tetracycline in doses of 25 mg/kg every 6 hours. This reaction was shown to be reversible when the drug was discontinued.

Tetracyclines are present in the milk of lactating women who are taking a drug in this class.

Precautions: As with other antibiotic preparations, use of this drug may result in overgrowth of nonsusceptible organisms, including fungi. If superinfection occurs, the antibiotic should be discontinued and appropriate therapy instituted.

In venereal diseases when coexistent syphilis is suspected, a dark field examination should be done before treatment is started and the blood serology repeated monthly for at least 4 months.

Because tetracyclines have been shown to depress plasma prothrombin activity, patients who are on anticoagulant therapy may require downward adjustment of their anticoagulant dosage.

In long term therapy, periodic laboratory evaluation of organ systems, including hematopoietic, renal and hepatic studies should be performed.

All infections due to Group A beta-hemolytic streptococci should be treated for at least 10 days. Since bacteriostatic drugs may interfere with the bactericidal action of penicillin, it is advisable to avoid giving tetracycline in conjunction with penicillin.

Adverse Reactions: Gastrointestinal: anorexia, nausea, vomiting, diarrhea, glossitis, dysphagia, enterocolitis, and inflammatory lesions (with monilial overgrowth) in the anogenital region. These reactions have been caused by both the oral and parenteral administration of tetracyclines. Rare instances of esophagitis and esophageal ulcerations have been reported in patients receiving capsule and tablet forms of drugs in the tetracycline class. Most of these patients took medications immediately before going to bed. (See Dosage and Administration.)

Skin: maculopapular and erythematous rashes. Exfoliative dermatitis has been reported but is uncommon. Photosensitivity is discussed above. (See "Warnings.")

Renal toxicity: Rise in BUN has been reported and is apparently dose related. (See "Warnings.")

Hypersensitivity reactions: Urticaria, angioneurotic edema, anaphylaxis, axaphylactoid purpura, pericarditis and exacerbation of systemic lupus erythematosus.

Bulging fontanels in infants and benign intracranial hypertension in adults have been reported in individuals receiving full therapeutic dosages. These conditions disappeared rapidly when the drug was discontinued.

Blood: Hemolytic anemia, thrombocytopenia, neutropenia and eosinophilia have been reported. When given over prolonged periods, tetracyclines have been reported to produce brown-black microscopic discoloration of thyroid glands. No abnormalities of thyroid function studies are known to occur.

Dosage and Administration:
Oral: Capsules:
Adults: Usual daily dose, 1–2 g divided in four equal doses, depending on the severity of the infection.

Film-coated Tablets only:
Adults: A dosage schedule providing 2 tablets initially, then 1 tablet every six hours, is the usual average dose. In severe infections a larger dose (2 to 4 grams daily) may be indicated.

The total daily dose should be administered in four equal portions given at six hour intervals.

All Oral Forms:
For children above eight years of age: Usual daily dose, 10–20 mg per pound (25–50 mg/kg) of body weight divided in four equal doses.

Therapy should be continued for at least 24–48 hours after symptoms and fever have subsided.

For treatment of brucellosis, 500 mg oxytetracycline four times daily for 3 weeks should be accompanied by streptomycin, 1 gram intramuscularly twice daily the first week, and once daily the second week.

For treatment of uncomplicated gonorrhea, when penicillin is contraindicated, tetracycline may be used for the treatment of both males and females in the following dividend dosage schedule: 1.5 grams initially followed by 0.5 gram q.i.d. for a total of 9.0 grams.

For treatment of syphilis, a total of 30–40 grams in equally divided doses over a period of 10–15 days should be given. Close follow-up, including laboratory tests, is recommended.

Administration of adequate amounts of fluid along with capsule and tablet forms of drugs in the tetracycline class is recommended to wash down the drugs and reduce the risk of esophageal irritation and ulceration. (See Adverse Reactions.)

Concomitant therapy: Antacids containing aluminum, calcium, or magnesium impair absorption and should not be given to patients taking oral tetracyclines.

Food and some dairy products also interfere with absorption. Oral forms of tetracyclines should be given 1 hours before or 2 hours after meals. Pediatric oral dosage forms should not be given with milk formulas and should be given at least 1 hour prior to feeding.

In patients with renal impairment: (See "Warnings.") Total dosage should be decreased by reduction of recommended individual doses and/or by extending time intervals between doses.

In the treatment of streptococcal infections, a therapeutic dose of oxytetracycline should be administered for at least 10 days.

How Supplied:
Oral: Terramycin (oxytetracycline HCl) Capsules are available as opaque, yellow, hard gelatin capsules which contain oxytetracycline HCl equivalent to 250 mg of oxytetracycline, and glucosamine hydrochloride (imprinted with code number 073): bottles of 16, 100, and 500 and unit dose pack of 100 (10 × 10's).

Terramycin (oxytetracycline) Tablets are available as:

250 mg film-coated tablets (imprinted with code number 084): bottles of 100.

Capsule Shown in Product Identification Section, page 426

(Capsule)   60-0755-00-6
(Film-coated Tablets)   23-1127-00-2

TERRAMYCIN®
(oxytetracycline)
INTRAMUSCULAR SOLUTION*
FOR INTRAMUSCULAR USE ONLY
contains 2% lidocaine

Description: Oxytetracycline is a product of the metabolism of *Streptomyces rimosus* and is one of the family of tetracycline antibiotics.

Oxytetracycline diffuses readily through the placenta into the fetal circulation, into the pleural fluid and, under some circumstances, into the cerebrospinal fluid. It appears to be concentrated in the hepatic system and excreted in the bile, so that it appears in the feces, as well as in the urine, in a biologically active form.

Composition:
[See table left].

Actions: Oxytetracycline is primarily bacteriostatic and is thought to exert its antimicrobial effect by the inhibition of protein synthesis. Oxytetracycline is active against a wide range of gram-negative and gram-positive organisms.

The drugs in the tetracycline class have closely similar antimicrobial spectra, and cross resistance among them is common. Microorganisms may be

Terramycin Intramuscular

contents per ml (w/v)

Ingredient	2 ml Single Dose Ampules and isoject		10 ml/Vial Multidose
	100 mg/2 ml	250 mg/2 ml	50 mg/ml 10 ml (5 × 2 ml Doses)
oxytetracycline	50 mg	25 mg	50 mg
lidocaine	2.0%	2.0%	2.0%
magnesium chloride hexahydrate	2.5%	6.0%	2.5%
sodium formaldehyde sulfoxylate	0.5%	0.5%	0.3%
α-monothioglycerol	—	—	1.0%
monoethanolamine	approx. 1.7%	approx. 4.2%	approx. 2.6%
citric acid	—	—	1.0%
propyl gallate	—	—	0.02%
propylene glycol	75.2%	67.0%	74.1%
water	18.8%	16.8%	18.5%

considered susceptible if the M.I.C. (minimum inhibitory concentration) is not more than 4.0 mcg/ml and intermediate if the M.I.C. is 4.0 to 12.5 mcg/ml.

Susceptibility plate testing: A tetracycline disc may be used to determine microbial susceptibility to drugs in the tetracycline class. If the Kirby-Bauer method of disc susceptibility testing is used, a 30 mcg tetracycline disc should give a zone of at least 19 mm when tested against an oxytetracycline-susceptible bacterial strain.

Tetracyclines are readily absorbed and are bound to plasma proteins in varying degree. They are concentrated by the liver in the bile and excreted in the urine and feces at high concentrations and in a biologically active form.

Indications: Oxytetracycline is indicated in infections caused by the following microorganisms:

Rickettsiae (Rocky Mountain spotted fever, typhus fever and the typhus group, Q fever, rickettsialpox and tick fevers).

Mycoplasma pneumoniae (PPLO, Eaton agent),
Agents of psittacosis and ornithosis,
Agents of lymphogranuloma venereum and granuloma inguinale,
The spirochetal agent of relapsing fever *(Borrelia recurrentis)*.
The following gram-negative microorganisms:
Haemophilus ducreyi (chancroid),
Pasteurella pestis and *Pasteurella tularensis*,
Bartonella bacilliformis,
Bacteroides species,
Vibrio comma and *Vibrio fetus*,
Brucella species (in conjunction with streptomycin).

Because many strains of the following groups of microorganisms have been shown to be resistant to tetracyclines, culture and susceptibility testing are recommended.

Oxytetracycline is indicated for treatment of infections caused by the following gram-negative microorganisms, when bacteriologic testing indicates appropriate susceptibility to the drug:
Escherichia coli,
Enterobacter aerogenes (formerly *Aerobacter aerogenes)*,
Shigella species,
Mima species and *Herellea* species,
Haemophilus influenzae(respiratory infections),
Klebsiella species (respiratory and urinary infections).

Oxytetracycline is indicated for treatment of infections caused by the following gram-positive microorganisms when bacteriologic testing indicates appropriate susceptibility to the drug: Streptococcus species;

Up to 44 percent of strains of *Streptococcus pyogenes* and 74 percent of *Streptococcus faecalis* have been found to be resistant to tetracycline drugs. Therefore, tetracyclines should not be used for streptococcal disease unless the organism has been demonstrated to be sensitive.

For upper respiratory infections due to Group A beta-hemolytic streptococci, penicillin is the usual drug of choice, including prophylaxis of rheumatic fever.

Diplococcus pneumoniae,
Staphylococcus aureus, skin and soft tissue infections. Oxytetracycline is not the drug of choice in the treatment of any type of staphylococcal infections.

When penicillin is contraindicated, tetracyclines are alternative drugs in the treatment of infections due to:
Neisseria gonorrhoeae,
Treponema pallidum and *Treponema pertenue* (syphilis and yaws),
Listeria monocytogenes,
Clostridium species,
Bacillus anthracis,
Fusobacterium fusiforme (Vincent's infection),
Actinomyces species.

In acute intestinal amebiasis, the tetracyclines may be a useful adjunct to amebicides.

Tetracyclines are indicated in the treatment of trachoma, although the infectious agent is not always eliminated, as judged by immunofluorescence.

Inclusion conjunctivitis may be treated with oral tetracyclines or with a combination of oral and topical agents.

Contraindications: This drug is contraindicated in persons who have shown hypersensitivity to any of the tetracyclines.

Warnings: THE USE OF TETRACYCLINES DURING TOOTH DEVELOPMENT (LAST HALF OF PREGNANCY, INFANCY, AND CHILDHOOD TO THE AGE OF 8 YEARS) MAY CAUSE PERMANENT DISCOLORATION OF THE TEETH (YELLOW-GRAY-BROWN).

This adverse reaction is more common during long term use of the drugs but has been observed following repeated short term courses. Enamel hypoplasia has also been reported. *TETRACYCLINES, THEREFORE, SHOULD NOT BE USED IN THIS AGE GROUP UNLESS OTHER DRUGS ARE NOT LIKELY TO BE EFFECTIVE OR ARE CONTRAINDICATED.*

If renal impairment exists, even usual oral or parenteral doses may lead to excessive systemic accumulation of the drug and possible liver toxicity. Under such conditions, lower than usual total doses are indicated and, if therapy is prolonged, serum level determinations of the drug may be advisable. This hazard is of particular importance in the parenteral administration of tetracyclines to pregnant or postpartum patients with pyelonephritis. When used under these circumstances, the blood level should not exceed 15 mcg/ml and liver function tests should be made at frequent intervals. Other potentially hepatotoxic drugs should not be prescribed concomitantly.

(In the presence of renal dysfunction, particularly in pregnancy, intravenous tetracycline therapy in daily doses exceeding 2 grams has been associated with deaths due to liver failure.)

Photosensitivity manifested by an exaggerated sunburn reaction has been observed in some individuals taking tetracyclnes. Patients apt to be exposed to direct sunlight or ultraviolet light should be advised that this reaction can occur with tetracycline drugs, and treatment should be discontinued at the first evidence of skin erythema.

The antianabolic action of the tetracyclines may cause an increase in BUN. While this is not a problem in those with normal renal function, in patients with significantly impaired function, higher serum levels of this drug may lead to azotemia, hyperphosphatemia, and acidosis.

Usage in pregnancy. (See above "Warnings" about use during tooth development.)

Results of animal studies indicate that tetracyclines cross the placenta, are found in fetal tissues and can have toxic effects on the developing fetus (often related to retardation of skeletal development). Evidence of embryotoxicity has also been noted in animals treated early in pregnancy.

Usage in newborns, infants, and children. (See above "Warnings" about use during tooth deveopment).

All tetracyclines form a stable calcium complex in any bone-forming tissue. A decrease in the fibula growth rate has been observed in prematures given oral tetracyclne in doses of 25 mg/kg every 6 hours. This reaction was shown to be reversible when the drug was discontinued.

Tetracyclines are present in the milk of lactating women who are taking a drug in this class.

Precautions: As with all intramuscular preparations, Terramycin (oxytetracycline) Intramuscular Solution should be injected well within the body of a relatively large muscle. ADULTS: The preferred sites are the upper outer quadrant of the buttock, (i.e., gluteus maximus), and the mid-lateral thigh. CHILDREN: It is recommended that intramuscular injections be given preferably in the mid-lateral muscles of the thigh. In infants and small children the periphery of the upper outer quadrant of the gluteal region should be used only when necessary, such as in burn patients, in order to minimize the possibility of damage to the sciatic nerve.

The deltoid area should be used only if well developed such as in certain adults and older children, and then only with caution to avoid radial nerve injury. Intramuscular injections should not be made into the lower and mid-thirds of the upper arm. As with all intramuscular injections, aspiration is necessary to help avoid inadvertent injection into a blood vessel.

As with other antibiotic preparations, use of this drug may result in overgrowth of nonsusceptible organisms, including fungi. If superinfection occurs, the antibiotic should be discontinued and appropriate therapy instituted.

In venereal diseases when coexistent syphilis is suspected, a dark field examination should be done before treatment is started and the blood serology repeated monthly for at least 4 months.

Because tetracyclines have been shown to depress plasma prothrombin activity, patients who are on anticoagulant therapy may require downward adjustment of their anticoagulant dosage.

In long term terapy, periodic laboratory evaluation of organ systems, including hematopoietic, renal and hepatic studies should be performed.

All infections due to Group A beta-hemolytic streptococci should be treated for at least 10 days. Since bacteriostatic drugs may interfere with the bactericidal action of penicillin, it is advisable to avoid giving tetracycline in conjunction with penicillin.

Adverse Reactions: Local irritation may be present after intramuscular injection. The injection should be deep, with care taken not to injure the sciatic nerve nor inject intravascularly.

Gastrointestinal: anorexia, nausea, vomiting, diarrhea, glossitis, dyphagia, enterocolitis, and inflammatory lesions (with monilial overgrowth) in the anogenital region. These reactions have been caused by both the oral and parenteral administration of tetracyclines.

Skin: maculopapular and erythematous rashes. Exfoliative dermatitis has been reported but is uncommon. Photosensitivity is discussed above. (See "Warnings").

Renal toxicity: Rise in BUN has been reported and is apparently dose related. (See "Warnings").

Hypersensitivity reactions: Urticaria, angioneurotic edema, anaphylaxis, anaphylactoid purpura, pericarditis, and exacerbation of systemic lupus erythematosus.

Bulging fontanels in infants and benign intracranial hypertension in adults have been reported in individuals receiving full therapeutic dosages. These conditions disappeared rapidly when the drug was discontinued.

Blood: Hemolytic anemia, thrombocytopenia, neutropenia, and eosinophilia have been reported. When given over prolonged periods, tetracyclines have been reported to produce brown-black microscopic discoloration of thyroid glands. No abnormalities of thyroid function studies are known to occur.

Dosage and Administration:
Intramuscular Administration:
Adults: The usual daily dose is 250 mg administered once every 24 hours or 300 mg given in divided doses at 8 to 12 hour intervals.

For children above eight years of age: 15-25 mg/kg body weight up to a maximum of 250 mg per single daily injection. Dosage may be divided and given at 8 to 12 hour intervals.

Intramuscular therapy should be reserved for situations in which oral therapy is not feasible. The intramuscular administration of oxytetracycline produces lower blood levels than oral administration in the recommended dosages. Patients placed on intramuscular oxytetracycline should be changed to the oral dosage form as soon as possible. If rapid, high blood levels are needed, oxytetracycline should be administered intravenously. In patients with renal impairment: (See "Warnings") Total dosage should be decreased by reduction of recommended individual doses and/or by extending time intervals between doses.

How Supplied: Terramycin (oxytetracycline) Intramuscular Solution is available as follows:

Continued on next page

Pfipharmecs—Cont.

Potency of 250 mg/2 ml—in 2 ml pre-scored glass ampules, packages of 5 and 100.
 2 ml Isoject® disposable syringe, packages of 10.
Potency of 100 mg/2 ml in 2 ml pre-scored glass ampules, packages of 5 and 100.
 2 ml Isoject® disposable syringe, packages of 10.
Potency of 50 mg/ml in 10 ml multiple dose vials, packages of 5.
*U.S. Pat. Nos. 3,017,323 and 3,026,248

TERRAMYCIN® OINTMENT
(oxytetracycline hydrochloride topical ointment with polymyxin B sulfate)

How Supplied: Each gram contains oxytetracycline hydrochloride equivalent to 30 mg. of oxytetracycline; and also 10,000 units of polymyxin B sulfate.
Available in ½ ounce and one ounce tubes, both sizes sold in cartons of twelve. A prescription is *not* required.

TERRAMYCIN® ℞
(oxytetracycline HCl with polymyxin B sulfate)
OPHTHALMIC OINTMENT
STERILE

Description: Each gram of sterile ointment contains oxytetracycline HCl equivalent to 5 mg oxytetracycline, 10,000 units of polymyxin B sulfate, white petrolatum, and liquid petrolatum.
Actions: Terramycin® (oxytetracycline HCl) is a widely used antibiotic with clinically proved activity against gram-positive and gram-negative bacteria, rickettsiae, spirochetes, large viruses, and certain protozoa.
Polymyxin B Sulfate, one of a group of related antibiotics derived from *Bacillus polymyxa*, is rapidly bactericidal. This action is exclusively against gram-negative organisms. It is particularly effective against *Pseudomonas aeruginosa* (*B. pyocyaneus*) and Koch-Weeks bacillus, frequently found in local infections of the eye.
There is thus made available a particularly effective antimicrobial combination of the broad-spectrum antibiotic Terramycin as well as polymyxin B sulfate against primarily causative or secondarily infecting organisms.
Indications: The sterile preparation. Terramycin with Polymyxin B Sulfate Ophthalmic Ointment, is indicated for the treatment of superficial ocular infections involving the conjunctiva and/or cornea caused by Terramycin with Polymyxin B Sulfate-susceptible organisms.
It may be administered topically alone, or as an adjunct to systemic therapy.
It is effective in infections caused by susceptible strains of staphylococci, streptococci, pneumococci, *Hemophilus influenzae, Pseudomonas aeruginosa*, Koch-Weeks bacillus, and *Proteus.*
Contraindications: This drug is contraindicated in individuals who have shown hypersensitivity to any of its components.
Precautions: As with all antibiotic preparations, use of this drug may result in overgrowth of nonsusceptible organisms, including fungi. If super-infection occurs, the antibiotic should be discontinued and appropriate specific therapy should be instituted.
Adverse Reactions: Terramycin with Polymyxin B Sulfate Ophthalmic Ointment is well tolerated by the epithelial membranes and other tissues of the eye. Allergic or inflammatory reactions due to individual hypersensitivity are rare.
Dosage and Administration: Approximately ½ inch of the ointment is squeezed from the tube onto the lower lid of the affected eye two to four times daily.
The patient should be instructed to avoid contamination of the tip of the tube when applying the ointment.

How Supplied: Terramycin with Polymyxin B Sulfate Ophthalmic Ointment is supplied in ⅛ oz., (3.5 g) tubes.

VISTARIL® ℞
(hydroxyzine hydrochloride)
Intramuscular Solution
For Intramuscular Use Only

Chemistry: Hydroxyzine hydrochloride is designated chemically as 1-(p-chlorobenzhydryl) 4-[2-(2-hydroxyethoxy) ethyl] piperazine dihydrochloride.
Actions: VISTARIL (hydroxyzine hydrochloride) is unrelated chemically to phenothiazine, reserpine, and meprobamate. Hydroxyzine has demonstrated its clinical effectiveness in the chemotherapeutic aspect of the total management of neuroses and emotional disturbances manifested by anxiety, tension, agitation, apprehension or confusion.
Hydroxyzine has been shown clinically to be a rapid-acting true ataraxic with a wide margin of safety. It induces a calming effect in anxious, tense, psychoneurotic adults and also in anxious, hyperkinetic children without impairing mental alertness. It is not a cortical depressant, but its action may be due to a suppression of activity in certain key regions of the subcortical area of the central nervous system.
Primary skeletal muscle relaxation has been demonstrated experimentally.
Hydroxyzine has been shown experimentally to have antispasmodic properties, apparently mediated through interference with the mechanism that reponds to spasmogenic agents such as serotonin, acetylcholine, and histamine.
Antihistaminic effects have been demonstrated experimentally and confirmed clinically.
An antiemetic effect, both by the apomorphine test and the veriloid test, has been demonstrated. Pharmacological and clinical studies indicate that hydroxyzine in therapeutic dosage does not increase gastric secretion or acidity and in most cases provides mild antisecretory benefits.
Indications: The total management of anxiety, tension, and psychomotor agitation in conditions of emotional stress requires in most instances a combined approach of psychotherapy and chemotherapy. Hydroxyzine has been found to be particularly useful for this latter phrase of therapy in its ability to render the disturbed patient more amenable to psychotherapy in long term treatment of the psychoneurotic and psychotic, although it should not be used as the sole treatment of psychosis or of clearly demonstrated cases of depression.
Hydroxyzine is also useful in alleviating the manifestations of anxiety and tension as in the preparation for dental procedures and in acute emotional problems. It has also been recommended for the management of anxiety associated with organic disturbances and as adjunctive therapy in alcoholism and allergic conditions with strong emotional overlay, such as in asthma, chronic urticaria, and pruritus.
VISTARIL (hydroxyzine hydrochloride) Intramuscular Solution is useful in treating the following types of patients when intramuscular administration is indicated:
1. The acutely disturbed or hysterical patient.
2. The acute or chronic alcoholic with anxiety withdrawal symptoms or delirium tremens.
3. As pre- and postoperative and pre- and postpartum adjunctive medication to permit reduction in narcotic dosage, allay anxiety and control emesis.

VISTARIL (hydroxyzine hydrochloride) has also demonstrated effectiveness in controlling nausea and vomiting, excluding nausea and vomiting of pregnancy. (See Contraindications.)
In prepartum states, the reduction in narcotic requirement effected by hydroxyzine is of particular benefit to both mother and neonate.
Hydroxyzine benefits the cardiac patient by its ability to allay the associated anxiety and apprehension attendant to certain types of heart disease. Hydroxyzine is not known to interfere with the action of digitalis in any way and may be used concurrently with this agent.

The effectiveness of hydroxyzine in long term use, that is, more than 4 months, has not been assessed by systematic clinical studies. The physician should reassess periodically the usefulness of the drug for the individual patient.
Contraindications: Hydroxyzine hydrochloride intramuscular solution is intended only for intramuscular administration and should not, under any circumstances, be injected subcutaneously, intra-arterially, or intravenously.
This drug is contraindicated for patients who have shown a previous hypersensitivity to it.
Hydroxyzine, when administered to the pregnant mouse, rat, and rabbit, induced fetal abnormalities in the rat at doses substantially above the human therapeutic range. Clinical data in human beings are inadequate to establish safety in early pregnancy. Until such data are available, hydroxyzine is contraindicated in early pregnancy.
Precautions: THE POTENTIATING ACTION OF HYDROXYZINE MUST BE CONSIDERED WHEN THE DRUG IS USED IN CONJUNCTION WITH CENTRAL NERVOUS SYSTEM DEPRESSANTS SUCH AS NARCOTICS, BARBITURATES, AND ALCOHOL. Therefore when central nervous system depressants are administered concomitantly with hydroxyzine their dosage should be reduced up to 50 per cent. The efficacy of hydroxyzine as adjunctive pre- and postoperative sedative medication has also been well established, especially as regards its ability to allay anxiety, control emesis, and reduce the amount of narcotic required.
HYDROXYZINE MAY POTENTIATE NARCOTICS AND BARBITURATES, so their use in preanesthetic adjunctive therapy should be modified on an individual basis. Atropine and other belladonna alkaloids are not affected by the drug.
When hydroxyzine is used preoperatively or prepartum, narcotic requirements may be reduced as much as 50 per cent. Thus, when 50 mg of VISTARIL (hydroxyzine hydrochloride) Intramuscular Solution is employed, meperidine dosage may be reduced from 100 mg to 50 mg. The administration of meperidine may result in severe hypotension in the postoperative patient or any individual whose ability to maintain blood pressure has been compromised by a depleted blood volume. Meperidine should be used with great caution and in reduced dosage in patients who are receiving other pre- and/or postoperative medications and in whom there is a risk of respiratory depression, hypotension, and profound sedation or coma occurring. Before using any medications concomitant with hydroxyzine, the manufacturer's prescribing information should be read carefully.
Since drowsiness may occur with the use of this drug, patients should be warned of this possibility and cautioned against driving a car or operating dangerous machinery while taking this drug.
As with all intramuscular preparations, VISTARIL Intramuscular Solution should be injected well within the body of a relatively large muscle. Inadvertent subcutaneous injection may result in significant tissue damage.
ADULTS: The preferred site is the upper outer quadrant of the buttock, (i.e., gluteus maximus), or the mid-lateral thigh.
CHILDREN: It is recommended that intramuscular injections be given preferably in the midlateral muscles of the thigh. In infants and small children the periphery of the upper outer quadrant of the gluteal region should be used only when necessary, such as in burn patients, in order to minimize the possibility of damage to the sciatic nerve.
The deltoid area should be used only if well developed such as in certain adults and older children, and then only with caution to avoid radial nerve injury. Intramuscular injections should not be made into the lower and mid-third of the upper arm. As with all intramuscular injections, aspiration is necessary to help avoid inadvertent injection into a blood vessel.
Adverse Reactions: Therapeutic doses of hydroxyzine seldom produce impairment of mental alertness. However, drowsiness may occur; if so, it is usually transitory and may disappear in a few

days of continued therapy or upon reduction of the dose. Dryness of the mouth may be encountered at higher doses. Extensive clinical use has substantiated the absence of toxic effects on the liver or bone marrow when administered in the recommended doses for over four years of uninterrupted therapy. The absence of adverse effects has been further demonstrated in experimental studies in which excessively high doses were administered. Involuntary motor activity, including rare instances of tremor and convulsions, has been reported, usually with doses considerably higher than those recommended. Continuous therapy with over one gram per day has been employed in some patients without these effects having been encountered.

Dosage and Administration: The recommended dosages for VISTARIL (hydroxyzine hydrochloride) Intramuscular Solution are:

For adult psychiatric and emotional emergencies, including acute alcoholism.	I.M.: 50–100 mg stat., and q. 4–6h., p.r.n.
Nausea and vomiting excluding nausea and vomiting of pregnancy.	Adults: 25–100 mg I.M. Children: 0.5 mg/lb. body weight I.M.
Pre- and postoperative adjunctive medication.	Adults: 25–100 mg I.M. Children: 0.5 mg/lb. body weight I.M.
Pre- and postpartum adjunctive therapy.	25–100 mg I.M.

As with all potent medications, the dosage should be adjusted according to the patient's response to therapy.
FOR ADDITIONAL INFORMATION ON THE ADMINISTRATION AND SITE OF SELECTION SEE PRECAUTIONS SECTION. NOTE: VISTARIL (hydroxyzine hydrochloride) Intramuscular Solution may be administered without further dilution.
Patients may be started on intramuscular therapy when indicated. They should be maintained on oral therapy whenever this route is practicable.
Supply: Vistaril IM is an aqueous solution containing either 25 mg or 50 mg hydroxyzine HCl per ml, 0.9% benzyl alcohol and sodium hydroxide to adjust to optimum pH.
Multi-Dose Vials
  25 mg per ml, 10 ml vials
  50 mg per ml, 10 ml vials
Unit Dose Vials: Packages of 10 vials
  50 mg per vial, 1 ml fill
  75 mg per vial, 1.5 ml fill
  100 mg per vial, 2 ml fill

WART–OFF™   OTC

Active Ingredient: Salicylic Acid, U.S.P., 17%, in Flexible Collodion, U.S.P. Wart-Off™ Solution contains approx. 20.5% Alcohol and 54.2% Ether—small losses are unavoidable.
Indications: Removal of Warts
Warnings: Keep this and all medications out of reach of children to avoid accidental poisoning. Flammable—Do not use near fire or flame. For external use only. In case of accidental ingestion, contact a physician or a Poison Control Center immediately. Do not use near eyes or on mucous membranes. Diabetics or other people with impaired circulation should not use Wart-Off™. Do not use on moles, birthmarks or unusual warts with hair growing from them. If wart persists, see your physician. If pain should develop, consult your physician. **Do not apply to surrounding skin.**
Dosage and Administration: Instructions For Use: Read warning and enclosed instructional brochure. Do not apply to surrounding skin. Make sure that surrounding skin is protected from accidental application. Apply Wart-Off™ to warts only. Before applying, soak affected area in hot water for several minutes. If any tissue has been loosened, remove by rubbing surface of wart gently with special brush enclosed in Wart-Off™ package. Dry thoroughly. Warts are contagious, so don't share your towel. Apply once or twice daily. Using plastic applicator attached to cap, apply one drop at a time until entire wart is covered. Lightly cover with small adhesive bandage. Replace cap tightly. This treatment may be used daily for three to four weeks if necessary.

How Supplied: 0.5 fluid ounce bottle with pinpoint plastic applicator, special cleaning brush and instructional brochure.
Shown in Product Identification Section, page 426

Pfizer Laboratories Division
PFIZER INC.
235 EAST 42ND STREET
NEW YORK, NY 10017

Full prescribing information for all Pfizer Laboratories products is available from your Pfizer Laboratories representative.

Product Identification Codes

To provide quick and positive identification of Pfizer Laboratories Division products, we have imprinted the product identification number of the National Drug Code on all tablets and capsules.
In order that you may quickly identify a product by its code number, we have compiled below a numerical list of code numbers with their corresponding product names. We are also listing the code numbers by alphabetical order of products.

NUMERICAL PRODUCT INDEX

Product Identification Code	Product
072 & 073	Terramycin® (Oxytetracycline HCl) Capsules (see Pfipharmecs listing.)
084	Terramycin® (Oxytetracycline) Film Coated Tablets (See Pfipharmecs listing.)
094	Vibramycin® Hyclate (Doxycycline Hyclate) Capsules 50 mg.
095	Vibramycin® Hyclate (Doxycycline Hyclate) Capsules 100 mg.
099	Vibra-Tabs® (Doxycycline Hyclate) Film Coated Tablets 100 mg.
260	Procardia® (Nifedipine) Capsules 10 mg.
322	Feldene® (Piroxicam) Capsules 10 mg.
323	Feldene® (Piroxicam) Capsules 20 mg.
375	Renese® (Polythiazide) Tablets 1 mg.
376	Renese® (Polythiazide) Tablets 2 mg.
377	Renese® (Polythiazide) Tablets 4 mg.
393	Diabinese® (Chlorpropamide) Tablets 100 mg.
394	Diabinese® (Chlorpropamide) Tablets 250 mg.
430	Minizide® 1 Capsules (1 mg. Prazosin HCl and 0.5 mg. Polythiazide)
431	Minipress® (Prazosin HCl) Capsules 1 mg.
432	Minizide® 2 Capsules (2 mg. Prazosin HCl and 0.5 mg. Polythiazide)
436	Minizide® 5 Capsules (5 mg. Prazosin HCl and 0.5 mg. Polythiazide)
437	Minipress® (Prazosin HCl) Capsules 2 mg.
438	Minipress® (Prazosin HCl) Capsules 5 mg.
441	Moderil® (Rescinnamine) Tablets 0.25 mg.
442	Moderil® (Rescinnamine) Tablets 0.5 mg.
446	Renese®-R (Polythiazide 2.0 mg. and Reserpine 0.25 mg.) Tablets
541	Vistaril® (Hydroxyzine Pamoate) Capsules 25 mg.
542	Vistaril® (Hydroxyzine Pamoate) Capsules 50 mg.
543	Vistaril® (Hydroxyzine Pamoate) Capsules 100 mg.

ALPHABETICAL PRODUCT INDEX

Product	Product Identification Code
Diabinese® (Chlorpropamide) Tablets 100 mg.	393
Diabinese® (Chlorpropamide) Tablets 250 mg.	394

Product	Code
Feldene® (Piroxicam) Capsules 10 mg.	322
Feldene® (Piroxicam) Capsules 20 mg.	323
Minipress® (Prazosin HCl) Capsules 1 mg.	431
Minipress® (Prazosin HCl) Capsules 2 mg.	437
Minipress® (Prazosin HCl) Capsules 5 mg.	438
Minizide® 1 Capsules (1 mg. Prazosin HCl and 0.5 mg. Polythiazide)	430
Minizide® 2 Capsules (2 mg. Prazosin HCl and 0.5 mg. Polythiazide)	432
Minizide® 5 Capsules (5 mg. Prazosin HCl and 0.5 mg. Polythiazide)	436
Moderil® (Rescinnamine) Tablets 0.25 mg.	441
Moderil® (Rescinnamine) Tablets 0.5 mg.	442
Procardia® (Nifedipine) Capsules 10 mg.	260
Renese® (Polythiazide) Tablets 1 mg.	375
Renese® (Polythiazide) Tablets 2 mg.	376
Renese® (Polythiazide) Tablets 4 mg.	377
Renese®-R (Polythiazide 2.0 mg. and Reserpine 0.25 mg.) Tablets	446
Terramycin® (Oxytetracycline HCl) Capsules (See Pfipharmecs listing.)	072 073
Terramycin® (Oxytetracycline) Film Coated Tablets (See Pfipharmecs listing.)	084
Vibramycin® Hyclate (Doxycycline Hyclate) Capsules 50 mg.	094
Vibramycin® Hyclate (Doxycycline Hyclate) Capsules 100 mg.	095
Vibra-Tabs® (Doxycycline Hyclate) Film Coated Tablets 100 mg.	099
Vistaril® (Hydroxyzine Pamoate) Capsules 25 mg.	541
Vistaril® (Hydroxyzine Pamoate) Capsules 50 mg.	542
Vistaril® (Hydroxyzine Pamoate) Capsules 100 mg.	543

DIABINESE®   R
[dī-ab'in-ees]
(chlorpropamide)
Tablets, USP
For Oral Use

Description: DIABINESE (chlorpropamide), is an oral blood-glucose-lowering drug of the sulfonylurea class. Chlorpropamide is 1-[(p-Chlorophenyl)sulfonyl]-3-propylurea, $C_{10}H_{13}ClN_2O_3S$. Chlorpropamide is a white crystalline powder, that has a slight odor. It is practically insoluble in water at pH 7.3 (solubility at pH 6 is 2.2 mg/ml). It is soluble in alcohol and moderately soluble in chloroform. The molecular weight of chlorpropamide is 276.74. DIABINESE is available as 100 mg and 250 mg tablets.
Clinical Pharmacology: DIABINESE appears to lower the blood glucose acutely by stimulating the release of insulin from the pancreas, an effect dependent upon functioning beta cells in the pancreatic islets. The mechanism by which DIABINESE lowers blood glucose during long-term administration has not been clearly established. Extra-pancreatic effects may play a part in the mechanism of action of oral sulfonylurea hypoglycemic drugs. While chlorpropamide is a sulfonamide derivative, it is devoid of antibacterial activity.
DIABINESE may also prove effective in controlling certain patients who have experienced primary or secondary failure to other sulfonylurea agents.
A method developed which permits easy measurement of the drug in blood is available on request. Chlorpropamide does not interfere with the usual tests to detect albumin in the urine.
DIABINESE is absorbed rapidly from the gastrointestinal tract. Within one hour after a single oral dose, it is readily detectable in the blood, and the level reaches a maximum within two to four hours. It undergoes metabolism in humans and it is excreted in the urine as unchanged drug and as hydroxylated or hydrolyzed metabolites. The biological half-life of chlorpropamide averages about 36

Continued on next page

hours. Within 96 hours, 80–90% of a single oral dose is excreted in the urine. However, long-term administration of therapeutic doses does not result in undue accumulation in the blood, since absorption and excretion rates become stabilized in about 5 to 7 days after the initiation of therapy.

DIABINESE exerts a hypoglycemic effect in normal humans within one hour, becoming maximal at 3 to 6 hours and persisting for at least 24 hours. The potency of chlorpropamide is approximately six times that of tolbutamide. Some experimental results suggest that its increased duration of action may be the result of slower excretion and absence of significant deactivation.

Indications and Usage: DIABINESE is indicated as an adjunct to diet to lower the blood glucose in patients with non-insulin-dependent diabetes mellitus (type II) whose hyperglycemia cannot be controlled by diet alone.

In initiating treatment for non-insulin-dependent diabetes, diet should be emphasized as the primary form of treatment. Caloric restriction and weight loss are essential in the obese diabetic patient. Proper dietary management alone may be effective in controlling the blood glucose and symptoms of hyperglycemia. The importance of regular physical activity should also be stressed, and cardiovascular risk factors should be identified and corrective measures taken where possible.

If this treatment program fails to reduce symptoms and/or blood glucose, the use of an oral sulfonylurea or insulin should be considered. Use of DIABINESE must be viewed by both the physician and patient as a treatment in addition to diet, and not as a substitute for diet or as a convenient mechanism for avoiding dietary restraint. Furthermore, loss of blood glucose control on diet alone may be transient, thus requiring only short-term administration of DIABINESE.

During maintenance programs, DIABINESE should be discontinued if satisfactory lowering of blood glucose is no longer achieved. Judgments should be based on regular clinical and laboratory evaluations.

In considering the use of DIABINESE in asymptomatic patients, it should be recognized that controlling the blood glucose in non-insulin-dependent diabetes, has not been definitely established to be effective in preventing the long-term cardiovascular or neural complications of diabetes.

Contraindications: DIABINESE is contraindicated in patients with:

1. Known hypersensitivity to the drug.
2. Diabetic ketoacidosis, with or without coma. This condition should be treated with insulin.

Warnings: SPECIAL WARNING ON INCREASED RISK OF CARDIOVASCULAR MORTALITY

The administration of oral hypoglycemic drugs has been reported to be associated with increased cardiovascular mortality as compared to treatment with diet alone or diet plus insulin. This warning is based on the study conducted by the University Group Diabetes Program (UGDP), a long-term prospective clinical trial designed to evaluate the effectiveness of glucose-lowering drugs in preventing or delaying vascular complications in patients with non-insulin-dependent diabetes. The study involved 823 patients who were randomly assigned to one of four treatment groups (*Diabetes,* 19 (supp. 2): 747–830, 1970).

UGDP reported that patients treated for 5 to 8 years with diet plus a fixed dose of tolbutamide (1.5 grams per day) had a rate of cardiovascular mortality approximately 2½ times that of patients treated with diet alone. A significant increase in total mortality was not observed, but the use of tolbutamide was discontinued based on the increase in cardiovascular mortality, thus limiting the opportunity for the study to show an increase in over-all mortality. Despite controversy regarding the interpretation of these results, the findings of the UGDP study provide an adequate basis for this warning. The patient should be informed of the potential risks and advantages of DIABINESE and of alternative modes of therapy.

Although only one drug in the sulfonylurea class (tolbutamide) was included in this study, it is prudent from a safety standpoint to consider that this warning may also apply to other oral hypoglycemic drugs in this class, in view of their close similarities in mode of action and chemical structure.

Precautions:

General

Hypoglycemia: All sulfonylurea drugs are capable of producing severe hypoglycemia. Proper patient selection, dosage, and instructions are important to avoid hypoglycemic episodes. Renal or hepatic insufficiency may cause elevated blood levels of DIABINESE and the latter may also diminish gluconeogenic capacity, both of which increase the risk of serious hypoglycemic reactions. Elderly, debilitated or malnourished patients, and those with adrenal or pituitary insufficiency are particularly susceptible to the hypoglycemic action of glucose-lowering drugs. Hypoglycemia may be difficult to recognize in the elderly, and in people who are taking beta-adrenergic blocking drugs. Hypoglycemia is more likely to occur when caloric intake is deficient, after severe or prolonged exercise, when alcohol is ingested, or when more than one glucose-lowering drug is used.

Because of the long half-life of chlorpropamide, patients who become hypoglycemic during therapy require careful supervision of the dose and frequent feedings for at least 3 to 5 days. Hospitalization and intravenous glucose may be necessary.

Loss of control of blood glucose: When a patient stabilized on any diabetic regimen is exposed to stress such as fever, trauma, infection, or surgery, a loss of control may occur. At such times, it may be necessary to discontinue DIABINESE and administer insulin.

The effectiveness of any oral hypoglycemic drug, including DIABINESE, in lowering blood glucose to a desired level decreases in many patients over a period of time, which may be due to progression of the severity of the diabetes or to diminished responsiveness to the drug. This phenomenon is known as secondary failure, to distinguish it from primary failure in which the drug is ineffective in an individual patient when first given.

Information For Patients: Patients should be informed of the potential risks and advantages of DIABINESE and of alternative modes of therapy. They should also be informed about the importance of adherence to dietary instructions, of a regular exercise program, and of regular testing of urine and/or blood glucose.

The risks of hypoglycemia, its symptoms and treatment, and conditions that predispose to its development should be explained to patients and responsible family members. Primary and secondary failure should also be explained.

Patients should be instructed to contact their physician promptly if they experience symptoms of hypoglycemia or other adverse reactions.

Laboratory Tests: Blood and urine glucose should be monitored periodically. Measurement of glycosylated hemoglobin may be useful.

Drug Interactions: The hypoglycemic action of sulfonylurea may be potentiated by certain drugs including nonsteroidal anti-inflammatory agents and other drugs that are highly protein bound, salicylates, sulfonamides, chloramphenicol, probenecid, coumarins, monoamine oxidase inhibitors, and beta-adrenergic blocking agents. When such drugs are administered to a patient receiving DIABINESE, the patient should be observed closely for hypoglycemia. When such drugs are withdrawn from a patient receiving DIABINESE, the patient should be observed closely for loss of control.

Certain drugs tend to produce hyperglycemia and may lead to loss of control. These drugs include the thiazides and other diuretics, corticosteroids, phenothiazines, thyroid products, estrogens, oral contraceptives, phenytoin, nicotinic acid, sympathomimetics, calcium channel blocking drugs, and isoniazid. When such drugs are administered to a patient receiving DIABINESE, the patient should be closely observed for loss of control. When such drugs are withdrawn from a patient receiving DIABINESE, the patient should be observed closely for hypoglycemia.

Since animal studies suggest that the action of barbiturates may be prolonged by therapy with chlorpropamide, barbiturates should be employed with caution. In some patients, a disulfiram-like reaction may be produced by the ingestion of alcohol.

Carcinogenesis, Mutagenesis, Impairment of Fertility: Chronic toxicity studies have been carried out in dogs and rats. Dogs treated for 6, 13, or 20 months with doses of DIABINESE greater than 20 times the human dose, have not shown any gross histological or pathological abnormalities. After treatment with 100 mg/kg of DIABINESE for 20 months, a dog showed no histopathological liver changes.

Rats treated with continuous DIABINESE therapy for 6 to 12 months showed varying degrees of suppression of spermatogenesis at higher dosage levels (up to 125 mg/kg). The extent of suppression seemed to follow that of growth retardation associated with chronic administration of high-dose DIABINESE in rats.

Pregnancy

Teratogenic Effects:

Pregnancy Category C. Animal reproductive studies have not been conducted with DIABINESE. It is also not known whether DIABINESE can cause fetal harm when administered to a pregnant woman or can affect reproduction capacity. DIABINESE should be given to a pregnant woman only if clearly needed.

Because recent information suggests that abnormal blood glucose levels during pregnancy are associated with a higher incidence of congenital abnormalities, many experts recommend that insulin be used during pregnancy to maintain blood glucose levels as close to normal as possible.

Nonteratogenic Effects:

Prolonged severe hypoglycemia (4 to 10 days) has been reported in neonates born to mothers who were receiving a sulfonylurea drug at the time of delivery. This has been reported more frequently with the use of agents with prolonged half-lives. If DIABINESE is used during pregnancy, it should be discontinued at least one month before the expected delivery date.

Nursing Mothers: An analysis of a composite of two samples of human breast milk, each taken five hours after ingestion of 500 mg of chlorpropamide by a patient, revealed a concentration of 5 mcg/ml. For reference, the normal peak blood level of chlorpropamide after a single 250 mg dose is 30 mcg/ml. Therefore, it is not recommended that a woman breast feed while taking this medication.

Use in Children: Safety and effectiveness in children have not been established.

Adverse Reactions:

Hypoglycemia: See PRECAUTIONS and OVERDOSAGE sections.

Gastrointestinal Reactions: Cholestatic jaundice may occur rarely; DIABINESE should be discontinued if this occurs. Gastrointestinal disturbances are the most common reactions; nausea has been reported in less than 5% of patients, and diarrhea, vomiting, anorexia, and hunger in less than 2%. Other gastrointestinal disturbances have occurred in less than 1% of patients including proctocolitis. They tend to be dose related and may disappear when dosage is reduced.

Dermatologic Reactions: Pruritus has been reported in less than 3% of patients. Other allergic skin reactions, e.g., urticaria and maculopapular eruptions, have been reported in approximately 1% or less of patients. These may be transient and may disappear despite continued use of DIABINESE; if skin reactions persist the drug should be discontinued.

Porphyria cutanea tarda and photosensitivity reactions have been reported with sulfonylureas.

Skin eruptions rarely progressing to erythema multiforme and exfoliative dermatitis have also been reported.

Hermatologic Reactions: Leukopenia, agranulocytosis, thrombocytopenia, hemolytic anemia, aplastic anemia, pancytopenia, and eosinophilia have been reported with sulfonylureas.

Metabolic Reactions: Hepatic porphyria and disulfiram-like reactions have been reported with DIABINESE. See DRUG INTERACTIONS section.

Endocrine Reactions: On rare occasions, chlorpropamide has caused a reaction identical to the

How Supplied:

Strength	Tablet Description	Tablet Code	NDC	Package Size
DIABINESE (chlorpropamide) 100 mg	Blue, D-shaped, scored	393	0663-3930-66 0663-3930-73 0663-3930-41	100's 500's 100 (10 × 10) unit dose
DIABINESE (chlorpropamide) 250 mg	Blue, D-shaped, scored	394	0663-3940-66 0663-3940-71 0663-3940-82 0663-3940-41	100's 250's 1000's 100 (10 × 10) unit dose
DIABINESE (chlorpropamide) 250 mg	Blue, D-shaped, scored	394	0663-3940-28	28's D-Pak

syndrome of inappropriate antidiuretic hormone (ADH) secretion. The features of this syndrome result from excessive water retention and include hyponatremia, low serum osmolality, and high urine osmolity.

Overdosage: Overdose of sulfonylureas including DIABINESE can produce hypoglycemia. Mild hypoglycemic symptoms without loss of consciousness or neurologic findings should be treated aggressively with oral glucose and adjustments in drug dosage and/or meal patterns. Close monitoring should continue until the physician is assured that the patient is out of danger. Severe hypoglycemic reactions with coma, seizure, or other neurological impairment occur infrequently, but constitute medical emergencies requiring immediate hospitalization. If hypoglycemic coma is diagnosed or suspected, the patient should be given a rapid intravenous injection of concentrated (50%) glucose solution. This should be followed by a continuous infusion of a more dilute (10%) glucose solution at a rate that will maintain the blood glucose at a level above 100 mg/dL. Patients should be closely monitored for a minimum of 24 to 48 hours since hypoglycemia may recur after apparent clinical recovery.

Dosage and Administration: There is no fixed dosage regimen for the management of diabetes mellitus with DIABINESE or any other hypoglycemic agent. In addition to the usual monitoring of urinary glucose, the patient's blood glucose must also be monitored periodically to determine the minimum effective dose for the patient; to detect primary failure, i.e., inadequate lowering of blood glucose at the maximum recommended dose of medication; and to detect secondary failure, i.e., loss of an adequate blood glucose lowering response after an initial period of effectiveness. Glycosylated hemoglobin levels may also be of value in monitoring the patient's response to therapy.

Short-term administration of DIABINESE may be sufficient during periods of transient loss of control in patients usually controlled well on diet.

The total daily dosage is generally taken at a single time each morning with breakfast. Occasionally cases of gastrointestinal intolerance may be relieved by dividing the daily dosage. A LOADING OR PRIMING DOSE IS NOT NECESSARY AND SHOULD NOT BE USED.

Initial Therapy: 1. The mild to moderately severe, middle-aged, stable, non-insulin-dependent diabetic patient should be started on 250 mg daily. In elderly patients, debilitated or malnourished patients, and patients with impaired renal or hepatic function, the initial and maintenance dosing should be conservative to avoid hypoglycemic reactions (see PRECAUTIONS section). Older patients should be started on smaller amounts of DIABINESE, in the range of 100 to 125 mg daily.
2. No transition period is necessary when transferring patients from other oral hypoglycemic agents to DIABINESE. The other agent may be discontinued abruptly and chlorpropamide started at once. In prescribing chlorpropamide, due consideration must be given to its greater potency.

Many mild to moderately severe, middle-aged, stable non-insulin-dependent diabetic patients receiving insulin can be placed directly on the oral drug and their insulin abruptly discontinued. For patients requiring more than 40 units of insulin daily, therapy with DIABINESE may be initiated with a 50 per cent reduction in insulin for the first few days, with subsequent further reductions dependent upon the response.

During the initial period of therapy with chlorpropamide, hypoglycemic reactions may occasionally occur, particularly during the transition from insulin to the oral drug. Hypoglycemia within 24 hours after withdrawal of the intermediate or long-acting types of insulin will usually prove to be the result of insulin carry-over and not primarily due to the effect of chlorpropamide.

During the insulin withdrawal period, the patient should test his urine for sugar and ketone bodies at least three times daily and report the results frequently to his physician. If they are abnormal, the physician should be notified immediately. In some cases, it may be advisable to consider hospitalization during the transition period.

Five to seven days after the inital therapy, the blood level of chlorpropamide reaches a plateau. Dosage may subsequently be adjusted upward or downward by increments of not more than 50 to 125 mg at intervals of three to five days to obtain optimal control. More frequent adjustments are usually undesirable.

Maintenance Therapy: Most moderately severe, middle-aged, stable non-insulin-dependent diabetic patients are controlled by approximately 250 mg daily. Many investigators have found that some milder diabetics do well on daily doses of 100 mg or less. Many of the more severe diabetics may require 500 mg daily for adequate control. PATIENTS WHO DO NOT RESPOND COMPLETELY TO 500 MG DAILY WILL USUALLY NOT RESPOND TO HIGHER DOSES. MAINTENANCE DOSES ABOVE 750 mg DAILY SHOULD BE AVOIDED.

(See table above)

Recommended Storage: Store below 86°F (30°C).

Caution: Federal law prohibits dispensing without prescription.

(60-2141-37-6)

Literature Available: Yes.

Shown in Product Identification Section, page 426

FELDENE®
[fĕl' deen]
(piroxicam)
CAPSULES
For Oral Use

Description: FELDENE (piroxicam) is 4-Hydroxy-2-methyl-N-2-pyridinyl-$2H$-1,2- benzothiazine-3-carboxamide 1,1-dioxide, an oxicam. Members of the oxicam family are not carboxylic acids, but they are acidic by virtue of the enolic 4-hydroxy substituent. FELDENE occurs as a white crystalline solid, sparingly soluble in water, dilute acid and most organic solvents. It is slightly soluble in alcohols and in aqueous alkaline solution. It exhibits a weakly acidic 4-hydroxy proton (pKa 5.1) and a weakly basic pyridyl nitrogen (pKa 1.8).

Clinical Pharmacology: FELDENE has shown anti-inflammatory, analgesic and antipyretic properties in animals. Edema, erythema, tissue proliferation, fever, and pain can all be inhibited in laboratory animals by the administration of FELDENE. It is effective regardless of the etiology of the inflammation. The mode of action of FELDENE is not fully established at this time. However, a common mechanism for the above effects may exist in the ability of FELDENE to inhibit the biosynthesis of prostaglandins, known mediators of inflammation.

It is established that FELDENE does not act by stimulating the pituitary-adrenal axis.

FELDENE is well absorbed following oral administration. Drug plasma concentrations are proportional for 10 and 20 mg doses, generally peak within three to five hours after medication, and subsequently decline with a mean half-life of 50 hours (range of 30 to 86 hours, although values outside of this range have been encountered). This prolonged half-life results in the maintenance of relatively stable plasma concentrations throughout the day on once daily doses and to significant drug accumulation upon multiple dosing. A single 20 mg dose generally produces peak piroxicam plasma levels of 1.5 to 2 mcg/ml, while maximum drug plasma concentrations, after repeated daily ingestion of 20 mg FELDENE, usually stabilize at 3–8 mcg/ml. Most patients approximate steady state plasma levels within 7 to 12 days. Higher levels, which approximate steady state at two to three weeks, have been observed in patients in whom longer plasma half-lives of piroxicam occurred.

FELDENE and its biotransformation products are excreted in urine and feces, with about twice as much appearing in the urine as the feces. Metabolism occurs by hydroxylation at the 5 position of the pyridyl side chain and conjugation of this product; by cyclodehydration; and by a sequence of reactions involving hydrolysis of the amide linkage, decarboxylation, ring contraction, and N-demethylation. Less than 5% of the daily dose is excreted unchanged.

Concurrent administration of aspirin (3900 mg/day) and FELDENE (20 mg/day), resulted in a reduction of plasma levels of piroxicam to about 80% of their normal values. The use of FELDENE in conjunction with aspirin is not recommended because data are inadequate to demonstrate that the combination produces greater improvement than that achieved with aspirin alone and the potential for adverse reactions is increased. Concomitant administration of antacids had no effect on FELDENE plasma levels. The effects of impaired renal function or hepatic disease on plasma levels have not been established.

FELDENE, like salicylates and other nonsteroidal anti-inflammatory agents, is associated with symptoms of gastrointestinal tract irritation (see ADVERSE REACTIONS). However, in a study utilizing ^{51}Cr-tagged red blood cells, 20 mg of FELDENE administered as a single dose for four days did not result in a significant increase in fecal blood loss and did not detectably affect the gastric mucosa. In the same study a total daily dose of 3900 mg of aspirin, i.e., 972 mg q.i.d., caused a significant increase in fecal blood loss and mucosal lesions as demonstrated by gastroscopy.

In controlled clinical trials, the effectiveness of FELDENE (piroxicam) has been established for both acute exacerbations and long-term management of rheumatoid arthritis and osteoarthritis. The therapeutic effects of FELDENE are evident early in the treatment of both diseases with a progressive increase in response over several (8–12) weeks. Efficacy is seen in terms of pain relief and, when present, subsidence of inflammation.

Doses of 20 mg/day FELDENE display a therapeutic effect comparable to therapeutic doses of aspirin, with a lower incidence of minor gastrointestinal effects and tinnitus.

FELDENE has been administered concomitantly with fixed doses of gold and corticosteroids. The existence of a "steroid-sparing" effect has not been adequately studied to date.

Indications and Usage: FELDENE is indicated for acute or long-term use in the relief of signs and symptoms of the following:
1. osteoarthritis
2. rheumatoid arthritis

Dosage recommendations for use in children have

Continued on next page

not been established.

Contraindications: FELDENE should not be used in patients who have previously exhibited hypersensitivity to it, or in individuals with the syndrome comprised of bronchospasm, nasal polyps, and angioedema precipitated by aspirin or other nonsteroidal anti-inflammatory drugs.

Warnings: Peptic ulceration, perforation, and G.I. bleeding—sometimes severe, and, in some instances fatal—have been reported with patients receiving FELDENE. If FELDENE must be given to patients with a history of upper gastrointestinal tract disease, the patient should be under close supervision (see ADVERSE REACTIONS). In controlled clinical trials, incidence of peptic ulceration with the maximum recommended FELDENE capsule dose of 20 mg per day was 0.8%. The use of doses higher than the recommended dose is associated with an increase in the incidence of gastrointestinal irritation and ulcers.

Precautions: As with other anti-inflammatory agents, long-term administration to animals results in renal papillary necrosis and related pathology in rats, mice, and dogs.

Acute renal failure and hyperkalemia as well as reversible elevations of BUN and serum creatinine have been reported with FELDENE. The effect is thought to result from inhibition of renal prostaglandin synthesis resulting in a change in medullary and deep cortical blood flow with an attendant effect on renal function. Patients with impaired renal function and on diuretics as well as elderly patients who have decreased renal function are more at risk. Because of the extensive renal excretion of piroxicam and its biotransformation products (less than 5% of the daily dose excreted unchanged, see CLINICAL PHARMACOLOGY), lower doses of piroxicam shoud be anticipated in patients with impaired renal function and they should be carefully monitored. In addition to reversible changes in renal function, interstitial nephritis, glomerulitis, papillary necrosis and the nephrotic syndrome have been reported with FELDENE.

Although other nonsteroidal anti-inflammatory drugs do not have the same direct effects on platelets that aspirin does, all drugs inhibiting prostaglandin biosynthesis do interfere with platelet function to some degree; therefore, patients who may be adversely affected by such an action should be carefully observed when FELDENE is administered.

Because of reports of adverse eye findings with nonsteroidal anti-inflammatory agents, it is recommended that patients who develop visual complaints during treatment with FELDENE have ophthalmic evaluation.

As with other nonsteroidal anti-inflammatory drugs, borderline elevations of one or more liver tests may occur in up to 15% of patients. These abnormalities may progress, may remain essentially unchanged, or may be transient with continued therapy. The SGPT (ALT) test is probably the most sensitive indicator of liver dysfunction. Meaningful (3 times the upper limit of normal) elevations of SGPT or SGOT (AST) occurred in controlled clinical trials in less than 1% of patients. A patient with symptoms and/or signs suggesting liver dysfunction, or in whom an abnormal liver test has occurred, should be evaluated for evidence of the development of more severe hepatic reaction while on therapy with FELDENE. Severe hepatic reactions, including jaundice and cases of fatal hepatitis, have been reported with FELDENE. Although such reactions are rare, if abnormal liver tests persist or worsen, if clinical signs and symptoms consistent with liver disease develop, or if systemic manifestations occur (e.g. eosinophilia, rash, etc.), FELDENE should be discontinued. (See also ADVERSE REACTIONS.)

Although at the recommended dose of 20 mg/day of FELDENE increased fecal blood loss due to gastrointestinal irritation did not occur (see CLINICAL PHARMACOLOGY), in about 4% of the patients treated with FELDENE alone or concomitantly with aspirin, reductions in hemoglobin and hematocrit values were observed. Therefore, these values should be determined if signs or symptoms of anemia occur.

Peripheral edema has been observed in approximately 2% of the patients treated with FELDENE. Therefore, as with other nonsteroidal anti-inflammatory drugs, FELDENE should be used with caution in patients with heart failure, hypertension or other conditions predisposing to fluid retention, since its usage may be associated with a worsening of these conditions.

A combination of dermatological and/or allergic signs and symptoms suggestive of serum sickness have occasionally occurred in conjunction with the use of FELDENE. These include arthralgias, pruritus, fever, fatigue, and rash including vesiculo bullous reactions and exfoliative dermatitis.

Drug Interactions: FELDENE is highly protein bound, and, therefore, might be expected to displace other protein-bound drugs. Although this has not occurred in *in vitro* studies with coumarin-type anticoagulants, interactions with coumarin-type anticoagulants have been reported with FELDENE since marketing, therefore, physicians should closely monitor patients for a change in dosage requirements when administering FELDENE to patients on coumarin-type anticoagulants and other highly protein-bound drugs.

Plasma levels of piroxicam are depressed to approximately 80% of their normal values when FELDENE is administered in conjunction with aspirin (3900 mg/day), but concomitant administration of antacids has no effect on piroxicam plasma levels (see CLINICAL PHARMACOLOGY).

Nonsteroidal anti-inflammatory agents, including FELDENE, have been reported to increase steady state plasma lithium levels. It is recommended that plasma lithium levels be monitored when initiating, adjusting and discontinuing FELDENE.

Carcinogenesis, Chronic Animal Toxicity and Impairment of Fertility

Subacute and chronic toxicity studies have been carried out in rats, mice, dogs, and monkeys.

The pathology most often seen was that characteristically associated with the animal toxicology of anti-inflammatory agents; renal papillary necrosis (see PRECAUTIONS) and gastrointestinal lesions.

In classical studies in laboratory animals piroxicam did not show any teratogenic potential.

Reproductive studies revealed no impairment of fertility in animals.

Pregnancy and Nursing Mothers

Like other drugs which inhibit the synthesis and release of prostaglandins, piroxicam increased the incidence of dystocia and delayed parturition in pregnant animals when piroxicam administration was continued late into pregnancy. Gastrointestinal tract toxicity was increased in pregnant females in the last trimester of pregnancy compared to non-pregnant females or females in earlier trimesters of pregnancy.

FELDENE is not recommended for use in nursing mothers or in pregnant women because of the animal findings and since safety for such use has not been established in humans.

Use in Children

Dosage recommendations and indications for use in children have not been established.

Adverse Reactions: The incidence of adverse reactions to piroxicam is based on clinical trials involving approximately 2300 patients, about 400 of whom were treated for more than one year and 170 for more than two years. About 30% of all patients receiving daily doses of 20 mg of FELDENE experienced side effects. Gastrointestinal symptoms were the most prominent side effects—occurring in approximately 20% of the patients, which in most instances did not interfere with the course of therapy. Of the patients experiencing gastrointestinal side effects, approximately 5% discontinued therapy with an overall incidence of peptic ulceration of about 1%.

Other than the gastrointestinal symptoms, edema, dizziness, headache, changes in hematological parameters, and rash have been reported in a small percentage of patients. Routine ophthalmoscopy and slit-lamp examinations have revealed no evidence of ocular changes in 205 patients followed from 3 to 24 months while on therapy.

Incidence Greater than 1% The following adverse reactions occurred more frequently than 1 in 100.

Gastrointestinal: stomatitis, anorexia, epigastric distress*, nausea*, constipation, abdominal discomfort, flatulence, diarrhea, abdominal pain, indigestion

Hematological: decreases in hemoglobin* and hematocrit* (see PRECAUTIONS), anemia, leucopenia, eosinophilia

Dermatologic: pruritus, rash

Central Nervous System: dizziness, somnolence, vertigo

Urogenital: BUN and creatinine elevations (see PRECAUTIONS)

Body as a Whole: headache, malaise

Special Senses: tinnitus

Cardiovascular/Respiratory: edema (see PRECAUTIONS)

*Reactions occurring in 3% to 9% of patients treated with FELDENE. Reactions occurring in 1–3% of patients are unmarked.

Incidence Less Than 1%
(Causal Relationship Probable)

The following adverse reactions occurred less frequently than 1 in 100. The probability exists that there is a causal relationship between FELDENE and these reactions.

Gastrointestinal: liver function abnormalities, jaundice, hepatitis (see PRECAUTIONS), vomiting, hematemesis, melena, gastrointestinal bleeding, perforation and ulceration (see WARNINGS), dry mouth

Hematological: thrombocytopenia, petechial rash, ecchymosis, bone marrow depression including aplastic anemia, epistaxis

Dermatologic: sweating, erythema, bruising, desquamation, exfoliative dermatitis, erythema multiforme, toxic epidermal necrolysis, Stevens-Johnson syndrome, vesiculo bullous reaction, photoallergic skin reactions

Central Nervous System: depression, insomnia, nervousness

Urogenital: hematuria, proteinuria, interstitial nephritis, renal failure, hyperkalemia, glomerulitis, papillary necrosis, nephrotic syndrome (see PRECAUTIONS)

Body as a Whole: pain (colic), fever, flu-like syndrome (see PRECAUTIONS)

Special Senses: swollen eyes, blurred vision, eye irritations

Cardiovascular/Respiratory: hypertension, worsening of congestive heart failure (see PRECAUTIONS), exacerbation of angina

Metabolic: hypoglycemia, hyperglycemia, weight increase, weight decrease

Hypersensitivity: anaphylaxis, bronchospasm, urticaria/angioedema, vasculitis, "serum sickness" (see PRECAUTIONS)

Incidence Less Than 1%
(Causal Relationship Unknown)

Other adverse reactions were reported with a frequency of less than 1 in 100, but a causal relationship between FELDENE and the reaction could not be determined.

Gastrointestinal: pancreatitis

Dermatologic: onycholysis, loss of hair

Central Nervous System: akathisia, hallucinations, mood alterations, dream abnormalities, mental confusion, paresthesias

Urogenital System: dysuria

Body as a Whole: weakness

Cardiovascular/Respiratory: palpitations, dyspnea

Hypersensitivity: positive ANA

Overdosage: In the event treatment for overdosage is required the long plasma half-life (see CLINICAL PHARMACOLOGY) of piroxicam should be considered. The absence of experience with acute overdosage precludes characterization of sequelae and recommendation of specific antidotal efficacy at this time. It is reasonable to assume, however, that the standard measures of gastric evacuation and general supportive therapy would apply. In addition to supportive measures, the use of activated charcoal may effectively reduce the absorption and reabsorption of piroxicam. Experiments in dogs have demonstrated that the use of multiple-dose treatments with activated charcoal could reduce the half-life of piroxicam elimination from 27 hours (without charcoal) to 11 hours and reduce the systemic bioavailability of piroxicam by as much as 37% when activated charcoal is given as late as 6 hours after administration of piroxicam.

Administration and Dosage:
Rheumatoid Arthritis, Osteoarthritis
It is recommended that FELDENE therapy be initiated and maintained at a single daily dose of 20 mg. If desired the daily dose may be divided. Because of the long half-life of FELDENE, steady-state blood levels are not reached for 7–12 days. Therefore although the therapeutic effects of FELDENE are evident early in treatment, there is a progressive increase in response over several weeks and the effect of therapy should not be assessed for two weeks.

Dosage recommendations and indications for use in children have not been established.

How Supplied: FELDENE Capsules for oral administration
Bottles of 100:   10 mg (NDC 0663-3220-66) maroon and blue #322
                  20 mg (NDC 0663-3230-66) maroon #323
Bottles of 500:   20 mg (NDC 0663-3230-73) maroon #323
Unit dose packages of 100: 20 mg (NDC 0663-3230-41) maroon #323

© 1982, Pfizer Inc.   69-4100-37-7
Literature available: Yes.
Shown in Product Identification Section, page 426.

MINIPRESS® CAPSULES   R

[mĭn′ē-prĕs]
(prazosin hydrochloride)
For Oral Use

Description: MINIPRESS (prazosin hydrochloride), a quinazoline derivative, is the first of a new chemical class of antihypertensives. It is the hydrochloride salt of 1-(4-amino-6,7-dimethoxy-2-quinazolinyl)-4-(2-furoyl) piperazine.

It is a white, crystalline substance, slightly soluble in water and isotonic saline and has a molecular weight of 419.87. Each 1 mg capsule of MINIPRESS (prazosin hydrochloride) contains drug equivalent to 1 mg free base.

Actions: The exact mechanism of the hypotensive action of prazosin is unknown. Prazosin causes a decrease in total peripheral resistance and was originally thought to have a direct relaxant action on vascular smooth muscle. Recent animal studies, however, have suggested that the vasodilator effect of prazosin is also related to blockade of postsynaptic *alpha*-adrenoceptors. The results of dog forelimb experiments demonstrate that the peripheral vasodilator effect of prazosin is confined mainly to the level of the resistance vessels (arterioles). Unlike conventional *alpha*-blockers, the antihypertensive action of prazosin is usually not accompanied by a reflex tachycardia. Tolerance has not been observed to develop in long term therapy.

Hemodynamic studies have been carried out in man following acute single dose administration and during the course of long term maintenance therapy. The results confirm that the therapeutic effect is a fall in blood pressure unaccompanied by a clinically significant change in cardiac output, heart rate, renal blood flow and glomerular filtration rate. There is no measurable negative chronotropic effect.

In clinical studies to date, MINIPRESS (prazosin hydrochloride) has not increased plasma renin activity.

In man, blood pressure is lowered in both the supine and standing positions. This effect is most pronounced on the diastolic blood pressure.

Following oral administration, human plasma concentrations reach a peak at about three hours with a plasma half-life of two to three hours. The drug is highly bound to plasma protein. Bioavailability studies have demonstrated that the total absorption relative to the drug in a 20% alcoholic solution is 90%, resulting in peak levels approximately 65% of that of the drug in solution. Animal studies indicate that MINIPRESS (prazosin hydrochloride) is extensively metabolized, primarily by demethylation and conjugation, and excreted mainly via bile and feces. Less extensive human studies suggest similar metabolism and excretion in man.

MINIPRESS (prazosin hydrochloride) has been administered without any adverse drug interaction in limited clinical experience to date with the following: (1) cardiac glycosides—digitalis and digoxin; (2) hypoglycemics—insulin, chlorpropamide, phenformin, tolazamide, and tolbutamide; (3) tranquilizers and sedatives—chlordiazepoxide, diazepam, and phenobarbital; (4) antigout—allopurinol, colchicine, and probenecid; (5) antiarrhythmics—procainamide, propranolol (see WARNINGS however), and quinidine; and (6) analgesics, antipyretics and anti-inflammatories—propoxyphene, aspirin, indomethacin, and phenylbutazone.

Indications: MINIPRESS (prazosin hydrochloride) is indicated in the treatment of hypertension. As an antihypertensive drug, it is mild to moderate in activity. It can be used as the initial agent or it may be employed in a general treatment program in conjunction with a diuretic and/or other antihypertensive drugs as needed for proper patient response.

Warnings: **MINIPRESS (prazosin hydrochloride) may cause syncope with sudden loss of consciousness. In most cases this is believed to be due to an excessive postural hypotensive effect, although occasionally the syncopal episode has been preceded by a bout of severe tachycardia with heart rates of 120–160 beats per minute. Syncopal episodes have usually occurred within 30 to 90 minutes of the initial dose of the drug; occasionally they have been reported in association with rapid dosage increases or the introduction of another antihypertensive drug into the regimen of a patient taking high doses of MINIPRESS (prazosin hydrochloride). The incidence of syncopal episodes is approximately 1% in patients given an initial dose of 2 mg or greater. Clinical trials conducted during the investigational phase of this drug suggest that syncopal episodes can be minimized by limiting the initial dose of the drug to 1 mg, by subsequently increasing the dosage slowly, and by introducing any additional antihypertensive drugs into the patient's regimen with caution (see DOSAGE AND ADMINISTRATION). Hypotension may develop in patients given MINIPRESS who are also receiving a beta-blocker such as propranolol.**

If syncope occurs, the patient should be placed in the recumbent position and treated supportively as necessary. This adverse effect is self-limiting and in most cases does not recur after the initial period of therapy or during subsequent dose titration.

Patients should always be started on the 1 mg capsules of MINIPRESS (prazosin hydrochloride). The 2 and 5 mg capsules are not indicated for initial therapy.

More common than loss of consciousness are the symptoms often associated with lowering of the blood pressure, namely, dizziness and lightheadedness. The patient should be cautioned about these possible adverse effects and advised what measures to take should they develop. The patient should also be cautioned to avoid situations where injury could result should syncope occur during the initiation of MINIPRESS (prazosin hydrochloride) therapy.

Usage in Pregnancy:
Although no teratogenic effects were seen in animal testing, the safety of MINIPRESS (prazosin hydrochloride) in pregnancy has not been established. MINIPRESS (prazosin hydrochloride) is not recommended in pregnant women unless the potential benefit outweighs potential risk to mother and fetus.

Usage in Children:
No clinical experience is available with the use of MINIPRESS (prazosin hydrochloride) in children.

Drug/Laboratory Test Interactions:
In a study on five patients given from 12 to 24 mg of prazosin per day for 10 to 14 days, there was an average increase of 42% in the urinary metabolite of norepinephrine and an average increase in urinary VMA of 17%. Therefore, false positive results may occur in screening tests for pheochromocytoma in patients who are being treated with prazosin. If an elevated VMA is found prazosin should be discontinued and the patient retested after a month.

Adverse Reactions: The most common reactions associated with MINIPRESS (prazosin hydrochloride) therapy are: dizziness 10.3%, headache 7.8%, drowsiness 7.6%, lack of energy 6.9%, weakness 6.5%, palpitations 5.3%, and nausea 4.9%. In most instances side effects have disappeared with continued therapy or have been tolerated with no decrease in dose of drug.

The following reactions have been associated with MINIPRESS (prazosin hydrochloride), some of them rarely. (In some instances exact causal relationships have not been established).

Gastrointestinal: vomiting, diarrhea, constipation, abdominal discomfort and/or pain, liver function abnormalities, pancreatitis.

Cardiovascular: edema, dyspnea, syncope, tachycardia.

Central Nervous System: nervousness, vertigo, depression, paresthesia, hallucinations.

Dermatologic: rash, pruritus, alopecia, lichen planus.

Genitourinary: urinary frequency, incontinence, impotence, priapism.

EENT: blurred vision, reddened sclera, epistaxis, tinnitus, dry mouth, nasal congestion.

Other: diaphoresis, fever.

Single reports of pigmentary mottling and serous retinopathy, and a few reports of cataract development or disappearance have been reported. In these instances, the exact causal relationship has not been established because the baseline observations were frequently inadequate.

In more specific slit-lamp and funduscopic studies, which included adequate baseline examinations, no drug-related abnormal ophthalmological findings have been reported.

Dosage and Administration: The dose of MINIPRESS (prazosin hydrochloride) should be adjusted according to the patient's individual blood pressure response. The following is a guide to its administration:

Initial Dose:
1 mg two or three times a day. (See Warnings.)

Maintenance Dose:
Dosage may be slowly increased to a total daily dose of 20 mg given in divided doses. The therapeutic dosages most commonly employed have ranged from 6 mg to 15 mg daily given in divided doses. Doses higher than 20 mg usually do not increase efficacy, however a few patients may benefit from further increases up to a daily dose of 40 mg given in divided doses. After initial titration some patients can be maintained adequately on a twice daily dosage regimen.

Use With Other Drugs:
When adding a diuretic or other antihypertensive agent, the dose of MINIPRESS (prazosin hydrochloride) should be reduced to 1 mg or 2 mg three times a day and retitration then carried out.

Overdosage: Accidental ingestion of at least 50 mg of MINIPRESS (prazosin hydrochloride) in a two year old child resulted in profound drowsiness and depressed reflexes. No decrease in blood pressure was noted. Recovery was uneventful.

Should overdosage lead to hypotension, support of the cardiovascular system is of first importance. Restoration of blood pressure and normalization of heart rate may be accomplished by keeping the patient in the supine position. If this measure is inadequate, shock should first be treated with volume expanders. If necessary, vasopressors should then be used. Renal function should be monitored and supported as needed. Laboratory data indicate MINIPRESS (prazosin hydrochloride) is not dialysable because it is protein bound.

Toxicology: Testicular changes, necrosis and atrophy have occurred at 25 mg/kg/day (60 times the usual maximum recommended dose of 20 mg per day in humans) in long term (one year or more)

Continued on next page

studies in rats and dogs. No testicular changes were seen in rats or dogs at the 10 mg/kg/day level (24 times the usual maximum recommended dose of 20 mg per day in humans). In view of the testicular changes observed in animals, 105 patients on long term MINIPRESS (prazosin hydrochloride) therapy were monitored for 17-ketosteroid excretion and no changes indicating a drug effect were observed. In addition, 27 males on MINIPRESS (prazosin hydrochloride) alone for up to 51 months did not demonstrate changes in sperm morphology suggestive of drug effect.

How Supplied: MINIPRESS (prazosin hydrochloride) is available in 1 mg (white #431), 2 mg (pink and white #437) capsules in bottles of 250, 1000, and unit dose institutional packages of 100 (10 × 10's); and 5 mg (blue and white #438) capsules in bottles of 250, 500 and unit dose institutional packages of 100 (10×10's).

60-2318-37-8

Literature Available—Yes.
Shown in Product Identification Section, page 426

MINIZIDE® CAPSULES ℞
[min'ĕ-zīd]
(prazosin hydrochloride and polythiazide)
FOR ORAL ADMINISTRATION

> This fixed combination drug is not indicated for initial therapy of hypertension. Hypertension requires therapy titrated to the individual patient. If the fixed combination represents the dose so determined, its use may be more convenient in patient management. The treatment of hypertension is not static, but must be re-evaluated as conditions in each patient warrant.

Description: MINIZIDE is a combination of MINIPRESS® (prazosin hydrochloride) plus RENESE® (polythiazide).
MINIPRESS (prazosin hydrochloride), a quinazoline derivative, is the first of a new chemical class of antihypertensives. It is the hydrochloride salt of 1-(4-amino-6,7-dimethoxy-2-quinazolinyl)-4-(2-furoyl) piperazine.
It is a white, crystalline substance, slightly soluble in water and isotonic saline, and has a molecular weight of 419.87. Each 1 mg capsule of MINIPRESS (prazosin hydrochloride) contains drug equivalent to 1 mg free base.
RENESE (polythiazide) is an orally effective, nonmercurial diuretic, saluretic, and antihypertensive agent.
It is designated chemically as 2H-1,2,4-Benzothiadiazine-7-sulfonamide,6-chloro-3,4-dihydro-2-methyl-3-[[(2,2,2-trifluoroethyl)thio]methyl]-,1,1-dioxide.
It is a white, crystalline substance insoluble in water, but readily soluble in alkaline solution.

Clinical Pharmacology:
MINIZIDE (prazosin hydrochloride/polythiazide)
Minizide produces a more pronounced antihypertensive response than occurs after either prazosin hydrochloride or polythiazide alone in equivalent doses.

MINIPRESS (prazosin hydrochloride)
The exact mechanism of the hypotensive action of prazosin is unknown. Prazosin causes a decrease in total peripheral resistance and was originally thought to have a direct relaxant action on vascular smooth muscle. Recent animal studies, however, have suggested that the vasodilator effect of prazosin is also related to blockade of postsynaptic *alpha*-adrenoceptors. The results of dog forelimb experiments demonstrate that the peripheral vasodilator effect of prazosin is confined mainly to the level of the resistance vessels (arterioles). Unlike conventional *alpha*-blockers, the antihypertensive action of prazosin is usually not accompanied by a reflex tachycardia. Tolerance has not been observed to develop in long term therapy.
Hemodynamic studies have been carried out in man following acute single dose administration and during the course of long term maintenance therapy. The results confirm that the therapeutic effect is a fall in blood pressure unaccompanied by a clinically significant change in cardiac output, heart rate, renal blood flow, and glomerular filtration rate. There is no measurable negative chronotropic effect.
In clinical studies to date, MINIPRESS has not increased plasma renin activity.
In man, blood pressure is lowered in both the supine and standing positions. This effect is most pronounced on the diastolic blood pressure.
Following oral administration, human plasma concentrations reach a peak at about three hours with a plasma half-life of two to three hours. The drug is highly bound to plasma protein. Bioavailability studies have demonstrated that the total absorption relative to the drug in a 20% alcoholic solution is 90%, resulting in peak levels approximately 65% of that of the drug in solution. Animal studies indicate that MINIPRESS is extensively metabolized, primarily by demethylation and conjugation, and excreted mainly via bile and feces. Less extensive human studies suggest similar metabolism and excretion in man.
MINIPRESS has been administered without any adverse drug interaction in limited clinical experience to date with the following: (1) cardiac glycosides—digitalis and digoxin; (2) hypoglycemics—insulin, chlorpropamide, phenformin, tolazamide, and tolbutamide; (3) tranquilizers and sedatives—chlordiazepoxide, diazepam, and phenobarbital; (4) antigout—allopurinol, colchicine, and probenecid; (5) antiarrhythmics—procainamide, propranolol (see WARNINGS however), and quinidine; and (6) analgesics, antipyretics and anti-inflammatories—propoxyphene, aspirin, indomethacin, and phenylbutazone.

RENESE (polythiazide)
RENESE is a member of the benzothiadiazine (thiazide) family of diuretic/antihypertensive agents. Its mechanism of action results in an interference with the renal tubular mechanism of electrolyte reabsorption. At maximal therapeutic dosage all thiazides are approximately equal in their diuretic potency. The mechanism whereby thiazides function in the control of hypertension is unknown. Renese is well absorbed, giving peak human plasma concentrations about 5 hours after oral administration. Drug is removed slowly thereafter with a plasma elimination half-life of approximately 27 hours. One fifth of the drug is recovered unchanged in human urine; the remainder is cleared via feces and as metabolites. Animal studies indicate metabolism occurs by rupture of the thiadiazine ring and loss of the side chain.

Indications and Usage: MINIZIDE is indicated in the treatment of hypertension. (See box warning.)

Contraindications: RENESE (polythiazide) is contraindicated in patients with anuria, and in patients known to be sensitive to thiazides or to other sulfonamide derivatives.

Warnings:
MINIPRESS (prazosin hydrochloride)
MINIPRESS may cause syncope with sudden loss of consciousness. In most cases this is believed to be due to an excessive postural hypotensive effect, although occasionally the syncopal episode has been preceded by a bout of severe tachycardia with heart rates of 120–160 beats per minute. Syncopal episodes have usually occurred within 30 to 90 minutes of the initial dose of the drug; occasionally they have been reported in association with rapid dosage increases or the introduction of another antihypertensive drug into the regimen of a patient taking high doses of MINIPRESS. The incidence of syncopal episodes is approximately 1% in patients given an initial dose of 2 mg or greater. Clinical trials conducted during the investigational phase of this drug suggest that syncopal episodes can be minimized by limiting the initial dose of the drug to 1 mg, by subsequently increasing the dosage slowly, and by introducing any additional antihypertensive drugs into the patient's regimen with caution (see DOSAGE AND ADMINISTRATION). Hypotension may develop in patients given MINIPRESS who are also receiving a beta-blocker such as propranolol.
If syncope occurs, the patient should be placed in the recumbent position and treated supportively as necessary. This adverse effect is self-limiting and in most cases does not recur after the initial period of therapy or during subsequent dose titration.
Patients should always be started on the 1 mg capsules of MINIPRESS (prazosin hydrochloride). The 2 and 5 mg capsules are not indicated for initial therapy.
More common than loss of consciousness are the symptoms often associated with lowering of the blood pressure, namely, dizziness and lightheadedness. The patient should be cautioned about these possible adverse effects and advised what measures to take should they develop. The patient should also be cautioned to avoid situations where injury could result should syncope occur during the initiation of MINIPRESS therapy.

RENESE (polythiazide)
RENESE should be used with caution in severe renal disease. In patients with renal disease, thiazides may precipitate azotemia. Cumulative effects of the drug may develop in patients with impaired renal function.
Thiazides should be used with caution in patients with impaired hepatic function or progressive liver disease, since minor alterations of fluid and electrolyte balance may precipitate hepatic coma. Sensitivity reactions may occur in patients with a history of allergy or bronchial asthma.
The possibility of exacerbation or activation of systemic lupus erythematosus has been reported.
Thiazides may be additive or potentiative of the action of other antihypertensive drugs.
Potentiation occurs with ganglionic or peripheral adrenergic blocking drugs.
Periodic determinations of serum electrolytes to detect possible electrolyte imbalance should be performed at appropriate intervals.
All patients receiving thiazide therapy should be observed for clinical signs of fluid or electrolyte imbalance, namely, hyponatremia, hypochloremic alkalosis, and hypokalemia. Serum and urine electrolyte determinations are particularly important when the patient is vomiting excessively or receiving parenteral fluids. Medications such as digitalis may also influence serum electrolytes. Warning signs, irrespective of cause, are: dryness of mouth, thirst, weakness, lethargy, drowsiness, restlessness, muscle pains or cramps, muscular fatigue, hypotension, oliguria, tachycardia, and gastrointestinal disturbances such as nausea and vomiting.
Hypokalemia may develop with thiazides as with any potent diuretic, especially with brisk diuresis, when severe cirrhosis is present, or during concomitant use of corticosteroids or ACTH.
Interference with adequate oral electrolyte intake will also contribute to hypokalemia. Digitalis therapy may exaggerate the metabolic effects of hypokalemia, especially with reference to myocardial activity.
Any chloride deficit is generally mild and usually does not require specific treatment except under extraordinary circumstances (as in hepatic or renal disease). Dilutional hyponatremia may occur in edematous patients in hot weather; appropriate therapy is water restriction rather than administration of salt, except in rare instances when the hyponatremia is life-threatening. In actual salt depletion, appropriate replacement is the therapy of choice.
Hyperuricemia may occur or frank gout may be precipitated in certain patients receiving thiazide therapy.
Insulin requirements in diabetic patients may be either increased, decreased, or unchanged. Latent diabetes mellitus may become manifest during thiazide administration.
Thiazide drugs may increase responsiveness to tubocurarine.
The antihypertensive effects of the drug may be enhanced in the post-sympathectomy patient.
Thiazides may decrease arterial responsiveness to norepinephrine. This diminution is not sufficient to preclude effectiveness of the pressor agent for therapeutic use.
If progressive renal impairment becomes evident, as indicated by a rising nonprotein nitrogen or blood urea nitrogen, a careful reappraisal of therapy is necessary with consideration given to with-

holding or discontinuing diuretic therapy.
Thiazides may decrease serum protein-bound iodine levels without signs of thyroid disturbance.

Precautions:

Drug/Laboratory Test Interactions: In a study on five patients given from 12 to 24 mg of prazosin per day for 10 to 14 days, there was an average increase of 42% in the urinary metabolite of norepinephrine and an average increase in urinary VMA of 17%. Therefore, false positive results may occur in screening tests for pheochromocytoma in patients who are being treated with prazosin. If an elevated VMA is found, prazosin should be discontinued and the patient retested after a month.

Carcinogenesis, Mutagenesis, Impairment of Fertility: No carcinogenic or mutagenic studies have been conducted with MINIZIDE. However, no carcinogenic potential was demonstrated in 18 month studies in rats with either MINIPRESS or RENESE at dose levels more than 100 times the usual maximum human doses. MINIPRESS was not mutagenic in *in vivo* genetic toxicology studies.

MINIZIDE produced no impairment of fertility in male or female rats at 50 and 20 mg/kg/day of MINIPRESS and RENESE respectively. In chronic studies (one year or more) of MINIPRESS in rats and dogs, testicular changes consisting of atrophy and necrosis occurred at 25 mg/kg/day (60 times the usual maximum recommended human dose). No testicular changes were seen in rats or dogs at 10 mg/kg/day (24 times the usual maximum recommended human dose). In view of the testicular changes observed in animals, 105 patients on long term MINIPRESS therapy were monitored for 17-ketosteroid excretion and no changes indicating a drug effect were observed. In addition, 27 males on MINIPRESS alone for up to 51 months did not have changes in sperm morphology suggestive of drug effect.

Use in Pregnancy: Pregnancy Category C. MINIZIDE was not teratogenic in either rats or rabbits when administered in oral doses more than 100 times the usual maximum human dose. Studies in rats indicated that the combination of RENESE (40 times the usual maximum recommended human dose) and MINIPRESS (8 times the usual maximum recommended human dose) caused a greater number of stillbirths, a more prolonged gestation, and a decreased survival of pups to weaning than that caused by MINIPRESS alone. There are no adequate and well controlled studies in pregnant women. Therefore, MINIZIDE should be used in pregnancy only if the potential benefit justifies the potential risk to the fetus.

Nursing Mothers: It is not known whether MINIPRESS or RENESE are excreted in human milk. Thiazides appear in breast milk. Thus, if use of the drug is deemed essential the patient should stop nursing.

Pediatric Use: Safety and effectiveness in children has not been established.

Adverse Reactions:

MINIPRESS (prazosin hydrochloride)
The most common reactions associated with MINIPRESS therapy are: dizziness 10.3%, headache 7.8%, drowsiness 7.6%, lack of energy 6.9%, weakness 6.5%, palpitations 5.3%, and nausea 4.9%. In most instances side effects have disappeared with continued therapy or have been tolerated with no decrease in dose of drug.
The following reactions have been associated with MINIPRESS, some of them rarely. (In some instances exact causal relationships have not been established.)
- Gastrointestinal: vomiting, diarrhea, constipation, abdominal discomfort and/or pain, liver function abnormalities, pancreatitis.
- Cardiovascular: edema, dyspnea, syncope, tachycardia.
- Central Nervous System: nervousness, vertigo, depression, paresthesia, hallucinations.
- Dermatologic: rash, pruritus, alopecia, lichen planus.
- Genitourinary: urinary frequency, incontinence, impotence, priapism.
- EENT: blurred vision, reddened sclera, epistaxis, tinnitus, dry mouth, nasal congestion.

How Supplied:

STRENGTH	COMPONENTS	COLOR	CAPSULE CODE	PKG. SIZE
MINIZIDE 1	1 mg prazosin + 0.5 mg polythiazide	Blue-Green	430	100's
MINIZIDE 2	2 mg prazosin + 0.5 mg polythiazide	Blue-Green/Pink	432	100's
MINIZIDE 5	5 mg prazosin + 0.5 mg polythiazide	Blue-Green/Blue	436	100's

Other: diaphoresis, fever.
Single reports of pigmentary mottling and serous retinopathy, and a few reports of cataract development or disappearance have been reported. In these instances, the exact causal relationship has not been established because the baseline observations were frequently inadequate.
In more specific slit-lamp and funduscopic studies, which included adequate baseline examinations, no drug-related abnormal ophthalmological findings have been reported.

RENESE (polythiazide)
- Gastrointestinal: anorexia, gastric irritation, nausea, vomiting, cramping, diarrhea, constipation, jaundice (intrahepatic cholestatic jaundice), pancreatitis.
- Central Nervous System: dizziness, vertigo, paresthesia, headache, xanthopsia.
- Hematologic: leukopenia, agranulocytosis, thrombocytopenia, aplastic anemia.
- Dermatologic: purpura, photosensitivity, rash, urticaria, necrotizing angiitis, (vasculitis) (cutaneous vasculitis).
- Cardiovascular: Orthostatic hypotension may occur and be aggravated by alcohol, barbiturates, or narcotics.
- Other: hyperglycemia, glycosuria, hyperuricemia, muscle spasm, weakness, restlessness.

Overdosage:

MINIPRESS (prazosin hydrochloride)
Accidental ingestion of at least 50 mg of MINIPRESS in a two year old child resulted in profound drowsiness and depressed reflexes. No decrease in blood pressure was noted. Recovery was uneventful.
Should overdose lead to hypotension, support of the cardiovascular system is of first importance. Restoration of blood pressure and normalization of heart rate may be accomplished by keeping the patient in the supine position. If this measure is inadequate, shock should first be treated with volume expanders. If necessary, vasopressors should then be used. Renal function should be monitored and supported as needed. Laboratory data indicate that MINIPRESS is not dialysable because it is protein bound.

RENESE (polythiazide)
Should overdosage with RENESE occur, electrolyte balance and adequate hydration should be maintained. Gastric lavage is recommended, followed by supportive treatment. Where necessary, this may include intravenous dextrose and saline with potassium and other electrolyte therapy, administered with caution as indicated by laboratory testing at appropriate intervals.

Dosage and Administration:

MINIZIDE (prazosin hydrochloride/polythiazide)
Dosage: as determined by individual titration of MINIPRESS (prazosin hydrochloride) and RENESE (polythiazide). (See box warning.)
Usual MINIZIDE dosage is one capsule two or three times daily, the strength depending upon individual requirement following titration.
The following is a general guide to the administration of the individual components of MINIZIDE:

MINIPRESS (prazosin hydrochloride)
Initial Dose: 1 mg two or three times a day. (See Warnings.)
Maintenance Dose: Dosage may be slowly increased to a total daily dose of 20 mg given in divided doses. The therapeutic dosages most commonly employed have ranged from 6 mg to 15 mg daily given in divided doses. Doses higher than 20 mg usually do not increase efficacy, however a few patients may benefit from further increases up to a daily dose of 40 mg given in divided doses. After initial titration some patients can be maintained adequately on a twice daily dosage regimen.
Use With Other Drugs: When adding a diuretic or other antihypertensive agent, the dose of MINIPRESS should be reduced to 1 mg or 2 mg three times a day and retitration then carried out.

RENESE (polythiazide)
The usual dose of Renese for antihypertensive therapy is 2 to 4 mg daily.

MINIZIDE CAPSULES
prazosin HCl/polythiazide
[See table above].

69-2463-37-3

Literature Available: Yes.
Shown in Product Identification Section, page 426

MODERIL® ℞
[mō'dĕr-ĭl]
(rescinnamine)
TABLETS

Description: Rescinnamine is a pure crystalline alkaloid that has been identified chemically as the 3,4,5-trimethoxycinnamic acid ester of methyl reserpate. Pure rescinnamine occurs as white, needle-shaped crystals that are readily absorbed when ingested.
Moderil is available as oval, scored salmon tablets providing 0.5 mg. of crystalline rescinnamine or as oval, scored yellow tablets providing 0.25 mg. of crystalline rescinnamine.

Actions: Rescinnamine probably produces its antihypertensive effects through depletion of tissue stores of catecholamines (epinephrine and norepinephrine) from peripheral sites. By contrast, its sedative and tranquilizing properties are thought to be related to depletion of 5-hydroxytryptamine from the brain.
Rescinnamine is characterized by slow onset of action and sustained effect. Both its cardiovascular and central nervous system effects may persist following withdrawal of the drug.

Indications: Indicated in the treatment of mild essential hypertension.

Contraindications: Do not use in patients with known hypersensitivity, mental depression—especially with suicidal tendencies, active peptic ulcer, and ulcerative colitis. It is also contraindicated in patients receiving electroconvulsive therapy.

Warnings: Extreme caution should be exercised in treating patients with a history of mental depression. Discontinue the drug at the first sign of despondency, early morning insomnia, loss of appetite, impotence, or self-depreciation. Drug-induced depression may persist for several months after drug withdrawal and may be severe enough to result in suicide.

Usage in pregnancy: The safety of rescinnamine for use during pregnancy or lactation has not been established. Therefore, the drug should be used in pregnant patients or in women of child-bearing potential only when, in the judgment of the physician, its use is deemed essential to the welfare of the patient. Increased respiratory secretions, nasal congestion, cyanosis, and anorexia may occur in infants born to rescinnamine-treated mothers, since this preparation is known to cross the placental barrier, appearing in cord blood and breast milk.

Precautions: Because Rauwolfia preparations increase gastrointestinal motility and secretion, this drug should be used cautiously in patients with a history of peptic ulcer, ulcerative colitis, or gallstones where biliary colic may be precipitated.

Continued on next page

Pfizer—Cont.

Caution should be exercised when treating hypertensive patients with renal insufficiency since they adjust poorly to lowered blood pressure levels.

Use rescinnamine cautiously with digitalis and quinidine since cardiac arrhythmias have occurred with Rauwolfia preparations.

Preoperative withdrawal of rescinnamine does not assure that circulatory instability will not occur. It is important that the anesthesiologist be aware of the patient's drug intake and consider this in the over-all management, since hypotension has occurred in patients receiving Rauwolfia preparations. Anticholinergic and/or adrenergic drugs (metaraminol, norepinephrine) have been employed to treat adverse vagocirculatory effects.

Adverse Reactions: Rauwolfia preparations have caused gastrointestinal reactions including hypersecretion, nausea and vomiting, anorexia, and diarrhea; cardiovascular reactions including angina-like symptoms, arrhythmias particularly when used concurrently with digitalis or quinidine, and bradycardia; and central nervous system reactions including drowsiness, depression, nervousness, paradoxical anxiety, nightmares, rare parkinsonian syndrome, C.N.S. sensitization manifested by dull sensorium, deafness, glaucoma, uveitis, and optic atrophy. Nasal congestion is a frequent complaint; and pruritus, rash, dryness of mouth, dizziness, headache, dyspnea, purpura, impotence or decreased libido, dysuria, muscular aches, conjunctival injection, and weight gain have been reported. Extrapyramidal tract symptoms have also occurred. These reactions are usually reversible and disappear when the drug is discontinued.

Water retention with edema in patients with hypertensive vascular disease may occur rarely, but the condition generally clears with cessation of therapy, or with the administration of a diuretic agent.

Dosage and Administration: For adults the average initial dose is 0.5 mg. orally, twice daily. Increase dosage gradually, if necessary. Maintenance doses may vary from 0.25 mg. to 0.5 mg. daily. Higher doses should be used cautiously because serious mental depression and other side effects may be increased considerably.

Concomitant use of rescinnamine and ganglionic blocking agents, guanethidine, veratrum, hydralazine, methyldopa, chlorthalidone, or thiazides necessitates careful titration of dosage with each agent.

Supply:
0.25 mg. tablets, oval, scored, yellow (imprinted with code number 441): bottles of 100.
0.5 mg. tablets, oval, scored, salmon (imprinted with code number 442): bottles of 100.

(60-0695-00-7)
Shown in Product Identification Section, page 426

PROCARDIA® R
[*pro-car'dē-ă*]
(nifedipine)
CAPSULES
For Oral Use

Description: PROCARDIA (nifedipine) is an antianginal drug belonging to a new class of pharmacological agents, the calcium channel blockers. Nifedipine is 3,5-pyridinedicarboxylic acid, 1,4-dihydro-2,6-dimethyl-4-(2-nitrophenyl)-, dimethyl ester, $C_{17}H_{18}N_2O_6$.

Nifedipine is a yellow crystalline substance, practically insoluble in water but soluble in ethanol. It has a molecular weight of 346.3. PROCARDIA CAPSULES are formulated as soft gelatin capsules for oral administration each containing 10 mg nifedipine.

Clinical Pharmacology: PROCARDIA is a calcium ion influx inhibitor (slow channel blocker or calcium ion antagonist) and inhibits the transmembrane influx of calcium ions into cardiac muscle and smooth muscle. The contractile processes of cardiac muscle and vascular smooth muscle are dependent upon the movement of extracellular calcium ions into these cells through specific ion channels. PROCARDIA selectively inhibits calcium ion influx across the cell membrane of cardiac muscle and vascular smooth muscle without changing serum calcium concentrations.

Mechanism of Action
The precise means by which this inhibition relieves angina has not been fully determined, but includes at least the following two mechanisms:

1) Relaxation and prevention of coronary artery spasm
PROCARDIA dilates the main coronary arteries and coronary arterioles, both in normal and ischemic regions, and is a potent inhibitor of coronary artery spasm, whether spontaneous or ergonovine-induced. This property increases myocardial oxygen delivery in patients with coronary artery spasm, and is responsible for the effectiveness of PROCARDIA in vasospastic (Prinzmetal's or variant) angina. Whether this effect plays any role in classical angina is not clear, but studies of exercise tolerance have not shown an increase in the maximum exercise rate-pressure product, a widely accepted measure of oxygen utilization. This suggests that, in general, relief of spasm or dilation of coronary arteries is not an important factor in classical angina.

2) Reduction of oxygen utilization
PROCARDIA regularly reduces arterial pressure at rest and at a given level of exercise by dilating peripheral arterioles and reducing the total peripheral resistance (afterload) against which the heart works. This unloading of the heart reduces myocardial energy consumption and oxygen requirements and probably accounts for the effectiveness of PROCARDIA in chronic stable angina.

Pharmacokinetics and Metabolism
PROCARDIA is rapidly and fully absorbed after oral administration. The drug is detectable in serum 10 minutes after oral administration, and peak blood levels occur in approximately 30 minutes. It is highly bound by serum proteins. PROCARDIA is extensively converted to inactive metabolites and approximately 80 percent of PROCARDIA and metabolites are eliminated via the kidneys. The half-life of nifedipine in plasma is approximately two hours. There is no information on the effects of renal or hepatic impairment on excretion or metabolism of PROCARDIA.

Hemodynamics
Like other slow channel blockers, PROCARDIA exerts a negative inotropic effect on isolated myocardial tissue. This is rarely, if ever, seen in intact animals or man, probably because of reflex responses to its vasodilating effects. In man, PROCARDIA causes decreased peripheral vascular resistance and a fall in systolic and diastolic pressure, usually modest (5-10mm Hg systolic), but sometimes larger. There is usually a small increase in heart rate, a reflex response to vasodilation. Measurements of cardiac function in patients with normal ventricular function have generally found a small increase in cardiac index without major effects on ejection fraction, left ventricular end diastolic pressure (LVEDP) or volume (LVEDV). In patients with impaired ventricular function, most acute studies have shown some increase in ejection fraction and reduction in left ventricular filling pressure.

Electrophysiologic Effects
Although like other members of its class, PROCARDIA decreases sinoatrial node function and atrioventricular conduction in isolated myocardial preparations, such effects have not been seen in studies in intact animals or in man. In formal electrophysiologic studies, predominantly in patients with normal conduction systems, PROCARDIA has had no tendency to prolong atrioventricular conduction, prolong sinus node recovery time, or slow sinus rate.

Indications and Usage:

I. Vasospastic Angina
PROCARDIA (nifedipine) is indicated for the management of vasospastic angina confirmed by any of the following criteria: 1) classical pattern of angina at rest accompanied by ST segment elevation, 2) angina or coronary artery spasm provoked by ergonovine, or 3) angiographically demonstrated coronary artery spasm. In those patients who have had angiography, the presence of significant fixed obstructive disease is not incompatible with the diagnosis of vasospastic angina, provided that the above criteria are satisfied. PROCARDIA may also be used where the clinical presentation suggests a possible vasospastic component but where vasospasm has not been confirmed, e.g., where pain has a variable threshold on exertion or in unstable angina where electrocardiographic findings are compatible with intermittent vasospasm, or when angina is refractory to nitrates and/or adequate doses of beta blockers.

II. Chronic Stable Angina (Classical Effort-Associated Angina)
PROCARDIA is indicated for the management of chronic stable angina (effort-associated angina) without evidence of vasospasm in patients who remain symptomatic despite adequate doses of beta blockers and/or organic nitrates or who cannot tolerate those agents.

In chronic stable angina (effort-associated angina) PROCARDIA has been effective in controlled trials of up to eight weeks duration in reducing angina frequency and increasing exercise tolerance, but confirmation of sustained effectiveness and evaluation of long term safety in these patients are incomplete.

Controlled studies in small numbers of patients suggest concomitant use of PROCARDIA and beta blocking agents may be beneficial in patients with chronic stable angina, but available information is not sufficient to predict with confidence the effects of concurrent treatment, especially in patients with compromised left ventricular function or cardiac conduction abnormalities. When introducing such concomitant therapy, care must be taken to monitor blood pressure closely since severe hypotension can occur from the combined effects of the drugs. (See WARNINGS.)

Contraindications: Known hypersensitivity reaction to PROCARDIA.

Warnings:
Excessive Hypotension
Although in most patients, the hypotensive effect of PROCARDIA is modest and well tolerated, occasional patients have had excessive and poorly tolerated hypotension. These responses have usually occurred during initial titration or at the time of subsequent upward dosage adjustment, and may be more likely in patients on concomitant beta blockers.

Severe hypotension and/or increased fluid volume requirements have been reported in patients receiving PROCARDIA together with a beta blocking agent who underwent coronary artery bypass surgery using high dose fentanyl anesthesia. The interaction with high dose fentanyl appears to be due to the combination of PROCARDIA and a beta blocker, but the possibility that it may occur with PROCARDIA alone, with low doses of fentanyl, in other surgical procedures, or with other narcotic analgesics cannot be ruled out. In PROCARDIA treated patients where surgery using high dose fentanyl anesthesia is contemplated, the physician should be aware of these potential problems and, if the patient's condition permits, sufficient time (at least 36 hours) should be allowed for PROCARDIA to be washed out of the body prior to surgery.

Increased Angina
Occasional patients have developed well documented increased frequency, duration or severity of angina on starting PROCARDIA or at the time of dosage increases. The mechanism of this response is not established but could result from decreased coronary perfusion associated with decreased diastolic pressure with increased heart rate, or from increased demand resulting from increased heart rate alone.

Beta Blocker Withdrawal
Patients recently withdrawn from beta blockers may develop a withdrawal syndrome with increased angina, probably related to increased sensitivity to catecholamines. Initiation of PROCARDIA treatment will not prevent this occurrence and might be expected to exacerbate it by provoking reflex catecholamine release. There

have been occasional reports of increased angina in a setting of beta blocker withdrawal and PROCARDIA initiation. It is important to taper beta blockers if possible, rather than stopping them abruptly before beginning PROCARDIA.

Congestive Heart Failure
Rarely, patients, usually receiving a beta blocker, have developed heart failure after beginning PROCARDIA. Patients with tight aortic stenosis may be at greater risk for such an event, as the unloading effect of PROCARDIA would be expected to be of less benefit to these patients, owing to their fixed impedance to flow across the aortic valve.

Precautions:
General: Hypotension: Because PROCARDIA decreases peripheral vascular resistance, careful monitoring of blood pressure during the initial administration and titration of PROCARDIA is suggested. Close observation is especially recommended for patients already taking medications that are known to lower blood pressure. (See WARNINGS.)

Peripheral edema: Mild to moderate peripheral edema, typically associated with arterial vasodilation and not due to left ventricular dysfunction, occurs in about one in ten patients treated with PROCARDIA. This edema occurs primarily in the lower extremities and usually responds to diuretic therapy. With patients whose angina is complicated by congestive heart failure, care should be taken to differentiate this peripheral edema from the effects of increasing left ventricular dysfunction.

Laboratory tests: Rare, usually transient, but occasionally significant elevations of enzymes such as alkaline phosphatase, CPK, LDH, SGOT and SGPT have been noted. The relationship to PROCARDIA therapy is uncertain in most cases, but probable in some. These laboratory abnormalities have rarely been associated with clinical symptoms, however, cholestasis with or without jaundice has been reported. Rare instances of allergic hepatitis have been reported.

PROCARDIA, like other calcium channel blockers, decreases platelet aggregation *in vitro*. Limited clinical studies have demonstrated a moderate but statistically significant decrease in platelet aggregation and increase in bleeding time in some PROCARDIA patients. This is thought to be a function of inhibition of calcium transport across the platelet membrane. No clinical significance for these findings has been demonstrated.

Drug interactions: Beta-adrenergic blocking agents: (See INDICATIONS and WARNINGS.) Experience in over 1400 patients in a non-comparative clinical trial has shown that concomitant administration of PROCARDIA and beta-blocking agents is usually well tolerated, but there have been occasional literature reports suggesting that the combination may increase the likelihood of congestive heart failure, severe hypotension or exacerbation of angina.

Long acting nitrates: PROCARDIA may be safely co-administered with nitrates, but there have been no controlled studies to evaluate the antianginal effectiveness of this combination.

Digitalis: Administration of PROCARDIA with digoxin increased digoxin levels in nine of twelve normal volunteers. The average increase was 45%. Another investigator found no increase in digoxin levels in thirteen patients with coronary artery disease. In an uncontrolled study of over two hundred patients with congestive heart failure during which digoxin blood levels were not measured, digitalis toxicity was not observed. Since there have been isolated reports of patients with elevated digoxin levels, it is recommended that digoxin levels be monitored when initiating, adjusting, and discontinuing PROCARDIA to avoid possible over- or under-digitalization.

Coumarin anticoagulants: There have been rare reports of increased prothrombin time in patients taking coumarin anticoagulants to whom PROCARDIA was administered. However, the relationship to PROCARDIA therapy is uncertain.

Cimetidine: A study in six healthy volunteers has shown a significant increase in peak nifedipine plasma levels (80%) and area-under-the-curve (74%) after a one week course of cimetidine at 1000 mg per day and nifedipine at 40 mg per day. Ranitidine produced smaller, non-significant increases. The effect may be mediated by the known inhibition of cimetidine on hepatic cytochrome P-450, the enzyme system probably responsible for the first-pass metabolism of nifedipine. If nifedipine therapy is initiated in a patient currently receiving cimetidine, cautious titration is advised.

Carcinogenesis, mutagenesis, impairment of fertility: Nifedipine was administered orally to rats for two years and was not shown to be carcinogenic. When given to rats prior to mating, nifedipine caused reduced fertility at a dose approximately 30 times the maximum recommended human dose. *In vivo* mutagenicity studies were negative.

Pregnancy: Pregnancy category C. Nifedipine has been shown to be teratogenic in rats when given in doses 30 times the maximum recommended human dose. Nifedipine was embryotoxic (increased fetal resorptions, decreased fetal weight, increased stunted forms, increased fetal deaths, decreased neonatal survival) in rats, mice and rabbits at doses of from 3 to 10 times the maximum recommended human dose. In pregnant monkeys, doses ⅔ and twice the maximum recommended human dose resulted in small placentas and underdeveloped chorionic villi. In rats, doses three times maximum human dose and higher caused prolongation of pregnancy. There are no adequate and well controlled studies in pregnant women. PROCARDIA should be used during pregnancy only if the potential benefit justifies the potential risk to the fetus.

Adverse Reactions: In multiple-dose U.S. and foreign controlled studies in which adverse reactions were reported spontaneously, adverse effects were frequent but generally not serious and rarely required discontinuation of therapy or dosage adjustment. Most were expected consequences of the vasodilator effects of PROCARDIA.

Adverse Effect	PROCARDIA (%) (N = 226)	Placebo (%) (N = 235)
Dizziness, lightheadedness, giddiness	27	15
Flushing, heat sensation	25	8
Headache	23	20
Weakness	12	10
Nausea, heartburn	11	8
Muscle cramps, tremor	8	3
Peripheral edema	7	1
Nervousness, mood changes	7	4
Palpitation	7	5
Dyspnea, cough, wheezing	6	3
Nasal congestion, sore throat	6	8

There is also a large uncontrolled experience in over 2100 patients in the United States. Most of the patients had vasospastic or resistant angina pectoris, and about half had concomitant treatment with beta-adrenergic blocking agents. The most common adverse events were:

Incidence Approximately 10% *Cardiovascular:* peripheral edema
Central Nervous System: dizziness or lightheadedness
Gastrointestinal: nausea
Systemic: headache and flushing, weakness

Incidence Approximately 5% *Cardiovascular:* transient hypotension

Incidence 2% or Less *Cardiovascular:* palpitation
Respiratory: nasal and chest congestion, shortness of breath
Gastrointestinal: diarrhea, constipation, cramps, flatulence
Musculoskeletal: inflammation, joint stiffness, muscle cramps
Central Nervous System: shakiness, nervousness, jitteriness, sleep disturbances, blurred vision, difficulties in balance
Other: dermatitis, pruritus, urticaria, fever, sweating, chills, sexual difficulties.

Incidence Approximately 0.5% *Cardiovascular:* syncope. Syncopal episodes did not recur with reduction in the dose of PROCARDIA or concomitant antianginal medication.

Incidence Less Than 0.5% *Hematologic:* thrombocytopenia, anemia, leukopenia, purpura
Gastrointestinal: allergic hepatitis
Oral: gingival hyperplasia
Other: erythromelalgia

Several of these side effects appear to be dose related. Peripheral edema occurred in about one in 25 patients at doses less than 60 mg per day and in about one patient in eight at 120 mg per day or more. Transient hypotension, generally of mild to moderate severity and seldom requiring discontinuation of therapy, occurred in one of 50 patients at less than 60 mg per day and in one of 20 patients at 120 mg per day or more. Very rarely, introduction of PROCARDIA therapy was associated with an increase in anginal pain, possibly due to associated hypotension.

In addition, more serious adverse events were observed, not readily distinguishable from the natural history of the disease in these patients. It remains possible, however, that some or many of these events were drug related. Myocardial infarction occurred in about 4% of patients and congestive heart failure or pulmonary edema in about 2%. Ventricular arrhythmias or conduction disturbances each occurred in fewer than 0.5% of patients.

In a subgroup of over 1000 patients receiving PROCARDIA with concomitant beta blocker therapy, the pattern and incidence of adverse experiences was not different from that of the entire group of PROCARDIA treated patients. (See PRECAUTIONS.)

In a subgroup of approximately 250 patients with a diagnosis of congestive heart failure as well as angina, dizziness or lightheadedness, peripheral edema, headache or flushing each occurred in one in eight patients. Hypotension occurred in about one in 20 patients. Syncope occurred in approximately one patient in 250. Myocardial infarction or symptoms of congestive heart failure each occurred in about one patient in 15. Atrial or ventricular dysrhythmias each occurred in about one patient in 150.

Overdosage: Although there is no well documented experience with PROCARDIA overdosage, available data suggest that gross overdosage could result in excessive peripheral vasodilation with subsequent marked and probably prolonged systemic hypotension. Clinically significant hypotension due to PROCARDIA overdosage calls for active cardiovascular support including monitoring of cardiac and respiratory function, elevation of extremities, and attention to circulating fluid volume and urine output. A vasoconstrictor (such as norepinephrine) may be helpful in restoring vascular tone and blood pressure, provided that there is no contraindication to its use. Clearance of PROCARDIA would be expected to be prolonged in patients with impaired liver function. Since PROCARDIA is highly protein-bound, dialysis is not likely to be of benefit.

Dosage and Administration: The dosage of PROCARDIA needed to suppress angina and that can be tolerated by the patient must be established by titration. Excessive doses can result in hypotension.

The starting dose is one 10 mg capsule, swallowed whole, 3 times/day. The usual effective dose range is 10–20 mg three times daily. Some patients, especially those with evidence of coronary artery spasm, respond only to higher doses, more frequent administration, or both. In such patients, doses of 20–30 mg three or four times daily may be effective. Doses above 120 mg daily are rarely necessary. More than 180 mg per day is not recommended.

In most cases, PROCARDIA titration should proceed over a 7–14 day period so that the physician can assess the response to each dose level and mon-

Continued on next page

Pfizer—Cont.

itor the blood pressure before proceeding to higher doses.

If symptoms so warrant, titration may proceed more rapidly provided that the patient is assessed frequently. Based on the patient's physical activity level, attack frequency, and sublingual nitroglycerin consumption, the dose of PROCARDIA may be increased from 10 mg t.i.d to 20 mg t.i.d and then to 30 mg t.i.d over a three-day period.

In hospitalized patients under close observation, the dose may be increased in 10 mg increments over four to six-hour periods as required to control pain and arrhythmias due to ischemia. A single dose should rarely exceed 30 mg.

No "rebound effect" has been observed upon discontinuation of PROCARDIA. However, if discontinuation of PROCARDIA is necessary, sound clinical practice suggests that the dosage should be decreased gradually with close physician supervision.

Co-Administration with Other Antianginal Drugs
Sublingual nitroglycerin may be taken as required for the control of acute manifestations of angina, particularly during PROCARDIA titration. See Precautions, Drug Interactions, for information on co-administration of PROCARDIA with beta blockers or long acting nitrates.

How Supplied: Each orange, soft gelatin PROCARDIA CAPSULE (code #260) contains 10 mg of nifedipine. PROCARDIA Capsules are supplied in bottles of 100 (NDC 0069-2600-66), 300 (NDC 0069-2600-72), and unit dose (10 × 10) (NDC 0069-2600-41).

The capsules should be protected from light and moisture and stored at controlled room temperature 59° to 77°F (15° to 25°C) in the manufacturer's original container.

© 1982, Pfizer Inc. 65-4027-00-3
Literature Available: Yes
Shown in Product Identification Section, page 426

RENESE® ℞
[rĕ-nēs']
(polythiazide)
TABLETS
For Oral Administration

Description: Renese is designated generically as polythiazide, and chemically as 2H-1,2,4-Benzothiadiazine-7-sulfonamide, 6-chloro-3,4-dihydro-2-methyl-3[[(2, 2, 2-trifluoroethyl)thio]methyl]-,1,1-dioxide. It is a white crystalline substance, insoluble in water but readily soluble in alkaline solution.

Action: The mechanism of action results in an interference with the renal tubular mechanism of electrolyte reabsorption. At maximal therapeutic dosage all thiazides are approximately equal in their diuretic potency. The mechanism whereby thiazides function in the control of hypertension is unknown.

Indications: Renese is indicated as adjunctive therapy in edema associated with congestive heart failure, hepatic cirrhosis, and corticosteroid and estrogen therapy.

Renese has also been found useful in edema due to various forms of renal dysfunction as: Nephrotic syndrome; Acute glomerulonephritis; and Chronic renal failure.

Renese is indicated in the management of hypertension either as the sole therapeutic agent or to enhance the effectiveness of other antihypertensive drugs in the more severe forms of hypertension.

Usage in Pregnancy: The routine use of diuretics in an otherwise healthy woman is inappropriate and exposes mother and fetus to unnecessary hazard. Diuretics do not prevent development of toxemia of pregnancy, and there is no satisfactory evidence that they are useful in the treatment of developed toxemia.

Edema during pregnancy may arise from pathological causes or from the physiologic and mechanical consequences of pregnancy. Thiazides are indicated in pregnancy when edema is due to pathologic causes, just as they are in the absence of pregnancy (however, see Warnings, below). Dependent edema in pregnancy, resulting from restriction of venous return by the expanded uterus, is properly treated through elevation of the lower extremities and use of support hose; use of diuretics to lower intravascular volume in this case is illogical and unnecessary. There is hypervolemia during normal pregnancy which is harmful to neither the fetus nor the mother (in the absence of cardiovascular disease), but which is associated with edema, including generalized edema, in the majority of pregnant women. If this edema produces discomfort, increased recumbency will often provide relief. In rare instances, this edema may cause extreme discomfort which is not relieved by rest. In these cases, a short course of diuretics may provide relief and may be appropriate.

Contraindications: Anuria. Hypersensitivity to this or other sulfonamide derived drugs.

Warnings: Thiazides should be used with caution in severe renal disease. In patients with renal disease, thiazides may precipitate azotemia. Cumulative effects of the drug may develop in patients with impaired renal function.

Thiazides should be used with caution in patients with impaired hepatic function or progressive liver disease, since minor alterations of fluid and electrolyte balance may precipitate hepatic coma.

Thiazides may add to or potentiate the action of other antihypertensive drugs. Potentiation occurs with ganglionic or peripheral adrenergic blocking drugs.

Sensitivity reactions may occur in patients with a history of allergy or bronchial asthma.

The possibility of exacerbation or activation of systemic lupus erythematosus has been reported.

Usage in pregnancy. Thiazides cross the placental barrier and appear in cord blood. The use of thiazides in pregnant women requires that the anticipated benefit be weighed against possible hazards to the fetus. These hazards include fetal or neonatal jaundice, thrombocytopenia, and possibly other adverse reactions which have occurred in the adult.

Nursing Mothers. Thiazides appear in breast milk. If use of the drug is deemed essential, the patient should stop nursing.

Precautions: Periodic determination of serum electrolytes to detect possible electrolyte imbalance should be performed at appropriate intervals. All patients receiving thiazide therapy should be observed for clinical signs of fluid or electrolyte imbalance; namely, hyponatremia, hypochloremic alkalosis, and hypokalemia. Serum and urine electrolyte determinations are particularly important when the patient is vomiting excessively or receiving parenteral fluids. Medication such as digitalis may also influence serum electrolytes. Warning signs, irrespective of cause, are: dryness of mouth, thirst, weakness, lethargy, drowsiness, restlessness, muscle pains or cramps, muscular fatigue, hypotension, oliguria, tachycardia, and gastrointestinal disturbances such as nausea and vomiting.

Hypokalemia may develop with thiazides as with any other potent diuretic, especially with brisk diuresis, when severe cirrhosis is present, or during concomitant use of corticosteroids or ACTH. Interference with adequate oral electrolyte intake will also contribute to hypokalemia. Digitalis therapy may exaggerate metabolic effects of hypokalemia especially with reference to myocardial activity.

Any chloride deficit is generally mild and usually does not require specific treatment except under extraordinary circumstances (as in liver disease or renal disease). Dilutional hyponatremia may occur in edematous patients in hot weather; appropriate therapy is water restriction, rather than administration of salt except in rare instances when the hyponatremia is life threatening. In actual salt depletion, appropriate replacement is the therapy of choice.

Hyperuricemia may occur or frank gout may be precipitated in certain patients receiving thiazide therapy.

Insulin requirements in diabetic patients may be increased, decreased, or unchanged. Latent diabetes mellitus may become manifest during thiazide administration.

Thiazide drugs may increase the responsiveness to tubocurarine.

The antihypertensive effects of the drug may be enhanced in the postsympathectomy patient.

Thiazides may decrease arterial responsiveness to norepinephrine. This diminution is not sufficient to preclude effectiveness of the pressor agent for therapeutic use.

If progressive renal impairment becomes evident, as indicated by a rising nonprotein nitrogen or blood urea nitrogen, a careful reappraisal of therapy is necessary with consideration given to withholding or discontinuing diuretic therapy.

Thiazides may decrease serum PBI levels without signs of thyroid disturbance.

Adverse Reactions:
A. GASTROINTESTINAL SYSTEM REACTIONS
1. anorexia
2. gastric irritation
3. nausea
4. vomiting
5. cramping
6. diarrhea
7. constipation
8. jaundice (intrahepatic cholestatic jaundice)
9. pancreatitis

B. CENTRAL NERVOUS SYSTEM REACTIONS
1. dizziness
2. vertigo
3. paresthesias
4. headache
5. xanthopsia

C. HEMATOLOGIC REACTIONS
1. leukopenia
2. agranulocytosis
3. thrombocytopenia
4. aplastic anemia

D. DERMATOLOGIC–HYPERSENSITIVITY REACTIONS
1. purpura
2. photosensitivity
3. rash
4. urticaria
5. necrotizing angiitis (vasculitis) (cutaneous vasculitis)

E. CARDIOVASCULAR REACTION
Orthostatic hypotension may occur and may be aggravated by alcohol, barbiturates or narcotics.

F. OTHER
1. hyperglycemia
2. glycosuria
3. hyperuricemia
4. muscle spasm
5. weakness
6. restlessness

Whenever adverse reactions are moderate or severe, thiazide dosage should be reduced or therapy withdrawn.

Dosage and Administration: Therapy should be individualized according to patient response. This therapy should be titrated to gain maximal therapeutic response as well as the minimal dose possible to maintain that therapeutic response. The usual dosage of Renese tablets for diuretic therapy is 1 to 4 mg daily, and for antihypertensive therapy is 2 to 4 mg daily.

How Supplied: RENESE (polythiazide) Tablets are available as:

1 mg white, scored tablets (imprinted with code number 375) in bottles of 100 and 1000.
2 mg yellow, scored tablets (imprinted with code number 376) in bottles of 100 and 1000.
4 mg white, scored tablets (imprinted with code number 377) in bottles of 100 and 1000.

(69-1116-00-3)
Literature Available: Yes.
Shown in Product Identification Section, page 426

RENESE®-R ℞
[rĕ-nēs']
(polythiazide and reserpine)

Warning
This fixed combination drug is not indicated for initial therapy of hypertension. Hypertension requires therapy titrated to the individual patient. If the fixed combination represents the dosage so determined, its use may be more convenient in patient management. The treatment of hypertension is not static, but

must be reevaluated as conditions in each patient warrant.

RENESE-R tablets combine polythiazide and reserpine, two antihypertensive agents with complementary properties. Each blue, scored tablet of RENESE-R provides:

Renese (polythiazide) .... 2.0 mg
Reserpine .... 0.25 mg

Actions: RENESE (polythiazide) is a member of the benzothiadiazine (thiazide) family of diuretic/antihypertensive agents. RENESE (polythiazide) alone has demonstrated clinical effectiveness in lowering elevated blood pressure in patients without visible edema as well as in edematous hypertensive patients. This antihypertensive action probably comes about through depletion of sodium and fluid accumulation in the blood vessel wall. RENESE (polythiazide) is $2H$-1,2,4-Benzothiadiazine-7-sulfonamide, 6-chloro-3,4-dihydro-2-methyl-3-[[(2,2,2-trifluoroethyl)thio]methyl]-, 1, 1- dioxide.

Reserpine, an alkaloid of Rauwolfia serpentina has several complementary actions of benefit to the hypertensive patient, including a calming effect and a slowing of the pulse rate. Its ultimate effect in lowering blood pressure is thought to be due to vasodilatation unaccompanied by reduction in cardiac performance, probably as a result of depletion of norepinephrine from tissue receptor sites.

Since polythiazide reduces or eliminates the sodium and fluid retention frequently associated with hypertension, it enhances the efficacy of reserpine in lowering elevated blood pressure. RENESE-R often has been found to be more effective than equivalent doses of either agent alone. Both the cardiovascular and central nervous system effects may persist following withdrawal of the drug.

Indications: Hypertension (see box warning).
Contraindications:
A. Related to polythiazide:
 1. Advanced renal or hepatic failure.
 2. Hypersensitivity to this or other sulfonamide derivatives.
B. Related to reserpine:
 1. Demonstrated hypersensitivity.
 2. Mental depression.
 3. Demonstrated peptic ulcer or ulcerative colitis.

Warnings: Serum electrolyte determinations are especially indicated for patients with severe derangement of metabolic processes, e.g., surgery, vomiting, or parenteral fluid therapy. Electrolyte imbalance may be caused by certain diseases such as cirrhosis, or it may result from drug therapy, such as therapy with corticosteroids. Patients with cirrhosis who are continually receiving RENESE-R should be observed carefully for the development of hepatic precoma or coma. Indications of impending hepatic failure are tremor, confusion, drowsiness, and hepatic fetor.

Thiazides may precipitate kidney failure and uremia in patients with pre-existing renal pathology and impaired renal function.

Available information tends to implicate all oral dosage forms of potassium salts ingested in solid form with or without thiazides in the etiology of nonspecific, small bowel lesions consisting of ulceration with or without stenosis, causing obstruction, hemorrhage and perforation, and frequently requiring surgery. Deaths due to these complications have been reported. All oral dosage forms of potassium salts ingested in solid form should be used only when adequate dietary supplementation is not practical and should be discontinued immediately if abdominal pain, distention, nausea, vomiting or gastrointestinal bleeding occur.

RENESE-R does not itself contain enteric-coated potassium.

Electroshock therapy should not be given within one week of cessation of reserpine.

Usage in Pregnancy and the Childbearing Age.
Since thiazides appear in breast milk, the usage of polythiazide is contraindicated in nursing mothers. Thiazides cross the placental barrier and appear in cord blood. The safety of reserpine for use during pregnancy or lactation has not been established. When polythiazide and reserpine are used in women of childbearing age, the potential benefits of this drug combination should be weighed against the possible hazards to the fetus. The hazards include fetal or neonatal jaundice, thrombocytopenia, and possibly other adverse reactions which have occurred in the adult.

Precautions: Since all diuretic agents may reduce serum levels of sodium, chloride, and potassium, especially with brisk diuresis or when used concurrently with steroids, patients should be observed regularly for early signs of fluid or electrolyte imbalance and serum electrolyte studies should be performed periodically. Warning signs of possible electrolyte imbalance irrespective of cause include fatigue, muscle cramps, gastrointestinal disturbances, lethargy, oliguria, and tachycardia. In extreme cases, hypotension, shock, and coma may develop. Frequently, serum electrolyte levels do not correlate with signs or symptoms of electrolyte imbalance. Unduly restricted salt intake as well as concurrent administration of digitalis may exaggerate metabolic effects of hypokalemia. A favorable ratio of potassium to sodium excretion lessens the possibility of hypokalemia. However, should this occur or be suspected, foods with a high potassium content (bananas, apricots, citrus fruits, prune juice, etc.) should be given. When necessary, oral potassium supplements may be administered. If other antihypertensive agents are used concurrently, lower than usual doses of RENESE-R and of the other agents should be considered.

Like other thiazide diuretics, polythiazide may cause a rise in serum uric acid levels with or without overt symptoms of gout. Thiazides are known to disturb glucose tolerance in some individuals, even when there is no history of glucose intolerance or diabetes in the individual or his family. Likewise, thiazides may decrease PBI levels without signs of thyroid disturbances.

Thiazide drugs may augment the paralyzing actions of tubocurarine, and may decrease the arterial responsiveness to norepinephrine. Extra precautions may be necessary in patients who may require these drugs or their derivatives, as in surgery. The antihypertensive effects of the drug may be enhanced in the postsympathectomy patient.

Reserpine: Since reserpine may increase gastric acid secretion, it should be used cautiously in patients with a history of peptic ulcer or ulcerative colitis. Extreme caution is needed in patients with a history of mental depression, and reserpine should be discontinued at the first sign of depressive symptoms. Parkinsonism and confusion have been encountered, particularly in psychiatric patients, and constitute an indication for withdrawal of the drug. Caution should be exercised when treating patients with impairment of renal function, as lowered blood pressure may result in further decompensation and embarrassment of function. Reserpine should be used cautiously with digitalis or quinidine as the concurrent use may enhance the appearance of arrhythmias. Discontinue the drug one to two weeks prior to elective surgery since an unexpected degree of hypotension and bradycardia have been reported in patients receiving anesthetic agents concurrently with reserpine, probably due to a reduced responsiveness to norepinephrine. For emergency surgical procedures vagal blocking agents may be given parenterally to prevent or reverse hypotension and/or bradycardia. Reserpine may cause increased appetite and weight gain in some patients.

Animal tumorigenicity: Rodent studies have shown that reserpine is an animal tumorigen, causing an increased incidence of mammary fibroadenomas in female mice, malignant tumors of the seminal vesicles in male mice, and malignant adrenal medullary tumors in male rats. These findings arose in 2 year studies in which the drug was administered in the feed at concentrations of 5 and 10 ppm—about 100 to 300 times the usual human dose. The breast neoplasms are thought to be related to reserpine's prolactin-elevating effect. Several other prolactin-elevating drugs have also been associated with an increased incidence of mammary neoplasia in rodents.

The extent to which these findings indicate a risk to humans is uncertain. Tissue culture experiments show that about one-third of human breast tumors are prolactin-dependent *in vitro,* a factor of considerable importance if the use of the drug is contemplated in a patient with previously detected breast cancer. The possibility of an increased risk of breast cancer in reserpine users has been studied extensively; however, no firm conclusion has emerged. Although a few epidemiologic studies have suggested a slightly increased risk (less than twofold in all studies except one) in women who have used reserpine, other studies of generally similar design have not confirmed this. Epidemiologic studies conducted using other drugs (neuroleptic agents) that, like reserpine, increase prolactin levels and therefore would be considered rodent mammary carcinogens, have not shown an association between chronic administration of the drug and human mammary tumorigenesis. While long-term clinical observation has not suggested such an association, the available evidence is considered too limited to be conclusive at this time. An association of reserpine intake with pheochromocytoma or tumors of the seminal vesicles has not been explored.

Adverse Reactions: **Polythiazide:** Side effects such as nausea, vertigo, weakness, paresthesias, and fatigue occur but seldom require cessation of therapy. Most of these can be overcome by reducing the dose or taking measures to improve electrolyte imbalance. Maculopapular skin rash has been reported, as has reversible cholestatic jaundice. Leukopenia (neutropenia) and purpura, with or without thrombocytopenia, have been reported rarely, and agranulocytosis and aplastic anemia have been reported with the older thiazides but not as yet with the newer compounds such as polythiazide. Pancreatitis, photosensitivity reactions, gastrointestinal disturbances, headache, xanthopsia, necrotizing angiitis, orthostatic hypotension, and dizziness have all been reported following the use of the benzothiadiazine class of diuretics.

Reserpine: Gastrointestinal reactions include hypersecretion, nausea and vomiting, anorexia, and diarrhea. Cardiovascular reactions reported include angina-like symptoms, arrhythmias—particularly when used concurrently with digitalis or quinidine, flushing of the skin, and bradycardia. Central nervous system reactions range from drowsiness, depression, nervousness, paradoxical anxiety, nightmares, and a rare Parkinsonian syndrome to C.N.S. sensitization manifested by deafness, glaucoma, uveitis, and optic atrophy. Nasal congestion is a frequent complaint, and pruritus, rash, dryness of mouth, dizziness, headache, purpura, impotence or decreased libido, and miosis have been reported with use of this drug. These reactions are usually reversible and disappear when the drug is discontinued.

Dosage: As determined by individual titration (see box warning).

Initial dosages of the combination should conform to those dosages of the individual components established during titration.

Maintenance dosages range from $\frac{1}{2}$ tablet to 2 tablets daily. Dosage of other antihypertensive agents, particularly ganglionic blockers, that are used concomitantly should be reduced.

Supply: RENESE-R tablets (2 mg polythiazide-0.25 mg reserpine) are available as blue, scored tablets (imprinted with code number 446) in bottles of 100 and 1,000.

(69-1200-00-9)

Literature Available: Yes.

Shown in Product Identification Section, page 426

Continued on next page

Pfizer—Cont.

TERRAMYCIN® ℞
[tĕra-my'sĭn]
Capsules
(oxytetracycline HCl)
Syrup
(calcium oxytetracycline)
Film-coated Tablets
(oxytetracycline)

Terramycin® is manufactured by Pfizer Pharmaceuticals and distributed by the Pfipharmecs Division. Please refer to Pfipharmecs PRODUCT INFORMATION for a full product description. Terramycin® (oxytetracycline HCl) Capsules appear under Pfipharmecs, page 426 in the PRODUCT IDENTIFICATION section.

VIBRAMYCIN® Hyclate   ℞
[vī″bra-mī″sĭn]
CAPSULES
VIBRA-TABS®
[vī″ bra-tabs']
(doxycycline hyclate)
FILM COATED TABLETS
VIBRAMYCIN® Calcium
(doxycycline calcium oral suspension)
SYRUP
VIBRAMYCIN® Monohydrate
(doxycycline monohydrate)
FOR ORAL SUSPENSION

Description: Vibramycin is a broad-spectrum antibiotic synthetically derived from oxytetracycline, and is available as Vibramycin Monohydrate (doxycycline monohydrate), Vibramycin Hyclate and Vibra-Tabs (doxycycline hydrochloride hemiethanolate hemihydrate), and Vibramycin Calcium (doxycycline calcium). The chemical designation of this light-yellow crystalline powder is alpha-6-deoxy-5-oxytetracycline. Doxycycline has a high degree of lipoid solubility and a low affinity for calcium binding. It is highly stable in normal human serum. Doxycycline will not degrade into an epianhydro form.

Actions: Doxycycline is primarily bacteriostatic and is thought to exert its antimicrobial effect by the inhibition of protein synthesis. Doxycycline is active against a wide range of gram-positive and gram-negative organisms.

The drugs in the tetracycline class have closely similar antimicrobial spectra, and cross resistance among them is common. Microorganisms may be considered susceptible if the M.I.C. (minimum inhibitory concentration) is less than 4.0 mcg/ml and intermediate if the M.I.C. is 4.0 to 12.5 mcg/ml.

Susceptibility plate testing: If the Kirby-Bauer method of disc susceptibility testing is used, a 30 mcg doxycycline disc should give a zone of at least 16 mm when tested against a doxycycline-susceptible bacterial strain. A tetracycline disc may be used to determine microbial susceptibility. If the Kirby-Bauer method of disc susceptibility testing is used, a 30 mcg tetracycline disc should give a zone of at least 19 mm when tested against a tetracycline-susceptible bacterial strain.

Tetracyclines are readily absorbed and are bound to plasma proteins in varying degree. They are concentrated by the liver in the bile, and excreted in the urine and feces at high concentrations and in a biologically active form. Doxycycline is virtually completely absorbed after oral administration.

Following a 200 mg dose, normal adult volunteers averaged peak serum levels of 2.6 mcg/ml of doxycycline at 2 hours decreasing to 1.45 mcg/ml at 24 hours. Excretion of doxycycline by the kidney is about 40%/72 hours in individuals with normal function (creatinine clearance about 75 ml/min.). This percentage excretion may fall as low as 1-5%/72 hours in individuals with severe renal insufficiency (creatinine clearance below 10 ml/min.). Studies have shown no significant difference in serum half-life of doxycycline (range 18–22 hours) in individuals with normal and severely impaired renal function.

Hemodialysis does not alter serum half-life.

Indications: Doxycycline is indicated in infections caused by the following microorganisms:

Rickettsiae: Rocky Mountain spotted fever, typhus fever and the typhus group, Q fever, rickettsialpox, and tick fevers.

Mycoplasma pneumoniae (PPLO, Eaton agent),
Agents of psittacosis and ornithosis,
Agents of lymphogranuloma venereum and granuloma inguinale,
The spirochetal agent of relapsing fever (*Borrelia recurrentis*).

The following gram-negative microorganisms:
Haemophilus ducreyi (chancroid),
Pasteurella pestis, and *Pasteurella tularensis*,
Bartonella bacilliformis,
Bacteroides species,
Vibrio comma and *Vibrio fetus*,
Brucella species (in conjunction with streptomycin).

Because many strains of the following groups of microorganisms have been shown to be resistant to tetracyclines, culture and susceptibility testing are recommended.

Doxycycline is indicated for treatment of infections caused by the following gram-negative microorganisms, when bacteriologic testing indicates appropriate susceptibility to the drug:

Escherichia coli,
Enterobacter aerogenes (formerly *Aerobacter aerogenes*),
Shigella species,
Mima species and *Herellea* species,
Haemophilus influenzae (respiratory infections),
Klebsiella species (respiratory and urinary infections).

Doxycycline is indicated for treatment of infections caused by the following gram-positive microorganisms when bacteriologic testing indicates appropriate susceptibility to the drug:

Streptococcus species:

Up to 44 percent of strains of *Streptococcus pyogenes* and 74 percent of *Streptococcus faecalis* have been found to be resistant to tetracycline drugs. Therefore, tetracyclines should not be used for streptococcal disease unless the organism has been demonstrated to be sensitive.

For upper respiratory infections due to group A beta-hemolytic streptococci, penicillin is the usual drug of choice, including prophylaxis of rheumatic fever.

Diplococcus pneumoniae,
Staphylococcus aureus, respiratory, skin and soft-tissue infections. Tetracyclines are not the drug of choice in the treatment of any type of staphylococcal infection.

When penicillin is contraindicated, doxycycline is an alternative drug in the treatment of infections due to:

Treponema pallidum and *Treponema pertenue* (syphilis and yaws),
Listeria monocytogenes,
Clostridium species,
Bacillus anthracis,
Fusobacterium fusiforme (Vincent's infection),
Actinomyces species.

In acute intestinal amebiasis doxycycline may be a useful adjunct to amebicides.

In severe acne doxycycline may be useful adjunctive therapy.

Doxycycline is indicated in the treatment of trachoma, although the infectious agent is not always eliminated, as judged by immunofluorescence. Inclusion conjunctivitis may be treated with oral doxycycline alone, or with a combination of topical agents.

Doxycycline is indicated for the treatment of uncomplicated urethral, endocervical, or rectal infections in adults caused by *Chlamydia trachomatis*.[1]

Doxycycline is indicated for the treatment of nongonococcal urethritis caused by *Chlamydia trachomatis* and *Ureaplasma urealyticum* and for the treatment of acute epididymo-orchitis caused by *Chlamydia trachomatis*.[1]

Doxycycline is indicated for the treatment of uncomplicated gonococcal infections in adults (except for anorectal infections in men) and acute epididymo-orchitis caused by *N. gonorrhoeae*.[1]

Contraindications: This drug is contraindicated in persons who have shown hypersensitivity to any of the tetracyclines.

Warnings: THE USE OF DRUGS OF THE TETRACYCLINE CLASS DURING TOOTH DEVELOPMENT (LAST HALF OF PREGNANCY, INFANCY AND CHILDHOOD TO THE AGE OF 8 YEARS) MAY CAUSE PERMANENT DISCOLORATION OF THE TEETH (YELLOW-GRAY-BROWN). This adverse reaction is more common during long term use of the drugs but has been observed following repeated short term courses. Enamel hypoplasia has also been reported. TETRACYCLINE DRUGS, THEREFORE, SHOULD NOT BE USED IN THIS AGE GROUP UNLESS OTHER DRUGS ARE NOT LIKELY TO BE EFFECTIVE OR ARE CONTRAINDICATED.

Photosensitivity manifested by an exaggerated sunburn reaction has been observed in some individuals taking tetracyclines. Patients apt to be exposed to direct sunlight or ultraviolet light should be advised that this reaction can occur with tetracycline drugs, and treatment should be discontinued at the first evidence of skin erythema. The antianabolic action of the tetracyclines may cause an increase in BUN. Studies to date indicate that this does not occur with the use of doxycycline in patients with impaired renal function.

Usage in Pregnancy: (See above "Warnings" about use during tooth development.)

Results of animal studies indicate that tetracyclines cross the placenta, are found in fetal tissues, and can have toxic effects on the developing fetus (often related to retardation of skeletal development). Evidence of embryotoxicity has also been noted in animals treated early in pregnancy.

Usage in Newborns, Infants, and Children: (See above "Warnings" about use during tooth development.)

As with other tetracyclines, doxycycline forms a stable calcium complex in any bone-forming tissue. A decrease in the fibula growth rate has been observed in prematures given oral tetracycline in doses of 25 mg/kg every six hours. This reaction was shown to be reversible when the drug was discontinued.

Tetracyclines are present in the milk of lactating women who are taking a drug in this class.

Precautions: As with other antibiotic preparations, use of this drug may result in overgrowth of nonsusceptible organisms, including fungi. If superinfection occurs, the antibiotic should be discontinued and appropriate therapy should be instituted.

In venereal disease when coexistent syphilis is suspected, a dark field examination should be done before treatment is started and the blood serology repeated monthly for at least four months.

Because the tetracyclines have been shown to depress plasma prothrombin activity, patients who are on anticoagulant therapy may require downward adjustment of their anticoagulant dosage.

In long term therapy, periodic laboratory evaluation of organ systems, including hematopoietic, renal, and hepatic studies should be performed.

All infections due to group A beta-hemolytic streptococci should be treated for at least 10 days.

Since bacteriostatic drugs may interfere with the bactericidal action of penicillin, it is advisable to avoid giving tetracycline in conjunction with penicillin.

Adverse Reactions: Due to oral doxycycline's virtually complete absorption, side effects of the lower bowel, particularly diarrhea, have been infrequent. The following adverse reactions have been observed in patients receiving tetracyclines:

Gastrointestinal: anorexia, nausea, vomiting, diarrhea, glossitis, dysphagia, enterocolitis, and inflammatory lesions (with monilial overgrowth) in the anogenital region. These reactions have been caused by both the oral and parenteral administration of tetracyclines. Rare instances of esophagitis and esophageal ulcerations have been reported in patients receiving capsule and tablet forms of drugs in the tetracycline class. Most of these patients took medications immediately before going to bed. (See Dosage and Administration.)

Skin: maculopapular and erythematous rashes. Exfoliative dermatitis has been reported but is uncommon. Photosensitivity is discussed above (see "Warnings").

Renal toxicity: Rise in BUN has been reported and is apparently dose related. (See "Warnings.")

Hypersensitivity reactions: urticaria, angioneurotic edema, anaphylaxis, anaphylactoid purpura, pericarditis, and exacerbation of systemic lupus erythematosus.

Bulging fontanels in infants and benign intracranial hypertension in adults have been reported in individuals receiving full therapeutic dosages. These conditions disappeared rapidly when the drug was discontinued.

Blood: Hemolytic anemia, thrombocytopenia, neutropenia, and eosinophilia have been reported with tetracyclines.

When given over prolonged periods, tetracyclines have been reported to produce brown-black microscopic discoloration of thyroid glands. No abnormalities of thyroid function studies are known to occur.

Dosage and Administration: THE USUAL DOSAGE AND FREQUENCY OF ADMINISTRATION OF DOXYCYCLINE DIFFERS FROM THAT OF THE OTHER TETRACYCLINES. EXCEEDING THE RECOMMENDED DOSAGE MAY RESULT IN AN INCREASED INCIDENCE OF SIDE EFFECTS.

Adults: The usual dose of oral doxycycline is 200 mg on the first day of treatment (administered 100 mg every 12 hours) followed by a maintenance dose of 100 mg/day. The maintenance dose may be administered as a single dose or as 50 mg every 12 hours. In the management of more severe infections (particularly chronic infections of the urinary tract), 100 mg every 12 hours is recommended.

For children above eight years of age: The recommended dosage schedule for children weighing 100 pounds or less is 2 mg/lb. of body weight divided into two doses on the first day of treatment, followed by 1 mg/lb. of body weight given as a single daily dose or divided into two doses, on subsequent days. For more severe infections up to 2 mg/lb. of body weight may be used. For children over 100 lbs. the usual adult dose should be used.

Uncomplicated gonococcal infections in adults (except anorectal infections in men): 100 mg, by mouth, twice a day for 7 days.[1]

As an alternate single visit dose, administer 300 mg stat followed in one hour by a second 300 mg dose. The dose may be administered with food, including milk or carbonated beverage, as required.

Acute epididymo-orchitis caused by *N. gonorrhoeae:* 100 mg, by mouth, twice a day for at least 10 days.[1]

Primary and secondary syphilis: 300 mg a day in divided doses for at least 10 days.

The therapeutic antibacterial serum activity will usually persist for 24 hours following recommended dosage.

When used in streptococcal infections, therapy should be continued for 10 days.

Administration of adequate amounts of fluid along with capsule and tablet forms of drugs in the tetracycline class is recommended to wash down the drugs and reduce the risk of esophageal irritation and ulceration. (See Adverse Reactions.)

If gastric irritation occurs, it is recommended that doxycycline be given with food or milk. The absorption of doxycycline is not markedly influenced by simultaneous ingestion of food or milk.

Uncomplicated urethral, endocervical, or rectal infection in adults caused by *Chlamydia trachomatis:* 100 mg, by mouth, twice a day for at least 7 days.[1]

Nongonococcal urethritis caused by *C. trachomatis* and *U. urealyticum:* 100 mg, by mouth, twice a day for at least 7 days.[1]

Acute epididymo-orchitis caused by *C. trachomatis:* 100 mg, by mouth, twice a day for at least 10 days.[1]

Concomitant therapy: Antacids containing aluminum, calcium, or magnesium impair absorption and should not be given to patients taking oral doxycycline.

Studies to date have indicated that administration of doxycycline at the usual recommended doses does not lead to excessive accumulation of the antibiotic in patients with renal impairment.

How Supplied: Vibramycin Hyclate (doxycycline hyclate) is available in capsules containing doxycycline hyclate equivalent to:

50 mg doxycycline (imprinted with code number 094)
bottles of 50
unit-dose pack of 100 (10 x 10's)
X-pack of 50 (5 x 10's)
100 mg doxycycline (imprinted with code number 095)
bottles of 50 and 500
unit-dose pack of 100 (10 x 10's)
V-pack of 25 (5 x 5's)
Nine-Paks (10 x 9's)

Vibra-Tabs (doxycycline hyclate) is available in film coated tablets (imprinted with code number 099) containing doxycycline hyclate equivalent to:

100 mg of doxycycline
bottles of 50 and 500
unit-dose pack of 100 (10 x 10's)

Vibramycin Calcium Syrup (doxycycline calcium oral suspension) is available as a raspberry-apple flavored oral suspension. Each teaspoonful (5 ml) contains doxycycline calcium equivalent to 50 mg of doxycycline: bottles of 1 oz. (30 ml) and 1 Pint (473 ml).

Vibramycin Monohydrate (doxycycline monohydrate) for Oral Suspension is available as a pleasant tasting, raspberry flavored, dry powder for oral suspension. When reconstituted, each teaspoonful (5 ml) contains doxycycline monohydrate equivalent to 25 mg of doxycycline: 2 oz. (60 ml) bottles.

Reference:
1. CDC Sexually Transmitted Diseases Treatment Guidelines 1982.

69-1680-00-7

Literature Available: Yes.

Shown in Product Identification Section, page 426

VIBRAMYCIN® Hyclate ℞
[vĭ" bra-mī' sin]
(doxycycline hyclate for injection)
INTRAVENOUS
For Intravenous Use Only

Description: Vibramycin (doxycycline hyclate for injection) Intravenous is a broad-spectrum antibiotic synthetically derived from oxytetracycline, and is available as Vibramycin Hyclate (doxycycline hydrochloride hemiethanolate hemihydrate). The chemical designation of this light-yellow crystalline powder is alpha-6-deoxy-5-oxytetracycline. Doxycycline has a high degree of lipoid solubility and a low affinity for calcium binding. It is highly stable in normal human serum.

Actions: Doxycycline is primarily bacteriostatic and thought to exert its antimicrobial effect by the inhibition of protein synthesis. Doxycycline is active against a wide range of gram-positive and gram-negative organisms.

The drugs in the tetracycline class have closely similar antimicrobial spectra and cross resistance among them is common. Microorganisms may be considered susceptible to doxycycline (likely to respond to doxycycline therapy) if the minimum inhibitory concentration (M.I.C.) is not more than 4.0 mcg/ml. Microorganisms may be considered intermediate (harboring partial resistance) if the M.I.C. is 4.0 to 12.5 mcg/ml and resistant (not likely to respond to therapy) if the M.I.C. is greater than 12.5 mcg/ml.

Susceptibility plate testing: If the Kirby-Bauer method of disc susceptibility testing is used, a 30 mcg doxycycline disc should give a zone of at least 16 mm when tested against a doxycycline-suscepti-

ble bacterial strain. A tetracycline disc may be used to determine microbial susceptibility. If the Kirby-Bauer method of disc susceptibility testing is used, a 30 mcg tetracycline disc should give a zone of at least 19 mm when tested against a tetracycline-susceptible bacterial strain.

Tetracyclines are readily absorbed and are bound to plasma proteins in varying degree. They are concentrated by the liver in the bile, and excreted in the urine and feces at high concentrations and in a biologically active form.

Following a single 100 mg dose administered in a concentration of 0.4 mg/ml in a one-hour infusion, normal adult volunteers average a peak of 2.5 mcg/ml, while 200 mg of a concentration of 0.4 mg/ml administered over two hours averaged a peak of 3.6 mcg/ml.

Excretion of doxycycline by the kidney is about 40 percent/72 hours in individuals with normal function (creatinine clearance about 75 ml/min.). This percentage excretion may fall as low as 1-5 percent/72 hours in individuals with severe renal insufficiency (creatinine clearance below 10 ml/min.). Studies have shown no significant difference in serum half-life of doxycycline (range 18-22 hours) in individuals with normal and severely impaired renal function.

Hemodialysis does not alter this serum half-life of doxycycline.

Indications: Doxycycline is indicated in infections caused by the following microorganisms:
Rickettsiae (Rocky Mountain spotted fever, typhus fever, and the typhus group, Q fever, rickettsialpox and tick fevers).
Mycoplasma pneumoniae (PPLO, Eaton Agent).
Agents of psittacosis and ornithosis.
Agents of lymphogranuloma venereum and granuloma inguinale.
The spirochetal agent of relapsing fever (*Borrelia recurrentis*).

The following gram-negative microorganisms:
Haemophilus ducreyi (chancroid),
Pasteurella pestis and *Pasteurella tularensis,*
Bartonella bacilliformis,
Bacteroides species,
Vibrio comma and *Vibrio fetus,*
Brucella species (in conjunction with streptomycin).

Because many strains of the following groups of microorganisms have been shown to be resistant to tetracyclines, culture and susceptibility testing are recommended.

Doxycycline is indicated for treatment of infections caused by the following gram-negative microorganisms when bacteriologic testing indicates appropriate susceptibility to the drug:
Escherichia coli,
Enterobacter aerogenes (formerly *Aerobacter aerogenes),*
Shigella species,
Mima species and *Herellea* species,
Haemophilus influenzae (respiratory infections),
Klebsiella species (respiratory and urinary infections).

Doxycycline is indicated for treatment of infections caused by the following gram-positive microorganisms when bacteriologic testing indicates appropriate susceptibility to the drug:
Streptococcus species:
Up to 44 percent of strains of *Streptococcus pyogenes* and 74 percent of *Streptococcus faecalis* have been found to be resistant to tetracycline drugs. Therefore, tetracyclines should not be used for streptococcal disease unless the organism has been demonstrated to be sensitive.

For upper respiratory infections due to group A beta-hemolytic streptococci, penicillin is the usual drug of choice, including prophylaxis of rheumatic fever.

Diplococcus pneumoniae,
Staphylococcus aureus, respiratory, skin and soft tissue infections. Tetracyclines are not the drugs of choice in the treatment of any type of staphylococcal infections.

Continued on next page

Pfizer—Cont.

When penicillin is contraindicated, doxycycline is an alternative drug in the treatment of infections due to:

Neisseria gonorrhoeae and *N. meningitidis*,
Treponema pallidum and *Treponema per-tenue* (syphilis and yaws),
Listeria monocytogenes,
Clostridium species,
Bacillus anthracis,
Fusobacterium fusiforme (Vincent's infection),
Actinomyces species.

In acute intestinal amebiasis, doxycycline may be a useful adjunct to amebicides.

Doxycycline is indicated in the treatment of trachoma, although the infectious agent is not always eliminated, as judged by immunofluorescence.

Contraindications: This drug is contraindicated in persons who have shown hypersensitivity to any of the tetracyclines.

Warnings: THE USE OF DRUGS OF THE TETRACYCLINE CLASS DURING TOOTH DEVELOPMENT (LAST HALF OF PREGNANCY, INFANCY AND CHILDHOOD TO THE AGE OF 8 YEARS) MAY CAUSE PERMANENT DISCOLORATION OF THE TEETH (YELLOW-GRAY-BROWN). This adverse reaction is more common during long-term use of the drugs but has been observed following repeated short-term courses. Enamel hypoplasia has also been reported. *TETRACYCLINE DRUGS, THEREFORE, SHOULD NOT BE USED IN THIS AGE GROUP UNLESS OTHER DRUGS ARE NOT LIKELY TO BE EFFECTIVE OR ARE CONTRAINDICATED.*

Photosensitivity manifested by an exaggerated sunburn reaction has been observed in some individuals taking tetracyclines. Patients apt to be exposed to direct sunlight or ultraviolet light should be advised that this reaction can occur with tetracycline drugs, and treatment should be discontinued at the first evidence of skin erythema.

The antianabolic action of the tetracyclines may cause an increase in BUN. Studies to date indicate that this does not occur with the use of doxycycline in patients with impaired renal function.

Usage in Pregnancy
(See above "Warnings" about use during tooth development.)
Vibramycin (doxycycline hyclate for injection) Intravenous has not been studied in pregnant patients. It should not be used in pregnant women unless, in the judgment of the physician, it is essential for the welfare of the patient.
Results of animal studies indicate that tetracyclines cross the placenta, are found in fetal tissues and can have toxic effects on the developing fetus (often related to retardation of skeletal development). Evidence of embryotoxicity has also been noted in animals treated early in pregnancy.

Usage in Children
The use of Vibramycin Intravenous in children under 8 years is not recommended because safe conditions for its use have not been established. (See above "Warnings" about use during tooth development.)
As with other tetracyclines, doxycycline forms a stable calcium complex in any bone-forming tissue. A decrease in the fibula growth rate has been observed in prematures given oral tetracycline in doses of 25 mg/kg every 6 hours. This reaction was shown to be reversible when the drug was discontinued.
Tetracyclines are present in the milk of lactating women who are taking a drug in this class.

Precautions: As with other antibiotic preparations, use of this drug may result in overgrowth of nonsusceptible organisms, including fungi. If superinfection occurs, the antibiotic should be discontinued and appropriate therapy instituted.
In venereal diseases when coexistent syphilis is suspected, a dark field examination should be done before treatment is started and the blood serology repeated monthly for at least 4 months.
Because tetracyclines have been shown to depress plasma prothrombin activity, patients who are on anticoagulant therapy may require downward adjustment of their anticoagulant dosage.
In long-term therapy, periodic laboratory evaluation of organ systems, including hematopoietic, renal, and hepatic studies should be performed.
All infections due to group A beta-hemolytic streptococci should be treated for at least 10 days.
Since bacteriostatic drugs may interfere with the bactericidal action of penicillin, it is advisable to avoid giving tetracycline in conjunction with penicillin.

Adverse Reactions: Gastrointestinal: anorexia, nausea, vomiting, diarrhea, glossitis, dysphagia, enterocolitis, and inflammatory lesions (with monilial overgrowth) in the anogenital region. These reactions have been caused by both the oral and parenteral administration of tetracyclines.

Skin: maculopapular and erythematous rashes. Exfoliative dermatitis has been reported but is uncommon. Photosensitivity is discussed above. (See "Warnings.")

Renal toxicity: Rise in BUN has been reported and is apparently dose related. (See "Warnings.")

Hypersensitivity reactions: urticaria, angioneurotic edema, anaphylaxis, anaphylactoid purpura, pericarditis and exacerbation of systemic lupus erythematosus.

Bulging fontanels in infants and benign intracranial hypertension in adults have been reported in individuals receiving full therapeutic dosages. These conditions disappeared rapidly when the drug was discontinued.

Blood: Hemolytic anemia, thrombocytopenia, neutropenia and eosinophilia have been reported.

When given over prolonged periods, tetracyclines have been reported to produce brown-black microscopic discoloration of thyroid glands. No abnormalities of thyroid function studies are known to occur.

Dosage and Administration: Note: Rapid administration is to be avoided. Parenteral therapy is indicated only when oral therapy is not indicated. Oral therapy should be instituted as soon as possible. If intravenous therapy is given over prolonged periods of time, thrombophlebitis may result.

THE USUAL DOSAGE AND FREQUENCY OF ADMINISTRATION OF VIBRAMYCIN I.V. (100-200 MG/DAY) DIFFERS FROM THAT OF THE OTHER TETRACYCLINES (1-2 G/DAY). EXCEEDING THE RECOMMENDED DOSAGE MAY RESULT IN AN INCREASED INCIDENCE OF SIDE EFFECTS.

Studies to date have indicated that Vibramycin at the usual recommended doses does not lead to excessive accumulation of the antibiotic in patients with renal impairment.

Adults: The usual dosage of Vibramycin (doxycycline hyclate for injection) I.V. is 200 mg on the first day of treatment administered in one or two infusions. Subsequent daily dosage is 100 to 200 mg depending upon the severity of infection, with 200 mg administered in one or two infusions.

In the treatment of primary and secondary syphilis, the recommended dosage is 300 mg daily for at least 10 days.

For children above eight years of age: The recommended dosage schedule for children weighing 100 pounds or less is 2 mg/lb. of body weight on the first day of treatment, administered in one or two infusions. Subsequent daily dosage is 1 to 2 mg/lb. of body weight given as one or two infusions, depending on the severity of the infection. For children over 100 pounds the usual adult dose should be used. (See "Warning" Section for Usage in Children.)

General: The duration of infusion may vary with the dose (100 to 200 mg per day), but is usually one to four hours. A recommended minimum infusion time for 100 mg of a 0.5 mg/ml solution is one hour. Therapy should be continued for at least 24-48 hours after symptoms and fever have subsided. The therapeutic antibacterial serum activity will usually persist for 24 hours following recommended dosage.

Intravenous solutions should not be injected intramuscularly or subcutaneously. Caution should be taken to avoid the inadvertent introduction of the intravenous solution into the adjacent soft tissue.

Preparation of Solution: To prepare a solution containing 10 mg/ml, the contents of the vial should be reconstituted with 10 ml (for the 100 mg/vial container) or 20 ml (for the 200 mg/vial container) of Sterile Water for Injection or any of the ten intravenous infusion solutions listed below. Each 100 mg of Vibramycin (i.e., withdraw entire solution from the 100 mg vial) is further diluted with 100 ml to 1000 ml of the intravenous solutions listed below. Each 200 mg of Vibramycin (i.e., withdraw entire solution from the 200 mg vial) is further diluted with 200 ml to 2000 ml of the following intravenous solutions:

1. Sodium Chloride Injection, USP
2. 5% Dextrose Injection, USP
3. Ringer's Injection, USP
4. Invert Sugar, 10% in Water
5. Lactated Ringer's Injection, USP
6. Dextrose 5% in Lactated Ringer's
7. Normosol-M® in D5-W (Abbott)
8. Normosol-R® in D5-W (Abbott)
9. Plasma-Lyte® 56 in 5% Dextrose (Travenol)
10. Plasma-Lyte® 148 in 5% Dextrose (Travenol)

This will result in desired concentrations of 0.1 to 1.0 mg/ml. Concentrations lower than 0.1 mg/ml or higher than 1.0 mg/ml are not recommended.

Stability:
When diluted with Sodium Chloride Injection, USP, or 5% Dextrose Injection, USP, or Ringer's Injection, USP, or Invert Sugar, 10% in Water, or Normosol-M® in D5-W (Abbott), or Normosol-R® in D5-W (Abbott), or Plasma-Lyte® 56 in 5% Dextrose (Travenol), or Plasma-Lyte® 148 in 5% Dextrose (Travenol), infusion of the solution (ca. 1.0 mg/ml) or lower concentrations (not less than 0.1 mg/ml) must be completed within 12 hours after reconstitution to ensure adequate stability. During infusion, the solution must be protected from direct sunlight. Reconstituted solutions (1.0 to 0.1 mg/ml) may also be stored up to 72 hours prior to start of infusion, if refrigerated and protected from sunlight and artificial light. Again, infusion must then be completed within 12 hours. Solutions must be used within these time periods or discarded.

When diluted with Lactated Ringer's Injection, USP, or Dextrose 5% in Lactated Ringer's, infusion of the solution (ca. 1.0 mg/ml) or lower concentrations (not less than 0.1 mg/ml) must be completed within six hours after reconstitution to ensure adequate stability. During infusion, the solution must be protected from direct sunlight. Solutions must be used within this time period or discarded.

Solutions of Vibramycin (doxycycline hyclate for injection) at a concentration of 10 mg/ml in Sterile Water for Injection, when frozen immediately after reconstitution are stable for 8 weeks when stored at −20°C. If the product is warmed, care should be taken to avoid heating it after the thawing is complete. Once thawed the solution should not be refrozen.

How Supplied: Vibramycin (doxycycline hyclate for injection) Intravenous is available as a sterile powder in a vial containing doxycycline hyclate equivalent to 100 mg of doxycycline with 480 mg of ascorbic acid, packages of 5; and in individually packaged vials containing doxycycline hyclate equivalent to 200 mg of doxycycline with 960 mg of ascorbic acid.

(23-1940-00-8)

Literature Available: Yes.

VISTARIL®
[vĭs'tăr-ĭl]
(hydroxyzine pamoate)
Capsules and Oral Suspension

Description: Hydroxyzine pamoate is designated chemically as 1-(p-chlorobenzhydryl) 4-[2-(2-hydroxyethoxy) ethyl] diethylenediamine salt of 1,1'-methylene bis (2 hydroxy-3-naphthalene carboxylic acid).

Clinical Pharmacology: Vistaril (hydroxyzine pamoate) is unrelated chemically to the phenothiazines, reserpine, meprobamate, or the benzodiazepines.

Vistaril is not a cortical depressant, but its action may be due to a suppression of activity in certain key regions of the subcortical area of the central nervous system. Primary skeletal muscle relaxation has been demonstrated experimentally. Bronchodilator activity, and antihistaminic and analgesic effects have been demonstrated experimentally and confirmed clinically. An antiemetic effect, both by the apomorphine test and the veriloid test, has been demonstrated. Pharmacological and clinical studies indicate that hydroxyzine in therapeutic dosage does not increase gastric secretion or acidity and in most cases has mild antisecretory activity. Hydroxyzine is rapidly absorbed from the gastrointestinal tract and Vistaril's clinical effects are usually noted within 15 to 30 minutes after oral administration.

Indications: For symptomatic relief of anxiety and tension associated with psychoneurosis and as an adjunct in organic disease states in which anxiety is manifested.

Useful in the management of pruritus due to allergic conditions such as chronic urticaria and atopic and contact dermatoses, and in histamine-mediated pruritus.

As a sedative when used as premedication and following general anesthesia, **Hydroxyzine may potentiate meperidine (Demerol®) and barbiturates,** so their use in pre-anesthetic adjunctive therapy should be modified on an individual basis. Atropine and other belladonna alkaloids are not affected by the drug. Hydroxyzine is not known to interfere with the action of digitalis in any way and it may be used concurrently with this agent. The effectiveness of hydroxyzine as an antianxiety agent for long term use, that is more than 4 months, has not been assessed by systematic clinical studies. The physician should reassess periodically the usefulness of the drug for the individual patient.

Contraindications: Hydroxyzine, when administered to the pregnant mouse, rat, and rabbit, induced fetal abnormalities in the rat and mouse at doses substantially above the human therapeutic range. Clinical data in human beings are inadequate to establish safety in early pregnancy. Until such data are available, hydroxyzine is contraindicated in early pregnancy.

Hydroxyzine pamoate is contraindicated for patients who have shown a previous hypersensitivity to it.

Warnings: Nursing Mothers: It is not known whether this drug is excreted in human milk. Since many drugs are so excreted, hydroxyzine should not be given to nursing mothers.

Precautions: THE POTENTIATING ACTION OF HYDROXYZINE MUST BE CONSIDERED WHEN THE DRUG IS USED IN CONJUNCTION WITH CENTRAL NERVOUS SYSTEM DEPRESSANTS SUCH AS NARCOTICS, NON-NARCOTIC ANALGESICS AND BARBITURATES. Therefore, when central nervous system depressants are administered concomitantly with hydroxyzine their dosage should be reduced. Since drowsiness may occur with use of the drug, patients should be warned of this possibility and cautioned against driving a car or operating dangerous machinery while taking Vistaril (hydroxyzine pamoate). Patients should be advised against the simultaneous use of other CNS depressant drugs, and cautioned that the effect of alcohol may be increased.

Adverse Reactions: Side effects reported with the administration of Vistaril are usually mild and transitory in nature.

Anticholinergic: Dry mouth.

Central Nervous System: Drowsiness is usually transitory and may disappear in a few days of continued therapy or upon reduction of the dose. Involuntary motor activity including rare instances of tremor and convulsions has been reported, usually with doses considerably higher than those recommended. Clinically significant respiratory depression has not been reported at recommended doses.

Overdosage: The most common manifestation of overdosage of Vistaril is hypersedation. As in the management of overdosage with any drug, it should be borne in mind that multiple agents may have been taken.

If vomiting has not occurred spontaneously, it should be induced. Immediate gastric lavage is also recommended. General supportive care, including frequent monitoring of the vital signs and close observation of the patient, is indicated. Hypotension, though unlikely, may be controlled with intravenous fluids and Levophed® (levarterenol) or Aramine® (metaraminol). Do not use epinephrine as Vistaril counteracts its pressor action. Caffeine and Sodium Benzoate Injection, U.S.P., may be used to counteract central nervous system depressant effects.

There is no specific antidote. It is doubtful that hemodialysis would be of any value in the treatment of overdosage with hydroxyzine. However, if other agents such as barbiturates have been ingested concomitantly, hemodialysis may be indicated. There is no practical method to quantitate hydroxyzine in body fluids or tissue after its ingestion or administration.

Dosage: For symptomatic relief of anxiety and tension associated with psychoneurosis and as an adjunct in organic disease states in which anxiety is manifested: in adults, 50–100 mg q.i.d.; children under 6 years, 50 mg daily in divided doses and over 6 years, 50–100 mg daily in divided doses.

For use in the management of pruritus due to allergic conditions such as chronic urticaria and atopic and contact dermatoses, and in histamine-mediated pruritus: in adults, 25 mg t.i.d. or q.i.d.; children under 6 years, 50 mg daily in divided doses and over 6 years, 50–100 mg daily in divided doses.

As a sedative when used as a premedication and following general anesthesia: 50–100 mg in adults, and 0.6 mg/kg in children.

When treatment is initiated by the intramuscular route of administration, subsequent doses may be administered orally.

As with all medications, the dosage should be adjusted according to the patient's response to therapy.

Supply:
Vistaril Capsules (hydroxyzine pamoate equivalent to hydroxyzine hydrochloride)

- 25 mg: 100's and 500's, and unit dose (10 × 10's)—two-tone green capsules (imprinted with code number 541).
- 50 mg: 100's and 500's, and unit dose (10 × 10's)—green and white capsules (imprinted with code number 542).
- 100 mg: 100's and 500's, and unit dose (10 × 10's)—green and gray capsules (imprinted with code number 543).

Vistaril Oral Suspension (hydroxyzine pamoate equivalent to 25 mg hydroxyzine hydrochloride per teaspoonful-5 ml): 1 pint bottles and 4 ounce (120 ml) bottles in packages of 4.

Bibliography: Available on request.

(60-0846-00-9)

Shown in Product Identification Section, page 427

VISTARIL® ℞
[vĭs'tăr-ĭl]
(hydroxyzine hydrochloride)
Intramuscular Solution
For Intramuscular Use Only

Vistaril® Intramuscular Solution is manufactured by Pfizer Pharmaceuticals and distributed by the Pfipharmecs Division. Please refer to Pfipharmecs PRODUCT INFORMATION for a full product description of Vistaril® Intramuscular Solution.

EDUCATIONAL MATERIAL

Booklets—free
The *Learning to Live With. . . .* series of patient information booklets on the symptoms of specific diseases, preventive measures, techniques for changing lifestyle habits, adherence to diet and drug regimens. This ongoing series includes booklets on angina, osteoarthritis and diabetes.
Address requests to:
Communications Program Coordination
Pfizer Pharmaceuticals
235 East 42nd Street
New York, N.Y. 10017

Pharmacia Laboratories
Division of Pharmacia Inc.
800 CENTENNIAL AVENUE
PISCATAWAY, NJ 08854

AZULFIDINE® (sulfasalazine USP)   ℞
[ă-zul'fĭ-dēn"]
Tablets
AZULFIDINE® (sulfasalazine USP)   ℞
EN-tabs®
AZULFIDINE® (sulfasalazine USP)   ℞
Oral Suspension

Description: AZULFIDINE Tablets contain sulfasalazine U.S.P., 500 mg/tablet. AZULFIDINE EN-tabs contain sulfasalazine U.S.P., 500 mg/enteric-coated tablet. AZULFIDINE EN-tabs are film coated with cellulose acetate phthalate to prevent disintegration of the tablet in the stomach and thus reduce possible irritation of the gastric mucosa. Cellulose acetate phthalate coatings disintegrate due to the hydrolytic effect of the intestinal esterases, even when the intestinal contents are acid.

AZULFIDINE Oral Suspension is an aqueous solution of sulfasalazine U.S.P. (250 mg/5 ml) with microcrystalline cellulose, Xanthan Gum, polysorbate 80, sodium benzoate, sucrose, and flavor.

Sulfasalazine is synthesized by the diazotization of sulfapyridine and the coupling of the diazonium salt with salicylic acid. Further processing results in a bright orange colored substance that chemically is designated: 5-[p-(2-Pyridylsulfamoyl) phenyl] azo] salicylic acid. Reductive splitting of the azo linkage yields sulfapyridine and 5-aminosalicylic acid.

Actions: After oral administration, AZULFIDINE is partially absorbed and extensively metabolized, as described below.

About one-third of a given dose of sulfasalazine (SS) is absorbed from the small intestine. The remaining two-thirds pass to the colon where the compound is split (presumably by intestinal bacteria) into its components, 5-aminosalicylic acid (5-ASA) and sulfapyridine (SP). Most of the SP thus liberated is absorbed, whereas only about one-third of the 5-ASA is absorbed, the remainder being excreted in the feces. The distribution, metabolism and excretion of SS and its two components are as follows:

AZULFIDINE Tablets:

Sulfasalazine (SS): Detectable serum concentrations of SS have been found in healthy subjects within 90 minutes after the ingestion of a single 2 g dose of AZULFIDINE Tablets. Maximum concentrations of SS occur between 1.5 and 6 hours, with the mean peak concentrations (14 mcg/ml) occurring at 3 hours. Small amounts of SS are excreted unchanged in the urine.

Sulfapyridine (SP): Following absorption and distribution, SP is acetylated and hydroxylated in the liver, and then conjugated with glucuronic acid. After ingestion of a single 2 g dose of AZULFIDINE Tablets by healthy subjects, SP and its various metabolites appear in the serum within 3 to 6 hours. Maximum concentrations of total SP occur between 6 and 24 hours, with the mean peak concentration (21 mcg/ml) occurring at 12 hours. The total recovery of SS and its SP metabolites from the urine of healthy subjects 3 days after the

Continued on next page

Pharmacia—Cont.

administration of a single 2 g dose of AZULFIDINE Tablets averaged 91%.

Mean serum concentrations of total SP, i.e., SP + its metabolites, tend to be significantly greater in patients with a slow acetylator phenotype than in those with a fast acetylator phenotype. SP serum concentrations greater than 50 mcg/ml appear to be associated with adverse reactions.

5-Aminosalicylic Acid (5-ASA): The serum concentration of 5-ASA in patients with ulcerative colitis was found to range from 0 to 4 mcg/ml, and to exist mainly in the form of free 5-ASA. The urinary recovery of this compound was mostly in the acetylated form.

AZULFIDINE EN-tabs

Sulfasalazine (SS): Detectable serum concentrations of SS have been found in healthy subjects within 90 minutes after the ingestion of a single 2 g dose of AZULFIDINE EN-tabs. Maximum concentrations of SS occur between 3 and 12 hours, with the mean peak concentrations (6 mcg/ml) occurring at 6 hours. Small amounts of SS are excreted unchanged in the urine.

Sulfapyridine (SP): Following absorption and distribution, SP is acetylated and hydroxylated in the liver, and then conjugated with glucuronic acid. After ingestion of a single 2 g dose of AZULFIDINE EN-tabs by healthy subjects, peak concentrations of SP and its various metabolites appear in the serum between 12 and 24 hours, with the peak concentration (13 mcg/ml) occurring at 12 and lasting until 24 hours. The total recovery of SS and its SP metabolites from the urine of healthy subjects 3 days after the administration of a single 2 g dose of AZULFIDINE EN-tabs averaged 81%.

Mean serum concentrations of total SP, i.e., SP + its metabolites, tend to be significantly greater in patients with a slow acetylator phenotype than in those with a fast acetylator phenotype. SP serum concentrations greater than 50 mcg/ml appear to be associated with adverse reactions.

5-Aminosalicylic Acid (5-ASA): The serum concentration of 5-ASA in patients with ulcerative colitis was found to range from 0 to 4 mcg/ml, and to exist mainly in the form of free 5-ASA. The urinary recovery of this compound was mostly in the acetylated form.

AZULFIDINE Oral Suspension

Sulfasalazine (SS): Detectable serum concentrations of SS have been found in healthy subjects within 90 minutes after the injection of a single 2 g dose of AZULFIDINE Oral Suspension. Maximum concentrations of SS occur between 1.5 and 6 hours, with the mean peak concentration (20 mcg/ml) occurring at 3 hours. Small amounts of SS are excreted unchanged in the urine.

Sulfapyridine (SP): Following absorption and distribution, SP is acetylated and hydroxylated in the liver, and then conjugated with glucuronic acid. After ingestion of a single 2 g dose of AZULFIDINE Oral Suspension by healthy subjects, SP and its various metabolites appear in the serum within 3 to 6 hours. Maximum concentrations of total SP occur between 9 and 24 hours with the mean peak concentration (19 mcg/ml) occurring at 12 hours. The total recovery of SS and its SP metabolites from the urine of healthy subjects 3 days after the administration of a single 2 g dose of AZULFIDINE Oral Suspension averaged 75%.

Mean serum concentrations of total SP, i.e., SP + its metabolites, tend to be significantly greater in patients with a slow acetylator phenotype than in those with a fast acetylator phenotype. SP serum concentrations greater than 50 mcg/ml appear to be associated with adverse reactions.

5-Aminosalicylic Acid (5-ASA): The serum concentrations of 5-ASA in normal subjects was found to range from 0 to 4 mcg/ml, and to exist mainly in the form of free 5-ASA. The urinary recovery of this compound was mostly in the acetylated form. The mode of action of AZULFIDINE is still under investigation. It may be related to the immunosuppressant properties that have been observed in animal and in vitro models, to its affinity for connective tissue, and/or to the relatively high concentration it reaches in serous fluids, the liver and intestinal wall, as demonstrated in autoradiographic studies in animals. AZULFIDINE has also been described as a highly efficient vehicle for carrying its principal metabolites, SP and 5-ASA, to the colon, where a local action for both of them has been postulated.

Indications: AZULFIDINE is indicated in the treatment of mild to moderate ulcerative colitis, and as adjunctive therapy in severe ulcerative colitis.

AZULFIDINE EN-tabs are particularly indicated in patients who cannot take the regular AZULFIDINE tablet because of gastrointestinal intolerance, and in whom there is evidence that this intolerance is not primarily due to high blood levels of sulfapyridine and its metabolites, e.g. patients experiencing nausea, vomiting, etc., when taking the first few doses of the drug or patients in whom a reduction in dosage does not alleviate the gastrointestinal side effects.

Contraindications: Hypersensitivity to sulfonamides or salicylates. In infants under 2 years. Intestinal and urinary obstruction. Patients with porphyria should not receive sulfonamides, as these drugs have been reported to precipitate an acute attack.

Warnings:

Use in pregnancy: Teratology studies have been performed with AZULFIDINE in rats and rabbits at doses up to 6 times the maximum recommended human dose and have revealed no evidence of harm to the developing fetus. There are, however, no adequate and well-controlled studies in pregnant women.

Because animal reproduction studies are not always predictive of human response, this drug should be used during pregnancy only if clearly needed.

Nursing mothers: Sulfonamides are excreted in the milk. In the newborn, they compete with bilirubin for binding sites on the plasma proteins and may thus cause kernicterus. Insignificant amounts of uncleaved sulfasalazine have been found in milk, whereas the sulfapyridine levels in milk are about 30-60 percent of those in the serum. Sulfapyridine has been shown to have a poor bilirubin-displacing capacity.

Impairment of fertility: Oligospermia and infertility have been described in men treated with AZULFIDINE. Withdrawal of the drug appears to reverse these effects.

Other warnings: Only after critical appraisal should AZULFIDINE be used in patients with hepatic or renal damage or blood dyscrasias. Deaths associated with the administration of AZULFIDINE have been reported from hypersensitivity reactions, agranulocytosis, aplastic anemia, other blood dyscrasias, renal and liver damage, irreversible neuromuscular and CNS changes, and fibrosing alveolitis. The presence of clinical signs such as sore throat, fever, pallor, purpura, or jaundice may be indications of serious blood disorders. Complete blood counts as well as urinalysis with careful microscopic examination should be done frequently in patients receiving AZULFIDINE.

Precautions: AZULFIDINE should be given with caution to patients with severe allergy or bronchial asthma. Adequate fluid intake must be maintained in order to prevent crystalluria and stone formation. Patients with glucose-6-phosphate dehydrogenase deficiency should be observed closely for signs of hemolytic anemia. This reaction is frequently dose related. If toxic or hypersensitivity reactions occur, the drug should be discontinued immediately.

Isolated instances have been reported when AZULFIDINE EN-tabs have passed undisintegrated. This may be due to a lack of intestinal esterases in these patients (see description). If this is observed, the administration of AZULFIDINE EN-tabs should be discontinued immediately.

Adverse Reactions: Adverse reactions have been observed in 5 to 55% of patients included in clinical studies reported in the literature. Experience suggests that with daily dosage of 4 g or more adverse reactions tend to increase.

The most common adverse reactions associated with AZULFIDINE therapy are anorexia, nausea, vomiting, and gastric distress. The following adverse reactions have been reported to occur during therapy with AZULFIDINE.

Blood dyscrasias, Agranulocytosis, aplastic anemia, thrombocytopenia, leukopenia, hemolytic anemia. Heinz Body anemia, megaloblastic (macrocytic) anemia, purpura, hypoprothrombinemia, "cyanosis" and methemoglobinemia.

Hypersensitivity reactions: Generalized skin eruptions, erythema multiforme (Stevens-Johnson syndrome), parapsoriasis varioliformis acuta (Mucha-Haberman syndrome), exfoliative dermatitis, epidermal necrolysis (Lyell's syndrome) with corneal damage, pruritus, urticaria, photosensitization, anaphylaxis, serum sickness syndrome, chills, drug fever, periorbital edema, conjunctival and scleral injection, arthralgia; transient pulmonary changes with eosinophilia and decreased pulmonary function; allergic myocarditis; polyarteritis nodosa, L.E. syndrome, and hepatitis with immune complexes. Incidents of alopecia have also been reported.

Gastrointestinal reactions: Anorexia, nausea, emesis, abdominal pains, diarrhea, bloody diarrhea, impaired folic acid and digoxin absorption, stomatitis, pancreatitis, and hepatitis.

CNS reactions: Headache, vertigo, tinnitus, hearing loss, peripheral neuropathy, transient lesions of posterior spinal column, transverse myelitis, ataxia, convulsions, insomnia, mental depression, hallucinations and drowsiness.

Renal reactions: Crystalluria, hematuria, proteinuria, and nephrotic syndrome. Toxic nephrosis with oliguria and anuria.

The sulfonamides bear certain chemical similarities to some goitrogens, diuretics, (acetazolamide and the thiazides), and oral hypoglycemic agents. Goiter production, diuresis, and hypoglycemia have occurred rarely in patients receiving sulfonamides. Cross-sensitivity may exist with these agents.

Rats appear to be especially susceptible to the goitrogenic effects of sulfonamides and long-term administration has produced thyroid malignancies in this species.

AZULFIDINE produces an orange-yellow color when the urine is alkaline. Similar discoloration of the skin has also been reported.

Treatment of Overdosage and Sensitivity Reactions:

Overdosage: Gastric lavage or emesis plus catharsis as indicated. Alkalinize urine. If kidney function is normal, force fluids. If anuria is present, restrict fluids and salt, and treat for renal failure. Catheterization of the ureters may be indicated for complete renal blockage by crystals. For agranulocytosis discontinue the drug immediately, hospitalize the patient and institute appropriate therapy.

Sensitivity reactions: Discontinue treatment immediately. Urticaria, other skin rashes, and serum sickness-like reactions may be controlled with antihistamines and, if necessary, systemic corticosteriods. When in the physician's opinion, reinstitution of AZULFIDINE is warranted, regimens modeled upon desensitization procedures may be attempted approximately two weeks after AZULFIDINE has been discontinued and symptoms have disappeared (see Dosage and Administration).

Dosage and Administration: Dosage should be adjusted to each individual's response and tolerance. The drug should be given in evenly divided doses over each 24-hour period; intervals between nighttime doses should not exceed 8 hours, with administration after meals recommended when feasible. Experience suggests that with daily dosages of 4 g or more adverse reactions tend to increase; hence patients receiving these dosages should be carefully observed for the appearance of adverse effects. Various desensitization-like regimens have been reported to be effective in 34 of 53 patients[1], 7 of 8 patients[2] and 19 of 20 patients[3]. Upon reinstituting AZULFIDINE, such regimens comprise a total daily dose of 50 to 250 mg which, every 4 to 7 days thereafter, is doubled until the desired therapeutic level is achieved. Administration of small desensitizing doses of AZULFIDINE are achieved most easily through the use of AZULFIDINE Oral Suspension (250 mg/5 ml). If the symptoms of sensitivity recur, AZULFIDINE should be discontinued. Desensitization should not be attempted in patients who have a history of agranulocytosis or who have experienced an anaphylactoid reaction while on a previous course of AZULFIDINE therapy.

Usual Dosage:

AZULFIDINE Tablets and AZULFIDINE EN-tabs
Initial therapy: Adults: 3-4 g daily in evenly divided doses. In some cases it is advisable to initiate therapy with a small dosage, e.g. 1-2 g daily, to lessen adverse gastrointestinal effects. If daily doses up to 8 g are required to achieve desired effects, the increased risk of toxicity should be kept in mind. Children: 40-60 mg per kg body weight in each 24-hour period, divided into 3-6 doses.
Maintenance therapy: Adults: 2 g daily. Children: 30 mg per kg body weight in each 24-hour period, divided into 4 doses. Response to therapy and adjustment of dosage should be determined by periodic examination. It is often necessary to continue medication, even when clinical symptoms, including diarrhea, have been controlled. When endoscopic examination confirms satisfactory improvement, dosage is reduced to a maintenance level. If diarrhea recurs, dosage should be increased to previous effective levels.

If symptoms of gastric intolerance (anorexia, nausea, vomiting, etc.) occur after the first few doses of AZULFIDINE, they are probably due to mucosal irritation, and may be alleviated by distributing the total daily dose more evenly over the day or by giving enteric-coated EN-tabs. If such symptoms occur after the first few days of treatment with AZULFIDINE, they are probably due to increased serum levels of total sulfapyridine, and may be alleviated by halving the dose and subsequently increasing it gradually over several days. If symptoms continue, the drug should be stopped for 5-7 days, then reinstituted at a lower daily dose.

AZULFIDINE Oral Suspension
[Each 5 ml (one teaspoonful) contains 250 mg of sulfasalazine.]
Initial Therapy:
Adults: 3-4 g daily in evenly divided doses. In some cases it is advisable to initiate therapy with a smaller dosage, e.g. 1-2 g daily, to lessen adverse gastrointestinal effects. If daily doses up to 8 g are required to achieve desired effects, the increased risk of toxicity should be kept in mind.
Children: 40-60 mg per kg body weight in each 24-hour period, divided into 3-6 doses.
Maintenance Therapy:
Adults: 2 g daily.
Children: 30 mg per kg body weight in each 24-hour period, divided into 4 doses.
Response to therapy and adjustment of dosage should be determined by periodic examination. It is often necessary to continue medication, even when clinical symptoms including diarrhea, have been controlled. When endoscopic examination confirms satisfactory improvement, dosage is reduced to a maintenance level. If diarrhea recurs, dosage should be increased to previous effective levels.

How Supplied:
AZULFIDINE Tablets 500 mg 100's — NDC No. 0016-0101-01
AZULFIDINE Tablets 500 mg 500's — NDC No. 0016-0101-05
AZULFIDINE Unit Dose Tablets
 500 mg 100's — NDC No. 0016-0101-11
AZULFIDINE Unit Dose Tablets
 500 mg 1000's — NDC No. 0016-0101-10
AZULFIDINE EN-tabs 500 mg 100's — NDC No. 0016-0102-01
AZULFIDINE EN-tabs 500 mg 500's — NDC No. 0016-0102-05
AZULFIDINE Oral Suspension 250 mg/5 ml — 1 Pint (473 ml) — NDC No. 0016-0103-06
 Store at Room Temperature (15°-30°C/59°-86°F)
 Avoid Freezing
 Shake Well Before Using

References:
1. Korelitz B. et al: Gastroenterology 82: 1104, 1982.
2. Holdsworth, C.D.: Brit. Med. J. 282: 110, 1981.
3. Taffet, S.L. and Das, K.M.: Amer. J. Med., 73: 520–524, 1982.
Revised June 1983
Shown in Product Identification Section, page 427

HEALON® ℞
[he'lon]
(sodium hyaluronate)

Description: HEALON is a sterile, nonpyrogenic, viscoelastic preparation of a highly purified, noninflammatory, high molecular weight fraction of sodium hyaluronate.
HEALON contains 10 mg/ml of sodium hyaluronate, dissolved in physiological sodium chloride-phosphate buffer (pH 7.0–7.5). This high molecular weight polymer is made up of repeating disaccharide units of N-acetylglucosamine and sodium glucuronate linked by β1-3 and β1-4 glycosidic bonds.

Characteristics: Sodium hyaluronate is a physiological substance that is widely distributed in the extracellular matrix of connective tissues in both animals and man. For example, it is present in the vitreous and aqueous humor of the eye, the synovial fluid, the skin and the umbilical cord. Sodium hyaluronates prepared from various human and animal tissues are not chemically different from each other.
HEALON is a specific fraction of sodium hyaluronate developed as an ophthalmo-surgical aid for use in anterior segment and vitreous procedures. It is specific in that:
1. It has a high molecular weight.
2. It is reported to be nonantigenic[1,6]
3. It does not cause inflammatory[2] or foreign body reactions.
4. It has a high viscosity.
Furthermore, the 1% solution of HEALON is transparent, is reported to remain in the anterior chamber for less than 6 days, [3] protects corneal endothelial cells[4,5] and other ocular structures. HEALON does not interfere with epithelialization and normal wound healing.

Uses: HEALON is indicated for use as a surgical aid in cataract extraction (intra- and extra-capsular), IOL implantation, corneal transplant, glaucoma filtration and retinal attachment surgery.
In surgical procedures in the anterior segment of the eye, instillation of HEALON serves to maintain a deep anterior chamber during surgery, allowing for efficient manipulation with less trauma to the corneal endothelium and other surrounding tissues.
Furthermore, its viscoelasticity helps to push back the vitreous face and prevent formation of a postoperative flat chamber. In posterior segmant surgery HEALON serves as a surgical aid to gently separate, maneuver and hold tissues. HEALON creates a clear field of vision thereby facilitating intra- and postoperative inspection of the retina and photocoagulation.

Contraindications: At present there are no known contraindications to the use of HEALON when used as recommended.

Precautions: Those normally associated with the surgical procedure being performed. Overfilling the anterior or posterior segment of the eye with HEALON may cause increased intraocular pressure, glaucoma, or other ocular damage.
Postoperative intraocular pressure may also be elevated as a result of pre-existing glaucoma, compromised outflow, and by operative procedures and sequelae thereto, including enzymatic zonulysis, absence of an iridectomy, trauma to filtration structures, and by blood and lenticular remnants in the anterior chamber. Since the exact role of these factors is difficult to predict in any individual case, the following precautions are recommended:

—Don't overfill the eye chambers with HEALON (except in glaucoma surgery—see Application section).
—In posterior segment procedures in aphakic diabetic patients special care should be exercised to avoid using large amounts of HEALON.
—Remove some of the HEALON by irrigation and/or aspiration at the close of surgery (except in glaucoma surgery—see Application section).
—Carefully monitor intraocular pressure, especially during the immediate postoperative period. If significant rises are observed, treat with appropriate therapy.

Care should be taken to avoid trapping the air bubbles behind HEALON.
Because HEALON is a highly purified fraction extracted from avian tissues and is known to contain minute amounts of protein, the physician should be aware of potential risks of the type that can occur with the injection of any biological material.
Because of reports of an occasional release of minute rubber particles, presumably formed when the diaphragm is punctured, the physician should be aware of this potential problem. Express a small amount of HEALON from the syringe prior to use, and carefully examine the remainder as it is injected. Avoid reuse of cannulas. If reuse becomes necessary, rinse cannula thoroughly with sterile distilled water.
Use only if solution is clear.

Adverse Reactions:
HEALON is extremely well tolerated after injection into human eyes. A transient rise of intraocular pressure postoperatively has been reported in some cases. In posterior segment surgery intraocular pressure rises have been reported in some patients, especially in aphakic diabetics, after injection of large amounts of HEALON.
Rarely, postoperative inflammatory reactions (iritis, hypopyon) as well as incidents of corneal edema and corneal decompensation have been reported. Their relationship to HEALON has not been established.

Applications: Cataract surgery—IOL implantation
A sufficient amount of HEALON is slowly and carefully introduced (using a cannula or needle) into the anterior chamber.
Injection of HEALON can be performed either before or after delivery of the lens. Injection prior to lens delivery will, however, have the additional advantage of protecting the corneal endothelium from possible damage arising from the removal of the cataractous lens.[5] HEALON may also be used to coat surgical instruments and the IOL prior to insertion.
Additional HEALON can be injected during surgery to replace any HEALON lost during surgical manipulation (see Precautions section).

Glaucoma filtration surgery: In conjunction with the performance of the trabeculectomy, HEALON is injected slowly and carefully through a corneal paracentesis to reconstitute the anterior chamber. Further injection of HEALON can be continued to allow it to extrude into the subconjunctival filtration site through and around the sutured outer scleral flap.

Corneal transplant surgery: After removal of the corneal button, the anterior chamber is filled with HEALON. The donor graft can then be placed on top of the bed of HEALON and sutured in place. Additional HEALON may be injected to replace the HEALON lost as a result of surgical manipulation (see Precaution section). HEALON has also been used in the anterior chamber of the donor eye prior to trepanation to protect the corneal endothelial cells of the graft[5].

Retinal attachment surgery: HEALON is slowly introduced into the vitreous cavity. By directing the injection, HEALON can be used to separate membranes (e.g. epiretinal membranes) away from the retina for safe excision and release of traction. HEALON also serves to maneuver tissues into the desired position, e.g. to gently push back a detached retina or unroll a retinal flap, and

Continued on next page

Pharmacia—Cont.

aids in holding the retina against the sclera for reattachment.

How Supplied: HEALON is a sterile, nonpyrogenic, viscoelastic preparation supplied in disposable glass syringes, delivering 2.0 ml, 0.75 ml or 0.4 ml sodium hyaluronate (10 mg/ml) dissolved in physiological sodium chloride-phosphate buffer (pH 7.0–7.5). Each ml of HEALON contains 10 mg of sodium hyaluronate, 8.5 mg of sodium chloride, 0.28 mg of disodium hydrogen phosphate dihydrate, 0.04 mg of sodium dihydrogen phosphate hydrate and q.s. water for injection U.S.P. HEALON syringes are terminally sterilized and aseptically packaged.

Refrigerated HEALON should be allowed to attain room temperature (approximately 30 minutes) prior to use.

For intraocular use.
Store at 2–8°C.
Protect from freezing.
Protect from light.
References: See Full Product Information.
Caution: Federal law restricts this device to sale by or on the order of a physician.
Revised September 1984

HYSKON® Hysteroscopy Fluid ℞
[his'kon]
32% (W/V) dextran 70 in dextrose

Description: HYSKON Hysteroscopy Fluid is a clear, viscid, sterile, non-pyrogenic solution of dextran 70 (32% W/V) in dextrose (10% W/V). Dextran 70 is that fraction of dextran, a branched polysaccharide composed of glucose units, having a weight average molecular weight of 70,000. The fluid is electrolyte-free and non-conductive. At room temperature HYSKON Hysteroscopy Fluid has a viscosity of 220 cS.

HYSKON has a tendency to crystalize when subjected to temperature variations or when stored for long periods. If flakes of dextran are present, heat at 100°–110° C until complete dissolution is achieved.

Indications: HYSKON Hysteroscopy Fluid is indicated for use with the hysteroscope as an aid in distending the uterine cavity and in irrigating and visualizing its surfaces.

Contraindications: HYSKON Hysteroscopy Fluid should not be instilled in patients known to be hypersensitive to dextran. All other contraindications are those relative to the hysteroscopic procedure itself, such as pregnancy, endometrial carcinoma, etc.

Warnings: It is not known to what extent systemic absorption of dextran 70 occurs from the uterine and peritoneal cavities. Because of the possibility that absorption can occur, the physician should familiarize himself with the systemic effects of this drug. The most alarming are severe, sometimes fatal anaphylactoid reactions, which are quite rare. Other noteworthy effects include plasma volume expansion and transient prolongation of bleeding time.

Adverse Reactions: The physician should be mindful of the fact that adverse reactions are known to occur with the administration of dextran 70. Such reactions, some of which have also been reported with the use of HYSKON, have included: allergic phenomena (generalized itching, macular rash, anaphylactoid reactions, urticaria, nasal congestion, wheezing, tightness of chest and mild hypotension), nausea, vomiting, fever and joint pains.

Dosage and Administration: The amount of HYSKON Hysteroscopy Fluid required per patient depends on a number of factors, such as the type and length of the diagnostic procedure, whether or not manipulation or surgery is performed, etc. Most often, however, the amount of HYSKON instilled into the uterus will be between 50 and 100 milliliters.

HYSKON should be introduced into the uterine cavity through the cannula of a hysteroscope under low pressure (approximately 100 mm Hg) until the uterus is sufficiently distended to permit adequate visualization. During the hysteroscopic examination, HYSKON should be infused at a rate that keeps the cavity suitably distended. To avoid injection of the fluid into the tissues of the uterus and parametria and to avoid having unnecessary amounts of the fluid pass into the peritoneal cavity and backwards along the side of the hysteroscope, infusion pressures greater than 150 mm Hg should not be used.

How Supplied: HYSKON Hysteroscopy Fluid (32% W/V dextran 70 in 10% W/V dextrose) is available as a sterile, nonpyrogenic solution in 100 ml bottles packed 12 to a carton..........................
NDC No. 0016-0231-61
and 250 ml bottles packed 6 to a carton................
NDC No. 0016-0231-62
Keep from cold during transportation.
Caution: Federal law restricts this device to sale by or on the order of a physician.
Revised January 1983

MACRODEX® ℞
[mak'ro-dex]
(Plasma Volume Expander)

6% Dextran 70 in 5% Dextrose Injection. 500 ml.
6% Dextran 70 in 0.9% Sodium Chloride Injection. 500 ml.

RHEOMACRODEX® ℞
[re"o-mak'ro-dex]
(low molecular weight dextran)

10% Dextran 40 in 5% Dextrose Injection. 500 ml.
10% Dextran 40 in 0.9% Sodium Chloride Injection. 500 ml.

The following products which are manufactured by KabiVitrum AB, Stockholm, Sweden, are distributed in the U.S.A. by Pharmacia under license from KabiVitrum AB.
We will be pleased to answer all inquiries and send full prescribing information upon request.

CRESCORMON® ℞
[kres"kor'mon]
somatropin
Sterile powder 4 IU/vial

How Supplied:
Crescormon® is supplied as a 4 IU (approx. 2 mg) vial of lyophilized, sterile somatropin; no preservative is included. Each vial of Crescormon is accompanied by a 2 ml sterile ampule of Sodium Chloride Injection. Each carrier carton contains ten combined packages of Crescormon and Sodium Chloride Injection.
NDC No: 00016-8050-1
Revision date Jan. 1982

KABIKINASE® ℞
[kă'be-ki"nās]
(Streptokinase)

How Supplied: KABIKINASE® (streptokinase) is supplied as a lyophilized powder in 5 ml vials containing 250,000, 600,000, or 750,000 IU per vial of purified streptokinase, and shipped in cartons containing 10 vials.
In each vial there is a 10% overfill above that stated on the label. Each vial also contains 11.0 mg of Sodium L-Glutamate per 100,000 IU of streptokinase and 14.5 mg of Albumin Human per 100,000 IU of streptokinase as stabilizers.
250,000 IU **NDC** 00016-8025-2
600,000 IU **NDC** 00016-8026-2
750,000 IU **NDC** 00016-8027-2

SECRETIN-KABI ℞
[se-kre'tin ka'be]
secretin

How Supplied: Secretin-Kabi is supplied as a lyophilized sterile powder in 10 ml vials containing 75 CU. Each box contains 5 vials Secretin-Kabi 75 CU. Secretin-Kabi 75 CU should be stored at −20°C. (freezer). However, the biological activity of Secretin-Kabi will not be significantly decreased by storage at 25°C or below for up to 3 weeks. Expiration date is marked on the label.
NDC 00016-075-05
Revision date Jan. 1982

Pharmacraft Division
PENNWALT CORPORATION
755 JEFFERSON ROAD
ROCHESTER, NY 14623

ALLEREST®
[al'e-rest]
Tablets, Childrens Chewable Tablets, Headache Strength Tablets, Sinus Pain Formula Tablets, Eye Drops and Nasal Spray

(See PDR For Nonprescription Drugs)

ALLEREST®
[al'e-rest]
Timed Release Allergy Capsules

(See PDR For Nonprescription Drugs)

CaldeCORT®
[cal'de-cort]
Hydrocortisone Multi-Purpose Anti-Itch Cream and Spray

(See PDR For Nonprescription Drugs)

CALDESENE®
[cal'de-sēn]
Medicated Ointment

(See PDR For Nonprescription Drugs)

CALDESENE®
[cal'de-sēn]
Medicated Baby Powder

(See PDR For Nonprescription Drugs)

COLD FACTOR 12™
[kōld fak'ter twelv]
12-Hour Nasal Decongestant/Antihistamine Liquid and Capsules

(See PDR For Nonprescription Drugs)

CRUEX®
[cru'ex]
Antifungal Cream

(See PDR For Nonprescription Drugs)

CRUEX®
[cru'ex]
Antifungal Powder and Spray Powder

(See PDR For Nonprescription Drugs)

DESENEX®
[dess'i-nex]
Antifungal Cream, Ointment, Foam and Liquid

(See PDR For Nonprescription Drugs)

DESENEX®
[dess'i-nex]
Antifungal Powder and Spray Powder

(See PDR For Nonprescription Drugs)

SINAREST®
[sīn'a-rest]
Tablets, Extra Strength Tablets and Nasal Spray

(See PDR For Nonprescription Drugs)

Products are cross-indexed by
generic and chemical names in the
YELLOW SECTION

Pharmaderm
a division of Altana Inc.
60 BAYLIS ROAD
MELVILLE, NY 11747

BETAMETHASONE VALERATE ℞
Cream, USP 0.1%
Ointment, USP 0.1%
Lotion, 0.1%
for dermatologic use only—not for ophthalmic use

betamethasone valerate cream
Description: Betamethasone Valerate Cream contains Betamethasone Valerate U.S.P. (Pregna-1, 4-diene-3, 20-dione, 9-fluoro-11, 21-dihydroxy-16-methyl-17-[(1-oxopentyl)oxy]-,(11B, 16B)-); it has an empirical formula of $C_{27}H_{37}FO_6$ and a molecular weight of 476.58 (CAS Registry Number 2152-44-5).

Each gram of the 0.1% cream contains 1.2 mg Betamethasone Valerate (equivalent to 1.0 mg Betamethasone) in a soft, white, hydrophilic cream of Water, Mineral Oil, White Petrolatum, Polyethylene Glycol 1000 Monocetyl Ether, Cetostearyl Alcohol, Monobasic Sodium Phosphate and Phosphoric Acid or Sodium Hydroxide; Chlorocresol is present as a preservative. Betamethasone Valerate Cream contains no parabens.

betamethasone valerate ointment
Description: Betamethasone Valerate Ointment contains Betamethasone Valerate U.S.P. (Pregna-1, 4-diene-3, 20-dione, 9-fluoro-11, 21-dihydroxy-16-methyl-17-[(1-oxopentyl)oxy]-,(11B, 16B)-); it has an empirical formula of $C_{27}H_{37}FO_6$ and a molecular weight of 476.58 (CAS Registry Number 2152-44-5).

Each gram of the 0.1% ointment contains 1.2 mg Betamethasone Valerate (equivalent to 1.0 mg Betamethasone) in an ointment base of White Petrolatum and Mineral Oil. Betamethasone Valerate Ointment contains no parabens.

betamethasone valerate lotion
Description: Betamethasone Valerate Lotion contains Betamethasone Valerate U.S.P. (Pregna-1, 4-diene-3, 20-dione, 9-fluoro-11, 21-dihydroxy-16-methyl-17-[(1-oxopentyl)oxy]-,(11B, 16B)-); it has an empirical formula of $C_{27}H_{37}FO_6$ and a molecular weight of 476.58 (CAS Registry Number 2152-44-5).

Each gram of the 0.1% lotion contains 1.2 mg Betamethasone Valerate (equivlalent to 1.0 mg Betamethasone) in a vehicle of Isopropyl Alcohol and Water slightly thickened with Carbomer 934P. Phosphoric Acid or Sodium Hydroxide are used to adjust the pH.

Clinical Pharmacology: Topical corticosteroids share anti-inflammatory, anti-pruritic and vasoconstrictive actions. The mechanism of anti-inflammatory activity of the topical corticosteroids is unclear. Various laboratory methods, including vasoconstrictor assays, are used to compare and predict potencies and/or clinical efficacies of the topical corticosteroids. There is some evidence to suggest that a recognizable correlation exists between vasoconstrictor potency and therapeutic efficacy in man.

Pharmacokinetics: The extent of percutaneous absorption of topical corticosteroids is determined by many factors including the vehicle, the integrity of the epidermal barrier, and the use of occlusive dressings. Topical corticosteroids can be absorbed from normal intact skin. Inflammation and/or other disease processes in the skin increase percutaneous absorption. Occlusive dressings substantially increase the percutaneous absorption of topical corticosteroids. Thus, occlusive dressings may be a valuable therapeutic adjunct for treatment of resistant dermatoses (See DOSAGE AND ADMINISTRATION). Once absorbed through the skin, topical corticosteroids are handled through pharmacokinetic pathways similar to systemically administered corticosteroids. Corticosteroids are bound to plasma proteins in varying degrees. Corticosteroids are metabolized primarily in the liver and are then excreted by the kidneys. Some of the topical corticosteroids and their metabolites are also excreted into the bile.

Indications and Usage: Topical corticosteroids are indicated for the relief of the inflammatory and pruritic manifestations of corticosteroid-responsive dermatoses.

Contraindications: Topical corticosteroids are contraindicated in those patients with a history of hypersensitivity to any of the components of the preparation.

Precautions: General: Systemic absorption of topical corticosteroids has produced reversible hypothalmic-pituitary-adrenal (HPA) axis suppression, manifestation of Cushing's syndrome, hyperglycemia, and glucosuria in some patients. Conditions which augment absorption include the application of the more potent steroids, use over large surface areas, prolonged use, and the addition of occlusive dressings. Therefore, patients receiving a large dose of a potent topical steroid applied to a large surface area or under an occlusive dressing should be evaluated periodically for evidence of HPA axis suppression by using the urinary free cortisol and ACTH stimulation tests. If HPA axis suppression is noted, an attempt should be made to withdraw the drug, to reduce the frequency of application, or to substitute a less potent steroid. Recovery of HPA axis function is generally prompt and complete upon discontinuation of the drug. Infrequently, signs and symptoms of steroid withdrawal may occur, requiring supplemental systemic corticosteroids. Children may absorb proportionally larger amounts of topical corticosteroids and thus be more susceptible to systemic toxicity (See PRECAUTIONS-Pediatric use). If irritation develops, topical corticosteroids should be discontinued and appropriate therapy instituted in the presence of dermatological infections, the use of an appropriate anti-fungal or antibacterial agent should be instituted. If a favorable response does not occur promptly, the corticosteroid should be discontinued until the infection has been adequately controlled.

Information for the Patient: Patients using topical corticosteroids should receive the following information and instructions:

1. This medication is to be used as directed by the physician. It is for external use only. Avoid contact with the eyes.
2. Patients should be advised not to use this medication for any disorder other than for which it was prescribed.
3. The treated skin area should not be bandaged or otherwise covered or wrapped as to be occlusive unless directed by the physician.
4. Patients should report any signs of local adverse reactions especially under occlusive dressing.
5. Parents of pediatric patients should be advised not to use tight fitting diapers or plastic pants on a child being treated in the diaper area, as these garments may constitute occlusive dressings.

Laboratory Tests: The following tests may be helpful in evaluating the HPA axis suppression: Urinary free cortisol test; ACTH stimulation test.

Carcinogenesis, Mutagenesis, and Impairment of Fertility: Long-term animal studies have not been performed to evaluate the carcinogenic potential or the effect on fertility of topical corticosteroids. Studies to determine mutagenicity with prednisolone and hydrocortisone have revealed negative results.

Pregnancy Category C: Corticosteroids are generally teratogenic in laboratory animals when administered systemically at relatively low dosage levels. The more potent corticosteroids have been shown to be teratogenic after dermal application in laboratory animals. There are no adequate and well-controlled studies in pregnant women on teratogenic effects from topically applied corticosteroids. Therefore, topical corticosteroids should be used during pregnancy only if the potential benefit justifies the potential risk to the fetus. Drugs of this class should not be used extensively on pregnant patients, in large amounts or for prolonged periods of time.

Nursing Mothers: It is not known whether topical administration of corticosteroids could result in sufficient systemic absorption to produce detectable quantities in breast milk. Systemically administered corticosteroids are secreted into breast milk in quantities not likely to have a deleterious effect on the infant. Nevertheless, caution should be exercised when topical corticosteroids are administered to a nursing woman.

Pediatric Use: Pediatric patients may demonstrate greater susceptibility to topical corticosteroid-induced HPA axis suppression and Cushing's syndrome than mature patients because of larger skin surface area to body weight ratio. Hypothalamic-pituitary-adrenal (HPA) axis suppression, Cushing's syndrome, and intracranial hypertension have been reported in children receiving topical corticosteroids. Manifestations of adrenal suppression in children include linear growth retardation, delayed weight gain, low plasma cortisol levels, and absence of response to ACTH stimulation. Manifestations of intracranial hypertension include bulging fontanelles, headaches, and bilateral papilledema. Administration of topical corticosteroids to children should be limited to the least amount compatible with an effective therapeutic regimen. Chronic corticosteroid therapy may interfere with the growth and development of children.

Adverse Reactions: The following local adverse reactions are reported infrequently with topical corticosteroids, but may occur more frequently with the use of occlusive dressings. These reactions are listed in an approximate decreasing order of occurrence. Burning, Itching, Irritation, Dryness, Folliculitis, Hypertrichosis, Acneiform eruptions, Hypopigmentation, Perioral dermatitis, Allergic contact dermatitis, Maceration of the skin, Secondary infection, Skin Atrophy, Striae and Miliaria.

Overdosage: Topically applied corticosteroids can be absorbed in sufficient amounts to produce systemic effects. (See PRECAUTIONS).

Dosage and Administration: Topical corticosteroid ointments and creams are generally applied to the affected area as a thin film two or three times daily depending on the severity of the condition. Lotion: Apply a few drops of Betamethasone Valerate Lotion to the affected area two or three times daily depending on the severity of the condition and massage lightly until it disappears. Occlusive dressings may be used for the management of psoriasis or recalcitrant conditions. If an infection develops, the use of occlusive dressings should be discontinued and appropriate antimicrobial therapy instituted.

How Supplied: Betamethasone Valerate Cream U.S.P., 0.1% in 15 gram tubes, NDC 0462-0040-15 and 45 gram tubes, NDC 0462-0040-46.
Betamethasone Valerate Ointment U.S.P., 0.1% in 15 gram tubes, NDC 0462-0033-15 and 45 gram tubes, NDC 0462-0033-46.
Betamethasone Valerate Lotion U.S.P., 0.1% in 60 ml bottles, NDC 0462-0041-60.

Caution: Federal law prohibits dispensing without prescription.

Other ℞ items available from Pharmaderm are:

BETAMETHASONE DIPROPIONATE CREAM USP		
NDC 0462-0055-15	0.05%	15 gm tube
NDC 0462-0055-46		45 gm tube
BETAMETHASONE DIPROPIONATE OINTMENT USP		
NDC 0462-0056-15	0.05%	15 gm tube
NDC 0462-0056-60		45 gm tube
HYDROCORTISONE CREAM USP		
NDC 0462-0015-29	1%	20 gm tube
NDC 0462-0015-31		1 oz. tube
NDC 0462-0015-04		4 oz. tube
NDC 0462-0015-16		1 lb. jar
FLUOCINOLONE ACETONIDE CREAM USP		
NDC 0462-0058-15	0.01%	15 gm tube
NDC 0462-0058-60		60 gm tube
NDC 0462-0060-15	0.025%	15 gm tube
NDC 0462-0060-60		60 gm tube

Continued on next page

Pharmaderm—Cont.

FLUOCINOLONE ACETONIDE OINTMENT USP
NDC 0462-0064-15 0.025% 15 gm tube
NDC 0462-0064-60   60 gm tube

FLUOCINOLONE ACETONIDE TOPICAL SOLUTION USP
NDC 0462-0059-60 0.01% 60 ml bottle

ERYTHROMYCIN OPHTHALMIC OINTMENT
(See PDR for Ophthalmology)

NYSTATIN CREAM 100,000 U/g USP
NDC 0462-0054-15 15 gm tube
NDC 0462-0054-30 30 gm tube

NYSTATIN OINTMENT 100,000 U/g USP
NDC 0462-0007-15 15 gm tube

NYSTATIN VAGINAL TABLETS
NDC 0462-0031-15 15 tablets
NDC 0462-0031-30 30 tablets

TRIAMCINOLONE ACETONIDE CREAM USP
NDC 0462-0003-15 0.025% 15 gm tube
NDC 0462-0003-80   80 gm tube
NDC 0462-0003-16   1 lb. jar
NDC 0462-0004-15 0.1%   15 gm tube
NDC 0462-0004-80   80 gm tube
NDC 0462-0004-16   1 lb. jar
NDC 0462-0002-15 0.5%   15 gm tube

TRIAMCINOLONE ACETONIDE OINTMENT USP
NDC 0462-0005-15 0.025% 15 gm tube
NDC 0462-0005-80   80 gm tube
NDC 0462-0006-15 0.1%   15 gm tube
NDC 0462-0006-80   80 gm tube

TRIPLE SULFA VAGINAL CREAM
(With applicator)
NDC 0462-0018-33 2.75 oz. tube

Pharmafair, Inc.
110 KENNEDY DRIVE
HAUPPAUGE, NY 11788

NDC 24208   TOPICALS

-430- **BENZOYL PEROXIDE GEL 5%** OTC
1.5 oz. plastic tube

-435- **BENZOYL PEROXIDE GEL 10%** OTC
1.5 oz. plastic tube

-510- **CORTIFAIR** OTC
(Hydrocortisone Cream ½% USP)
½ ounce tube
1 ounce tube
1 pound jar

-515- **CORTIFAIR** R
(Hydrocortisone Cream 1% USP)
½ ounce tube
1 ounce tube
1 pound jar

-500- **CORTIFAIR** OTC
(Hydrocortisone Lotion ½% USP)
1 ounce
4 ounce

-445- **FLUOCINOLONE ACETONIDE TOPICAL CREAM 0.025%** R
15 gram tube
30 gram tube
45 gram tube
60 gram tube
120 gram jar
425 gram jar

-450- **FLUOCINOLONE ACETONIDE TOPICAL CREAM 0.01%** R
15 gram tube
30 gram tube
45 gram tube
60 gram tube
120 tube jar
425 gram jar

-455- **FLUOCINOLONE ACETONIDE TOPICAL OINTMENT 0.025%** R
15 gram tube
30 gram tube
60 gram tube
120 gram tube
425 gram jar

-465- **FLUOCINOLONE ACETONIDE TOPICAL SOLUTION USP 0.01%** R
20 ml squeeze bottle
60 ml squeeze bottle

-470- **GENTAFAIR DERMATOLOGICAL CREAM** R
(Gentamicin Sulfate Cream USP 0.1%)
15 gram tube

-475- **GENTAFAIR DERMATOLOGICAL OINTMENT** R
(Gentamicin Sulfate Ointment USP 0.1%)
15 gram tube

-525- **IODO-CORTIFAIR**
(Iodochlorhydroxyquin 3% with Hydrocortisone 1% Cream)
20 gram
½ ounce tube
1 ounce tube

-405- **STERILE LUBRICATING JELLY** OTC
4¼ ounce tube

-530- **TOPISPORIN** OTC
(Neomycin and Polymyxin B Sulfates and Bacitracin Zinc Ointment)
½ ounce tube
1 ounce

-650- **TRIAMCINAIR CREAM 0.025%** R
(Triamcinolone Acetonide Cream 0.025% USP)
15 gram tube
30 gram tube
1 pound jar

-655- **TRIAMCINAIR CREAM 0.1%** R
(Triamcinolone Acetonide Cream 0.1% USP)
15 gram tube
20 gram tube
30 gram tube
1 pound jar

-660- **TRIAMCINAIR CREAM 0.5%** R
(Triamcinolone Acetonide Cream 0.5% USP)
15 gram tube
30 gram tube
1 pound jar

OTICS

-895- **ANTIPYRINE and BENZOCAINE OTIC SOLUTION**
15 ml

-615- **BOROFAIR OTIC** R
(Acetic Acid 2% in a modified Burow's Solution Sterile)
2 fluid oz.

-630- **OCTICAIR OTIC SOLUTION** R
(Neomycin Sulfate and Polymyxin B Sulfate and Hydrocortisone Otic Solution-Sterile)
10 ml

-635- **OCTICAIR OTIC SUSPENSION** R
(Neomycin Sulfate and Polymyxin B Sulfate and Hydrocortisone Otic Suspension-Sterile)
10 ml

SYRUP

-890- **TRIPROLIDINE HCl and PSEUDOEPHEDRINE HCl SYRUP** OTC
4 ounce bottles
1 pint bottles

Please see **PDR FOR OPHTHALMOLOGY** for a complete list of our ophthalmic products

Philips Roxane Laboratories

(See ROXANE LABORATORIES)

Poythress Laboratories, Inc.
16 N. 22nd ST.
POST OFFICE BOX 26946
RICHMOND, VA 23261

ANTROCOL® R
[an-trō'cal]
TABLETS, CAPSULES AND ELIXIR

Composition: Each tablet or capsule contains atropine sulfate, 0.195 mg.; phenobarbital, 16 mg. (Warning: may be habit-forming). Each lcc of elixir contains atropine sulfate 0.039 mg.; phenobarbital 3 mg., (Warning: May be habit-forming) and 20% alcohol (V/V). Citrus flavored-artificially colored.

How Supplied: Uncoated tablets, green #4 capsules branded WMP and green liquid.
Bottles of 100 tablets .... NDC 0095-0040-01
Bottles of 500 tablets .... NDC 0095-0040-05
Bottles of 100 capsules .... NDC 0095-0041-01
Bottles of 1 fl. oz (30cc) Elixir NDC 0095-0042-01
Containing individually wrapped droppers Calibrated from 0.5 to lcc for Pediatric use.
Bottles of 16 fl. oz. (475cc)
Elixir .... NDC 0095-0042-16

BENSULFOID® LOTION OTC
[ben'sul-foid]

Composition: A greaseless, cosmetic lotion containing Bensulfoid, 6% (33% colloidal sulfur) Zinc Oxide, 6%; thymol, 0.5% as active ingredients. Also contains alcohol (V/V) 12%; methyl salicylate, 5%; perfume; cosmetic colors; preservatives, 0.1%.

How Supplied:
2 oz. bottles .... NDC 0095-0130-02

LODRANE™ R
[lo'drāne]
(theophylline anhydrous)
SUSTAINED RELEASE CAPSULES

Composition: Lodrane 130 and Lodrane 260: Each capsule contains 130 mg. or 260 mg. of theophylline anhydrous in a sustained release bead formulation.

How Supplied:
130 mg. green and white capsules
Bottles of 100 .... NDC 0095-0060-01
260 mg. red and white capsules
Bottles of 100 .... NDC 0095-0065-01
Mfg. for Poythress Laboratories, Inc.

MUDRANE® TABLETS R
[mu'drāne]

Composition: Each tablet contains potassium iodide, 195 mg.; aminophylline (anhydrous), 130 mg.; phenobarbital, 8 mg. (Warning: may be habit-forming); ephedrine HCl, 16 mg.

Indications: A bronchodilator-mucolytic, Mudrane gives prompt symptomatic relief in bronchial asthma, emphysema and asthmatic bronchitis. Mudrane dilates the bronchi, liquefies the mucus plugs. The stability of Mudrane has been achieved without coating the potassium iodide; thus all the components in the fast-disintegrating tablet begin their actions promptly. Mudrane is buffered for gastric tolerance.

Contraindications: *Aminophylline/theophylline* is contraindicated in the presence of severe cardiac arrhythmias in patients with massive myocardial damage. *Ephedrine* is contraindicated in the presence of severe heart disease, severe hypertension and in hyperthyroidism. *Phenobarbital* is contraindicated in porphyria and in patients with known phenobarbital sensitivity. *Potassium iodide* is contraindicated in pregnancy (to protect the fetus

against possible iodide-induced depression of thyroid activity), in tuberculosis (produces gumma dissolution), and in acne; also, in the presence of known iodide sensitivity.
Precautions: *Aminophylline/theophylline* should be avoided in patients with massive myocardial damage and/or severe cardiac arrhythmias, and severe agitation. *Ephedrine* should be used with caution in the presence of severe cardiac disease, particularly arrhythmias and angina pectoris, it should be avoided in hyperthyroidism and severe hypertension. *Phenobarbital* may be habit-forming. Avoid overdosage. *Potassium iodide:* Discontinue in the presence of skin rash, swelling of the eyelids, or severe frontal headache. Long use may cause goiter.
Adverse Reactions: *Aminophylline/theophylline* may cause cardiac arrhythmias and aggravate severe myocardial disease; may cause headaches and tachycardia; vomiting and dizziness are not uncommon. *Ephedrine* may cause nervousness, tachycardia, extrasystole and ventricular arrhythmias in patients hypersensitive to CNS stimulation. Also, ephedrine may cause urinary retention, especially in the presence of partial prostatic obstruction. Psychoneurosis may be aggravated. Pre-existing anginal pain will be aggravated. *Phenobarbital* may produce severe skin rash; avoid overdosage; may be habit-forming. *Potassium iodide* may cause nausea; over very long period of use, iodides may cause goiter. Discontinue if patient developes skin rash, eye irritation, eyelid swelling or severe frontal headache.
Dosage: One tablet with full glass of water, 3 or 4 times daily, as required. Divide tablet for child's dose.
How Supplied: Yellow scored tablet with I.D. #9550.
Bottles of 100 ....NDC 0095-0050-01
Bottles of 1000 ....NDC 0095-0050-10

MUDRANE®-2 TABLETS
[mu'drāne]
Composition: Each tablet contains potassium iodide 195 mg. aminophylline (anhydrous) 130 mg.
How Supplied: White scored tablets with I.D. #9532.
Bottles of 100 ....NDC 0095-0032-01

MUDRANE® GG TABLETS
[mu'drāne]
Compositions: Each tablet contains aminophylline (anhydrous), 130 mg.; ephedrine HCl, 16mg.; phenobarbital, 8 mg. (Warning: may be habit-forming); Guaifenesin, 100 mg.
Indications: Same as Mudrane, EXCEPT Guaifenesin, 100 mg. replaces potassium iodide as a mucolytic-expectorant. Mudrane GG should be prescribed when acne or tuberculosis co-exist, during pregnancy, or when iodide intolerance is present. In emphysema, requiring constant Mudrane therapy, Mudrane GG may be substituted every fourth week to reduce the prossibility of iodide sensitivity.
Contraindications: Precautions: Adverse Reactions: See under Mudrane tablets above as listed for aminophylline/theophylline, ephedrine HCl, and phenobarbital.
Dosage: One tablet with full glass of water, 3 or 4 times daily.
How Supplied: Yellow, mottled, GG embossed tablets with I.D. #9551.
Bottles of 100 ....NDC 0095-0051-01
Bottles of 1000 ....NDC 0095-0051-10

MUDRANE® GG-2 TABLETS
[mu'drāne]
Composition: Each tablet contains aminophylline (anhydrous), 130 mg.; Guaifenesin, 100 mg.
How Supplied: Green, mottled, GG embossed tablets with I.D. #9533.
Bottles of 100 ....NDC 0095-0033-01

MUDRANE® GG ELIXIR
[mu'drāne]
Composition: Each 5 ml teaspoonful contains theophylline, 20 mg.; ephedrine HCl, 4 mg.; phenobarbital 2.5 mg. (Warning: may be habit-forming); Guaifenesin, 26 mg. The theophylline in the Elixir is in solution. (The theophylline in the tablet is supplied by aminophylline for prompt solubility from the rapid-disintegrating, uncoated tablet. Preserved with 0.1% paraben. Contains 20% alcohol.
Indications: Mudrane GG Elixir is a sugar-free bronchodilator-mucolytic especially formulated for pediatric use. Mudrane GG Elixir supplies the active ingredients of Mudrane GG tablets for the relief of asthma and asthmatic bronchitis.
Contraindications: Precautions: Adverse Reactions: See under Mudrane tablets above, as listed for aminophylline/theophylline, ephedrine HCl, and phenobarbital.
Dosage: Children, 1 ml for each 10 lbs. of body weight; one teaspoonful for 50 lb. child. May be repeated 3 or 4 times daily. Adult, one tablespoonful, 3 or 4 times daily. All doses should be followed with water.
How Supplied: As a red liquid.
Bottles of 16 fl. ozs. (475 cc).....NDC 0095-0053-16
Bottles of 64 fl. ozs. (1900 cc)...NDC 0095-0053-64

PANALGESIC®
[pan'al-gesic]
Liniment and Creme
Composition: (Liniment) Methyl Salicylate, 55%; Camphor 3.1%; Menthol, 1.25%; mineral oil & color, 18.6%; alcohol, 22% by weight, (Cream) methyl salicylate, 35%; menthol, 4%.
How Supplied:
Green, non-staining, greaseless liniment.
4 fl. oz. bottles..........................NDC 0095-0120-04
16 fl. oz. bottles........................NDC 0095-0120-16
64 fl. oz. bottles........................NDC 0095-0120-14
White, non-staining, greaseless cream
4 oz. jars..................................NDC 0095-0021-04

SOLFOTON®
[sulfa-tōne]
TABLETS AND CAPSULES
Composition: Each tablet or capsule contains phenobarbital, 16 mg. (Warning: may be habit-forming).
How Supplied: Uncoated P embossed tablets with I.D. #9523. Brown and yellow #4.
Capsules branded WmP and I.D. #9525
Bottles of 100 Tablets................NDC 0095-0023-01
Bottles of 500 Tablets................NDC 0095-0023-05
Bottles of 100 Capsules ....NDC 0095-0025-01
Bottles of 500 Capsules ....NDC 0095-0025-05

URO-PHOSPHATE TABLETS
[urō'fos-fāt]
(Methenamine, Sodium biphosphate)
Description: Uro-Phosphate, a urinary antibacterial agent, is a combination of Methenamine (urinary antiseptic) 300 mg. and sodium biphosphate (urinary acidifier) (sodium phospate, monobasic) 500 mg.
Actions: Methenamine is readily absorbed from the gastrointestinal tract but remains essentially inactive until concentrated and excreted by the kidney in an acid urine where hydrolysation produces antibacterial formaldehyde. An acid urine is essential for the conversion of methenamine to antibacterial formaldehyde with the maximum efficacy occurring at pH 5.5 or less. Methenamine alone may be ineffective in some infections with Proteus vulgaris and urea-splitting strains of Pseudomonas aeruginosa and A. aerogenes as they may raise the pH of the urine inhibiting formaldehyde formation. Sodium biphosphate, a natural urine acidifier, generally provides urine pH at an acid level conducive to formaldehyde production. Results in any individual case will depend on dosage, underlying pathology and overall management.
Indications: Uro-Phosphate (methenamine and sodium biphosphate) is indicated for suppressive or prophylactic treatment of chronic bacteriuria associated with pyelonephritis, cystitis, significant residual urine accompanying some neurological diseases and with prolonged bladder catheterization. The safety and nonspecific bacteriacidal effect of formaldehyde does not lead to bacterial resistance to Uro-Phosphate.
Contraindications: Renal insufficiency, severe dehydration or acidosis. Methenamine preparations should not be given patients taking sulfonamides since formaldehyde may form an insoluble precipitate with some sulfonamides in urine.
Warning: Safe use in pregnancy is not established.
Precautions: Large doses of methenamine (8 grams daily for 3 to 4 weeks) have caused bladder irritation, painful and frequent micturition, albuminures and gross hematuria. Care should be taken to maintain an acid pH of the urine especially when treating infections due to urea-splitting pathogens such as Proteus and strains of Pseudomonas.
Adverse Reactions: Minor adverse reactions have been reported in fewer than 3.5% of patients treated. These reactions have included nausea, upset stomach, dysuria and rash.
Dosage and Administration: 1 or 2 tablets at 4 to 6 hour intervals is usually sufficient to maintain proper urine acidity. Two tablets on retiring will maintain comfort and lessen frequency when residual urine is present.
How Supplied: White sugar-coated tablets branded WmP and I.D. #9531.
Bottles of 100 ....NDC 0095-0031-01
Bottles of 1000 ....NDC 0095-0031-10
Protect from heat, store at room temperature 60°–75°F.
Manufactured for Poythress Laboratories Inc., Richmond, Virginia 23261

Procter & Gamble
P. O. BOX 171
CINCINNATI, OH 45201

CHILDREN'S CHLORASEPTIC® LOZENGES
Description: Each Children's Chloraseptic Lozenge contains 5 mg. benzocaine as anesthetic in a grape flavored base of sugar and corn syrup solids.
Indications: Children's Chloraseptic Lozenges provide prompt, temporary relief of minor sore throat pain which may accompany conditions such as tonsillitis, pharyngitis and in posttonsillectomy soreness, and discomfort of minor mouth and gum irritations.
Dosage and Administration: Allow one lozenge to dissolve slowly in the mouth. Repeat hourly if needed. Do not take more than 12 lozenges per day.
In addition, consumer labeling carries the following statement:
Warning: Consult physician promptly if sore throat is severe or lasts more than 2 days or is accompanied by high fever, headache, nausea, or vomiting. Not for children under 3 years unless directed by physician or dentist.
Active Ingredient: benzocaine (5 mg per lozenge).
STORE BELOW 86°F (30°C). PROTECT FROM MOISTURE.
KEEP ALL MEDICINES OUT OF REACH OF CHILDREN.
Packaging: Carton of 18 lozenges.

CHLORASEPTIC® LIQUID
(oral anesthetic, antiseptic)
Description: An alkaline solution containing phenol and sodium phenolate (total phenol 1.4%). In addition, Menthol Chloraseptic and Cherry

Continued on next page

Procter & Gamble—Cont.

Chloraseptic 1.5-oz. Aerosol Spray contain compressed nitrogen as a propellant.

Indications: Pleasant-tasting Chloraseptic is an anesthetic, antiseptic, deodorizing mouthwash and gargle. It is an alkaline solution designed specifically to maintain oral hygiene and to relieve local soreness and irritation without "caines." Chloraseptic may be used as a topical anesthetic while antibacterials are used systemically in the treatment of infection.

Chloraseptic acts promptly, often providing effective surface anesthesia in minutes. It is a valuable adjunct for temporary relief of pain and discomfort. Also, Chloraseptic will temporarily reduce oral bacterial flora.

Chloraseptic is indicated for prompt temporary relief of discomfort due to the following conditions: *Medical*—oropharyngitis and throat infections; acute tonsillitis; and posttonsillectomy soreness; *Dental*—minor irritation or injury of soft tissue of the mouth; minor oral surgery or extractions; irritation caused by dentures or orthodontic appliances; and aphthous ulcers.

Administration and Dosage: Chloraseptic Spray (Pump), Mouthwash and Gargle—*Irritated throat:* Spray 5 times (children 3–12 years of age, 3 times) and swallow. May be used as a gargle. Repeat every 2 hours if necessary. *After oral surgery:* Allow full-strength solution to run over affected areas for 15 seconds without swishing, then expel remainder. Repeat every 2 hours if necessary. *Adjunctive gingival therapy:* Rinse vigorously with full-strength solution for 15 seconds, working between teeth, then expel remainder. Repeat every 2 hours if necessary. *Daily deodorizing mouthwash and gargle:* Dilute with equal parts of water and rinse thoroughly, or spray full strength, then expel remainder.

Chloraseptic Aerosol Spray: *Irritated throat:* Spray throat about 2 seconds (children 3-12 years about 1 second) and swallow. Repeat every 2 hours if necessary. *After oral surgery:* Spray affected area for 1 to 2 seconds, allow solution to remain for 15 seconds without swishing, then expel remainder. Repeat every 2 hours if necessary. *Adjunctive gingival therapy:* Spray affected area for about 2 seconds, swish for 15 seconds working between teeth, then expel remainder. Repeat every 2 hours if necessary. *Daily deodorizing spray:* Spray, rinse thoroughly, and expel remainder.

Consumer labeling contains the following caution statement:

Caution: Severe or persistent sore throat or sore throat accompanied by high fever, headache, nausea or vomiting may be serious. Consult your physician. If sore throat persists more than 2 days consult physician. Do not administer to children under 3 years unless directed by physician or dentist.

Warning: For 1.5 oz. Aerosol Spray—Avoid spraying in eyes. Contents under pressure. Do not puncture or incinerate. (Do not burn or throw in fire, as can will burst). Do not store at temperature above 120°F. (Such high temperatures may cause bursting.) **KEEP ALL MEDICINES OUT OF REACH OF CHILDREN.**

To insure product quality, avoid excessive heat (over 104°F or 40°C). See bottom of can for expiration date and control number.

How Supplied: Available in menthol or cherry flavor—6 oz. size with sprayer, 12 oz. refill bottle, and 1.5 oz. nitrogen propelled aerosol spray.

CHLORASEPTIC® LOZENGES

Description: Each Chloraseptic Lozenge contains phenol, sodium phenolate (total phenol 32.5 mg).

Indications: Chloraseptic Lozenges provide temporary relief of discomfort due to minor sore throat and mouth and gum irritations. They also may be used for topical anesthesia as an adjunct to systemic antibacterial therapy. For prompt temporary relief of pain and discomfort associated with the following conditions: *Medical*—oropharyngitis and throat infections; acute tonsillitis; and posttonsillectomy soreness; *Dental*—minor irritation or injury of soft tissue of the mouth; minor oral surgery; and aphthous ulcers.

Administration and Dosage: Adults and children over 3 years of age: Dissolve 1 lozenge in the mouth every 2 hours. Children under 12 years, do not exceed 8 lozenges per day.

Consumer labeling contains the following caution statement:

Caution: Consult physician if sore throat is severe or lasts more than 2 days or is accompanied by high fever, headache, nausea or vomiting. Not for children under 3 unless directed by physician or dentist.

KEEP ALL MEDICINES OUT OF REACH OF CHILDREN.

Avoid excessive heat (over 104°F or 40°C).

How Supplied: Available in choice of menthol or cherry flavor—packages of 18 and 36 lozenges.

ENCAPRIN®
Arthritis Pain Reliever

Composition: Regular Strength Encaprin capsules contain 325 mg (5 grains) of aspirin. Maximum Strength Encaprin capsules contain 500 mg (7.7 grains) of aspirin.

Description: Each capsule contains hundreds of individually enteric-coated micrograins of aspirin. These enteric-coated micrograins are designed to pass through the stomach to the small intestine before dissolving. The small size of the micrograins enables them to pass readily through the pylorus. Encaprin enteric-coated micrograins are associated with significantly less gastric damage than plain or even buffered aspirin.

Indications: Encaprin is an excellent analgesic, antipyretic and anti-inflammatory agent, particularly where there is a need to protect the stomach from aspirin-induced damage during chronic aspirin regimens. Encaprin provides temporary relief from mild arthritis symptoms, headache, painful discomfort of colds and flu, fever, sore throat, muscular aches and pains, dental pain, and menstrual pain.

Usual Adult Dosage: The following dosages are the maximum daily doses recommended for self-medication.

Regular Strength: Two or three capsules with water every 4 hours. Do not exceed 12 capsules in 24 hours unless directed by a physician. Children under 12— as recommended by a physician.

Maximum Strength: Two capsules with water every 4 hours. Do not exceed 8 capsules in 24 hours unless directed by a physician. Children under 12— as recommended by a physician.

B.I.D. Dosage: Bioavailability and endoscopy studies conducted at 4 grams/day indicate Encaprin can be safely prescribed on a b.i.d. dosage regimen by the physician. Patients should be titrated gradually to a b.i.d. regimen to avoid exceeding the individual's maximum aspirin tolerance level.

Precautions: This aspirin product should not be used by persons allergic to aspirin or under medical care without consulting a physician. If pain persists more than 10 days or redness is present, or in arthritic or rheumatic conditions affecting children under 12, consult a physician immediately. Discontinue use if dizziness, ringing in ears, or impaired hearing occurs. KEEP THIS AND ALL MEDICINES OUT OF REACH OF CHILDREN. IN CASE OF ACCIDENTAL OVERDOSE, CONTACT A PHYSICIAN OR POISON CONTROL CENTER IMMEDIATELY. As with any drug, if you are pregnant or nursing a baby, seek the advice of a health professional before using this product.

How Supplied:
Regular Strength Encaprin 325 mg (5 grains):
NDC 37000-027-03 Bottle of 75 capsules
NDC 37000-027-04 Bottle of 150 capsules
Maximum Strength Encaprin 500 mg (7.7 grains):
NDC 37000-028-03 Bottle of 50 capsules
NDC 37000-028-04 Bottle of 100 capsules
NDC 37000-028-05 Bottle of 200 capsules
Easy opening cap available on Regular Strength 150's and Maximum Strength 200's for households without young children.

For further product information, contact Encaprin Professional Services Division, (513) 530-2153.

Shown in Product Identification Section, page 427

HEAD & CHEST™
DECONGESTANT/EXPECTORANT COLD MEDICINE

Active Ingredients:
Each TABLET and CAPSULE contains:
Phenylpropanolamine HCl .... 25 mg
Guaifenesin .... 200 mg
Each 5 ml (one teaspoonful) LIQUID contains:
Phenylpropanolamine HCl .... 12.5 mg
Guaifenesin .... 100 mg
Alcohol 5%

Indications: HEAD & CHEST is indicated in colds, sinusitis, bronchitis, and other respiratory conditions to reduce nasal congestion and promote drainage of bronchial passageways.

Actions: Phenylpropanolamine HCl is an effective vasoconstrictor that decongests swollen mucous membranes of the respiratory tract. The expectorant guaifenesin enhances the flow of respiratory tract fluid, promotes ciliary action and facilitates removal of viscous, inspissated mucus. As a result, sinus and bronchial drainage is improved, and dry, nonproductive coughs become more productive and less frequent.

Warnings: This product should not be taken by persons who are hypersensitive to any of its ingredients or those who have high blood pressure, heart disease, diabetes, thyroid disease or persistent or chronic cough such as occurs with smoking, asthma, or emphysema, or where cough is accompanied by excessive secretions, or by children under 2 years except under the advice and supervision of a physician. If symptoms do not improve within 7 days or are accompanied by fever, rash, or persistent headache, consult a physician before continuing use. Do not exceed recommended dosage because at higher doses nervousness, dizziness or sleeplessness are more likely to occur. Keep all medicines out of reach of children. In case of accidental overdose, seek professional assistance or contact a poison control center immediately. As with any drug, if you are pregnant or nursing a baby, seek the advice of a health professional before using the product.

Drug Interaction Precaution: Do not take this product if you are presently taking a prescription antihypertensive or antidepressant drug containing a monoamine oxidase inhibitor except under the advice and supervision of a physician.

Overdosage: Treatment of overdosage should be directed toward supporting the patient and reversing the effects of the drug.

Dosage:
Adults and children over 12 years—2 teaspoonfuls LIQUID or 1 TABLET or 1 CAPSULE
Children 6–12 years—1 teaspoonful LIQUID or ½ tablet
Children 2–6 years—½ teaspoonful LIQUID
Repeat above dosage every 4 hours as needed to maximum of 6 doses in 24 hours.

How Supplied: LIQUID, TABLETS, AND CAPSULES

HEAD & SHOULDERS®
Antidandruff Shampoo

(See PDR For Nonprescription Drugs)

PEPTO-BISMOL®
LIQUID AND TABLETS
For upset stomach, indigestion and nausea.
Controls common diarrhea.

Active Ingredient: Bismuth subsalicylate, 300 mg per tablet or 262 mg per 15 ml (tablespoonful). Contains no sugar.

Indications: Heartburn and indigestion—Pepto-Bismol soothes irritation with a protective coat-

for possible revisions

ing action, without constipating. Nausea and upset stomach—Pepto-Bismol brings fast sure relief from distress of queasiness and that bloated feeling. Diarrhea—controls diarrhea within 24 hours, relieving associated abdominal cramps. Keep all medicines out of reach of children.

Caution: This product contains salicylates. If taken with aspirin and ringing of the ears occurs, discontinue use. If taking medicines for anticoagulation (thinning the blood), diabetes, or gout, consult physician before taking this product. If diarrhea is accompanied by high fever or continues more than 2 days, consult a physician.

Warning: As with any drug, if you are pregnant or nursing a baby, seek the advice of a health professional before using this product. Avoid excessive heat (over 140°F or 40°C).

Dosage Directions
Liquid—Shake well before using
Adults: 2 tablespoonfuls
Children (according to age):
  9–12 years—1 tablespoonful
  6–9 years—2 teaspoonsful
  3–6 years—1 teaspoonful
  For children under 3 years, consult a physician. Repeat above dosage every ½ to 1 hour, if needed to a maximum of 8 doses in 24-hour period.
Note: The beneficial medication may cause a temporary darkening of the stool. This condition is harmless and temporary.

Tablets
Adults: 2 tablets
Children (according to age):
  9–12 years—1 tablet
  6–9 years—⅔ tablet
  3–6 years—⅓ tablet
  For children under 3 years, consult a physician. Chew or dissolve in mouth. Repeat every ½ to 1 hour as needed, to a maximum of 8 doses in 24-hour period. Each tablet dose is a full liquid dose in concentrated form.

How Supplied: Pepto-Bismol is available in Liquid and Tablets.

Professional Health Products, Inc.
3496 BREAKWATER COURT
HAYWARD, CA 94545

ADDED PROTECTION III™
Multi-Vitamin and Multi-Mineral Supplement

Description: Added Protection III™ is a high-potency multi-vitamin multi-mineral supplement. This carefully balanced, professional formula provides a daily supply of 30 vitamins and minerals, selected from only the best, natural sources.

Composition:

SIX TABLETS PROVIDE:		% U.S. RDA*
VITAMINS		
Vitamin A (Palmitate) (Water Dispersible)	10,000 I.U.	300
Beta-Carotene (Water Dispersible)	5,000 I.U.	
Vitamin D₃ (Fish Liver Oil)	200 I.U.	50
Vitamin E (d-alpha Tocopheryl Succinate)	400 I.U.	1333
Vitamin C (Ascorbic Acid, corn-free)	1,200 mg	2000
Vitamin B₁ (Thiamine Mononitrate)	100 mg	6666
Vitamin B₂ (Riboflavin)	50 mg	2940
Niacin	40 mg	200
Niacinamide	150 mg	750
Pantothenic Acid (d-Calcium Pantothenate)	500 mg	5000
Vitamin B₆ (Pyridoxine HCl)	100 mg	5000
Vitamin B₁₂ (On Ion Exchange Resin)	100 mcg	1666
Folic Acid	800 mcg	100†
Biotin	300 mcg	100
Choline Bitartrate	150 mg	**
Inositol	100 mg	***
Citrus Bioflavonoid Complex	100 mg	***
PABA (Para-Amino-Benzoic Acid)	50 mg	***
MINERALS		
Calcium (Oyster Shell, Micronized)	500 mg	50
Magnesium (Ascorbate Complex)	166 mg	41
Magnesium (Aspartate Complex)	183 mg	46
Magnesium (Oxide)	151 mg	38
Potassium (Aspartate Complex)	99 mg	**
Iron (Fumarate)****	20 mg	110
Zinc (Aspartate Complex)	30 mg	200
Copper**** (Aspartate Complex)	2 mg	100
Manganese (Aspartate Complex)	20 mg	**
Iodine (Kelp)	200 mcg	133
Chromium (Chromium Amino Acid Complex, Glucose Tolerance Component)	200 mcg	**
Selenium (Organic Selenium in Amino Acid Complex and Kelp)	200 mcg	**
Molybdenum (Amino Acid Complex)	100 mcg	**
Trace Elements (From Sea Vegetation and Oyster Shell) (approx.)	100 mg	***
FREE AMINO ACIDS		
L-Cysteine HCl	250 mg	
DL-Methionine	62.5 mg	

*Percentage of U.S. Recommended Daily Allowance.
**Need in human nutrition established, but U.S. RDA not yet determined.
***Need in human nutrition not determined.
****Added Protection III™ also comes in a **without copper** formula, and a **without iron and copper** formula.
†U.S. RDA for pregnant and lactating women.

Added Protection III™ formulas contain no yeast, corn, wheat, soya, sugar or sweeteners, chlorine, phenol, dairy products, coal tar, added salicylates, or artificial color, preservatives, or flavoring.

Actions and Uses: A convenient source of vitamins, minerals, and amino acids.

Administration and Dosage: Adults: 2 tablets 3 times daily.

Children: as directed by physician.
Side Effects: None reported.
How Supplied: Bottles of 180 tablets.
Literature Available: Samples and product sheet available to physicians.
Storage: In a cool, dry place, away from direct light.

CARDIOGUARD™
[kar″de-o-gahrd]
Natural Lipotropic Dietary Supplement

Description: Cardioguard™ Natural Lipotropic Dietary Supplement is a professional formula, designed to enhance lipid metabolism.

Composition:
Each tablet provides:
Lecithin granules .... 400 mg.
Polysaccharides .... 390 mg.
Elastomucoprotease .... 50 mg.
Lethicon (Choline)™* .... 50 mg.
Silicon dioxide .... 50 mg.
Papain .... 50 mg.
Niacin** .... 10 mg.

*Lethicon is a trademark of A. Natterman.
**Provides 50% of the U.S. Recommended Daily Allowance for adults and for children 4 or more years of age.

Actions and Uses: As a dietary supplement for patients with lipid metabolism dysfunctions.
Administration and Dosage: 2 to 4 tablets daily, or as recommended by physician.
Side Effects: None reported.
How Supplied: Bottles of 100 tablets.
Literature Available: Samples and product sheet available to physicians.

CARDIOGUARD™
[kar″de-o-gahrd]
Natural Lipotropic Dietary Supplement Powder

Description: Cardioguard™ Natural Lipotropic Dietary Supplement Powder is a professional formula, designed to enhance lipid metabolism.

Composition:
Each slightly heaping teaspoon (6 gms) provides:
Lecithin granules .... 2400 mg.
Polysaccharides .... 2340 mg.
Elastomucoprotease .... 300 mg.
Lethicon™* (Choline) .... 300 mg.
Silicon dioxide .... 300 mg.
Papain .... 300 mg.
Niacin** .... 60 mg.

*Lethicon™ is a trademark of A. Natterman.
**Provides 300% of the U.S. Recommended Daily Allowance for adults and for children 4 or more years of age.

Actions and Uses: As a dietary supplement for patients with lipid metabolism dysfunctions.
Administration and Dosage: 2 to 4 grams daily, or as recommended by physician.
Side Effects: None reported.
How Supplied: Bottles of 600 grams.
Literature Available: Samples and product sheet available to physicians.

The Purdue Frederick Company
100 CONNECTICUT AVENUE
NORWALK, CT 06856

BETADINE® AEROSOL SPRAY
[bā' tăh-dīn"]
(povidone-iodine)
Topical Antiseptic Germicide

Uses: Nitrogen pressurized spray is easy to apply over large areas; eliminates the use of a contact applicator on the tender site. Also used for pre- and postoperative prepping of operative site, treatment of burns, including third-degree burns, decubitus and stasis ulcers, as a spray on the skin to be covered with a cast, and as a general topical microbicide.
BETADINE Aerosol Spray is film-forming and may be applied with or without bandages.
Administration: Spray the affected area thoroughly as needed. The improved actuator permits spraying from any angle.
How Supplied: Aerosol, nitrogen propelled, 3 fl. oz. bottle.

BETADINE® Antiseptic Gel
[bā' tăh-dīn"]
(povidone-iodine, 10%)

Action and Uses: Applied at bedtime, BETADINE Antiseptic Gel works through the night to provide prompt, soothing symptomatic relief of minor vaginal irritation, itching and soreness. Its active ingredient — the broad-spectrum microbicide povidone-iodine — significantly and rapidly reduces the aerobic and anaerobic count, offering comfort on contact from annoying vaginal symptoms and odor. May also be used for preoperative degerming.
Advantages: Its gel formulation offers the advantage of prolonged contact with irritated vaginal tissue to help provide long-lasting relief. BETADINE Antiseptic Gel is gentle and virtually nonirritating to delicate vaginal tissue. It is nongreasy and nonsticky.
Directions for Use: Insert one applicatorful of BETADINE Antiseptic Gel. Leave medication in the vagina overnight. A sanitary napkin should be worn overnight. When external irritation is present, BETADINE Antiseptic Gel may be applied manually to the affected area. Treatment should be continued for seven days.
How Supplied: 18 g tubes and 3 oz. tubes, each packaged with a convenient, easy-to-use vaginal applicator.

BETADINE® DOUCHE
[bā' tăh-dīn"]
(povidone-iodine)

A pleasantly scented solution, BETADINE Douche is clinically effective in the treatment of vaginitis. Also for the prompt symptomatic relief of minor vaginal irritation and itching, and as a cleansing douche.
Advantages: Low surface tension, with uniform wetting action to assist penetration into vaginal crypts and crevices. Active in the presence of blood, pus, or vaginal secretions. Virtually nonirritating to vaginal mucosa. Will not stain skin or natural fabrics.
Directions for Use: As a Therapeutic Douche: Two (2) tablespoonfuls to a quart of lukewarm water once daily. As a Routine Cleansing Douche: One (1) tablespoonful to a quart of lukewarm water once or twice per week. As a douche for prompt symptomatic relief of minor vaginal irritation and itching: One (1) tablespoonful to a quart of lukewarm water once daily for five days. Treatment should continue for the full five days, even if symptoms are relieved earlier.
How Supplied: 1 oz. and 8 oz. plastic bottles. Disposable ½ oz. (1 tablespoonful) packettes.
Also Available: BETADINE Douche Kit and Disposable BETADINE Medicated Douche.

BETADINE® HĒLAFOAM® SOLUTION
[bā' tăh-dīn" hē' lăh-fōm"]
(povidone-iodine)
Topical Antiseptic Microbicide

Description: A unique, broad-spectrum microbicidal foam which helps prevent infection in burns and wounds. The light, protective foam may be applied directly from canister to burn site. BETADINE Hēlafoam Solution adheres to the site of the burn wound with virtually no run-off.
Action and Uses: For use as a microbicide of choice for disinfection of wounds and for antiseptic treatment of lacerations, abrasions, and first-, second- and third-degree burns. For use as a prophylactic anti-infective agent in hospital and office procedures, including postoperative application to incisions to protect against possible infection.
By helping to control bacterial proliferation, BETADINE Hēlafoam Solution aids in prevention of partial-thickness burns progressing to full-thickness burns. A lower incidence of burn wound sepsis may help reduce the need for grafting or permit earlier grafting and shorten hospital stay.
Dosage and Administration: Shake well. Hold can upright and firmly press release button on top of can. Apply directly to treatment site, spreading gently with sterile-gloved hand or with sterile tongue-depressor. Alternative methods of application are to dispense directly onto sterile-gloved hand and apply gently over the treatment site; or onto sterile gauze and cover the wound thoroughly with the impregnated gauze. Apply BETADINE Hēlafoam Solution liberally, as needed. May be bandaged or covered with gauze.
Warning: Contents under pressure. Do not puncture or incinerate. Do not expose to temperatures above 120° Fahrenheit. Store at controlled room temperature (59°–86°F).
Supplied: Aerosol, 9 oz. (250 gm.) canister.

BETADINE® OINTMENT
[bā' tăh-dīn"]
(povidone-iodine)

Action: BETADINE Ointment, in a water-soluble base, is a topical agent active against organisms commonly encountered in skin and wound infections. BETADINE Ointment kills gram-positive and gram-negative bacteria (including antibiotic-resistant strains), fungi, viruses, protozoa and yeasts.
The broad-spectrum activity of BETADINE Ointment provides microbicidal action against most commonly occurring skin bacteria. Its range of antibacterial activity encompasses many bacteria — including antibiotic-resistant forms.
The active ingredient in BETADINE Ointment substantially retains the broad-spectrum germicidal activity of iodine without the undesirable features or disadvantages of iodine. BETADINE Ointment is virtually nonirritating, does not block air from reaching the site of application, and washes easily off skin and natural fabrics. The site to which BETADINE Ointment is applied can be bandaged.
Indications: Therapeutically, BETADINE Ointment may be used as an adjunct to systemic therapy where indicated; for primary or secondary topical infections caused by iodine-susceptible organisms such as, infected burns, infected surgical incisions, infected decubitus or stasis ulcers, pyodermas, secondarily infected dermatoses, and infected traumatic lesions.
Prophylactically: BETADINE Ointment may be used to prevent microbial contamination in burns, incisions and other topical lesions; for degerming skin in hyperalimentation, catheter care, the umbilical area or circumcision. The use of BETADINE Ointment for abrasions, minor cuts, and wounds, may prevent the development of infections and permit wound healing.
Administration: Apply directly to affected area as needed. May be bandaged.
Supplied: $\frac{1}{32}$ oz. and $\frac{1}{8}$ oz. packettes; 1 oz. tubes; 16 oz. (1 lb.) and 5 lbs.

BETADINE® SKIN CLEANSER
[bā' tăh-dīn"]
(povidone-iodine)

BETADINE Skin Cleanser is a sudsing antiseptic liquid cleanser. It essentially retains the broad microbicidal spectrum of iodine, yet virtually without the undesirable features associated with iodine. BETADINE Skin Cleanser kills gram-positive and gram-negative bacteria (including antibiotic-resistant strains), fungi, viruses, protozoa and yeasts. It forms rich golden lather; virtually nonirritating; nonstaining to skin and natural fabrics.
Indications: BETADINE Skin Cleanser aids in degerming the skin of patients with common pathogens, including *Staphylococcus aureus*. To help prevent the recurrence of acute inflammatory skin infections caused by iodine-susceptible pyogenic bacteria. In pyodermas, as a topical adjunct to systemic antimicrobial therapy. To help prevent spread of infection in acne pimples. Also kills three organisms often associated with acne vulgaris: *Staph. epidermidis*, *Corynebacterium acnes* and Pityrosporon.
Directions for Use: Wet the skin and apply a sufficient amount of Skin Cleanser to work up a rich golden lather. Allow lather to remain about 3 minutes. Then rinse. Repeat 2-3 times a day or as needed.
Caution: In rare instances of local sensitivity, discontinue use by the individual.
How Supplied: 1 fl. oz. and 4 fl. oz. plastic bottles.
Note: Blue stains on starched linen will wash off with soap and water.

BETADINE® SOLUTION
[bā' tăh-dīn"]
(povidone-iodine)
Topical Antiseptic Microbicide

Action and Uses: For preoperative prepping of operative site, including the vagina, and as a general topical microbicide for: disinfection of wounds; emergency treatment of lacerations and abrasions; second– and third–degree burns; as a prophylactic anti-infective agent in hospital and office procedures, including postoperative application to incisions to help prevent infection; oral moniliasis (thrush); bacterial and mycotic skin infections; decubitus and stasis ulcers; preoperatively, in the mouth and throat, as a swab. BETADINE Solution is microbicidal, and not merely bacteriostatic. It *kills* gram-positive and gram-negative bacteria (including antibiotic-resistant strains), fungi, viruses, protozoa and yeasts.
Administration: Apply full strength as often as needed as a paint, spray, or wet soak. May be bandaged. Caution: In preoperative prepping, avoid "pooling" beneath the patient. Prolonged exposure to unabsorbed, wet solution may cause irritation.
How Supplied: ½ oz., 4 oz., 8 oz., 16 oz. (1 pt.), 32 oz. (1 qt.) and 1 gal. plastic bottles and 1 oz. packettes.
Also Available: BETADINE® Solution Swab Aid® Pads for degerming small areas of skin or mucous membranes prior to injections, aspirations, catheterization and surgery; boxes of 100 packettes. Also: disposable BETADINE Solution Swabsticks, in packettes of 1's and 3's.

BETADINE® SURGICAL SCRUB
[bā' tăh-dīn"]
(povidone-iodine)
Topical Antiseptic Germicide

Action and Uses: An antiseptic, germicidal, sudsing skin cleanser for pre- and postoperative scrubbing or washing by hospital operating room personnel; for preoperative use on patients; and general use as an antiseptic germicide in physician's office. Forms rich, golden lather, virtually nonirritating; nonstaining to skin and natural fabrics.
Caution: In rare instance of local irritation or sensitivity, discontinue use by individual.
Directions for Use:
A. For Preoperative Washing by Operating Personnel

1. Wet hands and forearms with water. Pour about 5 cc. (1 teaspoonful) of BETADINE Surgical Scrub on the palm of the hand and spread over both hands and forearms. Without adding more water, rub the Scrub thoroughly over all areas for about five minutes. Use a brush if desired. Clean thoroughly under fingernails. Add a little water and develop copious suds. Rinse thoroughly under running water.
2. Complete the wash by scrubbing with another 5 cc. of BETADINE Surgical Scrub in the same way.

B. For Preoperative Use on Patients
After the skin area is shaved, wet it with water. Apply BETADINE Surgical Scrub (1 cc. is sufficient to cover an area of 20-30 square inches), develop lather and scrub thoroughly for about five minutes. Rinse off by aid of sterile gauze saturated with water. The area may then be painted with BETADINE Solution or sprayed with BETADINE Aerosol Spray and allowed to dry.

C. For use in the Physician's Office
Use for washing whenever a germicidal detergent is required. For maximum degerming of the hands proceed as under (A). To prepare the patient's skin proceed as under (B).
Note: Blue stains on starched linen will wash off with soap and water.

Supplied: 16 oz. (1 pint) plastic bottle with and without pump, 32 oz. (1 quart) and 1 gal. plastic bottles, and ½ oz. packettes.

BETADINE® Viscous Formula
[bā′ tăh-dīn″]
Antiseptic Gauze Pad
(povidone-iodine)

Description: BETADINE Viscous Formula Antiseptic Gauze Pads are available as 3″ × 9″ gauze pads impregnated with BETADINE Solution (povidone-iodine) in a viscous base that is formulated to remain moist for an extended period of time.

Actions: The active ingredient in BETADINE Viscous Formula Antiseptic Gauze Pad kills both gram-positive and gram-negative bacteria (including antibiotic-resistant strains), viruses, fungi, protozoa and yeasts. It is rapidly effective against *Staphylococcus aureus*. It is microbicidal, not merely bacteriostatic... and maintains its activity in the presence of blood, pus and serum.

Actions and Uses: As a Topical Microbicidal Dressing to help prevent topical infection; for disinfection of wounds; for antiseptic treatment of lacerations, abrasions and first-, second- and third-degree burns; for use as a prophylactic anti-infective agent in hospital and office procedures; for postoperative application to incisions to help protect against possible infection; for antiseptic treatment of cutaneous ulcers.

Directions for use: To open, separate seam in either corner of packette and peel down. Remove the gauze pad and apply directly to affected area. Gauze pad may be bandaged.

Supplied: 3″ × 9″ in boxes of 12 and boxes of 50.
Also Available: BETADINE® Antiseptic Gauze Pad, impregnated with BETADINE Solution in a water-soluble base of polyethylene glycols.

CARDIOQUIN® TABLETS ℞
[car′dē″ ō-quin]
(quinidine polygalacturonate)

Description: Each scored CARDIOQUIN Tablet contains 275 mg quinidine polygalacturonate equivalent in quinidine content to 3 grains (200 mg) of quinidine sulfate.

Actions: The quinidine component slows conduction time, prolongs the refractory period, and depresses the excitability of heart muscle. Polygalacturonate slows ionization of the drug and protects the gastrointestinal tract by its demulcent effect.[1-3]

Indications: CARDIOQUIN Tablets are indicated as maintenance therapy after spontaneous and electrical conversion of atrial tachycardia, flutter or fibrillation and in the treatment of:
• Premature atrial and ventricular contractions.
• Paroxysmal atrial tachycardia.
• Paroxysmal A-V junctional rhythm.
• Atrial flutter.
• Paroxysmal atrial fibrillation.
• Established atrial fibrillation when therapy is appropriate.
• Paroxysmal ventricular tachycardia when not associated with complete heartblock.

Contraindications:
1. History of hypersensitivity to quinidine manifested by thrombocytopenia, skin eruptions, febrile reactions, etc.
2. Complete A-V block.
3. Complete bundle branch block or other severe intraventricular conduction defects exhibiting marked QRS widening or bizarre complexes.
4. Myasthenia gravis.
5. Arrhythmias associated with digitalis toxicity.

Warnings:
1. In the treatment of atrial fibrillation with rapid ventricular response, ventricular rate should be controlled with digitalis glycosides *prior* to administration of quinidine.
2. In the treatment of atrial flutter with quinidine, reversion to sinus rhythm may be preceded by progressive reduction in the degree of A-V block to a 1:1 ratio resulting in an extremely high ventricular rate. This potential hazard may be reduced by digitalization prior to administration of quinidine.

Recent reports have described increased, potentially toxic, digoxin plasma levels when quinidine is administered concurrently. When concurrent use is necessary, digoxin dosage should be reduced and plasma concentration should be monitored and patients observed closely for digitalis intoxication.

3. Quinidine cardiotoxicity may be manifested by increased P-R and Q-T intervals, 50% widening of QRS, and/or ventricular ectopic beats or tachycardia. Appearance of these toxic signs during quinidine administration mandates immediate discontinuation of the drug, and/or close clinical and electrocardiographic monitoring. Note: Quinidine effect is enhanced by potassium and reduced in the presence of hypokalemia.
4. Quinidine syncope may occur as a complication of long-term therapy. It is manifested by sudden loss of consciousness and by ventricular arrhythmias with bizarre QRS complexes. This syndrome does not appear to be related to dose or plasma levels but occurs more often with prolonged Q-T intervals.
5. Because quinidine antagonizes the effect of vagal excitation upon the atrium and the A-V node, the administration of parasympathomimetic drugs (choline esters) or the use of any other procedure to enhance vagal activity may fail to terminate paroxysmal supraventricular tachycardia in patients receiving quinidine.
6. Quinidine should be used with extreme caution in:
a) The presence of incomplete A-V block, since a complete block and asystole may result.
b) Quinidine may cause unpredictable abnormalities of rhythm in digitalized hearts. Therefore, it should be used with caution in the presence of digitalis intoxication (see 2 above).
c) Partial bundle branch block.
d) Severe congestive heart failure and hypotensive states due to the depressant effects of quinidine on myocardial contractility and arterial pressure.
e) Poor renal function, especially renal tubular acidosis, because of the potential accumulation of quinidine in plasma leading to toxic concentrations.

Precautions:
1. Test Dose—A preliminary test dose of a single tablet of quinidine *sulfate* should be administered prior to the initiation of treatment with CARDIOQUIN Tablets to determine whether the patient has an idiosyncrasy to the quinidine molecule.
2. Hypersensitivity—During the first weeks of therapy, hypersensitivity to quinidine, although rare, should be considered (e.g., angioedema, purpura, acute asthmatic episode, vascular collapse).
3. Long-Term Therapy— Periodic blood counts and liver and kidney function tests should be performed during long-term therapy, and the drug should be discontinued if blood dyscrasias or signs of hepatic or renal disorders occur.
4. Large Doses—ECG monitoring and determination of plasma quinidine levels are recommended when doses greater than 2.5 g/day are administered.
5. Usage in Pregnancy—The use of quinidine in pregnancy should be reserved only for those cases where the benefits outweigh the possible hazards to the patient and fetus.
6. Nursing Mothers—The drug should be used with extreme caution in nursing mothers because the drug is excreted in breast milk.
7. General—In patients exhibiting asthma, muscle weakness and infection with fever *prior* to quinidine administration, hypersensitivity reactions to the drug may be masked.

Drug Interactions:
1. Caution should be used when quinidine and its analogs are administered concurrently with coumarin anticoagulants. This combination may reduce prothrombin levels and cause bleeding.
2. Quinidine, a weak base, may have its half-life prolonged in patients who are concurrently taking drugs that can alkalize the urine, such as thiazide diuretics, sodium bicarbonate, and carbonic anhydrase inhibitors. Quinidine and drugs which alkalize the urine should be used together cautiously.
3. Quinidine exhibits a distinct anticholinergic activity in the myocardial tissues. An additive vagolytic effect may be seen when quinidine and drugs having anticholinergic blocking activity are used together. Drugs having cholinergic activity may be antagonized by quinidine.
4. Quinidine and other antiarrhythmic agents may produce additive cardiac depressant effects when administered together.
5. Quinidine interaction with cardiac glycosides (digoxin). See Warnings.
6. Antacids may delay absorption of quinidine but appear unlikely to cause incomplete absorption.
7. Phenobarbital and phenytoin may reduce plasma half-life of quinidine by 50%.
8. Quinidine may potentiate the neuromuscular blocking effect in ventilatory depression of patients receiving decamethonium, tubocurare or succinylcholine.

Adverse Reactions: Symptoms of cinchonism (ringing in the ears, headache, disturbed vision) may appear in sensitive patients after a single dose of the drug.

Gastrointestinal: The most common side-effects encountered with quinidine are referable to this system. Diarrhea frequently occurs, but it rarely necessitates withdrawal of the drug. Nausea, vomiting and abdominal pain also occur. Some of these effects may be minimized by administering the drug with meals.

Cardiovascular: Widening of QRS complex, cardiac asystole, ventricular ectopic beats, idioventricular rhythms including ventricular tachycardias and fibrillation; paradoxical tachycardia, arterial embolism and hypotension.

Hematologic: Acute hemolytic anemia, hypoprothrombinemia, thrombocytopenic purpura, agranulocytosis.

CNS: Headache, fever, vertigo, apprehension, excitement, confusion, delirium and syncope, disturbed hearing (tinnitus, decreased auditory acuity), disturbed vision (mydriasis, blurred vision, disturbed color perception, photophobia, diplopia, night blindness, scotomata); optic neuritis.

Dermatologic: Cutaneous flushing with intense pruritus.

Hypersensitivity Reactions: Angioedema, acute asthmatic episode, vascular collapse, respiratory arrest, hepatic dysfunction.

Continued on next page

Purdue Frederick—Cont.

Dosage and Administration:
Each CARDIOQUIN Tablet contains 275 mg quinidine polygalacturonate, equivalent to a 3-grain tablet of quinidine sulfate. Dosage must be adjusted to individual patient's needs, both for conversion and maintenance. An initial dose of 1 to 3 tablets may be used to terminate arrhythmia, and may be repeated in 3-4 hours. If normal sinus rhythm is not restored after 3 or 4 equal doses, the dose may be increased by $\frac{1}{2}$ to 1 tablet (137.5 or 275 mg) and administered three to four times before any further dosage increase. For maintenance, one tablet may be used two or three times a day; generally, one tablet morning and night will be adequate.
Overdosage: Cardiotoxic effects of quinidine may be reversed in part by molar sodium lactate; the hypotension may be reversed by vasoconstrictors and by catecholamines (since vasodilation is partly due to alpha-adrenergic blockage).
Supplied: Uncoated, scored tablets in bottles of 100.
References:
1. Schwartz, G.: *Angiology* 10:115 (Apr.) 1959.
2. Tricot, R., Nogrette, P.: *Presse med.* 68:1085 (June 4) 1960.
3. Shaftel, N., Halpern, A.: *Am. J. Med. Sci.* 236:184 (Aug.) 1958.

Shown in Product Identification Section, page 427

CERUMENEX® DROPS   ℞
[sĕ-rū' měn-ĕx"]
(triethanolamine polypeptide oleate-condensate)
Cerumenolytic agent for effective and easy removal of earwax
Composition: CERUMENEX Drops contain (10%) Triethanolamine polypeptide oleate-condensate in propylene glycol with chlorbutanol (0.5%), for effective, convenient cerumenolytic action and easy removal of earwax.
Among its properties are:
1. Aqueous-miscible solution—low surface tension and optimal viscosity.
2. Slightly acid pH range to approximate surface of normal ear canal.
3. Hygroscopic — helps absorb aqueous transudates.
4. Antiseptic protection against contamination.

Advantages:
- Usually effective with a single 15-30 minute treatment.
- Excellent results reported in over 90% of about 2,700 adult and pediatric patients.
- Helps avoid painful instrumentation.
- Simple and easy to administer.

Action: CERUMENEX Drops are specifically designed as a cerumenolytic agent, to emulsify and disperse excess or impacted earwax for easier removal without painful instrumentation. They are usually effective with a single 15-30 minute treatment, and are simple and easy to administer.
Indications: Removal of impacted cerumen—including prior to ear examination, prior to otologic therapy, and prior to audiometry.
Contraindications:
- A history of a previous untoward reaction to CERUMENEX Drops.
- A positive patch test (see "Precautions").
- Knowledge or suspicion of a perforated eardrum or otitis media may be considered as a relative contraindication.

Precautions:
It is recommended that the following precautions be observed in prescribing and administration of this agent:
1. Extreme caution is indicated in patients with demonstrable dermatologic idiosyncrasies or with history of allergic reactions in general.
2. In case of doubt, a patch test should be performed by placing a drop of CERUMENEX Drops on the flexor surface of the arm or forearm and covering it with a small Band-Aid® strip. The results are read and interpreted after 24 hours. Positive reaction indicates the probability of an allergic reaction following instillation in the ear.
3. Exposure of the ear canal to the CERUMENEX Drops should be limited to 15-30 minutes.
4. Patients must be instructed not to exceed the time of exposure, nor to use the medication more frequently than directed by the physician.
5. When administering CERUMENEX Drops, care must be taken to avoid undue exposure of the periaural skin during the instillation and the flushing out of the medication. If the medication comes in contact with the skin, the area should be washed with soap and water. Use of proper technique (see Dosage and Administration) will help avoid such undue exposure.
6. Although introduction of CERUMENEX Drops (triethanolamine polypeptide oleate-condensate) into the middle ear of animals with surgically perforated drums or into patients with ruptured drums has been accomplished without untoward reactions, the use of this medication should be avoided in the presence of underlying disease in the middle ear (otitis media, perforated drum) and it should be used only with caution in certain types of external otitis.
7. Patients should be advised to discontinue the use of the medication in case of a possible reaction and to consult their physician promptly.

Adverse Reactions:
Clinical Reactions of Possible Allergic Origin
Localized dermatitis reactions were reported in about 1% of 2,700 patients treated, ranging from a very mild erythema and pruritus of the external canal to a severe eczematoid reaction involving the external ear and periauricular tissue, generally with duration of 2-10 days. In all cases, complete and uneventful resolution occurred without residual sequelae, sometimes without supplemental therapy. Such therapy may consist of only symptomatic relief in mild cases and may include anti-inflammatory agents when indicated. Thus, while reactions of a possible allergic origin may occur, their incidence is minimal and usually not disproportionate to other commonly used dermatologic agents.
Dosage and Administration:
1. Fill ear canal with CERUMENEX Drops with the patient's head tilted at a 45° angle.
2. Insert cotton plug and allow to remain 15-30 minutes.
3. Then gently flush ear with lukewarm water, using soft rubber syringe (avoid excessive pressure). Avoid undue exposure of large skin areas to the drug. If a second application is necessary in unusually hard impactions, the procedure may be repeated.

How Supplied: 6 ml and 12 ml bottles with cellophane-wrapped, blunt-end dropper.

FIBERMED®
[fī' bĕr-mĕd"]
High–Fiber Supplements
Fruit Flavor/Original Flavor
Description: FIBERMED High-Fiber Supplements provide a measured quantity of natural dietary fiber in a palatable, ready-to-eat biscuit form. FIBERMED Supplements are standardized to provide concentrated dietary fiber in precise amounts—10 grams in two delicious biscuits. Original-Flavor FIBERMED contain natural dietary fiber from corn, wheat and oats. Fruit-Flavor FIBERMED contain natural dietary fiber from six sources: corn, oats, wheat, soy, apple and currants. Dietary fiber is an integral part of treatment for constipation, irritable bowel syndrome, diverticulosis, and hemorrhoids. Lack of fiber in the diet is a recognized cause of constipation. With adequate fiber, food wastes move through the body quickly, making elimination easier and more regular.
In a two-week clinical trial, patients suffering from constipation took two FIBERMED Supplements daily. There were highly significant improvements in number, consistency, and ease of passage of bowel movements. The mean number of bowel movements per week doubled—4.3 per week before FIBERMED; 8.0 after FIBERMED ($p < 0.001$).
Two FIBERMED High-Fiber Biscuits a day help provide the supplementary bulk that patients may need in their diet to avoid constipation. Many individuals can increase their fiber intake by 50% or more simply by eating two FIBERMED Supplements each day.
FIBERMED helps curb appetite. FIBERMED may help in weight control programs two ways. Fiber produces feelings of satiety and fullness, and can reduce one's desire for food. As a result, less calories are consumed. And, FIBERMED has a low calorie-to-fiber ratio—only 12 calories per gram of fiber.
FIBERMED can overcome patient problems often associated with other fiber sources—such as undetermined fiber content, inconvenience and monotonous taste. FIBERMED Supplements are superior to other fiber sources because of their uniform high-fiber content, convenience and good taste, qualities which encourage good patient compliance.
Ready-to-eat FIBERMED Supplements can be eaten any time, any place. Unlike most high-fiber foods or powdered bulks, FIBERMED Supplements require no preparation and no mixing. They can be eaten with milk, coffee, tea, juice, soup or fruit; or dunked in a beverage.

NUTRITION INFORMATION PER SERVING OF ORIGINAL-FLAVOR FIBERMED:
Serving Size .... 1 Supplement
Servings per package 14
Calories 60
Protein .... 1 g
Carbohydrate .... 14 g*
Fat .... 2 g

PERCENTAGE OF U.S. RECOMMENDED DAILY ALLOWANCES (% U.S. RDA):
Riboflavin (Vitamin B_2) 2
Niacin 2
Iron 4
Contains less than 2% of the U.S. RDA of Protein, Vitamin A, Vitamin C, Thiamine amd Calcium.
*Includes 4.6 g of simple carbohydrates (brown sugar) and 9.4 g of complex carbohydrates.
Ingredients: Corn Bran, Brown Sugar, Wheat Flour, Corn Starch, Wheat Bran, Oat Flakes, Corn Germ Meal, Vegetable Shortening (Partially Hydrogenated Soybean Oil), Sodium Bicarbonate, Vanilla Flavor, Peanut Butter Flavor, Ammonium Bicarbonate, Baking Acid, Sodium Propionate, Salt and Citric Acid.

NUTRITION INFORMATION PER SERVING OF FRUIT-FLAVOR FIBERMED:
Serving Size .... 1 Supplement
Servings per package 14
Calories 60
Protein .... 2 g
Carbohydrate .... 13 g*
Fat .... 2 g
Sodium .... 110 mg
Dietary Fiber .... 5 g

PERCENTAGE OF U.S. RECOMMENDED DAILY ALLOWANCES (% U.S. RDA):
Protein 2
Riboflavin (Vitamin B_2) 2
Niacin 4
Calcium 2
Iron 4
Contains less than 2% of the U.S. RDA of Vitamin A, Vitamin C, Thiamine.
*Includes 4.5 g of simple carbohydrates (brown sugar) and 8.5 g of complex carbohydrates.
Ingredients: Corn Bran, Brown Sugar, Whole Rolled Oats, Soy Flour, Vegetable Shortening (Partially Hydrogenated Soybean Oil), Currants, Wheat Bran, Dried Apple, Ammonium Bicarbonate, Baking Soda, Citric Acid, Apple Flavor, Salt, Vanilla, Coconut Flavor, Baking Acid, Calcium Propionate, Cinnamon.
Usage: FIBERMED Supplements are indicated for those conditions, including constipation, in which it is desirable to regulate gastrointestinal

transit time, increase stool weight and make elimination easier. Because of their taste and convenience, FIBERMED Supplements are the product of choice to significantly increase intake of dietary fiber in uniform amounts.

Two FIBERMED Supplements a day provide a high level of dietary fiber—10 grams—more dietary fiber than a serving of high-fiber cereal.

Directions: Two FIBERMED Biscuits per day provide the extra fiber required by most people. As with any healthful diet, adequate fluid intake is important.

Supplied: FIBERMED Supplements are available in Fruit Flavor, as well as in Original Flavor. FIBERMED Supplements are supplied in boxes of 14. For most individuals, 14 is a week's supply.

Shown in Product Identification Section, page 427

M S CONTIN®
(morphine sulfate)
30 mg
Controlled-Release Tablets
WARNING: May be habit forming.

Description: Each MS CONTIN Tablet contains 30 mg morphine sulfate in a controlled-release formulation. Chemically, morphine sulfate is 7,8-didehydro-4,5,α-epoxy-17-methyl-morphinan-3,6α-diol sulfate (2:1) (salt) pentahydrate and has the following structural formula.

[Structural formula: morphine • H_2SO_4 • $5H_2O$, with subscript 2]

Clinical Pharmacology: Morphine exerts its major effects on the central nervous system and the bowel. Like other opium derivatives, it acts as an agonist, interacting with stereospecific and saturable binding sites or receptors in various tissues, including the brain. Morphine acts directly on the CNS to produce analgesia, drowsiness, mental clouding, and altered mood. Cough suppression is mediated through direct effect on the medullary center. Respiratory depression results from reduced responsiveness of the respiratory center to carbon dioxide. Emesis is a consequence of direct stimulation of the chemoreceptor trigger zone. Biliary tract pressure may result from morphine induced spasm of the Sphincter of Oddi. Constipation is secondary to the narcotic action on bowel wall nerve plexuses.

Indications and Usage: MS Contin is indicated for the prolonged relief of severe pain.

Contraindications: Contraindications include hypersensitivity to morphine; respiratory depression or insufficiency; bronchial asthma (attack); severe CNS depression; cardiac failure secondary to chronic pulmonary disease; cardiac arrhythmias; increased cerebrospinal or intracranial pressure; head injuries; brain tumor; acute alcoholism; delirium tremens; convulsive disorders and suspected surgical abdomen. Morphine is also contraindicated after biliary tract surgery, following surgical anastomosis, and concomitantly with MAO inhibitors (or within 14 days of such treatment).

As with all oral morphine preparations MS Contin Tablets should be used with caution peri-operatively in abdominal surgery. Should paralytic ileus occur during or after administration of MS Contin Tablets, their use should be immediately discontinued. As with all morphine preparations, patients who are scheduled for cordotomy or other pain-relieving surgical procedures, should not receive MS Contin Tablets within 24 hours prior to surgery.

Warnings: Morphine may cause tolerance as well as psychological and physical dependence. Withdrawal symptoms can occur upon abrupt discontinuation, or on administration of a narcotic antagonist.

Interaction with Other CNS Depressants
Morphine should be used with caution, in reduced dosage, during concurrent administration of other narcotic analgesics, general anesthetics, phenothiazines or other tranquilizers, sedative-hypnotics, tricyclic antidepressants, and other CNS depressants (including alcohol). If not, respiratory depression, hypotension, and profound sedation or coma may result.

Precautions:
General
Head Trauma and Increased Intracranial Pressure: The respiratory depressant effects of morphine, and the drug's capacity to elevate cerebrospinal fluid pressure, may be greatly exaggerated in the presence of increased intracranial pressure. In addition, narcotics can produce side effects that may obscure the clinical course in case of head injury. In such patients, morphine must be used with caution and only if it is judged essential.

Asthma and Other Respiratory Disorders: Morphine must be used with caution during acute asthmatic attacks, in patients with chronic obstructive lung disease, or cor pulmonale, and in patients with substantially decreased respiratory reserve, preexisting depression, hypoxia, or hypercapnia. Even commonly prescribed therapeutic doses of narcotics may reduce respiratory drive while simultaneously raising airway resistance to the point of apnea.

Hypotensive Effect: Morphine administration may result in severe hypotension in patients whose ability to maintain adequate blood pressure is already compromised by diminished blood volume or concurrent administration of such drugs as phenothiazines or certain anesthetics.

Acute Abdominal Conditions: The administration of morphine or other narcotics may obscure the diagnosis or clinical course of patients with such conditions.

Special Risk Groups: Morphine should be administered with caution, and at a reduced initial dose, in the elderly or debilitated, in patients with impaired hepatic or renal function, and in those with Addison's disease, hypothyroidism, urethral stricture or prostatic hypertrophy.

Note: Morphine may suppress respiration in the elderly, the very ill, and those with respiratory problems. Therefore, lower doses may be required in these patients. Care must also be taken when patients are under the effect of other drugs which affect respiratory function, such as during the immediate period following anesthesia.

Information for Patients
Ambulatory Patients: Morphine may impair the abilities, mental and/or physical, needed for certain potentially hazardous activities, such as driving a car or operating machinery. The patient should be cautioned accordingly.

Like other narcotics, morphine may cause orthostatic hypotension in ambulatory patients.

Patients should also be cautioned about the combined effects of other CNS depressants with morphine, including those of alcohol and antihistamines.

Drug Interactions
Generally, effects of morphine may be antagonized by acidifying agents and potentiated by alkalizing agents. The analgesic effect of morphine is potentiated by chlorpromazine and methocarbamol. CNS depressants, such as other narcotics, anesthetics, sedatives, hypnotic agents, barbiturates, phenothiazines, chloral hydrate, and glutethimide may enhance the depressant effects of morphine. Monoamine oxidase inhibitors (including procarbazine hydrochloride), furazolidone, antihistamines, "beta blockers" such as propranolol, and alcohol may also enhance the depressant effects of morphine.

Morphine may increase the anticoagulant activity of coumarin and other anticoagulant drugs.

Carcinogenicity/Mutagenicity
No long-term studies of the carcinogenic/mutagenic potential of morphine are available.

Pregnancy Category C: Reproduction studies in animals have not been carried out with morphine. It is also not known whether morphine can cause fetal harm when administered to a pregnant woman or can affect the reproduction capacity. Morphine should be given to a pregnant woman only if clearly needed.

Labor and Delivery
Morphine readily crosses the placental barrier and its administration during labor may lead to respiratory depression in the newborn.

Use by Nursing Mothers
Morphine has been detected in human milk. Caution should therefore be exercised when this drug is administered to a nursing woman.

Pediatric Usage
The safety and effectiveness of morphine in children has not been established.

Adverse Reactions
THE MAJOR HAZARDS ASSOCIATED WITH MORPHINE, AS WITH OTHER NARCOTIC ANALGESICS, ARE RESPIRATORY DEPRESSION, AND TO A LESSER DEGREE, CIRCULATORY DEPRESSION: RESPIRATORY ARREST, SHOCK, AND CARDIAC ARREST HAVE OCCURRED FOLLOWING ORAL OR PARENTERAL USE OF MORPHINE.

Lightheadedness, sedation, dizziness, nausea, vomiting and excessive sweating are among the most frequently observed adverse reactions. These effects seem to be more prominent in ambulatory patients and in those not experiencing intense pain. In such cases, lower doses are advisable. Some adverse reactions may be alleviated in ambulatory patients if they lie down.

Other adverse reactions observed include the following:

CNS: Weakness, headache, insomnia, disorientation, visual disturbances, agitation, euphoria and dysphoria.

Cardiovascular: Palpitations, bradycardia, faintness/syncope and facial flushing.

Gastrointestinal: Constipation, anorexia, dry mouth and spasm of the biliary tract.

Genitourinary: Urinary retention or hesitancy, anti-diuretic effect, reduced libido and/or reduced sexual potency.

Allergic: Pruritus, skin rashes including urticaria, hemorrhagic urticaria (rarely), and edema.

Treatment of the Most Frequent Adverse Effects
Constipation: Ample fluid intake should be encouraged. Concomitant administration of a stool-softener combined with a peristaltic stimulant (e.g. standardized senna concentrate with docusate sodium) can be effective prophylaxis against morphine-induced constipation. If elimination does not occur for two days, an enema should be considered to prevent fecal impaction.

If diarrhea occurs, seepage around an impaction should be evaluated as a possible cause before anti-diarrheal measures are used.

Nausea and Vomiting: Phenothiazines or antihistaminic agents can be effective treatments for nausea of medullary or vestibular origin, respectively. However, concomitant therapy with these drugs may potentiate the side effects of morphine.

Sedation: Once pain control is achieved, undesirable drowsiness can be minimized by adjustment of dosage to a level that just maintains a pain-free state or a tolerable level of pain.

Drug Abuse and Dependence
The narcotic morphine sulfate is a Schedule II controlled substance under the Federal Controlled Substance Act. As with other narcotics, its administration may result in development of physical and psychological dependence by some patients. Such patients may increase dosage without consulting a physician and subsequently may develop a physical dependence on the drug. In cases of this type, abrupt discontinuance may precipitate typical withdrawal symptoms, including convulsions. The drug should therefore be withdrawn gradually from those known to be taking excessive dosages over a prolonged period.

In treating the terminally ill, the benefits of morphine administration may outweigh the risk of drug dependence. The chance of such dependence is substantially reduced under a scheduled nar-

Continued on next page

Purdue Frederick—Cont.

cotic administration program as compared to PRN dosage.

Overdosage

Signs and Symptoms: Serious morphine overdosage is characterized by respiratory depression (reduced respiratory rate and/or tidal volume; Cheyne-Stokes respiration; cyanosis; extreme somnolence progressing to stupor or coma, flaccidity of skeletal muscle, cold or clammy skin, and sometimes hypotension and bradycardia. Severe overdosage may result in apnea, circulatory collapse, cardiac arrest and death.

Treatment: Primary attention should be given to the re-establishment of adequate respiratory exchange through the provision of a patent airway and controlled or assisted ventilation. The narcotic antagonist naloxone hydrochloride is a specific antidote against respiratory depression due to overdosage or as a result of unusual sensitivity to narcotics, including morphine. An appropriate dose of naloxone hydrochloride should therefore be administered, preferably by the intravenous route; the usual initial i.v. adult dose is 0.4 mg. Concomitant efforts at respiratory resuscitation should be carried out. Since the duration of action of morphine may exceed that of the antagonist, the patient should be under continued surveillance and doses of the antagonist should be repeated as needed to maintain adequate respiration.

Do not administer an antagonist in the absence of clinically significant respiratory or cardiovascular depression.

Oxygen, intravenous fluids, vasopressor substances, and other supportive measures should be used as indicated.

Evacuation of gastric contents may be useful in removing unabsorbed drug.

Dosage and Administration

Usual Adult Oral Dose: One 30 mg MS Contin (morphine sulfate) Tablet every 12 hours, or as directed by physician. Patients established on an immediate-release oral morphine product may be transferred to MS Contin Tablets on a mg-for-mg basis, using the same total daily dose (24 hour) divided for b.i.d. administration. If converting a patient from another narcotic to morphine sulfate on the basis of standard equivalence tables, a 1 to 3 ratio of parenteral to oral morphine equivalence is suggested.

Dosage of morphine is a patient-dependent variable, which must be individualized according to the patient's metabolism and response to morphine. Clinical studies* confirm that the majority of patients are adequately maintained with MS Contin Tablets administered q.12 h. Other patients will require dosing q.8 h. Due to the long-acting characteristics of MS Contin Tablets, dosage is not recommended more frequently than q.8 h. Each patient should be maintained at the lowest dosage level that will produce acceptable analgesia. As the patient's well-being improves after successful relief of severe pain, periodic reduction of dosage and/or extension of dosing interval should be attempted to minimize exposure to morphine.

Caution

DEA Order Form Required.
Federal law prohibits dispensing without prescription.

How Supplied

NDC 0034-0515-50: MS Contin (morphine sulfate) Tablets, 30 mg are supplied in opaque plastic bottles, containing 50 tablets.

Each round, lavender-colored tablet bears the symbol PF on one side and M30 on the other side. Store tablets at controlled room temperature 15 to 30°C (59°–86°F).

*Data available on request.
9/28/84

Shown in Product Identification Section, page 427

PRIODERM® LOTION
[*prī'ō" dĕrm*]
(0.5% malathion)

Description: A pleasantly scented, clear liquid containing 0.5% malathion in 78% isopropyl alcohol, terpineol, dipentene and pine needle oil.

Clinical Pharmacology: Malathion is lousicidal and ovicidal *in vitro*. Louse eggs succumb to 3 seconds of exposure to 0.062% malathion in acetone and lice to about 0.003%, respectively. Resistance to malathion could not be induced.

Human safety studies included a 21-day cumulative irritancy and others undertaken to determine the potential for contact sensitization, phototoxicity, and photo-contact sensitization. Application of Prioderm Lotion showed no evidence of sensitization and a very low level of irritation.

Indications and Usage: Prioderm Lotion is indicated for the treatment of head lice and their ova.

Contraindications: Prioderm Lotion should not be used by individuals with known sensitivity to Prioderm Lotion or to any of its components.

> **WARNING: PRIODERM LOTION CONTAINS FLAMMABLE ALCOHOL. THE LOTION AND WET HAIR SHOULD NOT BE EXPOSED TO OPEN FLAME OR ELECTRIC HEAT, INCLUDING HAIR DRYERS. DO NOT SMOKE WHILE APPLYING LOTION, OR WHILE HAIR IS WET. ALLOW HAIR TO DRY NATURALLY AND UNCOVERED AFTER APPLICATION.**

Precautions: If accidentally placed in the eye, flush immediately with water.

Carcinogenesis, Mutagenesis and Fertility—Malathion is neither carcinogenic in male or female F344 rats after 2 years feeding with up to 4000 ppm (0.4%) nor is it tumorigenic in Osborn-Mendel rats or B6C3F1 mice after a similar feeding for 80 weeks with 8,000 ppm (0.8%) and 16,000 ppm (1.6%), respectively. Tests for mutagenicity have not been conducted.

Pregnancy Category B—There was no evidence of teratogenicity in studies utilizing single i.p. injections of malathion at 600 and 900 mg/kg in pregnant rats or oral dosing with up to 300 mg/kg on days 6 through 15 of gestation. A reproduction study in rats failed to show any gross fetal abnormalities attributable to feeding malathion up to 2,500 ppm in the diet during a three-generation evaluation period. These studies employed at least 50 to 70 times the adult human topical dose. Because animal reproduction studies are not always predictive of human response, this drug should be used during pregnancy only if clearly needed.

Nursing Mothers—Malathion in an acetone vehicle has been reported to be absorbed through human skin only to the extent of 8% of the applied dose. However, percutaneous absorption from the Prioderm Lotion formulation has not been studied, and it is not known whether malathion is excreted in human milk. Because many drugs are excreted in human milk, caution should be exercised when Prioderm Lotion is administered to the nursing mother.

Adverse Reactions: Irritation of the scalp has been reported.

Overdosage: Consideration should be given as part of the treatment program to the high concentration of isopropyl alcohol in the vehicle.

Malathion, although a weaker cholinesterase inhibitor and therefore safer than other organophosphates, may be expected to exhibit the same symptoms of cholinesterase depletion after accidental ingestion orally. Vomiting should be induced promptly or the stomach lavaged with 5% sodium bicarbonate solution.

Severe respiratory distress is the major and most serious symptom of organophosphate poisoning requiring artifical respiration and large doses of i.m. or i.v. atropine. The usual starting dose of atropine is 1 to 4 mg with supplementation hourly, as needed, to counteract the symptoms of cholinesterase depletion. Repeat analyses of serum and RBC cholinesterase assist in establishing the diagnosis and formulating a long-range prognosis.

Dosage and Administration: 1) Sprinkle Prioderm Lotion on **DRY** hair and rub gently until the hair and scalp are thoroughly moistened. Pay special attention to the back of the head and neck. 2) Allow to dry naturally—use no heat or hair dryer and leave uncovered. 3) After at least 8 hours, the hair should be shampooed. 4) Rinse and use a fine-toothed comb to remove dead lice and eggs. 5) If required, repeat with second application of Prioderm Lotion in 7 to 9 days.

Further treatment is generally not necessary. Other family members should be evaluated to determine if infested and if so, receive treatment.

Caution: Federal law prohibits dispensing without a prescription.

How Supplied: Prioderm Lotion (0.5% malathion) in bottles of 2 fl. oz. (59 ml).

SENOKOT® SYRUP
[*sĕn'ō-kŏt*]
(standardized extract of senna fruit)

Action and Uses: For relief of functional constipation and whenever gentle laxation is indicated. A deliciously flavored liquid laxative, predictably and reliably effective.

Contraindications: Acute surgical abdomen.

Administration and Dosage: Preferably at bedtime. Adults: 2 to 3 tsp. (maximum—3 tsp. b.i.d.). For older, debilitated, and OB/GYN patients, the physician may consider prescribing ½ the initial adult dose. Children 5-15 years: 1 to 2 tsp. (maximum—2 tsp. b.i.d.). 1-5 years: ½ to 1 tsp. (maximum—1 tsp. b.i.d.). 1 month to 1 year: ¼ to ½ tsp. (maximum—½ tsp. b.i.d.). If comfortable evacuation is not achieved by the second day, decrease or increase daily dosage (up to maximum) by one half the starting dose until optimum dose for evacuation is established.

How Supplied: Bottles of 2 and 8 fl. oz.

SENOKOT® TABLETS/GRANULES
[*sĕn'ō-kŏt*]
(standardized senna concentrate)

Action and Uses: Indicated for relief of functional constipation (chronic or occasional). SENOKOT Tablets/Granules contain a natural vegetable derivative, purified and standardized for uniform action. The current theory of the mechanism of action is that glycosides are transported to the colon, where they are changed to aglycones that stimulate Auerbach's plexus to induce peristalsis. This virtually colon-specific action is gentle, effective and predictable, usually inducing comfortable evacuation of well-formed stool within 8-10 hours. Found effective even in many previously intractable cases of functional constipation, SENOKOT preparations may aid in rehabilitation of the constipated patient by facilitating regular elimination. At proper dosage levels, SENOKOT preparations are virtually free of adverse reactions (such as loose stools or abdominal discomfort) and enjoy high patient acceptance. Numerous and extensive clinical studies show their high degree of effectiveness in varieties of functional constipation: chronic, geriatric, antepartum and postpartum, drug-induced, pediatric, as well as in functional constipation concurrent with heart disease or anorectal surgery.

Contraindications: Acute surgical abdomen.

Administration and Dosage: Preferably at bedtime. GRANULES (deliciously cocoa-flavored): Adults: 1 level tsp. (maximum—2 level tsp. b.i.d.). For older, debilitated, and OB/GYN patients, the physician may consider prescribing ½ the initial adult dose. Children above 60 lb.: ½ level tsp. (maximum—1 level tsp. b.i.d.). TABLETS: Adults: 2 tablets (maximum—4 tablets b.i.d.). For older, debilitated, and OB/GYN patients, the physician may consider prescribing ½ the initial dose. Children above 60 lb.: 1 tablet (maximum—2 tablets b.i.d.). To meet individual requirements, if comfortable bowel movement is not achieved by the second day, decrease or increase daily by ½ level tsp. or 1 tablet (up to maximum) until optimal dose for evacuation is established.

How Supplied: Granules: 2, 6, and 12 oz. plastic canisters. Tablets: Box of 20, bottles of 50, 100 and 1000.

SENOKOT Tablets Unit Strip Packs in boxes of 100 tablets; each tablet individually sealed in see-through pockets.

SENOKOT-S® Tablets
[sĕn'ō-kŏt-ĕs"]
(standardized senna concentrate and docusate sodium)
Natural Laxative/Stool Softener Combination

Action and Uses: SENOKOT-S Tablets are designed to relieve both aspects of functional constipation—bowel inertia and hard, dry stools. They provide a natural neuroperistaltic stimulant combined with a classic stool softener: standardized senna concentrate gently stimulates Auerbach's plexus in the colonic wall, while docusate sodium softens the stool for smoother and easier evacuation. This coordinated dual action of the two ingredients results in colon-specific, predictable laxative effect, usually in 8–10 hours. Administering the tablets at bedtime allows the patient an uninterrupted night's sleep, with a comfortable evacuation in the morning. Flexibility of dosage permits fine adjustment to individual requirements. At proper dosage levels, SENOKOT-S Tablets are virtually free from side effects. SENOKOT-S Tablets are highly suitable for relief of postsurgical and postpartum constipation, and effectively counteract drug-induced constipation. They facilitate regular elimination in impaction-prone and elderly patients, and are indicated in the presence of cardiovascular disease where straining must be avoided, as well as in the presence of hemorrhoids and anorectal disease.

Contraindications: Acute surgical abdomen.

Administration and Dosage: (preferably at bedtime) Recommended Initial Dosage: ADULTS—2 tablets (maximum dosage—4 tablets b.i.d.); CHILDREN (above 60 lbs.)—1 tablet (maximum dosage—2 tablets b.i.d.). For older or debilitated patients, the physician may consider prescribing half the initial adult dose. To meet individual requirements, if comfortable bowel movement is not achieved by the second day, dosage may be decreased or increased by 1 tablet, up to maximum, until the most effective dose is established.

Supplied: Bottles of 30, 60 and 1000 Tablets.

TRILISATE® TABLETS/LIQUID
[trĭl'ĭ-sāt"]
(choline magnesium trisalicylate)
500 mg, 750 mg or 1000 mg
salicylate content

Description: TRILISATE Tablets/Liquid are non-steroidal, anti-inflammatory preparations combining choline salicylate and magnesium salicylate in mixtures which are freely soluble in water.

TRILISATE Tablets are available in scored, pale pink 500 mg tablets; in scored, white, film-coated 750 mg tablets, and in scored, red, film-coated 1000 mg tablets. Trilisate Liquid is a cherry cordial-flavored liquid providing 500 mg salicylate content per teaspoonful (5 ml) for oral administration.

Each 500 mg tablet contains 293 mg of choline salicylate combined with 362 mg of magnesium salicylate to provide 500 mg salicylate content. Each 750 mg tablet contains 440 mg of choline salicylate combined with 544 mg of magnesium salicylate to provide 750 mg salicylate content. Each 1000 mg tablet contains 587 mg of choline salicylate combined with 725 mg of magnesium salicylate to provide 1000 mg salicylate content. TRILISATE Liquid contains 293 mg of choline salicylate combined with 362 mg of magnesium salicylate to provide 500 mg salicylate content per teaspoonful (5 ml) in a clear amber, cherry cordial-flavored vehicle.

Clinical Pharmacology: TRILISATE Tablets/Liquid contain salicylate with anti-inflammatory, analgesic, and antipyretic action. On ingestion of TRILISATE Tablets/Liquid, the salicylate moiety is absorbed rapidly and reaches peak blood levels within an average of one to two hours after single doses of the tablets or liquid. The primary route of excretion is renal: the excretion products are chiefly the glycine and glucuronide conjugates. TRILISATE preparations differ from other non-steroidal anti-arthritic agents and from aspirin in having a more selective action on the prostaglandin pathway.

The bioequivalence of TRILISATE Liquid and Tablets 500 mg/750 mg/1000 mg has been established. With the tablets, a steady-state condition is usually reached after 4 to 5 doses, and the half-life of elimination, on repeated administration of the tablets, is 9 to 17 hours. This permits a maintenance dosage schedule of once or twice daily. Unlike aspirin and certain other non-steroidal anti-inflammatory agents, such as arylpropionic acid derivatives and arylacetic acid derivatives, choline magnesium trisalicylate, at therapeutic dosage levels, does not affect platelet aggregation, as shown in *in-vitro* and *in-vivo* studies.

Indications and Usage: Osteoarthritis, Rheumatoid Arthritis and Painful Shoulder: Salicylates are considered the base therapy of choice in the arthritides; and TRILISATE preparations are indicated for the relief of the signs and symptoms of rheumatoid arthritis, osteoarthritis and other arthritides. TRILISATE Tablets or Liquid are indicated in the long-term management of these diseases and especially in the acute flare of rheumatoid arthritis. TRILISATE Tablets or Liquid are also indicated for the treatment of acute painful shoulder.

TRILISATE preparations are effective and generally well tolerated, and are logical choices whenever salicylate treatment is indicated. They are particularly suitable when a once-a-day or b.i.d. dosage regimen is important to patient compliance; when gastrointestinal intolerance to aspirin is encountered; when gastrointestinal microbleeding or hematologic effects of aspirin are considered a patient hazard; and when interference (or the risk of interference) with normal platelet function by aspirin or by propionic acid derivatives is considered to be clinically undesirable. Use of TRILISATE Liquid is appropriate when a liquid dosage form is preferred, as in the elderly patient.

The efficacy of TRILISATE preparations has not been studied in those patients who are designated by the American Rheumatism Association as belonging in Functional Class IV (incapacitated, largely or wholly bedridden or confined to a wheelchair, with little or no self-care). Analgesic and Antipyretic Action: TRILISATE Tablets/Liquid are also indicated for the relief of mild to moderate pain and for antipyresis. *In children*, TRILISATE preparations are indicated for conditions requiring anti-inflammatory, analgesic or antipyretic action—such as juvenile rheumatoid arthritis and other appropriate conditions. Used concomitantly with antibiotics, TRILISATE preparations are useful for analgesia and antipyresis in many bacterial or viral infections.

Contraindications: Patients who are hypersensitive to non-acetylated salicylates should not take TRILISATE Tablets or Liquid.

Precautions: Like other salicylates, TRILISATE preparations should be used with caution in patients with chronic renal insufficiency or with active erosive gastritis or peptic ulcer.

Reports indicate that when acetylated salicylates are given with steroids, the butazones, or alcohol, the risk of gastrointestinal ulceration is increased. Caution should be exercised in patients requiring coumarin or indandione anticoagulants, or heparin.

While salicylates are not known to be associated wih teratogenic potential in man, the usual care should be exercised in the administration of any drug during pregnancy. Because of the possible inhibition of prostaglandin with high doses of salicylates, the use of TRILISATE (choline magnesium trisalicylate) preparations immediately prior to the onset of labor is not recommended.

Adverse Reactions: Choline magnesium trisalicylate is generally well-tolerated at recommended dosage ranges, and has been shown to be particularly well-tolerated by the gastrointestinal system. Salicylism and/or salicylate intoxication may occur with large doses or with extended therapy. Tinnitus may be regarded as a therapeutic guide. Should it develop, reduction of dosage is recommended.

Dosage: ADULTS: In rheumatoid arthritis, osteoarthritis, the more severe arthritides, and acute painful shoulder, the recommended daily dosage is 3000 mg given once a day (h.s.) or 1500 mg b.i.d. Dosage should be adjusted in accordance with the patient's response.

For mild to moderate pain or for antipyresis, the usual dosage is 2000 mg to 3000 mg daily in divided doses (b.i.d.). Based on patient response or salicylate blood levels, dosage may be adjusted to achieve optimum therapeutic effect. Salicylate blood levels should be in the range of 15 to 30 mg/100 ml for anti-inflammatory effect and 5 to 15 mg/100 ml for analgesia and antipyresis.

Each 500 mg tablet or teaspoonful is equivalent in salicylate content to 10 gr of aspirin, each 750 mg tablet to 15 gr of aspirin, and each 1000 mg tablet to 20 gr of aspirin.

If the physician prefers, the recommended daily dosage may be administered on a t.i.d. schedule. As with other therapeutic agents, individual dosage adjustment is advisable, and a number of patients may require higher or lower dosages than those recommended. Certain patients require 2 to 3 weeks of therapy for optimal effect.

CHILDREN: *Usual total daily dose for children for anti-inflammatory, analgesic and antipyretic action:*

TRILISATE 500 mg Tablets/Liquid and TRILISATE 750 mg and 1000 mg Tablets 50 mg/kg

Weight	Total daily dose
12–13	500 mg
14–17	750 mg
18–22	1000 mg
23–27	1250 mg
28–32	1500 mg
33–37	1750 mg

Total daily doses should be administered in divided doses (b.i.d.). Doses of TRILISATE preparations are calculated as the total daily dose of 50 mg/kg/day for children of 37 kg body weight or less and 2250 mg/day for heavier children.

TRILISATE Liquid is available for greater convenience in treating younger patients. TRILISATE Liquid may be mixed with fruit juices just before drinking.

Caution: Federal law prohibits dispensing without a prescription.

How Supplied: 500 mg TRILISATE Tablets (pale pink, scored) in bottles of 100 tablets.

750 mg TRILISATE Tablets (off-white, scored) in bottles of 100 tablets.

1000 mg TRILISATE Tablets (scored, red, film-coated) in bottles of 60 tablets.

TRILISATE Liquid in bottles of 8 fl. oz. (237 ml).

U.S. Patent Numbers 3759980 and 4067974

E145   10/1/84   8752

Shown in Product Identification Section, page 427

UNIPHYL® Tablets
[ū'ni-fĭl]
(theophylline, anhydrous)
200 mg
UNICONTIN®
Controlled-Release System

Description: Uniphyl Tablets contain 200 mg anhydrous theophylline in a controlled-release system. The tablets are scored to facilitate dosage adjustment.

Theophylline anhydrous, a xanthine bronchodilator, is a white, odorless, crystalline powder having a bitter taste. Theophylline has a molecular weight of 180.18, represented by $C_7H_8N_4O_2$ and depicted as: (See next page)

Continued on next page

Purdue Frederick—Cont.

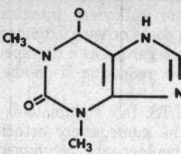

Clinical Pharmacology: Theophylline directly relaxes the smooth muscle of the bronchial airways and pulmonary blood vessels. The drug also produces other actions typical of the xanthine derivatives: coronary vasodilation, cardiac stimulation, diuresis, cerebral stimulation, and skeletal muscle stimulation. These actions may be mediated through inhibition of phosphodiesterase with a resultant increase in intracellular cyclic AMP. *In vitro,* theophylline has been shown to act synergistically with beta agonists that increase intracellular cyclic AMP through the stimulation of adenyl cyclase; but synergism has not been demonstrated in patient studies. More data are needed to determine if theophylline and beta agonists have a clinically important additive effect *in vivo.*

Pharmacokinetics: A single dose randomized cross-over bioavailability study in healthy male volunteers compared 200 mg Uniphyl Tablets with an approved controlled-release BID theophylline product. Uniphyl 200 mg tablets were found to be interchangeable on a mg basis according to average AUC (area under curve), Cmax (maximum theophylline concentration), T-max (time to maximum concentration), absorption rate and apparent elimination half-life.

In a multiple dose, steady-state study with Uniphyl Tablets, a single 400 mg dose produced a peak average serum level of 10.0 mcg/ml within 4 hours. The average trough level was 7.8 mcg/ml during steady-state indicating little fluctuation between Cmax and Cmin.

Newborns and neonates have extremely slow clearance rates compared to older infants (over 6 months) and children, and may also have a theophylline half-life of over 24 hours.

The half-life of theophylline in smokers averages 4 to 5 hours contrasted with 7 to 11 hours in nonsmokers. Following the cessation of smoking, the effects on theophylline pharmacokinetics may persist for 3 months to 2 years.

Theophylline Elimination Characteristics

	Theophylline Clearance Rates (mean±S.D.)	Half-Life Average (mean±S.D.)
Children (over 6 months of age)	1.45±0.58 ml/kg/min	3.7±1.1 hr
Adult nonsmokers with uncomplicated asthma	0.65±0.19 ml/kg/min	8.7±2.2 hr

Indications: Uniphyl Tablets are indicated for relief and/or prevention of symptoms of asthma and reversible bronchospasm associated with chronic bronchitis and emphysema.

Contraindications: This product is contraindicated in individuals who have shown hypersensitivity to theophylline.

Warnings: Status asthmaticus should be considered a medical emergency and is defined as that degree of bronchospasm which is not rapidly responsive to usual doses of conventional bronchodilators. Optimal therapy for such patients frequently requires both *additional medication,* parenterally administered, and *close monitoring,* preferably in an intensive care setting.

Excessive theophylline doses may be associated with toxicity. Determination of serum theophylline levels is recommended to assure maximum therapeutic benefit without excessive risk. The incidence of toxicity increases at serum levels greater than 20 mcg/ml.

Optimum therapeutic response occurs in most patients when the serum theophylline concentration is 10 to 20 mcg/ml. In other patients satisfactory results (as determined by both relief of symptoms and improvement in pulmonary function) may be obtained at lower levels. In still others, adequate response may require higher levels. The physician should adjust the desired serum concentration range to the patients' requirements, keeping in mind that *an increased probability of toxicity exists when levels exceed 20 mcg/ml.* Therefore, in order to assure maximum benefit without excessive risk, measurement of serum levels is highly recommended.

Reduced theophylline clearance may result in increased serum levels and potential toxicity in the following patient groups: (1) those with impaired renal or liver function, (2) those over 55 years of age, particularly males and those with chronic lung disease, (3) those with cardiac failure, (4) those receiving macrolide antibiotics or cimetidine, and (5) neonates. Decreased theophylline clearance may occur during active influenza infection or following immunization for influenza.

Less serious signs of theophylline toxicity, i.e. nausea and restlessness, may appear. Serious side effects such as ventricular arrhythmias, convulsions or even death may appear as the first sign of toxicity without any previous warning. *Serious toxicity is not reliably preceded by less severe side effects.*

Patients who require theophylline may exhibit tachycardia due to their underlying disease. The possible relationship of elevated serum theophylline concentration to tachycardia may not be recognized.

Theophylline products may cause arrhythmia and/or worsen pre-existing arrhythmia. Any significant change in rate and/or rhythm warrants monitoring and further investigation.

Precautions

General: Use with caution in patients with severe cardiac disease, severe hypoxemia, hypertension, hyperthyroidism, acute myocardial injury, cor pulmonale, liver disease, in the elderly (especially males) and in neonates. Particular caution should be used in giving theophylline to patients with congestive heart failure. Frequently, such patients have markedly prolonged theophylline serum levels with theophylline persisting in serum for long periods following discontinuation of the drug. Caution should be exercised in patients concurrently receiving other xanthine medications.

Some patients who are rapid metabolizers of theophylline, such as the young, smokers and some nonsmoking adults, may not be suitable candidates for once daily dosing. Dividing the total daily dose into two doses may be indicated for these patients, who may exhibit symptoms of bronchospasm repeatedly, especially near the end of a 24-hour dosing interval. Also, such individuals may have wider peak-to-trough differences than desired.

Theophylline half-life is shorter in smokers than in non-smokers. Therefore, smokers may require larger or more frequent doses.

Use theophylline cautiously in patients with history of peptic ulcer. Theophylline may occasionally act as a local irritant to the G.I. tract although gastrointestinal symptoms are more commonly centrally mediated and associated with serum drug concentrations over 20 mcg/ml.

Information for Patients: The physician should reinforce the importance of taking only the prescribed dose and observing the time interval between doses. All patients should be asked to report side effects which occur at any time, or recurrence of symptoms, especially toward the end of a dosing interval. Uniphyl Tablets are not to be chewed or crushed.

Drug Interactions: Toxic synergism with ephedrine has been documented and may occur with other sympathomimetic bronchodilators. Concomitant administration of theophylline with cimetidine, troleandomycin or erythromycin may lead to higher serum theophylline levels. Theophylline may increase the excretion of lithium carbonate and antagonize the effects of propranolol.

Drug-Laboratory Test Interactions: When plasma levels of theophylline are measured by spectrophotometric methods, coffee, tea, cola beverages, chocolate and acetaminophen contribute to falsely high values.

Carcinogenesis, Mutagenesis, and Impairment of Fertility: Long-term animal studies have not been performed to evaluate the carcinogenic potential, mutagenic potential or the effect on fertility of xanthine compounds.

Pregnancy: Category C—Animal reproduction studies have not been conducted with theophylline. It is not known whether theophylline can cause fetal harm when administered to a pregnant woman or can effect reproduction capacity. Xanthines should be given to a pregnant woman only if clearly needed.

Nursing Mothers: It has been reported that theophylline distributes readily into breast milk and may cause adverse effects in the infant. Caution must be used when prescribing xanthines to a mother who is nursing, taking into account the risk-benefit of this therapy.

Pediatric: Safety and effectiveness in children under six (6) years of age have not been established with 200 mg Uniphyl Tablets.

Adverse Reactions: The most consistent adverse reactions are usually due to overdose and are:

1. *Gastrointestinal:* nausea, vomiting, epigastric pain, hematemesis, diarrhea.
2. *Central Nervous System:* headaches, irritability, restlessness, insomnia, reflex hyperexcitability, muscle twitching, clonic and tonic generalized convulsions.
3. *Cardiovascular:* palpitation, tachycardia, extrasystole, flushing, hypotension, circulatory failure, ventricular arrhythmia.
4. *Respiratory:* tachypnea.
5. *Renal:* albuminuria, microhematuria, potentiation of diuresis.
6. *Others:* hyperglycemia; inappropriate ADH syndrome; rash.

Overdosage:

Management: If potential oral overdose is established and seizure has not occurred:
A. Induce vomiting. **B.** Administer a cathartic. This is particularly important with sustained-release drugs. **C.** Administer activated charcoal.
If patient is having a seizure:
A. Establish an airway. **B.** Administer oxygen. **C.** Treat the seizure with intravenous diazepam, 0.1 to 0.3 mg/kg up to 10 mg. **D.** Monitor vital signs, maintain blood pressure and provide adequate hydration.

Post Seizure Coma:

A. Maintain airway and oxygenation.
B. If a result of oral medication, follow above recommendations to prevent absorption of the drug, but intubation and lavage will have to be performed instead of inducing emesis, and the cathartic and charcoal will need to be introduced via a large bore gastric lavage tube.
C. Continue to provide full supportive care and adequate hydration while waiting for drug to be metabolized. In general, the drug is metabolized sufficiently rapidly so as not to warrant consideration of dialysis. However, if serum levels exceed 50 mcg/ml, charcoal hemoperfusion may be indicated.

Dosage and Administration: In chronic therapy, theophylline as found in Uniphyl Tablets is a treatment of first choice for the management of chronic asthma and other reversible obstructive pulmonary diseases to prevent and/or relieve symptoms and maintain patent airways.

Monitoring of clinical response and determining serum theophylline concentration is appropriate to guide dosing and minimize risk of toxicity due to overdosage. A serum level of 20 mcg/ml is an important safety reference point to reduce the possibility of toxicity.

There is considerable variation from patient to patient in the dosage required to achieve and maintain therapeutic and safe levels, primarily due to variable rates of elimination and the degree of bronchospasm present. Therefore, it is essential that dosage be individualized to the patients' clinical response and that serum levels be monitored before and after transfer to any sustained-release product.

Uniphyl, like other controlled-release theophylline products, is intended for patients with relatively continuous or recurring symptoms who have a need to maintain therapeutic serum levels of theophylline. It is not intended for patients experiencing an acute episode of bronchospasm (associated with asthma, chronic bronchitis or emphysema). Such patients require rapid relief of symptoms and should be treated with an immediate-release or intravenous theophylline preparation (or other bronchodilators) and not with controlled-release products.

Effective use of theophylline (i.e., the concentration of drug in the serum associated with optimal benefit and minimal risk of toxicity) is considered to occur when the theophylline concentration is maintained from 10 to 20 mcg/ml. The early studies from which these levels were derived were carried out in patients immediately after or shortly after recovery from acute exacerbations of their disease (some hospitalized with status asthmaticus).

Although the 20 mcg/ml level remains appropriate as a critical value (above which toxicity is more likely to occur) for safety purposes, additional data are now available which indicate that the serum theophylline concentrations required to produce maximum physiologic benefit may, in fact, fluctuate with the degree of bronchospasm present and are variable. Therefore, the physician should individualize the range appropriate to the patient's requirements, based on both symptomatic response and improvement in pulmonary function. It should be stressed that serum theophylline concentrations maintained at the upper level of the 10 to 20 mcg/ml range may be associated with potential toxicity when factors known to reduce theophylline clearance become operative. (See *Precautions* including *Drug Interactions*.)

Dosage guidelines are approximations only and the wide range of theophylline clearance between individuals (particularly those with concomitant disease) makes indiscriminate usage hazardous. Each patient should be titrated to establish the appropriate dosage, and serum theophylline levels used for any dosage adjustment after transfer to Uniphyl Tablets. As a practical consideration, it is not always possible to obtain serum level determinations. Under such conditions, restriction of the daily dose of Uniphyl Tablets (in otherwise healthy adults) to approximately 13 mg/kg/day (or up to 900 mg) will result in relatively few patients exceeding serum levels of 20 mcg/ml and the associated risk of toxicity.

Dosage Guidelines:
When appropriate, dosage should be calculated on the basis of lean body weight where mg/kg doses are to be prescribed since theophylline does not distribute into fatty tissue.

I *INITIATION OF THERAPY WITH UNIPHYL TABLETS*
a. *Stabilized Patients*
Individuals who are taking an immediate-release or controlled-release theophylline product may be transferred to twice-daily administration of 200 mg Uniphyl Tablets on a mg-for-mg basis. For example, a patient stablized on 400 mg twice daily (800 mg total daily dose) should be given two 200 mg Uniphyl Tablets q. 12 h.
It must be recognized that the peak and trough serum theophylline levels produced by the twice-daily dosing may vary from those produced by the previous product and/or regimen.
b. *Initiation of Theophylline Dosing*
Patients not currently receiving theophylline may be initiated on Uniphyl 200 mg Tablets as follows. THE AVERAGE INITIAL CHILDREN'S (15 TO 25 KG) DOSE IS ONE-HALF (100 MG) OF A UNIPHYL 200 MG TABLET q. 12 h.
THE AVERAGE INITIAL ADULT AND CHILDREN'S (OVER 25 KG) DOSE IS ONE UNIPHYL 200 MG TABLET q. 12 h.
If the desired response is not achieved with the above AVERAGE INITIAL DOSAGE recommendations, the dose may be adjusted as is described below.

II *TITRATION AND DOSE ADJUSTMENT*
a. *When Serum Levels Are Measured*
After 4 days therapy with Uniphyl Tablets, steady state should have been achieved, and peak serum theophylline concentration should be determined from blood samples obtained 8 to 12 hours after the morning dose. Trough concentration should be taken just prior to the administration of the next dose. It is important that the patient not have missed or added any dose during the previous 72 hours, and that the dosing intervals remain relatively constant. DOSAGE ADJUSTMENT BASED ON MEASUREMENTS WHEN THESE INSTRUCTIONS HAVE NOT BEEN FOLLOWED MAY RESULT IN TOXICITY.
Peak and trough theophylline serum concentration values allow: 1) maintaining the established dosage schedule if values are within the desired range and the dose is tolerated, 2) increasing the dose, or 3) decreasing the dose.
b. *When Serum Levels Are Not Measured*
In the absence of laboratory facilities for determining serum theophylline concentration levels, clinical judgment should be followed.
- The original total twice-daily dose should continue if it is well-tolerated and the clinical response is satisfactory.
- Minimal improvement with the initial dose usually requires increasing the dose as described below.
- If adverse reactions occur, decrease the dose as stated below.

c. *Increasing the Dose of Uniphyl Tablets*
If patient response with Uniphyl Tablets is unsatisfactory and/or the observed serum theophylline concentration range is too low, the dosage may be increased at recommended intervals as follows.

Serum Theophylline (mcg/ml)	Directions
7.5 to 10	Increase dose by about 25%* and recheck serum concentrations in 3 days
5 to 7.5	Increase dose by about 25% to the nearest dose increment and recheck serum theophylline for guidance in further dosage adjustment (another increase will probably be needed; but this provides a safety check).

d. *Decreasing the Dose of Uniphyl Tablets*
Serum theophylline values above 20 mcg/ml require decreasing the daily dose unless such dose is required to maintain the patient and is well-tolerated. Dosage may be reduced by adjustments as are described below. Peak and trough measurements should be taken 3 days after each decrease in dosage.

Serum Theophylline mcg/ml	Directions
20 to 25	Decrease dose by about 10%.*
25 to 30	Skip next dose and decrease subsequent doses by about 25%.
Over 30	Skip next 2 doses and decrease subsequent doses by 50%.

*Dividing the daily dose into 3 doses administered at 8-hour intervals may be indicated if symptoms occur repeatedly at the end of a dosing interval. Finer adjustments in dosage may be needed for some patients.

III *MAINTENANCE THERAPY*
Careful clinical titration is important to assure patient acceptance and safety of the medication. Patients when stabilized as established by serum theophylline concentration or respiratory function usually remain controlled without further dosage adjustment. It should be borne in mind, however, that for reasons stated in the Precautions and Warnings sections, dosage adjustments may be necessary. Serum theophylline levels should be measured periodically (at 6- to 12-month intervals) even in clincally controlled patients.
As with all sustained-release theophylline products, Uniphyl Tablets are for chronic or long-term use only and are not intended for initial treatment in a patient with acute symptoms.
Caution should be exercised for younger children who cannot complain of minor side effects. The elderly as well as patients with congestive heart failure, cor pulmonale, and/or liver disease may have unusually low dosage requirements and thus may experience toxicity even at the dosages recommended above.
It is important that no patient be maintained on any dosage that is not tolerated. In instructing patients to increase dosage according to the schedule above, they should be instructed not to take a subsequent dose if apparent side effects occur and to resume therapy at a lower dose once adverse effects have disappeared.
WARNING: DO NOT MAINTAIN ANY DOSE THAT IS NOT TOLERATED.
Caution: Federal law prohibits dispensing without prescription.
How Supplied: Uniphyl (theophylline, anhydrous) 200 mg scored Controlled-Release Tablets are supplied in white-opaque plastic bottles, containing 60 tablets or 240 tablets. Each round, white tablet bears the symbol PF on one side and is marked U200 on the other side.
Store tablets at controlled room temperature 15 to 30°C (59–86°F)
mfd. by The P.F. Laboratories, Inc., Totowa, N.J. 07512 for
THE PURDUE FREDERICK COMPANY, Norwalk, CT 06856, dist.
U.S. Patent Numbers 3965256 and 4235870
12-28-83   A 1494
Shown in Product Identification Section, page 427

UNIPHYL® Tablets   ℞
[ū'nĭ-fĭl]
(theophylline, anhydrous)
400 mg
UNICONTIN®
Controlled-Release System

Description: Uniphyl Tablets contain 400 mg anhydrous theophylline in a controlled-release system.
Theophylline anhydrous, a xanthine bronchodilator, is a white, odorless, crystalline powder having a bitter taste. Theophylline has a molecular weight of 180.18, represented by $C_7H_8N_4O_2$ and depicted as:

Clinical Pharmacology: Theophylline directly relaxes the smooth muscle of the bronchial airways and pulmonary blood vessels. The drug also produces other actions typical of the xanthine derivatives: coronary vasodilation, cardiac stimulation, diuresis, cerebral stimulation, and skeletal muscle stimulation. These actions may be mediated through inhibition of phosphodiesterase with a resultant increase in intracellular cyclic AMP.
In vitro, theophylline has been shown to act synergistically with beta agonists that increase intracellular cyclic AMP through the stimulation of adenyl cyclase; but synergism has not been demonstrated in patient studies. More data are needed to determine if theophylline and beta agonists have a clinically important additive effect *in vivo.*
Pharmacokinetics: A single-dose study in 15 normal male volunteers, whose theophylline inherent mean elimination half-life was verified by a liquid theophylline product to be 6.9 ± 2.5 (S.D.) hours were administered two or three 400 mg Uniphyl

Continued on next page

Purdue Frederick—Cont.

Tablets. Peak serum theophylline levels occurred at 6.9 ± 5.2 (S.D.) hours, with a normalized (to 800 mg) peak level being 6.2 ± 2.1 (S.D.). The apparent elimination half-life for the 400 mg Uniphyl Tablets was 17.2 ± 5.8 (S.D.) hours.

Steady-state pharmacokinetics were determined in a study in 12 patients with chronic reversible obstructive pulmonary disease. All were dosed with two 400 mg Uniphyl Tablets given once daily in the morning and a widely-used approved controlled-release B.I.D. product administered as two 200 mg tablets given 12 hours apart. The pharmacokinetic parameters obtained for Uniphyl Tablets given at doses of 800 mg once daily in the morning were virtually identical to the corresponding parameters for the reference drug when given as 400 mg B.I.D. In particular, the area-under-curve and highest and lowest mean serum theophylline levels, i.e., the AUC, Cmax and Cmin values, obtained in this study were as follows:

	Uniphyl Tablets 800 mg Q 24 h ± S.D.	Reference Drug 400 mg Q 12 h ± S.D.
AUC (0–24 hours). mcg·hr/ml	288.9 ± 21.5	283.5 ± 38.4
Cmax, mcg/ml	15.7 ± 2.8	15.2 ± 2.1
Cmin, mcg/ml	7.9 ± 1.6	7.8 ± 1.7
Cmax-Cmin diff.	7.7 ± 1.5	7.4 ± 1.5

Bioavailability was calculated to be $104 \pm 18\%$ (S.D.) for the 24-hour period with Uniphyl Tablets once daily as compared with the reference drug given twice daily, as shown above.

The AUC and Cmax are dose-dependent and will increase by upward dosage adjustment with Uniphyl Tablets. Patients who are fast theophylline metabolizers (clearance—greater than 5 L/hr) may not be suitable candidates for once-daily dosing. Those patients who are not well-maintained on recommended once-a-day therapy are likely to be better controlled when administered Uniphyl Tablets in divided doses.

The half-life of theophylline is prolonged in patients suffering from chronic alcoholism, impaired hepatic or renal function, congestive heart failure, and in patients receiving macrolide antibiotics and cimetidine. Older adults (over age 55) and patients with chronic obstructive pulmonary disease, with or without cor pulmonale, may also have slower clearance rates of theophylline with half-lives that exceed 24 hours. High fever for prolonged periods may reduce the rate of theophylline elimination. Newborns and neonates have extremely slow clearance rates compared to older infants (over 6 months) and children, and may also have a theophylline half-life of over 24 hours.

The half-life of theophylline in smokers averages 4 to 5 hours contrasted with 7 to 11 hours in nonsmokers. Following the cessation of smoking, the effects on theophylline pharmacokinetics may persist for 3 months to 2 years.

Theophylline Elimination Characteristics

	Theophylline Clearance Rates (mean ± S.D.)	Half-Life Average (mean ± S.D.)
Children (over 6 months of age)	1.45 ± 0.58 ml/kg/min	3.7 ± 1.1 hr.
Adult, nonsmokers with uncomplicated asthma	0.65 ± 0.19 ml/kg/min	8.7 ± 2.2 hr

Indications: Uniphyl Tablets are indicated for relief and/or prevention of symptoms of asthma and reversible bronchospasm associated with chronic bronchitis and emphysema.

Contraindications: This product is contraindicated in individuals who have shown hypersensitivity to theophylline.

Warnings: Status asthmaticus should be considered a medical emergency and is defined as that degree of bronchospasm which is not rapidly responsive to usual doses of conventional bronchodilators. Optimal therapy for such patients frequently requires both *additional medication*, parenterally administered, and *close monitoring*, preferably in an intensive-care setting.

Excessive theophylline doses may be associated with toxicity. Determination of serum theophylline levels is recommended to assure maximum therapeutic benefit without excessive risk. The incidence of toxicity increases at serum levels greater than 20 mcg/ml.

Optimum therapeutic response occurs in most patients when the serum theophylline concentration is 10 to 20 mcg/ml. In other patients satisfactory results (as determined by both relief of symptoms and improvement in pulmonary function) may be obtained at lower levels. In still others, adequate response may require higher levels. The physician should adjust the desired serum concentration range to the patients' requirements, keeping in mind that *an increased probability of toxicity exists when levels exceed 20 mcg/ml*. Therefore, in order to assure maximum benefit without excessive risk, measurement of serum levels is highly recommended.

Reduced theophylline clearance may result in increased serum levels and potential toxicity in the following patient groups: (1) those with impaired renal or liver function, (2) those over 55 years of age, particularly males and those with chronic lung disease, (3) those with cardiac failure, (4) those receiving macrolide antibiotics or cimetidine, and (5) neonates. Decreased theophylline clearance may occur during active influenza infection or following immunization for influenza.

Less serious signs of theophylline toxicity, i.e. nausea and restlessness, may appear. Serious side effects such as ventricular arrhythmias, convulsions or even death may appear as the first sign of toxicity without any previous warning. *Serious toxicity is not reliably preceded by less severe side effects.*

Patients who require theophylline may exhibit tachycardia due to their underlying disease. The possible relationship of elevated serum theophylline concentration to tachycardia may not be recognized.

Theophylline products may cause arrhythmia and/or worsen pre-existing arrhythmia. Any significant change in rate and/or rhythm warrants monitoring and further investigation.

Precautions

General: Use with caution in patients with severe cardiac disease, severe hypoxemia, hypertension, hyperthyroidism, acute myocardial injury, cor pulmonale, liver disease, in the elderly (especially males) and in neonates. Particular caution should be used in giving theophylline to patients with congestive heart failure. Frequently, such patients have markedly prolonged theophylline serum levels with theophylline persisting in serum for long periods following discontinuation of the drug. Caution should be exercised in patients concurrently receiving other xanthine medications.

Some patients who are rapid metabolizers of theophylline, such as the young, smokers and some nonsmoking adults, may not be suitable candidates for once daily dosing. Dividing the total daily dose into two doses may be indicated for these patients, who may exhibit symptoms of bronchospasm repeatedly, especially near the end of an 24-hour dosing interval. Also, such individuals may have wider peak-to-trough differences than desired.

Theophylline half-life is shorter in smokers than in non-smokers. Therefore, smokers may require larger or more frequent doses.

Use theophylline cautiously in patients with history of peptic ulcer. Theophylline may occasionally act as a local irritant to the G.I. tract although gastrointestinal symptoms are more commonly centrally mediated and associated with serum drug concentrations over 20 mcg/ml.

Information for Patients: The physician should reinforce the importance of taking only the prescribed dose and observing the time interval between doses. All patients should be asked to report side effects which occur at any time, or recurrence of symptoms, especially toward the end of a 24-hour dosing interval. Uniphyl Tablets are to be taken whole, and are not to be broken, chewed or crushed.

Drug Interactions: Toxic synergism with ephedrine has been documented and may occur with other sympathomimetic bronchodilators. Concomitant administration of theophylline with cimetidine, troleandomycin or erythromycin may lead to higher serum theophylline levels. Theophylline may increase the excretion of lithium carbonate and antagonize the effects of propranolol.

Drug-Laboratory Test Interactions: When plasma levels of theophylline are measured by spectrophotometric methods, coffee, tea, cola beverages, chocolate and acetaminophen contribute to falsely high values.

Carcinogenesis, Mutagenesis, and Impairment of Fertility: Long-term animal studies have not been performed to evaluate the carcinogenic potential, mutagenic potential or the effect on fertility of xanthine compounds.

Pregnancy: Category C—Animal reproduction studies have not been conducted with theophylline. It is not known whether theophylline can cause fetal harm when administered to a pregnant woman or can effect reproduction capacity. Xanthine should be given to a pregnant woman only if clearly needed.

Nursing Mothers: It has been reported that theophylline distributes readily into breast milk and may cause adverse effects in the infant. Caution must be used when prescribing xanthines to a mother who is nursing, taking into account the risk-benefit of this therapy.

Pediatric Use: Safety and effectiveness in children under 12 years of age have not been established with 400 mg Uniphyl Tablets.

Adverse Reactions: The most consistent adverse reactions are usually due to overdose and are:

1. *Gastrointestinal:* nausea, vomiting, epigastric pain, hematemesis, diarrhea.
2. *Central Nervous System:* headaches, irritability, restlessness, insomnia, reflex hyperexcitability, muscle twitching, clonic and tonic generalized convulsions.
3. *Cardiovascular:* palpitation, tachycardia, extrasystole, flushing, hypotension, circulatory failure, ventricular arrhythmia.
4. *Respiratory:* tachypnea.
5. *Renal:* albuminuria, microhematuria, potentiation of diuresis.
6. *Others:* hyperglycemia, inappropriate ADH syndrome, rash.

Overdosage:

Management: If potential oral overdose is established and seizure has not occurred:

A. Induce vomiting. **B.** Administer a cathartic. This is particularly important with sustained-release drugs. **C.** Administer activated charcoal. If patient is having a seizure:

A. Establish an airway. **B.** Administer oxygen. **C.** Treat the seizure with intravenous diazepam, 0.1 to 0.3 mg/kg up to 10 mg. **D.** Monitor vital signs, maintain blood presure and provide adequate hydration.

Post Seizure Coma:

A. Maintain airway and oxygenation. **B.** If a result of oral medication, follow above recommendations to prevent absorption of the drug, but intubation and lavage will have to be performed instead of inducing emesis, and the cathartic and charcoal will need to be introduced via a large bore gastric lavage tube. **C.** Continue to provide full supportive care and adequate hydration while waiting for drug to be metabolized. In general, the drug is metabolized sufficiently rapidly so as not to warrant consideration of dialysis. However, if serum levels

Product Information

exceed 50 mcg/ml, charcoal hemoperfusion may be indicated.

Dosage and Administration: In chronic therapy, theophylline as found in Uniphyl Tablets is a treatment of first choice for the management of chronic asthma and other reversible obstructive pulmonary diseases to prevent and/or relieve symptoms and maintain patent airways.

Monitoring of clinical response and determining serum theophylline concentration is appropriate to guide dosing and minimize risk of toxicity due to overdosing. A serum level of 20 mcg/ml is an important safety reference point to reduce the possibility of toxicity.

There is considerable variation from patient to patient in the dosage required to achieve and maintain therapeutic and safe levels, primarily due to variable rates of elimination and the degree of bronchospasm present. Therefore, it is essential that dosage be individualized to the patient's clinical response and that serum levels be monitored before and after transfer to any sustained-release product.

Uniphyl, like other controlled-release theophylline products, is intended for patients with relatively continuous or recurring symptoms who have a need to maintain therapeutic serum levels of theophylline. It is not intended for patients experiencing an acute episode of bronchospasm (associated with asthma, chronic bronchitis, or emphysema). Such patients require rapid relief of symptoms and should be treated with an immediate-release or intravenous theophylline preparation (or other bronchodilators) and not with controlled-release products.

Until additional data are available to evaluate the rate of absorption and/or clearance rates of theophylline from controlled-release dosage forms administered at night, it is not recommended that Uniphyl Tablets be administered at night when used on a once-daily schedule.

Effective use of theophylline (i.e., the concentration of drug in the serum associated with optimal benefit and minimal risk of toxicity) is considered to occur when the theophylline concentration is maintained from 10 to 20 mcg/ml. The early studies from which these levels were derived were carried out in patients immediately after or shortly after recovery from acute exacerbations of their disease (some hospitalized with status asthmaticus). Although the 20 mcg/ml level remains appropriate as a critical value (above which toxicity is more likely to occur) for safety purposes, additional data are now available which indicate that the serum theophylline concentrations required to produce maximum physiologic benefit may, in fact, fluctuate with the degree of bronchospasm present and are variable. Therefore, the physician should individualize the range appropriate to the patient's requirements, based on both symptomatic response and improvement in pulmonary function. It should be stressed that serum theophylline concentrations maintained at the upper level of the 10 to 20 mcg/ml range may be associated with potential toxicity when factors known to reduce theophylline clearance become operative. (See *Precautions,* including *Drug Interactions.*)

Uniphyl Tablets taken once daily in the morning at the recommended dosage may provide the required bronchodilation of patients who clear theophylline normally or relatively slowly, e.g. non-smokers. However, certain patients, such as the young, smokers and some non-smoking adults are likely to metabolize theophylline more rapidly and *may require dosing at 12-hour intervals.* Such patients may experience symptoms of bronchospasm toward the end of a once-daily dosing interval and/or require a high daily dose (higher than those recommended in labeling) and are more likely to experience relatively wide peak trough differences in serum theophylline concentrations.

Dosage guidelines are approximations only and the wide range of theophylline clearance between individuals (particularly those with concomitant disease) makes indiscriminate usage hazardous. Each patient should be titrated to establish the appropriate dosage, and serum theophylline levels used for any dosage adjustment after transfer to Uniphyl Tablets, especially on a once-a-day A.M. schedule. As a practical consideration, it is not always possible to obtain serum level determinations. Under such conditions, restriction of the daily dose of Uniphyl Tablets (in otherwise healthy adults), to approximately 13 mg/kg/day (or up to 900 mg) will result in relatively few patients exceeding serum levels of 20 mcg/ml and the associated risk of toxicity.

Dosage Guidelines:
Until additional bioavailability data are available, it is recommended that Uniphyl be taken as intact tablets only. When appropriate, dosage should be calculated on the basis of lean body weight where mg/kg doses are to be prescribed since theophylline does not distribute into fatty tissue.

I INITIATION OF THERAPY WITH UNIPHYL TABLETS

a. *Stabilized Patients* (12 years of age or older) Individuals who are taking an immediate-release or controlled-release theophylline product may be transferred to once-daily administration of 400 mg Uniphyl Tablets on a mg-for-mg basis. For example, a patient stabilized on 400 mg twice daily (800 mg total daily dose) should be given two 400 mg Uniphyl Tablets as a *single* A.M. daily dose of 800 mg.

It must be recognized that the peak and trough serum theophylline levels produced by the once-daily dosing may vary from those produced by the previous product and/or regimen.

b. *Initiation of Theophylline Dosing*
Adult patients and children 12 years of age and over not currently receiving theophylline may be titrated using an immediate- or sustained-release theophylline product, which can be adjusted in small dosage increments. Patients titrated to a total daily dose appproximating 400, 800, or 1200 mg, may be transferred to once-daily dosage with equivalent doses of 400 mg Uniphyl Tablets, as is described in (a) above.

II TITRATION AND DOSE ADJUSTMENT
a. *When Serum Levels Are Measured*
After 4 days therapy with Uniphyl Tablets, steady-state should have been achieved, and peak serum theophylline concentration should be determined from blood samples obtained 8 to 12 hours after the morning dose. Trough concentration should be taken just prior to the administration of the next dose. It is important that the patient not have missed or added any dose during the previous 72 hours, and that the dosing intervals remain relatively constant. DOSAGE ADJUSTMENT BASED ON MEASUREMENTS WHEN THESE INSTRUCTIONS HAVE NOT BEEN FOLLOWED MAY RESULT IN TOXICITY.
Peak and trough theophylline serum concentration values allow: 1) maintaining the established dosage schedule if values are within the desired range and the dose is tolerated, 2) increasing the dose, or 3) decreasing the dose.

b. *When Serum Levels Are Not Measured*
In the absence of laboratory facilities for determining serum theophylline concentration levels, clinical judgment should be followed.

- The original total once-daily dose should continue if it is well-tolerated and the clinical response is satisfactory.
- If adverse reactions occur, decrease the dose as stated below.
  If a patient is better controlled on another regimen than on a once-daily regimen, the patient should be maintained on the more effective regimen.

c. *Increasing the Dose of Uniphyl Tablets*
If patient response with Uniphyl Tablets is unsatisfactory and/or the observed serum theophylline concentration range is too low, the patient should be transferred to an immediate or controlled release (b.i.d.) theophylline schedule and dosage increased at recommended intervals as follows:

Serum Theophylline (mcg/ml)	Directions
7.5 to 10	Increase dose by about 25%* and recheck serum concentrations in 3 days.
5 to 7.5	Increase dose by about 25% to the nearest dose increment and recheck serum theophylline for guidance in further dosage adjustment (another increase will probably be needed, but this provides a safety check).

Patients titrated to a total daily dosage of 800 mg or 1200 mg on a twice-daily schedule, can be transferred to equivalent doses of once-daily A.M. dosing, using 400 mg Uniphyl Tablets.

d. *Decreasing the Dose of Uniphyl Tablets*
Serum theophylline values above 20 mcg/ml require decreasing the daily dose unless such dose is required to maintain the patient and is well-tolerated. Dosage may be reduced by transferring the patient to an immediate or controlled release (b.i.d.) theophylline product and making adjustments. Peak and trough measurements should be taken 3 days after each decrease in dosage.

Serum Theophylline (mcg/ml)	Directions
20 to 25	Decrease dose by about 10%.*
25 to 30	Skip next dose and decrease subsequent doses by about 25%.
Over 30	Skip next 2 doses and decrease subsequent doses by 50%.

* Dividing the daily dose into 3 doses administered at 8-hour intervals may be indicated if symptoms occur repeatedly at the end of a dosing interval.
Finer adjustments in dosage may be needed for some patients.

III MAINTENANCE THERAPY
Careful clinical titration is important to assure patient acceptance and safety of the medication. Patients when stabilized as established by serum theophylline concentration or respiratory function usually remain controlled without further dosage adjustment. It should be borne in mind, however, that for reasons stated in the Precautions and Warnings sections, dosage adjustments may be necessary. Serum theophylline levels should be measured periodically (at 6- to 12-month intervals) even in clinically controlled patients.
As with all sustained-release theophylline products, Uniphyl Tablets are for chronic or long-term use only and are not intended for initial treatment in a patient with acute symptoms.
Caution should be exercised for younger children who cannot complain of minor side effects. The elderly as well as patients with congestive heart failure, cor pulmonale, and/or liver disease may have unusually low dosage requirements and thus may experience toxicity even at the dosages recommended above.
It is important that no patient be maintained on any dosage that is not tolerated. In instructing patients to increase dosage according to the schedule above, they should be instructed not to take a subsequent dose if apparent side effects occur and to resume therapy at a lower dose once adverse effects have disappeared.
WARNING: *DO NOT MAINTAIN ANY DOSE THAT IS NOT TOLERATED.*
Caution: Federal law prohibits dispensing without prescription.
How Supplied: Uniphyl (theophylline, anhydrous) 400 mg scored Controlled-Release Tablets are supplied in white-opaque plastic bottles, containing 60 tablets or 240 tablets. Each round, white tablet bears the symbol PF on one side and is marked U400 on the other side.
Store tablets at controlled room temperature 15 to 30°C (59–86°F).

Continued on next page

Purdue Frederick—Cont.

mfd. by The P.F. Laboratories, Inc., Totowa, N.J. 07512 for
THE PURDUE FREDERICK COMPANY, Norwalk, CT 06856, dist.
U.S. Patent Numbers 3965256 and 4235870
12-22-83   B1374
Shown in Product Identification Section, page 427

RAM Laboratories Corp.
P. O. BOX 559071
MIAMI, FL 33255

ALGISIN Capsules   ℞
(chlorzoxazone 250 mg. + acetaminophen 300 mg.)

Supplied: Bottles of 60 capsules.

APETIL Liquid   ℞
(Therapeutic Vitamins–Minerals)

Supplied: Bottles 8 ounces.

DIGEPEPSIN   ℞
Enteric coated digestant tablets
(pepsin 250 mg. + pancreatin 300 mg. + bile salts 150 mg.)

Supplied: Bottles of 60 tablets.

GEROTON FORTE   OTC
Supplement—Stimulant tonic

Supplied: Bottles of 1 pint.

OTISAN Drops   ℞
Otic solution

Supplied: 10 ml. plastic dropper.

PASMOL Tablets   ℞
(Ethaverine Hydrochloride 100 mg.)

Supplied: Bottles 30 scored tablets.

ZINCVIT Capsules   ℞
Multivitamin and Multimineral Formula with 1 mg. folic acid and 120 mg. Zinc

Supplied: Bottles 60 capsules.

Reed & Carnrick
1 NEW ENGLAND AVENUE
PISCATAWAY, NJ 08854

ALPHOSYL®
Lotion, Cream

Description: Special crude coal tar extract 5.0% and allantoin 1.7% in synergistic combination in a greaseless, stainless vanishing cream base.
Actions: In the treatment of psoriasis and other chronic dermatoses with itching, scaling and erythema.
Precautions: ALPHOSYL is safe for use as directed. However, if irritation and/or redness occurs, discontinue use and consult physician. Alphosyl is for external use only; avoid contact with the eyes.
Directions for use: SHAKE WELL BEFORE USING.
1.) Apply ALPHOSYL Lotion to affected areas two to four times daily, morning and night, massaging thoroughly into the lesions.
2.) For persistent, long term cases, with heavy scaling and crusting, a hot daily bath is recommended to soften and facilitate removal of scales, prior to applying ALPHOSYL Lotion.
3.) MAINTENANCE THERAPY: Once the condition is under control, ALPHOSYL Lotion should be applied 2 to 3 times weekly to help prevent recurrence. Treatments may be repeated as directed by physician.

How Supplied: ALPHOSYL Lotion 8 fl. oz.; ALPHOSYL Cream 2 oz. tube.

CORTIFOAM®   ℞
(hydrocortisone acetate) 10%

Description: Contains hydrocortisone acetate 10% as the sole active ingredient in 20 g of a foam containing propylene glycol, emulsifying wax, steareth-10, cetyl alcohol, methylparaben and propylparaben, trolamine, water and inert propellants, dichlorodifluoromethane and dichlorotetrafluoroethane.
Each application delivers approximately 900 mg of foam containing 80 mg of hydrocortisone (90 mg of hydrocortisone acetate).
Clinical Pharmacology: CORTIFOAM provides effective topical administration of an anti-inflammatory corticosteroid as adjunctive therapy of ulcerative proctitis.
Indications: CORTIFOAM is indicated as adjunctive therapy in the topical treatment of ulcerative proctitis of the distal portion of the rectum in patients who cannot retain hydrocortisone or other corticosteroid enemas. Direct observations of methylene blue-containing foam have shown staining about 10 centimeters into the rectum.
Contraindications: Local contraindications to the use of intrarectal steroids include obstruction, abscess, perforation, peritonitis, fresh intestinal anastomoses, extensive fistulas and sinus tracts. Tuberculosis (active, latent or questionably healed), ocular herpes simplex and acute psychosis are usually considered absolute contraindications to the use of corticosteroids. Relative contraindications include active peptic ulcer, acute glomerulonephritis, myasthenia gravis, osteoporosis, diverticulitis, thrombophlebitis, psychic disturbances, pregnancy, diabetes, hyperthyroidism, acute coronary disease, hypertension, limited cardiac reserve, and local or systemic infections, including fungal or exanthematous diseases. Where these conditions exist, the expected benefits from steroid therapy must be weighed against the risks involved in its use. Pregnancy is a relative contraindication to corticosteroids, particularly during third trimester. If corticosteroids must be administered in pregnancy, watch newborn infant closely for signs of hypoadrenalism, and administer appropriate therapy if needed.
Warning: Do not insert any part of the aerosol container into the anus. Contents of the container are under pressure, but not flammable. Do not burn or puncture the aerosol container. Store at room temperature but not over 120° F. Because CORTIFOAM is not expelled, systemic hydrocortisone absorption may be greater from CORTIFOAM than from corticosteroid enema formulations. If there is no evidence of clinical or proctologic improvement within two or three weeks after starting CORTIFOAM therapy, or if the patient's condition worsens, discontinue the drug.
Precautions: Steroid therapy should be administered with caution in patients with severe ulcerative disease because these patients are predisposed to perforation of the bowel wall. Where surgery is imminent, it is hazardous to wait more than a few days for a satisfactory response to medical treatment. General precautions common to all corticosteroid therapy should be observed during treatment with CORTIFOAM. These include gradual withdrawal of therapy to allow for possible adrenal insufficiency and awareness to possible growth suppression in children. Patients should be kept under close observation, for, as with all drugs, rare individuals may react unfavorably under certain conditions. If severe reactions or idiosyncrasies occur, steroids should be discontinued immediately and appropriate measures instituted. Do not employ in immediate or early postoperative period following ileorectostomy.
Adverse Reactions: Corticosteroid therapy may produce side effects which include moon face, fluid retention, excessive appetite and weight gain, abnormal fat deposits, mental symptoms, hypertrichosis, acne, ecchymosis, increased sweating, pigmentation, dry scaly skin, thinning scalp hair, thrombophlebitis, decreased resistance to infection, negative nitrogen balance with delayed bone and wound healing, menstrual disorders, neuropathy, peptic ulcer, decreased glucose tolerance, hypopotassemia, adrenal insufficiency, necrotizing angiitis, hypertension, pancreatitis and increased intraocular pressure. In children, suppression of growth may occur. Increased intracranial pressure may occur and possibly account for headache, insomnia and fatigue. Subcapsular cataracts may result from prolonged usage. Long-term use of all corticosteroids results in catabolic effects characterized by negative protein and calcium balance. Osteoporosis, spontaneous fractures and aseptic necrosis of the hip and humerus may occur as part of this catabolic phenomenon. Where hypopotassemia and other symptoms associated with fluid and electrolyte imbalance call for potassium supplementation and salt poor or salt-free diets, these may be instituted and are compatible with diet requirements for ulcerative proctitis.
Administration and Dosage: Usual dose is one applicatorful once or twice daily for two or three weeks, and every second day thereafter, administered rectally. The patient directions packaged with the applicator describe how to use the aerosol container and applicator. Satisfactory response usually occurs within five to seven days marked by a decrease in symptoms. Symptomatic improvement in ulcerative proctitis should not be used as the sole criterion for evaluating efficacy. Sigmoidoscopy is also recommended to judge dosage adjustment, duration of therapy and rate of improvement.
Directions For Use:
1. Shake foam container vigorously for 5–10 seconds. <u>Do not remove cap.</u>
2. Withdraw applicator plunger past the fill line until it stops.
3. Place foam container upright on level surface, insert tip of cap into tip of applicator.
To fill applicator:
- Depress cap on foam container-RELEASE.
- Pause, a few seconds, allowing foam to enter and expand in applicator barrel.
- Repeat until foam rises to fill applicator to <u>Fill Line.</u>
4. Hold applicator by barrel and gently insert tip into anus. Once in place, push plunger to expel foam, then withdraw applicator.
Note: Pull applicator apart and wash thoroughly with warm water.
How Supplied: CORTIFOAM is supplied in an aerosol container with a special rectal applicator. Each applicator delivers approximately 900 mg of foam containing approximately 80 mg of hydrocortisone as 90 mg of hydrocortisone acetate. When used correctly the aerosol container will deliver a minimum of 14 applications.
Literature Available: Patient information available on request.
Shown in Product Identification Section, page 427

DILATRATE®-SR   ℞
[*dī' lă-trāt*]
(Isosorbide Dinitrate)
Sustained Release Capsules
40 mg

Description: Isosorbide dinitrate, an organic nitrate, is a vasodilator with effects on both arteries and veins. Isosorbide dinitrate is available as a 40 mg sustained release capsule. The chemical name for isosorbide dinitrate is 1,4,3,6-dianhydrosorbitol-2, 5-dinitrate and, the compound has the following structural formula:

Molecular Weight: 236.14
Isosorbide dinitrate is a white, crystalline, odorless compound which is stable in air and in solution,

has a melting point of 70°C and has an optical rotation of +134° (c=1.0, alcohol, 20°C). Isosorbide dinitrate is freely soluble in organic solvents such as acetone, alcohol, and ether, but is only sparingly soluble in water.

Clinical Pharmacology: The principal pharmacological action of isosorbide dinitrate is relaxation of vascular smooth muscle, producing a vasodilatory effect on both peripheral arteries and veins, with predominant effects on the latter. Dilation of the post-capillary vessels, including large veins, promotes peripheral pooling of blood and decreases venous return to the heart, thereby reducing left-ventricular end-diastolic pressure (preload). Arteriolar relaxation reduces systemic vascular resistance and arterial pressure (after-load). The mechanism by which isosorbide dinitrate relieves angina pectoris is not fully understood. Myocardial oxygen consumption or demand (as measured by the pressure-rate product, tension-time index, and stroke work index) is decreased by both the arterial and venous effects of isosorbide dinitrate and, presumably, a more favorable supply-demand ratio is achieved. While the large epicardial coronary arteries are also dilated by isosorbide dinitrate, the extent to which this contributes to relief of exertional angina is unclear.

Therapeutic doses of isosorbide dinitrate may reduce systolic, diastolic, and mean arterial blood pressures, especially in the upright posture. Effective coronary perfusion is usually maintained. The decrease in systemic blood pressure may result in reflex tachycardia, an effect which results in an unfavorable influence on myocardial oxygen demand. Hemodynamic studies indicate that isosorbide dinitrate may reduce the abnormally elevated left ventricular end-diastolic and pulmonary capillary wedge pressures that occur during an acute episode of angina pectoris.

Isosorbide dinitrate is metabolized by enzymatic denitration to the intermediate products isosorbide-2-mononitrate and isosorbide-5-mononitrate. Both metabolites have biological activity, especially the 5-mononitrate which is also the principal metabolite. The liver is a principal site of metabolism and isosorbide dinitrate is subject to a large first pass effect. The systemic clearance of the drug following intravenous infusion is about 3.4 liters/min. Since the clearance exceeds hepatic blood flow, considerable extra hepatic metabolism must also occur.

The average bioavailability of isosorbide dinitrate is 59 and 22 percent following sublingual and oral administration, respectively. The terminal half-life is about 20 minutes, 60 minutes, and 4 hours following IV, sublingual, and oral administration, respectively. The dependence of half-life on the route of administration is not understood. Over limited ranges of IV dosing, the pharmacokinetics of isosorbide dinitrate appear linear. However, both the 2- and 5-mononitrate metabolites have been shown to decrease the rate of disappearance of the dinitrate from the blood and the half-lives of isosorbide-5-mononitrate and isosorbide-2-mononitrate range from 4.0–5.6 and 1.5–3.1 hours, respectively.

The pharmacokinetics and/or bioavailability of isosorbide dinitrate during multiple dosing have not been well-studied. Because the metabolites influence the clearance of isosorbide dinitrate, prediction of blood levels of parent compound or metabolites from single-dose studies is uncertain.

Indications and Usage: Isosorbide dinitrate is indicated for the treatment and prevention of angina pectoris. Controlled clinical trials have demonstrated that the sublingual, chewable, immediate release, and controlled-release oral dosage forms of isosorbide dinitrate are effective in improving exercise tolerance in patients with angina pectoris. When single sublingual or chewable doses (5mg) of isosorbide dinitrate were administered prophylactically to patients with angina pectoris in various clinical studies, duration of exercise until chest pain or fatigue was significantly improved for at least 45 minutes (and as long as 2 hours in some studies) following dosing. Similar studies after single oral (15 to 120 mg) and oral controlled-released (40 to 80 mg) doses of isosorbide dinitrate have shown significant improvement in exercise tolerance for up to 8 hours following dosing. The exercise electrocardiographic evidence suggests that improved exercise tolerance with isosorbide dinitrate is not at the expense of greater myocardial ischemia. All dosage forms of isosorbide dinitrate may therefore be used prophylactically to decrease frequency and severity of anginal attacks and can be expected to decrease the need for sublingual nitroglycerin.

The sublingual and chewable forms of the drug are indicated for acute prophylaxis of angina pectoris when taken a few minutes before situations likely to provoke anginal attacks. Because of a slower onset of effect, the oral forms of isosorbide dinitrate are not indicated for acute prophylaxis.

In controlled clinical trials chewable and sublingual isosorbide dinitrate were effective in relieving an acute attack of angina pectoris. Relief occurred with a mean time of 2.9 and 3.4 minutes (chewable and sublingual respectively) compared to relief of angina with a mean time of 1.9 minutes following sublingual nitroglycerin. Because of the more rapid relief of chest pain with sublingual nitroglycerin, the use of sublingual or chewable isosorbide dinitrate for aborting an acute anginal attack should be limited to patients intolerant or unresponsive to sublingual nitroglycerin.

Contraindications: Isosorbide dinitrate is contraindicated in patients who have shown purported hypersensitivity or idiosyncrasy to it or other nitrates or nitrites.

Warnings: The benefits of isosorbide dinitrate during the early days of an acute myocardial infarction have not been established. If one elects to use organic nitrates in early infarction hemodynamic monitoring and frequent clinical assessment should be used because of the potential deleterious effects of hypotension.

Precautions:

General: Severe hypotensive response, particularly with upright posture, may occur with even small doses of isosorbide dinitrate. The drug should therefore be used with caution in subjects who may have blood volume depletion from diuretic therapy or in subjects who have low systolic blood pressure (e.g., below 90 mm Hg). Paradoxical bradycardia and increased angina pectoris may accompany nitrate-induced hypotension.

Nitrate therapy may aggravate the angina caused by hypertrophic cardiomyopathy. Tolerance to this drug and cross-tolerance to other nitrates and nitrites may occur.

Marked symptomatic, orthostatic hypotension has been reported when calcium channel blockers and organic nitrates were used in combination. Dose adjustment of either class of agents may be necessary.

Tolerance to the vascular and antianginal effects of isosorbide dinitrate or nitroglycerin has been demonstrated in clinical trials, experience through occupational exposure, and in isolated tissue experiments in the laboratory. The importance of tolerance to the appropriate use of isosorbide dinitrate in the management of patients with angina pectoris has not been determined. However, one clinical trial using treadmill exercise tolerance (as an endpoint) found an 8 hour duration of action of oral isosorbide dinitrate following the first dose (after a 2 week placebo washout) and only a 2 hour duration of effect of the same dose after 1 week of repetitive dosing a conventional dosing intervals. On the other hand, several trials have been able to differentiate isosorbide dinitrate from placebo after 4 weeks of therapy, and in open trials an effect seems detectable for as long as several months.

Tolerance clearly occurs in industrial workers continuously exposed to nitroglycerin. Moreover, physical dependence also occurs since chest pain, acute myocardial infarction, and even sudden death have occurred during temporary withdrawal of nitroglycerin from the workers. In clinical trials in angina patients, there are reports of anginal attacks being more easily provoked and of rebound in the hemodynamic effects soon after nitrate withdrawal. The relative importance of these observations to the routine, clinical use of isosorbide dinitrate is not known. However, it seems prudent to gradually withdraw patients from isosorbide dinitrate when the therapy is being terminated, rather than stopping the drug abruptly.

Information for Patients: Headache may occur during initial therapy with isosorbide dinitrate. Headache is usually relieved by the use of standard headache remedies, or by lowering the dose, and tends to disappear after the first week or two of use.

Drug Interactions: Alcohol may enhance any marked sensitivity to the hypotensive effect of nitrates. Isosorbide dinitrate acts directly on vascular smooth muscle; therefore, any other agent that depends on vascular smooth muscle as the final common path can be expected to have decreased or increased effect depending on the agent.

Carcinogenesis, Mutagenesis, Impairment of Fertility: No long-term studies in animals have been performed to evaluate the carcinogenic potential of this drug. A modified two-litter reproduction study in rats fed isosorbide dinitrate at 25 or 100 mg/kg/day did not reveal any effects on fertility or gestation or any remarkable growth pathology in any parent or offspring fed isosorbide dinitrate as compared with rats fed a basal controlled diet.

Pregnancy Category C: Isosorbide dinitrate has been shown to cause a dose-related increase in embryotoxicity (increase in mummified pups) in rabbits at oral doses 35 and 150 times the maximum recommended human daily dose.

There are no adequate and well-controlled studies in pregnant women. Isosorbide dinitrate should be used during pregnancy only if the potential benefit justifies the potential risk to the fetus.

Nursing Mothers: It is not known whether this drug is excreted in human milk. Because many drugs are excreted in human milk, caution should be exercised when isosorbide dinitrate is administered to a nursing woman.

Pediatric Use: The safety and effectiveness of isosorbide dinitrate in children has not been established.

Adverse Reactions: Adverse reactions, particularly headache and hypotension, are dose related. In clinical trials at various doses, the following have been observed.

Headache is the most common (reported incidence varies widely, apparently being dose related, with an average occurrence of about 25%) adverse reaction and may be severe and persistent. Cutaneous vasodilation wth flushing may occur. Transient episodes of dizziness and weakness, as well as other signs of cerebral ischemia associated with postural hypotension, may occasionally develop (the incidence of reported symptomatic hypotension ranges from 2% to 36%). An occasional individual will exhibit marked sensitivity to the hypotensive effects of nitrates and severe responses (nausea, vomiting, weakness, restlessness, pallor, perspiration, and collapse) may occur even with the usual therapeutic dose. Drug rash and/or exfoliative dermatitis may occasionally occur. Nausea and vomiting appear to be uncommon.

Overdosage:

Signs and Symptoms: These may include the following: a prompt fall in blood pressure, persistent and throbbing headache, vertigo, palpitation, visual disturbances, flushed and perspiring skin (later becoming cold and cyanotic), nausea and vomiting (possibly with colic and even bloody diarrhea), syncope (especially in the upright position), methemoglobinemia with cyanosis and anoxia, initial hyperpnea, dyspnea and slow breathing, slow pulse (dicrotic and intermittent), heart block, increased intracranial pressure with cerebral symptoms of confusion and moderate fever, paralysis and coma followed by clonic convulsions and possibly death due to circulatory collapse.

It is not known what dose of the drug is associated with symptoms of overdosing or what dose of the drug would be life-threatening. The acute oral LD50 of isosorbide dinitrate in rats was found to be approximately 1100 mg/kg of body weight. These

Continued on next page

Reed & Carnrick—Cont.

animal experiments indicate that approximately 500 times the usual therapeutic dose would be required to produce such toxic symptoms in humans. It is not known whether the drug is dialyzable.

Treatment of Overdosage: Prompt removal of the ingested material by gastric lavage is reasonable but not documented to be useful. Keep the patient recumbent in a shock position and comfortably warm. Passive movements of the extremities may aid venous return. Administer oxygen and artificial respiration if necessary. If methemoglobinemia is present, administer methylene blue (1% solution), 1 to 2 mg/kg intravenously.

Methemoglobin: Case reports of clinically significant methemoglobinemia are rare at conventional doses of organic nitrates. The formation of methemoglobin is dose related and in the case of genetic abnormalities of hemoglobin that favor methemoglobin formulation, even conventional doses of organic nitrate could produce harmful concentrations of methemoglobin.

Warning: Epinephrine is ineffective in reversing the severe hypotensive events associated with overdose. It and related compounds are contraindicated in this situation.

Dosage and Administration: For the treatment of angina pectoris the usual starting dose for sublingual isosorbide dinitrate is 2.5 to 5 mg; for chewable tablets, 5 mg; for oral (swallowed) tablets, 5 to 20 mg; and for controlled released forms, 40 mg.

Isosorbide dinitrate should be titrated upward until angina is relieved or side effects limit the dose. In ambulatory patients, the magnitude of the incremental dose increase should be guided by measurements of standing blood pressure.

The initial dosage of sublingual or chewable isosorbide dinitrate for prophylactic therapy in angina pectoris patients is generally 5 to 10 mg every 2 to 3 hours. Adequate, controlled clinical studies demonstrating the effectiveness of chronic maintenance therapy with these dosage forms have not been reported.

Isosorbide dinitrate in oral doses of 10 to 40 mg given every 6 hours (in oral controlled release doses of 40 to 80 mg given every 8 to 12 hours) is generally recommended. The extent to which development of tolerance should modify the dosage program has not been defined. The oral controlled release forms of isosorbide dinitrate should not be chewed.

How Supplied: Bottles of 100 (flesh cap and colorless body) capsules.

Storage: Store at controlled room temperature 15-30°C (59-86°F) in a dry place.

Warning: KEEP OUT OF REACH OF CHILDREN.

Caution: Federal law prohibits dispensing without prescription.

Manufactured for
Reed & Carnrick
by Phoenix Pharmaceuticals, Inc.
S. Hackensack, NJ 07606

Shown in Product Identification Section, page 427
Date of Revision
August 10, 1984

EPIFOAM® ℞
[ĕp'ē-fōm]
(hydrocortisone acetate 1% and pramoxine hydrochloride 1% topical aerosol)

Description: A topical corticosteroid aerosol foam containing hydrocortisone acetate 1% and pramoxine hydrochloride 1% in a base containing: propylene glycol, cetyl alcohol, glyceryl stearate, PEG-100 stearate, laureth-23, polyoxyl-40 stearate, methylparaben, propylparaben, trolamine or hydrochloric acid to adjust pH, purified water and propellants (inert): butane and propane.
EPIFOAM contains a synthetic steroid used as an anti-inflammatory and anti-pruritic agent, and a local anesthetic.

Molecular weight: Hydrocortisone acetate 404.51.
Solubility of hydrocortisone acetate in water: 1 mg/100 ml. Chemical name: Pregn-4-ene, 3,20-dione, 21-(acetyloxy)-11, 17-dihydroxy-, (11B).

Pramoxine Hydrochloride

Clinical Pharmacology: Topical corticosteroids share anti-inflammatory, anti-pruritic and vasoconstrictive actions.
The mechanism of anti-inflammatory activity of the topical corticosteroids is unclear. Various laboratory methods, including vasoconstrictor assays, are used to compare and predict potencies clinical efficacies of the topical corticosteroids. There is some evidence to suggest that a recognizable correlation exists between vasoconstrictor potency and therapeutic efficacy in man.

Pramoxine Hydrochloride: A surface or local anesthetic which is not chemically related to the "caine" types of local anesthetics. Its unique chemical structure is likely to minimize the danger of cross-sensitivity reactions in patients allergic to other local anesthetics.

Pharmacokinetics: The extent of percutaneous absorption of topical corticosteroids is determined by many factors including the vehicle, the integrity of the epidermal barrier, and the use of occlusive dressings.
Topical corticosteroids can be absorbed from normal intact skin. Inflammation and/or other disease processes in the skin increase the percutaneous absorption of topical corticosteroids. Occlusive dressings substantially increase the percutaneous absorption of topical corticosteroids. Thus, occlusive dressings may be a valuable therapeutic adjunct for treatment of resistant dermatoses. (See DOSAGE AND ADMINISTRATION.)
Once absorbed through the skin, topical corticosteroids are handled through pharmacokinetic pathways similar to systemically administered corticosteroids. Corticosteroids are bound to plasma proteins in varying degrees. Corticosteroids are metabolized primarily in the liver and are then excreted by the kidneys. Some of the topical corticosteroids and their metabolites are also excreted in the bile.

Indications and Usage: Topical corticosteroids are indicated for the relief of the inflammatory and pruritic manifestations of corticosteroid-responsive dermatoses.

Contraindications: Topical corticosteroid products are contraindicated in those patients with a history of hypersensitivity to any of the components of the preparation.

Warning: Not for prolonged use. If redness, pain, irritation or swelling persists, discontinue use and consult a physician. Contents of the container are under pressure, but not flammable. Do not burn or puncture the aerosol container. Store at temperatures below 120°F. Keep this and all medicines out of the reach of children.

Precautions: General: Systemic absorption of topical corticosteroids has produced reversible hypothalamic-pituitary-adrenal (HPA) axis suppression, manifestations of Cushing's syndrome, hyperglycemia and glucosuria in some patients. Conditions which augment systemic absorption include the application of the more potent steroids, use over large surface areas, prolonged use and the addition of occlusive dressings.

Therefore, patients receiving a large dose of a potent topical steroid applied to a large surface area or under an occlusive dressing should be evaluated periodically for evidence of HPA axis suppression by using the urinary hydrocortisone and ACTH stimulation tests. If HPA axis suppression is noted, an attempt should be made to withdraw the drug, to reduce the frequency of application, or to substitute a less potent steroid.
Recovery of HPA axis function is generally prompt and complete upon discontinuation of the drug. Infrequently, signs and symptoms of steroid withdrawal may occur, requiring supplemental systemic corticosteroids.
In children absorption may result in higher blood levels and thus more susceptibility to systemic toxicity. (See PRECAUTIONS—Pediatric Use.)
If irritation develops, topical corticosteroids should be discontinued and appropriate therapy instituted.
In the presence of dermatological infections, the use of an appropriate antifungal or antibacterial agent should be instituted. If a favorable response does not occur promptly, the corticosteroid should be discontinued until the infection has been adequately controlled.

Information for the Patient: Patients using topical corticosteroids should receive the following information and instructions:
1. This medication is to be used as directed by the physician. It is for external use only. Avoid contact with the eyes.
2. Do not use this medication for any disorder other than for which it was prescribed.
3. The treated skin area should not be bandaged or otherwise covered or wrapped as to be occlusive unless directed by physician.
4. Report any signs of local adverse reactions especially under occlusive dressings.
5. Do not use tight fitting diapers or plastic pants on a child being treated in the diaper area, as these garments may constitute occlusive dressings.

Laboratory Tests: The following test may be helpful in evaluating the HPA axis suppression:
Urinary hydrocortisone test
ACTH stimulation test

Carcinogenesis, Mutagenesis, and Impairment of Fertility: Long-term animal studies have not been performed to evaluate the carcinogenic potential or the effect on fertility of topical corticosteroids. Studies to determine mutagenicity with prednisolone and hydrocortisone have revealed negative results.

Pregnancy Category C: Corticosteroids are generally teratogenic in laboratory animals when administered systemically at relatively low dosage levels. The more potent corticosteroids have been shown to be teratogenic after dermal application in laboratory animals. There are no adequate and well-controlled studies in pregnant women of teratogenic effects from topically applied corticosteroids. Therefore, topical corticosteroids should be used during pregnancy only if the potential benefit justifies the potential risk to the fetus. Drugs of this class should not be used extensively on pregnant patients, in large amounts, or for prolonged periods of time.

Nursing Mothers: It is not known whether topical administration of corticosteroids could result in sufficient systemic absorption to produce detectable quantities in breast milk. Systemically administered corticosteroids are secreted into breast milk in quantities not likely to have a deleterious effect on the infant. Caution should be exercised when any topical corticosteroids are administered to a nursing woman.

Pediatric Use: Pediatric patients may demonstrate greater susceptibility to topical corticosteroid-induced HPA axis suppression and Cushing's syndrome than mature patients because of a larger skin surface area to body weight ratio. Hypothalamic-pituitary-adrenal (HPA) axis suppression, Cushing's syndrome and intracranial hypertension have been reported in children receiving topical corticosteroids. Manifestations of adrenal suppression in children include linear growth retardation, delayed weight gain, low plasma cortisone levels and absence of response to ACTH stimulation. Manifestations of intracranial hypertension include bulging fontanelles, headaches and bilateral papilladema.

Administration of topical corticosteroids to children should be limited to the least amount compatible with an effective therapeutic regimen. Chronic corticosteroid therapy may interfere with the growth and development of children.

Adverse Reactions: The following local adverse reactions are reported infrequently with topical corticosteroids, but may occur more frequently with the use of occlusive dressings. These reactions are listed in an approximately decreasing order of occurrence:

Burning
Itching
Irritation
Dryness
Folliculitis
Hypopigmentation
Perioral dermatitis
Allergic contact dermatitis
Maceration of the skin
Secondary infection
Skin atrophy
Striae
Miliaria

Overdosage: Topically applied corticosteroids can be absorbed in sufficient amounts to produce systemic effects. (See PRECAUTIONS.)

Dosage and Administration: Apply to affected area 3 or 4 times daily.

(NOTE: Refer to the enclosed Directions for Use.):

Directions For Use:
1. Shake foam container vigorously before use.
2. Hold container upright and dispense medication onto a pad by depressing the container cap several times. A small amount of foam is all that is needed on the pad. Apply to affected areas. Alternatively, the foam may be applied directly to affected areas.
3. The container and cap should be disassembled and rinsed with warm water after use.

NOTE: The aerosol container should never be inserted into the vagina or anus.

How Supplied: EPIFOAM (NDC-0021-0740-10) available in 10g pressurized cans.

Caution: FEDERAL LAW PROHIBITS DISPENSING WITHOUT PRESCRIPTION.

Reed & Carnrick
1 New England Avenue
Piscataway, NJ 08854

Revised 4/10/84
Shown in Product Identification Section, page 427

KWELL® Cream
[*kwel*]
(lindane) 1%

Description: Active ingredient lindane 1%. Inert ingredients: 99% in a non-greasy pleasantly scented water-dispersible cream, containing stearic acid, lanolin, glycerin, 2-amino-2-methyl-1-propanol, perfume and purified water.

Actions and Indications: KWELL Cream is an ectoparasiticide and ovacide indicated for the treatment of patients with Sarcoptes scabiei (scabies), as well as infestations of Pediculus capitis (head lice), Phthirus pubis (crab lice), and their ova.

Contraindications: KWELL Cream is contraindicated for individuals with known sensitivity to the product or to any of its components.

Warning: KWELL CREAM SHOULD BE USED WITH CAUTION, ESPECIALLY ON INFANTS, CHILDREN AND PREGNANT WOMEN. LINDANE PENETRATES HUMAN SKIN AND HAS THE POTENTIAL FOR CNS TOXICITY. STUDIES INDICATE THAT POTENTIAL TOXIC EFFECTS OF TOPICALLY APPLIED LINDANE ARE GREATER IN THE YOUNG. Seizures have been reported after the use of lindane, but a cause and effect relationship has not been established.

Simultaneous application of creams, ointments or oils may enhance the percutaneous absorption of lindane.

Precautions: If accidental ingestion occurs, prompt gastric lavage will rid the body of large amounts of the toxicant. However, since oils favor absorption, saline cathartics for intestinal evacuation should be given rather than oil laxatives. If central nervous system manifestations occur, they can be antagonized by the administration of pentobarbital or phenobarbital.

If accidental contact with the eyes occurs, flush with water. If irritation or sensitization occurs, discontinue use and consult a physician.

Adverse Reactions: Eczematous eruptions due to irritation from this product have been reported.

ADMINISTRATION
CAUTION: USE ONLY AS DIRECTED. DO NOT EXCEED RECOMMENDED DOSAGE.
NOTE: PLEASE READ CAREFULLY.

Directions for Use:
Pediculosis capitis (head lice)—KWELL Shampoo is the most convenient dosage form but the lotion and cream are also effective.

Apply a sufficient quantity to cover only the affected and adjacent hairy areas. The cream should be rubbed into scalp and hair, and left in place for 8–12 hours followed by a thorough washing (shower or bath).

Retreatment is usually not necessary. Demonstrable living lice after 7 days indicate that retreatment is necessary.

Pediculosis pubis (crab lice)—Apply a sufficient quantity to cover thinly the hair and skin of the pubic area, and if infested the thighs, trunk, and axillary regions. The medication should be rubbed into the skin and hair, and left in place for 8–12 hours followed by a thorough washing (shower or bath).

Retreatment is usually not necessary. Demonstrable living lice after 7 days indicate that retreatment is necessary. Sexual contacts should be treated simultaneously.

Scabies (Sarcoptes scabiei)—The cream should be applied to dry skin in a thin layer and rubbed in thoroughly. If crusted lesions are present, a warm bath preceding the medication is helpful. If a warm bath is used, allow the skin to dry and cool before applying the cream. Usually one ounce is sufficient for an adult. A total body application should be made from the neck down. Scabies rarely affects the head of children or adults but may occur in infants. The cream should be left on for 8–12 hours and should then be removed by a thorough washing (shower or bath).

ONE APPLICATION IS USUALLY CURATIVE. Many patients exhibit persistent pruritus after treatment; this is rarely a sign of treatment failure and is not an indication for retreatment, unless living mites can be demonstrated.

How Supplied: KWELL Cream in tubes of 2 oz (57G) and jars of 16 oz (454G).

Literature Available: Patient information and instruction pads with directions for use available on request.

KWELL® Lotion
[*kwel*]
(lindane) 1%

Description: Active ingredient lindane 1%. Inert ingredients: 99% in a non-greasy, pleasantly scented base, containing glyceryl monostearate, cetyl alcohol, stearic acid, trolamine, 2-amino-2-methyl-1-propanol, butyl p-hydrox- ybenzoate, methyl p-hydroxy-benzoate, Irish moss extract, perfume and purified water.

Actions and Indications: KWELL Lotion is an ectoparasiticide and ovacide indicated for the treatment of patients with Sarcoptes scabiei (scabies), as well as infestations of Pediculus capitis (head lice), Phthirus pubis (crab lice), and their ova.

Contraindications: KWELL Lotion is contraindicated for individuals with known sensitivity to the product or to any of its components.

Warning: KWELL LOTION SHOULD BE USED WITH CAUTION, ESPECIALLY ON INFANTS, CHILDREN AND PREGNANT WOMEN. LINDANE PENETRATES HUMAN SKIN AND HAS THE POTENTIAL FOR CNS TOXICITY. STUDIES INDICATE THAT POTENTIAL TOXIC EFFECTS OF TOPICALLY APPLIED LINDANE ARE GREATER IN THE YOUNG. Seizures have been reported after the use of lindane, but a cause and effect relationship has not been established.

Simultaneous application of creams, ointments or oils may enhance the percutaneous absorption of lindane.

Precautions: If accidental ingestion occurs, prompt gastric lavage will rid the body of large amounts of the toxicant. However, since oils favor absorption, saline cathartics for intestinal evacuation should be given rather than oil laxatives. If central nervous system manifestations occur, they can be antagonized by the administration of pentobarbital or phenobarbital.

If accidental contact with the eyes occurs, flush with water. If irritation or sensitization occurs, discontinue use and consult a physician.

Adverse Reactions: Eczematous eruptions due to irritation from this product have been reported.

ADMINISTRATION
CAUTION: USE ONLY AS DIRECTED. DO NOT EXCEED RECOMMENDED DOSAGE.
NOTE: PLEASE READ CAREFULLY.

Directions For Use:
Pediculosis capitis (head lice)—KWELL Shampoo is the most convenient dosage form but the lotion and cream are also effective.

Apply a sufficient quantity to cover only the affected and adjacent hairy areas. The lotion should be rubbed into scalp and hair, and left in place for 8–12 hours followed by a thorough washing (shower or bath).

Retreatment is usually not necessary. Demonstrable living lice after 7 days indicate that retreatment is necessary.

Pediculosis pubis (crab lice)—Apply a sufficient quantity to cover thinly the hair and skin of the pubic area, and if infested, the thighs, trunk, and axillary regions. The medication should be rubbed into the skin and hair and left in place for 8–12 hours followed by a thorough washing (shower or bath).

Retreatment is usually not necessary. Demonstrable living lice after 7 days indicate that retreatment is necessary. Sexual contacts should be treated simultaneously.

Scabies (Sarcoptes scabiei)—The lotion should be applied to dry skin in a thin layer and rubbed in thoroughly. If crusted lesions are present, a warm bath preceding the medication is helpful. If a warm bath is used, allow the skin to dry and cool before applying the lotion. Usually one ounce is sufficient for an adult. A total body application should be made from the neck down. Scabies rarely affects the head of children or adults but may occur in infants.

The lotion should be left on for 8–12 hours and should then be removed by a thorough washing (shower or bath). ONE APPLICATION IS USUALLY CURATIVE.

Many patients exhibit persistent pruritus after treatment; this is rarely a sign of treatment failure and is not an indication for retreatment, unless living mites can be demonstrated.

How Supplied: KWELL Lotion in bottles of 2 fl. oz (59ml), 16 fl. oz (472ml) and 1 gallon (3.8 L).

Literature Available: Patient information and instruction pads with directions for use available on request.

KWELL® Shampoo
[*kwel*]
(lindane) 1%

Description: Active ingredient lindane 1%. Inert ingredients: 99% in a cosmetically pleasant shampoo base, containing polyoxyethylene sorbitan monostearate, TEA-lauryl sulfate, acetone and purified water.

Actions and Indications: KWELL Shampoo is an ectoparasiticide and ovicide indicated for the treatment of infestations of Pediculus capitis

Continued on next page

Reed & Carnrick—Cont.

(head lice), Phthirus pubis (crab lice), and their nits.

Contraindications: KWELL Shampoo is contraindicated for individuals with known sensitivity to the product or to any of its components.

Warning: KWELL SHAMPOO SHOULD BE USED WITH CAUTION, ESPECIALLY ON INFANTS, CHILDREN AND PREGNANT WOMEN. LINDANE PENETRATES HUMAN SKIN AND HAS THE POTENTIAL FOR CNS TOXICITY. STUDIES INDICATE THAT POTENTIAL TOXIC EFFECTS OF TOPICALLY APPLIED LINDANE ARE GREATER IN THE YOUNG. Seizures have been reported after the use of lindane, but a cause and effect relationship has not been established.

Simultaneous application of creams, ointments or oils may enhance the percutaneous absorption of lindane.

Precautions: If accidental ingestion occurs, prompt gastric lavage will rid the body of large amounts of the toxicant. However, since oils favor absorption, saline cathartics for intestinal evacuation should be given rather than oil laxatives. If central nervous system manifestations occur, they can be antagonized by the administration of pentobarbital, or phenobarbital.

If accidental contact with the eyes occurs, flush with water. If irritation or sensitization occurs, discontinue use and consult a physician.

Adverse Reactions: Eczematous eruptions due to irritation from this product have been reported.

ADMINISTRATION
CAUTION: USE ONLY AS DIRECTED. DO NOT EXCEED RECOMMENDED DOSAGE.
NOTE: PLEASE READ CAREFULLY

Directions For Use:
Pediculosis capitis (head lice)—1) Apply a sufficient quantity of the shampoo to thoroughly wet the hair and skin of the infested and adjacent hairy areas. 2) Work thoroughly into the hair and allow to remain in place 4 minutes. 3) Add small quantities of water until a good lather forms. 4) Rinse thoroughly. Towel briskly. When the hair is dry, any remaining nits or nit shells may be removed by fine-tooth combing or with tweezers.

Retreatment is usually not necessary. Demonstrable living lice after 7 days indicate that retreatment is necessary.

Pediculosis pubis (crab lice)—1) Apply a sufficient quantity of the shampoo to thoroughly wet the hair and skin of the infested and adjacent, hairy areas. 2) Work thoroughly into the hair and allow to remain in place 4 minutes. 3) Add small quantities of water until a good lather forms. 4) Rinse thoroughly. Towel briskly. When the hair is dry, any remaining nits or nit shells may be removed by fine tooth combing or tweezers. 5) Sexual contacts should be examined and treated if necessary.

Retreatment is usually not necessary. Demonstrable living lice after 7 days indicate that retreatment is required. Sexual contacts should be treated simultaneously.

NOTE: KWELL Shampoo is intended only for head lice and crab lice infestations and should not be used as a routine shampoo. For other ectoparasitic infestations, such as scabies, the use of KWELL Cream or KWELL Lotion is recommended.

How Supplied: KWELL Shampoo in bottles of 2 fl. oz (59ml), 16 fl. oz (472ml) and 1 gallon (3.8L).

Literature Available: Patient information and instruction pads with directions for use available on request.

PHAZYME® Tablets
[fā'zīm]

Description: A pink coated two-phase tablet. The outer layer releases in the stomach: specially activated simethicone 20 mg. The enteric coated core releases in the small intestine: pancreatic enzymes (protease 3,000 USP units, lipase 240 USP units, amylase 2,000 USP units), and specially activated simethicone 40 mg.

Actions: PHAZYME is the only dual approach to the problem of gastrointestinal gas. Simethicone minimizes gas formation and relieves gas entrapment in both the stomach and the lower G.I. tract. This action combats pain, due to gastrointestinal gas. Pancreatic enzymes enhance the normal digestive process and help to reduce gas formation. Also, for relief of gas distress associated with other functional or organic conditions such as: diverticulitis, spastic colitis, hyperacidity, post-cholecystectomy syndrome and chronic cholecystitis.

Indications: PHAZYME is indicated for the relief of occasional or chronic pain caused by gas entrapped in the stomach or in the lower gastrointestinal tract—resulting from aerophagia, postoperative distention, dyspepsia and food intolerance.

Contraindications: A known sensitivity to any ingredient.

Dosage: One or two tablets with each meal and at bedtime or as required.

How Supplied: Pink coated two-phase tablet in bottles of 50, 100, and 1,000.

Shown in Product Identification Section, page 427

PHAZYME®-95 Tablets
[fā'zīm]

Description: A red coated two-phase tablet with the highest dose of simethicone available in a single tablet. The outer layer releases in the stomach: specially activated simethicone 25 mg. The enteric coated core releases in the small intestine: pancreatic enzymes (protease 6,000 USP units, lipase 480 USP units, amylase 4,000 USP units), and specially activated simethicone 70 mg.

Actions: PHAZYME is the only dual approach to the problem of gastrointestinal gas. Simethicone minimizes gas formation and relieves gas entrapment in both the stomach and the lower G.I. tract. This action combats pain due to gastrointestinal gas. Pancreatic enzymes enhance the normal digestive process and help to reduce gas formation. Also, for relief of gas distress associated with other functional or organic conditions such as: diverticulitis, spastic colitis, hyperacidity, post-cholecystectomy syndrome and chronic cholecystitis.

Indications: PHAZYME-95 is indicated for the relief of acute severe lower intestinal pain due to gas—resulting from aerophagia, postoperative distention, dyspepsia and food intolerance.

Contraindications: A known sensitivity to any ingredient.

Dosage: One tablet with each meal and at bedtime, or as required.

How Supplied: Red coated two-phase tablets, in bottles of 50, 100, and 1,000.

Shown in Product Identification Section, page 427

PHAZYME®-PB Tablets
[fā'zīm]

Description: A yellow coated two-phase tablet. The outer layer releases in the stomach: specially activated simethicone 20 mg and phenobarbital 15 mg, (WARNING: MAY BE HABIT FORMING). The enteric coated core releases in the small intestine: pancreatic enzymes (protease 3,000 USP units, lipase 240 USP units, amylase 2,000 USP units), and specially activated simethicone 40 mg.

Actions: PHAZYME-PB provides the same advantages of the PHAZYME formula (minimizes gas formation, relieves gas entrapment) and in addition, supplies the calming benefits of phenobarbital to control the emotional component of gastrointestinal gas pain. Also, for relief of gas distress associated with other functional or organic conditions such as: diverticulitis, spastic colitis, hyperacidity, post-cholecystectomy syndrome and chronic cholecystitis.

Indications: PHAZYME-PB is indicated for gas pain associated with anxiety-resulting in aerophagia, post-operative distention, dyspepsia and food intolerance.

Contraindications: Known sensitivity to barbiturates or to any ingredient.

Warning: May be habit forming.

Precautions: Excessive use may produce drowsiness.

Dosage: One or two tablets with each meal and at bedtime or as required.

How Supplied: Yellow coated two-phase tablets in bottles of 100 and 1000.

Shown in Product Identification Section, page 427

proctoFoam®/non-steroid
[prŏk' tō-fōm]
(pramoxine HCl 1%)

Description: proctoFoam is a foam for anal and perianal use containing pramoxine hydrochloride 1%, in a water-miscible mucoadhesive foam base of mineral oil.

Actions: proctoFoam is an anesthetic mucoadhesive foam which medicates the anorectal mucosa, and provides prompt temporary relief from itching and pain. Its lubricating action helps make bowel evacuations more comfortable.

Indications: Prompt, temporary relief of anorectal inflammation, pruritus and pain associated with hemorrhoids, proctitis, cryptitis, fissures, postoperative pain and pruritus ani.

Contraindications: Contraindicated in persons hypersensitive to any of the ingredients.

Warning: Not for prolonged use. Do not use more than four consecutive weeks. If redness, pain, irritation or swelling persists or rectal bleeding occurs, discontinue use and consult a physician. Keep this and all medicines out of the reach of children.

Caution: Do not insert any part of the aerosol container into the anus. Contents of the container are under pressure, but not flammable. Do not burn or puncture the aerosol container. Store at room temperature, not over 120° F.

Dosage:
One applicatorful two or three times daily and after bowel evacuation.

1. Shake foam container vigorously for 5–10 seconds. Do not remove cap.
2. Withdraw applicator plunger past the fill line until it stops.
3. Place foam container upright on level surface, insert tip of cap into tip of applicator.
   To fill applicator:
   - Depress cap on foam container—RELEASE.
   - Pause, a few seconds, allowing foam to enter and expand in applicator barrel.
   - Repeat until foam rises to fill applicator to Fill Line.
4. Hold applicator by barrel and gently insert tip into anus. Once in place, push plunger to expel foam, then withdraw applicator. Note: Pull applicator apart and wash thoroughly with water.

Note: To relieve itching place some foam on a tissue and apply externally.

How Supplied: Available in 15 g aerosol container, with special plastic applicator. When used correctly, the aerosol supplies approximately 18 applications.

Literature Available: Instruction pads with directions for use available upon request.

Shown in Product Identification Section, page 427

PROCTOFOAM®-HC
[prŏc' tō-fōm]
(hydrocortisone acetate) 1%

Description: PROCTOFOAM-HC contains as active ingredient: Hydrocortisone acetate 1% in a hydrophilic base containing: pramoxine hydrochloride, propylene glycol, ethoxylated cetyl and stearyl alcohol, steareth-10, cetyl alcohol, methylparaben, propylparaben, trolamine, purified water; propellant (inert) dichlorodifluoromethane and dichlorotetrafluoroethane.

Actions: Topical steroids are primarily effective because of their anti-inflammatory, anti-pruritic and vasoconstrictive actions.

Indications: For relief of the inflammatory manifestations of corticosteroid-responsive dermatoses of the anogenital area.

Contraindications: Topical steroids are contraindicated in those patients with a history of sensitivity to any of the components of the preparation.

Precautions: If irritation develops, the product should be discontinued and appropriate therapy instituted.

In the presence of an infection, the use of appropriate antifungal or antibacterial agents should be instituted. If a favorable response does not occur promptly, the corticosteroid should be discontinued until the infection has been adequately controlled.

If extensive areas are treated or if the occlusive technique is used, the possibility exists of increased systemic absorption of the corticosteroid and suitable precautions should be taken particularly in children and infants.

Although topical steroids have not been reported to have an adverse effect on human pregnancy, the safety of their use in pregnant women has not absolutely been established. In laboratory animals, increases in incidence of fetal abnormalities have been associated with exposure of gestating females to topical corticosteroids, in some cases at rather low dosage levels. Therefore, drugs of this class should not be used extensively on pregnant patients, in large amounts, or for prolonged periods of time.

This product is not for ophthalmic use.

Adverse Reactions: The following local adverse reactions have been reported with topical corticosteroids, especially under occlusive dressings: burning, itching, irritation, dryness, folliculitis, hypertrichosis, acneiform eruptions, hypopigmentation, allergic contact dermatitis, maceration of the skin, secondary infection, skin atrophy, striae, and miliaria.

Dosage and Administration: Apply to affected areas 3 or 4 times daily. Use the applicator supplied for rectal application. For perianal use, transfer a small quantity to a tissue and apply gently.

1. Shake foam container vigorously for 5–10 seconds. Do not remove cap.
2. Withdraw applicator plunger past the fill line until it stops.
3. Place foam container upright on level surface, insert tip of cap into tip of applicator.
Fill applicator by depressing cap on foam container:
 • Allow foam to enter applicator.
 • Release and allow foam to expand in applicator barrel.
 • Repeat until foam fills applicator to fill line.
4. Hold applicator by barrel and gently insert tip into anus. Once in place, push plunger to expel foam, then withdraw applicator. Note: Pull applicator apart and wash thoroughly with warm water.

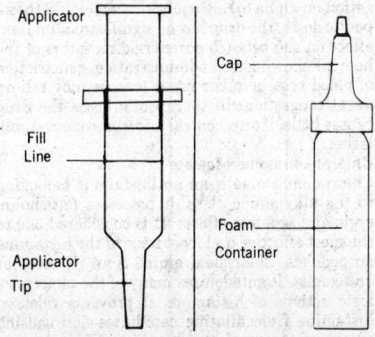

How Supplied: In aerosol container containing 10 g, with special rectal applicator. When used correctly, the aerosol supplies approximately 18 applications.

Literature Available: Instruction pads with directions for use available upon request.

[*Shown in Product Identification Section, page 427*]

PROXIGEL® Oral Cleanser
[prŏx′ĭ-jel]
(carbamide peroxide 10%)

Description: PROXIGEL is a cleansing aid for minor oral inflammations. Active ingredient: Carbamide peroxide 10% in a water free gel base.

Actions: PROXIGEL releases oxygen on contact with mouth tissues to provide cleansing effects. Unlike liquid preparations, PROXIGEL Oral Cleanser's unique viscous base adheres to affected areas for longer oxygenating and debriding action.

Indications: PROXIGEL is recommended for recurrent aphthous ulcerations (canker sores) and relief of minor inflammation of gums and other surfaces of the mouth and lips. PROXIGEL is also useful as adjunctive therapy in gingivitis, periodontitis, stomatitis, Vincent's infection and denture irritation. PROXIGEL helps to inhibit odor causing bacteria and helps soothe painful tissues.

Precautions: If condition persists or worsens, or irritation develops, discontinue use.

Dosage and Administration: Do not dilute. Use 4 times a day, or as directed. Apply directly with or without nozzle. Gently massage medication with finger or swab on affected area. Do not drink or rinse for 5 minutes. Always replace cap on nozzle after use. Store below 72°F (22°C).

How Supplied: Plastic tubes 1.2 oz. with special applicator top and guard cap.

R&C SPRAY® Lice Control Insecticide

Description: Active ingredients: 3-Phenoxybenzyl d-cis and trans 2,2-dimethyl-3-(2-meth-yl propenyl)

cyclopropanecarboxylate	0.382%
Other Isomers	0.018%
Petroleum Distillates	4.255%
Inert Ingredients:	95.345%
	100.000%

Actions: R&C SPRAY is specially formulated to kill lice and their nits on inanimate objects.

Indications: R&C SPRAY is recommended for use only on bedding, mattresses, furniture and other objects infested or possibly infested with lice which cannot be laundered or dry cleaned.

Warnings: Contents under pressure. Do not use or store near heat or open flame. Do not puncture or incinerate container. Exposure to temperatures above 130°F may cause bursting.

It is a violation of Federal law to use this product in a manner inconsistent with its labeling.
NOT FOR USE ON HUMANS OR ANIMALS.

Caution: Avoid spraying in eyes. Avoid breathing spray mist. Avoid contact with the skin. In case of contact, wash immediately with soap and water. Harmful if swallowed. Vacate room after treatment and ventilate before reoccupying. Avoid contamination of feed and foodstuffs.

Remove pets, birds and cover fish aquariums before spraying.

Directions: SHAKE WELL BEFORE AND OCCASIONALLY DURING USE. Spray on an inconspicuous area to test for possible staining or discoloration. Inspect after drying, then proceed to spray entire area to be treated.

Hold container upright with nozzle away from you. Depress valve and spray from a distance of 8 to 10 inches.

Spray each square foot for about three seconds. For mattresses, furniture, or similar objects (that cannot be laundered or dry cleaned): Spray thoroughly. Do not use article until spray is dry. Repeat treatment as necessary. Do not use in commercial food processing, preparation, storage or serving areas.

Storage: Store in a cool area away from heat or open flame.

Disposal: Wrap container and put in trash. Do not incinerate.

How Supplied: In 5 oz. and 10 oz. aerosol container.

EPA REG NO	36232-2
EPA EST NO	11598-CT-1
	11525-RI-1
	11525-IL-1
	5590-NJ-01
	13891-IN-1

TRICHOTINE® Powder Vaginal Douche
[trī′cō-tēn]

Description: A detergent, mucolytic, vaginal douche containing sodium lauryl sulfate, sodium perborate, sodium chloride, and aromatics.

Actions: Low surface tension enables TRICHOTINE to penetrate the rugal folds, remove mucous, debris, and vaginal discharge thereby making treatment of vaginitis more effective. TRICHOTINE deodorizes and affords prompt relief from itching and burning.

Indications: TRICHOTINE helps to establish a normal healthy mucosa as an adjunct in therapy of vaginitis. It may also be used in postmenstrual, postcoital or routine vaginal cleansing.

Contraindications: None reported.

Warning: For routine use, do not use more than twice weekly. May be used more frequently in concomitant use for treatment of vaginitis. Discontinue use if irritation develops.

Precautions: Use only in fresh solution— never use dry.

Side Effects: A transient localized sensation has been reported in rare instances.

Directions For Use: Dissolve one tablespoonful to each quart of warm water and mix thoroughly.

How Supplied: 5 oz., 12 oz., and 20 oz.

Literature Available: Instructions for the use of TRICHOTINE available in pads of 50 sheets.

TRICHOTINE® Liquid Vaginal Douche

Description: A detergent, mucolytic, vaginal douche containing sodium lauryl sulfate, sodium borate, with alcohol (SDA 23A) 8% and aromatics.

Actions: (See TRICHOTINE Powder above).

Indications: (See TRICHOTINE Powder above).

Contraindications: None reported.

Warning: For routine use, do not use more than twice weekly. May be used more frequently in concomitant use for treatment of vaginitis. Discontinue use if irritation develops.

Precautions: Use only fresh solution. Do not use full strength.

Side Effects: None reported.

Directions For Use: Two capfuls mixed well to each quart of warm water.

How Supplied: 4 and 8 fl. oz. plastic bottles.

Literature Available: Instructions for the use of TRICHOTINE are available in pads of 50 sheets.

Reid-Provident Laboratories Inc.

Executive Offices
640 TENTH STREET, N.W.
ATLANTA, GA 30318
Scientific Affairs and Manufacturing
25 FIFTH ST., N.W.
ATLANTA, GA 30308

COMPAL CAPSULES
[com′pal]

Description: Each light aqua and bluish-green capsule contains Dihydrocodeine Bitartrate 16 mg. (Warning: May be habit forming), Acetaminophen 356.4 mg., Caffeine 30 mg.

Clinical Pharmacology: Dihydrocodeine is a semi-synthetic narcotic analgesic related to codeine, with multiple actions qualitatively similar to those of codeine; the most prominent of these involve the central nervous system and organs with smooth muscle components. The principal action of therapeutic value is analgesia.

Compal also contains the nonopiate, non-salicylate antipyretic-analgesic, acetaminophen.

Indications: For the relief of moderate to moderately severe pain.

Contraindications: Hypersensitivity to dihydrocodeine, codeine, or acetaminophen.

Warnings:
Usage in Ambulatory Patients: Dihydrocodeine may impair the mental and/or physi-

Continued on next page

Reid-Provident—Cont.

cal abilities required for the performance of potentially hazardous tasks such as driving a car or operating machinery. The patient using Compal should be cautioned accordingly.

Interactions With Other Central Nervous System Depressants: Patients receiving other narcotic analgesias, general anesthetics, tranquilizers, sedative-hypnotics or other CNS depressants (including alcohol) concomitantly with Compal may exhibit an additive CNS depression. When such combined therapy is contemplated, the dose of one or both agents should be reduced.

Precautions:
General: Compal should be given with caution to certain patients such as the elderly or debilitated.
Drug Interactions: The CNS-depressant effects of dihydrocodeine bitartrate may be additive with that of other CNS depressants.
See "Warnings."
Usage in Pregnancy: Reproduction studies have not been performed in animals. There is no adequate information on whether this drug may affect fertility in human males and females or has a teratogenic potential or other adverse effect on the fetus.
Usage in Children: Since there is no experience in children who have received this drug, safety and efficacy in children have not been established.
Adverse Reactions: The most frequently observed reactions include lightheadedness, dizziness, drowsiness, sedation, nausea, vomiting, constipation, pruritus, and skin reactions.
Drug Abuse and Dependence: Compal is subject to the provisions of the Controlled Substance Act, and has been placed in Schedule III. Dihydrocodeine can produce drug dependence of the codeine type and therefore has the potential of being abused. Psychic dependence, physical dependence, and tolerance may develop upon repeated administration of dihydrocodeine, and it should be prescribed and administered with the same degree of caution appropriate to the use of other oral narcotic-containing medications.
Dosage and Administration: Dosage should be adjusted according to the severity of the pain and the response of the patient. Compal is given orally. The usual adult dose is two capsules every four (4) hours as needed for pain.
Management of Overdosage:
Dihydrocodeine:
Signs and Symptoms: Serious overdose with Compal is characterized by respiratory depression (a decrease in respiratory rate and/or tidal volume, Cheyne-Stokes respiration, cyanosis), extreme somnolence progressing to stupor or coma, skeletal muscle flaccidity, cold and clammy skin, and sometimes bradycardia and hypotension. In severe overdosage, apnea, circulatory collapse, cardiac arrest and death may occur.
Treatment: Primary attention should be given to the re-establishment of adequate respiratory exchange through provision of a patent airway and the institution of assisted or controlled ventilation. The narcotic antagonist naloxone is a specific antidote against respiratory depression which may result from overdosage or unusual sensitivity to narcotics, including codeine. Therefore, an appropriate dose of naloxone (usual initial adult dose: 0.4 mg.) should be administered, preferably by the intravenous route and simultaneously with efforts at respiratory resuscitation. Since the duration of action of dihydrocodeine may exceed that of the antagonist, the patient should be kept under continued surveillance and repeated doses of the antagonist should be administered as needed to maintain adequate respiration.
An antagonist should not be administered in the absence of clinically significant respiratory or cardiovascular depression.
Oxygen, intravenous fluids, vasopressors and other supportive measures should be employed as indicated.
Gastric emptying may be useful in removing unabsorbed drug.

Acetaminophen:
Signs and Symptoms: Acetaminophen in massive overdosage may cause hepatic toxicity in some patients. In all cases of suspected overdose, immediately call your reginal poison center or the Rocky Mountain Poison Center's toll-free number (800-525-6115) for assistance in diagnosis and for directions in the use of N-acetylcysteine as an antidote, a use currently restricted to investigational status. In adults, hepatic toxicity has rarely been reported with acute overdoses of less than 10 grams and fatalities with less than 15 grams. Importantly, young children seem to be more resistant than adults to the hepatotoxic effect of an acetaminophen overdose. Despite this, the measures outlined below should be initiated in any adult or child suspected of having ingested an acetaminophen overdose.
Early symptoms following a potentially hepatotoxic overdose may include: nausea, vomiting, diaphoresis and general malaise. Clincal and laboratory evidence of hepatic toxicity may not be apparent until 48 to 72 hours post-ingestion.
Treatment: The stomach should be emptied promptly by lavage or by induction of emesis with syrup of ipecac. Patients' estimates of the quantity of a drug ingested are notoriously unreliable. Therefore, if an acetaminophen overdose is suspected, a serum acetaminophen assay should be obtained as early as possible, but no sooner than four hours following ingestion. Liver function studies should be obtained initially and repeated at 24-hour intervals.
The antidote, N-acetylcysteine, should be administered as early as possible, and within 16 hours of the overdose ingestion for optimal results. Following recovery, there are no residual, structural or functional hepatic abnormalities.
How Supplied: Available in light aqua and bluish-green capsules imprinted with REID-PROVIDENT 1290 containing Dihydrocodeine Bitartrate 16 mg. (Warning: May be habit forming). Acetaminophen 356.4 mg., Caffeine 30 mg. Supplied in bottles of 100 capsules (NDC 0063-1290-06).
Storage: Store and dispense below 25°C (77°F) in tight, light-resistant containers as defined in the U.S.P.
Shown in Product Identification Section, page 427

CURRETAB® ℞
Medroxyprogesterone Acetate 10 mg tablets
How Supplied: Bottles of 50 (NDC 0063-1007-42).
Shown in Product Identification Section, page 427

ESTRATAB® ℞
[es'trah-tab]
Esterified Estrogens
0.3 mg., 0.625 mg. 1.25 mg. 2.5 mg.
How Supplied:
NDC 0063-1014-06 0.3 mg. Bottles of 100
NDC 0063-1022-06 0.625 mg. Bottles of 100
NDC 0063-1022-09 0.625 mg. Bottles of 1000
NDC 0063-1024-06 1.25 mg. Bottles of 100
NDC 0063-1024-09 1.25 mg. Bottles of 1000
NDC 0063-1025-06 2.5 mg. Bottles of 100
NDC 0063-1025-09 2.5 mg. Bottles of 1000
Shown in Product Identification Section, page 427

ESTRATEST® ℞
[es'trah-test]
ESTRATEST® H.S. (Half-Strength) ℞
Androgen–Estrogen Therapy
Description:
ESTRATEST® Oral Tablets
Each dark green tablet contains:
Esterified Estrogens, U.S.P. ....1.25 mg
Methyltestosterone, U.S.P. ....2.5 mg
ESTRATEST® H.S. (Half-Strength) Oral Tablets
Each light green tablet contains:
Esterified Estrogens, U.S.P. ....0.625 mg
Methyltestosterone, U.S.P. ....1.25 mg
How Supplied:
Estratest® NDC 0063-1026-06 bottles of 100
             NDC 0063-1026-09 bottles of 1000
Estratest® H.S. NDC 0063-1023-06 bottles of 100
Shown in Product Identification Section, page 427

HISTALET® Syrup ℞
HISTALET® DM Syrup
HISTALET® X Syrup (New Formula)
HISTALET® X Tablets (New Formula)
HISTALET® FORTE Tablets
[hist'ă-let for-tā]
for oral use only
[See table below].
Histalet® Forte Tablets:
Each tablet contains:
Phenylephrine HCl ....10 mg.
Phenylpropanolamine HCl ....50 mg.
Pyrilamine Maleate ....25 mg.
Chlorpheniramine Maleate ....4 mg.
Description: Each Histalet Forte tablet contains: Phenylpropanolamine HCl 50 mg, Pyrilamine Maleate 25 mg, Chlorpheniramine Maleate 4 mg and Phenlephrine HCl 10 mg.
Clinical Pharmacology:
Phenylpropanolamine Hydrochloride
The drug may directly stimulate adrenergic receptors, but probably indirectly stimulates both alpha (α) and beta (β) adrenergic receptors by releasing norepinephrine from its storage sites. Phenylpropanolamine increases heart rate, force of contraction and cardiac output, and excitability. It acts on alpha receptors in the mucosa of the respiratory tract, producing vasoconstriction which results in shrinkage of swollen mucous membranes, reduction of tissue, hyperemia, edema and nasal congestion, and an increase in nasal airway patency. Phenylpropanolamine causes CNS stimulation and reportedly has an anorexigenic effect.
Phenylephrine Hydrochloride
Phenylephrine acts predominantly by a direct action on alpha (α) adrenergic receptors. In therapeutic doses, the drug has no significant stimulant effect on the beta (β) adrenergic receptors of the heart. Following oral administration, constriction of blood vessels in the nasal mucosa may relieve nasal congestion. In therapeutic doses the drug causes little, if any, central nervous system stimulation.
Chlorpheniramine Maleate
Chlorpheniramine is an antihistamine belonging to the alkylamine class. It possesses anticholinergic and sedative effects. It is considered one of the most effective and least toxic of the histamine antagonists. Chlorpheniramine is an H_1 receptor antagonist. It antagonizes many of the pharmacologic actions of histamine. It prevents released histamine from dilating capillaries and causing edema of the respiratory mucosa. Chlorpheniramine has a duration of action of 4 to 6 hours in clinical studies.
Pyrilamine Maleate
Pyrilamine is an antihistamine belonging to the ethylenediamine class. Pyrilamine is a highly effective H_1 blocker. Pyrilamine is an especially active H_1 blocking drug which possesses local an-

DOSAGE SCHEDULE FOR HISTALET® FAMILY

Formula:	Per 5 ml:				Per tab
	Histalet® Syrup	Histalet® DM Syrup	Histalet® X Syrup (New Formula)		Histalet® X Tablets (New Formula)
Pseudoephedrine HCl	45 mg	45 mg	45 mg		120 mg
Chlorpheniramine Maleate	3 mg	3 mg			
Dextromethorphan HBr		15 mg			
Guaifenesin			200 mg		400 mg

esthetic activity. Pyrilamine antagonizes most of the smooth muscle stimulating actions of histamine on the H_1 receptors of the gastro-intestinal tract, blood vessels and bronchial muscle. It also antagonizes the actions of histamine that results in increased capillary permeability and the formation of edema. Pyrilamine has a duration of action of 4 to 6 hours in clinical studies.

Indications and Usage: Histalet Forte is indicated for symptomatic relief in allergic rhinitis, allergic bronchitis, bronchospasm, hay fever, common cold, sinusitis and skin allergies.

Contraindications: This preparation is contraindicated for individuals sensitive to phenylephrine HCl and antihistamines.

Precautions: General Precautions—Administer with caution to patients with hypertension, cardiac or peripheral vascular disease, hyperthyroidism or diabetes. **Information for Patients**—This medication may cause drowsiness. Patients should be advised not to drive a car or operate dangerous machinery while taking this medication.

Description: Each white with greenish dots, scored HISTALET® X Tablet contains: Pseudoephedrine HCl 120 mg, Guaifenesin 400 mg.

Each teaspoonful (5 ml) of HISTALET® X Syrup contains: Pseudoephedrine HCl 45 mg, Guaifenesin 200 mg, Alcohol 15%.

Clinical Pharmacology: Pseudoephedrine, a sympathomimetic amine, acts on alpha-adrenergic receptors in the mucosa of the respiratory tract, producing vasoconstriction. The medication shrinks swollen nasal mucous membranes, reduces tissue hyperemia, edema, and nasal congestion, and increases nasal airway patency. Also, drainage of sinus secretions is increased and obstructed eustachian ostia may be opened.

Guaifenesin has an expectorant action which increases the output of respiratory tract fluid by reducing adhesiveness and surface tension. The increased flow of less viscid secretions promotes ciliary action, lubricating irritated respiratory tract membranes, and facilitates removal of viscous, inspissated mucus. This changes a dry, unproductive cough to a cough that is more productiive and less frequent.

Indications: HISTALET® X Tablets and Syrup are indicated for the symptomatic relief of nasal congestion and dry non-productive cough in conditions such as: the common cold, acute bronchitis, allergic asthma, bronchiolitis, croup, emphysema and tracheobronchitis.

Contraindications: Contraindicated in patients with severe hypertension, severe coronary artery disease and in patients on monoamine oxidase (MAO) inhibitor therapy.

Nursing Mothers: Pseudoephedrine is contraindicated in nursing mothers because of the higher than usual risk for infants from sympathomimetic amines.

Hypersensitivity: This drug is contraindicated in patients with hypersensitivity or idiosyncrasy to its ingredients. Patient idiosyncrasy to adrenergic agents may be manifested by insomnia, dizziness, weakness, tremor or arrhythmias.

Warnings: HISTALET® X Tablets and Syrup should be used with considerable caution in patients with increased intraocular pressure (narrow angle glaucoma), symptomatic prostatic hypertrophy, bladder neck obstruction, hypertension, diabetes mellitus, ischemic heart disease, and hyperthyroidism.

Use in Children: As in adults, a sympathomimetic amine can elicit either mild stimulation or mild sedation.

Use in the Elderly (Approximately 60 years or older): The elderly are more likely to exhibit adverse reactions to sympathomimetics. At doses higher than the recommended dose, nervousness, dizziness, or sleeplessness may occur.

Precautions: General: DO NOT CRUSH OR CHEW HISTALET® X TABLETS BEFORE INGESTION. As with other sympathomimetic drugs, HISTALET® X Tablets and Syrup should be used with caution in the presence of hypertension, hyperthyroidism, diabetes, heart disease, glaucoma, and prostatic hypertrophy. Tricyclic antidepressants may antagonize the effects of pseudoephedrine.

Drug Interactions: Monoamine oxidase (MAO) inhibitors and beta adrenergic blockers may potentiate the effects of sympathomimetic amines. Sympathomimetic amines may reduce the antihypertensive effects of guanethidine, mecamylamine, methyldopa, reserpine, and veratrum alkaloids.

Drug/Laboratory Test Interations: Guaifenesin has been shown to produce a color interference with certain clinical laboratory determinations of 5-hydroxyindoleacetic acid (5-HIAA) and vanillylmandelic acid (VMA).

Usage in Pregnancy: Pregnancy Category C. Reproduction studies have not been performed in animals with HISTALET® X Tablets and Syrup. There is no adequate information on whether this drug may affect fertility in males and females or has a teratogenic potential or other adverse effect on the fetus.

Usage in Nursing Mothers: The components of HISTALET® X Tablets and Syrup are excreted in breast milk in small amounts, but the significance of their effect on nursing infants is not known. Because of the potential for serious adverse reactions to sympathomimetic amines in nursing infants from maternal ingestion of HISTALET® X Tablets and Syrup, a decision should be made whether to discontinue nursing or to discontinue the drug, taking into account the importance of the drug to the mother.

Adverse Reactions: Possible adverse reactions include nervousness, insomnia, restlessness, tachycardia, headache, nausea, weakness, dizziness, dry mouth, or urinary retention in patients with prostatic hypertrophy.

Dosage: Histalet® Syrup, Histalet® DM Syrup and Histalet® X Syrup—ADULTS—2 teaspoonfuls 4 times daily, CHILDREN (6–12)—1 teaspoonful 4 times daily, CHILDREN (2–6)—½ teaspoonful 4 times daily, CHILDREN (under 2)—only as directed by physician.

DO NOT EXCEED 4 DOSES IN 24 HOUR PERIOD

Histalet® X Tablets—ADULTS and Children Over 12—1 tablet every 12 hours, CHILDREN (6–12)—½ tablet every 12 hours. DO NOT EXCEED RECOMMENDED DOSAGE.

Histalet® Forte Tablets—ADULTS—1 tablet, 2-3 times daily, CHILDREN (6–12)—½ tablet 2-3 times daily.

Do not exceed recommended dosage.

How Supplied:
Histalet® Syrup NDC 0063-1035-12, pint bottles
Histalet® DM Syrup NDC 0063-1037-12, pint bottles
Histalet® X Syrup NDC 0063-1052-12, pint bottles
Histalet® X Tablets NDC 0063-1050-06, bottles of 100 tablets
Histalet® Forte Tablets NDC 0063-1039-06 bottles of 100 tablets
NDC 0063-1039-07 bottles of 250 tablets
Shown in Product Identification Section, page 428

MELFIAT®
[mel′ fē-aht]
Phendimetrazine Tartrate 35 mg tablets

How Supplied:
NDC 0063-1079-06 Bottles of 100
NDC 0063-1079-09 Bottles of 1000

MELFIAT®-105 UNICELLES®
[mel′ fē-aht 105 ūn′ i-sels]
(phendimetrazine tartrate) 105 mg.
Slow Release Capsules

Description: Chemical name: Phendimetrazine Tartrate (+) 3, 4 Dimethyl-2-phenylmorpholine tartrate. Phendimetrazine Tartrate is a white, odorless powder with a bitter taste. It is soluble in water, methanol and ethanol. It has a molecular weight of 341. The capsule is manufactured in a special base which is designed for prolonged release.

Clinical Pharmacology: Phendimetrazine Tartrate is a sympathomimetic amine with pharmacologic activity similar to the prototype of drugs of this class used in obesity, the amphetamines. Actions include central nervous system stimulation and elevation of blood pressure. Tachyphylaxis and tolerance have been demonstrated with all drugs of this class in which these phenomena have been looked for.

Drugs of this class used in obesity are commonly known as "anorectics" or "anorexigenics". It has not been established, however, that the action of such drugs in treating obesity is primarily one of appetite suppression. Other central nervous system actions, or metabolic effects, may be involved, for example. Adult obese subjects instructed in dietary management and treated with "anorectic" drugs, lose more weight on the average than those treated with placebo and diet, as determined in relatively short-term clinical trials.

The magnitude of increased weight loss of drug-treated patients over placebo-treated patients is only a fraction of a pound a week. The rate of weight loss is greatest in the first weeks of therapy for both drug and placebo subjects and tends to decrease in succeeding weeks. The possible origins of the increased weight loss due to the various drug effects are not established. The amount of weight loss associated with the use of an "anorectic" drug varies from trial to trial, and the increased weight loss appears to be related in part to variables other than the drug prescribed, such as the physician-investigator, the population treated, and the diet prescribed. Studies do not permit conclusions as to the relative importance of the drug and non-drug factors on weight loss.

The natural history of obesity is measured in years, whereas the studies cited are restricted to a few weeks duration; thus, the total impact of drug-induced weight loss over that of diet alone must be considered clinically limited.

The active drug, 105 mg. of Phendimetrazine Tartrate in each capsule of this special timed release dosage form approximates the action of three 35 mg. non-timed doses taken at four hour intervals. The major route of elimination is via the kidneys where most of the drug and metabolites are excreted. Some of the drug is metabolized to Phenmetrazine and also Phendimetrazine-N-oxide.

The average half-life of elimination when studied under controlled conditions is about 3.7 hours for both the timed and non-timed forms. The absorption half-life of the drug from conventional non-timed 35 mg. phendimetrazine tablets is appreciably more rapid than the absorption rate of the drug from the timed release formulation.

Indications and Usage: MELFIAT-105 (Phendimetrazine Tartrate) is indicated in the management of exogenous obesity as a short term adjunct (a few weeks) in a regimen of weight reduction based on caloric restriction. The limited usefulness of agents of this class (see CLINICAL PHARMACOLOGY) should be measured against possible risk factors inherent in their use such as those described below.

Contraindications: Advanced arteriosclerosis, symptomatic cardiovascular disease, moderate to severe hypertension, hyperthyroidism, known hypersensitivity, or idiosyncrasy to the sympathomimetic amines, glaucoma.

Agitated states.

Patients with a history of drug abuse.

During or within 14 days following the administration of monoamine oxidase inhibitors, (hypertensive crises may result).

Warnings: Tolerance to the anorectic effect usually develops within a few weeks. When this occurs, the recommended dose should not be exceeded in an attempt to increase the effect; rather, the drug should be discontinued. Phendimetrazine Tartrate may impair the ability of the patient to engage in potentially hazardous activities such as operating machinery or driving a motor vehicle; the patient should therefore be cautioned accordingly.

Continued on next page

Reid-Provident—Cont.

Drug Dependence: Phendimetrazine Tartrate is related chemically and pharmacologically to the amphetamines. Amphetamines and related stimulant drugs have been extensively abused, and the possibility of abuse of Phendimetrazine Tartrate should be kept in mind when evaluating the desirability of including a drug as part of a weight reduction program. Abuse of amphetamines and related drugs may be associated with intense psychological dependence and severe social dysfunction. There are reports of patients who have increased the dosage to many times that recommended. Abrupt cessation following prolonged high dosage administration results in extreme fatigue and mental depression; changes are also noted on the sleep EEG. Manifestations of chronic intoxication with anorectic drugs include severe dermatoses, marked insomnia, irritability, hyperactivity, and personality changes. The most severe manifestation of chronic intoxications is psychosis, often clinically indistinguishable from schizophrenia.

Usage in Pregnancy: The safety of phendimetrazine tartrate in pregnancy and lactation has not been established. Therefore, Phendimetrazine Tartrate should not be taken by women who are or may become pregnant.

Usage in Children: Phendimetrazine Tartrate is not recommended for use in children under 12 years of age.

Precaution: Caution is to be exercised in prescribing Phendimetrazine Tartrate for patients with even mild hypertension.
Insulin requirements in diabetes mellitus may be altered in association with the use of Phendimetrazine Tartrate and the concomitant dietary regimen. Phendimetrazine Tartrate may decrease the hypotensive effect of guanethidine. The least amount feasible should be prescribed or dispensed at one time in order to minimize the possibility of overdosage.

Adverse Reactions: Cardiovascular: Palpitation, tachycardia, elevation of blood pressure.
Central Nervous System: Overstimulation, restlessness, dizziness, insomnia, euphoria, dysphoria, tremor, headache; rarely psychotic episodes at recommended doses.
Gastrointestinal: Dryness of the mouth, unpleasant taste, diarrhea, constipation, other gastrointestinal disturbances.
Allergic: Urticaria.
Endocrine: Impotence, changes in libido.
Overdosage: Manifestations of acute overdosage with Phendimetrazine Tartrate include restlessness, tremor, hyperreflexia, rapid respiration, confusion, assaultiveness, hallucinations, panic states.
Fatigue and depression usually follow the central stimulation.
Cardiovascular effects include arrhythmias, hypertension or hypotension and circulatory collapse. Gastrointestinal symptoms include nausea, vomiting, diarrhea, and abdominal cramps. Fatal poisoning usually terminates in convulsions and coma. Management of acute Phendimetrazine Tartrate intoxication is largely symptomatic and includes lavage and sedation with a barbiturate. Experience with hemodialysis or peritoneal dialysis is inadequate to permit recommendation in this regard. Acidification of the urine increases Phendimetrazine Tartrate excretion. Intravenous phentolamine (Regitine) has been suggested for possible acute, severe hypertension, if this complicates Phendimetrazine Tartrate overdosage.

Dosage and Administration: Since MELFIAT-105 (Phendimetrazine Tartrate 105 mg.) is a slow release dosage form, limit to one slow release capsule in the morning.
MELFIAT-105 (Phendimetrazine Tartrate) is not recommended for use in children under 12 years of age.

How Supplied: Each orange and clear slow release capsule contains 105 mg. Phendimetrazine Tartrate in bottles of 100 (NDC 0063-1082-06).
Caution: Federal law prohibits dispensing without prescription.
Shown in Product Identification Section, page 428

P-V-TUSSIN® SYRUP
[p-v tŭs'in]
P-V-TUSSIN® TABLETS
Antitussive-Antihistamine-Expectorant
Liquid and Tablets

Description: Each teaspoonful (5 ml) of P-V-TUSSIN® Syrup contains: Hydrocodone Bitartrate 2.5 mg (WARNING: May be habit forming), Phenylephrine HCl 5 mg, Pyrilamine Maleate 6 mg, Chlorpheniramine Maleate 2 mg, Phenindamine Tartrate 5 mg, Ammonium Chloride 50 mg; Alcohol 5%
Each Scored P-V-TUSSIN® Tablet contains: Hydrocodone Bitartrate 5 mg (WARNING: May be habit forming), Phenindamine Tartrate 25 mg, Guaifenesin 200 mg.

Indications and Usage: For the symptomatic relief of cough and nasal congestion due to common cold, upper respiratory tract congestion associated with the common cold, influenza, bronchitis and sinusitis.
Contraindications: P-V-TUSSIN® Syrup and Tablets is contraindicated in patients with a known hypersensitivity to hydrocodone bitartrate, phenylephrine HCl, pyrilamine maleate, chlorpheniramine maleate, phenindamine tartrate, ammonium chloride, or guaifenesin.
Warning: Hydrocodone should be prescribed and administered with the same degree of caution as all oral medications containing a narcotic analgesic.
Precautions: General Precautions—Use with caution in the presence of hypertension, cardiovascular disease, hyperthyroidism, or diabetes.
Information for Patients—Patients should be cautioned against driving a car or engaging in mechanical operations which require alertness, until it is known that they do not respond to the drug by becoming drowsy or dizzy.
Drug Interactions—Hydrocodone may potentiate the effects of other narcotics, general anesthetics, tranquilizers, sedatives and hypnotics, tricyclic antidepressants, MAO inhibitors, alcohol and other CNS depressants.
Adverse Reactions: Adverse reactions, when they occur, include sedation, nausea, vomiting and constipation.
Drug Abuse and Dependence: Controlled Substance—P-V-Tussin® is a schedule III drug. Dependence—Continued use of hydrocodone may result in true addiction.
Dosage and Administration:
P-V-Tussin® Syrup:
Adults, 2 teaspoonfuls every 4 to 6 hours
Children 6 to 12, 1 teaspoonful every 4 to 6 hours
Children 3 to 6, ½ to 1 teaspoonful every 4 to 6 hours.
Children 1 to 3, ½ teaspoonful every 4 to 6 hours.
Dose for children should not be repeated more than 4 times in a 24 hour period.
P-V-Tussin® Tablets:
Adults and children over 12, 1 tablet 4 times daily or as directed by physician. Children 6 to 12, ½ tablet 4 times daily. Should be taken after meals and at bedtime, not less than 4 hours apart. Do not exceed the recommended dosage.
Caution: Federal law prohibits dispensing without prescription.
How Supplied:
P-V-Tussin® Syrup
NDC 0063-1087-12, pint bottles
NDC 0063-1087-13, gallon bottles
P-V-Tussin® Tablets
NDC 0063-1088-06, bottles of 100 tablets
Shown in Product Identification Section, page 428

RU-VERT-M®
[rū'vert-m"]
Description:
Each red film coated tablet contains:
Meclizine HCl..25 mg
How Supplied:
NDC 0063-7025-06, Bottles of 100
NDC 0063-7025-53, Bottles of 300
Shown in Product Identification Section, page 428

UNIPRES®
[ūn'ĭ-pres]
Formula: Each tablet contains:
Hydralazine Hydrochloride........................25 mg.
Hydrochlorothiazide...................................15 mg.
Reserprine..0.1 mg.
How Supplied:
NDC 0063-1132-06 Bottles of 100
NDC 0063-1132-09 Bottles of 1000
Shown in Product Identification Section, page 428

ZENATE PRENATAL TABLETS
[zē'nāt]
Film Coated)

Clinical Advantages: Each tablet contains iron that is specifically formulated to minimize gastric irritation.
[See table on left].
Indications and Uses: Vitamin-mineral dietary adjunct in nutritional stress associated with pregnancy and lactation.
Zenate is a phosphorous free[1] vitamin-mineral dietary supplement, specifically formulated for use during pregnancy and lactation. All ingredients covered by a warning or caution for usage in pregnancy have been formulated so as not to exceed maximum recommended strengths. The formulation includes essential vitamins and minerals, including 300 mg. of elemental calcium, 65 mg. of elemental iron and 20 mg. of elemental zinc. Zenate also offers 1 mg. of folic acid to aid in the prevention of megaloblastic anemia.
Precautions: Folic Acid in doses above 0.1 mg. daily may obscure pernicious anemia in that hematologic remission can occur while neurological manifestations remain progressive. Periodic laboratory studies are considered essential and are recommended. Allergic sensitization has been

ZENATE

Each tablet contains:	ZENATE	% U.S. RDA Pregnant or Lactating Women
VITAMINS:		
A (as palmitate)	5,000 I.U.	62.5
D (as calciferol)	400 I.U.	100
E (as dl-alpha tocopheryl acetate)	30 I.U.	100
C (ascorbic acid)	80 mg.	133
Folic Acid	1 mg.	125
Thiamine (as thiamine mononitrate Vitamin B_1)	3 mg.	176
Riboflavin (Vitamin B_2)	3 mg.	150
Niacin (as niacinamide)	20 mg.	100
B_6 (as pyridoxine hydrochloride)	10 mg.	400
B_{12} (cyanocobalamin)	12 mcg.	150
MINERALS:		
Calcium (from 833 mg. calcium carbonate)	300 mg.	23
Iodine (from 230 mcg. potassium iodide)	175 mcg.	117
Iron (from 198 mg. ferrous fumarate)	65 mg.	361
Magnesium (from 173 mg. magnesium oxide)	100 mg.	22
Zinc (from 25 mg. zinc oxide)	20 mg.	133

reported following both oral and parenteral administration of Folic Acid.
Dosage and Administration: As a dietary adjunct in nutritional stress associated with pregnancy and lactation. One tablet daily before the first meal, or as directed by physician.
How Supplied: Bottles of 100 baby blue film coated tablets.
NDC 0063-1146-06.
Caution: Federal Law Prohibits Dispensing Without Prescription.
Reference: 1. Pitkin, R.M.: Vitamins and Minerals in Pregnancy. *Clinics in Perinatology,* 2:221-232, 1975.
Shown in Product Identification Section, page 428

Rexar Pharmacal Corp.
396 ROCKAWAY AVENUE
VALLEY STREAM, NY 11581

PRODUCT Number	PRODUCT	
5432	OBETROL-10 BLUE TABLETS Dextroamphetamine Sulfate 2.5mg. Dextroamphetamine Saccharate 2.5mg. Amphetamine Sulfate 2.5mg. Amphetamine Aspartate 2.5mg.	℞ ©
5433	OBETROL-20 ORANGE TABLETS Dextroamphetamine Sulfate 5.0mg. Dextroamphetamine Saccharate 5.0mg. Amphetamine Sulfate 5.0mg. Amphetamine Aspartate 5.0mg.	℞ ©
5451	DEXTROAMPHETAMINE SULFATE 5mg. Scored Yellow Tablets	℞ ©
5452	DEXTROAMPHETAMINE SULFATE 10mg. Double Scored Yellow Tablets	℞ ©
5455	METHAMPHETAMINE HYDROCHLORIDE 5mg. Scored Pink Tablets	℞ ©
5456	METHAMPHETAMINE HYDROCHLORIDE 10mg. Double Scored Pink Tablets	℞ ©
5457	X-TROZINE TABLETS PHENDIMETRAZINE TARTRATE 35 mg. Colors: Blue; Green; Pink; Yellow	℞ ©
5463	X-TROZINE CAPSULES PHENDIMETRAZINE TARTRATE 35mg. Colors: Blue; Red/White; Black; Black/Orange	℞ ©
5462	X-TROZINE LA-105 PHENDIMETRAZINE TARTRATE 105mg. Long Acting Capsules— Color: Brown/Clear	℞ ©
5468	OBY-TRIM 30 CAPSULES PHENTERMINE HYDROCHLORIDE 30mg. Colors: Black; Yellow; Brown/White	℞ ©

IDENTIFICATION PROBLEM?
Consult PDR's
Product Identification Section
where you'll find over 1200
products pictured actual size
and in full color.

The following Riker products are available in Military and Veterans Administration depots:

Military Depot Items	National Stock Number
Disalcid® Tablets 500's	6505-01-067-2750
Duo-Medihaler® (aerosol) w/adapter 22.5 ml.	6505-00-071-7861
Medihaler-Iso® (aerosol) w/adapter 15 ml.	6505-00-023-6481
Medihaler-Iso® (aerosol) w/adapter 22.5 ml.	6505-00-014-8486
Norflex® Tablets 100's	6505-00-138-8462
Norgesic® Tablets 500's	6505-00-952-6762
Norgesic® Forte Tablets 500's	6505-01-029-9116
Tepanil® Ten-tab® (controlled-release tablet) 75 mg. 100's	6505-00-082-2684
Urex® Tablets 100's	6505-00-126-3207

Veterans Administration Depot Items	National Stock Number
Alu-Cap® Capsules 100's	6505-00-166-7844
Disalcid® Tablets 500's	6505-01-067-2750A
Duo-Medihaler® (aerosol) w/adapter 22.5 ml.	6505-00-071-7861A
Medihaler-Iso® (aerosol) w/adapter 22.5 ml.	6505-00-014-8486A
Norflex® Tablets 100's	6505-00-138-8462A
Norgesic® Tablets 500's	6505-00-952-6762A
Norgesic® Forte Tablets 500's	6505-01-029-9116A
Theolair™ Tablets 125 mg. 250's	6505-01-075-8307A
Theolair™ Tablets 250 mg. 250's	6505-01-075-8308A
Theolair™-SR Tablets 250 mg. 100's	6505-01-094-1613A
Urex® Tablets 500's	6505-00-443-4501

Riker Laboratories, Inc.
225-1S-07 3M CENTER
ST. PAUL, MN 55144

[See table above].

ALU-TAB® Tablets
and
ALU-CAP® Capsules

Description: Each green Alu-Tab "swallow" tablet contains dried aluminum hydroxide gel 600 mg. Each red and green Alu-Cap capsule contains dried aluminum hydroxide gel 475 mg.
Actions: Antacid actions include neutralization of gastric hyperacidity and mild astringent and absorbent properties. Aluminum hydroxide dried gel increases phosphate excretion in the bowel by the formation of non-absorbable salts.*
Indications: Treatment in uncomplicated peptic ulcer and gastric hyperacidity.
Precautions: Aluminum hydroxide is essentially a nontoxic compound. If constipation occurs, medication should be discontinued and a physician should be consulted. Aluminum hydroxide must be given with care to patients who have recently suffered massive upper gastrointestinal hemorrhage. Do not give this product to any patient presently taking a prescription antibiotic drug containing any form of tetracycline.
Directions: Three Alu-Tab "swallow" tablets three times a day or as prescribed by physician. Three Alu-Cap capsules three times a day or as prescribed by physician.
How Supplied: Bottles of 250 green film-coated Alu-Tab "swallow" tablets (NDC **0089-0107-25**). Bottles of 100 red and green Alu-Cap capsules (NDC **0089-0106-10**).
*Goodman, L.S., and Gilman, A.: *The Pharmacological Basis of Therapeutics,* 6th ed., Macmillan Publishing Co., Inc. New York, 1980, p. 990.

CALCIUM DISODIUM VERSENATE* ℞
(calcium disodium edetate injection, U.S.P.)
Injection

WARNING
Calcium Disodium Edetate is capable of producing toxic and potentially fatal effects. The dosage schedule should be followed and at no time should the recommended daily dose be exceeded. In lead encephalopathy avoid rapid infusion; intramuscular route is preferred.

Description: Calcium Disodium Versenate Injection (Calcium Disodium Edetate Injection, U.S.P.) is a sterile concentrated solution (20%) containing 200 mg. of calcium disodium edetate per ml. for intravenous infusion or intramuscular injection.
Clinical Pharmacology: The calcium in calcium disodium edetate is readily displaced by heavy metals, such as lead, to form stable complexes. Following parenteral injection, the chelate formed is excreted in the urine, with 50 percent appearing in the first hour after administration.
Indications and Usage: Calcium disodium edetate is indicated for the reduction of blood levels and depot stores of lead in lead poisoning (acute and chronic) and lead encephalopathy.
Contraindications: Calcium disodium edetate should not be given during periods of anuria.
Warnings: See box warning above.
Usage in pregnancy: The safe use of calcium disodium edetate has not been established with respect to possible adverse effects upon fetal development. Therefore, it should not be used in women of child-bearing potential and particularly during early pregnancy unless, in the judgment of the physician, the potential benefits outweigh the possible hazards.
Precautions: Severe acute lead poisoning by itself may cause proteinuria and microscopic hematuria. Calcium disodium edetate may produce the same signs of renal damage. Routine urinalysis should be done daily during each course of therapy to determine whether the proteinuria and hematuria is improving or the evidence of renal tubular injury is getting worse. The presence of large renal epithelial cells or increasing numbers of red blood cells in the urinary sediment or greater proteinuria call for immediate stopping of calcium disodium edetate administration. Evidence of renal impairment should be looked for by periodic blood urea nitrogen determinations before and during each course of therapy. The patient should also be monitored for irregularities of cardiac rhythm.
Adverse Reactions: The principal toxic effect is renal tubular necrosis.
Dosage and Administration: Calcium disodium edetate is equally effective whether administered intravenously, subcutaneously or intramuscularly. Because of convenience in administration and greater safety in treating symptomatic children, many physicians experienced in the treatment of lead poisoning prefer the intramuscular route which is recommended in patients with either overt or incipient lead encephalopathy. Rapid intravenous infusions may be lethal by suddenly increasing intracranial pressure in this group of patients with cerebral edema.
Note: In patients with lead encephalopathy and increased intracranial pressure, excess fluids must be avoided. In such case a 20 percent solution of calcium disodium edetate is mixed with procaine to give a final concentration of 0.5 percent of pro-

Continued on next page

Riker—Cont.

caine in the mixture which is administered intramuscularly.

Acutely ill individuals may be dehydrated from vomiting. Since calcium disodium edetate is excreted almost exclusively in the urine, it is very important to establish urine flow by intravenous infusion before the first dose of the chelating agent is given. Once urine flow is established further intravenous fluid is restricted to basal water and electrolyte requirements. Administration of calcium disodium edetate should be stopped whenever there is cessation of urine flow in order to avoid unduly high tissue levels of the drug.

Intravenous Administration: Dilute the 5 ml. (1 gram, 20% solution) from an ampule with 250-500 ml. of Solution Isotonic Sodium Chloride, USP, or sterile 5% dextrose solution in water. In asymptomatic adults, administer this diluted solution over a period of at least one hour. Such doses may be administered twice daily for periods up to 5 days. The therapy should then be interrupted for 2 days and followed by an additional 5 days of treatment, if indicated.

In mildy affected or asymptomatic individuals the dosage of 50 mg./kg. per day should not be exceeded.

In symptomatic adults, fluids should be kept to basal levels and the time of administration increased to two hours. A second daily infusion is to be given six or more hours after the first.

Intramuscular Administration: This is the route of choice for children. The dosage should not exceed 0.5 gram per 30 pounds of body weight twice daily (total, 1.0 gram/30 lbs./day). This is equivalent to 35 mg./kg. twice daily (total, approx. 75 mg./kg./day). In mild cases a dose of 50 mg./kg. per day should not be exceeded. For young children the total daily dose may be given in divided doses every 8 or 12 hours for 3 to 5 days. A second course may be given after a rest period of 4 or more days. Procaine to produce a concentration of 0.5% should be added to minimize pain at injection site. (1 ml. of 1% procaine solution for each ml. of concentrated Calcium Disodium Versenate solution, or crystalline procaine may be used to reduce volume.)

Regardless of method of administration, doses larger than those recommended should not be undertaken.

Lead Encephalopathy: This condition is relatively rare in adults but is quite common in children in whom the mortality rate has been high. Recent reports by Chisolm and by Coffin et al who employed a combination of BAL and calcium disodium edetate, suggest that this may be the preferred treatment, although calcium disodium edetate alone has been used over a longer period of time. Each group administered calcium disodium edetate intramuscularly concurrently with BAL in separate deep I.M. sites. Procaine was added to the 20% solution of calcium disodium edetate to give a procaine concentration of 0.5%. In the studies of Coffin and Chisolm, 125 children with acute lead encephalopathy have been treated with this combined therapy with only one death.

How Supplied: Calcium Disodium Versenate Injection, 5 ml. ampules containing 200 mg. of calcium disodium edetate per ml., boxes containing 6 ampules.
(NDC 0089-0510-06).

*Registered trademark of the Dow Chemical Company

CAL-SUP™
Calcium Supplement 300 mg

Composition: Each tablet contains 750 mg calcium carbonate (equivalent to 300 mg elemental calcium) with glycine.

Indications: For use in the prevention of calcium deficiency when needed or recommended by a physician.

Directions: Take three or four tablets daily, or as directed by your physician. Chew, swallow or melt in the mouth.

Three tablets daily provide:

Quantity	U.S. RDA†	
Calcium 900 mg	90%*	69%**

Four tablets daily provide:

Quantity	U.S. RDA†	
Calcium 1200 mg	120%*	92%**

† U.S. recommended daily allowance
* For adults and children 12 or more years of age
** For pregnant and lactating women

How Supplied: Bottles of 100 white tablets (NDC 0089-0110-10).

CIRCANOL®
(ergoloid mesylates)
TABLETS FOR SUBLINGUAL ADMINISTRATION

Description: Each white, round, sublingual 0.5 mg tablet contains dihydroergocornine 0.167 mg, dihydroergocristine 0.167 mg and dihydroergocryptine 0.167 mg (dihydro-alpha-ergocryptine and dihydro-beta-ergocryptine in the proportion of 2:1) as the methanesulfonates (mesylates), representing a total of 0.5 mg.

Each white, oval, sublingual 1.0 mg tablet contains dihydroergocornine 0.333 mg, dihydroergocristine 0.333 mg and dihydroergocryptine 0.333 mg (dihydro-alpha-ergocryptine and dihydro-beta-ergocryptine in the proportion of 2:1) as the methanesulfonates (mesylates), representing a total of 1.0 mg.

How Supplied: Circanol (ergoloid mesylates) sublingual tablets are supplied as 0.5 mg white round tablets in bottles of 100 (NDC 0089-0121-10) and 1,000 (NDC 0089-0121-80) and 1.0 mg white oval tablets in bottles of 1,000 (NDC 0089-0123-80) and 100 (NDC 0089-0123-10).

DISALCID®
(salsalate)
Tablets and Capsules

Description: DISALCID (salsalate) is a nonsteroidal anti-inflammatory agent for oral administration. Chemically, salsalate (salicylsalicylic acid or 2-hydroxy-benzoic acid 2-carboxyphenyl ester) is a dimer of salicylic acid.

Each round, aqua, film coated DISALCID tablet contains 500 mg salsalate. Each aqua and white DISALCID capsule contains 500 mg salsalate. Each capsule-shaped aqua, scored, film coated DISALCID tablet contains 750 mg salsalate. (See HOW SUPPLIED).

Clinical Pharmacology: DISALCID is insoluble in acid gastric fluids (<0.1 mg/ml at pH 1.0), but readily soluble in the small intestine where it is partially hydrolyzed to two molecules of salicylic acid. A significant portion of the parent compound is absorbed unchanged and undergoes rapid esterase hydrolysis in the body; its half-life is about one hour. About 13% is excreted through the kidneys as a glucuronide conjugate of the parent compound, the remainder as salicylic acid and its metabolites. Thus, the amount of salicylic acid available from DISALCID is about 15% less than from aspirin, when the two drugs are administered on a salicylic acid molar equivalent basis (3.6 g salsalate/5 g aspirin). Salicylic acid biotransformation is saturated at anti-inflammatory doses of DISALCID. Such capacity-limited biotransformation results in an increase in the half-life of salicylic acid from 3.5 to 16 or more hours. Thus, dosing with DISALCID twice a day will satisfactorily maintain blood levels within the desired therapeutic range (10 to 30 mg/100 ml) throughout the 12-hour intervals. Therapeutic blood levels continue for up to 16 hours after the last dose. The parent compound does not show capacity-limited biotransformation, nor does it accumulate in the plasma on multiple dosing. Food slows the absorption of all salicylates including DISALCID.

The mode of anti-inflammatory action of DISALCID and other nonsteroidal anti-inflammatory drugs is not fully defined. Although salicylic acid (the primary metabolite of DISALCID) is a weak inhibitor of prostaglandin synthesis in vitro, DISALCID appears to selectively inhibit prostaglandin synthesis in vivo, providing anti-inflammatory effect equivalent to aspirin, indomethacin, and ibuprofen. Unlike aspirin, DISALCID does not inhibit platelet aggregation.[1]

The usefulness of salicylic acid, the active in vivo product of DISALCID, in the treatment of arthritic disorders has been established.[2,3] In contrast to aspirin and the other nonsteroidal anti-inflammatory drugs, DISALCID does not cause gastrointestinal blood loss[4] or peptic disease.[5]

Indications and Usage: DISALCID is indicated for relief of the signs and symptoms of rheumatoid arthritis, osteoarthritis and related rheumatic disorders.

DISALCID can safely be given to aspirin-sensitive patients (and those sensitive to tartrazine, FD&C Yellow No. 5), since it does not induce asthma in such patients.[6]

Contraindications: DISALCID is contraindicated in patients hypersensitive to salsalate.

Warnings: See PRECAUTIONS.

Precautions:

General Precautions: Patients on long-term treatment with DISALCID should be warned not to take other salicylates so as to avoid potentially toxic concentrations. Great care should be exercised when DISALCID is prescribed in the presence of chronic renal insufficiency. Protein binding of salicylic acid can be influenced by nutritional status, competitive binding of other drugs, and fluctuations in serum proteins caused by disease (rheumatoid arthritis, etc.).

Laboratory Tests: Plasma salicylic acid concentrations should be periodically monitored during long-term treatment with DISALCID to aid maintenance of therapeutically effective levels: 10 to 30 mg/100 ml. Toxic manifestations are not usually seen until plasma concentrations exceed 30 mg/100 ml (see OVERDOSAGE). Urinary pH should also be regularly monitored: sudden acidification, as from pH 6.5 to 5.5, can double the plasma level, resulting in toxicity.

Drug Interactions: Salicylates antagonize the uricosuric action of drugs used to treat gout. Aspirin and other salicylate drugs will be additive to DISALCID and may increase plasma concentrations of salicylic acid to toxic levels. Drugs and foods that raise urine pH will increase renal clearance and urinary excretion of salicylic acid, thus lowering plasma levels; acidifying drugs or foods will decrease urinary excretion and increase plasma levels. Salicylates may competitively displace anticoagulant drugs from plasma protein binding sites and thereby predispose to systemic bleeding. Salicylates may enhance the hypoglycemic effect of oral antidiabetic drugs of the sulfonylurea class. Salicylate competes with a number of drugs for protein binding sites, notably penicillin, thiopental, thyroxine, triiodothyronine, phenytoin, sulfinpyrazone, naproxen, warfarin, methotrexate, and possibly corticosteroids.

Drug/Laboratory Test Interactions: Salicylate competes with thyroid hormone for binding to plasma proteins, which may be reflected in a depressed plasma T_4 value in some patients; thyroid function and basal metabolism are unaffected.

Carcinogenesis: No long-term animal studies have been performed with DISALCID to evaluate its carcinogenic potential; however, several such studies using aspirin and other salicylates have failed to demonstrate any association of these agents with cancerous cell changes.

Use in Pregnancy: Pregnancy Category C: Salsalate and salicylic acid have been shown to be teratogenic and embryocidal in rats when given in doses 4 to 5 times the usual human dose. These effects were not observed at doses twice as great as the usual human dose. There are no adequate and well-controlled studies in pregnant women. DISALCID should be used during pregnancy only if

for possible revisions   **Product Information**   **1643**

the potential benefit justifies the potential risk to the fetus.
Labor and Delivery: There exist no adequate and well-controlled studies in pregnant women. Although adverse effects on mother or infant have not been reported with DISALCID use during labor, caution is advised when anti-inflammatory dosage is involved. However, other salicylates have been associated with prolonged gestation and labor, maternal and neonatal bleeding sequelae, potentiation of narcotic and barbiturate effects (respiratory or cardiac arrest in the mother), delivery problems and stillbirth.
Nursing Mothers: It is not known whether salsalate per se is excreted in human milk; salicylic acid, the primary metabolite of DISALCID, has been shown to appear in human milk in concentrations approximating the maternal blood level. Thus the infant of a mother on DISALCID therapy might ingest in mother's milk 30 to 80% as much salicylate per kg body weight as the mother is taking. Accordingly, caution should be exercised when DISALCID is administered to a nursing woman.
Pediatric Use: Safety and effectiveness in children have not been established.
Adverse Reactions:
Auditory system: Tinnitus and temporary hearing loss can occur. Tinnitus probably represents blood salicylic acid levels reaching or exceeding the upper limit of the therapeutic range. It is therefore a helpful guide to dose titration. Temporary hearing loss disappears gradually upon discontinuation of the drug.
Gastrointestinal system: Nausea, dyspepsia and heartburn occur occasionally.
Drug Abuse and Dependence: Drug abuse and dependence have not been reported with DISALCID.
Overdosage: No deaths after overdosage have been reported for DISALCID. Death has followed ingestion of 10 to 30 g of other salicylates in adults, but much larger amounts have been ingested without fatal outcome.
The oral LD_{50} for DISALCID in rats is approximately 2000 mg/kg (sixty times the recommended maximum single dose for adults).
Symptoms: The usual symptoms of salicylism—tinnitus, vertigo, headache, confusion, drowsiness, sweating, hyperventilation, vomiting and diarrhea—will occur. More severe intoxication will lead to disruption of electrolyte balance and blood pH, and hyperthermia and dehydration.
Treatment: Further absorption of DISALCID from the G.I. tract should be prevented by emesis (syrup of ipecac) and, if necessary, by gastric lavage.
Fluid and electrolyte imbalance should be corrected by the administration of appropriate I.V. therapy. Adequate renal function should be maintained. Hemodialysis or peritoneal dialysis may be required in extreme cases.
Dosage and Administration:
Adults: The usual dosage is 3000 mg daily, given in divided doses as follows: 1) Two doses of two 750 mg tablets; 2) two doses of three 500 mg tablets/capsules; or 3) three doses of two 500 mg tablets/capsules. Dosage should be adjusted depending on individual response. Alleviation of symptoms is gradual, and full benefit may not be evident for 3 to 4 days, when plasma salicylate levels have achieved steady state. There is no evidence for development of tissue tolerance (tachyphylaxis), but salicylate therapy may induce increased activity of metabolizing liver enzymes, causing a greater rate of salicyluric acid production and excretion, with a resultant increase in dosage requirement for maintenance of therapeutic serum salicylate levels.
Children: DISALCID has not been evaluated in children. No dosage recommendations can, therefore, be made.
How Supplied:
750 mg tablets in bottles of 100 (NDC **0089-0151-10**)
750 mg tablets in bottles of 500 (NDC **0089-0151-50**)
500 mg tablets in bottles of 100 (NDC **0089-0149-10**)
500 mg tablets in bottles of 500 (NDC **0089-0149-50**)
500 mg capsules in bottles of 100 (NDC **0089-0148-10**)
References:
1. Estes D, Kaplan K: Lack of Platelet Effect With the Aspirin Analog, Salsalate. Arthritis and Rheumatism **23**: 1303, 1980.
2. Dick C, Dick PH, Nuki G, et al: Effect of Anti-inflammatory Drug Therapy on Clearance of ^{133}Xe from Knee Joints of Patients with Rheumatoid Arthritis. British Med. J. **3**:278–280, 1969.
3. Dick WC, Grayson MF, Woodburn A, et al: Indices of Inflammatory Activity. Ann. of the Rheum. Dis. **29**:643–648, 1970.
4. Cohen A: Fecal Blood Loss and Plasma Salicylate Study of Salicylsalicylic Acid and Aspirin. J. Clin. Pharmacol. **19**:242–247, 1979.
5. Voltin, RF: Safety of Salsalate in Peptic Disease. Scientific Exhibit, PANLAR, June 6–10, 1982.
6. Simon MR, Salberg DJ, Muller BF, et al: Lack of Adverse Reactions to Salsalate in Asthmatic Subjects. Data on file, Medical Department, Riker Laboratories, Inc.
Caution: Federal law prohibits dispensing without prescription.
Shown in Product Identification Section, page 428

DISIPAL®   ℞
(orphenadrine hydrochloride)
TABLETS
Description: Each round, green disipal tablet contains orphenadrine hydrochloride (2-dimethylaminoethyl 2-methylbenzhydryl ether hydrochloride) 50 mg.
How Supplied: Bottles of 100 Tablets (NDC 0089-0161-10) imprinted "RIKER" on one side and "161" on the other.

DUO-MEDIHALER®   ℞
(isoproterenol hydrochloride and phenylephrine bitartrate)
Description: Duo-Medihaler (isoproterenol hydrochloride and phenylephrine bitartrate) is an aerosol device which delivers micronized particles of isoproterenol hydrochloride and phenylephrine bitartrate suspended in an inert mixture of sorbitan trioleate, cetylpyridinium chloride with fluorochlorohydrocarbons as propellants. This drug-propellant system is contained in a hermetically sealed metal vial. Each valve actuation releases a uniform aerosolized dose of 0.16 mg. isoproterenol hydrochloride (equivalent to 0.137 mg. of isoproterenol base) and 0.24 mg. phenylephrine bitartrate (equivalent to 0.126 mg. of phenylephrine base).
How Supplied: *For long-term use:*
Initial Rx: Duo-Medihaler with adapter (450 doses, 22.5 ml.) NDC **0089-0732-21**.
Refill: Duo-Medihaler refill vial (450 doses, 22.5 ml.) NDC **0089-0732-11**.
For patients with less frequent need:
Initial Rx: Duo-Medihaler with adapter (300 doses, 15 ml.) NDC **0089-0735-21**.
Refill: Duo-Medihaler refill (300 doses, 15 ml.) NDC **0089-0735-11**.

MEDIHALER-EPI®
(epinephrine bitartrate)
FOR TEMPORARY RELIEF FROM ACUTE PAROXYSMS OF BRONCHIAL ASTHMA.
FOR ORAL INHALATION THERAPY ONLY
Each inhalation delivers 0.3 mg epinephrine bitartrate equivalent to 0.16 mg of epinephrine base.
How Supplied: 15 ml. size: Available as a combination package (vial with oral adapter) or as a refill (vial only).

MEDIHALER ERGOTAMINE®   ℞
(ergotamine tartrate)
Description: Medihaler Ergotamine (ergotamine tartrate) is an aerosol device which contains a fine particle suspension of 9.0 mg. ergotamine tartrate per ml. in an inert, nontoxic aerosol vehicle. Each depression of the valve delivers a measured dose of 0.36 mg. to the patient.
Action: Ergotamine exerts a constrictor action upon the cranial vessels.
Indications: As therapy to abort vascular headache, e.g., migraine, migraine variants, or so-called "histaminic cephalalgia."
Contraindications: Ergotamine tartrate should not be used in the presence of coronary artery disease, peripheral vascular disease, hypertension, impaired renal or hepatic function, infectious states or malnutrition.
Ergotamine tartrate is contraindicated in patients with a history of hypersensitivity reactions.
Pregnancy: Ergotamine tartrate is contraindicated in pregnancy.
Warnings: Patients who are being treated with Medihaler Ergotamine should be informed adequately of the symptoms of ergotism. Close medical supervision by the physician is recommended so that he may react appropriately should signs of ergotism develop. Six inhalations per day, if continued daily, entail the risk of vasospastic complications. Avoid prolonged administration or in excess of the recommended dosage because of the danger of ergotism and gangrene.
Pediatric Patients: Since there is no experience in children who have received this drug, safety and efficacy in children have not been established.
Nursing Mothers: Whether ergotamine tartrate is excreted in mothers' milk is not known. As a general rule, nursing should not be undertaken while a patient is on a drug (since many drugs are excreted in human milk).
Adverse Reactions: Ergotamine tartrate may cause nausea and vomiting. Patients with headaches may become nauseated and drug induced distress may be difficult to evaluate.
Ergotamine in large doses raises arterial pressure, produces coronary vasoconstriction and slows the heart both by direct action and its effect on the vagus. Under this condition, ergotamine also has oxytocic and spasmolytic properties. The above conditions are seen as a consequence of overdosage and may be manifested at the dosage recommended for control of headaches.
Vasoconstrictive complications, at times of a serious nature, may occur. These include pulselessness, weakness, muscle pains and paresthesias of the extremities and precordial distress and pain. Although these effects occur most commonly with long term therapy at relatively high doses, they have also been reported with short term or normal doses. Other adverse effects include transient tachycardia or bradycardia, nausea, vomiting, localized edema and itching.
Dosage and Administration:
Adults: A single inhalation at the first sign of headache or prodrome. Repeat this procedure in 5 minutes if relief is not obtained. Space any additional inhalations at no less than 5-minute intervals. No more than 6 inhalations should be administered in any 24-hour period, and no more than 15 in a one week period.
Children: A recommended dose for children has not been determined.
Directions For Use: Before each use, remove dust cap and shake Medihaler.
1. Breathe out fully and place mouthpiece well into the mouth, aimed at the back of the throat.
2. As you begin to breathe in deeply, press the vial firmly down into the adapter with the index finger. This releases one dose.
3. Release pressure on vial and remove unit from mouth. Hold the breath as long as possible, then breathe out slowly.
How Supplied: Metal vial (2.5 ml.) and adapter. Each depression of the valve delivers 0.36 mg. ergotamine tartrate. (NDC **0089-0762-21**).
Shown in Product Identification Section, page 428

Continued on next page

Riker—Cont.

MEDIHALER-ISO®
(isoproterenol sulfate)

℞

Description: Medihaler-Iso (isoproterenol sulfate) is an aerosol device which contains a fine particle suspension of 2.0 mg. per ml. isoproterenol sulfate in an inert propellant consisting of sorbitan trioleate and fluorochlorohydrocarbons. Each depression of the valve delivers a measured dose of 0.08 mg. to the patient.

How Supplied: Medihaler-Iso (isoproterenol sulfate) with oral adapter (300 doses 15 ml.) NDC **0089-0785-21**.
Medihaler-Iso (isoproterenol sulfate) refill vial only (300 doses 15 ml.) NDC **0089-0785-11**.
Medihaler-Iso (isoproterenol sulfate) with oral adapter (450 doses 22.5 ml.) NDC **0089-0782-21**.
Medihaler-Iso (isoproterenol sulfate) refill vial only (450 doses 22.5 ml.) NDC **0089-0782-11**.

NORFLEX®
(orphenadrine citrate)
Tablets and Injectable

℞

Description: Orphenadrine citrate is the citrate salt of orphenadrine (2-dimethyl aminoethyl 2-methylbenzhydryl ether citrate). It occurs as a white, crystalline powder having a bitter taste. It is practically odorless; sparingly soluble in water, slightly soluble in alcohol.

Actions: The mode of therapeutic action has not been clearly identified, but may be related to its analgesic properties. Orphenadrine citrate also possesses anti-cholinergic actions.

Indications: Orphenadrine citrate is indicated as an adjunct to rest, physical therapy, and other measures for the relief of discomfort associated with acute painful musculo skeletal conditions. The mode of action of the drug has not been clearly identified, but may be related to its analgesic properties. Orphenadrine citrate does not directly relax tense skeletal muscles in man.

Contraindications: Contraindicated in patients with glaucoma, pyloric or duodenal obstruction, stenosing peptic ulcers, prostatic hypertrophy or obstruction of the bladder neck, cardio-spasm (megaesophagus) and myasthenia gravis. Contraindicated in patients who have demonstrated a previous hypersensitivity to the drug.

Warnings: Some patients may experience transient episodes of light-headedness, dizziness or syncope. Norflex may impair the ability of the patient to engage in potentially hazardous activities such as operating machinery or driving a motor vehicle; ambulatory patients should therefore be cautioned accordingly.

Usage in Pregnancy: Safe use of orphenadrine has not been established with respect to adverse effects upon fetal development. Therefore, Norflex should be used in women of childbearing potential and particularly during early pregnancy only when in the judgment of the physician the potential benefits outweigh the possible hazards.

Usage in Children: Safety and effectiveness in children have not been established; therefore, this drug is not recommended for use in the pediatric age group.

Precautions: Confusion, anxiety and tremors have been reported in few patients receiving propoxyphene and orphenadrine concomitantly. As these symptoms may be simply due to an additive effect, reduction of dosage and/or discontinuation of one or both agents is recommended in such cases.
Orphenadrine citrate should be used with caution in patients with tachycardia, cardiac decompensation, coronary insufficiency, cardiac arrhythmias. Safety of continuous long-term therapy with orphenadrine has not been established. Therefore, if orphenadrine is prescribed for prolonged use, periodic monitoring of blood, urine and liver function values is recommended.

Adverse Reactions: Adverse effects of orphenadrine are mainly due to the mild anticholinergic action of orphenadrine, and are usually associated with higher dosage. Dryness of the mouth is usually the first adverse effect to appear. When the daily dose is increased, possible adverse effects include: tachycardia, palpitation, urinary hesitancy or retention, blurred vision, dilatation of pupils, increased ocular tension, weakness, nausea, vomiting, headache, dizziness, constipation, drowsiness, hypersensitivity reactions, pruritus, hallucinations, agitation, tremor, gastric irritation, and rarely urticaria and other dermatoses. Infrequently, an elderly patient may experience some degree of mental confusion. These adverse reactions can usually be eliminated by reduction in dosage. Very rare cases of aplastic anemia associated with the use of orphenadrine tablets have been reported. No causal relationship has been established.
Rare instances of anaphylactic reaction have been reported associated with the intramuscular injection of Norflex injectable.

Dosage and Administration: TABLETS: Adults—Two tablets per day; one in the morning and one in the evening.
INJECTABLE: Adults—One 2 ml. ampul (60 mg.) intravenously or intramuscularly; may be repeated every 12 hours. Relief may be maintained by 1 Norflex tablet twice daily.

How Supplied: TABLETS: Bottles of 100 (NDC **0089-0221-10**) and 500 (NDC **0089-0221-50**), each tablet containing 100 mg. of orphenadrine citrate.
INJECTABLE: Boxes of 6 (NDC **0089-0540-06**) and 50 (NDC **0089-0540-50**) 2 ml. ampuls, each ampul containing 60 mg. of orphenadrine citrate in aqueous solution, made isotonic with sodium chloride.

A.H.F.S. Category 12:08

Caution: Federal law prohibits dispensing without prescription.
Shown in Product Identification Section, page 428

NORGESIC®
and
NORGESIC® FORTE

℞
℞

Actions: Orphenadrine citrate is a centrally acting (brain stem) compound which in animals selectively blocks facilitatory functions of the reticular formation. Orphenadrine does not produce myoneural block, nor does it affect crossed extensor reflexes. Orphenadrine prevents nicotine-induced convulsions but not those produced by strychnine.
Chronic administration of Norgesic to dogs and rats has revealed no drug-related toxicity. No blood or urine changes were observed, nor were there any macroscopic or microscopic pathological changes detected. Extensive experience with combinations containing aspirin and caffeine has established them as safe agents. The addition of orphenadrine citrate does not alter the toxicity of aspirin and caffeine.
The mode of therapeutic action of orphenadrine has not been clearly identified, but may be related to its analgesic properties. Orphenadrine citrate also possesses anti-cholinergic actions.

Indications:
1. Symptomatic relief of mild to moderate pain of acute musculo-skeletal disorders.
2. The orphenadrine component is indicated as an adjunct to rest, physical therapy, and other measures for the relief of discomfort associated with acute painful musculo-skeletal conditions. The mode of action of orphenadrine has not been clearly identified, but may be related to its analgesic properties. Norgesic and Norgesic Forte do not directly relax tense skeletal muscles in man.

Contraindications: Because of the mild anticholinergic effect of orphenadrine, Norgesic or Norgesic Forte should not be used in patients with glaucoma, pyloric or duodenal obstruction, achalasia, prostatic hypertrophy or obstructions at the bladder neck. Norgesic or Norgesic Forte is also contraindicated in patients with myasthenia gravis and in patients known to be sensitive to aspirin or caffeine.
The drug is contraindicated in patients who have demonstrated a previous hypersensitivity to the drug.

Warnings: Norgesic Forte may impair the ability of the patient to engage in potentially hazardous activities such as operating machinery or driving a motor vehicle; ambulatory patients should therefore be cautioned accordingly.
Aspirin should be used with extreme caution in the presence of peptic ulcers and coagulation abnormalities.

Usage in Pregnancy: Since safety of the use of this preparation in pregnancy, during lactation, or in the childbearing age has not been established, use of the drug in such patients requires that the potential benefits of the drug be weighed against its possible hazard to the mother and child.

Usage in Children: The safe and effective use of this drug in children has not been established. Usage of this drug in children under 12 years of age is not recommended.

Precautions: Confusion, anxiety and tremors have been reported in few patients receiving propoxyphene and orphenadrine concomitantly. As these symptoms may be simply due to an additive effect, reduction of dosage and/or discontinuation of one or both agents is recommended in such cases.
Safety of continuous long term therapy with Norgesic Forte has not been established; therefore, if Norgesic Forte is prescribed for prolonged use, periodic monitoring of blood, urine and liver function values is recommended.

Adverse Reactions: Side effects of Norgesic or Norgesic Forte are those seen with aspirin and caffeine or those usually associated with mild anticholinergic agents. These may include tachycardia, palpitation, urinary hesitancy or retention, dry mouth, blurred vision, dilatation of the pupil, increased intraocular tension, weakness, nausea, vomiting, headache, dizziness, constipation, drowsiness, and rarely, urticaria and other dermatoses. Infrequently an elderly patient may experience some degree of confusion. Mild central excitation and occasional hallucinations may be observed. These mild side effects can usually be eliminated by reduction in dosage. One case of aplastic anemia associated with the use of Norgesic has been reported. No causal relationship has been established. Rare G.I. hemorrhage due to aspirin content may be associated with the administration of Norgesic or Norgesic Forte. Some patients may experience transient episodes of light-headedness, dizziness or syncope.

Dosage and Administration: Norgesic: Adults 1 to 2 tablets 3 to 4 times daily.
Norgesic Forte: Adults ½ to 1 tablet 3 to 4 times daily.

How Supplied: Norgesic tablets can be identified by their three layers colored light green, white and yellow. Each round tablet contains orphenadrine citrate (2-dimethylaminoethyl 2-methylbenzhydryl ether citrate) 25 mg., aspirin 385 mg., and caffeine 30 mg.
Norgesic Forte tablets are exactly twice the strength of Norgesic. They are identified by their scored capsule shape and by their three layers colored light green, white and yellow. Each capsule shaped tablet contains orphenadrine citrate 50 mg., aspirin 770 mg., and caffeine 60 mg.
Norgesic: Bottles of 100 (NDC **0089-0231-10**) and 500 tablets (NDC **0089-0231-50**).
Norgesic Forte: Bottles of 100 tablets (NDC **0089-0233-10**) and 500 tablets (NDC **0089-0233-50**).

Caution: Federal law prohibits dispensing without prescription.
Shown in Product Identification Section, page 428

RAUWILOID®
(alseroxylon)
tablets

℞

Description: Each tablet contains 2 mg. of the alseroxylon fraction of Rauwolfia serpentina, equivalent to not less than 0.15 mg. and not more than 0.20 mg. reserpine-rescinnamine group alkaloids expressed as reserpine.

for possible revisions **Product Information** 1645

How Supplied: Bottles of 100 (NDC 0089-0265-10) and 1000 (NDC 0089-0265-80) tablets.

TEPANIL®
(diethylpropion hydrochloride, U.S.P.)
TEPANIL® TEN-TAB®
(diethylpropion hydrochloride U.S.P.)
controlled release tablets

Description: Diethylpropion hydrochloride, a sympathomimetic agent, is 1-phenyl-2-diethylamino-1-propanone hydrochloride.
In Tepanil Ten-tab tablets, diethylpropion hydrochloride is dispersed in a hydrophilic matrix. On exposure to water the diethylpropion hydrochloride is released at a relatively uniform rate as a result of slow hydration of the matrix. The result is controlled release of the drug.
How Supplied: Tepanil 25 mg.: bottles of 100 (NDC 0089-0351-10) white tablets, Tepanil Ten-tab 75 mg.: bottles of 30 (NDC 0089-0353-03), 100 (NDC 0089-0353-10), and 250 (NDC 0089-0353-25) white tablets.
Shown Product Identification Section, page 428

THEOLAIR™
(theophylline)
TABLETS
THEOLAIR™
LIQUID
THEOLAIR™-SR
TABLETS

Description:
THEOLAIR Tablets contain 125 mg or 250 mg anhydrous theophylline.
THEOLAIR Liquid contains 80 mg theophylline per 15 ml (tablespoonful) in a nonalcoholic solution.
THEOLAIR-SR Tablets contain 200 mg, 250 mg, 300 mg or 500 mg anhydrous theophylline, in a sustained-release formulation.
How Supplied:
THEOLAIR Tablets:
  125 mg tablets—Bottles of 100 (NDC 0089-0342-10) and boxes of 250 unit-dose, aluminum foil, non-child-resistant strips (NDC 0089-0342-26). Each round, white, scored tablet imprinted with "RIKER" on one side and "342" on the other.
  250 mg tablets—Bottles of 100 (NDC 0089-0344-10) and boxes of 250 unit-dose, aluminum foil, non-child-resistant strips (NDC 0089-0344-26). Each capsule-shaped, white, scored tablet imprinted with "RIKER" on one side and "THEOLAIR 250" on the other.
  STORE AT CONTROLLED ROOM TEMPERATURE 15°–30° C (59°–86° F).
THEOLAIR Liquid:
  1 pint (NDC 0089-0960-16)
  STORE AT CONTROLLED ROOM TEMPERATURE 15°–30° C (59°–86° F).
THEOLAIR-SR Tablets:
  200 mg sustained-release tablets—Bottles of 100 (NDC 0089-0341-10). Each round white, scored tablet imprinted with "RIKER" on one side and "SR 200" on the other.
  250 mg sustained-release tablets—Bottles of 100 (NDC 0089-0345-10) and bottles of 250 (NDC 0089-0345-25). Each round, white, scored tablet imprinted with "RIKER" on one side and "SR 250" on the other.
  300 mg sustained-release tablets—Bottles of 100 (NDC 0089-0343-10). Each oval white, scored tablet imprinted with "RIKER" on one side and "SR 300" on the other.
  500 mg sustained-release tablets—Bottles of 100 (NDC 0089-0347-10) and bottles of 250 (NDC 0089-0347-25). Each capsule-shaped, white, scored tablet imprinted on one side with "RIKER" and "SR 500" on the other.
  STORE AT CONTROLLED ROOM TEMPERATURE 15°–30° C (59°–86° F).
Shown in Product Identification Section, page 428

THEOLAIR™–PLUS
TABLETS AND LIQUID

Description: Theolair-Plus contains anhydrous theophylline and guaifenesin and is available in two tablet strengths and as a pleasant tasting liquid.
Theolair-Plus 125—each tablet contains theophylline 125 mg and guaifenesin 100 mg.
Theolair-Plus 250—each tablet contains theophylline 250 mg and guaifenesin 200 mg.
Theolair-Plus Liquid—each 15 ml contains theophylline 125 mg and guaifenesin 100 mg.
How Supplied:
THEOLAIR-PLUS 125 tablets: Bottles of 100 (NDC 0089-0348-10).
THEOLAIR-PLUS 250 tablets: Bottles of 100 (NDC 0089-0349-10).
Shown in Product Identification Section, page 428
THEOLAIR-PLUS LIQUID—1 pint (NDC 0089-0962-16)

UREX®
(methenamine hippurate)

Description: Urex (methenamine hippurate) is the hippuric acid salt of methenamine (hexamethylenetetramine).
How Supplied: One gram scored, white tablets, bottles of 100 (NDC 0089-0371-10) and 500 (NDC 0089-0371-50).

The Robertson/Taylor Co.
A division of Intra-Medic Formulations, Inc.
1110 W. SUNRISE BLVD.
FORT LAUDERDALE, FL 33311

ANOREX–CCK   OTC
[*an'or-ex*]

Composition: A 1000 mg tablet consisting of bovine tissue (a natural source of cholecystokinin, using a patented production process), guar gum, carboxymethyl cellulose, and vegetable bran.
Actions and Usage: A powerful, non-chemical anorectic agent that elicits the full behavioral display of satiety and produces a dose-related reduction in meal size. CCK serves as a natural constituent messenger relaying satiety-induced signals along the gut-brain axis. CCK lessens food intake and shortens meal duration in obese and lean subjects, while producing a lasting satiety effect.
How Supplied: 126 Tablets, NDC 51729-8000-84.

INTRADERM–19
[*in'tra-derm*]
EMERGENCY ACNE STICK

Description: A convenient emergency drying stick that can be applied to blemishes. Intraderm-19 Emergency Acne Stick was specially formulated to fight bacteria and help control sebum production. It exhibits a cooling effect and should be used to treat conditions of irritation, inflammation and burns. Its stimulating effect on the circulation to the skin enhances cellular respiration and metabolism.
Composition: SDA 39 C Alcohol, Demineralized Water, Sulfidal, Zinc Oxide, Titanium Dioxide, Sodium Lauryl Ether Sulfate, Butylene Glycol, Camphor, Methylparaben.
Directions: Shake well before using. Apply to blemishes before bedtime and leave on overnight. Avoid contact with eyes and eye area.
How Supplied: .67 fl. oz., NDC 51729-1904-67

INTRADERM–19
[*in'tra-derm"*]
ORAL ACNE SUPPLEMENT

Description: An ultra potency formulation to be used in conjunction with Intraderm-19 Therapeutic Acne Scrub, Intraderm-19, Therapeutic Astringent Lotion, Intraderm-19 Emergency Acne Stick and Intraderm-19 Overnight Acne Masque. This supplement has been formulated for dermatologists to suggest as a powerful therapeutic weapon in the fight against acne.
Composition: Three (3) tablets contain: 10,000 I.U. Vitamin A (acetate), 5,000 I.U. Vitamin A palmitate (water soluble), 5,000 I.U. Beta Carotene (pro Vitamin A), 15 mg. Zinc elemental (from 150 mg. amino acid chelate), 200 mg. Citrus Pectin Cellulose, 250 mg. Vitamin C (ascorbic acid), 60 mg. Vitamin C (ascorbyl palmitate), 200 I.U. Vitamin E (natural) d. alpha tocopherol acid succinate, 50 mg. Vitamin F (essential fatty acids), 150 mg. Lactobacillus Acidophilus (freeze dried), 20 mg. Lipase (enteric coated), 1.5 mg. Vitamin B_1, 1.7 mg. Vitamin B_2, 20 mg. Niacin, 10 mg. Panthothenic Acid, 400 mcg. Folic Acid, 2 mg. Vitamin B_6, 300 mcg. Biotin, 6 mcg. Vitamin B_{12}.
Usage: Take one tablet three (3) times daily as a dietary supplement.
Caution: Keep out of reach of children. Store in a cool, dry place.
How Supplied: 45 Tablets, NDC 51729-1901-30.

INTRADERM–19
[*in'tra-derm"*]
OVERNIGHT ACNE MASQUE

Description: A powerful masque-forming gel designed specifically for the treatment of acne vulgaris. Intraderm-19 Overnight Acne Masque contains benzoyl peroxide and zinc phenosulfonate to fight bacteria, reduce blackheads and whiteheads and dry acne lesions. The product also contains moisturizers to minimize drying, and natural healing agents to reduce swelling and help eliminate red flareups.
Composition: Demineralized water, Isopropyl Alcohol, Benzoyl Peroxide, Butylene Glycol, Dimethicone Copolyol, Sodium PCA, Lantrol AWS, Zinc Phenolsulphonate, Allantoin, Bisabolol, Methyl Paraben.
Directions: Cleanse skin thoroughly and dry well. Apply masque with fingertips to produce a thin even layer. Leave on until dry—or overnight—peel off.
Caution: Persons with sensitive skin should not use this product which contains benzoyl peroxide. It should be tested on a small affected area for one or two days. If irritation or dryness occurs, reduce the frequency of use. If any excessive itching, redness or burning occurs, discontinue use.
How Supplied: 2 oz., NDC 51729-1900-02.

INTRADERM–19
[*in'tra-derm"*]
THERAPEUTIC ACNE SCRUB

Description: Intraderm-19 Therapeutic Acne Scrub is a specially formulated skin cleanser and stimulant—a powerful exfoliating agent for opening clogged pores and for removing excess oil. Intraderm-19 Therapeutic Acne Scrub is an effective but gentle supplemental cleanser.
Composition: Demineralized Water, Mineral Oil, Lanolin Alcohol, Butylene Glycol, Polyethelene, Glyceryl, Stearate, Magnesium Aluminum Silicate, Sodium Alkylauryl Ether Sulfonate, Eucalyptus Oil, Methylparaben, Propylparaben.
Usage: Use Intraderm-19 Therapeutic Acne Scrub sparingly as a supplemental cleanser for the exfoliation of problem skin. Wet the face with warm water. Put small amount of Intraderm-19 Therapeutic Acne Scrub onto fingertips and gently massage into the face. Continue scrubbing and adding water for about one minute, or until the face is thoroughly cleansed. Rinse thoroughly with warm water and dry. Use once daily or as directed by physician.
Caution: Avoid contact with eyes. If the particles get into the eyes, flush thoroughly with water and avoid rubbing eyes. If skin irritation and excessive dryness develops or increses, discontinue use and consult your physician.
How Supplied: 2 oz. jar, NDC 51729-1900-02.

Continued on next page

Robertson/Taylor—Cont.

INTRADERM-19
[in'tra-derm"]
THERAPEUTIC ASTRINGENT LOTION

Description: Intraderm-19 Therapeutic Astringent Lotion is a deep penetrating solution that cleans away dead skin cells and excess oil that clog pores and can cause acne flareups. Intraderm-19 Therapeutic Astringent Lotion contains moisturizers and healing agents, along with a natural compound rich in organic sulphur, which can help draw impurities from beneath the skin.

Composition: Aloe Vera Gel, Butylene Glycol, Witch Hazel, Sodium Lactate, Sodium PCA, Collagen, D-Arabohexulose, Urea, Niacinamide, Inositol, Sodium Benzoate, Ichthymnol, Lactic Acid, Burdock, Ivy, Lemon, Sage, Soapwart, Watercress Extracts, Neroli Oil, Polysorbate 80, Imidazolidinyl Urea, Methyl Paraben, Propylparaben, D-Alpha Tocopherol.

Actions and Usage: Intraderm-19 Therapeutic Astringent Lotion contains Ichthymnol—a natural ingredient rich in organic sulphur. It has great drawing properties which make it valuable for removing impurities from beneath the skin. Its bacteriostatic and analgesic properties are utilized for testing various skin conditions. After cleansing the skin thoroughly (with Intraderm Masque or other cleanser) squeeze Intraderm-19 Therapeutic Astringent Lotion onto a cotton ball and apply to the blemished areas of the face. Let dry and leave on. Use morning and evening.

How Supplied: 2 fl. oz., NDC 51729-1903-2.

L-2000™

Composition: A tablet consisting of 750 ml Thea Sinensis-Lapsang specially processed and pressed, coated to be easy to swallow.

Actions and Usage: Helps to restore mental alertness or wakefulness when experiencing fatigue, lethargy or drowsiness. Enhances mental process. Stimulates cerebrocortical areas involved with active mental processes. Take 2 tablets as needed. Do not exceed 6 tablets in any 24 hour period.

Warnings: Keep out of reach of children. For adult use only. Do not exceed recommended dose since side effects may occur which include increased nervousness, anxiety, irritability, difficulty in falling asleep. Do not give to children under 12 years of age. The recommended dose of this product contains about as much caffeine as a cup of coffee. Take this product with caution while taking caffeine contained in beverages such as coffee, tea or cola drinks because large doses of caffeine may cause side effects. As with any drug, if you are pregnant or nursing a baby, seek the advice of a health professional before using this product.

How Supplied:
60 Tablets, NDC-51729-2000-60.
90 Tablets, NDC-51729-2000-90.
120 Tablets, NDC-51729-2000-120.

MEDI-TEC 90™ Therapeutic Conditioner with Strengthening Agents

Composition: A concentrated liquid, lanolin free conditioning formula applied through the hair immediately following a thorough cleansing with Medi-Tec 90 Therapeutic Shampoo and Scalp Cleanser to condition and protect the hair shaft.
Contains: Deionized Water, Acetamide MEA, Stearalkonium Chloride, Emulsifying Wax, Cetyl Alcohol, Polysorbate 80, Keratin Amino Acid, Tocopherol Acetate, Niacin, D-Panthenol, PCA-Na, Biotin, Diazolidinyl Urea, Methyl/Propyl Parabens, Lactic Acid.

Actions and Usage: Medi-Tec 90 Therapeutic Conditioner with strengthening agents is a comprehensive, protective conditioning treatment that completes the total Medi-Tec 90 hair and scalp therapeutic program.
Specifically developed for dermatologists to recommend in cases where severe thinning of the scalp and excess hair fallout can be treated with the direct application of Medi-Tec 90 Formulations.

How Supplied:
240 ml. Medi-Tec 90 Therapeutic Conditioner with strengthening agents, NDC-51729-4290-08.
480 ml. Medi-Tec 90 Therapeutic Conditioner with strengthening agents, NDC-51729-4290-16.

MEDI-TEC 90™
NEW THERAPEUTIC OVERNIGHT CONCENTRATE

Composition: A powerful concentrated formula offering proven scalp vasodilation. An aqueous solution which is applied to the scalp and lightly massaged into the scalp for 60 seconds.
Contains: Extract of hops, rosemary, horsetail, pine cone and lemon, deionized water, niacin, niacinamide, butylene glycol, rosemary oil, diazolidinyl urea, isopropyl alcohol.

Actions and Usage: Specifically developed for dermatologists to recommend in cases where severe thinning of the hair and excess hair fallout can be treated with the direct application of Medi-Tec 90 formulations. Medi-Tec 90 New Therapeutic Overnight Concentrate contains non-chemical vasodilating agents and scalp cleansers. Apply 20–30 drops to the scalp before bedtime and lightly massage for 60 seconds. Shampoo thoroughly in the morning with Medi-Tec 90 Therapeutic Shampoo and Scalp Cleanser. Use in conjunction with daily application of Medi-Tec 90 Scalp Stimulant.

How Supplied: 30 ml, NDC-51729-4690-01.

MEDI-TEC 90™ Therapeutic Scalp Stimulant with Strengthening Agents

Composition: A pump-spray which is applied liberally onto the scalp 2 to 3 times daily. Before using Medi-Tec 90 Therapeutic Scalp Stimulant, cleanse hair and scalp daily (evening or morning) with lanolin free shampoo or Medi-Tec 90 Therapeutic Shampoo and Scalp Cleanser with strengthening agents.
Contains: Dionized Water, Quaternium-41, Acetamide MEA, Polysorbate 80, Niacin, D-Panthenol, Biotin, Oleth 3 Phosphate, Diazolidinyl Urea, Methyl Paraben, FD&C Blue #1.

Actions and Usage: Medi-Tec 90 Scalp Stimulant: An odorless, greaseless surfactant containing non-chemical vasodilators, proteins, and vitamin H along with a base formulation whose efficacy as a complete baldness treatment is now under study. Specifically developed for dermatologists to recommend in cases where severe thinning of the scalp and excess hair fallout can be treated with the direct application of Medi-Tec 90 Formulations.

How Supplied:
240 ml. Medi-Tec 90 Therapeutic Scalp Stimulant with Strengthening Agents, NDC-51729-4490-08.
480 ml. Medi-Tec 90 Therapeutic Scalp Stimulant with Strengthening Agents, NDC-51729-4490-16.

MEDI-TEC 90™ Therapeutic Shampoo and Scalp Cleanser with Strengthening Agents

Composition: An exclusive mild liquid surfactant which is liberally applied to the hair and scalp.
Contains: Deionized Water, Ammonium Lauryl Sulfate, Ammonium Laureth Sulfate, Lauramide DEA, Acetemide MEA, Quaternium-41, Polysorbate 80, Citric Acid, Niacin, D-Panthenol, Biotin, Diazolidinyl Urea, Methyl Paraben, FD&C Blue #1.

Actions and Usage: An effective lanolin free surfactant to be used alone or in conjunction with all Medi-Tec 90 Formulations. Medi-Tec 90 Therapeutic Shampoo and Scalp Cleanser cleans away debris and sebum while gently stimulating the scalp with non-chemical vasodilators.
Specifically developed for dermatologists to recommend in cases where severe thinning of the scalp and excess hair fallout can be treated with the direct application of Medi-Tec 90 Formulations.

How Supplied:
240 ml. Medi-Tec 90 Therapeutic Shampoo and Scalp Cleanser with Strengthening Agents, NDC-51729-4390-08.
480 ml. Medi-Tec 90 Therapeutic Shampoo and Scalp Cleanser with Strengthening Agents, NDC-51729-4390-16.

MEDI-TEC 90™ Vitamin-Mineral-Trace Mineral supplement for the hair and scalp

Composition: Formulated for dermatologists to recommend in cases where severe thinning or hair fallout can be helped by the ingestion of Medi-Tec 90 Oral Supplements.
Contains: Calcium Panthothenate, 100 mg., Choline Bitartrate, 125 mg., Inositol, 50 mg., Niacin, 35 mg., Para Amino Benzoic Acid, 30 mg., Folic Acid, 0.4, Cobalamin, 6 mcg., Iron (Ferrons Gluconate), 18 mg., Copper (Copper Gluconate), 2 mg., Iodine (Kelp), 0.15 mg., Manganese (Manganese Gluconate), 5 mg., Protein (from soy protein), 100 mg., Zinc (Zinc Gluconate), 15 mg.

Actions and Usage: Take one tablet daily to be used alone or in conjunction with all Medi-Tec 90 Formulations.

How Supplied:
30 Tablets, NDC-51729-4590-3.
60 Tablets, NDC-51729-4590-6.

METABOLITE 2050™
[mě-tab'o-līt"]

Composition: Metabolite 2050™ automatic weight-loss compound bonds with ingested food stuffs delaying gastric emptying time thereby increasing satiation and preventing additional caloric intake.
Contains: Specially prepared Cyamopsis Tetragonolobus, 750 mg.

Actions and Usage: Formulated specifically for beriatric physicians to recommend for use by the chronic overweight or by people who have been able to lose weight but have not been able to keep that weight off. Take 3 tablets in morning, 4 tablets in afternoon and 3 tablets in the evening.

How Supplied:
420 Tablets, NDC-51729-2100-420.

REVITALIN-SL 90™ Adult Supplement
[re-vīt"ă-lin']

Composition: An easy to swallow tablet. Each 2 tablets consists of Liver Extract, 50 mg., Water soluble B-12, 100 mg., Swedish Flower Pollen, 63 mg., Histidine, 20 mg., Carnitin, 20 mg., Arginine, 20 mg., Methionine, 20 mg., Glycine, 20 mg., Panthothenate, 50 mg., Thiamine, 50 mg., Riboflavin, 50 mg., Niacin, 75 mg., Pyridozine, 50 mg., L-Phenyalanine, 400 mg., Polysaccharide, 50 mg., Tillandsia Extract, 25 mg., Fresh veal bone, 25 mg., Defatted wheat germ, 50 mg., Pangamic Acid, 25 mg., Zinc Amino Acid Chelate, 100 mg.

Actions and Usage: A combination of herbs, nutrients, micro-nutrients, free-form amino acids and specific active portions of various roots, plants and flowers as a nutritional supplement to be recommended by physicians in cases where the specific action would be deemed helpful in alleviating stress, weaknesses (both mental and physical).
Recommended dosage: Take 2 tablets as needed.
Warnings: Keep out of reach of children. For adult use only. Do not take more than 2 tablets in any day. As with any drug, if you are pregnant or nursing a baby or are suffering from high blood pressure, kidney or liver problems, seek the advice of a health professional before using this product.

How Supplied:
30 Tablets, NDC-51729-9011-30.
60 Tablets, NDC-51729-9011-60.

TESTOREX-35™ Adult Male Supplement
[test'or-ex]

Composition: Contains specially prepared glandular material plus essential active nutrients, micronutrients and trace minerals to restore the production of testosterone to its maximum natural

intended limit which are typically lost through the aging process.
Contains: Testicular Extract, 10 mg., Cyanocobalamine, 12 mcg., D-Calcium Panthothenate, 10 mg., Niacin, 10 mg., Vitamin C, 60 mg., Folic Acid, 400 mcg., 250 mg. Zinc Amino Acid Chelate, Yielding 25 mg. Zinc Elemental, 500 mg. Dried Root of Smilax Aristolochiaefolia, Octocosanol, 5 mcg., Thea Sinensis, 20 mg., Vitamin A 1000 IU, D-Alpha Tocopherol 10 IU, Selenium (yeast) 10 mcg., Nicotinic Acid, 50 mg., in a base of Ginseng, Bee Pollen, Lecithin, Lysine, Calcium Supplier, Magnesium Gluconate, Manganese Sulfate, Kelp, L-Glutamine and Pituitary Gland Extract.
Actions and Usage: To be recommended for specific cases where nutrients and trace minerals would be beneficial in restoring testosterone production to its natural intended limit. Take one micro-tablet as a dietary supplement. Do not exceed one tablet in any 24 hour period.
How Supplied:
30 Tablets, NDC-51729-2935-30.

A. H. Robins Company
PHARMACEUTICAL DIVISION
1407 CUMMINGS DRIVE
RICHMOND, VA 23220

ALLBEE® WITH C CAPSULES
[all-be']
(See PDR For Nonprescription Drugs)

ALLBEE® C–800 TABLETS
ALLBEE® C–800 plus Iron tablets
[all-be']
(See PDR For Nonprescription Drugs)

DIMACOL® CAPSULES
DIMACOL® LIQUID
[di'mă-col]
(See PDR For Nonprescription Drugs)

DIMETANE EXTENTABS®
[di'mĕ-tāne eks"tĕn'tabs]
brand of Brompheniramine Maleate, USP
8 mg and 12 mg
(See PDR For Nonprescription Drugs)

DIMETANE®
[di'mĕ-tāne]
brand of Brompheniramine Maleate, USP
Tablets—4 mg
Elixir—2 mg/5 ml
  Alcohol, 3%
(See PDR For Nonprescription Drugs)

DIMETANE® DECONGESTANT ELIXIR
[di'mĕ-tāne]
DIMETANE® DECONGESTANT TABLETS
(See PDR For Nonprescription Drugs)

DIMETANE®-DC
COUGH SYRUP
(REPLACEMENT FORMULA FOR DIMETANE EXPECTORANT-DC)

Description: Dimetane-DC Cough Syrup is a bright red syrup with a raspberry flavor.
Each 5 ml (1 teaspoonful) contains:
Brompheniramine Maleate, USP..............2.0 mg
Phenylpropanolamine
  Hydrochloride, USP.........................12.5 mg
Codeine Phosphate, USP.....................10.0 mg
  (Warning: May be habit forming)
  Alcohol 0.95 percent
In a palatable aromatic vehicle.
Antihistamine/Nasal Decongestant/Antitussive syrup for oral administration.

Clinical Pharmacology: Brompheniramine maleate is a histamine antagonist, specifically an H_1-receptor-blocking agent belonging to the alkylamine class of antihistamines. Antihistamines appear to compete with histamine for receptor sites on effector cells. Brompheniramine also has anticholinergic (drying) and sedative effects. Among the antihistaminic effects, it antagonizes the allergic response (vasodilatation, increased vascular permeability, increased mucus secretion) of nasal tissue. Brompheniramine is well absorbed from the gastrointestinal tract, with peak plasma concentration after a single oral dose of 4 mg reached in 5 hours; urinary excretion is the major route of elimination, mostly as products of biodegradation; the liver is assumed to be the main site of metabolic transformation.
Phenylpropanolamine hydrochloride is a sympathomimetic drug which is readily absorbed from the gastrointestinal tract and produces nasal vasoconstriction (decongestion). Phenylpropanolamine stimulates both α and β-adrenergic receptors, similar to ephedrine. Part of its peripheral action is indirect and is due to the displacement of norepinephrine from storage sites, but it also has direct effect on the adrenergic receptors.
Codeine is an opiate analgesic and antitussive. Codeine calms the cough control center.
Indications and Usage: For relief of coughs and upper respiratory symptoms, including nasal congestion, associated with allergy or the common cold.
Contraindications: Hypersensitivity to any of the ingredients. Do not use in the newborn, in premature infants, in nursing mothers, in patients with severe hypertension or severe coronary artery disease, or in those receiving monoamine oxidase (MAO) inhibitors.
Antihistamines should not be used to treat lower respiratory tract conditions including asthma.
Warnings: Especially in infants and small children, antihistamines in overdosage may cause hallucinations, convulsions, death. Codeine may cause or aggravate constipation.
Antihistamines may diminish mental alertness. In the young child, they may produce excitation.
Precautions: *General:* Because of its antihistamine component, Dimetane-DC Cough Syrup should be used with caution in patients with a history of bronchial asthma, narrow angle glaucoma, gastrointestinal obstruction, or urinary bladder neck obstruction. Because of its sympathomimetic component, Dimetane-DC Cough Syrup should be used with caution in patients with diabetes, hypertension, heart disease, or thyroid disease.
Information for Patients: Patients should be warned about engaging in activities requiring mental alertness, such as driving a car or operating dangerous machinery.
Drug Interactions: Antihistamines have additive effects with alcohol and other CNS depressants (hypnotics, sedatives, tranquilizers, antianxiety agents, etc.). MAO inhibitors prolong and intensify the anticholinergic (drying) effects of antihistamines. MAO inhibitors may enhance the effect of phenylpropanolamine. Sympathomimetics may reduce the effects of antihypertensive drugs.
Carcinogenesis, Mutagenesis: Long-term studies in animals to evaluate carcinogenic and mutagenic potential have not been performed.
Pregnancy Category C: Animal reproduction studies have not been conducted with Dimetane-DC Cough Syrup. It is also not known whether Dimetane-DC Cough Syrup can cause fetal harm when administered to a pregnant woman or can affect reproduction capacity. Dimetane-DC Cough Syrup should be given to a pregnant woman only if clearly needed.
Reproduction studies of brompheniramine maleate (one of the components of the Dimetane formulations) in rats and mice at doses up to 16 times the maximum human dose have revealed no evidence of impaired fertility or harm to the fetus.
Nursing Mothers: Because of the higher risk of intolerance of antihistamines in small infants generally, and in newborns and prematures in particular, and the fact that codeine appears in human milk, Dimetane-DC Cough Syrup is contraindicated in nursing mothers.
Adverse Reactions: The most frequent adverse reactions to Dimetane-DC Cough Syrup are: sedation; dryness of mouth, nose and throat; thickening of bronchial secretions; dizziness. Other adverse reactions may include:
Dermatologic: Urticaria, drug rash, photosensitivity, pruritus.
Cardiovascular System: Hypotension, hypertension, cardiac arrhythmias.
CNS: Disturbed coordination, tremor, irritability, insomnia, visual disturbances, weakness, nervousness, convulsions, headache, euphoria, and dysphoria.
G. U. System: Urinary frequency, difficult urination.
G. I. System: Epigastric discomfort, anorexia, nausea, vomiting, diarrhea, constipation.
Respiratory System: Tightness of chest and wheezing, shortness of breath. At higher doses, codeine has most of the disadvantages of morphine including respiratory depression.
Hematologic System: Hemolytic anemia, thrombocytopenia, agranulocytosis.
Drug Abuse and Dependence: Codeine can produce drug dependence of the morphine type, and therefore has the potential for being abused. Psychic dependence, physical dependence and tolerance may develop upon repeated administration of this drug, and it should be prescribed and administered with the same degree of caution appropriate to the use of other oral narcotic medications.
Dimetane-DC Cough Syrup is subject to the Federal Controlled Substances Act (Schedule V).
Overdosage: *Signs and Symptoms:* Serious overdose with codeine is characterized by respiratory depression, extreme somnolence progressing to stupor or coma. In severe overdosage, apnea, circulatory collapse, cardiac arrest and death may occur. The central nervous system effects from overdosage of brompheniramine may vary from depression to stimulation. Anticholinergic effects may also occur. Overdosage of phenylpropanolamine may be associated with tachycardia, hypertension and cardiac arrhythmias.
Toxic Doses: Doses of 800 mg or more of codeine have caused partial loss of consciousness, delirium, restlessness, excitement, tremors, convulsions and collapse; or respiratory paralysis with such sequelae as mydriasis, marked vasodilatation, and finally death. A 2½-year-old child survived a dose of 300–900 mg of brompheniramine; the lethal dose of phenylpropanolamine is in the range of 50 mg/kg.
Treatment: Respiratory depression should be treated promptly. Oxygen, intravenous fluids, vasopressors and other supportive measures should be employed as indicated. If necessary, reestablishment of adequate respiratory exchange through provision of a patent airway and the institution of assisted or controlled ventilation must be provided. The narcotic antagonist, naloxone, is a specific antidote to codeine-induced respiratory depression, and should be administered by the intravenous route if appropriate (see package insert for naloxone). Since the duration of action of codeine may exceed that of the antagonist, the patient should be kept under constant surveillance.
Gastric emptying may be useful in removing unabsorbed drug, either by inducing emesis or lavage; precautions against aspiration must be taken. Stimulants or depressants should be used cautiously and only when specifically indicated. If marked excitement is present, one of the short-

Continued on next page

Prescribing information on A. H. Robins products listed here is based on official labeling in effect August 1, 1984, with Indications, Contraindications, Warnings Precautions, Adverse Reactions, and Dosage stated in full.

Robins—Cont.

acting barbiturates or chloral hydrate may be used.

Dosage and Administration: Adults and children 12 years of age and over: 2 teaspoonfuls every 4 hours. Children 6 to under 12 years: 1 teaspoonful every 4 hours. Children 2 to under 6 years: ½ teaspoonful every 4 hours. Children 6 months to under 2 years: Dosage to be established by physician.

Do not exceed 6 doses during a 24-hour period.

How Supplied: Dimetane-DC Cough Syrup is a bright red syrup containing in each 5 ml (1 teaspoonful): brompheniramine maleate 2 mg, phenylpropanolamine HCl 12.5 mg, and codeine phosphate 10 mg; available in pints (NDC 0031-1833-25) and gallons (NDC 0031-1833-29).

Store at controlled room temperature, between 15°C and 30°C (59°F and 86°F).

Dispense in tight, light-resistant container.

DIMETAPP® ELIXIR ℞
[di'mĕ-tap]

Each 5 ml (1 teaspoonful) contains:
Brompheniramine Maleate, USP .... 4 mg
Phenylephrine Hydrochloride, USP .... 5 mg
Phenylpropanolamine
 Hydrochloride, USP .... 5 mg
Alcohol, 2.3%

Actions: Dimetapp effectively reduces excessive nasopharyngeal secretions and diminishes inflammatory mucosal edema and congestion in the upper respiratory tract.

The antihistaminic action of brompheniramine maleate reduces or abolishes the allergic response of nasal tissue. It is complemented by the mild vasoconstrictor action of phenylephrine hydrochloride and phenylpropanolamine hydrochloride which provide a nasal decongestant effect.

Indications

Based on a review of this drug by the National Academy of Sciences—National Research Council and/or other information, FDA has classified the following indications as "probably effective" for Dimetapp Elixir: The symptomatic treatment of seasonal and perennial allergic rhinitis and vasomotor rhinitis; and "lacking substantial evidence of effectiveness as a fixed combination" for the following indications: Symptomatic relief of allergic manifestations of upper respiratory illnesses, acute sinusitis, nasal congestion, and otitis.

Final classification of the less-than-effective indications requires further investigation.

Contraindications: Hypersensitivity to antihistamines of the same chemical class. Dimetapp is contraindicated during pregnancy and in concurrent MAO inhibitor therapy. Because of its drying and thickening effect on the lower respiratory secretions, Dimetapp is not recommended in the treatment of bronchial asthma.

Warnings: *Use in children.* In infants and children particularly, antihistamines in overdosage may produce convulsions and death.

Precautions: Administer with care to patients with cardiac or peripheral vascular diseases, hypertension, diabetes or thyroid disease. Use cautiously in patients with a history of bronchial asthma, narrow angle glaucoma, gastrointestinal obstruction or urinary bladder neck obstruction. Until the patient's response has been determined, he should be cautioned against engaging in operations requiring alertness such as driving an automobile, operating machinery, etc. Patients receiving antihistamines should be warned against possible additive effects with CNS depressants such as alcohol, hypnotics, sedatives, tranquilizers, etc.

Adverse Reactions: Adverse reactions to Dimetapp may include hypersensitivity reactions such as rash, urticaria, leukopenia, agranulocytosis and thrombocytopenia; drowsiness, lassitude, giddiness, dryness of the mucous membranes, tightness of the chest, thickening of bronchial secretions, urinary frequency and dysuria, palpitation, hypotension/hypertension, headache, faintness, dizziness, tinnitus, incoordination, visual disturbances, mydriasis, CNS depressant and (less often) stimulant effect, increased irritability or excitement, anorexia, nausea, vomiting, diarrhea, constipation, and epigastric distress.

Dosage and Administration: Adults—1 to 2 teaspoonfuls 3 or 4 times daily.

Children (4 to 12 years)—1 teaspoonful 3 or 4 times daily; (2 to 4 years)—¾ teaspoonful 3 or 4 times daily; (7 months to 2 years)—½ teaspoonful 3 or 4 times daily; (1 to 6 months)—¼ teaspoonful 3 or 4 times daily.

How Supplied: Grape flavored Elixir in 4 fl. oz. (NDC 0031-2224-12), pints (NDC 0031-2224-25), gallons (NDC 0031-2224-29), and 5 ml Dis-Co® Unit Dose Packs (10 × 10s) (NDC 0031-2224-23).

DIMETAPP EXTENTABS® ℞
[di'mĕ-tap eks"tĕn'tabs]

Each Extentab contains:
Brompheniramine Maleate, USP .... 12 mg
Phenylephrine Hydrochloride, USP .... 15 mg
Phenylpropanolamine
 Hydrochloride, USP .... 15 mg
Extentabs provide a continuous release of medication which affords effects for ten to twelve hours.

Actions: Dimetapp Extentabs effectively reduce excessive nasopharyngeal secretions and diminish inflammatory mucosal edema and congestion in the upper respiratory tract.

The antihistaminic action of brompheniramine maleate reduces or abolishes the allergic response of nasal tissue. It is complemented by the mild vasoconstrictor action of phenylephrine hydrochloride and phenylpropanolamine hydrochloride which provide a nasal decongestant effect.

Indications

Based on a review of this drug by the National Academy of Sciences—National Research Council and/or other information, FDA has classified the following indications as "lacking substantial evidence of effectiveness as a fixed combination" for Dimetapp Extentabs: For the symptomatic treatment of seasonal and perennial allergic rhinitis and vasomotor rhinitis, allergic manifestations of upper respiratory illnesses, acute sinusitis, nasal congestion, and otitis.

Final classification of the less-than-effective indications requires further investigation.

Contraindications: Hypersensitivity to antihistamines of the same chemical class. Dimetapp Extentabs are contraindicated during pregnancy and in children under 12 years of age. Because of its drying and thickening effect on the lower respiratory secretions, Dimetapp is not recommended in the treatment of bronchial asthma. Also, Dimetapp Extentabs are contraindicated in concurrent MAO inhibitor therapy.

Warnings: *Use in Children.* In infants and children particularly, antihistamines in overdosage may produce convulsions and death.

Precautions: Administer with care to patients with cardiac or peripheral vascular diseases, hypertension, diabetes or thyroid disease. Use cautiously in patients with a history of bronchial asthma, narrow angle glaucoma, gastrointestinal obstruction or urinary bladder neck obstruction. Until the patient's response has been determined, he should be cautioned against engaging in operations requiring alertness such as driving an automobile, operating machinery, etc. Patients receiving antihistamines should be warned against possible additive effects with CNS depressants such as alcohol, hypnotics, sedatives, tranquilizers, etc.

Adverse Reactions: Adverse reactions to Dimetapp Extentabs may include hypersensitivity reactions such as rash, urticaria, leukopenia, agranulocytosis and thrombocytopenia; drowsiness, lassitude, giddiness, dryness of the mucous membranes, tightness of the chest, thickening of bronchial secretions, urinary frequency and dysuria, palpitation, hypotension/hypertension, headache, faintness, dizziness, tinnitus, incoordination, visual disturbances, mydriasis, CNS depressant and (less often) stimulant effect, increased irritability or excitement, anorexia, nausea, vomiting, diarrhea, constipation, and epigastric distress.

Dosage and Administration: Adults and Children 12 years and over. One Extentab morning and evening. If indicated, one Extentab every 8 hours may be given.

How Supplied: Light blue Extentabs monogrammed AHR and Dimetapp in bottles of 100 (NDC 0031-2274-63), 500 (NDC 0031-2274-70) and Dis-Co® unit dose packs of 100 (NDC 0031-2274-64).

Shown in Product Identification Section, page 428

DONNATAL® TABLETS ℞
DONNATAL® CAPSULES ℞
DONNATAL® ELIXIR ℞
[don'nă-tal]

Description: Each Donnatal tablet, capsule or 5 ml (teaspoonful) of elixir (23% alcohol) contains:
Phenobarbital, USP (¼ gr) .... 16.2 mg
 (Warning: May be habit forming)
Hyoscyamine Sulfate, USP .... 0.1037 mg
Atropine Sulfate, USP .... 0.0194 mg
Scopolamine Hydrobromide, USP .... 0.0065 mg

Actions: This drug combination provides natural belladonna alkaloids in a specific, fixed ratio combined with phenobarbital to provide peripheral anticholinergic/antispasmodic action and mild sedation.

Indications

Based on a review of this drug by the National Academy of Sciences—National Research Council and/or other information, FDA has classified the following indications as "possibly" effective:

For use as adjunctive therapy in the treatment of irritable bowel syndrome (irritable colon, spastic colon, mucous colitis) and acute enterocolitis.

May also be useful as adjunctive therapy in the treatment of duodenal ulcer. IT HAS NOT BEEN SHOWN CONCLUSIVELY WHETHER ANTICHOLINERGIC/ANTISPASMODIC DRUGS AID IN THE HEALING OF A DUODENAL ULCER, DECREASE THE RATE OF RECURRENCES OR PREVENT COMPLICATIONS.

Contraindications: Glaucoma, obstructive uropathy (for example, bladder neck obstruction due to prostatic hypertrophy); obstructive disease of the gastrointestinal tract (as in achalasia, pyloroduodenal stenosis, etc.); paralytic ileus, intestinal atony of the elderly or debilitated patient; unstable cardiovascular status in acute hemorrhage; severe ulcerative colitis especially if complicated by toxic megacolon; myasthenia gravis; hiatal hernia associated with reflux esophagitis.

Donnatal is contraindicated in patients with known hypersensitivity to any of the ingredients. Phenobarbital is contraindicated in acute intermittent porphyria and in those patients in whom phenobarbital produces restlessness and/or excitement.

Warnings: In the presence of a high environmental temperature, heat prostration can occur with belladonna alkaloids (fever and heatstroke due to decreased sweating).

Diarrhea may be an early symptom of incomplete intestinal obstruction, especially in patients with ileostomy or colostomy. In this instance treatment with this drug would be inappropriate and possibly harmful.

Donnatal may produce drowsiness or blurred vision. The patient should be warned, should these occur, not to engage in activities requiring mental alertness, such as operating a motor vehicle or other machinery, and not to perform hazardous work.

Phenobarbital may decrease the effect of anticoagulants, and necessitate larger doses of the anticoagulant for optimal effect. When the phenobarbital is discontinued, the dose of the anticoagulant may have to be decreased.

Phenobarbital may be habit forming and should not be administered to individuals known to be addiction prone or to those with a history of physical and/or psychological dependence upon drugs. Since barbiturates are metabolized in the liver, they should be used with caution and initial doses should be small in patients with hepatic dysfunction.

Precautions: Use with caution in patients with: autonomic neuropathy, hepatic or renal disease, hyperthyroidism, coronary heart disease, congestive heart failure, cardiac arrhythmias, tachycardia, and hypertension.

Belladonna alkaloids may produce a delay in gastric emptying (antral stasis) which would complicate the management of gastric ulcer.

Theoretically, with overdosage, a curare-like action may occur.

Carcinogenesis, mutagenesis. Long-term studies in animals have not been performed to evaluate carcinogenic potential.

Pregnancy Category C. Animal reproduction studies have not been conducted with Donnatal. It is not known whether Donnatal can cause fetal harm when administered to a pregnant woman or can affect reproduction capacity. Donnatal should be given to a pregnant woman only if clearly needed.

Nursing mothers. It is not known whether this drug is excreted in human milk. Because many drugs are excreted in human milk, caution should be exercised when Donnatal is administered to a nursing mother.

Adverse Reactions: Adverse reactions may include xerostomia; urinary hesitancy and retention; blurred vision; tachycardia; palpitation; mydriasis; cycloplegia; increased ocular tension; loss of taste sense, headache, nervousness; drowsiness; weakness; dizziness; insomnia; nausea; vomiting; impotence; suppression of lactation; constipation; bloated feeling; musculoskeletal pain; severe allergic reaction or drug idiosyncrasies, including anaphylaxis, urticaria and other dermal manifestations; and decreased sweating. Elderly patients may react with symptoms of excitement, agitation, drowsiness, and other untoward manifestations to even small doses of the drug.

Phenobarbital may produce excitement in some patients, rather than a sedative effect. In patients habituated to barbiturates, abrupt withdrawal may produce delirium or convulsions.

Dosage and Administration: The dosage of Donnatal should be adjusted to the needs of the individual patient to assure symptomatic control with a minimum of adverse effects.

Donnatal Tablets or Capsules. Adults: One or two Donnatal tablets or capsules three or four times a day according to condition and severity of symptoms.

Donnatal Elixir. Adults: One or two teaspoonfuls of elixir three or four times a day according to conditions and severity of symptoms.

Children (Elixir)—may be dosed every 4 or 6 hours.:

Body Weight	Starting Dosage q4h	q6h
10 lb (4.5 kg)	0.5 ml	0.75 ml
20 lb (9.1 kg)	1.0 ml	1.5 ml
30 lb (13.6 kg)	1.5 ml	2.0 ml
50 lb (22.7 kg)	½ tsp	¾ tsp
75 lb (34.0 kg)	¾ tsp	1 tsp
100 lb (45.4 kg)	1 tsp	1½ tsp

Overdosage: The signs and symptoms of overdose are headache, nausea, vomiting, blurred vision, dilated pupils, hot and dry skin, dizziness, dryness of the mouth, difficulty in swallowing, CNS stimulation. Treatment should consist of gastric lavage, emetics, and activated charcoal. If indicated, parenteral cholinergic agents such as physostigmine or bethanechol chloride, should be added.

How Supplied: *Donnatal Tablets.* White, compressed, embossed "R" on one side, scored and engraved 4250 on the reverse side; in bottles of 100 (NDC 0031-4250-63), 1000 (NDC 0031-4250-74) and Dis-Co® Unit Dose Packs of 100 (NDC 0031-4250-64).

Donnatal Capsules. Green and white, monogrammed "AHR" and "4207"; in bottles of 100 (NDC 0031-4207-63) and 1000 (NDC 0031-4207-74).

Donnatal Elixir. Green citrus flavored, in 4 fl. oz. (NDC 0031-4221-12), pints (NDC 0031-4221-25), gallons (NDC 0031-4221-29) and 5 ml Dis-Co® Unit Dose Packs (4 × 25s) (NDC 0031-4221-13).

Store at controlled room temperature, between 15°C and 30°C (59°F and 86°F).

Dispense in tight, light-resistant container.

Shown in Product Identification Section, page 428

DONNATAL EXTENTABS® ℞
[don'nă-tal ěks"těn'tabs]

Description: Each Donnatal Extentab contains:
Phenobarbital, USP (¾gr) ....48.6 mg
  (Warning: May be habit forming)
Hyoscyamine Sulfate, USP ....0.3111 mg
Atropine Sulfate, USP ....0.0582 mg
Scopolamine Hydrobromide,
  USP ....0.0195 mg

Each Donnatal Extentab contains the equivalent of three Donnatal tablets. The Extentab is designed to release the ingredients gradually to provide effects for up to twelve (12) hours.

Actions: Donnatal provides natural belladonna alkaloids in a specific, fixed ratio combined with phenobarbital to provide peripheral anticholinergic/antispasmodic action and mild sedation.

Indications
Based on a review of this drug by the National Academy of Sciences—National Research Council and/or other information, FDA has classified the following indications as "possibly" effective:

For use as adjunctive therapy in the treatment of irritable bowel syndrome (irritable colon, spastic colon, mucous colitis) and acute enterocolitis.

May also be useful as adjunctive therapy in the treatment of duodenal ulcer. IT HAS NOT BEEN SHOWN CONCLUSIVELY WHETHER ANTICHOLINERGIC/ANTISPASMODIC DRUGS AID IN THE HEALING OF A DUODENAL ULCER, DECREASE THE RATE OF RECURRENCES OR PREVENT COMPLICATIONS.

Contraindications: Glaucoma, obstructive uropathy (for example, bladder neck obstruction due to prostatic hypertrophy); obstructive disease of the gastrointestinal tract (as in achalasia, pyloroduodenal stenosis, etc.); paralytic ileus, intestinal atony of the elderly or debilitated patient; unstable cardiovascular status in acute hemorrhage; severe ulcerative colitis especially if complicated by toxic megacolon; myasthenia gravis, hiatal hernia associated with reflux esophagitis. Donnatal is contraindicated in patients with known hypersensitivity to any of the ingredients. Phenobarbital is contraindicated in acute intermittent porphyria and in those patients in whom phenobarbital produces restlessness and/or excitement.

Warnings: In the presence of a high environmental temperature, heat prostration can occur with belladonna alkaloids (fever and heatstroke due to decreased sweating).

Diarrhea may be an early symptom of incomplete intestinal obstruction, especially in patients with ileostomy or colostomy. In this instance treatment with this drug would be inappropriate and possibly harmful.

Donnatal may produce drowsiness or blurred vision. The patient should be warned, should these occur, not to engage in activities requiring mental alertness, such as operating a motor vehicle or other machinery, and not to perform hazardous work.

Phenobarbital may decrease the effect of anticoagulants and necessitate larger doses of the anticoagulant for optimal effect. When the phenobarbital is discontinued, the dose of the anticoagulant may have to be decreased.

Phenobarbital may be habit forming and should not be administered to individuals known to be addiction prone or to those with a history of physical and/or psychological dependence upon drugs. Since barbiturates are metabolized in the liver, they should be used with caution and initial doses should be small in patients with hepatic dysfunction.

Precautions: Use with caution in patients with: autonomic neuropathy, hepatic or renal disease, hyperthyroidism, coronary heart disease, congestive heart failure, cardiac arrhythmias, tachycardia, and hypertension.

Belladonna alkaloids may produce a delay in gastric emptying (antral stasis) which would complicate the management of gastric ulcer.

Theoretically, with overdosage, a curare-like action may occur.

Carcinogenesis, mutagenesis. Long-term studies in animals have not been performed to evaluate carcinogenic potential.

Pregnancy Category C. Animal reproduction studies have not been conducted with Donnatal. It is not known whether Donnatal can cause fetal harm when administered to a pregnant woman or can affect reproduction capacity. Donnatal should be given to a pregnant woman only if clearly needed.

Nursing mothers. It is not known whether this drug is excreted in human milk. Because many drugs are excreted in human milk, caution should be exercised when Donnatal is administered to a nursing mother.

Adverse Reactions: Adverse reactions may include xerostomia; urinary hesitancy and retention; blurred vision; tachycardia; palpitation; mydriasis; cycloplegia; increased ocular tension; loss of taste sense; headache; nervousness; drowsiness; weakness; dizziness; insomnia; nausea; vomiting; impotence; suppression of lactation; constipation; bloated feeling; musculoskeletal pain; severe allergic reaction or drug idiosyncrasies, including anaphylaxis, urticaria and other dermal manifestations; and decreased sweating. Elderly patients may react with symptoms of excitement, agitation, drowsiness, and other untoward manifestations to even small doses of the drug.

Phenobarbital may produce excitement in some patients, rather than a sedative effect. In patients habituated to barbiturates, abrupt withdrawal may produce delirium or convulsions.

Dosage and Administration: The dosage of Donnatal Extentabs should be adjusted to the needs of the individual patient to assure symptomatic control with a minimum of adverse reactions. The usual dose is one Extentab every twelve (12) hours. If indicated, one Extentab every eight (8) hours may be given.

Overdosage: The signs and symptoms of overdose are headache, nausea, vomiting, blurred vision, dilated pupils; hot and dry skin, dizziness, dryness of the mouth, difficulty in swallowing, CNS stimulation. Treatment should consist of gastric lavage, emetics, and activated charcoal. If indicated, parenteral cholinergic agents such as physostigmine or bethanechol chloride should be added.

How Supplied: Pale green, coated tablets, monogrammed AHR and Donnatal Extentab in bottles of 100 (NDC 0031-4235-63) and 500 (NDC 0031-4235-70); and Dis-Co® Unit Dose Packs of 100 (NDC 0031-4235-64).

Continued on next page

Prescribing information on A. H. Robins products listed here is based on official labeling in effect August 1, 1984, with Indications, Contraindications, Warnings Precautions, Adverse Reactions, and Dosage stated in full.

Robins—Cont.

Store at controlled room temperature, between 15°C and 30°C (59°F and 86°F).
Dispense in well-closed, light-resistant container.
Shown in Product Identification Section, page 428

DONNAZYME® TABLETS ℞
[don'nă" zīm]

Description: Donnazyme tablets are available for oral administration. Each tablet contains:
Pancreatin, USP equivalent ....300 mg
Pepsin ....150 mg
Bile Salts ....150 mg
Hyoscyamine Sulfate, USP ....0.0518 mg
Atropine Sulfate, USP ....0.0097 mg
Scopolamine Hydrobromide,
 USP ....0.0033 mg
Phenobarbital, USP (1/8 gr) ....8.1 mg
 (Warning: may be habit forming)

The combination of anticholinergic/antispasmodic/sedative components with natural digestive enzymes plus bile salts makes it useful for symptomatic relief of functional G.I. disorders.

Clinical Pharmacology: The outer layer of Donnazyme tablets is gastric-soluble and contains the belladonna alkaloids, phenobarbital and pepsin. These ingredients rapidly become available for absorption as the tablet begins disintegrating in the stomach. The pepsin supplements the stomach's digestive secretions by aiding the breakdown of proteins into proteoses and peptones. Spasmolysis and sedation are produced as the belladonna alkaloids and phenobarbital are absorbed.

The core of the tablet contains pancreatin and bile salts. It is designed to disintegrate in the alkaline medium of the duodenum where it releases the active enzyme components of pancreatin (trypsin, amylase and lipase), along with the bile salts. Trypsin breaks down larger protein fractions into peptides; amylase converts starch into maltose; lipase splits fat into fatty acids and glycerin; and bile salts enhance the fat-splitting action of the lipase and aid in the emulsification of fats and the absorption of fatty acids.

Indications and Usage: Donnazyme is indicated for the relief of symptoms associated with "nervous indigestion" and other functional G.I. disorders in the absence of organic pathology. Some of these conditions are chronic pancreatitis, chronic gastritis, postcholecystectomy syndrome, and chronic biliary disorders. Donnazyme may prove especially useful in patients with decreased digestive enzyme secretory activity, which is frequently suspect in older patients with visceral complaints.

Contraindications: Glaucoma, obstructive uropathy (for example, bladder neck obstruction due to prostatic hypertrophy); obstructive disease of the gastrointestinal tract (as in achalasia, pyloroduodenal stenosis, etc.); paralytic ileus, intestinal atony of the elderly or debilitated patient, unstable cardiovascular status in acute hemorrhage, severe ulcerative colitis especially if complicated by toxic megacolon; myasthenia gravis; hiatal hernia associated with reflux esophagitis.

Donnazyme is contraindicated in patients with known hypersensitivity to any of the ingredients. Phenobarbital is contraindicated in acute intermittent porphyria and in those patients in whom phenobarbital produces restlessness and/or excitement.

Warnings: In the presence of a high environmental temperature, heat prostration can occur with belladonna alkaloids (fever and heatstroke due to decreased sweating).

Diarrhea may be an early symptom of incomplete intestinal obstruction, especially in patients with ileostomy or colostomy. In this instance, treatment with this drug would be inappropriate and possibly harmful.

Donnazyme may produce drowsiness or blurred vision. The patient should be warned, should these occur, not to engage in activities requiring mental alertness, such as operating a motor vehicle or other machinery, and not to perform hazardous work.

Phenobarbital may decrease the effect of anticoagulants and necessitate larger doses of the anticoagulant for optimal effect. When the phenobarbital is discontinued, the dose of the anticoagulant may have to be decreased.

Phenobarbital may be habit forming and should not be administered to individuals known to be addiction prone or to those with a history of physical and/or psychological dependence upon drugs. Since barbiturates are metabolized in the liver, they should be used with caution and initial small doses in patients with hepatic dysfunction.

Precautions: *General.* Use with caution in patients with autonomic neuropathy, hepatic or renal disease, hyperthyroidism, coronary heart disease, congestive heart failure, cardiac arrhythmias, tachycardia, and hypertension.

Belladonna alkaloids may produce a delay in gastric emptying (antral stasis) which would complicate the management of gastric ulcer.

Theoretically, with overdosage, a curare-like action may occur.

Carcinogenesis, mutagenesis: Long-term studies in animals have not been performed to evaluate carcinogenic potential.

Pregnancy Category C. Animal reproduction studies have not been conducted with Donnazyme. It is not known whether Donnazyme can cause fetal harm when administered to a pregnant woman or can affect reproduction capacity. Donnazyme should be given to a pregnant woman only if clearly needed.

Nursing mothers: It is not known whether this drug is excreted in human milk. Because many drugs are excreted in human milk, caution should be exercised when Donnazyme is administered to a nursing mother.

Pediatric Use: Safety and effectiveness in children have not been established.

Adverse Reactions: Adverse reactions may include xerostomia; urinary hesitancy and retention; blurred vision; tachycardia; palpitation; mydriasis; cycloplegia; increased ocular tension; loss of taste sense; headache; nervousness; drowsiness; weakness, dizziness, insomnia; nausea; vomiting; impotence; suppression of lactation; constipation; bloated feeling; musculoskeletal pain; severe allergic reaction or drug idiosyncrasies, including "anaphylaxis, urticaria and other dermal manifestations; and decreased sweating." Elderly patients may react with symptoms of excitement, agitation, drowsiness, and other untoward manifestations to even small doses of the drug.

Phenobarbital may produce excitement in some patients, rather than a sedative effect. In patients habituated to barbiturates, abrupt withdrawal may produce delirium or convulsions.

Overdosage: The signs and symptoms of overdose are headache, nausea, vomiting, blurred vision, dilated pupils, hot and dry skin, dizziness, dryness of the mouth, difficulty in swallowing, CNS stimulation. Treatment should consist of gastric lavage, emetics, and activated charcoal. If indicated, parenteral cholinergic agents, such as physostigmine or bethanechol chloride, should be added.

Dosage and Administration: Adult dosage: Two tablets after each meal.

How Supplied: Kelly green tablets in bottles of 100 (NDC 0031-4649-63) and 500 (NDC 0031-4649-70). Store at controlled room temperature, between 15°C and 30°C (59°F and 86°F). Dispense in tight container.

Shown in Product Identification Section, page 428

DOPRAM® INJECTABLE ℞
[do'pram]
brand of Doxapram Hydrochloride Injection, USP

Description: Each 1 ml contains:
Doxapram Hydrochloride, USP ....20 mg.
Water for Injection, USP ....q.s.
Benzyl Alcohol, NF (as preservative) 0.9%

Actions: Doxapram hydrochloride produces respiratory stimulation mediated through the peripheral carotid chemoreceptors. As the dosage level is increased, the central respiratory centers in the medulla are stimulated with progressive stimulation of other parts of the brain and spinal cord.

The onset of respiratory stimulation following the recommended single intravenous injection of doxapram hydrochloride usually occurs in 20-40 seconds with peak effect at 1-2 minutes. The duration of effect may vary from 5-12 minutes.

The respiratory stimulant action is manifested by an increase in tidal volume associated with a slight increase in respiratory rate.

A pressor response may result following doxapram administration. Provided there is no impairment of cardiac function, the pressor effect is more marked in hypovolemic than in normovolemic states. The pressor response is due to the improved cardiac output rather than peripheral vasoconstriction. Following doxapram administration an increased release of catecholamines has been noted.

Although opiate induced respiratory depression is antagonized by doxapram, the analgesic effect is not affected.

Indications:
1. *Post-anesthesia.*
 a. When the possibility of airway obstruction and/or hypoxia have been eliminated, doxapram may be used to stimulate respiration in patients with drug-induced post-anesthesia respiratory depression or apnea other than that due to muscle relaxant drugs.
 b. To pharmacologically stimulate deep breathing in the so-called "stir-up" regimen in the postoperative patient. (Simultaneous administration of oxygen is desirable.)
2. *Drug-induced central nervous system depression.*
 Exercising care to prevent vomiting and aspiration, doxapram may be used to stimulate respiration, hasten arousal, and to encourage the return of laryngopharyngeal reflexes in patients with mild to moderate respiratory and CNS depression due to drug overdosage.
3. *Chronic pulmonary disease associated with acute hypercapnia.*
 Doxaram is indicated as a temporary measure in hospitalized patients with acute respiratory insufficiency superimposed on chronic obstructive pulmonary disease. Its use should be for a short period of time (approximately 2 hours) as an aid in the prevention of elevation of arterial CO₂ tension during the administration of oxygen. It should not be used in conjunction with mechanical ventilation. The adequacy of ventilation MUST be assessed by measurements of arterial blood gases as well as careful monitoring of the cardiovascular indices.

Contraindications:
1. *General Contraindications.*
 Doxapram is not recommended in the following conditions: epilepsy and other convulsive states; incompetence of the ventilatory mechanism due to muscle paresis, flail chest, pneumothorax, airway obstruction, and extreme dyspnea; severe hypertension and cerebrovascular accidents; hypersensitivity to doxapram; evidence of head injury.
2. *Contraindications in pulmonary disease.*
 Doxapram is not recommended in the following conditions: strongly suspected or confirmed pulmonary embolism, pneumothorax, acute bronchial asthma, respiratory failure due to neuromuscular disorders, and in restrictive respiratory diseases such as pulmonary fibrosis.
3. *Contraindications in cardiovascular disease.*
 Doxapram is not recommended in the following conditions: coronary artery disease, frank uncompensated heart failure.

Warnings:
1. *Warning in post-anesthetic use.*
 a. Doxapram is neither an antagonist to muscle relaxant drugs nor a specific narcotic antagonist. Adequacy of airway and oxygenation must be assured prior to doxapram administration.

b. Doxapram should be administered with great care and only under close supervision to patients with cerebral edema, history of bronchial asthma, severe tachycardia, cardiac arrhythmia, cardiac disease, hyperthyroidism, or pheochromocytoma.

c. Since narcosis may recur after stimulation with doxapram, care should be taken to maintain close observation until the patient has been fully alert for ½ to 1 hour.

2. *Warning in drug-induced CNS and respiratory depression.*

Doxapram alone may not stimulate adequate spontaneous breathing or provide sufficient arousal in patients who are *severely* depressed either due to respiratory failure or to CNS depressant drugs, but should be used as an adjunct to establish supportive measures and resuscitative techniques.

3. *Warning in chronic obstructive pulmonary disease.*

a. In an attempt to lower pCO_2, the rate of infusion of doxapram should not be increased in severely ill patients because of the associated increased work in breathing.

b. Doxapram should not be used in conjunction with mechanical ventilation.

4. *Warning in pregnancy.*

Clinically the safe use of doxapram in pregnancy has not been established. The physician must weigh the need against possible risks in using the drug in pregnant patients or in women of childbearing potential.

5. *Warning in children 12 years of age and under.*

Doxapram is not recommended for use in patients 12 years of age or under because studies to adequately evaluate its safety and efficacy have not been performed.

Precautions:

1. *General precautions.*

a. An adequate airway is essential.

b. Recommended dosages of doxapram should be employed and maximum total dosages should not be exceeded. In order to avoid side effects, it is advisable to use the minimum effective dosage.

c. Monitoring of the blood pressure and deep tendon reflexes is recommended to prevent overdosage.

d. Vascular extravasation or use of a single injection site over an extended period should be avoided since either may lead to thrombophlebitis or local skin irritation.

e. Rapid infusion may result in hemolysis.

f. Lowered pCO_2 induced by hyperventilation produces cerebral vasoconstriction and slowing of the cerebral circulation. This should be taken into consideration on an individual basis.

g. Intravenous short-acting barbiturates, oxygen and resuscitative equipment should be readily available to manage overdosage manifested by excessive central nervous system stimulation. Slow administration of the drug, careful observation of the patient during administration and for some time subsequently, are advisable. These precautions are to assure that the protective reflexes have been restored and to prevent possible posthyperventilation hypoventilation.

h. Doxapram should be administered cautiously to patients receiving sympathomimetic or monoamine oxidase inhibiting drugs, since an additive pressor effect may occur.

i. Blood pressure increases are generally modest but significant increases have been noted in some patients. Because of this doxapram is not recommended for use in severe hypertension (see Contraindications).

j. If sudden hypotension or dyspnea develops, doxapram should be stopped.

2. *Precautions in post-anesthetic use.*

a. In patients who have received muscle relaxants, doxapram may temporarily mask the residual effects of muscle relaxant drugs.

b. Since an increase in epinephrine release has been noted with doxapram, it is recommended that initiation of therapy be delayed for at least 10 minutes following the discontinuance of anesthetics known to sensitize the myocardium to catecholamines, such as halothane, cyclopropane and enflurane.

c. The same consideration to pre-existing disease states should be exercised as in non-anesthetized individuals. See Contraindications and Warnings covering use in hypertension, asthma, disturbances of respiratory mechanics including airway obstruction, CNS disorders including increased cerebrospinal fluid pressure, convulsive disorders, acute agitation, and profound metabolic disorders.

3. *Precautions in chronic obstructive pulmonary disease.*

a. Arrhythmias seen in some patients in acute respiratory failure secondary to chronic obstructive pulmonary disease are probably the result of hypoxia. Doxapram should be used with caution in these patients.

b. Arterial blood gases should be drawn prior to the initiation of doxapram infusion and oxygen administration, then at least every ½ hour. Doxapram administration does not diminish the need for careful monitoring of the patient or the need for supplemental oxygen in patients with acute respiratory failure. Doxapram should be stopped if the arterial blood gases deteriorate, and mechanical ventilation initiated.

Adverse Reactions: The following adverse reactions have been reported:

1. *Central and autonomic nervous systems.*

Headache, dizziness, apprehension, disorientation, pupillary dilatation, hyperactivity, involuntary movements, convulsions, muscle spasticity, increased deep tendon reflexes, clonus, bilateral Babinski; pyrexia, flushing, sweating; pruritus and paresthesia such as a feeling of warmth, burning, or hot sensation especially in the area of genitalia and perineum.

2. *Respiratory*

Cough, dyspnea, tachypnea, laryngospasm, bronchospasm, hiccough, and rebound hypoventilation.

3. *Cardiovascular.*

Phlebitis, variations in heart rate, lowered T-waves, arrhythmias, chest pain, tightness in chest. A mild to moderate increase in blood pressure is commonly noted. The elevation in blood pressure may be of concern only in hypertensive patients. (See Contraindications.)

4. *Gastrointestinal.*

Nausea, vomiting, diarrhea, desire to defecate.

5. *Genitourinary.*

Urinary retention, stimulation of urinary bladder with spontaneous voiding.

6. *Laboratory determinations.*

A decrease in hemoglobin, hematocrit, or red blood cell count has been observed in postoperative patients. In the presence of preexisting leukopenia, a further decrease in WBC has been observed following anesthesia and treatment with doxapram hydrochloride. Elevation of BUN and albuminuria have also been observed. As some of the patients cited above had received multiple drugs concomitantly, a cause and effect relationship could not be determined.

Dosage and Administration:

1. Doxapram hydrochloride is compatible with 5% and 10% dextrose in water or normal saline.

Table I. Dopram Injectable Dosage for post-anesthetic use—I.V.

I.V. Administration	Recommended dosage mg/kg	Recommended dosage mg/lb	Maximum dose per single injection mg/kg	Maximum dose per single injection mg/lb	Maximum total dose mg/kg	Maximum total dose mg/lb
Single Injection	0.5–1.0	0.25–0.5	1.5	0.70	1.5	0.70
Repeat Injections (5 min. intervals)	0.5–1.0	0.25–0.5	1.5	0.70	2.0	1.0
Infusion	0.5–1.0	0.25–0.5	—	—	4.0	2.0

ADMIXTURE OF DOXAPRAM WITH ALKALINE SOLUTIONS SUCH AS 2.5% THIOPENTAL SODIUM OR BICARBONATE WILL RESULT IN PRECIPITATION.

2. *In post-anesthetic use.*

a. By i.v. injection (see Table I. Dosage for post-anesthetic use—I.V.)

[See table above]

b. By infusion. The solution is prepared by adding 250 mg of doxapram (12.5 ml) to 250 ml of dextrose or saline solution. The infusion is initiated at a rate of approximately 5 mg/minute until a satisfactory respiratory response is observed, and maintained at a rate of 1–3 mg/minute. The rate of infusion should be adjusted to sustain the desired level of respiratory stimulation with a minimum of side effects. The recommended total dosage by infusion is 4 mg/kg (2.0 mg/lb), not to exceed 3 grams.

3. *In the management of drug-induced CNS depression.*

(See Table II. Dosage for drug-induced CNS depression.)

[See table on next page].

METHOD ONE

Using Single and/or Repeat Single I.V. *Injections.*

a. Give priming dose of 1.0 mg/lb (2.0 mg/kg) body weight and repeat in 5 minutes.

b. Repeat same dose q1-2h until patient wakens. Watch for relapse into unconsciousness or development of respiratory depression, since Dopram does not affect the metabolism of CNS-depressant drugs.

c. If relapse occurs, resume 1-2 hourly injections until arousal is sustained, or total maximum daily dose (3 grams) is given. Allow patient to sleep until 24 hours have elapsed from first injection of Dopram, using assisted or automatic respiration if necessary.

d. Repeat procedure until patient breathes spontaneously and sustains desired level of consciousness, or until maximum dosage (3 grams) is given.

e. Repetitive doses should be administered only to patients who have shown response to the initial dose.

f. Failure to respond appropriately indicates the need for neurologic evaluation for a possible central nervous system source of sustained coma.

METHOD TWO

By Intermittent I.V. *Infusion.*

a. Give priming dose as in Method One.

b. If patient wakens, watch for relapse; if no response, continue general supportive treatment for 1-2 hours and repeat Dopram. If some respiratory stimulation occurs, prepare I.V. infusion by adding 250 mg of Dopram (12.5 ml) to 250 ml of saline or dextrose solution. Deliver at rate of 1-3 mg/min (60-180 ml/hr) according to size of

Continued on next page

Prescribing information on A. H. Robins products listed here is based on official labeling in effect August 1, 1984, with Indications, Contraindications, Warnings, Precautions, Adverse Reactions, and Dosage stated in full.

Robins—Cont.

patient and depth of coma. Discontinue Dopram if patient begins to waken or at end of 2 hours.
c. Continue supportive treatment for ½ to 2 hours and repeat Step b.
d. Do not exceed 3 grams.

4. *Chronic obstructive pulmonary disease associated with acute hypercapnia.*
   a. One vial of doxapram (400 mg) should be mixed with 180 ml of the intravenous solution (concentration of 2.0 mg/ml). The infusion should be started at 1-2 mg/minute (½-1 ml/minute); if indicated, increase to a maximum of 3 mg/minute. Arterial blood gases should be determined prior to the onset of doxapram's administration and at least every half hour during the two hours of infusion to insure against the insidious development of CO_2-RETENTION AND ACIDOSIS. Alteration of oxygen concentration or flow rate may necessitate adjustment in the rate of doxapram infusion.
   b. Predictable blood gas patterns are more readily established with a continuous infusion of doxapram. If the blood gases show evidence of deterioration, the infusion of doxapram should be discontinued.
   c. ADDITIONAL INFUSIONS BEYOND THE SINGLE MAXIMUM TWO HOUR ADMINISTRATION PERIOD ARE NOT RECOMMENDED.

Overdosage: Excessive pressor effect, tachycardia, skeletal muscle hyperactivity, and enhanced deep tendon reflexes may be early signs of overdosage. Therefore, the blood pressure, pulse rate, and deep tendon reflexes should be evaluated periodically and the dosage or infusion rate adjusted accordingly. Convulsive seizures are unlikely at recommended dosages, but intravenous anticonvulsants, oxygen, and resuscitative equipment should be available.

How Supplied: Dopram Injectable (doxapram hydrochloride injection) is available in 20 ml multiple dose vials containing 20 mg of doxapram hydrochloride per ml, 20 mg/ml, with benzyl alcohol 0.9% as the preservative (NDC 0031-4849-83).
Additional literature available upon request.
Manufactured for Pharmaceutical Division, A. H. Robins Company, Richmond, Virginia 23220 by Elkins-Sinn, Inc., Cherry Hill, New Jersey 08034, a subsidiary of A. H. Robins Co.

Shown in Product Identification Section, page 428

ENTOZYME® TABLETS
[ĕn′ to-zīm]

Description: Entozyme tablets are available for oral administration. Each tablet contains:
Pancreatin, USP equivalent ....300 mg
Pepsin ....250 mg
Bile salts ....150 mg
Natural Digestive Enzymes

Construction: Entozyme is a specially constructed tablet. The outer layer dissolves in the stomach and releases pepsin. The "inner tablet" is protected by an enteric coating that disintegrates in the alkaline medium of the small intestine and releases pancreatin and bile salts, thus preserving the digestive potency of the pancreatin as it passes through the stomach.

Clinical Pharmacology: Entozyme should be considered a form of nutritional therapy since it is made up of naturally-occurring digestive enzymes. Entozyme enhances proteolysis by its peptic and tryptic activity, carbohydrate digestion by amylolytic activity, and fat emulsification and transport by lipolytic activity and the action of the bile salts. The components of six Entozyme tablets will digest 60 grams of fat, 48 grams of protein and 48 grams of carbohydrate, amounts of food that yield nearly 1,000 calories (one-third to one-half the daily caloric intake for many patients).

Indications and Usage: Entozyme is indicated for the relief of steatorrhea, pyrosis, flatulence, and belching associated with incomplete digestion of food due to a deficiency of digestive enzymes. By effectively supplementing the patient's secretion of digestive enzymes, Entozyme promotes more complete digestion of carbohydrates, proteins and fats.

Contraindications: Biliary tract obstruction or hypersensitivity to any of the ingredients.

Warnings: Do not administer to patients who are allergic to pork products.

Precautions: *Carcinogenesis, mutagenesis.* Long-term studies in animals have not been performed to evaluate carcinogenic potential.
Pregnancy Category C. Animal reproduction studies have not been conducted with Entozyme. It is not known whether Entozyme can cause fetal harm when administered to a pregnant woman or can affect reproduction capacity. Entozyme should be given to a pregnant woman only if clearly needed.
Nursing mothers. It is not known whether this drug is excreted in human milk. Because many drugs are excreted in human milk, caution should be exercised when Entozyme is administered to a nursing woman.
Pediatric Use. Safety and effectiveness in children have not been established.

Adverse Reactions: Skin rash is the most frequently reported adverse reaction to Entozyme, and appears to be associated with hypersensitivity to pork protein in the pancreatin. At high doses, a laxative effect may occur.

Overdosage: Excessive dosage may produce a laxative effect. Systemic toxicity does not occur.

Dosage and Administration: Two tablets with each meal and 1 or 2 tablets with each snack. The dose may be increased as necessary to achieve adequate digestion. Entozyme tablets should be swallowed whole and not crushed or chewed.

How Supplied: White coated tablets, monogrammed "AHR" and 5049 in bottles of 100 (NDC 0031-5049-63) and 500 (NDC 0031-5049-70).
Store at controlled room temperature, between 15°C and 30°C (59°F and 86°F). Dispense in tight container.

Shown in Product Identification Section, page 428

EXNA® TABLETS ℞
[ĕks′ nă]
brand of Benzthiazide Tablets, USP

Description: Each round, yellow scored Exna tablet contains benzthiazide 50 mg.

Action: The mechanism of action results in an interference with the renal tubular mechanism of electrolyte reabsorption. At maximal therapeutic dosage all thiazides are approximately equal in their diuretic potency. The mechanism whereby thiazides function in the control of hypertension is unknown.

Indications: Exna (benzthiazide) is indicated as adjunctive therapy in edema associated with congestive heart failure, hepatic cirrhosis and corticosteroid and estrogen therapy.
Exna has also been found useful in edema due to various forms of renal dysfunction as: nephrotic syndrome; acute glomerulonephritis; and chronic renal failure.
Exna is indicated in the management of hypertension either as the sole therapeutic agent or to enhance the effectiveness of other antihypertensive drugs in the more severe forms of hypertension.
Usage in Pregnancy. The routine use of diuretics in an otherwise healthy woman is inappropriate and exposes mother and fetus to unnecessary hazard. Diuretics do not prevent development of toxemia of pregnancy, and there is no satisfactory evidence that they are useful in the treatment of developed toxemia.
Edema during pregnancy may arise from pathological causes or from the physiologic and mechanical consequences of pregnancy. Thiazides are indicated in pregnancy when edema is due to pathologic causes, just as they are in the absence of pregnancy (however, see Warnings). Dependent edema in pregnancy, resulting from restriction of venous return by the expanded uterus, is properly treated through elevation of the lower extremities and use of support hose; use of diuretics to lower intravascular volume in this case is illogical and unnecessary. There is hypervolemia during normal pregnancy which is harmful to neither the fetus nor the mother (in the absence of cardiovascular disease), but which is associated with edema, including generalized edema, in the majority of pregnant women. If this edema produces discomfort, increased recumbency will often provide relief. In rare instances, this edema may cause extreme discomfort which is not relieved by rest. In these cases, a short course of diuretics may provide relief and may be appropriate.

Contraindications: Anuria. Hypersensitivity to this or other sulfonamide derived drugs.

Warnings: Thiazides should be used with caution in severe renal disease. In patients with renal disease, thiazides may precipitate azotemia. Cumulative effects of the drug may develop in patients with impaired renal function.
Thiazides should be used with caution in patients with impaired hepatic function or progressive liver disease, since minor alterations of fluid and electrolyte balance may precipitate hepatic coma.
Thiazides may add to or potentiate the action of other antihypertensive drugs. Potentiation occurs with ganglionic or peripheral adrenergic blocking drugs.
Sensitivity reactions may occur in patients with a history of allergy or bronchial asthma.
The possibility of exacerbation or activation of systemic lupus erythematosus has been reported.
Usage in Pregnancy: Thiazides cross the placental barrier and appear in cord blood. The use of thiazides in pregnant women requires that the anticipated benefit be weighed against possible hazards to the fetus. These hazards include fetal or neonatal jaundice, thrombocytopenia, and possibly other adverse reactions which have occurred in the adult.
Nursing Mothers: Thiazides appear in breast milk. If use of the drug is deemed essential, the patient should stop nursing.

Precautions: Periodic determination of serum electrolytes to detect possible electrolyte imbalance should be performed at appropriate intervals. All patients receiving thiazide therapy should be

---

Table II. Dopram Injectable Dosage for drug-induced CNS depression.

Level of Depression	METHOD ONE Priming dose single/repeat i.v. injection mg/kg	mg/lb	METHOD TWO Rate of intermittent i.v. infusion mg/kg/hr	mg/lb/hr
Mild*	1.0	0.5	1.0–2.0	0.5–1.0
Moderate†	2.0	1.0	2.0–3.0	1.0–1.5

*Mild Depression
Class 0: Asleep, but can be aroused and can answer questions.
Class 1: Comatose, will withdraw from painful stimuli, reflexes intact.

†Moderate Depression
Class 2: Comatose, will not withdraw from painful stimuli, reflexes intact.
Class 3: Comatose, reflexes absent, no depression of circulation or respiration.

observed for clinical signs of fluid or electrolyte imbalance; namely, hyponatremia, hypochloremic alkalosis, and hypokalemia. Serum and urine electrolyte determinations are particularly important when the patient is vomiting excessively or receiving parenteral fluids. Medication such as digitalis may also influence serum electrolytes. Warning signs, irrespective of cause, are: dryness of mouth, thirst, weakness, lethargy, drowsiness, restlessness, muscle pains or cramps, muscular fatigue, hypotension, oliguria, tachycardia, and gastrointestinal disturbances such as nausea and vomiting.

Hypokalemia may develop with thiazides as with any other potent diuretic especially with brisk diuresis, when severe cirrhosis is present or during concomitant use of corticosteroids or ACTH.

Interference with adequate oral electrolyte intake will also contribute to hypokalemia. Digitalis therapy may exaggerate metabolic effects of hypokalemia especially with reference to myocardial activity.

Any chloride deficit is generally mild and usually does not require specific treatment except under extraordinary circumstances (as in liver disease or renal disease). Dilutional hyponatremia may occur in edematous patients in hot weather; appropriate therapy is water restriction, rather than administration of salt except in rare instances when the hyponatremia is life threatening. In actual salt depletion, appropriate replacement is the therapy of choice.

Hyperuricemia may occur or frank gout may be precipitated in certain patients receiving thiazide therapy.

Insulin requirements in diabetic patients may be increased, decreased, or unchanged. Latent diabetes mellitus may become manifest during thiazide administration.

Thiazide drugs may increase the responsiveness to tubocurarine.

The antihypertensive effects of the drug may be enhanced in the postsympathectomy patient.

Thiazides may decrease arterial responsiveness to norepinephrine. This diminution is not sufficient to preclude effectiveness of the pressor agent for therapeutic use.

If progressive renal impairment becomes evident, as indicated by a rising nonprotein nitrogen or blood urea nitrogen, a careful reappraisal of therapy is necessary with consideration given to withholding or discontinuing diuretic therapy.

Thiazides may decrease serum PBI levels without signs of thyroid disturbance.

This product contains FD&C Yellow No. 5 (tartrazine) which may cause allergic-type reactions (including bronchial asthma) in certain susceptible individuals. Although the overall incidence of FD&C Yellow No. 5 (tartrazine) sensitivity in the general population is low, it is frequently seen in patients who have aspirin hypersensitivity.

Adverse Reactions: *Gastrointestinal System Reaction:* anorexia; gastric irritation; nausea; vomiting; cramping; diarrhea; constipation; jaundice (intrahepatic cholestatic jaundice); pancreatitis.
Central Nervous System Reactions: dizziness; vertigo; parasthesias; headache; xanthopsia.
Hematologic Reactions: leukopenia; agranulocytosis; thrombocytopenia; aplastic anemia.
Dermatologic-Hypersensitivity Reactions: purpura; photosensitivity; rash; urticaria; necrotizing angiitis (vasculitis) (cutaneous vasculitis).
Cardiovascular Reaction: Orthostatic hypotension may occur and may be aggravated by alcohol, barbiturates or narcotics.
Other: hyperglycemia; glycosuria; hyperuricemia; muscle spasm; weakness; restlessness.

Whenever adverse reactions are moderate or severe, thiazide dosage should be reduced or therapy withdrawn.

Dosage and Administration: Therapy should be individualized according to patient response. This therapy should be titrated to gain maximal therapeutic response as well as the minimal dose possible to maintain that therapeutic response.

	Diuretic	Antihypertensive
Benzthiazide	50 to 200 mg	50 to 200 mg

Edema: *Initiation of diuresis:* 50 to 200 mg daily should be used for several days, or until dry weight is attained. With 100 mg or more daily, it is generally preferable to administer benzthiazide in two doses, following morning and evening meals.
Maintenance of diuresis: 50 to 150 mg daily depending upon the patient's response. To maintain effectiveness, reduction to minimal effective dosage should be gradual.
Hypertension: *Initiation of antihypertensive therapy:* 50 to 100 mg daily is the average dose. It may be given in two doses of 25 mg or 50 mg each after breakfast and after lunch. This dosage may be continued until a therapeutic drop in blood pressure occurs.
Maintenance of antihypertensive therapy: Dosage should be adjusted according to the patient response, either upward to as much as 50 mg q.i.d., or downward to the minimal effective dosage level.
How Supplied: Exna (benzthiazide) is supplied in 50 mg yellow, scored monogramed AHR and 5449 tablets, packaged in bottles of 100 (NDC 0031-5449-63).

Shown in Product Identification Section, page 428

MICRO–K EXTENCAPS® ℞
MICRO–K 10 EXTENCAPS® ℞
brand of Potassium Chloride

Description: Micro-K Extencaps are pale orange, hard gelatin capsules, each containing 600 mg of dispersible small crystalline particles of potassium chloride (equivalent to 8 mEq K), monogrammed Micro-K and AHR/5720
Micro-K 10 Extencaps are pale orange and opaque white, hard gelatin capsules, each containing 750 mg of dispersible, small crystalline particles of potassium chloride (equivalent to 10 mEq K) monogrammed Micro-K 10 and AHR/5730. Each particle of potassium chloride (KCl) is microencapsulated by a patented process with a polymeric coating which allows for the controlled release of potassium and chloride ions over an eight- to ten-hour period. The dispersibility of the microcapsules and the controlled release of ions are intended to minimize the likelihood of high localized concentrations of potassium chloride and resultant mucosal ulceration within the gastrointestinal tract.

The polymeric coating forming the microcapsules functions as a water-permeable membrane. Fluids pass through the membrane and gradually dissolve the potassium chloride within the microcapsules. The resulting potassium chloride solution slowly diffuses outward through the membrane.

Actions: Potassium ion is the principal intracellular cation of most body tissues. Potassium ions participate in a number of essential physiological processes, including the maintenance of intracellular tonicity, the transmission of nerve impulses, the contraction of cardiac, skeletal, and smooth muscle and the maintenance of normal renal function.

Potassium depletion may occur whenever the rate of potassium loss through renal excretion and/or loss from the gastrointestinal tract exceeds the rate of potassium intake. Such depletion usually develops slowly as a consequence of prolonged therapy with oral diuretics, primary or secondary hyperaldosteronism, diabetic ketoacidosis, severe diarrhea, or inadequate replacement of potassium in patients on prolonged parenteral nutrition. Potassium depletion due to these causes is usually accompanied by a concomitant deficiency of chloride and is manifested by hypokalemia and metabolic alkalosis. Potassium depletion may produce weakness, fatigue, disturbances of cardiac rhythm (primarily ectopic beats), prominent U-waves in the electrocardiogram, and in advanced cases, flaccid paralysis and/or impaired ability to concentrate urine.

Potassium depletion associated with metabolic alkalosis is managed by correcting the fundamental causes of the deficiency whenever possible and administering supplemental potassium chloride, in the form of high potassium food or potassium chloride solution, capsules or tablets. In rare circumstances (e.g., patients with renal tubular acidosis) potassium depletion may be associated with metabolic acidosis and hyperchloremia. In such patients potassium replacement should be accomplished with potassium salts other than the chloride, such as potassium bicarbonate, potassium citrate, or potassium acetate.

INDICATIONS: BECAUSE OF REPORTS OF INTESTINAL AND GASTRIC ULCERATION AND BLEEDING WITH SLOW-RELEASE POTASSIUM CHLORIDE PREPARATIONS, THESE DRUGS SHOULD BE RESERVED FOR THOSE PATIENTS WHO CANNOT TOLERATE OR REFUSE TO TAKE LIQUID OR EFFERVESCENT POTASSIUM PREPARATIONS OR FOR PATIENTS IN WHOM THERE IS A PROBLEM OF COMPLIANCE WITH THESE PREPARATIONS.

1. For therapeutic use in patients with hypokalemia with or without metabolic alkalosis; in digitalis intoxication and in patients with hypokalemic familial periodic paralysis.

2. For prevention of potassium depletion when the dietary intake of potassium is inadequate in the following conditions: patients receiving digitalis and diuretics for congestive heart failure; hepatic cirrhosis with ascites; states of aldosterone excess with normal renal function; potassium-losing nephropathy, and certain diarrheal states.

3. The use of potassium salts in patients receiving diuretics for uncomplicated essential hypertension is often unnecessary when such patients have a normal dietary pattern. Serum potassium should be checked periodically, however, and, if hypokalemia occurs, dietary supplementation with potassium-containing foods may be adequate to control milder cases. In more severe cases, supplementation with potassium salts may be indicated.

Contraindications: Potassium supplements are contraindicated in patients with hyperkalemia since a further increase in serum potassium concentration in such patients can produce cardiac arrest. Hyperkalemia may complicate any of the following conditions: chronic renal failure, systemic acidosis such as diabetic acidosis, acute dehydration, extensive tissue breakdown as in severe burns, adrenal insufficiency, or the administration of a potassium-sparing diuretic (e.g., spironolactone, triamterene).

Wax-matrix potassium chloride preparations have produced esophageal ulceration in certain cardiac patients with esophageal compression due to an enlarged left atrium.

All solid dosage forms of potassium supplements are contraindicated in any patient in whom there is cause for arrest or delay in tablet passage through the gastrointestinal tract. In these instances, potassium supplementation should be with a liquid preparation.

Warnings: *Hyperkalemia.* In patients with impaired mechanisms for excreting potassium, the administration of potassium salts can produce hyperkalemia and cardiac arrest. This occurs most commonly in patients given potassium by the intravenous route but may also occur in patients given potassium orally. Potentially fatal hyperkalemia can develop rapidly and be asymptomatic. The use of potassium salts in patients with chronic renal disease, or any other condition which impairs potassium excretion, requires particularly careful monitoring of the serum potassium concentration and appropriate dosage adjustments.

Interaction with Potassium-Sparing Diuretics. Hypokalemia should not be treated by the concomi-

Continued on next page

Prescribing information on A. H. Robins products listed here is based on official labeling in effect August 1, 1984, with Indications, Contraindications, Warnings Precautions, Adverse Reactions, and Dosage stated in full.

Robins—Cont.

tant administration of potassium salts and a potassium-sparing diuretic (e.g., spironolactone or triamterene), since the simultaneous administration of these agents can produce severe hyperkalemia.

Gastrointestinal lesions. Potassium chloride tablets have produced stenotic and/or ulcerative lesions of the small bowel and deaths, in addition to upper gastrointestinal bleeding. These lesions are caused by a high localized concentration of potassium ion in the region of a rapidly dissolving tablet which injures the bowel wall and thereby produces obstruction, hemorrhage, or perforation.

Micro-K Extencaps contain microcapsules which disperse upon dissolution of the hard gelatin capsule. The microcapsules are formulated to provide a controlled release of potassium chloride. The dispersibility of the microcapsules and the controlled release of ions from the microcapsules are intended to minimize the possibility of a high local concentration near the gastrointestinal mucosa and the ability of the KCl to cause stenosis or ulceration. Other means of accomplishing this (e.g., incorporation of KCl into a wax matrix) have reduced the frequency of such lesions to less than one per 100,000 patient years (compared to 40-50 per 100,000 patient years with enteric-coated KCl), but have not eliminated them. The frequency of GI lesions with Micro-K Extencaps is, at present, unknown. Micro-K Extencaps should be discontinued immediately and the possibility of bowel obstruction or perforation considered if severe vomiting, abdominal pain, distention, or gastrointestinal bleeding occurs.

Metabolic Acidosis. Hypokalemia in patients with metabolic *acidosis* should be treated with an alkalinizing potassium salt such as potassium bicarbonate, potassium citrate, or potassium acetate.

Precautions: The diagnosis of potassium depletion is ordinarily made by demonstrating hypokalemia in a patient with a clinical history suggesting some cause for potassium depletion. In interpreting the serum potassium level, the physician should bear in mind that acute alkalosis per se can produce hypokalemia in the absence of a deficit in total body potassium, while acute acidosis per se can increase the serum potassium concentration into the normal range even in the presence of a reduced total body potassium. The treatment of potassium depletion, particularly in the presence of cardiac disease, renal disease, or acidosis, requires careful attention to acid-base balance and appropriate monitoring of serum electrolytes, the electrocardiogram, and the clinical status of the patient.

Adverse Reactions: The most common adverse reactions to oral potassium salts are nausea, vomiting, abdominal discomfort, and diarrhea. These symptoms are due to irritation of the gastrointestinal tract and may be minimized by taking the dose with meals or by reducing the dose.

Intestinal bleeding, ulceration, perforation and obstruction have been reported in patients treated with solid dosage forms of potassium salts and may occur with Micro-K Extencaps (see Contraindications and Warnings).

One of the most severe adverse effects of potassium supplementation is hyperkalemia (see Contraindicatons, Warnings, and Overdosage).

Skin rash has been reported rarely with potassium preparations.

Overdosage: The administration of oral potassium salts to persons with normal excretory mechanisms for potassium rarely causes serious hyperkalemia. However, if excretory mechanisms are impaired or if potassium is administered too rapidly intravenously, potentially fatal hyperkalemia can result (see Contraindications and Warnings). It is important to recognize that hyperkalemia is usually asymptomatic and may be manifested only by an increased serum potassium concentration and characteristic electrocardiogram changes (peaking of T-waves, loss of P-wave, depression of S-T segment, and prolongation of the QT interval). Late manifestations include muscle paralysis and cardiovascular collapse from cardiac arrest.

Treatment measures for hyperkalemia include the following: (1) elimination of foods and medications containing potassium and of potassium-sparing diuretics; (2) intravenous administration of 300 to 500 ml/hr of 10% dextrose solution containing 10–20 units of insulin per 1,000 ml; (3) correction of acidosis, if present, with intravenous sodium bicarbonate; (4) use of exchange resins, hemodialysis, or peritoneal dialysis.

In treating hyperkalemia, it should be recalled that in patients who have been stabilized on digitalis, too rapid a lowering of the serum potassium concentration can produce digitalis toxicity.

Dosage and Administration: The usual dietary intake of potassium by the average adult is 40 to 80 mEq per day. Potassium depletion sufficient to cause hypokalemia usually requires the loss of 200 or more mEq of potassium from the total body store.

Dosage must be adjusted to the individual needs of each patient, but typically is around 20 mEq per day for the prevention of hypokalemia and 40 to 100 mEq per day for the treatment of potassium depletion.

	For Prevention	For Treatment
Micro-K Extencaps (8 mEq K)	2 or 3 Extencaps/day (16–24 mEq K)	5 to 12 Extencaps/day (40–96 mEq K)
Micro-K 10 Extencaps (10 mEq K)	2 Extencaps/day (20 mEq K)	4 to 10 Extencaps/day (40–100 mEq K)

If more than 2 Micro-K Extencaps are prescribed per day, the total daily dosage should be divided into two or more separate doses. Those patients having difficulty swallowing the capsules may be advised to sprinkle the contents onto a spoonful of soft food to facilitate ingestion.

How Supplied: Micro-K Extencaps® are pale orange capsules monogrammed Micro-K and AHR/5720, each containing 600 mg microencapsulated potassium chloride (equivalent to 8 mEq K) in bottles of 100 (NDC 0031-5720-63), 500 (NDC 0031-5720-70) and Dis-Co® unit dose packs of 100 (NDC 0031-5720-64).

Micro-K 10 Extencaps® are pale orange and opaque white capsules monogrammed Micro-K 10 and AHR/5730, each containing 750 mg microencapsulated potassium chloride (equivalent to 10 mEq K) in bottles of 100 (NDC 0031-5730-63), 500 (NDC 0031-5730-70) and Dis-Co® unit dose packs of 100 (NDC 0031-5730-64).

Animal Toxicology: The ulcerogenic potential of microencapsulated KCl was studied in anesthetized cats by direct applications on exteriorized gastric mucosa. The microcapsules of KCl were found to be non-ulcerogenic and significantly less irritating than wax-matrix tablets and 20% solution of KCl.

In groups of monkeys (up to 8 monkeys per group) receiving different formulations of potassium chloride at equivalent daily dosage (2400 mg KCl) for four and one-half days, Micro-K Extencaps showed no tendency to cause intestinal ulceration (similar to liquid KCl and a wax-matrix preparation but in contrast to an enteric-coated KCl tablet) and minimal gastric irritation (less than a wax-matrix preparation).

Shown in Product Identification Section, page 428

MITROLAN® TABLETS
[mi' tro" lan]
brand of Calcium Polycarbophil

Each chewable tablet contains:
Calcium Polycarbophil (equivalent to 500 mg Polycarbophil, USP)

Actions: Mitrolan (calcium polycarbophil) is a hydrophilic agent. As a bulk laxative, Mitrolan retains free water within the lumen of the intestine, and indirectly opposes dehydrating forces of the bowel, promoting well-formed stools. In diarrhea, when the intestinal mucosa is incapable of absorbing water at normal rates, Mitrolan absorbs free fecal water, forming a gel and producing formed stools. Thus, in both diarrhea and constipation, the drug works by restoring a more normal moisture level and providing bulk in the patient's intestinal tract.

Indications: For the treatment of constipation or diarrhea, associated with conditions such as irritable bowel syndrome and diverticulosis. Also for the treatment of acute non-specific diarrhea. Restores normal stool consistency by regulating its water and bulk content.

Contraindications: As with all hydrophilic bulking agents, calcium polycarbophil should not be used in patients with signs of gastrointestinal obstruction.

Adverse Reactions: Abdominal fullness may be noted occasionally. An adjustment of the dosage schedule with smaller doses given more frequently but spaced evenly throughout the day may provide relief of this symptom during continued use of Mitrolan.

Drug Interaction: Antacids containing aluminum, calcium or magnesium impair absorption of tetracycline. Although Mitrolan is not an antacid, it releases free calcium after ingestion and should not be used by any patient who is taking a prescription antibiotic drug containing any form of tetracycline.

Caution: Caution should be exercised when prescribing this or any other medication for pregnant or nursing patients.

Directions of Use:
CHEW TABLETS BEFORE SWALLOWING.
Recommended dosage for OTC use: Adults— Chew and swallow 2 tablets 4 times a day, or as needed. Do not exceed 12 tablets in a 24-hour period. Children (6 to under 12 years)—Chew and swallow 1 tablet 3 times a day, or as needed. Do not exceed 6 tablets in a 24-hour period. Children (3 to under 6 years)—Chew and swallow 1 tablet 2 times a day, or as needed. Do not exceed 3 tablets in a 24-hour period.

For episodes of severe diarrhea, the dose may be repeated every ½ hour, but do not exceed the maximum daily dosage.

Dosage may be adjusted according to individual response.

When using as a laxative, patient should drink a full glass (8 fl. oz.) of water or other liquid with each dose.

Sodium Content: Less than 0.02 mEq (0.46 mg) per tablet.

How Supplied: *Chewable Tablets*—cartons of 36 individually packaged blister units (NDC 0031-1535-57), and bottles of 100 (NDC 0031-1535-63).

Shown in Product Identification Section, page 428

PABALATE® TABLETS
[păb' ah" lāt]

Description: Pabalate® tablets are intended for oral administration.

Each enteric-coated tablet contains:
Sodium Salicylate, USP ....0.3 g
Sodium Aminobenzoate ....0.3 g

Clinical Pharmacology: Sodium salicylate is a mild analgesic with antiinflammatory and antipyretic activity. Compared to aspirin, sodium salicylate has substantially less effect on platelet adhesiveness. In large doses, however, it has a hypoprothrombinemic effect. Sodium salicylate in conventional dosage form dissolves in the stomach and is absorbed as un-ionized salicylic acid. However, in Pabalate, the enteric coating delays release of the salicylate until the tablet reaches the alkaline medium of the intestine. After absorption, salicylic acid is extensively bound to plasma protein, and the bound portion is in equilibrium with the free salicylate in the plasma. The action of sodium aminobenzoate in this formulation has not been established.

Indications: Pabalate tablets are indicated for the temporary relief of mild to moderate pain.

Contraindications: Hypersensitivity to any of the ingredients. Presence of an active ulcer, hypoprothrombinemia, Vitamin K deficiency, severe hepatic or renal damage, or hemophilia. This product is not recommended for persons on a sodium-restricted diet.

Precautions:
General: Treatment with salicylates may interfere with blood clotting; therefore, salicylate therapy should be stopped at least one week prior to surgery.
Drug Interaction: This product contains sodium aminobenzoate, the aminobenzoic acid portion of which inhibits the bacteriostatic action of sulfonamides when the two are present concurrently.
Carcinogenesis, mutagenesis: Long-term studies in animals have not been performed to evaluate carcinogenic potential.
Pregnancy Category C: Animal reproduction studies have not been conducted with Pabalate. Safe use of Pabalate has not been established with regard to possible adverse effects upon fetal development. Therefore, Pabalate should not be used in women who are or may become pregnant and particularly during early pregnancy unless in the judgment of the physician the potential benefits outweigh the possible hazards.
Nursing Mothers: Salicylates appear in human milk in moderate amounts. They can produce a bleeding tendency by decreasing the amount of prothrombin in the infant's blood. As a general rule, nursing should not be undertaken while a patient is on this drug.
Pediatric Use: Safety and effectiveness in children below the age of 12 years have not been established.
Adverse Reactions: The most frequent adverse reactions to products such as Pabalate which contain salicylates are nausea and gastrointestinal upset. Fine rash with or without pruritus and urticaria occurs less frequently. The occasional occurrence of mild salicylism (diarrhea, tinnitus, dizziness) may require an adjustment in dosage.
Overdosage: Mild chronic overdosage, termed salicylism, may cause symptoms such as tinnitus, nausea, headache, hyperventilation, dizziness, drowsiness, mental confusion, dimness of vision, sweating, thirst and occasionally diarrhea. Withdrawal of salicylates and supportive therapy may be sufficient treatment.
A more severe degree of salicylate intoxication may occur with acute massive overdosage or the chronic administration of more moderate overdoses, especially in infants and children. CNS effects are more pronounced and may progress to delirium, hallucinations, gerneralized convulsions and coma. A variety of cutaneous lesions may be observed.
A most important feature of salicylate intoxication is a disturbance of acid-base balance and plasma electrolytes. Careful monitoring of these laboratory parameters along with plasma glucose concentration is essential. The type and quantity of repair solutions used will depend upon interpretation of the laboratory data. Bicarbonate solution should be administered IV in order to produce alkaline diuresis. Correction of hypoglycemia and ketosis by the administration of glucose is essential.
Since hyperthermia and dehydration are immediate threats to life, external sponging and the administration of adequate quantities of IV fluids are important first steps to correct these conditions and maintain adequate renal function.
If hemorrhagic phenomena (petechiae, thrombocytopenia) occur, whole blood transfusions and vitamin K may be necessary.
The gastrointestinal tract should be emptied either by emesis or purging to remove undissolved tablets in cases of acute ingestion of a large single dose. Since enteric coated tablets do not disintegrate in the stomach, they cannot be removed by lavage.
Rapid and immediate removal of salicylate from the body by alkaline diuresis is essential. In more severe cases, extrarenal measures such as peritoneal dialysis, hemodialysis, hemoperfusion or exchange transfusion may be required.
Dosage and Administration: The average adult dose is two tablets every 4 hours. Due to the enteric coating, tablets should not be taken within one hour of ingesting milk or antacids.

How Supplied: Yellow, enteric-coated tablets, monogrammed AHR and 5816 in bottles of 100 (NDC 0031-5816-63) and 500 (NDC 0031-5816-70). Store at Controlled Room Temperature, Between 15°C and 30°C (59°F and 86°F).
Shown in Product Identification Section, page 428

PABALATE®-SF TABLETS ℞
[păb'ah"lāt]

Description: Pabalate®-SF tablets are intended for oral administration.
Each enteric-coated tablet contains:
Potassium Salicylate .... 0.3 g
Potassium Aminobenzoate .... 0.3 g
Potassium content per tablet:
131.5 mg (3.4 mEq)
Analgesic Drug Product
Clinical Pharmacology: Potassium salicylate is a mild analgesic with antiinflammatory and antipyretic activity. Compared to aspirin, potassium salicylate has substantially less effect on platelet adhesiveness. In large doses, however, it has a hypoprothrombinemic effect. Potassium salicylate in conventional dosage form dissolves in the stomach and is absorbed as un-ionized salicylic acid. However, in Pabalate-SF, the enteric coating delays release of the salicylate until the tablet reaches the alkaline medium of the intestine. After absorption, salicylic acid is extensively bound to plasma protein, and the bound portion is in equilibrium with the free salicylate in the plasma. The action of potassium aminobenzoate in this formulation has not been established.
Indications: Pabalate-SF tablets are indicated for the temporary relief of mild to moderate pain complicated by conditions in which the restriction of sodium intake may be desirable, such as: congestive heart failure, essential hypertension and glomerulonephritis.
Contraindications: Hypersensitivity to any of the ingredients. Presence of an active ulcer, hypoprothrombinemia, Vitamin K deficiency, severe hepatic or renal damage, hemophilia, or hyperkalemia. Do not administer to patients who are receiving a potassium-sparing diuretic.
Warnings: There have been several reports, published and unpublished, concerning non-specific small bowel lesions consisting of stenosis with or without ulceration, associated with the administration of enteric-coated thiazides with potassium salts. These lesions may occur with enteric-coated potassium tablets alone or when they are used with nonenteric-coated thiazides, or certain other oral diuretics.
These small bowel lesions have caused obstruction, hemorrhage, and perforation. Surgery was frequently required and deaths have occurred. Based on a large survey of physicians and hospitals, both American and foreign, the incidence of these lesions is low, and a causal relationship in man has not been definitely established.
Available information tends to implicate enteric-coated potassium salts although lesions of this type also occur spontaneously. Therefore, coated potassium-containing formulations should be administered only when indicated, and should be discontinued immediately if abdominal pain, distension, nausea, vomiting, or gastrointestinal bleeding occur.
When prescribing Pabalate-SF for patients who are receiving concurrent potassium supplementation (e.g., to replace potassium excreted during thiazide therapy), it should be kept in mind that each Pabalate-SF tablet contains 131.5 mg (3.4 mEq) of potassium. A decrease in supplemental potassium dosage should be considered in order to avoid hyperkalemia.
The use of potassium salts in patients with chronic renal disease, or any other condition which impairs potassium excretion, requires particularly careful monitoring of the serum potassium concentration and appropriate dosage adjustment.
Precautions: *General:* Treatment with salicylates may interfere with blood clotting; therefore, salicylate therapy should be stopped at least one week prior to surgery.

Drug Interaction: This product contains aminobenzoic acid which inhibits the bacteriostatic action of sulfonamides when the two are administered concurrently.
Carcinogenesis, mutagenesis: Long-term studies in animals have not been performed to evaluate carcinogenic potential.
Pregnancy Category C: Animal reproduction studies have not been conducted with Pabalate-SF. Safe use of Pabalate-SF has not been established with regard to possible adverse effects upon fetal development. Therefore, Pabalate-SF should not be used in women who are or may become pregnant and particularly during early pregnancy unless in the judgment of the physician the potential benefits outweigh the possible hazards.
Nursing Mothers: Salicylates appear in human milk in moderate amounts. They can produce a bleeding tendency by decreasing the amount of prothrombin in the infant's blood. As a general rule, nursing should not be undertaken while a patient is on this drug.
Pediatric Use: Safety and effectiveness in children below the age of 12 have not been established.
Adverse Reactions: Hyperkalemia is a potential adverse effect (see Contraindications and Warnings). The most frequent adverse reactions to products such as Pabalate-SF which contain potassium and/or salicylates are nausea and gastrointestinal upset. Fine rash with or without pruritus and urticaria occur less frequently. The occasional occurrence of mild salicylism may require adjustment in dosage.
Overdosage: Overdose may cause symptoms of hyperkalemia and/or salicylate intoxication. Mild chronic overdosage, termed salicylism, may cause symptoms such as tinnitus, nausea, headache, hyperventilation, dizziness, drowsiness, mental confusion, dimness of vision, sweating, thirst, and occasionally diarrhea. Withdrawal of salicylates and supportive therapy may be sufficient treatment.
A more severe degree of salicylate intoxication may occur with acute massive overdosage or the chronic administration of more moderate overdoses, especially in infants and children. CNS effects are more pronounced and may progress to delirium, hallucinations, generalized convulsions and coma. A variety of cutaneous lesions may be observed.
A most important feature of salicylate intoxication is a disturbance of acid-base balance and plasma electrolytes. Careful monitoring of these laboratory parameters along with plasma glucose concentration is essential. The type and quantity of repair solutions used will depend upon interpretation of the laboratory data. Bicarbonate solution should be administered IV in order to produce alkaline diuresis. Correction of hypoglycemia and ketosis by the administration of glucose is essential.
Since hyperthermia and dehydration are immediate threats to life, external sponging and the administration of adequate quantities of IV fluids are important first steps to correct these conditions and maintain adequate renal function.
If hemorrhagic phenomena (petechiae, thrombocytopenia) occur, whole blood transfusions and vitamin K may be necessary.
The gastrointestinal tract should be emptied either by emesis or purging to remove undissolved tablets in cases of acute ingestion of a large single dose. Since enteric-coated tablets do not disintegrate in the stomach, they cannot be removed by lavage.
Rapid and immediate removal of salicylate from the body by alkaline diuresis is essential. In more severe cases, extrarenal measures such as perito-

Continued on next page

Prescribing information on A. H. Robins products listed here is based on official labeling in effect August 1, 1984, with Indications, Contraindications, Warnings Precautions, Adverse Reactions, and Dosage stated in full.

Robins—Cont.

neal dialysis, hemodialysis, hemoperfusion or exchange transfusion may be required.
Dosage and Administration: The average adult dose is two tablets every 4 hours. Due to the enteric coating, tablets should not be taken within one hour of ingesting milk or antacids.
How Supplied: Persian rose, enteric-coated tablets, monogrammed AHR and 5883 in bottles of 100 (NDC 0031-5883-63) and 500 (NDC 0031-5883-70).
Store at Controlled Room Temperature, Between 15°C and 30°C (59°F and 86°F).
Dispense in well-closed container.
Shown in Product Identification Section, page 428

PHENAPHEN® WITH CODEINE NO. 2
[fen'ah-fen"]

Codeine Phosphate, USP	15 mg
(Warning: May be habit forming)	
Acetaminophen, USP	325 mg

PHENAPHEN® WITH CODEINE NO. 3

Codeine Phosphate, USP	30 mg
(Warning: May be habit forming)	
Acetaminophen, USP	325 mg

PHENAPHEN® WITH CODEINE NO. 4

Codeine Phosphate, USP	60 mg
(Warning: May be habit forming)	
Acetaminophen, USP	325 mg

Description: Acetaminophen occurs as a white, odorless, crystalline powder possessing a slightly bitter taste. Codeine is an alkaloid, obtained from opium or prepared from morphine by methylation. Codeine occurs as colorless or white crystals, effloresces slowly in dry air and is affected by light.
Actions: Acetaminophen is a non-opiate, non-salicylate analgesic and antipyretic. Codeine is an opiate analgesic and antitussive. Codeine retains at least one-half of its analgesic activity when administered orally.
Indications and Usage: Phenaphen with Codeine No. 2 is indicated for the relief of mild to moderate pain.
Phenaphen with Codeine No. 3 is indicated for the relief of mild to moderately severe pain.
Phenaphen with Codeine No. 4 is indicated for the relief of moderate to moderately severe pain.
Contraindications: Hypersensitivity to acetaminophen or codeine.
Warnings: *Drug dependence.* Codeine can produce drug dependence of the morphine type, and, therefore, has the potential for being abused. Psychic dependence, physical dependence and tolerance may develop upon repeated administration of this drug and it should be prescribed and administered with the same degree of caution appropriate to the use of other oral narcotic medications. These acetaminophen with codeine dosage forms are subject to the Federal Controlled Substances Act (Schedule III).
Precautions: *General:*
Head injury and increased intracranial pressure. The respiratory depressant effects of narcotics and their capacity to elevate cerebrospinal fluid pressure may be markedly exaggerated in the presence of head injury, other intracranial lesions or a pre-existing increase in intracranial pressure. Furthermore, narcotics produce adverse reactions which may obscure the clinical course of patients with head injuries.
Acute abdominal condition. The administration of products containing codeine or other narcotics may obscure the diagnosis or clinical course in patients with acute abdominal conditions.
Special risk patients. Acetaminophen with codeine should be given with caution to certain patients such as the elderly or debilitated, and those with severe impairment of hepatic or renal function, hypothyroidism, Addison's disease, and prostatic hypertrophy or urethral stricture.

Information for Patients. Codeine may impair the mental and/or physical abilities required for the performance of potentially hazardous tasks such as driving a car or operating machinery. The patient taking this drug should be cautioned accordingly.
Drug Interactions. Patients receiving other narcotic analgesics, antipsychotics, antianxiety agents, or other CNS depressants (including alcohol) concomitantly with acetaminophen and codeine may exhibit additive CNS depression due to codeine component. When such therapy is contemplated, the dose of one or both agents should be reduced.
The use of monoamine oxidase inhibitors or tricyclic antidepressants with codeine preparations may increase the effect of either the antidepressant or codeine.
The concurrent use of anticholinergics with codeine may produce paralytic ileus.
Usage in Pregnancy. Safe use in pregnancy has not been established relative to possible adverse effects on fetal development. Therefore, acetaminophen and codeine should not be used in pregnant women unless, in the judgment of the physician, the potential benefits outweigh the possible hazards.
Nursing Mothers. It is not known whether the components of this drug are excreted in human milk. Because many drugs are excreted in human milk, caution should be exercised when acetaminophen with codeine is administered to a nursing woman.
Adverse Reactions: The most frequently observed adverse reactions include lightheadedness, dizziness, sedation; shortness of breath, nausea and vomiting. These effects seem to be more prominent in ambulatory than in nonambulatory patients, and some of these adverse reactions may be alleviated if the patient lies down.
Other adverse reactions include euphoria, dysphoria, constipation and pruritus. At higher doses, codeine has most of the disadvantages of morphine including respiratory depression.
Overdosage:
Acetaminophen:
Signs and Symptoms: Acetaminophen in massive overdosage may cause hepatic toxicity in some patients. In all cases of suspected overdose, immediately call your regional poison center or the Rocky Mountain Poison Center's toll-free number (800-525-6115) for assistance in diagnosis and for directions in the use of N-acetylcysteine as an antidote, a use currently restricted to investigational status.
In adults, hepatic toxicity has rarely been reported with acute overdoses of less than 10 grams and fatalities with less than 15 grams. Importantly, young children seem to be more resistant than adults to the hepatotoxic effect of an acetaminophen overdose. Despite this, the measures outlined below should be initiated in any adult or child suspected of having ingested an acetaminophen overdose.
Early symptoms following a potentially hepatotoxic overdose may include nausea, vomiting, diaphoresis and general malaise. Clinical and laboratory evidence of hepatic toxicity may not be apparent until 48 to 72 hours post-ingestion.
Treatment: The stomach should be emptied promptly by lavage or by induction of emesis with syrup of ipecac. Patient's estimates of the quantity of a drug ingested are notoriously unreliable. Therefore, if an acetaminophen overdose is suspected, a serum acetaminophen assay should be obtained as early as possible, but no sooner than four hours following ingestion. Liver function studies should be obtained initially and repeated at 24-hour intervals.
The antidote, N-acetylcysteine, should be administered as early as possible, and within 16 hours of the overdose ingestion for optimal results. Following recovery, there are no residual, structural or functional hepatic abnormalities.
Codeine:
Signs and Symptoms: Serious overdose with codeine is characterized by respiratory depression (a decrease in respiratory rate and/or tidal volume. Cheyne-Stokes respiration, cyanosis), extreme somnolence progressing to stupor or coma, skeletal muscle flaccidity, cold and clammy skin, and sometimes bradycardia and hypotension. In severe overdosage, apnea, circulatory collapse, cardiac arrest and death may occur.
Treatment: Primary attention should be given to the reestablishment of adequate respiratory exchange through provision of a patent airway and the institution of assisted or controlled ventilation. The narcotic antagonist naloxone is a specific antidote against respiratory depression which may result from overdosage or unusual sensitivity to narcotics, including codeine. Therefore, an appropriate dose of naloxone (see package insert) should be administered, preferably by the intravenous route, and simultaneously with efforts at respiratory resuscitation. Since the duration of action of codeine may exceed that of the antagonist, the patient should be kept under continued surveillance and repeated doses of the antagonist should be administered as needed to maintain adequate respiration.
An antagonist should not be administered in the absence of clinically significant respiratory or cardiovascular depression. Oxygen, intravenous fluids, vasopressors and other supportive measures should be employed as indicated.
Gastric emptying may be useful in removing unabsorbed drug.
Dosage and Administration: Dosage should be adjusted according to severity of pain and response of the patient. However, it should be kept in mind that tolerance to codeine can develop with continued use and that the incidence of untoward effects is dose related. This product is inappropriate even in high doses for severe or intractable pain. Adult doses of codeine higher than 60 mg fail to give commensurate relief of pain but merely prolong analgesia and are associated with an appreciably increased incidence of undesirable side effects. Equivalently high doses in children would have similar effects. The usual adult dose for Phenaphen with Codeine No. 2 and Phenaphen with Codeine No. 3 is one or two capsules every 4 hours as required. The usual adult dose for Phenaphen with Codeine No. 4 is one capsule every 4 hours as required.
How Supplied: Phenaphen with Codeine No. 2, black and yellow capsules in bottles of 100 (NDC 0031-6242-63) and 500 (NDC 0031-6242-70) and Dis-Co® Unit Dose Packs (4 × 25's) (6242-61).
Phenaphen with Codeine No. 3, black and green capsules in bottles of 100 (NDC 0031-6257-63) and 500 (NDC 0031-6257-70) and Dis-Co® Unit Dose Packs (4 × 25's) (6257-61) and (40 × 25's) (6257-72).
Phenaphen with Codeine No. 4, green and white capsules in bottles of 100 (NDC 0031-6274-63) and 500 (NDC 0031-6274-70) and Dis-Co® Unit Dose Packs (4 × 25's) (6274-61).
Store at controlled room temperature, between 15°C and 30°C (59°F and 86°F).
Dispense capsules in well-closed container.
Also available without codeine as Phenaphen® Capsules containing 325 mg of acetaminophen.
Shown in Product Identification Section, page 428

PHENAPHEN®-650 WITH CODEINE TABLETS
[fen'ah-fen"]

Description:
Each Phenaphen®-650 with Codeine tablet contains:

Codeine Phosphate, USP	30 mg
(Warning: May be habit forming)	
Acetaminophen, USP	650 mg

Acetaminophen occurs as a white, odorless, crystalline powder possessing a slightly bitter taste. Codeine is an alkaloid, obtained from opium or prepared from morphine by methylation. Codeine occurs as colorless or white crystals, effloresces slowly in dry air and is affected by light.
Actions: Acetaminophen is a non-opiate, non-salicylate analgesic and antipyretic. Codeine is an opiate analgesic and antitussive. Codeine retains

Robins—Cont.

appetite suppression. Other central nervous system actions or metabolic effects may be involved. Adult obese subjects instructed in dietary management and treated with "anorectic" drugs, lose more weight on the average than those treated with placebo and diet, as determined in relatively short-term trials.

The average magnitude of increased weight loss of drug-treated patients over placebo-treated is only a fraction of a pound a week. The rate of weight loss is greatest in the first weeks of therapy for both drug and placebo subjects and tends to decrease in succeeding weeks. The possible origins of the increased weight loss due to the various drug effects are not established. The average amount of weight loss associated with the use of an "anorectic" drug varies from trial to trial, and the increased weight loss appears to be related in part to variables other than the drug prescribed such as the physician-investigator, the population treated and the diet prescribed. Studies do not permit conclusions as to the relative importance of the drug and non-drug factors on weight loss.

The natural history of obesity is measured in years, whereas the studies cited are restricted to a few weeks duration; thus, the total impact of drug-induced weight loss over that of diet alone must be considered clinically limited.

Contraindications: Fenfluramine is contraindicated in patients with glaucoma or with hypersensitivity to fenfluramine or other sympathomimetic amines. Do not administer fenfluramine during or within 14 days following the administration of monoamine oxidase inhibitors, since hypertensive crises may result. Patients with a history of drug abuse should not receive the drug.

Do not administer fenfluramine to patients with alcoholism since psychiatric symptoms (paranoia, depression, psychosis) have been reported in a few such patients who had been administered this drug.

A fatal cardiac arrest has been reported shortly after the induction of anesthesia in a patient who had been taking fenfluramine prior to surgery. Fenfluramine may have a catecholamine-depleting effect when administered for prolonged periods of time; therefore, potent anesthetic agents should be administered with caution to patients taking fenfluramine. If general anesthesia cannot be avoided, full cardiac monitoring and facilities for instant resuscitative measures are a minimum necessity.

Warnings: When tolerance to the "anorectic" effect develops, the maximum recommended dose should not be exceeded in an attempt to increase the effect; rather, the drug should be discontinued.

Precautions: *General.* Fenfluramine differs in its pharmacological profile from other "anorectic" drugs with which the prescribing practitioner may be familiar. Correspondingly, there are possible adverse effects not associated with other "anorectics"; such effects include those of diarrhea, sedation, and depression. The possibility of these effects should be weighed against the possible advantage of decreased central nervous system stimulation and/or abuse potential.

Pulmonary hypertension has been reported in two female patients who had been taking fenfluramine (120 mg to 160 mg daily) for over 8 months for weight reduction. All symptoms and evidence of EKG changes associated with pulmonary hypertension disappeared in 3 to 6 weeks after discontinuation of treatment with fenfluramine. In one patient, evidence of pulmonary hypertension recurred after being rechallenged with fenfluramine (80 mg daily for 6 weeks). Patients taking fenfluramine should be advised to report immediately any deterioration in exercise tolerance.

Use only with caution in hypertension, with monitoring of blood pressure, since evidence is insufficient to rule out a possible adverse effect on blood pressure in some hypertensive patients. The drug is not recommended in severely hypertensive patients. The drug is not recommended for patients with symptomatic cardiovascular disease including arrhythmias.

Caution should be exercised in prescribing fenfluramine for patients with a history of mental depression. Further depression of mood may become evident while the patient is on fenfluramine or following withdrawal of fenfluramine. Symptoms of depression occurring immediately following abrupt withdrawal can be readily controlled by reinstituting Pondimin, followed by a gradual tapering off of the daily dose.

Information for Patients. Fenfluramine may impair the ability of the patient to engage in potentially hazardous activities such as operating machinery or driving a motor vehicle (see "Adverse Reactions"); the patient should be cautioned accordingly. Patient should also be advised to avoid alcoholic beverages while taking Pondimin.

Drug Interactions. Fenfluramine may increase slightly the effect of antihypertensive drugs, e.g., guanethidine, methyldopa, reserpine.

Other CNS depressant drugs should be used with caution in patients taking fenfluramine, since the effects may be additive.

Carcinogenesis, Mutagenesis. No carcinogenic studies or mutagenic studies have been undertaken with this drug.

Pregnancy Category C. Pondimin was shown to produce a questionable embryotoxic effect in rats and a reduced conception rate when given in a dose of 20 times the human dose. However, additional reproduction studies in rats, rabbits, mice, and monkeys at doses up to, respectively, 5 times, 20 times, 1 time, and 5 times the human dose yielded negative results.

There are no adequate and well-controlled studies in pregnant women. Pondimin should be used during pregnancy only if the potential benefit justifies the potential risk to the fetus.

Labor and Delivery. The effect of fenfluramine during labor or delivery on the mother and the fetus is unknown. The effect on later growth, development, and functional maturation of the child is unknown.

Nursing Mothers. It is not known whether this drug is excreted in human milk. Because many drugs are excreted in human milk, caution should be exercised when fenfluramine is administered to a nursing mother.

Pediatric Use. Safety and effectiveness in children below the age of 12 have not been established.

Adverse Reactions: The most common adverse reactions of fenfluramine are drowsiness, diarrhea, and dry mouth. Less frequent adverse reactions reported in association with fenfluramine are:

Central nervous system. Dizziness; confusion; incoordination; headache; elevated mood; depression; anxiety, nervousness, or tension; insomnia; weakness or fatigue; increased or decreased libido; agitation, dysarthria.

Gastrointestinal. Constipation; abdominal pain; nausea.

Autonomic. Sweating; chills; blurred vision.

Genitourinary. Dysuria; urinary frequency.

Cardiovascular. Palpitation; hypotension; hypertension; fainting; pulmonary hypertension.

Skin. Rash; urticaria; burning sensation.

Miscellaneous. Eye irritation; myalgia; fever; chest pain; bad taste.

Drug Abuse and Dependence: Pondimin (fenfluramine hydrochloride) is a controlled substance in Schedule IV. Fenfluramine is related chemically to the amphetamines, although it differs somewhat pharmacologically. The amphetamines and related stimulant drugs have been extensively abused and can produce tolerance and severe psychological dependence, as well as other adverse organic and mental changes. In this regard, there has been a report of abuse of fenfluramine by subjects with a history of abuse of other drugs. Abuse of 80 to 400 milligrams of the drug has been reported to be associated with euphoria, derealization, and perceptual changes. Fenfluramine did not produce signs of dependence in animals and appears to produce sedation more often than CNS stimulation at therapeutic doses. Its abuse potential appears qualitatively different from that of amphetamines. The possibility that fenfluramine may induce dependence should be kept in mind when evaluating the desirability of including the drug in the weight reduction programs of individual patients.

Overdosage: *Signs and Symptoms:* Only limited data have been reported concerning clinical effects and management of overdosage of fenfluramine.

Agitation and drowsiness, confusion, flushing, tremor (or shivering), fever, sweating, abdominal pain, hyperventilation, and dilated non-reactive pupils seem frequent in fenfluramine overdosage. Reflexes may be either exaggerated or depressed and some patients may have rotary nystagmus. Tachycardia may be present, but blood pressure may be normal or only slightly elevated. Convulsions, coma, and ventricular extrasystoles, culminating in ventricular fibrillation, and cardiac arrest, may occur at higher dosages.

Human Toxicity. Less than 5 mg/kg are toxic to humans. Five-ten mg/kg may produce coma and convulsions. Reported single overdoses have ranged from 300 to 2000 mg; the lowest reported fatal dose was a few hundred mg in a small child, and the highest reported nonfatal dose was 1800 mg in an adult. Most deaths were apparently due to respiratory failure and cardiac arrest.

Toxic effects will appear within 30 to 60 minutes and may progress rapidly to potentially fatal complications in 90 to 240 minutes. Symptoms may persist for extended periods depending upon the dose ingested.

Management. After overdosage, only a small percentage of the drug is excreted in the urine. Forced acid diuresis has been recommended only in extreme cases in which the patient survives the early hours of intoxication but fails to show decisive improvement from other measures. Hemodialysis and peritoneal dialysis are of theoretical advantage but have not been used clinically.

Reportedly the treatment of fenfluramine intoxication should include:

- *Gastric lavage* (but not drug-induced emesis because the patient may become unconscious at a very early stage.)
- In the event that gastric lavage is not feasible due to trismus, consult an anesthesiologist for endotracheal intubation after administration of muscle relaxants; only then gastric evacuation should be tried.
- Administration of activated charcoal after emesis or lavage may reduce absorption of drug.
- *Monitoring of vital functions.* If necessary, mechanical respiration, defibrillation, or "cardioversion" should be instituted.
- *Drug therapy.* Diazepam or phenobarbital for convulsions or muscular hyperactivity. In the presence of extreme trachycardia; propranolol; in the presence of ventricular extrasystoles; lidocaine; in the presence of hyperpyrexia; chlorpromazine.

Since fenfluramine has been shown to have a slight lowering effect on blood sugar in some patients, the theoretical possibility of hypoglycemia should be borne in mind although this effect has not been reported in cases of clinical overdosage.

Dosage and Administration: The usual dose is one 20 mg tablet three times daily before meals. Depending on the degree of effectiveness and side effects, the dosage may be increased at weekly intervals by one tablet (20 mg) daily until a maximum dosage of two tablets three times daily is attained. Total dosage of fenfluramine should not exceed 120 mg per day.

How Supplied: Pondimin is available in 20-mg orange, scored, compressed tablets monogrammed AHR and 6447, in bottles of 100 (NDC 0031-6447-63) and 500 (NDC 0031-6447-70). Store at controlled room temperature, between 15°C and 30°C (59°F and 86°F).

Dispense in well-closed container.

Shown in Product Identification Section, page 428

at least one-half of its analgesic activity when administered orally.

Indications and Usage: Phenaphen-650 with Codeine is indicated for the relief of mild to moderately severe pain.

Contraindications: Hypersensitivity to acetaminophen or codeine.

Warnings: *Drug dependence.* Codeine can produce drug dependence of the morphine type, and, therefore, has the potential for being abused. Psychic dependence, physical dependence and tolerance may develop upon repeated administration of this drug and it should be prescribed and administered with the same degree of caution appropriate to the use of other oral narcotic medications. This acetaminophen with codeine dosage form is subject to the Federal Controlled Substances Act (Schedule III).

Precautions: *General:*
Head Injury and increased intracranial pressure. The respiratory depressant effects of narcotics and their capacity to elevate cerebrospinal fluid pressure may be markedly exaggerated in the presence of head injury, other intracranial lesions or a pre-existing increase in intracranial pressure. Furthermore, narcotics produce adverse reactions which may obscure the clinical course of patients with head injuries.
Acute abdominal conditions. The administration of products containing codeine or other narcotics may obscure the diagnosis or clinical course in patients with acute abdominal conditions.
Special risk patients. Acetaminophen with codeine should be given with caution to certain patients such as the elderly or debilitated, and those with severe impairment of hepatic or renal function, hypothyroidism, Addison's disease, and prostatic hypertrophy or urethral stricture.
Information for Patients. Codeine may impair the mental and/or physical abilities required for the performance of potentially hazardous tasks such as driving a car or operating machinery. The patient taking this drug should be cautioned accordingly.
Drug Interactions. Patients receiving other narcotic analgesics, antipsychotics, antianxiety agents, or other CNS depressants (including alcohol) concomitantly with acetaminophen and codeine may exhibit additive CNS depression due to the codeine component. When such therapy is contemplated, the dose of one or both agents should be reduced.
The use of monoamine oxidase inhibitors or tricyclic antidepressants with codeine preparations may increase the effect of either the antidepressant or codeine.
The concurrent use of anticholinergics with codeine may produce paralytic ileus.
Usage in Pregnancy. Safe use in pregnancy has not been established relative to possible adverse effects on fetal development. Therefore, acetaminophen and codeine should not be used in pregnant women unless, in the judgment of the physician, the potential benefits outweigh the possible hazards.
Nursing Mothers. It is not known whether the components of this drug are excreted in human milk. Because many drugs are excreted in human milk, caution should be exercised when acetaminophen with codeine is administered to a nursing woman.
Adverse Reactions. The most frequently observed adverse reactions include lightheadedness, dizziness, sedation; shortness of breath, nausea and vomiting. These effects seem to be more prominent in ambulatory than in nonambulatory patients, and some of these adverse reactions may be alleviated if the patient lies down.
Other adverse reactions include euphoria, dysphoria, constipation and pruritus. At higher doses, codeine has most of the disadvantages of morphine including respiratory depression.

Overdosage:
Acetaminophen:
Signs and Symptoms: Acetaminophen in massive overdosage may cause hepatic toxicity in some patients. In all cases of suspected overdose, immediately call your regional poison center or the Rocky Mountain Poison Center's toll-free number (800-525-6115) for assistance in diagnosis and for directions in the use of N-acetylcysteine as an antidote, a use currently restricted to investigational status.

In adults, hepatic toxicity has rarely been reported with acute overdoses of less than 10 grams and fatalities with less than 15 grams. Importantly, young children seem to be more resistant than adults to the hepatotoxic effect of an acetaminophen overdose. Despite this, the measures outlined below should be initiated in any adult or child suspected of having ingested an acetaminophen overdose.
Early symptoms following a potentially hepatotoxic overdose may include: nausea, vomiting, diaphoresis and general malaise. Clinical and laboratory evidence of hepatic toxicity may not be apparent until 48 to 72 hours post-ingestion.
Treatment: The stomach should be emptied promptly by lavage or by induction of emesis with syrup of ipecac. Patient's estimates of the quantity of a drug ingested are notoriously unreliable. Therefore, if an acetaminophen overdose is suspected, a serum acetaminophen assay should be obtained as early as possible, but no sooner than four hours following ingestion. Liver function studies should be obtained initially and repeated at 24-hour intervals.
The antidote, N-acetylcysteine, should be administered as early as possible, and within 16 hours of the overdose ingestion for optimal results. Following recovery, there are no residual, structural or functional hepatic abnormalities.
Codeine:
Signs and Symptoms: Serious overdose with codeine is characterized by respiratory depression (a decrease in respiratory rate and/or tidal volume, Cheyne-Stokes respiration, cyanosis), extreme somnolence progressing to stupor or coma, skeletal muscle flaccidity, cold and clammy skin, and sometimes bradycardia and hypotension. In severe overdosage, apnea, circulatory collapse, cardiac arrest and death may occur.
Treatment: Primary attention should be given to the reestablishment of adequate respiratory exchange through provision of a patent airway and the institution of assisted or controlled ventilation. The narcotic antagonist naloxone is a specific antidote against respiratory depression which may result from overdosage or unusual sensitivity to narcotics, including codeine. Therefore, an appropriate dose of naloxone (see package insert) should be administered, preferably by the intravenous route, and simultaneously with efforts at respiratory resuscitation. Since the duration of action of codeine may exceed that of the antagonist, the patient should be kept under continued surveillance and repeated doses of the antagonist should be administered as needed to maintain adequate respiration.
An antagonist should not be administered in the absence of clinically significant respiratory or cardiovascular depression. Oxygen, intravenous fluids, vasopressors and other supportive measures should be employed as indicated.
Gastric emptying may be useful in removing unabsorbed drug.

Dosage and Administration: Dosage should be adjusted according to severity of pain and response of the patient. However, it should be kept in mind that tolerance to codeine can develop with continued use and that the incidence of untoward effects is dose related. This product is inappropriate even in high doses for severe or intractable pain. Adult doses of codeine higher than 60 mg fail to give commensurate relief of pain but merely prolong analgesia and are associated with an appreciably increased incidence of undesirable side effects. Equivalently high doses in children would have similar effects. The usual adult dose for Phenaphen-650 with Codeine is one tablet every four hours as required.

How Supplied: *Phenaphen-650 with Codeine* is available as a scored, white, capsule-shaped compressed tablet, engraved AHR and 6251 in bottles of 50 (NDC 0031-6251-60) and Dis-Co® Unit Dose Packs (4 × 25's) (6251-61).

Store at controlled room temperature, between 15°C and 30°C (59°F and 86°F).
Dispense tablets in well-closed container.
Shown in Product Identification Section, page 428

PONDIMIN® TABLETS ℞
[pŏn'dĭ-min]
brand of fenfluramine hydrochloride
Tablets—20 mg

Description: Pondimin (fenfluramine hydrochloride) is an anorectic drug for oral administration. Immediate release tablets containing 20 mg fenfluramine hydrochloride are orange, scored, compressed tablets engraved AHR and 6447.
Pondimin is a phenethylamine with the chemical name, N-ethyl-α-methyl-m-(trifluoro methyl) phenethylamine hydrochloride.

Clinical Pharmacology: Fenfluramine is a sympathomimetic amine, the pharmacologic activity of which differs somewhat from that of the prototype drugs of this class used in obesity, the amphetamines, in appearing to produce more central nervous system depression than stimulation. The mechanism of action of Pondimin is unclear but may be related to brain levels (or turnover rates) of serotonin or to increased glucose utilization. The antiappetite effects of Pondimin are suppressed by serotonin-blocking drugs and by drugs that lower brain levels of the amine. Furthermore, decreased serotonin levels produced by selective brain lesions suppress the action of Pondimin.
In a study of 20 normal males, fenfluramine increased glucose utilization, resulting in decreased blood glucose levels. Experimental work in animals suggested that increased glucose utilization activated the satiety center and decreased the activity of the feeding center. Perhaps by this mechanism Pondimin inhibits appetite. The relationship between glucose utilization and serotonin has not been clarified.
Fenfluramine is well-absorbed from the gastrointestinal tract, and a maximal anorectic effect is generally seen after 2 to 4 hours. In man, fenfluramine is de-ethylated to norfenfluramine which is subsequently oxidized to m-trifluoromethyl benzoic acid and excreted as the glycine conjugate, m-trifluoromethylhippuric acid. Other compounds found in the urine include unchanged fenfluramine and norfenfluramine.
The rate of excretion of fenfluramine is pH dependent, with much smaller amounts appearing in an alkaline than in an acid urine.
The half-life of fenfluramine is said to be about 20 hours, compared with 5 hours for amphetamines; however, if urinary excretion is rapid and the pH maintained in the acidic range (below pH 5), half-life can be reduced to 11 hours. Fenfluramine and norfenfluramine reach steady state concentrations in plasma within 3 to 4 days following chronic dosage.
The greatest weight loss is seen in those patients who maintain the highest levels of Pondimin. A 2-to-3-kg weight loss over 6 weeks is associated with a plasma level of 0.1 mcg/ml (or 10 mcg/100 ml).
Fenfluramine is widely distributed in almost all body tissues. It is soluble in lipids and crosses the blood-brain barrier. Fenfluramine crosses the placenta readily in monkeys.

Indications and Usage: Pondimin is indicated in the management of exogenous obesity as a short-term (a few weeks) adjunct in a regimen of weight reduction based on caloric restriction.
Drugs of this class used in obesity are commonly known as "anorectics" or "anorexigenics." It has not been established, however, that the action of such drug in treating obesity is primarily one of

Continued on next page

Prescribing information on A. H. Robins products listed here is based on official labeling in effect August 1, 1984, with Indications, Contraindications, Warnings Precautions, Adverse Reactions, and Dosage stated in full.

QUINIDEX EXTENTABS® ℞
[kwĭn'ĭ"dĕks ĕks"tĕn'tabs]
brand of Quinidine Sulfate, USP

Composition: Each Extentab (extended action tablet) contains 300 mg. Quinidine Sulfate, USP.

Description: Quinidex Extentabs (quinidine sulfate) are constructed to release one-third of their alkaloidal salt, quinidine sulfate (100 mg), on reaching the stomach, to begin absorption in the upper intestinal tract. The remaining two-thirds of the active drug (200 mg) is evenly distributed throughout a homogeneous core which slowly dissolves as it moves along the intestinal tract, releasing the quinidine sulfate for continuous absorption over an 8-12 hour period.

Action: The action of quinidine in preventing aberrant cardiac rhythms of atrial and ventricular origin resides in its ability to (a) depress excitability of cardiac muscle, (b) slow the rate of spontaneous rhythm, (c) decrease vagal tone, and (d) prolong conduction and effective refractory period.

Indications: Quinidex Extentabs are indicated in the treatment of:
Premature atrial and ventricular contractions.
Paroxysmal atrial tachycardia.
Paroxysmal A-V junctional rhythm.
Atrial flutter.
Paroxysmal atrial fibrillation.
Established atrial fibrillation when therapy is appropriate.
Paroxysmal ventricular tachycardia when not associated with complete heartblock.
Maintenance therapy after electrical conversion of atrial fibrillation and/or flutter.

Contraindications: Intraventricular conduction defects. A-V block. Idiosyncrasy or hypersensitivity.
Aberrant impulses and abnormal rhythms due to escape mechanisms should not be treated with quinidine.

Warning: In the treatment of atrial flutter, reversion to sinus rhythm may be preceded by a progressive reduction in the degree of A-V block to a 1:1 ratio and resulting extremely rapid ventricular rate.

Precautions: All the precautions applying to regular quinidine therapy apply to the Extentab form. Use with care in patients with severe congestive failure, renal insufficiency or with digitalis intoxication.
Patients should be carefully observed for signs of toxicity: e.g., (1) allergy or idiosyncrasy, such as febrile reactions, skin eruptions, and thrombocytopenia (extremely rare); (2) "cinchonism," such as tinnitus, blurred vision, dizziness, lightheadedness, and tremor; (3) G-I symptoms (nausea, vomiting, diarrhea, and colic); (4) cardiotoxic effects such as ventricular extrasystoles occurring at a rate of one or more every 6 normal beats, an increase of the QRS complex of 50% or more, a complete A-V block, or ventricular tachycardia.
NOTE: The development of "cinchonism" is not usually sufficient reason for terminating quinidine therapy. G-I symptoms can also be minimized by giving the drug with food.

Adverse Reactions: Cases of quinidine-induced hypoprothrombinemic hemorrhage in patients on chronic anticoagulant drug therapy have been reported.

Dosage: One or two tablets every 8 to 12 hours.

How Supplied: White sugar-coated Extentabs monogrammed Quinidex and AHR in bottles of 100 (NDC 0031-6649-63) and 250 (NDC 0031-6649-67).

Shown in Product Identification Section, page 428

REGLAN® ℞
[rĕg'lan]
(Metoclopramide Hydrochloride)
Tablets, Syrup and Injectable

Description: Reglan (metoclopramide hydrochloride) is available in both oral and parenteral forms. Reglan Tablets are pink, capsule-shaped tablets engraved Reglan on one side, scored and engraved AHR 10 on the opposite side.

Each tablet contains:
Metoclopramide base   **10 mg**
(as the monohydrochloride monohydrate)
Reglan Syrup is an orange-colored, palatable, aromatic, sugar-free liquid.
Each 5 ml (1 teaspoonful) contains:
Metoclopramide base   **5 mg**
(as the monohydrochloride monohydrate)
Reglan Injectable is a clear, colorless, sterile solution with a pH of 4.0–6.0 for intravenous or intramuscular administration.
2 ml and 10 ml **single dose** vials/ampuls; 30 ml **single dose** vial
Each **1 ml** contains:
Metoclopramide base   **5 mg**
(as the monohydrochloride monohydrate)
Sodium Chloride, USP 8.5 mg, Water for Injection, USP q.s.
pH adjusted, when necessary, with hydrochloric acid and/or sodium hydroxide.
CONTAINS NO PRESERVATIVE.
Metoclopramide hydrochloride is a white crystalline, odorless substance, freely soluble in water. Chemically, it is 4-amino-5-chloro-N-[2-(diethylamino)ethyl]-2-methoxy benzamide monohydrochloride monohydrate. Molecular weight: 354.3.

Clinical Pharmacology: Metoclopramide stimulates motility of the upper gastrointestinal tract without stimulating gastric, biliary, or pancreatic secretions. Its mode of action is unclear. It seems to sensitize tissues to the action of acetylcholine. The effect of metoclopramide on motility is not dependent on intact vagal innervation, but it can be abolished by anticholinergic drugs.
Metoclopramide increases the tone and amplitude of gastric (especially antral) contractions, relaxes the pyloric sphincter and the duodenal bulb, and increases peristalsis of the duodenum and jejunum resulting in accelerated gastric emptying and intestinal transit. It increases the resting tone of the lower esophageal sphincter. It has little, if any, effect on the motility of the colon or gallbladder.
In patients with gastroesophageal reflux and low LESP (lower esophageal sphincter pressure), single oral doses of metoclopramide produce dose-related increases in LESP. Effects begin at about 5 mg and increase through 20 mg (the largest dose tested). The increase in LESP from a 5 mg dose lasts about 45 minutes and that of 20 mg lasts between 2 and 3 hours. Increased rate of stomach emptying has been observed with single oral doses of 10 mg.
Like the phenothiazines and related drugs which are also dopamine antagonists, metoclopramide produces sedation and may produce extrapyramidal reactions, although these are comparatively rare (See Warnings). Metoclopramide inhibits the central and peripheral effects of apomorphine, induces release of prolactin and causes a transient increase in circulating aldosterone levels, which may be associated with transient fluid retention.
The onset of pharmacological action of metoclopramide is 1 to 3 minutes following an intravenous dose, 10 to 15 minutes following intramuscular administration, and 30 to 60 minutes following an oral dose; pharmacological effects persist for 1 to 2 hours.
Approximately 85% of the radioactivity of an orally administered radioactive dose appears in the urine within 72 hours. Of the 85% eliminated in the urine, about half was present as free or conjugated metoclopramide.

Indications and Usage: *Symptomatic gastroesophageal reflux.* Reglan Tablets are indicated as short-term (4 to 12 weeks) therapy for adults with symptomatic, documented gastroesophageal reflux who fail to respond to conventional therapy. The principal effect of metoclopramide is on symptoms of postprandial and daytime heartburn with less observed effect on nocturnal symptoms. If symptoms are confined to particular situations, such as following the evening meal, use of metoclopramide as single doses prior to the provocative situation should be considered, rather than using the drug throughout the day. Healing of ulcers and erosions has been endoscopically demonstrated at the end of a 12-week trial using doses of 15 mg q.i.d. As there is no documented correlation between symptoms and healing of esophageal lesions, patients with documented lesions should be monitored endoscopically.

Diabetic gastroparesis (diabetic gastric stasis). Reglan (metoclopramide hydrochloride) is indicated for the relief of symptoms associated with acute and recurrent diabetic gastric stasis. The usual manifestations of delayed gastric emptying (e.g., nausea, vomiting, heartburn, persistent fullness after meals and anorexia) appear to respond to Reglan within different time intervals. Significant relief of nausea occurs early and continues to improve over a three-week period. Relief of vomiting and anorexia may precede the relief of abdominal fullness by one week or more.

The prevention of nausea and vomiting associated with emetogenic cancer chemotherapy. Reglan Injectable is indicatd for the prophylaxis of vomiting associated with emetogenic cancer chemotherapy.

Small bowel intubation. Reglan Injectable may be used to facilitate small bowel intubation in adults and children in whom the tube does not pass the pylorus with conventional maneuvers.

Radiological examination. Reglan Injectable may be used to stimulate gastric emptying and intestinal transit of barium in cases where delayed emptying interferes with radiological examination of the stomach and/or small intestine.

Contraindications: Metoclopramide should not be used whenever stimulation of gastrointestinal motility might be dangerous, e.g., in the presence of gastrointestinal hemorrhage, mechanical obstruction, or perforation.
Metoclopramide is contraindicated in patients with pheochromocytoma because the drug may cause a hypertensive crisis, probably due to release of catecholamines from the tumor. Such hypertensive crises may be controlled by phentolamine.
Metoclopramide is contraindicated in patients with known sensitivity or intolerance to the drug. Metoclopramide should not be used in epileptics or patients receiving other drugs which are likely to cause extrapyramidal reactions, since the frequency and severity of seizures or extrapyramidal reactions may be increased.

Warnings: Extrapyramidal symptoms, manifested primarily as acute dystonic reactions, occur in approximately 1 in 500 patients treated with metoclopramide. These occur more frequently in children and young adults and are even more frequent at the higher doses used in prophylaxis of vomiting due to cancer chemotherapy. These symptoms may include involuntary movements of limbs and facial grimacing, torticollis, oculogyric crisis, rhythmic protrusion of tongue, bulbar type of speech, trismus, or dystonic reactions resembling tetanus. Rarely, dystonic reactions may present as stridor and dyspnea. If these symptoms should occur, inject 50 mg Benadryl® (diphenhydramine hydrochloride) intramuscularly, and they usually will subside. Parkinsonism as well as rare persistent dyskinesias have been reported. Depression bearing a temporal relationship to Reglan administration has been reported. The significance of this association is not known.

Precautions: *General.* Patients should be cautioned about engaging in activities requiring mental alertness for a few hours after the drug has been administered.

Diabetic Gastroparesis; Intubation and Radiology. Intravenous injections of metoclopramide should be made slowly over a 1- to 2-minute period, since a transient but intense feeling of anxiety and restlessness, followed by drowsiness, may occur with rapid administration.

Continued on next page

Prescribing information on A. H. Robins products listed here is based on official labeling in effect August 1, 1984, with Indications, Contraindications, Warnings Precautions, Adverse Reactions, and Dosage stated in full.

Robins—Cont.

Vomiting prophylaxis (cancer chemotherapy). Intravenous administration of Reglan Injectable diluted in one of the following large volume parenteral solutions should be made slowly over a period of not less than 15 minutes. The preferred large volume parenteral solution is Sodium Chloride Injection (normal saline), which when combined with Reglan Injectable, can be stored frozen for up to 4 weeks. Reglan Injectable is degraded when admixed and frozen with Dextrose–5% in Water. Reglan Injectable diluted in Sodium Chloride Injection, Dextrose–5% in Water, Dextrose–5% in 0.45% Sodium Chloride, Ringer's Injection or Lactated Ringer's Injection may be stored up to 48 hours (without freezing) ater preparation if protected from light. All dilutions may be stored unprotected from light under normal light conditions up to 24 hours after preparation.

Drug Interaction. The effects of metoclopramide on gastrointestinal motility are antagonized by anticholinergic drugs and narcotic analgesics. Additive sedative effects can occur when metoclopramide is given with alcohol, sedatives, hypnotics, narcotics or tranquilizers.

Absorption of drugs from the stomach may be diminished (e.g., digoxin) by metoclopramide, whereas absorption of drugs from the small bowel may be accelerated (e.g., acetaminophen, tetracycline, levodopa, ethanol).

Gastroparesis (gastric stasis) may be responsible for poor diabetic control in some patients. Exogenously administered insulin may begin to act before food has left the stomach and lead to hypoglycemia.

Because the action of metoclopramide will influence the delivery of food to the intestines and thus the rate of absorption, insulin dosage or timing of dosage may require adjustment.

Carcinogenesis, Mutagenesis, Impairment of Fertility: A 77-week study was conducted in rats in oral doses up to about 40 times the maximum recommended human daily doses. Metoclopramide elevates prolactin levels and the elevation persists during chronic administration. Tissue culture experiments indicate that approximately one-third of human breast cancers are prolactin-dependent *in vitro*, a factor of potential importance if the prescription of metoclopramide is contemplated in a patient with previously detected breast cancer. Although disturbances such as galactorrhea, amenorrhea, gynecomastia, and impotence have been reported wth prolactin-elevating drugs, the clinical significance of elevated serum prolactin levels is unknown for most patients. An increase in mammary neoplasms has been found in rodents after chronic administration of prolactin-stimulating neuroleptic drugs. Neither clinical studies nor epidemiologic studies conducted to date, however, have shown an association between chronic administration of these drugs and mammary tumorigenesis; the available evidence is too limited to be conclusive at this time.

An Ames mutagenicity test performed on metoclopramide was negative.

Pregnancy Category B. Reproduction studies performed in rats, mice, and rabbits by the i.v., i.m., s.c. and oral routes at maximum levels ranging from 12 to 250 times the human dose have demonstrated no impairment of fertility or significant harm to the fetus due to metoclopramide. There are, however, no adequate and well-controlled studies in pregnant women. Because animal reproduction studies are not always predictive of human response, this drug should be used during pregnancy only if clearly needed.

Nursing Mothers. Metoclopramide is excreted in human milk. Caution should be exercised when metoclopramide is administered to a nursing mother.

Adverse Reactions: The most frequent adverse reactions to metoclopramide are restlessness, drowsiness, fatigue and lassitude, which occur in approximately ten percent of patients receiving the most commonly prescribed dosage of 10 mg q.i.d.

A dose/duration related increase in the incidence of adverse reactions was suggested in clinical trials of 10 mg. 15 mg and 20 mg q.i.d. for periods lasting from 4 to 12 weeks.Because adverse effects are actively solicited in clinical trials and because each patient complaint, whether severe or trivial, lasting one minute or one week, is counted, the overall incidence (for both drug and placebo) is artificially high. Nevertheless, an increase in incidence of reported complaints with increased doses and increased durations of dosing, allows the conclusion that the actual ADR incidence correlates with the strength and duration of drug administration.

Shown in the tabulation below are the observed incidences of side effects in clinical trials of patients (GERD) and normal volunteers (SAFETY). [See table below].

Temporary dose reduction was sometimes necessary; in some of these cases, the original dose could be resumed.

Among patients receiving metoclopramide 10 mg q.i.d. in an open "compassionate" clinical trial, the drug was discontinued because of adverse reactions possibly/probably attributable to metoclopramide in 45 of the 1053 patients enrolled (4%). Less frequently, insomnia, headache, dizziness, nausea, bowel disturbances, rash, or extrapyramidal symptoms may occur. Rarely, depression and persistent dyskinesia have been reported (See Warnings and Precautions Sections).

A single insance of supraventricular tachycardia following intramuscular administration has been reported.

Transient alterations in blood pressure have been reported when metoclopramide was administered intravenously, primarily in association with the large doses used in preventing chemotherapy-induced emesis.

Overdosage: Symptoms of overdosage may include drowsiness, disorientation and extrapyramidal reactions. Anticholinergic or antiparkinson drugs or antihistamines with anticholinergic properties may be helpful in controlling the extrapyramidal reactions. Symptoms are self-limiting and usually disappear within 24 hours.

Literature reports describe methemoglobinemia in premature and full term neonates who were given metoclopramide intramucularly, 1–2 mg/kg/day for 3 or more days. Methemoglobinemia has not been reported in similar infants treated with 0.5 mg/kg/day in divided doses. Methemoglobinemia can be reversed by the intravenous administration of methylene blue.

Dosage and Administration: *For the relief of symptomatic gastroesophageal reflux:* Administer from 10 mg (1 tablet) to 15 mg (1½ tablets) up to q.i.d. 30 minutes before each meal and at bedtime, depending upon symptoms being treated and clinical response (see Clinical Pharmacology and Indications). If symptoms occur only intermittently or at specific times of the day, use of metoclopramide in single doses up to 20 mg prior to the provoking situation may be preferred rather than continuous treatment.

Experience with esophageal erosions and ulcerations is limited, but healing has thus far been documented in one controlled trial using q.i.d. therapy at 15 mg/dose, and this regimen should be used when lesions are present, so long as it is tolerated (see Adverse Reactions). Because of the poor correlation between symptoms and endoscopic appearance of the esophagus, therapy directed at esophageal lesions is best guided by endoscopic evaluation.

Therapy longer than 12 weeks has not been evaluated and cannot be recommended.

For the relief of symptoms associated with diabetic gastroparesis (diabetic gastric stasis): Administer 10 mg of metoclopramide 30 minutes before each meal and at bedtime for two to eight weeks, depending upon response and the likelihood of continued well-being upon drug discontinuation.

The initial route of administration should be determined by the severity of the presenting symptoms. If only the earliest manifestations of diabetic gastric stasis are present, oral administration of Reglan may be initiated. However, if severe symptoms are present, therapy should begin with Reglan Injectable (I.M. or I.V.). Doses of 10 mg may be administered slowly by the intravenous route over a 1-to-2 minute period.

Administration of Reglan Injectable up to 10 days may be required before symptoms subside, at which time oral administration may be instituted. Since diabetic gastric stasis is frequently recurrent, Reglan therapy should be reinstituted at the earliest manifestation.

For the prevention of nausea and vomiting associated with emetogenic cancer chemotherapy: For doses in excess of 10 mg. Reglan Injectable should be diluted in 50 ml of a large volume parenteral solution (Sodium Chloride Injection, Dextrose–5% in Water, Dextrose–5% in 0.45% Sodium Chloride, Ringer's Injection or Lactated Ringer's Injection). ***See Precautions section under subheading "Vomiting prophylaxis (cancer chemotherapy)."***

Intravenous infusions should be made slowly over a period of not less than 15 minutes, 30 minutes before beginning cancer chemotherapy and repeated every 2 hours for two doses, then every 3 hours for three doses.

The initial two doses should be 2 mg/kg if highly emetogenic drugs such as cisplatin or dacarbazine are used alone or in combination. For less emetogenic regimens, 1 mg/kg per dose may be adequate.

If extrapyramidal symptoms should occur, inject 50 mg Benadryl® (diphenhydramine hydrochloride) intramuscularly, and EPS usually will subside.

To facilitate small bowel intubation: If the tube has not passed the pylorus with conventional maneuvers in 10 minutes, a single dose (undiluted) may be administered slowly by the intravenous route over a 1- to 2-minute period.

The recommended single dose is: Adults—10 mg metoclopramide base (2 ml). Children (6-14 years of ag)—2.5 to 5 mg metoclopramide base (0.5 to 1 ml); (under 6 years of age)—0.1 mg/kg metoclopramide base.

To aid in radiological examinations: In patients where delayed gastric emptying interferes with radiological examination of the stomach and/or small intestine, a single dose may be administered slowly by the intravenous route over a 1- to 2-minute period.

For dosage, see intubation, above.

Parenteral drug products should be inspected visually for particulate matter and discoloration prior to administration, whenever solution and container permit.

Admixture Compatibilities. Reglan (metoclopramide hydrochloride) Injectable is compatible for mixing and injection with the following dosage forms to the extent indicated below:

Physically and Chemically Compatible up to 48 hours. Cimetidine Hydrochloride (SK&F), Mannitol, USP (Abbott), Potassium Acetate, USP (In-

			ADR INCIDENCE	
STUDY	DOSAGE	DURATION	METOCLOPRAMIDE	PLACEBO
GERD	10 mg qid	4-8 weeks	69%	65%
SAFETY	10 mg qid	12 weeks	89%	67%
*GERD	15 mg qid	12 weeks	81%	47%
SAFETY	20 mg qid	12 weeks	94%	67%

*One patient dropped out because of ADR

venex), Potassium Chloride, USP (ESI), Potassium Phosphate, USP (Invenex).

Physically Compatible up to 48 hours. Ascorbic Acid, USP (Abbott), Benztropine Mesylate, USP (MS&D), Cytarabine, USP (Upjohn), Dexamethasone Sodium Phosphate, USP (ESI, MS&D), Diphenhydramine Hydrochloride, USP (Parke-Davis), Doxorubicin Hydrochloride, USP (Adria), Heparin Sodium, USP (ESI), Hydrocortisone Sodium Phosphate (MS&D), Lidocaine Hydrochloride, USP (ESI), Magnesium Sulfate, USP (ESI), Multi-Vitamin Infusion (must be refrigerated-USV), Vitamin B Complex with Ascorbic Acid (Roche).

Physically Compatible up to 24 hours (Do not use if precipitation occurs). Aminophylline, USP (ESI), Clindamycin Phosphate, USP (Upjohn), Cyclophosphamide, USP (Mead-Johnson), Insulin, USP (Lilly), Methylprednisolone Sodium Succinate, USP (ESI).

Conditionally Compatible (Use Within one hour after mixing or may be infused directly into the same running IV line. Ampicillin Sodium, USP (Bristol), Calcium Gluconate, USP (ESI), Cisplatin (Bristol), Erythromycin Lactobionate, USP (Abbott), Methotrexate Sodium, USP (Lederle), Penicillin G Potassium, USP (Squibb), Tetracycline Hydrochloride, USP (Lederle).

Incompatible (Do Not Mix). Cephalothin Sodium, USP (Lilly), Chloramphenicol Sodium, USP (Parke-Davis), Sodium Bicarbonate, USP (Abbott).

How Supplied: Each pink, capsule-shaped, scored Reglan® Tablet contains 10 mg metoclopramide base (as the monohydrochloride monohydrate). Available in bottles of 100 (NDC 0031-6701-63), and 500 tablets (NDC 0031-6701-70) and Dis-Co® Unit Dose Packs of 100 tablets (NDC 0031-6701-64). Dispense tablets in tight container.

Reglan® Syrup, 5 mg metoclopramide base (as the monohydrochloride monohydrate) per 5 ml, available in pints (NDC 0031-6706-25) and 10 ml Dis-Co® Unit Dose Packs (10 × 10s) (NDC 0031-6706-26). Dispense syrup in well-closed container.

Reglan® Injectable, 5 mg metoclopramide base (as the monohydrochloride monohydrate) **per ml;** available in 2 ml single dose vials in cartons of 25 (NDC 0031-6702-72), 10 ml single dose vials in cartons of 25 (NDC 0031-6702-78); 30 ml single dose vials (NDC 0031-6702-85) and in cartons of 25 (NDC 0031-6702-24); 2 ml ampuls in cartons of 5 (NDC 0031-6702-90) and 25 (NDC 0031-6702-95); 10 ml ampuls in cartons of 25 (NDC 0031-6702-94).

Store vials/ampuls in carton until used. Do not store open vials/ampuls for later use, **as they contain no preservative.**

Dilutions may be stored unprotected from light under normal light conditions up to 24 hours after preparation.

TABLETS, SYRUP AND INJECTABLE SHOULD BE STORED AT CONTROLLED ROOM TEMPERATURE BETWEEN 15°C and 30°C (59°F and 86°F).

Reglan Injectable is manufactured for Pharmaceutical Division, A. H. Robins Company, Richmond, Virginia 23220 by Elkins-Sinn, Inc., Cherry Hill, NJ 08034, a subsidiary of A. H. Robins.

Tablet Shown in Product Identification Section, page 428

ROBAXIN® INJECTABLE   ℞
[ro″baks′in]
brand of Methocarbamol Injection, USP

Description: Robaxin Injectable is a parenteral dosage form.

Each ml contains:
Methocarbamol, USP 100 mg; Polyethylene Glycol 300, NF 0.5 ml; Water for Injection, USP q.s. pH adjusted, when necessary, with hydrochloric acid and/or sodium hydroxide.

AFTER MIXING WITH I.V. INFUSION FLUIDS, DO NOT REFRIGERATE.

Actions: The mechanism of action of methocarbamol in humans has not been established, but may be due to general central nervous system depression. It has no direct action on the contractile mechanism of striated muscle, the motor end plate or the nerve fiber.

Indications: The injectable form of methocarbamol is indicated as an adjunct to rest, physical therapy, and other measures for the relief of discomfort associated with acute, painful musculoskeletal conditions. The mode of action of this drug has not been clearly identified, but may be related to its sedative properties. Methocarbamol does not directly relax tense skeletal muscles in man.

Contraindications: Robaxin Injectable should not be administered to patients with known or suspected renal pathology. This caution is necessary because of the presence of polyethylene glycol 300 in the vehicle.

A much larger amount of polyethylene glycol 300 than is present in recommended doses of Robaxin Injectable is known to have increased pre-existing acidosis and urea retention in patients with renal impairment. Although the amount present in this preparation is well within the limits of safety, caution dictates this contraindication.

Robaxin Injectable is contraindicated in patients hypersensitive to any of the ingredients.

Warnings: Since methocarbamol may possess a general central nervous system depressant effect, patients receiving Robaxin Injectable (methocarbamol injection) should be cautioned about combined effects with alcohol and other CNS depressants.

Safe use of Robaxin Injectable has not been established with regard to possible adverse effects upon fetal development. Therefore, Robaxin Injectable should not be used in women who are or may become pregnant and particularly during early pregnancy unless in the judgment of the physician the potential benefits outweigh the possible hazards.

Precautions: As with other agents administered either intravenously or intramuscularly, careful supervision of dose and rate of injection should be observed. Rate of injection should not exceed 3 ml per minute—i.e., one 10 ml vial in approximately three minutes. Since Robaxin Injectable is hypertonic, vascular extravasation must be avoided. A recumbent position will reduce the likelihood of side reactions.

Blood aspirated into the syringe does not mix with the hypertonic solution. This phenomenon occurs with many other intravenous preparations. The blood may be safely injected with the methocarbamol, or the injection may be stopped when the plunger reaches the blood, whichever the physician prefers.

The total dosage should not exceed 30 ml (three vials) a day for more than three consecutive days except in the treatment of tetanus.

Caution should be observed in using the injectable form in suspected or known epileptic patients.

Safety and effectiveness in children below the age of 12 years have not been established except in tetanus. See special directions for use in tetanus.

It is not known whether this drug is secreted in human milk. As a general rule, nursing should not be undertaken while a patient is on a drug since many drugs are excreted in human milk.

Methocarbamol may cause a color interference in certain screening tests for 5-hydroxyindoleacetic acid (5-HIAA) and vanillylmandelic acid (VMA).

Adverse Reactions: Dizziness, lightheadedness, drowsiness, vertigo, fainting, syncope, hypotension, gastrointestinal upset, metallic taste, thrombophlebitis, sloughing at the site of injection, pain at the site of injection, anaphylactic reaction, urticaria, pruritus, rash, conjunctivitis with nasal congestion, flushing, nystagmus, diplopia, mild muscular incoordination, bradycardia, blurred vision, headache, fever. In most cases of syncope there was spontaneous recovery. In others, epinephrine, injectable steroids and/or injectable antihistamines were employed to hasten recovery. Certain of these complaints may have been due to any overly rapid rate of intravenous injection.

The onset of convulsive seizures during intravenous administration has been reported, including instances in known epileptics. The psychic trauma of the procedure may have been a contributing factor. Although several observers have reported success in terminating epileptiform seizures with Robaxin Injectable, its administration to patients with epilepsy is not recommended.

Dosage and Administration: *For Intravenous and Intramuscular Use Only.* Total adult dosage should not exceed 30 ml (3 vials) a day for more than 3 consecutive days except in the treatment of tetanus. A like course may be repeated after a lapse of 48 hours if the condition persists. Dosage and frequency of injection should be based on the severity of the condition being treated and therapeutic response noted.

For the relief of symptoms of moderate degree, 10 ml (one vial) may be adequate. Ordinarily this injection need not be repeated, as the administration of the oral form will usually sustain the relief initiated by the injection. For the severest cases or in postoperative conditions in which oral administration is not feasible, 20 to 30 ml (two to three vials) may be required.

Directions for Intravenous Use. Robaxin Injectable may be administered undiluted directly into the vein at a *maximum rate of three ml per minute.* It may also be added to an intravenous drip of Sodium Chloride Injection (Sterile Isotonic Sodium Chloride Solution for Parenteral Use) or five per cent Dextrose Injection (Sterile 5 per cent Dextrose Solution); one vial given as a single dose should not be diluted to more than 250 ml for I.V. infusion. Care should be exercised to avoid vascular extravasation of this hypertonic solution which may result in thrombophlebitis. It is preferable that the patient be in a recumbent position during and for at least 10 to 15 minutes following the injection.

Directions for Intramuscular Use. When the intramuscular route is indicated, not more than five ml (one-half vial) should be injected into each gluteal region. The injections may be repeated at eight hour intervals, if necessary. When satisfactory relief of symptoms is achieved, it can usually be maintained with tablets.

Not Recommended for Subcutaneous Administration.

Special Directions for Use in Tetanus: There is clinical evidence which suggests that methocarbamol may have a beneficial effect in the control of the neuromuscular manifestations of tetanus. It does not, however, replace the usual procedure of debridement, tetanus antitoxin, penicillin, tracheotomy, attention to fluid balance, and supportive care. Robaxin Injectable should be added to the regimen as soon as possible.

For adults: Inject one or two vials directly into the tubing of a previously inserted indwelling needle. An additional 10 ml or 20 ml may be added to the infusion bottle so that a total of up to 30 ml (three vials) is given as the initial dose (note Precautions). This procedure should be repeated every six hours until conditions allow for the insertion of a nasogastric tube. Crushed Robaxin (methocarbamol) tablets suspended in water or saline may then be given through this tube. Total daily oral doses up to 24 grams may be required as judged by patient response.

For children: A minimum initial dose of 15 mg/kg is recommended. This dosage may be repeated every six hours as indicated. The maintenance dosage may be given by injection into the tubing or by I.V. infusion with an appropriate quantity of fluid. See directions for I.V. use.

How Supplied: Robaxin Injectable—10 ml single dose vials in packages of 5 (NDC 0031-7409-87) and 25 (NDC 0031-7409-94).

Manufactured for PHARMACEUTICAL DIVISION, A. H. ROBINS CO., Richmond, VA 23220, by ELKINS-SINN, INC. Cherry Hill, NJ 08034, a subsidiary of A. H. Robins.

Shown in Product Identification Section, page 429

Continued on next page

Prescribing information on A. H. Robins products listed here is based on official labeling in effect August 1, 1984, with Indications, Contraindications, Warnings Precautions, Adverse Reactions, and Dosage stated in full.

Robins—Cont.

ROBAXIN® TABLETS
[ro″baks′ĭn]
brand of Methocarbamol Tablets, USP
500 mg per tablet

ROBAXIN®-750 TABLETS
brand of Methocarbamol Tablets, USP
750 mg per tablet

Actions: The mechanism of action of methocarbamol in humans has not been established, but may be due to general central nervous system depression. It has no direct action on the contractile mechanism of striated muscle, the motor end plate or the nerve fiber.

Indications: Robaxin (methocarbamol) is indicated as an adjunct to rest, physical therapy, and other measures for the relief of discomforts associated with acute, painful musculoskeletal conditions. The mode of action of this drug has not been clearly identified, but may be related to its sedative properties. Methocarbamol does not directly relax tense skeletal muscles in man.

Contraindications: Robaxin is contraindicated in patients hypersensitive to any of the ingredients.

Warnings: Since methocarbamol may possess a general central nervous system depressant effect, patients receiving Robaxin/Robaxin-750 (methocarbamol tablets) should be cautioned about combined effects with alcohol and other CNS depressants.

Safe use of methocarbamol has not been established with regard to possible adverse effects upon fetal development. Therefore, methocarbamol tablets should not be used in women who are or may become pregnant and particularly during early pregnancy unless in the judgment of the physician the potential benefits outweigh the possible hazards.

Precautions: Safety and effectiveness in children below the age of 12 years have not been established.

It is not known whether this drug is secreted in human milk. As a general rule, nursing should not be undertaken while a patient is on a drug since many drugs are excreted in human milk.

Methocarbamol may cause a color interference in certain screening tests for 5-hydroxyindoleacetic acid (5-HIAA) and vanilmandelic acid (VMA).

Adverse Reactions: Lightheadedness, dizziness, drowsiness, nausea, allergic manifestations such as urticaria, pruritus, rash, conjunctivitis with nasal congestion, blurred vision, headache, fever.

Dosage and Administration: Robaxin (methocarbamol), 500 mg—Adults: initial dosage, 3 tablets q.i.d.; maintenance dosage, 2 tablets q.i.d. Robaxin-750 (methocarbamol), 750 mg — Adults: initial dosage, 2 tablets q.i.d.; maintenance dosage, 1 tablet q.4h. or 2 tablets t.i.d.

Six grams a day are recommended for the first 48 to 72 hours of treatment. (For severe conditions 8 grams a day may be administered.) Thereafter, the dosage can usually be reduced to approximately 4 grams a day.

How Supplied: Robaxin—white, scored tablets monogrammed AHR and Robaxin in bottles of 100 (NDC 0031-7429-63), 500 (NDC 0031-7429-70), and Dis-Co® unit dose packs of 100 (NDC 0031-7429-64).

Robaxin-750—white capsule-shaped tablets monogrammed Robaxin 750 on one side, AHR on the reverse side in bottles of 100 (NDC 0031-7449-63), 500 (NDC 0031-7449-70), and Dis-Co® unit dose packs of 100 (NDC 0031-7449-64).

Shown in Product Identification Section, page 428

ROBAXISAL® TABLETS
[ro″baks′ĭ-sal″]

Description: For oral administration, Robaxisal is available as a pink and white laminated tablet containing:

Methocarbamol, USP ....400 mg
Aspirin, USP ....325 mg

Actions: Robaxisal provides a double approach to the management of discomforts associated with musculoskeletal disorders.

Methocarbamol. The mechanism of action of methocarbamol in humans has not been established, but may be due to general central nervous system depression. It has no direct action on the contractile mechanism of striated muscle, the motor end plate or the nerve fiber.

Aspirin. Aspirin is a mild analgesic with anti-inflammatory and antipyretic activity.

Indications: Robaxisal is indicated as an adjunct to rest, physical therapy, and other measures for the relief of discomfort associated with acute, painful musculoskeletal conditions. The mode of action of methocarbamol has not been clearly identified but may be related to its sedative properties. Methocarbamol does not directly relax tense skeletal muscles in man.

Contraindications: Hypersensitivity to methocarbamol or aspirin.

Warnings: Since methocarbamol may possess a general central nervous system depressant effect, patients receiving Robaxisal should be cautioned about combined effects with alcohol and other CNS depressants.

Precautions: Products containing aspirin should be administered with caution to patients with gastritis or peptic ulceration, or those receiving hypoprothrombinemic anticoagulants.

Methocarbamol may cause a color interference in certain screening tests for 5-hydroxyindoleacetic acid (5-HIAA) and vanilmandelic acid (VMA).

Pregnancy. Safe use of Robaxisal has not been established with regard to possible adverse effects upon fetal development. Therefore, Robaxisal should not be used in women who are or may become pregnant and particularly during early pregnancy unless in the judgment of the physician the potential benefits outweigh the possible hazards.

Nursing Mothers. It is not known whether methocarbamol is secreted in human milk; however, aspirin does appear in human milk in moderate amounts. It can produce a bleeding tendency either by interfering with the function of the infant's platelets or by decreasing the amount of prothrombin in the blood. The risk is minimal if the mother takes the aspirin just after nursing and if the infant has an adequate store of vitamin K. As a general rule, nursing should not be undertaken while a patient is on a drug.

Pediatric Use. Safety and effectiveness in children 12 years of age and below have not been established.

Use in Activities Requiring Mental Alertness. Robaxisal may rarely cause drowsiness. Until the patient's response has been determined, he should be cautioned against the operation of motor vehicles or dangerous machinery.

Adverse Reactions: The most frequent adverse reaction to methocarbamol is dizziness or lightheadedness and nausea. This occurs in about one in 20-25 patients. Less frequent reactions are drowsiness, blurred vision, headache, fever, allergic manifestations such as urticaria, pruritus, and rash.

Adverse reactions that have been associated with the use of aspirin include: nausea and other gastrointestinal discomfort, gastritis, gastric erosion, vomiting, constipation, diarrhea, angio-edema, asthma, rash, pruritus, urticaria.

Gastrointestinal discomfort may be minimized by taking Robaxisal with food.

Dosage and Administration: Adults and children over 12 years of age: Two tablets four times daily. Three tablets four times daily may be used in severe conditions for one to three days in patients who are able to tolerate salicylates. These dosage recommendations provide respectively 3.2 and 4.8 grams of methocarbamol per day.

Overdosage: Toxicity due to overdosage of methocarbamol is unlikely; however, acute overdosage of aspirin may cause symptoms of salicylate intoxication.

Treatment of Overdosage. Supportive therapy for 24 hours, as methocarbamol is excreted within that time. If salicylate intoxication occurs, especially in children, the hyperpnea may be controlled with sodium bicarbonate. Judicious use of 5% CO_2 with 95% O_2 may be of benefit. Abnormal electrolyte patterns should be corrected with appropriate fluid therapy.

How Supplied: Robaxisal® is supplied as pink and white laminated, compressed tablets monogrammed AHR and Robaxisal in bottles of 100 (NDC 0031-7469-63), 500 (NDC 0031-7469-70) and Dis-Co® Unit Dose Packs of 100 (NDC 0031-7469-64).

Shown in Product Identification Section, page 429

ROBINUL® TABLETS
[ro′bĭ-nul]
ROBINUL® FORTE TABLETS
brand of Glycopyrrolate Tablets, USP

Description: Robinul and Robinul Forte tablets contain the synthetic anticholinergic, glycopyrrolate. Glycopyrrolate is a quaternary ammonium compound with the following chemical name: 3-[(cyclopentylhydroxyphenylacetyl)oxy]-1,1-dimethylpyrrolidinium bromide.

Robinul tablets are scored, compressed pink tablets engraved AHR and 7824. Each tablet contains:
Glycopyrrolate, USP ....1 mg
Robinul Forte tablets are scored, compressed pink tablets engraved $\frac{AHR}{2}$ on one side and 7840 on the reverse side. Each tablet contains:
Glycopyrrolate, USP ....2 mg

Actions: Glycopyrrolate, like other anticholinergic (antimuscarinic) agents, inhibits the action of acetylcholine on structures innervated by postganglionic cholinergic nerves and on smooth muscles that respond to acetylcholine but lack cholinergic innervation. These peripheral cholinergic receptors are present in the autonomic effector cells of smooth muscle, cardiac muscle, the sinoatrial node, the atrioventricular node, exocrine glands, and, to a limited degree, in the autonomic ganglia. Thus, it diminishes the volume and free acidity of gastric secretions and controls excessive pharyngeal, tracheal, and bronchial secretions.

Glycopyrrolate antagonizes muscarinic symptoms (e.g., bronchorrhea, bronchospasm, bradycardia, and intestinal hypermotility) induced by cholinergic drugs such as the anticholinesterases.

The highly polar quaternary ammonium group of glycopyrrolate limits its passage across lipid membranes, such as the blood-brain barrier, in contrast to atropine sulfate and scopolamine hydrobromide, which are non-polar tertiary amines which penetrate lipid barriers easily.

Indications: For use as adjunctive therapy in the treatment of peptic ulcer.

Contraindications: Glaucoma; obstructive uropathy (for example, bladder neck obstruction due to prostatic hypertrophy); obstructive disease of the gastrointestinal tract (as in achalasia, pyloroduodenal stenosis, etc.); paralytic ileus; intestinal atony of the elderly or debilitated patient; unstable cardiovascular status in acute hemorrhage; severe ulcerative colitis; toxic megacolon complicating ulcerative colitis; myasthenia gravis. Robinul (glycopyrrolate) tablets are contraindicated in those patients with a hypersensitivity to glycopyrrolate.

Warnings: In the presence of a high environmental temperature, heat prostration (fever and heat stroke due to decreased sweating) can occur with use of Robinul.

Diarrhea may be an early symptom of incomplete intestinal obstruction, especially in patients with ileostomy or colostomy. In this instance treatment with this drug would be inappropriate and possibly harmful.

Robinul (glycopyrrolate) may produce drowsiness or blurred vision. In this event, the patient should be warned not to engage in activities requiring mental alertness such as operating a motor vehicle or other machinery, or performing hazardous work while taking this drug.

Theoretically, with overdosage a curare-like action may occur, i.e., neuromuscular blockade leading to muscular weakness and possible paralysis.

Pregnancy. The safety of this drug during pregnancy has not been established. The use of any drug during pregnancy requires that the potential benefits of the drug be weighed against possible hazards to mother and child. Reproduction studies in rats revealed no teratogenic effects from glycopyrrolate; however, the potent anticholinergic action of this agent resulted in diminished rates of conception and of survival at weaning, in a dose-related manner. Other studies in dogs suggest that this may be due to diminished seminal secretion which is evident at high doses of glycopyrrolate. Information on possible adverse effects in the pregnant female is limited to uncontrolled data derived from marketing experience. Such experience has revealed no reports of teratogenic or other fetus-damaging potential. No controlled studies to establish the safety of the drug in pregnancy have been performed.

Nursing Mothers. It is not known whether this drug is secreted in human milk. As a general rule, nursing should not be undertaken while a patient is on a drug since many drugs are excreted in human milk.

Pediatric Use. Since there is no adequate experience in children who have received this drug, safety and efficacy in children have not been established.

Precautions: Use Robinul with caution in the elderly and in all patients with:
- Autonomic neuropathy.
- Hepatic or renal disease.
- Ulcerative colitis—large doses may suppress intestinal motility to the point of producing a paralytic ileus and for this reason may precipitate or aggravate "toxic megacolon," a serious complication of the disease.
- Hyperthyroidism, coronary heart disease, congestive heart failure, cardiac tachyarrhythmias, tachycardia, hypertension and prostatic hypertrophy.
- Hiatal hernia associated with reflux esophagitis, since anticholinergic drugs may aggravate this condition.

Adverse Reactions: Anticholinergics produce certain effects, most of which are extensions of their fundamental pharmacological actions. Adverse reactions to anticholinergics in general may include xerostomia; decreased sweating; urinary hesitancy and retention; blurred vision; tachycardia, palpitations; dilatation of the pupil; cycloplegia; increased ocular tension; loss of taste; headaches; nervousness; mental confusion; drowsiness; weakness; dizziness; insomnia; nausea; vomiting; constipation; bloated feeling; impotence; suppression of lactation; severe allergic reaction or drug idiosyncrasies including anaphylaxis; urticaria and other dermal manifestations.

Robinul (glycopyrrolate) is chemically a quaternary ammonium compound; hence, its passage across lipid membranes, such as the blood-brain barrier, is limited in contrast to atropine sulfate and scopolamine hydrobromide. For this reason the occurrence of CNS related side effects is lower, in comparison to their incidence following administration of anticholinergics which are chemically tertiary amines that can cross this barrier readily.

Overdosage: The symptoms of overdosage of glycopyrrolate are peripheral in nature rather than central.
1. To guard against further absorption of the drug—use gastric lavage, cathartics and/or enemas.
2. To combat peripheral anticholinergic effects (residual mydriasis, dry mouth, etc.)—utilize a quaternary ammonium anticholinesterase, such as neostigmine methylsulfate.
3. To combat hypotension—use pressor amines (norepinephrine, metaraminol) i.v.; and supportive care.
4. To combat respiratory depression—administer oxygen; utilize a respiratory stimulant such as Dopram® i.v.; artificial respiration.

Dosage and Administration: *The dosage of Robinul or Robinul Forte should be adjusted to the needs of the individual patient to assure symptomatic control with a minimum of adverse reactions.*

The presently recommended maximum daily dosage of glycopyrrolate is 8 mg.

Robinul (glycopyrrolate, 1 mg) tablets. The recommended initial dosage of Robinul for adults is one tablet three times daily (in the morning, early afternoon, and at bedtime). Some patients may require two tablets at bedtime to assure overnight control of symptoms. For maintenance, a dosage of one tablet twice a day is frequently adequate.

Robinul Forte (glycopyrrolate, 2 mg) tablets. The recommended dosage of Robinul Forte for adults is one tablet two or three times daily at equally spaced intervals.

Robinul tablets are not recommended for use in children under the age of 12 years.

Drug Interactions: There are no known drug interactions.

How Supplied: Robinul (glycopyrrolate, 1 mg) tablets in bottles of 100 (NDC 0031-7824-63) and 500 (NDC 0031-7824-70).

Robinul Forte (glycopyrrolate, 2 mg) tablets in bottles of 100 (NDC 0031-7840-63) and 500 (NDC 0031-7840-70).

Shown in Product Identification Section, page 429

ROBINUL® INJECTABLE ℞
[ro'bĭ-nul]
brand of Glycopyrrolate Injection, USP

Description: Robinul (glycopyrrolate) is a synthetic anticholinergic agent. Each 1 ml contains:
Glycopyrrolate, USP .... 0.2 mg
Water for Injection, USP .... q.s.
Benzyl Alcohol, NF (preservative) 0.9%
pH adjusted, when necessary, with hydrochloric acid and/or sodium hydroxide.

For Intramuscular or Intravenous administration.

Unlike atropine, glycopyrrolate is completely ionized at physiological pH values.

Robinul Injectable is a clear, colorless, sterile liquid; pH 2.0–3.0.

Clinical Pharmacology: Glycopyrrolate, like other anticholinergic (antimuscarinic) agents, inhibits the action of acetylcholine on structures innervated by postganglionic cholinergic nerves and on smooth muscles that respond to acetylcholine but lack cholinergic innervation. These peripheral cholinergic receptors are present in the autonomic effector cells of smooth muscle, cardiac muscle, the sinoatrial node, the atrioventricular node, exocrine glands, and, to a limited degree, in the autonomic ganglia. Thus, it diminishes the volume and free acidity of gastric secretions and controls excessive pharyngeal, tracheal, and bronchial secretions.

Glycopyrrolate antagonizes muscarinic symptoms (e.g., bronchorrhea, bronchospasm, bradycardia, and intestinal hypermotility) induced by cholinergic drugs such as the anticholinesterases.

The highly polar quaternary ammonium group of glycopyrrolate limits its passage across lipid membranes, such as the blood-brain barrier, in contrast to atropine sulfate and scopolamine hydrobromide, which are non-polar tertiary amines which penetrate lipid barriers easily.

Peak effects occur approximately 30 to 45 minutes after intramuscular administration. The vagal blocking effects persist for 2 to 3 hours and the antisialagogue effects persist up to 7 hours, periods longer than for atropine. With intravenous injection, the onset of action is generally evident within one minute.

Indications and Usage:

In Anesthesia: Robinul (glycopyrrolate) Injectable is indicated for use as a preoperative antimuscarinic to reduce salivary, tracheobronchial, and pharyngeal secretions; to reduce the volume and free acidity of gastric secretions; and, to block cardiac vagal inhibitory reflexes during induction of anesthesia and intubation. When indicated, Robinul Injectable may be used intraoperatively to counteract drug-induced or vagal traction reflexes with the associated arrhythmias. Glycopyrrolate protects against the peripheral muscarinic effects (e.g., bradycardia and excessive secretions) of cholinergic agents such as neostigmine and pyridostigmine given to reverse the neuromuscular blockade due to nondepolarizing muscle relaxants.

In Peptic Ulcer: For use in adults as adjunctive therapy for the treatment of peptic ulcer when rapid anticholinergic effect is desired or when oral medication is not tolerated.

Contraindications: Known hypersensitivity to glycopyrrolate.

In addition, in the management of *peptic ulcer* patients, because of the longer duration of therapy, Robinul Injectable may be contraindicated in patients with concurrent glaucoma; obstructive uropathy (for example, bladder neck obstruction due to prostatic hypertrophy); obstructive disease of the gastrointestinal tract (as in achalasia, pyloroduodenal stenosis, etc.); paralytic ileus, intestinal atony of the elderly or debilitated patient; unstable cardiovascular status in acute hemorrhage; severe ulcerative colitis; toxic megacolon complicating ulcerative colitis; myasthenia gravis.

Warnings: This drug should be used with great caution, if at all, in patients with glaucoma or asthma.

In the ambulatory patient. Robinul (glycopyrrolate) may produce drowsiness or blurred vision. The patient should be cautioned regarding activities requiring mental alertness such as operating a motor vehicle or other machinery or performing hazardous work while taking this drug.

In addition, in the presence of a high environmental temperature, heat prostration (fever and heat stroke due to decreased sweating) can occur with use of Robinul (glycopyrrolate).

Diarrhea may be an early symptom of incomplete intestinal obstruction, expecially in patients with ileostomy or colostomy. In this instance treatment with Robinul (glycopyrrolate) would be inappropriate and possibly harmful.

Precautions: *General.*

Investigate any tachycardia before giving glycopyrrolate since an increase in the heart rate may occur.

Use with caution in patients with: coronary artery disease; congestive heart failure; cardiac arrhythmias; hypertension; hyperthyroidism.

In managing ulcer patients, use Robinul with caution in the elderly and in all patients with autonomic neuropathy, hepatic or renal disease, ulcerative colitis or hiatal hernia, since anticholinergic drugs may aggravate these conditions.

With overdosage, a curare-like action may occur.

Drug Interactions. The intravenous administration of any anticholinergic in the presence of cyclopropane anesthesia can result in ventricular arrhythmias; therefore, caution should be observed if Robinul (glycopyrrolate) Injectable is used during cyclopropane anesthesia. If the drug is given in small incremental doses of 0.1 mg or less, the likelihood of producing ventricular arrhythmias is reduced.

Carcinogenesis, mutagenesis, impairment of fertility. Long-term studies in animals have not been performed to evaluate carcinogenic potential. In the teratology studies, diminished rates of conception and of survival at weaning were observed in rats, in a dose-related manner. Studies in dogs suggest that this may be due to diminished seminal secretion which is evident at high doses of glycopyrrolate.

Pregnancy Category B. Reproduction studies have been performed in rats and rabbits up to 1000 times the human dose and have revealed no teratogenic effects from glycopyrrolate. There are, however, no adequate and well-controlled studies in pregnant women. Because animal reproduction studies are not always predictive of human response, this drug should be used during pregnancy only if clearly needed.

Continued on next page

Prescribing information on A. H. Robins products listed here is based on official labeling in effect August 1, 1984, with Indications, Contraindications, Warnings Precautions, Adverse Reactions, and Dosage stated in full.

Robins—Cont.

Nursing Mothers. It is not known whether this drug is excreted in human milk. Because many drugs are excreted in human milk, caution should be exercised when Robinul is administered to a nursing woman.

Pediatric Use. Safety and effectiveness in children below the age of 12 years have not been established for the management of peptic ulcer.

Adverse Reactions: Anticholinergics produce certain effects, most of which are extensions of their pharmacologic actions. Adverse reactions to anticholinergics in general may include dry mouth; urinary hesitancy and retention; blurred vision due to mydriasis; increased ocular tension; tachycardia; palpitation; decreased sweating; loss of taste; headache; nervousness; drowsiness; weakness; dizziness; insomnia; nausea; vomiting; impotence; suppression of lactation; constipation; bloated feeling; severe allergic reaction or drug idiosyncrasies incuding anaphylaxis; urticaria and other dermal manifestations; some degree of mental confusion and/or excitement, especially in elderly persons.

Robinul is chemically a quaternary ammonium compound; hence, its passage across lipid membranes, such as the blood-brain barrier is limited in contrast to atropine sulfate and scopolamine hydrobromide. For this reason the occurrence of CNS related side effects is lower, in comparison to their incidence following administration of anticholinergics which are chemically tertiary amines that can cross this barrier readily.

Overdosage: To combat peripheral anticholinergic effects, a quaternary ammonium anticholinesterase such as neostigmine methylsulfate (which does not cross the blood-brain barrier) may be given intravenously in increments of 0.25 mg in adults. This dosage may be repeated every five to ten minutes until anticholinergic over-activity is reversed or up to a maximum of 2.5 mg. Proportionately smaller doses should be used in children. Indication for repetitive doses of neostigmine should be based on close monitoring of the decrease in heart rate and the return of bowel sounds.

In the unlikely event that CNS symptoms (excitement, restlessness, convulsions, psychotic behavior) occur, physostigmine (which does cross the blood-brain barrier) should be used. Physostigmine 0.5 to 2 mg should be slowly administered intravenously and repeated as necessary up to a total of 5 mg in adults. Proportionately smaller doses should be used in children.

Fever should be treated symptomatically. In the event of a curare-like effect on respiratory muscles, artificial respiration should be instituted and maintained until effective respiratory action returns.

Dosage and Administration: Robinul (glycopyrrolate) Injectable may be administered intramuscularly, or intravenously, without dilution, in the following indications:

Adults: *Preanesthetic Medication.* The recommended dose of Robinul (glycopyrrolate) Injectable is 0.002 mg (0.01 ml) per pound of body weight by intramuscular injection, given 30 to 60 minutes prior to the anticipated time of induction of anesthesia or at the time the preanesthetic narcotic and/or sedative are administered.

Intraoperative Medication. Robinul (glycopyrrolate) Injectable may be used during surgery to counteract drug induced or vagal traction reflexes with the associated arrhythmias (e.g., bradycardia). It should be administered intravenously as single doses of 0.1 mg (0.5 ml) and repeated, as needed, at intervals of 2–3 minutes. The usual attempts should be made to determine the etiology of the arrhythmia, and the surgical or anesthetic manipulations necessary to correct parasympathetic imbalance should be performed.

Reversal of Neuromuscular Blockade. The recommended pediatric dose of Robinul (glycopyrrolate) Injectable is 0.2 mg (1.0 ml) for each 1.0 mg of neostigmine or 5.0 mg of pyridostigmine. In order to minimize the appearance of cardiac side effects, the drugs may be administered simultaneously by intravenous injection and may be mixed in the same syringe.

Children: *Preanesthetic Medication.* The recommended dose of Robinul (glycopyrrolate) Injectable in children to 12 years of age is 0.002 mg (0.01 ml) per pound of body weight intramuscularly, given 30 to 60 minutes prior to the anticipated time of induction of anesthesia or at the time the preanesthetic narcotic and/or sedative are administered.

Children under 2 years of age may require up to 0.004 mg (0.02 ml) per pound of body weight.

Intraoperative Medication. Because of the long duration of action of Robinul (glycopyrrolate) if used as preanesthetic medication, additional Robinul (glycopyrrolate) Injectable for anticholinergic effect intraoperatively is rarely needed; in the event it is needed the recommended pediatric dose is 0.002 mg (0.01 ml) per pound of body weight intravenously, not to exceed 0.1 mg (0.5 ml) in a single dose which may be repeated, as needed, at intervals of 2–3 minutes. The usual attempts should be made to determine the etiology of the arrhythmia, and the surgical or anesthetic manipulations necessary to correct parasympathetic imbalance should be performed.

Reversal of Neuromuscular Blockade. The recommended pediatric dose of Robinul (glycopyrrolate) Injectable is 0.2 mg (1.0 ml) for each 1.0 mg of neostigmine or 5.0 mg of pyridostigmine. In order to minimize the appearance of cardiac side effects, the drugs may be administered simultaneously by intravenous injection and may be mixed in the same syringe.

Adults: *Peptic Ulcer.* The usual recommended dose of Robinul Injectable is 0.1 mg (0.5 ml) administered at 4-hour intervals, 3 or 4 times daily intravenously or intramuscularly. Where more profound effect is required, 0.2 mg (1.0 ml) may be given. Some patients may need only a single dose, and frequency of administration should be dictated by patient response up to a maximum of four times daily.

Robinul Injectable is not recommended for peptic ulcers in children under 12 years of age. (See Precautions.)

NOTE: Parenteral drug products should be inspected visually for particulate matter and discoloration prior to administration whenever solution and container permit.

Admixture Compatibilities. Robinul (glycopyrrolate) Injectable is compatible for mixing and injection with the following injectable dosage forms: 5% and 10% glucose in water or saline; atropine sulfate, USP; Antilirium® (physostigmine salicylate); Benadryl® (diphenhydramine HCl); codeine phosphate, USP; Emete-Con® (benzquinamide HCl); hydromorphone HCl, USP; Inapsine® (droperidol); Innovar® (droperidol and fentanyl citrate); Largon® (propiomazine HCl); Levo-Dromoran® (levorphanol tartrate); lidocaine, USP; Mepergan® (meperidine and promethazine HCls); meperidine HCl, USP; Mestinon®/Regonol® (pyridostigmine bromide); morphine sulfate, USP; Nisentil® (alphaprodine HCl); Nubain® (nalbuphine HCl); Numorphan® (oxymorphone HCl); Pantopon® (opium alkaloids HCls); procaine HCl, USP; promethazine HCl, USP; Prostigmin® (neostigmine methylsulfate, USP); scopolamine HBr, USP; Sparine® (promazine HCl); Stadol® (butorphanol tartrate); Sublimaze® (fentanyl citrate); Talwin® (pentazocine lactate); Tigan® (trimethobenzamide HCl); Vesprin® (triflupromazine HCl); and Vistaril® (hydroxyzine HCl). Robinul Injectable may be administered via the tubing of a running infusion of physiological saline or lactated Ringer's solution.

Since the stability of glycopyrrolate is questionable above a pH of 6.0, do *not* combine Robinul Injectable in the same syringe with Brevital® (methohexital Na); Chloromycetin® (chloramphenicol Na succinate); Dramamine® (dimenhydrinate); Nembutal® (pentobarbital Na); Pentothal® (thiopental Na); Seconal® (secobarbital Na); sodium bicarbonate (Abbott); or Valium® (diazepam). A gas will evolve or a precipitate may form. Mixing with Decadron® (dexamethazone Na phosphate) or a buffered solution of lactated Ringer's solution will result in a pH higher than 6.0. Mixing chlorpromazine HCl, USP, or Compazine® (prochlorperazine) with other agents in a syringe is not recommended by the manufacturer, although the mixture with Robinul Injectable is physically compatible.

How Supplied: Robinul (glycopyrrolate) Injectable, 0.2 mg/ml, is available in 1 ml single dose vials packaged in 5's (NDC 0031-7890-87), and 25's (NDC 0031-7890-11), 2 ml single dose vials packaged in 25's (NDC 0031-7890-95), 5 ml multiple dose vials packaged individually (NDC 0031-7890-93) and in 25's (NDC 0031-7890-06), and 20 ml (NDC 0031-7890-83) multiple dose vials.

Store at controlled room temperature, between 15°C and 30°C (59°F and 86°F).

Manufactured for Pharmaceutical Division, A. H. Robins Company, Richmond, Virginia 23220 by Elkins-Sinn, Inc., Cherry Hill, NJ 08034, a subsidiary of A. H. Robins Co.

Shown in Product Identification Section, page 429

ROBITUSSIN®
[ro″ bĭ-tuss′ ĭn]
ROBITUSSIN-CF®
ROBITUSSIN-DM®
ROBITUSSIN-PE®

(See PDR For Nonprescription Drugs)

ROBITUSSIN A-C®
[ro″ bĭ-tuss′ ĭn]

Robitussin and codeine.
Each 5 ml (1 teaspoonful) contains:
Guaifenesin, USP .... 100 mg
Codeine Phosphate, USP .... 10 mg
(Warning: May be habit forming)
Alcohol 3.5 per cent
In a palatable, aromatic syrup

Actions: Robitussin A-C combines the expectorant, guaifenesin, with the cough suppressant, codeine. Guaifenesin enhances the output of lower respiratory tract fluid (RTF). The enhanced flow of less viscid secretions promotes ciliary action, and facilitates the removal of inspissated mucus. As a result, dry, unproductive coughs become more productive and less frequent.

Codeine phosphate is favored for its efficacy in low dosage. Robitussin A-C is especially useful when concurrent expectorant and cough suppressant actions are desired.

Indications: Robitussin A-C is useful in combating coughs associated with the common cold, bronchitis, laryngitis, tracheitis, pharyngitis, pertussis, influenza, and measles.

Contraindications: Hypersensitivity to any of the ingredients.

Warnings: Use this product with caution in children under 2 years or in children taking another drug. Prescribe cautiously for patients with persistent or chronic cough such as comes with smoking, asthma, emphysema, or where cough is accompanied by excessive secretions. In patients with chronic pulmonary disease or shortness of breath, this product should be administered with caution. This product may cause or aggravate constipation.

Note: Guaifenesin has been shown to produce a color interference with certain clinical laboratory determinations of 5-hydroxyindoleace- tic acid (5-HIAA) and vanillylmandelic acid (VMA).

Adverse Reactions: Rarely, nausea, gastrointestinal upset, constipation, and drowsiness may occur. No serious side effects from guaifenesin have been reported.

Dosage: Adults and children 12 years of age and over: 2 teaspoonfuls every four hours, not to exceed 12 teaspoonfuls in a 24 hour period; children 6 to under 12 years: 1 teaspoonful every four hours, not to exceed 6 teaspoonfuls in a 24 hour period; children 2 to under 6 years: ½ teaspoonful every four hours, not to exceed 3 teaspoonfuls in a 24 hour period; children under 2 years: use as directed by physician.

How Supplied: Bottles of 2 ounces (NDC 0031-8674-05), 4 ounces (NDC 0031-8674-12), one pint

ROBITUSSIN®-DAC
[ro"bĭ-tuss'in]

Each 5 ml (1 teaspoonful) contains:
Guaifenesin, USP .... 100 mg
Pseudoephedrine
  Hydrochloride, USP .... 30 mg
Codeine Phosphate, USP .... 10 mg
  (Warning: May be habit forming)
In a palatable, aromatic syrup
Alcohol 1.4 per cent

Indications: For the temporary relief of cough and nasal congestion as may occur with the common cold or with inhaled irritants.
Contains the expectorant, guaifenesin, which relieves irritated membranes in the respiratory passageways by preventing dryness through increased mucus flow. The nasal decongestant, pseudoephedrine, reduces the swelling of nasal passages. The antitussive, codeine, calms the cough control center and relieves coughing.
Contraindications: Hypersensitivity to any of the ingredients, marked hypertension, hyperthyroidism, or in patients who are receiving MAO inhibitors or antihypertensive medication.
Warnings: Use this product with caution in children under 2 years or in children taking another drug. Prescribe cautiously for patients with persistent or chronic cough such as comes with smoking, asthma, emphysema, or where cough is accompanied by excessive secretions. Caution should be taken in administering this drug to patients with high blood pressure, heart disease or diabetes. In patients with chronic pulmonary disease or shortness of breath, this product should be administered with caution. As with all products containing sympathomimetic amines, use with caution in patients with prostatic hypertrophy or glaucoma. Do not exceed recommended dosage because at higher doses nervousness, dizziness or sleeplessness may occur. May cause or aggravate constipation.
Note: Guaifenesin has been shown to produce a color interference with certain clinical laboratory determinations of 5-hydroxyindoleace- tic acid (5-HIAA) and vanillylmandelic acid (VMA).
Adverse Reactions: Agitation, dizziness, insomnia, palpitations or nausea may occur. In such instances, reduction in frequency and/or quantity of dose is indicated.
Recommended Dosage: Adults and children 12 years of age and over: 1 or 2 teaspoonfuls every four hours, not to exceed 8 teaspoonfuls in a 24-hour period; children 6 to under 12 years: 1 teaspoonful every four hours, not to exceed 4 teaspoonfuls in a 24-hour period; children 2 to under 6 years: 1/2 teaspoonful every four hours, not to exceed 2 teaspoonfuls in a 24-hour period; children under 2 years: use as directed by physician.
How Supplied: Robitussin-DAC is available in pints (NDC 0031-8680-25).

VIOKASE®
[vi'o-kās]
(Pancrelipase, USP)
Tablets
Powder

Description: Viokase (Pancrelipase, USP) is a pancreatic enzyme concentrate of porcine origin containing standardized lipase, protease, and amylase as well as other pancreatic enzymes. Viokase is available in tablet and powder dosage form for oral administration.
The enzyme potencies of the tablets and powder are:

	Each Tablet	Each 0.7g powder (1/4 teaspoonful)
Lipase, USP Units	8,000	16,800
Protease, USP Units	30,000	70,000
Amylase, USP Units	30,000	70,000

Clinical Pharmacology: The natural digestive enzymes in Viokase, hydrolyze fats into fatty acids

(NDC 0031-8674-25), and one gallon (NDC 0031-8674-29).

and glycerol, split protein into amino acids, and convert carbohydrates to dextrins and short chain sugars.
Under conditions of the USP test method (in vitro) Viokase has the following total digestive capacity:

	Each Tablet	Each 0.7g powder
Dietary Fat, grams	28	59
Dietary Protein, grams	30	70
Dietary Starch, grams	30	70

Viokase Tablets are not enteric coated.
The digestive capacity of a pancreatic enzyme concentrate depends on the amount that passes through the stomach unchanged and is available at the site of action in the small intestine.
Indications: Viokase (Pancrelipase, USP) is indicated as a digestive aid in the treatment of exocrine pancreatic insufficiency as associated with but not limited to cystic fibrosis, chronic pancreatitis, pancreatectomy, or obstruction of the pancreas ducts.
Contraindications: Do not use in patients hypersensitive to pork protein.
Precautions: *General:* Individuals previously sensitized to trypsin, pancreatin or pancrelipase may have allergic manifestations.
Information for patients: Viokase should not be held in the mouth as the proteolytic action may cause irritation of the mucosa.
Avoid inhalation of the powder when administering Viokase.
Carcinogenesis, Mutagenesis, Impairment of fertility: Long-term studies in animals have not been performed to evaluate carcinogenic potential.
Pregnancy Category C. Animal reproduction studies have not been conducted with Viokase. It is also not known whether Viokase can cause fetal harm when administered to a pregnant woman or can affect reproduction capacity. Viokase should be given to a pregnant woman only if clearly needed.
Nursing Mothers: It is not known whether this drug is excreted in human milk. Because many drugs are excreted in human milk, caution should be exercised when Viokase is administered to a nursing mother.
Adverse Reactions: The dust or finely powdered pancreatic enzyme concentrate is irritating to the nasal mucosa and the respiratory tract. It has been documented that inhalation of the airborne powder can precipitate an asthma attack. The literature also contains several references to asthma due to inhalation in patients sensitized to pancreatic enzyme concentrates. Extremely high doses of exogenous pancreatic enzymes have been associated with hyperuricemia and hyperuricosuria. Overdosage of pancreatic enzyme concentrate may cause diarrhea or transient intestinal upset.
Overdosage: Acute toxicity determinations in animals have not been possible since the maximum dose that could be given orally produced no toxic reaction. In chronic feeding tests. rats developed swollen salivary glands. This is believed due to the proteolytic activity and the mucosal irritation caused by tissue digestion.
No acute toxic reactions have been reported.
Dosage and Administration: *Powder:* Dosage for patients with cystic fibrosis—1/4 teaspoonful (0.7 grams) with meals.
Tablets: Dosage for patients with cystic fibrosis or chronic pancreatitis—1 to 3 tablets with meals or as directed by physician. As a digestive aid in patients with pancreatectomy or obstruction of pancreatic ducts—1 to 2 tablets taken at 2-hour intervals or as directed by physician.
How Supplied: *Tablets*—Tan, round, compressed tablets engraved Viokase/AHR on one side and 9111 on the other side in bottles of 100 (NDC 0031-9111-63) and 500 (NDC 0031-9111-70).
Powder—Tan powder in bottles of 4 oz. (113.5 grams) NDC 0031-9115-12) and 8 oz. (227 grams) (NDC 0031-9115-25).
Store in tightly closed container in a dry place at a temperature not exceeding 25°C (77°F).
Dispense tablets and powder in tight container, preferably with a desiccant.

Clinical Studies: The effectiveness of Viokase as a digestive aid in the treatment of patients with exocrine pancreatic insufficiency has been documented in the literature as follows:
1. Regan, PT, Malagelada J-R, DiMagno EP, Glanzman SL., Go VLW: Comparative effects of antacids, cimetidine and enteric coating on the therapeutic response to oral enzymes in severe pancreatic insufficiency. N. Engl. J. Med. 297-854-8, 1977.
2. Graham DY: Enzyme replacement therapy of exocrine pancreatic insufficiency in man. N. Engl. J. Med. 296:1314-7, 1977.

Z-BEC®
[zē'běk]
(See PDR For Nonprescription Drugs)

Roche Laboratories
Division of Hoffmann-La Roche Inc.
NUTLEY, NJ 07110

ACCUTANE®
[acc'u-tane]
(isotretinoin/Roche)
CAPSULES

The following text is complete prescribing information based on official labeling in effect August 1, 1984.

> **Contraindication:** Accutane must not be used by females who are pregnant or who intend to become pregnant while undergoing treatment.
> **Major human fetal abnormalities related to Accutane administration have been reported, including hydrocephalus, microcephalus, abnormalities of the external ear (micropinna, small or absent external auditory canals), microphthalmia and cardiovascular abnormalities.**
> Women of childbearing potential should not be given Accutane until pregnancy is excluded. It is strongly recommended that a pregnancy test be performed within two weeks prior to Accutane therapy. An effective form of contraception should be used for at least one month before and also throughout Accutane therapy. It is recommended that contraception be continued for one month following discontinuation of Accutane therapy.
> Females should be fully counseled on the serious risk to the fetus should they become pregnant while undergoing treatment. If pregnancy does occur during treatment, the physician and patient should discuss the desirability of continuing the pregnancy.

Description: Accutane (isotretinoin/Roche), a retinoid which inhibits sebaceous gland function and keratinization, is available in 10-mg, 20-mg and 40-mg soft gelatin capsules for oral administration. Chemically, isotretinoin is 13-*cis*-retinoic acid and is related to both retinoic acid and retinol (vitamin A). It is a yellow-orange to orange crystalline powder with a molecular weight of 300.44.
Clinical Pharmacology: The exact mechanism of action of Accutane is unknown.
Cystic Acne: Clinical improvement in cystic acne patients occurs in association with a reduction in sebum secretion. The decrease in sebum secretion is temporary and is related to the dose and duration of treatment with Accutane, and reflects a reduction in sebaceous gland size and an inhibition of sebaceous gland differentiation.[1]
Clinical Pharmacokinetics: The pharmacokinetic profile of isotretinoin is predictable and can be described using linear pharmacokinetic theory. After oral administration of 80 mg (two 40-mg capsules), peak blood concentrations ranged from

Continued on next page

Roche Labs.—Cont.

167 to 459 ng/ml (mean 256 ng/ml) and mean time to peak was 3.2 hours in normal volunteers, while in acne patients peak concentrations ranged from 98 to 535 ng/ml (mean 262 ng/ml) with a mean time to peak of 2.9 hours. The drug is 99.9% bound in human plasma almost exclusively to albumin. The terminal elimination half-life of isotretinoin ranged from 10 to 20 hours in volunteers and patients. Following an 80-mg liquid suspension oral dose of ^{14}C-isotretinoin, ^{14}C-activity in blood declined with a half-life of 90 hours. Relatively equal amounts of radioactivity were recovered in the urine and feces with 65% to 83% of the dose recovered.

The major identified metabolite in blood is 4-*oxo*-isotretinoin. Tretinoin and 4-*oxo*-tretinoin were also observed. The terminal elimination of 4-*oxo*-isotretinoin is formation rate limited and therefore the apparent half-life of the 4-*oxo*-metabolite is similar to isotretinoin following Accutane administration. After two 40-mg capsules of isotretinoin, maximum concentrations of the metabolite of 87 to 399 ng/ml occurred at 6 to 20 hours. The blood concentration of the major metabolite generally exceeded that of isotretinoin after six hours.

The mean ± SD minimum steady-state blood concentration of isotretinoin was 160 ± 19 ng/ml in ten patients receiving 40-mg *b.i.d.* doses. After single and multiple doses, the mean ratio of areas under the blood concentration:time curves of 4-*oxo*-isotretinoin to isotretinoin was 3 to 3.5.

Tissue Distribution in Animals: Tissue distribution of ^{14}C-isotretinoin in rats after oral dosing revealed high concentrations of radioactivity in many tissues after 15 minutes, with a maximum in one hour, and declining to nondetectable levels by 24 hours in most tissues. After seven days, however, low levels of radioactivity were detected in the liver, ureter, adrenal, ovary and lacrimal gland.

Indications and Usage: *Cystic Acne:* Accutane is indicated for the treatment of severe recalcitrant cystic acne, and a single course of therapy has been shown to result in complete and prolonged remission of disease in many patients.[1–3] If a second course of therapy is needed, it should not be initiated until at least eight weeks after completion of the first course, since experience has shown that patients may continue to improve while off drug.

Because of significant adverse effects associated with its use, Accutane should be reserved for patients with severe cystic acne who are unresponsive to conventional therapy, including systemic antibiotics.

Contraindications: **Pregnancy: Category X. See boxed Contraindication.**

Accutane should not be given to patients who are sensitive to parabens, which are used as preservatives in the gelatin capsule.

Warnings:

> *Pseudotumor cerebri:* Accutane use has been associated with a number of cases of pseudotumor cerebri (benign intracranial hypertension). Early signs and symptoms of pseudotumor cerebri include papilledema, headache, nausea and vomiting, and visual disturbances. Patients with these symptoms should be screened for papilledema and, if present, they should be told to discontinue Accutane immediately and be referred to a neurologist for further diagnosis and care.

Corneal opacities: Corneal opacities have occured in patients receiving Accutane for acne and more frequently when higher drug dosages were used in patients with disorders of keratinization. All Accutane patients experiencing visual difficulties should discontinue the drug and have an ophthalmological examination. The corneal opacities that have been observed in patients treated with Accutane have either completely resolved or were resolving at follow-up six to seven weeks after discontinuation of the drug. See ADVERSE REACTIONS.

Inflammatory Bowel Disease: Accutane has been temporally associated with inflammatory bowel disease (including regional ileitis) in patients without a prior history of intestinal disorders. Patients experiencing abdominal pain, rectal bleeding or severe diarrhea should discontinue Accutane immediately.

Lipids: Blood lipid determinations should be performed before Accutane is given and then at intervals until the lipid response to Accutane is established, which usually occurs within four weeks. See PRECAUTIONS.

Approximately 25% of patients receiving Accutane experienced an elevation in plasma triglycerides. Approximately 15% developed a decrease in high density lipoproteins and about 7% showed an increase in cholesterol levels. These effects on triglycerides, HDL and cholesterol were reversible upon cessation of Accutane therapy.

Patients with increased tendency to develop hypertriglyceridemia include those with diabetes mellitus, obesity, increased alcohol intake and familial history.

The cardiovascular consequences of hypertriglyceridemia are not well understood, but may increase the patient's risk status. In addition, elevation of serum triglycerides in excess of 800 mg/dl has been associated with acute pancreatitis. Therefore, every attempt should be made to control significant triglyceride elevation.

Some patients have been able to reverse triglyceride elevation by reduction in weight, restriction of dietary fat and alcohol, and reduction in dose while continuing Accutane.[4]

An obese male patient with Darier's disease developed elevated triglycerides and subsequent eruptive xanthomas.[5]

Hyperostosis: In clinical trials of disorders of keratinization with a mean dose of 2.24 mg/kg/day, a high prevalence of skeletal hyperostosis was noted. Two children showed x-ray findings suggestive of premature closure of the epiphysis. Additionally, skeletal hyperostosis was noted in six of eight patients in a prospective study of disorders of keratinization. These x-ray changes occurred between six and twelve months of therapy.

Animal Studies: In rats given 32 or 8 mg/kg/day of isotretinoin for 18 months or longer, the incidences of focal calcification, fibrosis and inflammation of the myocardium, calcification of coronary, pulmonary and mesenteric arteries and metastatic calcification of the gastric mucosa were greater than in control rats of similar age. Focal endocardial and myocardial calcifications associated with calcification of the coronary arteries were observed in two dogs after approximately six to seven months of treatment with isotretinoin at a dosage of 60 to 120 mg/kg/day.

In dogs given isotretinoin chronically at a dosage of 60 mg/kg/day, corneal ulcers and corneal opacities were encountered at a higher incidence than in control dogs. In general, these ocular changes tended to revert toward normal when treatment with isotretinoin was stopped, but did not completely clear during the observation period.

In rats given isotretinoin at a dosage of 32 mg/kg/day for approximately 15 weeks, long bone fracture has been observed.

Precautions: *Information for Patients:* Women of childbearing potential should be instructed that they must not be pregnant when Accutane therapy is initiated, and that they should use an effective form of contraception while taking Accutane and for one month after Accutane has been stopped. See boxed Contraindication.

Because of the relationship of Accutane to vitamin A, patients should be advised against taking vitamin supplements containing vitamin A to avoid additive toxic effects.

Patients should be informed that transient exacerbation of acne has been seen, generally during the initial period of therapy.

Laboratory Tests: The incidence of hypertriglyceridemia is 1 patient in 4 on Accutane therapy. Pretreatment and follow-up blood lipids should be obtained under fasting conditions. After consumption of alcohol at least 36 hours should elapse before these determinations are made. It is recommended that these tests be performed at weekly or biweekly intervals until the lipid response to Accutane is established.

Carcinogenesis, Mutagenesis, Impairment of Fertility: In Fischer 344 rats given isotretinoin at dosages of 32 or 8 mg/kg/day for greater than 18 months, there was an increased incidence of pheochromocytoma. The incidence of adrenal medullary hyperplasia was also increased at the higher dosage. The relatively high level of spontaneous pheochromocytomas occurring in the Fischer 344 rat makes it a poor model for study of this tumor, since the increase in adrenal medullary proliferative lesions following chronic treatment with relatively high dosages of isotretinoin may be an accentuation of a genetic predisposition in the Fischer 344 rat, and its relevance to the human population is not clear. In addition, a decreased incidence of liver adenomas, liver angiomas and leukemia was noted at the dose levels of 8 and 32 mg/kg/day.

The Ames test was conducted in two laboratories. The results of the tests in one laboratory were completely negative, while in the second laboratory a weakly positive (less than 1.6 x background) was seen with S. typhimurium TA100. No dose-response effect was seen and all other strains were negative. Additionally, other mutagenicity tests (Chinese hamster cells, mouse micronucleus test and S. cerevisiae) were also negative.

No adverse effects on gonadal function, fertility, conception rate, gestation or parturition were observed at dose levels of 2, 8 or 32 mg/kg/day in male and female rats.

In dogs, testicular atrophy was noted after treatment with isotretinoin for approximately 30 weeks at dosages of 60 or 20 mg/kg/day. In general, there was microscopic evidence for appreciable depression of spermatogenesis but some sperm were observed in all testes examined and in no instance were completely atrophic tubules seen. In studies in 66 human males, 30 of whom were patients with cystic acne, no significant changes were noted in the count or motility of spermatozoa in the ejaculate. Studies further evaluating this in humans are being conducted.

Pregnancy: **Category X. See boxed Contraindication.**

Nursing Mothers: It is not known whether this drug is excreted in human milk. Because of the potential for adverse effects, nursing mothers should not receive Accutane.

Adverse Reactions: *Clinical:* The percentages of adverse reactions listed below reflect the total experience in Accutane studies, including investigational studies of disorders of keratinization, with the exception of those pertaining to dry skin and mucous membranes. These latter reflect the experience only in patients with cystic acne because reactions relating to dryness are more commonly recognized as adverse reactions in this disease. Included in this category are dry skin, pruritus, epistaxis, dry nose and dry mouth, which may be seen in up to 80% of cystic acne patients.

The most frequent adverse reaction to Accutane is cheilitis, which occurs in over 90% of patients. A less frequent reaction was conjunctivitis (about two patients in five).

Approximately 16% of patients treated with Accutane developed musculoskeletal symptoms during treatment. In general, these were mild to moderate and have occasionally required discontinuation of drug. These symptoms generally cleared rapidly after discontinuation of Accutane.

In less than one patient in ten—rash, temporary thinning of hair.

In approximately one patient in twenty—peeling of palms and soles, skin infections, nonspecific urogenital findings, nonspecific gastrointestinal symptoms, fatigue, headache and increased susceptibility to sunburn.

Accutane has been associated with a number of cases of pseudotumor cerebri, some of which involved concomitant use of tetracyclines. See WARNINGS.

The following reactions have been reported in less than 1% of patients and may bear no relationship to therapy—changes in skin pigment (hypo- and hyperpigmentation), urticaria, bruising, disseminated herpes simplex, edema, hair problems (other than thinning), respiratory infections, weight loss, paresthesias, erythema nodosum, paronychia, dizziness and abnormal menses.

In Accutane studies to date, of 72 patients who had normal pretreatment ophthalmological examinations, five developed corneal opacities while on Accutane (all five patients had a disorder of keratinization). Corneal opacities have also been reported in cystic acne patients treated with Accutane. See WARNINGS.

Accutane has been temporally associated with inflammatory bowel disease. See WARNINGS.

As may be seen with healing cystic acne lesions, an occasional exaggerated healing response, manifested by exuberant granulation tissue with crusting, has also been reported in patients receiving therapy with Accutane.

Laboratory: Accutane therapy induces change in serum lipids in a significant number of treated subjects. Approximately 25% of patients had elevation of plasma triglycerides. Five out of 135 patients treated for cystic acne and 32 out of 298 total subjects treated for all diagnoses showed an elevation of triglycerides above 500 mg percent. About 16% of patients showed a mild to moderate decrease in serum high density lipoprotein (HDL) levels while receiving treatment with Accutane and about 7% of patients experienced minimal elevations of serum cholesterol during treatment. Abnormalities of serum triglycerides, HDL and cholesterol were reversible upon cessation of Accutane therapy.

Approximately 40% of patients receiving Accutane developed elevated sedimentation rates, often from elevated baseline values.

From one in ten to one in five patients showed decreases in red blood cell parameters and white blood cell counts, elevated platelet counts, white cells in the urine, increased alkaline phosphatase, SGOT, SGPT or LDH.

Less than one in ten patients showed proteinuria, red blood cells in the urine, elevated fasting blood sugar, elevated CPK or hyperuricemia.

Dose Relationship and Duration: Most adverse reactions appear to be dose related, with the more pronounced effects occurring at doses above 1.0 mg/kg/day. Adverse reactions in cystic acne patients were reversible when therapy was discontinued.

Overdosage: The oral LD$_{50}$ of isotretinoin is greater than 4000 mg/kg in rats and mice and is approximately 1960 mg/kg in rabbits. There has been no experience with acute overdosage in human beings.

Dosage and Administration: In general, the initial dose of Accutane should be individualized according to the patient's weight and severity of the disease. After two or more weeks of treatment, the dose should be adjusted according to the appearance of clinical side effects and the response of the disease.

The recommended course of therapy is one to two mg/kg, given in two divided doses daily for fifteen to twenty weeks. If the total cyst count has been reduced by more than 70% prior to this time period, the drug may be discontinued. After a period of two months off therapy, and if warranted by persistent severe cystic acne, a second course of therapy may be initiated. Patients whose disease is primarily manifest on the chest and back instead of the face, as well as patients who weigh more than 70 kg, may require doses at the higher end of the range.

ACCUTANE DOSING BY BODY WEIGHT

Body Weight		Total Mg/Day	
kilograms	pounds	1 mg/kg	2 mg/kg
40	88	40	80
50	110	50	100
60	132	60	120
70	154	70	140
80	176	80	160
90	198	90	180
100	220	100	200

How Supplied: Soft gelatin capsules, 10 mg (light pink), imprinted ACCUTANE 10 ROCHE; bottles of 100 (NDC-0004-0155-01).

Soft gelatin capsules, 20 mg (maroon), imprinted ACCUTANE 20 ROCHE; bottles of 100 (NDC-0004-0169-01).

Soft gelatin capsules, 40 mg (yellow), imprinted ACCUTANE 40 ROCHE; bottles of 100 (NDC-0004-0156-01).

References:
1. Peck, GL, Olsen, TG, Yoder, FW, Strauss, JS, Downing, DT, Pandya, M, Butkus, D, Arnaud-Battandier, J: Prolonged remissions of cystic and conglobate acne with 13-*cis*-retinoic acid. *N Engl J Med 300*:329–333, 1979. 2. Farrell, LN, Strauss, JS, Stranieri, AM: The treatment of severe cystic acne with 13-*cis*-retinoic acid. Evaluation of sebum production and the clinical response in a multiple-dose trial. *J Am Acad Dermatol 3*:602–611, 1980, 3. Jones, H, Blanc, D, Cunliffe, WJ: 13-*cis*-retinoic acid and acne. *Lancet 2*:1048–1049, 1980. 4. Katz, RA, Jorgensen, H, Nigra, TP: Elevation of serum triglyceride levels from oral isotretinoin in disorders of keratinization. *Arch Dermatol 116*:1369–1372, 1980. 5. Dicken, CH, Connolly, SM: Eruptive xanthomas associated with isotretinoin (13-*cis*-retinoic acid). *Arch Dermatol 116*:951–952, 1980.

Shown in Product Identification Section, page 429.

ALURATE® ELIXIR
[al'u-rate]
(aprobarbital/Roche)

The following text is complete prescribing information based on official labeling in effect August 1, 1984.

The following sections contain information specifically applicable to Alurate as well as information pertinent to other barbiturates. The information pertinent to other barbiturates should be considered when administering Alurate.

Description: Alurate (aprobarbital/Roche) is an intermediate-acting barbiturate which is used as a sedative-hypnotic. As with other barbiturates, it acts as a CNS depressant. Alurate is available for oral administration as a red elixir providing 40 mg of aprobarbital per teaspoonful (5 ml) in a vehicle containing 20 percent alcohol. Chemically, aprobarbital is 5-allyl-5-isopropylbarbituric acid. It is a bitter, white crystalline powder with an empirical formula of $C_{10}H_{14}N_2O_3$ and a molecular weight of 210.23.

Clinical Pharmacology: Barbiturates are capable of producing all levels of CNS mood alteration from excitation to mild sedation, hypnosis and deep coma. Overdosage can produce death. In high enough therapeutic doses, barbiturates induce anesthesia.

Barbiturates depress the sensory cortex, decrease motor activity, alter cerebellar function and produce drowsiness, sedation and hypnosis.

Barbiturate-induced sleep differs from physiological sleep. Sleep laboratory studies have demonstrated that barbiturates reduce the amount of time spent in the rapid eye movement (REM) phase of sleep or dreaming stage. Also, Stages III and IV sleep are decreased. Patients may experience markedly increased dreaming, nightmares and/or insomnia if barbiturates are prescribed for a period of time and then abruptly withdrawn. It is recommended that dosage be reduced gradually over a period of 5 or 6 days to lessen REM rebound and disturbed sleep (for example, decrease the dose from 3 to 2 doses a day for 1 week).

In studies, secobarbital sodium and pentobarbital sodium have been found to lose most of their effectiveness for both inducing and maintaining sleep by the end of 2 weeks of continued drug administration, even with the use of multiple doses. Other barbiturates might also be expected to lose their effectiveness for inducing and maintaining sleep after about 2 weeks. Therefore, as sleep medications, the barbiturates are of limited value beyond short-term use.

Barbiturates have little analgesic action at subanesthetic doses. Rather, they may increase the reaction to painful stimuli. All barbiturates exhibit anticonvulsant activity in anesthetic doses; however, only phenobarbital, mephobarbital and metharbital are effective as oral anticonvulsants in subhypnotic doses.

Barbiturates are respiratory depressants; the degree of depression is dose-dependent. With hypnotic doses, respiratory depression produced by barbiturates is similar to that which occurs during physiologic sleep. Hypnotic doses also cause a slight decrease in blood pressure and heart rate. Studies in laboratory animals have shown that barbiturates cause reduction in the tone and contractility of the uterus, ureters and urinary bladder. However, concentrations of the drugs required to produce this effect in humans are not reached with sedative-hypnotic doses.

Barbiturates do not impair normal hepatic function, but have been shown to induce liver microsomal enzymes, thus altering the metabolism of certain other drugs. (See Precautions — Drug Interactions section.)

Pharmacokinetics: Barbiturates are absorbed in varying degrees following oral administration. The onset of action for oral barbiturate administration varies from 20 to 60 minutes. Duration of action, which is related to the rate at which the barbiturates are redistributed throughout the body, varies among persons and in the same person from time to time. Aprobarbital, which is an intermediate-acting barbiturate, has a duration of action ranging from 6 to 8 hours.

Barbiturates are weak acids that are absorbed and rapidly distributed to all tissues and fluids, with high concentrations in the brain, liver and kidneys. Lipid solubility of the barbiturates is the dominant factor in their distribution throughout the body. Barbiturates are bound to plasma and tissue proteins to a varying degree, with the degree of binding increasing directly as a function of lipid solubility. Aprobarbital is approximately 20 percent plasma protein-bound.

The half-life of aprobarbital ranges from 14 to 34 hours with a mean half-life of 24 hours.

Barbiturates are metabolized primarily by the hepatic microsomal enzyme system; the metabolic products are excreted in the urine and, less commonly, in the feces. Approximately 13 to 24 percent of aprobarbital is eliminated unchanged in the urine. The inactive metabolites of the barbiturates are excreted as conjugates of glucuronic acid.

Indications and Usage: Alurate is indicated for sedation and induction of sleep, on a short-term basis, in conditions requiring a sedative-hypnotic.

Contraindications: Barbiturates are contraindicated in patients with known barbiturate sensitivity. Barbiturates are also contraindicated in patients with a history of manifest or latent porphyria.

Warnings: *Habit forming:* Barbiturates may be habit forming. Tolerance and psychological and physical dependence may occur with continued use. (See Drug Abuse and Dependence section.) Patients who have a psychological dependence on barbiturates may increase the dosage or decrease the dosage interval without consulting a physician and may subsequently develop a physical dependence. To minimize the possibility of overdosage or the development of dependence, the quantity of sedative-hypnotic barbiturates prescribed or dispensed should be limited to the amount required between appointments. Abrupt cessation after prolonged use may result in withdrawal symptoms, including delirium, convulsions and possibly death.

Barbiturates should be withdrawn gradually from any patient known to be taking excessive doses over long periods of time.

Continued on next page

Roche Labs.—Cont.

Acute or chronic pain: Caution should be exercised when barbiturates are administered to patients with acute or chronic pain, because paradoxical excitement may be induced or important symptoms may be masked.

Use in pregnancy: Barbiturates can cause fetal damage when administered to a pregnant woman. Retrospective case-controlled studies have suggested a connection between maternal consumption of barbiturates and a higher than expected incidence of fetal abnormalities. Following oral administration, barbiturates readily cross the placental barrier and are distributed throughout the placenta and fetal tissues, with highest concentrations found in the liver and brain.

Withdrawal symptoms occur in infants born to mothers who receive barbiturates throughout the last trimester of pregnancy. (See Drug Abuse and Dependence section.) If this drug is used during pregnancy, or if the patient becomes pregnant while taking this drug, the patient should be apprised of the potential hazard to the fetus.

Synergistic effects: The concomitant use of alcohol or other CNS depressants may produce additive CNS-depressant effects.

Precautions: *General:* Barbiturates may be habit forming. Tolerance and psychological and physical dependence may occur with continued use. (See Drug Abuse and Dependence section.) Barbiturates should be administered with caution, if at all, to patients who are mentally depressed, have suicidal tendencies, or a history of drug abuse. Elderly or debilitated patients may react to barbiturates with marked excitement, depression and confusion. In some persons, barbiturates repeatedly produce excitement rather than depression. In patients with hepatic damage, barbiturates should be administered with caution, and initially in reduced doses. Barbiturates should not be administered to patients showing the premonitory signs of hepatic coma.

Information for Patients: The use of barbiturates carries with it an associated risk of psychological and/or physical dependence. The patient should be warned against increasing the dose of the drug without consulting a physician.

Barbiturates may impair mental and/or physical abilities required for the performance of potentially hazardous tasks, such as driving a car or operating machinery.

Alcohol should not be consumed while taking barbiturates. Concurrent use of barbiturates with other CNS depressants (*e.g.,* alcohol, narcotics, tranquilizers, antihistamines) may result in additional CNS depressant effects.

Laboratory Tests: Prolonged therapy with barbiturates should be accompanied by periodic laboratory evaluation of organ systems, including hematopoietic, renal and hepatic systems.

Drug Interactions: Most reports of clinically significant drug interactions occurring with the barbiturates have involved phenobarbital. However, the application of these data to other barbiturates appears valid and warrants serial blood level determinations of the relevant drugs when there are multiple therapies.

1. *Anticoagulants.* Phenobarbital lowers the plasma levels of dicumarol (name previously used: bishydroxycoumarin) and causes a decrease in anticoagulant activity as measured by the prothrombin time. Barbiturates can induce hepatic microsomal enzymes resulting in increased metabolism of and decreased anticoagulant response to oral anticoagulants (*e.g.,* warfarin, acenocoumarol, dicumarol and phenprocoumon). Patients stabilized on anticoagulant therapy may require dosage adjustments if barbiturates are added to or withdrawn from their dosage regimen.

2. *Corticosteroids.* Barbiturates appear to enhance the metabolism of exogenous corticosteroids, probably through the induction of hepatic microsomal enzymes. Patients stabilized on corticosteroid therapy may require dosage adjustments if barbiturates are added to or withdrawn from their dosage regimen.

3. *Griseofulvin.* Phenobarbital appears to interfere with the absorption of orally administered griseofulvin, thus decreasing its blood level. This effect on therapeutic response has not been established; however, it would be preferable to avoid concomitant administration of these drugs.

4. *Doxycycline.* Phenobarbital has been shown to shorten the half-life of doxycycline for as long as two weeks after discontinuance of the barbiturate therapy. This action is probably the result of induction of hepatic microsomal enzymes that metabolize the antibiotic. If phenobarbital and doxycycline are administered concurrently, the clinical response to doxycycline should be monitored closely.

5. *Phenytoin, sodium valproate, valproic acid.* The effect of barbiturates on the metabolism of phenytoin appears to be variable. Some investigators report an accelerating effect, while others report no effect. Because the effect is not predictable, phenytoin and barbiturate blood levels should be monitored more frequently if these drugs are given concurrently. Sodium valproate and valproic acid appear to decrease barbiturate metabolism; therefore, barbiturate blood levels should be monitored and appropriate dosage adjustments made.

6. *Central nervous system depressants.* The concomitant use of other central nervous system depressants, including other sedatives or hypnotics, antihistamines, tranquilizers or alcohol, may produce additive effects.

7. *Monoamine oxidase inhibitors (MAOI).* MAOI prolong the effects of barbiturates, probably because metabolism of the barbiturates is inhibited.

8. *Estradiol, estrone, progesterone and other steroidal hormones.* Pretreatment with or concurrent administration of phenobarbital may decrease the effect of estradiol by increasing its metabolism. There have been reports of patients treated with antiepileptic drugs (*e.g.,* phenobarbital) who became pregnant while taking oral contraceptives. An alternate contraceptive method might be suggested to women taking phenobarbital.

Carcinogenesis: 1. Animal data. Phenobarbital sodium is carcinogenic in mice and rats after lifetime administration. In mice, it produced benign and malignant liver cell tumors. In rats, benign liver cell tumors were observed very late in life.

2. Human data. In a 29-year epidemiological study of 9136 patients who were treated on an anticonvulsant protocol which included phenobarbital sodium, results indicated a higher than normal incidence of hepatic carcinoma. Previously, some of these patients were treated with Thorotrast, a drug which is known to produce hepatic carcinomas. Thus, this study did not provide sufficient evidence that phenobarbital sodium is carcinogenic in humans.

A retrospective study of 84 children with brain tumors matched to 73 normal controls and 78 cancer controls (malignant disease other than brain tumors) suggested an association between exposure to barbiturates prenatally and an increased incidence of brain tumors.

Pregnancy: 1. Teratogenic Effects. Pregnancy Category D. See Warnings section.

2. Nonteratogenic Effects. Reports of infants suffering from long-term barbiturate exposure *in utero* include the acute withdrawal syndrome of seizures and hyperirritability from birth. A delayed onset of the symptoms may be seen for up to 14 days. (See Drug Abuse and Dependence section.)

Labor and Delivery: Hypnotic doses of barbiturates do not appear to significantly impair uterine activity during labor. Full anesthetic doses of barbiturates decrease the force and frequency of uterine contractions. Administration of sedative-hypnotic barbiturates to the mother during labor may result in respiratory depression in the newborn. Premature infants are particularly susceptible to the depressant effects of barbiturates. If barbiturates are used during labor and delivery, resuscitation equipment should be available.

Data are not currently available to evaluate the effect of these barbiturates when forceps delivery or other intervention is necessary. Also, data are not available to determine the effect of these barbiturates on the later growth, development and functional maturation of the child.

Nursing mothers: Small amounts of barbiturates are excreted in the human milk. Because of the potential for serious adverse reactions in nursing infants from barbiturates, a decision should be made whether to discontinue nursing or to discontinue the drug, taking into account the importance of the drug to the mother.

Pediatric use: Safety and effectiveness in children have not been established.

Adverse Reactions: The following adverse reactions have been reported following the use of Alurate in an incidence of less than 1 in 100 patients.

Nervous system: Dizziness, nervousness.
Digestive system: Nausea and vomiting.
Other reported reactions: Headache, hypersensitivity reactions (skin rashes) and purpura.

Although the following adverse reactions have not been reported with Alurate, they have been compiled from surveillance of thousands of hospitalized patients receiving barbiturates and should be considered when administering Alurate:

More than 1 in 100 patients. The most common adverse reaction estimated to occur at a rate of 1 to 3 patients per 100 is:
Nervous system: Somnolence.

Less than 1 in 100 patients. Adverse reactions estimated to occur at a rate of less than 1 in 100 patients are listed below, grouped by organ system and by decreasing order of occurrence:

Nervous system: Agitation, confusion, hyperkinesia, ataxia, CNS depression, nightmares, psychiatric disturbances, hallucinations, insomnia, anxiety, thinking abnormality.
Respiratory system: Hypoventilation, apnea.
Cardiovascular system: Bradycardia, hypotension, syncope.
Digestive system: Constipation.
Other reported reactions: Hypersensitivity reactions (angioedema, exfoliative dermatitis), fever, liver damage, megaloblastic anemia following chronic phenobarbital use.

Drug Abuse and Dependence: Alurate is subject to Class III control under the Federal Controlled Substances Act.

Barbiturates may be habit forming. Tolerance, psychological dependence and physical dependence may occur especially following prolonged use of high doses of barbiturates. Daily administration in excess of 400 mg of pentobarbital or secobarbital for approximately 90 days is likely to produce some degree of physical dependence. A dosage of from 600 to 800 mg taken for at least 35 days is sufficient to produce withdrawal seizures. The average daily dose for the barbiturate addict is usually about 1.5 grams. As tolerance to barbiturates develops, the amount needed to maintain the same level of intoxication increases; tolerance to fatal dosage, however, does not increase more than twofold. As this occurs, the margin between an intoxicating dosage and fatal dosage becomes smaller.

Symptoms of acute intoxication with barbiturates include unsteady gait, slurred speech and sustained nystagmus. Mental signs of chronic intoxication include confusion, poor judgment, irritability, insomnia and somatic complaints.

Symptoms of barbiturate dependence are similar to those of chronic alcoholism. If an individual appears to be intoxicated with alcohol to a degree that is radically disproportionate to the amount of alcohol in his or her blood, the use of barbiturates should be suspected. The lethal dose of a barbiturate is far less if alcohol is also ingested.

The symptoms of barbiturate withdrawal can be severe and may cause death. Minor withdrawal symptoms may appear 8 to 12 hours after the last dose of a barbiturate. These symptoms usually appear in the following order: anxiety, muscle twitching, tremor of hands or fingers, progressive weakness, dizziness, distortion in visual perception, nausea, vomiting, insomnia and orthostatic hypotension. Major withdrawal symptoms (convulsions and delirium) may occur within 16 hours and last up to 5 days after abrupt cessation of these drugs. Intensity of withdrawal symptoms gradually declines over a period of approximately 15 days. Individuals susceptible to barbiturate abuse and dependence include alcoholics and opiate abusers, as well as other sedative-hypnotic and amphetamine abusers.

Drug dependence to barbiturates arises from repeated administration of a barbiturate or an agent with barbiturate-like effect on a continuous basis, generally in amounts exceeding therapeutic dosage levels. The characteristics of drug dependence to barbiturates include: (a) a strong desire or need to continue taking the drug; (b) a tendency to increase the dose; (c) a psychic dependence on the effects of the drug related to subjective and individual appreciation of those effects; and (d) a physical dependence on the effects of the drug requiring its presence for maintenance of homeostasis and resulting in a definite, characteristic and self-limited abstinence syndrome when the drug is withdrawn.

Treatment of barbiturate dependence consists of cautious and gradual withdrawal of the drug. Barbiturate-dependent patients can be withdrawn by using a number of different withdrawal regimens. In all cases withdrawal takes an extended period of time. One method involves substituting 30 mg of phenobarbital for each 100 mg of the short-acting barbiturate which the patient has been taking. The total daily amount of phenobarbital is then administered in 4 divided doses, not to exceed 600 mg daily. Should signs of withdrawal occur on the first day of treatment, a loading dose of 200 mg of phenobarbital may be administered IM, and the daily oral dosage increased. After stabilization with phenobarbital is achieved, the total daily dose of phenobarbital is decreased by 30 mg a day as long as withdrawal is proceeding smoothly. An alternative method of treatment is to decrease the daily dosage of the barbiturate which the patient has been taking by 10 percent/day, if tolerated by the patient.

Infants physically dependent on barbiturates may be given phenobarbital 3 to 10 mg/kg/day. After withdrawal symptoms (hyperactivity, disturbed sleep, tremors, hyperreflexia) are relieved, the dosage of phenobarbital should be gradually decreased and completely withdrawn over a 2-week period.

Overdosage: The toxic dose of barbiturates varies considerably. In general, an oral dose of 1 gram of most barbiturates produces serious poisoning in an adult. Death commonly occurs after ingestion of 2 to 10 grams of barbiturate. Barbiturate intoxication may be confused with alcoholism, bromide intoxication and with various neurological disorders.

Acute overdosage with barbiturates is manifested by CNS and respiratory depression which may progress to Cheyne-Stokes respiration, areflexia, constriction of the pupils to a slight degree (though in severe poisoning they may show paralytic dilation), oliguria, tachycardia, hypotension, lowered body temperature and coma. Typical shock syndrome (apnea, circulatory collapse, respiratory arrest and death) may occur.

In extreme overdose, all electrical activity in the brain may cease, in which case the EEG may be "flat," which does not necessarily indicate clinical death. This effect is fully reversible unless hypoxic damage occurs. Consideration should be given to the possibility of barbiturate intoxication even in situations that appear to involve trauma.

Complications such as pneumonia, pulmonary edema, cardiac arrhythmias, congestive heart failure and renal failure may occur. Uremia may increase CNS sensitivity to barbiturates if renal function is impaired. Differential diagnosis should include hypoglycemia, head trauma, cerebrovascular accidents, convulsive states and diabetic coma. Blood levels from acute overdosage for some barbiturates are listed in the accompanying table. [See table above].

Treatment of overdosage is mainly supportive and consists of the following:

Concentration of Barbiturate in the Blood Versus Degree of CNS Depression

Barbiturate	Onset/duration	Degree of depression in nontolerant persons*				
		1	2	3	4	5
		Barbiturate blood levels in ppm (mcg/ml)				
Pentobarbital	Fast/short	≤2	0.5 to 3	10 to 15	12 to 25	15 to 40
Secobarbital	Fast/short	≤2	0.5 to 5	10 to 15	15 to 25	15 to 40
Amobarbital	Intermediate/intermediate	≤3	2 to 10	30 to 40	30 to 60	40 to 80
Butabarbital	Intermediate/intermediate	≤5	3 to 25	40 to 60	50 to 80	60 to 100
Phenobarbital	Slow/long	≤10	5 to 40	50 to 80	70 to 120	100 to 200

*Categories of degree of depression in nontolerant persons:
1. Under the influence and appreciably impaired for purposes of driving a motor vehicle or performing tasks requiring alertness and unimpaired judgment and reaction time.
2. Sedated, therapeutic range, calm, relaxed, and easily aroused.
3. Comatose, difficult to arouse, significant depression of respiration.
4. Compatible with death in aged or ill persons or in presence of obstructed airway, other toxic agents, or exposure to cold.
5. Usual lethal level, the upper end of the range includes those who received some supportive treatment.

1. Maintenance of an adequate airway, with assisted respiration and oxygen administration as necessary.
2. Monitoring of vital signs and fluid balance.
3. If the patient is conscious and has not lost the gag reflex, emesis may be induced with ipecac. Care should be taken to prevent pulmonary aspiration of vomitus. After completion of vomiting, 30 grams activated charcoal, in a glass of water, may be administered.
4. If emesis is contraindicated, gastric lavage may be performed with a cuffed endotracheal tube in place with the patient in the face down position. Activated charcoal may be left in the emptied stomach and a saline cathartic administered.
5. Fluid therapy and other standard treatment for shock, if needed.
6. If renal function is normal, forced diuresis may aid in the elimination of the barbiturate. *Alkalinization of the urine increases renal excretion of some barbiturates, especially* phenobarbital, *aprobarbital* and mephobarbital (which is metabolized to phenobarbital).
7. Although not recommended as a routine procedure, hemodialysis may be used in severe barbiturate intoxication or if the patient is anuric or in shock.
8. Patient should be rolled from side to side every 30 minutes.
9. Antibiotics should be given if pneumonia is suspected.
10. Appropriate nursing care to prevent hypostatic pneumonia, decubiti, aspiration and other complications in patients with altered states of consciousness.

Dosage and Administration: *Usual Adult Dosage:* As a sedative, one 5-ml teaspoonful (40 mg) three times daily; for mild insomnia, one to two 5-ml teaspoonfuls before retiring; for pronounced insomnia, two to four 5-ml teaspoonfuls before retiring.

Special Patient Population: Dosage should be reduced in the elderly or debilitated because these patients may be more sensitive to barbiturates. Dosage should be reduced for patients with impaired renal function or hepatic disease.

How Supplied: Elixir (red) providing 40 mg of aprobarbital/Roche per 5 ml in a vehicle containing 20 percent alcohol — bottles of 16 oz (1 pint) (NDC 0004-1000-28).

ANCOBON®
[an'co-bon]
(flucytosine/Roche)

The following text is complete prescribing information based on official labeling in effect August 1, 1984.

WARNING
Use with extreme caution in patients with impaired renal function. Close monitoring of hematologic, renal and hepatic status of all patients is essential. These instructions should be thoroughly reviewed before administration of Ancobon.

Description: Flucytosine, an antifungal agent, is a fluorinated pyrimidine chemically related to fluorouracil and floxuridine. Chemically, it is 5-fluorocytosine, a white to off-white crystalline powder, with a molecular weight of 129.1.

Actions: Flucytosine has *in vitro* and *in vivo* activity against Candida and Cryptococcus. The exact mode of action against these fungi is not known. Ancobon is not metabolized significantly when given orally to man.

SUSCEPTIBILITY:

Cryptococcus: Most strains initially isolated from clinical material have shown flucytosine minimal inhibitory concentrations (MIC's) ranging from .46 to 7.8 mcg/ml. Any isolate with an MIC greater than 12.5 mcg/ml is considered resistant. *In vitro* resistance has developed in originally susceptible strains during therapy. It is recommended that clinical cultures for susceptibility testing be taken initially and at weekly intervals during therapy. The initial culture should be reserved as a reference in susceptibility testing of subsequent isolates.

Candida: As high as 40 to 50 percent of the pretreatment clinical isolates of Candida have been reported to be resistant to flucytosine. It is recommended that susceptibility studies be performed as early as possible and be repeated during therapy. An MIC value greater than 100 mcg/ml is considered resistant.

Interference with *in vitro* activity of flucytosine occurs in complex or semisynthetic media. In order to rely upon the recommended *in vitro* interpretations of susceptibility, it is essential that the broth medium and the testing procedure used be that described by Shadomy.[1]

Indications: Ancobon is indicated only in the treatment of serious infections caused by susceptible strains of Candida and/or Cryptococcus. Candida: septicemia, endocarditis and urinary system infections have been effectively treated with flucytosine. Limited trials in pulmonary infections justify the use of flucytosine. Cryptococcus: meningitis and pulmonary infections have been treated effectively. Studies in septicemias and urinary tract infections are limited, but good responses have been reported.

Contraindications: Patients with a known hypersensitivity to the drug.

Continued on next page

Roche Labs.—Cont.

Warnings: Ancobon must be given with extreme caution to patients with impaired renal function. Since Ancobon is excreted primarily by the kidneys, renal impairment may lead to accumulation of the drug. Assays for blood levels of Ancobon should be done in order to determine the adequacy of renal excretion in such patients.[1]

Ancobon must be given with extreme caution to patients with bone marrow depression. Patients may be more prone to depression of bone marrow function if they: 1) have a hematologic disease, 2) are being treated with radiation or drugs which depress bone marrow, or 3) have a history of treatment with such drugs or radiation. Frequent monitoring of hepatic function and of the hematopoietic system is indicated during therapy.

Usage in Pregnancy: Safe use of Ancobon in pregnancy has not been established. NOTE: Teratogenic effects have been seen in rats which metabolize flucytosine to fluorouracil. Use of Ancobon in pregnancy, lactation and in women of childbearing age requires that the potential benefits of therapy be weighed against its possible hazards.

Precautions: Before therapy with Ancobon is instituted, the hematologic and renal status of the patient should be determined (see WARNINGS), and close monitoring of the patient is essential. Liver enzyme levels (alkaline phosphatase, SGOT, SGPT) should be determined at frequent intervals during therapy, as indicated.

Adverse Reactions: Nausea, vomiting, diarrhea, rash, anemia, leukopenia, thrombopenia, and elevation of hepatic enzymes, BUN and creatinine have been reported. Less frequently reported were confusion, hallucinations, headache, sedation and vertigo.

Dosage and Administration: The usual dosage is 50 to 150 mg/kg/day at 6-hour intervals. Nausea or vomiting may be reduced or avoided if the capsules are given a few at a time over a 15-minute period. If the BUN or the serum creatinine is elevated, or if there are other signs of renal impairment, the initial dose should be at the lower level (see WARNINGS).

How Supplied: Capsules, containing 250 mg flucytosine/Roche, green and gray; containing 500 mg flucytosine/Roche, white and gray; bottles of 100.

Reference:
1. Shadomy, S.: *Appl. Microbiol.*, 17:871, 1969.

Shown in Product Identification Section, page 429

ARFONAD®
[ar'fo-nad] ℞
(trimethaphan camsylate/Roche)
Ampuls

The following text is complete prescribing information based on official labeling in effect August 1, 1984.

Description: A thiophanium derivative, Arfonad is a vasodepressor agent used for inducing controlled hypotension. Chemically, trimethaphan camsylate is (+)-1,3-dibenzyldecahydro-2-oxoimidazo[4,5-c]thieno [1,2-a]- thiolium 2-oxo-10-bornanesulfonate. It has a molecular weight of 596.80.

Arfonad is stable under refrigeration; it should not be frozen, to avoid ampul breakage which may result from ice formation. Each 10-ml ampul contains 500 mg trimethaphan camsylate/Roche compounded with 0.013% sodium acetate and pH adjusted to approximately 5.2 with hydrochloric acid.

Actions: Arfonad is primarily a ganglionic blocking agent. It blocks transmission in autonomic ganglia without producing any preceding or concomitant change in the membrane potentials of the ganglion cells. It does not modify the conduction of impulses in the preganglionic or postganglionic neurones and does not prevent the release of acetylcholine by preganglionic impulses. Arfonad produces ganglionic blockade by occupying receptor sites on the ganglion cells and by stabilizing the postsynaptic membranes against the action of acetylcholine liberated from the presynaptic nerve endings.

In addition to ganglionic blocking, Arfonad may also exert a direct peripheral vasodilator effect. By inducing vasodilation, it causes pooling of blood in the dependent periphery and the splanchnic system. The vasodilation results in a lowering of the blood pressure. Arfonad liberates histamine.

Indications: Arfonad is indicated for the production of controlled hypotension during surgery; for the short term (acute) control of blood pressure in hypertensive emergencies; in the emergency treatment of pulmonary edema in patients with pulmonary hypertension associated with systemic hypertension.

Contraindications: Arfonad is contraindicated in those conditions where hypotension may subject the patient to undue risk, e.g., uncorrected anemia, hypovolemia, shock (both incipient and frank), asphyxia, or uncorrected respiratory insufficiency. Inadequate availability of fluids and inability to replace blood for technical reasons may also constitute contraindications.

Warnings: Arfonad is a powerful hypotensive drug and should always be diluted before use. It is recommended that the use of Arfonad to produce hypotension in surgical or medical indications be limited to physicians with proper training in this technique. Adequate facilities, equipment and personnel should be available for vigilant monitoring of the circulation since Arfonad is an extremely potent hypotensive agent. Adequate oxygenation must be assured throughout the treatment period, especially in regard to coronary and cerebral circulation.

Arfonad should be used with extreme caution in patients with arteriosclerosis, cardiac disease, hepatic or renal disease, degenerative disease of the central nervous system, Addison's disease, diabetes and patients who are under treatment with steroids.

Usage in Pregnancy: Induced hypotension may have serious consequences upon the fetus.

Precautions: Arfonad should be used with care in patients who have been receiving antihypertensive drugs, since an additive hypotensive effect may occur. It should be used with caution with anesthetic agents, especially spinal anesthetics, which themselves may produce hypotension. Also, use with great caution in the elderly or debilitated, or in children. Because Arfonad liberates histamine, it should be used with caution in allergic individuals. Concomitant therapy with other drugs can modify materially the dose of Arfonad necessary to achieve the desired response.

Diuretic agents may enhance markedly the responses evoked by ganglionic-blocking drugs.
NOTE: Pupillary dilation does not necessarily indicate anoxia or the depth of anesthesia, since Arfonad appears to have a specific effect on the pupil.

Some animal studies indicate that aggressive dosage administration may result in respiratory arrest. Rare cases of respiratory arrest in humans have been reported, although a causal relationship has not been established. It is recommended that the patient's respiratory status be monitored closely, particularly if large doses of Arfonad are used.

Dosage and Administration: Arfonad must always be diluted and administered by intravenous infusion. Solutions should be freshly prepared and any unused portions discarded. For this purpose a 0.1 per cent (1 mg/ml) concentration of Arfonad in 5% Dextrose Injection USP should be employed. Use of other diluents is not recommended, since experience with them has not been reported. The infusion fluid used for administration of Arfonad should not be employed as a vehicle for the simultaneous administration of any other drugs. One (1) ampul of Arfonad—10 ml, 50 mg/ml—should be diluted to 500 ml. Since individual response varies, the rate of administration must be adjusted to the requirements of each patient.

The patient should be positioned so as to avoid cerebral anoxia and, when used in surgery, adequate anesthesia established. Intravenous drip with Arfonad is started at an average rate of 3 to 4 ml (3 to 4 mg) per minute (see chart below). The rate of administration is then adjusted to maintain the desired level of hypotension. Since there is a marked variation of individual response, **frequent blood pressure determinations are essential to maintain proper control.** Rates from as low as 0.3 ml (0.3 mg) per minute to rates exceeding 6 ml (6 mg) per minute have been found necessary in the experience of clinical investigators of Arfonad.

0.1% (1 mg/ml) CONCENTRATION OF ARFONAD

Delivery System Drops/ml	Drops/Min to Obtain 3–4 ml (3–4 mg) Arfonad
10	30–40
15	45–60
60	180–240

For surgical use, administration of Arfonad should be stopped prior to wound closure in order to permit blood pressure to return to normal. A systolic pressure of 100 mm will usually be attained within 10 minutes after stopping Arfonad.

Overdosage: Vasopressor agents may be used to correct undesirable low pressures during surgery or to effect a more rapid return to normotensive levels. Phenylephrine HCl or mephentermine sulfate should be tried initially and nonepinephrine should be reserved for refractory cases.

How Supplied: Ampuls, 10 ml, boxes of 10.

AZO GANTANOL® ℞
[a"zo gan'tan-ol]

The following text is complete prescribing information based on official labeling in effect August 1, 1984.

Composition: Each tablet contains 0.5 Gm sulfamethoxazole/Roche and 100 mg phenazopyridine hydrochloride.

Description: Azo Gantanol combines the antibacterial effectiveness of sulfamethoxazole/Roche (Gantanol®) with the local urinary analgesic activity of phenazopyridine hydrochloride.

Gantanol (sulfamethoxazole/Roche) is an intermediate-dosage sulfonamide. Sulfamethoxazole is an almost white, odorless, tasteless compound. Chemically, it is N^1-(5-methyl-3-isoxazolyl) sulfanilamide.

Phenazopyridine hydrochloride is a urinary analgesic. Chemically, it is 3-phenylazo-2,6-diaminopyridine hydrochloride.

Sulfonamides exist in the blood as free, conjugated (acetylated and possibly other forms) and protein-bound forms. The "free" form is considered to be the therapeutically active form. It has been shown that approximately 70 per cent of Gantanol is protein bound in the blood;[1] of the unbound portion 80 to 90 per cent is in the nonacetylated form.[2,3] Excretion of sulfonamides is chiefly by the kidneys with glomerular filtration as the primary mechanism.

Actions: The systemic sulfonamides are bacteriostatic agents. The spectrum of activity is similar for all. Sulfonamides competitively inhibit bacterial synthesis of folic acid (pteroylglutamic acid) from para-aminobenzoic acid. Resistant strains are capable of utilizing folic acid precursors or preformed folic acid.

Phenazopyridine hydrochloride has a specific analgesic effect in the urinary tract, promptly relieving pain and burning.

Indications: For the initial treatment of uncomplicated urinary tract infections caused by susceptible strains of the following microorganisms: *Escherichia coli, Klebsiella* species, *Enterobacter* species, *Proteus mirabilis, Proteus vulgaris* and *Staphylococcus aureus* when relief of symptoms of pain, burning or urgency is needed during the first 2 days of therapy. Treatment with Azo Gantanol should not exceed 2 days. There is a lack of evidence that the combination of sulfamethoxazole and phenazopyridine hydrochloride provides greater benefit than sulfamethoxazole alone after 2 days. Treatment beyond 2 days should only be continued with Gantanol (sulfamethoxazole/Roche). (See DOSAGE AND ADMINISTRATION section.)

Important note. In vitro sulfonamide sensitivity tests are not always reliable. The test must be carefully coordinated with bacteriologic and clinical response. When the patient is already taking sulfonamides, follow-up cultures should have aminobenzoic acid added to the culture media.

Currently, the increasing frequency of resistant organisms is a limitation of the usefulness of antibacterial agents including the sulfonamides.

Wide variation in blood levels may result with identical doses. Blood levels should be measured in patients receiving sulfonamides for serious infections. Free sulfonamide blood levels of 5 to 15 mg per 100 ml may be considered therapeutically effective for most infections, with blood levels of 12 to 15 mg per 100 ml optimal for serious infections; 20 mg per 100 ml should be the maximum total sulfonamide level, as adverse reactions occur more frequently above this level.

Contraindications: Children below age 12. Hypersensitivity to sulfonamides. Pregnancy at term and during the nursing period, because sulfonamides pass the placenta and are excreted in the milk and may cause kernicterus.

Because Azo Gantanol contains phenazopyridine hydrochloride it is contraindicated in glomerulonephritis, severe hepatitis, uremia, and pyelonephritis of pregnancy with gastrointestinal disturbances.

Warnings: *Usage in Pregnancy:* The safe use of sulfonamides in pregnancy has not been established. The teratogenicity potential of most sulfonamides has not been thoroughly investigated in either animals or humans. However, a significant increase in the incidence of cleft palate and other bony abnormalities of offspring has been observed when certain sulfonamides of the short, intermediate and long-acting types were given to pregnant rats and mice at high oral doses (7 to 25 times the human therapeutic dose).

Deaths associated with the administration of sulfonamides have been reported from hypersensitivity reactions, hepatocellular necrosis, agranulocytosis, aplastic anemia and other blood dyscrasias. The presence of clinical signs such as sore throat, fever, pallor, purpura or jaundice may be early indications of serious blood disorders. Complete blood counts should be done frequently in patients receiving sulfonamides.

The frequency of renal complications is considerably lower in patients receiving the more soluble sulfonamides. Urinalysis with careful microscopic examination should be obtained frequently in patients receiving sulfonamides.

Precautions: Sulfonamides should be given with caution to patients with impaired renal or hepatic function and to those with severe allergy or bronchial asthma. In glucose-6-phosphate dehydrogenase-deficient individuals, hemolysis may occur. This reaction is frequently dose-related. Adequate fluid intake must be maintained in order to prevent crystalluria and stone formation.

Carcinogenesis: Azo Gantanol has not undergone adequate trials relating to carcinogenicity; each component, however, has been evaluated separately. Rats appear to be especially susceptible to the goitrogenic effects of sulfonamides, and long-term administration of sulfonamides has resulted in thyroid malignancies in this species. Long-term administration of phenazopyridine hydrochloride has induced neoplasia in rats (large intestine) and mice (liver). Although no association between phenazopyridine hydrochloride and human neoplasia has been reported, adequate epidemiological studies have not been conducted.

Adverse Reactions: *Blood dyscrasias:* Agranulocytosis, aplastic anemia, thrombocytopenia, leukopenia, hemolytic anemia, purpura, hypoprothrombinemia and methemoglobinemia.

Allergic reactions: Erythema multiforme (Stevens-Johnson syndrome), generalized skin eruptions, epidermal necrolysis, urticaria, serum sickness, pruritus, exfoliative dermatitis, anaphylactoid reactions, periorbital edema, conjunctival and scleral injection, photosensitization, arthralgia and allergic myocarditis.

Gastrointestinal reactions: Nausea, emesis, abdominal pains, hepatitis, hepatocellular necrosis, diarrhea, anorexia, pancreatitis and stomatitis.

C.N.S. reactions: Headache, peripheral neuritis, mental depression, convulsions, ataxia, hallucinations, tinnitus, vertigo and insomnia.

Miscellaneous reactions: Drug fever, chills, and toxic nephrosis with oliguria and anuria. Polyarteritis nodosa and L.E. phenomenon have occurred. The sulfonamides bear certain chemical similarities to some goitrogens, diuretics (acetazolamide and the thiazides) and oral hypoglycemic agents. Goiter production, diuresis and hypoglycemia have occurred rarely in patients receiving sulfonamides. Cross-sensitivity may exist with these agents.

Dosage and Administration: Azo Gantanol is intended for the acute, painful phase of urinary tract infections. The usual dosage in adults is 4 tablets initially followed by 2 tablets morning and evening for up to 2 days. Treatment with Azo Gantanol should not exceed 2 days. Treatment beyond 2 days should only be continued with Gantanol (sulfamethoxazole/Roche).

NOTE: Patients should be told that the orange-red dye (phenazopyridine HCl) will color the urine soon after ingestion of the medication.

How Supplied: Tablets, red, film-coated, each containing 0.5 Gm sulfamethoxazole/Roche and 100 mg phenazopyridine HCl—bottles of 100 and 500.

References:
1. Struller, T.: *Antibiot. Chemother.*, *14:* 179, 1968.
2. Boger, W. P., and Gavin, J. J.: *Antibiotics and Chemother.*, *10:*572, 1960.
3. Brandman, O., and Engelberg, R.: *Curr. Therap. Res.*, *2:*364, 1960.

Shown in Product Identification Section, page 429

AZO GANTRISIN® R
[a″zo gan′tris-in]

The following text is complete prescribing information based on official labeling in effect August 1, 1984.

Description: Azo Gantrisin is a combination containing 0.5 Gm of the antibacterial sulfisoxazole/Roche and 50 mg of the urinary analgesic phenazopyridine hydrochloride per tablet for oral administration.

Gantrisin® (sulfisoxazole/Roche), a rapid-acting sulfonamide, is N^1-(3,4-dimethyl-5-isoxazolyl)sulfanilamide. It is a white to slightly yellowish, odorless, slighty bitter, crystalline powder which is soluble in alcohol and very slightly soluble in water. Sulfisoxazole has an empirical formula of $C_{11}H_{13}N_3O_3S$, and a molecular weight of 267.30. Phenazopyridine hydrochloride, a local urinary analgesic, is 2,6-diamino-3-(phenylazo)-pyridine monohydrochloride. It is a light or dark red to dark violet, odorless, slightly bitter, crystalline powder with an empirical formula of $C_{11}H_{11}N_5 \cdot HCl$, and a molecular weight of 249.70.

Clinical Pharmacology: An oral dose of sulfisoxazole is rapidly and completely absorbed. Sulfonamides are present in the blood as free, conjugated (acetylated and possibly other forms) and protein-bound forms. The amount present as "free" drug is considered to be the therapeutically active form. Approximately 85% of a dose of sulfisoxazole is bound to plasma proteins.

Following a single 2.0-Gm dose of sulfisoxazole, the mean time of peak plasma concentration was 2.5 hours; the mean peak plasma concentration was 169 μg/ml, ranging from 127 to 211 μg/ml. Of the 97% of the original dose excreted in the urine within 0 to 48 hours, 52% was free sulfisoxazole and 45% was the metabolite N^4-acetyl sulfisoxazole. The mean elimination half-life was 5.8 hours, ranging from 4.6 to 7.8 hours.

Sulfonamides are excreted primarily by the kidneys through glomerular filtration. The drug diffuses across the placenta into the fetus and crosses the blood-brain barrier.

Phenazopyridine hydrochloride has a specific local analgesic effect in the urinary tract, promptly relieving pain and burning. No pharmacokinetic data are available on this drug.

Microbiology: The systemic sulfonamides are bacteriostatic agents. The spectrum of activity is similar for all. Sulfonamides competitively inhibit bacterial synthesis of folic acid (pteroylglutamic acid) from *para*-aminobenzoic acid. Resistant strains are capable of utilizing folic acid precursors or preformed folic acid.

Indications: For the initial treatment of uncomplicated urinary tract infections caused by susceptible strains of the following microorganisms: *Escherichia coli*, *Klebsiella* species, *Enterobacter* species, *Proteus mirabilis*, *Proteus vulgaris* and *Staphylococcus aureus* when relief of symptoms of pain, burning or urgency is needed during the first 2 days of therapy. Treatment with Azo Gantrisin should not exceed 2 days. There is a lack of evidence that the combination of sulfisoxazole and phenazopyridine hydrochloride provides greater benefit than sulfisoxazole alone after 2 days. Treatment beyond 2 days should only be continued with Gantrisin (sulfisoxazole/Roche). (See DOSAGE AND ADMINISTRATION section.)

Important Note: In vitro sensitivity tests for sulfonamides are not always reliable, and must be carefully coordinated with bacteriologic and clinical response. When the patient is already taking sulfonamides, follow-up cultures should have aminobenzoic acid added to the culture media.

Currently, the increasing frequency of resistant organisms is a limitation of the usefulness of antibacterial agents, including the sulfonamides.

Wide variation in blood levels may result with identical doses of a sulfonamide. Blood levels should be measured in patients receiving these drugs for serious infections. Free sulfonamide blood levels of 5 to 15 mg/100 ml may be considered therapeutically effective for most infections, with blood levels of 12 to 15 mg/100 ml being optimal for serious infections. The maximum sulfonamide level should be 20 mg/100 ml, since adverse reactions occur more frequently above this concentration.

Contraindications: Azo Gantrisin is contraindicated in patients with a known sensitivity to either of its components; in children younger than 12 years; and in pregnancy *at term* and during the nursing period, because sulfonamides pass the placenta and are excreted in the milk and may cause kernicterus.

Azo Gantrisin, because it contains phenazopyridine hydrochloride, is also contraindicated in glomerulonephritis, severe hepatitis, uremia, and pyelonephritis of pregnancy with gastrointestinal disturbances.

Warnings: Sulfonamides are bacteriostatic and resistance is frequent in organisms responsible for common infections. Sulfa drugs will not eradicate group A streptococci and have not been demonstrated, in these infections, to prevent sequelae such as rheumatic fever and glomerulonephritis. Deaths associated with the administration of sulfonamides have been reported from hypersensitivity reactions, hepatocellular necrosis, agranulocytosis, aplastic anemia and other blood dyscrasias. The presence of clinical signs such as sore throat, fever, pallor, purpura or jaundice may be early indications of serious blood disorders. Blood counts and renal function tests are recommended during treatment.

Precautions: *General:* Sulfonamides should be given with caution to patients with impaired renal or hepatic function and to those with severe allergy or bronchial asthma. In glucose-6-phosphate dehydrogenase-deficient individuals, hemolysis may occur; this reaction is frequently dose-related. The frequency of renal complications is considerably lower in patients receiving the more soluble sulfonamides. Adequate fluid intake must be maintained in order to prevent crystalluria and stone formation.

Continued on next page

Roche Labs.—Cont.

Information for Patients: Patients should maintain an adequate fluid intake. Patients should also be told that soon after ingestion of this medication, the phenazopyridine HCl component will produce reddish-orange discoloration of the urine.

Laboratory Tests: Urinalysis with careful microscopic examination should be performed at least once a week for patients receiving sulfonamides. Blood counts should be performed regularly in patients receiving sulfonamide therapy for longer than two weeks. Blood levels of a sulfonamide should be measured in patients receiving these drugs for serious infection (see INDICATIONS section).

Drug Interactions: It has been reported that some sulfonamides may displace oral anticoagulants from plasma protein binding sites and thereby increase the anticoagulant effect. Sulfonamides can also displace methotrexate from plasma protein binding sites.

Drug/Laboratory Test Interactions: Both components of Azo Gantrisin have been reported to affect results of liver function tests in isolated cases of hepatitis.

Carcinogenesis, Mutagenesis, Impairment of Fertility:
Carcinogenesis: Azo Gantrisin has not undergone adequate trials relating to carcinogenicity; each component, however, has been evaluated separately. Rats appear to be especially susceptible to the goitrogenic effects of sulfonamides, and long-term administration of sulfonamides has resulted in thyroid malignancies in this species. Long-term administration of phenazopyridine hydrochloride has induced neoplasia in rats (large intestine) and mice (liver). Although no association between phenazopyridine hydrochloride and human neoplasia has been reported, adequate epidemiological studies have not been conducted.
Mutagenesis: There are no studies available that evaluate the mutagenic potential of Azo Gantrisin or either of its components.
Impairment of Fertility: Azo Gantrisin has not undergone adequate trials relating to impairment of fertility; each component, however, has been studied in laboratory animals. In a reproduction study of rats given 800 mg/kg/day sulfisoxazole, no effects were observed regarding mating behavior, conception rate or fertility index (percent pregnant). No effects on fertility were demonstrated in a two-litter reproduction study of rats given 50 mg/kg/day phenazopyridine.

Pregnancy:
Teratogenic Effects: Pregnancy Category C. Each component of Azo Gantrisin has been evaluated in reproduction studies in laboratory animals. At dosages of 800 mg/kg/day, sulfisoxazole was not teratogenic in either rats or rabbits, and had no perinatal or postnatal effects in rats. However, in two other teratogenicity studies, cleft palates developed in both rats and mice after administration of 500 to 1000 mg/kg/day sulfisoxazole (8 to 16 times the therapeutic dose for an individual weighing 143 lbs). In regard to phenazopyridine, no congenital malformations developed in rats given 50 mg/kg/day.
There are no adequate or well-controlled studies of Azo Gantrisin in either laboratory animals or in pregnant women. It is not known whether Azo Gantrisin can cause fetal harm when administered to a pregnant woman or can affect reproduction capacity. Azo Gantrisin should be used during pregnancy only if the potential benefit justifies the potential risk to the fetus.
Nonteratogenic Effects: See **Contraindications** section.

Nursing Mothers: See **Contraindications** section.

Pediatric Use: See **Contraindications** section.

Adverse Reactions: Included in the listing that follows are adverse reactions that have not been reported with this specific drug; however, the pharmacologic similarities among the sulfonamides require that each of the reactions be considered with Azo Gantrisin administration.

Allergic: Anaphylaxis, generalized allergic reactions, angioneurotic edema, arteritis and vasculitis, myocarditis, serum sickness, conjunctival and scleral injection. In addition, periarteritis nodosa and systemic lupus erythematosus have been reported.

Cardiovascular: Tachycardia, palpitations, syncope and cyanosis.

Dermatologic: Rash, urticaria, pruritus, erythema multiforme, Stevens-Johnson syndrome, toxic epidermal necrolysis, exfoliative dermatitis and photosensitivity.

Endocrine: The sulfonamides bear certain chemical similarities to some goitrogens, diuretics (acetazolamide and the thiazides) and oral hypoglycemic agents. Cross-sensitivity may exist with these agents. Goiter production, diuresis and hypoglycemia have occurred rarely in patients receiving sulfonamides.

Gastrointestinal: Nausea, emesis, abdominal pain, anorexia, diarrhea, glossitis, stomatitis, flatulence, salivary gland enlargement, G.I. hemorrhage, pseudomembranous enterocolitis, melena and pancreatitis. Hepatic dysfunction, jaundice and hepatocellular necrosis have also been reported following the use of sulfonamides.

Genitourinary: Crystalluria, hematuria, BUN and creatinine elevation, nephritis and toxic nephrosis with oliguria and anuria. Acute renal failure and urinary retention have also been reported.

Hematologic: Leukopenia, agranulocytosis, aplastic anemia, thrombocytopenia, purpura, hemolytic anemia, anemia, eosinophilia, clotting disorders including hypoprothrombinemia and hypofibrinogenemia, sulfhemoglobinemia and methemoglobinemia.

Musculoskeletal: Arthralgia, chest pain and myalgia.

Neurologic: Headache, dizziness, peripheral neuritis, paresthesia, convulsions, tinnitus, vertigo, ataxia and intracranial hypertension.

Psychiatric: Psychosis, hallucinations, disorientation, depression and anxiety.

Miscellaneous: Edema (including periorbital), pyrexia, drowsiness, weakness, fatigue, lassitude, rigors, flushing, hearing loss, insomnia and pneumonitis.

Overdosage: Signs and symptoms of overdosage with Azo Gantrisin include anorexia, colic, nausea, vomiting, dizziness, drowsiness, and even unconsciousness. Pyrexia, hematuria and crystalluria may be noted. Blood dyscrasias and jaundice are potential late manifestations of overdosage.
General principles of treatment include instituting gastric lavage or emesis; forcing oral fluids; and administering intravenous fluids if urine output is low and renal function is normal. The patient should be monitored with blood counts and appropriate blood chemistries, including electrolytes. If the patient becomes cyanotic, the possibility of methemoglobinemia should be considered and, if present, the condition should be treated appropriately with intravenous 1% methylene blue. If a significant blood dyscrasia or jaundice occurs, specific therapy should be instituted for these complications.
The oral LD_{50} of Azo Gantrisin in mice is 4317 mg/kg.

Dosage and Administration: Azo Gantrisin is intended for the acute, painful phase of urinary tract infections. The recommended dosage in adults is 4 to 6 tablets initially, followed by 2 tablets four times daily for up to 2 days. Treatment with Azo Gantrisin should not exceed 2 days. Treatment beyond 2 days should only be continued with Gantrisin (sulfisoxazole/Roche).

How Supplied: Each red, film-coated tablet contains 0.5 Gm sulfisoxazole/Roche and 50 mg phenazopyridine HCl. Azo Gantrisin is available in bottles of 100 tablets (NDC-0004-0012-01) and 500 tablets (NDC-0004-0012-14).
Imprint on tablets: AZO GANTRISIN® ROCHE.
Shown in Product Identification Section, page 429

BACTRIM™ I.V. INFUSION ℞
[*bac' trim*]
(trimethoprim and sulfamethoxazole/Roche)

The following text is complete prescribing information based on official labeling in effect August 1, 1984.

Description: Bactrim I.V. Infusion, a sterile solution for intravenous infusion only, is a synthetic antibacterial combination product. Each 5 ml contains 80 mg trimethoprim (16 mg/ml) and 400 mg sulfamethoxazole (80 mg/ml) compounded with 40% propylene glycol, 10% ethyl alcohol and 0.3% diethanolamine; 1% benzyl alcohol and 0.1% sodium metabisulfite as preservatives; water for injection; and pH adjusted to approximately 10 with sodium hydroxide.
Trimethoprim is 2,4-diamino-5-(3,4,5-trimethoxybenzyl)pyrimidine. It is a white to light yellow, odorless, bitter compound with a molecular weight of 290.3.
Sulfamethoxazole is N^1-(5-methyl-3-isoxazolyl) sulfanilamide. It is an almost white in color, odorless, tasteless compound with a molecular weight of 253.28.

Clinical Pharmacology: Following a one-hour intravenous infusion of a single dose of 160 mg trimethoprim plus 800 mg sulfamethoxazole to 11 patients whose weight ranged from 105 lb to 165 lb (mean, 143 lb), the mean plasma concentrations of trimethoprim and sulfamethoxazole were 3.4 ± 0.3 μg/ml and 46.3 ± 2.7 μg/ml, respectively. Following repeated intravenous administration of the same dose at eight-hour intervals, the mean plasma concentrations just prior to and immediately after each infusion at steady state were 5.6 ± 0.6 μg/ml and 8.8 ± 0.9 μg/ml for trimethoprim and 70.6 ± 7.3 μg/ml and 105.6 ± 10.9 μg/ml for sulfamethoxazole. The mean plasma half-life was 11.3 ± 0.7 hours for trimethoprim and 12.8 ± 1.8 hours for sulfamethoxazole. All of these 11 patients had normal renal function, and their ages ranged from 17 to 78 years (median, 60 years).[1]
Pharmacokinetic studies in children and adults suggest an age-dependent half-life of trimethoprim, as indicated in the following table.[2]

Age (years)	No. of Patients	Mean TMP Half-life (hours)
<1	2	7.67
1-10	9	5.49
10-20	5	8.19
20-63	6	12.82

Sulfamethoxazole exists in the blood as free, conjugated and protein-bound forms; trimethoprim is present as free and protein-bound and metabolized forms. The free forms are considered to be the therapeutically active forms. Approximately 44 percent of trimethoprim and 70 percent of sulfamethoxazole are protein-bound in blood. The presence of 10 mg percent sulfamethoxazole in plasma decreases the protein binding of trimethoprim to an insignificant degree; trimethoprim does not influence the protein binding of sulfamethoxazole.
Excretion of Bactrim is chiefly by the kidneys through both glomerular filtration and tubular secretion. Urine concentrations of both sulfamethoxazole and trimethoprim are considerably higher than are concentrations in the blood. When administered together as in Bactrim, neither sulfamethoxazole nor trimethoprim affects the urinary excretion pattern of the other.

Microbiology:
Sulfamethoxazole inhibits bacterial synthesis of dihydrofolic acid by competing with *para*-aminobenzoic acid. Trimethoprim blocks the production of tetrahydrofolic acid from dihydrofolic acid by binding to and reversibly inhibiting the required enzyme, dihydrofolate reductase. Thus, Bactrim blocks two consecutive steps in the biosynthesis of nucleic acids and proteins essential to many bacteria.
In vitro studies have shown that bacterial resistance develops more slowly with Bactrim than with trimethoprim or sulfamethoxazole alone.

In vitro serial dilution tests have shown that the spectrum of antibacterial activity of Bactrim includes common bacterial pathogens with the exception of *Pseudomonas aeruginosa*. The following organisms are usually susceptible: *Escherichia coli, Klebsiella-Enterobacter, Proteus mirabilis*, indole-positive *Proteus* species, *Haemophilus influenzae* (including ampicillin-resistant strains), *Streptococcus pneumoniae, Shigella flexneri* and *Shigella sonnei*. It should be noted, however, that there are little clinical data on the use of intravenous Bactrim in serious systemic infections due to *H. influenzae* and *S. pneumoniae*.
[See table right].

The recommended quantitative disc susceptibility method may be used for estimating the susceptibility of bacteria to Bactrim.[3,4] With this procedure, a report from the laboratory of "Susceptible to trimethoprim-sulfamethoxazole" indicates that the infection is likely to respond to therapy with Bactrim. If the infection is confined to the urine, a report of "Intermediate susceptibility to trimethoprim-sulfamethoxazole" also indicates that the infection is likely to respond to therapy with Bactrim. A report of "Resistant to trimethoprim-sulfamethoxazole" indicates that the infection is unlikely to respond to therapy with Bactrim.

Indications and Usage:
PNEUMOCYSTIS CARINII PNEUMONITIS: Bactrim I.V. Infusion is indicated in the treatment of *Pneumocystis carinii* pneumonitis in children and adults.

SHIGELLOSIS: Bactrim I.V. Infusion is indicated in the treatment of enteritis caused by susceptible strains of *Shigella flexneri* and *Shigella sonnei* in children and adults.

URINARY TRACT INFECTIONS: Bactrim I.V. Infusion is indicated in the treatment of severe or complicated urinary tract infections due to susceptible strains of *Escherichia coli, Klebsiella-Enterobacter* and *Proteus* species when oral administration of Bactrim is not feasible and when the organism is not susceptible to single agent antibacterials effective in the urinary tract.

Although appropriate culture and susceptibility studies should be performed, therapy may be started while awaiting the results of these studies.

Contraindications:
Hypersensitivity to trimethoprim or sulfonamides. Documented megaloblastic anemia due to folate deficiency.

Pregnancy at term and during the nursing period, because sulfonamides pass the placenta and are excreted in the milk and may cause kernicterus. Infants less than two months of age.

Warnings:
BACTRIM I.V. INFUSION SHOULD NOT BE USED IN THE TREATMENT OF STREPTOCOCCAL PHARYNGITIS. Clinical studies have documented that patients with group A β-hemolytic streptococcal tonsillopharyngitis have a greater incidence of bacteriologic failure when treated with Bactrim than do those patients treated with penicillin, as evidenced by failure to eradicate this organism from the tonsillopharyngeal area.

Deaths associated with the administration of sulfonamides have been reported from hypersensitivity reactions, hepatocellular necrosis, agranulocytosis, aplastic anemia and other blood dyscrasias. Experience with trimethoprim alone is much more limited, but it has been reported to interfere with hematopoiesis in occasional patients. In elderly patients concurrently receiving certain diuretics, primarily thiazides, an increased incidence of thrombopenia with purpura has been reported.

The presence of clinical signs such as sore throat, fever, pallor, purpura or jaundice may be early indications of serious blood disorders.

Precautions:
i) *General:* Bactrim should be given with caution to patients with impaired renal or hepatic function, to those with possible folate deficiency and to those with severe allergy or bronchial asthma. In glucose-6-phosphate dehydrogenase-deficient individuals, hemolysis may occur. This reaction is frequently dose-related. Adequate fluid intake must be maintained in order to prevent crystalluria and stone formation.

REPRESENTATIVE MINIMUM INHIBITORY CONCENTRATION VALUES FOR BACTRIM-SUSCEPTIBLE ORGANISMS (MIC—μg/ml)

Bacteria	Trimethoprim alone	Sulfamethoxazole alone	TMP/SMX (1:20) TMP	TMP/SMX (1:20) SMX
Escherichia coli	0.05 – 1.5	1.0 – 245	0.05 – 0.5	0.95 – 9.5
Proteus spp. indole positive	0.5 – 5.0	7.35 – 300	0.05 – 1.5	0.95 – 28.5
Proteus mirabilis	0.5 – 1.5	7.35 – 30	0.05 – 0.15	0.95 – 2.85
Klebsiella-Enterobacter	0.15 – 5.0	2.45 – 245	0.05 – 1.5	0.95 – 28.5
Haemophilus influenzae	0.15 – 1.5	2.85 – 95	0.015 – 0.15	0.285 – 2.85
Streptococcus pneumoniae	0.15 – 1.5	7.35 – 24.5	0.05 – 0.15	0.95 – 2.85
Shigella flexneri	<0.01 – 0.04	<0.16 – >320	<0.002 – 0.03	0.04 – 0.625
Shigella sonnei	0.02 – 0.03	0.625 – >320	0.004 – 0.06	0.08 – 1.25

Local irritation and inflammation due to extravascular infiltration of the infusion have been observed. If these occur, the infusion should be discontinued and restarted at another site.

ii) *Laboratory tests:* Appropriate culture and susceptibility studies should be performed before and throughout treatment. Complete blood counts should be done frequently in patients receiving Bactrim. If a significant reduction in the count of any formed blood element is noted, Bactrim should be discontinued. Urinalyses with careful microscopic examination and renal function tests should be performed during therapy, particularly for those patients with impaired renal function.

iii) *Drug interactions:* It has been reported that Bactrim may prolong the prothrombin time in patients who are receiving the anticoagulant warfarin. This interaction should be kept in mind when Bactrim is given to patients already on anticoagulant therapy, and the coagulation time should be reassessed.

iv) *Carcinogenesis, mutagenesis, impairment of fertility:*
Carcinogenesis: Long-term studies in animals to evaluate carcinogenic potential have not been conducted with Bactrim I.V. Infusion.
Mutagenesis: Bacterial mutagenic studies have not been performed with sulfamethoxazole and trimethoprim in combination. Trimethoprim was demonstrated to be nonmutagenic in the Ames assay. No chromosomal damage was observed in human leukocytes cultured *in vitro* with sulfamethoxazole and trimethoprim alone or in combination; the concentrations used exceeded blood levels of these compounds following therapy with Bactrim. Observations of leukocytes obtained from patients treated with Bactrim revealed no chromosomal abnormalities.
Impairment of Fertility: Bactrim I.V. Infusion has not been studied in animals for evidence of impairment of fertility. However, studies in rats at oral dosages as high as 70 mg/kg trimethoprim plus 350 mg/kg sulfamethoxazole daily showed no adverse effects on fertility or general reproductive performance.

v) *Pregnancy:* Teratogenic Effects: Pregnancy Category C. In rats, oral doses of 533 mg/kg sulfamethoxazole or 200 mg/kg trimethoprim produced teratological effects manifested mainly as cleft palates. The highest dose which did not cause cleft palates in rats was 512 mg/kg sulfamethoxazole or 192 mg/kg trimethoprim when administered separately. In two studies in rats, no teratology was observed when 512 mg/kg of sulfamethoxazole was used in combination with 128 mg/kg of trimethoprim. However, in one study, cleft palates were observed in one litter out of nine when 355 mg/kg of sulfamethoxazole was used in combination with 88 mg/kg of trimethoprim.

In some rabbit studies, an overall increase in fetal loss (dead and resorbed and malformed conceptuses) was associated with doses of trimethoprim six times the human therapeutic dose.

While there are no large, well-controlled studies on the use of trimethoprim plus sulfamethoxazole in pregnant women, Brumfitt and Pursell[5] reported the outcome of 186 pregnancies during which the mother received either placebo or oral trimethoprim in combination with sulfamethoxazole.

The incidence of congenital abnormalities was 4.5% (3 of 66) in those who received placebo and 3.3% (4 of 120) in those receiving trimethoprim plus sulfamethoxazole. There were no abnormalities in the 10 children whose mothers received the drug during the first trimester. In a separate survey, Brumfitt and Pursell also found no congenital abnormalities in 35 children whose mothers had received oral trimethoprim plus sulfamethoxazole at the time of conception or shortly thereafter.

Because trimethoprim plus sulfamethoxazole may interfere with folic acid metabolism, Bactrim I.V. Infusion should be used during pregnancy only if the potential benefit justifies the potential risk to the fetus.

Nonteratogenic Effects: See "CONTRAINDICATIONS" section.

vi) *Nursing mothers:* See "CONTRAINDICATIONS" section.

Adverse Reactions:
The most frequently reported adverse reactions to Bactrim I.V. Infusion are nausea and vomiting, thrombocytopenia and rash. These occur in less than one-twentieth of patients. Local reaction, pain and slight irritation on I.V. administration are infrequent; thrombophlebitis has been observed rarely.

For completeness, all major reactions to sulfonamides and to trimethoprim are included below, even though they may not have been reported with Bactrim I.V. Infusion.

Allergic Reactions: Generalized skin eruptions, pruritus, urticaria, erythema multiforme, Stevens-Johnson syndrome, epidermal necrolysis, serum sickness, exfoliative dermatitis, anaphylactoid reactions, periorbital edema, conjunctival and scleral injection, photosensitization, arthralgia and allergic myocarditis.

Blood Dyscrasias: Megaloblastic anemia, hemolytic anemia, purpura, thrombocytopenia, leukopenia, agranulocytosis, aplastic anemia, hypoprothrombinemia and methemoglobinemia.

Gastrointestinal Reactions: Glossitis, stomatitis, nausea, emesis, abdominal pains, hepatitis, hepatocellular necrosis, diarrhea, pseudomembranous colitis and pancreatitis.

C.N.S. Reactions: Headache, peripheral neuritis, mental depression, ataxia, convulsions, hallucinations, tinnitus, vertigo, insomnia, apathy, fatigue, muscle weakness and nervousness.

Continued on next page

Roche Labs.—Cont.

Miscellaneous Reactions: Drug fever, chills, and toxic nephrosis with oliguria and anuria. Periarteritis nodosa and L.E. phenomenon have occurred. The sulfonamides bear certain chemical similarities to some goitrogens, diuretics (acetazolamide and the thiazides) and oral hypoglycemic agents. Cross-sensitivity may exist with these agents. Diuresis and hypoglycemia have occurred rarely in patients receiving sulfonamides.

Overdosage: Since there has been no extensive experience in humans with single doses of Bactrim I.V. Infusion in excess of 25 ml (400 mg trimethoprim and 2000 mg sulfamethoxazole), the maximum tolerated dose in humans is unknown.

Use of Bactrim I.V. Infusion at high doses and/or for extended periods of time may cause bone marrow depression manifested as thrombocytopenia, leukopenia and/or megaloblastic anemia. If signs of bone marrow depression occur, the patient should be given leucovorin 3 to 6 mg intramuscularly daily for three days, or as required to restore normal hematopoiesis.

Peritoneal dialysis is not effective and hemodialysis is only moderately effective in eliminating trimethoprim and sulfamethoxazole.

The Bactrim I.V. Infusion LD_{50} in mice is 700 mg/kg or 7.3 ml/kg; in rats and rabbits the LD_{50} is > 500 mg/kg or > 5.2 ml/kg. The vehicle produced the same LD_{50} in each of these species as the active drug.

The signs and symptoms noted in mice, rats and rabbits with Bactrim I.V. Infusion or its vehicle at the high I.V. doses used in acute toxicity studies included ataxia, decreased motor activity, loss of righting reflex, tremors or convulsions, and/or respiratory depression.

Dosage and Administration: CONTRAINDICATED IN INFANTS LESS THAN TWO MONTHS OF AGE. CAUTION—BACTRIM I.V. INFUSION MUST BE DILUTED IN 5% DEXTROSE IN WATER SOLUTION PRIOR TO ADMINISTRATION. DO NOT MIX BACTRIM I.V. INFUSION WITH OTHER DRUGS OR SOLUTIONS. RAPID INFUSION OR BOLUS INJECTION MUST BE AVOIDED.

Dosage:
Children and Adults:
Pneumocystis carinii Pneumonitis: Total daily dose is 15 to 20 mg/kg (based on the trimethoprim component), given in three or four equally divided doses q 6 to 8 hours for up to 14 days. One investigator noted that a total daily dose of 10 to 15 mg/kg was sufficient in ten adult patients with normal renal function.[6]

Severe Urinary Tract Infections and Shigellosis: Total daily dose is 8 to 10 mg/kg (based on the trimethoprim component), given in two to four equally divided doses q 6, 8 or 12 hours for up to 14 days for severe urinary tract infections and five days for shigellosis.

For Patients with Impaired Renal Function: When renal function is impaired, a reduced dosage should be employed using the following table:

Creatinine Clearance (ml/min)	Recommended Dosage Regimen
Above 30	Usual standard regimen
15-30	½ the usual regimen
Below 15	Use not recommended

Method of Preparation: Bactrim I.V. Infusion must be diluted. Each 5 ml should be added to 125 ml of 5% dextrose in water. After diluting with 5% dextrose in water, the solution should not be refrigerated and should be used within six hours. If upon visual inspection there is cloudiness or evidence of precipitation after mixing, the solution should be discarded and a fresh solution prepared.

The following infusion sets have been tested and found satisfactory: unit-dose glass containers (McGaw Laboratories, Cutter Laboratories, Inc., and Abbott Laboratories); unit-dose plastic containers (Viaflex from Travenol Laboratories and Accumed from McGaw Laboratories). No other systems have been tested and therefore no others can be recommended.

Dilution: EACH 5 ML OF BACTRIM I.V. INFUSION SHOULD BE ADDED TO 125 ML OF 5% DEXTROSE IN WATER.
NOTE: IN THOSE INSTANCES WHERE FLUID RESTRICTION IS DESIRABLE, each 5 ml may be added to 75 ml of 5% dextrose in water. Under these circumstances the solution should be mixed just prior to use and should be administered within two hours. If upon visual inspection there is cloudiness or evidence of crystallization after mixing, the solution should be discarded and a fresh solution prepared.
DO NOT MIX BACTRIM I.V. INFUSION – 5% DEXTROSE IN WATER WITH OTHER DRUGS OR SOLUTIONS.
Administration: The solution should be given by intravenous drip over a period of 60 to 90 minutes. Rapid infusion or bolus injection must be avoided. Bactrim I.V. Infusion should not be used intramuscularly.

How Supplied: 5-ml *ampuls,* containing 80 mg trimethoprim (16 mg/ml) and 400 mg sulfamethoxazole (80 mg/ml) for infusion with 5% dextrose in water. Boxes of 10 (NDC-0004-1943-06).
5-ml *vials,* containing 80 mg trimethoprim (16 mg/ml) and 400 mg sulfamethoxazole (80 mg/ml) for infusion with 5% dextrose in water. Boxes of 10 (NDC-0004-1956-01).
10-ml *vials,* containing 160 mg trimethoprim (16 mg/ml) and 800 mg sulfamethoxazole (80 mg/ml) for infusion with 5% dextrose in water. Boxes of 10 (NDC-0004-1955-01).
30-ml *multidose vials,* each 5 ml containing 80 mg trimethoprim (16 mg/ml) and 400 mg sulfamethoxazole (80 mg/ml) for infusion with 5% dextrose in water. Boxes of 1 (NDC-0004-1958-01).
STORE AT ROOM TEMPERATURE (15° – 30°C or 59° – 86°F). DO NOT REFRIGERATE.
Bactrim is also available as *DS (double strength) Tablets,* containing 160 mg trimethoprim and 800 mg sulfamethoxazole—bottles of 100 and 500; Tel-E-Dose® packages of 100; Prescription Paks of 20.
Tablets, containing 80 mg trimethoprim and 400 mg sulfamethoxazole—bottles of 100 and 500; Tel-E-Dose® packages of 100; Prescription Paks of 40.
Pediatric Suspension, containing 40 mg trimethoprim and 200 mg sulfamethoxazole per teaspoonful (5 ml); cherry flavored—bottles of 100 ml and 16 oz (1 pint).
Suspension, containing 40 mg trimethoprim and 200 mg sulfamethoxazole per teaspoonful (5 ml); fruit-licorice flavored—bottles of 16 oz (1 pint).

References:
1. Grose WE, Bodey GP, Loo TL: Clinical Pharmacology of Intravenously Administered Trimethoprim-Sulfamethoxazole. *Antimicrob Agents Chemother 15*:447-451, Mar 1979.
2. Siber GR, Gorham C, Durbin W, Lesko L, Levin MJ: Pharmacology of Intravenous Trimethoprim-Sulfamethoxazole in Children and Adults. *Current Chemotherapy and Infectious Diseases,* American Society for Microbiology, Washington, D.C., 1980, Vol. 1, pp. 691-692.
3. Bauer AW, Kirby WMM, Sherris JC, Turck M: Antibiotic Susceptibility Testing by a Standardized Single Disk Method. *Am J Clin Pathol 45*:493-496, Apr 1966.
4. Approved Standard ASM-2 Performance Standards for Antimicrobial Disc Susceptibility Test: National Committee for Clinical Laboratory Standards, 771 East Lancaster Avenue, Villanova, Pennsylvania 19085.
5. Brumfitt W and Pursell R: Trimethoprim/Sulfamethoxazole in the Treatment of Bacteriuria in Women. *J Infect Dis 128* (Suppl): S657-S663, Nov 1973.
6. Winston DJ, Lau WK, Gale RP, Young LS: Trimethoprim-Sulfamethoxazole for the Treatment of *Pneumocystis carinii* pneumonia. *Ann Intern Med 92*:762-769, June 1980.

BACTRIM™ ℞

[*bac′ trim*]
(trimethoprim and sulfamethoxazole/Roche)
Tablets, Suspension,
Pediatric Suspension,
DS (double strength) Tablets

The following text is complete prescribing information based on official labeling in effect August 1, 1984.

Description: Bactrim is a synthetic antibacterial combination product, available in DS (double strength), notched, capsule-shaped, white tablets, each containing 160 mg trimethoprim and 800 mg sulfamethoxazole; in scored, light-green tablets, each containing 80 mg trimethoprim and 400 mg sulfamethoxazole; as a pink, cherry-flavored pediatric suspension and as a pink, fruit-licorice flavored suspension, both forms containing in each teaspoonful (5 ml) 40 mg trimethoprim and 200 mg sulfamethoxazole, compounded with 0.3% alcohol. Trimethoprim is 2,4-diamino-5-(3,4,5-trimethoxybenzyl) pyrimidine. It is a white to light yellow, odorless, bitter compound with a molecular weight of 290.3.

Sulfamethoxazole is N^1-(5-methyl-3-isoxazolyl) sulfanilamide. It is an almost white in color, odorless, tasteless compound with a molecular weight of 253.28.

Actions: *Clinical Pharmacology:* Bactrim is rapidly absorbed following oral administration. The blood levels of trimethoprim and sulfamethoxazole are similar to those achieved when each component is given alone. Peak blood levels for the individual components occur one to four hours after oral administration. The half-lives of sulfamethoxazole (10 hours) and trimethoprim (8 to 10 hours) are relatively the same regardless of whether these compounds are administered as individual components or as Bactrim. Detectable amounts of trimethoprim and sulfamethoxazole are present in the blood 24 hours after drug administration. Free sulfamethoxazole and trimethoprim blood levels are proportionately dose-dependent. On repeated administration, the steady-state ratio of trimethoprim to sulfamethoxazole levels in the blood is about 1:20.

Sulfamethoxazole exists in the blood as free, conjugated and protein-bound forms; trimethoprim is present as free, protein-bound and metabolized forms. The free forms are considered to be the therapeutically active forms. Approximately 44 percent of trimethoprim and 70 percent of sulfamethoxazole are protein-bound in the blood. The presence of 10 mg percent sulfamethoxazole in plasma decreases the protein binding of trimethoprim to an insignificant degree; trimethoprim does not influence the protein binding of sulfamethoxazole.

Excretion of Bactrim is chiefly by the kidneys through both glomerular filtration and tubular secretion. Urine concentrations of both sulfamethoxazole and trimethoprim are considerably higher than are the concentrations in the blood. When administered together as in Bactrim, neither sulfamethoxazole nor trimethoprim affects the urinary excretion pattern of the other.

Microbiology: Sulfamethoxazole inhibits bacterial synthesis of dihydrofolic acid by competing with *para*-aminobenzoic acid. Trimethoprim blocks the production of tetrahydrofolic acid from dihydrofolic acid by binding to and reversibly inhibiting the required enzyme, dihydrofolate reductase. Thus, Bactrim blocks two consecutive steps in the biosynthesis of nucleic acids and proteins essential to many bacteria.

In vitro studies have shown that bacterial resistance develops more slowly with Bactrim than with trimethoprim or sulfamethoxazole alone.

In vitro serial dilution tests have shown that the spectrum of antibacterial activity of Bactrim includes the common urinary tract pathogens with the exception of *Pseudomonas aeruginosa.* The following organisms are usually susceptible: *Escherichia coli, Klebsiella-Enterobacter, Proteus mirabilis* and indole-positive proteus species.

In addition, the usual spectrum of antimicrobial activity of Bactrim includes the following bacterial pathogens isolated from middle ear exudate and from bronchial secretions: *Haemophilus influenzae*, including ampicillin-resistant strains, and *Streptococcus pneumoniae*.

Shigella flexneri and *Shigella sonnei* are also usually susceptible.

[See table on right].

The recommended quantitative disc susceptibility method (*Federal Register, 37*:20527–20529, 1972; Bauer AW, Kirby WMM, Sherris JC, Turck M: Antibiotic Susceptibility Testing by a Standardized Single Disc Method, *Am J Clin Pathol, 45*:493–496, 1966) may be used for estimating the susceptibility of bacteria to Bactrim. With this procedure, a report from the laboratory of "Susceptible to trimethoprim-sulfamethoxazole" indicates that the infection is likely to respond to therapy with Bactrim. If the infection is confined to the urine, a report of "Intermediate susceptibility to trimethoprim-sulfamethoxazole" also indicates that the infection is likely to respond. A report of "Resistant to trimethoprim-sulfamethoxazole" indicates that the infection is unlikely to respond to therapy with Bactrim.

Indications and Usage:
URINARY TRACT INFECTIONS: For the treatment of urinary tract infections due to susceptible strains of the following organisms: *Escherichia coli, Klebsiella-Enterobacter, Proteus mirabilis, Proteus vulgaris* and *Proteus morganii*. It is recommended that initial episodes of uncomplicated urinary tract infections be treated with a single effective antibacterial agent rather than the combination.

Note: Currently, the increasing frequency of resistant organisms is a limitation of the usefulness of all antibacterial agents, especially in the treatment of these urinary tract infections.

ACUTE OTITIS MEDIA: For the treatment of acute otitis media in children due to susceptible strains of *Haemophilus influenzae* or *Streptococcus pneumoniae* when in the judgment of the physician Bactrim offers some advantage over the use of other antimicrobial agents. To date, there are limited data on the safety of repeated use of Bactrim in children under two years of age. Bactrim is not indicated for prophylactic or prolonged administration in otitis media at any age.

ACUTE EXACERBATIONS OF CHRONIC BRONCHITIS IN ADULTS: For the treatment of acute exacerbations of chronic bronchitis due to susceptible strains of *Haemophilus influenzae* or *Streptococcus pneumoniae* when in the judgment of the physician Bactrim offers some advantage over the use of a single antimicrobial agent.

SHIGELLOSIS: For the treatment of enteritis caused by susceptible strains of *Shigella flexneri* and *Shigella sonnei* when antibacterial therapy is indicated.

PNEUMOCYSTIS CARINII PNEUMONITIS: Bactrim is also indicated in the treatment of documented *Pneumocystis carinii* pneumonitis.

Contraindications: Hypersensitivity to trimethoprim or sulfonamides. Patients with documented megaloblastic anemia due to folate deficiency. Pregnancy at term and during the nursing period because sulfonamides pass the placenta and are excreted in the milk and may cause kernicterus. Infants less than two months of age.

Warnings: BACTRIM SHOULD NOT BE USED IN THE TREATMENT OF STREPTOCOCCAL PHARYNGITIS. Clinical studies have documented that patients with group A β-hemolytic streptococcal tonsillopharyngitis have a greater incidence of bacteriologic failure when treated with Bactrim than do those patients treated with penicillin, as evidenced by failure to eradicate this organism from the tonsillopharyngeal area.

Deaths associated with the administration of sulfonamides have been reported from hypersensitivity reactions, hepatocellular necrosis, agranulocytosis, aplastic anemia and other blood dyscrasias. Experience with trimethoprim alone is much more limited, but it has been reported to interfere with hematopoiesis in occasional patients. In elderly patients concurrently receiving certain diuretics, primarily thiazides, an increased incidence of thrombopenia with purpura has been reported.

REPRESENTATIVE MINIMUM INHIBITORY CONCENTRATION VALUES FOR BACTRIM-SUSCEPTIBLE ORGANISMS
(MIC—mcg/ml)

Bacteria	Trimethoprim Alone	Sulfamethoxazole Alone	TMP/SMX (1:20) TMP	TMP/SMX (1:20) SMX
Escherichia coli	0.05 – 1.5	1.0 – 245	0.05 – 0.5	0.95 – 9.5
Proteus spp. indole positive	0.5 – 5.0	7.35 – 300	0.05 – 1.5	0.95 – 28.5
Proteus mirabilis	0.5 – 1.5	7.35 – 30	0.05 – 0.15	0.95 – 2.85
Klebsiella-Enterobacter	0.15 – 5.0	2.45 – 245	0.05 – 1.5	0.95 – 28.5
Haemophilus influenzae	0.15 – 1.5	2.85 – 95	0.015 – 0.15	0.285 – 2.85
Streptococcus pneumoniae	0.15 – 1.5	7.35 – 24.5	0.05 – 0.15	0.95 – 2.85
Shigella flexneri	<0.01 – 0.04	<0.16 – >320	<0.002 – 0.03	0.04 – 0.625
Shigella sonnei	0.02 – 0.03	0.625 – >320	0.004 – 0.06	0.08 – 1.25

The presence of clinical signs such as sore throat, fever, pallor, purpura or jaundice may be early indications of serious blood disorders. Complete blood counts should be done frequently in patients receiving Bactrim. If a significant reduction in the count of any formed blood element is noted, Bactrim should be discontinued.

Precautions: *General:* Bactrim should be given with caution to patients with impaired renal or hepatic function, to those with possible folate deficiency and to those with severe allergy or bronchial asthma. In glucose-6-phosphate dehydrogenase-deficient individuals, hemolysis may occur. This reaction is frequently dose-related. Adequate fluid intake must be maintained in order to prevent crystalluria and stone formation. Urinalyses with careful microscopic examination and renal function tests should be performed during therapy, particularly for those patients with impaired renal function.

It has been reported that Bactrim may prolong the prothrombin time of patients who are receiving the anticoagulant warfarin. This interaction should be kept in mind when Bactrim is given to patients already on anticoagulant therapy, and the coagulation time should be reassessed.

Pregnancy: Teratogenic Effects: Pregnancy Category C. In rats, doses of 533 mg/kg sulfamethoxazole or 200 mg/kg trimethoprim produced teratological effects manifested mainly as cleft palates. The highest dose which did not cause cleft palates in rats was 512 mg/kg sulfamethoxazole or 192 mg/kg trimethoprim when administered separately. In two studies in rats, no teratology was observed when 512 mg/kg of sulfamethoxazole was used in combination with 128 mg/kg of trimethoprim. In one study, however, cleft palates were observed in one litter out of 9 when 355 mg/kg of sulfamethoxazole was used in combination with 88 mg/kg of trimethoprim.

In some rabbit studies, an overall increase in fetal loss (dead and resorbed and malformed conceptuses) was associated with doses of trimethoprim 6 times the human therapeutic dose.

While there are no large well-controlled studies on the use of trimethoprim plus sulfamethoxazole in pregnant women, Brumfitt and Pursell (Trimethoprim/Sulfamethoxazole in the Treatment of Bacteriuria in Women. *J Infect Dis 128* (Suppl): S657–S663, 1973) reported the outcome of 186 pregnancies during which the mother received either placebo or trimethoprim in combination with sulfamethoxazole. The incidence of congenital abnormalities was 4.5% (3 of 66) in those who received placebo and 3.3% (4 of 120) in those receiving trimethoprim plus sulfamethoxazole. There were no abnormalities in the 10 children whose mothers received the drug during the first trimester. In a separate survey, Brumfitt and Pursell also found no congenital abnormalities in 35 children whose mothers had received trimethoprim plus sulfamethoxazole at the time of conception or shortly thereafter.

Because trimethoprim plus sulfamethoxazole may interfere with folic acid metabolism, Bactrim should be used during pregnancy only if the potential benefit justifies the potential risk to the fetus.

Nonteratogenic Effects: See "Contraindications" section.

Nursing Mothers: See "Contraindications" section.

Adverse Reactions: For completeness, all major reactions to sulfonamides and to trimethoprim are included below, even though they may not have been reported with Bactrim.

Blood dyscrasias: Agranulocytosis, aplastic anemia, megaloblastic anemia, thrombopenia, leukopenia, hemolytic anemia, purpura, hypoprothrombinemia and methemoglobinemia.

Allergic reactions: Erythema multiforme, Stevens-Johnson syndrome, generalized skin eruptions, epidermal necrolysis, urticaria, serum sickness, pruritus, exfoliative dermatitis, anaphylactoid reactions, periorbital edema, conjunctival and scleral injection, photosensitization, arthralgia and allergic myocarditis.

Gastrointestinal reactions: Glossitis, stomatitis, nausea, emesis, abdominal pains, hepatitis, hepatocellular necrosis, diarrhea, pseudomembranous colitis and pancreatitis.

C.N.S. reactions: Headache, peripheral neuritis, mental depression, convulsions, ataxia, hallucinations, tinnitus, vertigo, insomnia, apathy, fatigue, muscle weakness and nervousness.

Miscellaneous reactions: Drug fever, chills, and toxic nephrosis with oliguria and anuria. Periarteritis nodosa and L. E. phenomenon have occurred. The sulfonamides bear certain chemical similarities to some goitrogens, diuretics (acetazolamide and the thiazides) and oral hypoglycemic agents. Goiter production, diuresis and hypoglycemia have occurred rarely in patients receiving sulfonamides. Cross-sensitivity may exist with these agents. Rats appear to be especially susceptible to the goitrogenic effects of sulfonamides, and long-term administration has produced thyroid malignancies in the species.

Dosage and Administration: Not recommended for use in infants less than two months of age.

URINARY TRACT INFECTIONS AND SHIGELLOSIS IN ADULTS AND CHILDREN, AND ACUTE OTITIS MEDIA IN CHILDREN:

Adults: The usual adult dosage in the treatment of urinary tract infections is one Bactrium DS (double strength) tablet, two Bactrim tablets or four teaspoonfuls (20 ml) of Bactrim Pediatric Suspension or Bactrim Suspension every 12 hours for 10 to 14 days. An identical daily dosge is used for 5 days in the treatment of shigellosis.

Continued on next page

Roche Labs.—Cont.

Children: The recommended dose for children with urinary tract infections or acute otitis media is 8 mg/kg trimethoprim and 40 mg/kg sulfamethoxazole per 24 hours, given in two divided doses every 12 hours for 10 days. An identical daily dosage is used for 5 days in the treatment of shigellosis. The following table is a guideline for the attainment of this dosage:

Children two months of age or older:

Weight		Dose—every 12 hours	
lb	kg	Teaspoonfuls	Tablets
22	10	1 teasp. (5 ml)	—
44	20	2 teasp. (10 ml)	1 tablet
66	30	3 teasp. (15 ml)	1½ tablets
88	40	4 teasp. (20 ml)	2 tablets or 1 DS tablet

For patients with renal impairment:

Creatinine Clearance (ml/min)	Recommended Dosage Regimen
Above 30	Usual standard regimen
15–30	½ the usual regimen
Below 15	Use not recommended

ACUTE EXACERBATIONS OF CHRONIC BRONCHITIS IN ADULTS:
The usual adult dosage in the treatment of acute exacerbations of chronic bronchitis is one Bactrim DS (double strength) tablet, two Bactrim tablets or four teaspoonfuls (20 ml) of Bactrim Pediatric Suspension or Bactrim Suspension every 12 hours for 14 days.

PNEUMOCYSTIS CARINII PNEUMONITIS:
The recommended dosage for patients with *Pneumocystis carinii* pneumonitis is 20 mg/kg trimethoprim and 100 mg/kg sulfamethoxazole per 24 hours given in equally divided doses every 6 hours for 14 days. The following table is a guideline for the attainment of this dosage in children:

Weight		Dose—every six hours	
lb	kg	Teaspoonfuls	Tablets
18	8	1 teasp. (5 ml)	—
35	16	2 teasp. (10 ml)	1 tablet
53	24	3 teasp. (15 ml)	1½ tablets
70	32	4 teasp. (20 ml)	2 tablets or 1 DS tablet

How Supplied: *DS (double strength) Tablets,* containing 160 mg trimethoprim and 800 mg sulfamethoxazole—bottles of 100 and 500; Tel-E-Dose® packages of 100; Prescription Paks of 20. *Tablets,* containing 80 mg trimethoprim and 400 mg sulfamethoxazole—bottles of 100 and 500; Tel-E-Dose® packages of 100; Prescription Paks of 40. *Pediatric Suspension,* containing 40 mg trimethoprim and 200 mg sulfamethoxazole per teaspoonful (5 ml); cherry flavored—bottles of 100 ml and 16 oz (1 pint).
Suspension, containing 40 mg trimethoprim and 200 mg sulfamethoxazole per teaspoonful (5 ml); fruit-licorice flavored—bottles of 16 oz (1 pint).
Shown in Product Identification Section, page 429

BEROCCA® ℞
[ber-o'ka]
PARENTERAL NUTRITION
Injectable
Vitamins for Addition to
Intravenous Fluids

The following text is complete prescribing information based on official labeling in effect August 1, 1984.
Description: Berocca Parenteral Nutrition is a sterile injectable solution of nine water-soluble and three fat-soluble vitamins for addition to intravenous fluids. Each duplex package contains Solution 1 and Solution 2 in either ampuls or vials. When the contents of both containers are combined, 2 ml of the resulting parenteral multivitamin solution will provide eight B-complex vitamins and vitamins C, A, D and E at levels recommended by the American Medical Association.*

* Multivitamin Preparations for Parenteral Use: A Statement by the Nutrition Advisory Group. American Medical Association Department of Foods and Nutrition, 1975. JPEN 3:258–269, Jul-Aug 1979.

Each ml of Berocca Parenteral Nutrition Solution 1 provides:
Thiamine hydrochloride (B_1) .... 3 mg
d-Biotin .... 60 mcg
Riboflavin (as riboflavin 5'-phosphate sodium) (B_2) .... 3.6 mg
Niacinamide .... 40 mg
Pyridoxine hydrochloride (B_6) ...... 4 mg
Dexpanthenol .... 15 mg
Ascorbic Acid (C) .... 100 mg
compounded with propylene glycol 40%, gentisic acid ethanolamide 2%, disodium edetate 0.01%, and benzyl alcohol 1% as stabilizers and preservatives; and sodium hydroxide to adjust pH to approximately 5.

Each ml of Berocca Parenteral Nutrition Solution 2 provides:
Vitamin A palmitate .... 3300 USP units
Vitamin E (*dl*-alpha tocopherol) 10 USP units
Vitamin D_2 (ergocalciferol) .... 200 USP units
Folic acid .... 400 mcg
Cyanocobalamin (B_{12}) .... 5 mcg
compounded with polyoxyethylated vegetable oil 10% as solubilizer for vitamins A, D, E; propylene glycol 10%, ethyl alcohol 10%, gentisic acid ethanolamide 2%, sodium citrate 1.7%, benzyl alcohol 1%, and disodium edetate 0.01% as stabilizers and preservatives; and sodium hydroxide and citric acid to adjust pH to approximately 6.5.

Clinical Pharmacology: Vitamins are essential for maintenance of normal metabolic functions including hematopoiesis: The water-soluble vitamins play vital roles in the conversion of carbohydrate, protein and fat into tissue and energy. *Thiamine (B_1)* acts as a coenzyme in carbohydrate metabolism. *Riboflavin (B_2)* functions as a coenzyme in the electron transport system associated with conversion of tissue oxidations into usable energy. *Niacin* serves as a coenzyme in oxidation-reduction reactions in tissue respiration. *Pyridoxine hydrochloride (B_6)* is essential for the metabolism of amino acids. *Pantothenic acid* functions as a coenzyme in various metabolic acetylation reactions and *biotin* in specific carboxylation reactions in lipid metabolism. *Folic acid* and *cyanocobalamin (B_{12})* are metabolically interrelated. They are essential to nucleic acid synthesis and normal maturation of red blood cells. *Ascorbic acid (C)* performs a vital function in the process of cellular respiration, and is involved in both carbohydrate and amino acid metabolism. It is essential for collagen formation and tissue repair.
Vitamin A is necessary for proper functioning of the retina; it appears to be essential to the integrity of epithelial cells. *Vitamin D* is necessary for the absorption of calcium and for the maintenance of bone structure. *Vitamin E* is an antioxidant which preserves essential cellular constituents, including those of the red blood cell. It also serves as protection against lipid peroxidation.

Berocca Parenteral Nutrition provides, in a 2 ml dose, the daily requirements of twelve essential vitamins for nutritional rehabilitation and maintenance of optimal nutritional status in conditions for which parenteral vitamin nutrition is indicated.

Indications: Berocca Parenteral Nutrition is indicated for adults and children 11 years of age or older as a daily maintenance dosage of multivitamins when parenteral nutrition is required. This formulation, along with intermittent injections of vitamin K, is especially useful as a supplement in patients on long-term total parenteral nutrition (TPN).

Berocca Parenteral Nutrition is also indicated in other conditions only when oral administration of multivitamins is not feasible. Such conditions may include disorders which can affect oral intake, gastrointestinal absorption or utilization. For example: comatose states, persistent vomiting, prolonged fever, severe infectious diseases, major surgery, extensive burns, fractures and other traumas, cancer chemo- or radiotherapy, chronic alcoholism, maxillofacial surgery, esophageal burns or strictures, stenosis of the gastrointestinal tract, bowel obstruction, blind loop syndrome, diarrhea, steatorrheas, granulomatous bowel disease, small bowel fistula, pancreatic disease, or hepatic failure.

The physician should not await the development of clinical signs of vitamin deficiency before initiating therapy as there are few specific or pathognomonic signs of early vitamin deficiencies.

Contraindications: Berocca Parenteral Nutrition is contraindicated in patients known to be hypersensitive to any of its components and in those with a preexisting hypervitaminosis.

Warnings: Allergic reactions, including anaphylaxis, may occur in patients hypersensitive to thiamine or other components of the product.

Patients who have early Leber's disease (hereditary optic nerve atrophy) have been found to suffer severe, acute optic atrophy when treated with vitamin B_{12}. Pyridoxine can decrease the efficacy of levodopa in the treatment of patients with parkinsonism. Folic acid may alter patient response to methotrexate therapy. These facts should be considered before prescribing Berocca Parenteral Nutrition for such patients.

Folic acid in doses above 0.1 mg daily may obscure pernicious anemia. Berocca Parenteral Nutrition is not intended for treatment of pernicious anemia or other megaloblastic anemias where vitamin B_{12} is deficient. Neurologic involvement may develop or progress, despite temporary remission of anemia, in patients with vitamin B_{12} deficiency who receive supplemental folic acid and who are inadequately treated with B_{12}. This product should not be used as primary treatment for specific vitamin deficiencies such as beriberi, pellagra, scurvy, and riboflavin or pyridoxine deficiency.

Precautions: Because fat-soluble vitamins can accumulate in the body, toxicity from vitamins A and D is possible, especially if patients are inadvertently administered oral vitamin supplementation in addition to the parenteral regimen.

Berocca Parenteral Nutrition does not contain vitamin K. Supplements of vitamin K may be necessary to meet patients' individual requirements. Patients routinely receiving fat emulsion as part of the total parenteral regimen may have increased requirements for vitamin E.

Most antibiotics, methotrexate and pyrimethamine invalidate diagnostic microbiological blood assays for folic acid and cyanocobalamin.

Safety and effectiveness in children under the age of 11 have not been established.

Adverse Reactions: Allergic sensitization has been reported following parenteral administration of folic acid and thiamine. Hepatomegaly, leukopenia and projectile vomiting have been reported in the literature as vitamin A toxicity symptoms; elevated serum calcium and multiple areas of tissue calcification have been reported with hypervitaminosis D.

Dosage and Administration: For addition to intravenous fluids. Berocca Parenteral Nutrition should not be given as a direct bolus or by direct undiluted intravenous injection as histamine-like reactions have been observed in dogs after bolus injection.

The recommended daily dose is 2 ml of Berocca Parenteral Nutrition (1 ml of Solution 1 and 1 ml of Solution 2) added to intravenous infusion fluids. Berocca Parenteral Nutrition should be infused over a period of at least two hours.

IMPORTANT: DIRECTIONS FOR RECONSTITUTION, ADDITION TO INTRAVENOUS INFUSION SOLUTIONS AND STORAGE:
Ampuls: To prepare solution for single dose administration, mix 1 ml of Berocca Parenteral Nutrition Solution 1 with 1 ml of Berocca Parenteral Nutrition Solution 2. The reconstituted product is ready for addition to intravenous infusion fluids. Or, add the contents of each ampul directly to the

for possible revisions

Product Information

intravenous infusion fluid. *Multiple dose vials:* To prepare solution for 10 doses, add 10 ml of Berocca Parenteral Nutrition Solution 2 to 10 ml of Berocca Parenteral Nutrition Solution 1 (20 ml vial, 10 ml fill). To administer single doses, add 2 ml of the reconstituted product to intravenous infusion fluids. Or, add 1 ml of Solution 1 and 1 ml of Solution 2 directly to the intravenous infusion fluid.

BEROCCA PARENTERAL NUTRITION CAN BE USED WITH COMPATIBLE INTRAVENOUS INFUSION SOLUTIONS: 0.9% sterile saline, 5% or 10% sterile glucose or dextrose, lactated Ringer's solution. Two ml of Berocca Parenteral Nutrition (1 ml of Solution 1 and 1 ml of Solution 2) should be added to at least 250 ml of the intravenous infusion solution. Either glass or plastic containers can be used.

Berocca Parenteral Nutrition, like other parenteral vitamins, should not be added to I.V. fluids containing sodium bisulfite as this causes rapid degradation of vitamin B_1 (thiamine). If Berocca Parenteral Nutrition is added to I.V. fluids which do contain the preservative sodium bisulfite, a separate supplemental injection of thiamine should be administered.

Store unreconstituted product in refrigerator (2°–8°C, 36°–46°F). PROTECT FROM LIGHT. DO NOT STORE AT ROOM TEMPERATURE.

Store reconstituted (mixed) product for no longer than 14 days in refrigerator (2°–8°C, 36°–46°F). PROTECT FROM LIGHT.

Store intravenous fluids with added Berocca Parenteral Nutrition in refrigerator (2°–8°C, 36°–46°F) for no longer than 24 hours. PROTECT FROM LIGHT.

Note: Berocca Parenteral Nutrition contains a soluble form of riboflavin which permits use of a large dose and minimizes pain on injection. This form of riboflavin may result in darkening of the solution and the color change is intensified on prolonged storage. However, the darkening of the solution in no way affects the safety and therapeutic efficacy of the preparation.

Parenteral drug products should be inspected visually for particulate matter prior to administration, whenever solution and container permit.

How Supplied: *Ampuls:* Duplex packages, each containing a 1-ml ampul of Solution 1 and a 1-ml ampul of Solution 2; boxes of 25.

Vials: Duplex packages, each containing a 20-ml vial (10-ml fill) of Solution 1 and a 10-ml vial (10-ml fill) of Solution 2; boxes of 1.

Each Berocca® tablet contains:	Quantity	U.S. RDA—Adults and children 4 or more years of age	U.S. RDA—Pregnant or lactating women
Vitamin C (ascorbic acid)	500 mg	60 mg	60 mg
Vitamin B_1 (as thiamine mononitrate)	15 mg	1.5 mg	1.7 mg
Vitamin B_2 (riboflavin)	15 mg	1.7 mg	2 mg
Niacin (as niacinamide)	100 mg	20 mg	20 mg
Vitamin B_6 (as pyridoxine HCl)	4 mg	2 mg	2.5 mg
Pantothenic acid (as calcium *d*-pantothenate)	18 mg	10 mg	10 mg
Folic acid	0.5 mg	0.4 mg	0.8 mg
Vitamin B_{12} (cyanocobalamin)	5 mcg	6 mcg	8 mcg

BEROCCA® TABLETS
[ber-o'ka]

The following text is complete prescribing information based on official labeling in effect August 1, 1984.
[See table above].

Description: Berocca is a prescription-only oral multivitamin tablet specially formulated for prophylactic or therapeutic nutritional supplementation in conditions requiring water-soluble vitamins.

Berocca tablets supply *therapeutic* levels of ascorbic acid, vitamins B_1, B_2, B_6, niacin and pantothenic acid and a *supplemental* level of vitamin B_{12}. Berocca tablets also supply a supplemental level of folic acid for pregnant or lactating women and a therapeutic level for adults and children four or more years of age.

Clinical Pharmacology: Vitamins are essential for normal metabolic functions including hematopoiesis. The B-complex vitamins are necessary for the conversion of carbohydrate, protein and fat into tissue and energy.

Ascorbic acid (C) is involved in collagen formation and tissue repair.

The water-soluble vitamins (B-complex and C) are not significantly stored by the body; excess quantities are excreted in the urine. They must be replenished regularly through diet or other means to maintain essential tissue levels. Thus, these vitamins are rapidly depleted in conditions interfering with their intake or absorption.

Indications and Usage: Berocca is indicated for supportive nutritional supplementation in conditions in which water-soluble vitamins are required prophylactically or therapeutically. These include:

Conditions causing depletion, or reduced absorption or bioavailability of water-soluble vitamins— Gastrointestinal disorders, chronic alcoholism, febrile illnesses, prolonged or wasting diseases, hyperthyroidism or poorly controlled diabetes.

Conditions resulting in increased needs for water-soluble vitamins— Pregnancy, severe burns, recovery from surgery.

Contraindications: Berocca is contraindicated in patients known to be hypersensitive to any of its components.

Warnings: Berocca is not intended for treatment of pernicious anemia or other megaloblastic anemias where vitamin B_{12} is deficient. Neurologic involvement may develop or progress, despite temporary remission of anemia, in patients with vitamin B_{12} deficiency who receive supplemental folic acid and who are inadequately treated with B_{12}.

Precautions: *General:* Certain conditions listed above may require additional nutritional supplementation. During pregnancy, for instance, supplementation with fat-soluble vitamins and minerals may be required according to the dietary habits of the individual. Berocca is not intended for treatment of severe specific deficiencies.

Information for the Patient: Because toxic reactions have been reported with injudicious use of certain vitamins, urge patients to follow your specific instructions regarding dosage regimen. As with any medication, advise patients to keep Berocca out of reach of children.

Drug and Treatment Interactions: As little as 5 mg pyridoxine daily can decrease the efficacy of levodopa in the treatment of parkinsonism. Therefore, Berocca is not recommended for patients undergoing such therapy.

Adverse Reactions: Adverse reactions have been reported with specific vitamins, but generally at levels substantially higher than those in Berocca. However, allergic and idiosyncratic reactions are possible at lower levels.

Dosage and Administration: Usual adult dosage: one tablet daily.

Berocca is available on prescription only.

How Supplied: Light green, capsule-shaped tablets—bottles of 100 (NDC 0004-0020-01) and 500 (NDC 0004-0020-14).

Imprint on tablets: BEROCCA®
ROCHE

Shown in Product Identification Section, page 429

BEROCCA® PLUS TABLETS
[ber-o'ka]

The following text is complete prescribing information based on official labeling in effect August 1, 1984.
[See table below].

Description: Berocca Plus is a prescription-only oral multivitamin/mineral tablet specially formulated for prophylactic or therapeutic nutritional supplementation in physiologically stressful conditions.

Berocca Plus supplies: *therapeutic* levels of water-soluble vitamins (ascorbic acid and all B-complex vitamins except biotin); *supplemental* levels of biotin, fat-soluble vitamins (A and E) and minerals (iron, chromium, manganese, copper and zinc); plus magnesium.

Clinical Pharmacology: Vitamins and minerals are essential for normal metabolic functions including hematopoiesis. The B-complex vitamins are necessary for the conversion of carbohydrate, protein and fat into tissue and energy. Ascorbic

Each Berocca® Plus tablet contains:	Quantity	U.S. RDA—Adults and children 4 or more years of age	U.S. RDA—Pregnant or lactating women
Fat-Soluble Vitamins			
Vitamin A (as vitamin A acetate)	5000 IU	5000 IU	8000 IU
Vitamin E (as *dl*-alpha tocopheryl acetate)	30 IU	30 IU	30 IU
Water-Soluble Vitamins			
Vitamin C (ascorbic acid)	500 mg	60 mg	60 mg
Vitamin B_1 (as thiamine mononitrate)	20 mg	1.5 mg	1.7 mg
Vitamin B_2 (riboflavin)	20 mg	1.7 mg	2 mg
Niacin (as niacinamide)	100 mg	20 mg	20 mg
Vitamin B_6 (as pyridoxine HCl)	25 mg	2 mg	2.5 mg
Biotin	0.15 mg	0.30 mg	0.30 mg
Pantothenic acid (as calcium pantothenate)	25 mg	10 mg	10 mg
Folic acid	0.8 mg	0.4 mg	0.8 mg
Vitamin B_{12} (cyanocobalamin)	50 mcg	6 mcg	8 mcg
Minerals			
Iron (as ferrous fumarate)	27 mg	18 mg	18 mg
Chromium (as chromium nitrate)	0.1 mg	0.05–0.2 mg*	
Magnesium (as magnesium oxide)	50 mg	400 mg	450 mg
Manganese (as manganese dioxide)	5 mg	2.5–5 mg*	
Copper (as cupric oxide)	3 mg	2 mg	2 mg
Zinc (as zinc oxide)	22.5 mg	15 mg	15 mg

*Not established. Estimated by NAS/NRC as safe and adequate daily dietary intake for adults.

Continued on next page

Roche Labs.—Cont.

acid is involved in tissue repair and collagen formation. Vitamin A is necessary for proper functioning of the retina; it appears to be essential to the integrity of epithelial cells. Vitamin E is an antioxidant which preserves essential cellular constituents. Magnesium is a structural component of body tissues; iron, chromium, manganese, copper and zinc serve as catalysts in enzyme systems which perform vital cellular functions.

Water-soluble vitamins (B-complex and C) are not significantly stored by the body and must be replaced continually to maintain essential tissue levels; excess quantities are excreted in urine. These vitamins are rapidly depleted in conditions interfering with their intake or absorption. Berocca Plus supplies therapeutic levels of vitamin C and all B-complex vitamins (except biotin). Fat-soluble vitamins and several trace minerals, however, can accumulate in the body and do not need replacement as frequently. Therefore, Berocca Plus supplies more conservative levels of vitamins A and E and various essential minerals. Specifically, Berocca Plus contains an adequate level of vitamin B_6 (25 mg) to normalize the tryptophan metabolism disturbance which has been associated with the use of estrogenic oral contraceptives or other estrogen therapy. It provides zinc (22.5 mg) which facilitates wound healing, the level of folic acid (0.8 mg) recommended during pregnancy, and ascorbic acid (500 mg) which has been demonstrated to improve the absorption of inorganic iron.

Indications: Berocca Plus is indicated for prophylactic or therapeutic nutritional supplementation in physiologically stressful conditions. These include:

Conditions causing depletion, or reduced absorption or bioavailability of essential vitamins and minerals—
Inadequate intake due to highly restricted or unbalanced diets such as those frequently associated with anorexic conditions and other states of severe malnutrition.
Gastrointestinal disorders, chronic alcoholism, chronic or acute infections (especially those involving febrile illness), prolonged or wasting disease, congestive heart failure, hyperthyroidism, poorly controlled diabetes or other physiologic stress.
Also, patients on estrogenic oral contraceptives or other estrogen therapy, antibacterials which affect intestinal microflora, or other interfering drugs.

Certain conditions resulting from severe B-vitamin or ascorbic acid deficiency—
Cheilosis, gingivitis, stomatitis and certain other classic water-soluble vitamin deficiency syndromes.

Conditions resulting in increased needs for essential vitamins and minerals—
Recovery from surgery or trauma involving severe burns, fractures or other extensive tissue damage. Also, pregnant women and those with heavy menstrual bleeding.

Contraindications: Berocca Plus is contraindicated in patients hypersensitive to any of its components.

Warnings: Not intended for treatment of pernicious anemia or other megaloblastic anemias where vitamin B_{12} is deficient. Neurologic involvement may develop or progress, despite temporary remission of anemia, in patients with vitamin B_{12} deficiency who receive supplemental folic acid and who are inadequately treated with B_{12}.

Precautions: *General:* Certain conditions listed above may require additional nutritional supplementation. During pregnancy, for instance, supplementation with vitamin D and calcium may be required according to the dietary habits of the individual. Berocca Plus is not intended for treatment of severe specific deficiencies.

Information for the Patient: Because toxic reactions have been reported with injudicious use of certain vitamins and minerals, urge patients to follow your specific instructions regarding dosage regimen. Advise patients to keep Berocca Plus out of reach of children.

Drug and Treatment Interactions: As little as 5 mg pyridoxine daily can decrease the efficacy of levodopa in the treatment of parkinsonism. Therefore, Berocca Plus is not recommended for patients undergoing such therapy.

Adverse Reactions: Adverse reactions have been reported with specific vitamins and minerals, but generally at levels substantially higher than those in Berocca Plus. However, allergic and idiosyncratic reactions are possible at lower levels. Iron, even at the usual recommended levels, has been associated with gastrointestinal intolerance in some patients.

Dosage and Administration: Usual adult dosage: one tablet daily. Not recommended for children. *Berocca Plus is available on prescription only.*

How Supplied: Golden yellow, capsule-shaped tablets—bottles of 100.
Imprint on tablets: (front) BEROCCA PLUS; (back) ROCHE.
Shown in Product Identification Section, page 429

BEROCCA®-C
BEROCCA®-C 500
[ber-o'ka]

The following text is complete prescribing information based on official labeling in effect August 1, 1984.

Description: Berocca-C provides generous amounts of six important B-complex vitamins plus an ample dose of vitamin C (ascorbic acid) in readily absorbable form.

Each 2 ml of Berocca-C contains:
Thiamine HCl (B_1)	10 mg
Riboflavin (B_2) (as riboflavin 5'-phosphate sodium)	10 mg
Niacinamide	80 mg
Pyridoxine HCl (B_6)	20 mg
Dexpanthenol (equivalent to 23.2 mg calcium pantothenate)	20 mg
d-biotin	0.2 mg
Ascorbic acid (C)	100 mg

compounded with 1% benzyl alcohol as preservative and pH adjusted with sodium hydroxide (to approximately 4.2 with the vial, 5.1 with the ampul).

Berocca-C 500 is a duplex package containing one 2-ml ampul of Berocca-C and a separate 2-ml ampul of 400 mg of Vitamin C Sodium Injectable compounded with 0.2% parabens (methyl and propyl) as preservatives, and pH adjusted to 5.5—7.0 with sodium bicarbonate. When the contents of both ampuls are aspirated into the same syringe, the resulting solution (4 ml) will contain equal amounts of the vitamins listed above, with the exception of vitamin C which increases to 500 mg.
Note: the formula of Berocca-C contains a soluble form of riboflavin which permits use of a larger dose and minimizes pain upon injection. While this form of riboflavin causes darkening of the solution which may intensify on prolonged storage, this in no way affects the safety and therapeutic efficacy of the preparation. Berocca-C ampuls are ready for immediate use, are stable for at least 18 months (the vials are stable for 15 months) and need not be refrigerated.

Indications: Disorders requiring parenteral administration of water-soluble vitamins. Pre- and postoperative treatment; when requirements are increased, as in fever, severe burns, increased metabolism, hyperthyroidism, pregnancy; gastrointestinal disorders interfering with intake or absorption of water-soluble vitamins; prolonged or wasting diseases; alcoholism. In addition to these states indicated above, Berocca-C 500 is particularly useful in severe burns, shock, trauma or other instances when the need for vitamin C is increased out of proportion to that for other vitamins.

Precautions: Occasional sensitivity to thiamine hydrochloride has been reported. When not diluted with infusion fluids, Berocca-C should be injected SLOWLY. Intramuscular administration may cause transient pain.

Side Effects: Occasional hypersensitivity reactions to thiamine hydrochloride have been encountered, principally after repeated intravenous injections of concentrated solutions. Consequently, if the patient has previously received thiamine, subsequent injections should be given with care, and administration discontinued if untoward reactions develop. Pain on intramuscular injection has rarely been reported.

Dosage and Administration: Berocca-C is preferably administered by addition to parenteral infusion fluids—amino acids, glucose solutions, physiologic saline or electrolyte replacement fluids. From 2 ml to 20 ml of Berocca-C per liter of infusion fluid may be added to such solutions.
The contents of a duplex package of Berocca-C 500 (1 ampul of Berocca-C and 1 ampul of Vitamin C Sodium Injectable) should be aspirated into the same syringe—preferably shortly before administration. This preparation may then be added to parenteral infusion fluids—amino acids, glucose solutions, physiologic saline or electrolyte replacement fluids. Four ml of Berocca-C 500 per liter of infusion fluid are usually adequate. If desired, further amounts of vitamin C may be added to such solutions.
A dose of no more than 2 ml of Berocca-C or 4 ml of Berocca-C 500 may also be given undiluted by SLOW intravenous or intramuscular injection. Intravenous injection is usually preferable, since intramuscular administration may cause temporary pain.
Berocca-C may be administered until it is possible to replace it with oral vitamin supplementation.

How Supplied: Berocca-C ampuls: 2 ml, boxes of 10. Vials: 20 ml, boxes of 1. Berocca-C 500 Duplex Package: Contains one 2-ml ampul of Berocca-C and one 2-ml ampul containing 400 mg ascorbic acid—boxes of 10.

BUMEX®
[bu'mex]
(bumetanide/Roche)
TABLETS
INJECTION

The following text is complete prescribing information based on official labeling in effect August 1, 1984.

> **Warning:** Bumex (bumetanide/Roche) is a potent diuretic which, if given in excessive amounts, can lead to a profound diuresis with water and electrolyte depletion. Therefore, careful medical supervision is required, and dose and dosage schedule have to be adjusted to the individual patient's needs. (See DOSAGE AND ADMINISTRATION.)

Description: Bumex® (bumetanide/Roche) is a loop diuretic, available as scored tablets, 0.5 mg (light green) and 1 mg (yellow) for oral administration; and as 2-ml ampuls (0.25 mg/ml) for intravenous or intramuscular injection as a sterile solution, each 2 ml of which contains 0.5 mg (0.25 mg/ml) bumetanide compounded with 0.85% sodium chloride and 0.4% ammonium acetate as buffers; 0.01% disodium edetate; 1% benzyl alcohol as preservative, and pH adjusted to approximately 7 with sodium hydroxide.
Chemically, bumetanide is 3-(butylamino)-4-phenoxy-5-sulfamoylbenzoic acid. It is a practically white powder having a calculated molecular weight of 364.41.

Clinical Pharmacology: Bumex is a loop diuretic with a rapid onset and short duration of action. Pharmacological and clinical studies have shown that 1 mg Bumex has a diuretic potency equivalent to approximately 40 mg furosemide. The major site of Bumex action is the ascending limb of the loop of Henle.
The mode of action has been determined through various clearance studies in both humans and experimental animals. Bumex inhibits sodium reabsorption in the ascending limb of the loop of Henle, as shown by marked reduction of free-water clearance (CH_2O) during hydration and tubular free-

water reabsorption (T^CH_2O) during hydropenia. Reabsorption of chloride in the ascending loop is also blocked by Bumex, and Bumex is somewhat more chloruretic than natriuretic.

Potassium excretion is also increased by Bumex, in a dose-related fashion.

Bumex may have an additional action in the proximal tubule. Since phosphate reabsorption takes place largely in the proximal tubule, phosphaturia during Bumex-induced diuresis is indicative of this additional action. This is further supported by the reduction in the renal clearance of Bumex by probenecid, associated with diminution in the natriuretic response. This proximal tubular activity does not seem to be related to an inhibition of carbonic anhydrase. Bumex does not appear to have a noticeable action on the distal tubule.

Bumex decreases uric acid excretion and increases serum uric acid. Following oral administration of Bumex the onset of diuresis occurs in 30 to 60 minutes. Peak activity is reached between 1 and 2 hours. At usual doses (1 to 2 mg) diuresis is largely complete within 4 hours; with higher doses, the diuretic action lasts for 4 to 6 hours. Diuresis starts within minutes following an intravenous injection and reaches maximum levels within 15 to 30 minutes.

Several pharmacokinetic studies have shown that Bumex, administered orally or parenterally, is eliminated rapidly in humans, with a half-life of between 1 and 1½ hours. Plasma protein-binding is in the range of 94% to 96%.

Oral administration of carbon-14 labeled Bumex to human volunteers revealed that 81% of the administered radioactivity was excreted in the urine, 45% of it as unchanged drug. Urinary and biliary metabolites identified in this study were formed by oxidation of the N-butyl side chain. Biliary excretion of Bumex amounted to only 2% of the administered dose.

Indications and Usage: Bumex is indicated for the treatment of edema associated with congestive heart failure, hepatic and renal disease, including the nephrotic syndrome.

Almost equal diuretic response occurs after oral and parenteral administration of Bumex. Therefore, if impaired gastrointestinal absorption is suspected or oral administration is not practical, Bumex should be given by the intramuscular or intravenous route.

Successful treatment with Bumex following instances of allergic reactions to furosemide suggests a lack of cross-sensitivity.

Contraindications: Bumex is contraindicated in anuria. Although Bumex can be used to induce diuresis in renal insufficiency, any marked increase in blood urea nitrogen or creatinine, or the development of oliguria during therapy of patients with progressive renal disease, is an indication for discontinuation of treatment with Bumex. Bumex is also contraindicated in patients in hepatic coma or in states of severe electrolyte depletion until the condition is improved or corrected. Bumex is contraindicated in patients hypersensitive to this drug.

Warnings:

1. Volume and electrolyte depletion. The dose of Bumex should be adjusted to the patient's need. Excessive doses or too frequent administration can lead to profound water loss, electrolyte depletion, dehydration, reduction in blood volume and circulatory collapse with the possibility of vascular thrombosis and embolism, particularly in elderly patients.

2. Hypokalemia. Hypokalemia can occur as a consequence of Bumex administration. Prevention of hypokalemia requires particular attention in the following conditions: patients receiving digitalis and diuretics for congestive heart failure, hepatic cirrhosis and ascites, states of aldosterone excess with normal renal function, potassium-losing nephropathy, certain diarrheal states, or other states where hypokalemia is thought to represent particular added risks to the patient, i.e., history of ventricular arrhythmias.

In patients with hepatic cirrhosis and ascites, sudden alterations of electrolyte balance may precipitate hepatic encephalopathy and coma. Treatment in such patients is best initiated in the hospital with small doses and careful monitoring of the patient's clinical status and electrolyte balance. Supplemental potassium and/or spironolactone may prevent hypokalemia and metabolic alkalosis in these patients.

3. Ototoxicity. In cats, dogs and guinea pigs, Bumex has been shown to produce ototoxicity. In these test animals Bumex was 5 to 6 times more potent than furosemide and, since the diuretic potency of Bumex is about 40 to 60 times furosemide, it is anticipated that blood levels necessary to produce ototoxicity will rarely be achieved. The potential exists, however, and must be considered a risk of intravenous therapy, especially at high doses, repeated frequently in the face of renal excretory function impairment. Potentiation of aminoglycoside ototoxicity has not been tested for Bumex. Like other members of this class of diuretics, Bumex probably shares this risk.

4. Allergy to sulfonamides. Patients allergic to sulfonamides may show hypersensitivity to Bumex.

Precautions: *General:* Serum potassium should be measured periodically and potassium supplements or potassium-sparing diuretics added if necessary. Periodic determinations of other electrolytes are advised in patients treated with high doses or for prolonged periods, particularly in those on low salt diets.

Hyperuricemia may occur; it has been asymptomatic in cases reported to date. Reversible elevations of the BUN and creatinine may also occur, especially in association with dehydration and particularly in patients with renal insufficiency. Bumex may increase urinary calcium excretion with resultant hypocalcemia.

Laboratory Tests: Studies in normal subjects receiving Bumex revealed no adverse effects on glucose tolerance, plasma insulin, glucagon and growth hormone levels, but the possibility of an effect on glucose metabolism exists. Periodic determinations of blood sugar should be done, particularly in patients with diabetes or suspected latent diabetes.

Patients under treatment should be observed regularly for possible occurrence of blood dyscrasias, liver damage or idiosyncratic reactions, which have been reported occasionally in foreign marketing experience. The relationship of these occurrences to Bumex use is not certain.

Drug Interactions:

1. Drugs with ototoxic potential (see WARNINGS): Especially in the presence of impaired renal function, the use of parenterally administered Bumex in patients to whom aminoglycoside antibiotics are also being given should be avoided, except in life-threatening conditions.

2. Drugs with nephrotoxic potential: There has been no experience on the concurrent use of Bumex with drugs known to have a nephrotoxic potential. Therefore, the simultaneous administration of these drugs should be avoided.

3. Lithium: Lithium should generally not be given with diuretics (such as Bumex) because they reduce its renal clearance and add a high risk of lithium toxicity.

4. Probenecid: Pretreatment with probenecid reduces both the natriuresis and hyperreninemia produced by Bumex. This antagonistic effect of probenecid on Bumex natriuresis is not due to a direct action on sodium excretion but is probably secondary to its inhibitory effect on renal tubular secretion of bumetanide. Thus, probenecid should not be administered concurrently with Bumex.

5. Indomethacin: Indomethacin blunts the increases in urine volume and sodium excretion seen during Bumex treatment and inhibits the bumetanide-induced increase in plasma renin activity. Concurrent therapy with Bumex is thus not recommended.

6. Antihypertensives: Bumex may potentiate the effect of various antihypertensive drugs, necessitating a reduction in the dosage of these drugs.

7. Digoxin: Interaction studies in humans have shown no effect on digoxin blood levels.

8. Anticoagulants: Interaction studies in humans have shown Bumex to have no effect on warfarin metabolism or on plasma prothrombin activity.

Carcinogenesis, Mutagenesis, Impairment of Fertility: Bumex was devoid of mutagenic activity in various strains of *Salmonella typhimurium* when tested in the presence or absence of an *in vitro* metabolic activation system. An 18-month study showed an increase in mammary adenomas of questionable significance in female rats receiving oral doses of 60 mg/kg/day (2000 times a 2-mg human dose). A repeat study at the same doses failed to duplicate this finding.

Reproduction studies were performed to evaluate general reproductive performance and fertility in rats at oral dose levels of 10, 30, 60 or 100 mg/kg/day. The pregnancy rate was slightly decreased in the treated animals; however, the differences were small and not statistically significant.

Pregnancy: Teratogenic Effects: Pregnancy Category C. Bumex is neither teratogenic nor embryocidal in mice when given in doses up to 3400 times the maximum human therapeutic dose.

Bumex has been shown to be nonteratogenic, but it has a slight embryocidal effect in rats when given in doses of 3400 times the maximum human therapeutic dose and in rabbits at doses of 3.4 times the maximum human therapeutic dose. In one study, moderate growth retardation and increased incidence of delayed ossification of sternebrae were observed in rats at oral doses of 100 mg/kg/day, 3400 times the maximum human therapeutic dose. These effects were associated with maternal weight reductions noted during dosing. No such adverse effects were observed at 30 mg/kg/day (1000 times the maximum human therapeutic dose). No fetotoxicity was observed at 1000 to 2000 times the human therapeutic dose.

In rabbits, a dose-related decrease in litter size and an increase in resorption rate were noted at oral doses of 0.1 and 0.3 mg/kg/day (3.4 and 10 times the maximum human therapeutic dose). A slightly increased incidence of delayed ossification of sternebrae occurred at 0.3 mg/kg/day; however, no such adverse effects were observed at the dose of 0.03 mg/kg/day. The sensitivity of the rabbit to Bumex parallels the marked pharmacologic and toxicologic effects of the drug in this species.

Bumex was not teratogenic in the hamster at an oral dose of 0.5 mg/kg/day (17 times the maximum human therapeutic dose). Bumex was not teratogenic when given intravenously to mice and rats at doses up to 140 times the maximum human therapeutic dose.

There are no adequate and well-controlled studies in pregnant women. A small investigational experience in the United States and marketing experience in other countries to date have not indicated any evidence of adverse effects on the fetus, but these data do not rule out the possibility of harmful effects. Bumex should be given to a pregnant woman only if the potential benefit justifies the potential risk to the fetus.

Nursing Mothers: It is not known whether this drug is excreted in human milk. As a general rule, nursing should not be undertaken while the patient is on Bumex since it may be excreted in human milk.

Pediatric Use: Safety and effectiveness in children below the age of 18 have not been established.

Adverse Reactions: The most frequent clinical adverse reactions considered probably or possibly related to Bumex are muscle cramps (seen in 1.1% of treated patients), dizziness (1.1%), hypotension (0.8%), headache (0.6%), nausea (0.6%), and encephalopathy (in patients with preexisting liver disease) (0.6%). One or more of these adverse reactions have been reported in approximately 4.1% of Bumex-treated patients.

Less frequent clinical adverse reactions to Bumex are impaired hearing (0.5%), pruritus (0.4%), electrocardiogram changes (0.4%), weakness (0.2%), hives (0.2%), abdominal pain (0.2%), arthritic pain (0.2%), musculoskeletal pain (0.2%), rash (0.2%)

Continued on next page

Roche Labs.—Cont.

and vomiting (0.2%). One or more of these adverse reactions have been reported in approximately 2.9% of Bumex-treated patients.

Other clinical adverse reactions, which have each occurred in approximately 0.1% of patients, are vertigo, chest pain, ear discomfort, fatigue, dehydration, sweating, hyperventilation, dry mouth, upset stomach, renal failure, asterixis, itching, nipple tenderness, diarrhea, premature ejaculation and difficulty maintaining an erection.

Laboratory abnormalities reported have included hyperuricemia (in 18.4% of patients tested), hypochloremia (14.9%), hypokalemia (14.7%), azotemia (10.6%), hyponatremia (9.2%), increased serum creatinine (7.4%), hyperglycemia (6.6%), and variations in phosphorus (4.5%), CO_2 content (4.3%), bicarbonate (3.1%) and calcium (2.4%). Although manifestations of the pharmacologic action of Bumex, these conditions may become more pronounced by intensive therapy.

Diuresis induced by Bumex may also rarely be accompanied by changes in LDH (1.0%), total serum bilirubin (0.8%), serum proteins (0.7%), SGOT (0.6%), SGPT (0.5%), alkaline phosphatase (0.4%), cholesterol (0.4%) and creatinine clearance (0.3%). Also reported have been deviations in hemoglobin (0.8%), prothrombin time (0.8%), hematocrit (0.6%), WBC (0.3%), platelet counts (0.2%) and differential counts (0.1%). Increases in urinary glucose (0.7%) and urinary protein (0.3%) have also been seen.

Overdosage: Overdosage can lead to acute profound water loss, volume and electrolyte depletion, dehydration, reduction of blood volume and circulatory collapse with a possibility of vascular thrombosis and embolism. Electrolyte depletion may be manifested by weakness, dizziness, mental confusion, anorexia, lethargy, vomiting and cramps. Treatment consists of replacement of fluid and electrolyte losses by careful monitoring of the urine and electrolyte output and serum electrolyte levels.

Dosage and Administration: Dosage should be individualized with careful monitoring of patient response.

Oral Administration: The usual total daily dosage of Bumex is 0.5 to 2.0 mg and in most patients is given as a single dose.

If the diuretic response to an initial dose of Bumex is not adequate, in view of its rapid onset and short duration of action, a second or third dose may be given at 4- to 5-hour intervals up to a maximum daily dose of 10 mg. An intermittent dose schedule, whereby Bumex is given on alternate days or for 3 to 4 days with rest periods of 1 to 2 days in between, is recommended as the safest and most effective method for the continued control of edema. In patients with hepatic failure, the dosage should be kept to a minimum, and if necessary, dosage increased very carefully.

Because cross-sensitivity with furosemide has rarely been observed, Bumex can be substituted at approximately a 1:40 ratio of Bumex to furosemide in patients allergic to furosemide.

Parenteral Administration: Bumex may be administered parenterally (IV or IM) to patients in whom gastrointestinal absorption may be impaired or in whom oral administration is not practical.

Parenteral treatment should be terminated and oral treatment instituted as soon as possible.

The usual initial dose is 0.5 to 1.0 mg intravenously or intramuscularly. Intravenous administration should be given over a period of 1 to 2 minutes. If the response to an initial dose is deemed insufficient, a second or third dose may be given at intervals of 2 to 3 hours, but should not exceed a daily dosage of 10 mg.

Miscibility and Parenteral Solutions: The compatibility tests of Bumex injection (0.25 mg/ml, 2-ml ampuls) with 5% dextrose in water, 0.9% sodium chloride, and lactated Ringer's solution in both glass and plasticized PVC (Viaflex) containers have shown no significant absorption effect with either containers, nor a measurable loss of potency due to degradation of the drug. However, solutions should be freshly prepared and used within 24 hours.

Parenteral drug products should be inspected visually for particulate matter and discoloration prior to administration whenever solution and container permit.

How Supplied: *Tablets,* 0.5 mg (light green) and 1 mg (yellow), bottles of 100 and 500; Prescription Paks of 30; Tel-E-Dose® cartons of 100. Imprint on tablets: 0.5 mg—ROCHE BUMEX 0.5; 1 mg—ROCHE BUMEX 1.

Ampuls, 2 ml, 0.25 mg/ml, boxes of ten.

Shown in Product Identification Section, page 429

CLONOPIN®
[clon'o-pin]
(clonazepam/Roche)

The following text is complete prescribing information based on official labeling in effect August 1, 1984.

Description: Chemically, clonazepam is 5-(2-chlorophenyl) -1, 3- dihydro-7-nitro-2H-1,4-benzodiazepin-2-one. It is a light yellow crystalline powder. It has a molecular weight of 315.7.

Actions: In laboratory animals, Clonopin exhibits several pharmacologic properties which are characteristic of the benzodiazepine class of drugs. Convulsions produced in rodents by pentylenetetrazol or electrical stimulation are antagonized, as are convulsions produced by photic stimulation in susceptible baboons. A taming effect in aggressive primates, muscle weakness and hypnosis are likewise produced by Clonopin. In humans it is capable of suppressing the spike and wave discharge in absence seizures (petit mal) and decreasing the frequency, amplitude, duration and spread of discharge in minor motor seizures.

Single oral dose administration of Clonopin to humans gave maximum blood levels of drug, in most cases, within one to two hours. The half-life of the parent compound varied from approximately 18 to 50 hours, and the major route of excretion was in the urine. In humans, five metabolites have been identified. In general, the biotransformation of clonazepam followed two pathways: oxidative hydroxylation at the C-3 position and reduction of the 7-nitro function to form 7-amino and/or 7-acetyl-amino derivatives.

Indications: Clonopin is useful alone or as an adjunct in the treatment of the Lennox-Gastaut syndrome (petit mal variant), akinetic and myoclonic seizures. In patients with absence seizures (petit mal) who have failed to respond to succinimides, Clonopin may be useful.

In some studies, up to 30% of patients have shown a loss of anticonvulsant activity, often within three months of administration. In some cases, dosage adjustment may reestablish efficacy.

Contraindications: Clonopin should not be used in patients with a history of sensitivity to benzodiazepines, nor in patients with clinical or biochemical evidence of significant liver disease. It may be used in patients with open angle glaucoma who are receiving appropriate therapy, but is contraindicated in acute narrow angle glaucoma.

Warnings: Since Clonopin produces CNS depression, patients receiving this drug should be cautioned against engaging in hazardous occupations requiring mental alertness, such as operating machinery or driving a motor vehicle. They should also be warned about the concomitant use of alcohol or other CNS-depressant drugs during Clonopin therapy (see Drug Interactions).

Usage in Pregnancy: The effects of Clonopin in human pregnancy and nursing infants are unknown.

Recent reports suggest an association between the use of anticonvulsant drugs by women with epilepsy and an elevated incidence of birth defects in children born to these women. Data are more extensive with respect to diphenylhydantoin and phenobarbital, but these are also the most commonly prescribed anticonvulsants; less systematic or anecdotal reports suggest a possible similar association with the use of all known anticonvulsant drugs.

The reports suggesting an elevated incidence of birth defects in children of drug-treated epileptic women cannot be regarded as adequate to prove a definite cause and effect relationship. There are intrinsic methodologic problems in obtaining adequate data on drug teratogenicity in humans; the possibility also exists that other factors, *e.g.,* genetic factors or the epileptic condition itself, may be more important than drug therapy in leading to birth defects. The great majority of mothers on anticonvulsant medication deliver normal infants. It is important to note that anticonvulsant drugs should not be discontinued in patients in whom the drug is administered to prevent seizures because of the strong possibility of precipitating status epilepticus with attendant hypoxia and threat to life. In individual cases where the severity and frequency of the seizure disorder are such that the removal of medication does not pose a serious threat to the patient, discontinuation of the drug may be considered prior to and during pregnancy, although it cannot be said with any confidence that even mild seizures do not pose some hazards to the developing embryo or fetus.

These considerations should be weighed in treating or counseling epileptic women of childbearing potential.

Use of Clonopin in women of childbearing potential should be considered only when the clinical situation warrants the risk. Mothers receiving Clonopin should not breast feed their infants.

In a two-generation reproduction study with Clonopin given orally to rats at 10 or 100 mg/kg/day, there was a decrease in the number of pregnancies and a decrease in the number of offspring surviving until weaning. When Clonopin was administered orally to pregnant rabbits at 0.2, 1.0, 5.0 or 10.0 mg/kg/day, a nondose-related incidence of cleft palates, open eyelids, fused sternebrae and limb defects was observed at the 0.2 and 5.0 mg/kg/day levels. Nearly all of the malformations were seen from one dam in each of the affected dosages.

Usage in Children: Because of the possibility that adverse effects on physical or mental development could become apparent only after many years, a benefit-risk consideration of the long-term use of Clonopin is important in pediatric patients.

Physical and Psychological Dependence: Withdrawal symptoms similar in character to those noted with barbiturates and alcohol have occurred following abrupt discontinuance of benzodiazepine drugs. These symptoms include convulsions, tremor, abdominal and muscle cramps, vomiting and sweating. Addiction-prone individuals, such as drug addicts or alcoholics, should be under careful surveillance when receiving benzodiazepines because of the predisposition of such patients to habituation and dependence.

Precautions: When used in patients in whom several different types of seizure disorders coexist, Clonopin may increase the incidence or precipitate the onset of generalized tonic-clonic seizures (grand mal). This may require the addition of appropriate anticonvulsants or an increase in their dosages. The concomitant use of valproic acid and clonazepam may produce absence status.

Periodic blood counts and liver function tests are advisable during long-term therapy with Clonopin.

The abrupt withdrawal of Clonopin, particularly in those patients on long-term, high-dose therapy, may precipitate status epilepticus. Therefore, when discontinuing Clonopin, gradual withdrawal is essential. While Clonopin is being gradually withdrawn, the simultaneous substitution of another anticonvulsant may be indicated. Metabolites of Clonopin are excreted by the kidneys; to avoid their excess accumulation, caution should be exercised in the administration of the drug to patients with impaired renal function.

Clonopin may produce an increase in salivation. This should be considered before giving the drug to patients who have difficulty handling secretions.

Because of this and the possibility of respiratory

depression, Clonopin should be used with caution in patients with chronic respiratory diseases.
Adverse Reactions: The most frequently occurring side effects of Clonopin are referable to CNS depression. Experience to date has shown that drowsiness has occurred in approximately 50% of patients and ataxia in approximately 30%. In some cases, these may diminish with time; behavior problems have been noted in approximately 25% of patients. Others, listed by system, are:
Neurologic: Abnormal eye movements, aphonia, choreiform movements, coma, diplopia, dysarthria, dysdiadochokinesis, "glassy-eyed" appearance, headache, hemiparesis, hypotonia, nystagmus, respiratory depression, slurred speech, tremor, vertigo.
Psychiatric: Confusion, depression, forgetfulness, hallucinations, hysteria, increased libido, insomnia, psychosis, suicidal attempt (the behavior effects are more likely to occur in patients with a history of psychiatric disturbances).
Respiratory: Chest congestion, rhinorrhea, shortness of breath, hypersecretion in upper respiratory passages.
Cardiovascular: Palpitations.
Dermatologic: Hair loss, hirsutism, skin rash, ankle and facial edema.
Gastrointestinal: Anorexia, coated tongue, constipation, diarrhea, dry mouth, encopresis, gastritis, hepatomegaly, increased appetite, nausea, sore gums.
Genitourinary: Dysuria, enuresis, nocturia, urinary retention.
Musculoskeletal: Muscle weakness, pains.
Miscellaneous: Dehydration, general deterioration, fever, lymphadenopathy, weight loss or gain.
Hematopoietic: Anemia, leukopenia, thrombocytopenia, eosinophilia.
Hepatic: Transient elevations of serum transaminases and alkaline phosphatase.
Drug Interactions: The CNS-depressant action of the benzodiazepine class of drugs may be potentiated by alcohol, narcotics, barbiturates, nonbarbiturate hypnotics, antianxiety agents, the phenothiazines, thioxanthene and butyrophenone classes of antipsychotic agents, monoamine oxidase inhibitors and the tricyclic antidepressants, and by other anticonvulsant drugs.
Overdosage: Symptoms of Clonopin overdosage, like those produced by other CNS depressants, include somnolence, confusion, coma and diminished reflexes. Treatment includes monitoring of respiration, pulse and blood pressure, general supportive measures and immediate gastric lavage. Intravenous fluids should be administered and an adequate airway maintained. Hypotension may be combated by the use of levarterenol or metaraminol. Methylphenidate or caffeine and sodium benzoate may be given to combat CNS depression. Dialysis is of no known value.
Dosage and Administration: *Infants and Children:* Clonopin is administered orally. In order to minimize drowsiness, the initial dose for infants and children (up to 10 years of age or 30 kg of body weight) should be between 0.01 to 0.03 mg/kg/day but not to exceed 0.05 mg/kg/day given in two or three divided doses. Dosage should be increased by no more than 0.25 to 0.5 mg every third day until a daily maintenance dose of 0.1 to 0.2 mg/kg of body weight has been reached unless seizures are controlled or side effects preclude further increase. Whenever possible, the daily dose should be divided into three equal doses. If doses are not equally divided, the largest dose should be given before retiring.
Adults: The initial dose for adults should not exceed 1.5 mg/day divided into three doses. Dosage may be increased in increments of 0.5 to 1 mg every three days until seizures are adequately controlled or until side effects preclude any further increase. Maintenance dosage must be individualized for each patient depending upon response. Maximum recommended daily dose is 20 mg.
The use of multiple anticonvulsants may result in an increase of depressant adverse effects. This should be considered before adding Clonopin to an existing anticonvulsant regimen.

How Supplied: Scored tablets—0.5 mg, orange; 1 mg, blue; 2 mg, white—Prescription Paks of 100.
Shown in Product Identification Section, page 429

EFUDEX® ℞
[ef' u-dex]
(fluorouracil/Roche)

The following text is complete prescribing information based on official labeling in effect August 1, 1984.
Description: Efudex solutions and cream are topical preparations containing the fluorinated pyrimidine 5-fluorouracil, an antineoplastic antimetabolite.
Efudex Solution consists of 2% or 5% fluorouracil/Roche on a weight/weight basis, compounded with propylene glycol, tris(hydroxymethyl) aminomethane, hydroxypropyl cellulose, parabens (methyl and propyl) and disodium edetate.
Efudex Cream contains 5% fluorouracil/Roche in a vanishing cream base consisting of white petrolatum, stearyl alcohol, propylene glycol, polysorbate 60 and parabens (methyl and propyl).
Actions: There is evidence that the metabolism of fluorouracil in the anabolic pathway blocks the methylation reaction of deoxyuridylic acid to thymidylic acid. In this fashion fluorouracil interferes with the synthesis of deoxyribonucleic acid (DNA) and to a lesser extent inhibits the formation of ribonucleic acid (RNA). Since DNA and RNA are essential for cell division and growth, the effect of fluorouracil may be to create a thymine deficiency which provokes unbalanced growth and death of the cell. The effects of DNA and RNA deprivation are most marked on those cells which grow more rapidly and which take up fluorouracil at a more rapid pace. The catabolic metabolism of fluorouracil results in degradative products (e.g., CO_2, urea, α-fluoro-β-alanine) which are inactive.
Studies in man with topical application of ^{14}C-labeled Efudex demonstrated insignificant absorption as measured by ^{14}C content of plasma, urine and respiratory CO_2.
Indications: Efudex is recommended for the topical treatment of multiple actinic or solar keratoses. In the 5% strength it is also useful in the treatment of superficial basal cell carcinomas, when conventional methods are impractical, such as with multiple lesions or difficult treatment sites. The diagnosis should be established prior to treatment, since this new method has not been proven effective in other types of basal cell carcinomas. With isolated, easily accessible lesions, conventional techniques are preferred since success with such lesions is almost 100% with these methods. The success rate with Efudex cream and solution is approximately 93%. This 93% success rate is based on 113 lesions in 54 patients. Twenty-five lesions treated with the solution produced one failure and 88 lesions treated with the cream produced 7 failures.
Contraindications: Efudex is contraindicated in patients with known hypersensitivity to any of its components.
Warnings: If an occlusive dressing is used, there may be an increase in the incidence of inflammatory reactions in the adjacent normal skin. A porous gauze dressing may be applied for cosmetic reasons without increase in reaction.
Prolonged exposure to ultraviolet rays should be avoided while under treatment with Efudex because the intensity of the reaction may be increased.
Usage in Pregnancy: Safety for use in pregnancy has not been established.
Precautions: If Efudex is applied with the fingers, the hands should be washed immediately afterward. Efudex should be applied with care near the eyes, nose and mouth. Solar keratoses which do not respond should be biopsied to confirm the diagnosis. Patients should be forewarned that the reaction in the treated areas may be unsightly during therapy, and, in some cases, for several weeks following cessation of therapy.
Follow-up biopsies should be performed as indicated in the management of superficial basal cell carcinoma.

Adverse Reactions: The most frequently encountered local reactions are pain, pruritus, hyperpigmentation and burning at the site of application. Other local reactions include dermatitis, scarring, soreness, tenderness, suppuration, scaling and swelling.
Also reported are insomnia, stomatitis, irritability, medicinal taste, photosensitivity, lacrimation and telangiectasia, although a causal relationship is remote.
Laboratory abnormalities reported are leukocytosis, thrombocytopenia, toxic granulation and eosinophilia.
Dosage and Administration: When Efudex is applied to a lesion, a response occurs with the following sequence: erythema, usually followed by vesiculation, erosion, ulceration, necrosis and epithelization.
Actinic or solar keratosis: Apply cream or solution twice daily in an amount sufficient to cover the lesions. Medication should be continued until the inflammatory response reaches the erosion, necrosis and ulceration stage, at which time use of the drug should be terminated. The usual duration of therapy is from two to four weeks. Complete healing of the lesions may not be evident for one to two months following cessation of Efudex therapy.
Superficial basal cell carcinomas: **Only the 5% strength is recommended.** Apply cream or solution twice daily in an amount sufficient to cover the lesions. Treatment should be continued for at least three to six weeks. Therapy may be required for as long as 10 to 12 weeks before the lesions are obliterated. As in any neoplastic condition, the patient should be followed for a reasonable period of time to determine if a cure has been obtained.
How Supplied: Efudex Solution, 10-ml drop dispensers—containing 2% or 5% fluorouracil/Roche on a weight/weight basis, compounded with propylene glycol, tris(hydroxymethyl)aminomethane, hydroxypropyl cellulose, parabens (methyl and propyl) and disodium edetate.
Efudex Cream, 25-Gm tubes—containing 5% fluorouracil/Roche in a vanishing cream base consisting of white petrolatum, stearyl alcohol, propylene glycol, polysorbate 60 and parabens (methyl and propyl).

EMCYT® ℞
[em' sit]
(estramustine phosphate sodium/Roche)
CAPSULES

The following text is complete prescribing information based on official labeling in effect August 1, 1984.
Description: Estramustine phosphate sodium, an antineoplastic agent, is an off-white powder readily soluble in water. Emcyt is available as white opaque capsules, each containing estramustine phosphate sodium equivalent to 140 mg estramustine phosphate, for oral administration.
Chemically, estramustine phosphate sodium is estra-1, 3, 5(10)-triene -3, 17β- diol-3[bis-(2-chloroethyl)carbamate] 17-(dihydrogen phosphate), disodium salt. It is also referred to as estradiol 3-bis(2-chloroethyl)carbamate 17-(dihydrogen phosphate), disodium salt.
Estramustine phosphate sodium has an empiric formula of $C_{23}H_{30}Cl_2NNa_2O_6P$ and a calculated molecular weight of 582.4.
Clinical Pharmacology: Estramustine phosphate is a molecule combining estradiol and nornitrogen mustard by a carbamate link. The molecule is phosphorylated to make it water soluble.
Estramustine phosphate taken orally is readily dephosphorylated during absorption, and the major metabolites in plasma are estramustine, the estrone analog, estradiol and estrone.
Prolonged treatment with estramustine phosphate produces elevated total plasma concentrations of estradiol that fall within ranges similar to the elevated estradiol levels found in prostatic cancer patients given conventional estradiol therapy. Estrogenic effects, as demonstrated by

Continued on next page

Roche Labs.—Cont.

changes in circulating levels of steroids and pituitary hormones, are similar in patients treated with either estramustine phosphate or conventional estradiol.

The metabolic urinary patterns of the estradiol moiety of estramustine phosphate and estradiol itself are very similar, although the metabolites derived from estramustine phosphate are excreted at a slower rate.

Indications and Usage: Emcyt is indicated in the palliative treatment of patients with metastatic and/or progressive carcinoma of the prostate.

Contraindications: Emcyt should not be used in patients with any of the following conditions:
1) Known hypersensitivity to either estradiol or to nitrogen mustard.
2) Active thrombophlebitis or thromboembolic disorders, except in those cases where the actual tumor mass is the cause of the thromboembolic phenomenon and the physician feels the benefits of therapy may outweigh the risks.

Warnings: It has been shown that there is an increased risk of thrombosis, including nonfatal myocardial infarction, in men receiving estrogens for prostatic cancer. Emcyt should be used with caution in patients with a history of thrombophlebitis, thrombosis or thromboembolic disorders, especially if they were associated with estrogen therapy. Caution should also be used in patients with cerebral vascular or coronary artery disease.

Glucose Tolerance—Because glucose tolerance may be decreased, diabetic patients should be carefully observed while receiving Emcyt.

Elevated Blood Pressure—Because hypertension may occur, blood pressure should be monitored periodically.

Precautions: *General:* Fluid Retention—Exacerbation of preexisting or incipient peripheral edema or congestive heart disease has been seen in some patients receiving Emcyt therapy. Other conditions which might be influenced by fluid retention, such as epilepsy, migraine or renal dysfunction, require careful observation.

Emcyt may be poorly metabolized in patients with impaired liver function and should be administered with caution in such patients.

Because Emcyt may influence the metabolism of calcium and phosphorus, it should be used with caution in patients with metabolic bone diseases that are associated with hypercalcemia or in patients with renal insufficiency.

Information for the Patient: Because of the possibility of mutagenic effects, patients should be advised to use contraceptive measures.

Laboratory Tests: Certain endocrine and liver function tests may be affected by estrogen-containing drugs. Abnormalities of hepatic enzymes and of bilirubin have occurred in patients receiving Emcyt, but have seldom been severe enough to require cessation of therapy. Such tests should be done at appropriate intervals during therapy and repeated after the drug has been withdrawn for two months.

Food/Drug Interaction: Limited data now indicate that milk may impair the absorption of Emcyt. Therefore, consideration should be given to taking Emcyt at least one hour before or two hours after ingestion of milk.

Carcinogenesis, Mutagenesis, Impairment of Fertility: Long-term continuous administration of estrogens in certain animal species increases the frequency of carcinomas of the breast and liver. Compounds structurally similar to Emcyt are carcinogenic in mice. Carcinogenic studies of Emcyt have not been conducted in man. Although testing by the Ames method failed to demonstrate mutagenicity for estramustine phosphate sodium, it is known that both estradiol and nitrogen mustard are mutagenic. For this reason and because some patients who had been impotent while on estrogen therapy have regained potency while taking Emcyt, the patient should be advised to use contraceptive measures.

Adverse Reactions: In a randomized, double-blind trial comparing therapy with Emcyt in 93 patients (11.5 to 15.9 mg/kg/day) or diethylstilbestrol (DES) in 93 patients (3.0 mg/day), the following adverse effects were reported:

	EMCYT n=93	DES n=93
CARDIOVASCULAR–RESPIRATORY		
Cardiac Arrest	0	2
Cerebrovascular Accident	2	0
Myocardial Infarction	3	1
Thrombophlebitis	3	7
Pulmonary Emboli	2	5
Congestive Heart Failure	3	2
Edema	19	17
Dyspnea	11	3
Leg Cramps	8	11
Upper Respiratory Discharge	1	1
Hoarseness	1	0
GASTROINTESTINAL		
Nausea	15	8
Diarrhea	12	11
Minor Gastrointestinal Upset	11	6
Anorexia	4	3
Flatulence	2	0
Vomiting	1	1
Gastrointestinal Bleeding	1	0
Burning Throat	1	0
Thirst	1	0
INTEGUMENTARY		
Rash	1	4
Pruritus	2	2
Dry Skin	2	0
Pigment Changes	0	3
Easy Bruising	3	0
Flushing	1	0
Night Sweats	0	1
Fingertip–Peeling Skin	1	0
Thinning Hair	1	1
BREAST CHANGES		
Tenderness	66	64
Enlargement		
Mild	60	54
Moderate	10	16
Marked	0	5
MISCELLANEOUS		
Lethargy Alone	4	3
Depression	0	2
Emotional Lability	2	0
Insomnia	3	0
Headache	1	1
Anxiety	1	0
Chest Pain	1	1
Hot Flashes	0	1
Pain in Eyes	0	1
Tearing of Eyes	1	1
Tinnitus	0	1
LABORATORY ABNORMALITIES		
Hematologic		
Leukopenia	4	2
Thrombopenia	1	2
Hepatic		
Bilirubin Alone	1	5
Bilirubin and LDH	0	1
Bilirubin and SGOT	2	1
Bilirubin, LDH and SGOT	2	0
LDH and/or SGOT	31	28
Miscellaneous		
Hypercalcemia—Transient	0	1
	EMCYT n=93	DES n=93

Overdosage: Although there has been no experience with overdosage to date, it is reasonable to expect that such episodes may produce pronounced manifestations of the known adverse reactions. In the event of overdosage, the gastric contents should be evacuated by gastric lavage and symptomatic therapy should be initiated. Hematologic and hepatic parameters should be monitored for at least six weeks after overdosage of Emcyt.

Dosage and Administration: The recommended daily dose is 14 mg per kg of body weight (*i.e.*, one 140 mg capsule for each 10 kg or 22 lb of body weight), given in 3 or 4 divided doses. Most patients in studies in the United States have been treated at a dosage range of 10 to 16 mg per kg per day.

Patients should be treated for 30 to 90 days before the physician determines the possible benefits of continued therapy. Therapy should be continued as long as the favorable response lasts. Some patients have been maintained on therapy for more than three years at doses ranging from 10 to 16 mg per kg of body weight per day.

How Supplied: White opaque capsules, each containing estramustine phosphate sodium equivalent to 140 mg estramustine phosphate—bottles of 100 (NDC 0004-0132-02).

Note: Emcyt should be stored in the refrigerator at 36° to 46°F (2° to 8°C).

Shown in Product Identification Section, page 429

FANSIDAR® ℞
[fan'sid-ar]
(sulfadoxine and pyrimethamine/Roche)
TABLETS

The following text is complete prescribing information based on official labeling in effect August 1, 1984.

Description: Fansidar is an antimalarial agent, each tablet containing 500 mg N^1-(5,6-dimethoxy-4-pyrimidinyl) sulfanilamide (sulfadoxine) and 25 mg 2,4-diamino-5-(p-chlorophenyl)-6-ethylpyrimidine (pyrimethamine).

Clinical Pharmacology: Fansidar is an antimalarial agent which acts by reciprocal potentiation of its two components, achieved by a sequential blockade of two enzymes involved in the biosynthesis of folinic acid within the parasites.

Both the sulfadoxine and the pyrimethamine of Fansidar are absorbed orally and are excreted mainly by the kidney. Following a single tablet administration, sulfadoxine peak plasma concentrations of 51 to 76 mcg/ml were achieved in 2.5 to 6 hours and the pyrimethamine peak plasma concentrations of 0.13 to 0.4 mcg/ml were achieved in 1.5 to 8 hours. The apparent half-life of elimination of sulfadoxine ranged from 100 to 231 hours with a mean of 169 hours, whereas pyrimethamine half-lives ranged from 54 to 148 hours with a mean of 111 hours. Both drugs appear in breast milk of nursing mothers.

Fansidar is effective against certain plasmodia strains that are resistant to chloroquine. Fansidar susceptibility of plasmodia may vary by locations and time.

Fansidar is compatible with other antimalarial drugs, particularly quinine, and with antibiotics. It does not interfere with antidiabetic agents.

Indications and Usage: Fansidar is indicated for the treatment of malaria due to susceptible strains of plasmodia. The drug is also indicated for prophylaxis using a weekly or biweekly regimen.

Contraindications: Hypersensitivity to pyrimethamine or sulfonamides. Patients with documented megaloblastic anemia due to folate deficiency. Infants less than two months of age. Pregnancy at term and during the nursing period because sulfonamides pass the placenta and are excreted in the milk and may cause kernicterus.

Warnings: Deaths associated with the administration of sulfonamides have been reported from hypersensitivity reactions, hepatocellular necrosis, agranulocytosis, aplastic anemia and other blood dyscrasias. Fansidar prophylaxis should be discontinued if a significant reduction in the count of any formed blood element is noted or at the occurrence of active bacterial or fungal infections. Fansidar prophylactic regimen has been reported to cause leukopenia during a treatment of two months or longer. This leukopenia is generally mild and reversible.

Precautions:
1. *General:* Fansidar should be given with caution to patients with impaired renal or hepatic function, to those with possible folate deficiency and to those with severe allergy or bronchial asthma. As with some sulfonamide drugs, in glucose-6-phosphate dehydrogenase-deficient individuals, hemolysis may occur. Urinalysis with microscopic examination and renal function tests should

be performed during therapy of those patients who have impaired renal function.

2. *Information for the patient:* Adequate fluid intake must be maintained in order to prevent crystalluria and stone formation.

The patient should be warned that the appearance of sore throat, fever, pallor, purpura, jaundice or glossitis may be early indications of serious disorders which require prophylactic treatment to be stopped and medical treatment to be sought.

Females should be cautioned against becoming pregnant and should not breast feed their infants during Fansidar therapy or prophylactic treatment.

Patients should be warned to keep Fansidar out of reach of children.

3. *Laboratory tests:* Periodic blood counts and analysis of urine for crystalluria are desirable during prolonged prophylaxis.

4. *Drug interactions:* Antifolic drugs such as sulfonamides or trimethoprim-sulfamethoxazole combinations should not be used while the patient is receiving Fansidar for antimalarial prophylaxis. If signs of folic acid deficiency develop, Fansidar should be discontinued. Folinic acid (leucovorin) may be administered in doses of 3 mg to 9 mg intramuscularly daily, for 3 days or longer, for depressed platelet or white blood cell counts in patients with drug-induced folic acid deficiency when recovery is too slow.

5. *Carcinogenesis, mutagenesis, impairment of fertility:* Pyrimethamine was not found carcinogenic in female mice or in male and female rats. The carcinogenic potential of pyrimethamine in male mice could not be assessed from the study because of markedly reduced life-span. Pyrimethamine was found to be mutagenic in laboratory animals and also in human bone marrow following 3 or 4 consecutive daily doses totaling 200 mg to 300 mg. Pyrimethamine was not found mutagenic in the Ames test.

6. *Pregnancy:* Teratogenic effects: Pregnancy Category C. Fansidar has been shown to be teratogenic in rats when given in weekly doses approximately 12 times the weekly human prophylactic dose. Teratology studies with pyrimethamine plus sulfadoxine (1:20) in rats showed the minimum oral teratogenic dose to be approximately 0.9 mg/kg pyrimethamine plus 18 mg/kg sulfadoxine. In rabbits, no teratogenic effects were noted at oral doses as high as 20 mg/kg pyrimethamine plus 400 mg/kg sulfadoxine.

There are no adequate and well-controlled studies in pregnant women.

Because pyrimethamine plus sulfadoxine may interfere with folic acid metabolism, Fansidar therapy should be used during pregnancy only if the potential benefit justifies the potential risk to the fetus.

Nonteratogenic effects: See "CONTRAINDICATIONS" section.

7. *Nursing mothers:* See "CONTRAINDICATIONS" section.

8. *Pediatric use:* Fansidar should not be given to infants less than two months of age because of inadequate development of the glucuronide-forming enzyme system.

Adverse Reactions: For completeness, all major reactions to sulfonamides and to pyrimethamine are included below, even though they may not have been reported with Fansidar.

Blood dyscrasias: Agranulocytosis, aplastic anemia, megaloblastic anemia, thrombopenia, leukopenia, hemolytic anemia, purpura, hypoprothrombinemia and methemoglobinemia.

Allergic reactions: Erythema multiforme, Stevens-Johnson syndrome, generalized skin eruptions, epidermal necrolysis, urticaria, serum sickness, pruritus, exfoliative dermatitis, anaphylactoid reactions, periorbital edema, conjunctival and scleral injection, photosensitization, arthralgia and allergic myocarditis.

Gastrointestinal reactions: Glossitis, stomatitis, nausea, emesis, abdominal pains, hepatitis, hepatocellular necrosis, diarrhea and pancreatitis.

C.N.S. reactions: Headache, peripheral neuritis, mental depression, convulsions, ataxia, hallucinations, tinnitus, vertigo, insomnia, apathy, fatigue, muscle weakness and nervousness.

Miscellaneous reactions: Drug fever, chills, and toxic nephrosis with oliguria and anuria. Periarteritis nodosa and L. E. phenomenon have occurred. The sulfonamides bear certain chemical similarities to some goitrogens, diuretics (acetazolamide and the thiazides) and oral hypoglycemic agents. Diuresis and hypoglycemia have occurred rarely in patients receiving sulfonamides. Cross-sensitivity may exist with these agents. Rats appear to be especially susceptible to the goitrogenic effects of sulfonamides, and long-term administration has produced thyroid malignancies in the species.

Overdosage: Acute intoxication may be manifested by anorexia, vomiting and central nervous system stimulation (including convulsions), followed by megaloblastic anemia, leukopenia, thrombocytopenia, glossitis and crystalluria. In acute intoxication, emesis and gastric lavage followed by purges may be of benefit. The patient should be adequately hydrated to prevent renal damage. The renal and hematopoietic systems should be monitored for at least one month after an overdosage. If the patient is having convulsions, the use of a parenteral barbiturate is indicated. For depressed platelet or white blood cell counts, folinic acid (leucovorin) should be administered in a dosage of 3 mg to 9 mg intramuscularly daily for 3 days or longer.

Dosage and Administration:
(a) *Curative treatment of acute malaria*
For the treatment of acute attacks with a single dose of Fansidar, the following number of tablets is used either in sequence with quinine or primaquine, or alone:

Adults	2 to 3 tablets
9 to 14 years	2 tablets
4 to 8 years	1 tablet
Under 4 years	½ tablet

For acute attacks of malaria due to *Plasmodium vivax* and *Plasmodium malaria*, a single dose of Fansidar followed by primaquine for two weeks has been used to prevent relapse.

(b) *Prophylaxis management*
For malaria prophylaxis, Fansidar may be used alone. The first dose of Fansidar should be taken one or two days before departure to an endemic area; administration should be continued during the stay and for four to six weeks after return, and should be followed by a regimen of primaquine.

	Once Weekly	Once Every Two Weeks
Adults	1 tablet	2 tablets
9 to 14 years	¾ tablet	1½ tablets
4 to 8 years	½ tablet	1 tablet
Under 4 years	¼ tablet	½ tablet

How Supplied: Scored tablets, containing 500 mg sulfadoxine and 25 mg pyrimethamine—boxes of 25 (NDC-0004-0161-03).

Shown in Product Identification Section, page 429

FLUOROURACIL ℞
[flu″ro-u′ra-sil]
(5-fluorouracil/Roche)
INJECTABLE

The following text is complete prescribing information based on official labeling in effect August 1, 1984.

WARNING
It is recommended that FLUOROURACIL be given only by or under the supervision of a qualified physician who is experienced in cancer chemotherapy and who is well versed in the use of potent antimetabolites. Because of the possibility of severe toxic reactions, it is recommended that patients be hospitalized at least during the initial course of therapy. These instructions should be thoroughly reviewed before administration of Fluorouracil.

Description: FLUOROURACIL (5-fluorouracil/Roche), an antineoplastic antimetabolite, is a sterile nonpyrogenic injectable solution available in 10-ml ampuls for intravenous administration. Each 10-ml ampul contains 500 mg of 5-fluorouracil; pH is adjusted to approximately 9.0 with sodium hydroxide.

5-Fluorouracil is a fluorinated pyrimidine belonging to the category of antimetabolites. Fluorouracil resembles the natural uracil molecule in structure, except that a hydrogen atom has been replaced by a fluorine atom in the 5 position.

Actions: There is evidence that the metabolism of fluorouracil in the anabolic pathway blocks the methylation reaction of deoxyuridylic acid to thymidylic acid. In this fashion 5-fluorouracil interferes with the synthesis of deoxyribonucleic acid (DNA) and to a lesser extent inhibits the formation of ribonucleic acid (RNA). Since DNA and RNA are essential for cell division and growth, the effect of fluorouracil may be to create a thymine deficiency which provokes unbalanced growth and death of the cell. The effects of DNA and RNA deprivation are most marked on those cells which grow more rapidly and which take up fluorouracil at a more rapid pace. The catabolic metabolism of fluorouracil results in degradative products (e.g., CO_2, urea, α-fluoro-β-alanine) which are inactive. Following an intravenous injection, no intact drug can be detected in the plasma after three hours. Approximately 15 percent is excreted intact in the urine in six hours, of which over 90 percent is excreted in the first hour. Of the injected intravenous dose 60 to 80 percent is excreted as respiratory CO_2 in 8 to 12 hours.

Indications: Fluorouracil is effective in the palliative management of carcinoma of the colon, rectum, breast, stomach and pancreas in patients who are considered incurable by surgery or other means.

Contraindications: Fluorouracil therapy is contraindicated for patients in a poor nutritional state, those with depressed bone marrow function or those with potentially serious infections.

Warnings: THE DAILY DOSE OF FLUOROURACIL IS NOT TO EXCEED 800 MG. IT IS RECOMMENDED THAT PATIENTS BE HOSPITALIZED DURING THEIR FIRST COURSE OF TREATMENT.

Fluorouracil should be used with extreme caution in poor risk patients with a history of high-dose pelvic irradiation, previous use of alkylating agents or who have a widespread involvement of bone marrow by metastatic tumors or impaired hepatic or renal function. The drug is not intended as an adjuvant to surgery. Although severe toxicity is more likely in poor risk patients, fatalities may be encountered occasionally even in patients in relatively good condition.

Usage in Pregnancy: Safe use of Fluorouracil has not been established with respect to adverse effects on fetal development. Therefore, this drug should not be used during pregnancy, particularly in the first trimester, unless in the judgment of the physician the potential benefits to the patient outweigh the hazards.

Because the risk of mutagenesis has not been evaluated, such possible effects on males and females must be considered.

Combination Therapy: Any form of therapy which adds to the stress of the patient, interferes with nutrition or depresses bone marrow function will increase the toxicity of Fluorouracil.

Precautions: Fluorouracil is a highly toxic drug with a narrow margin of safety. Therefore, patients should be carefully supervised, since therapeutic response is unlikely to occur without some evidence of toxicity. Patients should be informed of expected toxic effects, particularly oral manifestations. White blood counts with differential are recommended before each dose. Severe hematological toxicity, gastrointestinal hemorrhage and even death may result from the use of Fluorouracil despite meticulous selection of patients and careful adjustment of dosage.

Therapy is to be discontinued promptly whenever one of the following signs of toxicity appears:
Stomatitis or *esophagopharyngitis*, At the first visible sign.

Continued on next page

Roche Labs.—Cont.

Leukopenia (WBC under 3500), or a *rapidly falling white blood count.*
Vomiting, Intractable.
Diarrhea, Frequent bowel movements or watery stools.
Gastrointestinal ulceration and bleeding.
Thrombocytopenia, Platelets under 100,000.
Hemorrhage from any site.

Adverse Reactions: Stomatitis and esophagopharyngitis (which may lead to sloughing and ulceration), diarrhea, anorexia, nausea and emesis are commonly seen during therapy.

Leukopenia usually follows every course of adequate therapy with Fluorouracil. The lowest white blood cell counts are commonly observed between the 9th and 14th days after the first course of treatment, although uncommonly the maximal depression may be delayed for as long as 20 days. By the 30th day the count has usually returned to the normal range.

Alopecia and dermatitis may be seen in a substantial number of cases. Patients should be alerted to the possibility of alopecia as a result of therapy and should be informed that it is a transient effect. The dermatitis most often seen is a pruritic maculopapular rash usually appearing on the extremities and less frequently on the trunk. It is generally reversible and usually responsive to symptomatic treatment. Dry skin and fissuring have also been noted. Photosensitivity, as manifested by erythema or increased pigmentation of the skin, has been observed on occasion. Also noted were photophobia, lacrimation, epistaxis, euphoria, acute cerebellar syndrome (which may persist following discontinuation of treatment) and nail changes, including loss of nails. Myocardial ischemia has also been reported.

Dosage and Administration: *General Instructions:* Administration of Fluorouracil Injectable should be done only intravenously, using care to avoid extravasation. No dilution is required.

All dosages are based on the patient's actual weight. However, the estimated lean body mass (dry weight) is used if the patient is obese or if there has been a spurious weight gain due to edema, ascites or other forms of abnormal fluid retention.

It is recommended that prior to treatment each patient be carefully evaluated in order to estimate as accurately as possible the optimum initial dosage of Fluorouracil.

Dosage: Twelve mg/kg are given intravenously once daily for four successive days. The daily dose should not be more than 800 mg. *If no toxicity is observed,* 6 mg/kg are given on the 6th, 8th, 10th and 12th days unless toxicity occurs. No therapy is given on the 5th, 7th, 9th or 11th days. *Therapy is to be discontinued at the end of the 12th day, even if no toxicity has become apparent.* (See CONTRAINDICATIONS and WARNINGS.)

Poor risk patients or those who are not in an adequate nutritional state (see CONTRAINDICATIONS and WARNINGS) should receive 6 mg/kg/day for three days. *If no toxicity is observed,* 3 mg/kg may be given on the 5th, 7th and 9th days *unless toxicity occurs.* No therapy is given on the 4th, 6th or 8th days. The daily dose should not exceed 400 mg.

A sequence of injections on either schedule constitutes a "course of therapy."

Maintenance Therapy: In instances where toxicity has not been a problem, it is recommended that therapy be continued using either of the following schedules:

1. Repeat dosage of first course every 30 days after the last day of the previous course of treatment.
2. When toxic signs resulting from the initial course of therapy have subsided, administer a maintenance dosage of 10 to 15 mg/kg/week as a single dose. Do not exceed 1 Gm per week.

The amount of the drug to be used should take into account the patient's reaction to the previous course and should be adjusted accordingly. Some patients have received from 9 to 45 courses of treatment during periods which ranged from 12 to 60 months.

How Supplied: *Injectable:* 10-ml ampuls (for intravenous use) containing 500 mg 5-fluorouracil in a colorless to faint yellow aqueous solution, with pH adjusted to approximately 9.0 with sodium hydroxide. Boxes of 10.

Note: Although Fluorouracil ampul solution may discolor slightly during storage, the potency and safety are not adversely affected.

Store at room temperature (59° to 86°F). Protect from light. If a precipitate occurs due to exposure to low temperatures, resolubilize by heating to 140°F with vigorous shaking; allow to cool to body temperature before using.

FUDR
[ef-u-dee-are]
(floxuridine/Roche) ℞

The following text is complete prescribing information based on official labeling in effect August 1, 1984.

FOR INTRA-ARTERIAL INFUSION ONLY

WARNING
It is recommended that FUDR be given only by or under the supervision of a qualified physician who is experienced in cancer chemotherapy and intra-arterial drug therapy. Because of the possibility of severe toxic reactions, all patients should be hospitalized for initiation of treatment.

Description: Floxuridine is a fluorinated pyrimidine belonging to the category of antimetabolites. It is a white to off-white odorless solid, soluble in alcohol and freely soluble in water. The 2% aqueous solution has a pH of 4.0 to 5.5. Chemically, floxuridine is 2'-deoxy-5-fluorouridine with a molecular weight of 246.19.

Actions: When FUDR is given by intra-arterial injection it is apparently rapidly catabolized to 5-fluorouracil. Thus, rapid injection of FUDR produces the same toxic and antimetabolic effects as does 5-fluorouracil. The primary effect is to interfere with the synthesis of deoxyribonucleic acid (DNA) and to a lesser extent inhibit the formation of ribonucleic acid (RNA). However, when FUDR is given by continuous intra-arterial infusion its direct anabolism to FUDR-monophosphate is enhanced, thus increasing the inhibition of DNA.

Indications: FUDR is effective in the palliative management of gastrointestinal adenocarcinoma metastatic to the liver, when given by continuous regional intra-arterial infusion in carefully selected patients who are considered incurable by surgery or other means. Patients with known disease extending beyond an area capable of infusion via a single artery should, except in unusual circumstances, be considered for systemic therapy with other chemotherapeutic agents.

Contraindications: FUDR therapy is contraindicated for patients in a poor nutritional state, those with depressed bone marrow function, or those with potentially serious infections.

Warnings: IT IS IMPERATIVE THAT ALL PATIENTS BE HOSPITALIZED FOR INITIATION OF TREATMENT.

FUDR should be used with extreme caution in poor risk patients with impaired hepatic or renal function or a history of high-dose pelvic irradiation or previous use of alkylating agents. The drug is not intended as an adjuvant to surgery.

Usage in Pregnancy: Safe use of FUDR has not been established with respect to adverse effects on fetal development. Therefore, this drug should not be used during pregnancy, particularly in the first trimester, unless in the judgment of the physician the potential benefits to the patient outweigh the hazards.

Because teratogenicity and mutagenicity have been demonstrated in animals, such possible effects on men and women must be considered.

Combination Therapy: Any form of therapy which adds to the stress of the patient, interferes with nutrition, or depresses bone marrow function will increase the toxicity of FUDR (floxuridine).

Therapy is to be discontinued promptly whenever one of the following signs of toxicity appears:
Stomatitis or esophagopharyngitis, At the first visible sign.
Leukopenia (WBC under 3500), or a rapidly falling white blood count.
Vomiting, Intractable.
Diarrhea, Frequent bowel movements or watery stools.
Gastrointestinal ulceration and bleeding.
Thrombocytopenia, Platelets under 100,000.
Hemorrhage from any site.

Precautions: FUDR is potentially a highly toxic drug with a narrow margin of safety. Therefore, patients should be carefully supervised since therapeutic response is unlikely to occur without some evidence of toxicity. Patients should be informed of expected toxic effects, particularly oral manifestations. Careful monitoring of the white blood count and platelet count is recommended. Severe hematological toxicity, gastrointestinal hemorrhage and even death may result from the use of FUDR despite meticulous selection of patients and careful adjustment of dosage. Although severe toxicity is more likely in poor risk patients, fatalities may be encountered occasionally even in patients in relatively good condition.

Adverse Reactions: The adverse reactions to the arterial infusion of FUDR are generally related to the drug-infused area and can be grouped under the following categories: functional gastrointestinal, mucosal gastrointestinal, hematologic, dermatologic, miscellaneous clinical reactions, laboratory abnormalities and procedural complications of regional arterial infusion.

The more common adverse reactions are nausea, vomiting, diarrhea, enteritis, stomatitis and localized erythema. The more common laboratory abnormalities are anemia, leukopenia, and elevations of alkaline phosphatase, serum transaminase, serum bilirubin and lactic dehydrogenase. Other adverse reactions are:

Functional gastrointestinal: anorexia, cramps and pain.
Mucosal gastrointestinal: duodenal ulcer, duodenitis, gastritis, gastroenteritis, glossitis and pharyngitis.
Dermatological: alopecia, dermatitis, nonspecific skin toxicity and rash.
Other clinical reactions: fever, lethargy, malaise, and weakness.
Laboratory abnormalities: BSP, prothrombin, total proteins, sedimentation rate and thrombopenia.
Procedural complications of regional arterial infusion: arterial aneurysm, arterial ischemia, arterial thrombosis, bleeding at catheter site, catheter blocked, displaced or leaking, embolism, fibromyositis, infection at catheter site, abscesses and thrombophlebitis.

Dosage and Administration: The recommended therapeutic dose schedule of FUDR by continuous arterial infusion is 0.1 to 0.6 mg/kg/day. The higher dose ranges (0.4 to 0.6 mg) are usually employed for hepatic artery infusion because the liver metabolizes the drug, thus reducing the potential for systemic toxicity. Therapy can be given until adverse reactions appear. When these side effects have subsided, therapy may be resumed. The patient should be maintained on therapy as long as response to FUDR continues. The administration of FUDR is best achieved with the use of an appropriate pump to overcome pressure in large arteries and to ensure a uniform rate of infusion.

How Supplied: 500 mg FUDR (floxuridine/Roche) sterile powder, in a 5-ml vial. This is reconstituted with 5 ml sterile water. Reconstituted vials should be stored under refrigeration (36° to 46°F.) for not more than two weeks.

Clinical Studies: In 349 evaluable patients treated with continuous arterial infusion of FUDR, 144 obtained significant objective response associated with clinical benefit for at least one month, and an additional 14 patients had objective and subjective benefits for at least one year.

GANTANOL®
[gan'tan-ol]
(sulfamethoxazole/Roche)
**TABLETS • SUSPENSION •
DS (double strength) TABLETS**

The following text is complete prescribing information based on official labeling in effect August 1, 1984.

Description: Gantanol is an intermediate-dosage sulfonamide. Sulfamethoxazole is an almost white, odorless, tasteless compound. Chemically, it is N^1-(5-methyl-3-isoxazolyl)sulfanilamide.

In a single dose study using two grams of drug, levels of free sulfamethoxazole achieved in the plasma with the tablet and suspension dosage forms were compared in a group of 19 normal subjects. There was no significant difference between the plasma levels obtained with the two dosage forms. The mean concentration of free sulfamethoxazole in plasma after administration of tablets was:

1½ hours	8.38 mg%
3 hours	12.08 mg%
6 hours	9.82 mg%
9 hours	7.9 mg%
12 hours	6.45 mg%

Administration of Gantanol at the adult recommended dosage of 2 Gm initially followed by 1 Gm every 12 hours for 4 days produced average blood concentrations of 5.8 mg% total sulfonamide and 5.1 mg% free sulfonamide 6 hours following the last dose.

Sulfonamides exist in the blood as free, conjugated (acetylated and possibly other forms) and protein-bound forms. The "free" form is considered to be the therapeutically active form. It has been shown that approximately 70 per cent of Gantanol is protein bound in the blood; of the unbound portion 80 to 90 per cent is in the nonacetylated form. Excretion of sulfonamides is chiefly by the kidneys with glomerular filtration as the primary mechanism.

Actions: The systemic sulfonamides are bacteriostatic agents. The spectrum of activity is similar for all. Sulfonamides competitively inhibit bacterial synthesis of folic acid (pteroylglutamic acid) from para-aminobenzoic acid. Resistant strains are capable of utilizing folic acid precursors or preformed folic acid.

Indications: Acute, recurrent or chronic urinary tract infections (primarily pyelonephritis, pyelitis and cystitis) due to susceptible organisms (usually *E. coli, Klebsiella-Aerobacter,* staphylococcus, *Proteus mirabilis,* and, less frequently, *Proteus vulgaris*) in the absence of obstructive uropathy or foreign bodies.

Meningococcal meningitis prophylaxis when sulfonamide-sensitive group A strains are known to prevail in family groups or larger closed populations. (The prophylactic usefulness of sulfonamides when group B or C infections are prevalent is not proven and in closed population groups may be harmful.)

In acute otitis media due to *Haemophilus influenzae* when used concomitantly with adequate doses of penicillin.

Trachoma. Inclusion conjunctivitis. Nocardiosis. Chancroid. Toxoplasmosis as adjunctive therapy with pyrimethamine. Malaria due to chloroquine-resistant strains of *Plasmodium falciparum,* when used as adjunctive therapy.

Important note. *In vitro* sulfonamide sensitivity tests are not always reliable. The test must be carefully coordinated with bacteriologic and clinical response. When the patient is already taking sulfonamides, follow-up cultures should have aminobenzoic acid added to the culture media.

Currently, the increasing frequency of resistant organisms is a limitation of the usefulness of antibacterial agents including the sulfonamides, especially in the treatment of chronic and recurrent urinary tract infections.

Wide variation in blood levels may result with identical doses. Blood levels should be measured in patients receiving sulfonamides for serious infections. Free sulfonamide blood levels of 5 to 15 mg per 100 ml may be considered therapeutically effective for most infections, with blood levels of 12 to 15 mg per 100 ml optimal for serious infections; 20 mg per 100 ml should be the maximum total sulfonamide level, as adverse reactions occur more frequently above this level.

Contraindications: Hypersensitivity to sulfonamides. Infants less than 2 months of age (except in the treatment of congenital toxoplasmosis as adjunctive therapy with pyrimethamine). Pregnancy at term and during the nursing period, because sulfonamides pass the placenta and are excreted in the milk and may cause kernicterus.

Warnings: *Usage in Pregnancy:* The safe use of sulfonamides in pregnancy has not been established. The teratogenicity potential of most sulfonamides has not been thoroughly investigated in either animals or humans. However, a significant increase in the incidence of cleft palate and other bony abnormalities of offspring has been observed when certain sulfonamides of the short, intermediate and long-acting types were given to pregnant rats and mice at high oral doses (7 to 25 times the human therapeutic dose).

The sulfonamides should not be used for the treatment of Group A beta-hemolytic streptococcal infections. In an established infection, they will not eradicate the streptococcus, and therefore will not prevent sequelae such as rheumatic fever and glomerulonephritis.

Deaths associated with the administration of sulfonamides have been reported from hypersensitivity reactions, hepatocellular necrosis, agranulocytosis, aplastic anemia and other blood dyscrasias. The presence of clinical signs such as sore throat, fever, pallor, purpura or jaundice may be early indications of serious blood disorders. Complete blood counts should be done frequently in patients receiving sulfonamides.

The frequency of renal complications is considerably lower in patients receiving the more soluble sulfonamides. Urinalysis with careful microscopic examination should be obtained frequently in patients receiving sulfonamides. At the present time there are insufficient clinical data on prolonged or recurrent therapy in chronic renal diseases of children under 6 years.

Precautions: Sulfonamides should be given with caution to patients with impaired renal or hepatic function and to those with severe allergy or bronchial asthma. In glucose-6-phosphate dehydrogenase-deficient individuals, hemolysis may occur. This reaction is frequently dose-related. Adequate fluid intake must be maintained in order to prevent crystalluria and stone formation.

Adverse Reactions: *Blood dyscrasias:* Agranulocytosis, aplastic anemia, thrombocytopenia, leukopenia, hemolytic anemia, purpura, hypoprothrombinemia and methemoglobinemia.

Allergic reactions: Erythema multiforme (Stevens-Johnson syndrome), generalized skin eruptions, epidermal necrolysis, urticaria, serum sickness, pruritus, exfoliative dermatitis, anaphylactoid reactions, periorbital edema, conjunctival and scleral injection, photosensitization, arthralgia and allergic myocarditis.

Gastrointestinal reactions: Nausea, emesis, abdominal pains, hepatitis, hepatocellular necrosis, diarrhea, anorexia, pancreatitis and stomatitis.

C.N.S. reactions: Headache, peripheral neuritis, mental depression, convulsions, ataxia, hallucinations, tinnitus, vertigo and insomnia.

Miscellaneous reactions: Drug fever, chills, and toxic nephrosis with oliguria and anuria. Periarteritis nodosa and L.E. phenomenon have occurred. The sulfonamides bear certain chemical similarities to some goitrogens, diuretics (acetazolamide and the thiazides) and oral hypoglycemic agents. Goiter production, diuresis and hypoglycemia have occurred rarely in patients receiving sulfonamides. Cross-sensitivity may exist with these agents.

Rats appear to be especially susceptible to the goitrogenic effects of sulfonamides, and long-term administration has produced thyroid malignancies in the species.

Dosage and Administration: Systemic sulfonamides are contraindicated in infants under 2 months of age, except in the treatment of congenital toxoplasmosis as adjunctive therapy with pyrimethamine.

The usual dosage schedule is as follows:

Children

Infants (2 Months or Older) and Children	Initial Dose (50-60 mg/kg)	Dose Morning and Evening Daily Thereafter (25-30 mg/kg)
20 lbs	1 tablet or 1 teasp. (0.5 Gm)	½ tablet or ½ teasp. (0.25 Gm)
40 lbs	2 tablets or 2 teasp. (1 Gm)	1 tablet or 1 teasp. (0.5 Gm)
60 lbs	3 tablets or 3 teasp. (1.5 Gm)	1½ tablets or 1½ teasp. (0.75 Gm)
80 lbs	2 DS (double strength) tablets or 4 tablets or 4 teasp. (2 Gm)	1 DS (double strength) tablet or 2 tablets or 2 teasp. (1 Gm)

The maximum dose for children should not exceed 75 mg/kg/24 hours.

Adults

Mild to Moderate Infections	2 DS (double strength) tablets or 4 tablets or 4 teasp. (2 Gm)	1 DS (double strength) tablet or 2 tablets or 2 teasp. (1 Gm)

Note: One teaspoonful equals 5 ml.

Severe Infections: 2 DS (double strength) tablets, or 4 tablets, or 4 teasp. (2 Gm) initially, followed by 1 DS (double strength) tablet, or 2 tablets, or 2 teasp. (1 Gm) three times daily thereafter.

How Supplied: DS (double strength) tablets, light orange, scored, each containing 1 Gm sulfamethoxazole/Roche—bottles of 100.

Tablets, green, scored, each containing 0.5 Gm sulfamethoxazole/Roche—bottles of 100 and 500; Tel-E-Dose® packages of 100.

Suspension, 10%, 0.5 Gm sulfamethoxazole/Roche per teaspoonful (5 ml), cherry-flavored—bottles of 16 oz (1 pint).

Shown in Product Identification Section, page 429

GANTRISIN®
[gan'tris-in]
(sulfisoxazole diolamine/Roche)
**OPHTHALMIC SOLUTION
OPHTHALMIC OINTMENT**

The following text is complete prescribing information based on official labeling in effect August 1, 1984.

Description: GANTRISIN Ophthalmic Ointment and Solution are sulfonamide preparations specifically for topical ophthalmic use. The solution is a sterile, isotonic preparation containing 4% (40 mg/ml) sulfisoxazole/Roche in the form of the diolamine salt and phenylmercuric nitrate 1:100,000 added as a preservative. It has a physiologic pH, and does not cause significant stinging or burning on application. The ointment is a sterile preparation containing 4% sulfisoxazole in the form of the diolamine salt compounded with white petrolatum, mineral oil and phenylmercuric nitrate 1:50,000 added as a preservative. Both dosage forms are stable at room temperature and do not require refrigeration.

Actions: Sulfonamides exert a bacteriostatic effect against a wide range of gram-positive and gram-negative microorganisms by restricting, through competition with para-aminobenzoic acid, the synthesis of folic acid which bacteria require for growth.

Indications: For the treatment of conjunctivitis, corneal ulcer, and other superficial ocular infections due to susceptible microorganisms, and as an adjunct in systemic sulfonamide therapy of trachoma.

Continued on next page

Roche Labs.—Cont.

Contraindications: Hypersensitivity to sulfonamide preparations.
Precautions: Gantrisin Ophthalmic Solution and Ointment are incompatible with silver preparations. Ophthalmic ointments may retard corneal healing. Nonsusceptible organisms, including fungi, may proliferate with the use of these preparations. Sulfonamides are inactivated by the para-aminobenzoic acid present in purulent exudates. Should undesirable reactions occur, discontinue administration immediately.
Dosage and Administration: Solution: Instill two to three drops in the eye three or more times daily. Care should be taken not to touch dropper tip to any surface, as contamination of solution may result. Ointment: Instill small amount in the lower conjunctival sac one to three times daily and at bedtime.
How Supplied: Solution: ½-oz bottles with dropper. Ointment: ⅛-oz tubes.

GANTRISIN® ℞
[gan'tris-in]
(sulfisoxazole/Roche) Tablets
GANTRISIN® ℞
(acetyl sulfisoxazole/Roche)
Pediatric Suspension and Syrup
LIPO GANTRISIN® ℞
(acetyl sulfisoxazole/Roche)
GANTRISIN® ℞
(sulfisoxazole diolamine/Roche)
Injectable

The following text is complete prescribing information based on official labeling in effect August 1, 1984.
Description: Sulfisoxazole is a white to slightly yellowish, odorless, slightly bitter, crystalline powder. It is soluble in alcohol and very slightly soluble in water. Chemically, it is N^1-(3,4-dimethyl-5-isoxazolyl)sulfanilamide. Acetyl sulfisoxazole, the tasteless form of sulfisoxazole, is N^1-acetyl sulfisoxazole and must be differentiated from the N^4-acetyl sulfisoxazole which is a metabolite of sulfisoxazole. The injectable form is the 2,2'-iminodiethanol salt of N^1-(3,4-dimethyl-5-isoxazolyl)sulfanilamide.
N^1-acetyl sulfisoxazole is believed to be metabolized to sulfisoxazole by digestive enzymes in the gastrointestinal tract and this enzymatic splitting is presumed responsible for the delayed absorption and attainment of blood levels.[1] With continued administration of N^1-acetyl sulfisoxazole, blood levels approximate those of sulfisoxazole.[1]
Sulfonamides exist in the blood as free, conjugated (acetylated and possibly other forms) and protein-bound forms. The "free" form is considered to be the therapeutically active form.
The concentrations of free and total sulfonamide in the blood with oral doses of 1 Gm sulfisoxazole every 4 hours have been reported as 5.85 mg% and 9.17 mg% respectively, at 24 hours.[2] In adults, doses of 3 Gm of the N^1-acetyl sulfisoxazole every 4 hours produced average blood levels of 8.7 mg%.[3] With Lipo Gantrisin (acetyl sulfisoxazole/Roche in lipid emulsion), administration of 100 mg/kg every 12 hours produced mean blood levels of free sulfonamide ranging between 8.8 and 16.6 mg% over a 24-hour period; continued administration yielded mean levels of between 11.7 and 16.8 mg% free sulfonamide.[4]
With a dosage schedule of 2 Gm intravenously every 8 hours, average blood levels of 11.7 mg/100 ml free and 16.7 mg/100 ml total were obtained.[2] With subcutaneous injection of 200 mg/kg sulfisoxazole, the average blood level at 12 hours was 10.4 mg% and at 24 hours, 7.1 mg%.[5] With single intramuscular dosage of 2 Gm, the plasma levels peaked from 1 to 4 hours, with average levels of 13.8 mg% of free sulfisoxazole[6] and 16.0 mg% total sulfisoxazole[7] obtained at 2 hours.
Approximately 85% of sulfisoxazole is protein bound in the blood;[8] of the unbound portion 65 to 72% is in the nonacetylated form.[1]

In normal subjects cerebrospinal fluid levels of sulfisoxazole have been reported to range from 8 to 57% of blood levels.[3,9] Higher cerebrospinal fluid levels are found in patients with inflamed meninges.[9]
Excretion of sulfonamides is chiefly by the kidneys with glomerular filtration as the primary mechanism.
Actions: The systemic sulfonamides are bacteriostatic agents. The spectrum of activity is similar for all. Sulfonamides competitively inhibit bacterial synthesis of folic acid (pteroylglutamic acid) from para-aminobenzoic acid. Resistant strains are capable of utilizing folic acid precursors or preformed folic acid.
Indications: Injectable sulfonamides should be used only when oral administration is impractical. Gantrisin is indicated for acute, recurrent or chronic urinary tract infections (primarily cystitis, pyelitis and pyelonephritis) due to susceptible organisms (usually *E. coli, Klebsiella-Aerobacter,* staphylococcus, *Proteus mirabilis,* and, less frequently, *Proteus vulgaris*) in the absence of obstructive uropathy or foreign bodies.
Meningococcal meningitis where the organism has been demonstrated to be susceptible. *Haemophilus influenzae* meningitis as adjunctive therapy with parenteral streptomycin.
Meningococcal meningitis prophylaxis when sulfonamide-sensitive group A strains are known to prevail in family groups or larger closed populations. (The prophylactic usefulness of sulfonamides when group B or C infections are prevalent is not proven and in closed population groups may be harmful.)
In acute otitis media due to *Haemophilus influenzae* when used concomitantly with adequate doses of penicillin or erythromycin (see appropriate erythromycin labeling for prescribing information).
Trachoma. Inclusion conjunctivitis. Nocardiosis. Chancroid. Toxoplasmosis as adjunctive therapy with pyrimethamine. Malaria due to chloroquine-resistant strains of *Plasmodium falciparum,* when used as adjunctive therapy.
Important note. In vitro sulfonamide sensitivity tests are not always reliable. The test must be carefully coordinated with bacteriologic and clinical response. When the patient is already taking sulfonamides, follow-up cultures should have aminobenzoic acid added to the culture media.
Currently, the increasing frequency of resistant organisms is a limitation of the usefulness of antibacterial agents including the sulfonamides, especially in the treatment of chronic and recurrent urinary tract infections.
Wide variation in blood levels may result with identical doses. Blood levels should be measured in patients receiving sulfonamides for serious infections. Free sulfonamide blood levels of 5 to 15 mg per 100 ml may be considered therapeutically effective for most infections, with blood levels of 12 to 15 mg per 100 ml optimal for serious infections; 20 mg per 100 ml should be the maximum total sulfonamide level, as adverse reactions occur more frequently above this level.
Contraindications: Hypersensitivity to sulfonamides. Infants less than 2 months of age (except in the treatment of congenital toxoplasmosis as adjunctive therapy with pyrimethamine). Pregnancy at term and during the nursing period, because sulfonamides pass the placenta and are excreted in the milk and may cause kernicterus.
Warnings: *Usage in Pregnancy:* The safe use of sulfonamides in pregnancy has not been established. The teratogenicity potential of most sulfonamides has not been thoroughly investigated in either animals or humans. However, a significant increase in the incidence of cleft palate and other bony abnormalities of offspring has been observed when certain sulfonamides of the short, intermediate and long-acting types were given to pregnant rats and mice at high oral doses (7 to 25 times the human therapeutic dose).
The sulfonamides should not be used for the treatment of Group A beta-hemolytic streptococcal infections. In an established infection, they will not eradicate the streptococcus, and therefore will not prevent sequelae such as rheumatic fever and glomerulonephritis.

Deaths associated with the administration of sulfonamides have been reported from hypersensitivity reactions, hepatocellular necrosis, agranulocytosis, aplastic anemia and other blood dyscrasias. The presence of clinical signs such as sore throat, fever, pallor, purpura or jaundice may be early indications of serious blood disorders. Complete blood counts should be done frequently in patients receiving sulfonamides.
The frequency of renal complications is considerably lower in patients receiving the more soluble sulfonamides. Urinalysis with careful microscopic examination should be obtained frequently in patients receiving sulfonamides.
Occasional severe systemic reactions may follow rapid intravenous administration.
Precautions: Sulfonamides should be given with caution to patients with impaired renal or hepatic function and to those with severe allergy or bronchial asthma. In glucose-6-phosphate dehydrogenase-deficient individuals, hemolysis may occur. This reaction is frequently dose-related. Adequate fluid intake must be maintained in order to prevent crystalluria and stone formation.
Adverse Reactions: *Blood dyscrasias:* Agranulocytosis, aplastic anemia, thrombocytopenia, leukopenia, hemolytic anemia, purpura, hypoprothrombinemia and methemoglobinemia.
Allergic reactions: Erythema multiforme (Stevens-Johnson syndrome), generalized skin eruptions, epidermal necrolysis, urticaria, serum sickness, pruritus, exfoliative dermatitis, anaphylactoid reactions, periorbital edema, conjunctival and scleral injection, photosensitization, arthralgia and allergic myocarditis.
Gastrointestinal reactions: Nausea, emesis, abdominal pains, hepatitis, hepatocellular necrosis, diarrhea, anorexia, pancreatitis and stomatitis.
C.N.S. reactions: Headache, peripheral neuritis, mental depression, convulsions, ataxia, hallucinations, tinnitus, vertigo and insomnia.
Miscellaneous reactions: Drug fever, chills and toxic nephrosis with oliguria and anuria. Periarteritis nodosa and L.E. phenomenon have occurred. Local reaction may occur with intramuscular injection.
The sulfonamides bear certain chemical similarities to some goitrogens, diuretics (acetazolamide and the thiazides) and oral hypoglycemic agents. Goiter production, diuresis and hypoglycemia have occurred rarely in patients receiving sulfonamides. Cross-sensitivity may exist with these agents.
Rats appear to be especially susceptible to the goitrogenic effects of sulfonamides, and long-term administration has produced thyroid malignancies in the species.
Dosage and Administration: Systemic sulfonamides are contraindicated in infants under 2 months of age, except in the treatment of congenital toxoplasmosis as adjunctive therapy with pyrimethamine. Injectable sulfonamides should be used only when oral administration is impractical.
<u>TABLETS, PEDIATRIC SUSPENSION AND SYRUP</u> (0.5 Gm sulfisoxazole per tablet or the equivalent in each 5-ml teaspoonful of the suspension or syrup)—
Usual dose for infants over 2 months of age and children:
Initial dose: One-half of the 24-hour dose.
Maintenance dose: 150 mg/kg/24 hours or 4 Gm/M²/24 hours—dose to be divided into 4 to 6 doses/24 hours with maximum of 6 Gm/24 hours.
Usual adult dose:
Initial dose: 2 to 4 Gm.
Maintenance dose: 4 to 8 Gm/24 hours, divided into 4 to 6 doses/24 hours.
<u>LIPO GANTRISIN</u> (containing the equivalent of 1 Gm sulfisoxazole in each 5-ml teaspoonful)—
Usual dose for infants over 2 months of age and children:
Initial dose: 60 to 75 mg/kg.
Maintenance dose: 60 to 75 mg/kg twice daily. The maximum dose should not exceed 6 Gm/24 hours.

for possible revisions

Usual adult dose:
4 to 5 Gm every twelve hours.

INJECTABLE: For subcutaneous and intravenous administration the 40% solution must be diluted to a concentration of 5% (combine a 5-ml ampul with 35 ml of water for injection USP).
Administration of the drug in combination with parenteral fluids is not recommended. The use of diluents other than water for injection USP may cause precipitation.
Injectable Gantrisin may be given intramuscularly without dilution.

Usual dose for infants over 2 months of age, children and adults:
Initial dose: One-half of the 24-hour dose. Maintenance dose: 100 mg/kg/24 hours or 2.25 Gm/M^2/24 hours, administered in a 5% solution—
a. Subcutaneous administration, divided into 3 doses/24 hours.
b. Intravenous administration, divided into 4 doses/24 hours. (Administer by slow injection or intravenous drip.)
For example—give 1 ml/kg of 5% solution as an initial dose. This should be followed by 0.50 ml/kg of 5% solution four times daily for intravenous administration or 0.66 ml/kg t.i.d. for subcutaneous administration.
c. Intramuscular administration, divided into 2 or 3 doses/24 hours. Up to 10 ml can be given, but not more than 5 ml in any one site. For children, the volume given intramuscularly in any one site should be correspondingly less than in adults.

How Supplied: *Tablets*, containing 0.5 Gm sulfisoxazole/Roche, white, scored—bottles of 100, 500 and 1000; Tel-E-Dose® packages of 100; Prescription Paks of 100.
Pediatric Suspension, containing, in each teaspoonful (5 ml), the equivalent of approximately 0.5 Gm sulfisoxazole in the form of acetyl sulfisoxazole/Roche; raspberry flavored—bottles of 4 oz and 16 oz (1 pint).
Syrup, containing, in each teaspoonful (5 ml), the equivalent of approximately 0.5 Gm sulfisoxazole in the form of acetyl sulfisoxazole/ Roche; chocolate flavored—bottles of 16 oz (1 pint).
Lipo Gantrisin — the long-acting form—containing, in each teaspoonful (5 ml), the equivalent of 1 Gm sulfisoxazole in the form of acetyl sulfisoxazole/Roche in a homogenized mixture containing a readily digestible vegetable oil; vanilla-mint flavored—bottles of 16 oz (1 pint).
Injectable, 5-ml ampuls, containing 2 Gm sulfisoxazole/Roche in the form of the diolamine salt. Each ml of solution contains 400 mg sulfisoxazole/Roche in the form of the diolamine salt compounded with 2 mg sodium metabisulfite. Packages of 10.

References:
1. Randall, L.O., *et al: Antibiot Chemother 4*:877-885, Aug. 1954.
2. Svec, F.A., Rhodes, P.S., Rohr, J.H.: *Arch Intern Med 85*:83-90, Jan. 1950.
3. Flake, R.E., *et al: J Lab Clin Med 44*:582-588, Oct. 1954.
4. Krugman, S.: *Ann NY Acad Sci 69*:399-403, Aug. 1957.
5. Price, P.C., Hansen, A.E.: *Texas Rep Biol Med 9*:764-769, Winter 1951.
6. Kaplan, S.A., *et al: J Pharm Sci 61*:773-778, May 1972.
7. Data on file, Hoffmann-La Roche Inc., Nutley, N.J.
8. Struller, T.: *Antibiot Chemother 14*:179-215, 1968.
9. Sarnoff, S.J.: *Proc Soc Exp Biol Med 68*:23-26, May 1948.

Shown in Product Identification Section, page 429

KONAKION® ℞
[*ko-nak'e-on*]
(phytonadione/Roche)
INJECTABLE
FOR INTRAMUSCULAR USE ONLY

The following text is complete prescribing information based on official labeling in effect August 1, 1984.

Product Information

Description: Konakion is an essentially clear, aqueous dispersion of vitamin K$_1$, available for injection by the intramuscular route only. Slight opalescence may occur in the 10 mg ampuls. However, this does not affect the potency, safety or usefulness of the preparation.
The ingredients are as follows: *0.5-ml ampuls:* Each 0.5 ml contains 1 mg phytonadione (vitamin K$_1$) compounded with 10 mg polysorbate 80, 0.45% phenol as preservative, 10.4 mg propylene glycol, 0.17 mg sodium acetate and 0.00002 ml glacial acetic acid.
1-ml ampuls: Each ml contains 10 mg phytonadione (vitamin K$_1$) compounded with 40 mg polysorbate 80, 20.7 mg propylene glycol, 0.8 mg sodium acetate and 0.00006 ml glacial acetic acid.

Actions: Konakion possesses the same type and degree of activity as does naturally occurring vitamin K, which is necessary for the synthesis in the liver of prothrombin (factor II), proconvertin (factor VII), plasma thromboplastin component (factor IX), and Stuart factor (factor X).
The prothrombin test is sensitive to the levels of factors II, VII and X. The mechanism by which vitamin K promotes formation of these clotting factors in the liver is not known.
The action of the aqueous dispersion when administered parenterally is generally detectable within an hour or two, and hemorrhage is usually controlled within 3 to 6 hours. A normal prothrombin level may often be obtained in 12 to 14 hours.
In the prophylaxis and treatment of hemorrhagic disease of the newborn, Konakion has demonstrated a greater margin of safety than that of the water-soluble vitamin K analogs.

Indications:
• anticoagulant-induced prothrombin deficiency;
• prophylaxis and therapy of hemorrhagic disease of the newborn;
• hypoprothrombinemia due to oral antibacterial therapy;
• hypoprothrombinemia secondary to factors limiting absorption or synthesis of vitamin K, *e.g.*, obstructive jaundice, biliary fistula, sprue, ulcerative colitis, celiac disease, intestinal resection, cystic fibrosis of the pancreas and regional enteritis;
• other drug-induced hypoprothrombinemia (such as that due to salicylates) where it is definitely shown that the result is due to interference with vitamin K metabolism.

Contraindications: Parenteral use in persons who are hypersensitive to the drug.

Warnings: Konakion promotes the synthesis of prothrombin by the liver and does not directly counteract the effects of the oral anticoagulants; it takes up to two hours for vitamin K to promote prothrombin synthesis. Fresh plasma or blood transfusions may be required for severe blood loss or lack of response to vitamin K. Phytonadione will not counteract the anticoagulant action of heparin.
When vitamin K$_1$ is used to correct excessive anticoagulant-induced hypoprothrombinemia, anticoagulant therapy still being indicated, the patient is again faced with the clotting hazards existing prior to starting the anticoagulant therapy. Phytonadione is not a clotting agent, but overzealous therapy with vitamin K may restore conditions which originally permitted thromboembolic phenomena. Dosage, therefore, should be kept as low as possible, and prothrombin time should be checked periodically as clinical conditions indicate. Repeated large doses of vitamin K are not warranted in liver disease if the response to initial use of the vitamin is unsatisfactory (Koller test). Failure to respond to vitamin K may indicate the presence of a coagulation defect or that the condition being treated is unresponsive to vitamin K.
Effects on reproduction have not been studied in animals. There is no adequate information on whether this drug may affect fertility in human males or females or have a teratogenic potential or other adverse effects on the fetus.

Precautions: Store in a dark place and protect from light at all times.
Temporary resistance to prothrombin-depressing anticoagulants may result, especially when larger doses of phytonadione are used. If relatively large doses have been employed, it may be necessary when reinstituting anticoagulant therapy to use somewhat larger doses of the prothrombin-depressing anticoagulant or to use one which acts on a different principle, such as heparin.

Adverse Reactions: Pain, swelling and tenderness at the injection site have occurred rarely. The possibility of allergic sensitivity, including an anaphylactoid reaction, should be kept in mind.
Although Konakion has a greater margin of safety than the water-soluble vitamin K analogs, hyperbilirubinemia has been reported in the newborn, particularly in prematures when used at 5 to 10 times the recommended dosage. This effect, with its possibility of attendant kernicterus, should be borne in mind if such dosages are deemed necessary.

Dosage and Administration: The human minimum daily requirements for vitamin K have not been established officially. Minimal daily requirements have been estimated at 1 to 5 micrograms per kilogram of body weight for infants and 0.03 micrograms per kilogram for adults. The dietary abundance of vitamin K satisfies the requirements normally except for the neonatal period of 5 to 8 days.

INFANTS
Neonatal hemorrhage due to hypoprothrombinemia:
• *Prophylactic*—1 to 2 mg intramuscularly, immediately after birth.
• *Control*—1 to 2 mg intramuscularly, daily.

ADULTS
Hypoprothrombinemia due to:
• *Anticoagulant therapy* (except of heparin type)—5 to 10 mg I.M. initially; up to 20 mg, if necessary.
• *Antibacterial therapy*—5 to 20 mg I.M.
• *Factors limiting absorption or synthesis*—2 to 20 mg I.M.
• *Other drugs* (*e.g.*, salicylates)—2 to 20 mg I.M.

In older children and adults, injection of Konakion should be in the upper outer quadrant of the buttocks. In infants and young children, the anterolateral aspect of the thighs or the deltoid region is preferred so that danger of sciatic nerve injury is avoided.

Storage: Konakion is stable in the air, but is photosensitive, decomposing with loss of potency on exposure to light. Therefore, it should be stored in a dark place and protected from light at all times. Konakion need not be refrigerated. Store at 59° to 86°F.

How Supplied: Ampuls, 0.5 ml (boxes of 10).
Ampuls, 1 ml (boxes of 10).

LAROBEC® TABLETS ℞
[*lar'o-bek*]

The following text is complete prescribing information based on official labeling in effect August 1, 1984.

Each Larobec® tablet contains:	Quantity	U.S. RDA— Adults and children 4 or more years of age
Water-Soluble Vitamins		
Vitamin C (ascorbic acid)	500 mg	60 mg
Vitamin B$_1$ (as thiamine mononitrate)	15 mg	1.5 mg
Vitamin B$_2$ (riboflavin)	15 mg	1.7 mg
Niacin (as niacinamide)	100 mg	20 mg
Pantothenic acid (as calcium *d*-pantothenate)	18 mg	10 mg
Folic acid	0.5 mg	0.4 mg

Continued on next page

Roche Labs.—Cont.

Vitamin B$_{12}$ .... 5 mcg   6 mcg
(cyanocobalamin)

Description: Larobec is a prescription-only oral multivitamin tablet specially formulated for patients who require prophylactic or therapeutic nutritional supplementation of water-soluble vitamins and are receiving levodopa therapy for Parkinson's disease and syndrome. Larobec provides *therapeutic* levels of ascorbic acid, vitamins B$_1$, B$_2$, niacin, pantothenic acid and folic acid and a *supplemental* level of vitamin B$_{12}$ *without* pyridoxine (vitamin B$_6$), which has been reported to reduce the clinical benefits of levodopa therapy.

Clinical Pharmacology: Vitamins are essential for maintenance of normal metabolic functions including hematopoiesis. The water-soluble vitamins play vital roles in the conversion of carbohydrate, protein and fat into tissue and energy. *Thiamine (B$_1$)* acts as a coenzyme in carbohydrate metabolism. *Riboflavin (B$_2$)* functions as a coenzyme in the electron transport system associated with conversion of tissue oxidations into usable energy. *Niacin* serves as a coenzyme in oxidation-reduction reactions in tissue respiration. *Pantothenic acid* functions as a coenzyme in various metabolic acetylation reactions. *Folic acid* and *cyanocobalamin (B$_{12}$)* are metabolically interrelated. They are essential to nucleic acid synthesis and normal maturation of red blood cells. *Ascorbic acid (C)* performs a vital function in the process of cellular respiration, and is involved in both carbohydrate and amino acid metabolism. It is essential for collagen formation and tissue repair.

The water-soluble vitamins (B-complex and C) are not significantly stored by the body; excess quantities are excreted in the urine. They must be replenished regularly through diet or other means to maintain essential tissue levels. Thus these vitamins are rapidly depleted in conditions interfering with their intake or absorption.

Indications and Usage: Larobec is indicated for supportive nutritional supplementation when a water-soluble vitamin formulation (without pyridoxine) is required prophylactically or therapeutically in patients who are undergoing treatment with levodopa.

Contraindications: Larobec is contraindicated in patients known to be hypersensitive to any of its components.

Warnings: Administration of vitamin B$_6$ may be required if signs of pyridoxine deficiency develop. Folic acid in doses above 0.1 mg daily may obscure pernicious anemia. Larobec is not intended for treatment of pernicious anemia or other megaloblastic anemias where vitamin B$_{12}$ is deficient. Neurologic involvement may develop or progress, despite temporary remission of anemia, in patients with vitamin B$_{12}$ deficiency who receive supplemental folic acid and who are inadequately treated with B$_{12}$.

Precautions: *General:* Certain patients may require additional nutritional supplementation with fat-soluble vitamins and minerals according to the dietary habits of the individual. Larobec is not intended for treatment of severe specific vitamin deficiencies.

Information for the Patient: Because toxic reactions have been reported with injudicious use of certain vitamins, urge patients to follow your specific instructions regarding dosage regimen. As with any medication, advise patients to keep Larobec out of reach of children.

Adverse Reactions: Adverse reactions have been reported with specific vitamins, but generally at levels substantially higher than those in Larobec. However, allergic and idiosyncratic reactions are possible at lower levels.

Dosage and Administration: Usual adult dosage: one tablet daily.

Larobec is available on prescription only.

How Supplied: Orange-colored, capsule-shaped tablets—bottles of 100 (NDC 0004-0073-01).

Imprint on tablets: LAROBEC®
ROCHE
Shown in Product Identification Section, page 429

LARODOPA® ℞
[lar″o-do′pa]
(levodopa/Roche)

The following text is complete prescribing information based on official labeling in effect August 1, 1984.

> In order to reduce the high incidence of adverse reactions, it is necessary to individualize the therapy and to gradually increase the dosage to the desired therapeutic level.

Description: Chemically, levodopa is (−)-3-(3,4-dihydroxyphenyl)-*L*-alanine. It is a colorless, crystalline compound, slightly soluble in water and insoluble in alcohol, with a molecular weight of 197.2.

Actions: Evidence indicates that the symptoms of Parkinson's disease are related to depletion of striatal dopamine. Since dopamine apparently does not cross the blood-brain barrier, its administration is ineffective in the treatment of Parkinson's disease. However, levodopa, the levo-rotatory isomer of dihydroxyphenylalanine (dopa) which is the metabolic precursor of dopamine, does cross the blood-brain barrier. Presumably it is converted into dopamine in the basal ganglia. This is generally thought to be the mechanism whereby oral levodopa acts in relieving the symptoms of Parkinson's disease.

The major urinary metabolites of levodopa in man appear to be dopamine and homovanillic acid (HVA). In 24-hour urine samples, HVA accounts for 13 to 42 percent of the ingested dose of levodopa.

Indications: Larodopa is indicated in the treatment of idiopathic Parkinson's disease (Paralysis Agitans), postencephalitic parkinsonism, symptomatic parkinsonism which may follow injury to the nervous system by carbon monoxide intoxication, and manganese intoxication. It is indicated in those elderly patients believed to develop parkinsonism in association with cerebral arteriosclerosis.

Contraindications: Monoamine oxidase (MAO) inhibitors and Larodopa should not be given concomitantly and these inhibitors must be discontinued two weeks prior to initiating therapy with Larodopa. Larodopa is contraindicated in patients with known hypersensitivity to the drug and in narrow angle glaucoma.

Because levodopa may activate a malignant melanoma, it should not be used in patients with suspicious, undiagnosed skin lesions or a history of melanoma.

Warnings: Larodopa should be administered cautiously to patients with severe cardiovascular or pulmonary disease, bronchial asthma, renal, hepatic or endocrine disease.

Care should be exercised in administering Larodopa to patients with a history of myocardial infarction who have residual atrial, nodal or ventricular arrhythmias. If Larodopa is necessary in this type of patient, it should be used in a facility with a coronary care unit or an intensive care unit. One must be on the alert for the possibility of upper gastrointestinal hemorrhage in those patients with a past history of active peptic ulcer disease.

All patients should be carefully observed for the development of depression with concomitant suicidal tendencies. Psychotic patients should be treated with caution.

Pyridoxine hydrochloride (vitamin B$_6$) in oral doses of 10 to 25 mg rapidly reverses the toxic and therapeutic effects of Larodopa. This should be considered before recommending vitamin preparations containing pyridoxine hydrochloride (vitamin B$_6$).

Usage in Pregnancy: The safety of Larodopa in women who are or who may become pregnant has not been established; hence it should be given only when the potential benefits have been weighed against possible hazards to mother and child. Studies in rodents have shown that levodopa at dosages in excess of 200 mg/kg/day has an adverse effect on fetal and postnatal growth and viability.

Larodopa should not be used in nursing mothers.

Usage in Children: The safety of Larodopa under the age of 12 has not been established.

Precautions: Periodic evaluations of hepatic, hematopoietic, cardiovascular and renal function are recommended during extended therapy in all patients.

Patients with chronic wide angle glaucoma may be treated cautiously with Larodopa, provided the intraocular pressure is well controlled and the patient monitored carefully for changes in intraocular pressure during therapy.

Postural hypotensive episodes have been reported as adverse reactions. Therefore, Larodopa should be administered to patients on antihypertensive drug cautiously (for patients receiving pargyline, see note on MAO inhibitors contraindications), and it may be necessary to adjust the dosage of the antihypertensive drugs.

Adverse Reactions: The most serious adverse reactions associated with the administration of Larodopa having frequent occurrences are: adventitious movements such as choreiform and/or dystonic movements. Other serious adverse reactions with a lower incidence are: cardiac irregularities and/or palpitations, orthostatic hypotensive episodes, bradykinetic episodes (the "on-off" phenomena), mental changes including paranoid ideation and psychotic episodes, depression with or without the development of suicidal tendencies, dementia, and urinary retention.

Rarely, gastrointestinal bleeding, development of duodenal ulcer, hypertension, phlebitis, hemolytic anemia, agranulocytosis, and convulsions have been observed. (The causal relationship between convulsions and Larodopa has not been established.)

Adverse reactions of a less serious nature having a relatively frequent occurrence are the following: anorexia, nausea and vomiting with or without abdominal pain and distress, dry mouth, dysphagia, sialorrhea, ataxia, increased hand tremor, headache, dizziness, numbness, weakness and faintness, bruxism, confusion, insomnia, nightmares, hallucinations and delusions, agitation and anxiety, malaise, fatigue and euphoria. Occurring with a lesser order of frequency are the following: muscle twitching and blepharospasm (which may be taken as an early sign of overdosage; consideration of dosage reduction may be made at this time), trismus, burning sensation of the tongue, bitter taste, diarrhea, constipation, flatulence, flushing, skin rash, increased sweating, bizarre breathing patterns, urinary incontinence, diplopia, blurred vision, dilated pupils, hot flashes, weight gain or loss, dark sweat and/or urine.

Rarely, oculogyric crises, sense of stimulation, hiccups, development of edema, loss of hair, hoarseness, priapism and activation of latent Horner's syndrome have been observed.

Elevations of blood urea nitrogen, SGOT, SGPT, LDH, bilirubin, alkaline phosphatase or protein-bound iodine have been reported; and the significance of this is not known. Occasional reductions in WBC, hemoglobin, and hematocrit have been noted.

Leukopenia has occurred and requires cessation, at least temporarily, of Larodopa administration. The Coombs test has occasionally become positive during extended therapy. Elevations of uric acid have been noted when colorimetric method was used but not when uricase method was used.

Overdosage: For acute overdosage general supportive measures should be employed, along with immediate gastric lavage. Intravenous fluids should be administered judiciously and an adequate airway maintained.

Electrocardiographic monitoring should be instituted and the patient carefully observed for the possible development of arrhythmias; if required, appropriate antiarrhythmic therapy should be given. Consideration should be given to the possibility of multiple drug ingestion by the patient. To date, no experience has been reported with dialysis; hence its value in Larodopa overdosage is not known. Although pyridoxine hydrochloride (vitamin B₆) has been reported to reverse the antiparkinson effects of Larodopa, its usefulness in the management of acute overdosage has not been established.

Dosage and Administration: The optimal daily dose of Larodopa, *i.e.,*the dose producing maximal improvement with tolerated side effects, must be determined and *carefully titrated for each individual patient.* The usual initial dosage is 0.5 to 1 Gm daily, divided in two or more doses with food.

The total daily dosage is then increased gradually in increments not more than 0.75 Gm every three to seven days as tolerated. The usual optimal therapeutic *dosage should not exceed 8 Gm.* The exceptional patient may carefully be given more than 8 Gms as required. In some patients, a significant therapeutic response may not be obtained until six months of treatment.

In the event general anesthesia is required, Larodopa therapy may be continued as long as the patient is able to take fluids and medication by mouth. If therapy is temporarily interrupted, the usual daily dosage may be administered as soon as the patient is able to take oral medication. Whenever therapy has been interrupted for longer periods, dosage should again be adjusted gradually; however, in many cases the patient can be rapidly titrated to his previous therapeutic dosage.

How Supplied: Tablets, pink, scored, each containing levodopa/Roche 0.1 Gm, bottles of 100; 0.25 Gm or 0.5 Gm—bottles of 100 and 500.

Capsules, each containing levodopa/Roche 0.1 Gm (pink and scarlet)—bottles of 100; 0.25 Gm (pink and beige) or 0.5 Gm (pink)—bottles of 100 and 500.

Shown in Product Identification Section, page 429

LEVO-DROMORAN®
[lee″ vo dro′ mo-ran]
(levorphanol tartrate/Roche)
Ampuls • Vials • Tablets

The following text is complete prescribing information based on official labeling in effect August 1, 1984.

Action: Levo-Dromoran (levorphanol tartrate/Roche) is a highly potent synthetic analgesic with properties and actions similar to those of morphine. It produces a degree of analgesia at least equal to that of morphine and greater than that of meperidine at far smaller doses than either. It is longer acting than either; from 6 to 8 hours of pain relief can be expected with Levo-Dromoran whether given orally or by injection. It is almost as effective orally as it is parenterally. Its safety margin is about equal to that of morphine, but it is less likely to produce nausea, vomiting and constipation.

Indications: Levo-Dromoran is recommended whenever a narcotic-analgesic is required. It is recommended for the relief of pain whether moderate or severe. For example, it may be used in alleviating pain due to biliary and renal colic, myocardial infarction, and severe trauma; intractable pain due to cancer and other tumors; and for postoperative pain relief. Used preoperatively, it allays apprehension, provides prolonged analgesia, reduces thiopental requirements and shortens recovery-room time. Levo-Dromoran is compatible with a wide range of anesthetic agents. It is a useful supplement to nitrous oxide-oxygen anesthesia. It has been given by slow intravenous injection for special indications.

Contraindications: As with the use of morphine, Levo-Dromoran is contraindicated in acute alcoholism, bronchial asthma, increased intracranial pressure, respiratory depression and anoxia.

Warning: May be habit forming. Levo-Dromoran is a narcotic with an addiction liability similar to that of morphine, and for this reason the same precautions should be taken in administering the drug as with morphine. As with all narcotics, Levo-Dromoran should be used in early pregnancy only when expected benefits outweigh risks.

Precautions: To prevent or to counteract narcotic-induced respiratory depression (particularly in parturients and neonates, or during nitrous oxide-oxygen anesthesia with narcotic supplementation), Levo-Dromoran combined with Lorfan® (levallorphan tartrate/Roche)—a narcotic antagonist—is recommended. In appropriate combination [1 part Lorfan to 10 parts Levo-Dromoran] respiratory depression is usually prevented without significantly reducing the pain relief provided by Levo-Dromoran. Lorfan usually acts within 1 minute and its action lasts for 2 to 5 hours.

Adverse Reactions: As is true with the use of any narcotic-analgesic, nausea, emesis and dizziness are not uncommon in the ambulatory patient. Respiratory depression, hypotension, urinary retention and various cardiac arrhythmias have been infrequently reported following the use of Levo-Dromoran, primarily in surgical patients. Occasional allergic reactions in the form of skin rash or urticaria have been reported. Pruritus or sweating are rarely observed.

Dosage and Administration: Good medical practice dictates that the dose of any narcotic-analgesic be appropriate to the degree of pain to be relieved. This is especially important during the postoperative period because (a) residual CNS-depressant effects of anesthetic agents may still be present, and (b) later, gradual lessening of pain may not warrant full narcotizing doses. The average adult dose is 2 mg orally or subcutaneously. The dosage may be increased to 3 mg, if necessary. When Levo-Dromoran is used in combination with the narcotic antagonist Lorfan, the following dosage ratio is recommended: Levo-Dromoran/Lorfan (subcutaneous or I.V.)—10:1 [*e.g.*, 2 mg Levo-Dromoran and 0.2 mg Lorfan].

Antidote for Overdosage: In the event of overdosage of the narcotic, Lorfan is a quick and effective antidote. When the narcotic dosage is of unknown magnitude, Lorfan 1 mg intravenously is usually adequate. If required, one or two additional 0.5 mg doses may be given at 3-minute intervals.

How Supplied: *Ampuls,* 1 ml (boxes of 10). Each ml of solution contains 2 mg levorphanol tartrate/Roche (WARNING: May be habit forming) compounded with 0.2% parabens (methyl and propyl) as preservatives, and sodium hydroxide to adjust pH to approximately 4.3.

Multiple Dose Vials, 10 ml, 2 mg/ml (boxes of 10). Each ml of solution contains 2 mg levorphanol tartrate/Roche (WARNING: May be habit forming) compounded with 0.45% phenol as preservative, and sodium hydroxide to adjust pH to approximately 4.3.

Oral Tablets, 2 mg, scored (bottles of 100). Each tablet contains 2 mg levorphanol tartrate/Roche (WARNING: May be habit forming).
Narcotic order required.

Shown in Product Identification Section, page 429

LORFAN®
[lor′ fan]
(levallorphan tartrate/Roche)
ampuls • vials

The following text is complete prescribing information based on official labeling in effect August 1, 1984.

Description: Chemically, levallorphan tartrate is (−)-*N*-allyl-3-hydroxymorphinan tartrate. It is chemically related to levorphanol tartrate from which it differs in the replacement of the methyl group on the nitrogen atom by an allyl group. Levallorphan tartrate is a white or practically white, odorless, crystalline powder; it is soluble in water and sparingly soluble in alcohol.

Each ml contains 1 mg levallorphan tartrate/Roche. The pH is adjusted to approximately 4.3 with sodium hydroxide. The solution in ampuls is compounded with 0.2% methyl and propyl parabens and that in vials is compounded with 0.45% phenol as preservatives.

Actions: Lorfan acts as a narcotic antagonist in the presence of a strong narcotic effect. If used in the absence of such a narcotic effect, Lorfan may cause respiratory depression and other undesirable effects.

Indications: For use in the treatment of significant narcotic-induced respiratory depression.

Contraindications: Mild respiratory depression. Narcotic addicts in whom it may produce withdrawal symptoms.

Warnings: Lorfan is ineffective against respiratory depression due to barbiturates, anesthetics, other nonnarcotic agents or pathologic causes, and may increase it.

Precautions: If used in the absence of a narcotic, Lorfan may cause respiratory depression. Artificial respiration with oxygen and other supportive measures should be employed in conjunction with Lorfan in the treatment of significant narcotic-induced respiratory depression. Lorfan does not counteract mild respiratory depression and may increase it. Repeated doses of Lorfan result in decreasing effectiveness and may eventually produce respiratory depression equal to or greater than that produced by narcotics.

Adverse Reactions: Dysphoria, miosis, pseudoptosis, lethargy, dizziness, drowsiness, gastric upset and sweating. Pallor, nausea and a sense of heaviness in the limbs may occur.

In high dosage Lorfan may produce psychotomimetic manifestations such as weird dreams, visual hallucinations, disorientation and feelings of unreality.

In *asphyxia neonatorum,* irritability and a tendency to increased crying may occur.

Dosage and Administration: Administration of Lorfan should be accompanied by the use of other resuscitative measures, such as oxygen or artificial respiration.

Adults: To reverse respiratory depression from narcotic overdosage—1 mg Lorfan intravenously; may be followed, if required, by one or two additional doses of 0.5 mg at 10 to 15 minute intervals. The initial dose should not exceed 1 mg if there is doubt as to whether a narcotic produced the respiratory depression. The total dose should not exceed 3 mg. This regimen may also be employed to overcome narcotic-induced respiratory depression in the parturient woman.

Neonates: To decrease respiratory depression secondary to narcotic administration to the mother, inject 0.05 to 0.1 mg Lorfan (approximately one-tenth the adult dose) into the umbilical cord vein immediately after delivery. If this vein cannot be used, injection may be made intramuscularly or subcutaneously.

Overdosage: Assisted respiration, including a patent airway, the administration of oxygen, and other supportive measures, should be used.

How Supplied: Ampuls, 1 ml, boxes of 10; vials, 10 ml, boxes of 10. Each ml contains 1 mg levallorphan tartrate/Roche.

MARPLAN® TABLETS
[mar′ plan]
(isocarboxazid/Roche)

The following text is complete prescribing information based on official labeling in effect August 1, 1984.

Description: Marplan (isocarboxazid/Roche) is an amine-oxidase inhibitor. Chemically, isocarboxazid is 5-methyl-3-isoxazolecarboxylic acid 2-benzylhydrazide.

Isocarboxazid is a colorless, crystalline substance with very little taste.

Actions: Isocarboxazid, a potent inhibitor of amine-oxidase, exhibits antidepressant activity. *In vivo* and *in vitro* studies demonstrated inhibition of amine-oxidase in the brain, heart and liver.

The oral LD_{50} in mice was 171 mg/kg and in rats, 270 mg/kg. In rats administered 120 mg/kg daily for 6 weeks, isocarboxazid produced a reduction of growth rate and appetite. In chronic tolerance studies of 24 weeks duration, hyperexcitability and depression of growth rate occurred in male rats given oral doses of 5 mg/kg/day and in both sexes of this species given 10 mg/kg/day orally. The relevance of these findings to the clinical use of Marplan is not known. No hematologic changes were observed.

Continued on next page

Roche Labs.—Cont.

Dogs given 15 mg/kg/day for 2 weeks showed emetic effects and a slight lowering of hemoglobin and hematocrit. No adverse effects were noted, however, at doses of 10 mg/kg/day for 6 weeks. Given as successively increasing daily oral doses to a dog, isocarboxazid was tolerated up to 40 mg/kg. Monkeys given 20 mg/kg/day orally for 2 weeks tolerated the drug with no apparent adverse effects.

Reproduction studies were carried out in rats given 0.5 and 5 mg/kg/day of isocarboxazid as a dietary mixture for 10 weeks prior to mating and continuing through two mating cycles to the weaning of the second litter. The parent animals remained in good condition throughout the test period. Litters of the treated groups compared favorably with those of the controls. No evidence of teratogenic effects was seen in any of the young.

INDICATIONS: Based on a review of this drug by the National Academy of Sciences—National Research Council and/or other information, FDA has classified the indications as follows:
"Probably" effective for the treatment of depressed patients who are refractory to tricyclic antidepressants or electroconvulsive therapy and depressed patients in whom tricyclic antidepressants are contraindicated.
Final classification of the less-than-effective indications requires further investigation.

Careful selection of candidates for Marplan— with due regard to the symptomatology of the patient and to the properties of the compound —will result in more effective therapy. Complete review of the package insert is advised before initiating treatment.

Contraindications: Marplan is contraindicated in patients with known hypersensitivity to the drug, severe impairment of liver or renal function, congestive heart failure or pheochromocytoma.
The potentiation of sympathomimetic substances by MAO inhibitors may result in *hypertensive crisis;* therefore, patients taking Marplan should not be given *sympathomimetic drugs* (including amphetamines, methyldopa, levodopa, dopamine, and tryptophan as well as epinephrine and norepinephrine) nor *foods with a high concentration of tryptophan* (broad beans) or *tyramine* (cheese, beers, wines, pickled herring, chicken livers, yeast extract). Excessive amounts of caffeine can also cause hypertensive reactions.
These hypertensive crises can be fatal, due to circulatory collapse or intracranial bleeding. Hypertensive crises are characterized by some or all of the following symptoms: occipital headache which may radiate frontally, neck stiffness or soreness, nausea, vomiting, photophobia, dilated pupils, sweating (sometimes with fever and sometimes with cold, clammy skin) and palpitations. Either tachycardia or bradycardia may be present, and can be associated with constricting chest pain. These crises usually occur within several hours after the ingestion of a contraindicated substance. Marplan should be discontinued immediately upon the occurrence of palpitations or frequent headaches.

Recommended treatment in hypertensive crisis: Marplan should be discontinued and therapy to lower blood pressure should be started immediately. A successful method of treatment is with an alpha-adrenergic blocking agent such as phentolamine, 5 mg, I.V., or pentolinium, 3 mg, subcutaneously. These drugs should be administered slowly to avoid excessive hypotension. Fever should be managed by external cooling.

Marplan should not be administered together with or immediately following other MAO inhibitors or dibenzazepines. Such combinations can produce hypertensive crisis, fever, marked sweating, excitation, delirium, tremor, twitching, convulsions, coma, and circulatory collapse. At least 10 days should elapse between the discontinuation of Marplan and the institution of another antidepressant, or the discontinuation of another MAO inhibitor and the institution of Marplan.
Some other amine-oxidase inhibitors commonly used in this country include: pargyline HCl, phenelzine sulfate and tranylcypromine.
Some antidepressants (dibenzazepine derivatives) commonly used in this country include amitriptyline HCl, desipramine HCl, imipramine HCl, nortriptyline HCl and protriptyline HCl.
Patients taking Marplan should not undergo elective surgery requiring general anesthesia. Should spinal anesthesia be essential, consideration should be given to possible combined hypotensive effects of Marplan and the blocking agent. Also, they should not be given cocaine or local anesthetic solutions containing sympathomimetic vasoconstrictors. Marplan should be discontinued at least 10 days prior to elective surgery.
Marplan should not be used in combination with CNS depressants such as narcotics and ethanol (see PRECAUTIONS for barbiturates). Circulatory collapse and death have been reported from the combination of amine-oxidase inhibitors and a single dose of meperidine. In addition, serious hyperpyrexia can occur following administration of this combination. It is thought that this latter reaction may be mediated by release of 5-hydroxytryptamine, as it does not occur in experimental animals pretreated with inhibitors of 5-HT synthesis.

Warnings: Because the most serious reactions to Marplan relate to effects on blood pressure, it is not advisable to use this drug in elderly or debilitated patients or in the presence of hypertension, cardiovascular or cerebrovascular disease. Patients with severe or frequent headaches should not be considered as candidates for therapy with Marplan because headaches during therapy may be the first symptom of a hypertensive reaction to the drug.
Marplan should be used with caution in combination with antihypertensive drugs including thiazide diuretics since hypotension may result.
In patients who may be suicidal risks, no single form of treatment, such as Marplan, electroshock or other therapy, should be relied on as a sole therapeutic measure. The strictest supervision, and preferably hospitalization, are advised.

Warning to patient: All patients taking Marplan should be warned against self-medication with proprietary cold, hay fever or reducing preparations, since most of these contain sympathomimetic agents. They should be warned against eating the foods previously mentioned that contain high concentrations of tyramine or tryptophan. Beverages containing caffeine should be used in moderation. Patients should be instructed to report promptly the occurrence of headache or other unusual symptoms.

Use in Children: Marplan is not recommended for use in patients under 16 years of age since there are no controlled studies of safety or efficacy in this group.

Use in Pregnancy: Safe use of Marplan during pregnancy or lactation has not yet been established. Before prescribing Marplan in pregnancy, lactation, or in women of childbearing age, the potential benefit of the drug should be weighed against its possible hazard to mother and child. (See ACTIONS.)

Precautions: Concomitant use of Marplan and other psychotropic agents is not recommended because of possible potentiating effects and decreased margin of safety. This is especially true in patients who may subject themselves to an overdosage of drugs. If combination therapy is indicated, careful consideration should be given to the pharmacology of all agents to be employed. The effects of Marplan may persist for a substantial period after discontinuation of the drug, and this should be borne in mind when another drug is prescribed following Marplan. To avoid potentiation, the physician wishing to terminate treatment with Marplan and begin therapy with another agent should allow for an interval of 10 days.
Marplan should be used cautiously in hyperactive or agitated patients, as well as schizophrenic patients, because it may cause excessive stimulation. Characteristically, in manic-depressive states there may be a tendency for patients to swing from a depressive to a manic phase. If such a swing should occur during Marplan therapy, brief discontinuation of the drug, followed by resumption of therapy at a reduced dosage, is advised.
Clinical evidence indicates only a low incidence of altered liver function or jaundice in patients treated with Marplan. It is difficult to differentiate most cases of drug-induced hepatocellular jaundice from viral hepatitis since they are histopathologically and biochemically indistinguishable. Moreover, many of the clinical signs and symptoms are identical. While some of the few cases of jaundice reported during Marplan therapy may have been drug-induced, the reaction is rare. Nevertheless, Marplan is an amine-oxidase inhibitor and, as with the use of all these agents, it is advisable to watch for hepatic complications. It is suggested that periodic liver function tests, such as bilirubins, alkaline phosphatase or transaminases, be performed during Marplan therapy; use of the drug should be discontinued at the first sign of hepatic dysfunction or jaundice. In patients with impaired renal function, Marplan should be used cautiously to prevent accumulation.
Marplan appears to have varying effects in epileptic patients; while some have a decrease in frequency of seizures, others have more seizures. Appropriate consideration must be given to the latter possibility if Marplan is prescribed for such patients.
All patients taking Marplan should be watched for symptoms of postural hypotension. If such hypotension occurs, the dose should be reduced or the drug discontinued.
Since the MAO inhibitors, including Marplan, potentiate hexobarbital hypnosis in animals, the dose of barbiturates if given concomitantly should be reduced.
Since the MAO inhibitors inhibit the destruction of serotonin, which is believed to be released from tissue stores by rauwolfia alkaloids, caution should be exercised when these drugs are used together.
There is conflicting evidence as to whether MAO inhibitors affect glucose metabolism or potentiate hypoglycemic agents. This should be considered if Marplan is used in diabetics.

Adverse Reactions: Marplan is a potent therapeutic agent with a relatively low incidence of adverse reactions. Since Marplan affects many enzyme systems of the body, a variety of side effects may be anticipated. The most frequently noted have been orthostatic hypotension, associated in some patients with falling, disturbances in cardiac rate and rhythm, complaints of dizziness and vertigo, constipation, headache, overactivity, hyperreflexia, tremors and muscle twitching, mania, hypomania, jitteriness, confusion and memory impairment, insomnia, peripheral edema, weakness, fatigue, dryness of the mouth, blurred vision, hyperhidrosis, anorexia and body weight changes, gastrointestinal disturbances, and minor sensitivity reactions such as skin rashes. Isolated cases of akathisia, ataxia, black tongue, coma, dysuria, euphoria, hematologic changes, incontinence, neuritis, photosensitivity, sexual disturbances, spider telangiectases and urinary retention have been reported. These side effects sometimes necessitate discontinuation of therapy. In rare instances, hallucinations have been reported with high dosages, but they have disappeared upon reduction of dosage or discontinuation of therapy. Toxic amblyopia was reported in one psychiatric patient who had received isocarboxazid for about a year; no causal relationship to isocarboxazid was established. Impaired water excretion compatible with the syndrome of inappropriate secretion of antidiuretic hormone (SIADH) has been reported.

Dosage and Administration: As with other potent drugs, for maximum therapeutic effect the dosage of Marplan must be individually adjusted on the basis of careful observation of the patient. The usual starting dose is 30 mg daily, to be given in single or divided doses. Marplan has a cumulative effect; therefore, as soon as clinical improvement is observed, the dosage should be reduced to a maintenance level of 10 to 20 mg daily (or less). Since daily doses larger than 30 mg may cause an increase in the incidence or severity of side effects, it is recommended that this dosage generally not be exceeded. Many patients may show a favorable response to Marplan therapy within a week or less; however, since Marplan acts by directly affecting enzyme metabolism, a beneficial effect may not be seen in some patients for three or four weeks. If no response is obtained by then, continued administration is unlikely to help.

Management of Overdosage: The lethal dose of Marplan in man is not known. There has been one report of a fatality in a patient who ingested 400 mg of Marplan together with an unspecified amount of another drug. Major overdosage may be evidenced by symptoms such as tachycardia, hypotension, coma, convulsions, respiratory depression, sluggish reflexes, pyrexia and diaphoresis; these signs may persist for 8 to 14 days. General supportive measures should be employed, along with immediate gastric lavage or emetics. If the latter are given, the danger of aspiration must be borne in mind. An adequate airway should be maintained, with supplemental oxygen if necessary. The mechanism by which amine-oxidase inhibitors produce hypotension is not fully understood, but there is evidence that these agents block the vascular bed response. Thus it is suggested that plasma may be of value in the management of this hypotension. Administration of pressor amines such as Levophed® (levarterenol bitartrate) may be of limited value (note that their effects may be potentiated by Marplan). Continue treatment for several days until homeostasis is restored. Liver function studies are recommended during the 4 to 6 weeks after recovery, as well as at the time of overdosage. As with the management of intentional overdosage with any drug, it should be borne in mind that multiple agents may have been ingested.

How Supplied: Tablets, 10 mg isocarboxazid/Roche each, peach-colored, scored—bottles of 100.
Shown in Product Identification Section, page 430

MATULANE®
[mat'u-lane]
(procarbazine hydrochloride/Roche)

The following text is complete prescribing information based on official labeling in effect August 1, 1984.

WARNING
It is recommended that MATULANE be given only by or under the supervision of a physician experienced in the use of potent antineoplastic drugs. Adequate clinical and laboratory facilities should be available to patients for proper monitoring of treatment.
The enclosed instructions should be thoroughly reviewed before administration of MATULANE.

Description: Matulane (procarbazine hydrochloride/Roche) has demonstrated an antineoplastic effect against Hodgkin's disease. The mode of cytotoxic action of Matulane has not yet been clearly defined; however, there is evidence that the drug may act by inhibition of protein, RNA and DNA synthesis. No cross-resistance with other chemotherapeutic agents, radiotherapy or steroids has been demonstrated.

Clinical studies, in which the duration of response is at least a month, show an over-all response rate of approximately 50 per cent. This includes both objective regression of disease and associated clinical benefit. These observations have been made in patients who have had prior treatment with radiotherapy and other antineoplastic agents.

The number of patients with malignant diseases other than Hodgkin's disease who have received Matulane therapy is inadequate at this time for any definitive statement regarding efficacy. Therefore, the use of this drug should be limited to Hodgkin's disease.

Chemistry: Procarbazine hydrochloride is N-isopropyl-α-(2-methylhydrazino)-p-toluamide monohydrochloride. It is a white to pale yellow crystalline substance, soluble but unstable in water or aqueous solutions. The molecular weight is 257.76.

Actions: In laboratory studies, procarbazine hydrochloride produced a variety of biologic effects. Among these have been immunosuppression, teratogenesis, carcinogenesis, cytotoxicity with mitotic suppression and chromatin derangement, and an antineoplastic effect against a spectrum of transplanted tumors in mice and rats. The major drug toxicities in acute and chronic animal studies were hematologic with granulocyte depression, thrombocyte depression and anemia. Reticuloendothelial system lymphocytic depletion, marrow cell depression, testicular atrophy and mucous membrane ulceration were further evidence of *in vivo* cytotoxicity.

Distribution of the drug in body fluids, studied in dog and man, showed rapid equilibration between plasma and cerebrospinal fluid after oral administration. Pharmacological studies indicated excellent gastrointestinal absorption. The major portion of drug was excreted in the urine as N-isopropylterephthalamic acid with approximately 25 to 42 per cent appearing during the first 24 hours after administration.

Leukemia and pulmonary tumors in mice, and mammary adenocarcinomas in rats, have been observed subsequent to procarbazine hydrochloride administration in high doses. The oral LD_{50} of procarbazine hydrochloride in mice and rats was determined to be 1320 ± 66 mg/kg and 785 ± 34 mg/kg respectively. In rabbits the oral LD_{50} was 147 ± 11.5 mg/kg.

Indication: Matulane is recommended for the palliative management of generalized Hodgkin's disease and in those patients who have become resistant to other forms of therapy. Although prolongation of survival time may not be evident, amelioration of the disease symptoms and regression of tumors have been demonstrated frequently. The drug should be used as an adjunct to standard modalities of therapy.

Contraindications: Matulane is contraindicated in patients with 1) known hypersensitivity to the drug, or 2) inadequate marrow reserve as demonstrated by bone marrow aspiration. Due consideration of this possible state should be given to each patient who has leukopenia, thrombocytopenia or anemia.

Warnings: To minimize CNS depression and possible synergism, barbiturates, antihistamines, narcotics, hypotensive agents or phenothiazines should be used with caution. Ethyl alcohol should not be used since there may be an Antabuse (disulfiram)-like reaction. Because Matulane exhibits some amine oxidase inhibitory activity, sympathomimetic drugs, tricyclic antidepressant drugs (*e.g.,* amitriptyline HCl, imipramine HCl), and other drugs and foods with known high tyramine content, such as ripe cheese and bananas, should be avoided. A further phenomenon of toxicity common to many hydrazine derivatives is hemolysis and the appearance of Heinz-Ehrlich inclusion bodies in erythrocytes.

Use In Pregnancy: Teratogenicity has been reported in animals. Use of any drug in pregnancy, lactation or in women of childbearing age requires that the potential benefit of the drug be weighed against its possible hazard to mother and child.

Precautions: Undue toxicity may occur if Matulane is used in patients with known impairment of renal and/or hepatic function. When appropriate, hospitalization for the initial course of treatment should be considered.

If radiation or a chemotherapeutic agent known to have marrow-depressant activity has been used, an interval of one month or longer without such therapy is recommended before starting treatment with Matulane. The length of this interval may also be determined by evidence of bone marrow recovery based on successive bone marrow studies.

Adverse Reactions: Leukopenia, anemia and thrombopenia occur frequently. Nausea and vomiting are the most commonly reported side effects. Other less frequent gastrointestinal complaints include anorexia, stomatitis, dry mouth, dysphagia, diarrhea and constipation. Pain, including myalgia and arthralgia, chills and fever, sweating, weakness, fatigue, lethargy and drowsiness are often noted. Intercurrent infections, effusion, edema, cough, and pneumonitis have been reported. Bleeding tendencies such as petechiae, purpura, epistaxis, hemoptysis, hematemesis and melena have not been rare. Dermatitis, pruritus, herpes, hyperpigmentation, flushing, alopecia and jaundice have also been noted. Paresthesias and neuropathies, headache, dizziness, depression, apprehension, nervousness, insomnia, nightmares, hallucinations, falling, unsteadiness, ataxia, footdrop, decreased reflexes, tremors, coma, confusion and convulsions have been less common. Hoarseness, tachycardia, retinal hemorrhage, nystagmus, photophobia, photosensitivity, genitourinary symptoms, hypotension and fainting have been rare. Isolated instances of diplopia, inability to focus, papilledema, altered hearing and slurred speech have occurred. Coincidental onset of leukemia during Matulane therapy has been reported in rare instances.

Dosage and Administration:

General Instructions: Baseline laboratory data should be obtained prior to initiation of therapy. The hematologic status as indicated by hemoglobin, hematocrit, white blood count (WBC), differential, reticulocytes and platelets should be monitored closely—at least every 3 or 4 days. Bone marrow depression often occurs 2 to 8 weeks after the start of treatment. If leukopenia occurs, hospitalization of the patient may be needed for appropriate treatment to prevent systemic infection.

Hepatic and renal evaluation are indicated prior to beginning therapy. Urinalysis, transaminase, alkaline phosphatase and blood urea nitrogen should be repeated at least weekly.

Prompt cessation of therapy is recommended if any one of the following occurs:

- Central nervous system signs or symptoms such as paresthesias, neuropathies or confusion.
- Leukopenia (white blood count under 4000).
- Thrombocytopenia (platelets under 100,000).
- Hypersensitivity reaction.
- Stomatitis—The first small ulceration or persistent spot soreness around the oral cavity is a signal for cessation of therapy.
- Diarrhea—Frequent bowel movements or watery stools.
- Hemorrhage or bleeding tendencies.

Therapy may be resumed, at the discretion of the physician, after toxic side effects have cleared on clinical evaluation and appropriate laboratory studies. Adjustment to a lower dosage schedule is recommended.

Dosage:

General Instructions: All dosages are based on the patient's actual weight. However, the estimated lean body mass (dry weight) is used if the patient is obese or if there has been a spurious weight gain due to edema, ascites or other forms of abnormal fluid retention.

Adults—To minimize nausea and vomiting experienced by a high percentage of patients beginning Matulane therapy, single or divided doses of 2 to 4 mg/kg/day (to the nearest 50 mg) for the first week are recommended. Daily dosage should then be maintained at 4 to 6 mg/kg/day until the white blood count falls below 4000 per cmm or the platelets fall below 100,000 per cmm or until maximum response is obtained. Upon evidence of hematologic toxicity the drug should be discontinued until there has been satisfactory recovery. Treatment may then be resumed at 1 to 2 mg/kg/day. When maximum response is obtained, the dose may be maintained at 1 to 2 mg/kg/day.

Children—Use of Matulane in children has been quite limited. Very close clinical monitoring is mandatory. Undue toxicity, evidenced by tremors, coma and convulsions, has occurred in a few cases. Dosage, therefore, must be highly individualized.

Continued on next page

Roche Labs.—Cont.

The following dosage schedule is provided as a guideline only.

50 mg daily is recommended for the first week. Daily dosage should then be maintained at 100 mg per square meter of body surface (to the nearest 50 mg) until leukopenia or thrombocytopenia occurs or maximum response is obtained. Upon evidence of hematologic toxicity the drug should be discontinued until there has been satisfactory recovery. Treatment may then be resumed at 50 mg per day. When maximum response is attained, the dose may be maintained at 50 mg daily.

How Supplied: *Capsules:* containing the equivalent of 50 mg procarbazine as the hydrochloride, ivory; bottles of 100.

Shown in Product Identification Section, page 430

MESTINON® INJECTABLE ℞
[mes'tin-on]
(pyridostigmine bromide/Roche)

The following text is complete prescribing information based on official labeling in effect August 1, 1984.

Description: Mestinon Injectable is an active cholinesterase inhibitor. Chemically, pyridostigmine bromide is 3-hydroxy-1-methylpyridinium bromide dimethylcarbamate.

Each ml contains 5 mg pyridostigmine bromide/Roche compounded with 0.2% parabens (methyl and propyl) as preservatives, 0.02% sodium citrate and pH adjusted to approximately 5.0 with citric acid and, if necessary, sodium hydroxide.

Actions: Mestinon facilitates the transmission of impulses across the myoneural junction by inhibiting the destruction of acetylcholine by cholinesterase. Pyridostigmine is an analog of neostigmine (Prostigmin®) but differs from it clinically by having fewer side effects. Currently available data indicate that pyridostigmine may have a significantly lower degree and incidence of bradycardia, salivation and gastrointestinal stimulation. Animal studies using the injectable form of pyridostigmine and human studies using the oral preparation have indicated that pyridostigmine has a longer duration of action than does neostigmine measured under similar circumstances.

Indications: Mestinon Injectable is useful in the treatment of myasthenia gravis and as a reversal agent or antagonist to nondepolarizing muscle relaxants such as curariform drugs and gallamine triethiodide.

Contraindications: Known hypersensitivity to anticholinesterase agents; intestinal and urinary obstructions of mechanical type.

Warnings: Mestinon Injectable should be used with particular caution in patients with bronchial asthma or cardiac dysrhythmias. Transient bradycardia may occur and be relieved by atropine sulfate. Atropine should also be used with caution in patients with cardiac dysrhythmias. When large doses of Mestinon are administered, as during reversal of muscle relaxants, the prior or simultaneous injection of atropine sulfate is advisable. Because of the possibility of hypersensitivity in an occasional patient, atropine and antishock medication should always be readily available.

As is true of all cholinergic drugs, overdosage of Mestinon may result in cholinergic crisis, a state characterized by increasing muscle weakness which, through involvement of the muscles of respiration, may lead to death. Myasthenic crisis due to an increase in the severity of the disease is also accompanied by extreme muscle weakness and thus may be difficult to distinguish from cholinergic crisis on a symptomatic basis. Such differentiation is extremely important, since increases in doses of Mestinon or other drugs in this class in the presence of cholinergic crisis or of a refractory or "insensitive" state could have grave consequences. Osserman and Genkins[1] indicate that the two types of crisis may be differentiated by the use of Tensilon® (edrophonium chloride) as well as by clinical judgment. The treatment of the two conditions obviously differs radically. Whereas the presence of *myasthenic crisis* requires more intensive anticholinesterase therapy, *cholinergic crisis,* according to Osserman and Genkins,[1] calls for the prompt withdrawal of all drugs of this type. The immediate use of atropine in cholinergic crisis is also recommended. A syringe containing 1 mg of atropine sulfate should be immediately available to be given in aliquots intravenously to counteract severe cholinergic reactions.

Atropine may also be used to abolish or obtund gastrointestinal side effects or other muscarinic reactions; but such use, by masking signs of overdosage, can lead to inadvertent induction of cholinergic crisis.

For detailed information on the management of patients with myasthenia gravis, the physician is referred to one of the excellent reviews such as those by Osserman and Genkins,[2] Grob[3] or Schwab.[4,5]

When used as an antagonist to nondepolarizing muscle relaxants, adequate recovery of voluntary respiration and neuromuscular transmission must be obtained prior to discontinuation of respiratory assistance and there should be continuous patient observation. Satisfactory recovery may be defined by a combination of clinical judgment, respiratory measurements and observation of the effects of peripheral nerve stimulation. If there is any doubt concerning the adequacy of recovery from the effects of the nondepolarizing muscle relaxant, artificial ventilation should be continued until all doubt has been removed.

Usage in Pregnancy: The safety of Mestinon during pregnancy or lactation in humans has not been established. Therefore, use of Mestinon in women who may become pregnant requires weighing the drug's potential benefits against its possible hazards to mother and child.

Adverse Reactions: The side effects of Mestinon are most commonly related to overdosage and generally are of two varieties, muscarinic and nicotinic. Among those in the former group are nausea, vomiting, diarrhea, abdominal cramps, increased peristalsis, increased salivation, increased bronchial secretions, miosis and diaphoresis. Nicotinic side effects are comprised chiefly of muscle cramps, fasciculation and weakness. Muscarinic side effects can usually be counteracted by atropine, but for reasons shown in the preceding section the expedient is not without danger. As with any compound containing the bromide radical, a skin rash may be seen in an occasional patient. Such reactions usually subside promptly upon discontinuance of the medication. Thrombophlebitis has been reported subsequent to intravenous administration.

Dosage and Administration:
For Myasthenia Gravis—To supplement oral dosage, pre- and postoperatively, during labor and postpartum, during myasthenic crisis, or whenever oral therapy is impractical, approximately 1/30th of the oral dose of Mestinon may be given parenterally, either by intramuscular or *very slow* intravenous injection. *The patient must be closely observed for cholinergic reactions, particularly if the intravenous route is used.*

For details regarding the management of myasthenic patients who are to undergo major surgical procedures, see the article by Foldes.[6]

Neonates of myasthenic mothers may have transient difficulty in swallowing, sucking and breathing. Injectable Mestinon may be indicated—by symptomatology and use of the Tensilon® (edrophonium chloride) test—until Mestinon Syrup can be taken. To date the world literature consists of less than 100 neonate patients.[7] Of these only 5 were treated with injectable pyridostigmine, with the vast majority of the remaining neonates receiving neostigmine. Dosage requirements of Mestinon Injectable are minute, ranging from 0.05 mg to 0.15 mg/kg of body weight given intramuscularly. It is important to differentiate between cholinergic and myasthenic crises in neonates. (See WARNINGS.)

Mestinon given parenterally one hour before completion of second stage labor enables patients to have adequate strength during labor and provides protection to infants in the immediate postnatal state. For further information on the use of Mestinon Injectable in neonates of myasthenic mothers, see the article by Namba.[7]

NOTE: For information on a diagnostic test for myasthenia gravis, and on the evaluation and stabilization of therapy, please see product information on Tensilon® (edrophonium chloride/Roche).

For Reversal of Nondepolarizing Muscle Relaxants: When Mestinon Injectable is given intravenously to reverse the action of muscle relaxant drugs, it is recommended that atropine sulfate (0.6 to 1.2 mg) also be given intravenously immediately prior to the Mestinon. Side effects, notably excessive secretions and bradycardia, are thereby minimized. Usually 10 or 20 mg of Mestinon will be sufficient for antagonism of the effects of the nondepolarizing muscle relaxants. Although full recovery may occur within 15 minutes in most patients, others may require a half hour or more. Satisfactory reversal can be evident by adequate voluntary respiration, respiratory measurements and use of a peripheral nerve stimulator device. It is recommended that the patient be well ventilated and a patent airway maintained until complete recovery of normal respiration is assured. Once satisfactory reversal has been attained, recurarization has not been reported. For additional information on the use of Mestinon for antagonism of nondepolarizing muscle relaxants see the article by Katz[8] and McNall.[9]

Failure of Mestinon Injectable to provide prompt (within 30 minutes) reversal may occur, *e.g.,* in the presence of extreme debilitation, carcinomatosis, or with concomitant use of certain broad spectrum antibiotics or anesthetic agents, notably ether. Under these circumstances ventilation must be supported by artificial means until the patient has resumed control of his respiration.

How Supplied: Mestinon is available in 2-ml ampuls (boxes of 10).

References:
1. K. E. Osserman and G. Genkins, *J.A.M.A. 183:*97, 1963.
2. K. E. Osserman and G. Genkins, *New York State J. Med., 61:*2076, 1961.
3. D. Grob, *Arch. Intern. Med., 108:*615, 1961.
4. R. S. Schwab, *New Eng. J. Med., 268:*596, 1963.
5. R. S. Schwab, *New Eng. J. Med., 268:*717, 1963.
6. F. F. Foldes and P. McNall, *Anesthesiology, 23:*837, 1962.
7. T. Namba et al., *Pediatrics, 45:*488, 1970.
8. R. L. Katz, *Anesthesiology, 28:*528, 1967.
9. P. McNall et al., *Anesthesia and Analgesia, 48:*1026, 1969.

MESTINON® ℞
[mes'tin-on]
(pyridostigmine bromide/Roche)
TABLETS and SYRUP
TIMESPAN® TABLETS

The following text is complete prescribing information based on official labeling in effect August 1, 1984.

Description: Mestinon is an orally active cholinesterase inhibitor. Chemically, pyridostigmine bromide is 3-hydroxy-1-methylpyridinium bromide dimethylcarbamate.

Actions: Mestinon inhibits the destruction of acetylcholine by cholinesterase and thereby permits freer transmission of nerve impulses across the neuromuscular junction. Pyridostigmine is an analog of neostigmine (Prostigmin®), but differs from it in certain clinically significant respects; for example, pyridostigmine is characterized by a longer duration of action and fewer gastrointestinal side effects.

Indication: Mestinon is useful in the treatment of myasthenia gravis.

Contraindications: Mestinon is contraindicated in mechanical intestinal or urinary obstruction, and particular caution should be used in its administration to patients with bronchial asthma. Care should be observed in the use of atropine for counteracting side effects, as discussed below.

Warnings: Although failure of patients to show clinical improvement may reflect underdosage, it can also be indicative of overdosage. As is true of all cholinergic drugs, overdosage of Mestinon may result in cholinergic crisis, a state characterized by increasing muscle weakness which, through involvement of the muscles of respiration, may lead to death. Myasthenic crisis due to an increase in the severity of the disease is also accompanied by extreme muscle weakness, and thus may be difficult to distinguish from cholinergic crisis on a symptomatic basis. Such differentiation is extremely important, since increases in doses of Mestinon or other drugs of this class in the presence of cholinergic crisis or of a refractory or "insensitive" state could have grave consequences. Osserman and Genkins[1] indicate that the differential diagnosis of the two types of crisis may require the use of Tensilon® (edrophonium chloride/Roche) as well as clinical judgment. The treatment of the two conditions obviously differs radically. Whereas the presence of myasthenic crisis suggests the need for more intensive anticholinesterase therapy, the diagnosis of cholinergic crisis, according to Osserman and Genkins,[1] calls for the prompt *withdrawal* of all drugs of this type. The immediate use of atropine in cholinergic crisis is also recommended.

Atropine may also be used to abolish or obtund gastrointestinal side effects or other muscarinic reactions; but such use, by masking signs of overdosage, can lead to inadvertent induction of cholinergic crisis.

For detailed information on the management of patients with myasthenia gravis, the physician is referred to one of the excellent reviews such as those by Osserman and Genkins,[2] Grob[3] or Schwab.[4,5]

Usage in Pregnancy: The safety of Mestinon during pregnancy or lactation in humans has not been established. Therefore, use of Mestinon in women who may become pregnant requires weighing the drug's potential benefits against its possible hazards to mother and child.

Adverse Reactions: The side effects of Mestinon are most commonly related to overdosage and generally are of two varieties, muscarinic and nicotinic. Among those in the former group are nausea, vomiting, diarrhea, abdominal cramps, increased peristalsis, increased salivation, increased bronchial secretions, miosis and diaphoresis. Nicotinic side effects are comprised chiefly of muscle cramps, fasciculation and weakness. Muscarinic side effects can usually be counteracted by atropine, but for reasons shown in the preceding section the expedient is not without danger. As with any compound containing the bromide radical, a skin rash may be seen in an occasional patient. Such reactions usually subside promptly upon discontinuance of the medication.

Dosage and Administration: Mestinon is available in three dosage forms:

Syrup—raspberry-flavored, containing 60 mg pyridostigmine bromide per teaspoonful (5 ml). This form permits accurate dosage adjustment for children and "brittle" myasthenic patients who require fractions of 60-mg doses. It is more easily swallowed, especially in the morning, by patients with bulbar involvement.

Conventional tablets—each containing 60 mg pyridostigmine bromide.

Timespan tablets—each containing 180 mg pyridostigmine bromide. This form provides uniformly slow release, hence prolonged duration of drug action; it facilitates control of myasthenic symptoms with fewer individual doses daily. The immediate effect of a 180-mg Timespan tablet is about equal to that of a 60-mg conventional tablet; however, its duration of effectiveness, although varying in individual patients, averages 2½ times that of a 60-mg dose.

Dosage: The size and frequency of the dosage must be adjusted to the needs of the individual patient.

Syrup and conventional tablets—The average dose is ten 60-mg tablets or ten 5-ml teaspoonfuls daily, spaced to provide maximum relief when maximum strength is needed. In severe cases as many as 25 tablets or teaspoonfuls a day may be required, while in mild cases one to six tablets or teaspoonfuls a day may suffice.

Timespan tablets—One to three 180-mg tablets, once or twice daily, will usually be sufficient to control symptoms; however, the needs of certain individuals may vary markedly from this average. The interval between doses should be at least six hours. For optimum control, it may be necessary to use the more rapidly acting regular tablets or syrup in conjunction with Timespan therapy.

Note: For information on a diagnostic test for myasthenia gravis, and for the evaluation and stabilization of therapy, please see product literature on Tensilon® (edrophonium chloride/Roche).

How Supplied: *Syrup,* 60 mg pyridostigmine bromide per teaspoonful (5 ml) and 5% alcohol—bottles of 16 fluid ounces (1 pint).

Tablets, scored, 60 mg pyridostigmine bromide each—bottles of 100 and 500.

Timespan tablets, scored, 180 mg pyridostigmine bromide each—bottles of 100.

Note: Because of the hygroscopic nature of the Timespan tablets, mottling may occur. This does not affect their efficacy.

References:
1. K. E. Osserman and G. Genkins, *J.A.M.A.,* 183:97, 1963.
2. K. E. Osserman and G. Genkins, *New York State J. Med.,* 61:2076, 1961.
3. D. Grob, *Arch. Int. Med.,* 108:615, 1961.
4. R. S. Schwab, *New England J. Med.,* 268:596, 1963.
5. R. S. Schwab, *New England J. Med.,* 268:717, 1963.

Shown in Product Identification Section, page 430

NIPRIDE® ℞
[ny'pryde]
(sodium nitroprusside/Roche)

The following text is complete prescribing information based on official labeling in effect August 1, 1984.

> Nipride is only to be used as an infusion with sterile 5% dextrose in water. Not for direct injection.
> Nipride should be used only when the necessary facilities and equipment for continuous monitoring of blood pressure are available.
> If at infusion rates of up to 10 μg/kg/minute, an adequate reduction of blood pressure is not obtained within ten minutes, administration of Nipride should be terminated.
> The instructions included herein should be reviewed thoroughly before administration of Nipride.

Description: Nipride (sodium nitroprusside/Roche) in injectable form contains the equivalent of 50 mg of sodium nitroprusside dihydrate (sodium nitrosylpentacyanoferrate [III]) in a 5-ml amber-colored, rubber-stoppered vial. Chemically, sodium nitroprusside is $Na_2Fe(CN)_5NO \cdot 2H_2O$. It is a reddish-brown powder which is soluble in water. In aqueous solution, it is photosensitive and should be protected from light.

Actions: Nipride is a potent, immediate acting, intravenous hypotensive agent. This action is probably due to the nitroso (NO) group. Its effect is almost immediate and ends when the IV infusion is stopped. Generally, Nipride is rapidly metabolized to cyanide and subsequently converted to thiocyanate through the mediation of a hepatic enzyme, rhodanase. The rate of conversion from cyanide to thiocyanate is dependent on the availability of sulfur, usually thiosulfate. The hypotensive effect is augmented by ganglionic blocking agents, volatile liquid anesthetics (such as halothane and enflurane) and by most other circulatory depressants.

The hypotensive effects of Nipride are caused by peripheral vasodilatation as a result of a direct action on the blood vessels, independent of autonomic innervation. No relaxation is seen in the smooth muscle of the uterus or duodenum *in situ* in animals.

Indications: Nipride is indicated for the immediate reduction of blood pressure of patients in hypertensive crises. Concomitant oral antihypertensive medication should be started while the hypertensive emergency is being brought under control with Nipride. There is no contraindication in using Nipride simultaneously with oral antihypertensive medications.

Nipride is also indicated for producing controlled hypotension during anesthesia in order to reduce bleeding in surgical procedures where surgeon and anesthesiologist deem it appropriate.

Contraindications: Nipride should not be used in the treatment of compensatory hypertension, *e.g.,* arteriovenous shunt or coarctation of the aorta.

The use of Nipride to produce controlled hypotension during surgery is contraindicated in patients with known inadequate cerebral circulation. Nipride is not intended for use during emergency surgery in moribund patients (A.S.A. Class 5E).

Warnings:

> If excessive amounts of Nipride are used and/or sulfur—usually thiosulfate—supplies are depleted, cyanide toxicity can occur. (See OVERDOSAGE.)
> If sodium nitroprusside infusion is to be extended, particularly if renal impairment is present, close attention should be given to not exceeding the recommended maximum infusion rate of 10 micrograms/kg/min. If in the course of therapy increased tolerance to the drug (as shown by the need for higher infusion rate) develops, it is essential to monitor blood acid-base balance, as metabolic acidosis is the earliest and most reliable evidence of cyanide toxicity. If signs of metabolic acidosis appear, Nipride should be discontinued and an alternate drug administered.
> Serum thiocyanate levels do not reflect cyanide toxicity. However, serum thiocyanate levels should be monitored daily if treatment is to be extended, especially in patients with renal dysfunction. Thiocyanate accumulation and toxicity may manifest itself as tinnitus, blurred vision, delirium.

Since cyanide is converted into thiocyanate through the mediation of a hepatic enzyme, rhodanase, Nipride should be used with caution in patients with hepatic insufficiency.

Since thiocyanate inhibits both the uptake and binding of iodine, caution should be exercised in using Nipride in patients with hypothyroidism or severe renal impairment.

The following Warnings apply to use of Nipride for controlled hypotension during anesthesia:

1. Tolerance to blood loss, anemia and hypovolemia may be diminished. If possible, pre-existing anemia and hypovolemia should be corrected prior to employing controlled hypotension.

2. Hypotensive anesthetic techniques may alter pulmonary ventilation perfusion ratio. Patients intolerant of additional dead air space at ordinary oxygen partial pressure may benefit from higher oxygen partial pressure.

3. Extreme caution should be exercised in patients who are especially poor surgical risks (A.S.A. Class 4 and 4E).

Nipride is only to be used as an infusion with sterile 5% dextrose in water. Not for direct injection.

Infusion rates greater than 10 μg/kg/minute are rarely required. If, at this rate, an adequate reduction in blood pressure is not obtained within 10 minutes, administration of Nipride should be stopped.

Hypertensive patients are more sensitive to the intravenous effect of sodium nitroprusside than are normotensive subjects. Patients who are receiving concomitant antihypertensive medications are more sensitive to the hypotensive effect of sodium nitroprusside and the dosage of Nipride should be adjusted accordingly.

Continued on next page

Roche Labs.—Cont.

Usage in Pregnancy: The safety of Nipride in women who are or who may become pregnant has not been established; hence, it should be given only when the potential benefits have been weighed against possible hazard to mother and child.

Precautions: Adequate facilities, equipment and personnel should be available for frequent and vigilant monitoring of blood pressure, since the hypotensive effect of Nipride occurs rapidly. When the infusion is slowed or stopped, blood pressure usually begins to rise immediately and returns to pretreatment levels within one to ten minutes. It should be used with caution and initially in low doses in elderly patients, since they may be more sensitive to the hypotensive effects of the drug. Young, vigorous males may require somewhat larger than ordinary doses of sodium nitroprusside for hypotensive anesthesia; however, the infusion rate of 10 µg/kg/minute should not be exceeded. Deepening of anesthesia, if indicated, might permit satisfactory conditions to exist within the recommended dosage range.

Because of the rapid onset of action and potency of Nipride, it should preferably be administered with the use of an infusion pump, micro-drip regulator, or any similar device that would allow precise measurement of the flow rate.

Once dissolved in solution, Nipride tends to deteriorate in the presence of light. Therefore, it should be protected from light by wrapping the container of the prepared solution with aluminum foil or other opaque materials. Solutions of Nipride should not be kept or used longer than twenty-four hours, while protected from light.

Nipride in aqueous solution yields the nitroprusside ion which reacts with even minute quantities of a wide variety of inorganic and organic substances to form usually highly colored reaction products (blue, green or dark red). If this occurs the infusion should be replaced.

Adverse Reactions: Nausea, retching, diaphoresis, apprehension, headache, restlessness, muscle twitching, retrosternal discomfort, palpitations, dizziness and abdominal pain have been noted with too rapid reduction in blood pressure, but these symptoms rapidly disappeared with slowing of the rate of the infusion or temporary discontinuation of infusion and did not reappear with continued slower rate of administration. Irritation at the infusion site may occur.

One case of hypothyroidism following prolonged therapy with intravenous sodium nitroprusside has been reported. A patient with severe hypertension with uremia received 3900 mg of sodium nitroprusside intravenously over a period of 21 days. This is one of the longest reported intravenous uses of this agent. There was no tachyphylaxis, but the patient developed evidence of hypothyroidism, together with retention of thiocyanate (9.5 mg/100 ml). With peritoneal dialysis the thiocyanate level diminished and the signs of hypothyroidism subsided.

Dosage and Administration: The contents of a 50-mg Nipride vial should be dissolved in 2 to 3 ml of dextrose in water. No other diluent should be used. Depending on the desired concentration, all of the prepared stock solution should be diluted in 250 to 1000 ml of 5 percent dextrose in water and promptly wrapped in aluminum foil or other opaque materials affording protection from light. Both the stock solution and the infusion solution should be freshly prepared and any unused portion discarded. The freshly prepared solution for infusion has a very faint brownish tint. If it is highly colored, it should be discarded (see PRECAUTIONS). *Once prepared, the solution should not be kept or used longer than 24 hours, while protected from light. The infusion fluid used for the administration of Nipride should not be employed as a vehicle for simultaneous administration of any other drug.*

In patients who are not receiving antihypertensive drugs, the average dose of Nipride for both adults and children is 3 µg/kg/minute (range of 0.5 to 10 µg/kg/minute). Usually, at 3 µg/kg/minute, blood pressure can be lowered by about 30 to 40 percent below the pretreatment diastolic levels and maintained. In hypertensive patients receiving concomitant antihypertensive medications, smaller doses are required. In order to avoid excessive levels of thiocyanate and lessen the possibility of a precipitous drop in blood pressure, infusion rates greater than 10 µg/kg/minute should rarely be used. If, at this rate, an adequate reduction of blood pressure is not obtained within 10 minutes, administration of Nipride should be stopped.

1 Vial (50 mg) Nipride in 1000 ml 5% DW (50 µg/ml)
1 Vial (50 mg) Nipride in 500 ml 5% DW (100 µg/ml)
1 Vial (50 mg) Nipride in 250 ml 5% DW (200 µg/ml)

Dose	µg/kg/min
Average	3
Range	0.5 to 10

The intravenous infusion of Nipride should be administered by an infusion pump, micro-drip regulator or any similar device that will allow precise measurement of the flow rate. Care should be taken to avoid extravasation. The rate of administration should be adjusted to maintain the desired antihypertensive or hypotensive effect, as determined by frequent blood pressure determinations. It is recommended that the blood pressure should not be allowed to drop at a too rapid rate and the systolic pressure not be lowered below 60 mmHg. In hypertensive emergencies Nipride infusion may be continued until the patient can safely be treated with oral antihypertensive medications alone.

How Supplied: Nipride injectable is supplied in 5-ml amber-colored vials containing the equivalent of 50 mg sodium nitroprusside dihydrate for reconstitution with dextrose in water—boxes of 1.

Human Pharmacology: Sodium nitroprusside administered intravenously to hypertensive and normotensive patients produced a marked lowering of the arterial blood pressure, slight increase in heart rate, a mild decrease in cardiac output and a moderate diminution in calculated total peripheral vascular resistance.

The decrease in calculated total peripheral vascular resistance suggests arteriolar vasodilatation. The decreases in cardiac and stroke index noted may be due to the peripheral vascular pooling of blood.

In hypertensive patients, moderate depressor doses induce renal vasodilatation roughly equivalent to the decrease in pressure without an appreciable increase in renal blood flow or a decrease in glomerular filtration.

In normotensive subjects, acute reduction of mean arterial pressure to 60 to 75 mmHg by infusion of sodium nitroprusside caused a significant increase in renin activity of renal venous plasma in correlation with the degree of reduction in pressure. Renal response to reduction in pressure was more striking in renovascular hypertensive patients, with significant increase in renin release occurring from the involved kidney at mean arterial pressures ranging from 90 to 137 mmHg. Furthermore, the magnitude of renin release from the involved kidney was significantly greater when compared with that in normotensive subjects, while in the contralateral, uninvolved kidney, no significant release of renin was detected during the reduction of pressure.

Overdosage: The first signs of sodium nitroprusside overdosage are those of profound hypotension. As with instances of depletion of thiosulfate supplies, overdosage may lead to cyanide toxicity. Metabolic acidosis and increasing tolerance to the drug are early indications of overdosage. These may be associated with or followed by dyspnea, headache, vomiting, dizziness, ataxia and loss of consciousness. Sodium nitroprusside should then be immediately discontinued. Other signs of cyanide poisoning are coma, imperceptible pulse, absent reflexes, widely dilated pupils, pink color, distant heart sounds, and shallow breathing. Oxygen alone will not provide relief. Nitrites should be administered to induce methemoglobin formation. Methemoglobin, in turn, combines with cyanide bound to cytochrome oxidase to liberate cytochrome oxidase and form a non-toxic complex, cyanmethemoglobin. Cyanide then gradually dissociates from the latter and is converted by administration of thiosulfate to sodium thiocyanate in the presence of rhodanase.

Treatment: In cases of massive overdosage when signs of cyanide toxicity are present use the following regimen:
1. Discontinue administration of Nipride.
2. Administer amyl nitrite inhalations for 15 to 30 seconds each minute until 3% sodium nitrite solution can be prepared for I.V. administration.
3. Sodium nitrite 3% solution should be injected intravenously at a rate not exceeding 2.5 to 5.0 ml/minute up to a total dose of 10 to 15 ml with careful monitoring of the blood pressure.
4. Following the above steps, inject sodium thiosulfate intravenously, 12.5 Gm in 50 ml of 5% dextrose in water over a ten-minute period.
5. Since signs of overdosage may reappear, the patient must be observed for several hours.
6. If signs of overdosage reappear, sodium nitrite and sodium thiosulfate injections are repeated in one-half of the above doses.
7. During the administration of nitrites and later when thiocyanate formation is taking place, blood pressure may drop but can be corrected with vasopressor agents.

NISENTIL®
[ny′sen-til]
(alphaprodine HCl/Roche)
INJECTABLE

The following text is complete prescribing information based on official labeling in effect August 1, 1984.

WARNINGS
- Nisentil should be used with great caution and in reduced dosage in patients who are receiving other narcotic analgesics, general anesthetics, tranquilizers (including phenothiazines), sedative-hypnotics (including barbiturates), tricyclic antidepressants, MAO inhibitors and other CNS depressants, including alcohol. The depressant effects of Nisentil are potentiated in the presence of such drugs. *Fatalities, severe cerebral damage, respiratory depression, hypotension and profound sedation or coma may result.*
- The DOSAGE AND ADMINISTRATION section should be strictly adhered to and careful attention should be given to the OVERDOSAGE section, particularly for treatment of respiratory depression.
- Nisentil should be used only when resuscitative equipment and personnel trained in such use are immediately available.
- Narcan (naloxone hydrochloride) should be immediately available when Nisentil use is contemplated. If clinically necessary, narcotic reversal with an agent such as Narcan should be performed following procedures in which Nisentil has been administered and the patient closely monitored by trained personnel familiar with such use. (See manufacturer's product information for full details of use.)
- Nisentil should be administered by intravenous, subcutaneous or submucosal routes only. (See DOSAGE AND ADMINISTRATION section.) Nisentil should *never* be administered intramuscularly because absorption is too unpredictable.

Description: Nisentil (alphaprodine hydrochloride/Roche), a synthetic narcotic analgesic, is a sterile aqueous solution for intravenous, subcutaneous or submucosal administration.

Alphaprodine hydrochloride, a white powder which is freely soluble in water, has a calculated molecular weight of 297.82. Chemically, alphaprodine hydrochloride, a piperidine derivative, is (±)-1,3-dimethyl-4-phenyl-4-piperidinol propionate (ester) hydrochloride.

Clinical Pharmacology: Nisentil is a rapid-acting narcotic analgesic with a short duration of action. Except for its more rapid onset and shorter duration of analgesic action, the pharmacologic properties of Nisentil are similar to those of morphine or meperidine. Also, Nisentil is more potent than meperidine. Nisentil acts principally on the central nervous system and on organs composed of smooth muscle. Nisentil is metabolized and probably detoxified by the liver. There is evidence that Nisentil enters the fetal circulation.

In man, the half-life of Nisentil has been reported to be 131 minutes following intravenous administration.

The onset of action following intravenous administration is 1 to 2 minutes; the duration of analgesic action is 30 to 90 minutes. Subcutaneous administration provides analgesic effects usually within 10 minutes (ranging from 2 to 30 minutes). The duration of action following subcutaneous administration of Nisentil lasts from 1 hour to over 2 hours, depending upon the dosage administered, as compared to the duration of action of meperidine, which is 2 to 4 hours.

Indications and Usage: Nisentil is indicated for obstetric analgesia; for urologic examinations and procedures—particularly cystoscopy; preoperatively in major surgery; in minor surgery where rapid analgesia of brief duration is desirable—particularly in children requiring analgesia during dental procedures. Nisentil is indicated in children only for analgesia during dental procedures.

Contraindications: Nisentil is contraindicated in patients with a known hypersensitivity to this drug or to other opiates.

Warnings: (See WARNINGS box.) *Drug Dependence.* Nisentil may be habit forming. Nisentil can produce drug dependence of the morphine type and has the potential for being abused. Psychological and physical dependence and tolerance may develop upon repeated administration of Nisentil; it should be prescribed and administered with the same degree of caution appropriate to the use of morphine.

Intravenous Use: When Nisentil is given intravenously, special attention should be given to the possibility of respiratory depression. Such depression is especially likely in patients with pulmonary disease and in the elderly or debilitated. The patient should be lying down when the drug is administered, and Narcan (naloxone hydrochloride), a narcotic antagonist, and facilities for assisted or controlled respiration should be immediately available.

Hypotensive Effects: The administration of Nisentil may result in severe hypotension in the postoperative patient or in any individual whose ability to maintain blood pressure has been compromised by a depleted blood volume or by the administration of drugs, such as the phenothiazines or certain anesthetics. Narcotics may produce orthostatic hypotension in ambulatory patients.

Head Injury: The respiratory depressant effects of Nisentil may be markedly exaggerated in the presence of head injury or other intracranial lesions. Furthermore, narcotics produce adverse reactions which may obscure the clinical course of patients with head injuries. In such patients, Nisentil must be used with extreme caution and only if its use is deemed essential.

Asthma and Other Respiratory Conditions: Nisentil should be used with extreme caution in patients with bronchial asthma, chronic obstructive pulmonary disease or cor pulmonale. Similarly, it should be used with extreme caution in patients having a decreased respiratory reserve or with preexisting respiratory depression, hypoxia or hypercapnia. In such patients, usual therapeutic doses of narcotics may decrease respiratory drive while simultaneously increasing airway resistance to the point of apnea.

Chronic Pain: Nisentil should not be used for relief of chronic pain because its short duration of action would require more frequent administration and might increase the possibility of physical dependence.

Precautions: *General:* The administration of Nisentil or other narcotics may obscure the diagnosis or clinical course in patients with acute abdominal conditions. Nisentil should be administered with caution and the initial dose should be reduced in patients who are elderly or debilitated, and in those patients with acute alcoholism, severe CNS depression, delirium tremens, severe impairment of hepatic or renal function, hypothyroidism, Addison's disease, toxic psychosis and prostatic hypertrophy or urethral stricture.

Nisentil should be used with caution in patients with atrial flutter and other supraventricular tachycardias because of a possible vagolytic action which may produce a significant increase in the ventricular response rate.

Nisentil may aggravate preexisting convulsions in patients with convulsive disorders. If dosage is escalated substantially above recommended levels because of tolerance development, convulsions may occur in individuals without a history of convulsive disorders.

Information for Patients: When Nisentil is administered to ambulatory patients, they should be cautioned against engaging in hazardous occupations requiring complete mental alertness such as operating machinery or driving a motor vehicle following drug administration.

Drug Interactions: (See WARNINGS box.)

Carcinogenesis, Mutagenesis, Impairment of Fertility: There have been no studies performed with Nisentil to permit an evaluation of its carcinogenic or mutagenic potential. Studies have not been performed to determine the effect of Nisentil on fertility or reproduction.

Pregnancy: Teratogenic Effects: Pregnancy Category C. There are no adequate or well-controlled studies of Nisentil in either laboratory animals or in pregnant women. While the safety and efficacy of Nisentil as an analgesic agent in obstetrics have been established, it is not known whether the drug can cause fetal harm when administered earlier in pregnancy. Nisentil should be used prior to the labor period only if it is clearly needed.

Nonteratogenic Effects: Animal studies have demonstrated that Nisentil depresses fetal respiratory movement and maternal respiratory rate in the rabbit and that it depresses both fetal and maternal cerebral oxygen availability in the guinea pig. (Also see *Labor and Delivery* section.)

Labor and Delivery: When used as an obstetric analgesic, Nisentil passes into the fetal circulation, which may produce depression of respiration and physiologic functions in the newborn. Narcan Neonatal should be used to reverse respiratory depression in the newborn. Resuscitation may be required. (See OVERDOSAGE section.) It has been reported that Nisentil may shorten the duration of labor; however, other studies have reported that Nisentil does not decrease the duration of labor. One study showed that in 9.6% of patients, Nisentil interfered with the mechanism of labor by decreasing the frequency and duration of uterine contractions. A possible explanation of this occurrence is that the drug was administered too early in labor. There are no long-term follow-up studies available on the growth, development and functional maturation of the child.

Nursing Mothers: It is not known whether alphaprodine is excreted in human milk. Because many drugs are excreted in human milk, caution should be exercised when alphaprodine is administered to a nursing woman.

Pediatric Use: Use of Nisentil in children for indications other than pediatric dentistry cannot be recommended because safety and effectiveness have not been established.

Adverse Reactions: Note: Included in this listing are adverse reactions which have not been reported with this specific drug; however, the pharmacologic similarities among the narcotics require that each of the reactions be considered with Nisentil administration.

Deaths and cerebral damage have been reported, especially when Nisentil has been given concomitantly with other CNS depressants. (See WARNINGS box.)

The major hazard of Nisentil administration, as with other narcotic analgesics, is respiratory depression which has led to respiratory arrest. This has also been reported following the administration of Nisentil preoperatively and during labor. The severity of respiratory depression may warrant active measures, particularly in neonatal situations. It is recommended that Narcan (naloxone hydrochloride) be administered in such cases. (See OVERDOSAGE section.) Circulatory depression, shock and cardiac arrest have also been reported following the administration of narcotic analgesics.

Other adverse reactions include:

Neurologic: Pinpoint pupils, visual disturbances, coma, sedation, dizziness, lightheadedness, headache, tremors, uncoordinated muscle movements.
Psychiatric: Euphoria, dysphoria, weakness, agitation, disorientation, confusion, hallucinations.
Cardiovascular: Hypotension, collapse, tachycardia, bradycardia, palpitation, syncope, phlebitis.
Dermatologic: Rash, urticaria (both local and generalized), pruritus, wheal and flare over the vein with intravenous injection.
Gastrointestinal: Nausea, emesis, constipation, dry mouth, biliary tract spasm.
Genitourinary: Urinary retention.
Miscellaneous: Diaphoresis, flushing, pain at the site of injection, allergic and anaphylactoid reactions, local tissue irritation and induration following subcutaneous injection.

Drug Abuse and Dependence: Nisentil is subject to Schedule II control under the Federal Controlled Substances Act of 1970. A narcotic order is required. This drug can produce drug dependence of the morphine type, and therefore has the potential for being abused. Psychological and physical dependence and tolerance may develop upon repeated administration of Nisentil, and consequently the same precautions should be taken in administering the drug as with morphine.

Overdosage: Serious overdosage with Nisentil is characterized by respiratory depression (a decrease in respiratory rate and/or tidal volume, Cheyne-Stokes respiration, cyanosis), extreme somnolence progressing to stupor or coma, skeletal muscle flaccidity, cold and clammy skin, and sometimes bradycardia and hypotension. In severe overdosage, apnea, circulatory collapse, cardiac arrest and death may occur. The triad of coma, pinpoint pupils and depressed respiration strongly suggests opioid poisoning.

Primary attention should be given to the reestablishment of adequate respiratory exchange through provision of a patent airway and through the institution of assisted or controlled ventilation. The narcotic antagonist Narcan (naloxone hydrochloride) is a specific antidote against respiratory depression resulting from narcotic overdosage or unusual sensitivity to narcotics. An appropriate dose of this antagonist should be administered simultaneously, preferably by the intravenous route, with efforts at respiratory resuscitation.

Oxygen, intravenous fluids, vasopressors and other supportive measures should be employed if needed.

Management of Respiratory Depression in Neonates: As in the case of adults, primary attention should be given to the reestablishment of adequate respiratory exchange through provision of a patent airway and through the institution of assisted or controlled ventilation. Administer Narcan (naloxone hydrochloride) at an initial dose of 0.01 mg/kg body weight by I.M., I.V., or S.C. routes. This dose may be repeated at 2- to 3-minute intervals, if necessary, until adequate narcotic reversal is accomplished. Oxygen, intravenous fluids, vasopressors or other supportive measures should be employed.

Note: The administration of the usual dose of a narcotic antagonist will precipitate an acute with-

Continued on next page

Roche Labs.—Cont.

drawal syndrome in patients physically dependent on narcotics. The severity of this syndrome will depend on the degree of physical dependence and the dose of the antagonist administered.

The use of narcotic antagonists in such patients should be avoided if possible. If a narcotic antagonist must be used in physically-dependent patients to treat serious respiratory depression, the antagonist should be administered with extreme care using only $\frac{1}{5}$ to $\frac{1}{10}$ the usual initial dose.

Death, cerebral damage and respiratory arrest have been reported when Nisentil has been administered within recommended dosages but concomitantly with other CNS depressants or administered intramuscularly. (See WARNINGS box.) Death and cerebral damage have been reported in children administered $2\frac{1}{2}$ to $7\frac{1}{2}$ times the recommended dosage of Nisentil.

The acute toxicity of Nisentil is as follows:

Species	Route	LD_{50} (mg/kg)
Mouse	I.V.	51.5 ± 4.0
Rat	I.V.	25.0 ± 6.8
	S.C.	50.0 ± 17.7
	P.O.	90.0 ± 18.7
Rabbit	I.V.	22.0 ± 2.9
Dog	I.V.	36.2 ± 18.3

Dosage and Administration: The dosages suggested are the usual amounts employed in adults; however, as with any other narcotic analgesic, good medical practice dictates the use of the minimal effective dose. If dosage is escalated substantially above recommended levels because of tolerance development, convulsions may occur. *The usual dosage is in the range of 0.4 to 0.6 mg/kg intravenously or 0.4 to 1.2 mg/kg subcutaneously.* Initially, the lower dosage range is recommended in order to evaluate the patient's response. Thus, *the initial intravenous dose should not exceed 30 mg, nor should the initial subcutaneous dose exceed 60 mg.* The total dose administered by any route should not be more than 240 mg in 24 hours. Whenever this drug is given intravenously, a narcotic antagonist and facilities for resuscitation should be available.

Subcutaneous administration provides analgesic effects usually within 10 minutes, lasting from 1 to over 2 hours. If required, an additional ¼ dose may be given 30 minutes after the initial dose. The *intravenous* route is recommended when more rapid onset (1 to 2 minutes) and shorter duration (½ to 1½ hours) of action are desired. An additional amount of ¼ the initial dose may be injected after 15 minutes, if required.

Obstetrics: Initially, 40 to 60 mg subcutaneously after cervical dilation has begun, repeated as required at two-hour intervals. Nisentil may be combined with scopolamine or atropine, and may be used in conjunction with nerve block or inhalation anesthesia as required. (See WARNINGS box on use with CNS depressants.)

Urologic Procedures, e.g., Cystoscopy: Initially, 20 to 30 mg intravenously.

Preoperatively in Major Surgery: Initially, 20 to 40 mg subcutaneously or 10 to 20 mg intravenously.

Minor Surgery: Initially, 40 mg subcutaneously or 20 mg intravenously.

Pediatric Dentistry: The usual recommended dose is 0.3 to 0.6 mg/kg by submucosal route only. If clinically necessary, narcotic reversal with an agent such as Narcan (naloxone hydrochloride) should be performed following procedures in which Nisentil has been administered and the patient closely monitored by trained personnel familiar with such use. (See manufacturer's product information for full details of use.) **Nisentil should be used with great caution and in reduced dosage in pediatric dental patients who are receiving other narcotic analgesics, general anesthetics, tranquilizers (including phenothiazines), sedative-hypnotics (including barbiturates), tricyclic antidepressants, MAO inhibitors and other CNS depressants. The depressant effects of Nisentil are potentiated in the presence of such drugs.** Fatalities, severe cerebral damage, respiratory depression, hypotension and profound sedation or coma may result. *Use of Nisentil in children for indications other than pediatric dentistry cannot be recommended due to limited experience.*

Parenteral drug products should be inspected visually for particulate matter and discoloration prior to administration, whenever possible.

How Supplied: Nisentil is supplied in:

1-ml ampuls—each ml contains 40 mg/ml alphaprodine hydrochloride compounded with 0.0875% citric acid and sodium citrate to adjust pH to approximately 4.6—boxes of 10 (NDC 0004-1915-06).

10-ml vials—each ml contains 60 mg/ml alphaprodine hydrochloride compounded with 0.45% phenol as preservative, 0.0875% citric acid and sodium citrate to adjust pH to approximately 4.6—boxes of 10 (NDC 0004-1917-01).

Narcotic order required.

NOLUDAR® 300
[nol′u-dar]
(methyprylon/Roche)
CAPSULES

NOLUDAR®
(methyprylon/Roche)
TABLETS

The following text is complete prescribing information based on official labeling in effect August 1, 1984.

Description: Noludar (methyprylon/Roche), a hypnotic, is available in three dosage forms for oral use: capsules containing 300 mg of methyprylon (Noludar® 300), tablets containing 200 mg of methyprylon and tablets containing 50 mg of methyprylon.

Chemically, methyprylon, a piperidine derivative, is 3,3-diethyl-5-methyl-2,4-piperidinedione. Methyprylon is a white crystalline powder, freely soluble in water, with a molecular weight of 183.25.

Clinical Pharmacology: In animal studies, methyprylon has been shown to increase the threshold of the arousal centers in the brainstem. In humans, when taken at bedtime, Noludar usually induces sleep within 45 minutes and provides sleep for 5 to 8 hours.

Methyprylon is rapidly absorbed following oral administration and is approximately 60% bound to plasma proteins. Mean peak plasma concentrations of methyprylon in six subjects following a single 650-mg dose occurred at one to two hours postadministration at concentrations of 5.7 to 10.0 mcg/ml. The concentrations declined to 3.3 to 7.9 mcg/ml at 4 hours. Trace amounts of the dihydrometabolite were detected in the one- to four-hour plasma specimens. Following administration of 400 mg of Noludar, less than 1% of the dose was recovered as intact drug and approximately 23% as identified metabolites in the 0- to 72-hour urine specimens. Identified metabolites include the dihydro-metabolite, the 6-oxo, the 5-hydroxymethyl and the 5-carboxyl derivatives. Methyprylon is metabolized by two pathways: dehydrogenation with subsequent oxidation to form the alcohol and corresponding acid, and oxidation to form 6-oxymethyprylon.

Therapeutic blood concentrations are approximately 1 mg%. Serum concentrations in excess of 30 mg/l are generally consistent with unconsciousness in the acutely poisoned patient.

Indications and Usage: Noludar is indicated for use as a hypnotic. In the sleep laboratory it has been objectively determined that Noludar is effective for at least 7 consecutive nights of drug administration. Since insomnia is often transient and intermittent, the prolonged use of hypnotics is usually not indicated and should only be undertaken concomitantly with appropriate evaluation of the patient.

Contraindications: Noludar is contraindicated in patients with known hypersensitivity to the drug.

Warnings: *Synergistic effects:* The concomitant use of alcohol or other CNS depressants may produce additive CNS depressant effects.

Precautions: *General:* Total daily intake should not exceed 400 mg, as greater amounts do not significantly increase hypnotic effects. Caution should be exercised in treating patients with impaired renal or hepatic function. In view of isolated reports associating methyprylon with exacerbation of porphyria, caution should be exercised in prescribing methyprylon to patients suffering from this disease.

Information for patients: Patients receiving Noludar should be cautioned about possible combined effects with alcohol and other CNS depressants. Since Noludar is an effective hypnotic agent, patients should also be cautioned against engaging in hazardous occupations requiring complete mental alertness, such as operating machinery or driving a motor vehicle shortly after ingesting the drug.

Laboratory tests: If Noludar is used repeatedly or over prolonged periods of time, periodic blood counts should be made.

Drug interactions: Noludar stimulates the hepatic microsomal enzyme system. (Also see WARNINGS section.)

Carcinogenesis, mutagenesis, impairment of fertility: Studies sufficient to evaluate the carcinogenic or mutagenic potential of Noludar have not been performed. Noludar had no adverse effects on the reproductive process in rats when administered at dose levels of 5 and 50 mg/kg/day.

Pregnancy: Teratogenic effects: Pregnancy Category B. Reproduction studies have been performed in rats and in rabbits at doses up to approximately 9 times the maximum recommended human dose and have revealed no evidence of teratogenic effects on the fetus due to Noludar. There are, however, no adequate or well-controlled studies in pregnant women. Because animal reproduction studies are not always predictive of human response, this drug should be used in pregnancy only if clearly needed.

Nonteratogenic effects: At a dose of 50 mg/kg/day, Noludar caused an increased incidence of resorptions in the rabbit.

Nursing mothers: It is not known whether this drug is excreted in human milk. Because many drugs are excreted in human milk, caution should be exercised when Noludar is administered to a nursing woman.

Pediatric use: Safety and effectiveness in children below the age of 12 have not been established.

Adverse Reactions: *Neurologic:* Convulsions, hallucinations, ataxia, EEG changes, pyrexia, morning drowsiness, headache, dizziness, vertigo. *Psychiatric:* Acute brain syndrome and confusion (particularly in elderly patients), paradoxical excitation, anxiety, depression, nightmares, dreaming. *Hematologic:* Aplastic anemia, thrombocytopenic purpura, neutropenia. *Cardiovascular:* Hypotension, syncope. *Ophthalmic:* Diplopia, blurred vision. *Gastrointestinal:* Esophagitis, vomiting, nausea, diarrhea, constipation. *Allergic:* Generalized allergic reactions. *Dermatologic:* Pruritus, rash. *Miscellaneous:* Hangover effect.

Drug Abuse and Dependence: Noludar is subject to Schedule III control under the Federal Controlled Substances Act of 1970. Physical and psychological dependence have been reported in patients receiving Noludar therapy. Withdrawal symptoms, when they occur, tend to resemble those associated with the withdrawal of barbiturates and should be treated in a similar fashion. Caution must be exercised in administering Noludar to individuals known to be addiction-prone or to those whose history suggests that they may increase the dosage on their own initiative. As with all hypnotic agents, good medical practice suggests the desirability of limiting repeated prescriptions without adequate medical supervision.

Overdosage: Manifestations of Noludar overdosage include somnolence, confusion, coma, shock, constricted pupils, respiratory depression, hypotension, tachycardia, edema and hepatic dysfunction. Blood concentrations of methyprylon associated with serious toxic symptoms in humans have been reported to range from 3 to 6 mg%. Blood concentrations of methyprylon that have been reported to cause death range from 5.3 to 114 mg%. A fatality occurred after ingestion of 6 grams of the drug. Respiration, pulse and blood pressure should be monitored, as in all cases of drug overdosage. General supportive measures should be employed, along with immediate gastric lavage with precautions to prevent pulmonary aspiration. Appropriate intravenous fluids should be administered and an adequate airway maintained. Hypotension may be combated by the use of Levophed® (norepinephrine bitartrate), Aramine (metaraminol bitartrate) or other accepted antihypotensive measures. Several reports clearly indicate that hemodialysis is of value. Therefore, its use should be considered, especially in those cases where supportive measures are failing and adequate urinary output cannot be maintained. There have been occasional reports of excitation and convulsions in patients following methyprylon overdosage, almost invariably during the recovery phase. Should these occur, barbiturates may be used, but only with great caution. As with the management of intentional overdosage of any drug, it should be borne in mind that multiple agents may have been ingested.

The acute toxicity of Noludar is as follows:

Species	Route	$LD_{50} \pm$ S.E. (mg/kg)
Mouse	P.O.	1000 ± 45
Rat	P.O.	400 ± 32
Rabbit	P.O.	340 ± 78

Dosage and Administration: The dosage should be individualized for maximum beneficial effects. The usual adult dosage is one capsule (300 mg) or one or two tablets of 200 mg (200 or 400 mg) before retiring.

Noludar is not recommended for use in children under 12 years of age. In children over 12 years, the effective dosage of Noludar varies greatly and, therefore, should also be individualized. Treatment may be initiated with one 50-mg tablet at bedtime, and increased up to 200 mg, if required.

How Supplied: Noludar is available as amethyst and white 300-mg capsules in bottles of 100 (NDC 0004-0019-01) and in bottles of 500 (NDC 0004-0019-14); as 50-mg white, scored tablets in bottles of 100 (NDC 0004-0016-01); and as 200-mg white, scored tablets in bottles of 100 (NDC 0004-0017-01). Imprints on all dosage forms of Noludar are as follows: Noludar 300—NOLUDAR® 300 Roche; Noludar 50-mg tablets—ROCHE 16; Noludar 200-mg tablets—ROCHE 17.

Shown in Product Identification Section, page 430

PANTOPON®
[pan'to-pon]
(hydrochlorides of opium alkaloids/Roche)

The following text is complete prescribing information based on official labeling in effect August 1, 1984.

Description: Pantopon (hydrochlorides of opium alkaloids), a narcotic analgesic, is a sterile injectable preparation for intramuscular and subcutaneous administration. It contains all the alkaloids of opium in a highly purified form free from inert matter and in approximately the same proportions as they occur in nature.

Hydrochlorides of opium alkaloids is a yellowish-gray powder which is freely soluble in water. The approximate composition of Pantopon is as follows: anhydrous morphine — 50 percent, and bases of secondary opium alkaloids — 29.9 to 34.2 percent. One part of Pantopon is equivalent to five parts of opium, U.S.P.

One ml of Pantopon contains 20 mg hydrochlorides of opium alkaloids compounded with 6% alcohol, 136 mg glycerin, 0.2% parabens (methyl and propyl) as preservatives, and either acetic acid, sodium hydroxide, or both, as necessary to adjust pH to approximately 3.3.

Clinical Pharmacology: The action of Pantopon is essentially that of opium. Pantopon, therefore, exhibits not only the action of morphine but also the actions of codeine, papaverine and other alkaloids present in opium. The other alkaloids in Pantopon enhance the sedative and analgesic effects of morphine and tend to minimize its undesirable side effects. Pharmacokinetic data on Pantopon are not available, however, data are available on morphine, the major component of Pantopon. Morphine acts as an agonist interacting with stereospecific receptors in the brain and other tissues; the receptor sites are distributed throughout the CNS and are present in highest concentrations in the limbic system, thalamus, striatum, hypothalamus, midbrain and spinal cord. Morphine is well absorbed after subcutaneous and intramuscular administration. When therapeutic concentrations of morphine are present in plasma, approximately one-third of the drug is protein bound. Unbound morphine accumulates in parenchyma tissues (such as lung, liver, kidney and spleen) and skeletal muscle; however, 24 hours following the last dose, concentrations of the drug in these tissues are quite low.

The half-life of morphine in plasma is about 2.5 to 3 hours in young adults; in older patients, the half-life may be more prolonged. The major metabolic pathway for the drug is conjugation with glucuronic acid and the major route of elimination is through glomerular filtration. Ninety percent of the total excretion takes place during the first 24 hours after administration, although traces of the drug are detectable in the urine for well over 48 hours. About 7 to 10% of administered morphine eventually appears in the feces.

Indications and Usage: Pantopon is indicated in conditions in which the analgesic, sedative-hypnotic or narcotic effect of an opiate is needed. It is recommended for the relief of severe pain in place of morphine.

Contraindications: Pantopon is contraindicated in patients with a known hypersensitivity to this drug or to other opiates.

Warnings: *Drug Dependence. Pantopon may be habit forming.* Pantopon can produce drug dependence of the morphine type and has the potential for being abused. Psychological and physical dependence and tolerance may develop upon repeated administration of Pantopon; it should be prescribed and administered with the same degree of caution appropriate to the use of morphine.

Intravenous Use: Pantopon should not be administered intravenously. Rapid intravenous injection of narcotic analgesics increases the incidence of adverse reactions; severe respiratory depression, apnea, hypotension, peripheral circulatory collapse and cardiac arrest have occurred.

Interaction with Other Central Nervous System Depressants: Pantopon should be used with great caution and in reduced dosage in patients who are concurrently receiving other narcotic analgesics, general anesthetics, tranquilizers (including phenothiazines), sedative-hypnotics (including barbiturates), tricyclic antidepressants, MAO inhibitors and other CNS depressants, including alcohol. Respiratory depression, hypotension and profound sedation or coma may result.

Hypotensive Effects: The administration of Pantopon may result in severe hypotension in the postoperative patient or in any individual whose ability to maintain blood pressure has been compromised by a depleted blood volume or by the administration of drugs, such as phenothiazines or certain anesthetics.

Head Injury: The respiratory depressant effects of Pantopon may be markedly exaggerated in the presence of head injury or other intracranial lesions. Furthermore, narcotics produce adverse reactions which may obscure the clinical course of patients with head injuries. In such patients Pantopon must be used with extreme caution and only if its use is deemed essential.

Asthma and Other Respiratory Conditions: Pantopon should be used with extreme caution in patients with bronchial asthma, chronic obstructive pulmonary disease or *cor pulmonale*. Similarly, it should be used with extreme caution in patients having a decreased respiratory reserve or with pre-existing respiratory depression, hypoxia or hypercapnia. In such patients, usual therapeutic doses of narcotics may decrease respiratory drive while simultaneously increasing airway resistance to the point of apnea.

Precautions: *General:* The administration of Pantopon or other narcotics may obscure the diagnosis or clinical course in patients with acute abdominal conditions. Pantopon should be administered with caution and the initial dose should be reduced in patients who are elderly or debilitated and in those patients with severe impairment of hepatic or renal function, hypothyroidism, Addison's disease, toxic psychosis, and prostatic hypertrophy or urethral stricture.

Information for Patients: In the unlikely event that Pantopon would be administered to ambulatory patients, they should be cautioned that Pantopon may impair the mental and/or physical abilities required for the performance of potentially hazardous tasks such as driving a car or operating machinery.

Drug Interactions: See WARNINGS section.

Carcinogenesis, mutagenesis, impairment of fertility: There have been no studies performed with Pantopon to permit an evaluation of its carcinogenic or mutagenic potential. Studies have not been performed to determine the effect of Pantopon on fertility and reproduction.

Pregnancy:
Teratogenic Effects. Pregnancy Category C. Animal studies have demonstrated the teratogenicity of morphine, the major component of Pantopon, in rats, mice and hamsters.

There are no adequate or well-controlled studies of Pantopon in either laboratory animals or in pregnant women. It is also not known whether Pantopon can cause fetal harm when administered to a pregnant woman or if it can affect reproductive capacity. Pantopon should be used during pregnancy only if the potential benefit justifies the potential risk to the fetus.

Nursing Mothers: It has been reported that morphine is excreted in human milk in microgram amounts. Because of the potential for serious adverse reactions from Pantopon in nursing infants, a decision should be made whether to discontinue nursing or to discontinue the drug, taking into account the importance of the drug to the mother.

Pediatric Use: Safety and effectiveness in children have not been established.

Adverse Reactions:
Note: Included in this listing are adverse reactions which have not been reported with this specific drug; however, the pharmacologic similarities among the narcotics require that each of the reactions be considered with Pantopon administration.

Neurologic: Respiratory depression and arrest, pinpoint pupils, visual disturbances, coma, sedation, dizziness, headache, tremors, uncoordinated muscle movements. Inadvertent injection in close proximity to a nerve may result in a sensory-motor paralysis which is usually, though not always, transitory.

Psychiatric: Delirium, euphoria, dysphoria, weakness, agitation, hallucinations.

Cardiovascular: Hypotension, collapse, tachycardia, bradycardia, palpitation.

Dermatologic: Rash, urticaria (local and generalized), pruritus.

Gastrointestinal: Nausea, emesis, constipation, dry mouth, biliary tract spasm.

Genitourinary: Urinary retention.

Miscellaneous: Diaphoresis, flushing, pain at the site of injection, anaphylactoid reactions.

Drug Abuse and Dependence: Pantopon is subject to Schedule II control under the Federal Controlled Substances Act of 1970. This drug can produce drug dependence of the morphine type and, therefore, has the potential for being abused. Psychological and physical dependence and tolerance may develop upon repeated administration of Pantopon, and consequently the same precautions should be taken in administering the drug as with morphine. A narcotic order is required.

Overdosage: Serious overdosage with Pantopon is characterized by respiratory depression (a decrease in respiratory rate and/or tidal volume, Cheyne-Stokes respiration, cyanosis), extreme somnolence progressing to stupor or coma, skeletal muscle flaccidity, cold and clammy skin, and sometimes bradycardia and hypotension. In severe

Continued on next page

Roche Labs.—Cont.

overdosage, apnea, circulatory collapse, cardiac arrest and death may occur. The triad of coma, pinpoint pupils and depressed respiration strongly suggests opioid poisoning.

Primary attention should be given to the reestablishment of adequate respiratory exchange through provision of a patent airway and through the institution of assisted or controlled ventilation. The narcotic antagonist, naloxone hydrochloride (Narcan), is a specific antidote against respiratory depression resulting from narcotic overdosage or unusual sensitivity to narcotics. An appropriate dose of this antagonist should be administered, preferably by the intravenous route, simultaneously with efforts at respiratory resuscitation. Levallorphan tartrate (Lorfan®) is also a narcotic antagonist which may be used in these cases. Administration is by the intravenous route, in an initial dose of 1 mg, followed at 10 to 15 minute intervals by additional doses of 0.5 mg as needed. An antagonist should not be administered in the absence of clinically significant respiratory or cardiovascular depression.

Oxygen, intravenous fluids, vasopressors and other supportive measures should be employed if needed.

Note: The administration of the usual dose of a narcotic antagonist will precipitate an acute withdrawal syndrome in patients physically dependent on narcotics. The severity of this syndrome will depend on the degree of physical dependence and the dose of the antagonist administered. The use of narcotic antagonists in such patients should be avoided if possible. If a narcotic antagonist must be used in physically dependent patients to treat serious respiratory depression, the antagonist should be administered with extreme care using only one-fifth to one-tenth the usual initial dose.

The intravenous LD_{50} of Pantopon in mice is 96 to 99 mg/kg.

Dosage and Administration: One-third grain (20 mg) of Pantopon with a morphine content of $\frac{1}{6}$ grain (10 mg) is therapeutically equivalent to and is usually administered where $\frac{1}{4}$ grain (15 mg) of morphine is indicated.

Usual Adult Dosage:

5 to 20 mg ($\frac{1}{12}$ to $\frac{1}{3}$ grain) approximately every 4 to 5 hours according to the individual needs and severity of pain. Administer only by intramuscular or subcutaneous injection.

Parenteral drug products should be inspected visually for particulate matter and discoloration prior to administration, whenever solution and container permit.

How Supplied: Pantopon is supplied in 1-ml ampuls each containing 20 mg (1/3 grain) hydrochlorides of opium alkaloids/Roche — boxes of 10 (NDC 0004-1918-06).

PROSTIGMIN®
[pro-stig' min]
(neostigmine methylsulfate/Roche)
INJECTABLE

The following text is complete prescribing information based on official labeling in effect August 1, 1984.

Description: Prostigmin (neostigmine methylsulfate/Roche) Injectable, an anticholinesterase agent, is a sterile aqueous solution intended for intramuscular, intravenous or subcutaneous administration.

Prostigmin Injectable is available in the following concentrations:

Prostigmin 1:2000 Ampuls — each ml contains 0.5 mg neostigmine methylsulfate compounded with 0.2% parabens (methyl and propyl) as preservatives and sodium hydroxide to adjust pH to approximately 5.9.

Prostigmin 1:4000 Ampuls — each ml contains 0.25 mg neostigmine methylsulfate compounded with 0.2% parabens (methyl and propyl) as preservatives and sodium hydroxide to adjust pH to approximately 5.9.

Prostigmin 1:1000 Multiple Dose Vials — each ml contains 1 mg neostigmine methylsulfate compounded with 0.45% phenol as preservative, 0.2 mg sodium acetate, and acetic acid and sodium hydroxide to adjust pH to approximately 5.9.

Prostigmin 1:2000 Multiple Dose Vials — each ml contains 0.5 mg neostigmine methylsulfate compounded with 0.45% phenol as preservative, 0.2 mg sodium acetate, and acetic acid and sodium hydroxide to adjust pH to approximately 5.9.

Chemically, neostigmine methylsulfate is (m-hydroxyphenyl)trimethylammonium methylsulfate dimethylcarbamate. It has a molecular weight of 334.39.

Clinical Pharmacology: Neostigmine inhibits the hydrolysis of acetylcholine by competing with acetylcholine for attachment to acetylcholinesterase at sites of cholinergic transmission. It enhances cholinergic action by facilitating the transmission of impulses across neuromuscular junctions. It also has a direct cholinomimetic effect on skeletal muscle and possibly on autonomic ganglion cells and neurons of the central nervous system. Neostigmine undergoes hydrolysis by cholinesterase and is also metabolized by microsomal enzymes in the liver. Protein binding to human serum albumin ranges from 15 to 25 percent.

Following intramuscular administration, neostigmine is rapidly absorbed and eliminated. In a study of five patients with myasthenia gravis, peak plasma levels were observed at 30 minutes, and the half-life ranged from 51 to 90 minutes. Approximately 80 percent of the drug was eliminated in urine within 24 hours; approximately 50 percent as the unchanged drug, and 30 percent as metabolites. Following intravenous administration, plasma half-life ranges from 47 to 60 minutes have been reported with a mean half-life of 53 minutes.

The clinical effects of neostigmine usually begin within 20 to 30 minutes after intramuscular injection and last from 2.5 to 4 hours.

Indications and Usage: Prostigmin is indicated for:

— the symptomatic control of myasthenia gravis when oral therapy is impractical.
— the prevention and treatment of postoperative distention and urinary retention after mechanical obstruction has been excluded.
— reversal of effects of nondepolarizing neuromuscular blocking agents (*e.g.*, tubocurarine, metocurine, gallamine, or pancuronium) after surgery.

Contraindications: Prostigmin is contraindicated in patients with known hypersensitivity to the drug. It is also contraindicated in patients with peritonitis or mechanical obstruction of the intestinal or urinary tract.

Warnings: Prostigmin should be used with caution in patients with epilepsy, bronchial asthma, bradycardia, recent coronary occlusion, vagotonia, hyperthyroidism, cardiac arrhythmias or peptic ulcer. When large doses of Prostigmin are administered, the prior or simultaneous injection of atropine sulfate may be advisable. Separate syringes should be used for the Prostigmin and atropine. Because of the possibility of hypersensitivity in an occasional patient, atropine and antishock medication should always be readily available.

Precautions: *General:* It is important to differentiate between myasthenic crisis and cholinergic crisis caused by overdosage of Prostigmin. Both conditions result in extreme muscle weakness but require radically different treatment. (See OVERDOSAGE section.)

Drug Interactions: Prostigmin does not antagonize, and may in fact prolong, the Phase I block of *depolarizing* muscle relaxants such as succinylcholine or decamethonium. Certain antibiotics, especially neomycin, streptomycin and kanamycin, have a mild but definite nondepolarizing blocking action which may accentuate neuromuscular block. These antibiotics should be used in the myasthenic patient only where definitely indicated, and then careful adjustment should be made of the anticholinesterase dosage. Local and some general anesthetics, antiarrhythmic agents and other drugs that interfere with neuromuscular transmission should be used cautiously, if at all, in patients with myasthenia gravis; the dose of Prostigmin may have to be increased accordingly.

Carcinogenesis, Mutagenesis and Impairment of Fertility: There have been no studies with Prostigmin which would permit an evaluation of its carcinogenic or mutagenic potential. Studies on the effect of Prostigmin on fertility and reproduction have not been performed.

Pregnancy:

Teratogenic Effects: Pregnancy Category C. There are no adequate or well-controlled studies of Prostigmin in either laboratory animals or in pregnant women. It is not known whether Prostigmin can cause fetal harm when administered to a pregnant woman or can affect reproductive capacity. Prostigmin should be given to a pregnant woman only if clearly needed.

Nonteratogenic Effects: Anticholinesterase drugs may cause uterine irritability and induce premature labor when given intravenously to pregnant women near term.

Nursing Mothers: It is not known whether Prostigmin is excreted in human milk. Because many drugs are excreted in human milk and because of the potential for serious adverse reactions from Prostigmin in nursing infants, a decision should be made whether to discontinue nursing or to discontinue the drug, taking into account the importance of the drug to the mother.

Pediatric Use: Safety and effectiveness in children have not been established.

Adverse Reactions: Side effects are generally due to an exaggeration of pharmacological effects of which salivation and fasciculation are the most common. Bowel cramps and diarrhea may also occur.

The following additional adverse reactions have been reported following the use of either neostigmine bromide or neostigmine methylsulfate:

Allergic: Allergic reactions and anaphylaxis.

Neurologic: Dizziness, convulsions, loss of consciousness, drowsiness, headache, dysarthria, miosis and visual changes.

Cardiovascular: Cardiac arrhythmias (including bradycardia, tachycardia, A-V block and nodal rhythm) and nonspecific EKG changes have been reported, as well as cardiac arrest, syncope and hypotension. These have been predominantly noted following the use of the injectable form of Prostigmin.

Respiratory: Increased oral, pharyngeal and bronchial secretions, dyspnea, respiratory depression, respiratory arrest and bronchospasm.

Dermatologic: Rash and urticaria.

Gastrointestinal: Nausea, emesis, flatulence and increased peristalsis.

Genitourinary: Urinary frequency.

Musculoskeletal: Muscle cramps and spasms, arthralgia.

Miscellaneous: Diaphoresis, flushing and weakness.

Overdosage: Overdosage of Prostigmin can cause cholinergic crisis, which is characterized by increasing muscle weakness, and through involvement of the muscles of respiration, may result in death. Myasthenic crisis, due to an increase in the severity of the disease, is also accompanied by extreme muscle weakness and may be difficult to distinguish from cholinergic crisis on a symptomatic basis. However, such differentiation is extremely important because increases in the dose of Prostigmin or other drugs in this class, in the presence of cholinergic crisis or of a refractory or "insensitive" state, could have grave consequences. The two types of crises may be differentiated by the use of Tensilon® (edrophonium chloride/Roche) as well as by clinical judgment.

Treatment of the two conditions differs radically. Whereas the presence of *myasthenic crisis* requires more intensive anticholinesterase therapy, *cholinergic crisis* calls for the prompt withdrawal of all drugs of this type. The immediate use of atropine in cholinergic crisis is also recommended. Atropine may also be used to abolish or minimize gastrointestinal side effects or other muscarinic reactions; but such use, by masking signs of overdose, can lead to inadvertent induction of cholinergic crisis.

The LD_{50} of neostigmine methylsulfate in mice is 0.3 ± 0.02 mg/kg intravenously, 0.54 ± 0.03 mg/kg subcutaneously, and 0.395 ± 0.025 mg/kg intramuscularly; in rats the LD_{50} is 0.315 ± 0.019 mg/kg intravenously, 0.445 ± 0.032 mg/kg subcutaneously, and 0.423 ± 0.032 mg/kg intramuscularly.

Dosage and Administration: *Symptomatic control of myasthenia gravis:* One ml of the 1:2000 solution (0.5 mg) subcutaneously or intramuscularly. Subsequent doses should be based on the individual patient's response. In most patients, however, oral treatment with Prostigmin (neostigmine bromide) tablets, 15 mg each, is adequate for control of symptoms.

Prevention of postoperative distention and urinary retention: One ml of the 1:4000 solution (0.25 mg) subcutaneously or intramuscularly as soon as possible after operation; repeat every 4 to 6 hours for two or three days.

Treatment of postoperative distention: One ml of the 1:2000 solution (0.5 mg) subcutaneously or intramuscularly, as required.

Treatment of urinary retention: One ml of the 1:2000 solution (0.5 mg) subcutaneously or intramuscularly. If urination does not occur within an hour, the patient should be catheterized. After the patient has voided, or the bladder has been emptied, continue the 0.5 mg injections every three hours for at least 5 injections.

Reversal of Effects of Nondepolarizing Neuromuscular Blocking Agents: When Prostigmin is administered intravenously, it is recommended that atropine sulfate (0.6 to 1.2 mg) also be given intravenously using separate syringes. Some authorities have recommended that the atropine be injected several minutes before the Prostigmin rather than concomitantly. The usual dose is 0.5 to 2 mg Prostigmin given by *slow* intravenous injection, repeated as required. Only in exceptional cases should the total dose of Prostigmin exceed 5 mg. It is recommended that the patient be well ventilated and a patent airway maintained until complete recovery of normal respiration is assured. The optimum time for administration of the drug is during hyperventilation when the carbon dioxide level of the blood is low. It should never be administered in the presence of high concentrations of halothane or cyclopropane. In cardiac cases and severely ill patients, it is advisable to titrate the exact dose of Prostigmin required, using a peripheral nerve stimulator device. In the presence of bradycardia, the pulse rate should be increased to about 80/minute with atropine before administering Prostigmin.

Parenteral drug products should be inspected visually for particulate matter and discoloration prior to administration, whenever solution and container permit.

How Supplied:
Prostigmin 1:2000 (0.5 mg neostigmine methylsulfate/ml), 1-ml ampuls — boxes of 10 (NDC 0004-1919-06).

Prostigmin 1:4000 (0.25 mg neostigmine methylsulfate/ml), 1-ml ampuls — boxes of 10 (NDC 0004-1920-06).

Prostigmin 1:1000 (1 mg neostigmine methylsulfate/ml), 10-ml multiple dose vials — boxes of 10 (NDC 0004-1921-06).

Prostigmin 1:2000 (0.5 mg neostigmine methylsulfate/ml), 10-ml multiple dose vials — boxes of 10 (NDC 0004-1922-06).

PROSTIGMIN® ℞
[*pro-stig'min*]
(neostigmine bromide/Roche)
TABLETS

The following text is complete prescribing information based on official labeling in effect August 1, 1984.

Description: Prostigmin (neostigmine bromide/Roche), an anticholinesterase agent, is available for oral administration in 15-mg tablets. Chemically, neostigmine bromide is (*m*-hydroxyphenyl)trimethylammonium bromide dimethylcarbamate. It is a white, crystalline, bitter powder, soluble 1:1 in water, with a molecular weight of 303.20.

Clinical Pharmacology: Neostigmine inhibits the hydrolysis of acetylcholine by competing with acetylcholine for attachment to acetylcholinesterase at sites of cholinergic transmission. It enhances cholinergic action by facilitating the transmission of impulses across neuromuscular junctions. It also has a direct cholinomimetic effect on skeletal muscle and possibly on autonomic ganglion cells and neurons of the central nervous system. Neostigmine undergoes hydrolysis by cholinesterase and is also metabolized by microsomal enzymes in the liver. Protein binding to human serum albumin ranges from 15 to 25 percent.

Neostigmine bromide is poorly absorbed from the gastrointestinal tract following oral administration. As a rule, 15 mg of neostigmine bromide orally is equivalent to 0.5 mg of neostigmine methylsulfate parenterally, due to poor absorption of the tablet from the intestinal tract. In a study in fasting myasthenic patients, the extent of absorption was estimated to be 1 to 2 percent of the ingested 30-mg single oral dose. Peak concentrations in plasma occurred 1 to 2 hours following drug ingestion, with considerable individual variations. The half-life ranged from 42 to 60 minutes with a mean half-life of 52 minutes.

Indications and Usage: Prostigmin is indicated for the symptomatic treatment of myasthenia gravis. Its greatest usefulness is in prolonged therapy where no difficulty in swallowing is present. In acute myasthenic crisis where difficulty in breathing and swallowing is present, the parenteral form (neostigmine methylsulfate) should be used. The patient can be transferred to the oral form as soon as it can be tolerated.

Contraindications: Prostigmin is contraindicated in patients with known hypersensitivity to the drug. Because of the presence of the bromide ion, it should not be used in patients with a previous history of reaction to bromides. It is contraindicated in patients with peritonitis or mechanical obstruction of the intestinal or urinary tract.

Warnings: Prostigmin should be used with caution in patients with epilepsy, bronchial asthma, bradycardia, recent coronary occlusion, vagotonia, hyperthyroidism, cardiac arrhythmias or peptic ulcer. As a rule, 15 mg of neostigmine bromide orally is equivalent to 0.5 mg of neostigmine methylsulfate parenterally, due to poor absorption of the tablet from the intestinal tract. Large doses should be avoided in situations where there might be an increased absorption rate from the intestinal tract. It should be used with caution when co-administered with anticholinergic drugs, in order to avoid reduction of intestinal motility.

Precautions: *General:* It is important to differentiate between myasthenic crisis and cholinergic crisis caused by overdosage of Prostigmin. Both conditions result in extreme muscle weakness but require radically different treatment. (See OVERDOSAGE section.)

Drug Interactions: Certain antibiotics, especially neomycin, streptomycin and kanamycin, have a mild but definite nondepolarizing blocking action which may accentuate neuromuscular block. These antibiotics should be used in the myasthenic patient only where definitely indicated, and then careful adjustment should be made of adjunctive anticholinesterase dosage.

Local and some general anesthetics, antiarrhythmic agents and other drugs that interfere with neuromuscular transmission should be used cautiously, if at all, in patients with myasthenia gravis; the dose of Prostigmin may have to be increased accordingly.

Carcinogenesis, Mutagenesis and Impairment of Fertility: There have been no studies with Prostigmin which would permit an evaluation of its carcinogenic or mutagenic potential. Studies on the effect of Prostigmin on fertility and reproduction have not been performed.

Pregnancy:
Teratogenic Effects: Pregnancy Category C. There are no adequate or well-controlled studies of Prostigmin in either laboratory animals or in pregnant women. It is not known whether Prostigmin can cause fetal harm when administered to a pregnant woman or can affect reproductive capacity. Prostigmin should be given to a pregnant woman only if clearly needed.

Nonteratogenic Effects: Anticholinesterase drugs may cause uterine irritability and induce premature labor when given intravenously to pregnant women near term.

Nursing Mothers: It is not known whether Prostigmin is excreted in human milk. Because many drugs are excreted in human milk and because of the potential for serious adverse reactions from Prostigmin in nursing infants, a decision should be made whether to discontinue nursing or to discontinue the drug, taking into account the importance of the drug to the mother.

Pediatric Use: Safety and effectiveness in children have not been established.

Adverse Reactions: Side effects are generally due to an exaggeration of pharmacological effects of which salivation and fasciculation are the most common. Bowel cramps and diarrhea may also occur.

The following additional adverse reactions have been reported following the use of either neostigmine bromide or neostigmine methylsulfate.

Allergic: Allergic reactions and anaphylaxis.
Neurologic: Dizziness, convulsions, loss of consciousness, drowsiness, headache, dysarthria, miosis and visual changes.
Cardiovascular: Cardiac arrhythmias (including bradycardia, tachycardia, A-V block and nodal rhythm) and nonspecific EKG changes have been reported, as well as cardiac arrest, syncope and hypotension. These have been predominantly noted following the use of the injectable form of Prostigmin.
Respiratory: Increased oral, pharyngeal and bronchial secretions, and dyspnea. Respiratory depression, respiratory arrest and bronchospasm have been reported following the use of the injectable form of Prostigmin.
Dermatologic: Rash and urticaria.
Gastrointestinal: Nausea, emesis, flatulence and increased peristalsis.
Genitourinary: Urinary frequency.
Musculoskeletal: Muscle cramps and spasms, arthralgia.
Miscellaneous: Diaphoresis, flushing and weakness.

Overdosage: Overdosage of Prostigmin can cause cholinergic crisis, which is characterized by increasing muscle weakness, and through involvement of the muscles of respiration, may result in death. Myasthenic crisis, due to an increase in the severity of the disease, is also accompanied by extreme muscle weakness and may be difficult to distinguish from cholinergic crisis on a symptomatic basis. However, such differentiation is extremely important because increases in the dose of Prostigmin or other drugs in this class, in the presence of cholinergic crisis or of a refractory or "insensitive" state, could have grave consequences. The two types of crises may be differentiated by the use of Tensilon® (edrophonium chloride/Roche) as well as by clinical judgment.

Treatment of the two conditions differs radically. Whereas the presence of *myasthenic crisis* requires more intensive anticholinesterase therapy, *cholinergic crisis* calls for the prompt withdrawal of all drugs of this type. The immediate use of atropine in cholinergic crisis is also recommended. Atropine may also be used to abolish or minimize gastrointestinal side effects or other muscarinic reactions; but such use, by masking signs of overdosage, can lead to inadvertent induction of cholinergic crisis.

The LD_{50} of neostigmine methylsulfate in mice is 0.3 ± 0.02 mg/kg intravenously, 0.54 ± 0.03 mg/kg subcutaneously, and 0.395 ± 0.025 mg/kg intramuscularly; in rats the LD_{50} is 0.315 ± 0.019 mg/kg intravenously, 0.445 ± 0.032 mg/kg subcutaneously, and 0.423 ± 0.032 mg/kg intramuscularly.

Continued on next page

Roche Labs.—Cont.

Dosage and Administration: The onset of action of Prostigmin given orally is slower than when given parenterally, but the duration of action is longer and the intensity of action more uniform. Dosage requirements for optimal results vary from 15 mg to 375 mg per day. In some instances it may be necessary to exceed these dosages, but the possibility of cholinergic crisis must be recognized. The average dose is 10 tablets (150 mg) administered over a 24-hour period. The interval between doses is of paramount importance. The dosage schedule should be adjusted for each patient and changed as the need arises. Frequently, therapy is required day and night. Larger portions of the total daily dose may be given at times when the patient is more prone to fatigue (afternoon, mealtimes, etc.). The patient should be encouraged to keep a daily record of his or her condition to assist the physician in determining an optimal therapeutic regimen.

How Supplied: Scored, white tablets containing 15 mg neostigmine bromide — bottles of 100 (NDC 0004-0035-01) and 1000 (NDC 0004-0035-13). Imprint on tablets: Roche 35.

Shown in Product Identification Section, page 430

ROCALTROL® ℞
[ro-cal'trol]
(calcitriol/Roche)
CAPSULES

The following text is complete prescribing information based on official labeling in effect August 1, 1984.

Description: Rocaltrol (calcitriol/Roche) is a synthetic vitamin D analog which is active in the regulation of the absorption of calcium from the gastrointestinal tract and its utilization in the body. Calcitriol is a colorless, crystalline compound which occurs naturally in humans. It has a calculated molecular weight of 416.65 and is soluble in organic solvents but relatively insoluble in water. Chemically, calcitriol is 9,10-seco(5Z,7E)-5,7,10(19)-cholestatriene-1α, 3β,25-triol.

The other names frequently used for calcitriol are 1α,25-dihydroxycholecalciferol, 1,25-dihydroxyvitamin D_3, 1,25-DHCC, 1,25(OH)$_2$D$_3$ and 1,25-diOHC.

Rocaltrol is available as 0.25-mcg and 0.5-mcg soft gelatin capsules for oral administration.

Clinical Pharmacology: Man's natural supply of vitamin D depends mainly on exposure to the ultraviolet rays of the sun for conversion of 7-dehydrocholesterol in the skin to vitamin D_3 (cholecalciferol). Vitamin D_3 must be metabolically activated in the liver and the kidney before it is fully active as a regulator of calcium and phosphorus metabolism at target tissues. The initial transformation of vitamin D_3 is catalyzed by a vitamin D_3-25-hydroxylase enzyme (25-OHase) present in the liver, and the product of this reaction is 25-hydroxyvitamin D_3 [25-(OH)D$_3$]. Hydroxylation of 25-(OH)D$_3$ occurs in the mitochondria of kidney tissue, activated by the renal 25-hydroxyvitamin D_3-1 alpha-hydroxylase (alpha-OHase), to produce 1,25-(OH)$_2$D$_3$ (calcitriol), the active form of vitamin D_3. Two metabolic pathways for calcitriol seem to have been identified: conversion to 1,24,25-(OH)$_3$D$_3$ and to an unknown substance with a loss of a side chain at the C26 or C27 position.

The two known sites of action of calcitriol are intestine and bone. A calcitriol receptor-binding protein appears to exist in the mucosa of human intestine. Additional evidence suggests that calcitriol may also act on the kidney and the parathyroid glands. Calcitriol is the most active known form of vitamin D_3 in stimulating intestinal calcium transport. In acutely uremic rats calcitriol has been shown to stimulate intestinal calcium absorption. It has been suggested that a vitamin D-resistant state exists in uremic patients because of the failure of the kidney to adequately convert precursors to the active compound, calcitriol.

Calcitriol is rapidly absorbed from the intestine. Peak serum concentrations (above basal values) were reached within 3 to 6 hours following oral administration of single doses of 0.25 to 1.0 mcg of Rocaltrol. The half-life of calcitriol elimination from serum was found to range from 3 to 6 hours. Following a single oral dose of 0.5 mcg, mean serum concentrations of calcitriol rose from a baseline value of 40.0 $\pm$ 4.4 (S.D.) pg/ml to 60.0 $\pm$ 4.4 pg/ml at 2 hours, and declined to 53.0 $\pm$ 6.9 at 4 hours, 50 $\pm$ 7.0 at 8 hours, 44 $\pm$ 4.6 at 12 hours and 41.5 $\pm$ 5.1 at 24 hours. The duration of pharmacologic activity of a single dose of calcitriol is about 3 to 5 days.

Calcitriol and other vitamin D metabolites are transported in blood, bound to specific plasma proteins. Enterohepatic recycling and biliary excretion of calcitriol occurs. Following intravenous administration of radiolabeled calcitriol in normal subjects, approximately 27% and 7% of the radioactivity appeared in the feces and urine, respectively, within 24 hours. When a 1-mcg oral dose of radiolabeled calcitriol was administered to normals, approximately 10% of the total radioactivity appeared in urine within 24 hours. Cumulative excretion of radioactivity on the sixth day following intravenous administration of radiolabeled calcitriol averaged 16% in urine and 49% in feces. There is evidence that maternal calcitriol may enter the fetal circulation. It is not known if calcitriol is excreted in human milk.

Indications and Usage: Rocaltrol is indicated in the management of hypocalcemia in patients undergoing chronic renal dialysis. In studies to date, it has been shown to reduce elevated parathyroid hormone levels in some of these patients. Rocaltrol is also indicated in the management of hypocalcemia and its clinical manifestations in patients with postsurgical hypoparathyroidism, idiopathic hypoparathyroidism, and pseudohypoparathyroidism.

Contraindications: Rocaltrol should not be given to patients with hypercalcemia or evidence of vitamin D toxicity.

Warnings: Since Rocaltrol is the most potent metabolite of vitamin D available, pharmacologic doses of vitamin D and its derivatives should be withheld during Rocaltrol treatment to avoid possible additive effects and hypercalcemia.

Aluminum carbonate or hydroxide gel should be used to control serum phosphate levels in patients undergoing dialysis.

Magnesium-containing antacids and Rocaltrol should not be used concomitantly in patients on chronic renal dialysis because such use may lead to the development of hypermagnesemia.

Overdosage of any form of vitamin D is dangerous (see also OVERDOSAGE). Progressive hypercalcemia due to overdosage of vitamin D and its metabolites may be so severe as to require emergency attention. Chronic hypercalcemia can lead to generalized vascular calcification, nephrocalcinosis and other soft-tissue calcification. **The serum calcium times phospate (Ca $\times$ P) product should not be allowed to exceed 70.** Radiographic evaluation of suspect anatomical regions may be useful in the early detection of this condition.

Precautions: *General:* Excessive dosage of Rocaltrol induces hypercalcemia and in some instances hypercalciuria; therefore, early in treatment during dosage adjustment, serum calcium should be determined twice weekly. In dialysis patients, a fall in serum alkaline phosphatase levels usually antedates the appearance of hypercalcemia and may be an indication of impending hypercalcemia. Should hypercalcemia develop, the drug should be discontinued immediately. Rocaltrol should be given cautiously to patients on digitalis, because hypercalcemia in such patients may precipitate cardiac arrhythmias.

In patients with normal renal function, chronic hypercalcemia may be associated with an increase in serum creatinine. While this is usually reversible, it is important in such patients to pay careful attention to those factors which may lead to hypercalcemia. Rocaltrol therapy should always be started at the lowest possible dose and should not be increased without careful monitoring of the serum calcium. An estimate of daily dietary calcium intake should be made and the intake adjusted when indicated.

Patients with normal renal function taking Rocaltrol should avoid dehydration. Adequate fluid intake should be maintained.

Information for the patient: The patient and his or her parents or spouse should be informed about compliance with dosage instructions, adherence to instructions about diet and calcium supplementation and avoidance of the use of unapproved nonprescription drugs. Patients should also be carefully informed about the symptoms of hypercalcemia (see ADVERSE REACTIONS section).

Laboratory tests: For dialysis patients, serum calcium, phosphorus, magnesium and alkaline phosphatase should be determined periodically. For hypoparathyroid patients, serum calcium, phosphorus and 24-hour urinary calcium should be determined periodically.

Drug interactions: Cholestyramine has been reported to reduce intestinal absorption of fat-soluble vitamins; as such it may impair intestinal absorption of Rocaltrol. (Also see WARNINGS and PRECAUTIONS [General] sections.)

Carcinogenesis, mutagenesis, impairment of fertility: Long-term studies in animals have not been conducted to evaluate the carcinogenic potential of Rocaltrol. There was no evidence of mutagenicity as studied by the Ames method. No significant effects of Rocaltrol on fertility and/or general reproductive performances were reported.

Pregnancy: Teratogenic effects: Pregnancy Category C. Rocaltrol has been found to be teratogenic in rabbits when given in doses 4 and 15 times the dose recommended for human use. All 15 fetuses in 3 litters at these doses showed external and skeletal abnormalities. However, none of the other 23 litters (156 fetuses) showed significant abnormalities compared with controls. Teratogenicity studies in rats showed no evidence of teratogenic potential. There are no adequate and well-controlled studies in pregnant women. Rocaltrol should be used during pregnancy only if the potential benefit justifies the potential risk to the fetus. Nonteratogenic effects: In the rabbit, dosages of 0.3 mcg/kg/day administered on days 7 to 18 of gestation resulted in 19% maternal mortality, a decrease in mean fetal body weight and a reduced number of newborn surviving to 24 hours. A study of peri- and postnatal development in rats resulted in hypercalcemia in the offspring of dams given Rocaltrol at doses of 0.08 or 0.3 mcg/kg/day, hypercalcemia and hypophosphatemia in dams at doses of 0.08 or 0.3 mcg/kg/day, and increased serum urea nitrogen in dams given Rocaltrol at a dose of 0.3 mcg/kg/day. In another study in rats, maternal weight gain was slightly reduced at a dose of 0.3 mcg/kg/day administered on days 7 to 15 of gestation.

The offspring of a woman administered 17 to 36 mcg/day of Rocaltrol (17 to 144 times the recommended dose) during pregnancy manifested mild hypercalcemia in the first two days of life which returned to normal at day 3.

Nursing mothers: It is not known whether calcitriol is excreted in human milk. Because many drugs are excreted in human milk and because of the potential for serious adverse reactions from Rocaltrol in nursing infants, a mother should not nurse while taking this drug.

Pediatric use: Safety and efficacy of Rocaltrol in children undergoing dialysis have not been established.

Adverse Reactions: Since Rocaltrol is believed to be the active hormone which exerts vitamin D activity in the body, adverse effects are, in general, similar to those encountered with excessive vitamin D intake. The early and late signs and symptoms of vitamin D intoxication associated with hypercalcemia include:

Early: Weakness, headache, somnolence, nausea, vomiting, dry mouth, constipation, muscle pain, bone pain and metallic taste.

Late: Polyuria, polydipsia, anorexia, weight loss, nocturia, conjunctivitis (calcific), pancreatitis, photophobia, rhinorrhea, pruritus, hyperthermia, decreased libido, elevated BUN, albuminuria, hy-

percholesterolemia, elevated SGOT and SGPT, ectopic calcification, hypertension, cardiac arrhythmias and, rarely, overt psychosis.
In clinical studies on hypoparathyroidism and pseudohypoparathyroidism, hypercalcemia was noted on at least one occasion in about 1 in 3 patients and hypercalciuria in about 1 in 7. Elevated serum creatinine levels were observed in about 1 in 6 patients (approximately one half of whom had normal levels at baseline).
One case of erythema multiforme was confirmed by rechallenge.
Overdosage: Administration of Rocaltrol to patients in excess of their daily requirements can cause hypercalcemia, hypercalciuria and hyperphosphatemia. High intake of calcium and phosphate concomitant with Rocaltrol may lead to similar abnormalities. High levels of calcium in the dialysate bath may contribute to the hypercalcemia.
Treatment of Hypercalcemia and Overdosage: General treatment of hypercalcemia (greater than 1 mg/dl above the upper limit of the normal range) consists of immediate discontinuation of Rocaltrol therapy, institution of a low calcium diet and withdrawal of calcium supplements. Serum calcium levels should be determined daily until normocalcemia ensues. Hypercalcemia frequently resolves in two to seven days. When serum calcium levels have returned to within normal limits, Rocaltrol therapy may be reinstituted at a dose of 0.25 mcg/day less than prior therapy. Serum calcium levels should be obtained at least twice weekly after all dosage changes and subsequent dosage titration. In dialysis patients, persistent or markedly elevated serum calcium levels may be corrected by dialysis against a calcium-free dialysate.
Treatment of Accidental Overdosage of Rocaltrol: The treatment of acute accidental overdosage of Rocaltrol should consist of general supportive measures. If drug ingestion is discovered within a relatively short time, induction of emesis or gastric lavage may be of benefit in preventing further absorption. If the drug has passed through the stomach, the administration of mineral oil may promote its fecal elimination. Serial serum electrolyte determinations (especially calcium), rate of urinary calcium excretion and assessment of electrocardiographic abnormalities due to hypercalcemia should be obtained. Such monitoring is critical in patients receiving digitalis. Discontinuation of supplemental calcium and a low calcium diet are also indicated in accidental overdosage. Due to the relatively short duration of the pharmacological action of calcitriol, further measures are probably unnecessary. Should, however, persistent and markedly elevated serum calcium levels occur, there are a variety of therapeutic alternatives which may be considered, depending on the patient's underlying condition. These include the use of drugs such as phosphates and corticosteroids as well as measures to induce an appropriate forced diuresis. The use of peritoneal dialysis against a calcium-free dialysate has also been reported.
The oral toxicity of calcitriol is as follows:

Species	LD_{50} (mg/kg)
mouse	2.0
rat	>5.0

Dosage and Administration: The optimal daily dose of Rocaltrol must be carefully determined for each patient.
The effectiveness of Rocaltrol therapy is predicated on the assumption that each patient is receiving an adequate daily intake of calcium. The U.S. RDA for calcium in adults is 800 to 1200 mg. To ensure that each patient receives an adequate daily intake of calcium, the physician should either prescribe a calcium supplement or instruct the patient in proper dietary measures.
Dialysis patients: The recommended initial dose of Rocaltrol is 0.25 mcg/day. If a satisfactory response in the biochemical parameters and clinical manifestations of the disease state is not observed, dosage may be increased by 0.25 mcg day at four- to eight-week intervals. During this titration period, serum calcium levels should be obtained at least twice weekly, and if hypercalcemia is noted, the drug should be immediately discontinued until normocalcemia ensues.
Patients with normal or only slightly reduced serum calcium levels may respond to Rocaltrol doses of 0.25 mcg every other day. Most patients undergoing hemodialysis respond to doses between 0.5 and 1 mcg/day.
Hypoparathyroidism: The recommended initial dose of Rocaltrol is 0.25 mcg/day given in the morning. If a satisfactory response in the biochemical parameters and clinical manifestations of the disease is not observed, the dose may be increased at two- to four-week intervals. During the dosage titration period, serum calcium levels should be obtained at least twice weekly and, if hypercalcemia is noted, Rocaltrol should be immediately discontinued until normocalcemia ensues. Careful consideration should also be given to lowering the dietary calcium intake.
Most adult patients and pediatric patients age 6 years and older have responded to dosages in the range of 0.5 to 2 mcg daily. Pediatric patients in the 1–5 year age group with hypoparathyroidism have usually been given 0.25 to 0.75 mcg daily. The number of treated patients with pseudohypoparathyroidism less than 6 years of age is too small to make dosage recommendations.
How Supplied: The recommended initial dose of Rocaltrol is 0.25 mcg calcitriol/Roche in soft gelatin, light orange, oval capsules, imprinted (front) HLR, (back) 143; bottles of 30, (NDC 0004-0143-23), and bottles of 100, (NDC 0004-0143-01). 0.5 mcg calcitriol/Roche in soft gelatin, dark orange, oblong capsules, imprinted (front) ROCHE, (back) 144; bottles of 100, (NDC 0004-0144-01).
Rocaltrol should be protected from heat and light.
Shown in Product Identification Section, p. 430.

SOLATENE® ℞
[sol′a-teen]
(beta-carotene/Roche)
capsules

The following text is complete prescribing information based on official labeling in effect August 1, 1984.
Description: Solatene (beta-carotene), precursor of vitamin A, is supplied in 30-mg capsules for oral administration. Beta-carotene is a carotenoid pigment occurring naturally in green and yellow vegetables. Chemically, beta-carotene has the empirical formula $C_{40}H_{56}$ and a calculated molecular weight of 536.85. Trans-beta-carotene is a red, crystalline compound which is insoluble in water.
Clinical Pharmacology: Beta-carotene, a provitamin A, belongs to the class of carotenoid pigments. In terms of its vitamin activity, 6 μg of dietary beta-carotene is considered equivalent to 1 μg of vitamin A (retinol). Bioavailability of beta-carotene depends on the presence of fat in the diet to act as a carrier, and bile in the intestinal tract for its absorption. Beta-carotene is metabolized, primarily in the intestine, to vitamin A at a rate of approximately 50% to 60% of normal dietary intake and falls off rapidly as intake goes up. In humans, an appreciable amount of unchanged beta-carotene is absorbed and stored in various tissues, especially the depot fat. Small amounts may be converted to vitamin A in the liver. The vitamin A derived from beta-carotene follows the same metabolic pathway as that from dietary sources. The major route of elimination is fecal excretion. Excessive ingestion of carotenes is not harmful, but it may cause yellow coloration of the skin, which disappears upon reduction or cessation of intake.
Indications and Usage: Solatene is used to reduce the severity of photosensitivity reactions in patients with erythropoietic protoporphyria (EPP).
Contraindications: Solatene is contraindicated in patients with known hypersensitivity to the drug.
Warnings: Solatene has not been shown to be effective as a sunscreen.
Precautions: *General:* Solatene should be used with caution in patients with impaired renal or hepatic function because safe use in the presence of these conditions has not been established.
Information for Patients: Patients receiving Solatene should be advised against taking supplementary vitamin A since Solatene administration will fulfill normal vitamin A requirements. They should be cautioned to continue sun protection, and forewarned that their skin may appear slightly yellow while receiving Solatene.
Carcinogenesis, Mutagenesis, Impairment of Fertility: Long-term studies in animals to determine carcinogenesis have not been completed. *In vitro* and *in vivo* studies to evaluate mutagenic potential were negative. No effects on fertility in male rats were observed at doses as high as 500 mg/kg/day (100 times the recommended human dose).
Pregnancy: Teratogenic Effects: Pregnancy Category C. Beta-carotene has been shown to be fetotoxic (i.e., cause an increase in resorption rate), but not teratogenic when given to rats at doses 300 to 400 times the maximum recommended human dose. No such fetotoxicity was observed at 75 times the maximum recommended human dose or less. A three-generation reproduction study in rats receiving beta-carotene at a dietary concentration of 0.1% (1000 ppm) has revealed no evidence of impaired fertility or effect on the fetus. There are no adequate and well-controlled studies in pregnant women. Solatene should be used during pregnancy only if the potential benefit justifies the potential risk to the fetus.
Nursing Mothers: It is not known whether this drug is excreted in human milk. Because many drugs are excreted in human milk, caution should be exercised when Solatene is administered to a nursing mother.
Adverse Reactions: Some patients may have occasional loose stools while taking Solatene. This reaction is sporadic and may not require discontinuance of medication. Other reactions which have been reported rarely are ecchymoses and arthralgia.
Overdosage: There are no reported cases of overdosage. The oral LD_{50} of beta-carotene (suspended in 5% gum acacia solution) in mice and rats is greater than 20,000 mg/kg. No lethality was observed in mice following administration of 30-mg beadlet capsules (ground and suspended in 5% gum acacia) at a dose of 1200 mg/kg beta-carotene.
Dosage and Administration: Solatene may be administered either as a single daily dose or in divided doses, preferably with meals.
Usage in Children: The usual dosage for children under 14 is 30 to 150 mg (1 to 5 capsules) per day. Capsules may be opened and the contents mixed in orange juice or tomato juice to aid administration.
Usage in Adults: The usual adult dosage is 30 to 300 mg (1 to 10 capsules) per day.
Dosage should be adjusted depending on the severity of the symptoms and the response of the patient. Several weeks of therapy are necessary to accumulate enough Solatene in the skin to exert its effect. Patients should be instructed not to increase exposure to sunlight until they appear carotenemic (first seen as yellowness of palms and soles). This usually occurs after two to six weeks of therapy. Exposure to the sun may then be increased gradually. The protective effect is not total and each patient should establish his or her own limits of exposure.
How Supplied: Solatene is available in blue and green capsules, each containing 30 mg of beta-carotene—bottles of 100 (NDC 0004-0115-01). Imprint on capsules: SOLATENE ROCHE.
Shown in Product Identification Section, page 430

SYNKAYVITE® ℞
(menadiol sodium diphosphate/Roche)
INJECTABLE

The following text is complete product information based on official labeling in effect August 1, 1984.

Continued on next page

Roche Labs.—Cont.

Description: Synkayvite (menadiol sodium diphosphate/Roche) Injectable, a synthetic water-soluble derivative of menadione (vitamin K_3), is a sterile aqueous solution intended for intramuscular, intravenous or subcutaneous administration. Synkayvite Injectable is available in the following concentrations:

1-ml Ampuls, 5 mg/ml—each ml contains 5 mg menadiol sodium diphosphate compounded with 2.5 mg sodium metabisulfite, 0.45% phenol as preservative, 0.4% sodium chloride for isotonicity and sodium hydroxide to adjust pH to approximately 8.0.

1-ml Ampuls, 10 mg/ml—each ml contains 10 mg menadiol sodium diphosphate compounded with 2.5 mg sodium metabisulfite, 0.45% phenol as preservative, 0.4% sodium chloride for isotonicity and sodium hydroxide to adjust pH to approximately 8.0.

2-ml Ampuls, 75 mg/2 ml—each 2 ml contains 75 mg menadiol sodium diphosphate compounded with 5 mg sodium metabisulfite, 0.45% phenol as preservative, 0.4% sodium chloride for isotonicity and sodium hydroxide to adjust pH to approximately 8.0.

Chemically, menadiol sodium diphosphate is 2-methyl-1,4-naphthalenediol bis (dihydrogen phosphate) tetrasodium salt, hexahydrate. It is a white to pink hygroscopic powder with a characteristic odor and is very soluble in water and insoluble in alcohol. It has a molecular weight of 530.18.

Clinical Pharmacology: Synkayvite is converted *in vivo* to menadione (vitamin K_3). Its potency is approximately one-half that of menadione. Synkayvite is similar in activity to naturally occurring vitamin K, which is necessary for the synthesis in the liver of blood coagulation factors prothrombin (factor II), proconvertin (factor VII), thromboplastin (factor IX) and Stuart factor (factor X). The prothrombin test is sensitive to the concentrations of factors II, VII and X. The mechanism by which vitamin K_1 promotes formation of these clotting factors is not known, but animal data suggest that it acts as an enzyme or catalyst upon a substrate within the liver or combines with an apoenzyme (AE) to form an active enzyme (AE-K) which then is involved in prothrombin synthesis.

Pharmacokinetic data are unavailable because there is no acceptable assay procedure for the determination of menadiol in biological specimens. The physiochemical properties of menadiol sodium diphosphate indicate a negligible potential for absorption problems. The action of menadiol sodium diphosphate is generally detectable within one to two hours following parenteral administration; the prothrombin time often returns to normal in 8 to 24 hours. Vitamin K appears to pass through the placenta.

Indications and Usage: Synkayvite Injectable is indicated for the treatment of hypoprothrombinemia secondary to factors limiting absorption or synthesis of vitamin K, *e.g.*, obstructive jaundice, biliary fistula, sprue, ulcerative colitis, celiac disease, intestinal resection, cystic fibrosis of the pancreas, regional enteritis and antibacterial therapy. It is also indicated in hypoprothrombinemia secondary to administration of salicylates.

Synkayvite Injectable may also be used as a liver function test, although newer methods are available.

Contraindications: Vitamin K, or any of its synthetic analogs, should not be administered to the mother during the *last few weeks of pregnancy* as a prophylactic measure against physiologic hypoprothrombinemia or hemorrhagic disease of the newborn.

Synkayvite is contraindicated in patients with known hypersensitivity to the drug.

Warnings: Synkayvite Injectable should not be used in the prophylaxis and treatment of hemorrhagic disease of the newborn, because phytonadione/Roche (Konakion®) is safer than the water-soluble vitamin K analogs.

Synkayvite and other water-soluble vitamin K analogs are ineffective in the treatment of oral anticoagulant-induced hypoprothrombinemia and, therefore, should not be used in its treatment. Synkayvite will not counteract the anticoagulant action of heparin.

Precautions: *General:* Temporary resistance to prothrombin-depressing anticoagulants may result, especially when larger doses of Synkayvite are used. If relatively large doses have been employed, it may be necessary when reinstituting anticoagulant therapy to use somewhat larger doses of prothrombin-depressing anticoagulant or one which has a different mode of action, such as heparin.

Since the liver is the site of metabolic synthesis of prothrombin, hypoprothrombinemia resulting from hepatocellular damage is not corrected by administration of vitamin K. Repeated large doses of vitamin K are not warranted in liver disease if the response to initial use of the vitamin is unsatisfactory (Koller test).

Failure to respond to vitamin K may indicate that a coagulation defect is present or that the condition being treated is unresponsive to vitamin K.

Laboratory Tests: The dose, route and frequency of administration and duration of treatment depend on the severity of the prothrombin deficiency and should be regulated by repeated determinations of prothrombin time.

Drug Interactions: Patients being treated with coumarin and indandione derivative anticoagulants are extremely sensitive to changes in available vitamin K. Therefore, large doses of menadione or menadiol sodium diphosphate may decrease patient sensitivity to oral anticoagulants, although these vitamin K analogs are ineffective in treating anticoagulant overdosage.

Drug/Laboratory Test Interactions: Menadione has been reported to interfere with the modified Reedy, Jenkins, Thorn procedure for determining urinary 17-hydroxycorticosteroids, producing falsely elevated levels.

Carcinogenesis, Mutagenesis and Impairment of Fertility: Synkayvite has not undergone adequate animal testing to evaluate carcinogenic potential. The mutagenicity of Synkayvite has not been evaluated in the Ames test. Synkayvite has not been evaluated for effects on fertility.

Pregnancy: Teratogenic Effects: Pregnancy Category C. Segment II reproduction studies have not been conducted with menadiol. However, menadione (vitamin K_3) was nonteratogenic in rats at doses of 15 and 150 mg/day. The 150 mg/day dose in rats is approximately 872 times the maximum human therapeutic dose of 30 mg daily for the treatment of hypoprothrombinemia and 350 times the human dose of 75 mg for the liver function test. It is not known whether Synkayvite can cause fetal harm when administered to a pregnant woman or can affect reproductive capacity. Synkayvite should be given to a pregnant woman only if clearly needed.

Nonteratogenic effects: Retardation of skeletal ossification and an increase in fetal resorptions have been reported in rats with menadione (vitamin K_3).

Menadione and its derivatives have been implicated in producing hemolytic anemia, hyperbilirubinemia and kernicterus in the newborn, especially in premature infants, when administered to the mother prior to delivery or to the newborn. A marked hyperbilirubinemia has been reported in premature infants of mothers given menadione 2 to 112 hours prior to delivery. Synkayvite given parenterally during labor caused an elevation in prothrombin levels in 16 of 22 infants. (Also see **Contraindications** section.)

Nursing Mothers: A study has shown that vitamin K is excreted in human milk. This should be considered if it is necessary to administer Synkayvite to a nursing mother.

Pediatric Use: See **Warnings** section.

Adverse Reactions: In adults, bromsulfalein retention and prolongation of prothrombin time have been reported after maximum doses of vitamin K analogs. In infants (particularly premature babies), excessive doses of vitamin K analogs may cause increased bilirubinemia in the first few days of life. This, in turn, may result in kernicterus, which may lead to brain damage or even death. Immaturity is apparently an important factor in the appearance of toxic reactions to vitamin K analogs as full-term and larger premature infants demonstrate greater tolerance than smaller premature infants. (Also see **Warnings** section.)

Menadione can induce erythrocyte hemolysis in persons having a genetic deficiency of glucose-6-phosphate dehydrogenase in their red blood cells.

In patients with severe hepatic disease, large doses of menadione may further depress liver function. Paradoxically, the administration of excessive doses of vitamin K or its analogs in an attempt to correct the hypoprothrombinemia associated with severe hepatitis or cirrhosis may actually result in a further depression of the concentration of prothrombin. (Also see **Precautions**, *General*, section.)

Occasional allergic reactions, such as skin rash and urticaria, have been reported.

Overdosage: There are no data available on overdosage of Synkayvite in man. The administration of large doses of menadione and its derivatives to animals has resulted in the production of anemia, polycythemia, splenomegaly, renal and hepatic damage and death.

The acute intravenous toxicity of Synkayvite is as follows:

	$LD_{50} \pm S.D.$
Mouse	500 ± 55 mg/kg
Rat	400 ± 65 mg/kg

Dosage and Administration: The U.S. Recommended Daily Allowances for vitamin K in humans have not been established officially. The adequate daily dietary intake of vitamin K for adults has been estimated to be 70 to 140 mcg; for infants 10 to 20 mcg; for children and adolescents 15 to 100 mcg. The dietary abundance of vitamin K normally satisfies the requirements except for the neonatal period of 5 to 8 days.

Synkayvite may be injected subcutaneously, intramuscularly or intravenously. The response after intravenous administration may be more prompt, but more sustained action follows intramuscular or subcutaneous use.

Duration of treatment and frequency of dosage should be governed by blood prothrombin-time determination. In the absence of impaired liver function, a single dose usually corrects hypoprothrombinemia in 8 to 24 hours. Injections should be repeated in 12 hours if tests at this time show no evidence of improvement.

Following are the usual recommended dosages:

	ADULTS	CHILDREN
For treatment of hypoprothrombinemia	5 to 15 mg once or twice daily	5 to 10 mg once or twice daily
For liver function test	75 mg intravenously	

Parenteral drug products should be inspected visually for particulate matter and discoloration prior to administration, whenever solution and container permit. Synkayvite Injectable is incompatible with protein hydrolysate.

How Supplied: *1-ml Ampuls* (5 mg menadiol sodium diphosphate/ml)—boxes of 10 (NDC 0004-1923-06).

1-ml Ampuls (10 mg menadiol sodium diphosphate/ml)—boxes of 10 (NDC 0004-1924-06).

2-ml Ampuls (75 mg menadiol sodium diphosphate/2 ml)—boxes of 10 (NDC 0004-1925-06).

Store at room temperature (15° to 30°C or 59° to 86°F).

Synkayvite need not be refrigerated.

SYNKAYVITE®
(menadiol sodium diphosphate/Roche) ℞
TABLETS

The following text is complete product information based on official labeling in effect August 1, 1984.

Description: Synkayvite (menadiol diphosphate/Roche), a synthetic, water-soluble derivative of menadione (vitamin K$_3$), is available for oral administration in 5-mg tablets. Chemically, it is 2-methyl-1,4-naphthalenediol bis (dihydrogen phosphate) tetrasodium salt, hexahydrate. It is a white to pink hygroscopic powder with a characteristic odor and is very soluble in water and insoluble in alcohol. It has a molecular weight of 530.18.

Clinical Pharmacology: Synkayvite is converted *in vivo* to menadione (vitamin K$_3$). Its potency is approximately one-half that of menadione. Synkayvite is similar in activity to naturally occurring vitamin K, which is necessary for the synthesis in the liver of blood coagulation factors prothrombin (factor II), proconvertin (factor VII), thromboplastin (factor IX) and Stuart factor (factor X). The prothrombin test is sensitive to the concentrations of factors II, VII and X. The mechanism by which vitamin K$_1$ promotes formation of these clotting factors is not known, but animal data suggest that it acts as an enzyme or catalyst upon a substrate within the liver or combines with an apoenzyme (AE) to form an active enzyme (AE-K) which then is involved in prothrombin synthesis.

Pharmacokinetic data are unavailable because there is no acceptable assay procedure for the determination of menadiol in biological specimens. The physiochemical properties of menadiol sodium diphosphate indicate a negligible potential for absorption problems. The onset and duration of action following oral administration are not known. Vitamin K appears to pass through the placenta.

Indications and Usage: Synkayvite Tablets are indicated for:
— vitamin K deficiency secondary to the administration of antibacterial therapy;
— hypoprothrombinemia secondary to obstructive jaundice and biliary fistulas;
— hypoprothrombinemia secondary to administration of salicylates.

Contraindications: Vitamin K, or any of its synthetic analogs, should not be administered to the mother *during the last few weeks of pregnancy* as a prophylactic measure against physiologic hypoprothrombinemia or hemorrhagic disease of the newborn.

Synkayvite is contraindicated in patients with known hypersensitivity to the drug.

Warnings: Synkayvite and other water-soluble vitamin K analogs are ineffective in the treatment of oral anticoagulant-induced hypoprothrombinemia and should, therefore, not be used in its treatment. Synkayvite will not counteract the anticoagulant action of heparin.

Precautions: *General:* Temporary resistance to prothrombin-depressing anticoagulants may result, especially when larger doses of Synkayvite are used. If relatively large doses have been employed, it may be necessary when reinstituting anticoagulant therapy to use somewhat larger doses of the prothrombin-depressing anticoagulant or one which has a different mode of action, such as heparin.

Since the liver is the site of metabolic synthesis of prothrombin, hypoprothrombinemia resulting from hepatocellular damage is not corrected by administration of vitamin K. Repeated large doses of vitamin K are not warranted in liver disease if the response to initial use of the vitamin is unsatisfactory (Koller test).

Failure to respond to vitamin K may indicate that a coagulation defect is present or that the condition being treated is unresponsive to vitamin K.

Information for Patients: To assure safe and effective use of this drug, the following information and instructions should be given to the patient:
1. Take this medication exactly as directed by your doctor. Do not increase or decrease the prescribed dosage, or take it more often, or take it for a longer period of time than instructed.
2. If you miss a dose, take it as soon as possible, and then continue with your normal dosing schedule. Do not take the missed dose if it is almost time for your next dose; continue on your normal schedule and inform your doctor about any doses that you miss. If you have any questions about this, ask your doctor or pharmacist.
3. Inform all doctors and pharmacists that you are taking this medication; other medicines may affect the way this medicine works.
4. Before starting or stopping any other medications, including nonprescription drugs such as aspirin, check with your doctor or pharmacist.
5. A blood test should be performed at regular intervals to determine how this medicine is working. This will help your doctor decide the best dosing schedule for you.
6. Inform your doctor if you are pregnant or become pregnant while using this drug, even though vitamin K has not been shown to cause birth defects or other problems. Also inform your doctor if you are nursing.

Laboratory Tests: The dose, route and frequency of administration and duration of treatment depend on the severity of the prothrombin deficiency and should be regulated by repeated determinations of prothrombin time.

Drug Interactions: Patients being treated with coumarin and indandione derviative anticoagulants are extremely sensitive to changes in available vitamin K. Therefore, large doses of menadione or menadiol sodium diphosphate may decrease patient sensitivity to oral anticoagulants, although these vitamin K analogs are ineffective in treating anticoagulant overdosage.

Drug/Laboratory Test Interactions: Menadione has been reported to interfere with the modified Reddy, Jenkins, Thorn procedure for determining urinary 17-hydroxycorticosteroids, producing falsely elevated levels.

Carcinogenesis, Mutagenesis and Impairment of Fertility: Synkayvite has not undergone adequate animal testing to evaluate carcinogenic potential. The mutagenicity of Synkayvite has not been evaluated in the Ames test. Synkayvite has not been evaluated for effects on fertility.

Pregnancy: Teratogenic Effects: Pregnancy Category C. Segment II reproduction studies have not been conducted with menadiol. However, menadione (vitamin K$_3$) was nonteratogenic in rats at doses of 15 and 150 mg/day. The 150 mg/day dose in rats is approximately 2640 times the maximum human therapeutic dose of 10 mg daily. It is not known whether Synkayvite can cause fetal harm when administered to a pregnant woman or can affect reproductive capacity. Synkayvite should be given to a pregnant woman only if clearly needed. Nonteratogenic Effects: Retardation of skeletal ossification and an increase in fetal resorptions have been reported in rats with menadione (vitamin K$_3$).

Menadione and its derivatives have been implicated in producing hemolytic anemia, hyperbilirubinemia and kernicterus in the newborn, especially in premature infants, when administered to the mother prior to delivery or to the newborn. A marked hyperbilirubinemia has been reported in premature infants of mothers given menadione 2 to 112 hours prior to delivery. Synkayvite given parenterally during labor caused an elevation in prothrombin levels in 16 of 22 infants. (Also see **Contraindications** section.)

Nursing Mothers: A study has shown that vitamin K is excreted in human milk. This should be considered if it is necessary to administer Synkayvite to a nursing mother.

Adverse Reactions: Bromsulfalein retention and prolongation of prothrombin time have been reported after maximum doses of vitamin K analogs.

Menadione can induce erythrocyte hemolysis in persons having a genetic deficiency of glucose-6-phosphate dehydrogenase in their red blood cells.

In patients with severe hepatic disease, large doses of menadione may further depress liver function. Paradoxically, the administration of excessive doses of vitamin K or its analogs in an attempt to correct the hypoprothrombinemia associated with severe hepatitis or cirrhosis may actually result in a further depression of the concentration of prothrombin. (Also see **Precautions**, *General*, section.)

Occasional allergic reactions, such as skin rash and urticaria, have been reported. There have also been minor instances of gastric disturbance.

Overdosage: There are no data on overdosage of Synkayvite in man. The administration of large doses of menadione and its derivatives to animals has resulted in the production of anemia, polycythemia, splenomegaly, renal and hepatic damage and death.

The acute oral toxicity of Synkayvite is as follows:

	LD$_{50}$ ± S.D.
Mouse	6172 ± 966 mg/kg
Rat	5250 ± 740 mg/kg

Dosage and Administration: The U.S. Recommended Daily Allowances for vitamin K in humans have not been established officially. The adequate daily dietary intake of vitamin K for adults has been estimated to be 70 to 140 mcg. The dietary abundance of vitamin K normally satisfies these requirements.

Following are the usual recommended dosages:

For hypoprothrombinemia secondary to obstructive jaundice and biliary fistulas	5 mg daily
For hypoprothrombinemia secondary to the administration of antibacterials or salicylates	5 to 10 mg daily

How Supplied: White tablets containing 5 mg menadiol sodium diphosphate—bottls of 100 (NDC 0004-0037-01). Imprint on tablets: ROCHE 37.

Note: Slight pink discoloration of tablets does not affect the safety and efficacy of Synkayvite. Store at room temperature (15° to 30° C or 59° to 86° F).

Shown in Product Identification Section, page 430

TARACTAN® TABLETS ℞
[*tar-ac'tan*]
(chlorprothixene/Roche)
TARACTAN® CONCENTRATE ℞
(chlorprothixene lactate and HCl/Roche)
TARACTAN® AMPULS ℞
(chlorprothixene HCl/Roche)

The following text is complete prescribing information based on official labeling in effect August 1, 1984.

Description: Tablets—each containing 10 mg, 25 mg, 50 mg or 100 mg chlorprothixene. Concentrate—100 mg/5 ml as the lactate and hydrochloride, fruit flavored. Ampuls—25 mg/2 ml as the hydrochloride, with 0.2% parabens (methyl and propyl) added as preservatives and pH adjusted to approximately 3.4 with HCl.

Taractan is a thioxanthene derivative. Chemically, it is the alpha isomer of 2-chloro-*N,N*-dimethylthioxanthene-Δ^9, γ-propylamine. In chemical structure chlorprothixene resembles the phenothiazines; however, in place of the nitrogen (N) in the phenothiazine ring, chlorprothixene carries a carbon atom with a double bond to a side chain.

Actions: EEG changes following the injection of Taractan into cats suggest that it acts on the brain stem. Effects demonstrated were the synchronization of the EEG tracings during rest, a shortening of cortical activation obtained by stimulation of the reticular formation, and modifications of elicited potentials.

Indications: Taractan is indicated for the management of manifestations of psychotic disorders. Taractan has not been shown effective in the management of behavioral complications in patients with mental retardation.

Contraindications: Circulatory collapse, comatose states due to central depressant drugs (alcohol, hypnotics, opiates, etc.) and known sensitivity to the drug are contraindications.

Warnings: *Usage in Pregnancy:* The safety of Taractan during pregnancy or lactation in humans has not been established. Therefore, use of Taractan in women who may become pregnant requires weighing the drug's potential benefits against its possible hazards to mother and child. For the results of reproductive and teratogenic

Continued on next page

Roche Labs.—Cont.

studies in rats and rabbits see ANIMAL PHARMACOLOGY AND TOXICOLOGY.

This drug may impair the mental and/or physical abilities required for the performance of hazardous tasks such as operating machinery or driving a motor vehicle; therefore, the patient should be cautioned accordingly.

As in the case of other CNS-acting drugs, patients receiving Taractan should be cautioned about possible combined effects with alcohol.

The safety and efficacy of Taractan have not been established for oral administration in children under age 6 or for parenteral use in those under age 12.

Precautions: Because of its structural similarity to the phenothiazines, all of the precautions associated with phenothiazine therapy should be considered when patients receive Taractan. Therefore, Taractan should be used with caution in patients who:

— are receiving barbiturates or narcotics, because of additive effects of central nervous system depressants. The dosage of the narcotic or barbiturate should be reduced when given concomitantly with Taractan.
— are receiving atropine or related drugs, because of additive anticholinergic effects.
— have a history of epilepsy. When necessary, Taractan may be used concomitantly with anticonvulsant drugs. However, use of Taractan may lower the convulsive threshold; therefore, an adequate dosage of the anticonvulsant should be maintained.
— are exposed to extreme heat or phosphorous insecticides.
— have cardiovascular disease.
— have respiratory impairment due to acute pulmonary infections or chronic respiratory disorders such as severe asthma or emphysema.

The concurrent use of Taractan and electroshock treatment should be reserved for those patients for whom it is essential, but the hazards may be increased.

Taractan may augment or interfere with the absorption, metabolism or therapeutic activity of other psychotropic drugs and vice versa.

The appearance of signs of blood dyscrasias requires immediate discontinuance of the drug and the institution of appropriate therapy.

The possibility of liver damage, variations in thyroid function, pigmentary retinopathy, lenticular or corneal deposits and development of irreversible dyskinesias should be kept in mind when patients are on prolonged therapy.

When used in the treatment of agitated states accompanying depression, the usual precautions indicated with such patients are necessary, particularly the recognition that a suicidal tendency may be present and protective measures necessary.

Taractan tablets contain FD&C Yellow No. 5 (tartrazine) which may cause allergic-type reactions (including bronchial asthma) in certain susceptible individuals. Although the overall incidence of FD&C Yellow No. 5 (tartrazine) sensitivity in the general population is low, it is frequently seen in patients who also have aspirin hypersensitivity.

Abrupt Withdrawal: Taractan is not known to produce physical dependence. However, gastritis, nausea and vomiting, dizziness and tremulousness have been reported following abrupt cessation of high-dose therapy.

Neuroleptic drugs elevate prolactin levels; the elevation persists during chronic administration. Tissue culture experiments indicate that approximately one-third of human breast cancers are prolactin-dependent *in vitro,* a factor of potential importance if the prescription of these drugs is contemplated in a patient with a previously detected breast cancer. Although disturbances such as galactorrhea, amenorrhea, gynecomastia and impotence have been reported, the clinical significance of elevated serum prolactin levels is unknown for most patients. An increase in mammary neoplasms has been found in rodents after chronic administration of neuroleptic drugs. Neither clinical studies nor epidemiologic studies conducted to date, however, have shown an association between chronic administration of these drugs and mammary tumorigenesis; the available evidence is considered too limited to be conclusive at this time.

Adverse Reactions: Not all of the following adverse reactions have been reported with Taractan; however, pharmacological similarities to the various phenothiazine derivatives require that each be considered.

Note: *Sudden death* has occasionally been reported in patients who have received phenothiazines. In some cases death was apparently due to cardiac arrest, in others the cause appeared to be asphyxia due to failure of the cough reflex. In some patients the cause could not be determined nor could it be established that death was due to the phenothiazine.

Drowsiness: May occur particularly during the first or second week, after which it generally disappears. If troublesome, dosage may be lowered.
Jaundice: Incidence is low. It usually occurs between the second and fourth weeks and is regarded as a sensitivity reaction. The clinical picture resembles infectious hepatitis with laboratory features of obstructive jaundice. It is usually reversible; however, chronic jaundice has been reported.
Hematological Disorders: Agranulocytosis, eosinophilia, leukopenia, hemolytic anemia, thrombocytopenic purpura and pancytopenia.
Agranulocytosis: Most cases have occurred between the fourth and tenth weeks of therapy. Patients should be watched closely during that period for the sudden appearance of sore throat or other signs of infection. If white blood count and differential show significant cellular depression, discontinue the drug and start appropriate therapy. However, a slightly lowered white count is not in itself an indication to discontinue the drug.
Cardiovascular: Postural hypotension, tachycardia (especially with sudden marked increase in dosage), bradycardia, cardiac arrest, faintness and dizziness. Occasionally the hypotensive effect may produce a shock-like condition. In the event a vasoconstrictor is required, levarterenol and phenylephrine are the most suitable. Other pressor agents, including epinephrine, should not be used, as a paradoxical further lowering of the blood pressure may ensue.
ECG changes, nonspecific, usually reversible, have been observed in some patients receiving phenothiazine tranquilizers. Their relationship to myocardial damage has not been confirmed.
CNS Effects: Neuromuscular (Extrapyramidal) Reactions: These are usually dosage-related and take three forms: (1) pseudoparkinsonism, (2) akathisia (motor restlessness) and (3) dystonias. Dystonias include spasms of the neck muscles, extensor rigidity of back muscles, carpopedal spasm, eyes rolled back, convulsions, trismus and swallowing difficulties. These resemble serious neurological disorders but usually subside within 48 hours. Management of the extrapyramidal symptoms, depending upon the type and severity, includes sedation, injectable diphenhydramine and the use of antiparkinsonism agents. In rare instances, persistent dyskinesias usually involving the face, tongue and jaw have been reported to last months, even years, particularly in elderly patients with previous brain damage.
Hyperreflexia has been reported in the newborn when a phenothiazine was used during pregnancy.
Adverse Behavioral Effects: Paradoxical exacerbation of psychotic symptoms.
Other CNS Effects: Cerebral edema. Abnormality of cerebrospinal fluid proteins. Convulsive seizures, particularly in patients with EEG abnormalities or a history of such disorders. Hyperpyrexia.
Allergic Reactions: Urticaria, itching, erythema, photosensitivity (avoid undue exposure to the sun), eczema. Severe reactions including exfoliative dermatitis (rare); contact dermatitis in nursing personnel administering the drug; asthma, laryngeal edema, angioneurotic edema, anaphylactoid reactions.
Endocrine Disorders: Lactation and moderate breast engorgement in females and gynecomastia in males on large doses, changes in libido, false-positive pregnancy tests, amenorrhea, hyperglycemia, hypoglycemia, glycosuria.
Autonomic Reactions: Dry mouth, nasal congestion, constipation, adynamic ileus, myosis, mydriasis, urinary retention.
Special Considerations in Long-Term Therapy: After prolonged administration of high doses, pigmentation of the skin has occurred chiefly in the exposed areas, especially in females on large doses. Ocular changes consisting of deposition of fine particulate matter in the cornea and lens, progressing in more severe cases to star-shaped lenticular opacities; epithelial keratopathies; pigmentary retinopathy.
Persistent Tardive Dyskinesia: As with all antipsychotic agents, tardive dyskinesia may appear in some patients on long-term therapy or may occur after drug therapy has been discontinued. The risk seems to be greater in elderly patients on high-dose therapy, especially females. The symptoms are persistent and in some patients appear to be irreversible. The syndrome is characterized by rhythmical involuntary movements of the tongue, face, mouth, or jaw (*e.g.,* protrusion of tongue, puffing of cheeks, puckering of mouth, chewing movements). Sometimes these may be accompanied by involuntary movements of extremities.
There is no known effective treatment for tardive dyskinesia; antiparkinsonism agents usually do not alleviate the symptoms of this syndrome. It is suggested that all antipsychotic agents be discontinued if these symptoms appear. Should it be necessary to reinstitute treatment, or increase the dosage of the agent, or switch to a different antipsychotic agent, the syndrome may be masked.
It has been reported that fine vermicular movements of the tongue may be an early sign of the syndrome and if the medication is stopped at that time the syndrome may not develop.
Other Adverse Reactions: Enlargement of the parotid gland; increases in appetite and weight; peripheral edema.
The occurrence of a systemic lupus erythematosus-like syndrome has been related to phenothiazine therapy.

Dosage and Administration: Dosage should be individually adjusted according to diagnosis and severity of the condition. In general, small doses should be used initially, and increased to the optimal effective level as rapidly as possible based on therapeutic response. When higher dosage is required, greater sedation may be encountered; therefore, patients should be closely supervised. Lethargy and drowsiness are readily controlled by dosage reduction. Initially, lower doses (10 to 25 mg three or four times daily) should be used for elderly or debilitated patients.
For convenience in prescribing and dispensing, all recommended dosages are expressed as strengths of the active moiety, chlorprothixene.
Taractan may be administered orally as tablets or concentrate. The concentrate, containing 100 mg of the drug per 5 ml teaspoonful, is pleasantly flavored and may be administered alone or in milk, water, fruit juices, coffee and carbonated beverages.

	Average Daily Dose
Oral	
Adults:	Initially, 25 to 50 mg three or four times daily; to be increased as needed. Dosages exceeding 600 mg daily are rarely required.
Children (over 6 years of age):	10 to 25 mg three or four times daily.
Parenteral	
Not to be used in children under the age of 12.	25 to 50 mg I.M. up to three or four times daily.

Pain or induration at the site of injection is minimal. Since postural hypotension may occur in some patients, injection should be given with the patient seated or recumbent. If hypotension does occur, recovery is usually spontaneous; however, the patient should be observed until symptoms of weakness or dizziness pass.

As soon as the acutely agitated patient is brought under control, oral medication should be instituted. The changeover should be made gradually, with oral and parenteral doses being given alternately on the same day, then oral doses only, adjusted to the required maintenance level.

Overdosage: Taractan can be fatal in overdosage in the range of 2.5 to 4 Gm or above. Manifestations of overdosage are drowsiness, coma, respiratory depression, hypotension (which may appear after a delay of several hours and may persist for two to three days), tachycardia, pyrexia and constricted pupils. Convulsions, hyperactivity and hematuria may be seen in the recovery period. Treatment is essentially symptomatic. Early gastric lavage is recommended, along with supportive measures such as I.V. fluids and the maintenance of an adequate airway. Severe hypotension usually responds to the use of levarterenol or metaraminol. Should coma be prolonged, caffeine and sodium benzoate, or ethamivan may be used, but the possibility must be borne in mind that these may lead to a convulsive episode. Should convulsions occur, the judicious use of sodium amytal is recommended. **Epinephrine must not be used in these patients.**

How Supplied: Tablets—10 mg, chlorprothixine — bottles of 100; 25 mg, 50 mg or 100 mg chlorprothixene—bottles of 100 and 500.

Concentrate—containing, in each teaspoonful, chlorprothixene 100 mg base (as the lactate and hydrochloride)—bottles of 16 fluid ounces (1 pint). Ampuls—containing chlorprothixene 25 mg/2 ml as the hydrochloride—boxes of 10.

Animal Pharmacology and Toxicology: In mice, the oral LD_{50} of the two oral dosage forms of chlorprothixene were 350 ± 27 mg/kg (as the 2 per cent concentrate) and 220 ± 24 mg/kg (as the tablet form ground and suspended in 5 per cent gum acacia). For the injectable form the intramuscular LD_{50} in mice was greater than 125 mg/kg.

Reproduction Studies: Reproductive and teratological studies in rats and rabbits were performed at levels of 12 and 24 mg/kg. In the rats, a decreased conception rate and an increased incidence of stillborns was noted at both levels. An increased number of resorptions was noted only at the high dose level. There was a decrease in the number of implantation sites at both doses. The number of live fetuses per litter and the mean fetal body weights were reduced slightly at 12 mg/kg and more so at 24 mg/kg. No teratological effects were observed. No deleterious effects on reproduction were seen in rabbits nor were any teratological findings noted.

Shown in Product Identification Section, page 430

TEL-E-DOSE®

Tel-E-Dose is a unit package designed by Roche for convenience in dispensing medications in the hospital and nursing home. Each unit, sealed against contamination and moisture, is clearly identified by product name and strength and carries the control number and expiration date.

Currently available in this package form are the following products: Bactrim™ (80 mg trimethoprim and 400 mg sulfamethoxazole) tablets; Bactrim™ DS (160 mg trimethoprim and 800 mg sulfamethoxazole) tablets; Bumex® (bumetanide HCl) tablets, 0.5 mg, 1 mg; Gantanol® (sulfamethoxazole) tablets, 0.5 Gm; Gantrisin® (sulfisoxazole) tablets, 0.5 Gm; Trimpex® (trimethoprim) tablets, 100 mg.

Shown in Product Identification Section, page 430

TENSILON® ℞
[ten'sil-on]
(edrophonium chloride/Roche)
Injectable Solution
ampuls • vials

The following text is complete prescribing information based on official labeling in effect August 1, 1984.

Description: Tensilon is a short and rapid-acting cholinergic drug. Chemically, edrophonium chloride is ethyl (*m*-hydroxyphenyl)dimethylammonium chloride.

10-ml vials: Each ml contains, in a sterile solution, 10 mg edrophonium chloride/Roche compounded with 0.45% phenol and 0.2% sodium sulfite as preservatives, buffered with sodium citrate and citric acid, and pH adjusted to approximately 5.4.

1-ml ampuls: Each ml contains, in a sterile solution, 10 mg edrophonium chloride/Roche compounded with 0.2% sodium sulfite, buffered with sodium citrate and citric acid, and pH adjusted to approximately 5.4.

Actions: Tensilon is an anticholinesterase drug. Its pharmacological action is due primarily to the inhibition or inactivation of acetylcholinesterase at sites of cholinergic transmission. Its effect is manifest within 30 to 60 seconds after injection and lasts an average of 10 minutes.

Indications: Tensilon is recommended for the differential diagnosis of myasthenia gravis and as an adjunct in the evaluation of treatment requirements in this disease. It may also be used for evaluating emergency treatment in myasthenic crises. Because of its brief duration of action, it is not recommended for maintenance therapy in myasthenia gravis.

Tensilon is also useful whenever a curare antagonist is needed to reverse the neuromuscular block produced by curare, tubocurarine, gallamine triethiodide or dimethyl-tubocurarine. It is *not* effective against decamethonium bromide and succinylcholine chloride. It may be used adjunctively in the treatment of respiratory depression caused by curare overdosage.

Contraindications: Known hypersensitivity to anticholinesterase agents; intestinal and urinary obstructions of mechanical type.

Warnings: Whenever anticholinesterase drugs are used for testing, a syringe containing 1 mg of atropine sulfate should be immediately available to be given in aliquots intravenously to counteract severe cholinergic reactions which may occur in the hypersensitive individual, whether he is normal or myasthenic. Tensilon should be used with caution in patients with bronchial asthma or cardiac dysrhythmias. The transient bradycardia which sometimes occurs can be relieved by atropine sulfate. Isolated instances of cardiac and respiratory arrest following administration of Tensilon have been reported. It is postulated that these are vagotonic effects.

Usage in Pregnancy: The safety of Tensilon during pregnancy or lactation in humans has not been established. Therefore, use of Tensilon in women who may become pregnant requires weighing the drug's potential benefits against its possible hazards to mother and child.

Precautions: Patients may develop "anticholinesterase insensitivity" for brief or prolonged periods. During these periods the patients should be carefully monitored and may need respiratory assistance. Dosages of anticholinesterase drugs should be reduced or withheld until patients again become sensitive to them.

Adverse Reactions: Careful observation should be made for severe cholinergic reactions in the hyperreactive individual. The myasthenic patient in crisis who is being tested with Tensilon should be observed for bradycardia or cardiac standstill and cholinergic reactions if an overdose is given. The following reactions common to anticholinesterase agents may occur, although not all of these reactions have been reported with the administration of Tensilon, probably because of its short duration of action and limited indications: **Eye:** Increased lacrimation, pupillary constriction, spasm of accommodation, diplopia, conjunctival hyperemia. **CNS:** Convulsions, dysarthria, dysphonia, dysphagia. **Respiratory:** Increased tracheobronchial secretions, laryngospasm, bronchiolar constriction, paralysis of muscles of respiration, central respiratory paralysis. **Cardiac:** Arrhythmias (especially bradycardia), fall in cardiac output leading to hypotension. **G.I.:** Increased salivary, gastric and intestinal secretion, nausea, vomiting, increased peristalsis, diarrhea, abdominal cramps. **Skeletal Muscle:** Weakness, fasciculations. **Miscellaneous:** Increased urinary frequency and incontinence, diaphoresis.

Dosage and Administration: *Tensilon Test in the Differential Diagnosis of Myasthenia Gravis:*[1-8] *Intravenous Dosage (Adults):* A tuberculin syringe containing 1 ml (10 mg) of Tensilon is prepared with an intravenous needle, and 0.2 ml (2 mg) is injected intravenously within 15 to 30 seconds. The needle is left *in situ. Only* if no reaction occurs after 45 seconds is the remaining 0.8 ml (8 mg) injected. If a cholinergic reaction (muscarinic side effects, skeletal muscle fasciculations and increased muscle weakness) occurs after injection of 0.2 ml (2 mg), the test is discontinued and atropine sulfate 0.4 mg to 0.5 mg is administered intravenously. After one-half hour the test may be repeated.

Intramuscular Dosage (Adults): In adults with inaccessible veins, dosage for intramuscular injection is 1 ml (10 mg) of Tensilon. Subjects who demonstrate hyperreactivity to this injection (cholinergic reaction), should be retested after one-half hour with 0.2 ml (2 mg) of Tensilon intramuscularly to rule out false-negative reactions.

Dosage (Children): The intravenous testing dose of Tensilon in children weighing up to 75 lbs is 0.1 ml (1 mg); above this weight, the dose is 0.2 ml (2 mg). If there is no response after 45 seconds, it may be titrated up to 0.5 ml (5 mg) in children under 75 lbs, given in increments of 0.1 ml (1 mg) every 30 to 45 seconds and up to 1 ml (10 mg) in heavier children. In infants, the recommended dose is 0.05 ml (0.5 mg). Because of technical difficulty with intravenous injection in children, the intramuscular route may be used. In children weighing up to 75 lbs, 0.2 ml (2 mg) is injected intramuscularly. In children weighing more than 75 lbs, 0.5 ml (5 mg) is injected intramuscularly. All signs which would appear with the intravenous test appear with the intramuscular test except that there is a delay of two to ten minutes before a reaction is noted.

Tensilon Test for Evaluation of Treatment Requirements in Myasthenia Gravis: The recommended dose is 0.1 ml to 0.2 ml (1 mg to 2 mg) of Tensilon, administered intravenously one hour after oral intake of the drug being used in treatment.[1-5] Response will be myasthenic in the undertreated patient, adequate in the controlled patient, and cholinergic in the overtreated patient. Responses to Tensilon in myasthenic and nonmyasthenic individuals are summarized in the accompanying chart.[2]

[See table on bottom next page].

Tensilon Test in Crisis: The term *crisis* is applied to the myasthenic whenever severe respiratory distress with objective ventilatory inadequacy occurs and the response to medication is not predictable. This state may be secondary to a sudden increase in severity of myasthenia gravis (myasthenic crisis), or to overtreatment with anticholinesterase drugs (cholinergic crisis).

When a patient is apneic, controlled ventilation must be secured immediately in order to avoid cardiac arrest and irreversible central nervous system damage. No attempt is made to test with Tensilon until respiratory exchange is adequate. *Dosage used at this time is most important:* If the patient is cholinergic, Tensilon will cause increased oropharyngeal secretions and further weakness in the muscles of respiration. If the crisis is myasthenic, the test clearly improves respiration and the patient can be treated with longer-acting intravenous anticholinesterase medication. When the test is performed, there should not be

Continued on next page

Roche Labs.—Cont.

more than 0.2 ml (2 mg) Tensilon in the syringe. An intravenous dose of 0.1 ml (1 mg) is given initially. The patient's heart action is carefully observed. If, after an interval of one minute, this dose does not further impair the patient, the remaining 0.1 ml (1 mg) can be injected. If no clear improvement of respiration occurs after 0.2 ml (2 mg) dose, it is usually wisest to discontinue all anticholinesterase drug therapy and secure controlled ventilation by tracheostomy with assisted respiration.[5]

For Use as a Curare Antagonist: Tensilon should be administered by intravenous injection in 1 ml (10 mg) doses given slowly over a period of 30 to 45 seconds so that the onset of cholinergic reaction can be detected. This dosage may be repeated whenever necessary. The maximal dose for any one patient should be 4 ml (40 mg). Because of its brief effect, Tensilon should not be given prior to the administration of curare, tubocurarine, gallamine triethiodide or dimethyl-tubocurarine; it should be used at the time when its effect is needed. When given to counteract curare overdosage, the effect of each dose on the respiration should be carefully observed before it is repeated, and assisted ventilation should always be employed.

Drug Interactions: Care should be given when administering this drug to patients with symptoms of myasthenic weakness who are also on anticholinesterase drugs. Since symptoms of anticholinesterase overdose (cholinergic crisis) may mimic underdosage (myasthenic weakness), their condition may be worsened by the use of this drug. (See OVERDOSAGE section for treatment.)

Overdosage: With drugs of this type, muscarine-like symptoms (nausea, vomiting, diarrhea, sweating, increased bronchial and salivary secretions and bradycardia) often appear with overdosage (cholinergic crisis). An important complication that can arise is obstruction of the airway by bronchial secretions. These may be managed with suction (especially if tracheostomy has been performed) and by the use of atropine. Many experts have advocated a wide range of dosages of atropine *(for Tensilon, see atropine dosage below)*, but if there are copious secretions, up to 1.2 mg intravenously may be given initially and repeated every 20 minutes until secretions are controlled. Signs of atropine overdosage such as dry mouth, flush and tachycardia should be avoided as tenacious secretions and bronchial plugs may form. A total dose of atropine of 5 to 10 mg or even more may be required. The following steps should be taken in the management of overdosage of Tensilon:

1. Adequate respiratory exchange should be maintained by assuring an open airway, and the use of assisted respiration augmented by oxygen.
2. Cardiac function should be monitored until complete stabilization has been achieved.
3. Atropine sulfate in doses of 0.4 to 0.5 mg should be administered intravenously. This may be repeated every 3 to 10 minutes. Because of the short duration of action of Tensilon the total dose required will seldom exceed 2 mg.
4. Pralidoxime chloride (a cholinesterase reactivator) may be given intravenously at the rate of 50 to 100 mg per minute; usually the total dose does not exceed 1000 mg. Extreme caution should be exercised in the use of pralidoxime chloride when the cholinergic symptoms are induced by double-bond phosphorous anticholinesterase drugs.[9]
5. If convulsions or shock is present, appropriate measures should be instituted.

How Supplied: *Multiple Dose Vials,* 10 ml, boxes of 10. *Ampuls,* 1 ml, boxes of 10.

References:
1. Osserman, K.E. and Kaplan, L.I., *J.A.M.A., 150:*265, 1952.
2. Osserman, K.E., Kaplan, L.I. and Besson, G., *J. Mt. Sinai Hosp., 20:*165, 1953.
3. Osserman, K.E. and Kaplan, L.I., *Arch. Neurol. & Psychiat., 70:*385, 1953.
4. Osserman, K.E. and Teng, P., *J.A.M.A., 160:*153, 1956.
5. Osserman, K.E. and Genkins, G., *Ann. N.Y. Acad. Sci., 135:*312, 1966.
6. Tether, J.E., Second International Symposium Proceedings, Myasthenia Gravis, 1961, p. 444.
7. Tether, J.E., in H.F. Conn: *Current Therapy 1960,* Philadelphia, W. B. Saunders Company, p. 551.
8. Tether, J.E., in H.F. Conn: *Current Therapy 1965,* Philadelphia, W. B. Saunders Company, p. 556.
9. Grob, D. and Johns, R.J., *J.A.M.A., 166:*1855, 1958.

TRIMPEX® ℞
[*trim'pex*]
(trimethoprim/Roche)
TABLETS

The following text is complete prescribing information based on official labeling in effect August 1, 1984.

Description: Trimpex (trimethoprim/Roche) is a synthetic antibacterial available as 100-mg tablets for oral administration.

Trimethoprim is 2,4-diamino-5-(3,4,5-trimethoxybenzyl)pyrimidine. It is a white to light yellow, odorless, bitter compound with a molecular weight of 290.3.

Clinical Pharmacology: Trimethoprim is rapidly absorbed following oral administration. It exists in the blood as unbound, protein-bound and metabolized forms. Ten to twenty percent of trimethoprim is metabolized, primarily in the liver; the remainder is excreted unchanged in the urine. The principal metabolites of trimethoprim are the 1- and 3-oxides and the 3'- and 4'-hydroxy derivatives. The free form is considered to be the therapeutically active form. Approximately 44% of trimethoprim is bound to plasma proteins.

Mean peak plasma concentrations of approximately 1.0 mcg/ml occur 1 to 4 hours after oral administration of a single 100-mg dose. A single 200-mg dose will result in plasma concentrations approximately twice as high. The half-life of trimethoprim ranges from 8 to 10 hours. However, patients with severely impaired renal function exhibit an increase in the half-life of trimethoprim, which requires either dosage regimen adjustment or not using the drug in such patients (see DOSAGE AND ADMINISTRATION section). During a 13-week study of trimethoprim administered at a dosage of 50 mg *q.i.d.*, the mean minimum steady-state concentration of the drug was 1.1 mcg/ml. Steady-state concentrations were achieved within 2 to 3 days of chronic administration and were maintained throughout the experimental period.

Excretion of trimethoprim is primarily by the kidneys through glomerular filtration and tubular secretion. Urine concentrations of trimethoprim are considerably higher than are the concentrations in the blood. After a single oral dose of 100 mg, urine concentrations of trimethoprim ranged from 30 to 160 mcg/ml during the 0- to 4-hour period and declined to approximately 18 to 91 mcg/ml during the 8- to 24-hour period. A 200-mg single oral dose will result in trimethoprim urine concentrations approximately twice as high. After oral administration, 50% to 60% of trimethoprim is excreted in urine within 24 hours, approximately 80% of this being unmetabolized trimethoprim.

Since normal vaginal and fecal flora are the source of most pathogens causing urinary tract infections, it is relevant to consider the distribution of trimethoprim into these sites. Concentrations of trimethoprim in vaginal secretions are consistently greater than those found simultaneously in the serum, being typically 1.6 times the concentrations of simultaneously obtained serum samples. Sufficient trimethoprim is excreted in the feces to markedly reduce or eliminate trimethoprim-susceptible organisms from the fecal flora. The dominant non-*Enterobacteriaceae* fecal organisms, *Bacteroides* spp. and *Lactobacillus* spp., are not susceptible to trimethoprim concentrations obtained with the recommended dosage.

Trimethoprim also passes the placental barrier and is excreted in breast milk.

Microbiology: Trimpex blocks the production of tetrahydrofolic acid from dihydrofolic acid by binding to and reversibly inhibiting the required enzyme, dihydrofolate reductase. This binding is very much stronger for the bacterial enzyme than for the corresponding mammalian enzyme. Thus, Trimpex selectively interferes with bacterial biosynthesis of nucleic acids and proteins.

In vitro serial dilution tests have shown that the spectrum of antibacterial activity of Trimpex includes the common urinary tract pathogens with the exception of *Pseudomonas aeruginosa*.
[See table above].

The recommended quantitative disc susceptibility method[1,2] may be used for estimating the susceptibility of bacteria to Trimpex. With this procedure,

Representative Minimum Inhibitory Concentrations for Trimethoprim-Susceptible Organisms

Bacteria	Trimethoprim MIC—mcg/ml (Range)
Escherichia coli	0.05—1.5
Proteus mirabilis	0.5—1.5
Klebsiella pneumoniae	0.5—5.0
Enterobacter species	0.5—5.0
Staphylococcus species (coagulase-negative)	0.15—5.0

Responses to Tensilon in Myasthenic and Nonmyasthenic Individuals

	Myasthenic*	Adequate**	Cholinergic***
Muscle Strength ... (ptosis, diplopia, dysphonia, dysphagia, dysarthria, respiration, limb strength)	Increased	No change	Decreased
Fasciculations ... (orbicularis oculi, facial muscles, limb muscles)	Absent	Present or absent	Present or absent
Side reactions ... (lacrimination, diaphoresis, salivation, abdominal cramps, nausea, vomiting, diarrhea)	Absent	Minimal	Severe

*Myasthenic Response—occurs in untreated myasthenics and may serve to establish diagnosis; in patients under treatment, indicates that therapy is inadequate.

**Adequate Response—observed in treated patients when therapy is stabilized; a typical response in normal individuals. In addition to this response in nonmyasthenics, the phenomenon of forced lid closure is often observed in psychoneurotics.[1]

***Cholinergic Response—seen in myasthenics who have been overtreated with anticholinesterase drugs.

reports from the laboratory giving results using the 5-mcg trimethoprim disc should be interpreted according to the following criteria: Organisms producing zones of 16 mm or greater are classified as susceptible, whereas those producing zones of 11 to 15 mm are classified as having intermediate susceptibility. A report from the laboratory of "Susceptible to trimethoprim" or "Intermediate susceptibility to trimethoprim" indicates that the infection is likely to respond when, as in uncomplicated urinary tract infections, effective therapy is dependent upon the urine concentration of trimethoprim. Organisms producing zones of 10 mm or less are reported as resistant, indicating that other therapy should be selected.

Dilution methods for determining susceptibility are also used, and results are reported as the minimum drug concentration inhibiting microbial growth (MIC).[3] If the MIC is 8 mcg per ml or less, the microorganism is considered "susceptible." If the MIC is 16 mcg per ml or greater, the microorganism is considered "resistant."

Indications and Usage: For the treatment of initial episodes of uncomplicated urinary tract infections due to susceptible strains of the following organisms: *Escherichia coli, Proteus mirabilis, Klebsiella pneumoniae, Enterobacter* species and coagulase-negative *Staphylococcus* species, including *S. saprophyticus.*

Cultures and susceptibility tests should be performed to determine the susceptibility of the bacteria to trimethoprim. Therapy may be initiated prior to obtaining the results of these tests.

Contraindications: Trimpex is contraindicated in individuals hypersensitive to trimethoprim and in those with documented megaloblastic anemia due to folate deficiency.

Warnings: Experience with trimethoprim alone is limited, but it has been reported rarely to interfere with hematopoiesis, especially when administered in large doses and/or for prolonged periods. The presence of clinical signs such as sore throat, fever, pallor or purpura may be early indications of serious blood disorders.

Precautions: *General:* Trimethoprim should be given with caution to patients with possible folate deficiency. Folates may be administered concomitantly without interfering with the antibacterial action of trimethoprim. Trimethoprim should also be given with caution to patients with impaired renal or hepatic function. If any clinical signs of a blood disorder are noted in a patient receiving trimethoprim, a complete blood count should be obtained and the drug discontinued if a significant reduction in the count of any formed blood element is found.

Drug interactions: Trimpex may inhibit the hepatic metabolism of phenytoin. Trimethoprim, given at a common clinical dosage, increased the phenytoin half-life by 51% and decreased the phenytoin metabolic clearance rate by 30%. When administering these drugs concurrently, one should be alert for possible excessive phenytoin effect.

Drug/laboratory test interactions: Trimethoprim can interfere with a serum methotrexate assay as determined by the competitive binding protein technique (CBPA) when a bacterial dihydrofolate reductase is used as the binding protein. No interference occurs, however, if methotrexate is measured by a radioimmunoassay (RIA).

The presence of trimethoprim may also interfere with the Jaffé alkaline picrate reaction assay for creatinine resulting in overestimations of about 10% in the range of normal values.

Carcinogenesis, mutagenesis, impairment of fertility:

Carcinogenesis: Long-term studies in animals to evaluate carcinogenic potential have not been conducted with trimethoprim.

Mutagenesis: Trimethoprim was demonstrated to be nonmutagenic in the Ames assay. No chromosomal damage was observed in human leukocytes cultured *in vitro* with trimethoprim; the concentration used exceeded blood levels following therapy with Trimpex.

Impairment of fertility: No adverse effects on fertility or general reproductive performance were observed in rats given trimethoprim in oral dosages as high as 70 mg/kg/day for males and 14 mg/kg/day for females.

Pregnancy: Teratogenic effects: Pregnancy Category C. Trimethoprim has been shown to be teratogenic in the rat when given in doses 40 times the human dose. In some rabbit studies, the overall increase in fetal loss (dead and resorbed and malformed conceptuses) was associated with doses 6 times the human therapeutic dose.

While there are no large well-controlled studies on the use of trimethoprim in pregnant women, Brumfitt and Pursell,[4] in a retrospective study, reported the outcome of 186 pregnancies during which the mother received either placebo or trimethoprim in combination with sulfamethoxazole. The incidence of congenital abnormalities was 4.5% (3 of 66) in those who received placebo and 3.3% (4 of 120) in those receiving trimethoprim plus sulfamethoxazole. There were no abnormalities in the 10 children whose mothers received the drug during the first trimester. In a separate survey, Brumfitt and Pursell also found no congenital abnormalities in 35 children whose mothers had received trimethoprim plus sulfamethoxazole at the time of conception or shortly thereafter.

Because trimethoprim may interfere with folic acid metabolism, Trimpex should be used during pregnancy only if the potential benefit justifies the potential risk to the fetus.

Nonteratogenic effects: The oral administration of trimethoprim to rats at a dose of 70 mg/kg/day commencing with the last third of gestation and continuing through parturition and lactation caused no deleterious effects on gestation or pup growth and survival.

Nursing mothers: Trimethoprim is excreted in human milk. Because trimethoprim may interfere with folic acid metabolism, caution should be exercised when Trimpex is administered to a nursing woman.

Pediatric use: The safety of trimethoprim in infants under two months of age has not been demonstrated. The effectiveness of trimethoprim has not been established in children under 12 years of age.

Adverse Reactions: The adverse effects encountered most often with trimethoprim were rash and pruritus. Other adverse effects reported involved the gastrointestinal and hematopoietic systems.

Dermatologic reactions: Rash, pruritus and exfoliative dermatitis. At the recommended dosage regimens of 100 mg *b.i.d.* or 200 mg *q.d.*, each for 10 days, the incidence of rash is 2.9% to 6.7%. In clinical studies which employed high doses of Trimpex, an elevated incidence of rash was noted. These rashes were maculopapular, morbilliform, pruritic and generally mild to moderate, appearing 7 to 14 days after the initiation of therapy.

Gastrointestinal reactions: Epigastric distress, nausea, vomiting and glossitis.

Hematologic reactions: Thrombocytopenia, leukopenia, neutropenia, megaloblastic anemia and methemoglobinemia.

Miscellaneous reactions: Fever, elevation of serum transaminase and bilirubin, and increases in BUN and serum creatinine levels.

Overdosage:

Acute: Signs of acute overdosage with trimethoprim may appear following ingestion of 1 gram or more of the drug and include nausea, vomiting, dizziness, headaches, mental depression, confusion and bone marrow depression (see CHRONIC OVERDOSAGE).

Treatment consists of gastric lavage and general supportive measures. Acidification of the urine will increase renal elimination of trimethoprim. Peritoneal dialysis is not effective and hemodialysis only moderately effective in eliminating the drug.

Chronic: Use of trimethoprim at high doses and/or for extended periods of time may cause bone marrow depression manifested as thrombocytopenia, leukopenia and/or megaloblastic anemia. If signs of bone marrow depression occur, trimethoprim should be discontinued and the patient should be given leucovorin, 3 to 6 mg intramuscularly daily for three days, or as required to restore normal hematopoiesis.

Dosage and Administration: The usual oral dosage is 100 mg every 24 hours or 200 mg every 24 hours, each for 10 days. The use of trimethoprim in patients with a creatinine clearance of less than 15 ml/min is not recommended. For patients with a creatinine clearance of 15 to 30 ml/min, the dose should be 50 mg every 12 hours.

The effectiveness of trimethoprim has not been established in children under 12 years of age.

How Supplied: *100-mg tablets* (white, elliptical, scored)—bottles of 100 (NDC 0004-0127-01); Tel-E-Dose® packages of 100 (NDC 0004-0127-49). Imprint on tablets: TRIMPEX 100 ROCHE.

References:

1. Bauer AW, Kirby WMM, Sherris JC, Turck M: Antibiotic Susceptibility Testing by Standardized Single Disk Method, *Am J Clin Pathol* 45:493–496, 1966.

2. Approved Standard ASM-2 Performance Standards for Antimicrobial Disc Susceptibility Test; National Committee for Clinical Laboratory Standards, 771 East Lancaster Avenue, Villanova, Pennsylvania 19085.

3. Ericsson HM, Sherris JC: Antibiotic Sensitivity Testing. Report of an International Collaborative Study. *Acta Pathol Microbiol Scand* [B] (Suppl 217): 1–90, 1971.

4. Brumfitt W, Pursell R: Trimethoprim/Sulfamethoxazole in the Treatment of Bacteriuria in Women, *J Infect Dis 128*(Suppl): S657–S663, 1973.

Shown in Product Identification section, page 430

VALRELEASE®
[val′re-lease]
(diazepam/Roche)
CAPSULES
A slow-release dosage form of
Valium® (diazepam/Roche)

The following text is complete prescribing information based on official labeling in effect August 1, 1984.

Description: Diazepam is a benzodiazepine derivative developed through original Roche research. Chemically, diazepam is 7-chloro-1,3- dihydro-1-methyl-5-phenyl-2H-1, 4-benzodiazepin -2- one. It is a colorless crystalline compound, insoluble in water and has a molecular weight of 284.74. Valrelease capsules provide the actions of Valium® (diazepam/Roche) in a slow-release dosage form.

Pharmacology: In animals, diazepam appears to act on parts of the limbic system, the thalamus and hypothalamus, and induces calming effects. Diazepam, unlike chlorpromazine and reserpine, has no demonstrable peripheral autonomic blocking action, nor does it produce extrapyramidal side effects; however, animals treated with diazepam do have a transient ataxia at higher doses. Diazepam was found to have transient cardiovascular depressor effects in dogs. Long-term experiments in rats revealed no disturbances of endocrine function.

Oral LD$_{50}$ of diazepam is 720 mg/kg in mice and 1240 mg/kg in rats. Intraperitoneal administration of 400 mg/kg to a monkey resulted in death on the sixth day.

Reproduction Studies: A series of rat reproduction studies was performed with diazepam in oral doses of 1, 10, 80 and 100 mg/kg. At 100 mg/kg there was a decrease in the number of pregnancies and surviving offspring in these rats. Neonatal survival of rats at doses lower than 100 mg/kg was within normal limits. Several neonates in these rat reproduction studies showed skeletal or other defects. Further studies in rats at doses up to and including 80 mg/kg/day did not reveal teratological effects on the offspring.

In humans, measurable blood levels of diazepam were obtained in maternal and cord blood, indicating placental transfer of the drug.

The administration of one 15-mg Valrelease capsule results in blood levels of diazepam over a 24-

Continued on next page

Roche Labs.—Cont.

hour period which are comparable to those of 5-mg Valium tablets given three times daily.

The mean time to maximum plasma diazepam concentrations after administration of 15-mg Valrelease capsules to eleven fasted subjects was 5.3 hours. The harmonic mean half-life of diazepam was 36 hours. The range of average minimum steady-state plasma diazepam concentrations during once daily administration of 15-mg Valrelease capsules to eleven normal subjects was 196 to 341 ng/ml.

Indications: Valrelease is indicated for the management of anxiety disorders or for the short-term relief of the symptoms of anxiety. Anxiety or tension associated with the stress of everyday life usually does not require treatment with an anxiolytic.

In acute alcohol withdrawal, Valrelease may be useful in the symptomatic relief of acute agitation, tremor, impending or acute delirium tremens and hallucinosis.

Valrelease is a useful adjunct for the relief of skeletal muscle spasm due to reflex spasm to local pathology (such as inflammation of the muscles or joints, or secondary to trauma); spasticity caused by upper motor neuron disorders (such as cerebral palsy and paraplegia); athetosis; and stiff-man syndrome.

Valrelease may be used adjunctively in convulsive disorders, although it has not proved useful as the sole therapy.

The effectiveness of diazepam in long-term use, that is, more than 4 months, has not been assessed by systematic clinical studies. The physician should periodically reassess the usefulness of the drug for the individual patient.

Contraindications: Valrelease is contraindicated in patients with a known hypersensitivity to this drug and, because of lack of sufficient clinical experience, in children under 6 months of age. It may be used in patients with open angle glaucoma who are receiving appropriate therapy, but is contraindicated in acute narrow angle glaucoma.

Warnings: Valrelease is not of value in the treatment of psychotic patients and should not be employed in lieu of appropriate treatment. As is true of most preparations containing CNS-acting drugs, patients receiving Valrelease should be cautioned against engaging in hazardous occupations requiring complete mental alertness such as operating machinery or driving a motor vehicle.

As with other agents which have anticonvulsant activity, when Valrelease is used as an adjunct in treating convulsive disorders, the possibility of an increase in the frequency and/ or severity of grand mal seizures may require an increase in the dosage of standard anticonvulsant medication. Abrupt withdrawal of Valrelease in such cases may also be associated with a temporary increase in the frequency and/ or severity of seizures.

Since Valrelease has a central nervous system depressant effect, patients should be advised against the simultaneous ingestion of alcohol and other CNS-depressant drugs during Valrelease therapy.

Physical and Psychological Dependence: Withdrawal symptoms (similar in character to those noted with barbiturates and alcohol) have occurred following abrupt discontinuance of diazepam (convulsions, tremor, abdominal and muscle cramps, vomiting and sweating). These were usually limited to those patients who had received excessive doses over an extended period of time. Although infrequently seen, milder withdrawal symptoms have also been reported following abrupt discontinuance of benzodiazepines taken continuously, generally at higher therapeutic levels, for at least several months. Consequently, after extended therapy, abrupt discontinuation should be generally avoided and a gradual tapering in dosage followed. Particularly addiction-prone individuals (such as drug addicts or alcoholics) should be under careful surveillance when receiving diazepam or other psychotropic agents because of the predisposition of such patients to habituation and dependence.

Usage in Pregnancy: An increased risk of congenital malformations associated with the use of minor tranquilizers (diazepam, meprobamate and chlordiazepoxide) during the first trimester of pregnancy has been suggested in several studies. Because use of these drugs is rarely a matter of urgency, their use during this period should almost always be avoided. The possibility that a woman of childbearing potential may be pregnant at the time of institution of therapy should be considered. Patients should be advised that if they become pregnant during therapy or intend to become pregnant they should communicate with their physicians about the desirability of discontinuing the drug.

Management of Overdosage: Manifestations of diazepam overdosage include somnolence, confusion, coma and diminished reflexes. Respiration, pulse and blood pressure should be monitored, as in all cases of drug overdosage, although, in general, these effects have been minimal following overdosage. General supportive measures should be employed, along with immediate gastric lavage. Intravenous fluids should be administered and an adequate airway maintained. Hypotension may be combated by the use of Levophed® (levarterenol) or Aramine (metaraminol). Dialysis is of limited value. As with the management of intentional overdosage with any drug, it should be borne in mind that multiple agents may have been ingested.

Precautions: If Valrelease is to be combined with other psychotropic agents or anticonvulsant drugs, careful consideration should be given to the pharmacology of the agents to be employed—particularly with known compounds which may potentiate the action of diazepam, such as phenothiazines, narcotics, barbiturates, MAO inhibitors and other antidepressants. The usual precautions are indicated for severely depressed patients or those in whom there is any evidence of latent depression; particularly the recognition that suicidal tendencies may be present and protective measures may be necessary. The usual precautions in treating patients with impaired renal or hepatic function should be observed.

In elderly and debilitated patients, it is recommended that the dosage be limited to the smallest effective amount to preclude the development of ataxia or oversedation (2 mg to 2½ mg once or twice daily, initially, to be increased gradually as needed and tolerated).

The clearance of Valium and certain other benzodiazepines can be delayed in association with Tagamet (cimetidine) administration. The clinical significance of this is unclear.

Adverse Reactions: Side effects most commonly reported were drowsiness, fatigue and ataxia. Infrequently encountered were confusion, constipation, depression, diplopia, dysarthria, headache, hypotension, incontinence, jaundice, changes in libido, nausea, changes in salivation, skin rash, slurred speech, tremor, urinary retention, vertigo and blurred vision. Paradoxical reactions such as acute hyperexcited states, anxiety, hallucinations, increased muscle spasticity, insomnia, rage, sleep disturbances and stimulation have been reported; should these occur, use of the drug should be discontinued.

Because of isolated reports of neutropenia and jaundice, periodic blood counts and liver function tests are advisable during long-term therapy. Minor changes in EEG patterns, usually low-voltage fast activity, have been observed in patients during and after diazepam therapy and are of no known significance.

Dosage and Administration: Dosage should be individualized for maximum beneficial effect. While the usual daily dosages given below will meet the needs of most patients, there will be some who may require higher doses. In such cases dosage should be increased cautiously to avoid adverse effects.

Whenever oral Valium® (diazepam/Roche), 5 mg t.i.d., would be considered the appropriate dosage, one 15-mg Valrelease capsule daily may be used.

Note: If 1 mg or 2½ mg is the desired dose, scored Valium (diazepam/Roche) tablets should be used.

Valrelease 15-mg capsules are recommended for elderly or debilitated patients and children only when it has been determined that 5 mg oral Valium t.i.d. is the optimal daily dose. Oral Valium is not recommended for children under 6 months of age.

Adults:	USUAL DAILY DOSE
Management of Anxiety Disorders and Relief of Symptoms of Anxiety.	Depending upon severity of symptoms—1 or 2 (15 to 30 mg) capsules once daily
Symptomatic Relief in Acute Alcohol Withdrawal	2 capsules (30 mg) the first 24 hours, followed by 1 capsule (15 mg) daily as needed.
Adjunctively for Relief of Skeletal Muscle Spasm.	1 or 2 capsules (15 to 30 mg) once daily
Adjunctively in Convulsive Disorders.	1 or 2 capsules (15 to 30 mg) once daily

How Supplied: For oral administration, Valrelease (diazepam/Roche) capsules—15 mg (yellow and blue)—bottles of 100; Tel-E-Dose® packages of 100; Prescription Paks of 30.

Shown in Product Identification Section, page 430

VI-PENTA® F CHEWABLES ℞
[vy-pen′ ta]

The following text is complete prescribing information based on official labeling in effect August 1, 1984.

Description: Vi-Penta F Chewables is a prescription-only chewable multivitamin tablet containing eleven vitamins and dietary fluoride. Vi-Penta F Chewables is specially formulated to provide daily nutritional support and aid in the prevention of tooth decay in children three years of age and older. Each fruit-flavored tablet contains less than one calorie and will not interfere with the appetite.

Each chewable tablet contains:

Fat-Soluble Vitamins
Vitamin A (as vitamin A acetate) .... 5000 IU
Vitamin D_2 (ergocalciferol) .... 400 IU
Vitamin E (as *dl*-alpha-tocopheryl
 acetate) .... 2 IU

Water-Soluble Vitamins
Vitamin C (as ascorbic acid and
 sodium ascorbate) .... 60 mg
Vitamin B_1 (as thiamine
 mononitrate) .... 1.2 mg
Vitamin B_2 (riboflavin) .... 1.5 mg
Niacin (as niacinamide) .... 10 mg
Vitamin B_6 (as pyridoxine HCl) .... 1 mg
d-biotin .... 40 mcg
Pantothenic acid (as calcium
 d-pantothenate) .... 9 mg
Vitamin B_{12} (cyanocobalamin) .... 3 mcg

Trace Elements
Fluoride (as sodium fluoride) .... 1 mg

Clinical Pharmacology: Vitamins are necessary for maintenance of normal metabolic functions including hematopoiesis. *Vitamin A* is necessary for proper functioning of the retina; it appears to be essential to the integrity of epithelial cells. *Vitamin D* is necessary for the absorption of calcium and for the proper development and maintenance of bone structure. *Vitamin E* is an antioxidant which preserves essential cellular constituents, including those of the red blood cell. It also serves as protection against lipid peroxidation.

The water-soluble vitamins play vital roles in the conversion of carbohydrate, protein and fat into tissue and energy. *Thiamine (B_1)* acts as a coenzyme in carbohydrate metabolism. *Riboflavin (B_2)* functions as a coenzyme in the electron transport system associated with conversion of tissue oxidations into usable energy. *Niacin* serves as a coenzyme in oxidation-reduction reactions in tissue respiration. *Pyridoxine (B_6)* is essential for the metabolism of amino acids. *Pantothenic acid* functions as a coenzyme in various metabolic acetylation reactions and *biotin* in specific carboxylation reactions in lipid metabolism. *Cyanocobalamin (B_{12})* is essential to nucleic acid synthesis and normal maturation of red blood cells. *Ascorbic acid (C)* performs a vital function in the process of cellular respiration, and is involved in both carbohydrate and amino acid metabolism. It is essential for collagen formation and tissue repair.

Fluorine is an essential trace element that renders the dentine and enamel of teeth more resistant to acid.

There is ample evidence that the fluoridation of drinking water leads to a substantial decrease in the incidence of dental caries in childhood. This effect is greatest when fluoride is ingested during the first 9 to 10 years of life when teeth are developing. However, in areas where drinking water is devoid of natural or artificially controlled fluoride, or where fluoridation is not feasible, a single daily dose of fluoride as a dietary supplement is recommended as an effective substitute.

Recognizing the merits of dietary fluoride supplements, the Council on Dental Therapeutics of the American Dental Association strongly urges: "*Such administration should be consistent and continuous over long periods of time if substantial benefit is to be anticipated.*"

Indications and Usage: Vi-Penta F Chewable Tablets are indicated for supportive nutritional supplementation and as an aid in the prevention of tooth decay in children three years of age and older who reside in areas where the fluoride content of drinking water is known to be less than 0.7 parts per million.

Contraindications: Vi-Penta F Chewables is contraindicated in patients known to be hypersensitive to any of its components.

Warnings: This preparation should not be used in areas where the fluoride content of drinking water is known to be 0.7 parts per million or greater. The recommended dose of Vi-Penta F Chewables should not be exceeded, since dental fluorosis may result from continued ingestion of excessive amounts of fluoride.

Precautions: *General:* Certain patients may require nutritional supplementation with folic acid as well as other nutrients according to the dietary needs of the individual. Vi-Penta F Chewables is not intended for treatment of pernicious anemia or other severe specific vitamin deficiencies.

Information for the Patient: Because dental fluorosis may result from continued ingestion of excessive amounts of fluoride and toxic reactions have been reported with injudicious use of certain vitamins, urge patients to follow your specific instructions regarding dosage regimen. As with any medication, advise patients to keep Vi-Penta F Chewables out of reach of children.

Adverse Reactions: Adverse reactions have been reported with specific vitamins, but generally at levels substantially higher than those in Vi-Penta F Chewables. However, allergic and idiosyncratic reactions are possible at lower levels.

Dosage and Administration: Usual dosage for children three years of age and over: one tablet daily, chewed or crushed.

Vi-Penta F Chewables is available on prescription only.

How Supplied: Green, yellow, pink, purple and orange shield-shaped, biconvex tablets, engraved ROCHE 51—bottles of 100 chewable tablets (NDC 0004-0051-01).

Shown in Product Identification Section, page 430

VI-PENTA® F INFANT DROPS ℞
[*vy-pen′ ta*]

The following text is complete prescribing information based on official labeling in effect August 1, 1984.

Description: Vi-Penta F Infant Drops is a prescription-only liquid multivitamin preparation containing ascorbic acid, dietary fluoride and fat-soluble vitamins A, D and E. It is specially formulated to provide daily nutritional support and aid in the prevention of tooth decay in infants from birth. Vi-Penta F Infant Drops is a fruit-flavored, liquid preparation in an aqueous nonalcoholic vehicle that may be administered by dropping directly on the tongue or mixing with liquids or food.

Each 0.6 ml provides:
Fat-Soluble Vitamins
Vitamin A (as vitamin A palmitate) .... 5000 IU
Vitamin D_2 (ergocalciferol) .... 400 IU
Vitamin E (as *dl*-alpha-tocopheryl acetate) .... 2 IU
Water-Soluble Vitamins
Vitamin C (ascorbic acid) .... 50 mg
Trace Elements
Fluoride (as sodium fluoride) .... 0.5 mg

Clinical Pharmacology: Vitamins are necessary for maintenance of normal metabolic functions including hematopoiesis. *Vitamin A* is necessary for proper functioning of the retina; it appears to be essential to the integrity of epithelial cells. *Vitamin D* is necessary for the absorption of calcium and for the proper development and maintenance of bone structure. *Vitamin E* is an antioxidant which preserves essential cellular constituents, including those of the red blood cell. It also serves as protection against lipid peroxidation. *Vitamin C* performs a vital function in the process of cellular respiration, and is involved in both carbohydrate and amino acid metabolism. It is essential for collagen formation and tissue repair.

Fluorine is an essential trace element that renders the dentine and enamel of teeth more resistant to acid.

There is ample evidence that the fluoridation of drinking water leads to a substantial decrease in the incidence of dental caries in childhood. This effect is greatest when fluoride is ingested during the first 9 to 10 years of life when teeth are developing. However, in areas where drinking water is devoid of natural or artificially controlled fluoride, or where fluoridation is not feasible, a single daily dose of fluoride as a dietary supplement is recommended as an effective substitute.

Recognizing the merits of dietary fluoride supplements, the Council on Dental Therapeutics of the American Dental Association strongly urges: "*Such administration should be consistent and continuous over long periods of time if substantial benefit is to be anticipated.*"

Indications and Usage: Vi-Penta F Infant Drops is indicated for supportive nutritional supplementation and as an aid in the prevention of tooth decay in infants from birth who reside in areas where the fluoride content of drinking water is known to be less than 0.7 parts per million.

Contraindications: Vi-Penta F Infant Drops is contraindicated in patients known to be hypersensitive to any of its components.

Warnings: This preparation should not be used in areas where the fluoride content of drinking water is known to be 0.7 parts per million or greater. The recommended dose of Vi-Penta F Infant Drops should not be exceeded, since dental fluorosis may result from continued ingestion of excessive amounts of fluoride.

Precautions: *General:* Certain patients may require nutritional supplementation with the B-complex vitamins as well as other nutrients according to the dietary needs of the individual. Vi-Penta F Infant Drops is not intended for treatment of severe specific vitamin deficiencies.

Information for the Patient: Because dental fluorosis may result from continued ingestion of excessive amounts of fluoride and toxic reactions have been reported with injudicious use of certain vitamins, urge patients to follow your specific instructions regarding dosage regimen. As with any medication, advise patients to keep Vi-Penta F Infant Drops out of reach of children. Vi-Penta F Infant Drops should be stored under refrigeration.

Adverse Reactions: Adverse reactions have been reported with specific vitamins, but generally at levels substantially higher than those in Vi-Penta F Infant Drops. However, allergic and idiosyncratic reactions are possible at lower levels.

Dosage and Administration: Usual dosage for infants from birth: 0.6 ml daily, as measured by the dropper. Vi-Penta F Infant Drops may be administered by dropping directly on the tongue or mixing with liquids or food.

Vi-Penta F Infant Drops is available on prescription only.

How Supplied: Fruit-flavored liquid in bottle of 30 ml, packaged with a calibrated dropper (NDC 0004-1012-23).

NOTE TO THE PHARMACIST: Vi-Penta F Infant Drops should be dispensed in the original special plastic containers, since contact with glass leads to instability and precipitation. Preparation should be stored under refrigeration.

VI-PENTA® F ℞
[*vy-pen′ ta*]
MULTIVITAMIN DROPS

The following text is complete prescribing information based on official labeling in effect August 1, 1984.

Description: Vi-Penta F Multivitamin Drops is a prescription-only liquid multivitamin preparation containing ten vitamins and dietary fluoride. It is specially formulated to provide daily nutritional support and aid in the prevention of tooth decay in infants and children. Vi-Penta F Multivitamin Drops is a fruit-flavored, liquid preparation in an aqueous nonalcoholic vehicle that may be administered by dropping directly on the tongue or mixing with liquids or food.

Each 0.6 ml provides:
Fat-Soluble Vitamins
Vitamin A (as vitamin A palmitate) ... 5000 IU
Vitamin D_2 (ergocalciferol) .... 400 IU
Vitamin E (as *dl*-alpha-tocopheryl acetate)... 2 IU
Water-Soluble Vitamins
Vitamin C (ascorbic acid)........................ 50 mg
Vitamin B_1 (as thiamine HCl)............... 1 mg
Vitamin B_2 (as riboflavin-5′-phosphate sodium)... 1 mg
Niacin (as niacinamide).......................... 10 mg
Vitamin B_6 (as pyridoxine HCl) .... 0.8 mg
d-Biotin .... 30 mcg
Pantothenic acid (as dexpanthenol) .... 10 mg
Trace Elements
Fluoride (as sodium fluoride).................. 0.5 mg

Clinical Pharmacology: Vitamins are necessary for maintenance of normal metabolic functions including hematopoiesis. *Vitamin A* is necessary for proper functioning of the retina; it appears to be essential to the integrity of epithelial cells. *Vitamin D* is necessary for the absorption of calcium and for the proper development and maintenance of bone structure. *Vitamin E* is an antioxidant which preserves essential cellular constituents, including those of the red blood cell. It also serves as protection against lipid peroxidation.

The water-soluble vitamins play vital roles in the conversion of carbohydrate, protein and fat into tissue and energy. *Thiamine (B_1)* acts as a coenzyme in carbohydrate metabolism. *Riboflavin (B_2)* functions as a coenzyme in the electron transport system associated with conversion of tissue oxidations into usable energy. *Niacin* serves as a coenzyme in oxidation-reduction reactions in tissue respiration. *Pyridoxine (B_6)* is essential for the metabolism of amino acids. *Pantothenic acid* functions as a coenzyme in various metabolic acetylation reactions and *biotin* in specific carboxylation reactions in lipid metabolism. *Ascorbic acid (C)* performs a vital function in the process of cellular respiration, and is involved in both carbohydrate and amino acid metabolism. It is essential for collagen formation and tissue repair.

Fluorine is an essential trace element that renders the dentine and enamel of teeth more resistant to acid.

There is ample evidence that the fluoridation of drinking water leads to a substantial decrease in the incidence of dental caries in childhood. This effect is greatest when fluoride is ingested during the first 9 to 10 years of life when teeth are devel-

Continued on next page

Roche Labs.—Cont.

oping. However, in areas were drinking water is devoid of natural or artificially controlled fluoride, or where fluoridation is not feasible, a single daily dose of fluoride as a dietary supplement is recommended as an effective substitute.

Recognizing the merits of dietary fluoride supplements, the Council on Dental Therapeutics of the American Dental Association strongly urges: "*Such administration should be consistent and continuous over long periods of time if substantial benefit is to be anticipated.*"

Indications and Usage: Vi-Penta F Multivitamin Drops is indicated for supportive nutritional supplementation and as an aid in the prevention of tooth decay in infants and children who reside in areas where the fluoride content of drinking water is known to be less than 0.7 parts per million.

Contraindications: Vi-Penta F Multivitamin Drops is contraindicated in patients known to be hypersensitive to any of its components.

Warnings: This preparation should not be used in areas where the fluoride content of drinking water is known to be 0.7 parts per million or greater. The recommended dose of Vi-Penta F Multivitamin Drops should not be exceeded, since dental fluorosis may result from continued ingestion of excessive amounts of fluoride.

Precautions: *General:* Certain patients may require nutritional supplementation with folic acid and vitamin B_{12} as well as other nutrients according to the dietary needs of the individual. Vi-Penta F Multivitamin Drops is not intended for treatment of severe specific vitamin deficiencies.

Information for the Patient: Because dental fluorosis may result from continued ingestion of excessive amounts of fluoride and toxic reactions have been reported with injudicious use of certain vitamins, urge patients to follow your specific instructions regarding dosage regimen. As with any medication, advise patients to keep Vi-Penta F Multivitamin drops out of reach of children. Vi-Penta F Multivitamin Drops should be stored under refrigeration.

Adverse Reactions: Adverse reactions have been reported with specific vitamins, but generally at levels substantially higher than those in Vi-Penta F Multivitamin Drops. However, allergic and idiosyncratic reactions are possible at lower levels.

Dosage and Administration: Usual dosage for infants and children: 0.6 ml daily, as measured by the dropper. Vi-Penta F Multivitamin Drops may be administered by dropping directly on the tongue or mixing with liquids or food.

Vi-Penta F Multivitamin Drops is available on prescription only.

How Supplied: Fruit-flavored liquid in bottles of 30 ml, packaged with a calibrated dropper (NDC 0004-1014-23).

NOTE TO THE PHARMACIST: Vi-Penta F Multivitamin Drops should be dispensed in the original special plastic containers, since contact with glass leads to instability and precipitation. Preparation should be stored under refrigeration.

VI-PENTA® INFANT DROPS
VI-PENTA® MULTIVITAMIN DROPS
[*vy-pen' ta*]

The following text is complete prescribing information based on official labeling in effect August 1, 1984.

Composition: Vi-Penta Infant Drops and Vi-Penta Multivitamin Drops are designed to fill the vitamin needs of specific age groups. (See Composition Table below.)

Action and Uses: Vi-Penta Drops are water miscible and can be mixed with food or infant formula, or placed directly on the tongue.

Vi-Penta Infant Drops—a selective formula for prevention of vitamin deficiencies in infants and young children. *Vi-Penta Multivitamin Drops*—a comprehensive formula for daily nutritional support in adults as well as children of all ages. It is an especially convenient dosage form when a small volume liquid vitamin supplement is desired, such as to supplement the diets of those patients with conditions which permanently or temporarily impair their ability to swallow, chew or consume normal amounts and/or kinds of food.

Dosage: The average daily dose is 0.6 cc; therapeutic doses should be given according to the needs of the patient.

How Supplied: Vi-Penta Infant Drops and Vi-Penta Multivitamin Drops—fruit flavored, 50-cc bottles packaged with calibrated dropper.

EDUCATIONAL MATERIAL

Videos:
COMMUNICATION FOR HOSPITAL PHARMACISTS: A WORKSHOP
  Vignettes showing techniques in interactive communication
  Free to Pharmacists
  ACPE accreditation
PATIENT EDUCATION IN ACTION
  Techniques for successfully handling commonly encountered patient education opportunities
  Free to Pharmacists
  ACPE accreditation

Vi-Penta Composition Table

Each 0.6 cc of Vi-Penta Infant Drops Provides:		% minimum daily requirements (MDR)	
		Infants (under 1 year)	Young Children (1–6 years)
Vitamin A (as the palmitate)	5000 U.S.P. Units	333%	166%
Vitamin D_2	400 U.S.P. Units	100%	100%
Vitamin C	50 mg	500%	250%
Vitamin E (as *dl*-α-tocopheryl acetate)	2 Int. Units	*	*

Each 0.6 cc of Vi-Penta Multivitamin Drops provides:		% minimum daily requirements (MDR)		
		Infants (under 1 year)	Children (1–6 years)	(6–12 years)
Vitamin A (as the palmitate)	5000 U.S.P. Units	333%	166%	166%
Vitamin D_2	400 U.S.P. Units	100%	100%	100%
Vitamin C	50 mg	500%	250%	250%
Vitamin B_1 (as hydrochloride)	1 mg	400%	200%	133%
Vitamin B_2 (as riboflavin-5'-phosphate sodium)	1 mg	166%	111%	111%
Vitamin B_6	1 mg	*	*	*
Vitamin E (as *dl*-α-tocopheryl acetate)	2 Int. Units	*	*	*
d-Biotin	30 mcg	†	†	†
Niacinamide	10 mg	*	200%	133%
Dexpanthenol (equiv. to 11.6 mg calcium pantothenate)	10 mg	†	†	†

*MDR for these vitamins has not been determined.
†The need for these vitamins in human nutrition has not been established.

Self-Assessment Home Study:
THE PATHOGENESIS CLASSIFICATION AND TREATMENT OF ACNE WITH EMPHASIS ON ISOTRETINOIN
  Free to Pharmacists
  ACPE accreditation
VITAMINS AND MINERALS RELATED TO ILLNESS
  Free to Pharmacists
  ACPE accreditation
Available through the Roche representative. For additional C.E. information, (201) 235-3707

Roche Products Inc.
MANATI, PUERTO RICO 00701

DALMANE®
[*dal' mane*]
(flurazepam hydrochloride/Roche)
Capsules

The following text is complete prescribing information based on official labeling in effect August 1, 1984.

Description: Flurazepam hydrochloride is chemically 7-chloro-1-[2-(diethylamino)ethyl]-5-(*o*-fluorophenyl)-1,3-dihydro-2*H*-1, 4-benzodiazepin-2-one dihydrochloride. It is a pale yellow, crystalline compound, freely soluble in U.S.P. alcohol and very soluble in water. It has a molecular weight of 460.826.

Clinical Pharmacology: Flurazepam hydrochloride is rapidly absorbed from the G.I. tract. Flurazepam is rapidly metabolized and is excreted primarily in the urine. Following a single oral dose, peak flurazepam plasma concentrations ranging from 0.5 to 4.0 ng/ml occur at 30 to 60 minutes post-dosing. The harmonic mean apparent half-life of flurazepam is 2.3 hours. The blood level profile of flurazepam and its major metabolites was determined in man following the oral administration of 30 mg daily for 2 weeks. The N_1-hydroxyethyl-flurazepam was measurable only during the early hours after a 30 mg dose and was not detectable after 24 hours. The major metabolite in blood was N_1-desalkyl-flurazepam, which reached steady-state (plateau) levels after 7 to 10 days of dosing, at levels approximately five- to sixfold greater than the 24-hour levels observed on Day 1. The half-life of elimination of N_1-desalkyl-flurazepam ranged from 47 to 100 hours. The major urinary metabolite is conjugated N_1-hydroxyethyl-flurazepam which accounts for 22 to 55 percent of the dose. Less than 1% of the dose is excreted in the urine as N_1-desalkyl-flurazepam. This pharmacokinetic profile may be responsible for the clinical observation that flurazepam is increasingly effective on the second or third night of consecutive use and that for one or two nights after the drug is discontinued both sleep latency and total wake time may still be decreased.

Indications: Dalmane is a hypnotic agent useful for the treatment of insomnia characterized by difficulty in falling asleep, frequent nocturnal awakenings, and/or early morning awakening. Dalmane can be used effectively in patients with recurring insomnia or poor sleeping habits, and in acute or chronic medical situations requiring restful sleep. Sleep laboratory studies have objectively determined that Dalmane is effective for at least 28 consecutive nights of drug administration. Since insomnia is often transient and intermittent, short-term use is usually sufficient. Prolonged use of hypnotics is usually not indicated and should only be undertaken concomitantly with appropriate evaluation of the patient.

Contraindications: Dalmane is contraindicated in patients with known hypersensitivity to the drug.

Usage in Pregnancy: Benzodiazepines may cause fetal damage when administered during pregnancy. An increased risk of congenital malformations associated with the use of diazepam and chlordiazepoxide during the first trimester of pregnancy has been suggested in several studies.

Dalmane is contraindicated in pregnant women. Symptoms of neonatal depression have been reported; a neonate whose mother received 30 mg of Dalmane nightly for insomnia during the 10 days prior to delivery appeared hypotonic and inactive during the first four days of life. Serum levels of N_1-desalkyl-flurazepam in the infant indicated transplacental circulation and implicate this long-acting metabolite in this case. If there is a likelihood of the patient becoming pregnant while receiving flurazepam, she should be warned of the potential risks to the fetus. Patients should be instructed to discontinue the drug prior to becoming pregnant. The possibility that a woman of childbearing potential may be pregnant at the time of institution of therapy should be considered.

Warnings: Patients receiving Dalmane should be cautioned about possible combined effects with alcohol and other CNS depressants. Also, caution patients that an additive effect may occur if alcoholic beverages are consumed during the day following the use of Dalmane for nighttime sedation. The potential for this interaction continues for several days following discontinuance of flurazepam, until serum levels of psychoactive metabolites have declined.

Patients should also be cautioned about engaging in hazardous occupations requiring complete mental alertness such as operating machinery or driving a motor vehicle after ingesting the drug, including potential impairment of the performance of such activities which may occur the day following ingestion of Dalmane.

Usage in Children: Clinical investigations of Dalmane have not been carried out in children. Therefore, the drug is not currently recommended for use in persons under 15 years of age.

Physical and Psychological Dependence: Physical and psychological dependence have not been reported or observed in persons taking recommended doses of Dalmane. Withdrawal symptoms have been reported following abrupt discontinuance of anxiolytic benzodiazepines taken continuously, generally at higher therapeutic levels, for at least several months. These have not been specifically reported for Dalmane. However, if it is determined that a patient has been taking Dalmane for a prolonged period of time, particularly at excessive doses, abrupt discontinuation should generally be avoided and a gradual tapering of dosage followed. Also, as with any hypnotic, caution must be exercised in administering Dalmane to individuals known to be addiction-prone or those whose history suggests they may increase the dosage on their own initiative.

Precautions: Since the risk of the development of oversedation, dizziness, confusion and/or ataxia increases substantially with larger doses in elderly and debilitated patients, it is recommended that in such patients the dosage be limited to 15 mg. If Dalmane is to be combined with other drugs having known hypnotic properties or CNS-depressant effects, due consideration should be given to potential additive effects.

The usual precautions are indicated for severely depressed patients or those in whom there is any evidence of latent depression; particularly the recognition that suicidal tendencies may be present and protective measures may be necessary. The usual precautions should be observed in patients with impaired renal or hepatic function and chronic pulmonary insufficiency.

Adverse Reactions: Dizziness, drowsiness, light-headedness, staggering, ataxia and falling have occurred, particularly in elderly or debilitated persons. Severe sedation, lethargy, disorientation and coma, probably indicative of drug intolerance or overdosage, have been reported.

Also reported were headache, heartburn, upset stomach, nausea, vomiting, diarrhea, constipation, gastrointestinal pain, nervousness, talkativeness, apprehension, irritability, weakness, palpitations, chest pains, body and joint pains and genitourinary complaints. There have also been rare occurrences of leukopenia, granulocytopenia, sweating, flushes, difficulty in focusing, blurred vision, burning eyes, faintness, hypotension, shortness of breath, pruritus, skin rash, dry mouth, bitter taste, excessive salivation, anorexia, euphoria, depression, slurred speech, confusion, restlessness, hallucinations, and elevated SGOT, SGPT, total and direct bilirubins, and alkaline phosphatase. Paradoxical reactions, *e.g.,* excitement, stimulation and hyperactivity, have also been reported in rare instances.

Dosage and Administration: Dosage should be individualized for maximal beneficial effects. The usual adult dosage is 30 mg before retiring. In some patients, 15 mg may suffice. In elderly and/or debilitated patients, 15 mg is usually sufficient for a therapeutic response and it is therefore recommended that therapy be initiated with this dosage.

Overdosage: Manifestations of Dalmane overdosage include somnolence, confusion and coma. Respiration, pulse and blood pressure should be monitored as in all cases of drug overdosage. General supportive measures should be employed, along with immediate gastric lavage. Intravenous fluids should be administered and an adequate airway maintained. Hypotension and CNS depression may be combated by judicious use of appropriate therapeutic agents. The value of dialysis has not been determined. If excitation occurs in patients following Dalmane overdosage, barbiturates should not be used. As with the management of intentional overdosage with any drug, it should be borne in mind that multiple agents may have been ingested.

How Supplied: Dalmane (flurazepam hydrochloride/Roche) capsules—15 mg, orange and ivory; 30 mg, red and ivory—bottles of 100 and 500; Tel-E-Dose® packages of 100, available in boxes containing 10 strips of 10, in trays of 4 boxes each containing a reverse-numbered roll of 25 and in boxes of 4 reverse-numbered cards of 25; Prescription Paks of 30, available in trays of 10.

Shown in Product Identification Section, page 429

ENDEP® ℞
[en'dep]
(amitriptyline HCl/Roche)
TABLETS

The following text is complete prescribing information based on official labeling in effect August 1, 1984.

Description: Endep (amitriptyline HCl/Roche), a tricyclic antidepressant, is available as 10-mg, 25-mg, 50-mg, 75-mg, 100-mg and 150-mg tablets for oral administration. Amitriptyline HCl, a dibenzocycloheptadiene derivative, is a white crystalline compound that is readily soluble in water. It is designated chemically as 10, 11-dihydro-N,N-dimethyl-5H-dibenzo[a,d]cycloheptene-$\Delta^{5,\gamma}$-propylamine hydrochloride. The molecular weight is 313.87. The empirical formula is $C_{20}H_{23}N \cdot HCl$.

Clinical Pharmacology: Endep is an antidepressant with sedative effects. Its mechanism of action in man is not known. It is not a monoamine oxidase inhibitor, and it does not act primarily by stimulation of the central nervous system.

Amitriptyline inhibits the membrane pump mechanism responsible for uptake of norepinephrine and serotonin in adrenergic and serotonergic neurons. Pharmacologically this action may potentiate or prolong neuronal activity, since reuptake of these biogenic amines is important physiologically in terminating its transmitting activity. This interference with reuptake of norepinephrine and/or serotonin is believed by some to underlie the antidepressant activity of amitriptyline.

Amitriptyline undergoes extensive metabolism primarily through N-demethylation to nortriptyline, an active metabolite, followed by extensive hydroxylation to their respective 10-hydroxy metabolites which are eliminated as glucuronide conjugates.

Following a single oral dose of 75 mg of amitriptyline HCl, the mean maximum plasma concentrations of 39.4 ng/ml of amitriptyline and 16.1 ng/ml of nortriptyline were reached in approximately 4 and 10 hours, respectively. The average minimum steady-state plasma concentrations in patients receiving 50 mg of amitriptyline HCl, three times a day for an average of 32 days, were 81 ng/ml for amitriptyline, 71 ng/ml for nortriptyline, 12 ng/ml for 10-hydroxyamitriptyline, 91 ng/ml for conjugated 10-hydroxyamitriptyline, 82 ng/ml for 10-hydroxynortriptyline and 176 ng/ml for conjugated 10-hydroxynortriptyline. Steady-state plasma concentrations are usually reached by day 14. The mean apparent half-life of elimination of amitriptyline is 22.4 hours and the apparent half-life of elimination of nortriptyline is 26.0 hours. Amitriptyline is approximately 96% bound to plasma proteins.

Amitriptyline has been shown to cross the blood-brain barrier in cats, mice and rats. It has also been shown to pass the placental barrier and to enter fetal circulation in mice after intramuscular and intravenous administration. Amitriptyline is excreted in human breast milk.

Indications and Usage: Endep is indicated for the relief of symptoms of depression. Endogenous depression is more likely to be alleviated than are other depressive states.

Contraindications: Endep is contraindicated in patients who have shown prior hypersensitivity to this agent; cross-sensitivity to other tricyclic antidepressants can occur.

Endep is not recommended for use during the acute recovery phase following myocardial infarction.

Endep should not be given concomitantly with a monoamine oxidase inhibitor. Hyperpyretic crises, severe convulsions and deaths have occurred in patients receiving tricyclic antidepressant and monoamine oxidase inhibiting drugs simultaneously. When it is desired to replace a monoamine oxidase inhibitor with Endep, a minimum of 14 days should be allowed to elapse after the former is discontinued. Endep should then be initiated cautiously with gradual increase in dosage until optimum response is achieved.

Warnings: Endep should be used with caution in patients with a history of seizures and, because of its atropine-like action, in patients with a history of urinary retention, angle-closure glaucoma or increased intraocular pressure.

In patients with angle-closure glaucoma, even average doses may precipitate an attack.

Patients with cardiovascular disorders should be watched closely. Tricyclic antidepressant drugs, including Endep, particularly when given in high doses, have been reported to produce arrhythmias, sinus tachycardia and prolongation of the conduction time. Myocardial infarction and stroke have been reported with drugs of this class.

Close supervision is required when Endep is given to hyperthyroid patients or those receiving thyroid medication.

Amitriptyline HCl may enhance the response to alcohol and the effects of barbiturates and other CNS depressants. In patients who may use alcohol excessively, it should be borne in mind that the potentiation may increase the danger inherent in any suicide attempt or overdosage.

Precautions: *General:* Schizophrenic patients may develop increased symptoms of psychosis; patients with paranoid symptomatology may have an exaggeration of such symptoms; manic depressive patients may experience a shift to the manic phase. In these circumstances, the dose of Endep may be reduced or a major tranquilizer such as perphenazine may be administered concurrently. The possibility of suicide in depressed patients remains during treatment and until significant remission occurs. Potentially suicidal patients should not have access to large quantities of this drug. Prescriptions should be written for the smallest amount feasible.

Concurrent administration of Endep and electroshock therapy may increase the hazards associated with such therapy. Such treatment should be limited to patients for whom it is essential.

Amitriptyline HCl should be used with caution in patients with impaired liver function.

Both elevation and lowering of blood sugar levels have been reported.

Continued on next page

Roche Products—Cont.

The drug should be discontinued several days before elective surgery, if possible.

Information for Patients: Patients should be cautioned about engaging in hazardous occupations requiring complete mental alertness such as operating machinery or driving a motor vehicle after ingesting the drug.

Patients receiving amitriptyline HCl should also be cautioned about the possible combined effects with alcohol, barbiturates and other CNS depressants.

Drug Interactions: MAO inhibitors—see CONTRAINDICATIONS section. Thyroid medications; alcohol, barbiturates and other CNS depressants—see WARNINGS section.

Endep may block the antihypertensive action of guanethidine or similarly acting compounds.

When Endep is given with anticholinergic agents or sympathomimetic drugs, including epinephrine combined with local anesthetics, close supervision and careful adjustment of dosages are required.

Paralytic ileus may occur in patients taking tricyclic antidepressants in combination with anticholinergic-type drugs.

Caution is advised if patients receive large doses of ethchlorvynol concurrently. Transient delirium has been reported in patients who were treated with one gram of ethchlorvynol and 75 to 150 mg of amitriptyline HCl.

Carcinogenesis, Mutagenesis, Impairment of Fertility: Carcinogenesis: Amitriptyline HCl has not been adequately studied in animals to permit an evaluation of its carcinogenic potential. However, in a study during which relatively small numbers of rats received amitriptyline HCl as a dietary admixture at dosages up to 100 mg/kg/day for 78 weeks, no increase in the incidence of any tumor was reported.

Mutagenesis: Amitriptyline HCl was tested in a bacterial mutagenesis assay (Ames test) in the presence and absence of activating enzymes. No evidence for mutagenicity was found using *Salmonella* tester strains TA 1535, TA 100, TA 98 and TA 1537 at concentrations up to 5000 mcg/plate.

Impairment of Fertility: Amitriptyline HCl was studied in a Segment I fertility and general reproduction study in rats at dosages up to 20 mg/kg/day. There were no adverse effects on fertility, fetal growth and development, litter size, pup survival or pup growth. Similarly, no adverse effects were reported in a rat litter test in which amitriptyline HCl was administered at dosages up to 20 mg/kg/day.

Pregnancy: Teratogenic Effects: Pregnancy Category C. Animal reproduction studies have been inconclusive, and clinical experience has been limited. Amitriptyline HCl was tested in rats and in rabbits for teratogenic potential at dosages up to 20 mg/kg/day. Although stunting and increased neonatal mortality were observed in rabbits, there was no evidence for teratogenicity in either rats or rabbits. In a brief report, amitriptyline HCl was shown to be teratogenic in the hamster at dosages up to 100 mg/kg administered intraperitoneally on day 8 of gestation. In a more detailed study, amitriptyline HCl was shown to produce malformations in the rabbit at dosages of 15 to 60 mg/kg/day and in the mouse at dosages of 14 to 56 mg/kg/day. In another study, amitriptyline HCl was shown to be teratogenic in JBT/Jd and JBT/Ju strains of mice at dosages of 60 to 65 mg/kg, respectively; these dosages are near the litter LD_{50}. The dosages which were teratogenic in animals ranged from 10.5 to 70 times the maximum recommended adult maintenance dosage of 100 mg/day of Endep and from 3.5 to 23 times the maximum recommended initial dosage for hospitalized patients (300 mg/day).

There are no adequate or well-controlled studies of Endep in pregnant women. Endep should be used during pregnancy only if the potential benefit justifies the potential risk to the fetus.

Nonteratogenic Effects: Amitriptyline HCl was tested in rats in a Segment II study at dosages up to 20 mg/kg/day. No significant adverse effects were observed in the peri- or postnatal development and growth of pups.

Nursing Mothers: Amitriptyline and its metabolite, nortriptyline, are excreted in breast milk. Because of the potential for serious adverse reactions from Endep in nursing infants, a decision should be made whether to discontinue nursing or to discontinue the drug, taking into account the importance of the drug to the mother.

Pediatric Use: Safety and effectiveness in children below the age of 12 have not been established.

Adverse Reactions: *Note:* Included in this listing which follows are a few adverse reactions which have not been reported with this specific drug. However, pharmacological similarities among the tricyclic antidepressant drugs require that each of the reactions be considered when Endep is administered.

Cardiovascular: Hypotension, hypertension, tachycardia, palpitation, myocardial infarction, arrhythmias, heart block, stroke.

CNS and Neuromuscular: Confusional states; disturbed concentration; disorientation; delusions; hallucinations; excitement; anxiety; restlessness; insomnia; nightmares; numbness; tingling and paresthesias of the extremities; peripheral neuropathy; incoordination; ataxia; tremors; seizures; alteration in EEG patterns; extrapyramidal symptoms; tinnitus.

Anticholinergic: Dry mouth, blurred vision, disturbance of accommodation, constipation, paralytic ileus, urinary retention, dilatation of urinary tract.

Allergic: Skin rash, urticaria, photosensitization, edema of face and tongue.

Hematologic: Bone marrow depression including agranulocytosis, leukopenia, eosinophilia, purpura, thrombocytopenia.

Gastrointestinal: Nausea, epigastric distress, vomiting, anorexia, stomatitis, peculiar taste, diarrhea, parotid swelling, black tongue. Rarely, hepatitis (including altered liver function and jaundice).

Endocrine: Testicular swelling and gynecomastia in the male, breast enlargement and galactorrhea in the female, increased or decreased libido, elevation and lowering of blood sugar levels, syndrome of inappropriate ADH (antidiuretic hormone) secretion.

Other: Dizziness, weakness, fatigue, headache, weight gain or loss, increased perspiration, urinary frequency, mydriasis, drowsiness, alopecia.

Withdrawal Symptoms: Abrupt cessation of treatment after prolonged administration may produce nausea, headache and malaise. These are not indicative of addiction.

Overdosage: *Manifestations:* High doses may cause temporary confusion, disturbed concentration or transient visual hallucinations. Overdosage may cause drowsiness; hypothermia; tachycardia and other arrhythmic abnormalities, such as bundle branch block; ECG evidence of impaired conduction; congestive heart failure; dilated pupils; convulsions; severe hypotension, stupor and coma. Other symptoms may be agitation, hyperactive reflexes, muscle rigidity, vomiting, hyperpyrexia or any of those listed in the ADVERSE REACTIONS section.

Treatment: **All patients suspected of having taken an overdosage should be admitted to a hospital as soon as possible.** Treatment is symptomatic and supportive. Empty the stomach as quickly as possible by emesis followed by gastric lavage upon arrival at the hospital. Following gastric lavage, activated charcoal may be administered. Twenty to 30 Gm of activated charcoal may be given every four to six hours during the first 24 to 48 hours after ingestion. An ECG should be taken and close monitoring of cardiac function instituted if there is any sign of abnormality. Maintain an open airway and adequate fluid intake; regulate body temperature.

The intravenous administration of 1 to 3 mg of physostigmine salicylate has been reported to reverse the symptoms of tricyclic antidepressant poisoning. Because physostigmine is rapidly metabolized, the dosage of physostigmine should be repeated as required, particularly if life-threatening signs such as arrhythmias, convulsions and deep coma recur or persist after the initial dosage of physostigmine. Because physostigmine itself may be toxic, it is not recommended for routine use.

Standard measures should be used to manage circulatory shock and metabolic acidosis. Cardiac arrhythmias may be treated with neostigmine, pyridostigmine or propranolol. Should cardiac failure occur, the use of digitalis should be considered. Close monitoring of cardiac function for not less than five days is advisable. Anticonvulsants may be given to control convulsions. Amitriptyline increases the CNS depressant action but not the anticonvulsant action of barbiturates; therefore, an inhalation anesthetic, diazepam or paraldehyde is recommended for control of convulsions. Dialysis is of no value because of low plasma concentrations of the drug.

Since overdosage is often deliberate, patients may attempt suicide by other means during the recovery phase.

Deaths by deliberate or accidental overdosage have occurred with this class of drugs.

The acute oral toxicity of amitriptyline HCl is as follows:

Species	$LD_{50} \pm$ S.E. (mg/kg)
Mouse	260 ± 16
Rat	617 ± 50
Rabbit	446 ± 32
Dog ~	~ 290

Dosage and Administration: *Oral Dosage:* Dosage should be initiated at a low level and increased gradually, noting carefully the clinical response and any evidence of intolerance.

Initial Dosage for Adults: Twenty-five mg 3 times a day usually is satisfactory for outpatients. If necessary, this may be increased to a total of 150 mg a day. Increases are made preferably in the late afternoon and/or bedtime doses. A sedative effect may be apparent before the antidepressant effect is noted, but an adequate therapeutic effect may take as long as 30 days to develop.

An alternative method of initiating therapy in outpatients is to begin with 50 to 100 mg amitriptyline HCl at bedtime. This may be increased by 25 to 50 mg as necessary in the bedtime dose to a total of 150 mg per day.

Hospitalized patients may require 100 mg a day initially. This can be increased gradually to 200 mg a day if necessary. A small number of hospitalized patients may need as much as 300 mg a day.

Adolescent and Elderly Patients: In general, lower dosages are recommended for these patients. Ten mg 3 times a day with 20 mg at bedtime may be satisfactory in adolescent and elderly patients who do not tolerate higher dosages.

Maintenance: The usual maintenance dosage of amitriptyline HCl is 50 to 100 mg per day. In some patients 40 mg per day is sufficient. For maintenance therapy the total daily dosage may be given in a single dose preferably at bedtime. When satisfactory improvement has been reached, dosage should be reduced to the lowest amount that will maintain relief of symptoms. It is appropriate to continue maintenance therapy 3 months or longer to lessen the possibility of relapse.

Usage in Children: In view of the lack of experience in children, this drug is not recommended at the present time for patients under 12 years of age.

How Supplied: 10-mg tablets, orange, round, film-coated, scored—bottles of 100 (NDC 0140-0106-01); Tel-E-Dose® packages of 100 (NDC 0140-0106-49). Imprint on tablets: ENDEP 10 ROCHE.

25-mg tablets, orange, round, film-coated, scored—bottles of 100 (NDC 0140-0107-01) and 500 (NDC 0140-0107-14); Tel-E-Dose® packages of 100 (NDC 0140-0107-49). Imprint on tablets: ENDEP 25 ROCHE.

50-mg tablets, orange, round, film-coated, scored—bottles of 100 (NDC 0140-0109-01) and 500 (NDC 0140-0109-14); Tel-E-Dose® packages of 100 (NDC 0140-0109-49). Imprint on tablets: ENDEP 50 ROCHE.

75-mg tablets, yellow, round, film-coated, scored—bottles of 100 (NDC 0140-0114-01); Tel-E-Dose®

packages of 100 (NDC 0140-0114-49). Imprint on tablets: ENDEP 75 ROCHE.
100-mg tablets, peach, round, film-coated, scored—bottles of 100 (NDC 0140-0116-01); Tel-E-Dose® packages of 100 (NDC 0140-0116-49). Imprint on tablets: ENDEP 100 ROCHE.
150-mg tablets, salmon, round, film-coated, scored—bottles of 100 (NDC 0140-0124-01). Imprint on tablets: ENDEP 150 ROCHE.
Shown in Product Identification Section, page 429

LIBRAX®
[lib'rax]

The following text is complete prescribing information based on official labeling in effect August 1, 1984.

Composition: Each capsule contains 5 mg chlordiazepoxide hydrochloride (Librium®) and 2.5 mg clidinium bromide (Quarzan®).

Description: Librax combines in a single capsule formulation the antianxiety action of Librium (chlordiazepoxide hydrochloride/Roche) and the anticholinergic/spasmolytic effects of Quarzan (clidinium bromide/Roche), both exclusive developments of Roche research.
Librium (chlordiazepoxide hydrochloride/Roche) is a versatile therapeutic agent of proven value for the relief of anxiety and tension. It is indicated when anxiety, tension or apprehension are significant components of the clinical profile. It is among the safer of the effective psychopharmacologic compounds.
Chlordiazepoxide hydrochloride is 7-chloro-2-methylamino-5-phenyl- 3 H -1, 4-benzodiazepine 4-oxide hydrochloride. A colorless, crystalline substance, it is soluble in water. It is unstable in solution and the powder must be protected from light. The molecular weight is 336.22.
Quarzan (clidinium bromide/Roche) is a synthetic anticholinergic agent which has been shown in experimental and clinical studies to have a pronounced antispasmodic and antisecretory effect on the gastrointestinal tract.

Animal Pharmacology: Chlordiazepoxide hydrochloride has been studied extensively in many species of animals and these studies are suggestive of action on the limbic system of the brain,[1,2,3] which recent evidence indicates is involved in emotional responses.[4,5]
Hostile monkeys were made tame by oral drug doses which did not cause sedation. Chlordiazepoxide hydrochloride revealed a "taming" action with the elimination of fear and aggression.[6] The taming effect of chlordiazepoxide hydrochloride was further demonstrated in rats made vicious by lesions in the septal area of the brain. The drug dosage which effectively blocked the vicious reaction was well below the dose which caused sedation in these animals.[6]
The oral LD$_{50}$ of single doses of chlordiazepoxide hydrochloride, calculated according to the method of Miller and Tainter,[7] is 720 ± 51 mg/kg as determined in mice observed over a period of five days following dosage.
Clidinium bromide is an effective anticholinergic agent with activity approximating that of atropine sulfate against acetylcholine-induced spasms in isolated intestinal strips. On oral administration in mice it proved an effective antisialagogue in preventing pilocarpine-induced salivation. Spontaneous intestinal motility in both rats and dogs is reduced following oral dosing with 0.1 to 0.25 mg/kg. Potent cholinergic ganglionic blocking effects (vagal) are produced with intravenous usage in anesthetized dogs.
Oral doses of 2.5 mg/kg to dogs produced signs of nasal dryness and slight pupillary dilation. In two other species, monkeys and rabbits, doses of 5 mg/kg, p.o., given three times daily for 5 days did not produce apparent secretory or visual changes.
The oral LD$_{50}$ of single doses of clidinium bromide is 860±57 mg/kg as determined in mice observed over a period of 5 days following dosage; the calculations were made according to the method of Miller and Tainter.[7]
Effects on Reproduction: Reproduction studies in rats fed chlordiazepoxide hydrochloride, 10, 20 and 80 mg/kg daily, and bred through one or two matings showed no congenital anomalies, nor were there adverse effects on lactation of the dams or growth of the newborn. However, in another study at 100 mg/kg daily there was noted a significant decrease in the fertilization rate and a marked decrease in the viability and body weight of offspring which may be attributable to sedative activity, thus resulting in lack of interest in mating and lessened maternal nursing and care of the young.[8,9] One neonate in each of the first and second matings in the rat reproduction study at the 100 mg/kg dose exhibited major skeletal defects. Further studies are in progress to determine the significance of these findings.
Two series of reproduction experiments with clidinium bromide were carried out in rats, employing dosages of 2.5 and 10 mg/kg daily in each experiment. In the first experiment clidinium bromide was administered for a 9-week interval prior to mating; no untoward effect on fertilization or gestation was noted. The offspring were taken by caesarean section and did not show a significant incidence of congenital anomalies when compared to control animals. In the second experiment adult animals were given clidinium bromide for ten days prior to and through two mating cycles. No significant effects were observed on fertility, gestation, viability of offspring or lactation, as compared to control animals, nor was there a significant incidence of congenital anomalies in the offspring derived from these experiments.
A reproduction study of Librax was carried out in rats through two successive matings. Oral daily doses were administered in two concentrations: 2.5 mg/kg chlordiazepoxide hydrochloride with 1.25 mg/kg clidinium bromide, or 25 mg/kg chlordiazepoxide hydrochloride with 12.5 mg/kg clidinium bromide. In the first mating no significant differences were noted between the control or the treated groups, with the exception of a slight decrease in the number of animals surviving during lactation among those receiving the highest dosage. As with all anticholinergic drugs, an inhibiting effect on lactation may occur. In the second mating similar results were obtained except for a slight decrease in the number of pregnant females and in the percentage of offspring surviving until weaning. No congenital anomalies were observed in both matings in either the control or treated groups. Additional animal reproduction studies are in progress.

Indications: Based on a review of this drug by the National Academy of Sciences—National Research Council and/or other information, FDA has classified the indications as follows:
"Possibly" effective: as adjunctive therapy in the treatment of peptic ulcer and in the treatment of the irritable bowel syndrome (irritable colon, spastic colon, mucous colitis) and acute enterocolitis.
Final classification of the less-than-effective indications requires further investigation.

Contraindications: Librax is contraindicated in the presence of glaucoma (since the anticholinergic component may produce some degree of mydriasis) and in patients with prostatic hypertrophy and benign bladder neck obstruction. It is contraindicated in patients with known hypersensitivity to chlordiazepoxide hydrochloride and/or clidinium bromide.

Warnings: As in the case of other preparations containing CNS-acting drugs, patients receiving Librax should be cautioned about possible combined effects with alcohol and other CNS depressants. For the same reason, they should be cautioned against hazardous occupations requiring complete mental alertness such as operating machinery or driving a motor vehicle.
Physical and Psychological Dependence: Physical and psychological dependence have rarely been reported in persons taking recommended doses of Librium (chlordiazepoxide hydrochloride/Roche). However, caution must be exercised in administering Librium to individuals known to be addiction-prone or those whose history suggests they may increase the dosage on their own initiative. Withdrawal symptoms following discontinuation of chlordiazepoxide hydrochloride have been reported.[10] These symptoms (including convulsions) are similar to those seen with barbiturates.
Usage in Pregnancy: **An increased risk of congenital malformations associated with the use of minor tranquilizers (chlordiazepoxide, diazepam and meprobamate) during the first trimester of pregnancy has been suggested in several studies. Because use of these drugs is rarely a matter of urgency, their use during this period should almost always be avoided. The possibility that a woman of childbearing potential may be pregnant at the time of institution of therapy should be considered. Patients should be advised that if they become pregnant during therapy or intend to become pregnant they should communicate with their physicians about the desirability of discontinuing the drug.**
As with all anticholinergic drugs, an inhibiting effect on lactation may occur. (See Animal Pharmacology.)
Management of Overdosage: Manifestations of Librium (chlordiazepoxide hydrochloride/Roche) overdosage include somnolence, confusion, coma and diminished reflexes. Respiration, pulse and blood pressure should be monitored, as in all cases of drug overdosage, although, in general, these effects have been minimal following Librium overdosage.
While the signs and symptoms of Librax overdosage may be produced by either of its components, usually such symptoms will be overshadowed by the anticholinergic actions of Quarzan (clidinium bromide/Roche). The symptoms of overdosage of Quarzan are excessive dryness of mouth, blurring of vision, urinary hesitancy and constipation.
General supportive measures should be employed, along with immediate gastric lavage. Administer physostigmine (Antilirium) 0.5 to 2 mg at a rate of no more than 1 mg per minute. This may be repeated in 1 to 4 mg doses if arrhythmias, convulsions or deep coma recur. Intravenous fluids should be administered and an adequate airway maintained. Hypotension may be combated by the use of Levophed® (levarterenol) or Aramine (metaraminol). Ritalin (methylphenidate) or caffeine and sodium benzoate may be given to combat CNS-depressive effects. Dialysis is of limited value. Should excitation occur, barbiturates should not be used. As with the management of intentional overdosage with any drug, it should be borne in mind that multiple agents may have been ingested.
Precautions: In elderly and debilitated patients, it is recommended that the dosage be limited to the smallest effective amount to preclude the development of ataxia, oversedation, or confusion (not more than two Librax capsules per day initially, to be increased gradually as needed and tolerated). In general, the concomitant administration of Librax and other psychotropic agents is not recommended. If such combination therapy seems indicated, careful consideration should be given to the pharmacology of the agents to be employed—particularly when the known potentiating compounds such as the MAO inhibitors and phenothiazines are to be used. The usual precautions in treating patients with impaired renal or hepatic function should be observed.
Paradoxical reactions to chlordiazepoxide hydrochloride, *e.g.*, excitement, stimulation and acute rage, have been reported in psychiatric patients and should be watched for during Librax therapy. The usual precautions are indicated when chlordiazepoxide hydrochloride is used in the treatment of anxiety states where there is any evidence of impending depression; it should be borne in mind that suicidal tendencies may be present and protective measures may be necessary. Although clinical studies have not established a cause and effect

Continued on next page

Roche Products—Cont.

relationship, physicians should be aware that variable effects on blood coagulation have been reported very rarely in patients receiving oral anticoagulants and Librium.

Adverse Reactions:[11] No side effects or manifestations not seen with either compound alone have been reported with the administration of Librax. However, since Librax contains chlordiazepoxide hydrochloride and clidinium bromide, the possibility of untoward effects which may be seen with either of these two compounds cannot be excluded. When chlordiazepoxide hydrochloride has been used alone the necessity of discontinuing therapy because of undesirable effects has been rare.[12] Drowsiness,[13] ataxia[14] and confusion[9] have been reported in some patients—particularly the elderly and debilitated.[9] While these effects can be avoided in almost all instances by proper dosage adjustment, they have occasionally been observed at the lower dosage ranges. In a few instances syncope has been reported.[15]
Other adverse reactions reported during therapy with Librium (chlordiazepoxide hydrochloride/Roche) include isolated instances of skin eruptions,[13] edema,[16] minor menstrual irregularities,[13] nausea and constipation,[17] extrapyramidal symptoms,[9] as well as increased and decreased libido. Such side effects have been infrequent and are generally controlled with reduction of dosage. Changes in EEG patterns (low-voltage fast activity) have been observed in patients during and after Librium treatment.[18]
Blood dyscrasias,[11] including agranulocytosis,[19] jaundice and hepatic dysfunction[20] have occasionally been reported during therapy with Librium. When Librium treatment is protracted, periodic blood counts and liver function tests are advisable.
Adverse effects reported with use of *Librax* are those typical of anticholinergic agents, *i.e.*, dryness of the mouth, blurring of vision, urinary hesitancy and constipation. Constipation has occurred most often when Librax therapy has been combined with other spasmolytic agents and/or a low residue diet.

Dosage: Because of the varied individual responses to tranquilizers and anticholinergics, the optimum dosage of Librax varies with the diagnosis and response of the individual patient. The dosage, therefore, should be individualized for maximum beneficial effects. The usual maintenance dose is 1 or 2 capsules, 3 or 4 times a day administered before meals and at bedtime.

How Supplied: Librax is available in green capsules, each containing 5 mg chlordiazepoxide hydrochloride (Librium®) and 2.5 mg clidinium bromide (Quarzan®)—bottles of 100 and 500; Tel-E-Dose® packages of 100.

References:
1. Schallek, W., *et al:* Arch. Int. Pharmacodyn. *149:*467-483, 1964.
2. Himwich, H. E., *et al:* J. Neuropsych. *3* (Suppl. 1):S15-S26, August 1962.
3. Morillo, A., *et al:* Psychopharmacologia *3* (No. 5):386-394, 1962.
4. MacLean, P. D.: Psychosomatic Med. *17:*355-366, September 1955.
5. Morgan, C. T.: Physiological Psychology, 3rd Ed.; New York, McGraw-Hill, 1965.
6. Randall, L. O. *et al:*J. Pharm. Exper. Therap. *129:*163-171, June 1960.
7. Miller, L. C. and Tainter, M. C.: Proc. Soc. Exp. Biol. Med. 57:261, 1944.
8. Zbinden, G., *et al:* Toxicology and Applied Pharmacology *3:*619-637, November 1961.
9. Data on file, Hoffmann-La Roche Inc., Nutley, New Jersey.
10. Hollister, L. E., *et al:* Psychopharmacologia *2:*63-68, 1961.
11. Bibliography and References available on request from Roche Laboratories.
12. Rickels, K. *et al:* Med. Times *93:*238-245, March 1965.
13. Tobin, J. M. *et al:* J. Amer. Med. Assoc. *174:*1242-1249, November 1960.
14. Jenner, F. A., *et al:* J. Ment. Sci. *107:*575-582, May 1961.
15. Robinson, R. C. V.: Dis. Nerv. System *21:*43-45, March 1960.
16. Rose, J. T.: Amer. J. Psychiat. *120:*899-900, March 1964.
17. Hines, L. R.: Curr. Therap. Res. *2:*227-236, June 1960.
18. Gibbs, F. A. and Gibbs, E. L.: J. Neuropsych., 3 (Suppl. 1):S73-S78, August 1962.
19. Kaelbling, R., *et al:* J. Amer. Med. Assoc. *174:*1863-1865, December 1960.
20. Cacioppo, J., *et al:* Amer. J. Psychiat. *117:*1040-1041, May 1961.

Shown in Product Identification Section, page 430

LIBRIUM® CAPSULES ℞
[lib′ ree-um]
(chlordiazepoxide HCl/Roche)
LIBRITABS® ℞
[lib′ rit-abs]
(chlordiazepoxide/Roche)

The following text is complete prescribing information based on official labeling in effect August 1, 1984.

Description: Librium (the original chlordiazepoxide HCl) and Libritabs (the original chlordiazepoxide), prototypes for the benzodiazepine compounds, were synthesized and developed at Hoffmann-La Roche Inc. They are versatile therapeutic agents of proven value for the relief of anxiety, and are among the safer of the effective psychopharmacologic compounds available, as demonstrated by extensive clinical evidence.

Chlordiazepoxide hydrochloride is 7-chloro-2-(methylamino) 5-phenyl-3H-1,4-benzodiazepine 4-oxide hydrochloride. A white to practically white crystalline substance, it is soluble in water. It is unstable in solution and the powder must be protected from light. The molecular weight is 336.22.
Chlordiazepoxide is 7-chloro-2-(methylamino)-5-phenyl-3H-1,4-benzodiazepine 4-oxide. A yellow crystalline substance, it is insoluble in water. The powder must be protected from light. The molecular weight is 299.76.

Actions: Librium (chlordiazepoxide HCl/Roche) and Libritabs (chlordiazepoxide/Roche) have antianxiety, sedative, appetite-stimulating and weak analgesic actions. The precise mechanism of action is not known. The drugs block EEG arousal from stimulation of the brain stem reticular formation. It takes several hours for peak blood levels to be reached and the half-life of the drugs is between 24 and 48 hours. After Librium or Libritabs is discontinued plasma levels decline slowly over a period of several days. Chlordiazepoxide is excreted in the urine, with 1 to 2% unchanged and 3 to 6% as a conjugate.

Indications: Librium and Libritabs are indicated for the management of anxiety disorders or for the short-term relief of symptoms of anxiety, withdrawal symptoms of acute alcoholism, and preoperative apprehension and anxiety. Anxiety or tension associated with the stress of everyday life usually does not require treatment with an anxiolytic.
The effectiveness of Librium or Libritabs in long-term use, that is, more than 4 months, has not been assessed by systematic clinical studies. The physician should periodically reassess the usefulness of the drug for the individual patient.

Contraindications: Librium and Libritabs are contraindicated in patients with known hypersensitivity to the drug.

Warnings: Chlordiazepoxide HCl and chlordiazepoxide may impair the mental and/or physical abilities required for the performance of potentially hazardous tasks such as driving a vehicle or operating machinery. Similarly, they may impair mental alertness in children. The concomitant use of alcohol or other central nervous system depressants may have an additive effect. PATIENTS SHOULD BE WARNED ACCORDINGLY.
Physical and Psychological Dependence: Physical and psychological dependence have rarely been reported in persons taking recommended doses of chlordiazepoxide HCl or chlordiazepoxide. However, caution must be exercised in administering chlordiazepoxide HCl or chlordiazepoxide to individuals known to be addiction-prone or those whose histories suggest they may increase the dosage on their own initiative. Withdrawal symptoms following abrupt discontinuation of chlordiazepoxide HCl or chlordiazepoxide have been reported in patients receiving excessive doses over extended periods of time. These symptoms (including convulsions) are similar to those seen with barbiturates. Although infrequently seen, milder withdrawal symptoms have also been reported following abrupt discontinuance of benzodiazepines taken continuously, generally at higher therapeutic levels, for at least several months. Consequently, after extended therapy, abrupt discontinuation should generally be avoided and a gradual tapering in dosage followed.

Usage in Pregnancy: An increased risk of congenital malformations associated with the use of minor tranquilizers (chlordiazepoxide, diazepam and meprobamate) during the first trimester of pregnancy has been suggested in several studies. Because use of these drugs is rarely a matter of urgency, their use during this period should almost always be avoided. The possibility that a woman of childbearing potential may be pregnant at the time of institution of therapy should be considered. Patients should be advised that if they become pregnant during therapy or intend to become pregnant they should communicate with their physicians about the desirability of discontinuing the drug.

Precautions: In elderly and debilitated patients, it is recommended that the dosage be limited to the smallest effective amount to preclude the development of ataxia or oversedation (10 mg or less per day initially, to be increased gradually as needed and tolerated). In general, the concomitant administration of Librium or Libritabs and other psychotropic agents is not recommended. If such combination therapy seems indicated, careful consideration should be given to the pharmacology of the agents to be employed — particularly when the known potentiating compounds such as the MAO inhibitors and phenothiazines are to be used. The usual precautions in treating patients with impaired renal or hepatic function should be observed.
Paradoxical reactions, *e.g.,* excitement, stimulation and acute rage, have been reported in psychiatric patients and in hyperactive aggressive children, and should be watched for during Librium or Libritabs therapy. The usual precautions are indicated when Librium or Libritabs is used in the treatment of anxiety states where there is any evidence of impending depression; it should be borne in mind that suicidal tendencies may be present and protective measures may be necessary. Although clinical studies have not established a cause and effect relationship, physicians should be aware that variable effects on blood coagulation have been reported very rarely in patients receiving oral anticoagulants and Librium or Libritabs. In view of isolated reports associating chlordiazepoxide HCl and chlordiazepoxide with exacerbation of porphyria, caution should be exercised in prescribing these agents to patients suffering from this disease.

Adverse Reactions: The necessity of discontinuing therapy because of undesirable effects has been rare. Drowsiness, ataxia and confusion have been reported in some patients — particularly the elderly and debilitated. While these effects can be avoided in almost all instances by proper dosage adjustment, they have occasionally been observed at the lower dosage ranges. In a few instances syncope has been reported.
Other adverse reactions reported during therapy include isolated instances of skin eruptions, edema, minor menstrual irregularities, nausea and constipation, extrapyramidal symptoms, as well as increased and decreased libido. Such side effects have been infrequent and are generally controlled with reduction of dosage. Changes in EEG patterns (low-voltage fast activity) have been

observed in patients during and after Librium or Libritabs treatment.

Blood dyscrasias (including agranulocytosis), jaundice and hepatic dysfunction have occasionally been reported during therapy. When Librium or Libritabs treatment is protracted, periodic blood counts and liver function tests are advisable.

Dosage and Administration: Because of the wide range of clinical indications for Librium and Libritabs, the optimum dosage varies with the diagnosis and response of the individual patient. The dosage, therefore, should be individualized for maximum beneficial effects.

ADULTS	Usual Daily Dose
Relief of mild and moderate anxiety disorders and symptoms of anxiety	5 mg or 10 mg, 3 or 4 times daily
Relief of severe anxiety disorders and symptoms of anxiety	20 mg or 25 mg, 3 or 4 times daily
Geriatric patients, or in the presence of debilitating disease	5 mg, 2 to 4 times daily

Preoperative apprehension and anxiety:
On days preceding surgery, 5 to 10 mg orally, 3 or 4 times daily. If used as preoperative medication, 50 to 100 mg I.M.* one hour prior to surgery.

CHILDREN	Usual Daily Dose
Because of the varied response of children to CNS-acting drugs, therapy should be initiated with the lowest dose and increased as required.	5 mg, 2 to 4 times daily (may be increased in some children to 10 mg, 2 or 3 times daily)

Since clinical experience in children under 6 years of age is limited, the use of the drug in this age group is not recommended.

For the relief of withdrawal symptoms of acute alcoholism, the parenteral form* is usually used initially. If the drug is administered orally, the suggested initial dose is 50 to 100 mg, to be followed by repeated doses as needed until agitation is controlled — up to 300 mg per day. Dosage should then be reduced to maintenance levels.

* See package insert for injectable Librium (chlordiazepoxide HCl/Roche).

Management of Overdosage: Manifestations of Librium or Libritabs overdosage include somnolence, confusion, coma and diminished reflexes. Respiration, pulse and blood pressure should be monitored, as in all cases of drug overdosage, although, in general, these effects have been minimal following Librium or Libritabs overdosage. General supportive measures should be employed, along with immediate gastric lavage. Intravenous fluids should be administered and an adequate airway maintained. Hypotension may be combated by the use of Levophed® (levarterenol) or Aramine (metaraminol). Dialysis is of limited value. There have been occasional reports of excitation in patients following chlordiazepoxide HCl or chlordiazepoxide overdosage; if this occurs barbiturates should not be used. As with the management of intentional overdosage with any drug, it should be borne in mind that multiple agents may have been ingested.

How Supplied: Librium (chlordiazepoxide HCl/Roche) capsules — 5 mg, green and yellow; 10 mg, green and black; 25 mg, green and white — bottles of 100 and 500; Tel-E-Dose® packages of 100, available in trays of 4 reverse-numbered cards of 25, and in boxes containing 10 strips of 10.

Libritabs (chlordiazepoxide/Roche) tablets — 5 mg or 10 mg or— bottles of 100 and 500; 25 mg—bottles of 100.

Shown in Product Identification Section, page 430

LIBRIUM® INJECTABLE
[lib'ree-um]
(chlordiazepoxide HCl/Roche)

Librium Injectable is manufactured by Hoffmann-La Roche Inc., Nutley, N.J. 07110 and distributed by Roche Products Inc., Manati, P.R. 00701.

The following text is complete prescribing information based on official labeling in effect August 1, 1984.

Description: Librium is a versatile therapeutic agent of proven value for the relief of anxiety and tension.

Librium is the first of a new class, unrelated chemically and pharmacologically to other types of tranquilizers. Librium promptly relieves anxiety and is among the safer of the effective psychopharmacologic compounds available.

Chlordiazepoxide HCl is 7-chloro-2-methylamino-5-phenyl-3H-1,4-benzodiazepine 4-oxide hydrochloride. A colorless, crystalline substance, it is soluble in water. It is unstable in solution and the powder must be protected from light. The molecular weight is 336.22.

Animal Pharmacology: The drug has been studied extensively in many species of animals and these studies are suggestive of action on the limbic system of the brain, which recent evidence indicates is involved in emotional responses.

Hostile monkeys were made tame by oral drug doses which did not cause sedation. Librium revealed a "taming" action with the elimination of fear and aggression. The taming effect of Librium was further demonstrated in rats made vicious by lesions in the septal area of the brain. The drug dosage which effectively blocked the vicious reaction was well below the dose which caused sedation in these animals.

The LD_{50} of parenterally administered chlordiazepoxide HCl was determined in mice (72 hours) and rats (5 days), and calculated according to the method of Miller and Tainter, with the following results: mice, I.V., 123 ± 12 mg/kg; mice, I.M., 366 ± 7 mg/kg; rats, I.V., 120 ± 7 mg/kg; rats, I.M., > 160 mg/kg.

Effects on Reproduction: Reproduction studies in rats fed 10, 20 and 80 mg/kg daily and bred through one or two matings showed no congenital anomalies, nor were there adverse effects on lactation of the dams or growth of the newborn. However, in another study at 100 mg/kg daily there was noted a significant decrease in the fertilization rate and a marked decrease in the viability and body weight of offspring which may be attributable to sedative activity, thus resulting in lack of interest in mating and lessened maternal nursing and care of the young. One neonate in each of the first and second matings in the rat reproduction study at the 100 mg/kg dose exhibited major skeletal defects. Further studies are in progress to determine the significance of these findings.

Indications: Injectable Librium is indicated for the management of anxiety disorders or for the short-term relief of symptoms of anxiety, withdrawal symptoms of acute alcoholism, and preoperative apprehension and anxiety. Anxiety or tension associated with the stress of everyday life usually does not require treatment with an anxiolytic.

Contraindications: Librium is contraindicated in patients with known hypersensitivity to the drug.

Warnings: As in the case of other CNS-acting drugs, patients receiving Librium should be cautioned about possible combined effects with alcohol and other CNS depressants.

As is true of all preparations containing CNS-acting drugs, patients receiving Librium should be cautioned against hazardous occupations requiring complete mental alertness such as operating machinery or driving a motor vehicle.

Physical and Psychological Dependence: Physical and psychological dependence have rarely been reported in persons taking recommended doses of Librium. However, caution must be exercised in administering Librium to individuals known to be addiction-prone or those whose history suggests they may increase the dosage on their own initiative. Withdrawal symptoms following abrupt discontinuation of chlordiazepoxide HCl have been reported in patients receiving excessive doses over extended periods of time. These symptoms (including convulsions) are similar to those seen with barbiturates. Although infrequently seen, milder withdrawal symptoms have also been reported following abrupt discontinuance of benzodiazepines taken continuously, generally at higher therapeutic levels, for at least several months. Consequently, after extended therapy, abrupt discontinuation should generally be avoided and a gradual tapering in dosage followed.

Usage in Pregnancy: An increased risk of congenital malformations associated with the use of minor tranquilizers (chlordiazepoxide, diazepam and meprobamate) during the first trimester of pregnancy has been suggested in several studies. Because use of these drugs is rarely a matter of urgency, their use during this period should almost always be avoided. The possibility that a woman of childbearing potential may be pregnant at the time of institution of therapy should be considered. Patients should be advised that if they become pregnant during therapy or intend to become pregnant they should communicate with their physicians about the desirability of discontinuing the drug.

Management of Overdosage: Manifestations of Librium overdosage include somnolence, confusion, coma and diminished reflexes. Respiration, pulse and blood pressure should be monitored, as in all cases of drug overdosage, although, in general, these effects have been minimal following Librium overdosage. General supportive measures should be employed, along with immediate gastric lavage. Intravenous fluids should be administered and an adequate airway maintained. Hypotension may be combated by the use of Levophed® (levarterenol) or Aramine (metaraminol). Dialysis is of limited value. There have been occasional reports of excitation in patients following Librium overdosage; if this occurs barbiturates should not be used. As with the management of intentional overdosage with any drug, it should be borne in mind that multiple agents may have been ingested.

Precautions: Injectable Librium (intramuscular or intravenous) is indicated primarily in acute states, and patients receiving this form of therapy should be kept under observation, preferably in bed, for a period of up to three hours. Ambulatory patients should not be permitted to operate a vehicle following an injection. Injectable Librium should not be given to patients in shock or comatose states. Reduced dosage (usually 25 to 50 mg) should be used for elderly or debilitated patients, and for children age twelve or older. In general, the concomitant administration of Librium and other psychotropic agents is not recommended. If such combination therapy seems indicated, careful consideration should be given to the pharmacology of the agents to be employed—particularly when the known potentiating compounds such as the MAO inhibitors and phenothiazines are to be used. The usual precautions in treating patients with impaired renal or hepatic function should be observed.

Paradoxical reactions, *e.g.*, excitement, stimulation and acute rage, have been reported in psychiatric patients and in hyperactive aggressive children, and should be watched for during Librium therapy. The usual precautions are indicated when Librium is used in the treatment of anxiety states where there is any evidence of impending depression; it should be borne in mind that suicidal tendencies may be present and protective measures may be necessary. Although clinical studies have not established a cause and effect relationship, physicians should be aware that variable effects on blood coagulation have been reported very rarely in patients receiving oral anticoagulants and Librium. In view of isolated reports associating chlordiazepoxide with exacerbation of porphyria, caution should be exercised in

Continued on next page

Roche Products—Cont.

prescribing chlordiazepoxide to patients suffering from this disease.

Adverse Reactions: The necessity of discontinuing therapy because of undesirable effects has been rare. Drowsiness, ataxia and confusion are more commonly seen in the elderly and debilitated.

Other adverse reactions reported during therapy include isolated instances of syncope, hypotension, tachycardia, skin eruptions, edema, minor menstrual irregularities, nausea and constipation, extrapyramidal symptoms, blurred vision, as well as increased and decreased libido. Such side effects have been infrequent and are generally controlled with reduction of dosage. Similarly, hypotension associated with spinal anesthesia has occurred. Pain following intramuscular injection has been reported. Changes in EEG patterns (low-voltage fast activity) have been observed in patients during and after Librium treatment.

Blood dyscrasias (including agranulocytosis), jaundice and hepatic dysfunction, have occasionally been reported during therapy. When Librium treatment is protracted, periodic blood counts and liver function tests are advisable.

Preparation and Administration of Solutions: Solutions of Librium for intramuscular or intravenous use should be prepared aseptically. Sterilization by heating should not be attempted.

Intramuscular: Add 2 ml of *Special Intramuscular Diluent* to contents of 5-ml dry-filled amber ampul of Librium Sterile Powder (100 mg). Avoid excessive pressure in injecting this special diluent into the ampul containing the powder since bubbles will form on the surface of the solution. Agitate gently until completely dissolved. Solution should be prepared immediately before administration. Any unused solution should be discarded. Deep intramuscular injection should be given *slowly* into the upper outer quadrant of the gluteus muscle.

Caution: Although the Librium preparation made with the intramuscular diluent has been given intravenously without untoward effects, such administration is not recommended because of the air bubbles which form when the intramuscular diluent is added to the Librium powder. Do not use diluent solution if it is opalescent or hazy.

Intravenous: In most cases, intramuscular injection is the preferred route of administration of Injectable Librium since beneficial effects are usually seen within 15 to 30 minutes. When, in the judgment of the physician, even more rapid action is mandatory, Injectable Librium may be administered intravenously. A suitable solution for intravenous administration may be prepared as follows: Add 5 ml of *sterile physiological saline* or *sterile water for injection* to contents of 5-ml dry-filled amber ampul of Librium Sterile Powder (100 mg). Agitate gently until thoroughly dissolved. Solution should be prepared immediately before administration. Any unused portion should be discarded. *Intravenous injection should be given slowly over a one-minute period.*

Caution: Librium solution made with physiological saline or sterile water for injection should not be given intramuscularly because of pain on injection.

Dosage: Dosage should be individualized according to the diagnosis and the response of the patient. While 300 mg may be given during a 6-hour period, this dose should not be exceeded in any 24-hour period.

INDICATION	ADULT DOSAGE*
Withdrawal Symptoms of Acute Alcoholism	50 to 100 mg I.M. or I.V. initially; repeat in 2 to 4 hours, if necessary
Acute or Severe Anxiety Disorders or Symptoms of Anxiety	50 to 100 mg I.M. or I.V. initially; then 25 to 50 mg 3 or 4 times daily, if necessary
Preoperative Apprehension and Anxiety	50 to 100 mg I.M. one hour prior to surgery

* Lower doses (usually 25 to 50 mg) should be used for elderly or debilitated patients, and for older children. Since clinical experience in children under 12 years of age is limited, the use of the drug in this age group is not recommended.

In most cases, acute symptoms may be rapidly controlled by parenteral administration so that subsequent treatment, if necessary, may be given orally. (See package insert for Oral Librium.)

How Supplied: For Parenteral Administration: Ampuls—Duplex package consisting of a 5-ml dry-filled ampul containing 100 mg chlordiazepoxide HCl in dry crystalline form, and a 2-ml ampul of Special Intramuscular Diluent (for intramuscular administration) compounded with 1.5% benzyl alcohol, 4% polysorbate 80, 20% propylene glycol, 1.6% maleic acid and sodium hydroxide to adjust pH to approximately 3.0. Boxes of 10.

Caution: Before preparing solution for intramuscular or intravenous administration, please read instructions for PREPARATION AND ADMINISTRATION OF SOLUTIONS.

LIMBITROL® TABLETS
[lim'bit-roll]

LIMBITROL 10–25
Each tablet contains 10 mg chlordiazepoxide and 25 mg amitriptyline in the form of the hydrochloride salt.

LIMBITROL 5–12.5
Each tablet contains 5 mg chlordiazepoxide and 12.5 mg amitriptyline in the form of the hydrochloride salt.

The following text is complete prescribing information based on official labeling in effect August 1, 1984.

Description: Limbitrol combines in a tablet for oral administration, chlordiazepoxide, an agent for the relief of anxiety and tension, and amitriptyline, an antidepressant.

Chlordiazepoxide is a benzodiazepine with the formula 7-chloro-2-(methylamino)-5-phenyl-3H-1,4-benzodiazepine 4-oxide. It is a slightly yellow crystalline material and is insoluble in water. The molecular weight is 299.76.

Amitriptyline is a dibenzocycloheptadiene derivative. The formula is 10,11-dihydro-N,N-dimethyl-5H-dibenzo [a, d] cycloheptene-$\Delta^{5,\gamma}$-propylamine hydrochloride. It is a white or practically white crystalline compound that is freely soluble in water. The molecular weight is 313.87.

Actions: Both components of Limbitrol exert their action in the central nervous system. Extensive studies with chlordiazepoxide in many animal species suggest action in the limbic system. Recent evidence indicates that the limbic system is involved in emotional response. Taming action was observed in some species. The mechanism of action of amitriptyline in man is not known, but the drug appears to interfere with the reuptake of norepinephrine into adrenergic nerve endings. This action may prolong the sympathetic activity of biogenic amines.

Indications: Limbitrol is indicated for the treatment of patients with moderate to severe depression associated with moderate to severe anxiety. The therapeutic response to Limbitrol occurs earlier and with fewer treatment failures than when either amitriptyline or chlordiazepoxide is used alone.

Symptoms likely to respond in the first week of treatment include: insomnia, feelings of guilt or worthlessness, agitation, psychic and somatic anxiety, suicidal ideation and anorexia.

Contraindications: Limbitrol is contraindicated in patients with hypersensitivity to either benzodiazepines or tricyclic antidepressants. It should not be given concomitantly with a monoamine oxidase inhibitor. Hyperpyretic crises, severe convulsions and deaths have occurred in patients receiving a tricyclic antidepressant and a monoamine oxidase inhibitor simultaneously. When it is desired to replace a monoamine oxidase inhibitor with Limbitrol, a minimum of 14 days should be allowed to elapse after the former is discontinued. Limbitrol should then be initiated cautiously with gradual increase in dosage until optimum response is achieved.

This drug is contraindicated during the acute recovery phase following myocardial infarction.

Warnings: Because of the atropine-like action of the amitriptyline component, great care should be used in treating patients with a history of urinary retention or angle-closure glaucoma. In patients with glaucoma, even average doses may precipitate an attack. Severe constipation may occur in patients taking tricyclic antidepressants in combination with anticholinergic-type drugs.

Patients with cardiovascular disorders should be watched closely. Tricyclic antidepressant drugs, particularly when given in high doses, have been reported to produce arrhythmias, sinus tachycardia and prolongation of conduction time. Myocardial infarction and stroke have been reported in patients receiving drugs of this class.

Because of the sedative effects of Limbitrol, patients should be cautioned about combined effects with alcohol or other CNS depressants. The additive effects may produce a harmful level of sedation and CNS depression.

Patients receiving Limbitrol should be cautioned against engaging in hazardous occupations requiring complete mental alertness, such as operating machinery or driving a motor vehicle.

Usage in Pregnancy: Safe use of Limbitrol during pregnancy and lactation has not been established. Because of the chlordiazepoxide component, please note the following:

An increased risk of congenital malformations associated with the use of minor tranquilizers (chlordiazepoxide, diazepam and meprobamate) during the first trimester of pregnancy has been suggested in several studies. Because use of these drugs is rarely a matter of urgency, their use during this period should almost always be avoided. The possibility that a woman of childbearing potential may be pregnant at the time of institution of therapy should be considered. Patients should be advised that if they become pregnant during therapy or intend to become pregnant they should communicate with their physicians about the desirability of discontinuing the drug.

Physical and Psychological Dependence: Experience with Limbitrol is as yet too limited to reasonably assess the combination's potential for physical and psychological dependence. However, since physical and psychological dependence to chlordiazepoxide have been reported rarely, caution must be exercised in administering Limbitrol to individuals known to be addiction-prone or to those whose history suggests they may increase the dosage on their own initiative.

In the so far limited experience with Limbitrol withdrawal symptoms have not been reported. However, withdrawal symptoms following abrupt cessation of prolonged therapy with either component alone have been reported. With amitriptyline, these have been noted to consist of nausea, headache and malaise; for chlordiazepoxide, the symptoms (including convulsions) are similar to those seen with barbiturates.

Precautions: *General:* Use with caution in patients with a history of seizures.

Close supervision is required when Limbitrol is given to hyperthyroid patients or those on thyroid medication.

The usual precautions should be observed when treating patients with impaired renal or hepatic function.

Patients with suicidal ideation should not have easy access to large quantities of the drug. The possibility of suicide in depressed patients remains until significant remission occurs.

Essential Laboratory Tests: Patients on prolonged treatment should have periodic liver function tests and blood counts.

Drug and Treatment Interactions: Because of its amitriptyline component, Limbitrol may block the antihypertensive action of guanethidine or compounds with a similar mechanism of action.

The effects of concomitant administration of Limbitrol and other psychotropic drugs have not been evaluated. Sedative effects may be additive.
The drug should be discontinued several days before elective surgery.
Concurrent administration of ECT and Limbitrol should be limited to those patients for whom it is essential.
Pregnancy: See WARNINGS section.
Nursing Mothers: It is not known whether this drug is excreted in human milk. As a general rule, nursing should not be undertaken while a patient is on a drug, since many drugs are excreted in human milk.
Pediatric Use: Safety and effectiveness in children below the age of 12 years have not been established.
Elderly Patients: In elderly and debilitated patients it is recommended that dosage be limited to the smallest effective amount to preclude the development of ataxia, oversedation, confusion or anticholinergic effects.
Adverse Reactions: Adverse reactions to Limbitrol are those associated with the use of either component alone. Most frequently reported were drowsiness, dry mouth, constipation, blurred vision, dizziness and bloating. Other side effects occurring less commonly included vivid dreams, impotence, tremor, confusion and nasal congestion. Many symptoms common to the depressive state, such as anorexia, fatigue, weakness, restlessness and lethargy, have been reported as side effects of treatment with both Limbitrol and amitriptyline.
Granulocytopenia, jaundice and hepatic dysfunction of uncertain etiology have also been observed rarely with Limbitrol. When treatment with Limbitrol is prolonged, periodic blood counts and liver function tests are advisable.
Note: Included in the listing which follows are adverse reactions which have not been reported with Limbitrol. However, they are included because they have been reported during therapy with one or both of the components or closely related drugs.
Cardiovascular: Hypotension, hypertension, tachycardia, palpitations, myocardial infarction, arrhythmias, heart block, stroke.
Psychiatric: Euphoria, apprehension, poor concentration, delusions, hallucinations, hypomania and increased or decreased libido.
Neurologic: Incoordination, ataxia, numbness, tingling and paresthesias of the extremities, extrapyramidal symptoms, syncope, changes in EEG patterns.
Anticholinergic: Disturbance of accommodation, paralytic ileus, urinary retention, dilatation of urinary tract.
Allergic: Skin rash, urticaria, photosensitization, edema of face and tongue, pruritus.
Hematologic: Bone marrow depression including agranulocytosis, eosinophilia, purpura, thrombocytopenia.
Gastrointestinal: Nausea, epigastric distress, vomiting, anorexia, stomatitis, peculiar taste, diarrhea, black tongue.
Endocrine: Testicular swelling and gynecomastia in the male, breast enlargement, galactorrhea and minor menstrual irregularities in the female, elevation and lowering of blood sugar levels, and syndrome of inappropriate ADH (antidiuretic hormone) secretion.
Other: Headache, weight gain or loss, increased perspiration, urinary frequency, mydriasis, jaundice, alopecia, parotid swelling.
Overdosage: There has been limited experience with Limbitrol overdosage *per se;* the manifestations of overdosage and recommendations for treatment are based on clinical experience with its components. Primary concern should be with the dangers associated with amitriptyline overdosage. Deaths by deliberate or accidental overdosage have occurred with this class of drugs.
All patients suspected of having an overdosage of Limbitrol should be admitted to a hospital as soon as possible.
Manifestations: High doses may cause drowsiness, temporary confusion, disturbed concentration or transient visual hallucinations. Overdosage may cause hypothermia, tachycardia and other arrhythmias, ECG evidence of impaired conduction (such as bundle branch block), congestive heart failure, dilated pupils, convulsions, severe hypotension, stupor and coma. Other symptoms may be agitation, hyperactive reflexes, muscle rigidity, vomiting, hyperpyrexia or any of those listed under Adverse Reactions.
Treatment: Empty the stomach as quickly as possible by emesis or lavage. In the comatose patient a cuff endotracheal tube should be placed in position prior to either of these measures. The instillation of activated charcoal into the stomach also should be considered. If the patient is stuporous but responds to stimuli, only close observation and nursing care may be required. It is essential to maintain an adequate airway and fluid intake. Body temperature should be watched closely and appropriate measures taken should deviations occur.
The intramuscular or slow intravenous administration of 1 to 3 mg in adults (or 0.5 mg in children) of physostigmine salicylate (Antilirium)[1-3] has been reported to reverse the manifestations of amitriptyline overdosage. Because of its relatively short half-life, additional doses may be needed at intervals of 30 minutes to 2 hours.
Convulsions may be treated by the use of an inhalation anesthetic rather than the use of barbiturates. Cardiac monitoring is advisable, and the cautious use of digitalis or other antiarrhythmic agents should be considered if serious cardiovascular abnormalities occur. Serum potassium levels should be monitored and kept within normal limits by the use of appropriate I.V. fluids. Standard measures including oxygen, I.V. fluids, plasma expanders and corticosteroids may be used to control circulatory shock.
Dialysis is unlikely to be of value, as it has not proven useful in overdosages of either amitriptyline or chlordiazepoxide. Since many suicidal attempts involve multiple drugs including barbiturates, the possibility of dialysis being beneficial for removal of other drugs should not be overlooked.
Treatment should be continued for at least 48 hours, along with cardiac monitoring in patients who do not respond to therapy promptly. Since relapses are frequent, patients should be hospitalized until their conditions remain stable without physostigmine for at least 24 hours.
Since overdosage is often deliberate, patients may attempt suicide by other means during the recovery phase.
References:
1. Granacher RP, Baldessarini RJ: Physostigmine: Its use in acute anticholinergic syndrome with antidepressant and antiparkinson drugs. *Arch Gen Psychiatry* 32:375–380, March 1975.
2. Burks JS, Walker JE, Rumack BH, Ott JE: Tricyclic antidepressant poisoning: Reversal of coma, choreoathetosis, and myoclonus by physostigmine. *JAMA* 230:1405–1407, Dec. 9, 1974.
3. Snyder BD, Blonde L, McWhirter WR: Reversal of amitriptyline intoxication by physostigmine. *JAMA* 230:1433–1434, Dec. 9, 1974.
Dosage and Administration: Optimum dosage varies with the severity of the symptoms and the response of the individual patient. When a satisfactory response is obtained, dosage should be reduced to the smallest amount needed to maintain the remission. The larger portion of the total daily dose may be taken at bedtime. In some patients, a single dose at bedtime may be sufficient. In general, lower dosages are recommended for elderly patients.
Limbitrol 10–25 is recommended in an initial dosage of three or four tablets daily in divided doses; this may be increased to six tablets daily as required. Some patients respond to smaller doses and can be maintained on two tablets daily.
Limbitrol 5–12.5 in an initial dosage of three or four tablets daily in divided doses may be satisfactory in patients who do not tolerate higher doses.
How Supplied: White, film-coated tablets, each containing 10 mg chlordiazepoxide and 25 mg amitriptyline (as the hydrochloride salt) and blue, film-coated tablets, each containing 5 mg chlordiazepoxide and 12.5 mg amitriptyline (as the hydrochloride salt)—bottles of 100 and 500; Tel-E-Dose® packages of 100; Prescription Paks of 50.
Shown in Product Identification Section, page 430

MENRIUM® 5–2 ℞
[men'ree-um]
Each tablet contains 5 mg chlordiazepoxide and 0.2 mg water-soluble esterified estrogens.
MENRIUM® 5–4
Each tablet contains 5 mg chlordiazepoxide and 0.4 mg water-soluble esterified estrogens.
MENRIUM® 10–4
Each tablet contains 10 mg chlordiazepoxide and 0.4 mg water-soluble esterified estrogens.

The following text is complete prescribing information based on official labeling in effect August 1, 1984.

Since estrogens are a component of Menrium, please note:
1. ESTROGENS HAVE BEEN REPORTED TO INCREASE THE RISK OF ENDOMETRIAL CARCINOMA.

Three independent case control studies have shown an increased risk of endometrial cancer in postmenopausal women exposed to exogenous estrogens for prolonged periods.[1-3] This risk was independent of the other known risk factors for endometrial cancer. These studies are further supported by the finding that incidence rates of endometrial cancer have increased sharply since 1969 in eight different areas of the United States with population-based cancer reporting systems, an increase which may be related to the rapidly expanding use of estrogens during the last decade.[4] The three case control studies reported that the risk of endometrial cancer in estrogen users was about 4.5 to 13.9 times greater than in nonusers. The risk appears to depend on both duration of treatment[1] and on estrogen dose.[3] In view of these findings, when estrogens are used for the treatment of menopausal symptoms, the lowest dose that will control symptoms should be utilized and medication should be discontinued as soon as possible. When prolonged treatment is medically indicated, the patient should be reassessed on at least a semiannual basis to determine the need for continued therapy. Although the evidence must be considered preliminary, one study suggests that cyclic administration of low doses of estrogen may carry less risk than continuous administration;[3] it therefore appears prudent to utilize such a regimen.

Close clinical surveillance of all women taking estrogens is important. In all cases of undiagnosed persistent or recurring abnormal vaginal bleeding, adequate diagnostic measures should be undertaken to rule out malignancy.

There is no evidence at present that "natural" estrogens are more or less hazardous than "synthetic" estrogens at equiestrogenic doses.

2. ESTROGENS SHOULD NOT BE USED DURING PREGNANCY

The use of female sex hormones, both estrogens and progestogens, during early pregnancy may seriously damage the offspring. It has been shown that females exposed in utero to diethylstilbestrol, a non-steroidal estrogen, have an increased risk of developing, in later life, a form of vaginal or cervical cancer that is ordinarily extremely rare.[5,6] This risk has been estimated as not greater than 4 per 1000 exposures.[7] Furthermore, a high percentage of such exposed women (from 30 to 90 percent) have been found to have vaginal adenosis,[8-12] epithelial changes of the vagina and cervix.

Continued on next page

Roche Products—Cont.

Although these changes are histologically benign, it is not known whether they are precursors of malignancy. Although similar data are not available with the use of other estrogens, it cannot be presumed they would not induce similar changes.

Several reports suggest an association between intrauterine exposure to female sex hormones and congenital anomalies, including congenital heart defects and limb reduction defects.[13-16] One case control study[16] estimated a 4.7 fold increased risk of limb reduction defects in infants exposed in utero to sex hormones (oral contraceptives, hormone withdrawal tests for pregnancy, or attempted treatment for threatened abortion). Some of these exposures were very short and involved only a few days of treatment. The data suggest that the risk of limb reduction defects in exposed fetuses is somewhat less than 1 per 1,000. In the past, female sex hormones have been used during pregnancy in an attempt to treat threatened or habitual abortion. There is considerable evidence that estrogens are ineffective for these indications, and there is no evidence from well-controlled studies that progestogens are effective for these uses.

If Menrium is used during pregnancy, or if the patient becomes pregnant while taking this drug, she should be apprised of the potential risks to the fetus, and the advisability of pregnancy continuation.

Description: Menrium affords in a single formulation the psychotropic action of Librium® (chlordiazepoxide/Roche) and hormonal replacement in the form of water-soluble esterified estrogens (expressed in terms of sodium estrone sulfate) to provide comprehensive management of the menopausal syndrome or the climacteric.

Librium (chlordiazepoxide/Roche) is a versatile therapeutic agent of proven value for the relief of anxiety and tension. It is indicated when anxiety, tension or apprehension are significant components of the clinical profile. It is among the safer of the effective psychopharmacologic compounds.

Chlordiazepoxide is 7-chloro-2-methylamino-5-phenyl-3H-1, 4-benzodiazepine 4-oxide. It is a slightly yellow, crystalline material and is insoluble in water. The molecular weight is 299.75.

Water-soluble esterified estrogens provide hormonal replacement in the menopausal patient, the need for which is widely recognized and accepted. Esterified estrogens is a mixture of the sodium salts of the sulfate esters of the estrogenic substances, principally estrone, that are of the type excreted by pregnant mares. It is a white-to buff-colored, amorphous powder, odorless or having a slight, characteristic odor.

Clinical Pharmacology: The estrogenic component of Menrium is water-soluble esterified estrogens—steroidal compounds—which occur naturally. The action of this substance is substantially equal to the action of both conjugated estrogens, also naturally occurring, and synthetic estrogenic substances.

Menopausal changes, such as atrophic changes of the genital tract and breasts due to a slow decline in estrogen secretion, may be reversed by substitution therapy with estrogenic substances.

Estrogens are, in general, completely absorbed following oral administration. Estrogens are detoxified by the liver, and excretion occurs by way of the urine and the feces.

Librium (chlordiazepoxide HCl/Roche) has antianxiety and sedative actions. The drug has been studied extensively in many species of animals and these studies are suggestive of action on the limbic system of the brain, which recent evidence indicates is involved in emotional responses. However, the precise mechanism of action in man is not known. The drug blocks EEG arousal from stimulation of the brain stem reticular formation. The mean $\pm$S.E. plasma peak time is 1.4 ($\pm$0.3) hours, and the half-life ranges between 7.1 to 19.8 hours with a mean $\pm$S.E. half-life of 12.0 ($\pm$0.7) hours. After the drug is discontinued, plasma levels are usually at the lowest quantitatively detectable amounts by 48-72 hours. Chlordiazepoxide HCl is excreted in urine with 1% or less unchanged and 12 to 34% recoverable as conjugates.

Indications: Menrium is indicated in the management of the manifestations generally associated with the menopausal syndrome—anxiety and tension, vasomotor complaints and hormonal deficiency states.

MENRIUM HAS NOT BEEN SHOWN TO BE EFFECTIVE FOR ANY PURPOSE DURING PREGNANCY AND ITS USE MAY CAUSE SEVERE HARM TO THE FETUS (SEE BOXED WARNING).

Contraindications: Menrium is contraindicated in patients with known hypersensitivity to chlordiazepoxide and/or esterified estrogens.

Estrogens should not be used in women (or men) with any of the following conditions:

1. Known or suspected cancer of the breast except in appropriately selected patients being treated for metastatic disease.
2. Known or suspected estrogen-dependent neoplasia.
3. Known or suspected pregnancy. (See Boxed Warning.)
4. Undiagnosed abnormal genital bleeding.
5. Active thrombophlebitis or thromboembolic disorders.
6. A past history of thrombophlebitis, thrombosis, or thromboembolic disorders associated with previous estrogen use.

Warnings:

1. *Induction of malignant neoplasms.* Long term continuous administration of natural and synthetic estrogens in certain animal species increases the frequency of carcinomas of the breast, cervix, vagina, and liver. There is now evidence that estrogens increase the risk of carcinoma of the endometrium in humans. (See Boxed Warning.)

At the present time there is no satisfactory evidence that estrogens given to postmenopausal women increase the risk of cancer of the breast,[17] although a recent long-term followup of a single physician's practice has raised this possibility.[18] Because of the animal data, there is a need for caution in prescribing estrogens for women with a strong family history of breast cancer or who have breast nodules, fibrocystic disease, or abnormal mammograms.

2. *Gall bladder disease.* A recent study has reported a 2- to 3-fold increase in the risk of surgically confirmed gall bladder disease in women receiving postmenopausal estrogens,[17] similar to the 2-fold increase previously noted in users of oral contraceptives.[19,24] In the case of oral contraceptives the increased risk appeared after two years of use.[24]

3. *Effects similar to those caused by estrogen-progestogen oral contraceptives.* There are several serious adverse effects of oral contraceptives, most of which have not, up to now, been documented as consequences of postmenopausal estrogen therapy. This may reflect the comparatively low doses of estrogen used in postmenopausal women. It would be expected that the larger doses of estrogen used to treat prostatic or breast cancer or postpartum breast engorgement are more likely to result in these adverse effects, and, in fact, it has been shown that there is an increased risk of thrombosis in men receiving estrogens for prostatic cancer and women for postpartum breast engorgement.[20-23]

a. *Thromboembolic disease.* It is now well established that users of oral contraceptives have an increased risk of various thromboembolic and thrombotic vascular diseases, such as thrombophlebitis, pulmonary embolism, stroke, and myocardial infarction.[24-31] Cases of retinal thrombosis, mesenteric thrombosis, and optic neuritis have been reported in oral contraceptive users. There is evidence that the risk of several of these adverse reactions is related to the dose of the drug.[32,33] An increased risk of postsurgery thromboembolic complications has also been reported in users of oral contraceptives.[34,35] If feasible, estrogen should be discontinued at least 4 weeks before surgery of the type associated with an increased risk of thromboembolism, or during periods of prolonged immobilization.

While an increased rate of thromboembolic and thrombotic disease in postmenopausal users of estrogens has not been found,[17,36] this does not rule out the possibility that such an increase may be present or that subgroups of women who have underlying risk factors or who are receiving relatively large doses of estrogens may have increased risk. Therefore, estrogens should not be used in persons with active thrombophlebitis or thromboembolic disorders, and they should not be used in persons with a history of such disorders in association with estrogen use. They should be used with caution in patients with cerebral vascular or coronary artery disease and only for those in whom estrogens are clearly needed.

Large doses of estrogen (5 mg conjugated estrogens per day), comparable to those used to treat cancer of the prostate and breast, have been shown in a large prospective clinical trial in men[37] to increase the risk of nonfatal myocardial infarction, pulmonary embolism and thrombophlebitis. When estrogen doses of this size are used, any of the thromboembolic and thrombotic adverse effects associated with oral contraceptive use should be considered a clear risk.

b. *Hepatic adenoma.* Benign hepatic adenomas appear to be associated with the use of oral contraceptives.[38-40] Although benign, and rare, these may rupture and may cause death through intraabdominal hemorrhage. Such lesions have not yet been reported in association with other estrogen or progestogen preparations but should be considered in estrogen users having abdominal pain and tenderness, abdominal mass, or hypovolemic shock. Hepatocellular carcinoma has also been reported in women taking estrogen-containing oral contraceptives.[39] The relationship of this malignancy to these drugs is not known at this time.

c. *Elevated blood pressure.* Increased blood pressure is not uncommon in women using oral contraceptives. There is now a report that this may occur with the use of estrogens in the menopause[41] and blood pressure should be monitored with estrogen use, especially if high doses are used.

d. *Glucose tolerance.* A worsening of glucose tolerance has been observed in a significant percentage of patients on estrogen-containing oral contraceptives. For this reason, diabetic patients should be carefully observed while receiving estrogen.

4. *Hypercalcemia.* Administration of estrogens may lead to severe hypercalcemia in patients with breast cancer and bone metastases. If this occurs, the drug should be stopped and appropriate measures taken to reduce the serum calcium level.

As in the case of other preparations containing CNS-acting drugs, patients receiving Menrium should be cautioned about possible combined effects with alcohol and other CNS depressants. Other causes of manifestations of the menopausal syndrome, such as pregnancy, should be excluded. As is true of all preparations containing CNS-acting drugs, patients receiving Menrium should be cautioned against hazardous occupations requiring complete mental alertness such as operating machinery or driving a motor vehicle.

Physical and Psychological Dependence: Withdrawal symptoms have not been observed in more than 1300 subjects during clinical trials with Menrium. Physical and psychological dependence have rarely been reported in persons taking recommended doses of Librium (chlordiazepoxide/Roche). However, caution must be exercised in administering Librium to individuals known to be addiction-prone or those whose history suggests they may increase the dosage on their own initiative. Withdrawal symptoms following discontinuation of chlordiazepoxide hydrochloride have been reported. These symptoms (including convulsions) are similar to those seen with barbiturates.

Precautions:

A. General Precautions.

1. A complete medical and family history should be taken prior to the initiation of any estrogen therapy. The pretreatment and periodic physical examinations should include special reference to blood pressure, breasts, abdomen, and pelvic organs, and should include a Papanicolaou smear. As a general rule, estrogen should not be prescribed for longer than one year without another physical examination being performed.

2. Fluid retention—Because estrogens may cause some degree of fluid retention, conditions which might be influenced by this factor such as epilepsy, migraine, and cardiac or renal dysfunction, require careful observation.

3. Certain patients may develop undesirable manifestations of excessive estrogenic stimulation, such as abnormal or excessive uterine bleeding, mastodynia, etc.

4. Oral contraceptives appear to be associated with an increased incidence of mental depression.[24] Although it is not clear whether this is due to the estrogenic or progestogenic component of the contraceptive, patients with a history of depression should be carefully observed.

5. Preexisting uterine leiomyomata may increase in size during estrogen use.

6. The pathologist should be advised of estrogen therapy when relevant specimens are submitted.

7. Patients with a past history of jaundice during pregnancy have an increased risk of recurrence of jaundice while receiving estrogen-containing oral contraceptive therapy. If jaundice develops in any patient receiving estrogen, the medication should be discontinued while the cause is investigated.

8. Estrogens may be poorly metabolized in patients with impaired liver function and they should be administered with caution in such patients.

9. Because estrogens influence the metabolism of calcium and phosphorus, they should be used with caution in patients with metabolic bone diseases that are associated with hypercalcemia or in patients with renal insufficiency.

10. Because of the effects of estrogens on epiphyseal closure, they should be used judiciously in young patients in whom bone growth is not complete.

11. Certain endocrine and liver function tests may be affected by estrogen-containing oral contraceptives. The following similar changes may be expected with larger doses of estrogen:

a. Increased sulfobromophthalein retention.

b. Increased prothrombin and factors VII, VIII, IX, and X; decreased antithrombin 3; increased norepinephrine-induced platelet aggregability.

c. Increased thyroid binding globulin (TBG) leading to increased circulating total thyroid hormone, as measured by PBI, T4 by column, or T4 by radioimmunoassay. Free T3 resin uptake is decreased, reflecting the elevated TBG; free T4 concentration is unaltered.

d. Impaired glucose tolerance.

e. Decreased pregnanediol excretion.

f. Reduced response to metyrapone test.

g. Reduced serum folate concentration.

h. Increased serum triglyceride and phospholipid concentration.

B. Information for the Patient.

See Text of Patient Package Insert which follows below.

WHAT YOU SHOULD KNOW ABOUT ESTROGENS

Estrogens are female hormones produced by the ovaries. The ovaries make several different kinds of estrogens. In addition, scientists have been able to make a variety of synthetic estrogens. As far as we know, all these estrogens have similar properties and therefore much the same usefulness, side effects, and risks. This leaflet is intended to help you understand what estrogens are used for, the risks involved in their use, and how to use them as safely as possible.

This leaflet includes the most important information about estrogens, but not all the information. If you want to know more, you can ask your doctor or pharmacist to let you read the package insert prepared for the doctor.

Uses of Estrogen: Estrogens are prescribed by doctors for a number of purposes, including:

1. To provide estrogen during a period of adjustment when a woman's ovaries no longer produce it, in order to prevent certain uncomfortable symptoms of estrogen deficiency. (All women normally stop producing estrogens, generally between the ages of 45 and 55; this is called the menopause.)

2. To prevent symptoms of estrogen deficiency when a woman's ovaries have been removed surgically before the natural menopause.

3. To prevent pregnancy. (Estrogens are given along with a progestogen, another female hormone; these combinations are called oral contraceptives or birth control pills. Patient labeling is available to women taking oral contraceptives and they will not be discussed in this leaflet.)

4. To treat certain cancers in women and men.

5. To prevent painful swelling of the breasts after pregnancy in women who choose not to nurse their babies.

THERE IS NO PROPER USE OF ESTROGENS IN A PREGNANT WOMAN.

Estrogens in the Menopause: In the natural course of their lives, all women eventually experience a decrease in estrogen production. This usually occurs between ages 45 and 55 but may occur earlier or later. Sometimes the ovaries may need to be removed before natural menopause by an operation, producing a "surgical menopause."

When the amount of estrogen in the blood begins to decrease, many women may develop typical symptoms: Feelings of warmth in the face, neck, and chest or sudden intense episodes of heat and sweating throughout the body (called "hot flashes" or "hot flushes"). These symptoms are sometimes very uncomfortable. A few women eventually develop changes in the vagina (called "atrophic vaginitis") which cause discomfort, especially during and after intercourse.

Estrogens can be prescribed to treat these symptoms of the menopause. It is estimated that considerably more than half of all women undergoing the menopause have only mild symptoms or no symptoms at all and therefore do not need estrogens. Other woman may need estrogens for a few months, while their bodies adjust to lower estrogen levels. Sometimes the need will be for periods longer than six months. In an attempt to avoid overstimulation of the uterus (womb), estrogens are usually given cyclically during each month of use, that is three weeks of pills followed by one week without pills.

Sometimes women experience nervous symptoms or depression during menopause. There is no evidence that estrogens are effective for such symptoms and they should not be used to treat them, although other treatment may be needed.

You may have heard that taking estrogens for long periods (years) after the menopause will keep your skin soft and supple and keep you feeling young. There is no evidence that this is so, however, and such long-term treatment carries important risks.

Estrogens to Prevent Swelling of the Breasts After Pregnancy: If you do not breast feed your baby after delivery, your breasts may fill up with milk and become painful and engorged. This usually begins about 3 to 4 days after delivery and may last for a few days to up to a week or more. Sometimes the discomfort is severe, but usually it is not and can be controlled by pain relieving drugs such as aspirin and by binding the breasts up tightly. Estrogens can be used to try to prevent the breasts from filling up. While this treatment is sometimes successful, in many cases the breasts fill up to some degree in spite of treatment. The dose of estrogens needed to prevent pain and swelling of the breasts is much larger than the dose needed to treat symptoms of the menopause and this may increase your chances of developing blood clots in the legs or lungs (see below). Therefore, it is important that you discuss the benefits and the risks of estrogen use with your doctor if you have decided not to breast feed your baby.

The Dangers of Estrogens:

1. *Cancer of the uterus.* If estrogens are used in the postmenopausal period for more than a year, there is an increased risk of *endometrial cancer* (cancer of the uterus). Women taking estrogens have roughly 5 to 10 times as great a chance of getting this cancer as women who take no estrogens. To put this another way, while a postmenopausal woman not taking estrogens has 1 chance in 1,000 each year of getting cancer of the uterus, a woman taking estrogens has 5 to 10 chances in 1,000 each year. For this reason *it is important to take estrogens only when you really need them.*

The risk of this cancer is greater the longer estrogens are used and also seems to be greater when larger doses are taken. For this reason *it is important to take the lowest dose of estrogen that will control symptoms and to take it only as long as it is needed.* If estrogens are needed for longer periods of time, your doctor will want to reevaluate your need for estrogens at least every six months.

Women using estrogens should report any irregular vaginal bleeding to their doctors; such bleeding may be of no importance, but it can be an early warning of cancer of the uterus. If you have undiagnosed vaginal bleeding, you should not use estrogens until a diagnosis is made and you are certain there is no cancer of the uterus.

If you have had your uterus completely removed (total hysterectomy), there is no danger of developing cancer of the uterus.

2. *Other possible cancers.* Estrogens can cause development of other tumors in animals, such as tumors of the breast, cervix, vagina, or liver, when given for a long time. At present there is no good evidence that women using estrogen in the menopause have an increased risk of such tumors, but there is no way yet to be sure they do not; and one study raises the possibility that use of estrogens in the menopause may increase the risk of breast cancer many years later. This is a further reason to use estrogens only when clearly needed. While you are taking estrogens, it is important that you go to your doctor at least once a year for a physical examination. Also, if members of your family have had breast cancer or if you have breast nodules or abnormal mammograms (breast x-rays), your doctor may wish to carry out more frequent examinations of your breasts.

3. *Gall bladder disease.* Women who use estrogens after menopause are more likely to develop gall bladder disease needing surgery as women who do not use estrogens. Birth control pills have a similar effect.

4. *Abnormal blood clotting.* Oral contraceptives increase the risk of blood clotting in various parts of the body. This can result in a stroke (if the clot is in the brain), a heart attack (clot in a blood vessel of the heart), or a pulmonary embolus (a clot which forms in the legs or pelvis, then breaks off and travels to the lungs). Any of these can be fatal. At this time use of estrogens in the menopause is not known to cause such blood clotting, but this has not been fully studied and there could still prove to be such a risk. It is recommended that if you have had clotting in the legs or lungs or a heart attack or stroke while you were using estrogens or birth control pills, you should not use estrogens (unless they are being used to treat cancer of the breast or prostate). If you have had a stroke or heart attack or if you have angina pectoris, estrogens should be used with great caution and only if clearly needed (for example, if you have severe symptoms of the menopause).

The larger doses of estrogen used to prevent swelling of the breasts after pregnancy have been reported to cause clotting in the legs and lungs.

Special Warning About Pregnancy: You should not receive estrogen if you are pregnant. If this should occur, there is a greater than usual chance that the developing child will be born with a birth defect, although the possibility remains fairly small. A female child may have an increased

Continued on next page

Roche Products—Cont.

risk of developing cancer of the vagina or cervix later in life (in the teens or twenties). Every possible effort should be made to avoid exposure to estrogens during pregnancy. If exposure occurs, see your doctor.

Other Effects of Estrogens: In addition to the serious known risks of estrogens described above, estrogens have the following side effects and potential risks:

1. *Nausea and vomiting.* The most common side effect of estrogen therapy is nausea. Vomiting is less common.
2. *Effects on breasts.* Estrogens may cause breast tenderness or enlargement and may cause the breasts to secrete a liquid. These effects are not dangerous.
3. *Effects on the uterus.* Estrogens may cause benign fibroid tumors of the uterus to get larger. Some women will have menstrual bleeding when estrogens are stopped. But if the bleeding occurs on days you are still taking estrogens you should report this to your doctor.
4. *Effects on liver.* Women taking oral contraceptives develop on rare occasions a tumor of the liver which can rupture and bleed into the abdomen. So far, these tumors have not been reported in women using estrogens in the menopause, but you should report any swelling or unusual pain or tenderness in the abdomen to your doctor immediately.
Women with a past history of jaundice (yellowing of the skin and white parts of the eyes) may get jaundice again during estrogen use. If this occurs, stop taking estrogens and see your doctor.
5. *Other effects.* Estrogens may cause excess fluid to be retained in the body. This may make some conditions worse, such as epilepsy, migraine, heart disease, or kidney disease.

Summary: Estrogens have important uses, but they have serious risks as well. You must decide, with your doctor, whether the risks are acceptable to you in view of the benefits of treatment. Except where your doctor has prescribed estrogens for use in special cases of cancer of the breast or prostate, you should not use estrogens if you have cancer of the breast or uterus, are pregnant, have undiagnosed abnormal vaginal bleeding, clotting in the legs or lungs, or have had a stroke, heart attack or angina, or clotting in the legs or lungs in the past while you were taking estrogens.

You can use estrogens as safely as possible by understanding that your doctor will require regular physical examinations while you are taking them and will try to discontinue the drug as soon as possible and use the smallest dose possible. Be alert for signs of trouble including:
1. Abnormal bleeding from the vagina.
2. Pains in the calves or chest or sudden shortness of breath, or coughing blood (indicating possible clots in the legs, heart, or lungs).
3. Severe headache, dizziness, faintness, or changes in vision (indicating possible developing clots in the brain or eye).
4. Breast lumps (you should ask your doctor how to examine your own breasts).
5. Jaundice (yellowing of the skin).
6. Mental depression.

Based on his or her assessment of your medical needs, your doctor has prescribed this drug for you. Do not give the drug to anyone else.

C. Pregnancy: See Contraindications and Box Warning.
D. Nursing Mothers: As a general principle, the administration of any drug to nursing mothers should be done only when clearly necessary since many drugs are excreted in human milk.
In elderly and debilitated patients, it is recommended that the dosage be limited to the smallest effective amount to preclude the development of ataxia or oversedation (10 mg chlordiazepoxide or less per day initially, to be increased gradually as needed and tolerated). In general, the concomitant administration of Menrium and other psychotropic agents is not recommended. If such combination therapy seems indicated, careful consideration should be given to the pharmacology of the agents to be employed—particularly when the known potentiating compounds such as the MAO inhibitors and phenothiazines are to be used. The usual precautions in treating patients with impaired renal or hepatic function should be observed.

Paradoxical reactions to chlordiazepoxide, e.g., excitement, stimulation and acute rage, have been reported in psychiatric patients and should be watched for during Menrium therapy. The usual precautions are indicated when chlordiazepoxide is used in the treatment of anxiety states where there is any evidence of impending depression; it should be borne in mind that suicidal tendencies may be present and protective measures may be necessary. Although clinical studies have not established a cause and effect relationship, physicians should be aware that variable effects on blood coagulation have been reported very rarely in patients receiving oral anticoagulants and Librium (chlordiazepoxide/Roche).

Adverse Reactions: No side effects or manifestations not seen with either compound alone have been reported with the administration of Menrium. However, since Menrium contains chlordiazepoxide and water-soluble esterified estrogens, the possibility of untoward effects which may be seen with either of these two compounds cannot be excluded.

(See Warnings regarding induction of neoplasia, adverse effects on the fetus, increased incidence of gall bladder disease, and adverse effects similar to those of oral contraceptives, including thromboembolism.) The following additional adverse reactions have been reported with estrogenic therapy, including oral contraceptives:

1. *Genitourinary system.*
Breakthrough bleeding, spotting, change in menstrual flow.
Dysmenorrhea.
Premenstrual-like syndrome.
Amenorrhea during and after treatment.
Increase in size of uterine fibromyomata.
Vaginal candidiasis.
Change in cervical eversion and in degree of cervical secretion.
Cystitis-like syndrome.
2. *Breasts.*
Tenderness, enlargement, secretion.
3. *Gastrointestinal.*
Nausea, vomiting.
Abdominal cramps, bloating.
Cholestatic jaundice.
4. *Skin.*
Chloasma or melasma which may persist when drug is discontinued.
Erythema multiforme.
Erythema nodosum.
Hemorrhagic eruption.
Loss of scalp hair.
Hirsutism.
5. *Eyes.*
Steepening of corneal curvature.
Intolerance to contact lenses.
6. *CNS.*
Headache, migraine, dizziness.
Mental depression.
Chorea.
7. *Miscellaneous.*
Increase or decrease in weight.
Reduced carbohydrate tolerance.
Aggravation of porphyria.
Edema.
Changes in libido.

When chlordiazepoxide has been used alone the necessity of discontinuing therapy because of undesirable effects has been rare. Drowsiness, ataxia and confusion have been reported in some patients—particularly the elderly and debilitated. While these effects can be avoided in almost all instances by proper dosage adjustment, they have occasionally been observed at the lower dosage ranges. In a few instances syncope has been reported.

Other adverse reactions reported during therapy include isolated instances of skin eruptions, edema, minor menstrual irregularities, nausea and constipation, extrapyramidal symptoms, as well as increased and decreased libido. Such side effects have been infrequent and are generally controlled with reduction of dosage. Changes in EEG patterns (low-voltage fast activity) have been observed in patients during and after Librium (chlordiazepoxide/Roche) treatment.

Blood dyscrasias, including agranulocytosis, jaundice and hepatic dysfunction have occasionally been reported during therapy. When Librium treatment is protracted, periodic blood counts and liver function tests are advisable.

Management of Overdosage: Numerous reports of ingestion of large doses of estrogen-containing oral contraceptives by young children indicate that serious ill effects do not occur. Overdosage of estrogen may cause nausea, and withdrawal bleeding may occur in females. Manifestations of Librium (chlordiazepoxide/Roche) overdosage include somnolence, confusion, coma and diminished reflexes. Respiration, pulse and blood pressure should be monitored, as in all cases of drug overdosage, although, in general, these effects have been minimal following Librium overdosage. General supportive measures should be employed, along with immediate gastric lavage. Intravenous fluids should be administered and an adequate airway maintained. Hypotension may be combated by the use of Levophed® (levarterenol) or Aramine (metaraminol). Dialysis is of limited value. There have been occasional reports of excitation in patients following chlordiazepoxide overdosage; if this occurs barbiturates should not be used. As with the management of intentional overdosage with any drug, it should be borne in mind that multiple agents may have been ingested.

Dosage: The lowest dose that will control symptoms should be chosen and medication should be discontinued as promptly as possible.

MENRIUM 5-2—for the majority of patients with the menopausal syndrome or the climacteric having anxiety and tension and hormonal deficiency states requiring estrogen replacement—One tablet, t.i.d.

MENRIUM 5-4—for patients with the menopausal syndrome or the climacteric with anxiety and tension and more severe vasomotor manifestations —One tablet, t.i.d.

MENRIUM 10-4—for patients with the menopausal syndrome or the climacteric with pronounced anxiety and tension and marked vasomotor complaints—One tablet, t.i.d.

Therapy should be continued for 21-day courses, followed by one-week rest periods. While these dosage schedules will prove generally satisfactory, individual adjustment of dosage is desirable, since some patients may obtain satisfactory relief with as little as one tablet daily of Menrium 5-2.

Treated patients with an intact uterus should be monitored closely for signs of endometrial cancer and appropriate diagnostic measures should be taken to rule out malignancy in the event of persistent or recurring abnormal vaginal bleeding.

How Supplied: Menrium 5-2, light green tablets—each tablet contains 5 mg chlordiazepoxide and 0.2 mg water-soluble esterified estrogens—bottles of 100; Menrium 5-4, dark green tablets—each tablet contains 5 mg chlordiazepoxide and 0.4 mg water-soluble esterified estrogens—bottles of 100; Menrium 10-4, purple tablets—each tablet contains 10 mg chlordiazepoxide and 0.4 mg water-soluble esterified estrogens—bottles of 100.

Physician References:
1. Ziel HK, Finkel WD: *N Engl J Med* 293:1167–1170, 1975
2. Smith DC, et al: *N Engl J Med* 293:1164–1167, 1975
3. Mack TM, et al: *N Engl J Med* 294:1262–1267, 1976
4. Weiss NS, Szekely DR, Austin DF: *N Engl J Med* 294:1259–1262, 1976
5. Herbst AL, Ulfelder H, Poskanzer DC: *N Engl J Med* 284:878–881, 1971
6. Greenwald P, et al: *N Engl J Med* 285:390–392, 1971
7. Lanier A, et al: *Mayo Clin Proc* 48:793–799, 1973

8. Herbst A, Kurman R, Scully R: *Obstet Gynecol* 40:287-298, 1972
9. Herbst A, et al: *Am J Obstet Gynecol* 118:607-615, 1974
10. Herbst, A, et al: *N Engl J Med* 292:334-339, 1975
11. Stafl A, et al: *Obstet Gynecol* 43:118-128, 1974
12. Sherman AI, et al: *Obstet Gynecol* 44:531-545, 1974
13. Gal I, Kirman B, Stern J: *Nature* 216:83, 1967
14. Levy EP, Cohen A, Fraser FC: *Lancet* 1:611, 1973
15. Nora J, Nora A: *Lancet* 1:941-942, 1973
16. Janerich DT, Piper JM, Glebatis DM: *N Engl J Med* 291:697-700, 1974
17. Boston Collaborative Drug Surveillance Program: *N Engl J Med* 290:15-19, 1974
18. Hoover R, et al: *N Engl J Med* 295:401-405, 1976
19. Boston Collaborative Drug Surveillance Program: *Lancet* 1:1399-1404, 1973
20. Daniel DG, Campbell H, Turnbull AC: *Lancet* 2:287-289, 1967
21. The Veterans Administration Cooperative Urological Research Group: *J Urol* 98:516-522, 1967
22. Bailar JC: *Lancet* 2:560, 1967
23. Blackard C, et al: *Cancer* 26:249-256, 1970
24. Royal College of General Practitioners: *J Coll Gen Pract* 13:267-279, 1967
25. Inman WHW, Vessey MP: *Br Med J* 2:193-199, 1968
26. Vessey MP, Doll R: *Br Med J* 2:651-657, 1969
27. Sartwell PE, et al: *Am J Epidemiol* 90:365-380, 1969
28. Collaborative Group for the Study of Stroke in Young Women: *N Engl J Med* 288:871-878, 1973
29. Collaborative Group for the Study of Stroke in Young Women: *JAMA* 231:718-722, 1975
30. Mann JI, Inman WHW: *Br Med J* 2:245-248, 1975
31. Mann JI, et al: *Br Med J* 2:241-245, 1975
32. Inman WHW, et al: *Br Med J* 2:203-209, 1970
33. Stolley PD, et al: *Am J Epidemiol* 102:197-208, 1975
34. Vessey MP, et al: *Br Med J* 3:123-126, 1970
35. Greene GR, Sartwell PE: *Am J Public Health* 62:680-685, 1972
36. Rosenberg L, Armstrong MB, Jick H: *N Engl J Med* 294:1256-1259, 1976
37. Coronary Drug Project Research Group: *JAMA* 214:1303-1313, 1970
38. Baum J, et al: *Lancet* 2:926-928, 1973
39. Mays ET, et al: *JAMA* 235:730-732, 1976
40. Edmondson HA, Henderson B, Benton B: *N Engl J Med* 294:470-472, 1976
41. Pfeffer RI, Van Den Noort S: *Am J Epidemiol* 103:445-456, 1976

Shown in Product Identification Section, page 430

QUARZAN® ℞
[kwar'zan]
(clidinium bromide/Roche)
CAPSULES

The following text is complete prescribing information based on official labeling in effect August 1, 1984.
Description: Clidinium bromide is 3-hydroxy-1-methylquinuclidinium bromide benzilate. A white or nearly white crystalline compound, it is soluble in water and has a calculated molecular weight of 432.36.
Clidinium bromide is a quaternary ammonium compound with anticholinergic and antispasmodic activity. Quarzan is available as green and red opaque capsules each containing 2.5 mg clidinium bromide, and green and grey opaque capsules each containing 5 mg clidinium bromide.
Actions: Quarzan inhibits gastrointestinal motility and diminishes gastric acid secretion. Its anticholinergic activity approximates that of atropine sulfate and propantheline bromide.
Indications: Quarzan is effective as adjunctive therapy in peptic ulcer disease. **Quarzan has not been shown to be effective in contributing to the healing of peptic ulcer, decreasing the rate of recurrence or preventing complications.**
Contraindications: Known hypersensitivity to clidinium bromide or to other anticholinergic drugs, glaucoma, obstructive uropathy (for example, bladder neck obstruction due to prostatic hypertrophy), obstructive disease of the gastrointestinal tract (for example, pyloroduodenal stenosis), paralytic ileus, intestinal atony of the elderly or debilitated patient, unstable cardiovascular status in acute hemorrhage, severe ulcerative colitis, toxic megacolon complicating ulcerative colitis, myasthenia gravis.
Warnings: Quarzan may produce drowsiness or blurred vision. The patient should be cautioned regarding activities requiring mental alertness such as operating a motor vehicle or other machinery or performing hazardous work while taking this drug. In the presence of high environmental temperature, heat prostration (fever and heat stroke) may occur with the use of anticholinergics due to decreased sweating. Diarrhea may be an early symptom of incomplete intestinal obstruction, especially in patients with ileostomy or colostomy. Use of anticholinergics in patients with suspected intestinal obstruction would be inappropriate and possibly harmful. With overdosage, a curare-like action may occur, *i.e.,* neuromuscular blockade leading to muscular weakness and possible paralysis.
Usage in Pregnancy: No controlled studies in humans have been performed to establish the safety of the drug in pregnancy. Uncontrolled data derived from clinical usage have failed to show abnormalities attributable to its use. Reproduction studies in rats have failed to show any impaired fertility or abnormality in the fetuses that might be associated with the use of Quarzan. Use of any drug in pregnancy or in women of childbearing potential requires that the pontential benefit of the drug be weighed against the possible hazards to mother and fetus.
Nursing Mothers: As with all anticholinergic drugs, Quarzan may be secreted in human milk and may inhibit lactation. As a general rule, nursing should not be undertaken while a patient is on Quarzan, or the drug should not be used by nursing mothers.
Pediatric Use: Since there is no adequate experience in children who have received this drug, safety and efficacy in children have not been established.
Precautions: Use Quarzan with caution in the elderly and in all patients with autonomic neuropathy, hepatic or renal disease, ulcerative colitis—large doses may suppress intestinal motility to the point of producing a paralytic ileus and for this reason precipitate or aggravate "toxic megacolon," a serious complication of the disease; hyperthyroidism; coronary heart disease; congestive heart failure; cardiac tachy-arrhythmias; tachycardia; hypertension; prostatic hypertrophy; hiatal hernia associated with reflux esophagitis, since anticholinergic drugs may aggravate this condition.
Adverse Reactions: As with other anticholinergic drugs, the most frequently reported adverse effects are dryness of mouth, blurring of vision, urinary hesitancy and constipation. Other adverse effects reported with the use of anticholinergic drugs include decreased sweating, urinary retention, tachycardia, palpitations, dilatation of the pupils, cycloplegia, increased ocular tension, loss of taste, headaches, nervousness, mental confusion, drowsiness, weakness, dizziness, insomnia, nausea, vomiting, bloated feeling, impotence, suppression of lactation and severe allergic reactions or drug idiosyncrasies including anaphylaxis, urticaria and other dermal manifestations.
Overdosage: The symptoms of overdosage with Quarzan progress from an intensification of the usual side effects to CNS disturbances (from restlessness and excitement to psychotic behavior), circulatory changes (flushing, tachycardia, fall in blood pressure, circulatory failure), respiratory failure, paralysis and coma.
Treatment should consist of: *General measures*—(1) gastric lavage, (2) maintenance of adequate airway, using artificial respiration if needed, (3) administration of i.v. fluids, and (4) for fever: alcohol sponging or ice packs.
Specific measures—(1) Antidotes: physostigmine (Antilirium) 0.5 to 2 mg, i.v., repeated as needed up to a total of 5 mg; or pilocarpine, 5 mg, s.c. at intervals until mouth is moist; neostigmine may also be useful. (2) Against excitement: sodium pentothal 2% may be given i.v. or chloral hydrate (100 to 200 ml, 2% solution) *rectally.* (3) Against hypotension and circulatory collapse: levarterenol (Levophed®) or metaraminol (Aramine) infusions. (4) Against CNS depression: caffeine and sodium benzoate.
The usefulness of dialysis is not known.
Dosage and Administration: For maximum efficacy, dosage should be individualized according to severity of symptoms and occurrence of side effects. The usual dosage is 2.5 to 5 mg three or four times daily before meals and at bedtime. Dosage in excess of 20 mg daily is usually not required to obtain maximum effectiveness. For the aged or debilitated, one 2.5-mg capsule three times daily before meals is recommended. The desired pharmacological effect of the drug is unlikely to be attained without occasional side effects.
Drug Interactions: No specific drug interactions are known.
How Supplied: Opaque capsules, 2.5 mg, green and red; 5 mg, green and grey—bottles of 100.
Shown in Product Identification Section, page 430

TEL-E-DOSE®

Tel-E-Dose is a unit package designed by Roche for convenience in dispensing medications in the hospital and nursing home. Each unit, sealed against contamination and moisture, is clearly identified by product name and strength and carries the control number and expiration date.
Currently available in this package form are the following products: Dalmane® (flurazepam HCl) capsules, 15 mg, 30 mg; Endep® (amitriptyline HCl) tablets, 10 mg, 25 mg, 50 mg, 75 mg, 100 mg; Librax® (5 mg chlordiazepoxide HCl and 2.5 mg clidinium Br) capsules; Librium® (chlordiazepoxide HCl) capsules, 5 mg, 10 mg, 25 mg; Limbitrol® (chlordiazepoxide and amitriptyline HCl) tablets, 10-25, 5-12.5; Valium® (diazepam) tablets, 2 mg, 5 mg, 10 mg.
Shown in Product Identification Section, page 430

VALIUM® Injectable ℞
[val'ee-um]
(diazepam/Roche)

Valium Injectable is manufactured by Hoffmann-La Roche Inc., Nutley, N.J. 07110 and distributed by Roche Products Inc., Manati, P.R. 00701.
The following text is complete prescribing information based on official labeling in effect August 1, 1984.
Description: Each ml contains 5 mg diazepam/Roche compounded with 40% propylene glycol, 10% ethyl alcohol, 5% sodium benzoate and benzoic acid as buffers, and 1.5% benzyl alcohol as preservative.
Diazepam is a benzodiazepine derivative developed through original Roche research. Chemically, diazepam is 7-chloro-1, 3-dihydro-1-methyl-5-phenyl-2H-1,4-benzodiazepin-2-one. It is a colorless crystalline compound, insoluble in water and has a molecular weight of 284.74.
Actions: In animals, diazepam appears to act on parts of the limbic system, the thalamus and hypothalamus, and induces calming effects. Diazepam, unlike chlorpromazine and reserpine, has no demonstrable peripheral autonomic blocking action, nor does it produce extrapyramidal side effects; however, animals treated with diazepam do have a transient ataxia at higher doses. Diazepam was found to have transient cardiovascular depressor effects in dogs. Long-term experiments in rats revealed no disturbances of endocrine function. Injections into animals have produced localized irritation of tissue surrounding injection sites and some thickening of veins after intravenous use.

Continued on next page

Roche Products—Cont.

Indications: Valium is indicated for the management of anxiety disorders or for the short-term relief of the symptoms of anxiety. Anxiety or tension associated with the stress of everyday life usually does not require treatment with an anxiolytic.

In acute alcohol withdrawal, Valium may be useful in the symptomatic relief of acute agitation, tremor, impending or acute delirium tremens and hallucinosis.

As an adjunct prior to endoscopic procedures if apprehension, anxiety or acute stress reactions are present, and to diminish the patient's recall of the procedures. (See WARNINGS.)

Valium is a useful adjunct for the relief of skeletal muscle spasm due to reflex spasm to local pathology (such as inflammation of the muscles or joints, or secondary to trauma); spasticity caused by upper motor neuron disorders (such as cerebral palsy and paraplegia); athetosis; stiff-man syndrome; and tetanus.

Injectable Valium is a useful adjunct in status epilepticus and severe recurrent convulsive seizures.

Valium is a useful premedication (the I.M. route is preferred) for relief of anxiety and tension in patients who are to undergo surgical procedures. Intravenously, prior to cardioversion for the relief of anxiety and tension and to diminish the patient's recall of the procedure.

Contraindications: Injectable Valium is contraindicated in patients with a known hypersensitivity to this drug; acute narrow angle glaucoma; and open angle glaucoma unless patients are receiving appropriate therapy.

Warnings: *When used intravenously, the following procedures should be undertaken to reduce the possibility of venous thrombosis, phlebitis, local irritation, swelling, and, rarely, vascular impairment: the solution should be injected slowly, taking at least one minute for each 5 mg (1 ml) given; do not use small veins, such as those on the dorsum of the hand or wrist; extreme care should be taken to avoid intra-arterial administration or extravasation.*

Do not mix or dilute Valium with other solutions or drugs in syringe or infusion flask. If it is not feasible to administer Valium directly I.V., it may be injected slowly through the infusion tubing as close as possible to the vein insertion.

Extreme care must be used in administering Injectable Valium, particularly by the I.V. route, to the elderly, to very ill patients and to those with limited pulmonary reserve because of the possibility that apnea and/or cardiac arrest may occur. Concomitant use of barbiturates, alcohol or other central nervous system depressants increases depression with increased risk of apnea. Resuscitative equipment including that necessary to support respiration should be readily available.

When Valium is used with a narcotic analgesic, the dosage of the narcotic should be reduced by at least one-third and administered in small increments. In some cases the use of a narcotic may not be necessary.

Injectable Valium should not be administered to patients in shock, coma, or in acute alcoholic intoxication with depression of vital signs. As is true of most CNS-acting drugs, patients receiving Valium should be cautioned against engaging in hazardous occupations requiring complete mental alertness, such as operating machinery or driving a motor vehicle.

Tonic status epilepticus has been precipitated in patients treated with I.V. Valium for petit mal status or petit mal variant status.

Physical and Psychological Dependence: Withdrawal symptoms (similar in character to those noted with barbiturates and alcohol) have occurred following abrupt discontinuance of diazepam (convulsions, tremor, abdominal and muscle cramps, vomiting and sweating). These were usually limited to those patients who had received excessive doses over an extended period of time. Although infrequently seen, milder withdrawal symptoms have also been reported following abrupt discontinuance of benzodiazepines taken continuously, generally at higher therapeutic levels, for at least several months. Consequently, after extended therapy, abrupt discontinuation should generally be avoided and a gradual tapering in dosage followed. Particularly addiction-prone individuals (such as drug addicts or alcoholics) should be under careful surveillance when receiving diazepam or other psychotropic agents because of the predisposition of such patients to habituation and dependence.

Usage in Pregnancy: **An increased risk of congenital malformations associated with the use of minor tranquilizers (diazepam, meprobamate and chlordiazepoxide) during the first trimester of pregnancy has been suggested in several studies. Because use of these drugs is rarely a matter of urgency, their use during this period should almost always be avoided. The possibility that a woman of childbearing potential may be pregnant at the time of institution of therapy should be considered. Patients should be advised that if they become pregnant during therapy or intend to become pregnant they should communicate with their physicians about the desirability of discontinuing the drug.**

In humans, measurable amounts of diazepam were found in maternal and cord blood, indicating placental transfer of the drug. Until additional information is available, Valium Injectable is not recommended for obstetrical use.

Use in Children: Efficacy and safety of parenteral Valium has not been established in the neonate (30 days or less of age).

Prolonged central nervous system depression has been observed in neonates, apparently due to inability to biotransform Valium into inactive metabolites.

In pediatric use, in order to obtain maximal clinical effect with the minimum amount of drug and thus to reduce the risk of hazardous side effects, such as apnea or prolonged periods of somnolence, it is recommended that the drug be given slowly over a three-minute period in a dosage not to exceed 0.25 mg/kg. After an interval of 15 to 30 minutes the initial dosage can be safely repeated. If, however, relief of symptoms is not obtained after a third administration, adjunctive therapy appropriate to the condition being treated is recommended.

Precautions: Although seizures may be brought under control promptly, a significant proportion of patients experience a return to seizure activity, presumably due to the short-lived effect of Valium after I.V. administration. The physician should be prepared to re-administer the drug. However, Valium is not recommended for maintenance, and once seizures are brought under control, consideration should be given to the administration of agents useful in longer term control of seizures. If Valium is to be combined with other psychotropic agents or anticonvulsant drugs, careful consideration should be given to the pharmacology of the agents to be employed—particularly with known compounds which may potentiate the action of Valium, such as phenothiazines, narcotics, barbiturates, MAO inhibitors and other antidepressants. In highly anxious patients with evidence of accompanying depression, particularly those who may have suicidal tendencies, protective measures may be necessary. The usual precautions in treating patients with impaired hepatic function should be observed. Metabolites of Valium are excreted by the kidney; to avoid their excess accumulation, caution should be exercised in the administration to patients with compromised kidney function.

Since an increase in cough reflex and laryngospasm may occur with peroral endoscopic procedures, the use of a topical anesthetic agent and the availability of necessary countermeasures are recommended.

Until additional information is available, injectable diazepam is not recommended for obstetrical use.

Injectable Valium has produced hypotension or muscular weakness in some patients particularly when used with narcotics, barbiturates or alcohol. Lower doses (usually 2 mg to 5 mg) should be used for elderly and debilitated patients.

The clearance of Valium and certain other benzodiazepines can be delayed in association with Tagamet (cimetidine) administration. The clinical significance of this is unclear.

Adverse Reactions: Side effects most commonly reported were drowsiness, fatigue and ataxia; venous thrombosis and phlebitis at the site of injection. Other adverse reactions less frequently reported include: *CNS:* confusion, depression, dysarthria, headache, hypoactivity, slurred speech, syncope, tremor, vertigo. *G.I.:* constipation, nausea. *G.U.:* incontinence, changes in libido, urinary retention. *Cardiovascular:* bradycardia, cardiovascular collapse, hypotension. *EENT:* blurred vision, diplopia, nystagmus. *Skin:* urticaria, skin rash. *Other:* hiccups, changes in salivation, neutropenia, jaundice. Paradoxical reactions such as acute hyperexcited states, anxiety, hallucinations, increased muscle spasticity, insomnia, rage, sleep disturbances and stimulation have been reported; should these occur, use of the drug should be discontinued. Minor changes in EEG patterns, usually low-voltage fast activity, have been observed in patients during and after Valium therapy and are of no known significance.

In peroral endoscopic procedures, coughing, depressed respiration, dyspnea, hyperventilation, laryngospasm and pain in throat or chest have been reported.

Because of isolated reports of neutropenia and jaundice, periodic blood counts and liver function tests are advisable during long-term therapy.

Dosage and Administration: Dosage should be individualized for maximum beneficial effect. The usual recommended dose in older children and adults ranges from 2 mg to 20 mg I.M. or I.V., depending on the indication and its severity. In some conditions, e.g., tetanus, larger doses may be required. (See dosage for specific indications.) In acute conditions the injection may be repeated within one hour although an interval of 3 to 4 hours is usually satisfactory. Lower doses (usually 2 mg to 5 mg) and slow increase in dosage should be used for elderly or debilitated patients and when other sedative drugs are administered. (See WARNINGS and ADVERSE REACTIONS.)

For dosage in infants above the age of 30 days and children, see the specific indications below. When intravenous use is indicated, facilities for respiratory assistance should be readily available.

Intramuscular: Injectable Valium should be injected deeply into the muscle.

Intravenous use: (See WARNINGS, particularly for use in children.) The solution should be injected slowly, taking at least one minute for each 5 mg (1 ml) given. Do not use small veins, such as those on the dorsum of the hand or wrist. Extreme care should be taken to avoid intra-arterial administration or extravasation. Do not mix or dilute Valium with other solutions or drugs in syringe or infusion flask. If it is not feasible to administer Valium directly I.V., it may be injected slowly through the infusion tubing as close as possible to the vein insertion.

[See table on top next page].

Once the acute symptomatology has been properly controlled with Injectable Valium, the patient may be placed on oral therapy with Valium if further treatment is required.

Management of Overdosage:

Manifestations of Valium overdosage include somnolence, confusion, coma, and diminished reflexes. Respiration, pulse and blood pressure should be monitored, as in all cases of drug overdosage, although, in general, these effects have been minimal. General supportive measures should be employed, along with intravenous fluids, and an adequate airway maintained. Hypotension may be combated by the use of Levophed® (levarterenol) or Aramine (metaraminol). Dialysis is of limited value.

How Supplied: Ampuls, 2 ml, boxes of 10; Vials, 10 ml, boxes of 1; Tel-E-Ject® (disposable syringes), 2 ml, boxes of 10.

Animal Pharmacology: Oral LD$_{50}$ of diazepam is 720 mg/kg in mice and 1240 mg/kg in rats. Intraperitoneal administration of 400 mg/kg to a monkey resulted in death on the sixth day.

Reproduction Studies: A series of rat reproduction studies was performed with diazepam in oral doses of 1, 10, 80 and 100 mg/kg given for periods ranging from 60–228 days prior to mating. At 100 mg/kg there was a decrease in the number of pregnancies and surviving offspring in these rats. These effects may be attributable to prolonged sedative activity, resulting in lack of interest in mating and lessened maternal nursing and care of the young. Neonatal survival of rats at doses lower than 100 mg/kg was within normal limits. Several neonates, both controls and experimentals, in these rat reproduction studies showed skeletal or other defects. Further studies in rats at doses up to and including 80 mg/kg/day did not reveal significant teratological effects on the offspring. Rabbits were maintained on doses of 1, 2, 5 and 8 mg/kg from day 6 through day 18 of gestation. No adverse effects on reproduction and no teratological changes were noted.

Shown in Product Identification Section, page 430

VALIUM® TABLETS
[val'ee-um]
(diazepam/Roche)

The following text is complete prescribing information based on official labeling in effect August 1, 1984.

Description: Valium (diazepam/Roche) is a benzodiazepine derivative developed through original Roche research. Chemically, diazepam is 7-chloro - 1,3 - dihydro - 1 - methyl - 5 - phenyl - 2H-1,4-benzodiazepin-2-one. It is a colorless crystalline compound, insoluble in water and has a molecular weight of 284.74.

Pharmacology: In animals Valium appears to act on parts of the limbic system, the thalamus and hypothalamus, and induces calming effects. Valium, unlike chlorpromazine and reserpine, has no demonstrable peripheral autonomic blocking action, nor does it produce extrapyramidal side effects; however, animals treated with Valium do have a transient ataxia at higher doses. Valium was found to have transient cardiovascular depressor effects in dogs. Long-term experiments in rats revealed no disturbances of endocrine function.

Oral LD$_{50}$ of diazepam is 720 mg/kg in mice and 1240 mg/kg in rats. Intraperitoneal administration of 400 mg/kg to a monkey resulted in death on the sixth day.

Reproduction Studies: A series of rat reproduction studies was performed with diazepam in oral doses of 1, 10, 80 and 100 mg/kg. At 100 mg/kg there was a decrease in the number of pregnancies and surviving offspring in these rats. Neonatal survival of rats at doses lower than 100 mg/kg was within normal limits. Several neonates in these rat reproduction studies showed skeletal or other defects. Further studies in rats at doses up to and including 80 mg/kg/day did not reveal teratological effects on the offspring.

In humans, measurable blood levels of Valium were obtained in maternal and cord blood, indicating placental transfer of the drug.

Indications: Valium is indicated for the management of anxiety disorders or for the short-term relief of the symptoms of anxiety. Anxiety or tension associated with the stress of everyday life usually does not require treatment with an anxiolytic.

In acute alcohol withdrawal, Valium may be useful in the symptomatic relief of acute agitation, tremor, impending or acute delirium tremens and hallucinosis.

Valium is a useful adjunct for the relief of skeletal muscle spasm due to reflex spasm to local pathology (such as inflammation of the muscles or joints, or secondary to trauma); spasticity caused by upper motor neuron disorders (such as cerebral palsy and paraplegia); athetosis; and stiff-man syndrome.

Oral Valium may be used adjunctively in convulsive disorders, although it has not proved useful as the sole therapy.

The effectiveness of Valium in long-term use, that is, more than 4 months, has not been assessed by systematic clinical studies. The physician should periodically reassess the usefulness of the drug for the individual patient.

Contraindications: Valium is contraindicated in patients with a known hypersensitivity to this

RECOMMENDED DOSAGE FOR *INJECTABLE VALIUM*® (diazepam/Roche)

	USUAL ADULT DOSAGE	DOSAGE RANGE IN CHILDREN (I.V. administration should be made slowly)
Moderate Anxiety Disorders and Symptoms of Anxiety	2 mg to 5 mg, I.M. or I.V. Repeat in 3 to 4 hours, if necessary.	
Severe Anxiety Disorders and Symptoms of Anxiety	5 mg to 10 mg, I.M. or I.V. Repeat in 3 to 4 hours, if necessary.	
Acute Alcohol Withdrawal: As an aid in symptomatic relief of acute agitation, tremor, impending or acute delirium tremens and hallucinosis.	10 mg, I.M. or I.V. initially, then 5 mg to 10 mg in 3 to 4 hours, if necessary.	
Endoscopic Procedures: Adjunctively, if apprehension, anxiety or acute stress reactions are present prior to endoscopic procedures. Dosage of narcotics should be reduced by at least a third and in some cases may be omitted. See *Precautions* for peroral procedures.	Titrate I.V. dosage to desired sedative response, such as slurring of speech, with slow administration immediately prior to the procedure. Generally 10 mg or less is adequate, but up to 20 mg I.V. may be given, particularly when concomitant narcotics are omitted. If I.V. cannot be used, 5 mg to 10 mg I.M. approximately 30 minutes prior to the procedure.	
Muscle Spasm: Associated with local pathology, cerebral palsy, athetosis, stiff-man syndrome or tetanus.	5 mg to 10 mg, I.M. or I.V. initially, then 5 mg to 10 mg in 3 to 4 hours, if necessary. For tetanus, larger doses may be required.	For tetanus in infants over 30 days of age, 1 mg to 2 mg I.M. or I.V., slowly, repeated every 3 to 4 hours as necessary. In children 5 years or older, 5 mg to 10 mg repeated every 3 to 4 hours may be required to control tetanus spasms. Respiratory assistance should be available.
Status Epilepticus and Severe Recurrent Convulsive Seizures: In the convulsing patient, the I.V. route is by far preferred. This injection should be administered slowly. However, if I.V. administration is impossible, the I.M. route may be used.	5 mg to 10 mg initially (I.V. preferred). This injection may be repeated if necessary at 10 to 15 minute intervals up to a maximum dose of 30 mg. If necessary, therapy with Valium (diazepam) may be repeated in 2 to 4 hours; however, residual active metabolites may persist, and readministration should be made with this consideration. Extreme caution must be exercised with individuals with chronic lung disease or unstable cardiovascular status.	Infants over 30 days of age and children under 5 years, 0.2 mg to 0.5 mg slowly every 2 to 5 minutes up to a maximum of 5 mg (I.V. preferred). Children 5 years or older, 1 mg every 2 to 5 minutes up to a maximum of 10 mg (slow I.V. administration preferred). Repeat in 2 to 4 hours if necessary. EEG monitoring of the seizure may be helpful.
Preoperative Medication: To relieve anxiety and tension. (If atropine, scopolamine or other premedications are desired, they must be administered in separate syringes.)	10 mg, I.M. (preferred route), before surgery.	
Cardioversion: To relieve anxiety and tension and to reduce recall of procedure.	5 mg to 15 mg, IV., within 5 to 10 minutes prior to the procedure.	

Continued on next page

Roche Products—Cont.

drug and, because of lack of sufficient clinical experience, in children under 6 months of age. It may be used in patients with open angle glaucoma who are receiving appropriate therapy, but is contraindicated in acute narrow angle glaucoma.

Warnings: Valium is not of value in the treatment of psychotic patients and should not be employed in lieu of appropriate treatment. As is true of most preparations containing CNS-acting drugs, patients receiving Valium should be cautioned against engaging in hazardous occupations requiring complete mental alertness such as operating machinery or driving a motor vehicle.

As with other agents which have anticonvulsant activity, when Valium is used as an adjunct in treating convulsive disorders, the possibility of an increase in the frequency and/or severity of grand mal seizures may require an increase in the dosage of standard anticonvulsant medication. Abrupt withdrawal of Valium in such cases may also be associated with a temporary increase in the frequency and/or severity of seizures.

Since Valium has a central nervous system depressant effect, patients should be advised against the simultaneous ingestion of alcohol and other CNS-depressant drugs during Valium therapy.

Physical and Psychological Dependence: Withdrawal symptoms (similar in character to those noted with barbiturates and alcohol) have occurred following abrupt discontinuance of diazepam (convulsions, tremor, abdominal and muscle cramps, vomiting and sweating). These were usually limited to those patients who had received excessive doses over an extended period of time. Although infrequently seen, milder withdrawal symptoms have also been reported following abrupt discontinuance of benzodiazepines taken continuously, generally at higher therapeutic levels, for at least several months. Consequently, after extended therapy, abrupt discontinuation should generally be avoided and a gradual tapering in dosage followed. Particularly addiction-prone individuals (such as drug addicts or alcoholics) should be under careful surveillance when receiving diazepam or other psychotropic agents because of the predisposition of such patients to habituation and dependence.

Usage in Pregnancy: An increased risk of congenital malformations associated with the use of minor tranquilizers (diazepam, meprobamate and chlordiazepoxide) during the first trimester of pregnancy has been suggested in several studies. Because use of these drugs is rarely a matter of urgency, their use during this period should almost always be avoided. The possibility that a woman of childbearing potential may be pregnant at the time of institution of therapy should be considered. Patients should be advised that if they become pregnant during therapy or intend to become pregnant they should communicate with their physicians about the desirability of discontinuing the drug.

Management of Overdosage: Manifestations of Valium overdosage include somnolence, confusion, coma and diminished reflexes. Respiration, pulse and blood pressure should be monitored, as in all cases of drug overdosage, although, in general, these effects have been minimal following overdosage. General supportive measures should be employed, along with immediate gastric lavage. Intravenous fluids should be administered and an adequate airway maintained. Hypotension may be combated by the use of Levophed® (levarterenol) or Aramine (metaraminol). Dialysis is of limited value. As with the management of intentional overdosage with any drug, it should be borne in mind that multiple agents may have been ingested.

Precautions: If Valium is to be combined with other psychotropic agents or anticonvulsant drugs, careful consideration should be given to the pharmacology of the agents to be employed—particularly with known compounds which may potentiate the action of Valium, such as phenothiazines, narcotics, barbiturates, MAO inhibitors and other antidepressants. The usual precautions are indicated for severely depressed patients or those in whom there is any evidence of latent depression; particularly the recognition that suicidal tendencies may be present and protective measures may be necessary. The usual precautions in treating patients with impaired renal or hepatic function should be observed.

In elderly and debilitated patients, it is recommended that the dosage be limited to the smallest effective amount to preclude the development of ataxia or oversedation (2 mg to 2½ mg once or twice daily, initially, to be increased gradually as needed and tolerated).

The clearance of Valium and certain other benzodiazepines can be delayed in association with Tagamet (cimetidine) administration. The clinical significance of this is unclear.

Adverse Reactions: Side effects most commonly reported were drowsiness, fatigue and ataxia. Infrequently encountered were confusion, constipation, depression, diplopia, dysarthria, headache, hypotension, incontinence, jaundice, changes in libido, nausea, changes in salivation, skin rash, slurred speech, tremor, urinary retention, vertigo and blurred vision. Paradoxical reactions such as acute hyperexcited states, anxiety, hallucinations, increased muscle spasticity, insomnia, rage, sleep disturbances and stimulation have been reported; should these occur, use of the drug should be discontinued.

Because of isolated reports of neutropenia and jaundice, periodic blood counts and liver function tests are advisable during long-term therapy. Minor changes in EEG patterns, usually low-voltage fast activity, have been observed in patients during and after Valium therapy and are of no known significance.

Dosage and Administration: Dosage should be individualized for maximum beneficial effect. While the usual dosages given below will meet the needs of most patients, there will be some who may require higher doses. In such cases dosage should be increased cautiously to avoid adverse effects.

	USUAL DAILY DOSE
Adults: Management of Anxiety Disorders and Relief of Symptoms of Anxiety	Depending upon severity of symptoms —2 mg to 10 mg, 2 to 4 times daily
Symptomatic Relief in Acute Alcohol Withdrawal.	10 mg, 3 or 4 times during the first 24 hours, reducing to 5 mg, 3 or 4 times daily as needed
Adjunctively for Relief of Skeletal Muscle Spasm.	2 mg to 10 mg, 3 or 4 times daily
Adjunctively in Convulsive Disorders.	2 mg to 10 mg, 2 to 4 times daily
Geriatric Patients, or in the presence of debilitating disease.	2 mg to 2½ mg, 1 or 2 times daily initially; increase gradually as needed and tolerated
Children: Because of varied responses to CNS-acting drugs, initiate therapy with lowest dose and increase as required. Not for use in children under 6 months.	1 mg to 2½ mg, 3 or 4 times daily initially; increase gradually as needed and tolerated

How Supplied: For oral administration, round, scored tablets with a cut out "V" design—2 mg, white; 5 mg, yellow; 10 mg, blue—bottles of 100 and 500; Prescription Paks of 50, available in trays of 10. Tel-E-Dose® packages of 100, available in cards of 4 reverse-numbered cards of 25, and in boxes containing 10 strips of 10.
Imprint on tablets:
2 mg:
2 VALIUM® (front)
ROCHE (scored side)
5 mg:
5 VALIUM® (front)
ROCHE (scored side)
10 mg:
10 VALIUM® (front)
ROCHE (scored side)

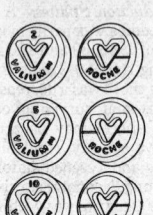

Shown in Product Identification Section, page 430

Products are cross-indexed

by product classifications

in the

BLUE SECTION

IDENTIFICATION PROBLEM?
Consult PDR's
Product Identification Section
where you'll find over 1200 products pictured actual size and in full color.

Important Notice
Before prescribing or administering any product described in PHYSICIANS' DESK REFERENCE always consult the PDR Supplement for possible new or revised information

Roerig
A division of Pfizer Pharmaceuticals
235 EAST 42nd STREET
NEW YORK, NY 10017

Product Identification Codes

To provide quick and positive identification of Roerig Division products, we have imprinted the product identification number of the National Drug Code on most tablets and capsules.
In order that you may quickly identify a product by its code number, we have compiled below a numerical list of code numbers with their corresponding product names. We are also listing the code numbers by alphabetical order of products.

Numerical Listing

Product Ident. Number	Product
035	Spectrobid® (bacampicillin HCl) Tablets, 400 mg., equivalent to 280 mg. ampicillin
092	Urobiotic®-250 (oxytetracycline HCl 250 mg. with sulfamethizole 250 mg. and phenazopyridine 50 mg.) Capsules
143	Geocillin® (carbenicillin indanyl sodium) Tablets, equivalent to 382 mg. carbenicillin
159	TAO® (troleandomycin) Capsules, 250 mg.
210	Antivert® (meclizine HCl) Tablets, 12.5 mg.
211	Antivert® /25 (meclizine HCl) Tablets, 25 mg.
212	Antivert® /25 (meclizine HCl) Chewable Tablets
214	Antivert® /50 (meclizine HCl) Tablets, 50 mg.
220	Sustaire® (theophylline [anhydrous]) Tablets, 100 mg.
221	Sustaire® (theophylline [anhydrous]) Tablets, 300 mg.
254	Marax® (ephedrine sulfate, 25 mg; theophylline, 130 mg; and Atarax® [hydroxyzine HCl], 10 mg) Tablets
411	Glucotrol® (glipizide) Tablets, 5 mg.
412	Glucotrol® (glipizide) Tablets, 10 mg.
504	Heptuna® plus (iron plus vitamins and minerals), Capsules.
534	Sinequan® (doxepin HCl) Capsules 10 mg.
535	Sinequan® (doxepin HCl) Capsules 25 mg.
536	Sinequan® (doxepin HCl) Capsules 50 mg.
537	Sinequan® (doxepin HCl) Capsules 150 mg.
538	Sinequan® (doxepin HCl) Casules 100 mg.
539	Sinequan® (doxepin HCl) Capsules 75 mg.
214	Antivert® /50 (meclizine HCl) Tablets, 50 mg.
560	Atarax® (hydroxyzine HCl) Tablets, 10 mg.
561	Atarax® (hydroxyzine HCl) Tablets, 25 mg.
562	Atarax® (hydroxyzine HCl) Tablets, 50 mg.
563	Atarax® (hydroxyzine HCl) Tablets, 100 mg.
571	Navane® (thiothixene) Capsules, 1 mg.
572	Navane® (thiothixene) Capsules, 2 mg.
573	Navane® (thiothixene) Capsules, 5 mg.
574	Navane® (thiothixene) Capsules, 10 mg.
577	Navane® (thiothixene) Capsules, 20 mg.

Alphabetical Listing

Prod. Ident. Number	Product
210	Antivert® (meclizine HCl) Tablets, 12.5 mg.
211	Antivert® /25 (meclizine HCl) Tablets, 25 mg.
212	Antivert® /25 (meclizine HCl) Chewable Tablets
214	Antivert® /50 (meclizine HCl) Tablets, 50 mg.
560	Atarax® (hydroxyzine HCl) Tablets, 10 mg.
561	Atarax® (hydroxyzine HCl) Tablets, 25 mg.
562	Atarax® (hydroxyzine HCl) Tablets, 50 mg.
563	Atarax® (hydroxyzine HCl) Tablets, 100 mg.
143	Geocillin® (carbenicillin indanyl sodium) Tablets equivalent to 382 mg. carbenicillin
411	Glucotrol® (glipizide) Tablets, 5 mg.
412	Glucotrol® (glipizide) Tablets, 10 mg.
504	Heptuna® plus (iron plus vitamins and minerals), Capsules.
254	Marax® (ephedrine sulfate, 25 mg; theophylline, 130 mg; and Atarax® [hydroxyzine HCl], 10 mg) Tablets
571	Navane® (thiothixene) Capsules, 1 mg.
572	Navane® (thiothixene) Capsules, 2 mg.
573	Navane® (thiothixene) Capsules, 5 mg.
574	Navane® (thiothixene) Capsules, 10 mg.
577	Navane® (thiothixene) Capsules, 20 mg.
534	Sinequan® (doxepin HCl) Capsules 10 mg.
535	Sinequan® (doxepin HCl) Capsules 25 mg.
536	Sinequan® (doxepin HCl) Capsules 50 mg.
539	Sinequan® (doxepin HCl) Capsules 75 mg.
538	Sinequan® (doxepin HCl) Capsules 100 mg.
537	Sinequan® (doxepin HCl) Capsules 150 mg.
035	Spectrobid® (bacampicillin HCl) Tablets, 400 mg., equivalent to 280 mg. ampicillin
220	Sustaire® (theophylline [anhydrous]) Tablets, 100 mg.
221	Sustaire® (theophylline [anhydrous]) Tablets, 300 mg.
159	TAO® (troleandomycin) Capsules, 250 mg.
092	Urobiotic®-250 (oxytetracycline HCl 250 mg. with sulfamethizole 250 mg. and phenazopyridine 50 mg.) Capsules

ANTIVERT® TABLETS ℞
[ăn'tĭ-vert"]
(12.5 mg. meclizine HCl)
ANTIVERT®/25 TABLETS ℞
(25 mg. meclizine HCl)
ANTIVERT®/25 CHEWABLE TABLETS ℞
(25 mg. meclizine HCl)
ANTIVERT®/50 TABLETS ℞
(50 mg. meclizine HCl)

Description: Chemically, Antivert (meclizine HCl) is 1-(p-chloro-α-phenylbenzyl)-4-(m-methylbenzyl) piperazine dihydrochloride monohydrate.
Actions: Antivert is an antihistamine which shows marked protective activity against nebulized histamine and lethal doses of intravenously injected histamine in guinea pigs. It has a marked effect in blocking the vasodepressor response to histamine, but only a slight blocking action against acetylcholine. Its activity is relatively weak in inhibiting the spasmogenic action of histamine on isolated guinea pig ileum.

INDICATIONS
Based on a review of this drug by the National Academy of Sciences-National Research Council and/or other information, FDA has classified the indications as follows:
Effective: Management of nausea and vomiting, and dizziness associated with motion sickness.
Possibly Effective: Management of vertigo associated with diseases affecting the vestibular system.
Final classification of the less than effective indications requires further investigation.

Contraindications: Meclizine HCl is contraindicated in individuals who have shown a previous hypersensitivity to it.
Warnings: Since drowsiness may, on occasion, occur with use of this drug, patients should be warned of this possibility and cautioned against driving a car or operating dangerous machinery. Patients should avoid alcoholic beverages while taking the drug. Due to its potential anticholinergic action, this drug should be used with caution in patients with asthma, glaucoma, or enlargement of the prostate gland.
USAGE IN CHILDREN:
Clinical studies establishing safety and effectiveness in children have not been done; therefore, usage is not recommended in children under 12 years of age.
USAGE IN PREGNANCY:
Pregnancy Category B. Reproduction studies in rats have shown cleft palates at 25–50 times the human dose. Epidemiological studies in pregnant women, however, do not indicate that meclizine increases the risk of abnormalities when administered during pregnancy. Despite the animal findings, it would appear that the possibility of fetal harm is remote. Nevertheless, meclizine, or any other medication, should be used during pregnancy only if clearly necessary.
Adverse Reactions: Drowsiness, dry mouth and, on rare occasions, blurred vision have been reported.
Dosage and Administration:
Vertigo:
For the control of vertigo associated with diseases affecting the vestibular system, the recommended dose is 25 to 100 mg. daily, in divided dosage, depending upon clinical response.
Motion Sickness:
The initial dose of 25 to 50 mg. of Antivert should be taken one hour prior to embarkation for protection against motion sickness. Thereafter, the dose may be repeated every 24 hours for the duration of the journey.
How Supplied:
Antivert—12.5 mg. tablets: Bottles of 100, 1000 and unit dose 100's.
Antivert/25—25 mg. tablets: Bottles of 100, 1000 and unit dose 100's.
Antivert/25 Chewable Tablets—25 mg. pink scored tablets: Bottles of 100 and 500.
Antivert/50—50 mg. tablets: Bottles of 100.
69-2148-37-6
Shown in Product Identification Section, page 431

ATARAX® ℞
[ăt'ā-raks"]
(hydroxyzine hydrochloride)
TABLETS AND SYRUP

Description: Hydroxyzine hydrochloride is designated chemically as 1-(p-chlorobenzhydryl) 4-[2-(2-hydroxyethoxy)-ethyl] piperazine dihydrochloride.

Continued on next page

Roerig—Cont.

Clinical Pharmacology: Atarax is unrelated chemically to the phenothiazines, reserpine, meprobamate, or the benzodiazepines.

Atarax is not a cortical depressant, but its action may be due to a suppression of activity in certain key regions of the subcortical area of the central nervous system. Primary skeletal muscle relaxation has been demonstrated experimentally. Bronchodilator activity, and antihistaminic and analgesic effects have been demonstrated experimentally and confirmed clinically. An antiemetic effect, both by the apomorphine test and the veriloid test, has been demonstrated. Pharmacological and clinical studies indicate that hydroxyzine in therapeutic dosage does not increase gastric secretion or acidity and in most cases has mild antisecretory activity. Hydroxyzine is rapidly absorbed from the gastrointestinal tract and Atarax's clinical effects are usually noted within 15 to 30 minutes after oral administration.

Indications: For symptomatic relief of anxiety and tension associated with psychoneurosis and as an adjunct in organic disease states in which anxiety is manifested.

Useful in the management of pruritus due to allergic conditions such as chronic urticaria and atopic and contact dermatoses, and in histamine-mediated pruritus.

As a sedative when used as premedication and following general anesthesia. **Hydroxyzine may potentiate meperidine (Demerol®) and barbiturates**, so their use in pre-anesthetic adjunctive therapy should be modified on an individual basis. Atropine and other belladonna alkaloids are not affected by the drug. Hydroxyzine is not known to interfere with the action of digitalis in any way and it may be used concurrently with this agent. The effectiveness of hydroxyzine as an antianxiety agent for long term use, that is more than 4 months, has not been assessed by systematic clinical studies. The physician should reassess periodically the usefulness of the drug for the individual patient.

Contraindications: Hydroxyzine, when administered to the pregnant mouse, rat, and rabbit, induced fetal abnormalities in the rat and mouse at doses substantially above the human therapeutic range. Clinical data in human beings are inadequate to establish safety in early pregnancy. Until such data are available, hydroxyzine is contraindicated in early pregnancy.

Hydroxyzine is contraindicated for patients who have shown a previous hypersensitivity to it.

Warnings:
Nursing Mothers: It is not known whether this drug is excreted in human milk. Since many drugs are so excreted, hydroxyzine should not be given to nursing mothers.

Precautions: THE POTENTIATING ACTION OF HYDROXYZINE MUST BE CONSIDERED WHEN THE DRUG IS USED IN CONJUNCTION WITH CENTRAL NERVOUS SYSTEM DEPRESSANTS SUCH AS NARCOTICS, NON-NARCOTIC ANALGESICS AND BARBITURATES. Therefore when central nervous system depressants are administered concomitantly with hydroxyzine their dosage should be reduced.

Since drowsiness may occur with use of this drug, patients should be warned of this possibility and cautioned against driving a car or operating dangerous machinery while taking Atarax. Patients should be advised against the simultaneous use of other CNS depressant drugs, and cautioned that the effect of alcohol may be increased.

Adverse Reactions: Side effects reported with the administration of Atarax (hydroxyzine hydrochloride) are usually mild and transitory in nature.

Anticholinergic: Dry mouth.
Central Nervous System: Drowsiness is usually transitory and may disappear in a few days of continued therapy or upon reduction of the dose. Involuntary motor activity including rare instances of tremor and convulsions have been reported, usually with doses considerably higher than those recommended. Clinically significant respiratory depression has not been reported at recommended doses.

Overdosage: The most common manifestation of Atarax overdosage is hypersedation. As in the management of overdosage with any drug, it should be borne in mind that multiple agents may have been taken.

If vomiting has not occurred spontaneously, it should be induced. Immediate gastric lavage is also recommended. General supportive care, including frequent monitoring of the vital signs and close observation of the patient, is indicated. Hypotension, though unlikely, may be controlled with intravenous fluids and Levophed® (levarterenol), or Aramine® (metaraminol). Do not use epinephrine as Atarax counteracts its pressor action.

There is no specific antidote. It is doubtful that hemodialysis would be of any value in the treatment of overdosage with hydroxyzine. However, if other agents such as barbiturates have been ingested concomitantly, hemodialysis may be indicated. There is no practical method to quantitate hydroxyzine in body fluids or tissue after its ingestion or administration.

Dosage: For symptomatic relief of anxiety and tension associated with psychoneurosis and as an adjunct in organic disease states in which anxiety is manifested: in adults, 50–100 mg q.i.d.: children under 6 years, 50 mg daily in divided doses and over 6 years, 50–100 mg daily in divided doses.

For use in the management of pruritus due to allergic conditions such as chronic urticaria and atopic and contact dermatoses, and in histamine-mediated pruritus: in adults, 25 mg t.i.d. or q.i.d.; children under 6 years, 50 mg daily in divided doses and over 6 years, 50–100 mg daily in divided doses.

As a sedative when used as a premedication and following general anesthesia: 50–100 mg in adults, and 0.6 mg/kg in children.

When treatment is initiated by the intramuscular route of administration, subsequent doses may be administered orally.

As with all medications, the dosage should be adjusted according to the patient's response to therapy.

Supply:
Atarax Tablets
10 mg: 100's (NDC 0049-5600-66), 500's (NDC 0049-5600-73), Unit Dose 10 × 10's (NDC 0049-5600-41), and Unit of Use 40's (NDC 0049-5600-43)—orange tablets

25 mg: 100's (NDC 0049-5610-66), 500's (NDC 0049-5610-73), Unit Dose 10 × 10's (NDC 0049-5610-41), and Unit of Use 40's (NDC 0049-5610-43)—green tablets
50 mg: 100's (NDC 0049-5620-66), 500's (NDC 0049-5620-73), and Unit Dose 10 × 10's (NDC 0049-5620-41)—yellow tablets
Atarax 100 Tablets
100 mg: 100's (NDC 0049-5630-66), and Unit Dose 10 × 10's (NDC 0049-5630-41)—red tablets
Atarax Syrup
10 mg per teaspoon (5 ml): 1 pint bottles (NDC 0049-5590-93)
Alcohol Content—Ethyl Alcohol—0.5% v/v
Bibliography: Available on request.

60-0618-00-2

Shown in Product Identification Section, page 431

CEFOBID®   ℞
[sĕf' ō-bĭd″]
(cefoperazone sodium)
For Intravenous or Intramuscular Use

Description: CEFOBID (cefoperazone sodium) is a sterile, semisynthetic, broad-spectrum, parenteral cephalosporin antibiotic for intravenous or intramuscular administration. It is the sodium salt of 7-[D(-)-α-(4-ethyl-2,3-dioxo-1-piperazinecarboxamido)-α-(4-hydroxyphenyl) acetamido]-3-[(1-methyl-1H-tetrazol-5-yl)thiomethyl]-3-cephem-4-carboxylic acid. Its chemical formula is $C_{25}H_{26}N_9NaO_8S_2$ with a molecular weight of 667.65. The structural formula is given below:

CEFOBID contains 34 mg sodium (1.5 mEq) per gram. CEFOBID is a white powder which is freely soluble in water. The pH of a 25% (w/v) freshly reconstituted solution varies between 4.5–6.5 and the solution ranges from colorless to straw yellow depending on the concentration.

Clinical Pharmacology: High serum and bile levels of CEFOBID are attained after a single dose of the drug. Table 1 demonstrates the serum concentrations of CEFOBID in normal volunteers following either a single 15-minute constant rate intravenous infusion of 1, 2, 3 or 4 grams of the drug, or a single intramuscular injection of 1 or 2 grams of the drug.
[See table below].
The mean serum half-life of CEFOBID is approximately 2.0 hours, independent of the route of administration.

In vitro studies with human serum indicate that the degree of CEFOBID reversible protein binding varies with the serum concentration from 93% at 25 mcg/ml of CEFOBID to 90% at 250 mcg/ml and 82% at 500 mcg/ml.

CEFOBID achieves therapeutic concentrations in the following body tissues and fluids:

Tissue or Fluid	Dose	Concentration
Ascitic Fluid	2 g	64 mcg/ml
Cerebrospinal Fluid (in patients with inflamed meninges)	50 mg/kg	1.8 mcg/ml to 8.0 mcg/ml
Urine	2 g	3,286 mcg/ml
Sputum	3 g	6.0 mcg/ml
Endometrium	2 g	74 mcg/g
Myometrium	2 g	54 mcg/g
Palatine Tonsil	1 g	8 mcg/g
Sinus Mucous Membrane	1 g	8 mcg/g
Umbilical Cord Blood	1 g	25 mcg/ml
Amniotic Fluid	1 g	4.8 mcg/ml
Lung	1 g	28 mcg/g
Bone	2 g	40 mcg/g

CEFOBID is excreted mainly in the bile. Maximum bile concentrations are generally obtained between one and three hours following drug ad-

TABLE 1. Cefoperazone Serum Concentrations

Dose/Route	Mean Serum Concentrations (mcg/ml)						
	0*	0.5 hr	1 hr	2 hr	4 hr	8 hr	12 hr
1 g IV	153	114	73	38	16	4	0.5
2 g IV	252	153	114	70	32	8	2
3 g IV	340	210	142	89	41	9	2
4 g IV	506	325	251	161	71	19	6
1 g IM	32**	52	65	57	33	7	1
2 g IM	40**	69	93	97	58	14	4

*Hours post-administration, with 0 time being the end of the infusion.
**Values obtained 15 minutes post-injection.

ministration and exceed concurrent serum concentrations by up to 100 times. Reported biliary concentrations of CEFOBID range from 66 mcg/ml at 30 minutes to as high as 6000 mcg/ml at 3 hours after an intravenous bolus injection of 2 grams.

Following a single intramuscular or intravenous dose, the urinary recovery of CEFOBID over a 12-hour period averages 20–30%. No significant quantity of metabolites has been found in the urine. Urinary concentrations greater than 2200 mcg/ml have been obtained following a 15-minute infusion of a 2 g dose. After an IM injection of 2 g, peak urine concentrations of almost 1000 mcg/ml have been obtained, and therapeutic levels are maintained for 12 hours.

Repeated administration of CEFOBID at 12-hour intervals does not result in accumulation of the drug in normal subjects. Peak serum concentrations, areas under the curve (AUC's), and serum half-lives in patients with severe renal insufficiency are not significantly different from those in normal volunteers. In patients with hepatic dysfunction, the serum half-life is prolonged and urinary excretion is increased. In patients with combined renal and hepatic insufficiencies, CEFOBID may accumulate in the serum.

CEFOBID has been used in pediatrics, but the safety and effectiveness in children have not been established. The half-life of CEFOBID in serum is 6–10 hours in low birth-weight neonates.

Microbiology
CEFOBID is active *in vitro* against a wide range of aerobic and anaerobic, gram-positive and gram-negative pathogens. The bactericidal action of CEFOBID results from the inhibition of bacterial cell wall synthesis. CEFOBID has a high degree of stability in the presence of beta-lactamases produced by most gram-negative pathogens. CEFOBID is usually active against organisms which are resistant to other beta-lactam antibiotics because of beta-lactamase production. CEFOBID is usually active against the following organisms *in vitro* and in clinical infections:

Gram-Positive Aerobes:
Staphylococcus aureus, penicillinase and non-penicillinase-producing strains
Staphylococcus epidermidis
Streptococcus pneumoniae (formerly *Diplococcus pneumoniae*)
Streptococcus pyogenes (Group A beta-hemolytic streptococci)
Streptococcus agalactiae (Group B beta-hemolytic streptococci)
Enterococcus (*Streptococcus faecalis*, *S. faecium* and *S. durans*)

Gram-Negative Aerobes:
Escherichia coli   *Providencia stuartii*
Klebsiella species   *Providencia rettgeri*
  (including   (formerly *Proteus rettgeri*)
  K. pneumoniae)
Enterobacter species
Citrobacter species   *Serratia marcescens*
Haemophilus influenzae   *Pseudomonas aeruginosa*
Proteus mirabilis   *Pseudomonas* species
Proteus vulgaris   Some strains of *Acinetobacter calcoaceticus*
Morganella morganii   *Neisseria gonorrhoeae*
  (formerly *Proteus morganii*)

Anaerobic Organisms:
Gram-positive cocci (including *Peptococcus* and *Peptostreptococcus*)
Clostridium species
Bacteroides fragilis
Other *Bacteroides* species
CEFOBID is also active *in vitro* against a wide variety of other pathogens although the clinical significance is unknown. These organisms include: *Salmonella* and *Shigella* species, *Serratia liquefaciens*, *N. meningitidis*, *Bordetella pertussis*, *Yersinia enterocolitica*, *Clostridium difficile*, *Fusobacterium* species, *Eubacterium* species and beta-lactamase producing strains of *H. influenzae* and *N. gonorrhoeae*.

Susceptibility Testing:
Diffusion Technique. For the disk diffusion method of susceptibility testing, a 75 mcg CEFOBID diffusion disk should be used. Organisms should be tested with the CEFOBID 75 mcg disk since CEFOBID has been shown *in vitro* to be active against organisms which are found to be resistant to other beta-lactam antibiotics.
Tests should be interpreted by the following criteria:

Zone Diameter	Interpretation
Greater than or equal to 21 mm	Susceptible
16–20 mm	Moderately Susceptible
Less than or equal to 15 mm	Resistant

Quantitative procedures that require measurement of zone diameters give the most precise estimate of susceptibility. One such method which has been recommended for use with the CEFOBID 75 mcg disk is the NCCLS approved standard. (Performance Standards for Antimicrobic Disc Susceptibility Tests. Second Information Supplement Vol. 2 No. 2 pp. 49–69. Publisher—National Committee for Clinical Laboratory Standards, Villanova, Pennsylvania.)

A report of "susceptible" indicates that the infecting organism is likely to respond to CEFOBID therapy and a report of "resistant" indicates that the infecting organism is not likely to respond to therapy. A "moderately susceptible" report suggests that the infecting organism will be susceptible to CEFOBID if a higher than usual dosage is used or if the infection is confined to tissues and fluids (e.g., urine or bile) in which high antibiotic levels are attained.

Dilution Techniques. Broth or agar dilution methods may be used to determine the minimal inhibitory concentration (MIC) of CEFOBID. Serial twofold dilutions of CEFOBID should be prepared in either broth or agar. Broth should be inoculated to contain 5×10^5 organisms/ml and agar "spotted" with 10^4 organisms.

MIC test results should be interpreted in light of serum, tissue, and body fluid concentrations of CEFOBID. Organisms inhibited by CEFOBID at 16 mcg/ml or less are considered susceptible, while organisms with MIC's of 17–63 mcg/ml are moderately susceptible. Organisms inhibited at CEFOBID concentrations of greater than or equal to 64 mcg/ml are considered resistant, although clinical cures have been obtained in some patients infected by such organisms.

Indications and Usage: CEFOBID is indicated for the treatment of the following infections when caused by susceptible organisms:

Respiratory Tract Infections caused by *S. pneumoniae*, *H. influenzae*, *S. aureus* (penicillinase and non-penicillinase producing strains), *S. pyogenes* (Group A beta-hemolytic streptococci), *P. aeruginosa*, *Klebsiella pneumoniae*, *E. coli*, *Proteus* species (indole-positive and indole-negative), and *Enterobacter* species.

Peritonitis and Other Intra-abdominal Infections caused by *E. coli*, *P. aeruginosa*, enterococci, anaerobic gram-positive cocci, and anaerobic gram-positive and gram-negative bacilli (including *Bacteroides fragilis*).

Bacterial Septicemia caused by *S. pneumoniae*, *S. pyogenes*, *S. agalactiae*, *S. aureus*, enterococci, *H. influenzae*, *Pseudomonas aeruginosa*, *E. coli*, *Klebsiella* spp., *Proteus* species (indole-positive and indole-negative), *Clostridium* spp. and anaerobic gram-positive cocci.

Infections of the Skin and Skin Structures caused by *S. aureus* (penicillinase and non-penicillinase producing strains), *S. pyogenes* and *P. aeruginosa*.

Pelvic Inflammatory Disease, Endometritis, and Other Infections of the Female Genital Tract caused by *N. gonorrhoeae*, *S. aureus* and *S. epidermidis*, *S. agalactiae*, *E. coli*, *Clostridium* spp., *Bacteroides* species (including *Bacteroides fragilis*) and anaerobic gram-positive cocci.

Urinary Tract Infections caused by *Enterococcus*, *Escherichia coli*, and *Pseudomonas aeruginosa*.

Susceptibility Testing
Before instituting treatment with CEFOBID, appropriate specimens should be obtained for isolation of the causative organism and for determination of its susceptibility to the drug. Treatment may be started before results of susceptibility testing are available.

Combination Therapy
Synergy between CEFOBID and aminoglycosides has been demonstrated with many gram-negative bacilli. However, such enhanced activity of these combinations is not predictable. If such therapy is considered, *in vitro* susceptibility tests should be performed to determine the activity of the drugs in combination, and renal function should be monitored carefully. (See PRECAUTIONS, and DOSAGE AND ADMINISTRATION sections).

Contraindications: CEFOBID is contraindicated in patients with known allergy to the cephalosporin-class of antibiotics.

Warnings: BEFORE THERAPY WITH CEFOBID IS INSTITUTED, CAREFUL INQUIRY SHOULD BE MADE TO DETERMINE WHETHER THE PATIENT HAS HAD PREVIOUS HYPERSENSITIVITY REACTIONS TO CEPHALOSPORINS, PENICILLINS OR OTHER DRUGS. THIS PRODUCT SHOULD BE GIVEN CAUTIOUSLY TO PENICILLIN-SENSITIVE PATIENTS. ANTIBIOTICS SHOULD BE ADMINISTERED WITH CAUTION TO ANY PATIENT WHO HAS DEMONSTRATED SOME FORM OF ALLERGY, PARTICULARLY TO DRUGS. SERIOUS ACUTE HYPERSENSITIVITY REACTIONS MAY REQUIRE THE USE OF SUBCUTANEOUS EPINEPHRINE AND OTHER EMERGENCY MEASURES.

PSEUDOMEMBRANOUS COLITIS HAS BEEN REPORTED WITH THE USE OF CEPHALOSPORINS (AND OTHER BROAD-SPECTRUM ANTIBIOTICS); THEREFORE, IT IS IMPORTANT TO CONSIDER ITS DIAGNOSIS IN PATIENTS WHO DEVELOP DIARRHEA IN ASSOCIATION WITH ANTIBIOTIC USE.

Treatment with broad-spectrum antibiotics alters normal flora of the colon and may permit overgrowth of clostridia. Studies indicate a toxin produced by *Clostridium difficile* is one primary cause of antibiotic-associated colitis. Cholestyramine and colestipol resins have been shown to bind the toxin *in vitro*.

Mild cases of colitis may respond to drug discontinuance alone.

Moderate to severe cases should be managed with fluid, electrolyte, and protein supplementation as indicated.

When the colitis is not relieved by drug discontinuance or when it is severe, oral vancomycin is the treatment of choice for antibiotic-associated pseudomembranous colitis produced by *C. difficile*. Other causes of colitis should also be considered.

Precautions: Although transient elevations of the BUN and serum creatinine have been observed, Cefobid alone does not appear to cause significant nephrotoxicity. However, concomitant administration of aminoglycosides and other cephalosporins has caused nephrotoxicity.

CEFOBID is extensively excreted in bile. The serum half-life of CEFOBID is increased 2–4 fold in patients with hepatic disease and/or biliary obstruction. In general, total daily dosage above 4 g should not be necessary in such patients. If higher dosages are used, serum concentrations should be monitored.

Because renal excretion is not the main route of elimination of CEFOBID (see CLINICAL PHARMACOLOGY), patients with renal failure require no adjustment in dosage when usual doses are administered. When high doses of CEFOBID are used, concentrations of drug in the serum should be monitored periodically. If evidence of accumulation exists, dosage should be decreased accordingly.

The half-life of CEFOBID is reduced slightly during hemodialysis. Thus, dosing should be scheduled to follow a dialysis period. In patients with both hepatic dysfunction and significant renal disease, CEFOBID dosage should not exceed 1–2 g

Continued on next page

Roerig—Cont.

	Cefoperazone Concentration	Volume of Diluent to be Added	Withdrawable Volume*
1 g vial	333 mg/ml	2.8 ml	3 ml
	250 mg/ml	3.8 ml	4 ml
2 g vial	333 mg/ml	5.6 ml	6 ml
	250 mg/ml	7.8 ml	8 ml

* There is sufficient excess present to allow for withdrawal of the stated volume.
† Final lidocaine concentration is approximately 0.5%.

daily without close monitoring of serum concentrations.
As with other antibiotics, vitamin K deficiency has occurred rarely in patients treated with CEFOBID. The mechanism is most probably related to the suppression of gut flora which normally synthesize this vitamin. Those at risk include patients with a poor nutritional status, malabsorption states (e.g., cystic fibrosis), alcoholism, and patients on prolonged hyper-alimentation regimens (administered either intravenously or via a naso-gastric tube). Prothrombin time should be monitored in these patients and exogenous vitamin K administered as indicated.
A disulfiram-like reaction characterized by flushing, sweating, headache, and tachycardia has been reported when alcohol (beer, wine) was ingested within 72 hours after CEFOBID administration. Patients should be cautioned about the ingestion of alcoholic beverages following the administration of CEFOBID. A similar reaction has been reported with other cephalosporins.
Prolonged use of CEFOBID may result in the overgrowth of nonsusceptible organisms. Careful observation of the patient is essential. If superinfection occurs during therapy, appropriate measures should be taken.
CEFOBID should be prescribed with caution in individuals with a history of gastrointestinal disease, particularly colitis.

Drug Laboratory Test Interactions
A false-positive reaction for glucose in the urine may occur with Benedict's or Fehling's solution.

Carcinogenesis, Mutagenesis, Impairment of Fertility
The maximum duration of CEFOBID animal toxicity studies is six months. In none of the *in vivo* or *in vitro* genetic toxicology studies did CEFOBID show any mutagenic potential at either the chromosomal or subchromosomal level. CEFOBID produced no impairment of fertility and had no effects on general reproductive performance or fetal development when administered subcutaneously at daily doses up to 500 to 1000 mg/kg prior to and during mating, and to pregnant female rats during gestation. These doses are 10 to 20 times the estimated usual single clinical dose.

Usage in Pregnancy
Pregnancy Category B: Reproduction studies have been performed in mice, rats, and monkeys at doses up to 10 times the human dose and have revealed no evidence of impaired fertility or harm to the fetus due to CEFOBID. There are, however, no adequate and well controlled studies in pregnant women. Because animal reproduction studies are not always predictive of human response, this drug should be used during pregnancy only if clearly needed.

Usage in Nursing Mothers
Only low concentrations of CEFOBID are excreted in human milk. Although CEFOBID passes poorly into breast milk of nursing mothers, caution should be exercised when CEFOBID is administered to a nursing woman.

Pediatric Use
Safety and effectiveness in children have not been established.

Adverse Reactions: In clinical studies the following adverse effects were observed and were considered to be related to CEFOBID therapy or of uncertain etiology.
Hypersensitivity: As with all cephalosporins, hypersensitivity manifested by skin reactions (1 patient in 45), drug fever (1 in 260), or a change in Coombs' test (1 in 60) has been reported. These reactions are more likely to occur in patients with a history of allergies, particularly to penicillin.
Hematology: As with other beta-lactam antibiotics, reversible neutropenia may occur with prolonged administration. Slight decreases in neutrophil count (1 patient in 50) have been reported. Decreased hemoglobins (1 in 20) or hematocrits (1 in 20) have been reported, which is consistent with published literature on other cephalosporins. Transient eosinophilia has occurred in 1 patient in 10.
Hepatic: Of 1285 patients treated with cefoperazone in clinical trials, one patient with a history of liver disease developed significantly elevated liver function enzymes during CEFOBID therapy. Clinical signs and symptoms of nonspecific hepatitis accompanied these increases. After CEFOBID therapy was discontinued, the patient's enzymes returned to pre-treatment levels and the symptomatology resolved. As with other antibiotics that achieve high bile levels, mild transient elevations of liver function enzymes have been observed in 5–10% of the patients receiving CEFOBID therapy. The relevance of these findings, which were not accompanied by overt signs or symptoms of hepatic dysfunction, has not been established.
Gastrointestinal: Diarrhea or loose stools has been reported in 1 in 30 patients. Most of these experiences have been mild or moderate in severity and self-limiting in nature. In all cases, these symptoms responded to symptomatic therapy or ceased when cefoperazone therapy was stopped. Nausea and vomiting have been reported rarely. Symptoms of pseudomembranous colitis can appear during or for several weeks subsequent to antibiotic therapy (see WARNINGS).
Renal Function Tests: Transient elevations of the BUN (1 in 16) and serum creatinine (1 in 48) have been noted.
Local Reactions: CEFOBID is well tolerated following intramuscular administration. Occasionally, transient pain (1 in 140) may follow administration by this route. When CEFOBID is administered by intravenous infusion some patients may develop phlebitis (1 in 120) at the infusion site.
Dosage and Administration: The usual adult daily dose of CEFOBID is 2 to 4 grams per day administered in equally divided doses every 12 hours. In severe infections or infections caused by less sensitive organisms, the total daily dose and/or frequency may be increased. Patients have been successfully treated with a total daily dosage of 6–12 grams divided into 2, 3 or 4 administrations ranging from 1.5 to 4 grams per dose.
In a pharmacokinetic study, a total daily dose of 16 grams was administered to severely immunocompromised patients by constant infusion without complications. Steady state serum concentrations were approximately 150 mcg/ml in these patients. When treating infections caused by *Streptococcus pyogenes*, therapy should be continued for at least 10 days.
If combination therapy with CEFOBID and an aminoglycoside is contemplated (see INDICATIONS), these drugs should be given at separate sites since there is a physical incompatibility between them. *In vitro* testing of the effectiveness of drug combination(s) is recommended.
Reconstitution: The following diluents may be used for reconstitution of CEFOBID sterile powder and used for intravenous infusion:
5% Dextrose Injection (USP)
5% Dextrose and Lactated Ringer's Injection
5% Dextrose and 0.9% Sodium Chloride Injection (USP)
5% Dextrose and 0.2% Sodium Chloride Injection (USP)
10% Dextrose Injection (USP)
Lactated Ringer's Injection (USP)
0.9% Sodium Chloride Injection (USP)
Normosol® M and 5% Dextrose Injection
Normosol® R
The following diluents may be used for reconstitution of CEFOBID sterile powder for intramuscular injection:
Bacteriostatic Water for Injection [Benzyl Alcohol or Parabens] (USP)
Lidocaine Hydrochloride Injection (USP) (See directions for "Preparation for Intramuscular Injection" below.)
Sterile Water for Injection
Preparations containing Benzyl Alcohol should not be used in neonates.

General Reconstitution Procedures
CEFOBID sterile powder for intravenous or intramuscular use may be reconstituted with any compatible solution for infusion mentioned above. Solutions should be allowed to stand after reconstitution to allow any foaming to dissipate to permit visual inspection for complete solubilization. Vigorous and prolonged agitation may be necessary to solubilize CEFOBID in higher concentrations (above 333 mg cefoperazone/ml). The maximum solubility of CEFOBID sterile powder is approximately 475 mg cefoperazone/ml of compatible diluent.

Preparation For Intramuscular Injection
Any suitable diluent listed above may be used to prepare solutions for intramuscular injection. When concentrations of 250 mg/ml or more are to be administered, a lidocaine solution should be used. These solutions should be prepared using Sterile Water for Injection and 2% Lidocaine Hydrochloride Injection (USP) to provide an approximately 0.5% Lidocaine Hydrochloride Solution. A two-step dilution process as follows is recommended. First, add the required amount of Sterile Water for Injection and agitate until CEFOBID powder is completely dissolved. Second, add the required amount of 2% Lidocaine and mix.
[See table below].
When a diluent other than Lidocaine HCl Injection (USP) is used reconstitute as follows:
[See table above].

Preparation For Intravenous Use
In general, CEFOBID concentrations of between 2 mg/ml and 50 mg/ml are recommended for intravenous administration. Vials of CEFOBID sterile powder may be initially reconstituted with a minimum of 2.8 ml per gram of cefoperazone of any compatible diluent listed above appropriate for intravenous administration. For ease of reconstitution the use of 5 ml of compatible diluent per gram of CEFOBID is recommended. The entire quantity of the resulting solution should then be withdrawn for further dilution and administration via intravenous administration system in one of the following manners:
Intermittent Infusion: Reconstituted CEFOBID should be further diluted in 20 ml to 40 ml of diluent per gram of cefoperazone and administered over a 15–30 minute time period.

	Final Cefoperazone Concentration	Step 1 Volume of Sterile Water	Step 2 Volume of 2% Lidocaine	Withdrawable Volume* †
1 g vial	333 mg/ml	2.2 ml	0.6 ml	3 ml
	250 mg/ml	2.8 ml	1.0 ml	4 ml
2 g vial	333 mg/ml	4.2 ml	1.4 ml	6 ml
	250 mg/ml	5.8 ml	2.0 ml	8 ml

Continuous Infusion: CEFOBID can be used for continuous infusion after dilution to a final concentration of between 2 and 25 mg cefoperazone per ml.

Stability: CEFOBID sterile powder is to be stored protected from light and refrigerated (2°–8°C/36°–46°F) prior to reconstitution. After reconstitution, protection from light is not necessary. The following parenteral diluents and approximate concentrations of CEFOBID provide stable solutions under the following conditions for the indicated time periods. (After the indicated time periods, unused portions of solutions should be discarded.)

Controlled Room Temperature (15°–25°C/59°–77°F)

24 Hours	Approximate Concentrations
Bacteriostatic Water for Injection [Benzyl Alcohol or Parabens] (USP)	300 mg/ml
5% Dextrose Injection (USP)	2 mg to 50 mg/ml
5% Dextrose and Lactated Ringer's Injection	2 mg to 50 mg/ml
5% Dextrose and 0.9% Sodium Chloride Injection (USP)	2 mg to 50 mg/ml
5% Dextrose and 0.2% Sodium Chloride Injection (USP)	2 mg to 50 mg/ml
10% Dextrose Injection (USP)	2 mg to 50 mg/ml
Lactated Ringer's Injection (USP)	2 mg/ml
0.5% Lidocaine Hydrochloride Injection (USP)	300 mg/ml
0.9% Sodium Chloride Injection (USP)	2 mg to 300 mg/ml
Normosol® M and 5% Dextrose Injection	2 mg to 50 mg/ml
Normosol® R	2 mg to 50 mg/ml
Sterile Water for Injection	300 mg/ml

Reconstituted CEFOBID solutions may be stored in glass or plastic syringes, or in glass or flexible plastic parenteral solution containers.

Refrigerator Temperature (2°–8°C/36°–46°F)

5 Days	Approximate Concentrations
Bacteriostatic Water for Injection [Benzyl Alcohol or Parabens] (USP)	300 mg/ml
5% Dextrose Injection (USP)	2 mg to 50 mg/ml
5% Dextrose and 0.9% Sodium Chloride Injection (USP)	2 mg to 50 mg/ml
5% Dextrose and 0.2% Sodium Chloride Injection (USP)	2 mg to 50 mg/ml
Lactated Ringer's Injection (USP)	2 mg/ml
0.5% Lidocaine Hydrochloride Injection (USP)	300 mg/ml
0.9% Sodium Chloride Injection (USP)	2 mg to 300 mg/ml
Normosol® M and 5% Dextrose Injection	2 mg to 50 mg/ml
Normosol® R	2 mg to 50 mg/ml
Sterile Water for Injection	300 mg/ml

Reconstituted CEFOBID solutions may be stored in glass or plastic syringes, or in glass or flexible plastic parenteral solution containers.

Freezer Temperature (−20° to −10°C/−4° to 14°F)

3 Weeks	Approximate Concentrations
5% Dextrose Injection (USP)	50 mg/ml
5% Dextrose and 0.9% Sodium Chloride Injection (USP)	2 mg/ml
5% Dextrose and 0.2% Sodium Chloride Injection (USP)	2 mg/ml

5 Weeks	
0.9% Sodium Chloride Injection (USP)	300 mg/ml
Sterile Water for Injection	300 mg/ml

Reconstituted CEFOBID solutions may be stored in plastic syringes, or in flexible plastic parenteral solution containers.

Frozen samples should be thawed at room temperature before use. After thawing, unused portions should be discarded. Do not refreeze.

How Supplied: CEFOBID sterile powder is available in 1 gram (NDC 0049-1201-28) and 2 gram (NDC 0049-1202-28) vials for either intramuscular or intravenous administration.

60-4163-00-1

EMETE-CON®
[ă-mĕt'ă-kŏn"]
(benzquinamide hydrochloride)
For Intramuscular and Intravenous Use

Description: Benzquinamide is a non-amine-depleting benzoquinolizine derivative, chemically unrelated to the phenothiazines and to other antiemetics.

Chemically, Emete-con (benzquinamide hydrochloride) is N,N-diethyl-1,3,4,6,7,11b-hexahydro-2-hydroxy-9, 10-dimethoxy-2H-benzo[a]quinolizine-3-carboxamide acetate hydrochloride. The empirical formula is $C_{22}H_{32}N_2O_5 \cdot HCl$ and the molecular weight is 441.

Emete-con for injection contains benzquinamide hydrochloride equivalent to 50 mg/vial of benzquinamide. When reconstituted with 2.2 ml of proper diluent, each vial yields 2 ml of a solution containing benzquinamide hydrochloride equivalent to 25 mg/ml of benzquinamide. When reconstituted this product maintains its potency for 14 days at room temperature.

Actions: Benzquinamide HCl exhibited antiemetic, antihistaminic, mild anticholinergic and sedative action in animals. Studies conducted in dogs and human volunteers have demonstrated suppression of apomorphine-induced vomiting; however, relevance to clinical efficacy has not been established. The mechanism of action in humans is unknown. The onset of antiemetic activity in humans usually occurs within 15 minutes.

Benzquinamide metabolism has been studied in animals and in man. In both species, 5-10% of an administered dose is excreted unchanged in the urine. The remaining drug undergoes metabolic transformation in the liver by at least three pathways to a spectrum of metabolites which are excreted in the urine and in the bile, from which the more polar metabolites are not reabsorbed but are excreted in the feces. The half-life in plasma of Emete-con is about 40 minutes. More than 95% of an administered dose was excreted within 72 hours in animal studies using C14-labeled benzquinamide. In blood, benzquinamide is about 58% bound to plasma protein.

Indications: Emete-con is indicated for the prevention and treatment of nausea and vomiting associated with anesthesia and surgery.

Since the incidence of postoperative and postanesthetic vomiting has decreased with the adoption of modern techniques and agents, the prophylactic use of Emete-con should be restricted to those patients in whom emesis would endanger the results of surgery or result in harm to the patient.

Contraindications: Emete-con is contraindicated in individuals who have demonstrated hypersensitivity to the drug.

Warnings:
Use in Pregnancy
No teratogenic effects of benzquinamide were demonstrated in reproduction studies in chick embryos, mice, rats and rabbits. The relevance of these data to the human is not known. However, safe use of this drug in pregnancy has not been established and its use in pregnancy is not recommended.

Use in Children
As the data available at present are insufficient to establish proper dosage in children, the use of Emete-con in children is not recommended.

Intravenous use
Sudden increase in blood pressure and transient arrhythmias (premature ventricular and auricular contractions) have been reported following intravenous administration of benzquinamide. Until a more predictable pattern of the effect of intravenous benzquinamide has been established, the intramuscular route of administration is considered preferable. The intravenous route of administration should be restricted to patients without cardiovascular disease and receiving no preanesthetic and/or concomitant cardiovascular drugs.

If patients receiving pressor agents or epinephrine-like drugs are also given benzquinamide, the latter should be given in fractions of the normal dose. Blood pressure should be monitored. Safeguards against hypertensive reactions are particularly important in hypertensive patients.

Precautions: Benzquinamide, like other antiemetics, may mask signs of overdosage of toxic drugs or may obscure diagnosis of such conditions as intestinal obstruction and brain tumor.

Adverse Reactions: The following adverse reactions have been reported in subjects who have received benzquinamide. However, drowsiness appears to be the most common reaction. One case of pronounced allergic reaction has been encountered, characterized by pyrexia and urticaria.

System Affected
Autonomic Nervous System: Dry mouth, shivering, sweating, hiccoughs, flushing, salivation, blurred vision.
Cardiovascular System: Hypertension, hypotension, dizziness, atrial fibrillation, premature auricular and ventricular contractions.
Hypertensive episodes have occurred after IM and IV administration.
Central Nervous System: Drowsiness, insomnia, restlessness, headache, excitement, nervousness.
Gastrointestinal System: Anorexia, nausea.
Musculoskeletal System: Twitching, shaking/tremors, weakness.
Skin: Hives/rash.
Other Systems: Fatigue, shaking chills, increased temperature.

Dosage and Administration:
Intramuscular: 50 mg (0.5 mg/kg–1.0 mg/kg)
First dose may be repeated in one hour with subsequent doses every 3-4 hours, as necessary. The precautions applicable to all intramuscular injections should be observed. Emete-con should be injected well within the mass of a larger muscle. The deltoid area should be used only if well developed. Injections should not be made into the lower and mid-thirds of the upper arm. Aspiration of the syringe should be carried out to avoid inadvertent intravascular injection.

Therapeutic blood levels and demonstrable antiemetic activity appear within fifteen minutes of intramuscular administration. When the objective of therapy is the prevention of nausea and vomiting, intramuscular administration is recommended at least fifteen minutes prior to emergence from anesthesia.

Intravenous: 25 mg (0.2 mg/kg–0.4 mg/kg as a single dose) administered slowly (1 ml per 0.5 to 1 minute). Subsequent doses should be given intramuscularly.

The intravenous route of administration should be restricted to patients without cardiovascular disease (See WARNINGS). If it is necessary to use Emete-con intravenously in elderly or debilitated patients, benzquinamide should be administered cautiously and the lower dose range is recommended.

This preparation must be initially reconstituted with 2.2 ml of Sterile Water for Injection, Bacteriostatic Water for Injection with benzyl alcohol or with methylparaben and propylparaben. This procedure yields 2 ml of a solution equivalent to 25 mg benzquinamide/ml, which maintains its potency for 14 days at room temperature.

Overdosage:
Manifestations: On the basis of acute animal toxicology studies, gross Emete-con overdosage in humans might be expected to manifest itself as a combination of Central Nervous System stimulant and depressant effects. This speculation is derived from experimental studies in which intravenous doses of benzquinamide, at least 150 times the human therapeutic dose, were administered to dogs.

Continued on next page

Roerig—Cont.

Treatment: There is no specific antidote for Emete-con overdosage. General supportive measures should be instituted, as indicated. Atropine may be helpful. Although there has been no direct experience with dialysis, it is not likely to be of value, since benzquinamide is extensively bound to plasma protein.

How Supplied: Emete-con for IM/IV use is available in a vial containing benzquinamide HCl equivalent to 50 mg of benzquinamide in packages of 10 vials.

Caution: Federal law prohibits dispensing without prescription.

60-1787-00-4

GEOCILLIN® ℞
[gē'ō-sĭl-ĭn]
(carbenicillin indanyl sodium)
TABLETS
For Oral Use

Description: Geocillin (carbenicillin indanyl sodium), a semisynthetic penicillin, is the sodium salt of the indanyl ester of Geopen® (carbenicillin disodium). Geocillin is acid stable and well absorbed following oral administration.

Actions:
Microbiology
The antibacterial activity of Geocillin is due to its rapid conversion to carbenicillin by hydrolysis. Though Geocillin provides substantial *in vitro* activity against a variety of both gram-positive and gram-negative microorganisms, the most important aspect of its profile is in its antipseudomonal and antiproteus activity. Because of the high urine levels obtained following administration, Geocillin has demonstrated clinical efficacy in urinary infections due to susceptible strains of:

Escherichia coli
Proteus mirabilis
Proteus morgani
Proteus rettgeri
Proteus vulgaris
Pseudomonas
Enterobacter
Enterococci

In addition, *in vitro* data, not substantiated by clinical studies, indicate the following pathogens to be usually susceptible to Geocillin:

Staphylococcus (non-penicillinase producing)
Streptococcus

Most *Klebsiella* species are often resistant to the action of Geocillin. Some strains of *Pseudomonas* have developed resistance to carbenicillin.

Susceptibility Testing
Geopen (carbenicillin disodium) Susceptibility Powder or 100 mcg. Geopen Susceptibility Discs may be used to determine microbial susceptibility to Geocillin.

Geocillin	DOSE	Mean Urine Concentration of Carbenicillin mcg/ml Hours After Initial Dose		
DRUG	DOSE	0–3	3–6	6–24
Geocillin	1 tablet q.6 hr.	1130	352	292
Geocillin	2 tablets q.6 hr.	1428	789	809

Mean serum concentrations of carbenicillin in this study for these dosages are:

DRUG	DOSE	1/2	1	2	4	6	24	25	26	28
Geocillin	1 tablet q.6 hr.	5.1	6.5	3.2	1.9	0.0	0.4	8.8	5.4	0.4
Geocillin	2 tablets q.6 hr.	6.1	9.6	7.9	2.6	0.4	0.8	13.2	12.8	3.8

Mean Serum Concentration mcg/ml Hours After Initial Dose

Interpretations:
[See table below].
Interpretations of susceptible, intermediate, and resistant correlate zone size diameters with MIC values. A laboratory report of "susceptible" indicates that the suspected causative microorganism most likely will respond to therapy with carbenicillin. A laboratory report of "resistant" indicates that the infecting microorganism most likely will not respond to therapy. A laboratory report of "intermediate" indicates that the microorganism is most likely susceptible if a high dosage of carbenicillin is used, or if the infection is such that high levels of carbenicillin may be attained as in urine.

Pharmacology
Geocillin is acid stable and well absorbed following oral administration. After absorption, Geocillin is rapidly hydrolyzed to carbenicillin, which is primarily excreted in the urine. In a study utilizing volunteers with normal renal function, the following mean urine levels of carbenicillin were achieved:
[See table above].

Indications: Geocillin (carbenicillin indanyl sodium) is indicated in the treatment of acute and chronic infections of the upper and lower urinary tract and in asymptomatic bacteriuria due to susceptible strains of the following organisms:

Escherichia coli
Proteus mirabilis
Proteus morgani
Proteus rettgeri
Proteus vulgaris
Pseudomonas
Enterobacter
Enterococci

Geocillin is also indicated in the treatment of prostatitis due to susceptible strains of the following organisms:

Escherichia coli
Enterococcus (S. faecalis)
Proteus mirabilis
Enterobacter sp.

WHEN HIGH RAPID BLOOD AND URINE LEVELS OF ANTIBIOTIC ARE INDICATED, THERAPY WITH GEOPEN (CARBENICILLIN DISODIUM) SHOULD BE INITIATED BY PARENTERAL ADMINISTRATION FOLLOWED, AT THE PHYSICIAN'S DISCRETION, BY ORAL THERAPY.

NOTE: Susceptibility testing should be performed prior to and during the course of therapy to detect the possible emergence of resistant organisms which may develop.

Contraindications: Geocillin is ordinarily contraindicated in patients who have a known penicillin allergy.

Warnings: Serious and occasionally fatal hypersensitivity (anaphylactic) reactions have been reported in patients on oral penicillin therapy. These reactions are more apt to occur in individuals with a history of sensitivity to multiple allergens.

There have been reports of individuals with a history of penicillin hypersensitivity who have experienced severe hypersensitivity reactions when treated with a cephalosporin, and vice versa. Therefore, before therapy with a penicillin, careful inquiry should be made concerning previous hypersensitivity reactions to penicillins, cephalosporins, and other allergens.

SERIOUS ANAPHYLACTOID REACTIONS REQUIRE IMMEDIATE EMERGENCY TREATMENT WITH EPINEPHRINE. OXYGEN, INTRAVENOUS STEROIDS AND AIRWAY MANAGEMENT, INCLUDING INTUBATION, SHOULD ALSO BE ADMINISTERED AS INDICATED.

Usage in Children: Since only limited clinical data is available to date in children, the safety of Geocillin administration in this age group has not yet been established.

Usage in Pregnancy: Safety for use in pregnancy has not been established.

Precautions: Periodic assessment of organ system function including renal, hepatic and hematopoietic systems is recommended during prolonged therapy.

Long term use of Geocillin may result in the overgrowth of nonsensitive organisms. If superinfection occurs during therapy, appropriate measures should be taken.

Since carbenicillin is excreted by the kidney, patients with severe renal impairment (creatinine clearance of less than 10 ml/min.) will not achieve therapeutic urine levels of carbenicillin.

Adverse Reactions: The following adverse reactions may occur during therapy with Geocillin:

Geocillin	Susceptible	Intermediate	Resistant
Pseudomonas aeruginosa and Enterococci			
Inhibition Zone	17 mm or greater*	16 mm–14 mm	13 mm or less
MIC	125 mcg/ml or less	greater than 125 mcg/ml less than 250 mcg/ml	250 mcg/ml or greater
Escherichia coli, Proteus species, and *Enterobacter*.			
Inhibition Zone	23 mm or greater	22 mm–18 mm	17 mm or less
MIC	15 mcg/ml or less	greater than 20 mcg/ml less than 40 mcg/ml	greater than 40 mcg/ml

*Zone diameter interpretations apply only to results obtained by the Bauer, Kirby, Sherris and Turck method of Susceptibility Testing Am. J. Clin. Path. 45:493, 1966.

Gastrointestinal Disturbances: Nausea, vomiting, and diarrhea.
Hypersensitivity Reactions: Skin rashes, urticaria, or pruritus have been reported infrequently.
Blood, Hepatic and Renal Studies: As with other penicillins, anemia, thrombocytopenia, leukopenia, neutropenia, and eosinophilia may occur.
Mild SGOT elevations have been observed following Geocillin administration.
Other reactions that have been reported are flatulence, dry mouth, furry tongue, vaginitis, and abdominal cramps.
Dosage and Administration:
Geocillin is available as a coated tablet, to be administered orally.

Usual Adult Dose

URINARY TRACT INFECTIONS	
Escherichia coli, *Proteus* species, and *Enterobacter*	1-2 tablets 4 times daily
Pseudomonas and Enterococci	2 tablets 4 times daily
PROSTATITIS	
Escherichia coli, *Proteus mirabilis*, *Enterobacter* and Enterococcus	2 tablets 4 times daily

How Supplied: Geocillin is available as filmcoated tablets in bottles of 100's, and unit-dose packages of 100 (10 × 10s). Each tablet contains carbenicillin indanyl sodium equivalent to 382 mg of carbenicillin.

69-1970-00-7
Shown in Product Identification Section, page 431

GEOPEN® ℞
[gē'ō-pen"]
sterile carbenicillin disodium
For Intramuscular and Intravenous Use

Description: Geopen (carbenicillin disodium) is a new semisynthetic injectable penicillin.
Geopen is a benzylpenicillin derivative with substitution by an ionizable functional group in the alpha position.
Actions:
Microbiology
Though Geopen has substantial *in vitro* activity against a variety of both gram-positive and gram-negative microorganisms the most important aspect of its profile is in its antipseudomonal and antiproteus effect.
Organisms found to be susceptible to Geopen *in vitro* include the following:
Staphylococcus aureus
(Non-penicillinase producing)
Staphylococcus albus
Diplococcus pneumoniae
Beta-hemolytic Streptococci
Streptococcus faecalis
Hemophilus influenzae
Neisseria species
Enterobacter species
Proteus mirabilis
Proteus morgani
Proteus rettgeri
Proteus vulgaris
Escherichia coli
Salmonella species
Pseudomonas aeruginosa
Anaerobic bacteria, including:
  Bacteroides species
  Peptostreptococcus species
  Peptococcus species
  Clostridium species
  Fusobacterium species
In vitro synergism between Geopen and gentamicin sulfate in certain strains of *Pseudomonas aeruginosa* has been demonstrated.
Geopen is not stable in the presence of penicillinase.
Most *Klebsiella* species are resistant to the action of Geopen.

CARBENICILLIN BLOOD LEVELS AND URINARY EXCRETION

Geopen

Dosage	ROUTE	SERUM LEVELS mcg/ml								Urinary excretion of administered dose
		¼ hr.	½ hr.	1 hr.	2 hr.	3 hr.	4 hr.	6 hr.	8 hr.	0–9 hours
500 mg.	IM	8	10	13	9.8	6.5	3.2	0	—	85%
1000 mg.	IM	—	13	18	15	12	7.5	1.7	0.7	74.6%*
2000 mg.	IM	26	38	47	37	25	15	5.9	1.2	79%
1000 mg.	IV	71	45	31	14	8.2	3	0	—	73%
1000 mg.+ 1 Gm. probenecid	IV Oral	72	55	40	26	17	12	6.5	2.0	74%

*0–24 hr. collection

Some of the newly emerging pathogenic strains of such microorganisms as *Herellea*, *Mima*, *Citrobacter* and *Serratia* have shown susceptibility to Geopen.
Some strains of *Pseudomonas* have developed resistance to Geopen fairly rapidly.
Pharmacology
Geopen is not absorbed orally, hence, it must be administered by the intramuscular or intravenous routes.
Following intramuscular injection, peak blood levels are obtained within 1–2 hours. The administration of probenecid results in somewhat higher and more prolonged serum levels as noted in the table (above).
The **MIC** for many strains of *Pseudomonas* and *Bacteroides fragilis* is relatively high; serum levels of 100 mcg./ml. or greater are required. However, the low degree of toxicity of carbenicillin permits the use of doses large enough to achieve adequate levels for these strains.
Other susceptible organisms usually require serum levels in the range of 10-25 mcg/ml.
Geopen is not highly bound to serum proteins and is excreted unchanged in high concentrations in the urine. After a 0.5 to 2 grams I.M. dose, a urine concentration of 1,000 to 5,000 mcg/ml may be achieved.

Indications: Geopen is primarily indicated in the treatment of infections due to susceptible *Pseudomonas aeruginosa*, *Proteus* species (particularly indole positive strains) and certain strains of *Escherichia coli*.
By virtue of the very high urinary levels achieved, Geopen is particularly effective in urinary tract infections due to one or more of the above mentioned organisms.
Clinical studies have demonstrated the effectiveness of Geopen in the following infections when due to these organisms:
1. Severe systemic infections and septicemia including meningitis due to *Hemophilus influenzae* and *Streptococcus pneumoniae*. Although Geopen possesses *in vitro* activity against many ampicillin-resistant *H. influenzae*, clinical data are insufficient to recommend its use for treatment of meningitis due to ampicillin-resistant strains.
2. Genitourinary tract infections including those due to *Neisseria gonorrhoeae*, *Enterobacter* and *Streptococcus faecalis* (enterococcus).
3. Acute and chronic respiratory infections. Though clinical improvement has been shown, bacteriologic cures cannot be expected in patients with chronic respiratory disease and cystic fibrosis.
4. Soft tissue infections.
Geopen is also indicated in the treatment of the following infections due to susceptible an- aerobic bacteria:
1. Septicemia.
2. Lower respiratory tract infections such as empyema, anaerobic pneumonitis and lung abscess.
3. Intra-abdominal infections such as peritonitis and intra-abdominal abscess. (Typically resulting from anaerobic organisms resident in the normal gastrointestinal tract.)
4. Infections of the female pelvis and genital tract such as endometritis, pelvic inflammatory disease, pelvic abscess and salpingitis.
5. Skin and soft tissue infections.
Although Geopen (carbenicillin disodium) is indicated primarily in gram-negative infections, its activity against gram-positive organisms should be kept in mind when both gram-positive and gram-negative organisms are isolated (see Actions).
In the treatment of infections due to certain susceptible strains of *Pseudomonas aeruginosa*, clinical efficacy may be enhanced by the use of combined therapy with Geopen (carbenicillin disodium) and gentamicin sulfate in full therapeutic dosages. For additional prescribing information, see the gentamicin sulfate package insert.
NOTE: During therapy, sensitivity testing should be repeated frequently to detect the possible emergence of resistant organisms which may develop, particularly if a suboptimal dose regimen is used.
Contraindications: Geopen is ordinarily contraindicated in patients who have a known penicillin allergy.
Warnings: Serious and occasional fatal hypersensitivity (anaphylactic) reactions have been reported in patients on penicillin therapy. These reactions are more apt to occur in individuals with a history of sensitivity to multiple allergens.
Patients with renal impairment should be observed for bleeding manifestations. Such patients should be dosed strictly according to recommendations (see Dosage and Administration section). If bleeding manifestations appear, the antibiotic should be discontinued and appropriate therapy be instituted.
There have been reports of individuals with a history of penicillin hypersensitivity reactions who have experienced severe hypersensitivity reactions when treated with a cephalosporin. Before therapy with a penicillin, careful inquiry should be made concerning previous hypersensitivity reactions to penicillins, cephalosporins, and other allergens. If an allergic reaction occurs, appropriate therapy should be instituted and discontinuance of carbenicillin therapy considered, unless, in the opinion of the physician the condition being treated is life threatening and amenable only to carbenicillin therapy. The usual agents (antihistamines, pressor amines and corticosteroids) should be readily available.
SERIOUS ANAPHYLACTOID REACTIONS REQUIRE IMMEDIATE EMERGENCY TREATMENT WITH EPINEPHRINE. OXYGEN AND INTRAVENOUS CORTICOSTEROIDS SHOULD ALSO BE ADMINISTERED AS INDICATED.
Usage in Pregnancy
Safety for use in pregnancy has not been established.
Precautions: While Geopen exhibits the characteristic low toxicity of the penicillin group of antibiotics, as with any other potent agent, it is advisable to check periodically for organ system dysfunction, including renal, hepatic and hematopoietic systems, during prolonged therapy.

Continued on next page

Roerig—Cont.

Emergence of resistant organisms, such as *Klebsiella spp.*, and *Serratia spp.*, which may cause superinfection, should be kept in mind.

Geopen is a disodium salt of carboxybenzylpenicillin and hence each gram of Geopen contains 4.7 mEq. of sodium. In patients where sodium restriction is necessary, such as cardiac patients, periodic electrolyte determinations and monitoring of cardiac status should be made.

In a few patients receiving high doses of Geopen, hypokalemia has been reported. Periodic serum potassium determinations should be made and corrective measures should be implemented when necessary.

As with any penicillin preparation, an allergic response, including anaphylaxis, may occur particularly in a hypersensitive individual.

Cases of gonorrhea with a suspected primary lesion of syphilis should have dark field examinations before treatment. In all other cases where concomitant syphilis is suspected, monthly serological tests should be made for a minimum of 4 months.

Adverse Reactions: The following adverse reactions may occur:

Hypersensitivity reactions: Skin rashes, pruritus, urticaria, drug fever, and anaphylactic reactions.

Gastrointestinal disturbances: Nausea

Hemic and Lymphatic Systems: As with other penicillins, anemia, thrombocytopenia, leukopenia, neutropenia, and eosinophilia may occur.

Blood, Hepatic and Renal Studies: As with other semisynthetic penicillins, SGOT and SGPT elevations have been observed after Geopen administration (particularly in children). In all studies to date, no clinical manifestations of hepatic or renal disorders have been demonstrated.

CNS: As with other penicillins, convulsions or neuromuscular irritability could occur with excessively high serum levels.

Other: Pain at the site of injection after intramuscular and intravenous administration has been reported but is rarely accompanied by induration. Several uremic patients receiving high doses (24 grams/day) have developed hemorrhagic manifestations associated with abnormalities of coagulation tests such as clotting time and prothrombin time. On withdrawal of the antibiotic, the bleeding ceased. The exact relationship of these findings to carbenicillin therapy is not clear.

Vein Irritation and Phlebitis have been reported occasionally, particularly when undiluted solution was directly injected into the vein.

Dosage and Administration:
[See table right].

NEONATES: In the neonate, for severe systemic infections (sepsis) due to susceptible strains of *Pseudomonas, Proteus,* and *E. coli, H. influenzae* and *S. pneumoniae,* the following Geopen (carbenicillin disodium) dosages may be given I.M. or by fifteen (15) minute I.V. infusion:

Infants under 2000 g body weight.
  Initial dose: 100 mg/kg.
  Subsequent doses during first week: 75 mg/kg./8 hrs (225 mg/kg./day)
  After 7 days of age: 100 mg/kg./6 hrs (400 mg/kg./day)

Infants over 2000 g body weight.
  Initial dose: 100 mg/kg.
  Subsequent doses during first 3 days: 75 mg/kg./6 hrs (300 mg/kg./day)
  After 3 days of age: 100 mg/kg./6 hrs (400 mg/kg./day)

NOTE: This dosage schedule should give maximum serum levels of approximately 150-175 mcg/ml and minimum levels of approximately 50-75 mcg/ml of Geopen.

Gentamicin may be used concurrently with carbenicillin for initial therapy until results of culture and susceptibility studies are known.

Seriously ill patients should receive the higher doses. GEOPEN has proved to be useful in infections in which protective mechanisms are impaired, such as in acute leukemia and during therapy with immunosuppressive or oncolytic drugs.

GEOPEN

Dosage and Administration: Indication: Clinical experience indicates that in serious urinary tract and systemic infections intravenous therapy in the higher doses should be used. The recommended maximum dose is 40 g per day. Intramuscular injections should not exceed 2 g per injection.

ADULTS:	*Pseudomonas*	*Proteus and E. coli*	*Enterobacter and S. faecalis*	*Anaerobes*	*H. influenzae and S. pneumoniae*
Urinary Tract Infections					
Serious	200 mg/kg/day by I.V. drip	200 mg/kg/day by I.V. drip	200 mg/kg/day by I.V. drip		
Uncomplicated	1–2 g I.M. or I.V. every 6 hours	1–2 g I.M. or I.V. every 6 hours	1–2 g I.M. or I.V. every 6 hours		
Severe Systemic Infections Septicemia Respiratory Infections Soft Tissue Infections	400–500 mg/kg/day (30–40 grams) I.V. in divided doses or continuously	300–400 mg/kg/day (20–30 grams) I.V. in divided doses or continuously			400–500 mg/kg/day (30–40 grams) I.V. in divided doses or continuously
Infections complicated by renal insufficiency (Creatinine clearance less than 5 ml/min)		2 g. I.V.[1] every 8–12 hours			

ADULTS:	*Pseudomonas*	*Proteus and E. coli*	*Enterobacter and S. faecalis*	*Anaerobes*	*H. influenzae and S. pneumoniae*
Meningitis					400-500 mg/kg day (30-40 grams) I.V. in divided doses or continuously
During peritoneal dialysis		2 g I.V. every 6 hours			
During hemodialysis		2 g I.V. every 4 hours			

(1) The serum half-life of Geopen in patients with severe renal failure is 12.5 hours. As a consequence 2 grams of Geopen administered intravenously to these patients every 8–12 hours will give Geopen serum levels of approximately 100 mcg/ml, a level notably free of any untoward effects while adequate for treatment of a majority of the infections amenable to Geopen therapy.

Treatment of gonorrhea[2]; acute uncomplicated ano-genital and urethral infections due to *N. gonorrhoeae.*

SINGLE 4 g I.M. injection, divided between 2 sites.

(2) Probenecid in a dosage of 1 gram may be administered orally about 30 minutes prior to the I.M. treatment of acute gonorrhoeal infections. For complete information and dosage of probenecid, refer to manufacturer's product information.

CHILDREN:	*Pseudomonas*	*Proteus and E. coli*	*Enterobacter and S. faecalis*	*Anaerobes*	*H. influenzae and S. pneumoniae*
Urinary Tract Infections	50–200 mg/kg/day in divided doses every 4–6 hours I.M. or I.V.	50–100 mg/kg/day in divided doses every 4–6 hours I.M. or I.V.	50–200 mg/kg/day in divided doses every 4–6 hours I.M. or I.V.		
Severe Systemic Infections Septicemia Respiratory Infections Soft Tissue Infections	400–500 mg/kg/day I.V. in divided doses or by continuous drip	300–400 mg/kg/day I.M. or I.V. in divided doses			400–500 mg/kg/day I.V. in divided doses or by continuous drip
Infections complicated by renal insufficiency (Creatinine clearance less than 5 ml/min)		Clinical data is insufficient to recommend an optimum dose			
Meningitis					400-500 mg/kg day in divided doses or by continuous drip

Intramuscular Use

As with all intramuscular preparations, Geopen (carbenicillin disodium) should be injected well within the body of a relatively large muscle.

Product Information

Adults: The preferred site is the upper outer quadrant of the buttock (i.e., gluteus maximus), or the mid-lateral thigh.

Children: It is recommended that intramuscular injections be given preferably in the midlateral muscles of the thigh. In infants and small children the periphery of the upper outer quadrant of the gluteal region should be used only when necessary, such as in burn patients, in order to minimize the possibility of damage to the sciatic nerve.

The deltoid area should be used only if well developed such as in certain adults and older children, and then only with caution to avoid radial nerve injury. Intramuscular injections should not be made into the lower and mid-third of the upper arm. As with all intramuscular injections, aspiration is necessary to help avoid inadvertent injection into a blood vessel.

Intravenous Use

As with all intravenous administrations, particular attention should be directed to insure that the drug is injected only into a vein (including aspiration and proper anatomical site selection) to avoid either intra-arterial injection or extravasation.

Preparation of Solution:

For Intramuscular Use—The 1 g vial should be reconstituted with 2.0 ml of Sterile Water for Injection. In order to facilitate reconstitution, up to 3.6 ml. of Sterile Water for Injection can be used.

Amount of Diluent to be added to the 1 g Vial	Volume to be Withdrawn for a 1 g Dose
2.0 ml	2.5 ml
2.5 ml	3.0 ml
3.6 ml	4.0 ml

The 2 g vial should be reconstituted with 4.0 ml. of Sterile Water for Injection. In order to facilitate reconstitution, up to 7.2 ml. of Sterile Water for Injection can be used.

Amount of Diluent to be added to the 2 g Vial	Volume to be Withdrawn for a 1 g Dose
4.0 ml	2.5 ml
5.0 ml	3.0 ml
7.2 ml	4.0 ml

The 5 g vial should be reconstituted with 7 ml. of Sterile Water for Injection. In order to facilitate reconstitution, up to 17 ml. of Sterile Water for Injection can be used.

Amount of Diluent to be added to the 5 g Vial	Volume to be Withdrawn for a 1 g Dose
7.0 ml	2.0 ml
9.5 ml	2.5 ml
12.0 ml	3.0 ml
17.0 ml	4.0 ml

After reconstitution, no significant loss of potency occurs for 24 hours at room temperature, and for 72 hours if refrigerated. Any of these unused solutions should be discarded.

For Direct Intravenous Injection—Following reconstitution, each gram should be further diluted by no less than 5 ml of Sterile Water for Injection. In order to avoid vein irritation, the solution should be administered as slowly as possible.

For Intravenous Infusion—Following reconstitution according to directions, Geopen (carbenicillin disodium) may be added to the desired volume of usual intravenous infusion solutions.

WHEN USING THE 2 g, 5 g, AND 10 g PIGGYBACK UNITS OR BULK PHARMACY PACK FOR...

Intravenous Use

As with all intravenous administrations, particular attention should be directed to insure that the drug is injected only into a vein (including aspiration and proper anatomical site selection) to avoid either intra-arterial injection or extravasation.

For Direct Intravenous Injection

The 2 gram vial should be reconstituted with a minimum of 20 ml. Sterile Water for Injection.

Amount of Diluent	Concentration of Solution
100 ml	1 g/50 ml
50 ml	1 g/25 ml
20 ml	1 g/10 ml

The 5 gram vial should be reconstituted with a minimum of 50 ml. of Sterile Water for Injection.

Amount of Diluent	Concentration of Solution
100 ml	1 g/20 ml
50 ml	1 g/10 ml

The 10 gram vial should be reconstituted with a minimum of 95 ml of Sterile Water for Injection.

Amount of Diluent	Concentration of Solution
95 ml	1 g/10 ml

In order to avoid vein irritation, the solution should be administered as slowly as possible. A dilution of 1 g/20 ml or more will further reduce the incidence of vein irritation.

After reconstitution, no significant loss of potency occurs for 24 hours at room temperature and for 72 hours if refrigerated. Any of these unused solutions should be discarded.

Bulk Pharmacy Package

The 30 gram vial should be reconstituted by adding 80 ml of water in two separate 40 ml aliquots. Add 40 ml, shake 25 seconds and add the last 40 ml aliquot and shake for final solution. The resulting solution will contain 300 mg/ml of carbenicillin. Transfer recommended dosage to appropriate intravenous infusion solution.

> Reconstituted bulk solution should not be used for direct infusion.

After reconstitution, no significant loss of potency occurs for 24 hours at room temperature and for 72 hours if refrigerated. Any of these unused solutions should be discarded.

For Continuous Intravenous Infusion

After reconstitution as directed, Geopen (carbenicillin disodium) may be added to the desired volume of usual intravenous infusion solutions.

Studies of Geopen at concentrations of 10 mg/ml and 100 mg/ml in the following intravenous infusion diluents indicate no significant loss of potency when stored at room temperature and under refrigeration (5°C) for the time periods stated: [See table above].

It is recommended that Geopen and gentamicin sulfate not be mixed together in the same IV solution due to the gradual inactivation of gentamicin sulfate under these circumstances. The therapeutic effect of the two drugs remains unimpaired when administered separately.

For Intramuscular Use Only:

Geopen for intramuscular injection ONLY may be diluted with one of the following:
1. 0.5% Lidocaine Hydrochloride (without epinephrine).
2. Bacteriostatic Water containing 0.9% Benzyl Alcohol.

For reconstitution of Geopen with these diluents for intramuscular use ONLY, follow the directions for the amount of diluent in the **PREPARATION OF SOLUTION, For Intramuscular Use** section.

Geopen may be diluted with these solutions and stored for 24 hours at room temperature or for 72 hours when refrigerated. Discard unused solutions stored longer than these time periods.

For full product information, refer to the package insert for Lidocaine Hydrochloride (without epinephrine).

GEOPEN
Intravenous Solution — **Stability**

	Room Temperature	Refrigerated
Sterile water for injection	72 hours	14 days
Sodium chloride injection, USP	72 hours	14 days
Dextrose injection, USP (5%)	72 hours	14 days
Ringer's injection, USP	72 hours	14 days
Dextrose 5% with 0.255% sodium chloride	24 hours	3 days
Lactated Ringer's injection, USP	24 hours	3 days
5% dextrose with electrolyte #48	24 hours	3 days
5% Levugen (fructose) with electrolyte #75	24 hours	3 days
Invert sugar 10% in water	24 hours	3 days
Dextrose 5% and 0.45% sodium chloride, USP	24 hours	3 days
5% alcohol, 5% dextrose in water	24 hours	3 days
5% alcohol, 5% dextrose in 0.9% sodium chloride	24 hours	3 days
5% dextrose in alcohol	24 hours	3 days
Maintenance electrolyte solution (electrolyte #75)	24 hours	3 days
Pediatric maintenance electrolyte solution (electrolyte #48)	24 hours	3 days

Discard any unused solutions after the time periods outlined above.

How Supplied: Geopen is available in 1 g, 2 g, and 5 g vials for intramuscular/intravenous use. Geopen is available in 2 g, 5 g, 10 g Piggyback Units, and 30 g Bulk Pharmacy Pack for intravenous use.

60-1856-00-6

GLUCOTROL® ℞
[glu' kă-trōl]
(glipizide)
TABLETS
For Oral Use

Description: GLUCOTROL (glipizide) is an oral blood-glucose-lowering drug of the sulfonylurea class.

The Chemical Abstracts name of glipizide is 1-cyclohexyl-3-[[p-[2-(5-methylpyrazinecarboxamido)ethyl]phenyl]sulfonyl]urea. The molecular formula is $C_{21}H_{27}N_5O_4S$; the molecular weight is 445.55; the structural formula is shown below:

Glipizide is a whitish, odorless powder with a melting point of 201–207°C (dec.) and a pKa of 5.9. It is insoluble in water and alcohols, but soluble in 0.1 N NaOH; it is freely soluble in dimethylformamide. GLUCOTROL tablets for oral use are available in 5 and 10 mg strengths.

Clinical Pharmacology:

Mechanism of Action: The primary mode of action of GLUCOTROL in experimental animals appears to be the stimulation of insulin secretion from the beta cells of pancreatic islet tissue and is thus dependent on functioning beta cells in the pancreatic islets. In humans GLUCOTROL appears to lower the blood glucose acutely by stimulating the release of insulin from the pancreas, an effect dependent upon functioning beta cells in the pancreatic islets. The mechanism by which GLUCOTROL lowers blood glucose during long-term administration has not been clearly established. In man, stimulation of insulin secretion by GLUCOTROL in response to a meal is undoubtedly of major importance. Fasting insulin levels are not elevated even on long-term GLUCOTROL administration, but the postprandial insulin response continues to be enhanced after at least 6 months of treatment. The insulinotropic response to a meal occurs within 30 minutes after an oral dose of GLUCOTROL in diabetic patients, but elevated insulin levels do not persist beyond the time of the meal challenge. Extrapancreatic effects may play a part in the mechanism of action of oral sulfonylurea hypoglycemic drugs.

Blood sugar control persists in some patients for up to 24 hours after a single dose of GLUCOTROL,

Continued on next page

Roerig—Cont.

even though plasma levels have declined to a small fraction of peak levels by that time (see Pharmacokinetics below).

Some patients fail to respond initially, or gradually lose their responsiveness to sulfonylurea drugs, including GLUCOTROL. Alternatively, GLUCOTROL may be effective in some patients who have not responded or have ceased to respond to other sulfonylureas.

Other Effects: It has been shown that GLUCOTROL therapy was effective in controlling blood sugar without deleterious changes in the plasma lipoprotein profiles of patients treated for NIDDM.

In a placebo-controlled, crossover study in normal volunteers, GLUCOTROL had no anti-diuretic activity, and, in fact, led to a slight increase in free water clearance.

Pharmacokinetics: Gastrointestinal absorption of GLUCOTROL in man is uniform, rapid, and essentially complete. Peak plasma concentrations occur 1–3 hours after a single oral dose. The half-life of elimination ranges from 2–4 hours in normal subjects, whether given intravenously or orally. The metabolic and excretory patterns are similar with the two routes of administration, indicating that first-pass metabolism is not significant. GLUCOTROL does not accumulate in plasma on repeated oral administration. Total absorption and disposition of an oral dose was unaffected by food in normal volunteers, but absorption was delayed by about 40 minutes. Thus GLUCOTROL was more effective when administered about 30 minutes before, rather than with, a test meal in diabetic patients. Protein binding was studied in serum from volunteers who received either oral or intravenous GLUCOTROL and found to be 98–99% one hour after either route of administration. The apparent volume of distribution of GLUCOTROL after intravenous administration was 11 liters, indicative of localization within the extracellular fluid compartment. In mice no GLUCOTROL or metabolites were detectable autoradiographically in the brain or spinal cord of males or females, nor in the fetuses of pregnant females. In another study, however, very small amounts of radioactivity were detected in the fetuses of rats given labelled drug.

The metabolism of GLUCOTROL is extensive and occurs mainly in the liver. The primary metabolites are inactive hydroxylation products and polar conjugates and are excreted mainly in the urine. Less than 10% unchanged GLUCOTROL is found in the urine.

Indications and Usage: GLUCOTROL is indicated as an adjunct to diet for the control of hyperglycemia and its associated symptomatology in patients with non-insulin-dependent diabetes mellitus (NIDDM; type II), formerly known as maturity-onset diabetes, after an adequate trial of dietary therapy has proved unsatisfactory.

In initiating treatment for non-insulin-dependent diabetes, diet should be emphasized as the primary form of treatment. Caloric restriction and weight loss are essential in the obese diabetic patient. Proper dietary management alone may be effective in controlling the blood glucose and symptoms of hyperglycemia. The importance of regular physical activity should also be stressed, and cardiovascular risk factors should be identified, and corrective measures taken where possible.

If this treatment program fails to reduce symptoms and/or blood glucose, the use of an oral sulfonylurea or insulin should be considered. Use of GLUCOTROL must be viewed by both the physician and patient as a treatment in addition to diet, and not as a substitute for diet or as a convenient mechanism for avoiding dietary restraint. Furthermore, loss of blood glucose control on diet alone may be transient, thus requiring only short-term administration of GLUCOTROL.

During maintenance programs, GLUCOTROL should be discontinued if satisfactory lowering of blood glucose is no longer achieved. Judgments should be based on regular clinical and laboratory evaluations.

In considering the use of GLUCOTROL in asymptomatic patients, it should be recognized that controlling blood glucose in non-insulin-dependent diabetes has not been definitely established to be effective in preventing the long-term cardiovascular or neural complications of diabetes.

Contraindications: GLUCOTROL is contraindicated in patients with:
1. Known hypersensitivity to the drug.
2. Diabetic ketoacidosis, with or without coma. This condition should be treated with insulin.

Warnings:
SPECIAL WARNING ON INCREASED RISK OF CARDIOVASCULAR MORTALITY: The administration of oral hypoglycemic drugs has been reported to be associated with increased cardiovascular mortality as compared to treatment with diet alone or diet plus insulin. This warning is based on the study conducted by the University Group Diabetes Program (UGDP), a long-term prospective clinical trial designed to evaluate the effectiveness of glucose-lowering drugs in preventing or delaying vascular complications in patients with non-insulin-dependent diabetes. The study involved 823 patients who were randomly assigned to one of four treatment groups (*Diabetes*, 19, supp. 2: 747-830, 1970).

UGDP reported that patients treated for 5 to 8 years with diet plus a fixed dose of tolbutamide (1.5 grams per day) had a rate of cardiovascular mortality approximately 2½ times that of patients treated with diet alone. A significant increase in total mortality was not observed, but the use of tolbutamide was discontinued based on the increase in cardiovascular mortality, thus limiting the opportunity for the study to show an increase in overall mortality. Despite controversy regarding the interpretation of these results, the findings of the UGDP study provide an adequate basis for this warning. The patient should be informed of the potential risks and advantages of GLUCOTROL and of alternative modes of therapy.

Although only one drug in the sulfonylurea class (tolbutamide) was included in this study, it is prudent from a safety standpoint to consider that this warning may also apply to other oral hypoglycemic drugs in this class, in view of their close similarities in mode of action and chemical structure.

Precautions:
General
Renal and Hepatic Disease: The metabolism and excretion of GLUCOTROL may be slowed in patients with impaired renal and/or hepatic function. If hypoglycemia should occur in such patients, it may be prolonged and appropriate management should be instituted.

Hypoglycemia: All sulfonylurea drugs are capable of producing severe hypoglycemia. Proper patient selection, dosage, and instructions are important to avoid hypoglycemic episodes. Renal or hepatic insufficiency may cause elevated blood levels of GLUCOTROL and the latter may also diminish gluconeogenic capacity, both of which increase the risk of serious hypoglycemic reactions. Elderly, debilitated or malnourished patients, and those with adrenal or pituitary insufficiency are particularly susceptible to the hypoglycemic action of glucose-lowering drugs. Hypoglycemia may be difficult to recognize in the elderly, and in people who are taking beta-adrenergic blocking drugs. Hypoglycemia is more likely to occur when caloric intake is deficient, after severe or prolonged exercise, when alcohol is ingested, or when more than one glucose-lowering drug is used.

Loss of Control of Blood Glucose: When a patient stabilized on any diabetic regimen is exposed to stress such as fever, trauma, infection, or surgery, a loss of control may occur. At such times, it may be necessary to discontinue GLUCOTROL and administer insulin.

The effectiveness of any oral hypoglycemic drug, including GLUCOTROL, in lowering blood glucose to a desired level decreases in many patients over a period of time, which may be due to progression of the severity of the diabetes or to diminished responsiveness to the drug. This phenomenon is known as secondary failure, to distinguish it from primary failure in which the drug is ineffective in an individual patient when first given.

Laboratory Tests: Blood and urine glucose should be monitored periodically. Measurement of glycosylated hemoglobin may be useful.

Information for Patients: Patients should be informed of the potential risks and advantages of GLUCOTROL and of alternative modes of therapy. They should also be informed about the importance of adhering to dietary instructions, of a regular exercise program, and of regular testing of urine and/or blood glucose.

The risks of hypoglycemia, its symptoms and treatment, and conditions that predispose to its development should be explained to patients and responsible family members. Primary and secondary failure should also be explained.

Drug Interactions: The hypoglycemic action of sulfonylureas may be potentiated by certain drugs including nonsteroidal anti-inflammatory agents and other drugs that are highly protein bound, salicylates, sulfonamides, chloramphenicol, probenecid, coumarins, monoamine oxidase inhibitors, and beta-adrenergic blocking agents. When such drugs are administered to a patient receiving GLUCOTROL, the patient should be observed closely for hypoglycemia. When such drugs are withdrawn from a patient receiving GLUCOTROL, the patient should be observed closely for loss of control. *In vitro* binding studies with human serum proteins indicate that GLUCOTROL binds differently than tolbutamide and does not interact with salicylate or dicumarol. However, caution must be exercised in extrapolating these findings to the clinical situation and in the use of GLUCOTROL with these drugs.

Certain drugs tend to produce hyperglycemia and may lead to loss of control. These drugs include the thiazides and other diuretics, corticosteroids, phenothiazines, thyroid products, estrogens, oral contraceptives, phenytoin, nicotinic acid, sympathomimetics, calcium channel blocking drugs, and isoniazid. When such drugs are administered to a patient receiving GLUCOTROL, the patient should be closely observed for loss of control. When such drugs are withdrawn from a patient receiving GLUCOTROL, the patient should be observed closely for hypoglycemia.

Carcinogenesis, Mutagenesis, Impairment of Fertility: A twenty month study in rats and an eighteen month study in mice at doses up to 75 times the maximum human dose revealed no evidence of drug-related carcinogenicity. Bacterial and *in vivo* mutagenicity tests were uniformly negative. Studies in rats of both sexes at doses up to 75 times the human dose showed no effects on fertility.

Pregnancy: Pregnancy Category C: GLUCOTROL (glipizide) was found to be mildly fetotoxic in rat reproductive studies at all dose levels (5–50 mg/kg). This fetotoxicity has been similarly noted with other sulfonylureas, such as tolbutamide and tolazamide. The effect is perinatal and believed to be directly related to the pharmacologic (hypoglycemic) action of GLUCOTROL. In studies in rats and rabbits no teratogenic effects were found. There are no adequate and well controlled studies in pregnant women. GLUCOTROL should be used during pregnancy only if the potential benefit justifies the potential risk to the fetus.

Because recent information suggests that abnormal blood glucose levels during pregnancy are associated with a higher incidence of congenital abnormalities, many experts recommend that insulin be used during pregnancy to maintain blood glucose levels as close to normal as possible.

Nonteratogenic Effects: Prolonged severe hypoglycemia (4 to 10 days) has been reported in neonates born to mothers who were receiving a sulfonylurea drug at the time of delivery. This has been reported more frequently with the use of agents with prolonged half-lives. If GLUCOTROL is used during pregnancy, it should be discontinued at least one month before the expected delivery date.

Nursing Mothers: Although it is not known whether GLUCOTROL is excreted in human milk, some sulfonylurea drugs are known to be excreted in human milk. Because the potential for hypoglycemia in nursing infants may exist, a decision should be made whether to discontinue nursing or to discontinue the drug, taking into account the importance of the drug to the mother. If the drug is discontinued and if diet alone is inadequate for controlling blood glucose, insulin therapy should be considered.

Pediatric Use: Safety and effectiveness in children have not been established.

Adverse Reactions: In U.S. and foreign controlled studies, the frequency of serious adverse reactions reported was very low. Of 702 patients, 11.8% reported adverse reactions and in only 1.5% was GLUCOTROL discontinued.

Hypoglycemia: See PRECAUTIONS and OVERDOSAGE sections.

Gastrointestinal: Gastrointestinal disturbances are the most common reactions. Gastrointestinal complaints were reported with the following approximate incidence: nausea and diarrhea, one in seventy; constipation and gastralgia, one in one hundred. They appear to be dose-related and may disappear on division or reduction of dosage. Cholestatic jaundice may occur rarely with sulfonylureas: GLUCOTROL should be discontinued if this occurs.

Dermatologic: Allergic skin reactions including erythema, morbilliform or maculopapular eruptions, urticaria, pruritus, and eczema have been reported in about one in seventy patients. These may be transient and may disappear despite continued use of GLUCOTROL; if skin reactions persist, the drug should be discontinued. Porphyria cutanea tarda and photosensitivity reactions have been reported with sulfonylureas.

Hematologic: Leukopenia, agranulocytosis, thrombocytopenia, hemolytic anemia, aplastic anemia, and pancytopenia have been reported with sulfonylureas.

Metabolic: Hepatic porphyria and disulfiram-like reactions have been reported with sulfonylureas. In the mouse, GLUCOTROL pretreatment did not cause an accumulation of acetaldehyde after ethanol administration. Clinical experience to date has shown that GLUCOTROL has an extremely low incidence of disulfiram-like alcohol reactions.

Miscellaneous: Dizziness, drowsiness, and headache have each been reported in about one in fifty patients treated with GLUCOTROL. They are usually transient and seldom require discontinuance of therapy.

Laboratory Tests: The pattern of laboratory test abnormalities observed with GLUCOTROL was similar to that for other sulfonylureas. Occasional mild to moderate elevations of SGOT, LDH, alkaline phosphatase, BUN and creatinine were noted. One case of jaundice was reported. The relationship of these abnormalities to GLUCOTROL is uncertain, and they have rarely been associated with clinical symptoms.

Overdosage: There is no well documented experience with GLUCOTROL overdosage. The acute oral toxicity was extremely low in all species tested (LD_{50} greater than 4 g/kg).

Overdosage of sulfonylureas including GLUCOTROL can produce hypoglycemia. Mild hypoglycemic symptoms without loss of consciousness or neurologic findings should be treated aggressively with oral glucose and adjustments in drug dosage and/or meal patterns. Close monitoring should continue until the physician is assured that the patient is out of danger. Severe hypoglycemic reactions with coma, seizure, or other neurological impairment occur infrequently, but constitute medical emergencies requiring immediate hospitalization. If hypoglycemic coma is diagnosed or suspected, the patient should be given a rapid intravenous injection of concentrated (50%) glucose solution. This should be followed by a continuous infusion of a more dilute (10%) glucose solution at a rate that will maintain the blood glucose at a level above 100 mg/dL. Patients should be closely monitored for a minimum of 24 to 48 hours since hypoglycemia may recur after apparent clinical recovery. Clearance of GLUCOTROL from plasma would be prolonged in persons with liver disease. Because of the extensive protein binding of GLUCOTROL, dialysis is unlikely to be of benefit.

Dosage and Administration: There is no fixed dosage regimen for the management of diabetes mellitus with GLUCOTROL or any other hypoglycemic agent. In addition to the usual monitoring of urinary glucose, the patient's blood glucose must also be monitored periodically to determine the minimum effective dose for the patient; to detect primary failure, i.e., inadequate lowering of blood glucose at the maximum recommended dose of medication; and to detect secondary failure, i.e., loss of an adequate blood-glucose-lowering response after an initial period of effectiveness. Glycosylated hemoglobin levels may also be of value in monitoring the patient's response to therapy.

Short-term administration of GLUCOTROL may be sufficient during periods of transient loss of control in patients usually controlled well on diet. In general, GLUCOTROL should be given approximately 30 minutes before a meal to achieve the greatest reduction in postprandial hyperglycemia.

Initial Dose: The recommended starting dose is 5 mg, given before breakfast. Geriatric patients or those with liver disease may be started on 2.5 mg.

Titration: Dosage adjustments should ordinarily be in increments of 2.5-5 mg, as determined by blood glucose response. At least several days should elapse between titration steps. If response to a single dose is not satisfactory, dividing that dose may prove effective. The maximum recommended once daily dose is 15 mg. Doses above 15 mg should ordinarily be divided and given before meals of adequate caloric content. The maximum recommended total daily dose is 40 mg.

Maintenance: Some patients may be effectively controlled on a once-a-day regimen, while others show better response with divided dosing. Total daily doses above 15 mg should ordinarily be divided. Total daily doses above 30 mg have been safely given on a b.i.d. basis to long-term patients. In elderly patients, debilitated or malnourished patients, and patients with impaired renal or hepatic function, the initial and maintenance dosing should be conservative to avoid hypoglycemic reactions (see PRECAUTIONS section).

Patients Receiving Insulin: As with other sulfonylurea-class hypoglycemics, many stable non-insulin-dependent diabetic patients receiving insulin may be safely placed on GLUCOTROL. When transferring patients from insulin to GLUCOTROL, the following general guidelines should be considered:

For patients whose daily insulin requirement is 20 units or less, insulin may be discontinued and GLUCOTROL therapy may begin at usual dosages. Several days should elapse between GLUCOTROL titration steps.

For patients whose daily insulin requirement is greater than 20 units, the insulin dose should be reduced by 50% and GLUCOTROL therapy may begin at usual dosages. Subsequent reductions in insulin dosage should depend on individual patient response. Several days should elapse between GLUCOTROL titration steps.

During the insulin withdrawal period, the patient should test urine samples for sugar and ketone bodies at least three times daily. Patients should be instructed to contact the prescriber immediately if these tests are abnormal. In some cases, especially when patient has been receiving greater than 40 units of insulin daily, it may be advisable to consider hospitalization during the transition period.

Patients Receiving Other Oral Hypoglycemic Agents: As with other sulfonylurea-class hypoglycemics, no transition period is necessary when transferring patients to GLUCOTROL. Patients should be observed carefully (1-2 weeks) for hypoglycemia when being transferred from longer half-life sulfonylureas (e.g., chlorpropamide) to GLUCOTROL due to potential overlapping of drug effect.

How Supplied: GLUCOTROL is available as white, dye-free, scored diamond-shaped tablets imprinted as follows: 5 mg tablet—Pfizer 411 (NDC 5 mg 0049-4110-66) Bottles of 100; 10 mg tablet—Pfizer 412 (NDC 10 mg 0049-4120-66) Bottles of 100.

Recommended Storage: Store below 86°F (30°C).

Caution: Federal law prohibits dispensing without prescription.

65-4227-00-0

Shown in Product Identification Section, page 431

HEPTUNA® PLUS ℞
[*hep-tū'na*]
CAPSULES
(Hard Gelatin)
Fortified Oral Hematopoietic Formulation

Each capsule contains:

HEMATOPOIETIC FACTORS

Ferrous Sulfate, dried, U.S.P. (provides 100 mg of elemental iron)	311 mg
Desiccated Liver (undefatted)	50 mg
Vitamin B_{12}, cobalamin concentrate NF (as Stablets®)	5 mcg
With intrinsic factor concentrate (non-inhibitory)	25 mg

VITAMINS

B_1 (thiamine mononitrate, U.S.P.)	3.1 mg
B_2 (riboflavin, U.S.P.)	2 mg
B_6 (pyridoxine hydrochloride, U.S.P.)	1.6 mg
Vitamin C (from sodium ascorbate)	150 mg
Niacin (niacinamide, U.S.P.)	15 mg
Pantothenic Acid (calcium pantothenate, U.S.P.)	0.9 mg

MINERALS

Copper (from copper sulfate)	1 mg
Molybdenum (from sodium molybdate)	0.2 mg
Calcium (from dibasic calcium phosphate)	37.4 mg
Iodine (from potassium iodide)	0.05 mg
Manganese (from manganese sulfate)	0.033 mg
Magnesium (from magnesium sulfate)	2 mg
Phosphorus (from dibasic calcium phosphate)	29 mg
Potassium (from potassium sulfate)	1.7 mg

Stablets® U.S. Pat. No. 2,830,933

Indications: Heptuna Plus is a multicomponent preparation effective in the treatment of those anemias amenable to oral hematinic therapy. These include pernicious anemia and other megaloblastic anemias, and also iron deficiency anemia. Heptuna Plus also contains balanced amounts of vitamin B complex, vitamin C, and minerals as nutritional supplements.

Clinical Pharmacology:

Hematopoietic Factors

Vitamin B_{12}: Exogenous sources of B_{12} are required for normal growth and maintenance of normal erythropoiesis as well as nucleo-protein synthesis, myelin synthesis, and cell reproduction. Vitamin B_{12} is irregularly absorbed from the intact gastrointestinal tract. Free vitamin B_{12} is bound to intrinsic factor which is normally secreted by the gastric mucosal tissue, and acts as a carrier protein for active transport through the gastrointestinal tract. This normal active transport system is usually saturated by 1.5 to 3 mg of vitamin B_{12}. Under conditions of functional or anatomical derangements of the stomach or ileum, where secretion of intrinsic factor is abnormally low, absorption of vitamin B_{12} will proceed poorly, if at all. Megaloblastic anemias may develop after gastrectomy, in Addinsonian permicious anemia, and in fish tapeworm (*Diphyllobothrium latum*) infection; treatment to free the host of competing bacteria and parasites is required. Other causes of B_{12} deficiency are strict vegetarianism, surgical compromise of gastric or ileum activity, gastric atrophy due to multiple sclerosis or iron deficiency or malabsorption syndromes of various etiologies; in this last case parenteral therapy or oral therapy with massive doses of vitamin B_{12} may be necessary for successful treatment. The megaloblastic anemias of malabsorption syndromes may be due to a deficiency of folate—which is not contained in Heptuna Plus, as well as to B_{12} deficiency, and combined therapy may be warranted.

Continued on next page

Roerig—Cont.

Desiccated Liver: Desiccated Liver is an extract of mammalian livers used in Heptuna Plus as a source of naturally occurring riboflavin, nicotinic acid, and choline as a nutritional supplement. Desiccated liver (undefatted) 50 mg. provides approximately 2.5 mcg riboflavin, 12.5 mcg nicotinic acid, and 0.5 mg choline.

Ferrous Sulfate: As compared to other sources of iron, ferrous sufate provides the highest amounts of elemental iron for utilization in patients with hypochronic anemias. Iron is a constituent of hemoglobin and its administration usually corrects erythropoietic abnormalities, and may reverse esophageal and gastrointestinal tissue changes associated with iron deficiency.

Approximately 25% of an orally administered dose of ferrous sulfate will be utilizable iron. The primary sites of iron absorption are the duodenum, the jejunum, the stomach, and the proximal portion of the ileum. The ferrous species of iron is the most readily absorbed fraction. While the exact mechanism of absorption is not known, the absorption, metabolism, and excretion of iron appear to be related to body requirements for this mineral. The excretion of iron as ferritin is by way of epithelial cells sloughed from the skin and gastrointestinal tract. There may be trace losses in bile, and cell-free sweat.

Vitamins

Vitamin C: It is known that an acidic environment favors the maintenance of iron in the ferrous state, retards formation of insoluble complexes of iron with food or other substrates, and will thus promote gastric absorption of ferrous iron. The vitamin C content of Heptuna Plus, in addition to contributing to the overall acidic environment of gastric fluids, may also be useful as a supplement to deficiency states. Prolonged and severe vitamin C deficiency is associated with an anemia which is usually hypochronic but occasionally megaloblastic. Vitamin C is also utilized in intracellular reactions such as conversion of folic acid and carbohydrate synthesis.

Vitamin B Complex (B_1, B_2, B_6, Niacin, Pantothenic Acid): These are provided in Heptuna Plus as nutritional supplements. Vitamin B complex is essential for the metabolism of carbohydrates and protein. Administration of these water-soluble vitamins may be useful in deficiency states associated with febrile diseases, severe burns, gastrointestinal disorders interfering with absorption of these vitamins, in prolonged or wasting diseases, or in nutritional deficiency.

One capsule of Heptuna Plus provides the following approximate percentage of the U.S. Recommended Adult Daily Allowances (U.S. RDA):

	% U.S. RDA
B_1	221.4
B_2	125
B_6	80
Vitamin C	333.3
Niacin	83.3
Pantothenic Acid	9

Minerals

One capsule of Heptuna Plus provides the following approximate percentages of U.S. Recommended Adult Daily Allowances (U.S. RDA):

	% U.S. RDA
Copper	50
Molybdenum	*
Calcium	4.25
Iodine	38.46
Manganese	*
Magnesium	0.57
Phosphorous	3.63
Potassium	*

*U.S. RDA not yet established.

The precise role of minerals in human nutritional maintenance has yet to be defined. However, several trace elements (including copper, molybdenum, calcium, iodine, manganese) have been identified as being essential for animal life.

Copper: Copper has been identified as a component of several amine oxidases. Copper depletion in experimental animals results in failure to utilize ferritin iron and is accompanied by increases in hepatic iron concentration sometimes with clear evidence of hemosiderosis. Copper-dependent enzyme systems may be intimately involved in tissue iron mobilization.

Molybdenum: Molybdenum has been identified as a component of xanthine oxidase (involved in purine oxidation and possibly in the release of iron from ferritin), aldehydeoxidase, and sulfite oxidase.

Calcium: In addition to this element's well known important roles in maintenance of bone, neurologic, and muscular tissue integrity, calcium may also play a role in maintaining the integrity of cell membrane structures.

Iodine: As the central element of thyroid activity, iodine intake may influence carbohydrate and cholesterol metabolism, functions of the central nervous system, catecholamine secretion, and skeletal growth and maturation. Its exact role in the hematopoietic process, if any, has not been determined.

Manganese: The main manifestations of manganese deficiency in laboratory animals are impaired growth, disturbed or depressed reproductive function, skeletal abnormalities, and nervous disorders. Its exact role in the hematopoietic process, if any, has not been determined.

Magnesium: Magnesium plays a fundamental role in most reactions that include phosphate transfer, and it is believed to be essential for the structural stabilization of nucleic acids. Magnesium depletion has been known to impair homeostasis of potassium and calcium. Deficiency of magnesium almost always occurs as a consequence of some underlying disease, including malabsorption syndromes.

Phosphorus: Hypophosphatemia may cause a marked decrease in erythrocytic concentrations of ATP and of 2,3 diphosphoglycerate. Acute hemolytic-type anemia may develop in severe deficiency states.

Potassium: Potassium is an essential mineral in electrolyte maintenance and in maintaining electrical excitability of cells and acid-base homeostasis. Its exact role in the hematopoietic process, if any, has not been determined.

Contraindications: Hemachromatosis and hemosiderosis are contraindications to iron therapy. Previous hypersensitivity to any of the components of Heptuna Plus contraindicates its use.

Precautions: Anemia is a manifestation of an underlying disease process. While Heptuna Plus provides components useful in the management of certain anemias, appropriate attention should be directed to an etiological diagnosis and treatment of the underlying causes of the anemia.

Resistance to the effects of exogenous intrinsic factor has been reported. Local intestinal antibodies which render exogenous intrinsic factor inactive have been noted to develop in approximately 50% of patients treated within one year of continuous oral therapy. If resistance develops, parenteral therapy or oral therapy with large doses of vitamin B_{12} may be necessary to circumvent normal active transport mechanisms and adequately treat the patient.

Although this product contains vitamin B_{12} (as Stablets®) with intrinsic factor concentrate (noninhibitory) and desiccated liver, it is not as reliable as parenterally administered cyanocobalamin (vitamin B_{12}) in the management of pernicious anemia. Some patients with pernicious anemia may not respond to orally ingested cobalamin concentrate (vitamin B_{12}). There is no known way to predict which patients will respond or which patients may cease to respond.

Information for Patients: As Heptuna Plus contains substantial amounts of iron, patients should be advised that gastrointestinal reactions such as diarrhea or constipation may occur with usage. Patients should be cautioned against concomitant usage of Heptuna Plus and tetracycline, or its analogs, so as to avoid a chelation interaction which would reduce the amounts of antibiotic and iron or divalent ions available for gastrointestinal absorption.

Laboratory Tests: Periodic clinical and laboratory monitoring are considered essential to proper use of hematopoietics. The following laboratory tests may be useful in evaluating patients' response to therapy: peripheral blood smears, reticulocyte count, serum iron, iron binding capacity, serum B_{12}, serum folic acid, hemoglobin and hematocrit, mean corpuscular volume.

Drug Interactions: The following drug/drug interactions may occur with the use of Heptuna Plus.

Agent	Interaction
Tetracycline and derivatives	Complexation of antibiotic and iron or divalent ions (such as calcium) decrease availability of component for gastric absorption. This may be avoided by administration of Heptuna Plus at least one hour before tetracycline-type agent.
Levodopa	Doses of pyridoxine of approximately 5 mg (three capsules Heptuna Plus provide 4.8 mg B_6) or more per day may reduce the beneficial effects of levodopa in parkinsonian disease. This is thought to be due to increased transamination of levodopa. Patients receiving this combination should be carefully observed for unwanted variations in parkinson control.
Lithium	The presence of iodine in Heptuna Plus may enhance the hypothyroid and goiterogenic potential of these two components. Patients receiving lithium and Heptuna Plus should have baseline and periodic thyroid status checks.

Laboratory Interactions: Heptuna Plus contains iodine 0.05 mg (as potassium iodide) as an active component and the iodinated dye tetraiodofluorescein (FD and C#3) in the capsule shell. These agents may interfere with I^{131} or other diagnostic radioiodine neucleotide testing procedures. Other than changes induced from the therapeutic effects of the components of Heptuna Plus, no other interferences with laboratory testing procedures have been identified.

Carcinogenesis, Mutagenesis, Impairment of Fertility: The potential for Heptuna Plus to impair fertility or act as a carcinogen or a mutagen has not been studied in vivo or in vitro.

Use in Pregnancy

Category C: Animal reproductive studies have not been conducted with Heptuna Plus. It is also not known whether Heptuna Plus can cause fetal harm when administered to a pregnant woman or can affect reproductive capacity. Heptuna Plus should be given to a pregnant woman only if clearly needed.

Nursing Mothers: It is not known whether this drug is excreted in human milk. Because many drugs are excreted in human milk, caution should be exercised when Heptuna Plus is administered to a nursing woman.

Pediatric Use: Safety and effectiveness in children have not been established.

Adverse Reactions:

Ferrous Sulfate: The most frequent adverse reactions to Heptuna Plus are those associated with oral iron therapy. An incidence of gastrointestinal discomfort in 19.5% to 27% of patients receiving "iron placebo" tablets has been reported. The gastrointestinal complaints usually noted are diarrhea, constipation, nausea, epigastric pain, ructus, vomiting, and black staining of stools. Reduction in dosage or administration with meals may minimize these effects.

In extremely rare instances, skin rash suggesting allergy has been noted following the oral administration of desiccated liver preparations.

Iodine: Allergic reactions, including angioedema, rashes, lymphadenopathy, eosinophilia, arteritis, and febrile reactions have been reported with iodine usage. Also, acne, swelling of salivary glands, iodine coryza, and stomach upsets have been reported. Iodine use may precipitate hypo- or hyperthyroid activity and goiter.

B Complex Vitamins: Adverse reactions to these water-soluble vitamins are rare:

—Thiamine; Hypersensitivity reactions are rare and have been reported mostly with parenteral administration.

—Pyridoxine; Allergic reactions have been reported, but are rare.

—Cyanocobalamine/Cobalamine; Mild forms of polycythemia, and peripheral vascular thrombosis during recovery from pernicious anemia treated with B_{12} have been observed. Use of high dose oral vitamin B_{12} has been associated with the appearance of acne.

Minerals: No adverse reactions other than those specified for iodine have been reported with orally administered minerals as supplied in Heptuna Plus.

Overdosage:

Acute Toxicity: Toxicity may result from overdosage due to ingestion of ferrous sulfate. In young children 300 mg of elemental iron may be fatal. The remainder of the ingredients are essentially nontoxic (water-soluble vitamins) or present in such small amounts as to be nontoxic even with overdosage.

Symptoms: Symptoms may occur 30 to 60 minutes after ingestion. Danger may exist for 24-48 hours. Acute gastroenteritis, vomiting, diarrhea, dehydration, collapse, and coma ending in death may occur. A severe acidosis may also be present. The diarrhea may initially be watery, becoming bloody and then tarry.

Dialyzability: It is known that iron, magnesium, potassium, iodide, and phosphate are dialyzable. Dialysis may not be effective in removing vitamin B_{12} or copper. The effect of dialysis on the other components in Heptuna Plus is not certain.

Management: Management should be directed primarily at the treatment of iron toxicity. Acute toxicity may occur in young children after ingestion of 1 gram of ferrous sulfate (equivalent to 3 capsules of Heptuna Plus). In adults iron toxicity is rare and is most likely to occur only after ingestion of more than 50 grams of ferrous sulfate (equivalent to 150 capsules of Heptuna Plus). Treatment involves gastric lavage and/or use of absorbents. A 1% sodium bicarbonate lavage fluid may be useful to prevent further iron absorption. Lavage must be performed with caution after the first hour of an overdosage because of the potential for gastric necrosis and perforation. Shock and acid-base imbalances should be treated with standard methods. Serum iron levels should be monitored and deferoxamine mesylate therapy initiated if necessary. Other chelating agents should be used only if deferoxamine mesylate is not available or otherwise contraindicated, as it may form toxic complexes with iron.

Dosage and Administration: For many patients one capsule of Heptuna Plus daily will provide sufficient amounts of hematopoietic factors for therapeutic results. If the severity and etiology of the anemia so indicate, 1 capsule three times a day (approximately every six hours) may be prescribed. Therapy with Heptuna Plus may be continued until patient response indicates discontinuation of therapy.

How Supplied: Heptuna Plus capsules are available as red and white gelatin capsules, in bottles of 100.

68-0331-00-7

Shown in Product Identification Section, page 431

MARAX® ℞
[mā'rax]
(ephedrine sulfate, theophylline, hydroxyzine HCl)
TABLETS AND DF SYRUP

Contents:

	Each Tablet Contains:	Each Teaspoon (5 ml.) Syrup Contains:
Ephedrine Sulfate	25 mg.	6.25 mg.
Theophylline	130 mg.	32.50 mg.
Atarax® (hydroxyzine HCl)	10 mg.	2.5 mg.
Alcohol (Ethyl Alcohol)		5% v/v.

Actions: The action of ephedrine as a vasoconstrictor is well known. It is therefore of significant benefit in symptomatic relief of the congestion occurring in bronchial asthma. As a bronchodilator, it has a slower onset but longer duration of action than does epinephrine, which, in contrast to ephedrine, is not effective upon oral administration.

The diverse actions of theophylline—bronchospasmolytic, cardiovascular, and diuretic—are well established, and make it a particularly useful drug in the treatment of bronchial asthma, both in the acute attack and in the prophylactic therapy of the disease.

Atarax (hydroxyzine HCl) modifies the central stimulatory action of ephedrine preventing excessive excitation in patients on Marax therapy.

In animal studies Atarax (hydroxyzine HCl) has demonstrated antiserotonin activity and antispasmodic potency of a nonspecific nature.

Marax-DF Syrup produces an expectorant action wherein the tenacity of the sputum is decreased and the ease of expectoration is increased.

Indications

Based on a review of this drug by the National Academy of Sciences-National Research Council and/or other information, FDA has classified the indications as follows:

"Possibly" Effective: For controlling bronchospastic disorders.

Final classification of the less than effective indication requires further investigation.

Contraindications: Because of the ephedrine, Marax is contraindicated in cardiovascular disease, hyperthyroidism, and hypertension. This drug is contraindicated in individuals who have shown hypersensitivity to the drug or its components.

Hydroxyzine, when administered to the pregnant mouse, rat, and rabbit induced fetal abnormalities in the rat at doses substantially above the human therapeutic range. Clinical data in human beings are inadequate to establish safety in early pregnancy. Until such data are available, hydroxyzine is contraindicated in early pregnancy.

Precautions: Because of the ephedrine component this drug should be used with caution in elderly males or those with known prostatic hypertrophy.

The potentiating action of hydroxyzine, although mild, must be taken into consideration when the drug is used in conjunction with central nervous system depressants; and when other central nervous system depressants are administered concomitantly with hydroxyzine their dosage should be reduced. Patients should be cautioned that hydroxyzine can increase the effect of alcohol.

Patients should be warned—because of the hydroxyzine component—of the possibility of drowsiness occurring and cautioned against driving a car or operating dangerous machinery while taking this drug.

Adverse Reactions: With large doses of ephedrine, excitation, tremulousness, insomnia, nervousness, palpitation, tachycardia, precordial pain, cardiac arrhythmias, vertigo, dryness of the nose and throat, headache, sweating, and warmth may occur. Because ephedrine is a sympathomimetic agent some patients may develop vesical sphincter spasm and resultant urinary hesitation, and occasionally acute urinary retention. This should be borne in mind when administering preparations containing ephedrine to elderly males or those with known prostatic hypertrophy. At the recommended dose for Marax, a side effect occasionally reported is palpitation, and this can be controlled with dosage adjustment, additional amounts of concurrently administered Atarax (hydroxyzine HCl), or discontinuation of the medication. When ephedrine is given three or more times daily patients may develop tolerance after several weeks of therapy.

Theophylline when given on an empty stomach frequently causes gastric irritation accompanied by upper abdominal discomfort, nausea, and vomiting. Administration of the medication after meals will serve to minimize this side effect. Theophylline may cause diuresis and cardiac stimulation. The amount of Atarax (hydroxyzine HCl) present in Marax has not resulted in disturbing side effects. When used alone specifically as a tranquilizer in the normal dosage range (25 to 50 mg. three or four times a day), side effects are infrequent; even at these higher doses, no serious side effects have been reported and confirmed to date. Those which do occasionally occur when Atarax (hydroxyzine HCl) is used alone are drowsiness, xerostomia and, at extremely high doses, involuntary motor activity, unsteadiness of gait, neuromuscular weakness, all of which may be controlled by reduction of the dosage or discontinuation of the medication.

With the relatively low dose of Atarax (hydroxyzine HCl) in Marax, these effects are not likely to occur. In addition, the ataractic action of Atarax (hydroxyzine HCl) may modify the cardiac stimulatory action of ephedrine, and concurrently, increasing the amount of Atarax (hydroxyzine HCl) may control or abolish this undesirable effect of ephedrine.

Dosage and Administration: The dosage of Marax should be adjusted according to the severity of complaints, and the patient's individual toleration.

Tablets: In general, an adult dose of 1 tablet, 2 to 4 times daily, should be sufficient. Some patients are controlled adequately with ½ to 1 tablet at bedtime. The time interval between doses should not be shorter than four hours. The dosage for children over 5 years of age and for adults who are sensitive to ephedrine, is one-half the usual adult dose. Clinical experience to date has been confined to ages above 5 years.

Syrup: The dose for children over 5 years of age is 1 teaspoon (5 ml.), 3 to 4 times daily. Dosage for children 2 to 5 years of age is ½ to 1 teaspoon (2.5-5 ml.), 3 to 4 times daily. Not recommended for children under 2 years of age.

How Supplied: Marax Tablets are available as scored, dye free, m-shaped tablets in bottles of 100 and 500.

Marax-DF Syrup is available in pints and gallons as a colorless syrup free of all coal tar dyes, and should be dispensed in tight, light-resistant containers (USP).

67-0928-00-6
65-2265-00-3

Shown in Product Identification Section, page 431

NAVANE® ℞
[nah'van]
(thiothixene) CAPSULES
NAVANE®
(thiothixene hydrochloride) CONCENTRATE

Description: Navane (thiothixene) is a thioxanthene derivative. Specifically, it is the *cis* isomer of N,N-dimethyl-9-[3-(4-methyl-1-piperazinyl)-propylidene] thioxanthene-2-sulfonamide.

The thioxanthenes differ from the phenothiazines by the replacement of nitrogen in the central ring with a carbon-linked side chain fixed in space in a rigid structural configuration. An N,N-dimethyl

Continued on next page

Roerig—Cont.

sulfonamide functional group is bonded to the thioxanthene nucleus.

Actions: Navane is a psychotropic agent of the thioxanthene series. Navane possesses certain chemical and pharmacological similarities to the piperazine phenothiazines and differences from the aliphatic group of phenothiazines.

Indications: Navane is effective in the management of manifestations of psychotic disorders. Navane has not been evaluated in the management of behavioral complications in patients with mental retardation.

Contraindications: Navane is contraindicated in patients with circulatory collapse, comatose states, central nervous system depression due to any cause, and blood dyscrasias. Navane is contraindicated in individuals who have shown hypersensitivity to the drug. It is not known whether there is a cross sensitivity between the thioxanthenes and the phenothiazine derivatives, but this possibility should be considered.

Warnings:

Usage in Pregnancy—Safe use of Navane during pregnancy has not been established. Therefore, this drug should be given to pregnant patients only when, in the judgment of the physician, the expected benefits from the treatment exceed the possible risks to mother and fetus. Animal reproduction studies and clinical experience to date have not demonstrated any teratogenic effects.

In the animal reproduction studies with Navane, there was some decrease in conception rate and litter size, and an increase in resorption rate in rats and rabbits. Similar findings have been reported with other psychotropic agents. After repeated oral administration of Navane to rats (5 to 15 mg/kg/day), rabbits (3 to 50 mg/kg/day), and monkeys (1 to 3 mg/kg/day) before and during gestation, no teratogenic effects were seen.

Usage in Children—The use of Navane in children under 12 years of age is not recommended because safe conditions for its use have not been established.

As is true with many CNS drugs, Navane may impair the mental and/or physical abilities required for the performance of potentially hazardous tasks such as driving a car or operating machinery, especially during the first few days of therapy. Therefore, the patient should be cautioned accordingly.

As in the case of other CNS-acting drugs, patients receiving Navane (thiothixene) should be cautioned about the possible additive effects (which may include hypotension) with CNS depressants and with alcohol.

Precautions: An antiemetic effect was observed in animal studies with Navane; since this effect may also occur in man, it is possible that Navane may mask signs of overdosage of toxic drugs and may obscure conditions such as intestinal obstruction and brain tumor.

In consideration of the known capability of Navane and certain other psychotropic drugs to precipitate convulsions, extreme caution should be used in patients with a history of convulsive disorders or those in a state of alcohol withdrawal, since it may lower the convulsive threshold. Although Navane potentiates the actions of the barbiturates, the dosage of the anticonvulsant therapy should not be reduced when Navane is administered concurrently.

Though exhibiting rather weak anticholinergic properties, Navane should be used with caution in patients who might be exposed to extreme heat or who are receiving atropine or related drugs.

Use with caution in patients with cardiovascular disease.

Caution as well as careful adjustment of the dosages is indicated when Navane is used in conjunction with other CNS depressants.

Also, careful observation should be made for pigmentary retinopathy, and lenticular pigmentation (fine lenticular pigmentation has been noted in a small number of patients treated with Navane for prolonged periods). Blood dyscrasias (agranulocytosis, pancytopenia, thrombocytopenic purpura), and liver damage (jaundice, biliary stasis), have been reported with related drugs.

Neuroleptic drugs elevate prolactin levels; the elevation persists during chronic administration. Tissue culture experiments indicate that approximately one-third of human breast cancers are prolactin dependent *in vitro*, a factor of potential importance if the prescription of these drugs is contemplated in a patient with a previously detected breast cancer. Although disturbances such as galactorrhea, amenorrhea, gynecomastia, and impotence have been reported, the clinical significance of elevated serum prolactin levels is unknown for most patients. An increase in mammary neoplasms has been found in rodents after chronic administration of neuroleptic drugs. Neither clinical studies nor epidemiologic studies conducted to date, however, have shown an association between chronic administration of these drugs and mammary tumorigenesis; the available evidence is considered too limited to be conclusive at this time.

Adverse Reactions:

NOTE: Not all of the following adverse reactions have been reported with Navane. However, since Navane has certain chemical and pharmacologic similarities to the phenothiazines, all of the known side effects and toxicity associated with phenothiazine therapy should be borne in mind when Navane is used.

Cardiovascular effects: Tachycardia, hypotension, lightheadedness, and syncope. In the event hypotension occurs, epinephrine should not be used as a pressor agent since a paradoxical further lowering of blood pressure may result. Nonspecific EKG changes have been observed in some patients receiving Navane. These changes are usually reversible and frequently disappear on continued Navane therapy. The incidence of these changes is lower than that observed with some phenothiazines. The clinical significance of these changes is not known.

CNS effects: Drowsiness, usually mild, may occur although it usually subsides with continuation of Navane therapy. The incidence of sedation appears similar to that of the piperazine group of phenothiazines but less than that of certain aliphatic phenothiazines. Restlessness, agitation and insomnia have been noted with Navane. Seizures and paradoxical exacerbation of psychotic symptoms have occurred with Navane infrequently.

Hyperreflexia has been reported in infants delivered from mothers having received structurally related drugs.

In addition, phenothiazine derivatives have been associated with cerebral edema and cerebrospinal fluid abnormalities.

Extrapyramidal symptoms, such as pseudo-parkinsonism, akathisia and dystonia have been reported. Management of these extrapyramidal symptoms depends upon the type and severity. Rapid relief of acute symptoms may require the use of an injectable antiparkinson agent. More slowly emerging symptoms may be managed by reducing the dosage of Navane and/or administering an oral antiparkinson agent.

Persistent Tardive Dyskinesia: As with all antipsychotic agents tardive dyskinesia may appear in some patients on long term therapy or may occur after drug therapy has been discontinued. The risk seems to be greater in elderly patients on high-dose therapy, especially females. The symptoms are persistent and in some patients appear to be irreversible. The syndrome is characterized by rhythmical involuntary movements of the tongue, face, mouth or jaw (e.g., protrusion of tongue, puffing of cheeks, puckering of mouth, chewing movements). Sometimes these may be accompanied by involuntary movements of extremities.

There is no known effective treatment for tardive dyskinesia; antiparkinsonism agents usually do not alleviate the symptoms of this syndrome. It is suggested that all antipsychotic agents be discontinued if these symptoms appear.

Should it be necessary to reinstitute treatment, or increase the dosage of the agent, or switch to a different antipsychotic agent, the syndrome may be masked.

It has been reported that fine vermicular movements of the tongue may be an early sign of the syndrome and if the medication is stopped at that time, the syndrome may not develop.

Hepatic effects: Elevations of serum transaminase and alkaline phosphatase, usually transient, have been infrequently observed in some patients. No clinically confirmed cases of jaundice attributable to Navane have been reported.

Hematologic effects: As is true with certain other psychotropic drugs, leukopenia and leucocytosis, which are usually transient, can occur occasionally with Navane. Other antipsychotic drugs have been associated with agranulocytosis, eosinophilia, hemolytic anemia, thrombocytopenia and pancytopenia.

Allergic reactions: Rash, pruritus, urticaria, photosensitivity and rare cases of anaphylaxis have been reported with Navane. Undue exposure to sunlight should be avoided. Although not experienced with Navane, exfoliative dermatitis and contact dermatitis (in nursing personnel), have been reported with certain phenothiazines.

Endocrine disorders: Lactation, moderate breast enlargement and amenorrhea have occurred in a small percentage of females receiving Navane (thiothixene). If persistent, this may necessitate a reduction in dosage or the discontinuation of therapy. Phenothiazines have been associated with false positive pregnancy tests, gynecomastia, hypoglycemia, hyperglycemia and glycosuria.

Autonomic effects: Dry mouth, blurred vision, nasal congestion, constipation, increased sweating, increased salivation and impotence have occurred infrequently with Navane therapy. Phenothiazines have been associated with miosis, mydriasis, and adynamic ileus.

Other adverse reactions: Hyperpyrexia, anorexia, nausea, vomiting, diarrhea, increase in appetite and weight, weakness or fatigue, polydipsia, and peripheral edema.

Although not reported with Navane, evidence indicates there is a relationship between phenothiazine therapy and the occurrence of a systemic lupus erythematosus-like syndrome.

NOTE: Sudden deaths have occasionally been reported in patients who have received certain phenothiazine derivatives. In some cases the cause of death was apparently cardiac arrest or asphyxia due to failure of the cough reflex. In others, the cause could not be determined nor could it be established that death was due to phenothiazine administration.

Dosage and Administration: Dosage of Navane should be individually adjusted depending on the chronicity and severity of the condition. In general, small doses should be used initially and gradually increased to the optimal effective level, based on patient response.

Some patients have been successfully maintained on once-a-day Navane therapy.

The use of Navane in children under 12 years of age is not recommended because safe conditions for its use have not been established.

In milder conditions, an initial dose of 2 mg. three times daily. If indicated, a subsequent increase to 15 mg./day total daily dose is often effective.

In more severe conditions, an initial dose of 5 mg. twice daily.

The usual optimal dose is 20 to 30 mg. daily. If indicated, an increase to 60 mg./day total daily dose is often effective. Exceeding a total daily dose of 60 mg. rarely increases the beneficial response.

Overdosage: Manifestations include muscular twitching, drowsiness and dizziness. Symptoms of gross overdosage may include CNS depression, rigidity, weakness, torticollis, tremor, salivation, dysphagia, hypotension, disturbances of gait, or coma.

Treatment: Essentially symptomatic and supportive. Early gastric lavage is helpful. Keep patient under careful observation and maintain an open airway, since involvement of the extrapyramidal system may produce dysphagia and respiratory difficulty in severe overdosage. If hypotension occurs, the standard measures for managing circulatory shock should be used (I.V. fluids and/or vasoconstrictors).

If a vasoconstrictor is needed, levarterenol and phenylephrine are the most suitable drugs. Other pressor agents, including epinephrine, are not recommended, since phenothiazine derivatives may reverse the usual pressor action of these agents and cause further lowering of blood pressure.

If CNS depression is present, recommended stimulants include amphetamine, dextroamphetamine, or caffeine and sodium benzoate. Stimulants that may cause convulsions (e. g. picrotoxin or pentylenetetrazol) should be avoided. Extrapyramidal symptoms may be treated with antiparkinson drugs.

There are no data on the use of peritoneal or hemodialysis, but they are known to be of little value in phenothiazine intoxication.

How Supplied: Navane (thiothixene) is available as capsules containing 1 mg, 2 mg, 5 mg, and 10 mg of thiothixene in bottles of 100, 1,000 and unit-dose pack of 100 (10 × 10's). Navane (thiothixene) is also available as capsules containing 20 mg of thiothixene in bottles of 100, 500 and unit-dose pack of 100 (10 × 10's).

Navane (thiothixene hydrochloride) Concentrate is available in 120 ml (4 oz.) bottles with an accompanying dropper calibrated at 2 mg, 3 mg, 4 mg, 5 mg, 6 mg, 8 mg, and 10 mg and in 30 ml (1 oz.) bottles with an accompanying dropper calibrated at 2 mg, 3 mg, 4 mg, and 5 mg. Each ml. contains thiothixene hydrochloride equivalent to 5 mg. of thiothixene. Contains alcohol, U.S.P. 7.0% v/v. (small loss unavoidable).

23-1655-00-2

Shown in Product Identification Section, page 431

NAVANE® R
[nah'vān]
(thiothixene hydrochloride)
Intramuscular
2 mg./ml. 5 mg./ml. †

Description: Navane (thiothixene hydrochloride) is a thioxanthene derivative. Specifically, it is the *cis* isomer of N,N-dimethyl-9-[3-(4-methyl-1-piperazinyl)-propylidene] thioxanthene-2-sulfonamide.

The thioxanthenes differ from the phenothiazines by the replacement of nitrogen in the central ring with a carbon-linked side chain fixed in space in a rigid structural configuration. An N,N-dimethyl sulfonamide functional group is bonded to the thioxanthene nucleus. †Navane Intramuscular contains in each ml. thiothixene HCl equivalent to 2 mg. of thiothixene, dextrose 5% w/v, benzyl alcohol 0.9% w/v, and propyl gallate 0.02% w/v.

Navane (thiothixene hydrochloride) Intramuscular For Injection, when reconstituted with 2.2 ml of Sterile Water For Injection, contains in each ml thiothixene hydrochloride equivalent to 5 mg of thiothixene, and 59.6 mg of mannitol.

Actions: Navane is a psychotropic agent of the thioxanthene series. Navane possesses certain chemical and pharmacological similarities to the piperazine phenothiazines and differences from the aliphatic group of phenothiazines. Navane's mode of action has not been clearly established.

Indications: Navane is effective in the management of manifestations of psychotic disorders. Navane has not been evaluated in the management of behavioral complications in patients with mental retardation.

Contraindications: Navane is contraindicated in patients with circulatory collapse, comatose states, central nervous system depression due to any cause, and blood dyscrasias. Navane is contraindicated in individuals who have shown hypersensitivity to the drug. It is not known whether there is a cross sensitivity between the thioxanthenes and the phenothiazine derivatives, but this possibility should be considered.

Warnings: Usage in Pregnancy—Safe use of Navane during pregnancy has not been established. Therefore, this drug should be given to pregnant patients only when, in the judgment of the physician, the expected benefits from treatment exceed the possible risks to mother and fetus. Animal reproductive studies and clinical experience to date have not demonstrated any teratogenic effects.

In the animal reproduction studies with Navane, there was some decrease in conception rate and litter size, and an increase in resorption rate in rats and rabbits, changes which have been similarly reported with other psychotropic agents. After repeated oral administration of Navane to rats (5 to 15 mg./kg./day), rabbits (3 to 50 mg./kg./day), and monkeys (1 to 3 mg./kg./day) before and during gestation, no teratogenic effects were seen. (See Precautions.)

Usage in Children—The use of Navane in children under 12 years of age is not recommended because safety and efficacy in the pediatric age group have not been established.

As is true with many CNS drugs, Navane may impair the mental and/or physical abilities required for the performance of potentially hazardous tasks such as driving a car or operating machinery, especially during the first few days of therapy. Therefore, the patient should be cautioned accordingly.

As in the case of other CNS-acting drugs, patients receiving Navane should be cautioned about the possible additive effects (which may include hypotension) with CNS depressants and with alcohol.

Precautions: An antiemetic effect was observed in animal studies with Navane (thiothixene hydrochloride); since this effect may also occur in man, it is possible that Navane may mask signs of overdosage of toxic drugs and may obscure conditions such as intestinal obstruction and brain tumor.

In consideration of the known capability of Navane and certain other psychotropic drugs to precipitate convulsions, extreme caution should be used in patients with a history of convulsive disorders, or those in a state of alcohol withdrawal since it may lower the convulsive threshold. Although Navane potentiates the actions of the barbiturates, the dosage of the anticonvulsant therapy should not be reduced when Navane is administered concurrently.

Caution as well as careful adjustment of the dosage is indicated when Navane is used in conjunction with other CNS depressants other than anticonvulsant drugs.

Though exhibiting rather weak anticholinergic properties, Navane should be used with caution in patients who are known or suspected to have glaucoma, or who might be exposed to extreme heat, or who are receiving atropine or related drugs.

Use with caution in patients with cardiovascular disease.

Also, careful observation should be made for pigmentary retinopathy, and lenticular pigmentation (fine lenticular pigmentation has been noted in a small number of patients treated with Navane for prolonged periods). Blood dyscrasias (agranulocytosis, pancytopenia, thrombocytopenic purpura), and liver damage (jaundice, biliary stasis), have been reported with related drugs.

Undue exposure to sunlight should be avoided. Photosensitive reactions have been reported in patients on Navane.

As with all intramuscular preparations, Navane Intramuscular should be injected well within the body of a relatively large muscle. The preferred sites are the upper outer quadrant of the buttock (i.e., gluteus maximus) and the mid-lateral thigh. The deltoid area should be used only if well developed such as in certain adults and older children, and then only with caution to avoid radial nerve injury. Intramuscular injections should not be made into the lower and mid-thirds of the upper arm. As with all intramuscular injections, aspiration is necessary to help avoid inadvertent injection into a blood vessel.

Neuroleptic drugs elevate prolactin levels; the elevation persists during chronic administration. Tissue culture experiments indicate that approximately one-third of human breast cancers are prolactin dependent *in vitro*, a factor of potential importance if the prescription of these drugs is contemplated in a patient with a previously detected breast cancer. Although disturbances such as galactorrhea, amenorrhea, gynecomastia, and impotence have been reported, the clinical significance of elevated serum prolactin levels is unknown for most patients. An increase in mammary neoplasms has been found in rodents after chronic administration of neuroleptic drugs. Neither clinical studies nor epidemiologic studies conducted to date, however, have shown an association between chronic administration of these drugs and mammary tumorigenesis; the available evidence is considered too limited to be conclusive at this time.

Adverse Reactions:

NOTE: Not all of the following adverse reactions have been reported with Navane. However, since Navane has certain chemical and pharmacologic similarities to the phenothiazines, all of the known side effects and toxicity associated with phenothiazine therapy should be borne in mind when Navane is used.

Cardiovascular effects: Tachycardia, hypotension, lightheadedness, and syncope. In the event hypotension occurs, epinephrine should not be used as a pressor agent since a paradoxical further lowering of blood pressure may result. Nonspecific EKG changes have been observed in some patients receiving Navane. These changes are usually reversible and frequently disappear on continued Navane therapy. The clinical significance of these changes is not known.

CNS effects: Drowsiness, usually mild, may occur although it usually subsides with continuation of Navane therapy. The incidence of sedation appears similar to that of the piperazine group of phenothiazines, but less than that of certain aliphatic phenothiazines. Restlessness, agitation and insomnia have been noted with Navane. Seizures and paradoxical exacerbation of psychotic symptoms have occurred with Navane infrequently. Hyperreflexia has been reported in infants delivered from mothers having received structurally related drugs.

In addition, phenothiazine derivatives have been associated with cerebral edema and cerebrospinal fluid abnormalities.

Extrapyramidal symptoms, such as pseudo-parkinsonism, akathisia, and dystonia have been reported. Management of these extrapyramidal symptoms depends upon the type and severity. Rapid relief of acute symptoms may require the use of an injectable antiparkinson agent. More slowly emerging symptoms may be managed by reducing the dosage of Navane and/or administering an oral antiparkinson agent.

Persistent Tardive Dyskinesia: As with all antipsychotic agents tardive dyskinesia may appear in some patients on long term therapy or may occur after drug therapy has been discontinued. The risk seems to be greater in elderly patients on high-dose therapy, especially females. The symptoms are persistent and in some patients appear to be irreversible. The syndrome is characterized by rhythmical involuntary movements of the tongue, face, mouth or jaw (e.g., protrusion of tongue, puffing of cheeks, puckering of mouth, chewing movements). Sometimes these may be accompanied by involuntary movements of extremities.

There is no known effective treatment for tardive dyskinesia; antiparkinsonism agents usually do not alleviate the symptoms of this syndrome. It is suggested that all antipsychotic agents be discontinued if these symptoms appear.

Should it be necessary to reinstitute treatment, or increase the dosage of the agent, or switch to a different antipsychotic agent, the syndrome may be masked.

It has been reported that fine vermicular movements of the tongue may be an early sign of the syndrome and if the medication is stopped at that time, the syndrome may not develop.

Hepatic effects: Elevations of serum transaminase and alkaline phosphatase, usually transient, have been infrequently observed in some patients. No clinically confirmed cases of jaundice attributable to Navane (thiothixene hydrochloride) have been reported.

Continued on next page

Roerig—Cont.

Hematologic effects: As is true with certain other psychotropic drugs, leukopenia and leucocytosis, which are usually transient, can occur occasionally with Navane. Other antipsychotic drugs have been associated with agranulocytosis, eosinophilia, hemolytic anemia, thrombocytopenia and pancytopenia.

Allergic reactions: Rash, pruritus, urticaria, and rare cases of anaphylaxis have been reported with Navane. Undue exposure to sunlight should be avoided. Although not experienced with Navane, exfoliative dermatitis, contact dermatitis (in nursing personnel), have been reported with certain phenothiazines.

Endocrine disorders: Lactation, moderate breast enlargement and amenorrhea have occurred in a small percentage of females receiving Navane. If persistent, this may necessitate a reduction in dosage or the discontinuation of therapy. Phenothiazines have been associated with false positive pregnancy tests, gynecomastia, hypoglycemia, hyperglycemia, and glycosuria.

Autonomic effects: Dry mouth, blurred vision, nasal congestion, constipation, increased sweating, increased salivation, and impotence have occurred infrequently with Navane therapy. Phenothiazines have been associated with miosis, mydriasis, and adynamic ileus.

Other adverse reactions: Hyperpyrexia, anorexia, nausea, vomiting, diarrhea, increase in appetite and weight, weakness or fatigue, polydipsia and peripheral edema.

Although not reported with Navane, evidence indicates there is a relationship between phenothiazine therapy and the occurrence of a systemic lupus erythematosus-like syndrome.

NOTE: Sudden deaths have occasionally been reported in patients who have received certain phenothiazine derivatives. In some cases the cause of death was apparently cardiac arrest or asphyxia due to failure of the cough reflex. In others, the cause could not be determined nor could it be established that death was due to phenothiazine administration.

Dosage and Administration:
Preparation
Navane (thiothixene hydrochloride) Intramuscular Solution is ready for use as supplied.
Navane (thiothixene hydrochloride) Intramuscular For Injection must be reconstituted with 2.2 ml of Sterile Water for Injection.

For Intramuscular Use Only
Dosage of Navane should be individually adjusted depending on the chronicity and severity of the condition. In general, small doses should be used initially and gradually increased to the optimal effective level, based on patient response.
Usage in children under 12 years of age is not recommended.
Where more rapid control and treatment of acute behavior is desirable, the intramuscular form of Navane may be indicated. It is also of benefit where the very nature of the patient's symptomatology, whether acute or chronic, renders oral administration impractical or even impossible.
For treatment of acute symptomatology or in patients unable or unwilling to take oral medication, the usual dose is 4 mg. of Navane Intramuscular administered 2 to 4 times daily. Dosage may be increased or decreased depending on response. Most patients are controlled on a total daily dosage of 16 to 20 mg. The maximum recommended dosage is 30 mg./day. An oral form should supplant the injectable form as soon as possible. It may be necessary to adjust the dosage when changing from the intramuscular to oral dosage forms. Dosage recommendations for Navane Capsules and Concentrate can be found in the Navane oral package insert.

Overdosage: Manifestations include muscular twitching, drowsiness, and dizziness. Symptoms of gross overdosage may include CNS depression, rigidity, weakness, torticollis, tremor, salivation, dysphagia, hypotension, disturbances of gait, or coma.

Treatment: Essentially symptomatic and supportive. Keep patient under careful observation and maintain an open airway, since involvement of the extrapyramidal system may produce dysphagia and respiratory difficulty in severe overdosage. If hypotension occurs, the standard measures for managing circulatory shock should be used (I.V. fluids and/or vasoconstrictors).

If a vasoconstrictor is needed, levarterenol and phenylephrine are the most suitable drugs. Other pressor agents, including epinephrine, are not recommended, since phenothiazine derivatives may reverse the usual pressor elevating action of these agents and cause further lowering of blood pressure.

If CNS depression is present and specific therapy is indicated, recommended stimulants include amphetamine, dextroamphetamine, or caffeine and sodium benzoate. Picrotoxin or pentylenetetrazol should be avoided. Extrapyramidal symptoms may be treated with antiparkinson drugs.
There are no data on the use of peritoneal or hemodialysis, but they are known to be of little value in phenothiazine intoxication.

How Supplied: Navane (thiothixene hydrochloride) Intramuscular Solution is available in a 2 ml. amber glass vial in packages of 10 vials. Each ml. contains thiothixene hydrochloride equivalent to 2 mg. of thiothixene, dextrose 5% w/v, benzyl alcohol 0.9% w/v, and propyl gallate 0.02% w/v.
Navane (thiothixene hydrochloride) Intramuscular For Injection is available in amber glass vials in packages of 10 vials. When reconstituted with 2.2 ml of Sterile Water for Injection, each ml contains thiothixene hydrochloride equivalent to 5 mg of thiothixene, and 59.6 mg of mannitol. The reconstituted solution of Navane Intramuscular For Injection may be stored for 48 hours at room temperature before discarding.

23-1865-00-9
23-4177-00-0

SINEQUAN® ℞
[sin'a-kwon]
(doxepin HCl)
Capsules
Oral Concentrate

Description: SINEQUAN (doxepin hydrochloride) is one of a class of psychotherapeutic agents known as dibenzoxepin tricyclic compounds. The molecular formula of the compound is $C_{19}H_{21}NO \cdot HCl$ having a molecular weight of 316. It is a white crystalline solid readily soluble in water, lower alcohols and chloroform.

Chemistry: SINEQUAN (doxepin HCl) is a dibenzoxepin derivative and is the first of a family of tricyclic psychotherapeutic agents. Specifically, it is an isomeric mixture of 1-Propanamine, 3-dibenz[b,e]oxepin-11(6H)ylidene-N,N-dimethyl-, hydrochloride.

Actions: The mechanism of action of SINEQUAN (doxepin HCl) is not definitely known. It is not a central nervous system stimulant nor a monoamine oxidase inhibitor. The current hypothesis is that the clinical effects are due, at least in part, to influences on the adrenergic activity at the synapses so that deactivation of norepinephrine by reuptake into the nerve terminals is prevented. Animal studies suggest that doxepin HCl does not appreciably antagonize the antihypertensive action of guanethidine. In animal studies anticholinergic, antiserotonin and antihistamine effects on smooth muscle have been demonstrated. At higher than usual clinical doses, norepinephrine response was potentiated in animals. This effect was not demonstrated in humans. At clinical dosages up to 150 mg per day, SINEQUAN can be given to man concomitantly with guanethidine and related compounds without blocking the antihypertensive effect. At dosages above 150 mg per day blocking of the antihypertensive effect of these compounds has been reported.

Sinequan is virtually devoid of euphoria as a side effect. Characteristic of this type of compound, Sinequan has not been demonstrated to produce the physical tolerance or psychological dependence associated with addictive compounds.

Indications: SINEQUAN is recommended for the treatment of:
1. Psychoneurotic patients with depression and/or anxiety.
2. Depression and/or anxiety associated with alcoholism (not to be taken concomitantly with alcohol).
3. Depression and/or anxiety associated with organic disease (the possibility of drug interaction should be considered if the patient is receiving other drugs concomitantly).
4. Psychotic depressive disorders with associated anxiety including involutional depression and manic-depressive disorders.

The target symptoms of psychoneurosis that respond particularly well to SINEQUAN include anxiety, tension, depression, somatic symptoms and concerns, sleep disturbances, guilt, lack of energy, fear, apprehension and worry.

Clinical experience has shown that SINEQUAN is safe and well-tolerated even in the elderly patient. Owing to lack of clinical experience in the pediatric population, SINEQUAN is not recommended for use in children under 12 years of age.

Contraindications: SINEQUAN is contraindicated in individuals who have shown hypersensitivity to the drug. Possibility of cross sensitivity with other dibenzoxepines should be kept in mind. SINEQUAN is contraindicated in patients with glaucoma or a tendency to urinary retention. These disorders should be ruled out, particularly in older patients.

Warnings: The once-a-day dosage regimen of SINEQUAN in patients with intercurrent illness or patients taking other medications should be carefully adjusted. This is especially important in patients receiving other medications with anticholinergic effects.

Usage in Geriatrics
The use of SINEQUAN on a once-a-day dosage regimen in geriatric patients should be adjusted carefully based on the patient's condition.

Usage in Pregnancy
Reproduction studies have been performed in rats, rabbits, monkeys and dogs and there was no evidence of harm to the animal fetus. The relevance to humans is not known. Since there is no experience in pregnant women who have received this drug, safety in pregnancy has not been established. There are no data with respect to the secretion of the drug in human milk and its effect on the nursing infant.

Usage in Children
The use of SINEQUAN in children under 12 years of age is not recommended because safe conditions for its use have not been established.

Drug Interactions:
MAO Inhibitors
Serious side effects and even death have been reported following the concomitant use of certain drugs with MAO inhibitors. Therefore, MAO inhibitors should be discontinued at least two weeks prior to the cautious initiation of therapy with SINEQUAN. The exact length of time may vary and is dependent upon the particular MAO inhibitor being used, the length of time it has been administered, and the dosage involved.

Cimetidine
Cimetidine has been reported to produce clinically significant fluctuations in steady-state serum concentrations of various tricyclic antidepressants. Serious anticholinergic symptoms (i.e., severe dry mouth, urinary retention and blurred vision) have been associated with elevations in the serum levels of tricyclic antidepressant when cimetidine therapy is initiated. Additionally, higher than expected tricyclic antidepressant levels have been observed when they are begun in patients already taking cimetidine. In patients who have been reported to be well controlled on tricyclic antidepressants receiving concurrent cimetidine therapy, discontinuation of cimetidine has been reported to decrease established steady-state serum tricyclic antidepressant levels and compromise their therapeutic effects.

Alcohol
It should be borne in mind that alcohol ingestion may increase the danger inherent in any intentional or unintentional SINEQUAN overdosage. This is especially important in patients who may use alcohol excessively.

Precautions: Since drowsiness may occur with the use of this drug, patients should be warned of the possibility and cautioned against driving a car or operating dangerous machinery while taking the drug. Patients should also be cautioned that their response to alcohol may be potentiated.

Since suicide is an inherent risk in any depressed patient and may remain so until significant improvement has occurred, patients should be closely supervised during the early course of therapy. Prescriptions should be written for the smallest feasible amount.

Should increased symptoms of psychosis or shift to manic symptomatology occur, it may be necessary to reduce dosage or add a major tranquilizer to the dosage regimen.

Adverse Reactions:
NOTE: Some of the adverse reactions noted below have not been specifically reported with SINEQUAN use. However, due to the close pharmacological similarities among the tricyclics, the reactions should be considered when prescribing SINEQUAN (doxepin HCl).

Anticholinergic Effects: Dry mouth, blurred vision, constipation, and urinary retention have been reported. If they do not subside with continued therapy, or become severe, it may be necessary to reduce the dosage.

Central Nervous System Effects: Drowsiness is the most commonly noticed side effect. This tends to disappear as therapy is continued. Other infrequently reported CNS side effects are confusion, disorientation, hallucinations, numbness, paresthesias, ataxia, and extrapyramidal symptoms and seizures.

Cardiovascular: Cardiovascular effects including hypotension and tachycardia have been reported occasionally.

Allergic: Skin rash, edema, photosensitization, and pruritus have occasionally occurred.

Hematologic: Eosinophilia has been reported in a few patients. There have been occasional reports of bone marrow depression manifesting as agranulocytosis, leukopenia, thrombocytopenia, and purpura.

Gastrointestinal: Nausea, vomiting, indigestion, taste disturbances, diarrhea, anorexia, and aphthous stomatitis have been reported. (See anticholinergic effects.)

Endocrine: Raised or lowered libido, testicular swelling, gynecomastia in males, enlargement of breasts and galactorrhea in the female, raising or lowering of blood sugar levels have been reported with tricyclic administration.

Other: Dizziness, tinnitus, weight gain, sweating, chills, fatigue, weakness, flushing, jaundice, alopecia, and headache have been occasionally observed as adverse effects.

Withdrawal Symptoms: The possibility of development of withdrawal symptoms upon abrupt cessation of treatment after prolonged Sinequan administration should be borne in mind. These are not indicative of addiction and gradual withdrawal of medication should not cause these symptoms.

Dosage and Administration: For most patients with illness of mild to moderate severity, a starting daily dose of 75 mg is recommended. Dosage may subsequently be increased or decreased at appropriate intervals and according to individual response. The usual optimum dose range is 75 mg/day to 150 mg/day.

In more severely ill patients higher doses may be required with subsequent gradual increase to 300 mg/day if necessary. Additional therapeutic effect is rarely to be obtained by exceeding a dose of 300 mg/day.

In patients with very mild symptomatology or emotional symptoms accompanying organic disease, lower doses may suffice. Some of these patients have been controlled on doses as low as 25-50 mg/day.

The total daily dosage of SINEQUAN may be given on a divided or once-a-day dosage schedule. If the once-a-day schedule is employed the maximum recommended dose is 150 mg/day. This dose may be given at bedtime. **The 150 mg capsule strength is intended for maintenance therapy only and is not recommended for initiation of treatment.**

Anti-anxiety effect is apparent before the antidepressant effect. Optimal antidepressant effect may not be evident for two to three weeks.

Overdosage:
A. Signs and Symptoms
 1. Mild: Drowsiness, stupor, blurred vision, excessive dryness of mouth.
 2. Severe: Respiratory depression, hypotension, coma, convulsions, cardiac arrhythmias and tachycardias.
 Also: urinary retention (bladder atony), decreased gastrointestinal motility (paralytic ileus), hyperthermia (or hypothermia), hypertension, dilated pupils, hyperactive reflexes.
B. Management and Treatment
 1. Mild: Observation and supportive therapy is all that is usually necessary.
 2. Severe: Medical management of severe SINEQUAN overdosage consists of aggressive supportive therapy. If the patient is conscious, gastric lavage, with appropriate precautions to prevent pulmonary aspiration, should be performed even though SINEQUAN is rapidly absorbed. The use of activated charcoal has been recommended, as has been continuous gastric lavage with saline for 24 hours or more. An adequate airway should be established in comatose patients and assisted ventilation used if necessary. EKG monitoring may be required for several days, since relapse after apparent recovery has been reported. Arrhythmias should be treated with the appropriate anti-arrhythmic agent. It has been reported that many of the cardiovascular and CNS symptoms of tricyclic antidepressant poisoning in adults may be reversed by the slow intravenous administration of 1 mg to 3 mg of physostigmine salicylate. Because physostigmine is rapidly metabolized, the dosage should be repeated as required. Convulsions may respond to standard anticonvulsant therapy, however, barbiturates may potentiate any respiratory depression. Dialysis and forced diuresis generally are not of value in the management of overdosage due to high tissue and protein binding of SINEQUAN.

Supply:
SINEQUAN is available as capsules containing doxepin HCl equivalent to: 10 mg, 75 mg, and 100 mg doxepin; bottles of 100, 1000, and unit-dose packages of 100 (10 × 10's).

25 mg and 50 mg doxepin: bottles of 100, 1000, 5000, and unit-dose packages of 100 (10 × 10's).

150 mg doxepin: bottles of 50, 500, and unit-dose packages of 100 (10 × 10's).

SINEQUAN Oral Concentrate is available in 120 ml bottles with an accompanying dropper calibrated at 5 mg, 10 mg, 15 mg, 20 mg, and 25 mg. Each ml contains doxepin HCl equivalent to 10 mg doxepin. Just prior to administration, SINEQUAN Oral Concentrate should be diluted with approximately 120 ml of water, whole or skimmed milk, or orange, grapefruit, tomato, prune or pineapple juice. SINEQUAN Oral Concentrate is not physically compatible with a number of carbonated beverages. For those patients requiring antidepressant therapy who are on methadone maintenance, SINEQUAN Oral Concentrate and methadone syrup can be mixed together with Gatorade®, lemonade, orange juice, sugar water, Tang®, or water; but not with grape juice. Preparation and storage of bulk dilutions is not recommended.

Literature Available: Yes.

69-2135-37-3
Shown in Product Identification Section, page 431

SPECTROBID®
[spek'trō-bid]
(bacampicillin HCl)
TABLETS and POWDER
for ORAL SUSPENSION

Description: SPECTROBID (bacampicillin HCl) is a member of the ampicillin class of semi-synthetic penicillins derived from the basic penicillin nucleus: 6-aminopenicillanic acid. SPECTROBID, as well as ampicillin and other ampicillin analogues, is acid resistant and suitable for oral administration.

SPECTROBID is the hydrochloride salt of 1-ethoxycarbonyloxyethyl ester of ampicillin, available either as tablets or as a microencapsulated oral suspension. During the process of absorption from the gastrointestinal tract, SPECTROBID is hydrolyzed rapidly to ampicillin, a well characterized and effective antibacterial agent. Each 400 mg tablet of SPECTROBID is chemically equivalent to 280 mg of ampicillin, and 125 mg/5 ml of the oral suspension is chemically equivalent to 87.5 mg of ampicillin.

Chemically, SPECTROBID is 1'-ethoxycarbonyloxyethyl-6-(D-α aminophenylacetamide)-penicillinate hydrochloride. It has a molecular weight of 501.96.

Actions:
Clinical Pharmacology
SPECTROBID is characterized by its more complete and more rapid absorption from the GI tract than ampicillin. SPECTROBID tablets of 400 mg, 800 mg, and 1600 mg have provided ampicillin peak serum concentrations of 7.9, 12.9, and 20.1 mcg/ml. These peak levels are approximately three times the levels obtained with administration of equivalent amounts of ampicillin. The areas-under-the-serum-concentration curves obtained during the first 6 hours were 24.8 and 12.9 mcg/ml/hr., when bacampicillin HCl 800 mg and ampicillin 500 mg were administered to adults. (See Graph 1.) Graph 2 shows the serum ampicillin curves following a 28 mg/kg dose of bacampicillin HCl and a 25 mg/kg dose of ampicillin in infants and young children. The areas-under-the-serum-concentration-curves were 28.2 and 13.1 respectively.

The absorption of the SPECTROBID oral suspension was shown to be equivalent to that of the 400 mg tablet in fasting adult volunteers. A 400 mg dose of suspension gave a peak serum ampicillin concentration of 7.6 mcg/ml and the tablet gave a peak of 7.2 mcg/ml. In fasting pediatric patients a 12.5 mg/kg dose provided a peak of 8.4 mcg/ml. After oral administration of SPECTROBID tablet or suspension, ampicillin activity in serum peaks at 0.7–0.9 hours (compared to 1.5–2.0 hours after administration of ampicillin). Serum ampicillin half-life is 1.1 hours after either SPECTROBID or ampicillin administration.

Peak tissue and body fluid ampicillin concentrations also are higher after administration of SPECTROBID. Utilizing a special skin window technique to determine ampicillin levels, therapeutic levels in the interstitial fluid were higher and more prolonged after SPECTROBID than after ampicillin administration. SPECTROBID is stable in the presence of gastric acid. SPECTROBID oral suspension absorption is affected by food. Food does not retard absorption of SPECTROBID tablets which may be given without regard to meals. SPECTROBID has been shown to be rapidly and well absorbed after oral administration, with about 75% of a given dose being recoverable in the urine as active ampicillin within 8 hours of administration. Urinary excretion can be delayed by concurrent administration of probenecid. The active moiety of SPECTROBID (i.e., ampicillin) diffuses readily into most body tissues and fluids. In serum, ampicillin is only 20% protein-bound, compared to 60–90% for other penicillins.

Microbiology
SPECTROBID per se has no *in vitro* antibacterial activity and owes its *in vivo* bactericidal activity to the parent compound, ampicillin. The ampicillin

Continued on next page

Roerig—Cont.

class of penicillins (including SPECTROBID) has a broad spectrum of activity against many gram-negative and gram-positive bacteria. Like other penicillins, the ampicillin class of penicillins inhibits the synthesis of cell wall mucopeptide.
Ampicillin class antibiotics are inactivated by β-lactamases produced by certain strains of *Enterobacter, Citrobacter, Haemophilus infuenzae,* and *Escherichia coli,* and by most strains of staphylococci and indole-positive *Proteus* spp. Ampicillin class antibiotics are not active against *Pseudomonas, Klebsiella,* or *Serratia* spp.

Susceptibility Testing:
Elution Technique: For the automated method of susceptibility testing (i.e., Autobac™), gram-negative organisms should be tested with the 4.5 mcg ampicillin elution disk, while gram-positive organisms should be tested with the 0.22 mcg disk.
Diffusion Technique: For the Kirby-Bauer method of susceptibility testing, a 10 mcg ampicillin diffusion disk should be used. With this procedure, a laboratory report of "susceptible" indicates that the infecting organism is likely to respond to SPECTROBID therapy, and a report of "resistant" indicates that the infecting organism is not likely to respond to therapy. An "intermediate susceptibility" report suggests that the infecting organism would be susceptible to SPECTROBID if a high dosage is used or if the infection is confined to tissues and fluids (e.g., urine) in which high antibiotic levels are attained.
Dilution Techniques: Broth or agar dilution methods may be used to determine the minimal inhibitory concentration (MIC) value for susceptibility of bacterial isolates to SPECTROBID. Since SPECTROBID per se has no *in vitro* activity, ampicillin powder should be used in a twofold concentration series of the antibiotic prepared in either broth (in tubes) or agar (in petri plates). Tubes should be inoculated to contain 10^4 to 10^5 organisms/ml or plates "spotted" with 10^3 to 10^4 organisms.

Indications and Usage:
SPECTROBID is indicated for the treatment of the following infections when caused by ampicillin-susceptible organisms:
1. Upper and Lower Respiratory Tract Infections (including acute exacerbations of chronic bronchitis) due to streptococci (β-hemolytic streptococci, *Streptococcus pyogenes*), pneumococci (*Streptococcus pneumoniae*), nonpenicillinase-producing staphylococci and *H. influenzae;*
2. Urinary Tract Infections due to *E. coli, Proteus mirabilis,* and *Streptococcus faecalis* (enterococci);
3. Skin and Skin Structure Infections due to streptococci and susceptible staphylococci;
4. Gonorrhea (acute uncomplicated urogenital infections) due to *Neisseria gonorrhoeae.*

Bacteriological studies to determine the causative organisms and their suspectibility to SPECTROBID (i.e., ampicillin) should be performed. Therapy may be instituted prior to obtaining results of susceptibility testing. Indicated surgical procedures should be performed.

Contraindications:
The use of ampicillin class antibiotics is contraindicated in individuals with a history of an allergic reaction to any of the penicillin antibiotics and/or cephalosporins.

Warnings: Serious and occasional fatal hypersensitivity (anaphylactic) reactions have been reported in patients on penicillin therapy. Although anaphylaxis is more frequent following parenteral therapy, it has occurred in patients on oral penicillins. These reactions are more apt to occur in individuals with a history of penicillin hypersensitivity and/or hypersensitivity to multiple allergens.
There have been reports of individuals with a history of penicillin hypersensitivity who have experienced severe reactions when treated with cephalosporins. Before therapy with a penicillin, careful inquiry should be made concerning previous hypersensitivity reactions to penicillins, cephalosporins, and other allergens.
IF AN ALLERGIC REACTION OCCURS, THE DRUG SHOULD BE DISCONTINUED AND THE APPROPRIATE THERAPY INSTITUTED. SERIOUS ANAPHYLACTOID REACTIONS REQUIRE IMMEDIATE EMERGENCY TREATMENT WITH EPINEPHRINE. OXYGEN, INTRAVENOUS STEROIDS, AND AIRWAY MANAGEMENT, INCLUDING INTUBATION, SHOULD ALSO BE ADMINISTERED AS INDICATED.

Precautions:
1. General: The possibility of superinfections with mycotic or bacterial pathogens should be kept in mind during therapy. If superinfections occur (usually involving *Aerobacter, Pseudomonas,* or *Candida*), the drug should be discontinued and appropriate therapy instituted.
As with any potent agent, it is advisable to check periodically for organ system dysfunction during prolonged therapy. This includes renal, hepatic, and hematopoietic systems and is particularly important in prematures, neonates, and patients with liver or renal impairments.
A high percentage of patients with mononucleosis who receive ampicillin develop a skin rash. Thus, ampicillin class antibiotics should not be administered to patients with mononucleosis.
2. Clinically Significant Drug Interactions: The concurrent administration of allopurinol and ampicillin increases substantially the incidence of rashes in patients receiving both drugs as compared to patients receiving ampicillin alone. It is not known whether this potentiation of ampicillin rashes is due to allopurinol or the hyperuricemia present in these patients. There are no data available on the incidence of rash in patients treated concurrently with SPECTROBID (bacampicillin HCl) and allopurinol. SPECTROBID should not be co-administered with Antabuse (disulfiram).
3. Drug and Laboratory Test Interactions: When testing for the presence of glucose in urine using Clinitest™, Benedict's Solution, or Fehling's Solution, high urine concentrations of ampicillin may result in false-positive reactions. Therefore, it is recommended that glucose tests based on enzymatic glucose oxidase reactions (such as Clinistix™ or Testape™) be used.
Following administration of ampicillin to pregnant women a transient decrease in plasma concentration of total conjugated estriol, estriol-glucuronide, conjugated estrone and estradiol, has been noted.
4. Pregnancy Category B: Reproduction studies have been performed in mice and rats at SPECTROBID doses of up to 750 mg/kg (more than 25 times the human dose) and have revealed no evidence of impaired fertility or harm to the fetus due to SPECTROBID.
There are, however, no adequate and well controlled studies in pregnant women. Because animal reproduction studies are not always predictive of human response, this drug should be used during pregnancy only if clearly needed.
5. Carcinogenesis, Mutagenesis, Impairment of Fertility: No carcinogenicity or mutagenicity studies were conducted. No impairment of fertility and no significant effect on general reproductive performance was observed in rats administered oral doses of up to 750 mg/kg of bacampicillin HCl per day prior to and during mating and gestation. In addition, bacampicillin HCl caused no drug-related effects on the reproductive organs of rats or dogs receiving daily oral doses of up to 800 and 650 mg/kg respectively for 6 months.
6. Labor and Delivery: Oral ampicillin class antibiotics are generally poorly absorbed during labor. Studies in guinea pigs showed that intravenous administration of ampicillin decreased the uterine tone, frequency of contractions, height of contractions, and duration of contractions. However, it is not known whether use of SPECTROBID in humans during labor or delivery has immediate or delayed adverse effects on the fetus, prolongs the duration of labor, or increases the likelihood that forceps delivery or other obstetrical intervention or resuscitation of the newborn will be necessary.
7. Nursing Mothers: Ampicillin class antibiotics are excreted in milk; therefore, caution should be exercised when ampicillin class antibiotics are administered to a nursing woman.
8. Pediatric Use: SPECTROBID tablets are indicated for children weighing 25 kg or more. The SPECTROBID oral suspension is indicated for children and infants weighing less than 25 kg or in those children not able to swallow a tablet.

Adverse Reactions: As with other penicillins, it may be expected that untoward reactions will be essentially limited to sensitivity phenomena. They are more likely to occur in individuals who have previously demonstrated hypersensitivity to penicillins and in those with a history of allergy, asthma, hay fever, or urticaria.
In well controlled clinical trials conducted in the U.S. the most frequent adverse reactions to SPECTROBID were epigastric upset (2%) and diarrhea (2%). Increased dosage may result in an increased incidence of diarrhea. In the same clinical trials the most frequent adverse effects for amoxicillin were diarrhea (4%) and nausea (2%). The following adverse reactions have been reported for ampicillin.
Gastrointestinal: diarrhea, gastritis, stomatitis, nausea, vomiting, glossitis, black "hairy" tongue, enterocolitis, and pseudomembranous colitis.
Hypsersensitivity Reactions: skin rashes, urticaria, erythema multiforme, and an occasional case of exfoliative dermatitis. These reactions may be controlled with antihistamines and, if necessary, systemic corticosteroids. Whenever such reactions occur, the drug should be discontinued, unless the opinion of the physician dictates otherwise.
Serious and occasional fatal hypersensitivity (anaphylactic) reactions can occur with oral penicillins. (See Warnings.)
Liver: A moderate rise in serum glutamic oxaloacetic transaminase (SGOT) has been noted in some ampicillin treated patients, but the significance of this finding is unknown. In well controlled clinical trials no difference was noted between ampicillin and SPECTROBID with regard to the incidence of liver function test abnormalities.
Hemic and Lymphatic Systems: Anemia, thrombocytopenia, thrombocytopenic purpura, eosinophilia, leukopenia, and agranulocytosis have been reported during therapy with penicillins. These reactions are usually reversible on discontinuation of therapy and are believed to be hypersensitivity phenomena.

Dosage and Administration: SPECTROBID tablets may be given without regard to meals. SPECTROBID oral suspension should be administered to fasting patients.
UPPER RESPIRATORY TRACT INFECTIONS (including otitis media) due to streptococci, pneumococci, nonpenicillinase-producing staphylococci and *H. influenzae;*
URINARY TRACT INFECTIONS due to *E. coli, Proteus mirabilis,* and *Streptococcus faecalis;*
SKIN AND SKIN STRUCTURES INFECTIONS due to streptococci and susceptible staphylococci;
Usual Dosage
Adults: 1 × 400 mg tablets every 12 hours (for patients weighing 25 kg or more).
Children: 25 mg/kg per day in 2 equally divided doses at 12 hour intervals.
IN SEVERE INFECTIONS OR THOSE CAUSED BY LESS SUSCEPTIBLE ORGANISMS:
Usual Dosage
Adults: 2 × 400 mg tablets every 12 hours (for patients weighing 25 kg or more).
Children: 50 mg/kg per day in 2 equally divided doses at 12 hour intervals.
LOWER RESPIRATORY TRACT INFECTIONS due to streptococci, pneumococci, nonpenicillinase-producing staphylococci, and *H. influenzae:*
Usual Dosage
Adults: 2 × 400 mg tablets every 12 hours (for patients weighing 25 kg or more).
Children: 50 mg/kg per day in 2 equally divided doses at 12 hour intervals.

GONORRHEA—acute uncomplicated urogenital infections due to *N. gonorrhoeae* (males and females):
1.6 grams (4 × 400 mg tablet plus 1 gram probenecid) as a single oral dose.
No pediatric dosage has been established.
Cases of gonorrhea with a suspected lesion of syphilis should have dark field examination before receiving SPECTROBID and monthly serological tests for a minimum of four months. Larger doses may be required for stubborn or severe infections. It should be recognized that in the treatment of chronic urinary tract infections, frequent bacteriological and clinical appraisals are necessary. Smaller doses than those recommended above should not be used. In stubborn infections, therapy may be required for several weeks. It may be necessary to continue clinical and/or bacteriological follow-up for several months after cessation of therapy. Except for gonorrhea, treatment should be continued for a minimum of 48 to 72 hours beyond the time that the patient becomes asymptomatic or evidence of bacterial eradication has been obtained.
IT IS RECOMMENDED THAT THERE BE AT LEAST 10 DAYS' TREATMENT FOR ANY INFECTION CAUSED BY HEMOLYTIC STREPTOCOCCI TO PREVENT THE OCCURRENCE OF ACUTE RHEUMATIC FEVER OR GLOMERULONEPHRITIS.

Directions for Mixing Oral Suspension:
Prepare suspension at the time of dispensing as follows:
Prior to reconstitution, tap bottle to thoroughly loosen powder. Add the required amount (see table below) of water to the contents of the bottle in approximately two equally divided portions and SHAKE WELL after each addition. Let stand at least 30 minutes and SHAKE WELL just prior to administering each dose. Each level teaspoon (5 ml) will contain 125 mg of bacampicillin HCl.

Final Volume after reconstitution	Amount of Water Required for reconstitution
70 ml	53 ml
100 ml	75 ml

Reconstituted suspension *must be stored under refrigeration and discarded after 10 days.*

GRAPH 1.
Comparison of Bacampicillin HCl 800 mg, Ampicillin 500 mg, and Amoxicillin 500 mg

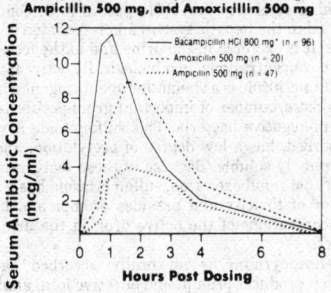

*800 mg Bacampicillin HCl is chemically equivalent to 560 mg of Ampicillin

GRAPH 2.
Crossover Comparison of Bacampicillin HCl Oral Suspension (28 mg/kg)* with Ampicillin Oral Suspension (25 mg/kg) in Fasted Infants and Children (n = 7).

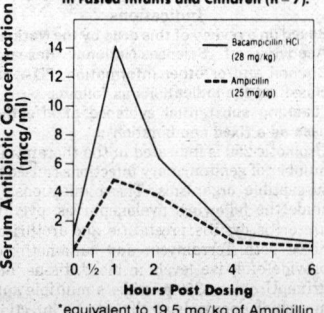

*equivalent to 19.5 mg/kg of Ampicillin

How Supplied:
SPECTROBID (bacampicillin HCl) Tablets 400 mg (NDC 0049-0350-66): white, film-coated, oblong, unscored are available in bottles of 100.
SPECTROBID (bacampicillin HCl) Powder for Oral Suspension.
Each 5 ml of reconstituted suspension contains 125 mg of bacampicillin HCl.
Bottles containing the following volumes are available: 70 ml (NDC 0049-0357-37), 100 ml (NDC 0049-0357-44).

67-4092-00-3
Shown in Product Identification Section, page 431

SUSTAIRE® ℞
[sus'tār]
theophylline (anhydrous)
SUSTAINED RELEASE TABLETS

Description: SUSTAIRE Sustained Release Tablets contain anhydrous theophylline, with no color additives. SUSTAIRE is available in two strengths: 100 mg and 300 mg; each tablet is scored for flexibility of dose. Theophylline, a xanthine compound, is a white, odorless crystalline powder, having a bitter taste.
Actions: The pharmacologic actions of theophylline are as a bronchodilator, pulmonary vasodilator, and smooth muscle relaxant since the drug directly relaxes the smooth muscle of the bronchial airways and pulmonary blood vessels. Theophylline also possesses other actions typical of the xanthine derivatives: coronary vasodilator, diuretic, cardiac stimulant, and skeletal muscle stimulant. The actions of theophylline may be mediated through inhibition of phosphodiesterase and a resultant increase in intracellular cyclic AMP which could mediate smooth muscle relaxation.
No development of tolerance appears to occur with chronic use of theophylline. The half-life is shortened with cigarette smoking and prolonged in alcoholism, reduced hepatic or renal function, congestive heart failure, and in patients receiving certain antibiotics (see DRUG INTERACTIONS). High fever for prolonged periods may decrease theophylline elimination. Children over six months of age have rapid clearances with average half-lives of approximately 3–5 hours. Newborn infants have extremely slow clearances and half-lives exceeding 24 hours. Older adults with chronic obstructive pulmonary disease, any patients with cor pulmonale or other causes of heart-failure, and patients with liver pathology may have much lower clearances with half-lives that exceed 24 hours. The half-life in non-smokers averages 7–9 hours.
In single dose studies, SUSTAIRE, administered at 8 mg/kg body weight, produced mean peak theophylline blood levels of 7.5 ± 1.9 mcg/ml at 9.2 ± 1.9 hours following administration. In the multiple dose, steady-state, 3 and 5 day studies, SUSTAIRE achieved remarkably constant intra-subject theophylline levels with an average peak-trough difference of only 4 mcg/ml. This is indicative of smooth and stable maintenance therapeutic theophylline levels throughout a q12h dosing interval.
Indications: Symptomatic relief and/or prevention of asthma and reversible bronchospasm associated with chronic bronchitis and emphysema.
Contraindications: SUSTAIRE is contraindicated in individuals who have shown hypersensitivity to any of its components or xanthine derivatives.
Warnings: Excessive theophylline doses may be associated with toxicity; serum theophylline levels should be monitored to assure maximum benefit with minimum risk. Incidence of toxicity increases at serum levels greater than 20 mcg/ml. High blood levels of theophylline resulting from conventional doses are correlated with clinical manifestations of toxicity in patients with lowered body plasma clearances, patients with liver dysfunction or chronic obstructive lung disease, and patients who are older than 55 years of age—particularly males. There are often no early signs of less serious theophylline toxicity such as nausea and restlessness, which may be the first signs of toxicity. Many patients who have higher theophylline serum levels exhibit a tachycardia. Theophylline products may worsen pre-existing arrhythmias.
Usage in Pregnancy: Safe use in pregnancy has not been established relative to possible adverse effects on fetal development, but neither have adverse effects on fetal development been established. This is, unfortunately, true for most antiasthmatic medications. Therefore, use of theophylline in pregnant women should be balanced against the risk of uncontrolled asthma.
Precautions: SUSTAIRE TABLETS SHOULD NOT BE CHEWED OR CRUSHED.
Theophylline should not be administered concurrently with other xanthine medications. It should be used with caution in patients with severe cardiac disease, severe hypoxemia, hypertension, hyperthyroidism, acute myocardial injury, cor pulmonale, congestive heart failure, liver disease, in the elderly (particularly males), and in neonates. Great caution should be used in giving theophylline to patients in congestive heart failure since these patients show markedly prolonged theophylline blood level curves. Use theophylline cautiously in patients with history of peptic ulcer. Theophylline may occasionally act as a local irritant to the G.I. tract although gastrointestinal symptoms are more commonly central and associated with high serum concentrations above 20 mcg/ml.
Adverse Reactions: The most consistent adverse reactions are usually due to overdose and are:
Gastrointestinal: nausea, vomiting, epigastric pain, hematemesis, diarrhea.
Central Nervous System: headaches, irritability, restlessness, insomnia, reflex hyperexcitability, muscle twitching, clonic and tonic generalized convulsions.
Cardiovascular: palpitation, tachycardia, extrasystoles, flushing, hypotension, circulatory failure, life threatening ventricular arrhythmias.
Respiratory: tachypnea
Renal: albuminuria, increased excretion of renal tubular cells and red blood cells; potentiation of diuresis.
Others: hyperglycemia and inappropriate ADH syndrome.
Drug Interactions:

Drug	Effect
Theophylline with Furosemide	Increased diuresis
Theophylline with Hexamethonium	Decreased chronotropic effect
Theophylline with Reserpine	Tachycardia
Theophylline with Cyclamycin, TAO® (troleandomycin) Erythromycin or Lincomycin	Increased theophylline blood levels

Overdosage:
Management
A. If potential oral overdose is established and seizure has not occurred:
 1) Induce vomiting.
 2) Administer a cathartic. (This is particularly important if sustained release preparations have been taken.)
 3) Administer activated charcoal.
B. Patient is having a seizure:
 1) Establish an airway.
 2) Administer O₂
 3) Treat the seizure with intravenous diazepam: 0.1 to 0.3 mg/kg up to 10 mg.
 4) Monitor vital signs. Maintain blood pressure and provide adequate hydration.

Continued on next page

Roerig—Cont.

C. Post Seizure Coma:
1) Maintain airway and oxygenation.
2) If a result of oral medication, follow above recommendations to prevent absorption of drug; but intubation and lavage will have to be performed instead of inducing emesis, and the cathartic and charcoal will need to be introduced via a large bore gastric lavage tube.
3) Continue to provide full supportive care and adequate hydration while waiting for drug to be metabolized. In general, the drug is metabolized sufficiently rapidly so as to not warrant consideration of dialysis.

Dosage and Administration: Therapeutic serum levels associated with optimal likelihood for benefit and minimal risk of toxicity are considered to be between 10 and 20 mcg/ml. There is a great variation from patient to patient in dosage needed in order to achieve a therapeutic blood level due to variable rates of elimination. Because of this wide variation from patient to patient, and the relatively narrow therapeutic range, dosage must be individualized.

THE AVERAGE INITIAL CHILDREN'S (UNDER 9 YEARS OF AGE) DOSE IS ONE SUSTAIRE 100 mg TABLET q12h.
THE AVERAGE INITIAL CHILDREN'S (AGES 9-12) DOSE IS ONE HALF (150 mg) OF A SUSTAIRE 300 mg TABLET q12h.
THE AVERAGE INITIAL ADOLESCENT (AGES 12-16) DOSE IS TWO SUSTAIRE 100 mg TABLETS q12h.
THE AVERAGE INITIAL ADULT DOSE IS ONE SUSTAIRE 300 mg TABLET q12h.
If the desired response is not achieved with the above AVERAGE INITIAL DOSAGE recommendations and there are no adverse reactions, the dose may be safely increased by 2-3 mg/kg body weight per day at 3 day intervals until the following MAXIMUM DOSE WITHOUT MEASUREMENT OF SERUM CONCENTRATION or a maximum of 900 mg in any 24 hour period, whichever is less, is attained:
[See table below].
If doses higher than those contained in the above MAXIMUM DOSE WITHOUT MEASUREMENT OF SERUM CONCENTRATION are necessary, it is recommended that serum theophylline levels be monitored. Check serum theophylline levels between 3 and 8 hours after a dose. It is important that the patient will have missed *no* doses during the previous 72 hours and that dosing intervals will have been reasonably typical with *no* added doses during that period of time. DOSAGE ADJUSTMENT BASED ON SERUM THEOPHYLLINE MEASUREMENTS WHEN THESE INSTRUCTIONS HAVE NOT BEEN FOLLOWED, MAY RESULT IN RECOMMENDATIONS THAT PRESENT RISK OF TOXICITY TO THE PATIENT.

How Supplied: SUSTAIRE 100 mg and 300 mg Sustained Release Tablets are available in bottles of 100, and Unit-dose packages of 100 (10 × 10's).
Storage Conditions: Keep tightly closed. Store at controlled room temperature 15–30° C (59–86° F).

67-3091-00-3
Shown in Product Identification Section, page 431

Sustaire
Maximum Dose Without Measurement Of Serum Concentration

	mg per kg body weight*	dose per interval
Children (under 9)	24 mg per day	12 mg q12h**
Children (9–12)	20 mg per day	10 mg q12h
Adolescents (12–16)	18 mg per day	9 mg q12h
Adults	13 mg per day	6.5 mg q12h

*Use ideal body weight for obese patients.
**Some children under 9 may require 8 mg q8h.

TAO®
[tā′ō]
(troleandomycin)
Capsules and Oral Suspension

Description: TAO (troleandomycin) is a synthetically derived acetylated ester of oleandomycin, an antibiotic elaborated by a species of *Streptomyces antibioticus*. It is a white crystalline compound, insoluble in water, but readily soluble and stable in the presence of gastric juice. The compound has a molecular weight of 814 and corresponds to the empirical formula $C_{41}H_{67}NO_{15}$.

Actions: TAO is an antibiotic shown to be active *in vitro* against the following gram-positive organisms:
Streptococcus pyogenes
Diplococcus pneumoniae
Susceptibility plate testing: If the Kirby-Bauer method of disc sensitivity is used, a 15 mcg. oleandomycin disc should give a zone of over 18 mm. when tested against a troleandomycin sensitive bacterial strain.

Indications:
Diplococcus pneumoniae
 Pneumococcal pneumonia due to susceptible strains.
Streptococcus pyogenes
 Group A beta-hemolytic streptococcal infections of the upper respiratory tract.
Injectable benzathine penicillin G is considered by the American Heart Association to be the drug of choice in the treatment and prevention of streptococcal pharyngitis and in long term prophylaxis of rheumatic fever.
Troleandomycin is generally effective in the eradication of streptococci from the nasopharynx. However, substantial data establishing the efficacy of TAO in the subsequent prevention of rheumatic fever are not available at present.

Contraindications: Troleandomycin is contraindicated in patients with known hypersensitivity to this antibiotic.

Warnings: Usage in Pregnancy: Safety for use in pregnancy has not been established.
The administration of troleandomycin has been associated with an allergic type of cholestatic hepatitis. Some patients receiving troleandomycin for more than two weeks or in repeated courses have shown jaundice accompanied by right upper quadrant pain, fever, nausea, vomiting, eosinophilia, and leukocytosis. The changes have been reversible on discontinuance of the drug. Liver function tests should be monitored in patients on such dosage, and the drug discontinued if abnormalities develop. Reports in the literature have suggested that the concurrent use of ergotamine-containing drugs and troleandomycin may induce ischemic reactions. Therefore, the concurrent use of ergotamine-containing drugs and troleandomycin should be avoided. Troleandomycin should be administered with caution to patients concurrently receiving estrogen containing oral contraceptives.
Studies in chronic asthmatic patients have suggested that the concurrent use of theophylline and troleandomycin may result in elevated serum concentrations of theophylline. Therefore, it is recommended that patients receiving such concurrent therapy be observed for signs of theophylline toxicity, and that therapy be appropriately modified if such signs develop.

Precautions: Troleandomycin is principally excreted by the liver.
Caution should be exercised in administering the antibiotic to patients with impaired hepatic function.

Adverse Reactions: The most frequent side effects of troleandomycin preparations are gastrointestinal, such as abdominal cramping and discomfort, and are dose related. Nausea, vomiting, and diarrhea occur infrequently with usual oral doses. During prolonged or repeated therapy, there is a possibility of overgrowth of nonsusceptible bacteria or fungi. If such infections occur, the drug should be discontinued and appropriate therapy instituted.
Mild allergic reactions such as urticaria and other skin rashes have occurred. Serious allergic reactions, including anaphylaxis, have been reported.

Dosage and Administration: Clinical judgment based on the type of infection and its severity should determine dosage within the below listed ranges.
Adults: 250 to 500 mg. 4 times a day
Children: 125 to 250 mg. (3-5 mg./lb. or 6.6 to 11 mg./kg.) every 6 hours
When used in streptococcal infection, therapy should be continued for ten days.

How Supplied:
TAO is supplied as:
Capsules 250 mg.: Each capsule contains troleandomycin equivalent to 250 mg. of oleandomycin; bottle of 100 capsules.

69-1800-00-6
Shown in Product Identification Section, page 431

UROBIOTIC®-250
[u″rō-bī-ot′iks]

Each capsule contains
Oxytetracycline hydrochloride equivalent to 250 mg. oxytetracycline
Sulfamethizole ....250 mg.
Phenazopyridine hydrochloride ....50 mg.

CAPSULES

Actions: Urobiotic-250 is a product designed for use specifically in urinary tract infections. Terramycin (oxytetracycline HCl) is a widely used antibiotic with clinically proved activity against gram-positive and gram-negative bacteria, rickettsiae, spirochetes, large viruses, and certain protozoa. Terramycin is well tolerated and well absorbed after oral administration. It diffuses readily through the placenta and is present in the fetal circulation. It diffuses into the pleural fluid, and under some circumstances, into the cerebrospinal fluid. Oxytetracycline HCl appears to be concentrated in the hepatic system and is excreted in the bile. It is excreted in the urine and in the feces, in high concentrations, in a biologically active form.
Sulfamethizole is a chemotherapeutic agent active against a number of important gram-positive and gram-negative bacteria. This sulfonamide is well absorbed, has a low degree of acetylation, and is extremely soluble. Because of these features and its rapid renal excretion, sulfamethizole has a low order of toxicity and provides prompt and high concentrations of the active drug in the urinary tract.
Phenazopyridine is an orally absorbed agent which produces prompt and effective local analgesia and relief of urinary symptoms by virtue of its rapid excretion in the urinary tract. These effects are confined to the genitourinary system and are not accompanied by generalized sedation or narcosis.

Indications
Based on a review of this drug by the National Academy of Sciences-National Research Council and/or other information, FDA has classified the indications as follows:
"Lacking substantial evidence of effectiveness as a fixed combination":
Urobiotic-250 is indicated in the therapy of a number of genitourinary infections caused by susceptible organisms. These infections include the following: pyelonephritis, pyelitis, ureteritis, cystitis, prostatitis, and urethritis. Since both Terramycin and sulfamethizole provide effective levels in blood, tissue, and urine, Urobiotic-250 provides a multiple antimicrobial approach at the site of infection.

Both antibacterial components are active against the most common urinary pathogens, including *Escherichia coli, Pseudomonas aeruginosa, Aerobacter aerogenes, Streptococcus faecalis, Streptococcus hemolyticus,* and *Micrococcus pyogenes*. Urobiotic-250 is particularly useful in the treatment of infections caused by bacteria more sensitive to the combination than to either component alone. The combination is also of value in those cases with mixed infections, and in those instances where the causative organism is unknown pending laboratory isolation.

Final classification of the less than effective indications require further investigation. Clinical studies to substantiate the efficacy of Urobiotic-250 are ongoing. Completion of these ongoing studies will provide data for final classification of these indications.

Contraindications: This drug is contraindicated in individuals who have shown hypersensitivity to any of its components.

This drug, because of the sulfonamide component, should not be used in patients with a history of sulfonamide sensitivities, and in pregnant females at term.

Warnings: If renal impairment exists, even usual oral or parenteral doses may lead to excessive systemic accumulation of the drug and possible liver toxicity. Under such conditions, lower than usual doses are indicated and if therapy is prolonged, tetracycline serum level determinations may be advisable.

Oxytetracycline HCl, which is one of the ingredients of Urobiotic-250, may form a stable calcium complex in any bone-forming tissue with no serious harmful effects reported thus far in humans. However, use of oxytetracycline during tooth development (last trimester of pregnancy, neonatal period and early childhood) may cause discoloration of the teeth (yellow-grey-brownish). This effect occurs mostly during long term use of the drug but it also has been observed in usual short treatment courses.

Because of its sulfonamide content, this drug should be used only after critical appraisal in patients with liver damage, renal damage, urinary obstruction, or blood dyscrasias. Deaths have been reported from hypersensitivity reactions, agranulocytosis, aplastic anemia, and other blood dyscrasias associated with sulfonamide administration. When used intermittently, or for a prolonged period, blood counts and liver and kidney function tests should be performed.

Certain hypersensitive individuals may develop a photodynamic reaction precipitated by exposure to direct sunlight during the use of this drug. This reaction is usually of the photoallergic type which may also be produced by other tetracycline derivatives. Individuals with a history of photosensitivity reactions should be instructed to avoid exposure to direct sunlight while under treatment with this or other tetracycline drugs, and treatment should be discontinued at first evidence of skin discomfort.
NOTE: Reactions of a photoallergic nature are exceedingly rare with Terramycin (oxytetracycline HCl). Phototoxic reactions are not believed to occur with Terramycin.

Precautions: As with all antibiotic preparations, use of this drug may result in overgrowth of nonsusceptible organisms, including fungi. If superinfection occurs, the antibiotic should be discontinued and appropriate specific therapy should be instituted. This drug should be used with caution in persons having histories of significant allergies and/or asthma.

Adverse Reactions: Glossitis, stomatitis, proctitis, nausea, diarrhea, vaginitis, and dermatitis, as well as reactions of an allergic nature, may occur during oxytetracycline HCl therapy, but are rare. If adverse reactions, individual idiosyncrasy, or allergy occur, discontinue medication. Rare instances of esophagitis and esophageal ulcerations have been reported in patients receiving capsule forms of drugs in the tetracycline class. Most of these patients took medications immediately before going to bed. (See Dosage and Administration.)

With oxytetracycline therapy bulging fontanels in infants and benign intracranial hypertension in adults have been reported in individuals receiving full therapeutic dosages. These conditions disappeared rapidly when the drug was discontinued. As in all sulfonamide therapy, the following reactions may occur: nausea, vomiting, diarrhea, hepatitis, pancreatitis, blood dyscrasias, neuropathy, drug fever, skin rash, injection of the conjunctiva and sclera, petechiae, purpura, hematuria and crystalluria. The dosage should be decreased or the drug withdrawn, depending upon the severity of the reaction.

Dosage and Administration: Urobiotic-250 is recommended in adults only. A dose of 1 capsule four times daily is suggested. In refractory cases 2 capsules four times a day may be used.

Therapy should be continued for a minimum of seven days or until bacteriologic cure in acute urinary tract infections.

Administration of adequate amounts of fluid along with capsule forms of drugs in the tetracycline class is recommended to wash down the drugs and reduce the risk of esophageal irritation and ulceration. (See Adverse Reactions.)

To aid absorption of the drug, it should be given at least one hour before or two hours after eating. Aluminum hydroxide gel given with antibiotics has been shown to decrease their absorption and is contraindicated.

Supply: Urobiotic-250 capsules: bottles of 50, and unit dose packages of 100 (10 x 10's).
Literature Available: Yes.

23-1636-00-6
Shown in Product Identification Section, page 431

ROERIG EDUCATIONAL MATERIALS

Interactive Videodiscs
1. "Nephrostolithotomy—The Percutaneous Route" Free to physicians.
2. "Urodynamics in Clinical Practice" Free to physicians.

Audiotapes
"Dialogues in Urology." Free to physicians.

Samples
Antivert (meclizine HCl) Tablets—25 mg, 50 mg
Atarax (hydroxyzine HCl) Tablets—10 mg, 25 mg
Atarax Syrup
Geocillin (carbenicillin indanyl sodium) Tablets (equivalent to 382 mg carbenicillin)
Glucotrol (glipizide) Tablets—5 mg
Navane (thiothixene) Capsules—2 mg, 5 mg, 10 mg, 20 mg
Navane Oral Concentrate
Sinequan (doxepin HCl) Capsules—25 mg, 50 mg, 75 mg
Spectrobid (bacampicillin HCl) Tablets—400 mg (equivalent to 280 mg ampicillin)

William H. Rorer, Inc.
500 VIRGINIA DRIVE
FORT WASHINGTON, PA 19034

ASCRIPTIN® Tablets
(See PDR For Nonprescription Drugs)

ASCRIPTIN® A/D Tablets
(See PDR For Nonprescription Drugs)

ASCRIPTIN® WITH CODEINE ℞
[*a-scrip' tin*"]
for the relief of severe pain...
with the protection of Maalox®

Description—Tablets for Oral Use:
Ascriptin® with Codeine No. 2. Each white tablet contains aspirin 325 mg; codeine phosphate 15 mg and Maalox® (magnesium hydroxide and dried aluminum hydroxide) 150 mg.

Ascriptin® with Codeine No. 3. Each white tablet contains aspirin 325 mg; codeine phosphate 30 mg and Maalox® (magnesium hydroxide and dried aluminum hydroxide) 150 mg.

Ascriptin® with Codeine is an analgesic, antipyretic, and anti-inflammatory designed to give effective relief from severe pain with minimal aspirin-induced gastric distress.

Aspirin, a salicylate, occurs as a white odorless, crystalline powder which possesses a slightly bitter taste. Aspirin is an analgesic, anti-inflammatory and antipyretic.

Codeine is an alkaloid obtained from opium (or prepared from morphine by methylation) and occurs as colorless or white crystals. Codeine effloresces slowly in dry air and is affected by light. Codeine is an analgesic and an antitussive.

In addition, Maalox® is added to the formula to help reduce gastric distress caused by aspirin. Studies show that the addition of Maalox® has no effect on the bioavailability of the two active drugs.

Clinical Pharmacology: Aspirin alleviates pain both centrally and peripherally. Orally ingested salicylates are absorbed rapidly, partly from the stomach but mostly from the small intestine. Appreciable concentrations are found in plasma in less than 30 minutes; after a single dose, a peak value is reached in about 2 hours and then gradually declines. Rate of absorption is determined by many factors, particularly the disintegration and dissolution rates if tablets are given, the pH at the mucosal surfaces, and gastric emptying time.

In man, the absorption half-time for unbuffered aspirin is about 30 minutes, for buffered aspirin about 20 minutes, and for an aspirin solution only slightly less. What differences do exist probably have no therapeutic significance, since the rate-limiting factor in the onset of effects is accumulation of these drugs at their sites of action. The presence of food delays absorption of salicylates.

The biotransformation of aspirin takes place mainly in the liver and normally follows first-order kinetics. Salicylates are excreted mainly by the kidney. Codeine is a narcotic analgesic. Once absorbed, it is metabolized by the liver and excreted chiefly in the urine, largely in inactive forms. A small fraction (approximately 10%) of administered codeine is demethylated to form morphine, and both free and conjugated morphine can be found in the urine after therapeutic doses of codeine. Codeine has an exceptionally low affinity for the opioid receptor, and the analgesic effect of codeine may be due to its conversion to morphine. The half-life of codeine in plasma is 2.5 to 3 hours. Maalox® provides neutralization of gastric acid, thus increasing the likelihood of G.I. tolerance with the aspirin component.

Indications: Ascriptin® with Codeine No. 2 and Ascriptin® with Codeine No. 3 are indicated for the relief of pain of all degrees of severity up to that which requires morphine.

Contraindications: Hypersensitivity or allergy to aspirin or codeine.

Warnings: Usage in ambulatory patients. Ascriptin® with Codeine may impair the mental and/or physical abilities required for the performance of potentially hazardous tasks such as driving a car or operating machinery. The patient using this drug should be cautioned accordingly.
Interaction with other central nervous system depressants. Patients receiving other narcotic analgesics, general anesthetics, phenothiazines, tranquilizers, sedative-hynotics or other CNS depressants (including alcohol) concomitantly with Ascriptin® with Codeine may exhibit an additive CNS depression. When such combined therapy is contemplated, the dose of one or both agents should be reduced.

Continued on next page

This product information was prepared in August 1984. Information concerning these products may be obtained by addressing William H. Rorer, Inc., 500 Virginia Drive, Fort Washington, PA 19034.

Rorer—Cont.

Do not use if patient is taking a tetracycline antibiotic.

Precautions: Usage in pregnancy. PREGNANCY CATEGORY C—Animal reproduction studies have not been conducted with **Ascriptin® with Codeine**. It is also not known whether **Ascriptin® with Codeine** can cause fetal harm when administered to pregnant women or can affect reproduction capacity. **Ascriptin® with Codeine** should be given to a pregnant woman only if clearly needed. It is not known whether this drug is excreted in human milk. Because many drugs are excreted in human milk, caution should be exercised when **Ascriptin® with Codeine** is administered to nursing women.

Head injury and increased intracranial pressure: The respiratory depressant effects of narcotics and their capability to elevate cerebrospinal fluid pressure may be markedly exaggerated in the presence of head injury, other intracranial lesions or a pre-existing increase in intracranial pressure. Furthermore, narcotics produce adverse reactions which may obscure the clinical course of patients with head injuries.

Acute abdominal conditions: The administration of **Ascriptin® with Codeine** or other narcotics may obscure the diagnosis or clinical course in patients with acute abdominal conditions.

History of allergy: Patients who have a history of allergies may also be hypersensitive or intolerant to aspirin. A history of reaction to other chemicals, asthma or the occurrence of nasal polyps are warning signs. Epinephrine is the drug of choice to treat a reaction should one occur.

Special risk patients: Codeine should be given with caution to certain patients such as the elderly or debilitated and those with severe impairment of hepatic or renal function, hypothyroidism, Addison's disease, and prostatic hypertrophy or urethral stricture. Long-term animal studies to determine carcinogenicity of the ingredients in **Ascriptin® with Codeine** have not been carried out. Safety and effectiveness in children under 12 years of age, have not been established.

Adverse Reactions: The most frequently observed adverse reactions to codeine include lightheadedness, dizziness, sleepiness, nausea and vomiting. These effects seem to be more prominent in ambulatory than in nonambulatory patients, and some of these adverse reactions may be alleviated if the patient lies down.

Less frequent adverse reactions include euphoria, dysphoria, constipation and pruritus.

The most frequently observed reactions to aspirin include headache, vertigo, ringing in the ears, mental confusion, drowsiness, sweating, thirst, nausea, and vomiting. Occasionally, patients experience gastric irritation and bleeding with aspirin. Some patients are unable to take salicylates without developing nausea and vomiting. Hypersensitivity may be manifested by a skin rash or even an anaphylactic reaction. Most of the side effects of aspirin occur only after repeated administration of large doses.

Drug Abuse and Dependence: Codeine can produce drug dependence of the morphine type, and therefore, has the potential for being abused. Psychic dependence, physical dependence and tolerance may develop upon repeated administration of this drug and it should be prescribed and administered with the same degree of caution appropriate to the user of other oral narcotic-containing medications. Like other narcotic-containing medications, the drug is subject to the Federal Controlled Substances Act.

Management of Overdosage: Signs and Symptoms: Serious overdose with **Ascriptin® with Codeine** is characterized by respiratory depression (a decrease in respiratory rate and/or tidal volume, Cheyne-Stokes respiration, cyanosis), extreme somnolence progressing to stupor or coma, skeletal muscle flaccidity, cold and clammy skin, and sometimes bradycardia and hypotension. In severe overdosage, apnea, circulatory collapse, cardiac arrest and death may occur. The ingestion of very large amounts of this drug may, in addition, result in acute hepatic toxicity.

Treatment: Primary attention should be given to the reestablishment of adequate respiratory exchange through provision of a patent airway and the institution of assisted or controlled ventilation. The narcotic antagonist, naloxone, is a specific antidote against respiratory depression which may result from overdosage or unusual sensitivity to narcotics, including codeine. Therefore, an appropriate dose of naloxone (usual initial adult dose: 0.4 mg) should be administered, preferably by the intravenous route, and simultaneously with efforts at respiratory resuscitation. Since the duration of action of codeine may exceed that of the antagonist, the patient should be kept under continued surveillance and repeated doses of the antagonist should be administered as needed to maintain adequate respiration.

An antagonist should not be administered in the absence of clinically significant respiratory or cardiovascular depression.

Oxygen, intravenous fluids, vasopressors and other supportive measures should be employed as indicated.

Gastric emptying may be useful in removing unabsorbed drug.

Salicylate poisoning represents an acute medical emergency. The treatment is largely symptomatic. From 10 to 30 g of aspirin has caused death in adults, but much larger amounts (130 g of aspirin, in one case) have been ingested without fatal outcome.

Initial therapy must be directed to correction of hyperthermia, dehydration and maintenance of adequate renal function. Intravenous fluids should be administered promptly, the type and amount based on interpretation of laboratory data on acid-base balance.

Measures to rid the body rapidly of salicylate should be immediately undertaken. Sodium bicarbonate administration is effective and rapid, if an alkaline urine can be produced. Forced diuresis with alkalinizing solution appears to be better than alkali alone; acetazolamide can be added to this combination if a more rapid effect is necessary and only if systemic acidosis is avoided. Potassium should be administered with the bicarbonate to prevent further depletion of intracellular potassium.

In severe intoxication, extrarenal measures such as exchange transfusion, peritoneal dialysis, hemodialysis, and hemoperfusion are the most effective measures available for the removal of salicylate. Hemodialysis in adults and older children and exchange transfusion or peritoneal dialysis in infants should be considered seriously in all salicylate-intoxicated patients whose clinical condition is deteriorating despite otherwise appropriate therapy and in those who have associated serious disease.

Dosage and Administration: Dosage should be adjusted according to the severity of the pain and the response of the patient. It may occasionally be necessary to exceed the usual dosage recommended below in cases of more severe pain or in those patients who have become tolerant to the analgesic effect of narcotics.

Ascriptin® with Codeine is given orally.

Usual Adult Dose: Ascriptin® with Codeine No. 2—two tablets every 3 to 4 hours when necessary. **Ascriptin® with Codeine No. 3**—one or two tablets every 3 to 4 hours as necessary.

Drug Interactions: The CNS depressant effect of **Ascriptin® with Codeine** may be additive with that of other CNS depressants. See WARNINGS. Keep this and all drugs out of the reach of children. In case of accidental overdose, seek professional assistance or contact a poison control center immediately.

Ascriptin® with Codeine No. 2: (Aspirin 325 mg, Maalox® 150 mg, codeine phosphate 15 mg) is available in bottles of 100 tablets. Tablets are marked on one side with the name Rorer and the Identification Number 142; the other side displays the number 2. (NDC 0067-0142-68)

Ascriptin® with Codeine No. 3: (Aspirin 325 mg, Maalox® 150 mg, codeine phosphate 30 mg) in bottles of 100 tablets. Tablets are marked on one side with the name Rorer and the Identification Number 143; the other side displays the number 3. (NDC 0067-0143-68)

DEA number required.

Shown in Product Identification Section, page 431

AZMACORT™ ℞
[ăz'ma-kort]
(triamcinolone acetonide)
inhaler

For Oral Inhalation Only

Description: Azmacort™ (triamcinolone acetonide) is an anti-inflammatory steroid having the chemical name 9α-fluoro-11β, 21-dihydroxy-16α, 17α-isopropylidenedioxy-1, 4-pregnadiene-3, 20-dione ($C_{24}H_{31}FO_6$).

Azmacort™ inhaler is a metered-dose aerosol unit containing a microcrystalline suspension of triamcinolone acetonide in the propellant dichlorodifluoromethane and dehydrated alcohol USP 1% w/w. Each canister contains 60 mg triamcinolone acetonide. Each actuation releases approximately 200 mcg triamcinolone acetonide, of which approximately 100 mcg are delivered from the unit (*in vitro* testing). There are at least 240 oral inhalations in one Azmacort™ inhaler canister. The device should not be used after 240 inhalations, since the amount delivered thereafter per actuation may be less than consistent.

Clinical Pharmacology: The precise mechanism of the action of the inhaled drug is unknown. However, use of the inhaler makes it possible to provide effective local steroid activity with minimal systemic effect.

Triamcinolone acetonide is a very potent derivative of triamcinolone. Although triamcinolone itself is 1–2 times as potent as prednisone in animal models of inflammation, triamcinolone acetonide is much more potent.

Pharmacokinetic studies with radiolabeled triamcinolone acetonide have been carried out by the oral route and intravenous route in several species. The pharmacokinetic behavior of the triamcinolone acetonide was similar in all species within each route of administration. The major portion of the dose was eliminated in the feces irrespective of route of administration with only one species (rabbit) showing significant urinary excretion of radioactivity.

The results of studies in which triamcinolone acetonide was administered as an aerosol showed rapid disappearance of radioactivity from the lungs comparable to that observed following oral administration with peak blood levels occurring in one to two hours. Virtually no radioactivity was present in the lung and trachea 24 hours after dosing.

Three metabolites of triamcinolone acetonide have been identified. They are: 6β-hydroxy-triamcinolone acetonide, 21-carboxy-triamcinolone acetonide, and 21-carboxy-6β-hydroxytriamcinolone acetonide. There appeared to be some quantitative differences in the metabolites among species. No differences were detected in metabolic pattern related to route of administration.

Indications: Azmacort™ (triamcinolone acetonide) inhaler is indicated only for patients who require chronic treatment with corticosteroids for the control of the symptoms of bronchial asthma. Such patients would include those already receiving systemic corticosteroids and selected patients who are inadequately controlled on a non-steroid regimen and in whom steroid therapy has been withheld because of concern over potential adverse effects.

Azmacort™ inhaler is *NOT* indicated:
1. For relief of asthma which can be controlled by bronchodilators and other non-steroid medications.
2. In patients who require systemic corticosteroid treatment infrequently.
3. In the treatment of non-asthmatic bronchitis.

Contraindications: **Azmacort™** inhaler is contraindicated in the primary treatment of status asthmaticus or other acute episodes of asthma where intensive measures are required.

Hypersensitivity to any of the ingredients of this preparation contraindicates its use.

Warnings:
Particular care is needed in patients who are transferred from systemically active corticosteroids to **Azmacort™** inhaler because deaths due to adrenal insufficiency have occurred in asthmatic patients during and after transfer from systemic corticosteroids to aerosolized steroids in recommended doses. After withdrawal from systemic corticosteroids, a number of months is usually required for recovery of hypothalamic-pituitary-adrenal (HPA) function. For some patients who have received large doses of oral steroids for long periods of time before therapy with **Azmacort™** inhaler is initiated, recovery may be delayed for one year or longer. During this period of HPA suppression, patients may exhibit signs and symptoms of adrenal insufficiency when exposed to trauma, surgery or infections, particularly gastroenteritis or other conditions with acute electrolyte loss. Although **Azmacort™** inhaler may provide control of asthmatic symptoms during these episodes, in recommended doses it supplies only normal physiological amounts of corticosteroid systemically and does NOT provide the increased systemic steroid which is necessary for coping with these emergencies.

During periods of stress or a severe asthmatic attack, patients who have been recently withdrawn from systemic corticosteroids should be instructed to resume systemic steroids (in large doses) immediately and to contact their physician for further instruction. These patients should also be instructed to carry a warning card indicating that they may need supplementary systemic steroids during periods of stress or a severe asthma attack.

Localized infections with *Candida albicans* have occurred infrequently in the mouth and pharynx. These areas should be examined by the treating physician at each patient visit. The percentage of positive mouth and throat cultures for *Candida albicans* did not change during a year of continuous therapy. The incidence of clinically apparent infection is low (2.5%). These infections may disappear spontaneously or may require treatment with appropriate antifungal therapy or discontinuance of treatment with **Azmacort™** inhaler.

Azmacort™ inhaler is not to be regarded as a bronchodilator and is not indicated for rapid relief of bronchospasm.

Patients should be instructed to contact their physician immediately when episodes of asthma which are not responsive to bronchodilators occur during the course of treatment with **Azmacort™** inhaler. During such episodes, patients may require therapy with systemic corticosteroids.

There is no evidence that control of asthma can be achieved by the administration of **Azmacort™** inhaler in amounts greater than the recommended doses, which appear to be the therapeutic equivalent of approximately 10 mg/day of oral prednisone.

Theoretically, the use of inhaled corticosteroids with alternate day prednisone oral therapy should be accompanied by more HPA suppression than a therapeutically equivalent regimen of either alone.

Transfer of patients from systemic steroid therapy to **Azmacort™** inhaler may unmask allergic conditions previously suppressed by the systemic steroid therapy, e.g., rhinitis, conjunctivitis, and eczema.

Precautions: During withdrawal from oral steroids, some patients may experience symptoms of systemically active steroid withdrawal, e.g., joint and/or muscular pain, lassitude and depression, despite maintenance or even improvement of respiratory function (See DOSAGE AND ADMINISTRATION for details). Although steroid withdrawal effects are usually transient and not severe, severe and even fatal exacerbation of asthma can occur if the previous daily oral corticosteroid requirement had significantly exceeded 10 mg/day of prednisone or equivalent.

In responsive patients, inhaled corticosteroids will often permit control of asthmatic symptoms with less suppression of HPA function than therapeutically equivalent oral doses of prednisone. Since triamcinolone acetonide is absorbed into the circulation and can be systemically active, the beneficial effects of **Azmacort™** inhaler in minimizing or preventing HPA dysfunction may be expected only when recommended dosages are not exceeded.

Suppression of HPA function has been reported in volunteers who received 4000 mcg daily of triamcinolone acetonide. In addition, suppression of HPA function has been reported in some patients who have received recommended doses for as little as 6–12 weeks. Since the response of HPA function to inhaled corticosteroids is highly individualized, the physician should consider this information when treating patients.

Because of the possibility of systemic absorption of inhaled corticosteroids, patients treated with these drugs should be observed carefully for any evidence of systemic corticosteroid effects including suppression of growth in children. Particular care should be taken in observing patients postoperatively or during periods of stress for evidence of a decrease in adrenal function.

The long-term effects of triamcinolone acetonide inhaler in human subjects are not completely known, although patients have received **Azmacort™** inhaler on a continuous basis for periods of two years or longer. While there has been no clinical evidence of adverse experiences, the local effects of the agent on developmental or immunologic processes in the mouth, pharynx, trachea and lung are also unknown.

The potential effects of **Azmacort™** inhaler on acute, recurrent, or chronic pulmonary infections, including active or quiescent tuberculosis, are not known. For this reason, since systemic administration of corticosteroids may mask some signs of fungal, bacterial, or viral infection, the same caution should be observed when treating patients with **Azmacort™** inhaler. The potential effects of long-term administration of **Azmacort™** inhaler on lung or other tissues are unknown. However, pulmonary infiltrates with eosinophilia have occurred in patients receiving other inhaled corticosteroids.

Pregnancy: Pregnancy Category D. **Azmacort™** (triamcinolone acetonide) has been shown to be teratogenic in rats and rabbits when given in doses comparable to the highest dose recommended for human use (approximately 0.032 mg/kg/day). Administration of aerosol inhalation to pregnant rats and rabbits produced embryotoxic and fetotoxic effects which were comparable to those produced by administraton by other routes.

Teratogenic effects in both species included a low incidence of cleft palate and/or internal hydrocephaly and axial skeletal defects. These findings represent known effects of glucocorticoids in laboratory animals.

There are no well-controlled studies in pregnant women. Experience with other dosage forms of triamcinolone acetonide does not include any positive evidence of adverse effects on the fetus. However, since such experience cannot exclude possibility of fetal damage, **Azmacort™** inhaler should be used during pregnancy only if the benefit clearly justifies the potential risk to the fetus. Infants born to mothers who have received substantial doses of corticosteroids during pregnancy should be carefully observed for hypoadrenalism.

Nursing mothers: It is not known whether this drug is excreted in human milk. Because of the potential for tumorigenicity shown for triamcinolone acetonide in animal studies, a decision should be made whether to discontinue nursing or to discontinue the drug, taking into account the importance of the drug to the mother.

Adverse Reactions: A few cases of oral candidiasis have been reported (see WARNINGS). In addition, some patients receiving **Azmacort™** inhaler have experienced hoarseness, dry throat, irritated throat and dry mouth. Increased wheezing and cough have been reported infrequently as has facial edema. These adverse effects have generally been mild and transient.

Dosage and Administration: All patients should be instructed that the **Azmacort™** inhaler must be used on a regular basis rather than prn. Reliable dosage delivery cannot be assured after 240 actuations and patients should be cautioned against longer use of individual cannisters.

Good oral hygiene including rinsing of the mouth after inhalation is recommended.

Adults: The usual dosage is two inhalations (approximately 200 mcg) given three to four times a day. The maximal daily intake should not exceed 16 inhalations (1600 mcg) in adults. Higher initial doses (12–16 inhalations per day) may be advisable in patients with more severe asthma, the dosage then being adjusted downward according to the response of the patient. In some patients maintenance can be accomplished when the total daily dose is given on a twice a day schedule.

Children 6 to 12 years of age: The usual dosage is one or two inhalations (100 to 200 mcg) given three to four times a day according to the response of the patient. The maximal daily intake should not exceed 12 inhalations (1200 mcg) in children 6 to 12 years of age. Insufficient clinical data exist with respect to the administration of **Azmacort™** inhaler in children below the age of 6. The long term effects of inhaled steroids on growth are still under evaluation.

Patients receiving bronchodilators by inhalation should be advised to use the bronchodilator before **Azmacort™** inhaler in order to enhance penetration of triamcinolone acetonide into the bronchial tree. After use of an aerosol bronchodilator, several minutes should elapse before use of the **Azmacort™** inhaler to reduce the potential toxicity from the inhaled fluorocarbon propellants in the two aerosols.

Different considerations must be given to the following groups of patients in order to obtain the full therapeutic benefit of **Azmacort™** inhaler:

Patients not receiving systemic steroids: The use of **Azmacort™** inhaler is straightforward in patients who are inadequately controlled with non-steroid medications but in whom systemic steroid therapy has been withheld because of concern over potential adverse reactions. In patients who respond to **Azmacort™**, an improvement in pulmonary functon is usually apparent within one to two weeks after the start of **Azmacort™** inhaler.

Patients receiving systemic steroids: In those patients dependent on systemic steroids, transfer to **Azmacort™** inhaler and subsequent management may be more difficult because recovery from impaired adrenal function is usually slow. Such suppression has been known to last for up to 12 months or longer. Clinical studies, however, have demonstrated that **Azmacort™** inhaler may be effective in the management of these asthmatic patients and may permit replacement or signifi-

Continued on next page

This product information was prepared in August 1984. Information concerning these products may be obtained by addressing William H. Rorer, Inc., 500 Virginia Drive, Fort Washington, PA 19034.

Rorer—Cont.

cant reduction in the dosage of systemic corticosteroids.

The patient's asthma should be reasonably stable before treatment with **Azmacort**™ inhaler is started. Initially the inhaler should be used concurrently with the patient's usual maintenance dose of systemic steroid. After approximately one week, gradual withdrawal of the systemic steroid is started by reducing the dose. The next reduction is made after an interval of one or two weeks, depending on the response of the patient. Generally, these decrements should not exceed 2.5 mg of prednisone or its equivalent. A slow rate of withdrawal cannot be overemphasized. During withdrawal, some patients may experience symptoms of systemically active steroid withdrawal, e.g., joint and/or muscular pain, lassitude and depression, despite maintenance or even improvement of respiratory function. Such patients should be encouraged to continue with the inhaler but should be watched carefully for objective signs of adrenal insufficiency, such as hypotension and weight loss. If evidence of adrenal insufficiency occurs, the systemic steroid dose should be boosted temporarily and thereafter further withdrawal should continue more slowly. No clinical studies have been conducted evaluating **Azmacort**™ with alternate day prednisone regimens. However, based on the results of such a study with another inhaled corticosteroid, inhaled corticosteroids generally are not recommended for chronic use with alternate day prednisone regimens (see warnings).

During periods of stress or a severe asthma attack, transfer patients will require supplementary treatment with systemic steroids. Exacerbations of asthma which occur during the course of treatment with **Azmacort**™ inhaler should be treated with a short course of systemic steroid which is gradually tapered as these symptoms subside. There is no evidence that control of asthma can be achieved by administration of **Azmacort**™ inhaler in amounts greater than the recommended doses.

Directions for Use: An illustrated leaflet of patient instructions for proper use accompanies each package of **Azmacort**™ inhaler.

Contents Under Pressure: Do not puncture. Do not use or store near heat or open flame. Exposure to temperatures above 120°F may cause bursting. Never throw container into fire or incinerator. Keep out of reach of children.

How Supplied: **Azmacort**™ inhaler contains 60 mg triamcinolone acetonide in a 20 gram package which delivers at least 240 oral inhalations. It is supplied with an oral adapter and patient's leaflet of instructions: box of one.

NDC 0067-0060-37

Caution: Federal law prohibits dispensing without prescription.

Shown in Product Identification Section, page 431

CALCIFEROL™ ℞
[kal-si'fur-ol]
(Ergocalciferol, Vitamin D₂)
50,000 USP Unit Tablets
500,000 USP Units/cc in Oil
8,000 USP Units/cc in Propylene Glycol

Description: CALCIFEROL™, also known as ergocalciferol or Vitamin D₂ is a Vitamin D analog. It occurs as white crystals and is insoluble in water and soluble in alcohol and in fatty oils. CALCIFEROL Tablets contain 1.25 mg (50,000 USP units) of Ergocalciferol (Vitamin D₂). CALCIFEROL In Oil Injection is a sterile solution of Vitamin D₂ in sesame oil for intramuscular use only. Each cc of CALCIFEROL In Oil contains 500,000 USP units of Ergocalciferol. CALCIFEROL Drops, oral solution, contains 8,000 USP units of Vitamin D₂ in Propylene Glycol, per ml (200 USP units per drop).

Pharmacology: CALCIFEROL in its activated form (1,25-dihydroxy ergocalciferol) along with parathyroid hormone and calcitonin, regulates calcium metabolism. Vitamin D deficiency leads to rickets in children and osteomalacia in adults. The administration of Vitamin D completely reverses the symptoms of nutritional rickets or osteomalacia unless permanent deformities have already occurred. In humans, activated CALCIFEROL functions primarily to increase intestinal absorption of calcium and phosphorus. It is also required for normal mineralization of bone and stimulates resorption of bone matrix.

CALCIFEROL is readily absorbed from the gastrointestinal tract if fat absorption is normal. The presence of bile is necessary for absorption of Vitamin D and its analogs. In patients with hepatic, biliary, or GI disease, the absorption of Vitamin D may decrease. Once absorbed, ergocalciferol appears in chylomicrons of lymph and then associates primarily with a specific alphaglobulin and with albumin. The plasma half-life of ergocalciferol is approximately 24 hours. Ergocalciferol is stored in the liver, fat, and muscle for prolonged periods.

Indications and Uses: CALCIFEROL is indicated for use in the treatment of hypoparathyroidism and refractory rickets. CALCIFEROL is used to increase serum calcium concentration to prevent or treat rickets or osteomalacia. Patients with gastrointestinal, liver or biliary disease associated with malabsorption of Vitamin D require intramuscular administration of Vitamin D.

Contraindications: CALCIFEROL should not be given to patients with hypercalcemia or evidence of Vitamin D toxicity.

Warning: Overdosage of any form of Vitamin D is dangerous. Progressive hypercalcemia due to overdosage of Vitamin D and its metabolites may be so severe as to require emergency attention. Chronic hypercalcemia can lead to generalized vascular calcification, nephrocalcinosis and other soft tissue calcification. Radiographic evaluation of suspect anatomical regions may be useful in the early detection of this condition.

Precautions: Treatment of patients with coronary disease, impaired renal function, and arteriosclerosis, especially in the elderly, should be cautious.

Large doses of Vitamin D are potentially dangerous; therefore, early in treatment or during dosage adjustment, serum calcium should be determined twice weekly. Similarly, phosphate, magnesium, and alkaline phosphatase and 24 hour urinary calcium and phosphate should be determined periodically. A fall in serum alkaline phosphatase levels usually precedes the appearance of hypercalcemia and may be an indication of impending hypercalcemia. Should hypercalcemia develop, the drug should be discontinued immediately.

Adverse Reactions: Excessive Vitamin D intake can produce vitamin toxicity. The early and late signs and symptoms of Vitamin D intoxication associated with hypercalcemia may include weakness and headache, vomiting, muscle pain, bone pain, anorexia, weight loss, hypertension, and cardiac arrhythmias.

Drug Abuse and Dependence: The information on drug abuse and dependence is limited to an existent literature survey and marketing experience. Such experience has revealed no evidence of drug abuse and dependence associated with use of CALCIFEROL.

Overdosage: Use of CALCIFEROL in excessive quantities in patients can cause hypercalcemia, hypercalciuria and hyperphosphatemia. High intake of calcium and phosphate concomitant with CALCIFEROL can lead to similar abnormalities. Treatment of Vitamin D intoxication consists of withdrawal of the drug and calcium supplements, administration of low-calcium diet, oral or parenteral fluids, and if needed, glucocorticoids or other drugs to decrease serum calcium levels. When serum calcium levels have returned to within normal limits, CALCIFEROL therapy may be reinstituted at a dose lower than prior therapy. Serum calcium levels should be determined at least twice weekly after all dosage changes and subsequent dosage titration. Persistent or markedly elevated serum calcium levels may be corrected by dialysis against a calcium free dialysate.

Dosage and Administration: The optimal daily dose of CALCIFEROL must be carefully determined for each patient. Patients with refractory rickets may need 50,000 to 500,000 units per day. After oral therapy with CALCIFEROL is instituted, normal serum calcium and phosphate levels may be observed within 2 weeks. Roentgenographic evidence of healing of bone may be seen within 4 weeks after administration of a fixed maintenance dose. During therapy with CALCIFEROL, the dosage must be individualized and carefully adjusted to avoid hypercalcemia. Determinations of serum calcium, phosphate, alkaline phosphatase, total protein, creatine and BUN should be made every two weeks or more frequently as needed. Until the condition stabilizes, monthly radiographic evaluation is helpful. In treatment of hypoparathyroidism, 50,000 to 400,000 units per day are recommended. In recommending CALCIFEROL, it is assumed that each patient is receiving an adequate daily intake of calcium. The recommended daily allowance for calcium in adults is 1 gram.

How Supplied: 50,000 USP unit tablets, bottles of 100 (NDC 0091-3150-01).
CALCIFEROL in Oil Injection is supplied in 1cc ampuls containing 500,000 USP units per cc in oil. Packaged in boxes of 5 (NDC 0091-1150-05).
CALCIFEROL Drops, oral solution, contains 8,000 USP units/ml in 60 ml bottle (NDC 0091-4150-60).

Shown in Product Identification Section, page 431

CAMALOX® Suspension and Tablets
(See PDR For Nonprescription Drugs)

CHARDONNA®-2 ℞
[char'dona]
brand of belladonna extract with phenobarbital

REFORMULATED WITHOUT CHARCOAL

Description: Each Chardonna-2 tablet contains: phenobarbital 15 mg (WARNING: may be habit forming) and belladonna extract 15 mg.

Actions: Chardonna-2 tablets produce antispasmodic, antisecretory and sedative effects. Belladonna acts to inhibit gastric secretion and gastrointestinal motility. The sedative action of phenobarbital allays anxiety accompanying functional gastrointestinal disorders.

> **Indications:** Based on a review of similar drugs by the National Academy of Sciences-National Research Council and/or other information, FDA has classified the indications as follows:
> "Possibly effective" as adjunctive therapy in the treatment of peptic ulcer and "possibly effective" in the treatment of irritable bowel syndrome (irritable colon, spastic colon, mucous colitis) and acute enterocolitis.
> Final classification of less-than-effective indications requires further investigation.

Contraindications: Chardonna-2 is contraindicated in persons with a known intolerance to any of the ingredients, a history of porphyria or marked impairment of hepatic or renal function, respiratory disease in the presence of dyspnea or obstruction, glaucoma or obstructive uropathy.

Precautions: Use with caution in patients with increased intraocular pressure, prostatic hypertrophy or moderate hepatic or renal disease. Barbiturates are known to stimulate hepatic microsomal enzymes and alter metabolism of certain drugs. Therefore, Chardonna-2 should be used with caution in patients on anticoagulant or corticosteroid therapy. Elderly or debilitated persons may react to barbiturates with marked excitement or depression. Patients should also be warned about the combined effects of central nervous system depressant drugs and alcohol.

Adverse Reactions: Blurred vision, dry mouth, vertigo, tachycardia, urinary retention, flushing

or dryness of the skin, drowsiness, lethargy, headache, skin eruptions, nausea and vomiting.
Adult Dosage: Usually given one-half hour before meals and at bedtime. One or two tablets, q.i.d.
Warning: Keep this and all drugs out of the reach of children. In case of accidental overdose, seek professional assistance or contact a poison control center immediately.
Supplied: Bottles of 100 (NDC 0067-0202-68).
Shown in Product Identification Section, page 431

EMETROL® Solution

(See PDR For Nonprescription Drugs)

FEDAHIST® GYROCAPS®, SYRUP TABLETS, EXPECTORANT
[*fed'a-hist*]

Description: Fedahist® is a combination of pseudoephedrine hydrochloride (1-phenyl-2 methylaminopropan-1-ol hydrochloride) and chlorpheniramine maleate (2-[p-chloro-a(2-dimethylaminoethyl) benzyl] pyridine maleate 1:1) as an oral antihistamine-decongestant.

FEDAHIST® GYROCAPS® (timed release capsules) ℞

Each white and yellow capsule contains:
Pseudoephedrine Hydrochloride ....65 mg
Chlorpheniramine Maleate ....10 mg
in a special base that provides for a prolonged, therapeutic effect.

FEDAHIST® EXPECTORANT (NONALCOHOLIC)

Each 5 ml (teaspoonful) contains:
Guaifenesin ....100 mg
Pseudoephedrine Hydrochloride ....30 mg
Chlorpheniramine Maleate ....2 mg
in pleasant-tasting, cherry-flavored syrup.

FEDAHIST® TABLETS (SCORED, DYE-FREE)

Each tablet contains:
Pseudoephedrine Hydrochloride ....60 mg
Chlorpheniramine Maleate ....4 mg

FEDAHIST® SYRUP (NONALCOHOLIC)

Each 5 ml (teaspoonful) contains:
Pseudoephedrine Hydrochloride ....30 mg
Chlorpheniramine Maleate ....2 mg
in pleasant-tasting, grape-flavored syrup.

Clinical Pharmacology: Fedahist® provides the antihistaminic activity of chlorpheniramine maleate with the vasoconstrictive actions of pseudoephedrine hydrochloride.
At the recommended oral dosage, pseudoephedrine has little or no pressor effects in normotensive adults, and is not known to produce drowsiness. Chlorpheniramine is an antihistamine which acts on H_1 receptors as an antagonist. It is well absorbed and has a duration of 4 to 6 hours. (The Gyrocaps® formulation provides for a longer therapeutic effect up to 12 hours.) Plasma half-life is approximately 22 hours. Degradation products of chlorpheniramine's metabolic transformation by the liver are almost completely excreted in 24 hours via the kidney. The alkylamines, of which chlorpheniramine is the prototype, are among the most potent H_1 blockers. Although not so prone as others to cause drowsiness, a significant proportion of patients do experience this effect. CNS stimulation is more common in chlorpheniramine than in other groups of H_1 blockers.
Pseudoephedrine is a sympathomimetic amine with peripheral effects similar to epinephrine and central effects similar to, but less intense than, amphetamines. Therefore, it has the potential for excitatory side effects. Pseudoephedrine at the recommended oral dosage has little or no pressor effect in normotensive adults.
Pseudoephedrine is an orally effective nasal decongestant. Patients taking pseudoephedrine orally have not been reported to experience the rebound congestion sometimes experienced with frequent repeated use of topical decongestants.
Indications and Usage: Fedahist® is indicated for the symptomatic relief of seasonal and perennial allergic rhinitis, and eustachian tube congestion.

Contraindications:
Use in Newborn or Premature Infants: This drug should not be used in newborn or premature infants.
Antihistamines are contraindicated in the following conditions: hypersensitivity to chlorpheniramine maleate and other antihistamines of similar chemical structure; monoamine oxidase inhibitor therapy (see Drug Interactions Section).
Fedahist® is also contraindicated in patients with hypersensitivity or idiosyncrasy to sympathomimetic amines. Sympathomimetic amines are contraindicated in patients with severe hypertension, severe coronary artery disease, and in patients on MAO inhibitor therapy. Patient idiosyncrasy to adrenergic agents may be manifested by insomnia, dizziness, weakness, tremor or arrhythmias.
Warnings: Antihistamines should be used with considerable caution in patients with: narrow angle glaucoma; stenosing peptic ulcer; pyloroduodenal obstruction; symptomatic prostatic hypertrophy; bladder neck obstruction.
Use in Children: In infants and children especially, antihistamines in **overdosage** may cause hallucinations, convulsions or death.
As in adults, antihistamines may diminish mental alertness in children. In the young child particularly, they may produce excitation.
Use with CNS Depressants: Chlorpheniramine maleate has additive effects with alcohol and other CNS depressants (hypnotics, sedatives, tranquilizers, etc.).
Use in Activities Requiring Mental Alertness: Patients should be warned about engaging in activities requiring mental alertness, such as driving a car or operating appliances, machinery, etc.
Use in the Elderly (approximately 60 years or older): Antihistamines are more likely to cause dizziness, sedation, hypotension in elderly patients.
The elderly are more likely to have adverse reactions to sympathomimetics. Overdosage of sympathomimetics in this age group may cause hallucinations, convulsions, CNS depression, and death. Therefore, safe use of a short-acting sympathomimetic should be demonstrated in the individual elderly patient before considering the use of a sustained-action formulation.
Sympathomimetic amines should be used judiciously and sparingly in patients with hypertension, diabetes mellitus, ischemic heart disease, increased intraocular pressure, hyperthyroidism, and prostatic hypertrophy. Sympathomimetics may produce central nervous system stimulation with convulsions or cardiovascular collapse with accompanying hypotension.
Do not exceed recommended dosage.
Precautions:
General: Chlorpheniramine maleate has an atropine-like action and therefore should be used with caution in patients with: a history of bronchial asthma, increased intraocular pressure, hyperthyroidism, cardiovascular disease and hypertension.
Pseudoephedrine should be used with caution in patients with diabetes, hypertension, cardiovascular disease and hyper-reactivity to ephedrine.
Drug Interactions: MAO inhibitors prolong and intensify the anticholinergic (drying) effects of antihistamines. MAO inhibitors and beta adrenergic blockers increase the effects of pseudoephedrine (sympathomimetics).
Sympathomimetics may reduce the antihypertensive effects of methyldopa, mecamylamine, reserpine and veratrum alkaloids.
Carcinogenicity: Studies show that the ingredients in Fedahist® have no carcinogenic effects on animals or humans.
Use in Pregnancy: The safety of the ingredients in Fedahist® for use during pregnancy has not been established.
Pregnancy Category C: Animal reproduction studies have not been conducted with Fedahist®. It is also not known whether Fedahist® can cause fetal harm when administered to a pregnant woman or can affect reproduction capacity.
There have been no reports that pseudoephedrine increases the risk of fetal abnormalities if administered during pregnancy. If this drug is used during pregnancy, the possibility of fetal harm appears remote. Because studies cannot rule out the possibility of harm, however, Fedahist® should be used during pregnancy only if clearly needed.
Nonteratogenic Effects
Nursing Mothers: Because of the potential for serious adverse reactions in nursing infants from Fedahist® a decision should be made whether to discontinue nursing or to discontinue the drug, taking into account the importance of the drug to the mother.
Adverse Reactions: Slight to moderate drowsiness occurs relatively infrequently with chlorpheniramine maleate. Other possible side effects common to antihistamines in general include:
General: Urticaria, drug rash, anaphylactic shock, photosensitivity, excessive perspiration, chills, dryness of mouth, nose, and throat.
Cardiovascular System: hypotension, headache, palpitations, tachycardia, extrasystoles.
Hematologic System: hemolytic anemia, thrombocytopenia, agranulocytosis.
Nervous System: sedation, dizziness, disturbed coordination, fatigue, confusion, restlessness, excitation, nervousness, tremor, irritability, insomnia, euphoria, paresthesias, blurred vision, diplopia, vertigo, tinnitus, acute labyrinthitis, hysteria, neuritis, convulsions.
Gastrointestinal System: epigastric distress, anorexia, nausea, vomiting, diarrhea, constipation.
Genitourinary System: urinary frequency, difficult urination, urinary retention, early menses.
Respiratory System: thickening of bronchial secretions, tightness of chest and wheezing, nasal stuffiness.
Individuals hyper-reactive to pseudoephedrine may display reactions such as tachycardia, palpitations, headache, dizziness or nausea. Sympathomimetic drugs have been associated with certain untoward reactions including fear, anxiety, tenseness, restlessness, tremor, weakness, pallor, respiratory difficulty, dysuria, insomnia, hallucinations, convulsions, CNS depression, arrhythmias, and cardiovascular collapse with hypotension.
Overdosage: In the event of overdosage, emergency treatment should be started immediately. Manifestations of antihistamine overdosage may vary from central nervous system depression (sedation, apnea, cardiovascular collapse) to stimulation (insomnia, hallucinations, tremors or convulsions). Other signs and symptoms may be dizziness, tinnitus, ataxia, blurred vision and hypotension. Stimulation is particularly likely in children, as are atropine-like signs and symptoms (dry mouth; fixed, dilated pupils; flushing, hyperthermia and gastrointestinal symptoms).
Treatment: The patient should be induced to vomit, even if emesis has occurred spontaneously. Pharmacologic vomiting by the administration of ipecac syrup is a preferred method. However, vomiting should not be induced in patients with impaired consciousness. The action of ipecac is facilitated by physical activity and by the administration of eight to twelve fluid ounces of water. If emesis does not occur within fifteen minutes, the dose of ipecac should be repeated. Precautions against aspiration must be taken, especially in infants and children. Following emesis, any drug remaining in the stomach may be absorbed by activated charcoal administered as a slurry with water. If vomiting is unsuccessful, or contraindicated, gastric lavage should be performed. Isotonic and one-half isotonic saline are the lavage solutions of choice. Saline cathartics, such as milk of magnesia, draw water into the bowel by osmosis and, therefore, may be valuable for their action in rapid dilution of bowel content. After emergency treatment the patient should continue to be medically moni-

Continued on next page

This product information was prepared in August 1984. Information concerning these products may be obtained by addressing William H. Rorer, Inc., 500 Virginia Drive, Fort Washington, PA 19034.

Rorer—Cont.

tored. Treatment of the signs and symptoms of overdosage is symptomatic and supportive.
Stimulants (analeptic agents) should not be used. Vasopressors may be used to treat hypotension. Short-acting barbiturates, diazepam or paraldehyde may be administered to control seizures. Hyperpyrexia, especially in children, may require treatment with tepid water sponge baths or a hypothermic blanket. Apnea is treated with ventilatory support.

Dosage and Administration:
FEDAHIST® GYROCAPS® (Timed Release Capsules)
Dosage: Adults and children 12 years and older: one capsule twice a day. Not recommended for children under 12 years.
FEDAHIST® EXPECTORANT (NONALCOHOLIC)
Dosage: Adults and children 12 years and over: two teaspoonfuls every 6 hours not to exceed 8 teaspoonfuls in 24 hours.
Children 6 to 12 years: one teaspoonful every 6 hours not to exceed 4 teaspoonfuls in 24 hours.
Children 2 to under 6 years: one-half teaspoonful every 6 hours not to exceed 2 teaspoonfuls in 24 hours.
Do not give to children under 6 years except under the advice and supervision of a physician.
FEDAHIST® TABLETS (SCORED, DYE-FREE)
Dosage: Adults and children 12 and over: one tablet every 6 hours not to exceed 4 tablets in 24 hours.
Children 6 to under 12 years: one-half tablet every 6 hours not to exceed 2 tablets in 24 hours.
Do not give to children under 6 years except under the advice and supervision of a physician.
FEDAHIST® SYRUP (NONALCOHOLIC)
Dosage: Adults and children 12 years and over: two teaspoonfuls every 6 hours not to exceed 8 teaspoonfuls in 24 hours.
Children 6 to under 12 years: one teaspoonful every 6 hours not to exceed 4 teaspoonfuls in 24 hours.
Children 2 to under 6 years: one-half teaspoonful every 6 hours not to exceed 2 teaspoonfuls in 24 hours.
Do not give to children under 6 years except under the advice and supervision of a physician.
KEEP THIS AND ALL MEDICATION OUT OF THE REACH OF CHILDREN. In case of accidental overdose, seek professional assistance or contact a poison control center immediately.
Supplied:
FEDAHIST® GYROCAPS® ℞: Available in bottles of 100 (NDC 0067-1053-68).
FEDAHIST® TABLETS: Available in bottles of 100 (NDC 0067-0050-68).
FEDAHIST® SYRUP: Available in 4 oz bottles (NDC 0067-0052-60).
FEDAHIST® EXPECTORANT: Available in 4 oz bottles (NDC 0067-0054-60).

Fedahist® Gyrocaps®
Manufactured by
Cord Laboratories, Inc.
Broomfield, CO 80020
For
William H. Rorer, Inc.

Fedahist® Gyrocaps® and Tablets Shown in Product Identification Section, page 431

FERMALOX® Tablets
(See PDR For Nonprescription Drugs)

GEMNISYN™ Tablets
(See PDR For Nonprescription Drugs)

KUDROX® Suspension
(See PDR For Nonprescription Drugs)

KUTRASE® CAPSULES ℞
[qū' trās″]

Description: KUTRASE® is a unique formulation containing 4 digestive enzymes, an antispasmodic-anticholinergic agent and a non-barbiturate sedative.
Each green and white capsule contains:

STANDARDIZED ENZYMES
Amylolytic	30 mg.
Proteolytic	6 mg.
Lipolytic	75 mg.
Cellulolytic	2 mg.

Phenyltoloxamine citrate .... 15 mg.
LEVSIN (Hyoscyamine Sulfate) 0.0625 mg.

Clinical Pharmacology: Diminution of secretions from exocrine glands is often a result of normal aging process. KUTRASE provides a balanced combination of natural proteolytic, amylolytic, cellulolytic and lipolytic enzymes to enhance digestion of proteins, starch and fat in the gastrointestinal tract. These enzymes do not exert any systemic pharmacologic effects. KUTRASE should be considered an enzyme supplement and not an enzyme replacement therapy. Enzymes in KUTRASE are basically derived from vegetable sources and possess a broad spectrum of pH activity. Enzymes are promptly released from the capsule and are bioavailable for digestion of food in the stomach and intestines. LEVSIN (Hyoscyamine Sulfate) provides a potent spasmolytic effect in reducing gastrointestinal hypermotility and intestinal spasm. A mild sedative effect is provided by Phenyltoloxamine Citrate.

Indications and Usage: KUTRASE is indicated for the relief of the symptoms of functional indigestion devoid of organic pathology commonly referred to as nervous indigestion and colloquially as "butterflies". The symptoms are bloating, gas, and fullness.

Contraindications: Glaucoma, obstructive uropathy, obstructive disease of the gastrointestinal tract (as in achalasia, pyloroduodenal stenosis); paralytic ileus, intestinal atony of the elderly or debilitated patients; unstable cardiovascular status in acute hemorrhage; severe ulcerative colitis; toxic megacolon, complicating ulcerative colitis; myasthenia gravis, or a hypersensitivity to any of the ingredients.

Warnings: In the presence of high environmental temperature, heat prostration can occur with drug use (fever and heat stroke due to decreased sweating). Diarrhea may be an early symptom of incomplete intestinal obstruction, especially in patients with ileostomy or colostomy. In this instance, treatment with this drug would be inappropriate. KUTRASE may produce drowsiness or blurred vision. In this event, the patient should be warned not to engage in activities requiring mental alertness such as operating a motor vehicle or other machinery or to perform hazardous work while taking this drug.

Precautions: Use with caution in patients with autonomic neuropathy, hyperthyroidism, coronary heart disease, congestive heart failure, cardiac arrhythmias, and hypertension. Investigate any tachycardia before giving any anticholinergic drugs since they may increase the heart rate. Use with caution in patients with hiatal hernia associated with reflux esophagitis.
Carcinogenesis, mutagenesis — Long-term studies in animals have not been performed to evaluate carcinogenic potential.
Pregnancy Category C—Animal reproduction studies have not been conducted with KUTRASE. It is not known whether KUTRASE can cause fetal harm when administered to a pregnant woman or can affect reproduction capacity. KUTRASE should be given to a pregnant woman only if clearly needed.

Adverse Reactions: Occasionally a slight looseness of the stools may be noticed. Other adverse reactions may include dryness of the mouth; urinary hesitancy and retention; blurred vision and tachycardia; palpitations; mydriasis; cycloplegia; increased ocular tension; headache; nervousness; drowsiness; weakness; suppression of lactation, and allergic reactions or drug idiosyncrasies, urticaria and other dermal manifestations and decreased sweating.

Drug Abuse and Dependence: The information on drug abuse and dependence is limited to uncontrolled data derived from marketing experience. Such experience has revealed no evidence of drug abuse and dependence associated with KUTRASE.

Overdosage: The signs and symptoms of overdose are headache, nausea, vomiting, blurred vision, dilated pupils, hot dry skin, dizziness, dryness of the mouth, difficulty in swallowing. Measures to be taken are immediate lavage of the stomach and injection of physostigmine 0.5 to 2 mg intravenously and repeated as necessary up to a total of 5 mg. Fever may be treated symptomatically. Excitement to a degree which demands attention may be managed with sodium thiopental 2% solution given slowly intravenously. In the event of paralysis of the respiratory muscles, artificial respiration should be instituted.

Administration and Dosage: The dosage of KUTRASE should be adjusted to the needs of the individual patient to assure symptomatic control with a minimum of adverse effects. The usual dose is one or two capsules at meal times, preferably taken during the course of the meal.

Supplied: KUTRASE capsules are green and white with a "Kremers-Urban 475" imprint.
Bottles of 100 capsules   NDC 0091-3475-01
Bottles of 500 capsules   NDC 0091-3475-05
Store at controlled room temperature, between 15°C and 30°C (59°F and 86°F).
Dispense in tight container.

Shown in Product Identification Section, page 431

KU-ZYME® CAPSULES ℞
[qū' zīm″]

Description: KU-ZYME® is a digestive aid containing 4 digestive enzymes which are highly purified, accurately standardized and potent.
Each yellow and white capsule contains:

STANDARDIZED ENZYMES
Amylolytic	30 mg.
Proteolytic	6 mg.
Lipolytic	75 mg.
Cellulolytic	2 mg.

Clinical Pharmacology: Diminution of secretions from exocrine glands is often a result of normal aging process. KU-ZYME provides a balanced combination of natural proteolytic, amylolytic, cellulolytic and lipolytic enzymes to enhance digestion of proteins, starch and fat in the gastrointestinal tract. These enzymes do not exert any systemic pharmacologic effects. KU-ZYME should be considered an enzyme supplement and not an enzyme replacement therapy. Enzymes in KU-ZYME are basically derived from vegetable sources and possess a broad spectrum of pH activity. Enzymes are promptly released from the capsule and are bioavailable for digestion of food in the stomach and intestines.

Indications and Usage: For the relief of functional indigestion when due to enzyme deficiency or imbalance. KU-ZYME relieves symptoms due to faulty digestion including the sensation of fullness after meals, dyspepsia, flatulence, abdominal distention and intolerance to certain foods.

Contraindications: There are no known contraindications to the administration of digestive enzymes. These enzymes do not attack living tissues and do not present any danger to the patient with ulceration or inflammation in the digestive tract.

Warnings: Do not administer to patients who are allergic to pork products.

Precautions: Long-term studies in animals have not been performed to evaluate carcinogenic potential.
Pregnancy Category C—Animal reproduction studies have not been conducted with KU-ZYME. It is not known whether KU-ZYME can cause fetal harm when administered to a pregnant woman or can affect reproduction capacity. KU-ZYME should be given to a pregnant woman only if clearly needed.

Adverse Reactions: Virtually unknown. Occasionally a slight looseness of stools may be noticed. If so, dosage should be reduced.

Overdosage: No systemic toxicity occurs. Excessive dosage may, however produce a laxative effect.

Dosage and Administration: For most patients, one capsule of KU-ZYME taken during the course of a meal will relieve symptoms due to a digestive deficiency. In patients (especially children) who experience difficulty in swallowing the capsule, it may be opened and the contents sprinkled on the food. In a few cases, where enzyme deficiency is marked (e.g. following gastrectomy, pancreatitis) the dosage may be doubled.

Supplied: KU-ZYME capsules are yellow and white with a "Kremers-Urban 522" imprint.
Bottles of 100 capsules
(NDC 0091-3522-01)
Bottles of 500 capsules
(NDC 0091-3522-05)

Store at controlled room temperature, between 15°C and 30°C (59°F and 86°F).
Dispense in tight container.
Shown in Product Identification Section, page 431

KU-ZYME® HP   ℞
[qū' zīm]
(Pancrelipase Capsules USP)

Description: KU-ZYME HP (Pancrelipase USP) is a standardized concentrate of pancreatic enzymes. Each white capsule contains:

Lipase	8,000 USP units
Protease	30,000 USP units
Amylase	30,000 USP units

Clinical Pharmacology: Pancrelipase USP is a pancreatic enzyme concentrate, which hydrolyzes fats to glycerol and fatty acids, changes protein into proteases and derived substances, and converts starch into dextrins and sugars. The administration of Pancrelipase reduces the fat and nitrogen content in the stool. Pancreatic enzymes are normally secreted in great excess. Generally, steatorrhea and malabsorption occur only after a 90 percent or greater reduction in secretion of lipase and proteolytic enzymes. It has been estimated that approximately 8,000 units of lipase per hour should be delivered into the duodenum postprandially. Even if all the enzymes taken orally reached the proximal intestine in active form, ingestion of 24,000 units of lipase (8,000 units per hour) for 3 postprandial hours would be required. If one could deliver sufficient pancreatic enzymes to the small intestine, malabsorption could be corrected. It is rarely possible to achieve complete relief of steatorrhea although major improvement in fat absorption can be achieved in most patients.

Indications: KU-ZYME HP is effective in patients with deficient exocrine pancreatic secretions. Thus, KU-ZYME HP may be used as enzyme replacement therapy in cystic fibrosis, chronic pancreatitis, post pancreatectomy, in ductal obstructions caused by cancer of the pancreas, pancreatic insufficiency and for steatorrhea of malabsorption syndrome and post gastrectomy (Billroth II and Total). May also be used as a presumptive test for pancreatic function, especially in pancreatic insufficiency due to chronic pancreatitis.

Contraindications: There are no known contraindications for the use of pancrelipase although sensitivity to pork protein may preclude its use.

Warnings: Pancreatic exocrine replacement therapy should not delay or supplant treatment of the primary disorder. Use with caution in patients known to be hypersensitive to pork or enzymes.

Precautions: Drug interactions—The serum iron response to oral iron may be decreased by concomitant administration of pancreatic extracts.

Carcinogenicity, Mutagenicity, and Impairment of Fertility—There have been no studies in animals to evaluate the carcinogenic, mutagenic or impairment of fertility potential of pancrelipase.

Adverse Reactions: High doses may cause nausea, abdominal cramps and/or diarrhea in certain patients.

Dosage and Administration: Dosage should be adjusted to individual patient needs. 1 to 3 capsules with meals and 1 capsule with any food between meals. In severe deficiencies, the dose may be increased to 8 capsules with meals or the frequency of administration may increase to hourly intervals if nausea, cramps and/or diarrhea do not occur.

Caution: Federal law prohibits dispensing without prescription.

Supplied: White capsules with a "Kremers-Urban 525" imprint, bottles of 100.
NDC 0091-3525-01
Shown in Product Identification Section, page 431

LACTRASE™
(See PDR For Nonprescription Drugs)

LEVSIN® Products   ℞
[lev'sin]
(Hyoscyamine Sulfate)

LEVSIN® Tablets
LEVSIN® Injection
LEVSIN® Elixir
LEVSIN® Drops (Oral Solution)
LEVSINEX™ TIMECAPS™

Description: LEVSIN® Tablets contain Hyoscyamine Sulfate 0.125 mg, are white, scored tablets with K-U logo and 531 imprint.

LEVSIN® Injection contains 0.5 mg/ml of Hyoscyamine Sulfate.

LEVSIN® Elixir contains Hyoscyamine Sulfate 0.125 mg/5 ml (Teaspoonful), it is orange colored and flavored and contains alcohol 20%.

LEVSIN® Drops contain Hyoscyamine Sulfate 0.125 mg/cc, orange colored and flavored and contain alcohol 5%. Supplied in a dropper bottle.

LEVSINEX™ TIMECAPS™ contain Hyoscyamine Sulfate 0.375 mg in a sustained release formulation designed for b.i.d. dosage, are brown and clear capsules containing brown and white beadlets.

Clinical Pharmacology: LEVSIN® is chemically pure Hyoscyamine Sulfate, one of the principal anticholinergic/antispasmodic components of Belladonna alkaloids. LEVSIN® inhibits specifically the actions of acetylcholine on structures innervated by postganglionic cholinergic nerves and on smooth muscles that respond to acetylcholine but lack cholinergic innervation. These peripheral cholinergic receptors are present in the autonomic effector cells of the smooth muscle, cardiac muscle, the sinoatrial node, the atrioventricular node and exocrine glands. It is completely devoid of any action in the autonomic ganglia. LEVSIN® inhibits gastrointestinal propulsive motility and decreases gastric acid secretion. LEVSIN® also controls excessive pharyngeal, tracheal, and bronchial secretions. LEVSIN® is absorbed totally and completely by sublingual administration as well as oral administration. Once absorbed, LEVSIN® disappears rapidly from the blood and is distributed throughout the entire body. The half-life of LEVSIN® is 3½ hours and the majority of drug is excreted in the urine unchanged within the first 12 hours. Only traces of this drug are found in breast milk.

Indications and Usage: LEVSIN® is effective as adjunctive therapy in the treatment of peptic ulcer. It can also be used to control gastric secretion, visceral spasm and hypermotility in spastic colitis, spastic bladder, cystitis, pylorospasm, and associated abdominal cramps. May be used in functional intestinal disorders to reduce symptoms such as those seen in mild dysenteries and diverticulitis. For use as adjunctive therapy in the treatment of irritable bowel syndrome (irritable colon, spastic colon, mucous colitis, and functional gastrointestinal disorders) and acute enterocolitis. Also as adjunctive therapy in the treatment of neurogenic bowel disturbances (including the splenic flexure syndrome and neurogenic colon). Also used in the treatment of infant colic (elixir and drops). LEVSIN® is indicated along with morphine and other narcotics in symptomatic relief of biliary and renal colic; as a "drying agent"

in the relief of symptoms of acute rhinitis; in the therapy of parkinsonism to reduce rigidity and tremors and to control associated sialorrhea, and hyperhydrosis. May be used in the therapy of poisoning of anticholinesterase agents.

Contraindications: Glaucoma; obstructive uropathy (for example, bladder neck obstruction due to prostatic hypertrophy); obstructive disease of the gastrointestinal tract (as in achalasia, pyloroduodenal stenosis); paralytic ileus; intestinal atony of the elderly or debilitated patients; unstable cardiovascular status in acute hemorrhage; severe ulcerative colitis; toxic megacolon complicating ulcerative colitis; myasthenia gravis.

Warnings: In the presence of high environmental temperature, heat prostration can occur with drug use (fever and heat stroke due to decreased sweating). Diarrhea may be an early symptom of incomplete intestinal obstruction, especially in patients with ileostomy or colostomy. In this instance, treatment with this drug would be inappropriate and possibly harmful. Like other anticholinergic agents, LEVSIN® may produce drowsiness or blurred vision. In this event, the patient should be warned not to engage in activities requiring mental alertness such as operating a motor vehicle or other machinery or to perform hazardous work while taking this drug.

Precautions: Use with caution in patients with autonomic neuropathy, hyperthyroidism, coronary heart disease, congestive heart failure, cardiac arrhythmias, and hypertension. Investigate any tachycardia before giving any anticholinergic drugs since they may increase the heart rate. Use with caution in patients with hiatal hernia associated with reflux esophagitis.

Adverse Reactions: Adverse reactions may include dryness of the mouth; urinary hesitancy and retention; blurred vision and tachycardia; palpitations; mydriasis; cycloplegia; increased ocular tension; headache; nervousness; drowsiness; weakness; suppression of lactation; allergic reactions or drug idiosyncrasies; urticaria and other dermal manifestations; and decreased sweating.

Drug Abuse and Dependence: The information on drug abuse and dependence is limited to uncontrolled data derived from marketing experience. Such experience has revealed no evidence of drug abuse and dependence associated with LEVSIN®.

Overdosage: The signs and symptoms of overdose are headache, nausea, vomiting, blurred vision, dilated pupils, hot/dry skin, dizziness, dryness of the mouth, difficulty in swallowing. Overdosage may be treated with immediate lavage of the stomach and injection of physostigmine 0.5 to 2 mg intravenously and repeated as necessary up to a total of 5 mg. Fever may be treated symptomatically (alcohol sponging, icepacks). Excitement to a degree which demands attention may be managed with sodium thiopental 2% solution given slowly intravenously or chloral hydrate (100/200 ml of a 2% solution) by rectal infusion. In the event of progression of the curare-like effect to paralysis of the respiratory muscles, artificial respiration should be instituted and maintained until effective respiratory action returns.

Dosage and Administration: The dosage of LEVSIN® products should be adjusted to the needs of the individual patient to assure symptomatic control with a minimum of adverse effects.

LEVSIN® Tablets: One or two tablets three to four times a day according to condition and severity of symptoms. May be taken orally or sublingually.

LEVSIN® Elixir: Adults, one or two teaspoonfuls of elixir three to four times a day according to conditions and severity of symptoms.

Continued on next page

This product information was prepared in August 1984. Information concerning these products may be obtained by addressing William H. Rorer, Inc., 500 Virginia Drive, Fort Washington, PA 19034.

Rorer—Cont.

Children (Elixir)

Body Weight	Starting Dosage
10 lb.	0.5 ml to 0.75 ml
20 lb.	1.25 ml (¼ tsp) to 2.0 ml
30 lb.	2.5 ml (½ tsp)
50 lb.	¾ tsp to 1 tsp
75–80 lb.	1 tsp to 1½ tsp

Doses may be repeated every 4 hours as needed; dosage adjustment may be necessary.

LEVSIN® Drops:
Infants

Body Weight	Starting Dosage (in drops)
5 lb.	3
7.5 lb.	4
10 lb.	6
15 lb.	7
20 lb.	9

Children 1-10 years: ½–1 cc
Adults: 1-2 cc

Doses may be repeated every 4 hours as needed; dosage adjustment may be necessary according to conditions and severity of symptoms.

LEVSIN® Injection may be administered subcutaneously, intramuscularly, or intravenously without dilution. The usual recommended dose of LEVSIN® in the treatment of gastrointestinal disorders is 0.5 to 1.0 ml (0.25 to 0.5 mg) administered at four hour intervals three to four times daily. Some patients may need only a single dose, others may require administration 2, 3, or 4 times a day. For hypotonic duodenography, LEVSIN® Injection may be used five to ten minutes prior to the diagnostic procedure. The usual dose is 0.5 to 1.0 ml (0.25 mg to 0.5 mg).

IN ANESTHESIA: As pre-anesthetic medication, the recommended dose of LEVSIN® Injection is 5 μg/kg of body weight, given thirty to sixty minutes prior to the anticipated time of induction of anesthesia, or at the time the pre-anesthetic narcotic or sedatives are administered. In intraoperative medication, LEVSIN® Injectable may be used during surgery to counteract drug induced bradycardia. It should be administered intravenously in increments of 0.25 ml and repeated as needed. To achieve reversal of neuromuscular blockage, the recommended dose of LEVSIN® Injectable is 0.2 mg for each 1 mg of neostigmine or the equivalent dose of physostigmine and pyridostigmine.

LEVSINEX™ TIMECAPS™:
Adults
The usual dose is one TIMECAPS™ every 12 hours. For patients requiring higher anticholinergic therapy, the dosage may be increased to two TIMECAPS™ every 12 hours or one TIMECAPS™ every 8 hours.

Children over 2 years
One capsule every 12 hours. Dosage may be increased to one capsule every 8 hours if needed.

How Supplied:
LEVSIN® Tablets (0.125 mg. Hyoscyamine Sulfate tablets) white, scored tablets; bottles of 100 (NDC 0091-3531-01), bottles of 500 (NDC 0091-3531-05).
LEVSIN® Elixir (0.125 mg Hyoscyamine Sulfate per 5 cc) orange colored and flavored; pints. (NDC 0091-4532-16).
LEVSIN® DROPS (0.125 mg Hyoscyamine Sulfate per cc), orange colored and flavored, 15 cc (NDC 0091-4538-15).
LEVSIN® Injection (0.5 mg Hyoscyamine Sulfate per ml) single dose ampuls, boxes of 5. (NDC 0091-1536-05); and 10 ml vials (NDC 0091-1536-10).
LEVSINEX™ TIMECAPS™ (0.375 mg Hyoscyamine Sulfate) brown and white sustained release beadlets in brown and clear capsules; bottles of 100. (NDC 0091-3537-01).

Shown in Product Identification Section, page 432

MAALOX® Suspension and Tablets
(See PDR For Nonprescription Drugs)

MAALOX® PLUS Suspension and Tablets
(See PDR For Nonprescription Drugs)

MAALOX® TC Suspension and Tablets
(See PDR For Nonprescription Drugs)

MILKINOL®
(See PDR For Nonprescription Drugs)

NITROL® OINTMENT ℞
[*nī' trōl*]
2% nitroglycerin ointment

Description: NITROL Ointment contains 2% nitroglycerin and lactose in a special absorptive lanolin and white petrolatum base formulated to provide a controlled release of the active ingredient. Each inch, as squeezed from the tube, contains approximately 15 mg of nitroglycerin.

Action: When the ointment is spread on the skin, the active ingredient (nitroglycerin) is continuously absorbed through the skin into the circulation, thus exerting prolonged vasodilator effect. Nitroglycerin ointment is effective in the control of angina pectoris when applied to the trunk or to the proximal parts of extremities.
Nitroglycerin relaxes smooth muscles, principally in the smaller blood vessels and dilates the arterioles and capillaries, especially in the coronary circulation. NITROL Ointment reduces the workload of the heart by virtue of its smooth muscle relaxation. This results predominantly in peripheral venous dilatation which reduces preload, but also to a lesser degree in peripheral arteriolar dilatation which reduces afterload. These hemodynamic effects have been advanced as explanations for the beneficial actions of nitroglycerin ointment in angina pectoris. Nitroglycerin exerts a favorable influence on myocardial oxygen consumption, resulting in increased myocardial efficiency and significant improvement in left ventricular function. Computerized digital plethysmographic studies have shown the duration of action of NITROL Ointment (2 inches applied to the chest) to be eight hours in comparison to placebo; the onset of action occurred within thirty minutes of administration. Controlled clinical studies have demonstrated that nitroglycerin ointment increased measured exercise tolerance in patients with angina pectoris up to three hours after application (the maximal time interval studied).

Indications:

> This drug product has been conditionally approved by the FDA for the prevention and treatment of angina pectoris due to coronary artery disease. The conditional approval reflects a determination that the drug may be marketed pending FDA evaluation of data submitted in support of its effectiveness. A final evaluation of the effectiveness of the product will be announced by the FDA.

Contraindications: In patients known to be intolerant of the organic nitrate drugs.

Warnings: In acute myocardial infarction or congestive heart failure, NITROL Ointment should be used under careful clinical and/or hemodynamic monitoring.

Precautions: NITROL Ointment should not be used for treatment of acute anginal attacks. Symptoms of hypotension, particularly when suddenly arising from the recumbent position, are signs of overdosage. When they occur, the dosage should be reduced.

Adverse Reactions: Transient headaches are the most common side effect, especially at higher dosages. Headaches should be treated with mild analgesics and NITROL Ointment continued. Only with untreatable headaches should the dosage be reduced. Although uncommon, hypotension, an increase in heart rate, faintness, flushing, dizziness, and nausea may occur. These are all attributable to the pharmacologic effects of nitroglycerin on the cardiovascular system, and are symptoms of overdosage. When they occur and persist, the dosage should be reduced. Occasionally, contact dermatitis has been reported with continuous use of topical nitroglycerin. Such incidences may be reduced by changing the site of application.

Management of Overdosage: Severe hypotension may result from overdosage of nitroglycerin ointment. Should hypotension develop, quickly remove the ointment. The patient should be placed in a recumbent position with the legs elevated. In case of persistent hypotension, an IV infusion of 5% dextrose should be started.

Dosage and Administration:
Using Conventional Appli-Rulers™ When applying the ointment, use the Appli-Ruler™ dose determining applicator supplied with the package and squeeze the necessary amount of ointment from the tube onto the applicator. Then place the applicator with the ointment side down onto the desired area of skin, usually the chest (although other areas can be used). Spread the ointment over at least a 2¼ × 3½ inch area in a thin uniform layer using the applicator. Cover the area with plastic wrap which can be held in place by adhesive tape. The Appli-Ruler allows the patient to measure the necessary amount of ointment and to spread it without being absorbed through the fingers while applying it to the skin surface.
Using TSAR™ Kit (Tape-Surrounded Appli-Rulers™) Measure the desired dosage of NITROL Ointment onto the Tape-Surrounded Appli-Ruler™. Spread the ointment by carefully folding the Tape-Surrounded Appli-Ruler™. Be careful not to spread any ointment onto the outer lined border. Bend the Tape-Surrounded Appli-Ruler™ at the star, peel off and discard the outer lined border. Apply the Tape-Surrounded Appli-Ruler™ to the desired body area and press the adhesive border firmly to the skin. To assure proper ointment contact, gently press the entire Tape-Surrounded Appli-Ruler™ surface area.
The usual therapeutic dose is 1 to 2 inches (2.5 to 5.0 cm) applied every eight hours, although some patients may require as much as 4 to 5 inches (10 to 12.5 cm) and/or application every four hours. Start at ½ inch (1.25 cm) every eight hours and increase the dose by ½ inch (1.25 cm) with each successive application to achieve the desired clinical effects. The optimal dosage should be selected based upon the clinical responses, side effects and the effects of therapy upon blood pressure. The greatest attainable decrease in resting blood pressure which is not associated with clinical symptoms of hypotension especially during orthostasis indicates the optimal dosage. To decrease adverse reactions, the dose and frequency of application should be tailored to the individual patient's needs.
The three gram titratable unit dose is a convenient hospital package. The tube has the same orifice as that of a larger NITROL tube and any prescribed dose up to four inches may be dispensed from the tube using the instructions described above.
Keep tube tightly closed and store at room temperature 59° to 86°F (15° to 30°C).

How Supplied:

(NDC 0091-5617-31)	30 gram tube
(NDC 0091-5617-02)	60 gram tube
(NDC 0091-5617-61)	30 gram 6 Pack
(NDC 0091-5617-62)	60 gram 6 Pack
(NDC 0091-5617-53)	Titratable Unit Dose—50 × 3g Tubes

NITROL Ointment TSAR™ Kits (Packages include a supply of Tape-Surrounded Appli-Rulers™ for convenient application)

(NDC 0091-5617-33)	30 gram tube TSAR™ Kit
(NDC 0091-5617-66)	60 gram tube TSAR™ Kit
(NDC 0091-5617-55)	Titratable Unit Dose—50 × 3g tubes TSAR™ Kit

Shown in Product Identification Section, page 432

PAREPECTOLIN®
Antidiarrheal

Contains opium (¼ grain) 15 mg. per fluid ounce. *(Warning: may be habit forming.)*
Formula: Each fluid ounce of creamy white suspension contains:
Paregoric (equivalent) .... 3.7 ml
Pectin.. 162 mg
Kaolin.. 5.5 g
(Alcohol 0.69%).

Indications: For symptomatic relief of diarrhea.
Action: The kaolin adsorbs irritants and forms a protective coating on intestinal mucosa. Pectin acts to consolidate the stool. Paregoric is very useful in diarrhea because it has a soothing action and allays griping pains.
Advantages: Because Parepectolin contains paregoric (equivalent), it effectively controls both diarrhea and colicky cramps. It is a stable suspension that tastes good.
Usual Adult Dose: One or two tablespoonfuls after each loose bowel movement for no more than four doses in twelve hours.
Usual Children's Dose: One or two teaspoonfuls after each loose bowel movement for no more than four doses in twelve hours.
Pediatric Dosage:

One year	½ teaspoonful
Three years	1½ teaspoonfuls
Six years	2 teaspoonfuls

after each loose bowel movement for no more than four doses in twelve hours.
Warning: Keep this and all drugs out of the reach of children. In case of accidental overdose, seek professional assistance or contact a poison control center immediately.
Supplied: Bottles of 4 (118 ml) (NDC 0067-0660-60) and 8 (237 ml) (NDC 0067-0660-66) fluid ounces.

PERDIEM® Granules

(See PDR For Nonprescription Drugs)

PERDIEM® PLAIN Granules

(See PDR For Nonprescription Drugs)

PRE-PEN®
[prē'pen]
(Benzylpenicilloyl-polylysine)
Skin Test Antigen

Description: PRE-PEN® is a sterile solution of benzylpenicilloyl-polylysine in a concentration of 6.0×10^{-5}M. (penicilloyl) in 0.01 M phosphate buffer and 0.15 M sodium chloride. The benzylpenicilloyl-polylysine in PRE-PEN® is a derivative of poly-l-lysine, where the epsilon amino groups are substituted with benzylpenicilloyl groups (50-70%) forming benzylpenicilloyl alpha amide. Each single dose ampule contains 0.25 ml of PRE-PEN®.
Action: PRE-PEN® (benzylpenicilloyl-polylysine) reacts specifically with benzylpenicilloyl skin sensitizing antibodies (reagins: IgE class) to initiate release of chemical mediators which produce an immediate wheal and flare reaction at a skin test site. All individuals exhibiting a positive skin test to PRE-PEN® possess reagins against the benzylpenicilloyl group which is a haptene. A haptene is a low molecular weight chemical which, when conjugated to a carrier, e.g., poly-l-lysine, has the properties under appropriate conditions of an antigen with the haptene's specificity.

It is to be noted that individuals who have previously received therapeutic penicillin may have positive skin test reactions to PRE-PEN® as well as to a number of other non-benzylpenicilloyl haptenes. The latter are designated as minor determinants, in that they are present in lesser amounts than the major determinant, benzylpenicilloyl. The minor determinants may nevertheless be associated with examples of significant clinical hypersensitivity.

Virtually everyone who receives penicillin develops specific antibodies to the drug as measured by hemagglutination studies, but (a) positive skin tests to various penicillin and penicillin-derived reagents become positive in less than 10% of patients who have tolerated penicillin in the past and (b) allergic responses are infrequent (less than 1%).

Many individuals reacting positively to PRE-PEN® will not develop a systemic allergic reaction on subsequent exposure to therapeutic penicillin. Thus, the PRE-PEN® skin test facilitates assessing the local allergic skin reactivity of a patient to benzylpenicilloyl.

Indications: PRE-PEN® is useful as an adjunct in assessing the risk of administering penicillin (benzylpenicillin or penicillin G) when it is the preferred drug of choice in adult patients who have previously received penicillin and have a history of clinical penicillin hypersensitivity. In this situation, a negative skin test to PRE-PEN® is associated with an incidence of allergic reactions of less than 5% after the administration of therapeutic penicillin, whereas the incidence may be more than 20% in the presence of a positive skin test to PRE-PEN®.

These allergic reactions are predominantly dermatologic. Because of the extremely low incidence of anaphylactic reactions, there are insufficient data at present to document that a decreased incidence of anaphylactic reactions following the administration of penicillin will occur in patients with a negative skin test to PRE-PEN®. Similarly, when deciding the risk of proposed penicillin treatment, there are not enough data at present to permit relative weighting in individual cases of a history of clinical penicillin hypersensitivity as compared to positive skin tests to PRE-PEN® and/or minor penicillin determinants.

It should be borne in mind that no reagent, test, or combination of tests will completely assure that a reaction to penicillin therapy will not occur.

Contraindications: PRE-PEN® is contraindicated in those patients who have exhibited either a systemic or marked local reaction to its previous administration. Patients known to be extremely hypersensitive to penicillin should not be skin tested.

Warnings: There are insufficient data to assess the potential danger of sensitization to penicillin from repeated skin testing with PRE-PEN®.

Rarely, a systemic allergic reaction (see below) may follow a skin test with PRE-PEN®. This can be avoided by making the first application by scratch test and very carefully following the instructions below in administering the intradermal test, using the intradermal route only if the scratch test has been entirely negative.

Skin testing with penicillin and/or other penicillin-derived reagents should not be performed simultaneously.

No controlled studies have been made of the safety of PRE-PEN® skin testing in pregnant women and therefore, the hazard of skin testing of such patients should be weighed against the hazards of penicillin therapy without skin testing.

Precautions: There are insufficient data derived from well-controlled studies to determine the value of the PRE-PEN® skin test as a means of assessing the risk of administering therapeutic penicillin (when penicillin is the preferred drug of choice) in the following situations:
(1) Adult patients who give no history of clinical penicillin hypersensitivity.
(2) Pediatric patients.

In addition, there are no data at present to assess the clinical value of PRE-PEN® where exposure to penicillin is suspected as a cause of a drug reaction and in patients who are undergoing routine allergy evaluation.

Furthermore, there are no data relating the clinical value of PRE-PEN® skin tests to the risk of administering semi-synthetic penicillins (phenoxymethyl penicillin, ampicillin, carbenicillin, dicloxacillin, methicillin, nafcillin, oxacillin, phenethicillin) and cephalosporin-derived antibiotics.

Recognition that the following clinical outcomes are possible makes it imperative for the physician to weigh risk to benefit in every instance where the decision to administer or not to administer penicillin is based in part on a PRE-PEN® skin test.

(1) An allergic reaction to therapeutic penicillin may occur in a patient with a negative skin test to PRE-PEN®.
(2) It is possible for a patient to have an anaphylactic reaction to therapeutic penicillin in the presence of a negative PRE-PEN® skin test and a negative history of clinical penicillin hypersensitivity.
(3) If penicillin is the absolute drug of choice in a life-threatening situation, successful desensitization with therapeutic penicillin may be possible irrespective of a positive skin test and/or a positive history of clinical penicillin hypersensitivity.

Adverse Reactions: Occasionally, patients may develop an intense local inflammatory response at the skin test site. Rarely, patients will develop a systemic allergic reaction, manifested by generalized erythema, pruritus, angioneurotic edema, urticaria, dyspnea, and/or hypotension. The usual methods of treating a skin test antigen induced reaction—the application of a venous occlusion tourniquet proximal to the skin test site and administration of epinephrine (and, at times, an injection of an antihistamine) — are recommended and will usually control the reaction. As a rule, systemic allergic reactions following skin test procedures are of short duration and controllable, but the patient should be kept under observation for several hours.

Skin Testing Dosage and Technique:
SCRATCH TESTING
Skin testing is usually performed on the inner volar aspect of the forearm. The skin test material should **always** be applied first by the scratch technique. After preparing the skin surface, a sterile 20 gauge needle should be used to make a 3–5 mm scratch of the epidermis. Very little pressure is required to break the epidermal continuity. If bleeding occurs, prepare a second site and scratch more lightly with the needle—sufficient to produce a non-bleeding scratched surface. Apply a small drop of PRE-PEN® solution to the scratch and rub gently with an applicator, toothpick, or the side of the needle. Observe for the appearance of a wheal, erythema, and the occurrence of itching at the test site during the succeeding 15 minutes at which time the solution over the scratch is wiped off. A positive reaction is unmistakable and consists of the development within 10 minutes of a pale wheal, usually with pseudopods, surrounding the scratch site and varying in diameter from 5 to 15 mm (or more). This wheal may be surrounded by a variable diameter of erythema, and accompanied by a variable degree of itching. The most sensitive individuals develop itching almost instantly, and the wheal and erythema are prompt in their appearance. As soon as a positive response as defined above is clearly evident, the solution over the scratch should be immediately wiped off. If the scratch test is either negative or equivocally positive (less than 5 mm wheal and little or no erythema, and no itching), an intradermal test may be performed.

THE INTRADERMAL TEST
Using a tuberculin syringe with a ⅜" to ⅝" long, 26 to 30 gauge, short bevel needle, withdraw the contents of the ampule. Prepare a sterile skin test area on the upper, outer arm, sufficiently below the deltoid muscle to permit proximal application of a tourniquet later, if necessary. Be sure to eject all air from the syringe through the needle, then insert the needle, bevel up immediately below the skin surface. Inject an amount of PRE-PEN® sufficient to raise the smallest possible perceptible bleb. This volume will be between 0.01 and 0.02 ml. Using a separate syringe and needle, inject a like amount of saline as a control at least 1½ inches removed from the test site. Most skin reactions

Continued on next page

This product information was prepared in August 1984. Information concerning these products may be obtained by addressing William H. Rorer, Inc., 500 Virginia Drive, Fort Washington, PA 19034.

Rorer—Cont.

will develop within 5–15 minutes and response to the skin test is read as follows:

(—) Negative response—no increase in size of original bleb and/or no greater reaction than the control site.

(±) Ambiguous response—wheal being only slightly larger than initial injection bleb, with or without accompanying erythematous flare and larger than the control site.

(+) Positive response—itching and marked increase in size of original bleb. Wheal may exceed 20 mm in diameter and exhibit pseudopodia.

The control site should be completely reactionless. If it exhibits a wheal greater than 2–3 mm, repeat the test, and if the same reaction is observed, a physician experienced with allergy skin testing should be consulted.

How Supplied: PRE-PEN® is supplied in ampules containing 0.25 ml and packaged in boxes of 5 (NDC 0091-1640-05).

PRE-PEN® is stable only when kept under refrigeration. It is, therefore, recommended that test materials subjected to ambient temperatures for over a day be discarded.

SLO-BID™ ℞
[slō'bid″]
(theophylline, anhydrous, Rorer)
50 mg, 100 mg, 200 mg, and 300 mg
Gyrocaps®
Timed Release Capsules

Description: Slo-bid™ Gyrocaps® contain 50 mg, 100 mg, 200 mg, or 300 mg theophylline anhydrous in the form of long-acting beads within a dye-free hard gelatin capsule and are intended for oral administration.

Theophylline is a bronchodilator and is a member of the xanthine class of chemical compounds related to both theobromine and caffeine.

Theophylline is a white, odorless, crystalline powder having a bitter taste. Slo-bid™ has been specially formulated to provide therapeutic serum concentrations when administered every 12 hours, and to minimize the peaks and valleys of serum concentration commonly found with shorter acting theophylline products.

Clinical Pharmacology: Theophylline directly relaxes the smooth muscle of the bronchial airways and pulmonary blood vessels with consequent bronchodilatation and pulmonary vasodilatation. Like other xanthines, the pharmacologic actions of theophylline also include cardiac stimulation (both inotropic and chronotropic), coronary vasodilation, stimulation of skeletal muscle, CNS stimulation, relaxation of smooth muscles including those in the bronchi and blood vessels (other than cerebral vessels), and diuresis. The mechanism of action is not clearly established but may include inhibition of phosphodiesterase with subsequent increase in intracellular cyclic AMP, direct inhibition of adenosine receptors, translocation of intracellular calcium, and others. The main use of theophylline has been in the treatment of reversible airway obstruction. No tolerance develops with chronic use.

In-vitro, theophylline has been shown to act synergistically with beta agonists that increase intracellular cyclic AMP through the stimulation of adenyl cyclase but synergism has not been demonstrated in patient studies. More data are needed to determine if the theohylline and beta agonists have a clinically important additive effect *in vivo*. Apparently no development of tolerance occurs with chronic use of theophylline.

Theophylline is, under usual conditions, rapidly and completely absorbed. Excretion, principally as inactive (1,3-dimethyluric acid, 1-methyluric acid) and active (3-methylxanthine) metabolites occurs primarily via the kidney. The half-life of theophylline varies widely among individuals (See Table).

Theophylline half-life is frequently shorter in cigarette smokers and in children over six months of age, but it is frequently prolonged in alcoholism, reduced hepatic or renal function, congestive heart failure and in patients receiving other concurrent drugs such as the antibiotics troleandomycin and erythromycin and the H_2 antagonist cimetidine. High fever for prolonged periods and certain viral illnesses may decrease theophylline elimination. Newborn and neonate infants have extremely slow clearances and theophylline half-lives frequently exceed 24 hours.

The half-life of theophylline in smokers (1 to 2 packs/day) averages 4-5 hours, much shorter than the half-life in non-smokers which averages 7-9 hours. The increase in theophylline clearance caused by smoking is probably the result of induction of drug-metabolizing enzymes that do not readily normalize after cessation of smoking. It appears that between 3 months and 2 years may be necessary for normalization of the effect of smoking on theophylline pharmacokinetics.

Older adults (over age 55) and patients with chronic obstructive pulmonary disease, with or without cor pulmonale, may also have much slower clearance rates. For such patients, the theophylline half-life may exceed 24 hours.

Preliminary pharmacokinetic data in pregnant patients suggest that the volume of distribution of theophylline increases with duration of pregnancy while clearance remains constant. This implies that the mg/kg theophylline dosage may be unchanged during pregnancy but the absolute dosage may increase during the latter part of pregnancy.

Representative Theophylline Serum Half-Lives	Half-Life (hours)
Adults	
non-smokers	7–9
smokers	4–5
congestive heart failure	24
Children (6-16 years)	3–5

Therapeutic theophylline serum levels usually range from 10 to 20 μg/ml with considerable interindividual variation.

Binding to plasma proteins is approximately 56% but is decreased in neonates and patients with cirrhosis. Theophylline is not preferentially taken up by any particular organ. Placental transfer of theophylline occurs and cord serum levels are very similar to maternal levels at delivery. Symptoms of irritability and tachycardia have been reported in neonates whose mothers were receiving theophylline. Since the half-life of theophylline is prolonged in neonates and since decreased protein binding may result in increased free and pharmacologically active drug at any given serum concentration, infants born to mothers on theophylline should be monitored for the pharmacologic actions of theophylline.

In single dose bioavailability studies in normal volunteers, 300 mg sustained release Slo-bid™ Gyrocaps® produced mean peak serum concentrations of 3.51±0.66 μg/ml at a mean time of 7.77±1.77 hours after dosing. At steady state in multiple dose bioavailability studies with q12h dosing, the mean peak-trough variation was 3.52±0.93 μg/ml.

Indications and Usage: For relief and/or prevention of reversible bronchospasm associated with such conditions as bronchial asthma, chronic bronchitis, and emphysema.

Contraindications: Slo-bid™ is contraindicated in individuals who have shown hypersensitivity to any of its components or to xanthine derivatives.

Warnings: Status asthmaticus should be considered a medical emergency and is defined as that degree of bronchospasm which is not rapidly responsive to usual doses of conventional bronchodilators. Optimal therapy for such patients frequently requires both *additional medication*, parenterally administered, and *close monitoring*, preferably in an intensive care setting.

Although increasing the dose of theophylline may bring about relief, such treatment may be associated with toxicity. The likelihood of such toxicity developing increases significantly when the serum theophylline concentration exceeds 20 μg/ml. Therefore, determination of serum theophylline levels is recommended to assure maximal benefit without excessive risk. Serum levels above 20 μg/ml are rarely found after appropriate administration of the recommended doses. However, in individuals in whom theophylline plasma clearance is reduced *for any reason*, even conventional doses may result in increased serum levels and potential toxicity. Reduced theophylline clearance has been documented in the following readily identifiable groups:

1) patients with impaired renal or liver function; 2) patients over 55 years of age, particularly males and those with chronic lung disease; 3) those with cardiac failure from any cause; 4) neonates; and 5) those patients taking certain drugs (macrolide antibiotics and cimetidine). Decreased clearance of theophylline may be associated with either influenza immunization or active infection with influenza.

Reduction of dosage and laboratory monitoring is especially appropriate in the above individuals. Less serious signs of theophylline toxicity, i.e. nausea and restlessness, may appear in up to 50% of patients.

Unfortunately, however, serious side effects such as ventricular arrhythmias, convulsions or even death may appear as the first signs of toxicity without any previous warning. Stated differently, *serious toxicity is not reliably preceded by less severe side effects*.

Many patients who require theophylline may exhibit tachycardia due to their underlying disease process so that the cause/effect relationship to elevated serum theophylline concentrations may not be appreciated.

Theophylline products may cause dysrhythmia and/or worsen pre-existing arrhythmias and any significant change in rate and/or rhythm warrants monitoring and further investigation.

The occurrence of arrhythmias and sudden death (with histological evidence of necrosis of the myocardium) has been recorded in laboratory animals (minipigs, rodents, and dogs) when theophylline and beta agonists were administered concomitantly, although not when either was administered alone. The significance of these findings when applied to human usage is currently unknown.

Precautions: Mean half-life in smokers is shorter than non-smokers. Therefore, smokers may require larger doses of theophylline.

Theophylline should not be administered with other xanthine preparations.

Use with caution in patients with severe cardiac disease, severe hypoxemia, hypertension, hyperthyroidism, acute myocardial injury, cor pulmonale, congestive heart failure, alcoholism, liver disease, and in the elderly, especially males, and neonates. Great caution should be used in giving theophylline to patients with congestive heart failure. Such patients have shown markedly prolonged theophylline blood levels with theophylline persisting in serum for long periods following discontinuation of the drug. Use theophylline cautiously in patients with a history of peptic ulcer. Theophylline may occasionally act as a local gastrointestinal irritant, although GI symptoms are more commonly centrally mediated and associated with high serum concentrations.

Information For Patients:
The physician should reinforce the importance of taking only the prescribed dose at the prescribed time intervals.

Patients should be advised of the need to individualize dosages. No dosage should be maintained which is not tolerated. Adverse effects are most commonly gastrointestinal but may also frequently be central nervous system or cardiovascular in nature. Patients should also be cautioned regarding the potentiating effects of other xanthines, especially caffeine, and of other drug interactions (see DRUG INTERACTIONS). Patients with low clearance and prolonged elimination (see CLINICAL PHARMACOLOGY and WARNINGS) should be advised to use theophylline with particular caution especially during the drug titration period. If necessary, taking the drug with food may help avoid local irritation of the G.I. tract.

Drug Interactions:

Drug	Effect
Aminophyline with lithium carbonate	Increased excretion of lithium carbonate
Aminophylline with propranolol	Mutual antagonism of therapeutic effects
Theophylline with furosemide	Increased diuresis
Theophylline with hexamethonium	Decreased hexamethonium-induced chronotropic effect
Theophylline with reserpine	Tachycardia
Theophylline with troleandomycin or erythromycin	Increased theophylline serum concentrations
Theophylline with chlordiazepoxide	Chlordiazepoxide-induced fatty acid metabolism
Theophylline with cimetidine	Increased theophylline serum concentrations

Toxic synergism with ephedrine has been documented and may occur with some other sympathomimetic bronchodilators.

Drug/Laboratory Test Interactions:
Theophylline may interfere with the assay of uric acid, especially by the phosphotungstate method. Serum uric acid concentrations may be overestimated. Theophylline-containing products may increase the plasma concentrations of free fatty acids and the urinary levels of epinephrine and norepinephrine.
When plasma levels of theophylline are measured by spectrophotometric methods, coffee, tea, cola beverages, chocolate, and acetaminophen contribute falsely high values.

Carcinogenesis, Mutagenesis, Impairment of Fertility:
Long-term animal studies have not been performed to evaluate the carcinogenic potential, mutagenic potential, or the effect of xanthine compounds on fertility.

Pregnancy:
Pregnancy Category C
Although xanthine derivatives have been implicated as teratogens, adequate animal reproduction studies have not been conducted with theophylline. It is not known whether theophylline can cause fetal harm when administered to a pregnant woman or can affect reproduction capacity. Theophylline should be given to a pregnant woman only if clearly needed.
Although theophylline has been reported to inhibit uterine contractions, labor is apparently not prolonged in asthmatic women receiving theophylline.
Placental transfer of theophylline occurs (see CLINICAL PHARMACOLOGY).
The effect of theophylline on later growth, development, and functional maturation of the child is not known.

Nursing Mothers:
Theophylline is excreted in the breast milk. The average milk/serum concentration ratio has been reported as about 0.7 and milk concentrations parallel the time course of serum concentrations. Caution should be exercised when theophylline is administered to a nursing mother.

Pediatric Use:
Drug elimination may be prolonged in premature infants and neonates (see CLINICAL PHARMACOLOGY and WARNINGS). Marked variation in theophylline metabolism is present in infants under six months of age.

Adverse Reactions: The frequency of adverse reactions is generally related to serum theophylline concentrations, particularly those in excess of 20 μg/ml. Gastrointestinal reactions are most frequently followed by central nervous system and cardiovascular reactions.
Gastrointestinal: hematemesis, epigastric pain, diarrhea, vomiting and nausea.
Central Nervous System: clonic and tonic generalized convulsions, reflex hyperexcitabity, muscle twitching, headaches, irritability, restlessness, insomnia.
Cardiovascular: life-threatening ventricular arrhythmias, circulatory failure, hypotension, tachycardia, extrasystoles, palpitation, flushing.
Respiratory: tachypnea.
Renal: albuminuria, increased excretion of renal tubular cells and red blood cells, potentiation of diuresis.
Other: hyperglycemia, inappropriate ADH syndrome, and rash.

Overdosage: Signs and Symptoms
Nervousness, agitation, headache, insomnia, nausea, vomiting, tachycardia, extrasystoles, tachypnea, hyperreflexia, fasciculation, and tonic/clonic convulsions. Children may be particularly prone to restlessness and hyperactivity which may proceed to convulsions.
Ingestion of an oral dose exceeding 10 mg/kg may require prompt emergency treatment. Measurement of serum theophylline concentrations is recommended. Patients with excessive concentrations should be monitored in an intensive care unit.
Charcoal hemoperfusion can rapidly remove theophylline and may be indicated where the serum concentration is very high (>40 μg/ml). However, the decision to dialyze must be individualized based on the clinical condition of the patient and the risks of charcoal hemoperfusion.
Peritoneal dialysis and other extracorporeal methods are inadequate in theophylline overdose.
Serious adverse effects are rare at serum theophylline concentrations below 20 μg/ml. Between 20 and 40 μg/ml sinus tachycardia and cardiac arrhythmias occur with increasing frequency. Above 40 μg/ml seizures and cardiorespiratory arrest can occur. However, convulsions and death have resulted at serum concentrations as low as 25 μg/ml.
A. If potential overdose is established and seizure has not occurred
 1. Induce vomiting
 2. Administer a cathartic (this is particularly important if sustained-release preparations have been taken)
 3. Administer activated charcoal
 4. Monitor vital signs, maintain blood pressure and provide adequate hydration
B. If patient is having seizure
 1. Establish an airway
 2. Administer oxygen
 3. Treat the seizure with intravenous diazepam 0.1 to 0.3 mg/kg up to a total dose of 10 mg
 4. Monitor vital signs, maintain blood pressure and provide adequate hydration
C. Post-Seizure Coma
 1. Maintain airway and oxygenation
 2. Follow above recommendations to prevent absorption of drug, but intubation and lavage will have to be performed instead of inducing emesis and the cathartic and charcoal will need to be introduced via a large bore gastric lavage tube
 3. Continue to provide full supportive care and adequate hydration while waiting for drug to be metabolized. In general, the drug is metabolized sufficiently rapidly so as to not warrant consideration of dialysis.

Dosage and Administration: For most patients, *effective use* of theophylline, i.e., associated with optimal likelihood of benefit combined with minimal risk of toxicity, is considered to occur when serum levels are maintained between 10 and 20 μg/ml. Levels above 20 μg/ml may produce toxicity, and in a small number of patients, toxicity may even be seen with serum levels between 15-20 μg/ml, particularly during initiation of therapy.
There is considerable variation from patient to patient in the dosage required to achieve and maintain therapeutic and safe levels, primarily due to variable rates of elimination. Therefore, it is essential that not only must dosage be individualized, but titration and monitoring of serum levels be utilized where available. When serum concentration cannot be obtained, restriction of dosage to the amounts and intervals recommended in the guidelines listed below becomes essential. Dosage should be calculated on the basis of lean (ideal) body weight where mg/kg doses are presented. Theophylline does not distribute into fatty tissue. Giving theophylline with food may prevent some local gastric irritation and though absorption is slower, it is still complete.
Frequency of Dosing: When immediate release products with rapid absorption (such as tablets or liquid) are used, dosing to maintain serum levels generally requires administration every 6 hours. This is particularly true in children, but dosing intervals up to 8 hours may be satisfactory in adults since they eliminate the drug at a slower rate. Some children, and adults requiring higher than average doses (those having rapid rates of clearance, e.g., half-lives of under 6 hours) may benefit and be more effectively controlled during chronic therapy when given products with sustained-release characteristics since these provide longer dosing intervals and/or less fluctuation in serum concentration between dosing. Those sustained-release products which provide flexibility in dosage through formulations of varying strengths are also helpful in controlling serum levels. Dosage guidelines are approximations only and the wide range of theophylline clearance between individuals (particularly those with concomitant disease) makes indiscriminate usage hazardous.
As a practical consideration, it is not always possible to obtain serum level determinations. Under such conditions, restriction of the daily dose (*in otherwise healthy adults*) to not greater than 16 mg/kg/day (of anhydrous theophylline) in divided doses will result in relatively few patients exceeding serum levels of 20 μg/ml and the resultant risk of toxicity.

Dosage Guidelines:
I. Acute Symptoms of Asthma Requiring Rapid Theophyllinization: Sustained-release products are not the treatment of choice for acute symptoms of asthma requiring rapid theophyllinization.

II. Chronic Therapy
Theophylline administration is a treatment of first choice for the management of chronic asthma (to prevent symptoms and maintain patent airways). Slow clinical titration is generally preferred to assure acceptance and safety of the medications.

Initial Dose: 16 mg/kg/24 hours or 400 mg/24 hours (whichever is less) of anhydrous theophylline in 2 or 3 divided doses at 8- or 12-hour intervals.
 THE AVERAGE INITIAL CHILDRENS' (15 to 20 kg) DOSE IS ONE Slo-bid™ Gyrocaps® 100 mg q12h.
 THE AVERAGE INITIAL CHILDRENS' (20 to 25 kg) DOSE IS ONE Slo-bid™ Gyrocaps® 100 mg AND ONE Slo-bid™ Gyrocaps® 50 mg q12h.
 THE AVERAGE INITIAL ADULT AND CHILDRENS' (over 25 kg) DOSE IS ONE Slo-bid™ Gyrocaps® 200 mg q12h.

Increasing Dose: The above dosage may be increased in approximately 25-percent increments at 2- to 3-day intervals so long as the drug is tolerated, until the maximum dose indicated in section III (below) is reached.
III. Maximum Dose of Theophylline Where the Serum Concentration is Not Measured:

WARNING: DO NOT ATTEMPT TO MAINTAIN ANY DOSE THAT IS NOT TOLERATED.
Not to exceed the following:
[See table on bottom next page].

Continued on next page

This product information was prepared in August 1984. Information concerning these products may be obtained by addressing William H. Rorer, Inc., 500 Virginia Drive, Fort Washington, PA 19034.

Rorer—Cont.

MAXIMUM DOSE WITHOUT MEASUREMENT OF SERUM CONCENTRATION

	Dose Per Interval
Children (15-20 kg)	150 mg q12h
Children (20-25 kg)	200 mg q12h
Children (25-35 kg)	250 mg q12h
Adults and Children (over 35 kg)	300 mg q12h

MINIMUM DOSE REQUIRING MEASUREMENT OF SERUM CONCENTRATION

	Dose Per Interval
Children (15-20 kg)	200 mg q12h
Children (20-30 kg)	250 mg q12h
Children (30-35 kg)	300 mg q12h
Children (35-40 kg)	350 mg q12h
Adults and Children (over 40 kg)	400 mg q12h

IV. Measurement of Serum Theophylline Concentrations During Chronic Therapy:

If the above doses are to be maintained or exceeded, serum theophylline measurement is recommended. The serum sample should be obtained at the time of peak absorption, 1 to 2 hours after administration for immediate release products and 3 to 8 hours after dosing for most sustained-release formulations. It is important that the patient will have missed *no* doses during the previous 48 hours and that dosing intervals will have been reasonably typical with no added doses during that period of time. DOSAGE ADJUSTMENT BASED ON SERUM THEOPHYLLINE MEASUREMENTS WHEN THESE INSTRUCTIONS HAVE NOT BEEN FOLLOWED MAY RESULT IN RECOMMENDATIONS THAT PRESENT RISK OF TOXICITY TO THE PATIENT.

V. Final adjustment of Dosage:
[See table above].

From the *Journal of Respiratory Diseases* 2(7):16, 1981

Caution should be exercised for younger children who cannot complain of minor side effects.

Older adults, those with cor pulmonale, congestive heart failure, and/or liver disease may have unusually low dosage requirements and thus may experience toxicity at the maximal dosage recommended above.

It is important that no patient be maintained on any dosage that is not tolerated. In instructing the patients to increase dosage according to the schedule above, they should be instructed not to take a subsequent dose if apparent side effects occur and to resume therapy at a lower dose once adverse effects have disappeared.

How Supplied: Slo-bid™ Gyrocaps® 50 mg are available in bottles of 100 (NDC 0067-0057-68), Slo-bid™ Gyrocaps® 100 mg are available in bottles of 100 (NDC 0067-0100-68) and unit dose 10 × 10 (NDC 0067-0100-01), Slo-bid™ Gyrocaps® 200 mg are available in bottles of 100 (NDC 0067-0200-68) and unit dose 10 × 10 (NDC 0067-0200-01), and Slo-bid™ Gyrocaps® 300 mg are available in bottles of 100 (NDC 0067-0300-68) and unit dose 10 × 10 (NDC 0067-0300-01).

Slo-bid™ Gyrocaps® are identified as follows:
50 mg—Clear (cap) and opaque white (body) capsule with WHR 50 mg printed in red on cap and body
100 mg—Clear capsule with WHR 100 printed in red on cap and body
200 mg—Opaque white (cap) and clear (body) capsule with WHR 200 printed in red on cap and body

Table 1—Dosage adjustment after serum theophylline measurement

If serum theophylline is:		Directions:
Within normal limits	10 to 20 μg/ml	Maintain dosage if tolerated. Recheck serum theophylline concentration at 6- to 12-month intervals.*
Too high	20 to 25 μg/ml	Decrease doses by about 10%. Recheck serum theophylline concentration at 6- to 12-month intervals.*
	25 to 30 μg/ml	Skip next dose and decrease subsequent doses by about 25%.
	Over 30 μg/ml	Skip next 2 doses and decrease subsequent doses by 50%. Recheck serum theophylline.
Too low	7.5 to 10 μg/ml	Increase dose by about 25%.** Recheck serum theophylline concentration at 6- to 12-month intervals.*
	5 to 7.5 μg/ml	Increase dose by about 25% to the nearest dose increment and recheck serum theophylline for guidance in further dosage adjustment (another increase will probably be needed, but this provides a safety check).

*Finer adjustments in dosage may be needed for some patients.
**The total daily dose may need to be administered at more frequent intervals if symptoms occur repeatedly at the end of a dosing interval.

300 mg—Opaque white capsule with WHR 300 printed in red on cap and body

Storage Conditions:
Store at room temperature. Protect from excessive heat, light, and moisture.
Caution: Federal law prohibits dispensing without a prescription.
Keep this and all medications out of the reach of children. Slo-bid™ Gyrocaps®.
Shown in Product Identification Section, page 432

SLO-PHYLLIN® ℞
(theophylline, anhydrous) SYRUP, TABLETS,
(immediate release)
GYROCAPS® (timed release capsules)
[slō″fil′in]

Description: Slo-Phyllin® Gyrocaps® contain 60 mg, 125 mg, or 250 mg theophylline, anhydrous, USP in the form of long acting dye-free beads with a hard gelatin capsule and are intended for oral administration.
Slo-Phyllin® Tablets (theophylline, anhydrous) are scored, dye-free tablets providing 100 mg or 200 mg of theophylline, anhydrous, U.S.P.
Slo-Phyllin® 80 mg Syrup (theophylline, anhydrous) is a nonalcoholic, sugar-free solution containing per 15 ml theophylline, anhydrous, U.S.P., 80 mg with sodium benzoate, N.F., 18 mg, and methylparaben, N.F., 3 mg added as preservatives. Theophylline is a bronchodilator and is a member of the xanthine class of chemical compounds related to both theobromine and caffeine.
Theophylline is a white odorless crystalline powder having a bitter taste.
Theophylline is 3,7-dihydro-1,3-dimethyl-1H-Purine-2,6-dione represented by the following structural formula:

Age	Dose per 8 hours	Dose per 12 hours
Age <9 years	24 mg/kg/day	8.0 mg/kg	12.0 mg/kg
Age 9-12 years	20 mg/kg/day	6.7 mg/kg	10.0 mg/kg
Age 12-16 years	18 mg/kg/day	6.0 mg/kg	9.0 mg/kg
Age >16 years	13 mg/kg/day	4.3 mg/kg	6.5 mg/kg
	OR 900 mg		
	(Whichever is less)		

Clinical Pharmacology: Theophylline directly relaxes the smooth muscle of the bronchial airways and pulmonary blood vessels, thus acting mainly as a bronchodilator and smooth muscle relaxant. The drug also produces other actions typical of the xanthine derivatives: cardiac stimulation, coronary vasodilatation, stimulation of skeletal muscle, cerebral stimulation, and diuresis. The action of theophylline may be mediated through inhibition of phosphodiesterase and a resultant increase in intracellular cyclic AMP. [*In vitro*, theophylline has been shown to act synergistically with beta agonists that increase intracellular cyclic AMP through the stimulation of adenyl cyclase but synergism has not been demonstrated in patient studies. More data are needed to determine if theophylline and beta agonists have a clinically important additive effect *in vivo*. Apparently, no development of tolerance occurs with chronic use of theophylline.

Pharmacokinetics: The half-life of theophylline is influenced by a number of known variables. It is prolonged in patients suffering from chronic alcoholism, impaired hepatic or renal function, congestive heart failure, and in patients receiving macrolide antibiotics and cimetidine. Older adults (over age 55) and patients with chronic obstructive pulmonary disease, with or without cor pulmonale, may also have much slower clearance rates. For such patients, the theophylline half-life may exceed 24 hours.

Newborns and neonates have extremely slow clearance rates compared to older infants (over 6 months) and children, and may also have a theophylline half-life of over 24 hours. High fever for prolonged periods may also reduce the rate of theophylline elimination.

Representative Theophylline Serum Half-Lives

	Half-Life (hours)
Adults	
non-smokers	7-9
smokers	4-5
congestive heart failure	24
Children (6 months-16 years)	3-5

The half-life of theophylline in smokers (1 to 2 packs/day) averages 4-5 hours, much shorter than the half-life in non-smokers which averages 7-9 hours. The increase in theophylline clearance caused by smoking is probably the result of induction of drug-metabolizing enzymes that do not readily normalize after cessation of smoking. It appears that between 3 months and 2 years may be necessary for normalization of the effect of smoking on theophylline pharmacokinetics.

In single-dose bioavailability studies in normal volunteers, 300 mg Slo-Phyllin® Syrup produced mean peak serum concentrations of 7.90 ± 1.67 µg/ml at a mean time of 1.43 ± 0.87 hours after dosing. At steady state in multiple dose bioavailability studies with four times a day dosing (600-1000 mg/day), the mean peak-trough variation was 4.39 ± 0.77 µg/ml.

In a single-dose bioavailability study in 20 normal subjects, sustained-release Slo-Phyllin® Gyrocaps® were compared to the immediate-release Slo-Phyllin® 80 Syrup. A dose of 250 mg Slo-Phyllin® Gyrocaps® produced a mean peak serum concentration of 4.0 ± 0.8 µg/ml at a mean time of 4.8 hours after dosing. At steady state in a multiple dose bioavailability study, Slo-Phyllin® Gyrocaps® were compared to Slo-Phyllin® 80 Syrup. Doses of 2.6 to 5.6 mg/kg (mean dose of 4.2 mg/kg) of Slo-Phyllin® Gyrocaps® were administered q8h in 17 normal subjects. The mean peak serum concentration was 17.4 ± 0.9 µg/ml and the mean trough was 10.4 ± 0.7 µg/ml. In both of these studies, subjects fasted overnight before dosing and four hours after the first dose.

A mulitple-dose bioequivalence study with 14 asthmatic children comparing Slo-Phyllis® Gyrocaps® administered as intact capsules and as the beaded contents sprinkled on applesauce with q8h dosing (125-250 mg/day) indicated no significant differences in maximum and minimum theophylline concentrations, time to achieve peak concentration, and peak-trough differences. The bioavailability as measured by comparing area under the curves (AUC$_{0-8\ hours}$ granules/AC$_{0-8\ hours}$ capsules) was 0.999 ± 0.324.

Indications and Use: For relief and/or prevention of symptoms from asthma and reversible bronchospasm associated with chronic bronchitis and emphysema.

Contraindications: Slo-Phyllin® Tablets, Syrup, and Gyrocaps® are contraindicated in individuals who have shown hypersensitivity to any of their components.

Warnings: Status asthmaticus should be considered a medical emergency and is defined as that degree of bronchospasm which is not rapidly responsive to usual doses of conventional bronchodilators. Optimal therapy for such patients frequently requires both *additional medication*, parenterally administered, and *close monitoring*, preferably in an intensive care setting. Although increasing the dose of theophylline may bring about relief, such treatment may be associated with toxicity. The likelihood of such toxicity developing increases significantly when the serum theophylline concentration exceeds 20 µg/ml. Therefore, determination of serum theophylline levels is recommended to assure maximal benefit without excessive risk.

Serum levels above 20 µg/ml are rarely found after appropriate administration of the recommended doses. However, in individuals in whom theophylline plasma clearance is reduced *for any reason*, even conventional doses may result in increased serum levels and potential toxicity. Reduced theophylline clearance has been documented in the following readily identifiable groups: 1) patients with impaired renal or liver function, 2) patients over 55 years of age, particularly males and those with chronic lung disease, 3) those with cardiac failure from any cause, 4) neonates, and 5) those patients taking certain drugs (macrolide antibiotics and cimetidine). Decreased clearance of theophylline may be associated with either influenza immunization or active infection with influenza.

Reduction of dosage and laboratory monitoring is especially appropriate in the above individuals. Less serious signs of theophylline toxicity, i.e. nausea and restlessness, may appear in up to 50% of patients.

Unfortunately, however, serious side effects such as ventricular arrhythmias, convulsions, or even death may appear as the first sign of toxicity without any previous warning. Stated differently, *serious toxicity is not reliably preceded by less severe side effects*.

Many patients who require theophylline may exhibit tachycardia due to their underlying disease process so that the cause/effect relationship to elevated serum theophylline concentrations may not be appreciated.

Theophylline products may cause dysrhythmia and/or worsen preexisting arrhythmias and any significant change in rate and/or rhythm warrants monitoring and further investigation.

The occurrence of arrhythmias and sudden death (with histological evidence of necrosis of the myocardium) has been recorded in laboratory animals (minipigs, rodents, and dogs) when theophylline and beta agonists were administered concomitantly, although not when either was administered alone. The significance of these findings when applied to human usage is currently unknown.

Precautions:
General: Mean half-life in smokers is shorter than non-smokers. Therefore, smokers may require larger or more frequent doses of theophylline. Morphine and curare should be used with caution in patients with airway obstruction as they may suppress respiration and stimulate histamine release. Alternative drugs shoud be used when possible.

Theophylline should not be administered concurrently with other xanthine preparations. Use with caution in patients with severe cardiac disease, severe hypoxemia, hypertension, hyperthyroidism, acute myocardial injury, cor pulmonale, congestive heart failure, alcoholism, liver disease, and in the elderly, especially males, and neonates. Great caution should be used in giving theophylline to patients with congestive heart failure. Frequently such patients have shown markedly prolonged theophylline blood levels with theophylline persisting in serum for long periods following discontinuation of the drug. Use theophylline cautiously in patients with a history of peptic ulcer. Theophylline may occasionally act as a local gastrointestinal irritant, although GI symptoms are more commonly centrally mediated and associated with serum drug concentrations over 20 µg/ml.

Information for Patients: The physician should reinforce the importance of taking only the prescribed dose at the prescribed time intervals. The patient should alert the physician if symptoms occur repeatedly, especially near the end of a dosing interval.

Drug Interactions: Drug-Drug: Toxic synergism with ephedrine has been documented and may occur with some other sympathomimetic bronchodilators. In addition, the following drug interactions have been demonstrated:

DRUG	EFFECT
Aminophylline with lithium carbonate	Increased excretion of lithium carbonate
Aminophylline with propranolol	Increased theophylline serum concentrations. Antagonism of propranolol effects
Theophylline with troleandomycin or erythromycin	Increased theophylline serum concentrations
Theophylline with cimetidine	Increased theophylline serum concentrations

Drug-Food: Slo-Phyllin® Gyrocaps® has not been adequately studied to determine whether its bioavailability is altered when it is given with food.

Available data suggest that drug administration at the time of food ingestion may influence the absorption characteristics of some or all theophylline controlled-release products resulting in serum values different from those found after administration in the fasting state.

A drug-food effect, if any, would likely have its greatest clinical significance when high theophylline serum levels are being maintained and/or when large single doses (greater than 13 mg/kg or 900 mg) of a controlled-release product are given. The influence of the type and amount of food on performance of controlled-release theophylline products is under study at this time.

Drug/Laboratory Test Interactions: When plasma levels of theophylline are measured by spectrophotometric methods, coffee, tea, cola beverages, chocolate, and acetaminophen contribute falsely high values.

Carcinogenesis, Mutagenesis, Impairment of Fertility: Long-term animal studies have not been performed to evaluate the carcinogenic potential, mutagenic potential, or the effect on fertility of xanthine compounds.

Pregnancy: Pregnancy Category C—Animal reproduction studies have not been conducted with theophylline. It is not known whether theophylline can cause fetal harm when administered to a pregnant woman or can affect reproduction capacity. Theophylline should be given to a pregnant woman only if clearly needed.

Nursing Mothers: It has been reported that theophylline distributes readily into breast milk and may cause adverse effects in the infant. Caution must be used if prescribing xanthines to a mother who is nursing, taking into account the risk-benefit of this therapy.

Pediatric Use: Due to the marked variation in theophylline metabolism in infants under 6 months of age, theophylline is not recommended for this age group.

Safety and effectiveness in children under 6 years of age have not been established with controlled-release theophylline products.

Adverse Reactions: The most consistent adverse reactions are usually due to overdose and are:

Gastrointestinal: nausea, vomiting, epigastric pain, hematemesis, diarrhea.

Central nervous system: headaches, irritability, restlessness, insomnia, reflex hyperexcitability, muscle twitching, clonic and tonic generalized convulsions.

Cardiovascular: palpitation, tachycardia, extrasystoles, flushing, hypotension, circulatory failure, and ventricular arrhythmias.

Respiratory: tachypnea.

Renal: albuminuria, increased excretion of renal tubular cells and red blood cells potentiation of diuresis.

Other: hyperglycemia and inappropriate ADH syndrome and rash.

Overdosage:
Management: A. If potential oral overdose is established and seizure has not occurred
1. Induce vomiting
2. Administer a cathartic (this is particularly important if sustained release preparations have been taken)
3. Administer activated charcoal
4. Monitor vital signs, maintain blood pressure, and provide adequate hydration
B. If patient is having a seizure:
1. Establish an airway
2. Administer oxygen
3. Treat the seizure with intravenous diazepam 0.1 to 0.3 mg/kg up to a total dose of 10 mg
4. Monitor vital signs, maintain blood pressure and provide adequate hydration
C. Post-seizure Coma:
1. Maintain airway and oxygenation
2. If a result of oral medication, follow above recommendations to prevent absorption of drug, but intubation and lavage will have to be performed instead of inducing emesis and the ca-

Continued on next page

This product information was prepared in August 1984. Information concerning these products may be obtained by addressing William H. Rorer, Inc., 500 Virginia Drive, Fort Washington, PA 19034.

Rorer—Cont.

thartic and charcoal will need to be introduced via a large bore gastric lavage tube.
3. Continue to provide full supportive care and adequate hydration while waiting for drug to be metabolized. In general, the drug is metabolized sufficiently rapidly so as to not warrant consideration of dialysis. However, if serum levels exceed 50 µg/ml, charcoal hemoperfusion may be indicated.

Dosage and Administration: Studies to determine the bioavailability of Slo-Phyllin® Gyrocaps® when administered with food are being initiated. (See PRECAUTIONS, Drug-Food Interactions.)

For most patients, *effective use* of theophylline, i.e. associated with optimal likelihood of benefit combined with minimal risk of toxicity, is considered to occur when serum levels are maintained between 10 and 20 µg/ml. Levels above 20 µg/ml may produce toxicity, and in a small number of patients, toxicity may even be seen with serum levels between 15–20 µg/ml, particularly during initiation of therapy.

There is considerable variation from patient to patient in the dosage required to achieve and maintain therapeutic and safe levels, primarily due to variable rates of elimination. Therefore, it is essential that not only must dosage be individualized, but titration and monitoring of serum levels be utilized where available. When serum concentration cannot be obtained, restriction of dosage to the amounts and intervals recommended in the guidelines listed below becomes essential. Dosage should be calculated on the basis of lean (ideal) body weight where mg/kg doses are presented. Theophylline does not distribute into fatty tissue. Giving immediate-release theophylline with food may prevent some local gastric irritation and though absorption is slower, it is still complete.

Frequency of Dosing: When immediate-release products with rapid absorption (such as tablets or liquid) are used, dosing to maintain serum levels generally requires administration every 6 hours. This is particularly true in children, but dosing intervals up to 8 hours may be satisfactory in adults since they eliminate the drug at a slower rate. Some children, and adults requiring higher than average doses (those having rapid rates of clearance, e.g. half-lifes of under 6 hours) may benefit and be more effectively controlled during chronic therapy when given products with sustained-release characteristics since these provide longer dosing intervals and/or less fluctuation in serum concentration between dosing. Those sustained release products which provide flexibility in dosage through formulations of varying strengths are also helpful in controlling serum levels. Dosage guidelines are approximations only and the wide range of theophylline clearance between individuals (particularly those with concomitant disease) make indiscriminate usage hazardous.

As a practical consideration, it is not always possible to obtain serum level determinations. Under such conditions, restriction of the daily dose (*in otherwise healthy adults*) to not greater than 13 mg/kg/day (or up to 900 mg) of anhydrous theophylline in divided doses will result in relatively few patients exceeding serum levels of 20 µg/ml and the resultant risk of toxicity.

Warning: do not attempt to maintain any dose that is not tolerated. Not to exceed the following:

Age			Dose per 8 hours	Dose per 12 hours
Age	6–9 years	24 mg/kg/day	8.0 mg/kg	12.0 mg/kg
Age	9–12 years	20 mg/kg/day	6.7 mg/kg	10.0 mg/kg
Age	12–16 years	18 mg/kg/day	6.0 mg/kg	9.0 mg/kg
Age	over 16 years	13 mg/kg/day OR 900 mg (WHICHEVER IS LESS)	4.3 mg/kg	6.5 mg/kg

Dosage Guidelines:
Slo-Phyllin® Gyrocaps®

I. Acute Symptoms

Slo-Phyllin® Gyrocaps® are not intended for patients experiencing an acute episode of bronchospasm (associated with asthma, chronic bronchitis, or emphysema). Such patients require *rapid* relief of symptoms and should be treated with an immediate-release or intravenous theophylline preparation (or other bronchodilators) and not with controlled release products.

II. Chronic Therapy

A. Initiating Therapy with an Immediate-Release Product

It is recommended that the appropriate dosage be established using an immediate-release preparation. Children weighing less than 25 kg should have their daily dosage requirements established with Slo-Phyllin® 80 Syrup to permit small dosage increments. Slow clinical titration is generally preferred to help assure acceptance and safety of the medication. Then, if the total 24-hour dose can be given by use of the sustained-release product, the patient can usually be switched to Slo-Phyllin® Gyrocaps®, giving one-third of the daily dose at 8-hour intervals or one-half the daily dose at 12-hour intervals. Patients who metabolize theophylline rapidly, such as the young, smokers, and some non-smoking adults are the most likely candidates for dosing at 8-hour intervals. Such patients can generally be identified as having trough serum concentrations lower than desired, or repeatedly exhibiting symptoms near the end of a dosing interval.

B. Initiating Therapy with Slo-Phyllin® Gyrocaps®

Alternatively, therapy can be initiated with Slo-Phyllin® Gyrocaps® since they are available in dosage strengths which permit titration and adjustments of dosage (in adults and older children).

Initial Dose:

16 mg/kg/24 hours of 400 mg/24 hours (whichever is less) of anhydrous theophylline in 2- or 3-divided doses at 8- or 12-hour intervals.

Increasing Dose:

The above dosage may be increased in approximately 25-percent increments at 3-day intervals so long as the drug is tolerated, until the maximum dose indicated in section III (below) is reached.

C. Sprinkling Contents on Food

Slo-Phyllin® Gyrocaps® may be administered by carefully opening the capsule and sprinkling the beaded contents on a spoonful of soft food such as applesauce; the soft food should be swallowed immediately without chewing and followed with a glass of cool water or juice to ensure complete swallowing of the beads. It is recommended that the food used should not be hot and should be soft enought to be swallowed without chewing. Any bead/food mixture should be used immediately and not stored for future use. Until additional bioavailability data are available, it is recommended that dosing using the sprinkling technique be at intervals up to 8 hours. It is recommended that dosing not take place at mealtime until a study is completed to show the effect of taking Slo-Phyllin® Gyrocaps® with food as compared to the fasting state.

III. Maximum Dose of Theophylline Where the Serum Concentration is Not Measured:
[See table below].

Slo-Phyllis® Tablets and Syrup

1. Acute Symptoms of Asthma Requiring Rapid Theophyllinization.

A. Patients not currently receiving theophylline products. Dosage recommendations are for theophylline anhydrous.

	Oral Loading:	Followed By:	Maintenance:
Children 6 months to 9 years	6 mg/kg	4 mg/kg q4 hrs × 3 doses	4 mg/kg q6 hrs
Children age 9–16 years and young adult smokers	6 mg/kg	3 mg/kg q4 hrs × 3 doses	3 mg/kg q9 hrs
Otherwise healthy non-smoking adults	6 mg/kg	3 mg/kg q6 hrs × 2 doses	3 mg/kg q8 hrs
Older patients and patients with cor pulmonale	6 mg/kg	2 mg/kg q6 hrs × 2 doses	2 mg/kg q8 hrs
Patients with congestive heart failure	6 mg/kg	2 mg/kg q8 hrs × 2 doses	1–2 mg/kg q12 hrs

B. Patients currently receiving theophylline products:

Determine, where possible, the time, amount, dosage form, and route of administration of the patient's last dose.

The loading dose for theophylline is based on the principle that each 0.5 mg/kg of theophylline administered as a loading dose will result in a 1.0 µg/ml increase in serum theophylline concentration. Ideally, the loading dose should be deferred if a serum theophylline concentration can be obtained rapidly.

If this is not possible, the clinician must exercise his judgment in selecting a dose based on the potential for benefit and risk. Where there is sufficient respiratory distress to warrant a small risk, then 2.5 mg/kg of theophylline administered in rapidly absorbed form is likely to increase serum concentration by approximately 5 µg/ml. If the patient is not experiencing theophylline toxicity, this is likely to result in dangerous adverse affects. Subsequent to the decision regarding modification of the loading dose for this group of patients, the maintenance dosage recommendations are the same as those described above.

II. Chronic Therapy

Theophylline administration is a treatment of first choice for the management of chronic asthma (to prevent symptoms and maintain patent airways). Slow clinical titration is generally preferred to assure acceptance and safety of the medications.

Initial Dose: 16 mg/kg/24 hours or 400 mg/24 hours (whichever is less) of anhydrous theophylline in 3- to 4-divided doses at 6- or 8-hour intervals.

Increasing Dose: The above dosage may be increased in approximately 25-percent increments at 2- to 3-day intervals so long as the drug is tolerated, until the maximum dose indicated in section III (below) is reached.

III. Maximum Dose of Theophylline Where the Serum Concentration is Not Measured:

WARNING: DO NOT ATTEMPT TO MAINTAIN ANY DOSE THAT IS NOT TOLERATED.

Not to exceed the following:

		Dose per 6 hours	Dose per 8 hours
Age <9 years	24 mg/kg/day	6.0 mg/kg	8.0 mg/kg
Age 9–12 years	20 mg/kg/day	5.0 mg/kg	6.7 mg/kg
Age 12–16 years	18 mg/kg/day	4.5 mg/kg	6.0 mg/kg

Age >16
years 13 mg/kg/day   3.5 mg/kg   4.3 mg/kg
OR 900 mg
(WHICHEVER IS LESS)

Measurement of Serum Theophylline Concentrations During Chronic Therapy:
If the above maximum doses are to be maintained or exceeded, serum theophylline measurement is recommended. The serum sample should be obtained at the time of peak absorption, 1 to 2 hours after administration for immediate-release Slo-Phyllin® products and 4 hours after dosing for Slo-Phyllin® Gyrocaps®. It is important that the patient will have missed *no* doses during the previous 48 hours and that dosing intervals will have been reasonably typical with no added doses during that period of time. DOSAGE ADJUSTMENT BASED ON SERUM THEOPHYLLINE MEASUREMENTS WHEN THESE INSTRUCTIONS HAVE NOT BEEN FOLLOWED MAY RESULT IN RECOMMENDATIONS THAT PRESENT RISK OF TOXICITY TO THE PATIENT.

Final Adjustment of Dosage: (see Table 1)
Table 1—Dosage adjustment after serum theophylline measurement

If serum theophylline is:		Directions:
Within normal limits	10 to 20 µg/ml	Maintain dosage if tolerated. Recheck serum theophylline concentration at 6- to 12-month intervals.*
Too high	20 to 25 µg/ml	Decrease doses by about 10%. Recheck serum theophylline concentration at 6- to 12-month intervals.*
	25 to 30 µg/ml	Skip next dose and decrease subsequent doses by about 25%.
	Over 30 µg/ml	Skip next 2 doses and decrease subsequent doses by 50%. Recheck serum theophylline.
Too low	7.5 to 10 µg/ml	Increase dose by about 25%.** Recheck serum theophylline concentration at 6- to 12-month intervals.*
	5 to 7.5 µg/ml	Increase dose by about 25% to the nearest dose increment and recheck serum theophylline for guidance in future dosage adjustment (another increase will probably be needed, but this provides a safety check)

*Finer adjustments in dosage may be needed for some patients
**The total daily dose may need to be administered at more frequent intervals if symptoms occur repeatedly at the end of dosing interval.
† From the *Journal of Respiratory Diseasees* 2(7):16, 1981

Caution should be exercised for younger children who cannot complain of minor side effects. Older adults, those with cor pulmonale, congestive heart failure, and/or liver disease may have unusually low dosage requirements and thus may experience toxicity at the maximal dosage recommended above. It is important that no patient be maintained on any dosage that is not tolerated. In instructing the patients to increase dosage according to the schelule above, they should be instructed not to take a subsequent dose if apparent side effects occur and to resume therapy at a lower dose once adverse effects have disappeared.

How Supplied: Slo-Phyllin® 100 mg Tablets (theophylline, anhydrous) scored, dye-free, white, round, convex tablet, imprinted "WHR 351" in bottles of 100 (NDC-0067-0351-68) and 1000 (NDC-0067-0351-82), and in unit dose packages of 100 tablets (NDC-0067-0351-01).
Slo-Phyllin® 200 mg Tablets (theophylline, anhydrous), scored, dye-free, white, flat faced tablet, imprinted "WHR 352" in bottles of 100 (NDC-0067-0352-68) and 1000 (NDC-0067-0352-82), and in unit dose packages of 100 tablets (NDC 0067-0352-01).
Slo-Phyllin® 80 mg Syrup theophylline, anhydrous 80 mg per 15 ml nonalcoholic, orange color in 4 fl oz (NDC-0067-0354-60), pint (NDC-0067-0354-16) and gallon (NDC-0067-0354-28) bottles, and 15 ml unit dose cups (NDC-0067-0354-15).
Slo-Phyllin® Gyrocaps® 60 mg are available in bottles of 100 (NDC-0067-1354-68) and 1000 (NDC-0067-1354-82). Slo-Phyllin® Gyrocaps® 125 mg are available in bottles of 100 (NDC-0067-1355-68), 1000 (NDC-0067-1355-82) and unit dose strip packages (NDC-0067-1355-01). Slo-Phyllin® Gyrocaps® 250 mg are available in bottles of 100 (NDC-0067-1356-68), 1000 (NDC-0067-1356-82) and unit dose strip packages (NDC-0067-1356-01).
Slo-Phyllin® Gyrocaps® are identified as follows:
60 mg—white capsule with WHR 1354 printed in black on body and cap, containing dye-free beads
125 mg—brown capsule with WHR 1355 printed in white on body and cap, containing dye-free beads.
250 mg—purple capsule with WHR 1356 printed in white on body and cap, containing dye-free beads.

Storage Conditions: Store at room temperature. Protect from excessive heat, light, and moisture.
Caution: Federal law prohibits dispensing without prescription.
Keep this and all medications out of the reach of children.
Slo-Phyllin® Gyrocaps® are manufactured by
CORD LABORATORIES, INC.
Broomfield, CO 80020
For
WILLIAM H. RORER, INC.
Fort Washington, PA 19034
Slo-Phyllin® Tablets and Syrup are manufactured by
WILLIAM H. RORER, INC.
Fort Washington, PA 19034
Shown in Product Identification Section, page 432

SLO–PHYLLIN® GG CAPSULES, ℞
SYRUP, Rorer
[slō″ fil′ in]
(theophylline, anhydrous with guaifenesin)

Description: Each **Slo-Phyllin® GG** soft gelatin capsule or tablespoonful (15 ml) of liquid contains 150 mg of theophylline (anhydrous) and 90 mg of guaifenesin, as an oral bronchodilator-expectorant. Theophylline (1, 3-dimethylxanthine), a xanthine compound, is a white, odorless crystalline powder, having a bitter taste.
Guaifenesin (3-[2-methoxyphenoxy] 1,2-propanediol), a guaiacol compound, is a white to slightly yellow crystalline powder with a bitter, aromatic taste.

Slo-Phyllin GG
Theophylline Elimination Characteristics

	Theophylline Clearance Rates (mean±S.D.)	Half-life Average (mean±S.D.)
Children (over 6 months of age):	1.45±.58 ml/kg/min	3.7±1.1 hours
Adult non-smokers with uncomplicated asthma:	.65±.19 ml/kg/min	8.7±2.2 hours

Clinical Pharmacology:
Theophylline: Theophylline directly relaxes the smooth muscle of the bronchial airways and pulmonary blood vessels, thus acting mainly as a bronchodilator, pulmonary vasodilator and smooth muscle relaxant. The drug also possesses other actions typical of the xanthine derivatives: coronary vasodilator, diuretic, cardiac stimulant, cerebral stimulant, and skeletal muscle stimulant. The actions of theophylline may be mediated through inhibition of phosphodiesterase and a resultant increase in intracellular cyclic AMP, which could mediate smooth muscle relaxation. At concentrations higher than attained in vivo, theophylline also inhibits the release of histamine by mast cells.
In vitro, theophylline has been shown to react synergistically with beta agonists that increase intracellular cyclic AMP through the stimulation of adenyl cyclase (isoproterenol), but synergism has not been demonstrated in patient studies and more data are needed to determine if theophylline and beta agonists have clinically important additive effects **in vivo**. Apparently, no development of tolerance occurs with chronic use of theophylline. The half-life is shortened with cigarette smoking. The half-life is prolonged in alcoholism, reduced hepatic or renal function, congestive heart failure, and in patients receiving antibiotics such as TAO (troleandomycin), erthromycin and clindamycin. High fever for prolonged periods may decrease theophylline elimination.
[See table above].
Newborn infants have extremely slow clearances and theophylline half-lives exceeding 24 hours which approach those seen for older children after about 3-6 months. Older adults with chronic obstructive pulmonary disease, any patients with cor pulmonale or other causes of heart failure, and patients with liver pathology may have much lower clearances with half-lives that may exceed 24 hours.
The half-life of theophylline in smokers (1 to 2 packs/day) averaged 4 to 5 hours among various studies, much shorter than the half-life in non-smokers who averaged about 7 to 9 hours. The increase in theophylline clearance caused by smoking is probably the result of induction of drug-metabolizing enzymes that do not readily normalize after cessation of smoking. It appears that between 3 months and 2 years may be necessary for normalization of the effect of smoking on theophylline pharmacokinetics.
Guaifenesin: Guaifenesin increases respiratory tract secretions, possibly by stimulating the Goblet cells. Guaifenesin appears to be well absorbed, but its pharmacokinetics have not been thoroughly studied.
Indications and Usage: For relief and/or prevention of symptoms of asthma and reversible bronchospasm associated with chronic bronchitis and emphysema.
Contraindications: In individuals who have shown hypersensitivity to any of its components.
Warnings: Status asthmaticus is a medical emergency. Optimal therapy frequently requires additional medication including corticosteroids

Continued on next page

This product information was prepared in August 1984. Information concerning these products may be obtained by addressing William H. Rorer, Inc., 500 Virginia Drive, Fort Washington, PA 19034.

Rorer—Cont.

when the patient is not rapidly responsive to bronchodilators.

Excessive theophylline doses may be associated with toxicity. Therefore, monitoring of serum theophylline levels is recommended to assure maximal benefit without excessive risk. Incidence of toxicity increases at levels greater than 20 μg/ml. Morphine, curare, and stilbamidine should be used with caution in patients with airflow obstruction since they stimulate histamine release and can induce asthmatic attacks. They may also suppress respiration leading to respiratory failure. Alternative drugs should be chosen whenever possible.

There is an excellent correlation between high blood levels of theophylline resulting from conventional doses and associated clinical manifestations of toxicity in (1) patients with lowered body plasma clearances (due to transient cardiac decompensation), (2) patients with liver dysfunction or chronic obstructive lung disease, (3) patients who are older than 55 years of age, particularly males.

There are often no early signs of less serious theophylline toxicity such as nausea and restlessness, which may appear in up to 50 percent of patients prior to onset of convulsions. Ventricular arrhythmias or seizures may be the first signs of toxicity.

Many patients who have higher theophylline serum levels exhibit tachycardia.

Theophylline products may worsen pre-existing arrhythmias.

Precautions:
General: Theophylline.

Mean half-life in smokers is shorter than non-smokers, therefore, smokers may require larger doses of theophylline. Theophylline should not be administered concurrently with other xanthine medications. Use with caution in patients with severe cardiac disease, severe hypoxemia, hypertension, hyperthyroidism, acute myocardial injury, cor pulmonale, congestive heart failure, liver disease, and in the'elderly (especially males) and in neonates. Great caution should especially be used in giving theophylline to patients in congestive heart failure. Such patients have shown markedly prolonged theophylline blood level curves with theophylline persisting in serum for long periods following discontinuation of the drug.

Use theophylline cautiously in patients with history of peptic ulcer. Theophylline may occasionally act as a local irritant to the G.I. tract although gastrointestinal symptoms are more commonly central and associated with serum concentrations over 20 μg/ml.

Drug Interactions: Toxic synergism with ephedrine has been documented and may occur with some other sympathomimetic bronchodilators.

DRUG	EFFECT
Aminophylline with lithium carbonate	Increased excretion of lithium carbonate
Aminophylline with propranolol	Antagonism of propranolol effect
Theophylline with Cimetidine	Increased theophylline blood levels
Theophylline with furosemide	Increased diuresis of furosemide
Theophylline with hexamethonium	Decreased hexamethonium-induced chronotropic effect
Theophylline with reserpine	Reserpine-induced tachycardia
Theophylline with chlordiazepoxide	Chlordiazepoxide-induced fatty acid mobilization
Theophylline with Cyclamycin (TAO= troleandomycin): erythromycin, clindamycin, lincomycin	Increased theophylline plasma levels

Drug Laboratory Test Interactions: Theophylline may increase uric acid levels and urinary catecholamines. Metabolites of guaifenesin may contribute to increased urinary 5-hydroxy-indoleacetic acid readings, when determined with nitrosonaphthol reagent.

Carcinogenicity:
Studies have shown that theophylline exhibits no carcinogenic effects on animals or humans.

Usage in Pregnancy:
Teratogenic effects:
Pregnancy Category C—Animal reproduction studies have not been conducted with **Slo-Phyllin® GG**. It is also not known whether **Slo-Phyllin® GG** can cause fetal harm when administered to a pregnant woman or can affect reproduction capacity. Therefore, it should be given to a pregnant woman only if clearly needed.

Nonteratogenic effects:
Theophylline may be excreted in the milk and cause irritability in the nursing infant. Therefore, caution should be exercised when **Slo-Phyllin® GG** is administered to a nursing mother.

Adverse Reactions: The frequency of adverse reactions is related to serum theophylline levels and is usually not a problem at levels below 20 μg/ml. The most consistent adverse reactions are usually due to overdosage, and while all have not been reported with **Slo-Phyllin® GG**, the following reactions may be considered when theophylline is administered. Central nervous system: clonic and tonic generalized convulsions, muscle twitching, reflex hyperexcitability, headaches, insomnia, restlessness, and irritability. Cardiovascular: circulatory failure, life threatening ventricular arrhythmias, hypotension, extrasystoles, tachycardia, palpitation, and flushing. Gastrointestinal: hematemesis, vomiting, diarrhea, epigastric pain, and nausea. Renal: increased excretion of renal tubular cells and red blood cells, albuminuria, and potentiation of diuresis. Respiratory: tachypnea. Others: hyperglycemia and inappropriate ADH syndrome.

Overdosage:
Symptoms
Nervousness, agitation, headache, insomnia, vomiting, tachycardia, extrasystoles, hyper-reflexia, fasciculations and clonic and tonic convulsions. Children may be particularly prone to restlessness and hyperactivity that can proceed to convulsions.

Management
A. If potential oral overdose is established and seizure has not occurred.
  1. Induce vomiting.
  2. Administer a cathartic (this is particularly important if sustained release preparations have been taken).
  3. Administer activated charcoal.
  4. Monitor vital signs, maintain blood pressure and provide adequate hydration.
B. If patient is having a seizure.
  1. Establish an airway.
  2. Administer O_2.
  3. Treat the seizure with intravenous diazepam 0.1 to 0.3 mg/kg up to 10 mg.
  4. Monitor vital signs, maintain blood pressure and provide adequate hydration.
C. Post-seizure coma.
  1. Maintain airway and oxygenation.
  2. If a result of oral medication, follow above recommendations to prevent absorption of drug, but intubation and lavage will have to be performed instead of inducing emesis and the cathartic and charcoal will need to be introduced via a large bore gastric lavage tube.
  3. Continue to provide full supportive care and adequate hydration while waiting for drug to be metabolized. In general, the drug is metabolized sufficiently rapidly enough so as to not warrant consideration of dialysis.
D. Animal studies suggest that phenobarbital may decrease theophylline toxicity. There are as yet, however, insufficient data to recommend pretreatment of an overdosage with phenobarbital.

General
The oral LD_{50} of the theophylline in mice is 350 mg/kg. The oral LD_{50} of guaifenesin in mice is 1725 mg/kg. In humans, adverse reactions often occur when serum theophylline levels exceed 20 μg/ml. Information of physiological variables which influence excretion of theophylline can be found under the heading "Clinical Pharmacology."

Dosage and Administration:
General
Therapeutic serum levels associated with optimal likelihood for benefit and minimal risk of toxicity are considered to be between 10 μg/ml and 20 μg/ml. Levels above 20 μg/ml may produce toxic effects. There is great variation from patient to patient in dosage needed in order to achieve a therapeutic blood level because of variable rates of elimination. Because of this wide variation from patient to patient and the relatively narrow therapeutic blood level range, dosage must be individualized and monitoring of serum theophylline levels is highly recommended.

Dosage should be calculated on the basis of lean (ideal) body weight where mg/kg doses are stated. Theophylline does not distribute into fatty tissue. Giving theophylline with food may prevent the rare case of stomach irritation and, although absorption may be slower, it is still complete.

When rapidly absorbed products such as solutions and soft gelatin capsules with rapid dissolution are used, dosing to maintain "around the clock" blood levels generally requires administration every 6 hours to obtain the greatest efficacy for clinical use in children; dosing intervals up to 8 hours may be satisfactory for adults because of their slower elimination. Children and adults requiring higher than average doses may benefit from products with slower absorption which may allow longer dosing intervals and/or less fluctuation in serum concentration over a dosing interval during chronic therapy.

Acute symptoms of asthma requiring rapid theophyllinization
Note: Due to their slower rate of absorption, sustained release theophylline products are not designed for use in conditions requiring rapid theophyllinization.
I. Not currently receiving theophylline products. [See table left]
II. Those currently receiving theophylline prod-

Slo-Phyllin GG Group	Oral Loading Dose (Theophylline)	Maintenance Dose for Next 12 hrs. (Theophylline)	Maintenance Dose Beyond 12 hrs. (Theophylline)
1. Children 6 months to 9 years	6 mg/kg	4 mg/kg q4hrs.	4 mg/kg q6hrs
2. Children 9–16 and young adult smokers	6 mg/kg	3 mg/kg q4hrs.	3 mg/kg q6hrs
3. Otherwise healthy non-smoking adults	6 mg/kg	3 mg/kg q6hrs	3 mg/kg q8hrs
4. Older patients and patients with cor pulmonale	6 mg/kg	2 mg/kg q6hrs	2 mg/kg q8hrs
5. Patients with congestive heart failure, liver failure	6 mg/kg	2 mg/kg q8hrs	1–2 mg/kg q12hrs

Body Weight		Dosage of Slo-Phyllin® GG Syrup Calculated at Approximately:		
Expressed in Kilos	Lbs	3mg Per Kilo	4mg Per Kilo	5mg Per Kilo
9	20	½ tsp	¾ tsp	1 tsp
18	40	1 tsp	1½ tsp	2 tsp
27	60	1½ tsp	2 tsp	2¾ tsp
36	79	2 tsp	3 tsp	3½ tsp
45	99	2¾ tsp	3½ tsp	4½ tsp
54	118	3¼ tsp	4½ tsp	5½ tsp

Administered every six (6) hours.

ucts: Determine, where possible, the time, amount, route of administration and form of the patient's last dose.

The loading dose for theophylline will be based on the principle that each .5 mg/kg of theophylline administered as a loading dose will result in a 1 µg/ml increase in serum theophylline concentration. Ideally, then, the loading dose should be deferred if a serum theophylline concentration can be rapidly obtained. If this is not possible, the clinician must exercise his judgment in selecting a dose based on the potential of benefit to risk. When there is sufficient respiratory distress to warrant a small risk, 2.5 mg/kg of theophylline is likely to increase the serum concentration when administered as a loading dose in rapidly absorbed form by only about 5 µg/ml. If the patient is not already experiencing theophylline toxicity, this is unlikely to result in dangerous adverse effects.

Once the determination is made regarding the loading dose in this group of patients, subsequent maintenance dosage recommendations are the same as those described above.

Comments: To achieve optimal therapeutic theophylline dosage, it is recommended that serum theophylline concentrations be monitored. However, it is not always possible or practical to obtain a serum theophylline level. Patients should be closely monitored for signs of toxicity. The present data suggest that the above dosage recommendations will achieve therapeutic serum concentrations with minimal risk of toxicity for most patients.

However, some risk of toxic serum concentration is still present. Adverse reactions to theophylline often occur when serum theophylline levels exceed 20 µg/ml.

Chronic Asthma: Theophyllinization is a treatment of first choice for the management of chronic asthma (to prevent symptoms and maintain patent airways). Slow clinical titration is generally preferred to assure acceptance and safety of the medication.

Initial dose: 16 mg/kg/day or 400 mg/day (whichever is lower) in 3 to 4 divided doses at 6 to 8 hour intervals for the Syrup and Capsules.

Increased dose: The above dosage may be increased in approximately 25 percent increments at 2 to 3 day intervals so long as no intolerance is observed, until the maximum indicated below is reached.

Maximum dose without measurement of serum concentration:
Not to exceed the following: (WARNING: DO NOT ATTEMPT TO MAINTAIN ANY DOSE THAT IS NOT TOLERATED.)
Age 6 months to 9 years .... 24 mg/kg/day
Age 9 to 12 years .... 20 mg/kg/day
Age 12 to 16 years .... 18 mg/kg/day
Age > 16 years .... 13 mg/kg/day or 900 mg/day (WHICHEVER IS LESS)

Note: Use ideal body weight for obese patients.

Measurement of serum theophylline concentration during chronic therapy:
If the above maximum doses are to be maintained or exceeded, serum theophylline measurement is recommended. This should be obtained at the approximate time of peak absorption during chronic therapy for the product used (1 to 2 hours for liquids, soft gelatin capsules, and plain uncoated tablets that undergo rapid dissolution, 3 to 5 hours for sustained release preparations). It is important that the patient will have missed no doses during the previous 48 hours and that dosing intervals will have been reasonably typical with no added doses during that period of time. **DOSAGE ADJUSTMENT BASED ON SERUM THEOPHYLLINE MEASUREMENTS WHEN THESE INSTRUCTIONS HAVE NOT BEEN FOLLOWED MAY RESULT IN RECOMMENDATIONS THAT PRESENT RISK OF TOXICITY TO THE PATIENT.**

Final Dosage Adjustment: Caution should be exercised for younger children who cannot complain of minor side effects. Older adults, those with cor pulmonale, congestive heart failure, and/or liver disease may have unusually low dosage requirements and thus may experience toxicity at the maximal dosage recommended above.

It is important that no patient be maintained on any dosage that he is not tolerating. In instructing patients to increase dosage according to the schedule above, they should be instructed not to take a subsequent dose if apparent side effects occur and to resume therapy at a lower dose once adverse effects have disappeared.

[See table above].

KEEP THIS AND ALL MEDICATION OUT OF THE REACH OF CHILDREN. In case of accidental overdose, seek professional assistance or contact a poison control center immediately.

Supplied:
Slo-Phyllin® GG Syrup is lemon-vanilla flavored, nonalcoholic, dye-free, and each 15 ml tablespoonful contains theophylline, anhydrous 150 mg and guaifenesin 90 mg. Available in 16 oz. bottles (NDC 0067-0357-16).

Slo-Phyllin® GG Capsules are white, liquid filled, and each soft gelatin capsule contains theophylline, anhydrous 150 mg and guaifenesin 90 mg. Available in bottles of 100 capsules (NDC 0067-2358-68).

Slo-Phyllin® GG Capsules
Manufactured by
R. P. Scherer Corporation
Detroit, MI 48226
For
William H. Rorer, Inc.

Slo-Phyllin® GG Capsules Shown in Product Identification Section, page 432

Ross Laboratories
COLUMBUS, OH 43216

ADVANCE®
[ad-vans¹]
Nutritional Beverage

Usage: As a fortified milk/soy-based feeding more appropriate than 2% lowfat milk for feeding older babies and toddlers.

Availability:
Concentrated Liquid: 13-fl-oz cans; 12 per case; No. 3313.
Ready To Feed: 32-fl-oz cans; 6 per case; No. 3301.
Preparation: Standard dilution (16 Cal/fl oz) is one part Concentrated Liquid to one part water. Ready To Feed requires no dilution.
For hospital use, prebottled ADVANCE is available in the Ross Hospital Formula System.
Composition: Concentrated Liquid
Ingredients: ⒹD Water, corn syrup, nonfat milk, soy oil, soy protein isolate, corn oil, mono- and diglycerides, soy lecithin, minerals (calcium phosphate tribasic, potassium citrate, magnesium chloride, ferrous sulfate, zinc sulfate, cupric sulfate, manganese sulfate), vitamins (ascorbic acid, alpha-tocopheryl acetate, niacinamide, calcium pantothenate, vitamin A palmitate, thiamine chloride hydrochloride, pyridoxine hydrochloride, riboflavin, folic acid, phylloquinone, vitamin D₃, cyanocobalamin), carrageenan and taurine.

Nutrients (wt/liter):	Concentrated		Standard Dilution*	
Protein	40.0	g	20.0	g
Fat	54.0	g	27.0	g
Carbohydrate	110.0	g	55.0	g
Minerals (Ash)	7.0	g	3.5	g
Calcium	1020	mg	510	mg
Phosphorus	780	mg	390	mg
Magnesium	128	mg	64	mg
Iron	24	mg	12	mg
Iodine	120	mcg	60	mcg
Zinc	10	mg	5.0	mg
Copper	1.2	mg	0.6	mg
Manganese	68	mcg	34	mcg
Sodium	460	mg	230	mg
Potassium	1800	mg	900	mg
Chloride	1040	mg	520	mg
Water	843	g	920	g
Crude Fiber	0	g		
Calories per fl oz	32		16	
Calories per liter	1080		540	

Vitamins Per Liter (Standard Dilution*)
Vitamin A	2000	I.U.
Vitamin D	400	I.U.
Vitamin E	20	I.U.
Vitamin K₁	55	mcg
Vitamin C	50	mg
Thiamine (Vit. B₁)	0.75	mg
Riboflavin (Vit. B₂)	0.90	mg
Vitamin B₆	0.60	mg
Vitamin B₁₂	2.5	mcg
Niacin	10	mg
Folic Acid	100	mcg
Pantothenic Acid	4.0	mg

*Standard dilution is equal amounts Concentrated Liquid and water.
(FAN 341-01)

Composition: Ready To Feed
Ingredients: ⒹD Water, corn syrup, nonfat milk, soy oil, soy protein isolate, corn oil, mono- and diglycerides, soy lecithin, minerals (calcium phosphate tribasic, potassium citrate, magnesium chloride, ferrous sulfate, zinc sulfate, cupric sulfate, manganese sulfate), vitamins (ascorbic acid, alpha-tocopheryl acetate, niacinamide, calcium pantothenate, vitamin A palmitate, thiamine chloride hydrochloride, pyridoxine hydrochloride, riboflavin, folic acid, phylloquinone, vitamin D₃, cyanocobalamin), carrageenan and taurine.

Nutrients (wt/liter):		
Protein	20.0	g
Fat	27.0	g
Carbohydrate	55.0	g
Minerals (Ash)	3.5	g
Calcium	510	mg
Phosphorus	390	mg
Magnesium	64	mg
Iron	12	mg
Iodine	60	mcg
Zinc	5.0	mg
Copper	0.6	mg
Manganese	34	mcg
Sodium	230	mg
Potassium	900	mg
Chloride	520	mg
Water	920	g
Crude Fiber	0	g
Calories per fl oz	16	
Calories per liter	540	

Vitamins Per Liter:
Vitamin A	2000	I.U.

Continued on next page

Ross—Cont.

Vitamin D	400	I.U.
Vitamin E	20	I.U.
Vitamin K$_1$	55	mcg
Vitamin C	50	mg
Thiamine (Vit. B$_1$)	0.75	mg
Riboflavin (Vit. B$_2$)	0.90	mg
Vitamin B$_6$	0.60	mg
Vitamin B$_{12}$	2.5	mcg
Niacin	10	mg
Folic Acid	100	mcg
Pantothenic Acid	4.0	mg

The addition of iron to this beverage conforms to the recommendation of the Committee on Nutrition of the American Academy of Pediatrics.
(FAN 341-01)

CLEAR EYES®   OTC
Eye Drops

Description: Clear Eyes is a sterile isotonic buffered solution containing naphazoline hydrochloride 0.012%, boric acid, sodium borate, and water. Edetate disodium 0.1% and benzalkonium chloride 0.01% are added as preservatives. (Contains vasoconstrictor.)

Indications: Clear Eyes is a decongestant ophthalmic solution specially designed to soothe as it removes redness from eyes irritated due to swimming, plant allergies (pollen), overindulgence, colds, smog, sun glare, wind, dust, wearing contact lenses, and eyestrain from reading, driving, TV and close work. Clear Eyes contains laboratory tested, and scientifically blended ingredients including an effective vasoconstrictor which narrows swollen blood vessels and rapidly whitens reddened eyes in a formulation which produces a refreshing, soothing effect. Clear Eyes is a sterile, isotonic solution compatible with the natural fluids of the eye.

Warning: Clear Eyes should only be used for minor eye irritations.
Clear Eyes should not be used by individuals with glaucoma and serious eye diseases. In some instances redness or inflammation may be due to serious eye conditions such as acute iritis, acute glaucoma, or corneal trauma. When redness, pain, or blurring persist, discontinue use. A physician should be consulted at once.

Dosage and Administration: One or two drops in eye(s) up to 4 times daily or as directed by physician. Do not touch bottle tip to any surface, since this may contaminate the solution. Remove contact lenses before using. Keep this and all other medicines out of the reach of children. Replace cap after using.

How Supplied: In 0.5 fl oz and 1.5 fl oz plastic dropper bottle.

EAR DROPS BY MURINE   OTC
See Murine Ear Wax Removal System/Murine Ear Drops

ENRICH™
[*en-rich*]
Liquid Nutrition with Fiber

Usage: As a high-fiber liquid food providing complete, balanced nutrition. The fiber level in Enrich helps maintain normal bowel function, and is useful for patients who have intolerance to low residue feedings. Enrich can be used as a full liquid diet, liquid supplement or tube-feeding.

Features:
- Complete, balanced nutrition—Enrich can be used as a sole source of nutrition. Caloric distribution: 14.5% protein, 30.5% fat, 55.0% carbohydrate (includes soy polysaccharide, a source of dietary fiber). 1530 Calories meets or surpasses 100% of the U.S. RDA for vitamins and minerals.
- Calorie-to-nitrogen ratio of 173:1—Assures that protein will be spared for tissue restoration and growth.
- High in dietary fiber—One serving provides 3.3 g of dietary fiber. Six servings provide 20 g of dietary fiber, a level comparable to a typical self-selected diet.
- High-quality protein—Amino acid profile meets the standard of high-quality proteins set by the National Academy of Sciences.
- Good nutrient absorption—Nitrogen balance, fat absorption and mineral balance (in the normally functioning gut) are not compromised by fiber.
- Lactose free—Enrich will not contribute to lactose-associated diarrhea.
- Low osmolality (480 mOsm/kg water)—Will not contribute to osmotically induced diarrhea.
- Good taste—Pleasant flavor is readily accepted by most patients. Ready To Use Enrich is available in Vanilla and Chocolate flavors. In addition, Vari-Flavors® Flavor Pacs (Pecan, Cherry, Strawberry, Lemon, Orange) mix easily with vanilla to offer patients a greater variety of flavors.

Dosage and Administration:
Ready to Use: Shake well. Enrich is ready to use and does not require dilution with water. Enrich may be stored (unopened) and fed at room temperature. Once opened, any unused Enrich should be covered and refrigerated; discard if not used within 48 hours.
Oral Feeding: Enrich may be used for total nutrition, or with and between meals for added nutritional support. Enrich is delicious when chilled.
Tube Feeding: Follow physician's instructions. When initiating feeding, the flow rate, volume and dilution are dependent on patient condition and tolerance. Care should be taken to avoid contamination of this product during preparation and administration. Lower temperatures increase the viscosity of Enrich. Therefore, the product should be at room temperature for tube-feeding.
Additional fluid requirements should be met by giving water orally with or after feedings, or when flushing the feeding tube.
Enrich is not recommended for situations requiring a low-residue feeding.
Under no circumstances should Enrich be administered parenterally. [See table below].

Availability:
Ready To Use:
8-fl-oz cans; 4 six-packs per case; Vanilla, No. 759; Chocolate, No. 756.

Composition: Ready To Use Vanilla (Chocolate flavor has similar composition. For specific information, see product label.)

Ingredients: Ⓤ Water, hydrolyzed corn starch, sucrose, sodium and calcium caseinates, corn oil, soy polysaccharide (a source of dietary fiber), minerals (potassium citrate, magnesium chloride, calcium phosphate tribasic, sodium citrate, potassium chloride, zinc sulfate, ferrous sulfate, manganese sulfate, cupric sulfate), soy protein isolate, natural and artificial flavor, soy lecithin and vitamins (choline chloride, ascorbic acid, alpha-tocopheryl acetate, niacinamide, calcium pantothenate, thiamine chloride hydrochloride, pyridoxine hydrochloride, riboflavin, vitamin A palmitate, folic acid, biotin, phylloquinone, cyanocobalamin, vitamin D$_3$).

Approximate Analysis (g/8 fl oz): Protein, 9.4; Fat, 8.8; Carbohydrate, 38.3†; Minerals (Ash), 1.9; Moisture, 196. Calories per fl oz, 32.5; Calories per ml, 1.10.

† Contains 5 g soy polysaccharide/8 fl oz (a source of dietary fiber) which contributes 10 Calories per 8 fl oz.

Vitamin/Mineral Content of Enrich (Ready To Use)

Vitamins/Minerals	Per 8 Fl Oz		Percent U.S. RDA* (Per 8 Fl Oz)
Vitamin A	850	I.U.	17
Vitamin D	68	I.U.	17
Vitamin E	7.5	I.U.	25
Vitamin K$_1$	12	mcg	**
Vitamin C	30	mg	50
Folic Acid	100	mcg	25
Thiamine (Vit. B$_1$)	0.38	mg	25
Riboflavin (Vit. B$_2$)	0.43	mg	25
Vitamin B$_6$	0.50	mg	25
Vitamin B$_{12}$	1.5	mcg	25
Niacin	5.0	mg	25
Choline	0.13	g	**
Biotin	75	mcg	25
Pantothenic Acid	2.5	mg	25
Sodium	200	mg	**
Potassium	370	mg	**
Chloride	340	mg	**
Calcium	0.17	g	17
Phosphorus	0.17	g	17
Magnesium	68	mg	17
Iodine	26	mcg	17
Manganese	0.83	mg	**
Copper	0.34	mg	17
Zinc	3.8	mg	25
Iron	3.1	mg	17

*For adults and children 4 or more years of age.
**U.S. RDA not established.
(FAN 292)

Sample Administration Schedule for ENRICH

Continuous Drip Schedule

Day	Time	Strength	Rate (mL/h)	Volume (mL)	Calories
1	1st 8 hours	Full	50	400	440
	2nd 8 hours	Full	75	600	660
	3rd 8 hours	Full	100	800	880
					1980 *Total Calories*
2	24 hours	Full	100–125	2400–3000	2640–3300 *Total Calories*

Intermittent Drip Schedule

Day	Time	Strength	Rate (5–10 mL/min)	Volume (mL)	Calories
1	7AM–11PM	Full	100 mL q 2 h (7AM, 9AM)	200	220
			150 mL q 2 h (11AM, 1PM, 3PM)	450	495
			200 mL q 2 h (5PM, 7PM, 9PM, 11PM)	800	880
					1595 *Total Calories*
2	7AM–11PM	Full	250 mL q 2 h (8 feedings) up to	2000	2200 *Total Calories*
			400 mL q 3 h (5 feedings)	2000	2200 *Total Calories*

- Always tube-feed the product at room temperature.
- When gavage feeding, use a size 10 French or large tube. Smaller tubes can be used for pump delivery.
- Check gastric residuals before every intermittent feeding or every 2–4 hours during continuous feeding.
- If intolerance develops (such as nausea, abdominal cramps, severe distention or diarrhea), return to previously tolerated rate.
- Rinsing the tube with water (eg, 25–100 mL) after each intermittent feeding or every 3 to 6 hours during continuous feeding will help avoid clogging and provide additional water.

ENSURE®
[en-shur']
Liquid Nutrition

Usage: For complete, balanced nutrition. Ensure can be used as a full liquid diet, liquid supplement or tube feeding (nasogastric, nasoduodenal, jejunal). Ensure is useful whenever the patient's medical, surgical or psychological state precludes normal food intake and/or leads to inadequate nutrition. Two quarts (2000 Calories) of Ensure meets or surpasses 100% of the U.S.RDA for vitamins and minerals for adults and children 4 or more years of age.

Features:
- Complete, balanced nutrition—1.06 Calories per ml, 250 Calories per 8-fl-oz feeding, 1000 Calories per quart from a balanced distribution of protein, fat, and carbohydrate (caloric distribution: protein, 14.0%; fat, 31.5%; carbohydrate, 54.5%).
- High biologic value protein—Ensure provides high-quality protein (sodium and calcium caseinates and soy protein isolate) at a level appropriate for most hospitalized patients. Ensure provides 14% of the total calories as protein.
- Lactose free—Ensure will not contribute to lactose-associated diarrhea. Hydrolyzed corn starch and sucrose are carbohydrate sources.
- Fat source—A good source of essential fatty acids. Cholesterol is low (<20 mg/L). The fat source is polyunsaturated corn oil.
- Low-residue liquid feeding—The amount of fecal residue produced by Ensure is comparable to that produced by a chemically defined, elemental diet. Therefore, Ensure is appropriate for use in situations where low residue is the primary consideration.
- Low osmolality (450 mOsm/kg water)—The osmolality of Ensure is low and will not contribute to osmotically induced diarrhea when proper feeding techniques are used.
- Good taste—Pleasant flavors are readily accepted by most patients. Ready To Use Ensure is available in a variety of flavors (Vanilla, Chocolate, Black Walnut, Coffee, Strawberry and Eggnog). In addition, Vari-Flavors® Flavor Pacs (Pecan, Cherry, Strawberry, Lemon, Orange) mix easily with Ensure Vanilla to offer patients a greater variety of flavors.
- Convenient—Available as a Ready To Use Liquid and Easy To Mix Powder. Ensure Powder mixes readily with water.

Dosage and Administration:
Ready To Use: Shake well. Do not add water for a standard 1 Calorie/ml feeding. Ensure may be stored (unopened) and fed at room temperature. Once opened, any unused Ensure should be covered and refrigerated; discard if not used within 48 hours.
Powder: To prepare an 8-fl-oz glassful: Put ¾ cup of cold water in a glass. Gradually stir in ½ cup Ensure Powder and mix until dissolved. Reconstituted Ensure should be used promptly or covered, refrigerated and used within 24 hours. Once can of Ensure Powder has been opened, contents should be used within 3 weeks. Opened can should be covered with overcap and stored in a cool, dry place, but not refrigerated.
- **Oral Feeding:** Ensure may be used for total nutrition, or with and between meals for added nutritional support. Ensure is delicious when chilled.
- **Tube Feeding:** Follow physician's instructions. When initiating feeding, the flow rate, volume and dilution are dependent on patient condition and tolerance. Care should be taken to avoid contamination of this product during preparation and administration.

Additional fluid requirements should be met by giving water orally with or after feedings, or when flushing the gavage tube.

Under no circumstances should Ensure be administered parenterally.

Table 1
Sample Administration Schedule For ENSURE

Continuous Drip Schedule

Day	Time	Strength	Rate (mL/hr)	Volume (mL)	Calories
1	1st 8 hours	Full	50	400	400
	2nd 8 hours	Full	75	600	600
	3rd 8 hours	Full	100	800	800
					1800 Total Calories
2	24 hours	Full	100–125	2400–3000	2400–3000 Total Calories

Intermittent Drip Schedule

Day	Time	Strength	Rate (5–10 mL/min)	Volume (mL)	Calories
1	7am–11pm	Full	100 mL q 2 hr (7am, 9am)	200	200
			150 mL q 2 hr (11am, 1pm, 3pm)	450	450
			200 mL q 2 hr (5pm, 7pm, 9pm, 11pm)	800	800
					1450 Total Calories
2	7am–11pm	Full	250 mL q 2 hr (8 feedings) up to	2000	2000 Total Calories
			400 mL q 3 hr (5 feedings)	2000	2000 Total Calories

- Check gastric residuals before every intermittent feeding or every 2–4 hours during continuous feeding.
- If intolerance develops (such as nausea, abdominal cramps, distention or diarrhea), switch to full strength OSMOLITE or feed ENSURE at half strength. After tolerance to half strength ENSURE is established, continue feeding schedule using half strength ENSURE until desired rate is achieved. Then switch to full strength. Do not alter rate and strength at the same time.
- Rinsing the tube with water (eg, 25–100 mL) after each intermittent feeding or every 3 to 6 hours during continuous feeding will help avoid clogging and provide additional water.

See Table 1
Availability:
Ready To Use:
8-fl-oz bottles; 24 per case; Vanilla, No. 708.
8-fl-oz cans; 4 six-packs per case; Chocolate, No. 701; Black Walnut, No. 703; Coffee, No. 704; Strawberry, No. 705; Eggnog, No. 710; Vanilla, No. 711.
32-fl-oz cans; 6 per case; Vanilla, No. 733.
Powder:
14-oz (400 g) cans; 6 per case; Vanilla, No. 750.
Composition: Ready To Use Vanilla (Other Ready To Use flavors and Vanilla Powder at standard dilution have similar composition and nutrient values. For specific information, see product labels.)
Ingredients: ⓊWater, hydrolyzed corn starch, sucrose, sodium and calcium caseinates, corn oil, minerals (potassium citrate, magnesium chloride, calcium phosphate tribasic, potassium chloride, sodium citrate, zinc sulfate, ferrous sulfate, manganous chloride, cupric sulfate), soy protein isolate, soy lecithin, natural and artificial flavor, vitamins (choline chloride, ascorbic acid, alpha-tocopheryl acetate, niacinamide, calcium pantothenate, thiamine chloride hydrochloride, pyridoxine hydrochloride, riboflavin, vitamin A palmitate, folic acid, biotin, phylloquinone, cyanocobalamin, vitamin D_3) and carrageenan.
Approximate Analysis (g/8 fl oz): Protein, 8.8; Fat, 8.8; Carbohydrate, 34.3; Ash, 1.4; Moisture, 199.5. Calories per ml, 1.06; Calories per fl oz, 31.8. [See table on bottom next page].
(FAN 340-01)

ENSURE® HN
[en-shur']
High Nitrogen Liquid Nutrition

Usage: As an all-purpose, high-nitrogen, low-residue liquid food, Ensure HN provides complete, balanced nutritional support for the stressed patient with an increase in RME (resting metabolic expenditure) of greater than 30%. Ensure HN can be used as a full liquid diet, liquid supplement or tube feeding (nasogastric, nasoduodenal, jejunal).

Features:
- Complete, balanced nutrition—1.06 Calories per ml, 250 Calories per 8 fl oz, 1000 Calories per quart from a balanced distribution of protein, fat and carbohydrate (caloric distribution: protein, 16.7%; fat, 30.1%; carbohydrate, 53.2%). 1400 Calories of Ensure HN provide at least 100% of the U.S. RDA for vitamins and minerals for adults and children 4 or more years of age.
- High levels of nitrogen—Ensure HN has a total calorie-to-nitrogen ratio of 150:1, indicated for the stressed patient because of increased nitrogen losses.
- High biologic value protein—Ensure HN provides high quality protein at a level appropriate for the stressed patient—10.5g/8 fl oz (1.68g nitrogen/8 fl oz). 16.7% of the total calories of Ensure HN are protein.
- Lactose-free—Ensure HN will not contribute to lactose-associated diarrhea. Hydrolyzed corn starch and sucrose are the carbohydrate sources.
- Low-residue feeding—Ensure HN is appropriate in situations in which low residue is a consideration.
- Low osmolality (470 mOsm/kg water)—Ensure HN will decrease the risk of osmotically induced diarrhea when proper feeding techniques are used.

Dosage and Administration:
Ready To Use: Ensure HN is ready to use and does not require dilution with water. Ensure HN may be stored (unopened) and fed at room temperature. Once opened, remaining Ensure HN should be covered, refrigerated and discarded if not used within 48 hours.
- **Oral Feeding:** Ensure HN may be used for total nutrition, or with and between meals for added

Continued on next page

Ross—Cont.

nutritional support. Ensure HN is delicious when chilled.
- **Tube Feeding:** Follow physician's instructions. When initiating feeding, the flow rate, volume and dilution are dependent on patient condition and tolerance. Care should be taken to avoid contamination of this product during preparation and administration.

Additional fluid requirements should be met by giving water orally with or after feedings, or when flushing feeding tube.

Under no circumstances should Ensure HN be administered parenterally.
[See table right].

Availability:
Ready To Use:
8-fl-oz cans; 4 six-packs per case; Chocolate, No. 712; Vanilla, No. 719.
32-fl-oz cans; 6 per case; Vanilla, No. 732.
Composition: Ready To Use Vanilla (Other flavors have similar composition. For specific information, see product labels.)
Ingredients: Ⓤ Water, hydrolyzed corn starch, sodium and calcium caseinates, sucrose, corn oil, minerals (magnesium chloride, potassium citrate, calcium phosphate tribasic, sodium citrate, potassium phosphate dibasic, potassium chloride, zinc sulfate, ferrous sulfate, manganese sulfate, cupric sulfate), soy protein isolate, soy lecithin, natural and artificial flavor, vitamins (choline chloride, ascorbic acid, alpha-tocopheryl acetate, niacinamide, calcium pantothenate, thiamine chloride hydrochloride, pyridoxine hydrochloride, riboflavin, vitamin A palmitate, folic acid, biotin, phylloquinone, cyanocobalamin, vitamin D_3) and carrageenan.

Approximate Analysis (g/8 fl oz): Protein, 10.5; Fat, 8.4; Carbohydrate, 33.4; Minerals (Ash), 1.9; Moisture, 199. Calories per ml, 1.06; Calories per fl oz, 31.3.
[See table on top next page].
(FAN 283)

ENSURE PLUS®
[en-shur']
High Calorie Liquid Nutrition

Usage: As a high-calorie liquid food providing complete, balanced nutrition. Caloric density is 1500 Calories per liter, 50% greater than most other liquid feedings. Ensure Plus is intended for use when extra calories and correspondingly higher concentrations of protein and most other nutrients are needed to achieve a required calorie intake in a limited volume. When utilized to provide total nutrition, Ensure Plus can deliver the high-calorie intakes required by patients who are nutritionally depleted, and who may not be able to tolerate large-volume intakes. As a dietary supplement, Ensure Plus can supply extra calories and protein for those patients unable or unwilling to consume adequate nutrition.

Features:
- Complete Nutrition—1.5 Cal per ml, 355 Cal per 8 fl oz, from a balanced distribution of protein, fat and carbohydrate (caloric distribution: protein, 14.7%; fat, 32.0%; carbohydrate, 53.3%). 2400 Cal (1.7 quarts) of Ensure Plus meets or surpasses 100% of the U.S. RDA for vitamins and minerals for adults and children 4 or more years of age.
- 1500 Calories per liter—The use of Ensure Plus will reduce the volume necessary to meet the caloric needs of debilitated patients.
  55 grams of protein per liter—Ensure Plus provides sufficient protein to meet demands of the nutritionally compromised patient. Appropriate levels of carbohydrate and fat are provided to spare protein for anabolic purposes, tissue synthesis and repair.
- Lactose free—Ensure Plus will not contribute to lactose-associated diarrhea. Hydrolyzed corn starch and sucrose are carbohydrate sources.
- Moderate osmolality (600 mOsm/kg water)—The osmolality of Ensure Plus is moderate, even though caloric density is 50% greater than standard liquid feedings. Ensure Plus will not contribute to osmotic diarrhea when proper feeding techniques are used.
- Good Taste—Pleasant flavor is readily accepted by most patients. Ready To Use Ensure Plus is available in a variety of flavors (Vanilla, Chocolate, Coffee, Strawberry and Eggnog). In addition, Vari-Flavors® Flavor Pacs (Pecan, Cherry, Strawberry, Lemon, Orange) mix easily with Ensure Plus Vanilla to offer patients a greater variety of flavors.
- Convenient—Ensure Plus is ready to use. Potential for contamination during preparation is reduced. Unopened, Ensure Plus can be stored at room temperature.

Dosage and Administration: Shake well. Ensure Plus is ready to use and does not require dilution with water. Ensure Plus may be stored (unopened) and fed at room temperature. Once opened, remaining Ensure Plus should be covered, refrigerated and discarded if not used within 48 hours.
- **Oral Feeding:** Ensure Plus may be used for total nutrition, or with and between meals for added nutritional support. Ensure Plus is delicious when chilled.
- **Tube Feeding:** Follow physician's instructions. When initiating feeding, the flow rate, volume and dilution are dependent on patient condition and tolerance. Care should be taken to avoid contamination of this product during preparation and administration.

Sample Administration Schedule For ENSURE HN

Continuous Drip Schedule

Day	Time	Strength	Rate (mL/h)	Volume (mL)	Calories
1	1st 8 hours	Full	50	400	400
	2nd 8 hours	Full	75	600	600
	3rd 8 hours	Full	100	800	800
					1800 Total Calories
2	24 hours	Full	100-125	2400-3000	2400-3000 Total Calories

Intermittent Drip Schedule

Day	Time	Strength	Rate (5-10 mL/min)	Volume (mL)	Calories
1	7am-11pm	Full	100 mL q 2 h (7am, 9am)	200	200
			150 mL q 2 h (11am, 1pm, 3pm)	450	450
			200 mL q 2 h (5pm, 7pm, 9pm, 11pm)	800	800
					1450 Total Calories
2	7am-11pm	Full	250 mL q 2 h (8 feedings) up to	2000	2000 Total Calories
			400 mL q 3 h (5 feedings)	2000	2000 Total Calories

- Check gastric residuals before every intermittent feeding or every 2–4 hours during continuous feeding.
- If intolerance develops, switch to full strength OSMOLITE® HN or feed ENSURE® HN at half strength. After tolerance to half strength ENSURE® HN is established, continue feeding schedule using half strength ENSURE® HN until desired rate is achieved. Then switch to full strength. Do not alter rate and strength at the same time.
- Rinsing the tube with water (eg, 25–100 mL) after each intermittent feeding or every 3 to 6 hours during continuous feeding will help avoid clogging and provide additional water.

Vitamin/Mineral Content of Ensure (Ready To Use)

Vitamins/Minerals	Per 8 Fl Oz		Percent U.S. RDA* (Per 8 Fl Oz)
Vitamin A	625	I.U.	12.5
Vitamin D	50	I.U.	12.5
Vitamin E	5.7	I.U.	19.0
Vitamin K_1	9	mcg	**
Vitamin C	38	mg	62.5
Folic Acid	50	mcg	12.5
Thiamine (Vit. B_1)	0.38	mg	25.0
Riboflavin (Vit. B_2)	0.43	mg	25.0
Vitamin B_6	0.50	mg	25.0
Vitamin B_{12}	1.5	mcg	25.0
Niacin	5.0	mg	25.0
Choline	0.13	g	**
Biotin	38	mcg	12.5
Pantothenic Acid	1.25	mg	12.5
Sodium	0.20	g	**
Potassium	0.37	g	**
Chloride	0.34	g	**
Calcium	0.13	g	12.5
Phosphorus	0.13	g	12.5
Magnesium	50	mg	12.5
Iodine	19	mcg	12.5
Manganese	0.50	mg	**
Copper	0.25	mg	12.5
Zinc	3.75	mg	25.0
Iron	2.25	mg	12.5

*For adults and children 4 or more years of age.
**U.S. RDA not established.

Product Information

Additional fluid requirements should be met by giving water orally with or after feedings, or when flushing the gavage tube.

Under no circumstances should Ensure Plus be administered parenterally.
(See table below)

Availability: 8-fl-oz bottles; 24 per case; Vanilla, No. 741.

8-fl-oz cans; 4 six-packs per case; Chocolate, No. 702; Vanilla, No. 707; Eggnog, No. 716; Coffee, No. 717; Strawberry, No. 718.

Composition: Ready To Use Vanilla (Other flavors have similar composition. For specific information, see product labels.)

Ingredients: Ⓤ Water, hydrolyzed corn starch, sodium and calcium caseinates, corn oil, sucrose, minerals (magnesium chloride, potassium citrate, calcium phosphate tribasic, sodium citrate, potassium chloride, zinc sulfate, ferrous sulfate, manganous chloride, cupric sulfate), soy protein isolate, soy lecithin, vitamins (choline chloride, ascorbic acid, alpha-tocopheryl acetate, niacinamide, calcium pantothenate, thiamine chloride hydrochloride, pyridoxine hydrochloride, riboflavin, vitamin A palmitate, folic acid, biotin, phylloquinone, cyanocobalamin, vitamin D_3), natural and artificial flavor and carrageenan.

Approximate Analysis (g/8 fl oz): Protein, 13.0; Fat, 12.6; Carbohydrate, 47.3; Ash, 2.2; Moisture, 182.0. Calories per ml, 1.5; Calories per fl oz, 44.4. [See table on top next page].
(FAN 340–01)

Vitamin/Mineral Content of Ensure HN (Ready To Use)

Vitamins/Minerals	Per 8 Fl Oz		Percent U.S. RDA* (Per 8 Fl Oz)
Vitamin A	900	I.U.	18
Vitamin D	72	I.U.	18
Vitamin E	8.1	I.U.	27
Vitamin K_1	13	mcg	**
Vitamin C	33	mg	55
Folic Acid	0.11	mg	27
Thiamine (Vit. B_1)	0.41	mg	27
Riboflavin (Vit B_2)	0.46	mg	27
Vitamin B_6	0.55	mg	27
Vitamin B_{12}	1.7	mcg	28
Niacin	5.4	mg	27
Choline	0.14	g	**
Biotin	82	mcg	27
Pantothenic Acid	2.7	mg	27
Sodium	220	mg	**
Potassium	370	mg	**
Chloride	340	mg	**
Calcium	0.18	g	18
Phosphorus	0.18	g	18
Magnesium	72	mg	18
Iodine	27	mcg	18
Manganese	0.90	mg	**
Copper	0.36	mg	18
Zinc	4.1	mg	27
Iron	3.3	mg	18

*For adults and children 4 or more years of age.
**U.S. RDA not established.

Sample Administration Schedule For ENSURE PLUS

Continuous Drip Schedule

Day	Time	Strength	Rate (mL/hr)	Volume (mL)	Calories
1	1st 8 hours	½	50	400	300
	2nd 8 hours	½	75	600	450
	3rd 8 hours	½	100	800	600
					1350 *Total Calories*
2	1st 8 hours	½	125	1000	750
	2nd 8 hours	Full	100–125	800–1000	1200–1500
	3rd 8 hours	Full	100–125	800–1000	1200–1500
					3150–3750 *Total Calories*
3	24 hours	Full	100–125	2400–3000	3600–4500 *Total Calories*

Intermittent Drip Schedule

Day	Time	Strength	Rate (5–10 mL/min)	Volume (mL)	Calories
1	7am–11pm	½	100 mL q 2 hr (7am, 9am)	200	150
		½	150 mL q 2 hr (11am, 1pm, 3pm)	450	338
		½	200 mL q 2 hr (5pm, 7pm, 9pm, 11pm)	800	600
					1088 *Total Calories*
2	7am–11pm	½	250 mL q 2 hr (7am, 9am, 11am)	750	563
		Full	250 mL q 2 hr (1pm, 3pm, 5pm, 7pm, 9pm, 11pm)	1500	2250
					2813 *Total Calories*
3	7am–11pm	Full	250 mL q 2 hr (8 feedings) up to	2000	3000 *Total Calories*
			400 mL q 3 hr (5 feedings)	2000	3000 *Total Calories*

- Check gastric residuals before every intermittent feeding or every 2–4 hours during continuous feeding.
- If intolerance develops (such as nausea, abdominal cramps, distention, or diarrhea), return to previously tolerated strength and rate. When tolerance is again established, proceed with feeding schedule as indicated. Do not alter rate and strength at the same time.
- Rinsing the tube with water (eg, 25–100 mL) after each intermittent feeding or every 3 to 6 hours during continuous feeding will help avoid clogging and provide additional water.

ENSURE PLUS® HN
[*en-shur'*]
High Calorie, High Nitrogen Liquid Nutrition

Usage: As a high-calorie, high-nitrogen liquid food, Ensure Plus HN provides complete, balanced nutrition. It is most appropriate for the stressed patient ($\geq$ 30% increase in resting metabolic expenditure) with extraordinary caloric needs, or for those patients whose volume intake is limited. Ensure Plus HN can be used as a full liquid diet, liquid supplement or tube feeding (nasogastric or nasoduodenal).

Features:
- Complete, balanced nutrition—1.5 Calories per ml, 355 Calories per 8 fl oz, 1500 Calories per liter from a balanced distribution of protein, fat and carbohydrate (caloric distribution: protein, 16.7%; fat, 30.0%; and carbohydrate, 53.3%). 1420 Calories of Ensure Plus HN meets or surpasses 100% of the U.S. RDA for vitamins and minerals for adults and children 4 or more years of age.
- High levels of nitrogen—Ensure Plus HN has a total calorie-to-nitrogen ratio of 150:1, indicated for the stressed patient because of increased nitrogen losses.
- Concentrated nutrition—Ensure Plus HN will reduce the volume necessary to meet the protein and caloric needs of the debilitated patient (62.6 g of protein per liter, 1500 Calories per liter).
- Lactose-free—Ensure Plus HN will not contribute to lactose-associated diarrhea. Hydrolyzed cornstarch and sucrose are the carbohydrate sources.
- Moderate osmolality (650 mOsm/kg water)—Ensure Plus HN will decrease the potential for osmotically induced diarrhea.

Dosage and Administration:
Ready To Use: Ensure Plus HN is ready to use and does not require dilution with water. Ensure Plus HN may be stored (unopened) and fed at room temperature. Once opened, remaining Ensure Plus HN should be covered, refrigerated and discarded if not used within 48 hours.

- **Oral Feeding:** Ensure Plus HN may be used for total nutrition, or with and between meals for added nutritional support. Ensure Plus HN is delicious when chilled.

Continued on next page

Ross—Cont.

- **Tube Feeding:** Follow physician's instructions. When initiating feeding, the flow rate, volume and dilution are dependent on patient condition and tolerance. Care should be taken to avoid contamination of this product during preparation and administration.

Additional fluid requirements should be met by giving water orally with or after feedings, or when flushing feeding tube.

Under no circumstances should Ensure Plus HN be administered parenterally.
[See table on top next page].

Availability:
Ready To Use:
8-fl-oz cans; 4 six-packs per case; Vanilla, No. 721.

Composition: Ready To Use Vanilla
Ingredients: Water, hydrolyzed corn starch, sodium and calcium caseinates, corn oil, sucrose, minerals (magnesium chloride, calcium phosphate tribasic, potassium citrate, sodium citrate, ferrous sulfate, zinc sulfate, cupric sulfate, manganese sulfate), soy protein isolate, soy lecithin, vitamins (choline chloride, ascorbic acid, alpha-tocopheryl acetate, niacinamide, calcium pantothenate, thiamine chloride hydrochloride, pyridoxine hydrochloride, riboflavin, vitamin A palmitate, folic acid, biotin, phylloquinone, cyanocobalamin, vitamin D_3), natural and artificial flavor, and carrageenan.

Approximate Analysis (g/8 fl oz): Protein, 14.8; Fat, 11.8; Carbohydrate, 47.3; Minerals (Ash), 2.3; Moisture, 181.9. Calories per fl oz, 44.4; Calories per 8 fl oz, 355.
[See table below].
(FAN 283)

FLEXIFLO® ENTERAL DELIVERY SYSTEM
[*fleks'ă-flō*″]
A complete delivery system specially designed for enteral feeding.

FLEXIFLO® Enteral Feeding Tube
8 French (45″ length)
Tungsten/C-FLEX weighted bolus

Usage: For administration of enteral feedings via the nasogastric or nasoenteric route.

Availability: Enteral feeding tube; 12 individually packed tubes per case; No. 53.

Vitamin/Mineral Content of Ensure Plus (Ready To Use)

Vitamins/Minerals	Per 8 Fl Oz		Percent U.S. RDA* (Per 8 Fl Oz)
Vitamin A	890	I.U.	17.8
Vitamin D	70	I.U.	17.5
Vitamin E	7.8	I.U.	26.0
Vitamin K_1	13	mcg	**
Vitamin C	38	mg	62.5
Folic Acid	75	mcg	18.8
Thiamine (Vit. B_1)	0.63	mg	41.3
Riboflavin (Vit. B_2)	0.65	mg	37.5
Vitamin B_6	0.75	mg	37.5
Vitamin B_{12}	2.25	mcg	37.5
Niacin	7.5	mg	37.5
Biotin	56	mcg	18.7
Choline	125	mg	**
Pantothenic Acid	2.0	mg	20
Sodium	0.27	g	**
Potassium	0.55	g	**
Chloride	0.47	g	**
Calcium	0.15	g	15
Phosphorus	0.15	g	15
Magnesium	75	mg	18.8
Manganese	0.50	mg	**
Iodine	25	mcg	16.3
Copper	0.38	mg	18.8
Iron	3.38	mg	18.8
Zinc	5.63	mg	37.5

*For adults and children 4 or more years of age.
**U.S. RDA not established.

FLEXIFLO® Enteral Feeding Tube
8 French w/Stylet (45″ length)
Tungsten/C-FLEX Weighted bolus

Usage: For administration of enteral feedings via the nasogastric or nasoenteric route.

Availability: Enteral feeding tube; 12 individually packed tubes per case; No. 54.

FLEXIFLO® Enteral Feeding Tube
12 French (36″ length)

Usage: For administration of enteral feedings via the nasogastric route.

Availability: Enteral feeding tube; 12 individually packed tubes per case; No. 55.

FLEXIFLO® Enteral Nutrition Pump
Peristaltic pump with constant-speed motor allows accurate flow control from 50 to 200 ml/hr (25-ml increments). The Flexiflo Pump, designed for enteral feeding, is simple to operate, reliable, and cost effective.

Availability: Pump; 1 pump per case; retail unit, No. 64; lease unit, No. 72.

FLEXIFLO® Enteral Pump Set
Usage: For use with the Flexiflo Enteral Nutrition Pump, Nos. 64 and 72. The set has a specially formulated insert, sight chamber, color coded flow regulation tabs and a tip adapter compatible with most indwelling feeding tubes.

Availability: Pump set; 24 individually packed sets per case; No. 65.

FLEXIFLO® Pump Set with Piercing Pin
Usage: For use with the Flexiflo Enteral Nutrition Pump, Nos. 64 and 72.

Availability: Pump set; 24 individually packed sets per case; No. 60.

FLEXIFLO®–II Portable Enteral Nutrition Pump
Usage: Provides maximum versatility for the delivery of enteral feedings.

Features:
- Flow rates of 20, 30, 40, 50, 60, 75, 100, 125, 150, 175, 200, 250 ml/hr.
- Portable with a battery life of at least 8 hours. Alarm override system prevents disturbing alarms when patient is ambulating.
- Ideal for the ambulatory patient, especially when used with shoulder strap. Lightweight. Expensive IV stand not necessary, but can be used if desired.
- Safety—Visual and audible alarm system signals tube occlusion, empty container and low battery.

Availability:
Pump; 1 pump per case; retail unit, No. 51; lease unit, No. 58.

FLEXIFLO®–II Enteral Pump Set
Usage: For use with the Flexiflo-II Portable Enteral Nutrition Pump, Nos. 51 and 58. The set has a specially formulated insert, sight chamber, and a tip adapter compatible with most indwelling feeding tubes.

Availability: Pump set; 24 individually packaged sets per case; No. 66.

FLEXIFLO®–II Pump Set with Piercing Pin
Usage: For use with the Flexiflo-II Portable Enteral Nutrition Pump, Nos. 51 and 58.

Availability: Pump set; 24 individually packed sets per case; No. 57.

Vitamin/Mineral Content of Ensure Plus HN (Ready To Use)

Vitamins/Minerals	Per 8 Fl Oz		Percent U.S. RDA* (Per 8 Fl Oz)
Vitamin A	1250	I.U.	25
Vitamin D	100	I.U.	25
Vitamin E	11.3	I.U.	37
Vitamin K_1	18	mcg	**
Vitamin C	60	mg	100
Folic Acid	0.20	mg	50
Thiamine (Vit. B_1)	0.75	mg	50
Riboflavin (Vit. B_2)	0.85	mg	50
Vitamin B_6	1.0	mg	50
Vitamin B_{12}	3.0	mcg	50
Niacin	10	mg	50
Choline	0.13	g	**
Biotin	150	mcg	50
Pantothenic Acid	5.0	mg	50
Sodium	280	mg	**
Potassium	430	mg	**
Chloride	380	mg	**
Calcium	0.25	g	25
Phosphorus	0.25	g	25
Magnesium	100	mg	25
Iodine	38	mcg	25
Manganese	0.50	mg	**
Copper	0.50	mg	25
Zinc	3.8	mg	25
Iron	4.5	mg	25

* For adults and children 4 or more years of age.
** U.S. RDA not established.

Product Information

FLEXIFLO®-III Enteral Nutrition Pump

Usage: For controlled, accurate delivery of enteral feedings. Microprocessor controlled rotary peristaltic pump. Flow rates of 1-300 ml/hr in 1 ml increments. Battery life of at least 8 hours. Visual and audible alarm system to signal tube occlusion, empty bag, low battery, dose complete.
Availability: Pump; 1 pump per case; retail unit, No. 76; lease unit, No. 82.

FLEXIFLO®-III Enteral Pump Set

Usage: For use with the Flexiflo-III Enteral Nutrition Pump, Nos. 76 and 82.
Availability: Pump set; 24 individually packed sets per case; No. 77.

FLEXIFLO®-III Pump Set with Piercing Pin

Usage: For use with the Flexiflo-III Enteral Nutrition Pump, Nos. 76 and 82.
Availability: Pump set; 24 individually packed sets per case; No. 78.

FLEXIFLO® Gravity Gavage Set

Usage: For use with the Flexitainer Enteral Nutrition Container, Flexitainer 500 Enteral Nutrition Container, or with 8-fl-oz bottles for controlled enteral feeding. Set is composed of a feeding cap, clear plastic sight chamber, air vent protected by bacteria-retentive filter, flow regulator (roller clamp), and tip adapter compatible with most indwelling feeding tubes.
Availability: Gavage set; 24 individually packed sets per case; No. 61.

FLEXIFLO® Gravity Feeding Set with Piercing Pin

Usage: For use with a variety of enteral nutrition containers with spike ports.
Availability: Gavage set; 24 individually packed sets per case; No. 59.

FLEXITAINER® Enteral Nutrition Container

Ready-to-use, large-volume, one-liter container combining the best features of a bottle and a bag... collapsible with a rigid neck and a large opening for easy filling, and graduated measurements for both filling and delivery.
Availability: Container; 24 per case; No. 69.

FLEXITAINER® 500 Enteral Nutrition Container

Usage: For convenient administration of small-volume enteral feedings.
Availability: Container; 24 per case; No. 68.

Sample Administration Schedule For ENSURE PLUS HN

Continuous Drip Schedule

Day	Time	Strength	Rate (mL/h)	Volume (mL)	Calories
1	1st 8 hours	½	50	400	300
	2nd 8 hours	½	75	600	450
	3rd 8 hours	½	100	800	600
					1350 Total Calories
2	1st 8 hours	½	125	1000	750
	2nd 8 hours	Full	100-125	800-1000	1200-1500
	3rd 8 hours	Full	100-125	800-1000	1200-1500
					3150-3750 Total Calories
3	24 hours	Full	100-125	2400-3000	3600-4500 Total Calories

Intermittent Drip Schedule

Day	Time	Strength	Rate (5-10 mL/min)	Volume (mL)	Calories
1	7am-11pm	½	100 mL q 2 h (7am, 9am)	200	150
		½	150 mL q 2 h (11am, 1pm, 3pm)	450	338
		½	200 mL q 2 h (5pm, 7pm, 9pm, 11pm)	800	600
					1088 Total Calories
2	7am-11pm	½	250 mL q 2 h (7am, 9am, 11am)	750	563
		Full	250 mL q 2 h (1pm, 3pm, 5pm, 7pm, 9pm, 11pm)	1500	2250
					2813 Total Calories
3	7am-11pm	Full	250 mL q 2 h (8 feedings)	2000	3000 Total Calories
			up to 400 mL q 3 h (5 feedings)	2000	3000 Total Calories

- Check gastric residuals before every intermittent feeding or every 2-4 hours during continuous feeding.
- If intolerance develops, return to previously tolerated strength and rate. When tolerance is again established, proceed with feeding schedule as indicated. Do not alter rate and strength at the same time.
- Rinsing the tube with water (eg, 25-100 mL) after each intermittent feeding or every 3 to 6 hours during continuous feeding will help avoid clogging and provide additional water.

FORTA® PUDDING
[fort′a]

Usage: To provide balanced nutrition in a delicious, easy-to-eat form. Each 5-oz serving provides at least 17% of the U.S. RDA for vitamins and minerals for adults and children 4 or more years of age.
Features:
- High caloric density—50 Cal/oz provides 250 Calories per 5-oz serving.
- Balanced caloric distribution—high-quality protein plus appropriate levels of fat and carbohydrate.
- Low sodium content—240 mg per serving of Vanilla Forta Pudding — appropriate for diets allowing moderate sodium intake.
- Easy-open 5-oz cans are ready to serve—at room temperature or chilled.
- Four delicious flavors (Vanilla, Chocolate, Butterscotch, Tapioca) satisfy each patient's preference—and provide taste and texture variety.
- Colorful label design brightens the meal tray.

Availability:
Ready To Eat: 5-oz cans; 12 four-packs per case; Chocolate, No. 790; Vanilla, No. 792; Tapioca, No. 794; Butterscotch, No. 798.
Composition: Vanilla (Other flavors have similar composition. For specific information, see product packaging.)

Ingredients: Water, nonfat milk, sucrose, partially hydrogenated soybean oil, modified food starch, minerals (magnesium sulfate, sodium phosphate dibasic, ferrous sulfate, zinc sulfate, manganous chloride, cupric sulfate), sodium stearoyl lactylate, artificial flavor, vitamins (ascorbic acid, alpha-tocopheryl acetate, choline chloride, niacinamide, calcium pantothenate, vitamin D_3, vitamin A palmitate, pyridoxine hydrochloride, thiamine chloride hydrochloride, biotin, folic acid, riboflavin, phylloquinone, cyanocobalamin) and FD&C yellow #5.

Approximate Analysis (per 5-oz serving): Protein, 6.8 g; Fat, 9.7 g; Carbohydrate, 34.0 g; Minerals (Ash), 0.6 g; Moisture, 90.6 g. Calories per serving, 250.
[See table left].
(FAN 242)

Vitamin/Mineral Content of Forta Pudding

Vitamins/Minerals	Per Can (5 oz)		Percent U.S. RDA* 250 Calories
Vitamin A	833	I.U.	17
Vitamin D	67	I.U.	17
Vitamin E	5.0	I.U.	17
Vitamin K_1	10	mcg	**
Vitamin C	15	mg	25
Folic Acid	67	mcg	17
Thiamine (Vit. B_1)	0.25	mg	17
Riboflavin (Vit. B_2)	0.28	mg	17
Vitamin B_6	0.33	mg	17
Vitamin B_{12}	1.0	mcg	17
Niacin	3.3	mg	17
Choline	25	mg	**
Biotin	50	mcg	17
Pantothenic Acid	1.66	mg	17
Sodium	240	mg	**
Potassium	330	mg	**
Chloride	220	mg	**
Calcium	0.20	g	20
Phosphorus	0.20	g	20
Magnesium	67	mg	17
Iodine	60	mcg	40
Manganese	0.66	mg	**
Copper	0.33	mg	17
Zinc	3.0	mg	20
Iron	3.0	mg	17

*For adults and children 4 or more years of age.
**U.S. RDA not established.

Continued on next page

Ross—Cont.

ISOMIL®
[ī′sō-mil]
Soy Protein Formula

Usage: As a beverage for infants, children and adults with an allergy or sensitivity to cow milk. A feeding for patients with disorders where lactose should be avoided: lactase deficiency, lactose intolerance and galactosemia. A feeding following diarrhea.

Availability:
Powder: 14-oz cans; measuring scoop enclosed; 6 per case; No. 00107. 1.07-oz packets; 12 four-packet cartons per case; No. 00219.
Concentrated Liquid: 13-fl-oz cans; 24 per case; No. 02110.
Ready To Feed: (Prediluted, 20 Cal/fl oz) 32-fl-oz cans; 6 per case; No. 00230.
8-fl-oz cans; 4 six-packs per case; No. 00173.
For hospital use, prebottled Isomil is available in the Ross Hospital Formula System.

Preparation:
Powder: Standard dilution (20 Cal/fl oz) is 1 level scoop of Isomil Powder for each 2 fl oz of warm water; or, 1 packet (1.07 oz) for each 7 fl oz of warm water.
Concentrated Liquid: Standard dilution (20 Cal/fl oz) is one part Concentrated Liquid to one part water.
Note: All forms of Isomil should be shaken well before feeding.
Composition: Powder
Ingredients: (Pareve, Ⓤ) 30.7% corn syrup solids, 20.5% sucrose, 16.1% soy protein isolate, 14.0% corn oil, 14.0% coconut oil, minerals (1.6% calcium phosphate tribasic, 0.9% potassium citrate, 0.3% potassium chloride, 0.3% magnesium chloride, 0.2% sodium chloride, calcium carbonate, ferrous sulfate, zinc sulfate, cupric sulfate, manganese sulfate, potassium iodide), vitamins (ascorbic acid, choline chloride, alpha-tocopheryl acetate, niacinamide, calcium pantothenate, vitamin A palmitate, thiamine chloride hydrochloride, riboflavin, pyridoxine hydrochloride, phylloquinone, folic acid, biotin, vitamin D₃, cyanocobalamin), L-methionine, taurine and L-carnitine.

Nutrients:	Powder (wt/100 g)	Standard Dilution* (wt/liter)
Protein	13.7 g	18.0 g
Fat	28.1 g	36.9 g
Carbohydrate	51.7 g	68.0 g
Minerals (Ash)	3.5 g	4.6 g
Calcium	530 mg	700 mg
Phosphorus	380 mg	500 mg
Magnesium	38 mg	50 mg
Iron	9.1 mg	12 mg
Iodine	80 mcg	100 mcg
Zinc	3.8 mg	5.0 mg
Copper	0.38 mg	0.50 mg
Manganese	150 mcg	200 mcg
Sodium	240 mg	320 mg
Potassium	580 mg	770 mg
Chloride	450 mg	590 mg
Moisture	2.5 g	902 g
Crude Fiber	0 g	
Calories	513	676
Calories per fl oz		20

Vitamins Per Liter (Standard Dilution*):

Vitamin A	2000	I.U.
Vitamin D	400	I.U.
Vitamin E	17	I.U.
Vitamin K₁	100	mcg
Vitamin C	55	mg
Thiamine (Vit. B₁)	0.40	mg
Riboflavin (Vit. B₂)	0.60	mg
Vitamin B₆	0.40	mg
Vitamin B₁₂	3.0	mcg
Niacin	9.0	mg
Folic Acid	100	mcg
Pantothenic Acid	5.0	mg
Biotin	30	mcg
Choline	53	mg
Inositol	32	mg

* Standard dilution is 1 level scoop of Isomil Powder for each 2 fl oz of warm water; or, 1 packet (1.07 oz) for each 7 fl oz of warm water. (FAN 360-04)

Composition: Concentrated Liquid
Ingredients: (Pareve, Ⓤ) 74% water, 7.2% corn syrup, 5.8% sucrose, 4.1% soy oil, 3.8% soy protein isolate, 2.7% coconut oil, 1.0% modified corn starch, minerals (calcium phosphate tribasic, potassium citrate, potassium chloride, magnesium chloride, sodium chloride, ferrous sulfate, zinc sulfate, cupric sulfate, manganese sulfate, potassium iodide), mono- and diglycerides, soy lecithin, vitamins (ascorbic acid, choline chloride, alpha-tocopheryl acetate, niacinamide, calcium pantothenate, vitamin A palmitate, thiamine chloride hydrochloride, riboflavin, pyridoxine hydrochloride, phylloquinone, folic acid, biotin, vitamin D₃, cyanocobalamin), L-methionine, carrageenan, taurine and L-carnitine.

Nutrients (wt/liter):	Concentrated	Standard Dilution*
Protein	36.0 g	18.0 g
Fat	73.8 g	36.9 g
Carbohydrate	136.0 g	68.0 g
Minerals (Ash)	7.5 g	3.8 g
Calcium	1400 mg	700 mg
Phosphorus	1000 mg	500 mg
Magnesium	100 mg	50 mg
Iron	24 mg	12 mg
Iodine	200 mcg	100 mcg
Zinc	10 mg	5.0 mg
Copper	1.0 mg	0.50 mg
Manganese	400 mcg	200 mcg
Sodium	640 mg	320 mg
Potassium	1540 mg	770 mg
Chloride	1180 mg	590 mg
Water	806 g	902 g
Crude Fiber	0 g	
Calories per fl oz	40	20
Calories per liter	1352	676

Vitamins Per Liter (Standard Dilution*):

Vitamin A	2000	I.U.
Vitamin D	400	I.U.
Vitamin E	20	I.U.
Vitamin K₁	100	mcg
Vitamin C	55	mg
Thiamine (Vit. B₁)	0.40	mg
Riboflavin (Vit. B₂)	0.60	mg
Vitamin B₆	0.40	mg
Vitamin B₁₂	3.0	mcg
Niacin	9.0	mg
Folic Acid	100	mcg
Pantothenic Acid	5.0	mg
Biotin	30	mcg
Choline	53	mg
Inositol	32	mg

*Standard dilution is equal amounts Isomil Concentrated Liquid and water. (FAN 360-03)
Composition: Ready To Feed
Ingredients: (Pareve, Ⓤ) 86.4% water, 4.1% corn syrup, 3.2% sucrose, 2.1% soy oil, 2.0% soy protein isolate, 1.4% coconut oil, minerals (calcium citrate, calcium phosphate tribasic, potassium phosphate monobasic, potassium chloride, potassium citrate, magnesium chloride, potassium phosphate dibasic, sodium chloride, ferrous sulfate, zinc sulfate, cupric sulfate, manganese sulfate, potassium iodide), mono- and diglycerides, soy lecithin, vitamins (ascorbic acid, choline chloride, alpha-tocopheryl acetate, niacinamide, calcium pantothenate, vitamin A palmitate, thiamine chloride hydrochloride, riboflavin, pyridoxine hydrochloride, phylloquinone, folic acid, biotin, Vitamin D₃, cyanocobalamin), carrageenan, L-methionine, taurine and L-carnitine.

Nutrients (wt/liter):

Protein	18.0	g
Fat	36.9	g
Carbohydrate	68.0	g
Minerals (Ash)	3.8	g
Calcium	700	mg
Phosphorus	500	mg
Magnesium	50	mg
Iron	12	mg
Iodine	100	mcg
Zinc	5.0	mg
Copper	0.50	mg
Manganese	200	mcg
Sodium	320	mg
Potassium	950	mg
Chloride	430	mg
Water	902	g
Crude Fiber	0	g
Calories per fl oz	20	
Calories per liter	676	

Vitamins Per Liter:

Vitamin A	2000	I.U.
Vitamin D	400	I.U.
Vitamin E	20	I.U.
Vitamin K₁	100	mcg
Vitamin C	55	mg
Thiamine (Vit. B₁)	0.40	mg
Riboflavin (Vit. B₂)	0.60	mg
Vitamin B₆	0.40	mg
Vitamin B₁₂	3.0	mcg
Niacin	9.0	mg
Folic Acid	100	mcg
Pantothenic Acid	5.0	mg
Biotin	30	mcg
Choline	53	mg
Inositol	32	mg

The addition of iron to this formula conforms to the recommendation of the Committee on Nutrition of the American Academy of Pediatrics. (FAN 360-03)

ISOMIL® SF
[ī′so-mil]
Sucrose-Free Soy Protein Formula

Usage: As a beverage for infants, children and adults with an allergy or sensitivity to cow milk protein or an intolerance to sucrose. A feeding for patients following acute diarrhea. A feeding for patients with disorders where lactose and sucrose should be avoided.

Availability:
Concentrated Liquid: 13-fl-oz cans; 12 per case; No. 00119.
Ready To Feed: (Prediluted, 20 Cal/fl oz) 32-fl-oz cans; 6 per case; No. 00128.
For hospital use, prebottled Isomil SF is available in the Ross Hospital Formula System.

Preparation:
Concentrated Liquid: Standard dilution (20 Cal/fl oz) is one part Isomil SF Concentrated Liquid to one part water.
Note: All forms of Isomil SF should be shaken well before feeding.
Composition: Concentrated Liquid
Ingredients: (Pareve, Ⓤ) 75.7% water, 13.2% corn syrup solids, 4.2% soy protein isolate, 4.0% soy oil, 2.6% coconut oil, minerals (calcium phosphate tribasic, potassium citrate, potassium chloride, magnesium chloride, calcium carbonate, sodium chloride, ferrous sulfate, zinc sulfate, cupric sulfate, manganese sulfate, potassium iodide), mono- and diglycerides, soy lecithin, vitamins (ascorbic acid, choline chloride, alpha-tocopheryl acetate, niacinamide, calcium pantothenate, vitamin A palmitate, thiamine chloride hydrochloride, riboflavin, pyridoxine hydrochloride, phylloquinone, folic acid, biotin, vitamin D₃, cyanocobalamin), L-methionine, taurine and L-carnitine.

Nutrients (wt/liter):	Concentrated	Standard Dilution*
Protein	40.0 g	20.0 g
Fat	72.0 g	36.0 g
Carbohydrate	136.0 g	68.0 g
Minerals (Ash)	7.5 g	3.8 g
Calcium	1400 mg	700 mg
Phosphorus	1000 mg	500 mg
Magnesium	100 mg	50 mg
Iron	24 mg	12 mg
Iodine	200 mcg	100 mcg

Zinc	10	mg	5.0	mg
Copper	1.0	mg	0.50	mg
Manganese	400	mcg	200	mcg
Sodium	640	mg	320	mg
Potassium	1540	mg	770	mg
Chloride	1180	mg	590	mg
Water	806	g	902	g
Crude Fiber	0	g		
Calories per fl oz	40		20	
Calories per liter	1352		676	

Vitamins Per Liter (Standard Dilution*):

Vitamin A	2000	I.U.
Vitamin D	400	I.U.
Vitamin E	20	I.U.
Vitamin K$_1$	100	mcg
Vitamin C	55	mg
Thiamine (Vit. B$_1$)	0.40	mg
Riboflavin (Vit. B$_2$)	0.60	mg
Vitamin B$_6$	0.40	mg
Vitamin B$_{12}$	3.0	mcg
Niacin	9.0	mg
Folic Acid	100	mcg
Pantothenic Acid	5.0	mg
Biotin	30	mcg
Choline	53	mg
Inositol	32	mg

* Standard dilution is equal amounts Isomil SF Concentrated Liquid and water. (FAN 360-02)

Composition: Ready To Feed
Ingredients: (Pareve, Ⓤ) 87.3% water, 6.7% corn syrup solids, 2.3% soy protein isolate, 2.0% soy oil, 1.4% coconut oil, minerals (calcium phosphate dibasic, potassium citrate, calcium carbonate, potassium chloride, calcium phosphate monobasic, magnesium chloride, ferrous sulfate, sodium chloride, zinc sulfate, cupric sulfate, manganese sulfate, potassium iodide), mono- and diglycerides, soy lecithin, vitamins (ascorbic acid, choline chloride, alpha-tocopheryl acetate, niacinamide, calcium pantothenate, vitamin A palmitate, thiamine chloride hydrochloride, riboflavin, pyridoxine hydrochloride, phylloquinone, folic acid, biotin, vitamin D$_3$, cyanocobalamin), carrageenan, L-methionine, taurine and L-carnitine.

Nutrients (wt/liter):

Protein	20.0	g
Fat	36.0	g
Carbohydrate	68.0	g
Minerals (Ash)	3.8	g
Calcium	700	mg
Phosphorus	500	mg
Magnesium	50	mg
Iron	12	mg
Iodine	100	mcg
Zinc	5.0	mg
Copper	0.50	mg
Manganese	200	mcg
Sodium	320	mg
Potassium	770	mg
Chloride	590	mg
Water	902	g
Crude Fiber	0	
Calories per fl oz	20	
Calories per liter	676	

Vitamins Per Liter:

Vitamin A	2000	I.U.
Vitamin D	400	I.U.
Vitamin E	20	I.U.
Vitamin K$_1$	100	mcg
Vitamin C	55	mg
Thiamine (Vit. B$_1$)	0.40	mg
Riboflavin (Vit. B$_2$)	0.60	mg
Vitamin B$_6$	0.40	mg
Vitamin B$_{12}$	3.0	mcg
Niacin	9.0	mg
Folic Acid	100	mcg
Pantothenic Acid	5.0	mg
Biotin	30	mcg
Choline	53	mg
Inositol	32	mg

The addition of iron to this formula conforms to the recommendation of the Committee on Nutrition of the American Academy of Pediatrics. (FAN 360-02)

MURINE® REGULAR FORMULA   OTC
[myur-ēn']
Eye Drops

Description: Murine Regular Formula is a sterile isotonic buffered solution containing glycerin, potassium chloride, sodium chloride, sodium phosphate (monobasic and dibasic), and water. Edetate disodium 0.05% and benzalkonium chloride 0.01% are added as preservatives. (No vasoconstrictor.)

Indications: Murine is a non-staining, clear solution formulated to closely match the natural fluid of the eye for gentle, soothing relief from minor eye irritation. Use whenever desired to cleanse or refresh the eyes and to relieve minor irritation due to smog, sun glare, wind, dust, wearing contact lenses and eyestrain from reading, driving, TV and close work.

Warning: Murine Regular Formula should only be used for minor eye irritations. If irritation persists or increases, discontinue use and consult your physician.

Dosage and Administration: Two or three drops into each eye as needed. Do not touch bottle tip to any surface since this may contaminate solution. Remove contact lenses before using. Keep this and all medications out of the reach of children. Replace cap after using.

How Supplied: In 0.5 fl oz and 1.5 fl oz plastic dropper bottle.

MURINE® PLUS
[myur-ēn']
Eye Drops

Description: Murine Plus is a sterile isotonic buffered solution containing tetrahydrozoline hydrochloride 0.05%, boric acid, sodium borate and water. Edetate disodium 0.1% and benzalkonium chloride 0.01% are added as preservatives. (Contains vasoconstrictor.)

Indications: Murine Plus is a sterile, isotonic decongestant ophthalmic solution, compatible with the natural fluids of the eye. Its primary ingredient is a sympathomimetic agent, tetrahydrozoline hydrochloride, which produces local vasoconstriction in the eye. Thus, the drug effectively narrows swollen blood vessels locally and provides symptomatic relief of edema and hyperemia of conjunctival tissues due to eye allergies, minor local irritations and catarrhal (or "nonspecific") conjunctivitis. The formula of the solution includes other ingredients designed to produce a refreshing, soothing effect in addition to decongestion. Desirable effects comprise attenuation of burning, irritant and itching sensations, redness, and excessive lacrimation (tearing). Eyes reddened by swimming, plant allergies (pollen), overindulgence, colds, smog, sun glare, wind, dust, wearing contact lenses and eyestrain from reading, driving, TV and close work are quickly whitened by the vasoconstrictor action noted above. Its effect is prompt (apparent within minutes) and sustained. Although other vasoconstrictors may dilate the pupil (mydriasis) or result in rebound hyperemia, the use of tetrahydrozoline in Murine Plus is not known to cause either of these effects.

Warning: Murine Plus should only be used for minor eye irritations. Murine Plus should not be used by individuals with glaucoma and serious eye diseases. In some instances redness or inflammation may be due to serious eye conditions such as acute iritis, acute glaucoma, or corneal trauma. Murine Plus Eye Drops have been shown by various studies to be both safe and efficacious for minor eye irritations. When redness, pain or blurring persist, its use should be discontinued and a physician should be consulted at once.

Dosage and Administration: One or two drops in eye(s) up to 4 times daily or as directed by physician. Do not touch bottle tip to any surface, since this may contaminate the solution. Remove contact lenses before using. Keep this and all other medicines out of the reach of children. Replace cap after using.

How Supplied: In 0.5 fl oz and 1.5 fl oz plastic dropper bottle.

MURINE® EAR WAX REMOVAL   OTC
SYSTEM/MURINE® EAR DROPS
[myur-ēn']

Description: Carbamide peroxide 6.5% in anhydrous glycerin and a 1.0 fl oz soft rubber bulb ear washer. The Murine Ear Wax Removal System is the only self-treatment method on the market for ear wax removal. Application of carbamide peroxide drops followed by warm water irrigation is an effective, medically recommended way to help loosen hardened ear wax.

Actions: The carbamide peroxide formula in Murine Ear Drops is an aid in the removal of hardened cerumen from the ear canal. Anhydrous glycerin penetrates and softens ear wax while the release of oxygen from carbamide peroxide provides a mechanical action resulting in the loosening of the softened wax accumulation. It is usually necessary to remove the loosened wax by gentle irrigation with warm water using the soft rubber bulb ear washer provided.

Indications: The Murine Ear Wax Removal System is indicated as an aid in the removal of hardened or tightly packed cerumen from the ear canal or as an aid in the prevention of ceruminosis.

Caution: If redness, tenderness, pain, dizziness or ear drainage are present or develop, the medication should not be used or continued until a physician is seen. Do not use if ear drum is known to be perforated.

Dosage and Administration: For wax removal—Adults and children over 12 years: Tilt head sideways and place 5 to 10 drops into ear. Tip of bottle should not enter ear canal. Keep drops in ear for several minutes by keeping head tilted or placing cotton in ear. Wax remaining after treatment may be removed by gently flushing ear with warm water, using soft rubber bulb ear washer placed on edge of ear canal. Use twice daily, up to 4 days if needed, or as directed by a doctor. Children under 12 years: Consult a doctor.
The ear canal can be kept free from accumulated hardened cerumen by regular usage of the Murine Ear Wax Removal System.

How Supplied: The Murine Ear Wax Removal System contains 0.5 fl oz drops and a 1.0 fl oz soft rubber bulb ear washer.
Also available in 0.5 fl oz drops only, Murine Ear Drops.

OSMOLITE®
[oz' mō-līt]
Isotonic Liquid Nutrition

Usage: As an isotonic liquid food providing complete, balanced nutrition. Osmolite has been designed for patients particularly sensitive to hyperosmotic feedings. Osmolite may be used as a tube feeding (nasogastric, nasoduodenal or jejunal) or as an oral feeding. Two quarts (2000 Calories) of Osmolite meets or surpasses 100% of the U.S. RDA for vitamins and minerals for adults and children 4 or more years of age.

Features:
• Complete, balanced nutrition—1.06 Calories per ml, 250 Calories per 8-fl oz feeding, 1000 Calories per quart from a balanced distribution of protein, fat and carbohydrate (caloric distribution: protein, 14.0%; fat, 31.4%; carbohydrate, 54.6%).
• Isotonic formulation—The osmolality is 300 mOsm/kg water, equaling the osmotic pressure of plasma.
• Carbohydrate source—Osmolite is lactose-free and will not contribute to lactose-associated diarrhea. Polycose® Glucose Polymers is the carbohydrate source, which is a readily available and easily digested source of calories.

Continued on next page

Ross—Cont.

- **High biologic value protein**—Osmolite provides a full complement of amino acids to meet the National Research Council's profile for high quality proteins and has a Calorie-to-nitrogen ratio of 178:1.
- **Fat source**—Osmolite contains a high level of essential fatty acids from corn and soy oils, as well as medium-chain triglycerides as 15% of total calories (50% of fat calories) to facilitate rapid, effective absorption of fat calories.
- **Low-residue feeding**—The amount of fecal residue produced by Osmolite is comparable to that produced by a chemically defined, elemental diet. Therefore, Osmolite is appropriate for use in situations where low residue is a primary consideration.
- **Low electrolyte levels**—Osmolite is appropriate for use with moderate electrolyte-restricted diets, yet provides electrolyte levels adequate for most hospitalized patients.
- **Unflavored**—The mild, acceptable taste makes Osmolite particularly appropriate for use with patients experiencing altered or heightened taste perceptions (eg, individuals undergoing radiation or chemotherapy treatment).
- **Convenient**—Osmolite is ready to use. No mixing is required. Potential for contamination during preparation is reduced.

Dosage and Administration: Shake well. Dilution is not required. Osmolite may be stored (unopened) and fed at room temperature. Once opened, Osmolite should be covered and refrigerated. Any unused portion should be discarded if not used within 48 hours.

Oral Feeding: Osmolite may be used as a sole source of nutrition, or with and between meals for added nutritional support.

Tube Feeding: Follow physician's instructions. When initiating feeding, the flow rate, volume and dilution are dependent on patient condition and tolerance. Care should be taken to avoid contamination of this product during preparation and administration.

Additional fluid requirements should be met by giving water orally with or after feedings, or when flushing the feeding tube.

Under no circumstances should Osmolite be administered parenterally.
[See table below].

Availability:
Ready To Use:
8-fl-oz bottles; 24 per case; No. 715.
8-fl-oz cans; 4 six-packs per case; No. 709.
32-fl-oz cans; 6 per case; No. 738.

Composition:
Ingredients: (U) Water, hydrolyzed corn starch, sodium and calcium caseinates, medium-chain triglycerides (fractionated coconut oil), corn oil, soy protein isolate, minerals (potassium citrate, calcium phosphate tribasic, magnesium sulfate, magnesium chloride, zinc sulfate, ferrous sulfate, manganous chloride, cupric sulfate), soy oil, soy lecithin, vitamins (choline chloride, ascorbic acid, alpha-tocopheryl acetate, niacinamide, calcium pantothenate, thiamine chloride hydrochloride, pyridoxine hydrochloride, riboflavin, vitamin A palmitate, folic acid, biotin, phylloquinone, cyanocobalamin, vitamin D_3) and carrageenan.

Approximate Analysis (g/8 fl oz): Protein, 8.8; Fat, 9.1; Carbohydrate, 34.3; Ash, 1.3; Moisture, 199.1. Calories per ml, 1.06; Calories per fl oz, 31.3. [See table above].
(FAN 340-01)

Vitamin/Mineral Content of Osmolite Ready To Use

Vitamins/Minerals	Per 8 Fl Oz		Percent U.S. RDA* (Per 8 Fl Oz)
Vitamin A	625	I.U.	12.5
Vitamin D	50	I.U.	12.5
Vitamin E	5.7	I.U.	19.0
Vitamin K_1	9	mcg	**
Vitamin C	38	mg	62.5
Folic Acid	50	mcg	12.5
Thiamine (Vit. B_1)	0.38	mg	25.0
Riboflavin (Vit. B_2)	0.43	mg	25.0
Vitamin B_6	0.50	mg	25.0
Vitamin B_{12}	1.5	mcg	25.0
Niacin	5.0	mg	25.0
Choline	0.13	g	**
Biotin	38	mcg	12.5
Pantothenic Acid	1.25	mg	12.5
Sodium	0.13	g	**
Potassium	0.24	g	**
Chloride	0.20	g	**
Calcium	0.13	g	12.5
Phosphorus	0.13	g	12.5
Magnesium	50	mg	12.5
Iodine	19	mcg	12.5
Manganese	0.50	mg	**
Copper	0.25	mg	12.5
Zinc	3.7	mg	25.0
Iron	2.2	mg	12.5

*For adults and children 4 or more years of age.
**U.S. RDA not established.

Sample Administration Schedule for OSMOLITE

Continuous Drip Schedule

Day	Time	Strength	Rate (mL/hr)	Volume (mL)	Calories
1	1st 8 hours	Full	50	400	400
	2nd 8 hours	Full	75	600	600
	3rd 8 hours	Full	100	800	800
					1800 Total Calories
2	24 hours	Full	100–125	2400–3000	2400–3000 Total Calories

Intermittent Drip Schedule

Day	Time	Strength	Rate (5–10 mL/min)	Volume (mL)	Calories
1	7am–11pm	Full	100 mL q 2 hr (7am, 9am)	200	200
		Full	150 mL q 2 hr (11am, 1pm, 3pm)	450	450
		Full	200 mL q 2 hr (5pm, 7pm, 9pm, 11pm)	800	800
					1450 Total Calories
2	7am–11pm	Full	250 mL q 2 hr (8 feedings) up to	2000	2000 Total Calories
			400 mL q 3 hr (5 feedings)	2000	2000 Total Calories

- Check gastric residuals before every intermittent feeding or every 2–4 hours during continuous feeding.
- If intolerance develops (such as nausea, abdominal cramps, distention, or diarrhea) return to previously tolerated rate, or dilute formula to half strength. After tolerance to half strength OSMOLITE is established, continue feeding schedule using half strength OSMOLITE until desired rate is achieved. Then switch to full strength. Do not alter strength and volume at the same time.
- Rinsing the tube with water (eg, 25–100 mL) after each intermittent feeding or every 3 to 6 hours during continuous feeding will help avoid clogging and provide additional water.

OSMOLITE® HN
[*oz'mō-lit*]
High Nitrogen Isotonic Liquid Nutrition

Usage: As a high-nitrogen, isotonic liquid food providing complete, balanced nutrition. Osmolite HN is most appropriate in moderately to severely stressed patients (≥ 30% increase in resting metabolic expenditure) with intolerance to hyperosmolar feedings or with fat maldigestion/malabsorption. Osmolite HN may be used as a tube feeding (nasogastric, nasoduodenal, or jejunal) or as an oral feeding.

Features:
- Complete, balanced nutrition—1.06 Calories per ml, 250 Calories per 8 fl oz, 1000 Calories per quart from a balanced distribution of protein, fat and carbohydrate (caloric distribution: protein, 16.7%; fat, 30.0%; carbohydrate, 53.3%). 1400 Calories of Osmolite HN meets or surpasses 100% of the U.S. RDA for vitamins and minerals for adults and children 4 or more years of age.
- High protein level—10.5 g high-quality protein per 8-fl-oz serving (1.68 g nitrogen/8 fl oz).
- Total calorie-to-nitrogen ratio of 150:1—appropriate for the stressed patient.
- Lactose-free—Osmolite HN will not contribute to lactose-associated diarrhea. Hydrolyzed corn starch is the carbohydrate source.
- Isotonic formulation—The osmolality is 310 mOsm/kg water.
- Fat source—Osmolite contains a high level of essential fatty acids from corn and soy oils, as

well as medium-chain triglycerides as 15% of total calories (50% of fat) to facilitate rapid, effective absorption of fat calories.

- Low-residue feeding—Osmolite HN is appropriate for use in situations where low residue is a consideration.
- Unflavored—The mild, acceptable taste makes Osmolite HN particularly appropriate for use with patients experiencing altered or heightened taste perceptions (eg, individuals undergoing radiation or chemotherapy treatment).
- Convenient—Osmolite HN is ready to use. No mixing is required. Potential for contamination during preparation is reduced.

Dosage and Administration:
Ready To Use: Shake well. Dilution is not required. Osmolite HN may be stored (unopened) and fed at room temperature. Once opened, Osmolite HN should be covered and refrigerated. Any unused portion should be discarded if not used within 48 hours.
Enteral Feeding: Follow physician's instructions. When initiating feeding, the flow rate, volume and dilution are dependent on patient condition and tolerance. Care should be taken to avoid contamination of this product during preparation and administration. Additional fluid requirements should be met by giving water orally with or after feedings, or when flushing the feeding tube.
Under no circumstances should Osmolite HN be administered parenterally.
[See table right].

Availability:
Ready To Use:
8-fl-oz bottles; 24 per case; No. 736.
8-fl-oz cans; 4 six-packs per case; No. 735.
32-fl-oz cans; 6 per case; No. 739.

Composition:
Ingredients: Ⓤ Water, hydrolyzed cornstarch, sodium and calcium caseinates, medium-chain triglycerides (fractionated coconut oil), corn oil, minerals (calcium phosphate tribasic, potassium citrate, magnesium chloride, magnesium sulfate, sodium citrate, potassium chloride, zinc sulfate, ferrous sulfate, manganese sulfate, cupric sulfate), soy protein isolate, soy oil, soy lecithin, vitamins (choline chloride, ascorbic acid, alpha-tocopheryl acetate, niacinamide, calcium pantothenate, thiamine chloride hydrochloride, pyridoxine hydrochloride, riboflavin, vitamin A palmitate, folic acid, biotin, phylloquinone, cyanocobalamin, vitamin D_3) and carrageenan.
Approximate Analysis (g/8 fl oz): Protein, 10.5; Fat, 8.7; Carbohydrate, 33.4; Minerals (Ash), 1.9;

Sample Administration Schedule For OSMOLITE HN

Continuous Drip Schedule

Day	Time	Strength	Rate (mL/h)	Volume (mL)	Calories
1	1st 8 hours	Full	50	400	400
	2nd 8 hours	Full	75	600	600
	3rd 8 hours	Full	100	800	800
					1800 Total Calories
2	24 hours	Full	100-125	2400-3000	2400-3000 Total Calories

Intermittent Drip Schedule

Day	Time	Strength	Rate (5-10 mL/min)	Volume (mL)	Calories
1	7am-11pm	Full	100 mL q 2 h (7am, 9am)	200	200
		Full	150 mL q 2 h (11am, 1pm, 3pm)	450	450
		Full	200 mL q 2 h (5pm, 7pm, 9pm, 11pm)	800	800
					1450 Total Calories
2	7am-11pm	Full	250 mL q 2 h (8 feedings) up to	2000	2000 Total Calories
			400 mL q 3 h (5 feedings)	2000	2000 Total Calories

- Check gastric residuals before every intermittent feeding or every 2-4 hours during continuous feeding.
- If intolerance develops, return to previously tolerated rate, or dilute formula to half strength. After tolerance to half strength OSMOLITE HN is established, continue feeding schedule using half strength OSMOLITE HN until desired rate is achieved. Then switch to full strength. Do not alter strength and volume at the same time.
- Rinsing the tube with water (eg, 25-100 mL) after each intermittent feeding or every 3 to 6 hours during continuous feeding will help avoid clogging and provide additional water.

Moisture, 199. Calories per ml, 1.06; Calories per fl oz, 31.3.
[See table below].
(FAN 283)

PEDIAFLOR® Drops ℞
[pē′ dē-e-flor″]
Sodium Fluoride Oral Solution, USP
Description:
One dropperful (1.0 ml) provides:
Fluoride (as sodium fluoride).........................0.5 mg
Indications and Usage: As an aid in the prevention of dental caries in infants and children.
Contraindications: Should be used only where the fluoride content of the drinking water supply is known to be 0.7 parts per million or less.

Precautions: The recommended dosage should not be exceeded since chronic overdosage of fluoride may result in mottling of tooth enamel and osseous changes.
Overdosage: In children, acute ingestion of 10 to 20 mg of sodium fluoride may cause excessive salivation and gastrointestinal disturbances; 500 mg may be fatal. Oral and/or intravenous fluids containing calcium may be indicated.
Dosage and Administration: Daily dosage —under 2 years of age, one-half dropperful or less daily; 2 years of age, one dropperful daily; 3 years of age or older, two dropperfuls or less daily; or as directed by physician or dentist.
Availability: 50-ml bottles, calibrated dropper enclosed; Rx; **NDC** 0074-0101-50.

PEDIALYTE®
[pe″de-e-līt]
Oral Electrolyte Maintenance Solution
Usage: For maintenance of water and electrolytes during mild or moderate diarrhea in infants and children; for maintenance of water and electrolytes following corrective parenteral therapy for severe diarrhea.
Features:
- Ready to use—no mixing or dilution necessary.
- Balanced electrolytes to replace usual stool losses and provide maintenance requirements.
- Provides glucose to promote sodium and water absorption.
- Fruit-flavored form available to enhance compliance in older infants.
- No coloring added.
- Widely available.

Availability: 32-fl-oz cans; 6 per case; Unflavored, No. 236—NDC 0074-6470-32; Fruit-flavored, No. 165—NDC 0074-6471-32.
8-fl-oz bottles; 4 six-packs per case; Unflavored, No. 160—NDC 0074-6470-08. For hospital use, prebottled PEDIALYTE is available in the Ross Hospital Formula System.
Dosage: Administration Guide for Maintenance of Body Water and Electrolytes Frequently Lost in Mild or Moderate Diarrhea (Pedialyte® or Fruit-Flavored Pedialyte®) and Management of Moderate to Severe Diarrhea Associated with Dehydration (Pedialyte® RS).

Vitamin/Mineral Content of Osmolite HN (Ready To Use)

Vitamins/Minerals	Per 8 Fl Oz		Percent U.S. RDA* (Per 8 Fl Oz)
Vitamin A	900	I.U.	18
Vitamin D	72	I.U.	18
Vitamin E	8.1	I.U.	27
Vitamin K_1	13	mcg	**
Vitamin C	33	mg	55
Folic Acid	0.11	mg	27
Thiamine (Vit. B_1)	0.41	mg	27
Riboflavin (Vit. B_2)	0.46	mg	27
Vitamin B_6	0.55	mg	27
Vitamin B_{12}	1.7	mcg	28
Niacin	5.4	mg	27
Choline	0.14	g	**
Biotin	82	mcg	27
Pantothenic Acid	2.7	mg	27
Sodium	220	mg	**
Potassium	370	mg	**
Chloride	340	mg	**
Calcium	0.18	g	18
Phosphorus	0.18	g	18
Magnesium	72	mg	18
Iodine	27	mcg	18
Manganese	0.90	mg	**
Copper	0.36	mg	18
Zinc	4.1	mg	27
Iron	3.3	mg	18

*For adults and children 4 or more years of age.
**U.S. RDA not established.

Continued on next page

Ross—Cont.

Pedialyte, Fruit-Flavored Pedialyte or Pedialyte RS should be offered frequently in amounts tolerated. Total daily intake should be adjusted to meet individual needs based on thirst and response to therapy. The suggested intakes for maintenance below are based on water requirements for ordinary energy expenditure.[1] The suggested intakes for replacement and maintenance are based on fluid losses of 5% or 10% of body weight including maintenance requirement.
[See table below].

Composition: Unflavored Pedialyte (Flavored Pedialyte has similar composition and nutrient values. For specific information, see product label.
Ingredients: (Pareve, Ⓤ) Water, dextrose, potassium citrate, sodium chloride and sodium citrate.

Provides:	Per 8 Fl Oz	Per Liter	Per 32 Fl Oz
Sodium (mEq)	10.6	45	42.4
Potassium (mEq)	4.7	20	18.8
Chloride (mEq)	8.3	35	33.2
Citrate (mEq)	7.1	30	28.4
Dextrose (grams)	5.9	25	23.6
Calories (FAN 328)	24	100	96

PEDIALYTE® RS
Oral Electrolyte Rehydration Solution

Usage: For replacement of water and electrolytes during moderate to severe diarrhea.
Features:
- Ready to use—no mixing or dilution necessary.
- Safe, economical alternative to IV therapy.
- 75 mEq of sodium per liter for effective replacement of fluid deficits.
- 2½% glucose solution to promote sodium and water absorption and provide energy.
- Widely available in pharmacies.

Availability:
8-fl-oz bottles; 4 six-packs per case; No. 162; NDC 0074-6472-08.

Dosage: (See chart below)
Ingredients: (Pareve, Ⓤ) Water, dextrose, sodium chloride, potassium citrate and sodium citrate.

Provides:	Per 8 Fl Oz	Per Liter
Sodium (mEq)	17.7	75
Potassium (mEq)	4.7	20
Chloride (mEq)	15.4	65
Citrate (mEq)	7.1	30
Dextrose (grams)	5.9	25
Calories (FAN 328)	24	100

PEDIAMYCIN®
[pē″dē-e-mī′san]
erythromycin ethylsuccinate

Description: Erythromycin is produced by a strain of *Streptomyces erythraeus* and belongs to the macrolide group of antibiotics. It is basic and readily forms salts with acids. The base, the stearate salt and the esters are poorly soluble in water. Erythromycin ethylsuccinate is an ester of erythromycin suitable for oral administration. The premixed suspension, granules and drops for oral administration are intended primarily for pediatric use but can also be used in adults.

Pediamycin 400 (erythromycin ethylsuccinate oral suspension), 400 mg erythromycin activity per teaspoonful (5 ml), is a premixed suspension with an appealing cherry flavor, supplied in pint (16 fl oz) bottles. Its form and flavor make it especially suitable for older children unwilling or unable to swallow capsules or tablets.

Pediamycin Liquid (erythromycin ethylsuccinate oral suspension), 200 mg erythromycin activity per teaspoonful (5 ml), is a premixed suspension with an appealing cherry flavor, supplied in pint (16 fl oz) bottles. Its form and flavor make it especially suitable for infants and children, and for older children unwilling or unable to swallow capsules or tablets.

Pediamycin Suspension and *Pediamycin Drops* (erythromycin ethylsuccinate for oral suspension), 200 mg erythromycin activity per teaspoonful (5 ml), 100 mg erythromycin activity per dropperful (2.5 ml), are pleasant-tasting cherry-flavored oral suspensions, dispensed as granules of erythromycin ethylsuccinate reconstituted with water. Pediamycin granules are packaged in 100-ml and 150-ml (Suspension), and 50-ml (Drops) bottles. A calibrated dropper is supplied with the 50-ml bottles.

Actions:
Microbiology
Biochemical tests demonstrate that erythromycin inhibits protein synthesis of the pathogen without directly affecting nucleic acid synthesis. Antagonism has been demonstrated between clindamycin and erythromycin.
NOTE: Many strains of *Hemophilus influenzae* are resistant to erythromycin alone but are susceptible to erythromycin and sulfonamides together. Staphylococci resistant to erythromycin may emerge during a course of erythromycin therapy. Culture and susceptibility testing should be performed.

Disc Susceptibility Tests
Quantitative methods that require measurement of zone diameters give the most precise estimates of antibiotic susceptibility. One recommended procedure (21 CFR section 460.1) uses erythromycin class discs for testing susceptibility; interpretations correlate zone diameters of this disc test with MIC values for erythromycin. With this procedure, a report from the laboratory of "susceptible" indicates that the infective organism is likely to respond to therapy. A report of "resistant" indicates that the infective organism is not likely to respond to therapy. A report of "intermediate susceptibility" suggests that the organism would be susceptible if higher doses were used.

Clinical Pharmacology: Erythromycin binds to the 50 S ribosomal subunits of susceptible bacteria and suppresses protein synthesis.
Orally administered erythromycin ethylsuccinate suspensions are readily and reliably absorbed. Comparable serum levels of erythromycin are achieved in the fasting and the nonfasting states. Erythromycin diffuses readily into most body fluids. Only low concentrations are normally achieved in the spinal fluid, but passage of the drug across the blood-brain barrier increases in meningitis. In the presence of normal hepatic function, erythromycin is concentrated in the liver and excreted in the bile; the effect of hepatic dysfunction on excretion of erythromycin by the liver into the bile is not known. Less than 5 percent of the orally administered dose of erythromycin is excreted in active form in the urine.
Erythromycin crosses the placental barrier and is excreted in breast milk.

Indications: *Streptococcus pyogenes* (Group A beta-hemolytic streptococcus): Upper and lower respiratory tract, skin, and soft tissue infections of mild to moderate severity.
Injectable benzathine penicillin G is considered by the American Heart Association to be the drug of choice in the treatment and prevention of streptococcal pharyngitis and in long-term prophylaxis of rheumatic fever.
When oral medication is preferred for treatment of the above conditions, penicillin G or V, or erythromycin is the alternate drug of choice.
When oral medication is given, the importance of strict adherence by the patient to the prescribed dosage regimen must be stressed. A therapeutic dose should be administered for at least 10 days.
Alpha-hemolytic streptococci (viridans group): Although no controlled clinical efficacy trials have been conducted, oral erythromycin has been suggested by the American Heart Association and American Dental Association for use in a regimen for prophylaxis against bacterial endocarditis in patients hypersensitive to penicillin who have congenital heart disease, or rheumatic or other acquired valvular heart disease when they undergo dental procedures and surgical procedures of the upper respiratory tract.[1] Erythromycin is not suitable prior to genitourinary or gastrointestinal tract surgery. NOTE: When selecting antibiotics for the prevention of bacterial endocarditis the physician or dentist should read the full joint

Pedialyte, Pedialyte RS Dosage

For Infants and Young Children

Age	2 Weeks	3 Months	6 Months	9 Months	1	1½	2	2½ Years	3	3½	4
Approximate Weight[2] (lb)	7	13	17	21	23	25	28	30	32	35	38
(kg)	3.2	6.0	7.8	9.2	10.2	11.4	12.6	13.6	14.6	16.0	17.0
PEDIALYTE or FRUIT-FLAVORED PEDIALYTE oz/day for Maintenance	13 to 16	28 to 32	34 to 40	38 to 44	41 to 46	45 to 50	48 to 53	51 to 56	54 to 58	56 to 60	57 to 62
PEDIALYTE RS oz/day for Replacement for 5% Dehydration (including Maintenance)	18 to 21	38 to 42	47 to 53	53 to 59	58 to 63	64 to 69	69 to 74	74 to 79	78 to 82	83 to 87	85 to 90
PEDIALYTE RS oz/day for Replacement for 10% Dehydration (including Maintenance)	23 to 26	48 to 52	60 to 66	68 to 74	75 to 80	83 to 88	90 to 95	97 to 102	102 to 106	110 to 114	113 to 118

Above administration guide does not apply to infants less than 1 week of age. For children over 4 years, maintenance intakes may exceed 2 quarts daily.

1. Extrapolated from Barness L: Nutrition and nutritional disorders, Behrman RE, Vaughan VC III *Nelson Textbook of Pediatrics*, ed 12 Philadelphia: WB Saunders Co, 1983, pp 136-38
2. Based on the 50th percentile of weight for age of the National Center for Health Statistics (NCHS) reference growth data: Hamill PVV, Drizd TA, Johnson CL, Reed RB, Roche AF, Moore WM: Physical growth: National Center for Health Statistics percentiles. *Am J Clin Nutr* 32: 607-629, 1979.

statement of the American Heart Association and the American Dental Association.[1]
Staphylococcus aureus: Acute infections of skin and soft tissue of mild to moderate severity. Resistant organisms may emerge during treatment.
Streptococcus (Diplococcus) pneumoniae: Upper respiratory tract infections (e.g., otitis media, pharyngitis) and lower respiratory tract infections (e.g., pneumonia) of mild to moderate degree.
Mycoplasma pneumoniae(Eaton agent, PPLO): For respiratory infections due to this organism.
Hemophilus influenzae: For upper respiratory tract infections of mild to moderate severity when used concomitantly with adequate doses of sulfonamides. (See sulfonamide labeling for appropriate prescribing information.) The concomitant use of the sulfonamides is necessary since not all strains of *Hemophilus influenzae* are susceptible to erythromycin at the concentrations of the antibiotic achieved with usual therapeutic doses.
Chlamydia trachomatis: For the treatment of urethritis in adult males due to *Chlamydia trachomatis.*
Ureaplasma urealyticum: For the treatment of urethritis in adult males due to *Ureaplasma urealyticum.*
Treponema pallidum: Erythromycin is an alternate choice of treatment for primary syphilis in patients allergic to the penicillins. In treatment of primary syphilis, spinal fluid examinations should be done before treatment and as part of follow-up after therapy.
Corynebacterium diphtheriae: As an adjunct to antitoxin, to prevent establishment of carriers, and to eradicate the organism in carriers.
Corynebacterium minutissimum: For the treatment of erythrasma.
Entamoeba histolytica: In the treatment of intestinal amebiasis only. Extra-enteric amebiasis requires treatment with other agents.
Listeria monocytogenes: Infections due to this organism.
Bordetella pertussis: Erythromycin is effective in eliminating the organism from the nasopharynx of infected individuals, rendering them non-infectious. Some clinical studies suggest that erythromycin may be helpful in the prophylaxis of pertussis in exposed susceptible individuals.
Legionnaire's Disease: Although no controlled clinical efficacy studies have been conducted, *in vitro* and limited preliminary clinical data suggest that erythromycin may be effective in treating Legionnaire's Disease.
Contraindications: Erythromycin is contraindicated in patients with known hypersensitivity to this antibiotic.
Precautions: Erythromycin is principally excreted by the liver. Caution should be exercised in administering the antibiotic to patients with impaired hepatic function. There have been reports of hepatic dysfunction, with or without jaundice occurring in patients receiving oral erythromycin products.
Areas of localized infection may require surgical drainage in addition to antibiotic therapy.
Recent data from studies of erythromycin reveal that its use in patients who are receiving high doses of theophylline may be associated with an increase of serum theophylline levels and potential theophylline toxicity. In case of theophylline toxicity and/or elevated serum theophylline levels, the dose of theophylline should be reduced while the patient is receiving concomitant erythromycin therapy.
Usage during pregnancy and lactation: The safety of erythromycin for use during pregnancy has not been established.
Erythromycin crosses the placental barrier. Erythromycin also appears in breast milk.
Adverse Reactions: The most frequent side effects of oral erythromycin preparations are gastrointestinal, such as abdominal cramping and discomfort, and are dose related. Nausea, vomiting and diarrhea occur infrequently with usual oral doses.
During prolonged or repeated therapy, there is a possibility of overgrowth of nonsusceptible bacteria or fungi. If such infections occur, the drug should be discontinued and appropriate therapy instituted.
Allergic reactions ranging from urticaria and mild skin eruptions to anaphylaxis have occurred.
There have been isolated reports of reversible hearing loss occurring chiefly in patients with renal insufficiency and in patients receiving high doses of erythromycin.
Dosage and Administration: Erythromycin ethylsuccinate suspensions may be administered without regard to meals.
Children: Age, weight and severity of the infection are important factors in determining the proper dosage. In mild to moderate infections the usual dosage of erythromycin ethylsuccinate for children is 30 to 50 mg/kg/day in equally divided doses. For more severe infections this dosage may be doubled.
Adults: 400 mg erythromycin ethylsuccinate every 6 hours is the usual dose. Dosage may be increased up to 4 g per day according to the severity of the infections.
If twice-a-day dosage is desired in either adults or children, one-half of the total daily dose may be given every 12 hours. Doses may also be given three times daily if desired by administering one-third of the total daily dose every 8 hours.
The following approximate dosage schedule is suggested for using *Pediamycin Liquid* (erythromycin ethylsuccinate oral suspension), *Pediamycin Suspension* and *Pediamycin Drops* (erythromycin ethylsuccinate for oral suspension) in the treatment of mild to moderate infections by susceptible organisms.

Body Weight	Dose	Frequency	Approximate Daily Dosage
Under 10 lbs (4.5 kg)	40 mg/kg/day (20 mg/lb/day) in divided doses		
10–15 lbs (4.5 to 6.8 kg)	½ dropperful (50 mg) or 1 dropperful (100 mg)	4 times/day 2 times/day	200 mg
15–25 lbs (6.8 to 11.3 kg)	1 dropperful (100 mg) ½ teaspoonful (100 mg) or 2 dropperfuls (200 mg) 1 teaspoonful (200 mg)	4 times/day 2 times/day	400 mg
25–50 lbs (11.3 to 22.7 kg)	1 teaspoonful (200 mg) or 2 teaspoonfuls (400 mg)	4 times/day 2 times/day	800 mg
50–100 lbs (22.7 to 45.4 kg)	1½ teaspoonfuls (300 mg) or 3 teaspoonfuls (600 mg)	4 times/day 2 times/day	1200 mg
over 100 lbs (45.4 kg)	2 teaspoonfuls (400 mg) or 4 teaspoonfuls (800 mg)	4 times/day 2 times/day	1600 mg

The following approximate dosage schedule is suggested for using *Pediamycin 400* (erythromycin ethylsuccinate oral suspension) in the treatment of mild to moderate infections by susceptible organisms.

Body Weight	Dose	Frequency	Approximate Daily Dosage
25–50 lbs (11.3 to 22.7 kg)	1 teaspoonful (400 mg)	2 times/day	800 mg
50–100 lbs (22.7 to 45.4 kg)	1½ teaspoonfuls (600 mg)	2 times/day	1200 mg
over 100 lbs (45.4 kg)	2 teaspoonfuls (800 mg)	2 times/day	1600 mg

The total daily dosage must be administered in equally divided doses.
In the treatment of streptococcal infections, a therapeutic dosage of erythromycin ethylsuccinate should be administered for at least 10 days. In continuous prophylaxis against recurrences of streptococcal infections in persons with a history of rheumatic heart disease, the usual dosage is 400 mg twice a day.
For prophylaxis against bacterial endocarditis[1] in patients with congenital heart disease, or rheumatic or other acquired valvular heart disease when undergoing dental procedures or surgical procedures of the upper respiratory tract, give 1.6 g (20 mg/kg for children) orally 1½ to 2 hours before the procedure, and then, 800 mg (10 mg/kg for children) orally every 6 hours for 8 doses.
For treatment of urethritis due to *C. trachomatis* or *U. urealyticum:* 800 mg three times a day for 7 days.
For treatment of primary syphilis: Adults: 48 to 64 g given in divided doses over a period of 10 to 15 days.
For intestinal amebiasis: Adults: 400 mg four times daily for 10 to 14 days. Children: 30 to 50 mg/kg/day in divided doses for 10 to 14 days.
For use in pertussis: Although optimal dosage and duration have not been established, doses of erythromycin utilized in reported clinical studies were 40 to 50 mg/kg/day, given in divided doses for 5 to 14 days.
For treatment of Legionnaire's Disease: Although optimal doses have not been established, doses utilized in reported clinical data were 1.6 to 4 g daily in divided doses.
(.3821)
How Supplied: *Pediamycin 400* (erythromycin ethylsuccinate oral suspension, USP) is supplied in 1 pint bottles (**NDC** 0074-0211-16). It provides erythromycin ethylsuccinate equivalent to 400 mg erythromycin per teaspoonful (5 ml).
Pediamycin Liquid (erythromycin ethylsuccinate oral suspension, USP) is supplied in 1 pint bottles (**NDC** 0074-0202-16). It provides erythromycin ethylsuccinate equivalent to 200 mg erythromycin per teaspoonful (5 ml).
Pediamycin Suspension (erythromycin ethylsuccinate for oral suspension, USP) is available for teaspoon dosage in 100-ml (**NDC** 0074-0206-13) and 150-ml (**NDC** 0074-0206-09) bottles, in the form of granules to be reconstituted with 77 ml and 115 ml of water, respectively. It provides erythromycin ethylsuccinate equivalent to 200 mg erythromycin per teaspoonful (5 ml).
Pediamycin Drops (erythromycin ethylsuccinate for oral suspension, USP) is available for dropper dosage in 50-ml bottles (**NDC** 0074-0207-50), in the form of granules to be reconstituted with 38 ml of water, providing 100 mg of erythromycin activity per dropperful (2.5 ml). Dropper marked for 100 mg (dropperful), 75 mg and 50 mg (half dropperful) doses is enclosed in the carton.
Pediamycin Liquid and *Pediamycin 400* require refrigeration to preserve taste. Refrigeration by patient is not required if used within 14 days.

Continued on next page

Ross—Cont.

Reference:
1. American Heart Association, 1977. Prevention of bacterial endocarditis. Circulation 56:139A-143A.

PEDIAZOLE® ℞
[pē'dē-e-zōl"]
erythromycin ethylsuccinate and sulfisoxazole acetyl for oral suspension

Description: Pediazole is a combination of erythromycin ethylsuccinate, USP and sulfisoxazole acetyl, USP. When reconstituted with water as directed on the label, the granules form a white, strawberry-banana flavor suspension which provides 200 mg erythromycin activity and the equivalent of 600 mg of sulfisoxazole per teaspoonful (5 ml).

Erythromycin is produced by a strain of *Streptomyces erythraeus* and belongs to the macrolide group of antibiotics. It is basic and readily forms salts and esters. Erythromycin ethylsuccinate is an ester of erythromycin.

Sulfisoxazole acetyl or N^1-acetyl sulfisoxazole is an ester of sulfisoxazole. Chemically, sulfisoxazole is N^1-(3,4-dimethyl-5-isoxazolyl) sulfanilamide.

Actions:
Clinical Pharmacology: Orally administered erythromycin ethylsuccinate suspension is reliably and readily absorbed and serum levels are comparable when administered to patients in either the fasting or non-fasting state. After absorption, erythromycin diffuses readily into most body fluids. In the presence of normal hepatic function, erythromycin is concentrated in the liver and excreted in the bile; the effect of hepatic dysfunction on excretion of erythromycin by the liver into the bile is not known. After oral administration, less than 5 percent of the activity of the administered dose can be recovered in the urine.

Erythromycin crosses the placental barrier but fetal plasma levels are generally low.

Sulfisoxazole acetyl is deacetylated by enzymatic hydrolysis in the gastrointestinal tract from which it is readily absorbed as sulfisoxazole. Sulfisoxazole exists in the blood primarily bound to serum proteins as well as conjugated and in the active or free form. Metabolic pathways include N^4-acetylation and oxidation with approximately 80 percent of an administered dose being excreted by the kidney within 24 hours.

Serum half-life for total erythromycin and free sulfisoxazole is about 1.5 and 6 hours, respectively.
Microbiology: Pediazole has been formulated to contain sulfisoxazole for concomitant use with erythromycin. The mode of action of erythromycin is by inhibition of protein synthesis without affecting nucleic acid synthesis. Sulfonamides, including sulfisoxazole, possess bacteriostatic activity. This bacteriostatic agent acts by means of competitively inhibiting bacterial synthesis of folic acid (pteroylglutamic acid) from para-aminobenzoic acid. Resistance to erythromycin blood levels ordinarily achieved has been demonstrated by some strains of *Hemophilus influenzae*. Pediazole is usually active against *Hemophilus influenzae in vitro*, including ampicillin-resistant strains.

Quantitative methods that require measurements of zone diameters give the most precise estimates of antibiotic susceptibility. One such standardized procedure, the ASM-2 method published by the National Committee for Clinical Laboratory Standards (NCCLS), has been recommended for use with discs to test susceptibility to erythromycin and sulfisoxazole. Interpretation involves correlation of the diameters obtained in the disc test with Minimal Inhibitory Concentrations (MIC) values for erythromycin and sulfisoxazole.

If the standardized ASM-2 procedure of disc susceptibility is used, a 15 mcg erythromycin disc should give a zone diameter of at least 18 mm when tested against an erythromycin-susceptible bacterial strain and a 250-300 mcg sulfisoxazole disc should give a zone diameter of at least 17 mm when tested against a sulfisoxazole-susceptible bacterial strain.

In vitro sulfonamide sensitivity tests are not always reliable because media containing excessive amounts of thymidine are capable of reversing the inhibitory effect of sulfonamides which may result in false resistant reports. The tests must be carefully coordinated with bacteriological and clinical responses. When the patient is already taking sulfonamides, follow-up cultures should have aminobenzoic acid added to the isolation media but not to subsequent susceptibility test media.

Indication: For treatment of ACUTE OTITIS MEDIA in children that is caused by susceptible strains of *Hemophilus influenzae*.

Contraindications: Known hypersensitivity to either erythromycin or sulfonamides.
Infants less than 2 months of age.
Pregnancy at term and during the nursing period, because sulfonamides pass into the placental circulation and are excreted in human breast milk and may cause kernicterus in the infant.

Warnings: FATALITIES ASSOCIATED WITH THE ADMINISTRATION OF SULFONAMIDES, ALTHOUGH RARE, HAVE OCCURRED DUE TO SEVERE REACTIONS INCLUDING STEVENS-JOHNSON SYNDROME, TOXIC EPIDERMAL NECROLYSIS, FULMINANT HEPATIC NECROSIS, AGRANULOCYTOSIS, APLASTIC ANEMIA, AND OTHER BLOOD DYSCRASIAS.
Clinical signs such as sore throat, fever, pallor, rash, purpura, or jaundice may be early indications of serious reactions.
PEDIAZOLE SHOULD BE DISCONTINUED AT THE FIRST APPEARANCE OF SKIN RASH OR ANY SIGN OF ADVERSE REACTION. In some instances a skin rash may be followed by a more severe reaction, such as Stevens-Johnson syndrome, toxic epidermal necrolysis, hepatic necrosis and serious blood disorders.
COMPLETE BLOOD COUNT SHOULD BE DONE FREQUENTLY IN PATIENTS RECEIVING SULFONAMIDES.
Usage in Pregnancy (SEE ALSO: CONTRAINDICATIONS): The safe use of erythromycin or sulfonamides in pregnancy has not been established. The teratogenic potential of most sulfonamides has not been thoroughly investigated in either animals or humans. However, a significant increase in the incidence of cleft palate and other bony abnormalities of offspring has been observed when certain sulfonamides of the short, intermediate and long-acting types were given to pregnant rats and mice at high oral doses (7 to 25 times the human therapeutic dose).
The frequency of renal complications is considerably lower in patients receiving the most soluble sulfonamides such as sulfisoxazole. Urinalysis with careful microscopic examination should be obtained frequently in patients receiving sulfonamides.

Precautions: Erythromycin is principally excreted by the liver. Caution should be exercised in administering the antibiotic to patients with impaired hepatic function. There have been reports of hepatic dysfunction, with or without jaundice occurring in patients receiving oral erythromycin products.
Recent data from studies of erythromycin reveal that its use in patients who are receiving high doses of theophylline may be associated with an increase of serum theophylline levels and potential theophylline toxicity. In case of theophylline toxicity and/or elevated serum theophylline levels, the dose of theophylline should be reduced while the patient is receiving concomitant erythromycin therapy.
Surgical procedures should be performed when indicated.
Sulfonamide therapy should be given with caution to patients with impaired renal or hepatic function and in those patients with a history of severe allergy or bronchial asthma. In the presence of a deficiency in the enzyme glucose-6-phosphate dehydrogenase, hemolysis may occur. This reaction is frequently dose-related. Adequate fluid intake must be maintained in order to prevent crystalluria and renal stone formation.

Adverse Reactions: The most frequent side effects of oral erythromycin preparations are gastrointestinal, such as abdominal cramping and discomfort, and are dose-related. Nausea, vomiting and diarrhea occur infrequently with usual oral doses. During prolonged or repeated therapy, there is a possibility of overgrowth of nonsusceptible bacteria or fungi. If such infections occur, the drug should be discontinued and appropriate therapy instituted. The overall incidence of these latter side effects reported for the combined administration of erythromycin and a sulfonamide is comparable to those observed in patients given erythromycin alone. Mild allergic reactions such as urticaria and other skin rashes have occurred. Serious allergic reactions, including anaphylaxis, have been reported with erythromycin.

There have been isolated reports of reversible hearing loss occurring chiefly in patients with renal insufficiency and in patients receiving high doses of erythromycin.

The following untoward effects have been associated with the use of sulfonamides:
Blood Dyscrasias: Agranulocytosis, aplastic anemia, thrombocytopenia, leukopenia, hemolytic anemia, purpura, hypoprothrombinemia and methemoglobinemia.
Allergic Reactions: Erythema multiforme (Stevens-Johnson syndrome), generalized skin eruptions, epidermal necrolysis, urticaria, serum sickness, pruritus, exfoliative dermatitis, anaphylactoid reactions, periorbital edema, conjunctival and scleral injection, photosensitization, arthralgia and allergic myocarditis.
Gastrointestinal Reactions: Nausea, emesis, abdominal pains, hepatitis, diarrhea, anorexia, pancreatitis and stomatitis.
CNS Reactions: Headache, peripheral neuritis, mental depression, convulsions, ataxia, hallucinations, tinnitus, vertigo and insomnia.
Miscellaneous Reactions: Drug fever, chills and toxic nephrosis with oliguria or anuria. Periarteritis nodosa and LE phenomenon have occurred.
The sulfonamides bear certain chemical similarities to some goitrogens, diuretics (acetazolamide and the thiazides) and oral hypoglycemic agents. Goiter production, diuresis and hypoglycemia have occurred rarely in patients receiving sulfonamides. Cross-sensitivity may exist with these agents.
Rats appear to be especially susceptible to the goitrogenic effects of sulfonamides, and long-term administration has produced thyroid malignancies in the species.

Dosage and Administration: PEDIAZOLE SHOULD NOT BE ADMINISTERED TO INFANTS UNDER 2 MONTHS OF AGE BECAUSE OF CONTRAINDICATIONS OF SYSTEMIC SULFONAMIDES IN THIS AGE GROUP.
For Acute Otitis Media in Children: The dose of Pediazole can be calculated based on the erythromycin component (50 mg/kg/day) or the sulfisoxazole component (150 mg/kg/day to a maximum of 6 g/day). Pediazole should be administered in equally divided doses four times a day for 10 days. It may be administered without regard to meals. The following approximate dosage schedule is recommended for using Pediazole:
Children: Two months of age or older

Weight	Dose—every 6 hours
Less than 8 kg (less than 18 lb)	Adjust dosage by body weight
8 kg (18 lb)	½ teaspoonful (2.5 ml)
16 kg (35 lb)	1 teaspoonful (5 ml)
24 kg (53 lb)	1½ teaspoonfuls (7.5 ml)
Over 45 kg (over 100 lb)	2 teaspoonfuls (10 ml)

How Supplied: Pediazole Suspension is available for teaspoon dosage in 100-ml (NDC 0074-8030-13), 150-ml (NDC 0074-8030-43) and 200-ml (NDC 0074-8030-53) bottles, in the form of granules to be reconstituted with water. The suspension provides erythromycin ethylsuccinate equivalent to 200 mg erythromycin activity and sulfisox-

Product Information

azole acetyl equivalent to 600 mg sulfisoxazole per teaspoonful (5 ml).
(.3821)

POLYCOSE®
[pol'ē-kōs]
Glucose Polymers

Usage: As a source of calories (derived solely from carbohydrate) for persons with increased caloric needs or those unable to meet their caloric needs with their normal diet. Polycose is particularly useful in supplying carbohydrate calories for protein-, electrolyte- and fat-restricted diets.

Features:
- Mixes readily with most foods and beverages.
- Minimal sweetness increases patient acceptance.
- Absorbed as rapidly as glucose.
- Low electrolyte levels.
- Low osmolality, as compared to other carbohydrate sources (900 mOsm/kg water), Polycose Liquid helps reduce potential for osmotic diarrhea.

Dosage and Administration: Polycose may be added to tube feeding formulas and most foods and beverages, or mixed in water, in amounts determined by taste, caloric requirement and tolerance. Small, frequent feedings are more desirable than large amounts given infrequently. Polycose may be used for extended periods with diets containing all other essential nutrients, or as an oral adjunct to intravenous administration of nutrients.
Polycose is not a balanced diet and should not be used as a sole source of nutrition. Undiluted Polycose should not be fed to comatose patients without physician supervision.
Refrigerate dissolved Polycose Powder and opened Polycose Liquid and discard unused portion after 24 hours. Concentrated solutions become more viscous when cold; thus serving Polycose at room temperature is advised.
NOT FOR PARENTERAL USE.

Precaution (For Infant Use): Not to be fed undiluted. Use only as directed by a physician.

Availability:
Powder: 12.3 oz (350g) cans; 6 per case; No. 746.
Liquid: (43% w/w aqueous solution): 4-fl-oz bottles; 48 per case; No. 749.

Composition:
Powder: (Pareve, Ⓤ) Glucose polymers derived from controlled hydrolysis of corn starch.

Approximate Analysis (per 100 grams):

Carbohydrate		94	g
Moisture		6	g
Calcium	Does not exceed	30	mg
		(1.5	mEq)
Sodium	Does not exceed	110	mg
		(4.8	mEq)
Potassium	Does not exceed	10	mg
		(0.3	mEq)
Chloride	Does not exceed	223	mg
		(6.3	mEq)
Phosphorus	Does not exceed	5	mg

Approximate Caloric Equivalents:
1 level teaspoonful (2 g) = 8 Calories; 1 level tablespoonful (6 g) = 23 Calories; 1/4 cup (25 g) = 95 Calories; 1/3 cup (33 g) = 125 Calories; 1/2 cup (50 g) = 190 Calories; 1 cup (100 g) = 380 Calories. (FAN 323)

Composition:
Liquid: Ⓤ (43% w/w aqueous solution): Water and glucose polymers derived from controlled hydrolysis of corn starch.

Approximate Analysis (per 100 ml):

Carbohydrate		50	g
Moisture		70	g
Minerals (Ash)	Does not exceed	0.25	g
Calcium	Does not exceed	20	mg
		(1.0	mEq)
Sodium	Does not exceed	70	mg
		(3.0	mEq)
Potassium	Does not exceed	6	mg
		(0.15	mEq)
Chloride		Does not exceed	140 mg
			(3.9 mEq)
Phosphorus	Does not exceed	3	mg

Approximate Caloric Equivalents:
1 ml = 2 Calories; 1 fl oz = 60 Calories; 100 ml = 200 Calories.
(FAN 298)

PRAMET® FA ℞
[pram'et]
Vitamin/Mineral Prescription
For Expectant and
New Mothers

Description: Each Pramet FA Filmtab® Film-Sealed oral tablet provides:

Vitamins

Vitamin A (as acetate and palmitate) 1.2 mg	4000	I.U.
Vitamin D (cholecalciferol, 10 mcg)	400	I.U.
Vitamin C (ascorbic acid)	100	mg
Folic Acid	1	mg
Vitamin B_1 (thiamine mononitrate)	3	mg
Vitamin B_2 (riboflavin)	2	mg
Niacinamide	10	mg
Vitamin B_6 (pyridoxine hydrochloride)	5	mg
Vitamin B_{12} (cyanocobalamin)	3	mcg
Pantothenic Acid (as calcium pantothenate)	0.92	mg

Minerals

Calcium (as calcium carbonate)	250	mg
Iodine (as calcium iodate)	100	mcg
Elemental Iron* (300 mg ferrous sulfate USP)	60	mg
Copper (as cupric chloride)	0.15	mg

* In controlled-release form—Gradumet®

Indications and Usage: To help prevent vitamin and mineral deficiencies during and after pregnancy and for treatment of megaloblastic anemias. One mg of folic acid has been found to be effective therapy for megaloblastic anemias of pregnancy and lactation.

Warning: Folic acid alone is improper therapy in the treatment of pernicious anemia and other megaloblastic anemias where vitamin B_{12} is deficient.

Precaution: Folic acid may mask the presence of pernicious anemia in that hematologic remission may occur while neurologic manifestations remain progressive.

Adverse Reaction: Allergic sensitization has been reported following both oral and parenteral administration of folic acid.

Overdosage: Acute overdosage of iron may cause nausea and vomiting and, in severe cases, cardiovascular collapse and death. The estimated lethal dose of orally ingested elemental iron is 300 mg per kg body weight. Serum iron and total iron-binding capacity may be used as guides for use of chelating agents such as deferoxamine.

Dosage and Administration: One tablet daily, or as directed by physician.

How Supplied: 100-tablet bottles; ℞ NDC 0074-0147-01.

Shown in Product Identification Section, page 432

PRAMILET® FA ℞
[pram'e-let"]
Prenatal
Vitamin/Mineral Preparation

Description: Each Pramilet FA Filmtab® Film-Sealed oral tablet provides:

Vitamins

Vitamin A (as acetate and palmitate) 1.2 mg	4000	I.U.
Vitamin D (cholecalciferol, 10 mcg)	400	I.U.
Vitamin C (as sodium ascorbate)	60	mg
Folic Acid	1	mg
Vitamin B_1 (thiamine mononitrate)	3	mg
Vitamin B_2 (riboflavin)	2	mg
Niacinamide	10	mg
Vitamin B_6 (pyridoxine hydrochloride)	3	mg
Vitamin B_{12} (cyanocobalamin)	3	mcg
Calcium Pantothenate	1	mg

Minerals

Calcium (as calcium carbonate)	250	mg
Iodine (as calcium iodate)	100	mcg
Elemental Iron (as ferrous fumarate)	40	mg
Magnesium (as magnesium oxide)	10	mg
Copper (as cupric chloride)	0.15	mg
Zinc (as zinc oxide)	0.085	mg

Indications and Usage: To help prevent vitamin and mineral deficiencies during and after pregnancy and for treatment of megaloblastic anemias. One mg of folic acid has been found to be effective therapy for megaloblastic anemias of pregnancy and lactation.

Warning: Folic acid alone is improper therapy in the treatment of pernicious anemia and other megaloblastic anemias where vitamin B_{12} is deficient.

Precaution: Folic acid may mask the presence of pernicious anemia in that hematologic remission may occur while neurologic manifestations remain progressive.

Adverse Reaction: Allergic sensitization has been reported following both oral and parenteral administration of folic acid.

Overdosage: Acute overdosage of iron may cause nausea and vomiting and, in severe cases, cardiovascular collapse and death. The estimated lethal dose of orally ingested elemental iron is 300 mg per kg body weight. Serum iron and total iron-binding capacity may be used as guides for use of chelating agents such as deferoxamine.

Dosage and Administration: One tablet daily, or as directed by physician.

How Supplied: 100-tablet bottles; ℞ NDC 0074-0121-01.

Shown in Product Identification Section, page 432

RCF®
Ross Carbohydrate Free
Soy Protein Formula Base

Usage: For use in the dietary management of persons unable to tolerate the type or amount of carbohydrate in milk or conventional infant formulas; many of these patients have intractable diarrhea and are not able to tolerate other formulas. This product has been formulated to contain no carbohydrates, which must be added before feeding.

Availability:
Concentrated Liquid only: 13-fl-oz cans; 12 per case; No. 108.

Preparation:
RCF is for use only under the direction of a physician. Physician's instructions must include the type and amount of carbohydrate and the amount of water to be added to RCF.
Standard dilution is one part Formula Base to one part prescribed carbohydrate and water solution. A full-strength formula, 20 Calories per fluid ounce, may be prepared with one of the following typical carbohydrates:
[See table on next page.]

Composition: Concentrated Liquid
Ingredients: (Pareve, Ⓤ) 87% water, 4.4% soy protein isolate, 4.2% soy oil, 2.8% coconut oil, minerals (calcium phosphates [mono- and tribasic], potassium citrate, potassium chloride, magnesium chloride, calcium carbonate, sodium chloride, zinc sulfate, cupric sulfate), carrageenan, mono- and diglycerides, soy lecithin, vitamins (ascorbic acid, choline chloride, alpha-tocopheryl acetate, niacinamide, calcium pantothenate, vitamin A palmitate, riboflavin, thiamine chloride hydrochloride, pyridoxine hydrochloride, phylloquinone, biotin, folic acid, vitamin D_3, cyanocobalamin), L-methionine, taurine and L-carnitine.

Nutrients (wt/liter):	Concentrated	Standard Dilution†
Protein	40.0 g	20.0 g
Fat	72.0 g	36.0 g
Carbohydrate	0.1 g	*
Minerals (Ash)	7.5 g	3.8 g
Calcium	1400 mg	700 mg
Phosphorus	1000 mg	500 mg

Continued on next page

Ross—Cont.

Magnesium	100	mg	50	mg
Iron	3.0	mg	1.5	mg

(This product is deficient in iron; an additional 5.3 mg iron per liter should be supplied from other sources.)

Iodine	200	mcg	100	mcg
Zinc	10	mg	5.0	mg
Copper	1.0	mg	0.50	mg
Manganese	400	mcg	200	mcg
Sodium	640	mg	320	mg
Potassium	1540	mg	770	mg
Chloride	1180	mg	590	mg
Water	885	g	*	
Crude Fiber	0	g		
Calories per fl oz	24		*	
Calories per liter	810		*	

Vitamins Per Liter (Standard Dilution†):

Vitamin A	2000	I.U.
Vitamin D	400	I.U.
Vitamin E	20	I.U.
Vitamin K$_1$	100	mcg
Vitamin C	55	mg
Thiamine (Vit. B$_1$)	0.40	mg
Riboflavin (Vit. B$_2$)	0.60	mg
Vitamin B$_6$	0.40	mg
Vitamin B$_{12}$	3.0	mcg
Niacin	9.0	mg
Folic Acid	100	mcg
Pantothenic Acid	5.0	mg
Biotin	30	mcg
Choline	53	mg
Inositol	32	mg

*Varies depending on quantity of carbohydrate and water used. If carbohydrate is not added to this product, a 1:1 dilution with water provides approximately 12 Cal/fl oz (40.5 Cal/100 ml).
†Standard dilution is one part Formula Base to one part prescribed carbohydrate and water solution.
(FAN 360-02)

RONDEC® Oral Drops ℞
[ron'dek]
RONDEC® Syrup ℞
RONDEC® Tablet ℞
RONDEC-TR® Tablet ℞

Description: Antihistamine/Decongestant for oral use.
For infants
RONDEC® Oral Drops
Each dropperful (1 ml) contains carbinoxamine maleate, 2 mg; pseudoephedrine hydrochloride, 25 mg.
For young children
RONDEC® Syrup
Each teaspoonful (5 ml) contains carbinoxamine maleate, 4 mg; pseudoephedrine hydrochloride, 60 mg.
For adults and children 6 years and over
RONDEC® Tablet
Each Filmtab® tablet contains carbinoxamine maleate, 4 mg; pseudoephedrine hydrochloride, 60 mg.
For adults and children 12 years and over
RONDEC-TR® Tablet
Each timed-release Filmtab tablet contains carbinoxamine maleate, 8 mg; pseudoephedrine hydrochloride, 120 mg.

RCF

Carbohydrate Source	Amount of Carbohydrate	Water	RCF Formula
Table Sugar (sucrose)	4 level tablespoonfuls*	12 fl oz	one 13-fl-oz can
Dextrose Powder (hydrous)	6 level tablespoonfuls*	12 fl oz	one 13-fl-oz can
Polycose® Glucose Polymers Powder	See Polycose label*	12 fl oz	one 13-fl-oz can

* Approximately the 52 grams needed for 20 Cal/fl oz formula.

Carbinoxamine maleate (2-[p-Chloro-α-[2-(dimethylamino) ethoxy] benzyl] pyridine maleate) is one of the ethanolamine class of H$_1$ antihistamines.
Pseudoephedrine hydrochloride (Benzenemethanol, α-[1-(methylamino)ethyl]-, [S-(R*, R*)]-, hydrochloride) is the hydrochloride of pseudoephedrine, a naturally occurring dextrorotatory stereoisomer of ephedrine.
Clinical Pharmacology: Antihistaminic and decongestant actions.
Carbinoxamine maleate possesses H$_1$ antihistaminic activity and mild anticholinergic and sedative effects. Serum half-life for carbinoxamine is estimated to be 10 to 20 hours. Virtually no intact drug is excreted in the urine.
Pseudoephedrine hydrochloride is an oral sympathomimetic amine which acts as a decongestant to respiratory tract mucous membranes. While its vasoconstrictor action is similar to that of ephedrine, pseudoephedrine has less pressor effect in normotensive adults. Serum half-life for pseudoephedrine is 6 to 8 hours. Acidic urine is associated with faster elimination of the drug. About one half of the administered dose is excreted in the urine.
Indications and Usage: For symptomatic relief of seasonal and perennial allergic rhinitis and vasomotor rhinitis.
Rondec Oral Drops, Rondec Syrup and Rondec Tablet are immediate-release dosage forms allowing titration of dose up to four times a day.
Rondec-TR Tablet utilizes a gradual-release mechanism providing approximately a 12-hour therapeutic effect, thus allowing twice-daily dosage.
Contraindications: Patients with hypersensitivity or idiosyncrasy to any ingredients, patients taking monoamine oxidase (MAO) inhibitors, patients with narrow-angle glaucoma, urinary retention, peptic ulcer, severe hypertension or coronary artery disease, or patients undergoing an asthmatic attack.
Warnings:
Use in Pregnancy: Safety for use during pregnancy has not been established.
Nursing Mothers: Use with caution in nursing mothers.
Special Risk Patients: Use with caution in patients with hypertension or ischemic heart disease, and persons over 60 years.
Precautions: Use with caution in patients with hypertension, heart disease, asthma, hyperthyroidism, increased intraocular pressure, diabetes mellitus and prostatic hypertrophy.
Information for Patients: Avoid alcohol and other CNS depressants while taking these products. Patients sensitive to antihistamines may experience moderate to severe drowsiness. Patients sensitive to sympathomimetic amines may note mild CNS stimulation. While taking these products, exercise care in driving or operating appliances, machinery, etc.
Drug Interactions: Antihistamines may enhance the effects of tricyclic antidepressants, barbiturates, alcohol, and other CNS depressants. MAO inhibitors prolong and intensify the anticholinergic effects of antihistamines. Sympathomimetic amines may reduce the antihypertensive effects of reserpine, veratrum alkaloids, methyldopa and mecamylamine. Effects of sympathomimetics are increased with MAO inhibitors and beta-adrenergic blockers.
Pregnancy Category C.: Animal reproduction studies have not been conducted with these products. It is also not known whether these products can cause fetal harm when administered to a pregnant woman or affect reproduction capacity. Give to pregnant women only if clearly needed.
Adverse Reactions: Antihistamines: Sedation, dizziness, diplopia, vomiting, dry mouth, headache, nervousness, nausea, anorexia, heartburn, weakness, polyuria and dysuria and, rarely, excitability in children.
Sympathomimetic Amines: Convulsions, CNS stimulation, cardiac arrhythmias, respiratory difficulty, increased heart rate or blood pressure, hallucinations, tremors, nervousness, insomnia, weakness, pallor and dysuria.
Overdosage: No information is available as to specific results of an overdose of these products. The signs, symptoms and treatment described below are those of H$_1$ antihistamine and ephedrine overdose.
Symptoms: Should antihistamine effects predominate, central action constitutes the greatest danger. In the small child, symptoms include excitation, hallucination, ataxia, incoordination, tremors, flushed face and fever. Convulsions, fixed and dilated pupils, coma and death may occur in severe cases. In the adult, fever and flushing are uncommon; excitement leading to convulsions and postictal depression is often preceded by drowsiness and coma. Respiration is usually not seriously depressed; blood pressure is usually stable.
Should sympathomimetic symptoms predominate, central effects include restlessness, dizziness, tremor, hyperactive reflexes, talkativeness, irritability and insomnia. Cardiovascular and renal effects include difficulty in micturition, headache, flushing, palpitation, cardiac arrhythmias, hypertension with subsequent hypotension and circulatory collapse. Gastrointestinal effects include dry mouth, metallic taste, anorexia, nausea, vomiting, diarrhea and abdominal cramps.
Treatment: a) Evacuate stomach as condition warrants. Activated charcoal may be useful. b) Maintain a nonstimulating environment. c) Monitor cardiovascular status. d) Do not give stimulants. e) Reduce fever with cool sponging. f) Support respiration. g) Use sedatives or anticonvulsants to control CNS excitation and convulsions. h) Physostigmine may reverse anticholinergic symptoms. i) Ammonium chloride may acidify the urine to increase excretion of pseudoephedrine. j) Further care is symptomatic and supportive.
Dosage and Administration:
Dosage:
Rondec Oral Drops
for oral use only

Age	Dose*	Frequency*
1–3 months	¼ dropperful (¼ml)	q.i.d.
3–6 months	½ dropperful (½ml)	q.i.d.
6–9 months	¾ dropperful (¾ml)	q.i.d.
9–18 months	1 dropperful (1 ml)	q.i.d.

Rondec Syrup and
Rondec Tablet
18 months–
6 years   ½ teaspoonful (2.5 ml)   q.i.d.
adults and
children   1 teaspoonful (5 ml)   q.i.d.
6 years and
over   or
                1 tablet
Rondec-TR Tablet
adults and children
12 years and over   1 tablet   b.i.d.
*In mild cases or in particularly sensitive patients, less frequent or reduced doses may be adequate.
How Supplied: Rondec Drops, berry-flavored, in 30-ml bottles for dropper dosage, **NDC** 0074-5783-30. Calibrated shatterproof dropper enclosed in each carton. Container meets safety closure requirements. Avoid exposure to excessive heat.
Rondec Syrup, berry-flavored, in 16-fl-oz (1-pint) bottles, **NDC** 0074-5782-16; and 4-fl-oz bottles, **NDC** 0074-5782-04. Dispense in USP tight glass container. Avoid exposure to excessive heat.
Rondec Tablet, Filmtab tablets, in bottles of 100, **NDC** 0074-5726-13; and bottles of 500, **NDC** 0074-5726-53. Each orange-colored tablet marked with Ross "R" and the number 5726 for professional identification. Dispense in USP tight container.

[Shown in Product Identification Section]
Rondec-TR Tablet, Filmtab tablets, in bottles of 100, **NDC** 0074-6240-13. Each blue-colored tablet marked with Ross "R" and the number 6240 for professional identification. Dispense in USP tight container.
(.4821)

Shown in Product Identification Section, page 432

RONDEC®–DM Syrup ℞
[ron′dek]
RONDEC®–DM Oral Drops ℞

Description:
Antihistamine/Decongestant/Antitussive for oral use.
Rondec®-DM Syrup
Each teaspoonful (5 ml) contains carbinoxamine maleate, 4 mg; pseudoephedrine hydrochloride, 60 mg; dextromethorphan hydrobromide, 15 mg; less than 0.6% alcohol.
Rondec®-DM Oral Drops
Each dropperful (1 ml) contains carbinoxamine maleate, 2 mg; pseudoephedrine hydrochloride, 25 mg; dextromethorphan hydrobromide, 4 mg; less than 0.6% alcohol.
Carbinoxamine maleate (2-[p-Chloro-α-[2-(dimethylamino) ethoxy]benzyl]pyridine maleate) is one of the ethanolamine class of H_1 antihistamines.
Pseudoephedrine hydrochloride (Benzenemethanol,α-[1-(methylamino) ethyl]-, [S-(R*, R*)]-, hydrochloride) is the hydrochloride of pseudoephedrine, a naturally occurring dextrorotatory stereoisomer of ephedrine.
Dextromethorphan hydrobromide (Morphinan, 3-methoxy-17-methyl-, (9α, 13α, 14α)-, hydrobromide, monohydrate) is the hydrobromide of d-form racemethorphan.

Clinical Pharmacology: Antihistaminic, decongestant and antitussive actions.
Carbinoxamine maleate possesses H_1 antihistaminic activity and mild anticholinergic and sedative effects. Serum half-life for carbinoxamine is estimated to be 10 to 20 hours. Virtually no intact drug is excreted in the urine.
Pseudoephedrine hydrochloride is an oral sympathomimetic amine which acts as a decongestant to respiratory tract mucous membranes. While its vasoconstrictor action is similar to that of ephedrine, pseudoephedrine has less pressor effect in normotensive adults. Serum half-life for pseudoephedrine is 6 to 8 hours. Acidic urine is associated with faster elimination of the drug. About one half of the administered dose is excreted in the urine.
Dextromethorphan hydrobromide is a nonnarcotic antitussive with effectiveness equal to codeine. It acts in the medulla oblongata to elevate the cough threshold. Dextromethorphan does not produce analgesia or induce tolerance, and has no potential for addiction. At usual doses, it will not depress respiration or inhibit ciliary activity. Dextromethorphan is rapidly metabolized, with trace amounts of the parent compound in blood and urine. About one half of the administered dose is excreted in the urine as conjugated metabolites.

Indications and Usage: For symptomatic relief of the common cold, nasopharyngitis with postnasal drip, bronchitis and related respiratory conditions.

Contraindications: Patients with hypersensitivity or idiosyncrasy to any ingredients, patients taking monoamine oxidase (MAO) inhibitors, patients with narrow-angle glaucoma, urinary retention, peptic ulcer, severe hypertension or coronary artery disease, or patients undergoing an asthmatic attack.

Warnings:
Use in Pregnancy: Safety for use during pregnancy has not been established.
Nursing Mothers: Use with caution in nursing mothers.
Special Risk Patients: Use with caution in patients with hypertension or ischemic heart disease, and persons over 60 years.

Precautions: Before prescribing medication to suppress or modify cough, identify and provide therapy for the underlying cause of cough.

Use with caution in patients with hypertension, heart disease, asthma, hyperthyroidism, increased intraocular pressure, diabetes mellitus and prostatic hypertrophy.

Information for Patients: Avoid alcohol and other CNS depressants while taking these products. Patients sensitive to antihistamines may experience moderate to severe drowsiness. Patients sensitive to sympathomimetic amines may note mild CNS stimulation. While taking these products, exercise care in driving or operating appliances, machinery, etc.

Drug Interactions: Antihistamines may enhance the effects of tricyclic antidepressants, barbiturates, alcohol, and other CNS depressants. MAO inhibitors prolong and intensify the anticholinergic effects of antihistamines. Sympathomimetic amines may reduce the antihypertensive effects of reserpine, veratrum alkaloids, methyldopa and mecamylamine. Effects of sympathomimetics are increased with MAO inhibitors and beta-adrenergic blockers. The cough suppressant action of dextromethorphan and narcotic antitussives are additive.

Pregnancy Category C.: Animal reproduction studies have not been conducted with Rondec-DM. It is also not known whether these products can cause fetal harm when administered to a pregnant woman or affect reproduction capacity. Give to pregnant women only if clearly needed.

Adverse Reactions:
Antihistamines: Sedation, dizziness, diplopia, vomiting, dry mouth, headache, nervousness, nausea, anorexia, heartburn, weakness, polyuria and dysuria and, rarely, excitability in children.
Sympathomimetic Amines: Convulsions, CNS stimulation, cardiac arrhythmias, respiratory difficulty, increased heart rate or blood pressure, hallucinations, tremors, nervousness, insomnia, weakness, pallor and dysuria.
Dextromethorphan: Drowsiness and GI disturbance.

Overdosage: No information is available as to specific results of an overdose of these products. The signs, symptoms and treatment described below are those of H_1 antihistamine, ephedrine and dextromethorphan overdose.

Symptoms: Should antihistamine effects predominate, central action constitutes the greatest danger. In the small child, predominant symptoms are excitation, hallucination, ataxia, incoordination, tremors, flushed face and fever. Convulsions, fixed and dilated pupils, coma, and death may occur in severe cases. In the adult, fever and flushing are uncommon; excitement leading to convulsions and postictal depression is often preceded by drowsiness and coma. Respiration is usually not seriously depressed; blood pressure is usually stable.
Should sympathomimetic symptoms predominate, central effects include restlessness, dizziness, tremor, hyperactive reflexes, talkativeness, irritability and insomnia. Cardiovascular and renal effects include difficulty in micturition, headache, flushing, palpitation, cardiac arrhythmias, hypertension with subsequent hypotension and circulatory collapse. Gastrointestinal effects include dry mouth, metallic taste, anorexia, nausea, vomiting, diarrhea and abdominal cramps.
Dextromethorphan may cause respiratory depression with a large overdose.

Treatment: a) Evacuate stomach as condition warrants. Activated charcoal may be useful. b) Maintain a nonstimulating environment. c) Monitor cardiovascular status. d) Do not give stimulants. e) Reduce fever with cool sponging. f) Treat respiratory depression with naloxone if dextromethorphan toxicity is suspected. g) Use sedatives or anticonvulsants to control CNS excitation and convulsions. h) Physostigmine may reverse anticholinergic symptoms. i) Ammonium chloride may acidify the urine to increase urinary excretion of pseudoephedrine. j) Further care is symptomatic and supportive.

Dosage and Administration:
Dosage:

Age	Dose*	Frequency*
Rondec-DM Syrup		
18 months–6 years	½ teaspoonful (2.5 ml)	q.i.d.
adults and children 6 years and over	1 teaspoonful (5 ml)	q.i.d.
Rondec-DM Oral Drops for oral use only		
1–3 months	¼ dropperful (¼ ml)	q.i.d.
3–6 months	½ dropperful (½ ml)	q.i.d.
6–9 months	¾ dropperful (¾ ml)	q.i.d.
9–18 months	1 dropperful (1 ml)	q.i.d.

*In mild cases or in particularly sensitive patients, less frequent or reduced doses may be adequate.

How Supplied: Rondec-DM Syrup, grape-flavored, in 16-fl-oz (1-pint) bottles, **NDC** 0074-5640-16; and 4-fl-oz bottles, **NDC** 0074-5640-04. Dispense in USP tight, light-resistant, glass container. Avoid exposure to excessive heat.
Rondec-DM Oral Drops, grape-flavored, in 30-ml bottles for dropper dosage. Calibrated, shatterproof dropper enclosed in each carton. Container meets safety closure requirements. **NDC** 0074-5639-30. Avoid exposure to excessive heat.
(.4821)

ROSS HOSPITAL FORMULA SYSTEM
Similac® infant formula products for hospital nursery use

SIMILAC® 13, Ready To Feed, 13 Cal/fl oz
Availability:
 4-fl-oz nursing bottles; 48 per case; No. 408.
SIMILAC® 20, Ready To Feed, 20 Cal/fl oz
Availability:
 4-fl-oz nursing bottles; 48 per case; No. 415.
 8-fl-oz nursing bottles; 24 per case; No. 841.
SIMILAC® 24, Ready To Feed, 24 Cal/fl oz
Availability:
 4-fl-oz nursing bottles; 48 per case; No. 404.
SIMILAC® 24 LBW, Ready To Feed, 24 Cal/fl oz
Availability:
 4-fl-oz nursing bottles; 48 per case; No. 422.
SIMILAC® 27, Ready To Feed, 27 Cal/fl oz
Availability:
 4-fl-oz nursing bottles; 48 per case; No. 427.
SIMILAC® WITH IRON 13, Ready To Feed, 13 Cal/fl oz
Availability:
 4-fl-oz nursing bottles; 48 per case; No. 413.
SIMILAC® WITH IRON 20, Ready To Feed, 20 Cal/fl oz
Availability:
 4-fl-oz nursing bottles; 48 per case; No. 426.
 8-fl-oz nursing bottles; 24 per case; No. 858.
SIMILAC® WITH IRON 24, Ready To Feed, 24 Cal/fl oz
Availability:
 4-fl-oz nursing bottles; 48 per case; No. 403.
SIMILAC® WITH WHEY + IRON 20, Ready To Feed, 20 Cal/fl oz
Availability:
 4-fl-oz nursing bottles; 48 per case; No. 442.
 8-fl-oz nursing bottles; 24 per case; No. 822.
SIMILAC® PM 60/40, Ready To Feed, 20 Cal/fl oz
Availability:
 4-fl-oz nursing bottles; 48 per case; No. 424.
SIMILAC® SPECIAL CARE™ 20, Ready To Feed, 20 Cal/fl oz
Availability:
 4-fl-oz nursing bottles; 48 per case; No. 439.
SIMILAC® SPECIAL CARE™ 24, Ready To Feed, 24 Cal/fl oz
Availability:
 4-fl-oz nursing bottles; 48 per case; No. 433.
ISOMIL® 20, Ready To Feed, 20 Cal/fl oz
Availability:
 4-fl-oz nursing bottles; 48 per case; No. 406.
 8-fl-oz nursing bottles; 24 per case; No. 871.
ISOMIL® SF 20, Ready To Feed, 20 Cal/fl oz
Availability:
 8-fl-oz nursing bottles; 24 per case; No. 801.

Continued on next page

Ross—Cont.

PEDIALYTE®, Ready To Use; unflavored; NDC 0074-6470-08
Availability:
8-fl-oz nursing bottles; 24 per case; No. 806.

ADVANCE®, Ready To Feed
Availability:
8-fl-oz nursing bottles; 24 per case; No. 804.

5% GLUCOSE WATER, Ready To Feed
Availability:
4-fl-oz nursing bottles; 48 per case; No. 405.

10% GLUCOSE WATER, Ready To Feed
Availability:
4-fl-oz nursing bottles; 48 per case; No. 410.

STERILIZED WATER, Ready To Feed
Availability:
4-fl-oz nursing bottles; 48 per case; No. 432.
8-fl-oz nursing bottles; 24 per case; No. 879.

VOLU-FEED®, Ross Volumetric Feeding System
Availability:
Volu-Feed Nursers; 100 per case; No. 080.
Volu-Feed Dispensing Caps; 250 per case; No. 081.

Component Nipple System
Availability:
Regular Nipple; 250 per case; No. 079.
Premature Nipple; 250 per case; No. 094.
Special Care Nipple; 250 per case; No. 095.
NUK® Nipple; 350 per case; No. 098.

Ross Cleft Palate Assembly
Availability:
Cleft Palate Nipple; supplied in packets of 3 nipple assemblies; No. 00070.

ROSS SLD™
Surgical Liquid Diet

Usage: A low-residue formula for patients requiring a clear liquid diet (ie, pre- and post-surgery, prior to diagnostic testing), that provides calories, high-quality protein, vitamins and minerals in a delicious-tasting, fruit punch flavor; and as a low fat diet.

Features:
- Provides 100% of the U.S. RDA for protein, vitamins and minerals in 840 Calories—A concentrated source of nutrients to better meet the needs of patients restricted to clear liquid diets.
- Low residue—Ross SLD is appropriate for use in situations where low-residue is the primary consideration.
- Total calorie/nitrogen ratio of 117:1—A protein-sparing caloric distribution.
- High-quality protein from egg white solids—45 g (6 servings) meets 100% of the U.S. RDA.
- Small, frequent servings enhance patient compliance—Each 6½-fl oz serving of Ross SLD helps improve nutrient intake yet avoids unnecessary waste.
- Low fat—Provides a concentrated source of nutrients for patients with maldigestion/malabsorption of fat.
- Lactose free/Gluten free—Appropriate for use in a variety of patient populations without the risk of intolerance commonly associated with lactose or gluten.
- Good taste—Delicious fruit-punch flavor enhances patient acceptance.

Dosage and Administration:
Instructions for Use: Mixes readily. Pour 6 fl oz (¾ cup) water into a container. Empty contents of one packet into the container and stir until powder dissolves. Use within 6 hours or store covered in refrigerator and use within 48 hours. Stir before use. Store unopened powder in a cool, dry place.
ROSS SLD is a lowfat product that should be used only under medical supervision. Not intended for infants.
Under no circumstances should ROSS SLD be administered parenterally.

Availability: 1.3 oz (37.8 g) packets of water-soluble Powder (artificial fruit-punch flavor); 6 packets per carton; 4 cartons per case; No. 673.
Composition: Powder
Ingredients: ⓤ Sugar (sucrose), egg white solids, hydrolyzed corn starch, minerals (calcium glycerophosphate, magnesium carbonate, ammonium phosphate dibasic, potassium citrate, sodium citrate, potassium chloride, ferrous sulfate, zinc sulfate, manganese glycerophosphate, copper gluconate, potassium iodide), citric acid, vitamins (choline bitartrate, ascorbic acid, alpha-tocopheryl acetate, niacinamide, calcium pantothenate, pyridoxine hydrochloride, vitamin A palmitate, thiamine mononitrate, riboflavin, folic acid, biotin, phylloquinone, vitamin D_3, cyanocobalamin), natural and artificial flavor, and artificial color.

Nutrients:	Per 140 Calories (1 packet)	Per 840 Calories (6 packets)
Protein, g	7.5	45
Fat, g	0.1	0.6
Carbohydrate, g	27.3	163.8
Minerals (Ash), g	1.4	8.4
Moisture, g	1.5	9.0

	Per 140 Calories (1 packet)	Per 840 Calories (6 packets)	Percent U.S. RDA* (840 Calories)
Vitamins/Minerals			
Vitamin A, IU	834	5000	100
Vitamin D, IU	67	400	100
Vitamin E, IU	7.5	45	150
Vitamin K_1, mcg	6	36	**
Vitamin C, mg	15	90	150
Folic Acid, mcg	100	600	150
Thiamine (Vit. B_1), mg	0.39	2.3	150
Riboflavin (Vit. B_2), mg	0.43	2.6	150
Vitamin B_6, mg	0.50	3.0	150
Vitamin B_{12}, mcg	1.5	9.0	150
Niacin, mg	5	30	150
Biotin, mcg	75	450	150
Pantothenic Acid, mg	2.5	15	150
Choline, mg	75	450	**
Calcium, mg	167	1000	100
Phosphorus, mg	167	1000	100
Sodium, mg	167	1000	**
Potassium, mg	167	1000	**
Chloride, mg	200	1200	**
Magnesium, mg	67	400	100
Iodine, mcg	25	150	100
Manganese, mg	0.84	5	**
Copper, mg	0.33	2	100
Zinc, mg	3.8	23	150
Iron, mg	3.0	18	100

*For adults and children 4 or more years of age.
**U.S. RDA not established.
(FAN 344-01)

SELSUN BLUE®   OTC
[sel'sen blü]
(selenium sulfide)
Dandruff Shampoo

Selsun Blue is a non-prescription anti-dandruff shampoo containing a 1% concentration of selenium sulfide in a freshly scented, pH balanced formula to leave hair clean and manageable. Available in formulations for dry, oily or normal hair types.
Clinical testing has shown it to be safe and more effective than other leading shampoos in helping control dandruff symptoms with regular use.
Directions: Shake well before using. Lather, rinse thoroughly and repeat. Use regularly, once or twice weekly, for effective dandruff control.
Caution: For external use only. Keep out of eyes—if this happens, rinse thoroughly with water. If used before or after bleaching, tinting or permanent waving, rinse hair for at least five minutes in cool running water. If irritation occurs, discontinue use.

Warning: Keep out of the reach of children.
How Supplied: 4, 7 and 11 fl oz plastic bottles.

SIMILAC®
[sim'e-lak]
Infant Formula

Usage: When an infant formula is needed if the decision is made to discontinue breast-feeding before age 1 year, if a supplement to breast-feeding is needed, or as a routine feeding if breast-feeding is not adopted.
Availability:
Powder: 1-lb cans, measuring scoop enclosed; 6 per case; No. 03139.
1.06-oz packets; 12 four-packet cartons per case; No. 00231.
Concentrated Liquid: 13-fl-oz cans; 24 per case; No. 00264.
Ready To Feed: (Prediluted, 20 Cal/fl oz)
32-fl-oz cans; 6 per case; No. 00232.
8-fl-oz cans; 4 six-packs per case; No. 00177.
4-fl-oz nursing bottles; 6 per carry-home carton, 8 cartons per case; No. 00480.
8-fl-oz nursing bottles; 6 per carry-home carton, 4 cartons per case; No. 00880.
For hospital use, Similac in disposable nursing bottles is available in the Ross Hospital Formula System.
Preparation:
Powder: Standard dilution (20 Cal/fl oz) is 1 level, unpacked scoop Powder (8.74 g) for each 2 fl oz water; or, 1 packet (30.1 g) for each 7 fl oz water.
Concentrated Liquid: Standard dilution (20 Cal/fl oz) is 1 part Concentrated Liquid to 1 part water.
Composition: Powder
Ingredients: ⓤ-D Nonfat milk, lactose, corn oil, coconut oil, vitamins (ascorbic acid, alpha-tocopheryl acetate, niacinamide, calcium pantothenate, vitamin A palmitate, thiamine chloride hydrochloride, pyridoxine hydrochloride, riboflavin, folic acid, phylloquinone, vitamin D_3, cyanocobalamin) minerals (zinc sulfate, ferrous sulfate, cupric sulfate, manganese sulfate) and taurine.

Nutrients:	Powder (wt/100 g)	Standard Dilution* (wt/liter)
Protein	11.4 g	15.0 g
Fat	27.6 g	36.3 g
Carbohydrate	54.9 g	72.3 g
Minerals (Ash)	3.1 g	4.1 g
Calcium	390 mg	510 mg
Phosphorus	300 mg	390 mg
Magnesium	31 mg	41 mg
Iron	1.1 mg	1.5 mg

(This product, like milk, is deficient in iron; an additional 5.3 mg iron per liter should be supplied from other sources.)

Iodine	76 mcg	100 mcg
Zinc	3.8 mg	5.0 mg
Copper	0.46 mg	0.60 mg
Manganese	26 mcg	34 mcg
Sodium	170 mg	230 mg
Potassium	610 mg	800 mg
Chloride	380 mg	500 mg
Water	2.0 g	902 g
Crude Fiber	0 g	
Calories	513	676
Calories per fl oz		20

Vitamins Per Liter (Standard Dilution*):

Vitamin A	2000	I.U.
Vitamin D	400	I.U.
Vitamin E	17	I.U.
Vitamin K_1	55	mcg
Vitamin C	55	mg
Thiamine (Vit. B_1)	0.65	mg
Riboflavin (Vit. B_2)	1.0	mg
Vitamin B_6	0.40	mg
Vitamin B_{12}	1.5	mcg
Niacin	7.0	mg
Folic Acid	100	mcg
Pantothenic Acid	3.0	mg

*Standard dilution is one level scoop of Powder for each 2 fluid ounces of warm water or 131.7 g of Powder diluted to one liter.
(FAN 341-02)

Composition: Concentrated Liquid
Ingredients: Ⓤ-D Water, nonfat milk, lactose, soy oil, coconut oil, mono- and diglycerides, soy lecithin, vitamins (ascorbic acid, alpha-tocopheryl acetate, niacinamide, calcium pantothenate, vitamin A palmitate, thiamine chloride hydrochloride, pyridoxine hydrochloride, riboflavin, folic acid, phylloquinone, vitamin D_3, cyanocobalamin), carrageenan, minerals (zinc sulfate, ferrous sulfate, cupric sulfate, manganese sulfate) and taurine.

Nutrients (wt/liter):	Concentrated		Standard Dilution*	
Protein	30.0	g	15.0	g
Fat	72.6	g	36.3	g
Carbohydrate	144.6	g	72.3	g
Minerals (Ash)	6.6	g	3.3	g
Calcium	1.0	g	510	mg
Phosphorus	0.78	g	390	mg
Magnesium	82	mg	41	mg
Iron	3.0	mg	1.5	mg

(This product, like milk, is deficient in iron; an additional 5.3 mg iron per liter should be supplied from other sources.)

Iodine	200	mcg	100	mcg
Zinc	10	mg	5.0	mg
Copper	1.2	mg	0.60	mg
Manganese	68	mcg	34	mcg
Sodium	460	mg	230	mg
Potassium	1600	mg	800	mg
Chloride	1000	mg	500	mg
Water	806	g	902	g
Crude Fiber	0	g		
Calories per fl oz	40		20	
Calories per liter	1352		676	

Vitamins Per Liter (Standard Dilution*):

Vitamin A	2000	I.U.
Vitamin D	400	I.U.
Vitamin E	20	I.U.
Vitamin K_1	55	mcg
Vitamin C	55	mg
Thiamine (Vit. B_1)	0.65	mg
Riboflavin (Vit. B_2)	1.0	mg
Vitamin B_6	0.40	mg
Vitamin B_{12}	1.5	mcg
Niacin	7.0	mg
Folic Acid	100	mcg
Pantothenic Acid	3.0	mg

*Standard dilution is equal parts Similac Concentrated Liquid and water.
(FAN 341-02)

Composition: Ready To Feed
Ingredients: Ⓤ-D Water, nonfat milk, lactose, soy oil, coconut oil, mono- and diglycerides, soy lecithin, vitamins (ascorbic acid, alpha-tocopheryl acetate, niacinamide, calcium pantothenate, vitamin A palmitate, thiamine chloride hydrochloride, pyridoxine hydrochloride, riboflavin, folic acid, phylloquinone, vitamin D_3, cyanocobalamin), carrageenan, minerals (zinc sulfate, ferrous sulfate, cupric sulfate, manganese sulfate) and taurine.

Nutrients (wt/liter):

Protein	15.0	g
Fat	36.3	g
Carbohydrate	72.3	g
Minerals (Ash)	3.3	g
Calcium	510	mg
Phosphorus	390	mg
Magnesium	41	mg
Iron	1.5	mg

(This product, like milk, is deficient in iron; an additional 5.3 mg iron per liter should be supplied from other sources.)

Iodine	100	mcg
Zinc	5.0	mg
Copper	0.60	mg
Manganese	34	mcg
Sodium	230	mg
Potassium	800	mg
Chloride	500	mg
Water	902	g
Crude Fiber	0	g
Calories per fl oz	20	
Calories per liter	676	

Vitamins Per Liter:

Vitamin A	2000	I.U.
Vitamin D	400	I.U.
Vitamin E	20	I.U.
Vitamin K_1	55	mcg
Vitamin C	55	mg
Thiamine (Vit. B_1)	0.65	mg
Riboflavin (Vit. B_2)	1.0	mg
Vitamin B_6	0.40	mg
Vitamin B_{12}	1.5	mcg
Niacin	7.0	mg
Folic Acid	100	mcg
Pantothenic Acid	3.0	mg

(FAN 341-01)

SIMILAC® PM 60/40
[sim'e-lak]
Infant Formula

Usage: For infants in the lower range of homeostatic capacity; for those who are problem feeders; those who are predisposed to hypocalcemia; and those whose renal, digestive or cardiovascular functions would benefit from lowered mineral levels.

Availability: Powder only: 1-lb cans, measuring scoop enclosed; 6 per case; No. 00850.
For hospital use, Ready To Feed Similac PM 60/40 in disposable nursing bottles is available in the Ross Hospital Formula System. (Ready To Feed has similar composition and nutrient values as Powder. For specific information see bottle tray.)

Preparation: Standard dilution (20 Cal/fl oz) is one level, unpacked scoop (8.56 g) Powder for each 2 fl oz of water.
Higher caloric feedings are prepared by adding 8.56 g (1 level, unpacked scoopful) of Similac PM 60/40 to the following amounts of water:

For:	Water:	Yields:
24 Cal/oz	48 ml	55 ml (1.8 fl oz)
27 Cal/oz	42 ml	49 ml (1.6 fl oz)
30 Cal/oz	37 ml	44 ml (1.5 fl oz)

Ingredients: Ⓤ-D Lactose, corn oil, coconut oil, whey protein concentrate, sodium caseinate, minerals (calcium phosphate tribasic, potassium citrate, potassium chloride, magnesium chloride, sodium chloride, calcium carbonate, zinc sulfate, ferrous sulfate, cupric sulfate, manganese sulfate), vitamins (m-inositol, ascorbic acid, choline chloride, alpha-tocopheryl acetate, niacinamide, calcium pantothenate, vitamin A palmitate, thiamine chloride hydrochloride, riboflavin, pyridoxine hydrochloride, folic acid, phylloquinone, vitamin D_3, biotin, cyanocobalamin) and taurine.

Nutrients:	Powder (wt/100 g)		Standard Dilution* (wt/liter)	
Protein (Lactalbumin and Lactoglobulin 60%, Casein 40%)	11.4	g	15.0	g
Fat	28.7	g	37.8	g
Carbohydrate	52.4	g	69.0	g
Minerals (Ash)	1.7	g	2.2	g
Calcium	304	mg	400	mg
Phosphorus	152	mg	200	mg
Magnesium	32	mg	42	mg
Iron	1.1	mg	1.5	mg

(This product, like milk, is deficient in iron; an additional 5.3 mg iron per liter should be supplied from other sources.)

Iodine	32	mcg	42	mcg
Zinc	3.8	mg	5.0	mg
Copper	0.46	mg	0.60	mg
Manganese	26	mcg	34	mcg
Sodium	121	mg	160	mg
Potassium	440	mg	580	mg
Chloride	304	mg	400	mg
Water	2.5	g	905	g
Crude Fiber	0	g		
Calories	513		676	
Calories per fl oz			20	

Vitamins Per Liter (Standard Dilution*):

Vitamin A	2000	I.U.
Vitamin D	400	I.U.
Vitamin E	17	I.U.
Vitamin K_1	55	mcg
Vitamin C	55	mg
Thiamine (Vit. B_1)	0.65	mg
Riboflavin (Vit. B_2)	1.0	mg
Vitamin B_6	0.40	mg
Vitamin B_{12}	1.5	mcg
Niacin	7.3	mg
Folic Acid	100	mcg
Pantothenic Acid	3.0	mg
Biotin	30	mcg
Choline	82	mg
Inositol	165	mg

*Standard dilution is 1 level scoop of Powder for each 2 fl oz water or 131.7 g of Powder diluted to 1 liter.

Precautions: In conditions where the infant is losing abnormal quantities of one or more electrolytes, it may be necessary to supply electrolytes from sources other than the formula. With premature infants weighing less than 1500 g at birth, it may be necessary to supply an additional source of sodium, calcium and phosphorus during the period of very rapid growth.
(FAN 341-01)

SIMILAC® WITH IRON
[sim'e-lak]
Infant Formula

Usage: When an iron-containing infant formula is needed if the decision is made to discontinue breast-feeding before age one, if a supplement to breast-feeding is needed, or as a routine feeding if breast-feeding is not adopted.

Availability:
Powder: 1-lb cans, measuring scoop enclosed; 6 per case; No. 03360.
1.06-oz packets; 12 four-packet cartons per case; No. 00235.
Concentrated Liquid: 13-fl oz cans; 24 cans per case; No. 00414.
Ready To Feed: (Prediluted, 20 Cal/fl oz)
32-fl oz cans; 6 per case; No. 00241.
8-fl oz cans; 4 six-packs per case; No. 00179.
4-fl oz nursing bottles; 6 per carry-home carton, 8 cartons per case; No. 06201.
8-fl oz nursing bottles; 6 per carry-home carton, 4 cartons per case; No. 06202.
For hospital use, prebottled Similac With Iron in disposable nursing bottles is available in the Ross Hospital Formula System.

Preparation:
Powder: Standard dilution (20 Cal/fl oz) is 1 level, unpacked scoop Powder (8.74 g) for each 2 fl oz of water; or, 1 packet (30.1 g) for each 7 fl oz water.
Concentrated Liquid: Standard dilution (20 Cal/fl oz) is one part Concentrated Liquid to one part water.
Composition: Powder
Ingredients: Ⓤ-D Nonfat milk, lactose, corn oil, coconut oil, vitamins (ascorbic acid, alpha-tocopheryl acetate, niacinamide, calcium pantothenate, vitamin A palmitate, thiamine chloride hydrochloride, pyridoxine hydrochloride, riboflavin, folic acid, phylloquinone, vitamin D_3, cyanocobalamin), minerals (ferrous sulfate, zinc sulfate, cupric sulfate, manganese sulfate) and taurine.

Nutrients:	Powder (wt/100 g)		Standard Dilution* (wt/liter)	
Protein	11.4	g	15.0	g
Fat	27.6	g	36.3	g
Carbohydrate	54.9	g	72.3	g
Minerals (Ash)	3.1	g	4.1	g

Continued on next page

Ross—Cont.

Calcium	390	mg	510	mg
Phosphorus	300	mg	390	mg
Magnesium	31	mg	41	mg
Iron	9.1	mg	12	mg
Iodine	76	mcg	100	mcg
Zinc	3.8	mg	5.0	mg
Copper	0.46	mg	0.60	mg
Manganese	26	mcg	34	mcg
Sodium	170	mg	230	mg
Potassium	610	mg	800	mg
Chloride	380	mg	500	mg
Water	2.0	g	902	g
Crude Fiber	0	g		
Calories	513		676	
Calories per fl oz			20	

Vitamins Per Liter (Standard Dilution*):

Vitamin A	2000	I.U.
Vitamin D	400	I.U.
Vitamin E	17	I.U.
Vitamin K$_1$	55	mcg
Vitamin C	55	mg
Thiamine (Vit. B$_1$)	0.65	mg
Riboflavin (Vit. B$_2$)	1.0	mg
Vitamin B$_6$	0.40	mg
Vitamin B$_{12}$	1.5	mcg
Niacin	7.0	mg
Folic Acid	100	mcg
Pantothenic Acid	3.0	mg

*Standard dilution is one level scoop of Powder for each 2 fluid ounces of warm water or 131.7 g of Powder diluted to 1 liter. (FAN 341-02)
Composition: Concentrated Liquid
Ingredients: Ⓤ-D Water, nonfat milk, lactose, soy oil, coconut oil, mono- and diglycerides, soy lecithin, vitamins (ascorbic acid, alpha-tocopheryl acetate, niacinamide, calcium pantothenate, vitamin A palmitate, thiamine chloride hydrochloride, pyridoxine hydrochloride, riboflavin, folic acid, phylloquinone, vitamin D$_3$, cyanocobalamin), carrageenan, minerals (ferrous sulfate, zinc sulfate, cupric sulfate, manganese sulfate) and taurine.

Nutrients (wt/liter):	Concentrated		Standard Dilution*	
Protein	30.0	g	15.0	g
Fat	72.6	g	36.3	g
Carbohydrate	144.6	g	72.3	g
Minerals (Ash)	6.6	g	3.3	g
Calcium	1.0	g	510	mg
Phosphorus	0.78	g	390	mg
Magnesium	82	mg	41	mg
Iron	24	mg	12	mg
Iodine	200	mcg	100	mcg
Zinc	10	mg	5.0	mg
Copper	1.2	mg	0.60	mg
Manganese	68	mcg	34	mcg
Sodium	460	mg	230	mg
Potassium	1600	mg	800	mg
Chloride	1000	mg	500	mg
Water	806	g	902	g
Crude Fiber	0			
Calories per fl oz	40		20	
Calories per liter	1352		676	

Vitamins Per Liter (Standard Dilution*):

Vitamin A	2000	I.U.
Vitamin D	400	I.U.
Vitamin E	20	I.U.
Vitamin K$_1$	55	mcg
Vitamin C	55	mg
Thiamine (Vit. B$_1$)	0.65	mg
Riboflavin (Vit. B$_2$)	1.0	mg
Vitamin B$_6$	0.40	mg
Vitamin B$_{12}$	1.5	mcg
Niacin	7.0	mg
Folic Acid	100	mcg
Pantothenic Acid	3.0	mg

*Standard dilution is equal amounts Similac With Iron Concentrated Liquid and water.
(FAN 341-02)
Composition: Ready To Feed
Ingredients: Ⓤ-D Water, nonfat milk, lactose, soy oil, coconut oil, mono- and diglycerides, soy lecithin, vitamins (ascorbic acid, alpha-tocopheryl acetate, niacinamide, calcium pantothenate, vitamin A palmitate, thiamine chloride hydrochloride, pyridoxine hydrochloride, riboflavin, folic acid, phylloquinone, vitamin D$_3$, cyanocobalamin), carrageenan, minerals (ferrous sulfate, zinc sulfate, cupric sulfate, manganese sulfate) and taurine.

Nutrients (wt/liter):

Protein	15.0	g
Fat	36.3	g
Carbohydrate	72.3	g
Minerals (Ash)	3.3	g
Calcium	510	mg
Phosphorus	390	mg
Magnesium	41	mg
Iron	12	mg
Iodine	100	mcg
Zinc	5.0	mg
Copper	0.60	mg
Manganese	34	mcg
Sodium	230	mg
Potassium	800	mg
Chloride	500	mg
Water	902	g
Crude Fiber	0	g
Calories per fl oz	20	
Calories per liter	676	

Vitamins Per Liter:

Vitamin A	2000	I.U.
Vitamin D	400	I.U.
Vitamin E	20	I.U.
Vitamin K$_1$	55	mcg
Vitamin C	55	mg
Thiamine (Vit. B$_1$)	0.65	mg
Riboflavin (Vit. B$_2$)	1.0	mg
Vitamin B$_6$	0.40	mg
Vitamin B$_{12}$	1.5	mcg
Niacin	7.0	mg
Folic Acid	100	mcg
Pantothenic Acid	3.0	mg

The addition of iron to this formula conforms to the recommendation of the Committee on Nutrition of the American Academy of Pediatrics.
(FAN 341-01)

SIMILAC® WITH WHEY + IRON
[sim′e-lak]
Infant Formula
Usage: When an iron-fortified, whey-predominant-protein formula is desired for feeding term infants if the decision is made to discontinue breast-feeding before age 1 year, if a supplement to breast-feeding is needed, or as a routine feeding if breast-feeding is not adopted.
Availability:
Powder: 1-lb cans, measuring scoop enclosed; 6 per case; No. 00372.
Concentrated Liquid: 13-fl-oz cans; 12 per case; No. 00352.
Ready To Feed: (prediluted, 20 Cal/fl oz) 32-fl-oz cans; 6 per case; No. 00312.
For hospital use, Similac With Whey + Iron in disposable nursing bottles is available in the Ross Hospital Formula System.
Preparation:
Powder: Standard dilution (20 Cal/fl oz) is 1 level, unpacked scoop Powder (8.74 g) for each 2 fl oz of water.
Concentrated Liquid: Standard dilution (20 Cal/fl oz) is one part Concentrated Liquid to one part water.
Composition: Powder
Ingredients: Ⓤ-D Nonfat milk, lactose, corn oil, coconut oil, whey protein concentrate, minerals (calcium phosphate tribasic, sodium chloride, magnesium chloride, potassium citrate, ferrous sulfate, zinc sulfate, cupric sulfate, manganese sulfate) vitamins (ascorbic acid, alpha-tocopheryl acetate, niacinamide, calcium pantothenate, vitamin A palmitate, thiamine chloride hydrochloride, riboflavin, pyridoxine hydrochloride, folic acid, phylloquinone, vitamin D$_3$, biotin, cyanocobalamin) and taurine.

Nutrients:	Powder (wt/100 g)		Standard Dilution* (wt/liter)	
Protein	11.4	g	15.0	g
(Lactoglobulin and Lactalbumin 60%, Casein 40%)				
Fat	27.6	g	36.3	g
Carbohydrate	54.9	g	72.3	g
Minerals (Ash)	2.6	g	3.4	g
Calcium	300	mg	400	mg
Phosphorus	230	mg	300	mg
Magnesium	38	mg	50	mg
Iron	9.1	mg	12	mg
Iodine	76	mcg	100	mcg
Zinc	3.8	mg	5.0	mg
Copper	0.46	mg	0.60	mg
Manganese	26	mcg	34	mcg
Sodium	175	mg	230	mg
Potassium	570	mg	750	mg
Chloride	325	mg	430	mg
Water	2.5	g	902	g
Crude Fiber	0	g		
Calories	513		676	
Calories per fl oz			20	

Vitamins Per Liter (Standard Dilution*):

Vitamin A	2000	I.U.
Vitamin D	400	I.U.
Vitamin E	17	I.U.
Vitamin K$_1$	55	mcg
Vitamin C	55	mg
Thiamine (Vit. B$_1$)	0.65	mg
Riboflavin (Vit. B$_2$)	1.0	mg
Vitamin B$_6$	0.40	mg
Vitamin B$_{12}$	1.5	mcg
Niacin	7.0	mg
Folic Acid	100	mcg
Pantothenic Acid	3.0	mg
Biotin	11	mcg

*Standard dilution is one level scoop of Powder for each 2 fluid ounces of warm water or 131.7 g of Powder diluted to 1 liter.
(FAN 341-02)
Composition: Concentrated Liquid
Ingredients: Ⓤ-D Water, nonfat milk, lactose, soy oil, coconut oil, whey protein concentrate, minerals (calcium phosphate tribasic, sodium chloride, potassium citrate, ferrous sulfate, magnesium chloride, zinc sulfate, cupric sulfate, manganese sulfate), soy lecithin, mono- and diglycerides, vitamins (ascorbic acid, alpha-tocopheryl acetate, niacinamide, calcium pantothenate, vitamin A palmitate, thiamine chloride hydrochloride, pyridoxine hydrochloride, folic acid, phylloquinone, vitamin D$_3$, biotin, cyanocobalamin), carrageenan and taurine.

Nutrients (wt/liter):	Concentrated		Standard Dilution*	
Protein	30.0	g	15.0	g
(Lactoglobulin and Lactalbumin 60%, Casein 40%)				
Fat	72.6	g	36.3	g
Carbohydrate	144.6	g	72.3	g
Minerals (Ash)	6.8	g	3.4	g
Calcium	800	mg	400	mg
Phosphorus	600	mg	300	mg
Magnesium	100	mg	50	mg
Iron	24	mg	12	mg
Iodine	200	mcg	100	mcg
Zinc	10	mg	5.0	mg
Copper	1.2	mg	0.60	mg
Manganese	68	mcg	34	mcg
Sodium	460	mg	230	mg
Potassium	1500	mg	750	mg
Chloride	860	mg	430	mg
Water	806	g	902	g

Product Information

Crude Fiber	0	g
Calories per fl oz	40	20
Calories per liter	1352	676

Vitamins Per Liter (Standard Dilution*):

Vitamin A	2000	I.U.
Vitamin D	400	I.U.
Vitamin E	20	I.U.
Vitamin K$_1$	55	mcg
Vitamin C	55	mcg
Thiamine (Vit. B$_1$)	0.65	mg
Riboflavin (Vit. B$_2$)	1.0	mg
Vitamin B$_6$	0.40	mg
Vitamin B$_{12}$	1.5	mcg
Niacin	7.0	mg
Folic Acid	100	mcg
Pantothenic Acid	3.0	mg
Biotin	11	mcg

*Standard dilution is equal amounts Similac With Whey + Iron Concentrated Liquid and water. (FAN 341-01)

Composition: Ready To Feed
Ingredients: Ⓤ-D Water, nonfat milk, lactose, soy oil, coconut oil, whey protein concentrate, minerals (calcium phosphate tribasic, sodium chloride, potassium citrate, ferrous sulfate, magnesium chloride, zinc sulfate, cupric sulfate, manganese sulfate), soy lecithin, mono- and diglycerides, vitamins (ascorbic acid, alpha-tocopheryl acetate, niacinamide, calcium pantothenate, vitamin A palmitate, thiamine chloride hydrochloride, riboflavin, pyridoxine hydrochloride, folic acid, phylloquinone, vitamin D$_3$, biotin, cyanocobalamin), carrageenan and taurine.

Nutrients (wt/liter):

Protein	15.0	g
(Lactoglobulin and Lactalbumin 60%, Casein 40%)		
Fat	36.3	g
Carbohydrate	72.3	g
Minerals (Ash)	3.4	g
Calcium	400	mg
Phosphorus	300	mg
Magnesium	50	mg
Iron	12	mg
Iodine	100	mcg
Zinc	5.0	mg
Copper	0.60	mg
Manganese	34	mcg
Sodium	230	mg
Potassium	750	mg
Chloride	430	mg
Water	902	g
Crude Fiber	0	g
Calories per fl oz	20	
Calories per liter	676	

Vitamins Per Liter:

Vitamin A	2000	I.U.
Vitamin D	400	I.U.
Vitamin E	20	I.U.
Vitamin K$_1$	55	mcg
Vitamin C	55	mcg
Thiamine (Vit. B$_1$)	0.65	mg
Riboflavin (Vit. B$_2$)	1.0	mg
Vitamin B$_6$	0.40	mg
Vitamin B$_{12}$	1.5	mcg
Niacin	7.0	mg
Folic Acid	100	mcg
Pantothenic Acid	3.0	mg
Biotin	11	mcg

The addition of iron to this formula conforms to the recommendation of the Committee on Nutrition of the American Academy of Pediatrics. (FAN 341-01)

TRONOLANE™   OTC
[*tron′e-lān*]
Cream:
(pramoxine hydrochloride)
Suppositories:
(pramoxine and pramoxine HCl)

Description: Tronolane contains a surface anesthetic agent, chemically unrelated to the benzoate esters of the "caine" type, which is chemically designated as a 4-n-butoxyphenyl gammamorpholinopropyl- ether hydrochloride.

Indications: Tronolane is indicated for use as a topical anesthetic to relieve pain, burning, itching and discomfort that accompanies hemorrhoids. It also has a soothing, lubricant action on mucous membranes.

Tronolane contains an excellent rapidly acting topical anesthetic with surface analgesia that lasts up to 5 hours. It fills a conspicuous gap among anesthetics by combining: prompt and potent relief from surface pain or itching, with almost complete freedom from toxicity and sensitization. Since the drug is chemically unrelated to other anesthetics, cross-sensitization is unlikely. Patients who are already sensitized to the "caine" drugs or other anesthetics can generally use Tronolane with excellent results. Tronolane cream and suppositories provide a desirable combination of properties—low toxicity, low sensitization, and structural individuality, together with prompt and adequate anesthetic effect.

Tronolane provides adjunctive therapy for the symptomatic relief of pain and discomfort in external and internal hemorrhoids.

The special emollient/emulsion base of the cream provides soothing lubrication making bowel movements easier and more comfortable. Tronolane cream is a bland, non-toxic, well balanced formula in a non-drying base which is nongreasy and non-staining to undergarments.

Warnings: If bleeding is present, consult physician. Certain persons can develop allergic reactions to ingredients in this product. During treatment, if condition worsens or persists 7 days, consult physician. For children under 12 years, use only as directed by physician.

Dosage and Administration: CREAM: Apply up to five times daily, especially morning, night and after bowel movements or as directed by physician.

External—Apply liberally to affected area. **Intrarectal**—Remove cap from tube and attach clean applicator. Squeeze tube gently to lubricate applicator. Gently insert applicator into rectum and squeeze tube. Thoroughly cleanse applicator after use.

Dosage and Administration: SUPPOSITORIES: Use up to five times daily, especially morning, night, and after bowel movements, or as directed by physician. Detach one suppository from pack. Tear notch at pointed end and remove wrapper before insertion. Insert suppository into the rectum, pointed end first.

How Supplied: Tronolane is available in 1-oz and 2-oz cream tubes and 10 and 20 count suppository boxes.

TWOCAL™ HN
[*tü′kal*]
High Nitrogen Liquid Nutrition

Usage: As a high-calorie, high-nitrogen liquid food, TwoCal HN delivers 100% of the U.S. RDA for vitamins and minerals in only 950 milliliters (1 quart). TwoCal HN is most appropriate for use in severely hypermetabolic and fluid-restricted patients. As a concentrated source of nutrition, TwoCal HN is an excellent dietary supplement when voluntary food intake is inadequate to meet nutrient needs.

Features:
- Complete, balanced nutrition—2.0 Calories per ml, 475 Calories per 8 fl oz, 2000 Calories per liter from a balanced distribution of protein, fat and carbohydrate (caloric distribution: protein, 16.7%; fat, 40.1%; and carbohydrate, 43.2%). 1900 Calories of TwoCal HN provide at least 100% of the U.S. RDA for vitamins and minerals for adults and children 4 or more years of age.
- High nitrogen—TwoCal HN has a total calorie-to-nitrogen ratio of 150:1, indicated for the stressed patient to meet increased nitrogen needs.
- Concentrated nutrition—TwoCal HN will reduce the volume necessary to meet the protein and calorie needs of the hypermetabolic or fluid-restricted patient (83.7g of protein per liter, 2000 Calories per liter).
- Lactose free—TwoCal HN will not contribute to lactose-associated diarrhea. Hydrolyzed corn starch and sucrose are the carbohydrate sources.

Dosage and Administration:
Ready To Use: Shake well. TwoCal HN is ready to use and does not require dilution with water. TwoCal HN may be stored (unopened) and fed at room temperature. Once opened, remaining TwoCal HN should be covered, refrigerated and discarded if not used within 48 hours.

Oral Feeding: TwoCal HN may be used for total nutrition, or as a supplement for added nutritional support. Serve TwoCal HN chilled for oral feeding.

Tube Feeding: Follow physician's instructions. When initiating feeding, the flow rate, volume and dilution are dependent on patient condition and tolerance. Care should be taken to avoid contamination of this product during preparation and administration.

When used as a sole source of nutrition, products containing 2 Cal/ml do not meet the water requirements of most patients. Monitor hydration status and provide additional water by enteral or parenteral routes as needed.

Under no circumstances should TwoCal HN be administered parenterally.
[See table on next page].

Availability:
Ready To Use: 8-fl-oz cans; 4 six-packs per case; Vanilla, No. 729.
Composition: Ready To Use Vanilla
Ingredients: Ⓤ-D Water, hydrolyzed corn starch, corn oil, sodium caseinate, sucrose, sodium calcium caseinate, medium-chain triglycerides (fractionated coconut oil), minerals (potassium citrate, magnesium chloride, calcium phosphate tribasic, sodium citrate, zinc sulfate, ferrous sulfate, manganous chloride, cupric sulfate), soy protein isolate, natural and artificial flavors, soy lecithin and vitamins (choline chloride, ascorbic acid, alpha-tocopheryl acetate, niacinamide, calcium pantothenate, pyridoxine hydrochloride, vitamin A palmitate, thiamine chloride hydrochloride, riboflavin, folic acid, biotin, phylloquinone, vitamin D$_3$, cyanocobalamin).

Nutrients (grams/8 fl oz): Protein, 19.8; Fat, 21.5; Carbohydrate, 51.4; Minerals (Ash), 2.4; Moisture, 168.5. Calories per ml, 2.0; Calories per fl oz, 59.4.

Vitamin/Mineral Content of TwoCal HN (Ready To Use)

Vitamins/Minerals	Per 8 Fl Oz		Percent U.S. RDA* (Per 8 Fl Oz)
Vitamin A	1250	I.U.	25
Vitamin D	100	I.U.	25
Vitamin E	11.4	I.U.	38
Vitamin K$_1$	18	mcg	**
Vitamin C	45	mg	75
Folic Acid	0.16	mg	40
Thiamine (Vit. B$_1$)	0.60	mg	40
Riboflavin (Vit. B$_2$)	0.68	mg	40
Vitamin B$_6$	0.80	mg	40
Vitamin B$_{12}$	2.4	mcg	40
Niacin	8.0	mg	40
Choline	0.19	g	**
Biotin	0.12	mg	40
Pantothenic Acid	4.0	mg	40
Sodium	250	mg	**
Potassium	550	mg	**
Chloride	370	mg	**
Calcium	0.25	g	25
Phosphorus	0.25	g	25

Continued on next page

Ross—Cont.

Magnesium	100	mg	25
Iodine	38	mcg	25
Manganese	1.5	mg	**
Copper	0.50	mg	25
Zinc	5.7	mg	38
Iron	4.5	mg	25

*For adults and children 4 or more years of age.
**U.S. RDA not established.
(FAN 348-02)

VARI-FLAVORS® Flavor Pacs
[var'ē-flā" verz]

Usage: To provide flavor variety for patients receiving full liquid diets and liquid supplements.

Features:
- Five flavors (Pecan, Cherry, Lemon, Orange, Strawberry) offer patients variety and encourage acceptance of liquid diets and liquid supplements.
- Vari-Flavors Flavor Pacs mix readily with Ross Medical Nutritional products to suit individual flavor preferences.
- Flavor Pacs may be stored for use in the dietary department, at nursing stations or by patient's bedside.

Availability:
One-gram packets; 24 per dispenser carton; Pecan, No. 720; Cherry, No. 722; Lemon, No. 724; Orange, No. 726; Strawberry, No. 728; Assorted flavors, No. 730.

Instructions for Use: Tap Pac lightly to shake contents to bottom. Tear off corner of packet. Pour contents into suitable dry serving container. Add 8 ounces of one of the Ross Medical Nutritional products. Allow flavor to dissolve for a few seconds. Stir until flavor is mixed and serve.

Composition: Dextrose, artificial flavor and color (Strawberry, Cherry, Orange). Dextrose and artificial flavor (Pecan). Dextrose, artificial flavor and FD & C Yellow #5 (Lemon).

When used as directed, Vari-Flavors contribute trace amounts of minerals and less than 1 gram of dextrose. The addition of a single Vari-Flavors Pac (1 gram) to one of the Ross Medical Nutritional products increases total calories per 8-oz serving by approximately 4 Calories.
(FAN 242)

VI-DAYLIN® ADC Drops
[vī" dā' lin]
Dietary Supplement of Vitamins A, D and C

Description: One dropperful (1.0 ml) provides:

Vitamins		% U.S. RDA*	% U.S. RDA**
Vitamin A	1500 I.U.	100	60
Vitamin D	400 I.U.	100	100
Vitamin C	35 mg	100	87

Ingredients: Propylene glycol, polysorbate 80, ascorbic acid, methylparaben (preservative), vitamin A palmitate, propylparaben (preservative), and ergocalciferol in a glycerin-water vehicle with added artificial pineapple-fruit flavoring and caramel coloring. Contains only a trace (less than 1/2%) of alcohol.

*% U.S. Recommended Daily Allowance for infants.
**% U.S. Recommended Daily Allowance for children under 4 years of age.

Indications and Usage: Dietary supplement of vitamins A, D and C for infants and children under 4 years of age.

Dosage and Administration: One dropperful daily, or as directed by physician.

How Supplied:
50-ml bottles, calibrated dropper enclosed; OTC; NDC 0074-0105-04.

VI-DAYLIN® Drops
[vī" dā' lin]
Multivitamin Supplement

Description: One dropperful (1.0 ml) provides:

Vitamins		% U.S. RDA*	% U.S. RDA**
Vitamin A	1500 I.U.	100	60
Vitamin D	400 I.U.	100	100
Vitamin E	5 I.U.	100	50
Vitamin C	35 mg	100	87
Thiamine (Vitamin B_1)	0.5 mg	100	71
Riboflavin (Vitamin B_2)	0.6 mg	100	75
Niacin	8 mg	100	88
Vitamin B_6	0.4 mg	100	57
Vitamin B_{12}	1.5 mcg	75	50

Ingredients: Ascorbic acid, d-alpha tocopheryl acid succinate, niacinamide, benzoic acid (preservative), ferric ammonium citrate (stabilizer), vitamin A palmitate, riboflavin-5'-phosphate sodium, methylparaben (preservative), thiamine hydrochloride, pyridoxine hydrochloride, ergocalciferol, disodium edetate (stabilizer) and cyanocobalamin in a glycerin-water vehicle with added artificial flavoring. Contains only a trace (less than 1/2%) of alcohol.

*% U.S. Recommended Daily Allowance for infants.
**% U.S. Recommended Daily Allowance for children under 4 years of age.

Indications and Usage: Multivitamin supplement for infants and children under 4 years of age.

Dosage and Administration: One dropperful daily, or as directed by physician.

How Supplied:
50-ml bottles, calibrated dropper enclosed; OTC; NDC 0074-0103-04.

VI-DAYLIN®/F ADC Drops ℞
[vī" dā' lin]
ADC Vitamins/Fluoride

Description: One dropperful (1.0 ml) provides:
Fluoride 0.25 mg

Vitamins		% U.S. RDA*	% U.S. RDA**
Vitamin A	1500 I.U.	100	60
Vitamin D	400 I.U.	100	100
Vitamin C	35 mg	100	87

Ingredients: Ascorbic acid, vitamin A palmitate, sodium fluoride, ergocalciferol. Alcohol, approximately 0.3%.

*% U.S. Recommended Daily Allowance for infants.
**% U.S. Recommended Daily Allowance for children under 4 years of age.

Indications and Usage: As an aid in the prevention of dental caries in infants and children, and in the prophylaxis of vitamin A, D and C deficiencies.

Contraindications: Should be used only where the fluoride content of the drinking water supply is known to be 0.7 parts per million or less.

Precautions: The recommended dosage should not be exceeded since chronic overdosage of fluoride may result in mottling of tooth enamel and osseous changes.

Overdosage: In children, acute ingestion of 10 to 20 mg of sodium fluoride may cause excessive salivation and gastrointestinal disturbances; 500 mg may be fatal. Oral and/or intravenous fluids containing calcium may be indicated.

Dosage and Administration: One dropperful daily, or as directed by physician or dentist.

How Supplied:
50-ml bottles, calibrated dropper enclosed; Rx; NDC 0074-1106-50.

VI-DAYLIN®/F ADC + IRON Drops ℞
[vī" dā' lin]
ADC Vitamins/Fluoride/Iron Supplement

Description: One dropperful (1.0 ml) provides:
Fluoride 0.25 mg

Vitamins		% U.S. RDA*	% U.S. RDA**
Vitamin A	1500 I.U.	100	60
Vitamin D	400 I.U.	100	100
Vitamin C	35 mg	100	87
Minerals			
Iron	10 mg	66	100

Ingredients: Ascorbic acid, ferrous sulfate, vitamin A palmitate, sodium fluoride, ergocalciferol.

*% U.S. Recommended Daily Allowance for infants.
**% U.S. Recommended Daily Allowance for children under 4 years of age.

Sample Administration Schedule for TwoCal HN

Continuous Drip Schedule

Day	Time	Strength	Rate (mL/hr)	Volume (mL)	Calories
1	1st 8 hours	1/2	50	400	400
	2nd 8 hours	1/2	50	400	400
	3rd 8 hours	1/2	75	600	600
					1400 Total Calories
2	1st 8 hours	1/2	75–100	600–800	600–800
	2nd 8 hours	1/2	75–100	600–800	600–800
	3rd 8 hours	1/2	75–100	600–800	600–800
					1800–2400 Total Calories
3	24 hours	Full	75–100	1800–2400	3600–4800 Total Calories

Intermittent Drip Schedule

Day	Time	Strength	Rate (5–10 mL/min)	Volume (mL)	Calories
1	7am–11pm	1/2	100 mL q 2 hr (7am, 9am)	200	200
		1/2	150 mL q 2 hr (11am, 1pm, 3pm)	450	450
		1/2	200 mL q 2 hr (5pm, 7pm, 9pm, 11pm)	800	800
					1450 Total Calories
2	7am–10pm	1/2	250 mL q 2 hr (7am, 9am, 11am)	750	750
		Full	250 mL q 3 hr (1pm, 4pm, 7pm, 10pm)	1000	2000
					2750 Total Calories
3	7am–10pm	Full	250 mL q 3 hr* in 5–8 feedings/day	1250–2000	2500–4000 Total Calories

*Preferable to q 2 hr
- Check gastric residuals before every intermittent feeding or every 2–4 hours during continuous feeding.
- If intolerance develops, return to previously tolerated strength and rate. When tolerance is again established, proceed with feeding schedule as indicated. Do not alter rate and strength at the same time.
- Rinsing the tube with water (eg, 25–100 mL) after each intermittent feeding or every 3 to 6 hours during continuous feeding will help avoid clogging and provide additional water.

Indications and Usage: As an aid in the prevention of dental caries in infants and children, and in the prophylaxis of iron and vitamin A, D and C deficiencies.

Contraindications: Should be used only where the fluoride content of the drinking water supply is known to be 0.7 parts per million or less.

Precautions: The recommended dosage should not be exceeded since chronic overdosage of fluoride may result in mottling of tooth enamel and osseous changes. In infants, oral iron-containing preparations may cause temporary darkening of the membrane covering the teeth.

Overdosage: In children, acute ingestion of 10 to 20 mg of sodium fluoride may cause excessive salivation and gastrointestinal disturbances; 500 mg may be fatal. Oral and/or intravenous fluids containing calcium may be indicated.

Acute overdosage of iron may cause nausea and vomiting and, in severe cases, cardiovascular collapse and death. The estimated lethal dose of orally ingested elemental iron is 300 mg per kg body weight. Serum iron and total iron-binding capacity may be used as guides for use of chelating agents such as deferoxamine.

Dosage and Administration: One dropperful daily, or as directed by physician or dentist.

How Supplied: 50-ml bottles, calibrated dropper enclosed; ℞; NDC 0074-8929-50.

VI-DAYLIN®/F Drops
[vī″dā′lin]
Multivitamins/Fluoride

Description: One dropperful (1.0 ml) provides:
Fluoride 0.25 mg

Vitamins			% U.S. RDA*	% U.S. RDA**
Vitamin A	1500	I.U.	100	60
Vitamin D	400	I.U.	100	100
Vitamin E	5	I.U.	100	50
Vitamin C	35	mg	100	87
Thiamine (Vitamin B$_1$)	0.5	mg	100	71
Riboflavin (Vitamin B$_2$)	0.6	mg	100	75
Niacin	8	mg	100	88
Vitamin B$_6$	0.4	mg	100	57

Ingredients: Ascorbic acid, niacinamide, d-alpha tocopheryl acid succinate, riboflavin-5′-phosphate sodium, sodium fluoride, vitamin A palmitate, thiamine hydrochloride, pyridoxine hydrochloride and ergocalciferol. No artificial sweeteners. Alcohol content less than 0.1%.

*% U.S. Recommended Daily Allowance for infants.
**% U.S. Recommended Daily Allowance for children under 4 years of age.

Indications and Usage: As an aid in the prevention of dental caries in infants and children, and in the prophylaxis of certain vitamin deficiencies.

Contraindications: Should be used only where the fluoride content of the drinking water supply is known to be 0.7 parts per million or less.

Precautions: The recommended dosage should not be exceeded since chronic overdosage of fluoride may result in mottling of tooth enamel and osseous changes.

Overdosage: In children, acute ingestion of 10 to 20 mg of sodium fluoride may cause excessive salivation and gastrointestinal disturbances; 500 mg may be fatal. Oral and/or intravenous fluids containing calcium may be indicated.

Dosage and Administration: One dropperful daily, or as directed by physician or dentist.

How Supplied: 50-ml bottles, calibrated dropper enclosed; Rx; NDC 0074-1104-50.

Vi-Daylin/F + Iron Chewable

Vitamins			% U.S. RDA*	% U.S. RDA**
Vitamin A (as palmitate, 0.75 mg)	2500	I.U.	100	50
Vitamin D (as cholecalciferol, 10 mcg)	400	I.U.	100	100
Vitamin E (as dl-alpha tocopheryl acetate)	15	I.U.	150	50
Vitamin C (as sodium ascorbate, 40 mg; ascorbic acid, 20 mg)	60	mg	150	100
Folic Acid	0.3	mg	150	75
Vitamin B$_1$ (as thiamine mononitrate)	1.05	mg	150	70
Vitamin B$_2$ (as riboflavin)	1.2	mg	150	70
Niacin (as niacinamide)	13.5	mg	150	67
Vitamin B$_6$ (as pyridoxine hydrochloride)	1.05	mg	150	52
Vitamin B$_{12}$ (as cyanocobalamin)	4.5	mcg	150	75
Minerals				
Iron (as ferrous fumarate)	12	mg	120	66

*% U.S. Recommended Daily Allowance for children under 4 years of age.
**% U.S. Recommended Daily Allowance for adults and children 4 or more years of age.

VI-DAYLIN®/F + IRON Chewable
[vī″dā′lin]
Multivitamins/Fluoride/Iron

Description: Each chewable tablet provides:
Fluoride (as sodium fluoride) 1 mg
[See table above].

Indications and Usage: As an aid in the prevention of dental caries in children, and in the prophylaxis of iron and certain vitamin deficiencies.

Contraindications: Should be used only where the fluoride content of the drinking water supply is known to be 0.7 parts per million or less.

Precautions: The recommended dosage should not be exceeded since chronic overdosage of fluoride may result in mottling of tooth enamel and osseous changes.

Dosage and Administration: Children 3 years of age or older, one chewable tablet daily; age 2-3 years, ½ chewable tablet daily; or as directed by physician or dentist.

Overdosage: In children, acute ingestion of 10 to 20 mg of sodium fluoride may cause excessive salivation and gastrointestinal disturbances; 500 mg may be fatal. Oral and/or intravenous fluids containing calcium may be indicated.

Acute overdosage of iron may cause nausea and vomiting and, in severe cases, cardiovascular collapse and death. The estimated lethal dose of orally ingested elemental iron is 300 mg per kg body weight. Serum iron and total iron-binding capacity may be used as guides for use of chelating agents such as deferoxamine.

How Supplied: 100-tablet bottles; ℞; NDC 0074-7621-13.

Shown in Product Identification Section, page 432

VI-DAYLIN®/F + IRON Drops
[vī″dā′lin]
Multivitamins/Fluoride/Iron Supplement

Description: One dropperful (1.0 ml) provides:
Fluoride 0.25 mg

Vitamins			% U.S. RDA*	% U.S. RDA**
Vitamin A	1500	I.U.	100	60
Vitamin D	400	I.U.	100	100
Vitamin E	5	I.U.	100	50
Vitamin C	35	mg	100	87
Thiamine (Vitamin B$_1$)	0.5	mg	100	71
Riboflavin (Vitamin B$_2$)	0.6	mg	100	75
Niacin	8	mg	100	88
Vitamin B$_6$	0.4	mg	100	57
Minerals				
Iron	10	mg	66	100

Ingredients: Ascorbic acid, ferrous sulfate, niacinamide, d-alpha tocopheryl acid succinate, vitamin A palmitate, riboflavin-5′-phosphate sodium, thiamine hydrochloride, sodium fluoride, pyridoxine hydrochloride and ergocalciferol. Alcohol content less than 0.1%.

*% U.S. Recommended Daily Allowance for infants.
**% U.S. Recommended Daily Allowance for children under 4 years of age.

Indications and Usage: As an aid in the prevention of dental caries in infants and children, and in the prophylaxis of iron and certain vitamin deficiencies.

Contraindications: Should be used only where the fluoride content of the drinking water supply is known to be 0.7 parts per million or less.

Precautions: The recommended dosage should not be exceeded since chronic overdosage of fluoride may result in mottling of tooth enamel and osseous changes. In infants, oral iron-containing preparations may cause temporary darkening of the membrane covering the teeth.

Overdosage: In children, acute ingestion of 10 to 20 mg of sodium fluoride may cause excessive salivation and gastrointestinal disturbances; 500 mg may be fatal. Oral and/or intravenous fluids containing calcium may be indicated.

Acute overdosage of iron may cause nausea and vomiting and, in severe cases, cardiovascular collapse and death. The estimated lethal dose of orally ingested elemental iron is 300 mg per kg body weight. Serum iron and total iron-binding capacity may be used as guides for use of chelating agents such as deferoxamine.

Dosage and Administration: One dropperful daily, or as directed by physician or dentist.

How Supplied: 50-ml bottles, calibrated dropper enclosed; ℞; NDC 0074-8928-50.

VI-DAYLIN® PLUS IRON Drops
[vī″dā′lin]
Multivitamin/Iron Supplement

Description: One dropperful (1 ml) provides:

Vitamins			% U.S. RDA*	% U.S. RDA**
Vitamin A	1500	I.U.	100	60
Vitamin D	400	I.U.	100	100
Vitamin E	5	I.U.	100	50
Vitamin C	35	mg	100	87
Thiamine (Vitamin B$_1$)	0.5	mg	100	71
Riboflavin (Vitamin B$_2$)	0.6	mg	100	75
Niacin	8	mg	100	88
Vitamin B$_6$	0.4	mg	100	57
Minerals				
Iron	10	mg	66	100

Ingredients: Ferrous sulfate, ascorbic acid, d-alpha-tocopheryl acid succinate, niacinamide, vitamin A palmitate, benzoic acid (preservative), riboflavin-5′-phosphate sodium, thiamine hydrochloride, methylparaben (preservative), pyridoxine hydrochloride, and ergocalciferol in a glycerin-water vehicle with added artificial coloring and flavoring. Contains only a trace (less than ½%) of alcohol.

*% U.S. Recommended Daily Allowance for infants.
**% U.S. Recommended Daily Allowance for children under 4 years of age.

Indications and Usage: Multivitamin supplement with iron for infants and children under 4 years of age.

Administration and Dosage: One dropperful daily, or as directed by physician.

Continued on next page

Ross—Cont.

How Supplied: 50-ml bottles, calibrated dropper enclosed; OTC; **NDC** 0074-0116-01.

VI-DAYLIN® PLUS IRON ADC Drops
[vī″dā′lin]
Dietary Supplement of Vitamins A, D and C with Iron

Description: One dropperful (1.0 ml) provides:

Vitamins		% U.S. RDA*	% U.S. RDA**
Vitamin A	1500 I.U.	100	60
Vitamin D	400 I.U.	100	100
Vitamin C	35 mg	100	87
Minerals			
Iron	10 mg	66	100

Ingredients: Polysorbate 80, ferrous sulfate, ascorbic acid, vitamin A palmitate, benzoic acid (preservative), methylparaben (preservative), and ergocalciferol in a glycerin-water vehicle with added artificial flavoring and coloring.
*% U.S. Recommended Daily Allowance for infants.
**% U.S. Recommended Daily Allowance for children under 4 years of age.
Indications and Usage: Dietary supplement of vitamins A, D and C with iron for infants and children under 4 years of age.
Dosage and Administration: One dropperful daily, or as directed by physician.
How Supplied: 50-ml bottles; calibrated dropper enclosed; OTC; **NDC** 0074-0117-01.

VI-DAYLIN® Chewable
[vī″dā′lin]
Multivitamin Supplement

Description: Each chewable tablet provides:

Vitamins			% U.S. RDA*	% U.S. RDA**
Vitamin A	2500	I.U.	100	50
Vitamin D	400	I.U.	100	100
Vitamin E	15	I.U.	150	50
Vitamin C	60	mg	150	100
Folic Acid	0.3	mg	150	75
Thiamine (Vitamin B_1)	1.05	mg	150	70
Riboflavin (Vitamin B_2)	1.2	mg	150	70
Niacin	13.5	mg	150	67
Vitamin B_6	1.05	mg	150	52
Vitamin B_{12}	4.5	mcg	150	75

Ingredients: Sucrose and dextrins, sodium ascorbate, niacinamide, dl-alpha tocopheryl acetate, ascorbic acid, vitamin A palmitate, riboflavin, pyridoxine hydrochloride, thiamine mononitrate, cholecalciferol, folic acid and cyanocobalamin. Made with natural sweeteners, artificial flavoring and artificially colored with natural ingredients.
*% U.S. Recommended Daily Allowance for children under 4 years of age.
**% U.S. Recommended Daily Allowance for adults and children 4 or more years of age.
Indications and Usage: Multivitamin supplement for children and adults.
Dosage and Administration: One chewable tablet daily, or as directed by physician.
How Supplied: 100-tablet bottles; OTC; **NDC** 0074-4519-13.
Shown in Product Identification Section, page 432

VI-DAYLIN®/F Chewable ℞
[vī″dā′lin]
Multivitamins/Fluoride

Description: Each chewable tablet provides:
Fluoride (as sodium fluoride) 1 mg

Vitamins			%U.S. RDA*	%U.S. RDA**
Vitamin A (as palmitate, 0.75 mg)	2500	I.U.	100	50
Vitamin D (cholecalciferol, 10 mcg)	400	I.U.	100	100
Vitamin E (dl-alpha tocopheryl acetate)	15	I.U.	150	50
Vitamin C (as sodium ascorbate, 40 mg; ascorbic acid, 20 mg)	60	mg	150	100
Folic Acid	0.3	mg	150	75
Vitamin B_1 (as thiamine mononitrate)	1.05	mg	150	70
Vitamin B_2 (as riboflavin)	1.2	mg	150	70
Niacin (as niacinamide)	13.5	mg	150	67
Vitamin B_6 (as pyridoxine hydrochloride)	1.05	mg	150	52
Vitamin B_{12} (as cyanocobalamin)	4.5	mcg	150	75

*% U.S. Recommended Daily Allowance for children under 4 years of age.
**% U.S. Recommended Daily Allowance for adults and children 4 or more years of age.
Indications and Usage: As an aid in the prevention of dental caries in children, and in the prophylaxis of certain vitamin deficiencies.
Contraindications: Should not be used where the fluoride content of the drinking water supply is known to be greater than 0.7 parts per million.
Precautions: The recommended use and dosage of Vi-Daylin/F Chewable should not be exceeded, since chronic overdosage of fluoride may result in mottling of tooth enamel and osseous changes.
Overdosage: In children, acute ingestion of 10 to 20 mg of sodium fluoride may cause excessive salivation and gastrointestinal disturbances; 500 mg may be fatal. Oral and/or intravenous fluids containing calcium may be indicated.
Dosage and Administration: Children 3 years of age or older, 1 chewable tablet daily; age 2 to 3 years, ½ chewable tablet daily; or as directed by physician or dentist.
How Supplied: 100-tablet bottles; Rx; NDC 0074-7626-13.
Shown in Product Identification Section, page 432

VI-DAYLIN® + IRON Chewable
[vī″dā′lin]
Multivitamin/Iron Supplement

Description: Each chewable tablet provides:

Vitamins			% U.S. RDA*	% U.S. RDA**
Vitamin A	2500	I.U.	100	50
Vitamin D	400	I.U.	100	100
Vitamin E	15	I.U.	150	50
Vitamin C	60	mg	150	100
Folic Acid	0.3	mg	150	75
Thiamine (Vitamin B_1)	1.05	mg	150	70
Riboflavin (Vitamin B_2)	1.2	mg	150	70
Niacin	13.5	mg	150	67
Vitamin B_6	1.05	mg	150	52
Vitamin B_{12}	4.5	mcg	150	75
Minerals				
Iron	12	mg	120	66

Ingredients: Sucrose and dextrins, mannitol, sodium ascorbate, niacinamide, ferrous fumarate, dl-alpha tocopheryl acetate, ascorbic acid, vitamin A palmitate, riboflavin, pyridoxine hydrochloride, thiamine mononitrate, cholecalciferol, folic acid and cyanocobalamin. Made with natural sweeteners, artificial flavoring and coloring.
*% U.S. Recommended Daily Allowance for children under 4 years of age.
**% U.S. Recommended Daily Allowance for adults and children 4 or more years of age.
Indications and Usage: Multivitamin supplement with iron for children and adults.
Dosage and Administration: One tablet daily, or as directed by physician.
How Supplied: 100-tablet bottles; OTC; **NDC** 0074-4520-13.
Shown in Product Identification Section, page 432

VI-DAYLIN® Liquid
[vī″dā′lin]
Multivitamin Supplement

Description: One teaspoonful (5.0 ml) provides:

Vitamins			% U.S. RDA*	% U.S. RDA**
Vitamin A	2500	I.U.	100	50
Vitamin D	400	I.U.	100	100
Vitamin E	15	I.U.	150	50
Vitamin C	60	mg	150	100
Thiamine (Vitamin B_1)	1.05	mg	150	70
Riboflavin (Vitamin B_2)	1.2	mg	150	70
Niacin	13.5	mg	150	68
Vitamin B_6	1.05	mg	150	50
Vitamin B_{12}	4.5	mcg	150	75

This product does not contain the essential vitamin folic acid.
*% U.S. Recommended Daily Allowance for children under 4 years of age.
**% U.S. Recommended Daily Allowance for adults and children 4 or more years of age.
Ingredients: Glucose, sucrose, ascorbic acid, polysorbate 80, d-alpha tocopheryl acetate, niacinamide, acacia, cysteine hydrochloride (stabilizer), benzoic acid (preservative), vitamin A palmitate, methylparaben (preservative), pyridoxine hydrochloride, riboflavin, thiamine hydrochloride, ergocalciferol and cyanocobalamin in an aqueous vehicle with added natural citrus flavoring and added color. Contains only a trace of alcohol (not more than ½%).
Indications and Usage: Multivitamin supplement for children and adults.
Dosage and Administration: One teaspoonful daily, or as directed by physician.
How Supplied:
16-fl-oz (pint) bottles; OTC; **NDC** 0074-3606-03.
8-fl-oz bottles; OTC; **NDC** 0074-3606-02.

VI-DAYLIN® PLUS IRON Liquid
[vī″dā′lin]
Multivitamin/Iron Supplement

Description: One teaspoonful (5.0 ml) provides:

Vitamins			% U.S. RDA*	% U.S. RDA**
Vitamin A	2500	I.U.	100	50
Vitamin D	400	I.U.	100	100
Vitamin E	15	I.U.	150	50
Vitamin C	60	mg	150	100
Thiamine (Vitamin B_1)	1.05	mg	150	70
Riboflavin (Vitamin B_2)	1.2	mg	150	70
Niacin	13.5	mg	150	68
Vitamin B_6	1.05	mg	150	50
Vitamin B_{12}	4.5	mcg	150	75
Minerals				
Iron	10	mg	100	55

This product does not contain the essential vitamin folic acid.
*% U.S. Recommended Daily Allowance for children under 4 years of age.
**% U.S. Recommended Daily Allowance for adults and children 4 or more years of age.
Ingredients: Glucose, sucrose, ascorbic acid, ferrous gluconate, polysorbate 80, d-alpha tocopheryl acetate, niacinamide, acacia, cysteine hydrochloride (stabilizer), benzoic acid (preservative), methylparaben (preservative), vitamin A palmitate, riboflavin-5′-phosphate sodium, pyridoxine hydrochloride, thiamine hydrochloride, propylparaben (preservative), ergocalciferol and cyanocobalamin in an aqueous vehicle with added natural citrus flavoring and added coloring. Contains only a trace of alcohol (not more than ½%).
Indications and Usage: Multivitamin supplement with iron for children and adults.
Dosage and Administration: One teaspoonful daily, or as directed by physician.
How Supplied:
16-fl-oz (pint) bottles; OTC; **NDC** 0074-6992-03.
8-fl-oz bottles; OTC; **NDC** 0074-6992-02.

VITAL® HIGH NITROGEN
[vīʹ tel]
Nutritionally Complete
Partially Hydrolyzed Diet

Usage: As a source of total or supplemental nutrition for patients with impaired gastrointestinal function (limited digestion/absorption). VITAL HIGH NITROGEN may be used as a tube feeding (nasogastric, nasoduodenal or jejunal) or as an oral feeding. Five servings (1500 Calories) meets or surpasses 100% of the daily U.S. RDA for vitamins and minerals for adults and children 4 or more years of age.

Features:
- Complete nutrition—In standard dilution, Vital High Nitrogen provides 1 Calorie per ml and 300 Calories per serving (1 packet). Caloric distribution: protein, 16.7%; fat, 9.4%; carbohydrate, 73.9%.
- High levels of nitrogen—Vital High Nitrogen provides 62.5 g of protein (10 g nitrogen) in 1500 Calories, with a total Calorie-to-nitrogen ratio of 150:1. Vital High Nitrogen provides partially hydrolyzed whey and meat, and soy fortified with essential amino acids, designed to maximize nitrogen absorption.
- Good taste—Vital High Nitrogen is significantly more palatable and acceptable than diets composed solely of crystalline amino acids. The mild, appealing vanilla flavor assures better patient acceptance of an elemental feeding with no disturbing aftertaste.
- High fat absorption—45% of fat from medium-chain triglycerides.
- Low osmolality—The osmolality of Vital High Nitrogen (460 mOsm/kg water) may help to avoid the gastrointestinal distress and dumping syndrome commonly associated with elemental feedings.
- Low fecal residue—The fecal residue produced by Vital High Nitrogen is comparable to that produced by traditional elemental diets.
- Low electrolyte levels—The electrolyte levels are appropriate for diets moderately restricted in electrolytes, yet adequate for most hospitalized patients.

Dosage and Administration:
Mixing Instructions: For standard dilution of 1 Calorie per ml. pour 255 ml (8.5 fl oz) of cold water into a container. Empty contents of one packet into container and mix until powder dissolves. Yields approximately 300 ml. Prepare only the amount intended for a single day's serving. Refrigerate after preparation. Discard if not used within 24 hours. Shake before use. Store unopened powder in a cool, dry place. UNDER NO CIRCUMSTANCES SHOULD VITAL HIGH NITROGEN BE ADMINISTERED PARENTERALLY.
Additional fluid requirements should be met by giving water orally with or after feedings, or by flushing the gavage tube.

Dilution Schedule*

Dilution Cal/mL	Vital Pouch (79 g)	Water mL	Total Volume mL
.50	1	555	600
.75	1	355	400
1.00	1	255	300
1.50	1	155	200
2.00	1	105	150

*Controlling the flow rate of viscous dilutions is facilitated by an enteral feeding pump.
- **Tube Feeding:** Follow physician's instructions. Flow rate, volume and dilution of feeding depend on patient's nutritional needs and tolerance for tube feedings. Care should be taken to avoid contamination of this product during preparation and administration.
[See table above].
- **Oral Feeding:** Serving Vital High Nitrogen chilled or with Vari-Flavors may enhance its flavor and increase palatability. Servings may provide total nutrition or supplemental nutrition with and between meals.

Availability: 2.79-oz (79 g) packets of water-soluble Powder (Vanilla flavor); 24 packets per case; No. 766.

Composition:
Ingredients: Hydrolyzed corn starch, protein components (partially hydrolyzed whey and meat, and soy), sucrose, minerals (potassium phosphate dibasic, calcium phosphate tribasic, magnesium sulfate, magnesium chloride, sodium chloride, ferrous sulfate, zinc sulfate, manganous chloride, cupric sulfate), safflower oil, amino acids (L-tyrosine, L-leucine, L-valine, L-isoleucine, L-phenylalanine, L-histidine, L-methionine, L-threonine, L-tryptophan, medium-chain triglycerides (fractionated coconut oil), artificial and natural flavor, vitamins (choline chloride, ascorbic acid, alpha-tocopheryl acetate, niacinamide, calcium pantothenate, vitamin A palmitate, riboflavin, pyridoxine hydrochloride, thiamine chloride hydrochloride, folic acid, biotin, phylloquinone, vitamin D_3, cyanocobalamin), mono- and diglycerides, and soy lecithin.

Sample Administration Schedule VITAL High Nitrogen
Continuous Drip Schedule (See dilution rates below)

Day	Time	Strength	Rate (mL/hr)	Volume (mL)	Calories
1	1st 8 hours	½	50	400	200
	2nd 8 hours	½	75	600	300
	3rd 8 hours	½	100	800	400
					900 Total Calories
2	1st 8 hours	¾	100	800	600
	2nd 8 hours	¾	100	800	600
	3rd 8 hours	¾	100	800	600
					1800 Total Calories
3	1st 8 hours	Full	100	800	800
	2nd 8 hours	Full	100–125	800–1000	800–1000
	3rd 8 hours	Full	100–125	800–1000	800–1000
					2400–2800 Total Calories

Intermittent Drip Schedule (See dilution rates below)

Day	Time	Strength	Rate (5–10 mL/min)	Volume (mL)	Calories
1	7am–11pm	½	100 mL q 2 hr (7am, 9am, 11am)	300	150
		½	200 mL q 2 hr (1pm, 3pm, 5pm)	600	300
		½	300 mL q 2 hr (7pm, 9pm, 11pm)	900	450
					900 Total Calories
2	7am–11pm	¾	300 mL q 2 hr (7am, 9am, 11am, 1pm, 3pm, 5pm, 7pm, 9pm, 11pm)	2700	2025 Total Calories
3	7am–11pm	Full	300 mL q 3 hr (5 feedings) up to 300 mL q 2 hr (8 feedings)	1500–2400	1500–2400 Total Calories

- Check gastric residuals before every intermittent feeding or every 2–4 hours during continuous feeding.
- If intolerance develops, return to previously tolerated rate and strength. When tolerance is again established, proceed with feeding schedule as indicated. Do not alter rate and strength at the same time.
- Rinsing the tube with water (eg, 25–100 mL) periodically or after intermittent feedings will help avoid clogging and provide additional water.

Approximate Analysis: (grams)	Per 300 Calories* (1 packet)	Per 1500 Calories* (5 packets)
Protein	12.5	62.5
Fat	3.25	16.25
Carbohydrate	55.4	277
Minerals (Ash)	1.6	8.0
Moisture (Max)	5.2	26.0

* In standard dilution (79 g of Vital High Nitrogen Vanilla Powder mixed in 255 ml of water).

Vitamins/ Minerals	Per 300 Calories	Per 1500 Calories	Percent U.S. RDA** 1500 Calories
Vitamin A, (I.U.)	1000	5000	100
Vitamin D, (I.U.)	80	400	100
Vitamin E, (I.U.)	9	45	150
Vitamin K_1, mcg	14	70	***
Vitamin C, mg	18	90	150
Folic Acid, mg	0.08	0.4	100
Thiamine (Vit. B_1), mg	0.3	1.5	100
Riboflavin (Vit. B_2), mg	0.34	1.7	100
Vitamin B_6, mg	0.44	2.2	100
Vitamin B_{12}, mcg	1.2	6	100
Niacin, mg	4	20	100
Biotin, mg	0.06	0.3	100
Pantothenic Acid, mg	2	10	100
Choline, mg	40	200	***
Calcium, mg	200	1000	100
Phosphorus, mg	200	1000	100
Sodium, mg	140	700	***
Potassium, mg	400	2000	***
Chloride, mg	270	1350	***
Magnesium, mg	80	400	100

Continued on next page

Ross—Cont.

Iodine, mcg	30	150	100
Manganese, mg	0.75	3.75	***
Copper, mg	0.4	2	100
Zinc, mg	3	15	100
Iron, mg	3.6	18	100

** For adults and children 4 or more years of age.
*** U.S. RDA not established.
(FAN 283)

EDUCATIONAL MATERIAL

A complete program of educational services for health professionals and patients is available. Contact your local Ross representative.

Rowell Laboratories, Inc.
**210 MAIN STREET W.
BAUDETTE, MN 56623**

CHENIX® ℞
[ke'nix]
Chenodiol Tablets 250 mg

SPECIAL NOTE

Because of the potential hepatotoxicity of chenodiol, poor response rates in some subgroups of chenodiol-treated patients, and an increased rate of a need for cholecystectomy in other chenodiol-treated subgroups, chenodiol is not an appropriate treatment for many patients with gallstones. Chenodiol should be reserved for carefully selected patients and treatment must be accompanied by systematic monitoring for liver function alterations. Aspects of patient selection, response rates and risks versus benefits are given in the insert.

Description: CHENIX® is chenodiol, the nonproprietary name for chenodeoxycholic acid, a naturally occurring human bile acid. It is a bitter-tasting white powder consisting of crystalline and amorphous particles freely soluble in methanol, acetone and acetic acid and practically insoluble in water. Its chemical name is $3\alpha,7\alpha$-dihydroxy-5β-cholan-24-oic acid ($C_{24}H_{40}O_4$), it has a molecular weight of 392.58, and its structure is shown below:

Clinical Pharmacology: At therapeutic doses, chenodiol suppresses hepatic synthesis of both cholesterol and cholic acid, gradually replacing the latter and its metabolite, deoxycholic acid, in an expanded bile acid pool. These actions contribute to biliary cholesterol desaturation and gradual dissolution of radiolucent cholesterol gallstones in the presence of a gallbladder visualized by oral cholecystography. Chenodiol has no effect on radiopaque (calcified) gallstones or on radiolucent bile pigment stones.

Chenodiol is well absorbed from the small intestine and taken up by the liver, where it is converted to its taurine and glycine conjugates and secreted in bile. Owing to 60% to 80% first-pass hepatic clearance, the body pool of chenodiol resides mainly in the enterohepatic circulation; serum and urinary bile acid levels are not significantly affected during chenodiol therapy.

At steady-state, an amount of chenodiol near the daily dose escapes to the colon and is converted by bacterial action to lithocholic acid. About 80% of the lithocholate is excreted in the feces; the remainder is absorbed and converted in the liver to its poorly absorbed sulfolithocholyl conjugates. During chenodiol therapy there is only a minor increase in biliary lithocholate, while fecal bile acids are increased three- to fourfold.

Lithocholic acid is a known hepatotoxin and in species that are unable to form sulfate conjugates, lithocholic acid produces dose-related hepatotoxicity ranging from barely detectable to death of the animal due to hepatic failure. The hepatotoxicity of lithocholic acid is characterized biochemically and morphologically as cholestatic.

Man has the capacity to form sulfate conjugates of lithocholic acid. Variation in this capacity among individuals has not been well established and a recent published report suggests that patients who develop chenodiol-induced serum aminotransferase elevations are poor sulfators of lithocholic acid (see **WARNINGS** and **ADVERSE REACTIONS**).

General Clinical Results: Both the desaturation of bile and the clinical dissolution of cholesterol gallstones are dose-related. In the National Cooperative Gallstone Study (NCGS) involving 305 patients in each treatment group, placebo and chenodiol dosages of 375 mg and 750 mg per day were associated with complete stone dissolution in 0.8%, 5.2% and 13.5%, respectively, of enrolled subjects over 24 months of treatment. Uncontrolled clinical trials using higher doses than those used in the NCGS have shown complete dissolution rates of 28 to 38% of enrolled patients receiving body weight doses of from 13 to 16 mg/kg/day for up to 24 months. In a prospective trial using 15 mg/kg/day, 31% enrolled surgical-risk patients treated more than six months (n=86) achieved complete confirmed dissolutions.

Observed stone dissolution rates achieved with chenodiol treatment are higher in subgroups having certain pretreatment characteristics. In the NCGS, patients with small (less than 15 mm in diameter) radiolucent stones, the observed rate of complete dissolution was approximately 20% on 750 mg/day. In the uncontrolled trials using 13 to 16 mg/kg/day doses of chenodiol, the rates of complete dissolution for small radiolucent stones ranged from 42% to 60%. Even higher dissolution rates have been observed in patients with small floatable stones. (See **Floatable versus Nonfloatable Stones,** below.) Some obese patients and occasional normal weight patients fail to achieve bile desaturation even with doses of chenodiol up to 19 mg/kg/day for unknown reasons.

Although dissolution is generally higher with increased dosage of chenodiol, doses that are too low are associated with increased cholecystectomy rates (see **ADVERSE REACTIONS**).

Stones have recurred within five years in about 50% of patients following complete confirmed dissolutions. Although retreatment with chenodiol has proven successful in dissolving some newly formed stones, the indications for and safety of retreatment are not well defined. Serum aminotransferase elevations and diarrhea have been notable in all clinical trials and are dose-related (refer to **ADVERSE REACTIONS** and **WARNINGS** sections for full information).

Floatable versus Nonfloatable Stones: A major finding in clinical trials was a difference between floatable and nonfloatable stones, with respect to both natural history and response to chenodiol. Over the two-year course of the National Cooperative Gallstone Study (NCGS), placebo-treated patients with floatable stones (n=47) had significantly higher rates of biliary pain and cholecystectomy than patients with nonfloatable stones (n=258) (47% versus 27% and 19% versus 4%, respectively). Chenodiol treatment (750 mg/day) compared to placebo was associated with a significant reduction in both biliary pain and the cholecystectomy rate in the group with floatable stones (27% versus 47% and 1.5% versus 19%, respectively). In an uncontrolled clinical trial using 15 mg/kg/day, 70% of the patients with small (less than 15 mm) floatable stones (n=10) had complete confirmed dissolutions.

In the NCGS in patients with nonfloatable stones, chenodiol produced no reduction in biliary pain and showed a tendency to increase the cholecystectomy rate (8% versus 4%). This finding was more pronounced with doses of chenodiol below 10 mg/kg. The subgroup of patients with nonfloatable stones and a history of biliary pain had the highest rates of cholecystectomy and aminotransferase elevations during chenodiol treatment. Except for the NCGS subgroup with pretreatment biliary pain, dose-related aminotransferase elevations and diarrhea have occurred with equal frequency in patients with floatable or nonfloatable stones. In the uncontrolled clinical trial mentioned above, 27% of the patients with nonfloatable stones (n=59) had complete confirmed dissolutions, including 35% with small (less than 15 mm) (n=40) and only 11% with large, nonfloatable stones (n=19).

Of 916 patients enrolled in NCGS, 17.8% had stones seen in upright films (horizontal X-ray beam) to float in the dye-laden bile during oral cholecystography using iopanoic acid. Other investigators report similar findings. Floatable stones are not detected by ultrasonography in the absence of dye. Chemical analysis has shown floatable stones to be essentially pure cholesterol.

Other Radiographic and Laboratory Features: Radiolucent stones may have rims or centers of opacity representing calcification. Pigment stones and partially calcified radiolucent stones do not respond to chenodiol. Subtle calcification can sometimes be detected in flat film X-rays, if not obvious in the oral cholecystogram. Among nonfloatable stones, cholesterol stones are more apt than pigment stones to be smooth-surfaced, less than 0.6 cm in diameter, and to occur in numbers less than 10. As stone size, number and volume increase, the probability of dissolution within 24 months decreases. Hemolytic disorders, chronic alcoholism, biliary cirrhosis and bacterial invasion of the biliary system predispose to pigment gallstone formation. Pigment stones of primary biliary cirrhosis should be suspected in patients with elevated alkaline phosphatase, especially if positive antimitochondrial antibodies are present. The presence of microscopic cholesterol crystals in aspirated gallbladder bile, and demonstration of cholesterol supersaturation by bile lipid analysis, increase the likelihood that the stones are cholesterol stones.

Patient Selection

Evaluation of Surgical Risk: Surgery offers the advantage of immediate and permanent stone removal, but carries a fairly high risk in some patients. About 5% of cholecystectomized patients have residual symptoms or retained common duct stones. The spectrum of surgical risk varies as a function of age and the presence of disease other than cholelithiasis. Selected tabulation of results from the National Halothane Study (**JAMA, 1966, 197:775–778**) is shown below; the study included 27,600 cholecystectomies.

Mortality per Operation
(Smoothed rates with denominators adjusted to one death.)

		Cholecystectomy	& Common Duct Exploration
Low Risk Patients*			
Women	0–49 yrs	1/1851	1/469
	50–69 yrs	1/357	1/99
Men	0–49 yrs	1/961	1/243
	50–69 yrs	1/185	1/52
High Risk patients**			
Women	0–49 yrs	1/79	1/21
	50–69 yrs	1/58	1/17
Men	0–49 yrs	1/41	1/11
	50–69 yrs	1/30	1/9

* Includes those with good health or moderate systemic disease, with or without emergency surgery.
** Severe or extreme systemic disease, with or without emergency surgery.

Women in good health, or having only moderate systemic disease, under 49 years of age have the lowest rate (0.054%); men in all categories have a surgical mortality rate twice that of women; common duct exploration quadruples the rates in all categories; the rates rise with each decade of life and increase tenfold or more in all categories with severe or extreme systemic disease.

Relatively young patients requiring treatment might be better treated by surgery than with CHENIX, because treatment with chenodiol, even if successful, is associated with a high rate of recurrence. The long-term consequences of repeated courses of chenodiol in terms of liver toxicity, neoplasia and elevated cholesterol levels are not known.

Watchful waiting has the advantage that no therapy may ever be required. For patients with silent or minimally symptomatic stones, the rate of moderate to severe symptoms or gallstone complications is estimated to be between 2% and 6% per year, leading to a cumulative rate of 7% and 27% in five years. Presumably the rate is higher for patients already having symptoms.

Indications and Usage: CHENIX is indicated for patients with radiolucent stones in well-opacifying gallbladders, in whom elective surgery would be undertaken except for the presence of increased surgical risk due to systemic disease or age. The likelihood of successful dissolution is far greater if the stones are floatable or small. For patients with nonfloatable stones, dissolution is less likely and added weight should be given to the risk that more emergency surgery might result from a delay due to unsuccessful treatment. Safety of use beyond 24 months is not established. CHENIX will not dissolve calcified (radiopaque) or radiolucent bile pigment stones.

Contraindications: Chenodiol is contraindicated in the presence of known hepatocyte dysfunction or the bile ductal abnormalities such as intrahepatic cholestasis, primary biliary cirrhosis or sclerosing cholangitis (see **WARNINGS**); a gallbladder confirmed as nonvisualizing after two consecutive single doses of dye; radiopaque stones; or gallstone complications or compelling reasons for gallbladder surgery including unremitting acute cholecystitis, cholangitis, biliary obstruction, gallstone pancreatitis, or biliary gastrointestinal fistula.

Pregnancy Category X:
Chenodiol may cause fetal harm when administered to a pregnant woman. Serious hepatic, renal and adrenal lesions occurred in fetuses of female Rhesus monkeys given 60 to 90 mg/kg/day (4 to 6 times the maximum recommended human dose, MRHD) from day 21 to day 45 of pregnancy. Hepatic lesions also occurred in neonatal baboons whose mothers had received 18 to 38 mg/kg (1 to 2 times the MRHD), all during pregnancy. Fetal malformations were not observed. Neither fetal liver damage nor fetal abnormalities occurred in reproduction studies in rats and hamsters. No human data are available at this time. Chenodiol is contraindicated in women who are or may become pregnant. If this drug is used during pregnancy or if the patient becomes pregnant while taking this drug, the patient should be apprised of the potential hazard to the fetus.

Warnings: Safe use of chenodiol depends upon selection of patients without preexisting liver disease and upon faithful monitoring of serum aminotransferase levels to detect drug-induced liver toxicity.

Aminotransferase elevations over three times the upper limit of normal have required discontinuation of chenodiol in 2% to 3% of patients.

Although clinical and biopsy studies have not shown fulminant lesions, the possibility remains that an occasional patient may develop serious hepatic disease.

Three patients with biochemical and histologic pictures of chronic active hepatitis while on chenodiol, 375 mg/day or 750 mg/day, have been reported. The biochemical abnormalities returned spontaneously to normal in two of the patients within 13 and 17 months; and after 17 months' treatment with prednisone in the third. Followup biopsies were not done; and the causal relationship of the drug could not be determined. Another biopsied patient was terminated from therapy because of elevated aminotransferase levels and a liver biopsy was interpreted as showing active drug hepatitis.

One patient with sclerosing cholangitis, biliary cirrhosis and a history of jaundice died during chenodiol treatment for hepatic duct stones. Before treatment, serum aminotransferase and alkaline phosphatase levels were over twice the upper limit of normal; within one month they rose to over 10 times normal. Chenodiol was discontinued at seven weeks when the patient was hospitalized with advanced hepatic failure and E. coli peritonitis; death ensued at the eighth week. A contribution of chenodiol to the fatal outcome could not be ruled out.

Epidemiologic studies suggest that bile acids might contribute to human colon cancer, but direct evidence is lacking. Bile acids, including chenodiol and lithocholic acid, have no carcinogenic potential in animal models, but have been shown to increase the number of tumors when administered with certain known carcinogens. The possibility that chenodiol therapy might contribute to colon cancer in otherwise susceptible individuals cannot be ruled out.

Precautions
Information for Patients: Patients should be counseled on the importance of periodic visits for liver function tests and oral cholecystograms (or ultrasonograms) for monitoring stone dissolution; they should be made aware of the symptoms of gallstone complications and be warned to report immediately such symptoms to the physician. Patients should be instructed on ways to facilitate faithful compliance with the dosage regimen throughout the usual long term of therapy, and on temporary dose reduction if episodes of diarrhea occur.

Drug Interactions: Bile acid sequestering agents, such as cholestyramine and colestipol, may interfere with the action of CHENIX by reducing its absorption. Aluminum-based antacids have been shown to adsorb bile acids *in vitro* and may be expected to interfere with CHENIX in the same manner as the sequestering agents. Estrogens, oral contraceptives and clofibrate (and perhaps other lipid-lowering drugs) increase biliary cholesterol secretion, and the incidence of cholesterol gallstones hence may counteract the effectiveness of CHENIX.

Carcinogenesis, Mutagenesis, and Impairment of Fertility: A two-year oral study of chenodiol in rats failed to show a carcinogenic potential at the tested levels of 15 to 60 mg/kg/day (1 to 4 times the maximum recommended human dose, (MRHD). It has been reported that chenodiol given in long-term studies at oral doses up to 600 mg/kg/day (40 times the MRHD) to rats and 1000 mg/kg/day (65 times the MRHD) to mice induced benign and malignant liver cell tumors in female rats and cholangiomata in female rats and male mice. Two-year studies of lithocholic acid (a major metabolite of chenodiol) in mice (125 to 250 mg/kg/day) and rats (250 and 500 mg/kg/day) found it not to be carcinogenic. The dietary administration of lithocholic acid to chickens is reported to cause hepatic adenomatous hyperplasia.

Pregnancy Category X: See **CONTRAINDICATIONS.**
Nursing Mothers: It is not known whether chenodiol is excreted in human milk. Because many drugs are excreted in human milk, caution should be exercised when chenodiol is administered to a nursing mother.

Pediatric Use: The safety and effectiveness of chenodiol in children have not been established.

Adverse Reactions
Hepatobiliary: Dose-related serum aminotransferase (mainly SGPT) elevations, usually not accompanied by rises in alkaline phosphatase or bilirubin, occurred in 30% or more of patients treated with the recommended dose of CHENIX. In most cases, these elevations were minor (1½ to 3 times the upper limit of laboratory normal) and transient, returning to within the normal range within six months despite continued administration of the drug. In 2% to 3% of patients, SGPT levels rose to over three times the upper limit of laboratory normal, recurred on rechallenge with the drug, and required discontinuation of chenodiol treatment. Enzyme levels have returned to normal following withdrawal of chenodiol (see **WARNINGS** section).

Morphologic studies of liver biopsies taken before and after 9 and 24 months' treatment with chenodiol have shown that 63% of the patients prior to chenodiol treatment had evidence of intrahepatic cholestasis. Almost all pretreatment patients had electron microscopic abnormalities. By the ninth month of treatment, reexamination of two-thirds of the patients showed an 89% incidence of the signs of intrahepatic cholestasis. Two of 89 patients at the ninth month had lithocholate-like lesions in the canalicular membrane, although there were no clinical enzyme abnormalities in the face of continued treatment and no change in Type 2 light microscopic parameters.

Increased Cholecystectomy Rates: NCGS patients with a history of biliary pain prior to treatment had higher cholecystectomy rates during the study if assigned to low dosage chenodiol (375 mg/day) than if assigned to either placebo or high dosage chenodiol (750 mg/day). The association with low dosage chenodiol, though not clearly a causal one, suggests that patients unable to take higher doses of chenodiol may be at greater risk of cholecystectomy.

Gastrointestinal: Dose-related diarrhea has been encountered in 30% to 40% of chenodiol-treated patients and may occur at any time during treatment, but is most commonly encountered when treatment is initiated. Usually, the diarrhea is mild, transient, well-tolerated and does not interfere with therapy. Dose reduction has been required in 10% to 15% of patients, and in a controlled trial about half of these required a permanent reduction in dose. Anti-diarrheal agents have proven useful in some patients.

Discontinuation of chenodiol because of failure to control diarrhea is to be expected in approximately 3% of patients treated. Steady epigastric pain with nausea typical of lithiasis (biliary colic) usually is easily distinguishable from the crampy abdominal pain of drug-induced diarrhea.

Other, less frequent, gastrointestinal side effects reported include urgency, cramps, heartburn, constipation, nausea and vomiting, anorexia, epigastric distress, dyspepsia, flatulence and nonspecific abdominal pain.

Serum Lipids: Serum total cholesterol and low-density lipoprotein (LDL) cholesterol may rise 10% or more during administration of chenodiol; no change has been seen in the high-density lipoprotein (HDL) fraction; small decreases in serum triglyceride levels for females have been reported.

Hematologic: Decreases in white cell count, never below 3000, have been noted in a few patients treated with chenodiol; the drug was continued in all patients without incident.

Overdosage: Accidental or intentional overdoses of chenodiol have not been reported. One patient tolerated 4 gm/day (58 mg/kg/day) for six months without incident.

Dosage and Administration: The recommended dose range for CHENIX is 13 to 16 mg/kg/day in two divided doses, morning and night, starting with 250 mg b.i.d. the first two weeks and increasing by 250 mg/day each week thereafter until the recommended or maximum tolerated dose is reached. If diarrhea occurs during dosage buildup or later in treatment, it usually can be controlled by temporary dosage adjustment until symptoms abate, after which the previous dose usually is tolerated. Dosage less than 10 mg/kg usually is ineffective and may be associated with increased risk of cholecystectomy, so is not recommended.

Weight/Dosage Guide

Body Weight		Recommended Tablets	Dose Range
lb	kg	/Day	mg/kg
100–130	45–58	3	17–13
131–165	59–75	4	17–13
166–200	76–90	5	16–14
201–235	91–107	6	16–14
236–275	108–125	7	16–14

The optimal frequency of monitoring liver function tests is not known. It is suggested that serum aminotransferase levels should be monitored monthly for the first three months and every three months thereafter during CHENIX administra-

Continued on next page

Rowell—Cont.

tion. Under NCGS guidelines, if a minor, usually transient, elevation (1½ to 3 times the upper limit of normal) persisted longer than three to six months, chenodiol was discontinued and resumed only after the aminotransferase level returned to normal; however, allowing the elevations to persist over such an interval is not known to be safe. Elevations over three times the upper limit of normal require immediate discontinuation of CHENIX, and usually reoccur on challenge.

Serum cholesterol should be monitored at six-month intervals. It may be advisable to discontinue CHENIX if cholesterol rises above the acceptable age-adjusted limit for a given patient.

Oral cholecystograms or ultrasonograms are recommended at six- to nine-month intervals to monitor response. Complete dissolutions should be confirmed by a repeat test after one to three months' continued CHENIX administration. Most patients who eventually achieve complete dissolution will show partial (or complete) dissolution at the first on-treatment test. If partial dissolution is not seen by nine to 12 months, the likelihood of success of treating longer is greatly reduced; CHENIX should be discontinued if there is no response by 18 months. Safety of use beyond 24 months is not established.

Stone recurrence can be expected within five years in 50% of cases. After confirmed dissolution, treatment generally should be stopped. Serial cholecystograms or ultrasonograms are recommended to monitor for recurrence, keeping in mind that radiolucency and gallbladder function should be established before starting another course of CHENIX. A prophylactic dose is not established; reduced doses cannot be recommended; stones have recurred on 500 mg/day. Low cholesterol or carbohydrate diets, and dietary bran, have been reported to reduce biliary cholesterol; maintenance of reduced weight is recommended to forestall stone recurrence.

Caution: Federal law prohibits dispensing without prescription.

How Supplied: CHENIX brand chenodiol is available as white, film-coated, 250-mg tablets imprinted "ROWELL 7720," in bottles of 100. NDC 0032-7720-01.

VIO-BEC FORTE™   R
Therapeutic B-Complex with Folic Acid, C, E, Zinc and Copper

Composition: Each film-coated tablet contains: Thiamine Mononitrate (B-1) 25 mg., Riboflavin (B-2) 25 mg., Pyridoxine Hydrochloride (B-6) 25 mg., Ascorbic Acid (C) 500 mg., Calcium Pantothenate 40 mg., Niacinamide 100 mg., dl-alpha Tocopheryl Acetate N.F. (E) 30 I.U., Cyanocobalamin (B-12) 5 mcg., Folic Acid 0.5 mg., Zinc 25 mg. (from Zinc Sulfate), Copper 3 mg. (from Copper Sulfate).

Warnings: Folic acid alone is inappropriate in therapy of pernicious anemia and other megaloblastic anemias where vitamin B-12 is deficient and oral vitamin B-12 is therapeutically ineffective.

Precautions: Folic acid, especially in doses above 1.0 mg./day, may obscure pernicious anemia by temporary hematologic remission while neurologic involvement remains progressive.

Adverse Reactions: Allergic sensitization has been reported after administration of folic acid.

Dosage: As indicated by clinical need, usually 1 tablet daily.

How Supplied: Capsule shaped tablet (film-coated brown and imprinted "ROWELL 1218") in bottles of 100 and unit-dose boxes of 100.

Products are cross-indexed by generic and chemical names in the **YELLOW SECTION**

Roxane Laboratories, Inc.
P.O. 16532
COLUMBUS, OH 43216

HOSPITAL UNIT DOSE

Hospital Unit Dose—Roxane, was developed to aid in improved drug distribution and administration. With Hospital Unit Dose, each single unit of medication moves from our quality controlled production lines to the patient's bedside in tamper resistant containers, labeled for positive identification, thus protecting dosage integrity to the point of administration.

The following products are currently available in Hospital Unit Dose:

Acetaminophen Elixir USP 160mg/5ml, 325mg/10.15ml, 650mg/20.3ml
Acetaminophen Elixir USP (cherry) 160mg/5ml, 325mg/10.15ml, 650mg/20.3ml
Acetaminophen Suppositories 120mg, 650mg
Acetaminophen Tablets USP 325mg, 650mg, 500 mg
Acetaminophen 300 mg with Codeine Phosphate 30 mg tablets
Acetaminophen 300 mg with Codeine Phosphate 60 mg tablets
Aluminum Hydroxide Gel USP (Flavored) 30ml
Aluminum Hydroxide, Concentrate, 20 ml, 30 ml
Aluminum Hydroxide Tablets 500 mg
Aluminum and Magnesium Hydroxides with Simethicone I 15ml, 30ml
Aluminum and Magnesium Hydroxides with Simethicone II 15ml, 30 ml
Aminophylline Tablets USP 100mg, 200mg
Amitriptyline Hydrochloride Tablets USP 10mg, 25mg, 50mg, 75mg, 100mg, 150mg
Aminophylline Oral Solution 210mg/10ml, 315mg/15ml
Aromatic Cascara Fluidextract USP 5ml
Ascorbic Acid Tablets USP 250mg, 500mg
Aspirin Suppositories USP 300mg, 600mg
Bisacodyl Suppositories USP 10mg
Bisacodyl Tablets USP 5mg
Bisacodyl Patient Pack
Calcium Carbonate Tablets USP 1250 mg
Calcium Carbonate Oral Suspension 1250 mg/5 ml
Calcium Gluconate Tablets USP 500 mg
Castor Oil USP 30ml, 60ml
Castor Oil Flavored 30ml, 60ml
Chloral Hydrate Syrup USP 500mg/10ml, 1g/10ml
Chloral Hydrate Capsules USP 500mg
Chlordiazepoxide Hydrochloride Capsules USP 10mg, 25mg
Chlorpheniramine Maleate Tablets USP 4mg
Cocaine Hydrochloride Topical Solution 4%/4 ml, 10%/4 ml
Codeine Phosphate Oral Solution 30 mg/10 ml, 60 mg/20 ml
Codeine Sulfate Tablets USP 30mg, 60mg
Dexamethasone Oral Solution 0.5 mg/5 ml, 2 mg/20 ml
Dexamethasone Tablets USP 0.5 mg, 0.75mg, 1 mg, 1.5mg, 2mg, 4mg, 6mg
Dihydrotachysterol Tablets USP 0.125mg, 0.2mg
Diluent (Flavored) for Oral Use 15 ml
Diphenhydramine Hydrochloride Elixir USP 25mg/10ml
Diphenhydramine Hydrochloride Capsules USP 50mg
Diphenoxylate Hydrochloride 2.5mg and Atropine Sulfate 0.025mg Tablets USP
Diphenoxylate Hydrochloride and Atropine Sulfate Oral Solution USP 4 ml, 10 ml
Docusate Sodium Capsules USP 50mg, 100mg, 250mg
Docusate Sodium Syrup USP 50mg/15ml, 100mg/30ml
Docusate Sodium 100mg with Casanthranol 30mg Capsules
Ferrous Sulfate Liquid 300mg/5ml
Ferrous Sulfate Tablets USP 300mg
Guaifenesin Syrup USP 100mg/5ml, 200mg/10ml, 300mg/15ml
Hydrochlorothiazide Tablets USP 25mg, 50mg
Hydrochlorothiazide Oral Solution 50 mg/5 ml
Imipramine Hydrochloride Tablets USP 10mg, 25mg, 50mg
Ipecac Syrup USP 15ml, 30ml
Isoetharine Hydrochloride 0.1%, 2.5ml
Isoetharine Hydrochloride 0.125%, 4ml
Isoetharine Hydrochloride 0.167%, 3ml
Isoetharine Hydrochloride 0.2%, 2.5ml
Isoetharine Hydrochloride 0.25%, 2ml
Isoxsuprine Hydrochloride Tablets USP 10mg, 20mg
Kaolin-Pectin Suspension 30ml
Kaolin-Pectin Suspension Concentrated 20ml
Lithium Carbonate Capsules USP 300mg
Lithium Carbonate Tablets USP 300mg
Lithium Citrate Syrup 8 mEq per 5 ml, 16 mEq per 10 ml
Magnesia and Alumina Oral Suspension USP 30ml
Methocarbamol Tablets USP 500 mg, 750 mg
Milk of Magnesia USP 15ml, 30ml
Milk of Magnesia Concentrated Flavored 10ml, 15ml, 20ml
Milk of Magnesia—Cascara Suspension Concentrated 15 ml
Milk of Magnesia—Mineral Oil Emulsion 30ml
Milk of Magnesia—Mineral Oil Emulsion (Flavored) 30ml
Mineral Oil-Light Sterile 10ml, 30ml
Mineral Oil USP 30ml
Morphine Sulfate Tablets 15mg, 30mg
Morphine Sulfate Oral Solution 10mg/5ml, 20mg/10ml
Neomycin Sulfate Tablets USP 500 mg
Niacin Tablets USP 50mg, 100mg
Oxycodone Hydrochloride Tablets 5mg
Oxycodone Hydrochloride 5mg and Acetaminophen 325mg Tablets
Oxycodone Hydrochloride 4.5mg, Oxycodone Terephthalate 0.38mg and Aspirin 325mg Tablets
Papaverine Hydrochloride Prolonged Release Capsules 150mg
Paregoric USP 5ml
Phenobarbital Elixir USP 20mg/5ml
Phenobarbital Tablets USP 15mg, 30mg, 60mg, 100mg
Potassium Chloride Oral Solution USP 5% (20mEq/30ml)
Potassium Chloride Oral Solution USP 10% (15mEq/11.25ml)
Potassium Chloride Oral Solution USP 10% (20mEq/15ml)
Potassium Chloride Oral Solution USP 10% (30mEq/22.5ml)
Potassium Chloride Oral Solution USP 10% (40mEq/30ml)
Potassium Chloride for Oral Solution USP 20mEq/4g
Potassium Chloride USP Powder Unflavored 20mEq/1.5g
Potassium Gluconate Elixir USP 20mEq/15ml
Potassium Iodide Liquid 500mg/15ml
Potassium Phosphates Oral Solution, 30ml
Prednisolone Tablets USP 5mg
Prednisone Tablets USP 1mg, 2.5mg, 5mg, 10mg, 20mg, 25mg, 50mg
Propantheline Bromide Tablets USP 15mg
Propoxyphene Hydrochloride Capsules USP 65 mg
Pseudoephedrine Hydrochloride Tablets USP 30mg, 60mg
Pseudoehedrine Hydrochloride Syrup USP 60mg/10ml
Quinidine Gluconate Sustained Release Tablets 324mg
Quinidine Sulfate Tablets USP 200mg, 300mg
Quinine Sulfate Capsules USP 200mg, 325mg
Sodium Chloride Inhalation USP (Normal Saline) Sterile 0.9% 3ml, 5ml
Sodium Phosphates Oral Solution USP 30ml
Sodium Polystyrene Sulfonate Suspension 60ml
Sulfisoxazole Tablets USP 500mg
Terpin Hydrate and Codeine Elixir USP 5ml
Theophylline Elixir 80mg/15ml, 160mg/30ml
Thioridazine Hydrochloride Tablets USP 10 mg, 25 mg, 50 mg

Triprolidine 2.5 mg and Pseudoephedrine Hydrochlorides 60 mg Tablets USP
Triprolidine Hydrochloride 2.5 mg and Pseudoephedrine Hydrochloride 60 mg/10 ml syrup
As research continues, new Roxane Laboratories' products will be available in Hospital Unit Dose packages.

DHT™
Dihydrotachysterol Tablets USP

Description: Each tablet contains:
Dihydrotachysterol ..... 0.125 mg, 0.2 mg; or 0.4 mg
Dihydrotachysterol is a synthetic reduction product of tachysterol, a close isomer of vitamin D. Chemically Dihydrotachysterol is $9,10$-Secoergosta-$5,7,22$-tri-en-3β - ol.
Dihydrotachysterol acts as a blood calcium regulator.

Clinical Pharmacology: Dyhydrotachysterol is hydroxylated in the liver to 25-hydroxydihydrotachysterol, which is the major circulating active form of the drug. It does not undergo further hydroxylation by the kidney and therefore is the analogue of 1,25-dihydroxyvitamin D. Dihydrotachysterol is effective in the elevation of serum calcium by stimulating intestinal calcium absorption and mobilizing bone calcium in the absence of parathyroid hormone and of functioning renal tissue. Dihydrotachysterol also increases renal phosphate excretion. In contrast to parathyroid extract, Dihydrotachysterol is active when taken orally, exerts a slow but persistent effect, and may be used for long periods without increasing the dosage or causing tolerance. Dihydrotachysterol is faster-acting than pharmacologic doses of vitamin D and is less persistent after cessation of treatment, thus decreasing the risk of accumulation and of hypercalcemia.

Indications and Usage: Dihydrotachysterol is indicated for the treatment of acute, chronic, and latent forms of postoperative tetany, idiopathic tetany, and hypoparathyroidism.

Contraindications: Contraindicated in patients with hypercalcemia, abnormal sensitivity to the effects of vitamin D, and hypervitaminosis D.

Precautions:
General: The difference between therapeutic dose and intoxicating dose may be small in any patient and therefore dosage must be individualized and periodically reevaluated.
In patients with renal osteodystrophy accompanied by hyperphosphatemia, maintenance of a normal serum phosphorus level by dietary phosphate restriction and/or administration of aluminum gels as intestinal phosphate binders is essential to prevent metastatic calcification.
Because of its effect on serum calcium, Dihydrotachysterol should be administered to pregnant patients or to patients with renal stones only when, in the judgment of the physician, the potential benefits outweigh the possible hazards.
Laboratory tests: To prevent hypercalcemia, treatment should always be controlled by regular determinations of blood calcium level, which should be maintained within the normal range.
Drug interactions: Administration of thiazide diuretics to hypoparathyroid patients who are concurrently being treated with Dihydrotachysterol may cause hypercalcemia.
Pregnancy: Teratogenic effects—Pregnancy Category C: Animal reproduction studies have shown fetal abnormalities in several species associated with hypervitaminosis D. These are similar to the supravalvular aortic stenosis syndrome described in infants by Black in England (1963). This syndrome was characterized by supravalvular aortic stenosis, elfin facies, and mental retardation.
There are no adequate and well-controlled studies in pregnant women. Dihydrotachysterol should be used during pregnancy only if the potential benefit justifies the potential risk to the fetus.
Nursing mothers: It is not known whether this drug is excreted in human milk. Because many drugs are excreted in human milk, caution should be exercised when Dihydrotachysterol is administered to a nursing woman.

Overdosage: The effects of Dihydrotachysterol can persist for up to one month after cessation of treatment.
Manifestations: Toxicity associated with Dihydrotachysterol is similar to that seen with large doses of vitamin D. Overdosage is manifested by symptoms of hypercalcemia, i.e., weakness, headache, anorexia, nausea, vomiting, abdominal cramps, diarrhea, constipation, vertigo, tinnitus, ataxia, hypotonia, lethargy, depression, amnesia, disorientation, hallucinations, syncope, and coma. Impairment of renal function may result in polyuria, polydipsia, and albuminuria. Widespread calcification of soft tissues, including heart, blood vessels, kidneys, and lungs, can occur. Death can result from cardiovascular or renal failure.
Treatment: Treatment of overdosage consists of withdrawal of Dihydrotachysterol, bed rest, liberal intake of fluids, a low-calcium diet, and administration of a laxative. Hypercalcemic crisis with dehydration, stupor, coma, and azotemia requires more vigorous treatment. The first step should be hydration of the patient. Intravenous saline may quickly and significantly increast urinary calcium excretion. A loop diuretic (furosemide or ethacrynic acid) may be given with the saline infusion to further increase renal calcium excretion. Other reported therapeutic measures include dialysis or the administration of citrates, sulfates, phosphates, corticosteroids, EDTA (ethylenediaminetetraacetic acids), and mithramycin via appropriate regimens.

Dosage and Administration: The dosage depends on the nature and seriousness of the disorder and should be adapted to each individual patient. Serum calcium levels should be maintained between 9 to 10 mg per 100 ml.
The following dosage schedule will serve as a guide:
Initial dose: 0.8 mg to 2.4 mg daily for several days.
Maintenance dose: 0.2 mg to 1.0 mg daily as required for normal serum calcium levels. The average maintenance dose is 0.6 mg daily. This dose may be supplemented with 10 to 15 grams of calcium lactate or gluconate by mouth daily.

How Supplied:
0.125 mg white tablets.
NDC 0054-8172-25: Unit dose, 10 tablets per strip, 10 strips per shelf pack, 10 shelf packs per shipper.
NDC 0054-4190-19: Bottles of 50 tablets.
0.2 mg pink tablets.
NDC 0054-8182-25: Unit dose, 10 tablets per strip, 10 strips per shelf pack, 10 shelf packs per shipper.
NDC 0054-4189-25: Bottles of 100 tablets.
0.4 mg white tablets.
NDC 0054-4191-19: Bottles of 50 tablets.
Oral Solution 0.2 mg/5 ml
NDC 0054-3171-63: 500 ml
Intensol 0.2 mg/ml
NDC 0054-3170-44: Bottles of 30 ml with calibrated dropper (graduated 0.25 ml to 1.0 ml)

LITHIUM CARBONATE
CAPSULES AND TABLETS USP, 300 mg

> **WARNING**
> Lithium toxicity is closely related to serum lithium levels, and can occur at doses close to therapeutic levels. Facilities for prompt and accurate serum lithium determinations should be available before initiating therapy.

Description: Each capsule or tablet for oral administration contains:
Lithium Carbonate .... 300 mg
Lithium Carbonate is a white, light alkaline powder with molecular formula Li_2CO_3 and molecular weight 73.89. Lithium is an element of the alkali-metal group with atomic number 3, atomic weight 6.94 and an emission line at 671 nm on the flame photometer. Lithium acts as an antimanic.

Clinical Pharmacology: Preclinical studies have shown that lithium alters sodium transport in nerve and muscle cells and effects a shift toward intraneuronal metabolism of catecholamines, but the specific biochemical mechanism of lithium action in mania is unknown.

Indications and Usage: Lithium carbonate is indicated in the treatment of manic episodes of Bipolar Disorder. Bipolar Disorder, Manic (DSM-III) is equivalent to Manic Depressive illness, Manic, in the older DSM-II terminology.
Lithium is also indicated as a maintenance treatment for individuals with a diagnosis of Bipolar Disorder. Maintenance therapy reduces the frequency of manic episodes and diminishes the intensity of those episodes which may occur.
Typical symptoms of mania include pressure of speech, motor hyperactivity, reduced need for sleep, flight of ideas, grandiosity, or poor judgment, aggressiveness, and possibly hostility. When given to a patient experiencing a manic episode, lithium may produce a normalization of symptomatology within 1 to 3 weeks.

Contraindications: Lithium should generally not be given to patients with significant renal or cardiovascular disease, severe debilitation or dehydration, or sodium depletion, and to patients receiving diuretics, since the risk of lithium toxicity is very high in such patients. If the psychiatric indication is life-threatening, and if such a patient fails to respond to other measures, lithium treatment may be undertaken with extreme caution, including daily serum lithium determinations and adjustment to the usualy low doses ordinarily tolerated by these individuals. In such instances, hospitlization is a necessity.

Warnings: Lithium may cause fetal harm when administered to a pregnant woman. There have been reports of lithium having adverse effects on nidation in rats, embryo viability in mice, and metabolism in-vitro of rat testis and human spermatozoa have been attributed to lithium, as have teratogenicity in submammalian species and cleft palates in mice. Studies in rats, rabbits and monkeys have shown no evidence of lithium-induced teratology. Data from lithium birth registries suggest an increase in cardiac and other anomalies, especially Ebstein's anomaly. If the patient becomes pregnant while taking lithium, she should be apprised of the potential risk to the fetus. If possible, lithium should be withdrawn for at least the first trimester unless it is determined that this would seriously endanger the mother.
Chronic lithium therapy may be associated with diminution of renal concentrating ability, occasionally presenting as nephrogenic diabetes insipidus, with polyuria and polydipsia. Such patients should be carefully managed to avoid dehydration with resulting lithium retention and toxicity. This condition is usually reversible when lithium is discontinued.
Morphologic changes with glomerular and interstitial fibrosis and nephron-atrophy have been reported in patients on chronic lithium therapy. Morphologic changes have been seen in bipolar patients never exposed to lithium. The relationship between renal functional and morphologic changes and their association with lithium therapy has not been established. To date, lithium in therapeutic doses has not been reported to cause end-stage renal disease.
When kidney function is assessed, for baseline data prior to starting lithium therapy or thereafter, routine urinalysis and other tests may be used to evaluate tubular function (e.g., urine specific gravity or osmolality following a period of water deprivation, or 24-hour urine volume) and glomerular function (e.g., serum creatinine or creatinine clearance). During lithium therapy, progressive or sudden changes in renal function, even within the normal range, indicate the need for reevaluation of treatment.
Lithium toxicity is closely related to serum lithium levels, and can occur at doses close to therapeutic levels (see DOSAGE AND ADMINISTRATION).

Precautions:
General: The ability to tolerate lithium is greater during the acute manic phase and decreases when

Continued on next page

Roxane—Cont.

manic symptoms subside (See DOSAGE AND ADMINISTRATION).

The distribution space of lithium approximates that of total body water. Lithium is primarily excreted in urine with insignificant excretion in feces. Renal excretion of lithium is proportional to its plasma concentration. The half-life of elimination of lithium is approximately 24 hours. Lithium decreases sodium reabsorption by the renal tubules which could lead to sodium depletion. Therefore, it is essential for the patient to maintain a normal diet, including salt, and an adequate fluid intake (2500-3000 ml) at least during the initial stabilization period. Decreased tolerance to lithium has been reported to ensue from protracted sweating or diarrhea and, if such occur, supplemental fluid and salt should be administered.

In addition to sweating and diarrhea, concomitant infection with elevated temperatures may also necessitate a temporary reduction or cessation of medication.

Previously existing underlying thyroid disorders do not necessarily constitute a contraindication to lithium treatment; where hypothyroidism exists, careful monitoring of thyroid function during lithium stabilization and maintenance allows for correction of changing thyroid parameters, if any. Where hypothyroidism occurs during lithium stabilization and maintenance, supplemental thyroid treatment may be used.

Information for the patients: Outpatients and their families should be warned that the patient must discontinue lithium therapy and contact his physician if such clinical signs of lithium toxicity as diarrhea, vomiting, tremor, mild ataxia, drowsiness, or muscular weakness occur.

Lithium may impair mental and/or physical abilities. Caution patients about activities requiring alertness (e.g., operating vehicles or machinery).

Drug interactions: Combined use of *haloperidol and lithium:* An encephalopathic syndrome (characterized by weakness, lethargy, fever, tremulousness and confusion, extrapyramidal symptoms, leucocytosis, elevated serum enzymes, BUN and FBS) followed by irreversible brain damage has occurred in a few patients treated with lithium plus haloperidol. A causal relationship between these events and the concomitant administration of lithium and haloperidol has not been established; however, patients receiving such combined therapy should be monitored closely for early evidence of neurological toxicity and treatment discontinued promptly if such signs appear.

The possibility of similar adverse interactions with other antipsychotic medication exists.

Lithium may prolong the effects of neuromuscular blocking agents. Therefore, neuromuscular blocking agents should be given with caution to patients receiving lithium.

Indomethacin (50 mg t.i.d.) has been reported to increase steady state plasma lithium levels from 30 to 59 percent. There is also evidence that other non-steroidal, anti-inflammatory agents may have a similar effect. When such combinations are used, increased plasma lithium level monitoring is recommended.

Pregnancy: Teratogenic effects—Pregnancy Category D, See "Warnings" section.

Nursing mothers: Lithium is excreted in human milk. Nursing should not be undertaken during lithium therapy except in rare and unusual circumstances where, in the view of the physician, the potential benefits to the mother outweigh possible hazards to the child.

Pediatric use: Since information regarding the safety and effectiveness of lithium in children under 12 years of age is not available, its use in such patients is not recommended at this time.

Adverse Reactions:
Lithium toxicity: The likelihood of toxicity increases with increasing serum lithium levels. Serum lithium levels greater than 1.5 mEq/l carry a greater risk than lower levels. However, patients sensitive to lithium may exhibit toxic signs at serum levels below 1.5 mEq/l.

Diarrhea, vomiting, drowsiness, muscular weakness and lack of coordination may be early signs of lithium toxicity, and can occur at lithium levels below 2.0 mEq/l. At higher levels, giddiness, ataxia, blurred vision, tinnitus and a large output of dilute urine may be seen. Serum lithium levels above 3.0 mEq/l may produce a complex clinical picture involving multiple organs and organ systems. Serum lithium levels should not be permitted to exceed 2.0 mEq/l during the acute treatment phase.

Fine hand tremor, polyuria and mild thirst may occur during initial therapy for the acute manic phase, and may persist throughout treatment. Transient and mild nausea and general discomfort may also appear during the first few days of lithium administration.

These side effects are an inconvenience rather than a disabling condition, and usually subside with continued treatment or a temporary reduction or cessation of dosage. If persistent, a cessation of dosage is indicated.

The following adverse reactions have been reported and do not appear to be directly related to serum lithium levels.

Neuromuscular: tremor, muscle hyperirritability (fasciculations, twitching, clonic movements of whole limbs), ataxia, choreo-athetotic movements, hyperactive deep tendon reflexes.

Central Nervous System: blackout spells, epileptiform seizures, slurred speech, dizziness, vertigo, incontinence of urine or feces, somnolence, psychomotor retardation, restlessness, confusion, stupor, coma.

Cardiovascular: cardiac arrhythmia, hypotension, peripheral circulatory collapse.

Gastrointestinal: anorexia, nausea, vomiting, diarrhea.

Genitourinary: albuminuria, oliguria, polyuria, glycosuria.

Dermatologic: drying and thinning of hair, anesthesia of skin, chronic folliculitis, xerosis cutis, alopecia and exacerbation of psoriasis.

Autonomic Nervous System: blurred vision, dry mouth.

Miscellaneous: fatigue, lethargy, tendency to sleep, dehydration, weight loss, transient scotomata.

Thyroid Abnormalities: euthyroid goiter and/or hypothyroidism (including myxedema) accompanied by lower T_3 and T_4. Iodine 131 uptake may be elevated. (See PRECAUTIONS). Paradoxically, rare cases of hyperthyroidism have been reported.

EEG Changes: diffuse slowing, widening of frequency spectrum, potentiation and disorganization of background rhythm.

EKG Changes: reversible flattening, isoelectricity or inversion of T-waves.

Miscellaneous: fatigue, lethargy, transient scotomata, dehydration, weight loss, tendency to sleep.

Miscellaneous reactions unrelated to dosage are: transient electroencephalographic and electrocardiographic changes, leucocytosis, headache, diffuse nontoxic goiter with or without hypothyroidism, transient hyperglycemia, generalized pruritis with or without rash, cutaneous ulcers, albuminuria, worsening of organic brain syndromes, excessive weight gain, edematous swelling of ankles or wrists, and thirst or polyuria, sometimes resembling diabetes insipidus, and metallic taste.

A single report has been received of the development of painful discoloration of fingers and toes and coldness of the extremities within one day of the starting of treatment of lithium. The mechanism through which these symptoms (resembling Raynaud's Syndrome) developed is not known. Recovery followed discontinuance.

Overdosage: The toxic levels for lithium are close to the therapeutic levels. It is therefore important that patients and their families be cautioned to watch for early symptoms and to discontinue the drug and inform the physician should they occur. Toxic symptoms are listed in detail under ADVERSE REACTIONS.

Treatment: No specific antidote for lithium poisoning is known. Early symptoms of lithium toxicity can usually be treated by reduction or cessation of dosage of the drug and resumption of the treatment at a lower dose after 24 to 48 hours. In severe cases of lithium poisoning, the first and foremost goal of treatment consists of elimination of this ion from the patient.

Treatment is essentially the same as that used in barbiturate poisoning: 1) gastric lavage, 2) correction of fluid and electrolyte imbalance and 3) regulation of kidney functioning. Urea, mannitol, and aminophylline all produce significant increases in lithium excretion. Hemodialysis is an effective and rapid means of removing the ion from the severely toxic patient. Infection prophylaxis, regular chest X-rays, and preservation of adequate respiration are essential.

Dosage and Administration:
Acute Mania: Optimal patient response to Lithium Carbonate usually can be established and maintained with 600 mg t.i.d. Such doses will normally produce an effective serum lithium level ranging between 1.0 and 1.5 mEq/l. Dosage must be individualized according to serum levels and clinical response. Regular monitoring of the patient's clinical state and of serum lithium levels is necessary. Serum levels should be determined twice per week during the acute phase, and until the serum level and clinical condition of the patient have been stabilized.

Long-term Control: The desirable serum lithium levels are 0.6 to 1.2 mEq/l. Dosage will vary from one individual to another, but usually 300 mg t.i.d. or q.i.d. will maintain this level. Serum lithium levels in uncomplicated cases receiving maintenance therapy during remission should be monitored at least every two months.

Patients abnormally sensitive to lithium may exhibit toxic signs at serum levels of 1.0 to 1.5 mEq/l. Elderly patients often respond to reduced dosage, and may exhibit signs of toxicity at serum levels ordinarily tolerated by other patients.

N.B.: Blood samples for serum lithium determination should be drawn immediately prior to the next dose when lithium concentrations are relatively stable (i.e., 8–12 hours after the previous dose.) Total reliance must not be placed on serum levels alone. Accurate patient evaluation requires both clinical and laboratory analysis.

How Supplied:
300 mg flesh-colored capsules.
NDC 0054-8527-25: Unit dose, 10 capsules per strip, 10 strips per shelf pack, 10 shelf packs per shipper.
NDC 0054-2527-25: Bottles of 100 capsules.
NDC 0054-2527-31: Bottles of 1000 capsules.
300 mg white, scored tablets.
NDC 0054-8528-25: Unit dose, 10 tablets per strip, 10 strips per shelf pack, 10 shelf packs per shipper. (For Institutional Use Only.)
NDC 0054-4527-25: Bottles of 100 tablets.
NDC 0054-4527-31: Bottles of 1000 tablets.

LITHIUM CITRATE SYRUP USP ℞
8 mEq of Lithium per 5 ml
SUGAR FREE
FOR ORAL ADMINISTRATION ONLY

Description: Lithium Citrate Syrup is a palatable oral dosage form of lithium ion. Lithium citrate is prepared in solution from lithium hydroxide and citric acid in a ratio approximating di-lithium citrate:

Each 5 ml of Lithium Citrate Syrup contains 8 mEq of lithium ion (Li+), equivalent to the amount of lithium in 300 mg of lithium carbonate and alcohol 0.3% v/v. Lithium is an element of the alkali-metal group with atomic number 3, atomic weight 6.94, and an emission line at 671nm on the flame photometer.

How Supplied:
Lithium Citrate Syrup, 8 mEq per 5 ml
NDC 0054-8529-04: Unit dose Patient Cup™ filled to deliver 5 ml, ten 5 ml Patient Cups™ per shelf pack, ten shelf packs per shipper. (For Institutional Use Only).
NDC 0054-3527-63: Bottles of 500 ml.
Refer to Lithium Carbonate Capsules and Tablets heading for complete text.

METHADONE HYDROCHLORIDE ORAL SOLUTION USP

(WARNING: May be habit forming)

CONDITIONS FOR DISTRIBUTION AND USE OF METHADONE PRODUCTS: Code of Federal Regulations, Title 21, Sec. 291.505

METHADONE PRODUCTS, WHEN USED FOR TREATMENT OF NARCOTIC ADDICTION IN DETOXIFICATION OR MAINTENANCE PROGRAMS, SHALL BE DISPENSED ONLY BY APPROVED HOSPITAL PHARMACIES, APPROVED COMMUNITY PHARMACIES, AND MAINTENANCE PROGRAMS APPROVED BY THE FOOD AND DRUG ADMINISTRATION AND THE DESIGNATED STATE AUTHORITY.

APPROVED MAINTENANCE PROGRAMS SHALL DISPENSE AND USE METHADONE IN ORAL FORM ONLY AND ACCORDING TO THE TREATMENT REQUIREMENTS STIPULATED IN THE FEDERAL METHADONE REGULATIONS (21 CFR 291.505).

FAILURE TO ABIDE BY THE REQUIREMENTS IN THESE REGULATIONS MAY RESULT IN CRIMINAL PROSECUTION, SEIZURE OF THE DRUG SUPPLY, REVOCATION OF THE PROGRAM APPROVAL, AND INJUNCTION PRECLUDING OPERATION OF THE PROGRAM.

A METHADONE PRODUCT, WHEN USED AS AN ANALGESIC, MAY BE DISPENSED IN ANY LICENSED PHARMACY.

Description: Each 5 ml of Methadone Hydrochloride Oral Solution contains:
Methadone Hydrochloride .... 5 mg or 10 mg
(Warning: May be habit forming)
Alcohol 8%

Chemically, Methadone Hydrochloride is 3-Heptanone, 6-(dimethylamino)-4,4-diphenyl-, hydrochloride, which can be represented by the following structural formula:

Methadone Hydrochloride acts as a narcotic analgesic.

Clinical Pharmacology: Methadone Hydrochloride is a synthetic narcotic analgesic with multiple actions quantitatively similar to those of morphine, the most prominent of which involve the central nervous system and organs composed of smooth muscle. The principal actions of therapeutic value are analgesia and sedation and detoxication or temporary maintenance in narcotic addiction. The methadone abstinence syndrome, although qualitatively similar to that of morphine, differs in that the onset is slower, the course is more prolonged, and the symptoms are less severe. When administered orally, methadone is approximately one-half as potent as when given parenterally. Oral administration results in a delay of the onset, a lowering of the peak, and an increase in the duration of analgesic effect.

Indications and Usage: Methadone Hydrochloride is indicated for relief of severe pain, for detoxification treatment of narcotic addiction, and for temporary maintenance treatment of narcotic addiction.

Note
If methadone is administered for treatment of heroin dependence for more than three weeks, the procedure passes from treatment of the acute withdrawal syndrome (detoxification) to maintenance therapy. Maintenance treatment is permitted to be undertaken only by approved methadone programs. This does not preclude the maintenance treatment of an addict who is hospitalized for medical conditions other than addiction and who requires temporary maintenance during the critical period of his stay or whose enrollment has been verified in a program which has approval for maintenance treatment with methadone.

Contraindications: Hypersensitivity to methadone.

Warnings: Methadone Hydrochloride, a narcotic, is a Schedule II controlled substance under the Federal Controlled Substances Act.

DRUG DEPENDENCE — METHADONE CAN PRODUCE DRUG DEPENDENCE OF THE MORPHINE TYPE AND, THEREFORE, HAS THE POTENTIAL FOR BEING ABUSED. PSYCHIC DEPENDENCE, PHYSICAL DEPENDENCE, AND TOLERANCE MAY DEVELOP UPON REPEATED ADMINISTRATION OF METHADONE, AND IT SHOULD BE PRESCRIBED AND ADMINISTERED WITH THE SAME DEGREE OF CAUTION APPROPRIATE TO THE USE OF MORPHINE.

Interaction with Other Central-Nervous-System Depressants—Methadone should be used with caution and in reduced dosage in patients who are concurrently receiving other narcotic analgesics, general anesthetics, phenothiazines, other tranquilizers, sedative-hypnotics, tricyclic antidepressants, and other C.N.S. depressants (including alcohol). Respiratory depression, hypotension, and profound sedation or coma may result.

Anxiety—Since methadone, as used by tolerant subjects at a constant maintenance dosage, is not a tranquilizer, patients who are maintained on this drug will react to life problems and stresses with the same symptoms of anxiety as do other individuals. The physician should not confuse such symptoms with those of narcotic abstinence and should not attempt to treat anxiety by increasing the dosage of methadone. The action of methadone in maintenance treatment is limited to the control of narcotic symptoms and is ineffective for relief of general anxiety.

Head Injury and Increased Intracranial Pressure—The respiratory depressant effects of methadone and its capacity to elevate cerebrospinal-fluid pressure may be markedly exaggerated in the presence of increased intracranial pressure. Furthermore, narcotics produce side effects that may obscure the clinical course of patients with head injuries. In such patients, methadone must be used with caution and only if it is deemed essential.

Asthma and Other Respiratory Conditions—Methadone should be used with caution in patients having an acute asthmatic attack, in those with chronic obstructive pulmonary disease or cor pulmonale, and in individuals with a substantially decreased respiratory reserve, preexisting respiratory depression, hypoxia, or hypercapnia. In such patients, even usual therapeutic doses of narcotics may decrease respiratory drive while simultaneously increasing airway resistance to the point of apnea.

Hypotensive Effect—The administration of methadone may result in severe hypotension in an individual whose ability to maintain his blood pressure has already been compromised by a depleted blood volume or concurrent administration of such drugs as the phenothiazines or certain anesthetics.

Use in Ambulatory Patients—Methadone may impair the mental and/or physical abilities required for the performance of potentially hazardous tasks, such as driving a car or operating machinery. The patient should be cautioned accordingly.

Methadone, like other narcotics, may produce orthostatic hypotension in ambulatory patients.

Use in Pregnancy—Safe use in pregnancy has not been established in relation to possible adverse effects on fetal development. Therefore, methadone should not be used in pregnant women unless, in the judgment of the physician, the potential benefits outweigh the possible hazards.

Methadone is not recommended for obstetric analgesia because its long duration of action increases the probability of respiratory depression in the newborn.

Use in Children—Methadone is not recommended for use as an analgesic in children, since documented clinical experience has been insufficient to establish a suitable dosage regimen for the pediatric age group.

Precautions:

Interaction with Pentazocine—Patients who are addicted to heroin or who are on the methadone maintenance program may experience withdrawal symptoms when given pentazocine.

Interaction with Rifampin—The concurrent administration of rifampin may possibly reduce the blood concentration of methadone. The mechanism by which rifampin may decrease blood concentrations of methadone is not fully understood, although enhanced microsomal drug-metabolized enzymes may influence drug disposition.

Acute Abdominal Conditions—The administration of methadone or other narcotics may obscure the diagnosis or clinical course in patients with acute abdominal conditions.

Interaction with Monoamine Oxidase (MAO) Inhibitors—Therapeutic doses of meperidine have precipitated severe reactions in patients concurrently receiving monoamine oxidase inhibitors or those who have received such agents within 14 days. Similar reactions thus far have not been reported with methadone; but if the use of methadone is necessary in such patients, a sensitivity test should be performed in which repeated small incremental doses are administered over the course of several hours while the patient's condition and vital signs are under careful observation.

Special-Risk Patients—Methadone should be given with caution and the initial dose should be reduced in certain patients, such as the elderly or debilitated and those with severe impairment of hepatic or renal function, hypothyroidism, Addison's disease, prostatic hypertrophy, or urethral stricture.

Adverse Reactions: THE MAJOR HAZARDS OF METHADONE, AS OF OTHER NARCOTIC ANALGESICS, ARE RESPIRATORY DEPRESSION AND, TO A LESSER DEGREE, CIRCULATORY DEPRESSION. RESPIRATORY ARREST, SHOCK, AND CARDIAC ARREST HAVE OCCURRED.

The most frequently observed adverse reactions include lightheadedness, dizziness, sedation, nausea, vomiting, and sweating. These effects seem to be more prominent in ambulatory patients and in those who are not suffering severe chronic pain. In such individuals, lower doses are advisable. Some adverse reactions may be alleviated in the ambulatory patient if he lies down.

Other adverse reactions include the following:

Central Nervous System—Euphoria, dysphoria, weakness, headache, insomnia, agitation, disorientation, and visual disturbances.

Gastrointestinal—Dry mouth, anorexia, constipation, and biliary tract spasm.

Cardiovascular—Flushing of the face, bradycardia, palpitation, faintness, and syncope.

Genitourinary—Urinary retention or hesitancy, antidiuretic effect, and reduced libido and/or potency.

Allergic—Pruritus, urticaria, other skin rashes, edema, and, rarely, hemorrhagic urticaria.

Administration and Dosage:

For relief of Severe Chronic Pain—Dosage should be adjusted according to the severity of the pain and the response of the patient. Occasionally it may be necessary to exceed the usual dosage

Continued on next page

Roxane—Cont.

recommended in cases of exceptionally severe chronic pain or in those patients who have become tolerant to the analgesic effect of narcotics.

The usual adult dosage is 5 mg to 20 mg every six to eight hours.

For Detoxification Treatment—THE DRUG SHALL BE ADMINISTERED DAILY UNDER CLOSE SUPERVISION AS FOLLOWS:

A detoxification treatment course shall not exceed 21 days and may not be repeated earlier than four weeks after completion of the preceding course.

The oral form of administration is preferred. However, if the patient is unable to ingest oral medication, he may be started on the parenteral form initially.

In detoxification, the patient may receive methadone when there are significant symptoms of withdrawal. The dosage schedules indicated below are recommended but could be varied in accordance with clinical judgment. Initially, a single dose of 15 to 20 mg of methadone will often be sufficient to suppress withdrawal symptoms. Additional methadone may be provided if withdrawal symptoms are not suppressed or if symptoms reappear. When patients are physically dependent on high doses, it may be necessary to exceed these levels. Forty mg per day in single or divided doses will usually constitute an adequate stabilizing dosage level. Stabilization can be continued for two to three days, and then the amount of methadone normally will be gradually decreased. The rate at which methadone is decreased will be determined separately for each patient. The dose of methadone can be decreased on a daily basis or at two-day intervals, but the amount of intake shall always be sufficient to keep withdrawal symptoms at a tolerable level. In hospitalized patients, a daily reduction of 20 percent of the total dose may be tolerated and may cause little discomfort. In ambulatory patients, a somewhat slower schedule may be needed. If methadone is administered for more than three weeks, the procedure is considered to have progressed from detoxification or treatment of the acute withdrawal syndrome to maintenance treatment, even though the goal and intent may be eventual total withdrawal.

Overdosage:

Symptoms—Serious overdosage of methadone is characterized by respiratory depression (a decrease in respiratory rate and/or tidal volume, Cheyne-Stokes respiration, cyanosis), extreme somnolence progressing to stupor or coma, maximally constricted pupils, skeletal-muscle flaccidity, cold and clammy skin, and sometimes, bradycardia and hypotension. In severe overdosage, particularly by the intravenous route, apnea, circulatory collapse, cardiac arrest, and death may occur.

Treatment—Primary attention should be given to the reestablishment of adequate respiratory exchange through provision of a patent airway and institution of assisted or controlled ventilation. If a nontolerant person, especially a child, takes a large dose of methadone, effective narcotic antagonists are available to counteract the potentially lethal respiratory depression. **The physician must remember, however, that methadone is a long-acting depressant (36 to 48 hours), whereas the antagonists act for much shorter periods (one to three hours).** The patient must, therefore, be monitored continuously for recurrence of respiratory depression and treated repeatedly with the narcotic antagonist as needed. If the diagnosis is correct and respiratory depression is due only to overdosage of methadone, the use of other respiratory stimulants is not indicated.

An antagonist should not be administered in the absence of clinically significant respiratory or cardiovascular depression. Intravenously administered narcotic antagonists (naloxone, nalorphine, and levallorphan) are the drugs of choice to reverse signs of intoxication. These agents should be given repeatedly until the patient's status remains satisfactory. The hazard that the narcotic agent will further depress respiration is less likely with the use of naloxone.

Oxygen, intravenous fluids, vasopressors, and other supportive measures should be employed as indicated.

> **Note**
> IN AN INDIVIDUAL PHYSICALLY DEPENDENT ON NARCOTICS, THE ADMINISTRATION OF THE USUAL DOSE OF A NARCOTIC ANTAGONIST WILL PRECIPITATE AN ACUTE WITHDRAWAL SYNDROME. THE SEVERITY OF THIS SYNDROME WILL DEPEND ON THE DEGREE OF PHYSICAL DEPENDENCE AND THE DOSE OF THE ANTAGONIST ADMINISTERED. THE USE OF A NARCOTIC ANTAGONIST IN SUCH A PERSON SHOULD BE AVOIDED IF POSSIBLE. IF IT MUST BE USED TO TREAT SERIOUS RESPIRATORY DEPRESSION IN THE PHYSICALLY DEPENDENT PATIENT, THE ANTAGONIST SHOULD BE ADMINISTERED WITH EXTREME CARE AND BY TITRATION WITH SMALLER THAN USUAL DOSES OF THE ANTAGONIST.

How Supplied:
Methadone Hydrochloride Oral Solution USP
5 mg per 5 ml
NDC 0054-3555-63: Bottles of 500 ml.
10 mg per 5 ml
NDC 0054-3556-63: Bottles of 500 ml.
Methadone Hydrochloride Tablets USP
5 mg white, scored tablets
NDC 0054-4570-25 Bottle of 100
NDC 0054-8553-11 Reverse Number 25 Control Pack, Unit Dose
10 mg white, scored tablets
NDC 0054-4571-25 Bottle of 100
NDC 0054-8554-11 Reverse Number 25 Control Pack, Unit Dose
Caution: Federal law prohibits dispensing without prescription.

MORPHINE SULFATE ORAL SOLUTION ⓒ
(WARNING: May be habit forming.)
MORPHINE SULFATE TABLETS ⓒ
(WARNING: May be habit forming.)

Description:
Each 5 ml of Morphine Sulfate Oral Solution contains:
Morphine Sulfate 108 .... 10 or 20 mg
(WARNING: May be habit forming.)
Alcohol 10%
Each tablet for oral administration contains:
Morphine Sulfate .... 15 or 30 mg
(WARNING: May be habit forming.)
How Supplied:
Morphine Sulfate Oral Solution
(Unflavored.)
10 mg per 5 ml.
NDC 0054-8585-04: Unit dose Patient Cup™ filled to deliver 5 ml (10 mg Morphine Sulfate), ten 5 ml Patient Cups™ per shelf pack, ten shelf packs per shipper.
NDC 0054-8586-04: Unit dose Patient Cup™ filled to deliver 10 ml (20 mg Morphine Sulfate), ten 10 ml Patient Cups™ per shelf pack, ten shelf packs per shipper.
NDC 0054-3785-49: 100 ml "Unit of use" calibrated bottle.
NDC 0054-3785-63: Bottles of 500 ml.
20 mg per 5 ml.
NDC 0054-3786-63: Bottles of 500 ml.
Tablets
15 mg white scored, identified (54/733) tablets.
NDC 0054-4582-11: Unit dose, 25 tablets per card (reverse numbered), 10 cards per shipper.
NDC 0054-4582-25: Bottles of 100 tablets.
30 mg white scored, identified (54/262) tablets.
NDC 0054-4583-11: Unit dose, 25 tablets per card (reverse numbered), 10 cards per shipper.
NDC 0054-4583-25: Bottles of 100 Tablets.
DEA Order Form Required
Caution: Federal law prohibits dispensing without prescription.

OXYCODONE HYDROCHLORIDE ⓒ
TABLET AND ORAL SOLUTION
[ox-ē-cō-dōn]

Description:
Each tablet contains:
Oxycodone Hydrochloride .... 5 mg
(WARNING: May be habit forming)
Each 5 ml Oral Solution contains:
Oxycodone Hydrochloride .... 5 mg
(WARNING: May be habit forming)
Oxycodone is 14-hydroxydihydrocodeinone, a white odorless crystalline powder which is derived from the opium alkaloid, thebaine.

Actions: The analgesic ingredient, oxycodone, is a semisynthetic narcotic with multiple actions qualitatively similar to those of morphine; the most prominent of these involve the central nervous system and organs composed of smooth muscle. The principal actions of therapeutic value of oxycodone are analgesia and sedation.

Oxycodone is similar to codeine and methadone in that it retains at least one half of its analgesic activity when administered orally.

Indications: For the relief of moderate to moderately severe pain.

Contraindications: Hypersensitivity to oxycodone.

Warnings:

Drug Dependence: Oxycodone can produce drug dependence of the morphine type, and therefore, has the potential for being abused. Psychic dependence, physical dependence and tolerance may develop upon repeated administration of this drug, and it should be prescribed and administered with the same degree of caution appropriate to the use of other oral narcotic-containing medications. Like other narcotic-containing medications, this drug is subject to the Federal Controlled Substances Act.

Usage in ambulatory patients: Oxycodone may impair the mental and/or physical abilities required for the performance of potentially hazardous tasks such as driving a car or operating machinery. The patient using this drug should be cautioned accordingly.

Interaction with other central nervous system depressants: Patients receiving other narcotic analgesics, general anesthetics, phenothiazines, other tranquilizers, sedative-hypnotics or other CNS depressants (including alcohol) concomitantly with oxycodone hydrochloride may exhibit an additive CNS depression. When such combined therapy is contemplated, the dose of one or both agents should be reduced.

Usage in pregnancy: Safe use in pregnancy has not been established relative to possible adverse effects on fetal development. Therefore, this drug should not be used in pregnant women unless, in the judgment of the physician, the potential benefits outweigh the possible hazards.

Usage in children: This drug should not be administered to children.

Precautions:

Head injury and increased intracranial Pressure: The respiratory depressant effects of narcotics and their capacity to elevate cerebrospinal fluid pressure may be markedly exaggerated in the presence of head injury, other intracranial lesions or a preexisting increase in intracranial pressure. Furthermore, narcotics produce adverse reactions which may obscure the clinical course of patients with head injuries.

Acute abdominal conditions: The administration of this drug or other narcotics may obscure the diagnosis or clinical course in patients with acute abdominal conditions.

Special risk patients: This drug should be given with caution to certain patients such as the elderly, or debilitated, and those with severe impairment of hepatic or renal function, hypothyroidism, Addison's disease and prostatic hypertrophy or urethral stricture.

Adverse Reactions: The most frequently observed adverse reactions include light headedness, dizziness, sedation, nausea and vomiting. These effects seem to be more prominent in ambulatory than in nonambulatory patients, and some of these adverse reactions may be alleviated if the patient lies down.

Other adverse reactions include euphoria, dysphoria, constipation, skin rash and pruritus.

Dosage and Administration: Dosage should be adjusted to the severity of the pain and the response of the patient. It may occasionally be necessary to exceed the usual dosage recommended below in cases of more severe pain or in those patients who have become tolerant to the analgesic effects of narcotics. This drug is given orally. The usual adult dose is one 5 mg tablet or 5 ml every 6 hours as needed for pain.

Drug Interactions: The CNS depressant effects of oxycodone hydrochloride may be additive with that of other CNS depressants. See WARNINGS.

Management of Overdosage:
Signs and Symptoms: Serious overdose of oxycodone hydrochloride is characterized by respiratory depression (a decrease in respiratory rate and/or tidal volume, Cheyne-Stokes respiration, cyanosis), extreme somnolence progessing to stupor or coma, skeletal muscle flaccidity, cold and clammy skin, and sometimes bradycardia and hypotension. In severe overdosage, apnea, circulatory collapse, cardiac arrest and death may occur.

Treatment: Primary attention should be given to the reestablishment of adequate respiratory exchange through provision of a patent airway and the institution of assisted or controlled ventilation. The narcotic antagonist naloxone is a specific antidote against respiratory depression which may result from overdosage or unusual sensitivity to narcotics, including oxycodone. Therefore, an appropriate dose of naloxone (usual initial adult dose: 0.4 mg) should be administered, preferably by the intravenous route, simultaneously with efforts at respiratory resuscitation. Since the duration of action of oxycodone may exceed that of the antagonist, the patient should be kept under continued surveillance and repeated doses of the antagonist should be administered as needed to maintain adequate respiration.

An antagonist should not be administered in the absence of clinically significant respiratory or cardiovascular depression.

Oxygen, intravenous fluids, vasopressors and other supportive measures should be employed as indicated.

Gastric emptying may be useful in removing unabsorbed drug.

How Supplied:
5 mg white scored tablets. (Identified 54 582).
NDC 0054-8657-11: Unit dose, 25 tablets per card (reverse numbered), 10 cards per shipper.
NDC 0054-4657-25: Bottles of 100 tablets.
5 mg per 5 ml oral solution.
NDC 0054-3682-63: Bottles of 500 ml.
DEA Order Form Required
Caution: Federal law prohibits dispensing without prescription.

POTASSIUM CHLORIDE ORAL SOLUTION USP, POTASSIUM CHLORIDE POWDER USP, and POTASSIUM CHLORIDE for ORAL SOLUTION USP

Description:
Potassium Chloride Oral Solution: 5, 10 or 20%:
Each 30 ml 5% solution contains potassium 20 mEq and chloride 20 mEq
Each 30 ml 10% solution contains potassium 40 mEq and chloride 40 mEq
Each 30 ml 20% solution contains potassium 80 mEq and chloride 80 mEq
The 5% and 10% solutions are cocoanut flavored, and the 20% solution is grapefruit flavored. Alcohol 5%.

Potassium Chloride Powder, 1.5 g packet (for oral solution); Potassium Chloride for Oral Solution (Cherry Flavored), 4 g packet:

Each packet contains potassium 20 mEq and chloride 20 mEq
Potassium Chloride is chemically KCl. Potassium Chloride is an electrolyte replenisher.

How Supplied:
POTASSIUM CHLORIDE ORAL SOLUTION USP, 5%
20 mEq of potassium per 30 ml
NDC 0054-8715-04: Unit dose Patient Cups™ filled to deliver 30 ml, ten 30 ml Patient Cups™ per shelf pack, ten shelf packs per shipper.
NDC 0054-3715-63: Bottles of 500 ml.
NDC 0054-3715-75: Bottles of 5 liter.
POTASSIUM CHLORIDE ORAL SOLUTIION USP, 10%
15 mEq of potassium per 11.25 ml
NDC 0054-8711-04: Unit dose Patient Cups™ filled to deliver 11.25 ml, ten 11.25 ml Patient Cups™ per shelf pack, ten shelf packs per shipper.
20 mEq of potassium per 15 ml
NDC 0054-8714-04: Unit dose Patient Cups™ filled to deliver 15ml, ten 15ml patient Cups™ per shelf pack, ten shelf packs per shipper.
30 mEq of potassium per 22.5 ml
NDC 0054-8712-04: Unit dose Patient Cups™ filled to deliver 22.5 ml, ten 22.5 ml Patient Cups™ per shelf pack, ten shelf packs per shipper.
40 mEq potassium pr 30 ml
NDC 0054-8713-04: Unit dose Patient Cups™ filled to deliver 30ml, ten 30ml Patient Cups™ per shelf pack, ten shelf packs per shipper.
NDC 0054-3716-54: Bottles of 180 ml.
NDC 0054-3716-63: Bottles of 500 ml.
NDC 0054-3716-68: Bottles of 1 liter.
NDC 0054-3716-75: Bottles of 5 liter.
POTASSIUM CHLORIDE ORAL SOLUTION USP, 20%
80 mEq of potassium per 30 ml
NDC 0054-3714-54: Bottles of 180 ml.
NDC 0054-3714-63: Bottles of 500 ml.
NDC 0054-3714-68: Bottles of 1 liter.
NDC 0054-3714-75: Bottles of 5 liter.
POTASSIUM CHLORIDE POWDER USP
20 mEq of potassium per 1.5 g (unflavored)
NDC 0054-8490-13: Unit dose, 1.5 g packets, 30 packets per carton.
NDC 0054-8490-25: Unit dose, 1.5 g packets, 100 packets per carton.
POTASSIUM CHLORIDE for ORAL SOLUTION USP
20 mEq of potassium per 4 g (cherry flavored)
NDC 0054-8716-13: Unit dose, 4 g packets, 30 packets per carton.
NDC 0054-8716-25: Unit dose, 4 g packets 100 packets per carton.

PREDNISONE TABLETS USP ℞
1 mg, 2.5 mg, 5 mg, 10 mg, 20 mg, 25 mg, or 50 mg

How Supplied:
1 mg white, scored tablets.
NDC 0054-8739-25: Unit dose, 10 tablets per strip, 10 strips per shelf pack, ten shelf packs per shipper.
NDC 0054-4741-25: Bottles of 100 tablets.
NDC 0054-4741-31: Bottles of 1000 tablets.
2.5 mg white, scored tablets.
NDC 0054-8740-25: Unit dose, 10 tablets per strip, 10 strips per shelf pack, 10 shelf packs per shipper.
NDC 0054-4742-25: Bottles of 100 tablets.
NDC 0054-4742-31: Bottles of 1000 tablets.
5 mg white, scored tablets.
NDC 0054-8724-25: Unit dose, 10 tablets per strip, 10 strips per shelf pack, ten shelf packs per shipper.
NDC 0054-4728-25: Bottles of 100 tablets.
NDC 0054-4728-31: Bottles of 1000 tablets.
10 mg white, scored tablets.
NDC 0054-8725-25: Unit dose, 10 tablets per strip, 10 strips per shelf pack, 10 shelf packs per shipper.
NDC 0054-4730-25: Bottles of 100 tablets.
NDC 0054-4730-29: Bottles of 500 tablets.
20 mg white, scored tablets.
NDC 0054-8726-25: Unit dose, 10 tablets per strip, 10 strips per shelf pack, 10 shelf packs per shipper.

NDC 0054-4729-25: Bottles of 100 tablets.
NDC 0054-4729-29: Bottles of 500 tablets.
25 mg white, scored tablets.
NDC 0054-8747-25: Unit dose, 10 tablets per strip, 10 strips per shelf pack, 10 shelf packs per shipper.
NDC 0054-4747-25: Bottles of 100 tablets.
50 mg white, scored tablets.
NDC 0054-8729-25: Unit dose, 10 tablets per strip, 10 strips per shelf pack, 10 shelf packs per shipper.
NDC 0054-4733-25: Bottles of 100 tablets.

ROXANOL™ ©
[rok'sĕ-nŭl]
Morphine Sulfate Intensified Oral Solution
20 mg per ml

(WARNING: May be habit forming.)

Description: Each ml of Roxanol™ contains:
Morphine Sulfate .... 20 mg
(Warning: May be habit forming.)
Chemically, Morphine Sulfate is, Morphinan3,6-diol, 7,8-didehydro-4,5-epoxy-17-methyl-, (5α,6α)-, sulfate (2:1) (salt), pentahydrate, which can be represented by the following structural formula:

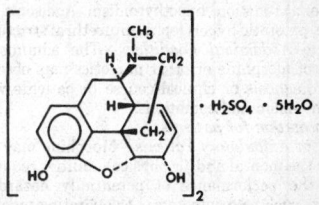

Morphine Sulfate acts as a narcotic analgesic.
Clinical Pharmacology: The major effects of morphine are on the central nervous system and the bowel. Opioids act as agonists, interacting with stereospecific and saturable binding sites or receptors in the brain and other tissues.

Morphine is about two-thirds absorbed from the gastrointestinal tract with the maximum analgesic effect occurring 60 minutes post administration.

Indications and Usage: Morphine is indicated for the relief of severe acute and severe chronic pain.

Contraindications: Hypersensitivity to morphine; respiratory insufficiency or depression; severe CNS depression; attack of bronchial asthma; heart failure secondary to chronic lung disease; cardiac arrhythmias; increased intracranial or cerebrospinal pressure; head injuries; brain tumor; acute alcoholism; delirium tremens; convulsive disorders; after biliary tract surgery; suspected surgical abdomen; surgical anastomosis; concomitantly with MAO inhibitors or within 14 days of such treatment.

Warnings: Morphine can cause tolerance, psychological and physical dependence. Withdrawal will occur on abrupt discontinuation or administration of a narcotic antagonist.

Interaction with Other Central-Nervous-System Depressants—Morphine should be used with caution and in reduced dosage in patients who are concurrently receiving other narcotic analgesics, general anesthetics, phenothiazines, other tranquilizers, sedative-hypnotics, tricyclic antidepressants, and other CNS depressants (including alcohol). Respiratory depression, hypotension, and profound sedation or coma may result.

Precautions:
General:
Head Injury and Increased Intracranial Pressure—The respiratory depressant effects of morphine and its capacity to elevate cerebrospinal-fluid pressure may be markedly exaggerated in the presence of increased intracranial pressure. Furthermore, narcotics produce side effects that

Continued on next page

Roxane—Cont.

may obscure the clinical course of patients with head injuries. In such patients, morphine must be used with caution and only if it is deemed essential.

Asthma and Other Respiratory Conditions—Morphine should be used with caution in patients having an acute asthmatic attack, in those with chronic obstructive pulmonary disease or cor pulmonale, and in individuals with a substantially decreased respiratory reserve, preexisting respiratory depression, hypoxia, or hypercapnia. In such patients, even usual therapeutic doses of narcotics may decrease respiratory drive while simultaneously increasing airway resistance to the point of apnea.

Hypotensive Effect—The administration of morphine may result in severe hypotension in an individual whose ability to maintain his blood pressure has already been compromised by a depleted blood volume or concurrent administration of such drugs as the phenothiazines or certain anesthetics.

Special-Risk Patients—Morphine should be given with caution and the initial dose should be reduced in certain patients, such as the elderly or debilitated and those with severe impairment of hepatic or renal function, hypothyroidism, Addison's disease, prostatic hypertrophy, or urethral stricture.

Acute Abdominal Conditions—The administration of morphine or other narcotics may obscure the diagnosis or clinical course in patients with acute abdominal conditions.

Information for patients:

Use in Ambulatory Patients—Morphine may impair the mental and/or physical abilities required for the performance of potentially hazardous tasks, such as driving a car or operating machinery. The patient should be cautioned accordingly. Morphine, like other narcotics, may produce orthostatic hypotension in ambulatory patients. Patients should be cautioned about the combined effects of alcohol or other central nervous system depressants with morphine.

Drug interactions:

Generally, effects of morphine may be potentiated by alkalizing agents and antagonized by acidifying agents. Analgesic effect of morphine is potentiated by chlorpromazine and methocarbamol. CNS depressants such as anaesthetics, hypnotics, barbiturates, phenothiazines, chloral hydrate, glutethimide, sedatives, MAO inhibitors (including procarbazine hydrochloride), antihistamines, β-blockers (propranolol), alcohol, furazolidone and other narcotics may enhance the depressant effects of morphine.

Morphine may increase anticoagulant activity of coumarin and other anticoagulants.

Carcinogenicity/Mutagenicity:

Long-term studies to determine the carcinogenic and mutagenic potential of morphine are not available.

Pregnancy:

Teratogenic Effects—Pregnancy Category C: Animal production studies have not been conducted with morphine. It is also not known whether morphine can cause fetal harm when administered to a pregnant woman or can affect reproduction capacity. Morphine should be given to a pregnant woman only if clearly needed.

Labor and Delivery:

Morphine readily crosses the placental barrier and, if administered during labor, may lead to respiratory depression in the neonate.

Nursing Mothers:

Morphine has been detected in human milk. For this reason, caution should be exercised when morphine is administered to a nursing woman.

Pediatric Usage:

Safety and effectiveness in children have not been established.

Adverse Reactions:

THE MAJOR HAZARDS OF MORPHINE AS OF OTHER NARCOTIC ANALGESICS, ARE RESPIRATORY DEPRESSION AND, TO A LESSER DEGREE, CIRCULATORY DEPRESSION, RESPIRATORY ARREST, SHOCK, AND CARDIAC ARREST HAVE OCCURRED.

The most frequently observed adverse reactions include lightheadedness, dizziness, sedation, nausea, vomiting, and sweating. These effects seem to be more prominent in ambulatory patients and in those who are not suffering severe pain. In such individuals, lower doses are advisable. Some adverse reactions may be alleviated in the ambulatory patient if he lies down.

Other adverse reactions include the following:

Central Nervous System—Euphoria, dysphoria, weakness, headache, insomnia, agitation, disorientation, and visual disturbances.

Gastrointestinal—Dry mouth, anorexia, constipation, and biliary tract spasm.

Cardiovascular—Flushing of the face, bradycardia, palpitation, faintness, and syncope.

Genitourinary—Urinary retention or hesitancy, anti-diuretic effect, and reduced libido and/or potency.

Allergic—Pruritus, urticaria, other skin rashes, edema, and, rarely hemorrhagic urticaria.

Treatment of the most frequent adverse reactions:

Constipation—Ample intake of water or other liquids should be encouraged. Concomittant administration of a stool softener and a peristaltic stimulant with the narcotic analgesic can be an effective preventive measure for those patients in need of therapeutics. If elimination does not occur for two days, an enema should be administered to prevent impaction.

In the event diarrhea occurs, seepage around a fecal impaction is a possible cause to consider before antidiarrheal measures are employed.

Nausea and Vomiting—Phenothiazines and antihistamines can be effective treatments for nausea of the medullary and vestibular sources respectively. However, these drugs may potentiate the side effects of the narcotics or the antinauseant.

Drowsiness (sedation)—Once pain control is achieved, undesirable sedation can be minimized by titrating the dosage to a level that just maintains a tolerable pain or pain free state.

Drug Abuse and Dependence: Morphine Sulfate, narcotic, is a Schedule II controlled substance under the Federal Controlled Substance Act. As with other narcotics, some patients may develop a physical and psychological dependence on morphine. They may increase dosage without consulting a physician and subsequently may develop a physical dependence on the drug. In such cases, abrupt discontinuance may precipitate typical withdrawal symptoms, including convulsions. Therefore the drug should be withdrawn gradually from any patient known to be taking excessive dosages over a long period of time.

In treating the terminally ill patient the benefit of pain relief may outweigh the possibility of drug dependence. **The chance of drug dependence is substantially reduced when the patient is placed on scheduled narcotic programs instead of a "pain to relief-of-pain" cycle typical of a PRN regimen.**

Overdosage:

Signs and Symptoms: Serious overdose with morphine is characterized by respiratory depression (a decrease in respiratory rate and/or tidal volume, Cheyne-Stokes respiration, cyanosis), extreme somnolence progressing to stupor or coma, skeletal muscle flaccidity, cold or clammy skin, and sometimes bradycardia and hypotension. In severe overdosage, apnea, circulatory collapse, cardiac arrest and death may occur.

Treatment: Primary attention should be given to the re-establishment of adequate respiratory exchange through provision of a patent airway and the institution of assisted or controlled ventilation. The narcotic antagonist naloxone is a specific antidote against respiratory depression which may result from overdosage or unusual sensitivity to narcotics, including morphine. Therefore, an appropriate dose of naloxone (usual initial adult dose: 0.4 mg) should be administered, preferably by the intravenous route and simultaneously with efforts at respiratory resuscitation. Since the duration of action of morphine may exceed that of the antagonist, the patient should be kept under continued surveillance and repeated doses of the antagonist should be administered as needed to maintain adequate respiration.

An antagonist should not be administered in the absence of clinically significant respiratory or cardiovascular depression.

Oxygen, intravenous fluids, vasopressors and other supportive measures should be employed as indicated.

Gastric emptying may be useful in removing unabsorbed drug.

Dosage and Administration:

ROXANOL™—Usual Adult Oral Dose: 10 to 30 mg every 4 hours or as directed by physician. Dosage is a patient dependent variable, therefore increased dosage may be required to achieve adequate analgesia.

For control of chronic, agonizing pain in patients with certain terminal disease, this drug should be administered on a regularly scheduled basis, every 4 hours, at the lowest dosage level that will achieve adequate analgesia.

Note: Medication may suppress respiration in the elderly, the very ill, and those patients with respiratory problems, therefore lower doses may be required.

Morphine Dosage Reduction: During the first two to three days of effective pain relief, the patient may sleep for many hours. This can be misinterpreted as the effect of excessive analgesic dosing rather than the first sign of relief in a pain exhausted patient. The dose, therefore, should be maintained for at least three days before reduction, if respiratory activity and other vital signs are adequate.

Following successful relief of severe pain, periodic attempts to reduce the narcotic dose should be made. Smaller doses or complete discontinuation of the narcotic analgesic may become feasible due to a physiologic change or the improved mental state of the patient.

How Supplied:

Roxanol™
(Morphine Sulfate Intensified Oral Solution)
20 mg per ml
NDC 0054-3751-44: Bottle of 30 ml with calibrated dropper.
NDC 0054-3751-50: Bottle of 120 ml with calibrated dropper.

DEA Order Form Required

Caution: Federal law prohibits dispensing without prescription.

SODIUM POLYSTYRENE SULFONATE SUSPENSION ℞

Description: Each 60 ml contains:
Sodium Polystyrene Sulfonate USP .... 15 g
Sorbitol Solution USP .... 21.5 ml
Alcohol 0.3%

The suspension is cherry-flavored and also contains propylene glycol USP, Veegum®, sodium saccharin USP, methylparaben NF, propylparaben NF, flavors, and purified water USP.

This concentration of resin gives a sodium content of 1.5 g (65 mEq) per 60 ml. It is a brown, slightly viscous suspension which has an exchange capacity of approximately 3 mEq of potassium per 4 ml (per gram of resin) of suspension in vitro. This product may be administered either orally or rectally.

Action: The action of this product is to partially release sodium ions from the resin, and replace them by potassium ions as the resin passes along the intestine or is retained in the colon after administration by enema. For the most part, this action occurs in the large intestine, which excretes potassium ions to a greater degree than does the small intestine. The efficiency of this process is limited and unpredictably variable. It commonly approximates the order of 33%, but the range is so large that definitive indices of electrolyte balance must be clearly monitored. Frequent serum potassium determinations, at least once every 24 hours, should be done in order to adjust the individual dosage. The action of this product can be accomplished by either oral administration or by retention enema.

Indication: Sodium Polystyrene Sulfonate suspension is indicated for treatment of hyperkalemia.

Warnings: Since the effective lowering of serum potassium with this product may take hours to days, treatment with this drug alone may be insufficient to rapidly correct severe hyperkalemia associated with states of rapid tissue breakdown (e.g., burns and renal failure) or hyperkalemia so marked as to constitute a medical emergency. Therefore, other definitive measures, including dialysis, should always be considered and may be imperative. Serious potassium deficiency can occur from Sodium Polystyrene Sulfonate therapy. The effect must be carefully controlled by frequent serum potassium determinations within each 24 hour period. Since intracellular potassium deficiency is not always reflected by serum potassium levels, the level at which treatment with this product should be discontinued must be determined individually for each patient. Important aids in making this determination are the patient's clinical condition and electrocardiogram. Early clinical signs of severe hypokalemia include a pattern of irritable confusion and delayed thought processes. Electrocardiographically, severe hypokalemia is often associated with a lengthened Q-T interval, widening, flattening, or inversion of the T wave, and prominant U waves. Also, cardiac arrhythmias may occur, such as premature atrial, nodal, and ventricular contractions, and supraventricular and ventricular tachycardias. The toxic effects of digitalis are likely to be exaggerated. Marked hypokalemia can also be manifested by severe muscle weakness, at times extending into frank paralysis.

Like all cation-exchange resins, Sodium Polystyrene Sulfonate is not totally selective (for potassium) in its actions, and small amounts of other cations such as magnesium and calcium can also be lost during treatment. Accordingly, patients receiving the product should be monitored for all applicable electrolyte disturbances. Systemic alkalosis has been reported after cation-exchange resins were administered orally in combination with nonabsorbable cation-donating antacids and laxatives such as magnesium hydroxide and aluminum carbonate. Magnesium hydroxide should not be administered with the product. One case of grand mal seizure has been reported in a patient with chronic hypocalcemia of renal failure who was given Sodium Polystyrene Sulfonate with magnesium hydroxide as a laxative. Also, the simultaneous oral administration of the product with nonabsorbable cation-donating antacids and laxatives may reduce the resin's potassium exchange capacity.

Precautions: Caution is advised when the product is administered to patients who cannot tolerate even a small increase in sodium loads (i.e., severe congestive heart failure, severe hypertension, or marked edema). In such instances compensatory restriction of sodium intake from other sources may be indicated.

If constipation occurs, patients should be treated with sorbital (from 10 to 20 ml of 70% syrup every 2 hours or as needed to produce 1 or 2 watery stools daily), a measure which also reduces any tendency to fecal impaction.

Adverse Reactions: The product may cause some degree of gastric irritation. Anorexia, nausea, vomiting, and constipation may occur especially if high doses are given. Also, hypokalemia, hypocalcemia, and significant sodium retention may occur. Occasionally diarrhea develops. Large doses in elderly individuals may cause fecal impaction (see Precautions). This effect may be obviated through usage of the resin in enemas as described under Dosage and Administration. Intestinal obstruction due to concretions of aluminum hydroxide, when used in combination with the product, has been reported.

Dosage and Administration: The recommended oral adult dose is 60 ml (4 tablespoonfuls) of suspension (15 g of resin) given one to four times a day. This should be accompanied by frequent serum potassium determinations.

A lower dose of the resin is recommended for children.

The suspension may also be given as a retention enema, but due to less effective potassium exchange, it is recommended that 120 to 180 ml of suspension be used (30 to 45 g of resin). The suspension should be administered following a cleansing enema. The suspension is administered at body temperature, into the sigmoid colon by the use of a tipped rubber tube and left in the colon for several hours, if possible. The hip may be elevated on pillows to prevent back leakage if necessary. The colon is then irrigated with a nonsodium containing solution at body temperature to remove the resin. The returns are drained through a Y-tube connection with as much as two quarts of flushing solution possibly needed.

The length of treatment will depend on the determined serum potassium levels in the individual patient.

The product should not be heated, for to do so may alter the exchange properties of the resin.

How Supplied: NDC 0054-8814-11: Unit dose bottle filled to deliver 60 ml, 10 bottles per shipper. NDC 0054-3084-63: 500 ml bottle

Store at Controlled Room Temperature
15°-30°C (59°-86°F)
Dispense in a tight container as defined
in the USP/NF.

Caution: Federal law prohibits dispensing without prescription.

EDUCATIONAL MATERIAL

Booklets
"Cancer Pain Management—A Dialogue," Selections from Opioid Analgesics in the Management of Clinical Pain, free to Physicians and Pharmacists
"Oral Morphine in Advanced Cancer," Robert G. Twycross and Sylvia A. Lack, Practical guidelines on the considerations which must be taken into account when initiating oral morphine therapy, free to Physicians and Pharmacists
Brochures
"Potassium Iodide Oral Solution USP—Thyroid Blocking in a Radiation Emergency," Information for professionals and consumers, free to Physicians, Pharmacists, and Patients

---

Rydelle Laboratories, Inc.
Subsidiary of S. C. Johnson & Son, Inc.
**1525 HOWE STREET
RACINE, WI 53403**

FIBERALL™ Natural Flavor
[fi'ber-al]

Description: Fiberall is a bulk forming non-irritant laxative which contains no sugar. The active ingredient is refined hydrophilic mucilloid, a recognized dietary fiber, extracted from the seed husk of blond psyllium seed (Plantago ovata). The smooth gelatinous bulk formed by Fiberall encourages peristaltic activity and a more normal elimination of the bowel contents.

The recommended dose of one slightly rounded teaspoonful (5g) contains 3.4g of psyllium hydrophillic mucilloid, wheat bran, less than 10mg of sodium, less than 60mg of potassium, and provides less than 6 calories.

Indications: Fiberall is indicated for the management of chronic constipation, temporary constipation caused by illness or pregnancy, in irritable bowel syndrome, and for constipation related to duodenal ulcer or diverticulosis. Fiberall is also indicated for stool softening in patients with hemorrhoids after anorectal surgery.

Actions: The homogenous, high fiber formula of Fiberall is readily dispersed in liquids and acts without irritants or stimulants in the gastrointestinal tract.

Dosage and Administration: The recommended daily dosage for adults is one slightly rounded teaspoonful (5g) stirred into an 8 oz. glass of cool water or other liquid and taken orally one to three times daily according to the individual response. An additional glass of liquid is recommended and generally provides optimal response. Maximum benefits are usually obtained after two or three days of regular use of Fiberall.

Contraindications: fecal impaction or intestinal obstruction.

How Supplied: Powder, in 5, 10, and 15 oz. containers.

FIBERALL™ Orange Flavor
[fi'ber-al]

Description: Fiberall is a bulk forming non-irritant laxative which contains no sugar. The active ingredient is refined hydrophillic mucilloid, a recognized dietary fiber, extracted from the seed husk of blond psyllium seed (Plantago ovata). The smooth gelatinous bulk formed by Fiberall encourages peristaltic activity and a more normal elimination of the lower bowel contents.

The recommended dose of one slightly rounded teaspoonful (5.9g) contains 3.4g of psyllium hydrophillic mucilloid, wheat bran, natural and artificial flavor, less than 40mg of saccharin, citric acid, yellow #6 Lake and beta-carotene (coloring agents) less than 10mg of sodium, less than 60mg of potassium, and provides less than 8 calories (calculated).

Indications: Fiberall is indicated for the management of chronic constipation, temporary constipation caused by illness or pregnancy, in irritable bowel syndrome, and for constipation related to duodenal ulcer or diverticulosis. Fiberall is also indicated for stool softening in patients with hemorrhoids after anorectal surgery.

Actions: The homogenous, high fiber formula of Fiberall is readily dispersed in liquids and acts without irritants or stimulants in the gastrointestinal tract.

Dosage and Administration: The recommended daily dosage for adults is one slightly rounded teaspoonful (5.9g) stirred into an 8 oz. glass of cool water or other liquid and taken orally one to three times daily according to the individual response. An additional glass of liquid is recommended and generally provides optimal response. Maximum benefits are usually obtained after two or three days of regular use of Fiberall.

Contraindications: fecal impaction or intestinal obstruction.

How Supplied: Powder, in 5, 10, and 15 oz. containers.

Rystan Company, Inc.
**47 CENTER STREET
P.O. BOX 214
LITTLE FALLS, NJ 07424**

CHLORESIUM®
[klor-eez'ium]
Ointment and Solution
Healing and Deodorizing Agent

Composition: Ointment: 0.5% water-soluble chlorophyll derivatives (Rystan brand, 100% concentration) in a hydrophilic base. Solution: 0.2% chlorophyll derivatives in isotonic saline solution.

Actions and Uses: To promote normal healing, relieve pain and inflammation and reduce malodors in wounds, burns, surface ulcers, cuts, abrasions and skin irritations.

Administration and Dosage: Ointment: Apply generously and cover with gauze, linen or other appropriate dressing. Dressings preferably changed no more often than every 48 to 72 hours. Solution: Apply full strength as continuous wet dressing, or instill directly into sinus tracts, fistulae, deep ulcers or cavities. As a mouthwash, use half strength.

Side Effects: CHLORESIUM Ointment and Solution are soothing and nontoxic. Sensitivity

Continued on next page

Rystan—Cont.

reactions are extremely rare, and only a few instances of slight itching or irritation have been reported.
How Supplied: Ointment: 1 oz. and 4 oz. tubes, 1 lb. jars. Solution: 8 oz. and 32 oz. bottles.

DERIFIL® Tablets and Powder
[der'ah-fil]
Fecal and Urinary Deodorizer

Composition: 100 mg. water-soluble chlorophyll derivatives (Rystan brand, 100% concentration) per tablet or per teaspoonful of prepared solution.
Actions and Uses: Oral tablet or solution for control of fecal and urinary odors in colostomy, ileostomy or incontinence; also to deodorize certain necrotic, ulcerative lesions such as decubitus ulcers; also urinary and fecal fistulas and certain breath and body odors not related to faulty hygiene.
Administration and Dosage: In incontinence, one tablet by mouth (or one teaspoonful of solution prepared by dissolving 1 oz. of powder in 1 pint of water) daily at mealtime or any other convenient time. For other conditions, the effective dosage varies with the severity of the odor problem (ordinarily within the range of one to three tablets daily) and is best determined by trial and error.
NOTE: Deodorizing effect is cumulative, may require up to seven days to reach maximum. If preferred, tablets may be placed directly in the ostomy appliance.
Side Effects: No toxic effects have been reported from use of DERIFIL, even at high dosage levels for extended periods. A temporary, mild laxative effect may be noted, and the stool is commonly stained dark green. Isolated instances of stomach discomfort or cramps have been reported on high dosages of DERIFIL.
How Supplied: Bottles of 30, 100 and 1000 tablets; 1 oz. and 10 oz. bottles of powder.

PANAFIL® Ointment   ℞
[pan'ah-fil]
PANAFIL®—White Ointment   ℞

Composition: PANAFIL contains standardized papain 10%; urea, U.S.P. 10%; and water-soluble chlorophyll derivatives, 0.5% in a hydrophilic base. PANAFIL—White is identical except that the chlorophyll derivatives are omitted.
Action and Uses: For enzymatic debridement and promotion of normal healing (and deodorization, with regular PANAFIL) of surface lesions, particularly where healing is retarded by necrotic tissue, fibrinous or purulent debris, or eschar.
Administration and Dosage: Apply directly to lesion once or twice daily and cover with gauze. At each redressing, irrigate lesion with mild cleansing solution (*not* hydrogen peroxide solution which may inactivate papain) to remove any accumulation of liquefied necrotic material.
Side Effects: An occasional itching or stinging sensation is sometimes associated with the first application of proteolytic enzymes.
Precautions: Not to be used in eyes.
How Supplied: PANAFIL—1 oz. tubes, 1 lb. jars. PANAFIL—White—1 oz. tubes.

PROPHYLLIN®
[pro-fil'in]
Wet Dressing Powder and Ointment

Composition: Each 2.3 gm. powder packet (or teaspoonful of bulk powder) in 8 ounces of water makes a solution containing 1% sodium propionate and 0.0025% water-soluble chlorophyll derivatives (Rystan brand, 100% concentration). Ointment: 5% sodium propionate and 0.0125% chlorophyll derivatives in an emollient base.
Action and Uses: Antifungal, antibacterial, antipruritic, antiinflammatory. Solution is nonastringent, nonirritating (even around eyes). Useful in dermatophytosis, contact dermatoses, eczemas, vulvovaginitis, minor burns.
Administration and Dosage: Use solution as wet dressing, soak, mouthwash or douche. Half-strength solution (one packet in 16 oz. water) may be preferred for footbath or in severe inflammation. Ointment: Apply liberally several times daily and on retiring.
How Supplied: Powder: Cartons of 12 packets and in 4 oz. jars. Ointment: 1 oz. tubes.

Sandoz, Inc.
Pharmaceutical Division
ROUTE 10
EAST HANOVER, NJ 07936

ASBRON G® ELIXIR and   ℞
[az'bron]
ASBRON G® INLAY-TABS®

The following prescribing information is based on official labeling in effect on November 1, 1984.
Description: Each ASBRON G INLAY-TAB and tablespoonful (15 ml) of ASBRON G Elixir contains: theophylline sodium glycinate 300 mg (equivalent to 150 mg theophylline), guaifenesin 100 mg. The elixir supplies the active ingredients in a solution containing 15% alcohol. ASBRON G contains a bronchodilator and an expectorant.
Theophylline sodium glycinate, a methylxanthine, is a white crystalline powder that is freely soluble in water, has a slight ammoniacal odor and a bitter taste. It is an equimolar mixture of theophylline sodium and glycine buffered by an additional mole of the essential amino acid, glycine.
The expectorant component is guaifenesin (formerly called glyceryl guaiacolate) which helps loosen and thus clear the bronchial passageways of bothersome, thickened mucus. Guaifenesin, 3-(o-methoxyphenoxy)-1,2-propanediol, occurs as a fine, white powder having a bitter, aromatic taste and a slight odor of guaiacol. The powder tends to become lumpy on storage. It is freely soluble in alcohol and soluble in water.
Clinical Pharmacology: Theophylline sodium glycinate is more stable in the presence of hydrochloric acid due to the buffering action of glycine with subsequent reduction of the chance of theophylline precipitation in the stomach. This and the high solubility of the product are suggested as the reasons why this product has better gastric tolerance than aminophylline.
Theophylline, the active ingredient of theophylline sodium glycinate, accounts for 50% of the weight of this compound. Theophylline sodium glycinate is highly effective in relaxing the smooth muscle of the bronchioles and the pulmonary blood vessels, thus acting primarily as a bronchodilator, pulmonary vasodilator and smooth muscle relaxant. Like other xanthines, theophylline sodium glycinate is a coronary vasodilator, a diuretic, a cerebral, cardiac and skeletal muscle stimulant.
Theophylline acts by inhibiting phosphodiesterase which causes an increase in intracellular cyclic AMP. This action produces smooth muscle relaxation and inhibits the release of histamine and other bronchoconstricting mediators from mast cells.
In vitro, using human white blood cells, theophylline has been shown to react synergistically with beta agonists to increase intracellular cyclic AMP. More data is required to clearly establish if theophylline and the beta agonists are synergistic or additive in vivo.
Even after prolonged therapy, it has not been possible to demonstrate the development of tolerance to theophylline sodium glycinate.
The half-life of theophylline varies from individual to individual. Since effective bronchodilatation depends upon maintaining serum theophylline levels between 10-20 mg/dl (10-20 mcg/ml), the determination of serum theophylline can be of value.
The half-life of theophylline is prolonged in alcoholism, in patients with reduced hepatic or renal function, congestive heart failure and in patients receiving antibiotics such as triacetyloleandomycin, erythromycin, clindamycin and lincomycin. Fever can also prolong theophylline half-life.
Cigarette smoking (1-2 packs per day) enhances theophylline elimination. The half-life of theophylline is shortened with cigarette smoking. This effect is probably related to the induction of enzymes and requires between three months and two years to normalize after stopping tobacco usage.
By increasing respiratory tract fluid, guaifenesin reduces the viscosity of tenacious secretions and acts as an expectorant. The drug is effective in productive as well as nonproductive cough, but is of particular value in dry, nonproductive cough which tends to injure the mucous membranes of the air passages.
[See table below].
Indications and Usage: For relief of acute bronchial asthma and for reversible bronchospasm associated with chronic bronchitis and emphysema.
Contraindications: ASBRON G INLAY-TABS and ASBRON G Elixir are contraindicated in individuals who have shown hypersensitivity to any of the components.
Warnings: There is an excellent correlation between high theophylline blood levels and the clinical manifestations of toxicity in (1) patients with lowered body plasma clearances (due to transient cardiac decompositions), (2) chronic obstructive lung disease or patients with liver dysfunction, (3) patients who are older than 55 years of age, particularly males.
There are often no early signs of theophylline toxicity such as nausea and restlessness which may appear in up to 50% of patients. Convulsions or ventricular arrhythmias may be the first signs of toxicity.
Excessive doses of theophylline sodium glycinate may be expected to be toxic and serum theophylline levels are recommended to monitor therapy. The incidence of toxicity increases significantly at levels greater than 20 mcg/ml. Many patients who have higher theophylline serum levels exhibit tachycardia. Theophylline products often worsen preexisting arrhythmias.
ASBRON G INLAY-TABS, ASBRON G Elixir and other oral theophylline compounds should never be used to treat status asthma.
Precautions:
General: Theophylline should be used with caution in patients with severe cardiovascular disease, severe hypoxemia, hypertension, hyperthyroidism, acute myocardial injury, obstructive lung disease, liver disease, in the elderly and in neonates.
Great caution should be used in giving theophylline to patients in congestive heart failure. Such

ASBRON G — THEOPHYLLINE ELIMINATION CHARACTERISTICS

Group	Theophylline Renal Clearance Rates	Half-Life Average
Children	1.4 ml/kg/min	3.5 hours
Adults with uncomplicated asthma	1.2 ml/kg/min	7 hours
Older adults with chronic obstructive pulmonary disease	0.6 ml/kg/min	up to 24 hours
Adults with chronic obstructive pulmonary disease and cor pulmonale or other causes of heart failure and liver pathology	0.6 ml/kg/min and less	may exceed 24 hours
Young smokers	Not available	4.3 hours

patients have markedly prolonged theophylline blood levels which have persisted for long periods after discontinuation of the drug.

Smokers have a shorter mean half-life of theophylline than nonsmokers and may require larger doses of theophylline.

Theophylline sodium glycinate should not be administered concurrently with other theophylline containing products.

Theophylline should be given with caution to patients with a history of peptic ulcer. Theophylline may act as a local irritant in the gastrointestinal tract.

Information for Patients: The importance of adherence to the prescribed dosage regimen should be stressed. Patients should be informed of symptoms associated with theophylline toxicity such as nausea and restlessness.

Laboratory Tests: There is great patient-to-patient variation in the serum half-life of theophylline. Therefore, when possible, serum theophylline levels should be measured to assist in titration of dosage.

Drug Interactions: The use of theophylline sodium glycinate with ephedrine and other sympathomimetic bronchodilators may result in a significant increase in side effects.
[See table above].

Drug/Laboratory Test Interactions
Theophylline has been shown to increase the urinary excretion of catecholamines. The VMA test for catechols may be falsely elevated by guaifenesin. Theophylline may increase the apparent serum uric acid in certain manual or automated chemical procedures by being treated as if it were uric acid. Guaifenesin may increase renal clearance for urate and thereby lower the serum uric acid. It may also falsely elevate the level of urinary 5H1AA in certain serotonin metabolite chemical tests.

Carcinogenesis, Mutagenesis, Impairment of Fertility: No data are available on the long-term potential for carcinogenicity, mutagenicity or impairment of fertility in animals or humans.

Pregnancy: *Pregnancy Category C*—Animal reproduction studies have not been conducted with ASBRON-G. Safe use in pregnancy has not been established relative to possible adverse effects on fetal development. Therefore, theophylline should not be used in pregnant patients unless, in the judgment of the physician, the potential benefits outweigh possible hazards.

Nursing Mothers: It is not known whether this drug is excreted in human milk. Because many drugs are excreted in human milk, caution should be observed when ASBRON G INLAY-TABS or ASBRON-G Elixir is administered to a nursing mother.

Pediatric Use: See Dosage and Administration Section for mg/kg dosage in pediatric patients.

Drug	Effect
Aminophylline with Lithium Carbonate	Increased excretion of Lithium Carbonate
Aminophylline with Propranolol	Antagonism of Propranolol effect
Theophylline with Furosemide	Increased Diuresis
Theophylline with Hexamethonium	Decreased Hexamethonium-induced chronotropic effect
Theophylline with Reserpine	Reserpine-induced Tachycardia
Theophylline with Cimetidine	Increased theophylline blood levels
Theophylline with clindamycin, troleandomycin, erythromycin, lincomycin	Increased theophylline blood levels

Adverse Reactions: Included in this listing which follows are adverse reactions, some of which may have been reported with theophylline sodium glycinate. However, pharmacological similarities among the xanthine drugs require that each of the reactions be considered when theophylline is administered. The most consistent adverse reactions are usually due to overdosage of theophylline sodium glycinate and are:

Gastrointestinal: nausea, vomiting, epigastric pain, hematemesis, diarrhea.

Central Nervous System: headaches, irritability, restlessness, insomnia, reflex hyperexcitability, muscle twitching, clonic and tonic generalized convulsions.

Cardiovascular: palpitation, tachycardia, extrasystoles, flushing hypotension, circulatory failure, life-threatening ventricular arrhythmias.

Respiratory: tachypnea.

Renal: albuminuria, increased excretion of renal tubular cells and red blood cells; potentiation of diuresis.

Others: hyperglycemia and inappropriate ADH syndrome.

Overdosage (Management):
If potential oral overdose is established and seizure has not occurred: (1) induce vomiting and resort to gastric lavage if the patient fails to vomit within 20-30 minutes; (2) administer a cathartic (this is particularly important if sustained-release preparations have been taken) and activated charcoal after successful vomiting has been induced or adequate gastric lavage performed.

If patient is having a seizure: (1) establish an airway; (2) administer O_2; (3) treat the seizure with intravenous diazepam 0.1 to 0.3 mg/kg up to 10 mg; (4) monitor vital signs, maintain blood pressure and provide adequate hydration.

Postseizure Coma: (1) maintain airway and oxygenation; (2) if a result of oral medication, follow above recommendations to prevent absorption of drug, but tracheal intubation and lavage will have to be performed instead of inducing emesis, and the cathartic and charcoal will need to be introduced via a large bore gastric lavage tube; (3) continue to provide full supportive care and adequate hydration while waiting for drug to be metabolized. In general, the drug is metabolized sufficiently rapidly so as to not warrant consideration of dialysis.

Dosage and Administration: Therapeutic serum levels associated with optimal likelihood for benefit and minimal risk of toxicity are between 10-20 mcg/ml. There is great variation from patient to patient in the dosage of theophylline needed to achieve a therapeutic blood level because of variable rates of elimination. Because of this and because of the relatively narrow therapeutic blood level range associated with optimal results, the monitoring of serum theophylline levels is highly recommended. (See Laboratory Tests)

Usual Dosage: Adults—1 or 2 tablets or tablespoonfuls (15-30 ml), 3 or 4 times daily. Children 6 to 12—2 or 3 teaspoonfuls (10-15 ml), 3 or 4 times daily. Children 3 to 6—1 to 1½ teaspoonfuls (5-7.5 ml), 3 or 4 times daily. Children 1 to 3—½ to 1 teaspoonful (2.5-5 ml), 3 or 4 times daily.

Dosage Titration:
FOR PATIENTS NOT CURRENTLY RECEIVING THEOPHYLLINE PRODUCTS:
[See table below].
FOR PATIENTS CURRENTLY RECEIVING THEOPHYLLINE PRODUCTS: Determine, where possible, the time, amount, route of administration and form of the patient's last dose of theophylline.

The loading dose of theophylline will be based on the principle that each 0.5 mg/kg of theophylline administered as a loading dose will result in a 1 mcg/ml increase in serum theophylline concentration. Ideally, then, the loading dose should be deferred if a serum theophylline concentration can be rapidly obtained. If this is not possible, the clinician must exercise his judgment in selecting a dose based on the potential for benefit and risk. When there is sufficient respiratory distress to warrant a small risk, 2.5 mg/kg of theophylline is likely to increase the serum concentration when administered as a loading dose in rapidly absorbed form by only about 5 mcg/ml. If the patient is not already experiencing theophylline toxicity, this is unlikely to result in dangerous adverse effects.

Measurement of serum theophylline concentration during chronic therapy:
Blood for peak theophylline determinations should be obtained 1-2 hours after a dose of theophylline sodium glycinate. When determining theophylline serum concentrations in patients who have received chronic therapy, it is essential to establish that no doses were omitted in the 48 hours prior to the determination. Missed doses could result in recommendations of future doses that would cause serious toxicity due to overdosage.

DOSAGE ADJUSTMENT BASED ON SERUM THEOPHYLLINE MEASUREMENTS WHEN THESE INSTRUCTIONS HAVE NOT BEEN FOLLOWED MAY RESULT IN RECOMMENDATIONS THAT PRESENT RISK OF TOXICITY TO THE PATIENT.

PATIENTS SHOULD NEVER BE MAINTAINED ON A DOSAGE OF THEOPHYLLINE THAT IS NOT WELL TOLERATED. Patients experiencing toxic side effects should be instructed to skip the next regular dose and to resume theophylline therapy at a lower dosage when all side effects have disappeared.

ASBRON G

	Oral Loading Dose (Theophylline Sodium Glycinate)	Maintenance Dose For Next 12 Hours (Theophylline Sodium Glycinate)	Maintenance Dose Beyond 12 Hours (Theophylline Sodium Glycinate)
Infants	8 mg/kg *(4 mg/kg)	3-8 mg/kg q6h *(1.5-4.0 mg/kg q6h)	4-6 mg/kg q6h *(2-3 mg/kg q6h)
Children 6 months to 9 years	12 mg/kg *(6 mg/kg)	8 mg/kg q4h *(4 mg/kg q4h)	8 mg/kg q6h *(4 mg/kg q6h)
Children age 9-16 and young adult Smokers	12 mg/kg *(6 mg/kg)	6 mg/kg q4h *(3 mg/kg q4h)	6 mg/kg q6h *(3 mg/kg q6h)
Otherwise healthy nonsmoking adults	12 mg/kg *(6 mg/kg)	6 mg/kg q6h *(3 mg/kg q6h)	6 mg/kg q8h *(3 mg/kg q8h)
Older patients and patients with cor pulmonale	12 mg/kg *(6 mg/kg)	4 mg/kg q6h *(2 mg/kg q6h)	4 mg/kg q8h *(2 mg/kg q8h)
Patients with congestive heart failure, liver failure	12 mg/kg *(6 mg/kg)	4 mg/kg q8h *(2 mg/kg q8h)	2-4 mg/kg q12h *(1-2 mg/kg q12h)

Equivalent theophylline dosage indicated in parenthesis and marked with an asterisk (*).
** PEDIATRICS, Vol. 55, No. 5, May 1975.

Continued on next page

Sandoz—Cont.

Maximum Dose Without Measurement of Serum Concentration: Not to exceed the following: (WARNING: DO NOT ATTEMPT TO MAINTAIN ANY DOSAGE THAT IS NOT WELL TOLERATED.)
[See table below].
Use ideal (lean) body weight for obese patients in computing dosage.
Dosage should always be calculated on the basis of ideal (lean) body weight when mg/kg doses are stated. Theophylline does not distribute into fatty tissues. NEVER ATTEMPT TO MAINTAIN A DOSAGE THAT IS NOT WELL TOLERATED BY THE PATIENT.
How Supplied: ASBRON G INLAY-TABS (green with white inlay) in bottles of 100. ASBRON G Elixir (green) in pint bottles.
Company's Product Identification Mark(s): Tablets imprinted "Asbron G" on one side, "78–202" on the other.
[ASB-Z1 Issued July 1, 1982]
Shown in Product Identification Section, page 432

BELLADENAL® Tablets ℞
[bel-ad'in-ol]
BELLADENAL-S® Tablets

The following prescribing information is based on official labeling in effect on November 1, 1984.
Composition: Each Belladenal® Tablet and Belladenal-S® Tablet contains 0.25 mg Bellafoline® (levorotatory alkaloids of belladonna, as malates), and 50 mg phenobarbital, USP. (Warning: May be habit forming.)
Properties and Therapeutics: Superior antispasmodic/anticholinergic. The natural levorotatory alkaloids of belladonna (Bellafoline) in Belladenal give the antispasmodic-anticholinergic action of belladonna with only minimal central side effects. One Belladenal Tablet or Belladenal-S Tablet has the antispasmodic-anticholinergic action of 27 minims of tincture belladonna. Both Belladenal Tablets and Belladenal-S Tablets are scored to permit dosage adjustments necessary for optimal control of symptoms.

Indications
Based on a review of this drug by the National Academy of Sciences—National Research Council and/or other information, FDA has classified the indications as follows:
"Possibly" effective: As adjunctive therapy in the treatment of peptic ulcer and in the treatment of the irritable bowel syndrome (irritable colon, spastic colon, mucous colitis) and acute enterocolitis.
Final classification of the less-than-effective indications requires further investigation.

Contraindications: Glaucoma, elevated intraocular pressure, advanced hepatic or renal disease. Hypersensitivity to any of the components.
Precautions: Due to presence of barbiturate, may be habit forming. Caution is advised in the elderly.
Belladenal-S Tablets contain FD&C Yellow No. 5 (tartrazine) which may cause allergic-type reactions (including bronchial asthma) in certain susceptible individuals. Although the overall incidence of FD&C Yellow No. 5 (tartrazine) sensitivity in the general population is low, it is frequently seen in patients who also have aspirin hypersensitivity.
Side Effects: Urinary retention, blurred vision, dry mouth, flushing or drowsiness may occur.
Usual Dosage: Belladenal Tablets— Adults: 2 to 4 tablets per day, in divided dose of $\frac{1}{4}$ to $\frac{1}{2}$ tablet. Children: $\frac{1}{4}$ to $\frac{1}{2}$ tablet one to four times daily, according to age. Tablets are scored so that they can be divided easily.
Belladenal-S Tablets—Adults: One tablet in the morning and one at night.
Supplied: Belladenal Tablets (compressed, white, scored) in bottles of 100. Belladenal-S Tablets (compressed, scored tablets of tri-colored pattern: salmon pink, emerald green and white) in bottles of 100.
Company's Product Identification Mark(s): Belladenal Tablets embossed 78-28 on one side and scored on reverse side. Belladenal-S Tablets embossed 78-27 on one side and scored on reverse side.
[BED-Z13 Issued April 25, 1983]
Shown in Product Identification Section, page 432

BELLERGAL® Tablets and ℞
[bel'er-gal]
BELLERGAL-S® Tablets

The following prescribing information is based on official labeling in effect on November 1, 1984.
Description: Each BELLERGAL® Tablet contains: phenobarbital, USP, central sedative (Warning: May be habit forming), 20 mg; Gynergen® (ergotamine tartrate, USP) sympathetic inhibitor, 0.3 mg; Bellafoline® (levorotatory alkaloids of belladonna, as malates) parasympathetic inhibitor, 0.1 mg. Each BELLERGAL-S® Tablet contains: phenobarbital, USP, central sedative (Warning: May be habit forming), 40 mg; Gynergen (ergotamine tartrate, USP) sympathetic inhibitor, 0.6 mg; Bellafoline (levorotatory alkaloids of belladonna, as malates) parasympathetic inhibitor, 0.2 mg.
Clinical Pharmacology: Based on the concept that functional disorders frequently involve hyperactivity of both the sympathetic and parasympathetic nervous systems, the ingredients in BELLERGAL are combined to provide a balanced preparation designed to correct imbalance of the autonomic nervous system. The integrated action of BELLERGAL is effected through the combined administration of ergotamine and the levorotatory alkaloids of belladonna, specific inhibitors of the sympathetic and parasympathetic respectively, reinforced by the synergistic action of phenobarbital in dampening the cortical centers. It should be noted that on a weight basis the levorotatory alkaloids of belladonna have approximately twice the pharmacological effect as do the usual racemic mixtures.
Indications and Usage: BELLERGAL is employed in the management of disorders characterized by nervous tension and exaggerated autonomic response: *Menopausal disorders* with hot flushes, sweats, restlessness and insomnia. *Cardiovascular disorders* with palpitation, tachycardia, chest oppression and vasomotor disturbances. *Gastrointestinal disorders* with hypermotility, hypersecretion, "nervous stomach," and alternately diarrhea and constipation.
Interval treatment of *recurrent, throbbing headache*.
Contraindications: Peripheral vascular disease, coronary heart disease, hypertension, impaired hepatic or renal function, sepsis, pregnancy, nursing mothers and glaucoma. The concomitant administration of ergotamine and dopamine should be avoided, due to the increased potential for ischemic vasoconstriction. Phenobarbital is contraindicated in patients with a history of manifest or latent porphyria. Phenobarbital is contraindicated in those patients in whom the drug produces restlessness and/or excitement. BELLERGAL is contraindicated in patients with a demonstrated hypersensitivity to any of the components.
Warnings: Total weekly dosage of ergotamine tartrate should not exceed 10 mg. (This dosage corresponds to 33 BELLERGAL Tablets or 16 BELLERGAL-S Tablets). Due to presence of a barbituate, may be habit forming.
Precautions: Even though the ergotamine tartrate content of this product is low and untoward effects have been rare and of minor significance, caution should be exercised if large or prolonged dosage is contemplated, and physicians should be alert to possible peripheral vascular complications in patients sensitive to ergot. Due to the presence of the anticholinergic agent, special caution should be excerised in the use of this drug in patients with bronchial asthma or obstructive uropathy.
BELLERGAL-S contains FD&C Yellow No. 5 (tartrazine) which may cause allergic-type reactions (including bronchial asthma) in certain susceptible individuals. Although the overall incidence of FD&C Yellow No. 5 (tartrazine) sensitivity in the general population is low, it is frequently seen in patients who also have aspirin hypersensitivity.
Information for patients: Patients on large or prolonged dosage should be asked to report numbness or tingling of extremities, claudication or other symptoms of peripheral vasoconstriction.
Drug Interactions:
1. *Oral Anticoagulants:* Phenobarbital may lower the plasma levels of dicumarol (name previously used: bishydroxycoumarin) and may cause a decrease in anticoagulant activity as measured by the prothrombin time. More frequent monitoring of prothrombin time responses is indicated whenever phenobarbital is initiated or discontinued, and the dosage of anticoagulants should be adjusted accordingly.
2. *CNS depressants:* Combined administration of phenobarbital and CNS depressants such as alcohol, tricyclic antidepressants, phenothiazines and narcotic analgesics may result in a potentiation of the depressant action.
3. *Beta adrenergic blocking agents:* Although proof is lacking, several reports in the literature suggest a possible interaction between ergot alkaloids and beta adrenergic blocking agents. This interaction may result in excessive vasoconstriction. Although many patients can apparently take propranolol and ergot alkaloids without ill effects, there is enough evidence of an interaction to dictate closer surveillance of patients so treated.
4. *Hepatic metabolism:* Through the mechanism of enzyme induction caused by phenobarbital, a number of substances have been shown to be metabolized at an increased rate. In these cases, clinical responses should be closely monitored and appropriate dosage adjustments made. Included are such substances as griseofulvin, quinidine, doxycycline and estrogen. Although the meaning of published reports regarding the effects of phenobarbital on estrogen metabolism are unclear at this time, if avoidance of pregnancy is critical, consideration should be given to alternative methods of contraception.
5. *Phenytoin, sodium valproate, valproic acid:* The effect of barbiturates on the metabolism of phenytoin appears to be variable. Some investigators report an accelerating effect, while others report no effect. Because the effect of barbiturates on the metabolism of phenytoin is not predictable, phenytoin and barbiturate blood levels should be monitored more frequently if these drugs are given concurrently. Sodium valproate and valproic acid appear to decrease barbiturate metabolism; therefore, barbiturate blood levels should be monitored and appropriate dosage adjustments made as indicated.

ASBRON G Age	Theophylline Sodium Glycinate	Equivalent Theophylline
Under 9 years	48 mg/kg/day	24 mg/kg/day
9-12 years	40 mg/kg/day	20 mg/kg/day
12-16 years	36 mg/kg/day	18/mg/kg/day
Over 16 years	26 mg/kg/day or 1800 mg/day (WHICHEVER IS LESS)	13 mg/kg/day or 900 mg/day (WHICHEVER IS LESS)

6. *Tricyclic antidepressants:* Due to the presence of levorotatory alkaloids of belladonna, concomitant administration of tricyclic antidepressants may result in additive anticholinergic effects.

Carcinogenesis: No data are available on the long-term potential for carcinogenicity in animals or humans.

Pregnancy: *Pregnancy Category X*—due to the potential uterotonic effects of the ergot alkaloids, the use of BELLERGAL® during pregnancy is contraindicated. See "Contraindications" section.

Nursing Mothers: A number of ergot alkaloids inhibit the secretion of prolactin. Therefore, BELLERGAL is contraindicated in nursing mothers. See "Contraindications" section.

Pediatric Use: Safety and effectiveness in children have not been established.

Adverse Reactions: Tingling and other paresthesias of the extremities, blurred vision, palpitations, dry mouth, decreased sweating, decreased gastrointestinal motility, urinary retention, tachycardia, flushing, drowsiness occur rarely.

Drug Abuse and Dependence: Barbiturates may be habit-forming. Tolerance, psychological dependence, and physical dependence may occur especially following prolonged use of high doses. Daily administration in excess of 400 mg of pentobarbital or secobarbital for approximately 90 days is likely to produce some degree of physical dependence. By way of comparison, the phenobarbital component of BELLERGAL and BELLERGAL-S® at the highest recommended daily dosage amounts to 120 mg and 80 mg respectively.

Overdosage:

Management of Overdosage: While severe symptoms of overdosage with BELLERGAL have not been reported, theoretically they could occur. It is imperative to note that overdosage symptoms with BELLERGAL may be attributable to any one or more of the three active ingredients. Which toxic manifestation might predominate in any individual case would be impossible to predict but one should be alert to the various possibilities. When anticholinergic/antispasmodic drugs are taken in sufficient overdose to produce such severe symptoms, prompt treatment should be instituted. Gastric lavage and other measures to limit intestinal absorption should be initiated without delay.

Cholinesterase inhibitors administered parenterally may be necessary for treatment of the serious manifestations of anticholinergic overdosage. Additionally, symptomatic therapy, including oxygen, sedatives and control of hyperthermia may be necessary.

Acute barbiturate overdosage symptoms with BELLERGAL, while possible, have not been reported. While the usual procedures for handling barbiturate poisoning should be employed, keep in mind the possibility of anticholinergic overdosing effects.

Acute ergot overdosage symptoms with BELLERGAL, while possible, have not been reported. The usual procedures for handling ergot overdosage include the administration of a peripheral vasodilator to counteract the vasospasm.

Dosage and Administration: BELLERGAL Tablets: Four tablets daily (one in the morning, one at noon and two at bedtime) is the dose usually employed. In more resistant cases begin with six tablets daily, then gradually reduce dosage at weekly intervals according to response. Where required, continue with the smallest effective dose to maintain the improved status of the patient. BELLERGAL-S® Tablets: One in the morning and one in the evening.

How Supplied: BELLERGAL® Tablets round, shell pink, sugar-coated in bottles of 100 and 1000. BELLERGAL-S Tablets, compressed tablets of tricolored pattern: dark green, orange and light lemon yellow, in bottles of 100.

Company's Product Identification Mark(s): BELLERGAL Tablets printed triangle "S" on one side and "78-32" on the other.

BELLERGAL-S Tablets scored on one side, embossed "78-31" other side.

[BEG-Z9 Issued May 7, 1984]
Shown in Product Identification Section, page 432.

CAFERGOT® ℞
[kaf′er-got]
(ergotamine tartrate and caffeine) tablets, USP
(ergotamine tartrate and caffeine) suppositories, USP
CAFERGOT® P-B
Tablets and Suppositories
FOR NON-NARCOTIC RELIEF OF ENTIRE MIGRAINE SYNDROME AND OTHER VASCULAR HEADACHES

The following prescribing information is based on official labeling in effect on November 1, 1984.

Description: Each Cafergot® Tablet contains: 1 mg Gynergen® (ergotamine tartrate, USP) and 100 mg caffeine, USP. Each Cafergot Suppository contains: 2 mg Gynergen® (ergotamine tartrate, USP); 100 mg caffeine, USP; tartaric acid, NF; cocoa butter, NF.

Each Cafergot P-B Tablet contains: 1 mg Gynergen® (ergotamine tartrate, USP); 100 mg caffeine, USP; 0.125 mg Bellafoline® (levorotatory alkaloids of belladonna, as malates); 30 mg pentobarbital sodium, USP, (*Warning:* May be habit forming). Each Cafergot P-B Suppository contains: 2 mg Gynergen® (ergotamine tartrate, USP); 100 mg caffeine, USP; 0.25 mg Bellafoline® (levorotatory alkaloids of belladonna, as malates); 60 mg pentobarbital, USP. (*Warning:* May be habit forming); tartaric acid, NF; malic acid, lactose, USP; cocoa butter, NF.

Cafergot Suppositories and Cafergot P-B Suppositories are *sealed* in foil to afford protection from cocoa butter leakage. If an unavoidable period of exposure to heat softens the suppository, it should be chilled in ice-cold water to solidify it before removing the foil.

Actions: Ergotamine is an alpha adrenergic blocking agent with a direct stimulating effect on the smooth muscle of peripheral and cranial blood vessels and produces depression of central vasomotor centers. The compound also has the properties of serotonin antagonism. In comparison to hydrogenated ergotamine, the adrenergic blocking actions are less pronounced and vasoconstrictive actions are greater.

Caffeine, also a cranial vasoconstrictor, is added to further enhance the vasoconstrictive effect without the necessity of increasing ergotamine dosage. For individuals experiencing excessive nausea and vomiting during migraine attacks the further addition of the anticholinergic and antiemetic alkaloids of belladonna and pentobarbital for reduction of nervous tension has been provided.

Many migraine patients experience excessive nausea and vomiting during attacks, making it impossible for them to retain any oral medication. In such cases, therefore, the only practical means of medication is through the rectal route where medication may reach the cranial vessels directly, evading the splanchnic vasculature and the liver.

Indications:
Cafergot
Indicated as therapy to abort or prevent vascular headache, e.g., migraine, migraine variants, or so-called "histaminic cephalalgia".

Cafergot P-B
Indicated as therapy to abort or prevent vascular headache complicated by tension and gastrointestinal disturbances.

Contraindications: Peripheral vascular disease, coronary heart disease, hypertension, impaired hepatic or renal function, sepsis and pregnancy. Hypersensitivity to any of the components.

Precautions: Although signs and symptoms of ergotism rarely develop even after long term intermittent use of the orally or rectally administered drugs, care should be exercised to remain within the limits of recommended dosage.

Adverse Reactions: Vasoconstrictive complications, at times of a serious nature, may occur. These include pulselessness, weakness, muscle pains and paresthesias of the extremities and precordial distress and pain. Although these effects occur most commonly with long-term therapy at relatively high doses, they have also been reported with short-term or normal doses. Other adverse effects include transient tachycardia or bradycardia, nausea, vomiting, localized edema and itching.

Drowsiness may occur with Cafergot P-B.

Dosage and Administration: Procedure: For the best results, dosage should start at the first sign of an attack. Adults: *Orally*—2 tablets at start of attack; 1 additional tablet every ½ hour, if needed for full relief (maximum 6 tablets per attack, 10 per week). *Rectally*—1 suppository at start of attack; second suppository after 1 hour, if needed for full relief (maximum 2 suppositories per attack, 5 per week).

Maximum Adult Dosage:

Orally: Total dose for any one attack should not exceed 6 tablets.

Rectally: Two suppositories is the maximum dose for an individual attack.

Total weekly dosage should not exceed 10 tablets or 5 suppositories.

In carefully selected patients, with due consideration of maximum dosage recommendations, administration of the drug at bedtime may be an appropriate short-term preventive measure.

Overdosage: The toxic effects of an acute overdosage of Cafergot® (ergotamine tartrate and caffeine) are due primarily to the ergotamine component. The amount of caffeine is such that its toxic effects will be overshadowed by those of ergotamine. Symptoms include vomiting; numbness, tingling, pain and cyanosis of the extremities associated with diminished or absent peripheral pulses; hypertension or hypotension; drowsiness, stupor, coma, convulsions and shock. A case has been reported of reversible bilateral papillitis with ring scotomata in a patient who received five times the recommended daily adult dose over a period of 14 days.

Treatment consists of removal of the offending drug by induction of emesis, gastric lavage, and catharsis. Maintenance of adequate pulmonary ventilation, correction of hypotension, and control of convulsions are important considerations. Treatment of peripheral vasospasm should consist of warmth, but not heat, and protection of the ischemic limbs. Vasodilators may be used with benefit but caution must be exercised to avoid aggravating an already existent hypotension.

How Supplied: Cafergot Tablets shell pink colored, sugar coated. Bottles of 250 and cartons of three SigPak® (dispensing unit) packages, each containing 30 tablets in individual blisters. Cafergot Suppositories (sealed in fuchsia-colored aluminum foil) in boxes of 12. Cafergot P-B Tablets bright green, sugar coated. Bottles of 250 and cartons of three SigPak® (dispensing unit) packages, each containing 30 tablets in individual blisters. Cafergot P-B Suppositories (sealed in blue aluminum foil) in boxes of 12.

Company's Product Identification Mark(s): Cafergot Tablets imprinted "CAFERGOT" on one side, triangle (S) other side.

Cafergot P-B Tablets imprinted "78-36" on one side, triangle (S) other side.

Cafergot Suppositories imprinted "triangle (S) CAFERGOT SUPPOSITORY 78-33 SANDOZ".

Cafergot P-B Suppositories imprinted "triangle (S) CAFERGOT P-B SUPPOSITORY 78-35 SANDOZ".

[CAF-Z20 Issued April 23, 1984]
Shown in Product Identification Section, page 432

CEDILANID®-D ℞
[sĕ-de-lan′id]
(deslanoside) injection, USP

The following prescribing information is based on official labeling in effect on November 1, 1984.

Description: The cardiac (or digitalis) glycosides are a closely related group of drugs having in common specific and powerful effects on the myocardium. These drugs are found in a number of plants. The term "digitalis" is used to designate the whole group. Typically, the glycosides are composed of three portions, a steroid nucleus, a lactone ring, and a sugar (hence "glycosides").

Cedilanid-D (deslanoside) is provided as ampul solution containing the cardioactive glycoside, desacetyl lanatoside C. This agent is prepared by controlled alkaline hydrolysis of lanatoside C, a glycoside obtained from digitalis lanata.

Continued on next page

Sandoz—Cont.

Supplied in ampuls of 2 ml. Each 2 ml contains:
deslanoside, USP .... 0.4 mg
citric acid, USP, q.s. to...................... pH 6.2±0.3
sodium phosphate, USP .... 10.6 mg
alcohol, USP... 9.8% by vol.
glycerin, USP... 15% by wt.
water for injection, USP, q.s. to 2 ml

Action: The digitalis glycosides have qualitatively the same therapeutic effect on the heart. They (1) increase the force of myocardial contraction, (2) increase the refractory period of the atrioventricular (A-V) node, and (3) to a lesser degree, affect the sinoatrial (S-A) node and conduction system via the parasympathetic and sympathetic nervous systems.

Cedilanid-D (deslanoside) has its onset of action in about 5 minutes after intravenous administration and reaches peak effect in 2-4 hours. Therapeutic action persists for 2 to 5 days.

Indications:
1. "Congestive heart failure," all degrees, is the primary indication. The increased cardiac output results in diuresis and general amelioration of the disturbances characteristic of right (venous congestion, edema) and left (dyspnea, orthopnea, cardiac asthma) heart failure.
   Digitalis, generally, is most effective in "low output" and less effective in "high output" (bronchopulmonary insufficiency, infection, hyperthyroidism) heart failure.
   Digitalis should be continued after failure is abolished unless some known precipitating factor is corrected.
2. "Atrial fibrillation"— especially when the ventricular rate is elevated. Digitalis rapidly reduces ventricular rates and eliminates the pulse deficit. Palpitation, precordial distress or weakness are relieved and any concomitant congestive failure ameliorated.
   Digitalis is continued in doses necessary to maintain the desired ventricular rate and other clinical effects.
3. "Atrial flutter" digitalis slows the heart and regular sinus rhythm may appear. Frequently the flutter is converted to atrial fibrillation with a slow ventricular rate. Stopping digitalis at this point may be followed by restoration of sinus rhythm, especially if the flutter was of the paroxysmal type. It is preferable, however, to continue digitalis if failure ensues or if atrial flutter is a frequent occurrence.
4. "Paroxysmal atrial tachycardia" digitalis may be used, especially if it is resistant to lesser measures. Depending on the urgency, a more rapid acting parenteral preparation may be preferable to initiate digitalization, although if failure has ensued or paroxysms recur frequently, digitalis is maintained by oral administration.
   Digitalis is not indicated in sinus tachycardia or premature systoles in the absence of heart failure.

"Cardiogenic shock"—the value of digitalis is not established, but the drug is often employed, especially when the condition is accompanied by pulmonary edema. Digitalis seems to adversely affect shock due to infections.

Contraindications: The presence of toxic effects (See "Overdosage") induced by any digitalis preparation is an absolute contraindication to all of the glycosides.

"Allergy," though rare, does occur. It may not extend to all preparations and another may be tried.

"Ventricular Fibrillation"

"Ventricular tachycardia," unless congestive failure supervenes after a protracted episode not itself due to digitalis.

Warnings: Many of the arrhythmias for which digitalis is advised are identical with those reflecting digitalis intoxication. If the possibility of digitalis intoxication cannot be excluded, cardiac glycosides should be temporarily withheld if permitted by the clinical situation.

The patient with congestive heart failure may complain of nausea and vomiting. These symptoms may also be indications of digitalis intoxication. A clinical determination of the cause of these symptoms must be attempted before further drug administration.

Precautions: "Potassium depletion" sensitizes the myocardium to digitalis and toxicity is apt to develop even with usual dosage. Hypokalemia also tends to reduce the positive inotropic effect of digitalis.

Potassium wastage may result from diuretic, corticosteroid, hemodialysis and other therapy. It is apt to accompany malnutrition, old age and long-standing congestive heart failure.

"Acute myocardial infarction," severe pulmonary disease, or far advanced heart failure are apt to be more sensitive to digitalis and more prone to disturbances of rhythm.

"Calcium" affects contractility and excitability of the heart in a manner similar to that of digitalis. Calcium may produce serious arrhythmias in digitalized patients.

"Myxedema"—Digitalis requirements are less because excretion rate is decreased and blood levels are significantly higher.

"Incomplete AV block," especially patients subject to Stokes Adams attacks, may develop advanced or complete heart block. Heart failure in these patients can usually be controlled by other measures and by increasing the heart rate.

"Chronic constrictive pericarditis," is apt to respond unfavorably.

"Idiopathic hypertrophic subaortic stenosis" must be managed extremely carefully. Unless cardiac failure is severe it is doubtful whether digitalis should be employed.

"Renal insufficiency" delays the excretion of digitalis and dosage must be adjusted accordingly in patients with renal disease.

NOTE: This applies also to potassium administration should it become necessary.

Electrical conversion of arrhythmias may require adjustment of digitalis dosage.

Adverse Reactions: Gynecomastia, uncommon.

Overdosage, Toxic Effects: "Gastrointestinal" anorexia, nausea, vomiting, diarrhea—are the most common early symptoms of overdosages in the adult.

Uncontrolled heart failure may also produce such symptoms.

"Central Nervous System"—headache, weakness, apathy, visual disturbances.

"Cardiac Disturbances"—
Arrhythmias —"ventricular premature beats" is the most common.

Paroxysmal and nonparoxysmal nodal rhythms, atrioventricular (inference) dissociation and paroxysmal atrial tachycardia (PAT) with block are also common arrhythmias due to digitalis overdosage.

Conduction Disturbances—excessive slowing of the pulse is a clinical sign of digitalis overdosage. Atrioventricular block of increasing degree, may proceed to complete heart block.

NOTE: The electrocardiogram is fundamental in determining the presence and nature of these toxic disturbances. Digitalis may also induce other changes (as of the ST segment), but these provide no measure of the degree of digitalization.

TREATMENT OF TOXIC ARRHYTHMIAS: Digitalis is discontinued until after all signs of toxicity are abolished. This may be all that is necessary if toxic manifestations are not severe and appear after the time for peak effect of the drug.

Potassium salts are commonly used. Potassium chloride in divided doses totaling 4 to 6 gm. for adults provided renal function is adequate.

When correction of the arrhythmia is urgent, potassium is administered intravenously in a solution of 5 percent dextrose in water, a total of 40-100 mEq. (40 mEq. per 500 ml.) at the rate of 40 mEq. per hour unless limited by pain due to local irritation.

Additional amounts may be given if the arrhythmia is uncontrolled and the potassium well tolerated.

Electrocardiographic monitoring is indicated to avoid potassium toxicity, e.g. peaking of T waves.

CAUTION: Potassium should not be used and may be dangerous for severe or complete heart block due to digitalis and not related to any tachycardia.

Chelating agents to bind calcium may also be used to counteract the arrhythmia effect of digitalis toxicity, hypokalemia and of elevated serum calcium which may also precipitate digitalis toxicity. Four grams (0.8 percent solution) of the disodium salt of EDTA is dissolved in 500 ml of 5 percent dextrose in water (50 mg per ml) and administered over a period of 2 hours unless the arrhythmia is controlled before the infusion is completed.

A continuous electrocardiogram should be observed so that the infusion may be promptly stopped when the desired effect is achieved.

Other counteracting agents are: Quinidine, procainamide, and beta adrenergic blocking agents.

Dosage and Administration: "Parenteral" administration should be used only when the drug cannot be taken orally, or rapid digitalization is very urgent.

Parenteral digitalization can be obtained within 12 hours by giving 8 ml (1.6 mg) *either intramuscularly* or *intravenously*. By the I.V. route the dose may be given as one injection or in portions of 4 ml each. By I.M. route, 4 ml portions are injected at each of 2 sites.

After parenteral digitalization with Cedilanid-D (deslanoside) maintenance therapy may be accomplished by starting administration of an oral preparation, within 12 hours.

How Supplied:
Ampuls, 2 ml size (2 ml contains 0.4 mg deslanoside, USP) Boxes of 20 ampuls.

Being chemically pure and of constant potency, deslanoside, USP is standardized by weight; the ampul solution of Cedilanid-D (deslanoside) contains in each 2 ml:
deslanoside, USP .... 0.4 mg
citric acid, USP q.s. to...................... pH 6.2±0.3
sodium phosphate, USP .... 10.6 mg
alcohol, USP... 9.8% by vol.
glycerin, USP... 15% by wt.
water for injection, USP, q.s. to 2 ml
[CED-Z17 Issued March 26, 1984]

D.H.E. 45® Injection ℞
(dihydroergotamine mesylate) injection, USP

The following prescribing information is based on official labeling in effect on November 1, 1984.

Description: DHE45® is hydrogenated ergotamine as the mesylate. It is a clear, colorless, stable ampul solution containing per ml:
dihydroergotamine
  mesylate, USP .... 1 mg
methanesulfonic acid/sodium
  hydroxide .... q.s. to pH 3.75±0.5
alcohol, USP... 6.1% by vol.
glycerin, USP... 15% by wt.
water for injection, USP, q.s. to...................... 1 ml

Actions: Dihydroergotamine is an alpha adrenergic blocking agent with a direct stimulating effect on the smooth muscle of peripheral and cranial blood vessels, and produces depression of central vasomotor centers. The compound also has the properties of serotonin antagonism. In comparison to ergotamine, the adrenergic blocking actions are more pronounced, the vasoconstrictive actions somewhat less pronounced, and there is reduced incidence and degree of nausea and vomiting.

Onset of action occurs in 15 to 30 minutes following intramuscular administration and persists for 3-4 hours.

Repeated dosage at 1 hour intervals up to 3 hours may be required to obtain maximal effect.

Indications: As therapy to abort or prevent vascular headache, e.g., migraine, migraine variants, or so-called "histaminic cephalalgia" when rapid control is desired or when other routes of administration are not feasible.

Contraindications: Peripheral vascular disease, coronary heart disease, hypertension, impaired hepatic or renal function, sepsis and pregnancy. Hypersensitivity.

Adverse Reactions: Numbness and tingling of fingers and toes, muscle pains in the extremities, weakness in the legs, precordial distress and pain, transient tachycardia or bradycardia, nausea, vomiting, localized edema and itching.

Dosage and Administration: *For vascular headache,* 1 ml intramuscularly at first warning sign of headache, repeated at 1 hour intervals to a total of 3 ml. Optimal results are obtained by titrating the dose for several headaches to find the minimal effective dose for each patient and this dose should then be employed at onset of subsequent attacks. Where more rapid effect is desired, the intravenous route may be employed to a maximum of 2 ml. Total weekly dosage should not exceed 6 ml.

Overdosage: Failure to observe the upper limits of repeated parenteral dosage may result in eventual onset of the peripheral toxic signs and symptoms of ergotism. Treatment includes discontinuance of the drug, warmth, vasodilators, and good nursing care to prevent tissue damage.

How Supplied: As a clear, colorless and stable solution in ampuls containing:

dihydroergotamine
 mesylate, USP .... 1 mg
methanesulfonic acid/sodium
 hydroxide .... q.s. to pH 3.75±0.5
alcohol, USP.. 6.1% by vol.
glycerin, USP.. 15% by wt.
water for injection, USP, q.s. to..................... 1 ml

Ampuls, 1 ml size—boxes of 20.
To assure constant potency, protect the ampuls from light and heat. In the event the ampul solution becomes discolored, it should not be used.

[D.H.E.-Z16 Issued February 1, 1983]

DIAPID® Nasal Spray
[dī'a-pid"]
(lypressin)
nasal solution, USP

The following prescribing information is based on official labeling in effect on November 1, 1984.

Description: Diapid® (lypressin) Nasal Spray contains synthetic lysine-8-vasopressin with an activity of 50 USP Posterior Pituitary (Pressor) Units per ml (0.185 mg/ml). Lysine-8-vasopressin is a polypeptide and is one of the two known naturally occurring molecular forms of mammalian posterior pituitary antidiuretic hormone. This synthetic polypeptide is present as a protein-free substance in Diapid Nasal Spray. Unlike preparations of posterior pituitary antidiuretic hormone of animal origin, Diapid Nasal Spray is completely free of oxytocin and foreign proteins. The molecular formula of lysine-8-vasopressin is $C_{46}H_{65}N_{13}O_{12}S_2$.

Action: The principal pharmacologic action of lysine-8-vasopressin, the active ingredient of Diapid (lypressin) Nasal Spray, is similar to that of arginine-8-vasopressin, the posterior pituitary antidiuretic hormone occurring in man. Diapid Nasal Spray increases the rate of reabsorption of solute free water from the distal renal tubules, without significantly modifying the rate of glomerular filtration, producing a fall in free water clearance and an increase in urinary osmolality. The rates of solute and creatinine excretion noted with therapeutic doses of Diapid Nasal Spray suggest that sodium clearance and glomerular filtration rates are essentially unaltered by this hormone. Diapid Nasal Spray is relatively free of oxytocic activity when used within the recommended therapeutic dose levels.

It possesses little pressor activity, the ratio of pressor to antidiuretic activity being in the range of 1:1000.

The antidiuretic effect produced by Diapid Nasal Spray begins rapidly and usually reaches a peak within 30 to 120 minutes. Its usual duration of action is 3 to 8 hours.

Indications: Diapid Nasal Spray is indicated for the control or prevention of the symptoms and complications of diabetes insipidus due to deficiency of endogenous posterior pituitary antidiuretic hormone. These symptoms and complications include polydipsia, polyuria, and dehydration. It is particularly useful in patients with diabetes insipidus who have become unresponsive to other forms of therapy or who experience various types of local and/or systemic reactions, allergic reactions, or other undesirable effects (e.g., excessive fluid retention) from preparations of posterior pituitary antidiuretic hormone of animal origin.

Contraindications: There are no known contraindications to the use of Diapid (lypressin) Nasal Spray.

Warnings: The safety of this drug in pregnancy has not been established. The possibility of risk to the mother and unborn child should be weighed against potential benefits before the drug is administered to women of child-bearing age.

Precautions: Cardiovascular pressor effects with Diapid Nasal Spray are minimal or absent when it is administered as a nasal spray in therapeutic doses. Nevertheless, it should be used with caution in patients for whom such effects would not be desirable because mild blood pressure elevation has been noted in unanesthetized subjects who received lypressin intravenously. Large doses intranasally may cause coronary artery constriction and caution should be observed in treating patients with coronary artery disease.

The effectiveness of Diapid (lypressin) Nasal Spray may be lessened in patients with nasal congestion, allergic rhinitis, and upper respiratory infections because these conditions may interfere with absorption of the drug by the nasal mucosa. In this event, larger doses of Diapid Nasal Spray, or adjunctive therapy, may be needed.

Patients with a known sensitivity to anti-diuretic hormone should be tested for sensitivity to Diapid Nasal Spray.

Adverse Reactions: With clinical use of Diapid (lypressin) Nasal Spray, adverse reactions have been infrequent and mild. To date, such reactions have included rhinorrhea, nasal congestion, irritation and pruritus of the nasal passages, nasal ulceration, headache, conjunctivitis, heartburn secondary to excessive nasal administration with drippage into the pharynx, and abdominal cramps and increased bowel movements. Periorbital edema with itching has been reported. Inadvertent inhalation of Diapid Nasal Spray has resulted in substernal tightness, coughing, and transient dyspnea. In one patient, an overdose of Diapid Nasal Spray caused marked, but transient, fluid retention. Tolerance or tachyphylaxis to Diapid Nasal Spray has not been reported to date.

Hypersensitivity manifested by a positive skin test.

Dosage and Administration: Patients should be instructed to administer 1 or 2 sprays of Diapid® (lypressin) Nasal Spray to one or both nostrils whenever frequency of urination becomes increased or significant thirst develops. (One spray provides approximately 2 USP Posterior Pituitary [Pressor] Units.) The usual dosage for adults and children is 1 or 2 sprays in each nostril 4 times daily. An additional dose at bedtime is often helpful to eliminate nocturia, if it is not controlled with the regular daily dosage. For patients requiring more than 2 sprays per nostril every 4 to 6 hours, it is recommended that the time interval between doses be reduced rather than increasing the number of sprays at each dose. (More than 2 or 3 sprays in each nostril usually results in wastage because the unabsorbed excess will drain posteriorly, by way of the nasopharynx, into the digestive tract where it will be inactivated.)

Diapid Nasal Spray permits individualization of dosage necessary to control the symptoms of diabetes insipidus. Patients quickly learn to regulate their dosage in accordance with their degree of polyuria and thirst, and once determined, daily requirements remain fairly stable for months or years. Although most patients require 1 or 2 sprays of Diapid (lypressin) Nasal Spray in each nostril 4 times daily, dosage has ranged from 1 spray per day at bedtime to 10 sprays in each nostril every 3-4 hours. Requirements of the larger doses may represent greater severity of disease or other phenomena, such as poor nasal absorption. A seeming requirement for large doses of lypressin may be due to the presence of mixed hypothalamic-hypophyseal and nephrogenic diabetes insipidus, the latter condition being unresponsive to administration of antidiuretic hormone.

Diapid (lypressin) Nasal Spray is conveniently administered, from a compact and portable, plastic squeeze bottle, by inserting the nozzle of the bottle into the nostril and squeezing once firmly to deliver each short spray.

NOTE: To assure that a uniform, well-diffused spray is delivered, the bottle of Diapid Nasal Spray should be held upright and the patient should be in a vertical position with head upright.

Supplied: Diapid Nasal Spray is supplied in a plastic bottle that contains 8 ml of solution. Each ml of solution contains lypressin (0.185 mg) equivalent to 50 USP Posterior Pituitary (Pressor) Units and the following: propylparaben, NF, methylparaben, NF, sodium phosphate, USP, citric acid, USP, sodium chloride, USP, sorbitol solution, USP, glycerin, USP, sodium acetate, USP, acetic acid, NF, chlorobutanol, NF, (0.1%-0.002%), purified water, USP.

This product has an expiration date of 36 months.
[DIA-Z12 Issued March 1, 1983]

FIOGESIC® Tablets
[fē-ō-je'zik]

The following prescribing information is based on official labeling in effect on November 1, 1984.

Composition: Each Tablet contains Calurin® (calcium carbaspirin) 382 mg, equivalent to 300 mg aspirin; phenylpropanolamine hydrochloride, USP 25 mg; pheniramine maleate 12.5 mg; pyrilamine maleate, USP 12.5 mg.

Actions and Uses: For prompt, temporary relief of headache, sinus and nasal congestion, pain and fever due to sinusitis, common cold, or influenza. FIOGESIC® promotes sinus and nasal decongestion and drainage with phenylpropanolamine, an orally used alpha adrenergic sympathomimetic approximately equal in potency to ephedrine but with less CNS stimulation, plus two antihistamines, pheniramine maleate and pyrilamine maleate. Calurin®, a freely soluble aspirin complex, alleviates pain and fever.

Contraindications: Sensitivity to any of the ingredients.

Caution: Not for children under 6. Individuals with high blood pressure, heart disease, diabetes, or thyroid disease should use only as directed by a physician. This preparation may cause drowsiness. Do not drive or operate machinery while taking this medication.

Side Effects: Drowsiness, blurred vision, cardiac palpitations, flushing, dizziness, nervousness, or gastrointestinal upsets may occur occasionally.

Dosage: Adults—Two tablets followed by one or two tablets every four hours, up to six per day. Children (6 to 12 years)—one-half to one tablet every four hours up to four tablets per day.

Supplied: Fiogesic Oblong Inlay-Tablets (white with yellow inlay) in bottles of 100.

Company's Product Identification Mark(s): Tablets embossed FIOGESIC on one side, SANDOZ other side.

Shown in Product Identification Section, page 432

FIORINAL®
[fē-ōr'i-nol]
Tablets and Capsules

PHENACETIN-FREE

The following prescribing information is based on official labeling in effect on November 1, 1984.

Description: Each Fiorinal® tablet or capsule for oral administration contains: Sandoptal® (butalbital, USP), 50 mg (Warning: May be habit forming); aspirin, USP, 325 mg; caffeine, USP, 40 mg.

Continued on next page

Sandoz—Cont.

Butalbital, 5-allyl-5-isobutyl-barbituric acid, a white odorless crystalline powder; is a short- to intermediate-acting barbiturate.

Actions: Pharmacologically, Fiorinal combines the analgesic properties of aspirin with the anxiolytic and muscle relaxant properties of Sandoptal.

The clinical effectiveness of Fiorinal in tension headache has been established in double-blind, placebo-controlled, multi-clinic trials. A factorial design study compared Fiorinal with each of its major components. This study demonstrated that each component contributes to the efficacy of Fiorinal in the treatment of the target symptoms of tension headache (headache pain, psychic tension, and muscle contraction in the head, neck and shoulder region). For each symptom and the symptom complex as a whole, Fiorinal was shown to have significantly superior clinical effects to either component alone.

Indications: Fiorinal is indicated for the relief of the symptom complex of tension (or muscle contraction) headache.

Contraindications: Hypersensitivity to aspirin, caffeine, or barbiturates. Patients with porphyria.

Warnings:

Drug Dependency: Prolonged use of barbiturates can produce drug dependence, characterized by psychic dependence, and less frequently, physical dependence and tolerance. The abuse liability of Fiorinal is similar to that of other barbiturate-containing drug combinations. Caution should be exercised when prescribing medication for patients with a known propensity for taking excessive quantities of drugs, which is not uncommon in patients with chronic tension headache.

Use in Ambulatory Patients: Fiorinal may impair the mental and/or physical abilities required for the performance of potentially hazardous tasks, such as driving a car or operating machinery. The patient should be cautioned accordingly. Central Nervous System depressant effects of butalbital may be additive with those of other CNS depressants. Concurrent use with other sedative-hypnotics or alcohol should be avoided. When such combined therapy is necessary, the dose of one or more agents may need to be reduced.

Use in Pregnancy: Adequate studies have not been performed in animals to determine whether this drug affects fertility in males or females, has teratogenic potential, or has other adverse effects on the fetus. While there are no well-controlled studies in pregnant women, over twenty years of marketing and clinical experience does not include any positive evidence of adverse effects on the fetus. Although there is no clearly defined risk, such experience cannot exclude the possibility of infrequent or subtle damage to the human fetus. Fiorinal should be used in pregnant women only when clearly needed.

Nursing Mothers: The effects of Fiorinal on infants of nursing mothers are not known. Salicylates and barbiturates are excreted in the breast milk of nursing mothers. The serum levels in infants are believed to be insignificant with therapeutic doses.

Precautions: Salicylates should be used with extreme caution in the presence of peptic ulcer or coagulation abnormalities.

Pediatric Use: Safety and effectiveness in children below the age of 12 have not been established.

Adverse Reactions: The most frequent adverse reactions are drowsiness and dizziness. Less frequent adverse reactions are lightheadedness and gastrointestinal disturbances including nausea, vomiting, and flatulence.

Overdosage: The toxic effects of acute overdosage of Fiorinal are attributable mainly to its barbiturate component, and, to a lesser extent, aspirin. Because toxic effects of caffeine occur in very high dosages only, the possibility of significant caffeine toxicity from Fiorinal overdosage is unlikely. Symptoms attributable to *acute barbiturate poisoning* include drowsiness, confusion, and coma; respiratory depression; hypotension; shock. Symptoms attributable to *acute aspirin poisoning* include hyperpnea; acid-base disturbances with development of metabolic acidosis; vomiting and abdominal pain; tinnitus; hyperthermia; hypoprothrombinemia; restlessness; delirium; convulsions. *Acute caffeine poisoning* may cause insomnia, restlessness, tremor, and delirium; tachycardia and extrasystoles. *Treatment* consists primarily of management of barbiturate intoxication and the correction of the acid-base imbalance due to salicylism. Vomiting should be induced mechanically or with emetics in the conscious patient. Gastric lavage may be used if the pharyngeal and laryngeal reflexes are present and if less than four hours have elapsed since ingestion. A cuffed endotracheal tube should be inserted before gastric lavage of the unconscious patient and when necessary to provide assisted respiration. Diuresis, alkalinization of the urine, and correction of electrolyte disturbances should be accomplished through administration of intravenous fluids such as 1% sodium bicarbonate in 5% dextrose in water. Meticulous attention should be given to maintaining adequate pulmonary ventilation. Correction of hypotension may require the administration of levarterenol bitartrate or phenylephrine hydrochloride by intravenous infusion. In severe cases of intoxication, peritoneal dialysis, hemodialysis, or exchange transfusion may be lifesaving. Hypoprothrombinemia should be treated with Vitamin K, intravenously.

Dosage and Administration: One or two tablets or capsules every four hours. Total daily dose should not exceed six tablets or capsules.

How Supplied: Fiorinal® Capsules: Color is bright Kelly green and lime green, in packages of 100 and 500. Also available in ControlPak® package, 25 capsules (continuous reverse numbered roll of sealed blisters). Fiorinal Tablets: White, compressed tablet 11 mm diameter, 5.5 mm thickness, in packages of 100 and 1000.

Company's Product Identification Mark(s): Tablets imprinted "FIORINAL" on one side, "SANDOZ"on other side, and Capsules imprinted "FIORINAL 78–103" on each half of capsule.

[FIO-ZZ20 Issued December 15, 1982]
Shown in Product Identification Section, page 433

FIORINAL® with CODEINE
[fē-or' i-nol]
Capsules
No. 1, 2 and 3

PHENACTIN-FREE

The following prescribing information is based on official labeling in effect on November 1, 1984.

Composition: Each Fiorinal® with Codeine *Capsule* contains: 50 mg Sandoptal® (butalbital, USP), (Warning: May be habit forming.) 40 mg caffeine, USP; and 325 mg aspirin, USP.

In addition, Fiorinal with Codeine #1, #2, #3 also contain, respectively, codeine phosphate, USP 7.5 mg (⅛ gr), 15 mg (¼ gr) and 30 mg (½ gr). (Warning: May be habit forming.)

Indications: "Fiorinal with Codeine" raises the threshold of pain and discomfort and can be used in a great variety of painful conditions short of those which require morphine.

Actions and Uses: Analgesic, antitussive, and antipyretic. The analgesic-sedative action of Fiorinal complements and increases the time-tested action of codeine. This enhanced analgesic-sedative effect is particularly well-suited for acute, short-range periods of pain and discomfort frequently seen in office practice.

The formulation of "Fiorinal with Codeine" provides additional benefits for patients who have developed a cycle of pain, anxiety, tension which reinforces the pain experienced by the patients.

"Fiorinal with Codeine" is indicated for all types of pain associated with medical and surgical aftercare, postpartum pain, dysmenorrhea, neuritis, pleurisy, sciatica, neuralgia, sinusitis, pharyngitis, tonsillitis, otitis, febrile diseases, dental pain following extractions, headache, bursitis, arthritis, rheumatism, low back pain, dislocations, strains, sprains, fractures, etc.

The analgesic, antitussive-antipyretic action of this product makes it particularly well-suited for the patient with upper respiratory infections such as acute colds, bronchitis, influenza, and pneumonia.

Contraindications: Hypersensitivity to any of the components.

Precautions: May be habit forming due to presence of codeine and barbiturate.

Side Effects: Nausea, vomiting, constipation, dizziness, skin rash, drowsiness, and miosis are possible side effects. Overdosage is primarily manifested by drowsiness.

Adult Dosage: 1 or 2 capsules, repeated if necessary up to 6 capsules per day, or as directed by physician.

Supplied: Fiorinal with Codeine: 7.5 mg (⅛ gr) imprinted "triangle (S) F-C #1" on one half, "SANDOZ 78-105" other half, color is red and yellow; 15 mg (¼ gr) imprinted "triangle (S) F-C #2" on one half, "SANDOZ 78-106" other half, color is gray and yellow; 30 mg (½ gr) imprinted "triangle (S) F-C #3" on one half; "SANDOZ 78-107" other half, color is blue and yellow. In bottles of 100.

Fiorinal with Codeine No. 3 (½ gr) also in ControlPak® package, 25 capsules (continuous reverse numbered roll of sealed blisters) and in bottles of 500.

Company's Product Identification Mark(s): All capsules imprinted triangle (S) with F-C #1, 2 and 3 on one half, SANDOZ plus NDC number other half.

[FWC-Z16 Issued May 14, 1984]
Shown in Product Identification Section, page 433

HYDERGINE®
[hī' der-jĕn]
(ergoloid mesylates) tablets, USP (ORAL)
(ergoloid mesylates) tablets, USP (SUBLINGUAL)
(ergoloid mesylates) liquid

HYDERGINE® LC
(ergoloid mesylates) liquid capsules

The following prescribing information is based on official labeling in effect on November 1, 1984.

Description and Type:

Hydergine® tablet 1 mg, Hydergine sublingual tablet 1 mg and Hydergine LC (liquid capsule) 1 mg, each contains ergoloid mesylates USP as follows: dihydroergocornine mesylate 0.333 mg, dihydroergocristine mesylate 0.333 mg, and dihydroergocryptine (dihydro-alpha-ergocryptine and dihydro-beta-ergocryptine in the proportion of 2:1) mesylate 0.333 mg, representing a total of 1 mg.

Hydergine sublingual tablet 0.5 mg, each contains ergoloid mesylates USP as follows: dihydroergocornine mesylate 0.167 mg, dihydroergocristine mesylate 0.167 mg, and dihydroergocryptine (dihydro-alpha-ergocryptine and dihydro-beta-ergocryptine in the proportion of 2:1) mesylate 0.167 mg, representing a total of 0.5 mg.

Hydergine liquid 1 mg/ml, each ml contains ergoloid mesylates USP as follows: dihydroergocornine mesylate 0.333 mg, dihydroergocristine mesylate 0.333 mg, and dihydroergocryptine (dihydro-alpha-ergocryptine and dihydro-beta-ergocryptine in the proportion of 2:1) mesylate 0.333 mg, representing a total of 1 mg; alcohol, USP, 30% by volume.

Pharmacokinetic Properties

Pharmacokinetic studies have been performed in normal volunteers with the help of radiolabelled drug as well as employing a specific radioimmunoassay technique. From the urinary excretion quotient of orally and intravenously administered tritium-labelled Hydergine (ergoloid mesylates) the absorption of ergoloid was calculated to be 25%. Following oral administration, peak levels of 0.5 ng Eq/ml/mg were achieved within 1.5-3 hr. Bioavailability studies with the specific radioimmunoassay confirm that ergoloid is rapidly absorbed from the gastrointestinal tract, with mean peak levels of 0.05-0.13 ng/ml/mg (with extremes of 0.03 and 0.18 ng/ml/mg) achieved within 0.6-1.3

hr. (with extremes of 0.4 and 2.8 hrs.). The finding of lower peak levels of ergoloid compared to the total drug-metabolite composite is consistent with a considerable first pass liver metabolism, with less than 50% of the therapeutic moiety reaching the systemic circulation. The elimination of radioactivity, representing ergoloid plus metabolites bearing the radiolabel, was biphasic with half-lives of 4 and 13 hr. The mean half-life of unchanged ergoloid in plasma is about 2.6-5.1 hr; after 3 half-lives ergoloid plasma levels are less than 10% of radioactivity levels, and by 24 hr no ergoloid is detectable.

Bioequivalence studies were performed comparing Hydergine oral tablets (administered orally) with Hydergine sublingual tablets (administered sublingually), Hydergine oral tablets with Hydergine liquid and Hydergine oral tablets with Hydergine (liquid capsules). The oral tablet, sublingual tablet and liquid capsule oral forms were shown to be bioequivalent. Within the bioequivalence limits, the liquid capsule showed a statistically significant (12%) greater bioavailability than the oral tablet. In the study comparing the oral tablet and liquid forms, both forms tested showed an equivalent rate of absorption and an equivalent peak plasma concentration (C_{max}).

Actions: There is no specific evidence which clearly establishes the mechanism by which Hydergine (ergoloid mesylates) preparations produce mental effects, nor is there conclusive evidence that the drug particularly affects cerebral arteriosclerosis or cerebrovascular insufficiency.

Indications: A proportion of individuals over sixty who manifest signs and symptoms of an idiopathic decline in mental capacity (i.e., cognitive and interpersonal skills, mood, self-care, apparent motivation) can experience some symptomatic relief upon treatment with Hydergine (ergoloid mesylates) preparations. The identity of the specific trait(s) or condition(s), if any, which would usefully predict a response to Hydergine (ergoloid mesylates) therapy is not known. It appears, however, that those individuals who do respond come from groups of patients who would be considered clinically to suffer from some ill-defined process related to aging or to have some underlying dementing condition (i.e., primary progressive dementia, Alzheimer's dementia, senile onset, multi-infarct dementia).

Before prescribing Hydergine (ergoloid mesylates), the physician should exclude the possibility that the patient's signs and symptoms arise from a potentially reversible and treatable condition. Particular care should be taken to exclude delirium and dementiform illness secondary to systemic disease, primary neurological disease, or primary disturbance of mood. Hydergine (ergoloid mesylates) preparations are not indicated in the treatment of acute or chronic psychosis, regardless of etiology (see CONTRAINDICATIONS section).

The decision to use Hydergine ®(ergoloid mesylates) in the treatment of an individual with a symptomatic decline in mental capacity of unknown etiology should be continually reviewed since the presenting clinical picture may subsequently evolve sufficiently to allow a specific diagnosis and a specific alternative treatment. In addition, continued clinical evaluation is required to determine whether any initial benefit conferred by Hydergine (ergoloid mesylates) therapy persist with time.

The efficacy of Hydergine (ergoloid mesylates) was evaluated using a special rating scale known as the SCAG (Sandoz Clinical Assessment-Geriatric). The specific items on this scale on which modest but statistically significant changes were observed at the end of twelve weeks include: mental alertness, confusion, recent memory, orientation, emotional lability, self-care, depression, anxiety/fears, cooperation, sociability, appetite, dizziness, fatigue, bothersome(ness), and an overall impression of clinical status.

Contraindications: Hydergine (ergoloid mesylates) preparations are contraindicated in individuals who have previously shown hypersensitivity to the drug. Hydergine (ergoloid mesylates) preparations are also contraindicated in patients who have psychosis, acute or chronic, regardless of etiology.

Precautions: *Practitioners are advised that because the target symptoms are of unknown etiology, careful diagnosis should be attempted before prescribing Hydergine (ergoloid mesylates) preparations.*

Adverse Reactions: Hydergine (ergoloid mesylates) preparations have not been found to produce serious side effects. Some sublingual irritation with the sublingual tablets, transient nausea, and gastric disturbances have been reported. Hydergine (ergoloid mesylates) preparations do not possess the vasoconstrictor properties of the natural ergot alkaloids.

Dosage and Administration: 1 mg three times daily.

Alleviation of symptoms is usually gradual and results may not be observed for 3-4 weeks.

How Supplied:
Hydergine tablets (for oral use):
1 mg, round, white, embossed "HYDERGINE 1" on one side, triangle (S) other side. Packages of 100 and 500.
Hydergine sublingual tablets:
1 mg, oval, white, packages of 100 and 1000.
0.5 mg, round, white, packages of 100 and 1000.
Hydergine liquid:
1 mg/ml. Bottles of 100 ml with an accompanying dropper graduated to deliver 1 mg.
Hydergine LC (liquid capsule):
1 mg, oblong, off white, packages of 100 and 500. (Encapsulated by R. P. Scherer, N.A., Clearwater, Florida 33518)
Company's Product Identification Mark(s):
Hydergine Tablets (for oral use): embossed "HYDERGINE" on one side, triangle (S) other side.
Hydergine Sublingual Tablets: 1 mg, embossed "HYDERGINE" on one side, "78-77" other side. 0.5 mg., embossed "HYDERGINE 0.5" on one side, triangle (S) other side.
Hydergine LC (liquid capsules): branded "HYDERGINE LC 1 mg" on one side, triangle (S) other side.
[HYD-ZZ24 Issued June 15, 1984]
Shown in Product Identification Section, page 433

KLORVESS® EFFERVESCENT GRANULES, and ℞
[klor′ves″]
KLORVESS® (potassium chloride) 10% LIQUID

The following prescribing information is based on official labeling in effect on November 1, 1984.
Description: KLORVESS® EFFERVESCENT GRANULES: Each packet (2.8 g) contains 20 mEq each of potassium and chloride supplied by potassium chloride 1.125 g, potassium bicarbonate 0.5 g, L-lysine monohydrochloride 0.913 g in a sodium-, sugar- and carbohydrate-free effervescent formulation. Dissolution of the packet contents in water provides the potassium and chloride available for oral ingestion as potassium chloride, potassium bicarbonate, potassium citrate and L-lysine monohydrochloride.

KLORVESS (potassium chloride) 10% LIQUID: Each tablespoonful (15 ml) contains 20 mEq of potassium chloride (provided by potassium chloride 1.5 g), in a palatable, cherry and pit flavored vehicle, alcohol 0.75%.

Indications: For the prevention and treatment of potassium depletion and hypokalemic-hypochloremic alkalosis. Deficits of body potassium and chloride can occur as a consequence of therapy with potent diuretic agents and adrenal corticosteroids.

Contraindications: Severe renal impairment characterized by azotemia or oliguria, untreated Addison's disease, Familial Periodic Paralysis, acute dehydration, heat cramps, patients receiving aldosterone-inhibiting or potassium-sparing diuretic agents, or hyperkalemia from any cause.

Precautions: In response to a rise in the concentration of body potassium, renal excretion of the ion is increased. In the presence of normal renal function and hydration, it is difficult to produce potassium intoxication by oral potassium salt supplements.

Since the extent of potassium deficiency cannot be accurately determined, it is prudent to proceed cautiously in undertaking potassium replacement. Periodic evaluations of the patient's clinical status, serum electrolytes and the EKG should be carried out when replacement therapy is undertaken. This is particularly important in patients with cardiac disease and those patients receiving digitalis.

High serum concentrations of potassium may cause death through cardiac depression, arrhythmia or cardiac arrest.

To minimize gastrointestinal irritation associated with potassium chloride preparations, patients should dissolve the packet contents of KLORVESS EFFERVESCENT GRANULES in 3 to 4 ounces of cold water, fruit juice, or other liquid, or dilute each tablespoonful of KLORVESS (potassium chloride) 10% LIQUID in 3 to 4 ounces of cold water. Both of these solutions should be ingested slowly with or immediately after meals.

Adverse Reactions: Abdominal discomfort, diarrhea, nausea and vomiting may occur with the use of potassium salts.

The symptoms and signs of potassium intoxication include paresthesias, heaviness, muscle weakness and flaccid paralysis of the extremities. Potassium intoxication can produce listlessness, mental confusion, a fall in blood pressure, shock, cardiac arrhythmias, heart block and cardiac arrest.

The EKG picture of hyperkalemia is characterized by the early appearance of tall, peaked T waves. The R wave is decreased in amplitude and the S wave deepens; the QRS complex widens progressively. The P wave widens and decreases in amplitude until it disappears. Occasionally, an apparent elevation of the RS-T junction and a cove plane RS-T segment and T wave will be noted in AVL.

Dosage and Administration: KLORVESS EFFERVESCENT GRANULES: Adults—One packet (20 mEq each of potassium and chloride) completely dissolved in 3 to 4 ounces of cold water, fruit juice or other liquid 2 to 4 times daily depending upon the requirements of the patient.

KLORVESS (potassium chloride) 10% LIQUID: Adults—One tablespoonful (15 ml) of KLORVESS Liquid (20 mEq of potassium chloride) completely diluted in 3 to 4 ounces of cold water 2 to 4 times daily depending upon the requirements of the patient.

Both of these solutions should be ingested slowly with meals or immediately after eating. Deviations from these recommended dosages may be indicated in certain cases of hypokalemia based upon the patient's status. The average total daily dosage must be governed by the patient's response as determined by frequent evaluation of serum electrolytes, EKG and clinical status.

Overdosage: Potassium intoxication may result from overdosage of potassium or from therapeutic dosage in conditions stated under "Contraindications." Hyperkalemia, when detected, must be treated immediately because lethal levels can be reached in a few hours.

Treatment of Hyperkalemia:
1. Dextrose solution, 10 or 25% containing 10 units of crystalline insulin per 20 g dextrose, given IV in a dose of 300 to 500 ml in an hour.
2. Adsorption and exchange of potassium using sodium or ammonium cycle cation exchange resins, orally and as retention enema. (Caution: Ammonium compounds should not be used in patients with hepatic cirrhosis.)
3. Hemodialysis and peritoneal dialysis.
4. The use of potassium-containing foods or medicaments must be eliminated.

In digitalized patients too rapid a lowering of plasma potassium concentration can cause digitalis toxicity.

How Supplied: KLORVESS® EFFERVESCENT GRANULES—packages of 30 packets (2.8 g each). KLORVESS (potassium chloride) 10% LIQUID (dark red) – as a cherry and pit flavored liquid in pint bottles.
[KLO-Z3 Issued February 20, 1984]

KLORVESS® ℞
[klor′ves″]
EFFERVESCENT TABLETS

The following prescribing information is based on official labeling in effect on November 1, 1984.

Continued on next page

Sandoz—Cont.

Description: Each dry, sodium- and sugar-free effervescent tablet contains 20 mEq each of potassium and chloride supplied by potassium chloride 1.125 g, potassium bicarbonate 0.5 g, L-lysine monohydrochloride 0.913 g. Dissolution of the tablet in water provides the potassium and chloride available for oral ingestion as potassium chloride, potassium bicarbonate, potassium citrate and L-lysine monohydrochloride.

Indications: For the prevention and treatment of potassium depletion and hypokalemic-hypochloremic alkalosis. Deficits of body potassium and chloride can occur as a consequence of therapy with potent diuretic agents and adrenal corticosteroids.

Contraindications: Severe renal impairment characterized by azotemia or oliguria, untreated Addison's disease, Familial Periodic Paralysis, acute dehydration, heat cramps, patients receiving aldosterone-inhibiting or potassium-sparing diuretic agents, or hyperkalemia from any cause.

Precautions: In response to a rise in the concentration of body potassium, renal excretion of the ion is increased. In the presence of normal renal function and hydration, it is difficult to produce potassium intoxication by oral potassium salt supplements.

Since the extent of potassium deficiency cannot be accurately determined, it is prudent to proceed cautiously in undertaking potassium replacement. Periodic evaluations of the patient's clinical status, serum electrolytes and the EKG should be carried out when replacement therapy is undertaken. This is particularly important in patients with cardiac disease and those patients receiving digitalis.

High serum concentrations of potassium may cause death through cardiac depression, arrhythmia or cardiac arrest.

To minimize gastrointestinal irritation associated with potassium chloride preparations, patients should dissolve each Klorvess® Tablet in 3 or 4 ounces of water or fruit juice. This solution should be ingested slowly with or immediately after meals.

Adverse Reactions: Abdominal discomfort, diarrhea, nausea and vomiting may occur with the use of potassium salts.

The symptoms and signs of potassium intoxication include paresthesias, heaviness, muscle weakness and flaccid paralysis of the extremities. Potassium intoxication can produce listlessness, mental confusion, a fall in blood pressure, shock, cardiac arrhythmias, heart block and cardiac arrest.

The EKG picture of hyperkalemia is characterized by the early appearance of tall, peaked T waves. The R wave is decreased in amplitude and the S wave deepens; the QRS complex widens progressively. The P wave widens and decreases in amplitude until it disappears. Occasionally, an apparent elevation of the RS-T junction and a cove-plane RS-T segment and T wave will be noted in AVL.

Dosage and Administration: Adults—One Klorvess Effervescent Tablet (20 mEq each of potassium and chloride) completely dissolved in 3 to 4 ounces of cold water or fruit juice 2 to 4 times daily depending upon the requirements of the patient.

The solution should be ingested slowly with meals or immediately after eating. Deviations from these recommended dosages may be indicated in certain cases of hypokalemia based upon the patient's status. The average total daily dosage must be governed by the patient's response as determined by frequent evaluation of serum electrolytes, EKG and clinical status.

Overdosage: Potassium intoxication may result from overdosage of potassium or from therapeutic dosage in conditions stated under "Contraindications." Hyperkalemia, when detected, must be treated immediately because lethal levels can be reached in a few hours.

Treatment of Hyperkalemia:
1. Dextrose solution, 10 or 25% containing 10 units of crystalline insulin per 20 g dextrose, given I.V. in a dose of 300 to 500 ml in an hour.
2. Adsorption and exchange of potassium using sodium or ammonium cycle cation exchange resins, orally and as retention enema. (Caution: Ammonium compounds should not be used in patients with hepatic cirrhosis.)
3. Hemodialysis and peritoneal dialysis.
4. The use of potassium-containing foods or medicaments must be eliminated.

In digitalized patients too rapid a lowering of plasma potassium concentration can cause digitalis toxicity.

How Supplied: Klorvess Effervescent Tablets (white)—60 tablets. Each tablet is individually foil wrapped. Klorvess® Tablets are also available in institutional packages of 30 and 1000 tablets.

[KLO-ZZ1 Issued April 29, 1983]
Shown in Product Identification Section, page 433

MELLARIL® ℞
[*mel′ah-ril″*]
(thioridazine) HCl tablets, USP
(thioridazine) HCl oral solution, USP
MELLARIL-S®
(thioridazine) oral suspension, USP

The following prescribing information is based on official labeling in effect on November 1, 1984.

Description: Mellaril® (thioridazine) is 2-methylmercapto -10- [2 - (N- methyl -2- piperidyl) ethyl] phenothiazine.*
*U.S. Patent No. 3,239,514

The presence of a thiomethyl radical (S-CH$_3$) in position 2, conventionally occupied by a halogen, is unique and could account for the greater toleration obtained with recommended doses of thioridazine as well as a greater specificity of psychotherapeutic action.

Clinical Pharmacology: Mellaril (thioridazine) is effective in reducing excitement, hypermotility, abnormal initiative, affective tension and agitation through its inhibitory effect on psychomotor functions. Successful modification of such symptoms is the prerequisite for, and often the beginning of, the process of recovery in patients exhibiting mental and emotional disturbances.

Thioridazine's basic pharmacological activity is similar to that of other phenothiazines, but certain specific qualities have come to light which support the observation that the clinical spectrum of this drug shows significant differences from those of the other agents of this class. Minimal antiemetic activity and minimal extrapyramidal stimulation, notably pseudoparkinsonism, are distinctive features of this drug.

Indications: For the management of manifestations of psychotic disorders.

For the short-term treatment of moderate to marked depression with variable degrees of anxiety in adult patients and for the treatment of multiple symptoms such as agitation, anxiety, depressed mood, tension, sleep disturbances, and fears in geriatric patients.

For the treatment of severe behavioral problems in children marked by combativeness and/or explosive hyperexcitable behavior (out of proportion to immediate provocations), and in the short-term treatment of hyperactive children who show excessive motor activity with accompanying conduct disorders consisting of some or all of the following symptoms: impulsivity, difficulty sustaining attention, aggressivity, mood lability, and poor frustration tolerance.

Contraindications: In common with other phenothiazines, Mellaril (thioridazine) is contraindicated in severe central nervous system depression or comatose states from any cause. It should also be noted that hypertensive or hypotensive heart disease of extreme degree is a contraindication of phenothiazine administration.

Warnings: It has been suggested in regard to phenothiazines in general, that people who have demonstrated a hypersensitivity reaction (e.g. blood dyscrasias, jaundice) to one may be more prone to demonstrate a reaction to others. Attention should be paid to the fact that phenothiazines are capable of potentiating central nervous system depressants (e.g. anesthetics, opiates, alcohol, etc.) as well as atropine and phosphorus insecticides. Physicians should carefully consider benefit versus risk when treating less severe disorders.

Reproductive studies in animals and clinical experience to date have failed to show a teratogenic effect with Mellaril (thioridazine). However, in view of the desirability of keeping the administration of all drugs to a minimum during pregnancy, Mellaril (thioridazine) should be given only when the benefits derived from treatment exceed the possible risks to mother and fetus.

Precautions: Leukopenia and/or agranulocytosis and convulsive seizures have been reported but are infrequent. Mellaril (thioridazine) has been shown to be helpful in the treatment of behavioral disorders in epileptic patients, but anticonvulsant medication should also be maintained. Pigmentary retinopathy, which has been observed primarily in patients taking larger than recommended doses, is characterized by diminution of visual acuity, brownish coloring of vision, and impairment of night vision; examination of the fundus discloses deposits of pigment. The possibility of this complication may be reduced by remaining within the recommended limits of dosage.

Where patients are participating in activities requiring complete mental alertness (e.g., driving) it is advisable to administer the phenothiazines cautiously and to increase the dosage gradually. Female patients appear to have a greater tendency to orthostatic hypotension than male patients. The administration of epinephrine should be avoided in the treatment of drug-induced hypotension in view of the fact that phenothiazines may induce a reversed epinephrine effect on occasion. Should a vasoconstrictor be required, the most suitable are levarterenol and phenylephrine.

Neuroleptic drugs elevate prolactin levels; the elevation persists during chronic administration. Tissue culture experiments indicate that approximately one-third of human breast cancers are prolactin dependent in vitro, a factor of potential importance if the prescription of these drugs is contemplated in a patient with a previously detected breast cancer. Although disturbances such as galactorrhea, amenorrhea, gynecomastia, and impotence have been reported, the clinical significance of elevated serum prolactin levels is unknown for most patients. An increase in mammary neoplasms has been found in rodents after chronic administration of neuroleptic drugs. Neither clinical studies nor epidemiologic studies conducted to date, however, have shown an association between chronic administration of these drugs and mammary tumorigenesis; the available evidence is considered too limited to be conclusive at this time.

It is recommended that a daily dose in excess of 300 mg. be reserved for use only in severe neuropsychiatric conditions.

Adverse Reactions: In the recommended dosage ranges with Mellaril® (thioridazine), most side effects are mild and transient.

Central Nervous System: Drowsiness may be encountered on occasion, especially where large doses are given early in treatment. Generally, this effect tends to subside with continued therapy or a reduction in dosage. Pseudoparkinsonism and other extrapyramidal symptoms may occur but are infrequent. Nocturnal confusion, hyperactivity, lethargy, psychotic reactions, restlessness and headache have been reported but are extremely rare.

Autonomic Nervous System: Dryness of mouth, blurred vision, constipation, nausea, vomiting, diarrhea, nasal stuffiness, and pallor have been seen.

Endocrine System: Galactorrhea, breast engorgement, amenorrhea, inhibition of ejaculation and peripheral edema have been described.

Skin: Dermatitis and skin eruptions of the urticarial type have been observed infrequently. Photosensitivity is extremely rare.

Cardiovascular System: ECG changes have been reported (see Phenothiazine Derivatives: Cardiovascular Effects).

Other: Rare cases described as parotid swelling have been reported following administration of Mellaril (thioridazine).

Phenothiazine Derivatives: It should be noted that efficacy, indications and untoward effects have varied with the different phenothiazines. It has been reported that old age lowers the tolerance for phenothiazines. The most common neurological side effects in these patients are parkinsonism and akathisia. There appears to be an increased risk of agranulocytosis and leukopenia in the geriatric population. The physician should be aware that the following have occurred with one or more phenothiazines and should be considered whenever one of these drugs is used:

Autonomic Reactions: Miosis, obstipation, anorexia, paralytic ileus.

Cutaneous Reactions: Erythema, exfoliative dermatitis, contact dermatitis.

Blood Dyscrasias: Agranulocytosis, leukopenia, eosinophilia, thrombocytopenia, anemia, aplastic anemia, pancytopenia.

Allergic Reactions: Fever, laryngeal edema, angioneurotic edema, asthma.

Hepatotoxicity: Jaundice, biliary stasis.

Cardiovascular Effects: Changes in the terminal portion of the electrocardiogram, including prolongation of the Q-T interval, lowering and inversion of the T-wave and appearance of a wave tentatively identified as a bifid T or a U wave have been observed in some patients receiving the phenothiazine tranquilizers, including Mellaril (thioridazine). To date, these appear to be due to altered repolarization and not related to myocardial damage. They appear to be reversible. While there is no evidence at present that these changes are in any way precursors of any significant disturbance of cardiac rhythm, it should be noted that several sudden and unexpected deaths apparently due to cardiac arrest have occurred in patients previously showing characteristic electrocardiographic changes while taking the drug. The use of periodic electrocardiograms has been proposed but would appear to be of questionable value as a predictive device. Hypotension, rarely resulting in cardiac arrest.

Extrapyramidal Symptoms: Akathisia, agitation, motor restlessness, dystonic reactions, trismus, torticollis, opisthotonus, oculogyric crises, tremor, muscular rigidity, akinesia.

Persistent Tardive Dyskinesia: As with all antipsychotic agents, tardive dyskinesia may appear in some patients on long-term therapy or may occur after drug therapy has been discontinued. This risk seems to be greater in elderly patients on high-dose therapy, especially females. The symptoms are presistent and in some patients appear to be irreversible. The syndrome is characterized by rhythmical involuntary movements of the tongue, face, mouth or jaw (e.g., protrusion of tongue, puffing of cheeks, puckering of mouth, chewing movements). Sometimes these may be accompanied by involuntary movements of extremities.

There is no known effective treatment for tardive dyskinesia; anti-parkinsonism agents usually do not alleviate the symptoms of this syndrome. It is suggested that all antipsychotic agents be discontinued if these symptoms appear.

Should it be necessary to reinstitute treatment, or increase the dosage of the agent, or switch to a different antipsychotic agent, the syndrome may be masked.

It has been reported that fine vermicular movements of the tongue may be an early sign of the syndrome and if the medication is stopped at that time, the syndrome may not develop.

Endocrine Disturbances: Menstrual irregularities, altered libido, gynecomastia, lactation, weight gain, edema. False positive pregnancy tests have been reported.

Urinary Disturbances: Retention, incontinence.

Others: Hyperpyrexia. Behavioral effects suggestive of a paradoxical reaction have been reported. These include excitement, bizarre dreams, aggravation of psychoses, and toxic confusional states. More recently, a peculiar skin-eye syndrome has been recognized as a side effect following long-term treatment with phenothiazines. This reaction is marked by progressive pigmentation of areas of the skin or conjunctiva and/or accompanied by discoloration of the exposed sclera and cornea. Opacities of the anterior lens and cornea described as irregular or stellate in shape have also been reported. Systemic lupus erythematosus-like syndrome.

Dosage: Dosage must be individualized according to the degree of mental and emotional disturbance. In all cases, the smallest effective dosage should be determined for each patient.

Adults: *Psychotic manifestations:* The usual starting dose is 50 to 100 mg. three times a day, with a gradual increment to a maximum of 800 mg. daily if necessary. Once effective control of symptoms has been achieved, the dosage may be reduced gradually to determine the minimum maintenance dose. The total daily dosage ranges from 200 to 800 mg, divided into two to four doses.

For the short-term treatment of moderate to marked depression with variable degrees of anxiety in adult patients and for the treatment of multiple symptoms such as agitation, anxiety, depressed mood, tension, sleep disturbances, and fears in geriatric patients: The usual starting dose is 25 mg three times a day. Dosage ranges from 10 mg two to four times a day in milder cases to 50 mg three or four times a day for more severely disturbed patients. The total daily dosage range is from 20 mg to a maximum of 200 mg.

Children: Mellaril (thioridazine) is not intended for children under 2 years of age. For children aged 2 to 12 the dosage of thioridazine hydrochloride ranges from 0.5 mg to a maximum of 3.0 mg/Kg per day. For children with moderate disorders 10 mg two or three times a day is the usual starting dose. For hospitalized, severely disturbed, or psychotic children, 25 mg two or three times daily is the usual starting dose. Dosage may be increased gradually until optimum therapeutic effect is obtained or the maximum has been reached.

Supplied:
MELLARIL (thioridazine) HCl
Tablets: 10 mg, 15 mg, 25 mg, 50 mg, 100 mg, 150 mg and 200 mg thioridazine hydrochloride, USP. Packages of 100 and 1000 tablets. (10 mg, 25 mg, 50 mg and 100 mg tablets are available in packages of 500). Also, for wholly tax-supported institutions only, packages of 4800 (48 × 100) and 5000 tablets.

Concentrate—30 mg/ml: Each ml contains 30 mg thioridazine hydrochloride, USP, alcohol, USP, 3.0% by volume. Immediate containers: Amber glass bottles of 4 fl. oz (118 ml) as follows:
4 fl. oz bottles, in cartons of 12 bottles, with an accompanying dropper graduated to deliver 10 mg, 25 mg and 50 mg of thioridazine hydrochloride, USP. Also, for wholly tax-supported institutions only, gallon cartons of 32 x 4 oz. bottles, each with the same dropper.

Concentrate—100 mg/ml: Each ml contains 100 mg thioridazine hydrochloride, USP, alcohol, 4.2% by volume, *4 fl. oz bottles,* in cartons of 12 bottles, with an accompanying dropper graduated to deliver 100 mg, 150 mg and 200 mg of thioridazine hydrochloride.

Remarks: Store and dispense: Below 86°F; tight, amber glass bottle.

The Concentrate may be diluted with distilled water, acidified tap water, or suitable juices. Each dose should be so diluted just prior to administration—preparation and storage of bulk dilutions is not recommended.

MELLARIL-S (thioridazine)
Suspension—25 mg/5 ml: Each 5 ml contains thioridazine, USP, equivalent to 25 mg thioridazine hydrochloride, USP. Buttermint-flavored in pint bottles.

Suspension—100 mg/5 ml: Each 5 ml contains thioridazine, USP, equivalent to 100 mg thioridazine hydrochloride, USP. Buttermint-flavored in pint bottles.

Company's Product Identification Mark(s): 10 mg and 15 mg tablets branded with NDC number on one side, triangle (S) other side. All other tablet strengths branded MELLARIL on one side, triangle (S) other side.

[MEL-Z36 Issued May 9, 1983]
Shown in Product Identification Section, page 433

MESANTOIN® Tablets ℞
[meh-san'toyn]
(mephenytoin) tablets, USP

The following prescribing information is based on official labeling in effect on November 1, 1984.

Description: Mesantoin® (mephenytoin) is 3-methyl 5,5-phenyl-ethyl-hydantoin. It may be considered to be the hydantoin homolog of the barbiturate mephobarbital.

Actions: Mephenytoin exhibits pharmacologic effects similar to both diphenylhydantoin and the barbiturates in antagonizing experimental seizures in laboratory animals. Mephenytoin produces behavioral and electroencephalographic effects in man which are similar to those produced by barbiturates.

Indications: For the control of grand mal, focal, Jacksonian, and psychomotor seizures in those patients who have been refractory to less toxic anticonvulsants.

Contraindications: Hypersensitivity to hydantoin products.

Warnings: Mephenytoin should be used only after safer anticonvulsants have been given an adequate trial and have failed.

As with all anticonvulsants, dose reduction must be gradual so as to minimize the risk of precipitating seizures.

Patients should be cautioned about possible additive effects of alcohol and other CNS depressants. Acute alcohol intoxication may increase the anticonvulsant effect due to decreased metabolic breakdown. Chronic alcohol abuse may result in decreased anticonvulsant effect due to enzyme induction.

Usage in Pregnancy: The effects of mephenytoin in human pregnancy and nursing infants are unknown.

Recent reports suggest an association between the use of anticonvulsant drugs by women with epilepsy and an elevated incidence of birth defects in children born to these women. Data are more extensive with respect to diphenylhydantoin and phenobarbital, but these are also the most commonly prescribed anticonvulsants; less systematic or anecdotal reports suggest a possible similar association with the use of all known anticonvulsant drugs.

The reports suggesting an elevated incidence of birth defects in children of drug-treated epileptic women cannot be regarded as adequate to prove a definite cause and effect relationship. There are intrinsic methodologic problems in obtaining adequate data on drug teratogenicity in humans; the possibility also exists that other factors, e.g., genetic factors or the epileptic condition itself, may be more important than drug therapy in leading to birth defects. The great majority of mothers on anticonvulsant medication deliver normal infants. It is important to note that anticonvulsant drugs should not be discontinued in patients in whom the drug is administered to prevent major seizures because of the strong possibility of precipitating status epilepticus with attendant hypoxia and threat to life. In individual cases where the severity and frequency of the seizure disorder are such that the removal of medication does not pose a serious threat to the patient, discontinuation of the drug may be considered prior to and during pregnancy, although it cannot be said with any confidence that even minor seizures do not pose some hazards to the developing embryo or fetus. The prescribing physician will wish to weigh these considerations in treating or counseling epileptic women of child-bearing potential.

Precautions: The patient taking Mesantoin (mephenytoin) must be kept under close medical supervision at all times since serious adverse reactions may emerge.

Because the primary site of degradation is the liver, it is recommended that screening tests of liver function precede introduction of the drug.

Continued on next page

Sandoz—Cont.

Some patients may show side reactions as the result of individual sensitivity. These reactions can be broken down into three types respectively according to severity: 1) blood dyscrasias; 2) skin and mucous membrane manifestations; and 3) central effects. The blood, skin and mucous membrane manifestations are the more important since they can be more serious in nature. Since mephenytoin has been reported to produce blood dyscrasia in certain instances, the patient must be instructed that in the event any unusual symptoms develop (e.g. sore throat, fever, mucous membrane bleeding, glandular swelling, cutaneous reaction), he must discontinue the drug and report for examination immediately. It is recommended that blood examinations be made (total white cell count and differential count) during the initial phase of administration. Such tests are best made: a) before starting medication; b) after 2 weeks on a low dosage; c) again after 2 weeks when full dosage is reached; d) thereafter, monthly for a year; e) from then on, every 3 months. If the neutrophils drop to between 2500 and 1600/cu.mm., counts are made every 2 weeks. Stop medication if the count drops to 1600.

Adverse Reactions: A number of side effects and toxic reactions have been reported with Mesantoin® (mephenytoin) as well as with other hydantoin compounds. Many of these appear to be dose related while others seem to be a manifestation of a hypersensitivity reaction to these drugs.

Blood Dyscrasias
Leukopenia, neutropenia, agranulocytosis, thrombocytopenia and pancytopenia have occurred. Eosinophilia, monocytosis, and leukocytosis have been described. Simple anemia, hemolytic anemia, megaloblastic anemia and aplastic anemia have occurred but are uncommon.

Skin and Mucous Membrane Manifestations
Maculopapular, morbilliform, scarlatiniform, urticarial, purpuric (associated with thrombocytopenia) and non-specific skin rashes have been reported. Exfoliative dermatitis, erythema multiforme (Stevens-Johnson Syndrome), toxic epidermal necrolysis and fatal dermatitides have been described on rare occasions. Skin pigmentation and rashes associated with a lupus erythematosus syndrome have also been reported.

Central Effects
Drowsiness is dose-related and may be reduced by a reduction in dose. Ataxia, diplopia, nystagmus, dysarthria, fatigue, irritability, choreiform movements, depression and tremor have been encountered.
Nervousness, nausea, vomiting, sleeplessness and dizziness may occur during the initial stages of therapy. Generally, these symptoms are transient, often disappearing with continued treatment.
Mental confusion and psychotic disturbances and increased seizures have been reported, but a definite causal relationship with the drug is uncertain.

Miscellaneous
Hepatitis, jaundice and nephrosis have been reported but a definite cause and effect relationship between the drug and these effects has not been established.
Alopecia, weight gain, edema, photophobia, conjunctivitis and gum hyperplasia have been encountered.
Polyarthropathy, pulmonary fibrosis, lupus erythematosus syndrome, and lymphadenopathy which simulates Hodgkin's Disease have also been observed.

Dosage and Administration: Dosage of antiepileptic therapy should be adjusted to the needs of the individual patient. Maintenance dosage is that smallest amount of antiepileptic necessary to suppress seizures completely or reduce their frequency. Optimum dosage is attained by starting with ½ or 1 tablet of Mesantoin (mephenytoin) per day during the first week and thereafter increasing the daily dose by ½ or 1 tablet at weekly intervals. No dose should be increased until it has been taken for at least one week.
The average dose of Mesantoin for adults ranges from 2 to 6 tablets (0.2 to 0.6 Gm.) daily. In some instances it may be necessary to administer as much as 8 tablets or more daily in order to obtain full seizure control. Children usually require from 1 to 4 tablets (0.1 Gm. to 0.4 Gm.) according to nature of seizures and age.
When the physician wishes to replace the anticonvulsant now being employed with Mesantoin (mephenytoin), he should give ½ or 1 tablet of Mesantoin daily during the first week and gradually increase the daily dose at weekly intervals while gradually reducing that of the drug being discontinued. The transition can be made smoothly over a period of three to six weeks. If seizures are not completely controlled with the dose so attained, the daily dose should then be increased by a one-tablet increment at weekly intervals to the point of maximum effect. If the patient had also been receiving phenobarbital, it is well to continue it until the transition is completed, at which time gradual withdrawal of the phenobarbital may be tried.

How Supplied: Each tablet contains 100 mg mephenytoin and is scored to permit half-tablet dosage. Packages of 100 and 1,000 tablets. (Pale pink, compressed, scored).

Company's Product Identification Mark(s):-
Tablets embossed 78-52 and scored on one side, triangle S SANDOZ other side.
[MES—Z14 Issued February 1, 1983]
Shown in Product Identification Section, page 433

METHERGINE® ℞
[*meth'er-gin*]
(methylergonovine maleate) injection, USP
(methylergonovine maleate) tablets, USP

The following prescribing information is based on official labeling in effect on November 1, 1984.
Description: Each Methergine® *Tablet* contains 0.2 mg (1/320 gr.) methylergonovine maleate, USP Methergine *Injection* contains per ml: 0.2 mg (1/320 gr.) methylergonovine maleate, USP; 0.25 mg tartaric acid, NF; 3 mg sodium chloride, USP; and water for injection, USP, q.s. to 1 ml.
Methergine (methylergonovine maleate) is the first semi-synthetic ergot alkaloid available for therapeutic application—the prevention and control of postpartum hemmorrhage.
Action: Methergine induces a rapid and sustained tetanic uterotonic effect which shortens the third stage of labor and reduces blood loss. The onset of action after i.v. administration is immediate; after i.m. administration, 2 to 5 minutes, and after oral administration, 5 to 10 minutes.
Indications: For routine management after delivery of the placenta; postpartum atony and hemorrhage; subinvolution. Under full obstetric supervision, it may be given in the second stage of labor following delivery of the anterior shoulder.
Contraindications: Hypertension; toxemia; pregnancy; and hypersensitivity.
Warning: This drug should not be administered i.v. routinely because of the possibility of inducing sudden hypertensive and cerebrovascular accidents. If i.v. administration is considered essential as a lifesaving measure, Methergine should be given slowly over a period of no less than 60 seconds with careful monitoring of blood pressure.
Precautions: Caution should be exercised in the presence of sepsis, obliterative vascular disease, hepatic or renal involvement.
Adverse Reactions: Nausea; vomiting; transient hypertension; dizziness; headache; tinnitus; diaphoresis and palpitation; temporary chest pain; and dyspnea.
Dosage and Administration: **Intramuscularly:** One ml, 0.2 mg (1/320 grain) after delivery of the anterior shoulder, after delivery of the placenta, or during the puerperium. May be repeated as required, at intervals of 2-4 hours. **Intravenously:** *SEE WARNING SECTION.* Dosage same as intramuscular.
Orally: One tablet, 0.2 mg (1/320 grain) 3 or 4 times daily in the puerperium for a maximum of 1 week.
Supplied: Tablets in packages of 100 and 1000; Injection in 1 ml ampuls, boxes of 20 and 100.
Remarks: Methergine injection is a clear and colorless solution. In the event the ampul solution becomes discolored, it should not be used.
Company's Product Identification Mark(s): Tablets imprinted 78-54 on one side, SANDOZ other side.
[Met-Z16 Issued March 1, 1984]
Shown in Product Identification Section, page 433

NEO-CALGLUCON® SYRUP
[*nē'ō cal"glū'kon*]
(glubionate calcium)
Palatable and Readily Absorbable Calcium Supplement.

The following prescribing information is based on official labeling in effect on November 1, 1984.
Description: Each teaspoonful (5 ml) of NEO-CALGLUCON® (glubionate calcium) Syrup contains: glubionate calcium 1.8 g (calcium content 115 mg—providing the same amount as 1.2 g calcium gluconate), benzoic acid, USP (as preservative) 5 mg.
Adequate calcium intake is particularly important during periods of bone growth in childhood and adolescence, during pregnancy and lactation. An adequate supply of calcium is considered necessary in adults, especially those over 40, to prevent a negative calcium balance which may contribute to the development of osteoporosis. The following are the US Government Recommended Daily Allowances (US RDA) of calcium.

Age Period	Calcium Requirements
Infants	0.6 g
Children under 4 years	0.8 g
Adults and children over 4	1.0 g
Pregnant and lactating women	1.3 g

Eight ounces of whole milk provide approximately 267 mg of calcium. One tablespoonful (15 ml) of NEO-CALGLUCON Syrup contains 345 mg of calcium.
Indications:
1. As a *dietary supplement* where calcium intake may be inadequate:
   a. childhood and adolescence
   b. pregnancy
   c. lactation
   d. postmenopausal females and in the aged
2. In the *treatment* of calcium deficiency states which may occur in diseases such as:
   a. tetany of the newborn*
   b. hypoparathyroidism, acute* and chronic
   c. pseudohypoparathyroidism
   d. postmenopausal and senile osteoporosis
   e. rickets and osteomalacia

*As a supplement to parenterally administered calcium.
Contraindications: Patients with renal calculi.
Warnings: Certain dietary substances interfere with the absorption of calcium. These include oxalic acid (found in large quantities in rhubarb and spinach), phytic acid (bran and whole cereals) and phosphorus (milk and other dairy products). Administration of corticosteroids may interfere with calcium absorption.
Precautions: When calcium is administered in therapeutic amounts for prolonged periods, hypercalcemia and hypercalciuria may result. This is most likely to occur in patients with hypoparathyroidism who are receiving high doses of Vitamin D. It can be avoided by frequent checks of plasma and urine calcium levels. Urine calcium levels may rise before plasma calcium levels. The former may be checked by determining 24-hour calcium excretion or by the Sulkowitch test.
[See table on next page].
Adverse Reactions: NEO-CALGLUCON (glubionate calcium) Syrup is exceptionally well tolerated. Gastrointestinal disturbances are exceedingly rare. A fatal case of hypercalcemia associated with an overdose of NEO-CALGLUCON Syrup has been reported in a two pound neonate. Symptoms of hypercalcemia include anorexia, nausea, vomiting, constipation, abdominal pain, dryness of the mouth, thirst and polyuria.

Dosage and Administration: NEO-CALGLUCON (glubionate calcium) Syrup should be administered before meals to enhance absorption. [See table below].
How Supplied: NEO-CALGLUCON Syrup (straw yellow) in pint bottles.

PAMELOR® ℞
[pam'ah-lar"]
(nortriptyline HCl), capsules, USP
(nortriptyline HCl) oral solution, USP

The following prescribing information is based on official labeling in effect on November 1, 1984.
Description: Pamelor® (nortriptyline HCl) is 5-(3-methylaminopropylidene)-10, 11-dihydro-5H-dibenzo [a,d] cycloheptene hydrochloride. Its molecular weight is 299.8, and its empirical formula is $C_{19}H_{21}N \cdot HCl$.
Actions: The mechanism of mood elevation by tricyclic antidepressants is at present unknown. Pamelor (nortriptyline HCl) is not a monoamine oxidase inhibitor. It inhibits the activity of such diverse agents as histamine, 5-hydroxytryptamine, and acetylcholine. It increases the pressor effect of norepinephrine but blocks the pressor response of phenethylamine. Studies suggest that Pamelor (nortriptyline HCl) interferes with the transport, release, and storage of catecholamines. Operant conditioning techniques in rats and pigeons suggest that Pamelor (nortriptyline HCl) has a combination of stimulant and depressant properties.
Indications: Pamelor (nortriptyline HCl) is indicated for the relief of symptoms of depression. Endogenous depressions are more likely to be alleviated than are other depressive states.
Contraindications: The use of Pamelor (nortriptyline HCl) or other tricyclic antidepressants concurrently with a monoamine oxidase (MAO) inhibitor is contraindicated. Hyperpyretic crises, severe convulsions, and fatalities have occurred when similar tricyclic antidepressants were used in such combinations. It is advisable to have discontinued the MAO inhibitor for at least two weeks before treatment with Pamelor (nortriptyline HCl) is started. Patients hypersensitive to Pamelor (nortriptyline HCl) should not be given the drug.
Cross-sensitivity between Pamelor (nortriptyline HCl) and other dibenzazepines is a possibility.

NEO-CALGLUCON

		Grams of Supplemental Calcium Provided Daily	Percentage of US Recommended Daily Allowance (US RDA)
I.	As a Dietary Supplement: Adults and children 4 or more years of age—1 tablespoonful 3 times daily.	1.0 g	104
	Pregnant or lactating women—1 tablespoonful 4 times daily.	1.4 g	106
	Children under 4 years of age—2 teaspoonfuls 3 times daily.	0.7 g	86
	Infants—1 teaspoonful 5 times daily (may be taken undiluted, mixed with infant's formula or fruit juice). (Part of need is supplied by diet)	0.6 g	96

NEO-CALGLUCON

II. In the treatment of Calcium Deficiency States:
Tetany of the Newborn (Tetany of the newborn appears to be a transient physiologic hypoparathyroidism related to the maturation of the parathyroid glands. Adequate parathyroid gland function usually occurs within one week after birth.)
Serum calcium should be determined before therapy is instituted. Hypocalcemia is defined as a serum calcium below 8 mg/100 ml or 4 mEq/liter. It is advisable to lower the solute and phosphorus loads in the feeding as well as to provide extra calcium. Intravenous administration of calcium solutions may be necessary for prompt relief of symptoms.
Dose: Infants with confirmed hypocalcemia may be benefited by the oral administration of calcium salts so as to provide ELEMENTAL CALCIUM in a dosage of 50 to 150 mg/kg/day divided into three or more doses. (NEO-CALGLUCON contains 115 mg ELEMENTAL CALCIUM per 5 ml teaspoon.)
The lower dosage range should be employed if calcium is also being provided by the parenteral route.
Whole milk formulas which are high in phosphorus should be eliminated in order to increase the calcium/phosphorus ratio. Supplemental oral calcium should be gradually reduced over a period of two or three weeks after the condition has completely stabilized.

Hypoparathyroidism

	Grams of Supplemental Ca Provided Daily
Acute — Intravenous administration of calcium solutions may be necessary for prompt correction of hypocalcemia. Supplementary calcium should be given orally as soon as possible.	See left-hand column
Dose: 1-3 tablespoonfuls 3 times daily	1.0–3.1
Chronic	
Dose: 1-3 tablespoonfuls daily	0.3–1.0
Pseudohypoparathyroidism	
Dose: 1-3 tablespoonfuls daily	0.3–1.0
Osteoporosis, postmenopausal and senile	
Dose: 1-2 tablespoonfuls 3 times daily	1.0–2.1

Rickets and Osteomalacia
Treatment of these disorders consists of the administration of Vitamin D orally. The addition of calcium to the therapeutic regimen may be desirable to provide calcium needed for remineralization and to avoid hypocalcemia which occurs not infrequently in the early days of treatment. Dosages should be those recommended above under Dietary Supplement.

Pamelor (nortriptyline HCl) is contraindicated during the acute recovery period after myocardial infarction.
Warnings: Patients with cardiovascular disease should be given Pamelor (nortriptyline HCl) only under close supervision because of the tendency of the drug to produce sinus tachycardia and to prolong the conduction time. Myocardial infarction, arrhythmia, and strokes have occurred. The antihypertensive action of guanethidine and similar agents may be blocked. Because of its anticholinergic activity, Pamelor (nortriptyline HCl) should be used with great caution in patients who have glaucoma or a history of urinary retention. Patients with a history of seizures should be followed closely when Pamelor (nortriptyline HCl) is administered, inasmuch as this drug is known to lower the convulsive threshold. Great care is required if Pamelor (nortriptyline HCl) is given to hyperthyroid patients or to those receiving thyroid medication, since cardiac arrhythmias may develop.
Pamelor (nortriptyline HCl) may impair the mental and/or physical abilities required for the performance of hazardous tasks, such as operating machinery or driving a car; therefore, the patient should be warned accordingly.
Excessive consumption of alcohol in combination with nortriptyline therapy may have a potentiating effect, which may lead to the danger of increased suicidal attempts or overdosage, especially in patients with histories of emotional disturbances or suicidal ideation.
Use in Pregnancy—Safe use of Pamelor (nortriptyline HCl) during pregnancy and lactation has not been established; therefore, when the drug is administered to pregnant patients, nursing mothers, or women of childbearing potential, the potential benefits must be weighed against the possible hazards. Animal reproduction studies have yielded inconclusive results.
Use in Children—This drug is not recommended for use in children, since safety and effectiveness in the pediatric age group have not been established.
Precautions: The use of Pamelor (nortriptyline HCl) in schizophrenic patients may result in an exacerbation of the psychosis or may activate latent schizophrenic symptoms. If the drug is given to overactive or agitated patients, increased anxiety and agitation may occur. In manic-depressive patients, Pamelor® (nortriptyline HCl) may cause symptoms of the manic phase to emerge. Administration of reserpine during therapy with a tricyclic antidepressant has been shown to produce a "stimulating" effect in some depressed patients.
Troublesome patient hostility may be aroused by the use of Pamelor (nortriptyline HCl). Epileptiform seizures may accompany its administration, as is true of other drugs of its class.
Close supervision and careful adjustment of the dosage are required when Pamelor (nortriptyline HCl) is used with other anticholinergic drugs and sympathomimetic drugs.
The patient should be informed that the response to alcohol may be exaggerated.
When it is essential, the drug may be administered

Continued on next page

Sandoz—Cont.

with electroconvulsive therapy, although the hazards may be increased. Discontinue the drug for several days, if possible, prior to elective surgery. The possibility of a suicidal attempt by a depressed patient remains after the initiation of treatment; in this regard, it is important that the least possible quantity of drug be dispensed at any given time.

Both elevation and lowering of blood sugar levels have been reported.

Adverse Reactions: Note: Included in the following list are a few adverse reactions that have not been reported with this specific drug. However, the pharmacologic similarities among the tricyclic antidepressant drugs require that each of the reactions be considered when nortriptyline is administered.

Cardiovascular—Hypotension, hypertension, tachycardia, palpitation, myocardial infarction, arrhythmias, heart block, stroke.

Psychiatric—Confusional states (especially in the elderly) with hallucinations, disorientation, delusions; anxiety, restlessness, agitation; insomnia, panic, nightmares; hypomania; exacerbation of psychosis.

Neurologic—Numbness, tingling, paresthesias of extremities; incoordination, ataxia, tremors; peripheral neuropathy; extrapyramidal symptoms; seizures, alteration in EEG patterns; tinnitus.

Anticholinergic—Dry mouth and, rarely, associated sublingual adenitis; blurred vision, disturbance of accommodation, mydriasis; constipation, paralytic ileus; urinary retention, delayed micturition, dilation of the urinary tract.

Allergic—Skin rash, petechiae, urticaria, itching, photosensitization (avoid excessive exposure to sunlight); edema (general or of face and tongue), drug fever, cross-sensitivity with other tricyclic drugs.

Hematologic—Bone-marrow depression, including agranulocytosis; eosinophilia; purpura; thrombocytopenia.

Gastrointestinal—Nausea and vomiting, anorexia, epigastric distress, diarrhea, peculiar taste, stomatitis, abdominal cramps, black-tongue.

Endocrine—Gynecomastia in the male, breast enlargement and galactorrhea in the female; increased or decreased libido, impotence; testicular swelling; elevation or depression of blood sugar levels; syndrome of inappropriate ADH (antidiuretic hormone) secretion.

Other—Jaundice (simulating obstructive); altered liver function; weight gain or loss; perspiration; flushing; urinary frequency, nocturia; drowsiness, dizziness, weakness, fatigue; headache, parotid swelling; alopecia.

Withdrawal Symptoms—Though these are not indicative of addiction, abrupt cessation of treatment after prolonged therapy may produce nausea, headache, and malaise.

Dosage and Administration: Pamelor (nortriptyline HCl) is not recommended for children.

Pamelor (nortriptyline HCl) is administered orally in the form of capsules or liquid. Lower than usual dosages are recommended for elderly patients and adolescents. Lower dosages are also recommended for outpatients than for hospitalized patients who will be under close supervision. The physician should initiate dosage at a low level and increase it gradually, noting carefully the clinical response and any evidence of intolerance. Following remission, maintenance medication may be required for a longer period of time at the lowest dose that will maintain remission.

If a patient develops minor side-effects, the dosage should be reduced. The drug should be discontinued promptly if adverse effects of a serious nature or allergic manifestations occur.

Usual Adult Dose—25 mg three or four times daily; dosage should begin at a low level and be increased as required. As an alternate regimen, the total daily dosage may be given once-a-day. When doses above 100 mg daily are administered, plasma levels of nortriptyline should be monitored and maintained in the optimum range of 50-150 ng/ml. Doses above 150 mg per day are not recommended.

Elderly and Adolescent Patients—30 to 50 mg per day, in divided doses, or the total daily dosage may be given once-a-day.

Overdosage: Toxic overdosage may result in confusion, restlessness, agitation, vomiting, hyperpyrexia, muscle rigidity, hyperactive reflexes, tachycardia, ECG evidence of impaired conduction, shock, congestive heart failure, stupor, coma, and C.N.S. stimulation with convulsions followed by respiratory depression. Deaths have occurred following overdosage with drugs of this class.

No specific antidote is known. General supportive measures are indicated, with gastric lavage. Respiratory assistance is apparently the most effective measure when indicated. The use of C.N.S. depressants may worsen the prognosis.

The administration of barbiturates for control of convulsions alleviates an increase in the cardiac work load but should be undertaken with caution to avoid potentiation of respiratory depression.

Intramuscular paraldehyde or diazepam provides anticonvulsant activity with less respiratory depression than do the barbiturates; diazepam seems to be preferred.

The use of digitalis and/or physostigmine may be considered in case of serious cardiovascular abnormalities or cardiac failure.

The value of dialysis has not been established.

How Supplied:

Solution: Pamelor® (nortriptyline HCl) USP, equivalent to 10 mg base per 5 ml is supplied in 16-fluid-ounce bottles. Alcohol content 4%.

Capsules: Pamelor (nortriptyline HCl) USP, equivalent to 10 mg, 25 mg and 75 mg base, are supplied in bottles of 100 and 500 and in boxes of 100 individually labeled blisters, each containing one capsule.

Company's Product Indentification Mark(s): 10 mg Capsules, branded "SANDOZ 78-86" on one half, "PAMELOR 10 mg" other half.

25 mg Capsules, branded "SANDOZ 78-87" on one half, "PAMELOR 25 mg" other half.

75 mg Capsules, branded "SANDOZ 78-79" one half, "PAMELOR 75 mg" other half.

[PAM-Z10 Issued November 15, 1984]

Shown in Product Identification Section, page 433

PARLODEL® ℞
[*par′ lō-del′*]
(bromocriptine mesylate) tablets, USP
(bromocriptine mesylate) capsules

The following prescribing information is based on official labeling in effect November 1, 1984.

Description: Parlodel® (bromocriptine mesylate) is a potent dopamine receptor agonist that inhibits prolactin secretion. This activity represents a new therapeutic use for specific peptide ergot alkaloid derivatives. Each Parlodel (bromocriptine mesylate) tablet for oral administration contains 2½ mg and each capsule contains 5 mg bromocriptine (as the mesylate). Parlodel (bromocriptine mesylate) is chemically designated as (1) Ergotaman-3′,6′,18-trione,2-bromo-12′-hydroxy-2′-(1-methylethyl) -5′- (2-methylpropyl)-, (5′α) monomethanesulfonate (salt); (2) 2-bromoergocryptine monomethanesulfonate (salt).*

*U.S. Pat. Nos. 3,752,814 and 3,752,888

Clinical Pharmacology: Parlodel (bromocriptine mesylate) is a dopamine receptor agonist, which activates post-synaptic dopamine receptors. The dopaminergic neurons in the tuberoinfundibular process modulate the secretion of prolactin from the anterior pituitary by secreting a prolactin inhibitory factor (thought to be dopamine); in the corpus striatum the dopaminergic neurons are involved in the control of motor function. Clinically, Parlodel (bromocriptine mesylate) has been shown to significantly reduce plasma levels of prolactin in patients with hyperprolactinemia. Pharmacologic experiments have demonstrated the efficacy and selectivity of bromocriptine in inhibiting prolactin secretion in several mammalian species under various experimental conditions. Studies have shown that bromocriptine suppresses physiological lactation in several species as well as galactorrhea in pathological hyperprolactinemic states at dose levels that do not affect other tropic hormones from the anterior pituitary. Experiments have demonstrated that bromocriptine induces long lasting stereotyped behavior in rodents and turning behavior in rats having unilateral lesions in the substantia nigra. These actions, characteristic of those produced by dopamine, are inhibited by dopamine antagonists and suggest a direct action of bromocriptine on striatal dopamine receptors.

Parlodel (bromocriptine mesylate) is a nonhormonal, nonestrogenic agent which inhibits the secretion of prolactin in humans, with little or no effect on other pituitary hormones, except in patients with acromegaly, where it lowers elevated blood levels of growth hormone.

In about 75% of cases of galactorrhea associated with amenorrhea, in the absence of demonstrable pituitary tumor, Parlodel (bromocriptine mesylate) therapy suppresses the galactorrhea completely, or almost completely, and reinitiates normal ovulatory menstrual cycles.

Menses are usually reinitiated prior to complete suppression of galactorrhea; the time for this on average is 6–8 weeks. However, some patients respond within a few days.

Galactorrhea may take longer to control depending on the degree of stimulation of the mammary tissue prior to therapy. At least a 75% reduction in secretion is usually observed after 8–12 weeks. Some patients may fail to respond even after 24 weeks of therapy.

Parlodel (bromocriptine mesylate), by virtue of its ability to inhibit prolactin secretion, acts to prevent physiological lactation in women when therapy is started after delivery and continued for two to three weeks. There is no evidence that Parlodel (bromocriptine mesylate) acts on the mammary tissues to prevent lactation, as is the case with estrogen-containing preparations.

Parlodel (bromocriptine mesylate) produces its therapeutic effect in the treatment of Parkinson's disease, a clinical condition characterized by a progressive deficiency in dopamine synthesis in the substantia nigra, by directly stimulating the dopamine receptors in the corpus striatum. In contrast, levodopa exerts its therapeutic effect only after conversion to dopamine by the neurons of the substantia nigra, which are known to be numerically diminished in this patient population.

Pharmacokinetics: The pharmacokinetics and metabolism of bromocriptine in human subjects were studied with the help of radioactively labeled drug. 28% of an oral dose was absorbed from the gastrointestinal tract. The blood levels following a 2½ mg dose were in the range of 2–3 ng equivalents/ml. Plasma levels were in the range of 4-6 ng equivalents/ml indicating that the red blood cells did not contain appreciable amounts of drug and/or metabolites. *In vitro* experiments showed that the drug was 90–96% bound to serum albumin. Bromocriptine was completely metabolized prior to excretion. The major route of excretion of absorbed drug was via the bile. Only 2.5–5.5% of the dose was excreted in the urine. Almost all (84.6%) of the administered dose was excreted in the feces in 120 hours.

Indications and Usage:
Amenorrhea/Galactorrhea

Parlodel® (bromocriptine mesylate), a dopamine receptor agonist, is indicated for the short-term treatment of amenorrhea/galactorrhea associated with hyperprolactinemia due to varied etiologies, excluding demonstrable pituitary tumors. It is not indicated in patients with normal prolactin levels.

Female Infertility

Parlodel (bromocriptine mesylate) tablets are indicated in the treatment of female infertility associated with hyperprolactinemia in the absence of a demonstrable pituitary tumor.

Prevention of Physiological Lactation

Parlodel (bromocriptine mesylate) tablets are indicated for the prevention of physiological lactation, (secretion, congestion, and engorgement) occurring:

1. After parturition when the mother elects not to breast feed the infant, or when breast feeding is contraindicated.

2. After stillbirth or abortion.

The physician should keep in mind that the incidence of significant painful engorgement is low and usually responsive to appropriate supportive therapy. In contrast with supportive therapy, Parlodel (bromocriptine mesylate) prevents the secretion of prolactin, thus inhibiting lactogenesis and the subsequent development of secretion, congestion and engorgement.

Once Parlodel (bromocriptine mesylate) therapy is stopped, 18% to 40% of patients experience rebound of breast secretion, congestion or engorgement, which is usually mild to moderate in severity.

Parkinson's Disease

Parlodel (bromocriptine mesylate) tablets or capsules are indicated in the treatment of the signs and symptoms of idiopathic or postencephalitic Parkinson's disease. As adjunctive treatment to levodopa (alone or with a peripheral decarboxylase inhibitor), Parlodel (bromocriptine mesylate) therapy may provide additional therapeutic benefits in those patients who are currently maintained on optimal dosages of levodopa, those who are beginning to deteriorate (develop tolerance) to levodopa therapy, and those who are experiencing "end of dose failure" on levodopa therapy. Parlodel (bromocriptine mesylate) may permit a reduction of the maintenance dose of levodopa and, thus may ameliorate the occurence and/or severity of adverse reactions associated with long-term levodopa therapy such as abnormal involuntary movements (e.g. dyskinesias) and the marked swings in motor function ("on-off" phenomenon). Continued efficacy of Parlodel (bromocriptine mesylate) during treatment of more than two years has not been established.

Data are insufficient to evaluate potential benefit from treating newly diagnosed Parkinson's disease with Parlodel (bromocriptine mesylate). Studies have shown, however, significantly more adverse reactions (notably nausea, hallucinations, confusion and hypotension) in Parlodel (bromocriptine mesylate) treated patients than in levodopa/carbidopa treated patients. Patients unresponsive to levodopa are poor candidates for Parlodel (bromocriptine mesylate) therapy.

Contraindications: Sensitivity to any ergot alkaloids.

Warnings: Symptomatic hypotension can occur in patients treated with Parlodel (bromocriptine mesylate) for any indication.

Since hyperprolactinemia with amenorrhea/galactorrhea and infertility has been found in patients with pituitary tumors (Forbes-Albright syndrome), a complete evaluation of the sella turcica is indicated before treatment with Parlodel (bromocriptine mesylate). Although Parlodel (bromocriptine mesylate) therapy will effectively lower plasma levels of prolactin in patients with pituitary tumors, this does not obviate the necessity of radiotherapy or surgical procedures where appropriate.

If pregnancy occurs during Parlodel (bromocriptine mesylate) administration, treatment should be discontinued immediately. Careful observation of these patients throughout pregnancy is mandatory. Small prolactin-secreting adenomas not detected previously may rapidly increase in size during pregnancy. Optic nerve compression may occur and emergency pituitary surgery or other appropriate measures may be necessary.

In postpartum studies with Parlodel (bromocriptine mesylate), decreases in supine systolic and diastolic pressures of greater than 20 mm and 10 mm Hg, respectively, have been observed in almost 30% of patients receiving Parlodel (bromocriptine mesylate). On occasion, the drop in supine systolic pressure was as much as 50–59 mm of Hg. Since decreases in blood pressure are frequently noted during the puerperium independent of drug therapy, it is likely that many of these decreases in blood pressure observed with Parlodel (bromocriptine mesylate) therapy were not drug induced. **However, Parlodel® (bromocriptine mesylate) is known to cause hypotension in some patients, and rarely may cause hypertension in selected patients; therefore, Parlodel® (bromocriptine mesylate) therapy for prevention of postpartum lactation should not be initiated until the vital signs have been stabilized and no sooner than four hours after delivery. Particular attention should be paid to patients with toxemia, and to those who have received within the preceding 24 hours other ergot alkaloids or other drugs which can alter the blood pressure.** Periodic monitoring of the blood pressure, particularly during the first few days of therapy, is advisable. Furthermore, care should be exercised when Parlodel (bromocriptine mesylate) is administered concomitantly with other medications known to lower blood pressure.

In clinical trials for the treatment of patients with amenorrhea/galactorrhea or for the prevention of postpartum lactation, dizziness (8–16%) and syncope (less than 1%) have been reported in patients receiving Parlodel (bromocriptine mesylate). Dizziness (9%) drowsiness (8%) and faintness/fainting (8%) have also been reported in patients treated with Parlodel (bromocriptine mesylate) for Parkinson's disease. Therefore, patients receiving this drug should be cautioned with regard to engaging in activities requiring rapid and precise responses, such as driving an automobile or operating machinery.

Long-term treatment (6–36 months) with Parlodel (bromocriptine mesylate) in doses ranging from 20–100 mg/day has been associated with pulmonary infiltrates, pleural effusion and thickening of the pleura in a few patients. In most instances in which Parlodel (bromocriptine mesylate) treatment was terminated, the changes slowly reverted towards normal.

Precautions: Safety and efficacy of Parlodel (bromocriptine mesylate) have not been established in patients with renal or hepatic disease. Phenothiazines should be avoided during Parlodel (bromocriptine mesylate) therapy. Care should be exercised when administering Parlodel (bromocriptine mesylate) therapy concomitantly with other medications known to lower blood pressure.

Amenorrhea/Galactorrhea

Treatment of women suffering from amenorrhea/galactorrhea with Parlodel (bromocriptine mesylate) may result in restoration of fertility. Therefore, patients who do not desire pregnancy should be advised to use contraceptive measures, other than the oral contraceptives, during treatment with Parlodel (bromocriptine mesylate). Since pregnancy may occur prior to reinitiation of menses, as an additional precaution, a pregnancy test is recommended at least every four weeks during the amenorrheic period, and, once menses are reinitiated, every time a patient misses a menstrual period.

Parlodel (bromocriptine mesylate) therapy has been demonstrated to be effective in the short-term management of amenorrhea/galactorrhea. Data are not available on the safety or effectiveness of its use in long-term continuous dosage, or in patients given repeated courses of treatment following recurrence of amenorrhea/galactorrhea after initial treatment. Recurrence rates are reportedly very high, ranging from 70 to 80% in domestic and foreign studies.

Female Infertility

Treatment of patients with Parlodel (bromocriptine mesylate) tablets should be discontinued as soon as the diagnosis of pregnancy has been established. Patients must be monitored closely throughout pregnancy for signs and symptoms which may develop if a previously undetected prolactin-secreting tumor enlarges.

Physiological Lactation

Decreases in blood pressure are common during the puerperium and, since Parlodel (bromocriptine mesylate) therapy is known to produce hypotension in some patients, the drug should not be administered until the vital signs have been stabilized.

Parkinson's Disease

Safety during long-term use for more than two years at the doses required for parkinsonism has not been established.

As with any chronic therapy, periodic evaluation of hepatic, hematopoietic, cardiovascular, and renal function is recommended. Symptomatic hypotension can occur and therefore caution should be exercised when treating patients receiving antihypertensive drugs.

High doses of Parlodel (bromocriptine mesylate) may be associated with confusion and mental disturbances. Since parkinsonian patients may manifest mild degrees of dementia, caution should be used when treating such patients.

Parlodel (bromocriptine mesylate) administered alone or concomitantly with levodopa may cause hallucinations (visual or auditory). Hallucinations usually resolve with dosage reduction; occasionally, discontinuation of Parlodel (bromocriptine mesylate) is required. Rarely, after high doses, hallucinations have persisted for several weeks following discontinuation of Parlodel® (bromocriptine mesylate).

As with levodopa, caution should be exercised when administering Parlodel (bromocriptine mesylate) to patients with a history of myocardial infarction who have a residual atrial, nodal, or ventricular arrhythmia.

Nursing Mothers

Since it prevents lactation, Parlodel (bromocriptine mesylate) should not be administered to mothers who elect to breast feed their offspring.

Pediatric Use

Safety and efficacy of Parlodel (bromocriptine mesylate) have not been established in children under the age of 15.

Use in Pregnancy

In human studies with Parlodel (bromocriptine mesylate) there have been 1276 reported pregnancies, which have yield 1109 live and 4 stillborn infants from women who took Parlodel (bromocriptine mesylate) during early pregnancy. Among the 1113 infants, 37 cases of congenital anomalies have been reported. There were 9 major malformations which included 3 limb reduction defects and 28 minor malformations which included 8 hip dislocations. The total incidence of malformations (3.3%) and the incidence of spontaneous abortions (11%) in this group of pregnancies does not exceed that generally reported for such occurrences in the population at large. There were three hydatidiform moles, two of which occurred in the same patient.

Adverse Reactions:

Amenorrhea/Galactorrhea/Female Infertility

The incidence of adverse effects is quite high (68%) but these are generally mild to moderate in degree. Therapy was discontinued in approximately 6% of patients because of adverse effects. These in decreasing order of frequency are: nausea 51%, headache 18%, dizziness 16%, fatigue 8%, abdominal cramps 7%, lightheadedness 6%, vomiting 5%, nasal congestion 5%, constipation 3% and diarrhea 3%.

A slight hypotensive effect may accompany Parlodel (bromocriptine mesylate) treatment. The occurence of adverse reactions may be lessened by temporarily reducing dosage to one-half tablet two or three times daily.

Physiological Lactation

23% of patients treated within the recommended dosage range for the prevention of physiological lactation had at least one side effect, but they were generally mild to moderate in degree. Therapy was discontinued in approximately 3% of patients. The most frequently occurring adverse reactions were: headache 10%, dizziness 8%, nausea 7%, vomiting 3%, fatigue 1.0%, syncope 0.7%, diarrhea 0.4% and cramps 0.4%. Decreases in blood pressure (≥ 20 mmHg systolic and ≥ 10 mmHg diastolic) occurred in 28% of patients at least once during the first three postpartum days; these were usually of a transient nature. Two reports of fainting in the puerperium may possibly be related to this effect. However, 6 cases of isolated hypertension, 3 cases of hypertension and stroke (including 1 fatal cerebral hemorrhage), 3 cases of hypertension and seizures, and 3 cases of isolated seizures have been reported. Some of these patients had toxemia (including postpartum eclampsia), and some received concomitantly other ergot alkaloids or other drugs which can raise the blood pressure, so that the relationship between these adverse reactions and Parlodel (bromocriptine mesylate) is not certain.

Parkinson's Disease

In clinical trials in which bromocriptine was administered with concomitant reduction in the dose

Continued on next page

Sandoz—Cont.

of levodopa/carbidopa, the most common newly appearing adverse reactions were: nausea, abnormal involuntary movements, hallucinations, confusion, "on-off" phenomenon, dizziness, drowsiness, faintness/fainting, vomiting, asthenia, abdominal discomfort, visual disturbance, ataxia, insomnia, depression, hypotension, shortness of breath, constipation, and vertigo.

Less common adverse reactions which may be encountered include: anorexia, anxiety, blepharospasm, dry mouth, dysphagia, edema of the feet and ankles, erythromelalgia, epileptiform seizure, fatigue, headache, lethargy, mottling of skin, nasal stuffiness, nervousness, nightmares, paresthesia, skin rash, urinary frequency, urinary incontinence, urinary retention, and rarely, signs and symptoms of ergotism such as tingling of fingers, cold feet, numbness, muscle cramps of feet and legs or exacerbation of Raynaud's syndrome.

Abnormalities in laboratory tests may include elevations in blood urea nitrogen, SGOT, SGPT, GGPT, CPK, alkaline phosphatase and uric acid, which are usually transient and not of clinical significance.

Dosage and Administration:
Amenorrhea/Galactorrhea
The therapeutic dosage of Parlodel (bromocriptine mesylate) is one 2½ mg tablet, two or three times daily, with meals. The duration of treatment should not exceed six months. It is recommended that treatment commence with one tablet daily, increasing to a therapeutic dosage within the first week, to reduce the possibility of adverse reactions.

Female Infertility
The therapeutic dosage of Parlodel® (bromocriptine mesylate) is one 2½ mg tablet, two or three times daily, with meals. It is recommended that treatment commence with one tablet daily, increasing to a therapeutic dosage within the first week, to reduce the possibility of adverse reactions. In order to reduce the likelihood of prolonged exposure to Parlodel (bromocriptine mesylate) in an unsuspected pregnancy, a mechanical contraceptive should be used in conjunction with Parlodel (bromocriptine mesylate) therapy until normal ovulatory menstrual cycles have been restored. Contraception should then be discontinued. If menstruation does not occur within 3 days of the expected date, Parlodel (bromocriptine mesylate) therapy should be discontinued and a pregnancy test performed.

Prevention of Physiological Lactation
Therapy should be started only after the patient's vital signs have been stabilized and no sooner than four hours after delivery. The recommended therapeutic dosage is one 2½ mg tablet of Parlodel (bromocriptine mesylate) twice daily with meals. The usual dosage range is from one 2½ mg tablet daily to one 2½ mg tablet three times daily with meals. Parlodel (bromocriptine mesylate) therapy should be continued for 14 days; however, therapy may be given for up to 21 days if necessary.

Parkinson's Disease
The basic principle of Parlodel (bromocriptine mesylate) therapy is to initiate treatment at a low dosage and, on an individual basis, increase the daily dosage slowly until a maximum therapeutic response is achieved. The dosage of levodopa during this introductory period should be maintained, if possible. The initial dose of Parlodel (bromocriptine mesylate) is one-half of a 2½ mg tablet twice daily with meals. Assessments are advised at two week intervals during dosage titration to ensure that the lowest dosage producing an optimal therapeutic response is not exceeded. If necessary, the dosage may be increased every 14 to 28 days by 2½ mg per day with meals. Should it be advisable to reduce the dosage of levodopa because of adverse reactions, the daily dosage of Parlodel (bromocriptine mesylate), if increased, should be accomplished gradually in small (2½ mg) increments.

The safety of Parlodel (bromocriptine mesylate) has not been demonstrated in dosages exceeding 100 mg per day.

How Supplied:
Tablets, 2½ mg
Round, white, scored tablets, each containing 2½ mg bromocriptine (as the mesylate) in packages of 30.

Capsules, 5 mg
Caramel and white capsules, each containing 5 mg bromocriptine (as the mesylate) in packages of 30 and 100.

Company's Product Identification Mark(s): Tablets embossed "PARLODEL 2½" on one side and scored on reverse side.

Capsules imprinted "PARLODEL 5 mg" on one half and triangle (S) on other half.

[PAR-Z10 Issues March 12, 1984]
Shown in Product Identification Section, page 433

RESTORIL®
[res'tah-ril"]
(temazepam) capsules

The following prescribing information is based on official labeling in effect on November 1, 1984.

Description: Restoril® (temazepam) is a benzodiazepine hypnotic agent. The chemical name is 7-chloro-1,3-dihydro-3-hydroxy-1-methyl-5-phenyl-2H-1,4-benzodiazepin-2-one.

Temazepam is a white, crystalline substance, very slightly soluble in water and sparingly soluble in alcohol USP. It has a molecular weight of 300.7. Restoril (temazepam) capsules, 15 mg and 30 mg, are for oral administration.

Clinical Pharmacology: Restoril (temazepam) improved sleep parameters in clinical studies. Residual medication effects ("hangover") were essentially absent. Early morning awakening, a particular problem in the geriatric patient, was significantly reduced.

In sleep laboratory studies, Restoril (temazepam) significantly improved sleep maintenance parameters [e.g., wake time after sleep onset, total sleep time and the number of nocturnal awakenings]. There was no significant reduction in sleep latency. REM sleep was essentially unchanged, slow wave sleep was decreased and no rebound effects occurred in these sleep stages. Transient sleep disturbance, mainly during the first night, occurred after withdrawal of the drug. In these studies, there was no evidence of tolerance when patients were given Restoril nightly for approximately one month.

A single and multiple dose absorption, distribution, metabolism and excretion (ADME) study using ^{3}H-labeled drug, as well as a bioavailability study, were carried out in normal volunteers. Absorption was complete and detectable blood levels were achieved at 20-40 minutes; peak concentration was reached at 2-3 hours. There was minimal (approximately 8%) first pass metabolism.

The only significant metabolite present in blood was the O-conjugate. The unchanged drug was 96% bound to plasma proteins. The blood level decline of the parent drug was biphasic with the short half-life ranging from 0.4-0.6 hours and the terminal half-life from 9.5-12.4 hours (mean: 10 hours), depending on the study population and method of determination. Metabolites were formed with a half-life of 10 hours and excreted with a half-life of approximately 2 hours. Thus, formation of the major metabolite is the rate limiting step in the biodisposition of temazepam. There is no accumulation of metabolites. The area under the blood concentration/time curve was directly proportional to the dose in the 0-45 mg range.

Temazepam was completely metabolized prior to excretion; 80-90% of the dose appeared in the urine. The major metabolite was the O-conjugate of temazepam (90%); the O-conjugate of N-demethyl temazepam was a minor metabolite (7%). There were no active metabolites.

At a dose of 30 mg once-a-day for 8 weeks, no evidence of enzyme induction was found in man. The steady state plasma concentration measured under therapeutic sleep laboratory conditions was 382 ± 192 ng/ml, 2.5 hours after a 30 mg dose, and 26 ng/ml at 24 hours. On a once-a-day regimen, steady state was attained on the third day.

Indications and Usage: Restoril (temazepam) is indicated for the relief of insomnia associated with the complaints of difficulty in falling asleep, frequent nocturnal awakenings, and/or early morning awakenings. In clinical trials there is a perception by patients that Restoril (temazepam) decreases sleep latency, but sleep laboratory studies have not confirmed such an effect when the drug was administered within 30 minutes of retiring.

Since insomnia is often transient and intermittent, the prolonged administration of Restoril (temazepam) is generally not necessary or recommended. Restoril (temazepam) has been employed for sleep maintenance for up to 35 consecutive nights of drug administration in sleep laboratory studies.

Since insomnia may be a symptom of several other disorders, the possibility that the complaint may be related to a condition for which there is more specific treatment should be considered.

Contraindications: Benzodiazepines may cause fetal damage when administered during pregnancy. An increased risk of congenital malformations associated with the use of diazepam and chlordiazepoxide during the first trimester of pregnancy has been suggested in several studies. Transplacental distribution has resulted in neonatal CNS depression following the ingestion of therapeutic doses of a benzodiazepine hypnotic during the last weeks of pregnancy.

Reproduction studies in animals with temazepam were performed in rats and rabbits. In a perinatal-postnatal study in rats, oral doses of 60 mg/kg/day resulted in increasing nursling mortality. Teratology studies in rats demonstrated increased fetal resorptions at doses of 30 and 120 mg/kg in one study and increased occurrence of rudimentary ribs, which were considered skeletal variants, in a second study at doses of 240 mg/kg or higher. In rabbits, occasional abnormalities such as exencephaly and fusion or asymmetry of ribs were reported without dose relationship. Although these abnormalities were not found in the concurrent control group, they have been reported to occur randomly in historical controls. At doses of 40 mg/kg or higher, there was an increased incidence of the 13th rib variant when compared to the incidence in concurrent and historical controls.

Restoril® (temazepam) is contraindicated in pregnant women. If there is a likelihood of the patient becoming pregnant while receiving temazepam, she should be warned of the potential risk to the fetus. Patients should be instructed to discontinue the drug prior to becoming pregnant. The possibility that a woman of childbearing potential may be pregnant at the time of institution of therapy should be considered.

Warnings: Patients receiving Restoril (temazepam) should be cautioned about possible combined effects with alcohol and other CNS depressants.

Precautions
General
Since the risk of the development of oversedation, dizziness, confusion and/or ataxia increases, substantially with larger doses of benzodiazepines in elderly and debilitated patients, 15 mg of Restoril (temazepam) is recommended as the initial dosage for such patients.

Restoril (temazepam) should be administered with caution in severely depressed patients or those in whom there is any evidence of latent depression; it should be recognized that suicidal tendencies may be present and protective measures may be necessary.

If Restoril (temazepam) is to be combined with other drugs having known hypnotic properties or CNS-depressant effects, consideration should be given to potential additive effects.

Information for Patients
Patients receiving Restoril (temazepam) should be cautioned about possible combined effects with alcohol and other CNS depressants. Patients should be cautioned not to operate machinery or drive a motor vehicle after ingesting the drug. Patients should also be advised that they may experience disturbed nocturnal sleep for the first or second night after discontinuing the drug.

Laboratory Tests
The usual precautions should be observed in patients with impaired renal or hepatic function. Abnormal liver function tests as well as blood dyscrasias have been reported with benzodiazepines.

Carcinogenesis, Impairment of Fertility
No carcinogenic potential was demonstrated in long-term studies in mice and rats. Fertility in male and female rats was not adversely affected by Restoril (temazepam).

Pregnancy
Pregnancy Category X. See Contraindications.

Nursing Mothers
It is not known whether this drug is excreted in human milk. Because many drugs are excreted in human milk, caution should be exercised when Restoril (temazepam) is administered to a nursing woman.

Pediatric Use
Safety and effectiveness in children below the age of 18 years have not been established.

Adverse Reactions: During clinical studies in which 795 patients received Restoril (temazepam), the drug was well tolerated. Side effects were usually mild and transient. These 795 patients included 175 subjects who received Restoril (temazepam) during daytime waking hours, sometimes in excess of recommended therapeutic dosage, in studies to evaluate dosage levels for safety and pharmacokinetic profiles.

The most common adverse reactions were drowsiness (17%), dizziness (7%), and lethargy (5%). Other side effects include confusion, euphoria and relaxed feeling (2-3%). Less commonly reported were weakness, anorexia and diarrhea (1-2%). Rarely reported were tremor, ataxia, lack of concentration, loss of equilibrium, falling and palpitations (less than 1%).

Hallucinations, horizontal nystagmus and paradoxical reactions, including excitement, stimulation and hyperactivity were rare (less than 0.5%).

Drug Abuse and Dependence
Controlled Substance
Restoril (temazepam) is a controlled substance in Schedule IV.

Abuse and Dependence
Withdrawal symptoms following abrupt discontinuation of benzodiazepines have been reported in patients receiving excessive doses over extended periods of time. These symptoms (including convulsions) are similar to those seen after barbiturate withdrawal. Although infrequently seen, milder withdrawal symptoms have also been reported following abrupt discontinuance of benzodiazepines taken continuously, generally at higher therapeutic levels, for at least several months. As with any hypnotic, caution must be exercised in administering Restoril® (temazepam) to individuals known to be addiction-prone or those whose history suggests they may increase the dosage on their own initiative. It is desirable to limit repeated prescriptions without adequate medical supervision.

Overdosage: Manifestations of acute overdosage of Restoril (temazepam) can be expected to reflect the CNS effects of the drug and include somnolence, confusion and coma, with reduced or absent reflexes, respiratory depression and hypotension. If the patient is conscious, vomiting should be induced mechanically or with emetics. Gastric lavage should be employed utilizing concurrently a cuffed endotracheal tube if the patient is unconscious to prevent aspiration and pulmonary complications. Maintenance of adequate pulmonary ventilation is essential. The use of pressor agents intravenously may be necessary to combat hypotension. Fluids should be administered intravenously to encourage diuresis. The value of dialysis has not been determined. If excitation occurs, barbiturates should not be used. It should be borne in mind that multiple agents may have been ingested.

The oral LD_{50} was 1963 mg/kg in mice, 1833 mg/kg in rats and > 2400 mg/kg in rabbits.

Dosage and Administration: The recommended usual adult dose is 30 mg before retiring. In some patients, 15 mg may be sufficient. As with all medications, dosage should be individualized for maximal beneficial effects. In elderly and/or debilitated patients it is recommended that therapy be initiated with 15 mg until individual responses are determined.

How Supplied: Restoril (temazepam) capsules-15 mg, maroon and pink, imprinted "RESTORIL 15 mg"; 30 mg, maroon and blue, imprinted "RESTORIL 30 mg". Packages of 30, 100, 500 and ControlPak® packages of 25 capsules (continuous reverse-numbered roll of sealed blisters).

Company's Product Information Mark(s): Restoril Capsules, 15 mg, imprinted "RESTORIL 15 mg" on each half.
Restoril Capsules, 30 mg, imprinted "RESTORIL 30 mg" on each half.

[RES-Z3 Issued March 15, 1983]
Shown in Product Identification Section, page 433

SANDIMMUNE® Oral Solution ℞
[san'di-mewn]
(cyclosporine)
SANDIMMUNE® I.V. ℞
(cyclosporine)

The following prescribing information is based on official labeling in effect on November 1, 1984.

WARNING

Only physicians experienced in immunosuppressive therapy and management of organ transplant patients should prescribe Sandimmune® (cyclosporine) Oral Solution and I.V. Patients receiving the drug should be managed in facilities equipped and staffed with adequate laboratory and supportive medical resources. The physician responsible for maintenance therapy should have complete information requisite for the follow-up of the patient.

Sandimmune (cyclosporine) Oral Solution and I.V. should be administered with adrenal corticosteroids but not with adrenal corticosteroids but not with other immunosuppressive agents. Increased susceptibility to infection and the possible development of lymphoma may result from immunosuppression.

The absorption of cyclosporine during chronic administration of Sandimmune Oral Solution was found to be erratic. It is recommended that patients taking the oral solution over a period of time be monitored at repeated intervals for cyclosporine blood levels and subsequent dose adjustments be made in order to avoid toxicity due to high levels and possible organ rejection due to low absorption of cyclosporine. This is of special importance in liver transplants. See Dosage and Administration section.

Description: Cyclosporine, the active principle in Sandimmune is a cyclic polypeptide immunosuppressant agent consisting of 11 amino acids. It is produced as a metabolite by the fungus species Tolypocladium inflatum Gams.

Chemically, cyclosporine is designated as [R-[R*,R*-(E)]]-cyclic-(L-alanyl-D-alanyl-N-methyl-L-leucyl-N-methyl-L-leucyl-N-methyl-L-valyl-3-hydroxy-N,4-dimethyl-L-2-amino-6-octenoyl-L-α-amino-butyryl-N-methylglycyl-N-methyl-L-leucyl-L-valyl-N-methyl-L-leucyl).

Sandimmune (cyclosporine) Oral Solution is available in 50 ml bottles.
Each ml contains:
cyclosporine .... 100 mg
alcohol, Ph. Helv. .... 12.5% by volume
dissolved in an olive oil, Ph. Helv./Labrafil® M 1944CS (polyoxyethylated oleic glycerides) vehicle which must be further diluted with milk, chocolate milk or orange juice before oral administration.
Sandimmune (cyclosporine) I.V. is available in a 5 ml sterile ampul for I.V. administration.
Each ml contains:
cyclosporine .... 50 mg
*Cremophor® EL .... 650 mg
(polyoxyethylated castor oil)
alcohol, Ph. Helv. .... 32.9% by volume
nitrogen .... qs
which must be diluted further with 0.9% Sodium Chloride Injection or 5% Dextrose Injection before use.

*Cremophor is the registered trademark of BASF Aktiengesellschaft.

Clinical Pharmacology: Sandimmune® (cyclosporine) is a potent immunosuppressive agent which in animals prolongs survival of allogeneic transplants involving skin, heart, kidney, pancreas, bone marrow, small intestine and lung. Sandimmune (cyclosporine) has been demonstrated to suppress some humoral immunity and to a greater extent, cell-mediated reactions such as allograft rejection, delayed hypersensitivity, experimental allergic encephalomyelitis, Freund's adjuvant arthritis and graft vs. host disease in many animal species for a variety of organs.

Successful kidney, liver and heart allogeneic transplants have been performed in man using Sandimmune (cyclosporine).

The exact mechanism of action of Sandimmune (cyclosporine) is not known. Experimental evidence suggests that the effectiveness of cyclosporine is due to specific and reversible inhibition of immunocompetent lymphocytes in the G_0 or G_1-phase of the cell cycle. T-lymphocytes are preferentially inhibited. The T-helper cell is the main target, although the T-suppressor cell may also be suppressed. Sandimmune (cyclosporine) also inhibits lymphokine production and release including interleukin-2 or T-cell growth factor (TCGF). No functional effects on phagocytic (changes in enzyme secretions not altered, chemotactic migration of granulocytes, macrophage migration, carbon clearance *in vivo*) or tumor cells (growth rate, metastasis) can be detected in small animals. Sandimmune (cyclosporine) does not cause bone marrow suppression in animal models or man.

The absorption of cyclosporine from the gastrointestinal tract is incomplete and variable. Peak concentrations (C_{max}) in blood and plasma are achieved at about 3.5 hours. C_{max} and area under the plasma or blood concentration/time curve (AUC) increase with the administered dose; for blood the relationship is curvilinear (parabolic) between 0 and 1400 mg. As determined by a specific assay, C_{max} is approximately 1.0 ng/mL/mg of dose for plasma and 2.7 to 1.4 ng/mL/mg of dose for blood (for low to high doses). Compared to an intravenous infusion, the absolute bioavailability of the oral solution is approximately 30% based upon the results in two patients.

Cyclosporine is distributed largely outside the blood volume. In blood the distribution is concentration dependent. Approximately 33–47% is in plasma, 4–9% in lymphocytes, 5–12% in granulocytes and 41–58% in erythrocytes. At high concentrations, the uptake by leukocytes and erythrocytes becomes saturated. In plasma, approximately 90% is bound to proteins, primarily lipoproteins.

The disposition of cyclosporine from blood is biphasic with a terminal half-life of approximately 19 hours (range: 10–27 hours). Elimination is primarily biliary with only 6% of the dose excreted in the urine.

Cyclosporine is extensively metabolized but there is no major metabolic pathway. Only 0.1% of the dose is excreted in the urine as unchanged drug. Of 15 metabolites characterized in human urine, 7 have been assigned structures. The major pathways consist of hydroxylation of the Cγ-carbon of two of the leucine residues, Cn-carbon hydroxylation and cyclic ether formation (with oxidation of the double bond) in the side chain of the amino acid 3-hydroxyl-N,4-dimethyl-L-2-amino-6-octenoic acid and N-demethylation of N-methyl leucine residues. Hydrolysis of the cyclic peptide chain or conjugation of the above metabolites do not appear to be important biotransformation pathways.

Indications and Usage: Sandimmune (cyclosporine) Oral Solution and I.V. are indicated for the prophylaxis of organ rejection in kidney, liver and heart allogeneic transplants. They are always to be used with adrenal corticosteroids. The drug may also be used in the treatment of chronic rejec-

Continued on next page

Sandoz—Cont.

tion in patients previously treated with other immunosuppressive agents.

Because of the risk of anaphylaxis, Sandimmune I.V. should be reserved for patients who are unable to take the oral solution.

Contraindications: Sandimmune (cyclosporine) I.V. is contraindicated in patients with a hypersensitivity to cyclosporine and/or Cremophor® EL (polyoxyethylated castor oil).

Warnings: SEE BOXED WARNINGS ABOVE
Sandimmune (cyclosporine), when used in high doses, can cause hepatotoxicity and nephrotoxicity.

It is not unusual for serum creatinine and BUN levels to be elevated during Sandimmune (cyclosporine) therapy. These elevations in renal transplant patients do not necessarily indicate rejection, and each patient must be fully evaluated before dosage adjustment is initiated.

Nephrotoxicity has been noted in 25% of cases of renal transplantation, 38% of cases of cardiac transplantation and 37% of cases of liver transplantation. Mild nephrotoxicity was generally noted two to three months after transplant and consisted of an arrest in the fall of the pre-operative elevations of BUN and creatinine at a range of 35–45 mg/dl and 2.0–2.5 mg/dl respectively. These elevations were often responsive to dosage reduction.

More overt nephrotoxicity was seen early after transplantation and was characterized by a rapidly rising BUN and creatinine. Since these events are similar to rejection episodes care must be taken to differentiate between them. This form of nephrotoxicity is usually responsive to Sandimmune (cyclosporine) dosage reduction.

Impaired renal function at any time requires close monitoring, and frequent dosage adjustment may be indicated. In patients with persistent high elevations of BUN and creatinine who are unresponsive to dosage adjustments, consideration should be given to switching to other immunosuppressive therapy. In the event of severe and unremitting rejection, it is preferable to allow the kidney transplant to be rejected and removed rather than increase the Sandimmune (cyclosporine) dosage to a very high level in an attempt to reverse the rejection.

Hepatotoxicity has been noted in 4% of cases of renal transplantation, 7% of cases of cardiac transplantation and 4% of cases of liver transplantation. This was usually noted during the first month of therapy when high doses of Sandimmune (cyclosporine) were used and consisted of elevations of hepatic enzymes and bilirubin. The chemistry elevations usually decreased with a reduction in dosage.

Lymphomas have developed in patients receiving Sandimmune® (cyclosporine) and other forms of immunosuppressive therapy after transplantation though no causal relationship has been established. With Sandimmune (cyclosporine), some patients have developed a lymphoproliferative disorder which regresses when the drug is discontinued.

Rarely (approximately 1 in 1000), patients receiving Sandimmune (cyclosporine) I.V. have experienced anaphylactic reactions. Although the exact cause of these reactions is unknown, it is believed to be due to the Cremophor® EL (polyoxyethylated castor oil) used as the vehicle for the I.V. formulation. These reactions have consisted of flushing of the face and upper thorax, acute respiratory distress with dyspnea and wheezing, blood pressure changes and tachycardia. One patient died after respiratory arrest and aspiration pneumonia. In some cases, the reaction subsided after the infusion was stopped.

Patients receiving Sandimmune I.V. should be under continuous observation for at least the first 30 minutes following start of the infusion and at frequent intervals thereafter. If anaphylaxis occurs, the infusion should be stopped. An aqueous solution of epinephrine 1:1000 should be available at the bedside as well as a source of oxygen.

Anaphylactic reactions have not been reported with the Oral Solution which lacks Cremophor® EL. In fact, patients experiencing anaphylactic reactions have been treated subsequently with the Oral Solution without incident.

Sandimmune (cyclosporine) Oral Solution and I.V. should not be used concomitantly with other immunosuppressive agents except adrenal corticosteroids. Immunosuppression can lead to increased susceptibility to infection and the possible development of lymphoma. [See Boxed Warning.] Care should be taken in using Sandimmune (cyclosporine) with nephrotoxic drugs. [See Precautions.]

Precautions:
General: Patients with malabsorption may have difficulty in achieving therapeutic levels with Sandimmune (cyclosporine) Oral Solution.

Hypertension is a fairly common side effect of Sandimmune therapy (see Adverse Reactions). In some patients with cardiac transplants antihypertensive therapy was required.

Information for Patients: Patients should be informed of the necessity of repeated laboratory tests while they are receiving the drug. They should be given careful dosage instructions, advised of the potential risks during pregnancy and informed of the increased risk of neoplasia.

Laboratory Tests: Renal and liver functions should be assessed repeatedly by measurement of BUN, serum creatinine, serum bilirubin and liver enzymes.

Drug Interactions: Care should be taken using Sandimmune (cyclosporine) with nephrotoxic drugs since potential synergies of nephrotoxicity may occur. Drugs which have been reported to increase the hepatic metabolism of cyclosporine and *decrease* its plasma levels include rifampin, phenytoin, phenobarbital and I.V. sulfatrimethoprim; drugs which have been reported to *increase* the plasma concentration of cyclosporine by decreasing its metabolism include cimetidine, and the antifungal agents, ketoconazole and amphotericin B. Monitoring of plasma or blood levels of cyclosporine and appropriate dosage adjustment are essential when these drugs are used concomitantly.

Carcinogenesis, Mutagenesis and Impairment of Fertility: Cyclosporine gave no evidence of mutagenic or teratogenic effects in appropriate test systems. Only at dose levels toxic to dams, were adverse effects seen in reproduction studies in rats. [See Pregnancy.]

Carcinogenicity studies were carried out in male and female rats and mice. In the 78 week mouse study, at doses of 1, 4 and 16 mg/kg/day, evidence of a statistically significant trend was found for lymphocytic lymphomas in females, and the incidence of hepatocellular carcinomas in mid-dose males significantly exceeded the control value. In the 24 month rat study, conducted at 0.5, 2 and 8 mg/kg/day, pancreatic islet cell adenomas significantly exceeded the control rate in the low dose level. The hepatocellular carcinomas and pancreatic islet cell adenomas were not dose related.

No impairment in fertility was demonstrated in studies in male and female rats.

Pregnancy: Pregnancy Category C. Sandimmune (cyclosporine) Oral Solution has been shown to be embryo- and fetotoxic in rats and rabbits when given in doses 2–5 times the human dose. At toxic doses (rats at 30 mg/kg/day and rabbits at 100 mg/kg/day), Sandimmune (cyclosporine) Oral Solution was embryo- and fetotoxic as indicated by increased pre- and postnatal mortality and reduced fetal weight together with related skeletal retardations. In the well-tolerated dose range (rats at up to 17 mg/kg/day and rabbits at up to 30 mg/kg/day), Sandimmune ® (cyclosporine) Oral Solution proved to be without any embryolethal or teratogenic effects.

There are no adequate and well-controlled studies in pregnant women. Sandimmune (cyclosporine) should be used during pregnancy only if the potential benefit justifies the potential risk to the fetus.

Nursing Mothers: Since Sandimmune (cyclosporine) is excreted in human milk, nursing should be avoided.

Pediatric Use: Although no adequate and well-controlled studies have been conducted in children, patients as young as 6 months of age have received the drug with no unusual adverse effects.

Adverse Reactions: The principal adverse reactions of Sandimmune (cyclosporine) therapy are renal dysfunction, tremor, hirsutism, hypertension and gum hyperplasia.

The following reactions occurred in 3% or greater of 892 patients involved in clinical trials of kidney, heart and liver transplants:
[See table below].

The following reactions occurred in 2% or less of patients: allergic reactions, anemia, anorexia,

Body System Adverse Reaction	Randomized Kidney Patients Sandimmune (N=227) %	Randomized Kidney Patients Azathioprine (N=228) %	All Sandimmune Patients Kidney (N=705) %	All Sandimmune Patients Heart (N=112) %	All Sandimmune Patients Liver (N=75) %
Genitourinary					
Renal Dysfunction	32	6	25	38	37
Cardiovascular					
Hypertension	26	18	13	53	27
Cramps	4	<1	2	<1	0
Skin					
Hirsutism	21	<1	21	28	45
Acne	6	8	2	2	1
Central Nervous System					
Tremor	12	0	21	31	55
Convulsions	3	1	1	4	5
Headache	2	<1	2	15	4
Gastrointestinal					
Gum Hyperplasia	4	0	9	5	16
Diarrhea	3	<1	3	4	8
Nausea/Vomiting	2	<1	4	10	4
Hepatotoxicity	<1	<1	4	7	4
Abdominal Discomfort	<1	0	<1	7	0
Autonomic Nervous System					
Paresthesia	3	0	1	2	1
Flushing	<1	0	4	0	4
Hematopoietic					
Leukopenia	2	19	<1	6	0
Lymphoma	<1		1	6	1
Respiratory					
Sinusitis	<1	0	4	3	7
Miscellaneous					
Gynecomastia	<1	0	<1	4	3

confusion, conjunctivitis, edema, fever, brittle fingernails, gastritis, hearing loss, hiccups, hyperglycemia, muscle pain, peptic ulcer, thrombocytopenia, tinnitus.

The following reactions occurred rarely: anxiety, chest pain, constipation, depression, hair breaking, hematuria, joint pain, lethargy, mouth sores, myocardial infarction, night sweats, pancreatitis, pruritus, swallowing difficulty, tingling, upper GI bleeding, visual disturbance, weakness, weight loss.

[See table above].

Cremophor® EL is known to cause hyperlipemia and electrophoretic abnormalities of lipoproteins. These effects are reversible upon discontinuation of treatment but are usually not a reason to stop treatment.

Overdosage: There is a minimal experience with overdosage. Because of the slow absorption of Sandimmune®(cyclosporine) Oral Solution, forced emesis would be of value up to 2 hours after administration. Transient hepatotoxicity and nephrotoxicity may occur which should resolve following drug withdrawal. General supportive measures and symptomatic treatment should be followed in all cases of overdosage. Sandimmune (cyclosporine) is not dialyzable to any great extent, nor is it cleared well by charcoal hemoperfusion. The oral LD_{50} is 2329 mg/kg in mice, 1480 mg/kg in rats, and > 1000 mg/kg in rabbits. The I.V. LD_{50} is 148 mg/kg in mice, 104 mg/kg in rats, and 46 mg/kg in rabbits.

Dosage and Administration:

Sandimmune Oral Solution: The initial dose of Sandimmune (cyclosporine) Oral Solution should be given 4–12 hours prior to transplantation as a single dose of 15 mg/kg per day (14–18 mg/kg per day were used in most clinical trials). This daily single dose is continued postoperatively for one or two weeks and then tapered by 5% per week to a maintenance level of 5–10 mg/kg per day. In pediatric usage, the same dose and dosing regimen may be used.

In one large controlled study in renal transplantation, a lower initial dose of 10 mg/kg/day was used after a preoperative oral dose of 20 mg/kg. In this study, however, dosage was adjusted to achieve specific *plasma* levels as determined by radioimmunoassay (RIA). During the first few weeks after transplant, trough *plasma* levels of 150–250 ng/ml were sought. By three months post-transplant, trough *plasma* levels of 50–150 ng/ml were sought. These values correspond to trough *whole blood* levels of 450–750 ng/ml and 150–450 ng/ml. Overt nephrotoxicity was uncommon in that trial (although BUN and creatinine were somewhat increased on the average), perhaps because of the lower dose. Such a dose should not be considered, however, unless cyclosporine level monitoring can be obtained.

Adjunct steroid therapy is to be used. Study centers used prednisone in different tapering schedules with seemingly similar results. One center started with 2.0 mg/kg/day for days 0–4, tapered to 1.0 mg/kg/day by 1 week, 0.6 mg/kg/day by 2 weeks, 0.3 mg/kg/day by 1 month and reached a maintenance dose of 0.15 mg/kg/day by 2 months. Another center started with a 200 mg dose initially, tapered by 40 mg/day until reaching 20 mg/day and continued at this level for 60 days. A further reduction to 10 mg/day was made during the following months. In all centers adjustments in dosage were made according to the clinical situation.

To make Sandimmune (cyclosporine) Oral Solution more palatable, the oral solution should be diluted with milk, chocolate milk, or orange juice preferably at room temperature.

Take the prescribed amount of Sandimmune (cyclosporine) from the container using the pipette supplied, after removal from the protective cover, and transfer the solution to a glass of milk, chocolate milk, or orange juice. Stir well and drink at once. Do not allow to stand before drinking. It is best to use a glass container and rinse it with more diluent to ensure that the total dose is taken.

RENAL TRANSPLANT PATIENTS IN WHOM THERAPY WAS DISCONTINUED

Reason for Discontinuation	Randomized Patients Sandimmune (N=227) %	Azathioprine (N=228) %	All Sandimmune Patients (N=705) %
Renal Toxicity	5.7	0	5.4
Infection	0	0.4	0.9
Lack of Efficacy	2.6	0.9	1.4
Acute Tubular Necrosis	2.6	0	1.0
Lymphoma/Lymphoproliferative Disease	0.4	0	0.3
Hypertension	0	0	0.3
Hematological Abnormalities	0	0.4	0
Other	0	0	0.7

Sandimmune® (cyclosporine) was discontinued on a temporary basis and then restarted in 18 additional patients.

INFECTIOUS COMPLICATIONS IN THE RANDOMIZED RENAL TRANSPLANT PATIENTS

Complication	Cyclosporine Treatment N=227 % of Complications	Standard Treatment* N=228 % of Complications
Septicemia	5.3	4.8
Abcesses	4.4	5.3
Systemic Fungal Infection	2.2	3.9
Local Fungal Infection	7.5	9.6
Cytomegalovirus	4.8	12.3
Other Viral Infections	15.9	18.4
Urinary Tract Infections	21.1	20.2
Wound and Skin Infections	7.0	10.1
Pneumonia	6.2	9.2

* Some patients also received ALG.

Sandimmune I.V. Note: Anaphylactic reactions have occurred with Sandimmune (cyclosporine) I.V. See WARNINGS above.

Patients unable to take Sandimmune (cyclosporine) Oral Solution pre- or postoperatively may be treated with the I.V. concentrate. **Sandimmune I.V. concentrate is administered at one third the oral dose.** The initial dose of Sandimmune (cyclosporine) I.V. should be given 4–12 hours prior to transplantation as a single I.V. dose of 5–6 mg/kg per day. This daily single dose is continued postoperatively until the patient can tolerate the oral solution. Patients should be switched to Sandimmune (cyclosporine) Oral Solution as soon as possible after surgery. In pediatric usage, the same dose and dosing regimen may be used.

Adjunct steroid therapy is to be used. (See above.) Immediately before use, the I.V. concentrate should be diluted 1 ml Sandimmune®(cyclosporine) I.V. in 20 ml to 100 ml 0.9% Sodium Chloride Injection or 5% Dextrose Injection and given in a slow intravenous infusion over approximately 2 to 6 hours.

The Cremophor® EL contained in the concentrate for intravenous infusion can cause phthalate stripping from PVC.

Parenteral drug products should be inspected visually for particulate matter and discoloration prior to administration, whenever solution and container permit.

Blood Level Monitoring: Several study centers have found blood level monitoring of cyclosporine useful in patient management. While no fixed relationships have yet been established, 24 hour trough values of 250–800 ng/ml (whole blood, RIA) or 50–300 ng/ml (plasma, RIA) appear to minimize side effects and rejection events.

How Supplied:

Sandimmune (cyclosporine) Oral Solution is supplied in 50 ml bottles containing 100 mg of cyclosporine per ml (NDC 0078-0110-22). A graduated pipette for dispensing is provided. Sandimmune (cyclosporine) Oral Solution should be stored and dispensed in the original container at temperatures below 86°F (30°C). Do not store in the refrigerator. Once opened, the contents must be used within 2 months.

Sandimmune (cyclosporine) I.V. for intravenous infusion is supplied as a 5 ml sterile ampul containing 50 mg of cyclosporine per ml (NDC 0078-0109-01). Sandimmune I.V. should be stored at temperatures below 86°F (30°C) and protected from light.

Manufactured by SANDOZ Ltd.
Basle, Switzerland for
SANDOZ, Inc.
East Hanover, N.J. 07936
[SDI-Z4 Issued June 1, 1984]

IMMUNE GLOBULIN INTRAVENOUS SANDOGLOBULIN®
[san'dō-glob"ū-lin]
Lyophilized Preparation

The following prescribing information is based on official labeling in effect on November 1, 1984.

Description: Immune Globulin Intravenous* (Sandoglobulin®) is a polyvalent antibody product containing in concentrated form all the IgG antibodies which regularly occur in the donor population. This immunoglobulin preparation is produced by cold alcohol precipitation from large pools of human venous plasma. Before pooling, the single donor units of plasma have been found nonreactive for hepatitis B surface antigen (HBsAg) using test procedures of third-generation sensitivity. Sandoglobulin (IGIV) is made suitable for intravenous use by treatment at acid pH in the presence of trace amounts of pepsin (1, 2). The preparation contains at least 96% of IgG and upon reconstitution has a pH of 6.6 ± 0.2. Most of the immunoglobulins are monomeric (7 S) IgG; the remainder consists of dimeric IgG and a small amount of polymeric IgG, traces of IgA and IgM and immunoglobulin fragments (3). The distribution of the IgG subclasses corresponds to that of normal serum (4, 5, 6). Final container lyophilized units are prepared so as to contain 1, 3 or 6 g protein and 1.67, 5 or 10 g sucrose, respectively, as well as small quantities of NaCl. The lyophilized powder reconstitutes with 0.9% saline to a sterile 3% or 6% protein solution containing 5% or 10% sucrose, devoid of any preservatives.

*Herein after referred to as IGIV.

Clinical Pharmacology: This product contains a broad spectrum of antibody specificities against bacterial and viral antigens, that are capable of both opsonization and neutralization of microbes and toxins. The 3 week half-life of Immune Globulin Intravenous (Sandoglobulin) corresponds to

Continued on next page

Sandoz—Cont.

that of immune serum globulin for intramuscular use, although individual variations in half-time have been observed (7, 8). Appropriate doses of Sandoglobulin (IGIV) restore abnormally low immunoglobulin G levels to the normal range. 100% of the infused dose is available in the recipient's circulation immediately after infusion. After approximately 6 days an equilibrium is reached between the intra- and extravascular compartments. This is distributed approximately 50% intravascular and 50% extravascular. In comparison, after the intramuscular injection of an intramuscular immune globulin, the IgG requires 2–5 days to reach its maximum concentration in the intravascular compartment. This concentration corresponds to about 40% of the injected dose (8).

While Sandoglobulin (IGIV) has been shown to be effective in some cases of idiopathic thrombocytopenic purpura (ITP) (see INDICATIONS AND USAGE), the mechanism of action in ITP has not been fully elucidated.

Toxicity from overdose has not been observed on regimens of 0.4 g per kg body weight each day for 5 days (9, 10, 11). Sucrose is added to Sandoglobulin (IGIV) for reasons of stability, solubility and safety.

The intravenous administration of the sucrose used for stabilizing Immune Globulin Intravenous (Sandoglobulin) is considered to be innocuous (12). Because sucrose is excreted unchanged in the urine when given intravenously, Sandoglobulin (IGIV) may be given to diabetics, without compensatory changes in insulin dosage regimen.

Indications and Usage:
Immunodeficiency:
Sandoglobulin (IGIV) is indicated for the substitution treatment of patients who are unable to produce sufficient amounts of IgG antibodies, e.g. in common variable immunodeficiency (10, 13, 14, 15). Sandoglobulin (IGIV) is preferable to intramuscular immune serum globulin preparations in treating patients who require an immediate and high increase in the intravascular immunoglobulin level (8), in patients with limited muscle mass, and in patients with bleeding tendencies for whom intramuscular injections are contraindicated. The infusions must be repeated at regular intervals. Sandoglobulin (IGIV) may also be used in severe combined immunodeficiency and in primary immunoglobulin deficiency syndromes such as X-linked agammaglobulinemia.

Idiopathic Thrombocytopenic Purpura
A controlled study was performed in which Sandoglobulin (IGIV) was compared with steroids for the treatment of acute (defined as less than 6 months duration) ITP in patients aged 13 years and younger. In this study, Sandoglobulin (IGIV) was as effective as steroids in increasing the platelet count (9, 17). However, it should be noted that many cases of acute ITP in childhood resolve spontaneously. The use of immune globulin in the treatment of acute ITP in patients 14 years of age or older has not been subjected to prospectively controlled clinical trials (19, 21, 22).

Some children and adults with chronic (defined as greater than 6 months duration) ITP have also shown an increase (albeit temporary) in platelet counts upon administration of Immune Globulin Intravenous (Sandoglobulin®) (18, 20, 23). Therefore, in situations that require a rapid, temporary rise in platelet count, for example prior to surgery or in control of excessive bleeding, use of Sandoglobulin (IGIV) should be considered. However, it should be noted that not all patients will respond. Even in those patients who do respond, this treatment should not be considered to be curative.

Contraindications:
As with all blood products containing IgA, Sandoglobulin (IGIV) is contraindicated in patients with selective IgA deficiency, who possess antibody to IgA. It may also be contraindicated in patients who have had severe systemic reactions to the intravenous or intramuscular administration of human immune globulin.

Warnings: Patients with agamma- or extreme hypogammaglobulinemia who have never before received immunoglobulin substitution treatment or whose time from last treatment is greater than 8 weeks, may be at risk of developing inflammatory reactions on rapid infusion of Sandoglobulin (IGIV) (over 20 drops [1 ml] per minute). These reactions are manifested by a rise in temperature, chills, nausea and vomiting. The patient's vital signs should be monitored continuously and he should be carefully observed throughout the infusion, since these reactions on rare occasions may lead to shock. Epinephrine should be available for treatment of an acute anaphylactic reaction. Particular care should be exercised when Immune Globulin Intravenous (Sandoglobulin is administered to patients with paraproteins (15).

Precautions: It is generally advisable not to dilute plasma derivatives with other infusable drugs. Sandoglobulin (IGIV) should be given by a separate infusion line. No other medications or fluids should be mixed with the Sandoglobulin (IGIV) preparation.

Pregnancy: Pregnancy Category C. Animal reproduction studies have not been conducted with Sandoglobulin (IGIV). It is also not known whether Sandoglobulin (IGIV) can cause fetal harm when administered to a pregnant woman or can affect reproduction capacity. Sandoglobulin (IGIV) should be given to a pregnant woman only if clearly needed (22).

Pediatric use: High dose administration of Sandoglobulin (IGIV) in children with acute or chronic idiopathic thrombocytopenic purpura or in preterm neonates did not reveal any pediatric-specific hazard (9, 16).

Adverse Reactions: Adverse reactions to Sandoglobulin (IGIV) are rare and occur in less than 1% of patients who are not immunodeficient. Agammaglobulinemic and hypogammaglobulinemic patients who have never received immunoglobulin substitution therapy before or whose time from last treatment is greater than 8 weeks may show adverse reactions if the initial infusion flow rate exceeds 20 drops (1 ml) per minute. This occurs in approximately 10% of the cases.

These reactions, which generally become apparent only 30 minutes to one hour after the beginning of the infusion, are as follows: flushing of the face, feelings of tightness in the chest, chills, fever, dizziness, nausea, diaphoresis and hypotension. In such cases the infusion should be temporarily stopped until the symptoms have subsided. Immediate anaphylactoid and hypersensitivity reactions due to previous sensitization of the recipient to certain antigens, most commonly IgA, may be observed in exceptional cases, described under CONTRAINDICATIONS (10, 11, 24).

Dosage and Administration:
Adult and child substitution therapy: The usual dose of Immune Globulin Intravenous (Sandoglobulin) in immunodeficiency syndromes is 0.2 g per kg of body weight administered once a month by intravenous infusion. If the clinical response is inadequate or the level of serum IgG achieved is insufficient (minimum serum level of 300 mg per dl), the dose may be increased to 0.3 g per kg of body weight or the infusion may be repeated more frequently than once a month (10, 13, 14, 15).

The first infusion of Sandoglobulin (IGIV) in previously untreated agammaglobulinemic or hypogammaglobulinemic patients must be given as a 3% immunoglobulin solution (use the total volume of fluid provided to reconstitute the lyophilized product). Start with a flow rate of 10 to 20 drops (0.5 to 1.0 ml) per minute. After 15–30 minutes the rate of infusion may be further increased to 30 to 50 drops (1.5 to 2.5 ml) per minute. Subsequent infusions may be administered at a rate of 40 to 50 drops (2.0 to 2.5 ml) per minute.

If high doses have to be administered repeatedly after the first dose, a 6% solution may be used (use half the volume of fluid provided to reconstitute the lyophilized product). In this case the initial rate of infusion should be 20 to 30 drops (1.0 to 1.5 ml) per minute, increased after 15–30 minutes to a maximum of 50 drops (2.5 ml) per minute.

Recent investigations confirm that Immune Globulin Intravenous (Sandoglobulin®) is well tolerated and not likely to produce side effects when infused at these rates (11). However, the first infusion of Sandoglobulin (IGIV) in previously untreated agammaglobulinemic and hypogammaglobulinemic patients may lead to systemic side effects. Some of the effects may occur as a result of the reaction between the antibodies administered and free antigens in the blood and tissues of the immunodeficient recipient (11, 24). When free antigen is no longer present, further administration of Sandoglobulin (IGIV) to immunodeficient patients as well as to normal individuals usually does not cause further untoward side effects.

Therapy of idiopathic thrombocytopenic purpura (ITP): 0.4 g per kg of body weight on 5 consecutive days.

Reconstitution: Preparation of a 3% or 6% solution
For a 3% solution:
1. Tear off the protective caps from the bottles containing the solvent and the Sandoglobulin (IGIV). Disinfect both rubber stoppers with alcohol.
2. Remove the protective cover from one end of the transfer set and insert the needle through the rubber stopper into the bottle containing the solvent.
3. Remove the cover from the other needle and plunge the inverted Sandoglobulin (IGIV) bottle onto it, as shown in 3.
4. Invert the two bottles, so that the solvent flows into the Sandoglobulin (IGIV) bottle.
5. Discard the empty solvent bottle and the transfer set.

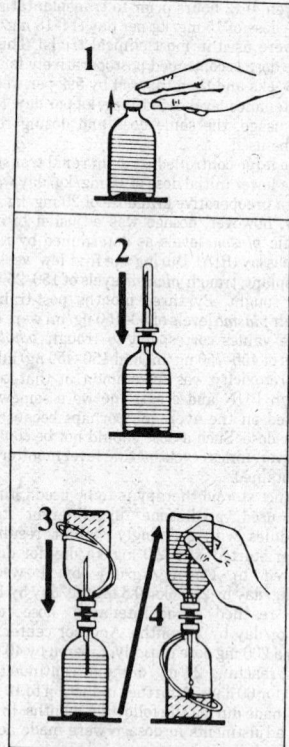

For a 6% solution*:
1. Follow steps 1–3 above.
2. Invert the two bottles, so that the solvent flows into the Immune Globulin Intravenous (Sandoglobulin) bottle. Use half the solvent by removing the solvent bottle with transfer needle as soon as the fluid reaches the 6% mark printed on the Sandoglobulin (IGIV) label.

*Note: The 6% mark is printed on the label only to provide general guidance in preparing a solution containing approximately 6 g protein per 100 ml. If an exact dosage of a 6% solution is

required, reconstitute with diluent by using a hypodermic needle and syringe; e.g.,
for 1 g vial use 16.5 ml diluent,
for 3 g vial use 50 ml diluent,
for 6 g vial use 100 ml diluent.
3. Discard any unused solvent and the transfer set. Sandoglobulin (IGIV) normally dissolves within a few minutes, though in exceptional cases it may take up to 20 minutes.

DO NOT SHAKE!
Any undissolved particles should respond to careful rotation of the bottle. Avoid frothing.
PROCEED WITH INFUSION ONLY IF SOLUTION IS CLEAR AND AT APPROXIMATELY BODY TEMPERATURE!
Parenteral drug products should be inspected visually for particulate matter and discoloration prior to administration, whenever solution and container permit.

How Supplied: Immune Globulin Intravenous Sandoglobulin is supplied as a kit containing the lyophilized preparation, sterile Sodium Chloride Injection USP, one double-ended spike for reconstitution and complete directions for use.
Sandoglobulin (IGIV) is available in three package sizes:
- 1 g Sandoglobulin (IGIV) and 33 ml reconstitution fluid
- 3 g Sandoglobulin (IGIV) and 100 ml reconstitution fluid
- 6 g Sandoglobulin (IGIV) and 200 ml reconstitution fluid

Storage:—Sandoglobulin (IGIV) should be stored at a temperature not exceeding 20°C (68°F).
The preparation should not be used after the expiration date printed on the label.
—Begin administration promptly after reconstitution.
—Partially used vials should be discarded.

Caution: U.S. Federal law prohibits dispensing without prescription.

References:
1. Römer, J., Morgenthaler, J.J., Scherz, R., and F. Skvaril: Characterization of various Immunoglobulin-Preparations for intravenous Application. I. Protein composition and antibody content. Vox. Sang. 42:62–73 (1982).
2. Römer, J., Späth, P.J., Skvaril, F., and U.E. Nydegger: Characterization of various Immunoglobulin Preparations for intravenous Application. II. Complement Activation and Binding to Staphylococcus Protein A. Vox. Sang. 42:74–80 (1982).
3. Römer, J. and P.J. Späth: Molecular Composition of Immunoglobulin Preparations and its Relation to Complement Activation. In Nydegger, U.E. (Editor): Immunohemotherapy: A Guide to Immunoglobulin Prophylaxis and Therapy. Academic Press, London, p. 123 (1981).
4. Skvaril, F., Roth-Wicky, B., and S. Barandun: IgG Subclasses in Human-γ-Globulin Preparations for Intravenous Use and their Reactivity with Staphylococcus Protein A. Vox. Sang. 38:147 (1980).
5. Skvaril, F.: Qualitative and Quantitative Aspects of IgG Subclasses in i.v. Immunoglobulin Preparations. In Nydegger, U.E. (Editor): Immunohemotherapy: A Guide to Immunoglobulin Prophylaxis and Therapy. Academic Press, London p. 113 (1981).
6. Skvaril, F., and S. Barandun: In vitro Characterization of Immunoglobulins for Intravenous Use. In: Immunoglobulins: Characteristics and Uses of Intravenous Preparations. Alving, B.M. and J.S. Finlayson (Eds.). DHHS Publication No. (FDA)-80-9005, Washington, pp. 201–206.
7. Morell, A., and F. Skvaril: Struktur und biologische Eigenschaften von Immunoglobulinen und γ-Globulin-Präparaten. II. Eigenschaften von γ-Globulin-Präparaten. Schweiz. Med. Wschr. 110:80 (1980).
8. Morell, A., Schürch, B., Ryser, D., Hofer, F., Skvaril, F., and S. Barandun: In vivo Behaviour of Gamma Globulin Preparations. Vox. Sang. 38:272 (1980).
9. Imbach, P., Barandun, S., d'Apuzzo, V., Baumgartner, C., Hirt, A., Morell, A., Rossi, E., Schöni, M., Vest, M., and H.P. Wagner: High-dose Intravenous Gammaglobulin for Idiopathic Thrombocytopenic Purpura in Childhood. The Lancet, June 6: 1228 (1981).
10. Barandun, S., Morell, A., and F. Skvaril: Clinical Experiences with Immunoglobulin for Intravenous Use. In: Immunoglobulins: Characteristics and Uses of Intravenous Preparations. Alving, B.M., and J.S. Finlayson (Eds.). DHHS Publication No. (FDA)-80-9005, Washington: U.S. Government Printing Office, 1980, pp. 31–35.
11. Barandun, S., and A. Morell: Adverse Reactions to Immunoglobulin Preparations. In Nydegger, U.E. (Editor): Immunohemotherapy: A Guide to Immunoglobulin Prophylaxis and Therapy. Academic Press, London, p. 223 (1981).
12. Martindale: The Extra Pharmacopoeia, 27th Edition, ed. by Wade, A., p. 65 (1979). The Pharmaceutical Press, London.
13. Joller, P.W., Barandun, S., and W.H. Hitzig: Neue Möglichkeiten der Immunoglobulin-Ersatztherapie bei Antikörpermangel. Syndrom. Schweiz. Med. Wschr. 110:1451 (1980).
14. Barandun, S., Imbach, P., Morell, A., and H.P. Wagner: Clinical Indications for Immunoglobulin Infusion. In Nydegger, U.E. (Editor): Immunohemotherapy: A Guide to Immunoglobulin Prophylaxis and Therapy. Academic Press, London, p. 275 (1981).
15. Cunningham-Rundles, C., Smithwick, E.M., Siegal, F.P., Day, N.K. et al.: Treatment of Primary Humoral Immunodeficiency Disease with Intravenous (pH 4.0 Treated) Gammaglobulin. In: Nydegger, U.E. (Editor): Immunohemotherapy: A Guide to Immunoglobulin Prophylaxis and Therapy. Academic Press, London, p. 283 (1981).
16. Von Muralt, G., and D. Sidiropoulos: Intravenous IgG Substitution Therapy in the Treatment of Septicemia in Preterm Neonates. In: Nydegger, U.E. (Editor): Immunohemotherapy: A Guide to Immunoglobulin Prophylaxis and Therapy. Academic Press, London, p. 313 (1981).
17. Imbach, P.: A Comparison of Intravenous Immunoglobulin and Oral Corticosteroids in the Treatment of Acute Idiopathic Thrombocytopenia (ITP): A Cooperative, Randomized Study at Swiss and German Paediatric Hospitals/Hospital Departments. Data on File, Sandoz, Inc., East Hanover, N.J.
18. Bussel, J.B., Kimberly, R. P., Inman, R. D., Schulman, I., Cunningham-Rundles, C., Smithwick, E.M., O'Malley, J., Barandun, S., Polk, J.R., Cheung, N., and M.W. Hilgartner: Intravenous Gammaglobulin for Chronic Idiopathic Thrombocytopenic Purpura. Blood 62(2):480–486(Aug) 1983.
19. Fehr, J., Hofmann, V., and U. Kappeler: Transient Reversal of Thrombocytopenia in Idiopathic Thrombocytopenic Purpura by High-Dose Intravenous Gamma Globulin. N. Engl. J. Med. 306:1254 (1982).
20. Abe, T., Matsuda, J., Kawasugi, K., Joshimuro, Y., Kinoshita, T., and M. Kazama: Clinical Effect of Intravenous Immunoglobulin in Chronic Idiopathic Thrombocytopenic Purpura. Blut 47 (2):69–75 (Aug) 1983.
21. Mueller-Eckhardt, C., Küenzlen, E., Thilo-Körner, D., and H. Pralle: High-Dose Intravenous Immunoglobulin for Posttransfusion Purpura. N. Engl. J. Med. 308 (5):287 (Feb. 3) 1983.
22. Wenske, G., Gaedicke, G., Küenzlen, E. Heyes, H., Mueller-Eckhardt, C., Kleihauer, E., and G. Lauritzen: Treatment of Idiopathic Thrombocytopenic Purpura in Pregnancy by High-Dose Intravenous Immunoglobulin. Blut 46:347–353 (1983).
23. Newland, A.C., Treleaven, J.G., Minchinton, B., and A.H. Waters: High-Dose Intravenous IgG in Adults with Autoimmune Thrombocytopenia. Lancet I :84–87 (Jan. 15) 1983.
24. Cunningham-Rundles, C., Day, N.K., Wahn, V., Smithwick, E.M., Siegal, F.P., Gupta, S., and R.A. Good: Reactions To Intravenous Gammaglobulin Infusions And Immune Complex Formation. In Nydegger, U.E. (Editor): Immunohemotherapy: A Guide to Immunoglobulin Prophylaxis and Therapy. Academic Press, London, p. 447 (1981).

Manufactured by:
CENTRAL LABORATORY
BLOOD TRANSFUSION SERVICE
SWISS RED CROSS
Wankdorfstrasse 10
3000 Berne 22
Switzerland
U.S. License No. 647
Distributed by:
SANDOZ, Inc.
East Hanover, N.J. 07936
[SGL-Z1 Issued: FEBRUARY 1, 1984]

SANOREX®
[san'ō-rex"]
(mazindol) tablets, USP

The following prescribing information is based on official labeling in effect on November 1, 1984.
Description: Sanorex®(mazindol) is an imidazoisoindole anorectic agent. It is chemically designated as 5-p-chloro-phenyl-5-hydroxy-2, 3-dihydro-5H-imidazo (2,1-a) isoindole, a tautomeric form of 2-[2'-(p-chlorobenzoyl) phenyl]-2-imidazoline.

Actions: Sanorex, (mazindol), although an isoindole, has pharmacologic activity similar in many ways to the prototype drugs used in obesity, the amphetamines. Actions include central nervous system stimulation in humans and animals, as well as such amphetamine-like effects in animals as the production of stereotyped behavior. Animal experiments also suggest certain differences from phenethylamine anorectic drugs, e.g., amphetamine, with respect to site and mechanism of action; for example, mazindol appears to exert its primary effects on the limbic system. The significance of these differences for humans is uncertain. It does not cause brain norepinephrine depletion in animals; on the other hand, it does appear to inhibit storage site uptake of norepinephrine as is suggested by its marked potentiation of the effect of exogenous norepinephrine on blood pressure in dogs (see WARNINGS) and on smooth muscle contraction in vitro.
Tolerance has been demonstrated with all drugs of this class in which this phenomenon has been studied.
Drugs used in obesity are commonly known as "anorectics" or "anorexigenics." It has not been established, however, that the action of such drugs in treating obesity is exclusively one of appetite suppression. Other central nervous system actions, or metabolic effects may be involved as well.
Adult obese subjects instructed in dietary management and treated with anorectic drugs, lose more weight on the average than those treated with placebo and diet, as determined in relatively short-term clinical trials.
The average magnitude of increased weight loss of drug-treated patients over placebo-treated patients in studies of anorectics in general is ordinarily only a fraction of a pound a week. The rate of weight loss is greatest in the first weeks of therapy for both drug and placebo subjects and tends to decrease in succeeding weeks.
The amount of weight loss associated with the use of Sanorex (mazindol), as with other anorectic drugs, varies from trial to trial, and the increased weight loss appears to be related in part to variables other than the drugs prescribed, such as the interaction between physician-investigator and the patient, the population treated, and the diet prescribed. The importance of non-drug factors in such weight loss has not been elucidated.
The natural history of obesity is measured in years, whereas, most studies cited are restricted to a few weeks' duration; thus, the total impact of drug-induced weight loss over that of diet alone must be considered clinically limited.
Indication: Sanorex (mazindol) is indicated in the management of exogenous obesity as a short-term (a few weeks) adjunct in a regimen of weight reduction based on caloric restriction. The limited usefulness of agents of this class (see ACTIONS) should be measured against possible risk factors

Continued on next page

Sandoz—Cont.

inherent in their use, such as those described below.

Contraindications: Glaucoma; hypersensitivity or idiosyncrasy to Sanorex (mazindol).
Agitated states.
Patients with a history of drug abuse.
During or within 14 days following the administration of monoamine oxidase inhibitors, (hypertensive crises may result).

Warnings: Tolerance to the effect of many anorectic drugs may develop within a few weeks; if this occurs, the recommended dose should not be exceeded in an attempt to increase the effect; rather, the drug should be discontinued.

Sanorex (mazindol) may impair the ability of the patient to engage in potentially hazardous activities such as operating machinery or driving a motor vehicle; the patient should therefore be cautioned accordingly.

Drug Interactions: Sanorex (mazindol) may decrease the hypotensive effect of guanethidine; patients should be monitored accordingly.
Sanorex (mazindol) may markedly potentiate the pressor effect of exogenous catecholamines. If it should be necessary to give a pressor amine agent (e.g., levarterenol or isoproterenol) to a patient in shock (e.g., from a myocardial infarction) who has recently been taking Sanorex® (mazindol) extreme care should be taken in monitoring blood pressure at frequent intervals and initiating pressor therapy with a low initial dose and careful titration.

Drug Dependence: Sanorex (mazindol) shares important pharmacologic properties with amphetamines. Amphetamines and related stimulant drugs have been extensively abused and can produce tolerance and severe psychologic dependence. In this regard, the manifestations of chronic overdosage or withdrawal of Sanorex® (mazindol) have not been determined in humans. Abstinence effects have been observed in dogs after abrupt cessation for prolonged periods. There was some self-administration of the drug in monkeys. EEG studies and "liking" scores in human subjects yielded equivocal results. While the abuse potential of Sanorex (mazindol) has not been further defined, the possibility of dependence should be kept in mind when evaluating the desirability of including Sanorex (mazindol) as part of a weight reduction program.

Usage in Pregnancy: Sanorex (mazindol) was studied in reproduction experiments in rats and rabbits and an increase in neonatal mortality and a possible increased incidence of rib anomalies in rats were observed at relatively high doses.
Although these studies have not indicated important adverse effects, use of mazindol by women who are or may become pregnant requires that the potential benefit be weighed against the possible hazard to mother and infant.

Usage in Children: Sanorex (mazindol) is not recommended for use in children under 12 years of age.

Precautions: Insulin requirements in diabetes mellitus may be altered in association with the use of mazindol and the concomitant dietary regimen. The least amount feasible should be prescribed or dispensed at one time in order to minimize the possibility of overdosage.
Use only with caution in hypertension with monitoring of blood pressure, since evidence is insufficient to rule out a possible adverse effect on blood pressure in some hypertensive patients. The drug is not recommended in severely hypertensive patients. The drug is not recommended for patients with symptomatic cardiovascular disease including arrhythmias.

Adverse Reactions: The most common adverse effects of Sanorex (mazindol) are dry mouth, tachycardia, constipation, nervousness and insomnia.
Cardiovascular: Palpitation, tachycardia.
Central Nervous System: Overstimulation, restlessness, dizziness, insomnia, dysphoria, tremor, headache, depression, drowsiness, weakness.

Gastrointestinal: Dryness of the mouth, unpleasant taste, diarrhea, constipation, nausea, other gastrointestinal disturbances.
Skin: Rash, excessive sweating, clamminess.
Endocrine: Impotence, changes in libido have rarely been observed with Sanorex (mazindol).
Eye: Treatment of dogs with high doses of Sanorex (mazindol) for long periods resulted in some corneal opacities, reversible on cessation of medication. No such effect has been observed in humans.

Dosage and Administration: Usual dosage is 1 mg three times daily, one hour before meals, or 2 mg once daily, one hour before lunch. The lowest effective dose should be used. To determine the lowest effective dose, therapy with Sanorex (mazindol) may be initiated at 1 mg once a day, and adjusted to the need and response of the patient. Should G.I. discomfort occur, Sanorex (mazindol) may be taken with meals.

Overdosage: There are no data as yet on acute overdosage with Sanorex (mazindol) in humans. Manifestations of acute overdosage with amphetamines and related substances include restlessness, tremor, rapid respiration, dizziness. Fatigue and depression may follow the stimulatory phase of overdosage. Cardiovascular effects include tachycardia, hypertension and circulatory collapse. Gastrointestinal symptoms include nausea, vomiting and abdominal cramps. While similar manifestations of overdosage may be seen with Sanorex (mazindol), their exact nature has yet to be determined. The management of acute intoxication is largely symptomatic. Data are not available on the treatment of acute intoxication with Sanorex (mazindol) by hemodialysis or peritoneal dialysis, but the substance is poorly soluble except at very acid pH.

How Supplied: Sanorex (mazindol) is available in 1 mg elliptical, white tablets and in 2 mg round, white scored tablets, in packages of 100.

Company's Product Indentification Mark(s): 1 mg tablets embossed SANOREX on one side, 78-71 other side. 2 mg tablets scored 78-66 on one side, SANDOZ other side.

[SNX-Z11 Issued June 15, 1983]
Shown in Product Identification Section, page 433

SANSERT®
[san'surt]
(methysergide maleate) tablets, USP

The following prescribing information is based on official labeling in effect on November 1, 1984.

WARNING
Retroperitoneal Fibrosis, Pleuropulmonary Fibrosis and Fibrotic Thickening of Cardiac Valves May Occur in Patients Receiving Long-term Methysergide Maleate Therapy. Therefore, This Preparation Must be Reserved for Prophylaxis in Patients Whose Vascular Headaches Are Frequent and/or Severe and Uncontrollable and Who Are Under Close Medical Supervision.
(*See Also "Warnings" Section.*)

Composition: Each Sansert tablet contains 2 mg methysergide maleate, USP.

Actions: Sansert (methysergide maleate) has been shown, *in vitro* and *in vivo*, to inhibit or block the effects of serotonin, a substance which may be involved in the mechanism of vascular headaches. Serotonin has been variously described as a central neurohumoral agent or chemical mediator, as a "headache substance" acting directly or indirectly to lower pain threshold (others in this category include tyramine; polypeptides, such as bradykinin; histamine; and acetylcholine), as an intrinsic "motor hormone" of the gastrointestinal tract, and as a "hormone" involved in connective tissue reparative processes. Suggestions have been made by investigators as to the mechanism whereby methysergide produces its clinical effects, but this has not been finally established.

Indications: For the prevention or reduction of intensity and frequency of vascular headaches in the following kinds of patients:

1. Patients suffering from one or more severe vascular headaches per week.
2. Patients suffering from vascular headaches that are uncontrollable or so severe that preventive therapy is indicated regardless of the frequency of the attack.

Contraindications: Pregnancy, peripheral vascular disease, severe arteriosclerosis, severe hypertension, coronary artery disease, phlebitis or cellulitis of the lower limbs, pulmonary disease, collagen diseases or fibrotic processes, impaired liver or renal function, valvular heart disease, debilitated states and serious infections.

Warnings: With long-term, uninterrupted administration, retroperitoneal fibrosis or related conditions—pleuropulmonary fibrosis and cardiovascular disorders with murmurs or vascular bruits have been reported. Patients must be warned to report immediately the following symptoms: cold, numb, and painful hands and feet; leg cramps on walking; any type of girdle, flank, or chest pain, or any associated symptomatology. Should any of these symptoms develop, methysergide should be discontinued. Continuous administration should not exceed 6 months. There must be a drug-free interval of 3-4 weeks after each 6-month course of treatment. The dosage should be reduced gradually during the last 2-3 weeks of each treatment course to avoid "headache rebound."

The drug is not recommended for use in children.

Precautions: All patients receiving Sansert (methysergide maleate) should remain under constant supervision of the physician and be examined regularly for the development of fibrotic or vascular complications. (See Adverse Reactions).
The manifestations of retroperitoneal fibrosis, pleuropulmonary fibrosis, and vascular shutdown have shown a high incidence of regression once Sansert (methysergide maleate) is withdrawn. These facts should be borne in mind to avoid unnecessary surgical intervention. Cardiac murmurs, which may indicate endocardial fibrosis, have shown varying degrees of regression, with complete disappearance in some and persistence in others.

Sansert (methysergide maleate) has been specifically designed for the prophylaxis of vascular headache and has no place in the management of the acute attack.

Sansert tablets contain FD&C Yellow No. 5 (tartrazine) which may cause allergic-type reactions (including bronchial asthma) in certain susceptible individuals. Although the overall incidence of FD&C Yellow No. 5 (tartrazine) sensitivity in the general population is low, it is frequently seen in patients who also have aspirin hypersensitivity.

Adverse Reactions: Within the recommended dose levels, the following side effects have been reported:

1) Fibrotic Complications
Fibrotic changes have been observed in the retroperitoneal, pleuropulmonary, cardiac, and other tissues, either singly or, very rarely, in combination.

Retroperitoneal Fibrosis: This non-specific fibrotic process is usually confined to the retroperitoneal connective tissue above the pelvic brim and may present clinically with one or more symptoms such as general malaise, fatigue, weight loss, backache, low grade fever (elevated sedimentation rate), urinary obstruction (girdle or flank pain, dysuria, polyuria, oliguria, elevated BUN), vascular insufficiency of the lower limbs (leg pain, Leriche syndrome, edema of legs, thrombophlebitis). The single most useful diagnostic procedure in suspected cases of retroperitoneal fibrosis is intravenous pyelography. Typical deviation and obstruction of one or both ureters may be observed.

Pleuropulmonary Complications: A similar nonspecific fibrotic process, limited to the pleural and immediately subjacent pulmonary tissues, usually presents clinically with dyspnea, tightness and pain in the chest, pleural friction rubs, and pleural effusion. These findings may be confirmed by chest X-ray.

Cardiac Complications: Nonrheumatic fibrotic thickenings of the aortic root and of the aortic and

for possible revisions   **Product Information**   1817

mitral valves usually present clinically with cardiac murmurs and dyspnea.

Other Fibrotic Complications: Several cases of fibrotic plaques, simulating Peyronie's disease have been described.

2) Cardiovascular Complications

Encroachment of retroperitoneal fibrosis on the aorta, inferior vena cava and their common iliac branches may result in vascular insufficiency of the lower limbs, the presenting features of which are mentioned under retroperitoneal fibrosis.

Intrinsic vasoconstriction of large and small arteries, involving one or more vessels or merely a segment of a vessel, may occur at any stage of therapy. Depending on the vessel involved, this complication may present with chest pain, abdominal pain, or cold, numb, painful extremities with or without paresthesias and diminished or absent pulses. Progression to ischemic tissue damage has rarely been reported. Prompt withdrawal of the drug at the first signs of impaired circulation is recommended (See Warnings) to obviate such effects.

Postural hypotension and tachycardia have also been observed.

3) Gastrointestinal Symptoms

Nausea, vomiting, diarrhea, heartburn, abdominal pain. These effects tend to appear early and can frequently be obviated by gradual introduction of the medication and by administration of the drug with meals.

Constipation and elevation of gastric HCl have also been reported.

4) CNS Symptoms

Insomnia, drowsiness, mild euphoria, dizziness, ataxia, lightheadedness, hyperesthesia, unworldly feelings (described variously as "dissociation," "hallucinatory experiences," etc.). Some of these symptoms may be associated with vascular headaches, per se, and may, therefore, be unrelated to the drug.

5) Dermatological Manifestations

Facial flush, telangiectasia, and nonspecific rashes have rarely been reported. Increased hair loss may occur, but in many instances the tendency has abated despite continued therapy.

6) Edema

Peripheral edema, and more rarely, localized brawny edema may occur.

Dependent edema has responded to lowered doses, salt restriction, or diuretics.

7) Weight Gain

Weight gain may be a reason to caution patients regarding their caloric intake.

8) Hematological Manifestations

Neutropenia, eosinophilia.

9) Miscellaneous

Weakness, arthralgia, myalgia.

Dosage and Administration: Usual adult dose 4 to 8 mg daily. Tablets to be given with meals.

Note: There must be a medication-free interval of 3-4 weeks after every 6-month course of treatment (see WARNINGS).

No pediatric dosage has been established.

If, after a 3-week trial period, efficacy has not been demonstrated, longer administration of Sansert (methysergide maleate) is unlikely to be of benefit.

How Supplied: Bottles of 100 tablets, each tablet containing 2 mg of methysergide maleate, USP.

Company's Product Identification Mark(s): Imprinted 78-58 on one side, SANDOZ other side.

[SAN-Z19 Issued January 16, 1984]

Shown in Product Identification Section, page 433

SYNTOCINON® INJECTION   ℞
[sin″tō′si-non]
(oxytocin injection, USP)

The following prescribing information is based on official labeling in effect on November 1, 1984.

Description: Syntocinon® (oxytocin) injection is a synthetic nonapeptide. Its commercial synthesis was first achieved in the Research Laboratories of Sandoz Ltd.

For intravenous or intramuscular administration.

Each 1 ml of Syntocinon solution contains 10 USP or International Units of oxytocin and the following inactive ingredients:

sodium acetate, USP ....1 mg
sodium chloride, USP ....0.017 mg
chlorobutanol, NF 0.5%
alcohol, USP ....0.61% by vol.
acetic acid, NF, qs to ....pH 4 ± .3
water for injection, USP, qs to ....1 ml

The Syntocinon solution in each ampul is sterile.

Syntocinon (oxytocin) is an oxytocic agent that, when given in appropriate doses during pregnancy, is capable of eliciting graded increases in uterine motility from a moderate increase in the rate and force of spontaneous motor activity to sustained tetanic contraction.

Syntocinon (oxytocin) is a cyclic (1→6) nonapeptide with the following chemical name.

Glycinamide, L-cysteinyl-L-tyrosyl-L-isoleucyl-L-glutaminyl-L-asparaginyl-L-cysteinyl-L-prolyl-L-leucyl-, cyclic (1→6)-disulfide

Its Chemical Abstract Registry number is: 50-56-6; and its chemical formula is shown below.

$$\underset{4}{Glu(NH_2)} - \underset{5}{Asp(NH_2)} - \underset{6}{Cys} - \underset{7}{Pro} - \underset{8}{Leu} - \underset{9}{Gly(NH_2)}$$
$$\underset{3}{Ileu} - \underset{2}{Tyr} - \underset{1}{Cys}$$

oxytocin

Action: The pharmacologic and clinical properties of Syntocinon (oxytocin) are identical with the naturally occurring oxytocic principle of the posterior lobe of the pituitary. Syntocinon (oxytocin) injection does not contain the amino acids characteristic of vasopressin, and therefore lacks cardiovascular effects. Syntocinon (oxytocin) exerts a selective action on the smooth musculature of the uterus, particularly toward the end of pregnancy, during labor and immediately following delivery. Oxytocin stimulates rhythmic contractions of the uterus, increases the frequency of existing contractions, and raises the tone of the uterine musculature.

Indications:

IMPORTANT NOTICE

Syntocinon (oxytocin) injection is indicated for the medical rather than the elective induction of labor. Available data and information are inadequate to define the benefits to risks considerations in the use of the drug product for elective induction. Elective induction of labor is defined as the initiation of labor for convenience in an individual with a term pregnancy who is free of medical indications.

Antepartum: Syntocinon (oxytocin) is indicated for the initiation or improvement of uterine contractions, where this is desirable and considered suitable, in order to achieve early vaginal delivery for fetal or maternal reasons. It is indicated for (1) induction of labor in patients with a medical indication for the initiation of labor, such as Rh problems, maternal diabetes, pre-eclampsia at or near term, when delivery is in the best interest of mother and fetus or when membranes are prematurely ruptured and delivery is indicated; (2) stimulation or reinforcement of labor, as in selected cases of uterine inertia; (3) as adjunctive therapy in the management of incomplete or inevitable abortion. In the first trimester currettage is generally considered primary therapy. In the second trimester abortion, oxytocin infusion will often be successful in emptying the uterus. Other means of therapy, however, may be required in such cases.

Postpartum: Syntocinon (oxytocin) injection is indicated to produce uterine contractions during the third stage of labor and to control postpartum bleeding or hemorrhage.

Contraindications: Syntocinon (oxytocin) injection is contraindicated in any of the following conditions: Significant cephalopelvic disproportion; unfavorable fetal positions or presentations which are undeliverable without conversion prior to delivery, i.e., (transverse lies); in obstetrical emergencies where the benefit-to-risk ratio for either the fetus or the mother favors surgical intervention; in cases of fetal distress where delivery is not imminent; prolonged use in uterine inertia or severe toxemia; hypertonic uterine patterns; patients with hypersensitivity to the drug; induction or augmentation of labor in those cases where vaginal delivery is contraindicated, such as cord presentation or prolapse, total placenta previa, and vasa previa.

Warnings: Syntocinon® (oxytocin) when given for induction or stimulation of labor, must be administered only by the intravenous route and with adequate medical supervision in a hospital.

Precautions:

1. All patients receiving intravenous oxytocin must be under continuous observation by trained personnel with a thorough knowledge of the drug and qualified to identify complications. A physician qualified to manage any complications should be immediately available.

2. When properly administered, oxytocin should stimulate uterine contractions similar to those seen in normal labor. Overstimulation of the uterus by improper administration can be hazardous to both mother and fetus. Even with proper administration and adequate supervision, hypertonic contractions can occur in patients whose uteri are hypersensitive to oxytocin.

3. Except in unusual circumstances, oxytocin should not be administered in the following conditions: prematurity, borderline cephalopelvic disproportion, previous major surgery on the cervix or uterus including cesarean section, over-distention of the uterus, grand multiparity, or invasive cervical carcinoma. Because of the variability of the combinations of factors which may be present in the conditions listed above, the definition of "unusual circumstances" must be left to the judgment of the physician. The decision can only be made by carefully weighing the potential benefits which oxytocin can provide in a given case against rare but definite potential for the drug to produce hypertonicity or tetanic spasm.

4. Maternal deaths due to hypertensive episodes, subarchnoid hemorrhage, rupture of the uterus, and fetal deaths due to various causes have been reported associated with the use of parental oxytocic drugs for induction of labor or for augmentation in the first and second stages of labor.

5. Oxytocin has been shown to have an intrinsic antidiuretic effect, acting to increase water reabsorption from the glomerular filtrate. Consideration should, therefore, be given to the possibility of water intoxication, particularly when oxytocin is administered continuously by infusion and the patient is receiving fluids by mouth.

Adverse reactions: The following adverse reactions have been reported: Fetal bradycardia, neonatal jaundice, anaphylactic reaction, postpartum hemorrhage, cardiac arrhythmia, fatal afibrinogenemia, nausea, vomiting, premature ventricular contractions and pelvic hematoma.

Excessive dosage or hypersensitivity to the drug may result in uterine hypertonicity, spasm, tetanic contraction, or rupture of the uterus.

The possibility of increased blood loss and afibrinogenemia should be kept in mind when administering the drug.

Severe water intoxication with convulsions and coma has occurred, associated with a slow oxytocin infusion over a 24-hour period. Maternal death due to oxytocin-induced water intoxication has been reported.

Dosage and Administration: Dosage of oxytocin is determined by uterine response. The following dosage information is based upon the various regimens and indications in general use.

A. Induction or Stimulation of Labor

Intravenous infusion (drip method) is the only acceptable method of administration for the induction or stimulation of labor.

Accurate control of the rate of infusion flow is essential. An infusion pump or other such device and frequent monitoring of strength of contractions and fetal heart rate are necessary for the safe administration of oxytocin for the induction or stimulation of labor. If uterine contractions become too

Continued on next page

Sandoz—Cont.

powerful, the infusion can be abruptly stopped, and oxytocic stimulation of the uterine musculature will soon wane.

1. An intravenous infusion of non-oxytocin containing solution should be started. Physiologic electrolyte solution should be used except under unusual circumstances.

2. To prepare the usual solution for infusion, the contents of one 1-ml ampul is combined aseptically with 1,000 ml of nonhydrating diluent. The combined solution, rotated in the infusion bottle to insure thorough mixing contains 10 mU/ml. Add the container with dilute oxytocic solution to the system through use of a constant infusion pump or other such device, to control accurately the rate of infusion.

3. The initial dose should be no more than 1–2 mU/min. The dose may be gradually increased in increments of no more than 1 to 2 mU/min. until a contraction pattern has been established, which is similar to normal labor.

4. The fetal heart rate, resting uterine tone, and the frequency, duration, and force of contractions should be monitored.

5. The oxytocin infusion should be discontinued immediately in the event of uterine hyperactivity or fetal distress. Oxygen should be administered to the mother. The mother and the fetus must be evaluated by the responsible physician.

B. Control of Postpartum Uterine Bleeding

1. *Intravenous Infusion (Drip Method):* To control postpartum bleeding, 10 to 40 units of oxytocin may be added to 1,000 ml of a nonhydrating diluent and run at a rate necessary to control uterine atony.

2. *Intramuscular Administration:* 1 ml (10 units) of oxytocin can be given after delivery of the placenta.

C. Treatment of Incomplete or Inevitable Abortion

Intravenous infusion with physiologic saline solution, 500 ml, or 5% dextrose in physiologic saline solution to which 10 units of Syntocinon® (oxytocin) have been added should be infused at a rate of 20 to 40 drops per minute.

How Supplied: Syntocinon (oxytocin) injection, ampuls, 1 ml (10 USP units) size, boxes of 20 and 100.

Store and dispense: Below 77°F; DO NOT FREEZE

[SYT-Z18 Issued March 12, 1984]

SYNTOCINON® NASAL SPRAY ℞
[sin″ tō′ si-non]
(oxytocin nasal solution, USP)

The following prescribing information is based on official labeling in effect on November 1, 1984.

Description: Each ml. contains 40 USP Units (International Units) Syntocinon® (oxytocin) and the following: dried sodium phosphate, USP, citric acid, USP, sodium chloride, USP, glycerin, USP, sorbitol solution, USP, methylparaben, NF, propylparaben, NF, chlorobutanol, NF max. 0.05%, purified water, USP.

Oxytocin is one of the polypeptide hormones of the posterior lobe of the pituitary gland. The pharmacologic and clinical properties of Syntocinon (oxytocin) are identical with *the oxytocic and the galactokinetic* principle of the natural hormone. Syntocinon was synthesized on a commercial scale by Sandoz, and was introduced for clinical use in 1957.

Since oxytocin, a polypeptide, is subject to inactivation by the proteolytic enzymes of the alimentary tract, it is *not absorbed from the gastrointestinal tract.* Intranasal application of the spray preparation, however, is a practical and effective method of administration.

Action: Syntocinon Nasal Spray acts specifically on the myoepithelial elements surrounding the alveoli of the breast, causing them to contract and thus force milk into the larger ducts where it is more readily available to the baby.

Indication: Initial milk let-down.
Contraindications: Pregnancy; hypersensitivity.
Dosage and Administration: One spray into one or both nostrils 2 to 3 minutes before nursing or pumping of breasts.

Note: The squeeze bottle should be held in upright position when administering drug to the nose and patient should be in a sitting position rather than lying down. If preferred, the solution can be instilled in drop form by inverting the squeeze bottle and exerting very gentle pressure on its walls.

Supplied: Syntocinon (oxytocin) Nasal Spray in squeeze bottles containing 2 ml oxytocin solution or 5 ml oxytocin solution.

[SYT-ZZ11 Issued June 15, 1983]

TAVIST-1® (clemastine fumarate) ℞
[tav′ ist]
TABLETS 1.34 mg
TAVIST® (clemastine fumarate)
TABLETS 2.68 mg

The following prescribing information is based on official labeling in effect on November 1, 1984.

Description: TAVIST (clemastine fumarate) belongs to the benzhydryl ether group of antihistaminic compounds. The chemical name is (+)-2-[2-[(p-chloro-α-methyl-α-phenylbenzyl) oxy]ethyl]-1-methylpyrrolidine* hydrogen fumarate.
*U.S. Patent No. 3,097,212.

Actions: TAVIST is an antihistamine with anticholinergic (drying) and sedative side effects. Antihistamines appear to compete with histamine for cell receptor sites on effector cells. The inherently long duration of antihistaminic effects of TAVIST has been demonstrated in wheal and flare studies. In normal human subjects who received histamine injections over a 24-hour period, the antihistaminic activity of TAVIST reached a peak at 5–7 hours, persisted for 10–12 hours and, in some cases, for as long as 24 hours. Pharmacokinetic studies in man utilizing ^{3}H and ^{14}C labeled compound demonstrates that: TAVIST (clemastine fumarate) is rapidly and nearly completely absorbed from the gastrointestinal tract, peak plasma concentrations are attained in 2–4 hours, and urinary excretion is the major mode of elimination.

Indications: TAVIST-1 Tablets 1.34 mg are indicated for the relief of symptoms associated with allergic rhinitis such as sneezing, rhinorrhea, pruritus and lacrimation.

TAVIST Tablets 2.68 mg are indicated for the relief of symptoms associated with allergic rhinitis such as sneezing, rhinorrhea, pruritus, and lacrimation. TAVIST Tablets 2.68 mg are also indicated for the relief of mild, uncomplicated allergic skin manifestations of urticaria and angioedema. It should be noted that TAVIST (clemastine fumarate) is indicated for the dermatologic indications at the 2.68 mg dosage level only.

Contraindications: *Use in Nursing Mothers:* Because of the higher risk of antihistamines for infants generally and for newborns and prematures in particular, antihistamine therapy is contraindicated in nursing mothers.

Use in Lower Respiratory Disease: Antihistamines should not be used to treat lower respiratory tract symptoms including asthma.

Antihistamines are also contraindicated in the following conditions:

Hypersensitivity to TAVIST (clemastine fumarate) or other antihistamines of similar chemical structure.

Monamine oxidase inhibitor therapy (see Drug Interaction Section).

Warnings: Antihistamines should be used with considerable caution in patients with: narrow angle glaucoma, stenosing peptic ulcer, pyloroduodenal obstruction, symptomatic prostatic hypertrophy, and bladder neck obstruction.

Use in Children: Safety and efficacy of TAVIST have not been established in children under the age of 12.

Use in Pregnancy: Experience with this drug in pregnant women is inadequate to determine whether there exists a potential for harm to the developing fetus.

Use with CNS Depressants: TAVIST has additive effects with alcohol and other CNS depressants (hypnotics, sedatives, tranquilizers, etc.)

Use in Activities Requiring Mental Alertness: Patients should be warned about engaging in activities requiring mental alertness such as driving a car or operating appliances, machinery, etc.

Use in the Elderly (approximately 60 years or older): Antihistamines are more likely to cause dizziness, sedation, and hypotension in elderly patients.

Precautions: TAVIST (clemastine fumarate) should be used with caution in patients with: history of bronchial asthma, increased intraocular pressure, hyperthyroidism, cardiovascular disease, and hypertension.

Drug Interactions: MAO inhibitors prolong and intensify the anticholinergic (drying) effects of antihistamines.

Adverse Reactions: Transient drowsiness, the most common adverse reaction associated with TAVIST (clemastine fumarate), occurs relatively frequently and may require discontinuation of therapy in some instances.

Antihistaminic Compounds: It should been noted that the following reactions have occurred with one or more antihistamines and, therefore, should be kept in mind when prescribing drugs belonging to this class, including TAVIST. The most frequent adverse reactions are underlined.

1. *General:* Urticaria, drug rash, anaphylactic shock, photosensitivity, excessive perspiration, chills, dryness of mouth, nose, and throat.
2. *Cardiovascular System:* Hypotension, headache, palpitations, tachycardia, extrasystoles.
3. *Hematologic System:* Hemolytic anemia, thrombocytopenia, agranulocytosis.
4. *Nervous System:* Sedation, sleepiness, dizziness, disturbed coordination, fatigue, confusion, restlessness, excitation, nervousness, tremor, irritability, insomnia, euphoria, paresthesias, blurred vision, diplopia, vertigo, tinnitus, acute labyrinthitis, hysteria, neuritis, convulsions.
5. *GI System:* Epigastric distress, anorexia, nausea, vomiting, diarrhea, constipation.
6. *GU System:* Urinary frequency, difficult urination, urinary retention, early menses.
7. *Respiratory System:* Thickening of bronchial secretions, tightness of chest and wheezing, nasal stuffiness.

Overdosage: Antihistamine overdosage reactions may vary from central nervous system depression to stimulation. Stimulation is particularly likely in children. Atropine-like signs and symptoms: dry mouth; fixed, dilated pupils; flushing; and gastrointestinal symptoms may also occur.

If vomiting has not occurred spontaneously the conscious patient should be induced to vomit. This is best done by having him drink a glass of water or milk after which he should be made to gag. Precautions against aspiration must be taken, especially in infants and children.

If vomiting is unsuccessful gastric lavage is indicated within 3 hours after ingestion and even later if large amounts of milk or cream were given beforehand. Isotonic and ½ isotonic saline is the lavage solution of choice.

Saline cathartics, such as milk of magnesia, by osmosis draw water into the bowel and therefore, are valuable for their action in rapid dilution of bowel content.

Stimulants should *not* be used.

Vasopressors may be used to treat hypotension.

Dosage and Administration: DOSAGE SHOULD BE INDIVIDUALIZED ACCORDING TO THE NEEDS AND RESPONSE OF THE PATIENT.

TAVIST-1 Tablets 1.34 mg: The recommended starting dose is one tablet twice daily. Dosage may be increased as required, but not to exceed six tablets daily.

TAVIST Tablets 2.68 mg: The maximum recommended dosage is one tablet three times daily. Many patients respond favorably to a single dose which may be repeated as required, but not to exceed three tablets daily.

How Supplied: TAVIST-1 Tablets: 1.34 mg clemastine fumarate. White, oval compressed, scored tablet, packages of 100.

TAVIST Tablets: 2.68 mg clemastine fumarate. White, round compressed tablet, packages of 100.

Company's Product Identification Mark(s):
Tavist-1 Tablets: 1.34 mg, embossed "78-75" on one side, "TAVIST-1" on the other.
Tavist Tablets: 2.68 mg, embossed "78/72" and scored on one side, "TAVIST" on the other.
[TAV-Z1 Issued September 15, 1982]
Shown in Product Identification Section, page 433

TAVIST–D®
[*tav'ist*]
(clemastine fumarate/ phenylpropanolamine HCl) Tablets

The following prescribing information is based on official labeling in effect on November 1, 1984.

Description: Each TAVIST-D (clemastine fumarate/phenylpropanolamine HCl) Tablet contains 1.34 mg clemastine fumarate (equivalent to 1 mg of the free base) and 75 mg phenylpropanolamine hydrochloride. The clemastine fumarate is in the outer shell of the tablet and is immediately released upon dissolution. The tablet's core is a sustained-release matrix which releases the phenylpropanolamine hydrochloride over a 12-hour period at a rate that produces blood levels bioequivalent to those obtained by the administration of 25 mg standard release tablets of phenylpropanolamine hydrochloride every four hours for three doses. Clemastine fumarate belongs to the benzhydryl ether group of antihistaminic compounds. The chemical name is (+)-2-[-2-[(p-chloro-α-methyl-α-phenyl benzyl) oxy] ethyl]-1-methylpyrrolidine hydrogen fumarate.

Phenylpropanolamine hydrochloride is a sympathomimetic, orally effective nasal decongestant. Sympathomimetic compounds, whether catecholamines or noncatecholamines, can be regarded as compounds produced by substitution on the phenylethylamine nucleus common to all these sympathomimetic products, whether their action is on the Alpha receptors of the sympathetic nervous system or on Beta-1 or Beta-2 receptors. The chemical name for phenylpropanolamine hydrochloride is α-(1-Aminoethyl)benzenemethanol hydrochloride.

Clinical Pharmacology: Clemastine fumarate is an antihistamine with anticholinergic (drying) and sedative side effects. Antihistamines appear to compete with histamine for cell receptor sites on effector cells. The inherently long duration of antihistaminic effects of clemastine fumarate has been demonstrated in wheal and flare studies. In normal human subjects who received intradermal histamine injections over a 24-hour period, the antihistaminic activity of clemastine fumarate, as demonstrated by inhibition of the wheal and flare reaction, reached a peak at 5–7 hours, persisted for 10–12 hours and, in some cases, for as long as 24 hours. Pharmacokinetic studies in man utilizing ^{3}H and ^{14}C labeled compound demonstrate that clemastine fumarate is rapidly and nearly completely absorbed from the gastrointestinal tract, peak plasma concentrations are attained in 2–4 hours, and urinary excretion is the major mode of elimination.

Phenylpropanolamine hydrochloride is an Alpha adrenergic stimulator producing nasal decongestion by constriction of arterioles and precapillary arterioles in the nasal mucosa. Phenylpropanolamine hydrochloride is one of the most widely used oral nasal decongestants; it is similar in action to ephedrine, but produces less central nervous system stimulation.

In adult subjects who were given one TAVIST-D (clemastine fumarate/phenylpropanolamine HCl) Tablet, the average peak plasma concentration of phenylpropanolamine was 85.4 ng/ml ± 13.1 (S.D.) which occurred at about 4.3 hours. In this crossover study these same subjects were given a 25 mg phenylpropanolamine hydrochloride tablet every 4 hours for 3 consecutive doses plus a single dose of a TAVIST-1 Tablet (clemastine fumarate 1.34 mg). The average peak concentration of phenylpropanolamine was found to be 67.6 ng/ml ± 11.6 (S.D.) which occurred at about 8.2 hours.

In another study, adult subjects received TAVIST-D Tablets every 12 hours for 4 consecutive days. The average peak concentration of phenylpropanolamine was found to be 117.29 ng/ml ± 14.52 (S.D.) which occurred at about 6.2 hours after the morning dose. In this crossover study these same subjects received a 25 mg phenylpropanolamine hydrochloride tablet every 4 hours for 4 consecutive days. In addition they received a TAVIST-1 Tablet (clemastine fumarate 1.34 mg) every 12 hours for 4 consecutive days. The average peak concentration of phenylpropanolamine was found to be 107.92 ng/ml ± 15.97 (S.D.) which occurred at about 4.8 hours after the first dose in the morning.

Indications and Usage: TAVIST-D (clemastine fumarate/phenylpropanolamine HCl) Tablets are indicated for the relief of symptoms associated with allergic rhinitis such as sneezing, rhinorrhea, pruritus of the eyes, nose or throat, lacrimation and nasal congestion.

Contraindications: Tavist-D Tablets are contraindicated in patients hypersensitive to any of the components. Antihistamines should not be used in newborn or premature infants or in nursing mothers. Antihistamines should not be used to treat lower respiratory tract symptoms including asthma. Tavist-D Tablets are contraindicated in patients receiving monoamine oxidase inhibitors (see PRECAUTIONS—Drug Interactions) and in patients with severe hypertension or severe coronary artery disease.

Warnings: Antihistamines such as clemastine fumarate should be used with considerable caution in patients with narrow angle glaucoma, stenosing peptic ulcer, pyloroduodenal obstruction, symptomatic prostatic hypertrophy, and bladder neck obstruction. Sympathomimetic drugs such as phenylpropanolamine hydrochloride should be used with caution in hypertension, cardiovascular disease, diabetes mellitus, and uncontrolled hyperthyroidism.

Use with CNS Depressants: Antihistamines have additive effects with alcohol and other CNS depressants (hypnotics, sedatives, tranquilizers, etc.).

Use in Activities Requiring Mental Alertness: Patients should be warned about engaging in activities requiring mental alertness such as driving a car or operating appliances, machinery, etc.

Use in the Elderly (approximately 60 years or older): Antihistamines are more likely to cause dizziness, sedation and hypotension in elderly patients. Overdosages of sympathomimetics in this age group may cause hallucinations, convulsions, CNS depression and death in elderly patients.

Use in Children: Safety and effectiveness of TAVIST-D (clemastine fumarate/phenylpropanolamine HCl) have not been established in children under the age of 12. In infants and children, especially, antihistamines in *overdosage* may cause hallucinations, convulsions or death. As in adults antihistamines may diminish mental alertness, but they may also produce excitation, particularly in young children.

Precautions:
General: TAVIST-D (clemastine fumarate/phenylpropanolamine HCl) Tablets should be used with caution in patients with: History of bronchial asthma, increased intraocular pressure, hyperthyroidism, cardiovascular disease, hypertension, diabetes mellitus, and prostate disease. (See WARNINGS.)

Information for Patients: Patients should be informed of the potential for sedation or drowsiness and warned about driving or operating machinery. The concomitant consumption of alcoholic beverages or other sedative drugs should be avoided.

Due to the inherently long-acting nature of clemastine fumarate and due to the sustained-release of phenylpropanolamine hydrochloride from the tablet's core, TAVIST-D Tablets provide prolonged symptomatic relief (10–14 hours).

Drug Interactions:
(1) Monoamine oxidase inhibitors; MAO inhibitors prolong and intensify the anticholinergic effects of antihistamines and potentiate the pressor effects of sympathomimetics.

(2) Alcohol and CNS depressants: These agents potentiate the sedative effects of antihistamines.

(3) Certain antihypertensives: Sympathomimetics may reduce the antihypertensive effects of methyldopa, mecamylamine, reserpine and veratrum alkaloids.

Carcinogenesis and Mutagenesis: Carcinogenic studies have not been conducted on the drug combination of clemastine fumarate/phenylpropanolamine hydrochloride. In a two-year oral study in the rat at a dose of 84 mg/Kg (about 1500 times the human dose) and an 85-week oral study in the mouse at 206 mg/Kg (about 3800 times the human dose), clemastine fumarate showed no evidence of carcinogenesis.

No mutagenic studies have been conducted with clemastine fumarate, phenylpropanolamine hydrochloride or the drug combination.

Inpairment of Fertility: Oral doses of clemastine fumarate alone in the rat produced a decrease in mating ability of the male at 933 times the human dose. This effect was not found at 466 times the human dose.

Pregnancy—*Pregnancy Category B:* Oral reproduction studies performed with clemastine fumarate alone in rats and rabbits at doses up to 933 and 560 times the human dose, respectively, have revealed no evidence of teratogenic effects. Reproduction studies have not been conducted with phenylpropanolamine hydrochloride alone.

Oral reproduction studies on the drug combination in a ratio of 1 part of clemastine fumarate to 49 parts of phenylpropanolamine hydrochloride in rats and rabbits at doses up to 100 and 67 times the human dose, respectively, have revealed no evidence of teratogenic effects. Adverse reactions attributed to the pharmacological effects of phenylpropanolamine were as follows: Rats—Impaired weight gain and deaths in dams at 33 times the human dose and a slight increase in pre-implantation loss and prenatal deaths, and reduced fetal weights at 100 times the human dose. Rabbits—Increased maternal deaths at 20 times the human dose, and increased maternal deaths and weight loss plus a slight increase in prenatal deaths (within normal limits) at 67 times the human dose. There are no adequate and well controlled studies of TAVIST-D (clemastine fumarate/phenylpropanolamine HCl) Tablets in pregnant women. Because animal reproduction studies are not always predictive of human response, this drug should be used in pregnancy only if clearly needed.

Nursing Mothers: See CONTRAINDICATIONS:

Adverse Reactions:
Antihistaminic Compounds: It should be noted that the following reactions have occurred with one or more antihistamines and, therefore, should be kept in mind when prescribing drugs belonging to this class, including clemastine fumarate. The most frequent adverse reactions reported with clemastine fumarate are underlined.

1. *General:* Urticaria, drug rash, anaphylactic shock, photosensitivity, excessive perspiration, chills, dryness of mouth, nose and throat.
2. *Cardiovascular System:* Hypotension, headache, palpitations, tachycardia, extrasystoles.
3. *Hematologic System:* Hemolytic anemia, thrombocytopenia, agranulocytosis.
4. *Nervous System:* Sedation, sleepiness, dizziness, disturbed coordination, fatigue, confusion, restlessness, excitation, nervousness, tremor, irritability, insomnia, euphoria, paresthesias, blurred vision, diplopia, vertigo, tinnitus, acute labyrinthitis, hysteria, neuritis, convulsions.
5. *GI System:* Epigastric distress, anorexia, nausea, vomiting, diarrhea, constipation.
6. *GU System:* Urinary frequency, difficult urination, urinary retention, early menses.
7. *Respiratory System:* Thickening of bronchial secretions, tightness of chest and wheezing, nasal stuffiness.

Continued on next page

Sandoz—Cont.

Sympathomimetic Compounds:
Nervous System: At higher doses may cause drowsiness, dizziness, nervousness, or sleeplessness, and especially in children may cause excitability. Phenylpropanolamine hydrochloride may cause elevated blood pressure and tachyarrhythmias, especially in hyperthyroid patients.

Overdosage: Antihistamine overdosage reactions may vary from central nervous system depression to stimulation. Stimulation is particularly likely in children. Atropine-like signs and symptoms: dry mouth; fixed, dilated pupils; flushing; and gastrointestinal symptoms may also occur.

Overdosage of the phenylpropanolamine hydrochloride may produce tachycardia, pupillary dilatation, excitation and arrhythmias.

If vomiting has not occurred spontaneously the conscious patient should be induced to vomit. This is best done by having the patient drink a glass of water or milk along with an appropriate amount of Syrup of Ipecac. Precautions against aspiration must be taken, especially in infants and children.

If vomiting is unsuccessful in 20 minutes, gastric lavage is indicated within 3 hours after ingestion and even later if large amounts of milk or cream were given beforehand. Isotonic and ½ isotonic saline is the lavage solution of choice.

Saline cathartics, such as milk of magnesia, by osmosis draw water into the bowel and therefore are valuable for their action in rapid dilution of bowel content.

Stimulants should *not* be used.

Activated charcoal has been demonstrated to interfere with phenylpropanolamine absorption.

The value of dialysis has not been established.

The concentration of phenylpropanolamine hydrochloride or clemastine fumarate in biological fluids associated with toxicity is not known.

The amount of TAVIST-D in single doses associated with significant signs of overdose or death is now known.

The oral LD_{50} for a mixture containing 50 mg phenylpropanolamine hydrochloride and 1.34 mg clemastine fumarate is 1277 mg/Kg in mice, 602 mg/Kg in rats and 634 mg/Kg in rabbits.

Dosage and Administration: Adults and children twelve years and over: One tablet swallowed whole every twelve hours.

How Supplied: TAVIST-D (clemastine fumarate/phenylpropanolamine HCl) Tablets: containing 1.34 mg clemastine fumarate (equivalent to 1 mg of the free base) and 75 mg phenylpropanolamine hydrochloride. White, round, film-coated multiple compressed tablet, embossed "TAVIST-D" on one side and "78-221" on the other. Packages of 100 (NDC 0078-0221-05). TAVIST-D Tablets should be stored and dispensed below 86°F in a tight, light-resistant container.

Company's Product Identification Mark(s): Tavist-D Tablets embossed "TAVIST-D" on one side and "78-221" on the other.

[TAD-Z2 issued April 1984]

Shown in Product Identification Section, page 433

VISKEN® ℞

[*vis' kin*]

(pindolol) tablets

The following prescribing information is based on official labeling in effect on November 1, 1984.

Description: Visken® (pindolol), a synthetic beta-adrenergic receptor blocking agent with intrinsic sympathomimetic activity is 4-(2-hydroxy-3-isopropylaminopropoxy)-indole.

Clinical Pharmacology: Visken (pindolol) is a non-selective beta-adrenergic antagonist (beta-blocker) which possesses intrinsic sympathomimetic activity (ISA) in therapeutic dosage ranges but does not possess quinidine-like membrane stabilizing activity.

Pharmacodynamics: In standard pharmacologic tests in man and animals, Visken (pindolol) attenuates increases in heart rate, systolic blood pressure, and cardiac output resulting from exercise and isoproterenol administration, thus confirming its beta-blocking properties. The ISA or partial agonist activity of Visken (pindolol) is mediated directly at the adrenergic receptor sites and may be blocked by other beta-blockers. In catecholamine depleted animal experiments, ISA is manifested as an increase in the inotropic and chronotropic activity of the myocardium. In man, ISA is manifested by a smaller reduction in the resting heart rate (4–8 beats/min) than is seen with drugs lacking ISA. There is also a smaller reduction in resting cardiac output. The clinical significance of this observation has not been evaluated and there is no evidence, or reason to believe, that exercise cardiac output is less affected by Visken (pindolol).

Visken (pindolol) has been shown in controlled, double-blind clinical studies to be an effective antihypertensive agent when used as monotherapy, or when added to therapy with thiazide-type diuretics. Divided dosages in the range of 10 mg—60 mg daily have been shown to be effective. As monotherapy, Visken (pindolol) is as effective as propranolol, α-methyldopa, hydrochlorothiazide and chlorthalidone in reducing systolic and diastolic blood pressure. The effect on blood pressure is not orthostatic, i.e. Visken (pindolol) was equally effective in reducing the supine and standing blood pressure.

In open, long term studies up to four (4) years, no evidence of diminution of the blood pressure lowering response was observed.

An average 3 pound increase in body weight has been noted in patients treated with Visken (pindolol) alone, a larger increase than was observed with propranolol or placebo. The weight gain appeared unrelated to blood pressure response and was not associated with an increased risk of heart failure, although edema was more common than in control patients. Visken (pindolol) does not have a consistent effect on plasma renin activity.

The mechanism of the antihypertensive effects of beta-blocking agents has not been established, but several mechanisms have been postulated: 1) an effect on the central nervous system resulting in a reduced sympathetic outflow to the periphery, 2) competitive antagonism of catecholamines at peripheral (especially cardiac) adrenergic receptor sites, leading to decreased cardiac output, 3) an inhibition of renin release. These mechanisms appear less likely for pindolol than other beta-blockers in view of the modest effect on resting cardiac output and renin.

Beta-blockade therapy is useful when it is necessary to suppress the effects of beta-adrenergic agonists in order to achieve therapeutic goals. However, in certain clinical situations, (e.g., cardiac failure, heart block, bronchospasm) the preservation of an adequate sympathetic tone may be necessary to maintain vital functions. Although a beta-antagonist with ISA such as Visken (pindolol) does not eliminate sympathetic tone entirely, there is no controlled evidence that it is safer than other beta-blockers in such conditions as heart failure, heart block, or bronchospasm or is less likely to cause those conditions. In single dose studies of the effects of beta-blockers on FEV_1, Visken (pindolol) was indistinguishable from other non-cardioselective agents in its reduction of FEV_1, and its reduction in the effectiveness of an exogenous beta agonist.

Exacerbation of angina and, in some cases, myocardial infarction and ventricular dysrhythmias have been reported after abrupt discontinuation of therapy with beta-adrenergic blocking agents in patients with coronary artery disease. Abrupt withdrawal of these agents in patients without coronary artery disease has resulted in transient symptoms, including tremulousness, sweating, palpitation, headache, and malaise. Several mechanisms have been proposed to explain these phenomena, among them increased sensitivity to catecholamines because of increased numbers of beta receptors.

Pharmacokinetics and Metabolism: Visken (pindolol) is rapidly and reproducibly absorbed (greater than 95%), achieving peak plasma concentrations within one hour of drug administration. Visken (pindolol) has no significant first-pass effect. The blood concentrations are proportional in a linear manner to the administered dose in the range of 5–20 mg. Upon repeated administration to the same subject, variation is minimal. After a single dose, intersubject variation for peak plasma concentrations was about 4 fold (e.g. 45–167 ng/ml for a 20 mg dose). Upon multiple dosing, intersubject variation decreased to 2–2.5 fold. Visken (pindolol) is only 40% bound to plasma proteins and is evenly distributed between plasma and red cells. The volume of distribution in healthy subjects is about 2 L/kg.

Visken (pindolol) undergoes extensive metabolism in animals and man. In man, 35–40% is excreted unchanged in the urine and 60–65% is metabolized primarily to hydroxy-metabolites which are excreted as glucuronides and ethereal sulfates. The polar metabolites are excreted with a half-life of approximately 8 hours and thus multiple dosing therapy (q.8H) results in a less than 50% accumulation in plasma. About 6–9% of an administered intravenous dose is excreted by the bile into the feces.

The disposition of Visken (pindolol) after oral administration is monophasic with a half-life in healthy subjects or hypertensive patients with normal renal function of approximately 3–4 hours. Following t.i.d. administration (q.8H), no significant accumulation of Visken (pindolol) is observed.

In elderly hypertensive patients with normal renal function the half-life of Visken (pindolol) is more variable, averaging about 7 hours, but with values as high as 15 hours.

In hypertensive patients with renal diseases, the half-life is within the range expected for healthy subjects. However, a significant decrease (50%) in volume of distribution (V_D) is observed in uremic patients and V_D appears to be directly correlated to creatinine clearance. Therefore, renal drug clearance is significantly reduced in uremic patients, resulting in a significant decrease in urinary excretion of unchanged drug. Uremic patients with a creatinine clearance of less than 20 ml/min generally excreted less than 15% of the administered dose unchanged in the urine.

In patients with histologically diagnosed cirrhosis of the liver, the elimination of Visken (pindolol) was more variable in rate and generally significantly slower than in healthy subjects. The total body clearance of Visken (pindolol) in cirrhotic patients ranged from about 50 ml/min to 300 ml/min and was directly correlated to antipyrine clearance. The half-life ranged from 2.5 hours to greater than 30 hours. These findings strongly suggest that caution should be exercised in dosage adjustments of Visken (pindolol) in such patients.

The bioavailability of Visken (pindolol) is not significantly affected by co-administration of food, hydralazine, hydrochlorothiazide or aspirin. Visken (pindolol) has no effect on warfarin activity or the clinical effectiveness of digoxin, although small transient decreases in plasma digoxin concentrations were noted.

Indications and Usage: Visken (pindolol) is indicated in the management of hypertension. It may be used alone or concomitantly with other antihypertensive agents, particularly with a thiazide type diuretic.

Contraindications: Visken (pindolol) is contraindicated in: 1) bronchial asthma; 2) overt cardiac failure; 3) cardiogenic shock; 4) second and third degree heart block; 5) severe bradycardia; (see Warnings).

Warnings:

Cardiac Failure: Sympathetic stimulation may be a vital component supporting circulatory function in patients with congestive heart failure, and its inhibition by beta-blockade may precipitate more severe failure. Although beta-blockers should be avoided in overt congestive heart failure, if necessary, Visken (pindolol) can be used with caution in patients with a history of failure who are well-compensated, usually with digitalis and diuretics. Beta-adrenergic blocking agents do not abolish the inotropic action of digitalis on heart muscle.

In Patients Without A History of Cardiac Failure: In patients with latent cardiac insufficiency, continued depression of the myocardium with beta-blocking agents over a period of time can in some cases lead to cardiac failure. At the first sign or symptom of impending cardiac failure, patients should be fully digitalized and/or be given a diuretic, and the response observed closely. If cardiac failure continues, despite adequate digitalization and diuretic, Visken (pindolol) therapy should be withdrawn (gradually if possible).

Exacerbation of Ischemic Heart Disease Following Abrupt Withdrawal: Hypersensitivity to catecholamines has been observed in patients withdrawn from beta-blocker therapy; exacerbation of angina and, in some cases, myocardial infarction have occurred after *abrupt* discontinuation of such therapy. When discontinuing chronically administered Visken® (pindolol), particularly in patients with ischemic heart disease, the dosage should be gradually reduced over a period of one to two weeks and the patient should be carefully monitored. If angina markedly worsens or acute coronary insufficiency develops, Visken (pindolol) administration should be reinstituted promptly, at least temporarily, and other measures appropriate for the management of unstable angina should be taken. Patients should be warned against interruption or discontinuation of therapy without the physician's advice. Because coronary artery disease is common and may be unrecognized, it may be prudent not to discontinue Visken (pindolol) therapy abruptly even in patients treated only for hypertension.

Nonallergic Bronchospasm (e.g., chronic bronchitis, emphysema)—Patients with Bronchospastic Diseases Should in General Not Receive Beta-Blockers: Visken (pindolol) should be administered with caution since it may block bronchodilation produced by endogenous or exogenous catecholamine stimulation of beta$_2$ receptors.

Major Surgery: Because beta blockade impairs the ability of the heart to respond to reflex stimuli and may increase the risks of general anesthesia and surgical procedures, resulting in protracted hypotension or low cardiac output, it has generally been suggested that such therapy should be withdrawn several days prior to surgery. Recognition of the increased sensitivity to catecholamines of patients recently withdrawn from beta-blocker therapy, however, has made this recommendation controversial. If possible, beta-blockers should be withdrawn well before surgery takes place. In the event of emergency surgery, the anesthesiologist should be informed that the patient is on beta-blocker therapy. The effects of Visken (pindolol) can be reversed by administration of beta-receptor agonists such as isoproterenol, dopamine, dobutamine, or levarterenol. Difficulty in restarting and maintaining the heart beat has also been reported with beta-adrenergic receptor blocking agents.

Diabetes and Hypoglycemia: Beta-adrenergic blockade may prevent the appearance of premonitory signs and symptoms (e.g., tachycardia and blood pressure changes) of acute hypoglycemia. This is especially important with labile diabetics. Beta-blockade also reduces the release of insulin in response to hyperglycemia; therefore, it may be necessary to adjust the dose of antidiabetic drugs.

Thyrotoxicosis: Beta-adrenergic blockade may mask certain clinical signs (e.g., tachycardia) of hyperthyroidism. Patients suspected of developing thyrotoxicosis should be managed carefully to avoid abrupt withdrawal of beta-blockade which might precipitate a thyroid crisis.

Precautions:

Impaired Renal or Hepatic Function: Beta-blocking agents should be used with caution in patients with impaired hepatic or renal function. Poor renal function has only minor effects on Visken (pindolol) clearance, but poor hepatic function may cause blood levels of Visken (pindolol) to increase substantially.

Information for Patients: Patients, especially those with evidence of coronary artery insufficiency, should be warned against interruption or discontinuation of Visken (pindolol) therapy without the physician's advice. Although cardiac failure rarely occurs in properly selected patients, patients being treated with beta-adrenergic blocking agents should be advised to consult the physician at the first sign or symptom of impending failure.

Body System/Adverse Reaction	Visken (pindolol) (N = 322) %	Active Controls* (N = 188) %	Placebo (N = 78) %
Central Nervous System			
Anxiety	4	<1	1
Bizarre or Many Dreams	8	3	8
Dizziness	17	23	8
Fatigue	15	19	12
Hallucinations	1	0	0
Insomnia	19	8	12
Lethargy	3	6	4
Nervousness	11	5	9
Weakness	7	5	4
Autonomic Nervous System			
Paresthesia	5	2	8
Visual Disturbances	4	3	4
Cardiovascular			
Dyspnea	9	8	9
Edema	11	9	3
Heart Failure	2	<1	0
Palpitations	2	2	0
Weight Gain	3	5	0
Musculo-Skeletal			
Chest Pain	5	3	5
Joint Pain	11	6	8
Muscle Cramps	8	2	0
Muscle Pain	12	12	9
Gastrointestinal			
Abdominal Discomfort	7	7	5
Nausea	7	4	1
Skin			
Pruritus	2	<1	0
Rash	2	3	3

*Active Controls: Patients received either propranolol, α-methyldopa or a diuretic (hydrochlorothiazide or chlorthalidone).

Drug Interactions: Catecholamine-depleting drugs (e.g., reserpine) may have an additive effect when given with beta-blocking agents. Patients receiving Visken (pindolol) plus a catecholamine depleting agent should, therefore, be closely observed for evidence of hypotension and/or marked bradycardia which may produce vertigo, syncope, or postural hypotension.

Visken (pindolol) has been used with a variety of antihypertensive agents, including hydrochlorothiazide, hydralazine, and guanethidine without unexpected adverse interactions.

Carcinogenesis, Mutagenesis, Impairment of Fertility: In chronic oral toxicologic studies (one to two years) in mice, rats, and dogs, Visken (pindolol) did not produce any significant toxic effects. In two-year oral carcinogenicity studies in rats and mice in doses as high as 59 mg/kg/day and 124 mg/kg/day (50 and 100 times the maximum recommended human dose), respectively, Visken (pindolol) did not produce any neoplastic, preneoplastic, or nonneoplastic pathologic lesions. In fertility and general reproductive performance studies in rats, Visken (pindolol) caused no adverse effects at a dose of 10 mg/kg.

In the male fertility and general reproductive performance test in rats, definite toxicity characterized by mortality and decreased weight gain was observed in the group given 100 mg/kg/day. At 30 mg/kg/day, decreased mating was associated with testicular atrophy and/or decreased spermatogenesis. This response is not clearly drug related, however, as there was no dose response relationship within this experiment and no similar effect on testes of rats administered Visken® (pindolol) as a dietary admixture for 104 weeks. There appeared to be an increase in prenatal mortality in males given 100 mg/kg but development of offspring was not impaired.

In females administered Visken (pindolol) prior to mating through day 21 of lactation, mating behavior was decreased at 100 mg/kg and 30 mg/kg. At these dosages there also was increased mortality of offspring. Prenatal mortality was increased at 10 mg/kg but there was not a clear dose response relationship in this experiment. There was an increased resorption rate at 100 mg/kg observed in females necropsied on the 15th day of gestation.

Pregnancy—Category B: Studies in rats and rabbits exceeding 100 times the maximum recommended human doses, revealed no embryotoxicity or teratogenicity. Since there are no adequate and well-controlled studies in pregnant women, and since animal reproduction studies are not always predictive of human response, Visken (pindolol), as with any drug, should be employed during pregnancy only if the potential benefit justifies the potential risk to the fetus.

Nursing Mothers: Since Visken (pindolol) is secreted in human milk, nursing should not be undertaken by mothers receiving the drug.

Pediatric Use: Safety and effectiveness in children have not been established.

Clinical Laboratory: Minor persistent elevations in serum transaminases (SGOT, SGPT) have been noted in 7% of patients during Visken (pindolol) administration, but progressive elevations were not observed and liver injury has not been reported in the medical literature over a ten (10) year period of marketing. Alkaline phosphatase, lactic acid dehydrogenase (LDH) and uric acid are also elevated on rare occasions. The significance of these findings is unknown.

Adverse Reactions: Most adverse reactions have been mild. The incidences listed in the following table are derived from 12 week comparative double-blind, parallel design trials in hypertensive patients given Visken (pindolol) as monotherapy, given various active control drugs as monotherapy, or given placebo. Data for Visken (pindolol) and the positive controls were pooled from several trials because no striking differences were seen in the individual studies, with one exception. The frequency of edema was noticeably higher in positive control trials (16% Visken (pindolol) vs 9% positive control) than in placebo controlled trials (6% Visken (pindolol) vs 3% placebo). The table includes adverse reactions reported in greater than 2% of Visken (pindolol) patients and other selected important reactions.
(See table above)

The following selected (potentially important) adverse reactions were seen in 2% or fewer pa-

Continued on next page

Sandoz—Cont.

tients and their relationship to Visken® (pindolol) is uncertain. AUTONOMIC NERVOUS SYSTEM: hyperhidrosis; CARDIOVASCULAR: bradycardia, claudication, cold extremities, heart block, hypotension, syncope, tachycardia; GASTROINTESTINAL: diarrhea, vomiting; RESPIRATORY: wheezing; UROGENITAL: impotence, pollakiuria; MISCELLANEOUS: eye discomfort or burning eyes.

Potential Adverse Effects: In addition, other adverse effects not listed above have been reported with other beta-adrenergic blocking agents and should be considered potential adverse effects of Visken (pindolol).

Central Nervous System: Reversible mental depression progressing to catatonia; an acute reversible syndrome characterized by disorientation for time and place, short-term memory loss, emotional lability, slightly clouded sensorium, and decreased performance on neuropsychometrics.

Cardiovascular: Intensification of AV block. See CONTRAINDICATIONS.

Allergic: Erythematous rash; fever combined with aching and sore throat; laryngospasm; respiratory distress.

Hematologic: Agranulocytosis; thrombocytopenic and nonthrombocytopenic purpura.

Gastrointestinal: Mesenteric arterial thrombosis; ischemic colitis.

Miscellaneous: Reversible alopecia; Peyronie's disease.

The oculomucocutaneous syndrome associated with the beta-blocker practolol has not been reported with Visken (pindolol) during investigational use and extensive foreign experience amounting to over 4 million patient-years.

Overdosage: No specific information on emergency treatment of overdosage is available. Therefore, on the basis of the pharmacologic actions of Visken (pindolol), the following general measures should be employed as appropriate in addition to gastric lavage:

Excessive Bradycardia: administer atropine; if there is no response to vagal blockade, administer isoproterenol cautiously.

Cardiac Failure: digitalize the patient and/or administer diuretic. It has been reported that glucagon may be useful in this situation.

Hypotension: administer vasopressors, e.g., epinephrine or levarterenol, with serial monitoring of blood pressure. (There is evidence that epinephrine may be the drug of choice.)

Bronchospasm: administer a beta$_2$ stimulating agent such as isoproterenol and/or a theophylline derivative.

A case of an acute overdosage has been reported with an intake of 500 mg of Visken (pindolol) by a hypertensive patient. Blood pressure increased and heart rate was ≥ 80 beat/ min. Recovery was uneventful. In another case 250 mg of Visken (pindolol) was taken with 150 mg diazepam and 50 mg nitrazepam, producing coma and hypotension. The patient recovered in 24 hours.

Dosage and Administration: The dosage of Visken (pindolol) should be individualized. The recommended initial dose of Visken (pindolol) is 5 mg b.i.d. alone or in combination with other antihypertensive agents. An antihypertensive response usually occurs within the first week of treatment. Maximal response, however, may take as long as or occasionally longer than two weeks. If a satisfactory reduction in blood pressure does not occur within 3–4 weeks, the dose may be adjusted in increments of 10 mg per day at these intervals up to a maximum of 60 mg per day.

How Supplied: White, round, scored tablets: 5 mg (NDC 0078-0111-05) and 10 mg (NDC 0078-0073-05), packages of 100.

Company's Product Identification Mark(s): 5 mg tablets embossed "VISKEN 5" on one side, and "78-111" and scored on other side.

10 mg tablets embossed "VISKEN 10" on one side, and "78-73" and scored on other side.

[VIS-Z3 Issued June 15, 1983]

Shown in Product Identification Section, page 433

Savage Laboratories
a division of Altana Inc.
60 BAYLIS ROAD
POST OFFICE BOX 2006
MELVILLE, NY 11747

ALPHATREX™ ℞
(betamethasone dipropionate)
Cream U.S.P. 0.05%
Ointment U.S.P., 0.05%
For Dermatologic Use Only–Not for Ophthalmic Use

Description: Alphatrex Cream and Ointment contain Betamethasone Dipropionate U.S.P. (Pregna-1, 4-diene-3, 20-dione, 9-fluoro-11-hydroxy-16-methyl-17, 21-bis (1-oxopropoxy)-(11B, 16B)-): it has an empirical formula of $C_{28}H_{37}FO_7$, and a molecular weight of 504.59 (CAS Registry Number 5593-20-4).

Each gram of the 0.05% Cream contains 0.64 mg Betamethasone Dipropionate (equivalent to 0.5 mg Betamethasone) in a soft, white, hydrophilic cream of Purified Water, Mineral Oil, White Petrolatum, Polyethylene Glycol 1000 Monocetyl Ether, Cetostearyl Alcohol, Monobasic Sodium Phosphate and Phosphoric Acid or Sodium Hydroxide; Chlorocresol is present as a preservative. Betamethasone Dipropionate Cream contains no parabens.

Each gram of the 0.05% Ointment contains 0.64 mg Betamethasone Dipropionate (equivalent to 0.5 mg Betamethasone) in an ointment base of Mineral Oil and White Petrolatum. Betamethasone Dipropionate Ointment contains no parabens.

Clinical Pharmacology: Topical corticosteroids share anti-inflammatory, anti-pruritic and vasoconstrictive actions. The mechanism of anti-inflammatory activity of the topical corticosteroids is unclear. Various laboratory methods, including vasoconstrictor assays, are used to compare and predict potencies and/or clinical efficacies of the topical corticosteroids. There is some evidence to suggest that a recognizable correlation exists between vasoconstrictor potency and therapeutic efficacy in man.

Pharmacokinetics: The extent of percutaneous absorption of topical corticosteroids is determined by many factors including the vehicle, the integrity of the epidermal barrier, and the use of occlusive dressings. Topical corticosteroids can be absorbed from normal intact skin. Inflammation and/or other disease processes in the skin increase percutaneous absorption. Occlusive dressings substantially increase the percutaneous absorption of topical corticosteroids. Thus, occlusive dressings may be a valuable therapeutic adjunct for treatment of resistant dermatoses (See DOSAGE AND ADMINISTRATION). Once absorbed through the skin, topical corticosteroids are handled through pharmacokinetic pathways similar to systemically administered corticosteroids. Corticosteroids are bound to plasma proteins in varying degrees. Corticosteroids are metabolized primarily in the liver and are then excreted by the kidneys. Some of the topical corticosteroids and their metabolites are also excreted into the bile.

Indications and Usage: Topical corticosteroids are indicated for the relief of the inflammatory and pruritic manifestations of corticosteroid-responsive dermatoses.

Contraindications: Topical corticosteroids are contraindicated in those patients with a history of hypersensitivity to any of the components of the preparation.

Precautions: General: Systemic absorption of topical corticosteroids has produced reversible hypothalamic-pituitary-adrenal (HPA) axis suppression, manifestations of Cushing's syndrome, hyperglycemia, and glucosuria in some patients. Conditions which augment systemic absorption include the application of the more potent steroids, use over large surface areas, prolonged use, and the addition of occlusive dressings. Therefore, patients receiving a large dose of a potent topical steroid applied to a large surface area or under an occlusive dressing should be evaluated periodically for evidence of HPA axis suppression by using the urinary free cortisol and ACTH stimulation tests. If HPA axis suppression is noted, an attempt should be made to withdraw the drug, to reduce the frequency of application, or to substitute a less potent steroid. Recovery of HPA axis function is generally prompt and complete upon discontinuation of the drug. Infrequently, signs and symptoms of steroid withdrawal may occur, requiring supplemental systemic corticosteroids. Children may absorb proportionally larger amounts of topical corticosteroids and thus be more susceptible to systemic toxicity (See PRECAUTIONS-Pediatric Use). If irritation develops topical corticosteroids should be discontinued and appropriate therapy instituted. In the presence of dermatological infections, the use of an appropriate anti-fungal or antibacterial agent should be instituted. If a favorable response does not occur promptly, the corticosteroid should be discontinued until the infection has been adequately controlled.

Information for the Patient: Patients using topical corticosteroids should receive the following information and instructions:

1. This medication is to be used as directed by the physician. It is for external use only. Avoid contact with the eyes.
2. Patients should be advised not to use this medication for any disorder other than for which it was prescribed.
3. The treated skin area should not be bandaged or otherwise covered or wrapped as to be occlusive unless directed by the physician.
4. Patients should report any signs of local adverse reactions especially under occlusive dressing.
5. Parents of pediatric patients should be advised not to use tight fitting diapers or plastic pants on a child being treated in the diaper area, as these garments may constitute occlusive dressings.

Laboratory Tests: The following tests may be helpful in evaluating the HPA axis suppression: Urinary free cortisol test; ACTH stimulation test.

Carcinogenesis, Mutagenesis, and Impairment of Fertility: Long-term animal studies have not been performed to evaluate the carcinogenic potential or the effect on fertility of topical corticosteroids. Studies to determine mutagenicity with prednisolone and hydrocortisone have revealed negative results.

Pregnancy Category C: Corticosteroids are generally teratogenic in laboratory animals when administered systemically at relatively low dosage levels. The more potent corticosteroids have been shown to be teratogenic after dermal application in laboratory animals. There are no adequate and well-controlled studies in pregnant women on teratogenic effects from topically applied corticosteroids. Therefore, topical corticosteroids should be used during pregnancy only if the potential benefit justifies the potential risk to the fetus. Drugs of this class should not be used extensively on pregnant patients, in large amounts, or for prolonged periods of time.

Nursing Mothers: It is not known whether topical administration of corticosteroids could result in sufficient systemic absorption to produce detectable quantities in breast milk. Systemically administered corticosteroids are secreted into breast milk in quantities not likely to have a deleterious effect on the infant. Nevertheless, caution should be exercised when topical corticosteroids are administered to a nursing woman.

Pediatric Use: Pediatric patients may demonstrate greater susceptibility to topical corticosteroid-induced HPA axis suppression and Cushing's syndrome than mature patients due to a larger skin surface area to body weight ratio. Hypothalamic-pituitary-adrenal (HPA) axis suppression, Cushing's syndrome, and intracranial hypertension have been reported in children receiving topical corticosteroids. Manifestations of adrenal suppression in children include linear growth retardation, delayed weight gain, low plasma cortisol levels, and absence of response to ACTH stimulation. Manifestations of intracranial hypertension include bulging fontanelles, headaches, and bilateral papilledema. Administration of topical corticosteroids to children should be limited to the least amount compatible with an effective therapeutic regimen. Chronic corticosteroid therapy may interfere with the growth and development of children.

Adverse Reactions: The following local adverse reactions are reported infrequently with topical corticosteroids, but may occur more frequently with the use of occlusive dressings. These reactions are listed in an approximate decreasing order of occurrence: Burning, Itching, Irritation, Dryness, Folliculitis, Hypertrichosis, Acneiform eruptions, Hypopigmentation, Perioral dermatitis, Allergic contact dermatitis, Maceration of the skin, Secondary infection, Skin Atrophy, Striae and Miliaria.

Overdosage: Topically applied corticosteroids can be absorbed in sufficient amounts to produce systemic effects (See PRECAUTIONS).

Dosage and Administration: Topical corticosteroids are generally applied to the affected area as a thin film two or three times daily or as directed by a physician depending on the severity of the condition. Occlusive dressings may be used for the management of psoriasis or recalcitrant conditions. If an infection develops, the use of occlusive dressings should be discontinued and appropriate antimicrobial therapy instituted.

How Supplied:
Alphatrex Cream U.S.P., 0.05%
  NDC 0281-0055-15, 15 gram tube
  NDC 0281-0055-46, 45 gram tube
Alphatrex Ointment U.S.P., 0.05%
  NDC 0281-0056-15, 15 gram tube
  NDC 0281-0056-46, 45 gram tube

Caution: Federal law prohibits dispensing without prescription.

BETATREX™
(betamethasone valerate)
Cream U.S.P., 0.1%
Ointment U.S.P., 0.1%
Lotion U.S.P., 0.1%
For Dermatologic Use Only—Not for Ophthalmic Use

Description: Betatrex Cream, Ointment and Lotion contain Betamethasone Valerate USP (Pregna-1, 4-diene-3, 20-dione, 9-fluoro-11, 21-dihydroxy-16-methyl-17-[(1-oxopentyl)oxy]-, (11B, 16B)-); it has an empirical formula of $C_{27}H_{37}FO_6$ and a molecular weight of 476.58 (CAS Registry Number 2152-44-5).

Each gram of the 0.1% cream contains 1.2 mg Betamethasone Valerate (equivalent to 1.0 mg Betamethasone) in a soft, white hydrophilic cream of Water, Mineral Oil, White Petrolatum, Polyethylene Glycol 1000 Monocetyl Ether, Cetostearyl Alcohol, Monobasic Sodium Phosphate and Phosphoric Acid or Sodium Hydroxide; Chlorocresol is present as a preservative. Betamethasone Valerate Cream contains no parabens.

Each gram of the 0.1% ointment contains 1.2 mg Betamethasone Valerate (equivalent to 1.0 mg Betamethasone) in an ointment base of White Petrolatum and Mineral Oil. Betamethasone Valerate Ointment contains no parabens.

Each gram of the 0.1% lotion contains 1.2 mg Betamethasone Valerate (equivalent to 1.0 mg Betamethasone) in a vehicle of Isopropyl Alcohol and Water slightly thickened with Carbomer 934P. Phosphoric Acid or Sodium Hydroxide are used to adjust the pH.

Clinical Pharmacology: Topical corticosteroids share anti-inflammatory, anti-pruritic and vasoconstrictive actions. The mechanism of anti-inflammatory activity of the topical corticosteroids is unclear. Various laboratory methods, including vasoconstrictor assays, are used to compare and predict potencies and/or clinical efficacies of the topical corticosteroids. There is some evidence to suggest that a recognizable correlation exists between vasoconstrictor potency and therapeutic efficacy in man.

Pharmacokinetics: The extent of percutaneous absorption of topical corticosteroids is determined by many factors including the vehicle, the integrity of the epidermal barrier, and the use of occlusive dressings. Topical corticosteroids can be absorbed from normal intact skin. Inflammation and/or other disease processes in the skin increase percutaneous absorption. Occlusive dressings substantially increase the percutaneous absorption of topical corticosteroids. Thus occlusive dressings may be a valuable therapeutic adjunct for treatment of resistant dermatoses (See DOSAGE AND ADMINISTRATION). Once absorbed through the skin, topical corticosteroids are handled through pharmacokinetic pathways similar to systemically administered corticosteroids. Corticosteroids are bound to plasma proteins in varying degrees. Corticosteroids are metabolized primarily in the liver and are then excreted by the kidneys. Some of the topical corticosteroids and their metabolites are also excreted into the bile.

Indications and Usage: Topical corticosteroids are indicated for the relief of the inflammatory and pruritic manifestations of corticosteroid-responsive dermatoses.

Contraindications: Topical corticosteroids are contraindicated in those patients with a history of hypersensitivity to any of the components of the preparation.

Precautions: General: Systemic absorption of topical corticosteroids has produced reversible hypothalamic-pituitary-adrenal (HPA) axis suppression, manifestations of Cushing's syndrome, hyperglycemia, and glucosuria in some patients. Conditions which augment systemic absorption include the application of the more potent steroids, use over large surface areas, prolonged use, and the addition of occlusive dressings. Therefore, patients receiving a large dose of a potent topical steroid applied to a large surface area or under an occlusive dressing should be evaluated periodically for evidence of HPA axis suppression by using the urinary free cortisol and ACTH stimulation tests. If HPA axis suppression is noted, an attempt should be made to withdraw the drug, to reduce the frequency of application, or to substitute a less potent steroid. Recovery of HPA axis function is generally prompt and complete upon discontinuation of the drug. Infrequently, signs and symptoms of steroid withdrawal may occur, requiring supplemental systemic corticosteroids. Children may absorb proportionally larger amounts of topical corticosteroids and thus be more susceptible to systemic toxicity (See PRECAUTIONS-Pediatric Use). If irritation develops, topical corticosteroids should be discontinued and appropriate therapy instituted. In the presence of dermatological infections, the use of an appropriate anti-fungal or antibacterial agent should be instituted. If a favorable response does not occur promptly, the corticosteroid should be discontinued until the infection has been adequately controlled.

Information for the Patient: Patients using topical corticosteroids should receive the following information and instructions:
1. This medication is to be used as directed by the physician. It is for external use only. Avoid contact with the eyes.
2. Patients should be advised not to use this medication for any disorder other than for which it was prescribed.
3. The treated skin area should not be bandaged or otherwise covered or wrapped as to be occlusive unless directed by the physician.
4. Patients should report any signs of local adverse reactions especially under occlusive dressing.
5. Parents of pediatric patients should be advised not to use tight fitting diapers or plastic pants on a child being treated in the diaper area, as these garments may constitute occlusive dressings.

Laboratory Tests: The following tests may be helpful in evaluating the HPA axis suppression: Urinary free cortisol test. ACTH stimulation test.

Carcinogenesis, Mutagenesis, and Impairment of Fertility: Long-term animal studies have not been performed to evaluate the carcinogenic potential or the effect on fertility of topical corticosteroids. Studies to determine mutagenicity with prednisolone and hydrocortisone have revealed negative results.

Pregnancy Category C: Corticosteroids are generally teratogenic in laboratory animals when administered systemically at relatively low dosage levels. The more potent corticosteroids have been shown to be teratogenic after dermal application in laboratory animals. There are no adequate and well-controlled studies in pregnant women on teratogenic effects from topically applied corticosteroids. Therefore, topical corticosteroids should be used during pregnancy only if the potential benefit justifies the potential risk to the fetus. Drugs of this class should not be used extensively on pregnant patients, in large amounts, or for prolonged periods of time.

Nursing Mothers: It is not known whether topical administration of corticosteroids could result in sufficient systemic absorption to produce detectable quantities in breast milk. Systemically administered corticosteroids are secreted into breast milk in quantities not likely to have a deleterious effect on the infant. Nevertheless, caution should be exercised when topical corticosteroids are administered to a nursing woman.

Pediatric Use: Pediatric patients may demonstrate greater susceptibility to topical corticosteroid-induced HPA axis suppression and Cushing's syndrome than mature patients because of a larger skin surface area to body weight ratio. Hypothalamic-pituitary-adrenal (HPA) axis suppression, Cushing's syndrome, and intracranial hypertension have been reported in children receiving topical corticosteroids. Manifestations of adrenal suppression in children include linear growth retardation, delayed weight gain, low plasma cortisol levels, and absence of response to ACTH stimulation. Manifestations of intracranial hypertension include bulging fontanelles, headaches, and bilateral papilledema. Administration of topical corticosteroids to children should be limited to the least amount compatible with an effective therapeutic regimen. Chronic corticosteroid therapy may interfere with the growth and development of children.

Adverse Reactions: The following local adverse reactions are reported infrequently with topical corticosteroids, but may occur more frequently with the use of occlusive dressings. These reactions are listed in an approximate decreasing order of occurrence: Burning, Itching, Irritation, Dryness, Folliculitis, Hypertrichosis, Acneiform eruptions, Hypopigmentation, Perioral dermatitis, Allergic contact dermatitis, Maceration of the skin, Secondary infection, Skin Atrophy, Striae and Miliaria.

Overdosage: Topically applied corticosteroids can be absorbed in sufficient amounts to produce systemic effects (See PRECAUTIONS)

Dosage and Administration:
Betatrex Cream: Apply a thin film of Betatrex Cream 0.1% to the affected area two or three times daily depending on the severity of the condition.
Betatrex Ointment: Apply a thin film of Betatrex Ointment 0.1% to the affected area two or three times daily depending on the severity of the condition.
Betatrex Lotion: Apply a few drops of Betatrex Lotion to the affected area two or three times daily depending on the severity of the condition.

How Supplied:
Betatrex Cream U.S.P., 0.1%
  NDC 0281-3510-44, 15 gram tube
  NDC 0281-3510-50, 45 gram tube
Betatrex Ointment U.S.P., 0.1%
  NDC 0281-3516-44, 15 gram tube
  NDC 0281-3516-50, 45 gram tube
Betatrex Lotion U.S.P., 0.1%
  NDC 0281-3519-46, 60 ml bottle

Caution: Federal law prohibits dispensing without prescription.

Continued on next page

Savage—Cont.

BREXIN® L.A. Capsules ℞

Description: A red and clear colored capsule containing red and blue colored beads. Each capsule for oral administration contains: chlorpheniramine maleate USP 8 mg, pseudoephedrine hydrochloride USP 120 mg, in a specially prepared base to provide prolonged action.

How Supplied: NDC 0281-1934-53, bottle of 100 capsules.

Shown in Product Identification Section, page 433

CHROMAGEN® CAPSULES ℞

Composition: Each maroon soft gelatin capsule contains ferrous fumarate USP 200 mg, ascorbic acid USP 250 mg, cyanocobalamin USP 10 mcg, desiccated stomach substance 100 mg.

Indications: For the treatment of all anemias responsive to oral iron therapy, such as hypochromic anemia associated with pregnancy, chronic or acute blood loss, dietary restriction, metabolic disease and post-surgical convalescence.

Administration and Dosage: Usual adult dose is 1 capsule daily.

Contraindications: Hemochromatosis and hemosiderosis are contraindications to iron therapy.

Side Effects: Average capsule doses in sensitive individuals or excessive dosage may cause nausea, skin rash, vomiting, diarrhea, precordial pain, or flushing of the face and extremities.

Supply:
NDC 0281-4285-53, bottle of 100
NDC 0281-4285-56, bottle of 500

Shown in Product Identification Section, page 433

CHROMAGEN OB® OTC

Description: A phosphorus-free pre-natal vitamin and mineral supplement for use during pregnancy and lactation.

Each 2 capsules contain:

		% U.S. R.D.A.*
Vitamin A (Palmitate)	8,000 IU	100%
Vitamin D (Ergocalciferol)	400 IU	100%
Vitamin E (dl-Alpha Tocopheryl Acetate)	30 IU	100%
Vitamin C (Ascorbic Acid and partially supplied by Sodium Ascorbate)	150 mg	250%
Folic Acid	800 mcg	100%
Thiamine (from Thiamine Mononitrate)	3 mg	176%
Riboflavin	3.4 mg	170%
Niacin (Niacinamide)	20 mg	100%
Vitamin B$_6$ (from Pyridoxine Hydrochloride)	10 mg	400%
Vitamin B$_{12}$ (from Cyanocobalamin)	12 mcg	150%
Calcium (from Calcium Carbonate)	250 mg	19%
Iodine (from Potassium Iodide)	300 mcg	200%
Iron (from Ferrous Fumarate)	66 mg	366%
Magnesium (from Magnesium Oxide)	25 mg	6%
Copper (from Copper Oxide)	2 mg	100%
Zinc (from Zinc Sulfate)	25 mg	166%
Docusate Sodium†	50 mg	—

* Percentage of U.S. Recommended Daily Allowance for Pregnant or lactating women.
† Added to counteract the constipating effect of iron.

Recommended daily dosage: 2 capsules or as prescribed by a physician.

Store at controlled room temperature 15° to 30° C (59°–86° F).

How Supplied: NDC 0281-0763-53 100 Capsules.

DILOR® Tablets ℞
(dyphylline)

Composition: Each blue, scored tablet contains dyphylline (dihydroxypropyl theophylline) 200 mg; each white scored tablet contains dyphylline (dihydroxypropyl theophylline) 400 mg.

Description: Dyphylline [7-(2,3-Dihydroxypropyl) theophylline] [$C_{10}H_{14}N_4O_4$] is a white, extremely bitter, amorphous solid, freely soluble in water and soluble to the extent of 2 gm in 100 ml alcohol.

Actions: As a xanthine derivative, dyphylline possesses the peripheral vasodilator and bronchodilator actions characteristic of theophylline. It has diuretic and myocardial stimulant effects, and is effective orally. Dyphylline may show fewer side effects than aminophylline, but its blood levels and possibly its activity are also lower.

Indications: For relief of acute bronchial asthma and for reversible bronchospasm associated with chronic bronchitis and emphysema.

Contraindications: In individuals who have shown hypersensitivity to any of its components. Dyphylline should not be administered concurrently with other xanthine preparations.

Warnings: Status asthmaticus is a medical emergency. Excessive doses may be expected to be toxic. In children treated with dyphylline elixir, the alcoholic vehicle of the drug product poses a truly significant factor of drug dependence including all three components of tolerance, physical dependence and compulsive abuse.

Usage in Pregnancy: Safe use in pregnancy has not been established relative to possible adverse effects on fetal development. Therefore, dyphylline should not be used in pregnant women unless, in the judgment of the physician, the potential benefits outweigh the possible hazards.

Precautions: Use with caution in patients with severe cardiac disease, hypertension, hyperthyroidism, or acute myocardial injury. Particular caution in dose administration must be exercised in patients with peptic ulcers, since the condition may be exacerbated. Chronic oral administration in high doses (500 to 1,000 mg.) is usually associated with gastrointestinal irritation. Great caution should be used in giving dyphylline to patients in congestive heart failure. Such patients have shown markedly prolonged blood level curves which have persisted for long periods following discontinuation of the drug.

Adverse Reactions: Note: Included in this listing which follows are a few adverse reactions which may not have been reported with this specific drug. However, pharmacological similarities among the xanthine drugs require that each of the reactions be considered when dyphylline is administered. The most consistent adverse reactions are: 1. Gastrointestinal irritation: nausea, vomiting, and epigastric pain, generally preceded by headache, hematemesis, diarrhea. 2. Central nervous system stimulation: irritability, restlessness, insomnia, reflex hyperexcitability, muscle twitching, clonic and tonic generalized convulsions, agitation. 3. Cardiovascular: palpitation, tachycardia, extra systoles, flushing, marked hypotension, and circulatory failure. 4. Respiratory: tachypnea, respiratory arrest. 5. Renal: albuminuria, increased excretion of renal tubule and red blood cells. 6. Others: fever, dehydration.

Overdosage:
Symptoms:
In infants and small children: agitation, headache, hyperreflexia, fasciculations, and clonic and tonic convulsions.
In adults: nervousness, insomnia, nausea, vomiting, tachycardia and extra systoles.
Therapy:
Discontinue drug immediately.
No specific treatment.
Ipecac syrup for oral ingestion.
Avoid sympathomimetics.
Supportive treatment for hypotension, seizure, arrhythmias and dehydration.
Sedatives such as short acting barbiturates will help control central nervous system stimulation.
Restore the acid-base balance with lactate or bicarbonate.
Oxygen and antibiotics provide supportive treatment as indicated.

Drug Interactions: Toxic synergism with ephedrine and other sympathomimetic bronchodilator drugs may occur.
Recent controlled studies suggest that the addition of ephedrine to adequate dosage regimens of dyphylline produces no increase in effectiveness over that of dyphylline alone, but does produce an increase in toxic effects.

Dosage and Administration: When administered orally it produces less nausea than aminophylline and other alkaline theophylline compounds. Absorption orally appears to be faster on an empty stomach; preferably the drug is to be given at six hour intervals. Adults: Usual Adult Dose: 15 mg/kg every 6 hours up to 4 times a day. The dosage should be individualized by titration to the condition and response of the patient.
Pulmonary functional measurements before and after a period of treatment allow an objective assessment of whether or not therapy should be continued in patients with chronic bronchitis and emphysema.

Supply: Tablets,
200 mg– NDC 0281-1115-53, Bottle of 100.
NDC 0281-1115-57, Bottle of 1000.
NDC 0281-1115-63, Unit dose, Box of 100
NDC 0281-1115-67, Unit dose, Box of 10 × 100
400 mg– NDC 0281-1116-53, Bottle of 100.
NDC 0281-1116-57, Bottle of 1000.
NDC 0281-1116-63, Unit dose, Box of 100
NDC 0281-1116-67, Unit dose, Box of 10 × 100

Also Available: Dilor Elixir, Dyphylline 160 mg/15 ml; and Dilor Injectable, dyphylline 250 mg/ml.

Shown in Product Identification Section, page 433

DILOR-G® ℞

Composition: Each pink, scored tablet contains dyphylline 200 mg, guaifenesin USP 200 mg; oral liquid: each teaspoonful (5 ml) contains dyphylline 100 mg, guaifenesin USP 100 mg.

Supply: Tablets, NDC 0281-1124-53, bottle of 100.

NDC 0281-1124-57, bottle of 1000.

NDC 0281-1124-63, unit dose, 1 × 100.
Liquid, NDC 0281-1127-74, pint.
NDC 0281-1127-76, gallon.

Shown in Product Identification Section, page 433

DITATE®–DS ℞
(testosterone enanthate USP and estradiol valerate USP injection)

Each ml contains: testosterone enanthate USP 180 mg, estradiol valerate USP 8 mg, benzyl alcohol NF 2%. In sesame oil NF.

How Supplied: NDC 0281-5807-32, box of ten 2 ml single-dose vials.
NDC 0281-5807-43, box of ten 2 ml single-dose syringes.

ESTROCON™ TABLETS ℞
(conjugated estrogens USP)

Description: Estrocon™ Tablets (conjugated estrogens) are a mixture of sodium salts of the sulfate esters of the estrogenic substances, principally estrone and equilin, that are of the type excreted by pregnant mares and are water soluble. Tablets are provided for oral administration.

How Supplied: NDC 0281-5182-53 Estrocon Tablets 0.625 mg. bottle of 100
NDC 0281-5185-53 Estrocon Tablets 1.25 mg. bottle of 100

R 9/83

Manufactured by
Zenith Laboratories, Inc.
Northvale, NJ 07647
Distributed by
Savage Laboratories
division of Altana Inc.

Melville, N.Y. 11747

Shown in Product Identification Section, page 433

HOMO-TET®

Description: Tetanus Immune Globulin (Human), Homo-Tet, is a sterile 10 to 18 percent solution of the immunoglobulin fraction of plasma from persons who have been hyperimmunized with tetanus toxoid.

How Supplied: Tetanus Immune Globulin (Human), Homo-Tet, is available in 250 unit prefilled disposable syringes and 250 unit single-dose vials.

Manufactured by
Hyland Therapeutics Division
Travenol Laboratories Inc.
Glendale, California 91202, U.S.A.
Distributed by
Savage Laboratories
division of Altana Inc.
Melville, New York 11747

IMMUGLOBIN®
(immune globulin USP)

Composition: Each ml. contains Gamma Globulin 16.5%±1.5%. Standardized for measles and polio antibody content.

Supply: NDC 0281-7770-16, 10 ml vial.

MYTREX™ Cream and Ointment
(nystatin neomycin gramicidin triamcinolone)

Description: Mytrex is available as a cream in an aqueous vanishing cream base and as an ointment in a polyethylene and mineral oil USP base. Each gram of the cream or ointment provides 100,000 units nystatin USP, neomycin sulfate USP equivalent to 2.5 mg neomycin base, 0.25 mg gramicidin NF, and 1 mg triamcinolone acetonide USP. The cream also contains polysorbate 60 NF, alcohol USP, aluminum hydroxide compressed gel, titanium dioxide USP, glyceryl monostearate, polyethylene glycol monostearate 400, simethicone, sorbic acid NF, propylene glycol USP, ethylenediamine USP, polyoxyethylene fatty alcohol ether, sorbitol solution USP, methyl paraben NF, propyl paraben NF, hydrochloric acid NF, white petrolatum USP, and purified water USP.

Actions: Triamcinolone acetonide is primarily effective because of its anti-inflammatory, antipruritic, and vasoconstrictive actions. Nystatin provides specific anticandidal activity and the two topical antibiotics, neomycin and gramicidin, provide antibacterial activity.

Indications
Based on a review of these drugs by the National Academy of Sciences-National Research Council and/or other information, FDA has classified the indications as follows:
Possibly effective: In
—cutaneous candidiasis
—superficial bacterial infections
—the following conditions when complicated by candidal and/or bacterial infection: atopic, eczematoid, stasis, nummular, contact, or seborrheic dermatitis; neuro-dermatitis and dermatitis venenata
—infantile eczema
—lichen simplex chronicus
—the Cream is also possibly effective in pruritus ani and pruritus vulvae
Final classification of the less-than-effective indications requires further investigation.

Contraindications: Topical steroids are contraindicated in viral diseases of the skin, such as vaccinia and varicella. The preparations are also contraindicated in fungal lesions of the skin except candidiasis, and in those patients with a history of hypersensitivity to any of their components.
The preparations are not for ophthalmic use nor should they be applied in the external auditory canal of patients with perforated eardrums. Topical steroids should not be used when circulation is markedly impaired.

Warnings: Because of the potential hazard of nephrotoxicity and ototoxicity, prolonged use or use of large amounts of these products should be avoided in the treatment of skin infections following extensive burns, trophic ulceration, and other conditions where absorption of neomycin is possible.

Usage in Pregnancy: Although topical steroids have not been reported to have an adverse effect on the fetus, the safety of topical steroid preparations during pregnancy has not been absolutely established; therefore, they should not be used extensively on pregnant patients, in large amounts, or for prolonged periods of time.

Precautions: As with any antibiotic preparation, prolonged use may result in over-growth of nonsusceptible organisms, including fungi other than Candida. Constant observation of the patient is essential. Should superinfection due to nonsusceptible organisms occur, suitable concomitant anti-microbial therapy must be administered. If a favorable response does not occur promptly, application of Mytrex Cream and Ointment should be discontinued until the infection is adequately controlled by other anti-infective measures.

If extensive areas are treated or if the occlusive technique is used, the possibility exists of increased systemic absorption of the corticosteroid and suitable precautions should be taken. If irritation develops, the product should be discontinued and appropriate therapy instituted.

Adverse Reactions: Hypersensitivity to nystatin is extremely uncommon. Sensitivity reactions following the topical use of gramicidin are rarely encountered. Hypersensitivity to neomycin has been reported and articles in the current medical literature indicate an increase in its prevalence.

The following local adverse reactions have been reported with topical corticosteroids either with or without occlusive dressings: burning sensations, itching, irritation, dryness, folliculitis, secondary infection, skin atrophy, striae, miliaria, hypertrichosis acneiform eruption, maceration of the skin and hypopigmentation. Contact sensitivity to a particular dressing material or adhesive may occur occasionally.

Ototoxicity and nephrotoxicity have been reported.

Dosage and Administration: Mytrex Cream—Rub into affected areas two to three times daily.
Mytrex Ointment—Apply a thin film to the affected areas two to three times daily.

Occlusive Dressing Technique:
Cream: Gently rub a small amount of the cream into the lesion until it disappears. Reapply the Cream leaving a thin coating on the lesion and cover with a pliable nonporous film. If needed, additional moisture may be provided by covering the lesion with a dampened clean cotton cloth before the plastic film is applied or by briefly soaking the affected area in water.
The frequency of changing dressings is best determined on an individual basis. Reapplication is essential at each dressing change.
Ointment: Apply the Ointment leaving a thin coating on the lesion and cover with a pliable nonporous film. If needed, additional moisture may be provided by covering the lesions with a dampened clean cotton cloth before the plastic film is applied or by briefly soaking the affected area in water. The frequency of changing dressings is best determined on an individual basis. Reapplication is essential at each dressing change.

How Supplied:
Cream: NDC 0281-3311-44, 15 gram tube.
         NDC 0281-3311-45, 30 gram tube.
         NDC 0281-3311-46, 60 gram tube.
         NDC 0281-3311-49, 120 gram jar.
Ointment: NDC 0281-3318-44, 15 gram tube.
          NDC 0281-3318-45, 30 gram tube.
          NDC 0281-3318-46, 60 gram tube.

Caution: Federal law prohibits dispensing without prescription.
FOR EXTERNAL USE ONLY

NYSTEX™
(nystatin cream USP and ointment USP)

Description: Nystatin Cream contains the antifungal antibiotic nystatin at a concentration of 100,000 units per gram in an aqueous, perfumed vanishing cream base containing polysorbate 60, aluminum hydroxide compressed gel, titanium dioxide, glyceryl monostearate, polyethylene glycol monostearate 400, simethicone, sorbic acid, propylene glycol, ethylenediamine, polyoxyethylene fatty alcohol ether, sorbitol solution, methyl paraben, propyl paraben, hydrochloric acid, white petrolatum, and purified water.
Nystatin Ointment contains 100,000 units nystatin per gram in a polyethylene and mineral oil base.

How Supplied:
Nystatin Cream
   NDC 0281-3208-44, 15 gram tube
   NDC 0281-3208-45, 30 gram tube
Nystatin Ointment
   NDC 0281-3212-44, 15 gram tube

NYSTEX™
(nystatin oral suspension U.S.P.)

Description: Nystatin is an antifungal antibiotic that is both fungistatic and fungicidal in vitro against a wide variety of yeasts and yeastlike fungi. It is a polyene antibiotic of undetermined structural formula that is obtained from *Streptomyces noursei*. Nystex Oral Suspension contains 100,000 units nystatin per ml in a vehicle containing 50% sucrose and not more than 1% alcohol by volume.

How Supplied: Nystex Oral Suspension (NDC 0281-0037-60) is available as a pleasant-tasting, ready-to-use suspension containing 100,000 units nystatin per ml in 60 ml bottles (each supplied with a calibrated dropper).

Storage: Store at room temperaure; avoid freezing.

SĀTRIC™ Tablets
(metronidazole USP)

WARNING: Sātric has been shown to be carcinogenic in mice and rats. (*See Warnings*). Unnecessary use of this drug should be avoided. Its use should be reserved for the conditions described in the *Indications And Usage* section below.

Description: Sātric is a 1-(β-hydroxyethyl)-2-methyl-5-nitroimidazole. Sātric is classified therapeutically as an antiprotozoal (Trichomonas), and antibacterial (antianaerobic) agent. It occurs as pale yellow crystals that are slightly soluble in water and alcohol. Metronidazole has the following structural formula:

$$O_2N \underset{N}{\overset{N}{\bigvee}} \begin{array}{c} CH_2CH_2OH \\ | \\ N \\ CH_3 \end{array}$$

Clinical Pharmacology: Metronidazole is usually well absorbed after oral administration, with peak plasma concentrations occurring between one and two hours. An average elimination half-life is 8 hours in healthy humans. Plasma concentrations of metronidazole are proportional to the administered dose. Oral administration of 250 mg., 500 mg., or 2,000 mg. produced peak plasma concentration of 6 mcg/ml, 12 mcg/ml, and 40 mcg/ml, respectively. Studies reveal no significant bioavailability differences between males and females, however, because of weight differences, the resulting plasma levels in males are generally lower.
Metronidazole is a major conponent appearing in the plasma, with lesser quantities of the 2-hydroxymethyl metabolite also being present.

Continued on next page

Savage—Cont.

Less than 20% of the circulating metronidazole is bound to plasma proteins. Both the parent compound and the metabolite possess in vitro trichomonacidal activity and in vitro bactericidal activity against most strains of anaerobic bacteria.

The major route of elimination of metronidazole and its metabolites is via the urine (60–80% of the dose), with fecal excretion accounting for 6–15% of the dose. The metabolites that appear in the urine result primarily from side-chain oxidation [1-(β-hydroxyethyl)-2-hydroxymethyl-5-nitroimidazole and 2-methyl-5-nitroimidazole-1-yl-acetic acid] and glucuronide conjugation, with unchanged metronidazole accounting for approximately 20% of the total. Renal clearance of metronidazole is approximately 10 ml/min/1.73 m².

Decreased renal function does not alter the single-dose pharmacokinetics of metronidazole. However, plasma clearance of metronidazole is decreased in patients with decreased liver function. Metronidazole appears in cerebrospinal fluid, saliva, and breast milk in concentrations similar to those found in plasma. Bactericidal concentrations of metronidazole have also been detected in pus from hepatic abscesses.

Microbiology: Metronidazole possesses direct trichomonacidal and amebacidal activity against *Trichomonas Vaginalis* and *Entamoeba Histolytica*. The in vitro minimal inhibitory concentration (MIC) for most strains of these organisms is 1 mcg/ml or less. Metronidazole's mechanism of antiprotozoal action is unknown.

Anaerobic Bacteria: Metronidazole is active in vitro against obligate anaerobes, but does not appear to possess any clinically relevant activity against facultative anaerobes or obligate aerobes. Against susceptible organisms, Metronidazole is generally bactericidal at concentrations equal to or slightly higher than the minimal inhibitory concentrations (MIC). Metronidazole has been shown to have in vitro and clinical activity against the following organisms:

Anaerobic gram-negative bacilli, including:
Bacteroides species, including the *Bacteroides fragilis* group (*B. fragilis, B. distasonis, B. ovatus, B. thetaiotaomicron, B. vulgatus*)
Fusobacterium species

Anaerobic gram-positive bacilli, including:
Clostridium species and susceptible strains of *Eubacterium*

Anaerobic gram-positive cocci, including:
Peptococcus species
Peptostreptococcus species

Susceptibility tests: Bacteriologic studies should be performed to determine the causative organisms and their susceptibility to metronidazole; however, the rapid, routine susceptibility testing of individual isolates of anaerobic bacteria is not always practical, and therapy may be started while awaiting these results.

Quantitative methods give the most precise estimates of susceptibility to antibacterial drugs. A standardized agar dilution method and a broth microdilution method are recommended.[1]

Control strains are recommended for standardized susceptibility testing. Each time the test is performed, one or more of the following strains should be included: *Clostridium perfringens* ATCC 13124, *Bacteroides fragilis* ATCC 25285, and *Bacteroides thetaiotaomicron* ATCC 29741. The mode metronidazole MIC's for those three strains are reported to be 0.25, 0.25, and 0.5 mcg/ml, respectively.

A clinical laboratory is considered under acceptable control if the results of the control strains are within one doubling dilution of the mode MIC's reported for metronidazole.

A bacterial isolate may be considered susceptible if the MIC value for Metronidazole is not more than 16 mcg/ml. An organism is considered resistant if the MIC is greater than 16 mcg/ml. A report of "resistant" from the laboratory indicates that the infecting organism is not likely to respond to therapy.

Indications and Usage:

Symptomatic Trichomoniasis: Sātric is indicated for the treatment of symptomatic trichomoniasis in females and males when the presence of trichomonad has been confirmed by appropriate laboratory procedures (wet smears and/or cultures).

Asymptomatic Trichomoniasis: Sātric is indicated in the treatment of asymptomatic females when the organism is associated with endocervicitis, cervicitis, or cervical erosion. Since there is evidence that presence of the trichomonad can interfere with accurate assessment of abnormal cytological smears, additional smears should be performed after eradication of the parasite.

Treatment of Asymptomatic Consorts: *T. vaginalis* infection is a venereal disease. Therefore, asymptomatic sexual partners of treated patients should be treated simultaneously if the organism has been found to be present in order to prevent reinfection of the partner. The decision as to whether to treat an asymptomatic male partner with a negative culture or one in whom no culture has been attempted is an individual one. In making this decision, it should be noted that there is evidence that women may become reinfected if the consort is not treated. Also, since there can be considerable difficulty in isolating the organism from the asymptomatic male carrier, negative smears and cultures cannot be relied upon in this regard. In any event, the consort should be treated with Sātric in cases of reinfection.

Amebiasis: Sātric is indicated in the treatment of acute intestinal amebiasis (amebic dysentery) and amebic liver abscess.

In amebic liver abscess, Sātric therapy does not obviate the need for aspiration or drainage of pus.

Anaerobic Bacterial Infections: Sātric is indicated in the treatment of serious infections caused by susceptible anaerobic bacteria. Indicated surgical procedures should be performed in conjunction with metronidazole therapy. In a mixed aerobic and anaerobic infection, antibiotics appropriate for the treatment of aerobic infection should be used in addition to metronidazole. In the treatment of most serious anaerobic infections the intravenous form of metronidazole is usually administered initially. This may be followed by oral therapy with metronidazole at the discretion of the physician.

INTRA-ABDOMINAL INFECTION, including peritonitis, intra-abdominal abscess, and liver abscess, caused by *Bacteroides* species including the *B. fragilis* group (*B. fragilis, B. distasonis, B. ovatus, B. thetaiotaomicron, B. vulgatus*), *Clostridium* species, *Eubacterium* species, *Peptococcus* species, and *Peptostreptococcus* species.

SKIN AND SKIN STRUCTURE INFECTIONS caused by *Bacteroides* species including the *B. fragilis* group, *Clostridium* species, *Peptococcus* species, *Peptostreptococcus* species, and *Fusobacterium* species.

GYNECOLOGIC INFECTIONS, including endometritis, endomyometritis, tubo-ovarian abscess, and post-surgical vaginal cuff infection, caused by *Bacteroides* species including the *B. fragilis* group, *Clostridium* species, *Peptococcus* species, and *Peptostreptococcus* species.

BACTERIAL SEPTICEMIA caused by *Bacteroides* species including the *B. fragilis* group, and *Clostridium* species.

BONE AND JOINT INFECTIONS, as adjunctive therapy, caused by *Bacteroides* species including the *B. fragilis* group.

CENTRAL NERVOUS SYSTEM (CNS) INFECTIONS, including meningitis and brain abscess, caused by *Bacteroides* species including the *B. fragilis* group.

LOWER RESPIRATORY TRACT INFECTIONS, including pneumonia, empyema, and lung abscess, caused by *Bacteroides* species including the *B. fragilis* group.

ENDOCARDITIS caused by *Bacteroides* species including the *B. fragilis* group.

Contraindications: Sātric is contraindicated in patients with a prior history of hypersensitivity to metronidazole, or other nitroimidazole derivatives. In patients with trichomoniasis, Sātric is contraindicated during the first trimester of pregnancy. (See Warnings).

Warnings:

Convulsive Seizures and Peripheral Neuropathy: Convulsive seizures and peripheral neuropathy, the latter characterized mainly by numbness or paresthesia of an extremity, have been reported in patients treated with metronidazole. The appearance of abnormal neurologic signs demands the prompt discontinuation of Sātric therapy. Sātric should be administered with caution to patients with central nervous system diseases.

Tumorigenicity Studies in Rodents: Metronidazole has shown evidence of carcinogenic activity in a number of studies involving chronic, oral administration in mice and rats.

Prominent among the effects in the mouse was the promotion of pulmonary tumorigenesis. This has been observed in all six reported studies in that species, including one study in which the animals were dosed on an intermittent schedule (administration during every fourth week only). At very high dose levels (approx. 500 mg/kg/day) there was a statistically significant increase in the incidence of malignant liver tumors in males. Also, the published results of one of the mouse studies indicated an increase in the incidence of malignant lymphomas as well as pulmonary neoplasms associated with lifetime feeding of the drug. All these effects are statistically significant.

Several long-term oral dosing studies in the rats have been completed. There was a statistically significant increase in the incidence of various neoplasms, particularly in mammary and hepatic tumors, among female rats administered metronidazole over those noted in the concurrent female control groups.

Two lifetime tumorigenicity studies in hamsters have been performed and reported to be negative.

Mutagenicity Studies: Although metronidazole has shown mutagenic activity in a number of in vitro assay systems, studies in mammals (in vivo) have failed to demonstrate a potential for genetic damage.

Precautions:

General: Patients with severe hepatic disease metabolize metronidazole slowly, with resultant accumulation of metronidazole and its metabolites in the plasma. Accordingly, for such patients, doses below those usually recommended should be administered cautiously.

Known or previously unrecognized candidiasis may present more prominent symptoms during therapy with Sātric and requires treatment with a candicidal agent.

Laboratory Tests: Sātric (metronidazole) is a nitroimidazole and should be used with care in patients with evidence of, or history of blood dyscrasia. A mild leukopenia has been observed during its administration; however, no persistent hematologic abnormalities attributable to metronidazole have been observed in clinical studies. Total and differential leukocyte counts are recommended before and after therapy for trichomoniasis and amebiasis, especially if a second course of therapy is necessary, and before and after therapy for anaerobic infection.

Drug Interactions: Metronidazole has been reported to potentiate the anticoagulant effect of coumarin and warfarin resulting in a prolongation of prothrombin time. This possible drug interaction should be considered when Sātric is prescribed for patients on this type of anti-coagulant therapy.

Alcoholic beverages should not be consumed during Sātric therapy because abdominal cramps, nausea, vomiting, headache, and flushing may occur.

Drug/Laboratory Test Interactions: Metronidazole may interfere with certain chemical analyses for serum glutamic oxalacetic transaminase, resulting in decreased values. Values of zero may be observed.

Carcinogenesis: (See Warnings.)

Pregnancy: *Teratogenic Effects—Pregnancy Category B:* Metronidazole crosses the placental barrier and enters the fetal circulation rapidly. Reproduction studies have been performed in rabbits and rats at doses up to five times the human dose and have revealed no evidence of impaired fertility or harm to the fetus due to Metronidazole. There are, however, no adequate and well-controlled studies in pregnant women. Because animal reproduction studies are not always predictive of human response, and because metronidazole is a carcinogen in rodents, this drug should be used during pregnancy only if clearly needed. *(See Contraindications).*

Use of Sātric for trichomoniasis in the second and third trimesters should be restricted to those in whom local palliative treatment has been inadequate to control symptoms.

Nursing Mothers: Because of the potential for tumorigenicity shown for metronidazole in mouse and rat studies, a decision should be made whether to discontinue nursing or to discontinue the drug, taking into account the importance of the drug to the mother. Metronidazole is secreted in breast milk in concentrations similar to those found in plasma.

Pediatric Use: Safety and effectiveness in children have not been established, except for the treatment of amebiasis.

Adverse Reactions: The two most serious adverse reactions reported in patients treated with metronidazole have been convulsive seizures and peripheral neuropathy, the latter characterized mainly by numbness or paresthesia of an extremity. Since persistent peripheral neuropathy has been reported in some patients receiving prolonged administration of metronidazole, patients should be specifically warned about these reactions and should be told to stop the drug and report immediately to their physicians if any neurologic symptoms occur.

The most common adverse reactions reported have been referable to the gastrointestinal tract, particularly nausea, sometimes accompanied by headache, anorexia, and occasionally vomiting; diarrhea; epigastric distress; and abdominal cramping. Constipation has also been reported.

The following reactions have also been reported during the treatment with metronidazole.

Mouth: A sharp, unpleasant metallic taste is not ununusual. Furry tongue, glossitis, and stomatitis have occurred; these may be associated with a sudden overgrowth of *Candida* which may occur during effective therapy.

Hematopoietic: Reversible neutropenia (leukopenia). Cardiovascular: Flattening of the T-wave may be seen in electrocardiographic tracings.

Central Nervous System: Convulsive seizures, peripheral neuropathy, dizziness, vertigo, incoordination, ataxia, confusion, irritability, depression, weakness, and insomnia.

Hypersensitivity: Urticaria, erythematous rash, flushing, nasal congestion, dryness of the mouth (or vagina or vulva) and fever.

Renal: Dysuria, cystitis, polyuria, incontinence, and a sense of pelvic pressure. Instances of darkened urine have been reported, and this manifestation has been the subject of a special investigation. Although the pigment which is probably responsible for this phenomenon has not been positively identified, it is almost certainly a metabolite of metronidazole and seems to have no clinical significance.

Other: Proliferation of *Candida* in the vagina, dyspareunia, decrease of libido, proctitis, and fleeting joint pains sometimes resembling "serum sickness." If patients receiving Sātric drink alcoholic beverages, they may experience abdominal distress, nausea, vomiting, flushing, or headache. A modification of the taste of alcoholic beverages has also been reported.

Overdosage: Single oral doses of metronidazole, up to 15 g. have been reported in suicide attempts and accidental overdoses. Symptoms reported include nausea, vomiting, and ataxia. Oral metronidazole has been studied as a radiation sensitizer in the treating of malignant tumors. Neurotoxic effects, including seizures and peripheral neuropathy, have been reported after 5 to 7 days of doses of 6 to 10.4 g every other day.

Treatment: There is no specific antidote for Sātric overdose; therefore, management of the patient should consist of symptomatic and supportive therapy.

Dosage and Administration:
Trichomoniasis: In the Female: One-day treatment—two grams of Sātric given either as a single dose or in two divided doses of one gram each given in the same day.

Seven-day course of treatment—250 mg three times daily for seven consecutive days. There is some indication from controlled comparative studies that cure rates as determined by vaginal smears, signs and symptoms, may be higher after a seven-day course of treatment than after a one-day treatment regimen.

The dosage regimen should be individualized. Single-dose treatment can assure compliance, especially if administered under supervision, in those patients who cannot be relied on to continue the seven-day regimen.

A seven-day course of treatment may minimize reinfection of the female long enough to treat sexual contacts. Further, some patients may tolerate one course of therapy better than the other. Pregnant patients should not be treated during the first trimester with either regimen. If treated during the second or third trimester, the one-day course of therapy should not be used, as it results in higher serum levels which reach the fetal circulation. *(See Contraindications and Precautions).*

When repeated courses of the drug are required, it is recommended that an interval of four to six weeks elapse between courses and that the presence of the trichomonad be reconfirmed by appropriate laboratory measures. Total and differential leukocyte counts should be made before and after treatment.

In the Male: Treatment should be individualized as for the female.

Amebiasis: Adults: For Acute Intestinal Amebiasis (Acute Amebic Dysentery): 750 mg orally 3 times daily for 5 to 10 days.

For Amebic Liver Abscess: 500 mg or 750 mg orally 3 times daily for 5 to 10 days.

Children: 35 to 50 mg/kg of body weight/24 hours divided into 3 doses, orally for 10 days.

Anaerobic Bacterial Infections:
In the treatment of most serious anaerobic infections the intravenous form of metronidazole is usually administered initially.

Following intravenous therapy, oral metronidazole may be used when conditions warrant based upon the severity of the disease and the response of the patient to intravenous treatment. The usual adult *oral* dosage is 7.5 mg/kg every six hours (approximately 500 mg for a 70 kg adult). A maximum of 4.0 g should not be exceeded during a 24 hour period.

The usual duration of therapy is 7 to 10 days; however, infections of the bone and joint, lower respiratory tract, and endocardium may require longer treatment.

Patients with severe hepatic disease metabolize metronidazole slowly, with resultant accumulation of metronidazole and its metabolites in the plasma. Accordingly, for such patients, doses below those usually recommended should be administered cautiously. Close monitoring of plasma metronidazole levels[2] and toxicity is recommended.

The dose of metronidazole should not be specifically reduced in anuric patients since accumulated metabolites may be rapidly removed by dialysis.

How Supplied: Available in tablets containing 250 mg and 500 mg of metronidazole USP. Each tablet of 250 mg is imprinted 3681. It is a white, to off-white round, convex tablet, packaged in bottles of 100 and 250 tablets. Each tablet of 500 mg is imprinted 3688. It is a white to off-white oblong, convex tablet, packaged in bottles of 60.
NDC **0281-3681-53**, bottle of 100
NDC **0281-3681-55**, bottle of 250
NDC **0281-3688-52**, bottle of 60
Dispense in well closed, light resistant containers as defined in the USP.

Store below 86°F (30°C).
Caution: Federal law prohibits dispensing without prescription.
1. Proposed standard: PSM-11—Proposed Reference Dilution Procedure for Antimicrobic Susceptibility Testing of Anaerobic Bacteria, National Committee for Clinical Laboratory Standards, and Sutter, et al: Collaborative Evaluation of a Proposed Reference Dilution Method of Susceptibility Testing of Anaerobic Bacteria, Antimicrob. Agents Chemother. 16:495–502 (Oct.) 1979; and Talley, et al: *In Vitro* Activity of Thienamycin, Antimicrob. Agents Chemother. 14:436–438 (Sept.) 1978.
2. Ralph, E.D. and Kirby, W.M.M.: Bioassay of Metronidazole With Either Anaerobic or Aerobic Incubation, J. Infect. Dis. 132:587–591 (Nov.) 175; or Gulaid, et al: Determination of Metronidazole and Its Major Metabolites in Biological Fluids by High Pressure Liquid Chromatography, Br. J. Clin. Pharmacol. 6:430–432, 1978.
Manufactured by R 11/82
Zenith Laboratories, Inc.
Northvale, New Jersey 07647
Distributed by
SAVAGE LABORATORIES
a division of Altana Inc.
Melville, NY 11747
Shown in Product Identification Section, page 433

TRYMEX™ ℞
triamcinolone acetonide
Cream U.S.P. and Ointment U.S.P.

Description: Trymex contains Triamcinolone Acetonide [Pregna-1, 4-diene-3, 20 dione, 9-fluoro-11, 21-dihydroxy-16, 17-[(1-methylethylidene) bis (oxy)]-, (11B, 16A)-], with the empirical formula $C_{24}H_{31}FO_6$ and molecular weight 434.50. CAS 76-25-5.

How Supplied:
Trymex Cream U.S.P., 0.025%
   NDC 0281-3622-44, 15 gram tube
   NDC 0281-3622-48, 80 gram tube
   NDC 0281-3622-87, 1 pound jar
Trymex Cream U.S.P., 0.1%
   NDC 0281-3625-44, 15 gram tube
   NDC 0281-3625-48, 80 gram tube
   NDC 0281-3625-87, 1 pound jar
Trymex Cream U.S.P., 0.5%
   NDC 0281-3627-44, 15 gram tube
Trymex Ointment U.S.P., 0.025%
   NDC 0281-3633-44, 15 gram tube
   NDC 0281-3633-48, 80 gram tube
Trymex Ointment U.S.P., 0.1%
   NDC 0281-3636-44, 15 gram tube
   NDC 0281-3636-48, 80 gram tube
Caution: Federal law prohibits dispensing without prescription.
FOR EXTERNAL USE ONLY

TRYSUL® ℞
(triple sulfa vaginal cream)

Description: Active Ingredients: sulfathiazole 3.42%, sulfacetamide 2.86%, sulfabenzamide 3.70% and urea 0.64%
In a Base Containing: Glyceryl monostearate, cetyl alcohol, stearic acid, lecithin, peanut oil, diethylaminoethyl steramide, phosphoric acid, propylene glycol, ethoxylated cholesterol, methyl paraben 0.15% and propyl paraben 0.05% as preservatives, and purified water.
How Supplied: NDC 0281-3790-47, 78 g tube with measured dose applicator.

Products are cross-indexed by
generic and chemical names
in the
YELLOW SECTION

Henry Schein, Inc.
5 HARBOR PARK DRIVE
PORT WASHINGTON, NY 11050

COMPREHENSIVE LIST OF SCHEIN GENERIC PRODUCTS

NDC 0364	PRODUCT
	Acetazolamide Tablets ℞
04-0001	250 mg, 100's
04-0002	250 mg, 1000's
	Allopurinol Tablets ℞
06-3201	100 mg, 100's
06-3202	100 mg, 1000's
06-3301	300 mg, 100's
06-3305	300 mg, 500's
	Aminophylline Oral Liquid ℞
73-4276	8 oz
	Aminophylline Suppositories ℞
71-1612	250 mg 12's
	Aminophylline Tablets ℞
00-0401	1½ gr C/T, 100's
00-0402	1½ gr C/T, 1000's
00-0501	3 gr C/T, 100's
00-0502	3 gr C/T, 1000's
	Amitriptyline HCl Tablets ℞
05-7301	10 mg, 100's
05-7302	10 mg, 1000's
05-7401	25 mg, 100's
05-7402	25 mg, 1000's
05-7501	50 mg, 100's
05-7502	50 mg, 1000's
05-7601	75 mg, 100's
05-7701	100 mg, 100's
05-7801	150 mg, 100's
	Amoxicillin Trihydrate Capsules ℞
20-4001	250 mg, 100's
20-4005	250 mg, 500's
20-4150	500 mg, 50's
	Amoxicillin Trihydrate Powder For Oral Suspension ℞
72-1560	125 mg, 80 ml
72-1561	125 mg, 100 ml
72-1562	125 mg, 150 ml
72-1660	250 mg, 80 ml
72-1661	250 mg, 100 ml
72-1662	250 mg, 150 ml
	Ampicillin Trihydrate Capsules ℞
20-0101	250 mg, 100's
20-0105	250 mg, 500's
20-0201	500 mg, 100's
20-0205	500 mg, 500's
	Ampicillin Trihydrate Powder For Oral Suspension ℞
20-0361	125 mg, 100 ml
20-0363	125 mg, 200 ml
20-0461	250 mg, 100 ml
20-0463	250 mg, 200 ml
	Antispasmodic Capsules ℞
06-6702	1000's
	Antispasmodic Elixir ℞
	(Atropine Derivatives, Hyoscyamine, Phenobarbital)
70-0216	Pt
70-0299	Gal
	Antispasmodic Tablets ℞
	(Atropine Derivatives, Hyoscyamine, Phenobarbital)
00-2002	1000's
00-2003	5000's
	Apap 300 mg with Codeine Tablets ℂ
03-2301	15 mg, 100's
03-2401	30 mg, 100's
03-2402	30 mg, 1000's
03-2601	60 mg, 100's
03-2602	60 mg, 1000's
	Apap with Codeine Elixir ℂ
72-0716	Pt
	Aspirin 325 mg with Codeine Tablets ℂ
05-4001	30 mg, 100's
05-4002	30 mg, 1000's
05-4101	60 mg, 100's
00-4102	**Azo-Sulfisoxazole Tablets** ℞ 1000's
	Bromanyl Expectorant ℂ
	(Bromodiphenhydramine HCl, Codeine Phosphate)
74-0516	Pt
74-0599	Gal
	Bromphen Compound Tablets ℞
	(Brompheniramine Maleate, Phenylephrine HCl, Phenylpropanolamine HCl)
05-8401	100's
05-8402	1000's
	Bromphen Compound Elixir - Sugar Free
	(Brompheniramine Maleate, Phenylephrine HCl, Phenylpropanolamine)
72-8116	Pt
72-8199	Gal
	Bromphen Expectorant ℞
	(Brompheniramine Maleate, Psuedoephedrine, HCl, Dextromethorphan HBr.)
73-8616	Pt
73-8699	Gal
	Bromphen DC Expectorant ℂ
	(Brompheniramine Maleate, Codeine Phosphate, Phenylpropanolamine)
73-8716	Pt
73-8799	Gal
	Butalbital Compound ℂ
	(Butalbital, Aspirin, Caffeine)
06-7701	100's
06-7702	1000's
	Cardec DM ℞
	(Carbinoxamine Maleate, Dextromethorphan Hydrobromide, Pseudoephedrine HCl)
72-7756	Drops, 30 ml
73-1816	Syrup, Pt
73-1899	Syrup, Gal
	Cafetrate-PB Suppositories ℞
	(Caffeine, Ergotamine Tartrate)
73-4910	10's
	Chloral Hydrate Capsules ℂ
00-6101	7½ gr, 100's
00-6102	7½ gr, 1000's
	Chloramphenicol Ophthalmic Solution 5% ℞
73-6172	15 cc
	Chlordiazepoxide HCl Capsules ℂ
04-3601	5 mg, 100's
04-3605	5 mg, 500's
04-3602	5 mg, 1000's
04-3701	10 mg, 100's
04-3705	10 mg, 500's
04-3702	10 mg, 1000's
04-3801	25 mg, 100's
04-3805	25 mg, 500's
	Chloroserpine - 250 Tablets ℞
	(Chlorothiazide, Reserpine)
04-2201	250 mg, 100's
04-2202	250 mg, 1000's
04-2301	500 mg, 100's
	Chlorothiazide Tablets ℞
03-8901	250 mg, 100's
03-8902	250 mg, 1000's
03-9001	500 mg, 100's
03-9002	500 mg, 1000's
	Chlorpromazine HCl Tablets ℞
03-8001	10 mg, 100's
03-8002	10 mg, 1000's
03-8101	25 mg, 100's
03-8102	25 mg, 1000's
03-8201	50 mg, 100's
03-8202	50 mg, 1000's
03-8301	100 mg, 100's
03-8302	100 mg, 1000's
03-8401	200 mg, 100's
03-8402	200 mg, 1000's
	Chlorthalidone Tablets ℞
05-9201	25 mg, 100's
05-9202	25 mg, 1000's
05-9301	50 mg, 100's
05-9302	50 mg, 1000's
	Chlorzone Forte Tablets ℞
	(Acetaminophen, Chlorzoxazone)
04-6201	100's
04-6202	1000's
	Clipoxide Capsules ℞
	(Chlordiazepoxide HCl, Clidinium Bromide)
05-5901	100's
05-5905	500's
	Cloxacillin Sodium Capsules ℞
20-6101	250 mg, 100's
20-6201	500 mg, 100's
	Conjugated Estrogens Tablets - Coated ℞
00-7801	.625 mg, 100's
00-7802	.625 mg, 1000's
00-7901	1.25 mg, 100's
00-7902	1.25 mg, 1000's
00-8001	2.5 mg, 100's
	Cyclandelate Capsules ℞
05-7001	200 mg, 100's
05-7002	200 mg, 1000's
05-7101	400 mg, 100's
05-7102	400 mg, 1000's
	Cyproheptadine HCl Syrup ℞
72-7216	Pt
72-7299	Gal
	Cyproheptadine HCl Tablets ℞
04-9901	4 mg, 100's
04-9905	4 mg, 500's
	Decongestant Elixir OTC
	(Chlorpheniramine, Menthol, Phenylpropanolamine)
72-2316	Pt
72-2399	Gal
	Decongestant Expectorant ℂ
	(Codeine Phosphate, Guaifenesin, Pseudoephedrine HCl)
73-8316	Pt
73-8399	Gal
	Decongestant-AT (Antitussive) Liquid ℂ
	(Chlorpheniramine Maleate, Codeine Phosphate, Pseudoephedrine HCl)
73-8416	Pt
73-8499	Gal
	Detussin Liquid ℂ
	(Hydrocodone Bitartrate, Pseudoephedrine)
72-5716	Pt
	Detussin Expectorant ℂ
	(Hydrocodone Bitartrate, Guaifenesin, Pseudoephedrine)
72-5816	Pt
	Dexamethasone Tablets - Pentagonal Shaped ℞
03-9701	.25 mg, 100's
03-9702	.25 mg, 1000's
03-9801	.50 mg, 100's
03-9802	.50 mg, 1000's
00-9801	.75 mg, 100's
00-9802	.75 mg, 1000's
03-9901	1.5 mg, 100's
06-8301	4 mg, 100's
	Dexamycin Ophthalmic ℞
73-7770	⅛ oz Ointment
73-9453	5 ml Solution
	Dexchlor Repeat Action Tablets ℞
	(Dexchlorpheniramine Maleate)
05-8501	4 mg, 100's
05-8601	6 mg, 100's
05-8602	6 mg, 1000's
	Dicloxacillin Sodium Capsules ℞
20-7001	250 mg, 100's
20-7101	500 mg, 100's
	Diethylpropion HCl Tablets ℂ
03-2901	25 mg, 100's
03-2902	25 mg, 1000's
	Diethylpropion HCl Timed Tablets ℂ
04-4001	75 mg, 100's
04-4004	75 mg, 250's

Product Information

Dihydrocodeine Compound Capsules ⓒ
(Dihydrocodeinone Bitartrate, Aspirin, Caffeine)
- 07-1801 100's Blue
- 07-1805 500's Blue
- 07-0101 100's (G/R)

Dioctocal Capsules OTC
Docusate Calcium USP
- 05-8901 240 mg, 100's

Diphenhydramine HCl Capsules ℞
- 01-1602 25 mg, 1000's
- 01-1702 50 mg, 1000's

Diphenoxylate & Atropine Tablets (DPXL) ⓒ
- 04-4901 100's
- 04-4905 500's
- 04-4902 1000's
- 73-3658 2 oz Liquid

Dipyridamole Tablets ℞
- 05-1101 25 mg, 100's
- 05-1102 25 mg, 1000's
- 05-9601 50 mg, 100's
- 05-9602 50 mg, 1000's
- 05-5201 75 mg, 100's
- 05-5205 75 mg, 500's

Disulfiram ℞
- 03-3601 250 mg, 100's
- 03-3750 500 mg, 50's

Doxycycline Hyclate Capsules ℞
- 20-3250 50 mg, 50's
- 20-3350 100 mg, 50's

Doxycycline Tablets ℞
- 20-6350 100 mg, 50's

Effervescent Potassium Tablets ℞
- 06-3530 25 meg, 30's

Erythromycin Estolate Capsules ℞
- 05-3001 250 mg, 100's

Erythromycin Estolate Suspension ℞
- 20-7816 125 mg, pints
- 20-7916 250 mg, pints

Erythromycin Ethylsuccinate ℞
- 20-5761 Granules 200 mg, 100 ml
- 20-6716 Suspension 200 mg, Pt
- 20-7016 Suspension 400 mg, Pt
- 20-7401 Tablets 400 mg, 100's

Erythromycin Stearate Tablets ℞
- 20-0501 250 mg, 100's
- 20-0505 250 mg, 500's
- 20-3801 500 mg, 100's

Erythromycin Tablets E/C ℞
- 20-3101 250 mg, 100's
- 20-3105 250 mg, 500's

Fluocinolone Acetonide Cream ℞
- 72-6272 0.01%, 15 gm
- 72-6258 0.01%, 60 gm
- 72-6372 0.025%, 15 gm
- 72-6358 0.025%, 60 gm
- 06-5901 100's

Furosemide Tablets ℞
- 05-6801 20 mg, 100's
- 05-6802 20 mg, 1000's
- 05-1401 40 mg, 100's
- 05-1402 40 mg, 1000's

Gentamicin 0.1% ℞
(Gentamicin Sulfate)
- 73-0572 Cream, 15 gm
- 73-3872 Ointment, 15 gm

Gentamicin Ophthalmic Ointment ℞
- 73-8770 3 mg, 1/8 oz Ointment
- 73-8853 3 mg, 5cc Solution

Glutethimide Tablets ⓒ
- 02-9601 0.5 gm, 100's
- 02-9602 0.5 gm, 1000's

Guiatuss Syrup OTC
(Guaifenesin)
- 70-2516 Pt
- 70-2599 Gal

Guiatuss A-C Syrup ⓒ
(Codeine Phosphate, Guaifenesin)
- 70-2616 Pt
- 70-2699 Gal

Guiatuss D-M Syrup OTC
(Dextromethorphan, Guaifenesin)
- 70-2716 Pt
- 70-2799 Gal

H-H-R Tablets ℞
(Hydralazine, Hydrochlorothiazide, Reserpine)
- 03-6101 100's
- 03-6102 1000's

Hydralazine HCl Tablets ℞
- 06-4701 10 mg, 100's
- 06-4702 10 mg, 1000's
- 01-4401 25 mg, 100's
- 01-4402 25 mg, 1000's
- 01-4501 50 mg, 100's
- 01-4502 50 mg, 1000's

Hydralazine-Thiazide Capsules ℞
- 06-1601 25/25, 100's
- 06-1701 50/50, 100's

Hydrochlorothiazide Tablets ℞
- 03-2201 25 mg, 100's
- 03-2202 25 mg, 1000's
- 03-2801 50 mg, 100's
- 03-2802 50 mg, 1000's
- 03-5302 50 mg (Y), 1000's
- 04-2101 100 mg, 100's
- 04-2102 100 mg, 1000's

Hydrocodone Syrup ⓒ
- 72-5416 Pt
- 72-5499 Gal

Hydro-Ergoloid Oral Tablets ℞
- 06-2201 1.0 mg, 100's
- 06-2205 1.0 mg, 500's

Hydro-Ergoloid Sublingual Tablets ℞
(Dihydroergocornine, Dihydroergocrystine, Dihydroergokryptine, Hydrogenated Ergot Alkaloids)
- 04-1501 0.5 mg, 100's
- 04-1502 0.5 mg, 1000's
- 04-4601 1.0 mg, 100's
- 04-4602 1.0 mg, 1000's

Hydroflumethiazide Tablets ℞
- 06-7401 50 mg, 100's

Hydro-Fluserpine Tablets #1 ℞
(Hydrofluomethiazide 25 mg, Reserpine 0.125 mg)
- 06-7501 100's
- 06-7505 500's

Hydro-Fluserpine Tablets #2 ℞
(Hydrofluomethiazide 50 mg, Reserpine 0.125 mg)
- 06-7601 100's
- 06-7602 1000's

Hydroserpine Tablets ℞
(Hydrochlorothiazide, Reserpine)
- 03-5401 #1 25 mg, 100's
- 03-5402 #1 25 mg, 1000's
- 03-5501 #2 5 mg, 100's
- 03-5502 #2 5 mg, 1000's

Hydroxyzine HCl Tablets ℞
- 04-9401 10 mg, 100's
- 04-9405 10 mg, 500's
- 04-9501 25 mg, 100's
- 04-9505 25 mg, 500's
- 04-9601 50 mg, 100's
- 04-9605 50 mg, 500's
- 72-7316 Syrup, Pt

Hydroxyzine Pamoate Capsules ℞
- 04-8301 25 mg, 100's
- 04-8305 25 mg, 500's
- 04-8401 50 mg, 100's
- 04-8405 50 mg, 500's

Imipramine HCl Tablets ℞
- 04-4301 10 mg, 100's
- 04-4302 10 mg, 1000's
- 04-0601 25 mg, 100's
- 04-0602 25 mg, 1000's
- 04-3501 50 mg, 100's
- 04-3502 50 mg, 1000's

Iophen-C Liquid ⓒ
(Chlorpheniramine Maleate, Codeine Phosphate, Iodinated Glycerol)
- 73-2816 Pt

Isosorbide Dinitrate Oral Tablets ℞
- 03-4001 5 mg, 100's
- 03-4002 5 mg, 1000's
- 03-4101 10 mg, 100's
- 03-4102 10 mg, 1000's
- 05-0901 20 mg, 100's
- 05-0902 20 mg, 1000's
- 06-2801 30 mg, 100's
- 06-2802 30 mg, 1000's

Isosorbide Dinitrate Sublingual Tablets ℞
- 03-6701 2.5 mg, 100's
- 03-6702 2.5 mg, 1000's
- 03-6801 5.0 mg, 100's
- 03-6802 5.0 mg, 1000's
- 06-2701 10 mg, 100's
- 06-2702 10 mg, 1000's

Isosorbide Dinitrate Timed Capsules ℞
- 03-4201 40 mg, 100's
- 03-4202 40 mg, 1000's

Isosorbide Dinitrate Timed Tablets ℞
- 04-0101 40 mg, 100's
- 04-0102 40 mg, 1000's

Isoxsuprine HCl Tablets ℞
- 03-9301 10 mg, 100's
- 03-9302 10 mg, 1000's
- 03-9401 20 mg, 100's
- 03-9402 20 mg, 1000's

Kaolin-Pectin Mixture OTC
- 70-3016 Pt
- 70-3099 Gal

Kaolin, Pectin, Belladonna Mixture OTC
- 70-3116 Pt
- 70-3199 Gal

Kaolin-Pectin PG Mixture ⓒ
- 72-6616 Pt
- 72-6699 Gal

Lidocaine HCl 2% Viscous Solution OTC
- 72-8261 100 ml

Lindane Lotion ℞
- 73-2658 2 oz
- 73-2616 Pt

Lindane Shampoo ℞
- 73-2758 2 oz
- 73-2716 Pt

Liothyronine Sodium Tablets ℞
- 06-2401 25 mcg, 100's
- 06-2501 50 mcg, 100's

Meclizine HCl MLT Tablets ℞
- 04-1101 12.5 mg, 100's
- 04-1102 12.5 mg, 1000's
- 04-1201 25 mg, 100's
- 04-1202 25 mg, 1000's

Meprobamate Tablets ⓒ
- 01-6001 200 mg, 100's
- 01-6002 200 mg, 1000's
- 01-6101 400 mg, 100's
- 01-6102 400 mg, 1000's

Mepro Compound Tablets ⓒ
(Aspirin, Meprobamate)
- 07-0201 100's
- 07-0205 500's

Methenamine Mandelate Tablets ℞
- 01-6502 0.5 mg, 1000's
- 01-6605 1.0 mg, 500's

Methenamine Mandelate Forte Suspension ℞
- 71-9416 Pt

Methocarbamol Tablets ℞
- 03-4601 500 mg, 100's
- 03-4605 500 mg, 500's
- 03-4701 750 mg, 100's
- 03-4705 750 mg, 500's

Methocarbamol w/Aspirin Tablets ℞
- 04-9201 100's
- 04-9205 500's

Methyclothiazide Tablets ℞
- 06-1901 2.5 mg, 100's
- 06-2001 5.0 mg, 100's
- 06-2002 5.0 mg, 1000's

Methylprednisolone Tablets ℞
- 04-6701 4 mg, 100's

Metronidazole Oral Tablets ℞
- 05-9501 250 mg, 100's
- 05-9504 250 mg, 250's

Continued on next page

Product Information

Always consult Supplement

Schein—Cont.

Code	Product
06-8750	500 mg, 50's
	Nitrofurantoin Tablets ℞
03-0901	50 mg, 100's
03-0902	50 mg, 1000's
03-1001	100 mg, 100's
03-1002	100 mg, 1000's
	Nitrofurantoin Capsules ℞
03-3101	50 mg, 100's
03-3105	50 mg, 500's
03-3201	100 mg, 100's
	Nitroglycerin Ointment 2% ℞
73-0656	30 gm
73-0658	60 gm
	Nitrolin Timed Capsules ℞
	(Nitroglycerin)
01-7401	2.5 mg, 100's
04-3201	6.5 mg, 100's
06-6406	9 mg, 60's
	Nylidrin HCl Tablets ℞
03-9101	6 mg, 100's
03-9102	6 mg, 1000's
03-9201	12 mg, 100's
03-9202	12 mg, 1000's
	Nystatin Cream ℞
72-1072	15 gm
	Nystatin Oral Tablets ℞
20-5101	500,000 uts, 100's
	Nystatin Vaginal Tablets ℞
72-0915	15's
72-0930	30's
	Nyst-olone Cream ℞
	(Gramicidin, Neomycin Sulfate, Nystatin, Triamcinolone Acetonide)
72-1472	15 gm
72-1456	30 gm
72-1458	60 gm
72-1416	1 lb
	Nyst-olone Ointment ℞
	(Gramicidin, Neomycin Sulfate, Nystatin, Triamcinolone Acetonide)
72-7672	15 gm
	Oxacillin Sodium Capsules ℞
20-5901	250 mg, 100's
20-6001	500 mg, 100's
	Oxacillin Sodium Powder For Oral Suspension ℞
20-6461	250 mg, 100 ml
	Oxytetracycline HCl Capsules ℞
20-0701	250 mg, 100's
20-0702	250 mg, 1000's
	Papaverine HCl Timed Capsules ℞
01-8101	150 mg, 100's
01-8102	150 mg, 1000's
	Penicillin VK Tablets ℞
20-2001	250 mg Rd, 100's
20-2002	250 mg Rd, 1000's
20-2101	250 mg Oval, 100's
20-2102	250 mg Oval, 1000's
20-2201	500 mg Rd, 100's
20-2202	500 mg Rd, 1000's
20-5801	500 mg Oval, 100's
20-5802	500 mg Oval, 1000's
	Penicillin VK Powder For Oral Suspension
20-2361	125 mg, 100 ml
20-2363	125 mg, 200 ml
20-2461	250 mg, 100 ml
20-2463	250 mg, 200 ml
	Pentaerythritol Tetranitrate Tablets (PETN) ℞
01-8402	10 mg, 1000's
01-8502	20 mg, 1000's
	Pentaerythritol Tetranitrate Timed Release ℞
01-8901	80 mg Capsules, 100's
01-8902	80 mg Capsules, 1000's
05-3101	80 mg Tablets, 100's
05-3102	80 mg Tablets, 1000's
	Phenobarbital Elixir ℭ
70-4616	Pt
70-4699	Gal
	Phenobarbital Tablets ℭ
02-0002	¼ gr, 1000's
02-0302	½ gr, 1000's
	1 gr, 1000's
02-0602	1½ gr, 1000's
	Phentermine HCl Capsules ℭ
03-3501	30 mg (Y), 100's
03-3502	30 mg (Y), 1000's
05-3802	30 mg (B/C), 1000's
	Phenylbutazone ℞
05-3701	100 mg Tablets, 100's
05-3702	100 mg Tablets, 1000's
06-3401	100 mg Capsules, 100's
06-3402	100 mg Capsules, 1000's
	Phenytoin Sodium Capsules - Prompt Action ℞
01-1902	100 mg, 1000's
	Polyvitamin-Fluoride Drops ℞
	(Sodium Fluoride, Vitamins)
71-7057	50 ml
	Polyvitamin-Fluoride Tablets ℞
	(Sodium Fluoride, Vitamins)
10-7501	100's
10-7502	1000's
	Potassium Chloride Liquid 10% Sugar Free ℞
70-4716	Pt
70-4799	Gal
	Potassium Chloride Concentrate 20% ℞
71-6616	Pt
71-6699	Gal
	Potassium Chloride Powder For Oral Solution ℞
73-7830	30 pkts/box
	Potassium Gluconate Elixir ℞
70-4816	Pt
70-4899	Gal
	Prednisolone Tablets ℞
02-1701	5 mg, 100's
02-1702	5 mg, 1000's
	Prednisone Tablets ℞
02-1801	5 mg, 100's
02-1802	5 mg, 1000's
04-6101	10 mg, 100's
04-6105	10 mg, 500's
04-4201	20 mg, 100's
04-4205	20 mg, 500's
05-5601	50 mg, 100's
	Primidone Tablets ℞
03-6601	250 mg, 100's
03-6602	250 mg, 1000's
	Probenecid Tablets ℞
03-1401	100's
03-1402	1000's
	Probenecid with Colchicine Tablets ℞
03-1501	100's
03-1502	1000's
	Procainamide HCl Capsules ℞
02-1901	250 mg, 100's
02-1902	250 mg, 1000's
03-4301	375 mg, 100's
03-4302	375 mg, 1000's
03-4401	500 mg, 100's
03-4402	500 mg, 1000's
	Prochlor-Iso Timed Release Capsules ℞
	(Isopropamide Iodide, Prochlorperazine)
04-7401	100's
04-7405	500's
	Propantheline Bromide Tablets ℞
03-0401	15 mg, 100's
03-0402	15 mg, 1000's
	Propoxyphene Compound 65 ℭ
	Propoxyphene HCl 65 mg, Aspirin 389 mg, Caffeine 32.4 mg)
06-6801	100's
06-6802	1000's
	Propoxyphene HCl Capsules ℭ
03-1201	65 mg, 100's
03-1205	65 mg, 500's
	Propoxyphene & Apap Tablets 65/650 ℭ
03-9601	100's
03-9605	500's
	Pseudoephedrine HCl Tablets
05-9801	30 mg, 100's OTC
02-2502	60 mg, 1000's ℞
	Pyrinyl Liquid OTC
	(Piperonyl Butoxide, Pyrethrins)
71-7858	2 oz
	Quadrahist Timed Release Tablets ℞
	(Chlorpheniramine, Phenylephrine, Phenylpropanolamine, Phenyltoloxamine)
05-8101	100's
05-8102	1000's
	Quadrahist Pediatric Syrup ℞
	(Chlorpheniramine, Phenylephrine, Phenylpropanolamine, Phenyltoloxamine)
73-3216	Pt
	Quadrahist Syrup ℞
	(Chlorpheniramine, Phenylephrine, Phenylpropanolamine, Phenyltoloxamine)
71-8116	Pt
71-8199	Gal
	Quinidine Gluconate Tablets ℞
06-0401	324 mg, 100's
06-0404	324 mg, 250's
	Quinidine Sulfate Tablets ℞
02-2901	200 mg, 100's
02-2902	200 mg, 1000's
02-8201	300 mg, 100's
	Quinine Sulfate Capsules ℞
02-3001	5 gr, 100's
02-3002	5 gr, 1000's
	Quinine Sulfate Tablets ℞
05-6001	260 mg, 100's
	Reserpine Tablets ℞
02-3402	0.25 mg, 1000's
02-3403	0.25 mg, 5000's
	Soprodol Tablets (Carisoprodol) ℞
04-7501	100's
04-7505	500's
	Spironazide Tablets ℞
	(Hydrochlorothiazide, Spironolactone)
05-1301	100's
05-1302	1000's
	Spironolactone Tablets ℞
05-1201	100's
05-1202	1000's
	Sulfasalazine Tablets ℞
04-4401	500 mg, 100's
04-4405	500 mg, 500's
06-8801	500 mg E/C, 100's
	Sulfatrim Tablets ℞
	(Trimethoprim, Sulfamethoxazole)
20-6801	100's
	Sulfatrim D/S Tablets ℞
	(Trimethoprim, Sulfamethoxazole)
20-6901	Oval Shaped, 100's
06-8601	Capsule Shaped, 100's
06-6905	Oval Shaped, 500's
06-8605	Capsule Shaped, 500's
	Sulfinpyrazone Tablets ℞
06-2601	100 mg, 100's
	Sulfisoxazole Tablets ℞
02-6502	0.5 gm, 1000's
	T-E-P Tablets ℞
	(Ephedrine, Theophylline, Phenobarbital)
02-6602	1000's
	Tetracycline HCl Capsules ℞
20-2601	250 mg O/Y, 100's
20-2602	250 mg O/Y, 1000's
20-2701	250 mg B/Y, 100's
20-2702	250 mg B/Y, 1000's
20-2901	500 mg Bk/Y, 100's
20-2902	500 mg Bk/Y, 1000's
	Tetracycline HCl Syrup ℞
20-3058	2 oz
20-3016	Pt
	Theophylline Anhydrous Tablets ℞
06-8001	100 mg, 100's
06-8101	200 mg, 100's
06-8105	200 mg, 500's
06-6001	300 mg, 100's
06-6005	300 mg, 500's
	Theophylline Elixir ℞
70-6016	Pt
70-6099	Gal

for possible revisions — **Product Information** — 1831

	Theophylline KI Elixir ℞	07-1001	60 mg, 100's		Tablets
72-6716	Pt		**Benztropine Mesylate Tablets** ℞		Tablets with Vitamin C
72-6799	Gal	07-0301	1 mg, 100's		**CORICIDIN®•** OTC
	Theozine Tablets ℞	07-0401	2 mg, 100's		Cough Syrup
	(Ephedrine Sulfate, Hydroxyzine HCl, Theophylline)		**Dexamethasone Tablets** ℞		D® Decongestant Tablets 871
		06-9550	6 mg, 50's		**DEMILETS®** Tablets
05-3501	100's		**Erythromycin Opth. Oint** ℞		**MEDILETS®** Tablets
05-3505	500's	73-9870	1/8 oz.		Nasal Mist
	Theozine Syrup - Dye Free ℞		**Indomethacin Capsules**		Sinus Headache Tablets
	(Ephedrine Sulfate, Hydroxyzine HCl, Theophylline)	06-9101	25 mg, 100's		(Extra Strength)
		06-9102	25 mg, 1000's		Tablets 171
72-4616	Pt	06-9201	50 mg, 100's		**CORILIN®** Infant Liquid† ℞
	Thioridazine Tablets ℞	06-9205	50 mg, 500's		**DEMAZIN®•** OTC
06-6101	10 mg, 100's		**Isoetharine HCl 1.0** ℞		Timed-Release Tablets 751
06-6102	10 mg, 1000's	74-1154	10 ml		Syrup
06-6901	15 mg	74-1156	30 ml		**DERMOLATE™•** OTC
06-6201	25 mg, 100's		**Methy-Deserpidine Tablets** ℞		hydrocortisone 0.5%
06-6202	25 mg, 1000's	06-9801	100's		Anti-Itch Cream
06-6301	50 mg, 100's		**Phentermine HCl 37.5 mg** ℂ		Anal-Itch Ointment
06-6302	50 mg, 1000's	07-0605	Capsules, 500's		Anti-Itch Spray
06-7001	100 mg, 100's	07-0705	Tablets, 500's		Scalp-Itch Lotion
	L-Thyroxine Tablets ℞		**Thylline Tablets** ℞		**DIPROLENE®** ℞
02-7702	0.1 mg, 1000's		(Dyphylline)		betamethasone dipropionate, USP
02-7802	0.2 mg, 1000's	07-1101	200 mg, 100's		Ointment 0.05%
	Tolbutamide Tablets ℞	07-1201	400 mg, 1100's		**DIPROSONE®** ℞
04-7701	0.5 gm, 100's		**Thylline—GG Tablets** ℞		betamethasone dipropionate, USP
04-7702	0.5 gm, 1000's		(Dyphylline, Guaifenesin)		Aerosol 0.1%
	Triafed OTC	07-1301	100's		Cream 0.05%
	(Pseudoephedrine, Triprolidine)				Lotion 0.05%
06-9401	Tablets, 100's				Ointment 0.05%
06-9402	Tablets, 1000's		**Schering Corporation**		**DISOPHROL®•** OTC
	Syrup, 4 oz		GALLOPING HILL ROAD		CHRONOTAB® Tablets 85-WMH/231
71-7216	Syrup, Pt		KENILWORTH, NJ 07033		
71-7299	Syrup, Gal				**DISOPHROL®†** WBS/866 OTC
	Triafed-C Expectorant ℂ		**Product Identification Codes**		Tablets
	(Codeine Phosphate, Guaifenesin, Pseudoephedrine HCl, Triprolidine HCl)		To provide quick and positive identification of Schering Products, we have imprinted the product identification number of the National Drug Code on most tablets and capsules. In some cases, identification letters also appear.		**DRIXORAL®•** Sustained-Action Tablets OTC
					EMKO®• OTC
71-7316	Pt				BECAUSE® Contraceptor®•
71-7399	Gal				PRE-FIL® Vaginal Contraceptive Foam
	Triamcinolone Acetonide Cream 0.025% ℞		For convenience, a complete list of all Schering products and their identification codes, where appropriate, follow:		Vaginal Contraceptive Foam
					ESTINYL® Tablets ℞
72-1172	15 gm				estinyl estradiol, USP
72-1160	80 gm		**Product Listing**		0.02 mg 298/ER
72-1116	1 lb		Product Code		0.05 mg 070/EM
	Triamcinolone Acetonide Cream 0.1% ℞		A&D™ Hand Cream* OTC		0.5 mg 150/EP
			A&D™ Ointment* OTC		**ETRAFON®** Tablets ℞
72-1272	15 gm		**AFRIN®•** OTC		perphenazine, USP-amitriptyline hydrochloride, USP
72-1260	80 gm		oxymetazoline HCl		
72-1216	1 lb		Nasal Spray 0.05%		Tablets (2–10) ANA/287
	Triamcinolone Acetonide Cream 0.5% ℞		Menthol Nasal Spray 0.05%		Tablets (2–25) ANC/598
			Nose Drops 0.05%		A Tablets (4–10) ANB/119
72-1372	15 gm		Pediatric Nose Drops 0.025%		Forte Tablets (4–25) ANE/720
	Triamcinolone Tablets ℞		**AFRINOL®•** OTC		**FULVICIN® P/G Tablets** ℞
03-5201	4 mg, 100's		pseudoephedrine sulfate		ultramicrosize griseofulvin, USP
03-5205	4 mg, 500's		Repetabs Tablets Long-Acting		125 mg 228
	Trichlormethiazide Tablets ℞		Nasal Decongestant 258		165 mg 654
03-0702	4 mg, 1000's		**AKRINOL®** Cream† ℞		250 mg 507
	Trifluoperazine Tablets ℞		acrisorcin, USP		330 mg 352
06-0001	1 mg, 100's		**CELESTONE®** ℞		**FULVICIN U/F®** Tablets ℞
06-0101	2 mg, 100's		betamethasone, USP		griseofulvin, (microsize), USP
06-0201	5 mg, 100's		Cream†		250 mg AUF/948
06-0301	10 mg, 100's		Phosphate Injection		500 mg AUG/496
	Trimethobenzamide HCl Suppositories ℞		Soluspan® Suspension		**GARAMYCIN®** Injectables ℞
			Syrup		gentamicin sulfate, USP
73-4710	100 mg, 10's		Tablets 0.6 mg 011/BDA		Disposable Syringes 1.5 ml (60 mg)
73-4810	200 mg, 10's		**CHLOR-TRIMETON®•** OTC		Disposable Syringes 2.0 ml (80 mg)
	Triple Sulfa Vaginal Cream ℞		chlorpheniramine maleate		Injectable 2 ml vial (80 mg)
	(Sulfabenzamide, Sulfacetamide Sulfathiazole)		Allergy Syrup		Injectable 20 ml vial (800 mg)
			Allergy Tablets 4 mg 080/TW		Intrathecal 2 ml (4 mg) ampul
72-8437	2.75 oz		Long-Acting Allergy Repetabs® Tablets 8 mg 374		Pediatric Injectable 2 ml vial (20 mg)
	Tri-Thalmic Ophthalmic Solution ℞				I.V. Piggyback Injection– 60 ml (60 mg), 80 ml (80 mg)
			12 mg Antihistamine Timed-Release Allergy Tablets 009/AAE		
	(Polymycin B Sulfate 10,000/cc, Neomycin Sulfate (equiv. to 1.75 mg as base), Gramicidin 0.025 mg)				**GARAMYCIN®** Topicals ℞
			CHLOR-TRIMETON®• OTC		gentamicin sulfate, USP
73-7554	10 cc		chlorpheniramine maleate/pseudoephedrine sulfate		Cream
	Tuss-Ade Timed Capsules ℞				Ointment
	(Caramiphen Edisylate, Phenylpropanolamine)		Decongestant Tablets 901		Ophthalmic Ointment
			Long-Acting Decongestant Repetabs® Tablets		Ophthalmic Solution
06-1405	500's				**GYNE-LOTRIMIN®** ℞
	Warfarin Sodium Tablets ℞		**CHLOR-TRIMETON®†** ℞		clotrimazole, USP
06-3901	2.5 mg, 100's		chlorpheniramine maleate, USP		
06-4001	5.0 mg, 100's		Injection 10 mg/ml		*Continued on next page*
06-4002	5.0 mg, 1000's		**COD LIVER OIL CONCENTRATE*** OTC		
	NEW PRODUCTS ADDITIONS		Capsules		Information on Schering products appearing on these pages is effective as of September 30, 1984.
	Apap 300 mg W/Codeine Caps ℂ				
07-0901	30 mg, 100's				

Schering—Cont.

Vaginal Cream 1%
Vaginal Tablets 100 mg 734
HYPERSTAT® I.V. Injection ℞
diazoxide, USP
LOTRIMIN® ℞
clotrimazole, USP
 Cream 1%
 Lotion 1%
 Solution 1%
LOTRISONE® Cream ℞
clotrimazole, USP, betamethasone and dipropionate, USP
METICORTEN® Tablets† ℞
prednisone, USP
 1 mg KEM/843
 5 mg ABB/172
METI-DERM® Cream†
prednisolone, USP
METIMYD® ℞
prednisolone acetate, USP/
sulfacetamide sodium, USP
 Ophthalmic Ointment
 Ophthalmic Solution
METRETON® Ophthalmic/Otic ℞
Solution
prednisolone sodium phosphate, USP
MIRADON® Tablets ℞
anisindione, USP
MOL-IRON® * OTC
 Chronosule® Capsules
 Tablets
 Tablets with Vitamin C
MY OWN® * OTC
 Feminine Deodorant Spray Mist
NAQUA® Tablets ℞
trichlormethiazide, USP
 2 mg AHG/822
 4 mg AHH/547
NAQUIVAL® Tablets ℞
trichlormethiazide,
USP/reserpine, USP AHT/394
NETROMYCIN® ℞
netilmicin sulfate
 Injection 100 mg/ml
 Pediatric Injection 25 mg/ml
 Neonatal Injection 10 mg/ml
NORMODYNE® ℞
labetalol HCl
 Tablets 200 mg 752
   300 mg 438
 Injection 5 mg/ml
OPTIMINE® Tablets ℞
azatadine maleate, USP 282
OPTIMYD® Ophthalmic Solution† ℞
prednisolone sodium phosphate, USP/
sulfacetamide sodium, USP
ORETON® ℞
methyltestosterone, USP
 Methyl Tablets 10 mg JD/311
       25 mg JE/499
 Methyl Buccal Tablets BE/970
OTOBIOTIC® Otic Solution ℞
polymyxin B sulfate, USP and
hydrocortisone, USP
PAXIPAM® Tablets ℞
halazepam
 20 mg 251
 40 mg 538
PERMITIL® ℞
fluphenazine hydrochloride, USP
 Oral Concentrate
 Tablets 0.25 mg WBK/122
   2.5 mg WDR/442
   5 mg WFF/550
   10 mg WFG/316
POLARAMINE® ℞
dexchlorpheniramine maleate, USP
 Expectorant†
 Repetabs® Tablets 4 mg AGA/095
       6 mg AGB/148
 Syrup
 Tablets 2 mg AGT/820
PROGLYCEM®
diazoxide, USP
 Capsules 50 mg PBA/205
 Suspension

PROVENTIL® ℞
albuterol
 Inhaler
PROVENTIL® ℞
albuterol sulfate
 Tablets 2 mg 252
   4 mg 573
RELA® Tablets† ℞
carisoprodol AHR/160
SEBIZON® Lotion† ℞
sodium sulfacetamide, USP 10%
SODIUM SULAMYD® ℞
sodium sulfacetamide, USP
 Ophthalmic Ointment 10%
 Ophthalmic Solution 10%
 Ophthalmic Solution 30% w/v
SOLGANAL® Suspension ℞
aurothioglucose, USP
SUNRIL® * Capsules OTC
THEOVENT® Long-Acting Capsules ℞
theophylline anhydrous, USP
 125 mg 402
 250 mg 753
TINACTIN® * OTC
tolnaftate, USP
 Cream 1%
 Jock Itch Cream
 Jock Itch Spray Powder
 Liquid 1% Aerosol
 Powder 1%
 Powder 1% Aerosol
 Solution 1%
TINDAL® Tablets† BBA/968 ℞
acetophenazine maleate, USP
TRILAFON® ℞
perphenazine, USP
 Concentrate
 Injection
 Repetabs® Tablets ADX/141
 Tablets 2 mg ADH/705
   4 mg ADK/940
   8 mg ADJ/313
   16 mg ADM/077
TRINALIN® Long-Acting ℞
Antihistamine/Decongestant
 Repetabs® Tablets 703
VALISONE® ℞
betamethasone valerate, USP
 Cream 0.1%
 Lotion 0.1%
 Ointment 0.1%
 Reduced Strength Cream 0.01%
VANCENASE® Nasal Inhaler ℞
beclomethasone dipropionate, USP
VANCERIL® Oral Inhaler ℞
beclomethasone dipropionate, USP

---

* For complete prescribing information see PDR for Nonprescription Drugs.
† For complete prescribing information contact the Schering Professional Services Department.

CELESTONE® ℞
[se-les'tōn]
brand of betamethasone
 Tablets, USP
 Syrup, USP

Description: Glucocorticoids are adrenocortical steroids, both naturally occurring and synthetic, that are readily absorbed from the gastrointestinal tract. A derivative of prednisolone, CELESTONE has a 16β-methyl group that enhances the anti-inflammatory action of the molecule and reduces the sodium- and water-retaining properties of the fluorine atom bound at carbon 9.
The formula for betamethasone is $C_{22}H_{29}FO_5$ and has a molecular weight of 392.47. Chemically, it is 9-fluoro-11β, 17,21-trihydroxy-16β-methylpregna-1,4-diene-3,20-dione.
Betamethasone is a white to practically white, odorless, crystalline powder. It melts at about 240°C with some decomposition. Betamethasone is sparingly soluble in acetone, alcohol, dioxane, and methanol; very slightly soluble in chloroform and ether; and is insoluble in water.

Each CELESTONE Tablet contains 0.6 mg betamethasone, USP.
CELESTONE Syrup contains 0.6 mg betamethasone, USP in each 5 ml and less than 1% alcohol.
Actions: Naturally occurring glucocorticoids (hydrocortisone and cortisone), which also have salt-retaining properties, are used as replacement therapy in adrenocortical deficiency states. Their synthetic analogs, such as betamethasone, are primarily used for their potent anti-inflammatory effects in disorders of many organ systems.
Glucocorticoids, such as betamethasone, cause profound and varied metabolic effects. In addition, they modify the body's immune response to diverse stimuli.
Indications:
Endocrine disorders: primary or secondary adrenocortical insufficiency (hydrocortisone or cortisone is the first choice; synthetic analogs may be used in conjunction with mineralocorticoids where applicable; in infancy mineralocorticoid supplementation is of particular importance).
congenital adrenal hyperplasia
nonsuppurative thyroiditis
hypercalcemia associated with cancer
Rheumatic disorders: as adjunctive therapy for short-term administration (to tide the patient over an acute episode or exacerbation) in:
psoriatic arthritis
rheumatoid arthritis, including juvenile rheumatoid arthritis (selected cases may require low-dose maintenance therapy)
ankylosing spondylitis
acute and subacute bursitis
acute nonspecific tenosynovitis
acute gouty arthritis
post-traumatic osteoarthritis
synovitis of osteoarthritis
epicondylitis
Collagen diseases: during an exacerbation or as maintenance therapy in selected cases of:
systemic lupus erythematosus
acute rheumatic carditis
Dermatologic diseases:
pemphigus
bullous dermatitis herpetiformis
severe erythema multiforme (Stevens-Johnson syndrome)
exfoliative dermatitis
mycosis fungoides
severe psoriasis
severe seborrheic dermatitis
Allergic states: control of severe or incapacitating allergic conditions intractable to adequate trials of conventional treatment:
seasonal or perennial allergic rhinitis
serum sickness
bronchial asthma
contact dermatitis
atopic dermatitis
drug hypersensitivity reactions
Ophthalmic diseases: severe acute and chronic allergic and inflammatory processes involving the eye and its adnexa, such as:
allergic conjunctivitis
keratitis
allergic corneal marginal ulcers
herpes zoster ophthalmicus
iritis and iridocyclitis
chorioretinitis
anterior segment inflammation
diffuse posterior uveitis and choroiditis
optic neuritis
sympathetic ophthalmia
Respiratory diseases:
symptomatic sarcoidosis
Loffler's syndrome not manageable by other means
berylliosis
fulminating or disseminated pulmonary tuberculosis when used concurrently with appropriate antituberculous chemotherapy
aspiration pneumonitis
Hematologic disorders:
idiopathic thrombocytopenic purpura in adults
secondary thrombocytopenia in adults
acquired (autoimmune) hemolytic anemia

erythroblastopenia (RBC anemia)
congenital (erythroid) hypoplastic anemia
Neoplastic diseases: for palliative management of:
leukemias and lymphomas in adults
acute leukemia of childhood
Edematous states: to induce a diuresis or remission of proteinuria in the nephrotic syndrome, without uremia, of the idiopathic type or that due to lupus erythematosus.
Gastrointestinal diseases: to tide the patient over a critical period of the disease in:
ulcerative colitis
regional enteritis
Miscellaneous: tuberculous meningitis with subarachnoid block or impending block when used concurrently with appropriate antituberculous chemotherapy; trichinosis with neurologic or myocardial involvement.
Contraindications: CELESTONE **Tablets** and **Syrup** are contraindicated in systemic fungal infections.
Warnings: In patients on corticosteroid therapy subjected to unusual stress, increased dosage of rapidly acting corticosteroids before, during, and after the stressful situation is indicated.
Corticosteroids may mask some signs of infection, and new infections may appear during their use. There may be decreased resistance and inability to localize infection when corticosteroids are used.
Prolonged use of corticosteroids may produce posterior subcapsular cataracts, glaucoma with possible damage to the optic nerves, and may enhance the establishment of secondary ocular infections due to fungi or viruses.
Average and large doses of hydrocortisone or cortisone can cause elevation of blood pressure, salt and water retention, and increased excretion of potassium. These effects are less likely to occur with the synthetic derivatives except when used in large doses. Dietary salt restrictions and potassium supplementation may be necessary. All corticosteroids increase calcium excretion.
While on corticosteroid therapy patients should not be vaccinated against smallpox. Other immunization procedures should not be undertaken in patients who are on corticosteroids, especially on high doses, because of possible hazards of neurological complications and a lack of antibody response.
The use of CELESTONE **Syrup** and **Tablets** in active tuberculosis should be restricted to those cases of fulminating or disseminated tuberculosis in which the corticosteroid is used for the management of the disease in conjunction with an appropriate antituberculous regimen.
If corticosteroids are indicated in patients with latent tuberculosis or tuberculin reactivity, close observation is necessary as reactivation of the disease may occur. During prolonged corticosteroid therapy, these patients should receive chemoprophylaxis.
Usage in pregnancy: Since adequate human reproduction studies have not been done with corticosteroids, the use of these drugs in pregnancy, nursing mothers or women of childbearing potential requires that the possible benefits of the drug be weighed against the potential hazards to the mother and embryo or fetus. Infants born of mothers who have received substantial doses of corticosteroids during pregnancy should be carefully observed for signs of hypoadrenalism.
Precautions: Drug-induced secondary adrenocortical insufficiency may be minimized by gradual reduction of dosage. This type of relative insufficiency may persist for months after discontinuation of therapy; therefore, in any situation of stress occurring during that period, hormone therapy should be reinstituted. Since mineralocorticoid secretion may be impaired, salt and/or a mineralocorticoid should be administered concurrently.
There is an enhanced effect of corticosteroids on patients with hypothyroidism and in those with cirrhosis.
Corticosteroids should be used cautiously in patients with ocular herpes simplex because of possible corneal perforation.
The lowest possible dose of corticosteroid should be used to control the condition under treatment, and when reduction in dosage is possible, the reduction should be gradual.
Psychic derangements may appear when corticosteroids are used, ranging from euphoria, insomnia, mood swings, personality changes, and severe depression to frank psychotic manifestations. Also, existing emotional instability or psychotic tendencies may be aggravated by corticosteroids.
Aspirin should be used cautiously in conjunction with corticosteroids in hypoprothrombinemia.
Steroids should be used with caution in nonspecific ulcerative colitis, if there is a probability of impending perforation, abscess or other pyogenic infection; diverticulitis; fresh intestinal anastomoses; active or latent peptic ulcer; renal insufficiency; hypertension; osteoporosis; and myasthenia gravis.
Growth and development of infants and children on prolonged corticosteroid therapy should be carefully observed.
Adverse Reactions:
Fluid and electrolyte disturbances: sodium retention, fluid retention, congestive heart failure in susceptible patients, potassium loss, hypokalemic alkalosis, hypertension.
Musculoskeletal: muscle weakness, steroid myopathy, loss of muscle mass, osteoporosis, vertebral compression fractures, aseptic necrosis of femoral and humeral heads, pathologic fracture of long bones; tendon rupture.
Gastrointestinal: peptic ulcer with possible perforation and hemorrhage, pancreatitis, abdominal distention, ulcerative esophagitis.
Dermatologic: impaired wound healing, thin fragile skin, petechiae and ecchymoses, facial erythema, increased sweating, may suppress reactions to skin tests.
Neurological: convulsions, increased intracranial pressure with papilledema (pseudotumor cerebri) usually after treatment, vertigo, headache.
Endocrine: menstrual irregularities; development of Cushingoid state; suppression of growth in children; secondary adrenocortical and pituitary unresponsiveness, particularly in times of stress, as in trauma, surgery or illness; decreased carbohydrate tolerance; manifestations of latent diabetes mellitus; increased requirements of insulin or oral hypoglycemic agents in diabetics.
Ophthalmic: posterior subcapsular cataracts, increased intraocular pressure, glaucoma, exophthalmos.
Metabolic: negative nitrogen balance due to protein catabolism.
Dosage and Administration: The initial dosage of CELESTONE may vary from 0.6 mg to 7.2 mg per day depending on the specific disease entity being treated. In situations of less severity lower doses will generally suffice, while in selected patients higher initial doses may be required. The initial dosage should be maintained or adjusted until a satisfactory response is noted. If after a reasonable period of time there is a lack of satisfactory clinical response, betamethasone should be discontinued and the patient transferred to other appropriate therapy. IT SHOULD BE EMPHASIZED THAT DOSAGE REQUIREMENTS ARE VARIABLE AND MUST BE INDIVIDUALIZED ON THE BASIS OF THE DISEASE UNDER TREATMENT AND THE RESPONSE OF THE PATIENT. After a favorable response is noted, the proper maintenance dosage should be determined by decreasing the initial drug dosage in small decrements at appropriate time intervals until the lowest dosage which will maintain an adequate clinical response is reached. It should be kept in mind that constant monitoring is needed in regard to drug dosage. Included in the situations which may make dosage adjustments necessary are changes in clinical status secondary to remissions or exacerbations in the disease process, the patient's individual drug responsiveness, and the effect of patient exposure to stressful situations not directly related to the disease entity under treatment; in this latter situation it may be necessary to increase the dosage of betamethasone for a period of time consistent with the patient's condition. If after long-term therapy the drug is to be stopped, it is recommended that it be withdrawn gradually rather than abruptly.
How Supplied: CELESTONE **Tablets,** 0.6 mg pink, compressed, scored tablets impressed with the Schering trademark and product identification letters, BDA, or numbers, 011; bottles of 100 (NDC 0085-0011-05) and 500 (NDC 0085-0011-07). Also available, CELESTONE Tablet Pack (For Six Day Therapy), 0.6 mg, 21 tablets (NDC 0085-0011-01) and CELESTONE **Syrup,** 0.6 mg per 5 ml, orange-red colored liquid; 4 oz. bottle (NDC 0085-0942-05).
Store **Tablets** between 2° and 30°C (36° and 86°F). Additionally, protect the **Tablet Pack** from excessive moisture.
Protect **Syrup** from light.
Store Syrup between 2° and 30° C (36° and 86° F).
Copyright © 1968, 1983, Schering Corporation. All rights reserved.
Revised 7/83
Shown in Product Identification Section, page 433

CELESTONE® Phosphate ℞
[*se-les'tōn*]
brand of betamethasone sodium phosphate, USP
Injection

Description: CELESTONE Phosphate Injection is a sterile, aqueous solution containing in each ml: 4.0 mg betamethasone sodium phosphate, USP equivalent to 3.0 mg betamethasone alcohol; 10 mg dibasic sodium phosphate; 0.1 mg edetate disodium; 3.2 mg sodium bisulfite; and 5.0 mg phenol as preservative. The pH is adjusted to approximately 8.5 with sodium hydroxide.
The formula for betamethasone sodium phosphate is $C_{22}H_{28}FNa_2O_8P$ and has a molecular weight of 516.41. Chemically, it is 9-fluoro-11β,17,21-trihydroxy-16β-methylpregna-1,4-diene-3,20-dione 21-(disodium phosphate).
Betamethasone sodium phosphate is a white to practically white, odorless powder, and is hygroscopic. Betamethasone sodium phosphate is freely soluble in water and methanol and is practically insoluble in acetone and chloroform.
Actions: Naturally occurring glucocorticoids (hydrocortisone), which also have salt-retaining properties, are used as replacement therapy in adrenocortical deficiency states. Their synthetic analogs are primarily used for their potent anti-inflammatory effects in disorders of many organ systems.
Glucocorticoids cause profound and varied metabolic effects. In addition, they modify the body's immune responses to diverse stimuli.
Indications: When oral therapy is not feasible and the strength, dosage form, and route of administration of the drug reasonably lend the preparation to the treatment of the condition, the **intravenous or intramuscular use** of CELESTONE Phosphate Injection is indicated as follows:
Endocrine disorders:
Primary or secondary adrenocortical insufficiency (hydrocortisone or cortisone is the drug of choice; synthetic analogs may be used in conjunction with mineralocorticoids where applicable; in infancy, mineralocorticoid supplementation is of particular importance).
Acute adrenocortical insufficiency (hydrocortisone or cortisone is the drug of choice; mineralocorticoid supplementation may be necessary, particularly when synthetic analogs are used).
Preoperatively and in the event of serious trauma or illness, in patients with known adrenal insufficiency or when adrenocortical reserve is doubtful.
Shock unresponsive to conventional therapy if adrenocortical insufficiency exists or is suspected.

Continued on next page

Information on Schering products appearing on these pages is effective as of September 30, 1984.

Schering—Cont.

Congenital adrenal hyperplasia.
Nonsuppurative thyroiditis.
Hypercalcemia associated with cancer.
Rheumatic disorders: As adjunctive therapy for short-term administration (to tide the patient over an acute episode or exacerbation) in:
Post-traumatic osteoarthritis.
Synovitis of osteoarthritis.
Rheumatoid arthritis, including juvenile rheumatoid arthritis (selected cases may require low-dose maintenance therapy).
Acute and subacute bursitis.
Epicondylitis.
Acute nonspecific tenosynovitis.
Acute gouty arthritis.
Psoriatic arthritis.
Ankylosing spondylitis.
Collagen diseases: During an exacerbation or as maintenance therapy in selected cases of:
Systemic lupus erythematosus.
Acute rheumatic carditis.
Dermatologic diseases:
Pemphigus.
Severe erythema multiforme (Stevens-Johnson syndrome).
Exfoliative dermatitis.
Bullous dermatitis herpetiformis.
Severe seborrheic dermatitis.
Severe psoriasis.
Mycosis fungoides.
Allergic states. Control of severe or incapacitating allergic conditions intractable to adequate trials of conventional treatment in:
Bronchial asthma.
Contact dermatitis.
Atopic dermatitis.
Serum sickness.
Seasonal or perennial allergic rhinitis.
Drug hypersensitivity reactions.
Urticarial transfusion reactions.
Acute noninfectious laryngeal edema (epinephrine is the drug of first choice).
Ophthalmic diseases: Severe, acute and chronic allergic and inflammatory processes involving the eye, such as:
Herpes zoster ophthalmicus.
Iritis, iridocyclitis.
Chorioretinitis.
Diffuse posterior uveitis and choroiditis.
Optic neuritis.
Sympathetic ophthalmia.
Anterior segment inflammation.
Allergic conjunctivitis.
Allergic corneal marginal ulcers.
Keratitis.
Gastrointestinal diseases: To tide the patient over a critical period of disease in:
Ulcerative colitis—(systemic therapy).
Regional enteritis—(systemic therapy).
Respiratory diseases:
Symptomatic sarcoidosis.
Berylliosis.
Fulminating or disseminated pulmonary tuberculosis when used concurrently with appropriate antituberculous chemotherapy.
Loffler's syndrome not manageable by other means.
Aspiration pneumonitis.
Hematologic disorders:
Acquired (autoimmune) hemolytic anemia.
Idiopathic thrombocytopenic purpura in adults (I.V. only; I.M. administration is contraindicated).
Secondary thrombocytopenia in adults.
Erythroblastopenia (RBC anemia).
Congenital (erythroid) hypoplastic anemia.
Neoplastic diseases: For palliative management of:
Leukemias and lymphomas in adults.
Acute leukemia of childhood.
Edematous states. To induce diuresis or remission of proteinuria in the nephrotic syndrome, without uremia, of the idiopathic type or that due to lupus erythematosus.

Miscellaneous:
Tuberculous meningitis with subarachnoid block or impending block when used concurrently with appropriate antituberculous chemotherapy.
Trichinosis with neurologic or myocardial involvement.
When the strength and dosage form of the drug lend the preparation to the treatment of the condition, the **intra-articular or soft tissue administration** of CELESTONE Phosphate Injection is indicated as adjunctive therapy for short-term administration (to tide the patient over an acute episode or exacerbation) in:
Synovitis of osteoarthritis.
Rheumatoid arthritis.
Acute and subacute bursitis.
Acute gouty arthritis.
Epicondylitis.
Acute nonspecific tenosynovitis.
Post-traumatic osteoarthritis.
When the strength and dosage form of the drug lend the preparation to the treatment of the condition, the **intralesional administration** of CELESTONE Phosphate Injection is indicated for:
Keloids.
Localized hypertrophic, infiltrated, inflammatory lesions of: lichen planus, psoriatic plaques, granuloma annulare, and lichen simplex chronicus (neurodermatitis).
Discoid lupus erythematosus.
Necrobiosis lipoidica diabeticorum.
Alopecia areata.
CELESTONE Phosphate injection may also be useful in cystic tumors of an aponeurosis or tendon (ganglia).

Contraindications: CELESTONE Phosphate Injection is contraindicated in systemic fungal infections.

Warnings: In patients on corticosteroid therapy subjected to any unusual stress, increased dosage of rapidly acting corticosteroids before, during, and after the stressful situation is indicated.
Corticosteroids may mask some signs of infection, and new infections may appear during their use. There may be decreased resistance and inability to localize infection when corticosteroids are used.
Prolonged use of corticosteroids may produce posterior subcapsular cataracts, glaucoma with possible damage to the optic nerves, and may enhance the establishment of secondary ocular infections due to fungi or viruses.
Average and large doses of cortisone or hydrocortisone can cause elevation of blood pressure, salt and water retention, and increased excretion of potassium. These effects are less likely to occur with the synthetic derivatives except when used in large doses. Dietary salt restriction and potassium supplementation may be necessary. All corticosteroids increase calcium excretion.
While on Corticosteroid Therapy Patients Should Not Be Vaccinated Against Smallpox. Other Immunization Procedures Should Not Be Undertaken in Patients Who are on Corticosteroids, Especially in High Doses, Because of Possible Hazards of Neurological Complications and Lack of Antibody Response.
The use of CELESTONE Phosphate Injection in active tuberculosis should be restricted to those cases of fulminating or disseminated tuberculosis in which the corticosteroid is used for the management of the disease in conjunction with appropriate antituberculous regimen.
If corticosteroids are indicated in patients with latent tuberculosis or tuberculin reactivity, close observation is necessary as reactivation of the disease may occur. During prolonged corticosteroid therapy, these patients should receive chemoprophylaxis.
Because rare instances of anaphylactoid reactions have occurred in patients receiving parenteral corticosteroid therapy, appropriate precautionary measures should be taken prior to administration, especially when the patient has a history of allergy to any drug.
Usage in pregnancy: Since adequate human reproduction studies have not been done with corticosteroids, the use of these drugs in pregnancy, nursing mothers, or women of childbearing potential requires that the possible benefits of the drug be weighed against the potential hazards to the mother and embryo or fetus. Infants born to mothers who have received substantial doses of corticosteroids during pregnancy should be carefully observed for signs of hypoadrenalism.

Precautions: Drug-induced secondary adrenocortical insufficiency may be minimized by gradual reduction of dosage. This type of relative insufficiency may persist for months after discontinuation of therapy; therefore, in any situation of stress occurring during that period, hormone therapy should be reinstituted. Since mineralocorticoid secretion may be impaired, salt and/or a mineralocorticoid should be administered concurrently.
There is an enhanced effect of corticosteroids in patients with hypothyroidism and in those with cirrhosis.
Corticosteroids should be used cautiously in patients with ocular herpes simplex for fear of corneal perforation.
The lowest possible dose of corticosteroid should be used to control the condition under treatment, and when reduction in dosage is possible, the reduction must be gradual.
Psychic derangements may appear when corticosteroids are used, ranging from euphoria, insomnia, mood swings, personality changes, and severe depression to frank psychotic manifestations. Also, existing emotional instability or psychotic tendencies may be aggravated by corticosteroids.
Aspirin should be used cautiously in conjunction with corticosteroids in hypoprothrombinemia.
Steroids should be used with caution in nonspecific ulcerative colitis, if there is a probability of impending perforation, abscess or other pyogenic infection, also in diverticulitis, fresh intestinal anastomoses, active or latent peptic ulcer, renal insufficiency, hypertension, osteoporosis, and myasthenia gravis. Growth and development of infants and children on prolonged corticosteroid therapy should be carefully followed.
The following additional precautions also apply for parenteral corticosteroids. Intra-articular injection of a corticosteroid may produce systemic as well as local effects.
Appropriate examination of any joint fluid present is necessary to exclude a septic process.
A marked increase in pain accompanied by local swelling, further restriction of joint motion, fever, and malaise are suggestive of septic arthritis. If this complication occurs and the diagnosis of sepsis is confirmed, appropriate antimicrobial therapy should be instituted.
Local injection of a steroid into a previously infected joint is to be avoided.
Corticosteroids should not be injected into unstable joints.
The slower rate of absorption by intramuscular administration should be recognized.

Adverse Reactions:
Fluid and electrolyte disturbances: sodium retention; fluid retention; congestive heart failure in susceptible patients; potassium loss; hypokalemic alkalosis; hypertension.
Musculoskeletal: muscle weakness; steroid myopathy; loss of muscle mass; osteoporosis; vertebral compression fractures; aseptic necrosis of femoral and humeral heads; pathologic fracture of long bones.
Gastrointestinal: peptic ulcer with possible subsequent perforation and hemorrhage; pancreatitis; abdominal distention; ulcerative esophagitis.
Dermatologic: impaired wound healing; thin fragile skin; petechiae and ecchymoses; facial erythema; increased sweating; may suppress reactions to skin tests.
Neurological: convulsions; increased intracranial pressure with papilledema (pseudotumor cerebri) usually after treatment; vertigo; headache.
Endocrine: menstrual irregularities; development of Cushingoid state; suppression of growth in children; secondary adrenocortical and pituitary unresponsiveness, particularly in times of stress, as in trauma, surgery or illness; decreased carbohydrate tolerance; manifestations of latent diabetes mellitus; increased requirements for insulin or oral hypoglycemic agents in diabetics.

Ophthalmic: posterior subcapsular cataracts; increased intraocular pressure; glaucoma; exophthalmos.
Metabolic: negative nitrogen balance due to protein catabolism.
The following *additional* adverse reactions are also related to parenteral corticosteroid therapy: rare instances of blindness associated with intralesional therapy around the face and head; hyperpigmentation or hypopigmentation; subcutaneous and cutaneous atrophy; sterile abscess; postinjection flare (following intra-articular use); charcot-like arthropathy.

Dosage and Administration: The initial dosage of parenterally administered betamethasone may vary up to 9.0 mg per day depending on the specific disease entity being treated. In situations of less severity, lower doses will generally suffice while in selected patients higher initial doses may be required. Usually the parenteral dosage ranges are one-third to one-half the 12-hourly oral dose. However, in certain overwhelming, acute, life-threatening situations, administration in dosages exceeding the usual dosages may be justified and may be in multiples of the oral dosages.
The initial dosage should be maintained or adjusted until a satisfactory response is noted. If after a reasonable period of time there is a lack of satisfactory clinical response, CELESTONE Phosphate Injection should be discontinued and the patient transferred to other appropriate therapy. *It Should Be Emphasized that Dosage Requirements are Variable and Must Be Individualized on the Basis of the Disease Under Treatment and the Response of the Patient.* After a favorable response is noted, the proper maintenance dosage should be determined by decreasing the initial drug dosage in small decrements at appropriate time intervals until the lowest dosage which will maintain an adequate clinical response is reached. It should be kept in mind that constant monitoring is needed in regard to drug dosage. Included in the situations which may make dosage adjustments necessary are changes in clinical status secondary to remissions or exacerbations in the disease process, the patient's individual drug responsiveness, and the effect of patient exposure to stressful situations not directly related to the disease entity under treatment; in this latter situation it may be necessary to increase dosage of CELESTONE Phosphate Injection for a period of time consistent with the patient's condition. If after long-term therapy the drug is to be stopped, it is recommended that it be withdrawn gradually rather than abruptly.

How Supplied: CELESTONE Phosphate Injection, 4.0 mg per ml (equivalent to 3.0 mg per ml betamethasone alcohol), 5 ml multiple-dose vials, box of one (NDC 0085-0879-05).
Protect from freezing.
Protect from light.
Copyright © 1973, 1983, Schering Corporation. All rights reserved.
Revised 7/83

CELESTONE® SOLUSPAN® *   ℞
[se-les'tōn]
Suspension
brand of sterile betamethasone sodium phosphate
and betamethasone acetate suspension, USP
6 mg per ml

Description: Each ml of CELESTONE SOLUSPAN* Suspension contains: 3.0 mg betamethasone as betamethasone sodium phosphate; 3.0 mg betamethasone acetate; 7.1 mg dibasic sodium phosphate; 3.4 mg monobasic sodium phosphate; 0.1 mg edetate disodium; and 0.2 mg benzalkonium chloride. It is a sterile, aqueous suspension with a pH between 6.8 and 7.2.
The formula for betamethasone sodium phosphate is $C_{22}H_{28}FNa_2O_8P$ with a molecular weight of 516.41. Chemically it is 9-Fluoro-11β, 17,21-trihydroxy-16β-methylpregna-1,4-diene-3,20-dione 21-(disodium phosphate).
The formula for betamethasone acetate is $C_{24}H_{31}FO_6$ with a molecular weight of 434.50. Chemically it is 9-Fluoro-11β,17,21-trihydroxy-16β-methylpregna-1, 4-diene-3, 20-dione 21-acetate.
Betamethasone sodium phosphate is a white to practically white, odorless powder, and is hygroscopic. It is freely soluble in water and in methanol, but is practically insoluble in acetone and in chloroform.
Betamethasone acetate is a white to creamy white, odorless powder that sinters and resolidifies at about 165°C, and remelts at about 200°C–220°C with decomposition. It is practically insoluble in water, but freely soluble in acetone, and is soluble in alcohol and in chloroform.
*brand of rapid and repository injectable.

Actions: Naturally occurring glucocorticoids (hydrocortisone), which also have salt-retaining properties, are used as replacement therapy in adrenocortical deficiency states. Their synthetic analogs are primarily used for their potent anti-inflammatory effects in disorders of many organ systems.
Betamethasone sodium phosphate, a soluble ester, provides prompt activity, while betamethasone acetate is only slightly soluble and affords sustained activity.
Glucocorticoids cause profound and varied metabolic effects. In addition, they modify the body's immune responses to diverse stimuli.

Indications: When oral therapy is not feasible and the strength, dosage form, and route of administration of the drug reasonably lend the preparation to the treatment of the condition, CELESTONE SOLUSPAN Suspension for **intramuscular use** is indicated as follows:
Endocrine disorders: Primary or secondary adrenocortical insufficiency (hydrocortisone or cortisone is the drug of choice; synthetic analogs may be used in conjunction with mineralocorticoids where applicable; in infancy, mineralocorticoid supplementation is of particular importance).
Acute adrenocortical insufficiency (hydrocortisone or cortisone is the drug of choice; mineralocorticoid supplementation may be necessary, particularly when synthetic analogs are used). Preoperatively and in the event of serious trauma or illness, in patients with known adrenal insufficiency or when adrenocortical reserve is doubtful. Shock unresponsive to conventional therapy if adrenocortical insufficiency exists or is suspected. Congenital adrenal hyperplasia. Nonsuppurative thyroiditis. Hypercalcemia associated with cancer.
Rheumatic disorders: As adjunctive therapy for short-term administration (to tide the patient over an acute episode or exacerbation) in: post-traumatic osteoarthritis; synovitis of osteoarthritis; rheumatoid arthritis; acute and subacute bursitis; epicondylitis; acute nonspecific tenosynovitis; acute gouty arthritis; psoriatic arthritis; ankylosing spondylitis; juvenile rheumatoid arthritis (selected cases may require low-dose maintenance therapy).
Collagen disease: During an exacerbation or as maintenance therapy in selected cases of: systemic lupus erythematosus; acute rheumatic carditis.
Dermatologic diseases: Pemphigus: severe erythema multiforme (Stevens-Johnson syndrome); exfoliative dermatitis; bullous dermatitis herpetiformis; severe seborrheic dermatitis; severe psoriasis; mycosis fungoides.
Allergic states: Control of severe or incapacitating allergic conditions intractable to adequate trials of conventional treatment in: bronchial asthma; contact dermatitis; atopic dermatitis; serum sickness; seasonal or perennial allergic rhinitis; drug hypersensitivity reactions; urticarial transfusion reactions; acute noninfectious laryngeal edema (epinephrine is the drug of first choice).
Ophthalmic diseases: Severe, acute and chronic allergic and inflammatory processes involving the eye, such as: herpes zoster ophthalmicus; iritis, iridocyclitis; chorioretinitis; diffuse posterior uveitis and choroiditis; optic neuritis; sympathetic ophthalmia; anterior segment inflammation; allergic conjunctivitis; allergic corneal marginal ulcer; keratitis.
Gastrointestinal diseases: To tide the patient over a critical period of disease in: ulcerative colitis—(systemic therapy); regional enteritis—(systemic therapy).
Respiratory diseases: Symptomatic sarcoidosis; berylliosis; fulminating or disseminated pulmonary tuberculosis, when concurrently with appropriate antituberculous chemotherapy; aspiration pneumonitis; Loffler's syndrome not manageable by other means.
Hematologic disorders: Acquired (autoimmune) hemolytic anemia. Secondary thrombocytopenia in adults. Erythroblastopenia (RBC anemia). Congenital (erythroid) hypoplastic anemia.
Neoplastic diseases: For palliative management of: leukemias and lymphomas in adults; acute leukemia of childhood.
Edematous state: To induce diuresis or remission of proteinuria in the nephrotic syndrome, without uremia, of the idiopathic type or that due to lupus erythematosus.
Miscellaneous: Tuberculous meningitis with subarachnoid block or impending block when used concurrently with appropriate antituberculous chemotherapy. Trichinosis with neurologic or myocardial involvement.
When the strength and dosage form of the drug lend the preparation to the treatment of the condition, the **intra-articular or soft tissue administration** of CELESTONE SOLUSPAN Suspension is indicated as adjunctive therapy for short-term administration (to tide the patient over an acute episode or exacerbation) in: synovitis of osteoarthritis; rheumatoid arthritis; acute and subacute bursitis; acute gouty arthritis; epicondylitis; acute nonspecific tenosynovitis; post-traumatic osteoarthritis.
When the strength and dosage form of the drug lend the preparation to the treatment of the condition, the **intralesional administration** of CELESTONE SOLUSPAN Suspension is indicated for: keloids; localized hypertrophic, infiltrated, inflammatory lesions of lichen planus, psoriatic plaques, granuloma annulare, and lichen simplex chronicus (neurodermatitis); discoid lupus erythematosus; necrobiosis lipoidica diabeticorum; alopecia areata.
CELESTONE SOLUSPAN Suspension may also be useful in cystic tumors of an aponeurosis or tendon (ganglia).

Contraindications:
CELESTONE SOLUSPAN Suspension is contraindicated in systemic fungal infections.

Warnings: CELESTONE SOLUSPAN should not be administered intravenously.
In patients on corticosteroid therapy subjected to any unusual stress, increased dosage of rapidly acting corticosteroids before, during, and after the stressful situation is indicated.
Corticosteroids may mask some signs of infection, and new infections may appear during their use. There may be decreased resistance and inability to localize infection when corticosteroids are used.
Prolonged use of corticosteroids may produce posterior subcapsular cataracts, glaucoma with possible damage to the optic nerves, and may enhance the establishment of secondary ocular infections due to fungi or viruses.
CELESTONE SOLUSPAN contains two betamethasone esters one of which, betamethasone sodium phosphate, disappears rapidly from the injection site. The potential for systemic effect produced by the soluble portion of CELESTONE SOLUSPAN should therefore be taken into account by the physician when using the drug.
Average and large doses of cortisone or hydrocortisone can cause elevation of blood pressure, salt and water retention, and increased excretion of potassium. These effects are less likely to occur with the synthetic derivatives except when used in large doses. Dietary salt restriction and potassium sup-

Continued on next page

Information on Schering products appearing on these pages is effective as of September 30, 1984.

Schering—Cont.

plementation may be necessary. All corticosteroids increase calcium excretion.

While on Corticosteroid Therapy Patients Should Not Be Vaccinated Against Smallpox. Other Immunization Procedures Should Not Be Undertaken in Patients Who Are on Corticosteroids, Especially in High Doses, Because of Possible Hazards of Neurological Complications and Lack of Antibody Response.

The use of CELESTONE SOLUSPAN Suspension in active tuberculosis should be restricted to those cases of fulminating or disseminated tuberculosis in which the corticosteroid is used for the management of the disease in conjunction with appropriate antituberculous regimen.

If corticosteroids are indicated in patients with latent tuberculosis or tuberculin reactivity, close observation is necessary as reactivation of the disease may occur. During prolonged corticosteroid therapy, these patients should receive chemoprophylaxis.

Because rare instances of anaphylactoid reactions have occurred in patients receiving parenteral corticosteroid therapy, appropriate precautionary measures should be taken prior to administration, especially when the patient has a history of allergy to any drug.

Usage in pregnancy: Since adequate human reproduction studies have not been done with corticosteroids, the use of these drugs in pregnancy, nursing mothers, or women of childbearing potential requires that the possible benefits of the drug be weighed against the potential hazards to the mother and embryo or fetus. Infants born of mothers who have received substantial doses of corticosteroids during pregnancy should be carefully observed for signs of hypoadrenalism.

Precautions: Drug-induced secondary adrenocortical insufficiency may be minimized by gradual reduction of dosage. This type of relative insufficiency may persist for months after discontinuation of therapy; therefore, in any situation of stress occurring during that period, hormone therapy should be reinstituted. Since mineralocorticoid secretion may be impaired, salt and/or a mineralocorticoid should be administered concurrently.

There is an enhanced effect of corticosteroids in patients with hypothyroidism and in those with cirrhosis.

Corticosteroids should be used cautiously in patients with ocular herpes simplex for fear of corneal perforation.

The lowest possible dose of corticosteroid should be used to control the condition under treatment, and when reduction in dosage is possible, the reduction must be gradual.

Psychic derangements may appear when corticosteroids are used, ranging from euphoria, insomnia, mood swings, personality changes, and severe depression to frank psychotic manifestations. Also, existing emotional instability or psychotic tendencies may be aggravated by corticosteroids.

Aspirin should be used cautiously in conjunction with corticosteroids in hypoprothrombinemia.

Steroids should be used with caution in nonspecific ulcerative colitis, if there is a probability of impending perforation, abscess or other pyogenic infection, also in diverticulitis, fresh intestinal anastomoses, active or latent peptic ulcer, renal insufficiency, hypertension, osteoporosis, and myasthenia gravis.

Growth and development of infants and children on prolonged corticosteroid therapy should be carefully followed.

The following additional precautions also apply for parenteral corticosteroids. **Intra-articular injection of a corticosteroid may produce systemic as well as local effects.**

Appropriate examination of any joint fluid present is necessary to exclude a septic process.

A marked increase in pain accompanied by local swelling, further restriction of joint motion, fever, and malaise are suggestive of septic arthritis. If this complication occurs and the diagnosis of sepsis is confirmed, appropriate antimicrobial therapy should be instituted.

Local injection of a steroid into a previously infected joint is to be avoided.

Corticosteroids should not be injected into unstable joints.

The slower rate of absorption by intramuscular administration should be recognized.

Adverse Reactions:

Fluid and electrolyte disturbances: sodium retention; fluid retention; congestive heart failure in susceptible patients; potassium loss; hypokalemic alkalosis; hypertension.

Musculoskeletal: muscle weakness; steroid myopathy; loss of muscle mass; osteoporosis; vertebral compression fractures; aseptic necrosis of femoral and humeral heads; pathologic fracture of long bones.

Gastrointestinal: peptic ulcer with possible subsequent perforation and hemorrhage; pancreatitis; abdominal distention; ulcerative esophagitis.

Dermatologic: impaired wound healing; thin fragile skin; petechiae and ecchymoses; facial erythema; increased sweating; may suppress reactions to skin tests.

Neurological: convulsions; increased intracranial pressure with papilledema (pseudotumor cerebri) usually after treatment; vertigo; headache.

Endocrine: menstrual irregularities; development of Cushingoid state; suppression of growth in children; secondary adrenocortical and pituitary unresponsiveness, particularly in times of stress, as in trauma, surgery, or illness; decreased carbohydrate tolerance; manifestations of latent diabetes mellitus; increased requirements for insulin or oral hypoglycemic agents in diabetics.

Ophthalmic: posterior subcapsular cataracts; increased intraocular pressure; glaucoma; exophthalmos.

Metabolic: negative nitrogen balance due to protein catabolism.

The following *additional* adverse reactions are related to parenteral corticosteroid therapy: rare instances of blindness associated with intralesional therapy around the face and head; hyperpigmentation or hypopigmentation; subcutaneous and cutaneous atrophy; sterile abscess; post-injection flare (following intra-articular use); charcot-like arthropathy.

Dosage and Administration: The initial dosage of CELESTONE SOLUSPAN Suspension may vary from 0.5 to 9.0 mg per day depending on the specific disease entity being treated. In situations of less severity, lower doses will generally suffice while in selected patients higher initial doses may be required. Usually the parenteral dosage ranges are one-third to one-half the oral dose given every 12 hours. However, in certain overwhelming, acute, life-threatening situations, administration in dosages exceeding the usual dosages may be justified and may be in multiples of the oral dosages.

The initial dosage should be maintained or adjusted until a satisfactory response is noted. If after a reasonable period of time there is a lack of satisfactory clinical response, CELESTONE SOLUSPAN Suspension should be discontinued and the patient transferred to other appropriate therapy. *It Should Be Emphasized That Dosage Requirements Are Variable and Must Be Individualized on the Basis of the Disease Under Treatment and the Response of the Patient.* After a favorable response is noted, the proper maintenance dosage should be determined by decreasing the initial drug dosage in small decrements at appropriate time intervals until the lowest dosage which will maintain an adequate clinical response is reached. It should be kept in mind that constant monitoring is needed in regard to drug dosage. Included in the situations which may make dosage adjustments necessary are changes in clinical status secondary to remissions or exacerbations in the disease process, the patient's individual drug responsiveness, and the effect of patient exposure to stressful situations not directly related to the disease entity under treatment; in this latter situation it may be necessary to increase the dosage of CELESTONE SOLUSPAN Suspension for a period of time consistent with the patient's condition. If after long-term therapy the drug is to be stopped, it is recommended that it be withdrawn gradually rather than abruptly.

If coadministration of a local anesthetic is desired, CELESTONE SOLUSPAN Suspension may be mixed with 1% or 2% lidocaine hydrochloride, using the formulations which do not contain parabens. Similar local anesthetics may also be used. Diluents containing methylparaben, propylparaben, phenol, etc., should be avoided since these compounds may cause flocculation of the steroid. The required dose of CELESTONE SOLUSPAN Suspension is first withdrawn from the vial into the syringe. The local anesthetic is then drawn in, and the syringe shaken briefly. **Do not inject local anesthetics into the vial of CELESTONE SOLUSPAN Suspension.**

Bursitis, tenosynovitis, peritendinitis. In acute subdeltoid, subacromial, olecranon, and prepatellar bursitis, one intrabursal injection of 1.0 ml CELESTONE SOLUSPAN Suspension can relieve pain and restore full range of movement. Several intrabursal injections of corticosteroids are usually required in recurrent acute bursitis and in acute exacerbations of chronic bursitis. Partial relief of pain and some increase in mobility can be expected in both conditions after one or two injections. Chronic bursitis may be treated with reduced dosage once the acute condition is controlled. In tenosynovitis and tendinitis, three or four local injections at intervals of one to two weeks between injections are given in most cases. Injections should be made into the affected tendon sheaths rather than into the tendons themselves. In ganglions of joint capsules and tendon sheaths, injection of 0.5 ml directly into the ganglion cysts has produced marked reduction in the size of the lesions. *Rheumatoid arthritis and osteoarthritis.* Following intra-articular administration of 0.5 to 2.0 ml of CELESTONE SOLUSPAN Suspension, relief of pain, soreness, and stiffness may be experienced. Duration of relief varies widely in both diseases. Intra-articular Injection—CELESTONE SOLUSPAN Suspension is well tolerated in joints and periarticular tissues. There is virtually no pain on injection, and the "secondary flare" that sometimes occurs a few hours after intra-articular injection of corticosteroids has not been reported with CELESTONE SOLUSPAN Suspension. Using sterile technique, a 20- to 24-gauge needle on an empty syringe is inserted into the synovial cavity, and a few drops of synovial fluid are withdrawn to confirm that the needle is in the joint. The aspirating syringe is replaced by a syringe containing CELESTONE SOLUSPAN Suspension and injection is then made into the joint.

Recommended Doses for Intra-articular Injection

Size of joint	Location	Dose (ml)
Very Large	Hip	1.0-2.0
Large	Knee, Ankle, Shoulder	1.0
Medium	Elbow, Wrist	0.5-1.0
Small (Metacarpophalangeal, interphalangeal) (Sternoclavicular)	Hand Chest	0.25-0.5

A portion of the administered dose of CELESTONE SOLUSPAN Suspension is absorbed systemically following intra-articular injection. In patients being treated concomitantly with oral or parenteral corticosteroids, especially those receiving large doses, the systemic absorption of the drug should be considered in determining intra-articular dosage. *Dermatologic conditions.* In intralesional treatment, 0.2 ml/sq. cm. of CELESTONE SOLUSPAN Suspension is injected intradermally (not subcutaneously) using a tuberculin syringe with a 25-gauge, ½-inch needle. Care should be taken to deposit a uniform depot of medication intradermally. A total of no more than 1.0 ml. at weekly intervals is recommended. *Disorders of the foot.* A tuberculin syringe with a 25-gauge, ¾-inch needle is suitable for most injections into the foot. The following doses are recommended at intervals of three days to a week.

Diagnosis	CELESTONE SOLUSPAN Suspension Dose (ml)
Bursitis	
under heloma durum or heloma molle	0.25-0.5
under calcaneal spur	0.5
over hallux rigidus or digiti quinti varus	0.5
Tenosynovitis, periostitis of cuboid	0.5
Acute gouty arthritis	0.5-1.0

How Supplied: CELESTONE SOLUSPAN Suspension, 5 ml multiple-dose vial, box of one (NDC-0085-0566-05). **Shake well before using. Store between 2° and 25°C (36° and 77°F). Protect from light.**
Revised 7/83
Copyright © 1969, 1983, Schering Corporation. All rights reserved.

DIPROLENE® ℞
[dī'pro-lēn]
brand of betamethasone dipropionate
Ointment, USP 0.05%
(potency expressed as betamethasone)

For Dermatologic Use Only–Not for Ophthalmic Use

Description: DIPROLENE Ointment contains betamethasone dipropionate, USP, a synthetic adrenocorticosteroid, for dermatologic use. Betamethasone, an analog of prednisolone, has a high degree of corticosteroid activity and a slight degree of mineralocorticoid activity. Betamethasone dipropionate is the 17,21-dipropionate ester of betamethasone.
Chemically, betamethasone dipropionate is 9-fluoro-11β, 17, 21-trihydroxy-16β-methyl-pregna-1,4-diene-3,20-dione 17,21-dipropionate, with the empirical formula $C_{28}H_{37}FO_7$, and a molecular weight of 504.6.
Betamethasone dipropionate is a white to creamy white, odorless crystalline powder, insoluble in water.
Each gram of DIPROLENE Ointment 0.05% contains: 0.64 mg betamethasone dipropionate, USP (equivalent to 0.5 mg betamethasone), in an improved ointment base of propylene glycol, propylene glycol stearate, white wax and white petrolatum.
Clinical Pharmacology: The corticosteroids are a class of compounds comprising steroid hormones secreted by the adrenal cortex and their synthetic analogs. In pharmacologic doses, corticosteroids are used primarily for their anti-inflammatory and/or immunosuppressive effects.
Topical corticosteroids, such as betamethasone dipropionate, are effective in the treatment of corticosteroid-responsive dermatoses primarily because of their anti-inflammatory, anti-pruritic, and vasoconstrictive actions. However, while the physiologic, pharmacologic, and clinical effects of the corticosteroids are well-known, the exact mechanisms of their actions in each disease are uncertain. Betamethasone dipropionate, a corticosteroid, has been shown to have topical (dermatologic) and systemic pharmacologic and metabolic effects characteristic of this class of drugs.
Pharmacokinetics: The extent of percutaneous absorption of topical corticosteroids is determined by many factors including the vehicle, the integrity of the epidermal barrier, and the use of occlusive dressings. (See **DOSAGE AND ADMINISTRATION** section.)

Topical corticosteroids can be absorbed from normal intact skin. Inflammation and/or other disease processes in the skin may increase percutaneous absorption. Occlusive dressings substantially increase the percutaneous absorption of topical corticosteroids. (See **DOSAGE AND ADMINISTRATION** section.)
Once absorbed through the skin, topical corticosteroids enter pharmacokinetic pathways similar to systemically administered corticosteroids. Corticosteroids are bound to plasma proteins in varying degrees. Corticosteroids are metabolized primarily in the liver and are then excreted by the kidneys. Some of the topical corticosteroids and their metabolites are also excreted into the bile.
At 14 g per day, DIPROLENE Ointment was shown to depress the plasma levels of adrenal cortical hormones following repeated application to diseased skin in patients with psoriasis. Adrenal depression in these patients was transient, and rapidly returned to normal upon cessation of treatment. At 7 g per day (3.5 g bid), DIPROLENE Ointment was shown to cause minimal inhibition of the hypothalamic-pituitary-adrenal (HPA) axis when applied two times daily for two to three weeks, in normal patients and in patients with psoriasis and eczematous disorders.
Indications and Usage: DIPROLENE Ointment is indicated for relief of the inflammatory and pruritic manifestations of corticosteroid-responsive dermatoses.
Contraindications: DIPROLENE Ointment is contraindicated in patients who are hypersensitive to betamethasone dipropionate, to other corticosteroids, or to any ingredient in this preparation.
Precautions: General: Systemic absorption of topical corticosteroids has produced reversible HPA axis suppression, manifestations of Cushing's syndrome, hyperglycemia, and glucosuria in some patients.
Conditions which augment systemic absorption include the application of the more potent corticosteroids, use over large surface areas, prolonged use, and the addition of occlusive dressings. (See **DOSAGE AND ADMINISTRATION** section.)
Therefore, patients receiving a large dose of a potent topical steroid applied to a large surface area should be evaluated periodically for evidence of HPA axis suppression by using the urinary free cortisol and ACTH stimulation tests. If HPA axis suppression is noted, an attempt should be made to withdraw the drug, to reduce the frequency of application, or to substitute a less potent steroid.
Recovery of HPA axis function is generally prompt and complete upon discontinuation of the drug. Infrequently, signs and symptoms of steroid withdrawal may occur, requiring supplemental systemic corticosteroids.
Children may absorb proportionally larger amounts of topical corticosteroids and thus be more susceptible to systemic toxicity. (See **PRECAUTIONS–Pediatric Use.**)
If irritation develops, topical corticosteroids should be discontinued and appropriate therapy instituted.
In the presence of dermatological infections, the use of an appropriate antifungal or antibacterial agent should be instituted. If a favorable response does not occur promptly, the corticosteroid should be discontinued until the infection has been adequately controlled.
Information for Patients: Patients using topical corticosteroids should receive the following information and instructions:
1. This medication is to be used as directed by the physician and should not be used longer than the prescribed time period. It is for external use only. Avoid contact with the eyes.
2. Patients should be advised not to use this medication for any disorder other than that for which it was prescribed.
3. The treated skin area should not be bandaged or otherwise covered or wrapped as to be occlusive. (See **DOSAGE AND ADMINISTRATION** section.)
4. Patients should report any signs of local adverse reactions.

Laboratory Tests: The following tests may be helpful in evaluating HPA axis suppression:
Urinary free cortisol test
ACTH stimulation test
Carcinogenesis, Mutagenesis, and Impairment of Fertility: Long-term animal studies have not been performed to evaluate the carcinogenic potential or the effect on fertility of topically applied corticosteroids.
Studies to determine mutagenicity with prednisolone have revealed negative results.
Pregnancy Category C: Corticosteroids are generally teratogenic in laboratory animals when administered systemically at relatively low dosage levels. The more potent corticosteroids have been shown to be teratogenic after dermal application in laboratory animals. There are no adequate and well-controlled studies of the teratogenic effects of topically applied corticosteroids in pregnant women. Therefore, topical corticosteroids should be used during pregnancy only if the potential benefit justifies the potential risk to the fetus. Drugs of this class should not be used extensively on pregnant patients, in large amounts, or for prolonged periods of time.
Nursing Mothers: It is not known whether topical administration of corticosteroids could result in sufficient systemic absorption to produce detectable quantities in breast milk. Systemically administered corticosteroids are secreted into breast milk in quantities not likely to have a deleterious effect on the infant. Nevertheless, caution should be exercised when topical corticosteroids are prescribed for a nursing woman.
Pediatric Use: Use of DIPROLENE Ointment in children under 12 years is not recommended.
<u>Pediatric patients may demonstrate greater susceptibility to topical corticosteroid-induced HPA axis suppression and Cushing's syndrome than mature patients because of a larger skin surface area to body weight ratio.</u>
Hypothalamic-pituitary-adrenal (HPA) axis suppression, Cushing's syndrome, and intracranial hypertension have been reported in children receiving topical corticosteroids. Manifestations of adrenal suppression in children include linear growth retardation, delayed weight gain, low plasma cortisol levels, and absence of response to ACTH stimulation. Manifestations of intracranial hypertension include bulging fontanelles, headaches, and bilateral papilledema.
Administration of topical corticosteroids to children should be limited to the least amount compatible with an effective therapeutic regimen. Chronic corticosteroid therapy may interfere with the growth and development of children.
Adverse Reactions: The local adverse reactions that were reported with DIPROLENE Ointment during clinical studies are as follows: folliculitis, 2 per 500 patients; erythema, 2 per 500 patients; pruritus, 1 per 500 patients; vesiculation, 1 per 500 patients.
The following local adverse reactions are reported infrequently when topical corticosteroids are used as recommended. These reactions are listed in an approximate decreasing order of occurrence: burning, itching, irritation, dryness, folliculitis, hypertrichosis, acneiform eruptions, hypopigmentation, perioral dermatitis, allergic contact dermatitis, maceration of the skin, secondary infection, skin atrophy, striae, miliaria.
Systemic absorption of topical corticosteroids has produced reversible HPA axis suppression, manifestations of Cushing's syndrome, hyperglycemia, and glucosuria in some patients.
Overdosage: Topically applied corticosteroids can be absorbed in sufficient amounts to produce systemic effects. (See **PRECAUTIONS.**)
Dosage and Administration: Apply a thin film of DIPROLENE Ointment to the affected skin areas twice daily, once in the morning and once at

Continued on next page

Information on Schering products appearing on these pages is effective as of September 30, 1984.

Schering—Cont.

night. Amounts greater than 45 g per week should not be used.
DIPROLENE Ointment is not to be used with occlusive dressings.
How Supplied: DIPROLENE Ointment 0.05% is supplied in 15-(NDC 0085-0575-02), and 45-gram (NDC 0085-0575-03) tubes; boxes of one.
Store between 2° and 30°C (36° and 86°F).
Revised 4/83
Copyright © 1983, Schering Corporation. All rights reserved.

DIPROSONE® ℞
[dĭ-pro'sŏn]
brand of betamethasone dipropionate
 Cream, USP 0.05%
 Ointment, USP 0.05%
 Lotion, USP 0.05% w/w
 Topical Aerosol, USP 0.1% w/w
 (potency expressed as betamethasone)
 For Dermatologic Use Only—
 Not for Ophthalmic Use

Description: DIPROSONE Cream, Ointment, Lotion, and Topical Aerosol contain betamethasone dipropionate, USP, a synthetic adrenocorticosteroid, for dermatologic use. Betamethasone, an analog of prednisolone, has high corticosteroid activity and slight mineralocorticoid activity. Betamethasone dipropionate is the 17,21-dipropionate ester of betamethasone.
Chemically, betamethasone dipropionate is 9-Fluoro-11β, 17, 21-trihydroxy-16β-methylpregna-1, 4-diene-3, 20-dione 17, 21-dipropionate, with the empirical formula $C_{28}H_{37}FO_7$, a molecular weight of 504.6.
Betamethasone dipropionate is a white to creamy white, odorless crystalline powder, insoluble in water.
Each gram of DIPROSONE **Cream** 0.05% contains: 0.64 mg betamethasone dipropionate, USP (equivalent to 0.5 mg betamethasone), in a hydrophilic emollient cream consisting of purified water, mineral oil, white petrolatum, polyethylene glycol 1000 monocetyl ether, cetearyl alcohol, monobasic sodium phosphate, and phosphoric acid; chlorocresol and propylene glycol as preservatives.
Each gram of DIPROSONE **Ointment** 0.05% contains: 0.64 mg betamethasone dipropionate, USP (equivalent to 0.5 mg betamethasone), in an ointment base of mineral oil and white petrolatum.
Each gram of DIPROSONE **Lotion** 0.05% w/w contains: 0.64 mg betamethasone dipropionate, USP (equivalent to 0.5 mg betamethasone), in a lotion base of isopropyl alcohol (46.8%) and purified water slightly thickened with carbomer 934P; the pH is adjusted to approximately 4.7 with sodium hydroxide.
DIPROSONE **Topical Aerosol** 0.1% w/w contains: 6.4 mg betamethasone dipropionate, USP (equivalent to 5.0 mg betamethasone), in a vehicle of mineral oil and caprylic/capric triglyceride; also containing 10% isopropyl alcohol and sufficient inert hydrocarbon (propane and isobutane) propellant to make 85 grams. The aerosol spray deposits betamethasone dipropionate equivalent to approximately 0.1% betamethasone in a nonvolatile, almost invisible film. A three-second spray delivers betamethasone dipropionate equivalent to approximately 0.06 mg betamethasone.
Clinical Pharmacology: The corticosteroids are a class of compounds comprising steroid hormones secreted by the adrenal cortex and their synthetic analogs. In pharmacologic doses corticosteroids are used primarily for their anti-inflammatory and/or immunosuppressive effects.
Topical corticosteroids, such as betamethasone dipropionate, are effective in the treatment of corticosteroid-responsive dermatoses primarily because of their anti-inflammatory, anti-pruritic, and vasoconstrictive actions. However, while the physiologic, pharmacologic, and clinical effects of the corticosteroids are well-known, the exact mechanisms of their actions in each disease are uncertain. Betamethasone dipropionate, a corticosteroid, has been shown to have topical (dermatologic) and systemic pharmacologic and metabolic effects characteristic of this class of drugs.
Pharmacokinetics: The extent of percutaneous absorption of topical corticosteroids is determined by many factors including the vehicle, the integrity of the epidermal barrier, and the use of occlusive dressings. (See **DOSAGE AND ADMINISTRATION** section.)
Topical corticosteroids can be absorbed from normal intact skin. Inflammation and/or other disease processes in the skin increase percutaneous absorption. Occlusive dressings substantially increase the percutaneous absorption of topical corticosteroids. (See **DOSAGE AND ADMINISTRATION** section.)
Once absorbed through the skin, topical corticosteroids are handled through pharmacokinetic pathways similar to systemically administered corticosteroids. Corticosteroids are bound to plasma proteins in varying degrees. Corticosteroids are metabolized primarily in the liver and are then excreted by the kidneys. Some of the topical corticosteroids and their metabolites are also excreted into the bile.
Indications and Usage: DIPROSONE Cream, Ointment, Lotion, and Topical Aerosol are indicated for relief of the inflammatory and pruritic manifestations of corticosteroid-responsive dermatoses.
Contraindications: DIPROSONE Cream, Ointment, Lotion, and Topical Aerosol are contraindicated in patients who are hypersensitive to betamethasone dipropionate, to other corticosteroids, or to any ingredient in these preparations.
Precautions: General: Systemic absorption of topical corticosteroids has produced reversible hypothalamic-pituitary-adrenal (HPA) axis suppression, manifestations of Cushing's syndrome, hyperglycemia, and glucosuria in some patients. Conditions which augment systemic absorption include the application of the more potent steroids, use over large surface areas, prolonged use, and the addition of occlusive dressings. (See **DOSAGE AND ADMINISTRATION** section.)
Therefore, patients receiving a large dose of a potent topical steroid applied to a large surface area should be evaluated periodically for evidence of HPA axis suppression by using the urinary free cortisol and ACTH stimulation tests. If HPA axis suppression is noted, an attempt should be made to withdraw the drug, to reduce the frequency of application, or to substitute a less potent steroid.
Recovery of HPA axis function is generally prompt and complete upon discontinuation of the drug. Infrequently, signs and symptoms of steroid withdrawal may occur, requiring supplemental systemic corticosteroids.
Children may absorb proportionally larger amounts of topical corticosteroids and thus be more susceptible to systemic toxicity. (See **PRECAUTIONS-Pediatric Use**.)
If irritation develops, topical corticosteroids should be discontinued and appropriate therapy instituted.
In the presence of dermatological infections, the use of an appropriate antifungal or antibacterial agent should be instituted. If a favorable response does not occur promptly, the corticosteroid should be discontinued until the infection has been adequately controlled.
Information for Patients: Patients using topical corticosteroids should receive the following information and instructions:
1. This medication is to be used as directed by the physician. It is for external use only. Avoid contact with the eyes.
2. Patients should be advised not to use this medication for any disorder other than for which it was prescribed.
3. The treated skin area should not be bandaged or otherwise covered or wrapped as to be occlusive. (See **DOSAGE AND ADMINISTRATION** section.)
4. Patients should report any signs of local adverse reactions.
5. Parents of pediatric patients should be advised not to use tight-fitting diapers or plastic pants on a child being treated in the diaper area, as these garments may constitute occlusive dressing. (See **DOSAGE AND ADMINISTRATION** section.)
6. When using DIPROSONE Topical Aerosol, the patient should be advised of the following:
 • the spray should be kept away from the eyes or other mucous membranes
 • avoid freezing tissues by not spraying for more than three seconds, at a distance of not less than six inches between the nozzle and the skin
 • use only as directed; intentional misuse by deliberately concentrating and inhaling the container contents can be harmful or fatal
 • the container contents are under pressure; do not puncture the container
 • the container mixture is flammable; do not use or store the container near heat or an open flame; exposure to temperatures above 120° Fahrenheit may cause bursting; never throw container into a fire or incinerator
 • keep out of the reach of children

Laboratory Tests: The following tests may be helpful in evaluating HPA axis suppression:
 Urinary free cortisol test
 ACTH stimulation test
Carcinogenesis, Mutagenesis, and Impairment of Fertility: Long-term animal studies have not been performed to evaluate the carcinogenic potential or the effect on fertility of topical corticosteroids. Studies to determine mutagenicity with prednisolone have revealed negative results.
Pregnancy Category C: Corticosteroids are generally teratogenic in laboratory animals when administered systemically at relatively low dosage levels. The more potent corticosteroids have been shown to be teratogenic after dermal application in laboratory animals. There are no adequate and well-controlled studies in pregnant women on teratogenic effects from topically applied corticosteroids. Therefore, topical corticosteroids should be used during pregnancy only if the potential benefit justifies the potential risk to the fetus. Drugs of this class should not be used extensively on pregnant patients, in large amounts, or for prolonged periods of time.
Nursing Mothers: It is not known whether topical administration of corticosteroids could result in sufficient systemic absorption to produce detectable quantities in breast milk. Systemically administered corticosteroids are secreted into breast milk in quantities not likely to have a deleterious effect on the infant. Nevertheless, caution should be exercised when topical corticosteroids are prescribed for a nursing woman.
Pediatric use: Pediatric patients may demonstrate greater susceptibility to topical corticosteroid-induced HPA axis suppression and Cushing's syndrome than mature patients because of a larger skin surface area to body weight ratio. Hypothalamic-pituitary-adrenal (HPA) axis suppression, Cushing's syndrome, and intracranial hypertension have been reported in children receiving topical corticosteroids. Manifestations of adrenal suppression in children include linear growth retardation, delayed weight gain, low plasma cortisol levels, and absence of response to ACTH stimulation. Manifestations of intracranial hypertension include bulging fontanelles, headaches, and bilateral papilledema.
Administration of topical corticosteroids to children should be limited to the least amount compatible with an effective therapeutic regimen. Chronic corticosteroid therapy may interfere with the growth and development of children.
Adverse Reactions: The following local adverse reactions are reported infrequently when DIPROSONE Products are used as recommended in the **DOSAGE AND ADMINISTRATION** section. These reactions are listed in an approximate decreasing order of occurrence: burning; itching; irritation; dryness; folliculitis; hypertrichosis; acneiform eruptions; hypopigmentation; perioral

dermatitis; allergic contact dermatitis; maceration of the skin; secondary infection; skin atrophy; striae; miliaria.

Systemic absorption of topical corticosteroids has produced reversible hypothalamic-pituitary-adrenal (HPA) axis suppression, manifestations of Cushing's syndrome, hyperglycemia, and glucosuria in some patients.

Overdosage: Topically applied corticosteroids can be absorbed in sufficient amounts to produce systemic effects. (See **PRECAUTIONS.**)

Dosage and Administration: DIPROSONE **Cream:** Apply a thin film of DIPROSONE **Cream** 0.05% to the affected skin areas once daily. In some cases, a twice daily dosage may be necessary.
DIPROSONE **Ointment:** Apply a thin film of DIPROSONE **Ointment** to the affected skin areas once daily. In some cases, a twice daily dosage may be necessary.
DIPROSONE **Lotion:** Apply a few drops of DIPROSONE **Lotion** to the affected area and massage lightly until it disappears. Apply twice daily, in the morning and at night. For the most effective and economical use, apply nozzle very close to affected area and gently squeeze bottle.
DIPROSONE **Topical Aerosol:** Apply sparingly to the affected skin area three times a day. The container may be held upright or inverted during use. The spray should be directed onto the affected area from a distance of not less than six inches and applied for only three seconds. For the most effective and economical use, a three-second spray is sufficient to cover an area about the size of the hand.
DIPROSONE Products are not to be used with occlusive dressings.

How Supplied: DIPROSONE Cream 0.05% is supplied in 15-gram (NDC-0085-0853-02), 45-gram (NDC-0085-0853-03).
DIPROSONE Lotion 0.05% w/w is available in 20 ml (18.7 g) (NDC-0085-0028-04); and 60 ml (56.2 g) (NDC-0085-0028-06) plastic squeeze bottles; boxes of one. **Protect from light. Store in carton until contents are used.**
DIPROSONE Ointment 0.05% is supplied in 15-gram (NDC 0085-0510-04) and 45- gram (NDC-0085-0510-06) tubes; boxes of one.
DIPROSONE Topical Aerosol 0.1% w/w is supplied as an 85-gram spray can.
(NDC-0085-0475-06)
Store all DIPROSONE preparations between 2° and 30°C (36° and 86°F).
Revised 12/83
Copyright © 1974, 1982, 1983, Schering Corporation.
All rights reserved.

ESTINYL® ℞
[*es'ti-nil*]
brand of ethinyl estradiol,
   Tablets, USP

BOXED WARNINGS

1. ESTROGENS HAVE BEEN REPORTED TO INCREASE THE RISK RATIO OF ENDOMETRIAL CARCINOMA.
Three independent case control studies have reported an increased risk ratio of endometrial cancer in postmenopausal women exposed to exogenous estrogens for prolonged periods.[1-3] This risk ratio was independent of the other risk factors for endometrial cancer. These studies are further supported by the report that incidence rates of endometrial cancer have increased sharply since 1969 in eight different areas of the United States with population-based cancer reporting systems, an increase which may be related to the rapidly expanding use of estrogens during the last decade.[4]
The three case control studies reported that the risk ratio of endometrial cancer in estrogen users was about 4.5 to 13.9 times greater than in nonusers. The risk ratio appears to depend on both duration of treatment[1] and on estrogen dose.[3] In view of these reports, when estrogens are used for the treatment of menopausal symptoms, the lowest dose that will control symptoms should be utilized and medication should be discontinued as soon as possible. When prolonged treatment is medically indicated, the patient should be reassessed on at least a semiannual basis to determine the need for continued therapy. Although the evidence must be considered preliminary, one study suggests that cyclic administration of low doses of estrogen may carry less risk than continuous administration[3]; it therefore appears prudent to utilize such a regimen.
Close clinical surveillance of all women taking estrogens is important. In all cases of undiagnosed persistent or recurring abnormal vaginal bleeding, adequate diagnostic measures should be undertaken to rule out malignancy.
There is no evidence at present that "natural" estrogens are more or less hazardous than "synthetic" estrogens at equiestrogenic doses.

2. ESTROGENS SHOULD NOT BE USED DURING PREGNANCY.
The use of estrogens during early pregnancy may seriously damage the offspring. It has been reported that females exposed in utero to diethylstilbestrol, a non-steroidal estrogen, may have an increased risk of developing in later life a form of vaginal or cervical cancer that is ordinarily extremely rare.[5,6] This risk has been estimated statistically as not greater than 4 per 1000 exposures.[7] In certain studies, a high percentage of such exposed women (from 30 to 90 percent) have been found to have vaginal adenosis,[8-11] epithelial changes of the vagina and cervix. Although these changes are histologically benign, it is not known whether they are precursors of malignancy. Although similar data are not available with the use of other estrogens, it cannot be presumed they would not induce similar changes.
Several reports suggest an association between intrauterine fetal exposure to female sex hormones and congenital anomalies, including congenital heart defects and limb reduction defects.[12-15] One case control study[15] estimated a 4.7 fold increased risk of limb reduction defects in infants exposed in utero to sex hormones (oral contraceptives, hormone withdrawal tests for pregnancy, or attempted treatment for threatened abortion). Some of these exposures were very short and involved only a few days of treatment. The data suggest that the risk of limb reduction defects in exposed fetuses is somewhat less than 1 per 1000.
In the past, estrogens have been used during pregnancy in an attempt to treat threatened or habitual abortion. There is considerable evidence that estrogens are ineffective for these indications.
If ESTINYL is used during pregnancy, or if the patient becomes pregnant while taking this drug, she should be apprised of the potential risks to the fetus, and the advisability of pregnancy continuation.

Description: ESTINYL Tablets contain ethinyl estradiol, a potent synthetic estrogen having the chemical name, 19-Nor-17α-pregna-1,3,5(10)-trien-20-yne-3,17-diol.
ESTINYL for oral administration is available in tablets containing 0.02, 0.05, or 0.5 mg. ethinyl estradiol, USP.
Clinical Pharmacology: Ethinyl estradiol promotes growth of the endometrium and thickening, stratification and cornification of the vagina. It causes growth of the ducts of the mammary gland, but inhibits lactation. It also inhibits the anterior pituitary and causes capillary dilatation, fluid retention and protein anabolism.
Indications: ESTINYL Tablets are indicated in the treatment of: 1) Moderate to severe *vasomotor* symptoms associated with the menopause. (There is no evidence that estrogens are effective for nervous symptoms or depression which might occur during menopause, and they should not be used to treat these conditions.) 2) Female hypogonadism. 3) Prostatic carcinoma—palliative therapy of advanced disease. 4) Breast cancer (for palliation only) in appropriately selected women, such as those who are more than 5 years postmenopausal with progressing inoperable or radiation-resistant disease.
ESTINYL HAS NOT BEEN SHOWN TO BE EFFECTIVE FOR ANY PURPOSE DURING PREGNANCY AND ITS USE MAY CAUSE SEVERE HARM TO THE FETUS (SEE BOXED WARNING ABOVE).
Contraindications: Estrogens should not be used in women (or men) with any of the following conditions:
1. Known or suspected cancer of the breast except in appropriately selected patients being treated for metastatic disease.
2. Known or suspected estrogen-dependent neoplasia.
3. Known or suspected pregnancy (See Boxed Warning).
4. Undiagnosed abnormal genital bleeding.
5. Active thrombophlebitis or thromboembolic disorders.
6. A past history of thrombophlebitis, thrombosis or thromboembolic disorders associated with previous estrogen use (except when used in treatment of breast or prostatic malignancy).
Warnings: 1. *Induction of malignant neoplasms.* Long-term continuous administration of natural and synthetic estrogens in certain animal species increases the frequency of carcinomas of the breast, cervix, vagina, and liver. There is now evidence that estrogens increase the risk of carcinoma of the endometrium in humans. (See Boxed Warning.)
At the present time there is no satisfactory evidence that estrogens given to postmenopausal women increase the risk of cancer of the breast,[16] although a recent long-term follow-up of a single physician's practice has raised this possibility.[17] Because of the animal data, there is a need for caution in prescribing estrogens for women with a strong family history of breast cancer or who have breast nodules, fibrocystic disease, or abnormal mammograms.
Estrogens have been reported to be associated with carcinoma of the male breast and suspicious lesions in males receiving estrogen therapy should be investigated accordingly.
2. *Gallbladder disease.* A recent study has reported a 2- to 3-fold increase in the risk of surgically confirmed gallbladder disease in women receiving postmenopausal estrogens,[16] similar to the 2-fold increase previously noted in users of oral contraceptives.[18,22] In the case of oral contraceptives, the increased risk appeared after two years of use.[22]
3. *Effects similar to those caused by estrogen-progestagen oral contraceptives.* There are several serious adverse effects of oral contraceptives, most of which have not, up to now, been documented as consequences of postmenopausal estrogen therapy. This may reflect the comparatively low doses of estrogen used in postmenopausal women. It would be expected that the larger doses of estrogen used to treat prostatic or breast cancer are more likely to result in these adverse effects, and, in fact, it has been shown that there is an increased risk of thrombosis in men receiving estrogens for prostatic cancer.[19-22]
a. *Thromboembolic disease* It is now well established that users of oral contraceptives have an increased risk of various thromboembolic and thrombotic vascular diseases, such as thrombophlebitis, pulmonary embolism, stroke and myocardial infarction.[22-29] Cases of retinal thrombo-

Continued on next page

Information on Schering products appearing on these pages is effective as of September 30, 1984.

Schering—Cont.

sis, mesenteric thrombosis, and optic neuritis have been reported in oral contraceptive users. There is evidence that the risk of several of these adverse reactions is related to the dose of the drug.[30,31] An increased risk of postsurgery thromboembolic complications has also been reported in users of oral contraceptives.[32,33] If feasible, estrogen should be discontinued at least 4 weeks before surgery of the type associated with an increased risk of thromboembolism, or during periods of immobilization.

While an increased rate of thromboembolic and thrombotic disease in postmenopausal users of estrogen has not been found,[16,34] this does not rule out the possibility that such an increase may be present or that subgroups of women who have underlying risk factors or who are receiving relatively large doses of estrogens may have increased risk. Therefore, estrogens should not be used in persons with active thrombophlebitis or thromboembolic disorders, and they should not be used (except in treatment of malignancy) in persons with a history of such disorders in association with estrogen use. They should be used with caution in patients with cerebral vascular or coronary artery disease and only for those in whom estrogens are clearly needed.

Large doses of estrogen (5 mg. conjugated estrogens per day), comparable to those used to treat cancer of the prostate and breast, have been shown in a large prospective clinical trial in men[35] to increase the risk of nonfatal myocardial infarction, pulmonary embolism and thrombophlebitis. When estrogen doses of this size are used, any of the thromboembolic and thrombotic adverse effects associated with oral contraceptive use should be considered a clear risk.

b. *Hepatic adenoma* Benign hepatic adenomas appear to be associated with the use of oral contraceptives.[36–38] Although benign, and rare, these may rupture and may cause death through intra-abdominal hemorrhage. Such lesions have not yet been reported in association with other estrogen or progestagen preparations but should be considered in estrogen users having abdominal pain and tenderness, abdominal mass, or hypovolemic shock. Hepatocellular carcinoma has also been reported in women taking estrogen-containing oral contraceptives.[37] The relationship of this malignancy to these drugs is not known at this time.

c. *Elevated blood pressure* Increased blood pressure is not uncommon in women using oral contraceptives. There is now a report that this may occur with use of estrogens in the menopause[39] and blood pressure should be monitored with estrogen use, especially if high doses are used.

d. *Glucose tolerance* A worsening of glucose tolerance has been observed in a significant percentage of patients on estrogen-containing oral contraceptives. For this reason, diabetic patients should be carefully observed while receiving estrogen.

4. *Hypercalcemia.* Administration of estrogens may lead to severe hypercalcemia in patients with breast cancer and bone metastases. If this occurs, the drug should be stopped and appropriate measures taken to reduce the serum calcium level.

Precautions:
General Precautions
1. A complete medical and family history should be taken prior to the initiation of any estrogen therapy. The pretreatment and periodic physical examinations should include special reference to blood pressure, breasts, abdomen, and pelvic organs, and should include a Papanicolaou smear. As a general rule, estrogen should not be prescribed for longer than one year without another physical examination being performed.
2. Fluid retention—Because estrogens may cause some degree of fluid retention, conditions which might be influenced by this factor, such as epilepsy, migraine, and cardiac or renal dysfunction, require careful observation.

3. Certain patients may develop undesirable manifestations of excessive estrogenic stimulation, such as abnormal or excessive uterine bleeding, mastodynia, etc.
4. Oral contraceptives appear to be associated with an increased incidence of mental depression.[22] Although it is not clear whether this is due to the estrogenic or progestagenic component of the contraceptive, patients with a history of depression should be carefully observed.
5. Preexisting uterine leiomyomata may increase in size during estrogen use.
6. The pathologist should be advised of estrogen therapy when relevant specimens are submitted.
7. Patients with a past history of jaundice during pregnancy have an increased risk of recurrence of jaundice while receiving estrogen-containing oral contraceptive therapy. If jaundice develops in any patient receiving estrogen, the medication should be discontinued while the cause is investigated.
8. Estrogens may be poorly metabolized in patients with impaired liver function and they should be administered with caution in such patients.
9. Because estrogens influence the metabolism of calcium and phosphorus, they should be used with caution in patients with metabolic bone diseases that are associated with hypercalcemia or in patients with renal insufficiency.
10. Because of the effects of estrogens on epiphyseal closure, they should be used judiciously in young patients in whom bone growth is not complete.
11. Certain endocrine and liver function tests may be affected by estrogen-containing oral contraceptives. The following similar changes may be expected with larger doses of estrogen:
Increased sulfobromophthalein retention; increased prothrombin and factors VII, VIII, IX, and X; decreased antithrombin 3; increased norepinephrine-induced platelet aggregation; increased thyroid binding globulin (TBG) leading to increased circulating total thyroid hormone, as measured by PBI, T4 by column, or T4 by radioimmunoassay. Free T3 resin uptake is decreased, reflecting the elevated TBG; free T4 concentration is unaltered; impaired glucose tolerance; decreased pregnanediol excretion; reduced response to metyrapone test; reduced serum folate concentration; increased serum triglyceride and phospholipid concentration.
12. ESTINYL Tablets, .02 mg. contain FD&C Yellow No. 5 (tartrazine) which may cause allergic-type reactions (including bronchial asthma) in certain susceptible individuals. Although the overall incidence of FD&C Yellow No. 5 (tartrazine) sensitivity in the general population is low, it is frequently seen in patients who also have aspirin hypersensitivity.
Information for the Patient: See text of Patient Package Insert.
Pregnancy Category X. See Contraindications and Boxed Warning above.
Nursing Mothers: As a general principle, the administration of any drug to nursing mothers should be done only when clearly necessary, since many drugs are excreted in human milk.
Adverse Reactions: (See Warnings regarding induction of neoplasia, adverse effects on the fetus, increased incidence of gallbladder disease, and adverse effects similar to those of oral contraceptives, including thromboembolism.) The following additional adverse reactions have been reported with estrogenic therapy, including oral contraceptives:
Genitourinary system: Breakthrough bleeding, spotting, change in menstrual flow; dysmenorrhea; premenstrual-like syndrome; amenorrhea during and after treatment; increase in size of uterine fibromyomata; vaginal candidiasis; change in cervical eversion and in degree of cervical secretion; cystitis-like syndrome.
Breasts: Tenderness, enlargement, secretion.
Gastrointestinal: Nausea, vomiting; abdominal cramps, bloating; cholestatic jaundice.
Skin: Chloasma or melasma which may persist when drug is discontinued; erythema multiforme;

erythema nodosum; hemorrhagic eruption; loss of scalp hair; hirsutism.
Eyes: Steepening of corneal curvature; intolerance to contact lenses.
CNS: Headache, migraine, dizziness; mental depression; chorea.
Miscellaneous: Increase or decrease in weight; reduced carbohydrate tolerance; aggravation of porphyria; edema; changes in libido.
Acute Overdosage: Numerous reports of ingestion of large doses of estrogen-containing oral contraceptives by young children indicate that serious ill effects do not occur. Overdosage of estrogen may cause nausea, and withdrawal bleeding may occur in females.
Dosage and Administration: 1. *Given cyclically for short-term use only.*
For treatment of moderate to severe *vasomotor* symptoms associated with the menopause: The lowest dose that will control symptoms should be chosen and medication should be discontinued as promptly as possible. Administration should be cyclic (e.g., 3 weeks on and 1 week off). Attempts to discontinue or taper medication should be made at 3- to 6-month intervals. The usual dosage range is one 0.02 mg. or 0.05 mg. tablet daily. In some instances, the effective dose may be as low as one 0.02 mg. tablet every other day. A useful dosage schedule for early menopause, while spontaneous menstruation continues, is 0.05 mg. once a day for twenty-one days and then a rest period for seven days. This can be continued cyclically indefinitely adding a progestational agent during the latter part of the cycle. For the initial treatment of the late menopause, the same regimen is indicated with the 0.02 mg. ESTINYL Tablet for the first few cycles, after which the 0.05 mg. dosage may be substituted. In more severe cases, such as those due to surgical and roentgenologic castration, one 0.05 mg. tablet may be administered three times daily at the start of treatment. With adequate clinical improvement, usually obtainable in a few weeks, the dosage may be reduced to one 0.05 mg. tablet daily and the patient continued thereafter on a maintenance dosage as in the average case. At the discretion of the physician, a progestational agent may be added during the latter part of a planned cycle.
2. *Given cyclically.*
Female hypogonadism: One 0.05 mg. tablet is given one to three times daily during the first two weeks of a theoretical menstrual cycle. This is followed by progesterone during the last half of the arbitrary cycle. This regimen is continued for three to six months. The patient is then allowed to go untreated for two months to determine whether or not she can maintain the cycle without hormonal therapy. If not, additional courses of therapy may be prescribed.
3. *Given chronically.*
Inoperable progressing prostatic cancer: From three 0.05 mg. to four 0.5 mg. tablets may be administered daily for palliation.
Inoperable progressing breast cancer in appropriately selected postmenopausal women (See Indications): Two 0.5 mg. tablets three times daily for palliation.
Treated patients with an intact uterus should be monitored closely for signs of endometrial cancer and appropriate diagnostic measures should be taken to rule out malignancy in the event of persistent or recurring abnormal vaginal bleeding.
How Supplied: ESTINYL Tablets 0.02 mg., beige, sugar-coated tablets branded in black with the Schering trademark and either product identification numbers, 298, or letters, ER; bottles of 100 and 250.
ESTINYL Tablets 0.05 mg., pink, sugar-coated tablets branded in black with the Schering trademark and either product identification numbers, 070, or letters, EM; bottles of 100 and 250.
ESTINYL Tablets 0.5 mg., peach-colored, compressed, scored tablets impressed with the Schering trademark and either product identification numbers, 150, or letters, EP; bottle of 100.

Store between 2° and 30° C (36° and 86° F).
Patient package inserts are being dispensed with this product. They are available to physicians upon request. Physician references available on request.
Copyright © 1968, 1980, Schering Corporation. All rights reserved.
Shown in Product Identification Section, page 434

ETRAFON® ℞
[ĕ′ trah-fon]
brand of perphenazine, USP—amitriptyline hydrochloride, USP
ETRAFON 2-10 TABLETS (2–10)
ETRAFON TABLETS (2–25)
ETRAFON-A TABLETS (4–10)
ETRAFON-FORTE TABLETS (4–25)

Description: ETRAFON Tablets contain perphenazine, USP and amitriptyline hydrochloride, USP. Perphenazine is a piperazinyl phenothiazine having the chemical formula, $C_{21}H_{26}ClN_3OS$. Amitriptyline hydrochloride is a dibenzocycloheptadiene derivative having the chemical formula, $C_{20}H_{23}N \cdot HCl$.
ETRAFON Tablets are available in multiple strengths to afford dosage flexibility for optimum management. They are available as ETRAFON 2-10 Tablets, 2 mg perphenazine and 10 mg amitriptyline hydrochloride; ETRAFON Tablets, 2 mg perphenazine and 25 mg amitriptyline hydrochloride. ETRAFON-A Tablets, 4 mg perphenazine and 10 mg amitriptyline hydrochloride; and ETRAFON-FORTE Tablets, 4 mg perphenazine and 25 mg amitriptyline hydrochloride.
Actions: ETRAFON combines the tranquilizing action of perphenazine with the antidepressant properties of amitriptyline hydrochloride. Perphenazine acts on the central nervous system and has a greater behavioral potency than other phenothiazine derivatives whose side chains do not contain a piperazine moiety. Amitriptyline hydrochloride is a tricyclic antidepressant. It is not a monoamine oxidase inhibitor, but its mechanism of action in man is not known.
Indications: ETRAFON Tablets are indicated for the treatment of patients with moderate to severe anxiety and/or agitation and depressed mood; patients with depression in whom anxiety and/or agitation are moderate or severe; patients with anxiety and depression associated with chronic physical disease; patients in whom depression and anxiety cannot be clearly differentiated. Schizophrenic patients who have associated symptoms of depression should be considered for therapy with ETRAFON.
Many patients presenting symptoms such as agitation, anxiety, insomnia, psychomotor retardation, functional somatic complaints, a feeling of tiredness, loss of interest, and anorexia have responded to therapy with ETRAFON Tablets.
Contraindications: ETRAFON Tablets are contraindicated in comatose or greatly obtunded patients and in patients receiving large doses of central nervous system depressants (barbiturates, alcohol, narcotics, analgesics, or antihistamines); in the presence of existing blood dyscrasias, bone marrow depression, or liver damage; and in patients who have shown hypersensitivity to ETRAFON Tablets, its components, or related compounds.
ETRAFON Tablets are also contraindicated in patients with suspected or established subcortical brain damage, with or without hypothalamic damage, since a hyperthermic reaction with temperatures in excess of 104°F may occur in such patients, sometimes not until 14 to 16 hours after drug administration. Total body ice-packing is recommended for such a reaction; antipyretics may also be useful.
ETRAFON should not be given concomitantly with a monoamine oxidase inhibiting compound. Hyperpyretic crises, severe convulsions and deaths have occurred in patients receiving tricyclic antidepressant and monoamine oxidase inhibiting drugs simultaneously. In patients who have been receiving a monoamine oxidase inhibitor, it is recommended that two weeks or longer elapse before the start of treatment with ETRAFON Tablets to permit recovery from the effects of the MAO inhibitor and to avoid possible potentiation. Treatment with ETRAFON Tablets should be initiated cautiously in such patients, with gradual increase in dosage until a satisfactory response is obtained.
Amitriptyline hydrochloride is not recommended for use during the acute recovery phase following myocardial infarction.
Warnings: Patients with cardiovascular disorders should be watched closely. Tricyclic antidepressant drugs, including amitriptyline hydrochloride, particularly when given in high doses, have been reported to produce arrhythmias, sinus tachycardia, and prolongation of the conduction time. Myocardial infarction and stroke have been reported with drugs of this class.
ETRAFON should not be given concomitantly with guanethidine or similarly acting compounds, since amitriptyline, like other tricyclic antidepressants, may block the antihypertensive effect of these compounds.
If hypotension develops, epinephrine should not be administered, since its action is blocked and partially reversed by perphenazine. If a vasopressor is needed, norepinephrine may be used. Severe, acute hypotension has occurred with the use of phenothiazines and is particularly likely to occur in patients with mitral insufficiency or pheochromocytoma. Rebound hypertension may occur in pheochromocytoma patients.
Perphenazine can lower the convulsive threshold in susceptible individuals; it should be used with caution in patients with convulsive disorders. If the patient is being treated with an anticonvulsant agent, increased dosage of that agent may be required when ETRAFON Tablets are used concomitantly.
Because of the anticholinergic activity of amitriptyline hydrochloride, ETRAFON should be used with caution in patients with glaucoma, increased ocular pressure, and those in whom urinary retention is present or anticipated. In patients with angle-closure glaucoma even average doses may precipitate an attack.
Close supervision is required when amitriptyline hydrochloride is given to hyperthyroid patients or those receiving thyroid medication.
ETRAFON Tablets may impair the mental and/or physical abilities required for the performance of potentially hazardous tasks, such as driving a car or operating machinery, the patient should be warned accordingly.
Usage in Children: Since a dosage for children has not been established, ETRAFON is not recommended for use in children.
Usage in Pregnancy: Safe use of ETRAFON Tablets during pregnancy and lactation has not been established; therefore, in administering the drug to pregnant patients, nursing mothers, or women who may become pregnant, the possible benefits must be weighed against the possible hazards to mother and child.
Precautions: The possibility of suicide in depressed patients remains during treatment and until significant remission occurs. This type of patient should not have easy access to large quantities of this drug.

Perphenazine
As with all phenothiazine compounds, perphenazine should not be used indiscriminately. Caution should be observed in giving it to patients who have previously exhibited severe adverse reactions to other phenothiazines. Some of the untoward actions of perphenazine tend to appear more frequently when high doses are used. However, as with other phenothiazine compounds, patients receiving perphenazine in any dosage should be kept under close supervision.
Neuroleptic drugs elevate prolactin levels; the elevation persists during chronic administration. Tissue culture experiments indicate that approximately one-third of human breast cancers are prolactin dependent *in vitro*, a factor of potential importance if the prescription of these drugs is contemplated in a patient with a previously detected breast cancer. Although disturbances such as galactorrhea, amenorrhea, gynecomastia, and impotence have been reported, the clinical significance of elevated serum prolactin levels is unknown for most patients. An increase in mammary neoplasms has been found in rodents after chronic administration of neuroleptic drugs. Neither clinical studies nor epidemiologic studies conducted to date, however, have shown an association between chronic administration of these drugs and mammary tumorigenesis; the available evidence is considered too limited to be conclusive at this time.
The antiemetic effect of perphenazine may obscure signs of toxicity due to overdosage of other drugs, or render more difficult the diagnosis of disorders such as brain tumors or intestinal obstruction.
A significant, not otherwise explained, rise in body temperature may suggest individual intolerance to perphenazine, in which case ETRAFON should be discontinued.
Patients on large doses of a phenothiazine drug who are undergoing surgery should be watched carefully for possible hypotensive phenomena. Moreover, reduced amounts of anesthetics or central nervous system depressants may be necessary. Since phenothiazines and central nervous system depressants (opiates, analgesics, antihistamines, barbiturates) can potentiate each other, less than the usual dosage of the added drug is recommended, and caution is advised, when they are administered concomitantly.
Use with caution in patients who are receiving atropine or related drugs because of additive anticholinergic effects and also in patients who will be exposed to extreme heat or organic phosphate insecticides.
The use of alcohol should be avoided, since additive effects and hypotension may occur. Patients should be cautioned that their response to alcohol may be increased while they are being treated with ETRAFON Tablets. The risk of suicide and the danger of overdose may be increased in patients who use alcohol excessively due to it potentiation of the drug's effect.
Blood counts and hepatic and renal functions should be checked periodically. The appearance of signs of blood dyscrasias requires the discontinuance of the drug and institution of appropriate therapy. If abnormalities in hepatic tests occur, phenothiazine treatment should be discontinued. Renal function in patients on long-term therapy should be monitored; if blood urea nitrogen (BUN) becomes abnormal, treatment with the drug should be discontinued.
The use of phenothiazine derivatives in patients with diminished renal function should be undertaken with caution.
Use with caution in patients suffering from respiratory impairment due to acute pulmonary infections, or in chronic respiratory disorders such as severe asthma or emphysema.
In general, phenothiazines do not produce psychic dependence. Gastritis, nausea and vomiting, dizziness, and tremulousness have been reported following abrupt cessation of high-dose therapy. Reports suggest that these symptoms can be reduced by continuing concomitant antiparkinson agents for several weeks after the phenothiazine is withdrawn.
The possibility of liver damage, corneal and lenticular deposits, and irreversible dyskinesias should be kept in mind when patients are on long-term therapy.
Because photosensitivity has been reported, undue exposure to the sun should be avoided during phenothiazine treatment.

Amitriptyline Hydrochloride
In manic-depressive psychosis, depressed patients may experience a shift toward the manic phase if they are treated with an antidepressant drug. Patients with paranoid symptomatology may have an exaggeration of such symptoms. The tranquiliz-

Continued on next page

Information on Schering products appearing on these pages is effective as of September 30, 1984.

Schering—Cont.

ing effect of ETRAFON has seemed to reduce the likelihood of this effect.

When amitriptyline hydrochloride is given with anticholinergic agents or sympathomimetic drugs, including epinephrine combined with local anesthetics, close supervision and careful adjustment of dosages are required.

Paralytic ileus may occur in patients taking tricyclic antidepressants in combination with anticholinergic-type drugs.

Concurrent use of large doses of ethchlorvynol should be used with caution, since transient delirium has been reported in patients receiving this drug in combination with amitriptyline hydrochloride.

This drug may enhance the response to alcohol and the effects of barbiturates and other CNS depressants.

Concurrent administration of amitriptyline hydrochloride and electroshock therapy may increase the hazards of therapy. Such treatment should be limited to patients for whom it is essential.

Discontinue the drug several days before elective surgery, if possible.

Both elevation and lowering of blood sugar levels have been reported.

The usefulness of amitriptyline in the treatment of depression has been amply demonstrated; however, it should be realized that abuse of amitriptyline among a narcotic-dependent population is not uncommon.

Adverse Reactions: Adverse reactions to ETRAFON Tablets are the same as those to its components, perphenazine and amitriptyline hydrochloride. There have been no reports of effects peculiar to the combination of these components in ETRAFON Tablets.

Perphenazine

Not all of the following adverse reactions have been reported with perphenazine; however, pharmacological similarities among various phenothiazine derivatives require that each be considered. With the piperazine group (of which perphenazine is an example), the extrapyramidal symptoms are more common, and others (e.g., sedative effects, jaundice, and blood dyscrasias) are less frequently seen.

CNS Effects: *Extrapyramidal reactions:* opisthotonus, trismus, torticollis, retrocollis, aching and numbness of the limbs, motor restlessness, oculogyric crisis, hyperreflexia, dystonia, including protrusion, discoloration, aching and rounding of the tongue, tonic spasm of the masticatory muscles, tight feeling in the throat, slurred speech, dysphagia, akathisia, dyskinesia, parkinsonism, and ataxia. Their incidence and severity usually increase with an increase in dosage, but there is considerable individual variation in the tendency to develop such symptoms. Extrapyramidal symptoms can usually be controlled by the concomitant use of effective antiparkinsonian drugs, such as benztropine mesylate, and/or by reduction in dosage.

In some instances, however, these extrapyramidal reactions may persist after discontinuation of treatment with perphenazine.

Persistent tardive dyskinesia: As with all antipsychotic agents, tardive dyskinesia may appear in some patients on long-term therapy or may appear after drug therapy has been discontinued. Although the risk appears to be greater in elderly patients on high-dose therapy, especially females it may occur in either sex and in children. The symptoms are persistent and in some patients appear to be irreversible. The syndrome is characterized by rhythmical, involuntary movements of the tongue, face, mouth or jaw (eg, protrusion of tongue, puffing of cheeks, puckering of mouth, chewing movements). Sometimes these may be accompanied by involuntary movements of the extremities. There is no known effective treatment for tardive dyskinesia; antiparkinsonism agents usually do not alleviate the symptoms of this syndrome. It is suggested that all antipsychotic agents be discontinued if these symptoms appear. Should it be necessary to reinstitute treatment, or increase the dosage of the agent, or switch to a different antipsychotic agent, the syndrome may be masked. It has been reported that fine, vermicular movements of the tongue may be an early sign of the syndrome, and if the medication is stopped at that time the syndrome may not develop.

Other CNS effects include cerebral edema; abnormality of cerebrospinal fluid proteins; convulsive seizures, particularly in patients with EEG abnormalities or a history of such disorders; and headaches.

Drowsiness may occur, particularly during the first or second week, after which it generally disappears. If troublesome, lower the dosage. Hypnotic effects appear to be minimal, especially in patients who are permitted to remain active.

Adverse behavioral effects include paradoxical exacerbation of psychotic symptoms, catatoniclike states, paranoid reactions, lethargy, paradoxical excitement, restlessness, hyperactivity, nocturnal confusion, bizarre dreams, and insomnia. Hyperreflexia has been reported in the newborn when a phenothiazine was used during pregnancy.

Autonomic Effects: dry mouth or salivation, nausea, vomiting, diarrhea, anorexia, constipation, obstipation, fecal impaction, urinary retention, frequency or incontinence, polyuria, bladder paralysis, nasal congestion, pallor, myosis, mydriasis, blurred vision, glaucoma, perspiration, hypertension, hypotension, and a change in pulse rate occasionally may occur. Significant autonomic effects have been infrequent in patients receiving less than 24 mg perphenazine daily.

Adynamic ileus occasionally occurs with phenothiazine therapy and if severe can result in complications and death. It is of particular concern in psychiatric patients, who may fail to seek treatment of the condition.

Allergic Effects: urticaria, erythema, eczema, exfoliative dermatitis, pruritus, photosensitivity, asthma, fever, anaphylactoid reactions, laryngeal edema, and angioneurotic edema; contact dermatitis in nursing personnel administering the drug; and in extremely rare instances, individual idiosyncrasy or hypersensitivity to phenothiazines has resulted in cerebral edema, circulatory collapse, and death.

Endocrine Effects: lactation, galactorrhea, moderate breast enlargement in females and gynecomastia in males on large doses, disturbances in the menstrual cycle, amenorrhea, changes in libido, inhibition of ejaculation, false positive pregnancy tests, hyperglycemia, hypoglycemia, glycosuria, syndrome of inappropriate ADH (antidiuretic hormone) secretion.

Cardiovascular Effects: Postural hypotension, tachycardia (especially with sudden marked increase in dosage), bradycardia, cardiac arrest, faintness, and dizziness. Occasionally the hypotensive effect may produce a shock-like condition. ECG changes, nonspecific, (quinidine-like effect) usually reversible, have been observed in some patients receiving phenothiazine tranquilizers.

Sudden death has occasionally been reported in patients who have received phenothiazines. In some cases the death was apparently due to cardiac arrest; in others the cause appeared to be asphyxia due to cardiac arrest; in others the cause appeared to be asphyxia due to failure of the cough reflex. In some patients, the cause could not be determined nor could it be established that the death was due to the phenothiazine.

Hematological Effects: agranulocytosis, eosinophilia, leukopenia, hemolytic anemia, thrombocytopenic purpura, and pancytopenia. Most cases of agranulocytosis have occurred between the fourth and tenth weeks of therapy. Patients should be watched closely especially during that period for the sudden appearance of sore throat or signs of infection. If white blood cell and differential cell counts show significant cellular depression, discontinue the drug and start appropriate therapy. However, a slightly lowered white count is not in itself an indication to discontinue the drug.

Other Effects: Special considerations in long-term therapy include pigmentation of the skin, occurring chiefly in the exposed areas; ocular changes consisting of deposition of fine particulate matter in the cornea and lens, progressing in more severe cases to starshaped lenticular opacities; epithelial keratopathies; and pigmentary retinopathy. Also noted: peripheral edema, reversed epinephrine effect, increase in PBI not attributable to an increase in thyroxine, parotid swelling (rare), hyperpyrexia, systemic lupus erythematosus-like syndrome, increases in appetite and weight, polyphagia, photophobia, and muscle weakness.

Liver damage (biliary stasis) may occur. Jaundice may occur, usually between the second and fourth weeks of treatment, and is regarded as a hypersensitivity reaction. Incidence is low. The clinical picture resembles infectious hepatitis but with laboratory features of obstructive jaundice. It is usually reversible; however, chronic jaundice has been reported.

Amitriptyline Hydrochloride

Although activation of latent schizophrenia has been reported with antidepressant drugs, including amitriptyline hydrochloride, it may be prevented with ETRAFON Tablets in some cases because of the antipsychotic effect of perphenazine. A few instances of epileptiform seizures have been reported in chronic schizophrenic patients during treatment with amitriptyline hydrochloride.

Note: Included in the listing which follows are a few adverse reactions which have not been reported with this specific drug. However, pharmacological similarities among the tricyclic antidepressant drugs require that each of the reactions be considered when amitriptyline hydrochloride is administered.

Allergic: Rash, pruritus, urticaria, photosensitization, edema of face and tongue.

Anticholinergic: Dry mouth, blurred vision, disturbance of accommodation, constipation, paralytic ileus, urinary retention, dilatation of urinary tract.

Cardiovascular: Hypotension, hypertension, tachycardia, palpitations, myocardial infarction, arrhythmias, heart block, stroke.

CNS and Neuromuscular: Confusional states, disturbed concentration, disorientation, delusions, hallucinations, excitement, jitteriness, anxiety, restlessness, insomnia, nightmares, numbness, tingling, and paresthesias of the extremities, peripheral neuropathy, incoordination, ataxia, tremors, seizures, alteration in EEG patterns, extrapyramidal symptoms, tinnitus.

Endocrine: Testicular swelling and gynecomastia in the male, breast enlargement and galactorrhea in the female, increased or decreased libido, elevation and lowering of blood sugar levels, syndrome of inappropriate ADH (antidiuretic hormone secretion).

Gastrointestinal: Nausea, epigastric distress, heartburn, vomiting, anorexia, stomatitis, peculiar taste, diarrhea, jaundice, parotid swelling, black tongue. Rarely hepatitis has occurred (including altered liver function and jaundice).

Hematologic: Bone marrow depression including agranulocytosis, leukopenia, eosinophilia, purpura, thrombocytopenia.

Other: Dizziness, weakness, fatigue, headache, weight gain or loss, increased perspiration, urinary frequency, mydriasis, drowsiness, alopecia.

Withdrawal Symptoms: Abrupt cessation of treatment after prolonged administration may produce nausea, headache, and malaise. These are not indicative of addiction.

Dosage and Administration:

Initial Dosage

In psychoneurotic patients whose anxiety and depression warrant combined therapy, one ETRAFON Tablet (2–25) or one ETRAFON-FORTE Tablet (4–25) three or four times a day is recommended.

In elderly patients, adolescents and other patients as indicated, one ETRAFON-A Tablet (4–10) may be administered three or four times a day as initial dosage. This dosage may be adjusted as required to produce an adequate response.

In more severely ill patients with schizophrenia, two ETRAFON-FORTE Tablets (4–25) three times a day are recommended as the initial dosage. If necessary, a fourth dose may be given at bedtime. The total daily dosage should not exceed eight tablets of any strength.

Maintenance Dosage

Depending on the condition being treated, the onset of therapeutic response may vary from a few days to a few weeks or even longer. After a satisfactory response is noted, dosage should be reduced to the smallest dose which is effective for relief of the symptoms for which ETRAFON Tablets are being administered. A useful maintenance dosage is one ETRAFON Tablet (2–25) or one ETRAFON-FORTE Tablet (4–25) two to four times a day. In some patients, maintenance dosage is required for many months.

ETRAFON 2-10 Tablets (2–10) and ETRAFON-A Tablets (4–10) can be used to increase flexibility in adjusting maintenance dosage to the lowest amount consistent with relief of symptoms.

Overdosage: In the event of overdosage, emergency treatment should be started immediately. All patients suspected of having taken an overdose should be hospitalized as soon as possible.

Manifestations: Overdosage of perphenazine primarily involves the extrapyramidal mechanism and produces the same side effects described under ADVERSE REACTIONS, but to a more marked degree. It is usually evidenced by stupor or coma; children may have convulsive seizures.

High doses may cause temporary confusion, disturbed concentration, or transient visual hallucinations. Overdosage may cause drowsiness; hypothermia; tachycardia and other arrhythmic abnormalities—for example, bundle branch block; ECG evidence of impaired conduction; congestive heart failure; dilated pupils; convulsions; severe hypotension; stupor; and coma. Other symptoms may be agitation, hyperactive reflexes, muscle rigidity, vomiting, hyperpyrexia, or any of the adverse reactions listed for perphenazine or amitriptyline hydrochloride.

Overdosage with tricyclic antidepressants (TCAs), such as imipramine, doxepin, or amitriptyline may result in plasma TCA levels of 1,000 ng/ml or higher. Such levels more accurately define patients who are at risk for major medical complications of overdosage than does the amount of drug ingested based on patient history. In one study, all patients with TCA levels of this magnitude had a QRS duration of 100 msec or more on a routine ECG within the first 24 hours following overdose. In the absence of TCA blood level determinations, a QRS of 100 msec or more suggests a greater likelihood of serious complications.

Oculomotor paresis (loss of conjugate movement in the so-called doll's eyes maneuver) as a manifestation of amitriptyline overdosage has been reported as being significant in the differential diagnosis of a patient in light coma.

Treatment: Treatment is symptomatic and supportive. There is no specific antidote. The patient should be induced to vomit even if emesis has occurred spontaneously. Pharmacologic vomiting by the administration of ipecac syrup is a preferred method. It should be noted that ipecac has a central mode of action in addition to its local gastric irritant properties, and the central mode of action may be blocked by the antiemetic effect of ETRAFON Tablets. Vomiting should not be induced in patients with impaired consciousness. The action of ipecac is facilitated by physical activity and by the administration of 8 to 12 fluid ounces of water. If emesis does not occur within 15 minutes, the dose of ipecac should be repeated. Precautions against aspiration must be taken, especially in infants and children. Following emesis, any drug remaining in the stomach may be adsorbed by activated charcoal administered as a slurry with water. If vomiting is unsuccessful or contraindicated, gastric lavage should be performed. Isotonic and one-half isotonic saline are the lavage solutions of choice. Saline cathartics, such as milk of magnesia, draw water into the bowel by osmosis and therefore may be valuable for their action in rapid dilution of bowel content.

Standard measures (oxygen, intravenous fluids, corticosteroids) should be used to manage circulatory shock or metabolic acidosis. An open airway and adequate fluid intake should be maintained. Body temperature should be regulated. Hypothermia is expected, but severe hyperthermia may occur and must be treated vigorously. (See CONTRAINDICATIONS.)

An electrocardiogram should be taken and close monitoring of cardiac function instituted if there is any sign of abnormality. Cardiac arrhythmias may be treated with neostigmine, pyridostigmine, or propranolol. Digitalis should be considered for cardiac failure. Close monitoring of cardiac function is advisable for not less than five days.

Vasopressors such as norepinephrine may be used to treat hypotension, but epinephrine should NOT be used.

The intravenous administration of 1 to 3 mg physostigmine salicylate has been reported to reverse the symptoms of tricyclic antidepressant poisoning and therefore, should be considered in the symptomatic treatment of the central anticholinergic effects due to overdosage with ETRAFON Tablets. Because physostigmine is rapidly metabolized, it should be re-administered as required, especially if life-threatening signs, such as arrhythmias, convulsions, or deep coma recur or persist.

Anticonvulsants (an inhalation anesthetic, diazepam, or paraldehyde) are recommended for control of convulsions, since perphenazine increases the central nervous system depressant action, but not the anticonvulsant action of barbiturates.

If acute parkinson-like symptoms result from perphenazine intoxication, benztropine mesylate or diphenhydramine may be administered.

Central nervous system depression may be treated with nonconvulsant doses of CNS stimulants. Avoid stimulants that may cause convulsions (e.g., picrotoxin and pentylenetetrazol).

Signs of arousal may not occur for 48 hours.

Dialysis is of no value because of low plasma concentrations of the drug.

Since overdosage is often deliberate, patients may attempt suicide by other means during the recovery phase. Deaths by deliberate or accidental overdosage have occurred with this class of drugs.

How Supplied: ETRAFON 2-10 Tablets (perphenazine 2 mg and amitriptyline hydrochloride 10 mg): deep yellow, sugar-coated tablets branded in blue-black with the Schering trademark and either product identification letters, ANA, or number, 287; bottles of 100 (NDC 0085-0287-04) and 500 (NDC 0085-0287-07) and box of 100 for unit-dose dispensing (10 strips of 10 tablets each) (NDC 0085-0287-08).

ETRAFON Tablets (perphenazine 2 mg and amitriptyline hydrochloride 25 mg): pink, sugar-coated tablets branded in red with the Schering trademark and either product identification letters, ANC or number, 598; bottles of 100 (NDC 0085-0598-04) and 500 (NDC 0085-0598-07) and box of 100 for unit-dose dispensing (10 strips of 10 tablets each) (NDC 0085-0598-08).

ETRAFON-A Tablets (perphenazine 4 mg and amitriptyline hydrochloride 10 mg): orange, sugar-coated tablets branded in blue-black with the Schering trademark ( ) and either product identification letters, ANB, or number, 119; bottles of 100 (NDC 0085-0119-04) and 500 (NDC 0085-0119-07) and box of 100 for unit-dose dispensing (10 strips of 10 tablets each) (NDC 0085-0119-08).

ETRAFON-FORTE Tablets (perphenazine 4 mg and amitriptyline hydrochloride 25 mg): red, sugar-coated tablets branded in blue with the Schering trademark and either product identification letters, ANE, or number, 720; bottles of 100 (NDC 0085-0720-04) and 500 (NDC 0085-0720-07) and box of 100 for unit-dose dispensing (10 strips of 10 tablets each) (NDC 0085-0720-08).

Store ETRAFON 2-10, 4-10, 2-25 and 4-25 Tablets between 2° and 30°C (36° and 86°F). In addition, protect unit-dose packages from excessive moisture.

Revised 12/83
Copyright © 1969, 1980, 1983 Schering Corporation. All rights Reserved.
Shown in Product Identification Section, page 434

FULVICIN® P/G ℞
[*ful' vĭ-sin*]
brand of ultramicrosize griseofulvin, USP Tablets

Description: FULVICIN P/G Tablets contain ultramicrosize crystals of griseofulvin, an antibiotic derived from a species of *Penicillium*. Griseofulvin crystals are partly dissolved in polyethylene glycol 6000 and partly dispersed throughout the tablet matrix.

Each FULVICIN P/G Tablet contains 125 mg or 250 mg griseofulvin ultramicrosize.

Actions: Microbiology Griseofulvin is fungistatic with *in vitro* activity against various species of *Microsporum*, *Epidermophyton*, and *Trichophyton*. It has no effect on bacteria or on other genera of fungi.

Human Pharmacology: Following oral administration, griseofulvin is deposited in the keratin precursor cells and has a greater affinity for diseased tissue. The drug is tightly bound to the new keratin which becomes highly resistant to fungal invasions.

The efficiency of gastrointestinal absorption of ultramicrocrystalline griseofulvin is approximately one and one-half times that of the conventional microsized griseofulvin. This factor permits the oral intake of two-thirds as much ultramicrocrystalline griseofulvin as the microsize form. However, there is currently no evidence that this lower dose confers any significant clinical differences with regard to safety and/or efficacy.

Indications: FULVICIN P/G Tablets are indicated for the treatment of ringworm infections of the skin, hair, and nails, namely: tinea corporis, tinea pedis, tinea cruris, tinea barbae, tinea capitis, tinea unguium (onychomycosis) when caused by one or more of the following genera of fungi: *Trichophyton rubrum*, *Trichophyton tonsurans*, *Trichophyton mentagrophytes*, *Trichophyton interdigitale*, *Trichophyton verrucosum*, *Trichophyton megninii*, *Trichophyton gallinae*, *Trichophyton crateriforme*, *Trichophyton sulphureum*, *Trichophyton schoenleinii*, *Microsporum audouinii*, *Microsporum canis*, *Microsporum gypseum*, and *Epidermophyton floccosum*.

Note: Prior to therapy, the type of fungi responsible for the infection should be identified.

The use of this drug is not justified in minor or trivial infections which will respond to topical agents alone.

Griseofulvin is not effective in the following: bacterial infections, candidiasis (moniliasis), histoplasmosis, actinomycosis, sporotrichosis, chromoblastomycosis, coccidioidomycosis, North American blastomycosis, cryptococcosis (torulosis), tinea versicolor, and nocardiosis.

Contraindications: This drug is contraindicated in patients with porphyria, hepatocellular failure, and in individuals with a history of hypersensitivity to griseofulvin.

Warnings: *Prophylactic Usage:* Safety and efficacy of griseofulvin for prophylaxis of fungal infections have not been established.

Animal Toxicology: Chronic feeding of griseofulvin, at levels ranging from 0.5–2.5% of the diet, resulted in the development of liver tumors in several strains of mice, particularly in males. Smaller particle sizes result in an enhanced effect. Lower oral dosage levels have not been tested. Subcutaneous administration of relatively small doses of griseofulvin once a week during the first three weeks of life has also been reported to induce hepatomata in mice. Thyroid tumors, mostly adenomas but some carcinomas, have been reported in male rats receiving griseofulvin at levels of 2.0%, 1.0%, and 0.2% of the diet, and in female

Continued on next page

Information on Schering products appearing on these pages is effective as of September 30, 1984.

Schering—Cont.

rats receiving the two higher dose levels. Although studies in other animal species have not yielded evidence of tumorigenicity, these studies were not of adequate design to form a basis for conclusions in this regard.

In subacute toxicity studies, orally administered griseofulvin produced hepatocellular necrosis in mice, but this has not been seen in other species. Disturbances in porphyrin metabolism have been reported in griseofulvin-treated laboratory animals. Griseofulvin has been reported to have a colchicine-like effect on mitosis and cocarcinogenicity with methylcholanthrene in cutaneous tumor induction in laboratory animals.

Usage in Pregnancy: The safety of this drug during pregnancy has not been established.

Animal Reproduction Studies: It has been reported in the literature that griseofulvin was found to be embryotoxic and teratogenic on oral administration to pregnant rats. Pups with abnormalities have been reported in the litters of a few bitches treated with griseofulvin.

Suppression of spermatogenesis has been reported to occur in rats, but investigation in man failed to confirm this.

Precautions: Patients on prolonged therapy with any potent medication should be under close observation. Periodic monitoring of organ system function, including renal, hepatic, and hematopoietic, should be done.

Since griseofulvin is derived from species of *Penicillium*, the possibility of cross-sensitivity with penicillin exists; however, known penicillin-sensitive patients have been treated without difficulty.

Since a photosensitivity reaction is occasionally associated with griseofulvin therapy, patients should be warned to avoid exposure to intense natural or artificial sunlight.

Lupus erythematosus or lupus-like syndromes have been reported in patients receiving griseofulvin.

Griseofulvin decreases the activity of warfarin-type anticoagulants so that patients receiving these drugs concomitantly may require dosage adjustment of the anticoagulant during and after griseofulvin therapy.

Barbiturates usually depress griseofulvin activity, and concomitant administration may require a dosage adjustment of the antifungal agent.

The effects of alcohol may be potentiated by griseofulvin, producing such effects as tachycardia and flush.

Adverse Reactions: When adverse reactions occur, they are most commonly of the hypersensitivity type, such as skin rashes, urticaria, and rarely, angioneurotic edema, and may necessitate withdrawal of therapy and appropriate countermeasures. Paresthesias of the hands and feet have been reported rarely after extended therapy. Other side effects reported occasionally are oral thrush, nausea, vomiting, epigastric distress, diarrhea, headache, fatigue, dizziness, insomnia, mental confusion, and impairment of performance of routine activities.

Proteinuria and leukopenia have been reported rarely. Administration of the drug should be discontinued if granulocytopenia occurs.

When rare, serious reactions occur with griseofulvin, they are usually associated with high dosages, long periods of therapy, or both.

Dosage and Administration: Accurate diagnosis of the infecting organism is essential. Identification should be made either by direct microscopic examination of a mounting of infected tissue in a solution of potassium hydroxide or by culture on an appropriate medium.

Medication must be continued until the infecting organism is completely eradicated as indicated by appropriate clinical or laboratory examination. Representative treatment periods are tinea capitis, 4 to 6 weeks; tinea corporis, 2 to 4 weeks; tinea pedis, 4 to 8 weeks; tinea unguium—depending on rate of growth—fingernails, at least 4 months; toenails, at least 6 months.

General measures in regard to hygiene should be observed to control sources of infection or reinfection. Concomitant use of appropriate topical agents is usually required particularly in treatment of tinea pedis. In some forms of athlete's foot, yeasts and bacteria may be involved as well as fungi. Griseofulvin will not eradicate the bacterial or monilial infection.

Adults: Daily administration of 375 mg (as a single dose or in divided amounts) will give a satisfactory response in most patients with tinea corporis, tinea cruris, and tinea capitis. For those fungus infections more difficult to eradicate, such as tinea pedis and tinea unguium, a divided daily dose of 750 mg is recommended.

Children: Approximately 3.3 mg per pound of body weight per day of ultramicrosize griseofulvin is an effective dose for most children. On this basis, the following dosage schedule is suggested: Children weighing 35 to 60 pounds—125 mg to 187.5 mg daily. Children weighing over 60 pounds—187.5 mg to 375 mg daily.

Children 2 years of age and younger—dosage has not been established.

Clinical experience with griseofulvin in children with tinea capitis indicates that a single daily dose is effective. Clinical relapse will occur if the medication is not continued until the infecting organism is eradicated.

How Supplied: FULVICIN P/G Tablets, 125 mg, white, compressed, scored tablets impressed with the Schering trademark and product identification numbers, 228; bottle of 100.

FULVICIN P/G Tablets, 250 mg, white, compressed, scored tablets impressed with the Schering trademark and product identification numbers, 507; bottle of 100.

Store at controlled room temperature 59°F to 86°F (15°C to 30°C).

Revised 2/82

Copyright © 1976, 1982, Schering Corporation. All rights reserved.

Shown in Product Identification Section, p. 434

FULVICIN® P/G 165 and 330 R
[ful' vĭ-sin]
brand of ultramicrosize griseofulvin
Tablets, USP

Description: FULVICIN P/G Tablets contain ultramicrosize crystals of griseofulvin, an antibiotic derived from a species of *Penicillium*. Griseofulvin crystals are partly dissolved in polyethylene glycol 8000 and partly dispersed throughout the tablet matrix.

Each FULVICIN P/G Tablet contains 165 mg or 330 mg ultramicrosize griseofulvin, USP.

Actions: Microbiology: Griseofulvin is fungistatic with *in vitro* activity against various species of *Microsporum, Epidermophyton,* and *Trichophyton.* It has no effect on bacteria or on other genera of fungi.

Human Pharmacology: Following oral administration, griseofulvin is deposited in the keratin precursor cells and has a greater affinity for diseased tissue. The drug is tightly bound to the new keratin which becomes highly resistant to fungal invasions.

The efficiency of gastrointestinal absorption of ultramicrocrystalline griseofulvin is approximately one and one-half times that of the conventional microsize griseofulvin. This factor permits the oral intake of two-thirds as much ultramicrocrystalline griseofulvin as the microsize form. However, there is currently no evidence that this lower dose confers any significant clinical differences with regard to safety and/or efficacy.

Indications: FULVICIN P/G Tablets are indicated for the treatment of ringworm infections of the skin, hair, and nails, namely: tinea corporis, tinea pedis, tinea cruris, tinea barbae, tinea capitis, tinea unguium (onychomycosis) when caused by one or more of the following genera of fungi: *Trichophyton rubrum, Trichophyton tonsurans, Trichophyton mentagrophytes, Trichophyton interdigitale, Trichophyton verrucosum, Trichophyton megninii, Trichophyton gallinae, Trichophyton crateriforme, Trichophyton sulphureum, Trichophyton schoenleinii, Microsporum audouinii, Microsporum canis, Microsporum gypseum,* and *Epidermophyton floccosum.*

Note: Prior to therapy, the type of fungi responsible for the infection should be identified.

The use of this drug is not justified in minor or trivial infections which will respond to topical agents alone.

Griseofulvin is not effective in the following: bacterial infections, candidiasis (moniliasis), histoplasmosis, actinomycosis, sporotrichosis, chromoblastomycosis, coccidioidomycosis, North American blastomycosis, cryptococcosis (torulosis), tinea versicolor, and nocardiosis.

Contraindications: This drug is contraindicated in patients with porphyria, hepatocellular failure, and in individuals with a history of hypersensitivity to griseofulvin.

Warnings: *Prophylactic Usage:* Safety and efficacy of griseofulvin for prophylaxis of fungal infections have not been established.

Animal Toxicology: Chronic feeding of griseofulvin, at levels ranging from 0.5–2.5% of the diet, resulted in the development of liver tumors in several strains of mice, particularly in males. Smaller particle sizes result in an enhanced effect. Lower oral dosage levels have not been tested. Subcutaneous administration of relatively small doses of griseofulvin once a week during the first three weeks of life has also been reported to induce hepatomata in mice. Thyroid tumors, mostly adenomas but some carcinomas, have been reported in male rats receiving griseofulvin at levels of 2.0%, 1.0%, and 0.2% of the diet, and in female rats receiving the two higher dose levels. Although studies in other animal species have not yielded evidence of tumorigenicity, these studies were not of adequate design to form a basis for conclusions in this regard.

In subacute toxicity studies, orally administered griseofulvin produced hepatocellular necrosis in mice, but this has not been seen in other species. Disturbances in porphyrin metabolism have been reported in griseofulvin-treated laboratory animals. Griseofulvin has been reported to have a colchicine-like effect on mitosis and cocarcinogenicity with methylcholanthrene in cutaneous tumor induction in laboratory animals.

Usage in Pregnancy: The safety of this drug during pregnancy has not been established.

Animal Reproduction Studies: It has been reported in the literature that griseofulvin was found to be embryotoxic and teratogenic on oral administration to pregnant rats. Pups with abnormalities have been reported in the litters of a few bitches treated with griseofulvin.

Suppression of spermatogenesis has been reported to occur in rats, but investigation in man failed to confirm this.

Precautions: Patients on prolonged therapy with any potent medication should be under close observation. Periodic monitoring of organ system function, including renal, hepatic, and hematopoietic, should be done.

Since griseofulvin is derived from species of *Penicillium*, the possibility of cross-sensitivity with penicillin exists; however, known penicillin-sensitive patients have been treated without difficulty.

Since a photosensitivity reaction is occasionally associated with griseofulvin therapy, patients should be warned to avoid exposure to intense natural or artificial sunlight.

Lupus erythematosus or lupus-like syndromes have been reported in patients receiving griseofulvin.

Griseofulvin decreases the activity of warfarin-type anticoagulants so that patients receiving these drugs concomitantly may require dosage adjustment of the anticoagulant during and after griseofulvin therapy.

Barbiturates usually depress griseofulvin activity, and concomitant administration may require a dosage adjustment of the antifungal agent.

The effects of alcohol may be potentiated by griseofulvin, producing such effects as tachycardia and flush.

Adverse Reactions: When adverse reactions occur, they are most commonly of the hypersensitivity type, such as skin rashes, urticaria, and rarely, angioneurotic edema, and may necessitate withdrawal of therapy and appropriate countermeasures. Paresthesias of the hands and feet have been reported rarely after extended therapy. Other side effects reported occasionally are oral thrush, nausea, vomiting, epigastric distress, diarrhea, headache, fatigue, dizziness, insomnia, mental confusion, and impairment of performance of routine activities.

Proteinuria and leukopenia have been reported rarely. Administration of the drug should be discontinued if granulocytopenia occurs.

When rare, serious reactions occur with griseofulvin, they are usually associated with high dosages, long periods of therapy, or both.

Dosage and Administration: Accurate diagnosis of the infecting organism is essential. Identification should be made either by direct microscopic examination of a mounting of infected tissue in a solution of potassium hydroxide or by culture on an appropriate medium.

Medication must be continued until the infecting organism is completely eradicated as indicated by appropriate clinical or laboratory examination. Representative treatment periods are tinea capitis, 4 to 6 weeks, tinea corporis, 2 to 4 weeks, tinea pedis, 4 to 8 weeks, tinea unguium—depending on rate of growth—fingernails, at least 4 months; toenails, at least 6 months.

General measures in regard to hygiene should be observed to control sources of infection or reinfection. Concomitant use of appropriate topical agents is usually required particularly in treatment of tinea pedis. In some forms of athlete's foot, yeasts and bacteria may be involved as well as fungi. Griseofulvin will not eradicate the bacterial or monilial infection.

Adults: Daily administration of 330 mg (as a single dose or in divided amounts) will give a satisfactory response in most patients with tinea corporis, tinea cruris, and tinea capitis. For those fungus infections more difficult to eradicate, such as tinea pedis and tinea unguium, a divided daily dosage of 660 mg is recommended.

Children: Approximately 3.3 mg per pound of body weight per day is an effective dose for most children. On this basis, the following dosage schedule is suggested: Children weighing 30 to 50 pounds—82.5 mg to 165 mg daily. Children weighing over 50 pounds—165 mg to 330 mg daily. Children 2 years of age and younger—dosage has not been established.

Clinical experience with griseofulvin in children with tinea capitis indicates that a single daily dose is effective. Clinical relapse will occur if the medication is not continued until the infecting organism is eradicated.

How Supplied: FULVICIN P/G 165 Tablets, 165 mg, off-white, oval, compressed, scored tablets impressed with the product name (FULVICIN P/G) and product identification numbers, 654; bottle of 100.

FULVICIN P/G 330 Tablets, 330 mg, off-white, oval, compressed, scored tablets impressed with the product name (FULVICIN P/G) and product identification numbers, 352; bottle of 100.

Store between 2° and 30°C (36° and 86°F).

Revised 9/83

Copyright © 1976, 1983, Schering Corporation. All rights reserved.

Shown in Product Identification Section, page 434

FULVICIN-U/F®   R
[ful' vĭ-sin]
brand of griseofulvin, USP
Tablets

Description: FULVICIN-U/F Tablets contain microsize crystals of griseofulvin, an antibiotic derived from a species of *Penicillium*.

Actions: Microbiology: Griseofulvin is fungistatic with *in vitro* activity against various species of *Microsporum*, *Epidermophyton*, and *Trichophyton*. It has no effect on bacteria or on other genera of fungi.

Human Pharmacology: Griseofulvin absorption from the gastrointestinal tract varies considerably among individuals mainly because of insolubility of the drug in aqueous media of the upper G.I. tract. The peak serum level found in fasting adults given 0.5 g occurs at about four hours and ranges between 0.5 to 1.5 mcg/ml. The serum level may be increased by giving the drug with a meal with a high fat content.

Griseofulvin is deposited in the keratin precursor cells and has a greater affinity for diseased tissue. The drug is tightly bound to the new keratin which becomes highly resistant to fungal invasions.

Indications: FULVICIN-U/F Tablets are indicated for the treatment of ringworm infections of the skin, hair, and nails, namely: tinea corporis, tinea pedis, tinea cruris, tinea barbae, tinea capitis, tinea unguium (onychomycosis) when caused by one or more of the following genera of fungi: *Trichophyton rubrum*, *Trichophyton tonsurans*, *Trichophyton mentagrophytes*, *Trichophyton interdigitale*, *Trichophyton verrucosum*, *Trichophyton megninii*, *Trichophyton gallinae*, *Trichophyton crateriforme*, *Trichophyton sulphureum*, *Trichophyton schoenleinii*, *Microsporum audouinii*, *Microsporum canis*, *Microsporum gypseum*, and *Epidermophyton floccosum*.

Note: Prior to therapy, the type of fungi responsible for the infection should be identified.

The use of this drug is not justified in minor or trivial infections which will respond to topical agents alone.

Griseofulvin is not effective in the following: bacterial infections, candidiasis (moniliasis), histoplasmosis, actinomycosis, sporotrichosis, chromoblastomycosis, coccidioidomycosis, North American blastomycosis, cryptococcosis (torulosis), tinea versicolor, and nocardiosis.

Contraindications: This drug is contraindicated in patients with porphyria, hepatocellular failure, and in individuals with a history of hypersensitivity to griseofulvin.

Warnings: Prophylactic usage: Safety and efficacy of griseofulvin for prophylaxis of fungal infections have not been established.

Animal toxicology: Chronic feeding of griseofulvin, at levels ranging from 0.5-2.5% of the diet, resulted in the development of liver tumors in several strains of mice, particularly in males. Smaller particle sizes result in an enhanced effect. Lower oral dosage levels have not been tested. Subcutaneous administration of relatively small doses of griseofulvin, once a week, during the first three weeks of life has also been reported to induce hepatomata in mice. Thyroid tumors, mostly adenomas but some carcinomas, have been reported in male rats receiving griseofulvin at levels of 2.0%, 1.0%, and 0.2% of the diet, and in female rats receiving the two higher dose levels. Although studies in other animal species have not yielded evidence of tumorigenicity, these studies were not of adequate design to form a basis for conclusions in this regard.

In subacute toxicity studies, orally administered griseofulvin produced hepatocellular necrosis in mice, but this has not been seen in other species. Disturbances in porphyrin metabolism have been reported in griseofulvin-treated laboratory animals. Griseofulvin has been reported to have a colchicine-like effect on mitosis and cocarcinogenicity with methylcholanthrene in cutaneous tumor induction in laboratory animals.

Usage in pregnancy: The safety of this drug during pregnancy has not been established.

Animal reproduction studies: It has been reported in the literature that griseofulvin was found to be embryotoxic and teratogenic on oral administration to pregnant rats. Pups with abnormalities have been reported in the litters of a few bitches treated with griseofulvin.

Suppression of spermatogenesis has been reported to occur in rats, but investigation in man failed to confirm this.

Precautions: Patients on prolonged therapy with any potent medication should be under close observation. Periodic monitoring of organ system functions, including renal, hepatic, and hematopoietic, should be done.

Since griseofulvin is derived from species of *Penicillium*, the possibility of cross sensitivity with penicillin exists; however, known penicillin-sensitive patients have been treated without difficulty. Since a photosensitivity reaction is occasionally associated with griseofulvin therapy, patients should be warned to avoid exposure to intense natural or artificial sunlight.

Lupus erythematosus or lupus-like syndromes have been reported in patients receiving griseofulvin.

Griseofulvin decreases the activity of warfarin-type anticoagulants so that patients receiving these drugs concomitantly may require dosage adjustment of the anticoagulant during and after griseofulvin therapy.

Barbiturates usually depress griseofulvin activity and concomitant administration may require a dosage adjustment of the antifungal agent.

The effects of alcohol may be potentiated by griseofulvin, producing such effects as tachycardia and flush.

Adverse Reactions: When adverse reactions occur, they are most commonly of the hypersensitivity type, such as skin rashes, urticaria, and rarely, angioneurotic edema, and may necessitate withdrawal of therapy and appropriate countermeasures. Paresthesias of the hands and feet have been reported rarely after extended therapy. Other side effects reported occasionally are oral thrush, nausea, vomiting, epigastric distress, diarrhea, headache, fatigue, dizziness, insomnia, mental confusion, and impairment of performance of routine activities.

Proteinuria and leukopenia have been reported rarely. Administration of the drug should be discontinued if granulocytopenia occurs.

When rare, serious reactions occur with griseofulvin, they are usually associated with high dosages, long periods of therapy, or both.

Dosage and Administration: Accurate diagnosis of the infecting organism is essential. Identification should be made either by direct microscopic examination of a mounting of infected tissue in a solution of potassium hydroxide or by culture on an appropriate medium.

Medication must be continued until the infecting organism is completely eradicated as indicated by appropriate clinical or laboratory examination. Representative treatment periods are for tinea capitis, four to six weeks; tinea corporis, two to four weeks; tinea pedis, four to eight weeks; tinea unguium, depending on the rate of growth, fingernails, at least four months; toenails, at least six months.

General measures in regard to hygiene should be observed to control sources of infection or reinfection. Concomitant use of appropriate topical agents is usually required, particularly in treatment of tinea pedis. In some forms of athlete's foot, yeasts and bacteria may be involved as well as fungi. Griseofulvin will not eradicate the bacterial or monilial infection.

Adults: Daily administration of 500 mg (as a single dose or in divided amounts), will give a satisfactory response in most patients with tinea corporis, tinea cruris, and tinea capitis.

For those fungus infections more difficult to eradicate, such as tinea pedis and tinea unguium, daily dosage of 1.0 g is recommended.

Children: Approximately 5 mg per pound of body weight per day is an effective dose for most children. On this basis the following dosage schedule for children is suggested:

Children weighing 30 to 50 pounds—125 mg to 250 mg daily.

Children weighing over 50 pounds—250 mg to 500 mg daily.

Clinical experience with griseofulvin in children with tinea capitis indicates that a single daily dose is effective. Clinical relapse will occur if the medication is not continued until the infecting organism is eradicated.

Continued on next page

Information on Schering products appearing on these pages is effective as of September 30, 1984.

Schering—Cont.

How Supplied: FULVCIN-U/F Tablets, 250 mg: white, compressed, scored tablets impressed with the Schering trademark and product identification letters, AUF, or numbers, 948; bottles of 60 and 250.
FULVICIN-U/F Tablets, 500 mg: white, compressed, scored tablets impressed with the Schering trademark and product identification letters, AUG, or numbers, 496; bottles of 60 and 250.
Store between 2° and 30° C (36° and 86° F).
Revised 8/80
Copyright © 1968, 1980, Schering Corporation. All rights reserved.
Shown in Product Identification Section, page 434

GARAMYCIN® ℞
[gar-ah-mī'sin]
brand of gentamicin sulfate
  Cream, USP 0.1%
  Ointment, USP 0.1%
For Dermatologic Use only
Not For Ophthalmic Use

Description: Each gram of GARAMYCIN Cream 0.1% contains 1.7 mg gentamicin sulfate, USP equivalent to 1.0 mg gentamicin base, with 1.0 mg methylparaben and 4.0 mg butylparaben as preservatives, in a bland emulsion-type vehicle composed of stearic acid, propylene glycol stearate, isopropyl myristate, propylene glycol, polysorbate 40, sorbitol solution and purified water.
Each gram of GARAMYCIN Ointment 0.1% contains 1.7 mg gentamicin sulfate, USP equivalent to 1.0 mg gentamicin base, with 0.5 mg methylparaben and 0.1 mg propylparaben as preservatives in a bland, unctuous petrolatum base.
Actions: GARAMYCIN, a wide-spectrum antibiotic, provides highly effective topical treatment in primary and secondary bacterial infections of the skin. GARAMYCIN may clear infections that have not responded to other topical antibiotic agents. In impetigo contagiosa and other primary skin infections, treatment three or four times daily with GARAMYCIN usually clears the lesions promptly. In secondary skin infections, GARAMYCIN facilitates the treatment of the underlying dermatosis by controlling the infection. Bacteria susceptible to the action of GARAMYCIN include sensitive strains of streptococci (group A beta-hemolytic, alpha-hemolytic), *Staphylococcus aureus* (coagulase-positive, coagulase-negative, and some penicillinase-producing strains), and the gram-negative bacteria, *Pseudomonas aeruginosa, Aerobacter aerogenes, Escherichia coli, Proteus vulgaris,* and *Klebsiella pneumoniae.*
Indications: *Primary skin infections:* Impetigo contagiosa, superficial folliculitis, ecthyma, furunculosis, sycosis barbae, and pyoderma gangrenosum. *Secondary skin infections:* Infectious eczematoid dermatitis, pustular acne, pustular psoriasis, infected seborrheic dermatitis, infected contact dermatitis (including poison ivy), infected excoriations, and bacterial superinfections of fungal or viral infections. Note: GARAMYCIN is a bactericidal agent that is not effective against viruses or fungi in skin infections. GARAMYCIN is useful in the treatment of infected skin cysts and certain other skin abscesses when preceded by incision and drainage to permit adequate contact between the antibiotic and the infecting bacteria. Good results have been obtained in the treatment of infected stasis and other skin ulcers, infected superficial burns, paronychia, infected insect bites and stings, infected lacerations and abrasions, and wounds from minor surgery. Patients sensitive to neomycin can be treated with gentamicin, although regular observation of patients sensitive to topical antibiotics is advisable when such patients are treated with any topical antibiotic.
GARAMYCIN Ointment helps retain moisture and has been useful in infection on dry eczematous or psoriatic skin. GARAMYCIN Cream is recommended for wet, oozing primary infections, and greasy, secondary infections, such as pustular acne or infected seborrheic dermatitis. If a water-washable preparation is desired, GARAMYCIN Cream is preferable. GARAMYCIN Ointment and Cream have been used successfully in infants over one year of age as well as in adults and children.
Contraindications: This drug is contraindicated in individuals with a history of sensitivity reactions to any of its components.
Precautions: Use of topical antibiotics occasionally allows overgrowth of nonsusceptible organisms, including fungi. If this occurs, or if irritation, sensitization, or superinfection develops, treatment with gentamicin should be discontinued and appropriate therapy instituted.
Adverse Reactions: In patients with dermatoses treated with gentamicin, irritation (erythema and pruritus) that did not usually require discontinuance of treatment has been reported in a small percentage of cases. There was no evidence of irritation or sensitization, however, in any of these patients patch-tested subsequently with gentamicin on normal skin. Possible photosensitization has been reported in several patients but could not be elicited in these patients by reapplication of gentamicin followed by exposure to ultraviolet radiation.
Dosage and Administration: A small amount of GARAMYCIN Cream or Ointment should be applied gently to the lesions three or four times daily. The area treated may be covered with a gauze dressing if desired. In impetigo contagiosa, the crusts should be removed before application of GARAMYCIN to permit maximum contact between the antibiotic and the infection. Care should be exercised to avoid further contamination of the infected skin. Infected stasis ulcers have responded well to GARAMYCIN under gelatin packing.
How Supplied: GARAMYCIN Cream 0.1% (NDC-0085-0008-05) and GARAMYCIN Ointment 0.1% (NDC-0085-0343-05), 15 g tubes.
Store between 2° and 30° C (36° and 86° F).
Revised 12/83
Copyright © 1966, 1981 Schering Corporation. All rights reserved.

GARAMYCIN® ℞
[gar-ah-mī'sin]
brand of gentamicin sulfate
  Ophthalmic Solution, USP—Sterile
  Ophthalmic Ointment, USP—Sterile
Each ml or gram contains gentamicin sulfate, USP equivalent to 3.0 mg gentamicin

Description: Gentamicin sulfate is a water-soluble antibiotic of the aminoglycoside group active against a wide variety of pathogenic gram-negative and gram-positive bacteria.
GARAMYCIN Ophthalmic Solution is a sterile, aqueous solution buffered to approximately pH 7 for use in the eye. Each ml. contains gentamicin sulfate, USP (equivalent to 3.0 mg. gentamicin), disodium phosphate, monosodium phosphate, sodium chloride, and benzalkonium chloride as a preservative.
GARAMYCIN Ophthalmic Ointment is a sterile ointment, each gram containing gentamicin sulfate, USP (equivalent to 3.0 mg. gentamicin) in a bland base of white petrolatum, with methylparaben and propylparaben as preservatives.
Actions: The gram-positive bacteria against which gentamicin sulfate is active include coagulase-positive and coagulase-negative staphylococci, including certain strains that are resistant to penicillin; Group A beta-hemolytic and non-hemolytic streptococci; and *Diplococcus pneumoniae.* The gram-negative bacteria against which gentamicin sulfate is active include certain strains of *Pseudomonas aeruginosa,* indole-positive and indole-negative *Proteus* species, *Escherichia coli, Klebsiella pneumoniae* (Friedlander's bacillus), *Haemophilus influenza* and *Haemophilus aegyptius* (Koch-Weeks bacillus), *Aerobacter aerogenes, Moraxella lacunata* (diplobacillus of Morax-Axenfeld), and *Neisseria* species, including *Neisseria gonorrhoeae.* Although significant resistant organisms have not been isolated from patients treated with gentamicin at the present time, this may occur in the future as resistance has been produced with difficulty *in vitro* by repeated exposures.
Indications: GARAMYCIN Ophthalmic Solution and Ointment are indicated in the topical treatment of infections of the external eye and its adnexa caused by susceptible bacteria. Such infections embrace conjunctivitis, keratitis and keratoconjunctivitis, corneal ulcers, blepharitis and blepharoconjunctivitis, acute meibomianitis, and dacryocystitis.
Contraindications: GARAMYCIN Ophthalmic Solution and Ointment are contraindicated in patients with known hypersensitivity to any of the components.
Warnings: GARAMYCIN Ophthalmic Solution is not for injection. It should never be injected subconjunctivally, nor should it be directly introduced into the anterior chamber of the eye.
Precautions: Prolonged use of topical antibiotics may give rise to overgrowth of nonsusceptible organisms, such as fungi. Should this occur, or if irritation or hypersensitivity to any component of the drug develops, discontinue use of the preparation and institute appropriate therapy.
Ophthalmic ointments may retard corneal healing.
Adverse Reactions: Transient irritation has been reported with the use of GARAMYCIN Ophthalmic Solution.
Occasional burning or stinging may occur with the use of GARAMYCIN Ophthalmic Ointment.
Dosage and Administration: GARAMYCIN Ophthalmic Solution: instill one or two drops into the affected eye every four hours. In severe infections, dosage may be increased to as much as two drops once every hour.
GARAMYCIN Ophthalmic Ointment: apply a small amount to the affected eye two to three times a day.
How Supplied: GARAMYCIN Ophthalmic Solution—Sterile, 5 ml. plastic dropper bottle, boxes of one and six.
GARAMYCIN Ophthalmic Ointment—Sterile, 3.5 g, boxes of one and six.
Store GARAMYCIN Ophthalmic Ointment and Solution between 2° and 30°C (36° and 86°F).
Revised 4/84
Copyright © 1969, 1981, Schering Corporation. All rights reserved.

GARAMYCIN® Injectable ℞
[gar-ah-mī'sin]
brand of gentamicin sulfate injection, USP
40 mg. per ml.
Each ml. contains gentamicin sulfate, USP equivalent to 40 mg. gentamicin.
For Parenteral Administration

WARNINGS

Patients treated with aminoglycosides should be under close clinical observation because of the potential toxicity associated with their use.
As with other aminoglycosides, GARAMYCIN Injectable is potentially nephrotoxic. The risk of nephrotoxicity is greater in patients with impaired renal function and in those who receive high dosage or prolonged therapy.
Neurotoxicity manifested by ototoxicity, both vestibular and auditory, can occur in patients treated with GARAMYCIN Injectable primarily in those with pre-existing renal damage and in patients with normal renal function treated with higher doses and/or for longer periods than recommended. Aminoglycoside-induced ototoxicity is usually irreversible. Other manifestations of neurotoxicity may include numbness, skin tingling, muscle twitching and convulsions.
Renal and eighth cranial nerve function should be closely monitored, especially in patients with known or suspected reduced renal function at onset of therapy and also in those whose renal function is initially normal but who develop signs of renal dysfunction

during therapy. Urine should be examined for decreased specific gravity, increased excretion of protein, and the presence of cells or casts. Blood urea nitrogen, serum creatinine, or creatinine clearance should be determined periodically. When feasible, it is recommended that serial audiograms be obtained in patients old enough to be tested, particularly high-risk patients. Evidence of ototoxicity (dizziness, vertigo, tinnitus, roaring in the ears or hearing loss) or nephrotoxicity requires dosage adjustment or discontinuance of the drug. As with the other aminoglycosides, on rare occasions changes in renal and eighth cranial nerve function may not become manifest until soon after completion of therapy.

Serum concentrations of aminoglycosides should be monitored when feasible to assure adequate levels and to avoid potentially toxic levels. When monitoring gentamicin peak concentrations, dosage should be adjusted so that prolonged levels above 12 mcg/ml are avoided. When monitoring gentamicin trough concentrations, dosage should be adjusted so that levels above 2 mcg/ml are avoided. Excessive peak and/or trough serum concentrations of aminoglycosides may increase the risk of renal and eighth cranial nerve toxicity. In the event of overdose or toxic reactions, hemodialysis may aid in the removal of gentamicin from the blood, especially if renal function is, or becomes, compromised. Removal of gentamicin by peritoneal dialysis is at a rate considerably less than by hemodialysis.

Concurrent and/or sequential systemic or topical use of other potentially neurotoxic and/or nephrotoxic drugs, such as cisplatin, cephaloridine, kanamycin, amikacin, neomycin, polymyxin B, colistin, paromomycin, streptomycin, tobramycin, vancomycin, and viomycin, should be avoided. Other factors which may increase patient risk of toxicity are advanced age and dehydration.

The concurrent use of gentamicin with potent diuretics, such as ethacrynic acid or furosemide, should be avoided, since certain diuretics by themselves may cause ototoxicity. In addition, when administered intravenously, diuretics may enhance aminoglycoside toxicity by altering the antibiotic concentration in serum and tissue.

Description: Gentamicin sulfate, USP, a water-soluble antibiotic of the aminoglycoside group, is derived from *Micromonospora purpurea*, an actinomycete. GARAMYCIN Injectable is a sterile, aqueous solution for parenteral administration. Each ml. contains gentamicin sulfate, USP equivalent to 40 mg. gentamicin base, 1.8 mg. methylparaben and 0.2 mg. propylparaben as preservatives, 3.2 mg. sodium bisulfite, and 0.1 mg. edetate disodium.

Clinical Pharmacology: After intramuscular administration of GARAMYCIN Injectable, peak serum concentrations usually occur between 30 and 60 minutes and serum levels are measurable for six to eight hours. When gentamicin is administered by intravenous infusion over a two-hour period, the serum concentrations are similar to those obtained by intramuscular administration.

In patients with normal renal function, peak serum concentrations of gentamicin (mcg/ml) are usually up to four times the single intramuscular dose (mg/kg); for example, a 1.0 mg/kg injection in adults may be expected to result in a peak serum concentration up to 4 mcg/ml; a 1.5 mg/kg dose may produce levels up to 6 mcg/ml. While some variation is to be expected due to a number of variables such as age, body temperature surface area and physiological differences, the individual patient given the same dose tends to have similar levels in repeated determinations. Gentamicin administered at 1.0 mg/kg every eight hours for the usual 7- to 10-day treatment period to patients with normal renal function does not accumulate in serum.

Gentamicin, like all aminoglycosides, may accumulate in the serum and tissues of patients treated with higher doses and/or for prolonged periods, particularly in the presence of impaired renal function. In adult patients, treatment with gentamicin dosages of 4 mg/kg/day or higher for seven to ten days may result in a slight, progressive rise in both peak and trough concentrations. In patients with impaired renal function, gentamicin is cleared from the body more slowly than in patients with normal renal function. The more severe the impairment, the slower the clearance. (Dosage must be adjusted.)

Since gentamicin is distributed in extracellular fluid, peak serum concentrations may be lower than usual in adult patients who have a large volume of this fluid. Serum concentrations of gentamicin in febrile patients may be lower than those in afebrile patients given the same dose. When body temperature returns to normal serum concentrations of the drug may rise. Febrile and anemic states may be associated with a shorter than usual serum half-life. (Dosage adjustment is usually not necessary.) In severely burned patients, the half-life may be significantly decreased and resulting serum concentrations may be lower than anticipated from the mg/kg dose.

Protein binding studies have indicated that the degree of gentamicin binding is low; depending upon the methods used for testing, this may be between 0 and 30%.

After initial administration to patients with normal renal function, generally 70% or more of the gentamicin dose is recoverable in the urine in 24 hours, concentrations in urine above 100 mcg/ml may be achieved. Little, if any, metabolic transformation occurs; the drug is excreted principally by glomerular filtration. After several days of treatment, the amount of gentamicin excreted in the urine approaches the daily dose administered. As with other aminoglycosides, a small amount of the gentamicin dose may be retained in the tissues, especially in the kidneys. Minute quantities of aminoglycosides have been detected in the urine weeks after drug administration was discontinued. Renal clearance of gentamicin is similar to that of endogenous creatinine.

In patients with marked impairment of renal function, there is a decrease in the concentration of aminoglycosides in urine and in their penetration into defective renal parenchyma. This decreased drug excretion, together with the potential nephrotoxicity of aminoglycosides, should be considered when treating such patients who have urinary tract infections.

Probenecid does not affect renal tubular transport of gentamicin.

The endogenous creatinine clearance rate and the serum creatinine level have a high correlation with the half-life of gentamicin in serum. Results of these tests may serve as guides for adjusting dosage in patients with renal impairment (see DOSAGE AND ADMINISTRATION).

Following parenteral administration, gentamicin can be detected in serum, lymph, tissues, sputum, and in pleural, synovial, and peritoneal fluids. Concentrations in renal cortex sometimes may be eight times higher than the usual serum levels. Concentrations in bile, in general, have been low and have suggested minimal biliary excretion. Gentamicin crosses the peritoneum as well as the placental membranes. Since aminoglycosides diffuse poorly into the subarachnoid space after parenteral administration, concentrations of gentamicin in cerebrospinal fluid are often low and dependent upon dose, rate of penetration, and degree of meningeal inflammation. There is minimal penetration of gentamicin into ocular tissues following intramuscular or intravenous administration.

Microbiology: *In vitro* tests have demonstrated that gentamicin is a bactericidal antibiotic which acts by inhibiting normal protein synthesis in susceptible microorganisms. It is active against a wide variety of pathogenic bacteria including *Escherichia coli*, *Proteus* species, (indole-positive and indole-negative), *Pseudomonas aeruginosa*, species of the *Klebsiella-Enterobacter-Serratia* group. *Citrobacter* species and *Staphylococcus* species (including penicillin- and methicillin-resistant strains). Gentamicin is also active *in vitro* against species of *Salmonella* and *Shigella*. The following bacteria are usually resistant to aminoglycoside: *Streptococcus pneumoniae*, most species of streptococci, particularly group D and anaerobic organisms, such as *Bacteroides* species or *Clostridium* species.

In vitro studies have shown that an aminoglycoside combined with an antibiotic that interferes with cell wall synthesis may act synergistically against some group D streptococcal strains. The combination of gentamicin and penicillin G has a synergistic bactericidal effect against virtually all strains of *Streptococcus faecalis* and its varieties (*S. faecalis* var. *liquifaciens*, *S. faecalis* var. *zymogenes*), *S. faecium* and *S. durans*. An enhanced killing effect against many of these strains has also been shown *in vitro* with combinations of gentamicin and ampicillin, carbenicillin, nafcillin, or oxacillin.

The combined effect of gentamicin and carbenicillin is synergistic for many strains of *Pseudomonas aeruginosa*. *In vitro* synergism against other gram-negative organisms has been shown with combinations of gentamicin and cephalosporins.

Gentamicin may be active against clinical isolates of bacteria resistant to other aminoglycosides. Bacteria resistant to one aminoglycoside may be resistant to one or more other aminoglycosides. Bacterial resistance to gentamicin is generally developed slowly.

Susceptibility Testing: If the disc method of susceptibility testing used is that described by Bauer et al. (*Am J Clin Path* 45:493, 1966; *Federal Register* 37:20525-20529, 1972), a disc containing 10 mcg of gentamicin should give a zone of inhibition of 15mm. or more to indicate susceptibility of the infecting organism. A zone of 12mm. or less indicates that the infecting organism is likely to be resistant. Zones greater than 12mm and less than 15mm indicate intermediate susceptibility. In certain conditions it may be desirable to do additional susceptibility testing by the tube or agar dilution method; gentamicin substance is available for this purpose.

Indications and Usage: GARAMYCIN Injectable is indicated in the treatment of serious infections caused by susceptible strains of the following microorganisms: *Pseudomonas aeruginosa*, *Proteus* species (indole-positive and indole-negative), *Escherichia coli*, *Klebsiella-Enterobacter-Serratia* species, *Citrobacter* species and *Staphylococcus* species (coagulase-positive and coagulase-negative).

Clinical studies have shown GARAMYCIN Injectable to be effective in bacterial neonatal sepsis; bacterial septicemia; and serious bacterial infections of the central nervous system (meningitis), urinary tract, respiratory tract, gastrointestinal tract (including peritonitis), skin, bone and soft tissue (including burns). Aminoglycosides, including gentamicin, are not indicated in uncomplicated initial episodes of urinary tract infections unless the causative organisms are susceptible to these antibiotics and are not susceptible to antibiotics having less potential for toxicity.

Specimens for bacterial culture should be obtained to isolate and identify causative organisms and to determine their susceptibility to gentamicin.

GARAMYCIN may be considered as initial therapy in suspected or confirmed gram-negative infections, and therapy may be instituted before obtaining results of susceptibility testing. The decision to continue therapy with this drug should be based on the results of susceptibility tests, the severity of the infection, and the important additional concepts contained in the "WARNINGS Box" above. If the causative organisms are resistant to gentamicin, other appropriate therapy should be instituted.

Continued on next page

Information on Schering products appearing on these pages is effective as of September 30, 1984.

Schering—Cont.

In serious infections when the causative organisms are unknown, GARAMYCIN may be administered as initial therapy in conjunction with a penicillin-type or cephalosporin-type drug before obtaining results of susceptibility testing. If anaerobic organisms are suspected as etiologic agents, consideration should be given to using other suitable antimicrobial therapy in conjunction with gentamicin. Following identification of the organism and its susceptibility, appropriate antibiotic therapy should then be continued.

GARAMYCIN has been used effectively in combination with carbenicillin for the treatment of life-threatening infections caused by *Pseudomonas aeruginosa*. It has also been found effective when used in conjunction with a penicillin-type drug for the treatment of endocarditis caused by group D streptococci.

GARAMYCIN Injectable has also been shown to be effective in the treatment of serious staphylococcal infections. While not the antibiotic of first choice, GARAMYCIN Injectable may be considered when penicillins or other less potentially toxic drugs are contraindicated and bacterial susceptibility tests and clinical judgment indicate its use. It may also be considered in mixed infections caused by susceptible strains of staphylococci and gram-negative organisms.

In the neonate with suspected bacterial sepsis or staphylococcal pneumonia, a penicillin-type drug is also usually indicated as concomitant therapy with gentamicin.

Contraindications: Hypersensitivity to gentamicin is a contraindication to its use. A history of hypersensitivity or serious toxic reactions to other aminoglycosides may contraindicate use of gentamicin because of the known cross-sensitivity of patients to drugs in this class.

Warnings: (See "WARNINGS Box" above.)

Precautions: Neurotoxic and nephrotoxic antibiotics may be absorbed in significant quantities from body surfaces after local irrigation or application. The potential toxic effect of antibiotics administered in this fashion should be considered.

Increased nephrotoxicity has been reported following concomitant administration of aminoglycoside antibiotics and cephalosporins.

Neuromuscular blockade and respiratory paralysis have been reported in the cat receiving high doses (40 mg/kg) of gentamicin. The possibility of these phenomena occurring in man should be considered if aminoglycosides are administered by any route to patients receiving anesthetics, or to patients receiving neuromuscular blocking agents, such as succinylcholine, tubocurarine, or decamethonium, or in patients receiving massive transfusions of citrate-anticoagulated blood. If neuromuscular blockade occurs, calcium salts may reverse it.

Aminoglycosides should be used with caution in patients with neuromuscular disorders, such as myasthenia gravis or parkinsonism, since these drugs may aggravate muscle weakness because of their potential curare-like effects on the neuromuscular junction.

Elderly patients may have reduced renal function which may not be evident in the results of routine screening tests, such as BUN or serum creatinine. A creatinine clearance determination may be more useful. Monitoring of renal function during treatment with gentamicin, as with other aminoglycosides, is particularly important in such patients.

Cross-allergenicity among aminoglycosides has been demonstrated.

Patients should be well hydrated during treatment.

Although the *in vitro* mixing of gentamicin and carbenicillin results in a rapid and significant inactivation of gentamicin, this interaction has not been demonstrated in patients with normal renal function who received both drugs by different routes of administration. A reduction in gentamicin serum half-life has been reported in patients with severe renal impairment receiving carbenicillin concomitantly with gentamicin.

Treatment with gentamicin may result in overgrowth of nonsusceptible organisms. If this occurs, appropriate therapy is indicated.

See "WARNINGS Box" regarding concurrent use of potent diuretics and regarding concurrent and/or sequential use of other neurotoxic and/or nephrotoxic antibiotics and for other essential information.

Usage in Pregnancy—Safety for use in pregnancy has not been established.

Adverse Reactions: *Nephrotoxicity:* Adverse renal effects, as demonstrated by the presence of casts, cells, or protein in the urine or by rising BUN, NPN, serum creatinine or oliguria, have been reported. They occur more frequently in patients with a history of renal impairment and in patients treated for longer periods or with larger dosage than recommended.

Neurotoxicity: Serious adverse effects on both vestibular and auditory branches of the eighth nerve have been reported, primarily in patients with renal impairment (especially if dialysis is required), and in patients on high doses and/or prolonged therapy. Symptoms include dizziness, vertigo, tinnitus, roaring in the ears and also hearing loss, which, as with the other aminoglycosides, may be irreversible. Hearing loss is usually manifested initially by diminution of high-tone acuity. Other factors which may increase the risk of toxicity include excessive dosage, dehydration and previous exposure to other ototoxic drugs.

Numbness, skin tingling, muscle twitching and convulsions have also been reported.

Note: The risk of toxic reactions is low in patients with normal renal function who do not receive GARAMYCIN Injectable at higher doses or for longer periods of time than recommended.

Other reported adverse reactions possibly related to gentamicin include: respiratory depression, lethargy, confusion, depression, visual disturbances, decreased appetite, weight loss, and hypotension and hypertension; rash, itching, urticaria, generalized burning, laryngeal edema, anaphylactoid reactions, fever, and headache, nausea, vomiting, increased salivation, and stomatitis; purpura, pseudotumor cerebri, acute organic brain syndrome, pulmonary fibrosis, alopecia, joint pain, transient hepatomegaly, and splenomegaly.

Laboratory abnormalities possibly related to gentamicin include: increased levels of serum transaminase (SGOT, SGPT), serum LDH and bilirubin; decreased serum calcium, magnesium, sodium and potassium; anemia, leukopenia, granulocytopenia, transient agranulocytosis, eosinophilia, increased and decreased reticulocyte counts, and thrombocytopenia.

While local tolerance of GARAMYCIN Injectable is generally excellent, there has been an occasional report of pain at the injection site. Subcutaneous atrophy or fat necrosis suggesting local irritation has been reported rarely.

Overdosage: In the event of overdose or toxic reactions, hemodialysis may aid in the removal of gentamicin from the blood, especially if renal function is, or becomes, compromised. Removal of gentamicin by peritoneal dialysis is at a rate considerably less than by hemodialysis.

Dosage and Administration: GARAMYCIN Injectable may be given intramuscularly or intravenously. The patient's pretreatment body weight should be obtained for calculation of correct dosage. The dosage of aminoglycosides in obese patients should be based on an estimate of the lean body mass. It is desirable to limit the duration of treatment with aminoglycosides to short term.

PATIENTS WITH NORMAL RENAL FUNCTION

Adults: The recommended dosage of GARAMYCIN Injectable for patients with serious infections and normal renal function is 3 mg/kg/day, administered in three equal doses every eight hours (Table I).

For patients with life-threatening infections, dosages up to 5 mg/kg/day may be administered in three or four equal doses. This dosage should be reduced to 3 mg/kg/day as soon as clinically indicated (Table I).

It is desirable to measure both peak and trough serum concentrations of gentamicin to determine the adequacy and safety of the dosage. When such measurements are feasible, they should be carried out periodically during therapy to assure adequate but not excessive drug levels. For example, the peak concentration (at 30 to 60 minutes after intramuscular injection) is expected to be in the range of 4 to 6 mcg/ml. When monitoring peak concentrations after intramuscular or intravenous administration, dosage should be adjusted so that prolonged levels above 12 mcg/ml are avoided. When monitoring trough concentrations (just prior to the next dose), dosage should be adjusted so that levels above 2 mcg/ml are avoided. Determination of the adequacy of a serum level for a particular patient must take into consideration the susceptibility of the causative organism, the severity of the infection, and the status of the patient's host-defense mechanisms.

In patients with extensive burns, altered pharmacokinetics may result in reduced serum concentrations of aminoglycosides. In such patients treated with gentamicin, measurement of serum concentrations is recommended as a basis for dosage adjustment.

TABLE I
DOSAGE SCHEDULE GUIDE FOR ADULTS WITH NORMAL RENAL FUNCTION
(Dosage at Eight-Hour Intervals)
40 mg. per ml.

Patient's Weight*		Usual Dose For Serious Infections 1 mg/kg q8h (3 mg/kg/day)		Dose for Life-Threatening Infections (Reduce as Soon as Clinically Indicated) 1.7 mg/kg q8h** (5 mg/kg/day)	
kg	(lb)	mg/dose q8h	ml/dose	mg/dose q8h	ml/dose
40	(88)	40	1.0	66	1.6
45	(99)	45	1.1	75	1.9
50	(110)	50	1.25	83	2.1
55	(121)	55	1.4	91	2.25
60	(132)	60	1.5	100	2.5
65	(143)	65	1.6	108	2.7
70	(154)	70	1.75	116	2.9
75	(165)	75	1.9	125	3.1
80	(176)	80	2.0	133	3.3
85	(187)	85	2.1	141	3.5
90	(198)	90	2.25	150	3.75
95	(209)	95	2.4	158	4.0
100	(220)	100	2.5	166	4.2

* The dosage of aminoglycosides in obese patients should be based on an estimate of the lean body mass.

** For q6h schedules, dosage should be recalculated.

Children: 6 to 7.5 mg/kg/day. (2.0 to 2.5 mg/kg administered every 8 hours.)

Infants and Neonates: 7.5 mg/kg/day. (2.5 mg/kg administered every 8 hours.)

Premature or Full-Term Neonates One Week of Age or Less: 5 mg/kg/day. (2.5 mg/kg administered every 12 hours).

For further information concerning the use of gentamicin in infants and children, see GARAMYCIN Pediatric Injectable Product Information.

The usual duration of treatment for all patients is seven to ten days. In difficult and complicated infections, a longer course of therapy may be necessary. In such cases monitoring of renal, auditory, and vestibular functions is recommended, since toxicity is more apt to occur with treatment extended for more than ten days. Dosage should be reduced if clinically indicated.

For Intravenous Administration

The intravenous administration of gentamicin may be particularly useful for treating patients with bacterial septicemia or those in shock. It may also be the preferred route of administration for some patients with congestive heart failure, hematologic disorders, severe burns, or those with reduced muscle mass. For intermittent intravenous administration in adults, a single dose of GARAMYCIN Injectable may be diluted in 50 to 200 ml. of sterile isotonic saline solution or in a sterile solution of dextrose 5% in water; in infants and children, the volume of diluent should be less. The solution may be infused over a period of one-half to two hours.

The recommended dosage for intravenous and intramuscular administration is identical.

GARAMYCIN Injectable should not be physically premixed with other drugs, but should be administered separately in accordance with the recommended route of administration and dosage schedule.

PATIENTS WITH IMPAIRED RENAL FUNCTION

Dosage must be adjusted in patients with impaired renal function. Whenever possible, serum concentrations of gentamicin should be monitored. One method of dosage adjustment is to increase the interval between administration of the usual doses. Since the serum creatinine concentration has a high correlation with the serum half-life of gentamicin, this laboratory test may provide guidance for adjustment of the interval between doses. The interval between doses (in hours) may be approximated by multiplying the serum creatinine level (mg/100 ml) by 8. For example, a patient weighing 60 kg. with a serum creatinine level of 2.0 mg/100 ml could be given 60 mg. (1 mg/kg) every 16 hours (2 × 8).

In patients with serious systemic infections and renal impairment, it may be desirable to administer the antibiotic more frequently but in reduced dosage. In such patients, serum concentrations of gentamicin should be measured so that adequate but not excessive levels result. A peak and trough concentration measured intermittently during therapy will provide optimal guidance for adjusting dosage. After the usual initial dose, a rough guide for determining reduced dosage at eight-hour intervals is to divide the normally recommended dose by the serum creatinine level (Table II). For example, after an initial dose of 60 mg. (1 mg/kg), a patient weighing 60 kg. with a serum creatinine level of 2.0 mg/100 ml could be given 30 mg. every eight hours (60÷2). It should be noted that the status of renal function may be changing over the course of the infectious process.

It is important to recognize that deteriorating renal function may require a greater reduction in dosage than that specified in the above guidelines for patients with stable renal impairment.

TABLE II
DOSAGE ADJUSTMENT GUIDE FOR PATIENTS WITH RENAL IMPAIRMENT
(Dosage at Eight-Hour Intervals After the Usual Initial Dose)

Serum Creatinine (mg %)	Approximate Creatinine Clearance Rate (ml/min/1.73M^2)	Percent of Usual Doses Shown in Table I
≤ 1.0	> 100	100
1.1–1.3	70–100	80
1.4–1.6	55–70	65
1.7–1.9	45–55	55
2.0–2.2	40–45	50
2.3–2.5	35–40	40
2.6–3.0	30–35	35
3.1–3.5	25–30	30
3.6–4.0	20–25	25
4.1–5.1	15–20	20
5.2–6.6	10–15	15
6.7–8.0	< 10	10

In adults with renal failure undergoing hemodialysis, the amount of gentamicin removed from the blood may vary depending upon several factors including the dialysis method used. An eight-hour hemodialysis may reduce serum concentrations of gentamicin by approximately 50%. The recommended dosage at the end of each dialysis period is 1 to 1.7 mg/kg depending upon the severity of infection. In children, a dose of 2 mg/kg may be administered.

The above dosage schedules are not intended as rigid recommendations but are provided as guides to dosage when the measurement of gentamicin serum levels is not feasible.

A variety of methods are available to measure gentamicin concentrations in body fluids; these include microbiologic, enzymatic and radioimmunoassay techniques.

How Supplied: GARAMYCIN Injectable, 40 mg. per ml., for parenteral administration, is supplied in 2 ml. (80 mg.) vials, boxes of 1 and 25; 20 ml. (800 mg) vials, box of 5; and in 1.5 ml. (60 mg.) and 2 ml. (80 mg.) disposable syringes, each in boxes of 1 and 10.

Also available, GARAMYCIN Pediatric Injectable, 10 mg. per ml., for parenteral administration, supplied in 2 ml. (20 mg) vials; box of one.

GARAMYCIN Injectable is a clear, stable solution that requires no refrigeration.

Store between 2° and 30°C (36° and 86°F).

Schering Pharmaceutical Corporation (PR)
Manati, Puerto Rico 00701
An Affiliate of Schering Corporation
Kenilworth, N.J. 07033
Copyright © 1968, 1983, Schering Corporation.
All rights reserved.
Revised 10/83

GARAMYCIN® PEDIATRIC   ℞
[gar-ah-mī'sin]
Injectable
brand of gentamicin sulfate injection, USP
10 mg. per ml.

Each ml. contains gentamicin sulfate, USP equivalent to 10 mg. gentamicin.
For Parenteral Administration

WARNINGS

Patients treated with aminoglycosides should be under close clinical observation because of the potential toxicity associated with their use.

As with other aminoglycosides, GARAMYCIN Pediatric Injectable is potentially nephrotoxic. The risk of nephrotoxicity is greater in patients with impaired renal function and in those who receive high dosage or prolonged therapy.

Neurotoxicity manifested by ototoxicity, both vestibular and auditory, can occur in patients treated with GARAMYCIN Pediatric Injectable, primarily in those with pre-existing renal damage and in patients with normal renal function treated with higher doses and/or for longer periods than recommended. Aminoglycoside-induced ototoxicity is usually irreversible. Other manifestations of neurotoxicity may include numbness, skin tingling, muscle twitching, and convulsions.

Renal and eighth cranial nerve function should be closely monitored, especially in patients with known or suspected reduced renal function at onset of therapy and also in those whose renal function is initially normal but who develop signs of renal dysfunction during therapy. Urine should be examined for decreased specific gravity, increased excretion of protein, and the presence of cells or casts. Blood urea nitrogen, serum creatinine, or creatinine clearance should be determined periodically. When feasible, it is recommended that serial audiograms be obtained in patients old enough to be tested, particularly high-risk patients. Evidence of ototoxicity (dizziness, vertigo, tinnitus, roaring in the ears or hearing loss) or nephrotoxicity requires dosage adjustment or discontinuance of the drug. As with the other aminoglycosides, on rare occasions changes in renal and eighth cranial nerve function may not become manifest until soon after completion of therapy.

Serum concentrations of aminoglycosides should be monitored when feasible to assure adequate levels and to avoid potentially toxic levels. When monitoring gentamicin peak concentrations, dosage should be adjusted so that prolonged levels above 12 mcg/ml are avoided. When monitoring gentamicin trough concentrations, dosage should be adjusted so that levels above 2 mcg/ml are avoided. Excessive peak and/or trough serum concentrations of aminoglycosides may increase the risk of renal and eighth cranial nerve toxicity. In the event of overdose or toxic reactions, hemodialysis may aid in the removal of gentamicin from the blood, especially if renal function is, or becomes, compromised. Removal of gentamicin by peritoneal dialysis is at a rate considerably less than by hemodialysis.

In the newborn infant, exchange transfusions may also be considered.

Concurrent and/or sequential systemic or topical use of other potentially neurotoxic and/or nephrotoxic drugs, such as cisplatin, cephaloridine, kanamycin, amikacin, neomycin, polymyxin B, colistin, paromomycin, streptomycin, tobramycin, vancomycin, and viomycin, should be avoided. Another factor which may increase patient risk of toxicity is dehydration.

The concurrent use of gentamicin with potent diuretics, such as ethacrynic acid or furosemide, should be avoided, since certain diuretics by themselves may cause ototoxicity. In addition, when administered intravenously, diuretics may enhance aminoglycoside toxicity by altering the antibiotic concentration in serum and tissue.

Description: Gentamicin sulfate, USP, a water-soluble antibiotic of the aminoglycoside group, is derived from *Micromonospora purpurea*, an actinomycete. GARAMYCIN Pediatric Injectable is a sterile, aqueous solution for parenteral administration. Each ml. contains gentamicin sulfate, USP equivalent to 10 mg. gentamicin base, 1.3 mg. methylparaben and 0.2 mg. propylparaben as preservatives, 3.2 mg. sodium bisulfite and 0.1 mg. edetate disodium.

Clinical Pharmacology: After intramuscular administration of GARAMYCIN Pediatric Injectable, peak serum concentrations usually occur between 30 and 60 minutes and serum levels are measurable for 6 to 12 hours. In infants, a single dose of 2.5 mg/kg usually provides a peak serum level in the range of 3 to 5 mcg/ml. When gentamicin is administered by intravenous infusion over a two-hour period, the serum concentrations are similar to those obtained by intramuscular administration. Age markedly affects the peak concentrations: in one report, a 1 mg/kg dose produced mean peak concentrations of 1.58, 2.03, and 2.81 mcg/ml in patients 6 months to 5 years old, 5 to 10 years old, and over 10 years old, respectively.

In infants one week to six months of age, the half-life is 3 to 3½ hours. In full-term and large premature infants less than one week old, the appropriate serum half-life of gentamicin is 5½ hours. In small premature infants, the half-life is inversely related to birth weight. In premature infants weighing less than 1500 grams, the half-life is 11½ hours; in those weighing 1500 to 2000 grams, the half-life is 8 hours; in those weighing over 2000 grams, the half-life is approximately 5 hours. While some variation is to be expected due to a number of variables such as age, body temperature, surface area and physiologic differences, the individual patient given the same dose tends to have similar levels in repeated determinations. Gentamicin, like all aminoglycosides, may accumulate in the serum and tissues of patients treated with higher doses and/or for prolonged periods,

Continued on next page

Information on Schering products appearing on these pages is effective as of September 30, 1984.

Schering—Cont.

particularly in the presence of impaired or immature renal function. In patients with immature or impaired renal function, gentamicin is cleared from the body more slowly than in patients with normal renal function. The more severe the impairment, the slower the clearance. (Dosage must be adjusted.)

Since gentamicin is distributed in extracellular fluid, peak serum concentrations may be lower than usual in patients who have a large volume of this fluid. Serum concentrations of gentamicin in febrile patients may be lower than those in afebrile patients given the same dose. When body temperature returns to normal, serum concentrations of the drug may rise. Febrile and anemic states may be associated with a shorter than usual serum half-life. (Dosage adjustment is usually not necessary.) In severly burned patients, the half-life may be significantly decreased and resulting serum concentrations may be lower than anticipated from the mg/kg/dose.

Protein binding studies have indicated that the degree of gentamicin binding is low, depending upon the methods used for testing, this may be between 0 and 30%.

In neonates less than 3 days old, approximately 10% of the administered dose is excreted in 12 hours; in infants 5 to 40 days old, approximately 40% is excreted over the same period. Excretion of gentamicin correlates with postnatal age and creatinine clearance. Thus, with increasing postnatal age and concomitant increase in renal maturity, gentamicin is excreted more rapidly. Little, if any metabolic transformation occurs; the drug is excreted principally by glomerular filtration. After several days of treatment, the amount of gentamicin excreted in the urine approaches, but does not equal, the daily dose administered. As with other aminoglycosides, a small amount of the gentamicin dose may be retained in the tissues, especially in the kidneys. Minute quantities of aminoglycosides have been detected in the urine of some patients weeks after drug administration was discontinued. Renal clearance of gentamicin is similar to that of endogenous creatinine.

In patients with marked impairment of renal function, there is a decrease in the concentration of aminoglycosides in urine and in their penetration into defective renal parenchyma. This decreased drug excretion, together with the potential nephrotoxicity of aminoglycosides, should be considered when treating such patients who have urinary tract infections.

Probenecid does not affect renal tubular transport of gentamicin.

The endogenous creatinine clearance rate and the serum creatinine level have a high correlation with the half-life of gentamicin in serum. Results of these tests may serve as guides for adjusting dosage in patients with renal impairment (see DOSAGE AND ADMINISTRATION).

Following parenteral administration, gentamicin can be detected in serum, lymph, tissues, sputum and in pleural, synovial, peritoneal fluids. Concentrations in renal cortex sometimes may be eight times higher than the usual serum levels. Concentrations in bile, in general, have been low and have suggested minimal biliary excretion. Gentamicin crosses the peritoneal as well as the placental membranes. Since aminoglycosides diffuse poorly into the subarachnoid space after parenteral administration, concentrations of gentamicin in cerebrospinal fluid are often low and dependent upon dose, rate of penetration, and degree of meningeal inflammation. There is minimal penetration of gentamicin into ocular tissues following intramuscular or intravenous administration.

Microbiology: *In vitro* tests have demonstrated that gentamicin is a bactericidal antibiotic which acts by inhibiting normal protein synthesis in susceptible microorganisms. It is active against a wide variety of pathogenic bacteria including *Escherichia coli*, *Proteus* species (indole-positive and indole-negative), *Pseudomonas aeruginosa*, species of *Klebsiella-Enterobacter-Serratia* group, *Citrobacter* species, and *Staphylococcus* species (including penicillin- and methicillin-resistant strains). Gentamicin is also active *in vitro* against species of *Salmonella* and *Shigella*. The following bacteria are usually resistant to aminoglycosides: *Streptococcus pneumoniae*, most species of streptococci, particularly group D and anaerobic organisms, such as *Bacteroides* species or *Clostridium* species. *In vitro* studies have shown that an aminoglycoside combined with an antibiotic that interferes with cell wall synthesis may act synergistically against some group D streptococcal strains. The combination of gentamicin and penicillin G has a synergistic bactericidal effect against virtually all strains of *Streptococcus faecalis* and its varieties (*S. faecalis* var. *liquifaciens, S. faecalis* var. *zymogenes), S. faecium* and *S. durans*. An enhanced killing effect against many of these strains has also been shown *in vitro* with combinations of gentamicin and ampicillin, carbenicillin, nafcillin, or oxacillin.

The combined effect of gentamicin and carbenicillin is synergistic for many strains of *Pseudomonas aeruginosa*. *In vitro* synergism against other gram-negative organisms has been shown with combinations of gentamicin and cephalosporins.

Gentamicin may be active against clinical isolates of bacteria resistant to other aminoglycosides. Bacteria resistant to one aminoglycoside may be resistant to one or more other aminoglycosides. Bacterial resistance to gentamicin is generally developed slowly.

Susceptibility Testing: If the disc method of susceptibility testing used is that described by Bauer et al (*Am J Clin Path* 45:493, 1966; *Federal Register* 37:20525–20529, 1972), a disc containing 10 mcg. of gentamicin should give a zone of inhibition of 15 mm or more to indicate susceptibility of the infecting organism. A zone of 12 mm or less indicates that the infecting organism is likely to be resistant. Zones greater than 12mm and less than 15mm indicate intermediate susceptibility. In certain conditions it may be desirable to do additional susceptibility testing by the tube or agar dilution method; gentamicin substance is available for this purpose.

Indications and Usage: GARAMYCIN Pediatric Injectable is indicated in the treatment of serious infections caused by susceptible strains of the following microorganisms: *Pseudomonas aeruginosa, Proteus* species (indole-positive and indole-negative), *Escherichia coli, Klebsiella-Enterobacter-Serratia* species, *Citrobacter* species, and *Staphyloccus* species (coagulase-positive and coagulase-negative).

Clinical studies have shown GARAMYCIN Pediatric Injectable to be effective in bacterial neonatal sepsis; bacterial septicemia; and serious bacterial infections of the central nervous system (meningitis), urinary tract, respiratory tract, gastrointestinal tract (including peritonitis), skin, bone and soft tissue (including burns).

Aminoglycosides, including gentamicin, are not indicated in uncomplicated initial episodes of urinary tract infections unless the causative organisms are susceptible to these antibiotics and are not susceptible to antibiotics having less potential for toxicity.

Specimens for bacterial culture should be obtained to isolate and identify causative organisms and to determine their susceptibility to gentamicin.

GARAMYCIN may be considered as initial therapy in suspected or confirmed gram-negative infections, and therapy may be instituted before obtaining results of susceptibility testing. The decision to continue therapy with this drug should be based on the results of susceptibility tests, the severity of the infection, and the important additional concepts contained in the "WARNINGS Box" above. If the causative organisms are resistant to gentamicin, other appropriate therapy should be instituted.

In serious infections when the causative organisms are unknown, GARAMYCIN may be administered as initial therapy in conjunction with a penicillin-type or cephalosporin-type drug before obtaining results of susceptibility testing. If anaerobic organisms are suspected as etiologic agents, consideration should be given to using other suitable antimicrobial therapy in conjunction with gentamicin. Following identification of the organism and its susceptibility, appropriate antibiotic therapy should then be continued.

GARAMYCIN has been used effectively in combination with carbenicillin for the treatment of life-threatening infections caused by *Pseudomonas aeruginosa*. It has also been found effective when used in conjunction with a penicillin-type drug for the treatment of endocarditis caused by group D streptococci.

GARAMYCIN Pediatric Injectable has also been shown to be effective in the treatment of serious staphylococcal infections. While not the antibiotic of first choice, GARAMYCIN Pediatric Injectable may be considered when penicillins or other less potentially toxic drugs are contraindicated and bacterial susceptibility tests and clinical judgment indicate its use. It may also be considered in mixed infections caused by susceptible strains of staphylococci and gram-negative organisms.

In the neonate with suspected bacterial sepsis or staphylococcal pneumonia, a penicillin-type drug is also usually indicated as concomitant therapy with gentamicin.

Contraindications: Hypersensitivity to gentamicin is a contraindication to its use. A history of hypersensitivity or serious toxic reactions to other aminoglycosides may contraindicate use of gentamicin because of the known cross-sensitivity of patients to drugs in this class.

Warnings: (See "WARNINGS Box" above.)

Precautions: Neurotoxic and nephrotoxic antibiotics may be absorbed in significant quantities from body surfaces after local irrigation or application. The potential toxic effect of antibiotics administered in this fashion should be considered.

Increased nephrotoxicity has been reported following concomitant administration of aminoglycoside antibiotics and cephalosporins.

Neuromuscular blockade and respiratory paralysis have been reported in the cat receiving high doses (40 mg/kg) of gentamicin. The possibility of these phenomena occurring in man should be considered if aminoglycosides are administered by any route to patients receiving anesthetics, or to patients receiving neuromuscular blocking agents, such as succinylcholine, tubocurarine, or decamethonium, or in patients receiving massive transfusions of citrate-anticoagulated blood. If neuromuscular blockade occurs, calcium salts may reverse it.

Aminoglycosides should be used with caution in patients with neuromuscular disorders, such as myasthenia gravis or parkinsonism, since these drugs may aggravate muscle weakness because of their potential curare-like effects on the neuromuscular junction.

Cross-allergenicity among aminoglycosides has been demonstrated.

Patients should be well hydrated during treatment.

Although the *in vitro* mixing of gentamicin and carbenicillin results in a rapid and significant inactivation of gentamicin, this interaction has not been demonstrated in patients with normal renal function who received both drugs by different routes of administration. A reduction in gentamicin serum half-life has been reported in patients with severe renal impairment receiving carbenicillin concomitantly with gentamicin.

Treatment with gentamicin may result in overgrowth of nonsusceptible organisms. If this occurs, appropriate therapy is indicated. See "WARNINGS Box" regarding concurrent use of potent diuretics and regarding concurrent and/or sequential use of other neurotoxic and/or nephrotoxic antibiotics and for other essential information.

Usage in Pregnancy—Safety for use in pregnancy has not been established.

Adverse Reactions: *Nephrotoxicity* Adverse renal effects, as demonstrated by the presence of casts, cells or protein in the urine or by rising BUN, NPN, serum creatinine or oliguria, have been reported. They occur more frequently in patients treated for longer periods or with larger dosages than recommended.

Neurotoxicity Serious adverse effects on both vestibular and auditory branches of the eighth nerve have been reported, primarily in patients with renal impairment (especially if dialysis is required), and in patients on high doses and/or prolonged therapy. Symptoms include dizziness, vertigo, tinnitus, roaring in the ears and also hearing loss, which, as with the other aminoglycosides, may be irreversible. Hearing loss is usually manifested initially by diminution of high-tone acuity. Other factors which may increase the risk of toxicity include excessive dosage, dehydration and previous exposure to other ototoxic drugs.

Numbness, skin tingling, muscle twitching and convulsions have also been reported.

Note: The risk of toxic reactions is low in neonates, infants and children with normal renal function who do not receive GARAMYCIN Pediatric Injectable at higher doses or for longer periods of time than recommended.

Other reported adverse reactions possibly related to gentamicin include: respiratory depression, lethargy, confusion, depression, visual disturbances, decreased appetite, weight loss and hypotension and hypertension; rash, itching, urticaria, generalized burning, laryngeal edema, anaphylactoid reactions, fever, and headache; nausea, vomiting, increased salivation, and stomatitis; purpura, pseudotumor cerebri, acute organic brain syndrome, pulmonary fibrosis, alopecia, joint pain, transient hepatomegaly, and splenomegaly.

Laboratory abnormalities possibly related to gentamicin include: increased levels of serum transaminase (SGOT, SGPT), serum LDH and bilirubin; decreased serum calcium, magnesium, sodium, and potassium; anemia, leukopenia, granulocytopenia, transient agranulocytosis, eosinophilia, increased and decreased reticulocyte counts, and thrombocytopenia.

While local tolerance of GARAMYCIN Pediatric Injectable is generally excellent, there has been an occasional report of pain at the injection site. Subcutaneous atrophy or fat necrosis suggesting local irritation has been reported rarely.

Overdosage: In the event of overdose or toxic reactions, hemodialysis may aid in the removal of gentamicin from the blood, especially if renal function is, or becomes, compromised. Removal of gentamicin by peritoneal dialysis is at a rate considerably less than by hemodialysis. In the newborn infant, exchange transfusions may also be considered.

Dosage and Administration: GARAMYCIN Pediatric Injectable may be given intramuscularly or intravenously. The patient's pretreatment body weight should be obtained for calculation of correct dosage. The dosage of aminoglycosides in obese patients should be based on an estimate of the lean body mass. It is desirable to limit the duration of treatment with aminoglycosides to short term.

PATIENTS WITH NORMAL RENAL FUNCTION

Children: 6 to 7.5 mg/kg/day. (2.0 to 2.5 mg/kg administered every 8 hours.)

Infants and Neonates: 7.5 mg/kg/day. (2.5 mg/kg administered every 8 hours.)

Premature or Full-Term Neonates One Week of Age or Less: 5 mg/kg/day. (2.5 mg/kg administered every 12 hours.)

It is desirable to measure both peak and trough serum concentrations of gentamicin to determine the adequacy and safety of the dosage. When such measurements are feasible, they should be carried out periodically during therapy to assure adequate but not excessive drug levels. For example, the peak concentration (at 30 to 60 minutes after intramuscular injection) is expected to be in the range of 3 to 5 mcg/ml. When monitoring peak concentrations after intramuscular or intravenous administration, dosage should be adjusted so that prolonged levels above 12 mcg/ml are avoided. When monitoring trough concentrations (just prior to the next dose), dosage should be adjusted so that levels above 2 mcg/ml are avoided.

Determination of the adequacy of a serum level for a particular patient must take into consideration the susceptibility of the causative organism, the severity of the infection, and the status of the patient's host-defense mechanisms.

In patients with extensive burns, altered pharmacokinetics may result in reduced serum concentrations of aminoglycosides. In such patients treated with gentamicin, measurement of serum concentrations is recommended as a basis for dosage adjustment.

The usual duration of treatment is seven to ten days. In difficult and complicated infections, a longer course of therapy may be necessary. In such cases monitoring of renal, auditory, and vestibular functions is recommended, since toxicity is more apt to occur with treatment extended for more than ten days. Dosage should be reduced if clinically indicated.

For Intravenous Administration

The intravenous administration of gentamicin may be particularly useful for treating patients with bacterial septicemia or those in shock. It may also be the preferred route of administration for some patients with congestive heart failure, hematologic disorders, severe burns, or those with reduced muscle mass.

For intermittent intravenous administration, a single dose of GARAMYCIN Pediatric Injectable may be diluted in sterile isotonic saline solution or in a sterile solution of dextrose 5% in water. The solution may be infused over a period of one-half to two hours.

The recommended dosage of intravenous and intramuscular administration is identical.

GARAMYCIN Pediatric Injectable should not be physically premixed with other drugs, but should be administered separately in accordance with the recommended route of administration and dosage schedule.

PATIENTS WITH IMPAIRED RENAL FUNCTION

Dosage must be adjusted in patients with impaired renal function. Whenever possible, serum concentrations of gentamicin should be monitored. One method of dosage adjustment is to increase the interval between administration of the usual doses. Since the serum creatinine concentration has a high correlation with the serum half-life of gentamicin, this laboratory test may provide guidance for adjustment of the interval between doses. In adults, the interval between doses (in hours) may be approximated by multiplying the serum creatinine level (mg/100 ml) by 8. For example, a patient weighing 60 kg. with a serum creatinine level of 2.0 mg/100 ml could be given 60 mg. (1 mg/kg) every 16 hours (2×8). These guidelines may be considered when treating infants and children with serious renal impairment.

In patients with serious systemic infections and renal impairment, it may be desirable to administer the antibiotic more frequently but in reduced dosage. In such patients, serum concentrations of gentamicin should be measured so that adequate but not excessive levels result.

A peak and trough concentration measured intermittently during therapy will provide optimal guidance for adjusting dosage. After the usual initial dose, a rough guide for determining reduced dosage at eight-hour intervals is to divide the normally recommended dose by the serum creatinine level (Table 1). For example, after an initial dose of 20 mg. (2.0 mg/kg), a child weighing 10 kg with a serum creatinine level of 2.0 mg/100 ml could be given 10 mg. every eight hours ($20 \div 2$). It should be noted that the status of renal function may be changing over the course of the infectious process. It is important to recognize that deteriorating renal function may require a greater reduction in dosage than that specified in the above guidelines for patients with stable renal impairment.

TABLE 1
DOSAGE ADJUSTMENT GUIDE FOR
PATIENTS WITH RENAL IMPAIRMENT
(Dosage at Eight-Hour Intervals
After the Usual Initial Dose)

Serum Creatinine (mg %)	Approximate Creatinine Clearance Rate (ml/min/1.73M^2)	Percent of Usual Doses Shown Above
≤ 1.0	> 100	100
1.1–1.3	70–100	80
1.4–1.6	55–70	65
1.7–1.9	45–55	55
2.0–2.2	40–45	50
2.3–2.5	35–40	40
2.6–3.0	30–35	35
3.1–3.5	25–30	30
3.6–4.0	20–25	25
4.1–5.1	15–20	20
5.2–6.6	10–15	15
6.7–8.0	< 10	10

In patients with renal failure undergoing hemodialysis, the amount of gentamicin removed from the blood may vary depending upon several factors including the dialysis method used. An eight-hour hemodialysis may reduce serum concentrations of gentamicin by approximately 50%. In children, the recommended dose at the end of each dialysis period is 2.0 to 2.5 mg/kg depending upon the severity of infection.

The above dosage schedules are not intended as rigid recommendations but are provided as guides to dosage when the measurement of gentamicin serum levels is not feasible.

A variety of methods are available to measure gentamicin concentrations in body fluids; these include microbiologic, enzymatic and radioimmunoassay techniques.

How Supplied: GARAMYCIN Pediatric Injectable, 10 mg. per ml., for parenteral administration, supplied in 2 ml. (20 mg.) vials; box of one.

Also available, GARAMYCIN Injectable, 40 mg. per ml., for parenteral administration, supplied in 2 ml. (80 mg.) vials, boxes of 1 and 25; 20 ml (800 mg) vials, box of 5; and in 1.5 ml. (60 mg.) and 2 ml. (80 mg.) disposable syringes, each in boxes of 1 and 10.

GARAMYCIN Pediatric Injectable is a clear, stable solution that requires no refrigeration.

Store between 2° and 30°C (36° and 86°F).

Schering Pharmaceutical Corporation (PR)
Manati, Puerto Rico 00701
An Affiliate of Schering Corporation
Kenilworth, N.J. 07033
Copyright © 1968, 1983, Schering Corporation. All rights reserved.
Revised 10/83

GARAMYCIN® I.V.   ℞
[*gar-ah-mi′sin*]
Piggyback Injection   Sterile
brand of gentamicin sulfate, USP
1 mg per ml
Each ml contains gentamicin sulfate, USP equivalent to 1 mg gentamicin.
For Intermittent Intravenous Infusion

Warnings: Patients treated with aminoglycosides should be under close clinical observation because of the potential toxicity associated with their use.

As with other aminoglycosides, gentamicin sulfate is potentially nephrotoxic. The risk of nephrotoxicity is greater in patients with impaired renal function and in those who receive high dosage or prolonged therapy.

Neurotoxicity manifested by ototoxicity, both vestibular and auditory, can occur in patients treated with gentamicin sulfate, primarily in those with preexisting renal damage and in patients with normal renal function treated with higher doses and/or for longer periods than recommended. Aminoglycoside-induced

Continued on next page

Information on Schering products appearing on these pages is effective as of September 30, 1984.

Schering—Cont.

ototoxicity is usually irreversible. Other manifestations of neurotoxicity may include numbness, skin tingling, muscle twitching and convulsions.

Renal and eighth cranial nerve function should be closely monitored, especially in patients with known or suspected reduced renal function at onset of therapy and also in those whose renal function is initially normal but who develop signs of renal dysfunction during therapy. Urine should be examined for decreased specific gravity, increased excretion of protein, and the presence of cells or casts. Blood urea nitrogen, serum creatinine, or creatinine clearance should be determined periodically. When feasible, it is recommended that serial audiograms be obtained in patients old enough to be tested, particularly high-risk patients. Evidence of ototoxicity (dizziness, vertigo, tinnitus, roaring in the ears or hearing loss) or nephrotoxicity requires dosage adjustment or discontinuance of the drug. As with the other aminoglycosides, on rare occasions changes in renal and eighth cranial nerve function may not become manifest until soon after completion of therapy.

Serum concentrations of aminoglycosides should be monitored when feasible to assure adequate levels and to avoid potentially toxic levels. When monitoring gentamicin peak concentrations, dosage should be adjusted so that prolonged levels above 12 mcg/ml are avoided. When monitoring gentamicin trough concentrations, dosage should be adjusted so that levels above 2 mcg/ml are avoided. Excessive peak and/or trough serum concentrations of aminoglycosides may increase the risk of renal and eighth cranial nerve toxicity. In the event of overdose or toxic reactions, hemodialysis may aid in the removal of gentamicin from the blood, especially if renal function is, or becomes, compromised. Removal of gentamicin by peritoneal dialysis is at a rate considerably less than by hemodialysis.

Concurrent and/or sequential systemic or topical use of other potentially neurotoxic and/or nephrotoxic drugs, such as cisplatin, cephaloridine, kanamycin, amikacin, neomycin, polymyxin B, colistin, paromomycin, tobramycin, vancomycin, and viomycin, should be avoided. Other factors which may increase patient risk of toxicity are advanced age and dehydration.

The concurrent use of gentamicin with potent diuretics, such as ethacrynic acid or furosemide, should be avoided, since certain diuretics by themselves may cause ototoxicity. In addition, when administered intravenously, diuretics may enhance aminoglycoside toxicity by altering the antibiotic concentration in serum and tissue.

Description: Gentamicin sulfate, USP, a water-soluble antibiotic of the aminoglycoside group, is derived from *Micromonospora purpurea*, an actinomycete. GARAMYCIN I.V. Piggyback Injection is a sterile, aqueous solution for intravenous infusion. Each ml contains gentamicin sulfate, USP, equivalent to 1 mg gentamicin base; and 8.9 mg sodium chloride. It does not contain preservatives.

Clinical Pharmacology: When gentamicin sulfate is administered by intravenous infusion over a two-hour period, the serum concentrations are similar to those obtained by intramuscular administration. Peak serum concentrations following intravenous administration occur 30 to 60 minutes following cessation of infusion. Serum levels are measurable for 6 to 8 hours.

In patients with normal renal function, peak serum concentrations of gentamicin (mcg/ml) are usually up to four times the single intramuscular dose (mg/kg); for example, a 1.0 mg/kg injection in adults may be expected to result in a peak serum concentration up to 4 mcg/ml; a 1.5 mg/kg dose may produce levels up to 6 mcg/ml. While some variation is to be expected due to a number of variables such as age, body temperature, surface area, and physiologic differences, the individual patient given the same dose tends to have similar levels in repeated determinations. Gentamicin administered at 1.0 mg/kg every eight hours for the usual 7- to 10-day treatment period to patients with normal renal function does not accumulate in the serum.

Gentamicin, like all aminoglycosides, may accumulate in the serum and tissues of patients treated with higher doses and/or for prolonged periods, particularly in the presence of impaired renal function. In adult patients, treatment with gentamicin dosages of 4 mg/kg/day or higher for seven to ten days may result in a slight, progressive rise in both peak and trough concentrations. In patients with impaired renal function, gentamicin is cleared from the body more slowly than in patients with normal renal function. The more severe the impairment, the slower the clearance. (Dosage must be adjusted.)

Since gentamicin is distributed in extracellular fluid, peak serum concentrations may be lower than usual in adult patients who have a large volume of this fluid. Serum concentrations of gentamicin in febrile patients may be lower than those in afebrile patients given the same dose. When body temperature returns to normal, serum concentrations of the drug may rise. Febrile and anemic states may be associated with a shorter than usual serum half-life. (Dosage adjustment is usually not necessary.) In severely burned patients, the half-life may be significantly decreased and resulting serum concentrations may be lower than anticipated from the mg/kg dose.

Protein binding studies have indicated that the degree of gentamicin binding is low; depending upon the methods used for testing, this may be between 0 and 30%.

After initial administration to patients with normal renal function, generally 70% or more of the gentamicin dose is recoverable in the urine in 24 hours; concentrations in urine above 100 mcg/ml may be achieved. Little, if any, metabolic transformation occurs; the drug is excreted principally by glomerular filtration. After several days of treatment, the amount of gentamicin excreted in the urine approaches the daily dose administered. As with other aminoglycosides, a small amount of the gentamicin dose may be retained in the tissues, especially in the kidneys. Minute quantities of aminoglycosides have been detected in the urine weeks after drug administration was discontinued. Renal clearance of gentamicin is similar to that of endogenous creatinine.

In patients with marked impairment of renal function, there is a decrease in the concentration of aminoglycosides in urine and in their penetration into defective renal parenchyma. This decreased drug excretion, together with the potential nephrotoxicity of aminoglycosides, should be considered when treating such patients who have urinary tract infections.

Probenecid does not affect renal tubular transport of gentamicin.

The endogenous creatinine clearance rate and the serum creatinine level have a high correlation with the half-life of gentamicin in serum. Results of these tests may serve as guides for adjusting dosage in patients with renal impairment (see DOSAGE AND ADMINISTRATION).

Following parenteral administration, gentamicin can be detected in serum, lymph, tissues, sputum, and in pleural, synovial, and peritoneal fluids. Concentrations in renal cortex sometimes may be eight times higher than the usual serum levels. Concentrations in bile, in general, have been low and have suggested minimal biliary excretion. Gentamicin crosses the peritoneal as well as the placental membranes. Since aminoglycosides diffuse poorly into the subarachnoid space after parenteral administration, concentrations of gentamicin in cerebrospinal fluid are often low and dependent upon dose, rate of penetration, and degree of meningeal inflammation. There is minimal penetration of gentamicin into ocular tissues following intramuscular or intravenous administration.

Microbiology: *In vitro* tests have demonstrated that gentamicin is a bactericidal antibiotic which acts by inhibiting normal protein synthesis in susceptible microorganisms. It is active against a wide variety of pathogenic bacteria including *Escherichia coli*, *Proteus* species (indole-positive and indole-negative), *Pseudomonas aeruginosa*, species of the *Klebsiella-Enterobacter-Serratia* group, *Citrobacter* species and *Staphylococcus* species (including penicillin- and methicillin-resistant strains). Gentamicin is also active *in vitro* against species of *Salmonella* and *Shigella*. The following bacteria are usually resistant to aminoglycosides: *Streptococcus pneumoniae*, most species of streptococci, particularly group D and anaerobic organisms, such as *Bacteroides* species or *Clostridium* species.

In vitro studies have shown that an aminoglycoside combined with an antibiotic that interferes with cell wall synthesis may act synergistically against some group D streptococcal strains. The combination of gentamicin and penicillin G has a synergistic bactericidal effect against virtually all strains of *Streptococcus faecalis* and its varieties (*S. faecalis* var. *liquifaciens*, *S. faecalis* var. *zymogenes*), *S. faecium* and *S. durans*. An enhanced killing effect against many of these strains has also been shown *in vitro* with combinations of gentamicin and ampicillin, carbenicillin, nafcillin, or oxacillin.

The combined effect of gentamicin and carbenicillin is synergistic for many strains of *Pseudomonas aeruginosa*. *In vitro* synergism against other gram-negative organisms has been shown with combinations of gentamicin and cephalosporins.

Gentamicin may be active against clinical isolates of bacteria resistant to other aminoglycosides.

Bacteria resistant to one aminoglycoside may be resistant to one or more other aminoglycosides. Bacterial resistance to gentamicin is generally developed slowly.

Susceptibility Testing: If the disc method of susceptibility testing used is that described by Bauer et al (*Am J Clin Path* 45:493, 1966; *Federal Register* 37:20525-20529, 1972), a disc containing 10 mcg of gentamicin should give a zone of inhibition of 15mm or more to indicate susceptibility of the infecting organism. A zone of 12mm or less indicates that the infecting organism is likely to be resistant. Zones greater than 12mm and less than 15mm indicate intermediate susceptibility. In certain conditions it may be desirable to do additional susceptibility testing by the tube or agar dilution method; gentamicin substance is available for this purpose.

Indications and Usage: GARAMYCIN I.V. Piggyback Injection is indicated in the treatment of serious infections caused by susceptible strains of the following microorganisms: *Pseudomonas aeruginosa*, *Proteus* species (indole-positive and indole-negative), *Escherichia coli*, *Klebsiella-Enterobacter-Serratia* species, *Citrobacter* species and *Staphylococcus* species (coagulase-postive and coagulase-negative).

Clinical studies have shown GARAMYCIN to be effective in bacterial neonatal sepsis; bacterial septicemia; and serious bacterial infections of the central nervous system (meningitis), urinary tract, respiratory tract, gastrointestinal tract (including peritonitis), skin, bone and soft tissue (including burns). Aminoglycosides, including gentamicin, are not indicated in uncomplicated initial episodes of urinary tract infections unless the causative organisms are susceptible to these antibiotics and are not susceptible to antibiotics having less potential for toxicity.

Specimens for bacterial culture should be obtained to isolate and identify causative organisms and to determine their susceptibility to gentamicin.

GARAMYCIN may be considered as initial therapy in suspected or confirmed gram-negative infections, and therapy may be instituted before obtaining results of susceptibility testing. The decision to continue therapy with this drug should be based on the results of susceptibility tests, the severity of the infection, and the important additional concepts contained in the "WARNINGS Box" above. If the causative organisms are resistant to gentamicin, other appropriate therapy should be instituted.

In serious infections when the causative organisms are unknown, GARAMYCIN may be administered as initial therapy in conjunction with a penicillin-type or cephalosporin-type drug before obtaining results of susceptibility testing. If anaerobic organisms are suspected as etiologic agents, consideration should be given to using other suitable antimicrobial therapy in conjunction with gentamicin. Following identification of the organism and its susceptibility, appropriate antibiotic therapy should then be continued. GARAMYCIN has been used effectively in combination with carbenicillin for the treatment of life-threatening infections caused by *Pseudomonas aeruginosa*. It has also been found effective when used in conjunction with a penicillin-type drug for the treatment of endocarditis caused by group D streptococci.

GARAMYCIN has also been shown to be effective in the treatment of serious staphylococcal infections. While not the antibiotic of first choice, GARAMYCIN may be considered when penicillins or other less potentially toxic drugs are contraindicated and bacterial susceptibility tests and clinical judgment indicate its use. It may also be considered in mixed infections caused by susceptible strains of staphylococci and gram-negative organisms.

In the neonate with suspected bacterial sepsis or staphylococcal pneumonia, a penicillin-type drug is also usually indicated as concomitant therapy with gentamicin.

Contraindications: Hypersensitivity to gentamicin is a contraindication to its use. A history of hypersensitivity or serious toxic reactions to other aminoglycosides may contraindicate use of gentamicin because of the known cross-sensitivity of patients to drugs in this class.

Warnings: (See "WARNINGS Box" above.)

Precautions: Neurotoxic and nephrotoxic antibiotics may be absorbed in significant quantities from body surfaces after local irrigation or application. The potential toxic effect of antibiotics administered in this fashion should be considered. Increased nephrotoxicity has been reported following concomitant administration of aminoglycoside antibiotics and cephalosporins. Neuromuscular blockade and respiratory paralysis have been reported in the cat receiving high doses (40 mg/kg) of gentamicin. The possibility of these phenomena occurring in man should be considered if aminoglycosides are administered by any route to patients receiving anesthetics, or to patients receiving neuromuscular blocking agents, such as succinylcholine, tubocurarine, or decamethonium, or in patients receiving massive transfusions of citrate-anticoagulated blood. If neuromuscular blockade occurs, calcium salts may reverse it. Aminoglycosides should be used with caution in patients with neuromuscular disorders, such as myasthenia gravis or parkinsonism, since these drugs may aggravate muscle weakness because of their potential curare-like effects on the neuromuscular junction.

Elderly patients may have reduced renal function which may not be evident in the results of routine screening tests, such as BUN or serum creatinine. A creatinine clearance determination may be more useful. Monitoring of renal function during treatment with gentamicin, as with other aminoglycosides, is particularly important in such patients.

Cross-allergenicity among aminoglycosides has been demonstrated.

Patients should be well hydrated during treatment.

Although the *in vitro* mixing of gentamicin and carbenicillin results in a rapid and significant inactivation of gentamicin, this interaction has not been demonstrated in patients with normal renal function who received both drugs by different routes of administration. A reduction in gentamicin serum half-life has been reported in patients with severe renal impairment receiving carbenicillin concomitantly with gentamicin.

Treatment with gentamicin may result in overgrowth of nonsusceptible organisms. If this occurs, appropriate therapy is indicated. See "WARNINGS Box" regarding concurrent use of potent diuretics and regarding concurrent and/or sequential use of other neurotoxic and/or nephrotoxic antibiotics and for other essential information.

Usage in Pregnancy—Safety for use in pregnancy has not been established.

Adverse Reactions: *Nephrotoxicity* Adverse renal effects, as demonstrated by the presence of casts, cells, or protein in the urine or by rising BUN, NPN, serum creatinine or oliguria, have been reported. They occur more frequently in patients with a history of renal impairment and in patients treated for longer periods or with larger dosage than recommended.

Neurotoxicity Serious adverse effects on both vestibular and auditory branches of the eighth nerve have been reported, primarily in patients with renal impairment (especially if dialysis is required), and in patients on high doses and/or prolonged therapy. Symptoms include dizziness, vertigo, tinnitus, roaring in the ears and also hearing loss, which, as with the other aminoglycosides, may be irreversible. Hearing loss is usually manifested initially by diminution of high-tone acuity. Other factors which may increase the risk of toxicity include excessive dosage, dehydration and previous exposure to other ototoxic drugs.

Numbness, skin tingling, muscle twitching and convulsions have also been reported.

Note: The risk of toxic reactions is low in patients with normal renal function who do not receive GARAMYCIN at higher doses or for longer periods of time than recommended. Other reported adverse reactions possibly related to gentamicin include: respiratory depression, lethargy, confusion, depression, visual disturbances, decreased appetite, weight loss, and hypotension and hypertension; rash, itching, urticaria, generalized burning, laryngeal edema, anaphylactoid reactions, fever, and headache; nausea, vomiting, increased salivation, and stomatitis; purpura, pseudotumor cerebri, acute organic brain syndrome, pulmonary fibrosis, alopecia, joint pain, transient hepatomegaly, and splenomegaly.

Laboratory abnormalities possibly related to gentamicin include: increased levels of serum transaminase (SGOT, SGPT), serum LDH and bilirubin; decreased serum calcium, magnesium, sodium and potassium; anemia, leukopenia, granulocytopenia, transient agranulocytosis, eosinophilia, increased and decreased reticulocyte counts, and thrombocytopenia.

While local tolerance of GARAMYCIN is generally excellent, there has been an occasional report of pain at the injection site. Subcutaneous atrophy or fat necrosis suggesting local irritation has been reported rarely.

Overdosage: In the event of overdose or toxic reactions, hemodialysis may aid in the removal of gentamicin from the blood, especially if renal function is, or becomes, compromised. Removal of gentamicin by peritoneal dialysis is at a rate considerably less than by hemodialysis.

Dosage and Administration: GARAMYCIN I.V. Piggyback Injection should only be administered intravenously. This product does not contain a preservative system; the contents must be used promptly after the seal is broken. Any unused portion must be discarded. DO NOT RETAIN FOR LATER USE.

It is desirable to limit the duration of treatment with aminoglycosides to short-term.

The usual duration of treatment for all patients is seven to ten days. In difficult and complicated infections, a longer course of therapy may be necessary. In such cases monitoring of renal, auditory, and vestibular functions is recommended, since toxicity is more apt to occur with treatment extended for more than ten days. Dosage should be reduced if clinically indicated.

The patient's pretreatment body weight should be obtained for calculation of correct dosage. The dosage of aminoglycosides in obese patients should be based on an estimate of the lean body mass.

In patients with extensive burns, altered pharmacokinetics may result in reduced serum concentrations of aminoglycosides. In such patients treated with gentamicin, measurement of serum concentrations is recommended as a basis for dosage adjustment.

It is desirable to measure both peak and trough serum concentrations of gentamicin to determine the adequacy and safety of the dosage. When such measurements are feasible, they should be carried out periodically during therapy to assure adequate but not excessive drug levels. For example, the peak concentrations (at 30 to 60 minutes following cessation of infusion) is expected to be in the range of 4 to 6 mcg/ml. When monitoring peak concentrations, dosage should be adjusted so that prolonged levels above 12 mcg/ml are avoided. When monitoring trough concentrations (just prior to the next dose), dosage should be adjusted so that levels above 2 mcg/ml are avoided. Determination of the adequacy of a serum level for a particular patient must take into consideration the susceptibility of the causative organism, the severity of the infection, and the status of the patient's host-defense mechanisms.

The intravenous administration of gentamicin may be particularly useful for treating patients with bacterial septicemia or those in shock. It may also be the preferred route of administration for some patients with congestive heart failure, hematologic disorders, severe burns, or those with reduced muscle mass. The solution may be infused over a period of one-half to two hours.

GARAMYCIN I.V. Piggyback Injection should not be physically premixed with other drugs but should be administered separately in accordance with the recommended route of administration and dosage schedule.

The dosage recommendations which follow are not intended as rigid schedules, but are provided as guides for initial therapy or when the measurement of gentamicin serum levels during therapy is not feasible.

PATIENTS WITH NORMAL RENAL FUNCTION

Adults: The recommended dosage of GARAMYCIN I.V. Piggyback Injection for patients with serious infections and normal renal function is 3 mg/kg/day, administered in three equal doses every eight hours (Table I).

For patients with life-threatening infections, dosages up to 5 mg/kg/day may be administered in three or four equal doses. This dosage should be reduced to 3 mg/kg/day as soon as clinically indicated (Table I).

[See table on next page].

Children: 6 to 7.5 mg/kg/day (2.0 to 2.5 mg/kg administered every 8 hours.)

Infants and Neonates: 7.5 mg/kg/day (2.5 mg/kg administered every 8 hours.)

Premature or Full-Term Neonates one week of age or less: 5 mg/kg/day (2.5 mg/kg administered every 12 hours.)

Note: For further information concerning the use of gentamicin in infants and children, see GARAMYCIN Pediatric Injectable Product Information.

PATIENTS WITH IMPAIRED RENAL FUNCTION

Dosage must be adjusted in patients with impaired renal function. Whenever possible, serum concentrations of gentamicin should be monitored. One method of dosage adjustment is to increase the interval between administration of the usual doses. Since the serum creatinine concentration has a high correlation with the serum half-life of gentamicin, this laboratory test may provide guidance for adjustment of the interval between doses. The interval between doses (in hours) may be ap-

Continued on next page

Information on Schering products appearing on these pages is effective as of September 30, 1984.

Schering—Cont.

proximated by multiplying the serum creatinine level (mg/100 ml) by 8. For example, a patient weighing 60 kg with a serum creatinine level of 2.0 mg/100 ml could be given 60 mg (1 mg/kg every 16 hours (2 × 8).

In patients with serious systemic infections and renal impairment, it may be desirable to administer the antibiotic more frequently but in reduced dosage. In such patients, serum concentrations of gentamicin should be measured so that adequate but not excessive levels result. A peak and trough concentration measured intermittently during therapy will provide optimal guidance for adjusting dosage. After the usual initial dose, a rough guide for determining reduced dosage at eight-hour intervals is to divide the normally recommended dose by the serum creatinine level (Table II). For example, after an initial dose of 60 mg (1 mg/kg), a patient weighing 60 kg with a serum creatinine level of 2.0 mg/100 ml could be given 30 mg every eight hours (60 ÷ 2). It should be noted that the status of renal function may be changing over the course of the infectious process. It is important to recognize that deteriorating renal function may require a greater reduction in dosage than that specified in the above guidelines for patients with stable renal impairment.
[See table above].

In adults with renal failure undergoing hemodialysis, the amount of gentamicin removed from the blood may vary depending upon several factors including the dialysis method used. An eight-hour hemodialysis may reduce serum concentrations of gentamicin by approximately 50%. The recommended dosage at the end of each dialysis period is 1 to 1.7 mg/kg depending upon the severity of infection. In children, a dose of 2 mg/kg may be administered.

A variety of methods are available to measure gentamicin concentrations in body fluids; these include microbiologic, enzymatic and radio-immunoassay techniques.

INSTRUCTIONS FOR THE ADMINISTRATION OF GARAMYCIN I.V. PIGGYBACK INJECTION
(For proper apparatus setup see accompanying Instruction Sheet.)

THIS PRODUCT IS IN A READY-TO-USE FORM AND IS INTENDED FOR USE ONLY AS AN I.V. PIGGYBACK.

If the prescribed dose is exactly 60 or 80 mg, use the appropriate unit; if the prescribed dose is higher or lower than that of the supplied unit, adjustments can be made in either piggyback unit. If the dose is higher that the contents of the 80 mg unit, the additional amount should be removed from a vial of GARAMYCIN Injectable (40 mg/ml) and added to the 80 mg piggyback unit. If the prescribed dose is less, decrements can be made by removing and discarding the appropriate amount from either unit. **It should be kept in mind that each ml of the piggyback unit contains 1 mg of gentamicin.**

The following are specific examples of dosage adjustment:
- to prepare a 90 mg dose, remove ¼ ml from a vial of GARAMYCIN Injectable (40 mg/ml) and add to the 80 mg piggyback unit.
- to prepare a 70 mg dose, either remove and discard 10 ml from the 80 mg piggyback unit or add the 10 ml from the 80 mg piggyback unit to the 60 mg piggyback unit.
- to prepare a 40 mg dose, remove and discard 20 ml from the 60 mg piggyback unit.

Observe all precautions for sterile technique when adding or removing contents of these units.

How Supplied: GARAMYCIN I.V. Piggyback Injection, 1 mg per ml for intravenous infusion, is supplied in 60 ml (60 mg) and 80 ml (80 mg) units; box of one.
Store between 2° and 30°C (36° and 86°F).
Also available, GARAMYCIN Injectable, 40 mg per ml, for parenteral administration, is supplied in 2 ml (80 mg) vials; boxes of 1 and 25; and 20 ml vials; box of 5; and in 1.5 ml (60 mg) and 2 ml (80 mg) disposable syringes, each in boxes of 1 and 10.
GARAMYCIN Pediatric Injectable, 10 mg per ml for parenteral administration, supplied in 2 ml (20 mg) vials; box of one.
GARAMYCIN Products are clear, stable solutions that require no refrigeration.

Schering Pharmaceutical
Corporation (P.R.),
Manati, Puerto Rico 00701
An Affiliate of Schering
Corporation, Kenilworth,
N.J. 07033

Revised 10/83
Copyright © 1968, 1983, Schering Corporation. All rights reserved.

GARAMYCIN® Intrathecal
[gar-ah-mī′sin]
brand of gentamicin sulfate, USP
Injection 2.0 mg/ml
FOR DIRECT ADMINISTRATION INTO THE CEREBROSPINAL FLUID SPACES OF THE CENTRAL NERVOUS SYSTEM

WARNINGS
GARAMYCIN Intrathecal Injection is intended as adjunctive therapy in patients with central nervous system infections. Since patients considered for treatment with GARAMYCIN Intrathecal Injection will usually be receiving concomitant treatment with intramuscular or intravenous gentamicin sulfate, all warnings and precautions for this or other concomitantly administered agents must be observed. Moreover, when the drug is administered by more than one route, additive effects must be considered. (See GARAMYCIN Injectable or GARAMYCIN Pediatric Injectable Product Information.) Laboratory studies in animals have shown that gentamicin sulfate, when administered directly into the central nervous system, has caused neurologic disturbances, including adverse effects on the eighth cranial nerve. The risk of direct administration of a potentially neurotoxic drug into the cerebrospinal fluid spaces of the central nervous system must be weighed against the potential benefit to be derived from this route of administration.

Description: Gentamicin sulfate, USP, a water-soluble antibiotic of the aminoglycoside group, is derived from *Micromonospora purpurea*, an actinomycete. GARAMYCIN Intrathecal Injection is a sterile, aqueous solution for direct administration into the cerebrospinal fluid spaces of the central nervous system. Each ml contains: gentamicin sulfate, USP equivalent to 2.0 mg gentamicin base; and 8.5 mg sodium chloride.

Clinical Pharmacology: Since gentamicin sulfate and other aminoglycosides diffuse poorly into

---

Garamycin I.V.
TABLE II
DOSAGE ADJUSTMENT GUIDE FOR PATIENTS WITH RENAL IMPAIRMENT
(Dosage at Eight-Hour Intervals After the Usual Initial Dose)

Serum Creatinine (mg %)	Approximate Creatinine Clearance Rate (ml/min/1.73M^2)	Percent of Usual Doses Shown in Table I
≤1.0	>100	100
1.1-1.3	70-100	80
1.4-1.6	55-70	65
1.7-1.9	45-55	55
2.0-2.2	40-45	50
2.3-2.5	35-40	40
2.6-3.0	30-35	35
3.1-3.5	25-30	30
3.6-4.0	20-25	25
4.1-5.1	15-20	20
5.2-6.6	10-15	15
6.7-8.0	<10	10

Garamycin I.V.
TABLE I
DOSAGE SCHEDULE GUIDE FOR ADULTS WITH NORMAL RENAL FUNCTION
(Dosage at Eight-Hour Intervals)
1 mg/ml

Patient's Weight* kg (lb)	Usual Dose for Serious Infections 1 mg/kg q8h (3 mg/kg/day) mg/dose	Dose for Life-Threatening Infections (Reduce As Soon As Clinically Indicated) 1.7 mg/kg q8h** (5 mg/kg/day) mg/dose
40 (88)	40	66
45 (99)	45	75
50 (110)	50	83
55 (121)	55	91
60 (132)	60	100
65 (143)	65	108
70 (154)	70	116
75 (165)	75	125
80 (176)	80	133
85 (187)	85	141
90 (198)	90	150
95 (209)	95	158
100 (220)	100	166

* The dosage of aminoglycosides in obese patients should be based on an estimate of the lean body mass.
** For q6h schedules, dosage should be recalculated.

the subarachnoid space after systemic administration, concentrations of these antibiotics in the lumbar or ventricular cerebrospinal fluid (CSF) are often low. Following intramuscular or intravenous administration of the usual doses, gentamicin concentrations in CSF in the absence of infection are usually less than 1 mcg/ml. In acute meningitis, slightly higher concentrations are obtained but these vary and are usually well below the peak serum concentration. CSF concentrations which are attained following intravenous or intramuscular administration of gentamicin sulfate tend to become lower as meningeal inflammation subsides. GARAMYCIN Intrathecal Injections are intended to increase the concentration of gentamicin in the CSF when used as part of the management of patients with central nervous system infections.

When GARAMYCIN Intrathecal Injection is given concomitantly with systemically administered gentamicin sulfate, the CSF levels are substantially increased depending upon the location of the injection. Peak CSF concentrations which follow intralumbar administration generally occur at 1 to 6 hours after injection.

Factors which affect the concentration of gentamicin in the CSF following injection into cerebrospinal fluid spaces are the dose administered, the site of the injection (intralumbar, intraventricular), the volume in which the dose is diluted, and the presence or absence of obstruction to the CSF flow. There appears to be considerable inter-patient variation.

The half-life of gentamicin in the CSF of adults who received intralumbar injections is approximately 5.5 hours; this is somewhat longer than that in serum.

In one pharmacokinetic study in adults, a 3 to 4 mg. intralumbar injection resulted in a mean CSF concentration of 6.2 mcg/ml 24 hours after injection. The mean CSF concentration was noted to decrease with time; during days 1 through 6 of treatment with GARAMYCIN Intrathecal Injection by the intralumbar route, the mean 24-hour concentration was 9.9 mcg/ml, while during days 7 through 13, the mean concentration was 3.7 mcg/ml.

In another study in adults, CSF levels were measured at varying intervals after intralumbar administration of gentamicin sulfate. During days 1 through 6 of treatment, a 4 mg. dose produced a mean CSF level of 2.4 mcg/ml 24 hours after injection, while during days 7 through 13, the same dose produced a mean 24-hour level of 0.5 mcg/ml. Following intralumbar administration there may be limited upward diffusion of the drug, presumably because of the direction of the CSF flow. Intraventricular administration produces high concentrations in the ventricles and throughout the central nervous system. Adequate levels will usually result from dosing every 24 hours, but it is desirable to manage each patient's infection with serial monitoring of gentamicin serum and CSF concentrations.

Microbiology: *In vitro* tests have demonstrated that gentamicin is a bactericidal antibiotic which acts by inhibiting normal protein synthesis in susceptible microorganisms. It is active against a wide variety of pathogenic bacteria including *Escherichia coli, Proteus* species (indole-positive and indole-negative), *Pseudomonas aeruginosa,* species of the *Klebsiella-Enterobacter-Serratia* group, *Citrobacter* species, and *Staphylococcus* species (including penicillin- and methicillin-resistant strains). Gentamicin is also active *in vitro* against species of *Salmonella* and *Shigella.* The following bacteria are usually resistant to aminoglycosides: *Streptococcus pneumoniae,* most species of streptococci, particularly group D and anaerobic organisms, such as *Bacteroides* species or *Clostridium* species.

In vitro studies have shown that an aminoglycoside combined with an antibiotic that interferes with cell wall synthesis may act synergistically against some group D streptococcal strains. The combination of gentamicin sulfate and penicillin G has a synergistic bactericidal effect against virtually all strains of *Streptococcus faecalis* and its varieties *(S. faecalis* var. *liquifaciens, S. faecalis* var. *zymogenes), S. faecium* and *S. durans.* An enhanced killing effect against many of these strains has also been shown *in vitro* with combinations of gentamicin and ampicillin, carbenicillin, nafcillin, or oxacillin.

The combined effect of gentamicin and carbenicillin is synergistic for many strains of *Pseudomonas aeruginosa.*

Gentamicin may be active against clinical isolates of bacteria resistant to other aminoglycosides. However, bacteria resistant to one aminoglycoside may be resistant to one or more other aminoglycosides.

Susceptibility Testing: If the disc method of susceptibility testing used is that described by Bauer *et al(Am J Clin Path* **45**:493, 1966; *Federal Register* **37**:20525–20529, 1972), a disc containing 10 mcg. of gentamicin, when tested against a bacterial strain susceptible to gentamicin, should give a zone of inhibition of $\geq$ 15 mm. A zone of $\leq$ 12 mm. indicates resistance. Zones greater than 12mm and less than 15mm indicate intermediate susceptibility. In certain conditions it may be desirable to do additional susceptibility testing by the broth or agar dilution method; gentamicin substance is available for this purpose.

Indications and Usage: GARAMYCIN Intrathecal Injection is indicated as adjunctive therapy to systemically administered gentamicin sulfate in the treatment of serious central nervous system infections (meningitis, ventriculitis) caused by susceptible *Pseudomonas* species.

Bacteriologic tests should be performed to determine that the causative organisms are *Pseudomonas* species susceptible to gentamicin.

Contraindications: Hypersensitivity to gentamicin sulfate is a contraindication to its use. A history of hypersensitivity or serious toxic reactions to aminoglycosides may also contraindicate use of gentamicin sulfate because of the known cross-sensitivity of patients to drugs in this class.

Warnings: (See "WARNINGS Box" above and the WARNINGS listed in the Product Information for GARAMYCIN Injectable and GARAMYCIN Pediatric Injectable.)

Precautions: (See PRECAUTIONS listed in the Product Information for GARAMYCIN Injectable and GARAMYCIN Pediatric Injectable.)

In a patient with a seven-year history of multiple sclerosis who was treated with gentamicin sulfate by intralumbar injection, disseminated microscopic lesions of the brain stem were reported at autopsy. Lesions observed were: tissue rarefaction with loss and marked swelling of axis cylinders with occasional calcification, loss of oligodendroglia and astroglia, and a poor inflammatory response.

Safety and efficacy in children below the age of three months have not been established.

Adverse Reactions: Local tolerance to GARAMYCIN Intrathecal Injection has been good. Local reactions of arachnoiditis or burning at the injection site have been reported rarely.

Because the recommended dosage of GARAMYCIN Intrathecal Injection is low, the potential for systemic adverse effects is minimal. However, GARAMYCIN Intrathecal Injection is recommended as adjunctive therapy with other antibiotics, such as parenteral gentamicin sulfate, which should be administered in full therapeutic dosages. Evidence of eighth nerve dysfunction, changes in renal function, leg cramps, rash, fever, convulsions, and an increase in cerebrospinal fluid protein have been reported in patients who were treated concomitantly with GARAMYCIN Intrathecal Injection and the parenteral preparation of gentamicin.

Administration of excessive (40 to 160 mg.) doses of the parenteral formulation of gentamicin sulfate (which contains a preservative agent) by the various intrathecal routes has been reported to produce neuromuscular disturbances, e.g., ataxia, paresis, and incontinence.

Dosage and Administration: GARAMYCIN Intrathecal Injection is intended for administration directly into the cerebrospinal fluid spaces of the central nervous system.

The dosage will vary depending upon factors, such as age and weight of the patient, site of injection, degree of obstruction to cerebrospinal fluid flow and the amount of cerebrospinal fluid estimated to be present. In general, the recommended dose for infants 3 months of age and older (see PRECAUTIONS) and children is 1 to 2 mg. once a day. For adults, 4 to 8 mg. may be administered once a day. Administration of GARAMYCIN Intrathecal Injection should be continued as long as sensitive organisms are demonstrated in the cerebrospinal fluid. Since the intralumbar or intraventricular dose is administered immediately after specimens are taken for laboratory study, treatment should usually be continued for at least one day after negative results have been obtained from CSF cultures and/or stained smears.

The suggested method for administering GARAMYCIN Intrathecal Injection into the lumbar area is as follows: the desired quantity of GARAMYCIN Intrathecal Injection is drawn up carefully from the ampule into a 5- or 10-ml. sterile syringe. After the lumbar puncture is performed and a specimen of the spinal fluid is removed for laboratory tests, the syringe containing GARAMYCIN Intrathecal Injection is inserted into the hub of the spinal needle. A quantity of cerebrospinal fluid (approximately 10% of the estimated total CSF volume) is allowed to flow into the syringe and mix with the GARAMYCIN Intrathecal Injection. The resultant solution is then injected over a period of 3 to 5 minutes with the bevel of the needle directed upward.

If the cerebrospinal fluid is grossly purulent, or if it is unobtainable, GARAMYCIN Intrathecal Injection may be diluted with sterile normal saline before injection.

GARAMYCIN Intrathecal Injection may also be administered directly into the subdural space or directly into the ventricles, including administration by use of an implanted reservoir.

How Supplied: GARAMYCIN Intrathecal Injection, 2.0 mg. per ml., is supplied in 2 ml. ampules; box of 25.

Store below 30°C (86°F).

NOTE: This preparation does not contain any preservative. Once opened, contents should be used immediately and unused portions should be discarded.

Animal Pharmacology and Toxicology: In dogs, an 8-hour perfusion of the ventriculosubarachnoid system with a solution containing 40 mcg/ml. (~5 mg. or ~0.3 mg/kg) gentamicin produced no seizure activity or change in vital signs during administration. No morphological changes were observed when the dogs were sacrificed at 10 and 90 days following infusion.

The effects of repeated intrathecal injections of gentamicin at 0.1 and 0.3 mg/kg were evaluated in tranquilized beagle puppies. Transient flaccid paralysis was observed on the first day when the drug was administered rapidly (i.e., in less than 5 seconds), but no adverse effects were observed thereafter when the drug was administered less rapidly (i.e., over a period of approximately 30 seconds). No drug-related changes were found on histological examination of the cerebellum, brain stem or cephalic cord. In cats, gentamicin administered intracisternally at one-hour intervals in doses of up to 50 mg/kg did not produce any abnormalities in the electroencephalogram. In another study in cats, gentamicin sulfate given daily by the intracisternal route for up to 7 days caused neurologic disturbances, including adverse effects on the eighth cranial nerve.

In rabbits intracisternal injection of gentamicin at doses 50 and 100 times the therapeutic dose produced peak CSF concentrations of 160 and 180 mcg/ml, respectively. These doses were associated with changes in the myelin sheath predominantly of the lateral columns of the upper cervical

Continued on next page

Information on Schering products appearing on these pages is effective as of September 30, 1984.

Schering—Cont.

cord, and some changes in glial cells and lesions in the medulla oblongata. In addition to a high incidence of mortality, the animals demonstrated weakness, ataxia and paralysis. At doses of one and ten times the therapeutic dose (providing peak levels of 16.5 and 40 mcg/ml CSF), no morphologic changes occurred and there were no drug-related symptoms identified.

Schering Pharmaceutical Corporation (PR)
Manati, Puerto Rico 00701
An Affiliate of Schering Corporation
Kenilworth, New Jersey 07033
Revised 7/83
Copyright © 1979, 1983, Schering Corporation.
All rights reserved.

GYNE–LOTRIMIN® ℞
[gī″ne-lo′trim-in]
brand of clotrimazole
Vaginal Tablets, USP
Vaginal Cream, USP 1%

Description: GYNE-LOTRIMIN is clotrimazole [1-(o-Chloro-α, α-diphenylbenzyl) imidazole], a synthetic antifungal agent having the chemical formula $C_{22}H_{17}ClN_2$.
Each GYNE-LOTRIMIN **Vaginal Tablet** contains 100 mg clotrimazole, USP dispersed in lactose, povidone, corn starch, and magnesium stearate.
Each applicatorful of GYNE-LOTRIMIN **Vaginal Cream** contains approximately 50 mg clotrimazole, USP dispersed in sorbitan monostearate, polysorbate 60, cetyl esters wax, cetearyl alcohol, 2-octyldodecanol, purified water, and as preservative, benzyl alcohol (1%).
Actions: Clotrimazole is a broad-spectrum antifungal agent that inhibits the growth of pathogenic yeasts. Clotrimazole exhibits fungicidal activity *in vitro* against *Candida albicans* and other species of the genus *Candida*.
No single-step or multiple-step resistance to clotrimazole has developed during successive passages of *Candida albicans*.
Indications: GYNE-LOTRIMIN **Vaginal Cream** and **Tablets** are indicated for the local treatment of patients with vulvovaginal candidiasis (moniliasis). The diagnosis should be confirmed by KOH smears and/or cultures. Other pathogens commonly associated with vulvovaginitis (*Trichomonas* and *Hemophilus vaginalis*) should be ruled out by appropriate laboratory methods.
The 3-day regimen of GYNE-LOTRIMIN **Vaginal Tablets** did not prove to be effective in pregnant patients.
Studies with clotrimazole cream have shown that women taking oral contraceptives had a cure rate similar to those not taking oral contraceptives.
Contraindications: GYNE-LOTRIMIN **Vaginal Tablets** and **Vaginal Cream** are contraindicated in women who have shown hypersensitivity to any of the components of the preparation.
Precautions: Laboratory Tests: If there is a lack of response to GYNE-LOTRIMIN, appropriate microbiological studies should be repeated to confirm the diagnosis and rule out other pathogens before instituting another course of antimycotic therapy.
Application of ^{14}C-labeled clotrimazole has shown negligible absorption (peak of 0.03 mcg/ml of serum 24 hours after insertion of a 100 mg tablet; peak serum level of 0.01 mcg/ml 24 hours after insertion of vaginal cream containing 50 mg of active drug) from both normal and inflamed human vaginal mucosa.
Usage in Pregnancy: While GYNE-LOTRIMIN **Vaginal Tablets** and **Cream** have not been studied in the first trimester of pregnancy, use in the second and third trimesters has not been associated with ill effects. Follow-up reports now available on 71 neonates of 177 pregnant patients treated with GYNE-LOTRIMIN **Vaginal Tablets** reveal no adverse effects or complications attributable to GYNE-LOTRIMIN therapy.
Adverse Reactions: Eighteen (1.6%) of the 1116 patients treated with GYNE-LOTRIMIN **Vaginal Tablets** in double-blind studies reported complaints during therapy that were possibly drug-related. Mild burning occurred in six patients while other complaints, such as skin rash, itching, vulval irritation, lower abdominal cramps and bloating, slight cramping, slight urinary frequency, and burning or irritation in the sexual partner, occurred rarely.
Three (0.5%) of the 653 patients treated with GYNE-LOTRIMIN **Vaginal Cream** reported complaints during therapy that were possibly drug-related. Vaginal burning occurred in one patient; erythema, irritation and burning in another, intercurrent cystitis was reported in the third.
Dosage and Administration: GYNE-LOTRIMIN **Vaginal Cream** has been found to be effective when used from seven to fourteen days; studies have shown that patients treated for fourteen days had a significantly higher cure rate. The recommended dose is one applicatorful of cream (approximately 5 grams) inserted intravaginally for seven to fourteen consecutive days, preferably at bedtime.
GYNE-LOTRIMIN **Vaginal Tablets**: Two tablets inserted intravaginally at bedtime for three nights or one tablet inserted intravaginally at bedtime for seven nights.
In the event of treatment failure, other pathogens commonly responsible for vaginitis should be ruled out before instituting another course of antimycotic therapy.
How Supplied: GYNE-LOTRIMIN **Vaginal Tablets**, 100 mg, white, uncoated tablets impressed with the trademark GYNE-LOTRIMIN and/or the Schering trademark and product identification number, 734; carton of six tablets for three-day treatment regimen and carton of seven tablets for seven-day treatment regimen; with plastic applicator and patient instructions.
Store between 2° and 30°C (36° and 86°F).
GYNE-LOTRIMIN **Vaginal Cream 1%** is supplied in 45-gram tubes with a measured-dose applicator; box of one for seven-day treatment; box of two for fourteen-day treatment.
Store between 2° and 30°C (36° and 86°F).
Copyright © 1976, 1982, Schering Corporation.
Revised 8/82
Shown in Product Identification Section, page 434

HYPERSTAT® I.V. ℞
[hi′per-stat]
brand of diazoxide, USP
Injection
For Intravenous Use In Hospitalized Patients Only

Description: HYPERSTAT I.V. Injection is a nondiuretic benzothiadiazine antihypertensive agent. Each ampule (20 ml) contains 300 mg diazoxide, USP, in a clear, colorless aqueous solution; the pH is adjusted to approximately 11.6 with sodium hydroxide.
Diazoxide is 7-chloro-3-methyl-2H-1,2,4-benzothiadiazine 1,1-dioxide, with the empirical formula $C_8H_7ClN_2O_2S$, and the molecular weight 230.7. It is a white crystalline powder practically insoluble to sparingly soluble in water.
Clinical Pharmacology: HYPERSTAT I.V. Injection produces a prompt reduction of blood pressure in man by relaxing smooth muscle in the peripheral arterioles. Cardiac output is increased as blood pressure is reduced. Studies in animals demonstrate that coronary blood flow is maintained, while renal blood flow is increased after an initial decrease.
Transient hyperglycemia occurs in the majority of patients treated with HYPERSTAT, but usually requires treatment only in patients with diabetes mellitus. It will respond to the usual management measures, including insulin.
Blood glucose levels should be monitored especially in patients with diabetes and in those requiring multiple injections of diazoxide. Cataracts have been observed in a few animals receiving repeated daily doses of intravenous diazoxide.
Since diazoxide causes sodium retention, repeated injections may precipitate edema and congestive heart failure. Increased volume of extracellular fluid may be a cause of treatment failure in nonresponsive patients. The increase in fluid volume characteristically responds to diuretic agents if adequate renal function exists. Concurrently administered thiazide diuretics may be expected to potentiate the antihypertensive and hyperuricemic actions of diazoxide. (See **Drug Interactions**.)
Diazoxide is extensively bound to serum protein (>90%). The plasma half-life is 28 ± 8.3 hours; however, the duration of its antihypertensive effect is variable, generally lasting less than 12 hours.
Indications and Usage: HYPERSTAT I.V. Injection is indicated for short-term use in the emergency reduction of blood pressure in severe, non-malignant and malignant hypertension in hospitalized adults; and in acute severe hypertension in hospitalized children, when prompt and urgent decrease of diastolic pressure is required. Treatment with orally effective antihypertensive agents should not be instituted until blood pressure has stabilized. The use of HYPERSTAT I.V. Injection for longer than 10 days is not recommended.
HYPERSTAT I.V. Injection is ineffective against hypertension due to pheochromocytoma.
Contraindications: HYPERSTAT I.V. Injection should not be used in the treatment of compensatory hypertension, such as that associated with aortic coarctation or arteriovenous shunt, and should not be used in patients hypersensitive to diazoxide, other thiazides, or other sulfonamide-derived drugs.
Warnings: <u>Rapid decrease of blood pressure</u> Caution must be observed when reducing severely elevated blood pressure. Diazoxide should only be administered utilizing the new 150 mg minibolus dosage. The use of a 300 mg intravenous dose of diazoxide has been associated with angina and with myocardial and cerebral infarction. One instance of optic nerve infarction was reported when a 100 mmHg reduction in diastolic pressure occurred over ten minutes following a single 300 mg bolus. In one prospective trial conducted in patients with severe hypertension and coexistent coronary artery disease, a 50% incidence of ischemic changes in the electrocardiogram was observed following single 300 mg bolus injections of diazoxide. The desired blood pressure lowering should therefore be achieved over as long a period of time as is compatible with the patient's status. At least several hours and preferably one or two days is tentatively recommended.
Improved safety with equal efficacy can be achieved by administering HYPERSTAT I.V. Injection as a mini-bolus dose (1 to 3 mg/kg every 5 to 15 minutes up to a maximum of 150 mg in a single injection) until a diastolic blood pressure below 100 mmHg is achieved. HYPERSTAT I.V. Injection should not be administered in a bolus dose of 300 mg since this mode of administration is less predictable and less controllable than the minibolus dosage. If hypotension severe enough to require therapy results from the reduction in blood pressure, it will usually respond to the Trendelenberg maneuver. If necessary, sympathomimetic agents such as dopamine or norepinephrine may be administered.
Special attention is required for patients with diabetes mellitus and those in whom retention of salt and water may present serious problems.
<u>Myocardial Lesions in Animals</u> Intravenous administration of diazoxide in dogs has induced subendocardial necrosis and necrosis of papillary muscles. These lesions, which are also produced by other vasodilator drugs (i.e., hydralazine, minoxidil) and by catecholamines, are presumed to be related to anoxia resulting from a combination of reflex tachycardia and decreased perfusion.
Precautions: General: HYPERSTAT (diazoxide) I.V. Injection is an effective antihypertensive agent requiring close monitoring of the patient's blood pressure at frequent intervals. Its administration may occasionally cause hypotension requiring treatment with sympathomimetic drugs. Therefore, HYPERSTAT, I.V. Injection should be used primarily in the hospital or where adequate facilities exist to treat such untoward responses.
HYPERSTAT I.V. Injection should be administered only into a peripheral vein. Because the al-

kalinity of the solution is irritating to tissue, avoid extravascular injection or leakage. Subcutaneous administration has produced inflammation and pain without subsequent necrosis. If leakage into subcutaneous tissue occurs, the area should be treated with warm compresses and rest.

HYPERSTAT I.V. Injection should be used with care in patients who have impaired cerebral or cardiac circulation, that is, patients in whom abrupt reduction in blood pressure might be detrimental or those in whom mild tachycardia or decreased blood perfusion may be deleterious (see **Warnings**). Prolonged hypotension should be avoided so as not to aggravate preexisting renal failure.

Information for Patients: During and immediately following intravenous, injection of HYPERSTAT I.V. Injection, the patient should remain supine.

Laboratory Tests: Diagnostic laboratory tests necessary to establish the patient's condition and status should be carried out prior to treatment with HYPERSTAT I.V. Injection. During and following treatment with HYPERSTAT I.V. Injection, laboratory tests to monitor the effects of treatment with this drug and the patient's condition should be done. Among the tests (not necessarily inclusive) are: hematologic (hematocrit, hemoglobin, white blood cell and platelet counts); metabolic (glucose, uric acid, total protein, albumin); electrolyte (sodium, potassium) and osmolality; renal function (creatinine, urine-protein); electrocardiogram.

Drug Interactions: Diazoxide is highly bound to serum protein. It can be expected to displace other substances which are also bound to protein, such as bilirubin or coumarin and its derivatives, resulting in higher blood levels of these substances. An undesirable hypotension may result when diazoxide is administered to patients who have received other antihypertensive medication within six hours.

One patient in a clinical study exhibited excessive hypotension after concomitant administration of HYPERSTAT with hydralazine and methyldopa. An episode of maternal hypotension and fetal bradycardia occurred in a patient in labor who received both reserpine and hydralazine prior to administration of diazoxide. Neonatal hyperglycemia following intrapartum administration of HYPERSTAT I.V. Injection has also been reported.

HYPERSTAT I.V. Injection should not be administered within six hours of the administration of hydralazine, reserpine, alphaprodine, methyldopa, beta-blockers, prazosin, minoxidil, the nitrites and other papaverine-like compounds.

Concomitant administration with thiazides or other commonly used diuretics may be expected to potentiate the hyperuricemic and antihypertensive effects of diazoxide.

Drug/Laboratory Test Interactions: The hyperglycemic and hyperuricemic effects of diazoxide preclude proper assessment of these metabolic states. Increased renin secretion, IgG concentrations and decreased cortisol secretion have also been noted. Diazoxide inhibits glucagon-stimulated insulin release and will cause a false-negative insulin response to glucagon. In the rat, dog and monkey, diazoxide increased serum free fatty acids and decreased plasma insulin levels.

Carcinogenesis, Mutagenesis, Impairment of Fertility: No long-term animal dosing study has been done to evaluate the carcinogenic potential of diazoxide. No laboratory studies of mutagenic potential or animal studies of effects on fertility have been done.

Pregnancy Category C: Diazoxide has been shown to reduce fetal and/or pup survival; and to reduce fetal growth in rats, rabbits, and dogs at daily doses of 30, 21, or 10 mg/kg, respectively. In rats treated at term, diazoxide, at doses of 10 mg/kg and above, prolonged parturition.

The safety of HYPERSTAT I.V. Injection in pregnancy has not been established.

Non-teratogenic Effects: Diazoxide crosses the placental barrier and appears in cord blood. When given to the mother prior to delivery the drug may produce fetal or neonatal hyperbilirubinemia, thrombocytopenia, altered carbohydrate metabolism, and possibly other side effects that have occurred in adults.

Labor and Delivery: HYPERSTAT I.V. Injection is not indicated for use in pregnancy. Intravenous administration of the drug during labor may cause cessation of uterine contractions, requiring administration of an oxytocic agent.

Nursing Mothers: Information is not available concerning the passage of HYPERSTAT in breast milk. Because many drugs are excreted in human milk and because of the potential for adverse reactions in nursing infants from diazoxide, a decision should be made whether to discontinue nursing or to discontinue the drug, taking into account the importance of the drug to the mother.

Pediatric Use: See **Indications and Usage**.

Adverse Reactions: It is reasonable to speculate that the currently recommended mini-bolus dosing regimen, which has replaced the 300 mg bolus dose in clinical practice, will result in adverse effects which are of similar character but of lesser frequency and severity.

In clinical experience with the rapid bolus administration of 300 mg, the most common adverse reactions reported were: hypotension (7%); nausea and vomiting (4%); dizziness and weakness (2%). Additional adverse reactions reported with bolus administration of 300 mg were as follows:

Cardiovascular: sodium and water retention after repeated injections, especially important in patients with impaired cardiac reserve; hypotension to shock levels; myocardial ischemia, usually transient and manifested by angina, atrial and ventricular arrhythmias, and marked electrocardiographic changes, but occasionally leading to myocardial infarction; optic nerve infarction following too rapid decrease in severely elevated blood pressure; supraventricular tachycardia and palpitation; bradycardia; chest discomfort or nonanginal "tightness in the chest."

Central Nervous System: cerebral ischemia, usually transient but occasionally leading to infarction and manifested by unconsciousness, convulsions, paralysis, confusion, or focal neurological deficit such as numbness of the hands; vasodilative phenomena, such as orthostatic hypotension, sweating, flushing, and generalized or localized sensations of warmth; various transient neurological findings secondary to alteration in regional blood flow to brain, such as headache (sometimes throbbing), dizziness, lightheadedness, sleepiness (also reported as lethargy, somnolence or drowsiness), euphoria or "funny feeling," ringing in the ears and momentary hearing loss, and weakness of short duration; apprehension or anxiety.

Gastrointestinal: rarely, acute pancreatitis; nausea, vomiting and/or abdominal discomfort, anorexia; alteration in taste, parotid swelling; salivation; dry mouth; lacrimation; ileus; constipation and diarrhea.

Other: hyperglycemia in diabetic patients, especially after repeated injections; hyperosmolar coma in an infant; transient hyperglycemia in nondiabetic patients; transient retention of nitrogenous wastes; various respiratory findings secondary to the relaxation of smooth muscle, such as dyspnea, cough and choking sensation; warmth or pain along the injected vein; cellulitis without sloughing and/or phlebitis at the injection site of extravasation; back pain and increased nocturia; hypersensitivity reactions, such as rash, leukopenia and fever; papilledema induced by plasma volume expansion secondary to the administration of diazoxide reported in a patient who had received eleven injections (300 mg/dose) over a 22-day period; malaise and blurred vision; transient cataract in an infant; hirsutism, and decreased libido.

Overdosage: Overdosage of HYPERSTAT I.V. Injection may cause an undesirable hypotension. Usually, this can be controlled with the Trendelenberg maneuver. If necessary, sympathomimetic agents, such as dopamine or norepinephrine, may be administered. Failure of blood pressure to rise in response to such agents suggests that the hypotension may have been caused by something other than diazoxide. Excessive hyperglycemia resulting from overdosage will respond to conventional therapy of hyperglycemia.

Diazoxide may be removed from the blood by peritoneal dialysis or hemodialysis.

Dosage and Administration: HYPERSTAT I.V. Injection was originally recommended for use by bolus administration of 300 mg. Recent studies have shown that minibolus administration of HYPERSTAT I.V. Injection i.e., doses of 1 to 3 mg/kg repeated at intervals of 5 to 15 minutes is as effective in reducing blood pressure. Minibolus administration usually provides a more gradual reduction in blood pressure and thus may be expected to reduce the circulatory and neurological risks associated with acute hypotension.

HYPERSTAT I.V. Injection is administered undiluted and rapidly by intravenous injections of 1 to 3 mg/kg up to a maximum of 150 mg in a single injection. This dose may be repeated at intervals of 5 to 15 minutes until a satisfactory reduction in blood pressure (diastolic pressure below 10 mmHg) has been achieved.

With the patient recumbent, the calculated dose of HYPERSTAT I.V. Injection is administered intravenously in 30 seconds or less.

HYPERSTAT I.V. Injection should only be given into a peripheral vein. Do no administer it intramuscularly, subcutaneously, or into body cavities. Avoid extravasation of the drug into subcutaneous tissues.

Following the use of HYPERSTAT I.V. Injection, the blood pressure should be monitored closely until it has stabilized. Thereafter, measurements taken hourly during the balance of the effect should indicate any unusual response. A further decrease in blood pressure 30 minutes or more after injection should be investigated for causes other than the action of HYPERSTAT I.V. Injection. It is preferable that the patient remain supine for at least one hour after injection. In ambulatory patients, the blood pressure should also be measured with the patient standing before surveillance is ended.

Repeated administration of HYPERSTAT I.V. Injection at intervals of 4 to 24 hours usually will maintain the blood pressure below pretreatment levels until a regimen of oral antihypertensive medication can be instituted. The interval between injections may be adjusted by the duration of the response to each injection. It is usually unnecessary to continue treatment with HYPERSTAT I.V. Injection for more than four to five days.

Since repeated administration of HYPERSTAT I.V. Injection can lead to sodium and water retention, administration of a diuretic may be necessary both for maximal blood pressure reduction and to avoid congestive heart failure. (See **Clinical Pharmacology**.)

How Supplied: HYPERSTAT I.V. Injection is supplied in a 20 ml. ampule, containing 300 mg diazoxide, in a clear, colorless aqueous solution; box of one ampule. (NDC 0085-0201-05).

Protect from light and freezing. Store between 36° and 86°F (2° and 30°C).

Revised 6/83

Copyright ©1972, 1984. Schering Corporation. All rights reserved.

LOTRIMIN® R

[*lo'trim-in*]
brand of clotrimazole
 Cream, USP 1%
 Lotion 1%
 Solution, USP 1%
For Dermatologic Use Only—
Not For Ophthalmic Use

Description: LOTRIMIN products contain clotrimazole, USP, a synthetic antifungal agent having the chemical name [1-(o-Chloro-α,α-diphenyl-

Continued on next page

Information on Schering products appearing on these pages is effective as of September 30, 1984.

Schering—Cont.

benzyl)imidazole]; the empirical formula, $C_{22}H_{17}ClN_2$; and a molecular weight of 344.84. Clotrimazole is an odorless, white crystalline substance. It is practically insoluble in water, sparingly soluble in ether and very soluble in polyethylene glycol 400, ethanol and chloroform.

Each gram of LOTRIMIN **Cream** contains 10 mg clotrimazole, USP in a vanishing cream base of sorbitan monostearate, polysorbate 60, cetyl esters wax, cetearyl alcohol, 2-octyldodecanol, purified water and, as preservative, benzyl alcohol (1%).

Each gram of LOTRIMIN **Lotion** contains 10 mg clotrimazole, USP dispersed in an emulsion vehicle composed of sorbitan monostearate, polysorbate 60, cetyl esters wax, cetearyl alcohol, 2-octyldodecanol, purified water; benzyl alcohol (1%) as preservative; sodium phosphate dibasic and sodium biphosphate to adjust pH.

Each ml of LOTRIMIN **Solution** contains 10 mg clotrimazole, USP in a nonaqueous vehicle of polyethylene glycol 400.

Clinical Pharmacology: Clotrimazole is a broad-spectrum antifungal agent that is used for the treatment of dermal infections caused by various species of pathogenic dermatophytes, yeasts, and *Malassezia furfur*. The primary action of clotrimazole is against dividing and growing organisms.

In vitro, clotrimazole exhibits fungistatic and fungicidal activity against isolates of *Trichophyton rubrum*, *Trichophyton mentagrophytes*, *Epidermophyton floccosum*, *Microsporum canis*, and *Candida* species, including *Candida albicans*. In general, the *in vitro* activity of clotrimazole corresponds to that of tolnaftate and griseofulvin against the mycelia of dermatophytes (*Trichophyton*, *Microsporum*, and *Epidermophyton*), and to that of the polyenes (amphotericin B and nystatin) against budding fungi (*Candida*). Using an *in vivo* (mouse) and an *in vitro* (mouse kidney homogenate) testing system, clotrimazole and miconazole were equally effective in preventing the growth of the pseudomycelia and mycelia of *Candida albicans*.

Strains of fungi having a natural resistance to clotrimazole are rare. Only a single isolate of *Candida guilliermondi* has been reported to have primary resistance to clotrimazole.

No single-step or multiple-step resistance to clotrimazole has developed during successive passages of *Candida albicans* and *Trichophyton mentagrophytes*. No appreciable change in sensitivity was detected after successive passages of isolates of *C. albicans*, *C. krusei*, or *C. pseudotropicalis* in liquid or solid media containing clotrimazole. Also, resistance could not be developed in chemically induced mutant strains of polyene-resistant isolates of *C. albicans*. Slight, reversible resistance was noted in three isolates of *C. albicans* tested by one investigator. There is a single report that records the clinical emergence of a *C. albicans* strain with considerable resistance to flucytosine and miconazole, and with cross-resistance to clotrimazole; the strain remained sensitive to nystatin and amphotericin B.

In studies of the mechanism of action, the minimum fungicidal concentration of clotrimazole caused leakage of intracellular phosphorus compounds into the ambient medium with concomitant breakdown of cellular nucleic acids and accelerated potassium efflux. Both these events began rapidly and extensively after addition of the drug. Clotrimazole appears to be well absorbed in humans following oral administration and is eliminated mainly as inactive metabolites. Following topical and vaginal administration, however, clotrimazole appears to be minimally absorbed.

Six hours after the application of radioactive clotrimazole 1% cream and 1% solution onto intact and acutely inflamed skin, the concentration of clotrimazole varied from 100 mcg/cm in the stratum corneum to 0.5 to 1 mcg/cm in the stratum reticulare, and 0.1 mcg/cm in the subcutis. No measurable amount of radioactivity (≤ 0.001 mcg/ml) was found in the serum within 48 hours after application under occlusive dressing of 0.5 ml of the solution or 0.8 g of the cream. Only 0.5% or less of the applied radioactivity was excreted in the urine.

Following intravaginal administration of 100 mg ^{14}C-clotrimazole vaginal tablets to nine adult females, an average peak serum level, corresponding to only 0.03 µg equivalents/ml of clotrimazole, was reached one to two days after application. After intravaginal administration of 5 g of 1% ^{14}C-clotrimazole vaginal cream, containing 50 mg active drug, to five subjects (one with candidal colpitis), serum levels corresponding to approximately 0.01 µg equivalents/ml were reached between 8 and 24 hours after application.

Indications and Usage: LOTRIMIN products are indicated for the topical treatment of the following dermal infections: tinea pedis, tinea cruris, and tinea corporis due to *Trichophyton rubrum*, *trichophyton mentagrophytes*, *Epidermophyton floccosum*, and *Microsporum canis;* candidiasis due to *Candida albicans;* and tinea versicolor due to *Malassezia furfur*.

Contraindications: LOTRIMIN products are contraindicated in individuals who have shown hypersensitivity to any of their components.

Warnings: LOTRIMIN products are not for ophthalmic use.

Precautions: General: If irritation or sensitivity develops with the use of clotrimazole, treatment should be discontinued and appropriate therapy instituted.

Information For Patients:
The patient should be advised to:
1. Use the medication for the full treatment time even though the symptoms may have improved. Notify the physician if there is no improvement after four weeks of treatment.
2. Inform the physician if the area of application shows signs of increased irritation (redness, itching, burning, blistering, swelling, oozing) indicative of possible sensitization.
3. Avoid the use of occlusive wrappings or dressings.
4. Avoid sources of infection or reinfection.

Laboratory Tests: If there is lack of response to clotrimazole, appropriate microbiological studies should be repeated to confirm the diagnosis and rule out other pathogens before instituting another course of antimycotic therapy.

Drug Interactions: Synergism or antagonism between clotrimazole and nystatin, or amphotericin B, or flucytosine against strains of *C. albicans* has not been reported.

Carcinogenesis, Mutagenesis, Impairment of Fertility: An 18-month oral dosing study with clotrimazole in rats has not revealed any carcinogenic effect.

In tests for mutagenesis, chromosomes of the spermatophores of Chinese hamsters which had been exposed to clotrimazole were examined for structural changes during the metaphase. Prior to testing, the hamsters had received five oral clotrimazole doses of 100 mg/kg body weight. The results of this study showed that clotrimazole had no mutagenic effect.

Usage in Pregnancy: Pregnancy Category B: The disposition of ^{14}C-clotrimazole has been studied in humans and animals. Clotrimazole is very poorly absorbed following dermal application or intravaginal administration to humans. (See **Clinical Pharmacology**.)

In clinical trials, use of vaginally applied clotrimazole in pregnant women in their second and third trimesters has not been associated with ill effects. There are, however, no adequate and well-controlled studies in pregnant women during the first trimester of pregnancy.

Studies in pregnant rats with intravaginal doses up to 100 mg/kg have revealed no evidence of harm to the fetus due to clotrimazole.

High oral doses of clotrimazole in rats and mice ranging from 50 to 120 mg/kg resulted in embryotoxicity (possibly secondary to maternal toxicity), impairment of mating, decreased litter size and number of viable young and decreased pup survival to weaning. However, clotrimazole was not teratogenic in mice, rabbits and rats at oral doses up to 200, 180 and 100 mg/kg, respectively. Oral absorption in the rat amounts to approximately 90% of the administered dose.

Because animal reproduction studies are not always predictive of human response, this drug should be used only if clearly indicated during the first trimester of pregnancy.

Nursing Mothers: It is not known whether this drug is excreted in human milk. Because many drugs are excreted in human milk, caution should be exercised when clotrimazole is used by a nursing woman.

Pediatric Use: Safety and effectiveness in children have been established for clotrimazole when used as indicated and in the recommended dosage.

Adverse Reactions: The following adverse reactions have been reported in connection with the use of clotrimazole: erythema, stinging, blistering, peeling, edema, pruritus, urticaria, burning, and general irritation of the skin.

Overdosage: Acute overdosage with topical application of clotrimazole is unlikely and would not be expected to lead to a life-threatening situation.

Dosage and Administration: Gently massage sufficient LOTRIMIN into the affected and surrounding skin areas twice a day, in the morning and evening.

Clinical improvement, with relief of pruritus, usually occurs within the first week of treatment with LOTRIMIN. If the patient shows no clinical improvement after four weeks of treatment with LOTRIMIN, the diagnosis should be reviewed.

How Supplied: LOTRIMIN **Cream** 1% is supplied in 15, 30, 45 and 90-g tubes (NDC 0085-0613-02, 05, 04, 03, respectively); boxes of one.

LOTRIMIN **Lotion** 1% is supplied in 30 ml bottles (NDC 0085-0707-02); boxes of one.

Shake well before using.

LOTRIMIN **Solution** 1% is supplied in 10 ml and 30 ml plastic bottles (NDC 0085-0182-02, 04, respectively); boxes of one.

Store LOTRIMIN products between 2° and 30°C (36° and 86°F).

Copyright © 1984. Schering Corporation.
All rights reserved. 3/84

LOTRISONE® ℞
[lō' trĭ - sōn]
brand of clotrimazole, USP and betamethasone dipropionate, USP Cream

**For Dermatologic Use Only—
Not for Ophthalmic Use**

Description: LOTRISONE Cream contains a combination of clotrimazole, USP, a synthetic antifungal agent, and betamethasone dipropionate, USP, a synthetic corticosteroid, for dermatologic use.

Chemically, clotrimazole is 1-(o-Chloro-α,α-diphenyl benzyl) imidazole, with the empirical formula $C_{22}H_{17}ClN_2$ and a molecular weight of 344.8.

Clotrimazole is an odorless, white crystalline powder, insoluble in water and soluble in ethanol.

Betamethasone dipropionate has the chemical name 9-Fluoro-11β, 17,21-trihydroxy-16β-methylpregna-1,4-diene-3,20-dione 17,21-dipropionate, with the empirical formula $C_{28}H_{37}FO_7$ and a molecular weight of 504.6.

Betamethasone dipropionate is a white to creamy white, odorless crystalline powder, insoluble in water.

Each gram of LOTRISONE Cream contains 10.0 mg clotrimazole, USP, and 0.64 mg betamethasone dipropionate, USP (equivalent to 0.5 mg betamethasone), in a hydrophilic emollient cream consisting of purified water, mineral oil, white petrolatum, cetearyl alcohol, ceteth 20, propylene glycol, sodium phosphate monobasic, and phosphoric acid; benzyl alcohol as preservative.

LOTRISONE is a smooth, uniform, white to off-white cream.

Clinical Pharmacology:
Clotrimazole
Clotrimazole is a broad-spectrum, antifungal agent that is used for the treatment of dermal infections caused by various species of pathogenic dermatophytes, yeasts, and *Malassezia furfur.* The primary action of clotrimazole is against dividing and growing organisms.

In vitro, clotrimazole exhibits fungistatic and fungicidal activity against isolates of *Trichophyton rubrum, Trichophyton mentagrophytes, Epidermophyton floccosum* and *Microsporum canis.* In general, the *in vitro* activity of clotrimazole corresponds to that of tolnaftate and griseofulvin against the mycelia of dermatophytes (*Trichophyton, Microsporum,* and *Epidermophyton*).

In vivo studies in guinea pigs infected with *Trichophyton mentagrophytes* have shown no measurable loss of clotrimazole activity due to combination with betamethasone dipropionate.

Strains of fungi having a natural resistance to clotrimazole have not been reported.

No single-step or multiple-step resistance to clotrimazole has developed during successive passages of *Trichophyton mentagrophytes.*

In studies of the mechanism of action in fungal cultures, the minimum fungicidal concentration of clotrimazole caused leakage of intracellular phosphorous compounds into the ambient medium with concomitant breakdown of cellular nucleic acids, and accelerated potassium efflux. Both of these events began rapidly and extensively after addition of the drug to the cultures.

Clotrimazole appears to be minimally absorbed following topical application to the skin. Six hours after the application of radioactive clotrimazole 1% cream and 1% solution onto intact and acutely inflamed skin, the concentration of clotrimazole varied from 100 mcg/cm^3 in the stratum corneum, to 0.5 to 1 mcg/cm^3 in the stratum reticulare, and 0.1 mcg/cm^3 in the subcutis. No measurable amount of radioactivity (<0.001 mcg/ml) was found in the serum within 48 hours after application under occlusive dressing of 0.5 ml of the solution or 0.8 g of the cream.

Betamethasone dipropionate
Betamethasone dipropionate, a corticosteroid, is effective in the treatment of corticosteroid-responsive dermatoses primarily because of its anti-inflammatory, antipruritic, and vasoconstrictive actions. However, while the physiologic, pharmacologic, and clinical effects of corticosteroids are well-known, the exact mechanisms of their actions in each disease are uncertain. Betamethasone dipropionate, a corticosteroid, has been shown to have topical (dermatologic) and systemic pharmacologic and metabolic effects characteristic of this class of drugs.

Pharmacokinetics: The extent of percutaneous absorption of topical corticosteroids is determined by many factors including the vehicle, the integrity of the epidermal barrier, and the use of occlusive dressings. (See **Dosage and Administration** section.)

Topical corticosteroids can be absorbed from normal intact skin. Inflammation and/or other disease processes in the skin increase percutaneous absorption. Occlusive dressings substantially increase the percutaneous absorption of topical corticosteroids. (See **Dosage and Administration** section.)

Once absorbed through the skin, topical corticosteroids are handled through pharmacokinetic pathways similar to systemically administered corticosteroids. Corticosteroids are bound to plasma proteins in varying degrees. Corticosteroids are metabolized primarily in the liver and are then excreted by the kidneys. Some of the topical corticosteroids and their metabolites are also excreted into the bile.

Clotrimazole and betamethasone dipropionate
In clinical studies of tinea corporis, tinea cruris and tinea pedis, patients treated with LOTRISONE Cream showed a better clinical response at the first return visit, than patients treated with clotrimazole cream. In tinea corporis and tinea cruris, the patient returned three days after starting treatment, and in tinea pedis, after one week.

Mycological cure rates observed in patients treated with LOTRISONE Cream were as good as or better than in those patients treated with clotrimazole cream.

In these same clinical studies, patients treated with LOTRISONE Cream showed statistically significantly better clinical responses and mycological cure rates when compared with patients treated with betamethasone dipropionate cream.

Indications and Usage: LOTRISONE Cream is indicated for the topical treatment of the following dermal infections: tinea pedis, tinea cruris, and tinea corporis due to *Trichophyton rubrum, Trichophyton mentagrophytes, Epidermophyton floccosum,* and *Microsporum canis.*

Contraindications: LOTRISONE Cream is contraindicated in patients who are sensitive to clotrimazole, betamethasone dipropionate, other corticosteroids or imidazoles, or to any ingredient in this preparation.

Precautions: General: Systemic absorption of topical corticosteroids has produced reversible hypothalamic-pituitary-adrenal (HPA) axis suppression, manifestations of Cushing's syndrome, hyperglycemia, and glucosuria in some patients. Conditions which augment systemic absorption include the application of the more potent steroids, use over large surface areas, prolonged use, and the addition of occlusive dressings. (See **Dosage and Administration** section.)

Therefore, patients receiving a large dose of a potent topical steroid applied to a large surface area should be evaluated periodically for evidence of HPA axis suppression by using the urinary free cortisol and ACTH stimulation tests. If HPA axis suppression is noted, an attempt should be made to withdraw the drug, to reduce the frequency of application, or to substitute a less potent steroid.

Recovery of HPA axis function is generally prompt and complete upon discontinuation of the drug. Infrequently, signs and symptoms of steroid withdrawal may occur, requiring supplemental systemic corticosteroids.

Children may absorb proportionally larger amounts of topical corticosteroids and thus be more susceptible to systemic toxicity. (See **Precautions-Pediatric Use.**)

If irritation or hypersensitivity develops with the use of LOTRISONE Cream, treatment should be discontinued and appropriate therapy instituted.

Information for Patients Patients using LOTRISONE Cream should receive the following information and instructions:

1. This medication is to be used as directed by the physician. It is for external use only. Avoid contact with the eyes.
2. The medication is to be used for the full prescribed treatment time, even though the symptoms may have improved. Notify the physician if there is no improvement after one week of treatment for tinea cruris or tinea corporis, or after two weeks for tinea pedis.
3. Patients should be advised not to use this medication for any disorder other than for which it was prescribed.
4. The treated skin areas should not be bandaged or otherwise covered or wrapped as to be occluded. (See **Dosage and Administration** section.)
5. When using this medication in the groin area, patients should be advised to use the medication for two weeks only, and to apply the cream sparingly. The physician should be notified if the condition persists after two weeks. Patients should also be advised to wear loose fitting clothing. (See **Dosage and Administration** section.)
6. Patients should report any signs of local adverse reactions.
7. Parents of pediatric patients should be advised not to use tight-fitting diapers or plastic pants on a child being treated in the diaper area, as these garments may constitute occlusive dressing. (See **Dosage and Administration** section.)
8. Patients should avoid sources of infection or reinfection.

Laboratory Tests: If there is a lack of response to LOTRISONE Cream, appropriate microbiological studies should be repeated to confirm the diagnosis and rule out other pathogens before instituting another course of antimycotic therapy.

The following tests may be helpful in evaluating HPA axis suppression due to the corticosteroid component:
 Urinary free cortisol test
 ACTH stimulation test

Carcinogenesis, Mutagenesis, Impairment of Fertility: There are no animal or laboratory studies with the combination clotrimazole and betamethasone dipropionate to evaluate carcinogenesis, mutagenesis or impairment of fertility.

An 18-month oral dosing study with clotrimazole in rats has not revealed any carcinogenic effect.

In tests for mutagenesis, chromosomes of the spermatophores of Chinese hamsters which have been exposed to clotrimazole were examined for structural changes during the metaphase. Prior to testing, the hamsters had received five oral clotrimazole doses of 100 mg/kg body weight. The results of this study showed that clotrimazole had no mutagenic effect.

Pregnancy Category C: There have been no teratogenic studies performed with the combination clotrimazole and betamethasone dipropionate.

Studies in pregnant rats with intravaginal doses up to 100 mg/kg have revealed no evidence of harm to the fetus due to clotrimazole.

High oral doses of clotrimazole in rats and mice ranging from 50 to 120 mg/kg resulted in embryotoxicity (possibly secondary to maternal toxicity), impairment of mating, decreased litter size and number of viable young and decreased pup survival to weaning. However, clotrimazole was not teratogenic in mice, rabbits and rats at oral doses up to 200, 180 and 100 mg/kg, respectively. Oral absorption in the rat amounts to approximately 90% of the administered dose.

Corticosteroids are generally teratogenic in laboratory animals when administered systemically at relatively low dosage levels. The more potent corticosteroids have been shown to be teratogenic after dermal application in laboratory animals.

There are no adequate and well-controlled studies in pregnant women on teratogenic effects from a topically applied combination of clotrimazole and betamethasone dipropionate. Therefore, LOTRISONE Cream should be used during pregnancy only if the potential benefit justifies the potential risk to the fetus.

Drugs containing corticosteroids should not be used extensively on pregnant patients, in large amounts, or for prolonged periods of time.

Nursing Mothers: It is not known whether this drug is excreted in human milk. Because many drugs are excreted in human milk, caution should be exercised when LOTRISONE Cream is used by a nursing woman.

Pediatric Use: Safety and effectiveness in children below the age of 12 have not been established with LOTRISONE Cream. However, dosage forms containing concentrations of clotrimazole and of betamethasone dipropionate found in LOTRISONE Cream have been demonstrated to be safe and effective when used as indicated and in the recommended dosages.

Pediatric patients may demonstrate greater susceptibility to topical corticosteroid-induced HPA axis suppression and Cushing's syndrome than mature patients because of a larger skin surface area to body weight ratio.

Hypothalamic-pituitary-adrenal (HPA) axis suppression, Cushing's syndrome, and intracranial hypertension have been reported in children receiving topical corticosteroids. Manifestations of adrenal suppression in children include linear growth retardation, delayed weight gain, low plasma cortisol levels, and absence of response to ACTH stimulation. Manifestations of intracranial hypertension include bulging fontanelles, headaches, and bilateral papilledema.

Continued on next page

Information on Schering products appearing on these pages is effective as of September 30, 1984.

Schering—Cont.

Administration of topical dermatologics containing a corticosteroid to children should be limited to the least amount compatible with an effective therapeutic regimen. Chronic corticosteroid therapy may interfere with the growth and development of children.

Adverse Reactions: The following adverse reactions have been reported in connection with the use of LOTRISONE Cream: paresthesia in 5 of 270 patients, maculopapular rash, edema, and secondary infection, each in 1 of 270 patients.

Adverse reactions reported with the use of clotrimazole are as follows: erythema, stinging, blistering, peeling, edema, pruritus, urticaria, and general irritation of the skin.

The following local adverse reactions are reported infrequently when topical corticosteroids are used as recommended. These reactions are listed in an approximate decreasing order of occurrence: burning, itching, irritation, dryness, folliculitis, hypertrichosis, acneiform eruptions, hypopigmentation, perioral dermatitis, allergic contact dermatitis, maceration of the skin, secondary infection, skin atrophy, striae, and miliaria.

Overdosage: Acute overdosage with topical application of LOTRISONE Cream is unlikely and would not be expected to lead to a life-threatening situation.

Topically applied corticosteroids can be absorbed in sufficient amounts to produce systemic effects. (See **Precautions**.)

Dosage and Administration: Gently massage sufficient LOTRISONE Cream into the affected and surrounding skin areas twice a day, in the morning and evening for two weeks in tinea cruris and tinea corporis, and for four weeks in tinea pedis. The use of LOTRISONE Cream for longer than four weeks is not recommended.

Clinical improvement, with relief of erythema and pruritus, usually occurs within three to five days of treatment. If a patient with tinea cruris and tinea corporis shows no clinical improvement after one week of treatment with LOTRISONE Cream, the diagnosis should be reviewed. In tinea pedis, the treatment should be applied for two weeks prior to making that decision.

Treatment with LOTRISONE Cream should be discontinued if the condition persists after two weeks in tinea cruris and tinea corporis, and after four weeks in tinea pedis. Alternate therapy may then be instituted with LOTRIMIN Cream, a product containing an antifungal only.

LOTRISONE Cream should not be used with occlusive dressings.

How Supplied: LOTRISONE Cream is supplied in 15-gram (NDC 0085-0924-01), and 45-gram tubes (NDC 0085-0924-02); boxes of one.

Store between 2° and 30°C (36° and 86°F).
4/84
Copyright © 1984, Schering Corporation. All rights reserved.

METIMYD® ℞
[met′ĭ-mid]
brand of prednisolone acetate, USP
and sulfacetamide sodium, USP
  Ophthalmic Suspension–Sterile
  Ophthalmic Ointment–Sterile

Description: METIMYD Ophthalmic Suspension is a steroid/anti-infective sterile preparation having a pH range of 7.0 to 7.4. Each ml contains: 5 mg prednisolone acetate, USP; 100 mg sulfacetamide sodium, USP; sodium phosphate dibasic, sodium phosphate monobasic, tyloxapol, sodium thiosulfate, edetate disodium, and purified water; 5 mg phenylethyl alcohol and 0.25 mg benzalkonium chloride as preservatives.

METIMYD Ophthalmic Ointment is a steroid/anti-infective sterile preparation containing in each gram: 5 mg prednisolone acetate, USP and 100 mg sulfacetamide sodium, USP; 0.5 mg methylparaben and 0.1 mg propylparaben as preservatives, in a bland, unctuous base of mineral oil and white petrolatum.

The empirical formula for prednisolone acetate, a 1-unsaturated analog of hydrocortisone acetate, is $C_{23}H_{30}O_6$. The molecular weight is 402.49. Chemically it is 11β,17,21-trihydroxypregna-1,4-diene-3,20-dione 21-acetate.

Prednisolone acetate is a nearly odorless, white to practically white, crystalline powder. It is slightly soluble in acetone, alcohol, and chloroform, and practically insoluble in water.

Sulfacetamide sodium, $C_8H_9N_2NaO_3S \cdot H_2O$, is a sulfonamide antibacterial agent with a molecular weight of 254.24. Chemically it is N-[(4-aminophenyl)sulfonyl]-, acetamide, monosodium salt, monohydrate.

Sulfacetamide sodium is an odorless, white, crystalline powder. It is freely soluble in water, sparingly soluble in alcohol and practically insoluble in benzene, chloroform, and ether.

Clinical Pharmacology: Corticosteroids suppress the inflammatory response to a variety of agents and they probably delay or slow healing. Since corticosteroids may inhibit the body's defense mechanism against infection, a concomitant antimicrobial drug may be used when this inhibition is considered to be clinically significant in a particular case.

The anti-infective component in the combination is included to provide action against specific organisms susceptible to it.

When a decision is made to administer both a corticoid and an antimicrobial, the administration of such drugs in combination has the advantages of greater patient compliance and convenience and added assurance that the appropriate dosage of both drugs is administered. There is also assured compatibility of ingredients when both types of drug are in the same formulation and, particularly, that the correct volume of drug is delivered and retained.

The relative potency of corticosteroids depends on the molecular structure, concentration, and release from the vehicle.

Indications and Usage: METIMYD Ophthalmic Suspension or Ointment is indicated for steroid-responsive inflammatory ocular conditions for which a corticosteroid is indicated and where bacterial infection or a risk of bacterial ocular infection exists.

Ocular steroids are indicated in inflammatory conditions of the palpebral and bulbar conjunctivae, cornea, and anterior segment of the globe where the inherent risk of steroid use in certain infective conjunctivitides is accepted to obtain a diminution in edema and inflammation. They are also indicated in chronic anterior uveitis and corneal injury from chemical, radiation, or thermal burns, or penetration of foreign bodies.

The use of a combination drug with an anti-infective component is indicated where the risk of infection is high or where there is an expectation that potentially dangerous numbers of bacteria will be present in the eye.

The particular anti-infective drug in this product is active against the following common bacterial eye pathogens: *Pseudomonas* species. *Hemophilus influenzae, Klebsiella* species, *Staphylococcus aureus, Streptococcus pneumoniae, Streptococcus* (Viridans group), *Escherichia coli,* and *Enterobacter* species.

This product does not provide adequate coverage against: *Neisseria* species and *Serratia marcescens*.

Contraindications: METIMYD is contraindicated in: epithelial herpes simplex keratitis (dendritic keratitis), vaccinia, varicella, and many other viral diseases of the cornea or conjunctiva; mycobacterial infection of the eye; and fungal diseases of ocular structures. METIMYD is contraindicated in individuals with known or suspected hypersensitivity to any of the ingredients of the preparation, or to other sulfonamides, or other corticosteroids. (Hypersensitivity to the antibacterial component occurs at a higher rate than for other components.) The use of these combinations is always contraindicated after uncomplicated removal of a corneal foreign body.

Warnings: Prolonged use may result in glaucoma, with damage to the optic nerve, defects in visual acuity and fields of vision, and in posterior subcapsular cataract formation. Prolonged use may suppress the host response and thus increase the hazard of secondary ocular infections. In those diseases causing thinning of the cornea or sclera, perforations have been known to occur with the use of topical steroids. In acute purulent conditions of the eye, steroids may mask infection or enhance existing infection. If these products are used for 10 days or longer, intraocular pressure should be routinely monitored even though this may be difficult in children and uncooperative patients.

Employment of steroid medication in the treatment of herpes simplex requires great caution.

A significant percentage of staphylococcal isolates are completely resistant to sulfonamides.

Precautions: The initial prescription and renewal of the medication order beyond 20 ml of METIMYD Ophthalmic **Suspension** or beyond 8 g of the Ointment should be made by a physician only after examination of the patient with the aid of magnification, such as slitlamp biomicroscopy and where appropriate, fluorescein staining.

The possibility of fungal infections of the cornea should be considered after prolonged steroid dosing.

Sensitization may recur when a sulfonamide is readministered irrespective of the route of administration and cross-sensitivity among different sulfonamides may occur. (See ADVERSE REACTIONS.) Cross-allergenicity among corticosteroids has been demonstrated. If signs of hypersensitivity or other untoward reactions occur, discontinue use of the preparation.

Adverse Reactions: Adverse reactions have occurred which can be attributed to the steroid component, the anti-infective component, or the combination. Exact incidence figures are not available since no denominator of treated patients is available.

Reactions occurring most often from the presence of the anti-infective ingredient are allergic sensitizations. Instances of Stevens-Johnson syndrome and systemic lupus erythematosus (in one case producing a fatal outcome) have been reported following the use of ophthalmic sulfonamide containing preparations.

The reactions due to the steroid component in decreasing order of frequency are: elevation of intraocular pressure (IOP) with possible development of glaucoma, and infrequent optic nerve damage; posterior subcapsular cataract formation; and delayed wound healing.

Corticosteroid-containing preparations can also cause acute anterior uveitis or perforation of the globe. Mydriasis, loss of accommodation, and ptosis have occasionally been reported following local use of corticosteroids.

Secondary Infection: The development of secondary infection has occurred after use of combinations containing steroids and antimicrobials. Fungal infections of the cornea are particularly prone to develop coincidentally with long-term applications of the steroid. The possibility of fungal invasion must be considered in any persistent corneal ulceration where steriod treatment has been used. Secondary bacterial ocular infection following suppression of host responses also occurs.

Dosage and Administration: METIMYD Ophthalmic Suspension: Two or three drops should be instilled into the conjunctival sac every one to two hours during the day and at bedtime until a favorable response is obtained.

METIMYD Ophthalmic Ointment: A thin film should be applied three or four times daily and once at bedtime until a favorable response is obtained.

The initial prescription of METIMYD Ophthalmic should *not* be more than 20 ml of the **Suspension** or 8 g of the **Ointment** and the prescription should not be refilled without further evaluation as outlined in PRECAUTIONS.

Dosage should be adjusted according to the specific needs of the patient. METIMYD Ophthalmic Suspension or Ointment dosage may be reduced, but care should be taken not to discontinue therapy prematurely. In chronic conditions, with-

drawal of treatment should be carried out by gradually decreasing the frequency of application.
How Supplied: METIMYD Ophthalmic Suspension, 5 ml dropper bottle; box of one. **Store between 2° and 30°C (36° and 86°F). Clumping may occur on long standing at high temperatures. Shake well before using. Protect from light.**
METIMYD Ophthalmic Ointment, 3.5 g applicator tube; box of one. **Store between 2° and 30°C (36° and 86°F).**
Revised 1/83
Copyright© 1969, 1983, Schering Corporation. All rights reserved.

METRETON®
[met'rĕ-ton]
brand of prednisolone sodium phosphate, USP
(0.5% prednisolone phosphate equivalent)
Ophthalmic/Otic Solution—Sterile

Description: METRETON Ophthalmic/Otic Solution is a clear, sterile, aqueous solution. Each ml contains 5.5 mg prednisolone sodium phosphate, USP (equivalent to 5.0 mg prednisolone phosphate), edetate disodium, monobasic sodium phosphate, dibasic sodium phosphate, tyloxapol, purified water, sodium hydroxide to adjust pH to approximately 7.8; benzalkonium chloride and phenylethyl alcohol are added as preservatives.
Actions: METRETON Ophthalmic/Otic Solution inhibits the inflammatory response to inciting agents of a mechanical, chemical or immunological nature. No generally accepted explanation of this steroid property has been advanced.
Indications: METRETON Ophthalmic/Otic Solution is indicated for the treatment of the following conditions.
Eye: steroid-responsive inflammatory conditions of the palpebral and bulbar conjunctiva, cornea and anterior segment of the globe, such as allergic conjunctivitis, acne rosacea, superficial punctate keratitis, herpes zoster keratitis, iritis, cyclitis, selected infective conjunctivitis when the inherent hazard of steroid use is accepted to obtain an advisable diminution in edema and inflammation; corneal injury from chemical or thermal burns or penetration of foreign bodies.
Ear: steroid-responsive inflammatory conditions of the external auditory canal, such as allergic otitis externa, selected purulent and nonpurulent infective otitis externa when the hazard of steroid use is accepted to obtain an advisable diminution in edema and inflammation.
Contraindications: Hypersensitivity to a component of this medication contraindicates its use.
Eye: METRETON Ophthalmic/Otic Solution should not be used in acute superficial herpes simplex keratitis or in other viral infections of the cornea and conjunctiva, such as vaccinia and varicella. It is also contraindicated in patients with tuberculosis of the eye or in those with fungal infections of ocular structures.
Ear: METRETON Ophthalmic/Otic Solution is contraindicated if the tympanic membrane is perforated or in those patients with fungal infections of external ear structures.
Warnings: *Eye:* METRETON Ophthalmic/Otic Solution is not effective in mustard gas keratitis and in Sjogren's keratoconjunctivitis.
Steroids should be used with great caution in the treatment of stromal herpes simplex; frequent slit-lamp microscopy is mandatory.
Prolonged use of this medication may result in glaucoma, damage to the optic nerve, defects in visual acuity and fields of vision, posterior subcapsular cataract formation, or may aid in the establishment of secondary ocular infections from pathogens liberated from ocular tissues.
In those diseases causing thinning of the cornea or sclera, perforation has been known to occur with the use of topical steriods.
Acute, purulent, untreated infection of the eye may be masked or activity enhanced by the presence of steroid medication.

Ear: Acute, purulent, untreated infection of the ear may be masked or activity enhanced by the presence of steroid medication.
Usage in Pregnancy The safety of intensive or protracted use of topical steroids during pregnancy has not been substantiated.
Precautions: *Eye:* Since fungal infections of the cornea are particularly prone to develop coincidentally with long-term local steroid applications, fungus invasion must be considered in any persistent corneal ulceration where a steroid is in use or has been used.
Intraocular pressure should be checked frequently.
Ear: If symptoms in the ear persist, the presence of a fungus infection must be considered.
Adverse Reactions: Glaucoma with optic nerve damage, visual acuity and field defects, posterior subcapsular cataract formation, secondary ocular infections from pathogens, including herpes simplex liberated from ocular tissues, perforation of the globe.
Rarely, stinging or burning may occur.
Dosage and Administration: The duration of treatment will vary with the type of lesion and may extend from a few days to several weeks, depending on therapeutic response. Relapses, more common in chronic, active lesions than in self-limited conditions, usually respond to retreatment.
Eye Instill one or two drops of METRETON Ophthalmic/Otic Solution into the conjunctival sac every hour during the day and every two hours during the night as initial therapy. When a favorable response is observed, reduce dosage to one drop every four hours. Later, further reduction in dosage to one drop three or four times daily may suffice to control symptoms.
Ear Clean the aural canal thoroughly and sponge dry. Instill the solution directly into the aural canal. A suggested initial dosage is three or four drops two or three times a day. When a favorable response is obtained, reduce dosage gradually and eventually discontinue.
If preferred, the aural canal may be packed with a gauze wick saturated with solution. Keep the wick moist with the preparation and remove from the ear after 12 to 24 hours. Treatment may be repeated as often as necessary at the discretion of the physician.
How Supplied: METRETON Ophthalmic/Otic Solution, 5-ml plastic dropper bottle, box of one. **Store between 2° and 30°C (36° and 86°F). Protect from light.**
Store in carton until contents are used.
Revised 7/80
Copyright© 1973, 1980. Schering Corporation. All rights reserved.

NAQUA®
[nak'wah]
brand of trichlormethiazide
Tablets, USP

Description: NAQUA Tablets contain trichlormethiazide, USP, an antihypertensive agent and diuretic of the benzothiadiazine series having the chemical formula, $C_8H_8Cl_3N_3O_4S_2$. Each NAQUA Tablet contains 2 or 4 mg trichlormethiazide, USP.
Actions: The mechanism of action results in an interference with the renal tubular mechanism of electrolyte reabsorption. At maximal therapeutic dosage all thiazides are approximately equal in their diuretic potency. The mechanism whereby thiazides function in the control of hypertension is unknown.
Indications: NAQUA Tablets are indicated as adjunctive therapy in edema associated with congestive heart failure, hepatic cirrhosis, and corticosteroid and estrogen therapy.
NAQUA Tablets have also been found useful in edema due to various forms of renal dysfunction, such as: nephrotic syndrome; acute glomerulonephritis; and chronic renal failure.
NAQUA Tablets are indicated in the management of hypertension either as the sole therapeutic agent or to enhance the effectiveness of other antihypertensive drugs in the more severe forms of hypertension.
Usage in Pregnancy The routine use of diuretics in an otherwise healthy woman is inappropriate and exposes the mother and fetus to unnecessary hazard. Diuretics do not prevent development of toxemia in pregnancy, and there is no satisfactory evidence that they are useful in the treatment of developed toxemia.
Edema during pregnancy may arise from pathological causes or from the physiologic and mechanical consequences of pregnancy. Thiazides are indicated in pregnancy when edema is due to pathologic causes, just as they are in the absence of pregnancy (however, see WARNINGS, below). Dependent edema in pregnancy, resulting from restriction of venous return by the expanded uterus, is properly treated through elevation of the lower extremities and use of support hose; use of diuretics to lower intravascular volume in this case is illogical and unnecessary. There is hypervolemia during normal pregnancy which is harmful to neither the fetus nor the mother (in the absence of cardiovascular disease), but which is associated with edema, including generalized edema, in the majority of pregnant women. If this edema produces discomfort, increased recumbency will often provide relief. In rare instances, this edema may cause extreme discomfort which is not relieved by rest. In these cases, a short course of diuretics may provide relief and may be appropriate.
Contraindications: NAQUA Tablets are contraindicated in patients with anuria.
Hypersensitivity to this or other sulfonamide-derived drugs is a contraindication to the use of this product.
Warnings: Thiazides should be used with caution in severe renal disease. In patients with renal disease, thiazides may precipitate azotemia. Cumulative effects of the drug may develop in patients with impaired renal function.
Thiazides should be used with caution in patients with impaired hepatic function or progressive liver disease, since minor alterations of fluid and electrolyte balance may precipitate hepatic coma.
Thiazides may add to or potentiate the action of other antihypertensive drugs. Potentiation occurs with ganglionic or peripheral adrenergic blocking drugs.
Hypersensitivity reactions may occur in patients with a history of allergy or bronchial asthma.
The possibility of exacerbation or activation of systemic lupus erythematosus has been reported.
Usage in Pregnancy Thiazides cross the placental barrier and appear in cord blood. The use of thiazides in pregnant women requires that the anticipated benefit be weighed against possible hazards to the fetus. These hazards include fetal or neonatal jaundice, thrombocytopenia, and possibly other adverse reactions which have occurred in the adult.
Nursing Mothers Thiazides appear in breast milk. If use of the drug is deemed essential, the patient should stop nursing.
Precautions: Periodic determination of serum electrolytes to detect possible electrolyte imbalance should be performed at appropriate intervals.
All patients receiving thiazide therapy should be observed for clinical signs of fluid or electrolyte imbalance, namely, hyponatremia, hypochloremic alkalosis, hypokalemia, hypomagnesemia, and changes in serum and urinary calcium. Serum and urine electrolyte determinations are particularly important when the patient is vomiting excessively or receiving parenteral fluids. Medications such as digitalis derivatives are sensitive to changes in serum electrolytes. Warning signs, irrespective of cause, are: dryness of mouth, thirst, weakness, lethargy, drowsiness, restlessness, muscle pains or cramps, muscular fatigue, hypoten-

Continued on next page

Information on Schering products appearing on these pages is effective as of September 30, 1984.

Schering—Cont.

sion, oliguria, tachycardia, and gastrointestinal disturbances such as nausea and vomiting.
Hypokalemia may develop with thiazides as with any other potent diuretic, especially with brisk diuresis, when severe cirrhosis is present, or during concomitant use of corticosteroids or ACTH. Interference with adequate oral electrolyte intake will also contribute to hypokalemia. Digitalis therapy may exaggerate metabolic effects of hypokalemia especially with reference to myocardial activity.
Any chloride deficit is generally mild and usually does not require specific treatment except under extraordinary circumstances (as in liver disease or renal disease). Dilutional hyponatremia may occur in edematous patients in hot weather; appropriate therapy is water restriction, rather than administration of salt, except in rare instances when the hyponatremia is life-threatening. In actual salt depletion, appropriate replacement is the therapy of choice.
Hyperuricemia may occur or frank gout may be precipitated in certain patients receiving thiazide therapy.
Insulin requirements in diabetic patients may be increased, decreased, or unchanged. Latent diabetes mellitus may become manifest during thiazide administration; diabetic complications such as reversible oculomotor paresis may occur.
Thiazide drugs may increase the responsiveness to tubocurarine.
The antihypertensive effects of the drug may be enhanced in the post-sympathectomy patient.
Thiazides may decrease arterial responsiveness to norepinephrine. This diminution is not sufficient to preclude effectiveness of the pressor agent for therapeutic use.
If progressive renal impairment becomes evident, as indicated by a rising nonprotein nitrogen or blood urea nitrogen, a careful reappraisal of therapy is necessary with consideration given to withholding or discontinuing diuretic therapy.
Thiazides may decrease serum PBI levels without signs of thyroid disturbance.
Adverse Reactions: *Gastrointestinal System Reactions:* anorexia; gastric irritation; nausea; vomiting; cramping; diarrhea; constipation; jaundice (intrahepatic cholestatic jaundice); pancreatitis.
Central Nervous System Reactions: dizziness; vertigo; paresthesias; headache; xanthopsia.
Hematologic Reactions: leukopenia; agranulocytosis; thrombocytopenia; aplastic anemia.
Dermatologic—Hypersensitivity Reactions: purpura; photosensitivity; rash; urticaria; necrotizing angiitis (vasculitis, cutaneous vasculitis).
Cardiovascular Reaction: Orthostatic hypotension may occur and may be aggravated by alcohol, barbiturates or narcotics.
Other: hyperglycemia; glycosuria; hyperuricemia; muscle spasm; weakness; restlessness. Whenever adverse reactions are moderate or severe, thiazide dosage should be reduced or therapy withdrawn.
Dosage and Administration: Therapy should be individualized according to patient response. This therapy should be titrated to gain maximal therapeutic response as well as the minimal dose possible to maintain that therapeutic response.
Edematous Conditions The usual dosage of NAQUA Tablets for diuretic effect is 1 to 4 mg daily.
Hypertension The usual dosage of NAQUA Tablets for antihypertensive effect is 2 to 4 mg daily.
How Supplied: NAQUA Tablets, 2 mg, pink, clover-shaped, compressed tablets impressed with the letter S and either product identification letters, AHG, or numbers 822; bottles of 100 (NDC 0085-0822-03) and 1000 (NDC 0085-0822-06).
NAQUA Tablets, 4 mg, aqua, clover-shaped, compressed tablets impressed with the letter S and either product identification letters, AHH, or numbers 547; bottles of 100 (NDC 0085-0547-03) and 1000 (NDC 0085-0547-06).

Revised 7/83
Copyright © 1968, 1983, Schering Corporation. All rights reserved.
Shown in Product Identification Section, page 434

NAQUIVAL® ℞
[nak'kwiv-al]
brand of trichlormethiazide, USP—reserpine, USP
Tablets

Warning
This fixed combination drug is not indicated for initial therapy of hypertension. Hypertension requires therapy titrated to the individual patient. If the fixed combination represents the dosage so determined, its use may be more convenient in patient management. The treatment of hypertension is not static, but must be re-evaluated as conditions in each patient warrant.

Description: Each NAQUIVAL Tablet contains 4 mg NAQUA® (brand of trichlormethiazide, USP) and 0.1 mg reserpine, USP. Trichlormethiazide is an antihypertensive agent and diuretic of the benzothiadiazine series having the chemical formula, $C_8H_8Cl_3N_3O_4S_2$. The antihypertensive agent, reserpine, is a rauwolfia alkaloid having the chemical formula, $C_{33}H_{40}N_2O_9$.
Actions: NAQUIVAL Tablets combine the antihypertensive and diuretic properties of trichlormethiazide with the antihypertensive actions of reserpine; maximum antihypertensive effects are achieved with minimal doses of each ingredient.
Indications: NAQUIVAL Tablets are indicated for the treatment of hypertension (see box warning).
Contraindications: NAQUIVAL Tablets are contraindicated in patients with anuria.
Hypersensitivity to this or other sulfonamide-derived drugs is a contraindication to the use of this product.
The routine use of diuretics in an otherwise healthy pregnant woman with or without mild edema is contraindicated and possibly hazardous.
The presence of an active peptic ulcer, ulcerative colitis, or severe depression contraindicates the use of reserpine.
Warnings: NAQUIVAL Tablets should be withdrawn at least three weeks prior to elective surgery or electroconvulsive therapy because of the reserpine activity.
If parenteral antihypertensive therapy is indicated for a patient receiving NAQUIVAL Tablets, the physician should be alert to the possible synergism of reserpine and trichlormethiazide with such drugs, especially those administered by rapid infusion, e.g., diazoxide.
Sympathomimetics should be used with caution in patients who are receiving reserpine, since its antihypertensive effects may be reduced.
NAQUIVAL Tablets should be used with caution in severe renal disease. In patients with renal disease, thiazides may precipitate azotemia. Cumulative effects of the drug may develop in patients with impaired renal function.
Thiazides should be used with caution in patients with impaired hepatic function or progressive liver disease, since minor alterations of fluid and electrolyte balance may precipitate hepatic coma.
Thiazides may be additive or potentiative of the action of other antihypertensive drugs. Potentiation occurs with ganglionic or peripheral adrenergic blocking drugs or vasodilators.
Hypersensitivity reactions may occur in patients with a history of allergy or bronchial asthma.
The possibility of exacerbation or activation of systemic lupus erythematosus has been reported.
Usage in Pregnancy Usage of thiazides in women of childbearing age requires that the potential benefits of the drug be weighed against its possible hazards to the fetus. These hazards include fetal or neonatal jaundice, thrombocytopenia, and possibly other adverse reactions which have occurred in the adult.

The safety of reserpine for use during pregnancy or lactation has not been established; therefore, it should be used in pregnant patients or in women of childbearing age only when, in the judgment of the physician, its use is deemed essential to the welfare of the patient.
Nursing Mothers Thiazides cross the placental barrier and appear in cord blood and breast milk.
Precautions: Periodic determination of serum electrolytes to detect possible electrolyte imbalance should be performed at appropriate intervals.
All patients receiving thiazide therapy should be observed for clinical signs of fluid or electrolyte imbalance, namely, hyponatremia, hypochloremic alkalosis, hypokalemia, hypomagnesemia, and changes in serum and urinary calcium. Serum and urine electrolyte determinations are particularly important when the patient is vomiting excessively or receiving parenteral fluids. Medications such as digitalis derivatives are sensitive to changes in serum electrolytes. Warning signs, irrespective of cause, are: dryness of mouth, thirst, weakness, lethargy, drowsiness, restlessness, muscle pains or cramps, muscular fatigue, hypotension, oliguria, tachycardia, and gastrointestinal disturbances such as nausea and vomiting.
Hypokalemia may develop with thiazides as with any other potent diuretic, especially with brisk diuresis, when severe cirrhosis is present, or during concomitant use of corticosteroids or ACTH. Interference with adequate oral electrolyte intake will also contribute to hypokalemia. Digitalis therapy may exaggerate metabolic effects of hypokalemia especially with reference to myocardial activity.
Any chloride deficit is generally mild and usually does not require specific treatment except under extraordinary circumstances (as in liver disease or renal disease). Dilutional hyponatremia may occur in edematous patients in hot weather; appropriate therapy is water restriction, rather than administration of salt, except in rare instances when the hyponatremia is life-threatening. In actual salt depletion, appropriate replacement is the therapy of choice.
Hyperuricemia may occur or frank gout may be precipitated in certain patients receiving thiazide therapy.
Insulin requirements in diabetic patients may be increased, decreased, or unchanged. Latent diabetes mellitus may become manifest during thiazide administration; diabetic complications such as reversible oculomotor paresis may occur.
Thiazide drugs may increase the responsiveness to tubocurarine.
The antihypertensive effects of the drug may be enhanced in the post-sympathectomy patient.
Thiazides may decrease arterial responsiveness to norepinephrine. This diminution is not sufficient to preclude effectiveness of the pressor agent for therapeutic use.
If progressive renal impairment becomes evident, as indicated by a rising nonprotein nitrogen or blood urea nitrogen, a careful reappraisal of therapy is necessary with consideration given to withholding or discontinuing diuretic therapy.
Thiazides may decrease serum PBI levels without signs of thyroid disturbance.
Reserpine may augment secretory and motor activity of the gastrointestinal tract, and gastric hyperacidity, peptic ulceration, and mucous colitis may develop. Patients undergoing emergency surgery should be watched for precipitous falls in blood pressure; vasopressor agents such as levarterenol should be available.
Reserpine may precipitate biliary colic in patients with gallstones.
Because of the decreased sympathetic tone caused by reserpine catecholamine depletion, special care should be exercised in treating patients with a history of bronchial asthma.
NAQUIVAL Tablets contain FD&C Yellow No. 5 (tartrazine) which may cause allergic-type reactions (including bronchial asthma) in certain susceptible individuals. Although the overall incidence of FD&C Yellow No. 5 (tartrazine) sensitivity in the general population is low, it is frequently

seen in patients who also have aspirin hypersensitivity.

Animal Tumorigenicity Rodent studies have shown that reserpine is an animal tumorigen, causing an increased incidence of mammary fibroadenomas in female mice, malignant tumors of the seminal vesicles in male mice, and malignant adrenal medullary tumors in male rats. These findings arose in 2 year studies in which the drug was administered in the feed at concentrations of 5 and 10 ppm-about 100 to 300 times the usual human dose. The breast neoplasms are thought to be related to reserpine's prolactin-elevating effect. Several other prolactin-elevating drugs have also been associated with an increased incidence of mammary neoplasia in rodents.

The extent to which these findings indicate a risk to humans is uncertain. Tissue culture experiments show that about one-third of human breast tumors are prolactin-dependent *in vitro*, a factor of considerable importance if the use of the drug is contemplated in a patient with previously detected breast cancer. The possibility of an increased risk of breast cancer in reserpine users has been studied extensively; however, no firm conclusion has emerged. Although a few epidemiologic studies have suggested a slightly increased risk (less than twofold in all studies except one) in women who have used reserpine, other studies of generally similar design have not confirmed this. Epidemiologic studies conducted using other drugs (neuroleptic agents) that, like reserpine, increase prolactin levels and therefore would be considered rodent mammary carcinogens, have not shown an association between chronic administration of the drug and human mammary tumorigenesis. While long-term clinical observation has not suggested such an association, the available evidence is considered too limited to be conclusive at this time. An association of reserpine intake with pheochromocytoma or tumors of the seminal vesicles has not been explored.

Adverse Reactions: *Autonomic Reactions:* nasal stuffiness; dryness of the mouth; blurred vision; flushing of the face.

Gastrointestinal System Reactions: anorexia; gastric irritation; nausea; vomiting; cramping; diarrhea; constipation; jaundice (intrahepatic cholestatic jaundice); pancreatitis.

Central Nervous System Reactions: dizziness; vertigo; paresthesias; headache; xanthopsia; depression; central nervous system sensitization manifested as dull sensorium, deafness, glaucoma, uveitis, and optic atrophy.

Hematologic Reactions: leukopenia; agranulocytosis; thrombocytopenia; aplastic anemia.

Dermatologic—Hypersensitivity Reactions: purpura; photosensitivity; rash; urticaria; necrotizing angiitis (vasculitis, cutaneous vasculitis).

Cardiovascular Reactions: Ectopic cardiac rhythms, particularly when used concurrently with digitalis; orthostatic hypotension may occur and may be aggravated by alcohol, barbiturates or narcotics.

Other: hyperglycemia; glycosuria; hyperuricemia; muscle spasm; weakness; restlessness; drowsiness; weight gain; dyspnea; dyskinesia; impotence and decreased libido; conjunctival injection.

Whenever adverse reactions are moderate or severe, NAQUIVAL dosage should be reduced or therapy withdrawn.

Dosage and Administration: The dosage of NAQUIVAL should be determined by individual titration (see box warning).

Initial dosage with NAQUIVAL is frequently one tablet twice a day, with reduction to maintenance levels as therapeutic benefits become manifest.

When NAQUIVAL is used with ganglionic blocking agents, careful downward adjustment of these drugs should be made to avoid precipitous blood pressure falls.

How Supplied: NAQUIVAL Tablets: peach-colored, scored, compressed tablets impressed with the Schering Trademark and product identification letters, AHT or numbers, 394; bottles of 100 (NDC 0085-0394-03) and 500 (NDC 0085-0394-06).

Store between 2° and 30°C (36° and 86°F).
Revised 6/83
Copyright © 1968, 1983, Schering Corporation. All rights reserved.
Shown in Product Identification Section, page 434

NETROMYCIN®   R
[ně″trō-mĭ sĭn]
brand of netilmicin sulfate
Injection, USP 100 mg/ml
Pediatric Injection, USP 25 mg/ml
Neonatal Injection, USP 10 mg/ml

WARNINGS

Patients treated with aminoglycosides should be under close clinical observation because of the potential toxicity associated with the use of these drugs.

Netilmicin has potent neuromuscular blocking potential. Neuromuscular blockade and respiratory paralysis have been reported in animals receiving netilmicin. The possibility of these phenomena occurring in man should be considered if aminoglycosides are administered by any route to patients receiving neuromuscular blocking agents, such as succinylcholine, tubocurarine, or decamethonium, or to patients receiving massive transfusions of citrate-anticoagulated blood. If neuromuscular blockade occurs, calcium salts may lessen it, but mechanical respiratory assistance may also be necessary.

As with other aminoglycosides, netilmicin sulfate injection is potentially nephrotoxic. The risk is greater in patients with impaired renal function, in those who receive high dosage or prolonged therapy, and in the elderly. Neurotoxicity manifested by ototoxicity, both vestibular and auditory, can occur in patients treated with netilmicin, primarily in those with preexisting renal damage and in patients, treated with higher doses and/or for longer periods than recommended. Aminoglycoside-induced ototoxicity is usually irreversible. Other manifestations of aminoglycoside-induced neurotoxicity include numbness, skin tingling, muscle twitching, and convulsions.

Renal and eighth cranial nerve function should be closely monitored, especially in patients with known or suspected impairment of renal function either at onset of therapy or during therapy. Urine should be examined for increased excretion of protein, the presence of cells or casts, and decreased specific gravity. Serum creatinine concentration or blood urea nitrogen should be determined periodically. A more precise measure of glomerular filtration rate is a carefully conducted determination of creatinine clearance rate or, often more practically, an estimate of creatinine clearance based on published nomograms or equations. (See DOSAGE AND ADMINISTRATION.) When feasible it is recommended that serial audiograms be obtained in patients old enough to be tested, particularly in high-risk patients. The dosage of netilmicin should be reduced or administration discontinued if evidence of drug-induced auditory or vestibular toxicity (vertigo, tinnitus, nystagmus, or hearing loss) develops during therapy. If evidence of nephrotoxicity occurs, dosage should be adjusted. (See DOSAGE AND ADMINISTRATION, Dosage for Impaired Renal Function.) As with the other aminoglycosides, on rare occasions changes in renal and eighth cranial nerve functions may not become manifest until soon after completion of therapy.

Serum concentrations of aminoglycosides should be monitored when feasible to assure adequate levels and to avoid potentially toxic levels. After administration of an appropriate dose of netilmicin, peak serum concentrations occur approximately 30 to 60 minutes after an intramuscular injection or at the end of a one hour intravenous infusion. Dosage should be adjusted so that prolonged peak serum concentrations above 16 mcg/ml are avoided.

When monitoring trough concentrations, dosage should be adjusted so that levels above 4 mcg/ml are avoided. Excessive peak and/or trough serum concentrations of aminoglycosides may increase the risk of renal and eighth cranial nerve toxicity. In the event of overdose or toxic reactions, hemodialysis may aid in removal of netilmicin from the blood, especially if renal function is, or becomes, compromised. Removal of netilmicin by peritoneal dialysis is at a rate considerably less than by hemodialysis.

Concurrent and/or sequential systemic or topical use of other potentially neurotoxic and/or nephrotoxic drugs, such as: cephaloridine, amphotericin B, streptomycin, kanamycin, gentamicin, tobramycin, amikacin, neomycin, vancomycin, bacitracin, polymyxin B, colistin, paromomycin, viomycin, or cisplatin should be avoided. The concurrent use of aminoglycosides with potent diuretics, such as ethacrynic acid or furosemide, should be avoided since certain diuretics by themselves may cause ototoxicity. In addition, when administered intravenously, diuretics may enhance aminoglycoside toxicity by altering the antibiotic concentration in the serum and tissues. Other factors which may increase patient risk of toxicity are advanced age and dehydration.

Description: NETROMYCIN Injection, NETROMYCIN Pediatric Injection, and NETROMYCIN Neonatal Injection contain netilmicin sulfate in clear, sterile aqueous solution with a pH range of 3.5 to 6.0 for intramuscular or intravenous administration. Netilmicin is a semisynthetic, water-soluble antibiotic of the aminoglycoside group, derived from sisomicin. Its chemical name is: O-3-Deoxy-4-C-methyl-3-(methylamino)-β-L-arabinopyranosyl(1→4)-O-[2,6-diamino-2,3,4,6-tetradeoxy-α-D-$glycero$-hex-4-enopyranosyl-(1→6)]-2-deoxy-N^3-ethyl-L-streptamine sulfate (2:5) (salt).

Each ml of NETROMYCIN Injection contains netilmicin sulfate equivalent to 100 mg netilmicin; 10 mg benzyl alcohol as a preservative; 0.1 mg edetate disodium; 2.4 mg sodium metabisulfite; 0.8 mg sodium sulfite; and water for injection, q.s. Each ml of NETROMYCIN Pediatric Injection contains netilmicin sulfate equivalent to 25 mg netilmicin; 0.2 mg propylparaben and 1.3 mg methylparaben as preservatives; 0.1 mg edetate disodium; 2.6 mg sodium sulfate; 2.1 mg sodium metabisulfite; 1.2 mg of sodium sulfite; and water for injection, q.s. NETROMYCIN Neonatal Injection contains in each ml netilmicin sulfate equivalent to 10 mg netilmicin; 2.4 mg sodium metabisulfite; 0.8 mg sodium sulfite; 6.5 mg sodium chloride; and water for injection, q.s.

Clinical Pharmacology: Netilmicin is rapidly and completely absorbed after intramuscular injection. Peak serum levels, after intramuscular injection, usually occur within 30 to 60 minutes and levels are measurable for 12 hours. In adult volunteers with normal renal function, peak serum concentrations of netilmicin in mcg/ml are usually about 3 to 3.5 times the single intramuscular dose in mg/kg. For example, a dose of 2.0 mg/kg may be expected to result in a peak serum concentration of approximately 7 mcg/ml. At eight or more hours after administration of a dose in the recommended range, serum levels are usually less than 3 mcg/ml. When a single dose of netilmicin is administered by 60-minute intravenous infusion, the peak serum concentrations are similar to those obtained by intramuscular administration. Following a rapid intravenous injection

Continued on next page

Information on Schering products appearing on these pages is effective as of September 30, 1984.

Schering—Cont.

of netilmicin, levels in serum may be transiently 2 to 3 times higher than those of the 60-minute infusion. Netilmicin rapidly distributes to tissues.

The half-life of netilmicin after single doses is usually 2 to 2.5 hours, a half-life which is very similar to that of gentamicin, and is independent of the route of administration. The half-life increases as the dose increases (e.g., 2.2 hours after a 1 mg/kg dose to 3 hours after a 3 mg/kg dose). Approximately 80% of the administered dose is excreted in the urine within 24 hours; the urine netilmicin concentration after a dose often exceeds 100 mcg/ml. There is no evidence of metabolic transformation of netilmicin. The drug is excreted principally by glomerular filtration. Probenecid does not affect tubular transport of aminoglycosides. The volume of distribution of netilmicin is approximately 20% of body weight; total body clearance is about 80 ml/min and renal clearance is about 60 ml/min. In multiple-dose studies in volunteers when the drug was administered every 12 hours at doses ranging from 1.0 to 4.0 mg/kg, steady-state levels were obtained by the second day.

The serum levels at steady-state were less than 20% higher than those of the first dose. As with other aminoglycosides, the half-life of netilmicin increases, and its renal clearance decreases with decreasing renal function.

The endogenous creatinine clearance rate and the serum creatinine level have a high correlation with the half-life of netilmicin. Results of these tests can serve as a guide for adjusting dosage in patients with renal impairment.

In patients with marked impairment of renal function, there is a decrease in the concentration of aminoglycosides in urine and in their penetration into defective renal parenchyma. This should be considered when treating patients with urinary tract infections. In one study of adults with renal failure undergoing hemodialysis, netilmicin serum levels were reduced by approximately 63% over an 8-hour dialysis session. Shorter dialysis sessions will remove less drug. No hemodialysis information is available for children. Aminoglycosides are also removed by peritoneal dialysis but at a rate considerably less than by hemodialysis.

Since netilmicin is distributed in extracellular fluid, peak serum concentrations may be lower than usual in patients whose extracellular fluid volume is expanded (e.g., patients with edema or ascites). Serum concentrations of aminoglycosides in febrile patients may be lower than those in afebrile patients given the same dose. When body temperature returns to normal, serum concentrations of the drug may rise. Both febrile and anemic states may be associated with a shorter than usual half-life. (Dosage adjustment is usually not necessary.)

In severely burned patients, the half-life of aminoglycosides may be significantly decreased, and serum concentrations resulting from a particular dose may be lower than anticipated.

The elimination half-life of netilmicin in neonates during the first week of life is inversely correlated with body weight, ranging from approximately 8 hours for neonates weighing 1.5 to 2.0 kg to approximately 4.5 hours for 3.0 to 4.0 kg neonates. The elimination half-life of infants and children 6 weeks of age and older is 1.5 to 2.0 hours.

Following parenteral administration, aminoglycosides can be detected in serum, tissues, and sputum and in pericardial, pleural, synovial, and peritoneal fluids. A variety of methods are available to measure netilmicin concentrations in body fluids; these include microbiologic, enzymatic, and radioimmunoassay techniques. Concentrations in renal cortex may be markedly higher than the usual serum levels.

Minute quantities of aminoglycosides have been detected in the urine for up to 30 days after discontinuing administration. Hepatic secretion is minimal. As with all aminoglycosides, netilmicin diffuses poorly into the subarachnoid space after parenteral administration. Concentrations of netilmicin in cerebrospinal fluid are often low and dependent upon dose and the degree of meningeal inflammation. Netilmicin crosses the placenta and has been detected in cord blood and in the fetus. Studies in nursing mothers indicate that small amounts of the drug are excreted in breast milk. Netilmicin is poorly absorbed from the intact gastrointestinal tract after oral administration. As with other aminoglycosides, the binding of netilmicin to serum proteins is low (0–30%).

Microbiology: Netilmicin is a rapidly acting, broad-spectrum bactericidal antibiotic which appears to act by inhibiting normal protein synthesis in susceptible microorganisms. Netilmicin is active *in vitro* against a wide variety of pathogenic bacteria, primarily gram-negative bacilli and also a few gram-positive organisms, including *Citrobacter, Enterobacter, Escherichia coli, Klebsiella* species, *Proteus mirabilis, Pseudomonas aeruginosa, Salmonella* species, *Shigella species,* and *Staphylococcus* species (penicillin- and methicillin-resistant strains).

Netilmicin is also active *in vitro* against some isolates of *Acinetobacter* and *Neisseria* species, indolepositive *Proteus* species, *Pseudomonas* and *Serratia* species. In addition, netilmicin is active *in vitro* against many strains which have acquired resistance to other aminoglycosides. Such resistance is usually caused by aminoglycoside modifying (inactivating) enzymes. In general, netilmicin is active against organisms which inactivate aminoglycosides by either phosphorylation or adenylation; it has variable activity against acetylating strains, depending on the specific type. For example, the susceptibility of *Serratia* species producing a combination of adenylating and acetylating enzymes varies according to the level of acetylating enzyme present. Netilmicin is active *in vitro* against certain strains of gram-negative bacteria resistant to gentamicin and tobramycin: *Citrobacter, Enterobacter* species, *Escherichia coli, Klebsiella, Proteus* (indole-positive), *Pseudomonas, Salmonella,* and *Shigella* species. Netilmicin is active *in vitro* against certain staphylococci resistant to amikacin and tobramycin. Like other aminoglycosides, netilmicin is not active against bacteria with reduced permeability to this class of antibiotics.

Most species of streptococci and anaerobic organisms, such as *Bacteroides* and *Clostridium* species, are resistant to aminoglycosides.

The effects of media pH, protein content, divalent cation concentration, and of inoculum size on the *in vitro* activity of netilmicin are similar to those of other aminoglycosides.

Netilmicin acts synergistically *in vitro* with members of the penicillin class of antibiotics against *Streptococcus faecalis.* It also acts synergistically with those pencillins which are active alone against many strains of *Pseudomonas.* In addition, many, but not all isolates of *Serratia* which are resistant to multiple antibiotics, are inhibited by synergistic combinations of netilmicin with carbenicillin, azlocillin, mezlocillin, cefamandole, cefotaxime, or moxalactam. Tests for antibiotic synergy are necessary.

Susceptibility Testing: Quantitative methods that require measurements of zone diameters give the most precise estimates of antibiotic susceptibility. One such procedure has been recommended for use with discs to test susceptibility to netilmicin. Interpretation involves correlation of the diameters obtained in the disc test with minimal inhibitory concentration (MIC) values for netilmicin.

Reports from the laboratory giving results of the standardized single disc susceptibility test (Bauer, et al. Am J Clin Path 1966; 45:493 and Federal Register 37:20525-20529, 1972), using a 30 mcg netilmicin disc should be interpreted according to the following criteria:

Organisms producing zones of 15 mm or greater, or MIC's of 8.0 mcg or less are considered susceptible, indicating that the tested organism is likely to respond to therapy.

Resistant organisms produce zones of 12 mm or less or MIC's of 16 mcg or greater. A report of "resistant" from the laboratory indicates that the infecting organism is not likely to respond to therapy.

Zones greater than 12 mm and less than 15 mm, or MIC's of greater than 8.0 mcg and less than 16 mcg, indicate intermediate susceptibility. A report of "intermediate" susceptibility suggests that the organism would be susceptible if the infection is confined to tissues and fluids (e.g., urine), in which high antibiotic levels are attained.

Control organisms are recommended for susceptibility testing. Each time the test is performed one or more of the following organisms should be included: *Escherichia coli* ATCC 25922, *Staphylococcus aureus* ATCC 25923, and *Pseudomonas aeruginosa* ATCC 27853. The control organisms should produce zones of inhibition within the following ranges:

Escherichia coli (ATCC 25922) 22–30 mm
Staphylococcus aureus (ATCC 25923) 22–31 mm
Pseudomonas aeruginosa (ATCC 27853) 17–23 mm

In certain circumstances, particularly with strains of *Pseudomonas aeruginosa,* it may be desirable to do additional susceptibility testing by the tube or agar dilution method. Netilmicin sulfate powder, a diagnostic reagent, is available for this purpose. The MIC values of netilmicin for the control strains are the following:

Escherichia coli (ATCC 25922)
0.25–0.5 mcg/ml
Staphylococcus aureus (ATCC 25923) 0.125–0.25 mcg/ml
Pseudomonas aeruginosa (ATCC 27853)
4–8 mcg/ml in media supplemented with calcium and magnesium.

Indications and Usage: Netilmicin sulfate injection is indicated for the short-term treatment of patients of all ages, including neonates, infants, and children with serious or life-threatening bacterial infections caused by susceptible strains of the designated microorganisms in the diseases listed below:

COMPLICATED URINARY TRACT infections caused by *Escherichia coli, Klebsiella pneumoniae, Pseudomonas aeruginosa, Enterobacter* species, *Proteus mirabilis, Proteus* species (indole-positive), *Serratia** and *Citrobacter* species, and *Staphylococcus aureus***.

SEPTICEMIA caused by *Escherichia coli, Klebsiella pneumoniae, Pseudomonas aeruginosa, Enterobacter* and *Serratia** species, and *Proteus mirabilis.*

SKIN AND SKIN STRUCTURE infections caused by *Escherichia coli, Klebsiella pneumoniae, Pseudomonas aeruginosa, Enterobacter* and *Serratia** species, *Proteus mirabilis, Proteus* species (indole-positive), and *Staphylococcus aureus*** (penicillinase- and non-penicillinase-producing strains).

INTRA-ABDOMINAL infections including peritonitis and intra-abdominal abscess caused by *Escherichia coli, Klebsiella pneumoniae, Psuedomonas aeruginosa, Enterobacter* species, *Proteus mirabilis, Proteus* species (indole-positive), and *Staphylococcus aureus*** (penicillinase- and non-penicillinase-producing strains).

LOWER RESPIRATORY TRACT infections caused by *Escherichia coli, Klebsiella pneumoniae, Pseudomonas aeruginosa, Enterobacter* and *Serratia** species, *Proteus mirabilis, Proteus* species (indole-positive), and *Staphylococcus aureus*** (penicillinase- and non-penicillinase-producing strains).

*(See **Microbiology** Section.)

**While not the antibiotic class of first choice, aminoglycosides, including netilmicin, may be considered for the treatment of serious staphylococcal infections when penicillins or other less potentially toxic drugs are contraindicated and bacterial susceptibility tests and clinical judgment indicate their use. They may also be considered in mixed infections caused by susceptible strains of staphylococci and gram-negative organisms.

Aminoglycosides are indicated for those infections for which less potentially toxic antimicrobial agents are ineffective or contraindicated. They are not indicated in the treatment of uncomplicated initial episodes of urinary tract infection unless the causative organisms are resistant to antimicrobial agents having less potential toxicity.

Netilmicin sulfate injection may be considered as initial therapy in suspected or confirmed gram-negative infections, and therapy may be instituted before obtaining results of susceptibility testing. The decision to continue therapy with netilmicin should be based on the results of susceptibility tests, the severity of the infection, and the important additional concepts contained in the "WARNINGS Box" above. If the causative organisms are resistant to netilmicin, other appropriate therapy should be instituted.

In serious infections when the causative organisms are unknown, netilmicin may be administered as initial therapy in conjunction, with a penicillin-type or cephalosporin-type drug before obtaining results of susceptibility testing. In neonates with suspected sepsis, a penicillin-type drug is also usually indicated as concomitant therapy with netilmicin. If anaerobic organisms are suspected as etiologic agents, other suitable antimicrobial therapy should also be given. Following identification of the organism and its susceptibility, appropriate antibiotic therapy should then be continued.

Netilmicin sulfate injection has been used effectively in combination with carbenicillin or ticarcillin for the treatment of life-threatening infections caused by *Pseudomonas aeruginosa*.

Clinical studies have shown that netilmicin has been effective in the treatment of serious infections caused by some organisms resistant to other aminoglycosides, *i.e.*, gentamicin, tobramycin, and/or amikacin.

Specimens for bacterial culture should be obtained to isolate and identify causative organisms and to determine their susceptibility to netilmicin.

Contraindication: Hypersensitivity to netilmicin or to any of the ingredients of the preparation is a contraindication to its use. See WARNINGS if patient is hypersensitive to another aminoglycoside.

Warnings: (See "WARNINGS Box" above.)

If the patient has a history of hypersensitivity or serious toxic reaction to another aminoglycoside, netilmicin should be used very cautiously, if at all, because cross-sensitivity to drugs in this class has been reported.

Aminoglycosides can cause fetal harm when administered to a pregnant woman. Aminoglycoside antibiotics cross the placenta and there have been several reports of total irreversible bilateral congenital deafness in children whose mothers received streptomycin during pregnancy. Although serious side effects to fetus or newborn have not been reported in the treatment of pregnant women with other aminoglycosides, the potential for harm exists. Reproduction studies of netilmicin have been performed in rats and rabbits using intramuscular and subcutaneous doses approximately 13–15 times the highest adult human dose and have revealed no evidence of impairment of fertility or harm to the fetus. Moreover, there was no evidence of ototoxicity in the offspring of rats treated subcutaneously with netilmicin throughout pregnancy and during the subsequent lactation period. However, if this drug is used during pregnancy, or if the patient becomes pregnant while taking this drug, the patient should be apprised of the potential hazard to the fetus.

Precautions: General: Neurotoxic and nephrotoxic antibiotics may be almost completely absorbed from body surfaces (except the urinary bladder) after local irrigation and after topical application during surgical procedures. The potential toxic effects of antibiotics administered in this fashion (neuromuscular blockade, respiratory paralysis, oto- and nephrotoxicity) should be considered. (See "WARNINGS Box".)

Increased nephrotoxicity has been reported following concomitant administration of aminoglycoside antibiotics with some cephalosporins.

Aminoglycosides should be used with caution in patients with neuromuscular disorders, such as myasthenia gravis, parkinsonism, or infant botulism, since these drugs may aggravate muscle weakness because of their potential curare-like effect on the neuromuscular junction.

Elderly patients may have reduced renal function which may not be evident in the results of routine screening tests, such as BUN or serum creatinine levels. Determination of creatinine clearance or an estimate based on published nomograms or equations may be more useful. Monitoring of renal function during treatment with netilmicin, as with other aminoglycosides, is particularly important in such patients.

Patients should be well hydrated during treatment.

Treatment with netilmicin may result in overgrowth of non-susceptible organisms. If this occurs, appropriate therapy is indicated.

Laboratory Tests: *Test of renal function:* Urine should be examined periodically for increased excretion of protein and the presence of cells and casts, keeping in mind the effects of the primary illness on these tests. One or more of the following laboratory measurements should be obtained at the onset of therapy, periodically during therapy, and at, or shortly after, the end of therapy;

- creatinine clearance rate (either carefully measured or estimated from published nomograms or equations based on the patient's age, sex, body weight, and serum creatinine concentration) (preferred over BUN);
- serum creatinine concentration (preferred over BUN);
- blood urea nitrogen (BUN).

More frequent testing is desirable if renal functon is changing.

See also "PRECAUTIONS, **General**" above regarding elderly patients.

Test of eighth cranial nerve function: Serial audiometric tests are suggested, particularly when renal function is impaired and/or prolonged aminoglycoside therapy is required; such tests should also be repeated periodically after treatment if there is evidence of a hearing deficit or vestibular abnormality before or during therapy, or when consecutive or concomitant use of other potentially ototoxic drugs is unavoidable.

Drug Interactions: *In vitro* mixing of an aminoglycoside with beta-lactam-type antibiotics (penicillins or cephalosporins) may result in a significant mutual inactivation. Even when an aminoglycoside and a penicillin-type drug are administered separately by different routes, a reduction in aminoglycoside serum half-life or serum levels has been reported in patients with impaired renal function and in some patients with normal renal function. Usually, such inactivation of the aminoglycoside is clinically significant only in patients with severely impaired renal function. (See also "Drug/Laboratory test interactions.") See "WARNINGS Box" regarding concurrent use of potent diuretics, concurrent and/or sequential use of other neurotoxic and/or nephrotoxic antibiotics, and for other essential information.

See also "PRECAUTIONS, **General**."

Drug/Laboratory test interactions: Concomitant cephalosporin therapy may spuriously elevate creatinine determinations.

The inactivation between aminoglycosides and beta-lactam antibiotics described in "Drug Interactions" may continue in specimens of body fluids collected for assay, resulting in inaccurate, false low aminoglycoside readings. Such specimens should be properly handled, *i.e.*, assayed promptly, frozen, or treated with beta-lactamase.

Carcinogenesis, mutagenesis, impairment of fertility: Lifetime carcinogenicity tests have been undertaken in the mouse and rat and no drug-related tumors were observed. Similarly, mutagenesis tests with netilmicin have proven negative, and no impairment in fertility has been observed in the rat.

Pregnancy Category D: (See WARNINGS Section.)

Nursing mothers: Clinical studies in nursing mothers indicate that small amounts of netilmicin are excreted in breast milk. Because of the potential for serious adverse reactions from aminoglycosides in nursing infants, a decision should be made whether to discontinue nursing or to discontinue the drug, taking into account the importance of the drug to the mother.

Pediatric Use: Aminoglycosides should be used with caution in prematures and neonates because of the renal immaturity of these patients and the resulting prolongation of serum half-life of these drugs.

Adverse Reactions: *Nephrotoxicity*—Adverse renal effects due to netilmicin were reported in 7 per 100 patients.

They were demonstrated by a rise in serum creatinine and may have been accompanied by oliguria; the presence of casts, cells or protein in the urine; by rising levels of BUN; or by decreasing creatinine clearance rates. These effects occurred more frequently in the elderly, in patients with a history of renal impairment, and in patients treated for longer periods or with larger doses than recommended. While permanent impairment of renal function may occur following aminoglycoside therapy, observed renal impairment associated with netilmicin was usually mild and reversible after treatment ended while the drug was being excreted.

Neurotoxicity—Adverse effects on both the auditory and vestibular branches of the eighth cranial nerve have been reported.

Audiometric changes associated with netilmicin occurred in approximately 4 per 100 patients. Subjective netilmicin-related hearing loss occurred in about 1 per 250 patients. Vestibular abnormalities related to netilmicin were seen in 1 per 150 patients. Factors which may increase the risk of aminoglycoside-induced ototoxicity include renal impairment (especially if hemodialysis is required), excessive dosage, dehydration, concomitant administration of ethacrynic acid or furosemide, or previous exposure to other ototoxic drugs. Symptoms include vertigo, tinnitus, nystagmus, and hearing loss. Aminoglycoside-induced ototoxicity is usually irreversible. Cochlear damage is usually manifested initially by small changes in audiometric test results at the higher frequencies and may not be associated with subjective hearing loss. Vestibular dysfunction is usually manifested by nystagmus, vertigo, nausea, vomiting, or acute Meniere's syndrome.

The risk of toxic reactions is low in patients with normal renal function who do not receive netilmicin injection at higher doses or for longer periods of time than recommended. Some patients who have had previous neurotoxic reactions to other aminoglycosides have been treated with netilmicin without further neurotoxicity.

Neuromuscular blockade manifested as acute muscular paralysis and apnea can occur following treatment with aminoglycosides. (See "WARNINGS Box".)

The approximate incidence of other reported adverse reactions to netilmicin injection follows: increased levels of serum transaminase (SGOT or SGPT), alkaline phosphatase, or bilirubin in 15 patients per 1000; rash or itching in 4 or 5 patients per 1000; eosinophilia in 4 patients per 1000; thrombocytosis in 2 patients per 1000; prolonged prothrombin time in 1 patient per 1000; fever in 1 patient per 1000.

Fewer than one patient per 1000 was reported to have netilmicin-related anemia, leukopenia, thrombocytopenia, leukemoid reaction, immature circulating white blood cells, hyperkalemia, vomiting, diarrhea, palpitations, hypotension, headache, disorientation, blurred vision, or paresthesias. Local tolerance to intramuscular injection and intravenous infusion of netilmicin is generally excellent, but approximately four patients per 1000 have had severe pain, and similar numbers had induration or hematomas.

Overdosage: In the event of overdosage or toxic reaction, netilmicin can be removed from the blood by hemodialysis, especially if renal function

Continued on next page

Information on Schering products appearing on these pages is effective as of September 30, 1984.

Schering—Cont.

is, or becomes compromised. Although there is no specific information concerning removal of netilmicin by peritoneal dialysis, other aminoglycosides are known to be removed by this method but at a rate considerably less than by hemodialysis.

Dosage and Administration: Netilmicin injection may be given intramuscularly or intravenously. (See CLINICAL PHARMACOLOGY.) The recommended dosage for both methods of administration is identical.

The patient's pretreatment body weight should be obtained for calculation of correct dosage. The dosage of aminoglycosides in obese patients should be based on an estimate of the lean body mass.

The status of renal function should be estimated by measurement of the serum creatinine concentration or calculation of the endogenous creatinine clearance rate. The blood urea nitrogen (BUN) level is much less reliable for this purpose. Reassessment of renal function should be made periodically during therapy.

In patients with extensive body surface burns, altered pharmacokinetics may result in reduced serum concentrations of aminoglycosides. Measurement of netilmicin serum concentrations is particularly important as a basis for dosage adjustment in such patients.

Duration of Treatment: It is desirable to limit the duration of treatment with aminoglycosides to short-term whenever feasible. The usual duration of treatment for all patients is seven to fourteen days. In complicated infections, a longer course of therapy may be necessary. Although prolonged courses of netilmicin injection have been well tolerated, it is particularly important that patients treated for longer than the usual period be carefully monitored for changes in renal, auditory, and vestibular functions. Dosage should be adjusted if clinically indicated.

Measurement of serum concentrations: It is desirable to measure both peak and trough serum concentrations of netilmicin to determine the adequacy and safety of the administered dosage. When such measurements are feasible, they should be carried out periodically during therapy. Peak serum concentrations are expected to range from 4 to 12 mcg/ml. Dosage should be adjusted to attain the desired peak and trough concentrations and to avoid prolonged peak serum concentrations above 16 mcg/ml. When monitoring trough concentrations (just prior to the next dose), dosage should be adjusted so that levels above 4 mcg/ml are avoided. Inter-patient variation of aminoglycoside serum concentrations occurs in patients with normal or abnormal renal function. Generally, desirable peak and trough concentrations will be in the range of 6–10 and 0.5–2 mcg/ml, respectively.

Determination of the adequacy of a serum level for a particular patient must take into consideration the susceptibility of the causative organism, the severity of the infection, and the status of the patient's host-defense mechanisms.

The dosage recommendations which follow are not intended as rigid schedules, but are provided as guides for initial therapy, or for when the measurement of netilmicin serum levels during therapy is not feasible.

DOSAGE FOR PATIENTS WITH NORMAL RENAL FUNCTION

Table I shows the recommended dosage of netilmicin injection for patients of various ages with normal renal function.
[See table below].

DOSAGE FOR PATIENTS WITH IMPAIRED RENAL FUNCTION

Dosage must be individualized in patients with impaired renal function to ensure therapeutic levels are attained. There are several methods of doing this; however, dosage adjustment based upon the measurement of serum drug concentrations during treatment is the most accurate.

If netilmicin serum concentrations are not available and renal function is stable, serum creatinine and creatinine clearance values are the most reliable, readily available indicators of the degree of renal impairment for use as a guide for dosage adjustment.

It is also important to recognize that deteriorating renal function may require a greater reduction in dosage than that specified in the guidelines given below for patients with stable renal impairment. The initial or loading dose is the same as that for a patient with normal renal function. A number of methods are available to adjust the total daily dosage for the degree of renal impairment. Three suggested methods are:

1) Divide the suggested dosage value for patients with normal renal function from Table I above by the serum creatinine level to obtain the adjusted size of each dose.
2) If the creatinine clearance rate is known or can be estimated from the serum creatinine levels using the formula given below; the adjusted daily dose of netilmicin may be determined by multiplying the dose given in Table I by:

$$\frac{\text{Patient's Creatinine Clearance Rate}}{\text{Normal Creatinine Clearance Rate}}$$

3) Alternatively, the following graph may be used to obtain the percentage of the dose selected from Table I, which should be administered at 8-hour intervals:

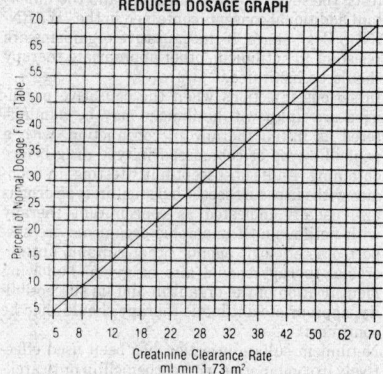

REDUCED DOSAGE GRAPH

Creatinine clearance can be estimated from serum creatinine levels by the following formula for adult males; multiply by 0.85 for adult females (Nephron, 1976; 16:31-41): Nephron, 1976; 16:31–41):

$$C_{cr} = \frac{(140 - \text{Age})(\text{Wt. Kg})}{72 \times S_{cr}\,(\text{mg}/100\,\text{ml})}$$

The adjusted total daily dose may be administered as one dose at 24-hour intervals, or as 2 or 3 equally divided doses at 12-hour or 8-hour intervals, respectively. Generally, each individual dose should not exceed 3.25 mg/kg. In adults with renal failure who are undergoing hemodialysis, the amount of netilmicin removed from the blood may vary depending upon the dialysis equipment and methods used. (See Clinical Pharmacology.) In adults, a dose of 2.0 mg/kg at the end of each dialysis period is recommended until the results of tests measuring netilmicin serum levels become available. Dosage should then be appropriately adjusted based on these tests.

ALTERNATE DOSING METHOD FOR PATIENTS WITH NORMAL OR IMPAIRED RENAL FUNCTION

An alternate method of determining dosage regimen (dose and dosing interval) applicable to all ages and all states of renal function (both normal and abnormal) is to employ pharmacokinetic parameters derived from measurements of serum concentrations.

Following the administration of an initial dose of netilmicin and the determination of drug serum concentrations in post-infusion blood samples, the drug's half-life and the patient's elimination rate constant and volume of distribution can be calculated. Desired peak and trough serum levels for a particular patient are then selected by taking into consideration the susceptibility of the causative organism, the severity of infection, and the status of the patient's host-defense mechanisms. The dosage regimen (dose and dosing interval) is then determined using standardized formulae and the appropriate computer program, and the dosage regimen can be adjusted to the nearest practical interval and amount.

ADDITION OF NETILMICIN SULFATE TO VARIOUS INTRAVENOUS PREPARATIONS

In adults, a single dose of netilmicin injection may be diluted in 50 to 200 ml of one of the parenteral solutions listed below. In infants and children, the volume of diluent should be less according to the fluid requirements of the patient. The solution may be infused over a period of one-half to two hours.

Tested at concentrations of 2.1 to 3.0 mg/ml, netilmicin sulfate has been shown to be stable in the following large volume parenteral solutions for up

TABLE I
Dosage Guide for Adults with Normal Renal Function

Patient's Weight* kg	(lb)	For Complicated Urinary Tract Infections, Give 3.0–4.0 mg/kg/day as 1.5–2.0 mg/kg EVERY 12 HOURS mg/dose	For Serious Systemic Infections Give 4.0–6.5 mg/kg/day as 1.3–2.2 mg/kg EVERY 8 HOURS mg/dose	or 2.0–3.25 mg/kg EVERY 12 HOURS mg/dose
40	(88)	60– 80	52– 88	80–130
45	(99)	68– 90	59– 99	90–146
50	(110)	75–100	65–110	100–163
55	(121)	83–110	72–121	110–179
60	(132)	90–120	78–132	120–195
65	(143)	98–130	85–143	130–211
70	(154)	105–140	91–154	140–228
75	(165)	113–150	98–165	150–244
80	(176)	120–160	104–176	160–260
85	(187)	128–170	111–187	170–276
90	(198)	135–180	117–198	180–293
95	(209)	143–190	124–209	190–309
100	(220)	150–200	130–220	200–325

*The dosage of aminoglycosides in obese patients should be based on an estimate of the lean body mass.
Neonates (less than 6 weeks): 4.0 to 6.5 mg/kg/day given as 2.0 to 3.25 mg/kg every 12 hours.
Infants and Children (6 weeks through 12 years): 5.5 to 8.0 mg/kg/day given either as 1.8 to 2.7 mg/kg every 8 hours, or as 2.7 to 4.0 mg/kg every 12 hours.

to 72 hours when stored in glass containers, both when refrigerated and at room temperature. Use after this time period is not recommended. [See table on right].

Parenteral drug products should be inspected visually for particulate matter and discoloration prior to administration, whenever solution and container permit.

How Supplied: NETROMYCIN Injection 100 mg/ml is supplied in 1.5 ml vials, box of 10 (NDC 0085-0264-02), and box of 25 (NDC 0085-0264-06); in 15 ml multiple-dose vials, box of 5 (NDC 0085-0264-04); and in 1.5 ml disposable syringes, box of 10 (NDC 0085-0264-05). **Store between 2° and 30°C (36° and 86°F).**

NETROMYCIN Pediatric Injection 25 mg/ml is supplied in 2.0-ml vial; box of 10 (NDC-0085-0459-02). **Store between 2° and 30°C (36° and 86°F). Protect from freezing.**

NETROMYCIN Neonatal Injection 10 mg/ml is supplied in 2.0-ml ampuls; box of 25 (NDC-0085-0743-03). **Store between 2° and 30°C (36° and 86°F).**

Animal Pharmacology and/or Animal Toxicology: Netilmicin sulfate, administered by the intravenous and intramuscular routes, has been compared to kanamycin, sisomicin, gentamicin, amikacin, and tobramycin in studies ranging in duration from two weeks to three months. Among the aminoglycosides, netilmicin is one of the more potent neuromuscular-blocking agents; however, in six different species, netilmicin sulfate has proven to be the least nephrotoxic and ototoxic of these aminoglycosides, using morphological as well as functional end-points.

In the clinical trials nephrotoxicity and ototoxicity occurred at about the same frequency in netilmicin-treated patients as in those treated with other aminoglycosides.

Schering Biochem Corporation
Manati, Puerto Rico 00701
An Affiliate of Schering Corporation,
Kenilworth, NJ 07033

Revised 11/83
Copyright © 1980, 1983, Schering Corporation, USA. All rights reserved.

NORMODYNE® R
[nŏr′ mō-dīn]
brand of labetalol hydrochloride Injection

Description: NORMODYNE (labetalol HCl) is an adrenergic receptor blocking agent that has both selective alpha$_1$- and nonselective beta-adrenergic receptor blocking actions in a single substance.

Labetalol HCl is 5-[1-hydroxy-2-[(1-methyl-3-phenylpropyl) amino]ethyl]salicylamide monohydrochloride.

Labetalol HCl has the empirical formula $C_{19}H_{24}N_2O_3 \cdot HCl$ and a molecular weight of 364.9. It has two asymmetric centers and therefore exists as a molecular complex of two diastereoisomeric pairs.

Labetalol HCl is a white or off-white crystalline powder, soluble in water.

NORMODYNE (labetalol HCl) Injection is a clear, colorless to light yellow aqueous sterile isotonic solution for intravenous injection. It has a pH range of 3.0 to 4.0. Each ml contains 5 mg labetalol HCl, 45 mg anhydrous dextrose, 0.10 mg edetate disodium; 0.80 mg methylparaben and 0.10 mg propylparaben as preservatives; citric acid monohydrate and sodium hydroxide, as necessary, to bring the solution into the pH range.

Clinical Pharmacology: NORMODYNE (labetalol HCl) combines both selective, competitive alpha$_1$-adrenergic blocking and nonselective, competitive beta-adrenergic blocking activity in a single substance. In man, the ratios of alpha- to beta-blockage have been estimated to be approximately 1:3 and 1:7 following oral and intravenous administration, respectively. Beta$_2$-agonist activity has been demonstrated in animals with minimal beta$_1$-agonist (ISA) activity detected. In animals, at doses greater than those required for alpha or beta-adrenergic blockade, a membrane stabilizing effect has been demonstrated.

TABLE II
LARGE VOLUME PARENTERAL SOLUTIONS IN WHICH NETILMICIN SULFATE IS STABLE

Products/Compositions Tested	Other Trade Names and Manufacturers
	(Solutions of Same Composition)
Sterile Water for Injection	
0.9% Sodium Chloride Injection alone or with 5% Dextrose	
5% or 10% Dextrose Injection in Water, or 5% Dextrose in Polysal Injection, or 5% Dextrose with Electrolyte #48 or #75	
Ringer's and Lactated Ringer's and Lactated Ringer's with 5% Dextrose Injection	
10% Travert with Electrolyte #2 or #3 Injection (Travenol)	Electrolyte #3 (Cooke & Crowley's Solution) with 10% Inverted Sugar Injection (Cutter)
Isolyte E, M, or P with 5% Dextrose Injection	
10% Dextran 40 or 6% Dextran 75 in 5% Dextrose Injection	
Plasma-Lyte 56 or 148 Injection with 5% Dextrose (Travenol)	Normosol-M or R in D5-W (Abbott), Isolyte H or S with 5% Dextrose (McGaw), Polyonic R-148 or M-56 with 5% Dextrose (Cutter)
Plasma-Lyte M Injection 5% Dextrose (Travenol)	Polysal M with 5% Dextrose (Cutter)
Ionosol B in D5-W	
5% Amigen Injection alone or with 5% Dextrose	
Normosol-R	Polyonic R-148 (Cutter), Isolyte S (McGaw), Plasma-Lyte 148 Injection in Water (Travenol)
Polysal (Plain)	
Aminosol 5% Injection	
Fre-Amine II 8.5% Injection	
Plasma-Lyte 148 Injection (approx. pH 7.4) (Travenol)	Normosol-R pH 7.4 (Abbott)
10% Fructose Injection	

Pharmacodynamics: The capacity of labetalol HCl to block alpha receptors in man has been demonstrated by attenuation of the pressor effect of phenylephrine and by a significant reduction of the pressor response caused by immersing the hand in ice-cold water ("cold-pressor test"). Labetalol HCl's beta$_1$-receptor blockade in man was demonstrated by a small decrease in the resting heart rate, attenuation of tachycardia produced by isoproterenol or exercise, and by attenuation of the reflex tachycardia to the hypotension produced by amyl nitrite. Beta$_2$-receptor blockade was demonstrated by inhibition of the isoproterenol-induced fall in diastolic blood pressure. Both the alpha- and beta-blocking actions of orally administered labetalol HCl contribute to a decrease in blood pressure in hypertensive patients. Labetalol HCl consistently, in dose related fashion, blunted increases in exercise-induced blood pressure and heart rate, and in their double product. The pulmonary circulation during exercise was not affected by labetalol HCl dosing.

Single oral doses of labetalol HCl administered in patients with coronary artery disease had no significant effect on sinus rate, intraventricular conduction, or QRS duration. The AV conduction time was modestly prolonged in 2 of 7 patients. In another study, intravenous labetalol HCl slightly prolonged AV nodal conduction time and atrial effective refractory period with only small changes in heart rate. The effects on AV nodal refractoriness were inconsistent.

Labetalol HCl produces dose-related falls in blood pressure without reflex tachycardia and without significant reduction in heart rate, presumably through a mixture of its alpha-blocking and beta-blocking effects. Hemodynamic effects are variable with small nonsignificant changes in cardiac output seen in some studies but not others, and small decreases in total peripheral resistance. Elevated plasma renins are reduced.

Doses of labetalol HCl that controlled hypertension did not affect renal function in mild to severe hypertensive patients with normal renal function. Due to the alpha$_1$-receptor blocking activity of labetalol HCl, blood pressure is lowered more in the standing than in the supine position, and symptoms of postural hypotension can occur. During dosing with intravenous labetalol HCl, the contribution of the postural component should be considered when positioning the patient for treatment, and the patient should not be allowed to move to an erect position unmonitored until their ability to do so is established.

In a clinical pharmacologic study in severe hypertensives, an initial 0.25 mg/kg injection of labetalol HCl administered to patients in the supine position, decreased blood pressure by an average of 11/7 mmHg. Additional injections of 0.5 mg/kg at 15 minute intervals up to a total cumulative dose of 1.75 mg/kg of labetalol HCl caused further dose related decreases in blood pressure. Some patients required cumulative doses of up to 3.25 mg/kg. The maximal effect of each dose level occurred within 5 minutes. Following discontinuation of intravenous treatment with labetalol HCl, the

Continued on next page

Information on Schering products appearing on these pages is effective as of September 30, 1984.

Schering—Cont.

blood pressure rose gradually and progressively, approaching pretreatment baseline values within an average of 16-18 hours in the majority of patients.

Similar results were obtained in the treatment of patients with severe hypertension requiring urgent blood pressure reduction with an initial dose of 20 mg (which corresponds to 0.25 mg/kg for an 80 kg patient) followed by additional doses of either 40 or 80 mg at 10 minute intervals to achieve the desired effect or up to a cumulative dose of 300 mg.

Labetalol HCl administered as a continuous intravenous infusion, with a mean dose of 136 mg (27 to 300 mg) over a period of 2 to 3 hours (mean of 2 hours and 39 minutes) lowered the blood pressure by an average of 60/35 mmHg.

Exacerbation of angina and, in some cases, myocardial infarction and ventricular dysrhythmias have been reported after abrupt discontinuation of therapy with beta-adrenergic blocking agents in patients with coronary artery disease. Abrupt withdrawal of these agents in patients without coronary artery disease has resulted in transient symptoms, including tremulousness, sweating, palpitation, headache, and malaise. Several mechanisms have been proposed to explain these phenomena, among them increased sensitivity to catecholamines because of increased numbers of beta receptors.

Although beta-adrenergic receptor blockade is useful in the treatment of angina and hypertension, there are also situations in which sympathetic stimulation is vital. For example, in patients with severely damaged hearts, adequate ventricular function may depend on sympathetic drive. Beta-adrenergic blockade may worsen AV block by preventing the necessary facilitating effects of sympathetic activity on conduction. Beta$_2$-adrenergic blockade results in passive bronchial constriction by interfering with endogenous adrenergic bronchodilator activity in patients subject to bronchospasm and may also interfere with exogenous bronchodilators in such patients.

Pharmacokinetics and Metabolism Following intravenous infusion, the elimination half-life is about 5.5 hours and the total body clearance is approximately 33 ml/min/kg. The plasma half-life of labetalol following oral administration is about six to eight hours. In patients with decreased hepatic or renal function, the elimination half-life of labetalol is not altered; however, the relative bioavailability in hepatically impaired patients is increased due to decreased "first-pass" metabolism.

The metabolism of labetalol is mainly through conjugation to glucuronide metabolites. These metabolites are present in plasma and are excreted in the urine and, via the bile, into the feces. Approximately 55 to 60% of a dose appears in the urine as conjugates or unchanged labetalol within the first 24 hours of dosing.

Labetalol has been shown to cross the placental barrier in humans. Only negligible amounts of the drug crossed the blood-brain barrier in animal studies. Labetalol is approximately 50% protein bound.

Indications and Usage: NORMODYNE (labetalol HCl) Injection is indicated for control of blood pressure in severe hypertension.

Contraindications: NORMODYNE (labetalol HCl) Injection is contraindicated in bronchial asthma, overt cardiac failure, greater than first degree heart block, cardiogenic shock, and severe bradycardia. (See **WARNINGS.**)

Warnings:

Cardiac Failure: Sympathetic stimulation is a vital component supporting circulatory function in congestive heart failure. Beta blockade carries a potential hazard of further depressing myocardial contractility and precipitating more severe failure. Although beta-blockers should be avoided in overt congestive heart failure, if necessary, labetalol HCl can be used with caution in patients with a history of heart failure who are well-compensated. Congestive heart failure has been observed in patients receiving labetalol HCl. Labetalol HCl does not abolish the inotropic action of digitalis on heart muscle.

In Patients Without a History of Cardiac Failure: In patients with latent cardiac insufficiency, continued depression of the myocardium with beta-blocking agents over a period of time can in some cases lead to cardiac failure. At the first sign or symptom of impending cardiac failure, patients should be fully digitalized and/or be given a diuretic, and the response observed closely. If cardiac failure continues, despite adequate digitalization and diuretic, NORMODYNE (labetalol HCl) therapy should be withdrawn (gradually if possible).

Ischemic Heart Disease: Angina pectoris has not been reported upon labetalol HCl discontinuation. However, following abrupt cessation of therapy with some beta-blocking agents in patients with coronary artery disease, exacerbations of angina pectoris and, in some cases, myocardial infarction have been reported. Therefore, such patients should be cautioned against interruption of therapy without the physician's advice. Even in the absence of overt angina pectoris, when discontinuation of NORMODYNE is planned, the patient should be carefully observed and should be advised to limit physical activity. If angina markedly worsens or acute coronary insufficiency develops, NORMODYNE (labetalol HCl) administration should be reinstituted promptly, at least temporarily, and other measures appropriate for the management of unstable angina should be taken.

Nonallergic Bronchospasm (e.g., chronic bronchitis and emphysema): Since NORMODYNE (labetalol HCl) Injection at the usual intravenous therapeutic doses has not been studied in patients with nonallergic bronchospastic disease, it should not be used in such patients.

Pheochromocytoma: Intravenous labetalol HCl has been shown to be effective in lowering the blood pressure and relieving symptoms in patients with pheochromocytoma; higher than usual doses may be required. However, paradoxical hypertensive responses have been reported in a few patients with this tumor; therefore, use caution when administering labetalol HCl to patients with pheochromocytoma.

Diabetes Mellitus and Hypoglycemia: Beta-adrenergic blockade may prevent the appearance of premonitory signs and symptoms (e.g., tachycardia) of acute hypoglycemia. This is especially important with labile diabetics. Beta-blockade also reduces the release of insulin in response to hyperglycemia; it may therefore be necessary to adjust the dose of antidiabetic drugs.

Major Surgery: The necessity or desirability of withdrawing beta-blocking therapy prior to major surgery is controversial. Protracted severe hypotension and difficulty in restarting or maintaining a heart beat have been reported with beta-blockers. The effect of labetalol HCl's alpha-adrenergic activity has not been evaluated in this setting.

A synergism between labetalol HCl and halothane anesthesia has been shown (see **Drug Interactions**).

Rapid Decreases of Blood Pressure: Caution must be observed when reducing severely elevated blood pressure. Although such findings have not been reported with intravenous labetalol HCl, a number of adverse reactions, including cerebral infarction, optic nerve infarction, angina and ischemic changes in the electrocardiogram, have been reported with other agents when severely elevated blood pressure was reduced over time courses of several hours to as long as one or two days. The desired blood pressure lowering should therefore be achieved over as long a period of time as is compatible with the patient's status.

Precautions:

General: *Impaired Hepatic Function* may diminish metabolism of NORMODYNE (labetalol HCl) Injection.

Hypotension: Symptomatic postural hypotension (incidence 58%) is likely to occur if patients are tilted or allowed to assume the upright position within 3 hours of receiving NORMODYNE (labetalol HCl) Injection. Therefore, the patient's ability to tolerate an upright position should be established before permitting any ambulation.

Jaundice or Hepatic Dysfunction: On rare occasions, oral labetalol HCl has been associated with jaundice (both hepatic and cholestatic). It is therefore recommended that treatment with labetalol HCl be stopped immediately, should a patient develop jaundice or laboratory evidence of liver injury. Both have been shown to be reversible on stopping therapy.

Information for Patients

The following information is intended to aid in the safe and effective use of this medication. It is not a disclosure of all possible adverse or intended effects. During and immediately following (for up to 3 hours) NORMODYNE Injection, the patient should remain supine. Subsequently, the patient should be advised on how to proceed gradually to become ambulatory, and should be observed at the time of first ambulation.

When the patient is started on NORMODYNE Tablets, following adequate control of blood pressure with NORMODYNE Injection, appropriate directions for titration of dosage should be provided. (See **DOSAGE AND ADMINISTRATION.**)

As with all drugs with beta-blocking activity, certain advice to patients being treated with labetalol HCl is warranted: While no incident of the abrupt withdrawal phenomenon (exacerbation of angina pectoris) has been reported with labetalol HCl, dosing with NORMODYNE Tablets should not be interrupted or discontinued without a physician's advice. Patients being treated with NORMODYNE Tablets should consult a physician at any sign of impending cardiac failure. Also, transient scalp tingling may occur, usually when treatment with NORMODYNE Tablets is initiated (see **ADVERSE REACTIONS**).

Laboratory Tests

Routine laboratory tests are ordinarily not required before or after intravenous labetalol HCl. In patients with concomitant illnesses, such as impaired renal function, appropriate tests should be done to monitor these conditions.

Drug Interactions

Since NORMODYNE (labetalol HCl) Injection may be administered to patients already being treated with other medications, including other antihypertensive agents, careful monitoring of these patients is necessary to detect and treat promptly any undesired effect from concomitant administration.

In one survey, 2.3% of patients taking labetalol HCl orally in combination with tricyclic antidepressants experienced tremor as compared to 0.7% reported to occur with labetalol HCl alone. The contribution of each of the treatments to this adverse reaction is unknown but the possibility of a drug interaction cannot be excluded.

Drugs possessing beta-blocking properties can blunt the bronchodilator effect of beta-receptor agonist drugs in patients with bronchospasm; therefore, doses greater than the normal antiasthmatic dose of beta-agonist bronchodilator drugs may be required.

Cimetidine has been shown to increase the bioavailability of labetalol HCl administered orally. Since this could be explained either by enhanced absorption or by an alteration of hepatic metabolism of labetalol HCl, special care should be used in establishing the dose required for blood pressure control in such patients.

Synergism has been shown between halothane anesthesia and intravenously administered labetalol HCl. During controlled hypotensive anesthesia using labetalol HCl in association with halothane, high concentrations (3% or above) of halothane should not be used because the degree of hypotension will be increased and because of the possibility of a large reduction in cardiac output and an increase in central venous pressure. The anesthesiologist should be informed when a patient is receiving labetalol HCl.

Labetalol HCl blunts the reflex tachycardia produced by nitroglycerin without preventing its hypotensive effect. If labetalol HCl is used with nitroglycerin in patients with angina pectoris, additional antihypertensive effects may occur.

Drug/Laboratory Test Interactions
The presence of a metabolite of labetalol in the urine may result in falsely increased levels of urinary catecholamines when measured by a nonspecific trihydroxyindole (THI) reaction. In screening patients suspected of having a pheochromocytoma and being treated with labetalol HCl, specific radioenzymatic or high performance liquid chromatography assay techniques should be used to determine levels of catecholamines or their metabolites.

Carcinogenesis, Mutagenesis, Impairment of Fertility
Long-term oral dosing studies with labetalol HCl for 18 months in mice and for 2 years in rats showed no evidence of carcinogenesis. Studies with labetalol HCl, using dominant lethal assays in rats and mice, and exposing microorganisms according to modified Ames tests, showed no evidence of mutagenesis.

Pregnancy Category C
Teratogenic studies have been performed with labetalol in rats and rabbits at oral doses up to approximately 6 and 4 times the maximum recommended human dose (MRHD), respectively. No reproducible evidence of fetal malformations was observed. Increased fetal resorptions were seen in both species at doses approximating the MRHD. There are no adequate and well-controlled studies in pregnant women. Labetalol should be used during pregnancy only if the potential benefit justifies the potential risk to the fetus.

Nonteratogenic Effects
Infants of mothers who were treated with labetalol HCl for hypertension during pregnancy did not appear to be adversely affected by the drug. Oral administration of labetalol to rats during late gestation through weaning at doses of 2 to 4 times the MRHD caused a decrease in neonatal survival.

Labor and Delivery
Labetalol HCl given to pregnant women with hypertension did not appear to affect the usual course of labor and delivery.

Nursing Mothers
Small amounts of labetalol (approximately 0.004% of the maternal dose) are excreted in human milk. Caution should be exercised when NORMODYNE (labetalol HCl) Injection is administered to a nursing woman.

Pediatric Use
Safety and effectiveness in children have not been established.

Adverse Reactions: NORMODYNE (labetalol HCl) Injection is usually well tolerated. Most adverse effects have been mild and transient and in controlled trials involving 92 patients did not require labetalol HCl withdrawal. Symptomatic postural hypotension (incidence 58%) is likely to occur if patients are tilted or allowed to assume the upright position within 3 hours of receiving NORMODYNE (labetalol HCl) Injection. Moderate hypotension occurred in 1 of 100 patients while supine. Increased sweating was noted in 4 of 100 patients, and flushing occurred in 1 of 100 patients.
The following also were reported with NORMODYNE Injection with the incidence per 100 patients as noted:
Cardiovascular System: Ventricular arrhythmia in 1.
Central and Peripheral Nervous Systems: Dizziness in 9; tingling of the scalp/skin 7; hypoesthesia (numbness), and vertigo 1 each.
Gastrointestinal System: Nausea in 13; vomiting 4; dyspepsia and taste distortion, 1 each.
Metabolic Disorders: Transient increases in blood urea nitrogen and serum creatinine levels occurred in 8 of 100 patients; these were associated with drops in blood pressure, generally in patients with prior renal insufficiency.
Psychiatric Disorders: Somnolence/yawning in 3.
Respiratory System: Wheezing in 1.
Skin: Pruritus in 1.
The incidence of adverse reactions depends upon the dose of labetalol HCl. The largest experience is with oral labetalol HCl (see NORMODYNE Tablet Product Information for details). Certain of the side effects increased with increasing oral dose as shown in the table below which depicts the entire U.S. therapeutic trials data base for adverse reactions that are clearly or possibly dose related.
[See table above].

Labetalol HCl Daily Dose (mg)	200	300	400	600	800	900	1200	1600	2400
Number of Patients	522	181	606	608	503	117	411	242	175
Dizziness (%)	2	3	3	3	5	1	9	13	16
Fatigue	2	1	4	4	5	3	7	6	10
Nausea	<1	0	1	2	4	0	7	11	19
Vomiting	0	0	<1	<1	<1	0	1	2	3
Dyspepsia	1	0	2	1	1	0	2	2	4
Paresthesias	2	0	2	2	1	1	2	5	5
Nasal Stuffiness	1	1	2	2	2	2	4	5	6
Ejaculation Failure	0	2	1	2	3	0	4	3	5
Impotence	1	1	1	1	2	4	3	4	3
Edema	1	0	1	1	1	0	1	2	2

The oculomucocutaneous syndrome associated with the beta-blocker practolol has not been reported with labetalol HCl during investigational use and extensive foreign marketing experience.

Clinical laboratory tests: Among patients dosed with NORMODYNE (labetalol HCl) Tablets, there have been reversible increases of serum transaminases in 4% of patients tested, and more rarely, reversible increases in blood urea.

Overdosage: Overdosage with NORMODYNE (labetalol HCl) Injection causes excessive hypotension which is posture sensitive, and sometimes, excessive bradycardia. Patients should be laid supine and their legs raised if necessary to improve the blood supply to the brain. The following additional measures should be employed if necessary: *Excessive bradycardia*—administer atropine (3.0 mg). If there is no response to vagal blockade, administer isoproterenol cautiously. *Cardiac failure*—administer a digitalis glycoside and a diuretic. *Hypotension*—administer vasopressors, e.g., norepinephrine. There is pharmacological evidence that norepinephrine may be the drug of choice. *Bronchospasm*—administer a beta$_2$-stimulating agent and/or a theophylline preparation.
If overdosage with labetalol HCl follows oral ingestion, gastric lavage or pharmacologically induced emesis (using syrup of ipecac) is useful for removal of the drug shortly after ingestion. Labetalol HCl can be removed from the general circulation by hemodialysis.
The oral LD$_{50}$ value of labetalol HCl in the mouse is approximately 600 mg/kg and in the rat is greater than 2 gm/kg. The intravenous LD$_{50}$ in these species is 50 to 60 mg/kg.

Dosage and Administration: NORMODYNE (labetalol HCl) Injection is intended for intravenous use in hospitalized patients. DOSAGE MUST BE INDIVIDUALIZED depending upon the severity of hypertension and the response of the patient during dosing.
Patients should always be kept in a supine position during the period of intravenous drug administration. A substantial fall in blood pressure on standing should be expected in these patients. The patient's ability to tolerate an upright position should be established before permitting any ambulation, such as using toilet facilities.
Either of two methods of administration of NORMODYNE Injection may be used: a) repeated intravenous injections, b) slow continuous infusion.
Repeated Intravenous Injection: Initially, NORMODYNE (labetalol HCl) Injection should be given in a dose of 20 mg labetalol HCl (which corresponds to 0.25 mg/kg for an 80 kg patient) by slow intravenous injection over a two-minute period. Immediately before the injection and at five and ten minutes after injection, supine blood pressure should be measured to evaluate response. Additional injections of 40 mg or 80 mg can be given at ten minute intervals until a desired supine blood pressure is achieved or a total of 300 mg labetalol HCl has been injected. The maximum effect usually occurs within 5 minutes of each injection.
Slow Continuous Infusion: NORMODYNE (labetalol HCl) Injection is prepared for intravenous continuous infusion by diluting the ampule contents with commonly used intravenous fluids (see below). Examples of two methods of preparing the infusion solution are:
The contents of two ampules (40 ml) are added to 160 ml of a commonly used intravenous fluid such that the resultant 200 ml of solution contains 200 mg of labetalol HCl, 1 mg/ml. The diluted solution should be administered at a rate of 2 ml/min to deliver 2 mg/min.
Alternatively, the contents of two ampules (40 ml) of NORMODYNE (labetalol HCl) Injection can be added to 250 ml of a commonly used intravenous fluid. The resultant solution will contain 200 mg of labetalol HCl, approximately 2 mg/3 ml. The diluted solution should be administered at a rate of 3 ml/min to deliver approximately 2 mg/min.
The rate of infusion of the diluted solution may be adjusted according to the blood pressure response, at the discretion of the physician. To facilitate a desired rate of infusion, the diluted solution can be infused using a controlled administration mechanism, e.g., graduated burette or mechanically driven infusion pump.
Since the half life of labetalol is 5 to 8 hours, steady-state blood levels (in the face of a constant rate of infusion) would not be reached during the usual infusion time period. The infusion should be continued until a satisfactory response is obtained and should then be stopped and oral labetalol HCl started (see below). The effective intravenous dose is usually in the range of 50 to 200 mg. A total dose of up to 300 mg may be required in some patients.
Blood Pressure Monitoring: The blood pressure should be monitored during and after completion of the infusion or intravenous injections. Rapid or excessive falls in either systolic or diastolic blood pressure during intravenous treatment should be avoided. In patients with excessive systolic hypertension, the decrease in systolic pressure should be used as an indicator of effectiveness in addition to the response of the diastolic pressure.
Initiation of Dosing with NORMODYNE (labetalol HCl) Tablets: Subsequent oral dosing with NORMODYNE (labetalol HCl) Tablets should begin when it has been established that the supine diastolic blood pressure has begun to rise. The recommended initial dose is 200 mg, followed in 6-12 hours by an additional dose of 200 or 400 mg, depending on the blood pressure response. Thereafter, *inpatient titration with NORMODYNE (labetalol HCl) Tablets* may proceed as follows:

Inpatient Titration Instructions

Regimen	Daily Dose*
200 mg bid	400 mg
400 mg bid	800 mg
800 mg bid	1600 mg
1200 mg bid	2400 mg

*If needed, the total daily dose may be given in three divided doses.
While in the hospital, the dosage of NORMODYNE Tablets may be increased at one day intervals to achieve the desired blood pressure reduction.
For subsequent outpatient titration or maintenance dosing see NORMODYNE Tablets Product

Continued on next page

Information on Schering products appearing on these pages is effective as of September 30, 1984.

Schering—Cont.

Information **DOSAGE AND ADMINISTRATION** for additional recommendations.

Compatibility with commonly used intravenous fluids

Parenteral drug products should be inspected visually for particulate matter and discoloration prior to administration, whenever solution and container permit.

NORMODYNE (labetalol HCl) Injection was tested for compatibility with commonly used intravenous fluids at final concentrations of 1.25 mg to 3.75 mg labetalol HCl per ml of the mixture. NORMODYNE Injection was found to be compatible with and stable (for 24 hours refrigerated or at room temperature) in mixtures with the following solutions:
Ringers Injection, USP
Lactated Ringers Injection, USP
5% Dextrose and Ringers Injection
5% Lactated Ringers and 5% Dextrose Injection
5% Dextrose Injection, USP
0.9% Sodium Chloride Injection, USP
5% Dextrose and 0.2% Sodium Chloride Injection, USP
2.5% Dextrose and 0.45% Sodium Chloride Injection, USP
5% Dextrose and 0.9% Sodium Chloride Injection, USP
5% Dextrose and 0.33% Sodium Chloride Injection, USP
NORMODYNE (labetalol HCl) Injection was NOT compatible with 5% Sodium Bicarbonate Injection, USP.

How Supplied: NORMODYNE (labetalol HCl) Injection, 5 mg/ml, is supplied in 20 ml (100 mg) ampules, box of 1; NDC-0085-0362-03.

Store between 2° and 30°C (36° and 86°F). Do not freeze.

Revised 6/84

Copyright © 1984, Schering Corporation. All rights reserved.

NORMODYNE®
[nōr' mō-dīn]
brand of labetalol hydrochloride
Tablets

Description: NORMODYNE (labetalol HCl) is an adrenergic receptor blocking agent that has both selective alpha$_1$- and nonselective beta-adrenergic receptor blocking actions in a single substance.

Labetalol HCl is 5-[1-hydroxy-2-[(1-methyl-3-phenylpropyl) amino] ethyl]salicylamide monohydrochloride.

Labetalol HCl has the empirical formula $C_{19}H_{24}N_2O_3$ HCl and a molecular weight of 364.9. It has two asymmetric centers and therefore exists as a molecular complex of two diastereoisomeric pairs.

Labetalol HCl is a white or off-white crystalline powder, soluble in water.

NORMODYNE Tablets contain 200 mg or 300 mg labetalol HCl and are taken orally.

Clinical Pharmacology: NORMODYNE (labetalol HCl) combines both selective, competitive alpha$_1$-adrenergic blocking and nonselective, competitive beta-adrenergic blocking activity in a single substance. In man, the ratios of alpha- to beta-blockade have been estimated to be approximately 1:3 and 1:7 following oral and intravenous administration, respectively. Beta$_2$-agonist activity has been demonstrated in animals with minimal beta$_1$-agonist (ISA) activity detected. In animals, at doses greater than those required for alpha or beta-adrenergic blockade, a membrane stabilizing effect has been demonstrated.

Pharmacodynamics: The capacity of labetalol HCl to block alpha receptors in man has been demonstrated by attenuation of the pressor effect of phenylephrine and by a significant reduction of the pressor response caused by immersing the hand in ice-cold water ("cold-pressor test"). Labetalol HCl's beta$_1$-receptor blockade in man was demonstrated by a small decrease in the resting heart rate, attenuation of tachycardia produced by isoproterenol or exercise, and by attenuation of the reflex tachycardia to the hypotension produced by amyl nitrite. Beta$_2$-receptor blockade was demonstrated by inhibition of the isoproterenol-induced fall in diastolic blood pressure. Both the alpha- and beta-blocking actions of orally administered labetalol HCl contribute to a decrease in blood pressure in hypertensive patients. Labetalol HCl consistently, in dose related fashion, blunted increases in exercise-induced blood pressure and heart rate, and in their double product. The pulmonary circulation during exercise was not affected by labetalol HCl dosing.

Single oral doses of labetalol HCl administered in patients with coronary artery disease had no significant effect on sinus rate, intraventricular conduction, or QRS duration. The AV conduction time was modestly prolonged in 2 of 7 patients. In another study, intravenous labetalol HCl slightly prolonged AV nodal conduction time and atrial effective refractory period with only small changes in heart rate. The effects on AV nodal refractoriness were inconsistent.

Labetalol HCl produces dose-related falls in blood pressure without reflex tachycardia and without significant reduction in the heart rate, presumably through a mixture of its alpha-blocking and beta-blocking effects. Hemodynamic effects are variable with small nonsignificant changes in cardiac output seen in some studies but not others, and small decreases in total peripheral resistance. Elevated plasma renins are reduced.

Doses of labetalol HCl that controlled hypertension did not affect renal function in mild to severe hypertensive patients with normal renal function. Due to the alpha$_1$-receptor blocking activity of labetalol HCl, blood pressure is lowered more in the standing that in the supine position, and symptoms of postural hypotension (2%), including rare instances of syncope, can occur. Following oral administration, when postural hypotension has occurred, it has been transient and is uncommon when the recommended starting dose and titration increments are closely followed (See **DOSAGE AND ADMINISTRATION**). Symptomatic postural hypotension is most likely to occur 2 to 4 hours after a dose, especially following the use of large initial doses or upon large changes in dose.

The peak effects of single oral doses of labetalol HCl occur within 2 to 4 hours. The duration of effect depends upon dose, lasting at least 8 hours following single oral doses of 100 mg and more than 12 hours following single oral doses of 300 mg. The maximum, steady-state blood pressure response upon oral, twice-a-day dosing occurs within 24 to 72 hours.

The antihypertensive effect of labetalol has a linear correlation with the logarithm of labetalol plasma concentration, and there is also a linear correlation between the reduction in exercise-induced tachycardia occurring at two hours after oral administration of labetalol HCl and the logarithm of the plasma concentration.

About 70% of the maximum beta-blocking effect is present for five hours after the administration of a single oral dose of 400 mg with suggestion that about 40% remains at eight hours.

The anti-anginal efficacy of labetalol HCl has not been studied. In 37 patients with hypertension and coronary artery disease, labetalol HCl did not increase the incidence or severity of angina attacks. Exacerbation of angina and, in some cases, myocardial infarction and ventricular dysrhythmias have been reported after abrupt discontinuation of therapy with beta-adrenergic blocking agents in patients with coronary artery disease. Abrupt withdrawal of these agents in patients without coronary artery disease has resulted in transient symptoms, including tremulousness, sweating, palpitation, headache, and malaise. Several mechanisms have been proposed to explain these phenomena, among them increased sensitivity to catecholamines because of increased numbers of beta receptors.

Although beta-adrenergic receptor blockade is useful in the treatment of angina and hypertension, there are also situations in which sympathetic stimulation is vital. For example, in patients with severely damaged hearts, adequate ventricular function may depend on sympathetic drive. Beta-adrenergic blockade may worsen AV block by preventing the necessary facilitating effects of sympathetic activity on conduction. Beta$_2$-adrenergic blockade results in passive bronchial constriction by interfering with endogenous adrenergic bronchodilator activity in patients subject to bronchospasm and may also interfere with exogenous bronchodilators in such patients.

Pharmacokinetics and Metabolism: Labetalol HCl is completely absorbed from the gastrointestinal tract with peak plasma levels occurring one to two hours after oral administration. The relative bioavailability of labetalol HCl tablets compared to an oral solution is 100%. The absolute bioavailability (fraction of drug reaching systemic circulation) of labetalol when compared to an intravenous infusion is 25%; this is due to extensive "first-pass" metabolism. Despite "first-pass" metabolism there is a linear relationship between oral doses of 100 to 3000 mg and peak plasma levels. The absolute bioavailability of labetalol is increased when administered with food.

The plasma half-life of labetalol following oral administration is about six to eight hours. Steady-state plasma levels of labetalol during repetitive dosing are reached by about the third day of dosing. In patients with decreased hepatic or renal function, the elimination half-life of labetalol is not altered; however, the relative bioavailability in hepatically impaired patients is increased due to decreased "first-pass" metabolism.

The metabolism of labetalol is mainly through conjugation to glucuronide metabolites. These metabolites are present in plasma and are excreted in the urine and, via the bile, into the feces. Approximately 55 to 60% of a dose appears in the urine as conjugates or unchanged labetalol within the first 24 hours of dosing.

Labetalol has been shown to cross the placental barrier in humans. Only negligible amounts of the drug crossed the blood-brain barrier in animal studies. Labetalol is approximately 50% protein bound.

Indications and Usage: NORMODYNE (labetalol HCl) Tablets are indicated in the management of hypertension. NORMODYNE Tablets may be used alone or in combination with other antihypertensive agents, especially thiazide and loop diuretics.

Contraindications: NORMODYNE (labetalol HCl) Tablets are contraindicated in bronchial asthma, overt cardiac failure, greater than first degree heart block, cardiogenic shock, and severe bradycardia. (See **WARNINGS**.)

Warnings:

Cardiac Failure: Sympathetic stimulation is a vital component supporting circulatory function in congestive heart failure. Beta blockade carries a potential hazard of further depressing myocardial contractility and precipitating more severe failure. Although beta-blockers should be avoided in overt congestive heart failure, if necessary, labetalol HCl can be used with caution in patients with a history of heart failure who are well-compensated. Congestive heart failure has been observed in patients receiving labetalol HCl. Labetalol HCl does not abolish the inotropic action of digitalis on heart muscle.

In Patients Without a History of Cardiac Failure: In patients with latent cardiac insufficiency, continued depression of the myocardium with beta-blocking agents over a period of time can in some cases lead to cardiac failure. At the first sign or symptom of impending cardiac failure, patients should be fully digitalized and/or be given a diuretic, and the response observed closely. If cardiac failure continues, despite adequate digitalization and diuretic, NORMODYNE (labetalol HCl) therapy should be withdrawn (gradually if possible).

Exacerbation of Ischemic Heart Disease Following Abrupt Withdrawal: Angina pectoris has not been reported upon labetalol HCl discontinuation. However, hypersensitivity to catecholamines has been observed in patients withdrawn from beta-blocker therapy; exacerbation of angina and, in some cases, myocardial infarction have occurred after *abrupt* discontinuation of such therapy. When discontinuing chronically administered NORMODYNE (labetalol HCl), particularly in patients with ischemic heart disease, the dosage should be gradually reduced over a period of one to two weeks and the patient should be carefully monitored. If angina markedly worsens or acute coronary insufficiency develops, NORMODYNE (labetalol HCl) administration should be reinstituted promptly, at least temporarily, and other measures appropriate for the management of unstable angina should be taken. Patients should be warned against interruption or discontinuation of therapy without the physician's advice. Because coronary artery disease is common and may be unrecognized, it may be prudent not to discontinue NORMODYNE (labetalol HCl) therapy abruptly even in patients treated only for hypertension.

Nonallergic Bronchospasm (e.g., chronic bronchitis and emphysema) Patients with bronchospastic disease should, in general, not receive beta-blockers. NORMODYNE may be used with caution, however, in patients who do not respond to, or cannot tolerate, other antihypertensive agents. It is prudent, if NORMODYNE is used, to use the smallest effective dose, so that inhibition of endogenous or exogenous beta-agonists is minimized.

Pheochromocytoma: Labetalol HCl has been shown to be effective in lowering the blood pressure and relieving symptoms in patients with pheochromocytoma. However, paradoxical hypertensive responses have been reported in a few patients with this tumor; therefore, use caution when administering labetalol HCl to patients with pheochromocytoma.

Diabetes Mellitus and Hypoglycemia: Beta-adrenergic blockade may prevent the appearance of premonitory signs and symptoms (e.g., tachycardia) of acute hypoglycemia. This is especially important with labile diabetics. Beta-blockade also reduces the release of insulin in response to hyperglycemia; it may therefore be necessary to adjust the dose of antidiabetic drugs.

Major Surgery: The necessity or desirability of withdrawing beta-blocking therapy prior to major surgery is controversial. Protracted severe hypotension and difficulty in restarting or maintaining a heart beat have been reported with beta-blockers. The effect of labetalol HCl's alpha-adrenergic activity has not been evaluated in this setting. A synergism between labetalol HCl and halothane anesthesia has been shown (See **Drug Interactions**).

Precautions:
General: Impaired Hepatic Function: NORMODYNE (labetalol HCl) Tablets should be used with caution in patients with impaired hepatic function since metabolism of the drug may be diminished.

Jaundice or Hepatic Dysfunction: On rare occasions, labetalol HCl has been associated with jaundice (both hepatic and cholestatic). It is therefore recommended that treatment with labetalol HCl be stopped immediately, should a patient develop jaundice or laboratory evidence of liver injury. Both have been shown to be reversible on stopping therapy.

Information for Patients
As with all drugs with beta-blocking activity, certain advice to patients being treated with labetalol HCl is warranted. This information is intended to aid in the safe and effective use of this medication. It is not a disclosure of all possible adverse or intended effects. While no incident of the abrupt withdrawal phenomenon (exacerbation of angina pectoris) has been reported with labetalol HCl, dosing with NORMODYNE Tablets should not be interrupted or discontinued without a physician's advice. Patients being treated with NORMODYNE Tablets should consult a physician at any sign of impending cardiac failure. Also, transient scalp tingling may occur, usually when treatment with NORMODYNE Tablets is initiated (See **ADVERSE REACTIONS**).

Laboratory Tests
As with any new drug given over prolonged periods, laboratory parameters should be observed over regular intervals. In patients with concomitant illnesses, such as impaired renal function, appropriate tests should be done to monitor these conditions.

Drug Interactions
In one survey, 2.3% of patients taking labetalol HCl in combination with tricyclic antidepressants experienced tremor as compared to 0.7% reported to occur with labetalol HCl alone. The contribution of each of the treatments to this adverse reaction is unknown but the possibility of a drug interaction cannot be excluded.

Drugs possessing beta-blocking properties can blunt the bronchodilator effect of beta-receptor agonist drugs in patients with bronchospasm; therefore, doses greater than the normal antiasthmatic dose of beta-agonist bronchodilator drugs may be required.

Cimetidine has been shown to increase the bioavailability of labetalol HCl. Since this could be explained either by enhanced absorption or by an alteration of hepatic metabolism of labetalol HCl, special care should be used in establishing the dose required for blood pressure control in such patients.

Synergism has been shown between halothane anesthesia and intravenously administered labetalol HCl. During controlled hypotensive anesthesia using labetalol HCl in association with halothane, high concentrations (3% or above) of halothane should not be used because the degree of hypotension will be increased and because of the possibility of a large reduction in cardiac output and an increase in central venous pressure. The anesthesiologist should be informed when a patient is receiving labetalol HCl.

Labetalol HCl blunts the reflex tachycardia produced by nitroglycerin without preventing its hypotensive effect. If labetalol HCl is used with nitroglycerin in patients with angina pectoris, additional antihypertensive effects may occur.

Drug/Laboratory Test Interactions
The presence of a metabolite of labetalol in the urine may result in falsely increased levels of urinary catecholamines when measured by a nonspecific trihydroxyindole (THI) reaction. In screening patients suspected of having a pheochromocytoma and being treated with labetalol HCl, specific radioenzymatic or high performance liquid chromatography assay techniques should be used to determine levels of catecholamines or their metabolites.

Carcinogenesis, Mutagenesis, Impairment of Fertility
Long-term oral dosing studies with labetalol HCl for 18 months in mice and for 2 years in rats showed no evidence of carcinogenesis. Studies with labetalol HCl, using dominant lethal assays in rats and mice, and exposing microorganisms according to modified Ames tests, showed no evidence of mutagenesis.

Pregnancy Category C
Teratogenic studies have been performed with labetalol in rats and rabbits at oral doses up to approximately 6 and 4 times the maximum recommended human dose (MRHD), respectively. No reproducible evidence of fetal malformations was observed. Increased fetal resorptions were seen in both species at doses approximating the MRHD. There are no adequate and well-controlled studies in pregnant women. Labetalol should be used during pregnancy only if the potential benefit justifies the potential risk to the fetus.

Nonteratogenic Effects
Infants of mothers who were treated with labetalol HCl for hypertension during pregnancy did not appear to be adversely affected by the drug. Oral administration of labetalol to rats during late gestation through weaning at doses of 2 to 4 times the MRHD caused a decrease in neonatal survival.

Labor and Delivery
Labetalol HCl given to pregnant women with hypertension did not appear to affect the usual course of labor and delivery.

Nursing Mothers
Small amounts of labetalol (approximately 0.004% of the maternal dose) are excreted in human milk. Caution should be exercised when NORMODYNE Tablets are administered to a nursing woman.

Pediatric Use
Safety and effectiveness in children have not been established.

Adverse Reactions: Most adverse effects are mild, transient and occur early in the course of treatment. In controlled clinical trials of 3 to 4 months duration, discontinuation of NORMODYNE (labetalol HCl) Tablets due to one or more adverse effect was required in 7% of all patients. In these same trials, beta-blocker control agents led to discontinuation in 8 to 10% of patients, and a centrally acting alpha-agonist in 30% of patients.

The incidence rates of adverse reactions listed in the following table were derived from multicenter controlled clinical trials, comparing labetalol HCl, placebo, metoprolol and propranolol, over treatment periods of 3 and 4 months. Where the frequency of adverse effects for labetalol HCl and placebo is similar, causal relationship is uncertain. The rates are based on adverse reactions considered probably drug-related by the investigator. If all reports are considered, the rates are somewhat higher (e.g., dizziness 20%, nausea 14%, fatigue 11%), but the overall conclusions are unchanged.

[See table on bottom next page].

The adverse effects were reported spontaneously and are representative of the incidence of adverse effects that may be observed in a properly selected hypertensive patient population, i.e., a group excluding patients with bronchospastic disease, overt congestive heart failure, or other contraindications to beta-blocker therapy.

Clinical trials also included studies utilizing daily doses up to 2400 mg in more severely hypertensive patients. Certain of the side effects increased with increasing dose as shown in the table below which depicts the entire U.S. therapeutic trials data base for adverse reactions that are clearly or possibly dose related.

[See table on top next page].

In addition, a number of other less common adverse events have been reported in clincal trials or the literature:

Cardiovascular: Syncope. *Central and Peripheral Nervous Systems:* Paresthesias, most frequently described as scalp tingling. In most cases, it was mild, transient and usually occurred at the beginning of treatment. *Collagen Disorders:* Systemic lupus erythematosus; positive antinuclear factor (ANF). *Eyes:* Dry eyes. *Immunological System:* Antimitochondrial antibodies. *Liver and Biliary System:* Cholestasis with or without jaundice. *Musculo-Skeletal System:* Muscle cramps; toxic myopathy. *Respiratory System:* Bronchospasm. *Skin and Appendages:* Rashes of various types, such as generalized maculo-papular; lichenoid; urticarial; bullous lichen planus; psoriaform; facial erythema; Peyronie's disease; reversible alopecia. *Urinary System:* Difficulty in micturition, including acute urinary bladder retention.

Following approval for marketing in the United Kingdom, a monitored release survey involving approximately 6,800 patients was conducted for further safety and efficacy evaluation of this product. Results of this survey indicate that the type, severity, and incidence of adverse effects were comparable to those cited above.

Continued on next page

Information on Schering products appearing on these pages is effective as of September 30, 1984.

Schering—Cont.

Potential Adverse Effects
In addition, other adverse effects not listed above have been reported with other beta-adrenergic blocking agents.

Central Nervous System: Reversible mental depression progressing to catatonia; an acute reversible syndrome characterized by disorientation for time and place, short-term memory loss, emotional lability, slightly clouded sensorium, and decreased performance on neuropsychometrics.

Cardiovascular: Intensification of AV block. See CONTRAINDICATIONS.

Allergic: Fever combined with aching and sore throat; laryngospasm; respiratory distress.

Hematologic: Agranulocytosis; thrombocytopenic or nonthrombocytopenic purpura.

Gastrointestinal: Mesenteric artery thrombosis; ischemic colitis.

The oculomucocutaneous syndrome associated with the beta-blocker practolol has not been reported with labetalol HCl.

Clinical laboratory tests: There have been reversible increases of serum transaminases in 4% of patients treated with labetalol HCl and tested, and more rarely, reversible increases in blood urea.

Overdosage: Overdosage with NORMODYNE (labetalol HCl) Tablets causes excessive hypotension which is posture sensitive, and sometimes, excessive bradycardia. Patients should be laid supine and their legs raised if necessary to improve the blood supply to the brain. The following additional measures should be employed if necessary. *Excessive bradycardia*—administer atropine (3.0 mg). If there is no response to vagal blockade, administer isoproterenol cautiously. *Cardiac failure*—administer a digitalis glycoside and a diuretic. *Hypotension*—administer vasopressors, e.g., norepinephrine. There is pharmacological evidence that norepinephrine may be the drug of choice. *Bronchospasm*—administer a beta$_2$-stimulating agent and/or a theophylline preparation.

Gastric lavage or pharmacologically induced emesis (using syrup of ipecac) is useful for removal of the drug shortly after ingestion. Labetalol HCl can be removed from the general circulation by hemodialysis.

The oral LD$_{50}$ value of labetalol HCl in the mouse is approximately 600 mg/kg and in the rat is greater than 2 gm/kg. The intravenous LD$_{50}$ in these species is 50 to 60 mg/kg.

Labetalol HCl

Daily Dose (mg)	200	300	400	600	800	900	1200	1600	2400
Number of Patients	522	181	606	608	503	117	411	242	175
Dizziness (%)	2	3	3	3	5	1	9	13	16
Fatigue	2	1	4	4	5	3	7	6	10
Nausea	<1	0	1	2	4	0	7	11	19
Vomiting	0	0	<1	<1	<1	0	1	2	3
Dyspepsia	1	0	2	1	1	0	2	2	4
Paresthesias	2	0	2	2	1	1	2	5	5
Nasal Stuffiness	1	1	2	2	2	2	4	5	6
Ejaculation Failure	0	2	1	2	3	0	4	3	5
Impotence	1	1	1	1	2	4	3	4	3
Edema	1	0	1	1	1	0	1	2	2

Dosage and Administration: DOSAGE MUST BE INDIVIDUALIZED. The recommended <u>initial</u> dose is 100 mg <u>twice</u> daily whether used alone or added to a diuretic regimen. After 2 or 3 days, using standing blood pressure as an indicator, dosage may be titrated in increments of 100 mg bid every 2 or 3 days. The usual <u>maintenance</u> dosage of labetalol HCl is between 200 and 400 mg <u>twice</u> daily.

Since the full antihypertensive effect of labetalol HCl is usually seen within the first one to three hours of the initial dose or dose increment, the assurance of a lack of an exaggerated hypotensive response can be clinically established in the office setting. The antihypertensive effects of continued dosing can be measured at subsequent visits, approximately 12 hours after a dose, to determine whether further titration is necessary.

Patients with severe hypertension may require from 1200 mg to 2400 mg per day, with or without thiazide diuretics. Should side effects (principally nausea or dizziness) occur with these doses administered bid, the same total daily dose administered tid may improve tolerability and facilitate further titration. Titration increments should not exceed 200 mg bid.

When a diuretic is added, an additive antihypertensive effect can be expected. In some cases this may necessitate a labetalol HCl dosage adjustment. As with most antihypertensive drugs, optimal dosages of NORMODYNE Tablets are usually lower in patients also receiving a diuretic.

When transferring patients from other antihypertensive drugs, NORMODYNE Tablets should be introduced as recommended and the dosage of the existing therapy progressively decreased.

How Supplied: NORMODYNE (labetalol HCl) Tablets, <u>200</u> mg, white, round, scored, film-coated tablets engraved on one side with Schering and product identification numbers 752, and on the other side the number 200 for the strength; bottles of 100 (NDC-0085-0752-04), 500 (NDC-0085-0752-05), box of 100 for unit-dose dispensing (NDC-0085-0752-08), and Patient Calendar Package of 56 (4 bottles of 14 tablets) (NDC-0085-0752-03).

NORMODYNE (labetalol HCl) Tablets, <u>300</u> mg, blue, round, film-coated tablets engraved on one side with Schering and product identification numbers 438, and on the other side the number 300 for the strength; bottles of 100 (NDC-0085-0438-03), 500 (NDC-0085-0438-05), box of 100 for unit-dose dispensing (NDC-0085-0438-06), and Patient Calendar Package of 56 (4 bottles of 14 tablets) (NDC-0085-0438-02).

NORMODYNE (labetalol HCl) Tablets should be stored between 2° and 30°C (36° and 86°F).

NORMODYNE (labetalol HCl) Tablets in the unit-dose boxes should be protected from excessive moisture.

Revised 6/84

Copyright © 1984, Schering Corporation. All rights reserved.

Shown in Product Identification Section, page 434

OPTIMINE®
[op′ tĭ-mēn] ℞
brand of azatadine maleate, USP
Tablets

Description: OPTIMINE Tablets contain azatadine maleate, an antihistamine having the empirical formula, $C_{20}H_{22}N_2 \cdot 2C_4H_4O_4$, the chemical name, 6,11-Dihydro-11-(1-methyl-4-piperidylidene)-5H-benzo[5,6]cyclohepta[1,2-β]pyridine maleate (1:2).

The molecular weight of azatadine maleate is 522.54. It is a white to off-white powder and is very soluble in water and soluble in alcohol.

Each OPTIMINE Tablet contains 1 mg azatadine maleate, USP.

Clinical Pharmacology: Azatadine maleate is an antihistamine related to cyproheptadine, with antiserotonin, anticholinergic (drying), and sedative effects.

Antihistamines competitively antagonize those pharmacological effects of histamine which are mediated through activation of histamine H$_1$-receptor sites on effector cells. Histamine-related allergic reactions and tissue injury are blocked or diminished in intensity. Antihistamines antagonize the vasodilator effect of endogenously released histamine, especially in small vessels, and mitigate the effect of histamine which results in increased capillary permeability and edema formation. As consequences of these actions, antihistamines antagonize the physiological manifestations of histamine release in the nose following antigen-antibody interactions, such as congestion related to vascular engorgement, mucosal edema, and profuse, watery secretion, and irritation and sneezing resulting from histamine action on afferent nerve terminals.

Pharmacokinetic studies in normal volunteers dosed orally with radio-labeled azatadine maleate show that the drug is readily absorbed with peak plasma levels at about four hours after dosing. Approximately 50% of the drug is excreted in the urine within five days after administration of a

	Labetalol HCl (N=227) %	Placebo (N=98) %	Propranolol (N=84) %	Metoprolol (N=49) %
Body as a whole				
fatigue	5	0	12	12
asthenia	1	1	1	0
headache	2	1	1	2
Gastrointestinal				
nausea	6	1	1	2
vomiting	<1	0	0	0
dyspepsia	3	1	1	0
abdominal pain	0	0	1	2
diarrhea	<1	0	2	0
taste distortion	1	0	0	0
Central and Peripheral Nervous Systems				
dizziness	11	3	4	4
paresthesias	<1	0	0	0
drowsiness	<1	2	0	2
Autonomic Nervous System				
nasal stuffiness	3	0	0	0
ejaculation failure	2	0	0	0
impotence	1	0	1	3
increased sweating	<1	0	0	0
Cardiovascular				
edema	1	0	0	0
postural hypotension	1	0	0	0
bradycardia	0	0	5	12
Respiratory				
dyspnea	2	0	1	2
Skin				
rash	1	0	0	0
Special Senses				
vision abnormality	1	0	0	0
vertigo	2	1	0	0

single dose, and no evidence of drug accumulation was seen after daily dosing for 30 days. The elimination half-life of azatadine maleate, based on plasma radioactivity, was approximately 9 hours. Approximately 20% of the drug is excreted unchanged and extensive conjugation of the drug and its metabolites occurs. Azatadine maleate is minimally bound to plasma protein.

While the antihistamines have not been studied for passage through the blood-brain and placental barriers, the occurrence of pharmacologic effects in the central nervous system and in the newborn indicate presence of the drug.

Indications and Usage: OPTIMINE Tablets are indicated for the treatment of perennial and seasonal allergic rhinitis and chronic urticaria.

Contraindications: Antihistamines *should NOT* be used to treat lower respiratory tract symptoms, including asthma.

Antihistamines, including azatadine maleate, are also contraindicated in patients hypersensitive to this medication and to other antihistamines of similar chemical structure, and in patients receiving monoamine oxidase inhibitor therapy. (See Drug Interactions.)

Warnings: Antihistamines should be used with caution in patients with narrow angle glaucoma, stenosing peptic ulcer; pyloroduodenal obstruction; and urinary bladder obstruction due to symptomatic prostatic hypertrophy and narrowing of the bladder neck.

Use with CNS Depressants: Antihistamines have additive effects with alcohol and other CNS depressants (hypnotics, sedatives, tranquilizers, etc.).

Use in Activities Requiring Mental Alertness: Patients should be warned about engaging in activities requiring mental alertness, such as driving a car or operating certain appliances, machinery, etc., until their response to this medication has been determined.

Use in Patients approximately 60 years or older: Antihistamines are more likely to cause dizziness, sedation, and hypotension in patients over 60 years of age.

Precautions: General: Azatadine maleate has an atropine-like action and therefore should be used with caution in patients with: a history of bronchial asthma; increased intraocular pressure; hyperthyroidism; cardiovascular disease; hypertension.

Information for Patients:
1. Antihistamines may cause drowsiness.
2. Patients taking antihistamines should not engage in activities requiring mental alertness, such as driving a car or operating machinery, certain appliances, etc., until their response to this medication has been determined.
3. Alcohol or other sedative drugs may enhance the drowsiness caused by antihistamines.
4. Patients should not take this medication if they are receiving a monoamine oxidase (MAO) inhibitor, or if they are receiving oral anticoagulants.
5. This medication should not be given to children less than 12 years of age.

Drug Interactions: MAO inhibitors prolong and intensify the anticholinergic and sedative effects of antihistamines. Additive effects may occur from the concomitant use of antihistamines with tricyclic antidepressants. (See also WARNINGS.) The action of oral anticoagulants may be diminished by antihistamines.

Drug/Laboratory Test Interaction: Antihistamines should be discontinued about four days prior to skin testing procedures since these drugs may prevent or diminish otherwise positive reactions to dermal reactivity indicators.

Carcinogenesis, Mutagenesis, and Impairment of Fertility: Long-term oral dosing studies with azatadine maleate in rats and mice showed no evidence of carcinogenesis. No mutagenic effect was seen in a dominant lethal assay study in mice dosed with azatadine maleate orally and intraperitoneally. There was no impairment of fertility in rats fed azatadine maleate at doses greater than 150 times the recommended human daily dose.

Pregnancy Category B: Reproduction studies have been performed in rats and rabbits at doses up to 188 times and 38 times, respectively, the human dose and have revealed no evidence of impaired fertility or harm to the fetus due to azatadine maleate. There are, however, no adequate and well-controlled studies in pregnant women. Because animal reproduction studies are not always predictive of human response, this drug should be used during pregnancy only if clearly needed. (See **Non-Teratogenic Effects**.)

Non-Teratogenic Effects: Antihistamines should not be used in the third trimester of pregnancy because newborns and premature infants may have severe reactions, such as convulsions, to them.

Nursing Mothers: It is not known whether this drug is excreted in human milk. However, certain antihistamines are known to be excreted in human milk in low concentration. Because of the higher risk of antihistamines for infants generally and for newborns and prematures in particular, a decision should be made whether to discontinue nursing or to discontinue the drug, taking into account the importance of the drug to the mother.

Pediatric Use: Safety and effectiveness in children below the age of 12 years have not been established.

Adverse Reactions: Slight to moderate drowsiness may occur with azatadine maleate. Other possible side effects common to antihistamines in general include: (the most frequent are underlined).

General: urticaria, drug rash, anaphylactic shock, photosensitivity, excessive perspiration, chills, dryness of mouth, nose, and throat.

Cardiovascular: hypotension, headache, palpitations, tachycardia, extrasystoles.

Hematologic: hemolytic anemia, hypoplastic anemia, thrombocytopenia, agranulocytosis.

Nervous: sedation, sleepiness, dizziness, vertigo, tinnitus, acute labyrinthitis, disturbed coordination, fatigue, confusion, restlessness, excitation, nervousness, tremor, irritability, insomnia, euphoria, paresthesias, blurred vision diplopia, hysteria, neuritis, convulsions.

Gastrointestinal: epigastric distress, anorexia, nausea, vomiting, diarrhea, constipation.

Genitourinary: urinary frequency, difficult urination, urinary retention, early menses.

Respiratory: thickening of bronchial secretions, tightness of chest and wheezing, nasal stuffiness.

Drug Abuse and Dependence: There is no information to indicate that abuse or dependency occurs with azatadine maleate.

Overdosage: In the event of overdosage, emergency treatment should be started immediately.

Manifestations: Antihistamine overdosage effects may vary from central nervous system depression (sedation, apnea, diminished mental alertness, cardiovascular collapse) to stimulation (insomnia, hallucinations, tremors or convulsions) to death. Other signs and symptoms may be dizziness, tinnitus, ataxia, blurred vision, and hypotension. Stimulation is particularly likely in children, as are atropine-like signs and symptoms (dry mouth; fixed, dilated pupils; flushing; hyperthermia; and gastrointestinal symptoms).

Treatment: The patient should be induced to vomit, even if emesis has occurred spontaneously. Pharmacologic vomiting by the administration of ipecac syrup is a preferred method. However, vomiting should not be induced in patients with impaired consciousness. The action of ipecac is facilitated by physical activity and by the administration of 8 to 12 fluid ounces of water. If emesis does not occur within fifteen minutes, the dose of ipecac should be repeated. Precautions against aspiration must be taken, especially in infants and children. Following emesis, any drug remaining in the stomach may be absorbed by activated charcoal administered as a slurry with water. If vomiting is unsuccessful or contraindicated, gastric lavage should be performed. Physiologic saline solution is the lavage solution of choice, particularly in children. In adults, tap water can be used; however, as much as possible of the amount administered should be removed before the next instillation. Saline cathartics, such as milk of magnesia, draw water into the bowel by osmosis and, therefore, may be valuable for their action in rapid dilution of bowel content. Dialysis is of little value in antihistamine poisoning. After emergency treatment, the patient should continue to be medically monitored.

Treatment of the signs and symptoms of overdosage is symptomatic and supportive. Stimulants (analeptic agents) should not be used. Vasopressors may be used to treat hypotension. Short acting barbiturates, diazepam, or paraldehyde may be administered to control seizures. Hyperpyrexia, especially in children, may require treatment with tepid water sponge baths or a hypothermic blanket. Apnea is treated with ventilatory support.

Dosage and Administration: DOSAGE SHOULD BE INDIVIDUALIZED ACCORDING TO THE NEEDS AND THE RESPONSE OF THE PATIENT.

OPTIMINE Tablets are not recommended for use in children under 12 years of age.

The usual adult dosage is 1 or 2 mg, twice a day.

How Supplied: OPTIMINE Tablets, 1 mg. white, compressed, scored tablets impressed with the Schering trademark and product identification numbers, 282; bottle of 100 (NDC 0085-0282-03).

Store between 2° and 30°C (36° and 86°F).

Revised 5/81

Copyright © 1973, 1981, Schering Corporation. All rights reserved.

Shown in Product Identification Section, page 434

ORETON® Methyl ℞
[or′e-ton]
brand of methyltestosterone
Tablets, USP
Buccal Tablets, USP

Description: ORETON Methyl Tablets and Buccal Tablets contain methyltestosterone, USP, a synthetic androgen. Androgens are steroids that develop and maintain primary and secondary male sex characteristics. ORETON Methyl Tablets are to be taken orally. ORETON Methyl Buccal Tablets are NOT to be swallowed but are to be placed in the lower or upper buccal pouches.

Androgens are derivatives of cyclopentanoperhydrophenanthrene. Endogenous androgens are C-19 steroids with a side chain at C-17, and with two angular methyl groups. Testosterone is the primary endogenous androgen. In their active form, all drugs in the class have a 17-beta-hydroxy group. 17-alpha alkylation (methyltestosterone) increases the pharmacologic activity per unit weight compared to testosterone when given orally.

Methyltestosterone is the 17α-methyl derivative of testosterone, the true testicular hormone. Chemically, methyltestosterone is 17β-Hydroxy-17-methylandrost-4-en-3-one, with the empirical formula $C_{20}H_{30}O_2$, a molecular weight of 302.5. Methyltestosterone is a white to creamy-white, odorless, slightly hygroscopic powder. It is practically insoluble in water, soluble in alcohol and other organic solvents.

ORETON Methyl Tablets contain either 10 mg or 25 mg of methyltestosterone, USP.

Each ORETON Methyl Buccal Tablet contains 10 mg methyltestosterone, USP.

Clinical Pharmacology: Endogenous androgens are responsible for the normal growth and development of the male sex organs and for maintenance of secondary sex characteristics. These effects include the growth and maturation of prostate, seminal vesicles, penis, and scrotum: the development of male hair distribution, such as beard, pubic, chest, and axillary hair; laryngeal enlargement, vocal chord thickening, alterations in body musculature, and fat distribution. Drugs in this class also cause retention of nitrogen, sodium, potassium, phosphorus, and decreased urinary excretion of calcium. Androgens have been reported to increase protein anabolism and decrease protein

Continued on next page

Information on Schering products appearing on these pages is effective as of September 30, 1984.

Schering—Cont.

catabolism. Nitrogen balance is improved only when there is sufficient intake of calories and protein.

Androgens are responsible for the growth spurt of adolescence and for the eventual termination of linear growth which is brought about by fusion of the epiphyseal growth centers. In children, exogenous androgens accelerate linear growth rates, but may cause a disproportionate advancement in bone maturation. Use over long periods may result in fusion of the epiphyseal growth centers and termination of the growth process. Androgens have been reported to stimulate the production of red blood cells by enhancing the production of erythropoietic stimulating factor.

During exogenous administration of androgens, endogenous testosterone release is inhibited through feedback inhibition of pituitary luteinizing hormone (LH). With large doses of exogenous androgens, spermatogenesis may also be suppressed through feedback inhibition of pituitary follicle stimulating hormone (FSH).

There is a lack of substantial evidence that androgens are effective in fractures, surgery, convalescence, and functional uterine bleeding.

Pharmacokinetics: Testosterone given orally is metabolized by the gut and 44 percent is cleared by the liver in the first pass. Oral doses as high as 400 mg per day are needed to achieve clinically effective blood levels for full replacement therapy. The synthetic androgen (methyltestosterone) is less extensively metabolized by the liver and has a longer half-life. It is more suitable than testosterone for oral administration. Additionally, buccal administration permits the methyltestosterone to be absorbed directly into the systemic venous return so that the unmetabolized hormone is carried directly to the tissues. The buccal tablets have approximately twice the potency of the orally ingested methyltestosterone.

Testosterone in plasma is 98 percent bound to a specific testosterone-estradiol binding globulin, and about one percent is free. Generally, the amount of this sex-hormone binding globulin in the plasma will determine the distribution of testosterone between free and bound forms, and the free testosterone concentration will determine its half-life.

About 90 percent of a dose of testosterone is excreted in the urine as glucuronic and sulfuric acid conjugates of testosterone and its metabolites; about 6 percent of a dose is excreted in the feces, mostly in the unconjugated form. Inactivation of testosterone occurs primarily in the liver. Testosterone is metabolized to various 17-keto steroids through two different pathways. As reported in the literature, the half-life of testosterone varies considerably, ranging from 10 to 100 minutes.

In many tissues the activity of testosterone appears to depend on reduction to dihydrotestosterone, which binds to cytosol receptor proteins. The steroid-receptor complex is transported to the nucleus where it initiates transcription events and cellular changes related to androgen action.

Indications and Usage: *In the male:* ORETON Methyl Tablets and Methyl Buccal Tablets are indicated for replacement therapy in conditions associated with a deficiency or absence of endogenous testosterone:

Primary hypogonadism (congenital or acquired) —testicular failure due to cryptorchidism, bilateral torsion, orchitis, vanishing testis syndrome; or orchidectomy.

Hypogonadotropic hypogonadism (congenital or acquired)—idopathic gonadotropin of LHRH deficiency, or pituitary-hypothalamic injury from tumors, trauma, or radiation.

If the above conditions occur prior to puberty, androgen replacement therapy will be needed during the adolescent years for development of secondary sexual characteristics. Prolonged androgen treatment will be required to maintain sexual characteristics in these and other males who develop testosterone deficiency after puberty.

Androgens may be used to stimulate puberty in carefully selected males with clearly delayed puberty. These patients usually have a familial pattern of delayed puberty that is not secondary to a pathological disorder; puberty is expected to occur spontaneously at a relatively late date. Brief treatment with conservative doses may occasionally be justified in these patients if they do not respond to psychological support. The potential adverse effect on bone maturation should be discussed with the patient and parents prior to androgen administration. An X-ray of the hand and wrist to determine bone age should be obtained every 6 months to assess the effect of treatment on the epiphyseal centers. (See WARNINGS.)

In the female: ORETON Methyl Tablets and Methyl Buccal Tablets may be used secondarily in women with advancing inoperable metastatic (skeletal) mammary cancer who are 1 to 5 years postmenopausal. Primary goals of therapy in these women include ablation of the ovaries. Other methods of counteracting estrogen activity are adrenalectomy, hypophysectomy, and/or antiestrogen therapy. This treatment has also been used in premenopausal women with breast cancer who have benefited from oophorectomy and are considered to have a hormone-responsive tumor. Judgment concerning androgen therapy should be made by an oncologist with expertise in this field. Androgens, such as methyltestosterone, have been used for the management of postpartum breast pain and engorgement.

Contraindications: ORETON Methyl and Methyl Buccal Tablets are contraindicated for use in men with carcinomas of the breast or with known or suspected carcinomas of the prostate, and in women who are or may become pregnant. When administered to pregnant women, androgens cause virilization of the external genitalia of the female fetus. This virilization includes clitoromegaly, abnormal vaginal development, and fusion of genital folds to form a scrotal-like structure. The degree of masculinization is related to the amount of drug given and to the age of the fetus, and is most likely to occur in the female fetus when the drugs are given in the first trimester. If the patient becomes pregnant while taking these drugs, she should be apprised of the potential hazard to the fetus.

Warnings: In patients with breast cancer, androgen therapy may cause hypercalcemia by stimulating osteolysis. In this case, the drugs should be discontinued.

Prolonged use of high doses of androgens has been associated with the development of peliosis hepatis and hepatic neoplasms including hepatocellular carcinoma. (See PRECAUTIONS:—Carcinogenesis, Mutagenesis, Impairment of Fertility.) Peliosis hepatis can be a life-threatening or fatal complication.

Cholestatic hepatitis and jaundice occur with 17-alpha-alkylandrogens (such as methyltestosterone) at a relatively low dose. If cholestatic hepatitis with jaundice appears or if liver function tests become abnormal, the androgen should be discontinued and the etiology should be determined. Drug-induced jaundice is reversible when the medication is discontinued.

Geriatric patients treated with androgens may be at an increased risk for the development of prostatic hypertrophy and prostatic carcinoma.

Edema with or without congestive heart failure may be a serious complication in patients with preexisting cardiac, renal, or hepatic disease. In addition to discontinuation of the drug, diuretic therapy may be required.

Gynecomastia frequently develops and occasionally persists in patients being treated for hypogonadism.

Androgen therapy should be used cautiously in healthy males with delayed puberty. The effect on bone maturation should be monitored by assessing bone age of the wrist and hand every 6 months. In children, androgen treatment may accelerate bone maturation without producing compensatory gain in linear growth. This adverse effect may result in compromised adult stature. The younger the child the greater the risk of compromising final mature height.

Precautions: General: Women should be observed for signs of virilization (deepening of the voice, hirsutism, acne, clitoromegaly and menstrual irregularities). Discontinuation of drug therapy at the time of evidence of mild virilism is necessary to prevent irreversible virilization. Such virilization is usual following androgen use at high doses. A decision may be made by the patient and the physician that some virilization will be tolerated during treatment for breast carcinoma.

Priapism or excessive sexual stimulation may develop. Males, especially the elderly, may become overstimulated. In treating males for symptoms of climacteric, avoid stimulation to the point of increasing the nervous, mental, and physical activities beyond the patient's cardiovascular capacity. Oligospermia and reduced ejaculatory volume may occur after prolonged administration or excessive dosage.

Information for the Patients: The physician should instruct patients to report any of the following side effects of androgens:

Adult or Adolescent Males: Too frequent or persistent erections of the penis.

Women: Hoarseness, acne, changes in menstrual periods, or more hair on the face.

All Patients: Any nausea, vomiting, changes in skin color or ankle swelling.

Any male adolescent patient receiving androgens for delayed puberty should have bone development checked every six months.

Patients should be instructed in the proper taking of ORETON Methyl Buccal Tablets. These tablets should **NOT** be swallowed. They should be placed in the space between the gum and cheek and allowed to dissolve, so that the medication enters the body through the lining of the cheek. Avoid eating, drinking, chewing, or smoking while the buccal tablet is in place. The mouth should be rinsed with water after the tablet has dissolved completely.

Laboratory Tests: Women with disseminated breast carcinomas should have frequent determination of urine and serum calcium levels during the course of androgen therapy. (See WARNINGS.)

Because of the hepatoxicity associated with the use of 17-alpha-alkylated androgens, liver function tests should be obtained periodically.

Periodic (every 6 months) X-ray examinations of bone age should be made during treatment of prepubertal males to determine the rate of bone maturation and the effects of androgen therapy on the epiphyseal centers.

Hemoglobin and hematocrit should be checked periodically for polycythemia in patients who are receiving high doses of androgens.

Drug Interactions: Anticoagulants C-17 substituted derivatives of testosterone, such as methandrostenolone, have been reported to decrease the anticoagulant requirements of patients receiving oral anticoagulants. Patients receiving oral anticoagulant therapy require close monitoring especially when androgens are started or stopped.

Oxyphenbutazone Concurrent administration of oxyphenbutazone and androgens may result in elevated serum levels of oxyphenbutazone.

Insulin In diabetic patients the metabolic effects of androgens may decrease blood glucose and insulin requirements.

Drug/Laboratory Test Interferences: Androgens may decrease levels of thyroxine-binding globulin, resulting in decreased total T_4 serum levels and increased resin uptake of T_3 and T_4. Free thyroid hormone levels remain unchanged, however, and there is no clinical evidence of thyroid dysfunction.

Carcinogenesis, Mutagenesis, Impairment of Fertility: *Animal Data:* Testosterone has been tested by subcutaneous injection and implantation in mice and rats. The implant induced cervical-uterine tumors in mice which metastasized in some cases. There is suggestive evidence that injection of testosterone into some strains of female mice increases their susceptibility to hepatoma. Testosterone is also known to increase the number of tumors and decrease the degree of differentiation of chemically induced carcinomas of the liver in rats.

Human Data: There are rare reports of hepatocellular carcinoma in patients receiving long-term therapy with androgens in high doses. Withdrawal of the drugs did not lead to regression of the tumors in all cases.

Geriatric patients treated with androgens may be at an increased risk for the development of prostatic hypertrophy and prostatic carcinoma. Information on mutagenesis is unknown.

Pregnancy: *Teratogenic Effects—Pregnancy Category X:* See CONTRAINDICATIONS.

Nursing Mothers: It is not known whether androgens are excreted in human milk. Because many drugs are excreted in human milk and because of the potential for serious adverse reactions in nursing infants from androgens, a decision should be made whether to discontinue nursing or to discontinue the drug, taking into account the importance of the drug to the mother.

Pediatric Use: Androgen therapy should be used very cautiously in children and only by specialists who are aware of the adverse effects on bone maturation. Skeletal maturation must be monitored every six months by an X-ray of the hand and wrist. (See INDICATIONS AND USAGE, and WARNINGS.)

Adverse Reactions: Endocrine and Urogenital: *Female:* The most common side effects of androgen therapy are amenorrhea and other menstrual irregularities, inhibition of gonadotropin secretion, and virilization, including deepening of the voice and clitoral enlargement. The latter usually is not reversible after androgens are discontinued. When administered to a pregnant woman, androgens cause virilization of external genitalia of the female fetus.

Male: Gynecomastia, and excessive frequency and duration of penile erections. Oligospermia may occur at high dosages. (See CLINICAL PHARMACOLOGY.)

Skin and appendages: Hirsutism, male pattern of baldness, and acne.

Fluid and Electrolyte Disturbances: Retention of sodium, chloride, water, potassium, calcium, and inorganic phosphates.

Gastrointestinal: Nausea, cholestatic jaundice, alterations in liver function tests, rarely hepatocellular neoplasms and peliosis hepatitis (See WARNINGS.)

Hematologic: Suppression of clotting factors, II, V, VII, and X, bleeding in patients on concomitant anticoagulant therapy, and polycythemia.

Nervous System: Increased or decreased libido, headache, anxiety, depression, and generalized paresthesiae.

Metabolic: Increased serum cholesterol.

Miscellaneous: Stomatitis with buccal preparations; rarely anaphylactoid reactions.

Overdosage: Overdose of medication may be reflected in the occurrence of the signs and symptoms associated with testosterone-anabolic drugs. Nausea and early appearance of the manifestations of edema should be looked for. However, there has been no report of acute overdosage with androgens.

Dosage and Administration: Dosage must be strictly individualized. The suggested dosage for androgens varies depending on the age, sex, and diagnosis of the individual patient. Adjustments and duration of dosage will depend upon the patient's response and the appearance of adverse reactions.

	Route	Dose	Frequency
ORETON Methyl Tablets			
breast cancer	oral	50–200 mg	daily
postpartum breast pain and engorgement	oral	80 mg	daily (3 to 5 days)
ORETON Methyl Buccal Tablets			
breast cancer	buccal	25–100 mg*	daily
postpartum breast pain and engorgement	buccal	40 mg*	daily (3 to 5 days)

* NOTE: ORETON Methyl Buccal Tablets have approximately twice the potency of the orally ingested ORETON Methyl Tablets.

	Route	Dose	Frequency
ORETON Methyl Tablets	Oral	10–50 mg	Daily
ORETON Methyl Buccal Tablets	Buccal	5–25 mg*	Daily

* NOTE: ORETON Methyl Buccal Tablets have approximately twice the potency of the orally ingested ORETON Methyl Tablets.

Males: In the androgen-deficient male the following guideline for replacement therapy indicates the usual initial dosages:
[See table above].

Various dosage regimens have been used to induce pubertal changes in hypogonadal males; some experts have advocated lower dosages initially, gradually increasing the dose as puberty progresses, with or without a decrease to maintenance levels. Other experts emphasize that higher dosages are needed to induce pubertal changes and lower dosages can be used for maintenance after puberty. The chronological and skeletal ages must be taken into consideration, both in determining the initial dose and in adjusting the dose.

Dosages used in delayed puberty generally are in the lower ranges of those given above, and are for limited duration, for example, 4 to 6 months.

Females: Women with metastatic breast carcinoma must be followed closely because androgen therapy occasionally appears to accelerate the disease. Thus, many experts prefer to use the shorter acting androgen preparations rather than those with prolonged activity for treating breast carcinoma particularly during the early stages of androgen therapy.

Guideline dosages of androgens for use in the palliative treatment of women with metastatic breast cancer and for the prevention of postpartum breast pain and engorgement are:
[See table below].

Administration of Buccal Tablets: ORETON Methyl Buccal Tablets should NOT be swallowed, since the hormone is meant to be absorbed through the oral mucous membranes. Place the buccal tablet in the upper or lower buccal pouch between the gum and cheek; let the tablet dissolve completely. Avoid eating, drinking, chewing, or smoking while the buccal tablet is in place. Proper oral hygienic measures (e.g., rinsing mouth with water) are particularly important after the use of buccal tablets.

How Supplied: ORETON Methyl Buccal Tablets, 10 mg, compressed, lavender-colored, oval tablets impressed with the Schering trademark and product identification letters, BE, or numbers, 970; bottle of 100 (NDC–0085–0970–06).

Store between 2° and 30°C (36° and 86°F).

NOTE: Color of tablets may fade; potency and effectiveness are not impaired.

ORETON Methyl Tablets, 10 mg, compressed, white, round tablets impressed with the Schering trademark and product identification letters, JD, or numbers 311; bottle of 100 (NDC–0085–0311–06).

ORETON Methyl Tablets, 25 mg, compressed, peach-colored, round tablets impressed with the Schering trademark and product identification letters, JE, or numbers, 499; bottle of 100 (NDC–0085–0499–06).

Revised 6/83

Copyright © 1968, 1982, 1983, Schering Corporation. All rights reserved.

Shown in Product Identification Section, page 434

OTOBIOTIC® R

[oʺto-bi-ahʹ tik]
brand of polymyxin B sulfate and hydrocortisone
Sterile Otic Solution, USP

Description: OTOBIOTIC Otic Solution is a sterile, antibacterial solution containing an anti-inflammatory agent for use in the external ear. Each ml contains polymyxin B sulfate, USP equivalent to 10,000 units polymyxin B and 5.0 mg hydrocortisone, USP in a propylene glycol, glycerin vehicle which also contains edetate disodium, sodium bisulfite, anhydrous sodium sulfite, and purified water; sulfuric acid used to adjust pH between 3.0 and 5.0.

Actions: Polymyxin B sulfate is effective against *Pseudomonas aeruginosa* and some other gram-negative organisms, including strains of *Escherichia,* that commonly cause otitis externa. The addition of hydrocortisone to the antibiotic affords an anti-inflammatory effect and relief against allergic manifestations and pruritus and reduces the possibility of hypersensitivity and tissue reaction.

Indications: OTOBIOTIC Otic Solution is indicated for the treatment of superficial bacterial infections of the external auditory canals caused by organisms susceptible to the action of the antibiotic.

Contraindications: OTOBIOTIC Otic Solution is contraindicated in those individuals who are hypersensitive to corticosteroids, polymyxin or colistin, or to any of its other components, and in infections due to herpes simplex, vaccinia, and zoster-varicella viruses or to fungi.

Perforated tympanic membranes are frequently considered a contraindication to the use of external ear canal medication.

Warnings: As with other antibiotic preparations, prolonged treatment with OTOBIOTIC Otic Solution may result in overgrowth of nonsusceptible organisms and fungi.

Infections of the external auditory canals can be of mixed microbial origin and occasionally may be caused by both bacteria and fungi. If the infection is not improved after one week, bacterial and fungal cultures and susceptibility tests should be done to verify the identity of the organism and to determine whether therapy should be changed.

Patients who prefer to warm the medication before using it should be cautioned against heating the solution above body temperature in order to avoid loss of potency.

Precautions: If sensitization or irritation occurs, treatment with OTOBIOTIC Otic Solution should be discontinued promptly. Treatment with OTOBIOTIC Otic Solution should not be continued for longer than ten days.

OTOBIOTIC Otic Solution is not for ophthalmic use.

Dosage and Administration: The external auditory canal should be thoroughly cleansed and dried with a sterile cotton applicator before administration of OTOBIOTIC Otic Solution.

For adults, four drops of the solution should be instilled into the affected ear three or four times a day. For infants and children, three drops, instilled into the affected ear three or four times a day, are suggested because of the smaller capacity of the ear canal.

The patient should lie with the affected ear upward and then the drops should be instilled. This position should be maintained for five minutes to

Continued on next page

Information on Schering products appearing on these pages is effective as of September 30, 1984.

Schering—Cont.

facilitate penetration of the drops into the ear canal. Repeat, if necessary, for the opposite ear.
Note: When placing the dropper in the bottle and during use, do not allow the dropper to touch affected area, fingers, or any other surface. This precaution is necessary to preserve the sterility of the solution.

How Supplied: OTOBIOTIC Otic Solution, 15 ml bottle with sterile dropper packaged separately; box of one.

Store between 2° and 30°C (36° and 86°F).
Copyright © 1981, 1982, Schering Corporation. All rights reserved.
Revised 11/82

PAXIPAM®
[pak'si-pam]
brand of halazepam
Tablets

Description: PAXIPAM Tablets contain halazepam, a benzodiazepine derivative having the chemical name, 7-chloro-1,3-dihydro-5-phenyl-1-(2,2,2-trifluoroethyl)-2H-1,4-benzodiazepin-2-one. Each PAXIPAM Tablet contains 20 mg or 40 mg halazepam. The compound is a white to light cream-colored powder with a molecular weight of 352.8.

Clinical Pharmacology: Central nervous system agents of the 1,4-benzodiazepine class presumably exert their effects by binding at stereo specific receptors at several sites within the central nervous system. Their exact mechanism of action is unknown. Clinically, all benzodiazepines cause a dose-related central nervous system depressant activity varying from mild impairment of task performance to hypnosis.

Halazepam is rapidly and well-absorbed and primarily excreted in the urine. Maximum plasma concentration of halazepam is achieved between one and three hours following oral administration. Studies involving 12 normal subjects indicate the median half-life of elimination of halazepam following a 40 mg dose is approximately 14 hours. The major active plasma metabolite of halazepam is N-desmethyldiazepam. Maximum plasma concentrations of N-desmethyldiazepam usually occur within three to six hours. This metabolite has a half-life of elimination of approximately 50 to 100 hours. Less than one percent of the dose is excreted in the urine as unchanged drug. The major metabolite of halazepam in the urine is a conjugate, 3-hydroxyhalazepam. As with other benzodiazepines, enterohepatic recycling of halazepam and its metabolites may occur in uremic patients.

The degree of plasma protein binding of benzodiazepines is high. Since binding is to serum albumin, the extent of binding is dependent on the albumin concentration. In chronic alcoholics, patients with cirrhosis, and newborns, reduced binding may occur. Protein binding may be greatly reduced in patients with renal insufficiency. Since hepatic biotransformation is the predominant route for the metabolism of benzodiazepines, the disposition of these drugs may be impaired in patients with chronic liver disease. Oral dosing of rats with halazepam for a brief period induced the synthesis of hepatic microsomal drug-metabolizing enzymes. As a result, assuming similar responses in humans, the metabolism of other drugs metabolized in the liver may be increased. The transplacental transfer of halazepam has not been studied. However, other benzodiazepines readily cross the placental barrier. Following administration of halazepam to lactating women, halazepam and its major metabolite, N-desmethyldiazepam, were present in the milk.

Indications and Usage: PAXIPAM Tablets are indicated for the management of anxiety disorders or the short-term relief of the symptoms of anxiety. Anxiety or tension associated with the stress of everyday life usually does not require treatment with an anxiolytic.

The effectiveness of PAXIPAM Tablets for long-term use, that is, more than *four* months, has not been established.
The physician should periodically reassess the usefulness of the drug for the individual patient.

Contraindications: PAXIPAM Tablets are contraindicated in patients with known sensitivity to this drug or other benzodiazepines. It may be used in patients with open angle glaucoma who are receiving appropriate therapy, but is contraindicated in acute narrow angle glaucoma.

Warnings: PAXIPAM Tablets are not of value in the treatment of psychotic patients and should not be employed in lieu of appropriate treatment for psychosis. PAXIPAM Tablets are also not recommended as the primary treatment for major depressive disorders. Because of its depressant CNS effects, patients receiving PAXIPAM Tablets should be cautioned against engaging in hazardous occupations requiring complete mental alertness, such as operating machinery or driving a motor vehicle. For the same reason, patients should be cautioned about the simultaneous ingestion of alcohol and other CNS depressant drugs during treatment with PAXIPAM Tablets.

Benzodiazepines can potentially cause fetal harm when administered to pregnant women. If PAXIPAM Tablets are used during pregnancy, or if the patient becomes pregnant while taking this drug, she should be apprised of the potential hazard to the fetus. Because of experience with other members of the benzodiazepine class, PAXIPAM Tablets are assumed to be capable of causing an increased risk of congenital abnormalities when administered to a pregnant woman during the first trimester. Because use of these drugs is rarely a matter of urgency, their use during the first trimester should almost always be avoided. The possibility that a woman of childbearing potential may be pregnant at the time of institution of therapy should be considered. Patients should be advised that if they become pregnant during therapy or intend to become pregnant, they should communicate with their physicians about the desirability of discontinuing the drug.

Precautions: General: If PAXIPAM Tablets are to be combined with other psychotropic agents or anticonvulsant drugs, careful consideration should be given to the pharmacology of the agents to be employed, particularly with compounds which might potentiate the action of benzodiazepines (See Drug Interactions section).
As with other psychotropic medications, the usual precautions with respect to administration of the drug and size of the prescription are indicated for severely depressed patients or those in whom there is reason to expect concealed suicidal ideation or plans.
In elderly and debilitated patients, it is recommended that the dosage be limited to the smallest effective amount to preclude the development of ataxia or oversedation (See DOSAGE AND ADMINISTRATION section). The usual precautions in treating patients with impaired renal or hepatic function should be observed.

Information for Patients: To assure safe and effective use of benzodiazepines, the following information and instructions should be given to the patient:
1. Inform your physician about any alcohol consumption and medicine you are taking now, including drugs you buy without a prescription. Alcohol should generally not be used during treatment with benzodiazepines.
2. Inform your physician if you are planning to become pregnant, if you are pregnant, or if you become pregnant while you are taking this medication.
3. Inform your physician if you are nursing.
4. Until you experience how this medicine affects you, do not drive a car or operate potentially dangerous machinery, etc.
5. If benzodiazepines are used in large doses and/or for an extended period of time, they produce habituation, emotional and physical dependence. Therefore, do not increase the dose even if you think that the drug "does not work anymore."
6. Do not stop taking the drug abruptly without consulting your physician, since withdrawal symptoms can occur.

Laboratory Tests: Laboratory tests are not ordinarily required in otherwise healthy patients.

Drug Interactions: The benzodiazepines, including PAXIPAM Tablets, produce additive CNS depressant effects when co-administered with other psychotropic medications, anticonvulsants, antihistaminics, ethanol, and other drugs which themselves produce CNS depression.
Pharmacokinetic interactions with benzodiazepines have been reported. For example, cimetidine has been reported to reduce diazepam clearance. However, it is not known at this time whether a similar interaction occurs with PAXIPAM Tablets.

Drug/Laboratory Test Interactions: Although interactions between benzodiazepines and commonly employed clinical laboratory tests have occasionally been reported, there is no consistent pattern for a specific drug or specific test.

Carcinogenesis, Mutagenesis, Impairment of Fertility: The results of oral oncogenicity studies in rats and mice treated at doses 5 to 50 times the usual 120 mg daily human dose revealed no evidence of carcinogenicity or other significant pathology. Studies regarding mutagenesis have not been done. Reproduction studies performed in rats have revealed no evidence of impaired fertility.

Pregnancy: Teratogenic Effects: Pregnancy Category D: (See WARNINGS section).

Nonteratogenic Effects: The child born of a mother who is on benzodiazepines may be at some risk for withdrawal symptoms from the drug during the postnatal period. Also, neonatal flaccidity has been reported in children born of mothers who had been receiving benzodiazepines.

Labor and Delivery: PAXIPAM Tablets have no established use in labor or delivery.

Nursing Mothers: Halazepam and its major metabolites are excreted in the milk of lactating postpartum women. Since neonates metabolize benzodiazepines more slowly than adults, and since accumulation of the drug and its metabolites to toxic levels is possible in neonates, the drug should not be given to nursing mothers.
For example, chronic administration of the closely related benzodiazepine, diazepam, to nursing mothers has been reported to cause their infants to become lethargic and lose weight.

Pediatric Use: Safety and effectiveness in children below the age of 18 years have not been established.

Adverse Reactions: Central Nervous System: The most frequent adverse reactions to PAXIPAM Tablets were CNS disturbances. The most common of these were drowsiness, which occurred in approximately 29 per 100 patients. Other CNS disturbances occurred in approximately 9 per 100 patients (e.g., headache, apathy, psychomotor retardation, disorientation, confusion, euphoria, dysarthria, depression, syncope). Less frequent CNS disturbances were: dizziness, which occurred in approximately 8 per 100 patients; ataxia which occurred in 5 per 100 patients; fatigue, which occurred in approximately 4 per 100 patients; and visual disturbances and paradoxical reaction, which occurred in 1 per 100 patients. Sleep disturbances, changes in libido, and auditory disturbances occurred in fewer than 1 per 100 patients.

Gastrointestinal: Less frequent adverse reactions were: gastrointestinal disturbances (e.g., sense of seasickness, nausea, constipation, increased salivation, difficulty in swallowing, vomiting, gastric disorder) which occurred in approximately 9 per 100 patients; change in appetite, which occurred in approximately 1 per 100 patients; and dry mouth, which occurred in approximately 3 per 100 patients.

Hematologic: Clinically unimportant fluctuations in the white blood and differential counts were reported in less than 5% of 761 patients.

Hepatic: Small to moderate elevations of the following hepatic enzymes were reported; alkaline phosphatase in 20 (2.8%) of 705 patients; SGOT in 35 (5.4%) of 647 patients; SGPT in 3 (<1%) of 336 patients. No serious abnormalities were seen.

The following adverse reactions were reported to occur rarely in those patients treated with PAXIPAM Tablets.

Cardiovascular: Cardiovascular disturbances (e.g., tachycardia, bradycardia, hypotension) were reported to occur in approximately 2 per 100 patients.

Musculoskeletal: Muscular disturbances were reported to occur in approximately 2 per 100 patients.

Other: The following adverse reactions occurred in fewer than 1 per 100 patients: allergic manifestations, genitourinary disturbance, paresthesias, and respiratory disturbance.

Adverse Reactions not reported with the use of PAXIPAM Tablets, but reported with the use of other benzodiazepines are: jaundice, agranulocytosis, edema, slurred speech, minor menstrual irregularities, dystonia, pruritus, incontinence, urinary retention, and diplopia.

Drug Abuse and Dependence: Physical and Psychological Dependence: Withdrawal symptoms (similar in character to those noted with barbiturates and alcohol) have occurred following abrupt discontinuance of benzodiazepines. These can range from mild dysphoria and insomnia to a major syndrome which may include abdominal and muscle cramps, vomiting, sweating, tremor, and convulsions. These signs and symptoms, especially the more serious ones, are generally more common in those patients who have received excessive doses over an extended period of time. However, withdrawal symptoms have also been reported following abrupt discontinuance of benzodiazepines taken continuously, at therapeutic levels, for several months. Consequently, after extended therapy, abrupt discontinuation should generally be avoided and a gradual tapering in dosage followed.

Patients with a history of seizures or epilepsy, regardless of their concomitant anti-seizure drug therapy, should not be abruptly withdrawn from any CNS depressant agent, including PAXIPAM Tablets. Addiction-prone individuals (such as drug addicts or alcoholics) should be under careful surveillance when receiving halazepam or other psychotropic agents because of the predisposition of such patients to habituation and dependence.

Controlled Substance Class: PAXIPAM is a controlled substance under the Controlled Substance Act and has been assigned by the Drug Enforcement Administration to Schedule IV.

Overdosage: Manifestations of PAXIPAM Tablets overdosage include somnolence, confusion, impaired coordination, diminished reflexes, and coma.

No delayed reactions (e.g., organ toxicity) or clinical laboratory abnormalities have been reported.

General Treatment Of Overdose: Overdosage reports with halazepam are limited. Respiration, pulse, and blood pressure should be monitored, as in all cases of drug overdosage. General supportive measures should be employed, along with immediate gastric lavage. Intravenous fluids should be administered and an adequate airway maintained. Hypotension may be combated by the use of Levophed® (levarterenol) or Aramine® (metaraminol). Dialysis is of limited value. Animal experiments have suggested that forced diuresis or hemodialysis are probably of little value in treating overdosage. As with the management of intentional overdosing with any drug, it should be borne in mind that multiple agents may have been ingested.

Dosage and Administration: Dosage should be individualized for maximum beneficial effect. While the usual daily dosages given below will meet the needs of most patients, there will be some who require higher doses. In such cases, dosage should be increased cautiously to avoid adverse effects.

PAXIPAM Tablets are administered orally in divided doses and the dosage should be individualized according to the severity of symptoms and response of the patient. To facilitate dosing, the tablets are scored. The usual recommended dose is 20 to 40 mg three or four times a day.

The response of the patient to several days of treatment will permit the physician to adjust the dose upward or downward. The optimal dosage usually ranges from 80 to 160 mg daily. In debilitated patients or the elderly (70 years or older), the initial recommended dosage is 20 mg once or twice a day. The dose should be adjusted as needed and tolerated.

If side effects occur with the starting dose, the dose should be lowered.

How Supplied: PAXIPAM Tablets, 20 mg, orange, compressed, scored tablets impressed with the Schering trademark and product identification numbers, 251; bottles of 100 (NDC-0085-0251-04).

PAXIPAM Tablets, 40 mg, white, compressed, scored tablets impressed with the Schering trademark and product identification numbers, 538; bottles of 100 (NDC-0085-0538-04).

Store between 2° and 30°C (36° and 86°F).

Animal Pharmacology and/or Animal Toxicology: In animal studies, the antianxiety activity of halazepam was demonstrated by its ability to induce calming effects in normally aggressive species, such as the monkey, and to alleviate suppressed behavior in animals placed in a conflict situation. Halazepam was also shown to block aggressive behavior invoked by stressful stimuli.

Halazepam has relatively little effect on autonomic function and unlike major tranquilizers such as chlorpromazine or haloperidol, it does not cause extrapyramidal side effects. As with other CNS depressants, halazepam at relatively high doses produces transient cardiovascular depressant effects, but no EKG disturbances were seen in dogs.

A battery of tests were performed in monkeys to evaluate the abuse potential of PAXIPAM. Although PAXIPAM did cause physical dependence and positive drug-seeking behavior, these effects were judged to be weaker than those caused by diazepam or chlordiazepoxide in each case. However, the abuse potential of PAXIPAM in man in comparison with that of diazepam or chlordiazepoxide remains to be established.

Revised 9/81

Copyright © 1981, Schering Corporation. All rights reserved.

Shown in Product Identification Section, page 434

PERMITIL® ℞
[per′ mĭ-til]
brand of fluphenazine hydrochloride
Tablets, USP
Oral Concentrate

Description: PERMITIL products are formulations of fluphenazine hydrochloride, USP, a phenothiazine of the piperazine group. It is available as Tablets, 0.25, 2.5, 5, and 10 mg and as an Oral Concentrate, 5 mg fluphenazine hydrochloride per ml and alcohol 1%.

Actions: Fluphenazine hydrochloride has actions at all levels of the central nervous system, as well as on other organ systems. However, the site and mechanism of action of therapeutic effect are not known.

Indications: PERMITIL **Tablets** and **Oral Concentrate** are indicated for the management of manifestations of psychotic disorders.

PERMITIL has not been shown effective in the management of behavioral complications in patients with mental retardation.

Contraindications: PERMITIL is contraindicated in comatose or greatly obtunded patients and in patients receiving large doses of central nervous system depressants (barbiturates, alcohol, narcotics, analgesics, or antihistamines); in the presence of existing blood dyscrasias, bone marrow depression, or liver damage; and in patients who have shown hypersensitivity to PERMITIL products, their components, or related compounds.

PERMITIL is also contraindicated in patients with suspected or established subcortical brain damage, with or without hypothalamic damage, since a hyperthermic reaction with temperatures in excess of 104° F may occur in such patients, sometimes not until 14 to 16 hours after drug administration. Total body ice-packing is recommended for such a reaction; antipyretics may also be useful.

Warnings: If hypotension develops, epinephrine should not be administered since its action is blocked and partially reversed by fluphenazine hydrochloride. If a vasopressor is needed, norepinephrine may be used. Severe, acute hypotension has occurred with the use of phenothiazines and is particularly likely to occur in patients with mitral insufficiency or pheochromocytoma. Rebound hypertension may occur in pheochromocytoma patients.

PERMITIL can lower the convulsive threshold in susceptible individuals; it should be used with caution in alcohol withdrawal and in patients with convulsive disorders. If the patient is being treated with an anticonvulsant agent, increased dosage of that agent may be required when PERMITIL is used concomitantly.

PERMITIL should be used with caution in patients with psychic depression.

Fluphenazine hydrochloride may impair the mental and/or physical abilities required for the performance of hazardous tasks such as driving a car or operating machinery; therefore, the patient should be warned accordingly.

Usage in Children Safety and effectiveness in children have not been established; therefore, PERMITIL is not recommended for use in children.

Usage in Pregnancy Safe use of fluphenazine hydrochloride during pregnancy and lactation has not been established; therefore, in administering the drug to pregnant patients, nursing mothers, or women who may become pregnant, the possible benefits must be weighed against the possible hazards to mother and child.

Precautions: The possibility of suicide in depressed patients remains during treatment and until significant remission occurs. This type of patient should not have access to large quantities of this drug.

As with all phenothiazine compounds, fluphenazine hydrochloride should not be used indiscriminately. Caution should be observed in giving it to patients who have previously exhibited severe adverse reactions to other phenothiazines. Some of the untoward actions of fluphenazine hydrochloride tend to appear more frequently when high doses are used. However, as with other phenothiazine compounds, patients receiving PERMITIL in any dosage should be kept under close supervision. Neuroleptic drugs elevate prolactin levels; the elevation persists during chronic administration. Tissue culture experiments indicate that approximately one-third of human breast cancers are prolactin dependent *in vitro*, a factor of potential importance if the prescription of these drugs is contemplated in a patient with a previously detected breast cancer. Although disturbances such as galactorrhea, amenorrhea, gynecomastia, and impotence have been reported, the clinical significance of elevated serum prolactin levels is unknown for most patients. An increase in mammary neoplasms has been found in rodents after chronic administration of neuroleptic drugs. Neither clinical studies nor epidemiologic studies conducted to date, however, have shown an association between chronic administration of these drugs and mammary tumorigenesis; the available evidence is considered too limited to be conclusive at this time. The antiemetic effect of fluphenazine hydrochloride may obscure signs of toxicity due to overdosage of other drugs, or render more difficult the diagnosis of disorders such as brain tumors or intestinal obstruction.

Adynamic ileus occasionally occurs with phenothiazine therapy and, if severe, can result in complications and death. It is of particular concern in psychiatric patients, who may fail to seek treatment of the condition.

Continued on next page

Information on Schering products appearing on these pages is effective as of September 30, 1984.

Schering—Cont.

A significant, not otherwise explained, rise in body temperature may suggest individual intolerance to fluphenazine hydrochloride in which case it should be discontinued.

Patients on large doses of a phenothiazine drug who are undergoing surgery should be watched carefully for possible hypotensive phenomena. Moreover, reduced amounts of anesthetics or central nervous system depressants may be necessary. Since phenothiazines and central nervous system depressants (opiates, analgesics, antihistamines, barbiturates) can potentiate each other, less than the usual dosage of the added drug is recommended; caution is advised when they are administered concomitantly.

Use with caution in patients who are receiving atropine or related drugs because of additive anticholinergic effects and also in patients who will be exposed to extreme heat or phosphorus insecticides.

The use of alcohol should be avoided since additive effects and hypotension may occur. Patients should be cautioned that their response to alcohol may be increased while they are being treated with PERMITIL. The risk of suicide and the danger of overdose may be increased in patients who use alcohol excessively due to its potentiation of the drug's effect.

Blood counts and hepatic and renal functions should be checked periodically. The appearance of signs of blood dyscrasias requires the discontinuance of the drug and institution of appropriate therapy. If abnormalities in hepatic tests occur, phenothiazine treatment should be discontinued. Renal function in patients on long-term therapy should be monitored: if blood urea nitrogen (BUN) becomes abnormal, treatment with the drug should be discontinued.

The use of phenothiazine derivatives in patients with diminished renal function should be undertaken with caution.

Use with caution in patients suffering from respiratory impairment due to acute pulmonary infections, or in chronic respiratory disorders such as severe asthma or emphysema.

In general, phenothiazines, including fluphenazine hydrochloride, do not produce psychic dependence. Gastritis, nausea and vomiting, dizziness, and tremulousness have been reported following abrupt cessation of high-dose therapy. Reports suggest that these symptoms can be reduced by continuing concomitant antiparkinson agents for several weeks after the phenothiazine is withdrawn.

The possibility of liver damage, corneal and lenticular deposits, and irreversible dyskinesias should be kept in mind when patients are on long-term therapy.

Because photosensitivity has been reported, undue exposure to the sun should be avoided during phenothiazine treatment.

PERMITIL Tablets 0.25 mg contain FD&C Yellow No. 5 (tartrazine) which may cause allergic-type reactions (including bronchial asthma) in certain susceptible individuals. Although the overall incidence of FD&C Yellow No. 5 (tartrazine) sensitivity in the general population is low, it is frequently seen in patients who also have aspirin hypersensitivity.

Adverse Reactions: Not all of the following adverse reactions have been reported with this specific drug; however, pharmacological similarities among various phenothiazine derivatives require that each be considered. In the case of the piperazine group (of which fluphenazine hydrochloride is an example), the extrapyramidal symptoms are more common, and others (e.g., sedative effects, jaundice, and blood dyscrasias) are less frequently seen.

CNS Effects: *Extrapyramidal reactions:* opisthotonus, trismus, torticollis, retrocollis, aching and numbness of the limbs, motor restlessness, oculogyric crisis, hyperreflexia, dystonia, including protrusion, discoloration, aching and rounding of the tongue, tonic spasm of the masticatory muscles, tight feeling in the throat, slurred speech, dysphagia, akathisia, dyskinesia, parkinsonism, and ataxia. Their incidence and severity usually increase with an increase in dosage, but there is considerable individual variation in the tendency to develop such symptoms. Extrapyramidal symptoms can usually be controlled by the concomitant use of effective antiparkinsonian drugs, such as benztropine mesylate, and/or by reduction in dosage.

Persistent tardive dyskinesia: As with all antipsychotic agents, tardive dyskinesia may appear in some patients on long-term therapy or may appear after drug therapy has been discontinued. Although the risk appears to be greater in elderly patients on high-dose therapy, especially females, it may occur in either sex and in children. The symptoms are persistent and in some patients appear to be irreversible. The syndrome is characterized by rhythmical, involuntary movements of the tongue, face, mouth or jaw (e.g., protrusion of tongue, puffing of cheeks, puckering of mouth, chewing movements). Sometimes these may be accompanied by involuntary movements of the extremities. There is no known effective treatment for tardive dyskinesia; antiparkisonism agents usually do not alleviate the symptoms of this syndrome. It is suggested that all antipsychotic agents be discontinued if these symptoms appear. Should it be necessary to reinstitute treatment, or increase the dosage of the agent, or switch to a different antipsychotic agent the syndrome may be masked. It has been reported that fine, vermicular movements of the tongue may be an early sign of the syndrome, and if the medication is stopped at that time the syndrome may not develop.

Other CNS effects include cerebral edema; abnormality of cerebrospinal fluid proteins; convulsive seizures, particularly in patients with EEG abnormalities or a history of such disorders; and headaches.

Drowsiness may occur, particularly during the first or second week, after which it generally disappears. If troublesome, lower the dosage. Hypnotic effects appear to be minimal, especially in patients who are permitted to remain active.

Adverse behavioral effects include paradoxical exacerbation of psychotic symptoms, catatonic-like states, paranoid reactions, lethargy, paradoxical excitement, restlessness, hyperactivity, nocturnal confusion, bizarre dreams, and insomnia.

Hyperreflexia has been reported in the newborn when a phenothiazine was used during pregnancy.

Autonomic Effects: dry mouth or salivation, nausea, vomiting, diarrhea, anorexia, constipation, obstipation, fecal impaction, urinary retention, frequency or incontinence, bladder paralysis, polyuria, nasal congestion, pallor, adynamic ileus, myosis, mydriasis, blurred vision, glaucoma, perspiration, hypertension, hypotension, and change in pulse rate occasionally may occur. Significant autonomic effects have been infrequent in patients receiving less than 6 mg fluphenazine hydrochloride daily.

Allergic Effects: urticaria, erythema, eczema, exfoliative dermatitis, pruritus, photosensitivity, asthma, fever, anaphylactoid reactions, laryngeal edema, and angioneurotic edema; contact dermatitis in nursing personnel administering the drug; and in extremely rare instances, individual idiosyncrasy or hypersensitivity to phenothiazines has resulted in cerebral edema, circulatory collapse, and death.

Endocrine Effects: lactation, galactorrhea, moderate breast enlargement in females and gynecomastia in males on large doses, disturbances in the menstrual cycle, amenorrhea, changes in libido, inhibition of ejaculation, syndrome of inappropriate ADH (antidiuretic hormone) secretion, false positive pregnancy tests, hyperglycemia, hypoglycemia, glycosuria.

Cardiovascular Effects: postural hypotension, tachycardia (especially with sudden marked increase in dosage), bradycardia, cardiac arrest, faintness, and dizziness. Occasionally the hypotensive effect may produce a shock-like condition. ECG changes, nonspecific, (quinidine-like effect) usually reversible, have been observed in some patients receiving phenothiazine tranquilizers. Sudden death has occasionally been reported in patients who have received phenothiazines. In some cases the death was apparently due to cardiac arrest; in others, the cause appeared to be asphyxia due to failure of the cough reflex. In some patients, the cause could not be determined nor could it be established that the death was due to the phenothiazine.

Hematological Effects: agranulocytosis, eosinophilia, leukopenia, hemolytic anemia, thrombocytopenic purpura, and pancytopenia. Most cases of agranulocytosis have occurred between the fourth and tenth weeks of therapy. Patients should be watched closely especially during that period for the sudden appearance of sore throat or signs of infection. If white blood cell and differential cell counts show significant cellular depression, discontinue the drug and start appropriate therapy. However, a slightly lowered white count is not in itself an indiction to discontinue the drug.

Other Effects: Special considerations in long-term therapy include pigmentation of the skin, occurring chiefly in the exposed area; ocular changes consisting of deposition of fine particulate matter in the cornea and lens, progressing in more severe cases to star-shaped lenticular opacities; epithelial keratopathies; and pigmentary retinopathy. Also noted: peripheral edema, reversed epinephrine effect, increase in PBI not attributable to an increase in thyroxine, parotid swelling (rare), hyperpyrexia, systemic lupus erythematosus-like syndrome, increases in appetite and weight, polyphagia, photophobia, and muscle weakness.

Liver damage (biliary stasis) may occur. Jaundice may occur usually between the second and fourth weeks of treatment and is regarded as a hypersensitivity reaction. Incidence is low. The clinical picture resembles infectious hepatitis but with laboratory features of obstructive jaundice. It is usually reversible; however, chronic jaundice has been reported.

Dosage and Administration: In all cases the smallest effective dose should be used. Doses should be initiated at a low level and increased gradually to determine clinical response. Patients who are acutely ill may respond to lower doses than those who are chronically ill. Acutely ill patients may require a rapid increase of dosage. Elderly and debilitated patients and adolescents may respond to low dosages. Outpatients should receive smaller dosages than are given to hospitalized patients who are under close supervision.

Adults: The total daily dose ranges from 0.5 mg to 10 mg and is usually administered in divided doses. In general, a daily dose in excess of 3 mg is rarely necessary. A dose in excess of 20 mg should be used with caution.

Administration of an adequate dose should be continued for sufficiently long periods in order to obtain maximum benefits. After maximum therapeutic response is obtained, dosage may be decreased gradually to a maintenance level.

Geriatric patients: Reduced dosage is usually recommended.

PERMITIL **Oral Concentrate** is a palatable liquid preparation, suitable for administration with the following diluents: water, saline, Seven-Up, homogenized milk, carbonated orange beverage, and pineapple, apricot, prune, orange, V-8, tomato, and grapefruit juices.

PERMITIL **Oral Concentrate** should not be mixed with beverages containing caffeine (coffee, cola) tannics (tea), or pectinates (apple juice) since physical incompatability may result.

Overdosage: In the event of overdosage, emergency treatment should be started immediately. All patients suspected of having taken an overdose should be hospitalized as soon as possible.

Manifestations: Overdosage of fluphenazine hydrochloride primarily involves the extrapyramidal mechanism and produces the same side effects described under ADVERSE REACTIONS, but to a more marked degree. It is usually evidenced by stupor or coma; children may have convulsive seizures.

Treatment: Treatment is symptomatic and supportive. There is no specific antidote. The patient should be induced to vomit even if emesis has occurred spontaneously. Pharmacologic vomiting by the administration of ipecac syrup is a preferred method. It should be noted that ipecac has a central mode of action in addition to its local gastric irritant properties, and the central mode of action may be blocked by the antiemetic effect of PERMITIL products.

Vomiting should not be induced in patients with impaired consciousness. The action of ipecac is facilitated by physical activity and by the administration of 8 to 12 fluid ounces of water. If emesis does not occur within 15 minutes, the dose of ipecac should be repeated. Precautions against aspiration must be taken, especially in infants and children. Following emesis, any drug remaining in the stomach may be adsorbed by activated charcoal administered as a slurry with water. If vomiting is unsuccessful or contraindicated, gastric lavage should be performed. Isotonic and one-half isotonic saline are the lavage solutions of choice. Saline cathartics, such as milk of magnesia, draw water into the bowel by osmosis and therefore may be valuable for their action in rapid dilution of bowel content.

Standard measures (oxygen, intravenous fluids, corticosteroids) should be used to manage circulatory shock or metabolic acidosis. An open airway and adequate fluid intake should be maintained. Body temperature should be regulated. Hypothermia is expected, but severe hyperthermia may occur and must be treated vigorously. (See CONTRAINDICATIONS.)

An electrocardiogram should be taken and close monitoring of cardiac function instituted if there is any sign of abnormality. Cardiac arthythmias may be treated with neostigmine, pyridostigmine, or propranolol. Digitalis should be considered for cardiac failure. Close monitoring of cardiac function is advisable for not less than five days. Vasopressors such as norepinephrine may be used to treat hypotension, but epinephrine should NOT be used.

Anticonvulsants (an inhalation anesthetic, diazepam or paraldehyde) are recommended for control of convulsions, since fluphenazine hydrochloride increases the central nervous system depressant action, but not the anticonvulsant action, of barbiturates.

If acute parkinson-like symptoms result from fluphenazine hydrochloride intoxication, benztropine mesylate or diphenhydramine may be administered.

Central nervous system depression may be treated with non-convulsant doses of CNS stimulants. Avoid stimulants that may cause convulsions (e.g., picrotoxin and pentylenetetrazol).

Signs of arousal may not occur for 48 hours.

Dialysis is of no value because of low plasma concentrations of the drug.

Since overdosage is often deliberate, patients may attempt suicide by other means during the recovery phase. Deaths by deliberate or accidental overdosage have occurred with this class of drugs.

How Supplied: PERMITIL **Tablets,** 0.25 mg, sugar-coated, bright green tablets branded in black with the Schering trademark and product identification letters, WBK, or numbers, 122; bottle of 100.

PERMITIL **Tablets,** 2.5 mg, compressed, scored, light orange, oval tablets impressed with the Schering trademark and product identification letters, WDR, or numbers, 442; bottle of 100.

PERMITIL **Tablets,** 5 mg, compressed, scored, purple-pink, oval tablets impressed with the Schering trademark and product identification letters WFF, or numbers, 550; bottle of 100.

PERMITIL **Tablets,** 10 mg, compressed, scored, light red, oval tablets impressed with the Schering trademark and product identification letters, WFG, or numbers, 316; bottle of 1000.

PERMITIL **Oral Concentrate,** 5 mg per ml, a straw-colored, unflavored syrup containing alcohol 1%; bottle of 4 fluid ounces (118 ml), with dropper calibrated both in mg of fluphenazine hydrochloride and in ml of concentrate. **Protect from light and dispense only in amber bottles. Store PERMITIL Tablets and Oral Concentrate between 2° and 30°C (36° and 86°F).**

Copyright © 1964, 1983, Schering Corporation. All rights reserved. Revised 7/83

Shown in Product Identification Section; page 434

POLARAMINE®

[*po-lar'ah-mēn*]
brand of dexchlorpheniramine maleate
REPETABS® Tablets
Tablets, USP
Syrup, USP

Description: POLARAMINE products contain dexchlorpheniramine maleate, USP, an antihistamine having the formula, $C_{16}H_{19}ClN_2 \cdot C_4H_4O_4$, and a molecular weight of 390.87. Chemically, it is (+)-2-[*p*- Chloro - α - [2 - (dimethylamino)ethyl] benzyl] pyridine maleate (1:1).

POLARAMINE REPETABS (brand of repeat-action tablets) **Tablets** (4 mg and 6 mg) contain respectively 2 or 3 mg dexchlorpheniramine maleate, USP in an outer layer for prompt effect and 2 or 3 mg in an inner core for release three to six hours after ingestion.

POLARAMINE **Tablets** contain 2 mg dexchlorpheniramine maleate, USP.

POLARAMINE **Syrup** contains 2 mg dexchlorpheniramine maleate, USP per 5 ml, in a pleasant-tasting vehicle containing 6% alcohol.

Dexchlorpheniramine maleate is a white, odorless, crystalline powder which in aqueous solution has a pH of between 4 and 5. It is freely soluble in water, soluble in alcohol and in chloroform, but only slightly soluble in benzene or ether.

Clinical Pharmacology: POLARAMINE (dexchlorpheniramine maleate) is an antihistamine with anticholinergic properties. It is capable of producing a slight to moderate sedative effect. Antihistamines appear to compete with histamine for receptor sites on effector cells and are of value clinically in the prevention and relief of many allergic manifestations.

In vitro and *in vivo* assays of the antihistamine potencies of the optically active isomers of chlorpheniramine demonstrate that the predominant activity is in the dextro-isomer. The dextro-isomer is approximately two times more active than the racemic compound. Since dexchlorpheniramine is the dextro-isomer and active moiety of chlorpheniramine, it can be assumed that experience with chlorpheniramine also applies to dexchlorpheniramine.

Chlorpheniramine maleate 4 mg given to fasting human volunteers produced prompt blood levels after oral administration. Peak blood levels were approximately 7 ng/ml at an average time of 3 hours after administration. The half-life of chlorpheniramine maleate ranged from 20 to 24 hours. Following a single dose of tritium-labeled chlorpheniramine maleate to humans, the drug was found to be extensively metabolized whether given orally or by intravenous administration. The drug and metabolites were primarily excreted in the urine, with 19% of the dose appearing in 24 hours and a total of 34% in 48 hours.

Another study in volunteers has demonstrated that a **REPETABS Tablet** containing 12 mg chlorpheniramine maleate gives essentially identical plasma levels of drug as 12 mg of chlorpheniramine given in divided doses.

In a study in normal volunteers, a high flow rate of acidic urine resulted in a high excretion rate of chlorpheniramine maleate. Over a concentration range of 0.28 to 1.24 mcg/ml of plasma, chlorpheniramine maleate was 72 to 69% bound to plasma protein, respectively.

Indications and Usage: POLARAMINE is indicated for the treatment of perennial and seasonal allergic rhinitis; vasomotor rhinitis; allergic conjunctivitis; mild, uncomplicated allergic skin manifestations of urticaria and angioedema; amelioration of allergic reactions to blood or plasma; and dermographism. They are also indicated as therapy for anaphylactic reactions adjunctive to epinephrine and other standard measures after the acute manifestations have been controlled.

Contraindications: Hypersensitivity to dexchlorpheniramine maleate or other antihistamines of similar chemical structure contraindicates the use of POLARAMINE.

Drug products containing dexchlorpheniramine maleate should not be used in newborn or premature infants because of the possibility of severe reactions such as convulsions.

Antihistamines *should not* be used to treat lower respiratory tract symptoms. Antihistamines are also contraindicated for use in conjunction with monoamine oxidase inhibitor therapy.

Warnings: Dexchlorpheniramine, as with all antihistamines, should be used with caution in patients with narrow angle glaucoma, stenosing peptic ulcer, pyloroduodenal obstruction, symptomatic prostatic hypertrophy, and bladder neck obstruction.

Overdoses of antihistamines may cause hallucinations, convulsions, or death, especially in infants and children.

Products containing dexchlorpheniramine maleate have additive effects with alcohol and other CNS depressants (hypnotics, sedatives, tranquilizers, etc.). Patients should not engage in activities requiring mental alertness, such as driving a car or operating machinery.

Antihistamines are more likely to cause dizziness, sedation, and hypotension in elderly patients (approximately 60 years or older).

Precautions: *General:* Dexchlorpheniramine maleate has an atropine-like action and therefore products containing it should be used with caution in patients with: a history of bronchial asthma; increased intraocular pressure; hyperthyroidism; cardiovascular disease; hypertension.

Information for Patients:
1. Dexchlorpheniramine may cause slight to moderate drowsiness.
2. Patients should not engage in activities requiring mental alertness, such as driving or operating machinery.
3. Alcohol or other sedative drugs may enhance the drowsiness caused by antihistamines.
4. Patients should not take POLARAMINE in conjunction with a monoamine oxidase inhibitor or oral anticoagulant.

Drug Interactions: Dexchlorpheniramine maleate may cause severe hypotension when given in conjunction with a monoamine oxidase inhibitor.

Alcohol and other sedative drugs will potentiate the sedative effects of dexchlorpheniramine. (See WARNINGS.)

The action of oral anticoagulants may be inhibited by antihistamines.

Carcinogenesis, Mutagenesis, Impairment of Fertility: Although there have been no oncogenic or mutagenic studies on dexchlorpheniramine, a 103-week oncogenic study in rats on the racemic mixture, chlorpheniramine, did not produce an increase in the incidence of tumors in the drug-treated groups, as compared with the controls.

An Ames mutagenicity test performed on chlorpheniramine and its nitrosation product was negative. An early study in rats with chlorpheniramine maleate revealed a reduction in fertility in female rats at doses approximately 67 times the human dose. More recent studies in rabbits and rats, using more appropriate methodology and doses up to approximately 50 and 85 times the human dose, showed no reduction in fertility in the animals.

Pregnancy Category B: Reproduction studies have been performed in rabbits and rats at doses up to 50 times and 85 times the human dose, respectively, and have revealed no evidence of harm to the fetus due to chlorpheniramine maleate. (See above, "*Impairment of Fertility*.") There are, however, no adequate and well-controlled studies in pregnant women. Because animal reproduction

Continued on next page

Information on Schering products appearing on these pages is effective as of September 30, 1984.

Schering—Cont.

studies are not always predictive of human response, this drug should be used during the first two trimesters of pregnancy only if clearly needed. Dexchlorpheniramine maleate should not be used in the third trimester of pregnancy because newborn and premature infants may have severe reactions to antihistamines. (See CONTRAINDICATIONS.)

Nonteratogenic Effects: Studies of chlorpheniramine maleate done in rats revealed a decrease in the postnatal survival rate of pups of animals dosed with 33 and 67 times the human dose.

Nursing Mothers: It is not known whether this drug is excreted in human milk. Because certain other antihistamines are known to be excreted in human milk, and because dexchlorpheniramine maleate is contraindicated in newborn and premature infants, caution should be exercised when it is administered to a nursing woman.

Pediatric Use: Safety and effectiveness of the 4 and 6 mg **REPETABS Tablets** in children below the ages of 6 and 12 years, respectively, have not been established. Safety and effectiveness of the **Tablets** and **Syrup** in children below the age of 2 years have not been established.

Adverse Reactions: Slight to moderate drowsiness is the most frequent side effect of dexchlorpheniramine maleate. Other possible side effects of antihistamines include:
General: urticaria, drug rash, anaphylactic shock, photosensitivity, excessive perspiration, chills, dryness of mouth, nose, and throat.
Cardiovascular System: headache, palpitations, tachycardia, extrasystoles, hypotension.
Hematologic System: hemolytic anemia, hypoplastic anemia, thrombocytopenia, agranulocytosis.
Nervous System: sedation, dizziness, vertigo, tinnitus, acute labyrinthitis, disturbed coordination, fatigue, confusion, restlessness, excitation, nervousness, tremor, irritability, insomnia, euphoria, paresthesias, blurred vision, hysteria, neuritis, convulsions.
Gastrointestinal System: epigastric distress, anorexia, nausea, vomiting, diarrhea, constipation.
Genitourinary System: urinary frequency, difficult urination, urinary retention, early menses.
Respiratory System: thickening of bronchial secretions, tightness of chest, wheezing, nasal stuffiness.

Overdosage: In the event of overdosage, emergency treatment should be started immediately.
Manifestations of antihistamine overdosage may vary from central nervous system depression (sedation, apnea, diminished mental alertness, cardiovascular collapse) to stimulation (insomnia, hallucinations, tremors, or convulsions) to death. Other signs and symptoms may be dizziness, tinnitus, ataxia, blurred vision, and hypotension. Stimulation is particularly likely in children, as are atropine-like signs and symptoms (dry mouth; fixed, dilated pupils; flushing; hyperthermia; and gastrointestinal symptoms).
Treatment—The patient should be induced to vomit, even if emesis has occurred spontaneously. Pharmacologic vomiting by the administration of ipecac syrup is a preferred method. However, vomiting should not be induced in patients with impaired consciousness. The action of ipecac is facilitated by physical activity and by the administration of eight to twelve fluid ounces of water. If emesis does not occur within fifteen minutes, the dose of ipecac should be repeated. Precautions against aspiration must be taken, especially in infants and children. Following emesis, any drug remaining in the stomach may be adsorbed by activated charcoal administered as a slurry with water. If vomiting is unsuccessful or contraindicated, gastric lavage should be performed. Isotonic and one-half isotonic saline are the lavage solutions of choice. Saline cathartics, such as milk of magnesia, draw water into the bowel by osmosis and therefore may be valuable for their action in rapid dilution of bowel content. Dialysis is of little value in antihistamine poisoning. After emergency treatment, the patient should continue to be medically monitored.
Treatment of the signs and symptoms of overdosage is symptomatic and supportive. *Stimulants* (analeptic agents) should *not* be used. Vasopressors may be used to treat hypotension. Short-acting barbiturates, diazepam, or paraldehyde may be administered to control seizures. Hyperpyrexia, especially in children, may require treatment with tepid water sponge baths or a hypothermic blanket. Apnea is treated with ventilatory support.
In mice, the oral LD$_{50}$ of dexchlorpheniramine is 258 mg/kg. In humans, the estimated lethal dose of racemic chlorpheniramine is 5 to 10 mg/kg. Thus a dose of 2.5 to 5 mg/kg of dexchlorpheniramine should be similarly regarded.

Dosage and Administration: DOSAGE SHOULD BE INDIVIDUALIZED ACCORDING TO THE NEEDS AND RESPONSE OF THE PATIENT.
POLARAMINE **REPETABS Tablets**—*Adults and children 12 years or older:* one 4 or 6 mg **REPETABS** Tablet at bedtime or every 8 to 10 hours during the day.
Children 6 to 12 years: one 4 mg **REPETABS** Tablet daily, taken preferably at bedtime.
POLARAMINE **Tablets**—*Adults and children 12 years of age and over:* one tablet every 4 to 6 hours. *Children 6 through 11 years:* one-half tablet every 4 to 6 hours. *Children 2 through 5 years:* one-quarter tablet every 4 to 6 hours.
POLARAMINE **Syrup**—*Adults and children 12 years of age and over:* 1 teaspoonful (2 mg) every 4 to 6 hours. *Children 6 through 11 years:* one-half teaspoonful (1 mg) every 4 to 6 hours. *Children 2 through 5 years:* one-quarter teaspoonful (½ mg) every 4 to 6 hours.

How Supplied: POLARAMINE **REPETABS Tablets**, 4 mg, light red, sugar-coated, oval tablets branded in blue-black with the Schering trademark and product identification letters, AGA, or numbers, 095; bottle of 100.
POLARAMINE **REPETABS Tablets**, 6 mg, bright red, sugar-coated, oval tablets branded in white with the Schering trademark and product identification letters, AGB, or numbers, 148; bottles of 100 and 1000.
POLARAMANE **Tablets**, 2 mg, red, compressed, oval tablets impressed with the Schering trademark and either product identification letters, AGT, or numbers, 820; bottle of 100.
POLARAMINE **Syrup**, 2 mg per 5 ml, red-orange-colored, orange-like flavored liquid; 16-fluid ounce (473 ml) bottle.

Store POLARAMINE between 2° and 30°C (36° and 86°F).
Copyright © 1968, 1980, Schering Corporation. All rights reserved.
Shown in Product Identification Section; page 434

PROGLYCEM® ℞
[*pro-gli'sem*]
brand of diazoxide
  Capsules
  Suspension, USP
FOR ORAL ADMINISTRATION

Description: PROGLYCEM (diazoxide) is a nondiuretic benzothiadiazine derivative taken orally for the management of symptomatic hypoglycemia. PROGLYCEM **Capsules** contain 50 mg diazoxide, USP. The **Suspension** contains 50 mg of diazoxide, USP in each milliliter and has a chocolate-mint flavor; alcohol content is approximately 7.25%.
Diazoxide is 7-chloro-3-methyl-2H-1,2,4-benzothiadiazine 1,1-dioxide with the empirical formula $C_8H_7ClN_2O_2S$ and the molecular weight 230.7. It is a white powder practically insoluble to sparingly soluble in water.

Clinical Pharmacology: Diazoxide administered orally produces a prompt dose-related increase in blood glucose level, due primarily to an inhibition of insulin release from the pancreas, and also to an extrapancreatic effect. The hyperglycemic effect begins within an hour and generally lasts no more than eight hours in the presence of normal renal function.
PROGLYCEM decreases the excretion of sodium and water, resulting in fluid retention which may be clinically significant.
The hypotensive effect of diazoxide on blood pressure is usually not marked with the oral preparation. This contrasts with the intravenous preparation of diazoxide (see ADVERSE REACTIONS).
Other pharmacologic actions of PROGLYCEM include increased pulse rate; increased serum uric acid levels due to decreased excretion; increased serum levels of free fatty acids; decreased chloride excretion; decreased para-aminohippuric acid (PAH) clearance with no appreciable effect on glomerular filtration rate.
The concomitant administration of a benzothiazide diuretic may intensify the hyperglycemic and hyperuricemic effects of PROGLYCEM. In the presence of hypokalemia, hyperglycemic effects are also potentiated.
PROGLYCEM-induced hyperglycemia is reversed by the administration of insulin or tolbutamide. The inhibition of insulin release by PROGLYCEM is antagonized by alpha-adrenergic blocking agents.
PROGLYCEM is extensively bound (more than 90%) to serum proteins, and is excreted in the kidneys. The plasma half-life following I.V. administration is 28±8.3 hours. Limited data on oral-administration revealed a half-life of 24 and 36 hours in two adults. In four children aged four months to six years, the plasma half-life varied from 9.5 to 24 hours on long-term oral administration. The half-life may be prolonged following overdosage, and in patients with impaired renal function.

Indications and Usage: PROGLYCEM (oral diazoxide) is useful in the management of hypoglycemia due to hyperinsulinism associated with the following conditions:
  Adults: Inoperable islet cell adenoma or carcinoma, or extrapancreatic malignancy.
  Infants and Children: Leucine sensitivity, islet cell hyperplasia, nesidioblastosis, estrapancreatic malignancy, islet cell adenoma, or adenomatosis. PROGLYCEM may be used preoperatively as a temporary measure, and postoperatively, if hypoglycemia persists.
PROGLYCEM should be used only after a diagnosis of hypoglycemia due to one of the above conditions has been definitely established. When other specific medical therapy or surgical management either has been unsuccessful or is not feasible, treatment with PROGLYCEM should be considered.

Contraindications: The use of PROGLYCEM for functional hypoglycemia is contraindicated. The drug should not be used in patients hypersensitive to diazoxide or to other thiazides unless the potential benefits outweigh the possible risks.

Warnings: The antidiuretic property of diazoxide may lead to significant fluid retention, which in patients with compromised cardiac reserve, may precipitate congestive heart failure. The fluid retention will respond to conventional therapy with diuretics.
It should be noted that concomitantly administered thiazides may potentiate the hyperglycemic and hyperuricemic actions of diazoxide (See DRUG INTERACTIONS and ANIMAL PHARMACOLOGY AND/OR TOXICOLOGY).
Ketoacidosis and nonketotic hyperosmolar coma have been reported in patients treated with recommended doses of PROGLYCEM usually during intercurrent illness. Prompt recognition and treatment are essential (See OVERDOSAGE), and prolonged surveillance following the acute episode is necessary because of the long drug half-life of approximately 30 hours. The occurrence of these serious events may be reduced by careful education of patients regarding the need for monitoring the urine for sugar and ketones and for prompt reporting of abnormal findings and unusual symptoms to the physician.
Transient cataracts occurred in association with hyperosmolar coma in an infant, and subsided on correction of the hyperosmolarity. Cataracts have

been observed in several animals receiving daily doses of intravenous or oral diazoxide.

Precautions: General: treatment with PROGLYCEM should be initiated under close clinical supervision with careful monitoring of blood glucose and clinical response until the patient's condition has stabilized. This usually requires several days. If not effective in two to three weeks, the drug should be discontinued.

Prolonged treatment requires regular monitoring of the urine for sugar and ketones, especially under stress conditions, with prompt reporting of any abnormalities to the physician. Additionally, blood sugar levels should be monitored periodically by the physician to determine the need for dose adjustment.

The effects of diazoxide on the hematopoietic system and the level of serum uric acid should be kept in mind; the latter should be considered particularly in patients with hyperuricemia or a history of gout.

In some patients, higher blood levels have been observed with the oral suspension than with the capsule formulation of PROGLYCEM. Dosage should be adjusted as necessary in individual patients if changed from one formulation to the other.

Since the plasma half-life of diazoxide is prolonged in patients with impaired renal function, a reduced dosage should be considered. Serum electrolyte levels should also be evaluated for such patients.

The antihypertensive effect of other drugs may be enhanced by PROGLYCEM, and this should be kept in mind when administering it concomitantly with antihypertensive agents.

Because of the protein binding, administration of PROGLYCEM with coumarin or its derivatives may require reduction in the dosage of the anticoagulant, although there has been no reported evidence of excessive anticoagulant effect. In addition, PROGLYCEM may possibly displace bilirubin from albumin; this should be kept in mind particularly when treating newborns with increased bilirubinemia.

Information for Patients: During treatment with PROGLYCEM the patient should be advised to consult regularly with the physician and to cooperate in the periodic monitoring of his condition by laboratory tests.

In addition, the patient should be advised:
—to take the drug on a regular schedule as prescribed, not to skip doses, not to take extra doses;
—not to use this drug with other medications unless this is done with the physician's advice;
—not to allow anyone else to take this medication;
—to follow dietary instructions;
—to report promptly any adverse effects (i.e., increased urinary frequency, increased thirst, fruity breath odor);
—to report pregnancy or to discuss plans for pregnancy.

Laboratory tests: The following procedures may be especially important in patient monitoring (not necessarily inclusive): blood glucose determinations (recommended at periodic intervals in patients taking diazoxide orally for treatment of hypoglycemia, until stabilized); blood urea nitrogen (BUN) determinations and creatinine clearance determinations; hematocrit determinations; platelet count determinations; total and differential leukocyte counts; serum aspartate aminotransferase (AST) level determinations; serum uric acid level determinations; and urine testing for glucose and ketones (in patients being treated with diazoxide for hypoglycemia, semi-quantitative estimation of sugar and ketones in serum performed by the patient and reported to the physician provides frequent and relatively inexpensive monitoring of the condition).

Drug Interactions: Since diazoxide is highly bound to serum proteins, it may displace other substances which are also bound to protein, such as bilirubin or coumarin and its derivatives, resulting in higher blood levels of these substances. Concomitant administration of oral diazoxide and diphenylhydantoin may result in a loss of seizure control. These potential interactions must be considered when administering PROGLYCEM Capsules or Suspension.

The concomitant administration of thiazides or other commonly used diuretics may potentiate the hyperglycemic and hyperuricemic effects of diazoxide.

Drug/Laboratory Test Interactions: The hyperglycemic and hyperuricemic effects of diazoxide preclude proper assessment of these metabolic states. Increased renin secretion, IgG concentrations and decreased cortisol secretion have also been noted. Diazoxide inhibits glucagon-stimulated insulin release and causes a false-negative insulin response to glucagon.

Carcinogenesis, mutagenesis, impairment of fertility: No long-term animal dosing study has been done to evaluate the carcinogenic potential of diazoxide. No laboratory study of mutagenic potential or animal study of effects on fertility has been done.

Pregnancy Category C: Reproduction studies using the oral preparation in rats have revealed increased fetal resorptions and delayed parturition, as well as fetal skeletal anomalies; evidence of skeletal and cardiac teratogenic effects in rabbits has been noted with intravenous administration. The drug has also been demonstrated to cross the placental barrier in animals and to cause degeneration of the fetal pancreatic beta cells (See ANIMAL PHARMACOLOGY AND/OR TOXICOLOGY). Since there are no adequate data on fetal effects of this drug when given to pregnant women, safety in pregnancy has not been established. When the use of PROGLYCEM is considered, the indications should be limited to those specified above for adults (See INDICATIONS AND USAGE), and the potential benefits to the mother must be weighed against possible harmful effects to the fetus.

Non-Teratogenic effects: Diazoxide crosses the placental barrier and appears in cord blood. When given to the mother prior to delivery of the infant, the drug may produce fetal or neonatal hyperbilirubinemia, thrombocytopenia, altered carbohydrate metabolism, and possibly other side effects that have occurred in adults.

Alopecia and hypertrichosis lanuginosa have occurred in infants whose mothers received oral diazoxide during the last 19 to 60 days of pregnancy.

Labor and delivery: Since *intravenous* administration of the drug during labor may cause cessation of uterine contractions, and administration of oxytocic agents may be required to reinstate labor, caution is advised in administering PROGLYCEM at that time.

Nursing mothers: Information is not available concerning the passage of diazoxide in breast milk. Because many drugs are excreted in human milk and because of the potential for adverse reactions from diazoxide in nursing infants, a decision should be made whether to discontinue nursing or to discontinue the drug, taking into account the importance of the drug to the mother.

Pediatric use: (See INDICATIONS AND USAGE).

Adverse Reactions *Frequent and Serious:* Sodium and fluid retention is most common in young infants and in adults and may precipitate congestive heart failure in patients with compromised cardiac reserve. It usually responds to diuretic therapy (See DRUG INTERACTIONS).

Infrequent but Serious: Diabetic ketoacidosis and hyperosmolar nonketotic coma may develop very rapidly. Conventional therapy with insulin and restoration of fluid and electrolyte balance is usually effective if instituted promptly. Prolonged surveillance is essential in view of the long half-life of PROGLYCEM (See OVERDOSAGE).

Other frequent adverse reactions: Hirsutism of the lanugo type, mainly on the forehead, back and limbs, occurs most commonly in children and women and may be cosmetically unacceptable. It subsides on discontinuation of the drug.

Hyperglycemia or glycosuria may require reduction in dosage in order to avoid progression to ketoacidosis or hyperosmolar coma.

Gastrointestinal intolerance may include anorexia, nausea, vomiting, abdominal pain, ileus, diarrhea, transient loss of taste. Tachycardia, palpitations, increased levels of serum uric acid are common.

Thrombocytopenia with or without purpura may require discontinuation of the drug. Neutropenia is transient, is not associated with increased susceptibility to infection, and ordinarily does not require discontinuation of the drug. Skin rash, headache, weakness, and malaise may also occur. Other adverse reactions which have been observed are:

Cardiovascular: hypotension occurs occasionally, which may be augmented by thiazide diuretics given concurrently. A few cases of transient hypertension, for which no explanation is apparent, have been noted. Chest pain has been reported rarely.

Hematologic: eosinophilia; decreased hemoglobin/hematocrit; excessive bleeding; decreased IgG.

Hepato-renal: increased AST, alkaline phosphatase; azotemia, decreased creatinine clearance, reversible nephrotic syndrome, decreased urinary output, hematuria, albuminuria. *Neurologic:* anxiety, dizziness, insomnia, polyneuritis, paresthesia, pruritus, extrapyramidal signs. *Ophthalmologic:* transient cataracts, subconjunctival hemorrhage, ring scotoma, blurred vision, diplopia, lacrimation. *Skeletal, integumentary:* monilial dermatitis, herpes, advance in bone age; loss of scalp hair. *Systemic:* fever, lymphadenopathy. *Other:* gout, acute pancreatitis/pancreatic necrosis, galactorrhea, enlargement of lump in breast.

Overdosage: An overdosage of PROGLYCEM causes marked hyperglycemia which may be associated with ketoacidosis. It will respond to prompt insulin administration and restoration of fluid and electrolyte balance. Because of the drug's long half-life (approximately 30 hours), the symptoms of overdosage require prolonged surveillance for periods up to seven days, until the blood sugar level stabilizes within the normal range. One investigator reported successful lowering of diazoxide blood levels by peritoneal dialysis in one patient and by hemodialysis in another.

Dosage and Administration: Patients should be under close clinical observation when treatment with PROGLYCEM is initiated. The clinical response and blood glucose level should be carefully monitored until the patient's condition has stabilized satisfactorily; in most instances, this may be accomplished in several days. If administration of PROGLYCEM is not effective after two or three weeks, the drug should be discontinued. The dosage of PROGLYCEM must be individualized based on the severity of the hypoglycemic condition and the blood glucose level and clinical response of the patient. The dosage should be adjusted until the desired clinical and laboratory effects are produced with the least amount of the drug. Special care should be taken to assure accuracy of dosage in infants and young children.

Adults and children: The usual daily dosage is 3 to 8 mg/kg, divided into two or three equal doses every 8 or 12 hours. In certain instances, patients with refractory hypoglycemia may require higher dosages. Ordinarily, an appropriate starting dosage is 3 mg/kg/day, divided into three equal doses every eight hours. Thus, an average adult would receive a starting dosage of approximately 200 mg daily.

Infants and newborns: The usual daily dosage is 8 to 15 mg/kg, divided into two or three equal doses every 8 to 12 hours. An appropriate starting dosage is 10 mg/kg/day, divided into three equal doses every eight hours.

How Supplied: PROGLYCEM Capsules, 50 mg, half opaque orange and half clear capsules, branded in black with the Schering trademark and

Continued on next page

Information on Schering products appearing on these pages is effective as of September 30, 1984.

Schering—Cont.

either product identification letters, PBA or numbers; 205; bottle of 100 (NDC 0085-0205-05).

PROGLYCEM Suspension, 50 mg/ml, a chocolate-mint flavored suspension; bottle of 30 ml (NDC 0085-0426-04), with dropper calibrated to deliver 10, 20, 30, 40, and 50 mg diazoxide. **Shake well before each use. Protect from light. Store in carton until contents are used. Store PROGLYCEM Capsules and Suspension between 2° and 30°C (36° and 86°F).**

Animal Pharmacology and/or Toxicology: Oral diazoxide in the mouse, rat, rabbit, dog, pig, and monkey produces a rapid and transient rise in blood glucose levels. In dogs, increased blood glucose is accompanied by increased free fatty acids, lactate, and pyruvate in the serum. In mice, a marked decrease in liver glycogen and an increase in the blood urea nitrogen level occur.

In acute toxicity studies the LD_{50} for oral diazoxide suspension is >5000 mg/kg in the rat, >522 mg/kg in the neonatal rat, between 1900 and 2572 mg/kg in the mouse, and 219 mg/kg in the guinea pig. Although the oral LD_{50} was not determined in the dog, a dosage of up to 500 mg/kg was well tolerated.

In subacute oral toxicity studies, diazoxide at 400 mg/kg in the rat produced growth retardation, edema, increases in liver and kidney weights, and adrenal hypertrophy. Daily dosages up to 1080 mg/kg for three months produced hyperglycemia, an increase in liver weight and an increase in mortality. In dogs given oral diazoxide at approximately 40 mg/kg/day for one month, no biologically significant gross or microscopic abnormalities were observed. Cataracts, attributed to markedly disturbed carbohydrate metabolism, have been observed in a few dogs given repeated daily doses of oral or intravenous diazoxide. The lenticular changes resembled those which occur experimentally in animals with increased blood glucose levels. In chronic toxicity studies, rats given a daily dose of 200 mg/kg diazoxide for 52 weeks had a decrease in weight gain and an increase in heart, liver, adrenal and thyroid weights. Mortality in drug-treated and control groups was not different. Dogs treated with diazoxide at dosages of 50, 100 and 200 mg/kg/day for 82 weeks had higher blood glucose levels than controls. Mild bone marrow stimulation and increased pancreas weights were evident in the drug-treated dogs; several developed inguinal hernias, one had a testicular seminoma, and another had a mass near the penis. Two females had inguinal mammary swellings. The etiology of these changes was not established. There was no difference in mortality between drug-treated and control groups. In a second chronic oral toxicity study, dogs given milled diazoxide at 50, 100, and 200 mg/kg/day had anorexia and severe weight loss, causing death in a few. Hematologic biochemical, and histologic examinations did not indicate any cause of death other than inanition. After one year of treatment, there is no evidence of herniation or tissue swelling in any of the dogs.

When diazoxide was administered at high dosages concomitantly with either chlorothiazide to rats or trichlormethiazide to dogs, increased toxicity was observed. In rats, the combination was nephrotoxic; epithelial hyperplasia was observed in the collecting tubules. In dogs, a diabetic syndrome was produced which resulted in ketosis and death. Neither of the drugs given alone produced these effects.

Although the data are inconclusive, reproduction and teratology studies in several species of animals indicate that diazoxide, when administered during the critical period of embryo formation, may interfere with normal fetal development, possibly through altered glucose metabolism. Parturition was occasionally prolonged in animals treated at term. Intravenous administration of diazoxide to pregnant sheep, goats, and swine produced in the fetus an appreciable increase in blood glucose level and degeneration of the beta cells of the Islets of Langerhans. The reversibility of these effects was not studied.

Copyright © 1972, 1983, Schering Corporation. All rights reserved.
Revised 6/83

PROVENTIL® Inhaler ℞
[pro-ven'til]
brand of albuterol
Bronchodilator Aerosol
FOR ORAL INHALATION ONLY

Description: The active component of PROVENTIL Inhaler is albuterol (α^1-[(tert-butylamino)methyl]-4-hydroxy-m-xylene-α,α'-diol), a relatively selective beta$_2$-adrenergic bronchodilator. Albuterol is the official generic name in the United States. The international generic name for the drug is salbutamol. The molecular weight of albuterol is 239.3.

PROVENTIL Inhaler is a metered-dose aerosol unit for oral inhalation. It contains a microcrystalline suspension of albuterol in propellants (trichloromonofluoromethane and dichlorodifluoromethane) with oleic acid. Each actuation delivers from the mouthpiece 90 mcg of albuterol. Each canister provides at least 200 inhalations.

Clinical Pharmacology: The prime action of beta-adrenergic drugs is to stimulate adenyl cyclase, the enzyme which catalyzes the formation of cyclic-3',5'-adenosine monophosphate (cyclic AMP) from adenosine triphosphate (ATP). The cyclic AMP thus formed mediates the cellular responses. By virtue of its relatively selective action on beta$_2$-adrenoceptors, albuterol relaxes smooth muscle of the bronchi, uterus, and vascular supply to skeletal muscle, but may have less cardiac stimulant effects than does isoproterenol.

Albuterol is longer acting than isoproterenol by any route of administration in most patients because it is not a substrate for the cellular uptake processes for catecholamines nor for catechol-O-methyl transferase.

Because of its gradual absorption from the bronchi, systemic levels of albuterol are low after inhalation of recommended doses. Studies undertaken with four subjects administered tritiated albuterol, resulted in maximum plasma concentrations occurring within two to four hours. Due to the sensitivity of the assay method, the metabolic rate and half-life of elimination of albuterol in plasma could not be determined. However, urinary excretion provided data indicating that albuterol has an elimination half-life of 3.8 hours. Approximately 72 percent of the inhaled dose is excreted within 24 hours in the urine, and consists of 28 percent of unchanged drug and 44 percent as metabolite.

Results of animal studies show that albuterol does not pass the blood-brain barrier.

The effects of rising doses of albuterol and isoproterenol aerosols were studied in volunteers and asthmatic patients. Results in normal volunteers indicated that albuterol is $\frac{1}{2}$ to $\frac{1}{4}$ as active as isoproterenol in producing increases in heart rate. In asthmatic patients similar cardiovascular differentiation between the two drugs was also seen.

Indications and Usage: PROVENTIL Inhaler is indicated for the relief of bronchospasm in patients with reversible obstructive airway disease.

In controlled clinical trials the onset of improvement in pulmonary function was within 15 minutes, as determined by both maximal midexpiratory flow rate (MMEF) and FEV_1. MMEF measurements also showed that near maximum improvement in pulmonary function generally occurs within 60 to 90 minutes following 2 inhalations of albuterol and that clinically significant improvement generally continues for 3 to 4 hours in most patients. In clinical trials, some patients with asthma showed a therapeutic response (defined by maintaining FEV_1 values 15 percent or more above base line) which was still apparent at 6 hours. Continued effectiveness of albuterol was demonstrated over a 13-week period in these same trials.

Contraindications: PROVENTIL Inhaler is contraindicated in patients with a history of hypersensitivity to any of its components.

Warnings: As with other adrenergic aerosols, the potential for paradoxical bronchospasm should be kept in mind. If it occurs, the preparation should be discontinued immediately and alternative therapy instituted.

Fatalities have been reported in association with excessive use of inhaled sympathomimetic drugs. The exact cause of death is unknown, but cardiac arrest following the unexpected development of a severe acute asthmatic crisis and subsequent hypoxia is suspected.

The contents of PROVENTIL Inhaler are under pressure. Do not puncture. Do not use or store near heat or open flame. Exposure to temperatures above 120°F may cause bursting. Never throw container into fire or incinerator. Keep out of reach of children.

Precautions: Although it has less effect on the cardiovascular system than isoproterenol at recommended dosages, albuterol is a sympathomimetic amine and as such should be used with caution in patients with cardiovascular disorders, including coronary insufficiency and hypertension, in patients with hyperthyroidism or diabetes mellitus, and in patients who are unusually responsive to sympathomimetic amines.

Large doses of intravenous albuterol have been reported to aggravate preexisting diabetes and ketoacidosis. The relevance of this observation to the use of PROVENTIL Inhaler is unknown, since the aerosol dose is much lower than the doses given intravenously.

Although there have been no reports concerning the use of PROVENTIL Inhaler during labor and delivery, it has been reported that high doses of albuterol administered intravenously inhibit uterine contractions. Although this effect is extremely unlikely as a consequence of aerosol use, it should be kept in mind.

Information For Patients: The action of PROVENTIL Inhaler may last up to six hours and therefore it should not be used more frequently than recommended. Do not increase the number or frequency of doses without medical consultation. If symptoms get worse, medical consultation should be sought promptly. While taking PROVENTIL Inhaler, other inhaled medicines should not be used unless prescribed.

See illustrated Patient Instructions For Use.

Drug Interactions: Other sympathomimetic aerosol bronchodilators or epinephrine should not be used concomitantly with albuterol.

Albuterol should be administered with caution to patients being treated with monoamine oxidase inhibitors or tricyclic antidepressants, since the action of albuterol on the vascular system may be potentiated.

Beta-receptor blocking agents and albuterol inhibit the effect of each other.

Carcinogenesis, Mutagenesis, and Impairment of Fertility: In a 2 year study in the rat, albuterol sulfate caused a significant dose-related increase in the incidence of benign leiomyomas of the mesovarium at doses corresponding to 111, 555, and 2,800 times the maximum human inhalational dose. The relevance of these findings to humans is not known. An 18-month study in mice revealed no evidence of tumorigenicity. Studies with albuterol revealed no evidence of mutagenesis. Reproduction studies in rats revealed no evidence of impaired fertility.

Teratogenic Effects — Pregnancy Category C: Albuterol has been shown to be teratogenic in mice when given in doses corresponding to 14 times the human dose. There are no adequate and well-controlled studies in pregnant women. Albuterol should be used during pregnancy only if the potential benefit justifies the potential risk to the fetus. A reproduction study in CD-1 mice with albuterol (0.025, 0.25, and 2.5 mg/kg, corresponding to 1.4, 14, and 140 times the maximum human inhalational dose) showed cleft palate formation in 5 of 111 (4.5 percent) fetuses at 0.25 mg/kg and in 10 of 108 (9.3 percent) fetuses at 2.5 mg/kg. None were observed at 0.025 mg/kg. Cleft palate also occurred in 22 of 72 (30.5 percent) fetuses treated with 2.5 mg/kg isoproterenol (positive control). A reproduction study in Stride Dutch rabbits revealed cranioschisis in 7 of 19 (37 percent) fetuses at 50 mg/kg, corresponding to 2,800 times the maximum human inhalational dose.

Nursing Mothers: It is not known whether this drug is excreted in human milk. Because of the potential for tumorigenicity shown for albuterol in animal studies, a decision should be made whether to discontinue nursing or to discontinue the drug, taking into account the importance of the drug to the mother.

Pediatric Use: Safety and effectiveness in children below the age of 12 years have not been established.

Adverse Reactions: The adverse reactions of albuterol are similar in nature to those of other sympathomimetic agents, although the incidence of certain cardiovascular effects is less with albuterol. A 13-week double-blind study compared albuterol and isoproterenol aerosols in 147 asthmatic patients. The results of this study showed that the incidence of cardiovascular effects was: palpitations, less than 10 per 100 with albuterol and less than 15 per 100 with isoproterenol; tachycardia, 10 per 100 with both albuterol and isoproterenol; and increased blood pressure, less than 5 per 100 with both albuterol and isoproterenol. In the same study, both drugs caused tremor or nausea in less than 15 patients per 100; dizziness or heartburn in less than 5 per 100 patients. Nervousness occurred in less than 10 per 100 patients receiving albuterol and in less than 15 per 100 patients receiving isoproterenol.

In addition, albuterol, like other sympathomimetic agents, can cause adverse reactions such as hypertension, angina, vomiting, vertigo, central stimulation, insomnia, headache, unusual taste, and drying or irritation of the oropharynx.

Overdosage: Exaggeration of the effects listed in ADVERSE REACTIONS can occur. Anginal pain and hypertension may result.

The oral LD_{50} in male and female rats and mice was greater than 2,000 mg/kg. The aerosol LD_{50} could not be determined.

Dialysis is not appropriate treatment for overdosage of PROVENTIL Inhaler. The judicious use of a cardioselective beta-receptor blocker, such as metoprolol tartrate, is suggested, bearing in mind the danger of inducing an asthmatic attack.

Dosage and Administration: The usual dosage for adults and children 12 years and older is 2 inhalations repeated every 4 to 6 hours; in some patients, 1 inhalation every 4 hours may be sufficient. More frequent administration or a larger number of inhalations is not recommended. The use of PROVENTIL Inhaler can be continued as medically indicated to control recurring bouts of bronchospasm. During this time most patients gain optimal benefit from regular use of the inhaler. Safe usage for periods extending over several years has been documented.

If a previously effective dosage regimen fails to provide the usual relief, medical advice should be sought immediately as this is often a sign of seriously worsening asthma which would require reassessment of therapy.

How Supplied: PROVENTIL Inhaler, 17.0 g canister; box of one. Each actuation delivers 90 mcg of albuterol from the mouthpiece. It is supplied with an oral adapter and patient's instructions (NDC-0085-0614-02). PROVENTIL Inhaler REFILL canister, 17.0g, with patient's instructions; box of one (NDC-0085-0614-03).

Store between 15° and 30°C (59° and 86°F). Shake well before using.

Copyright© 1981, 1982, Schering Corporation. All rights reserved.
Revised 11/82

Shown in Product Identification Section, page 435

PROVENTIL® ℞
[*pro-ven'til*]
brand of albuterol sulfate
Tablets

Description: PROVENTIL Tablets contain albuterol sulfate, a relatively selective beta$_2$-adrenergic bronchodilator. Albuterol sulfate has the chemical name α^1-[(*tert*-Butylamino) methyl]-4-hydroxy-*m*-xylene-α,α'-diol sulfate (2:1) (salt). Albuterol sulfate has a molecular weight of 576.7 and the empirical formula $(C_{13}H_{21}NO_3)_2 \cdot H_2SO_4$. Albuterol sulfate is a white crystalline powder, soluble in water and slightly soluble in ethanol. The international generic name for albuterol base is salbutamol.

Each PROVENTIL Tablet contains 2 or 4 mg of albuterol as 2.4 and 4.8 mg of albuterol sulfate, respectively.

Clinical Pharmacology: The prime action of beta-adrenergic drugs is to stimulate adenyl cyclase, the enzyme which catalyzes the formation of cyclic-3',5'-adenosine monophosphate (cyclic AMP) from adenosine triphosphate (ATP). The cyclic AMP thus formed mediates the cellular responses. Based on pharmacologic studies in animals, albuterol appears to exert direct and preferential action on beta$_2$-adrenoceptors including those of the bronchial tree and uterus, and may have less cardiac stimulant effect than isoproterenol, when given in the usual recommended dose.

Albuterol is longer acting than isoproterenol in most patients by any route of administration because it is not a substrate for the cellular uptake processes for catecholamines nor for catechol-*O*-methyl transferase.

In three normal volunteers given tablets containing 6 mg tritiated albuterol sulfate, the maximum plasma concentrations of albuterol occurred within 2.5 hours. In other studies, the analysis of peak plasma samples indicated that the metabolite of albuterol represented 80% of the radioactivity present. Albuterol was shown to have a plasma half-life ranging from 2.7 to 5.0 hours when administered orally. Analysis of urine samples showed that 76% of the dose was excreted over 3 days, with the majority of the dose being excreted within the first 24 hours. Sixty percent of this radioactivity was shown to be the metabolite. Feces collected over this period contained 4% of the administered dose.

Animal studies show that albuterol does not pass the blood-brain barrier.

Indications and Usage: PROVENTIL Tablets are indicated for the relief of bronchospasm in patients with reversible obstructive airway disease.

In controlled clinical trials in patients with asthma, the onset of improvement in pulmonary function, as measured by maximal midexpiratory flow rate, MMEF, was noted within 30 minutes after a dose of PROVENTIL Tablets with peak improvement occurring between 2 to 3 hours. In controlled clinical trials in which measurements were conducted for 6 hours, significant clinical improvement in pulmonary function (defined as maintaining a 15% or more increase in FEV_1 and a 20% or more increase in MMEF over baseline values) was observed in 60% of patients at 4 hours and in 40% at 6 hours. No decrease in the effectiveness of PROVENTIL Tablets has been reported in patients who received long-term treatment with the drug in uncontrolled studies for periods up to 6 months.

Contraindications: PROVENTIL Tablets are contraindicated in patients with a history of hypersensitivity to any of its components.

Precautions: General: Although albuterol usually has minimal effects on the beta$_1$-adrenoceptors of the cardiovascular system at the recommended dosage, occasionally the usual cardiovascular and CNS stimulatory effects common to all sympathomimetic agents have been seen with patients treated with albuterol necessitating discontinuation. Therefore, albuterol should be used with caution in patients with cardiovascular disorders, including coronary insufficiency and hypertension, in patients with hyperthyroidism or diabetes mellitus, and in patients who are unusually responsive to sympathomimetic amines.

Large doses of intravenous albuterol have been reported to aggravate preexisting diabetes mellitus and ketoacidosis. Additionally, albuterol and other beta agonists, when given intravenously, may cause a decrease in serum potassium, possibly through intracellular shunting. The decrease is usually transient, not requiring supplementation. The relevance of these observations to the use of PROVENTIL Tablets is unknown.

Information for Patients: The action of PROVENTIL Tablets may last for six hours or longer and therefore it should not be taken more frequently than recommended. Do not increase the dose or frequency of medication without medical consultation. If symptoms get worse, medical consultation should be sought promptly.

Drug Interactions: The concomitant use of PROVENTIL Tablets and other oral sympathomimetic agents is not recommended since such combined use may lead to deleterious cardiovascular effects. This recommendation does not preclude the judicious use of an aerosol bronchodilator of the adrenergic stimulant type in patients receiving PROVENTIL Tablets. Such concomitant use, however, should be individualized and not given on a routine basis. If regular coadministration is required, then alternative therapy should be considered.

Albuterol should be administered with extreme caution to patients being treated with monoamine oxidase inhibitors or tricyclic antidepressants, since the action of albuterol on the vascular system may be potentiated.

Beta-receptor blocking agents and albuterol inhibit the effect of each other.

Carcinogenesis, Mutagenesis, and Impairment of Fertility: Albuterol sulfate, like other agents in its class, caused a significant dose-related increase in the incidence of benign leiomyomas of the mesovarium in a 2-year study in the rat, at doses corresponding to 3, 16, and 78 times the maximum human oral dose. In another study this effect was blocked by the coadministration of propranolol. The relevance of these findings to humans is not known. An 18-month study in mice and a lifetime study in hamsters revealed no evidence of tumorigenicity. Studies with albuterol revealed no evidence of mutagenesis. Reproduction studies in rats revealed no evidence of impaired fertility.

Teratogenic Effects—Pregnancy Category C: Albuterol has been shown to be teratogenic in mice when given subcutaneously in doses corresponding to 0.4 times the maximum human oral dose. There are no adequate and well-controlled studies in pregnant women. Albuterol should be used during pregnancy only if the potential benefit justifies the potential risk to the fetus. A reproduction study in CD-1 mice with albuterol showed cleft palate formation in 5 of 111 (4.5%) fetuses at 0.25 mg/kg and in 10 of 108 (9.3%) fetuses at 2.5 mg/kg, none were observed at 0.025 mg/kg. Cleft palate also occurred in 22 of 72 (30.5%) fetuses treated with 2.5 mg/kg isoproterenol (positive control). A reproduction study in Stride Dutch rabbits revealed cranioschisis in 7 of 19 (37%) fetuses at 50 mg/kg, corresponding to 78 times the maximum human oral dose of albuterol.

Labor and Delivery: Oral albuterol has been shown to delay preterm labor in some reports. There are presently no well controlled studies which demonstrate that it will stop preterm labor or prevent labor at term. Therefore, cautious use of PROVENTIL Tablets is required in pregnant patients when given for relief of bronchospasm so as to avoid interference with uterine contractibility.

Nursing Mothers: It is not known whether this drug is excreted in human milk. Because of the potential for tumorigenicity shown for albuterol in animal studies, a decision should be made whether

Continued on next page

Information on Schering products appearing on these pages is effective as of September 30, 1984.

Schering—Cont.

to discontinue nursing or to discontinue the drug, taking into account the importance of the drug to the mother.

Pediatric Use: Safety and effectiveness in children below the age of 12 years have not been established.

Adverse Reactions: The adverse reactions to albuterol are similar in nature to those of other sympathomimetic agents. The most frequent adverse reactions to PROVENTIL Tablets were nervousness and tremor, with each occurring in approximately 20 of 100 patients. Other reported reactions were headache, 7 of 100 patients; tachycardia and palpitations, 5 of 100 patients; muscle cramps, 3 of 100 patients; insomnia, nausea, weakness, and dizziness, each occurred in 2 of 100 patients. Drowsiness, flushing, restlessness, irritability, chest discomfort, and difficulty in micturition each occurred in less than 1 of 100 patients.

In addition, albuterol, like other sympathomimetic agents, can cause adverse reactions such as hypertension, angina, vomiting, vertigo, central stimulation, unusual taste, and drying or irritation of the oropharynx.

The reactions are generally transient in nature, and it is usually not necessary to discontinue treatment with PROVENTIL Tablets. In selected cases, however, dosage may be reduced temporarily; after the reaction has subsided, dosage should be increased in small increments to the optimal dosage.

Overdosage: Manifestations of overdosage include anginal pain, hypertension, hypokalemia, and exaggeration of the effects listed in **ADVERSE REACTIONS.**

The oral LD$_{50}$ in rats and mice was greater than 2,000 mg/kg.

Dialysis is not appropriate treatment for overdosage of PROVENTIL Tablets. The judicious use of a cardioselective beta-receptor blocker, such as metoprolol tartrate, is suggested, bearing in mind the danger of inducing an asthmatic attack.

Dosage and Administration: The following dosages of PROVENTIL Tablets are expressed in terms of albuterol base.

Usual Dose: The usual starting dosage for adults and children 12 years and over is 2 mg or 4 mg three or four times a day.

Dosage Adjustment: Doses above 4 mg, four times a day should be used only when the patient fails to respond. If a favorable response does not occur with the 4 mg initial dosage, it should be cautiously increased step wise up to a maximum of 8 mg four times a day as tolerated.

Elderly Patients and Those Sensitive to Beta-Adrenergic Stimulators: An initial dosage of 2 mg three or four times a day is recommended for elderly patients and for those with a history of unusual sensitivity to beta-adrenergic stimulators. If adequate bronchodilatation is not obtained, dosage may be increased gradually to as much as 8 mg three or four times a day.

The total daily dose should not exceed 32 mg in adults and children 12 years and over.

How Supplied: PROVENTIL Tablets, 2 mg albuterol as the sulfate, white, round, compressed tablets, impressed with the product name (PROVENTIL) and the number 2 on one side, and product identification numbers, 252, and scored on the other; bottles of 100 (NDC 0085-0252-02) and 500 (NDC 0085-0252-03)

PROVENTIL Tablets, 4 mg albuterol as the sulfate, white, round, compressed tablets, impressed with the product name (PROVENTIL) and the number 4 on one side, and product identification numbers, 573, and scored on the other; bottles of 100 (NDC 0085-0573-02) and 500 (NDC 0085-0573-03).

Store between 2° and 30°C (36° and 86°F).
Copyright © 1982, 1984, Schering Corporation. All rights reserved.
Revised 6/84
Shown in Product Identification Section, page 435

Sodium SULAMYD®
[so′dē-um soo′lah-mid]
brand of sulfacetamide sodium
Ophthalmic Solution, USP 30%—Sterile
Ophthalmic Solution, USP 10%—Sterile
Ophthalmic Ointment, USP 10%—Sterile

Description: Sodium SULAMYD is available in three ophthalmic forms:

Ophthalmic Solution 30% contains in each ml of sterile aqueous solution 300 mg sulfacetamide sodium, USP, 1.5 mg sodium thiosulfate, with 0.5 mg methylparaben and 0.1 mg propylparaben added as preservatives, and sodium dihydrogen phosphate as buffer.

Ophthalmic Solution 10% contains in each ml of sterile aqueous solution 100 mg sulfacetamide sodium, USP, 3.1 mg sodium thiosulfate, and 5 mg methylcellulose, with 0.5 mg methylparaben and 0.1 mg propylparaben added as preservatives and sodium dihydrogen phosphate as buffer.

Ophthalmic Ointment 10% is a sterile ointment, each gram containing 100 mg sulfacetamide sodium, USP, with 0.5 mg methylparaben, 0.1 mg propylparaben and 0.25 mg benzalkonium chloride added as preservatives, and sorbitan monolaurate and water in a bland, unctuous, petrolatum base.

Actions: Sodium SULAMYD exerts a bacteriostatic effect against a wide range of gram-positive and gram-negative microorganisms by restricting, through competition with para-aminobenzoic acid, the synthesis of folic acid which bacteria require for growth.

Indications: Sodium SULAMYD is indicated for the treatment of conjunctivitis, corneal ulcer, and other superficial ocular infections due to susceptible microorganisms, and as adjunctive treatment in systemic sulfonamide therapy of trachoma.

Contraindications: Sodium SULAMYD is contraindicated in individuals with known or suspected sensitivity to sulfonamides or to any of the ingredients of the preparations.

Precautions: Sodium SULAMYD products are incompatible with silver preparations. Ophthalmic ointments may retard corneal healing. Nonsusceptible organisms, including fungi, may proliferate with the use of these preparations. Sulfonamides are inactivated by the para-aminobenzoic acid present in purulent exudates.

Sensitization may recur when a sulfonamide is re-administered irrespective of the route of administration, and cross sensitivity between different sulfonamides may occur. If signs of sensitivity or other untoward reactions occur, discontinue use of the preparation.

Adverse Reactions: Sulfacetamide sodium may cause local irritation. Transient stinging or burning has been reported with the 30% solution of sulfacetamide sodium.

Although sensitivity reactions to sulfacetamide sodium are rare, an isolated incident of Stevens-Johnson syndrome was reported in a patient who had experienced a previous bullous drug reaction to an orally administered sulfonamide and a single instance of local hypersensitivity was reported which progressed to a fatal syndrome resembling systemic lupus erythematosus.

Dosage and Administration: Sodium SULAMYD Ophthalmic Solution 30%. *For conjunctivitis or corneal ulcer:* instill one drop into lower conjunctival sac every two hours or less frequently according to severity of infection. *For trachoma:* Two drops every two hours; concomitant systemic sulfonamide therapy is indicated.

Sodium SULAMYD Ophthalmic Solution 10%. One or two drops into the lower conjunctival sac every two or three hours during the day and less often at night.

Sodium SULAMYD Ophthalmic Ointment 10%. Apply a small amount four times daily and at bedtime. The ointment may be used adjunctively with either of the solution forms.

How Supplied: Sodium SULAMYD Ophthalmic Ointment 10%, 3.5 g tube (NDC 0085-0066-03), box of one. **Store away from heat.**

Sodium SULAMYD Ophthalmic Solution 30%, 15 ml dropper bottle (NDC 0085-0717-06), box of one. **Store between 2° and 30°C (36° and 86°F).**
Sodium SULAMYD Ophthalmic Solution 10%, 5 ml dropper bottle (NDC 0085-0946-03), box of 25; 15 ml dropper bottle (NDC 0085-0946-06), box of one. **Store between 2° and 30°C (36° and 86°F).**
On long standing, sulfonamide solutions will darken in color and should be discarded.
Revised 5/84
Copyright © 1969, 1984, Schering Corporation. All rights reserved.

SOLGANAL®
[sol′gah-nal]
brand of sterile aurothioglucose Suspension, USP
FOR INTRAMUSCULAR
INJECTION ONLY—
NOT FOR INTRAVENOUS USE

WARNINGS

Physicians planning to use SOLGANAL Suspension should thoroughly familiarize themselves with its toxicity and its benefits. The possibility of toxic reactions should always be explained to the patient before starting therapy. Patients should be warned to report promptly any symptom suggesting toxicity. Before **each** injection of SOLGANAL Suspension, the physician should review the results of laboratory work and see the patient to determine the presence or absence of adverse reactions, since some of these can be severe or even fatal.

Description: SOLGANAL is a sterile suspension, for **intramuscular injection only.** SOLGANAL Suspension is an antiarthritic agent which is absorbed gradually following intramuscular injection, producing a therapeutically desired prolonged effect.

Each ml contains 50 mg of aurothioglucose, USP in sterile sesame oil with 2% aluminum monostearate; 1 mg propylparaben is added as preservative. Aurothioglucose contains approximately 50% gold by weight.

The empirical formula for aurothioglucose is $C_6H_{11}AuO_5S$; the molecular weight is 392.18. Chemically it is (1-Thio-D-glucopyranosato) gold. Aurothioglucose is a nearly odorless, yellow powder which is stable in air. An aqueous solution is unstable on long standing. Aurothioglucose is freely soluble in water but practically insoluble in acetone, in alcohol, in chloroform, and in ether.

Clinical Pharmacology: Although the mechanism of action is not well understood, gold compounds have been reported to decrease synovial inflammation and retard cartilage and bone destruction.

Gold is absorbed from injection sites, reaching peak concentration in blood in four to six hours. Following a single intramuscular injection of 50 mg SOLGANAL Suspension in each of two patients, peak serum levels were about 235 mcg/dl in one patient and 450 mcg/dl in the other. In plasma, 95% is bound to the albumin fraction. Approximately 70% of the gold is eliminated in the urine and approximately 30% in the feces. When a standard weekly treatment schedule is followed, approximately 40% of the administered dose is excreted each week, and the remainder is excreted over a longer period. The biological half-life of gold salts following a single 50 mg dose has been reported to range from 3 to 27 days. Following successive weekly doses, the half-life increases and may be 14 to 40 days after the third dose and up to 168 days after the eleventh weekly dose.

After the initial injection, the serum level of gold rises sharply and declines over the next week. Peak levels with aqueous preparations are higher and decline faster than those with oily preparations. Weekly administration produces a continuous rise in the basal value for several months, after which the serum level becomes relatively stable. After a standard weekly dose, considerable individual variation in the levels of gold has been found. A steady decline in gold levels occurs when the interval between injections is lengthened, and small amounts may be found in the serum for months after discontinuance of therapy. The incidence of toxic reactions is apparently unrelated to the plasma level of gold, but it may be related to the cumulative body content of gold.

Storage of gold in human tissues is dependent upon organ mass as well as upon the concentration of gold. Therefore, tissues having the highest gold levels (weight/weight) do not necessarily contain the greatest total amounts of gold. The major depots, in decreasing order of total gold content, are the bone marrow, liver, skin, and bone, accounting for approximately 85% of body gold. The highest concentrations of gold are found in the lymph nodes, adrenal glands, liver, kidneys, bone marrow, and spleen. Relatively small concentrations are found in articular structures.

Gold passes the blood-brain barrier in hamsters. Transfer of gold across the human placenta at the twentieth week of pregnancy has been documented. The placenta showed numerous gold deposits and smaller amounts were detected in the fetal liver and kidneys; other tissues provided no evidence of gold deposition.

Gold is excreted into human milk in significant amounts and trace amounts can be demonstrated in the blood of nursing infants. (See PRECAUTIONS, "*Nursing Mothers*.")

Indications and Usage: (SOLGANAL Suspension is indicated for the adjunctive treatment of early active rheumatoid arthritis (both of the adult and juvenile types) not adequately controlled by other anti-inflammatory agents and conservative measures. In chronic, advanced cases of rheumatoid arthritis, gold therapy is less valuable.

Antirheumatic measures such as salicylates and other anti-inflammatory drugs (both steroidal and non-steroidal) may be continued after initiation of gold therapy. After improvement commences, these measures may be discontinued slowly as symptoms permit.

See Precautions, "*Laboratory Tests*" and **Dosage and Administration.**

Contraindications: A history of known hypersensitivity to any component of SOLGANAL Suspension contraindicates its use. Gold therapy is contraindicated in patients with uncontrolled diabetes mellitus, severe debilitation, systemic lupus erythematosus, renal disease, hepatic dysfunction, uncontrolled congestive heart failure, marked hypertension, agranulocytosis, other blood dyscrasias, or hemorrhagic diathesis; or if there is a history of infectious hepatitis. Patients who recently have had radiation, and those who have developed severe toxicity from previous exposure to gold or other heavy metals should not receive SOLGANAL Suspension.

Urticaria, eczema, and colitis are also contraindications.

Gold therapy is usually contraindicated in pregnancy. (See PRECAUTIONS, "*Usage in Pregnancy*".)

Gold salts should not be used with penicillamine (See MANAGEMENT OF ADVERSE REACTIONS) or antimalarials. The safety of coadministration with immunosuppressive agents other than corticosteroids has not been established.

Warnings: The following signs should be considered danger signals of gold toxicity, and no additional injection should be given unless further studies reveal some other cause for their presence; rapid reduction of hemoglobin, leukopenia (WBC below 4000/cu mm), eosinophilia above 5%, platelet count below 100,000/cu mm, albuminuria, hematuria, pruritus, dermatitis, stomatitis, jaundice, and petechiae.

Effects that may occur immediately following an injection, or at any time during gold therapy, include: anaphylactic shock, syncope, bradycardia, thickening of the tongue, difficulty in swallowing and breathing, and angioneurotic edema. If such effects are observed, treatment with SOLGANAL Suspension should be discontinued.

Tolerance to gold usually decreases with advancing age. Diabetes mellitus or congestive heart failure should be under control before gold therapy is instituted.

SOLGANAL Suspension should be used with extreme caution in patients with: skin rash, hypersensitivity to other medications, or a history of renal or liver disease.

Precautions: *General:* Before **each** injection, the physician should personally check the patient for adverse reactions and inquiry should be made regarding pruritus, rash, sore mouth, indigestion, and metallic taste. The patient should be observed for at least 15 minutes following each injection. (See also "*Laboratory Tests*".)

Patients with HLA-D locus histocompatibility antigens DRw2 and DRw3 may have a genetic predisposition to develop certain toxic reactions, such as proteinuria, during treatment with gold or D-penicillamine.

SOLGANAL Suspension should be used with caution in patients with compromised cardiovascular or cerebral circulation.

Information for Patients:

1. Promptly report to the physician any unusual symptoms such as pruritus (itching), rash, sore mouth, indigestion, or metallic taste.
2. Increased joint pain may occur for one or two days after an injection and usually subsides after the first few injections.
3. Exposure to sunlight or artificial ultraviolet light should be minimized.
4. Careful oral hygiene is recommended in conjunction with therapy.
5. Patients should be aware of potential hazards if they become pregnant while receiving gold therapy. (See "*Usage in Pregnancy*".)

Laboratory Tests: Before treatment is started, a complete blood count, platelet count, and urinalysis should be done to serve as reference points. Since gold therapy is usually contraindicated in pregnant patients, pregnancy should be ruled out before treatment is started. Throughout the treatment period, urinalysis should be repeated prior to each injection, and complete blood cell and platelet counts should be performed every two weeks. A platelet count is indicated any time that purpura or ecchymosis occurs.

Drug Interactions: Drug interactions have not been reported. (See **Contraindications**.)

Carcinogenesis, Mutagenesis, and Impairment of Fertility: Renal adenomas developed in rats receiving an injectable gold product similar to SOLGANAL Suspension at doses of 2 mg/kg weekly for 46 weeks, followed by 6 mg/kg daily for 47 weeks. These doses were higher and administered more frequently than the recommended human doses. The adenomas were similar histologically to those produced by chronic administration of other gold compounds and heavy metals, such as lead or nickel.

Renal tubular cell neoplasia consisting of renal adenoma and adenocarcinoma were noted in a dose-response relationship in another study in rats using daily intramuscular doses of 3 mg/kg and 6 mg/kg for up to 2 years. These doses were higher and were administered more frequently than the recommended human doses. In this same study, sarcomas at the injection site occurred in some rats but their numbers were not sufficient to demonstrate a dose-response relationship.

No report of renal adenoma or sarcoma at the injection site in man in association with the use of SOLGANAL Suspension has been received.

Gold compounds have not been studied for evaluation of mutagenesis.

Gold sodium thiomalate given subcutaneously did not adversely affect fertility or reproductive performance.

Usage in Pregnancy: Gold therapy is usually contraindicated in pregnant patients. The patient should be warned about the hazards of becoming pregnant while on gold therapy. Rheumatoid arthritis frequently improves when the patient becomes pregnant, thereby eliminating the need for gold therapy. The potential nephrotoxicity of gold should not be superimposed on the increased renal burden which normally occurs in pregnancy and hence, gold therapy should be discontinued upon recognition of pregnancy unless continued use is required in an individual case. The slow excretion of gold and its persistence in body tissues after discontinuation of treatment should be kept in mind when a woman of child-bearing potential being treated with gold plans to become pregnant.

Pregnancy Category C: Gold sodium thiomalate administered subcutaneously, a route not used clinically, has been shown to be teratogenic during the organogenic period in rats and rabbits when given in doses 140 and 175 times, respectively, the usual human dose. Hydrocephalus and microphthalmia were the malformations observed in rats when gold sodium thiomalate was administered at a dose of 25 mg/kg/day from day 6 through day 15 of gestation. In rabbits, limb defects and gastroschisis were the malformations observed when gold sodium thiomalate was administered at doses of 20 to 45 mg/kg/day from day 6 through day 18 of gestation.

Gold compounds administered orally to rabbits from days 6 through 18 of pregnancy resulted in the occurrence of abdominal defects, such as gastroschisis and umbilical hernia; anomalies of the brain, heart, lung, and skeleton; and microphthalmia.

The administration of excessive doses of gold-containing compounds during pregnancy in the above studies was toxic to the mothers and their embryos; the embryotoxic effects probably were secondary to maternal toxicity. Therefore, the significance of these findings in relation to human use is unknown.

There are no adequate and well-controlled studies with SOLGANAL Suspension in pregnant women. Extensive clinical experience with SOLGANAL Suspension has not demonstrated human teratogenicity.

Nursing Mothers: Gold has been demonstated in the milk of lactating mothers. In one patient, a total dose of 135 mg of gold thioglucose was given during the postpartum period. Samples of the maternal milk and urine, and samples of red blood cells and serum of the mother and child were evaluated by atomic absorption spectrophotometry. Trace amounts of gold appeared in the serum and red blood cells of the nursing offspring. It has been postulated that this may be the cause of unexplained rashes, nephritis, hepatitis, and hematologic aberrations in the nursing infants of mothers treated with gold. Because of the potential for serious adverse reactions in nursing infants, a decision should be made whether to discontinue nursing or to discontinue the gold therapy, taking into account the importance of the drug to the mother. The slow excretion of gold and its persistence in the mother after discontinuation of treatment should be kept in mind.

Pediatric Use: Safety and effectiveness in children below the age of six years have not been established.

Adverse Reactions: Adverse reactions to gold therapy may occur at any time during treatment or many months after therapy has been discontinued. The incidence of toxic reactions is apparently unrelated to the plasma level of gold, but it may be related to the cumulative body content of gold. Higher than conventional dosage schedules may increase the occurrence and severity of toxicity. Severe effects are most common after 300 to 500 mg have been administered.

Cutaneous Reactions: Dermatitis is the most common reaction. Pruritus should be considered a warning signal of an impending cutaneous reaction. Erythema and occasionally the more severe reactions such as papular, vesicular, and exfoliative dermatitis leading to alopecia and shedding of the nails may occur. Chrysiasis (gray-to-blue pigmentation) has been reported, especially on photoexposed areas. Gold dermatitis may be aggravated

Continued on next page

Information on Schering products appearing on these pages is effective as of September 30, 1984.

Schering—Cont.

by exposure to sunlight, or an actinic rash may develop.

Mucous Membrane Reactions: Stomatitis is the second most common adverse reaction. Shallow ulcers on the buccal membranes, on the borders of the tongue and on the palate, diffuse glossitis, or gingivitis may be preceded by the sensation of metallic taste. Careful oral hygiene is recommended. Inflammation of the upper respiratory tract, pharyngitis, gastritis, colitis, tracheitis, and vaginitis have also been reported. Conjunctivitis is rare.

Renal Reactions: Nephrotic syndrome or glomerulitis with hematuria, which is usually relatively mild, subsides completely if recognized early and treatment is discontinued. These reactions become severe and chronic if gold therapy is continued after their onset. Therefore, it is important to perform a urinalysis before each injection and to discontinue treatment promptly if proteinuria or hematuria develops.

Hematologic Reactions: Although rare, blood dyscrasias, including granulocytopenia, agranulocytosis, thrombocytopenia with or without purpura, leukopenia, eosinophilia, panmyelopathy, hemorrhagic diathesis, and hypoplastic and aplastic anemia, have been reported. These reactions may occur separately or in combination.

Nitritoid and Allergic Reactions: These reactions, which may rarely occur with SOLGANAL Suspension and which resemble anaphylactoid effects, include flushing, fainting, dizziness, sweating, malaise, weakness, nausea, and vomiting.

Miscellaneous Reactions: On rare occasions, gastrointestinal symptoms, i.e., nausea, vomiting, colic, anorexia, abdominal cramps, diarrhea, ulcerative enterocolitis, and headache have been reported.

There have been rare reports of iritis and corneal ulcers. Transient, asymptomatic gold deposits in the cornea or conjunctiva may occur.

Other reported reactions include encephalitis, immunological destruction of the synovia, EEG abnormalities, intrahepatic cholestasis, hepatitis with jaundice, toxic hepatitis, acute yellow atrophy, peripheral neuritis, gold bronchitis, pulmonary injury manifested by interstitial pneumonitis or fibrosis, fever, and partial or complete hair loss.

Less common but more severe effects that may occur shortly after an injection or at any time during gold therapy include: anaphylactic shock, syncope, bradycardia, thickening of the tongue, difficulty in swallowing and breathing, and angioneurotic edema. If they are observed, treatment with SOLGANAL Suspension should be discontinued. Arthralgia may occur for one or two days after an injection and usually subsides after the first few injections. The mechanism of the transient increase in rheumatic symptoms after injection of gold (the so-called nonvasomotor postinjection reaction) is unknown. These reactions are usually mild but occasionally may be so severe that treatment is stopped prematurely.

Management of Adverse Reactions: In the event of toxic reactions, gold therapy should be discontinued immediately.

In the presence of mild reactions, it may be sufficient to discontinue the administration of SOLGANAL Suspension for a short period and then to resume treatment with smaller doses.

Dermatitis and pruritus may respond to soothing lotions, other appropriate antipruritic treatment, or topical glucocorticoids.

If dermatitis or stomatitis becomes severe or spreads, systemic glucocorticoid treatment may be indicated. For renal, hematologic, and most other adverse reactions, glucocorticoids may be required in larger doses and for a longer time than for dermatologic reactions. Often this treatment may be required for many months because of the slow elimination of gold from the body.

If severe adverse reactions do not improve with steroid treatment in patients who receive large doses of gold, a chelating agent, such as dimercaprol (BAL), may be used. In one case, it was reported that penicillamine was beneficial in the treatment of gold-induced thrombocytopenia. Adjunctive use of an anabolic steroid with other drugs (i.e., BAL, penicillamine, and corticosteroids) may contribute to recovery of bone marrow deficiency.

In the presence of severe or idiosyncratic reactions, treatment with SOLGANAL Suspension should not be reinstituted.

Overdosage: Overdosage resulting from too rapid increases in dosing with SOLGANAL Suspension will be manifested by rapid appearance of toxic reactions, particularly those relating to renal damage, such as hematuria, proteinuria, and to hematologic effects, such as thrombocytopenia and granulocytopenia. Other toxic effects, including fever, nausea, vomiting, diarrhea, and various skin disorders such as papulovesicular lesions, urticaria, and exfoliative dermatitis, all attended with severe pruritus, may develop. Treatment consists of prompt discontinuation of the medication, and early administration of dimercaprol. Specific supportive therapy should be given for the renal and hematologic complications. (See also MANAGEMENT OF ADVERSE REACTIONS above).

Dosage and Administration: Adults—The usual dosage schedule for the intramuscular administration of SOLGANAL is as follows: first dose, 10 mg; second and third doses, 25 mg; fourth and subsequent doses, 50 mg. The interval between doses is one week. The 50 mg dose is continued at weekly intervals until 0.8 to 1.0 g SOLGANAL has been given. If the patient has improved and has exhibited no sign of toxicity, the 50 mg dose may be continued many months longer, at three- to four-week intervals. A weekly dose above 50 mg is usually unnecessary and contraindicated; the tendency in gold therapy is toward lower dosage. With this in mind, it may eventually be established that a 25 mg dose is the one of choice. If no improvement has been demonstrated after a total administration of 1.0 g of SOLGANAL Suspension, the necessity for gold therapy should be reevaluated.

Children 6 to 12 years—one-fourth of the adult dose, governed chiefly by body weight, not to exceed 25 mg per dose.

SOLGANAL Suspension should be injected **intramuscularly**, (preferably intragluteally), **never intravenously**. The patient should be lying down and should remain recumbent for approximately 10 minutes after the injection. The vial should be thoroughly shaken in order to suspend all of the active material. Heating the vial to body temperature (by immersion in warm water) will facilitate drawing the suspension into the syringe. An 18-gauge, 1½-inch needle is recommended for depositing the preparation deep into the muscular tissue. For obese patients, an 18-gauge, 2-inch needle may be used. The site usually selected for injection is the upper outer quadrant of the gluteal region.

NOTE: Shake the vial in horizontal position before the dose is withdrawn. Needle and syringe must be dry. The patient should be observed for at least 15 minutes following each injection.

How Supplied: SOLGANAL Suspension is available in 10 ml multiple-dose vials containing 5% (50 mg/ml) aurothioglucose; box of one.

Shake well before using. Store between 0° and 30°C (32° and 86°F). Protect from light. Store in carton until contents are used.

Copyright © 1963, 1981, Schering Corporation. All rights reserved.

THEOVENT® ℞
[thē-ō-vĕnt]
brand of theophylline anhydrous, USP
Long-Acting Capsules

Description: THEOVENT Long-Acting Capsules are a specially formulated preparation of anhydrous theophylline which is gradually released for prolonged therapeutic effect after oral administration. The product is formulated so that most of the dose is released after leaving the stomach, thereby minimizing exposure of the gastric mucosa to the potentially irritating effects of theophylline. Each capsule contains either 125 mg or 250 mg of anhydrous theophylline, USP.

Anhydrous theophylline is 3,7-Dihydro-1,3-dimethyl-1H-purine-2,6-dione, anhydrous.

Anhydrous theophylline is a xanthine compound having the chemical formula, $C_7H_8N_4O_2$, with a molecular weight of 180.17. It is a white, odorless, crystalline powder which is stable in air and has a bitter taste. Theophylline is slightly soluble in water, freely soluble in solutions of alkali hydroxides and in ammonia, while only slightly soluble in alcohol, chloroform, or ether.

Clinical Pharmacology: Theophylline directly relaxes the smooth muscle of the bronchial airways and pulmonary blood vessels, thus acting mainly as a bronchodilator, pulmonary vasodilator, and smooth muscle relaxant. It produces an increase in vital capacity and counteracts the entrapment of residual air. Its bronchodilating action helps relieve wheezing, coughing, and other respiratory symptoms associated with reversible bronchospasm.

Theophylline also possesses other actions typical of the xanthine derivatives: coronary vasodilation; diuretic; and skeletal muscle, cardiac, and cerebral stimulation. Its actions may be mediated through inhibition of phosphodiesterase and a resultant increase in intracellular cyclic AMP which could mediate smooth muscle relaxation. Theophylline also inhibits the release of histamine by mast cells *in vitro* at concentrations higher than those usually attained clinically.

In vitro theophylline has been shown to react synergistically with appropriate beta agonists (e.g., isoproterenol), by increasing intracellular cyclic AMP through stimulation of adenyl cyclase, but therapeutic synergistic bronchodilation has not been demonstrated in clinical studies. More data are needed to determine if theophylline and beta agonists have clinically important therapeutic additive effects.

Tolerance (tachyphylaxis) does not appear to develop with prolonged use of theophylline.

The elimination characteristics of theophylline are as follows:

Patient Population	Theophylline Plasma Clearance Rates (mean ± S.D.)	Average Half-Life (mean ± S.D.)
Children (over 6 months of age)	1.45 ± .58 ml/kg/min	3.7 ± 1.1 hours
Adult non-smokers with uncomplicated asthma	.65 ± .19 ml/kg/min	8.7 ± 2.2 hours

The half-life is shortened by cigarette smoking and also by a low carbohydrate, high protein diet. Conversely, the half-life is prolonged by a high carbohydrate, low protein diet, and also in patients with alcoholism, reduced hepatic or renal functions, congestive heart failure, and in patients receiving certain antibiotics, such as troleandomycin, erythromycin, lincomycin, or clindamycin. High fever for prolonged periods may decrease theophylline elimination.

THEOVENT Long-Acting Capsules *are not indicated* for young children or infants. It should be noted that newborn infants have extremely slow theophylline clearances with a half-life exceeding 24 hours.

In infants 3 to 6 months old, these elimination characteristics are similar to those in older children.

Older adults with chronic obstructive pulmonary disease, patients with cor pulmonale or other causes of heart failure, and patients with liver disease may have much lower clearances with a half-life that may exceed 24 hours.

The half-life of the theophylline in smokers (of 1 to 2 packs of cigarettes per day) averaged 4 to 5 hours among various studies, much shorter than the half-life in non-smokers, which averaged about 7 to 9 hours. The increase in theophylline clearance caused by smoking is probably the result of induction of drug-metabolizing enzymes. After cessation of smoking, normalization of theophylline pharmacokinetics may not occur for 3 months to 2 years.

In a well-controlled study in normal adult males, a single dose of 500 mg THEOVENT Long-Acting Capsules, administered as 2 capsules each containing 250 mg, resulted in a mean peak serum concentration of 7.5 mcg/ml at 4.6 hours after administration. The relative bioavailability of THEOVENT Long-Acting Capsules was complete compared to that of a standard theophylline syrup. In a multiple-dose study in which asthmatic adults received 500 mg THEOVENT Long-Acting Capsules every 12 hours, therapeutic levels of theophylline were achieved by the second day of therapy and were maintained within the optimal therapeutic range of 10 to 20 mcg/ml from the second day through the last treatment day (day 4) of the study. In chronic therapy of patients requiring higher than average doses, the gradual absorption of theophylline from THEOVENT Long-Acting Capsules, as compared with that of non-sustained release theophylline products, may minimize the fluctuation (peaks and troughs) in serum concentrations and permit longer intervals between dosing.

Studies suggest that 1-demethylation of theophylline to 3-methylxanthine is the principal biotransformation pathway of theophylline elimination. Only 10% of an administered dose of theophylline appears unchanged in the urine. Principal metabolites are 3-methylxanthine, 1,3-dimethyluric acid, and 1-methyluric acid. Animal experiments have shown that theophylline enters the cerebrospinal fluid. The degree of protein binding (55% to 63%) of theophylline at the therapeutic serum concentration has little effect on theophylline distribution. Theophylline distributes well into breast milk; the average ratio of milk to serum concentration of the drug was approximately 0.7, and milk concentrations paralleled the time course of serum concentrations.

Indications and Usage: THEOVENT Long-Acting Capsules are indicated for relief and/or prevention of reversible bronchospasm associated with asthma, chronic bronchitis, or emphysema. Use of theophylline is a treatment of first choice for the management of chronic asthma to prevent symptoms and maintain patent airways.

Contraindications: This product is contraindicated in individuals who have shown hypersensitivity to any of its components, to aminophylline, or to other xanthines, e.g., theobromine or caffeine.

Warnings: Status asthmaticus is a medical emergency. When the patient is not rapidly responsive to bronchodilators, optimal therapy requires additional medication, including corticosteroids. Severe episodes of bronchospasm may require inhalant and/or parenteral therapy or a rapidly acting theophylline preparation.

Although early signs of theophylline toxicity, such as nausea and restlessness, are often seen, in some cases more serious signs such as ventricular arrhythmias or convulsions may be the first signs of toxicity. It is important to discontinue doses which are not tolerated. In situations where therapy is to be resumed, it should be at a lower dosage after all signs of toxicity have disappeared.

Patients with higher than the recommended therapeutic theophylline serum levels are more likely to experience tachycardia than patients whose levels are within the recommended therapeutic range. Theophylline products may worsen preexisting arrhythmias. (See *Drug Interactions* under Precautions.)

Precautions: *General:* Theophylline should not be administered concurrently with other xanthine medications such as aminophylline and caffeine. Use theophylline with caution in patients with severe cardiac disease, arrhythmias, acute myocardial injury, congestive heart failure, cor pulmonale, hypertension, severe hypoxemia, hyperthyroidism, liver or renal disease, dehydration, and in the elderly (especially males over 55 years of age). In patients with a peptic ulcer or a history of peptic ulcer, their condition may be exacerbated. Theophylline may occasionally act as a local gastrointestinal irritant, especially in high doses and during chronic use, but gastrointestinal symptoms are more commonly central and associated with serum concentrations exceeding 20 mcg/ml.

Factors known to influence body clearance of theophylline are:

Increased Clearance	Decreased Clearance
Cigarette smoking	Increasing age
	Congestive heart failure
	Liver disease
	Pulmonary edema
	Concurrent infection
	Concomitant use of any of the following: erythromycin troleandomycin clindamycin lincomycin

In the presence of any of the above factors, it is advisable to monitor theophylline serum levels periodically. Other circumstances in which it is advisable to monitor serum levels include: unexplained poor control of asthma; occurrence of toxic symptoms; addition or removal of other drugs from the therapeutic regimen which affect the metabolism of theophylline; use of unusually high doses.

Information for Patients:
1. Contact a physician immediately if vomiting, nausea, restlessness, convulsions, or irregular heartbeat occurs.
2. Take only the dosage which has been prescribed; especially do not take a larger dose, or take the drug more frequently, or for a longer time than directed.
3. Do not take other medicines, especially those for asthma or breathing problems, except under advice and supervision of a physician.
4. Avoid drinking large amounts of caffeine-containing beverages, such as tea, coffee (except decaffeinated), cocoa, and cola drinks or eating large amounts of chocolate while taking this medicine, since these products may add to the side effects of theophylline.

Laboratory Tests: Periodic measurement of theophylline serum levels is recommended to assure maximal benefit from the drug with minimal risk of toxicity. The incidence of toxicity increases sharply at serum levels greater than 20 mcg/ml. For purposes of monitoring serum theophylline concentrations, serum should be obtained at the time of peak drug absorption (2 to 5 hours after ingestion). In the preceding 48 hours, dosage should have been reasonably typical of the prescribed regimen and no doses should have been missed or added. INCREASING DOSAGE BASED ON SERUM THEOPHYLLINE MEASUREMENTS WHEN THESE INSTRUCTIONS HAVE NOT BEEN FOLLOWED MAY INCREASE THE RISK OF TOXICITY TO THE PATIENT. Generally, the optimum therapeutic serum levels of theophylline are between 10 and 20 mcg/ml; higher levels may produce toxic effects. There are wide interpatient and intrapatient variations in the dosage needed to achieve and maintain therapeutic serum levels. Because of these wide variations and the relatively narrow range between therapeutic and toxic serum levels, dosage must be individualized, and serum level monitoring is recommended, particularly when prolonged use is planned. (See also Clinical Pharmacology and Warnings sections).

High serum levels of theophylline in association with manifestations of toxicity may result from conventional doses in clinical situations such as: lowered body plasma clearances (due to transient cardiac decompensation); liver dysfunction or chronic obstructive lung disease; age of 55 years or more, particularly in males.

Further, in the presence of any of the factors discussed under PRECAUTIONS, *General*, it is especially advisable to monitor theophylline serum levels periodically. (See also DOSAGE AND ADMINISTRATION.)

Drug Interactions: (See also PRECAUTIONS, *General.*) Toxic synergism with ephedrine has been documented and may occur with some other sympathomimetic bronchodilators. Recent controlled studies suggest that the addition of ephedrine to dosage regimens of theophylline results in an increase in toxic effects, but not in efficacy, when compared to theophylline alone. The concurrent use of theophylline and sympathomimetic drugs is of particular concern in the presence of arrhythmias. Following is a list of other drugs and the effects seen from their interaction with theophylline:

DRUG	EFFECT
lithium carbonate	increased excretion of lithium carbonate
propranolol	antagonism of propranolol
furosemide	increased diuresis
reserpine	tachycardia
troleandomycin erythromycin lincomycin, or clindamycin	increased theophylline blood levels

Drug/Laboratory Test Interactions: Theophylline may increase the results of tests for urinary catecholamines, plasma free fatty acids, serum uric acid, bilirubin, and sedimentation rate. Theophylline may decrease the results of ^{131}I uptake tests.

Carcinogenesis, Mutagenesis, Impairment of Fertility: No long-term study of theophylline has been done in animals to evaluate carcinogenic potential. Theophylline has been reported to cause chromosomal breakage in human cells in culture at concentrations approximately 35 times the maximum therapeutic serum concentrations.

Pregnancy Category C: Theophylline has been shown to be teratogenic in mice when given in doses 30 times the adult human dose. It was not teratogenic when administered to Br46-Wistar II rats prior to mating and at various stages of gestation. As with most anti-asthmatic medications, there are no adequate and well-controlled studies in pregnant women. Theophylline should be used during pregnancy only if the potential benefits justify the potential risks to the fetus. To be considered in the benefit-risk assessment are the dangers of uncontrolled asthma in pregnant women and the reported presence of theophylline in cord serum.

Nonteratogenic Effects: Theophylline levels have been found in cord serum and there have been reports of slight tachycardia and jitteriness in neonates whose mothers received theophylline up to the time of delivery.

Nursing Mothers: It has been reported that theophylline distributes readily into breast milk. One nursing infant experienced mild symptoms of irritability, fretfulness, and insomnia on the days the mother took aminophylline. Four other asthmatic mothers receiving theophylline did not observe any irritability in their nursing children. Caution should be exercised when theophylline is administered to a nursing woman.

Pediatric Use: Safety and effectiveness of THEOVENT Long-Acting Capsules in children below the age of 6 years have not been established.

Adverse Reactions: Most adverse reactions are usually due to overdose and include:
Gastrointestinal: hematemesis, nausea, epigastric pain, vomiting, diarrhea.
Central Nervous System: clonic and tonic generalized convulsions, muscle twitching, headaches, irritability, restlessness, insomnia, reflex hyperexcitability.

Continued on next page

Information on Schering products appearing on these pages is effective as of September 30, 1984.

Schering—Cont.

Cardiovascular: life-threatening ventricular arrhythmias, circulatory failure, extrasystoles, hypotension, tachycardia, palpitations, flushing.
Respiratory: tachypnea.
Renal: albuminuria, increased excretion of renal tubular cells and red blood cells; potentiation of diuresis.
Others: hyperglycemia and inappropriate antidiuretic hormone syndrome. Methylxanthines may cause persistence of benign breast tumors.
Overdosage: ALTHOUGH EARLY EVIDENCE OF THEOPHYLLINE TOXICITY, SUCH AS NAUSEA AND RESTLESSNESS, IS OFTEN SEEN, IN SOME CASES MORE SERIOUS SIGNS, SUCH AS VENTRICULAR ARRHYTHMIAS OR CONVULSIONS, MAY BE THE FIRST MANIFESTATIONS OF TOXICITY.
Management: Emergency treatment should be started immediately.
A. If overdose is established and seizure has not occurred:
   1. Induce vomiting, even if emesis has occurred spontaneously; the administration of ipecac syrup is the preferred method. Emesis should not be induced in patients with impaired consciousness. The action of ipecac is facilitated by physical activity and the administration of 8 to 12 ounces of water. If emesis does not occur within 15 minutes, the dose of ipecac should be repeated. Precautions against aspiration must be taken, especially in infants and children. If vomiting is unsuccessful or contraindicated, gastric lavage should be performed.
   2. Administer a cathartic (this is particularly important if a sustained-release preparation has been taken).
   3. Administer activated charcoal.
B. If the patient is having a seizure:
   1. Establish an airway.
   2. Administer oxygen.
   3. Treat the seizure with intravenous diazepam 0.1 to 0.3 mg/kg up to 10 mg.
   4. Monitor vital signs, maintain blood pressure, and provide adequate hydration.
C. Post-Seizure Coma:
   1. Maintain airway and oxygenation.
   2. Follow above recommendations to prevent absorption of drug, but perform intubation and lavage instead of inducing emesis. Introduce the cathartic and charcoal via a large bore gastric lavage tube.
   3. Continue to provide full supportive care and adequate hydration while waiting for the drug to be metabolized, which generally occurs rapidly enough that dialysis is not necessary.
D. General:
   Treatment is symptomatic and supportive. *Stimulants (analeptic agents) should not be used.* If atrial arrhythmia occurs during treatment with theophylline, lidocaine should be administered with caution, since both drugs may produce accelerated atrioventricular conduction.
Intravenous fluids may be required to overcome dehydration, acid-base imbalance, and hypotension; the latter may also be treated with vasopressors. Apnea will require ventilatory support. Hyperpyrexia, especially in children, may be treated with tepid water sponge baths or a hypothermic blanket. Theophylline serum levels should be monitored until they fall below 20 mcg/ml. After emergency treatment, medical monitoring should be continued.
Theophylline is dialyzable; peritoneal and hemodialyses are effective means of removing theophylline and may be useful adjuncts in the management of overdosage. In one case of massive overdose, charcoal hemoperfusion over a 6-hour period rapidly removed theophylline from the serum with notable clinical improvement. Charcoal hemoperfusion should be considered in patients with severe theophylline intoxication as a possible means of preventing irreversible central nervous system damage.
Animal studies suggest that phenobarbital may decrease theophylline toxicity, but at present there are insufficient data to recommend it as a treatment for theophylline overdosage. Following the unsuccessful trial of the other preferable modalities of theophylline overdosage treatment mentioned above, phenobarbital should only be considered for trial in those patients who are awake.
The oral LD_{50} of theophylline is 100 mg/kg in cats and 300 to 400 mg/kg in rabbits.
Dosage and Administration: The usual initial dosage is: For adults 17 years and older—one or two 250 mg capsules every 12 hours.
For adolescents, 13 through 16 years—one 250 mg capsule every 12 hours.
For children, 9 through 12 years—one or two 125 mg capsules every 12 hours.
For children, 6 through 8 years—one 125 mg capsule every 12 hours.
Patients currently maintained on non-sustained release theophylline or aminophylline products: The total daily dose of a non-sustained release product may be replaced by administering one-half (½) of the equivalent amount of anhydrous theophylline given as THEOVENT Long-Acting Capsules, every 12 hours.
DOSAGE MUST BE ADJUSTED ACCORDING TO THE NEEDS AND RESPONSE OF THE PATIENT. In order to achieve optimal therapeutic dosage, especially if doses higher than those recommended above are required, monitoring of serum theophylline concentrations is recommended. (See PRECAUTIONS, *Laboratory Tests*.)
Dosage should be calculated on the basis of lean (ideal) body weight. Theophylline does not distribute into fatty tissue.
Giving theophylline with food may prevent stomach irritation; although absorption may be slower, it is still complete. If the desired response is not achieved with the recommended usual initial dosage and there are no adverse reactions, the dose may be increased by 2 to 3 mg/kg body weight per day at 3-day intervals, until the following MAXIMUM DOSE WITHOUT MEASUREMENT OF SERUM CONCENTRATION is attained, or until a maximum of 1000 mg is taken in any 24-hour period, whichever occurs first.

MAXIMUM DOSE WITHOUT MEASUREMENT OF SERUM CONCENTRATION

Age	Daily Dose* (mg/kg of body weight)	Dose per 12-hour Interval (mg/kg of body weight)
Adults	13	6.5
Adolescents 13–16 years	18	9
Children 9–12 years	20	10
Children 6–8 years	24	12†

* Use ideal body weight for obese patients
† Some children under 9 years may require 8 mpk q8h

How Supplied: THEOVENT Long-Acting Capsules, 125 mg, dark green and yellow capsules, branded in blue with the Schering trademark and product identification numbers, 402; bottle of 100 and 500.
THEOVENT Long-Acting Capsules, 250 mg, dark green and clear capsules, branded in blue with the Schering trademark and product identification numbers, 753; bottles of 100 and 500.
Store between 2° and 30°C (36° and 86°F).
Revised 11/80
Copyright © 1979, 1980, Schering Corporation. All rights reserved.
Shown in Product Identification Section, page 435

TRILAFON® ℞
[*tri' lah-fon*]
brand of perphenazine, USP
Tablets
REPETABS® Tablets
Concentrate
Injection

Description: TRILAFON products contain perphenazine, USP (4-[3-(2-chlorophenothiazin-10-yl)propyl)]-1-piperazineethanol), a piperazinyl phenothiazine having the chemical formula, $C_{21}H_{26}ClN_3OS$. It is available as **Tablets**, 2, 4, 8 and 16 mg; REPETABS (brand of repeat-action tablets) **Tablets**, 4 mg in an outer layer for immediate effect and 4 mg in an inner core for release three to six hours later; **Concentrate**, 16 mg perphenazine per 5 ml and alcohol less than 0.1%; and **Injection**, perphenazine 5 mg, disodium citrate 24.6 mg, sodium bisulfite 2 mg, and Water for Injection, USP, per 1 ml.
Actions: Perphenazine has actions at all levels of the central nervous system, particularly the hypothalamus. However, the site and mechanism of action are not known.
Indications: Perphenazine is indicated for use in the management of the manifestations of psychotic disorders; and for the control of severe nausea and vomiting in adults.
TRILAFON has not been shown effective in the management of behavioral complications in patients with mental retardation.
Contraindications: TRILAFON products are contraindicated in comatose or greatly obtunded patients and in patients receiving large doses of central nervous system depressants (barbiturates, alcohol, narcotics, analgesics, or antihistamines); in the presence of existing blood dyscrasias, bone marrow depression, or liver damage; and in patients who have shown hypersensitivity to TRILAFON products, their components, or related compounds.
TRILAFON products are also contraindicated in patients with suspected or established subcortical brain damage, with or without hypothalamic damage, since a hyperthermic reaction with temperatures in excess of 104°F may occur in such patients, sometimes not until 14 to 16 hours after drug administration. Total body ice-packing is recommended for such a reaction; antipyretics may also be useful.
Warnings: If hypotension develops, epinephrine should not be administered since its action is blocked and partially reversed by perphenazine. If a vasopressor is needed, norepinephrine may be used. Severe, acute hypotension has occurred with the use of phenothiazines and is particularly likely to occur in patients with mitral insufficiency or pheochromocytoma. Rebound hypertension may occur in pheochromocytoma patients.
TRILAFON products can lower the convulsive threshold in susceptible individuals; they should be used with caution in alcohol withdrawal and in patients with convulsive disorders. If the patient is being treated with an anticonvulsant agent, increased dosage of that agent may be required when TRILAFON products are used concomitantly.
TRILAFON products should be used with caution in patients with psychic depression.
Perphenazine may impair the mental and/or physical abilities required for the performance of hazardous tasks such as driving a car or operating machinery; therefore, the patient should be warned accordingly.
TRILAFON products are not recommended for children under 12 years of age.
Usage in Pregnancy: Safe use of TRILAFON during pregnancy and lactation has not been established; therefore, in administering the drug to pregnant patients, nursing mothers, or women who may become pregnant, the possible benefits must be weighed against the possible hazards to mother and child.
Precautions: The possibility of suicide in depressed patients remains during treatment and until significant remission occurs. This type of patient should not have access to large quantities of this drug.

As with all phenothiazine compounds, perphenazine should not be used indiscriminately. Caution should be observed in giving it to patients who have previously exhibited severe adverse reactions to other phenothiazines. Some of the untoward actions of perphenazine tend to appear more frequently when high doses are used. However, as with other phenothiazine compounds, patients receiving TRILAFON products in any dosage should be kept under close supervision.

Neuroleptic drugs elevate prolactin levels; the elevation persists during chronic administration Tissue culture experiments indicate that approximately one-third of human breast cancers are prolactin dependent *in vitro*, a factor of potential importance if the prescription of these drugs is contemplated in a patient with a previously detected breast cancer. Although disturbances such as galactorrhea, amenorrhea, gynecomastia, and impotence have been reported the clinical significance of elevated serum prolactin levels is unknown for most patients. An increase in mammary neoplasms has been found in rodents after chronic administration of neuroleptic drugs. Neither clinical studies nor epidemiologic studies conducted to date, however, have shown an association between chronic administration of these drugs and mammary tumorigenesis, the available evidence is considered too limited to be conclusive at this time.

The antiemetic effect of perphenazine may obscure signs of toxicity due to overdosage of other drugs, or render more difficult the diagnosis of disorders such as brain tumors or intestinal obstruction.

A significant, not otherwise explained, rise in body temprature may suggest individual intolerance to perphenazine, in which case it should be discontinued.

Patients on large doses of a phenothiazine drug who are undergoing surgery should be watched carefully for possible hypotensive phenomena. Moreover, reduced amounts of anesthetics or central nervous system depressants may be necessary. Since phenothiazines and central nervous system depressants (opiates, analgesics, antihistamines, barbiturates) can potentiate each other, less than the usual dosage of the added drug is recommended, and caution is advised, when they are administered concomitantly.

Use with caution in patients who are receiving atropine or related drugs because of additive anticholinergic effects and also in patients who will be exposed to extreme heat or phosphorus insecticides.

The use of alcohol should be avoided, since additive effects and hypotension may occur. Patients should be cautioned that their response to alcohol may be increased while they are being treated with TRILAFON products. The risk of suicide and the danger of overdose may be increased in patients who use alcohol excessively due to its potentiation of the drug's effect.

Blood counts and hepatic and renal functions should be checked periodically. The appearance of signs of blood dyscrasias requires the discontinuance of the drug and institution of appropriate therapy. If abnormalities in hepatic tests occur, phenothiazine treatment should be discontinued. Renal function in patients on long-term therapy should be monitored; if blood urea nitrogen (BUN) becomes abnormal, treatment with the drug should be discontinued.

The use of phenothiazine derivatives in patients with diminished renal function should be undertaken with caution.

Use with caution in patients suffering from respiratory impairment due to acute pulmonary infections, or in chronic respiratory disorders such as severe asthma or emphysema.

In general, phenothiazines, including perphenazine, do not produce psychic dependence. Gastritis, nausea and vomiting, dizziness, and tremulousness have been reported following abrupt cessation of high-dose therapy. Reports suggest that these symptoms can be reduced by continuing concomitant antiparkinson agents for several weeks after the phenothiazine is withdrawn.

The possiblity of liver damage, corneal and lenticular deposits, and irreversible dyskinesias should be kept in mind when patients are on long-term therapy.

Because photosensitivity has been reported, undue exposure to the sun should be avoided during phenothiazine treatment.

Adverse Reactions: Not all of the following adverse reactions have been reported with this specific drug; however, pharmacological similarities among various phenothiazine derivatives require that each be considered. In the case of the piperazine group (of which perphenazine is an example) the extrapyramidal symptoms are more common, and others (e.g., sedative effects, jaundice, and blood dyscrasias) are less frequently seen.

CNS Effects: *Extrapyramidal reactions:* opisthotonus, trismus, torticollis, retrocollis, aching and numbness of the limbs, motor restlessness, oculogyric crisis, hyperreflexia, dystonia, including protrusion, discoloration, aching and rounding of the tongue, tonic spasm of the masticatory muscles, tight feeling in the throat, slurred speech, dysphagia, akathisia, dyskinesia, parkinsonism, and ataxia. Their incidence and severity usually increase with an increase in dosage, but there is considerable individual variation in the tendency to develop such symptoms. Extrapyramidal symptoms can usually be controlled by the concomitant use of effective antiparkinsonian drugs. Such as benztropine mesylate, and/or by reduction in dosage. In some instances, however, these extrapyramidal reactions may persist after discontinuation of treatment with perphenazine.

Persistent tardive dyskinesia: As with all antipsychotic agents, tardive dyskinesia may appear in some patients on long-term therapy or may appear after drug therapy has been discontinued. Although the risk appears to be greater in elderly patients on high-dose therapy, especially females, it may occur in either sex and in children. The symptoms are persistent and in some patients appear to be irreversible. The syndrome is characterized by rhythmical, involuntary movements of the tongue, face, mouth, or jaw (e.g. protrusion of tongue, puffing of cheeks, puckering of mouth, chewing movements). Sometimes these may be accompanied by involuntary movements of the extremities. There is no known effective treatment for tardive dyskinesia; antiparkinsonism agents usually do not alleviate the symptoms of this syndrome. It is suggested that all antipsychotic agents be discontinued if these symptoms appear. Should it be necessary to reinstitute treatment, or increase the dosage of the agent, or switch to a different antipsychotic agent, the syndrome may be masked. It has been reported that fine, vermicular movements of the tongue may be an early sign of the syndrome, and if the medication is stopped at that time the syndrome may not develop.

Other CNS effects include cerebral edema; abnormality of cerebrospinal fluid proteins; convulsive seizures, particularly in patients with EEG abnormalities or a history of such disorders, and headaches.

Drowsiness may occur, particularly during the first or second week, after which it generally disappears. If troublesome, lower the dosage. Hypnotic effects appear to be minimal, especially in patients who are permitted to remain active.

Adverse behavioral effects include paradoxical exacerbation of psychotic symptoms, catatonic-like states, paranoid reactions, lethargy, paradoxical excitement, restlessness, hyperactivity, nocturnal confusion, bizarre dreams, and insomnia.

Hyperreflexia has been reported in the newborn when a phenothiazine was used during pregnancy.

Autonomic Effects: dry mouth or salivation, nausea, vomiting, diarrhea, anorexia, constipation, obstipation, fecal impaction, urinary retention, frequency or incontinence, bladder paralysis, polyuria, nasal congestion, pallor, myosis, mydriasis, blurred vision, glaucoma, perspiration, hypertension, hypotension, and change in pulse rate occasionally may occur. Significant autonomic effects have been infrequent in patients receiving less than 24 mg perphenazine daily.

Adynamic ileus occasionally occurs with phenothiazine therapy and if severe can result in complications and death. It is of particular concern in psychiatric patients, who may fail to seek treatment of this condition.

Allergic Effects: urticaria, erythema, eczema, exfoliative dermatitis, pruritus, photosensitivity, asthma, fever, anaphylactoid reactions, laryngeal edema, and angioneurotic edema; contact dermatitis in nursing personnel administering the drug, and in extremely rare instances, individual idiosyncrasy or hypersensitivity to phenothiazines has resulted in cerebral edema, circulatory collapse, and death.

Endocrine Effects: lactation, galactorrhea, moderate breast enlargement in females and gynecomastia in males on large doses, disturbances in the menstrual cycle, amenorrhea, changes in libido, inhibition of ejaculation, syndrome of inappropriate ADH (antidiuretic hormone) secretion, false positive pregnancy tests, hyperglycemia, hypoglycemia, glycosuria.

Cardiovascular Effects: postural hypotension, tachycardia (especially with sudden marked increase in dosage), bradycardia, cardiac arrest, faintness, and dizziness. Occasionally the hypotensive effect may produce a shock-like condition. ECG changes, nonspecific, (quindine-like effect) usually reversible, have been observed in some patients receiving phenothiazine tranquilizers.

Sudden death has occasionally been reported in patients who have received phenothiazines. In some cases the death was apparently due to cardiac arrest; in others, the cause appeared to be asphyxia due to failure of the cough reflex. In some patients, the cause could not be determined nor could it be established that the death was due to the phenothiazine.

Hematological Effects: agranulocytosis, eosinophilia, leukopenia, hemolytic anemia, thrombocytopenic purpura, and pancytopenia. Most cases of agranulocytosis have occurred between the fourth and tenth weeks of therapy. Patients should be watched closely especially during that period for the sudden appearance of sore throat or signs of infection. If white blood cell and differential cell counts show significant cellular depression, discontinue the drug and start appropriate therapy. However, a slightly lowered white count is not in itself an indication to discontinue the drug.

Other Effects: Special considerations in long-term therapy include pigmentation of the skin, occurring chiefly in the exposed areas, ocular changes consisting of deposition of fine particulate matter in the cornea and lens, progressing in more severe cases to star-shaped lenticular opacities; epithelial keratopathies; and pigmentary retinopathy. Also noted: peripheral edema, reversed epinephrine effect, increase in PBI not attributable to an increase in thyroxine, parotid swelling (rare), hyperpyrexia, systemic lupus erythematosus-like syndrome, increases in appetite and weight, polyphagia, photophobia, and muscle weakness.

Liver damage (biliary stasis) may occur. Jaundice may occur, usually between the second and fourth weeks of treatment and is regarded as a hypersensitivity reaction. Incidence is low. The clinical picture resembles infectious hepatitis but with laboratory features of obstructive jaundice. It is usually reversible; however, chronic jaundice has been reported.

Side effects with intramuscular TRILAFON Injection have been infrequent and transient. Dizziness or significant hypotension after treatment with TRILAFON Injection is a rare occurrence.

Dosage and Administration: Dosage must be individualized and adjusted according to the severity of the condition and the response obtained. As with all potent drugs, the best dose is the lowest

Continued on next page

Information on Schering products appearing on these pages is effective as of September 30, 1984.

Schering—Cont.

dose that will produce the desired clinical effect. Since extrapyramidal symptoms increase in frequency and severity with increased dosage, it is important to employ the lowest effective dose. These symptoms have disappeared upon reduction of dosage, withdrawal of the drug or administration of an anti-parkinsonian agent.

Prolonged administration of doses exceeding 24 mg daily should be reserved for hospitalized patients or patients under continued observation for early detection and management of adverse reactions. An antiparkinsonian agent, such as trihexyphenidyl hydrochloride or benztropine mesylate, is valuable in controlling drug-induced, extrapyramidal symptoms.

TRILAFON Tablets and REPETABS Tablets Suggested dosages for Tablets and REPETABS Tablets for various conditions follow:

Moderately disturbed non-hospitalized psychotic patients:
Tablets 4 to 8 mg t.i.d., or one or two REPETABS Tablets b.i.d., initially; reduce as soon as possible to minimum effective dosage.

Hospitalized psychotic patients: Tablets 8 to 16 mg b.i.d. to q.i.d. or one to four REPETABS Tablets b.i.d.; avoid dosages in excess of 64 mg daily.

Severe nausea and vomiting in adults: Tablets 8 to 16 mg daily in divided doses or one REPETABS Tablet b.i.d.; 24 mg occasionally may be necessary; early dosage reduction is desirable. Two REPETABS Tablets may be administered in acute cases.

TRILAFON INJECTION—Intramuscular Administration

The injection is used when rapid effect and prompt control of acute or intractable conditions is required or when oral administration is not feasible. TRILAFON Injection, administered by deep intramuscular injection, is well tolerated. The injection should be given with the patient seated or recumbent, and the patient should be observed for a short period after administration.

Therapeutic effect is usually evidenced in 10 minutes and is maximal in 1 to 2 hours. The average duration of effective action is 6 hours, occasionally 12 to 24 hours.

Pediatric dosage has not yet been established. Children over 12 years may receive the lowest limit of adult dosage.

The usual initial dose is 5 mg (1 ml). This may be repeated every 6 hours. Ordinarily, the total daily dosage should not exceed 15 mg in ambulatory patients or 30 mg in hospitalized patients. When required for satisfactory control of symptoms in severe conditions, an initial 10 mg intramuscular dose may be given. Patients should be placed on oral therapy as soon as practicable. Generally, this may be achieved within 24 hours. In some instances, however, patients have been maintained on injectable therapy for several months. It has been established that TRILAFON Injection is more potent than TRILAFON Tablets. Therefore, equal or higher dosage should be used when the patient is transferred to oral therapy after receiving the injection.

Psychotic conditions: While 5 mg of the Injection has a definite tranquilizing effect, it may be necessary to use 10 mg doses to initiate therapy in severely agitated states. Most patients will be controlled and amendable to oral therapy within a maximum of 24 to 48 hours. Acute conditions (hysteria, panic reaction) often respond well to a single dose whereas in chronic conditions, several injections may be required. When transferring patients to oral therapy, it is suggested that increased dosage be employed to maintain adequate clinical control. This should be followed by gradual reduction to the minimal maintenance dose which is effective.

Severe nausea and vomiting in adults: To obtain rapid control of vomiting, administer 5 mg (1 ml); in rare instances it may be necessary to increase the dosage to 10 mg, in general, higher dosage should be given only to hospitalized patients.

TRILAFON Injection—Intravenous Administration

The intravenous administration of TRILAFON Injection is seldom required. This route of administration should be used with particular caution and care and only when absolutely necessary to control severe vomiting, intractable hiccoughs, or acute conditions, such as violent retching during surgery. Its use should be limited to recumbent, hospitalized adults in doses not exceeding 5 mg. When employed in this manner, intravenous injection ordinarily should be given as a diluted solution by either fractional injection or a slow drip infusion. In the surgical patient, slow infusion of no more than 5 mg is preferred. When administered in divided doses, TRILAFON Injection should be diluted to 0.5 mg/ml (1 ml mixed with 9 ml of physiologic saline solution), and not more than 1 mg per injection given at not less than one-to two-minute intervals. Intravenous injection should be discontinued as soon as symptoms are controlled and should not exceed 5 mg. The possibility of hypotensive and extrapyramidal side effects should be considered and appropriate means for management kept available. Blood pressure and pulse should be monitored continuously during intravenous administration. Pharmacologic and clinical studies indicate that intravenous administration of norepinephrine should be useful in alleviating the hypotensive effect.

TRILAFON Concentrate

In hospitalized psychotic patients, the usual dosage range is 8 to 16 mg b.i.d. to q.i.d., depending on the severity of symptoms and individual response. Although a number of investigators have employed higher dosages, a total daily dose of more than 64 mg ordinarily is not required. The Concentrate should be diluted only with water, saline, Seven-Up, homogenized milk, carbonated orange drink and pineapple, apricot, prune, orange. V-8, tomato, and grapefruit juices. Trilafon Concentrate should not be mixed with beverages containing caffeine (coffee, cola) tannics (tea), or pectinates (apple juice) since physical incompatibility may result. Suggested dilution is approximately two fluid ounces of diluent for each 5 ml (16 mg) teaspoonful of TRILAFON Concentrate. For convenience in measuring smaller doses, a graduated dropper marked to measure 8 mg or 4 mg is supplied with each bottle.

Overdosage: In the event of overdosage, emergency treatment should be started immediately. All patients suspected of having taken an overdose should be hospitalized as soon as possible.

Manifestations: Overdosage of perphenazine primarily involves the extrapyramidal mechanism and produces the same side effects described under ADVERSE REACTIONS, but to a more marked degree. It is usually evidenced by stupor or coma; children may have convulsive seizures.

Treatment: Treatment is symptomatic and supportive. There is no specific antidote. The patient should be induced to vomit even if emesis has occurred spontaneously. Pharmacologic vomiting by the administration of ipecac syrup is a preferred method. It should be noted that ipecac has a central mode of action in addition to its local gastric irritant properties, and the central mode of action may be blocked by the antiemetic effect of TRILAFON products. Vomiting should not be induced in patients with impaired consciousness. The action of ipecac is facilitated by physical activity and by the administration of 8 to 12 fluid ounces of water. If emesis does not occur within 15 minutes, the dose of ipecac should be repeated. Precautions against aspiration must be taken, especially in infants and children. Following emesis, any drug remaining in the stomach may be adsorbed by activated charcoal administered as a slurry with water. If vomiting is unsuccessful or contraindicated, gastric lavage should be performed. Isotonic and one-half isotonic saline are the lavage solutions of choice. Saline cathartics, such as milk of magnesia, draw water into the bowel by osmosis and therefore may be valuable for their action in rapid dilution of bowel content.

Standard measures (oxygen, intravenous fluids, corticosteroids) should be used to manage circulatory shock or metabolic acidosis. An open airway and adequate fluid intake should be maintained. Body temperature should be regulated. Hypothermia is expected, but severe hyperthermia may occur and must be treated vigorously. (See CONTRAINDICATIONS.)

An electrocardiogram should be taken and close monitoring of cardiac function instituted if there is any sign of abnormality. Cardiac arrhythmias may be treated with neostigmine, pyridostigmine, or propranolol. Digitalis should be considered for cadiac failure. Close monitoring of cardiac function is advisable for not less than five days. Vasopressors such as norepinephrine may be used to treat hypotension, but epinephrine should NOT be used.

Anticonvulsants (an inhalation anesthetic, diazepam, or paraldehyde) are recommended for control of convulsions, since perphenazine increases the central nervous system depressant action, but not the anticonvulsant action, of barbiturates.

If acute parkinson-like symptoms result from perphenazine intoxication, benztropine mesylate or diphenydramine may be administered.

Central nervous system depression may be treated with non-convulsant doses of CNS stimulants. Avoid stimulants that may cause convulsions (e.g., picrotoxin and pentylenetetrazol).

Signs of arousal may not occur for 48 hours.

Dialysis is of no value because of low plasma concentrations of the drug.

Since overdosage is often deliberate, patients may attempt suicide by other means during the recovery phase. Deaths by deliberate or accidental overdosage have occurred with this class of drugs.

How Supplied: TRILAFON Tablets (2 mg): gray, sugar-coated tablets branded in black with the Schering trademark and either product identification letters, ADH, or numbers 705; bottles of 100 and 500.
TRILAFON Tablets (4 mg): gray, sugar-coated tablets branded in green with the Schering trademark and either product identification letters, ADK, or numbers, 940; bottles of 100 and 500.
TRILAFON Tablets (8 mg): gray, sugar-coated tablets branded in blue with the Schering trademark and either product identification letters, ADJ, or numbers 313; bottles of 100 and 500.
TRILAFON Tablets (16 mg): gray, sugar-coated tablets branded in red with the Schering trademark and either product identification letters, ADM, or numbers, 077; bottles of 100 and 500.
TRILAFON REPETABS Tablets (8 mg): white, sugar-coated tablets branded in gray with the Schering trademark and either product identification letters, ADX, or numbers, 141; bottle of 100.
TRILAFON Concentrate, 16 mg per 5 ml, 4 fluid ounce (118 ml) bottle with graduated dropper. The Concentrate is light-sensitive and should be dispensed in amber bottles. **Protect from light. Store in carton until contents are used. Shake well.**
TRILAFON Injection, 5 mg per ml, 1-ml ampul for intramuscular or intravenous use, box of 100. Keep package closed to protect from light. Exposure may cause discoloration. Slight yellowish discoloration will not alter potency or therapeutic efficacy; if markedly discolored, ampul should be discarded. **Protect from light. Store in carton until contents are used.**

Store all TRILAFON Tablets and TRILAFON Concentrate between 2° and 30°C (36° and 86°F).

Revised 2/82
Copyright©1969, 1982, Schering Corporation. All rights reserved.
Shown in Product Identification Section, page 435

TRINALIN™   ℞
[trin'a-lin]
brand of azatadine maleate USP and pseudoephedrine sulfate, USP
Long-Acting Antihistamine/Decongestant REPETABS® Tablets

Description: TRINALIN Long-Acting Antihistamine/Decongestant REPETABS (brand of repeat-action tablets) Tablets contain 1 mg azatadine maleate USP in the tablet coating and 120 mg pseudoephedrine sulfate, USP, equally distributed between the tablet coating and the barrier-coated core. Following ingestion, the two active components in the coating are quickly liberated; release of the decongestant in the core is delayed for several hours.

Azatadine maleate is an antihistamine having the empirical formula, $C_{20}H_{22}N_2 \cdot 2C_4H_4O_4$, the chemical name, 6,11-Dihydro-11-(1-methyl-4-piperidylidene)-5H-benzo[5,6]cyclohepta[1,2-b] pyridine maleate (1:2).

The molecular weight of azatadine maleate is 522.54. Azatadine maleate is a white to off-white powder and is very soluble in water and soluble in alcohol.

Pseudoephedrine sulfate, a sympathomimetic amine, is a salt of pseudoephedrine, one of the naturally occurring alkaloids obtained from various species of the plant *Ephedra*. The empirical formula for pseudoephedrine sulfate is $(C_{10}H_{15}NO)_2 \cdot H_2SO_4$; the chemical name is Benzenemethanol, α-[1-(methylamino)ethyl]-, [$S(R^*, R^*)$]-, sulfate (2:1) (salt).

The molecular weight of pseudoephedrine sulfate is 428.56. It is a white to off-white crystal or powder, very soluble in water, freely soluble in alcohol, and sparingly soluble in chloroform.

Clinical Pharmacology: Azatadine maleate is an antihistamine, related to cyproheptadine, with antiserotonin, anticholinergic (drying), and sedative effects. Antihistamines appear to compete with histamine for histamine H_1-receptor sites on effector cells. The antihistamines antagonize those pharmacological effects of histamine which are mediated through activation of H_1-receptor sites and thereby reduce the intensity of allergic reactions and tissue injury response involving histamine release. Antihistamines antagonize the vasodilator effect of endogenously released histamine, especially in small vessels, and mitigate the effect of histamine which results in increased capillary permeability and edema formation. As consequences of these actions, antihistamines antagonize the physiological manifestations of histamine release in the nose following antigen-antibody interaction, such as congestion related to vascular engorgement, mucosal edema, and profuse, watery secretion, and irritation and sneezing resulting from histamine action on afferent nerve terminals.

Pseudoephedrine sulfate (d-isoephedrine sulfate) is an orally effective nasal decongestant which appears to exert its sympathomimetic effect indirectly, predominantly through release of adrenergic mediators from post-ganglionic nerve terminals. In effective recommended oral dosage, pseudoephedrine sulfate produces minimal other sympathomimetic effects, such as pressor activity and CNS stimulation. Use of an orally administered vasoconstrictor for shrinkage of congested nasal mucosa has several advantages: a) it produces a gradual but sustained decongestant effect, causing little, if any "rebound" congestion; b) it facilitates shrinkage of swollen mucosa in upper respiratory areas that are relatively inaccessible to topically applied sprays or drops; c) it relieves nasal obstruction without the additional irritation that may result from local medication.

Pseudoephedrine passes through the blood-brain and placental barriers. While the antihistamines have not been studied systematically for passage through these barriers, the occurrence of pharmacologic effects in the central nervous system and in newborns indicate presence of the drug.

Following administration of the two drugs to normal volunteers in either a single TRINALIN REPETABS Tablet or similar doses in two conventional pseudoephedrine sulfate tablets and a conventional tablet of azatadine maleate, the blood levels of pseudoephedrine and the urinary excretion of azatadine showed that the TRINALIN REPETABS Tablets are bioequivalent to the conventional dosage forms. The apparent elimination half-life of pseudoephedrine in TRINALIN REPETABS Tablets was approximately 6½ hours. The apparent elimination half-life of azatadine maleate (available from the outer layer of the TRINALIN REPETABS Tablets or from the conventional azatadine maleate tablet) was approximately 12 hours.

Indications and Usage: TRINALIN Long-Acting Antihistamine/Decongestant REPETABS Tablets are indicated for the relief of the symptoms of upper respiratory mucosal congestion in perennial and allergic rhinitis, and for the relief of nasal congestion and eustachian tube congestion. Analgesics, antibiotics, or both may be administered concurrently, when indicated.

Contraindications: Antihistamines should not be used to treat lower respiratory tract symptoms, including asthma.

This product is contraindicated in patients with narrow-angle glaucoma or urinary retention, and in patients receiving monoamine oxidase (MAO) inhibitor therapy or within ten days of stopping such treatment. (See Drug Interactions section.) It is also contraindicated in patients with severe hypertension, severe coronary artery disease, hyperthyroidism, and in those who have shown hypersensitivity or idiosyncrasy to its components, to adrenergic agents, or to other drugs of similar chemical structures. Manifestations of patient idiosyncrasy to adrenergic agents include: insomnia, dizziness, weakness, tremor, or arrhythmias.

Warnings: TRINALIN REPETABS Tablets should be used with considerable caution in patients with: stenosing peptic ulcer, pyloroduodenal obstruction, urinary bladder obstruction due to symptomatic prostatic hypertrophy, or narrowing of the bladder neck. It should also be administered with caution to patients with cardiovascular disease, including hypertension or ischemic heart disease; increased intraocular pressure (See CONTRAINDICATIONS); diabetes mellitus, or in patients receiving digitalis or oral anticoagulants. Central nervous system stimulation and convulsions or cardiovascular collapse with accompanying hypotension may be produced by sympathomimetics.

Do not exceed recommended dosage.

Use in Activities Requiring Mental Alertness: Patients should be warned about engaging in activities requiring mental alertness, such as driving a car or operating appliances, machinery, etc.

Use in Patients Approximately 60 Years and Older: Antihistamines are more likely to cause dizziness, sedation, and hypotension in patients over 60 years of age. In these patients, sympathomimetics are also more likely to cause adverse reactions, such as confusion, hallucinations, convulsions, CNS depression, and death. For this reason, before considering the use of a repeat-action formulation, the safe use of a short-acting sympathomimetic in that particular patient should be demonstrated.

Precautions: General: Because of the atropine-like action of antihistamines, this product should be used with caution in patients with a history of bronchial asthma.

Information for Patients:
1. Products containing antihistamines may cause drowsiness.
2. Patients should not engage in activities requiring mental alertness, such as driving or operating machinery or appliances.
3. Alcohol or other sedative drugs may enhance the drowsiness caused by antihistamines.
4. Patients should not take TRINALIN REPETABS Tablets if they are receiving a monoamine oxidase inhibitor or within 10 days of stopping such treatment, or if they are receiving oral anticoagulants.
5. This medication should not be given to children less than 12 years of age.

Drug Interactions: MAO inhibitors prolong and intensify the effects of antihistamines. Concomitant use of antihistamines with alcohol, tricyclic antidepressants, barbiturates, or other central nervous system depressants may have an additive effect. The action of oral anticoagulants may be inhibited by antihistamines.

When sympathomimetic drugs are given to patients receiving monoamine oxidase inhibitors, hypertensive reactions, including hypertensive crises, may occur. The antihypertensive effects of methyldopa, mecamylamine, reserpine, and veratrum alkaloids may be reduced by sympathomimetics. Beta-adrenergic blocking agents may also interact with sympathomimetics. Increased ectopic pacemaker activity can occur when pseudoephedrine is used concomitantly with digitalis. Antacids increase the rate of absorption of pseudoephedrine, while kaolin decreases it.

Drug/Laboratory Test Interactions: The *in vitro* addition of pseudoephedrine to sera containing the cardiac isoenzyme MB of serum creatine phosphokinase progressively inhibits the activity of the enzyme. The inhibition becomes complete over six hours.

Carcinogenesis, Mutagenesis, and Impairment of Fertility: There is no animal or laboratory study of the mixture of azatadine maleate and pseudoephedrine sulfate to evaluate carcinogenesis or mutagenesis. Reproduction studies of this mixture in rats showed no evidence of impaired fertility.

Pregnancy Category C: Retarded fetal development and the presence of angulated hyoid wings were seen in the offspring of pregnant rabbits administered TRINALIN at about 12.5 times and 5 times the recommended human dosage, respectively; increased resorption was noted at about 25 times the human dosage. A decreased survival rate at day 21 was seen in rat pups born of mothers given TRINALIN during pregnancy at a dose about 12.5 times the human dosage. There are no adequate and well-controlled studies in pregnant women. TRINALIN REPETABS Tablets should be used during pregnancy only if the potential benefits to the mother justify the potential risks to the infant. (See Nonteratogenic Effects.)

Nonteratogenic Effects: Antihistamines should not be used in the third trimester of pregnancy, because newborns and premature infants may have severe reactions to them such as convulsions.

Nursing Mothers: It is not known whether these drugs are excreted in human milk. However, certain antihistamines and sympathomimetics are known to be excreted in human milk. Because of the higher risks of antihistamines for infants generally and for newborns and prematures in particular, a decision should be made whether to discontinue nursing or to discontinue the drug, taking into account the importance of the drug to the mother.

There is a report of irritability, excessive crying and disturbed sleeping patterns in a nursing infant whose mother had taken a product containing an antihistamine and pseudoephedrine.

Pediatric use: Safety and effectiveness in children below the age of 12 years have not been established.

Adverse Reactions: The following adverse reactions are associated with antihistamine and sympathomimetic drugs. (Those adverse reactions which occur most frequently with the antihistamines are underlined.)

General: Urticaria, drug rash, anaphylactic shock, photosensitivity, excessive perspiration, chills, dryness of mouth, nose, and throat.

Cardiovascular: Hypertension (see CONTRAINDICATIONS and WARNINGS), hypotension, arrhythmias and cardiovascular collapse, headache, palpitations, extrasystoles, tachycardia, angina.

Hematologic: Hemolytic anemia, hypoplastic anemia, thrombocytopenia, agranulocytosis.

Central Nervous System: Sedation, sleepiness, dizziness, vertigo, tinnitus, acute labyrinthitis, disturbed coordination, fatigue, mydriasis, confusion, restlessness, excitation, nervousness, tension, tremor, irritability, insomnia, euphoria, paresthesias, blurred vision, hysteria, neuritis, convulsions, fear, anxiety, hallucinations, CNS depression, weakness, pallor.

Gastrointestinal: Epigastric distress, anorexia, nausea, vomiting, diarrhea, constipation, abdominal cramps.

Genitourinary: Urinary frequency, urinary retention, dysuria, early menses.

Continued on next page

Information on Schering products appearing on these pages is effective as of September 30, 1984.

Schering—Cont.

Respiratory: Thickening of bronchial secretions, tightness of chest and wheezing, nasal stuffiness, respiratory difficulty.

Drug Abuse and Dependence: There is no information to indicate that abuse or dependency occurs with azatadine maleate.

Pseudoephedrine, like other central nervous system stimulants, has been abused. At high doses, subjects commonly experience an elevation of mood, a sense of increased energy and alertness, and decreased appetite. Some individuals become anxious, irritable, and loquacious. In addition to the marked euphoria, the user experiences a sense of markedly enhanced physical strength and mental capacity. With continued use, tolerance develops, the user increases the dose, and toxic signs and symptoms appear. Depression may follow rapid withdrawal.

Overdosage: In the event of overdosage, emergency treatment should be instituted immediately.
Manifestations of overdosage may vary from central nervous system depression (sedation, apnea, diminished mental alertness, cyanosis, coma, cardiovascular collapse) to stimulation (insomnia, hallucinations, tremors, or convulsions) to death. Other signs and symptoms may be euphoria, excitement, tachycardia, palpitations, thirst, perspiration, nausea, dizziness, tinnitus, ataxia, blurred vision, and hypertension or hypotension. Stimulation is particularly likely in children, as are atropine-like signs and symptoms (dry mouth; fixed, dilated pupils, flushing; hyperthermia; and gastrointestinal symptoms).

In large doses sympathomimetics may give rise to giddiness, headache, nausea, vomiting, sweating, thirst, tachycardia, precordial pain, palpitations, difficulty in micturition, muscular weakness and tenseness, anxiety, restlessness, and insomnia. Many patients can present a toxic psychosis with delusions and hallucinations. Some may develop cardiac arrhythmias, circulatory collapse, convulsions, coma, and respiratory failure.

The oral LD_{50} of the mixture of the two drugs in mature rats and mice was greater than 1700 mg/kg and 600 mg/kg, respectively.

Treatment—The patient should be induced to vomit, even if emesis has occurred spontaneously. Pharmacologically induced vomiting by the administration of ipecac syrup is a preferred method. However, vomiting should not be induced in patients with impaired consciousness. The action of ipecac is facilitated by physical activity and by the administration of eight to twelve fluid ounces of water. If emesis does not occur within fifteen minutes, the dose of ipecac should be repeated. Precautions against aspiration must be taken, especially in infants and children. Following emesis, any drug remaining in the stomach may be adsorbed by activated charcoal administered as a slurry with water. If vomiting is unsuccessful or contraindicated, gastric lavage should be performed. Isotonic and one-half isotonic saline are the lavage solutions of choice. Saline cathartics, such as milk of magnesia, draw water into the bowel by osmosis and therefore may be valuable for their action in rapid dilution of bowel content. Dialysis is of little value in antihistamine poisoning. After emergency treatment the patient should continue to be medically monitored.

Treatment of the signs and symptoms of overdosage is symptomatic and supportive. Stimulants (analeptic agents) should <u>not</u> be used. Vasopressors may be used to treat <u>hypotension</u>. Short-acting barbiturates, diazepam, or paraldehyde may be administered to control seizures. Hyperpyrexia, especially in children, may require treatment with tepid water sponge baths or a hypothermic blanket. Apnea is treated with ventilatory support.

Dosage and Administration: TRINALIN REPETABS Tablets ARE NOT INTENDED FOR USE IN CHILDREN UNDER 12 YEARS OF AGE. The usual adult dosage is one tablet twice a day.

How Supplied: TRINALIN REPETABS Tablets contain 1 mg azatadine maleate and 120 mg pseudoephedrine sulfate. TRINALIN REPETABS Tablets are coral-colored, sugar-coated tablets branded in black with the Schering trademark, or the product name and product identification numbers, 703; bottle of 100 (NDC-0085-0703-04).

Store between 2° and 30°C (36° and 86°F).
Copyright © 1981, Schering Corporation. All rights reserved.
Revised 11/81
Shown in Product Identification Section, page 435

VALISONE® ℞
[*val'ĭ-sōn*]
brand of betamethasone valerate
Cream, USP 0.1%
Ointment, USP 0.1%
Lotion, USP 0.1%
Reduced Strength Cream, USP 0.01%
(potency expressed as betamethasone)
For Dermatologic Use Only
Not for Ophthalmic Use

Description: VALISONE **Cream, Reduced Strength Cream, Ointment** and **Lotion** contain betamethasone valerate, USP, a synthetic adrenocorticoid for dermatologic use. Betamethasone, an analog of prednisolone, has a high degree of corticosteroid activity and a slight degree of mineralocorticosteroid activity. Betamethasone valerate is the 17-valerate ester of betamethasone. Chemically, betamethasone valerate is 9-Fluoro-11β,17,21-trihydroxy-16β,methylpregna-1,4-diene-3,20-dione 17-valerate, with the empirical formula $C_{27}H_{37}FO_6$, and a molecular weight of 476.58.

Betamethasone valerate is a white to practically white, odorless crystalline powder, and is practically insoluble in water, freely soluble in acetone and in chloroform, soluble in alcohol, and slightly soluble in benzene and in ether.

Each gram of VALISONE **Cream** 0.1% contains: 1.2 mg betamethasone valerate, USP (equivalent to 1.0 mg betamethasone), in an aqueous hydrophilic emollient cream consisting of mineral oil, white petrolatum, polyethylene glycol 1000 monocetyl ether, cetearyl alcohol, monobasic sodium phosphate, and phosphoric acid; chlorocresol and propylene glycol as preservatives.

Each gram of VALISONE **Ointment** 0.1% contains: 1.2 mg betamethasone valerate, USP (equivalent to 1.0 mg betamethasone), in an ointment base of mineral oil, white petrolatum, and hydrogenated lanolin.

Each gram of VALISONE **Lotion** 0.1% contains: 1.2 mg betamethasone valerate, USP (equivalent to 1.0 mg betamethasone) in a lotion base of isopropyl alcohol (47.5%) and water slightly thickened with carbomer 934P; the pH is adjusted to approximately 4.7 with sodium hydroxide.

Each gram of VALISONE **Reduced Strength Cream** 0.01% contains: 0.12 mg betamethasone valerate, USP (equivalent to 0.1 mg betamethasone), in an aqueous hydrophilic emollient cream consisting of mineral oil, white petrolatum, polyethylene glycol 1000 monocetyl ether, cetearyl alcohol, monobasic sodium phosphate, and phosphoric acid; chlorocresol and propylene glycol as preservatives.

Clinical Pharmacology: The corticosteroids are a class of compounds comprising steroid hormones secreted by the adrenal cortex and their synthetic analogs. In pharmacologic doses corticosteroids are used primarily for their anti-inflammatory and/or immunosuppressive effects.

Topical corticosteroids, such as betamethasone valerate, are effective in the treatment of corticosteroid-responsive dermatoses primarily because of their anti-inflammatory, anti-pruritic, and vasoconstrictive actions. However, while the physiologic, pharmacologic, and clinical effects of the corticosteroids are well-known, the exact mechanisms of their actions in each disease are uncertain. Betamethasone valerate, a corticosteroid, has been shown to have topical (dermatologic) and systemic pharmacologic and metabolic effects characteristic of this class of drugs.

Pharmacokinetics: The extent of percutaneous absorption of topical corticosteroids is determined by many factors including the vehicle, the integrity of the epidermal barrier, and the use of occlusive dressings.

Topical corticosteroids can be absorbed from normal intact skin. Inflammation and/or other disease processes in the skin increase percutaneous absorption. Occlusive dressings substantially increase the percutaneous absorption of topical corticosteroids. Thus, occlusive dressings may be a valuable therapeutic adjunct for treatment of resistant dermatoses.

Once absorbed through the skin, topical corticosteroids are handled through pharmacokinetic pathways similar to systemically administered corticosteroids. Corticosteroids are bound to plasma proteins in varying degrees. Corticosteroids are metabolized primarily in the liver and are then excreted by the kidneys. Some of the topical corticosteroids and their metabolites are also excreted into the bile.

Indications and Usage: VALISONE **Cream, Reduced Strength Cream, Ointment** and **Lotion** are indicated for relief of the inflammatory and pruritic manifestations of corticosteroid-responsive dermatoses.

Contraindications: VALISONE **Cream, Reduced Strength Cream, Ointment,** and **Lotion** are contraindicated in patients who are hypersensitive to betamethasone valerate, to other corticosteroids, or to any ingredient in this preparation.

Precautions: General: Systemic absorption of topical corticosteroids has produced reversible hypothalamic-pituitary-adrenal (HPA) axis suppression, manifestations of Cushing's syndrome, hyperglycemia, and glucosuria in some patients. Conditions which augment systemic absorption include the application of the more potent steroids, use over large surface areas, prolonged use, and the addition of occlusive dressings.

Therefore, patients receiving a large dose of a potent topical steroid applied to a large surface area or under an occlusive dressing should be evaluated periodically for evidence of HPA axis suppression by using the urinary free cortisol and ACTH stimulation tests. If HPA axis suppression is noted, an attempt should be made to withdraw the drug, to reduce the frequency of application, or to substitute a less potent steroid.

Recovery of HPA axis function is generally prompt and complete upon discontinuation of the drug. Infrequently, signs and symptoms of steroid withdrawal may occur, requiring supplemental systemic corticosteroids.

Children may absorb proportionally larger amounts of topical corticosteroids and thus be more susceptible to systemic toxicity. (See **PRECAUTIONS-Pediatric Use.**)

If irritation develops, topical corticosteroids should be discontinued and appropriate therapy instituted.

In the presence of dermatological infections, the use of an appropriate antifungal or antibacterial agent should be instituted. If a favorable response does not occur promptly, the corticosteroid should be discontinued until the infection has been adequately controlled.

Information for Patients: Patients using topical corticosteroids should receive the following information and instructions:

1. This medication is to be used as directed by the physician. It is for external use only. Avoid contact with the eyes.
2. Patients should be advised not to use this medication for any disorder other than for which it was prescribed.
3. The treated skin area should not be bandaged or otherwise covered or wrapped as to be occlusive unless directed by the physician.
4. Patients should report any signs of local adverse reactions especially under occlusive dressing.
5. Parents of pediatric patients should be advised not to use tight-fitting diapers or plastic pants on a child being treated in the diaper area, as these garments may constitute occlusive dressings.

Laboratory Tests: The following tests may be helpful in evaluating HPA axis suppression:

Urinary free cortisol test
ACTH stimulation test

Carcinogenesis, Mutagenesis, and Impairment of Fertility: Long-term animal studies have not been performed to evaluate the carcinogenic potential or the effect on fertility of topical corticosteroids. Studies to determine mutagenicity with prednisolone have revealed negative results.

Pregnancy Category C: Corticosteroids are generally teratogenic in laboratory animals when administered systemically at relatively low dosage levels. The more potent corticosteroids have been shown to be teratogenic after dermal application in laboratory animals. There are no adequate and well-controlled studies in pregnant women on teratogenic effects from topically applied corticosteroids. Therefore, topical corticosteroids should be used during pregnancy only if the potential benefit justifies the potential risk to the fetus. Drugs of this class should not be used extensively on pregnant patients, in large amounts, or for prolonged periods of time.

Nursing Mothers: It is not known whether topical administration of corticosteroids could result in sufficient systemic absorption to produce detectable quantities in breast milk. Systemically administered corticosteroids are secreted into breast milk in quantities not likely to have a deleterious effect on the infant. Nevertheless, caution should be exercised when topical corticosteroids are prescribed for a nursing woman.

Pediatric Use: Pediatric patients may demonstrate greater susceptibility to topical corticosteroid-induced HPA axis suppression and Cushing's syndrome than mature patients because of a larger skin surface area to body weight ratio. Hypothalamic-pituitary-adrenal (HPA) axis suppression, Cushing's syndrome, and intracranial hypertension, have been reported in children receiving topical corticosteroids. Manifestations of adrenal suppression in children include linear growth retardation, delayed weight gain, low plasma cortisol levels, and absence of response to ACTH stimulation. Manifestations of intracranial hypertension include bulging fontanelles, headaches, and bilateral papilledema.

Administration of topical corticosteroids to children should be limited to the least amount compatible with an effective therapeutic regimen. Chronic corticosteroid therapy may interfere with the growth and development of children.

Adverse Reactions: The following local adverse reactions have been reported with topical dermatologic corticosteroids, especially under occlusive dressings: burning; itching; irritation; dryness; folliculitis; hypertrichosis; acneiform eruptions; hypopigmentation; perioral dermatitis; allergic contact dermatitis; maceration of the skin; secondary infection; skin atrophy; striae; miliaria.

Systemic absorption of topical corticosteroids has produced reversible hypothalamic-pituitary-adrenal (HPA) axis suppression, manifestations of Cushing's syndrome, hyperglycemia, and glucosuria in some patients.

Overdosage: Topically applied corticosteroids can be absorbed in sufficient amounts to produce systemic effects (see PRECAUTIONS.)

Dosage and Administration: VALISONE Cream: Apply a thin film of VALISONE Cream 0.1% to the affected skin areas one to three times a day. Dosage once or twice a day is often effective.
VALISONE Ointment: Apply a thin film of VALISONE Ointment 0.1% to the affected skin areas one to three times a day. Dosage once or twice a day is often effective.
VALISONE Lotion: Apply a few drops of VALISONE Lotion 0.1% to the affected area and massage lightly until it disappears. Apply twice daily, in the morning and at night. Dosage may be increased in stubborn cases. Following improvement, apply once daily. For the most effective and economical use, apply nozzle very close to affected area and gently squeeze bottle.
VALISONE Reduced Strength Cream: Apply a thin film of VALISONE Reduced Strength Cream to the affected skin areas one to three times daily. Commonly, treatment twice a day is adequate. In some cases, treatment three times a day is necessary; in others, once a day suffices.

How Supplied: VALISONE Cream 0.1% is available in 15-gram (NDC 0085-0136-04), 45-gram (NDC 0085-0136-06), and 110-gram (NDC 0085-0136-07) tubes; boxes of one; and a 430-gram jar (NDC 0085-0136-08).
VALISONE Lotion 0.1% is available in 20 ml (18.7 g) (NDC 0085-0002-03), and 60 ml (56.2 g) (NDC 0085-0002-05) plastic squeeze bottles; boxes of one.
Protect from light. Store in carton until contents are used.
VALISONE Ointment 0.1% is supplied in 15-gram (NDC 0085-0898-04), and 45-gram (NDC 0085-0898-06) tubes; boxes of one.
VALISONE Reduced Strength Cream 0.01% is supplied in 15-gram (NDC 0085-0929-04), and 60-gram (NDC 0085-0929-08) tubes; boxes of one.
Store between 2° and 30°C (36° and 86°F).
Revised 4/84
Copyright© 1969, 1982, 1983, 1984, Schering Corporation. All rights reserved.

VANCENASE® Nasal Inhaler ℞
[van'sen-ās]
brand of beclomethasone dipropionate, USP
For Nasal Inhalation Only

Description: Beclomethasone dipropionate, USP, the active component of VANCENASE Nasal Inhaler, is an anti-inflammatory steroid having the chemical name, 9-Chloro-11β,17,21-trihydroxy-16β-methylpregna-1, 4-diene-3, 20-dione 17, 21-dipropionate.
Beclomethasone dipropionate is a white to creamy-white odorless powder with a molecular weight of 521.25. It is very slightly soluble in water; very soluble in chloroform; and freely soluble in acetone and in alcohol.
VANCENASE Nasal Inhaler is a metered-dose aerosol unit containing a microcrystalline suspension of beclomethasone dipropionate-trichloromonofluoromethane clathrate in a mixture of propellants (trichloromonofluoromethane and dichlorodifluoromethane) with oleic acid. Each canister contains beclomethasone dipropionate-trichloromonofluoromethane clathrate having a molecular proportion of beclomethasone dipropionate to trichloromonofluoromethane between 3:1 and 3:2. Each actuation delivers from the nasal adapter a quantity of clathrate equivalent to 42 mcg of beclomethasone dipropionate, USP. The contents of one canister provide at least 200 metered doses.

Clinical Pharmacology: Beclomethasone 17,21-dipropionate is a diester of beclomethasone, a synthetic corticosteroid which is chemically related to dexamethasone. Beclomethasone differs from dexamethasone only in having a chlorine at the 9-α position in place of a fluorine. Animal studies showed that beclomethasone dipropionte has potent glucocorticoid and weak mineralocorticoid activity. The mechanisms for the anti-inflammatory action of beclomethasone dipropionate are unknown. The precise mechanism of the aerosolized drug's action in the nose is also unknown. Biopsies of nasal mucosa obtained during clinical studies showed no histopathologic changes when beclomethasone dipropionate was administered intranasally.
The effects of beclomethasone dipropionate on hypothalamic-pituitary-adrenal (HPA) function have been evaluated in adult volunteers, by other routes of administration. Studies are currently being undertaken with beclomethasone dipropionate by the intranasal route, which may demonstrate that there is more or that there is less absorption by this route of administration. There was no suppression of early morning plasma cortisol concentrations when beclomethasone dipropionate was administered in a dose of 1000 mcg/day for one month as an oral aerosol or for three days by intramuscular injection. However, partial suppression of plasma cortisol concentration was observed when beclomethasone dipropionate was administered in doses of 2000 mcg/day either by oral aerosol or intramuscularly. Immediate suppression of plasma cortisol concentrations was observed after single doses of 4000 mcg of beclomethasone dipropionate. Suppression of HPA function (reduction of early morning plasma cortisol levels) has been reported in adult patients who received 1600 mcg daily doses of oral beclomethasone dipropionate for one month. In clinical studies using beclomethasone dipropionate intranasally, there was no evidence of decreased adrenal insufficiency.

Beclomethasone dipropionate is sparingly soluble. When given by nasal inhalation in the form of an aerosolized suspension, the drug is deposited primarily in the nasal passages. A portion of the drug is swallowed. Absorption occurs rapidly from all respiratory and gastrointestinal tissues. There is no evidence of tissue storage of beclomethasone dipropionate or its metabolites. *In vitro* studies, have shown that tissue other than the liver (lung slices) can rapidly metabolize beclomethasone dipropionate to beclomethasone 17-monopropionate and more slowly to free beclomethasone (which has very weak anti-inflammatory activity). However, irrespective of the route of entry, the principal route of excretion of the drug and its metabolites is the feces. In humans, 12% to 15% of an orally administered dose of beclomethasone dipropionate is excreted in the urine as both conjugated and free metabolites of the drug. The half-life of beclomethasone dipropionate in humans is approximately 15 hours.
Studies have shown that the degree of binding to plasma proteins is 87%.

Indications and Usage: VANCENASE Nasal Inhaler is indicated for the relief of the symptoms of seasonal or perennial rhinitis, in those cases poorly responsive to conventional treatment.
Clinical studies have shown that improvement is usually apparent within a few days. However, symptomatic relief may not occur in some patients for as long as two weeks. Although systemic effects are minimal at recommended doses, VANCENASE should not be continued beyond three weeks in the absence of significant symptomatic improvement. VANCENASE should not be used in the presence of untreated localized infection involving the nasal mucosa.

Contraindications: Hypersensitivity to any of the ingredients of this preparation contraindicates its use.

Warnings: The replacement of a systemic corticosteroid with VANCENASE Nasal Inhaler can be accompanied by signs of adrenal insufficiency.
When transferred to VANCENASE Nasal Inhaler, careful attention must be given to patients previously treated for prolonged periods with systemic corticosteroids. This is particularly important in those patients who have associated asthma or other clinical conditions, where too rapid a decrease in systemic corticosteroids may cause a severe exacerbation of their symptoms.
Studies have shown that the combined administration of alternate day prednisone systemic treatment and orally inhaled beclomethasone increased the likelihood of HPA suppression compared to a therapeutic dose of either one alone. Therefore, VANCENASE treatment should be used with caution in patients already on alternate day prednisone regimens for any disease.

Precautions: *General:* During withdrawal from oral steroids, some patients may experience symptoms of withdrawal, e.g., joint and/or muscular pain, lassitude, and depression.
In clinical studies with beclomethasone dipropionate administered intranasally, the development of localized infections of the nose and pharynx with *Candida albicans* has occurred only rarely. When such an infection develops, it may require treatment with appropriate local therapy or discontinuance of treatment with VANCENASE Nasal Inhaler.

Continued on next page

Information on Schering products appearing on these pages is effective as of September 30, 1984.

Schering—Cont.

Beclomethasone dipropionate is absorbed into the circulation. Use of excessive doses of VANCENASE Nasal Inhaler may suppress HPA function.

VANCENASE should be used with caution, if at all, in patients with active or quiescent tuberculous infections of the respiratory tract, or in untreated fungal, bacterial, systemic viral infections, or ocular herpes simplex.

Because of the inhibitory effect of corticosteroids on wound healing, patients who have experienced recent nasal septal ulcers, nasal surgery, or trauma should not use a nasal corticosteroid until healing has occurred.

Although systemic effects have been minimal with recommended doses, this potential increases with excessive doses. Therefore, larger than recommended doses should be avoided.

Information for Patients: Patients should use VANCENASE Nasal Inhaler at regular intervals since its effectiveness depends on its regular use. The patient should take the medication as directed. It is not acutely effective and the prescribed dosage should not be increased. Instead, nasal vasoconstrictors or oral antihistamines may be needed until the effects of VANCENASE Nasal Inhaler are fully manifested. One to two weeks may pass before full relief is obtained. The patient should contact the doctor if symptoms do not improve, or if the condition worsens, or if sneezing or nasal irritation occurs. For the proper use of this unit and to attain maximum improvement, the patient should read and follow the accompanying Patient's Instructions carefully.

Carcinogenesis, Mutagenesis, Impairment of Fertility: Treatment of rats for a total of 95-weeks, 13 weeks by inhalation and 82 weeks by the oral route, resulted in no evidence of carcinogenic activity. Mutagenic studies have not been performed.

Impairment of fertility, as evidenced by inhibition of the estrus cycle in dogs, was observed following treatment by the oral route. No inhibition of the estrus cycle in dogs was seen following treatment with beclomethasone dipropionte by the inhalation route.

Pregnancy Category C: Like other corticoids, parenteral (subcutaneous) beclomethasone dipropionate has been shown to be teratogenic and embryocidal in the mouse and rabbit when given in doses approximately ten times the human dose. In these studies beclomethasone was found to produce fetal resorption, cleft palate, agnathia, microstomia, absence of tongue, delayed ossification, and agenesis of the thymus. No teratogenic or embryocidal effects have been seen in the rat when beclomethasone dipropionate was administered by inhalation at ten times the human dose or orally at 1000 times the human dose. There are no adequate and well-controlled studies in pregnant women. Beclomethasone dipropionate should be used during pregnancy only if the potential benefit justifies the potential risk to the fetus.

Nonteratogenic effects: Hypoadrenalism may occur in infants born of mothers receiving corticosteroids during pregnancy. Such infants should be carefully observed.

Nursing Mothers: It is not known whether beclomethasone dipropionate is excreted in human milk. Because other corticosteroids are excreted in human milk, caution should be exercised when VANCENASE Nasal Inhaler is administered to nursing women.

Pediatric Use: Safety and effectiveness in children below the age of 12 years have not been established.

Adverse Reactions: In general, side effects in clinical studies have been primarily associated with the nasal mucous membranes. Adverse reactions reported in controlled clinical trials and long-term open studies in patients treated with VANCENASE are described below.

Sensations of irritation and burning in the nose (11 per 100 patients) following the use of VANCENASE Nasal Inhaler have been reported. Also, occasional sneezing attacks (10 per 100 patients) have occurred immediately following the use of the intranasal inhaler.

Localized infections of the nose and pharynx with *Candida albicans* have occurred rarely. (see PRECAUTIONS)

Less than 2 per 100 patients reported transient episodes of bloody discharge from the nose.

Ulceration of the nasal mucosa has been reported rarely. Systemic corticosteroid side effects were not reported during the controlled clinical trials. If recommended doses are exceeded, however, or if individuals are particularly sensitive, symptoms of hypercorticism, i.e., Cushing's syndrome could occur.

Dosage and Administration: *Adults and Children 12 years of age and over:* the usual dosage is one inhalation (42 mcg) in each nostril two to four times a day (total dose 168–336 mcg/day). Patients can often be maintained on a maximum dose of one inhalation in each nostril three times a day (252 mcg/day).

In patients who respond to VANCENASE Nasal Inhaler, an improvement of the symptoms of seasonal or perennial rhinitis usually becomes apparent within one to five days after the start of VANCENASE Inhaler therapy.

The therapeutic effects of corticosteroids, unlike those of decongestants are not immediate. This should be explained to the patient in advance in order to ensure cooperation and continuation of treatment with the prescribed dosage regimen.

VANCENASE Nasal Inhaler is **not** recommended for children below 12 years of age.

In the presence of excessive nasal mucus secretion or edema of the nasal mucosa, the drug may fail to reach the site of intended action. In such cases it is advisable to use a nasal vasoconstrictor during the first two to three days of VANCENASE Nasal Inhaler therapy.

Directions for Use: Illustrated PATIENT INSTRUCTIONS for proper use accompany each package of VANCENASE Nasal Inhaler.

CONTENTS UNDER PRESSURE. Do not puncture. Do not use or store near heat or open flame. Exposure to temperatures above 120°F may cause bursting. Never throw container into fire or incinerator. Keep out of reach of children.

Overdosage: When used at excessive doses, systemic corticosteroid effects such as hypercorticism and adrenal suppression may appear. If such symptoms appear, the dosage should be decreased.

The oral LD$_{50}$ of beclomethasone dipropionate is greater than 1 g/kg in rodents. One canister of VANCENASE Nasal Inhaler contains 8.4 mg of beclomethasone dipropionate, therefore acute overdosage is unlikely.

How Supplied: VANCENASE Nasal Inhaler, 16.8 g canister; box of one. Supplied with nasal adapter and PATIENT'S INSTRUCTIONS; (NDC 0085-0041-06).

Store between 2° and 30°C (36° and 86°F).

Revised 9/81

Copyright ©1981, Schering Corporation. All rights reserved.

Shown in Product Identification Section, page 435

VANCERIL® Inhaler ℞
[*van'ser-il*]
brand of beclomethasone dipropionate, USP
FOR ORAL INHALATION ONLY

Description: Beclomethasone dipropionate, USP, the active component of VANCERIL Inhaler, is an anti-inflammatory steroid having the chemical name 9-Chloro-11β,17-21-trihydroxy-16 β-methylpregna-1,4-diene-3, 20-dione 17,21-dipropionate.

VANCERIL Inhaler is a metered-dose aerosol unit containing a microcrystalline suspension of beclomethasone dipropionate-trichloromonofluoromethane clathrate in a mixture of propellants (trichloromonofluoromethane and dichlorodifluoromethane) with oleic acid. Each canister contains beclomethasone dipropionate-trichloromonofluoromethane clathrate having a molecular proportion of beclomethasone dipropionate to trichloromonofluoromethane between 3:1 and 3:2. Each actuation delivers from the mouthpiece a quantity of clathrate equivalent to 42 mcg. of beclomethasone dipropionate, USP. The contents of one canister provide at least 200 oral inhalations.

Clinical Pharmacology: Beclomethasone 17,21-dipropionate is a diester of beclomethasone, a synthetic corticosteroid which is chemically related to prednisolone. Beclomethasone differs from prednisolone only in having a chlorine at the 9-alpha and a methyl group at the 16-beta position in place of hydrogen. Animal studies showed that beclomethasone dipropionate has potent anti-inflammatory activity. When administered systemically to mice, the anti-inflammatory activity was accompanied by other typical features of glucocorticoid action including thymic involution, liver glycogen deposition, and pituitary-adrenal suppression. However, after systemic administration to rats, the anti-inflammatory action was associated with little or no effect on other tests of glucocorticoid activity.

Beclomethasone dipropionate is sparingly soluble and is poorly mobilized from subcutaneous or intramuscular injection sites. However, systemic absorption occurs after all routes of administration. When given to animals in the form of an aerosolized suspension of the trichloromonofluoromethane clathrate, the drug is deposited in the mouth and nasal passages, the trachea and principal bronchi, and in the lung; a considerable portion of the drug is also swallowed. Absorption occurs rapidly from all respiratory and gastrointestinal tissues, as indicated by the rapid clearance of radioactively labeled drug from local tissues and appearance of tracer in the circulation. There is no evidence of tissue storage of beclomethasone dipropionate or its metabolites. Lung slices can metabolize beclomethasone dipropionate rapidly to beclomethasone 17-monopropionate and more slowly to free beclomethasone (which has very weak anti-inflammatory activity). However, irrespective of the route of administration (injection, oral, or aerosol), the principal route of excretion of the drug and its metabolites is the feces. Less than 10% of the drug and its metabolites is excreted in the urine. In humans, 12% to 15% of an orally administered dose of beclomethasone dipropionate was excreted in the urine as both conjugated and free metabolites of the drug.

The mechanisms responsible for the anti-inflammatory action of beclomethasone dipropionate are unknown. The precise mechanism of the aerosolized drug's action in the lung is also unknown.

Indications: VANCERIL Inhaler is indicated only for patients who require chronic treatment with corticosteroids for control of the symptoms of bronchial asthma. Such patients would include those already receiving systemic corticosteroids, and selected patients who are inadequately controlled on a non-steroid regimen and in whom steroid therapy has been withheld because of concern over potential adverse effects.

VANCERIL Inhaler is NOT indicated:
1. For relief of asthma which can be controlled by bronchodilators and other non-steroid medications.
2. In patients who require systemic corticosteroid treatment infrequently.
3. In the treatment of non-asthmatic bronchitis.

Contraindications: VANCERIL Inhaler is contraindicated in the primary treatment of status asthmaticus or other acute episodes of asthma where intensive measures are required.

Hypersensitivity to any of the ingredients of this preparation contraindicates its use.

Warnings:

Particular care is needed in patients who are transferred from systemically active corticosteroids to VANCERIL Inhaler because deaths due to adrenal insufficiency have occurred in asthmatic patients during and after transfer from systemic corticosteroids to aerosol beclomethasone dipropionate. After withdrawal from systemic corticosteroids, a number of months are required for recovery of hypothalamic-pituitary-adrenal (HPA) function. During this period of HPA suppression, patients may exhibit signs and symptoms of adrenal insufficiency when exposed to trauma, surgery or infections, particularly gastroenteritis. Although VANCERIL Inhaler may provide control of asthmatic symptoms during these episodes, it does NOT provide the systemic steroid which is necessary for coping with these emergencies.

During periods of stress or a severe asthmatic attack, patients who have been withdrawn from systemic corticosteroids should be instructed to resume systemic steroids (in large doses) immediately and to contact their physician for further instruction. These patients should also be instructed to carry a warning card indicating that they may need supplementary systemic steroids during periods of stress or a severe asthma attack. To assess the risk of adrenal insuffficiency in emergency situations, routine tests of adrenal cortical function, including measurement of early morning resting cortisol levels, should be performed periodically in all patients. An early morning resting cortisol level may be accepted as normal only if it falls at or near the normal mean level.

Localized infections with *Candida albicans* or *Aspergillus niger* have occurred frequently in the mouth and pharynx and occasionally in the larynx. Positive cultures for oral *Candida* may be present in up to 75% of patients. Although the frequency of clinically apparent infection is considerably lower, these infections may require treatment with appropriate antifungal therapy or discontinuance of treatment with VANCERIL Inhaler.

VANCERIL Inhaler is not to be regarded as a bronchodilator and is not indicated for rapid relief of bronchospasm.

Patients should be instructed to contact their physician immediately when episodes of asthma which are not responsive to bronchodilators occur during the course of treatment with VANCERIL. During such episodes, patients may require therapy with systemic corticosteroids.

There is no evidence that control of asthma can be achieved by the administration of VANCERIL in amounts greater than the recommended doses.

Transfer of patients from systemic steroid therapy to VANCERIL Inhaler may unmask allergic conditions previously suppressed by the systemic steroid therapy, e.g., rhinitis, conjunctivitis, and eczema.

Precautions: During withdrawal from oral steroids, some patients may experience symptoms of systemically active steroid withdrawal, e.g., joint and/or muscular pain, lassitude and depression, despite maintenance or even improvement of respiratory function (See DOSAGE AND ADMINISTRATION for details).

In responsive patients, beclomethasone dipropionate may permit control of asthmatic symptoms without suppression of HPA function, as discussed below (See CLINICAL STUDIES). Since beclomethasone dipropionate is absorbed into the circulation and can be systemically active, the beneficial effects of VANCERIL Inhaler in minimizing or preventing HPA dysfunction may be expected only when recommended dosages are not exceeded.

The long-term effects of beclomethasone dipropionate in human subjects are still unknown. In particular, the local effects of the agent on developmental or immunologic processes in the mouth, pharynx, trachea, and lung are unknown. There is also no information about the possible long-term systemic effects of the agent.

The potential effects of VANCERIL on acute, recurrent, or chronic pulmonary infections, including active or quiescent tuberculosis, are not known. Similarly, the potential effects of long-term administration of the drug on lung or other tissues are unknown.

Pulmonary infiltrates with eosinophilia may occur in patients on VANCERIL Inhaler therapy. Although it is possible that in some patients this state may become manifest because of systemic steroid withdrawal when inhalational steroids are administered, a causative role for beclomethasone dipropionate and/or its vehicle cannot be ruled out.

Use in Pregnancy: Glucocorticoids are known teratogens in rodent species and beclomethasone dipropionate is no exception.

Teratology studies were done in rats, mice, and rabbits treated with subcutaneous beclomethasone dipropionate. Beclomethasone dipropionate was found to produce fetal resorptions, cleft palate, agnathia, microstomia, absence of tongue, delayed ossification and partial agenesis of the thymus. Well-controlled trials relating to fetal risk in humans are not available. Glucocorticoids are secreted in human milk. It is not known whether beclomethasone dipropionate would be secreted in human milk but it is safe to assume that it is likely. The use of beclomethasone dipropionate in pregnancy, nursing mothers, or women of childbearing potential requires that the possible benefits of the drug be weighed against the potential hazards to the mother, embryo, or fetus. Infants born of mothers who have received substantial doses of corticosteroids during pregnancy should be carefully observed for hypoadrenalism.

Adverse Reactions: Deaths due to adrenal insufficiency have occurred in asthmatic patients during and after transfer from systemic corticosteroids to aerosol beclomethasone dipropionate (See WARNINGS).

Suppression of HPA function (reduction of early morning plasma cortisol levels) has been reported in adult patients who received 1600 mcg. daily doses of VANCERIL for one month. A few patients on VANCERIL have complained of hoarseness or dry mouth. Bronchospasm and rash have been reported rarely.

Dosage and Administration: Adults: The usual dosage is two inhalations (84 mcg.) given three or four times a day. In patients with severe asthma, it is advisable to start with 12 to 16 inhalations a day and adjust the dosage downward according to the response of the patient. The maximal daily intake should not exceed 20 inhalations, 840 mcg. (0.84 mg.), in adults.

Children 6 to 12 years of age: The usual dosage is one or two inhalations (42 to 84 mcg.) given three or four times a day according to the response of the patient. The maximal daily intake should not exceed ten inhalations, 420 mcg. (0.42 mg.), in children 6 to 12 years of age. Insufficient clinical data exist with respect to the administration of VANCERIL Inhaler in children below the age of 6.

Rinsing the mouth after inhalation is advised.

Patients receiving bronchodilators by inhalation should be advised to use the bronchodilator before VANCERIL Inhaler in order to enhance penetration of beclomethasone dipropionate into the bronchial tree. After use of an aerosol bronchodilator, several minutes should elapse before use of the VANCERIL Inhaler to reduce the potential toxicity from the inhaled fluorocarbon propellants in the two aerosols.

Different considerations must be given to the following groups of patients in order to obtain the full therapeutic benefit of VANCERIL Inhaler.

Patients not receiving systemic steroids: The use of VANCERIL Inhaler is straightforward in patients who are inadequately controlled with nonsteroid medications but in whom systemic steroid therapy has been withheld because of concern over potential adverse reactions. In patients who respond to VANCERIL, an improvement in pulmonary function is usually apparent within one to four weeks after the start of VANCERIL Inhaler.

Patients receiving systemic steroids: In those patients dependent on systemic steroids, transfer to VANCERIL and subsequent management may be more difficult because recovery from impaired adrenal function is usually slow. Such suppression has been known to last for up to 12 months. Clinical studies, however, have demonstrated that VANCERIL may be effective in the management of these asthmatic patients and may permit replacement or significant reduction in the dosage of systemic corticosteroids.

The patient's asthma should be reasonably stable before treatment with VANCERIL Inhaler is started. Initially, the aerosol should be used concurrently with the patient's usual maintenance dose of systemic steroid. After approximately one week, gradual withdrawal of the systemic steroid is started by reducing the daily or alternate daily dose. The next reduction is made after an interval of one or two weeks, depending on the response of the patient. Generally, these decrements should not exceed 2.5 mg. of prednisone or its equivalent. A slow rate of withdrawal cannot be overemphasized. During withdrawal, some patients may experience symptoms of systemically active steroid withdrawal, e.g., joint and/or muscular pain, lassitude and depression, despite maintenance or even improvement of respiratory function. Such patients should be encouraged to continue with the Inhaler but should be watched carefully for objective signs of adrenal insufficiency, such as hypotension and weight loss. If evidence of adrenal insufficiency occurs, the systemic steroid dose should be boosted temporarily and thereafter further withdrawal should continue more slowly.

During periods of stress or a severe asthma attack, transfer patients will require supplementary treatment with systemic steroids. Exacerbations of asthma which occur during the course of treatment with VANCERIL Inhaler should be treated with a short course of systemic steroid which is gradually tapered as these symptoms subside. There is no evidence that control of asthma can be achieved by administration of VANCERIL in amounts greater than the recommended doses.

Directions for Use: Illustrated patient instructions for proper use accompany each package of VANCERIL Inhaler.

CONTENTS UNDER PRESSURE. Do not puncture. Do not use or store near heat or open flame. Exposure to temperatures above 120°F. may cause bursting. Never throw container into fire or incinerator. Keep out of reach of children.

How Supplied: VANCERIL Inhaler 16.8 g canister supplied with an oral adapter and patient's instructions; box of one. (NDC-0085-0736-04).

Store between 2° and 30°C (36° and 86°F).

Animal Pharmacology and Toxicology: Studies in a number of animal species including rats, rabbits, and dogs have shown no unusual toxicity during acute experiments. However, the effects of beclomethasone dipropionate in producing signs of glucocorticoid excess during chronic administration by various routes were dose related.

Clinical Studies: The effects of beclomethasone dipropionate on hypothalamic-pituitary-adrenal (HPA) function have been evaluated in adult volunteers. There was no suppression of early morning plasma cortisol concentrations when beclomethasone dipropionate was administered in a dose of 1000 mcg./day for one month as an aerosol or for three days by intramuscular injection. However, partial suppression of plasma cortisol concentration was observed when beclomethasone dipropionate was administered in doses of 2000 mcg./day either intramuscularly or by aerosol. Immediate suppression of plasma cortisol concentrations was observed after single doses of 4000 mcg. of beclomethasone dipropionate.

In one study, the effects of beclomethasone dipropionate on HPA function were examined in patients with asthma. There was no change in basal early morning plasma cortisol concentrations or in the cortisol responses to tetracosactrin (ACTH 1:24) stimulation after daily administration of 400, 800 or 1200 mcg. of beclomethasone dipropionate for 28 days. After daily administration of 1600 mcg. each day for 28 days, there was a slight reduction in basal cortisol concentrations and a statisti-

Continued on next page

Information on Schering products appearing on these pages is effective as of September 30, 1984.

Schering—Cont.

cally significant (p < .01) reduction in plasma cortisol responses to tetracosactrin stimulation. The effects of a more prolonged period of beclomethasone dipropionate administration on HPA function have not been evaluated. However, a number of investigators have noted that when systemic corticosteroid therapy in asthmatic subjects can be replaced with recommended doses of beclomethasone dipropionate, there is gradual recovery of endogenous cortisol concentrations to the normal range. There is still no documented evidence of recovery from other adverse systemic corticosteroid-induced reactions during prolonged therapy of patients with beclomethasone dipropionate.

Clinical experience has shown that some patients with bronchial asthma who require corticosteroid therapy for control of symptoms can be partially or completely withdrawn from systemic corticosteroid if therapy with beclomethasone dipropionate aerosol is substituted. Beclomethasone dipropionate aerosol is not effective for all patients with bronchial asthma or at all stages of the disease in a given patient.

The early clinical experience has revealed several new problems which may be associated with the use of beclomethasone dipropionate by inhalation for treatment of patients with bronchial asthma:

1. There is a risk of adrenal insufficiency when patients are transferred from systemic corticosteroids to aerosol beclomethasone dipropionate. Although the aerosol may provide adequate control of asthma during the transfer period, it does not provide the systemic steroid which is needed during acute stress situations. <u>Deaths due to adrenal insufficiency have occurred in asthmatic patients during and after transfer from systemic corticosteroids to aerosol beclomethasone dipropionate. (See WARNINGS.)</u>

2. Transfer of patients from systemic steroid therapy to beclomethasone dipropionate aerosol may unmask allergic conditions which were previously controlled by the systemic steroid therapy, e.g., rhinitis, conjunctivitis, and eczema.

3. Localized infections with *Candida albicans* or *Aspergillus niger* have occurred frequently in the mouth and pharynx and occasionally in the larynx. It has been reported that up to 75% of the patients who receive prolonged treatment with beclomethasone dipropionate have positive oral cultures for *Candida albicans*. The incidence of clinically apparent infection is considerably lower but may require therapy with appropriate antifungal agents or discontinuation of treatment with beclomethasone dipropionate aerosol.

The long-term effects of beclomethasone dipropionate in human subjects are still unknown. In particular, the local effects of the agent on developmental or immunologic processes in the mouth, pharynx, trachea and lung are unknown. There is also no information about the possible long-term systemic effects of the agent. The possible relevance of the data in animal studies to results in human subjects cannot be evaluated.

Revised 6/81
Copyright © 1973, 1980, 1981, Schering Corporation. All rights reserved.

Shown in Product Identification Section, page 435

Information on Schering products appearing on these pages is effective as of September 30, 1984.

Products are
listed alphabetically
in the
PINK SECTION.

Schmid Products Company
Division of Schmid Laboratories, Inc.
ROUTE 46 WEST
LITTLE FALLS, NJ 07424

RAMSES® Contraceptive Vaginal Jelly
[ram'sēz]

Composition: Active Ingredient: Nonoxynol-9, 5%.

Action and Uses: RAMSES® Contraceptive Vaginal Jelly is effective for birth control by jelly-alone technique or with a diaphragm. It is colorless, non-staining and contains a fast acting spermicide to instantly immobilize sperm. It is safe, will not liquify at body temperature, pleasantly scented, water soluble and acceptable to both partners. Store at room temperature.

Dosage and Administration: For complete instructions, please read pamphlet.

RAMSES® Jelly-Alone Technique
One applicatorful of RAMSES® Jelly is sufficient for one intercourse and should be inserted just prior to intercourse. Remove cap from tube and replace it with applicator, gently turning applicator until it is firmly attached. Squeeze tube from the bottom forcing the jelly into the applicator until the plunger is pushed out as far as it will go and the barrel is filled. After detaching from the tube, hold the filled applicator by the barrel and insert well into the vagina. Press the plunger completely thus depositing the correct amount of contraceptive jelly in front of the cervix.

Remove the applicator, holding it by the barrel while the plunger is still depressed.

One applicatorful of RAMSES® Jelly is sufficient for one act of intercourse only. An additional applicatorful is required each time intercourse is repeated.

RAMSES® Jelly With Diaphragm
For maximum protection, the combined use of a diaphragm and RAMSES® Jelly is recommended. Prior to inserting your diaphragm put about a teaspoonful of RAMSES® Jelly into the dome of the diaphragm and spread a small amount around the rim. This provides the proper lubrication for easy insertion and the jelly forms a seal and barrier to sperm. If intercourse occurs more than six hours after insertion, or if repeated intercourse takes place, an additional application of RAMSES® Jelly is necessary. Do not remove the diaphragm, just put more RAMSES® Jelly into the vagina with the applicator taking care not to dislodge the diaphragm.

It is important that the diaphragm remain in place for at least six hours after intercourse. Removal of the diaphragm before this time may increase the risk of becoming pregnant. If you wish, the diaphragm may be left in place for up to 24 hours.

Precaution: If your doctor advised against pregnancy for medical reasons you should discuss your birth control method with him so that both you and your doctor are satisfied that the method you have selected is right for you.

Side Effects: No significant side effects reported to date. If burning or irritation of the vagina or penis is experienced discontinue use and consult your physician.

Warning: Keep out of the reach of children.

VAGISEC PLUS® SUPPOSITORIES   B
[vaj'ĕ-sĕk"]
VAGISEC® MEDICATED DOUCHE LIQUID CONCENTRATE

Description: VAGISEC PLUS SUPPOSITORIES contain a combination of trichomonacidal and bactericidal agents and provide continued medication by gradual liquefaction. Each vaginal suppository contains the following ingredients:

9-aminoacridine HCl	6.00 mg.
Polyoxyethylene nonyl phenol	5.25 mg.
Sodium edetate	0.66 mg.
Sodium dioctyl sulfosuccinate	0.07 mg.

in a polyethylene glycol base containing glycerin and citric acid.

VAGISEC MEDICATED DOUCHE LIQUID CONCENTRATE contains a combination of polyoxyethylene nonyl phenol, sodium edetate, and sodium dioctyl sulfosuccinate, a complex proven to be effective trichomonacide when used as a vaginal douche (Vagisec Liquid).

Clinical Pharmacology: 9-aminoacridine is a broad-spectrum anti-infective of extensive medical acceptance for the topical treatment of bacterial infections. The combination of polyoxyethylene nonyl phenol, sodium edetate, and sodium dioctyl sulfosuccinate is a trichomonacide which when in solution and diluted disintegrates the flagellates through marked changes in surface tension.

Indications and Usage: The Vagisec Liquid/-Suppository regimen is indicated for the specific treatment, in adults, of vaginitis, as evidenced by pruritus, malodorous leukorrhea, erythema of the vaginal mucosa, dyspareunia, caused by Trichomonas vaginalis and mixed vaginal infections complicated by a bacterial moiety.

The presence of trichomonads can be established by a hanging drop mount preparation of the discharge from the posterior fornix and confirmed by cultures grown on STS medium; the atypical bacterial moiety can be identified by examination of gram-stained preparations of smeared vaginal secretions.

Contraindications: Douching is not recommended during pregnancy. VAGISEC Medicated Douche and VAGISEC PLUS Suppositories are spermicidal and should not be used when the patient is trying to conceive.

Precautions: *General:* The full course of therapy must be completed to eliminate the infecting micro-organisms from the vagina. It is generally desirable to continue treatment through the menses in order to guard against potential flare-ups since the presence of blood favors the rapid growth of Trichomonas. Recurrence of vaginitis often indicates extravaginal foci or infection in cervical, vestibular and urethral glands, etc. or reinfection by the sexual partner.

Information for Patients: During treatment, patient should refrain from intercourse, or the partner should wear a prophylactic. To prevent flare-ups after completion of therapy and for continued vaginal cleanliness, the patient is advised to continue with VAGISEC Liquid as a regular douche, but no more than twice weekly unless otherwise directed by physician.

Laboratory Tests: No patient should be considered cured until cultures on STS medium and gram-stained preparations of smeared vaginal secretions, taken at monthly intervals for 3 months following treatment, show absence of trichomonads and a return to the normal vaginal bacterial flora.

Adverse Reactions: No significant adverse reactions have been reported to date for Vagisec Plus Suppositories or Vagisec Liquid. Any minor irritation is generally relieved by discontinuance of douche for 24 hours.

Overdosage: *Antidote:* Copious use of water. The dilute Vagisec solution is non-toxic.

Dosage & Administration: *Office Treatment (Adult):* For the treatment of vaginal trichomoniasis and mixed vaginal infections, best results are obtained by scrubbing the vagina with VAGISEC Liquid, diluted 1:100 by the physician in the office: 3 scrubs the first week, 2 the second. A suppository is inserted after each office scrub in the Liquid/-Suppository regimen. Patient should be instructed to continue treatment at home. *Home Treatment:* The combination douche and suppositories (Liquid/Suppository regimen) is recommended for home use. The usual daily home treatment is VAGISEC Medicated Douche in the morning, followed by a VAGISEC PLUS Suppository inserted deep in the vagina, using tip of finger, and a second suppository inserted in like manner at bedtime for a period of 14 days. Treatment should be omitted the night and morning preceding an office visit. In chronic or stubborn cases, therapy may be repeated with no interval between courses. The Liquid/Suppository regimen may be continued throughout the menstrual cycle. It is advisable to continue treatment through two menstrual periods. Patients should be reexamined 3 days after home treatment has been discontinued. The full course of therapy must be completed to eliminate the infecting micro-organisms from the vagina. No patient should be considered cured until vaginal smears or cultures, taken at monthly intervals for 3 months following treatment, show absence of trichomonads and a return to the normal vaginal flora.

How Supplied: VAGISEC PLUS® SUPPOSITORIES—box of 28 plastic-wrapped 3 gram suppositories. VAGISEC® MEDICATED DOUCHE LIQUID CONCENTRATE—4 oz. plastic bottle with instructions for dilution and douching.

Caution: Federal law prohibits dispensing VAGISEC PLUS Suppositories without prescription.

Sclavo Inc.
5 MANSARD COURT
WAYNE, NJ 07470

COMPLETE INFORMATION FOR THE BELOW LISTED PRODUCTS IS FURNISHED IN THE PACKAGING.
ANTIRABIES SERUM (equine) USP ℞
CHOLERA VACCINE, USP ℞
DIPHTHERIA ANTITOXIN (equine) USP ℞
DIPHTHERIA TOXOID, USP ℞
DIPHTHERIA AND TETANUS ℞
 TOXOIDS ADSORBED, USP
 (For Pediatric Use)
SclavoTest®-PPD ℞
 Tuberculin Purified Protein
 Derivative (PPD)
 Multiple Puncture Device
 For product information, consult Diagnostic Product Information Section.
TETANUS ANTITOXIN (equine) USP ℞
TETANUS TOXOID, ADSORBED, USP ℞
TETANUS AND DIPHTHERIA ℞
 TOXOIDS ADSORBED, USP
 (For Adult Use)

EDUCATIONAL MATERIAL

Sclavo Test Brochure Free on Request to Physicians
"**Tuberculin Skin Testing: Mantoux or Multiple Puncture Device**" Paper by J. J. Piecoro, Jr., Pharm D, H. David Wilson, M.D. and Irene G. Melvin, M.S. Available on request to physicians free.

Scot-Tussin Pharmacal Co., Inc.
50 CLEMENCE STREET
CRANSTON, RI 02920-0217

S-T DECONGEST™ SUGAR-FREE & DYE-FREE ℞
Complete prescribing information is furnished in the packaging.
Composition: Each 5 ml (1 teaspoonful) contains:
Brompheniramine Maleate, USP ....4 mg
Phenylpropanolamine HCl, USP ....5 mg
Phenylephrine HCl, USP ....5 mg
Alcohol, 2.3 per cent
How Supplied: 8 fl. oz. (NDC 0372-0010-08), pint (NDC 0372-0010-16), and gallon (NDC 0372-0010-28) bottles.

S-T FORTE™ SUGAR-FREE ©
S-T FORTE™ Syrup
Complete prescribing information is furnished in the packaging.
Composition: Each 5 ml (1 teaspoonful) contains:

Hydrocodone Bitartrate, USP ....2.5 mg
 (**Warning:** May be habit forming)
Phenylephrine HCl, USP ....5 mg
Phenylpropanolamine HCl, USP ....5 mg
Pheniramine Maleate, USP ....13.33 mg
Guaifenesin, USP ....80 mg
Alcohol 5 per cent
How Supplied:
Syrup: Pints (NDC 0372-0004-16); Gallons (NDC 0372-0004-28).
Sugar-Free: Pints (NDC 0372-0005-16); Gallons (NDC 0372-0005-28).

SCOT-TUSSIN® SUGAR-FREE   OTC
COUGH & COLD MEDICINE
Composition: Each 5 ml (1 teaspoonful) contains:
Dextromethorphan HBr., USP .... 15 mg.
Chlorpheniramine Maleate, USP .... 2 mg.
How Supplied: Bottles of 4 fl. oz. (NDC 0372-0036-04)

SCOT-TUSSIN® SUGAR-FREE   OTC
EXPECTORANT
DYE-FREE & SODIUM-FREE COUGH FORMULA
Composition: Each 5 ml (1 teaspoonful) contains:
Guaifenesin, USP ....100 mg
Alcohol 3.5 per cent
How Supplied: Bottles of 4 fl. oz. (NDC 0372-0006-04).

TUSSIREX™ SUGAR-FREE   ©
TUSSIREX™ Syrup
Complete prescribing information is furnished in the packaging.
Composition: Each 5 ml (1 teaspoonful) contains:
Codeine Phosphate, USP ....10 mg
 (**Warning:** May be habit forming)
Pheniramine Maleate, USP ....13.33 mg
Phenylephrine HCl., USP ....4.17 mg
Sodium Citrate, USP ....83.33 mg
Sodium Salicylate, USP ....83.33 mg
Caffeine Citrate, USP ....25 mg
In a palatable, non-alcoholic vehicle.
How Supplied: Both Tussirex™ Sugar-Free (yellow, lemon flavor), and Tussirex™ Syrup (red, cherry-strawberry flavor) are available in pint (sugar-free NDC 0372-0018-16; syrup NDC 0372-0017-16), and gallon (sugar-free NDC 0372-0018-28; syrup NDC 0372-0017-28) bottles.

Seamless Hospital Products Co.
Div. of Dart Industries
P.O. BOX 828
BARNES INDUSTRIAL PARK, N. WALLINGFORD, CT 06492

ANTI-SEPT™
[an″ti-sept′]
(chloroxylenol)
Description: Anti-Sept™ surgical scrub is composed of a broad spectrum bactericidal, germacidal chloroxylenol formula. Anti-Sept™ is a high sudsing formula that assures maximum degermation of skin areas.
Action: For pre- and post operative scrubbing by hospital operating room personnel; a fast acting bactericide with persistent bacteriostatic properties that significantly reduces the number of microorganisms of the hands and forearms prior to patient care or surgery; for use as an antibacterial scrub in the physicians office. The formula produces a thick sudsing that is effective, non-irritating, and will not stain skin or fabrics. The range of pH, 5.6 to 5.8, optimizes the effectiveness of the product and assures compatability with normal skin pH.

The germicidal action of Anti-Sept™ reduces the possibility of cross contamination through control of possible skin infection.
Cautions: In the rare occurrence of local irritation the sensitive individual should discontinue use.
Direction For Use: A scrub for hospital personnel for pre- and post operative washing and for physician use.
Remove the premoistened scrub brush and pick from the package. Wet hands and forearms with water. Following a generally recognized effective scrub technique, use the Anti-Sept™ brush to clean the skin. Pay particular attention to the interdigital and finger nail areas. Use the pick to clean the nails during scrubbing. Develop a full lather over the hands and forearms to assure coverage for proper degermation and physical cleaning.
After scrubbing rinse off the Anti-Sept™ in running water.
How Supplied: Wet pack, Surgical Scrub Brush, with nail cleaner, ready to use.

Searle Pharmaceuticals Inc.
BOX 5110
CHICAGO, IL 60680

Searle Consumer Products*
Division of G. D. Searle & Co.
BOX 5110
CHICAGO, IL 60680

Searle & Co.†
SAN JUAN, PUERTO RICO 00936

Alphabetic Product Listing*
List#, Prod. ID# (NDC§), Form, Strength

46	†Aldactazide, 1011, Tablet, 25 mg/25 mg
649	†Aldactazide, 1021, Tablet, 50 mg/50 mg
39	†Aldactone, 1001, Tablet, 25 mg
916	†Aldactone, 1041, Tablet, 50 mg
134	†Aldactone, 1031, Tablet, 100 mg
96	Aminophyllin Injection, 1213, Ampul, 250 mg/10 ml
95	Aminophyllin Injection, 1223, Ampul, 500 mg/20 ml
18	†Aminophyllin, 1231, Tablet, 100 mg
44	†Aminophyllin, 1251, Tablet, 200 mg
43	†Anavar, 1401, Tablet, 2.5 mg
40	†Banthine, 1501, Tablet, 50 mg
563	Calan, 1853, Ampul, 5 mg/2 ml
207	Calan, 1958, Syringe, I.V., 5 mg/2 ml
221	Calan, 1968, Syringe, I.V., 10 mg/4 ml
626	†Calan, 1851, Tablet, 80 mg
632	†Calan, 1861, Tablet, 120 mg
584	Calan, 1864, Vial, I.V., 5 mg/2 ml
593	Calan, 1874, Vial, I.V., 10 mg/4 ml
511	Chlorthalidone, 531, Tablet, 25 mg
512	Chlorthalidone, 541, Tablet, 50 mg
152	Cu-7, 708, Unit
139	†Demulen 1/35-21, Compack, 151, Tablet, 1 mg/35 mcg
51	†Demulen 1/35-21, Refill, 151, Tablet, 1 mg/35 mcg
80	†Demulen 1/35-28, Compack, 151 (0161), Tablet, 1 mg/35 mcg
108	†Demulen 1/35-28, Refill, 151 (0161), Tablet, 1 mg/35 mcg
163	†Demulen 1/50-21, Compack, 71, Tablet, 1 mg/50 mcg

Continued on next page

Searle—Cont.

172	†Demulen 1/50-21, Refill, 71, Tablet, 1 mg/50 mcg	
156	†Demulen 1/50-28, Compack, 71 (0081), Tablet, 1 mg/50 mcg	
164	†Demulen 1/50-28, Refill, 71 (0081), Tablet, 1 mg/50 mcg	
251	Diulo, 501, Tablet, 2½ mg	
273	Diulo, 511, Tablet, 5 mg	
285	Diulo, 521, Tablet, 10 mg	
34	Dramamine Injection, 1703, Ampul, 50 mg/1 ml	
74	Dramamine Injection, 1724, Vial, 250 mg/5 ml	
	*Dramamine, 1736, Liquid, 12.5 mg/4 ml, 3 oz	
73	Dramamine, 1736, Liquid, 12.5 mg/4 ml, 16 oz	
	*Dramamine, 1701, Tablet, 50 mg (12s, 36s, 100s)	
72	Dramamine, 1701, Tablet, 50 mg (1,000s)	
112	Dramamine, 1701, Unit Dose, Tablet, 50 mg	
56	†Enovid, 51, Tablet, 5 mg/75 mcg	
67	†Enovid, 101, Tablet, 10 mg/(9.85 mg/0.15 mg)	
153	†Enovid-E 21, Compack, 131, Tablet, 2.5 mg/0.1 mg	
191	†Enovid-E 21, Refill, 131, Tablet, 2.5 mg/0.1 mg	
111	†Flagyl, 1831, Tablet, 250 mg	
155	†Flagyl, 500 (1821), Tablet, 500 mg	
270	Flagyl I.V., 1804, Vial (partial fill, lyoph. pwd.), 500 mg	
261	Flagyl I.V. RTU, 1844, Vial, 500 mg/100 ml	
661	Flagyl I.V. RTU, 1847, Plastic Container, 500 mg/100 ml	
639	Furosemide, 571, Tablet, 20 mg	
640	Furosemide, 581, Tablet, 40 mg	
81	†Lomotil, 61, Tablet, 2.5 mg/0.025 mg	
94	†Lomotil, Liquid, 66, 2.5 mg/0.025 mg per 5 ml	
154	Mark-7, 709, Unit	
	*Metamucil, 2209, Powder, Regular Flavor, 7 oz, 14 oz, 21 oz	
	*Metamucil, 2209, Powder, Regular Flavor, Unit Dose, Packets, 7 g, 100s	
	*Metamucil, 2319, Powder, Regular Flavor, Sugar Free, 3.7 oz, 7.4 oz, 11.1 oz	
	*Metamucil, 2319, Powder, Regular Flavor, Sugar Free, Unit Dose, Packers, 3.7 g, 100s	
	*Metamucil, 2229, Powder, Orange Flavor, 7 oz, 14 oz, 21 oz	
	*Metamucil, 2269, Powder, Strawberry Flavor, 7 oz, 14 oz, 21 oz	
	*Metamucil Instant Mix, 2219, Regular Flavor, Packets, 16s, 30s	
	*Metamucil Instant Mix, 2219, Regular Flavor, Unit Dose, Packets, 100s	
	*Metamucil Instant Mix, 2259, Orange Flavor, Packets, 16s, 30s	
580	Nitrodisc, 2058, Transcutaneous Disc, 5 mg/24 hr (8 cm^2)	
581	Nitrodisc, 2068, Transcutaneous Disc, 10 mg/24 hr (16 cm^2)	
123	†Norpace, 2752, Capsule, 100 mg	
906	†Norpace, 2762, Capsule, 150 mg	
256	†Norpace CR, 2732, Capsule, 100 mg	
278	†Norpace CR, 2742, Capsule, 150 mg	
129	†Ovulen-21, Compack, 401, Tablet, 1 mg/0.1 mg	
137	†Ovulen-21, Refill, 401, Tablet, 1 mg/0.1 mg	
130	†Ovulen-28, Compack, 401 (0421), Tablet, 1 mg/0.1 mg	
141	†Ovulen-28, Refill, 401 (0421), Tablet, 1 mg/0.1 mg	
28	†Pro-Banthine, 601, Tablet, 15 mg	
121	†Pro-Banthine, Unit Dose, 601, Tablet, 15 mg	
9	†Pro-Banthine, 611, Tablet, 7½ mg	
29	†Pro-Banthine w/Phenobarbital, 631, Tablet, 15 mg/15 mg	
132	†Pro-Banthine w/Phenobarbital, Unit Dose, 631, Tablet, 15 mg/15 mg	
	*Prompt, 2249, Powder, 2½ oz and 5 oz	
	*Prompt, 2249, Powder, Packets, 12s	
20	Tatum-T, 508, Unit	
587	†Theo-24, 2832, Capsule, 100 mg	
588	†Theo-24, 2842, Capsule, 200 mg	
589	†Theo-24, 2852, Capsule, 300 mg	

* Products of Searle Consumer Products (those not shown in this publication are included in the PDR for Nonprescription Drugs).

†Products of Searle & Co.

[Products without reference marks are Searle Pharmaceuticals Inc. products.]

§When the product ID# is not the same as the NDC#, the NDC# appears in parentheses.

Various educational materials are available for physicians, pharmacists, nurses, physicians' assistants, and patients (through the physician). Please ask your Searle representative for information about these materials.

Searle Pharmaceuticals Inc.
BOX 5110
CHICAGO, IL 60680

AMINOPHYLLIN INJECTION™ ℞
[am-in-off'i-lin]
(aminophylline injection USP)

Description: Aminophyllin Injection is a sterile solution of theophylline in water for injection prepared with the aid of ethylenediamine. Aminophyllin Injection contains anhydrous theophylline USP 19.7 mg/ml and ethylenediamine USP 3.6 mg/ml (equivalent to aminophylline dihydrate 25 mg/ml) in water for injection.

Aminophylline is a 2:1 complex of theophylline ($C_7H_8N_4O_2$), a bronchodilator, and ethylenediamine ($C_2H_8N_2$).

Aminophylline is white or slightly yellowish granules or powder, having a slight ammoniacal odor and a bitter taste.

Clinical Pharmacology: Theophylline directly relaxes the smooth muscle of the bronchial airways and pulmonary blood vessels, thus acting mainly as a bronchodilator and smooth muscle relaxant. The drug also possesses other actions typical of the xanthine derivatives: coronary vasodilation, cardiac stimulation, diuresis, cerebral stimulation, and skeletal muscle stimulation. The actions of theophylline may be mediated through inhibition of phosphodiesterase and a resultant increase in intracellular cyclic AMP. *In vitro*, theophylline inhibits the release of histamine by mast cells at concentrations generally higher than attained *in vivo*. *In vitro*, theophylline has been shown to act synergistically with beta agonists that increase intracellular cyclic AMP through the stimulation of adenyl cyclase. More data are needed to determine if theophylline and beta agonists have a clinically important additive effect *in vivo*.

Pharmacokinetics:

Theophylline Elimination Characteristics

	Theophylline Clearance Rates (mean ± S.D.)	Half-life Average (mean ± S.D.)
Children (over 6 months of age):	1.45 ± 0.58 ml/kg/min	3.7 ± 1.1 hr
Adult nonsmokers with uncomplicated asthma	0.65 ± 0.19 ml/kg/min	8.7 ± 2.2 hr

The half-life of theophylline is prolonged in patients with alcoholism, reduced hepatic or renal function, or congestive heart failure, and in patients receiving cimetidine or macrolide antibiotics such as troleandomycin and erythromycin. High fever for prolonged periods may reduce the rate of theophylline elimination.

Newborn infants have extremely slow theophylline clearance rates. The theophylline half-life in newborn infants may exceed 24 hours. Not until the age of 3 to 6 months do clearance rates approach those seen in older children.

Patients over age 55 and patients with chronic obstructive pulmonary disease, cardiac failure, or liver insufficiency may have much slower clearance rates with half-lives that exceed 24 hours.

The average half-life of theophylline in smokers (1 to 2 packs/day) is 4 to 5 hours; the average half-life in nonsmokers is 7 to 10 hours. The increase in theophylline clearance caused by smoking is probably the result of induction of drug-metabolizing enzymes. The effect of smoking on theophylline pharmacokinetics may persist for 3 months to 2 years after smoking is discontinued.

Tolerance does not appear to develop during long-term use of theophylline.

Indications and Usage: Aminophyllin Injection is indicated for relief of acute bronchial asthma and for reversible bronchospasm associated with chronic bronchitis and emphysema.

Contraindications: Patients with a history of hypersensitivity to aminophylline or its components (theophylline or ethylenediamine) should not be treated with Aminophyllin Injection (aminophylline).

Warnings: Status asthmaticus is a medical emergency. Optimal therapy frequently requires additional medication including corticosteroids when the patient is not rapidly responsive to bronchodilators.

Excessive theophylline doses may be associated with toxicity. The determination of theophylline serum levels is recommended to assure maximal benefit without excessive risk. Incidence of toxicity increases at theophylline serum levels greater than 20 mcg/ml.

Morphine and curare should be used with caution in patients with airflow obstruction because they stimulate histamine release and can induce asthmatic attacks. They may also suppress respiration leading to respiratory failure. Alternative drugs should be chosen whenever possible.

There is an excellent correlation between high serum levels of theophylline resulting from conventional doses and associated clinical manifestations of toxicity in (1) patients with lowered body plasma clearances (due to transient cardiac decompensation), (2) patients with liver dysfunction or chronic obstructive lung disease, (3) patients who are older than 55 years of age, particularly males.

Less serious signs of theophylline toxicity such as nausea and restlessness may appear in up to 50% of patients. However, serious side effects such as ventricular arrhythmias and convulsions may appear as the first signs of toxicity.

Many patients who have high theophylline serum levels exhibit tachycardia. Theophylline products may worsen preexisting arrhythmias.

Aminophyllin injection should not be injected rapidly (no more than 25 mg/min) or through a central venous catheter. Intravenous doses given too rapidly or excessive doses given by any route of administration may be expected to be toxic, causing gastrointestinal, central nervous system, cardiovascular, and/or respiratory symptoms (see *OVERDOSAGE*). Some children may be unusually sensitive to aminophylline. Toxic synergism with ephedrine and other sympathomimetic drugs may occur.

Caution should be used when aminophylline is given to patients with impaired liver function. Serum levels in such patients may persist longer than expected.

In minipigs, rodents, and dogs, arrhythmia and sudden death (with histological evidence of myocardial necrosis) have been observed when theophylline and beta agonists were administered concomitantly but not when either was administered alone. The significance of these findings for human use is unknown.

Precautions: General: Mean half-life in smokers is shorter than in nonsmokers; therefore smokers may require larger doses of aminophylline. Aminophylline should not be administered concomitantly with other xanthine medications. Use with caution in patients with severe cardiac disease, severe hypoxemia, hypertension, hyperthyroidism, acute myocardial injury, cor pulmonale, congestive heart failure, or liver disease, and in the elderly (especially males) and in neonates. Particular caution should be used in giving aminophylline to patients in congestive heart failure. Frequently, such patients have markedly prolonged theophylline serum levels with theophylline persisting in serum for long periods following discontinuation of the drug.

Convulsions may occur in patients with aminophylline overdosage with serum levels of 30 mcg/ml or higher. Aminophylline may lower the seizure threshold.

Methylxanthines are known to increase gastric acidity. Therefore, aminophylline should be used cautiously in patients with a history of peptic ulcer since the disease may be exacerbated. Theophylline may occasionally act as a local irritant to the gastrointestinal tract, although gastrointestinal symptoms are more commonly mediated through the central nervous system and are usually associated with serum drug concentrations over 20 mcg/ml.

Laboratory tests: The determination of serum theophylline levels is highly recommended.

Drug interactions: Elevated serum levels of theophylline may occur in patients treated concomitantly with theophylline preparations and cimetidine, troleandomycin, or erythromycin. Therefore, such patients should be watched carefully for signs of theophylline toxicity and the dose of aminophylline decreased if necessary. If ephedrine or other sympathomimetic drugs are given concomitantly with aminophylline, toxic synergism may occur.

Interaction	Effect
With lithium carbonate	Increased excretion of lithium carbonate
With propranolol	Antagonism of propranolol effect
With cimetidine	Increased theophylline serum levels
With troleandomycin or erythromycin	Increased theophylline serum levels

Drug/Laboratory test interactions: Consumption of coffee, tea, cola beverages, chocolate, or acetaminophen contributes to falsely high serum theophylline levels when theophylline is measured spectrophotometrically without previous isolation by chromatography.

Use in pregnancy: Safe use in pregnancy has not been established relative to possible adverse effects on fetal development, but neither have adverse effects on fetal development been established. This is true for most antiasthmatic medications. Use of aminophylline in pregnant women should be balanced against the risk of uncontrolled asthma.

Nursing mothers: Theophylline is secreted in breast milk and may cause adverse effects in the infant. Caution must be used when prescribing aminophylline to a nursing mother, taking into account the risk/benefit of this therapy.

Adverse Reactions: The most consistent adverse reactions are usually due to overdose and are:

1. Gastrointestinal: nausea, vomiting, epigastric pain, hematemesis, diarrhea.
2. Central nervous system: headaches, irritability, restlessness, insomnia, reflex hyperexcitability, muscle twitching, clonic and tonic generalized convulsions, coma.
3. Cardiovascular: palpitation, tachycardia, extrasystoles, flushing, hypotension, circulatory failure, ventricular arrhythmias.

A. Not currently receiving theophylline products:

Group	Loading Dose* (mg/kg)	Maintenance Dose for Next 12 Hours (mg/kg/hr)	Maintenance Dose Beyond 12 Hours (mg/kg/hr)
1. Children 6 months to 9 years	6 (5)†	1.2 (1.0)†	1.0 (0.8)†
2. Children age 9 to 16 and young adult smokers	6 (5)	1.0 (0.8)	0.8 (0.65)
3. Otherwise healthy nonsmoking adults	6 (5)	0.7 (0.6)	0.5 (0.4)
4. Older patients and patients with cor pulmonale	6 (5)	0.6 (0.5)	0.3 (0.24)
5. Patients with congestive heart failure, liver disease	6 (5)	0.5 (0.4)	0.1–0.2 (0.08–0.16)

* Administer slowly, no faster than 25 mg/min.
† Equivalent anhydrous theophylline indicated in parentheses.

4. Respiratory: tachypnea.
5. Renal: albuminuria, microhematuria, potentiation of diuresis.
6. Others: hyperglycemia and inappropriate ADH (antidiuretic hormone) syndrome; rash (ethylenediamine).

Overdosage:
Management of Toxic Symptoms:
1. Discontinue drug immediately.
2. There is no known specific antidote.
3. Treatment is supportive and symptomatic.
4. Avoid administration of sympathomimetic drugs.
5. Theophylline is dialyzable; charcoal hemoperfusion should be considered in severe theophylline toxic reactions.
6. Administer intravenous fluids, oxygen, and other supportive measures to prevent hypotension, correct dehydration and acid-base imbalance.
7. For hyperthermia, use a cooling blanket or give sponge baths as necessary.
8. Maintain patent airway and use artificial respiration (mechanical ventilation) in case of respiratory depression.
9. Control convulsions with appropriate parenteral medication(s) such as short-acting barbiturates, diazepam (0.1 to 0.3 mg/kg up to 10 mg), or phenytoin.
10. Monitor theophylline serum levels until below 20 mcg/ml.

Dosage and Administration: Therapeutic theophylline serum levels associated with optimal likelihood for benefit and minimal risk of toxicity are considered to be between 10 and 20 mcg/ml. Levels above 20 mcg/ml may produce toxic effects. There is great variation from patient to patient in dosage needed in order to achieve a therapeutic serum level because of variable rates of elimination. Because of this wide interpatient variation, and the relatively narrow therapeutic serum level range, dosage must be individualized. Monitoring of theophylline serum levels is highly recommended. Continuous cardiac monitoring may offer additional safety. Patients should be closely monitored for signs of toxicity. Dosage should be temporarily discontinued and resumed later at a lower dose if any signs of theophylline toxicity are present.

Dosage should be calculated on the basis of lean (ideal) body weight where mg/kg doses are stated. Theophylline does not distribute into fatty tissue. Due to the marked variation in theophylline metabolism in infants, this drug is not recommended for infants under 6 months of age.

Aminophylline Dosage for Patient Population: [See table above].
B. Currently receiving theophylline products: Determine, where possible, the time, amount, route of administration, and form of the patient's last dose.

The loading dose for theophylline is based on the principle that each 0.5 mg/kg of theophylline administered as a loading dose will result in a 1 mcg/ml increase in serum theophylline concentration. Ideally, the loading dose should be deferred if serum theophylline concentration can be rapidly obtained. If this is not possible, the clinician must exercise judgment in selecting a dose based on the potential for benefit and risk. When there is sufficient respiratory distress to warrant a small risk, 2.5 mg/kg of anhydrous theophylline (3.1 mg/kg of intravenous aminophylline) is likely to increase the serum concentration when administered as a loading dose in rapidly absorbed form by approximately 5 mcg/ml. If the patient is not already experiencing theophylline toxicity, this is unlikely to result in dangerous adverse effects.

Subsequent to the decision regarding modification of the loading dose in this group of patients, the maintenance dosage recommendations are the same as those described above.

Aminophyllin Injection in intravenous ampuls of 10 ml (250 mg) or 20 ml (500 mg) can either be injected very slowly by syringe or, more conveniently, may be infused in a small quantity (usually 100 or 200 ml) of 5% dextrose injection or 0.9% sodium chloride injection. This solution is sometimes given "piggyback" through an I.V. system already in place. Do not exceed the rate of 25 mg/min.

Thereafter, maintenance therapy can be administered by a large volume infusion to deliver the desired amount of drug each hour. Aminophyllin is compatible with most commonly used I.V. solutions.

Oral therapy should be substituted for intravenous aminophylline as soon as adequate improvement is achieved.

Parenteral drug products should be inspected visually for particulate matter and discoloration prior to administration, whenever solution and container permit. Use only if solution is clear and no crystals are present.

INTRAVENOUS ADMIXTURE INCOMPATIBILITY: Although there have been reports of aminophylline precipitating in acidic media, these reports do not apply to the dilute solutions found in intravenous infusions. Aminophyllin Injection (aminophylline) should not be mixed in a syringe with other drugs but should be added separately to the intravenous solution.

When an intravenous solution containing aminophylline is given "piggyback," the intravenous system already in place should be turned off while the aminophylline is infused if there is a potential problem with admixture incompatibility.

The following may be incompatible when mixed with aminophylline in intravenous fluids: anileridine HCl, ascorbic acid, chlorpromazine, codeine phosphate, dimenhydrinate, epinephrine HCl, erythromycin gluceptate, hydralazine HCl, insulin, levorphanol tartrate, meperidine HCl, methadone HCl, methicillin sodium, morphine sulfate, norepinephrine bitartrate, oxytetracycline HCl, penicillin G potassium, phenobarbital sodium, phenytoin sodium, prochlorperazine maleate, promazine HCl, promethazine HCl, tetracycline HCl, vancomycin HCl, vitamin B complex with C.

Continued on next page

Searle Pharm.—Cont.

How Supplied:
Aminophyllin Injection is available in 10-ml (250 mg) or 20-ml (500 mg) ampuls, aqueous solution, USP; cartons of 25 and boxes of 100.
Store below 86°F (30°C) and protect from light and from freezing.
Tablets Shown in Product Identification Section, page 435

CALAN®
[*cal'an*]
(verapamil hydrochloride)
For Intravenous Injection

Description: Calan (verapamil HCl) is a slow-channel inhibitor or calcium antagonist available as a sterile solution for intravenous injection in 5-mg ampuls and in 5-mg and 10-mg vials and syringes. Each form contains verapamil HCl 2.5 mg/ml and sodium chloride 8.5 mg/ml in water for injection. Hydrochloric acid and/or sodium hydroxide is used for pH adjustment. The pH of the solution is between 4.1 and 6.0.
The structural formula of verapamil HCl is given below:

$C_{27}H_{38}N_2O_4 \cdot HCl \quad M.W.=491.08$

Benzeneacetonitrile, α-[3-[[2-(3,4-dimethoxy-phenyl)ethyl]methylamino]propyl]-3, 4-dimethoxy-α-(l-methylethyl)hydrochloride

Verapamil HCl is an almost white, crystalline powder, practically free of odor, with a bitter taste. It is soluble in water, chloroform, and methanol. Verapamil HCl is not chemically related to other antiarrhythmic drugs.

Clinical Pharmacology:
Mechanism of Action: Calan (verapamil HCl) inhibits the calcium ion (and possibly sodium ion) influx through slow channels into conductile and contractile myocardial cells and vascular smooth muscle cells. The antiarrhythmic effect of Calan appears to be due to its effect on the slow channel in cells of the cardiac conductile system.
Electrical activity through the SA and AV nodes depends, to a significant degree, upon calcium influx through the slow channel. By inhibiting this influx, Calan slows AV conduction and prolongs the effective refractory period within the AV node in a rate-related manner, reducing elevated ventricular rate in patients with supraventricular tachycardia due to atrial flutter and/or atrial fibrillation. By interrupting reentry at the AV node, Calan can restore normal sinus rhythm in patients with paroxysmal supraventricular tachycardias (PSVT), including Wolff-Parkinson-White (W-P-W) syndrome. Calan has no effect on conduction across accessory bypass tracts. Calan does not alter the normal atrial action potential or intraventricular conduction time but depresses amplitude, velocity of depolarization, and conduction in depressed atrial fibers.
In the isolated rabbit heart, concentrations of Calan that markedly affect SA nodal fibers or fibers in the upper and middle regions of the AV node have very little effect on fibers in the lower AV node (NH region) and no effect on atrial action potentials or His bundle fibers.
Calan does not induce peripheral arterial spasm. Calan has a local anesthetic action that is 1.6 times that of procaine on an equimolar basis. It is not known whether this action is important at the doses used in man.
Calan does not alter total serum calcium levels.
Hemodynamics: In animals and man, Calan (verapamil HCl) reduces afterload and myocardial contractility. In most patients, including those with organic cardiac disease, the negative inotropic action of Calan is countered by reduction of afterload, and cardiac index is usually not reduced, but in patients with moderately severe to severe cardiac dysfunction (pulmonary wedge pressure above 20 mm Hg, ejection fraction less than 30%), acute worsening of heart failure may be seen. Peak therapeutic effects occur within 3 to 5 minutes after a bolus injection. The commonly used intravenous doses of 5-10 mg Calan produce transient, usually asymptomatic, reduction in normal systemic arterial pressure, systemic vascular resistance and contractility; left ventricular filling pressure is slightly increased.
Pharmacokinetics: Intravenously administered Calan (verapamil HCl) has been shown to be rapidly metabolized in both humans and animals. Following intravenous infusion in man, verapamil is eliminated bi-exponentially, with a rapid early distribution phase (half-life about 4 minutes) and a slower terminal elimination phase (half-life 2-5 hours). In healthy men, orally administered Calan undergoes extensive metabolism in the liver, with 12 metabolites having been identified, most in only trace amounts. The major metabolites have been identified as various N- and O-dealkylated products of Calan. Approximately 70% of an administered dose is excreted in the urine and 16% or more in the feces within 5 days. About 3% to 4% is excreted as unchanged drug.
Indications and Usage: Calan (verapamil HCl) is indicated for the treatment of supraventricular tachyarrhythmias, including:
• Rapid conversion to sinus rhythm of paroxysmal supraventricular tachycardias, including those associated with accessory bypass tracts (Wolff-Parkinson-White [W-P-W] and Lown-Ganong-Levine [L-G-L] syndromes). When clinically advisable, appropriate vagal maneuvers (eg, Valsalva maneuver) should be attempted prior to Calan administration.
• Temporary control of rapid ventricular rate in atrial flutter or atrial fibrillation.
In controlled studies in the United States, about 60% of patients with supraventricular tachycardia converted to normal sinus rhythm within 10 minutes after intravenous verapamil HCl. Uncontrolled studies reported in the world literature describe a conversion rate of about 80%. About 70% of patients with atrial flutter and/or fibrillation with a fast ventricular rate respond with a decrease in heart rate of at least 20%. Conversion of atrial flutter or fibrillation to sinus rhythm is uncommon (about 10%) after verapamil HCl and may reflect the spontaneous conversion rate, since the conversion rate after placebo was similar. The effect of a single injection lasts for 30–60 minutes when conversion to sinus rhythm does not occur.
Because a small fraction (<1.0%) of patients treated with verapamil HCl respond with life-threatening adverse responses (rapid ventricular rate in atrial flutter/fibrillation, marked hypotension, or extreme bradycardia/asystole—see *Warnings*), the initial use of intravenous verapamil HCl should, if possible, be in a treatment setting with monitoring and resuscitation facilities, including D.C.-cardioversion capability. As familiarity with the patient's response is gained, an office setting would be acceptable.
Contraindications:
Verapamil HCl is contraindicated in:
1. Severe hypotension or cardiogenic shock
2. Second- or third-degree AV block
3. Sick sinus syndrome (except in patients with a functioning artificial ventricular pacemaker)
4. Severe congestive heart failure (unless secondary to a supraventricular tachycardia amenable to verapamil therapy)
5. Patients receiving **intravenous** beta-adrenergic blocking drugs (eg, propranolol). **Intravenous** verapamil and **intravenous** beta-adrenergic blocking drugs should not be administered in close proximity to each other (within a few hours), since both may have a depressant effect on myocardial contractility and AV conduction.
6. Known hypersensitivity to verapamil HCl
Warnings:
CALAN SHOULD BE GIVEN AS A SLOW INTRAVENOUS INJECTION OVER AT LEAST A TWO-MINUTE PERIOD OF TIME. (See *Dosage and Administration*.)

Hypotension: Intravenous verapamil often produces a decrease in blood pressure below baseline levels that is usually transient and asymptomatic but may result in dizziness. Systolic pressure less than 90 mm Hg and/or diastolic pressure less than 60 mm Hg was seen in 5%–10% of patients in controlled U.S. trials in supraventricular tachycardia and in about 10% of the patients with atrial flutter/fibrillation. The incidence of symptomatic hypotension observed in studies conducted in the U.S. was approximately 1.5%. Three of the five symptomatic patients required pharmacologic treatment (norepinephrine bitartrate IV, metaraminol bitartrate IV, or 10% calcium gluconate IV). All recovered without sequelae.
Rapid ventricular response or ventricular fibrillation in atrial flutter/fibrillation: Patients with atrial flutter/fibrillation and an accessory AV pathway (eg, Wolff-Parkinson-White or Lown-Ganong-Levine syndromes) may develop increased antegrade conduction across the aberrant pathway bypassing the AV node, producing a very rapid ventricular response after receiving verapamil (or digitalis). This has been reported in 1% of the patients treated in controlled double-blind trials in the U.S. Treatment is usually D.C.-cardioversion. Cardioversion has been used safely and effectively after intravenous Calan. (See *Adverse Reactions* including suggested treatment of adverse reactions.)
Extreme bradycardia/asystole: Verapamil slows conduction across the AV node and rarely may produce second- or third-degree AV block, bradycardia, and, in extreme cases, asystole. This is more likely to occur in patients with a sick sinus syndrome (SA nodal disease), which is more common in older patients. Bradycardia associated with sick sinus syndrome was reported in 0.3% of the patients treated in controlled double-blind trials in the U.S. The total incidence of bradycardia (ventricular rate less than 60 beats/min) was 1.2% in these studies. Asystole in patients other than those with sick sinus syndrome is usually of short duration (few seconds or less), with spontaneous return to AV nodal or normal sinus rhythm. If this does not occur promptly, appropriate treatment should be initiated immediately. (See *Adverse Reactions* including suggested treatment of adverse reactions.)
Heart failure: When heart failure is not severe or rate related, it should be controlled with optimum digitalization and diuretics, as appropriate, before Calan is used.
In patients with moderately severe to severe cardiac dysfunction (pulmonary wedge pressure above 20 mm Hg, ejection fraction less than 30%), acute worsening of heart failure may be seen.
Concomitant antiarrhythmic therapy:
Digitalis: Intravenous verapamil has been used concomitantly with digitalis preparations without the occurrence of serious adverse effects. However, since both drugs slow AV conduction, patients should be monitored for AV block or excessive bradycardia.
Quinidine—procainamide: Intravenous verapamil has been administered to a small number of patients receiving oral quinidine and oral procainamide without the occurrence of serious adverse effects.
Beta-adrenergic blocking drugs: Intravenous verapamil has been administered to patients receiving **oral** beta blockers without the development of serious adverse effects. However, since both drugs may depress myocardial contractility or AV conduction, these possibilities should be considered. On rare occasions, the concomitant administration of **intravenous** beta blockers and **intravenous** verapamil has resulted in serious adverse reactions (see *Contraindications*), especially in patients with severe cardiomyopathy, congestive heart failure, or recent myocardial infarction.
Disopyramide: Until data on possible interactions between verapamil and all forms of disopyramide phosphate are obtained, disopyramide should not be administered within 48 hours before or 24 hours after verapamil administration.

Heart block: Calan prolongs AV conduction time. While high-degree AV block has not been observed in controlled clinical trials in the U.S., a low percentage (less than 0.5%) has been reported in the world literature. Development of second- or third-degree AV block or unifascicular, bifascicular, or trifascicular bundle branch block requires reduction in subsequent doses or discontinuation of verapamil and institution of appropriate therapy, if needed. (See *Adverse Reactions* and *Concomitant antiarrhythmic therapy*.)

Hepatic and renal failure: Significant hepatic and renal failure should not increase the effects of a single intravenous dose of Calan but may prolong its duration. Repeated injections of intravenous Calan in such patients may lead to accumulation and an excessive pharmacologic effect of the drug. There is no experience to guide use of multiple doses in such patients, and this generally should be avoided. If repeated injections are essential, blood pressure and PR interval should be closely monitored and smaller repeat doses should be utilized. Data on the clearance of verapamil by dialysis are not yet available.

Premature ventricular contractions: During conversion to normal sinus rhythm or marked reduction in ventricular rate, a few benign complexes of unusual appearance (sometimes resembling premature ventricular contractions) may be seen after treatment with verapamil. Similar complexes are seen during spontaneous conversion of supraventricular tachycardia and after D.C.-cardioversion or other pharmacologic therapy. These complexes appear to have no clinical significance.

Precautions:
Drug interactions: (See *Warnings: Concomitant antiarrhythmic therapy*.) Intravenous verapamil has been used concomitantly with other cardioactive drugs (especially digitalis and quinidine) without evidence of serious negative drug interactions, except, in rare instances, when patients with severe cardiomyopathy, congestive heart failure, or recent myocardial infarction were given **intravenous** beta-adrenergic blocking agents or disopyramide. Drug interaction studies are ongoing. As verapamil is highly bound to plasma proteins, it should be administered with caution to patients receiving other highly protein-bound drugs.

Pregnancy: Pregnancy Category B. Reproduction studies have been performed in rats and rabbits. At doses up to 2.5 and 1.5 times the human **oral** dose, respectively, no evidence of impaired fertility or harm to the fetus due to verapamil was revealed. There are, however, no adequate and well-controlled studies in pregnant women. Because animal reproduction studies are not always predictive of human response, this drug should be used during pregnancy only if clearly needed.

Labor and delivery: There have been few controlled studies to determine whether the use of verapamil during labor or delivery has immediate or delayed adverse effects on the fetus, or whether it prolongs the duration of labor or increases the need for forceps delivery or other obstetric intervention. Such adverse experiences have not been reported in the literature, despite a long history of use of intravenous Calan in Europe in the treatment of cardiac side effects of beta-adrenergic agonist agents used to treat premature labor.

Nursing mothers: It is not known whether this drug is excreted in human milk. Because many drugs are excreted in human milk and because of the potential for adverse reactions in nursing infants from verapamil, nursing should be discontinued while verapamil is administered.

Pediatric use: Controlled studies with verapamil have not been conducted in pediatric patients, but uncontrolled experience with intravenous administration in more than 250 patients, about half under 12 months of age and about 25% newborn, indicates that results of treatment are similar to those in adults. The most commonly used single doses in patients up to 12 months of age have ranged from 0.1 to 0.2 mg/kg of body weight, while in patients aged 1 to 15 years, the most commonly used single doses ranged from 0.1 to 0.3 mg/kg of body weight. Most of the patients received the lower dose of 0.1 mg/kg once, but in some cases, the dose was repeated once or twice every 10 to 30 minutes.

Adverse Reactions: The following reactions were reported with intravenous verapamil use in controlled U.S. clinical trials involving 324 patients:
Cardiovascular: Symptomatic hypotension (1.5%); bradycardia (1.2%); severe tachycardia (1.0%). The worldwide experience in open clinical trials in more than 7,900 patients was similar.
Central Nervous System Effects: Dizziness (1.2%); headache (1.2%).
Gastrointestinal: Nausea (0.9%); abdominal discomfort (0.6%).
The following reactions were reported in single patients: emotional depression, rotary nystagmus, sleepiness, vertigo, muscle fatigue, or diaphoresis. In rare cases of hypersensitivity, broncho/laryngeal spasm accompanied by itch and urticaria has been reported.

Suggested Treatment of Acute Cardiovascular Adverse Reactions*
The frequency of these adverse reactions was quite low, and experience with their treatment has been limited.
[See table above].

Overdosage: Treatment of overdosage should be supportive. Beta-adrenergic stimulation or parenteral administration of calcium solutions (calcium chloride) may increase calcium ion flux across the slow channel. These pharmacologic interventions have been effectively used in treatment of deliberate overdosage with oral verapamil. Clinically significant hypotensive reactions or high-degree AV block should be treated with vasopressor agents or cardiac pacing, respectively. Asystole should be handled by the usual measures including isoproterenol hydrochloride, other vasopressor agents, or cardiopulmonary resuscitation (see *Suggested Treatment of Acute Cardiovascular Adverse Reactions*).

Dosage and Administration: For intravenous use only. The recommended intravenous doses of Calan (verapamil HCl) are as follows:
Adult:
Initial dose—5–10 mg (0.075–0.15 mg/kg body weight) given as an intravenous bolus over 2 minutes.
Repeat dose—10 mg (0.15 mg/kg body weight) 30 minutes after the first dose if the initial response is not adequate.
Older Patients—The dose should be administered over at least 3 minutes to minimize the risk of untoward drug effects.
Pediatric:
Initial dose
0–1 year: 0.1–0.2 mg/kg body weight (usual single dose range: 0.75–2 mg) should be administered as an intravenous bolus over 2 minutes *under continuous ECG monitoring*.
1–15 years: 0.1–0.3 mg/kg body weight (usual single dose range: 2–5 mg) should be administered as an intravenous bolus over 2 minutes. *Do not exceed 5 mg.*
Repeat dose
0–1 year: 0.1–0.2 mg/kg body weight (usual single dose range: 0.75–2 mg) 30 minutes after the first dose if the initial response is not adequate *under continuous ECG monitoring*.
1–15 years: 0.1–0.3 mg/kg body weight (usual single dose range: 2–5 mg) 30 minutes after the first dose if the initial response is not adequate. *Do not exceed 10 mg as a single dose.*
NOTE: Parenteral drug products should be inspected visually for particulate matter and discoloration prior to administration, whenever solution and container permit. Use only if solution is clear and vial seal is intact. Unused amount of solution should be discarded immediately following withdrawal of any portion of contents.

How Supplied: All forms are individually packaged.

Size	NDC Number	Carton Size
5-mg (2 ml) ampul	0025-1853-10	10
5-mg (2 ml) vial	0025-1864-05	5
5-mg (2 ml) vial	0025-1864-10	10
10-mg (4 ml) vial	0025-1874-05	5
10-mg (4 ml) vial	0025-1874-10	10
5-mg (2 ml) syringe	0025-1958-05	5
10-mg (4 ml) syringe	0025-1968-05	5

Store at 59° to 86° F (15° to 30° C) and protect from light during storage.
Caution: Federal law prohibits dispensing without prescription.

Continued on next page

CALAN IV

Adverse Reaction	Proven Effective Treatment	Treatment With Good Theoretical Rationale	Supportive Treatment
1. Symptomatic hypotension requiring treatment	Calcium chloride IV Norepinephrine bitartrate IV Metaraminol bitartrate IV Isoproterenol HCl IV	Dopamine HCl IV Dobutamine HCl IV	Intravenous fluids Trendelenburg position
2. Bradycardia, AV block, Asystole	Isoproterenol HCl IV Calcium chloride IV Norepinephrine bitartrate IV Atropine sulfate IV Cardiac pacing	—	Intravenous fluids (slow drip)
3. Rapid ventricular rate (due to antegrade conduction in flutter/fibrillation with W-P-W or L-G-L syndromes)	D.C.-cardioversion (high energy may be required) Procainamide IV Lidocaine HCl IV	—	Intravenous fluids (slow drip)

*Actual treatment and dosage should depend on the severity of the clinical situation and the judgment and experience of the treating physician.

Searle Pharm.—Cont.

Calan ampuls and syringes are manufactured for Searle Pharmaceuticals Inc.
Shown in Product Identification Section, page 435

CU-7®
[*cē' ū-sev"en*]
(intrauterine copper contraceptive)

Description: The plastic component of the Cu-7 is composed of pharmaceutical grade polypropylene homopolymer with barium sulfate added to render it radiopaque. Its shape approximates the number 7. It is substantially smaller than previously available intrauterine devices; the vertical dimension measures 36 mm and the horizontal, 26 mm.

Coiled around the vertical limb is 89 mg of copper wire providing approximately 200 mm^2 of exposed copper surface area. A retrieval thread is fastened to the free end of the vertical limb of the Cu-7.

The Cu-7 is supplied with a simple tubular plastic inserter. All components are sterile.

[*The following sections apply to both Cu-7 and Tatum-T.*]

Clinical Pharmacology: Available data indicate that the contraceptive effectiveness of the Cu-7 or Tatum-T is enhanced by a minute quantity of copper released continuously from the coiled copper into the uterine cavity.

The exact mechanism by which metallic copper enhances the contraceptive effect of an IUD has not been conclusively demonstrated. Various hypotheses have been advanced, the most common being that copper placed in the uterus interferes with enzymatic or other processes that regulate blastocyst implantation.

Animal studies suggest that copper may play an additional role by reduction of sperm transport within the uterine environment.

Indication and Usage: The Cu-7 or Tatum-T is indicated for contraception.

Contraindications: The Cu-7 or Tatum-T should not be inserted when any of the following conditions exist: pregnancy or suspicion of pregnancy; abnormalities of the uterus resulting in distortion of the uterine cavity; acute pelvic inflammatory disease, a history of repeated or recent pelvic inflammatory disease, or a history of severe pelvic inflammatory disease; genital actinomycosis; postpartum endometritis or infected abortion in the past three months; known or suspected uterine or cervical disease such as hyperplasia or carcinoma including unresolved, abnormal Pap test; vaginal bleeding of unknown etiology; untreated acute cervicitis until infection is controlled; diagnosed Wilson's disease; known or suspected allergy to copper; previous ectopic pregnancy; significant anemia; and valvular heart disease, leukemia, or use of chronic corticosteroid therapy because of the increased susceptibility to infection with certain microorganisms which may possibly be introduced at the time of an IUD insertion.

Warnings:
1. *Pregnancy:* (a) *Long-term effects.* The long-term effects on the offspring of the presence of copper in the uterus when pregnancy occurs with the Cu-7 or Tatum-T are unknown.
(b) *Septic abortion.* Reports have indicated an increased incidence of septic abortion associated in some instances with septicemia, septic shock and death in patients becoming pregnant with an IUD in place. Most of these reports have been associated with the mid-trimester of pregnancy. In some cases, the initial symptoms have been insidious and not easily recognized. If pregnancy should occur with a Cu-7 or Tatum-T in situ, the Cu-7 or Tatum-T should be removed if the thread is visible or, if removal proves to be or would be difficult, interruption of the pregnancy should be considered and offered to the patient as an option, bearing in mind that the risks associated with an elective abortion increase with gestational age.
(c) *Continuation of pregnancy.* If the patient chooses to continue the pregnancy and the Cu-7 or Tatum-T remains in situ, she must be warned of the increased risk of spontaneous abortion and the increased risk of sepsis, including death. The patient must be closely observed and she must be advised to report immediately all abnormal symptoms, such as flu-like syndrome, fever, abdominal cramping and pain, bleeding, or vaginal discharge, because generalized symptoms of septicemia may be insidious.
2. *Ectopic pregnancy:* (a) A pregnancy which occurs with an IUD in situ is more likely to be ectopic than a pregnancy occurring without an IUD. Therefore, patients who become pregnant while using a Cu-7 or Tatum-T should be carefully evaluated for the possibility of an ectopic pregnancy.
(b) Special attention should be directed to patients with delayed menses, slight metrorrhagia and/or unilateral pelvic pain, and to those patients who wish to interrupt a pregnancy occurring in the presence of a Cu-7 or Tatum-T, to determine whether ectopic pregnancy has occurred.
3. *Pelvic infection:* An increased risk of pelvic inflammatory disease associated with the use of IUDs has been reported. While unconfirmed, this risk appears to be greatest for young women who are nulliparous and/or who have a multiplicity of sexual partners. Salpingitis can result in tubal damage and occlusion, thereby threatening future fertility. Therefore, it is recommended that patients be taught to look for symptoms of pelvic inflammatory disease. The decision to use an IUD in a particular case must be made by the physician and patient with the consideration of a possible deleterious effect on future fertility. This consideration is especially important for women who may wish to have children at a later date, particularly nulliparous women.

Pelvic infection may occur with a Cu-7 or Tatum-T in situ and at times result in the development of tubo-ovarian abscesses or general peritonitis. The symptoms of pelvic infection include: new development of menstrual disorders (prolonged or heavy bleeding), abnormal vaginal discharge, abdominal or pelvic pain, dyspareunia, fever. The symptoms are especially significant if they occur following the first two or three cycles after insertion. Appropriate aerobic and anaerobic bacteriologic studies should be done and antibiotic therapy initiated promptly. If the infection does not show marked clinical improvement within 24 to 48 hours, the Cu-7 or Tatum-T should be removed and the continuing treatment reassessed on the basis of the results of culture and sensitivity tests. Genital actinomycosis has been associated primarily with long-term IUD use. It has been reported with the use of copper-bearing IUDs as well. Treatment requires prompt removal of the IUD and appropriate antibiotic therapy.
4. *Embedment:* Partial penetration or lodging of the Cu-7 or Tatum-T in the endometrium or myometrium can result in a difficult removal. This may occur more frequently in smaller uteri. (See removal instructions.)
5. *Perforation:* Partial or total perforation of the uterine wall or cervix may occur with the use of the Cu-7 or Tatum-T, usually during insertions into patients sooner than two months after abortion or delivery, or in uterine cavities too small for the Cu-7 or Tatum-T. An increased risk of perforation has been reported to occur when an IUD is inserted into lactating women compared to non-lactating parous women. The possibility of perforation must be kept in mind during insertion and at the time of any subsequent examination. If perforation occurs, laparotomy or laparoscopy should be performed as soon as medically feasible and the Cu-7 or Tatum-T removed. Abdominal adhesions, intestinal penetration, intestinal obstruction, and local inflammatory reaction with abscess formation and erosion of adjacent viscera may result if the Cu-7 or Tatum-T is left in the peritoneal cavity.
6. *Medical diathermy:* The use of medical diathermy (shortwave and microwave) in a patient with a metal-containing IUD may cause heat injury to the surrounding tissue. Therefore, medical diathermy to the abdominal and sacral areas should not be used on patients using a Cu-7 or Tatum-T.
7. *Effects of copper:* Additional amounts of copper available to the body from the Cu-7 or Tatum-T may precipitate symptoms in women with undiagnosed Wilson's disease. The incidence of Wilson's disease is 1 in 200,000.

Malonaldehyde (MA) is a normal trace by-product of both prostaglandin biosynthesis and the oxidative breakdown of body fat, and occurs naturally in the human body. MA and related fat breakdown products have been reported to be mutagenic in a variety of test systems, and systemically carcinogenic when applied to the skin of mice at higher than naturally occurring levels. A study has reported that levels of MA were detected in the cervical mucus of women using copper-bearing IUDs, but not in controls. The author stated that increased levels of MA within the uterus represent an increased risk of carcinogenesis. The concentrations of MA reported to be mutagenic in bacterial or cell culture systems or carcinogenic in mice are higher than the concentration of MA observed in the cervical mucus of women using copper-bearing IUDs.

Precautions:
1. *Patient counseling.* Prior to the insertion the physician, nurse, or other trained health professional must provide the patient with the Patient Brochure. The patient should be given the opportunity to read the brochure and discuss fully any questions she may have concerning the Cu-7 or Tatum-T as well as other methods of contraception.
2. *Patient evaluation and clinical considerations.*
(a) A complete medical history should be obtained to determine conditions that might influence the selection of an IUD. A physical examination should include a pelvic examination, Pap test, gonorrhea culture, and, if indicated, appropriate tests for other forms of genital disease including genital actinomycosis, which usually can be detected by the Pap test. The physician should determine that the patient is not pregnant.
(b) The uterus should be carefully sounded prior to the insertion to determine the degree of patency of the endocervical canal and the internal os, and the direction and depth of the uterine cavity. Exercise care to avoid perforation with the sound. DO NOT USE THE Cu-7 OR Tatum-T INSERTION INSTRUMENT AS A SOUND. In occasional cases, severe cervical stenosis may be encountered. Do not use excessive force to overcome this resistance.
(c) The uterus usually sounds to a depth of 6 cm to 8 cm. Insertion of a Cu-7 or Tatum-T into a uterine cavity measuring less than 6.5 cm by sounding may increase the incidence of pain, bleeding, partial or complete expulsion, perforation, and possibly pregnancy.
(d) To reduce the possibility of insertion in the presence of an existing undetermined pregnancy, the optimal time for insertion is the latter part of the menstrual flow or one or two days thereafter. The Cu-7 or Tatum-T should not be inserted post partum or post abortion until involution of the uterus is complete. The incidence of perforation and expulsion is greater if involution is not complete.

It is, however, necessary to place the Cu-7 or Tatum-T as high as possible within the uterine cavity to help avoid partial or complete expulsion that could result in pregnancy.

Since the Cu-7 or Tatum-T represents a different design in intrauterine contraception, physicians are cautioned that it is imperative for them to become thoroughly familiar with the instructions for use before attempting placement of the Cu-7 or Tatum-T.
(e) IUDs should be used with caution in those patients who have an anemia or a history of menorrhagia or hypermenorrhea. Patients experiencing menorrhagia and/or metrorrhagia following IUD insertion may be at risk for the development of hypochromic microcytic anemia. Also, IUDs should be used with caution in patients receiving anticoagulants or having a coagulopathy.
(f) Syncope, bradycardia or other neurovascular episodes may occur during insertion or removal of IUDs, especially in patients with a previous disposition to these conditions.

(g) Patients with valvular or congenital heart disease are more prone to develop subacute bacterial endocarditis than patients who do not have valvular or congenital heart disease. Use of an IUD in these patients may represent a potential source of septic emboli. See *Contraindications*.

(h) Use of an IUD in those patients with acute cervicitis should be postponed until proper treatment has cleared up the infection.

(i) Since the Cu-7 or Tatum-T may be partially or completely expelled, patients should be reexamined and evaluated shortly after the first postinsertion menses, but definitely within three months after insertion. Thereafter annual examination with appropriate medical and laboratory evaluation, and a Pap test, including examination for *Actinomyces* organisms, should be carried out. The Cu-7 or Tatum-T should be replaced every three years.

(j) The patient should be told that some bleeding or cramping may occur during the first few weeks after insertion, but if these symptoms continue or are severe she should report them to her physician. She should be instructed on how to check after each menstrual period to make certain that the thread still protrudes from the cervix and cautioned that there is no contraceptive protection if the Cu-7 or Tatum-T has been expelled. She should also be cautioned not to dislodge the Cu-7 or Tatum-T by pulling on the thread. If a partial expulsion occurs, removal is indicated and a new Cu-7 or Tatum-T may be inserted. The patient should be told to return within three years for removal of the Cu-7 or Tatum-T and for replacement if desired.

(k) A copper-induced urticarial allergic skin reaction may develop in women using a copper-containing IUD. If symptoms of such an allergic response occur, the patient should be instructed to tell the consulting physician that a copper-containing device is being used.

(l) The Cu-7 or Tatum-T should be removed for the following medical reasons: menorrhagia and/or metrorrhagia producing significant anemia; uncontrolled pelvic infection; genital actinomycosis; intractable pain often aggravated by intercourse, dyspareunia; pregnancy, if the thread is visible; endometrial or cervical malignancy; uterine or cervical perforation; or any indication of partial expulsion.

(m) If the retrieval thread cannot be visualized it may have retracted into the uterus or have been broken off, or the Cu-7 or Tatum-T may have been expelled. Localization usually can be made by feeling with a probe; if not, contact hysteroscopy, x-ray, or sonography can be used. When the physician elects to recover a Cu-7 or Tatum-T with the thread not visible, the removal instructions should be considered.

(n) If any patient with a Cu-7 or Tatum-T suddenly develops overt clinical hepatitis or abnormal liver function tests, appropriate diagnostic procedures should be initiated.

(o) It has been reported that IUDs may be less effective in insulin-dependent diabetics.

Adverse Reactions: Perforations of uterus and cervix have occurred. Perforation into the abdomen has been followed by abdominal adhesions, intestinal penetration, intestinal obstruction, local inflammatory reaction with abscess formation and erosion of adjacent viscera. Pregnancy has occurred with the Cu-7 or Tatum-T in situ and when the Cu-7 or Tatum-T has been partially or completely expelled.

The incidence of spontaneous abortion, when conception occurs with intrauterine devices in situ, appears to be increased over that in unprotected women. Insertion cramping, usually of no more than a few seconds' duration, may occur; however, some women may experience residual cramping for several hours or even days. Intermenstrual spotting or bleeding, or prolonged or increased menstrual flow may occur.

Pelvic infection including salpingitis with tubal damage or occlusion has been reported. This may result in future infertility. Complete or partial expulsion of the Cu-7 or Tatum-T may sometimes occur, particularly in those patients with uteri measuring less than 6.5 cm by sounding. Urticarial allergic skin reaction may occur. The following complaints have also been reported with IUDs although their relation to the Cu-7 or Tatum-T has not been established: amenorrhea or delayed menses, backaches, cervical erosion, cystic masses in the pelvis, vaginitis, leg pain or soreness, erythema nodosum, weight loss or gain, nervousness, dyspareunia, cystitis, endometritis, septic abortion, mycotic chorioamnionitis, septicemia, leukorrhea, ectopic pregnancy, difficult removal, uterine embedment, anemia, pain, neurovascular episodes including bradycardia and syncope secondary to insertion, dysmenorrhea, and fragmentation of the IUD.

[*The following sections do not apply to Tatum-T. See* **Directions for Use, Clinical Studies, Procedure for Insertion, and Removal of the Tatum-T** *under that product's heading.*]

Directions for Use: The Cu-7 is to be placed within the uterine cavity. See the *Procedure for Insertion* that follows, which describes two insertion techniques.

The small diameter of the Cu-7 inserter tube facilitates easy insertion in nulligravidous and nulliparous, as well as parous, women. The optimal time of insertion is during the latter part of the menstrual flow or one or two days thereafter. The cervical canal is relatively more patent at this time, and there is little chance that the patient may be pregnant.

Present information indicates that efficacy is retained for 36 months. There is no evidence that contraceptive efficacy decreases with time up to three years of use, but unless new data support a longer period of efficacy and safety, the Cu-7 must be removed within 36 months from the date of insertion and a new one inserted if desired. If partial expulsion occurs, removal is indicated, and a new Cu-7 may be inserted. Removal of the Cu-7 may also be indicated in the event of heavy or persistent bleeding.

The physician should become thoroughly familiar with the instructions for use before attempting insertion or removal of the Cu-7.

Clinical Studies: Different event rates have been reported with the use of different intrauterine contraceptives. Inasmuch as these rates are usually derived from separate studies conducted by different investigators in several population groups, a comparison cannot be made with precision. Even in different studies with the same contraceptive, considerably different rates are likely to be obtained because of differing characteristics of the study population. Furthermore, event rates per unit of time tend to be lower as clinical experience is expanded, possibly due to retention in the clinical study of those patients who accept the treatment regimen, not having discontinued due to adverse reactions or pregnancy, so that those remaining in the study were those less susceptible. In clinical trials of the Cu-7 conducted by Searle, use effectiveness was determined as follows for parous and nulliparous women, as tabulated by the life table method. (Rates are expressed as cumulative events per 100 women through 12, 24, and 36 months of use.)

	12 Months Parous	12 Months Nulliparous	24 Months Parous	24 Months Nulliparous	36 Months Parous	36 Months Nulliparous
Pregnancy	1.9	1.7	3.0	2.6	3.5	3.1
Expulsion	5.6	7.8	6.7	9.0	7.2	9.4
Medical removal	10.9	13.7	18.3	20.9	24.8	28.7
Continuation	69.8	65.9	45.7	45.8	21.6	17.8

After elective removal of the Cu-7 for desire to become pregnant, 60% of the women conceived within three months and 75% had conceived within one year of removal.

Cu-7® Insertion Instrument

This experience encompasses 373,948 woman-months of use, including 12 months for 11,288 women, 24 months for 7,518, and 36 months for 3,371.

Cumulative rates were:
[See table above].

Procedure for Insertion

The Cu-7 may be inserted easily at any time during the menstrual cycle. It is *not* necessary to delay insertion until a menstrual flow is in progress; however, the possibility of existing undetermined pregnancy is lessened if insertion is made during or shortly following a menstrual period.

The cervix should be cleansed with antiseptic solution and its anterior lip grasped with a tenaculum prior to sounding the uterus and insertion of the Cu-7. Insertion of the Cu-7 into a severely anteverted or severely retroverted uterus may be difficult unless sufficient tension is applied to the tenaculum. Determination of the depth and direction of the uterine cavity should be made with a sound prior to insertion.

An aseptic technique should be employed. Sterile gloves are recommended; however, the sterile sheath covering the Cu-7 in the package may be used to avoid handling any part of the copper figure seven or the tube which will enter the cervical canal.

To load the Cu-7 into the tube, fold the transverse arm against the copper-clad stem and push it into the tube until only the mushroom tip protrudes. Center the dot (thread knot) on the stem of the plastic carrier with the long axis (horizontal plane) of the cervical stop.

Caution: DO NOT leave the Cu-7 folded in the tube longer than two minutes or the plastic will lose its "memory"; it will then fail to resume its original configuration within the uterus and thus invite loss of effectiveness and early expulsion.

DO NOT remove the thread-retaining clip from the insertion rod until after insertion has been made and you are ready to deposit the Cu-7 within the uterine cavity.

DO NOT force the insertion. It is generally believed that most perforations occur at the time of insertion, although the perforation may not be detected until some time later. The position of the uterus should be determined during the pre-insertion examination. Great care must be exercised during the pre-insertion sounding and subsequent insertion.

Note: If the uterine cavity measures under 6.5 cm, the incidence of pain, bleeding, partial or complete expulsion, perforation, and possibly pregnancy increases. Insertion is not recommended into a uterus that sounds under 5.5 cm.

Release Technique

Note: After sounding, the cervical stop should be set at the depth measured on the sound. *See Figure 1.* Load the Cu-7 into the tube and immediately

Continued on next page

Searle Pharm.—Cont.

begin the insertion. DO NOT leave the Cu-7 in the tube longer than 2 minutes.

1. Apply tension with the tenaculum and gently insert the loaded instrument through the cervical canal, *see Figure 2*, to the fundus, *see Figure 3*, at which time the cervical stop should be at the cervix. Pinch the thread-retaining clip to the tube-stop during insertion to prevent the tube from crimping. The end of the rod should be touching the end of the Cu-7 at all times. Keep the cervical stop in the horizontal plane until it reaches the cervix. DO NOT FORCE.

2. Hold the rod firmly with the cervical stop at the cervix and free the thread by pressing the thread-retaining clip from the rod. Release the Cu-7 into the uterine cavity by *withdrawing* the tube to ½ inch from the handle. (DO NOT PUSH ON THE HANDLE; perforation could result.) *See Figure 4*.

3. Hold the tube still (do not withdraw further) and gently push the rod all of the way into the tube to correctly seat the Cu-7 entirely within the uterine cavity. *See Figure 5*.

4. Withdraw the insertion instrument and cut the thread at least 2 in (5 cm) from the external os. DO NOT PULL OUT EXCESS THREAD BEFORE CUTTING. *See Figure 6*.

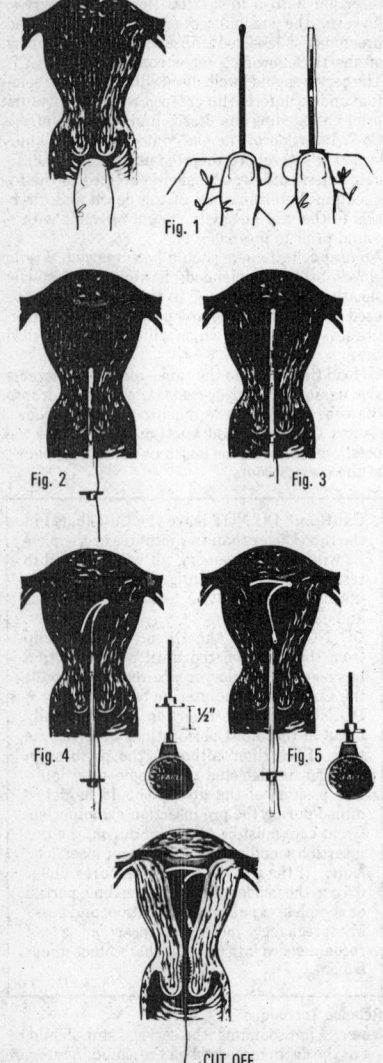

Push-In Technique

Note: The cervical stop has been preset on the tube at 34 mm from the proximal end. *See Figure 1*. This will allow proper placement of the Cu-7 in a uterus which sounds to 2¾ in (7.0 cm) using *this* insertion technique only. (Since the cervical stop may have moved during shipment, this measurement should be verified.) If the uterus sounds to a depth greater than 2¾ in (7.0 cm), the cervical stop should be moved farther from the end of the tube by that many inches (centimeters). If the uterus sounds to a depth less than 2¾ in (7.0 cm), the cervical stop should be moved that much closer to the end of the tube.

1. Apply tension with the tenaculum and gently insert the loaded instrument through the cervical canal to the cervical stop, *see Figure 2*. Pinch the thread-retaining clip to the tube-stop during insertion to prevent the tube from crimping. The end of the rod should be touching the end of the Cu-7 at all times. Keep the cervical stop in the horizontal plane until it reaches the cervix. DO NOT FORCE.

2. Hold the tube firmly; remove the thread-retaining clip by pressing it off the rod and gently push

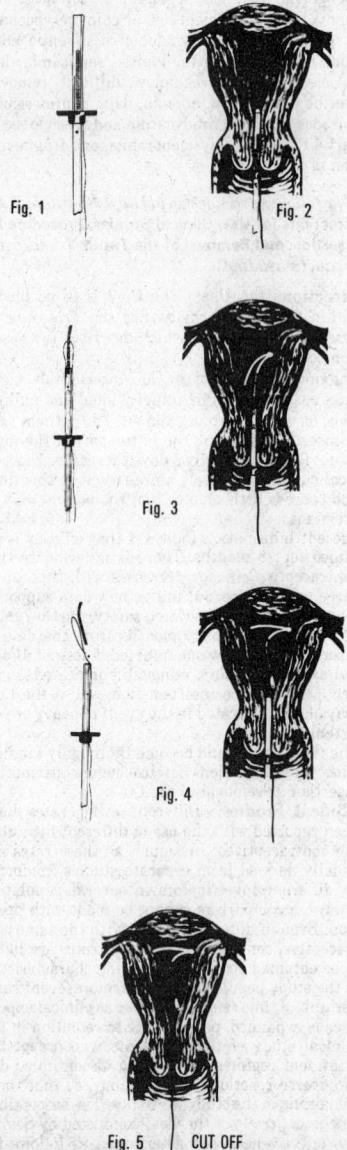

the rod, *see Figure 3*, all the way into the tube to correctly seat the Cu-7 entirely within the uterine cavity. *See Figure 4*.

3. Withdraw the insertion instrument and cut the thread at least 2 in (5 cm) from the external os. DO NOT PULL OUT EXCESS THREAD BEFORE CUTTING. *See Figure 5*.

Removal of the Cu-7

ROUTINE REMOVAL—THREAD VISIBLE:

1. DO NOT exert a sudden pull or jerk on the retrieval thread. Exert a firm, steady pull on the thread. A jerk may cause the thread to break.
2. A ring (sponge) forceps, with its smooth edges and minimal crushing force, is a good instrument with which to grasp the thread.
3. Other instruments may be used, but care must be exerted to avoid crushing or cutting the thread.
4. Avoid winding or angulating the thread about the jaws of the withdrawal instrument.
5. Utilize the minimum force needed to remove the Cu-7.
6. Should resistance be encountered, dislodge the Cu-7 by the aseptic use of a slim instrument (eg, uterine dressing forceps) before making further removal attempts.

THREAD NOT VISIBLE: If the Cu-7 is in the uterus and the thread is not visible, the following procedures should be considered when you elect to recover it:

1. Aseptic use of a slim instrument (eg, uterine dressing forceps) or contact hysteroscopy will frequently permit removal in the office.
2. Hysteroscopy under hospital conditions may be required.
3. D & C and also suction aspiration have been used as alternative measures.

NOTE: If intrauterine manipulative procedures are required, allow an appropriate healing period before inserting a new Cu-7.

How Supplied: Available in boxes of 10, 30, and 100 sterile units (Cu-7 with an inserter), and sufficient patient brochures and identification cards.

Shown in Product Identification Section, page 435

DIULO™ ℞
[*dī'ū-lō*]
(metolazone)

Description: Each Diulo tablet contains 2½, 5, or 10 mg of metolazone, a diuretic/saluretic/antihypertensive drug. Metolazone has the molecular formula $C_{16}H_{16}ClN_3O_3S$. The structural formula of the metolazone molecule is

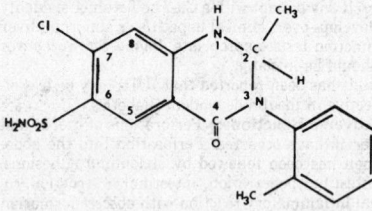

and its chemical name is 7-chloro-1, 2, 3, 4-tetrahydro-2-methyl-4-oxo-3-o-tolyl-6- quinazolinesulfonamide. Metolazone is only sparingly soluble in water, but more soluble in plasma, blood, alkali, and organic solvents.

Actions: Diulo (metolazone) is a diuretic/saluretic/antihypertensive drug whose action results in an interference with the renal tubular mechanism of electrolyte reabsorption. The mechanism of this action is unknown. Diulo acts primarily to inhibit sodium reabsorption at the cortical diluting site and in the proximal convoluted tubule. Sodium and chloride ions are excreted in approximately equivalent amounts. The increased delivery of sodium to the distal-tubular exchange site may result in increased potassium excretion.

Drug Interaction Studies: In animals pretreated with metolazone, the drug did not alter the characteristic effect of heparin on clotting time nor protamine antagonism; dicumarol on prothrombin time nor Vitamin K antagonism; the response of guanethidine, reserpine and hydralazine to cardiovascular parameters nor the pressor response of the subsequent dose of norepinephrine.

Metolazone and furosemide, administered concurrently have produced marked diuresis in some patients whose edema or ascites was refractory to treatment with maximum recommended doses of these or other diuretics administered alone. The mechanism of this interaction is not known.

In clinical usage, metolazone does not inhibit carbonic anhydrase. Its proximal action has been evidenced in humans by increased excretion of phosphate and magnesium ions, by markedly increased fractional excretion of sodium in patients with severely compromised glomerular filtration, and in animals by the results of micropuncture studies. Decrease in calcium ion excretion has not been noted.

At maximum therapeutic dosage Diulo is approximately equal to thiazide diuretics in its diuretic potency. However, Diulo may produce diuresis in patients with glomerular filtration rates below 20 ml/min.

When Diulo is given, diuresis and saluresis usually begin within one hour and persist for 12 to 24 hours depending on dosage. Maximum effect occurs about two hours after administration. At the higher recommended dosages, effect may be prolonged beyond 24 hours. *A single daily dose is recommended.* For most patients the duration of effect can be varied by adjusting the daily dose. The prolonged duration of action of Diulo is attributed to protein binding and enterohepatic recycling. A small amount of Diulo is metabolized and the fraction so changed is nontoxic. The primary route of excretion is renal.

The mechanism whereby diuretics function in the control of hypertension is unknown; both renal and extrarenal actions may be involved. An antihypertensive effect may be seen as early as three to four days after Diulo has been started. Administration for three to four weeks, however, is usually required for optimum antihypertensive effect.

Indications and Usage: Diulo (metolazone) is indicated in the management of hypertension either as the sole therapeutic agent or to enhance the effectiveness of other antihypertensive drugs in the more severe forms of hypertension.

Diulo (metolazone) is indicated for the treatment of salt and water retention including
— edema accompanying congestive heart failure
— edema accompanying renal diseases, including the nephrotic syndrome, and states of diminished renal function.

Usage in Pregnancy: The routine use of diuretics in an otherwise healthy woman is inappropriate and exposes mother and fetus to unnecessary hazard. Diuretics do not prevent development of toxemia of pregnancy, and there is no satisfactory evidence that they are useful in the treatment of developed toxemia.

Edema during pregnancy may arise from pathological causes or from the physiologic and mechanical consequences of pregnancy. Diulo is indicated in pregnancy when edema is due to pathologic causes, just as it is in the absence of pregnancy (however, see *Precautions,* below). Dependent edema in pregnancy, resulting from restriction of venous return by the expanded uterus, is properly treated through elevation of the lower extremities and use of support hose; use of diuretics to lower intravascular volume in this case is illogical and unnecessary. There is hypervolemia during normal pregnancy which is harmful to neither the fetus nor the mother (in the absence of cardiovascular disease), but which is associated with edema, including generalized edema, in the majority of pregnant women. If this edema produces discomfort, increased recumbency will often provide relief. In rare instances, this edema may cause extreme discomfort which is not relieved by rest. In these cases, a short course of diuretics may provide relief and may be appropriate.

Contraindications: Anuria.
Hepatic coma or pre-coma; known allergy or hypersensitivity to metolazone.

Warnings: While not reported to date, cross-allergy theoretically may occur when metolazone is given to patients known to be allergic to sulfonamide-derived drugs, thiazides, or quinethazone.

Hypokalemia may occur, with consequent weakness, cramps, and cardiac dysrhythmias. Hypokalemia is a particular hazard in digitalized patients; dangerous or fatal arrhythmias may be precipitated.

Azotemia and hyperuricemia may be noted or precipitated during the administration of metolazone. Infrequently, gouty attacks have been reported in persons with history of gout.

If azotemia and oliguria worsen during treatment of patients with severe renal disease, Diulo should be discontinued.

Until additional data have been obtained, Diulo is not recommended for patients in the pediatric age group.

Unusually large or prolonged effects on volume and electrolytes may result when metolazone and furosemide are administered concurrently. It is recommended that concurrent administration of these diuretics for treatment of resistant edema be started under hospital conditions in order to provide for adequate monitoring.

When Diulo is used with other antihypertensive drugs, particular care must be taken, especially during initial therapy. Dosage of other antihypertensive agents, especially the ganglionic blockers, should be reduced.

Diulo may be given with a potassium-sparing diuretic when indicated. In this circumstance, diuresis may be potentiated and dosages should be reduced. Potassium retention and hyperkalemia may result; the serum potassium should be determined frequently. Potassium supplementation is contraindicated when a potassium-sparing diuretic is given.

Precautions: Periodic determination of serum electrolytes to detect possible electrolyte imbalance should be performed at appropriate intervals. Blood urea nitrogen, uric acid, and glucose levels should be assessed at intervals during diuretic therapy.

All patients receiving Diulo (metolazone) therapy should be observed for clinical signs of fluid and/or electrolyte imbalance; namely, hyponatremia, hypochloremic alkalosis, and hypokalemia. Serum and urine electrolyte determinations are particularly important when the patient is vomiting excessively or receiving parenteral fluids. Medication such as digitalis may also influence serum electrolytes. Warning signs, irrespective of cause, are: dryness of mouth, thirst, weakness, lethargy, drowsiness, restlessness, muscle pains or cramps, muscular fatigue, hypotension, oliguria, tachycardia, and gastrointestinal disturbances such as nausea and vomiting.

The serum potassium should be determined at regular intervals, and potassium supplementation instituted whenever indicated. Hypokalemia will be more common in association with intensive or prolonged diuretic therapy, with concomitant steroid or ACTH therapy, and with inadequate electrolyte intake.

While not reported to date for metolazone, related diuretics have increased responsiveness to tubocurarine and decreased arterial responsiveness to norepinephrine. Accordingly, it may be advisable to discontinue Diulo three days before elective surgery.

Caution should be observed when administering Diulo to hyperuricemic or gouty patients. Diulo exerts minimal effects on glucose metabolism; insulin requirements may be affected in diabetics, and hyperglycemia and glycosuria may occur in patients with latent diabetes.

Chloride deficit and hypochloremic alkalosis may occur. In patients with severe edema accompanying cardiac failure or renal disease, a low-salt syndrome may be produced; hot weather and a low-salt diet will contribute.

Caution should be observed when administering Diulo to patients with severely impaired renal function. As most of the drug is excreted by the renal route, cumulative effects may be seen in this circumstance.

Orthostatic hypotension may occur; this may be potentiated by alcohol, barbiturates, narcotics, or concurrent therapy with other antihypertensive drugs.

While not reported for metolazone, use of other diuretics has been associated on rare occasions with pathological changes in the parathyroid glands and with hypercalcemia. This possibility should be kept in mind with clinical use of Diulo.

Usage in Pregnancy
Diulo crosses the placental barrier and appears in cord blood. The use of Diulo in pregnant women requires that the anticipated benefit be weighed against possible hazards to the fetus. These hazards include fetal or neonatal jaundice, thrombocytopenia, and possibly other adverse reactions which have occurred in the adult.

Nursing Mothers
Metolazone appears in breast milk. If use of the drug is deemed essential, the patient should stop nursing.

Adverse Reactions: Adverse reactions encountered during therapy with potent medications should be considered in two groups: those that represent extension of the expected pharmacologic actions of the drug, and those which are pharmacologically unexpected, idiosyncratic, specially toxic, due to allergy or hypersensitivity, or due to unexplained causes.

For Diulo (metolazone), adverse reactions constituting extensions of the expected pharmacologic actions of this potent diuretic/ saluretic/ antihypertensive drug may include:

Gastrointestinal reactions: constipation.
Central nervous system reactions: syncope, dizziness, drowsiness.
Cardiovascular reactions: orthostatic hypotension, excessive volume depletion, hemoconcentration, venous thrombosis.
Other reactions: dryness of the mouth, symptomatic and asymptomatic hypokalemia, hyponatremia, hypochloremia; hypochloremic alkalosis, hypophosphatemia, hyperuricemia, hyperglycemia, glycosuria, increase in BUN or creatinine, fatigue, muscle cramps or spasm, weakness, restlessness sometimes resulting in insomnia.

In the second classification, adverse reactions to Diulo may include:
Gastrointestinal reactions: nausea, vomiting, anorexia, diarrhea, abdominal bloating, epigastric distress, intrahepatic cholestatic jaundice, hepatitis.
Central nervous system reactions: vertigo, headache, paresthesias.
Hematologic reactions: leukopenia, aplastic anemia.
Dermatologic-hypersensitivity reactions: urticaria and other skin rashes, purpura, necrotizing angiitis (cutaneous vasculitis).
Cardiovascular reactions: palpitation, chest pain.
Other reactions: chills, acute gouty attacks, transient blurred vision.

Adverse reactions which have occurred with other diuretics include: pancreatitis, xanthopsia, agranulocytosis, thrombocytopenia, and photosensitivity. These reactions should be considered as possible occurrences with clinical usage of Diulo.

Whenever adverse reactions are moderate or severe, Diulo dosage should be reduced or therapy withdrawn.

Dosage and Administration: Therapy should be individualized according to patient response. Programs of therapy with Diulo (metolazone) should be titrated to gain a maximal initial therapeutic response, and to determine the minimal dose possible to maintain that therapeutic response.

Diulo is a potent drug with a prolonged, 12- to 24-hour duration of action. When an initially-desired

Continued on next page

Searle Pharm.—Cont.

therapeutic effect has been obtained, it is ordinarily advisable to reduce the dosage of Diulo to a lower maintenance level. The time interval required for the initial higher-dosage regimen may vary from days in edematous states to three or four weeks in the treatment of elevated blood pressure. The daily dosage depends on the severity of each patient's condition, sodium intake, and responsiveness. Therefore, dosage adjustment is usually necessary during the course of therapy. A decision to reduce the daily dosage of Diulo from a higher induction level to a lower maintenance level should be based on the results of thorough clinical and laboratory evaluations. If antihypertensive drugs or diuretics are given concurrently with Diulo, careful dosage adjustment may be necessary.

Usual Dosage
Suitable initial dosages will usually fall in the ranges given:
Edema of cardiac failure:
  Diulo 5–10 mg, once daily
Edema of renal disease:
  Diulo 5–20 mg, once daily
Mild to moderate essential hypertension:
  Diulo 2½–5 mg, once daily
For patients with congestive cardiac failure who tend to experience paroxysmal nocturnal dyspnea, it is usually advisable to employ a dosage near the upper end of the range, to ensure prolongation of diuresis and saluresis for a full 24-hour period.

How Supplied: Diulo (metolazone) is supplied as tablets containing 2½, 5, and 10 mg of metolazone.
Diulo 2½-mg tablets are round, pink tablets with SEARLE debossed on one side and 501 on the other side.
Diulo 5-mg tablets are round, blue tablets with SEARLE debossed on one side and 511 on the other side.
Diulo 10-mg tablets are round, yellow tablets with SEARLE debossed on one side and 521 on the other side.
Diulo 2½ mg, 5 mg, and 10 mg are available in bottles of 100 tablets.
Shown in Product Identification Section, page 435

DRAMAMINE® Liquid
[*dram'uh-meen*]
(dimenhydrinate syrup USP)
DRAMAMINE® Tablets
DRAMAMINE INJECTION™ B
(dimenhydrinate)

Description: Dimenhydrinate, an antinauseant/antiemetic, is the 8-chlorotheophylline (8-chloro-3, 7-dihydro-1, 3-dimethyl-1H-purine-2,6-dione) salt of diphenhydramine (2-diphenyl-methoxy-N,N-dimethylethanamine). The structural formula of dimenhydrinate is

Dimenhydrinate contains not less than 53% and not more than 56% of diphenhydramine, and not less than 44% and not more than 47% of 8-chlorotheophylline, calculated on the dried basis. Dramamine Injection ampuls and vials contain a sterile solution of dimenhydrinate 50 mg/ml in benzyl alcohol 5%, propylene glycol 50%, and water for injection.

Clinical Pharmacology: While the precise mode of action of dimenhydrinate is not known, it has a depressant action on hyperstimulated labyrinthine function.

Indications and Usage: Dramamine is indicated for the prevention and treatment of the nausea, vomiting, or vertigo of motion sickness.

Contraindications: Neonates and patients with a history of hypersensitivity to dimenhydrinate or its components (diphenhydramine or 8-chlorotheophylline) should be treated with Dramamine Injection.

Warnings: Caution should be used when Dramamine is given in conjunction with certain antibiotics that may cause ototoxicity, since Dramamine is capable of masking ototoxic symptoms and an irreversible state may be reached. As with any drug, pregnant or nursing women should seek the advice of a health professional before using this product.

This drug may impair the mental and/or physical abilities required for the performance of potentially hazardous tasks, such as driving a vehicle or operating machinery. The concomitant use of alcohol or other central nervous system depressants may have an additive effect. Therefore, patients should be warned accordingly.

Dimenhydrinate should be used with caution in patients having conditions which might be aggravated by anticholinergic therapy (ie, prostatic hypertrophy, stenosing peptic ulcer, pyloroduodenal obstruction, bladder neck obstruction, narrow-angle glaucoma, bronchial asthma, or cardiac arrhythmias).

This preparation should not be injected intra-arterially.

Usage in children: For infants and children especially, antihistamines in overdosage may cause hallucinations, convulsions, or death.
As in adults, antihistamines may diminish mental alertness in children. In the young child, particularly, they may produce excitation.

Precautions:
General: Drowsiness may be experienced by some patients, especially with high dosage. This condition frequently is not undesirable in conditions for which the drug is used.

Information for patients: Because of the potential for drowsiness, patients taking Dramamine should be cautioned against operating automobiles or dangerous machinery. See *Warnings*.

Carcinogenesis, mutagenesis, impairment of fertility: Mutagenicity screening tests performed with dimenhydrinate, diphenhydramine, and 8-chlorotheophylline produced positive results in the bacterial systems and negative results in the mammalian systems. There are no human data that indicate Dramamine is a carcinogen or mutagen or that it impairs fertility.

Pregnancy: Pregnancy Category B. Reproduction studies have been performed in rats at doses up to 20 times the human dose, and in rabbits at doses up to 25 times the human dose (on an mg/kg basis), and have revealed no evidence of impaired fertility or harm to the fetus due to Dramamine. There are no adequate and well-controlled studies in pregnant women. However, clinical studies in pregnant women have not indicated that Dramamine increases the risk of abnormalities when administered in any trimester of pregnancy. It would appear that the possibility of fetal harm is remote when the drug is used during pregnancy. Nevertheless, because the studies in humans cannot rule out the possibility of harm, Dramamine should be used during pregnancy only if clearly needed.

Nursing mothers: Small amounts of dimenhydrinate are excreted in breast milk. Because of the potential for adverse reactions in nursing infants from dimenhydrinate, a decision should be made whether to discontinue nursing or to discontinue the drug, taking into account the importance of the drug to the mother.

Adverse Reactions: The most frequent adverse reaction to Dramamine (dimenhydrinate) is drowsiness. Dizziness may also occur. Symptoms of dry mouth, nose and throat, blurred vision, difficult or painful urination, headache, anorexia, nervousness, restlessness or insomnia (especially in children), skin rash, thickening of bronchial secretions, tachycardia, epigastric distress, lassitude, excitation, and nausea have been reported.

Overdosage: Drowsiness is the usual clinical side effect. Convulsions, coma, and respiratory depression may occur with massive overdosage. No specific antidote is known. If respiratory depression occurs, mechanically assisted respiration should be initiated and oxygen administered. Convulsions should be treated with appropriate doses of diazepam. Phenobarbital (5 to 6 mg/kg) may be given to control convulsions in children.
The oral LD_{50} in mice and rats is 203 mg/kg and 1320 mg/kg, respectively. The intraperitoneal LD_{50} in mice is 149 mg/kg.

Dosage and Administration:
Dramamine Tablets: To prevent motion sickness, the first dose should be taken ½ to 1 hour before starting the activity. Additional medication depends on travel conditions. *Dosage: Adults:* Nausea or vomiting may be expected to be controlled for approximately 4 hours with 50 mg of Dramamine, and prevented by a similar dose every 4 hours. Its administration may be attended by some degree of drowsiness in some patients, and 100 mg every 4 hours may be given in conditions in which drowsiness is not objectionable or is even desirable. The usual adult dosage is 1 to 2 tablets every 4 to 6 hours, not to exceed 8 tablets in 24 hours. *Children 6 to 12 years:* ½ to 1 tablet every 6 to 8 hours, not to exceed 3 tablets in 24 hours. *Children 2 to 6 years:* Up to ½ tablet every 6 to 8 hours, not to exceed 1½ tablets in 24 hours. Children may also be given Dramamine (dimenhydrinate) cherry-flavored liquid in accordance with directions for use. Not for frequent or prolonged use except on advice of a physician. Do not exceed recommended dosage.

Dramamine Liquid: To prevent motion sickness, the first dose should be taken ½ to 1 hour before starting your activity. Additional medication depends on travel conditions. *Dosage: Adults:* 4 to 8 teaspoonfuls (4 ml per teaspoonful) every 4 to 6 hours, not to exceed 32 teaspoonfuls in 24 hours. *Children 6 to 12 years:* 2 to 4 teaspoonfuls (4 ml per teaspoonful) every 6 to 8 hours, not to exceed 12 teaspoonfuls in 24 hours. *Children 2 to 6 years:* 1 to 2 teaspoonfuls every 6 to 8 hours, not to exceed 6 teaspoonfuls in 24 hours. *Children under 2 years:* Only on advice of a physician.
Not for frequent or prolonged use except on advice of a physician. Do not exceed recommended dosage. Use of a measuring device is recommended for all liquid medication.

Dramamine Injection (dimenhydrinate injection) is indicated when the oral form is impractical.
Adults: Nausea or vomiting may be expected to be controlled for approximately 4 hours with 50 mg, and prevented by a similar dose every 4 hours. Its administration may be attended by some degree of drowsiness in some patients, and 100 mg every 4 hours may be given in conditions in which drowsiness is not objectionable or is even desirable.

For *intramuscular* administration, each milliliter (50 mg) of solution is injected as needed, but for *intravenous* administration, each milliliter (50 mg) of solution must be diluted in 10 ml of 0.9% Sodium Chloride Injection USP and injected over a period of 2 minutes.

Pediatric: For intramuscular administration, 1.25 mg/kg of body weight or 37.5 mg/m² of body surface area is administered four times daily. The maximum dose should not exceed 300 mg daily. Parenteral drug products should be inspected visually for particulate matter and discoloration prior to administration, whenever solution and container permit. Use only if solution is clear and vial seal is intact.

How Supplied: Dramamine (dimenhydrinate) is supplied in the following dosage forms and package sizes:
For oral use—scored white **tablets** of 50 mg, with SEARLE debossed on one side and 1701 on the other side; bottles of 36, 100, and 1,000, packets of 12 tablets, and cartons of 100 single-dose individually blister-sealed tablets; liquid, 12.5 mg/4 ml, ethyl alcohol 5%, bottles of 3 fl oz (OTC) and 16 fl oz.
Dramamine Injection (dimenhydrinate) is supplied in 1-ml ampuls, each containing 50 mg of dimenhydrinate, in cartons of 5, 25, and 100, and in 5-ml (50 mg/ml, 250 mg total) vials in cartons of 5, 25, and 100.

[*Please note: Dramamine Tablets and Liquid are also shown in the PDR For Nonprescription Drugs.*]
Tablets are shown in Product Identification Section, page 435

FLAGYL I.V.™ ℞
[*flaj'yl*]
(metronidazole hydrochloride)
FLAGYL I.V.™ RTU® ℞
(metronidazole) Ready-to-Use
Sterile
For Intravenous Infusion Only

> **Warning**
> Metronidazole has been shown to be carcinogenic in mice and rats (see *Warnings*). Its use, therefore, should be reserved for serious anaerobic infections where, in the judgment of the physician, the benefit outweighs the possible risk.

Description: Flagyl I.V., sterile (metronidazole hydrochloride), and Flagyl I.V. RTU, sterile (metronidazole), are parenteral dosage forms of the synthetic antibacterial agents 1-(β-hydroxyethyl)-2-methyl-5-nitroimidazole hydrochloride and 1-(β-hydroxyethyl)-2-methyl-5-nitroimidazole, respectively.

metronidazole hydrochloride

metronidazole

Each single-dose vial of lyophilized Flagyl I.V. contains sterile, nonpyrogenic metronidazole hydrochloride, equivalent to 500 mg metronidazole, and 415 mg mannitol.
Each Flagyl I.V. RTU 100-ml single-dose glass vial or plastic container contains a sterile, nonpyrogenic, isotonic, buffered solution of 500 mg metronidazole, 47.6 mg sodium phosphate, 22.9 mg citric acid, and 790 mg sodium chloride in Water for Injection USP. Flagyl I.V. RTU has a tonicity of 310 mOsm/L and a pH of 5 to 7. Each container contains 14 mEq of sodium.
The plastic container is fabricated from a specially formulated polyvinyl chloride plastic. Water can permeate from inside the container into the overwrap in amounts insufficient to affect the solution significantly. Solutions in contact with the plastic container can leach out certain of its chemical components in very small amounts within the expiration period, eg, di 2-ethylhexyl phthalate (DEHP), up to 5 parts per million. However, the safety of the plastic has been confirmed in tests in animals according to USP biological tests for plastic containers as well as by tissue culture toxicity studies.

Clinical Pharmacology: Metronidazole is a synthetic antibacterial compound. Disposition of metronidazole in the body is similar for both oral and intravenous dosage forms, with an average elimination half-life in healthy humans of eight hours.
The major route of elimination of metronidazole and its metabolites is via the urine (60–80% of the dose), with fecal excretion accounting for 6–15% of the dose. The metabolites that appear in the urine result primarily from side-chain oxidation [1-(β-hydroxyethyl)-2-hydroxymethyl-5-nitroimidazole and 2-methyl-5-nitroimidazole-1-yl-acetic acid] and glucuronide conjugation, with unchanged metronidazole accounting for approximately 20% of the total. Renal clearance of metronidazole is approximately 10 ml/min/1.73m².
Metronidazole is the major component appearing in the plasma, with lesser quantities of the 2-hydroxymethyl metabolite also being present. Less than 20% of the circulating metronidazole is bound to plasma proteins. Both the parent compound and the metabolite possess *in vitro* bactericidal activity against most strains of anaerobic bacteria.

Metronidazole appears in cerebrospinal fluid, saliva, and breast milk in concentrations similar to those found in plasma. Bactericidal concentrations of metronidazole have also been detected in pus from hepatic abscesses.
Plasma concentrations of metronidazole are proportional to the administered dose. An eight-hour intravenous infusion of 100–4,000 mg of metronidazole in normal subjects showed a linear relationship between dose and peak plasma concentration. In patients treated with Flagyl I.V., using a dosage regimen of 15 mg/kg loading dose followed six hours later by 7.5 mg/kg every six hours, peak steady-state plasma concentrations of metronidazole averaged 25 mcg/ml with trough (minimum) concentrations averaging 18 mcg/ml.
Decreased renal function does not alter the single-dose pharmacokinetics of metronidazole. However, plasma clearance of metronidazole is decreased in patients with decreased liver function. In one study newborn infants appeared to demonstrate diminished capacity to eliminate metronidazole. The elimination half-life, measured during the first three days of life, was inversely related to gestational age. In infants whose gestational ages were between 28 and 40 weeks, the corresponding elimination half-lives ranged from 109 to 22.5 hours.

Microbiology: Metronidazole is active *in vitro* against most obligate anaerobes, but does not appear to possess any clinically relevant activity against facultative anaerobes or obligate aerobes. Against susceptible organisms, metronidazole is generally bactericidal at concentrations equal to or slightly higher than the minimal inhibitory concentrations. Metronidazole has been shown to have *in vitro* and clinical activity against the following organisms:
Anaerobic gram-negative bacilli, including:
  Bacteroides species, including the *Bacteroides fragilis* group (*B. fragilis, B. distasonis, B. ovatus, B. thetaiotaomicron, B. vulgatus*)
  Fusobacterium species.
Anaerobic gram-positive bacilli, including:
  Clostridium species and susceptible strains of *Eubacterium*
Anaerobic gram-positive cocci, including:
  Peptococcus species
  Peptostreptococcus species

Susceptibility Tests: Bacteriologic studies should be performed to determine the causative organisms and their susceptibility to metronidazole; however, the rapid, routine susceptibility testing of individual isolates of anaerobic bacteria is not always practical, and therapy may be started while awaiting these results.
Quantitative methods give the most accurate estimates of susceptibility to antibacterial drugs. A standardized agar dilution method and a broth microdilution method are recommended.[1]
Control strains are recommended for standardized susceptibility testing. Each time the test is performed, one or more of the following strains should be included: *Clostridium perfringens* ATCC 13124, *Bacteroides fragilis* ATCC 25285, and *Bacteroides thetaiotaomicron* ATCC 29741. The mode metronidazole MICs for those three strains are reported to be 0.25, 0.25, and 0.5 mcg/ml, respectively.
A clinical laboratory test is considered under acceptable control if the results of the control strains are within one doubling dilution of the mode MICs reported for metronidazole.
A bacterial isolate may be considered susceptible if the MIC value for metronidazole is not more than 16 mcg/ml. An organism is considered resistant if the MIC is greater than 16 mcg/ml. A report of "resistant" from the laboratory indicates that the infecting organism is not likely to respond to therapy.

Indications and Usage: Flagyl I.V. (metronidazole hydrochloride) and Flagyl I.V. RTU (metronidazole) are indicated in the treatment of serious infections caused by susceptible anaerobic bacteria. Indicated surgical procedures should be performed in conjunction with Flagyl I.V. or Flagyl I.V. RTU therapy. In a mixed aerobic and anaerobic infection, antibiotics appropriate for the treatment of the aerobic infection should be used in addition to Flagyl I.V. or Flagyl I.V. RTU.
Flagyl I.V. and Flagyl I.V. RTU are effective in *Bacteroides fragilis* infections resistant to clindamycin, chloramphenicol, and penicillin.
INTRA-ABDOMINAL INFECTIONS, including peritonitis, intra-abdominal abscess, and liver abscess, caused by *Bacteroides* species including the *B. fragilis* group (*B. fragilis, B. distasonis, B. ovatus, B. thetaiotaomicron, B. vulgatus*), *Clostridium* species, *Eubacterium* species, *Peptococcus* species, and *Peptostreptococcus* species.
SKIN AND SKIN STRUCTURE INFECTIONS caused by *Bacteroides* species including the *B. fragilis* group, *Clostridium* species, *Peptococcus* species, *Peptostreptococcus* species, and *Fusobacterium* species.
GYNECOLOGIC INFECTIONS, including endometritis, endomyometritis, tubo-ovarian abscess, and postsurgical vaginal cuff infection, caused by *Bacteroides* species including the *B. fragilis* group, *Clostridium* species, *Peptococcus* species, and *Peptostreptococcus* species.
BACTERIAL SEPTICEMIA caused by *Bacteroides* species including the *B. fragilis* group, and *Clostridium* species.
BONE AND JOINT INFECTIONS, as adjunctive therapy, caused by *Bacteroides* species including the *B. fragilis* group.
CENTRAL NERVOUS SYSTEM (CNS) INFECTIONS, including meningitis and brain abscess, caused by *Bacteroides* species including the *B. fragilis* group.
LOWER RESPIRATORY TRACT INFECTIONS, including pneumonia, empyema, and lung abscess, caused by *Bacteroides* species including the *B. fragilis* group.
ENDOCARDITIS caused by *Bacteroides* species including the *B. fragilis* group.

Contraindications: Flagyl I.V. and Flagyl I.V. RTU are contraindicated in patients with a prior history of hypersensitivity to metronidazole or other nitroimidazole derivatives.

Warnings:
Convulsive Seizures and Peripheral Neuropathy: Convulsive seizures and peripheral neuropathy, the latter characterized mainly by numbness or paresthesia of an extremity, have been reported in patients treated with metronidazole. The appearance of abnormal neurologic signs demands the prompt evaluation of the benefit/risk ratio of the continuation of therapy.
Tumorigenicity in Rodents: Metronidazole has shown evidence of carcinogenic activity in studies involving chronic, oral administration in mice and rats, but similar studies in the hamster gave negative results. Also, metronidazole has shown mutagenic activity in a number of *in vitro* assay systems, but studies in mammals (*in vivo*) failed to demonstrate a potential for genetic damage.

Precautions:
General: Patients with severe hepatic disease metabolize metronidazole slowly, with resultant accumulation of metronidazole and its metabolites in the plasma. Accordingly, for such patients, doses below those usually recommended should be administered cautiously.
Administration of solutions containing sodium ions may result in sodium retention. Care should be taken when administering Flagyl I.V. RTU to patients receiving corticosteroids or to patients predisposed to edema.
Known or previously unrecognized candidiasis may present more prominent symptoms during therapy with Flagyl I.V. (metronidazole hydrochloride) or Flagyl I.V. RTU (metronidazole) and requires treatment with a candicidal agent.
Laboratory Tests: Metronidazole is a nitroimidazole, and Flagyl I.V. or Flagyl I.V. RTU should be used with care in patients with evidence of or history of blood dyscrasia. A mild leukopenia has been observed during its administration; however, no persistent hematologic abnormalities attributable to metronidazole have been observed in clini-

Continued on next page

Searle Pharm.—Cont.

cal studies. Total and differential leukocyte counts are recommended before and after therapy.
Drug Interactions: Metronidazole has been reported to potentiate the anticoagulant effect of warfarin and other oral coumarin anticoagulants, resulting in a prolongation of prothrombin time. This possible drug interaction should be considered when Flagyl I.V. or Flagyl I.V. RTU is prescribed for patients on this type of anticoagulant therapy.
The simultaneous administration of drugs that induce microsomal liver enzymes, such as phenytoin or phenobarbital, may accelerate the elimination of metronidazole, resulting in reduced plasma levels.
The simultaneous administration of drugs that decrease microsomal liver enzyme activity, such as cimetidine, may prolong the half-life and decrease plasma clearance of metronidazole.
Alcoholic beverages should not be consumed during metronidazole therapy because abdominal cramps, nausea, vomiting, headaches, and flushing may occur.
Drug/Laboratory Test Interactions: Metronidazole may interfere with certain types of determinations of serum chemistry values, such as, aspartate aminotransferase (AST, SGOT), alanine aminotransferase (ALT, SGPT), lactate dehydrogenase (LDH), triglycerides, and hexokinase glucose. Values of zero may be observed. All of the assays in which interference has been reported involve enzymatic coupling of the assay to oxidation-reduction of nicotine adenine dinucleotide (NAD+ ⇌ NADH). Interference is due to the similarity in absorbance peaks of NADH (340 nm) and metronidazole (322 nm) at pH 7.
Carcinogenesis: See *Warnings.*
Pregnancy: Teratogenic Effects—Pregnancy Category B. Metronidazole crosses the placental barrier and enters the fetal circulation rapidly. Reproduction studies have been performed in rats at doses up to five times the human dose and have revealed no evidence of impaired fertility or harm to the fetus due to metronidazole. Metronidazole administered intraperitoneally to pregnant mice at approximately the human dose caused fetotoxicity; administered orally to pregnant mice, no fetotoxicity was observed. There are, however, no adequate and well-controlled studies in pregnant women. Because animal reproduction studies are not always predictive of human response, and because metronidazole is a carcinogen in rodents, these drugs should be used during pregnancy only if clearly needed.
Nursing Mothers: Because of the potential for tumorigenicity shown for metronidazole in mouse and rat studies, a decision should be made whether to discontinue nursing or to discontinue the drug, taking into account the importance of the drug to the mother. Metronidazole is secreted in breast milk in concentrations similar to those found in plasma.
Pediatric Use: Safety and effectiveness in children have not been established.
Adverse Reactions: The two most serious adverse reactions reported in patients treated with Flagyl I.V. have been convulsive seizures and peripheral neuropathy, the latter characterized mainly by numbness or paresthesia of an extremity. Since persistent peripheral neuropathy has been reported in some patients receiving prolonged oral administration of Flagyl® (metronidazole), patients should be observed carefully if neurologic symptoms occur and a prompt evaluation made of the benefit/risk ratio of the continuation of therapy.
The following reactions have also been reported during treatment with Flagyl I.V. (metronidazole hydrochloride):
  Gastrointestinal: Nausea, vomiting, abdominal discomfort, diarrhea, and an unpleasant metallic taste.
  Hematopoietic: Reversible neutropenia (leukopenia).
  Dermatologic: Erythematous rash and pruritus.
  Central Nervous System: Headache, dizziness, and syncope.
  Local Reactions: Thrombophlebitis after intravenous infusion. This reaction can be minimized or avoided by avoiding prolonged use of indwelling intravenous catheters.
  Other: Fever. Instances of a darkened urine have also been reported, and this manifestation has been the subject of a special investigation. Although the pigment which is probably responsible for this phenomenon has not been positively identified, it is almost certainly a metabolite of metronidazole and seems to have no clinical significance.
The following adverse reactions have been reported during treatment with oral Flagyl (metronidazole):
  Gastrointestinal: Nausea, sometimes accompanied by headache, anorexia and occasionally vomiting; diarrhea, epigastric distress, abdominal cramping, and constipation.
  Mouth: A sharp, unpleasant metallic taste is not unusual. Furry tongue, glossitis, and stomatitis have occurred; these may be associated with a sudden overgrowth of *Candida* which may occur during effective therapy.
  Hematopoietic: Reversible neutropenia (leukopenia).
  Cardiovascular: Flattening of the T-wave may be seen in electrocardiographic tracings.
  Central Nervous System: Convulsive seizures, peripheral neuropathy, dizziness, vertigo, incoordination, ataxia, confusion, irritability, depression, weakness, and insomnia.
  Hypersensitivity: Urticaria, erythematous rash, flushing, nasal congestion, dryness of mouth (or vagina or vulva), and fever.
  Renal: Dysuria, cystitis, polyuria, incontinence, a sense of pelvic pressure, and darkened urine.
  Other: Proliferation of *Candida* in the vagina, dyspareunia, decrease of libido, proctitis, and fleeting joint pains sometimes resembling "serum sickness." If patients receiving metronidazole drink alcoholic beverages, they may experience abdominal distress, nausea, vomiting, flushing, or headache. A modification of the taste of alcoholic beverages has also been reported.
Overdosage: Use of dosages of Flagyl I.V. (metronidazole hydrochloride) higher than those recommended has been reported. These include the use of 27 mg/kg three times a day for 20 days, and the use of 75 mg/kg as a single loading dose followed by 7.5 mg/kg maintenance doses. No adverse reactions were reported in either of the two cases.
Single oral doses of metronidazole, up to 15 g, have been reported in suicide attempts and accidental overdoses. Symptoms reported include nausea, vomiting, and ataxia.
Oral metronidazole has been studied as a radiation sensitizer in the treatment of malignant tumors. Neurotoxic effects, including seizures and peripheral neuropathy, have been reported after 5 to 7 days of doses of 6 to 10.4 g every other day.
Treatment: There is no specific antidote for overdose; therefore, management of the patient should consist of symptomatic and supportive therapy.
Dosage and Administration: The recommended dosage schedule for *adults* is:
  Loading dose:
    15 mg/kg infused over one hour (approximately 1 g for a 70-kg adult).
  Maintenance Dose:
    7.5 mg/kg infused over one hour every six hours (approximately 500 mg for a 70-kg adult). The first maintenance dose should be instituted six hours following the initiation of the loading dose.
Parenteral therapy may be changed to oral Flagyl (metronidazole) when conditions warrant, based upon the severity of the disease and the response of the patient to Flagyl I.V. or Flagyl I.V. RTU (metronidazole) treatment. The usual adult oral dosage is 7.5 mg/kg every six hours.

A maximum of 4 g should not be exceeded during a 24-hour period.
Patients with severe hepatic disease metabolize metronidazole slowly, with resultant accumulation of metronidazole and its metabolites in the plasma. Accordingly, for such patients, doses below those usually recommended should be administered cautiously. Close monitoring of plasma metronidazole levels[2] and toxicity is recommended.
The dose of Flagyl I.V. or Flagyl I.V. RTU should not be specifically reduced in anuric patients since accumulated metabolites may be rapidly removed by dialysis.
The usual duration of therapy is 7 to 10 days; however, infections of the bone and joint, lower respiratory tract, and endocardium may require longer treatment.
CAUTION: Flagyl I.V. (metronidazole hydrochloride) or Flagyl I.V. RTU (metronidazole) is to be administered by slow intravenous drip infusion only, either as a continuous or intermittent infusion. I.V. admixtures containing metronidazole and other drugs should be avoided. Additives should not be introduced into the Flagyl I.V. RTU solution. If used with a primary intravenous fluid system, the primary solution should be discontinued during metronidazole infusion. DO NOT USE EQUIPMENT CONTAINING ALUMINUM (EG, NEEDLES, CANNULAE) THAT WOULD COME IN CONTACT WITH THE DRUG SOLUTION.

FLAGYL I.V.
Flagyl I.V. cannot be given by direct intravenous injection (I.V. bolus) because of the low pH (0.5 to 2.0) of the reconstituted product. FLAGYL I.V. MUST BE FURTHER DILUTED AND NEUTRALIZED FOR I.V. INFUSION.
Flagyl I.V. is prepared for use in two steps:
NOTE: ORDER OF MIXING IS IMPORTANT
A. Reconstitution.
B. Dilution in intravenous solution followed by pH neutralization with sodium bicarbonate injection into the dilution.
Reconstitution: To prepare the solution, add 4.4 ml of one of the following diluents and mix thoroughly: Sterile Water for Injection, USP; Bacteriostatic Water for Injection, USP; 0.9% Sodium Chloride Injection, USP; or Bacteriostatic 0.9% Sodium Chloride Injection, USP. The resultant approximate withdrawal volume is 5.0 ml with an approximate concentration of 100 mg/ml.
The pH of the reconstituted product will be in the range of 0.5 to 2.0. Reconstituted Flagyl I.V. is clear, and pale yellow to yellow-green in color.
Dilution in Intravenous Solutions: Properly reconstituted Flagyl I.V. may be added to a glass or plastic I.V. container not to exceed a concentration of 8 mg/ml. Any of the following intravenous solutions may be used: 0.9% Sodium Chloride Injection, USP; 5% Dextrose Injection, USP; or Lactated Ringer's Injection, USP.
NEUTRALIZATION IS REQUIRED PRIOR TO ADMINISTRATION
The final product should be mixed thoroughly and used within 24 hours.
Neutralization For Intravenous Infusion: Neutralize the intravenous solution containing Flagyl I.V. with approximately 5 mEq of sodium bicarbonate injection for each 500 mg of Flagyl I.V. used. Mix thoroughly. The pH of the neutralized intravenous solution will be approximately 6.0 to 7.0. Carbon dioxide gas will be generated with neutralization. It may be necessary to relieve gas pressure within the container.
Note: When the contents of one vial (500 mg) are diluted and neutralized to 100 ml, the resultant concentration is 5 mg/ml. Do not exceed an 8 mg/ml concentration of Flagyl I.V. in the neutralized intravenous solution, since neutralization will decrease the aqueous solubility and precipitation may occur. DO NOT REFRIGERATE NEUTRALIZED SOLUTIONS; otherwise, precipitation may occur.
Storage and Stability: Reconstituted vials of Flagyl I.V. are chemically stable for 96 hours when stored below 86°F (30°C) in room light.

Use diluted and neutralized intravenous solutions containing Flagyl I.V. within 24 hours of mixing.

FLAGYL I.V. RTU
Flagyl I.V. RTU is a ready-to-use isotonic solution. **NO DILUTION OR BUFFERING IS REQUIRED.** Do not refrigerate. Each container of Flagyl I.V. RTU contains 14 mEq of sodium.

Directions for use of plastic container:
CAUTION: Do not use plastic containers in series connections. Such use could result in air embolism due to residual air (approximately 15 ml) being drawn from the primary container before administration of the fluid from the secondary container is complete.

To open. Tear overwrap down side at slit and remove solution container. Check for minute leaks by squeezing inner bag firmly. If leaks are found discard solution as sterility may be impaired.

Preparation for administration:
1. Suspend container from eyelet support.
2. Remove plastic container from outlet port at bottom of container.
3. Attach administration set. Refer to complete directions accompanying set.

Parenteral drug products should be inspected visually for particulate matter and discoloration prior to administration, whenever solution and container permit. Do not use if cloudy or precipitated or if the seal is not intact.
Use sterile equipment. It is recommended that the intravenous administration apparatus be replaced at least once every 24 hours.

How Supplied:
FLAGYL I.V.
Flagyl I.V., sterile (metronidazole hydrochloride), is supplied in single-dose lyophilized vials each containing 500 mg metronidazole equivalent, individually packaged in cartons of 10 vials.
Flagyl I.V., prior to reconstitution, should be stored below 86°F (30°C) and protected from light.

FLAGYL I.V. RTU
In plastic container: Flagyl I.V. RTU, sterile (metronidazole), is supplied in 100-ml single-dose containers, each containing an isotonic, buffered solution of 500 mg metronidazole, individually packaged in boxes of 24.
In glass: Flagyl I.V. RTU, sterile (metronidazole), is supplied in 100-ml single-dose vials, each containing an isotonic, buffered solution of 500 mg metronidazole, individually packaged in cartons of 6 vials.
Flagyl I.V. RTU should be stored at controlled room temperature, 59° to 86° F (15° to 30°C), and protected from light during storage.

1. Proposed standard: PSM-11—Proposed Reference Dilution Procedure for Antimicrobic Susceptibility Testing of Anaerobic Bacteria, National Committee for Clinical Laboratory Standards, and Sutter, et al.: Collaborative Evaluation of a Proposed Reference Dilution Method of Susceptibility Testing of Anaerobic Bacteria, Antimicrob. Agents Chemother. 16:495-502 (Oct.) 1979; and Tally, et al: *In Vitro* Activity of Thienamycin, Antimicrob. Agents Chemother. 14:436-438 (Sept.) 1978.
2. Ralph, E.D., and Kirby, W.M.M.: Bioassay of Metronidazole With Either Anaerobic or Aerobic Incubation, J. Infect. Dis. 132:587-591 (Nov.) 1975; or Gulaid, et al.: Determination of Metronidazole and Its Major Metabolites in Biological Fluids by High Pressure Liquid Chromatography, Br. J. Clin. Pharmacol. 6:430-432, 1978.

Shown in Product Identification Section, page 436

NITRODISC® ℞
[nī' trō' disc]
(nitroglycerin)
5 mg/24 hr; 10 mg/24 hr

Description: Nitrodisc incorporates a patented Microseal Drug Delivery™ system consisting of a solid, nitroglycerin-impregnated polymer bonded to a flexible, non-sensitizing adhesive bandage. It is designed to be applied topically. Nitrodisc provides constant and controlled drug delivery over a uniform skin surface area for 24 hours.

Nitrodisc is available in two strengths which release either 5 mg or 10 mg of nitroglycerin during a 24-hour period. The 5 mg/24 hr system contains 16 mg nitroglycerin over an 8 cm^2 releasing surface. The 10 mg/24 hr system contains 32 mg nitroglycerin over a 16 cm^2 releasing surface (see *How Supplied* section).

Actions: When Nitrodisc is applied to the skin, nitroglycerin is absorbed continuously through the skin into the systemic circulation. This results in active drug reaching the target organs (heart and peripheral vasculature) before being inactivated by the liver. Nitroglycerin is a smooth muscle relaxant with vascular effects manifested predominantly by venous dilation and pooling. The major beneficial effect of nitroglycerin in angina pectoris is due to a reduction in myocardial oxygen consumption secondary to vascular smooth muscle relaxation and consequent reduced cardiac preload and afterload. In addition, a direct effect of nitroglycerin on the coronary vessels is recognized as well.

In normal volunteers, transdermal absorption of nitroglycerin from Nitrodisc occurred in a continuous and well-controlled manner for a minimum of 24 hours. Detectable plasma levels were attained within 1 hour after the application of the disc and remained at a similar level for 24 hours. Precise definition of "therapeutic plasma level" is not known, at this time. Plasma levels of nitroglycerin were still detectable 30 minutes after removal of the system.

The amount of nitroglycerin released (5 mg/24 hr or 10 mg/24 hr) represents the mean release rate of nitroglycerin from the disc as determined from healthy volunteers and, hence, the amount potentially available for absorption through the skin. Absorption will vary among individuals.

Indications and Usage:

> Nitrodisc has been conditionally approved by the FDA for the prevention and treatment of angina pectoris due to coronary artery disease. The conditional approval reflects a determination that the drug may be marketed while further investigation of its effectiveness is undertaken. A final evaluation of the effectiveness of the product will be announced by the FDA.

Contraindications: Nitrodisc (nitroglycerin) is contraindicated in patients known to be intolerant of organic nitrate drugs and in patients with marked anemia.

Warnings: In patients with acute myocardial infarction or congestive heart failure, Nitrodisc should be used under careful clinical and/or hemodynamic monitoring.
In terminating treatment of patients with angina, both the dosage and frequency of application must be gradually reduced over a period of 4 to 6 weeks to prevent potential withdrawal reactions, which are characteristic of all vasodilators in the nitrate class.

Precautions: Symptoms of hypotension, such as faintness, weakness, or dizziness, particularly orthostatic hypotension, may be due to overdosage. When these symptoms occur, the dosage should be reduced or use of the product discontinued.
Nitrodisc is not intended for immediate relief of anginal attacks. For this purpose, occasional use of sublingual preparations may be necessary.

Adverse Reactions: Transient headache is the most common side effect, especially when higher doses of the drug are used. These headaches should be treated with mild analgesics while Nitrodisc therapy is continued. When such headaches are unresponsive to treatment, the nitroglycerin dosage should be reduced or use of the product discontinued.
Adverse reactions reported less frequently include hypotension, increased heart rate, faintness, flushing, dizziness, nausea, vomiting, and dermatitis. With the exception of dermatitis, these symptoms are attributable to the known pharmacologic effects of nitroglycerin, but may be symptoms of overdosage. When they persist, Nitrodisc (nitroglycerin) dose should be reduced or use of the product discontinued.

Dosage and Administration: Nitrodisc should be applied once each day. To use Nitrodisc, follow the instructions on the package. Nitrodisc should be applied to an intact skin site free of hair and not subject to excessive movement. It should not be applied to the distal parts of the extremities. A suitable area should be shaved free of hair, if necessary. The application site should be changed slightly each time to avoid undue skin irritation. A new Nitrodisc should be applied if the product loosens.

The optimal dosage regimen should be selected based upon the clinical response, the side effects, and the effects of therapy upon blood pressure and heart rate. It is recommended that therapy be initiated with Nitrodisc 5 mg/24 hr, and that Nitrodisc 10 mg/24 hr be utilized when a greater response is desired. In the event that higher doses are necessary, multiple pads may be applied.

Patient Instructions for Application: These are provided with the product.

How Supplied:

Nitrodisc	5 mg/24 hr	10 mg/24 hr
Drug released per 24 hours	5 mg	10 mg
Total drug content	16 mg	32 mg
Drug releasing surface	8 cm^2	16 cm^2

Nitrodisc (nitroglycerin) is supplied in cartons of 30 discs. Store at a controlled room temperature of 59°-86°F (15°-30°C). **Do not refrigerate.** Extremes of temperature and humidity should be avoided.
Shown in Product Identification Section, page 436

TATUM-T® ℞
[tā' tum-tē'']
(intrauterine copper contraceptive)

Description: The plastic component of the Tatum-T (intrauterine copper contraceptive) is composed of polyethylene with barium sulfate added to render it radiopaque. Its shape approximates the letter T. The vertical dimension measures 36 mm and the horizontal, 32 mm.
Coiled around the vertical limb is 120 mg of copper wire providing approximately 210 mm^2 of exposed copper surface area. A retrieval thread is fastened to the free end of the vertical limb of the Tatum-T. The Tatum-T is supplied with a simple tubular plastic inserter. All components are sterile.

For **Clinical Pharmacology, Indications and Usage, Contraindications, Warnings, Precautions,** *and* **Adverse Reactions,** *see Cu-7 (intrauterine copper contraceptive) under this manufacturer.*

Directions for Use: The Tatum-T is to be placed within the uterine cavity. See the *Procedure for Insertion* for the insertion technique.
The optimal time of insertion is during the latter part of the menstrual flow or one or two days thereafter. The cervical canal is relatively more patent at this time, and there is little chance that the patient may be pregnant.
Present information indicates that efficacy is retained for 36 months. There is no evidence that contraceptive efficacy decreases within time up to three years of use, but unless new data support a longer period of efficacy and safety, the Tatum-T must be removed within 36 months from the date of insertion and a new one inserted if desired. If partial expulsion occurs, removal is indicated, and a new Tatum-T may be inserted. Removal of the

Continued on next page

Searle Pharm.—Cont.

Tatum-T may also be indicated in the event of heavy or persistent bleeding.

The physician should become thoroughly familiar with the instructions for use before attempting insertion or removal of the Tatum-T.

Clinical Studies: Different event rates have been reported with the use of different intrauterine contraceptives. Inasmuch as these rates are usually derived from separate studies conducted by different investigators in several population groups, a comparison cannot be made with precision. Even in clinical studies with the same contraceptive, considerably different rates are likely to be obtained because of differing characteristics of the study population. Furthermore, event rates per unit of time tend to be lower as clinical experience is expanded, possibly due to retention in the clinical study of those patients who accept the treatment regimen, not having discontinued due to adverse reactions or pregnancy, so that those remaining in the study were those less susceptible. In clinical trials of the Tatum-T conducted in the United States and Canada, use effectiveness was determined as follows for parous and nulliparous women, as tabulated by the life table method. (Rates are expressed as cumulative events per 100 women through 12, 24, and 36 months of use.)

This experience encompasses 236,060 woman-months of use, including 12 months for 8,232 women, 24 months for 4,247, and 36 months for 1,408.

Cumulative rates were:
[See table below].

Procedure for Insertion

Physicians are cautioned that it is imperative that they become thoroughly familiar with the instructions for insertion before attempting placement of the "T." The insertion technique is different in several respects from that employed with other intrauterine contraceptives currently available; particular attention should be paid to the illustrations and instructions.

The Tatum-T may be inserted easily at any time during the menstrual cycle. It is *not* necessary to delay insertion until a menstrual flow is in progress; however, the possibility of existing undetermined pregnancy is lessened if insertion is made during or shortly following a menstrual period.

The cervix should be cleansed with antiseptic solution and its anterior lip grasped with a tenaculum prior to sounding the uterus and insertion of the Tatum-T. Insertion of the Tatum-T into a severely anteverted or severely retroverted uterus may be difficult unless sufficient tension is applied to the tenaculum. Determination of the depth and direction of the uterine cavity should be made with a sound prior to insertion.

An aseptic technique should be employed. Sterile gloves are recommended; however, the package itself may be used to set the cervical stop and to load the "T" into the insertion tube. A small loading device is contained within the package to facilitate this step. Exercise care to avoid contaminating the "T" or that part of the tube which will enter the cervical canal.

Caution:
DO NOT load the "T" into the tube until after the cervical stop on the tube has been set to the sounded depth nor leave it loaded longer than 2 minutes. The plastic of the Tatum-T is soft and it will lose its "memory"; it will then fail to return to its "T" configuration within the uterus and thus invite loss of effectiveness and early expulsion.

DO NOT push the "T" into the tube so that less than $\frac{1}{4}$ in of the frame protrudes; placement may be improper; the arms may be damaged. If more than $\frac{1}{4}$ in protrudes, the risk of perforation is increased.

DO NOT remove the thread-retaining clip from the insertion rod until after insertion has been made and you are ready to deposit the Tatum-T within the uterine cavity. The thread-retaining clip on the rod prevents the "T" and/or rod from falling to a non-sterile surface. When held against the end of the tube during the loading procedure, it helps to keep the "T" from being pushed too far into the tube and prevents premature ejection of the "T" during the insertion procedure.

DO NOT force the insertion. It is generally believed that most perforations occur at the time of insertion, although the perforation may not be detected until some time later. The position of the uterus should be determined during the pre-insertion examination. Great care must be exercised during the pre-insertion sounding and subsequent insertion.

Note: If the uterine cavity measures under 6.5 cm, the incidence of pain, bleeding, partial or complete expulsion, perforation, and possibly pregnancy, increases. Insertion is not recommended into a uterus that sounds under 6.0 cm.

1. Sterile gloves are recommended for the insertion procedure. If sterile gloves are used, the instrument may be removed from the package when setting the cervical stop and loading it into the insertion tube. If sterile gloves are not used then the package containing the "T" should be used for these procedures. (The package should be torn open just over halfway.)

2. After sounding, adjust the $\frac{1}{4}$-in-thick blue cervical stop on the tube. The edge closer to the handle must be set at the sounded depth of the uterus, *see Figure 1*, because the "T" protrudes $\frac{1}{4}$ in from the end of the tube. If the package is being used to set the cervical stop, do not put the sound inside the package since it could contaminate the "T".

3. The plastic loading device affixed to the cardboard backing near the "T" will help facilitate loading the "T" into the tube. NOTE: It is easier to load the "T" when the sides of the loading device are not squeezed together. For this reason it is best to hold the cardboard backing and not the device. Free the insertion instrument from the cardboard mount. Holding the insertion instrument midway between the cervical stop and the handle, push the insertion rod and tube so that the arms of the "T" slide into the cul-de-sac of the loading device. *See Figure 2.* The arms of the "T" are now folded against the tube. Retract the tube and rod together until the tube clears the arms of the "T". Again push the insertion instrument towards the loading device, trapping the arms of the "T" in the tube until $\frac{1}{4}$ in ($\sim$0.6 cm) of the folded "T" protrudes and the end of the rod just touches the stem of the "T". *See Figure 3.* To release the "T" from the loading device, rotate the insertion instrument 90° and slide the inserter out. If the package is being used to maintain sterility, the insertion instrument should not be completely removed from the package until the cervical stop has been aligned. Align the folded arms of the "T" with the wings of the cervical stop. After the cervical stop has been aligned, open the package the rest of the way.

4. Immediately apply gentle traction on the uterus with a tenaculum and insert the Tatum-T through the cervical canal up to the fundus. *See*

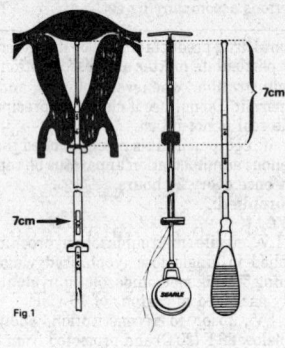

Fig 1

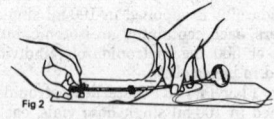

Fig 2

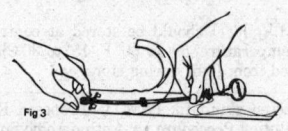

Fig 3

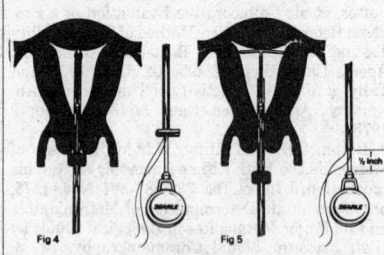

Fig 4   Fig 5

	12 Months		24 Months		36 Months	
	Parous	Nulliparous	Parous	Nulliparous	Parous	Nulliparous
Pregnancy	3.0	2.1	4.9	4.5	6.0	5.8
Expulsion	7.8	8.0	9.8	9.6	10.8	10.9
Medical removal	10.9	13.9	18.2	21.9	23.3	26.9
Continuation	73.4	71.4	55.0	53.9	41.9	40.1

It has been reported that the return of fertility (cumulative gross rate) after elective removal of the Tatum-T in women desiring pregnancy was 87% at one year after removal.

Tatum-T Placement Instrument

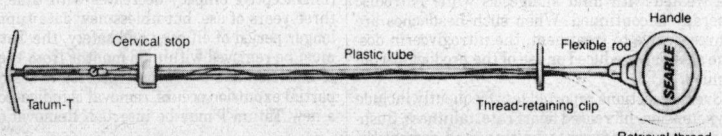

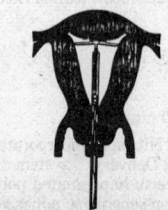

Fig 6

Figure 4. Maintain or align the cervical stop at the cervix in a horizontal plane.
5. Press the thread-retaining clip back toward the handle to free the thread. Hold the rod firmly, but without undue pressure against the stem of the "T," and withdraw the tube to about ½ in (1.3 cm) from the handle. This frees the arms of the "T" but still keeps the stem end in the tube. *See Figure 5. Push the tube back until the cervical stop touches the cervix. See Figure 6.* This holds the "T" near the fundus while the rod is removed.
6. Hold the tube still and withdraw the insertion rod.
7. Withdraw the tube, depositing the "T" in the uterus. Cut the thread about 2 in (5 cm) from the external os. DO NOT PULL OUT EXCESS THREAD BEFORE CUTTING.

Removal of the Tatum-T
ROUTINE REMOVAL—THREAD VISIBLE:
1. DO NOT exert a sudden pull or jerk on the retrieval thread. Exert a firm, steady pull on the thread. A jerk may cause the thread to break.
2. A ring (sponge) forceps, with its smooth edges and minimal crushing force, is a good instrument with which to grasp the thread.
3. Other instruments may be used, but care must be exerted to avoid crushing or cutting the thread.
4. Avoid winding or angulating the thread about the jaws of the withdrawal instrument.
5. Utilize the minimum force needed to remove the Tatum-T.
6. Should resistance be encountered, dislodge the Tatum-T with a probe or uterine sound before making further removal attempts.
THREAD NOT VISIBLE: If the Tatum-T is in the uterus and the thread is not visible, the following procedures should be considered when you elect to recover it:
1. Aseptic use of a slim instrument (eg, uterine dressing forceps) or contact hysteroscopy will frequently permit removal in the office.
2. Hysteroscopy under hospital conditions may be required.
3. D & C and also suction aspiration have been used as alternative measures.
NOTE: If intrauterine manipulative procedures are required, allow an appropriate healing period before inserting a new Tatum-T.
How Supplied: Available in boxes of 10 sterile units (Tatum-T with an inserter), and sufficient patient brochures and identification cards.
Shown in Product Identification Section, page 436

The preceding prescribing information for Searle Pharmaceuticals Inc. was current on November 15, 1984.

Searle Consumer Products
Division of G. D. Searle & Co.
BOX 5110
CHICAGO, IL 60680

DRAMAMINE®
[drăm'uh-meen]
(dimenhydrinate)

Product information for all forms of Dramamine is now shown under Searle Pharmaceuticals Inc. in this publication, and for the forms shown below in the PDR for Nonprescription Drugs.
The oral forms of Dramamine are available as follows:
How Supplied: *Tablets*—Scored, white tablets of 50 mg, with SEARLE debossed on one side and 1701 on the other side, in packets of 12 and bottles of 36 and 100 (OTC); also available in single-dose packets of 100 and in bottles of 1,000. *Liquid*—12.5 mg per 4 ml, ethyl alcohol 5%, bottles of 3 fl oz (OTC); also available in pint bottles.
Shown in Product Identification Section, page 435

Regular Flavor METAMUCIL®
[met"uh-mū'sil]
(psyllium hydrophilic mucilloid)

Description: Regular Flavor Metamucil is a bulk laxative containing refined hydrophilic mucilloid, a highly efficient dietary fiber derived from the husk of the psyllium seed *(Plantago ovata).* An equal amount of dextrose, a carbohydrate, is added as a dispersing agent. Each dose contains about 1 mg of sodium, 31 mg of potassium, and 14 calories. Carbohydrate content is approximately 3.5 g; psyllium mucilloid content is 3.4 g.
Actions: Metamucil provides a bland, nonirritating bulk and promotes normal elimination. It is uniform, instantly miscible, palatable, and nonirritative in the gastrointestinal tract.
Indications: Metamucil is indicated in the management of chronic constipation, in irritable bowel syndrome, as adjunctive therapy in the constipation of duodenal ulcer and diverticular disease, in the bowel management of patients with hemorrhoids, and for constipation during pregnancy, convalescence, and senility.
Contraindications: Intestinal obstruction, fecal impaction.
Dosage and Administration: The usual adult dosage is one rounded teaspoonful (7 g) stirred into a standard 8-oz glass of cool water or other suitable liquid and taken orally one to three times a day, depending on the need and response. It may require continuing use for 2 or 3 days to provide optimal benefit. Best results are observed if each dose is followed by an additional glass of liquid.
How Supplied: Powder, containers of 7 oz, 14 oz, and 21 oz (OTC); also available in cartons of 100 single-dose (7g) packets.
Is this product OTC: Yes. See also PDR for Nonprescription Drugs.

Sugar Free Regular Flavor METAMUCIL®
[met"uh-mū'sil]
(psyllium hydrophilic mucilloid)

Description: Sugar Free Regular Flavor Metamucil is a bulk laxative containing refined hydrophilic mucilloid, a highly efficient dietary fiber derived from the husk of the psyllium seed *(Plantago ovata),* which has been sweetened with NutraSweet® brand of aspartame. It contains no chemical stimulants or sugar. Each dose contains 3.4 g of psyllium mucilloid, less than 0.01 g of sodium, 0.006 g of phenylalanine, and about 1 calorie.
Actions: Metamucil provides a bland, nonirritating bulk and promotes normal elimination. It is uniform, instantly miscible, palatable, and nonirritative in the gastrointestinal tract.
Indications: Metamucil is indicated in the management of chronic constipation, in irritable bowel syndrome, as adjunctive therapy in the constipation of duodenal ulcer and diverticular disease, in the bowel management of patients with hemorrhoids, and for constipation during pregnancy, convalescence, and senility.
Contraindications: Intestinal obstruction, fecal impaction.
Warning: Phenylketonurics should be aware that Sugar Free Metamucil contains phenylalanine.
Dosage and Administration: The usual adult dosage is one rounded teaspoonful (3.7 g) stirred into a standard 8-oz glass of cool water or other suitable liquid and taken orally one to three times a day, depending on the need and response. It may require continuing use for 2 or 3 days to provide optimal benefit. Best results are observed if each dose is followed by an additional glass of liquid.
How Supplied: Powder, containers of 3.7 oz, 7.4 oz, and 11.1 oz (OTC); also available in cartons of 100 single-dose (3.7 g) packets.
Is this product OTC: Yes. See also PDR for Nonprescription Drugs.

Orange Flavor METAMUCIL®
Strawberry Flavor METAMUCIL®
[met"uh-mū'sil]
(psyllium hydrophilic mucilloid)

Description: Orange Flavor and Strawberry Flavor Metamucil are bulk laxatives containing refined hydrophilic mucilloid, a highly efficient dietary fiber derived from the husk of the psyllium seed *(Plantago ovata),* with sucrose (a carbohydrate) as a dispersing agent, citric acid, flavoring, and coloring. Each dose contains about 1 mg of sodium, 31 mg of potassium, and 28 calories. Carbohydrate content is approximately 7.1 g; psyllium mucilloid content is 3.4 g.
Actions: Metamucil provides a bland, nonirritating bulk and promotes normal elimination. It is uniform, instantly miscible, palatable, and nonirritative in the gastrointestinal tract.
Indications: Metamucil is indicated in the management of chronic constipation, in irritable bowel syndrome, as adjunctive therapy in the constipation of duodenal ulcer and diverticular disease, in the bowel management of patients with hemorrhoids, and for constipation during pregnancy, convalescence, and senility.
Contraindications: Intestinal obstruction, fecal impaction.
Dosage and Administration: The usual adult dose is one rounded tablespoonful (11 g) stirred into a standard 8-oz glass of cool water and taken orally one to three times a day, depending on the need and response. It may require continuing use for 2 or 3 days to provide optimal benefit. Best results are observed if each dose is followed by an additional glass of liquid.
How Supplied: Powder, containers of 7 oz, 14 oz, and 21 oz.
Is this product OTC: Yes. See also PDR for Nonprescription Drugs.

Regular Flavor INSTANT MIX METAMUCIL®
[met"uh-mū'sil]
(psyllium hydrophilic mucilloid)

Description: Regular flavor Instant Mix Metamucil is a bulk laxative containing refined hydrophilic mucilloid, a highly efficient dietary fiber derived from the husk of the psyllium seed *(Plantago ovata),* together with citric acid, sucrose (a carbohydrate), potassium bicarbonate, calcium carbonate, flavoring, and sodium bicarbonate. Each dose contains approximately 7 mg of sodium, 60 mg of calcium, 280 mg of potassium, and less than 4 calories. Carbohydrate content is 0.9 g; psyllium mucilloid content is 3.6 g.
Actions: Instant Mix Metamucil provides a bland, nonirritating bulk and promotes normal elimination. It is effervescent and requires no stirring, and it is uniform, instantly miscible, palatable, and nonirritative in the gastrointestinal tract.
Indications: Instant Mix Metamucil is indicated in the management of chronic constipation, in irritable bowel syndrome, as adjunctive therapy in the constipation of duodenal ulcer and diverticular disease, in the bowel management of patients with hemorrhoids, and for constipation during pregnancy, convalescence, and senility.
Contraindications: Intestinal obstruction, fecal impaction.
Dosage and Administration: The usual adult dosage is the contents of one packet (6.4 g) taken one to three times daily as follows: (1) Entire contents of a packet are poured into a standard 8-oz water glass. (2) The glass is slowly filled with cool water. (3) Entire contents are to be drunk immediately. (An additional glass of water may be taken for best results.)
How Supplied: Cartons of 16 and 30 single-dose (6.4 g) packets (OTC); also available in cartons of 100 single-dose (6.4 g) packets.
Is this product OTC: Yes. See also PDR for Nonprescription Drugs.

Continued on next page

Searle Consumer—Cont.

Orange Flavor
INSTANT MIX METAMUCIL®
[met"uh-mū'sil]
(psyllium hydrophilic mucilloid)

Description: Orange Flavor Instant Mix Metamucil is a bulk laxative containing refined hydrophilic mucilloid, a highly efficient dietary fiber derived from the husk of the psyllium seed (*Plantago ovata*), together with sucrose (a carbohydrate), citric acid, potassium bicarbonate, flavoring, coloring, and sodium bicarbonate. Each dose contains approximately 6 mg of sodium, 307 mg of potassium, and 4½ calories. Carbohydrate content is about 1.1 g; psyllium mucilloid content is 3.6 g.

Actions: Instant Mix Metamucil provides a bland, nonirritating bulk and promotes normal elimination. It is effervescent and requires no stirring, and it is uniform, instantly miscible, palatable, and nonirritative in the gastrointestinal tract.

Indications: Instant Mix Metamucil is indicated in the management of chronic constipation, in irritable bowel syndrome, as adjunctive therapy in the constipation of duodenal ulcer and diverticular disease, in the bowel management of patients with hemorrhoids, and for constipation during pregnancy, convalescence, and senility.

Contraindications: Intestinal obstruction, fecal impaction.

Dosage and Administration: The usual adult dosage is the contents of one packet (6.4 g) taken one to three times daily as follows: (1) Entire contents of a packet are poured into a standard 8-oz water glass. (2) The glass is slowly filled with cool water. (3) Entire contents are to be drunk immediately. (An additional glass of water may be taken for best results.)

How Supplied: Cartons of 16 and of 30 single-dose (6.4 g) packets.

Is this product OTC: Yes. See also PDR for Nonprescription Drugs.

PROMPT®
(psyllium hydrophilic mucilloid with sennosides)

Description: Prompt combines a natural-source stimulant laxative with bulk-producing dietary fiber for gentle overnight relief from constipation. Prompt contains no artificial chemicals. Each individual-dose packet or one rounded teaspoonful of bulk powder (6.5 g) contains psyllium hydrophilic mucilloid 3.5 g, and sennosides 12.4 mg, with sucrose.

Actions: Prompt provides gentle, effective stimulation to the colon, and additionally provides bland, nonirritating bulk to encourage normal elimination. The bulk in the bowel aids in the prevention of rebound constipation, thus helping to avoid a laxative habit.

Indication: Prompt is indicated for short-term relief of constipation. Onset of action is generally within 8 to 10 hours.

Contraindications: Intestinal obstruction, fecal impaction.

Warnings: Prompt or any laxative should not be taken when nausea, vomiting, or abdominal pain is present. Habitual use of laxatives may result in dependence on them. As with any drug, pregnant or nursing women should seek the advice of a health professional before using this product.

Drug Interactions: None known.

Symptoms and Treatment of Oral Overdosage: Treat symptomatically; there is no specific antidote.

Dosage and Administration: *Adults:* A single daily dose is usually taken at bedtime. Stir the contents of one to two packets, or one to two rounded teaspoonfuls of bulk powder, into an 8-oz glass of cold juice or water and drink immediately. *Children 6 to 12 years:* Use one-half of the adult dose.

How Supplied: Powder, containers of 2½ oz and 5 oz; single-dose packets, cartons of 12 (OTC); also available in cartons of 100 single-dose (6.5 g) packets.

Is this product OTC: Yes. See also PDR for Nonprescription Drugs.

The preceding prescribing information for Searle Consumer Products was current as of December 15, 1984.

Searle & Co.
SAN JUAN, PUERTO RICO 00936

ALDACTAZIDE®   ℞
[al-dac'tuh"zīde]
(spironolactone with hydrochlorothiazide)

Warning
Spironolactone, an ingredient of Aldactazide, has been shown to be a tumorigen in chronic toxicity studies in rats (see *Warnings*). Aldactazide should be used only in those conditions described under *Indications and Usage*. Unnecessary use of this drug should be avoided. Fixed-dose combination drugs are not indicated for initial therapy of edema or hypertension. Edema or hypertension requires therapy titrated to the individual patient. If the fixed combination represents the dosage so determined, its use may be more convenient in patient management. The treatment of hypertension and edema is not static, but must be reevaluated as conditions in each patient warrant.

Description:
Aldactazide oral tablets contain:
spironolactone .... 25 mg
hydrochlorothiazide .... 25 mg
    or
spironolactone .... 50 mg
hydrochlorothiazide .... 50 mg

Spironolactone (Aldactone®), an aldosterone antagonist, is 17-hydroxy-7α-mercapto-3-oxo-17α-pregn-4-ene-21-carboxylic acid γ-lactone acetate and has the following structure:

Spironolactone is practically insoluble in water, soluble in alcohol, and freely soluble in benzene and in chloroform.

Hydrochlorothiazide, a diuretic and antihypertensive, is 6-chloro-3,4-dihydro-2H-1,2,4-benzothiadiazine-7-sulfonamide 1,1-dioxide and has the following structure:

Hydrochlorothiazide is slightly soluble in water and freely soluble in sodium hydroxide solution.

Clinical Pharmacology: Aldactazide is a combination of two diuretic agents with different but complementary mechanisms and sites of action, thereby providing additive diuretic and antihypertensive effects. Additionally, the spironolactone component helps to minimize the potassium loss characteristically induced by the thiazide component.

The diuretic effect of spironolactone is mediated through its action as a specific pharmacologic antagonist of aldosterone, primarily by competitive binding of receptors at the aldosterone-dependent sodium-potassium exchange site in the distal convoluted renal tubule. Hydrochlorothiazide promotes the excretion of sodium and water primarily by inhibiting their reabsorption in the cortical diluting segment of the renal tubule.

Aldactazide is effective in significantly lowering the systolic and diastolic blood pressure in many patients with essential hypertension, even when aldosterone secretion is within normal limits.

Both spironolactone and hydrochlorothiazide reduce exchangeable sodium, plasma volume, body weight, and blood pressure. The diuretic and antihypertensive effects of the individual components are potentiated when spironolactone and hydrochlorothiazide are given concurrently.

In the human, the bioavailability of both spironolactone and hydrochlorothiazide from orally administered Aldactazide 25 mg/25 mg uncoated tablets and Aldactazide film-coated tablets has been evaluated in hypertensive subjects. Equivalent doses of the film-coated tablets, which contain microcrystalline spironolactone, showed 20% to 25% higher bioavailability of spironolactone compared to the uncoated Aldactazide tablets. Hydrochlorothiazide bioavailability was similar in the film-coated and uncoated tablets.

Spironolactone is rapidly and extensively metabolized. The primary metabolite is canrenone, which attains peak serum levels at two to four hours following single oral administration. Canrenone plasma concentrations decline in two distinct phases, being rapid in the first 12 hours and slower from 12 to 96 hours. The log-linear phase half-life of canrenone, following multiple doses of Aldactone (spironolactone), is between 13 and 24 hours. Both spironolactone and canrenone are more than 90% bound to plasma proteins. The metabolites of spironolactone are excreted primarily in urine, but also in bile.

Hydrochlorothiazide is rapidly absorbed following oral administration. Onset of action is observed within one hour and persists for 6 to 12 hours. Plasma concentrations attain peak levels at one to two hours and decline with a half-life of four to five hours. Hydrochlorothiazide undergoes only slight metabolic alteration and is excreted in urine. It is distributed throughout the extracellular space, with essentially no tissue accumulation except in the kidney.

Indications and Usage: Spironolactone, an ingredient of Aldactazide, has been shown to be a tumorigen in chronic toxicity studies in rats (see *Warnings* section). Aldactazide should be used only in those conditions described below. Unnecessary use of this drug should be avoided.

Aldactazide is indicated for:

Edematous conditions for patients with:

Congestive heart failure: For the management of edema and sodium retention when the patient is only partially responsive to, or is intolerant of, other therapeutic measures. The treatment of diuretic-induced hypokalemia in patients with congestive heart failure when other measures are considered inappropriate. The treatment of patients with congestive heart failure taking digitalis when other therapies are considered inadequate or inappropriate.

Cirrhosis of the liver accompanied by edema and/or ascites: Aldosterone levels may be exceptionally high in this condition. Aldactazide is indicated for maintenance therapy together with bed rest and the restriction of fluid and sodium.

The nephrotic syndrome: For nephrotic patients when treatment of the underlying disease, restriction of fluid and sodium intake, and the use of other diuretics do not provide an adequate response.

Essential hypertension
For patients with essential hypertension in whom other measures are considered inadequate or inappropriate. In hypertensive patients for the treatment of a diuretic-induced hypoka-

lemia when other measures are considered inappropriate.

Usage in Pregnancy. The routine use of diuretics in an otherwise healthy woman is inappropriate and exposes mother and fetus to unnecessary hazard. Diuretics do not prevent development of toxemia of pregnancy, and there is no satisfactory evidence that they are useful in the treatment of developing toxemia.

Edema during pregnancy may arise from pathologic causes or from the physiologic and mechanical consequences of pregnancy. Aldactazide is indicated in pregnancy when edema is due to pathologic causes just as it is in the absence of pregnancy (however, see *Warnings* section). Dependent edema in pregnancy, resulting from restriction of venous return by the expanded uterus, is properly treated through elevation of the lower extremities and use of support hose; use of diuretics to lower intravascular volume in this case is unsupported and unnecessary. There is hypervolemia during normal pregnancy which is harmful to neither the fetus nor the mother (in the absence of cardiovascular disease), but which is associated with edema, including generalized edema, in the majority of pregnant women. If this edema produces discomfort, increased recumbency will often provide relief. In rare instances, this edema may cause extreme discomfort which is not relieved by rest. In these cases, a short course of diuretics may provide relief and may be appropriate.

Contraindications: Aldactazide is contraindicated in patients with anuria, acute renal insufficiency, significant impairment of renal function, or hyperkalemia, and in patients who are allergic to thiazide diuretics or to other sulfonamide-derived drugs. Aldactazide may also be contraindicated in acute or severe hepatic failure.

Warnings: Potassium supplementation, either in the form of medication or as a diet rich in potassium, should not ordinarily be given in association with Aldactazide therapy. Excessive potassium intake may cause hyperkalemia in patients receiving Aldactazide (see *Precautions* section). Aldactazide should not be administered concurrently with other potassium-sparing diuretics.

Sulfonamide derivatives, including thiazides, have been reported to exacerbate or activate systemic lupus erythematosus.

Spironolactone has been shown to be a tumorigen in chronic toxicity studies performed in rats, with its proliferative effects manifested on endocrine organs and the liver. In one study using 25, 75, and 250 times the usual daily human dose (2 mg/kg) there was a statistically significant dose-related increase in benign adenomas of the thyroid and testes. In female rats there was a statistically significant increase in malignant mammary tumors at the mid-dose only. In male rats there was a dose-related increase in proliferative changes in the liver. At the highest dosage level (500 mg/kg), the range of effects included hepatocytomegaly, hyperplastic nodules, and hepatocellular carcinoma; the last was not statistically significant at a value of $p = 0.05$. A dose-related (above 20 mg/kg/day) incidence of myelocytic leukemia was observed in rats fed daily doses of potassium canrenoate for a period of one year. Canrenone and canrenoic acid are the major metabolites of potassium canrenoate. Spironolactone is also metabolized to canrenone. An increased incidence of leukemia was not observed in chronic rat toxicity studies conducted with spironolactone at doses up to 500 mg/kg/day.

Precautions: Patients receiving Aldactazide therapy should be carefully evaluated for possible disturbances of fluid and electrolyte balance. Hyperkalemia may occur in patients with impaired renal function or excessive potassium intake and can cause cardiac irregularities which may be fatal. Consequently, no potassium supplement should ordinarily be given with Aldactazide. Hyperkalemia can be treated promptly by the rapid intravenous administration of glucose (20% to 50%) and regular insulin, using 0.25 to 0.5 units of insulin per gram of glucose. This is a temporary measure to be repeated as required. Aldactazide should be discontinued and potassium intake (including dietary potassium) restricted.

Hypokalemia may develop as a result of profound diuresis, particularly when Aldactazide is used concomitantly with loop diuretics, glucocorticoids, or ACTH. Hypokalemia may exaggerate the effects of digitalis therapy. Potassium depletion may induce signs of digitalis intoxication at previously tolerated dosage levels.

Warning signs of possible fluid and electrolyte imbalance include dryness of the mouth, thirst, weakness, lethargy, drowsiness, restlessness, muscle pains or cramps, muscular fatigue, hypotension, oliguria, tachycardia, and gastrointestinal symptoms.

Aldactazide therapy may cause a transient elevation of BUN. This appears to represent a concentration phenomenon rather than renal toxicity, since the BUN returns to normal after Aldactazide is discontinued. Progressive elevation of BUN is suggestive of the presence of preexisting renal impairment.

Reversible hyperchloremic metabolic acidosis, usually in association with hyperkalemia, has been reported to occur in some patients with decompensated hepatic cirrhosis, even in the presence of normal renal function.

Dilutional hyponatremia, manifested by dryness of the mouth, thirst, lethargy, and drowsiness, and confirmed by a low serum sodium level, may be induced, especially when Aldactazide is administered in combination with other diuretics. A true low-salt syndrome may rarely develop with Aldactazide therapy and may be manifested by increasing mental confusion similar to that observed with hepatic coma. This syndrome is differentiated from dilutional hyponatremia in that it does not occur with obvious fluid retention. Its treatment requires that diuretic therapy be discontinued and sodium administered.

Gynecomastia may develop in association with the use of spironolactone, and physicians should be alert to its possible onset. The development of gynecomastia appears to be related to both dosage level and duration of therapy and is normally reversible when Aldactazide is discontinued. In rare instances some breast enlargement may persist.

Thiazides have been demonstrated to alter the metabolism of uric acid and carbohydrates, with possible development of hyperuricemia, gout, and decreased glucose tolerance. Thiazides may temporarily exaggerate abnormalities of glucose metabolism in diabetic patients or cause abnormalities to appear in patients with latent diabetes.

The antihypertensive effects of hydrochlorothiazide may be enhanced in patients who have undergone sympathectomy.

Pathologic changes in the parathyroid gland with hypercalcemia and hypophosphatemia have been observed in patients on prolonged thiazide therapy. Thiazides may also decrease serum PBI levels without evidence of alteration of thyroid function.

Both spironolactone and hydrochlorothiazide reduce the vascular responsiveness to norepinephrine. Therefore, caution should be exercised in the management of patients subjected to regional or general anesthesia while they are being treated with Aldactazide. Thiazides may also increase the responsiveness to tubocurarine.

Several reports of possible interference with digoxin radioimmunoassays by spironolactone, or its metabolites, have appeared in the literature. Neither the extent nor the potential clinical significance of its interference (which may be assay-specific) has been fully established.

Usage in Pregnancy. Spironolactone or its metabolites may, and hydrochlorothiazide does, cross the placental barrier. Therefore, the use of Aldactazide in pregnant women requires that the anticipated benefit be weighed against possible hazards to the fetus. These hazards include fetal or neonatal jaundice, thrombocytopenia, and possible other adverse reactions which have been reported in the adult.

Nursing Mothers. Canrenone, a metabolite of spironolactone, and hydrochlorothiazide appear in breast milk. If use of these drugs is deemed essential, an alternative method of infant feeding should be instituted.

Adverse Reactions: Gynecomastia is observed not infrequently. Other adverse reactions that have been reported in association with the use of spironolactone are: gastrointestinal symptoms including cramping and diarrhea, drowsiness, lethargy, headache, maculopapular or erythematous cutaneous eruptions, urticaria, mental confusion, drug fever, ataxia, inability to achieve or maintain erection, irregular menses or amenorrhea, postmenopausal bleeding, hirsutism, and deepening of the voice. Carcinoma of the breast has been reported in patients taking spironolactone, but a cause and effect relationship has not been established.

Adverse reactions reported in association with the use of thiazides include: gastrointestinal symptoms (anorexia, nausea, vomiting, diarrhea, abdominal cramps), purpura, thrombocytopenia, leukopenia, agranulocytosis, dermatologic symptoms (cutaneous eruptions, pruritus, erythema multiforme), paresthesia, acute pancreatitis, jaundice, dizziness, vertigo, headache, xanthopsia, photosensitivity, necrotizing angiitis, aplastic anemia, orthostatic hypotension, muscle spasm, weakness, and restlessness.

Adverse reactions are usually reversible upon discontinuation of Aldactazide.

Dosage and Administration: Optimal dosage should be established by individual titration of the components (see Box Warning).

Edema in adults (*congestive heart failure, hepatic cirrhosis, or nephrotic syndrome*). The usual maintenance dose of Aldactazide is 100 mg each of spironolactone and hydrochlorothiazide daily, administered in a single dose or in divided doses, but may range from 25 mg to 200 mg of each component daily depending on the response to the initial titration. In some instances it may be desirable to administer separate tablets of either Aldactone (spironolactone) or hydrochlorothiazide in addition to Aldactazide in order to provide optimal individual therapy.

The onset of diuresis with Aldactazide occurs promptly and, due to prolonged effect of the spironolactone component, persists for two to three days after Aldactazide is discontinued.

Edema in children. The usual daily maintenance dose of Aldactazide should be that which provides 0.75 to 1.5 mg of spironolactone per pound of body weight (1.65 to 3.3 mg/kg).

Essential hypertension. Although the dosage will vary depending on the results of titration of the individual ingredients, many patients will be found to have an optimal response to 50 mg to 100 mg each of spironolactone and hydrochlorothiazide daily, given in a single dose or in divided doses.

Concurrent potassium supplementation is not recommended when Aldactazide is used in the long-term management of hypertension or in the treatment of most edematous conditions, since the spironolactone content of Aldactazide is usually sufficient to minimize loss induced by the hydrochlorothiazide component.

How Supplied:
Aldactazide tablets containing 25 mg of spironolactone (Aldactone) and 25 mg of hydrochlorothiazide are round, tan, film coated, with SEARLE and 1011 debossed on one side and ALDACTAZIDE and 25 on the other side; bottles of 100, 500, 1,000, and 2,500, and cartons of 100 unit-dose individually blister-sealed tablets.

Aldactazide tablets containing 50 mg of spironolactone (Aldactone) and 50 mg of hydrochlorothiazide are oblong, tan, scored, film coated, with SEARLE and 1021 debossed on the scored side and ALDACTAZIDE and 50 on the other side; bottles of 100 and cartons of 100 unit-dose individually blister-sealed tablets.

Shown in Product Identification Section, page 435

Continued on next page

Searle & Co.—Cont.

ALDACTONE® ℞
[al-dac'tone]
(spironolactone)

> **Warning**
> Spironolactone has been shown to be a tumorigen in chronic toxicity studies in rats (see *Warnings*). Aldactone should be used only in those conditions described under *Indications and Usage*. Unnecessary use of this drug should be avoided.

Description: Aldactone oral tablets contain 25 mg, 50 mg, or 100 mg of the aldosterone antagonist spironolactone, 17-hydroxy-7α-mercapto-3-oxo-17α-pregn-4-ene-21-carboxylic acid γ-lactone acetate. The structural formula of spironolactone is:

Spironolactone is practically insoluble in water, soluble in alcohol, and freely soluble in benzene and in chloroform.

Clinical Pharmacology: Aldactone (spironolactone) is a specific pharmacologic antagonist of aldosterone, acting primarily through competitive binding of receptors at the aldosterone-dependent sodium-potassium exchange site in the distal convoluted renal tubule. Aldactone causes increased amounts of sodium and water to be excreted, while potassium is retained. Aldactone acts both as a diuretic and as an antihypertensive drug by this mechanism. It may be given alone or with other diuretic agents which act more proximally in the renal tubule.

Increased levels of the mineralocorticoid, aldosterone, are present in primary and secondary hyperaldosteronism. Edematous states in which secondary aldosteronism is usually involved include congestive heart failure, hepatic cirrhosis, and the nephrotic syndrome. By competing with aldosterone for receptor sites, Aldactone provides effective therapy for the edema and ascites in those conditions. Aldactone counteracts secondary aldosteronism induced by the volume depletion and associated sodium loss caused by active diuretic therapy.

Aldactone is effective in lowering the systolic and diastolic blood pressure in patients with primary hyperaldosteronism. It is also effective in most cases of essential hypertension, despite the fact that aldosterone secretion may be within normal limits in benign essential hypertension.

Through its action in antagonizing the effect of aldosterone, Aldactone inhibits the exchange of sodium for potassium in the distal renal tubule and helps to prevent potassium loss.

Aldactone has not been demonstrated to elevate serum uric acid, to precipitate gout, or to alter carbohydrate metabolism.

In the human, the bioavailability of spironolactone from orally administered Aldactone 25-mg and 100-mg film-coated tablets, which contain microcrystalline spironolactone, has been evaluated in hypertensive subjects. Equivalent doses showed 35% and 20% higher bioavailability of spironolactone from the 25-mg and 100-mg film-coated tablets, respectively, compared to the 25-mg uncoated Aldactone tablets.

Spironolactone is rapidly and extensively metabolized. The primary metabolite is canrenone, which attains peak serum levels at two to four hours following single oral administration. In the dose range of 25 mg to 200 mg, an approximately linear relationship exists between a single dose of spironolactone and plasma levels of canrenone. Plasma concentrations of canrenone decline in two distinct phases, the first phase lasting from 3 to 12 hours, being more rapid than the second phase lasting from 12 to 96 hours. Canrenone clearance data, following multiple doses of spironolactone, indicate that accumulation of canrenone in the body with 100 mg once a day would be lower than with 25 mg four times a day. Both spironolactone and canrenone are more than 90-percent bound to plasma proteins. The metabolites of spironolactone are excreted primarily in urine, but also in bile.

Indications and Usage: Aldactone (spironolactone) is indicated in the management of:

Primary hyperaldosteronism for:
Establishing the diagnosis of primary hyperaldosteronism by therapeutic trial.
Short-term preoperative treatment of patients with primary hyperaldosteronism.
Long-term maintenance therapy for patients with discrete aldosterone-producing adrenal adenomas who are judged to be poor operative risks or who decline surgery.
Long-term maintenance therapy for patients with bilateral micro- or macronodular adrenal hyperplasia (idiopathic hyperaldosteronism).

Edematous conditions for patients with:
Congestive heart failure: For the management of edema and sodium retention when the patient is only partially responsive to, or is intolerant of, other therapeutic measures. Aldactone is also indicated for patients with congestive heart failure taking digitalis when other therapies are considered inappropriate.

Cirrhosis of the liver accompanied by edema and/or ascites: Aldosterone levels may be exceptionally high in this condition. Aldactone is indicated for maintenance therapy together with bed rest and the restriction of fluid and sodium.

The nephrotic syndrome: For nephrotic patients when treatment of the underlying disease, restriction of fluid and sodium intake, and the use of other diuretics do not provide an adequate response.

Essential hypertension
Usually in combination with other drugs, Aldactone is indicated for patients who cannot be treated adequately with other agents or for whom other agents are considered inappropriate.

Hypokalemia
For the treatment of patients with hypokalemia when other measures are considered inappropriate or inadequate. Aldactone is also indicated for the prophylaxis of hypokalemia in patients taking digitalis when other measures are considered inadequate or inappropriate.

Usage in Pregnancy. The routine use of diuretics in an otherwise healthy woman is inappropriate and exposes mother and fetus to unnecessary hazard. Diuretics do not prevent development of toxemia of pregnancy, and there is no satisfactory evidence that they are useful in the treatment of developing toxemia.

Edema during pregnancy may arise from pathologic causes or from the physiologic and mechanical consequences of pregnancy.

Aldactone is indicated in pregnancy when edema is due to pathologic causes just as it is in the absence of pregnancy (however, see *Warnings* section). Dependent edema in pregnancy, resulting from restriction of venous return by the expanded uterus, is properly treated through elevation of the lower extremities and use of support hose; use of diuretics to lower intravascular volume in this case is unsupported and unnecessary. There is hypervolemia during normal pregnancy which is harmful to neither the fetus nor the mother (in the absence of cardiovascular disease), but which is associated with edema, including generalized edema, in the majority of pregnant women. If this edema produces discomfort, increased recumbency will often provide relief. In rare instances, this edema may cause extreme discomfort which is not relieved by rest. In these cases, a short course of diuretics may provide relief and may be appropriate.

Contraindications: Aldactone is contraindicated for patients with anuria, acute renal insufficiency, significant impairment of renal function, or hyperkalemia.

Warnings: Potassium supplementation, either in the form of medication or as a diet rich in potassium, should not ordinarily be given in association with Aldactone therapy. Excessive potassium intake may cause hyperkalemia in patients receiving Aldactone (see *Precautions* section). Aldactone should not be administered concurrently with other potassium-sparing diuretics.

Spironolactone has been shown to be a tumorigen in chronic toxicity studies performed in rats, with its proliferative effects manifested on endocrine organs and the liver. In one study using 25, 75, and 250 times the usual daily human dose (2 mg/kg) there was a statistically significant dose-related increase in benign adenomas of the thyroid and testes. In female rats there was a statistically significant increase in malignant mammary tumors at the mid-dose only. In male rats there was a dose-related increase in proliferative changes in the liver. At the highest dosage level (500 mg/kg) the range of effects included hepatocytomegaly, hyperplastic nodules, and hepatocellular carcinoma; the last was not statistically significant at a value of $p = 0.05$. A dose-related (above 20 mg/kg/day) incidence of myelocytic leukemia was observed in rats fed daily doses of potassium canrenoate for a period of one year. Canrenone and canrenoic acid are the major metabolites of potassium canrenoate. Spironolactone is also metabolized to canrenone. An increased incidence of leukemia was not observed in chronic rat toxicity studies conducted with spironolactone at doses up to 500 mg/kg/day.

Precautions: General: Because of the diuretic action of Aldactone (spironolactone), patients should be carefully evaluated for possible disturbances of fluid and electrolyte balance. Hyperkalemia may occur in patients with impaired renal function or excessive potassium intake and can cause cardiac irregularities which may be fatal. Consequently, no potassium supplement should ordinarily be given with Aldactone. Hyperkalemia can be treated promptly by the rapid intravenous administration of glucose (20% to 50%) and regular insulin, using 0.25 to 0.5 units of insulin per gram of glucose. This is a temporary measure to be repeated as required. Aldactone should be discontinued and potassium intake (including dietary potassium) restricted.

Reversible hyperchloremic metabolic acidosis, usually in association with hyperkalemia, has been reported to occur in some patients with decompensated hepatic cirrhosis, even in the presence of normal renal function.

Hyponatremia, manifested by dryness of the mouth, thirst, lethargy, and drowsiness, and confirmed by a low serum sodium level, may be caused or aggravated, especially when Aldactone is administered in combination with other diuretics.

Gynecomastia may develop in association with the use of spironolactone, and physicians should be alert to its possible onset. The development of gynecomastia appears to be related to both dosage level and duration of therapy and is normally reversible when Aldactone is discontinued. In rare instances some breast enlargement may persist. Aldactone therapy may cause a transient elevation of BUN, especially in patients with preexisting renal impairment. Aldactone may cause mild acidosis.

Drug interactions: When used in combination with other diuretics or antihypertensive agents Aldactone potentiates their effects. Therefore, the dosage of such drugs, particularly the ganglionic blocking agents, should be reduced by at least 50 percent when Aldactone is added to the regimen. Spironolactone reduces the vascular responsiveness to norepinephrine. Therefore, caution should be exercised in the management of patients subjected to regional or general anesthesia while they are being treated with Aldactone.

Drug/Laboratory test interactions: Several reports of possible interference with digoxin radioimmunoassays by spironolactone, or its metabolites, have appeared in the literature. Neither the extent nor the potential clinical significance of its interference (which may be assay-specific) has been fully established.

Usage in pregnancy: Spironolactone or its metabolites may cross the placental barrier. Therefore, the use of Aldactone in pregnant women requires that the anticipated benefit be weighed against possible hazard to the fetus.

Nursing mothers: Canrenone, a metabolite of spironolactone, appears in breast milk. If use of the drug is deemed essential, an alternative method of infant feeding should be instituted.

Adverse Reactions: Gynecomastia is observed not infrequently. Other adverse reactions that have been reported in association with Aldactone are: gastrointestinal symptoms including cramping and diarrhea, drowsiness, lethargy, headache, maculopapular or erythematous cutaneous eruptions, urticaria, mental confusion, drug fever, ataxia, inability to achieve or maintain erection, irregular menses or amenorrhea, postmenopausal bleeding, hirsutism, and deepening of the voice. Carcinoma of the breast has been reported in patients taking spironolactone, but a cause and effect relationship has not been established.

Adverse reactions are usually reversible upon discontinuation of the drug.

Dosage and Administration: Primary hyperaldosteronism. Aldactone may be employed as an initial diagnostic measure to provide presumptive evidence of primary hyperaldosteronism while patients are on normal diets.

Long test: Aldactone (spironolactone) is administered at a daily dosage of 400 mg for three to four weeks. Correction of hypokalemia and of hypertension provides presumptive evidence for the diagnosis of primary hyperaldosteronism.

Short test: Aldactone is administered at a daily dosage of 400 mg for four days. If serum potassium increases during Aldactone administration but drops when Aldactone is discontinued, a presumptive diagnosis of primary hyperaldosteronism should be considered.

After the diagnosis of hyperaldosteronism has been established by more definitive testing procedures, Aldactone may be administered in doses of 100 to 400 mg daily in preparation for surgery. For patients who are considered unsuitable for surgery, Aldactone may be employed for long-term maintenance therapy at the lowest effective dosage determined for the individual patient.

Edema in adults (*congestive heart failure, hepatic cirrhosis, or nephrotic syndrome*). An initial daily dosage of 100 mg of Aldactone administered in either single or divided doses is recommended, but may range from 25 to 200 mg daily. When given as the sole agent for diuresis, Aldactone should be continued for at least five days at the initial dosage level, after which it may be adjusted to the optimal therapeutic or maintenance level administered in either single or divided daily doses. If, after five days, an adequate diuretic response to Aldactone has not occurred, a second diuretic which acts more proximally in the renal tubule may be added to the regimen. Because of the additive effect of Aldactone when administered concurrently with such diuretics, an enhanced diuresis usually begins on the first day of combined treatment; combined therapy is indicated when more rapid diuresis is desired. The dosage of Aldactone should remain unchanged when other diuretic therapy is added.

Edema in children. The initial daily dosage should provide approximately 1.5 mg of Aldactone per pound of body weight (3.3 mg/kg) administered in either single or divided doses.

Essential hypertension. For adults, an initial daily dosage of 50 to 100 mg of Aldactone administered in either single or divided doses is recommended. Aldactone may also be given with diuretics which act more proximally in the renal tubule or with other antihypertensive agents. Treatment with Aldactone should be continued for at least two weeks, since the maximum response may not occur before this time. Subsequently, dosage should be adjusted according to the response of the patient.

Hypokalemia. Aldactone in a dosage ranging from 25 mg to 100 mg daily is useful in treating a diuretic-induced hypokalemia, when oral potassium supplements or other potassium-sparing regimens are considered inappropriate.

How Supplied:
Aldactone 25-mg tablets are round, light yellow, film coated, with SEARLE and 1001 debossed on one side and ALDACTONE and 25 on the other side; bottles of 100, 500, 1,000, and 2,500, and cartons of 100 unit-dose individually blister-sealed tablets.

Aldactone 50-mg tablets are oval, light orange, scored, film coated, with SEARLE and 1041 debossed on the scored side and ALDACTONE and 50 on the other side; bottles of 100 and cartons of 100 unit-dose individually blister-sealed tablets.

Aldactone 100-mg tablets are round, peach colored, scored, film coated, with SEARLE and 1031 debossed on the scored side and ALDACTONE and 100 on the other side; bottles of 100 and cartons of 100 unit-dose individually blister-sealed tablets.

Shown in Product Identification Section, page 435

AMINOPHYLLIN™ Tablets ℞
[*am-in-off"i-lin*]
(aminophylline)

Description: Each tablet contains 100 mg or 200 mg of aminophylline USP calculated as the dihydrate, which is equivalent to 79 mg and 158 mg of anhydrous theophylline, respectively. Aminophylline USP (anhydrous) is a soluble complex containing approximately 85% anhydrous theophylline and 15% ethylenediamine. Aminophylline is white or slightly yellowish granules or powder, having a slight ammoniacal odor and a bitter taste.

Actions: Aminophylline directly relaxes the smooth muscle of the bronchial airways and pulmonary blood vessels, thus acting mainly as a bronchodilator, pulmonary vasodilator, and smooth muscle relaxant. The drug also possesses other actions typical of the xanthine derivatives: coronary vasodilator, diuretic, cardiac stimulant, cerebral stimulant, and skeletal muscle stimulant.

Indications: Aminophyllin Tablets are indicated for the relief and/or prevention of symptoms from asthma and reversible bronchospasm associated with chronic bronchitis and emphysema.

Contraindications: Aminophylline should not be administered to patients with active peptic ulcer disease, since it may increase the volume and acidity of gastric secretions.

Patients with a history of hypersensitivity to aminophylline or theophylline should not be treated with the drug.

Aminophylline should not be administered with other xanthine preparations.

Warnings: Excessive doses may be expected to be toxic. Some children may be unusually sensitive to aminophylline. Toxic synergism with ephedrine and other sympathomimetic bronchodilator drugs may occur.

Usage in Pregnancy. Safe use in pregnancy has not been established relative to possible adverse effects on fetal development. Therefore, aminophylline should not be used in pregnant women unless, in the judgment of the physician, the potential benefits outweigh the possible hazards.

Precautions: Use with caution in patients with severe cardiac disease, hypertension, hyperthyroidism, or acute myocardial injury. Particular caution in dose administration must be exercised in patients with a history of peptic ulcer since the condition may be exacerbated. Chronic oral administration in high doses may be associated with gastrointestinal irritation.

Caution should be used in giving aminophylline to patients in congestive heart failure. Serum levels in such patients have persisted for long periods following discontinuation of the drug.

The addition of ephedrine or other sympathomimetic drugs to regimens of aminophylline increases the toxicity potential and may result in symptoms of overdosage, due to the additive pharmacological effects of these compounds.

Adverse Reactions: The most consistent adverse reactions observed with *therapeutic* amounts of aminophylline are:
1. Gastrointestinal: Nausea, vomiting, anorexia, bitter aftertaste, dyspepsia, heavy feeling in the stomach, and gastrointestinal distress.
2. Central nervous system: Dizziness, vertigo, light-headedness, headache, nervousness, insomnia, and agitation.
3. Cardiovascular: Palpitation, tachycardia, flushing, and extrasystoles.
4. Respiratory: Increase in respiratory rate.
5. Dermatologic: Urticaria.

Overdosage: The most consistent reactions observed with *toxic* overdoses of aminophylline are:
1. Gastrointestinal: Nausea, vomiting, epigastric pain, hematemesis, and diarrhea.
2. Central nervous system: In addition to those cited above, the patient may exhibit hyperreflexia, fasciculations, and clonic and tonic convulsions. These are especially prone to occur in cases of overdosage in infants and small children.
3. Cardiovascular: In addition to those outlined above, marked hypotension and circulatory failure may be manifest.
4. Respiratory: Tachypnea and respiratory arrest may occur.
5. Renal: Albuminuria and microhematuria may occur. Increased excretion of renal tubular cells has been observed.
6. General systemic effects: Syncope, collapse, fever, and dehydration.

Management of Toxic Symptoms:
1. Discontinue drug immediately.
2. There is no known specific antidote.
3. Gastric lavage.
4. Emetic medication may be of value.
5. Avoid administration of sympathomimetic drugs.
6. Intravenous fluids, oxygen, and other supportive measures to prevent hypotension and overcome dehydration.
7. Central nervous system stimulation and seizures may respond to short-acting barbiturates.
8. Monitor serum levels until below 20 mcg/ml.

Dosage and Administration: The oral dose for adults should be adjusted according to the need and response of the patient. Usually a daily dose in the range of 600 to 1600 mg, administered in 3 or 4 divided doses, will provide the desired therapeutic effect. Similarly, the dose for children should be adjusted according to the response. An oral dose of 12 mg/kg/24 hours, administered in four divided doses, will usually provide the desired therapeutic effect in children.

Therapeutic serum levels are considered to be between 10 mcg/ml and 20 mcg/ml. Levels above 20 mcg/ml may produce toxic effects. There is great variation from patient to patient in dosage needed to achieve a therapeutic serum level and in the duration of action of oral aminophylline. Because of these wide variations and the relatively narrow therapeutic serum-level range, dosage must be individualized with monitoring of theophylline serum levels, particularly when prolonged use is planned.

How Supplied: Aminophyllin Tablets are supplied as:
Round, white, scored tablets with 1231 debossed on the scored side and SEARLE on the other side, each tablet containing 100 mg of aminophylline; bottles of 100 and 1,000, and cartons of 100 unit-dose individually blister-sealed tablets.

Oval, white, scored tablets with 1251 debossed on the scored side and SEARLE on the other side, each tablet containing 200 mg of aminophylline; bottles of 100 and 1,000, and cartons of 100 unit-dose individually blister-sealed tablets.

Shown in Product Identification Section, page 435

Continued on next page

Searle & Co.—Cont.

ANAVAR® ℞
[an'uh-var]
(oxandrolone)

Description: Anavar oral tablets contain 2.5 mg of the anabolic steroid oxandrolone, a synthetic derivative of testosterone. Oxandrolone is 17β-hydroxy-17α-methyl-2-oxa-5α-androstan-3-one with the following structural formula:

Clinical Pharmacology: Anavar is used primarily for its protein anabolic effect and its catabolism-inhibiting effect on tissue. Nitrogen balance is improved by anabolic agents, but only when the intake of calories and protein is sufficient. It has not been established whether this positive nitrogen balance indicates a primary benefit in the utilization of protein-building dietary substances. Some clinical effects and adverse reactions reported demonstrate the androgenic properties of drugs of this class. Complete dissociation of anabolic from androgenic effects has not been achieved. The actions of anabolic steroids are therefore similar to those of male sex hormones with the possibility that serious disturbances of growth and sexual development may be caused if given to young children.

Use of androgens in children over long periods of time may result in fusion of the epiphyseal growth centers.

Anabolic steroids have been reported to increase low-density lipoproteins and decrease high-density lipoproteins. Serum lipid determination should be done periodically.

During exogenous administration of anabolic androgens, endogenous testosterone release is inhibited through inhibition of pituitary luteinizing hormone (LH). At large doses spermatogenesis may be suppressed through feedback inhibition of pituitary follicle-stimulating hormone (FSH).

Indications and Usage: Anavar is indicated as adjunctive therapy to promote weight gain after weight loss following extensive surgery, chronic infections, or severe trauma, and in some patients who without definite pathophysiologic reasons fail to gain or to maintain normal weight, to offset the protein catabolism associated with prolonged administration of corticosteroids, and for the relief of the bone pain frequently accompanying osteoporosis. (See *Dosage and Administration*.)

Contraindications:
1. Carcinoma of the prostate or male breast.
2. Carcinoma of the breast in some women.
3. Nephrosis or the nephrotic phase of nephritis.
4. Pregnancy, because of possible masculinization of the fetus. Anavar has been shown to cause embryotoxicity, fetotoxicity, infertility, and masculinization of female animal offspring when given in doses 9 times the human dose. No *in vitro* mutagenicity tests have been conducted.
5. Hypercalcemia.

Warnings:
ANABOLIC STEROIDS DO NOT ENHANCE ATHLETIC ABILITY.

Geriatric patients treated with anabolic/androgenic steroids may be at an increased risk for the development of prostatic hypertrophy and prostatic carcinoma.

There have been rare reports of hepatocellular neoplasms, including carcinoma, and peliosis hepatis in association with anabolic/androgenic steroid therapy.

Cholestatic hepatitis and jaundice may occur with 17-alpha-alkylated androgens at a relatively low dose. If cholestatic hepatitis with jaundice appears or if liver function tests become abnormal, Anavar should be discontinued and the etiology should be determined. Drug-induced jaundice is reversible when the medication is discontinued.

Hypercalcemia may develop both spontaneously and as a result of hormonal therapy in women with disseminated breast carcinoma. Anavar therapy should be discontinued if hypercalcemia occurs.

Edema with or without congestive heart failure may be a serious complication in patients with preexisting cardiac, renal, or hepatic disease. Therapy with Anavar may increase the edema.

In children, androgen therapy may accelerate bone maturation without producing compensatory gain in linear growth. The effect on bone maturation should be monitored. (See *Precautions/Laboratory tests*.)

Precautions:
General: Women should be observed for signs of virilization (deepening of the voice, hirsutism, acne, clitoromegaly, and menstrual irregularities). Discontinuation of drug therapy at the time of evidence of mild virilism is necessary to prevent irreversible virilization.

Suppression of clotting factors II, V, VII, and X has been observed.

Information for patients: The physician should instruct patients to report any of the following side effects of androgens:
Prepubertal males: Too frequent or persistent erections of the penis.
Females: Hoarseness, acne, changes in menstrual periods, or more facial hair.
All patients: Nausea, vomiting, changes in skin color, or ankle swelling.

Laboratory tests:
1. Women with disseminated breast carcinoma should have frequent determination of urine and serum calcium levels during the course of therapy (see *Warnings*).
2. Because of the hepatotoxicity associated with the use of 17-alpha-alkylated androgens, liver function tests should be obtained periodically.
3. Periodic (every 6 months) x-ray examinations of bone age should be made during treatment of prepubertal males to determine the rate of bone maturation and the effects of androgen therapy on the epiphyseal centers.
4. Serum lipid determinations should be done periodically as anabolic/androgenic steroids have been reported to increase low-density lipoproteins and decrease high-density lipoproteins.
5. Serum cholesterol levels may increase during therapy. Therefore, caution is required when administering these agents to patients with a history of myocardial infarction or coronary artery disease. Serial determinations of serum cholesterol should be made and therapy adjusted accordingly.

Drug interactions
Anticoagulants: C-17 substituted derivatives of testosterone have been reported to decrease the anticoagulant requirements of patients receiving oral anticoagulants. Patients receiving oral anticoagulant therapy require close monitoring, especially when androgens are started or stopped.
Insulin: In diabetic patients the metabolic effects of androgens may decrease blood glucose and insulin requirements.
Oral hypoglycemic agents: Anavar may inhibit the metabolism of oral hypoglycemic agents.
Adrenal steroids or ACTH: In patients with edema, concomitant administration with adrenal steroids or ACTH may increase the edema.
Drug/Laboratory test interactions: If thyroid function tests are performed, the physician should be aware that androgens may decrease levels of thyroxine-binding globulin, resulting in decreased total T_4 serum levels and increased resin uptake of T_3 and T_4. In addition, a decrease in PBI and radioactive iodine uptake may occur.

Alterations in the metyrapone test have occurred.

Carcinogenesis, mutagenesis, impairment of fertility
Animal data: In two-year chronic oral rat studies, a dose-related reduction of spermatogenesis and decreased organ weights (testes, prostate, seminal vesicles, ovaries, uterus, adrenals, and pituitary) were shown. Anavar has not been tested in laboratory animals for carcinogenic or mutagenic effects.

Human data: There are rare reports of hepatocellular carcinoma in patients receiving long-term therapy with anabolic/androgenic steroids in high doses. Withdrawal of the drugs did not lead to regression of the tumors in all cases.

Geriatric patients treated with androgens may be at an increased risk for the development of prostatic hypertrophy and prostatic carcinoma.

Pregnancy: Teratogenic effects; Pregnancy Category X. See *Contraindications*.

Nursing mothers: It is not known whether anabolic steroids are excreted in human milk. Because of the potential for serious adverse reactions in nursing infants from Anavar, a decision should be made whether to discontinue nursing or to discontinue the drug, taking into account the importance of the drug to the mother.

Pediatric use: Anabolic/androgenic steroid therapy should be used very cautiously in children and only by specialists who are aware of the effects on bone maturation. Skeletal maturation should be monitored every six months by an x-ray of hand and wrist. (See *Warnings*.)

Adverse Reactions: The following adverse reactions have been associated with use of anabolic steroids:
Endocrine: Masculinization of the fetus, increased or decreased libido, inhibition of gonadotropin secretion, and premature closure of epiphyses in children.
In *males*:
 Prepubertal
  Phallic enlargement
  Increased frequency or persistence of erections
 Postpubertal
  Inhibition of testicular function and oligospermia
  Gynecomastia
In *females*:
 Hirsutism, male-pattern baldness, deepening of the voice, and clitoral enlargement. (These changes are usually irreversible even after prompt discontinuance of therapy and are not prevented by concomitant use of estrogens.)
 Menstrual irregularities
 When administered to a pregnant woman, anabolic/androgenic steroids cause virilization of external genitalia of the female fetus.
Gastrointestinal: Nausea, abdominal fullness, loss of appetite, vomiting, and burning of the tongue.
Dermatologic: Acne (especially in females and prepubertal males).
Hepatic: Cholestatic jaundice, alterations in liver function tests and, rarely, hepatocellular neoplasms and peliosis hepatis (see *Warnings*).
General: Bleeding in patients on concomitant anticoagulant therapy.
Fluid and electrolyte disturbances: Retention of sodium, chloride, water, potassium, calcium, and inorganic phosphate.
Metabolism: Increased serum cholesterol.
Overdosage: No symptoms or signs associated with overdosage have been reported. It is possible that sodium and water retention may occur.

The oral LD_{50} of oxandrolone in mice and dogs is greater than 5,000 mg/kg. No specific antidote is known, but gastric lavage may be used.

Dosage and Administration: Therapy with anabolic steroids is adjunctive to and not a replacement for conventional therapy. The duration of therapy with Anavar (oxandrolone) will depend on the response of the patient and the possible appearance of adverse reactions. Therapy should be intermittent.

Adults. The *usual adult dosage* of Anavar is one 2.5-mg tablet two to four times daily. However, the response of individuals to anabolic steroids varies, and a daily dosage of as little as 2.5 mg or as much as 20 mg may be required to achieve the desired response. A course of therapy of two to four weeks is usually adequate. This may be repeated intermittently as indicated.

Children. For children the *total daily dosage* of Anavar is 0.25 mg per kilogram or 0.12 mg per

pound of body weight. This may be repeated intermittently as indicated.
How Supplied: Anavar 2.5-mg tablets are oval, white, and scored, with 1401 debossed on the scored side and SEARLE on the other side; bottles of 100.
Federal law prohibits dispensing without prescription.
Shown in Product Identification Section, page 435

CALAN® Tablets ℞
[*cal'an*]
(verapamil hydrochloride)
Description: Calan (verapamil HCl) is a calcium ion influx inhibitor (slow-channel blocker or calcium ion antagonist) available for oral administration in film-coated tablets containing 80 mg or 120 mg of verapamil hydrochloride.
The structural formula of verapamil HCl is:

$$CH_3O \underset{CH_3O}{} \underset{}{\bigcirc} \underset{}{\overset{CN}{\underset{C(CH_2)_3NCH_2CH_2}{\mid}}} \underset{CH(CH_3)_2}{} \underset{}{\bigcirc} \underset{}{\overset{OCH_3}{}} OCH_3 \cdot HCl$$

$C_{27}H_{38}N_2O_4 \cdot HCl \qquad M.W.= 491.08$

Benzeneacetonitrile, α-[3-[[2-(3, 4-dimethoxyphenyl) ethyl] methylamino] propyl]-3, 4- dimethoxy-α- (1-methylethyl) hydrochloride.
Verapamil HCl is an almost white, crystalline powder, practically free of odor, with a bitter taste. It is soluble in water, chloroform, and methanol. Verapamil HCl is not chemically related to other cardioactive drugs.
Clinical Pharmacology: Calan is a calcium ion influx inhibitor (slow-channel blocker or calcium ion antagonist) that exerts its pharmacologic effects by modulating the influx of ionic calcium across the cell membrane of the arterial smooth muscle as well as in conductile and contractile myocardial cells.
Mechanism of action: The precise mechanism of action of Calan as an antianginal agent remains to be fully determined, but includes the following two mechanisms:
1. *Relaxation and prevention of coronary artery spasm:* Calan dilates the main coronary arteries and coronary arterioles, both in normal and ischemic regions, and is a potent inhibitor of coronary artery spasm, whether spontaneous or ergonovine-induced. This property increases myocardial oxygen delivery in patients with coronary artery spasm and is responsible for the effectiveness of Calan in vasospastic (Prinzmetal's or variant) as well as unstable angina at rest. Whether this effect plays any role in classical effort angina is not clear, but studies of exercise tolerance have not shown an increase in the maximum exercise rate–pressure product, a widely accepted measure of oxygen utilization. This suggests that, in general, relief of spasm or dilation of coronary arteries is not an important factor in classical angina.
2. *Reduction of oxygen utilization:* Calan regularly reduces arterial pressure at rest and at a given level of exercise by dilating peripheral arterioles and reducing the total peripheral resistance (afterload) against which the heart works. This unloading of the heart reduces myocardial energy consumption and oxygen requirements and probably accounts for the effectiveness of Calan in chronic stable effort angina.
Electrical activity through the SA and AV nodes depends, to a significant degree, on calcium influx through the slow channel. By inhibiting this influx, Calan slows AV conduction and prolongs the effective refractory period within the AV node in a rate-related manner. It can interfere with sinus node impulse generation and induce sinus arrest in patients with sick sinus syndrome; it also can induce atrioventricular block, although this has been seen rarely in clinical use. Calan may shorten the antegrade effective refractory period of the accessory bypass tracts. Calan does not alter the normal atrial action potential or intraventricular conduction time, but depresses amplitude, velocity of depolarization, and conduction in depressed atrial fibers.
Calan (verapamil HCl) has a local anesthetic action that is 1.6 times that of procaine on an equimolar basis. It is not known whether this action is important at the doses used in man.
Calan does not alter total serum calcium levels.
Pharmacokinetics and metabolism: More than 90% of the orally administered dose of Calan is absorbed. Because of rapid biotransformation of verapamil during its first pass through the portal circulation, absolute bioavailability ranges from 20% to 35%. Peak plasma concentrations are reached between 1 and 2 hours after oral administration. Chronic oral administration of 120 mg of verapamil every 6 hours resulted in plasma levels of verapamil ranging from 125 to 400 ng/ml, with higher values reported occasionally. A close relationship exists between verapamil plasma concentration and prolongation of the PR interval. The mean elimination half-life in single-dose studies ranged from 2.8 to 7.4 hours. In these same studies, after repetitive dosing, the half-life increased to a range from 4.5 to 12.0 hours (after less than 10 consecutive doses given 6 hours apart). Half-life may increase during titration due to saturation of hepatic enzyme systems as plasma verapamil levels rise.
Verapamil is highly bound to plasma proteins. In healthy men, orally administered Calan undergoes extensive metabolism in the liver. Twelve metabolites have been identified in plasma; all except norverapamil are present in trace amounts only. Norverapamil can reach steady-state plasma concentrations approximately equal to those of verapamil itself. The major metabolites of verapamil have been identified as various N- and O-dealkylated products of verapamil. Approximately 70% of an administered dose is excreted as metabolites in the urine and 16% or more in the feces within 5 days. About 3% to 4% is excreted in the urine as unchanged drug. Approximately 90% is bound to plasma proteins. In patients with hepatic insufficiency, metabolism is delayed and elimination half-life prolonged up to 14 to 16 hours (see *Precautions*); the volume of distribution is increased and plasma clearance reduced to about 30% of normal. Verapamil clearance values suggest that patients with liver dysfunction may attain therapeutic verapamil plasma concentrations with one third of the oral daily dose required for patients with normal liver function.
Hemodynamics and myocardial metabolism: In animals and man, Calan (verapamil HCl) reduces afterload and myocardial contractility. In most patients, including those with organic cardiac disease, the negative inotropic action of Calan is countered by reduction of afterload, and cardiac index is usually not reduced. However, in patients with severe left ventricular dysfunction (eg, pulmonary wedge pressure above 20 mm Hg or ejection fraction less than 30%), or in patients taking beta-adrenergic blocking agents or other cardiodepressant drugs, deterioration of ventricular function may occur (see *Drug interactions*).
Pulmonary function: Calan does not induce bronchoconstriction and, hence, does not impair ventilatory function.
Indications and Usage: Calan tablets are indicated for the treatment of angina pectoris, including:
1. Angina at rest, including:
 • Vasospastic (Prinzmetal's variant) angina
 • Unstable (crescendo, preinfarction) angina
2. Chronic stable angina (classic effort-associated angina)
Contraindications:
Verapamil HCl is contraindicated in:
1. Severe left ventricular dysfunction (see *Warnings*)
2. Hypotension (systolic pressure less than 90 mm Hg) or cardiogenic shock
3. Sick sinus syndrome (except in patients with a functioning artificial ventricular pacemaker)
4. Second- or third-degree AV block
Warnings:
Heart failure: Verapamil has a negative inotropic effect, which in most patients is compensated by its afterload reduction (decreased peripheral vascular resistance) properties without a net impairment of ventricular performance. In clinical studies involving 1,166 patients, 11 (0.9%) developed congestive heart failure or pulmonary edema. Congestive heart failure/pulmonary edema led to discontinuation or reduction of dosage of verapamil in 6 patients (0.5%). Verapamil should be avoided in patients with severe left ventricular dysfunction (eg, ejection fraction less than 30%) or moderate to severe symptoms of cardiac failure and in patients with any degree of ventricular dysfunction if they are receiving a beta-blocker (see *Drug interactions*). Patients with milder ventricular dysfunction should, if possible, be controlled with optimum doses of digitalis and/or diuretics before verapamil treatment. **(Note interactions with digoxin under *Precautions*.)**
Hypotension: Occasionally, the pharmacologic action of verapamil may produce a decrease in blood pressure below normal levels, which may result in dizziness or symptomatic hypotension. Hypotension is usually asymptomatic, orthostatic, mild, and can be controlled by a decrease in the Calan (verapamil HCl) dose. The incidence of hypotension observed in 1,166 patients enrolled in clinical trials was 2.9%.
Elevated liver enzymes: Elevations of transaminases with and without concomitant elevations in alkaline phosphatase and bilirubin have been reported. Such elevations have sometimes been transient and may disappear even in the face of continued verapamil treatment. However, four cases of hepatocellular injury produced by verapamil have been proven by rechallenge; two of these four cases had clinical symptoms of malaise, fever, and/or right upper quadrant pain, in addition to elevation of SGOT, SGPT, and alkaline phosphatase. Periodic monitoring of liver function in patients receiving verapamil is therefore prudent.
Atrial flutter/fibrillation with accessory bypass tract: Patients with atrial flutter and/or fibrillation and an accessory AV pathway (eg, Wolff-Parkinson-White or Lown-Ganong-Levine syndromes) may develop increased antegrade conduction across the aberrant pathway bypassing the AV node, producing a very rapid ventricular response after receiving verapamil (or digitalis). Treatment is usually D.C.-cardioversion. Cardioversion has been used safely and effectively after oral Calan.
Atrioventricular block: The effect of verapamil on AV conduction and the SA node leads to first-degree AV block and transient bradycardia, sometimes accompanied by nodal escape rhythms, fairly commonly during the peaks of serum concentration. Higher degrees of AV block, however, were infrequently observed (0.8%). Marked first-degree block or progressive development to second- or third-degree AV block requires a reduction in dosage or, in rare instances, discontinuation of verapamil HCl and institution of appropriate therapy, depending on the clinical situation.
Patients with hypertrophic cardiomyopathy (IHSS): In 120 patients with hypertrophic cardiomyopathy (most of them refractory or intolerant to propranolol) who received therapy with verapamil at doses up to 720 mg/day, a variety of serious adverse effects was seen. Three patients died in pulmonary edema; all had a past history of severe left ventricular outflow obstruction and left ventricular dysfunction. Eight other patients had pulmonary edema and/or severe hypotension; abnormally high (greater than 20 mm Hg) pulmonary wedge pressure and a marked left ventricular outflow obstruction were present in most of these patients. Concomitant administration of quinidine preceded the severe hypotension in 3 of the 8 patients (2 of whom developed pulmonary edema). Sinus bradycardia occurred in 11% of the patients, second-degree AV block in 4%, and sinus arrest in 2%. It must be appreciated that this group of patients had a serious disease with a high mortality rate. Most adverse effects responded well to dose reduction, and only rarely did verapamil use have to be discontinued.

Continued on next page

Searle & Co.—Cont.

Precautions:
General
Use in patients with impaired hepatic function: Since verapamil is highly metabolized by the liver, it should be administered cautiously to patients with impaired hepatic function. Severe liver dysfunction prolongs the elimination half-life of verapamil to about 14 to 16 hours; hence, approximately 30% of the dose given to patients with normal liver function should be administered to these patients. Careful monitoring for abnormal prolongation of the PR interval or other signs of excessive pharmacologic effects (see *Overdosage*) should be carried out.

Use in patients with impaired renal function: About 70% of an administered dose of verapamil is excreted as metabolites in the urine. Until further data are available, verapamil should be administered cautiously to patients with impaired renal function. These patients should be carefully monitored for abnormal prolongation of the PR interval or other signs of overdosage (see *Overdosage*).

Drug interactions
Beta-blockers: Controlled studies in small numbers of patients suggest that the concomitant use of Calan (verapamil HCl) and beta-blocking agents may be beneficial in patients with chronic stable angina, but available information is not sufficient to predict with confidence the effects of concurrent treatment, especially in patients with left ventricular dysfunction or cardiac conduction abnormalities.

The combination can have adverse effects on cardiac function. In one study involving 15 patients treated with high doses of propranolol (median dose, 480 mg/day; range, 160 to 1,280 mg/day) for severe angina, with preserved left ventricular function (ejection fraction greater than 35%), the hemodynamic effects of additional therapy with verapamil HCl were assessed using invasive methods. The addition of verapamil to high-dose beta-blockers induced modest negative inotropic and chronotropic effects that were not severe enough to limit short-term (48 hours) combination therapy in this study. These modest cardiodepressant effects persisted for greater than 6 but less than 30 hours after abrupt withdrawal of beta-blockers and were closely related to plasma levels of propranolol. The primary verapamil/beta-blocker interaction in this study appeared to be hemodynamic rather than electrophysiologic.

In 3 other studies involving 51 patients, verapamil did not induce negative inotropic or chronotropic effects in patients with preserved left ventricular function receiving low or moderate doses of propranolol (less than or equal to 320 mg/day). Because of the still limited experience with combination therapy, verapamil should be used alone, if possible. If combined therapy is used, close surveillance of vital signs and clinical status should be carried out and the need for concomitant treatment with propranolol reassessed periodically. Combined therapy should usually be avoided in patients with atrioventricular conduction abnormalities and those with depressed left ventricular function.

Digitalis: Chronic verapamil treatment increases serum digoxin levels by 50% to 70% during the first week of therapy, and this can result in digitalis toxicity. Maintenance digitalization doses should be reduced when verapamil is administered and the patient should be carefully monitored to avoid over- or underdigitalization. Whenever overdigitalization is suspected, the daily dose of digoxin should be reduced or temporarily discontinued. On discontinuation of Calan (verapamil HCl) use, the patient should be monitored to avoid underdigitalization.

Antihypertensive agents: Verapamil administered concomitantly with oral antihypertensive agents (eg, vasodilators, diuretics) may have an additive effect on lowering blood pressure. Patients receiving these combinations should be appropriately monitored. In patients who have recently received drugs such as methyldopa, which attenuate alpha-adrenergic response, combined therapy of verapamil and propranolol should probably be avoided (severe hypotension may occur).

Disopyramide: Until data on possible interactions between verapamil and disopyramide are obtained, disopyramide should not be administered within 48 hours before or 24 hours after verapamil administration.

Quinidine: In a small number of patients with hypertrophic cardiomyopathy (IHSS), concomitant use of verapamil and quinidine resulted in significant hypotension. Until further data are obtained, combined therapy of verapamil and quinidine in patients with hypertrophic cardiomyopathy should probably be avoided.

Nitrates: Verapamil has been given concomitantly with short- and long-acting nitrates without any undesirable drug interactions. The pharmacologic profile of both drugs and the clinical experience suggest beneficial interactions.

Carcinogenesis, mutagenesis, impairment of fertility: Adequate animal carcinogenicity studies have not been performed with verapamil. An 18-month toxicity study in rats, at a low multiple (6-fold) of the maximum recommended human dose, and not the maximum tolerated dose, did not suggest a tumorigenic potential. A 2-year carcinogenicity study will be carried out in rats.

Verapamil was not mutagenic in the Ames test in 5 test strains at 3 mg per plate with or without metabolic activation.

Studies in female rats at daily dietary doses up to 5.5 times (55 mg/kg/day) the maximum recommended human dose did not show impaired fertility. Effects on male fertility have not been determined.

Pregnancy: Pregnancy Category C. Reproduction studies have been performed in rabbits and rats at oral doses up to 1.5 (15 mg/kg/day) and 6 (60 mg/kg/day) times the human oral daily dose, respectively, and have revealed no evidence of teratogenicity. In the rat, however, this multiple of the human dose was embryocidal and retarded fetal growth and development, probably because of adverse maternal effects reflected in reduced weight gains of the dams. This oral dose has also been shown to cause hypotension in rats. There are no adequate and well-controlled studies in pregnant women. Because animal reproduction studies are not always predictive of human response, this drug should be used during pregnancy only if clearly needed.

Labor and delivery: It is not known whether the use of verapamil during labor or delivery has immediate or delayed adverse effects on the fetus, or whether it prolongs the duration of labor or increases the need for forceps delivery or other obstetric intervention. Such adverse experiences have not been reported in the literature, despite a long history of use of verapamil in Europe in the treatment of cardiac side effects of beta-adrenergic agonist agents used to treat premature labor.

Nursing mothers: It is not known whether this drug is excreted in human milk. Because many drugs are excreted in human milk and because of the potential for adverse reactions in nursing infants from verapamil, nursing should be discontinued while verapamil is administered. Studies in rats at 2.5 times the maximum recommended human dose revealed no evidence of an effect of verapamil on lactation or weaning.

Animal pharmacology and/or animal toxicology: Chronic animal toxicology studies indicate that verapamil causes lenticular and/or suture line changes at 30 mg/kg/day or greater, and frank cataracts at 62.5 mg/kg/day or greater in the beagle dog but not in the rat. These effects are thought to be species specific. Development of cataracts due to verapamil has not been reported in man.

Adverse Reactions: Serious adverse reactions are rare when Calan (verapamil HCl) therapy is initiated with upward dose titration within the recommended single and total daily dose. The following reactions to orally administered verapamil were reported from clinical studies involving 1,166 patients with angina or arrhythmia. Adverse reactions occurred at a similar rate in controlled clinical trials and uncontrolled clinical experience.

Cardiovascular: Hypotension (2.9%), peripheral edema (1.7%), AV block: third-degree (0.8%), bradycardia: HR <50/min (1.1%), CHF or pulmonary edema (0.9%).

Central nervous system: Dizziness (3.6%), headache (1.8%), fatigue (1.1%).

Gastrointestinal: Constipation (6.3%), nausea (1.6%); elevations of liver enzymes have been reported (see *Warnings*).

The following reactions, reported in less than 0.5% of patients, occurred under circumstances where a causal relationship is not certain, and are therefore mentioned to alert the physician to a possible relationship: confusion, paresthesia, insomnia, somnolence, equilibrium disorders, blurred vision, syncope, muscle cramps, shakiness, claudication, hair loss, macular eruptions, spotty menstruation, ecchymosis, bruising, gynecomastia, and psychotic symptoms.

In addition, more serious adverse events were observed, not readily distinguishable from the natural history of the disease in these patients. Of the 1,166 patients evaluated, 16 (1.4%) had myocardial infarctions. Nine of these 16 patients had myocardial infarctions while being treated for unstable angina, 4 of these were receiving placebo, the remaining 5 received verapamil.

The daily dose of verapamil was reduced in 6.3% and discontinued in 5.5% of the 1,166 patients. In general, the highest incidence of adverse reactions was seen in the dose-titration periods in all the studies.

Treatment of acute cardiovascular adverse reactions: The frequency of cardiovascular adverse reactions that require therapy is rare; hence, experience with their treatment is limited. Whenever severe hypotension or complete AV block occur following oral administration of verapamil, the appropriate emergency measures should be applied immediately; eg, intravenously administered isoproterenol HCl, norepinephrine bitartrate, atropine sulfate (all in the usual doses), or calcium gluconate (10% solution). In patients with hypertrophic cardiomyopathy (IHSS), alpha-adrenergic agents (phenylephrine HCl, metaraminol bitartrate, or methoxamine HCl) should be used to maintain blood pressure and isoproterenol and norepinephrine should be avoided. If further support is necessary, dopamine HCl or dobutamine HCl may be administered. Actual treatment and dosage should depend on the severity of the clinical situation and the judgment and experience of the treating physician.

Overdosage: Treatment of overdosage should be supportive. Beta-adrenergic stimulation or parenteral administration of calcium solutions may increase calcium ion flux across the slow channel, and have been used effectively in treatment of deliberate overdosage with verapamil. Clinically significant hypotensive reactions or fixed high-degree AV block should be treated with vasopressor agents or cardiac pacing, respectively. Asystole should be handled by the usual measures, including cardiopulmonary resuscitation.

Dosage and Administration: The dose of verapamil must be individualized by titration. Calan (verapamil HCl) is available in 80-mg and 120-mg tablets. The usual initial dose is 80 mg every 6 to 8 hours. Dosage may be increased at daily (eg, patients with unstable angina) or weekly intervals until optimum clinical response is obtained. In general, maximum effects of any given dosage would be apparent during the first 24 to 48 hours of therapy, but note that between 24 and 48 hours, the half-life of verapamil increases; therefore, the maximum response may be delayed. The total daily dose ranges from 240 to 480 mg. The optimum daily dose for most patients ranges from 320 to 480 mg. The usefulness and safety of dosages exceeding 480 mg/day in angina pectoris have not been established.

How Supplied:
Calan 80-mg tablets are oval, peach colored, scored, film coated, with CALAN debossed on one side and 80 on the other, supplied as:

NDC Number	Size
0014-1851-31	bottle of 100
0014-1851-51	bottle of 500
0014-1851-52	bottle of 1,000
0014-1851-34	carton of 100 unit dose

Calan 120-mg tablets are oval, brown, scored, film coated, with CALAN 120 debossed on one side, supplied as:

NDC Number	Size
0014-1861-31	bottle of 100
0014-1861-51	bottle of 500
0014-1861-52	bottle of 1,000
0014-1861-34	carton of 100 unit dose

Store at 59° to 86°F (15° to 30°C).

Shown in Product Identification Section, page 435

SEARLE ORAL CONTRACEPTIVES
DEMULEN 1/35™-21 ℞
DEMULEN 1/35™-28 ℞
DEMULEN 1/50™-21 ℞
DEMULEN 1/50™-28 ℞
[dem′ū-len]
(ethynodiol diacetate with ethinyl estradiol)
OVULEN-21® ℞
OVULEN-28® ℞
[ov′ū-len]
(ethynodiol diacetate with mestranol)
ENOVID-E® 21 ℞
ENOVID® 5 mg ℞
ENOVID® 10 mg ℞
[ē-nov′id]
(norethynodrel with mestranol)

Description:
Demulen 1/35™-21 and Demulen 1/35™-28. Each white tablet contains 1 mg of ethynodiol diacetate and 35 mcg of ethinyl estradiol. Each blue tablet in the Demulen 1/35™-28 package is a placebo, containing no active ingredients.
Demulen 1/50™-21 and Demulen 1/50™-28. Each white tablet contains 1 mg of ethynodiol diacetate and 50 mcg of ethinyl estradiol. Each pink tablet in the Demulen 1/50™-28 package is a placebo containing no active ingredients.
Ovulen-21 and Ovulen-28. Each white tablet contains 1 mg of ethynodiol diacetate and 0.1 mg of mestranol. Each pink tablet in the Ovulen-28 package is a placebo containing no active ingredients.
Enovid-E 21. Each tablet contains 2.5 mg of norethynodrel and 0.1 mg of mestranol.
Enovid 5 mg. Each tablet contains 5 mg of norethynodrel and 75 mcg of mestranol.
Enovid 10 mg. Each tablet contains 9.85 mg of norethynodrel and 0.15 mg of mestranol.
The chemical name for norethynodrel is 17α-ethynyl-17-hydroxy-5(10)-estren-3-one, for mestranol it is 3-methoxy-19-nor-17α-pregna-1,3,5(10)-trien-20-yn-17-ol, for ethynodiol diacetate it is 19-nor-17α-pregn-4-en-20-yne-3β,17-diol diacetate, and for ethinyl estradiol it is 19-nor-17α-pregna-1, 3, 5(10)-trien-20-yne-3,17-diol. Their structural formulas are as follows:

ethynodiol diacetate

mestranol

ethinyl estradiol

norethynodrel

Therapeutic Class: Oral contraceptive (except for Enovid 10 mg). Estrogen-progestogen combination (Enovid 5 mg and 10 mg only).

Clinical Pharmacology: Combination oral contraceptives act primarily through the mechanism of gonadotropin suppression due to the estrogenic and progestational activity of their components. Although the primary mechanism of action is inhibition of ovulation, alterations in the genital tract, including changes in the cervical mucus (which reduce sperm penetration) and the endometrium (which reduce the likelihood of implantation) may also contribute to contraceptive effectiveness.
Enovid 5 mg or Enovid 10 mg, when used for the treatment of endometriosis, may be administered to induce changes in areas of endometriosis similar to those that occur during pregnancy. In many instances when Enovid 5 mg or Enovid 10 mg is taken continuously the areas of endometriosis develop a decidua-like response followed by necrosis, which may result in destruction of the abnormally located tissue and resolution of the lesions.

Indications and Usage: Demulen 1/35, Demulen 1/50, Ovulen, Enovid-E, and Enovid 5 mg are indicated for the prevention of pregnancy in women who elect to use oral contraceptives as a method of contraception.
Enovid 5 mg and Enovid 10 mg are indicated for the treatment of endometriosis, for the treatment of hypermenorrhea, and for the production of cyclic withdrawal bleeding.
NOTE: The contraindication, warning, precaution, and adverse reaction information in this monograph also applies when Enovid 5 mg is prescribed for indications other than contraception or when Enovid 10 mg is prescribed.
Oral contraceptives are highly effective. The pregnancy rate in women using conventional combination oral contraceptives (containing 35 mcg or more of ethinyl estradiol or 50 mcg or more of mestranol) is generally reported to be less than 1 pregnancy per 100 woman-years of use. Slightly higher rates (somewhat more than 1 pregnancy per 100 woman-years of use) are reported for some combination products containing 35 mcg or less of ethinyl estradiol, and rates on the order of 3 pregnancies per 100 woman-years are reported for the progestogen-only oral contraceptives.
These rates are derived from separate studies conducted by different investigators in several population groups; therefore, a precise comparison cannot be made. Furthermore, pregnancy rates tend to be lower as clinical studies are continued, possibly due to selective retention in the longer studies of those patients who accept the treatment regimen and do not discontinue as a result of adverse reactions, pregnancy, or other reasons. In Table 1 ranges of pregnancy rates as reported in the literature[1] are shown for other means of contraception. The efficacy of these means of contraception, except for the IUD, depends upon the degree of adherence to the method.
In clinical trials with Ovulen, 5,938 patients completed 83,463 cycles, and a total of 8 pregnancies were reported. This represents a pregnancy rate of 0.12 per 100 woman-years.
In clinical trials with Enovid-E, 1,657 patients completed 28,400 cycles, and a total of 8 pregnancies were reported. This represents a pregnancy rate of 0.34 per 100 woman-years.
In clinical trials with Demulen 1/50, 2,256 patients completed 30,409 cycles, and a total of 30 pregnancies were reported. This represents a pregnancy rate of 1.18 per 100 woman-years.
In clinical trials with Demulen 1/35, 1,231 patients completed 14,641 cycles, and a total of 15 pregnancies were reported. This represents a pregnancy rate of 1.23 per 100 woman-years.
In clinical trials with Demulen 1/35, the incidence of delayed or breakthrough bleeding was 44% at cycle 6. However, only 9.9% of the patients dropped out of the study due to bleeding.

Table 1
Pregnancies per 100 Woman-Years

Method	Range
IUD	<1 to 6
Diaphragm with spermicidal cream or gel	2 to 20
Condom	3 to 36
Spermicidal aerosol foams	2 to 29
Spermicidal gels and creams	4 to 36
Periodic abstinence (rhythm), all types	<1 to 47
1. Calendar method	14 to 47
2. Temperature method	1 to 20
3. Temperature method (intercourse only in post-ovulatory phase)	<1 to 7
4. Mucus method	1 to 25
No contraception	60 to 80

Dose-related Risk of Thromboembolism From Oral Contraceptives: Studies have shown a positive association between the dose of estrogens in oral contraceptives and the risk of thromboembolism[2,96,97] (see Warning No. 1). For this reason, it is prudent and in keeping with good principles of therapeutics to minimize exposure to estrogen. The oral contraceptive product prescribed for any given patient should be that product which contains the least amount of estrogen that is compatible with an acceptable pregnancy rate and patient acceptance. It is recommended that new users of oral contraceptives be started on preparations containing 50 mcg or less of estrogen.

Contraindications: Oral contraceptives should not be used in women with any of the following conditions:
1. Thrombophlebitis or thromboembolic disorders.
2. A past history of deep vein thrombophlebitis or thromboembolic disorders.
3. Cerebral vascular disease, myocardial infarction or coronary artery disease, or a past history of these conditions.
4. Known or suspected carcinoma of the breast.
5. Known or suspected estrogen-dependent neoplasia.
6. Undiagnosed abnormal genital bleeding.
7. Known or suspected pregnancy (see Warning No. 5).
8. Past or present, benign or malignant liver tumors among women who developed these tumors during the use of oral contraceptives or other estrogen-containing products (see Warning No. 4).

WARNINGS

Cigarette-smoking increases the risk of serious cardiovascular side effects from oral contraceptive use. This risk increases with age and with heavy smoking (15 or more cigarettes per day) and is quite marked in women over 35 years of age. Women who use oral contraceptives should be strongly advised not to smoke.

The use of oral contraceptives is associated with increased risk of several serious conditions including venous and arterial thromboembolism, thrombotic and hemorrhagic stroke, myocardial infarction, visual disorders, hepatic tumors, gallbladder disease, hypertension, and fetal abnormalities. Practi-

Continued on next page

tioners prescribing oral contraceptives should be familiar with the following information relating to these and other risks.

1. Thromboembolic Disorders and Other Vascular Problems. An increased risk of thromboembolic and thrombotic disease associated with the use of oral contraceptives is well established. One study in Great Britain[3] demonstrated an increased relative risk for fatal venous thromboembolism; several British[4,5,14,22,92] and U.S. [6–8,23,98–101,126] studies demonstrated an increased relative risk for nonfatal venous thromboembolism. U.S. studies[6,9,10,99,101–103] demonstrated an increased relative risk for stroke, which had not been shown in prior British studies.[3–5] In these studies it was estimated that users of oral contraceptives were 1.9 to 11 times more likely than nonusers to manifest these diseases without evident cause (Table 2). In a British study of idiopathic deep vein thrombosis and pulmonary embolism, the projected annual hospitalization rates for women aged 16–40 were 47 per 100,000 users and 5 for nonusers.[77] In one British mortality study,[3] overall excess mortality due to pulmonary embolism or stroke was on the order of 1.3 to 3.4 deaths annually per 100,000 users and increased with age.

Cerebrovascular Disorders: In a collaborative U.S. study[9,10] of cerebrovascular disorders in women with and without predisposing causes, it was estimated that the risk of hemorrhagic stroke was 2.0 times greater in users than in nonusers, and the risk of thrombotic stroke was 4.0[10] to 9.5[9] times greater in users than in nonusers (Table 2). Analysis of mortality trends in 21 countries indicates that, since oral contraceptives first became available, changes in mortality from nonrheumatic heart disease and hypertension, cerebrovascular disease, and all nonrheumatic cardiovascular disease among women aged 15 to 44 years have been associated with changes in the prevalence of oral contraceptive use in each country.[11]

Table 2. *Summary of Relative Risks of Thromboembolic Disorders and Other Vascular Problems in Oral Contraceptive Users Compared with Nonusers.*

Disorders	*Relative Risk*
Idiopathic thromboembolic disease	2 to 11 times greater
Postsurgery thromboembolic complications	4 to 7 times greater
Thrombotic stroke	4 to 9.5 times greater
Hemorrhagic stroke	2.0 to 2.3 times greater
Myocardial infarction	2 to 12 times greater

In May 1974 the Royal College of General Practitioners[12] issued an interim report of its continuing large-scale prospective study comparing a user group with a nonuser group. It stated: "A statistically significant higher rate of reporting of cerebrovascular accidents in Takers is evident, but the numbers are too small to justify an estimation of the degree of risk." A 1981 analysis of data from this study was reported[13] to show a 4-fold increased mortality from circulatory diseases, mainly from myocardial infarction and hemorrhagic stroke, in users. The excess mortality was associated with age and smoking in users. A 1983 analysis[138] of arterial diseases reported a significantly increased incidence of cerebrovascular disease among current oral contraceptive users. Risk appeared to increase with duration of use up to 8 years. Categories with a significantly increased incidence included cerebral thrombosis or embolism, and transient ischemic attacks, but not hemorrhagic strokes. Incidence of peripheral arterial thromboembolism, Raynaud's disease, and acute myocardial infarction was increased in current users. Women aged 30 years and older had appreciably higher rates of arterial disease than did younger women. Smoking increased the risk for older women in each usage group, the greatest risk being in current users aged 35 years and older who smoked. Expressed as the percentage of women diagnosed as having an arterial disease who died of that disease, the case-fatality rates were 2 to 3 times greater for users who smoked than for women in the other groups.

In October 1976 an interim report was issued on the long-term follow-up study of the British Family Planning Association.[14] There was a highly significant association between oral contraceptive use and stroke, although total numbers were small in this study also. The increase in risk of venous thrombosis and pulmonary embolism among users was about 4-fold and was statistically highly significant. In later reports[15] it was noted that mortality from nonrheumatic heart disease was greater in women who had ever used oral contraceptives. A 1984 report[147] on stroke found pill use to be a significant risk factor for nonhemorrhagic stroke, but not for subarachnoid hemorrhage. Smoking and hypertension were significant risk factors only for the latter.

In the Walnut Creek prospective study,[99,101,102] the risk of subarachnoid hemorrhage was associated with heavy smoking, age, and use of the pill.

Myocardial Infarction: An increased risk of myocardial infarction associated with the use of oral contraceptives has been reported in Great Britain,[16–19,136,138] confirming a previously suspected association.[3] The morbidity study[16,17] found that the greater the number of underlying risk factors for coronary artery disease (cigarette-smoking, hypertension, hypercholesterolemia, obesity, diabetes, history of preeclamptic toxemia), the higher the risk of developing myocardial infarction, regardless of whether the patient was an oral contraceptive user or not. Oral contraceptives were considered an additional risk factor.

The annual excess rate of fatal myocardial infarction in British oral contraceptive users was estimated to be approximately 3.5 cases per 100,000 women users in the 30- to 39-year age group and 20 per 100,000 women users in the 40- to 44-year age group.[19] (These estimates are based on British vital statistics, which show acute myocardial infarction death rates 2 to 3 times less than in the U.S. for women in these age groups. In an attempt to extrapolate these figures to U.S. women, it was estimated that the annual excess rates in users are 25.7 cases per 100,000 for women aged 30–39 with predisposing conditions versus 1.5 cases without; corresponding estimates for women aged 40–44 were 86.2 versus 5.1.[78]) The annual excess rate of hospitalization for nonfatal myocardial infarction in married British oral contraceptive users was estimated to be approximately 3.5 per 100,000 women users in the 30- to 39-year age group and 47 per 100,000 women users in the 40- to 44-year age group.[16]

Smoking is considered a major predisposing condition to myocardial infarction. In terms of relative risk, it has been estimated[20] that oral contraceptive users who do not smoke are about twice as likely to have a fatal myocardial infarction as nonusers who do not smoke. Oral contraceptive users who are also smokers have about a 5-fold increased risk of fatal infarction compared to users who do not smoke, but about a 10- to 12-fold increased risk compared to nonusers who do not smoke. Furthermore, the amount of smoking is also an important factor. In determining the importance of these relative risks, however, the baseline rates for various age groups, as shown in Table 3, must be given serious consideration. The importance of other predisposing conditions mentioned above in determining relative and absolute risks has not been quantified; it is likely that the same synergistic action exists, but perhaps to a lesser extent.

Similar findings relating nonfatal and fatal myocardial infarction, oral contraceptives, smoking, and age were subsequently published in the U.S.[91,99,104–108] and by the Royal College of General Practitioners in Great Britain. [13,138]

Risk of Dose: Reports of thromboembolism following the use of oral contraceptives containing 50 mcg or more of estrogen received by drug safety committees in Great Britain, Sweden, and Denmark were compared with the distribution expected from market research estimates of sales.[2] A positive correlation was found between the dose of estrogen and the reporting of thromboembolism, including coronary thrombosis, in excess of that predicted by sales estimates. Preparations containing 100 mcg or more of estrogen were associated with a higher risk of thromboembolism than those containing 50 to 80 mcg of estrogen. The authors' analysis did suggest, however, that the quantity of estrogen may not be the sole factor involved. Any influence on the part of the progestogens was not considered, which may have been responsible for certain discrepancies in the data. No significant differences were detected between preparations containing the same dose of estrogen nor between the two estrogens ethinyl estradiol and mestranol. A subsequent study of a similar nature in Great Britain found a positive association between the dose of progestogen or estrogen and certain thromboembolic conditions, [96] which is consistent with findings of the Royal College study. [12,92,135] Swedish authorities noted decreased reporting of thromboembolic episodes when higher estrogen preparations were no longer prescribed.[97] Careful epidemiologic studies to determine the degree of thromboembolic risk associated with progestogen-only oral contraceptives have not been performed. Cases of thromboembolic disease have been reported in women using these products, and they should not be presumed to be free of excess risk.

Table 3. *Estimated Annual Mortality Rate per 100,000 Women from Myocardial Infarction by Use of Oral Contraceptives, Smoking Habits, and Age in Years*[20]

	Myocardial infarction			
	Women aged 30–39		Women aged 40–44	
Smoking habits	Users	Non-users	Users	Non-users
All smokers	10.2	2.6	62.0	15.9
Heavy*	13.0	5.1	78.7	31.3
Light	4.7	0.9	28.6	5.7
Nonsmokers ...	1.8	1.2	10.7	7.4
Smokers and nonsmokers	5.4	1.9	32.8	11.7

*15 or more cigarettes per day

The relative risk of oral contraceptive use one month prior to hospitalization for various types of thromboembolism was calculated in a U.S. retrospective case-control study.[8] If no account is taken of the relative estrogenic potency of different estrogens and if any possible influence of the different progestogenic components is ignored, the products employed may be divided into those containing less than 100 mcg and those containing 100 mcg or more of estrogen. For all cases combined, the larger-dose category was associated with only a slightly higher relative risk; for the idiopathic subgroup, the relative risk was approximately doubled with the larger estrogen content, but the confidence limits overlapped considerably and the differences, therefore, were not statistically significant. Apparently there was less of an increased relative risk for the subgroup with predispositions to thromboembolism.[98]

In the British Family Planning Association study,[147] no nonhemorrhagic strokes occurred during 9,100 woman-years of current use of pills containing less than 50 mcg of estrogen, in contrast to 13 observed during 39,400 woman-years of current use of pills with higher doses.

The risk of thromboembolic and thrombotic disorders, both in users and in nonusers of oral contraceptives, increases with age. Oral contraceptives have been considered an independent risk factor for these events.

Persistence of Risk: A 1977 analysis[13a] of the mortality data from the prospective study of the Royal College of General Practitioners (RCGP) suggested that the risk of circulatory disease increases with the duration of oral contraceptive use and may persist after discontinuation. The ratio of the mortality rate from circulatory disease in former users to that in controls was 4.3 to 1 ($P < 0.01$), and was still 3.7 to 1 even after excluding the two deaths from malignant hypertension, where use was stopped because of the onset of hypertension. For the category of fatal subarachnoid hemorrhage, the rate ratio comparing former users to controls was also statistically significant.

In 1981, a new analysis of the RCGP mortality data[13] showed significantly increased risk ratios in former users for the categories of all nonrheumatic heart disease plus hypertension (4.6 to 1), cerebrovascular disease (3.6 to 1), as well as the subcategory of subarachnoid hemorrhage (4.5 to 1). Overall, the incidence of fatal circulatory disease for former users was 4.3 times that of the controls.

A 1983 analysis of the incidence of arterial disease in the RCGP study[138] showed that the incidence of all cerebrovascular disease, fatal and nonfatal, was significantly greater in former users than in controls (risk ratio = 2.6) and remained elevated for at least 6 years after discontinuation of oral contraceptives. Former users had significantly increased rates for cerebral thrombosis (4 vs 0), transient ischemic attacks (8.7 to 1), and "other" cerebrovascular disease (3.8 to 1).

In the Walnut Creek prospective study,[102] former use of oral contraceptives was significantly associated with increased risk of subarachnoid hemorrhage, the relative risk being 5.3.

In a U.S. hospital-based, case-control study,[137] when the duration of oral contraceptive use was considered, the data suggested that the rate of myocardial infarction is increased approximately 2- to 3-fold in older women who had used oral contraceptives for more than 10 years before discontinuation. The excess risk associated with long-term use was evident in subjects who had stopped less than 5 years previously, as well as in those who had stopped 5 to 9 years previously. Whether the excess risk persisted for more than 10 years after discontinuation could not be assessed because of a paucity of data.

In summary, persistence of risk after discontinuation of oral contraceptives has been reported for circulatory disease in general,[13,13a] for nonrheumatic heart disease,[13,137] and for cerebrovascular disease,[13,138] including subarachnoid hemorrhage,[13,13a,102] cerebral thrombosis,[138] and transient ischemic attacks.[138]

Estimate of Excess Mortality from Circulatory Diseases: A large prospective study[13] carried out in the U.K. provided estimates of the mortality rate per 100,000 women per year from diseases of the circulatory system for users and nonusers of oral contraceptives according to age, smoking habits, and duration of use. The overall annual excess death rate from circulatory diseases for oral contraceptive users was estimated at 23 per 100,000 for women of all ages. The rates for nonsmokers and smokers, respectively, were: ages 25–34, 2 and 10 per 100,000; ages 35–44, 15 and 48 per 100,000; and ages 45 and older, 41 and 179 per 100,000. The risk was statistically significant only in cigarette-smokers over age 34. The majority of deaths were due to subarachnoid hemorrhage or ischemic heart disease. Relative risk for women who had ever used oral contraceptives rose with increasing parity, a new observation that needs confirmation. The available data from a variety of sources have been analyzed[21] to estimate the risk of death associated with various methods of contraception. The estimates of risk of death for each method included the combined risk of the contraceptive method (eg, thromboembolic and thrombotic disease in the case of oral contraceptives) plus the risk attributable to pregnancy or abortion in the event of method failure. This latter risk varies with the effectiveness of the contraceptive method. The findings of this analysis are shown in Figure 1.[21] The study concluded that the mortality associated with all methods of birth control is low and below that associated with childbirth, except for that associated with oral contraceptives in women over 40 who smoke. (The rates given for pill only/smokers for each age group are for smokers as a class. For "heavy" smokers [more than 15 cigarettes a day], the rates given would be about double; for "light" smokers [less than 15 cigarettes a day], about 50 percent.[20]) The mortality associated with oral contraceptive use in nonsmokers over 40 is higher than with any other method of contracep-

tion in that age group. The lowest mortality is associated with the condom or diaphragm backed up by early legal abortion.

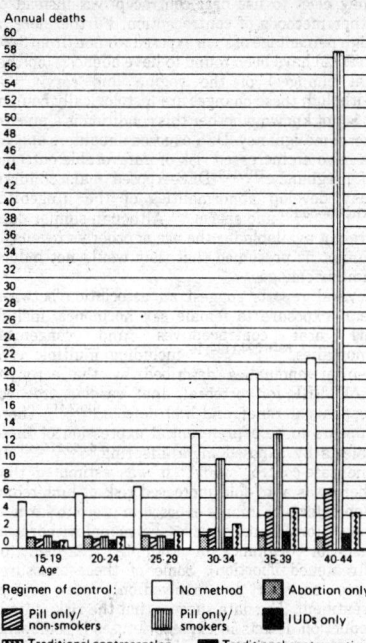

Figure 1 Estimated annual number of deaths associated with control of fertility and no control per 100,000 nonsterile women, by regimen of control and age of woman

The risk of thromboembolic and thrombotic disease associated with oral contraceptives increases with age after approximately age 30 and, for myocardial infarction, is further increased by hypertension, hypercholesterolemia, obesity, diabetes, or history of preeclamptic toxemia, and especially by cigarette-smoking.[20,78,79]

Based on the data currently available, the following table gives a gross estimate of the risk of death from circulatory disorders associated with the use of oral contraceptives:

Table 4. *Smoking Habits and Other Predisposing Conditions—Risk Associated with Use of Oral Contraceptives*

Age	Below 30	30–39	40+
Heavy smokers	C	B	A
Light smokers	D	C	B
Nonsmokers (no predisposing conditions)	D	C,D	C
Nonsmokers (other predisposing conditions)	C	C,B	B,A

A—Use associated with very high risk.
B—Use associated with high risk.
C—Use associated with moderate risk.
D—Use associated with low risk.

The physician and patient should be alert to the earliest manifestations of thromboembolic and thrombotic disorders (eg, thrombophlebitis, pulmonary embolism, cerebrovascular insufficiency, coronary artery disease or myocardial infarction, retinal thrombosis, and mesenteric thrombosis). Should any of these occur or be suspected, the drug should be discontinued immediately.

A 4- to 7-fold increased risk of postsurgery thromboembolic complications has also been reported in oral contraceptive users.[22,23] If feasible, oral contraceptives should be discontinued at least 4 weeks before elective surgery or during periods of pro-

longed immobilization. The decision as to when to resume oral contraception following major surgery or bed rest should balance the recognized risks of postsurgery thromboembolic complications with the need to reinstate contraceptive practices.

The Royal College of General Practitioners in a large prospective study reported a higher incidence of superficial and deep vein thrombosis in users, the former being correlated with the progestogen dose. The RCGP data suggest that the presence of varicose veins substantially increases the risk of superficial venous thrombosis of the leg, the risk depending upon the severity of the varicosities. The evidence suggests that the presence of varicose veins has little effect on the development of deep vein thrombosis in the leg.[92] Other prospective studies have also reported a higher incidence of venous thrombosis in users.[14,99–101,109]

2. *Ocular Lesions.* There have been reports of neuro-ocular lesions such as optic neuritis or retinal thrombosis associated with the use of oral contraceptives. Discontinue medication if there is unexplained, gradual or sudden, partial or complete loss of vision; proptosis or diplopia; papilledema; or any evidence of retinal vascular lesions. Appropriate diagnostic and therapeutic measures should be instituted.

3. *Carcinoma.* Long-term continuous administration of either natural or synthetic estrogens in certain animal species increases the frequency of certain carcinomas, and/or nonmalignant neoplasms, such as those of the breast, uterus, cervix, vagina, ovary, liver, and pituitary. Certain synthetic progestogens, none currently contained in oral contraceptives, have been noted to increase the incidence of mammary nodules, benign and malignant, in dogs.

There is now evidence that estrogens increase the risk of carcinoma of the endometrium in humans. In several independent, retrospective case-control studies,[24–28,80,93] an increased relative risk (2.2 to 13.9 times) was reported, associating endometrial carcinoma with the prolonged use of estrogens in postmenopausal women who took estrogen replacement medication to relieve menopausal symptoms. This risk was independent of the other known risk factors for endometrial cancer and appeared to depend both on duration of treatment[24,27,28] and on estrogen dose.[26–28] These findings are supported by the observation that incidence rates of endometrial cancer have increased sharply since 1969 in 8 different areas of the U.S. with population-based cancer-reporting systems, an increase which may be related to the rapidly expanding use of estrogens during the past decade.[29] There is no evidence at present that "natural" estrogens are more or less hazardous than "synthetic" estrogens at equiestrogenic doses.

One publication[30] reported on the first 30 cases submitted by physicians to a registry of cases of adenocarcinoma of the endometrium in women under 40 on oral contraceptives. Of the adenocarcinomas found in women without predisposing risk factors for adenocarcinoma of the endometrium (eg, irregular bleeding at the time oral contraceptives were first given, polycystic ovaries), nearly all occurred in women who had used a sequential oral contraceptive. These products are no longer marketed. No statistical association has been reported suggesting an increased risk of endometrial cancer in users of conventional combination or progestogen-only oral contraceptives, although individual cases have been reported. Several studies[7,31–35,99,121,122] have shown no increased risk of breast cancer to women taking oral contraceptives or estrogens. In one study,[36,37] however, while no overall increased risk of breast cancer was noted in women treated with oral contraceptives, a greater risk was suggested for the subgroups of oral contraceptive users with documented benign breast disease and for long-term (2–4 years) users. Another study[123,142] reported increased risk of breast cancer in women who had

Continued on next page

Searle & Co.—Cont.

used the pill for more than 4 years before their first full-term pregnancy. One other study[38] indicated an increasing risk of breast cancer in women taking menopausal estrogens, which increased with duration of follow-up. Several other studies have also shown oral contraceptives[127-129,133,140,141,144,146] or estrogens[130,145] to be associated with breast cancer, particularly in connection with other risk factors[127-129] (eg, family history, previous breast biopsy, late age of first delivery) and long duration of use.[127,128,130,146] A reduced occurrence of benign breast tumors in users of oral contraceptives has been well documented.[7,12,14,31,36,39,40,86,99]

Some epidemiologic studies[41,81-84,99,109,120,143] have suggested an increased risk of cervical dysplasia, erosion, and carcinoma in long-term pill users; however, cause and effect has not been established. There have been other reports of microglandular dysplasia of the cervix in users.

In summary, there is at present no consistent evidence from human studies of an increased risk of cancer associated with oral contraceptives.[42] Close clinical surveillance of all women taking oral contraceptives is, nevertheless, essential. In all cases of undiagnosed persistent or recurrent abnormal vaginal bleeding, nonfunctional causes should be borne in mind and appropriate diagnostic measures should be taken to rule out malignancy. Women who have a strong family history of breast cancer or who have breast nodules, fibrocystic disease, recurrent cystic mastitis, abnormal mammograms, or cervical dysplasia should be monitored with particular care if they elect to use oral contraceptives.

4. *Hepatic Lesions (adenomas, hepatomas, hamartomas, regenerating nodules, focal nodular hyperplasia, hemangiomas, hepatocellular carcinoma, etc).* Benign hepatic adenomas and other hepatic lesions have been associated with the use of oral contraceptives.[43-46,85] One study[46] reported that oral contraceptive formulations with high "hormonal potency" were associated with a higher risk than lower-potency formulations, as was age over 30 years. Although benign, these hepatic lesions may rupture and may cause death through intra-abdominal hemorrhage. This has been reported in short-term as well as long-term users of oral contraceptives. Two studies related risk with duration of use of the contraceptive, the risk being much greater after 4 or more years of oral contraceptive use.[45,46] Long-term users of oral contraceptives have an estimated annual incidence of hepatocellular adenoma of 3 to 4 per 100,000.[46] While such hepatic lesions are rare, they should be considered in women presenting with abdominal pain and tenderness, abdominal mass, or shock. Patients with liver tumors have demonstrated variable clinical features, which may make preoperative diagnosis difficult. About one quarter of the cases presented because of abdominal masses; up to one half had signs and symptoms of acute intraperitoneal hemorrhage. Routine radiologic and laboratory studies may not be helpful. Liver scans may clearly show a focal defect. Hepatic arteriography or computed tomography may be useful procedures in diagnosing primary liver neoplasms.

A few cases of hepatocellular carcinoma have been reported in women taking oral contraceptives.[44] The relationship of these drugs to this type of malignancy is not known at this time.

Oral contraceptives are contraindicated if there are past or present, benign or malignant liver tumors among women who developed these tumors during the use of oral contraceptives or other estrogen-containing products.

5. *Use In or Immediately Preceding Pregnancy, Birth Defects in Offspring, and Malignancy in Offspring.* The use of female sex hormones, both estrogens and progestogens, during early pregnancy may seriously damage the offspring. It has been reported that females exposed in utero to diethylstilbestrol and other nonsteroidal estrogens have an increased risk of developing in later life a form of vaginal or cervical cancer that is ordinarily extremely rare.[47,48] This risk has been estimated to be on the order of 1 in 1,000 exposures or less.[49,50] Although there is no evidence at the present time that oral contraceptives further enhance the risk of developing this type of malignancy, such patients should be monitored with particular care if they elect to use oral contraceptives instead of other methods of contraception. Furthermore, a high percentage of such exposed women (from 30% to 90%) have been found to have adenosis (epithelial changes) of the vagina and cervix.[51-55] Although these changes are histologically benign, it is not known whether this condition is a precursor of malignancy. DES-exposed daughters appear to have an increased risk of unfavorable outcome of pregnancy.[110-112] DES-exposed male children may develop abnormalities of the urogenital tract[56-58,131] and sperm.[131] Although similar data are not available for the use of other estrogens, it cannot be presumed that they would not induce similar changes.

Several reports suggest an association between fetal exposure to female sex hormones, including oral contraceptives, and congenital anomalies,[59-64,94,113-116] including multiple congenital anomalies described by the acronym VACTERL, for vertebral, anal, cardiac, tracheoesophageal, renal, and limb defects.[61,62,113] There appears to be a preferential expression of these defects by exposed male offspring.[63,65,115,121] In one case-control study[63] it was estimated that there was a 4.7-fold increased risk of limb-reduction defects in infants exposed in utero to sex hormones (oral contraceptives, hormonal withdrawal tests for pregnancy, or attempted treatment for threatened abortion). Some of these exposures were very short and involved only a few days of treatment. The data suggest that the risk of limb-reduction defects in exposed fetuses is somewhat less than 1 in 1,000 live births. In a large prospective study,[64] cardiovascular defects in children born to women who received female hormones, including oral contraceptives, during early pregnancy occurred at a rate of 18.2 per 1,000 births, compared to 7.8 per 1,000 for children not so exposed in utero. These results are statistically significant. The incidence of twin births may be increased for women who conceive shortly after discontinuing use of the pill.[14,63,117,118,124]

In the past, female sex hormones have been used during pregnancy in an attempt to treat threatened or habitual abortion. There is considerable evidence that estrogens are ineffective for these indications, and there is no evidence from well-controlled studies that progestogens are effective for these uses.

There is some evidence that triploidy and possibly other types of polyploidy are increased among abortuses from women who become pregnant soon after stopping oral contraceptives.[66] Embryos with these anomalies are virtually always aborted spontaneously. Whether there is an overall increase in spontaneous abortion of pregnancies conceived soon after stopping the oral contraceptives is unknown.

The safety of this product in pregnancy has not been demonstrated. Pregnancy should be ruled out before initiating or continuing the contraceptive regimen. Pregnancy should always be considered if withdrawal bleeding does not occur. It is recommended that for any patient who has missed 2 consecutive periods, pregnancy should be ruled out before continuing the contraceptive regimen. If the patient has not adhered to the prescribed schedule, the possibility of pregnancy should be considered at the time of the first missed period, and further use of oral contraceptives should be withheld until pregnancy has been ruled out. If pregnancy is confirmed, the patient should be apprised of the potential risks to the fetus, and the advisability of continuation of the pregnancy should be discussed in the light of these risks.

It is recommended that women who discontinue oral contraceptives with the intent of becoming pregnant use an alternative form of contraception for a period of time before attempting to conceive. Many clinicians recommend 3 months, although no precise information is available on which to base this recommendation.

The administration of progestogen-only or progestogen-estrogen combinations to induce withdrawal bleeding should not be used as a test of pregnancy.

6. *Gallbladder Disease.* Reports of studies[7,8,12,14,33] indicate an increased risk for surgically confirmed gallbladder disease in users of oral contraceptives or estrogens. In one study,[12] an increased risk appeared after 2 years of use and doubled after 4 or 5 years of use. In one of the other studies[7] an increased risk was apparent between 6 and 12 months of use.

7. *Carbohydrate and Lipid Metabolism.* A decrease in glucose tolerance has been observed in a significant percentage of patients on oral contraceptives. For this reason, prediabetic and diabetic patients should be carefully observed while receiving oral contraceptives. An increase in triglycerides and total phospholipids has been observed in patients receiving oral contraceptives.[67] The clinical significance of this finding remains to be defined.

8. *Elevated Blood Pressure.* An increase in blood pressure has been reported in patients receiving oral contraceptives.[12,69,109] There is evidence that the degree of hypertension may correlate directly with increasing dosage of progestogen.[86] In some women, hypertension may occur within a few months of beginning oral contraceptive use. The prevalence of hypertension in users is low in the first year of use, and may be no higher than that in a comparable group of nonusers. The prevalence in users increases, however, with longer exposure and, in the fifth year of use, is 2½ to 3 times the reported prevalence in the first year. Age is also strongly correlated with the development of hypertension in oral contraceptive users.

Women with a history of elevated blood pressure (hypertension), preexisting renal disease, a history of toxemia or elevated blood pressure during pregnancy, a familial tendency to hypertension or its consequences, or a history of excessive weight gain or fluid retention during the menstrual cycle may be more likely to develop elevation of blood pressure when given oral contraceptives and, therefore, should be monitored closely.[68] Even though elevated blood pressure may remain within the "normal" range, the clinical implications of elevations should not be ignored and close surveillance is indicated, particularly for women with other risk factors for cardiovascular disease or stroke.[69] High blood pressure may or may not persist after discontinuation of the oral contraceptive.

9. *Headache.* The onset or exacerbation of migraine or development of headache of a new pattern which is recurrent, persistent, or severe, requires discontinuation of oral contraceptives and evaluation of the cause.

10. *Bleeding Irregularities.* Breakthrough bleeding, spotting, and amenorrhea are frequent reasons for discontinuance of oral contraceptives. In breakthrough bleeding, as in all cases of irregular vaginal bleeding, nonfunctional causes should be borne in mind. In patients with undiagnosed persistent or recurrent abnormal vaginal bleeding, adequate diagnostic measures are indicated to rule out pregnancy or malignancy. If a pathologic basis has been excluded, passage of time or a change to another formulation may correct the bleeding problem. A change to an oral contraceptive with a higher estrogen content, while potentially useful in minimizing menstrual irregularity, should be made only when considered necessary since this may increase the risk of thromboembolic disease. Women with a past history of oligomenorrhea or secondary amenorrhea or young women who have not established regular cycles may have a tendency to remain anovulatory or to become amenorrheic after discontinuation of oral contraceptives. Women with these preexisting problems should be informed of these possibilities and encouraged to use other contraceptive methods. Post-use anovulation, possibly prolonged, may also occur in women without previous irregularities. A higher incidence of galactorrhea and of pituitary tumors (eg, adenomas) has been associated with amenorrhea in former users compared with nonusers.[87]

One study[70] reported a 16-fold increased prevalence of pituitary prolactin-secreting tumors among patients with postpill amenorrhea when galactorrhea was present.

11. *Ectopic Pregnancy.* Contraceptive failure may result in either ectopic or intrauterine pregnancy. In failures with combination-type oral contraceptives, the ratio of ectopic to intrauterine pregnancies is no higher than in women who are not receiving oral contraceptives.

12. *Breast Feeding.* Oral contraceptives given in the postpartum period may interfere with lactation. There may be a decrease in the quantity and quality of the breast milk. Furthermore, a small fraction of the hormonal agents in oral contraceptives has been identified in the milk of mothers receiving these drugs.[71,88,89] The effects, if any, on the breast-fed child have not been determined. If feasible, the use of oral contraceptives should be deferred until the infant has been weaned.

13. *Infertility.* There is evidence of fertility impairment in women discontinuing oral contraceptives in comparison with those discontinuing other methods.[14,90,132] The impairment appears to be independent of the duration of use. While the impairment diminishes with time, there is still an appreciable difference in the results in nulliparous women 30 months after discontinuation of birth control; the difference is negligible after 42 months. For parous women the difference is no longer apparent 30 months after cessation of contraception.

Precautions:
General. 1. A complete medical and family history should be taken and a thorough physical examination should be performed prior to the initiation of oral contraceptives. The pretreatment and periodic physical examinations should include special reference to blood pressure, breasts, abdomen, and pelvic organs, including a Pap smear and relevant laboratory tests. As a general rule, oral contraceptives should not be prescribed for longer than one year without the performance of another physical examination (see *Warnings*).

2. Preexisting uterine leiomyomata may increase in size during oral contraceptive use.

3. Oral contraceptives appear to be associated with an increased incidence of mental depression. Therefore, patients with a history of depression should be carefully observed and the drug discontinued if depression recurs to a serious degree. Patients becoming significantly depressed while taking oral contraceptives should stop the medication and use an alternative method of contraception in an attempt to determine whether the symptom is drug related.

4. Oral contraceptives may cause some degree of fluid retention. They should be prescribed with caution, and only with careful monitoring, in patients with conditions which might be aggravated by fluid retention, such as convulsive disorders, migraine syndrome, asthma, or cardiac, hepatic, or renal dysfunction.

5. Patients with a past history of jaundice during pregnancy have an increased risk of recurrence of jaundice and should be carefully observed while receiving oral contraceptives. If jaundice develops in any patient receiving such drugs, the medication should be discontinued while the cause is investigated. Cholestatic jaundice has been reported after combined treatment with oral contraceptives and troleandomycin.

6. Steroid hormones may be poorly metabolized in patients with impaired liver function and should be administered with caution in such patients.

7. Oral contraceptive users may have disturbances in normal tryptophan metabolism, which may result in a relative pyridoxine deficiency. The clinical significance of this is unknown, although megaloblastic anemia has been reported.

8. Serum folate levels may be depressed by oral contraceptive therapy. Since the pregnant woman is predisposed to folate deficiency and the incidence of folate deficiency increases with lengthening gestation, it is possible that if a woman becomes pregnant shortly after stopping oral contraceptives, she may have a greater chance of developing folate deficiency and complications attributable to this deficiency.

9. The pathologist should be advised of oral contraceptive therapy when relevant specimens are submitted.

10. Certain endocrine and liver function tests may be affected by estrogen-containing oral contraceptives. Therefore, it is recommended that any abnormal tests be repeated after the drug has been withdrawn for two months. The following alterations in laboratory results have been observed with the use of oral contraceptives:

a. Hepatic function: Increased sulfobromophthalein retention and other abnormalities in tests of liver function.

b. Coagulation tests: Increased prothrombin and coagulation factors VII, VIII, IX, and X; decreased antithrombin III; increased platelet aggregability.

c. Thyroid function: Increased thyroid-binding globulin (TBG) leading to increased circulating total thyroid hormone, as measured by protein-bound iodine (PBI) or T^4 by column or radioimmunoassay. Free T^3 resin uptake is decreased, reflecting the elevated TBG; free T^4 concentration is unaltered.

d. Decreased pregnanediol excretion.

e. Reduced response to metyrapone test.

f. Increased blood transcortin and corticosteroid levels.

g. Increased blood triglyceride and phospholipid concentrations.

h. Reduced serum folate concentration.

i. Impaired glucose tolerance.

j. Altered plasma levels of trace minerals (eg, increased ceruloplasmin).

11. The influence of prolonged oral contraceptive therapy on pituitary, ovarian, adrenal, hepatic, or uterine function, or on the immune response, has not been established.

12. Treatment with oral contraceptives may mask the onset of the climacteric. (See *Warnings* section regarding risks in this age group.)

Information for the Patient. See patient labeling printed at end.

Drug Interactions. Oral contraceptives may be rendered less effective and increased incidence of breakthrough bleeding may occur by virtue of drug interaction with rifampin, isoniazid, ampicillin, neomycin, penicillin V, tetracycline, chloramphenicol, sulfonamides, nitrofurantoin, griseofulvin, barbiturates, phenytoin, primidone, phenylbutazone, analgesics, tranquilizers, and antimigraine preparations.[72-74,95,125] Oral contraceptives may alter the effectiveness of other types of drugs, such as oral anticoagulants, anticonvulsants, tranquilizers (eg, diazepam), tricyclic antidepressants, antihypertensive agents (eg, guanethidine), theophylline, vitamins, hypoglycemic agents, clofibrate, glucocorticoids, and acetaminophen.[72,119,134,139] (See *Precaution* No. 5).

Carcinogenesis. See *Warnings* No. 3 and 4 for information on the carcinogenic potential of oral contraceptives.

Pregnancy. Pregnancy category X. See *Contraindication* No. 7 and *Warning* No. 5.

Nursing Mothers. See *Warning* No. 12.

Adverse Reactions: An increased risk of the following serious adverse reactions has been associated with the use of oral contraceptives (see *Warnings*):

Thrombophlebitis and thrombosis
Pulmonary embolism
Arterial thromboembolism
Raynaud's disease
Myocardial infarction and coronary thrombosis
Cerebral thrombosis
Cerebral hemorrhage
Hypertension
Gallbladder disease
Benign adenomas and other hepatic lesions, with or without intra-abdominal bleeding
Congenital anomalies

There is evidence of an association between the following conditions and the use of oral contraceptives, although confirmatory studies have not been done:

Mesenteric thrombosis
Budd-Chiari syndrome
Neuro-ocular lesions, (eg, retinal thrombosis and optic neuritis)

The following adverse reactions have been reported in patients receiving oral contraceptives and are believed to be drug related:

Nausea and vomiting (Usually the most common adverse reactions, occurring in approximately 10% or fewer patients during the first cycle. Other reactions, as a general rule, are seen much less frequently or only occasionally.)
Gastrointestinal symptoms (eg, abdominal cramps and bloating)
Breakthrough bleeding
Spotting
Change in menstrual flow
Dysmenorrhea
Amenorrhea during and after use
Infertility after discontinuation
Edema
Chloasma or melasma, which may persist when the drug is discontinued
Breast changes: tenderness, enlargement, and secretion
Change in weight (increase or decrease)
Change in cervical erosion and secretion
Endocervical hyperplasia
Possible diminution in lactation when given immediately post partum
Cholestatic jaundice
Migraine
Increase in size of uterine leiomyomata
Rash (allergic)
Mental depression
Reduced tolerance to carbohydrates
Vaginal candidiasis
Change in corneal curvature (steepening)
Intolerance to contact lenses

The following adverse reactions or conditions have been reported in users of oral contraceptives, and the association has been neither confirmed nor refuted:

Premenstrual-like syndrome
Cataracts
Changes in libido
Chorea
Changes in appetite
Cystitis-like syndrome
Headache
Paresthesia
Nervousness
Dizziness
Auditory disturbances
Rhinitis
Fatigue
Backache
Hirsutism
Loss of scalp hair
Erythema multiforme
Erythema nodosum
Hemorrhagic eruption
Hemolytic uremic syndrome
Malignant hypertension
Itching
Vaginitis
Porphyria
Impaired renal function
Acute renal failure, sometimes irreversible
Anemia
Pancreatitis
Hepatitis
Colitis
Gingivitis
Dry socket
Lupus erythematosus
Rheumatoid arthritis
Pituitary tumors (eg, adenoma) with amenorrhea and/or galactorrhea after OC use
Malignant melanoma
Endometrial, cervical, and breast carcinoma (see *Warning* No. 3)

Acute Overdosage: Serious ill effects have not been reported following the acute ingestion of large doses of oral contraceptives by young chil-

Continued on next page

Searle & Co.—Cont.

dren.[75,76] Overdosage may cause nausea, and withdrawal bleeding might occur in females.

Dosage and Administration:

Contraception: Demulen 1/35™-21, Demulen 1/35™-28, Demulen 1/50™-21, Demulen 1/50™-28, Ovulen-21, Ovulen-28, Enovid-E 21, and Enovid 5 mg.

To achieve maximum contraceptive effectiveness, oral contraceptives must be taken exactly as directed and at intervals of 24 hours.

IMPORTANT: The patient should be instructed to use an additional method of protection until after the first week of administration *in the initial cycle.* The possibility of ovulation and conception prior to initiation of use should be considered.

Enovid 5 mg 20-Tablet Dosage Schedule: The patient should take one tablet daily for twenty consecutive days beginning each 20-tablet course on day 5 of her menstrual cycle or eight days after taking the last pill from the previous cycle, whichever occurs first. The first day of menstruation is counted as day 1.

Demulen 1/35™-21, Demulen 1/35™-28, Demulen 1/50™-21, Demulen 1/50™-28, Ovulen-21, Ovulen-28, and Enovid-E 21 Dosage Schedules: The Demulen 1/35™-21, Demulen 1/50™-21, Ovulen-21, and Enovid-E 21 Compack® tablet dispensers contain 21 tablets arranged in three numbered rows of 7 tablets each. The Demulen 1/35™-28, Demulen 1/50™-28, and Ovulen-28 tablet dispensers contain 21 white active tablets arranged in three numbered rows of 7 tablets each, followed by a fourth row of 7 pink (blue for Demulen 1/35™-28) placebo tablets.

Days of the week are printed above the tablets, starting with Sunday on the left.

Two dosage schedules are described, one of which may be more convenient or suitable than the other for an individual patient.

Schedule #1: Sunday Start: The patient begins taking Demulen 1/35™-21, Demulen 1/35™-28, Demulen 1/50™-21, Demulen 1/50™-28, Ovulen-21, Ovulen-28, or Enovid-E 21, from the first row of her package, one tablet daily, starting on the first Sunday after the onset of menstruation. If the patient's period begins on a Sunday she takes her first tablet that very same day. The 21st tablet or the 28th tablet, depending on whether the patient is taking the 21- or 28-tablet course, will then be taken on a Saturday.

Subsequent Cycles:

21-tablet course—The patient begins a new 21-tablet course on the eighth day, Sunday, after taking her last tablet. All subsequent cycles will also begin on Sunday, one tablet being taken each day for three weeks followed by a week of no pill-taking.

28-tablet course—The patient begins a new 28-tablet course on the next day, Sunday, and all subsequent cycles will also begin on Sunday, one tablet being taken each and every day.

With a Sunday-start schedule, a woman whose period begins on the day of or one to four days before taking the first tablet should expect a diminution of flow and fewer menstrual days. The initial cycle will likely be shortened by from one to five days. Thereafter, cycles should be about 28 days in length.

Schedule #2: Day 5 Start: The patient begins taking Demulen 1/35™-21, Demulen 1/50™-21, Ovulen-21, or Enovid-E 21 from the first row of her package, one tablet daily, starting with the pill day which corresponds to day 5 of her menstrual cycle; the first day of menstruation is counted as day 1. After the last (Saturday) tablet in row #3 has been taken, if any remain in the first row, the patient completes her 21-tablet schedule starting with Sunday in row #1.

Subsequent Cycles: The patient begins a new 21-tablet course on the eighth day after taking her last tablet, again starting the same day of the week on which she began her first course. All subsequent cycles will also begin on that same day, one tablet being taken each day for three weeks followed by a week of no pill-taking.

Postpartum Administration. Ovulen-21 and Ovulen-28 oral contraceptives may be prescribed at the first postpartum examination regardless of whether or not the patient has experienced spontaneous menstruation. In non-nursing mothers, administration may be initiated immediately after delivery if desired or on the first Sunday after delivery. If preferred the tablets may be started on the day the patient leaves the hospital. (For nursing mothers, see *Warning* No. 12.)

Hypermenorrhea; Production of Cyclic Withdrawal Bleeding: Enovid 5 mg or 10 mg only. Most patients with hypermenorrhea may be expected to respond to Enovid 5-mg or 10-mg therapy within 24 to 48 hours. Regular withdrawal bleeding may then be induced by cyclic administration. Vaginal bleeding at times other than the regular menstrual period requires that a diagnosis be established prior to beginning therapy.

For emergency control of severe bleeding in patients with hypermenorrhea give 20 to 30 mg of Enovid daily until the bleeding is controlled, then reduce the daily dose to 10 mg and continue through day 24 of the cycle. Then discontinue Enovid and withdrawal flow usually will begin approximately two to three days later.

Cyclic withdrawal bleeding may be produced after treatment in this initial cycle by giving the patient 5 to 10 mg of Enovid 5 mg or 10 mg daily from day 5 through day 24 of the next two or three cycles. A new course of Enovid therapy should be started on day 5 of her menstrual cycle or eight days after the last pill from the previous cycle, whichever occurs first. The first day of menstruation is counted as day 1.

Endometriosis: Enovid 5 mg or 10 mg only. A daily dose of Enovid should be given for six to nine months or longer on the following schedule: 5 or 10 mg should be given for two weeks beginning on day 5 of a menstrual cycle. This daily dose should be given continuously (without cyclic interruption) and increased 5 or 10 mg at two-week intervals until the patient is receiving 20 mg daily. This dose of 20 mg should be continued for six to nine months and further increased (up to 40 mg daily) if breakthrough bleeding occurs.

Therapy may be discontinued after six months if the disease is mild and the lesions are no longer palpable. If the disorder is more severe continue treatment for nine months or longer.

When surgery is contemplated, prior administration of Enovid may facilitate the surgical procedure. (See *Warning* No. 1 concerning discontinuation prior to elective surgery.)

Special Notes: *Spotting or Breakthrough Bleeding.* If spotting (bleeding insufficient to require a pad) or breakthrough bleeding (heavier bleeding similar to a menstrual flow) occurs when these products are used for contraception the patient should continue taking her tablets as directed. The incidence of spotting or breakthrough bleeding is minimal, most frequently occurring in the first cycle. Ordinarily spotting or breakthrough bleeding will stop within a week. Usually the patient will begin to cycle regularly within two or three courses of tablet-taking. If breakthrough bleeding occurs while the patient is taking Enovid for hypermenorrhea she should immediately increase the daily dosage by 5 or 10 mg until bleeding has been controlled for three days, after which the original dosage usually may be resumed. In the event of spotting or breakthrough bleeding organic causes should be borne in mind. (See *Warning* No. 10.)

Missed Menstrual Periods. Withdrawal flow will normally occur two or three days after the last active tablet is taken. Failure of withdrawal bleeding ordinarily does not mean that the patient is pregnant, providing the dosage schedule has been correctly followed. (See *Warning* No. 5.)

If the patient has *not* adhered to the prescribed dosage regimen, the possibility of pregnancy should be considered after the first missed period, and oral contraceptives should be withheld until pregnancy has been ruled out.

If the patient has adhered to the prescribed regimen and misses two consecutive periods, pregnancy should be ruled out before continuing the contraceptive regimen.

The first intermenstrual interval after discontinuing the tablets is usually prolonged; consequently, a patient for whom a 28-day cycle is usual might not begin to menstruate for 35 days or longer. Ovulation in such prolonged cycles will occur correspondingly later in the cycle. Posttreatment cycles after the first one, however, are usually typical for the individual woman prior to taking tablets. (See *Warnings* No. 10 and 11.)

Missed Tablets (Contraception). If a woman misses taking one active tablet the missed tablet should be taken as soon as it is remembered. In addition, the next tablet should be taken at the usual time. If two consecutive active tablets are missed the dosage should be doubled for the next two days. The regular schedule should then be resumed, but an additional method of protection is recommended for the remainder of the cycle.

While there is little likelihood of ovulation if only one active tablet is missed, the possibility of spotting or breakthrough bleeding is increased and should be expected if two or more successive active tablets are missed. However, the possibility of ovulation increases with each successive day that scheduled active tablets are missed.

If one or more placebo tablets of Demulen 1/35™-28, Demulen 1/50™-28, or Ovulen-28 are missed, the Demulen 1/35™-28, Demulen 1/50™-28, or Ovulen-28 schedule should be resumed on the following Sunday (the eighth day after the last white tablet was taken). Omission of placebo tablets in the 28-tablet courses does not increase the possibility of conception provided that this schedule is followed.

How Supplied:

Demulen 1/35: Each white Demulen 1/35 tablet is round in shape, with a debossed SEARLE on one side and 151 and design on the other side, and contains 1 mg of ethynodiol diacetate and 35 mcg of ethinyl estradiol.

Demulen 1/35™-21 is packaged in cartons of 6 and 24 Compack tablet dispensers of 21 tablets each, and in cartons of 12 Compack refills of 21 tablets each.

Demulen 1/35™-28 is packaged in cartons of 6 and 24 Compack tablet dispensers and in cartons of 12 Compack refills. Each Compack and refill contains 21 white Demulen 1/35 tablets and 7 blue placebo tablets. (Placebo tablets have a debossed SEARLE on one side and a "P" on the other side.)

Demulen: 1/50: Each white Demulen 1/50 tablet is round in shape, with a debossed SEARLE on one side and 71 on the other side, and contains 1 mg of ethynodiol diacetate and 50 mcg of ethinyl estradiol.

Demulen 1/50™-21 is packaged in cartons of 6 and 24 Compack tablet dispensers of 21 tablets each, and in cartons of 12 Compack refills of 21 tablets each.

Demulen 1/50™-28 is packaged in cartons of 6 and 24 Compack tablet dispensers and in cartons of 12 Compack refills. Each Compack and refill contains 21 white Demulen 1/50 tablets and 7 pink placebo tablets. (Placebo tablets have a debossed SEARLE on one side and a "P" on the other side.)

Ovulen: Each white Ovulen tablet is pentagonal in shape, with a debossed SEARLE on one side and 401 on the other side, and contains 1 mg of ethynodiol diacetate and 0.1 mg of mestranol.

Ovulen-21 is packaged in cartons of 6 and 24 Compack tablet dispensers of 21 tablets each, and in cartons of 12 Compack refills of 21 tablets each.

Ovulen-28 is packaged in cartons of 6 Compack tablet dispensers and in cartons of 12 Compack refills. Each Compack and refill contains 21 white Ovulen tablets and 7 pink placebo tablets. (Placebo tablets have a debossed SEARLE on one side and a "P" on the other side.)

Enovid-E: Each Enovid-E tablet is pale pink, round in shape, with a debossed SEARLE E on one side and 131 on the other side, and contains 2.5 mg of norethynodrel and 0.1 mg of mestranol.

Enovid-E 21 is packaged in cartons of 6 Compack tablet dispensers of 21 tablets each, and in cartons of 12 Compack refills of 21 tablets each.

Enovid 5 mg: Each Enovid 5 mg tablet is pink, round in shape, with a debossed SEARLE 5 on one side and 51 on the other side, and contains 5 mg of norethynodrel and 75 mcg of mestranol. Enovid 5 mg is packaged in bottles of 100 tablets each.

Enovid 10 mg: Each Enovid 10 mg tablet is coral colored, round in shape, with a debossed SEARLE 10 on one side and 101 on the other side, and contains 9.85 mg of norethynodrel and 0.15 mg of mestranol. Enovid 10 mg is packaged in bottles of 50 tablets each.

References:

1. Population Reports, Series H, No. 2 (May) 1974; Series I, No. 1 (June) 1974; Series B, No. 3 (May) 1979; Series H, No. 3 (Jan.) 1975; Series H, No. 4 (Jan.) 1976; Population Information Program, Geo. Washington U. Medical Center, Washington, D.C. **2.** Inman, W. H. W., et al.: Br. Med. J. *2*:203 (April 25) 1970. **3.** Inman, W. H. W., et al.: Br. Med. J. *2*:193 (April 27) 1968. **4.** Royal College of General Practitioners: J. Coll. Gen. Pract. *13*:267 (May) 1967. **5.** Vessey, M. P., et al.: Br. Med. J. *2*:651 (June 14) 1969. **6.** Sartwell, P. E., et al.: Am. J. Epidemiol. *90*:365 (Nov.) 1969. **7.** Boston Collaborative Drug Surveillance Programme: Lancct *1*:1399 (June 23) 1973. **8.** Stolley, P.D., et al.: Am. J. Epidemiol. *102*:197 (Sept.) 1975. **9.** Collaborative Group for the Study of Stroke in Young Women: N. Engl. J. Med. *288*:871 (April 26) 1973.

10. Collaborative Group for the Study of Stroke in Young Women: J.A.M.A. *231*:718 (Feb. 17) 1975. **11.** Beral, V.: Lancet *2*:1047 (Nov. 13) 1976. **12.** Royal College of General Practitioners: Oral Contraceptives and Health, New York, Pitman Publ. Corp., May 1974. **13.** Layde, P., et al.: Lancet *1*:541 (March 7) 1981. **13a.** Beral, V., et al.: Lancet *2*:727 (Oct. 8) 1977. **14.** Vessey, M., et al.: J. Biosoc. Sci. *8*:373 (Oct.) 1976. **15.** Vessey, M., et al.: Lancet *2*:731 (Oct. 8) 1977; *1*:549 (March 7) 1981. **16.** Mann, J. I., et al.: Br. Med. J. *2*:241 (May 3) 1975. **17.** Mann, J. I., et al.: Br. Med. J. *3*:631 (Sept. 13) 1975. **18.** Mann, J. I., et al.: Br. Med. J. *2*:245 (May 3) 1975. **19.** Mann, J. I., et al.: Br. Med. J. *2*:445 (Aug. 21) 1976.

20. Jain, A. K.: Stud. Fam. Plann. *8*:50 (March) 1977. **21.** Tietze, C.: Fam. Plann. Perspect. *9*:74 (March-April) 1977. **22.** Vessey, M. P., et al.: Br. Med. J. *3*:123 (July 18) 1970. **23.** Greene, G. R., et al.: Am. J. Public Health *62*:680 (May) 1972. **24.** Ziel, H. K., et al.: N. Engl. J. Med. *293*:1167 (Dec. 4) 1975. **25.** Smith, D. C., et al.: N. Engl. J. Med. *293*:1164 (Dec. 4) 1975. **26.** Mack, T. M., et al.: N. Engl. J. Med. *294*:1262 (June 3) 1976. **27.** Gray, L. A., et al.: Obstet. Gynecol. *49*:385 (April) 1977. **28.** McDonald, T. W., et al.: Am. J. Obstet. Gynecol. *127*:572 (March 15) 1977. **29.** Weiss, N. S., et al.: N. Engl. J. Med. *294*:1259 (June 3) 1976.

30. Silverberg, S. G., et al.: Cancer *39*:592 (Feb.) 1977. **31.** Vessey, M. P., et al.: Br. Med. J. *3*:719 (Sept. 23) 1972. **32.** Vessey, M. P., et al.: Lancet *1*:941 (April 26) 1975. **33.** Boston Collaborative Drug Surveillance Program: N. Engl. J. Med. *290*:15 (Jan. 3) 1974. **34.** Arthes, F. G., et al.: Cancer *28*:1391 (Dec.) 1971. **35.** Casagrande, J., et al.: J. Natl. Cancer Inst. *56*:839 (April) 1976. **36.** Fasal, E., et al.: J. Natl. Cancer Inst. *55*:767 (Oct.) 1975. **37.** Paffenbarger, R. S., et al.: Cancer *49*:1887 (April Suppl.) 1977. **38.** Hoover, R., et al.: N. Engl. J. Med. *295*:401 (Aug. 19) 1976. **39.** Kelsey, J. L., et al.: Am. J. Epidemiol. *107*:236 (March) 1978.

40. Ory, H., et al.: N. Engl. J. Med. *294*:419 (Feb. 19) 1976. **41.** Stern, E., et al.: Science *196*:1460 (June 24) 1977. **42.** Population Reports, Series A, No. 4 (May) 1977: Population Information Program, Geo. Washington U. Medical Center, Washington, D.C. **43.** Baum, J. K., et al.: Lancet *2*:926 (Oct. 27) 1973. **44.** Mays, E. T., et al.: J.A.M.A. *235*:730 (Feb. 16) 1976. **45.** Edmondson, H. A., et al.: N. Engl. J. Med. *294*:470 (Feb. 26) 1976. **46.** Rooks, J. B., et al.: J.A.M.A. *242*:644 (Aug. 17) 1979. **47.** Herbst, A. L., et al.: N. Engl. J. Med. *284*:878 (April 22) 1971. **48.** Greenwald, P., et al.: N. Engl. J. Med. *285*:390 (Aug. 12) 1971. **49.** Lanier, A. P., et al.: Mayo Clin. Proc. *48*:793 (Nov.) 1973.

50. Herbst, A. L., et al.: Am. J. Obstet. Gynecol. *128*:43 (May 1) 1977. **51.** Herbst, A. L., et al.: Obstet. Gynecol. *40*:287 (Sept.) 1972. **52.** Herbst, A. L., et al.: Am. J. Obstet. Gynecol. *118*:607 (March 1) 1974. **53.** Herbst, A. L., et al.: N. Engl. J. Med. *292*:334 (Feb. 13) 1975. **54.** Stafl, A., et al.: Obstet. Gynecol. *43*:118 (Jan.) 1974. **55.** Sherman, A. I., et al.: Obstet. Gynecol. *44*:531 (Oct.) 1974. **56.** Bibbo, M., et al.: J. Reprod. Med. *15*:29 (July) 1975. **57.** Gill, W., et al.: J. Reprod. Med. *16*:147 (April) 1976. **58.** Henderson, B., et al.: Pediatrics *58*:505 (Oct.) 1976. **59.** Gal, I., et al.: Nature *240*:241 (Nov. 24) 1972.

60. Levy, E. P., et al.: Lancet *1*:611 (March 17) 1973. **61.** Nora, J. J., et al.: Lancet *1*:941 (April 28) 1973. **62.** Nora, A. H., et al.: Arch. Environ. Health *30*:17 (Jan.) 1975; Adv. Plann. Parent. *12*:156, 1978. **63.** Janerich, D. T., et al.: N. Engl. J. Med. *291*:697 (Oct. 3) 1974. **64.** Heinonen, O. P., et al.: N. Engl. J. Med. *296*:67 (Jan. 13) 1977. **65.** Nora, J. J., et al.: N. Engl. J. Med. *291*:731 (Oct. 3) 1974. **66.** Carr, D. H.: Can. Med. Assoc. J. *103*:343 (Aug. 15 & 29) 1970. **67.** Wynn, V., et al.: Lancet *2*:720 (Oct. 1) 1966. **68.** Laragh, J. H.: Am. J. Obstet. Gynecol. *126*:141 (Sept.) 1976. **69.** Fisch, I. R., et al.: J.A.M.A. *237*:2499 (June 6) 1977.

70. Van Campenhout, J., et al.: Fertil. Steril. *28*:728 (July) 1977. **71.** Laumas, K. R., et al.: Am. J. Obstet. Gynecol. *98*:411 (June 1) 1967. **72.** Stockley, I.: Pharmaceut. J. *216*:140 (Feb. 14) 1976. **73.** Hempel, E., et al.: Drugs *12*:442 (Dec.) 1976. **74.** Bessot, J.-C., et al.: Nouv. Presse Med. *6*:1568 (April 30) 1977. **75.** Francis, W. G., et al.: Can. Med. Assoc. J. *92*:191 (Jan. 23) 1965. **76.** Verhulst, H. L., et al.: J. Clin. Pharmacol. *7*:9 (Jan.-Feb.) 1967. **77.** Vessey, M. P., et al.: Br. Med. J. *2*:199 (April 27) 1968. **78.** Ory, H. W.: J.A.M.A. *237*:2619 (June 13) 1977. **79.** Jain, A. K.: Am. J. Obstet. Gynecol. *126*:301 (Oct. 1) 1976.

80. Ziel, H. K., et al.: Am. J. Obstet. Gynecol. *124*:735 (April 1) 1976. **81.** Peritz, E., et al.: Am. J. Epidemiol. *106*:462 (Dec.) 1977. **82.** Ory, H. W., et al.: in Garattini, S., and Berendes, H. (eds.), Pharmacology of Steroid Contraceptive Drugs, Raven Press, N.Y., 1977. **83.** Goldacre, M. J., et al.: Br. Med. J. *1*:748 (March 25) 1978. **84.** Meisels, A., et al.: Cancer *40*:3076 (Dec.) 1977. **85.** Klatskin, G.: Gastroenterology *73*:386 (Aug.) 1977. **86.** Kay, C. R.: Lancet *1*:624 (March 19) 1977. **87.** March, C. M., et al.: Fertil. Steril. *28*:346 (March) 1977. **88.** Saxena, B. N., et al.: Contraception *16*:605 (Dec.) 1977. **89.** Nilsson, S., et al.: Contraception *17*:131 (Feb.) 1978.

90. Vessey, M. P., et al.: Br. Med. J. *1*:265 (Feb. 4) 1978. **91.** Jick, H., et al.: J.A.M.A. *239*:1403, 1407 (April 3) 1978. **92.** Kay, C. R.: J. R. Coll. Gen. Pract. *28*:393 (July) 1978. **93.** Hoogerland, D. L., et al.: Gynecol. Oncol. *6*:451 (Oct.) 1978. **94.** Lorber, C. A., et al.: Fertil. Steril. *31*:21 (Jan.) 1979. **95.** Bacon, J. F., et al.: Br. Med. J. *280*:293 (Feb. 2) 1980. **96.** Meade, T. W., et al.: Br. Med. J. *280*:1157 (May 10) 1980. **97.** Böttiger, L. E., et al.: Lancet *1*:1097 (May 24) 1980. **98.** Maguire, M. G., et al.: Am. J. Epidemiol. *110*:188 (Aug.) 1979. **99.** Ramcharan, S., et al.: The Walnut Creek Contraceptive Drug Study, Vol. 3, U.S. Govt. Ptg. Off., 1981; J. Reprod. Med. *25*:346 (Dec.) 1980.

100. Petitti, D. B., et al.: Am. J. Epidemiol. *108*:480 (Dec.) 1978. **101.** Petitti, D. B., et al.: J.A.M.A. *242*:1150 (Sept. 14) 1979. **102.** Petitti, D. B., et al.: Lancet *2*:234 (July 29) 1978. **103.** Jick, H., et al.: Ann. Int. Med. *88*:58 (July) 1978. **104.** Jick, H., et al.: J.A.M.A. *240*:2548 (Dec. 1) 1978. **105.** Shapiro, S., et al.: Lancet *1*:743 (April 7) 1979. **106.** Rosenberg, L., et al.: Am. J. Epidemiol. *111*:59 (Jan.) 1980. **107.** Kreuger, D. E., et al.: Am. J. Epidemiol. *111*:655 (June) 1980. **108.** Arthes, F. G., et al.: Chest *70*:574 (Nov.) 1976. **109.** Hoover, R., et al.: Am. J. Public Health *18*:335 (April) 1978.

110. Herbst, A. L., et al.: J. Reprod. Med. *24*:62 (Feb.) 1980. **111.** Barnes, A. B., et al.: N. Engl. J. Med. *302*:609 (March 13) 1980. **112:** Cousins, L., et al.: Obstet. Gynecol. *56*:70 (July) 1980. **113.** Nora, J. J., et al.: J.A.M.A. *240*:837 (Sept. 1) 1978. **114.** Aarskog, D.: N. Engl. J. Med. *300*:75 (Jan. 11) 1979. **115.** Janerich, D. T., et al.: Am. J. Epidemiol. *112*:73 (July) 1980. **116.** Kasan, P. N., et al.: Br. J. Obstet. Gynaecol. *87*:545 (July) 1980. **117.** Rothman, K. J.: N. Engl. J. Med. *297*:468 (Sept. 1) 1977. **118.** Bracken, M. B.: Am. J. Obstet. Gynecol. *133*:432 (Feb. 15) 1979. **119.** De Teresa, E., et al.: Br. Med. J. *2*:1260 (Nov. 17) 1979.

120. Swan, S., et al.: Am. J. Obstet. Gynecol. *139*:52 (Jan. 1) 1981. **121.** Kay, C. R.: Br. Med. J. *282*:2089 (June 27) 1981. **122.** Vessey, M. P., et al.: Br. Med. J. *282*:2093 (June 27) 1981. **123.** Pike, M. C., et al.: Br. J. Cancer *43*:72 (Jan.) 1981. **124.** Harlap, S., et al.: Obstet. Gynecol. *55*:447 (April) 1980. **125.** Back, D. J., et al.: Drugs *21*:46 (Jan.) 1981. **126.** Porter, J. B., et al.: Obstet. Gynecol. *59*:229 (March) 1982. **127.** Lees, A.W., et al.: Int. J. Cancer *22*:700, 1978. **128.** Brinton, L. A., et al.: J. Natl. Cancer Inst. (JNCI) *62*:37 (Jan.) 1979. **129.** Black, M. M.: Pathol. Res. Pract. *166*:491. 1980; Cancer *46*:2747 (Dec.) 1980; Cancer *51*: 2147 (June 1) 1983.

130. Hoover, R., et al.; JNCI *67*:815 (Oct.) 1981. **131.** Gill, W. B., et al.: J. Urol. *122*:36 (July) 1979. **132.** Linn, S., et al.: J.A.M.A. *247*:629 (Feb. 5) 1982. **133.** Clavel, F., et al.: Bull. Cancer (Paris) *68*:449 (Dec.) 1981. **134.** Abernethy, D. R., et al.: N. Engl. J. Med. *306*:791 (April 1) 1982. **135.** Kay, C. R.: Am. J. Obstet. Gynecol. *142*:762 (March 15) 1982. **136.** Adam, S. A., et al.: Br. J. Obstet. Gynaecol. *88*:838 (Aug.) 1981. **137.** Slone, D., et al.: N. Engl. J. Med. *305*:420 (Aug. 20) 1981. **138.** Layde, P.M., et al.: J.R. Coll. Gen. Pract. *33*:75 (Feb.) 1983. **139.** Abernethy, D. R., et al.: Obstet. Gynecol. *60*:338 (Sept.) 1982.

140. Brinton, L.A., et al.: Int. J. Epidemiol. *11*:316, 1982. **141.** Harris, N.V., et al.: Am. J. Epidemiol. *116*:643 (Oct.) 1982. **142.** Pike, M.C., et al.: Lancet *2*:926 (Oct. 22) 1983. **143.** Vessey, M.P., et al.: Lancet *2*:930 (Oct. 22) 1983. **144.** Jick, H., et al.: Am. J. Epidemiol. *112*:577 (Nov.) 1980. **145.** Jick, H., et al.: Am. J. Epidemiol. *112*:586 (Nov.) 1980. **146.** McPherson, K., et al.: Lancet *2*:1414 (Dec. 17) 1983. **147.** Vessey, M.P., et al.: Br. Med. J. *289*:530 (Sept. 1) 1984.

Brief Summary of Patient Labeling

Cigarette-smoking increases the risk of serious adverse effects on the heart and blood vessels from oral contraceptive use. This risk increases with age and with heavy smoking (15 or more cigarettes per day) and is quite marked in women over 35 years of age. Women who use oral contraceptives should not smoke.

In the detailed leaflet, "What You Should Know About Oral Contraceptives," which you have received, the risks and benefits of oral contraceptives are discussed in much more detail. This leaflet also provides information on other forms of contraception. Please take time to read it carefully for it may have been recently revised.

If you have any questions or problems regarding this information, contact your doctor.

Oral contraceptives taken as directed are about 99% effective in preventing pregnancy. (The minipill, however, is somewhat less effective.) Forgetting to take your pills increases the chance of pregnancy.

Women who have or have had clotting disorders, cancer of the breast or sex organs, unexplained vaginal bleeding, stroke, heart attack, chest pains on exertion (angina pectoris), liver tumors associated with the use of the pill or with other estrogen-containing products, or who suspect they may be pregnant should not use oral contraceptives.

Most side effects of the pill are not serious. The most common side effects are nausea, vomiting, bleeding between menstrual periods, weight gain, and breast tenderness. However, proper use of oral contraceptives requires that they be taken under your doctor's continuing supervision, because they can be associated with serious side effects which may be fatal. Fortunately, these are very uncommon, but the risks may persist after use of the pill is discontinued. The serious side effects are:

Continued on next page

Searle & Co.—Cont.

1. Blood clots in the legs, arms, lungs, brain, heart, eyes, abdomen, or elsewhere in the body.
2. Bleeding in the brain (hemorrhage) as a result of bursting of a blood vessel.
3. Disorders of vision.
4. Liver tumors, which may rupture and cause severe bleeding.
5. Birth defects if the pill is taken during pregnancy.
6. High blood pressure.
7. Gallbladder disease.

The symptoms associated with these serious side effects are discussed in the detailed leaflet given you with your supply of pills. Notify your doctor if you notice any unusual physical disturbance while taking the pill.

Breast cancer and other cancers have developed in certain animals when given the estrogens in oral contraceptives for long periods. These findings suggest that oral contraceptives may also cause cancer in humans. However, studies to date in women taking currently marketed oral contraceptives have not confirmed that oral contraceptives cause cancer in humans.

Caution: Oral contraceptives are of no value in the prevention or treatment of venereal disease.

Various drugs, such as antibiotics, may also decrease the effectiveness of oral contraceptives.

Detailed Patient Labeling: What You Should Know About Oral Contraceptives

Oral contraceptives (the pill) are the most effective way (except for sterilization) to prevent pregnancy if you follow the directions for their use and are careful not to skip doses or take them irregularly. They are also convenient and, for most women, free of serious or unpleasant side effects. Oral contraceptives must always be taken under the continuing supervision of a doctor.

It is important that any woman who considers using an oral contraceptive understands the risks involved. Although the oral contraceptives have important advantages over other methods of contraception, they have certain risks that no other method has. Only you can decide whether the advantages are worth these risks. This leaflet will tell you about the most important risks. It will explain how you can help your doctor prescribe the pill as safely as possible by telling him/her about yourself and being alert for the earliest signs of trouble. And it will tell you how to use the pill properly, so that it will be as effective as possible.

THERE IS MORE DETAILED INFORMATION AVAILABLE IN THE LEAFLET PREPARED FOR DOCTORS. Your pharmacist can show you a copy; you may need your doctor's help in understanding parts of it.

Enovid 5 mg or 10 mg can be prescribed as a treatment for endometriosis and as a treatment for hypermenorrhea and regulating periods. If you are taking Enovid 5 mg or 10 mg for one of these other conditions besides contraception the warning information in this detailed leaflet also applies, so please read this leaflet.

Caution: Oral contraceptives are of no value in the prevention or treatment of venereal disease.

> Cigarette-smoking increases the risk of serious adverse effects on the heart and blood vessels from oral contraceptive use. This risk increases with age and with heavy smoking (15 or more cigarettes per day) and is quite marked in women over 35 years of age. Women who use oral contraceptives should not smoke.

Who Should Not Use Oral Contraceptives:

You should not use oral contraceptives:
A. If you have any of the following conditions:
1. Blood clots in the legs, lungs, or elsewhere in the body.
2. Chest pains on exertion (angina pectoris).
3. Known or suspected cancer of the breast or sex organs, such as the womb (uterus), vagina, or cervix.
4. Unusual vaginal bleeding that has not been diagnosed by your doctor.
5. Known or suspected pregnancy (one or more menstrual periods missed).

B. If you have had any of the following conditions:
1. Heart attack or stroke (clots or bleeding in the brain).
2. Blood clots in the legs, lungs, or elsewhere in the body.
3. Liver tumor associated with use of the pill or other estrogen-containing products.

C. If you have scanty or irregular periods or are a young woman without a regular cycle, you should use another method of contraception because, if you use the pill, you may have difficulty becoming pregnant or may fail to have menstrual periods after discontinuing the pill.

Deciding to Use Oral Contraceptives.

If you do not have any of the conditions listed above and are thinking about using oral contraceptives, to help you decide, you need information about the advantages and risks of oral contraceptives and of other contraceptive methods as well. This leaflet describes the advantages and risks of oral contraceptives. Except for sterilization, the intrauterine device (IUD), and abortion, which have their own specific risks, the only risks of other methods of contraception are those due to pregnancy should the method fail. Your doctor can answer questions you may have with respect to other methods of contraception, and further questions you may have on oral contraceptives after reading this leaflet.

1. *What Oral Contraceptives Are and How They Work.*

Oral contraceptives are of two types. The most common, often simply called "the pill," is a *combination* of an estrogen and a progestogen, the two kinds of female hormones. The amount of estrogen and progestogen can vary, but the amount of estrogen is more important because both the effectiveness and some of the dangers of oral contraceptives have been related to the amount of estrogen. This combination oral contraceptive works principally by preventing release of an egg from the ovary during the cycle in which the pills are taken. When the amount of estrogen is 50 micrograms or more, and the pill is taken as directed, oral contraceptives are more than 99% effective (that is, there would be less than 1 pregnancy in 100 women using the pill for one year). Pills that contain 20 to 35 micrograms of estrogen vary slightly in effectiveness, ranging from 98% to more than 99% effective.

The second type of oral contraceptive, often called the mini-pill, contains only a progestogen. It works in part by preventing release of an egg from the ovary, but also by keeping sperm from reaching the egg and by making the womb (uterus) less receptive to any fertilized egg that reaches it. The mini-pill is less effective than the combination oral contraceptive, about 97% effective. In addition, the mini-pill has a tendency to cause irregular bleeding, which may be quite inconvenient, or cessation of bleeding entirely. The mini-pill is used despite its lower effectiveness in the hope that it will prove not to have some of the serious side effects of the estrogen-containing pill, but it is not yet certain that the mini-pill does in fact have fewer serious side effects. The following discussion, while based mainly on information about the combination pills, should be considered to apply as well to the mini-pill.

2. *Other Nonsurgical Ways to Prevent Pregnancy.*

As this leaflet will explain, oral contraceptives have several serious risks. Other methods of contraception have lesser risks or none at all. They are also less effective than oral contraceptives, but, used properly, may be effective enough for many women. The following table gives reported pregnancy rates (the number of women out of 100 who would become pregnant in one year) for these methods:

Method	Pregnancies per 100 Women per Year Range
Intrauterine device (IUD)	less than 1 to 6
Diaphragm with spermicidal cream or jelly	2 to 20
Condom (rubber)	3 to 36
Spermicidal aerosol foams	2 to 29
Spermicidal jellies or creams	4 to 36
Periodic abstinence (rhythm), all types	less than 1 to 47
1. Calendar method	14 to 47
2. Temperature method	1 to 20
3. Temperature method (intercourse only in postovulatory phase)	less than 1 to 7
4. Mucus method	1 to 25
No contraception	60 to 80

These figures (except for the IUD) vary widely because people differ in how well they use each method. Very faithful users of the various methods obtain the best results, except for users of the periodic abstinence (rhythm) calendar method. Effective use of these methods, except for the IUD, requires somewhat more effort than simply taking a single pill every day, but it is an effort that many couples undertake successfully. Your doctor can tell you a great deal more about these methods of contraception and their effectiveness.

3. *The Dangers of Oral Contraceptives.*

a. *Circulatory Disorders (Blood Clots, Strokes, and Heart Attacks).* Blood clots occasionally form in the blood vessels of the body and, though rare, are the most common of the serious side effects of oral contraceptives. Clotting can result in a stroke (a clot in the brain), a heart attack (a clot in a blood vessel of the heart), or a pulmonary embolus (a clot that forms in the legs or abdominal region, then breaks off and travels to the lungs), or loss of a limb (a clot in a blood vessel in, or leading to, an arm or leg). Clots can also form in the blood vessels of the intestines or liver. Any of these events can be fatal (lead to death). Clots also occur rarely in the blood vessels of the eye, resulting in blindness or impairment of vision in that eye. There is some evidence that the risk of clotting may increase with higher estrogen doses. It is therefore important for your doctor to keep the dose of estrogen as low as possible, so long as the oral contraceptive used has an acceptable pregnancy rate and doesn't cause unacceptable changes in the menstrual pattern. Higher doses of progestogen have also been suggested as increasing the risk of clotting. Furthermore, cigarette-smoking by oral contraceptive users increases the risk of serious adverse effects on the heart and blood vessels. This risk increases with age and with heavy smoking (15 or more cigarettes per day) and begins to become quite marked in women over 35 years of age. For this reason, women who use oral contraceptives should not smoke.

The risk of abnormal clotting increases with age both in users and in nonusers of oral contraceptives, but the increased risk with the oral contraceptives appears to be present at all ages.

The risks of circulatory disorders may persist or continue after the pill is stopped. This has been reported for circulatory disorders in general, for heart disease or heart attacks, and for strokes caused either by a bursting blood vessel in the brain or by blood clots in the brain.

For oral contraceptive users in general, it has been estimated that in women between the ages of 25 and 34 the risk of death due to circulatory disorders in nonsmokers is about 1 in 23,000 per year. In contrast, for nonusers of the pill the risk is about 1 in 37,000 per year. Estimates of the risk of death due to circulatory disorders can be made, depending upon the woman's age, whether or not she uses oral contraceptives, and whether or not she smokes cigarettes. In the age group 25-34 years, women who use the pill have a risk of 1 in 7,000 (for smokers) to 1 in 23,000 (for nonsmokers) per year. This may be compared to the corresponding risk in women who have not used the pill: 1 in 24,000 (for smokers) to 1 in 37,000 (for nonsmokers) per year. The risks are greater in older women; thus, in the age group 35–44 years, women who use the pill have a risk of 1 in 1,600 (for smokers) to 1 in 4,700 (for nonsmokers) per year. The corresponding risk for women who have not used the pill is 1 in 6,600 (for smokers) to 1 in 16,000 (for nonsmokers) per year.

For women aged 16 to 40 it is estimated that about 1 in 2,000 using oral contraceptives will be hospitalized each year because of abnormal clotting in the veins or lungs. Among nonusers of the same age, about 1 in 20,000 would be hospitalized each year for these disorders.

Disease of the arteries characterized by paleness, numbness, or tingling in the fingers or toes has been reported to be more common in pill users. Strokes are caused by a bursting blood vessel in the brain (hemorrhage) or a loss of blood circulation to the brain due to blood clots. When they occur, paralysis of all or part of the body may result; death can result. The risk of strokes due to clots or hemorrhages in the brain has been reported to be increased in pill users when compared with nonusers.

It has been estimated that pill users are twice as likely as nonusers to have a stroke due to a bursting blood vessel in the brain. It has further been estimated that pill users are 4 to 10 times as likely as nonusers to have a stroke due to clotting in a blood vessel in or leading to the brain.

It has been reported that women using the pill may have a greater risk of heart attack than nonusers. Even without the pill the risk of having a heart attack increases with age and is also increased by additional risk factors such as high blood pressure, high blood cholesterol, obesity, diabetes, cigarette-smoking, or the occurrence during pregnancy of high blood pressure, swelling of the legs, or protein in the urine. Without any risk factors present, the use of oral contraceptives alone may double the risk of heart attack. However, the combination of cigarette-smoking, especially heavy smoking, and oral contraceptive use greatly increases the risk of heart attack. Oral contraceptive users who smoke are about five times more likely to have a heart attack than users who do not smoke, and about ten times more likely to have a heart attack than nonusers who do not smoke. It has been estimated that users between the ages of 30 and 39 who smoke have about a 1 in 10,000 chance each year of having a fatal heart attack compared to about a 1 in 50,000 chance in users who do not smoke, and about a 1 in 100,000 chance in nonusers who do not smoke. In the age group 40 to 44, the risk is about 1 in 1,700 per year for users who smoke compared to about 1 in 10,000 for users who do not smoke, and to about 1 in 14,000 per year for nonusers who do not smoke. Heavy smoking (about 15 cigarettes or more a day) further increases the risk. If you do not smoke and have none of the other heart attack risk factors described above, you will have a smaller risk than listed. If you have several heart attack risk factors, the risk may be considerably greater than listed. The above are average figures for Great Britain; comparable estimates for the U.S. have been higher.

Oral contraceptives should never be used at any age by women who have had a stroke, a heart attack, or chest pains on exertion (angina pectoris), or who have had blood clots in the legs, lungs, or elsewhere.

Anyone using the pill who has severe leg or chest pains, coughs up blood, has difficulty in breathing, severe headache or vomiting, dizziness or fainting, disturbances of vision or speech, weakness, numbness, or pain in an arm or leg should call her doctor immediately and stop taking the pill, and use another method of contraception.

b. *Formation of tumors.* When certain animals are given the female sex hormone estrogen (which is an ingredient in oral contraceptives) continuously for long periods, cancers may develop in organs such as the breast, cervix, vagina, liver, womb, ovary, and pituitary.

These findings suggest that oral contraceptives may cause cancer in humans. However, studies to date in women taking currently marketed oral contraceptives have not confirmed that oral contraceptives cause cancer in humans, but it remains possible they will be discovered in the future to do so. Several studies have found no increase in breast cancer in users, although it has been suggested that oral contraceptives might cause an increase in breast cancer in women who already have benign (noncancerous) breast disease (for example, cysts), in long-term (2–4 years) users, or in the presence of other risk factors (such as a family history of breast cancer, a previous breast biopsy, or delay in having the first child).

Women with a family history of breast cancer or who have breast nodules (lumps), fibrocystic disease (breast cysts), or abnormal mammograms (x-ray pictures of the breasts), or who were exposed to the estrogen diethylstilbestrol (DES) during their mother's pregnancy, or who have abnormal Pap smears should be followed very closely by their doctors if they choose to use oral contraceptives instead of another method of contraception. Many studies have shown that women taking oral contraceptives have less risk of getting benign (noncancerous) breast disease than those who have not used oral contraceptives. There is strong evidence that estrogens (one component of combination-type oral contraceptives), when given for periods of more than one year to women after the menopause (change-of-life), increase the risk of cancer of the womb (uterus). There is also some evidence that the sequential oral contraceptive, a kind of oral contraceptive that is no longer sold, may increase the risk of cancer of the womb. There is no evidence, however, that the oral contraceptives now available increase the risk of this type of cancer, although some individual cases have been reported. Cancer of the cervix may develop more readily in long-term users of the pill, particularly if they have had preexisting abnormal Pap smears. Cervical erosion and cell abnormalities have been reported to be more frequent in pill users.

Very rarely, oral contraceptive users may have a noncancerous tumor of the liver. These tumors do not spread, but they may rupture and cause internal bleeding, which may be fatal. This has been reported in short-term as well as long-term users, although increasing duration of use increases the risk. Long-term users have an estimated annual incidence of 3 to 4 per 100,000. One study reported that oral contraceptive products with a high "hormonal potency" were associated with a higher risk than lower-potency products, as was age over 30 years. A few cases of cancer of the liver have been reported in women using oral contraceptives, but it is not yet known whether the drug caused them. A type of skin cancer that has been linked to exposure to sunlight (malignant melanoma) has been reported to be more frequent among pill users. It was not possible to determine what the effect was of greater exposure to sunlight in users.

c. *Dangers to a developing baby if oral contraceptives are used in or immediately preceding pregnancy.* Oral contraceptives should not be taken by pregnant women because they may damage the developing baby. There is an increased risk to the baby of abnormalities of such parts of the body as the backbone, anus, heart, windpipe, esophagus, kidneys, arms, and legs. In addition, the developing female child whose mother has received DES, a synthetic estrogen, during pregnancy has a risk of getting cancer of the vagina or cervix in her teens or young adulthood. This risk is estimated to be about 1 in 1,000 exposures or less. DES-exposed daughters appear to have an increased risk of unfavorable outcome of pregnancy. Abnormalities of the urinary and sex organs and sperm have been reported in DES-exposed male babies as well. It is possible that other estrogens, such as the estrogens in oral contraceptives, could have the same effect in the baby if the mother takes them during pregnancy.

Occasionally women who are taking the pill miss periods. It has been reported to occur as frequently as several times each year in some women, depending on various factors such as age and prior his-

tory. (Your doctor is the best source of information about this.) The pill should not be used when you are pregnant or suspect you may be pregnant. Very rarely, women who are using the pill as directed become pregnant. The likelihood of becoming pregnant is higher if you occasionally miss one or two pills. Therefore, if you miss a period you should consult your physician before continuing to take the pill. If you miss a period, especially if you have not taken the pill regularly, you should use an alternative method of contraception until pregnancy has been ruled out; if you have missed more than one pill at any time, you should immediately start using an additional method of contraception and complete your pill cycle.

You should not attempt to become pregnant for at least three months after discontinuing oral contraceptives. Use another method of contraception during this period of time. The reason for this is that during this period there may be an increased risk of miscarriage and deformity to the baby, or an increased chance of having twins. Whether there is an overall increase in miscarriage in women who become pregnant soon after stopping the pill as compared with women who did not use the pill is not known, but it is possible that there may be.

If, however, you do become pregnant soon after stopping oral contraceptives, and do not have a miscarriage, there is no evidence that the baby has an increased risk of being abnormal.

d. *Gallbladder disease.* Women who use oral contraceptives have a greater risk than nonusers of having gallbladder disease requiring surgery. The increased risk may first appear within one year of use and may double after 4 or 5 years of use.

e. *Other side effects of oral contraceptives.* Some women using oral contraceptives experience unpleasant side effects from the pill which are not dangerous and are not likely to damage their health. Some of these side effects are similar to symptoms women experience in early pregnancy and may be temporary. Your breasts may feel tender, be enlarged, or have a discharge; nausea and vomiting or other stomach or intestinal problems may occur; you may gain or lose weight, and your ankles may swell. A spotty darkening of the skin, particularly of the face, is possible and may persist after the drug is discontinued. An allergic or other type of rash or vaginal yeast infection might occur. You may notice unexpected vaginal bleeding, change in discharge, or changes in your menstrual period. Irregular bleeding is frequently seen when the mini-pill or the combination oral contraceptives containing less than 50 micrograms of estrogen are used. These should all be reported to your doctor.

Other side effects include worsening of migraine, asthma, convulsive disorders (such as epilepsy), and kidney, liver, or heart disease because of a tendency for water to be retained in the body when oral contraceptives are used. Other side effects are painful periods, growth of preexisting fibroid tumors of the womb; mental depression; and liver problems with jaundice (yellowing of the whites of the eyes or of the skin). Your doctor may find that levels of sugar and fatty substances in your blood are elevated; the long-term effects of these changes are not known. Some women develop high blood pressure while taking oral contraceptives, which ordinarily, but not always, returns to the original levels when the oral contraceptive is stopped. The degree of blood pressure rise may be related to the amount of progestogen in the pill. Women with a history of increased blood pressure, kidney disease, or toxemia during pregnancy (increased blood pressure, swelling of the legs, protein in the urine, or convulsions), or a family tendency to high blood pressure or its consequences (stroke, heart disease, kidney disease, blood vessel problems), or a history of excessive weight gain or swelling of the legs during their menstrual cycle, may be more likely to develop increased blood pressure when given oral contraceptives; therefore, they should

Continued on next page

Searle & Co.—Cont.

have their blood pressure taken frequently. High blood pressure predisposes one to stroke, heart attacks, kidney disease, and other diseases of the blood vessels. The effect of prolonged use of oral contraceptives on several of your organs (pituitary, liver, ovaries, womb, and adrenals) or immune system is not known at this time.

Other conditions, although not proved to be caused by oral contraceptives, are occasionally reported. These include more frequent urination and some discomfort when urinating, kidney disease, nervousness, dizziness, hearing problems, inflammation of the nasal passages, loss of scalp hair, an increase in body hair, an increase or decrease in sex drive, appetite changes, gum disease, dry socket, cataracts, a need for a change in contact lens prescription or inability to use contact lenses, tiredness, backache, vaginal infections, itching, anemia, blood cell breakdown with kidney failure, headache, symptoms similar to those you get before a period; breast, womb, and cervical cancer; inflammation of the pancreas, liver, or colon; chorea (spasmodic movements), burning or prickly sensation, and rheumatoid arthritis.

After you stop using oral contraceptives, there may be a delay before you are able to become pregnant or before you resume having menstrual periods. This is especially true of women who had irregular menstrual cycles prior to the use of oral contraceptives.

One study showed that this delay in becoming pregnant can persist to 30 months after stopping the pill, especially if you have never had children, and does not depend on how long you have used the pill. Very rarely there may be secretions from the breast associated with the absence of periods, which might be due to a noncancerous tumor of the pituitary gland requiring surgery. This may occur more frequently in former users of the pill than in nonusers. As discussed previously, you should wait at least three months after stopping the pill before you try to become pregnant. During the first three months after stopping oral contraceptives, use another form of contraception. You should consult your doctor before resuming use of oral contraceptives after childbirth, especially if you plan to nurse your baby. Drugs in oral contraceptives are known to appear in the milk, and the long-range effect on babies is not known at this time. Furthermore, oral contraceptives may cause a decrease in your milk supply as well as in the quality of the milk.

4. *Comparison of the Risks of Oral Contraceptives and Other Contraceptive Methods.*

The many studies on the risks and effectiveness of oral contraceptives and other methods of contraception have been analyzed to estimate the risk of death associated with various methods of contraception. This risk has two parts: (a) the risk of the method itself (for example, the risk that oral contraceptives might cause death due to abnormal blood clotting), and (b) the risk of death due to pregnancy or abortion in the event the method should fail. The results of this analysis are shown in the following bar graph. The height of the bars indicates the number of deaths per 100,000 women each year. There are six sets of bars, each set referring to a specific age group of women. Within each set of bars, there is a single bar for each of the different contraceptive methods.

For oral contraceptives, there are two bars —one for smokers and the other for nonsmokers. The analysis is based on present knowledge and new information could, of course, alter it. The analysis shows that the risk of death from all methods of birth control is low and below that associated with the risks of childbirth, *except for oral contraceptives in women over 40 who smoke.* The risk of death associated with pill use in nonsmokers over 40 is higher than with any other method of contraception in that age group. It shows that the lowest risk of death is associated with the condom or diaphragm (traditional contraception) backed up by early legal abortion in case of failure of the condom or diaphragm to prevent pregnancy. Also, at any age, the risk of death (due to unexpected pregnancy) from use of traditional contraception, even without a backup of abortion, is generally the same as, or less than, that from use of oral contraceptives.

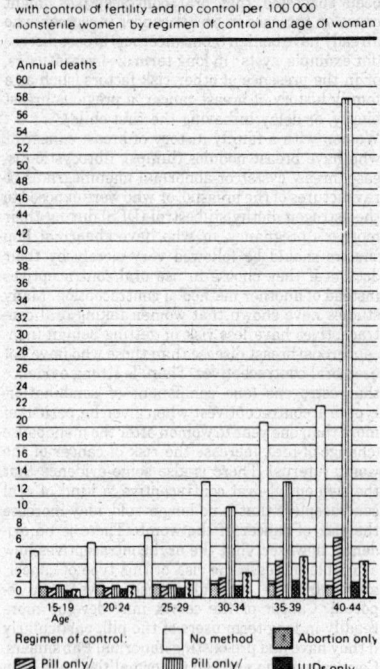

Figure 1 Estimated annual number of deaths associated with control of fertility and no control per 100 000 nonsterile women, by regimen of control and age of woman

How to Use Oral Contraceptives as Safely and Effectively as Possible, Once You Have Decided to Use Them:

1. *What to Tell Your Doctor.* You can make use of the pill as safe as possible, by telling your doctor if you have any of the following:
a. Conditions that mean you should not use oral contraceptives:
   If you *now* have any of the following:
   1. Blood clots in the legs, lungs, or elsewhere in the body.
   2. Chest pains on exertion (angina pectoris).
   3. Known or suspected cancer of the breast or sex organs, such as the womb (uterus), vagina, or cervix.
   4. Unusual vaginal bleeding that has not been diagnosed by your doctor.
   5. Known or suspected pregnancy (one or more menstrual periods missed).
   If you have *ever* had any of the following:
   1. Heart attack or stroke (clots or bleeding in the brain).
   2. Blood clots in the legs, lungs, or elsewhere in the body.
   3. Liver tumor associated with use of the pill or other estrogen-containing products.
b. Inform your doctor of the following conditions since s/he will want to watch them closely or they might cause him/her to suggest another method of contraception:
   A family history of breast cancer
   Breast nodules (lumps), fibrocystic disease (breast cysts), abnormal mammograms (x-ray pictures of the breasts), or abnormal Pap smears
   Diabetes
   High blood pressure
   High blood cholesterol
   Cigarette-smoking
   Migraine
   Heart or kidney disease
   Asthma
   Problems during a prior pregnancy
   Epilepsy
   Mental depression
   Fibroid tumors of the womb
   History of jaundice (yellowing of the whites of the eyes or of the skin)
   Gallbladder disease
   Varicose veins
   Tuberculosis
   Plans for elective surgery
   Previous problems with your periods (irregularities)
   Use of any of the following kinds of drugs, which might interact with the pill: antibiotics (such as rifampin, ampicillin, and tetracycline), sulfa drugs, drugs for epilepsy or migraine, painkillers, tranquilizers, sedatives or sleeping pills, blood-thinning drugs, cortisone-like drugs, vitamins, drugs being used for the treatment of depression, high blood pressure, high blood sugar (diabetes), elevated blood lipids, or asthma
c. Once you are using oral contraceptives, you should be alert for signs of a serious adverse effect and call your doctor immediately if any of these occur:
   Sharp pain in the chest, coughing up of blood, or sudden shortness of breath (indicating possible clots in the lungs).
   Pain in the calf (possible clot in the leg).
   Crushing chest pain or heaviness (indicating possible heart attack).
   Sudden severe headache or vomiting, dizziness or fainting, disturbance of vision or speech, or weakness or numbness in an arm or leg (indicating a possible stroke).
   Sudden partial or complete loss of vision (indicating a possible clot in the blood vessels of the eye).
   Abnormal vaginal bleeding.
   Breast discharge or lumps (you should ask your doctor to show you how to examine your own breasts).
   Severe and/or persistent pain or a mass in the abdomen (indicating a possible tumor of the liver, which might have ruptured).
   Severe depression.
   Yellowing of the whites of the eyes or of the skin (jaundice).
   Unusual swelling.
   Other unusual conditions.

2. *How to Take the Pill So That It Is Most Effective. Dosage Schedules.* See later sections in this leaflet concerning spotting, breakthrough bleeding, forgotten pills, and missed menstruation.

When you first begin to use the pill, you should use an additional method of protection until you have taken your first seven pills.

To remove a pill, press down on it. The pill will drop through a hole in the bottom of the Compack®.

The "20-pill" Schedule. Enovid® 5 mg may be prescribed on the 20-pill schedule.

Take a pill each day for 20 consecutive days, beginning each pill cycle on day 5 after your period starts, just as you did during the first pill cycle, or on the eighth day after having taken the last pill, whichever occurs first. Count the day you start to menstruate as day 1.

Continue this 20-pill schedule, cycle after cycle, regardless of whether your flow has or has not ceased when you start or whether you happen to spot or experience unexpected (breakthrough) bleeding during a cycle.

You will probably have your periods about every 27 days.

The Two "three weeks on—one week off" Schedules. Your Demulen 1/35™-21, Demulen 1/50™-21, Ovulen 21, or Enovid-E 21 Compack contains 21 tablets arranged in three numbered rows with the days of the week printed above them.

Day-5 Schedule. If you are to begin on day 5, count the day you start to menstruate as day 1 and determine which day to start. Start in row #1 with the pill under the day which corresponds to day 5 after your flow began. Continue to take one pill each day on consecutive days of the week.

After the last (Saturday) pill in row #3 has been taken, if any remain in the first row, complete your 21-pill schedule by taking one pill daily starting with Sunday in row #1. Then stop for one week before starting to take the pills again. Begin your next pill cycle on the same day of the week that you began the first cycle.

Sunday Schedule. Start taking the pills on the first Sunday after your period begins unless your period begins on Sunday. If your period begins on Sunday start taking the pill that very same day. Begin in row #1 and take your pills, one each day on consecutive days, for three weeks (21 days), then stop taking them for one week (7 days) before starting to take the pills again on Sunday.

Whether you begin on "day 5" or on Sunday, continue taking your pills as directed, month after month, regardless of whether your flow has or has not ceased or whether you may have experienced spotting or unexpected (breakthrough) bleeding during your pill cycle. You will probably have your period about every 28 days.

The "Pill-a-day" Schedule. Your Demulen 1/35™-28, Demulen 1/50™-28, or Ovulen-28 Compack contains 28 pills arranged in four numbered rows of seven pills each with the days of the week printed above them.

You must take your pills in order, one pill each day. Begin with the Sunday pill in row #1.

1—Start taking the pills on the first Sunday after your period begins unless your period begins on Sunday. *If your period begins on Sunday start taking the pills that very same day.*

2—Continue to take one pill each day on consecutive days of the week.

3—After the Saturday pill in row #1 has been taken begin taking pills in row #2, and so on, until the Saturday pill in row #4 has been taken.

4—Replace the Refill in your Compack at once, and begin a new pill cycle the next day, starting with the Sunday pill in row #1.

You will probably have your period about every 28 days, while you are taking the pink (blue for Demulen 1/35™-28) pills.

Continue your pill-a-day schedule, month after month, regardless of whether your flow ceases while you are taking the colored pills, or whether you experience spotting or unexpected (breakthrough) bleeding during a cycle.

Take your pill faithfully every "pill day"!

It is important that you take a pill without fail every pill day at intervals of 24 hours, for two reasons. First, your ovaries may release an egg and therefore you may become pregnant if you do not take your pills regularly. Second, you may spot or start to flow between your periods. This may be inconvenient.

Take your pill at the same time every day!

You are probably wondering why the same time of day is important. By taking your pill at the same time every day it becomes a good habit, and you are much less likely to forget. You may wish to keep your pills in the medicine cabinet near your toothbrush as a reminder to take them when you brush your teeth at night. The best time to take your daily pill may be either with your evening meal or at bedtime. You may find it helpful to associate your pill-taking with something else you do every day at a particular time.

Another very important reason for you to take your pills as "regular as clockwork" is that you are protected best when you take one every 24 hours; they are made to work that way. Just remember that once every day is not the same as once every 24 hours. Here is why: Suppose you were to take your Monday pill in the morning when you get up, and then not take your Tuesday pill till the evening before you go to bed. True, you will have taken a pill each day, on Monday and on Tuesday—but the time between pill-taking will probably have been more than 36 hours, or more than 1½ days! You might spot. Chances are you would still be protected and would not get pregnant, but why risk it when it is so easy to guarantee yourself maximal protection by taking your pill faithfully every pill day and at the same time every pill day? In summary, you should take the pills exactly as directed and at intervals of 24 hours in order to achieve maximum contraceptive effectiveness.

Spotting. This is a slight staining between your menstrual periods which may not even require a pad. Some women spot even though they take their pills exactly as directed. Many women spot although they have never taken the pills. Spotting does not mean that your ovaries are releasing an egg. Spotting may be the result of irregular pill-taking. Getting back on schedule will usually stop it.

If you should spot while taking the pills you should not be alarmed because spotting usually stops by itself within a few days. It seldom occurs after the first pill cycle. Consult your doctor if spotting persists for more than a few days or if it occurs after the second cycle.

Unexpected (Breakthrough) Bleeding. Unexpected (breakthrough) bleeding does not mean your ovaries have released an egg. It seldom occurs, but when it does happen it is most common in the first pill cycle. It is a flow much like a regular period, requiring the use of a pad or tampon.

If you experience breakthrough bleeding use a pad or tampon and continue with your schedule. Usually your periods will become regular within a few cycles. Breakthrough bleeding will seldom bother you again.

Consult your doctor if breakthrough bleeding does not stop within a week or if it occurs after the second cycle.

Forgotten Pills. There is little likelihood of your getting pregnant if only one active pill is missed; however, the possibility increases with each successive day that the scheduled active pills are missed. If you forget to take a pill one day, take two the next day—the one you forgot as soon as you remember and your regular pill at your usual time.

If you forget your pills (except the inactive colored pills in Demulen 1/35™-28, Demulen 1/50™-28, or Ovulen-28) on two consecutive days, do not be surprised if you spot or start to flow. You should take two pills each day for the next two days, and use an additional method of protection for the remainder of the cycle.

If you are using Demulen 1/35™-28, Demulen 1/50™-28, or Ovulen-28 and forget to take one or more colored pills, begin a new cycle on the next Sunday; use a new package and start taking the white pills. Missing the colored pills does not increase your chances of getting pregnant providing the white pill schedule has been followed.

Missed Menstruation. At times there may be no menstrual period after a cycle of pills. Therefore, if you miss one menstrual period but have taken the pills *exactly as you were supposed to*, continue as usual into the next cycle. You may wish to call your doctor. If you have not taken the pills correctly and miss a menstrual period, *you may be pregnant* and should stop taking oral contraceptives until your doctor determines whether or not you are pregnant. Until you can get to your doctor, use another form of contraception. If two consecutive menstrual periods are missed, you should stop taking the pills until it is determined whether you are pregnant. If you do become pregnant while using oral contraceptives, you should discuss the risks to the developing baby with your doctor.

3. *Periodic Examinations.* Your doctor will take a complete medical and family history before prescribing oral contraceptives. At that time and about once a year thereafter, s/he will generally examine your blood pressure, breasts, abdomen, and internal female organs (including a Pap smear test for cancer of the cervix) and perform certain laboratory tests. Certain health problems or conditions in your medical or family history may require that your doctor see you more frequently while you are taking the pill.

4. *Using Enovid for Purposes Other Than Contraception.* Since dosage schedules for these uses must be individualized for each patient, please follow the directions of your doctor.

Summary: Oral contraceptives are the most effective method, except sterilization, for preventing pregnancy. Other methods, when used conscientiously, are also very effective and have fewer risks. The serious side effects of oral contraceptives are uncommon, but the risk of experiencing them may persist after discontinuing the pill. The pill is a very convenient method for preventing pregnancy.

Women who use oral contraceptives should not smoke.

If you have certain conditions or have had these conditions in the past, you should not use oral contraceptives because of increased risk. These conditions are listed in this leaflet. If you do not have these conditions, and decide to use the pill, please read this leaflet carefully so that you can use the pill safely and effectively. Be certain to read new revisions of this leaflet.

Based on your doctor's assessment of your medical needs, this drug has been prescribed for you. Do not give it to anyone else.

See your doctor regularly, ask any questions you may have about the use of the pill, and report any special problems that may arise.

These products are shown in the Product Identification Section, pages 435 & 436

ENOVID-E® 21 ℞
[ē-nov'id-ē]
(norethynodrel with mestranol)

See Demulen products under Searle & Co. for Enovid-E 21 prescribing information.
Shown in Product Identification Section, page 436

ENOVID® 5 mg ℞
ENOVID® 10 mg ℞
[ē-nov'id]
(norethynodrel with mestranol)

See Demulen products under Searle & Co. for Enovid 5 mg and Enovid 10 mg prescribing information.
Shown in Product Identification Section, page 435

FLAGYL® Tablets ℞
[flaj'yl]
(metronidazole)

Warning

Metronidazole has been shown to be carcinogenic in mice and rats (see *Warnings*). Unnecessary use of the drug should be avoided. Its use should be reserved for the conditions described in the *Indications and Usage* section below.

Description: Flagyl (metronidazole) is an oral synthetic antiprotozoal and antibacterial agent, 1-(β-hydroxyethyl) - 2 - methyl - 5-nitroimidazole.

Clinical Pharmacology: Disposition of metronidazole in the body is similar for both oral and intravenous dosage forms, with an average elimination half-life in healthy humans of eight hours. The major route of elimination of metronidazole and its metabolites is via the urine (60–80% of the dose), with fecal excretion accounting for 6–15% of the dose. The metabolites that appear in the urine result primarily from side-chain oxidation [1-β-hydroxyethyl)- 2-hydroxymethyl-5-nitroimidazole and 2-methyl-5-nitroimidazole-1-yl-acetic acid] and glucuronide conjugation, with unchanged metronidazole accounting for approximately 20% of the total. Renal clearance of metronidazole is approximately 10 ml/min/1.73 m².

Metronidazole is the major component appearing in the plasma, with lesser quantities of the 2-hydroxymethyl metabolite also being present. Less than 20% of the circulating metronidazole is bound to plasma proteins. Both the parent compound and the metabolite possess *in vitro* bactericidal activity against most strains of anaerobic bacteria and *in vitro* trichomonacidal activity.

Continued on next page

Metronidazole appears in cerebrospinal fluid, saliva, and breast milk in concentrations similar to those found in plasma. Bactericidal concentrations of metronidazole have also been detected in pus from hepatic abscesses.

Following oral administration metronidazole is well absorbed, with peak plasma concentrations occurring between one and two hours after administration. Plasma concentrations of metronidazole are proportional to the administered dose. Oral administration of 250 mg, 500 mg, or 2,000 mg produced peak plasma concentrations of 6 mcg/ml, 12 mcg/ml, and 40 mcg/ml, respectively. Studies reveal no significant bioavailability differences between males and females; however, because of weight differences, the resulting plasma levels in males are generally lower.

Decreased renal function does not alter the single-dose pharmacokinetics of metronidazole. However, plasma clearance of metronidazole is decreased in patients with decreased liver function.

Microbiology: *Trichomonas vaginalis, Entamoeba histolytica.* Flagyl (metronidazole) possesses direct trichomonacidal and amebacidal activity against *T. vaginalis* and *E. histolytica*. The *in vitro* minimal inhibitory concentration (MIC) for most strains of these organisms is 1 mcg/ml or less.

Anaerobic Bacteria. Metronidazole is active *in vitro* against most obligate anaerobes, but does not appear to possess any clinically relevant activity against facultative anaerobes or obligate aerobes. Against susceptible organisms, metronidazole is generally bactericidal at concentrations equal to or slightly higher than the minimal inhibitory concentrations. Metronidazole has been shown to have *in vitro* and clinical activity against the following organisms:

Anaerobic gram-negative bacilli, including:
  Bacteroides species including the *Bacteroides fragilis* group (*B. fragilis, B. distasonis, B. ovatus, B. thetaiotaomicron, B. vulgatus*)
  Fusobacterium species
Anaerobic gram-positive bacilli, including:
  Clostridium species and susceptible strains of *Eubacterium*
Anaerobic gram-positive cocci, including:
  Peptococcus species
  Peptostreptococcus species

Susceptibility Tests: Bacteriologic studies should be performed to determine the causative organisms and their susceptibility to metronidazole; however, the rapid, routine susceptibility testing of individual isolates of anaerobic bacteria is not always practical, and therapy may be started while awaiting these results.

Quantitative methods give the most precise estimates of susceptibility to antibacterial drugs. A standardized agar dilution method and a broth microdilution method are recommended.[1]

Control strains are recommended for standardized susceptibility testing. Each time the test is performed, one or more of the following strains should be included: *Clostridium perfringens* ATCC 13124, *Bacteroides fragilis* ATCC 25285, and *Bacteroides thetaiotaomicron* ATCC 29741. The mode metronidazole MICs for those three strains are reported to be 0.25, 0.25, and 0.5 mcg/ml, respectively.

A clinical laboratory is considered under acceptable control if the results of the control strains are within one doubling dilution of the mode MICs reported for metronidazole.

A bacterial isolate may be considered susceptible if the MIC value for metronidazole is not more than 16 mcg/ml. An organism is considered resistant if the MIC is greater than 16 mcg/ml. A report of "resistant" from the laboratory indicates that the infecting organism is not likely to respond to therapy.

Indications and Usage:
Symptomatic Trichomoniasis. Flagyl is indicated for the treatment of symptomatic trichomoniasis in females and males when the presence of the trichomonad has been confirmed by appropriate laboratory procedures (wet smears and/or cultures).

Asymptomatic Trichomoniasis. Flagyl is indicated in the treatment of asymptomatic females when the organism is associated with endocervicitis, cervicitis, or cervical erosion. Since there is evidence that presence of the trichomonad can interfere with accurate assessment of abnormal cytological smears, additional smears should be performed after eradication of the parasite.

Treatment of Asymptomatic Consorts. *T. vaginalis* infection is a venereal disease. Therefore, asymptomatic sexual partners of treated patients should be treated simultaneously if the organism has been found to be present, in order to prevent reinfection of the partner. The decision as to whether to treat an asymptomatic male partner who has a negative culture or one for whom no culture has been attempted is an individual one. In making this decision, it should be noted that there is evidence that a woman may become reinfected if her consort is not treated. Also, since there can be considerable difficulty in isolating the organism from the asymptomatic male carrier, negative smears and cultures cannot be relied upon in this regard. In any event, the consort should be treated with Flagyl in cases of reinfection.

Amebiasis. Flagyl is indicated in the treatment of acute intestinal amebiasis (amebic dysentery) and amebic liver abscess.

In amebic liver abscess, Flagyl therapy does not obviate the need for aspiration or drainage of pus.

Anaerobic Bacterial Infections. Flagyl is indicated in the treatment of serious infections caused by susceptible anaerobic bacteria. Indicated surgical procedures should be performed in conjunction with Flagyl therapy. In a mixed aerobic and anaerobic infection, antibiotics appropriate for the treatment of the aerobic infection should be used in addition to Flagyl.

In the treatment of most serious anaerobic infections, Flagyl I.V.™ (metronidazole hydrochloride) or Flagyl I.V.™ RTU® (metronidazole) is usually administered initially. This may be followed by oral therapy with Flagyl (metronidazole) at the discretion of the physician.

INTRA-ABDOMINAL INFECTIONS, including peritonitis, intra-abdominal abscess, and liver abscess, caused by *Bacteroides* species including the *B. fragilis* group (*B. fragilis, B. distasonis, B. ovatus, B. thetaiotaomicron, B. vulgatus*), *Clostridium* species, *Eubacterium* species, *Peptococcus* species, and *Peptostreptococcus* species.

SKIN AND SKIN STRUCTURE INFECTIONS caused by *Bacteroides* species including the *B. fragilis* group, *Clostridium* species, *Peptococcus* species, *Peptostreptococcus* species, and *Fusobacterium* species.

GYNECOLOGIC INFECTIONS, including endometritis, endomyometritis, tubo-ovarian abscess, and postsurgical vaginal cuff infection, caused by *Bacteroides* species including the *B. fragilis* group, *Clostridium* species, *Peptococcus* species, and *Peptostreptococcus* species.

BACTERIAL SEPTICEMIA caused by *Bacteroides* species including the *B. fragilis* group, and *Clostridium* species.

BONE AND JOINT INFECTIONS, as adjunctive therapy, caused by *Bacteroides* species including the *B. fragilis* group.

CENTRAL NERVOUS SYSTEM (CNS) INFECTIONS, including meningitis and brain abscess, caused by *Bacteroides* species including the *B. fragilis* group.

LOWER RESPIRATORY TRACT INFECTIONS, including pneumonia, empyema, and lung abscess, caused by *Bacteroides* species including the *B. fragilis* group.

ENDOCARDITIS caused by *Bacteroides* species including the *B. fragilis* group.

Contraindications: Flagyl is contraindicated in patients with a prior history of hypersensitivity to metronidazole or other nitroimidazole derivatives. In patients with trichomoniasis, Flagyl is contraindicated during the first trimester of pregnancy. (See *Warnings.*)

Warnings: *Convulsive Seizures and Peripheral Neuropathy:* Convulsive seizures and peripheral neuropathy, the latter characterized mainly by numbness or paresthesia of an extremity, have been reported in patients treated with metronidazole. The appearance of abnormal neurologic signs demands the prompt discontinuation of Flagyl therapy. Flagyl should be administered with caution to patients with central nervous system diseases.

Tumorigenicity Studies in Rodents: Metronidazole has shown evidence of carcinogenic activity in a number of studies involving chronic, oral administration in mice and rats.

Prominent among the effects in the mouse was the promotion of pulmonary tumorigenesis. This has been observed in all six reported studies in that species, including one study in which the animals were dosed on an intermittent schedule (administration during every fourth week only). At very high dose levels (approx. 500 mg/kg/day) there was a statistically significant increase in the incidence of malignant liver tumors in males. Also, the published results of one of the mouse studies indicate an increase in the incidence of malignant lymphomas as well as pulmonary neoplasms associated with lifetime feeding of the drug. All these effects are statistically significant.

Several long-term, oral-dosing studies in the rat have been completed. There were statistically significant increases in the incidence of various neoplasms, particularly in mammary and hepatic tumors, among female rats administered metronidazole over those noted in the concurrent female control groups.

Two lifetime tumorigenicity studies in hamsters have been performed and reported to be negative.

Mutagenicity Studies: Although metronidazole has shown mutagenic activity in a number of *in vitro* assay systems, studies in mammals (*in vivo*) have failed to demonstrate a potential for genetic damage.

Precautions:
General: Patients with severe hepatic disease metabolize metronidazole slowly, with resultant accumulation of metronidazole and its metabolites in the plasma. Accordingly, for such patients, doses below those usually recommended should be administered cautiously.

Known or previously unrecognized candidiasis may present more prominent symptoms during therapy with Flagyl and requires treatment with a candicidal agent.

Information for Patients: Alcoholic beverages should be avoided while taking Flagyl and for at least one day afterward. See *Drug Interactions.*

Laboratory Tests: Flagyl (metronidazole) is a nitroimidazole and should be used with care in patients with evidence of or history of blood dyscrasia. A mild leukopenia has been observed during its administration; however, no persistent hematologic abnormalities attributable to metronidazole have been observed in clinical studies. Total and differential leukocyte counts are recommended before and after therapy for trichomoniasis and amebiasis, especially if a second course of therapy is necessary, and before and after therapy for anaerobic infection.

Drug Interactions: Metronidazole has been reported to potentiate the anticoagulant effect of warfarin and other oral coumarin anticoagulants, resulting in a prolongation of prothrombin time. This possible drug interaction should be considered when Flagyl is prescribed for patients on this type of anticoagulant therapy.

The simultaneous administration of drugs that induce microsomal liver enzymes, such as phenytoin or phenobarbital, may accelerate the elimination of metronidazole, resulting in reduced plasma levels.

The simultaneous administration of drugs that decrease microsomal liver enzyme activity, such as cimetidine, may prolong the half-life and decrease plasma clearance of metronidazole.

Alcoholic beverages should not be consumed during Flagyl therapy and for at least one day afterward because abdominal cramps, nausea, vomiting, headaches, and flushing may occur.

Drug/Laboratory Test Interactions: Metronidazole may interfere with certain types of determinations of serum chemistry values, such as aspartate aminotransferase (AST, SGOT), alanine aminotransferase (ALT, SGPT), lactate dehydrogenase (LDH), triglycerides, and hexokinase glucose. Values of zero may be observed. All of the assays in which interference has been reported involve enzymatic coupling of the assay to oxidation-reduction of nicotine adenine dinucleotide (NAD ⇌ NADH). Interference is due to the similarity in absorbance peaks of NADH (340 nm) and metronidazole (322 nm) at pH 7.

Carcinogenesis: See *Warnings.*

Pregnancy: Teratogenic Effects—Pregnancy Category B. Metronidazole crosses the placental barrier and enters the fetal circulation rapidly. Reproduction studies have been performed in rats at doses up to five times the human dose and have revealed no evidence of impaired fertility or harm to the fetus due to metronidazole. Metronidazole administered intraperitoneally to pregnant mice at approximately the human dose caused fetotoxicity; administered orally to pregnant mice, no fetotoxicity was observed. There are, however, no adequate and well-controlled studies in pregnant women. Because animal reproduction studies are not always predictive of human response, and because metronidazole is a carcinogen in rodents, this drug should be used during pregnancy only if clearly needed (see *Contraindications*).

Use of Flagyl for trichomoniasis in the second and third trimesters should be restricted to those in whom local palliative treatment has been inadequate to control symptoms.

Nursing Mothers: Because of the potential for tumorigenicity shown for metronidazole in mouse and rat studies, a decision should be made whether to discontinue nursing or to discontinue the drug, taking into account the importance of the drug to the mother. Metronidazole is secreted in breast milk in concentrations similar to those found in plasma.

Pediatric Use: Safety and effectiveness in children have not been established, except for the treatment of amebiasis.

Adverse Reactions: The two most serious adverse reactions reported in patients treated with Flagyl (metronidazole) have been convulsive seizures and peripheral neuropathy, the latter characterized mainly by numbness or paresthesia of an extremity. Since persistent peripheral neuropathy has been reported in some patients receiving prolonged administration of Flagyl, patients should be specifically warned about these reactions and should be told to stop the drug and report immediately to their physicians if any neurologic symptoms occur.

The most common adverse reactions reported have been referable to the gastrointestinal tract, particularly nausea reported by about 12% of patients, sometimes accompanied by headache, anorexia, and occasionally vomiting; diarrhea; epigastric distress; and abdominal cramping. Constipation has also been reported.

The following reactions have also been reported during treatment with Flagyl (metronidazole):

Mouth: A sharp, unpleasant metallic taste is not unusual. Furry tongue, glossitis, and stomatitis have occurred; these may be associated with a sudden overgrowth of *Candida* which may occur during effective therapy.

Hematopoietic: Reversible neutropenia (leukopenia).

Cardiovascular: Flattening of the T-wave may be seen in electrocardiographic tracings.

Central Nervous System: Convulsive seizures, peripheral neuropathy, dizziness, vertigo, incoordination, ataxia, confusion, irritability, depression, weakness, and insomnia.

Hypersensitivity: Urticaria, erythematous rash, flushing, nasal congestion, dryness of mouth (or vagina or vulva), and fever.

Renal: Dysuria, cystitis, polyuria, incontinence, and a sense of pelvic pressure. Instances of darkened urine have been reported by approximately one patient in 100,000. Although the pigment which is possibly responsible for this phenomenon has not been positively identified, it is almost certainly a metabolite of metronidazole and seems to have no clinical significance.

Other: Proliferation of *Candida* in the vagina, dyspareunia, decrease of libido, proctitis, and fleeting joint pains sometimes resembling "serum sickness." If patients receiving Flagyl drink alcoholic beverages, they may experience abdominal distress, nausea, vomiting, flushing, or headache. A modification of the taste of alcoholic beverages has also been reported.

Overdosage: Single oral doses of metronidazole, up to 15 g, have been reported in suicide attempts and accidental overdoses. Symptoms reported include nausea, vomiting, and ataxia.

Oral metronidazole has been studied as a radiation sensitizer in the treatment of malignant tumors. Neurotoxic effects, including seizures and peripheral neuropathy, have been reported after 5 to 7 days of doses of 6 to 10.4 g every other day.

Treatment: There is no specific antidote for Flagyl overdose; therefore, management of the patient should consist of symptomatic and supportive therapy.

Dosage and Administration:

Trichomoniasis:

In the Female:

One-day treatment—two grams of Flagyl, given either as a single dose or in two divided doses of one gram each given in the same day.

Seven-day course of treatment—250 mg three times daily for seven consecutive days. There is some indication from controlled comparative studies that cure rates as determined by vaginal smears, signs and symptoms, may be higher after a seven-day course of treatment than after a one-day treatment regimen.

The dosage regimen should be individualized. Single-dose treatment can assure compliance, especially if administered under supervision, in those patients who cannot be relied on to continue the seven-day regimen. A seven-day course of treatment may minimize reinfection of the female long enough to treat sexual contacts. Further, some patients may tolerate one course of therapy better than the other. Pregnant patients should not be treated during the first trimester with either regimen. If treated during the second or third trimester, the one-day course of therapy should not be used, as it results in higher serum levels which reach the fetal circulation. (See *Contraindications* and *Precautions.*)

When repeat courses of the drug are required, it is recommended that an interval of four to six weeks elapse between courses and that the presence of the trichomonad be reconfirmed by appropriate laboratory measures. Total and differential leukocyte counts should be made before and after re-treatment.

In the Male: Treatment should be individualized as for the female.

Amebiasis:

Adults:

For acute intestinal amebiasis (acute amebic dysentery): 750 mg orally three times daily for 5 to 10 days.

For amebic liver abscess: 500 mg or 750 mg orally three times daily for 5 to 10 days.

Children: 35 to 50 mg/kg/24 hours, divided into three doses, orally for 10 days.

Anaerobic Bacterial Infections: In the treatment of most serious anaerobic infections, Flagyl I.V.™ (metronidazole hydrochloride) or Flagyl I.V.™ RTU® (metronidazole) is usually administered initially.

The usual adult *oral* dosage is 7.5 mg/kg every six hours (approx. 500 mg for a 70-kg adult). A maximum of 4 g should not be exceeded during a 24-hour period.

The usual duration of therapy is 7 to 10 days; however, infections of the bone and joint, lower respiratory tract, and endocardium may require longer treatment.

Patients with severe hepatic disease metabolize metronidazole slowly, with resultant accumulation of metronidazole and its metabolites in the plasma. Accordingly, for such patients, doses below those usually recommended should be administered cautiously. Close monitoring of plasma metronidazole levels[2] and toxicity is recommended.

The dose of Flagyl should not be specifically reduced in anuric patients since accumulated metabolites may be rapidly removed by dialysis.

How Supplied:

Flagyl 250-mg tablets are round, blue, film coated, with SEARLE and 1831 debossed on one side and FLAGYL and 250 on the other side; bottles of 100, 250, 500, 1,000, and 2,500, and cartons of 100 unit-dose individually blister-sealed tablets.

Flagyl 500-mg tablets are oblong, blue, film coated, with FLAGYL debossed on one side and 500 on the other side; bottles of 100 and 500, and cartons of 100 unit-dose individually blister-sealed tablets.

Storage and Stability: Store below 86°F (30°C) and protect from light.

1. Proposed standard: PSM-11—Proposed Reference Dilution Procedure for Antimicrobic Susceptibility Testing of Anaerobic Bacteria, National Committee for Clinical Laboratory Standards, and Sutter, et al.: Collaborative Evaluation of a Proposed Reference Dilution Method of Susceptibility Testing of Anaerobic Bacteria, Antimicrob. Agents Chemother. 16:495-502 (Oct.) 1979; and Tally, et al.: *In Vitro* Activity of Thienamycin, Antimicrob. Agents Chemother. 14:436-438 (Sept.) 1978.

2. Ralph, E.D., and Kirby, W.M.M.: Bioassay of Metronidazole With Either Anaerobic or Aerobic Incubation, J. Infect. Dis. 132:587-591 (Nov.) 1975; or Gulaid, et al.: Determination of Metronidazole and Its Major Metabolites in Biological Fluids by High Pressure Liquid Chromatography, Br. J. Clin. Pharmacol. 6:430-432, 1978.

Shown in Product Identification Section, page 436

●**LOMOTIL®** Liquid   ℂ
●**LOMOTIL®** Tablets   ℂ
[lō-mō′til]
(diphenoxylate hydrochloride with atropine sulfate)

Description: Each Lomotil tablet and each 5 ml of Lomotil liquid for oral use contains:

diphenoxylate hydrochloride .... 2.5 mg
(Warning—May be habit forming.)
atropine sulfate .... 0.025 mg

Diphenoxylate hydrochloride, an antidiarrheal, is ethyl 1-(3-cyano-3,3-diphenylpropyl)-4-phenylisonipecotate monohydrochloride and has the following structure:

Atropine sulfate, an anticholinergic, is endo-(±)-α-(hydroxymethyl) benzeneacetic acid 8-methyl-8-azabicyclo[3.2.1] oct-3-yl ester sulfate (2:1) (salt) monohydrate and has the following structure:

Important Information: Lomotil is classified as a Schedule V controlled substance by federal law. Diphenoxylate hydrochloride is chemically related to the narcotic meperidine. Therefore, in case of overdosage, treatment is similar to that for meperidine or morphine intoxication, in which prolonged and careful monitoring is essential. Respiratory depression may be evidenced as late as 30 hours after ingestion and may recur in spite of an initial response to narcotic antagonists. A subtherapeutic amount of atropine sulfate is present to discourage deliberate overdosage. LOMOTIL IS *NOT* AN INNOCUOUS DRUG AND DOSAGE RECOMMENDATIONS SHOULD BE STRICTLY ADHERED TO, ESPECIALLY IN CHILDREN. KEEP THIS AND ALL MEDICATIONS OUT OF REACH OF CHILDREN.

Clinical Pharmacology: Diphenoxylate is rapidly and extensively metabolized in man by ester hydrolysis to diphenoxylic acid (difenoxine), which

Continued on next page

Searle & Co.—Cont.

is biologically active and the major metabolite in the blood. After a 5-mg oral dose of carbon-14 labeled diphenoxylate hydrochloride in ethanolic solution was given to three healthy volunteers, an average of 14% of the drug plus its metabolites was excreted in the urine and 49% in the feces over a four-day period. Urinary excretion of the unmetabolized drug constituted less than 1% of the dose, and diphenoxylic acid plus its glucuronide conjugate constituted about 6% of the dose. In a sixteen-subject cross-over bioavailability study, a linear relationship in the dose range of 2.5 to 10 mg was found between the dose of diphenoxylate hydrochloride (given as Lomotil liquid) and the peak plasma concentration, the area under the plasma concentration-time curve, and the amount of diphenoxylic acid excreted in the urine. In the same study the bioavailability of the tablet compared with an equal dose of the liquid was approximately 90%. The average peak plasma concentration of diphenoxylic acid following ingestion of four 2.5-mg tablets was 163 ng/ml at about 2 hours, and the elimination half-life of diphenoxylic acid was approximately 12 to 14 hours.

In dogs, diphenoxylate hydrochloride has a direct effect on circular smooth muscle of the bowel, that conceivably results in segmentation and prolongation of gastrointestinal transit time. The clinical antidiarrheal action of diphenoxylate hydrochloride may thus be a consequence of enhanced segmentation that allows increased contact of the intraluminal contents with the intestinal mucosa.

Indications and Usage: Lomotil is effective as adjunctive therapy in the management of diarrhea.

Contraindications: Lomotil is contraindicated in patients with
1. Known hypersensitivity to diphenoxylate or atropine.
2. Obstructive jaundice.
3. Diarrhea associated with pseudomembranous enterocolitis.

Warnings: LOMOTIL IS *NOT* AN INNOCUOUS DRUG AND DOSAGE RECOMMENDATIONS SHOULD BE STRICTLY ADHERED TO, ESPECIALLY IN CHILDREN. LOMOTIL IS NOT RECOMMENDED FOR CHILDREN UNDER 2 YEARS OF AGE. OVERDOSAGE MAY RESULT IN SEVERE RESPIRATORY DEPRESSION AND COMA, POSSIBLY LEADING TO PERMANENT BRAIN DAMAGE OR DEATH (SEE *OVERDOSAGE*). THEREFORE, KEEP THIS MEDICATION OUT OF THE REACH OF CHILDREN.
THE USE OF LOMOTIL SHOULD BE ACCOMPANIED BY APPROPRIATE FLUID AND ELECTROLYTE THERAPY, WHEN INDICATED. IF SEVERE DEHYDRATION OR ELECTROLYTE IMBALANCE IS PRESENT, LOMOTIL SHOULD BE WITHHELD UNTIL APPROPRIATE CORRECTIVE THERAPY HAS BEEN INITIATED. DRUG-INDUCED INHIBITION OF PERISTALSIS MAY RESULT IN FLUID RETENTION IN THE INTESTINE, WHICH MAY FURTHER AGGRAVATE DEHYDRATION AND ELECTROLYTE IMBALANCE.
LOMOTIL SHOULD BE USED WITH SPECIAL CAUTION IN YOUNG CHILDREN BECAUSE THIS AGE GROUP MAY BE PREDISPOSED TO DELAYED DIPHENOXYLATE TOXICITY AND BECAUSE OF THE GREATER VARIABILITY OF RESPONSE IN THIS AGE GROUP.

Antiperistaltic agents may prolong and/or worsen diarrhea associated with organisms that penetrate the intestinal mucosa (toxigenic *E. coli, Salmonella, Shigella*), and pseudomembranous enterocolitis associated with broad-spectrum antibiotics. Antiperistaltic agents should not be used in these conditions.

In some patients with acute ulcerative colitis, agents that inhibit intestinal motility or prolong intestinal transit time have been reported to induce toxic megacolon. Consequently, patients with acute ulcerative colitis should be carefully observed and Lomotil therapy should be discontinued promptly if abdominal distention occurs or if other untoward symptoms develop.

Since the chemical structure of diphenoxylate hydrochloride is similar to that of meperidine hydrochloride, the concurrent use of Lomotil with monoamine oxidase (MAO) inhibitors may, in theory, precipitate hypertensive crisis.

Lomotil should be used with extreme caution in patients with advanced hepatorenal disease and in all patients with abnormal liver function since hepatic coma may be precipitated.

Diphenoxylate hydrochloride may potentiate the action of barbiturates, tranquilizers, and alcohol. Therefore, the patient should be closely observed when any of these are used concomitantly.

Precautions:
General: Since a subtherapeutic dose of atropine has been added to the diphenoxylate hydrochloride, consideration should be given to the precautions relating to the use of atropine. In children, Lomotil should be used with caution since signs of atropinism may occur even with recommended doses, particularly in patients with Down's syndrome.

Information for patients: INFORM THE PATIENT (PARENT OR GUARDIAN) NOT TO EXCEED THE RECOMMENDED DOSAGE AND TO KEEP LOMOTIL OUT OF THE REACH OF CHILDREN AND IN A CHILD-RESISTANT CONTAINER. INFORM THE PATIENT OF THE CONSEQUENCES OF OVERDOSAGE, INCLUDING SEVERE RESPIRATORY DEPRESSION AND COMA, POSSIBLY LEADING TO PERMANENT BRAIN DAMAGE OR DEATH. Lomotil may produce drowsiness or dizziness. The patient should be cautioned regarding activities requiring mental alertness, such as driving or operating dangerous machinery. Potentiation of the action of alcohol, barbiturates, and tranquilizers with concomitant use of Lomotil should be explained to the patient. The physician should also provide the patient with other information in this labeling, as appropriate.

Drug interactions: Known drug interactions include barbiturates, tranquilizers, and alcohol. Lomotil may interact with MAO inhibitors (see *Warnings*).

In studies with male rats, diphenoxylate hydrochloride was found to inhibit the hepatic microsomal enzyme system at a dose of 2 mg/kg/day. Therefore, diphenoxylate has the potential to prolong the biological half-lives of drugs for which the rate of elimination is dependent on the microsomal drug metabolizing enzyme system.

Carcinogenesis, mutagenesis, impairment of fertility: No long-term study in animals has been performed to evaluate carcinogenic potential. Diphenoxylate hydrochloride was administered to male and female rats in their diets to provide dose levels of 4 and 20 mg/kg/day throughout a three-litter reproduction study. At 50 times the human dose (20 mg/kg/day), female weight gain was reduced and there was a marked effect on fertility as only 4 of 27 females became pregnant in three test breedings. The relevance of this finding to usage of Lomotil in humans is unknown.

Pregnancy: Pregnancy Category C. Diphenoxylate hydrochloride has been shown to have an effect on fertility in rats when given in doses 50 times the human dose (see above discussion). Other findings in this study include a decrease in maternal weight gain of 30% at 20 mg/kg/day and of 10% at 4 mg/kg/day. At 10 times the human dose (4 mg/kg/day), average litter size was slightly reduced.

Teratology studies were conducted in rats, rabbits, and mice with diphenoxylate hydrochloride at oral doses of 0.4 to 20 mg/kg/day. Due to experimental design and small numbers of litters, embryotoxic, fetotoxic, or teratogenic effects cannot be adequately assessed. However, examination of the available fetuses did not reveal any indication of teratogenicity.

There are no adequate and well-controlled studies in pregnant women. Lomotil should be used during pregnancy only if the anticipated benefit justifies the potential risk to the fetus.

Nursing mothers: Caution should be exercised when Lomotil is administered to a nursing woman, since the physicochemical characteristics of the major metabolite, diphenoxylic acid, are such that it may be excreted in breast milk and since it is known that atropine is excreted in breast milk.

Pediatric use: Lomotil may be used as an adjunct to the treatment of diarrhea but should be accompanied by appropriate fluid and electrolyte therapy, if needed. LOMOTIL IS NOT RECOMMENDED FOR CHILDREN UNDER 2 YEARS OF AGE. Lomotil should be used with special caution in young children because of the greater variability of response in this age group. See *Warnings* and *Dosage and Administration.* In case of accidental ingestion by children, see *Overdosage* for recommended treatment.

Adverse Reactions:
At *therapeutic* doses, the following have been reported; they are listed in decreasing order of severity, but not of frequency:

Nervous system: numbness of extremities, euphoria, depression, malaise/lethargy, confusion, sedation/drowsiness, dizziness, restlessness, headache.

Allergic: anaphylaxis, angioneurotic edema, urticaria, swelling of the gums, pruritus.

Gastrointestinal system: toxic megacolon, paralytic ileus, vomiting, nausea, anorexia, abdominal discomfort.

The following atropine sulfate effects are listed in decreasing order of severity, but not of frequency: hyperthermia, tachycardia, urinary retention, flushing, dryness of the skin and mucous membranes. These effects may occur especially in children.

THIS MEDICATION SHOULD BE KEPT IN A CHILD-RESISTANT CONTAINER AND OUT OF THE REACH OF CHILDREN SINCE AN OVERDOSAGE MAY RESULT IN SEVERE RESPIRATORY DEPRESSION AND COMA, POSSIBLY LEADING TO PERMANENT BRAIN DAMAGE OR DEATH.

Drug Abuse and Dependence:
Controlled substance: Lomotil is classified as a Schedule V controlled substance by federal regulation. Diphenoxylate hydrochloride is chemically related to the narcotic analgesic meperidine.

Drug abuse and dependence: In doses used for the treatment of diarrhea, whether acute or chronic, diphenoxylate has not produced addiction.

Diphenoxylate hydrochloride is devoid of morphine-like subjective effects at therapeutic doses. At high doses it exhibits codeine-like subjective effects. The dose which produces antidiarrheal action is widely separated from the dose which causes central nervous system effects. The insolubility of diphenoxylate hydrochloride in commonly available aqueous media precludes intravenous self-administration. A dose of 100 to 300 mg/day, which is equivalent to 40 to 120 tablets, administered to humans for 40 to 70 days, produced opiate withdrawal symptoms. Since addiction to diphenoxylate hydrochloride is possible at high doses, the recommended dosage should not be exceeded.

Overdosage:
RECOMMENDED DOSAGE SCHEDULES SHOULD BE STRICTLY FOLLOWED. THIS MEDICATION SHOULD BE KEPT IN A CHILD-RESISTANT CONTAINER AND OUT OF THE REACH OF CHILDREN, SINCE AN OVERDOSAGE MAY RESULT IN SEVERE, EVEN FATAL, RESPIRATORY DEPRESSION.

Diagnosis: Initial signs of overdosage may include dryness of the skin and mucous membranes, mydriasis, restlessness, flushing, hyperthermia, and tachycardia followed by lethargy or coma, hypotonic reflexes, nystagmus, pinpoint pupils, and respiratory depression. Respiratory depression may be evidenced as late as 30 hours after ingestion and may recur in spite of an initial response to narcotic antagonists. TREAT ALL POSSIBLE LOMOTIL OVERDOSAGES AS SERIOUS AND MAINTAIN MEDICAL OBSERVATION FOR AT LEAST 48 HOURS, PREFERABLY UNDER CONTINUOUS HOSPITAL CARE.

Product Information

Treatment: In the event of overdose, induction of vomiting, gastric lavage, establishment of a patent airway, and possibly mechanically assisted respiration are advised. *In vitro* and animal studies indicate that activated charcoal may significantly decrease the bioavailability of diphenoxylate. In non-comatose patients, a slurry of 100 g of activated charcoal can be administered immediately after the induction of vomiting or gastric lavage.

A pure narcotic antagonist (eg, naloxone) should be used in the treatment of respiratory depression caused by Lomotil. When a narcotic antagonist is administered intravenously, the onset of action is generally apparent within two minutes. It may also be administered subcutaneously or intramuscularly, providing a slightly less rapid onset of action but a more prolonged effect.

To counteract respiratory depression caused by Lomotil overdosage, the following dosage schedule for the narcotic antagonist naloxone hydrochloride should be followed:

Adult dosage: The usual initial adult dose of naloxone hydrochloride is 0.4 mg (1 ml) administered intravenously. If respiratory function does not adequately improve after the initial dose, the same I.V. dose may be repeated at two- to three-minute intervals.

Children: The usual initial dose of naloxone hydrochloride for children is 0.01 mg/kg of body weight administered intravenously and repeated at two- to three-minute intervals if necessary.

Following initial improvement of respiratory function, repeated doses of naloxone hydrochloride may be required to counteract recurrent respiratory depression. Supplemental intramuscular doses of naloxone hydrochloride may be utilized to produce a longer-lasting effect.

Since the duration of action of diphenoxylate hydrochloride is longer than that of naloxone hydrochloride, improvement of respiration following administration may be followed by recurrent respiratory depression. Consequently, continuous observation is necessary until the effect of diphenoxylate hydrochloride on respiration has passed. This effect may persist for many hours. The period of observation should extend over at least 48 hours, preferably under continuous hospital care. Although signs of overdosage and respiratory depression may not be evident soon after ingestion of diphenoxylate hydrochloride, respiratory depression may occur from 12 to 30 hours later.

Dosage and Administration:
DO NOT EXCEED RECOMMENDED DOSAGE.

Adults: The recommended initial dosage is two Lomotil tablets four times daily or 10 ml (two regular teaspoonfuls) of Lomotil liquid four times daily (20 mg per day). Most patients will require this dosage until initial control has been achieved, after which the dosage may be reduced to meet individual requirements. Control may often be maintained with as little as 5 mg (two tablets or 10 ml of liquid) daily.

Clinical improvement of acute diarrhea is usually observed within 48 hours. If clinical improvement of chronic diarrhea after treatment with a maximum daily dose of 20 mg of diphenoxylate hydrochloride is not observed within 10 days, symptoms are unlikely to be controlled by further administration.

Children: Lomotil is not recommended in children under 2 years of age and should be used with special caution in young children (see *Warnings* and *Precautions*). The nutritional status and degree of dehydration must be considered. In children under 13 years of age, use Lomotil liquid. Do not use Lomotil tablets for this age group.

Only the plastic dropper should be used when measuring Lomotil liquid for administration to children.

Dosage schedule for children. The recommended initial total daily dosage of Lomotil liquid for children is 0.3 to 0.4 mg/kg, administered in four divided doses. The following table provides an *approximate* initial daily dosage recommendation for children.

Age (years)	Approximate weight (kg)	(lb)	Dosage in ml (four times daily)
2	11–14	24–31	1.5–3.0
3	12–16	26–35	2.0–3.0
4	14–20	31–44	2.0–4.0
5	16–23	35–51	2.5–4.5
6–8	17–32	38–71	2.5–5.0
9–12	23–55	51–121	3.5–5.0

These pediatric schedules are the best approximation of an average dose recommendation which may be adjusted downward according to the overall nutritional status and degree of dehydration encountered in the sick child. Reduction of dosage may be made as soon as initial control of symptoms has been achieved. Maintenance dosage may be as low as one-fourth of the initial daily dosage. If no response occurs within 48 hours, Lomotil is unlikely to be effective.

KEEP THIS AND ALL MEDICATIONS OUT OF THE REACH OF CHILDREN.

How Supplied:
Tablets—round, white, with SEARLE debossed on one side and 61 on the other side and containing 2.5 mg of diphenoxylate hydrochloride and 0.025 mg of atropine sulfate, supplied as:

NDC Number	Size
0014-0061-31	bottle of 100
0014-0061-51	bottle of 500
0014-0061-52	bottle of 1,000
0014-0061-55	bottle of 2,500
0014-0061-34	carton of 100 unit dose

Liquid—containing 2.5 mg of diphenoxylate hydrochloride and 0.025 mg of atropine sulfate per 5 ml; bottles of 2 fl oz (NDC Number 0014-0066-02). A plastic dropper calibrated in increments of ½ ml (¼ mg) with a capacity of 2 ml (1 mg) accompanies each 2-oz bottle of Lomotil liquid. Only this plastic dropper should be used when measuring Lomotil liquid for administration to children.

Shown in Product Identification Section, page 436

NORPACE® Capsules ℞
[nor′ pāce]
(disopyramide phosphate)
NORPACE® CR Capsules ℞
(disopyramide phosphate)
Controlled-Release

Description:
Norpace (disopyramide phosphate) is an antiarrhythmic drug available for oral administration in immediate-release and controlled-release capsules containing 100 mg or 150 mg of disopyramide base, present as the phosphate. The base content of the phosphate salt is 77.6%. The structural formula of Norpace is:

α-[2-(diisopropylamino)ethyl]-α-phenyl-2-pyridineacetamide phosphate

Norpace is freely soluble in water, and the free base (pKa 10.4) has an aqueous solubility of 1 mg/ml. The chloroform: water partition coefficient of the base is 3.1 at pH 7.2.

Norpace is a racemic mixture of *d*- and *l*-isomers. This drug is not chemically related to other antiarrhythmic drugs.

Norpace CR (controlled-release) capsules are designed to afford a gradual and consistent release of disopyramide. Thus, for maintenance therapy, Norpace CR provides the benefit of less frequent dosing (every 12 hours) as compared with the every-6-hour dosage schedule of immediate-release Norpace capsules.

Clinical Pharmacology:
Mechanisms of Action
Norpace (disopyramide phosphate) is a Type 1 antiarrhythmic drug (ie, similar to procainamide and quinidine). *In animal studies* Norpace decreases the rate of diastolic depolarization (phase 4) in cells with augmented automaticity, decreases the upstroke velocity (phase 0) and increases the action potential duration of normal cardiac cells, decreases the disparity in refractoriness between infarcted and adjacent normally perfused myocardium, and has no effect on alpha- or beta-adrenergic receptors.

Electrophysiology
In man, Norpace at therapeutic plasma levels shortens the sinus node recovery time, lengthens the effective refractory period of the atrium, and has a minimal effect on the effective refractory period of the AV node. Little effect has been shown on AV-nodal and His-Purkinje conduction times or QRS duration. However, prolongation of conduction in accessory pathways occurs.

Hemodynamics
At recommended oral doses, Norpace rarely produces significant alterations of blood pressure in patients without congestive heart failure (see *Warnings*). With intravenous Norpace, either increases in systolic/diastolic or decreases in systolic blood pressure have been reported, depending on the infusion rate and the patient population. Intravenous Norpace may cause cardiac depression with an approximate mean 10% reduction of cardiac output, which is more pronounced in patients with cardiac dysfunction.

Anticholinergic Activity
The *in vitro* anticholinergic activity of Norpace is approximately 0.06% that of atropine; however, the usual dose for Norpace is 150 mg every 6 hours and for Norpace CR 300 mg every 12 hours, compared to 0.4–0.6 mg for atropine (see *Warnings* and *Adverse Reactions* for anticholinergic side effects).

Pharmacokinetics
Following oral administration of immediate-release Norpace, disopyramide phosphate is rapidly and almost completely absorbed, and peak plasma levels are usually attained within 2 hours. The usual therapeutic plasma levels of disopyramide base are 2–4 mcg/ml, and at these concentrations protein binding varies from 50–65%. Because of concentration-dependent protein binding, it is difficult to predict the concentration of the free drug when total drug is measured.

The mean plasma half-life of disopyramide in healthy humans is 6.7 hours (range of 4 to 10 hours). In six patients with impaired renal function (creatinine clearance less than 40 ml/min), disopyramide half-life values were 8 to 18 hours. In healthy men about 50% of a given dose of disopyramide is excreted in the urine as the unchanged drug, about 20% as the mono-N-dealkylated metabolite, and 10% as the other metabolites. The plasma concentration of the major metabolite is approximately one tenth that of disopyramide. Altering the urinary pH in man does not affect the plasma half-life of disopyramide.

In a crossover study in healthy subjects, the bioavailability of disopyramide from Norpace CR capsules was similar to that from the immediate-release capsules. With a single 300-mg oral dose, peak disopyramide plasma concentrations of 3.23 ± 0.75 mcg/ml (mean ± SD) at 2.5 ± 2.3 hours were obtained with two 150-mg immediate-release capsules and 2.22 ± 0.47 mcg/ml at 4.9 ± 1.4 hours with two 150-mg Norpace CR capsules. The elimination half-life of disopyramide was 8.31 ± 1.83 hours with the immediate-release capsules and 11.65 ± 4.72 hours with Norpace CR capsules. The amount of disopyramide and mono-N-dealkylated metabolite excreted in the urine in 48 hours was 128 and 48 mg, respectively, with the immediate-release capsules, and 112 and 33 mg, respectively, with Norpace CR capsules. The differences in the urinary excretion of either constituent were not statistically significant.

Continued on next page

Searle & Co.—Cont.

Following multiple doses, steady-state plasma levels of between 2 and 4 mcg/ml were attained following either 150 mg every-6-hour dosing with immediate-release capsules or 300 mg every-12-hour dosing with Norpace CR capsules.

Indications and Usage:
Norpace or Norpace CR should be prescribed only after appropriate electrocardiographic assessment.

Norpace and Norpace CR are indicated for suppression and prevention of recurrence of the following cardiac arrhythmias when they occur singly or in combination:
1. Unifocal premature (ectopic) ventricular contractions.
2. Premature (ectopic) ventricular contractions of multifocal origin.
3. Paired premature ventricular contractions (couplets).
4. Episodes of ventricular tachycardia (persistent ventricular tachycardia is ordinarily treated with D.C.-cardioversion).

In controlled trials of ambulatory patients, 150 mg of Norpace every 6 hours was as effective as 325 mg of quinidine every 6 hours in reducing the frequency of ventricular ectopic activity. Norpace was equally effective in digitalized and nondigitalized patients. Norpace is also equally effective in the treatment of primary cardiac arrhythmias and those which occur in association with organic heart disease, including coronary artery disease. Oral disopyramide phosphate has not been adequately studied in patients with acute myocardial infarction or in patients with persistent ventricular tachycardia or atrial arrhythmias.

Norpace CR should not be used initially if rapid establishment of disopyramide plasma levels is desired.

Type 1 antiarrhythmic drugs are usually not effective in treating arrhythmias secondary to digitalis intoxication and, therefore, Norpace or Norpace CR is not indicated for such cases.

The value of antiarrhythmic drugs in preventing sudden death in patients with serious ventricular ectopic activity has not been established.

Contraindications:
Norpace and Norpace CR are contraindicated in the presence of cardiogenic shock, preexisting second- or third-degree AV block (if no pacemaker is present), or known hypersensitivity to the drug.

Warnings:
Negative Inotropic Properties:
Heart Failure/Hypotension
Norpace or Norpace CR may cause or worsen congestive heart failure or produce severe hypotension as a consequence of its negative inotropic properties. Hypotension has been observed primarily in patients with primary cardiomyopathy or inadequately compensated congestive heart failure. Norpace or Norpace CR should not be used in patients with uncompensated or marginally compensated congestive heart failure or hypotension unless the congestive heart failure or hypotension is secondary to cardiac arrhythmia. Patients with a history of heart failure may be treated with Norpace or Norpace CR, but careful attention must be given to the maintenance of cardiac function, including optimal digitalization. If hypotension occurs or congestive heart failure worsens, Norpace or Norpace CR should be discontinued and, if necessary, restarted at a lower dosage only after adequate cardiac compensation has been established.

QRS Widening
Although it is unusual, significant widening (greater than 25%) of the QRS complex may occur during Norpace or Norpace CR administration; in such cases Norpace or Norpace CR should be discontinued.

Q-T Prolongation
As with other Type 1 antiarrhythmic drugs, prolongation of the Q-T interval (corrected) and worsening of the arrhythmia, including ventricular tachycardia and ventricular fibrillation, may occur. Patients who have evidenced prolongation of the Q-T interval in response to quinidine may be at particular risk. If a Q-T prolongation of greater than 25% is observed and if ectopy continues, the patient should be monitored closely, and consideration be given to discontinuing Norpace or Norpace CR.

Hypoglycemia
In rare instances significant lowering of blood glucose values has been reported during Norpace administration. The physician should be alert to this possibility, especially in patients with congestive heart failure, chronic malnutrition, hepatic, renal, or other diseases, or drugs (eg, beta adrenoceptor blockers, alcohol) which could compromise preservation of the normal glucoregulatory mechanisms in the absence of food. In these patients the blood glucose levels should be carefully followed.

Concomitant Antiarrhythmic Therapy
The concomitant use of Norpace or Norpace CR with other Type 1 antiarrhythmic agents (such as quinidine or procainamide) and/or propranolol should be reserved for patients with life-threatening arrhythmias who are demonstrably unresponsive to single-agent antiarrhythmic therapy. Such use may produce serious negative inotropic effects, or may excessively prolong conduction. This should be considered particularly in patients with any degree of cardiac decompensation or those with a prior history thereof. Patients receiving more than one antiarrhythmic drug must be carefully monitored.

Heart Block
If first-degree heart block develops in a patient receiving Norpace or Norpace CR, the dosage should be reduced. If the block persists despite reduction of dosage, continuation of the drug must depend upon weighing the benefit being obtained against the risk of higher degrees of heart block. Development of second- or third-degree AV block or unifascicular, bifascicular, or trifascicular block requires discontinuation of Norpace or Norpace CR therapy, unless the ventricular rate is adequately controlled by a temporary or implanted ventricular pacemaker.

Anticholinergic Activity
Because of its anticholinergic activity, disopyramide phosphate should not be used in patients with glaucoma, myasthenia gravis, or urinary retention unless adequate overriding measures are taken; these consist of the topical application of potent miotics (eg, pilocarpine) for patients with glaucoma, and catheter drainage or operative relief for patients with urinary retention. Urinary retention may occur in patients of either sex as a consequence of Norpace or Norpace CR administration, but males with benign prostatic hypertrophy are at particular risk. In patients with a family history of glaucoma, intraocular pressure should be measured before initiating Norpace or Norpace CR therapy. Disopyramide phosphate should be used with special care in patients with myasthenia gravis since its anticholinergic properties could precipitate a myasthenic crisis in such patients.

Precautions:
General
Atrial Tachyarrhythmias
Patients with atrial flutter or fibrillation should be digitalized prior to Norpace or Norpace CR administration to ensure that drug-induced enhancement of AV conduction does not result in an increase of ventricular rate beyond physiologically acceptable limits.

Conduction Abnormalities
Care should be taken when prescribing Norpace or Norpace CR for patients with sick sinus syndrome (bradycardia-tachycardia syndrome), Wolff-Parkinson-White syndrome (WPW), or bundle branch block. The effect of disopyramide phosphate in these conditions is uncertain at present.

Cardiomyopathy
Patients with myocarditis or other cardiomyopathy may develop significant hypotension in response to the usual dosage of disopyramide phosphate, probably due to cardiodepressant mechanisms. Therefore, a loading dose of Norpace should not be given to such patients and initial dosage and subsequent dosage adjustments should be made under close supervision (see *Dosage and Administration*).

Renal Impairment
More than 50% of disopyramide is excreted in the urine unchanged. Therefore Norpace dosage should be reduced in patients with impaired renal function (see *Dosage and Administration*). The electrocardiogram should be carefully monitored for prolongation of PR interval, evidence of QRS widening, or other signs of overdosage (see *Overdosage*).

Norpace CR is not recommended for patients with severe renal insufficiency (creatinine clearance 40 ml/min or less).

Hepatic Impairment
Hepatic impairment also causes an increase in the plasma half-life of disopyramide. Dosage should be reduced for patients with such impairment. The electrocardiogram should be carefully monitored for signs of overdosage (see *Overdosage*).

Patients with cardiac dysfunction have a higher potential for hepatic impairment; this should be considered when administering Norpace or Norpace CR.

Potassium Imbalance
Antiarrhythmic drugs may be ineffective in patients with hypokalemia, and their toxic effects may be enhanced in patients with hyperkalemia. Therefore, potassium abnormalities should be corrected before starting Norpace or Norpace CR therapy.

Drug Interactions
If phenytoin or other hepatic enzyme inducers are taken concurrently with Norpace or Norpace CR, lower plasma levels of disopyramide may occur. Monitoring of disopyramide plasma levels is recommended in such concurrent use to avoid ineffective therapy. Other antiarrhythmic drugs (eg, quinidine, procainamide, lidocaine, propranolol) have occasionally been used concurrently with Norpace but no specific drug interaction studies have been conducted (see *Warnings*). Excessive widening of the QRS complex and/or prolongation of the Q-T interval may occur in these situations. Norpace does not increase serum digoxin levels.

Pregnancy
Reproduction studies in rats and teratology studies performed both in rats and in rabbits have revealed minimal evidence of impaired fertility. No fetal anomalies were attributable to Norpace. Disopyramide has been found in human fetal blood. However, well-controlled studies of Norpace have not been performed in pregnant women and experience with Norpace during pregnancy is limited; therefore the possibility of damage to the fetus cannot be excluded. Norpace has been reported to stimulate contractions of the pregnant uterus. Norpace or Norpace CR should be used in pregnant women only when it is clearly indicated and the benefit/risk ratio has been carefully evaluated.

Labor and Delivery
It is not known whether the use of Norpace or Norpace CR during labor or delivery has immediate or delayed adverse effects on the fetus, or whether it prolongs the duration of labor or increases the need for forceps delivery or other obstetric intervention.

Nursing Mothers
Studies in rats have shown that the concentration of disopyramide and its metabolites is between one and three times greater in milk than it is in plasma. Following oral administration, disopyramide has been detected in human milk at a concentration not exceeding that in plasma. Therefore, if use of the drug is deemed essential, an alternative method of infant feeding should be instituted.

Adverse Reactions:
The adverse reactions which were reported in Norpace clinical trials encompass observations in 1,500 patients, including 90 patients studied for at least 4 years. The most serious adverse reactions are hypotension and congestive heart failure. The

most common adverse reactions, which are dose dependent, are associated with the anticholinergic properties of the drug. These may be transitory, but may be persistent or can be severe. Urinary retention is the most serious anticholinergic effect.

The following reactions were reported in 10–40% of patients:

Anticholinergic: dry mouth (32%), urinary hesitancy (14%), constipation (11%)

The following reactions were reported in 3–9% of patients:

Anticholinergic: blurred vision, dry nose/eyes/throat
Genitourinary: urinary retention, urinary frequency and urgency
Gastrointestinal: nausea, pain/bloating/gas
General: dizziness, general fatigue/muscle weakness, headache, malaise, aches/pains

The following reactions were reported in 1–3% of patients:

Genitourinary: impotence
Cardiovascular: hypotension with or without congestive heart failure, increased congestive heart failure (see *Warnings*), cardiac conduction disturbances (see *Warnings*), edema/weight gain, shortness of breath, syncope, chest pain
Gastrointestinal: anorexia, diarrhea, vomiting
Dermatologic: generalized rash/dermatoses, itching
Central nervous system: nervousness
Other: hypokalemia, elevated cholesterol/triglycerides

The following reactions were reported in less than 1%:

Depression, insomnia, dysuria, numbness/tingling, elevated liver enzymes, AV block, elevated BUN, elevated creatinine, decreased hemoglobin/hematocrit

Hypoglycemia has been reported in association with Norpace administration (see *Warnings*).

Infrequent occurrences of reversible cholestatic jaundice, fever, and respiratory difficulty have been reported in association with disopyramide therapy, as have rare instances of thrombocytopenia, reversible agranulocytosis, and gynecomastia. Rarely, acute psychosis has been reported following Norpace therapy, with prompt return to normal mental status when therapy was stopped. The physician should be aware of these possible reactions and should discontinue Norpace or Norpace CR therapy promptly if they occur.

Overdosage:
Symptoms
Deliberate or accidental overdose of oral disopyramide may be followed by apnea, loss of consciousness, cardiac arrhythmias, and loss of spontaneous respiration. Death has occurred following overdose.

Toxic plasma levels of disopyramide produce excessive widening of the QRS complex and Q-T interval, worsening of congestive heart failure, hypotension, varying kinds and degrees of conduction disturbance, bradycardia, and finally asystole. Obvious anticholinergic effects are also observed.

Treatment
Experience indicates that prompt and vigorous treatment of overdosage is necessary even in the absence of symptoms. Such treatment may be lifesaving. No specific antidote for disopyramide phosphate has been identified. Treatment should be symptomatic and may include induction of emesis or gastric lavage, administration of a cathartic followed by activated charcoal by mouth or stomach tube, intravenous administration of isoproterenol and dopamine, insertion of an intra-aortic balloon for counterpulsation, and mechanically assisted ventilation. Hemodialysis or, preferably, hemoperfusion with charcoal may be employed to lower serum concentration of the drug.

The electrocardiogram should be monitored, and supportive therapy with cardiac glycosides and diuretics should be given as required.

If progressive AV block should develop, endocardial pacing should be implemented. In case of any impaired renal function, measures to increase the glomerular filtration rate may reduce the toxicity (disopyramide is excreted primarily by the kidney).

The anticholinergic effects can be reversed with neostigmine at the discretion of the physician. Altering the urinary pH in humans does not affect the plasma half-life or the amount of disopyramide excreted in the urine.

Dosage and Administration:
The dosage of Norpace or Norpace CR must be individualized for each patient on the basis of response and tolerance. The usual adult dosage of Norpace or Norpace CR is 400 to 800 mg per day given in divided doses. The recommended dosage for most adults is 600 mg/day given in divided doses (either 150 mg every 6 hours for immediate-release Norpace or 300 mg every 12 hours for Norpace CR). For patients whose body weight is less than 110 pounds (50 kg), the recommended dosage is 400 mg/day given in divided doses (either 100 mg every 6 hours for immediate-release Norpace or 200 mg every 12 hours for Norpace CR).

For patients with cardiomyopathy or possible cardiac decompensation, a loading dose, as discussed below, should not be given and initial dosage should be limited to 100 mg of immediate-release Norpace every 6 hours. Subsequent dosage adjustments should be made gradually, with close monitoring for the possible development of hypotension and/or congestive heart failure (see *Warnings*).

For patients with moderate renal insufficiency (creatinine clearance greater than 40 ml/min) or hepatic insufficiency, the recommended dosage is 400 mg/day given in divided doses (either 100 mg every 6 hours for immediate-release Norpace or 200 mg every 12 hours for Norpace CR).

For patients with severe renal insufficiency (C_{cr} 40 ml/min or less) the recommended dosage regimen of immediate-release Norpace is 100 mg at intervals shown in the table below, with or without an initial loading dose of 150 mg.

IMMEDIATE-RELEASE NORPACE DOSAGE INTERVAL FOR PATIENTS WITH RENAL INSUFFICIENCY

Creatinine clearance (ml/min)	40–30	30–15	less than 15
Approximate maintenance-dosing interval	q 8 hr	q 12 hr	q 24 hr

The above dosing schedules are for Norpace immediate-release capsules; Norpace CR is not recommended for patients with severe renal insufficiency.

For patients in whom rapid control of ventricular arrhythmia is essential, an initial loading dose of 300 mg of immediate-release Norpace (200 mg for patients whose body weight is less than 110 pounds) is recommended, followed by the appropriate maintenance dosage. Therapeutic effects are usually attained 30 minutes to 3 hours after administration of a 300-mg loading dose. If there is no response or evidence of toxicity within 6 hours of the loading dose, 200 mg of immediate-release Norpace every 6 hours may be prescribed instead of the usual 150 mg. If there is no response to this dosage within 48 hours, either Norpace should then be discontinued or the physician should consider hospitalizing the patient for careful monitoring while subsequent immediate-release Norpace doses of 250 mg or 300 mg every 6 hours are given. A limited number of patients with severe refractory ventricular tachycardia have tolerated daily doses of Norpace up to 1600 mg per day (400 mg every 6 hours) resulting in disopyramide plasma levels up to 9 mcg/ml. If such treatment is warranted, it is essential that patients be hospitalized for close evaluation and continuous monitoring.

Norpace CR should not be used initially if rapid establishment of disopyramide plasma levels is desired.

Transferring to Norpace or Norpace CR
The following dosage schedule based on theoretical considerations rather than experimental data is suggested for transferring patients with normal renal function from either quinidine sulfate or procainamide therapy (Type 1 antiarrhythmic agents) to Norpace or Norpace CR therapy:

Norpace or Norpace CR should be started using the regular maintenance schedule **without a loading dose** 6–12 hours after the last dose of quinidine sulfate or 3–6 hours after the last dose of procainamide.

In patients in whom withdrawal of quinidine sulfate or procainamide is likely to produce life-threatening arrhythmias, the physician should consider hospitalization of the patient. When transferring a patient from immediate-release Norpace to Norpace CR, the maintenance schedule of Norpace CR may be started 6 hours after the last dose of immediate-release Norpace.

Pediatric Dosage
Controlled clinical studies have not been conducted in pediatric patients; however, the following suggested dosage table is based on published clinical experience.

Total daily dosage should be divided and equal doses administered orally every 6 hours or at intervals according to individual patient needs. Disopyramide plasma levels and therapeutic response must be monitored closely. Patients should be hospitalized during the initial treatment period, and dose titration should start at the lower end of the ranges provided below.

SUGGESTED TOTAL DAILY DOSAGE*

Age (years)	Disopyramide (mg/kg body weight/day)
Under 1	10 to 30
1 to 4	10 to 20
4 to 12	10 to 15
12 to 18	6 to 15

* Dosage is expressed in milligrams of disopyramide base. Since Norpace (disopyramide phosphate) 100-mg capsules contain 100 mg of disopyramide base, the pharmacist can readily prepare a 1-mg/ml to 10-mg/ml liquid suspension by adding the entire contents of Norpace capsules to cherry syrup, NF. The resulting suspension, when refrigerated, is stable for one month and should be thoroughly shaken before the measurement of each dose. The suspension should be dispensed in an amber glass bottle with a child-resistant closure.

Norpace CR capsules should not be used to prepare the above suspension.

How Supplied
Norpace (disopyramide phosphate) is supplied in hard gelatin capsules containing either 100 mg or 150 mg of disopyramide base, present as the phosphate.

Norpace 100-mg capsules are white and orange, with markings SEARLE, 2752, Norpace, and 100 MG.

Norpace 150-mg capsules are brown and orange, with markings SEARLE, 2762, Norpace, and 150 MG.

Available in bottles of 100, 500, and 1,000 capsules, and cartons of 100 unit-dose individually blister-sealed capsules.

Norpace CR (disopyramide phosphate) Controlled-Release is supplied as specially prepared controlled-release beads in hard gelatin capsules containing either 100 mg or 150 mg of disopyramide base, present as the phosphate.

Norpace CR 100-mg capsules are white and light green, with markings SEARLE, 2732, NORPACE CR, and 100 mg.

Norpace CR 150-mg capsules are brown and light green, with markings SEARLE, 2742, NORPACE CR, and 150 mg.

Available in bottles of 100 and 500 capsules, and cartons of 100 unit-dose individually blister-sealed capsules.

Continued on next page

Searle & Co.—Cont.

Certain manufacturing operations for Norpace CR have been performed by G. D. Searle & Co. LTD., Morpeth, England.

Shown in Product Identification Section, page 436

OVULEN-21®
OVULEN-28®
[*ov'ū-len*]
(ethynodiol diacetate with mestranol)

See Demulen products under Searle & Co. for Ovulen prescribing information.

Shown in Product Identification Section, page 436

PRO-BANTHĪNE® Tablets
[*prō-ban'thīne*]
(propantheline bromide USP)

Description: Pro-Banthīne oral tablets contain 15 mg or 7½ mg of the anticholinergic propantheline bromide, (2-hydroxyethyl)diisopropylmethylammonium bromide xanthene-9-carboxylate. The structural formula of Pro-Banthīne is:

Clinical Pharmacology: Pro-Banthīne inhibits gastrointestinal motility and diminishes gastric acid secretion. The drug also inhibits the action of acetylcholine at the postganglionic nerve endings of the parasympathetic nervous system.

Propantheline bromide is extensively metabolized in man primarily by hydrolysis to the inactive materials xanthene-9-carboxylic acid and (2-hydroxyethyl) diisopropylmethylammonium bromide. After a single 30-mg oral dose given as two 15-mg tablets the mean peak plasma concentration of propantheline was 21 ng/ml at one hour in six healthy subjects.

The plasma elimination half-life of propantheline is about 1.6 hours. Approximately 70% of the dose is excreted in the urine, mostly as metabolites. The urinary excretion of propantheline is about 3% after oral tablet administration.

Indications and Usage: Pro-Banthīne is effective as adjunctive therapy in the treatment of peptic ulcer.

Contraindications: Pro-Banthīne (propantheline bromide) is contraindicated in patients with:
1. Glaucoma, since mydriasis is to be avoided.
2. Obstructive disease of the gastrointestinal tract (pyloroduodenal stenosis, achalasia, paralytic ileus, etc).
3. Obstructive uropathy (eg, bladder-neck obstruction due to prostatic hypertrophy).
4. Intestinal atony of elderly or debilitated patients.
5. Severe ulcerative colitis or toxic megacolon complicating ulcerative colitis.
6. Unstable cardiovascular adjustment in acute hemorrhage.
7. Myasthenia gravis.

Warnings: In the presence of a high environmental temperature, heat prostration (fever and heat stroke due to decreased sweating) can occur with the use of Pro-Banthīne.

Diarrhea may be an early symptom of incomplete intestinal obstruction, especially in patients with ileostomy or colostomy. In this instance treatment with Pro-Banthīne would be inappropriate and possibly harmful.

With overdosage, a curare-like action may occur (ie, neuromuscular blockade leading to muscular weakness and possible paralysis).

Pro-Banthīne may cause increased heart rate and, therefore, should be used with caution in patients with heart disease.

Precautions: General: Pro-Banthīne (propantheline bromide) should be used with caution in the elderly and in all patients with autonomic neuropathy, hepatic or renal disease, hyperthyroidism, coronary heart disease, congestive heart failure, cardiac tachyarrhythmias, hypertension, or hiatal hernia associated with reflux esophagitis, since anticholinergics may aggravate this condition.

In patients with ulcerative colitis, large doses of Pro-Banthīne may suppress intestinal motility to the point of producing paralytic ileus and, for this reason, may precipitate or aggravate toxic megacolon, a serious complication of the disease.

Information for patients: Pro-Banthīne may produce drowsiness or blurred vision. The patient should be cautioned regarding activities requiring mental alertness, such as operating a motor vehicle or other machinery or performing hazardous work, while taking this drug.

Drug interactions: Anticholinergics may delay absorption of other medication given concomitantly.

Excessive cholinergic blockade may occur if Pro-Banthīne is given concomitantly with belladonna alkaloids, synthetic or semisynthetic anticholinergic agents, narcotic analgesics such as meperidine, Type 1 antiarrhythmic drugs (eg, disopyramide, procainamide, or quinidine), antihistamines, phenothiazines, tricyclic antidepressants, or other psychoactive drugs. Pro-Banthīne may also potentiate the sedative effect of phenothiazines. Increased intraocular pressure may result from concurrent administration of anticholinergics and corticosteroids.

Concurrent use of Pro-Banthīne with slow-dissolving tablets of digoxin may cause increased serum digoxin levels. This interaction can be avoided by using only those digoxin tablets that rapidly dissolve by USP standards.

Carcinogenesis, mutagenesis, impairment of fertility: No long-term fertility, carcinogenicity, or mutagenicity studies have been done with Pro-Banthīne.

Pregnancy. Pregnancy Category C. Animal reproduction studies have not been conducted with Pro-Banthīne. It is also not known whether Pro-Banthīne can cause fetal harm when administered to a pregnant woman or can affect reproduction capacity. Pro-Banthīne should be given to a pregnant woman only if clearly needed.

Nursing mothers: It is not known whether this drug is excreted in human milk. Because many drugs are excreted in human milk, caution should be exercised when Pro-Banthīne is administered to a nursing woman. Suppression of lactation may occur with anticholinergic drugs.

Pediatric use: Safety and effectiveness in children have not been established.

Adverse Reactions: Varying degrees of drying of salivary secretions may occur as well as decreased sweating. Ophthalmic side effects include blurred vision, mydriasis, cycloplegia, and increased ocular tension. Other reported adverse reactions include urinary hesitancy and retention, tachycardia, palpitations, loss of the sense of taste, headache, nervousness, mental confusion, drowsiness, weakness, dizziness, insomnia, nausea, vomiting, constipation, bloated feeling, impotence, suppression of lactation, and allergic reactions or drug idiosyncracies, including anaphylaxis, urticaria, and other dermal manifestations.

Overdosage: The symptoms of overdosage with Pro-Banthīne progress from an intensification of the usual side effects to CNS disturbances (from restlessness and excitement to psychotic behavior), circulatory changes (flushing, fall in blood pressure, circulatory failure), respiratory failure, paralysis, and coma.

Measures to be taken are (1) immediate induction of emesis or lavage of the stomach, (2) injection of physostigmine 0.5 to 2 mg intravenously, repeated as necessary up to a total of 5 mg, and (3) monitoring of vital signs and managing as necessary.

Fever may be treated symptomatically (cooling blanket or alcohol sponging). Excitement of a degree which demands attention may be managed with thiopental sodium 2% solution given slowly intravenously or diazepam, 5 to 10 mg intravenously or 10 mg intramuscularly. In the event of progression of the curare-like effect to paralysis of the respiratory muscles, mechanical respiration should be instituted and maintained until effective respiratory action returns.

Dosage and Administration: The usual initial adult dosage of Pro-Banthīne tablets is 15 mg taken 30 minutes before each meal and 30 mg at bedtime (a total of 75 mg daily). Subsequent dosage adjustment should be made according to the patient's individual response and tolerance. The administration of one 7½-mg tablet three times a day is convenient for patients with mild manifestations, for geriatric patients, and for those of small stature.

How Supplied:
Pro-Banthīne 15-mg tablets are round, peach colored, sugar coated, with SEARLE imprinted on one side and 601 on the other side; bottles of 100 and 500, and cartons containing 100 unit-dose, individually blister-sealed tablets.

Pro-Banthīne 7½-mg tablets are round, white, sugar coated, with SEARLE imprinted on one side and 611 on the other side; bottles of 100.

Shown in Product Identification Section, page 436

PRO-BANTHĪNE® with PHENOBARBITAL Tablets
[*pro-ban-thine with phē-nō-bar-bih-tal*]
(propantheline bromide with phenobarbital)

Description:
Pro-Banthīne with Phenobarbital oral tablets contain:
propantheline bromide............................ 15 mg
phenobarbital .... 15 mg
(Warning—May be habit forming.)

Propantheline bromide, an anticholinergic, is (2-hydroxyethyl) diisopropylmethylammonium bromide xanthene-9-carboxylate and has the following structure:

Phenobarbital, a sedative, is 5-ethyl-5-phenylbarbituric acid and has the following structure:

For *Clinical Pharmacology* see Pro-Banthīne Tablets.

Indications and Usage:

Based on a review of this drug by the National Academy of Sciences—National Research Council and/or other information, FDA has classified the indications as follows:
"Possibly" effective: as adjunctive therapy in the treatment of peptic ulcer and in the treatment of the irritable bowel syndrome (irritable colon, spastic colon, mucous colitis, acute enterocolitis, and functional gastrointestinal disorders).
Final classification of the less-than-effective indications requires further investigation.

Contraindications are the same as those shown for Pro-Banthīne, plus the following:
8. Porphyria.

Warnings are the same as those shown for Pro-Banthīne, plus the following fifth paragraph:

PHENOBARBITAL MAY BE HABIT FORMING.

Precautions are the same as those shown for Pro-Banthine, *plus the following:*

Under the **Drug Interactions** subsection, add the following fourth paragraph:
As phenobarbital is a potent microsomal enzyme inducer, it may decrease the prothrombin-time response to oral anticoagulants. More frequent monitoring of prothrombin-time responses is indicated whenever phenobarbital is initiated or discontinued, and the dosage of anticoagulants should be adjusted accordingly.

The **Pregnancy** *subsection should read as follows:*
Pregnancy: Pregnancy Category C. Animal reproduction studies have not been conducted with propantheline bromide. It is also not known whether propantheline bromide can cause fetal harm when administered to a pregnant woman or can affect reproduction capacity.
A reproductive study in rats concluded that the administration of phenobarbital given as a single daily subcutaneous dose of 40 mg/kg, from the twelfth to the nineteenth day of pregnancy, resulted in altered reproductive function in the female offspring, as evidenced by delayed onset of puberty, disorders in the estrous cycle, and infertility. An increased incidence of congenital malformations in humans has also been reported in response to phenobarbital exposure in utero. There are no adequate and well-controlled studies in pregnant women.
Pro-Banthine with Phenobarbital should be given to a pregnant woman only if clearly needed.

Adverse Reactions: With propantheline bromide, varying degrees of drying of salivary secretions may occur as well as decreased sweating. Ophthalmic side effects include blurred vision, mydriasis, cycloplegia, and increased ocular tension. Other reported adverse reactions include urinary hesitancy and retention, tachycardia, palpitations, loss of the sense of taste, headache, nervousness, mental confusion, drowsiness, weakness, dizziness, insomnia, nausea, vomiting, constipation, bloated feeling, impotence, suppression of lactation, and allergic reactions or drug idiosyncracies, including anaphylaxis, urticaria, and other dermal manifestations.
In some patients, phenobarbital may produce excitement rather than a sedative effect. Some patients may acquire a sensitivity to barbiturates.

The **Overdosage** *section is the same as shown for Pro-Banthine, plus the following fourth paragraph:*
While the usual procedures for handling anticholinergic poisoning should be employed, the possibility of barbiturate overdosing effects should be kept in mind.

Dosage and Administration: The usual adult dosage of Pro-Banthine with Phenobarbital is one or two tablets three or four times daily.

How Supplied: Pro-Banthine with Phenobarbital tablets containing 15 mg of propantheline bromide and 15 mg of phenobarbital are round, ivory colored, sugar coated, with SEARLE imprinted on one side and 631 on the other side; bottles of 100, and cartons containing 100 unit-dose, individually blister-sealed tablets.
Shown in Product Identification Section, page 436

THEO-24®
[thē'ō-24]
(theophylline anhydrous)

Description: Theo-24 oral capsules contain 100 mg, 200 mg, or 300 mg of anhydrous theophylline, a bronchodilator, in a controlled-release formulation which allows a 24-hour dosing interval for appropriate patients.
The structural formula of theophylline, 1,3-dimethylxanthine, is: (See next column)
Theophylline is a white, odorless, crystalline powder having a bitter taste.

Clinical Pharmacology: Theophylline directly relaxes the smooth muscle of the bronchial airways and pulmonary blood vessels, thus acting mainly as a bronchodilator and smooth muscle

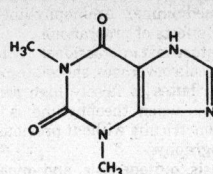

relaxant. The drug also possesses other actions typical of the xanthine derivatives: coronary vasodilation, cardiac stimulation, diuresis, cerebral stimulation, and skeletal muscle stimulation. The actions of theophylline may be mediated through inhibition of phosphodiesterase and a resultant increase in intracellular cyclic AMP. *In vitro*, theophylline also has been shown to act synergistically with beta agonists that increase intracellular cyclic AMP through the stimulation of adenyl cyclase. More data are needed to determine if theophylline and beta agonists have a clinically important additive effect *in vivo*.

Pharmacokinetics:

Theophylline Elimination Characteristics

	Theophylline Clearance Rates (mean ± S.D.)	Half-Life Average (mean ± S.D.)
Children (over 6 months of age)	1.45 ± 0.58 ml/kg/min	3.7 ± 1.1 hr
Adult nonsmokers with uncomplicated asthma	0.65 ± 0.19 ml/kg/min	8.7 ± 2.2 hr

The half-life of theophylline is prolonged in patients with alcoholism, reduced hepatic or renal function, or congestive heart failure, and in patients receiving cimetidine or macrolide antibiotics such as troleandomycin and erythromycin. High fever for prolonged periods may reduce the rate of theophylline elimination.
Newborn infants have extremely slow theophylline clearance rates. The theophylline half-life in newborn infants may exceed 24 hours. Not until the age of 3 to 6 months do clearance rates approach those seen in older children.
Patients over age 55 and patients with chronic obstructive pulmonary disease, cardiac failure, or liver insufficiency may have much slower clearance rates with half-lives that exceed 24 hours. The average half-life of theophylline in smokers (1 to 2 packs/day) is 4 to 5 hours; the average half-life in nonsmokers is 7 to 10 hours. The increase in theophylline clearance caused by smoking is probably the result of induction of drug-metabolizing enzymes. The effect of smoking on theophylline pharmacokinetics may persist for 3 months to 2 years after smoking is discontinued.
Tolerance does not appear to develop during long-term use of theophylline.
Theo-24 capsules contain hundreds of coated beads of theophylline. Each bead is an individual controlled-release delivery system. After dissolution of the capsules these beads are released and distributed throughout the gastrointestinal tract, thus minimizing the occurrence of high local concentrations of theophylline at any particular site. The beads have been designed to provide a prolonged and reproducible gastrointestinal transit time. As a result, Theo-24 provides theophylline serum levels for 24 hours with a single daily dose in appropriate patients.
Following the single-dose administration (8 mg/kg) of Theo-24 to 20 normal subjects who had fasted overnight and 2 hours after morning dosing, peak serum theophylline concentrations of 4.8 ± 1.5 (S.D.) mcg/ml were obtained at 13.3 ± 4.7 (S.D.) hours. The fraction of the amount of the dose absorbed was approximately 13% at 3 hours, 31% at 6 hours, 55% at 12 hours, 70% at 16 hours, and 88% at 24 hours. The extent of theophylline bioavailability from Theo-24 was comparable to the most widely used 12-hour controlled-release product when both products were administered every 12 hours.
In a 6-day multiple-dose study involving 18 subjects (with theophylline clearance rates between 0.57 and 1.02 ml/kg/min) who had fasted overnight and 2 hours after morning dosing, Theo-24 given once daily in a dose of 1500 mg produced serum theophylline levels that ranged between 5.7 mcg/ml and 22 mcg/ml. The mean minimum and maximum values were 11.6 mcg/ml and 18.1 mcg/ml, respectively, with an average peak-trough difference of 6.5 mcg/ml. A 24-hour single-dose study demonstrated an approximately proportional increase in serum levels as the dose was increased from 600 to 1500 mg.

Indications and Usage: Theo-24 is indicated for the relief and/or prevention of symptoms of bronchial asthma and for reversible bronchospasm associated with chronic bronchitis and emphysema.

Contraindications: Theo-24 (theophylline anhydrous) is contraindicated in patients who have shown hypersensitivity to theophylline.

Warnings: Status asthmaticus is a medical emergency and is defined as that degree of bronchospasm not rapidly responsive to recommended doses of usual bronchodilators. Oral theophylline alone is not appropriate treatment for status asthmaticus. Patients with status asthmaticus require *medication administered parenterally* and *close monitoring,* preferably in an intensive-care setting.
Optimum therapeutic response occurs in many patients when the serum theophylline concentration is 10 to 20 mcg/ml. In other patients satisfactory results (as determined by both relief of symptoms and improvement in pulmonary function) may be obtained at lower levels. In still others, adequate response may require higher levels. The physician should adjust the desired serum concentration range to the patients' requirements, keeping in mind that *an increased probability of toxicity exists when levels exceed 20 mcg/ml.* Therefore, in order to assure maximum benefit without excessive risk, measurement of serum levels is highly recommended.
Serum levels above 20 mcg/ml are rarely found after appropriate administration of the recommended doses. However, in individuals in whom theophylline plasma clearance is reduced *for any reason,* even conventional doses may result in increased serum levels with subsequent toxicity. Reduced theophylline clearance has been documented in the following readily identifiable groups:
1. Patients with impaired renal or liver function.
2. Patients over 55 years of age, particularly males and those with chronic lung disease.
3. Patients with cardiac failure from any cause.
4. Neonates.
5. Patients taking certain drugs (macrolide antibiotics or cimetidine).

Decreased clearance of theophylline may be associated with either influenza immunization or active influenza, and with other viral infections. Reduction of dosage and measurement of serum theophylline levels are especially appropriate in the above individuals.
Although the effects of theophylline are dose related, *serious toxicity is not reliably preceded by less severe side effects.* Ventricular arrhythmias, convulsions, or even death may appear as the first sign of toxicity without previous warning. Less serious signs of theophylline toxicity (ie, nausea and restlessness) may appear in up to 50% of these patients.
Patients who require theophylline may exhibit tachycardia due to the underlying disease process so that the cause/effect relationship to elevated serum theophylline concentrations will not be recognized.
Theophylline products may cause arrhythmia or worsen preexisting arrhythmia. Any significant change in cardiac rate and/or rhythm warrants monitoring and further investigation.

Continued on next page

Searle & Co.—Cont.

In minipigs, rodents, and dogs, arrhythmia and sudden death (with histological evidence of myocardial necrosis) have been observed when theophylline and beta agonists were administered concomitantly but not when either was administered alone. The significance of these findings for human use is unknown.

Precautions: General: Use with caution in patients with severe cardiac disease, hypertension, acute myocardial injury, congestive heart failure, cor pulmonale, severe hypoxemia, hyperthyroidism, hepatic impairment, or alcoholism, and in the elderly (especially males) and in neonates. Particular caution should be used in administering theophylline to patients with congestive heart failure. Reduced theophylline clearance in these patients may cause serum theophylline levels to persist long after the drug is discontinued.

Individuals who are rapid metabolizers of theophylline (such as the young, smokers, and some nonsmoking adults) may not be suitable candidates for once-a-day dosing. Dividing the daily dose into two doses may be indicated if symptoms of bronchospasm occur repeatedly, especially near the end of a 24-hour dosing interval, or if the patient exhibits wider peak-trough differences than desired.

Convulsions may occur in patients with theophylline overdosage when serum theophylline concentrations exceed 30 mcg/ml. Theophylline may lower the seizure threshold.

Theophylline should not be administered concomitantly with other xanthine medications.

Methylxanthines are known to increase gastric acidity. Therefore, theophylline should be used cautiously in patients with a history of peptic ulcer since the disease may be exacerbated. Theophylline may occasionally act as a local irritant to the gastrointestinal tract, although gastrointestinal symptoms are more commonly mediated through the central nervous system and are usually associated with serum drug concentrations over 20 mcg/ml.

Food effects: Taking Theo-24 (theophylline anhydrous) with food may result in a significant increase in peak serum level and in the extent of absorption of theophylline as compared to administration in the fasted state. In some cases (especially with once-daily doses of 900 mg or more taken with food) serum theophylline levels may exceed the 20 mcg/ml level, above which theophylline toxicity is more likely to occur.

Information for patients: Patients should be instructed to take this medication in the morning, at approximately the same time each day, and to not exceed the prescribed dose.

Patients should be informed of the potential effect of food on the absorption of theophylline from Theo-24. Patients taking Theo-24 in once-daily doses equal to or greater than 900 mg or 13 mg/kg (whichever is less) should take the drug after fasting overnight and approximately two hours before eating. If the patient cannot comply with this regimen, he/she should be placed on alternative therapy such as twice-daily dosing. Patients receiving once-daily doses of less than 900 mg should be closely monitored.

As with any controlled-release theophylline product the patient should alert the physician if symptoms occur repeatedly, especially near the end of a dosing interval.

Laboratory tests: The determination of serum theophylline levels is highly recommended.

Drug interactions: Elevated serum levels of theophylline may occur in patients treated concomitantly with theophylline and cimetidine, troleandomycin, or erythromycin. Therefore, such patients should be watched carefully for signs of theophylline toxicity and the dose of theophylline decreased if necessary. Increased toxicity may occur when ephedrine or other sympathomimetic drugs are given concomitantly with theophylline. The excretion of lithium carbonate is increased in patients receiving aminophylline (theophylline with ethylenediamine). Aminophylline may antagonize the effects of propranolol.

Drug/Laboratory test interactions: Consumption of coffee, tea, cola beverages, chocolate, or acetaminophen contributes to falsely high serum theophylline levels when theophylline is measured spectrophotometrically without previous isolation by chromatography.

Carcinogenesis, mutagenesis, and impairment of fertility: Long-term animal studies have not been performed with theophylline to evaluate carcinogenic potential, mutagenic potential, or effect on fertility.

Pregnancy: Pregnancy Category C. Animal reproduction studies have not been conducted with theophylline. It is not known whether theophylline can cause fetal harm when administered to a pregnant woman or can affect reproductive capacity. Xanthines should be given to a pregnant woman only if clearly needed.

Nursing mothers: Theophylline is secreted in breast milk and may cause adverse effects in the infant. Caution must be used when prescribing theophylline to a nursing mother, taking into account the risk/benefit of this therapy.

Pediatric use: Safety and effectiveness in children under 12 years of age have not been established with this product.

Adverse Reactions: The most consistent adverse reactions are usually due to overdose and are:
1. Gastrointestinal: nausea, vomiting, epigastric pain, hematemesis, diarrhea.
2. Central nervous system: headaches, irritability, restlessness, insomnia, reflex hyperexcitability, muscle twitching, clonic and tonic generalized convulsions, coma.
3. Cardiovascular: palpitation, tachycardia, extrasystoles, flushing, hypotension, circulatory failure, ventricular arrhythmias.
4. Respiratory: tachypnea.
5. Renal: albuminuria, microhematuria, potentiation of diuresis.
6. Other: hyperglycemia and inappropriate ADH (antidiuretic hormone) syndrome.

Overdosage: Management: If overdose following oral administration is suspected and a seizure has not occurred:
A. Induce vomiting or perform gastric lavage.
B. Administer activated charcoal.
C. Administer a cathartic, particularly if a controlled-release preparation has been taken.

If patient is having a seizure:
A. Establish an airway.
B. Administer oxygen.
C. Treat the seizure with intravenous diazepam, 0.1 to 0.3 mg/kg up to 10 mg.
D. Monitor vital signs, maintain blood pressure, and provide adequate hydration.

If patient is in post-seizure coma:
A. Maintain airway and oxygenation.
B. Gastric lavage must be performed and a cathartic and activated charcoal introduced via a large-bore tube.
C. Continue to provide full supportive care and adequate hydration while waiting for drug to be metabolized. The drug is metabolized rapidly enough by most patients so that dialysis is usually not needed. If serum levels exceed 50 mcg/ml, charcoal hemoperfusion may be indicated.

Dosage and Administration: Effective use of theophylline (ie, the concentration of drug in the serum associated with optimal benefit and minimal risk of toxicity) is considered to occur when the theophylline concentration is maintained from 10 to 20 mcg/ml. The early studies from which these levels were derived were carried out in patients immediately or shortly after recovery from acute exacerbations of their disease (some hospitalized with status asthmaticus).

Although the 20 mcg/ml level remains appropriate as a critical value (above which toxicity is more likely to occur) for safety purposes, additional data are now available which indicate that the serum theophylline concentrations required to produce maximum physiologic benefit may, in fact, fluctuate with the degree of bronchospasm present and are variable. Therefore, the physician should individualize the range appropriate to the patient's requirements, based on both symptomatic response and improvement in pulmonary function. It should be stressed that serum theophylline concentrations maintained at the upper level of the 10 to 20 mcg/ml range may be associated with potential toxicity when factors known to reduce theophylline clearance are operative. (See *Precautions*, including *Drug interactions*.)

Theo-24, like other controlled-release theophylline products, is intended for patients with relatively continuous or recurring symptoms who have a need to maintain therapeutic serum levels of theophylline. It is not intended for patients experiencing an acute episode of bronchospasm (associated with asthma, chronic bronchitis, or emphysema). Such patients require *rapid* relief of symptoms and should be treated with an immediate-release or intravenous theophylline preparation (or other bronchodilators) and not with controlled-release products.

Theo-24 administered on a once-daily dosage regimen is appropriate for patients who metabolize theophylline at a normal or a slow rate. Patients who metabolize theophylline rapidly (eg, the young, smokers, and some nonsmoking adults) and who have symptoms repeatedly at the end of a dosing interval, will require either increased doses given once a day or may need to be switched to a schedule of divided daily dosage. Those patients who require increased daily doses are more likely to experience relatively wide peak-trough differences and may be candidates for twice-a-day dosing with Theo-24.

Patients should be instructed to take this medication each morning at approximately the same time and not to exceed the prescribed dose.

Recent studies suggest that dosing of controlled-release theophylline products at night (after the evening meal) results in serum concentrations of theophylline which are not identical to those recorded during waking hours and may be characterized by early trough and delayed peak levels. This appears to occur whether the drug is given as an immediate-release, controlled-release, *or* intravenous product. To avoid this phenomenon when two doses per day are prescribed, it is recommended that the second dose be given 10 to 12 hours after the morning dose and before the evening meal.

Food and posture, along with changes associated with circadian rhythm, may influence the rate of absorption and/or clearance rates of theophylline from controlled-release dosage forms administered at night. The exact relationship of these and other factors to nighttime serum concentrations and the clinical significance of such findings require additional study. Therefore, it is not recommended that Theo-24 (when used as a once-a-day product) be administered at night.

Since there is a wide variation from patient to patient in the total dose of theophylline required to attain the desired level in the serum, it is essential that the dose be titrated and that serum levels be monitored before and after *transfer* to any sustained-release product.

When serum levels are not measured, the initial dosage should be restricted to the amount recommended below (see *Initiation of Therapy*).

As a practical consideration, it is not always possible to obtain serum level determinations. Under such conditions, restriction of the daily dose (in otherwise healthy adults) to not greater than 13 mg/kg/day (or 900 mg, whichever is lower) will result in relatively few patients exceeding serum levels of 20 mcg/ml, thereby reducing the risk of developing toxicity.

Dosage Guidelines

WARNING: DO NOT ATTEMPT TO MAINTAIN ANY DOSE THAT IS NOT TOLERATED. Dosage guidelines are approximations only, and the wide range of clearance of theophylline among individuals (particularly those with concomitant disease) makes indiscriminate usage hazardous.

Because food may significantly increase the peak level and extent of absorption of theophylline from Theo-24, patients receiving large single doses (ie, equal to or greater than 900 mg or 13 mg/kg, whichever is less) should be instructed to take their medication after fasting overnight and approximately two hours before eating. If the physician cannot be assured that the patient will follow this potentially difficult regimen, then the patient should be placed on alternative therapy such as twice-daily dosing.

For patients receiving lower once-daily single doses (less than 900 mg), very high peak levels are less likely to occur when Theo-24 (theophylline anhydrous) is taken with food. With close monitoring, patients less certain to observe the fasting requirements could be treated with once-daily dosing.

It is recommended that dosing be considered in three stages: (I) initiation of therapy with Theo-24, (II) titration and adjustment, and (III) chronic maintenance.

I. Initiation of Therapy with Theo-24

A. *Transfer of patients* already on established daily doses of theophylline (whether stabilized on immediate- or controlled-release products) can be accomplished by administering the total daily dosage as a single dose given in the morning (eg, 300 mg of an immediate-release product given t.i.d. should be given as 900 mg of Theo-24). The initial transfer should not be made at doses exceeding 900 mg/day or 13 mg/kg/day, whichever is less. Subsequent dose titration should be done on the basis of serum levels and with appropriate attention to the fasting recommendation made above.

It must be recognized that the peak and trough serum theophylline levels produced by once-daily dosing may vary (usually wider peak-trough differences) from those produced by the previous product and/or dosage regimen.

B. *For initiation of therapy with Theo-24* in patients who are not currently taking a theophylline product, the total daily dose, administered in the morning, must be established in accordance with the following guidelines:

Body Weight	Daily Dose
Children	
30 to 35 kg	300 mg
35 kg and above	400 mg
Adults	400 mg

Theophylline does not distribute into fatty tissue. Therefore, dosage should be calculated on the basis of lean (ideal) body weight where mg/kg doses are presented.

If appropriate serum theophylline concentrations or adequate improvement in pulmonary function is not obtained after 3 days, the instructions in Part II (below) should be followed.

II. Titration and Adjustment of Dose:

This phase of adjustment should be implemented either by the use of serum concentration measurements or by empirical principles when serum level determinations are not available.

A. *If serum levels can be measured:*

After 3 days' therapy with Theo-24, serum levels should be determined for peak concentration (sample obtained 12 hours after the morning dose) and trough concentration (24 hours after the morning dose). It is important that the patient has not missed or added any dose during the 72-hour period and that dosing intervals have been reasonably consistent. DOSE ADJUSTMENT BASED ON MEASUREMENTS WHEN THESE INSTRUCTIONS HAVE NOT BEEN FOLLOWED MAY RESULT IN TOXICITY.

Based on the results of the peak-trough values obtained, *three possibilities* exist:

1. The values of serum theophylline concentration fall within the desired range. If this result is obtained, the dosage should be maintained if it is tolerated.
2. If the serum theophylline concentration is too high, the dosage should be reduced as follows:

   a. If the values are between 20 and 25 mcg/ml, the daily dose may be reduced by about 10% and serum theophylline levels should be rechecked after 3 days.
   b. If the values are between 25 and 30 mcg/ml, the next dose should be skipped and the daily dose reduced by about 25%. The serum concentration should be rechecked after 3 days.
   c. If the values are over 30 mcg/ml, the next dose should be skipped and the daily dose reduced by 50%. The serum concentration should be rechecked after 3 days.

3. If the serum theophylline concentration is too low, the dosage should be increased at 3-day intervals by 100 mg or 200 mg (or 25% of the current dose), depending upon the desired goal. The serum concentration may be rechecked at appropriate intervals, but at least at the end of this adjustment period.

B. *If serum levels cannot be measured:*

1. If the clinical response is satisfactory then the total daily dose should be maintained.
2. If the response is unsatisfactory (due to persistence of symptoms or minimal improvement in measured function) after 3 days, then the dose may be increased by 100-mg increments. Reevaluation should be undertaken every 3 days.
3. If the response is still unsatisfactory and there are no adverse reactions, the dose may be cautiously adjusted upward in increments of 100 mg/day at 3- to 5-day intervals up to 900 mg (or 13 mg/kg/day, whichever is less).
4. If a response is accompanied by adverse reactions, then the next dose should be withheld or reduced by 25% depending on the severity of the reactions.

III. Chronic Maintenance

After the dose is established theophylline serum concentrations usually remain stable. However, as noted elsewhere (see *Precautions* and *Warnings*), certain exogenous and endogenous factors alter theophylline elimination (including concomitant disease and drug interactions) which require drug monitoring and adjustments in total daily dose requirements while such factors are operative.

Older adults, those with cor pulmonale, congestive heart failure, and/or liver disease may have unusually low dosage requirements and thus may experience toxicity at the minimal dosage recommended above.

If the patient's condition is otherwise clinically stable and none of the recognized factors which alter elimination are present, measurement of serum levels need be repeated only every 6 to 12 months.

How Supplied: Theo-24 (theophylline anhydrous) is supplied in controlled-release capsules containing 100, 200, or 300 mg of anhydrous theophylline.

Theo-24 100-mg capsules are gold and clear, with markings Theo-24, 100 mg, SEARLE, and 2832.

Theo-24 200-mg capsules are orange and clear, with markings Theo-24, 200 mg, SEARLE, and 2842.

Theo-24 300-mg capsules are red and clear, with markings Theo-24, 300 mg, SEARLE, and 2852.

Available in bottles of 100, and cartons of 100 unit-dose individually blister-sealed capsules.

Shown in Product Identification Section, page 436

The preceding prescribing information for Searle & Co. products was current on December 15, 1984.

SERES Laboratories, Inc.
3331 INDUSTRIAL DRIVE
BOX 470
SANTA ROSA, CA 95402

CANTHARONE® ℞
[*kan'tha-rone*]
(cantharidin collodion)
For External Use Only

Description: CANTHARONE, cantharidin collodion, is a topical liquid containing 0.7% cantharidin in a film-forming vehicle containing acetone, ethocel and flexible collodion. Ether 35%, alcohol 11%. The active ingredient, cantharidin, is a vesicant. The chemical name is Hexahydro-3aα, 7aα-dimethyl-4β, 7β-epoxyisobenzofuran-1, 3-dione. $C_{10}H_{12}O_4$

How Supplied: 7.5 mL bottles (NDC 50694-096-01). Close tightly immediately after use. Keep away from heat.
Revised Nov. 1983
Direct inquiries to Kathryn MacLeod, Ph.D.

CANTHARONE® PLUS ℞
[*kan'tha rone PLUS*]
For External Use Only

Description: CANTHARONE PLUS is a topical liquid containing 30% salicylic acid, 5% podophyllin, 1% cantharidin in a film-forming vehicle containing 0.5% octylphenylpolyethylene glycol, cellosolve, ethocel, collodion, castor oil and acetone. Salicylic acid is a deratolytic. The chemical name is 2-Hydroxybenzoic acid. Podophyllin is a caustic. It is an extract of the rhizomes and roots of Podophyllum peltatum. Cantharidin is a vesicant, the chemical name is Hexahydro-3aα, 7aα-dimethyl-4β, 7β-epoxyisobenzofuran-1, 3-dione.

How Supplied: 7.5 mL bottles (NDC 50694-097-01). Close tightly immediately after use. Keep away from heat. Do not refrigerate.
Revised Nov. 1983
Direct inquiries to Kathryn MacLeod, Ph.D.

NIGHT CAST™ Formula R
(Medicated Acne Mask)

Description: Contains 8% sulfur, 2% resorcinol and 29% alcohol in a non-comedogenic vehicle.
How Supplied: 8 fl. oz. in a plastic dispenser bottle.
(NDC 50694-010-01) Revised Oct. 1984
Direct inquiries to Kathryn MacLeod, Ph.D.

NIGHT CAST™ Formula S
(Medicated Acne Mask)

Description: Contains 4% sulfur, 1.5% salicylic acid and 30.5% alcohol in a non-comedogenic vehicle.
How Supplied: 8 fl. oz. in a plastic dispenser bottle.
(NDC 50694-011-01) Revised Oct. 1984
Direct inquiries to Kathryn MacLeod, Ph.D.

IDENTIFICATION PROBLEM?
Consult PDR's
Product Identification Section
where you'll find over 1200
products pictured actual size
and in full color.

Serono Laboratories, Inc.
280 POND STREET
RANDOLPH, MA 02368

Serono Laboratories, Inc. will be pleased to answer inquiries about the following products:

ASELLACRIN®
[a-sel'ah-crin]
(somatropin)

FOR SUBCUTANEOUS OR INTRAMUSCULAR INJECTION

Description: ASELLACRIN® (somatropin) is a sterile, lyophilized, purified somatropic hormone extracted from the human pituitary gland, the natural source of this hormone.

The potency of ASELLACRIN® is determined by in vitro radio-receptor assay.

The 5 ml vial contains 2 IU of somatropin and 20 mg of mannitol. The 10 ml vial contains 10 IU of somatropin and 40 mg of mannitol.

After reconstituting the 2 IU or 10 IU vial in 0.5 ml or 2.5 ml, respectively, for subcutaneous injection, each 0.5 ml of ASELLACRIN® contains 2 IU of somatropin and 20 mg or 8 mg, respectively, of mannitol, as well as other pituitary hormones as shown below. After reconstituting the 2 IU or 10 IU vial in 1 ml or 5 ml, respectively, for intramuscular injection, each 1.0 ml of ASELLACRIN® contains 2 IU of somatropin and 20 mg or 8 mg, respectively, of mannitol, as well as other pituitary hormones as shown below.

Follitropin (FSH)	less than 0.714 IU
Lutropin (LH)	less than or equal to 17.85 IU
Corticotropin (ACTH)	less than or equal to 0.014 IU
Thyrotropin (TSH)	less than 0.071 IU
Prolactin (PRL)	less than or equal to 2.86 IU

The pH is adjusted between 6 and 8 with sodium phosphate and sodium acid phosphate. The 2 IU vial contains 2.0 to 2.4 mg sodium phosphate and 0.3 to 0.4 mg sodium acid phosphate. The 10 IU vial contains 2.7 to 3.3 mg sodium phosphate and 0.4 to 0.5 mg sodium acid phosphate.

Clinical Pharmacology:

A. Skeletal Growth
ASELLACRIN® stimulates linear growth in patients with pituitary growth hormone deficiency. The measurable increase in growth (body length) after somatropin administration results from its effect on cartilaginous growth areas of the long bones. It is known that somatropin's effect is mediated by a sulfation factor, or somatomedin which permits the incorporation of sulfate into cartilage. Somatomedin is low in serum of the growth hormone deficient patients whose growth hormone deficiency is the result of hypopituitarism or hypophysectomy, whereas its presence can be demonstrated after somatropin therapy.

B. Cellular Growth
In addition to its effect on the skeleton, somatropin brings about an increase in the muscular and visceral mass. In muscle tissue the increase in mass is observed by a corresponding increase in number and dimension of muscular fiber cells.

C. Carbohydrate Metabolism
The diabetogenic effect of somatropin is well known in clinical medicine. Acromegalic patients often suffer from diabetes mellitus while hypopituitary children experience hypoglycemia. In healthy patients, very large doses of somatropin can interfere with glucose tolerance.

A simultaneous increase in the plasma insulin level is observed upon somatropin administration. The diabetogenic activity of somatropin is perhaps due to several concomitant factors:
 a. Reduced transport of glucose into peripheral tissues.
 b. Increased release of glucose from the liver.
 c. Reduced concentration of insulin at the muscular level.
 d. Reduced glycolysis resulting from the block of the enzyme triose phosphate dehydrogenase, mediated by non-esterified fatty acids.

D. Protein Metabolism
ASELLACRIN® is an anabolic agent that stimulates intracellular transport of amino acids and net retention of nitrogen, which can be quantitated by observing the decline in urinary nitrogen excretion and BUN. At the subcellular level, somatropin may stimulate the duplication of DNA, the synthesis of messenger ribonucleic acid (mRNA), the activation of cyclic AMP and the subsequent coupling of amino acids with their respective transfer RNA's. The increase of mRNA observed by some investigators may perhaps point to mRNA synthesis as the primary process in turn provoking protein synthesis.

E. Fat Metabolism
Somatropin stimulates intracellular lipolysis, increases the plasma concentration of free fatty acids and stimulates the oxidation of fatty acids. In the diabetic patient, somatropin has been shown to accentuate ketogenesis.

F. Connective Tissue Metabolism
Somatropin stimulates the synthesis of chondroitin sulfate and collagen as well as the urinary excretion of hydroxyproline.

G. Mineral Metabolism
Somatropin induces the net retention of phosphorus and potassium and to a lesser degree sodium. Somatropin induces the increased intestinal absorption of calcium and the increased renal tubular reabsorption of phosphorus with increased serum and inorganic phosphate. Increased serum alkaline phosphatase may also be observed during somatropin therapy.

Indications and Usage: Growth failure due to a deficiency of pituitary growth hormone is the only indication for ASELLACRIN® administration. The criteria for treatment are as follows:

1. Other causes for growth failure should be eliminated. Disorders of the pulmonary, cardiac, gastrointestinal and central nervous system and nutritional disorders which interfere with growth should be ruled out. There should be no evidence of a specific bone or cartilage disorder such as achondroplasia or other chondrodystrophy. The patient must not have psychosocial dwarfism. Primary hypothyroidism should be eliminated by appropriate laboratory testing. An abnormality of the X-chromosome should be ruled out by a karyotype in girls whenever indicated.
2. Patients must show significant short stature and/or a retarded growth rate. Patients with congenital growth hormone deficiency should be below the third percentile for height and growing at a rate of less than 5.0 cm/year over at least one year of continuous observation by the same physician. Height should be compared to appropriate standards for age. The most suitable are those compiled by the National Center for Health Statistics. Charts based on these standards are generally available. Patients with acquired growth hormone deficiency should also have grown less than 5.0 cm/year and should have been observed continuously by the same physician for at least 12 months.
3. Skeletal maturation should be compatible with a beneficial response to therapy. Epiphyseal maturation should be incomplete. In general, the response to therapy is diminished when the bone age is advanced beyond 13 to 14 years. While this is not a contraindication to the use of ASELLACRIN®, epiphyseal maturation should be below 12 to 13 years to increase the likelihood of a beneficial response.
4. The diagnosis of pituitary growth hormone deficiency should be confirmed by objective tests of growth hormone function. There must be failure to increase the serum concentration of growth hormone above 5 to 7 ng/ml in response to two standard stimuli. The stimuli which may be used are insulin-induced hypoglycemia, an intravenous infusion of arginine, oral L-DOPA, or subcutaneous or intramuscular glucagon. Suitable modifications of such procedures, such as pretreatment with estrogen or the administration of propranolol, may also be employed. Fasting serum growth hormone concentrations or the growth hormone response to exercise or sleep are not regarded as definitive tests for documentation of the diagnosis.
5. Tests of other pituitary hormone deficiencies should be carried out. Additional deficiencies should be recognized and treated where appropriate.

Deficiency of thyrotropin (TSH) must be treated before definitive testing for growth hormone deficiency can be performed. Patients must have been euthyroid for 4 to 8 weeks prior to testing. They must also have been observed for at least 6 months while euthyroid to determine whether the growth rate meets the criteria for treatment. Corticotropin (ACTH) deficiency should also be appropriately treated, as should deficiency of antidiuretic hormone. If indicated, gonadotropin deficiency may be treated concomitantly with ASELLACRIN® administration, but this may rapidly advance epiphyseal maturation and limit the long-term response to therapy.

Contraindications: ASELLACRIN® is ineffective, and should not be used, in patients with closed epiphyses.

ASELLACRIN® is contraindicated in the face of any progression of underlying intracranial lesion. Intracranial lesions must be inactive for 12 months prior to instituting therapy and ASELLACRIN® should be discontinued if there is evidence of recurrent activity.

Warnings: The possible appearance of hypothyroidism in the course of the disease, though unrelated to growth hormone therapy, must not go undiagnosed as this would jeopardize response to growth hormone.

In spite of rigorous requirements for the collection of pituitary glands used in the preparation of ASELLACRIN®, the risk of transmitting hepatitis cannot be excluded. The risk can be considered extremely small, as no cases have been reported.

Precautions: Because of its diabetogenic actions, which include the induction of hyperglycemia and ketosis, ASELLACRIN® should be used with caution in patients with diabetes mellitus or with a family history of diabetes mellitus. Regular urine testing for evidence of glycosuria should be carried out in all patients.

Local lipoatrophy or lipodystrophy resulting from subcutaneous administration may be avoided by rotating the injection site.

Bone age must be monitored annually during ASELLACRIN® administration especially in patients who are pubertal and/or receiving concomitant thyroid replacement therapy. Under these circumstances, epiphyseal maturation may progress rapidly to closure.

Concomitant glucocorticoid therapy may inhibit the response of ASELLACRIN® and should not exceed 10–15 mg hydrocortisone equivalent/M^2 body surface area during the administration of ASELLACRIN®.

Patients with growth hormone deficiency secondary to an intracranial lesion should be examined frequently for progression or recurrence of the underlying disease process.

Adverse Reactions: Antibodies to somatropin are formed in 30–40% of the patients who have received somatropin prepared by similar methods. In general, these antibodies are not neutralizing and do not interfere with the response to ASELLACRIN® administration. Approximately 5% of treated patients developed neutralizing antibodies and failed to respond to somatropin. Therefore, testing for anti-somatropin antibodies should be carried out in any patient with well-documented growth hormone deficiency who fails to respond to therapy.

Dosage and Administration: Although the 2 IU and 10 IU sizes are supplied with Sodium Chloride Injection (USP) as diluent, ASELLACRIN® may be reconstituted with either Sodium Chloride Injection (USP) or Bacteriostatic Water for Injection. ASELLACRIN® may be given subcutaneous or intramuscular injection.

Product Information

Subcutaneous Injection

ASELLACRIN® may be given subcutaneously by reconstituting the 2 IU vial with 0.5 ml of diluent. When using the enclosed 2 ml ampule of diluent, discard the remaining 1.5 ml of diluent. The reconstituted vial of ASELLACRIN® for subcutaneous injection contains 2 IU somatropin per 0.5 ml, 2 IU per vial.

For subcutaneous injection, reconstitute the 10 IU vial of ASELLACRIN® with 2.5 ml of diluent. When using the enclosed 10 ml vial of diluent, discard the remaining 7.5 ml of diluent. The reconstituted vial of ASELLACRIN® for subcutaneous injection contains 2 IU somatropin per 0.5 ml, 10 IU per vial.

Intramuscular Injection

ASELLACRIN® may be given intramuscularly by reconstituting the 2 IU vial with 1 ml of diluent. When using the enclosed 2 ml ampule of diluent, discard the remaining 1 ml of diluent. The reconstituted vial of ASELLACRIN® for intramuscular injection contains 2 IU somatropin per ml, 2 IU per vial.

For intramuscular injection, reconstitute the 10 IU vial of ASELLACRIN® with 5 ml of diluent. When using the enclosed 10 ml vial of diluent, discard the remaining 5 ml of diluent. The reconstituted vial of ASELLACRIN® for intramuscular injection contains 2 IU somatropin per ml, 10 IU per vial.

It is recommended that ASELLACRIN® be administered subcutaneously or intramuscularly at a dose of 0.06 to 0.10 IU/kg three times a week. The minimum dose should be 2 IU and the maximum dose should be 5 IU three times a week. At least 48 hours should elapse between injections. If at any time during the continuous ASELLACRIN® administration the growth rate does not exceed 2.5 cm (1 in) in a 6-month period the dose may be doubled for the next 6 months. This may be done with or without the presence of antibodies to ASELLACRIN®. If there is still no satisfactory response, ASELLACRIN® should be discontinued and the patient reinvestigated.

Treatment should be discontinued when the patient has reached a satisfactory adult height, when the epiphyses have fused, or when the patient ceases to respond to ASELLACRIN® administration.

Storage: Unreconstituted vials of ASELLACRIN® may be stored at room temperature (15°–30°C/59°–86°F).

Reconstituted vials must be refrigerated (2°–8°C/36°–46°F) and used within one month.

How Supplied: ASELLACRIN® is supplied in a sterile, lyophilized form in vials containing 2 IU or 10 IU somatropin. The following package combinations are available:

- 1 vial 2 IU ASELLACRIN® and 1 ampule 2 ml Sodium Chloride Injection (USP), NDC 44087-3002-1
- 1 vial 10 IU ASELLACRIN® and 1 vial 10 ml Sodium Chloride Injection (USP), NDC 44087-3010-1

©Serono Laboratories, Inc., 1984

PERGONAL® R
[per'go-nal]
(menotropins U.S.P.)

Description: Pergonal® (menotropins) is a purified preparation of gonadotropins extracted from the urine of postmenopausal women. Each ampule of Pergonal® contains 75 I.U. of follicle-stimulating hormone (FSH) activity and 75 I.U. of luteinizing hormone (LH) activity plus 10 mg lactose in a sterile, lyophilized form.

Pergonal® is biologically standardized for FSH and LH (ICSH) gonadotropin activities in terms of the Second International Reference Preparation for Human Menopausal Gonadotropins established in September, 1964, by the Expert Committee on Biological Standards of the World Health Organization.

Actions:
WOMEN:
Pergonal® administered for nine to twelve days produces ovarian follicular growth in women who do not have primary ovarian failure. Treatment with Pergonal® in most instances results only in follicular growth and maturation. In order to effect ovulation, hCG (human chorionic gonadotropin) must be given following the administration of Pergonal® when clinical assessment of the patient indicates that sufficient follicular maturation has occurred.

MEN:
Pergonal® administered concomitantly with human chorionic gonadotropin (hCG) for at least three months induces spermatogenesis in men with primary or secondary pituitary hypofunction who have achieved adequate masculinization with prior hCG therapy.

Indications:
WOMEN:
Pergonal® and human chorionic gonadotropin (hCG) given in a sequential manner are indicated for the induction of ovulation and pregnancy in the anovulatory infertile patient, in whom the cause of anovulation is functional and is not due to primary ovarian failure.

MEN:
Pergonal® with concomitant hCG is indicated for the stimulation of spermatogenesis in men who have primary or secondary hypogonadotropic hypogonadism.

Pergonal® with concomitant hCG has proven effective in inducing spermatogenesis in men with primary hypogonadotropic hypogonadism due to a congenital factor or prepubertal hypophysectomy and in men with secondary hypogonadotropic hypogonadism due to hypophysectomy, craniopharyngioma, cerebral aneurysm or chromophobe adenoma.

Selection of Patients:
WOMEN:
1. Before treatment with Pergonal® is instituted, a thorough gynecologic and endocrinologic evaluation must be performed. This should include a hysterosalpingogram (to rule out uterine and tubal pathology) and documentation of anovulation by means of basal body temperature, serial vaginal smears, examination of cervical mucus, determination of urinary pregnanediol and endometrial biopsy.
2. Primary ovarian failure should be excluded by the determination of gonadotropin levels.
3. Careful examination should be made to rule out the presence of an early pregnancy.
4. Patients in late reproductive life have a greater predilection to endometrial carcinoma as well as a higher incidence of anovulatory disorders. Cervical dilation and curettage should always be done for diagnosis before starting Pergonal® (menotropins) therapy in such patients.
5. Evaluation of the husband's fertility potential should be included in the workup.

MEN:
Patient selection should be made based on a documented lack of pituitary function. Prior to hormonal therapy, these patients will have low testosterone levels and low or absent gonadotropin levels. Patients with primary hypogonadotropic hypogonadism will have a subnormal development of masculinization, and those with secondary hypogonadotropic hypogonadism will have decreased masculinization.

Contraindications:
WOMEN:
1. A high gonadotropin level indicating primary ovarian failure.
2. The presence of overt thyroid and adrenal dysfunction.
3. An organic intracranial lesion such as a pituitary tumor.
4. The presence of any cause of infertility other than anovulation, as stated in the indications.
5. In patients with abnormal bleeding of undetermined origin.
6. In patients with ovarian cysts or enlargement not due to polycystic ovary syndrome.
7. Pregnancy.

MEN:
1. Normal gonadotropin levels indicating normal pituitary function.
2. Elevated gonadotropin levels indicating primary testicular failure.
3. Infertility disorders other than hypogonadotropic hypogonadism.

Warnings: Pergonal® is a drug that should only be used by physicians who are thoroughly familiar with infertility problems. It is a potent gonadotropic substance capable of causing mild to severe adverse reactions in women. In female patients it must be used with a great deal of care.

Precautions:
WOMEN:
1. Diagnosis Prior to Therapy
   Careful attention should be given to diagnosis in candidates for Pergonal® therapy. (See sections headed "Indications" and "Selection of Patients").
2. Overstimulation of the Ovary During Pergonal® Therapy
   In order to minimize the hazard associated with the occasional abnormal ovarian enlargement associated with Pergonal® -hCG therapy, the lowest dose consistent with expectation of good results should be used.
   Mild to moderate uncomplicated ovarian enlargement which may be accompanied by abdominal distension and/or abdominal pain occurs in approximately 20% of those treated with Pergonal® and hCG, and generally regresses without treatment within two or three weeks. The hyperstimulation syndrome characterized by sudden ovarian enlargement accompanied by ascites with or without pain and/ or pleural effusion occurs in approximately 0.4% of patients when the recommended dose is administered. In studies performed the overall incidence of the hyperstimulation syndrome was 1.3%.
   If hyperstimulation occurs, treatment should be stopped and the patient hospitalized. The hyperstimulation syndrome develops rapidly over a period of three to four days and generally occurs during the two week period immediately following treatment. The phenomenon of hemoconcentration associated with fluid loss in the abdominal cavity has been seen to occur and should be thoroughly assessed in the following manner: 1) fluid intake and output, 2) weight, 3) hematocrit, 4) serum and urinary electrolytes, and 5) urine specific gravity. These determinations are to be performed daily or more often if the need arises. Treatment is primarily symptomatic and would consist primarily of bed rest, fluid and electrolyte replacement and analgesics if needed. The ascitic fluid should never be removed because of the potential danger of injury to the ovary.
   Hemoperitoneum may occur from ruptured ovarian cysts. This is usually the result of pelvic examination. If this does occur, and if bleeding becomes such that surgery is required, the conservative approach with partial resection of the enlarged ovary or ovaries is generally adequate. Intercourse should be prohibited in those patients in whom significant ovarian enlargement occurs after ovulation because of the danger of hemoperitoneum resulting from ruptured ovarian cysts.
3. Arterial Thromboembolism
   Arterial thromboembolism following Pergonal® (menotropins) and hCG therapy has been reported in two patients, one of whom died (1).
4. Multiple Births
   Of the pregnancies following therapy with Pergonal® and hCG, 80% have resulted in single births and 20% in multiple births, most of which have been twins. Fifteen percent of the total pregnancies resulted in twins, of which 93% were viable (78 surviving infants from 43 sets of twins). Five per cent of the total pregnancies have resulted in three or more conceptuses, of which only 20% were viable (nine surviving infants from three sets of triplets, four surviving infants from four sets of quadruplets, and no surviving infants from four sets of quintuplets). The patient and her husband should be advised of the frequency and potential hazards of multiple pregnancy before starting treatment.

Continued on next page

Serono—Cont.

Adverse Reactions:
WOMEN:
1. Ovarian Enlargement
2. Hyperstimulation Syndrome
3. Hemoperitoneum
4. Arterial Thromboembolism (see "Precautions" above).
5. Sensitivity to Pergonal®
   Three patients experienced febrile reactions after the administration of Pergonal®. It is not clear whether or not these were pyrogenic responses or possibly allergic reactions.
6. Defects at Birth
   From 287 completed pregnancies following Pergonal®-hCG therapy, five incidents of birth defects have been reported. One infant had multiple congenital anomalies consisting of imperforate anus, aplasia of the sigmoid colon, third degree hypospadias, cecovesicle fistula, bifid scrotum, meningocele, bilateral internal tibial torsion, and right metatarsus adductus. Another infant was born with an imperforate anus and possible congenital heart lesions; another had a supernumerary digit; another was born with hypospadias and exstrophy of the bladder; and the fifth child had Down's syndrome. None of the investigators felt that these defects were drug-related.

MEN:
1. Gynecomastia may occur occasionally during Pergonal®-hCG therapy. This is a known effect of hCG treatment.
2. Erythrocytosis (hct 50% hgb 17.8 g%) was recorded in 1 patient.

Dosage and Administration for Intramuscular Administration
WOMEN:
1. Treatment for Induction of Ovulation
   Treatment with Pergonal® in most instances results only in follicular growth and maturation. In order to effect ovulation, hCG must be given following the administration of Pergonal® when clinical assessment of the patient indicates that sufficient follicular maturation has occurred. This is indirectly estimated by the estrogenic effect upon the target organs. These indices of estrogenic activity include:
   a) Changes in the vaginal smear
   b) Appearance and volume of the cervical mucus
   c) Spinnbarkeit, and
   d) Ferning of the cervical mucus.
   If available, the urinary excretion of estrogens is a more reliable index of follicular maturation.
   The clinical confirmation of ovulation, with the exception of pregnancy, is obtained by indirect indices of progesterone production. The indices most generally used are as follows:
   a) a rise in basal body temperature
   b) change of the cervical mucus from a "fern" pattern to a "cellular" pattern
   c) vaginal cytology characteristic of the luteal phase of the menstrual cycle
   d) increase in urinary pregnanediol, and
   e) menstruation following the shift in basal body temperature.
   Because of the subjectivity of the various tests for the determination of follicular maturation and ovulation, it cannot be over-emphasized that the physician should choose tests with which he is thoroughly familiar.
2. Dosage of Pergonal®
   The dose of Pergonal® to produce maturation of the follicle must be individualized for each patient. It is recommended that the initial dose to any patient should be 75 I.U. of FSH and 75 I.U. of LH (one ampule) per day, **ADMINISTERED INTRAMUSCULARLY**, for nine to twelve days followed by hCG, 10,000 I.U., one day after the last dose of Pergonal®. The hyperstimulation syndrome has never occurred with administration of 75 I.U. of FSH and 75 I.U. of LH (one ampule) per day for up to twelve days. Administration of Pergonal® should not exceed 12 days. The patient should be treated until indices of estrogenic activity, as indicated under Item 1 above, are equivalent to or greater than those of the normal individual. If urinary estrogen determinations are available, they may be useful as a guide to therapy. If the total estrogen excretion is less than 100 mcg/24 hours or the estriol excretion is less than 50 mcg/24 hours prior to hCG administration, the hyperstimulation syndrome is less likely to occur. If the estrogen values are greater than this it is not advisable to administer hCG because the hyperstimulation syndrome is more likely to occur. If the ovaries are abnormally enlarged on the last day of Pergonal® therapy, hCG should not be administered in this course of therapy; this will reduce the chances of development of the hyperstimulation syndrome. If there is evidence of ovulation but no pregnancy, repeat this dosage regime for at least two more courses before increasing the dose of Pergonal® to 150 I.U. of FSH and 150 I.U. of LH (two ampules) per day for nine to twelve days. As before, this dose should be followed by 10,000 I.U. of hCG one day after the last dose of Pergonal®. 150 I.U. of FSH and 150 I.U. of LH (two ampules) of Pergonal® per day has proven to be the most effective dose. If evidence of ovulation is present, but pregnancy does not ensue, repeat the same dose for two more courses. Doses larger than this are not recommended.
   During treatment with both Pergonal® and hCG and during a two-week post-treatment period, patients should be examined at least every other day for signs of excessive ovarian stimulation. It is recommended that Pergonal® administration be stopped if the ovaries become abnormally enlarged or abdominal pain occurs. Most of the ovarian hyperstimulation occurs after treatment has been discontinued and reaches its maximum at about seven to ten days post-ovulation. Patients should be followed for at least two weeks after hCG administration.
   The couple should be encouraged to have intercourse daily, beginning on the day prior to the administration of hCG until ovulation becomes apparent from the indices employed for the determination of progestational activity. Care should be taken to insure insemination. In the light of the foregoing indices and parameters mentioned, it should become obvious that, unless a physician is willing to devote considerable time to these patients and be familiar with and conduct the necessary laboratory studies, he should not use Pergonal® (menotropins).
3. How to Administer Pergonal®
   Dissolve the contents of one ampule of Pergonal® in one to two ml. of sterile saline and **ADMINISTER INTRAMUSCULARLY** immediately. Any unused reconstituted material should be discarded.

MEN:
1. Dosage of Pergonal®
   Prior to concomitant therapy with Pergonal® (hMG) and hCG, pretreatment with hCG alone (5000 IU three times a week) is required. Treatment should continue for a period sufficient to achieve serum testosterone levels within the normal range and masculinization as judged by the appearance of secondary sex characteristics. Such pretreatment may require four to six months, then the recommended dose of Pergonal® is one ampule **ADMINISTERED INTRAMUSCULARLY**, three times a week and the recommended dose of hCG is 2,000 IU twice a week. Therapy should be carried on for a minimum of four more months to insure detecting spermatozoa in the ejaculate, as it takes 74 ± 4 days in the human male for germ cells to reach the spermatozoa stage.
   In one clinical series consisting of nine patients, 4 patients produced 2 million sperm per ejaculate with a dosage of Pergonal® of 25 IU every other day concomitantly with 2,000 IU hCG three times a week. When 38 IU of Pergonal® every other day was administered, 7 of the 9 subjects produced at least 2 million sperm per ejaculate, and at the higher dose of 75 IU of Pergonal® every other day, 8 of the 9 subjects were sperm positive at 2 million per ejaculate. In this series, Pergonal® was administered concomitantly with 2,000 IU hCG three times a week, after achievement of adequate masculinization with prior hCG therapy. The non-responder had a history of surgical orchiopexy to repair bilateral cryptorchidism at the age of 12, and this may have complicated the response of his testes to gonadotropin replacement. The results obtained in this series are in keeping with very recent studies quantitating the production rate of FSH in the human as approximately 30 or 40 IU a day.
   If the patient has not responded with evidence of increased spermatogenesis at the end of four months therapy, treatment may continue with one ampule of Pergonal® three times a week, or the dose can be increased to two ampules (150 IU FSH and 150 IU LH) three times a week, with the hCG dose unchanged.
2. How to Administer Pergonal®
   Dissolve the contents of one ampule of Pergonal® in one to two ml of sterile saline and **ADMINISTER INTRAMUSCULARLY** immediately. Any unused reconstituted material should be discarded.

How Supplied: Each ampule of Pergonal® (menotropins) contains 75 I.U. of FSH and 75 I.U. of LH (ICSH). By biological assay, one I.U. of LH for the Second International Reference Preparation (2nd-IRP) for hMG is biologically equivalent to approximately ½ I.U. of human chorionic gonadotropin (hCG).
Lyophilized powder may be stored refrigerated or at room temperature, 3°C–30°C (37°–86°F).

Clinical Studies:
WOMEN:
The results of the clinical experience and effectiveness of the administration of Pergonal® (menotropins) to 1,286 patients in 3,002 courses of therapy are summarized below. The values include patients who were treated with other than the recommended dosage regime. The values for the presently recommended dosage regime are essentially the same, except for the fact that the hyperstimulation syndrome has not occurred with administration of 75 I.U. of Pergonal® per day for 9 to 12 days and the incidence of the hyperstimulation syndrome with administration of 150 I.U. of Pergonal® per day for 9 to 12 days has not exceeded 0.4%.

	%
Patients ovulating	75
Patients pregnant	25
Patients aborting	25*
Multiple pregnancies	20†
Twins	15†
Three or more conceptuses	5†
Fetal abnormalities	1.7†
Hyperstimulation syndrome	1.3

* Based on total pregnancies
† Based on total deliveries

Results by diagnosis group are summarized below. (These values include patients who were treated with other than the present recommended dosage regime).
[See table on next page].

MEN:
Clinical results of the treatment of men with primary or secondary hypogonadotropic hypogonadism are as follows:
In the Serono Cooperative study, with an adequate treatment period of 3 to 8 months, 60 of 70 men with primary hypogonadotropic hypogonadism and 8 of 11 men with secondary hypogonadotropic hypogonadism responded with mean increases in their sperm counts from less than 5 to 24 million spermatozoa per milliliter of ejaculate. Forty-one wives of 54 men with primary hypogonadotropic hypogonadism desiring offspring and 7 wives of men with secondary hypogonadotropic hypogonadism conceived. Patients treated with Pergonal® and hCG for less than 3 months or with Pergonal® alone did not respond to therapy.
A world-wide data search revealed that of 160 recorded pregnancies as the result of use of Per-

gonal® -hCG in men, there were 7 spontaneous abortions, one ectopic pregnancy and 3 congenital anomalies at birth (esophageal atresia in a female infant which was later corrected by surgery, unilateral cryptorchidism, inguinal hernia).

References:
1. Mozes, M., Bogokowsky, H., Antebi, E., et al.: Thromboembolic phenomena after ovarian stimulation with human gonadotropins, Lancet 2:1213-1215, 1965.

PROFASI® HP
[pro'fah-se]
(human chorionic gonadotropin, USP)
FOR INTRAMUSCULAR USE ONLY

Description: Human chorionic gonadotropin (HCG), a polypeptide hormone produced by the human placenta, is composed of an alpha and a beta sub-unit. The alpha sub-unit is essentially identical to the alpha sub-units of the human pituitary gonadotropins, luteinizing hormone (LH) and follicle-stimulating hormone (FSH), as well as to the alpha sub-unit of human thyroid-stimulating hormone (TSH). The beta sub-units of these hormones differ in amino acid sequence.

Chorionic Gonadotropin is a water soluble glycoprotein derived from human pregnancy urine. The sterile lyophilized powder is stable. When reconstituted the solution should be refrigerated and should be used within 60 days.

Each vial when reconstituted will contain:
Chorionic Gonadotropin: 5,000 USP Units or 10,000 USP Units; Mannitol: 100 mg with Dibasic Sodium Phosphate and Monobasic Sodium Phosphate to adjust pH.

In addition, when reconstituted with the diluent provided (Bacteriostatic Water for Injection, USP containing 0.9% v/v Benzyl Alcohol) each serum vial will contain Benzyl Alcohol 0.9%.

Clinical Pharmacology: The action of HCG is virtually identical to that of pituitary LH, although HCG appears to have a small degree of FSH activity as well. It stimulates production of gonadal steroid hormones by stimulating the interstitial cells (Leydig cells) of the testis to produce androgens and the corpus luteum of the ovary to produce progesterone. Androgen stimulation in the male leads to the development of secondary sex characteristics and may stimulate testicular descent when no anatomical impediment to descent is present. This descent is usually reversible when HCG is discontinued. During the normal menstrual cycle, LH participates with FSH in the development and maturation of the normal ovarian follicle, and the mid-cycle LH surge triggers ovulation. HCG can substitute for LH in this function.

During a normal pregnancy, HCG secreted by the placenta maintains the corpus luteum after LH secretion decreases, supporting continued secretion of estrogen and progesterone and preventing menstruation. HCG HAS NO KNOWN EFFECT ON FAT MOBILIZATION, APPETITE OR SENSE OF HUNGER, OR BODY FAT DISTRIBUTION.

Indications and Usage: HCG HAS NOT BEEN DEMONSTRATED TO BE EFFECTIVE ADJUNCTIVE THERAPY IN THE TREATMENT OF OBESITY. THERE IS NO SUBSTANTIAL EVIDENCE THAT IT INCREASES WEIGHT LOSS BEYOND THAT RESULTING FROM CALORIC RESTRICTION, THAT IT CAUSES A MORE ATTRACTIVE OR "NORMAL" DISTRIBUTION OF FAT, OR THAT IT DECREASES THE HUNGER AND DISCOMFORT ASSOCIATED WITH CALORIE-RESTRICTED DIETS.

1. Prepubertal cryptorchidism not due to anatomical obstruction. In general, HCG is thought to induce testicular descent in situations when descent would have occurred at puberty. HCG thus may help predict whether or not orchiopexy will be needed in the future. Although, in some cases descent following HCG administration is permanent, in most cases, the response is temporary. Therapy is usually instituted between the ages of 4 and 9.

Pergonal	% Pts. Ovul.	% Pts. Preg.	% Abort	% Multi Preg.	% Twins	% 3 or More Conceptuses	% Hyperstim. Syndr.
Primary Amenorrhea	62	22	14	25	25	0	0
Secondary Amenorrhea	61	28	24	28	18	10	1.9
Secondary Amen. with Galactorrhea	77	42	21	41	31	10	1.2
Polycystic Ovaries	76	26	39	17	17	0	1.1
Anovulatory Cycles	77	24	15	14	9	5	2.0
Miscellaneous	83	20	36	2	2	0	0.1

2. Selected cases of hypogonadotropic hypogonadism (hypogonadism secondary to a pituitary deficiency) in males.
3. Induction of ovulation and pregnancy in the anovulatory, infertile woman in whom the cause of anovulation is secondary and not due to primary ovarian failure, and who has been appropriately pre-treated with human menotropins.

Contraindications: Precocious puberty, prostatic carcinoma or other androgen-dependent neoplasm, prior allergic reaction to HCG.

Warnings: HCG should be used in conjunction with human menopausal gonadotropins only by physicians experienced with infertility problems who are familiar with the criteria for patient selection, contraindications, warnings, precautions, and adverse reactions described in the package insert for menotropins. The principal serious adverse reactions during this use are: (1) Ovarian hyperstimulation, a syndrome of sudden ovarian enlargement, ascites with or without pain, and/or pleural effusion, (2) Rupture of ovarian cysts with resultant hemoperitoneum, (3) Multiple births, and (4) Arterial thromboembolism.

Precautions:
1. Induction of androgen secretion by HCG may induce precocious puberty in patients treated for cryptorchidism. Therapy should be discontinued if signs of precocious puberty occur.
2. Since androgens may cause fluid retention, HCG should be used with caution in patients with cardiac or renal disease, epilepsy, migraine, or asthma.

Adverse Reactions: Headache, irritability, restlessness, depression, fatigue, edema, precocious puberty, gynecomastia, pain at the site of injection.

Dosage and Administration: (Intramuscular Use Only): The dosage regimen employed in any particular case will depend upon the indication for use, the age and weight of the patient, and the physician's preference. The following regimens have been advocated by various authorities.

Prepubertal cryptorchidism not due to anatomical obstruction:
1. 4,000 USP Units three times weekly for three weeks.
2. 5,000 USP Units every second day for four injections.
3. 15 injections of 500 to 1,000 USP Units over a period of six weeks.
4. 500 USP Units three times weekly for four to six weeks. If this course of treatment is not successful, another is begun one month later, giving 1,000 USP Units per injection.

Selected cases of hypogonadotropic hypogonadism in males:
1. 500 to 1,000 USP Units three times a week for three weeks, followed by the same dose twice a week for three weeks.
2. 4,000 USP Units three times weekly for six to nine months, following which the dosage may be reduced to 2,000 USP Units three times weekly for an additional three months.

Induction of ovulation and pregnancy in the anovulatory, unfertile woman in whom the cause of anovulation is secondary and not due to primary ovarian failure and who has been appropriately pre-treated with human menotropins (see prescribing information for menotropins for dosage and administration for that drug product):
5,000 to 10,000 USP Units one day following the last dose of menotropins (a dosage of 10,000 USP Units is recommended in the labeling for menotropins).

How Supplied: Regular 10 ml lyophilized multiple dose vial
5,000 USP Units per Vial—NDC 44087-8005-3
10,000 USP Units per Vial—NDC 44087-8010-3
with 10 ml vial Bacteriostatic Water for Injection, USP (containing Benzyl Alcohol 0.9% v/v).

Caution: Federal law prohibits dispensing without prescription.

Directions For Reconstitution: TWO-VIAL PACKAGE: Withdraw sterile air from lyophilized vial and inject into diluent vial. Remove 10 ml from diluent and add to lyophilized vial; agitate gently until solution is complete.

SEROPHENE®
[se"ro-fēn]
(clomiphene citrate tablets, U.S.P.)

Description: Each scored white tablet contains: Clomiphene Citrate USP 50 mg. Clomiphene citrate is designated chemically as 2-[p-(2-chloro-1,2-diphenylvinyl) phenoxy] triethylamine dihydrogen citrate and is represented structurally as:

$(C_2H_5)_2NCH_2CH_2O\text{—}C=C\text{—}C_6H_8O_7$

clomiphene citrate USP (Serophene)

As shown, one molecule of citric acid is chemically bound with one molecule of the organic base, clomiphene.

Clomiphene citrate is a chemical analog of other triarylethylene compounds such as chlorotrianisene and the cholesterol inhibitor, triparanol.

Actions: Clomiphene citrate, an orally-administered, non-steroidal agent, may induce ovulation in selected anovulatory women. It is a drug of considerable pharmacologic potency. Careful evaluation and selection of the patient and close attention to the timing of the dose is mandatory prior to treatment with clomiphene citrate. Conservative selection and management of the patient contribute to successful therapy of anovulation. Clomiphene citrate induces ovulation in most selected anovulatory patients. The various criteria for ovulation include: an ovulation peak of estrogen excretion followed by a biphasic basal body temperature curve; urinary excretion of pregnanediol at post-ovulatory levels and, endometrial histologic findings characteristic of the luteal phase.

A review of eleven publications appearing between 1964 and 1978 showed that pregnancy occurred in 35% of 5154 patients with ovulatory dysfunction who received clomiphene citrate.
[See table on next page].

Clomiphene citrate therapy appears to mediate ovulation through increased output of pituitary gonadotropins. These stimulate the maturation and endocrine activity of the ovarian follicle which is followed by the development and function of the corpus luteum. Increased urinary excretion of

Continued on next page

Serono—Cont.

gonadotropins and estrogen suggest involvement of the pituitary.

Studies with ^{14}C labeled clomiphene citrate have shown that it is readily absorbed orally in humans, and is excreted principally in the feces. An average of 51% of the administered dose was excreted after 5 days. After intravenous administration 37% was excreted in 5 days. The appearance of ^{14}C in the feces six weeks after administration suggests that the remaining drug and/or metabolites are slowly excreted from a sequestered enterohepatic recirculation pool.

Indications: Clomiphene citrate is indicated for the treatment of ovulatory failure in patients desiring pregnancy, and whose husbands are fertile and potent. Impediments to this goal must be excluded or adequately treated before beginning therapy. Administration of clomiphene citrate is indicated only in patients with demonstrated ovulatory dysfunction and in whom the following conditions apply:
1. Normal liver function.
2. Physiologic indications of normal endogenous estrogen (as estimated from vaginal smears, endometrial biopsy, assay of urinary estrogen, or from bleeding in response to progesterone). Reduced estrogen levels, while less favorable, do not prevent successful therapy.
3. Clomiphene citrate therapy is not effective for those patients with primary pituitary or ovarian failure. It cannot substitute for appropriate therapy of other disturbances leading to ovulatory dysfunction, e.g., diseases of the thyroid or adrenals.
4. Particularly careful evaluation prior to clomiphene citrate therapy should be done in patients with abnormal uterine bleeding. It is most important that neoplastic lesions are detected.

Contraindications:

Pregnancy

Although no direct effect of clomiphene citrate therapy on the human fetus has been seen, clomiphene citrate should not be administered in cases of suspected pregnancy as such effects have been reported in animals. To prevent inadvertent clomiphene citrate administration during early pregnancy, the basal body temperature should be recorded throughout all treatment cycles, and therapy should be discontinued if pregnancy is suspected. If the basal body temperature following clomiphene citrate is biphasic and is not followed by menses, the possibility of an ovarian cyst and/or pregnancy should be excluded. Until the correct diagnosis has been determined, the next course of therapy should be delayed.

Liver Disease

Patients with liver disease or a history of liver dysfunction should not receive clomiphene citrate therapy.

Abnormal Uterine Bleeding

Clomiphene citrate is contraindicated in patients with abnormal uterine bleeding.

Warnings:

Visual Symptoms

Patients should be warned that blurring and/or other visual symptoms may occur occasionally with clomiphene citrate therapy. These may make activities such as driving or operating machinery more hazardous than usual, particularly under conditions of variable lighting. While their significance is not yet understood (see ADVERSE REACTIONS), patients having any visual symptoms, should discontinue treatment and have a complete ophthalmologic evaluation.

Precautions:

Diagnosis Prior to Clomiphene Citrate Therapy

Careful evaluation should be given to candidates for clomiphene citrate therapy. A complete pelvic examination should be performed prior to treatment and repeated before each subsequent course. Clomiphene citrate should not be given to patients with an ovarian cyst, as further ovarian enlargement may result.

Since the incidence of endometrial carcinoma and of ovulatory disorders increases with age, endometrial biopsy should always exclude the former as causative in such patients. If abnormal uterine bleeding is present, full diagnostic measures are necessary.

Ovarian Overstimulation During Treatment with Clomiphene Citrate

To minimize the hazard associated with the occasional abnormal ovarian enlargement during clomiphene citrate therapy (see ADVERSE REACTIONS), the lowest dose producing good results should be chosen. Some patients with polycystic ovary syndrome are unusually sensitive to gonadotropin and may have an exaggerated response to usual doses of clomiphene citrate. Maximal enlargement of the ovary, whether abnormal or physiologic, does not occur until several days after discontinuation of clomiphene citrate. The patient complaining of pelvic pains after receiving clomiphene citrate should be examined carefully. If enlargement of the ovary occurs, clomiphene citrate therapy should be withheld until the ovaries have returned to pretreatment size, and the dosage or duration of the next course should be reduced. The ovarian enlargement and cyst formation following clomiphene citrate therapy regress spontaneously within a few days or weeks after discontinuing treatment. Therefore, unless a strong indication for laparotomy exists, such cystic enlargement always should be managed conservatively.

Multiple Pregnancy

In the reviewed publications, the incidence of multiple pregnancies was increased during those cycles in which clomiphene citrate was given. Among the 1803 pregnancies on which the outcome was reported, 90% were single and 10% twins. Less than 1% of the reported deliveries resulted in triplets or more.

Of these multiple pregnancies, 96-99% resulted in the births of live infants. The patient and her husband should be advised of the frequency and potential hazards of multiple pregnancy before starting treatment.

Adverse Reactions:

Symptoms

Side effects are not prominent at the recommended dosage of clomiphene citrate and infrequently interfere with treatment. Side effects tend to occur more frequently at higher doses and in the longer treatment courses used in some early studies. The more common side effects and the percent of patients experiencing them include vasomotor flushes (11%), abdominal discomfort (7.4%), abnormal uterine bleeding (0.5%), ovarian enlargement (14%), breast tenderness (2.1%), and visual symptoms (1.6%). The vasomotor symptoms resemble menopausal "hot flushes", and are not usually severe. They promptly disappear after treatment is discontinued. Abdominal discomfort may resemble ovulatory (mittelschmerz) or premenstrual phenomena, or that due to ovarian enlargement. In addition, nausea and vomiting (2.1%), nervousness and insomnia (1.9%), headache (1%), dizziness and lightheadedness (1%), increased urination (0.9%), depression and fatigue (0.8%), urticaria and allergic dermatitis (0.6%), weight gain (0.4%), and reversible hair loss (0.3%) have been reported.

When clomiphene citrate is administered at the recommended dose, abnormal ovarian enlargement (see PRECAUTIONS) is infrequent, although the usual cyclic variation in ovarian size may be exaggerated. Similarly, mid-cycle ovarian pain (mittelschmerz) may be accentuated. With prolonged or higher dosage, ovarian enlargement and cyst formation (usually luteal) may occur more often and the luteal phase of the cycle may be prolonged. Patients with polycystic ovary disease may be unusually sensitive to clomiphene therapy. Rare occurrences of massive ovarian enlargement have been reported, for example, in a patient with polycystic ovary syndrome whose clomiphene citrate therapy consisted of 100 mg daily for 14 days. Since abnormal ovarian enlargement usually regresses spontaneously, most of these patients should be treated conservatively.

The incidence of visual symptoms (see WARNINGS for further recommendations), usually described as "blurring" or spots or flashes (scintillating scotomata), correlates with increasing total dose. The symptoms disappear within a few days or weeks after clomiphene citrate is discontinued. This may be due to intensification and/or prolongation of after-images. Symptoms often appear first, or are accentuated, upon exposure to a more brightly lit environment. While measured visual acuity has not generally been affected, in one patient taking 200 mg daily, visual blurring developed on the seventh day of treatment, and progressed to severe diminution of visual acuity by the tenth day. No other abnormality was coincident, and the visual acuity was normal by the third day after treatment was stopped. Ophthalmologically definable scotomata and electroretinographic retinal function changes have also been reported.

BSP Laboratory Studies

Greater than 5% retention of sulfobromophthalein (BSP) has been reported in approximately 10 to 20% of patients in whom it was measured. Retention was usually minimal but was elevated during prolonged clomiphene citrate administration or with apparently unrelated liver disease. In some patients, pre-existing BSP retention decreased even though clomiphene citrate therapy was continued. Other liver function tests were usually normal.

Other Laboratory Studies

Clomiphene citrate has not been reported to cause a significant abnormality in hematologic or renal tests, in protein bound iodine, or in serum cholesterol levels.

Birth Defects

Of 1803 births following clomiphene citrate administration, 45 infants with birth defects were reported for a cumulative rate of 2.5%.

Six cases of Down's Syndrome, one neonatal death with multiple malformations and one case each of the following were reported: extropia, club foot, tibial torsion, blocked tear duct and hemangioma. The other congenital abnormalities were not described. The investigators did not report that these were presumed to be due to therapy. The cumulative rate of congenital abnormalities does not exceed that reported in the general population.

Serophene

PREGNANCIES FOLLOWING CLOMIPHENE CITRATE U.S.P.[a]

		(Range)
Number of Patients	= 5154	
Percent of Patients Ovulating[b]	= 75	(50-94)%
Percent of Ovulatory Cycles	= 53	(33-69)%
Percent of Patients Pregnant	= 35	(11-52)%
Percent Patients Pregnant	= 46	(22-61)%
Percent Patients Ovulating		
Percent Live Births	= 86	(74-99.8)%
Percent Abortions	= 14	(0.2-26)%
Percent of Single Births	= 90	(67-100)%
Percent Surviving	= 99	(98.2-100)%
Percent of Multiple Births	= 10	(0-33)%
Percent Surviving	= 96	(82-100)%

a) includes patients receiving other than recommended dosage regimen.
b) average from studies

Dosage and Administration:
General Considerations
Physicians experienced in managing gynecologic or endocrine disorders should supervise the work-up and treatment of candidate patients for clomiphene citrate therapy. Patients should be chosen for clomiphene citrate therapy only after careful diagnostic evaluation (see INDICATIONS). The plan of therapy should be outlined in advance. Impediments to achieving the goal of therapy must be excluded or adequately treated before beginning clomiphene citrate.

In determining a starting dose schedule, efficacy must be balanced against potential side effects. For example, the available data so far suggests that ovulation and pregnancy are slightly more attainable with 100 mg/day for 5 days than with 50 mg/day for 5 days. As the dosage is increased, however, ovarian overstimulation and other side effects may be expected to increase. Although the data do not yet establish a relationship between dose level and multiple births, it is reasonable that such a correlation exists on pharmacologic grounds.

For these reasons, treatment of the usual patient should initiate with a 50 mg daily dose for 5 days. The dose may be increased only in those patients who do not respond to the first course (see Recommended Dosage). Special treatment with lower dosage over shorter duration is particularly recommended if unusual sensitivity to pituitary gonadotropin is suspected, including patients with polycystic ovary syndrome (see PRECAUTIONS).

Recommended Dosage
The recommended dosage for the first course of clomiphene citrate is 50 mg (1 tablet) daily for 5 days. Therapy may be started at any time if the patient has had no recent uterine bleeding. If progestin-induced bleeding is intended, or if spontaneous uterine bleeding occurs prior to therapy, the regimen of 50 mg daily for 5 days should be started on or about the fifth day of the cycle. When ovulation occurs at this dosage, there is no advantage to increasing the dose in subsequent cycles of treatment.

If ovulation does not appear to have occurred after the first course of therapy, a second course of 100 mg daily (two 50 mg tablets given as a single daily dose) for 5 days may be started. This course may begin as early as 30 days after the previous one. Increasing the dosage or duration of therapy beyond 100 mg/day for 5 days should not be undertaken.

The majority of patients who respond do so during the first course of therapy, and 3 courses constitute an adequate therapeutic trial. If ovulatory menses do not occur, the diagnosis should be re-evaluated. Treatment beyond this is not recommended in the patient who does not exhibit evidence of ovulation.

Pregnancy
Properly timed coitus is very important for good results. For regularity of cyclic ovulatory response it is also important that each course of clomiphene citrate be started on or about the fifth day of the cycle, once ovulation has been established. As with other therapeutic modalities, Serophene® therapy follows the rule of diminishing returns, such that likelihood of conception diminishes with each succeeding course of therapy. If pregnancy has not been achieved after 3 ovulatory responses to Serophene, further treatment is not generally recommended. Before starting treatment patients should be advised of the possibility and potential hazards of multiple pregnancy if conception occurs following clomiphene citrate therapy.

Long-Term Cyclic Therapy—Not Recommended
Since the relative safety of long-term cyclic therapy has not yet been conclusively demonstrated, and since the majority of patients will ovulate following 3 courses, long-term cyclic therapy is not recommended.

How Supplied: Serophene is available as 50 mg scored white tablets, packaged in cartons of 30. Each carton contains 3 strips of 10 tablets, each in a 2 × 5 arrangement.

PRODUCT INFORMATION: AVAILABLE ONLY ON PRESCRIPTION

For additional information, please contact:
Serono Laboratories, Inc.
Medical Information Department
280 Pond Street
Randolph, MA 02368
800-225-5185 (Toll free, outside MA)
617-963-8154 (Inside MA)

Smith Kline & French Laboratories
Division of SmithKline Beckman Corporation
1500 SPRING GARDEN ST.
P.O. BOX 7929
PHILADELPHIA, PA 19101

SK&F Co.
Carolina, P.R. 00630
Subsidiary of SmithKline Beckman Corporation

SK&F Lab Co.
Carolina, P.R. 00630
Subsidiary of SmithKline Beckman Corporation

Menley & James Laboratories
A SmithKline Beckman Company
P.O. BOX 8082
PHILADELPHIA, PA 19101

SK&F PRODUCT CODE INDEX

Code	Product, Form and Strength
C44	'Compazine' *Spansule* capsules 10 mg.
C46	'Compazine' *Spansule* capsules 15 mg.
C47	'Compazine' *Spansule* capsules 30 mg.
C60	'Compazine' Suppositories 2 ½ mg.
C61	'Compazine' Suppositories 5 mg.
C62	'Compazine' Suppositories 25 mg.
C66	'Compazine' Tablets 5 mg.
C67	'Compazine' Tablets 10 mg.
C69	'Compazine' Tablets 25 mg.
D14	'Cytomel' Tablets 5 mcg.
D16	'Cytomel' Tablets 25 mcg.
D17	'Cytomel' Tablets 50 mcg.
D62	'Darbid' Tablets 5 mg.
E12	'Dexedrine' *Spansule* capsules 5 mg.
E13	'Dexedrine' *Spansule* capsules 10 mg.
E14	'Dexedrine' *Spansule* capsules 15 mg.
E19	'Dexedrine' Tablets 5 mg.
E33	'Dibenzyline' Capsules 10 mg.
J09	'Eskalith' Tablets 300 mg.
J10	'Eskalith' Controlled Release Tablets 450 mg.
120	'SK-Amitriptyline HCl' Tablets 10 mg.
121	'SK-Amitriptyline HCl' Tablets 25 mg.
123	'SK-Amitriptyline HCl' Tablets 50 mg.
124	'SK-Amitriptyline HCl' Tablets 75 mg.
131	'SK-Amitriptyline HCl' Tablets 100 mg.
132	'SK-Amitriptyline HCl' Tablets 150 mg.
101	'SK-Ampicillin' Capsules 250 mg.
102	'SK-Ampicillin' Capsules 500 mg.
494	'SK-APAP' with CODEINE Tablets 300 mg./15 mg.
496	'SK-APAP' with CODEINE Tablets 300 mg./30 mg.
497	'SK-APAP' with CODEINE Tablets 300 mg./60 mg.
133	'SK-Bamate' Tablets 200 mg.
134	'SK-Bamate' Tablets 400 mg.
176	'SK-Chloral Hydrate' Capsules 500 mg.
419	'SK-Chlorothiazide' Tablets 250 mg.
420	'SK-Chlorothiazide' Tablets 500 mg.
374	'SK-Dexamethasone' Tablets 0.5 mg.
376	'SK-Dexamethasone' Tablets 0.75 mg.
377	'SK-Dexamethasone' Tablets 1.5 mg.
423	'SK-Diphenoxylate' Tablets 2.5 mg./0.025 mg.
379	'SK-Dipyridamole' Tablets 25 mg.
380	'SK-Dipyridamole' Tablets 50 mg.
381	'SK-Dipyridamole' Tablets 75 mg.
347	'SK-Doxycycline Hyclate' Capsules 50 mg.
348	'SK-Doxycycline Hyclate' Capsules 100 mg.
367	'SK-Erythromycin' Tablets 250 mg.
369	'SK-Erythromycin' Tablets 500 mg.
340	'SK-Furosemide' Tablets 20 mg.
341	'SK-Furosemide' Tablets 40 mg.
363	'SK-Hydrochlorothiazide' Tablets 25 mg.
364	'SK-Hydrochlorothiazide' Tablets 50 mg.
441	'SK-Lygen' Capsules 5 mg.
442	'SK-Lygen' Capsules 10 mg.
443	'SK-Lygen' Capsules 25 mg.
426	'SK-Metronidazole' Tablets 250 mg.
319	'SK-Oxycodone' with Aspirin Tablets
320	'SK-Oxycodone' with Acetaminophen Tablets
111	'SK-Penicillin G' Tablets 400,000 units
112	'SK-Penicillin G' Tablets 800,000 units
116	'SK-Penicillin VK' Tablets 250 mg.
117	'SK-Penicillin VK' Tablets 500 mg.
136	'SK-Phenobarbital' Tablets 15 mg.
137	'SK-Phenobarbital' Tablets 30 mg.
321	'SK-Pramine' Tablets 10 mg.
322	'SK-Pramine' Tablets 25 mg.
323	'SK-Pramine' Tablets 50 mg.
339	'SK-Prednisone' Tablets 5 mg.
499	'SK-Probenecid' Tablets 500 mg.
310	'SK-Propantheline Bromide' Tablets 15 mg.
171	'SK-Quinidine Sulfate' Tablets 200 mg.
169	'SK-Reserpine' Tablets 0.25 mg.
463	'SK-65' Capsules 65 mg.
468	'SK-65 Compound' Capsules
474	'SK-65 APAP' Tablets
163	'SK-Soxazole' Tablets 500 mg.
126	'SK-Tetracycline HCl' Capsules 250 mg.
127	'SK-Tetracycline HCl' Capsules 500 mg.
371	'SK-Thioridazine HCl' Tablets 10 mg.
372	'SK-Thioridazine HCl' Tablets 25 mg.
373	'SK-Thioridazine HCl' Tablets 50 mg.
375	'SK-Thioridazine HCl' Tablets 100 mg.
409	'SK-Tolbutamide' Tablets 500 mg.
S03	*'Stelazine' Tablets 1 mg.
S04	*'Stelazine' Tablets 2 mg.
S06	*'Stelazine' Tablets 5 mg.
S07	*'Stelazine' Tablets 10 mg.
T01	'Temaril' *Spansule* capsules 5 mg.
T03	'Temaril' Tablets 2.5 mg.
T63	'Thorazine' *Spansule* capsules 30 mg.
T64	'Thorazine' *Spansule* capsules 75 mg.
T66	'Thorazine' *Spansule* capsules 150 mg.
T67	'Thorazine' *Spansule* capsules 200 mg.
T69	'Thorazine' *Spansule* capsules 300 mg.
T70	'Thorazine' Suppositories 25 mg.
T71	'Thorazine' Suppositories 100 mg.
T73	'Thorazine' Tablets 10 mg.
T74	'Thorazine' Tablets 25 mg.
T76	'Thorazine' Tablets 50 mg.
T77	'Thorazine' Tablets 100 mg.
T79	'Thorazine' Tablets 200 mg.

*A product of SK&F Co., Carolina, P.R. 00630, Subsidiary of SmithKline Beckman Corporation, Philadelphia, Pa.

ANCEF®
[*an-sef'*]
(brand of sterile cefazolin sodium and cefazolin sodium injection)

Description: Ancef (sterile cefazolin sodium, SK&F) is a semi-synthetic cephalosporin for parenteral administration. It is the sodium salt of 3-{[(5-methyl-1, 3, 4-thiadiazol-2-yl) thio]-methyl}-8-oxo -7- [2- (1H-tetrazol -1- yl) acetamido] -5- thia-1-azabicyclo [4.2.0] oct-2-ene-2-carboxylic acid.

The sodium content is 46 mg. per gram of cefazolin.

'Ancef' in lyophilized form is supplied in vials equivalent to 250 mg., 500 mg. or 1 gram of cefazolin, in "Piggyback" Vials for intravenous admixture equivalent to 500 mg. or 1 gram of cefazolin;

Continued on next page

Smith Kline & French—Cont.

and in Pharmacy Bulk Vials equivalent to 5 grams or 10 grams of cefazolin.

'Ancef', equivalent to 1 gram of cefazolin, is also supplied as a frozen, sterile, nonpyrogenic solution of cefazolin sodium in an iso-osmotic diluent in plastic containers. After thawing, the solution is intended for intravenous use.

The plastic container is fabricated from specially formulated polyvinyl chloride. Solutions in contact with the plastic container can leach out certain of its chemical components in very small amounts within the expiration period, e.g., di 2-ethylhexyl phthalate (DEHP), up to 5 parts per million. However, the safety of the plastic has been confirmed in tests in animals according to the USP biological tests for plastic containers as well as by tissue culture toxicity studies.

Clinical Pharmacology:
Human Pharmacology: The following tables demonstrate the blood levels and duration of cefazolin following the administration of 'Ancef'.

TABLE 1
Duration of Blood Levels of Cefazolin
250 mg. I.M. Dose (Figures are µg./ml.)

	Time After Injection in Hours			
	½	1	2	4	6
CEFAZOLIN	15.5	17.0	13.0	5.1	2.5

TABLE 2
500 mg. I.M. Dose (Figures are µg./ml.)

	Time After Injection in Hours				
	½	1	2	4	6	8
CEFAZOLIN	36.2	36.8	37.9	15.5	6.3	3.0

TABLE 3
1 gram I.M. Dose (Figures are µg./ml.)

	Time After Injection in Hours					
	½	1	2	4	6	8	10
CEFAZOLIN*	60.1	63.8	54.3	29.3	13.2	7.1	<4.1

*Average of the two studies

Clinical pharmacology studies in patients hospitalized with infections indicate that Ancef (sterile cefazolin sodium, SK&F) produces mean peak serum levels approximately equivalent to those seen in normal volunteers.

In a study (using normal volunteers) of constant intravenous infusion with dosages of 3.5 mg./kg. for 1 hour (approximately 250 mg.) and 1.5 mg./kg. the next two hours (approximately 100 mg.), 'Ancef' produced a steady serum level at the third hour of approximately 28 µg./ml. The following table shows the average serum concentration and average half life of cefazolin after I.V. injection of a single 1 gram dose of 'Ancef'.

TABLE 4
1 gram I.V. Dose (Figures are µg./ml.)

	Time After Injection, Min.			
	5	15	30	60
CEFAZOLIN	188.4	135.8	106.8	73.7

1 gram I.V. Dose (Figures are µg./ml.)

	Time After Injection, Min.		Peak	Half-life in Hours
	120	240		
CEFAZOLIN	45.6	16.5	190.0	1.4

Controlled studies on adult normal volunteers, receiving 1 gram 4 times a day for 10 days, monitoring CBC, SGOT, SGPT, bilirubin, alkaline phosphatase, BUN, creatinine, and urinalysis, indicated no clinically significant changes attributed to 'Ancef'.

'Ancef' is excreted unchanged in the urine. In the first six hours approximately 60% of the drug is excreted in the urine and this increases to 70%–80% within 24 hours. 'Ancef' achieves peak urine concentrations of approximately 2400 µg./ml. and 4000 µg./ml. respectively following 500 mg. and 1 gram intramuscular doses.

In patients undergoing peritoneal dialysis (2 l./hr.), 'Ancef' produced mean serum levels of approximately 10 and 30 µg./ml. after 24 hours' instillation of a dialyzing solution containing 50 mg./l. and 150 mg./l., respectively. Mean peak levels were 29 µg./ml. (range 13-44 µg./ml.) with 50 µg./l. (three patients), and 72 µg./ml. (range 26-142 µg./ml.) with 150 µg./l. (six patients). Intraperitoneal administration of 'Ancef' is usually well tolerated.

Bile levels in patients without obstructive biliary disease can reach or exceed serum levels by up to five times; however, in patients with obstructive biliary disease, bile levels of 'Ancef' are considerably lower than serum levels (<1.0 µg./ml.). In synovial fluid, the 'Ancef' level becomes comparable to that reached in serum at about four hours after drug administration. Studies of cord blood show prompt transfer of 'Ancef' across the placenta. 'Ancef' is present in very low concentrations in the milk of nursing mothers.

Microbiology: *In vitro* tests demonstrate that the bactericidal action of cephalosporins results from inhibition of cell wall synthesis. Ancef (sterile cefazolin sodium, SK&F) is active against the following organisms *in vitro* and in clinical infections:

Staphylococcus aureus (penicillin-sensitive and penicillin-resistant)
Staphylococcus epidermidis
Group A beta-hemolytic streptococci and other strains of streptococci (many strains of enterococci are resistant)
Streptococcus pneumoniae (formerly *D. pneumoniae*)
Escherichia coli
Proteus mirabilis
Klebsiella species
Enterobacter aerogenes
Hemophilus influenzae

Most strains of *Enterobacter cloacae* and indole positive Proteus (*P. vulgaris, P. morgani, P. rettgeri*) are resistant. Methicillin-resistant staphylococci, serratia, pseudomonas, mima, herellea species are almost uniformly resistant to cefazolin.

Disc Susceptibility Tests
Disc diffusion technique—Quantitative methods that require measurement of zone diameters give the most precise estimates of antibiotic susceptibility. One such procedure[1] has been recommended for use with discs to test susceptibility to cefazolin. Reports from a laboratory using the standardized single-disc susceptibility test[1] with a 30 mcg. cefazolin disc should be interpreted according to the following criteria:

Susceptible organisms produce zones of 18 mm. or greater, indicating that the tested organism is likely to respond to therapy.
Organisms of intermediate susceptibility produce zones 15 to 17 mm., indicating that the tested organism would be susceptible if high dosage is used or if the infection is confined to tissues and fluids (e.g., urine), in which high antibiotic levels are attained.
Resistant organisms produce zones of 14 mm. or less, indicating that other therapy should be selected.

For gram-positive isolates, a zone of 18 mm. is indicative of a cefazolin-susceptible organism when tested with either the cephalosporin-class disc (30 mcg. cephalothin) or the cefazolin disc (30 mcg. cefazolin).

Gram-negative organisms should be tested with the cefazolin disc (using the above criteria), since cefazolin has been shown by *in vitro* tests to have activity against certain strains of *Enterobacteriaceae* found resistant when tested with the cephalothin disc. Gram-negative organisms having zones of less than 18 mm. around the cephalothin disc may be susceptible to cefazolin.

Standardized procedures require use of control organisms. The 30 mcg. cefazolin disc should give zone diameter between 23 and 29 mm. for *E. coli* ATCC 25922 and between 29 and 35 mm. for *S. aureus* ATCC 25923.

The cefazolin disc should not be used for testing susceptibility to other cephalosporins.

Dilution techniques—A bacterial isolate may be considered susceptible if the minimal inhibitory concentration (MIC) for cefazolin is not more than 16 mcg. per ml. Organisms are considered resistant if the MIC is equal to or greater than 64 mcg. per ml.

The range of MIC's for the control strains are as follows:
S. aureus ATCC 25923, 0.25-1.0 mcg./ml.
E. coli ATCC 25922, 1.0-4.0 mcg./ml.

Indications and Usage: Ancef (sterile cefazolin sodium, SK&F) is indicated in the treatment of the following serious infections due to susceptible organisms:

RESPIRATORY TRACT INFECTIONS due to *Streptococcus pneumoniae* (formerly *D. pneumoniae*), *Klebsiella* species, *Hemophilus influenzae*, *Staphylococcus aureus* (penicillin-sensitive and penicillin-resistant), and group A beta-hemolytic streptococci.

Injectable benzathine penicillin is considered to be the drug of choice in treatment and prevention of streptococcal infections, including the prophylaxis of rheumatic fever.

'Ancef' is effective in the eradication of streptococci from the nasopharynx; however, data establishing the efficacy of 'Ancef' in the subsequent prevention of rheumatic fever are not available at present.

URINARY TRACT INFECTIONS due to *Escherichia coli, Proteus mirabilis, Klebsiella* species, and some strains of enterobacter and enterococci.
SKIN AND SKIN STRUCTURE INFECTIONS due to *Staphylococcus aureus* (penicillin-sensitive and penicillin-resistant), group A beta-hemolytic streptococci and other strains of streptococci.
BILIARY TRACT INFECTIONS due to *Escherichia coli*, various strains of streptococci, *Proteus mirabilis, Klebsiella* species and *Staphylococcus aureus*.
BONE AND JOINT INFECTIONS due to *Staphylococcus aureus*.
GENITAL INFECTIONS (i.e., prostatitis, epididymitis) due to *Escherichia coli, Proteus mirabilis, Klebsiella* species, and some strains of enterococci.
SEPTICEMIA due to *Streptococcus pneumoniae* (formerly *D. pneumoniae*), *Staphylococcus aureus* (penicillin-sensitive and penicillin-resistant), *Proteus mirabilis, Escherichia coli*, and *Klebsiella* species.
ENDOCARDITIS due to *Staphylococcus aureus* (penicillin-sensitive and penicillin-resistant) and group A beta-hemolytic streptococci.

Appropriate culture and susceptibility studies should be performed to determine susceptibility of the causative organism to 'Ancef'.

PERIOPERATIVE PROPHYLAXIS: The prophylactic administration of 'Ancef' preoperatively, intraoperatively, and postoperatively may reduce the incidence of certain postoperative infections in patients undergoing surgical procedures which are classified as contaminated or potentially contaminated (e.g., vaginal hysterectomy, and cholecystectomy in high-risk patients such as those over 70 years of age, with acute cholecystitis, obstructive jaundice, or common duct bile stones).

The perioperative use of 'Ancef' may also be effective in surgical patients in whom infection at the operative site would present a serious risk (e.g., during open-heart surgery and prosthetic arthroplasty.

The prophylactic administration of 'Ancef' should usually be discontinued within a 24-hour period after the surgical procedure. In surgery where the occurrence of infection may be particularly devastating (e.g., open-heart surgery and prosthetic arthroplasty), the prophylactic administration of 'Ancef' may be continued for 3 to 5 days following the completion of surgery.

If there are signs of infection, specimens for cultures should be obtained for the identification of the causative organism so that appropriate therapy may be instituted.
(See Dosage and Administration.)

Contraindications: ANCEF (STERILE CEFAZOLIN SODIUM, SK&F) IS CONTRAINDICATED IN PATIENTS WITH KNOWN ALLERGY TO THE CEPHALOSPORIN GROUP OF ANTIBIOTICS.

Warnings: BEFORE CEFAZOLIN THERAPY IS INSTITUTED, CAREFUL INQUIRY SHOULD BE MADE CONCERNING PREVIOUS HYPERSENSITIVITY REACTIONS TO CEPHALOSPORINS AND PENICILLIN. CEPHALOSPORIN C DERIVATIVES SHOULD BE GIVEN CAUTIOUSLY IN PENICILLIN-SENSITIVE PATIENTS.

SERIOUS ACUTE HYPERSENSITIVITY REACTIONS MAY REQUIRE EPINEPHRINE AND OTHER EMERGENCY MEASURES.

There is some clinical and laboratory evidence of partial cross-allergenicity of the penicillins and the cephalosporins. Patients have been reported to have had severe reactions (including anaphylaxis) to both drugs.

Any patient who has demonstrated some form of allergy, particularly to drugs, should receive antibiotics cautiously. No exception should be made with regard to 'Ancef'.

Pseudomembranous colitis has been reported with the use of cephalosporins (and other broad-spectrum antibiotics); therefore, it is important to consider its diagnosis in patients who develop diarrhea in association with antibiotic use.

Treatment with broad-spectrum antibiotics alters normal flora of the colon and may permit overgrowth of clostridia. Studies indicate a toxin produced by *Clostridium difficile* is one primary cause of antibiotic-associated colitis. Cholestyramine and colestipol resins have been shown to bind the toxin *in vitro*.

Mild cases of colitis may respond to drug discontinuance alone.

Moderate to severe cases should be managed with fluid, electrolyte and protein supplementation as indicated.

When the colitis is not relieved by drug discontinuance or when it is severe, oral vancomycin is the treatment of choice for antibiotic-associated pseudomembranous colitis produced by *C. difficile*. Other causes of colitis should also be considered.

Precautions:

General—Prolonged use of Ancef (sterile cefazolin sodium, SK&F) may result in the overgrowth of nonsusceptible organisms. Careful clinical observation of the patient is essential.

When 'Ancef' is administered to patients with low urinary output because of impaired renal function, lower daily dosage is required (see Dosage and Administration).

'Ancef', as with all cephalosporins, should be prescribed with caution in individuals with a history of gastrointestinal disease, particularly colitis.

Drug Interactions—Probenecid may decrease renal tubular secretion of cephalosporins when used concurrently, resulting in increased and more prolonged cephalosporin blood levels.

Drug/Laboratory Test Interactions—A false positive reaction for glucose in the urine may occur with Benedict's solution, Fehling's solution, or with Clinitest® tablets, but not with enzyme-based tests such as Clinistix® and Tes-Tape®.

Positive direct and indirect antiglobulin (Coombs) tests have occurred; these may also occur in neonates whose mothers received cephalosporins before delivery.

Carcinogenesis/Mutagenesis — Mutagenicity studies and long-term studies in animals to determine the carcinogenic potential of 'Ancef' have not been performed.

Pregnancy — Teratogenic Effects — Pregnancy Category B. Reproduction studies have been performed in rats, mice and rabbits at doses up to 25 times the human dose and have revealed no evidence of impaired fertility or harm to the fetus due to 'Ancef'. There are, however, no adequate and well-controlled studies in pregnant women. Because animal reproduction studies are not always predictive of human response, this drug should be used during pregnancy only if clearly needed.

Labor and Delivery—When cefazolin has been administered prior to caesarean section, drug levels in cord blood have been approximately one quarter to one third of maternal drug levels. The drug appears to have no adverse effect on the fetus.

Nursing Mothers—'Ancef' is present in very low concentrations in the milk of nursing mothers. Caution should be exercised when 'Ancef' is administered to a nursing woman.

Pediatric Use—Safety and effectiveness for use in prematures and infants under one month of age have not been established. See Dosage and Administration for recommended dosage in children over one month.

Adverse Reactions: The following reactions have been reported:

Gastrointestinal: Diarrhea, oral candidiasis (oral thrush), vomiting, nausea, stomach cramps, anorexia. Symptoms of pseudomembranous colitis can appear during antibiotic treatment. Nausea and vomiting have been reported rarely.

Allergic: Anaphylaxis, eosinophilia, itching, drug fever, skin rash.

Hematologic: Neutropenia, leukopenia, thrombocythemia.

Hepatic and Renal: Transient rise in SGOT, SGPT, BUN and alkaline phosphatase levels has been observed without clinical evidence of renal or hepatic impairment.

Local Reactions: Rare instances of phlebitis have been reported at site of injection. Pain at the site of injection after intramuscular administration has occurred infrequently. Some induration has occurred.

Other Reactions: Genital and anal pruritus (including vulvar pruritus, genital moniliasis, and vaginitis).

Dosage and Administration: Ancef (sterile cefazolin sodium, SK&F) may be administered intramuscularly or intravenously after reconstitution.

DILUTION TABLE*

Vial Size	Diluent to Be Added	Approximate Available Volume	Approximate Average Concentration
250 mg.	2.0 ml.	2.0 ml.	125 mg./ml.
500 mg.	2.0 ml.	2.2 ml.	225 mg./ml.
1 gram	2.5 ml.	3.0 ml.	330 mg./ml.

* See labeling on "Piggyback" Vials (500 mg. and 1 gram) and Pharmacy Bulk Vials (5 and 10 grams) for their reconstitution directions.

Intramuscular Administration—Reconstitute vials with Sterile Water for Injection, Bacteriostatic Water for Injection or Sodium Chloride Injection, according to the dilution table above. Shake well until dissolved. 'Ancef' should be injected into a large muscle mass. Pain on injection is infrequent with 'Ancef'. Reconstituted 'Ancef' is stable for 24 hours at room temperature or for 96 hours if stored under refrigeration. However, the solution is light sensitive and should be protected from light until used.

Intravenous Administration—Ancef (sterile cefazolin sodium, SK&F) may be administered by intravenous injection or by continuous or intermittent infusion. Total daily dosages are the same as with intramuscular injection.

Intermittent intravenous infusion: 'Ancef' can be administered along with primary intravenous fluid management programs in a volume control set or in a separate, secondary I.V. bottle. Reconstituted 500 mg. or 1 gram of 'Ancef' may be diluted in 50 to 100 ml. of one of the following intravenous solutions:

- Sodium Chloride Injection
- 5% or 10% Dextrose Injection
- 5% Dextrose in Lactated Ringer's Injection
- 5% Dextrose and 0.9% Sodium Chloride Injection (also may be used with 5% Dextrose and 0.45% or 0.2% Sodium Chloride Injection)
- Lactated Ringer's Injection
- Invert Sugar 5% or 10% in Sterile Water for Injection
- Ringer's Injection
- 5% Sodium Bicarbonate in Sterile Water for Injection

'Ancef' is stable in these intravenous fluids for 24 hours at room temperature or 96 hours if stored under refrigeration (5°C).

Direct intravenous injection: Reconstituted 500 mg. or 1 gram of 'Ancef' should be diluted with Sterile Water for Injection. The Sterile Water for Injection may be added to the 'Ancef' vial to achieve a total volume of 10 ml. Inject solution slowly over 3 to 5 minutes. May be administered directly into vein or through tubing for patient receiving the above parenteral fluids.

Parenteral drug products should be inspected visually for particulate matter and discoloration prior to administration, whenever solution and container permit.

Usual Adult Dosage

Type of Infection	Dose	Frequency
Moderate to severe infections	500 mg. to 1 gram	every 6 to 8 hrs.
Mild infections caused by susceptible gram + cocci	250 mg. to 500 mg.	every 8 hours
Acute, uncomplicated urinary tract infections	1 gram	every 12 hours
Pneumococcal pneumonia	500 mg.	every 12 hours
Severe, life-threatening infections (e.g., endocarditis, septicemia)*	1 gram to 1.5 grams	every 6 hours

* In rare instances, doses of up to 12 grams of 'Ancef' per day have been used.

Dosage Adjustment for Patients with Reduced Renal Function

'Ancef' may be used in patients with reduced renal function with the following dosage adjustments: Patients with a creatinine clearance of 55 ml./min. or greater or serum creatinine of 1.5 mg. % or less can be given full doses. Patients with creatinine clearance rates of 35 to 54 ml./min. or serum creatinine of 1.6 to 3.0 mg. % can also be given full doses but dosage should be restricted to at least 8 hour intervals. Patients with creatinine clearance rates of 11 to 34 ml./min. or serum creatinine of 3.1 to 4.5 mg. % should be given ½ the usual dose every 12 hours. Patients with creatinine clearance rates of 10 ml./min. or less or serum creatinine of 4.6 mg. % or greater should be given ½ the usual dose every 18 to 24 hours. All reduced dosage recommendations apply after an initial loading dose appropriate to the severity of the infection. Patients undergoing peritoneal dialysis: See Human Pharmacology.

DIRECTIONS FOR USE OF ANCEF (CEFAZOLIN SODIUM INJECTION, SK&F) PLASTIC CONTAINERS

'Ancef' supplied as a frozen, sterile, nonpyrogenic solution in plastic containers is to be administered either as a continuous or intermittent infusion. Thaw container at room temperature. After thawing, check for minute leaks by squeezing bag

Continued on next page

Smith Kline & French—Cont.

firmly. If leaks are found, discard solution as sterility may be impaired. Additives should not be introduced into this solution. Do not use if the solution is cloudy or precipitated or if the seal is not intact.

After thawing, the solution is stable for 24 hours at room temperature and 10 days if stored under refrigeration (5°C). DO NOT REFREEZE.

Use sterile equipment. It is recommended that the intravenous administration apparatus be replaced at least once every 48 hours.

CAUTION: Do not use plastic containers in series connections. Such use could result in air embolism due to residual air (approximately 15 ml.) being drawn from the primary container before administration of the fluid from the secondary container is complete.

Preparation for administration:
1. Suspend container from eyelet support.
2. Remove plastic protector from outlet port at bottom of container.
3. Attach administration set. Refer to complete directions accompanying set.

Perioperative Prophylactic Use
To prevent postoperative infection in contaminated or potentially contaminated surgery, recommended doses are:
 a. 1 gram I.V. or I.M. administered ½ hour to 1 hour prior to the start of surgery.
 b. For lengthy operative procedures (e.g., 2 hours or more), 500 mg. to 1 gram I.V. or I.M. during surgery (administration modified depending on the duration of the operative procedure).
 c. 500 mg. to 1 gram I.V. or I.M. every 6 to 8 hours for 24 hours postoperatively.

It is important that (1) the preoperative dose be given just (½ to 1 hour) prior to the start of surgery so that adequate antibiotic levels are present in the serum and tissues at the time of initial surgical incision; and (2) 'Ancef' be administered, if necessary, at appropriate intervals during surgery to provide sufficient levels of the antibiotic at the anticipated moments of greatest exposure to infective organisms.

In surgery where the occurrence of infection may be particularly devastating (e.g., open-heart surgery and prosthetic arthroplasty), the prophylactic administration of 'Ancef' may be continued for 3 to 5 days following the completion of surgery.

Pediatric Dosage
In children, a total daily dosage of 25 to 50 mg. per kg. (approximately 10 to 20 mg. per pound) of body weight, divided into three or four equal doses, is effective for most mild to moderately severe infections. Total daily dosage may be increased to 100 mg. per kg. (45 mg. per pound) of body weight for severe infections. Since safety for use in premature infants and in infants under one month has not been established, the use of 'Ancef' in these patients is not recommended.

Pediatric Dosage Guide

Weight		25 mg./kg./Day Divided into 3 Doses		25 mg./kg./Day Divided into 4 Doses	
Lbs.	Kg.	Approximate Single Dose mg./q8h	Vol. (ml.) needed with dilution of 125 mg./ml.	Approximate Single Dose mg./q6h	Vol. (ml.) needed with dilution of 125 mg./ml.
10	4.5	40 mg.	0.35 ml.	30 mg.	0.25 ml.
20	9.0	75 mg.	0.60 ml.	55 mg.	0.45 ml.
30	13.6	115 mg.	0.90 ml.	85 mg.	0.70 ml.
40	18.1	150 mg.	1.20 ml.	115 mg.	0.90 ml.
50	22.7	190 mg.	1.50 ml.	140 mg.	1.10 ml.

Weight		50 mg./kg./Day Divided into 3 Doses		50 mg./kg./Day Divided into 4 Doses	
Lbs.	Kg.	Approximate Single Dose mg./q8h	Vol. (ml.) needed with dilution of 225 mg./ml.	Approximate Single Dose mg./q6h	Vol. (ml.) needed with dilution of 225 mg./ml.
10	4.5	75 mg.	0.35 ml.	55 mg.	0.25 ml.
20	9.0	150 mg.	0.70 ml.	110 mg.	0.50 ml.
30	13.6	225 mg.	1.00 ml.	170 mg.	0.75 ml.
40	18.1	300 mg.	1.35 ml.	225 mg.	1.00 ml.
50	22.7	375 mg.	1.70 ml.	285 mg.	1.25 ml.

In children with mild to moderate renal impairment (creatinine clearance of 70 to 40 ml./min.), 60 percent of the normal daily dose given in equally divided doses every 12 hours should be sufficient. In patients with moderate impairment (creatinine clearance of 40 to 20 ml./min.), 25 percent of the normal daily dose given in equally divided doses every 12 hours should be adequate. Children with severe renal impairment (creatinine clearance of 20 to 5 ml./min.) may be given 10 percent of the normal daily dose every 24 hours. All dosage recommendations apply after an initial loading dose.

How Supplied: Ancef (sterile cefazolin sodium, SK&F)—supplied in vials equivalent to 250 mg., 500 mg. or 1 gram of cefazolin; in "Piggyback" Vials for intravenous admixture equivalent to 500 mg. or 1 gram of cefazolin; and in Pharmacy Bulk Vials equivalent to 5 grams or 10 grams of cefazolin.

Ancef (cefazolin sodium injection, SK&F) as a frozen, sterile, nonpyrogenic solution in plastic containers—supplied in 50 ml. single-dose containers equivalent to 1 gram of cefazolin in 5% Dextrose Injection (D5W). Do not store above −10°C.

'Ancef' supplied as a frozen, sterile, nonpyrogenic solution in plastic containers is manufactured for Smith Kline &French Laboratories by Travenol Laboratories, Inc., Deerfield, IL 60015.

Military—Vial, 5 gram, 100 ml., 10's, 6505-01-058-2046; 1 gram, 6505-01-010-0832; 500 mg., 6505-01-010-0833.

Veterans Administration—500 mg., 6505-00-431-7294; 1 gram, 6505-00-431-7290; 10 gram, 6505-00-008-3408.

1 Bauer, A.W.; Kirby, W.M.M.; Sherris, J.C., and Turck, M.: Antibiotic Testing by a Standardized Single Disc Method, Am. J. Clin. Path. 45:493, 1966. Standardized Disc Susceptibility Test, Federal Register 39:19182-19184, 1974.

AF:L34

ANSPOR® ℞
[an-spore']
(brand of cephradine)
Capsules, 250 mg. and 500 mg.
and
for Oral Suspension, 125 mg./5 ml. and 250 mg./5 ml.

('Anspor' is manufactured for Smith Kline &French Laboratories, Division of SmithKline Beckman Corporation, Philadelphia, Pa., by Squibb Manufacturing, Inc., Humacao, P.R., Subsidiary of E.R. Squibb & Sons, Inc.)

Description: Anspor (cephradine, SK&F) is a semisynthetic cephalosporin antibiotic chemically designated as (6R,7R)-7-[(R)-2-amino-2-(1,4-cyclohexadien-1-yl)acetamido]-3-methyl-8-oxo-5-thia-1-azabicyclo[4.2.0]oct-2-ene-2-carboxylic acid. Each Anspor (cephradine, SK&F) Capsule contains 250 mg. or 500 mg. of cephradine. 'Anspor' for Oral Suspension is available in bottles containing 2.5 grams or 5 grams of cephradine, which after reconstitution with 61 ml. of water, respectively, provides 125 mg. or 250 mg. of cephradine per 5 ml. teaspoonful.

Clinical Pharmacology:

Human Pharmacology: Anspor (cephradine, SK&F) is acid stable. It is rapidly absorbed after oral administration in the fasting state. Following doses of 250 mg. and 500 mg. in normal adult volunteers, average peak serum levels within one hour were approximately 9 and 16.5 mcg. per ml. respectively. The presence of food in the gastrointestinal tract delays the absorption but does not affect the total amount of cephradine absorbed. Over 90 percent of the drug is excreted unchanged in the urine within 6 hours. Peak urine concentrations are approximately 1600 mcg. per ml. following a 250 mg. dose and 3200 mcg. per ml. following a 500 mg. dose.

Microbiology: *In vitro* tests demonstrate that the cephalosporins are bactericidal because of their inhibition of cell-wall synthesis. Cephradine is active against the following organisms *in vitro* and in clinical infections:
Beta-hemolytic streptococci
Staphylococci, including coagulase-positive, coagulase-negative, and penicillinase-producing strains
Streptococcus pneumoniae (formerly *D. pneumoniae*)
Escherichia coli
Proteus mirabilis
Klebsiella sp.
Hemophilus influenzae

Note—Some strains of enterococci (*Streptococcus faecalis*) are resistant to cephradine. It is not active against most strains of *Enterobacter* sp., *Pr. morganii*, and *Pr. vulgaris*. It has no activity against *Pseudomonas* or *Herellea* species. When tested by *in vitro* methods, staphylococci exhibit cross-resistance between cephradine and methicillin-type antibiotics.

Disc Susceptibility Tests: Quantitative methods that require measurement of zone diameters give the most precise estimates of antibiotic susceptibility. One recommended procedure (21 CFR § 460.1) uses cephalosporin class discs for testing susceptibility; interpretations correlate zone diameters of this disc test with MIC values for cephradine. With this procedure, a report from the laboratory of "resistant" indicates that the infecting organism is not likely to respond to therapy. A report of "intermediate susceptibility" suggests that the organism would be susceptible if the infection is confined to the urinary tract, as high antibiotic levels can be obtained in the urine, or if high dosage is used in other types of infection.

Indications and Usage: Anspor (cephradine, SK&F) Capsules and 'Anspor' for Oral Suspension are indicated in the treatment of the following infections when caused by susceptible strains of designated microorganisms:

Infections of the respiratory tract (e.g., tonsillitis, pharyngitis, and lobar pneumonia) caused by group A beta-hemolytic streptococci and *Streptococcus pneumoniae* (formerly *D. pneumoniae*). (Penicillin is the usual drug of choice in the treatment and prevention of streptococcal infections, including the prophylaxis of rheumatic fever. 'Anspor' is generally effective in the eradication of streptococci from the nasopharynx; substantial data establishing the efficacy of 'Anspor' in the subsequent prevention of rheumatic fever are not available at present.)

Otitis media caused by group A beta-hemolytic streptococci, *Streptococcus pneumoniae* (formerly *D. pneumoniae*), *Hemophilus influenzae* and staphylococci.

Skin and skin structure infections caused by staphylococci (penicillin-susceptible and penicillin-resistant) and beta-hemolytic streptococci.

Infections of the urinary tract, including prostatitis, caused by *Escherichia coli*, *Pr. mirabilis*, and *Klebsiella* sp.

Note—Culture and susceptibility tests should be initiated prior to and during therapy. Renal function studies should be performed when indicated.

Contraindications: Cephradine is contraindicated in patients with known hypersensitivity to the cephalosporin group of antibiotics.

Warnings: BEFORE CEPHRADINE THERAPY IS INSTITUTED, CAREFUL INQUIRY SHOULD

BE MADE CONCERNING PREVIOUS HYPERSENSITIVITY REACTIONS TO CEPHALOSPORINS AND PENICILLIN. CEPHALOSPORIN C DERIVATIVES SHOULD BE GIVEN CAUTIOUSLY IN PENICILLIN-SENSITIVE PATIENTS.

SERIOUS ACUTE HYPERSENSITIVITY REACTIONS MAY REQUIRE EPINEPHRINE AND OTHER EMERGENCY MEASURES.

There is some clinical and laboratory evidence of partial cross-allergenicity of the penicillins and the cephalosporins. Patients have been reported to have had severe reactions (including anaphylaxis) to both drugs.

Any patient who has demonstrated some form of allergy, particularly to drugs, should receive antibiotics cautiously. No exception should be made with regard to Anspor (cephradine, SK&F).

Pseudomembranous colitis has been reported with the use of cephalosporins (and other broad-spectrum antibiotics); therefore, it is important to consider its diagnosis in patients who develop diarrhea in association with antibiotic use.

Treatment with broad-spectrum antibiotics alters normal flora of the colon and may permit overgrowth of clostridia. Studies indicate a toxin produced by *Clostridium difficile* is one primary cause of antibiotic-associated colitis. Cholestyramine and colestipol resins have been shown to bind the toxin *in vitro*.

Mild cases of colitis may respond to drug discontinuance alone.

Moderate to severe cases should be managed with fluid, electrolyte and protein supplementation as indicated.

When the colitis is not relieved by drug discontinuance or when it is severe, oral vancomycin is the treatment of choice for antibiotic-associated pseudomembranous colitis produced by *C. difficile*. Other causes of colitis should also be considered.

Precautions:
General—Patients should be followed carefully so that any side effects or unusual manifestations of drug idiosyncrasy may be detected. If a hypersensitivity reaction occurs, the drug should be discontinued and the patient treated with the usual agents, e.g., pressor amines, antihistamines, or corticosteroids.

Administer cephradine with caution in the presence of markedly impaired renal function. In patients with known or suspected renal impairment, careful clinical observation and appropriate laboratory studies should be made prior to and during therapy as cephradine accumulates in the serum and tissues. See DOSAGE AND ADMINISTRATION section for information on treatment of patients with impaired renal function.

Prolonged use of antibiotics may promote the overgrowth of nonsusceptible organisms. Should superinfection occur during therapy, appropriate measures should be taken.

Anspor (cephradine, SK&F), as with all cephalosporins, should be prescribed with caution in individuals with a history of gastrointestinal disease, particularly colitis.

Information for Patients—Cephradine may be taken without regard to meals, unless gastrointestinal irritation occurs.

Diabetic patients receiving 'Anspor' should be cautioned to check with physicians before changing diet or dosage of diabetes medication. A false positive reaction for glucose in the urine may occur with Benedict's solution, Fehling's solution, or with Clinitest® tablets, but not with enzyme-based tests such as Clinistix® and Tes-Tape®.

Laboratory Tests—In chronic urinary tract infections, frequent bacteriologic tests are necessary during drug therapy and may be necessary for several months afterwards.

Drug Interactions—Probenecid may decrease renal tubular secretion of cephalosporins when used concurrently, resulting in increased and more prolonged cephalosporin blood levels.

Drug/Laboratory Test Interactions—After treatment with cephradine, a false positive reaction for glucose in the urine may occur with Benedict's solution, Fehling's solution, or with Clinitest® tablets, but not with enzyme-based tests such as Clinistix® and Tes-Tape®.

A false positive direct Coombs test has been reported after treatment with other cephalosporins; therefore, it should be recognized that a positive Coombs test may be due to the drug.

Carcinogenesis/Mutagenesis — Mutagenicity studies and long-term studies in animals to determine the carcinogenic potential of Anspor (cephradine, SK&F) have not been performed.

Pregnancy—*Teratogenic Effects*—Pregnancy Category B. Reproduction studies have been performed in mice and rats receiving doses up to four times the maximum human dose and have revealed no evidence of impaired fertility or harm to the fetus due to cephradine. There are, however, no adequate and well-controlled studies in pregnant women. Because animal reproduction studies are not always predictive of human response, this drug should be used during pregnancy only if clearly needed.

Nursing Mothers—Cephradine is present in very low concentrations in the milk of nursing mothers. Caution should be exercised when cephradine is administered to a nursing woman.

Pediatric Use—Safety and effectiveness for use in infants under nine months of age have not been established. See DOSAGE AND ADMINISTRATION section for recommended dosage in children over nine months.

Adverse Reactions: As with other cephalosporins, untoward reactions are limited essentially to gastrointestinal disturbances and to hypersensitivity phenomena. The latter are more likely to occur in individuals who have previously demonstrated hypersensitivity and those with a history of allergy, asthma, hay fever, or urticaria.

The following adverse reactions have been reported following the use of cephradine:

Gastrointestinal: Diarrhea or loose stools, vomiting, glossitis, nausea, abdominal pain and heartburn.

Symptoms of pseudomembranous colitis can appear during antibiotic treatment.

Nausea and vomiting have been reported rarely.

Allergic: Anaphylaxis, mild urticaria or skin rash, pruritus, joint pains.

Hematologic: Mild, transient eosinophilia, leukopenia and neutropenia.

Liver: Transient mild rise of SGOT, SGPT, and total bilirubin has been observed with no evidence of hepatocellular damage.

Renal: Transitory rises in BUN have been observed in some patients treated with cephalosporins; their frequency increases in patients over 50 years old. In adults for whom serum creatinine determinations were performed, the rise in BUN was not accompanied by a rise in serum creatinine.

Other: Dizziness and tightness in the chest and candidal vaginitis.

Dosage and Administration: Anspor (cephradine, SK&F) may be given without regard to meals.

Adults: For skin and soft-tissue and respiratory tract infections (other than lobar pneumonia), the usual dose is 250 mg. every 6 hours or 500 mg. every 12 hours. For acute infections of the urinary tract, including prostatitis, and pneumococcal lobar pneumonia, the usual dose is 500 mg. every 6 hours or 1 gram every 12 hours. Severe or chronic infections may require larger doses.

Children: No adequate information is available on the efficacy of b.i.d. regimens in children under nine months of age. The usual dose in children over nine months of age is 25 to 50 mg./kg./day administered in equally divided doses every 6 or 12 hours. For otitis media due to *H. influenzae*, doses are from 75 to 100 mg./kg./day administered in equally divided doses every 6 or 12 hours. Doses for children should not exceed doses recommended for adults. The maximum dose should not exceed 4 grams per day.

All patients, regardless of age and weight: Larger doses (up to 1 gram, q.i.d.) may be given for severe or chronic infections.

As with antibiotic therapy generally, therapy should be continued for a minimum of 48 to 72 hours after the patient becomes asymptomatic or evidence of bacterial eradication has been obtained. In infections caused by group A beta-hemolytic streptococci, a minimum of 10 days of treatment is recommended to guard against the risk of rheumatic fever or glomerulonephritis. In the treatment of chronic urinary tract infection, frequent bacteriologic and clinical appraisal is necessary during therapy and may be necessary for several months afterwards. Persistent infections may require treatment for several weeks. Prolonged intensive therapy is recommended for prostatitis. Doses smaller than those indicated are not recommended.

Patients with Impaired Renal Function
Not on Dialysis: The following initial dosage schedule is suggested as a guideline based on creatinine clearance. Further modification in the dosage schedule may be required because of individual variations in absorption.

Creatinine Clearance	Dose	Time Interval
> 20 ml./min.	500 mg.	6 hours
5–20 ml./min.	250 mg.	6 hours
< 5 ml./min.	250 mg.	12 hours

On Chronic, Intermittent Hemodialysis:
250 mg. Start
250 mg. at 12 hours
250 mg. 36–48 hours (after start)

Children may require dosage modification proportional to their weight and severity of infection.

How Supplied: Anspor (cephradine, SK&F) is available as 'Anspor' Capsules in 250 mg. in bottles of 100 and in Single Unit Packages of 100 (intended for institutional use only); and in 500 mg. in bottles of 20 and 100 and in Single Unit Packages of 100 (intended for institutional use only). 'Anspor' is also available as 'Anspor' for Oral Suspension which, after reconstitution, provides 125 mg. or 250 mg. of cephradine per 5 ml. teaspoonful in a pleasant, fruit-flavored suspension in 100 ml. bottles.

Notes on Stability: Anspor (cephradine, SK&F) Capsules—Do not store above 86°F.; keep bottle tightly closed. 'Anspor' for Oral Suspension—Prior to reconstitution, do not store above 86°F. After reconstitution, suspensions retain their potency for seven days at room temperature and for 14 days if refrigerated.

Shown in Product Identification Section, page 436
AN:L13

CEFIZOX® B
[*sef' eh-zocks*]
(brand of sterile ceftizoxime sodium and ceftizoxime sodium injection)

Description: Cefizox (sterile ceftizoxime sodium, FSK) is a sterile, semisynthetic, broad-spectrum, beta-lactamase resistant cephalosporin antibiotic for parenteral (I.V., I.M.) administration. It is the sodium salt of [6R-[6α, 7 β(Z)]]-7-[[(2,3-dihydro-2-imino-4-thiazolyl) (methoxyimino) acetyl] amino]-8-oxo-5-thia-1-azabicyclo [4.2.0] oct-2-ene-2-carboxylic acid. Its sodium content is approximately 60 mg. (2.6 mEq.) per gram of ceftizoxime activity.

Sterile ceftizoxime sodium is a white to pale yellow crystalline powder.

'Cefizox' is supplied in vials equivalent to 1 gram or 2 grams of ceftizoxime, and the "Piggyback" Vials for intravenous admixture equivalent to 1 gram or 2 grams of ceftizoxime.

'Cefizox', equivalent to 1 gram or 2 grams of ceftizoxime, is also supplied as a frozen, sterile, nonpyrogenic solution of ceftizoxime sodium in an isoosmotic diluent in plastic containers. After thawing, the solution is intended for intravenous use. The plastic container is fabricated from specially formulated polyvinyl chloride. Solutions in contact with the plastic container can leach out certain of its chemical components in very small amounts within the expiration period, e.g., di 2-ethylhexyl phthalate (DEHP), up to 5 parts per million. However, the safety of the plastic has been confirmed in tests in animals according to the USP

Continued on next page

Smith Kline & French—Cont.

biological tests for plastic containers as well as by tissue culture toxicity studies.

Clinical Pharmacology: The table below demonstrates the serum levels and duration of Cefizox (sterile ceftizoxime sodium, FSK) following intramuscular administration of 500 mg. and 1.0 gram doses respectively to normal volunteers. [See table below].

Following intravenous administration of 1.0, 2.0 and 3.0 gram doses of 'Cefizox' to normal volunteers, the following serum levels were obtained: [See table above].

Serum Concentrations After Intravenous Administration
Serum Concentration (mcg./ml.)

Dose	5 mins.	10 mins.	30 mins.	1 hr.	2 hrs.	4 hrs.	8 hrs.
1.0 gram	ND	ND	60.5	38.9	21.5	8.4	1.4
2.0 grams	131.8	110.9	77.5	53.6	33.1	12.1	2.0
3.0 grams	221.1	174.0	112.7	83.9	47.4	26.2	4.8

ND = Not Done

A serum half-life of approximately 1.7 hours was observed after intravenous or intramuscular administration.

'Cefizox' is 30% protein bound.

'Cefizox' is not metabolized, and is excreted virtually unchanged by the kidneys in 24 hours. This provides a high urinary concentration. Concentrations greater than 6,000 mcg./ml. have been achieved in the urine by 2 hours after a 1 gram dose of 'Cefizox' intravenously. Probenecid slows tubular secretion and produces even higher serum levels, increasing the duration of measurable serum concentrations.

'Cefizox' achieves therapeutic levels in various body fluids, e.g., cerebrospinal fluid (in patients with inflamed meninges), bile, surgical wound fluid, pleural fluid, aqueous humor, ascitic fluid, peritoneal fluid, prostatic fluid and saliva, and the following body tissues: heart, gallbladder, bone, biliary, peritoneal, prostatic and uterine.

In clinical experience to date, no disulfiram-like reactions have been reported with Cefizox (sterile ceftizoxime sodium, FSK).

Microbiology

The bactericidal action of 'Cefizox' results from inhibition of cell-wall synthesis. 'Cefizox' is highly resistant to a broad spectrum of beta-lactamases (penicillinase and cephalosporinase), including Richmond types I, II, III, TEM, and IV, produced by both aerobic and anaerobic gram-positive and gram-negative organisms. 'Cefizox' is active against a wide range of gram-positive and gram-negative organisms, and is usually active against the following organisms *in vitro* and in clinical situations (see Indications and Usage):

Gram-Positive Aerobes:
Staphylococcus sp. including penicillinase and nonpenicillinase producing *S. aureus* and *S. epidermidis*. Note: Methicillin-resistant staphylococci are resistant to cephalosporins, including ceftizoxime.
Streptococcus sp. including *S. pneumoniae* (formerly *D. pneumoniae*) and *S. pyogenes*.
Note: 'Cefizox' is usually inactive *in vitro* against most strains of enterococci, e.g., *S. faecalis*.

Gram-Negative Aerobes:
Klebsiella sp. including *K. pneumoniae*
Escherichia coli
Proteus mirabilis
Proteus vulgaris
Morganella morganii (formerly *Proteus morganii*) and
Providencia rettgeri (formerly *Proteus rettgeri*)
Serratia sp. including *S. marcescens*
Enterobacter sp.
Pseudomonas sp. including *Ps. aeruginosa*
Haemophilus sp. including ampicillin-resistant strains of *H. influenzae*
Neisseria gonorrhoeae

Anaerobes:
Bacteroides sp. including *B. fragilis*
Anaerobic cocci including *Peptococcus* sp. *Peptostreptococcus* sp.

'Cefizox' is usually active against strains of *Acinetobacter* sp.

Cefizox (sterile ceftizoxime sodium, FSK) is usually active against the following organisms *in vitro*, but the clinical significance of these data has not been established.

Gram-Positive Aerobes:
Corynebacterium diphtheriae

Gram-Negative Aerobes:
Shigella sp.
Providencia stuartii
Salmonella sp.
Aeromonas hydrophila
Yersinia enterocolitica
Moraxella sp.
Pasteurella multocida
Neisseria meningitidis
Citrobacter sp.

Anaerobes:
Actinomyces sp.
Veillonella sp.
Eubacterium sp.
Clostridium sp.
Fusobacterium sp.
Bifidobacterium sp.
Propionibacterium sp.

(Note: Most strains of *C. difficile* are resistant.)

Susceptibility Testing

Quantitative methods that require measurement of zone diameters give the most precise estimate of antibiotic susceptibility. One such procedure* has been recommended for use with discs to test susceptibility to ceftizoxime.

Reports from the laboratory giving results of the standard single-disc susceptibility test with a 30 mcg. ceftizoxime disc should be interpreted according to the following criteria (with the exception of *Ps. aeruginosa*):

Susceptible organisms produce zones of 20 mm. or greater, indicating that the test organism is likely to respond to therapy.

Organisms that produce zones of 15 to 19 mm. are expected to be susceptible if high dosage is used or if the infection is confined to tissues and fluids (e.g., urine) in which high antibiotic levels are attained.

Resistant organisms produce zones of 14 mm. or less, indicating that other therapy should be selected.

Organisms should be tested with the 'Cefizox' disc, since 'Cefizox' has been shown by *in vitro* tests to be active against certain strains found resistant when other beta-lactam discs are used.

Susceptibility Testing for Pseudomonas in Urinary Tract Infections

Most strains of *Ps. aeruginosa* are moderately susceptible to Cefizox (sterile ceftizoxime sodium, FSK). 'Cefizox' achieves high levels in the urine (greater than 6,000 mcg./ml. at 2 hours with 1 gram I.V.) and therefore the following zone sizes should be used when testing 'Cefizox' for treatment of urinary tract infections caused by *Ps. aeruginosa*:

Susceptible organisms produce zones of 20 mm. or greater, indicating that the test organism is likely to respond to therapy.

Organisms that produce zones of 11 to 19 mm. are expected to be susceptible when the infection is confined to the urinary tract in which high antibiotic levels are attained.

Resistant organisms produce zones of 10 mm. or less, indicating that other therapy should be selected.

A bacterial isolate may be considered susceptible if the MIC value for 'Cefizox' is equal to or less than 16 mcg./ml. Organisms are considered moderately susceptible if the MIC is greater than 16 mcg./ml. but less than 64 mcg./ml. Organisms are considered resistant if the MIC is 64 mcg./ml. or greater. For most organisms the MBC value for 'Cefizox' is the same as the MIC value.

The standardized quality control procedure requires use of control organisms. The 30 mcg. ceftizoxime disc should give the zone diameters listed below for the quality control strains.

Organism	ATCC	Zone Size Range
E. coli	25922	30–36 mm.
S. aureus	25923	27–35 mm.
Ps. aeruginosa	27853	12–17 mm.

Indications and Usage: Cefizox (sterile ceftizoxime sodium, FSK) is indicated in the treatment of infections due to susceptible strains of the microorganisms listed below:

LOWER RESPIRATORY TRACT INFECTIONS caused by *Streptococcus* sp. including *S. pneumoniae* (formerly *D. pneumoniae*), but excluding enterococci; *Klebsiella* sp.; *Proteus mirabilis*; *Escherichia coli*; *Haemophilus influenzae* including ampicillin-resistant strains; *Staphylococcus aureus* (penicillinase and nonpenicillinase producing); *Serratia* sp.; *Enterobacter* sp.; and *Bacteroides* sp.

URINARY TRACT INFECTIONS caused by *Staphylococcus aureus* (penicillinase and nonpenicillinase producing); *Escherichia coli*; *Pseudomonas* sp. including *Ps. aeruginosa*; *Proteus mirabilis*; *P. vulgaris*; *Providencia rettgeri* (formerly *Proteus rettgeri*) and *Morganella morganii* (formerly *Proteus morganii*); *Klebsiella* sp.; *Serratia* sp. including *S. marcescens*; *Enterobacter* sp.

GONORRHEA. Uncomplicated cervical and urethral gonorrhea caused by *Neisseria gonorrhoeae*.

INTRA-ABDOMINAL INFECTIONS caused by *Escherichia coli*; *Staphylococcus epidermidis*; *Streptococcus* sp. (excluding enterococci); *Enterobacter* sp.; *Klebsiella* sp.; *Bacteroides* sp. including *B. fragilis*; and anaerobic cocci, including *Peptococcus* sp. and *Peptostreptococcus* sp.

SEPTICEMIA caused by *Streptococcus* sp. including *S. pneumoniae* (formerly *D. pneumoniae*), but excluding enterococci; *Staphylococcus aureus* (penicillinase and nonpenicillinase producing); *Escherichia coli*; *Bacteroides* sp. including *B. fragilis*; *Klebsiella* sp.; and *Serratia* sp.

SKIN AND SKIN STRUCTURE INFECTIONS caused by *Staphylococcus aureus* (penicillinase and nonpenicillinase producing); *Staphylococcus epidermidis*; *Escherichia coli*; *Klebsiella* sp.; *Streptococcus* sp. including *Streptococcus pyogenes* (group A beta-hemolytic), but excluding enterococci; *Proteus mirabilis*; *Serratia* sp.; *Enterobacter* sp.; *Bacteroides* sp. including *B. fragilis*; and anaerobic cocci, including *Peptococcus* sp. and *Peptostreptococcus* sp.

BONE AND JOINT INFECTIONS caused by *Staphylococcus aureus* (penicillinase and nonpenicillinase producing); *Streptococcus* sp. (excluding enterococci); *Proteus mirabilis*; *Bacteroides* sp.; and anaerobic cocci, including *Peptococcus* sp. and *Peptostreptococcus* sp.

MENINGITIS caused by *Haemophilus influenzae*. 'Cefizox' has also been used successfully in the treatment of a limited number of pediatric and adult cases of meningitis caused by *Streptococcus pneumoniae*.

Serum Concentrations After Intramuscular Administration
Serum Concentration (mcg./ml.)

Dose	½ hr.	1 hr.	2 hrs.	4 hrs.	6 hrs.	8 hrs.
500 mg.	13.3	13.7	9.2	4.8	1.9	0.7
1.0 gram	36.0	39.0	31.0	15.0	6.0	3.0

Product Information

'Cefizox' has been effective in the treatment of seriously ill, compromised patients, including those who were debilitated, immunosuppressed or neutropenic.

Infections caused by aerobic gram-negative and by mixtures of organisms resistant to other cephalosporins, aminoglycosides, or penicillins have responded to treatment with 'Cefizox'.

Because of the serious nature of some urinary tract infections due to *Ps. aeruginosa* and because many strains of *Pseudomonas* species are only moderately susceptible to 'Cefizox', higher dosage is recommended. Other therapy should be instituted if the response is not prompt.

Susceptibility studies on specimens obtained prior to therapy should be used to determine the response of causative organisms to 'Cefizox'. Therapy with 'Cefizox' may be initiated pending results of the studies; however, treatment should be adjusted according to study findings. In serious infections 'Cefizox' has been used concomitantly with aminoglycosides (see Precautions). Before using 'Cefizox' concomitantly with other antibiotics, the prescribing information for those agents should be reviewed for contraindications, warnings, precautions and adverse reactions. Renal function should be carefully monitored.

Contraindications: Cefizox (sterile ceftizoxime sodium, FSK) is contraindicated in patients who have known allergy to the drug.

Warnings: BEFORE THERAPY WITH CEFIZOX (STERILE CEFTIZOXIME SODIUM, FSK) IS INSTITUTED, CAREFUL INQUIRY SHOULD BE MADE TO DETERMINE WHETHER THE PATIENT HAS HAD PREVIOUS HYPERSENSITIVITY REACTIONS TO CEPHALOSPORINS, PENICILLINS, OR OTHER DRUGS. THIS PRODUCT SHOULD BE GIVEN CAUTIOUSLY TO PENICILLIN-SENSITIVE PATIENTS. ANTIBIOTICS SHOULD BE ADMINISTERED WITH CAUTION TO ANY PATIENT WHO HAS DEMONSTRATED SOME FORM OF ALLERGY, PARTICULARLY TO DRUGS. SERIOUS ACUTE HYPERSENSITIVITY REACTIONS MAY REQUIRE EPINEPHRINE AND OTHER EMERGENCY MEASURES.

Pseudomembranous colitis has been reported with the use of cephalosporins (and other broad-spectrum antibiotics); therefore, it is important to consider its diagnosis in patients who developed diarrhea in association with antibiotic use.

Treatment with broad-spectrum antibiotics alters normal flora of the colon and may permit overgrowth of *Clostridia*. Studies indicate a toxin produced by *Clostridium difficile* is one primary cause of antibiotic-associated colitis. Cholestyramine and colestipol resins have been shown to bind the toxin *in vitro*.

Mild cases of colitis may respond to drug discontinuance alone.

Moderate to severe cases should be managed with fluid, electrolyte and protein supplementation as indicated.

When the colitis is not relieved by drug discontinuance or when it is severe, oral vancomycin is the treatment of choice for antibiotic-associated pseudomembranous colitis produced by *C. difficile*. Other causes of colitis should also be considered.

Precautions:
General: As with all broad-spectrum antibiotics, Cefizox (sterile ceftizoxime sodium, FSK) should be prescribed with caution in individuals with a history of gastrointestinal disease, particularly colitis.

Although 'Cefizox' has not been shown to produce an alteration in renal function, renal status should be evaluated, especially in seriously ill patients receiving maximum dose therapy. As with any antibiotic, prolonged use may result in overgrowth of nonsusceptible organisms. Careful observation is essential; appropriate measures should be taken if superinfection occurs.

Drug Interactions: Although the occurrence has not been reported with 'Cefizox', nephrotoxicity has been reported following concomitant administration of other cephalosporins and aminoglycosides.

General Guidelines for Dosage of 'Cefizox'

Type of Infection	Daily Dose (Grams)	Frequency and Route
Uncomplicated Urinary Tract	1	500 mg. q12h I.M. or I.V.
Other Sites	2–3	1 gram q8–12h I.M. or I.V.
Severe or Refractory	3–6	1 gram q8h I.M. or I.V. 2 grams q8–12h I.M.* or I.V.
Life-Threatening†	9–12	3–4 grams q8h I.V.

*When administering 2 gram I.M. doses, the dose should be divided and given in different large muscle masses.
† In life-threatening infections dosages up to 2 grams every 4 hours have been given.

Pregnancy: (Category B.) Reproduction studies have been performed in rats and rabbits and have revealed no evidence of impaired fertility or harm to the fetus due to 'Cefizox'. There are, however, no adequate and well-controlled studies in pregnant women. Because animal reproduction studies are not always predictive of human response, this drug should be used during pregnancy only if clearly needed.

Labor and Delivery: Safety of 'Cefizox' use during labor and delivery has not been established.

Nursing Mothers: 'Cefizox' is excreted in human milk in low concentrations. Caution should be exercised when 'Cefizox' is administered to a nursing woman.

Infants and Children: Safety and efficacy in infants from birth to six months of age have not been established. In children six months of age and older, treatment with 'Cefizox' has been associated with transient elevated levels of eosinophils, SGOT, SGPT and CPK (creatine phosphokinase). The CPK elevation may be related to I.M. administration.

Adverse Reactions: Ceftizoxime is generally well tolerated. The *most* frequent adverse reactions (*greater than 1%* but less than 5%) are:
Hypersensitivity—Rash, pruritus, fever.
Liver—Transient elevation in SGOT, SGPT and alkaline phosphatase.
Blood—Transient eosinophilia, thrombocytosis. Some individuals have developed a positive Coombs test.
Local—Injection site—Burning, cellulitis, phlebitis with I.V. administration, pain, induration, tenderness, paresthesia.
The *less* frequent adverse reactions (*less than 1%*) are:
Renal—Transient elevations of BUN and creatinine have been occasionally observed with ceftizoxime.
Blood—Neutropenia, leukopenia and thrombocytopenia have been reported rarely.
Genitourinary—Vaginitis has rarely occurred.
Gastrointestinal—Diarrhea; nausea and vomiting have been reported occasionally.
Symptoms of pseudomembranous colitis can appear during or after antibiotic treatment. (See Warnings section.) Nausea and vomiting have been reported rarely.

Dosage and Administration: The usual adult dosage is 1 or 2 grams of Cefizox (sterile ceftizoxime sodium, FSK) every 8 to 12 hours. Proper dosage and route of administration should be determined by the condition of the patient, severity of the infection and susceptibility of the causative organisms.
[See table above].
Because of the serious nature of urinary tract infections due to *Ps. aeruginosa* and because many strains of *Pseudomonas* species are only moderately susceptible to 'Cefizox', higher dosage is recommended. Other therapy should be instituted if the response is not prompt.

A single, 1 gram I.M. dose is the usual dose for treatment of uncomplicated gonorrhea.

The intravenous route may be preferable for patients with bacterial septicemia, localized parenchymal abscesses (such as intra-abdominal abscess), peritonitis, or other severe or life-threatening infections.

In those with normal renal function, the intravenous dosage for such infections is 2 to 12 grams of Cefizox (sterile ceftizoxime sodium, FSK) daily. In conditions such as bacterial septicemia, 6 to 12 grams/day may be given initially by the intravenous route for several days, and the dosage may then be gradually reduced according to clinical response and laboratory findings.

Pediatric Dosage Schedule

	Unit Dose	Frequency
Children 6 months and older	50 mg./kg.	q6-8h

Dosage may be increased to a total daily dose of 200 mg./kg. (not to exceed the maximum adult dose for serious infection).

Impaired Renal Function
Modification of 'Cefizox' dosage is necessary in patients with impaired renal function. Following an initial loading dose of 500 mg.–1.0 gram I.M. or I.V., the maintenance dosing schedule shown below should be followed. Further dosing should be determined by therapeutic monitoring, severity of the infection and susceptibility of the causative organisms.

When only the serum creatinine level is available, creatinine clearance may be calculated from the following formula. The serum creatinine level should represent current renal function at the steady state.

Males
$$Clcr = \frac{Weight (kg.) \times (140 - age)}{72 \times serum\ creatinine\ (mg./100\ ml.)}$$
Females 0.85 of the above values

In patients undergoing hemodialysis no additional supplemental dosing is required following hemodialysis; however, dosing should be timed so that the patient receives the dose (according to the table below) at the end of the dialysis.

Dosage in Adults with Reduced Renal Function

Creatinine Clearance ml./min.	Renal Function	Less Severe Infections	Life-Threatening Infections
79–50	Mild impairment	500 mg. q8h	0.75 gram–1.5 grams q8h
49–5	Moderate to severe impairment	250 mg.–500 mg. q12h	0.5 gram–1.0 gram q12h
4–0	Dialysis patients	500 mg. q48h or 250 mg. q24h	0.5 gram–1.0 gram q48h or 0.5 gram q24h

Continued on next page

Smith Kline & French—Cont.

Preparation of Parenteral Solution
RECONSTITUTION

I.M. Administration: Reconstitute with Sterile Water for Injection. SHAKE WELL.

Vial Size	Diluent to Be Added	Approx. Avail. Vol.	Approx. Avg. Concentration
1 gram	3.0 ml.	3.7 ml.	270 mg./ml.
2 grams*	6.0 ml.	7.4 ml.	270 mg./ml.

*When administering 2 gram I.M. doses, the dose should be divided and given in different large muscle masses.

I.V. Administration: Reconstitute with Sterile Water for Injection. SHAKE WELL.

Vial Size	Diluent to Be Added	Approx. Avail. Vol.	Approx. Avg. Concentration
1 gram	10 ml.	10.7 ml.	95 mg./ml.
2 grams	20 ml.	21.4 ml.	95 mg./ml.

These solutions of Cefizox (sterile ceftizoxime sodium, FSK) are stable 8 hours at room temperature or 48 hours if refrigerated (5°C.).

Parenteral drug products should be inspected visually for particulate matter prior to administration. If particulate matter is evident in reconstituted fluids, then the drug solution should be discarded. Reconstituted solutions may range from yellow to amber without changes in potency.

"Piggyback" Vials: Reconstitute with 50 to 100 ml. of Sodium Chloride Injection or any other I.V. solution listed below. SHAKE WELL.
Administer with primary I.V. fluids, as a single dose. These solutions of 'Cefizox' are stable 8 hours at room temperature or 48 hours if refrigerated (5°C.).

A solution of 1 gram 'Cefizox' in 13 ml. Sterile Water for Injection is isotonic.

I.M. Injection: Inject well within the body of a relatively large muscle. Aspiration is necessary to avoid inadvertent injection into a blood vessel. When administering 2 gram I.M. doses, the dose should be divided and given in different large muscle masses.

I.V. Administration: Direct (bolus) injection, slowly over 3 to 5 minutes, directly or through tubing for patients receiving parenteral fluids (see list below). Intermittent or continuous infusion, dilute reconstituted 'Cefizox' in 50 to 100 ml. of one of the following solutions:

- Sodium Chloride Injection
- 5% or 10% Dextrose Injection
- 5% Dextrose and 0.9%, 0.45%, or 0.2% Sodium Chloride Injection
- Ringer's Injection
- Lactated Ringer's Injection
- Invert Sugar 10% in Sterile Water for Injection
- 5% Sodium Bicarbonate in Sterile Water for Injection
- 5% Dextrose in Lactated Ringer's Injection (only when reconstituted with 4% Sodium Bicarbonate Injection)

In these fluids 'Cefizox' is stable 8 hours at room temperature or 48 hours if refrigerated (5°C.).

DIRECTIONS FOR USE OF CEFIZOX (CEFTIZOXIME SODIUM INJECTION, FSK) PLASTIC CONTAINERS

'Cefizox' supplied as a frozen, sterile, nonpyrogenic solution in plastic containers is to be administered either as a continuous or intermittent infusion.

Thaw container at room temperature. After thawing, check for minute leaks by squeezing bag firmly. If leaks are found, discard solution as sterility may be impaired. Additives should not be introduced into this solution. Do not use if the solution is cloudy or precipitated or if the seal is not intact.

After thawing, the solution is stable for 24 hours at room temperature or 10 days if stored under refrigeration (5°C.). DO NOT REFREEZE.

Use sterile equipment. It is recommended that the intravenous administration apparatus be replaced at least once every 48 hours.

CAUTION: Do not use plastic containers in series connections. Such use could result in air embolism due to residual air being drawn from the primary container before administration of the fluid from the secondary container is complete.

Preparation for administration:
1. Suspend container from eyelet support.
2. Remove plastic protector from outlet port at bottom of container.
3. Attach administration set. Refer to complete directions accompanying set.

How Supplied: Cefizox (sterile ceftizoxime sodium, FSK)—supplied in vials equivalent to 1 gram or 2 grams of ceftizoxime; in "Piggyback" Vials for I.V. admixture equivalent to 1 gram or 2 grams of ceftizoxime.

Note: Unreconstituted Cefizox (sterile ceftizoxime sodium, FSK) should be protected from excessive light, and stored at controlled room temperature (59°–86°F.) in the original package until used.
Cefizox (ceftizoxime sodium injection, FSK) as a frozen, sterile, nonpyrogenic solution in plastic containers—supplied in 50 ml. single-dose containers equivalent to 1 gram or 2 grams of ceftizoxime in 5% Dextrose (D5W). Do not store above −20°C.
'Cefizox' supplied as a frozen, sterile, nonpyrogenic solution in plastic containers is manufactured for Fujisawa SmithKline Corporation by Travenol Laboratories, Inc., Deerfield, IL 60015.

* Am. J. Clin. Pathol. 45:493, 1966; Federal Register 39:19182–19184, 1974.

CF:L12

COMBID® SPANSULE® CAPSULES ℞
[kom′bid]

Description: Each 'Combid' *Spansule* capsule contains 10 mg. of prochlorperazine, as the maleate, and isopropamide iodide equivalent to 5 mg. of isopropamide.
The prochlorperazine component is so prepared that an initial dose is released promptly and the remaining medication is released gradually over a prolonged period. The isopropamide iodide component is not in sustained release form because it can provide 10 to 12 hours of antisecretory-antispasmodic action.

Actions: A single 'Combid' *Spansule* capsule b.i.d. (every 12 hours) can provide the following actions: (1) reduction of gastric secretion, (2) inhibition of spasm and motility, (3) relief of anxiety and tension, and (4) control of nausea and vomiting.

Indications
Based on a review of this drug by the National Academy of Sciences—National Research Council and/or other information, FDA has classified the indications as follows:
Possibly effective: As adjunctive therapy in peptic ulcer and in the irritable bowel syndrome (irritable colon, spastic colon, mucous colitis, functional gastrointestinal disorders); functional diarrhea.
Final classification of the less-than-effective indications requires further investigation.

Contraindications: Known hypersensitivity to prochlorperazine maleate and/or isopropamide iodide, existing drug-induced C.N.S. depression, glaucoma, pyloric obstruction, prostatic hypertrophy, bladder neck obstruction, obstructive intestinal lesions and/or ileus, intestinal atony of the elderly or debilitated patient, unstable cardiovascular status in acute hemorrhage, severe ulcerative colitis, toxic megacolon complicating ulcerative colitis; myasthenia gravis, bone marrow depression, jaundice, hepatic disease, blood dyscrasias.
Children under 12 years of age.
Because of the antiemetic action of the prochlorperazine component, 'Combid' *Spansule* capsules should not be used where nausea and vomiting are believed to be a manifestation of intestinal obstruction or brain tumor.

Warnings: Use cautiously in patients with a past history of jaundice, hepatic abnormality or blood dyscrasias. Because of possible additive effects, caution patients about concomitant use of alcohol and other C.N.S. depressants. Also, caution patients about activities requiring alertness (e.g., operating vehicles or machinery).
In patients with ulcerative colitis, large doses of isopropamide iodide may suppress intestinal motility to the point of producing paralytic ileus, and the use of this drug may precipitate or aggravate the serious complication of toxic megacolon.
In the presence of a high environmental temperature, heat prostration (fever and heat stroke due to decreased sweating) can occur. In patients with diarrhea due to incomplete intestinal obstruction (especially those with ileostomy or colostomy), treatment with isopropamide iodide would be inappropriate and possibly harmful. With overdosage, a curare-like action, due to the isopropamide iodide component, may occur.

Usage in Pregnancy: Use of any drug in pregnancy, lactation, or in women who may bear children requires that the potential benefit of the drug be weighed against its possible hazards to the mother and child. As with all anticholinergic drugs, an inhibiting effect on lactation may occur.
Nursing Mothers: There is evidence that phenothiazines are excreted in breast milk.
Precautions: Patients who have shown a sensitivity reaction to other drugs may be more liable to have such a reaction to prochlorperazine.
Since the iodine in isopropamide iodide may alter PBI test results and will suppress I^{131} uptake, it is suggested that 'Combid' *Spansule* capsules be discontinued one week prior to these tests. Also, iodine skin rash may occur rarely.
Use with caution in elderly patients and patients with autonomic neuropathy, hepatic or renal disease, hyperthyroidism, coronary heart disease, congestive heart failure, cardiac arrhythmia, hypertension and nonobstructive prostatic hypertrophy. Anticholinergic drugs may aggravate gastroesophageal reflux. Investigate any tachycardia before giving anticholinergic (atropine-like) drugs, since they may increase the heart rate.
Neuroleptic drugs elevate prolactin levels; the elevation persists during chronic administration. Tissue culture experiments indicate that approximately one-third of human breast cancers are prolactin-dependent in vitro, a factor of potential importance if the prescribing of these drugs is contemplated in a patient with a previously detected breast cancer. Although disturbances such as galactorrhea, amenorrhea, gynecomastia, and impotence have been reported, the clinical significance of elevated serum prolactin levels is unknown for most patients. An increase in mammary neoplasms has been found in rodents after chronic administration of neuroleptic drugs. Neither clinical nor epidemiologic studies conducted to date, however, have shown an association between chronic administration of these drugs and mammary tumorigenesis; the available evidence is considered too limited to be conclusive at this time.
Drugs which lower the seizure threshold, including phenothiazine derivatives, should not be used with 'Amipaque'.* 'Combid' should be discontinued at least 48 hours before myelography, should not be resumed for at least 24 hours postprocedure, and should not be used for the control of nausea and vomiting occurring either prior to myelography or postprocedure.
Long-Term Therapy: Long-term therapy with neuroleptic agents, including prochlorperazine, has been reported to result in the appearance of tardive dyskinesia in some patients. To lessen the likelihood of this adverse reaction related to cumulative drug effect, patients in whom long-term 'Combid' therapy is indicated should be evaluated periodically to determine whether the dosage could be lowered or drug therapy discontinued.
Adverse Reactions:
Isopropamide Iodide: Xerostomia (dry mouth); urinary hesitancy and retention; tachycardia; palpitations; mydriasis (dilatation of the pupils); cycloplegia; blurred vision; constipation; bloated feeling; nausea; dysphagia; fever; nasal congestion.

Other adverse reactions possible with anticholinergics include: increased ocular tension; loss of taste; headaches; nervousness; drowsiness; weakness; dizziness; insomnia; vomiting; impotence; suppression of lactation; severe allergic reaction or drug idiosyncrasies, including anaphylaxis; urticaria and other dermal manifestations; some degree of mental confusion and/or excitement, especially in elderly persons. Decreased sweating may occur. It should be noted that adrenergic innervation of the eccrine sweat glands on the palms and soles makes complete control of sweating impossible. An end point of complete anhidrosis cannot occur because large drug doses would be required, and this would produce severe side effects from parasympathetic paralysis.

Prochlorperazine or Other Phenothiazine Derivatives: Adverse reactions with different phenothiazines vary in type, frequency, and mechanism of occurrence, i.e., some are dose-related, while others involve individual patient sensitivity. Some adverse reactions may be more likely to occur, or occur with greater intensity, in patients with special medical problems, e.g., patients with mitral insufficiency or pheochromocytoma have experienced severe hypotension following recommended doses of certain phenothiazines.

Not all of the following adverse reactions have been observed with every phenothiazine derivative, but they have been reported with one or more and should be borne in mind when drugs of this class are administered.

Extrapyramidal symptoms (opisthotonos, oculogyric crisis, hyperreflexia, dystonia, akathisia, dyskinesia, pseudo-parkinsonism) have been reported. (These symptoms usually subside several hours after 'Combid' is discontinued; if troublesome to the patient, mild sedation or injectable 'Benadryl'† may be useful.) As with all antipsychotic agents, persistent or tardive dyskinesia may appear after long-term therapy—especially in elderly female patients on high doses. Symptoms are persistent and in some patients irreversible. The syndrome is characterized by rhythmical involuntary movements of the tongue, face, mouth or jaw, sometimes accompanied by involuntary movements of extremities. Fine vermicular movements of the tongue may be an early sign; if these appear, discontinuation of medication is suggested.

Other adverse reactions include drowsiness; dizziness; grand mal convulsions; altered cerebrospinal fluid proteins; cerebral edema; intensification and prolongation of the action of central nervous system depressants (opiates, analgesics, antihistamines, barbiturates, alcohol), atropine, heat, organophosphorus insecticides; autonomic reactions (dryness of mouth, nasal congestion, headache, nausea, constipation, obstipation, adynamic ileus, inhibition of ejaculation, priapism); reactivation of psychotic processes, catatonic-like states; hypotension (sometimes fatal); cardiac arrest; blood dyscrasias (pancytopenia, thrombocytopenic purpura, leukopenia, agranulocytosis, eosinophilia); liver damage (jaundice, biliary stasis); endocrine disturbances (lactation, galactorrhea, gynecomastia, menstrual irregularities, false positive pregnancy tests); skin disorders (photosensitivity, itching, erythema, urticaria, eczema up to exfoliative dermatitis); other allergic reactions (asthma, laryngeal edema, angioneurotic edema, anaphylactoid reactions); peripheral edema; reversed epinephrine effect; hyperpyrexia; a systemic lupus erythematosus-like syndrome; pigmentary retinopathy; with prolonged administration of substantial doses, skin pigmentation, epithelial keratopathy, and lenticular and corneal deposits.

EKG changes—particularly nonspecific, usually reversible Q and T wave distortions—have been observed in some patients receiving phenothiazine tranquilizers. Their relationship to myocardial damage has not been confirmed.

Although phenothiazines cause neither psychic nor physical dependence, sudden discontinuance in long-term psychiatric patients may cause temporary symptoms, e.g., nausea and vomiting, dizziness, tremulousness.

Rare occurrences of neuroleptic malignant syndrome (NMS) have been reported in patients receiving neuroleptic drugs. This syndrome is comprised of the symptom complex of hyperthermia, altered consciousness, muscular rigidity and autonomic dysfunction and is potentially fatal.

Note: There have been occasional reports of sudden death in patients receiving phenothiazines. In some cases, the cause appeared to be asphyxia due to failure of the cough reflex. In others, the cause could not be determined. There is not sufficient evidence to establish a relationship between such deaths and the administration of phenothiazines.

Dosage and Administration: *Adults and children over 12*—One 'Combid' *Spansule* capsule b.i.d. (every 12 hours). Some patients may require only one capsule every 24 hours (on arising). Only the exceptional patient will require two capsules in the morning and two at night.

Overdosage: (See also Adverse Reactions)
Symptoms of 'Combid' overdosage may be those of either isopropamide iodide or prochlorperazine overdosage.

Isopropamide Iodide: *Symptoms*—May include dryness of mouth, dysphagia, thirst, blurred vision, dilated pupils, photophobia, fever, rapid pulse and respiration, disorientation. Depression and circulatory collapse may result from severe overdosage.

Treatment—Gastric lavage, repeated several times.

Respiratory depression should be promptly treated by the use of oxygen and stimulants. If marked excitement is present, one of the short-acting barbiturates, chloral hydrate, or gas anesthesia may be used. Otherwise do not administer sedation. Hyperpyrexia may be treated with physical cooling measures. Force fluids by mouth or, if necessary, by intravenous administration.

While pilocarpine or similar drugs are sometimes recommended for the relief of dry mouth, many authorities feel that these drugs are not indicated, since they relieve the minor peripheral effect but do not influence the more serious central effects and, thus, may merely mask signs of drug activity. If photophobia occurs, the patient should be kept in a darkened room.

It is not known whether isopropamide is dialyzable.

Prochlorperazine: *Symptoms*—Primarily involvement of the extrapyramidal mechanism producing some of the dystonic reactions described above. Symptoms of central nervous system depression to the point of somnolence or coma. Agitation and restlessness may also occur. Other possible manifestations include convulsions, fever, and autonomic reactions such as hypotension, dry mouth and ileus.

Treatment—Essentially symptomatic and supportive. Early gastric lavage is helpful. Keep patient under observation and maintain an open airway, since involvement of the extrapyramidal mechanism may produce dysphagia and respiratory difficulty in severe overdosage. **Do not attempt to induce emesis because a dystonic reaction of the head or neck may develop that could result in aspiration of vomitus.** Extrapyramidal symptoms may be treated with barbiturates or 'Benadryl'.

If administration of a stimulant is desirable, amphetamine, dextroamphetamine, or caffeine with sodium benzoate is recommended. Stimulants that may cause convulsions (e.g., picrotoxin or pentylenetetrazol) should be avoided.

If hypotension occurs, the standard measures for managing circulatory shock should be initiated. If it is desirable to administer a vasoconstrictor, 'Levophed' and 'Neo-Synephrine'‡ are most suitable. Other pressor agents, including epinephrine, are not recommended because phenothiazine derivatives may reverse the usual elevating action of these agents and cause a further lowering of blood pressure.

Limited experience indicates that phenothiazines are *not* dialyzable.

Special note on 'Spansule' capsules—Since much of the 'Spansule' capsule medication is coated for gradual release, therapy directed at reversing the effects of the ingested drugs and at supporting the patient should be continued for as long as overdosage symptoms remain. Saline cathartics are useful for hastening evacuation of pellets that have not already released medication.

How Supplied: In bottles of 50 and 500; in Single Unit Packages of 100 (intended for institutional use only).

Military—Capsules, 500's, 6505-00-935-9817
Veterans Administration—Capsules, 500's, 6505-00-935-9817A

*Trademark Reg. U.S. Pat. Off.: 'Amipaque' for metrizamide, Winthrop Laboratories.
†Trademark Reg. U.S. Pat. Off.: 'Benadryl' for diphenhydramine hydrochloride, Parke-Davis.
‡'Levophed' and 'Neo-Synephrine' are the trademarks (Reg. U.S. Pat. Off.) of Winthrop Laboratories for its brands of levarterenol and phenylephrine respectively.

Shown in Product Identification Section, page 436
CB:L34

COMPAZINE® ℞
[komp'ah-zeen]
(brand of prochlorperazine)

Description: Tablets—Each tablet contains 5 mg., 10 mg., or, for severe neuropsychiatric conditions, 25 mg. of prochlorperazine as the maleate.
Spansule® sustained release capsules—Each 'Spansule' capsule contains 10 mg., 15 mg. or 30 mg. of prochlorperazine as the maleate, so prepared that an initial dose is released promptly and the remaining medication is released gradually over a prolonged period. (In general, dosage recommendations for other oral forms of the drug may be applied to 'Spansule' capsules on the basis of the total daily dose in milligrams.)
Ampuls, 2 ml. (5 mg./ml.)—Each ml. contains, in aqueous solution, 5 mg. prochlorperazine as the edisylate, 1 mg. sodium sulfite, 1 mg. sodium bisulfite, 8 mg. sodium phosphate and 12 mg. sodium biphosphate.
Multiple-dose Vials, 10 ml. (5 mg./ml.)—Each ml. contains, in aqueous solution, 5 mg. prochlorperazine as the edisylate, 5 mg. sodium biphosphate, 12 mg. sodium tartrate, 0.9 mg. sodium saccharin, and 0.75% benzyl alcohol as preservative.
Disposable Syringes, 2 ml. (5 mg./ml.)—Each ml. contains, in aqueous solution, 5 mg. prochlorperazine as the edisylate, 5 mg. sodium biphosphate, 12 mg. sodium tartrate, 0.9 mg. sodium saccharin, and 0.75% benzyl alcohol as preservative.
Suppositories—Each suppository contains 2½ mg., 5 mg., or 25 mg. of prochlorperazine; with glycerin, glyceryl monopalmitate, glyceryl monostearate, hydrogenated cocoanut oil fatty acids and hydrogenated palm kernel oil fatty acids.
Syrup—Each 5 ml. (one teaspoonful) contains 5 mg. of prochlorperazine as the edisylate.
Indications: For control of severe nausea and vomiting.

For management of the manifestations of psychotic disorders.

Compazine (prochlorperazine, SK&F) is effective for the short-term treatment of generalized non-psychotic anxiety. However, 'Compazine' is not the first drug to be used in therapy for most patients with non-psychotic anxiety, because certain risks associated with its use are not shared by common alternative treatments (e.g., benzodiazepines).

When used in the treatment of non-psychotic anxiety, 'Compazine' should not be administered at doses of more than 20 mg. per day or for longer than 12 weeks, because the use of 'Compazine' at higher doses or for longer intervals may cause persistent tardive dyskinesia that may prove irreversible. (See Warnings section.)

The effectiveness of 'Compazine' as treatment for non-psychotic anxiety was established in four-week clinical studies of outpatients with generalized anxiety disorder. This evidence does not predict that 'Compazine' will be useful in patients with other non-psychotic conditions in which anxiety, or signs that mimic anxiety, are found (e.g.,

Continued on next page

Smith Kline & French—Cont.

physical illness, organic mental conditions, agitated depression, character pathologies, etc.).
'Compazine' has not been shown effective in the management of behavioral complications in patients with mental retardation.

Contraindications: In comatose or greatly depressed states due to central nervous system depressants; and in the presence of bone marrow depression.

Do not use in pediatric surgery.

Do not use in children under 2 years of age or under 20 lbs. Do not use in children for conditions for which dosage has not been established.

Warnings: The extrapyramidal symptoms which can occur secondary to Compazine (prochlorperazine, SK&F) may be confused with the central nervous system signs of an undiagnosed primary disease responsible for the vomiting, e.g., Reye's syndrome or other encephalopathy. The use of 'Compazine' and other potential hepatotoxins should be avoided in children and adolescents whose signs and symptoms suggest Reye's syndrome.

Patients who have demonstrated a hypersensitivity reaction (e.g., blood dyscrasias, jaundice) with a phenothiazine should not be reexposed to any phenothiazine, including 'Compazine', unless in the judgment of the physician the potential benefits of treatment outweigh the possible hazard.

'Compazine' may impair mental and/or physical abilities, especially during the first few days of therapy. Therefore, caution patients about activities requiring alertness (e.g., operating vehicles or machinery).

Phenothiazines may intensify or prolong the action of central nervous system depressants (e.g., alcohol, anesthetics, narcotics).

Persistent Tardive Dyskinesia: Persistent tardive dyskinesia may appear in some patients on long-term therapy with antipsychotic agents or may appear after drug therapy has been discontinued. In some patients the symptoms appear to be irreversible. There is no known effective treatment for tardive dyskinesia. It is suggested that all antipsychotic agents be discontinued if symptoms of this syndrome appear. (See Adverse Reactions section.)

Usage in Pregnancy: Safety for the use of 'Compazine' during pregnancy has not been established. Therefore, 'Compazine' is not recommended for use in pregnant patients except in cases of severe nausea and vomiting that are so serious and intractable that, in the judgment of the physician, drug intervention is required and potential benefits outweigh possible hazards.

Nursing Mothers: There is evidence that phenothiazines are excreted in the breast milk of nursing mothers.

Precautions: The antiemetic action of 'Compazine' may mask the signs and symptoms of overdosage of other drugs and may obscure the diagnosis and treatment of other conditions such as intestinal obstruction, brain tumor and Reye's syndrome (See Warnings).

'Compazine' should be used cautiously with cancer chemotherapy drugs that cause vomiting at toxic levels because vomiting, as a sign of toxicity, may be obscured.

Because hypotension may occur, large doses and parenteral administration should be used cautiously in patients with impaired cardiovascular systems. To minimize the occurrence of hypotension after initial injection, keep patient lying down and observe for at least ½ hour. If hypotension occurs after parenteral or oral dosing, place patient in head-low position with legs raised. If a vasoconstrictor is required, 'Levophed' and 'Neo-Synephrine'* are suitable. Other pressor agents, including epinephrine, should not be used because they may cause a paradoxical further lowering of blood pressure.

Aspiration of vomitus has occurred in a few postsurgical patients who have received 'Compazine' as an antiemetic. Although no causal relationship has been established, this possibility should be borne in mind during surgical aftercare.

Deep sleep, from which patients can be aroused, and coma have been reported, usually with overdosage.

Neuroleptic drugs elevate prolactin levels; the elevation persists during chronic administration. Tissue culture experiments indicate that approximately one-third of human breast cancers are prolactin-dependent *in vitro*, a factor of potential importance if the prescribing of these drugs is contemplated in a patient with a previously detected breast cancer. Although disturbances such as galactorrhea, amenorrhea, gynecomastia and impotence have been reported, the clinical significance of elevated serum prolactin levels is unknown for most patients. An increase in mammary neoplasms has been found in rodents after chronic administration of neuroleptic drugs. Neither clinical nor epidemiologic studies conducted to date, however, have shown an association between chronic administration of these drugs and mammary tumorigenesis; the available evidence is considered too limited to be conclusive at this time.

As with all drugs which exert an anticholinergic effect, and/or cause mydriasis, prochlorperazine should be used with caution in patients with glaucoma.

Phenothiazines can diminish the effect of oral anticoagulants.

Phenothiazines can produce alpha-adrenergic blockade.

Concomitant administration of propranolol with phenothiazines results in increased plasma levels of both drugs.

Phenothiazines may lower the convulsive threshold; dosage adjustments of anticonvulsants may be necessary. Potentiation of anticonvulsant effects does not occur. However, it has been reported that phenothiazines may interfere with the metabolism of 'Dilantin'† and thus precipitate 'Dilantin' toxicity.

Long-Term Therapy: To lessen the likelihood of adverse reactions related to cumulative drug effect, patients with a history of long-term therapy with Compazine (prochlorperazine, SK&F) and/or other neuroleptics should be evaluated periodically to decide whether the maintenance dosage could be lowered or drug therapy discontinued.

Children with acute illnesses (e.g., chickenpox, C.N.S. infections, measles, gastroenteritis) or dehydration seem to be much more susceptible to neuromuscular reactions, particularly dystonias, than are adults. In such patients, the drug should be used only under close supervision.

'Compazine' *Spansule* capsules and tablets have been reformulated to remove FD&C Yellow #5 (tartrazine). However, until the transition process is complete, some lots of 'Compazine' *Spansule* capsules and tablets containing FD&C Yellow #5 (tartrazine) will still be in stock. FD&C Yellow #5 (tartrazine) may cause allergic-type reactions (including bronchial asthma) in certain susceptible individuals. Although the overall incidence of FD&C Yellow #5 (tartrazine) sensitivity in the general population is low, it is frequently seen in patients who also have aspirin sensitivity.

For specific information, contact Smith Kline &French Laboratories (outside Pa., call toll-free: 1-800-523-4835, ext. 4262; in Pa., call collect: 215-751-4262).

Drugs which lower the seizure threshold, including phenothiazine derivatives, should not be used with 'Amipaque'.†† As with other phenothiazine derivatives, 'Compazine' should be discontinued at least 48 hours before myelography, should not be resumed for at least 24 hours postprocedure, and should not be used for the control of nausea and vomiting occurring either prior to myelography or postprocedure.

Adverse Reactions: Drowsiness, dizziness, amenorrhea, blurred vision, skin reactions and hypotension may occur.

Cholestatic jaundice has occurred. If fever with grippe-like symptoms occurs, appropriate liver studies should be conducted. If tests indicate an abnormality, stop treatment. There have been a few observations of fatty changes in the livers of patients who have died while receiving the drug. No causal relationship has been established.

Leukopenia and agranulocytosis have occurred. Warn patients to report the sudden appearance of sore throat or other signs of infection. If white blood cell and differential counts indicate leukocyte depression, stop treatment and start antibiotic and other suitable therapy.

Neuromuscular (Extrapyramidal) Reactions
These symptoms are seen in a significant number of hospitalized mental patients. They may be characterized by motor restlessness, be of the dystonic type, or they may resemble parkinsonism.

Depending on the severity of symptoms, dosage should be reduced or discontinued. If therapy is reinstituted, it should be at a lower dosage. Should these symptoms occur in children or pregnant patients, the drug should be stopped and not reinstituted. In most cases barbiturates by suitable route of administration will suffice. (Or, injectable 'Benadryl'§ may be useful.) In more severe cases, the administration of an anti-parkinsonism agent, except levodopa, usually produces rapid reversal of symptoms. Suitable supportive measures such as maintaining a clear airway and adequate hydration should be employed.

Motor Restlessness: Symptoms may include agitation or jitteriness and sometimes insomnia. These symptoms often disappear spontaneously. At times these symptoms may be similar to the original neurotic or psychotic symptoms. Dosage should not be increased until these side effects have subsided.

If this phase becomes too troublesome, the symptoms can usually be controlled by a reduction of dosage or concomitant administration of a barbiturate.

Dystonias: Symptoms may include: spasm of the neck muscles, sometimes progressing to torticollis; extensor rigidity of back muscles, sometimes progressing to opisthotonos; carpopedal spasm, trismus, swallowing difficulty, oculogyric crisis and protrusion of the tongue.

These usually subside within a few hours, and almost always within 24 to 48 hours, after the drug has been discontinued.

In mild cases, reassurance or a barbiturate is often sufficient. *In moderate cases,* barbiturates will usually bring rapid relief. *In more severe adult cases,* the administration of an anti-parkinsonism agent, except levodopa, usually produces rapid reversal of symptoms. *In children,* reassurance and barbiturates will usually control symptoms. (Or, injectable 'Benadryl' may be useful. Note: See 'Benadryl' prescribing information for appropriate *children's* dosage.) If appropriate treatment with anti-parkinsonism agents or 'Benadryl' fails to reverse the signs and symptoms, the diagnosis should be reevaluated.

Pseudo-parkinsonism: Symptoms may include: mask-like facies; drooling; tremors; pillrolling motion; cogwheel rigidity; and shuffling gait. Reassurance and sedation are important. In most cases these symptoms are readily controlled when an anti-parkinsonism agent is administered concomitantly. Anti-parkinsonism agents should be used only when required. Generally, therapy of a few weeks to two or three months will suffice. After this time patients should be evaluated to determine their need for continued treatment. (Note: Levodopa has not been found effective in pseudo-parkinsonism.) Occasionally it is necessary to lower the dosage of 'Compazine' or to discontinue the drug.

Persistent Tardive Dyskinesia: As with all antipsychotic agents, tardive dyskinesia may appear in some patients on long-term therapy or may appear after drug therapy has been discontinued. This condition appears in all age groups. However, the risk appears to be greater in elderly patients on high-dose therapy, especially females. The symptoms are persistent and in some patients appear to be irreversible. The syndrome is characterized by rhythmical involuntary movements of the tongue, face, mouth or jaw (e.g., protrusion of tongue, puffing of cheeks, puckering of mouth, chewing movements). Sometimes these may be accompanied by involuntary movements of extremities. In rare instances, these involuntary movements of the extremities are the only manifestations of tardive dyskinesia.

There is no known effective treatment for tardive dyskinesia; anti-parkinsonism agents do not alleviate the symptoms of this syndrome. It is suggested that all antipsychotic agents be discontinued if these symptoms appear. Should it be necessary to reinstitute treatment, or increase the dosage of the agent, or switch to a different antipsychotic agent, the syndrome may be masked.

It has been reported that fine vermicular movements of the tongue may be an early sign of the syndrome and if the medication is stopped at that time the syndrome may not develop.

Contact Dermatitis: Avoid getting the Injection solution on hands or clothing because of the possibility of contact dermatitis.

Adverse Reactions Reported with Compazine (prochlorperazine, SK&F) or Other Phenothiazine Derivatives: Adverse reactions with different phenothiazines vary in type, frequency, and mechanism of occurrence, i.e., some are dose-related, while others involve individual patient sensitivity. Some adverse reactions may be more likely to occur, or occur with greater intensity, in patients with special medical problems, e.g., patients with mitral insufficiency or pheochromocytoma have experienced severe hypotension following recommended doses of certain phenothiazines.

Not all of the following adverse reactions have been observed with every phenothiazine derivative, but they have been reported with one or more and should be borne in mind when drugs of this class are administered: extrapyramidal symptoms (opisthotonos, oculogyric crisis, hyperreflexia, dystonia, akathisia, dyskinesia, parkinsonism) some of which have lasted months and even years—particularly in elderly patients with previous brain damage; grand mal and petit mal convulsions; altered cerebrospinal fluid proteins; cerebral edema; intensification and prolongation of the action of central nervous system depressants (opiates, analgesics, antihistamines, barbiturates, alcohol), atropine, heat, organophosphorus insecticides; autonomic reactions (dryness of mouth, nasal congestion, headache, nausea, constipation, obstipation, adynamic ileus, inhibition of ejaculation, priapism); reactivation of psychotic processes, catatonic-like states; hypotension (sometimes fatal); cardiac arrest; blood dyscrasias (pancytopenia, thrombocytopenic purpura, leukopenia, agranulocytosis, eosinophilia, hemolytic anemia, aplastic anemia); liver damage (jaundice, biliary stasis); endocrine disturbances (lactation, galactorrhea, gynecomastia, menstrual irregularities, false positive pregnancy tests); skin disorders (photosensitivity, itching, erythema, urticaria, eczema up to exfoliative dermatitis); other allergic reactions (asthma, laryngeal edema, angioneurotic edema, anaphylactoid reactions); peripheral edema; reversed epinephrine effect; hyperpyrexia; mild fever after large I.M. doses; increased appetite; increased weight; a systemic lupus erythematosus-like syndrome; pigmentary retinopathy; with prolonged administration of substantial doses, skin pigmentation, epithelial keratopathy, and lenticular and corneal deposits.

EKG changes—particularly nonspecific, usually reversible Q and T wave distortions—have been observed in some patients receiving phenothiazine tranquilizers. Their relationship to myocardial damage has not been confirmed.

Although phenothiazines cause neither psychic nor physical dependence, sudden discontinuance in long-term psychiatric patients may cause temporary symptoms, e.g., nausea and vomiting, dizziness, tremulousness.

Rare occurrences of neuroleptic malignant syndrome have been reported in patients receiving neuroleptic drugs. This syndrome is comprised of the symptom complex of hyperthermia, altered consciousness, muscular rigidity and autonomic dysfunction and is potentially fatal.

Note: There have been occasional reports of sudden death in patients receiving phenothiazines. In some cases, the cause appeared to be asphyxia due to failure of the cough reflex. In others, the cause could not be determined. There is not sufficient evidence to establish a relationship between such deaths and the administration of phenothiazines.

Dosage and Administration: Notes on Injection: *Stability*—This solution should be protected from light. Slight yellowish discoloration will not alter potency. If markedly discolored, solution should be discarded.

Compatibility—It is recommended that Compazine (prochlorperazine, SK&F) Injection not be mixed with other agents in the syringe. Do not dilute the contents of 'Compazine' ampuls with any diluent that contains parabens as a preservative.

Dosage and Administration—Adults:
(For children's dosage and administration, see below.) Dosage should be increased more gradually in debilitated or emaciated patients.

Elderly Patients: In general, dosages in the lower range are sufficient for most elderly patients. Since they appear to be more susceptible to hypotension and neuromuscular reactions, such patients should be observed closely. Dosage should be tailored to the individual, response carefully monitored, and dosage adjusted accordingly. Dosage should be increased more gradually in elderly patients.

1. **To Control Severe Nausea and Vomiting:** Adjust dosage to the response of the individual. Begin with the lowest recommended dosage.

Oral Dosage: Usually 5 or 10 mg. 3 or 4 times daily; by 'Spansule' capsule, usually one 15 mg. capsule on arising or one 10 mg. capsule q12h.

Rectal Dosage: 25 mg. twice daily.

I.M. Dosage: Initially 5 to 10 mg. (1–2 ml.) injected *deeply* into the upper outer quadrant of the buttock. If necessary, repeat every 3 or 4 hours. Total I.M. dosage should not exceed 40 mg. per day.

Subcutaneous administration is not advisable because of local irritation.

2. **Adult Surgery (for severe nausea and vomiting):** Total parenteral dosage should not exceed 40 mg. per day. Hypotension is a possibility if the drug is given by I.V. injection or infusion.

I.M. Dosage: 5 to 10 mg. (1–2 ml.) 1 to 2 hours before induction of anesthesia (repeat once in 30 minutes, if necessary), or to control acute symptoms during and after surgery (repeat once if necessary).

I.V. Injection: 5 to 10 mg. (1–2 ml.) 15 to 30 minutes before induction of anesthesia, or to control acute symptoms during or after surgery. Repeat once if necessary. 'Compazine' may be administered either undiluted or diluted in isotonic solution, but a single dose of the drug should not exceed 10 mg. The rate of administration should not exceed 5 mg./ml./min. When administered I.V., do not use bolus injection.

I.V. Infusion: 20 mg. (4 ml.) per liter of isotonic solution. Do not dilute in less than one liter of isotonic solution. Add to I.V. infusion 15 to 30 minutes before induction.

3. **In Adult Psychiatric Disorders:** Adjust dosage to the response of the individual and according to the severity of the condition. Begin with the lowest recommended dose. Although response ordinarily is seen within a day or two, longer treatment is usually required before maximal improvement is seen.

Oral Dosage: *Non-Psychotic Anxiety*—Usual dosage is 5 mg. 3 or 4 times daily: by 'Spansule' capsule, usually one 15 mg. capsule on arising or one 10 mg. capsule q12h. Do not administer in doses of more than 20 mg. per day or for longer than 12 weeks.

Psychotic Disorders—In relatively mild conditions, as seen in private psychiatric practice or in outpatient clinics, dosage is 5 or 10 mg. 3 or 4 times daily.

In moderate to severe conditions, for hospitalized or adequately supervised patients, usual starting dosage is 10 mg. 3 or 4 times daily. Increase dosage gradually until symptoms are controlled or side effects become bothersome. When dosage is increased by small increments every 2 or 3 days, side effects either do not occur or are easily controlled. Some patients respond satisfactorily on 50 to 75 mg. daily.

In more severe disturbances, optimum dosage is usually 100 to 150 mg. daily.

I.M. Dosage: For immediate control of severely disturbed adults, inject an initial dose of 10 to 20 mg. (2–4 ml.) *deeply* into the upper outer quadrant of the buttock. Many patients respond shortly after the first injection. If necessary, however, repeat the initial dose every 2 to 4 hours (or, in resistant cases, every hour) to gain control of the patient. More than 3 or 4 doses are seldom necessary. After control is achieved, switch patient to an oral form of the drug at the same dosage level or higher. If, in rare cases, parenteral therapy is needed for a prolonged period, give 10 to 20 mg. (2–4 ml.) every 4 to 6 hours. Pain and irritation at the site of injection have seldom occurred.

Subcutaneous administration is not advisable because of local irritation.

Dosage and Administration—Children:
Do not use in pediatric surgery.

Children seem more prone to develop extrapyramidal reactions, even on moderate doses. Therefore, use lowest effective dosage. Tell parents not to exceed prescribed dosage, since the possibility of adverse reactions increases as dosage rises.

Occasionally the patient may react to the drug with signs of restlessness and excitement; if this occurs, do not administer additional doses. Take particular precaution in administering the drug to children with acute illnesses or dehydration (see under Dystonias).

When writing a prescription for the $2\frac{1}{2}$ mg. size suppository, write "$2\frac{1}{2}$," not "2.5"; this will help avoid confusion with the 25 mg. adult size.

1. **Severe Nausea and Vomiting in Children:** Compazine (prochlorperazine, SK&F) should not be used in children under 20 pounds in weight or two years of age. It should not be used in conditions for which children's dosages have not been established. Dosage and frequency of administration should be adjusted according to the severity of the symptoms and the response of the patient. The duration of activity following intramuscular administration may last up to 12 hours. Subsequent doses may be given by the same route if necessary.

Oral or Rectal Dosage: More than one day's therapy is seldom necessary.

Weight	Usual Dosage	Not to Exceed
under 20 lbs.	not recommended	
20–29 lbs.	$2\frac{1}{2}$ mg. 1 or 2 times a day	7.5 mg. per day
30–39 lbs.	$2\frac{1}{2}$ mg. 2 or 3 times a day	10 mg. per day
40–85 lbs.	$2\frac{1}{2}$ mg. 3 times a day or 5 mg. 2 times a day	15 mg. per day

I.M. Dosage: Calculate each dose on the basis of 0.06 mg. of the drug per lb. of body weight; give by deep I.M. injection. Control is usually obtained with one dose.

2. **In Psychotic Children:**

Oral or Rectal Dosage: For children 2 to 12 years, starting dosage is $2\frac{1}{2}$ mg. 2 or 3 times daily. Do not give more than 10 mg. the first day. Then increase dosage according to patient's response.

FOR AGES 2–5, total daily dosage usually does not exceed 20 mg.

FOR AGES 6–12, total daily dosage usually does not exceed 25 mg.

I.M. Dosage: For ages under 12, calculate each dose on the basis of 0.06 mg. of Compazine (prochlorperazine, SK&F) per lb. of body weight; give by deep I.M. injection. Control is usually obtained with one dose. After control is achieved, switch the patient to an oral form of the drug at the same dosage level or higher.

Continued on next page

Smith Kline & French—Cont.

Overdosage: (See also Adverse Reactions.)
Symptoms—Primarily involvement of the extrapyramidal mechanism producing some of the dystonic reactions described above.
Symptoms of central nervous system depression to the point of somnolence or coma. Agitation and restlessness may also occur. Other possible manifestations include convulsions, EKG changes and cardiac arrhythmias, fever, and autonomic reactions such as hypotension, dry mouth and ileus.
Treatment—It is important to determine other medications taken by the patient since multiple dose therapy is common in overdosage situations. Treatment is essentially symptomatic and supportive. Early gastric lavage is helpful. Keep patient under observation and maintain an open airway, since involvement of the extrapyramidal mechanism may produce dysphagia and respiratory difficulty in severe overdosage. **Do not attempt to induce emesis because a dystonic reaction of the head or neck may develop that could result in aspiration of vomitus.** Extrapyramidal symptoms may be treated with anti-parkinsonism drugs, barbiturates, or 'Benadryl'. See prescribing information for these products. Care should be taken to avoid increasing respiratory depression.
If administration of a stimulant is desirable, amphetamine, dextroamphetamine, or caffeine with sodium benzoate is recommended. Stimulants that may cause convulsions (e.g., picrotoxin or pentylenetetrazol) should be avoided.
If hypotension occurs, the standard measures for managing circulatory shock should be initiated. If it is desirable to administer a vasoconstrictor, 'Levophed' and 'Neo-Synephrine' are most suitable. Other pressor agents, including epinephrine, are not recommended because phenothiazine derivatives may reverse the usual elevating action of these agents and cause a further lowering of blood pressure.
Limited experience indicates that phenothiazines are *not* dialyzable.
Special note on 'Spansule' capsules—Since much of the 'Spansule' capsule medication is coated for gradual release, therapy directed at reversing the effects of the ingested drug and at supporting the patient should be continued for as long as overdosage symptoms remain. Saline cathartics are useful for hastening evacuation of pellets that have not already released medication.
How Supplied:
Tablets—5 and 10 mg., in bottles of 100 and 1000; in Single Unit Packages of 100 (intended for institutional use only). For use in severe neuropsychiatric conditions, 25 mg., in bottles of 100 and 1000.
'Spansule' capsules—10, 15 and 30 mg., in bottles of 50 and 500; in Single Unit Packages of 100 (intended for institutional use only).
Ampuls—2 ml. (5 mg./ml.), in boxes of 10, 100 and 500.
Multiple-dose Vials—10 ml. (5 mg./ml.), in boxes of 1, 20 and 100.
Disposable Syringes—2 ml. (5 mg./ml.), individually packaged in boxes of 10 and 100.
Suppositories—2½ mg. (for young children), 5 mg. (for older children) and 25 mg. (for adults), in boxes of 12.
Syrup—5 mg./5 ml. (1 teaspoonful) in 4 fl. oz. bottles.
Veterans Administration—Injection, 10 ml., 100's, 6505-00-684-9630A; 'Spansule' Capsules, 15 mg., 500's, 6505-00-014-1188.
Military—Injection, 2 ml., 100's, 6505-00-656-1610; Suppositories, 2½ mg., 12's, 6505-00-133-5213; 25 mg., 12's, 6505-00-133-5214; Tablets, 5 mg., 1000's, 6505-00-022-1328, and S.U.P. 100's 6505-00-118-2563; 10 mg., 1000's, 6505-00-022-1329.

---

*'Levophed' and 'Neo-Synephrine' are the trademarks (Reg. U.S. Pat. Off.) of Winthrop Laboratories for its brands of levarterenol and phenylephrine respectively.
†Trademark Reg. U.S. Pat. Off.: 'Dilantin' for diphenylhydantoin, Parke-Davis.
††Trademark Reg. U.S. Pat. Off.: 'Amipaque' for metrizamide, Winthrop Laboratories.
§Trademark Reg. U.S. Pat. Off.: 'Benadryl' for diphenhydramine hydrochloride, Parke-Davis.
Shown in Product Identification Section, page 436
CZ:L62

CYTOMEL® ℞
[*sigh" toe' mel*]
**brand of liothyronine sodium
Tablets**

Description: Thyroid hormone drugs are natural or synthetic preparations containing tetraiodothyronine (T_4, levothyroxine) sodium or triiodothyronine (T_3, liothyronine) sodium or both. T_4 and T_3 are produced in the human thyroid gland by the iodination and coupling of the amino acid tyrosine. T_4 contains four iodine atoms and is formed by the coupling of two molecules of diiodotyrosine (DIT). T_3 contains three atoms of iodine and is formed by the coupling of one molecule of DIT with one molecule of monoiodotyrosine (MIT). Both hormones are stored in the thyroid colloid as thyroglobulin.
Thyroid hormone preparations belong to two categories: (1) natural hormonal preparations derived from animal thyroid, and (2) synthetic preparations. Natural preparations include desiccated thyroid and thyroglobulin. Desiccated thyroid is derived from domesticated animals that are used for food by man (either beef or hog thyroid), and thyroglobulin is derived from thyroid glands of the hog. The United States Pharmacopeia (USP) has standardized the total iodine content of natural preparations. Thyroid USP contains not less than (NLT) 0.17 percent and not more than (NMT) 0.23 percent iodine, and thyroglobulin contains not less than (NLT) 0.7 percent of organically bound iodine. Iodine content is only an indirect indicator of true hormonal biologic activity.
Cytomel (liothyronine sodium, SK&F) Tablets contain liothyronine (L-triiodothyronine or LT_3), a synthetic form of a natural thyroid hormone, and is available as the sodium salt.
Twenty-five mcg. of liothyronine is equivalent to approximately 1 grain of desiccated thyroid or thyroglobulin and 0.1 mg. of L-thyroxine.
Cytomel (liothyronine sodium, SK&F) is supplied in tablets for oral administration, containing liothyronine sodium equivalent to 5, 25 or 50 mcg. of liothyronine.
Clinical Pharmacology: The mechanisms by which thyroid hormones exert their physiologic action are not well understood. These hormones enhance oxygen consumption by most tissues of the body, increase the basal metabolic rate and the metabolism of carbohydrates, lipids and proteins. Thus, they exert a profound influence on every organ system in the body and are of particular importance in the development of the central nervous system.
Pharmacokinetics
Since liothyronine sodium (T_3) is not firmly bound to serum protein, it is readily available to body tissues. The onset of activity of liothyronine sodium is rapid, occurring within a few hours. Maximum pharmacologic response occurs within two or three days, providing early clinical response. The biological half-life is about 2-½ days.
T_3 is almost totally absorbed, 95 percent in four hours. The hormones contained in the natural preparations are absorbed in a manner similar to the synthetic hormones.
Liothyronine sodium has a rapid cutoff of activity which permits quick dosage adjustment and facilitates control of the effects of overdosage, should they occur.
The higher affinity of levothyroxine (T_4) for both thyroid-binding globulin and thyroid-binding prealbumin as compared to triiodothyronine (T_3) partially explains the higher serum levels and longer half-life of the former hormone. Both protein-bound hormones exist in reverse equilibrium with minute amounts of free hormone, the latter accounting for the metabolic activity.
Indications and Usage: Thyroid hormone drugs are indicated:

1. As replacement or supplemental therapy in patients with hypothyroidism of any etiology, except transient hypothyroidism during the recovery phase of subacute thyroiditis. This category includes cretinism, myxedema and ordinary hypothyroidism in patients of any age (children, adults, the elderly), or state (including pregnancy); primary hypothyroidism resulting from functional deficiency, primary atrophy, partial or total absence of thyroid gland, or the effects of surgery, radiation, or drugs, with or without the presence of goiter; and secondary (pituitary) or tertiary (hypothalamic) hypothyroidism (See WARNINGS).
2. As pituitary thyroid-stimulating hormone (TSH) suppressants, in the treatment or prevention of various types of euthyroid goiters, including thyroid nodules, subacute or chronic lymphocytic thyroiditis (Hashimoto's) and multinodular goiter.
3. As diagnostic agents in suppression tests to differentiate suspected mild hyperthyroidism or thyroid gland autonomy.

Cytomel (liothyronine sodium, SK&F) Tablets can be used in patients allergic to desiccated thyroid or thyroid extract derived from pork or beef.
Contraindications: Thyroid hormone preparations are generally contraindicated in patients with diagnosed but as yet uncorrected adrenal cortical insufficiency, untreated thyrotoxicosis and apparent hypersensitivity to any of their active or extraneous constituents. There is no well-documented evidence from the literature, however, of true allergic or idiosyncratic reactions to thyroid hormone.
Warnings:

> Drugs with thyroid hormone activity, alone or together with other therapeutic agents, have been used for the treatment of obesity. In euthyroid patients, doses within the range of daily hormonal requirements are ineffective for weight reduction. Larger doses may produce serious or even life-threatening manifestations of toxicity, particularly when given in association with sympathomimetic amines such as those used for their anorectic effects.

The use of thyroid hormones in the therapy of obesity, alone or combined with other drugs, is unjustified and has been shown to be ineffective. Neither is their use justified for the treatment of male or female infertility unless this condition is accompanied by hypothyroidism.
Thyroid hormones should be used with great caution in a number of circumstances where the integrity of the cardiovascular system, particularly the coronary arteries, is suspected. These include patients with angina pectoris or the elderly, in whom there is a greater likelihood of occult cardiac disease. In these patients, liothyronine sodium therapy should be initiated with low doses, with due consideration for its relatively rapid onset of action. Starting dosage of Cytomel (liothyronine sodium, SK&F) Tablets is 5 mcg. daily, and should be increased by no more than 5 mcg. increments at two-week intervals. When, in such patients, a euthyroid state can only be reached at the expense of an aggravation of the cardiovascular disease, thyroid hormone dosage should be reduced.
Morphologic hypogonadism and nephrosis should be ruled out before the drug is administered. If hypopituitarism is present, the adrenal deficiency must be corrected prior to starting the drug.
Myxedematous patients are very sensitive to thyroid; dosage should be started at a very low level and increased gradually.
Severe and prolonged hypothyroidism can lead to a decreased level of adrenocortical activity commensurate with the lowered metabolic state. When thyroid-replacement therapy is administered, the metabolism increases at a greater rate than adrenocortical activity. This can precipitate adrenocortical insufficiency. Therefore, in severe and prolonged hypothyroidism, supplemental adrenocortical steroids may be necessary.

In rare instances the administration of thyroid hormone may precipitate a hyperthyroid state or may aggravate existing hyperthyroidism.

Precautions:

General—Thyroid hormone therapy in patients with concomitant diabetes mellitus or insipidus or adrenal cortical insufficiency aggravates the intensity of their symptoms. Appropriate adjustments of the various therapeutic measures directed at these concomitant endocrine diseases are required.

The therapy of myxedema coma requires simultaneous administration of glucocorticoids.

Hypothyroidism decreases and hyperthyroidism increases the sensitivity to oral anticoagulants. Prothrombin time should be closely monitored in thyroid-treated patients on oral anticoagulants and dosage of the latter agents adjusted on the basis of frequent prothrombin time determinations. In infants, excessive doses of thyroid hormone preparations may produce craniosynostosis.

Information for the Patient—Patients on thyroid hormone preparations and parents of children on thyroid therapy should be informed that:

1. Replacement therapy is to be taken essentially for life, with the exception of cases of transient hypothyroidism, usually associated with thyroiditis, and in those patients receiving a therapeutic trial of the drug.
2. They should immediately report during the course of therapy any signs or symptoms of thyroid hormone toxicity, e.g., chest pain, increased pulse rate, palpitations, excessive sweating, heat intolerance, nervousness, or any other unusual event.
3. In case of concomitant diabetes mellitus, the daily dosage of antidiabetic medication may need readjustment as thyroid hormone replacement is achieved. If thyroid medication is stopped, a downward readjustment of the dosage of insulin or oral hypoglycemic agent may be necessary to avoid hypoglycemia. At all times, close monitoring of urinary glucose levels is mandatory in such patients.
4. In case of concomitant oral anticoagulant therapy, the prothrombin time should be measured frequently to determine if the dosage of oral anticoagulants is to be readjusted.
5. Partial loss of hair may be experienced by children in the first few months of thyroid therapy, but this is usually a transient phenomenon and later recovery is usually the rule.

Laboratory Tests—Treatment of patients with thyroid hormones requires the periodic assessment of thyroid status by means of appropriate laboratory tests besides the full clinical evaluation. The TSH suppression test can be used to test the effectiveness of any thyroid preparation, bearing in mind the relative insensitivity of the infant pituitary to the negative feedback effect of thyroid hormones. Serum T_4 levels can be used to test the effectiveness of all thyroid medications except products containing liothyronine sodium. When the total serum T_4 is low but TSH is normal, a test specific to assess unbound (free) T_4 levels is warranted. Specific measurements of T_4 and T_3 by competitive protein binding or radioimmunoassay are not influenced by blood levels of organic or inorganic iodine and have essentially replaced older tests of thyroid hormone measurements, i.e., PBI, BEI and T_4 by column.

Drug Interactions

Oral Anticoagulants—Thyroid hormones appear to increase catabolism of vitamin K-dependent clotting factors. If oral anticoagulants are also being given, compensatory increases in clotting factor synthesis are impaired. Patients stabilized on oral anticoagulants who are found to require thyroid replacement therapy should be watched very closely when thyroid is started. If a patient is truly hypothyroid, it is likely that a reduction in anticoagulant dosage will be required. No special precautions appear to be necessary when oral anticoagulant therapy is begun in a patient already stabilized on maintenance thyroid replacement therapy.

Insulin or Oral Hypoglycemics—Initiating thyroid replacement therapy may cause increases in insulin or oral hypoglycemic requirements. The effects seen are poorly understood and depend upon a variety of factors such as dose and type of thyroid preparations and endocrine status of the patient. Patients receiving insulin or oral hypoglycemics should be closely watched during initiation of thyroid replacement therapy.

Cholestyramine—Cholestyramine binds both T_4 and T_3 in the intestine, thus impairing absorption of these thyroid hormones. *In vitro* studies indicate that the binding is not easily removed. Therefore, four to five hours should elapse between administration of cholestyramine and thyroid hormones.

Estrogen, Oral Contraceptives—Estrogens tend to increase serum thyroxine-binding globulin (TBg). In a patient with a nonfunctioning thyroid gland who is receiving thyroid replacement therapy, free levothyroxine may be decreased when estrogens are started thus increasing thyroid requirements. However, if the patient's thyroid gland has sufficient function, the decreased free thyroxine will result in a compensatory increase in thyroxine output by the thyroid. Therefore, patients without a functioning thyroid gland who are on thyroid replacement therapy may need to increase their thyroid dose if estrogens or estrogen-containing oral contraceptives are given.

Tricyclic Antidepressants—Use of thyroid products with imipramine and other tricyclic antidepressants may increase receptor sensitivity and enhance antidepressant activity; transient cardiac arrhythmias have been observed. Thyroid hormone activity may also be enhanced.

Digitalis—Thyroid preparations may potentiate the toxic effects of digitalis. Thyroid hormonal replacement increases metabolic rate, which requires an increase in digitalis dosage.

Ketamine—When administered to patients on a thyroid preparation, this parenteral anesthetic may cause hypertension and tachycardia. Use with caution and be prepared to treat hypertension, if necessary.

Levarterenol—Thyroxine increases the adrenergic effect of catecholamines such as epinephrine and norepinephrine. Therefore, injection of these agents into patients receiving thyroid preparations increases the risk of precipitating coronary insufficiency, especially in patients with coronary artery disease. Careful observation is required.

Drug/Laboratory Test Interactions—The following drugs or moieties are known to interfere with laboratory tests performed in patients on thyroid hormone therapy: androgens, corticosteroids, estrogens, oral contraceptives containing estrogens, iodine-containing preparations and the numerous preparations containing salicylates.

1. Changes in TBg concentration should be taken into consideration in the interpretation of T_4 and T_3 values. In such cases, the unbound (free) hormone should be measured. Pregnancy, estrogens and estrogen-containing oral contraceptives increase TBg concentrations. TBg may also be increased during infectious hepatitis. Decreases in TBg concentrations are observed in nephrosis, acromegaly and after androgen or corticosteroid therapy. Familial hyper- or hypo-thyroxine-binding-globulinemias have been described. The incidence of TBg deficiency approximates 1 in 9000. The binding of thyroxine by thyroxine-binding prealbumin (TBPA) is inhibited by salicylates.
2. Medicinal or dietary iodine interferes with all *in vivo* tests of radioiodine uptake, producing low uptakes which may not be reflective of a true decrease in hormone synthesis.
3. The persistence of clinical and laboratory evidence of hypothyroidism in spite of adequate dosage replacement indicates either poor patient compliance, poor absorption, excessive fecal loss, or inactivity of the preparation. Intracellular resistance to thyroid hormone is quite rare.

Carcinogenesis, Mutagenesis and Impairment of Fertility—A reportedly apparent association between prolonged thyroid therapy and breast cancer has not been confirmed and patients on thyroid for established indications should not discontinue therapy. No confirmatory long-term studies in animals have been performed to evaluate carcinogenic potential, mutagenicity, or impairment of fertility in either males or females.

Pregnancy—Category A. Thyroid hormones do not readily cross the placental barrier. The clinical experience to date does not indicate any adverse effect on fetuses when thyroid hormones are administered to pregnant women. On the basis of current knowledge, thyroid replacement therapy to hypothyroid women should not be discontinued during pregnancy.

Nursing Mothers—Minimal amounts of thyroid hormones are excreted in human milk. Thyroid is not associated with serious adverse reactions and does not have a known tumorigenic potential. However, caution should be exercised when thyroid is administered to a nursing woman.

Pediatric Use—Pregnant mothers provide little or no thyroid hormone to the fetus. The incidence of congenital hypothyroidism is relatively high (1:4000) and the hypothyroid fetus would not derive any benefit from the small amounts of hormone crossing the placental barrier. Routine determinations of serum T_4 and/or TSH is strongly advised in neonates in view of the deleterious effects of thyroid deficiency on growth and development.

Treatment should be initiated immediately upon diagnosis and maintained for life, unless transient hypothyroidism is suspected, in which case, therapy may be interrupted for two to eight weeks after the age of three years to reassess the condition. Cessation of therapy is justified in patients who have maintained a normal TSH during those two to eight weeks.

Adverse Reactions: Adverse reactions, other than those indicative of hyperthyroidism because of therapeutic overdosage, either initially or during the maintenance period are rare (See OVERDOSAGE).

In rare instances, allergic skin reactions have been reported with Cytomel (liothyronine sodium, SK&F) Tablets.

Overdosage:

Signs and Symptoms—Headache, irritability, nervousness, sweating, tachycardia, increased bowel motility and menstrual irregularities. Angina pectoris or congestive heart failure may be induced or aggravated. Shock may also develop. Massive overdosage may result in symptoms resembling thyroid storm. Chronic excessive dosage will produce the signs and symptoms of hyperthyroidism.

Treatment of Overdosage—Dosage should be reduced or therapy temporarily discontinued if signs and symptoms of overdosage appear. Treatment may be reinstituted at a lower dosage. In normal individuals, normal hypothalamic-pituitary-thyroid axis function is restored in six to eight weeks after thyroid suppression.

Treatment of acute massive thyroid hormone overdosage is aimed at reducing gastrointestinal absorption of the drugs and counteracting central and peripheral effects, mainly those of increased sympathetic activity. Vomiting may be induced initially if further gastrointestinal absorption can reasonably be prevented and barring contraindications such as coma, convulsions, or loss of the gagging reflex. Treatment is symptomatic and supportive. Oxygen may be administered and ventilation maintained. Cardiac glycosides may be indicated if congestive heart failure develops. Measures to control fever, hypoglycemia, or fluid loss should be instituted if needed. Antiadrenergic agents, particularly propranolol, have been used advantageously in the treatment of increased sympathetic activity. Propranolol may be administered intravenously at a dosage of 1 to 3 mg. over a 10-minute period or orally, 80 to 160 mg./day, especially when no contraindications exist for its use.

Dosage and Administration: The dosage of thyroid hormones is determined by the indication

Continued on next page

Smith Kline & French—Cont.

and must in every case be individualized according to patient response and laboratory findings.
Thyroid hormones are given orally. In acute, emergency conditions, injectable levothyroxine sodium may be given intravenously when oral administration is not feasible or desirable, as in the treatment of myxedema coma or during total parenteral nutrition. Injectable liothyronine sodium is also available from Smith Kline &French Laboratories upon request, under investigational status, for the treatment of myxedema coma. Intramuscular administration of these two preparations is not advisable because of reported poor absorption.
With Cytomel (liothyronine sodium, SK&F) Tablets once-a-day dosage is recommended; although liothyronine sodium has a rapid cutoff, its metabolic effects persist for a few days following discontinuance.

Mild Hypothyroidism: Recommended starting dosage is 25 mcg. daily. Daily dosage then may be increased by 12.5 or 25 mcg. every one or two weeks. Usual maintenance dose is 25-75 mcg. daily. Smaller doses may be fully effective in some patients, while dosage of 100 mcg. daily may be required in others.

The rapid onset and dissipation of action of liothyronine sodium (T_3), as compared with levothyroxine sodium (T_4), has led some clinicians to prefer its use in patients who might be more susceptible to the untoward effects of thyroid medication. However, the wide swings in serum T_3 levels that follow its administration and the possibility of more pronounced cardiovascular side effects tend to counterbalance the stated advantages.

Cytomel (liothyronine sodium, SK&F) Tablets may be used in preference to levothyroxine (T_4) during radioisotope scanning procedures, since induction of hypothyroidism in those cases is more abrupt and can be of shorter duration. It may also be preferred when impairment of peripheral conversion of T_4 and T_3 is suspected.

Myxedema: Recommended starting dosage is 5 mcg. daily. This may be increased by 5 to 10 mcg. daily every one or two weeks. When 25 mcg. daily is reached, dosage may often be increased by 12.5 or 25 mcg. every one or two weeks. Usual maintenance dose is 50 to 100 mcg. daily.

Myxedema Coma: Myxedema coma is usually precipitated in the hypothyroid patient of long standing by intercurrent illness or drugs such as sedatives and anesthetics and should be considered a medical emergency. A 'Cytomel' Injection Kit for the emergency treatment of myxedema coma is available from Smith Kline &French Laboratories upon request, under investigational status. Instructions which accompany this kit provide information on administration.

Congenital Hypothyroidism: Recommended starting dosage is 5 mcg. daily, with a 5 mcg. increment every three to four days until the desired response is achieved. Infants a few months old may require only 20 mcg. daily for maintenance. At one year, 50 mcg. daily may be required. Above three years, full adult dosage may be necessary (See PRECAUTIONS, Pediatric Use).

Simple (non-toxic) Goiter: Recommended starting dosage is 5 mcg. daily. This dosage may be increased by 5 to 10 mcg. daily every one or two weeks. When 25 mcg. daily is reached, dosage may be increased every week or two by 12.5 or 25 mcg. Usual maintenance dosage is 75 mcg. daily.

In the elderly or in children, therapy should be started with 5 mcg. daily and increased only by 5 mcg. increments at the recommended intervals.

When switching a patient to Cytomel (liothyronine sodium, SK&F) Tablets from thyroid, L-thyroxine or thyroglobulin, discontinue the other medication, initiate 'Cytomel' at a low dosage, and increase gradually according to the patient's response. When selecting a starting dosage, bear in mind that this drug has a rapid onset of action, and that residual effects of the other thyroid preparation may persist for the first several weeks of therapy.

Thyroid Suppression Therapy: Administration of thyroid hormone in doses higher than those produced physiologically by the gland results in suppression of the production of endogenous hormone. This is the basis for the thyroid suppression test and is used as an aid in the diagnosis of patients with signs of mild hyperthyroidism in whom baseline laboratory tests appear normal or to demonstrate thyroid gland autonomy in patients with Graves' ophthalmopathy. ^{131}I uptake is determined before and after the administration of the exogenous hormone. A 50 percent or greater suppression of uptake indicates a normal thyroid-pituitary axis and thus rules out thyroid gland autonomy.

Cytomel (liothyronine sodium, SK&F) Tablets are given in doses of 75-100 mcg./day for seven days, and radioactive iodine uptake is determined before and after administration of the hormone. If thyroid function is under normal control, the radioiodine uptake will drop significantly after treatment. Cytomel (liothyronine sodium, SK&F) Tablets should be administered cautiously to patients in whom there is a strong suspicion of thyroid gland autonomy, in view of the fact that the exogenous hormone effects will be additive to the endogenous source.

How Supplied: Round, white tablets in three dosage strengths: 5 mcg. tablets in bottles of 100; 25 mcg. tablets (scored) in bottles of 100 and 1000; and 50 mcg. tablets (scored) in bottles of 100.
CY:L29
Shown in Product Identification Section, page 437

DARBID® TABLETS, 5 mg. ℞
[*dahr' bid*]
(brand of isopropamide iodide)

Description: Each tablet contains isopropamide iodide equivalent to 5 mg. of isopropamide. Chemically, Darbid (isopropamide iodide, SK&F) is (3-carbamoyl-3, 3-diphenylpropyl) diisopropylmethyl ammonium iodide.

Actions: Darbid (isopropamide iodide, SK&F) is a synthetic anticholinergic that produces 10- to 12-hour gastric acid antisecretory effect and gastrointestinal antispasmodic response in man.

Indications
Based on a review of this drug by the National Academy of Sciences—National Research Council and/or other information, FDA has classified the indications as follows:
Effective: As adjunctive therapy in peptic ulcer.
Probably effective: In the irritable bowel syndrome (irritable colon, spastic colon, mucous colitis, acute enterocolitis, and functional gastrointestinal disorders).
Final classification of the less-than-effective indications requires further investigation.

IT SHOULD BE NOTED AT THIS POINT IN TIME THAT THERE IS A LACK OF CONCURRENCE AS TO THE VALUE OF ANTICHOLINERGICS IN THE TREATMENT OF GASTRIC ULCER. IT HAS NOT BEEN SHOWN CONCLUSIVELY WHETHER ANTICHOLINERGIC DRUGS AID IN THE HEALING OF A PEPTIC ULCER, DECREASE THE RATE OF RECURRENCES, OR PREVENT COMPLICATION.
FUNCTIONAL DISORDERS ARE OFTEN RELIEVED BY VARYING COMBINATIONS OF SEDATIVES, REASSURANCE, PHYSICIAN INTEREST, AMELIORATION OF ENVIRONMENTAL FACTORS, ETC.
To be effective, dosage must be titrated to the individual patient's needs.

Contraindications: Glaucoma; obstructive uropathy (e.g., bladder neck obstruction due to prostatic hypertrophy); obstructive disease of the gastrointestinal tract (as in achalasia, pyloroduodenal stenosis, etc.); obstructive or paralytic ileus; intestinal atony of the elderly or debilitated patient; unstable cardiovascular status in acute hemorrhage; severe ulcerative colitis; toxic megacolon complicating ulcerative colitis; myasthenia gravis.

Warnings: In the presence of a high environmental temperature, heat prostration (fever and heat stroke due to decreased sweating) can occur.
In patients with diarrhea due to incomplete intestinal obstruction (especially those with ileostomy or colostomy), treatment with Darbid (isopropamide iodide, SK&F) would be inappropriate and possibly harmful.
'Darbid' may produce drowsiness or blurred vision. In this event, the patient should be warned not to engage in activities requiring mental alertness such as operating a motor vehicle or other machinery or perform hazardous work while taking this drug.

Usage in Pregnancy: In pregnancy, lactation, and in women who may bear children, the potential benefits of the drug must be weighed against possible hazards.

Precautions: Use cautiously in elderly patients. Since the iodine in isopropamide iodide may alter PBI test results and will suppress I^{131} uptake, it is suggested that therapy be discontinued one week prior to these tests. Also, iodine skin rash may occur rarely.
Use with caution in patients with:
Autonomic neuropathy.
Hepatic or renal disease.
Ulcerative colitis (large doses may suppress intestinal motility to the point of producing paralytic ileus, and the use of this drug may precipitate or aggravate the serious complication of toxic megacolon).
Hyperthyroidism, coronary heart disease, congestive heart failure, cardiac arrhythmia, hypertension and nonobstructing prostatic hypertrophy.
Hiatal hernia associated with reflux esophagitis (anticholinergic drugs may aggravate this condition).
It should be noted that the use of anticholinergic drugs in the treatment of gastric ulcer may produce a delay in gastric emptying time (antral stasis) and, thus, complicate therapy.
Do not rely on the use of the drug in the presence of complication of biliary tract disease.
Investigate any tachycardia before giving anticholinergic (atropine-like) drugs, since they may increase the heart rate.
With overdosage, a curare-like action may occur.

Adverse Reactions: Anticholinergics produce certain pharmacological effects which may be desirable or undesirable, depending upon the individual patient's response. The physician must delineate these.
Adverse reactions which have occurred with Darbid (isopropamide iodide, SK&F) include: xerostomia (dry mouth); urinary hesitancy and retention; blurred vision; tachycardia; palpitations; mydriasis (dilatation of the pupils); cycloplegia; constipation; bloated feeling; nausea; dysphagia; fever; and nasal congestion.
Other adverse reactions possible with anticholinergics include: increased ocular tension; loss of taste; headaches; nervousness; drowsiness; weakness; dizziness; insomnia; vomiting; impotence; suppression of lactation; severe allergic reaction or drug idiosyncrasies including anaphylaxis; urticaria and other dermal manifestations; some degree of mental confusion and/or excitement, especially in elderly persons. Decreased sweating may occur. It should be noted that adrenergic innervation of the eccrine sweat glands on the palms and soles makes complete control of sweating impossible. An end point of complete anhidrosis cannot occur because large doses of drug would be required, and this would produce severe side effects from parasympathetic paralysis.

Dosage and Administration: Not for use in children under 12. Adults and children over 12—Usual starting dose is one 5 mg. tablet b.i.d. (every 12 hours). Patients with severe symptoms may require two 5 mg. tablets b.i.d., or more. Dosage should be individualized and titrated to the patient's need for greatest therapeutic effect.

Overdosage: Involves the cardiovascular, respiratory, gastrointestinal, central and peripheral nervous systems.
SYMPTOMS—May include dryness of mouth, dysphagia, thirst, blurred vision, dilated pupils, photophobia, fever, rapid pulse and respiration, disorientation. Depression and circulatory collapse may result from severe overdosage. TREATMENT—Gastric lavage, repeated several times. Respiratory depression should be promptly treated by the use of oxygen and stimulants. If marked excitement is present, one of the short-acting barbiturates, chloral hydrate, or gas anesthesia may be used. Otherwise do not administer sedation. Hyperpyrexia may be treated with physical cooling measures. Force fluids by mouth or, if necessary, by intravenous administration.
While pilocarpine or similar drugs are sometimes recommended for the relief of dry mouth, many authorities feel that these drugs are not indicated, since they relieve the minor peripheral effect but do not influence the more serious central effects and, thus, may merely mask signs of drug activity. If photophobia occurs, the patient should be kept in a darkened room.
How Supplied: In bottles of 50.
Shown in Product Identification Section, page 436
DB:L15

DEXEDRINE®
[dex'eh-dreen]
(brand of dextroamphetamine sulfate)
SPANSULE® CAPSULES,
TABLETS and ELIXIR
Warning:

> AMPHETAMINES HAVE A HIGH POTENTIAL FOR ABUSE. THEY SHOULD THUS BE TRIED ONLY IN WEIGHT REDUCTION PROGRAMS FOR PATIENTS IN WHOM ALTERNATIVE THERAPY HAS BEEN INEFFECTIVE. ADMINISTRATION OF AMPHETAMINES FOR PROLONGED PERIODS OF TIME IN OBESITY MAY LEAD TO DRUG DEPENDENCE AND MUST BE AVOIDED. PARTICULAR ATTENTION SHOULD BE PAID TO THE POSSIBILITY OF SUBJECTS OBTAINING AMPHETAMINES FOR NON-THERAPEUTIC USE OR DISTRIBUTION TO OTHERS, AND THE DRUGS SHOULD BE PRESCRIBED OR DISPENSED SPARINGLY.

Description: Dexedrine (dextroamphetamine sulfate, SK&F) is the dextro isomer of the compound d,l-amphetamine sulfate, a sympathomimetic amine of the amphetamine group. Chemically, dextroamphetamine is d-alpha-methylphenethylamine, and is present in all forms of 'Dexedrine' as the neutral sulfate.
Spansule® sustained release capsules—Each 'Spansule' sustained release capsule for oral administration contains dextroamphetamine sulfate, 5 mg., 10 mg., or 15 mg., so prepared that an initial dose is released promptly and the remaining medication is released gradually over a prolonged period.
Tablets—Each tablet for oral administration contains dextroamphetamine sulfate, 5 mg.
Elixir—Each 5 ml. (one teaspoonful) contains dextroamphetamine sulfate, 5 mg., and alcohol, 10%.
Clinical Pharmacology: Amphetamines are non-catecholamine, sympathomimetic amines with CNS stimulant activity. Peripheral actions include elevations of systolic and diastolic blood pressures and weak bronchodilator and respiratory stimulant action.
There is neither specific evidence which clearly establishes the mechanism whereby amphetamines produce mental and behavioral effects in children, nor conclusive evidence regarding how these effects relate to the condition of the central nervous system.
Drugs of this class used in obesity are commonly known as "anorectics" or "anorexigenics." It has not been established, however, that the action of such drugs in treating obesity is primarily one of appetite suppression. Other central nervous system actions, or metabolic effects, may be involved, for example.
Adult obese subjects instructed in dietary management and treated with "anorectic" drugs lose more weight on the average than those treated with placebo and diet, as determined in relatively short-term clinical trials.
The magnitude of increased weight loss of drug-treated patients over placebo-treated patients is only a fraction of a pound a week. The rate of weight loss is greatest in the first weeks of therapy for both drug and placebo subjects and tends to decrease in succeeding weeks. The origins of the increased weight loss due to the various possible drug effects are not established. The amount of weight loss associated with the use of an "anorectic" drug varies from trial to trial, and the increased weight loss appears to be related in part to variables other than the drug prescribed, such as the physician-investigator, the population treated, and the diet prescribed. Studies do not permit conclusions as to the relative importance of the drug and nondrug factors on weight loss.
The natural history of obesity is measured in years, whereas the studies cited are restricted to a few weeks' duration; thus, the total impact of drug-induced weight loss over that of diet alone must be considered clinically limited.
Dexedrine (dextroamphetamine sulfate, SK&F) *Spansule* capsules are formulated to release the active drug substance *in vivo* in a more gradual fashion than the standard formulation, as demonstrated by blood levels. The formulation has not been shown superior in effectiveness over the same dosage of the standard, noncontrolled-release formulations given in divided doses.
Pharmacokinetics
Elixir—Ingestion of 10 mg. of dextroamphetamine sulfate in elixir form by healthy volunteers produced an average peak dextroamphetamine blood level of 33.2 ng./ml. The half-life was 11.75 hours. The average urinary recovery was 38% in 48 hours.
Tablet—The single ingestion of two 5 mg. tablets by healthy volunteers produced an average peak dextroamphetamine blood level of 29.2 ng./ml. at 2 hours post-administration. The average half-life was 10.25 hours. The average urinary recovery was 45% in 48 hours.
'Spansule' capsule—Ingestion of a 'Spansule' capsule containing 15 mg. radiolabeled dextroamphetamine sulfate by healthy volunteers produced a peak blood level of radioactivity, on the average, at 8-10 hours post-administration with peak urinary recovery seen at 12-24 hours.
Indications and Usage: Dexedrine (dextroamphetamine sulfate, SK&F) is indicated:
1. **In Narcolepsy.**
2. **In Attention Deficit Disorder with Hyperactivity,** as an integral part of a total treatment program which typically includes other remedial measures (psychological, educational, social) for a stabilizing effect in children with a behavioral syndrome characterized by the following group of developmentally inappropriate symptoms: moderate to severe distractibility, short attention span, hyperactivity, emotional lability, and impulsivity. The diagnosis of this syndrome should not be made with finality when these symptoms are only of comparatively recent origin. Nonlocalizing (soft) neurological signs, learning disability, and abnormal EEG may or may not be present, and a diagnosis of central nervous system dysfunction may or may not be warranted.
3. **In Exogenous Obesity,** as a short-term (a few weeks) adjunct in a regimen of weight reduction based on caloric restriction, for patients refractory to alternative therapy, e.g., repeated diets, group programs, and other drugs. The limited usefulness of amphetamines (see CLINICAL PHARMACOLOGY) should be weighed against possible risks inherent in use of the drug, such as those described below.

Contraindications: Advanced arteriosclerosis, symptomatic cardiovascular disease, moderate to severe hypertension, hyperthyroidism, known hypersensitivity or idiosyncrasy to the sympathomimetic amines, glaucoma.
Agitated states.
Patients with a history of drug abuse.
During or within 14 days following the administration of monoamine oxidase inhibitors (hypertensive crises may result).
Warning: When tolerance to the "anorectic" effect develops, the recommended dose should not be exceeded in an attempt to increase the effect; rather, the drug should be discontinued.
Precautions:
General: Caution is to be exercised in prescribing amphetamines for patients with even mild hypertension.
The least amount feasible should be prescribed or dispensed at one time in order to minimize the possibility of overdosage.
These products contain FD&C Yellow #5 (tartrazine), which may cause allergic-type reactions (including bronchial asthma) in certain susceptible individuals. Although the overall incidence of FD&C Yellow #5 (tartrazine) sensitivity in the general population is low, it is frequently seen in patients who also have aspirin hypersensitivity.
Information for Patients: Amphetamines may impair the ability of the patient to engage in potentially hazardous activities such as operating machinery or vehicles; the patient should therefore be cautioned accordingly.
Drug Interactions
Acidifying agents—Gastrointestinal acidifying agents (guanethidine, reserpine, glutamic acid HCl, ascorbic acid, fruit juices, etc.) lower absorption of amphetamines. Urinary acidifying agents (ammonium chloride, sodium acid phosphate, etc.) increase the concentration of the ionized species of the amphetamine molecule, thereby increasing urinary excretion. Both groups of agents lower blood levels and efficacy of amphetamines.
Adrenergic blockers—Adrenergic blockers are inhibited by amphetamines.
Alkalinizing agents—Gastrointestinal alkalinizing agents (sodium bicarbonate, etc.) increase absorption of amphetamines. Urinary alkalinizing agents (acetazolamide, some thiazides) increase the concentration of the non-ionized species of the amphetamine molecule, thereby decreasing urinary excretion. Both groups of agents increase blood levels and therefore potentiate the actions of amphetamines.
Antidepressants, tricyclic—Amphetamines may enhance the activity of tricyclic or sympathomimetic agents; d-amphetamine with desipramine or protriptyline and possibly other tricyclics cause striking and sustained increases in the concentration of d-amphetamine in the brain; cardiovascular effects can be potentiated.
MAO inhibitors—MAOI antidepressants, as well as a metabolite of furazolidone, slow amphetamine metabolism. This slowing potentiates amphetamines, increasing their effect on the release of norepinephrine and other monoamines from adrenergic nerve endings; this can cause headaches and other signs of hypertensive crisis. A variety of neurological toxic effects and malignant hyperpyrexia can occur, sometimes with fatal results.
Antihistamines—Amphetamines may counteract the sedative effect of antihistamines.
Antihypertensives—Amphetamines may antagonize the hypotensive effects of antihypertensives.
Chlorpromazine—Chlorpromazine blocks dopamine and norepinephrine reuptake, thus inhibiting the central stimulant effects of amphetamines, and can be used to treat amphetamine poisoning.
Ethosuximide—Amphetamines may delay intestinal absorption of ethosuximide.
Haloperidol—Haloperidol blocks dopamine and norepinephrine reuptake, thus inhibiting the central stimulant effects of amphetamines.
Lithium carbonate—The antiobesity and stimulatory effects of amphetamines may be inhibited by lithium carbonate.

Continued on next page

Smith Kline & French—Cont.

Meperidine—Amphetamines potentiate the analgesic effect of meperidine.
Methenamine therapy—Urinary excretion of amphetamines is increased, and efficacy is reduced, by acidifying agents used in methenamine therapy.
Norepinephrine—Amphetamines enhance the adrenergic effect of norepinephrine.
Phenobarbital—Amphetamines may delay intestinal absorption of phenobarbital; co-administration of phenobarbital may produce a synergistic anticonvulsant action.
Phenytoin—Amphetamines may delay intestinal absorption of phenytoin; co-administration of phenytoin may produce a synergistic anticonvulsant action.
Propoxyphene—In cases of propoxyphene overdosage, amphetamine CNS stimulation is potentiated and fatal convulsions can occur.
Veratrum alkaloids—Amphetamines inhibit the hypotensive effect of veratrum alkaloids.
Drug/Laboratory Test Interactions
- Amphetamines can cause a significant elevation in plasma corticosteroid levels. This increase is greatest in the evening.
- Amphetamines may interfere with urinary steroid determinations.

Carcinogenesis/Mutagenesis: Mutagenicity studies and long-term studies in animals to determine the carcinogenic potential of Dexedrine (dextroamphetamine sulfate, SK&F) have not been performed.
Pregnancy—Teratogenic Effects: Pregnancy Category C. 'Dexedrine' has been shown to have embryotoxic and teratogenic effects when administered to A/Jax mice and C57BL mice in doses approximately 41 times the maximum human dose. Embryotoxic effects were not seen in New Zealand white rabbits given the drug in doses 7 times the human dose nor in rats given 12.5 times the maximum human dose. There are no adequate and well-controlled studies in pregnant women. 'Dexedrine' should be used during pregnancy only if the potential benefit justifies the potential risk to the fetus.
Nonteratogenic Effects: Infants born to mothers dependent on amphetamines have an increased risk of premature delivery and low birth weight. Also, these infants may experience symptoms of withdrawal as demonstrated by dysphoria, including agitation, and significant lassitude.
Nursing Mothers: It is not known whether this drug is excreted in breast milk; efforts to measure amphetamines in breast milk have been unsuccessful. Because many drugs are excreted in human milk, caution should be exercised when 'Dexedrine' is administered to a nursing woman.
Pediatric Use: Long-term effects of amphetamines in children have not been well established. Amphetamines are not recommended for use as anorectic agents in children under 12 years of age, or in children under 3 years of age with Attention Deficit Disorder with Hyperactivity described under INDICATIONS AND USAGE.
Clinical experience suggests that in psychotic children, administration of amphetamines may exacerbate symptoms of behavior disturbance and thought disorder.
Amphetamines have been reported to exacerbate motor and phonic tics and Tourette's syndrome. Therefore, clinical evaluation for tics and Tourette's syndrome in children and their families should precede use of stimulant medications.
Data are inadequate to determine whether chronic administration of amphetamines may be associated with growth inhibition; therefore, growth should be monitored during treatment.
Drug treatment is not indicated in all cases of Attention Deficit Disorder with Hyperactivity and should be considered only in light of the complete history and evaluation of the child. The decision to prescribe amphetamines should depend on the physician's assessment of the chronicity and severity of the child's symptoms and their appropriateness for his/her age. Prescription should not depend solely on the presence of one or more of the behavioral characteristics.
When these symptoms are associated with acute stress reactions, treatment with amphetamines is usually not indicated.

Adverse Reactions:
Cardiovascular: Palpitations, tachycardia, elevation of blood pressure.
Central Nervous System: Psychotic episodes at recommended doses (rare), overstimulation, restlessness, dizziness, insomnia, euphoria, dyskinesia, dysphoria, tremor, headache, exacerbation of motor and phonic tics and Tourette's syndrome.
Gastrointestinal: Dryness of the mouth, unpleasant taste, diarrhea, constipation, other gastrointestinal disturbances. Anorexia and weight loss may occur as undesirable effects when amphetamines are used for other than the anorectic effect.
Allergic: Urticaria.
Endocrine: Impotence, changes in libido.
Drug Abuse and Dependence: Dextroamphetamine sulfate is a Schedule II controlled substance.
Amphetamines have been extensively abused. Tolerance, extreme psychological dependence, and severe social disability have occurred. There are reports of patients who have increased the dosage to many times that recommended. Abrupt cessation following prolonged high dosage administration results in extreme fatigue and mental depression; changes are also noted on the sleep EEG.
Manifestations of chronic intoxication with amphetamines include severe dermatoses, marked insomnia, irritability, hyperactivity, and personality changes. The most severe manifestation of chronic intoxication is psychosis, often clinically indistinguishable from schizophrenia. This is rare with oral amphetamines.
Overdosage: Individual patient response to amphetamines varies widely. While toxic symptoms occasionally occur as an idiosyncrasy at doses as low as 2 mg., they are rare with doses of less than 15 mg.; 30 mg. can produce severe reactions, yet doses of 400 to 500 mg. are not necessarily fatal.
In rats, the oral LD_{50} of dextroamphetamine sulfate is 96.8 mg./kg.
SYMPTOMS—Manifestations of acute overdosage with amphetamines include restlessness, tremor, hyperreflexia, rapid respiration, confusion, assaultiveness, hallucinations, panic states.
Fatigue and depression usually follow the central stimulation.
Cardiovascular effects include arrhythmias, hypertension or hypotension and circulatory collapse. Gastrointestinal symptoms include nausea, vomiting, diarrhea, and abdominal cramps. Fatal poisoning is usually preceded by convulsions and coma.
TREATMENT—Management of acute amphetamine intoxication is largely symptomatic and includes gastric lavage and sedation with a barbiturate. Experience with hemodialysis or peritoneal dialysis is inadequate to permit recommendation in this regard. Acidification of the urine increases amphetamine excretion. If acute, severe hypertension complicates amphetamine overdosage, administration of intravenous phentolamine (Regitine®, CIBA) has been suggested. However, a gradual drop in blood pressure will usually result when sufficient sedation has been achieved.
Chlorpromazine antagonizes the central stimulant effects of amphetamines and can be used to treat amphetamine intoxication.
Since much of the 'Spansule' capsule medication is coated for gradual release, therapy directed at reversing the effects of the ingested drug and at supporting the patient should be continued for as long as overdosage symptoms remain. Saline cathartics are useful for hastening the evacuation of pellets that have not already released medication.
Dosage and Administration: Regardless of indication, amphetamines should be administered at the lowest effective dosage and dosage should be individually adjusted. Late evening doses—particularly with the 'Spansule' capsule form—should be avoided because of the resulting insomnia.

Narcolepsy: Usual dose 5 to 60 milligrams per day in divided doses, depending on the individual patient response.
Narcolepsy seldom occurs in children under 12 years of age; however, when it does, Dexedrine (dextroamphetamine sulfate, SK&F) may be used. The suggested initial dose for patients aged 6–12 is 5 mg. daily; daily dose may be raised in increments of 5 mg. at weekly intervals until optimal response is obtained. In patients 12 years of age and older, start with 10 mg. daily; daily dosage may be raised in increments of 10 mg. at weekly intervals until optimal response is obtained. If bothersome adverse reactions appear (e.g., insomnia or anorexia), dosage should be reduced. 'Spansule' capsules may be used for once-a-day dosage wherever appropriate. With tablets or elixir, give first dose on awakening; additional doses (1 or 2) at intervals of 4 to 6 hours.
Attention Deficit Disorder with Hyperactivity: Not recommended for children under 3 years of age.
In children from 3 to 5 years of age, start with 2.5 mg. daily, by tablet or elixir; daily dosage may be raised in increments of 2.5 mg. at weekly intervals until optimal response is obtained.
In children 6 years of age and older, start with 5 mg. once or twice daily; daily dosage may be raised in increments of 5 mg. at weekly intervals until optimal response is obtained. Only in rare cases will it be necessary to exceed a total of 40 milligrams per day.
'Spansule' capsules may be used for once-a-day dosage wherever appropriate.
With tablets or elixir, give first dose on awakening; additional doses (1 or 2) at intervals of 4 to 6 hours.
Where possible, drug administration should be interrupted occasionally to determine if there is a recurrence of behavioral symptoms sufficient to require continued therapy.
Exogenous Obesity: Usual dosage is one 10 or 15 mg. 'Spansule' capsule daily, taken in the morning, or up to 30 mg. daily by tablets or elixir, taken in divided doses of 5 to 10 mg. 30 to 60 minutes before meals. Not recommended for this use in children under 12 years of age.
How Supplied:
'Spansule' capsules—gelatin capsules having a natural body and brown cap, filled with small, light orange, medium orange and dark orange pellets; 5 mg., in bottles of 50; 10 mg. and 15 mg., in bottles of 50 and 500.
Tablets—pastel orange, triangular-shaped, single scored, compressed tablets; 5 mg., in bottles of 100 and 1000.
Elixir—a clear, orange-colored, orange-flavored liquid, containing 5 mg./5 ml., in 16 fl. oz. (473 ml.) bottles.
Shown in Product Identification Section, page 436
DX:L33

DIBENZYLINE® Capsules ℞
[di-benz′eh-leen]
(brand of phenoxybenzamine hydrochloride)

Description: Each maroon capsule for oral administration contains phenoxybenzamine hydrochloride, 10 mg.
'Dibenzyline' is N-(2-Chloroethyl)-N-(1-methyl-2-phenoxyethyl) benzylamine hydrochloride.
Phenoxybenzamine hydrochloride is a colorless, crystalline powder with a molecular weight of 340.3 which melts between 136° and 141°C. It is soluble in water, alcohol and chloroform; insoluble in ether.
Actions: Dibenzyline (phenoxybenzamine hydrochloride, SK&F) is a long-acting, adrenergic, α-receptor blocking agent which can produce and maintain "chemical sympathectomy" by oral administration. It increases blood flow to the skin, mucosa and abdominal viscera, and lowers both supine and erect blood pressures. It has no effect on the parasympathetic system.
Indication: Pheochromocytoma, to control episodes of hypertension and sweating. If tachycardia is excessive, it may be necessary to use a beta-blocking agent concomitantly.

Contraindications: Conditions where a fall in blood pressure may be undesirable.

Warning: 'Dibenzyline'-induced *alpha*-adrenergic blockade leaves *beta*-adrenergic receptors unopposed. Compounds that stimulate both types of receptors may therefore produce an exaggerated hypotensive response and tachycardia.

Precautions: Phenoxybenzamine hydrochloride has shown *in vitro* mutagenic activity in the Ames test and in the mouse lymphoma assay; it has not shown mutagenic activity in the micronucleus test in mice. In rats and mice repeated intraperitoneal administration of phenoxybenzamine hydrochloride resulted in peritoneal sarcomas. Chronic oral dosing in rats has produced malignant tumors of the gastrointestinal tract.

The clinical significance of such test results is not established. Nevertheless, these results should be given consideration in determining the benefit-risk ratio as it applies to the individual patient. Administer with caution in patients with marked cerebral or coronary arteriosclerosis or renal damage. Adrenergic blocking effect may aggravate symptoms of respiratory infections.

Adverse Reactions: Nasal congestion, miosis, postural hypotension, tachycardia and inhibition of ejaculation may occur. These so-called "side effects" are actually evidence of adrenergic blockade and vary according to the degree of blockade. Furthermore, they tend to decrease as therapy is continued. Gastrointestinal irritation, drowsiness and fatigue have also been reported.

Dosage and Administration: The dosage should be adjusted to fit the needs of each patient. Small initial doses should be *slowly* increased until the desired effect is obtained or the side effects from blockade become troublesome. *After each increase, the patient should be observed on that level before instituting another increase.* The dosage should be carried to a point where symptomatic relief and/or objective improvement are obtained, but not so high that the side effects from blockade become troublesome.

Initially, 10 mg. of Dibenzyline (phenoxybenzamine hydrochloride, SK&F) twice a day. Dosage should be increased every other day, usually to 20 to 40 mg. two or three times a day, until an optimal dosage is obtained, as judged by blood pressure control.

Overdosage: *Symptoms*—These are largely the result of block of the sympathetic nervous system and of the circulating epinephrine. They may include postural hypotension resulting in dizziness or fainting; tachycardia, particularly postural; vomiting; lethargy; shock. *Treatment*—When symptoms and signs of overdosage exist, discontinue the drug. Treatment of circulatory failure, if present, is a prime consideration. In cases of mild overdosage, recumbent position with legs elevated usually restores cerebral circulation. In the more severe cases, the usual measures to combat shock should be instituted. Usual pressor agents are *not* effective. Epinephrine is contraindicated because it stimulates both α and β receptors; since α receptors are blocked, the net effect of epinephrine administration is vasodilation and a further drop in blood pressure (epinephrine reversal).

The patient may have to be kept flat for 24 hours or more in the case of overdose, as the effect of the drug is prolonged. Leg bandages and an abdominal binder may shorten the period of disability.

I.V. infusion of levarterenol bitartrate* may be used to combat severe hypotensive reactions, because it stimulates α receptors primarily. Although Dibenzyline (phenoxybenzamine hydrochloride, SK&F) is an α adrenergic blocking agent, a sufficient dose of levarterenol bitartrate will overcome this effect.

How Supplied: Dibenzyline (phenoxybenzamine hydrochloride, SK&F) is supplied in maroon gelatin capsules containing 10 mg. of phenoxybenzamine hydrochloride in bottles of 100.

---

*Available as Levophed® Bitartrate (brand of levarterenol bitartrate) from Winthrop Laboratories.

Shown in Product Identification Section, page 436
DI:L20

DYAZIDE® Capsules   ℞
[*dye-uh-zide'*]

('Dyazide' is a product of SK&F Co., Carolina, P.R. 00630, Subsidiary of SmithKline Beckman Corporation, Philadelphia, Pa.)

Warning:
This fixed combination drug is not indicated for initial therapy of edema or hypertension. Edema or hypertension requires therapy titrated to the individual patient. If the fixed combination represents the dosage so determined, its use may be more convenient in patient management. The treatment of hypertension and edema is not static, but must be reevaluated as conditions in each patient warrant.

Description: Each maroon and white 'Dyazide' capsule contains 50 mg. of Dyrenium® (brand of triamterene), a potassium-sparing agent, and 25 mg. of hydrochlorothiazide.

'Dyrenium' is 2, 4, 7-triamino-6-phenylpteridine. Hydrochlorothiazide is 6-chloro-3, 4-dihydro-2H-1, 2, 4-benzothiadiazine-7-sulfonamide 1, 1-dioxide. At 50°C., triamterene is practically insoluble in water (less than 0.1%). It is soluble in formic acid, sparingly soluble in methoxyethanol, and very slightly soluble in alcohol.

Hydrochlorothiazide is slightly soluble in water. It is soluble in dilute ammonia, dilute aqueous sodium hydroxide, and dimethylformamide. It is sparingly soluble in methanol.

Action: 'Dyazide' is a diuretic/antihypertensive drug product that combines the natriuretic, hydrochlorothiazide, and the potassium-sparing natriuretic, triamterene, each of which complements the action of the other. The hydrochlorothiazide component blocks the reabsorption of sodium and chloride ions, and thereby increases the quantity of sodium traversing the distal tubule and the volume of water excreted. A portion of the additional sodium presented to the distal tubule is exchanged there for potassium and hydrogen ions. With continued use of hydrochlorothiazide and depletion of sodium, compensatory mechanisms tend to increase this exchange and may produce excessive loss of potassium, hydrogen and chloride ions. Hydrochlorothiazide also decreases the excretion of calcium and uric acid, may increase the excretion of iodide and may reduce glomerular filtration rate. The exact mechanism of the antihypertensive effect of hydrochlorothiazide is not known.

The triamterene component of 'Dyazide' exerts its diuretic effect on the distal renal tubule to inhibit the reabsorption of sodium in exchange for potassium and hydrogen ions. Its natriuretic activity is limited by the amount of sodium reaching its site of action. Although it blocks the increase in this exchange that is stimulated by mineralocorticoids (chiefly aldosterone) it is not a competitive antagonist of aldosterone and its activity can be demonstrated in adrenalectomized rats and patients with Addison's disease. As a result the dose of triamterene required is not proportionally related to the level of mineralocorticoid activity, but is dictated by the response of the individual patient, and the kaliuretic effect of concomitantly administered drugs. By inhibiting the distal tubular exchange mechanism, triamterene maintains or increases the sodium excretion and reduces the excess loss of potassium, hydrogen, and chloride ions induced by hydrochlorothiazide. As with hydrochlorothiazide, triamterene may reduce glomerular filtration and renal plasma flow. Via this mechanism it may reduce uric acid excretion although it has no tubular effect on uric acid reabsorption or secretion. Triamterene does not affect calcium excretion. No predictable antihypertensive effect has been demonstrated for triamterene.

Duration of diuretic activity and effective dosage range of the hydrochlorothiazide and triamterene components of 'Dyazide' are similar. Onset of diuresis with 'Dyazide' takes place within one hour, peaks at two-three hours and tapers off during the subsequent seven to nine hours.

Indications: This combination drug finds its usefulness primarily in the treatment of edema. Any usefulness of triamterene when used with a thiazide in hypertension will derive from its potassium-sparing effect. Either its main diuretic effect or potassium-sparing effect when used with a thiazide drug should be determined by individual titration. (See box warning.)

When the fixed combination represents the dosage determined by titration, 'Dyazide' is indicated as adjunctive therapy in edema associated with congestive heart failure, hepatic cirrhosis and the nephrotic syndrome. It is also indicated in corticosteroid and estrogen induced edema and idiopathic edema.

When the potassium-sparing action of its Dyrenium (triamterene, SK&F CO.) component is warranted and the fixed combination represents the dosage determined by titration, 'Dyazide' is indicated in the management of hypertension as determined by individual dosage titration of all agents employed. (See box warning.)

Usage in Pregnancy. The routine use of diuretics in an otherwise healthy woman is inappropriate and exposes mother and fetus to unnecessary hazard. Diuretics do not prevent development of toxemia of pregnancy, and there is no satisfactory evidence that they are useful in the treatment of developed toxemia.

Edema during pregnancy may arise from pathological causes or from the physiologic and mechanical consequences of pregnancy. Diuretics are indicated in pregnancy when edema is due to pathologic causes, just as they are in the absence of pregnancy (however, see Warnings, below). Dependent edema in pregnancy, resulting from restriction of venous return by the expanded uterus, is properly treated through elevation of the lower extremities and use of support hose; use of diuretics to lower intravascular volume in this case is illogical and unnecessary. There is hypervolemia during normal pregnancy which is harmful to neither the fetus nor the mother (in the absence of cardiovascular disease), but which is associated with edema, including generalized edema, in the majority of pregnant women. If this edema produces discomfort, increased recumbency will often provide relief. In rare instances, this edema may cause extreme discomfort which is not relieved by rest. In these cases, a short course of diuretics may provide relief and may be appropriate.

Contraindications: 'Dyazide' should not be given to patients receiving other potassium-sparing agents such as spironolactone or amiloride. Two deaths have been reported in patients receiving concomitant spironolactone and Dyrenium (triamterene, SK&F CO.) or 'Dyazide'. In one case dosage recommendations were exceeded; in the other serum electrolytes were not properly monitored.

'Dyazide' is contraindicated for further use in patients who exhibit anuria or progressive renal dysfunction, including increasing oliguria or increasing azotemia or in patients who develop hyperkalemia while on the drug.

'Dyazide' should not be used in patients with pre-existing elevated serum potassium, as is sometimes seen in patients with impaired renal function. Increasing hepatic dysfunction in patients on 'Dyazide' contraindicates further use of the preparation. Hypersensitivity to either drug in the preparation or to other sulfonamide-derived drugs is a contraindication.

Warnings: Patients should not be placed on dietary potassium supplements, potassium salts, or potassium-containing salt substitutes in conjunction with 'Dyazide' unless they develop hypokalemia or their dietary intake of potassium is markedly impaired. Because of the potassium conserving effect of Dyrenium (triamterene, SK&F CO.), hypokalemia is an uncommon occurrence with the use of 'Dyazide'.

If the need for supplementary potassium is demonstrated by repeated low serum potassium determinations a form other than potassium tablets

Continued on next page

Smith Kline & French—Cont.

should be used since these have been implicated in the development of nonspecific small bowel lesions consisting of stenosis with or without ulceration. Abnormal elevation of serum potassium, though uncommon, is potentially the most severe electrolyte disturbance with 'Dyazide' therapy. Hyperkalemia has been reported and in some cases has been associated with cardiac irregularities. Hyperkalemia is more likely to occur in patients who are severely ill, with relatively small urine volumes (less than one liter per day), or in elderly or diabetic patients with confirmed or suspected renal insufficiency. Acute transient hyperkalemia has been observed during intravenous glucose tolerance testing of diabetics dosed with the Dyrenium (triamterene, SK&F CO.) component of 'Dyazide'. Fatalities due to hyperkalemia have been reported, accordingly no potassium supplements should ordinarily be given with 'Dyazide' therapy, and periodic determinations of serum potassium should be made. If hyperkalemia develops, withdraw 'Dyazide', substitute a thiazide alone, and restrict potassium intake.

If hyperkalemia is present or suspected, an electrocardiogram should be obtained. If the ECG shows no widening of the QRS or arrhythmia in the presence of hyperkalemia, it is usually sufficient to discontinue 'Dyazide' and any potassium supplementation and substitute a thiazide alone. Sodium polystyrene sulfonate (Kayexalate®, Winthrop) may be administered to enhance the excretion of excess potassium. **The presence of a widened QRS complex or arrhythmia in association with hyperkalemia requires prompt additional therapy.** For tachyarrhythmia, infuse 44 mEq. of sodium bicarbonate or 10 ml. of 10% calcium gluconate or calcium chloride over several minutes. For asystole, bradycardia or A-V block transvenous pacing is also recommended.

The effect of calcium and sodium bicarbonate is transient and repeated administration may be required. When indicated by the clinical situation, excess K+ may be removed by dialysis or oral or rectal administration of Kayexalate®. Infusion of glucose and insulin has also been used to treat hyperkalemia.

Sensitivity reactions may occur in patients with or without a history of allergy or bronchial asthma. The possibility of exacerbation or activation of systemic lupus erythematosus has been reported with thiazide diuretics.

Usage in Pregnancy. Thiazides cross the placental barrier and appear in cord blood. The use of thiazides in pregnant women requires that the anticipated benefit be weighed against possible hazards to the fetus. These hazards include fetal or neonatal jaundice, thrombocytopenia, and possibly other adverse reactions which have occurred in the adult.

Nursing Mothers. Thiazides appear and triamterene may appear in breast milk. If use of the drug product is deemed essential, the patient should stop nursing.

Usage in Children
Adequate information on the use of 'Dyazide' in children is not available.

Precautions: Electrolyte imbalance, often encountered in such conditions as heart failure, renal disease, or cirrhosis of the liver, may also be aggravated by diuretics, and should be considered during 'Dyazide' therapy when using high doses for prolonged periods or in patients on a salt-restricted diet. Serum determinations of electrolytes should be performed, and are particularly important if the patient is vomiting excessively or receiving fluids parenterally. Possible fluid and electrolyte imbalance may be indicated by such warning signs as: dry mouth, thirst, weakness, lethargy, drowsiness, restlessness, muscle pain or cramps, muscular fatigue, hypotension, oliguria, tachycardia, and gastrointestinal symptoms.

Because of the potassium-sparing characteristic of Dyrenium (triamterene, SK&F CO.), hypokalemia is uncommon with 'Dyazide' but may occur in some cases when the 'Dyrenium' component is unable to completely compensate for the potassium-wasting effect of the hydrochlorothiazide component or the disease. The myocardial effects of digitalis may be exaggerated in patients with hypokalemia. In these patients signs of digitalis intoxication may be produced by previously tolerated doses of digitalis.

Hypokalemia is uncommon with 'Dyazide' but should it develop, corrective measures should be taken such as potassium supplementation or increased dietary intake of potassium-rich foods. Institute such measures cautiously with frequent determinations of serum potassium levels. Discontinue corrective measures immediately if laboratory determinations reveal an abnormal elevation of serum potassium. Discontinue 'Dyazide' and substitute a thiazide diuretic alone until potassium levels return to normal.

Although any chloride deficit is generally mild and usually does not require specific treatment except under extraordinary circumstances (as in liver disease or renal disease), chloride replacement may be required in the treatment of metabolic alkalosis. Dilutional hyponatremia may occur in edematous patients in hot weather; appropriate therapy is water restriction, rather than administration of salt, except in rare instances when the hyponatremia is life threatening. In actual salt depletion, appropriate replacement is the therapy of choice.

'Dyazide' may produce an elevated blood urea nitrogen level, creatinine level, or both. This apparently is secondary to a reversible reduction of glomerular filtration rate or a depletion of intravascular fluid volume (prerenal azotemia) rather than renal toxicity; levels return to normal when 'Dyazide' is discontinued. Elevated levels are seldom seen with every-other-day therapy. If azotemia increases, discontinue 'Dyazide'. Cumulative effects of the drug may develop in patients with impaired renal function. Periodic BUN or serum creatinine determinations should be made, especially in elderly patients and in patients with suspected or confirmed renal insufficiency.

Triamterene has been found in renal stones in association with the other usual calculus components. Therefore, 'Dyazide' should be used with caution in patients with histories of stone formation.

A possible interaction resulting in acute renal failure has been reported in a few patients on 'Dyazide' when treated with indomethacin, a nonsteroidal anti-inflammatory agent. Caution is advised in administering nonsteroidal anti-inflammatory agents with 'Dyazide'.

Thiazides should be used with caution in patients with impaired hepatic function. They can precipitate hepatic coma in patients with severe liver disease. Potassium depletion induced by the thiazide may be important in this connection. Administer 'Dyazide' cautiously and be alert for such early signs of impending coma as confusion, drowsiness and tremor; if mental confusion increases discontinue 'Dyazide' for a few days. Attention must be given to other factors that may precipitate hepatic coma, such as blood in the gastrointestinal tract or preexisting potassium depletion.

Patients should be observed regularly for the possible occurrence of blood dyscrasias, liver damage, or other idiosyncratic reactions. There have been reports of blood dyscrasias in patients receiving 'Dyrenium'. Leukopenia, thrombocytopenia, agranulocytosis, and aplastic and hemolytic anemia have been reported with the thiazides. Cirrhotics with splenomegaly may have marked variations in their blood pictures—including thrombocyte and leukocyte levels—which are not related to drug therapy. Since the 'Dyrenium' component of 'Dyazide' is a weak folic acid antagonist, it may contribute to the appearance of megaloblastosis in cases where folic acid stores are depleted. Periodic blood studies in these patients are recommended. The antihypertensive effects of 'Dyazide' may be enhanced in the post-sympathectomy patient.

Diabetes mellitus which has been latent may become manifest during thiazide administration. Thiazides may cause hyperglycemia and glycosuria, and alter insulin requirements in diabetes. 'Dyazide' may have similar effects; concurrent use with chlorpropamide may increase the risk of severe hyponatremia. Hyperuricemia may be observed, with possible occurrence of gout. Dyrenium (triamterene, SK&F CO.) may cause a decreasing alkali reserve with the possibility of metabolic acidosis.

Thiazides may add to or potentiate the action of other antihypertensive drugs. See Dosage and Administration for concomitant use with other antihypertensive drugs.

Thiazides have been shown to decrease arterial responsiveness to norepinephrine (an effect attributed to loss of sodium). This diminution is not sufficient to preclude effectiveness of the pressor agent for therapeutic use. Thiazides have also been shown to increase the paralyzing effect of nondepolarizing muscle relaxants such as tubocurarine (an effect attributed to potassium loss); consequently caution should be observed in patients undergoing surgery.

Thiazides may decrease serum PBI levels without signs of thyroid disturbance.

Calcium excretion is decreased by thiazides. Pathologic changes in the parathyroid glands with hypercalcemia and hypophosphatemia have been observed in a few patients on prolonged thiazide therapy. The common complications of hyperparathyroidism such as renal lithiasis, bone resorption, and peptic ulceration have not been seen. Thiazides should be discontinued before carrying out tests for parathyroid function.

'Dyrenium' and quinidine have similar fluorescence spectra; thus, 'Dyazide' will interfere with the fluorescent measurement of quinidine.

Lithium generally should not be given with diuretics because they reduce its renal clearance and increase the risk of lithium toxicity. Read circulars for lithium preparations before use of such concomitant therapy with 'Dyazide'.

Concurrent use of hydrochlorothiazide with amphotericin B or corticosteroids or corticotropin (ACTH) may intensify electrolyte imbalance, particularly hypokalemia, although the presence of triamterene minimizes the hypokalemic effects.

The effects of oral anticoagulants may be decreased when used concurrently with hydrochlorothiazide; dosage adjustments may be necessary.

Adverse Reactions: Side effects observed in association with the use of 'Dyazide' include: muscle cramps, weakness, dizziness, headache and dry mouth; anaphylaxis, rash, urticaria, photosensitivity, purpura and other dermatological conditions; nausea and vomiting, diarrhea, constipation, and other gastrointestinal disturbances (such nausea can usually be prevented by giving the drug after meals). It should be noted that symptoms of nausea and vomiting can also be indicative of electrolyte imbalance (see Precautions). Postural hypotension (may be aggravated by alcohol, barbiturates, or narcotics). Impotence has been reported in a few patients on 'Dyazide', although a causal relationship has not been established.

Triamterene has been found in renal stones in association with the other usual calculus components (see Precautions).

Thiazides alone have been known to cause necrotizing vasculitis, paresthesias, icterus, pancreatitis, xanthopsia, and respiratory distress including pneumonitis and pulmonary edema, transient blurred vision, sialadenitis, and vertigo. Rare incidents of acute interstitial nephritis have been reported with the use of 'Dyazide'.

Newborn, whose mothers had received thiazides during pregnancy, in rare instances have developed thrombocytopenia or pancreatitis.

Dosage and Administration: As determined by individual titration. (See box warning.)

Adults:
The usual dose is one or two capsules twice daily after meals. Some patients may be maintained on one capsule daily or every other day. Maximum daily dose should not exceed four capsules, and at this dosage, the incidence of side effects may increase.

Since 'Dyazide' has an antihypertensive effect, hypotensive drugs used concomitantly should be added at reduced dosage—at least one half the usual dosage—particularly if it is a ganglionic or peripheral adrenergic blocking agent. Adjust dosage as indicated.

Children:
Adequate information on the use of 'Dyazide' in children is not available.

Note: Potassium supplementation used concurrently with other diuretics should be discontinued when titrating with Dyrenium (triamterene, SK&F CO.). They should not be reinstituted when the patient is placed on 'Dyazide' unless the triamterene component does not completely compensate for the potassium loss.

Overdosage: Electrolyte imbalance is the major concern (See Warnings section). Symptoms reported include: polyuria, nausea, vomiting, weakness, lassitude, fever, flushed face, and hyperactive deep tendon reflexes. If hypotension occurs, it may be treated with pressor agents such as levarterenol to maintain blood pressure. Carefully evaluate the electrolyte pattern and fluid balance. Induce immediate evacuation of the stomach through emesis or gastric lavage. There is no specific antidote.

Although triamterene is largely protein-bound (approximately 67%), there may be some benefit to dialysis in cases of overdosage.

How Supplied: 'Dyazide' is supplied in gelatin capsules having an opaque white body and maroon cap, with tapered ends, in bottles of 1000 capsules; in Single Unit Packages (unit-dose) of 100 (intended for institutional use only); in Patient-Pak™ unit-of-use bottles of 100.

Military—Capsules, 1000's, 6505-00-901-0043; 100's, 6505-00-901-0024.

Veterans Administration—Capsules, 100's, 6505-00-901-0024A; 100's, 6505-00-901-0043A; 100's (SUP), 6505-00-524-7060A.

Shown in Product Identification Section, page 437
DZ:L36

DYRENIUM® R
[di-ren'ee-um]
(brand of triamterene)

('Dyrenium' is a product of SK&F Co., Carolina, P.R. 00630, Subsidiary of SmithKline Beckman Corporation, Philadelphia, Pa.)

Description: Each capsule contains triamterene, 50 mg. or 100 mg.

Dyrenium (triamterene, SK&F CO.) is 2,4,7- triamino-6-phenylpteridine.

Action: Dyrenium (triamterene, SK&F CO.) has a unique mode of action; it inhibits the reabsorption of sodium ions in exchange for potassium and hydrogen ions at that segment of the distal tubule under the control of adrenal mineralocorticoids (especially aldosterone). This activity takes place through a direct effect on the renal tubule and not by competitive aldosterone antagonism; it is not directly related to the level of aldosterone secretion.

The fraction of filtered sodium reaching this distal tubular exchange site is relatively small, and the amount which is exchanged depends on the level of mineralocorticoid activity. Thus, the degree of natriuresis and diuresis produced by inhibition of the exchange mechanism is necessarily limited. Increasing the amount of available sodium and the level of mineralocorticoid activity by the use of more proximally-acting diuretics will increase the degree of diuresis and potassium conservation.

'Dyrenium' occasionally causes increases in serum potassium which, in some instances, can result in hyperkalemia. It does not produce alkalosis because it does not cause excessive excretion of titratable acid and ammonium.

Indications: Dyrenium (triamterene, SK&F CO.) is indicated in the treatment of edema associated with congestive heart failure, cirrhosis of the liver, and the nephrotic syndrome; also in steroid-induced edema, idiopathic edema, and edema due to secondary hyperaldosteronism.

'Dyrenium' may be used alone or with other diuretics either for its added diuretic effect or its potassium-conserving potential. It also promotes increased diuresis when patients prove resistant or only partially responsive to thiazides or other diuretics because of secondary hyperaldosteronism.

Usage in Pregnancy. The routine use of diuretics in an otherwise healthy woman is inappropriate and exposes mother and fetus to unnecessary hazard. Diuretics do not prevent development of toxemia of pregnancy, and there is no satisfactory evidence that they are useful in the treatment of developed toxemia.

Edema during pregnancy may arise from pathological causes or from the physiologic and mechanical consequences of pregnancy. Diuretics are indicated in pregnancy when edema is due to pathologic causes, just as they are in the absence of pregnancy (however, see Warnings, below). Dependent edema in pregnancy, resulting from restriction of venous return by the expanded uterus, is properly treated through elevation of the lower extremities and use of support hose; use of diuretics to lower intravascular volume in this case is illogical and unnecessary. There is hypervolemia during normal pregnancy which is harmful to neither the fetus nor the mother (in the absence of cardiovascular disease), but which is associated with edema, including generalized edema, in the majority of pregnant women. If this edema produces discomfort, increased recumbency will often provide relief. In rare instances, this edema may cause extreme discomfort which is not relieved by rest. In these cases, a short course of diuretics may provide relief and may be appropriate.

Contraindications: Dyrenium (triamterene, SK&F CO.) should not be given to patients receiving other potassium-sparing agents such as spironolactone or amiloride. Two deaths have been reported in patients receiving concomitant spironolactone and 'Dyrenium': In one case, dosage recommendations were exceeded; in the other, serum electrolytes were not properly monitored.

Anuria. Severe or progressive kidney disease or dysfunction with the possible exception of nephrosis. Severe hepatic disease. Hypersensitivity to the drug.

'Dyrenium' should not be used in patients with preexisting elevated serum potassium, as is sometimes seen in patients with impaired renal function or azotemia, or in patients who develop hyperkalemia while on the drug. Patients should not be placed on dietary potassium supplements, potassium salts, or potassium-containing salt substitutes in conjunction with 'Dyrenium'.

Warnings: Patients should be observed regularly for the possible occurrence of blood dyscrasias, liver damage, or other idiosyncratic reactions. There have been reports of blood dyscrasias in patients receiving Dyrenium (triamterene, SK&F CO.).

Periodic BUN and serum potassium determinations should be made to check kidney function, especially in patients with suspected or confirmed renal insufficiency. It is particularly important to make serum potassium determinations in elderly or diabetic patients receiving the drug; these patients should be observed carefully for possible adverse serum potassium increases.

Usage in Pregnancy. Triamterene has been shown to cross the placental barrier and appear in the cord blood of ewes; this may occur in humans. The use of 'Dyrenium' in pregnant women requires that the anticipated benefit be weighed against possible hazards to the fetus. These possible hazards include adverse reactions which have occurred in the adult.

Nursing Mothers. Triamterene appears in cow's milk; this may occur in humans. If use of the drug is deemed essential, the patient should stop nursing.

Precautions: Dyrenium (triamterene, SK&F CO.) tends to conserve potassium rather than to promote its excretion as do many diuretics and, occasionally, can cause increases in serum potassium which, in some instances, can result in hyperkalemia. In rare instances, hyperkalemia has been associated with cardiac irregularities.

Hyperkalemia will rarely occur in patients with adequate urinary output, but it is a possibility if large doses are used for considerable periods of time.* If hyperkalemia is observed, 'Dyrenium' should be withdrawn. Because 'Dyrenium' conserves potassium, it has been theorized that in patients who have received intensive therapy or been given the drug for prolonged periods, a rebound kaliuresis could occur upon abrupt withdrawal. In such patients withdrawal of 'Dyrenium' should be gradual.

Electrolyte imbalance often encountered in such diseases as congestive heart failure, renal disease, or cirrhosis may be aggravated or caused independently by any effective diuretic agent including 'Dyrenium'. The use of full doses of a diuretic when salt intake is restricted can result in a low-salt syndrome.

'Dyrenium' can cause mild nitrogen retention which is reversible upon withdrawal of the drug and is seldom observed with intermittent (every-other-day) therapy.

Triamterene has been found in renal stones in association with other usual calculus components. Therefore, 'Dyrenium' should be used with caution in patients with histories of stone formation.

By the very nature of their illness, cirrhotics with splenomegaly sometimes have marked variations in their blood pictures. Since 'Dyrenium' is a weak folic acid antagonist, it may contribute to the appearance of megaloblastosis in cases where folic acid stores have been depleted. Therefore, periodic blood studies in these patients are recommended.

Although 'Dyrenium' has not proved to be a consistent antihypertensive agent, the physician should be aware of a possible lowering of blood pressure. Concomitant use with antihypertensive drugs may result in an additive effect.

'Dyrenium' may cause a decreasing alkali reserve with the possibility of metabolic acidosis.

'Dyrenium' and quinidine have similar fluorescence spectra; thus, 'Dyrenium' will interfere with the fluorescent measurement of quinidine.

A possible interaction resulting in acute renal failure has been reported in a few subjects when indomethacin, a nonsteroidal anti-inflammatory agent, was given with triamterene. Caution is advised in administering nonsteroidal anti-inflammatory agents with triamterene.

Lithium generally should not be given with diuretics because they reduce its renal clearance and increase the risk of lithium toxicity. Read circulars for lithium preparations before use of such concomitant therapy with 'Dyrenium'.

Adverse Reactions: There have been occasional reports of diarrhea, nausea and vomiting, and other gastrointestinal disturbances. Such nausea can usually be prevented by giving the drug after meals. It should be noted that symptoms of nausea and vomiting can also be indicative of electrolyte imbalance (see Precautions). Weakness, headache, dry mouth, anaphylaxis, photosensitivity, and rash have also been reported. Only rarely has it been necessary to discontinue therapy because of these side effects.

Triamterene has been found in renal stones in association with the other usual calculus components. Rare occurrences of acute interstitial nephritis have been reported with use of triamterene.

Note on Gout and Diabetes: In special studies, investigators found that Dyrenium (triamterene, SK&F CO.) has little or no effect on serum uric acid levels or carbohydrate metabolism. However, it has elevated uric acid, especially in persons predisposed to gouty arthritis.

Dosage and Administration: Adult Dosage Dosage should be titrated to the needs of the individual patient. When used alone, the usual starting dose is 100 mg. twice daily after meals. When combined with another diuretic, the total daily dosage of each agent should usually be lowered initially, and then adjusted to the patient's needs. The total daily dosage should not exceed 300 mg.

Continued on next page

Smith Kline & French—Cont.

Onset of action is 2–4 hours after ingestion. Most patients will respond to Dyrenium (triamterene, SK&F CO.) during the first day of treatment. Maximum therapeutic effect, however, may not be seen for several days. Duration of diuresis depends on several factors, especially renal function, but it generally tapers off 7–9 hours after administration.

When 'Dyrenium' is added to other diuretic therapy or when patients are switched to 'Dyrenium' from other diuretics, all potassium supplementation should be discontinued.

Overdosage: In the event of overdosage it can be theorized that electrolyte imbalance would be the major concern, with particular attention to possible hyperkalemia. Other symptoms that might be seen would be nausea and vomiting, other g.i. disturbances, and weakness. It is conceivable that some hypotension could occur. As with an overdose of any drug, immediate evacuation of the stomach should be induced through emesis and gastric lavage. Careful evaluation of the electrolyte pattern and fluid balance should be made. There is no specific antidote.

Although triamterene is largely protein-bound (approximately 67%), there may be some benefit to dialysis in cases of overdosage.

How Supplied: 50 mg. capsules, in bottles of 100, in Single Unit Packages of 100 (intended for institutional use only). 100 mg. capsules in bottles of 100 and 1000, in Single Unit Packages of 100 (intended for institutional use only).

Military—Capsules 100 mg., 100's, 6505-00-982-9143.

Veterans Administration—Capsules 100 mg., 100's, 6505-00-982-9143A.

---

*In making laboratory checks, blood samples require careful handling to prevent hemolysis on standing with resulting false serum potassium readings.

Shown in Product Identification Section, page 437
DY:L26

ESKALITH® ℞
[ess-kah'lith]
(brand of lithium carbonate)
Capsules, 300 mg.
Tablets, 300 mg.

ESKALITH CR® ℞
(brand of lithium carbonate)
Controlled Release Tablets, 450 mg.

> **WARNING**
> Lithium toxicity is closely related to serum lithium levels, and can occur at doses close to therapeutic levels. Facilities for prompt and accurate serum lithium determinations should be available before initiating therapy (see DOSAGE AND ADMINISTRATION).

Description: 'Eskalith' contains lithium carbonate, a white, light alkaline powder with molecular formula Li_2CO_3 and molecular weight 73.89. Lithium is an element of the alkali-metal group with atomic number 3, atomic weight 6.94 and an emission line at 671 nm on the flame photometer. 'Eskalith CR' tablets 450 mg. are designed to release a portion of the dose initially and the remainder gradually; the release pattern of the controlled release tablets reduces the variability in lithium blood levels seen with the immediate release dosage forms.

Actions: Preclinical studies have shown that lithium alters sodium transport in nerve and muscle cells and effects a shift toward intraneuronal metabolism of catecholamines, but the specific biochemical mechanism of lithium action in mania is unknown.

Indications: Eskalith (lithium carbonate, SK&F) is indicated in the treatment of manic episodes of manic-depressive illness. Maintenance therapy prevents or diminishes the intensity of subsequent episodes in those manic-depressive patients with a history of mania.

Typical symptoms of mania include pressure of speech, motor hyperactivity, reduced need for sleep, flight of ideas, grandiosity, elation, poor judgment, aggressiveness, and possibly hostility. When given to a patient experiencing a manic episode, 'Eskalith' may produce a normalization of symptomatology within 1 to 3 weeks.

Warnings: Lithium should generally not be given to patients with significant renal or cardiovascular disease, severe debilitation or dehydration, or sodium depletion, and to patients receiving diuretics, since the risk of lithium toxicity is very high in such patients. If the psychiatric indication is life-threatening, and if such a patient fails to respond to other measures, lithium treatment may be undertaken with extreme caution, including daily serum lithium determinations and adjustment to the usually low doses ordinarily tolerated by these individuals. In such instances, hospitalization is a necessity.

Chronic lithium therapy may be associated with diminution of renal concentrating ability, occasionally presenting as nephrogenic diabetes insipidus, with polyuria and polydipsia. Such patients should be carefully managed to avoid dehydration with resulting lithium retention and toxicity. This condition is usually reversible when lithium is discontinued.

Morphologic changes with glomerular and interstitial fibrosis and nephron atrophy have been reported in patients on chronic lithium therapy. Morphologic changes have also been seen in manic-depressive patients never exposed to lithium. The relationship between renal functional and morphologic changes and their association with lithium therapy have not been established.

When kidney function is assessed, for baseline data prior to starting lithium therapy or thereafter, routine urinalysis and other tests may be used to evaluate tubular function (e.g., urine specific gravity or osmolality following a period of water deprivation, or 24-hour urine volume) and glomerular function (e.g., serum creatinine or creatinine clearance). During lithium therapy, progressive or sudden changes in renal function, even within the normal range, indicate the need for reevaluation of treatment.

An encephalopathic syndrome (characterized by weakness, lethargy, fever, tremulousness and confusion, extrapyramidal symptoms, leukocytosis, elevated serum enzymes, BUN and FBS) followed by irreversible brain damage has occurred in a few patients treated with lithium plus haloperidol. A causal relationship between these events and the concomitant administration of lithium and haloperidol has not been established; however, patients receiving such combined therapy should be monitored closely for early evidence of neurologic toxicity and treatment discontinued promptly if such signs appear. The possibility of similar adverse interactions with other antipsychotic medication exists.

Lithium toxicity is closely related to serum lithium levels, and can occur at doses close to therapeutic levels (see DOSAGE AND ADMINISTRATION).

Outpatients and their families should be warned that the patient must discontinue lithium carbonate therapy and contact his physician if such clinical signs of lithium toxicity as diarrhea, vomiting, tremor, mild ataxia, drowsiness, or muscular weakness occur.

Lithium carbonate may impair mental and/or physical abilities. Caution patients about activities requiring alertness (e.g., operating vehicles or machinery).

Lithium may prolong the effects of neuromuscular blocking agents. Therefore, neuromuscular blocking agents should be given with caution to patients receiving lithium.

Usage in Pregnancy: Adverse effects on implantation in rats, embryo viability in mice, and metabolism *in vitro* of rat testes and human spermatozoa have been attributed to lithium, as have teratogenicity in submammalian species and cleft palates in mice.

In humans, lithium carbonate may cause fetal harm when administered to a pregnant woman. Data from lithium birth registries suggest an increase in cardiac and other anomalies, especially Ebstein's anomaly. If this drug is used during pregnancy, or if a patient becomes pregnant while taking this drug, the patient should be apprised of the potential hazard to the fetus.

Usage in Nursing Mothers: Lithium is excreted in human milk. Nursing should not be undertaken during lithium therapy except in rare and unusual circumstances where, in the view of the physician, the potential benefits to the mother outweigh possible hazards to the child.

Usage in Children: Since information regarding the safety and effectiveness of lithium carbonate in children under 12 years of age is not available, its use in such patients is not recommended at this time.

Precautions: The ability to tolerate lithium is greater during the acute manic phase and decreases when manic symptoms subside (see DOSAGE AND ADMINISTRATION).

The distribution space of lithium approximates that of total body water. Lithium is primarily excreted in urine with insignificant excretion in feces. Renal excretion of lithium is proportional to its plasma concentration. The half-life of elimination of lithium is approximately 24 hours. Lithium decreases sodium reabsorption by the renal tubules which could lead to sodium depletion. Therefore, it is essential for the patient to maintain a normal diet, including salt, and an adequate fluid intake (2500–3000 ml.) at least during the initial stabilization period. Decreased tolerance to lithium has been reported to ensue from protracted sweating or diarrhea and, if such occur, supplemental fluid and salt should be administered.

In addition to sweating and diarrhea, concomitant infection with elevated temperatures may also necessitate a temporary reduction or cessation of medication.

Previously existing underlying thyroid disorders do not necessarily constitute a contraindication to lithium treatment; where hypothyroidism exists, careful monitoring of thyroid function during lithium stabilization and maintenance allows for correction of changing thyroid parameters, if any; where hypothyroidism occurs during lithium stabilization and maintenance, supplemental thyroid treatment may be used.

Indomethacin has been reported to increase steady state plasma lithium levels from 30 to 59 percent. There is also some evidence that other nonsteroidal anti-inflammatory agents may have a similar effect. When such combinations are used, increased plasma lithium level monitoring is recommended.

Adverse Reactions: Adverse reactions are seldom encountered at serum lithium levels below 1.5 mEq./l., except in the occasional patient unusually sensitive to lithium. Mild to moderate toxic reactions may occur at levels from 1.5 to 2.5 mEq./l., and moderate to severe reactions may be seen at levels from 2.0 to 2.5 mEq./l., depending upon the individual response to the drug.

Fine hand tremor, polyuria, and mild thirst may occur during initial therapy for the acute manic phase, and may persist throughout treatment. Transient and mild nausea and general discomfort may also appear during the first few days of lithium administration.

These side effects are an inconvenience rather than a disabling condition, and usually subside with continued treatment or a temporary reduction or cessation of dosage. If persistent, a cessation of dosage is indicated.

Diarrhea, vomiting, drowsiness, muscular weakness, and lack of coordination may be early signs of lithium intoxication, and can occur at lithium levels below 2.0 mEq./l. At higher levels, ataxia, giddiness, tinnitus, blurred vision, and a large output of dilute urine may be seen. Serum lithium levels above 3.0 mEq./l. may produce a complex clinical picture, involving multiple organs and

for possible revisions

organ systems. Serum lithium levels should not be permitted to exceed 2.0 mEq./l. during the acute treatment phase.
The following reactions have been reported and appear to be related to serum lithium levels, including levels within the therapeutic range: **Neuromuscular/Central Nervous System**—tremor, muscle hyperirritability (fasciculations, twitching, clonic movements of whole limbs), ataxia, choreo-athetotic movements, hyperactive deep tendon reflex, extrapyramidal symptoms, blackout spells, epileptiform seizures, slurred speech, dizziness, vertigo, incontinence of urine or feces, somnolence, psychomotor retardation, restlessness, confusion, stupor, coma, tongue movements, tics, tinnitus, hallucinations, poor memory, slowed intellectual functioning, startled response; **Cardiovascular**—cardiac arrhythmia, hypotension, peripheral circulatory collapse, bradycardia, sinus node dysfunction with severe bradycardia (which may result in syncope); **Gastrointestinal**—anorexia, nausea, vomiting, diarrhea, gastritis, salivary gland swelling, abdominal pain, excessive salivation, flatulence, indigestion; **Genitourinary**—albuminuria, oliguria, polyuria, glycosuria, decreased creatinine clearance; **Dermatologic**—drying and thinning of hair, alopecia, anesthesia of skin, chronic folliculitis, xerosis cutis, psoriasis or its exacerbation, itching, angioedema; **Autonomic**—blurred vision, dry mouth; **Thyroid Abnormalities**—euthyroid goiter and/or hypothyroidism (including myxedema) accompanied by lower T_3 and T_4, I^{131} uptake may be elevated. (See Precautions.) Paradoxically, rare cases of hyperthyroidism have been reported; **EEG Changes**—diffuse slowing, widening of the frequency spectrum, potentiation and disorganization of background rhythm; **EKG Changes**—reversible flattening, isoelectricity or inversion of T-waves; **Miscellaneous**—fatigue, lethargy, transient scotomata, dehydration, weight loss, tendency to sleep, transient electroencephalographic and electrocardiographic changes, leukocytosis, headache, diffuse nontoxic goiter with or without hypothyroidism, transient hyperglycemia, hypercalcemia, hyperparathyroidism, generalized pruritus with or without rash, cutaneous ulcers, albuminuria, worsening of organic brain syndromes, excessive weight gain, edematous swelling of ankles or wrists, thirst or polyuria, sometimes resembling diabetes insipidus, metallic taste, dysgeusia/taste distortion, salty taste, swollen lips, tightness in chest, impotence/sexual dysfunction, swollen and/or painful joints, fever, polyarthralgia, hypertoxicity, dental caries.
A few reports have been received of the development of painful discoloration of fingers and toes and coldness of the extremities within one day of the starting of treatment with lithium. The mechanism through which these symptoms (resembling Raynaud's syndrome) developed is not known. Recovery followed discontinuance.
Two cases of reversible papilledema without evidence of increased intracranial pressure have been reported.
Dosage and Administration: Immediate release capsules and tablets are usually given t.i.d. or q.i.d. Doses of controlled release tablets are usually given b.i.d. (approximately 12-hour intervals). When initiating therapy with immediate release or controlled release lithium, dosage must be individualized according to serum levels and clinical response.
When switching a patient from immediate release capsules or tablets to the 'Eskalith CR' Controlled Release Tablets, give the same total daily dose when possible. Most patients on maintenance therapy are stabilized on 900 mg. daily, e.g., 450 mg. 'Eskalith CR' b.i.d. When the previous dosage of immediate release lithium is not a multiple of 450 mg., for example, 1500 mg., initiate 'Eskalith CR' dosage at the multiple of 450 mg. nearest to, but *below*, the original daily dose, i.e., 1350 mg. When the two doses are unequal, give the larger dose in the evening. In the above example, with a total daily dosage of 1350 mg., generally 450 mg. 'Eskalith CR' should be given in the morning and 900 mg. 'Eskalith CR' in the evening. If desired,

Product Information

the total daily dosage of 1350 mg. can be given in three equal 450 mg. 'Eskalith CR' doses. These patients should be monitored at 1-2 week intervals, and dosage adjusted if necessary, until stable and satisfactory serum levels and clinical state are achieved.
When patients require closer titration than that available with 'Eskalith CR' doses in increments of 450 mg., immediate release capsules or tablets should be used.
Acute Mania—Optimal patient response to Eskalith (lithium carbonate, SK&F) can usually be established and maintained with 1800 mg. per day in divided doses. Such doses will normally produce the desired serum lithium level ranging between 1.0 and 1.5 mEq./l.
Dosage must be individualized according to serum levels and clinical response. Regular monitoring of the patient's clinical state and serum lithium levels is necessary. Serum levels should be determined twice per week during the acute phase, and until the serum level and clinical condition of the patient have been stabilized.
Long-Term Control—The desirable serum lithium levels are 0.6 to 1.2 mEq./l. Dosage will vary from one individual to another, but usually 900 mg. to 1200 mg. per day in divided doses will maintain this level. Serum lithium levels in uncomplicated cases receiving maintenance therapy during remission should be monitored at least every two months.
Patients abnormally sensitive to lithium may exhibit toxic signs at serum levels of 1.0 to 1.5 mEq./l. Elderly patients often respond to reduced dosage, and may exhibit signs of toxicity at serum levels ordinarily tolerated by other patients.
N.B.: Blood samples for serum lithium determinations should be drawn immediately prior to the next dose when lithium concentrations are relatively stable (i.e., 8-12 hours after the previous dose). Total reliance must not be placed on serum levels alone. Accurate patient evaluation requires both clinical and laboratory analysis.
Overdosage: The toxic levels for lithium are close to the therapeutic levels. It is therefore important that patients and their families be cautioned to watch for early toxic symptoms and to discontinue the drug and inform the physician should they occur. Toxic symptoms are listed in detail under ADVERSE REACTIONS.
Treatment
No specific antidote for lithium poisoning is known. Early symptoms of lithium toxicity can usually be treated by reduction or cessation of dosage of the drug and resumption of the treatment at a lower dose after 24 to 48 hours. In severe cases of lithium poisoning, the first and foremost goal of treatment consists of elimination of this ion from the patient. Treatment is essentially the same as that used in barbiturate poisoning: 1) gastric lavage, 2) correction of fluid and electrolyte imbalance, and 3) regulation of kidney function. Urea, mannitol, and aminophylline all produce significant increases in lithium excretion. Hemodialysis is an effective and rapid means of removing the ion from the severely toxic patient. Infection prophylaxis, regular chest X-rays, and preservation of adequate respiration are essential.
How Supplied:
ESKALITH (lithium carbonate, SK&F) Capsules available as 300 mg. yellow and gray capsules in bottles of 100 and 500.
ESKALITH (lithium carbonate, SK&F) Tablets available as 300 mg. round, gray, single scored tablets in bottles of 100.
ESKALITH CR (lithium carbonate, SK&F) Controlled Release Tablets available as 450 mg. round, buff, single scored tablets in bottles of 100.
Shown in Product Identification Section, page 437
EL:L28

HISPRIL® ℞
[hiss' prill]
(brand of diphenylpyraline hydrochloride)
SPANSULE® CAPSULES 5 mg.

Description: Hispril®, brand of diphenylpyraline HCl, is an antihistamine.

Each 'Spansule' capsule contains diphenylpyraline hydrochloride, 5 mg., so prepared that an initial dose is released promptly and the remaining medication is released gradually over a prolonged period.
Actions: Diphenylpyraline hydrochloride is an antihistamine with anticholinergic (drying) and sedative side effects. Antihistamines appear to compete with histamine for cell receptor sites on effector cells.
Indications: For the symptomatic treatment of perennial and seasonal allergic rhinitis; vasomotor rhinitis; allergic conjunctivitis due to inhalant allergens and foods; mild, uncomplicated allergic skin manifestations of urticaria and angioedema; amelioration of allergic reactions to blood or plasma; dermographism; and as therapy for anaphylactic reactions adjunctive to epinephrine and other standard measures after the acute manifestations have been controlled.
Contraindications:
Use in Newborn or Premature Infants—This drug should *not* be used in newborn or premature infants.
Use in Nursing Mothers—Because of the higher risk of antihistamines for infants generally and for newborns and prematures in particular, antihistamine therapy is contraindicated in nursing mothers.
Use in Lower Respiratory Disease—Antihistamines *should NOT* be used to treat lower respiratory tract symptoms including asthma.
Antihistamines are also contraindicated in the following conditions:
Hypersensitivity to diphenylpyraline hydrochloride and other antihistamines of similar chemical structure
Monoamine oxidase inhibitor therapy (See Drug Interactions section)
Warnings: Antihistamines should be used with considerable caution in patients with:
Narrow angle glaucoma
Stenosing peptic ulcer
Pyloroduodenal obstruction
Symptomatic prostatic hypertrophy
Bladder neck obstruction
Use in Children—In infants and children, especially, antihistamines in *overdosage* may cause hallucinations, convulsions, or death.
As in adults, antihistamines may diminish mental alertness in children. In the young child, particularly, they may produce excitation.
Use in Pregnancy—Experience with this drug in pregnant women is inadequate to determine whether there exists a potential for harm to the developing fetus.
Use with CNS Depressants—Diphenylpyraline hydrochloride has additive effects with alcohol and other CNS depressants (hypnotics, sedatives, tranquilizers, etc.).
Use in Activities Requiring Mental Alertness—Patients should be warned about engaging in activities requiring mental alertness as driving a car or operating appliances, machinery, etc.
Use in the Elderly (approximately 60 years or older)—Antihistamines are more likely to cause dizziness, sedation, and hypotension in the elderly than in younger patients.
Precautions: Diphenylpyraline hydrochloride has an atropine-like action and, therefore, should be used with caution in patients with:
History of bronchial asthma
Increased intraocular pressure
Hyperthyroidism
Cardiovascular disease
Hypertension
Drug Interactions—MAO inhibitors prolong and intensify the anticholinergic (drying) effects of antihistamines.
Adverse Reactions: The most frequent adverse reactions are underlined:
1. **General:** Urticaria, drug rash, anaphylactic shock, photosensitivity, excessive perspiration, chills, dryness of mouth, nose, and throat.

Continued on next page

Smith Kline & French—Cont.

2. **Cardiovascular System:** Hypotension, headache, palpitations, tachycardia, extrasystoles.
3. **Hematologic System:** Hemolytic anemia, thrombocytopenia, agranulocytosis.
4. **Nervous System:** Sedation, sleepiness, dizziness, disturbed coordination, fatigue, confusion, restlessness, excitation, nervousness, tremor, irritability, insomnia, euphoria, paresthesias, blurred vision, diplopia, vertigo, tinnitus, acute labyrinthitis, hysteria, neuritis, convulsions.
5. **G.I. System:** Epigastric distress, anorexia, nausea, vomiting, diarrhea, constipation.
6. **G.U. System:** Urinary frequency, difficult urination, urinary retention, early menses.
7. **Respiratory System:** Thickening of bronchial secretions, tightness of chest and wheezing, nasal stuffiness.

Overdosage: Antihistamine overdosage reactions may vary from central nervous system depression to stimulation. Stimulation is particularly likely in children. Atropine-like signs and symptoms—dry mouth; fixed, dilated pupils; flushing; and gastrointestinal symptoms may also occur. Marked cerebral irritation, resulting in jerking of muscles and possible convulsions, may be followed by deep stupor.

If vomiting has not occurred spontaneously the patient should be induced to vomit. This is best done by having him drink a glass of water or milk after which he should be made to gag. Precautions against aspiration must be taken, especially in infants and children.

If vomiting is unsuccessful gastric lavage is indicated within 3 hours after ingestion and even later if large amounts of milk or cream were given beforehand. Isotonic and $\frac{1}{2}$ isotonic saline is the lavage solution of choice.

Saline cathartics, as milk of magnesia, by osmosis draw water into the bowel and therefore are valuable for their action in rapid dilution of bowel content.

Do not treat CNS depression with analeptics which might precipitate convulsions. Use only short-acting depressants to treat convulsions.

Stimulants should *not* be used.

If a vasoconstrictor is required for hypotension, levarterenol bitartrate, USP, may be used. Other pressor agents, including epinephrine, should not be used as they may cause a paradoxical further lowering of blood pressure.

Special note on 'Spansule' capsules—Since much of the 'Spansule' capsule medication is coated for gradual release, therapy directed at reversing the effects of the ingested drug and at supporting the patient should be continued for as long as overdosage symptoms remain. Saline cathartics are useful for hastening evacuation of pellets that have not already released medication.

Dosage and Administration: DOSAGE SHOULD BE INDIVIDUALIZED ACCORDING TO THE NEEDS AND THE RESPONSE OF THE PATIENT.

Adults—One capsule (5 mg.), q12h.

Older Children (6–12 years)—One 5 mg. capsule daily is usually sufficient. The physician should bear in mind that in children a higher incidence and a greater degree of antihistaminic side effects may be encountered. Do not use in children under 6 years.

How Supplied: Bottles of 50 capsules.

Shown in Product Identification Section, page 437

HI:L18

Tissue and Body Fluid Levels

Tissue or Body Fluid	Dosage and Route (No. of Patients Sampled)	Time of Sampling After Dose	Average Tissue or Fluid Levels (mcg./g. or/ml.)
Bone	1 g. I.M. (7)	60–90 min.	6.8
	1 g. I.V. (10)	44–99 min.	14.0
Gallbladder	1 g. I.M. (10)	60–70 min.	15.5
Bile	1 g. I.M. (10)	60–70 min.	7.5
Prostate	1 g. I.M. (10)	50–115 min.	13.0
Uterine Tissue	1 g. I.M. (6)	60–90 min.	17.5
Wound Fluid	1 g. I.M. (10)	60–75 min.	37.7
Purulent Wound	1 g. I.M. (9)	60 min.	11.5
Adipose Tissue	1 g. I.M. (5)	60 min.	4.0
Atrial Appendage	1 g. I.M. (7)	77–170 min.	7.5
	2 g. I.M. (7)	105–170 min.	8.7
	15 mg./kg. I.V. (10)	53–160 min.	15.4

MONOCID®
[mon¹oh-sid]
brand of sterile cefonicid sodium (lyophilized)

Description: Monocid (sterile cefonicid sodium, SK&F), a sterile, lyophilized, semisynthetic, broad-spectrum cephalosporin antibiotic for intravenous and intramuscular administration, is 5-Thia-1-azabicyclo [4.2.0] oct-2-ene-2-carboxylic acid, 7-[(hydroxyphenylacetyl)-amino]-8-oxo-3-[[[1-(sulfomethyl)-1H-tetrazol-5-yl]thio] methyl]-disodium salt, [6R-[6α, 7β(R*)]].

Cefonicid sodium contains 85 mg. (3.7 mEq.) sodium per gram of cefonicid activity.

Clinical Pharmacology:
Human Pharmacology
The table below demonstrates the levels and duration of Monocid (sterile cefonicid sodium, SK&F) in serum following intravenous and intramuscular administration of 1 gram to normal volunteers. [See table below].

Serum half-life is approximately 4.5 hours with intravenous and intramuscular administration. 'Monocid' is highly (greater than 90%) and reversibly protein bound.

'Monocid' is not metabolized; 99% is excreted unchanged in the urine in 24 hours. A 500 mg. I.M. dose provides a high (384 mcg./ml.) urinary concentration at 6–8 hours. Probenecid, given concurrently with 'Monocid', slows renal excretion, produces higher peak serum levels and significantly increases the serum half-life of the drug (8.2 hours).

'Monocid' reaches therapeutic levels in the following tissues and fluids:
[See table above].

Note: Although 'Monocid' reaches therapeutic levels in bile, those levels are lower than those seen with other cephalosporins, and amounts of 'Monocid' released into the gastrointestinal tract are minute. This small amount of 'Monocid' in the gastrointestinal tract is thought to be the reason for the low incidence of gastrointestinal reactions following therapy with 'Monocid'.

No disulfiram-like reactions were reported in a crossover study conducted in healthy volunteers receiving 'Monocid' and alcohol.

Microbiology
The bactericidal action of Monocid (sterile cefonicid sodium, SK&F) results from inhibition of cell-wall synthesis. 'Monocid' is highly resistant to beta-lactamases produced by *Staphylococcus aureus*, *Hemophilus influenzae*, *Neisseria gonorrhoeae* and Richmond type I beta-lactamases. 'Monocid' is resistant to degradation by beta-lactamases from certain members of *Enterobacteriaceae*. Active against a wide range of gram-positive and gram-negative organisms, 'Monocid' is usually active against the following organisms *in vitro* and in clinical situations:

Gram-Positive Aerobes: *Staphylococcus aureus* (beta-lactamase producing and non-beta-lactamase producing) and *S. epidermidis* (Note: Methicillin-resistant staphylococci are resistant to cephalosporins, including cefonicid.); *Streptococcus pneumoniae, S. pyogenes* (Group A beta-hemolytic *Streptococcus*), and *S. agalactiae* (Group B *Streptococcus*).

Gram-Negative Aerobes: *Escherichia coli; Klebsiella pneumoniae; Proteus mirabilis* (indole-negative *Proteus*); and *Hemophilus influenzae* (ampicillin-sensitive and -resistant).

In addition to the preceding, 'Monocid' is usually active against the following organisms *in vitro*, but the clinical significance of these data has not been established:

Gram-Negative Aerobes: *Klebsiella oxytoca; Providencia rettgerii* (formerly *Proteus rettgerii*); *Enterobacter aerogenes; Neisseria gonorrhoeae* (penicillin-sensitive and -resistant); *Citrobacter freundii* and *C. diversus*.

Anaerobes: *Peptostreptococcus anaerobius, Propionibacterium acnes*.

'Monocid' is usually inactive *in vitro* against most strains of *Pseudomonas, Serratia, Enterococcus* and *Acinetobacter*. Most strains of *B. fragilis* are resistant.

Susceptibility Testing
Results from standardized single-disc susceptibility tests using a 30 mcg. 'Monocid' disc should be interpreted according to the following criteria:

Zones of 18 mm. or greater indicate that the tested organism is susceptible to 'Monocid' and is likely to respond to therapy.

Zones from 15 to 17 mm. indicate that the tested organism is of intermediate (moderate) susceptibility, and is likely to respond to therapy if a higher dosage is used or if the infection is confined to tissues and fluids in which high antibiotic levels are attained.

Zones of 14 mm. or less indicate that the organism is resistant.

Only the 'Monocid' disc should be used to determine susceptibility, since *in vitro* tests show that 'Monocid' has activity against certain strains not susceptible to other cephalosporins. The 'Monocid' disc should not be used for testing susceptibility to other cephalosporins.

A bacterial isolate may be considered susceptible if the MIC value for 'Monocid' is equal to or less than 8 mcg./ml. in accordance with NCCLS* guidelines. Organisms are considered resistant if the MIC is equal to or greater than 32 mcg./ml. For most organisms the MBC value for 'Monocid' is the same as the MIC value.

* National Committee for Clinical Laboratory Standards

The standardized quality control procedure requires use of control organisms. The 30 mcg. 'Monocid' disc should give the zone diameters listed below for the quality control strains.

Organism	ATCC	Zone Size Range
E. coli	25922	25–29 mm.
S. aureus	25923	22–28 mm.

Indications and Usage: Monocid (sterile cefonicid sodium, SK&F) is indicated in the treatment of infections due to susceptible strains of the microorganisms listed below:

Serum Concentrations After 1 Gram Administration (mcg./ml.)

Interval	5 min.	15 min.	30 min.	1 hr.	2 hr.	4 hr.	6 hr.	8 hr.	10 hr.	12 hr.	24 hr.
I.V.	221.3	176.4	147.6	124.2	88.9	61.4	40.0	29.3	20.6	15.2	2.6
I.M.	13.5	45.9	73.1	98.4	97.1	77.8	54.9	38.5	28.9	20.6	4.5

LOWER RESPIRATORY TRACT INFECTIONS, due to *Streptococcus pneumoniae* (formerly *D. pneumoniae*); *Klebsiella pneumoniae*; *Escherichia coli*; and *Hemophilus influenzae* (ampicillin-resistant and ampicillin-sensitive).

URINARY TRACT INFECTIONS, due to *Escherichia coli*; *Proteus mirabilis* (indole-negative *Proteus*); and *Klebsiella pneumoniae*.

SKIN AND SKIN STRUCTURE INFECTIONS, due to *Staphylococcus aureus* and *S. epidermidis*; *Streptococcus pyogenes* (Group A *Streptococcus*) and *S. agalactiae* (Group B *Streptococcus*).

SEPTICEMIA, due to *Streptococcus pneumoniae* (formerly *D. pneumoniae*) and *Escherichia coli*.

BONE AND JOINT INFECTIONS, due to *Staphylococcus aureus*.

SURGICAL PROPHYLAXIS
Administration of a single 1 gram dose of 'Monocid' before surgery may reduce the incidence of postoperative infections in patients undergoing surgical procedures classified as contaminated or potentially contaminated (e.g., colorectal surgery, vaginal hysterectomy, or cholecystectomy in high-risk patients), or in patients in whom infection at the operative site would present a serious risk (e.g., prosthetic arthroplasty, open heart surgery). Although cefonicid has been shown to be as effective as cefazolin in prevention of infection following coronary artery bypass surgery, no placebo-controlled trials have been conducted to evaluate any cephalosporin antibiotic in the prevention of infection following coronary artery bypass surgery or prosthetic heart valve replacement.

In cesarean section, the use of 'Monocid' (after the umbilical cord has been clamped) may reduce the incidence of certain postoperative infections.

When administered one hour prior to surgical procedures for which it is indicated, a single 1 gram dose of 'Monocid' provides protection from most infections due to susceptible organisms throughout the course of the procedure and for approximately 24 hours after administration. Intraoperative and postoperative administration of 'Monocid' is not necessary. Daily doses of 'Monocid' may be administered for two additional days in patients undergoing prosthetic arthroplasty or open heart surgery.

If there are signs of infection, the causative organisms should be identified and appropriate therapy determined through susceptibility testing.

Studies on specimens obtained prior to therapy should be used to determine the susceptibility of the causative organisms to 'Monocid'. Therapy with 'Monocid' may be initiated pending results of the studies; however, treatment should be adjusted according to study findings.

Before using 'Monocid' concomitantly with other antibiotics, the prescribing information for those agents should be reviewed for contraindications, warnings, precautions and adverse reactions. Renal function should be carefully monitored.

Contraindications: Monocid (sterile cefonicid sodium, SK&F) is contraindicated in persons who have shown hypersensitivity to cephalosporin antibiotics.

Warnings: BEFORE THERAPY WITH MONOCID (STERILE CEFONICID SODIUM, SK&F) IS INSTITUTED, CAREFUL INQUIRY SHOULD BE MADE TO DETERMINE WHETHER THE PATIENT HAS HAD PREVIOUS HYPERSENSITIVITY REACTIONS TO CEPHALOSPORINS, PENICILLINS, OR OTHER DRUGS. THIS PRODUCT SHOULD BE GIVEN CAUTIOUSLY TO PENICILLIN-SENSITIVE PATIENTS. ANTIBIOTICS SHOULD BE ADMINISTERED WITH CAUTION TO ANY PATIENT WHO HAS DEMONSTRATED SOME FORM OF ALLERGY, PARTICULARLY TO DRUGS. SERIOUS ACUTE HYPERSENSITIVITY REACTIONS MAY REQUIRE EPINEPHRINE AND OTHER EMERGENCY MEASURES.

Pseudomembranous colitis has been reported with the use of cephalosporins (and other broad-spectrum antibiotics); therefore, it is important to consider that diagnosis in patients who develop diarrhea in association with antibiotic use.

Treatment with broad-spectrum antibiotics alters normal flora of the colon and may permit overgrowth of Clostridia. Studies indicate a toxin produced by *Clostridium difficile* is one primary cause of antibiotic-associated colitis. Cholestyramine and colestipol resins have been shown to bind the toxin *in vitro*.

Mild cases of colitis may respond to drug discontinuance alone.

Moderate to severe cases should be managed with fluid, electrolyte and protein supplementation as indicated.

When the colitis is not relieved by drug discontinuance and when it is severe, oral vancomycin is the treatment of choice for antibiotic-associated pseudomembranous colitis produced by *C. difficile*. Other causes of colitis should also be considered.

Precautions:
General: With any antibiotic, prolonged use may result in overgrowth of nonsusceptible organisms. Careful observation is essential, and appropriate measures should be taken if superinfection occurs.

Drug Interactions: Nephrotoxicity has been reported following concomitant administration of other cephalosporins and aminoglycosides.

Pregnancy: (Category B.) Reproduction studies have been performed in mice, rabbits and rats at doses up to an equivalent of 40 times the usual adult human dose and have revealed no evidence of impaired fertility or harm to the fetus due to Monocid (sterile cefonicid sodium, SK&F). There are, however, no adequate and well-controlled studies in pregnant women. Because animal reproduction studies are not always predictive of human response, this drug should be used in pregnancy only if clearly needed.

Labor and Delivery: In cesarean section, 'Monocid' should be administered only after the umbilical cord has been clamped.

Nursing Mothers: 'Monocid' is excreted in human milk in low concentrations. Caution should be exercised when 'Monocid' is administered to a nursing woman.

Pediatric Use: Safety and effectiveness in children have not been established.

Adverse Reactions: Monocid (sterile cefonicid sodium, SK&F) is generally well tolerated and adverse reactions have occurred infrequently. The most common adverse reaction has been pain on I.M. injection. On-therapy conditions occurring in greater than 1% of 'Monocid'-treated patients were:

Injection Site Phenomena (5.7%): Pain and/or discomfort on injection; less often, burning, phlebitis at I.V. site.
Increased Platelets (1.7%).
Increased Eosinophils (2.9%).
Liver Function Test Alterations (1.6%): Increased alkaline phosphatase, increased SGOT, increased SGPT, increased GGTP, increased LDH.

Less frequent on-therapy conditions occurring in less than 1% of 'Monocid'-treated patients were:

Hypersensitivity Reactions: Fever, rash, pruritus, erythema, myalgia and anaphylactoid-type reactions have been reported.
Hematology: Decreased WBC, neutropenia, positive Coombs' test.
Diarrhea.

Dosage and Administration:
General
The usual adult dosage is 1 gram of Monocid (sterile cefonicid sodium, SK&F) given once every 24 hours, intravenously or by deep intramuscular injection. Doses in excess of 1 gram daily are rarely necessary; however, in exceptional cases dosage of up to 2 grams given once daily have been well tolerated. When administering 2 gram I.M. doses once daily, one-half the dose should be administered in different large muscle masses.

Surgical Prophylaxis
When administered one hour prior to appropriate surgical procedures (see INDICATIONS AND USAGE), a 1 gram dose of 'Monocid' provides protection from most infections due to susceptible organisms throughout the course of the procedure and for approximately 24 hours after administration. Intraoperative and postoperative administration of 'Monocid' is not necessary. Daily doses of 'Monocid' may be administered for two additional days in patients undergoing prosthetic arthroplasty or open heart surgery.

In cesarean section 'Monocid' should be administered only after the umbilical cord has been clamped.

General Guidelines for Dosage of 'Monocid', I.V. or I.M.

Type of Infection	Daily Dose (grams)	Frequency
Uncomplicated Urinary Tract	0.5	once every 24 hours
Mild to Moderate	1	once every 24 hours
Severe or Life-Threatening	2*	once every 24 hours
Surgical Prophylaxis	1	1 hour preoperatively

* When administering 2 gram I.M. doses once daily, one-half the dose should be administered in different large muscle masses.

Impaired Renal Function
Modification of Monocid (sterile cefonicid sodium, SK&F) dosage is necessary in patients with impaired renal function. Following an initial loading dosage of 7.5 mg./kg. I.M. or I.V., the maintenance dosing schedule shown below should be followed. Further dosing should be determined by therapeutic monitoring, severity of the infection and susceptibility of the causative organism.
[See table on next page].

Preparation of Parenteral Solution
Parenteral drug products should be SHAKEN WELL when reconstituted, and inspected visually for particulate matter prior to administration. If particulate matter is evident in reconstituted fluids, the drug solutions should be discarded.

RECONSTITUTION
Single-Dose Vials
For I.M. injection, I.V. direct (bolus) injection, or I.V. infusion, reconstitute with Sterile Water for Injection according to the following table. SHAKE WELL.

Vial Size	Diluent to Be Added	Approx. Avail. Volume	Approx. Avg. Concentration
500 mg.	2.0 ml.	2.2 ml.	220 mg./ml.
1 gram	2.5 ml.	3.1 ml.	325 mg./ml.

These solutions of Monocid (sterile cefonicid sodium, SK&F) are stable 24 hours at room temperature or 72 hours if refrigerated (5°C.). Slight yellowing does not affect potency.

For I.V. infusion, dilute reconstituted solution in 50 to 100 ml. of the parenteral fluids listed under ADMINISTRATION.

Pharmacy Bulk Vials (10 grams)
For I.M. injection, I.V. direct (bolus) injection or I.V. infusion, reconstitute with Sterile Water for Injection, Bacteriostatic Water for Injection, or Sodium Chloride Injection according to the following table:

Amount of Diluent	Approx. Concentration	Approx. Avail. Volume
25 ml.	1 gram/3 ml.	31 ml.
45 ml.	1 gram/5 ml.	51 ml.

These solutions of 'Monocid' are stable 24 hours at room temperature or 72 hours if refrigerated (5°C.). Slight yellowing does not affect potency.

For I.V. infusion add to parenteral fluids listed under ADMINISTRATION.

"Piggyback" Vials
Reconstitute with 50 to 100 ml. of Sodium Chloride Injection or other I.V. solution listed under ADMINISTRATION. Administer with primary I.V. fluids, as a single dose. These solutions of 'Monocid' are stable 24 hours at room temperature or 72

Continued on next page

Smith Kline & French—Cont.

hours if refrigerated (5°C.). Slight yellowing does not affect potency.

A solution of 1 gram of 'Monocid' in 18 ml. of Sterile Water for Injection is isotonic.

Administration:

I.M. Injection: Inject well within the body of a relatively large muscle. Aspiration is necessary to avoid inadvertent injection into a blood vessel. When administering 2 gram I.M. doses once daily, one-half the dose should be given in different large muscle masses.

I.V. Administration: For direct (bolus) injection, administer reconstituted 'Monocid' slowly over 3 to 5 minutes, directly or through tubing for patients receiving parenteral fluids (see list below). For infusion, dilute reconstituted 'Monocid' in 50 to 100 ml. of one of the following solutions:

- 0.9% Sodium Chloride Injection, USP
- 5% Dextrose Injection, USP
- 5% Dextrose and 0.9% Sodium Chloride Injection, USP
- 5% Dextrose and 0.45% Sodium Chloride Injection, USP
- 5% Dextrose and 0.2% Sodium Chloride Injection, USP
- 10% Dextrose Injection, USP
- Ringer's Injection, USP
- Lactated Ringer's Injection, USP
- 5% Dextrose and Lactated Ringer's Injection
- 10% Invert Sugar in Sterile Water for Injection
- 5% Dextrose and 0.15% Potassium Chloride Injection
- Sodium Lactate Injection, USP

In these fluids 'Monocid' is stable 24 hours at room temperature or 72 hours if refrigerated (5°C.). Slight yellowing does not affect potency.

How Supplied: Monocid (sterile cefonicid sodium, SK&F) is supplied in vials equivalent to 500 mg. and 1 gram of cefonicid; in "Piggyback" Vials for I.V. admixture equivalent to 1 gram of cefonicid; and in Pharmacy Bulk Vials equivalent to 10 grams of cefonicid.

Shown in Product Identification Section, page 436.

MC:L11

ORNADE® SPANSULE® CAPSULES ℞
[or'naid]

Description: Each 'Ornade' *Spansule* capsule contains 75 mg. of phenylpropanolamine hydrochloride and 12 mg. of chlorpheniramine maleate, so prepared that an initial dose is released promptly and the remaining medication is released gradually over a prolonged period.

A single capsule dose produces blood levels comparable to those produced by administration of three 25 mg. doses of phenylpropanolamine hydrochloride and three 4 mg. doses of chlorpheniramine maleate in conventional release form given at four-hour intervals.

Actions: Phenylpropanolamine hydrochloride is a decongestant that provides vasoconstriction similar to that of ephedrine, but with less CNS stimulation.

Chlorpheniramine maleate is an antihistamine with anticholinergic (drying) and sedative side effects. Antihistamines appear to compete with histamines for H_1 cell receptor sites on effector cells.

Indications

For symptomatic relief of nasal congestion, runny nose, sneezing, itchy nose or throat, and itchy and watery eyes as may occur with the common cold or in allergic rhinitis (e.g., hay fever).

N.B.: A final determination has not been made on the effectiveness of this drug combination in accordance with efficacy requirements of the 1962 Amendments to the Food, Drug and Cosmetic Act.

Contraindications: Hypersensitivity to either ingredient; severe hypertension; coronary artery disease; stenosing peptic ulcer; pyloroduodenal or bladder neck obstruction.

'Ornade' *Spansule* capsules should NOT be used to treat lower respiratory tract conditions, including asthma.

As with any product containing a sympathomimetic, 'Ornade' *Spansule* capsules should NOT be used in patients taking MAO inhibitors.

Because of the higher risk of antihistamine side effects in infants generally, and for newborns and prematures in particular, antihistamine therapy is contraindicated in nursing mothers. This drug product should NOT be used in newborn or premature infants.

Warnings: Caution patients about activities requiring alertness (e.g., operating vehicles or machinery). Patients should also be warned about the possible additive effects of alcohol and other CNS depressants (hypnotics, sedatives, tranquilizers, etc.).

Precautions: Use with caution in patients with narrow-angle glaucoma, hypertension, cardiovascular disease, prostatic hypertrophy, hyperthyroidism, or diabetes. Patients taking this medication should be cautioned not to take simultaneously other products containing phenylpropanolamine HCl or amphetamines.

Use in Children: In infants and children, antihistamines in *overdosage* may cause hallucinations, convulsions, or death.

As in adults, antihistamines may diminish mental alertness in children. In the young child, particularly, they may produce excitation.

Use in Pregnancy: Experience with this drug in pregnant women is inadequate to determine whether there exists a potential for harm to the developing fetus. Therefore, 'Ornade' *Spansule* capsules should be used in pregnant women only when clearly needed in the judgment of the physician.

Use in the Elderly (approximately 60 years or older): The risk of dizziness, sedation, and hypotension is greater in the elderly patient.

Adverse Reactions:

General: excessive dryness of nose, throat, or mouth; headache; rash; weakness.

Cardiovascular System: angina pain; palpitations; hypertension; hypotension.

Hematologic: thrombocytopenia; leukopenia; hemolytic anemia; agranulocytosis.

Nervous System: drowsiness; nervousness or insomnia; dizziness; irritability; incoordination; tremor; convulsions; visual disturbances.

GI System: nausea; vomiting; epigastric distress; diarrhea; abdominal pain; anorexia; constipation.

GU System: difficulty in urination; dysuria.

Respiratory System: tightness of chest.

Dosage and Administration: Adults and children over 12 years of age—one capsule every 12 hours.

'Ornade' *Spansule* capsules should not be used in children under 12.

Overdosage: Symptoms may vary from central nervous system depression to stimulation. Also, atropine-like signs and symptoms (dry mouth; fixed, dilated pupils; flushing, etc.) as well as gastrointestinal symptoms may occur. Marked cerebral irritation resulting in jerking of muscles and possible convulsions may be followed by deep stupor and respiratory failure. Acute hypertension or cardiovascular collapse with accompanying hypotension may occur.

Treatment of Overdosage: Immediate evacuation of the stomach should be induced by emesis and gastric lavage. Since much of the 'Spansule' capsule medication is coated for gradual release, saline cathartics should be administered to hasten evacuation of pellets that have not already released medication.

Respiratory depression should be treated promptly with oxygen. Do not treat respiratory or CNS depression with analeptics that might precipitate convulsions; if convulsions or marked CNS excitement occurs, only short-acting barbiturates or chloral hydrate should be used.

Supplied: In bottles of 50 and 500 capsules, and in Single Unit Packages of 100 capsules (intended for institutional use only).

Military—Capsules, 500's, 6505-01-108-9574.

Veterans Administration—Capsules, 500's, 6505-01-108-9574A.

Shown in Product Identification Section, page 437

DR:L31

PAREDRINE® 1% ℞
[pah-red'drin]
(brand of hydroxyamphetamine hydrobromide)
with BORIC ACID, OPHTHALMIC SOLUTION

Description: Hydroxyamphetamine hydrobromide, 1%, in distilled water. Made tear-isotonic with 2% boric acid, and preserved with thimerosal, 1:50,000.

Action: Dilates the pupil; probably by stimulating the dilator muscles of the iris.

Indication: To dilate the pupil; produces a pupillary dilatation which lasts for a few hours.

Contraindication: Narrow-angle glaucoma.

Precautions: Use with caution in patients with hypertension, hyperthyroidism and diabetes.

Adverse Reactions: With widely dilated pupils there will likely be increased intraocular pressure, photophobia and blurring of vision.

Dosage and Administration: Instil 1 or 2 drops into the conjunctival sac.

Overdosage: *Symptoms*—Dilatation of pupils. *Treatment*—Dilute pilocarpine (1%) may be administered if desired. Instil one drop at intervals. Repeat as necessary. **Accidental ingestion**—*Symptoms*—These may include marked rise in blood pressure, palpitation, cardiac arrhythmias, substernal discomfort, headache, sweating, nausea,

---

Dosage of 'Monocid' in Adults with Reduced Renal Function

(Monitor blood levels and adjust accordingly.)

Creatinine Clearance (ml./min. per 1.73 M²)	Dosage Regimen	
	Mild to Moderate Infections	Severe Infections
79–60	10 mg./kg. (every 24 hours)	25 mg./kg. (every 24 hours)
59–40	8 mg./kg. (every 24 hours)	20 mg./kg. (every 24 hours)
39–20	4 mg./kg. (every 24 hours)	15 mg./kg. (every 24 hours)
19–10	4 mg./kg. (every 48 hours)	15 mg./kg. (every 48 hours)
9–5	4 mg./kg. (every 3 to 5 days)	15 mg./kg. (every 3 to 5 days)
<5	3 mg./kg. (every 3 to 5 days)	4 mg./kg. (every 3 to 5 days)

Note: It is not necessary to administer additional dosage following dialysis.

vomiting and gastrointestinal irritation. *Treatment*—Sedation is indicated. Further treatment is symptomatic. Shock, if present, should be treated promptly. If hypertension is prominent, measures should be taken to lower blood pressure.
How Supplied: ½ fl. oz. (15 ml.) bottles.
PHO:L27

PARNATE® ℞
[pahr′naight]
(brand of tranylcypromine sulfate)

Before prescribing, the physician should be familiar with the entire contents of this prescribing information.
Description: Each tablet contains tranylcypromine sulfate equivalent to 10 mg. of tranylcypromine.
Chemically, tranylcypromine sulfate is (±)-*trans*-2-phenylcyclopropylamine sulfate (2:1).
Action: Tranylcypromine is a non-hydrazine monoamine oxidase inhibitor with a rapid onset of activity. It increases the concentration of epinephrine, norepinephrine, and serotonin in storage sites throughout the nervous system, and in theory, this increased concentration of monoamines in the brainstem is the basis for its antidepressant activity. When tranylcypromine is withdrawn, monoamine oxidase activity is recovered in 3 to 5 days, although the drug is excreted in 24 hours.

> **Indications**
> Based on a review of this drug by the National Academy of Sciences—National Research Council and/or other information, FDA has classified the indications as follows:
> Probably effective: For symptomatic relief of severe reactive or endogenous depression in hospitalized or closely supervised patients who have not responded to other antidepressant therapy.
> Final classification of the less-than-effective indications requires further investigation.

Summary of Contraindications: Parnate (tranylcypromine sulfate, SK&F) should not be administered in combination with any of the following: MAO inhibitors or dibenzazepine derivatives; sympathomimetics (including amphetamines); some central nervous system depressants (including narcotics and alcohol); antihypertensive, diuretic, antihistaminic, sedative or anesthetic drugs; cheese or other foods with a high tyramine content; or excessive quantities of caffeine.
Parnate (tranylcypromine sulfate, SK&F) should not be administered to any patient beyond 60 years of age or with a confirmed or suspected cerebrovascular defect or to any patient with cardiovascular disease, hypertension or history of headache.
(For complete discussion of contraindications and warnings, see below.)
Contraindications: Parnate (tranylcypromine sulfate, SK&F) is contraindicated:
1. In patients with cerebrovascular defects or cardiovascular disorders
Parnate (tranylcypromine sulfate, SK&F) should not be administered to any patient with a confirmed or suspected cerebrovascular defect or to any patient with cardiovascular disease or hypertension. The drug should also be withheld from individuals beyond the age of 60 because of the possibility of existing cerebral sclerosis with damaged vessels.
2. In the presence of pheochromocytoma
Parnate (tranylcypromine sulfate, SK&F) should not be used in the presence of pheochromocytoma since such tumors secrete pressor substances.
3. In combination with MAO inhibitors or with dibenzazepine-related entities
Parnate (tranylcypromine sulfate, SK&F) should not be administered together or in rapid succession with other MAO inhibitors or with dibenzazepine-related entities. Hypertensive crises or severe convulsive seizures may occur in patients receiving such combinations.

In patients being transferred to 'Parnate' from another MAO inhibitor or from a dibenzazepine-related entity, allow a medication-free interval of at least a week, then initiate 'Parnate' using half the normal starting dosage for at least the first week of therapy. Similarly, at least a week should elapse between the discontinuance of 'Parnate' and the administration of another MAO inhibitor or a dibenzazepine-related entity.
Other MAO inhibitors presently known to be marketed in this country:

Generic Name	Trademark
Isocarboxazid	'Marplan' (Roche Laboratories)
Pargyline HCl	'Eutonyl' (Abbott Laboratories)
Pargyline HCl and methyclothiazide	'Eutron' (Abbott Laboratories)
Phenelzine sulfate	'Nardil' (Warner-Chilcott Laboratories)

Dibenzazepine-related entities and other tricyclic drugs presently known to be marketed in this country:

Generic Name	Trademark
Amitriptyline HCl	'Elavil' (Merck Sharp & Dohme)
	'SK-Amitriptyline' (Smith Kline & French)
Perphenazine and amitriptyline HCl	'Etrafon' (Schering)
	'Triavil' (Merck Sharp & Dohme)
Desipramine HCl	'Norpramin' (Merrell-National)
	'Pertofrane' (USV)
Imipramine HCl	'Imavate' (Robins)
	'Presamine' (USV)
	'SK-Pramine' (Smith Kline & French)
	'Tofranil' (Geigy Pharmaceuticals)
Nortriptyline HCl	'Aventyl' (Eli Lilly & Co.)
	'Pamelor' (Sandoz)
Protriptyline HCl	'Vivactil' (Merck Sharp & Dohme)
Doxepin HCl	'Adapin' (Pennwalt)
	'Sinequan' (Pfizer)
Carbamazepine	'Tegretol' (Geigy Pharmaceuticals)
Cyclobenzaprine HCl	'Flexeril' (Merck Sharp & Dohme)
Amoxapine	'Asendin' (Lederle)
Maprotiline HCl	'Ludiomil' (CIBA)
Trimipramine maleate	'Surmontil' (Ives)

4. In combination with sympathomimetics
Parnate (tranylcypromine sulfate, SK&F) should not be administered in combination with sympathomimetics, including amphetamines, and over-the-counter drugs such as cold, hay fever or weight-reducing preparations that contain vasoconstrictors.
During 'Parnate' therapy, it appears that certain patients are particularly vulnerable to the effects of sympathomimetics when the activity of certain enzymes is inhibited. Use of sympathomimetics and compounds such as methyldopa, dopamine, levodopa and tryptophan with 'Parnate' may precipitate hypertension, headache, and related symptoms.
5. In combination with meperidine
Do not use meperidine concomitantly with MAO inhibitors or within two or three weeks following MAOI therapy. Serious reactions have been precipitated with concomitant use, including coma, severe hypertension or hypotension, severe respiratory depression, convulsions, malignant hyperpyrexia, excitation, peripheral vascular collapse and death. It is thought that these reactions may be mediated by accumulation of 5-HT (serotonin) consequent to MAO inhibition.
6. In combination with cheese or other foods with a high tyramine content
Hypertensive crises have sometimes occurred during Parnate (tranylcypromine sulfate, SK&F) therapy after ingestion of foods with a high tyramine content. In general, the patient should avoid protein foods in which aging or protein breakdown is used to increase flavor. In particular, patients should be instructed not to take foods such as cheese (particularly strong or aged varieties), sour cream, Chianti wine, sherry, beer, pickled herring, liver, canned figs, raisins, bananas or avocados (particularly if overripe), chocolate, soy sauce, the pods of broad beans (fava beans), yeast extracts, or meat prepared with tenderizers.
7. In patients undergoing elective surgery
Patients taking 'Parnate' should not undergo elective surgery requiring general anesthesia. Also, they should not be given cocaine or local anesthesia containing sympathomimetic vasoconstrictors. The possible combined hypotensive effects of 'Parnate' and spinal anesthesia should be kept in mind. 'Parnate' should be discontinued at least 10 days prior to elective surgery.
Additional Contraindications: In general, the physician should bear in mind the possibility of a lowered margin of safety when Parnate (tranylcypromine sulfate, SK&F) is administered in combination with potent drugs.
1. 'Parnate' should not be used in combination with some central nervous system depressants such as narcotics and alcohol, or with hypotensive agents. A marked potentiating effect on these classes of drugs has been reported.
2. Anti-parkinsonism drugs should be used with caution in patients receiving 'Parnate' since severe reactions have been reported.
3. 'Parnate' should not be used in patients with a history of liver disease or in those with abnormal liver function tests.
4. Excessive use of caffeine in any form should be avoided in patients receiving 'Parnate'.
Warning to Physicians: Parnate (tranylcypromine sulfate, SK&F) is a potent agent with the capability of producing serious side effects. 'Parnate' is not recommended in those severe endogenous depressions in which electroconvulsive therapy is the treatment of choice or in those depressive reactions where other antidepressant drugs may be effective. **It should be reserved for patients who are either hospitalized or under close supervision and who have not responded satisfactorily to other antidepressant therapy.**
Before prescribing, the physician should be completely familiar with the full material on dosage, side effects, and contraindications on these pages, with the principles of MAO inhibitor therapy and the side effects of this class of drugs. Also, the physician should be familiar with the symptomatology of mental depressions and alternate methods of treatment to aid in the careful selection of patients for 'Parnate' therapy. In depressed patients, the possibility of suicide should always be considered and adequate precautions taken.
Pregnancy Warning: Use of any drug in pregnancy, during lactation, or in women of childbearing age requires that the potential benefits of the drug be weighed against its possible hazards to mother and child. Animal reproductive studies show that Parnate (tranylcypromine sulfate, SK&F) passes through the placental barrier into the fetus of the rat. Also, it passes into milk of the lactating dog. The absence of a harmful action of 'Parnate' on fertility or on postnatal development by either prenatal treatment or from the milk of treated animals has not been demonstrated.
Warning to the Patient: Patients should be instructed to report promptly the occurrence of headache or other unusual symptoms.
Patients should be warned against eating the foods listed in Section 6 under Contraindications while on Parnate (tranylcypromine sulfate, SK&F) ther-

Continued on next page

Smith Kline & French—Cont.

apy. Also, they should be told not to drink alcoholic beverages.

Patients should be warned against self-medication with proprietary (over-the-counter) drugs such as cold, hay fever or weight-reducing preparations that contain pressor agents. They should be advised not to consume excessive amounts of caffeine in any form.

Warnings: Hypertensive Crises: The most important reaction associated with Parnate (tranylcypromine sulfate, SK&F) is the occurrence of hypertensive crises which have sometimes been fatal.

These crises are characterized by some or all of the following symptoms: occipital headache which may radiate frontally, palpitation, neck stiffness or soreness, nausea or vomiting, sweating (sometimes with fever and sometimes with cold, clammy skin) and photophobia. Either tachycardia or bradycardia may be present, and associated constricting chest pain and dilated pupils may occur. Intracranial bleeding, sometimes fatal in outcome, has been reported in association with the paradoxical increase in blood pressure.

In all patients taking 'Parnate' blood pressure should be followed closely to detect evidence of any pressor response. It is emphasized that full reliance should not be placed on blood pressure readings, but that the patient should also be observed frequently.

Therapy should be discontinued immediately upon the occurrence of palpitation or frequent headaches during 'Parnate' therapy. These signs may be prodromal of a hypertensive crisis.

Important: Recommended treatment in hypertensive crises

If a hypertensive crisis occurs, Parnate (tranylcypromine sulfate, SK&F) should be discontinued and therapy to lower blood pressure should be instituted immediately. Headache tends to abate as blood pressure is lowered. On the basis of present evidence, phentolamine (available as 'Regitine'*) is recommended. (The dosage reported for phentolamine is 5 mg. i.v.) Care should be taken to administer this drug slowly in order to avoid producing an excessive hypotensive effect. Fever should be managed by means of external cooling. Other symptomatic and supportive measures may be desirable in particular cases. Do not use parenteral reserpine.

Precautions: Hypotension—Hypotension has been observed during Parnate (tranylcypromine sulfate, SK&F) therapy. Symptoms of postural hypotension are seen more commonly but not exclusively in patients with pre-existent hypertension; blood pressure usually returns rapidly to pretreatment levels upon discontinuation of the drug. At doses above 30 mg. daily, postural hypotension is a major side effect and may result in syncope. Dosage increases should be made more gradually in patients showing a tendency toward hypotension at the beginning of therapy. Postural hypotension may be relieved by having the patient lie down until blood pressure returns to normal.

Also, when 'Parnate' is combined with those phenothiazine derivatives or other compounds known to cause hypotension, the possibility of additive hypotensive effects should be considered.

Other Precautions: There have been reports of drug dependency in patients using doses of tranylcypromine significantly in excess of the therapeutic range. Some of these patients had a history of previous substance abuse. The following withdrawal symptoms have been reported: restlessness, anxiety, depression, confusion, hallucinations, headache, weakness and diarrhea.

Drugs which lower the seizure threshold, including MAO inhibitors, should not be used with 'Amipaque'.† As with other MAO inhibitors, Parnate (tranylcypromine sulfate, SK&F) should be discontinued at least 48 hours before myelography and should not be resumed for at least 24 hours post-procedure.

In depressed patients, the possibility of suicide should always be considered and adequate precautions taken. Exclusive reliance on drug therapy to prevent suicidal attempts is unwarranted, as there may be a delay in the onset of therapeutic effect or an increase in anxiety and agitation. Also, of course, some patients fail to respond to drug therapy or may respond only temporarily.

MAO inhibitors may have the capacity to suppress anginal pain that would otherwise serve as a warning of myocardial ischemia. The usual precautions should be observed in patients with impaired renal function since there is a possibility of accumulative effects in such patients.

Although excretion of 'Parnate' is rapid, inhibition of MAO may persist up to 10 days following discontinuation.

Because the influence of 'Parnate' on the convulsive threshold is variable in animal experiments, suitable precautions should be taken if epileptic patients are treated.

Some MAO inhibitors have contributed to hypoglycemic episodes in diabetic patients receiving insulin or oral hypoglycemic agents. Therefore, 'Parnate' should be used with caution in diabetics using these drugs.

'Parnate' may aggravate coexisting symptoms in depression, such as anxiety and agitation.

Use 'Parnate' with caution in hyperthyroid patients because of their increased sensitivity to pressor amines.

'Parnate' should be administered with caution to patients receiving disulfiram (Antabuse®‡). In a single study, rats given high intraperitoneal doses of *d* or *l* isomers of tranylcypromine sulfate plus disulfiram experienced severe toxicity including convulsions and death. Additional studies in rats given high oral doses of racemic tranylcypromine sulfate ('Parnate') and disulfiram produced no adverse interaction.

Adverse Reactions: Overstimulation which may include increased anxiety, agitation and manic symptoms is usually evidence of excessive therapeutic action. Dosage should be reduced, or a phenothiazine tranquilizer should be administered concomitantly.

Patients may experience restlessness or insomnia; may notice some weakness, drowsiness, episodes of dizziness, or dry mouth; or may report nausea, diarrhea, abdominal pain, or constipation. Most of these effects can be relieved by lowering the dosage or by giving suitable concomitant medication. Tachycardia, significant anorexia, edema, palpitation, blurred vision, chills, and impotence have each been reported.

Headaches without blood pressure elevation have occurred.

Rare instances of hepatitis and skin rash have been reported.

Impaired water excretion compatible with the syndrome of inappropriate secretion of antidiuretic hormone (SIADH) has been reported.

Tinnitus, muscle spasm and tremors, paresthesia and urinary retention have been reported so rarely that the role of Parnate (tranylcypromine sulfate, SK&F) cannot be established.

Blood toxicity has not been reported.

Dosage and Administration: Dosage should be adjusted to the requirements of the individual patient. Improvement should be seen within 48 hours to three weeks after starting therapy.

1. Recommended starting dosage is 20 mg. per day—10 mg. in the morning and 10 mg. in the afternoon.
2. This dosage may be continued for two weeks.
3. If no signs of a response appear, dosage may be increased to 30 mg. daily—20 mg. in the morning and 10 mg. in the afternoon.
4. This dosage may be continued for a week. If no improvement occurs, continued administration is unlikely to be beneficial.
5. When a satisfactory response is obtained, dosage may usually be reduced to a maintenance level.
6. Some patients will be maintained on 20 mg. per day; many will need only 10 mg. daily.
7. Although dosages above 30 mg. daily have been used, the physician should bear in mind that the likelihood of side effects increases as dosage is raised.
8. When ECT is being administered concurrently, 10 mg. b.i.d. can usually be given during the series, then reduced to 10 mg. daily for maintenance therapy.

Dosage increases should be made in increments of 10 mg. per day and ordinarily at intervals of one to three weeks. It is important that the lowest effective dose be used.

Reduction from peak to maintenance dosage is desirable before withdrawal. If withdrawn prematurely, original symptoms will recur. Although no tendency to produce rebound depressions of greater intensity has been seen, this is a theoretical possibility.

Overdosage: *Symptoms:* The characteristic symptoms that may be caused by overdosage are usually those described in the preceding paragraphs.

However, an intensification of these symptoms and sometimes severe additional manifestations may be seen, depending on the degree of overdosage and on individual susceptibility. Some patients exhibit insomnia, restlessness and anxiety, progressing in severe cases to agitation, mental confusion and incoherence. Hypotension, dizziness, weakness and drowsiness may occur, progressing in severe cases to extreme dizziness and shock. A few patients have displayed hypertension with severe headache and other symptoms. Rare instances have been reported in which hypertension was accompanied by twitching or myoclonic fibrillation of skeletal muscles with hyperpyrexia, sometimes progressing to generalized rigidity and coma.

Treatment: Gastric lavage is helpful if performed early. Treatment should normally consist of general supportive measures, close observation of vital signs and steps to counteract specific symptoms as they occur, since MAO inhibition may persist. The management of hypertensive crises is described under Hypertensive Crises.

External cooling is recommended if hyperpyrexia occurs. Barbiturates have been reported to help relieve myoclonic reactions, but frequency of administration should be controlled carefully because Parnate (tranylcypromine sulfate, SK&F) may prolong barbiturate activity. When hypotension requires treatment, the standard measures for managing circulatory shock should be initiated. If pressor agents are used, the rate of infusion should be regulated by careful observation of the patient because an exaggerated pressor response sometimes occurs in the presence of MAO inhibition. Remember that the toxic effect of 'Parnate' may be delayed or prolonged following the last dose of the drug. Therefore, the patient should be closely observed for at least a week.

How Supplied: Tablets, containing tranylcypromine sulfate equivalent to 10 mg. of tranylcypromine, in bottles of 100 and 1000.

Clinical Studies: There have been only a small number of controlled studies (e.g., 1,2,3,4) of the effectiveness of Parnate (tranylcypromine sulfate, SK&F) in comparison to placebo or other antidepressant drugs, embracing comparatively few subjects. These and other studies disclose a remarkably high incidence, about 50 percent, of favorable placebo effect and a statistically significant but small superiority of 'Parnate' and other antidepressant drugs over placebo. No statistically significant superiority of 'Parnate' over other antidepressant drugs, including other MAO inhibitors, has been regularly demonstrated. However, clinical experience also indicates that some patients who fail to respond satisfactorily to one therapy may respond to another.

References:

1. Bartholomew, A.A.: An evaluation of tranylcypromine ('Parnate') in the treatment of depression, *M. J. Australia 1:*655 (May 5) 1962.
2. Khanna, J.L., et al.: A study of certain effects of tranylcypromine, a new antidepressant, *J. New Drugs 3:*227, 1963.
3. Spear, F.G., et al.: A comparison of subjective responses to imipramine and tranylcypromine, *Brit. J. Psychiat. 110:*53, 1964.

for possible revisions **Product Information** 1971

4. Janacek, J., et al.: Pargyline and tranylcypromine in the treatment of hospitalized depressed patients, *J. New Drugs* 3: 309, 1963.

---

*Trade Mark Reg. U.S. Pat. Off.: 'Regitine' for phentolamine mesylate, U.S.P., CIBA.
†Trademark Reg. U.S. Pat. Off.: 'Amipaque' for metrizamide, Winthrop Laboratories.
‡Trademark of Ayerst Laboratories.
Shown in Product Identification Section, page 437
PT:L45

SK-LINE®

SK-AMITRIPTYLINE HCl™ ℞
[am'eh-trip"teh'leen]
(amitriptyline hydrochloride, SK&F)

Tablets: 10 mg. (No. 120), 25 mg. (No. 121), 50 mg. (No. 123), 75 mg. (No. 124), 100 mg. (No. 131), 150 mg. (No. 132).

SK-AMPICILLIN® ℞
[amp'eh-sill'in]
(ampicillin, SK&F)

Capsules: 250 mg. (No. 101), 500 mg. (No. 102).
For Oral Suspension: 125 mg./5 ml. (No. 103), 250 mg./5 ml. (No. 104), 100 mg./ml. (No. 109).

SK-AMPICILLIN-N® ℞
[amp'eh-sill'in]
(sterile ampicillin sodium, SK&F)

Injection: 500 mg. (No. 106).

SK-APAP™ with CODEINE ©
[ay'pap]
(acetaminophen, codeine phosphate)

Tablets: 300 mg./15 mg. (No. 494), 300 mg./30 mg. (No. 496), 300 mg./60 mg. (No. 497).

SK-BAMATE™ ©
[bam'ate]
(meprobamate, SK&F)

Tablets: 200 mg. (No. 133), 400 mg. (No. 134).

SK-CHLORAL HYDRATE™ ©
(chloral hydrate, SK&F)

Capsules: 500 mg. (No. 176).

SK-CHLOROTHIAZIDE™ ℞
[klor'oh-thigh'ah-zide]
(chlorothiazide, SK&F)

Tablets: 250 mg. (No. 419), 500 mg. (No. 420).

SK-DEXAMETHASONE™ ℞
[dex'a-meth"a-soan]
(dexamethasone, SK&F)

Tablets: 0.5 mg. (No. 374), 0.75 mg. (No. 376), 1.5 mg. (No. 377).

SK-DIPHENOXYLATE™ ©
[di'fen-ox"il-ate]
(diphenoxylate HCl, atropine sulfate, SK&F)

Tablets: 2.5 mg./0.025 mg. (No. 423).

SK-DIPYRIDAMOLE™ ℞
[die-pie-rid'ah-mole]
(dipyridamole, SK&F)

Tablets: 25 mg. (No. 379), 50 mg. (No. 380), 75 mg. (No. 381).

SK-ERYTHROMYCIN™ ℞
(erythromycin stearate, SK&F)

Tablets: 250 mg. (No. 367), 500 mg. (No. 369).

SK-FUROSEMIDE™ ℞
[few-row"seh-mide']
(furosemide, SK&F)

Tablets: 20 mg. (No. 340), 40 mg. (No. 341).

SK-HYDROCHLOROTHIAZIDE™ ℞
[hi'drow-klor-oh-thigh'eh-zide]
(hydrochlorothiazide, SK&F)

Tablets: 25 mg. (No. 363), 50 mg. (No. 364).

SK-LYGEN® ©
[lye'gen]
(chlordiazepoxide hydrochloride, SK&F)

Capsules: 5 mg. (No. 441), 10 mg. (No. 442), 25 mg. (No. 443).

SK-METRONIDAZOLE™ ℞
[meh-troe-nigh'da-zoal]
(metronidazole, SK&F)

Tablets: 250 mg. (No. 426).

SK-OXYCODONE™
with ACETAMINOPHEN ©
[ox-e'co-doan]

Tablets: 5 mg. oxycodone hydrochloride; 325 mg. acetaminophen (No. 320).

SK-OXYCODONE™ with ASPIRIN ©
[ox-e'co-doan]

Tablets: 4.5 mg. oxycodone hydrochloride; 0.38 mg. oxycodone terephthalate; 325 mg. aspirin (No. 319).

SK-PENICILLIN G™ ℞
[penn'eh-sill"in]
(penicillin G potassium, SK&F)

Tablets: 400,000 units (No. 111), 800,000 units (No. 112).

SK-PENICILLIN VK™ ℞
[pen'eh-sill"in]
(penicillin V potassium, SK&F)

Tablets: 250 mg. (No. 116), 500 mg. (No. 117).
For Oral Solution: 125 mg./5 ml. (No. 118), 250 mg./5 ml. (No. 119).

SK-PHENOBARBITAL™ ©
[fee'no-bar'beh-tahl]
(phenobarbital, SK&F)

Tablets: 15 mg. (No. 136), 30 mg. (No. 137).

SK-PRAMINE™ ℞
[pram'een]
(imipramine hydrochloride, SK&F)

Tablets: 10 mg. (No. 321), 25 mg. (No. 322), 50 mg. (No. 323).

SK-PREDNISONE™ ℞
[pred-neh'soan]
(prednisone, SK&F)

Tablets: 5 mg. (No. 339).

SK-PROBENECID™ ℞
[pro-ben'eh-sid]
(probenecid, SK&F)

Tablets: 500 mg. (No. 499).

SK-PROPANTHELINE BROMIDE™ ℞
[pro-pan'theh-leen broh'mide]
(propantheline bromide, SK&F)

Tablets: 15 mg. (No. 310).

SK-QUINIDINE SULFATE™ ℞
[kwin'eh-deen sul-fate]
(quinidine sulfate, SK&F)

Tablets: 200 mg. (No. 171).

SK-RESERPINE™ ℞
[reh-sir'peen]
(reserpine, SK&F)

Tablets: 0.25 mg. (No. 169).

SK-65® ©
(propoxyphene hydrochloride, SK&F)

Capsules: 65 mg. (No. 463).

SK-65 APAP® ©
[ay'pap]

Each tablet: 65 mg. propoxyphene HCl, 650 mg. acetaminophen (No. 474).

SK-65® COMPOUND ©

Each capsule: 65 mg. propoxyphene HCl, 389 mg. aspirin, 32.4 mg. caffeine (No. 468).

SK-SOXAZOLE™ ℞
[socks'a-zole]
(sulfisoxazole, SK&F)

Tablets: 500 mg. (No. 163).

SK-TERPIN HYDRATE
and CODEINE ™ ©
[ter'pin hi'drate]
(terpin hydrate and codeine, SK&F)

Elixir: 85 mg./10 mg./5 ml. (No. 354).

SK-TETRACYCLINE HCl™ CAPSULES ℞
[tet-rah-sigh'clean]
(tetracycline hydrochloride, SK&F)

250 mg. (No. 126), 500 mg. (No. 127).

SK-TETRACYCLINE™ SYRUP ℞
[tet-rah-sigh'clean]
(tetracycline oral suspension, SK&F)

125 mg./5 ml. (No. 125).

SK-THIORIDAZINE HCl™ ℞
[thigh-oh-rid'a-zeen]
(thioridazine hydrochloride, SK&F)

Tablets: 10 mg. (No. 371), 25 mg. (No. 372), 50 mg. (No. 373), 100 mg. (No. 375).

SK-TOLBUTAMIDE™ ℞
[toll-bu'tah-mide]
(brand of tolbutamide)

Tablets: 500 mg. (No. 409).

STELAZINE® ℞
[stel'ah-zeen]
(brand of trifluoperazine hydrochloride)

('Stelazine' is a product of SK&F Co., Carolina, P.R. 00630, Subsidiary of SmithKline Beckman Corporation, Philadelphia, Pa.)
Description: Tablets—Each tablet contains trifluoperazine, 1 mg., 2 mg., 5 mg., or 10 mg., as the hydrochloride.
Multiple-dose Vials, 10 ml. (2 mg./ml.)—Each ml. contains, in aqueous solution, trifluoperazine, 2 mg., as the hydrochloride; sodium tartrate, 4.75 mg.; sodium biphosphate, 11.6 mg.; sodium saccharin, 0.3 mg.; benzyl alcohol, 0.75%, as preservative.
Concentrate (intended for institutional use only) —Each ml. contains trifluoperazine, 10 mg., as the hydrochloride.
N.B.: The Concentrate is for use in severe neuropsychiatric conditions when oral medication is preferred and other oral forms are considered impractical.
Indications: For the management of the manifestations of psychotic disorders.
Stelazine (trifluoperazine HCl, SK&F) has not been shown effective in the management of behavioral complications in patients with mental retardation.

Continued on next page

Smith Kline & French—Cont.

'Stelazine' is considered possibly effective in the treatment of non-psychotic anxiety. However, 'Stelazine' is not the first drug to be used in therapy for most patients with non-psychotic anxiety because certain risks associated with its use are not shared by common alternative treatments (e.g., benzodiazepines).

When used in the treatment of non-psychotic anxiety, 'Stelazine' should not be administered in doses of more than 5 mg. per day or for longer than 12 weeks because the use of 'Stelazine' at higher doses or for longer intervals may cause persistent tardive dyskinesia that may prove irreversible. (See Warnings section.)

Final classification by the FDA of the non-psychotic anxiety indication requires further investigation.

Contraindications: Comatose or greatly depressed states due to central nervous system depressants, and in cases of existing blood dyscrasias, bone marrow depression and pre-existing liver damage.

Warnings: Patients who have demonstrated a hypersensitivity reaction (e.g., blood dyscrasias, jaundice) with a phenothiazine should not be re-exposed to any phenothiazine, including Stelazine (trifluoperazine HCl, SK&F), unless in the judgment of the physician the potential benefits of treatment outweigh the possible hazard.

'Stelazine' may impair mental and/or physical abilities, especially during the first few days of therapy. Therefore, caution patients about activities requiring alertness (e.g., operating vehicles or machinery).

If agents such as sedatives, narcotics, anesthetics, tranquilizers, or alcohol are used either simultaneously or successively with the drug, the possibility of an undesirable additive depressant effect should be considered.

Persistent Tardive Dyskinesia: Persistent tardive dyskinesia may appear in some patients on long-term therapy with antipsychotic agents or may appear after drug therapy has been discontinued. In some patients the symptoms appear to be irreversible. There is no known effective treatment for tardive dyskinesia. It is suggested that all antipsychotic agents be discontinued if symptoms of this syndrome appear. (See Adverse Reactions section.)

Usage in Pregnancy: Animal reproductive studies and clinical experience to date have not demonstrated any teratogenic effect from Stelazine (trifluoperazine HCl, SK&F). However, as with any medication, it should be used in pregnant patients only when, in the judgment of the physician, it is necessary for the welfare of the patient.

Nursing Mothers: There is evidence that phenothiazines are excreted in the breast milk of nursing mothers.

Precautions: Thrombocytopenia and anemia have been reported in patients receiving the drug. Agranulocytosis and pancytopenia have also been reported—warn patients to report the sudden appearance of sore throat or other signs of infection. If white blood cell and differential counts indicate cellular depression, stop treatment and start antibiotic and other suitable therapy.

Jaundice of the cholestatic type of hepatitis or liver damage has been reported. If fever with grippe-like symptoms occurs, appropriate liver studies should be conducted. If tests indicate an abnormality, stop treatment.

One result of therapy may be an increase in mental and physical activity. For example, a few patients with angina pectoris have complained of increased pain while taking the drug. Therefore, angina patients should be observed carefully and, if an unfavorable response is noted, the drug should be withdrawn.

Because hypotension has occurred, large doses and parenteral administration should be avoided in patients with impaired cardiovascular systems. To minimize the occurrence of hypotension after initial injection, keep patient lying down and observe for at least ½ hour. If hypotension occurs from parenteral or oral dosing, place patient in head-low position with legs raised. If a vasoconstrictor is required, 'Levophed' and 'Neo-Synephrine'* are suitable. Other pressor agents, including epinephrine, should not be used as they may cause a paradoxical further lowering of blood pressure.

Since certain phenothiazines have been reported to produce retinopathy, the drug should be discontinued if ophthalmoscopic examination or visual field studies should demonstrate retinal changes. An antiemetic action of 'Stelazine' may mask the signs and symptoms of toxicity or overdosage of other drugs and may obscure the diagnosis and treatment of other conditions such as intestinal obstruction, brain tumor and Reye's syndrome.

With prolonged administration at high dosages, the possibility of cumulative effects, with sudden onset of severe central nervous system or vasomotor symptoms, should be kept in mind.

Neuroleptic drugs elevate prolactin levels; the elevation persists during chronic administration. Tissue culture experiments indicate that approximately one-third of human breast cancers are prolactin-dependent in vitro, a factor of potential importance if the prescribing of these drugs is contemplated in a patient with a previously detected breast cancer. Although disturbances such as galactorrhea, amenorrhea, gynecomastia and impotence have been reported, the clinical significance of elevated serum prolactin levels is unknown for most patients. An increase in mammary neoplasms has been found in rodents after chronic administration of neuroleptic drugs. Neither clinical nor epidemiologic studies conducted to date, however, have shown an association between chronic administration of these drugs and mammary tumorigenesis; the available evidence is considered too limited to be conclusive at this time.

As with all drugs which exert an anticholinergic effect, and/or cause mydriasis, trifluoperazine should be used with caution in patients with glaucoma.

Phenothiazines may diminish the effect of oral anticoagulants.

Phenothiazines can produce alpha-adrenergic blockade.

Concomitant administration of propranolol with phenothiazines results in increased plasma levels of both drugs.

Phenothiazines may lower the convulsive threshold; dosage adjustments of anticonvulsants may be necessary. Potentiation of anticonvulsant effects does not occur. However, it has been reported that phenothiazines may interfere with the metabolism of 'Dilantin'† and thus precipitate 'Dilantin' toxicity.

Drugs which lower the seizure threshold, including phenothiazine derivatives, should not be used with 'Amipaque'.‡ As with other phenothiazine derivatives, 'Stelazine' should be discontinued at least 48 hours before myelography, should not be resumed for at least 24 hours postprocedure, and should not be used for the control of nausea and vomiting occurring either prior to myelography or postprocedure.

Long-Term Therapy: To lessen the likelihood of adverse reactions related to cumulative drug effect, patients with a history of long-term therapy with Stelazine (trifluoperazine HCl, SK&F) and/or other neuroleptics should be evaluated periodically to decide whether the maintenance dosage could be lowered or drug therapy discontinued.

Adverse Reactions: Drowsiness, dizziness, skin reactions, rash, dry mouth, insomnia, amenorrhea, fatigue, muscular weakness, anorexia, lactation, blurred vision and neuromuscular (extrapyramidal) reactions.

Neuromuscular (Extrapyramidal) Reactions

These symptoms are seen in a significant number of hospitalized mental patients. They may be characterized by motor restlessness, be of the dystonic type, or they may resemble parkinsonism.

Depending on the severity of symptoms, dosage should be reduced or discontinued. If therapy is reinstituted, it should be at a lower dosage. Should these symptoms occur in children or pregnant patients, the drug should be stopped and not reinstituted. In most cases barbiturates by suitable route of administration will suffice. (Or, injectable 'Benadryl'§ may be useful.) In more severe cases, the administration of an anti-parkinsonism agent, except levodopa, usually produces rapid reversal of symptoms. Suitable supportive measures such as maintaining a clear airway and adequate hydration should be employed.

Motor Restlessness: Symptoms may include agitation or jitteriness and sometimes insomnia. These symptoms often disappear spontaneously. At times these symptoms may be similar to the original neurotic or psychotic symptoms. Dosage should not be increased until these side effects have subsided.

If this phase becomes too troublesome, the symptoms can usually be controlled by a reduction of dosage or concomitant administration of a barbiturate.

Dystonias: Symptoms may include: spasm of the neck muscles, sometimes progressing to torticollis; extensor rigidity of back muscles, sometimes progressing to opisthotonos; carpopedal spasm, trismus, swallowing difficulty, oculogyric crisis and protrusion of the tongue.

These usually subside within a few hours, and almost always within 24 to 48 hours, after the drug has been discontinued.

In mild cases, reassurance or a barbiturate is often sufficient. *In moderate cases,* barbiturates will usually bring rapid relief. *In more severe adult cases,* the administration of an anti-parkinsonism agent, except levodopa, usually produces rapid reversal of symptoms. Also, intravenous caffeine with sodium benzoate seems to be effective. *In children,* reassurance and barbiturates will usually control symptoms. (Or, injectable 'Benadryl' may be useful.) Note: See 'Benadryl' prescribing information for appropriate children's dosage. If appropriate treatment with anti-parkinsonism agents or 'Benadryl' fails to reverse the signs and symptoms, the diagnosis should be reevaluated.

Pseudo-parkinsonism: Symptoms may include: mask-like facies; drooling; tremors; pillrolling motion; cogwheel rigidity; and shuffling gait. Reassurance and sedation are important. In most cases these symptoms are readily controlled when an anti-parkinsonism agent is administered concomitantly. Anti-parkinsonism agents should be used only when required. Generally, therapy of a few weeks to two or three months will suffice. After this time patients should be evaluated to determine their need for continued treatment. (Note: Levodopa has not been found effective in pseudo-parkinsonism.) Occasionally it is necessary to lower the dosage of 'Stelazine' or to discontinue the drug.

Persistent Tardive Dyskinesia: As with all antipsychotic agents, tardive dyskinesia may appear in some patients on long-term therapy or may appear after drug therapy has been discontinued. This condition appears in all age groups. However, the risk appears to be greater in elderly patients on high-dose therapy, especially females. The symptoms are persistent and in some patients appear to be irreversible. The syndrome is characterized by rhythmical involuntary movements of the tongue, face, mouth or jaw (e.g., protrusion of tongue, puffing of cheeks, puckering of mouth, chewing movements). Sometimes these may be accompanied by involuntary movements of extremities. In rare instances, these involuntary movements of the extremities are the only manifestations of tardive dyskinesia.

There is no known effective treatment for tardive dyskinesia; anti-parkinsonism agents do not alleviate the symptoms of this syndrome. It is suggested that all antipsychotic agents be discontinued if these symptoms appear. Should it be necessary to reinstitute treatment, or increase the dosage of the agent, or switch to a different antipsychotic agent, the syndrome may be masked.

It has been reported that fine vermicular movements of the tongue may be an early sign of the syndrome and if the medication is stopped at that time the syndrome may not develop.

Adverse Reactions Reported with Stelazine (trifluoperazine HCl, SK&F) or Other Phenothiazine Derivatives: Adverse effects with different phenothiazines vary in type, frequency, and mechanism of occurrence, i.e., some are dose-related, while others involve individual patient sensitivity. Some adverse effects may be more likely to occur, or occur with greater intensity, in patients with special medical problems, e.g., patients with mitral insufficiency or pheochromocytoma have experienced severe hypotension following recommended doses of certain phenothiazines.

Not all of the following adverse reactions have been observed with every phenothiazine derivative, but they have been reported with one or more and should be borne in mind when drugs of this class are administered: extrapyramidal symptoms (opisthotonos, oculogyric crisis, hyperreflexia, dystonia, akathisia, dyskinesia, parkinsonism) some of which have lasted months and even years—particularly in elderly patients with previous brain damage; grand mal and petit mal convulsions; altered cerebrospinal fluid proteins; cerebral edema; intensification and prolongation of the action of central nervous system depressants (opiates, analgesics, antihistamines, barbiturates, alcohol), atropine, heat, organophosphorus insecticides; autonomic reactions (dryness of mouth, nasal congestion, headache, nausea, constipation, obstipation, adynamic ileus, priapism, inhibition of ejaculation); reactivation of psychotic processes, catatonic-like states; hypotension (sometimes fatal); cardiac arrest; blood dyscrasias (pancytopenia, thrombocytopenic purpura, leukopenia, agranulocytosis, eosinophilia, hemolytic anemia, aplastic anemia); liver damage (jaundice, biliary stasis); endocrine disturbances (lactation, galactorrhea, gynecomastia, menstrual irregularities, false positive pregnancy tests); skin disorders (photosensitivity, itching, erythema, urticaria, eczema up to exfoliative dermatitis); other allergic reactions (asthma, laryngeal edema, angioneurotic edema, anaphylactoid reactions); peripheral edema; reversed epinephrine effect; hyperpyrexia; mild fever after large I.M. doses; increased appetite; increased weight; a systemic lupus erythematosus-like syndrome; pigmentary retinopathy; with prolonged administration of substantial doses, skin pigmentation, epithelial keratopathy, and lenticular and corneal deposits.

EKG changes—particularly nonspecific, usually reversible Q and T wave distortions—have been observed in some patients receiving phenothiazine tranquilizers. Their relationship to myocardial damage has not been confirmed. Although phenothiazines cause neither psychic nor physical dependence, sudden discontinuance in long-term psychiatric patients may cause temporary symptoms, e.g., nausea and vomiting, dizziness, tremulousness.

Rare occurrences of neuroleptic malignant syndrome (NMS) have been reported in patients receiving neuroleptic drugs. This syndrome is comprised of the symptom complex of hyperthermia, altered consciousness, muscular rigidity and autonomic dysfunction and is potentially fatal.

Note: There have been occasional reports of sudden death in patients receiving phenothiazines. In some cases, the cause appeared to be asphyxia due to failure of the cough reflex. In others, the cause could not be determined. There is not sufficient evidence to establish a relationship between such deaths and the administration of phenothiazines.

Dosage and Administration: Dosage should be adjusted to the needs of the individual. The lowest effective dosage should always be used. Dosage should be increased more gradually in debilitated or emaciated patients. When maximum response is achieved, dosage may be reduced gradually to a maintenance level. Because of the inherent long action of the drug, patients may be controlled on convenient b.i.d. administration; some patients may be maintained on once-a-day administration. When Stelazine (trifluoperazine HCl, SK&F) is administered by intramuscular injection, equivalent oral dosage may be substituted once symptoms have been controlled.

Elderly Patients: In general, dosages in the lower range are sufficient for most elderly patients. Since they appear to be more susceptible to hypotension and neuromuscular reactions, such patients should be observed closely. Dosage should be tailored to the individual, response carefully monitored, and dosage adjusted accordingly. Dosage should be increased more gradually in elderly patients.

1. Adult Dosage

Oral (for office patients and outpatients): 1 or 2 mg. twice daily. It is seldom necessary to exceed 4 mg. a day except in patients with more severe conditions and in discharged mental patients.

Treatment of non-psychotic anxiety: Do not administer at doses of more than 5 mg. per day or for longer than 12 weeks.

Oral (for hospitalized patients or those under close supervision): Usual starting dosage is 2 mg. to 5 mg. b.i.d. (Small or emaciated patients should always be started on the lower dosage.)

Most patients will show optimum response on 15 mg. or 20 mg. daily, although a few may require 40 mg. a day or more. Optimum therapeutic dosage levels should be reached within two or three weeks.

When the Concentrate dosage form is to be used, it should be added to 60 ml. (2 fl. oz.) or more of diluent *just prior to administration* to insure palatability and stability. Vehicles suggested for dilution are: tomato or fruit juice, milk, simple syrup, orange syrup, carbonated beverages, coffee, tea, or water. Semisolid foods (soup, puddings, etc.) may also be used.

Intramuscular (for prompt control of severe symptoms): Usual dosage is 1 mg. to 2 mg. ($\frac{1}{2}$-1 ml.) by deep intramuscular injection q4-6h, p.r.n. More than 6 mg. within 24 hours is rarely necessary. Only in very exceptional cases should intramuscular dosage exceed 10 mg. within 24 hours. Injections should not be given at intervals of less than 4 hours because of a possible cumulative effect.

Note: Stelazine (trifluoperazine HCl, SK&F) Injection has been usually well tolerated and there is little, if any, pain and irritation at the site of injection.

The Injection should be protected from light. Exposure may cause discoloration. Slight yellowish discoloration will not alter potency or efficacy. If markedly discolored, the solution should be discarded.

2. Dosage for Psychotic Children

Dosage should be adjusted to the weight of the child and severity of the symptoms. These dosages are for children, ages 6 to 12, who are hospitalized or under close supervision.

Oral: The starting dosage is 1 mg. administered once a day or b.i.d. Dosage may be increased gradually until symptoms are controlled or until side effects become troublesome.

While it is usually not necessary to exceed dosages of 15 mg. daily, some older children with severe symptoms may require higher dosages.

Intramuscular: There has been little experience with the use of Stelazine (trifluoperazine HCl, SK&F) Injection in children. However, if it is necessary to achieve rapid control of severe symptoms, 1 mg. ($\frac{1}{2}$ ml.) of the drug may be administered intramuscularly once or twice a day.

Overdosage (See also under Adverse Reactions.):

Symptoms—Primarily involvement of the extrapyramidal mechanism producing some of the dystonic reactions described above. Symptoms of central nervous system depression to the point of somnolence or coma. Agitation and restlessness may also occur. Other possible manifestations include convulsions, EKG changes and cardiac arrhythmias, fever, and autonomic reactions such as hypotension, dry mouth and ileus.

Treatment—It is important to determine other medications taken by the patient since multiple dose therapy is common in overdosage situations. Treatment is essentially symptomatic and supportive. Early gastric lavage is helpful. Keep patient under observation and maintain an open airway, since involvement of the extrapyramidal mechanism may produce dysphagia and respiratory difficulty in severe overdosage. **Do not attempt to induce emesis because a dystonic reaction of the head or neck may develop that could result in aspiration of vomitus.** Extrapyramidal symptoms may be treated with anti-parkinsonism drugs, barbiturates, or 'Benadryl'. See prescribing information for these products. Care should be taken to avoid increasing respiratory depression. If administration of a stimulant is desirable, amphetamine, dextroamphetamine, or caffeine with sodium benzoate is recommended. Stimulants that may cause convulsions (e.g., picrotoxin or pentylenetetrazol) should be avoided.

If hypotension occurs, the standard measures for managing circulatory shock should be initiated. If it is desirable to administer a vasoconstrictor, 'Levophed' and 'Neo-Synephrine' are most suitable. Other pressor agents, including epinephrine, are not recommended because phenothiazine derivatives may reverse the usual elevating action of these agents and cause a further lowering of blood pressure.

Limited experience indicates that phenothiazines are *not* dialyzable.

How Supplied:

Tablets, 1 mg. and 2 mg., in bottles of 100 and 1000; in Single Unit Packages of 100 (intended for institutional use only).

For psychiatric patients who are hospitalized or under close supervision:

Tablets, 5 mg. and 10 mg., in bottles of 100 and 1000; in Single Unit Packages of 100 (intended for institutional use only).

Multiple-dose Vials, 10 ml. (2 mg./ml.), in boxes of 1 and 20.

Concentrate (intended for institutional use only)—10 mg./ml., in 2 fl. oz. bottles and in cartons of 12 bottles.

Each bottle is packaged with a graduated dropper. The Concentrate form is light-sensitive. For this reason, it should be protected from light and dispensed in amber bottles. *Refrigeration is not required.*

Note: Although there is little likelihood of contact dermatitis due to the drug, persons with known sensitivity to phenothiazine drugs should avoid direct contact.

Military—Tablets, 1 mg., 1000's, 6505-00-022-1336, and S.U.P. 100's, 6505-00-132-0132; 2 mg., 1000's, 6505-00-022-1337, and S.U.P. 100's, 6505-00-132-0143; 5 mg., 1000's, 6505-00-022-1338, and S.U.P. 100's, 6505-00-132-0144; 10 mg., 1000's, 6505-00-022-1343, and S.U.P. 100's, 6505-00-132-0188.

*'Levophed' and 'Neo-Synephrine' are the trademarks (Reg. U.S. Pat. Off.) of Winthrop Laboratories for its brands of levarterenol and phenylephrine respectively.

†Trademark Reg. U.S. Pat. Off.: 'Dilantin' for diphenylhydantoin, Parke-Davis.

‡Trademark Reg. U.S. Pat. Off.: 'Amipaque' for metrizamide, Winthrop Laboratories.

§Trademark Reg. U.S. Pat. Off.: 'Benadryl' for diphenhydramine hydrochloride, Parke-Davis.

Shown in Product Identification Section, page 437

SZ:L54

TAGAMET® ℞

[tag'ah-met]

(brand of cimetidine tablets
cimetidine hydrochloride liquid and
cimetidine hydrochloride injection)

('Tagamet' is a product of SK&F Lab Co., Carolina, P.R. 00630, Subsidiary of SmithKline Beckman Corporation, Philadelphia, Pa.)

Description: 'Tagamet' (brand of cimetidine) is a histamine H_2 receptor antagonist. Chemically it is N'''-cyano-N-methyl-N'-[2-[[(5-methyl-1H-imidazol-4-yl) methyl] thio]-ethyl]-guanidine. (The liquid and injection dosage forms contain cimetidine as the hydrochloride.)

Cimetidine has a bitter taste and characteristic odor.

Tablets: Each tablet contains 200 mg., 300 mg., or 400 mg. of cimetidine.

Continued on next page

Liquid: Each 5 ml. (1 teaspoonful) contains, in aqueous solution, cimetidine hydrochloride equivalent to cimetidine, 300 mg.; alcohol, 2.8%.

Vials: Each 2 ml. contains, in aqueous solution, cimetidine hydrochloride equivalent to cimetidine, 300 mg.; phenol, 10 mg.

Multiple-dose Vials: 8 ml. (300 mg./2 ml.): Each 2 ml. contains, in aqueous solution, cimetidine hydrochloride equivalent to cimetidine, 300 mg.; phenol, 10 mg.

Single-dose Prefilled Disposable Syringes: Each 2 ml. contains, in aqueous solution, cimetidine hydrochloride equivalent to cimetidine, 300 mg.; phenol, 10 mg.

Clinical Pharmacology: 'Tagamet' (brand of cimetidine) competitively inhibits the action of histamine at the histamine H_2 receptors of the parietal cells and thus represents a new class of pharmacological agents, the histamine H_2-receptor antagonists.

'Tagamet' is not an anticholinergic agent. Studies have shown that 'Tagamet' inhibits both daytime and nocturnal basal gastric acid secretion. 'Tagamet' also inhibits gastric acid secretion stimulated by food, histamine, pentagastrin, caffeine and insulin.

Antisecretory Activity

1) **Acid Secretion:** *Basal:* Oral 'Tagamet' 300 mg. inhibited basal gastric acid secretion by 100% for at least two hours and by at least 90% throughout the 4 hour study in fasting duodenal ulcer patients.

The gastric pH in all subjects was increased to 5.0 or greater for at least $2\frac{1}{4}$ hours.

Nocturnal: Nighttime basal secretion in fasting duodenal ulcer patients was inhibited by a 300 mg. dose of 'Tagamet' by 100% for at least one hour and by a mean of 89% over a seven hour period. Gastric pH was increased to 5.0 or greater in most of the patients for three to four hours.

'Tagamet' 300 mg. reduced non-stimulated acid concentration by 70-100% and the non-stimulated volume of gastric secretion by 20-50%.

Food Stimulated: During the first hour after a standard experimental meal, oral 'Tagamet' 300 mg. inhibited gastric acid secretion in duodenal ulcer patients by at least 50%. During the subsequent two hours 'Tagamet' inhibited gastric acid secretion by at least 75%.

The effect of a 300 mg. breakfast dose of 'Tagamet' continued for at least four hours and there was partial suppression of the rise in gastric acid secretion following the luncheon meal in duodenal ulcer patients. This suppression of gastric acid output was enhanced and could be maintained by another 300 mg. dose of 'Tagamet' given with lunch.

In another study, 'Tagamet' 300 mg. given with the meal increased gastric pH as compared with placebo.

	Mean Gastric pH	
	'Tagamet'	Placebo
1 hour	3.5	2.6
2 hours	3.1	1.6
3 hours	3.8	1.9
4 hours	6.1	2.2

The effects of oral 'Tagamet' 300 mg. and propantheline bromide on food-stimulated gastric acid secretion were compared in 7 duodenal ulcer patients. Propantheline bromide was titrated to maximally tolerated dosages—the average dose was 45 mg. 'Tagamet' 300 mg. reduced gastric acid output by 67% vs. 27% ($p < 0.05$) for propantheline bromide.

24-Hour Mean H^+ Activity: The 24-hour acid suppression provided by 'Tagamet' with the 400 mg. b.i.d. and 300 mg. q.i.d. regimens is similar (54% and 59%, respectively). However, the 300 mg. q.i.d. regimen produces greater daytime acid suppression, while the 400 mg. b.i.d. regimen results in greater suppression of nocturnal acid secretion. The exact degree and duration of acid suppression needed for healing ulcers are not known.

Chemically Stimulated: Oral 'Tagamet' (brand of cimetidine) significantly inhibited gastric acid secretion stimulated by betazole (an isomer of histamine), pentagastrin, caffeine and insulin as follows:

Stimulant	Stimulant Dose	'Tagamet'	% Inhibition
Betazole	1.5mg/kg (sc)	300mg (po)	85% at $2\frac{1}{2}$ hours
Pentagastrin	6mcg/kg/hr (iv)	100mg/hr (iv)	60% at 1 hour
Caffeine	5mg/kg/hr (iv)	300mg (po)	100% at 1 hour
Insulin	0.03 units/kg/hr (iv)	100mg/hr (iv)	82% at 1 hour

When food and betazole were used to stimulate secretion, inhibition of hydrogen ion concentration usually ranged from 45–75% and the inhibition of volume ranged from 30–65%.

2) **Pepsin:** Oral 'Tagamet' 300 mg. reduced total pepsin output as a result of the decrease in volume of gastric juice.

3) **Intrinsic Factor:** Intrinsic factor secretion was studied with betazole as a stimulant. Oral 'Tagamet' 300 mg. inhibited the rise in intrinsic factor concentration produced by betazole, but some intrinsic factor was secreted at all times.

Other

Lower Esophageal Sphincter Pressure and Gastric Emptying

'Tagamet' has no effect on lower esophageal sphincter (LES) pressure or the rate of gastric emptying.

Pharmacokinetics

'Tagamet' is rapidly absorbed after oral administration and peak levels occur in 45–90 minutes. The half-life of 'Tagamet' is approximately 2 hours. Both oral and parenteral (IV or IM) administration provide comparable periods of therapeutically effective blood levels; blood concentrations remain above that required to provide 80% inhibition of basal gastric acid secretion for 4–5 hours following a dose of 300 mg. The principal route of excretion of 'Tagamet' is the urine. Following parenteral administration, most of the drug is excreted as the parent compound; following oral administration, the drug is more extensively metabolized, the sulfoxide being the major metabolite. Following a single oral dose, 48% of the drug is recovered from the urine after 24 hours as the parent compound. Following IV or IM administration, approximately 75% of the drug is recovered from the urine after 24 hours as the parent compound.

Clinical Trials:

Duodenal Ulcer

'Tagamet' (brand of cimetidine) has been shown to be effective in the treatment of active duodenal ulcer and, at reduced dosage, in the prevention of recurrent ulcer.

Active Duodenal Ulcer: In worldwide double-blind clinical studies, endoscopically evaluated duodenal ulcer healing rates with 'Tagamet' were consistently higher than those of the placebo controls. In many of the studies, these differences were statistically significant.

Specifically, in various definitive, controlled studies conducted worldwide with daily doses of 'Tagamet' ranging from 800 mg. (400 mg. b.i.d.) to 1200 mg. (300 mg. q.i.d.), healing rates ranged from 36% to 90% at two weeks; 57% to 100% at four weeks; and 58% to 100% at six weeks in duodenal ulcer outpatients. The corresponding healing rates for placebo groups were 8% to 50% at two weeks; 14% to 78% at four weeks; and 23% to 67% at six weeks.

In these studies, 'Tagamet'-treated patients reported a general reduction in both daytime and nocturnal pain, and they also consumed less antacid than did placebo-treated patients. In trials comparing q.i.d. and b.i.d. regimens, there was a nonsignificant trend toward lower antacid use in the q.i.d. group.

While short-term treatment with 'Tagamet' (brand of cimetidine) can result in complete healing of the duodenal ulcer, acute therapy will not prevent ulcer recurrence after 'Tagamet' has been discontinued. Some follow-up studies have reported that the rate of recurrence once therapy was discontinued was slightly higher for patients healed on 'Tagamet' than for patients healed on other forms of therapy; however, the 'Tagamet'-treated patients generally had more severe disease.

Recurrent Duodenal Ulcer: Extended treatment with a reduced dose of 'Tagamet' has been shown to decrease the recurrence of duodenal ulcer.

In double-blind multicenter studies, 400 mg. of 'Tagamet', taken at bedtime, resulted in a significantly lower incidence of duodenal ulcer recurrence in patients treated for up to one year.

PERCENT RECURRING IN EACH QUARTER

Double-Blind Studies Conducted in the U.S.

Quarter	'Tagamet' 400 mg. h.s.	Placebo
I	7% (3/46)	22% (11/49)
II	7% (2/28)	46% (13/28)
III	6% (1/16)	10% (1/10)
IV	– (0/4)	33% (1/3)
Total	13% (6/46)	53% (26/49)

Double-Blind Studies Conducted in Europe

Quarter	'Tagamet' 400 mg. h.s.	Placebo
I	5% (8/179)	32% (108/333)
II	10% (14/143)	24% (45/184)
III	5% (4/78)	21% (17/82)
IV	5% (2/44)	20% (10/49)
Total	16% (28/179)	54% (180/333)

Active Benign Gastric Ulcer

'Tagamet' has been shown to be effective in the short-term treatment of active benign gastric ulcer.

In a multicenter, double-blind U.S. study, patients with endoscopically confirmed benign gastric ulcer were treated with 'Tagamet' 300 mg. four times a day or with placebo for six weeks. Patients were limited to those with ulcers ranging from 0.5-2.5 cm. in size. Endoscopically confirmed healing at six weeks was seen in significantly* more 'Tagamet'-treated patients than in patients receiving placebo, as shown below:

	'Tagamet'	Placebo
week 2	14/63 (22%)	7/63 (11%)
total at week 6	43/65 (66%)*	30/67 (45%)

*$p < 0.05$

Similarly, in worldwide double-blind clinical studies, endoscopically evaluated benign gastric ulcer healing rates were consistently higher with 'Tagamet' than with placebo.

Pathological Hypersecretory Conditions (such as Zollinger-Ellison Syndrome)

'Tagamet' significantly inhibited gastric acid secretion and reduced occurrence of diarrhea, anorexia and pain in patients with pathological hypersecretion associated with Zollinger-Ellison Syndrome, systemic mastocytosis and multiple endocrine adenomas. Use of 'Tagamet' was also followed by healing of intractable ulcers.

Indications:

'Tagamet' (brand of cimetidine) is indicated in:

(1) **Short-term treatment of active duodenal ulcer.** Since most patients heal within 6-8 weeks, there is rarely reason to use 'Tagamet' at full dosage for longer periods. Concomitant antacids should be given as needed for relief of pain. However, simultaneous administration of 'Tagamet' and antacids is not recommended, since antacids have been reported to interfere with the absorption of 'Tagamet'.

(2) **Prophylactic use in duodenal ulcer patients, at reduced dosage, to prevent ulcer recurrence in patients likely to need surgical treatment, e.g., as demonstrated by a history of recurrence or complications, and in patients with concomitant illness in whom surgery would constitute a greater than usual risk.** Limitation of use to this population is recommended because the consequences of very long-term use, i.e., beyond one year, of continuous 'Tagamet' therapy

are not known.
(3) **Short-term treatment of active benign gastric ulcer.** There is no information concerning usefulness of treatment periods of longer than 8 weeks.
(4) **The treatment of pathological hypersecretory conditions** (i.e., Zollinger-Ellison Syndrome, systemic mastocytosis, multiple endocrine adenomas).

Contraindications: There are no known contraindications to the use of 'Tagamet' (brand of cimetidine). However, the physician should refer to the Precautions section regarding usage in pregnant, nursing, or pediatric patients.

Precautions: 'Tagamet' (brand of cimetidine) has demonstrated a weak antiandrogenic effect. In animal studies this was manifested as reduced prostate and seminal vesicle weights. However, there was no impairment of mating performance or fertility, nor any harm to the fetus in these animals at doses 9 to 56 times the full therapeutic dose of 'Tagamet', as compared with controls. The cases of gynecomastia seen in patients treated for one month or longer may be related to this effect. In human studies, 'Tagamet' has been shown to have no effect on spermatogenesis, sperm count, motility, morphology or *in vitro* fertilizing capacity.

In a 24-month toxicity study conducted in rats, at dose levels of 150, 378 and 950 mg./kg./day (approximately 9 to 56 times the recommended human dose), there was a small increase in the incidence of benign Leydig cell tumors in each dose group; when the combined drug-treated groups and control groups were compared, this increase reached statistical significance. In a subsequent 24-month study, there were no differences between the rats receiving 150 mg./kg./day and the untreated controls. However, a statistically significant increase in benign Leydig cell tumor incidence was seen in the rats that received 378 and 950 mg./kg./day. These tumors were common in control groups as well as treated groups and the difference became apparent only in aged rats.

Rare instances of cardiac arrhythmias and hypotension have been reported following the rapid administration of 'Tagamet' HCl (brand of cimetidine hydrochloride) Injection by intravenous bolus.

Symptomatic response to 'Tagamet' therapy does not preclude the presence of a gastric malignancy. There have been rare reports of transient healing of gastric ulcers despite subsequently documented malignancy.

Reversible confusional states (see Adverse Reactions) have been observed on occasion, predominantly, but not exclusively, in severely ill patients. Advancing age (50 or more years) and preexisting liver and/or renal disease appear to be contributing factors. In some patients these confusional states have been mild and have not required discontinuation of 'Tagamet' therapy. In cases where discontinuation was judged necessary, the condition usually cleared within 3-4 days of drug withdrawal.

Drug Interactions: 'Tagamet', apparently through an effect on certain microsomal enzyme systems, has been reported to reduce the hepatic metabolism of warfarin-type anticoagulants, phenytoin, propranolol, chlordiazepoxide, diazepam, lidocaine and theophylline, thereby delaying elimination and increasing blood levels of these drugs.

Clinically significant effects have been reported with the warfarin anticoagulants; therefore, close monitoring of prothrombin time is recommended, and adjustment of the anticoagulant dose may be necessary when 'Tagamet' is administered concomitantly. Interaction with phenytoin, lidocaine and theophylline has also been reported to produce adverse clinical effects.

Dosage of the drugs mentioned above and other similarly metabolized drugs, particularly those of low therapeutic ratio or in patients with renal and/or hepatic impairment, may require adjustment when starting or stopping concomitantly administered 'Tagamet' to maintain optimum therapeutic blood levels.

Additional clinical experience may reveal other drugs affected by the concomitant administration of 'Tagamet'.

Decreased white blood cell counts, including agranulocytosis, have been reported in 'Tagamet'-treated patients who also received antimetabolites, alkylating agents or other drugs and/or treatment known to produce neutropenia.

Usage in Pregnancy: There has been no experience to date with the use of 'Tagamet' in pregnant patients. However, animal studies have demonstrated that 'Tagamet' crosses the placental barrier. Teratology studies (100–950 mg./kg./day) have shown no effects attributable to 'Tagamet' on litter parameters or early development of the young.

'Tagamet' should not be used in pregnant patients or women of childbearing potential unless, in the judgment of the physician, the anticipated benefits outweigh the potential risks.

Nursing Mothers: Cimetidine is secreted in human milk and, as a general rule, nursing should not be undertaken while a patient is on a drug.

Pediatric Use: Clinical experience in children is limited. Therefore, 'Tagamet' therapy cannot be recommended for children under 16, unless, in the judgment of the physician, anticipated benefits outweigh the potential risks. In very limited experience, doses of 20–40 mg./kg. per day have been used.

Adverse Reactions: Mild and transient diarrhea, dizziness, somnolence and rash have been reported in a small number of patients, e.g., approximately 1 in 100, during treatment with 'Tagamet' (brand of cimetidine). A few cases of headache, ranging from mild to severe, have been reported; these cleared on withdrawal of the drug. There have been rare reports of reversible arthralgia and myalgia; exacerbation of joint symptoms in patients with preexisting arthritis has also been reported. Such symptoms have usually been alleviated by a reduction in 'Tagamet' (brand of cimetidine) dosage. A few cases of polymyositis have been reported, but no causal relationship has been established.

Reversible confusional states, e.g., mental confusion, agitation, psychosis, depression, anxiety, hallucinations, disorientation, have been reported predominantly, but not exclusively, in severely ill patients. They have usually developed within 2-3 days of initiation of 'Tagamet' therapy and have cleared within 3-4 days of discontinuation of the drug.

Mild gynecomastia has been reported in patients treated for one month or longer. In patients being treated for pathological hypersecretory states, this occurred in about 4 percent of cases while in all others the incidence was 0.3% to 1% in various studies. No evidence of induced endocrine dysfunction was found, and the condition remained unchanged or returned toward normal with continuing 'Tagamet' treatment.

Reversible impotence has been reported in patients with pathological hypersecretory disorders, e.g., Zollinger-Ellison Syndrome, receiving 'Tagamet', particularly in high doses, for at least 12 months (range 12–79 months, mean 38 months). However, in large-scale surveillance studies at regular dosage, the incidence has not exceeded that commonly reported in the general population. Furthermore, in controlled long-term studies in patients receiving a single daily bedtime dose, the incidence of reversible impotence did not differ significantly between the 'Tagamet' and placebo groups.

Reversible alopecia has been reported very rarely.

Decreased white blood cell counts in 'Tagamet'-treated patients (approximately 1 per 100,000 patients), including agranulocytosis (approximately 3 per million patients), have been reported, including a few reports of recurrence on rechallenge. These patients generally had serious concomitant illnesses and received drugs and/or treatment known to produce neutropenia. Thrombocytopenia (approximately 3 per million patients) and a few cases of aplastic anemia have also been reported.

Regularly observed small increases in plasma creatinine and some increases in serum transaminase have been reported. These did not progress with continued therapy and disappeared at the end of therapy.

Rare cases of fever, interstitial nephritis and pancreatitis, which cleared on withdrawal of the drug, have been reported. Adverse hepatic effects have been reported rarely. These were reversible and cholestatic or mixed cholestatic-hepatocellular in nature. Because of the predominance of cholestatic features, severe parenchymal injury is considered highly unlikely.

There has been reported a single case of biopsy-proven periportal hepatic fibrosis in a patient receiving 'Tagamet'.

Dosage and Administration:

Duodenal Ulcer

Active Duodenal Ulcer: The recommended adult oral dosage regimen of 'Tagamet' for the routine treatment of duodenal ulcer is 300 mg. four times a day, with meals and at bedtime, the dosage regimen with which U.S. physicians have the most experience. European clinical trials have studied smaller daily dosages: 200 mg. three times a day with meals and 400 mg. at bedtime, as well as 400 mg. twice a day, in the morning and at bedtime. Although the advantages of one regimen over another for a particular patient population have yet to be demonstrated, the 400 mg. twice-a-day regimen may be particularly appropriate for those patients in whom dosing convenience is important.

Concomitant antacids should be given as needed for relief of pain. However, simultaneous administration of 'Tagamet' and antacids is not recommended, since antacids have been reported to interfere with the absorption of 'Tagamet' (brand of cimetidine).

While healing with 'Tagamet' often occurs during the first week or two, treatment should be continued for 4–6 weeks unless healing has been demonstrated by endoscopic examination.

Prophylaxis of Recurrent Duodenal Ulcer: In those patients in whom prophylactic use is indicated, one 400 mg. tablet or two 200 mg. tablets at bedtime is recommended. Prophylactic treatment with higher or more frequent doses does not improve effectiveness.

Active Benign Gastric Ulcer

The recommended adult oral dosage for short-term treatment of active benign gastric ulcer is 300 mg. four times a day with meals and at bedtime. Controlled clinical studies were limited to six weeks of treatment (see Clinical Trials). Symptomatic response to 'Tagamet' does not preclude the presence of a gastric malignancy. It is important to follow gastric ulcer patients to assure rapid progress to complete healing.

Pathological Hypersecretory Conditions (such as Zollinger-Ellison Syndrome)

Recommended adult oral dosage: 300 mg. four times a day with meals and at bedtime. In some patients it may be necessary to administer 'Tagamet' 300 mg. doses more frequently. Doses should be adjusted to individual patient needs, but should not usually exceed 2400 mg. per day and should continue as long as clinically indicated.

Parenteral Administration

In some hospitalized patients with pathological hypersecretory conditions or intractable ulcers, or in patients who are unable to take oral medication, 'Tagamet' may be administered parenterally according to the following recommendations:

Intramuscular injection: 300 mg. q 6 hours (no dilution necessary). Transient pain at the site of injection has been reported.

Intermittent intravenous infusion: 300 mg. q 6 hours. Dilute 'Tagamet' HCl Injection, 300 mg., in 100 ml. of Dextrose Injection (5%) or other compatible i.v. solution (see Stability of 'Tagamet' HCl Injection) and infuse over 15–20 minutes. In some patients it may be necessary to increase dosage. When this is necessary the increases should be made by more frequent administration of a 300 mg. dose, but should not

Continued on next page

Smith Kline & French—Cont.

exceed 2400 mg. per day. **Intravenous injection:** 300 mg. q 6 hours. Dilute 'Tagamet' HCl Injection, 300 mg., in Sodium Chloride Injection (0.9%) or other compatible i.v. solution (see Stability of 'Tagamet' HCl Injection) to a total volume of 20 ml. and inject over a period of not less than 2 minutes (see Precautions).

Dosage Adjustment for Patients with Impaired Renal Function

Patients with severely impaired renal function have been treated with 'Tagamet'. However, such usage has been very limited. On the basis of this experience the recommended dosage is 300 mg. q 12 hours orally or by intravenous injection. Should the patient's condition require, the frequency of dosing may be increased to q 8 hours or even further with caution. In severe renal failure accumulation may occur and the lowest frequency of dosing compatible with an adequate patient response should be used. When liver impairment is also present, further reductions in dosage may be necessary. Hemodialysis reduces the level of circulating 'Tagamet'. Ideally, the dosage schedule should be adjusted so that the timing of a scheduled dose coincides with the end of hemodialysis.

Stability of 'Tagamet' HCl Injection

'Tagamet' HCl (brand of cimetidine hydrochloride) Injection is stable for 48 hours at normal room temperature when added to or diluted with most commonly used intravenous solutions, e.g., Sodium Chloride Injection (0.9%), Dextrose Injection (5% or 10%), Lactated Ringer's Solution, 5% Sodium Bicarbonate Injection.

Overdosage: The usual measures to remove unabsorbed material from the gastrointestinal tract, clinical monitoring and supportive therapy should be employed. Studies in animals indicate that toxic doses are associated with respiratory failure and tachycardia which may be controlled by assisted respiration and the administration of a beta-blocker.

Human experience with gross overdosage is limited. However, in the few cases which have been reported, doses up to 10 grams have not been associated with any untoward effects.

How Supplied:

Pale Green Tablets: 200 mg. tablets in bottles of 100; 300 mg. tablets in bottles of 100 and Single Unit Packages of 100 (intended for institutional use only); and 400 mg. tablets in bottles of 60.

Liquid: 300 mg./5 ml., in 8 fl. oz. (237 ml.) amber glass bottles.

Injection: 300 mg./2 ml. in single-dose vials and in 8 ml. multiple-dose vials, in packages of 10, and in single-dose, prefilled disposable syringes.

Military—Tablets, 200 mg., 100's, 6505-01-103-6335; 300 mg., Individually Sealed, 100's, 6505-01-050-3546, and 300 mg., 100's, 6505-01-050-3547; Injection, 2 ml., 10's, 6505-01-051-4698; 8 ml., 10's, 6505-01-069-1661.

Veterans Administration—Tablets, 200 mg., 100's, 6505-01-103-6335A; 300 mg., 100's, 6505-01-050-3547A; 300 mg., SUP, 100's, 6505-01-050-3546A; 400 mg., 60's, 6505-01-176-0712; Liquid, 300 mg. 8 oz., 6505-01-119-0616A; Injection, 2 ml., 10's, 6505-01-051-4698B; 8 ml., 10's, 6505-01-069-1661B.

Shown in Product Identification Section, page 437

TG:L53

TEMARIL® ℞
[tem'ah-rill]
(brand of trimeprazine tartrate)
Tablets, Syrup and
Spansule® capsules

Description: 'Temaril', available as trimeprazine tartrate, a phenothiazine derivative, is 10-[3-(dimethylamino) -2-methylpropyl] -phenothiazine tartrate.

Trimeprazine tartrate is a white to off-white odorless, crystalline powder readily soluble in water.

Tablets—Each tablet contains trimeprazine tartrate equivalent to 2.5 mg. of trimeprazine.

Syrup—Each 5 ml. (one teaspoonful) contains trimeprazine tartrate equivalent to 2.5 mg. of trimeprazine, and alcohol, 5.7%.

Spansule® sustained release capsules — Each 'Spansule' capsule contains trimeprazine tartrate equivalent to 5 mg. of trimeprazine, so prepared that an initial dose is released promptly and the remaining medication is released gradually over a prolonged period.

Actions: Temaril (trimeprazine tartrate, SK&F), a phenothiazine, possesses antipruritic and antihistaminic properties with anticholinergic (drying) and sedative side effects.

Indications: Treatment of pruritic symptoms in urticaria. Relief of pruritic symptoms in a variety of allergic and non-allergic conditions including atopic dermatitis, neurodermatitis, contact dermatitis, pityriasis rosea, poison ivy dermatitis, eczematous dermatitis, pruritus ani and vulvae, and drug rash.

Contraindications: Temaril (trimeprazine tartrate, SK&F) is contraindicated: in comatose patients; in patients who have received large amounts of central nervous system depressants (alcohol, barbiturates, narcotics, etc.); in patients with bone marrow depression; in patients who have demonstrated an idiosyncrasy or hypersensitivity to 'Temaril' or other phenothiazines; in newborn or premature children; and in nursing mothers. It should not be used in children who are acutely ill and/or dehydrated, as there is an increased susceptibility to dystonias in such patients.

Warnings: Temaril (trimeprazine tartrate, SK&F) may impair the mental and/or physical ability required for the performance of potentially hazardous tasks, such as driving a vehicle or operating machinery. Similarly, it may impair mental alertness in children. The concomitant use of alcohol or other central nervous system depressants may have an additive effect. Patients should be warned accordingly.

'Temaril' should be used with extreme caution in patients with:
  Asthmatic attack
  Narrow-angle glaucoma
  Prostatic hypertrophy
  Stenosing peptic ulcer
  Pyloroduodenal obstruction
  Bladder neck obstruction
  Patients receiving monoamine oxidase inhibitors

Usage in Pregnancy: The safe use of 'Temaril' has not been established with respect to the possible adverse effects upon fetal development. Therefore, it should not be used in women of childbearing potential. Jaundice and prolonged extrapyramidal symptoms have been reported in infants whose mothers received phenothiazines during pregnancy.

Usage in Children: 'Temaril' should be used with caution in children who have a history of sleep apnea or a family history of sudden infant death syndrome (SIDS). It should also be used with caution in young children, in whom it may cause excitation.

Overdosage may produce hallucinations, convulsions and sudden death.

Usage in Elderly Patients (60 years or older): Elderly patients are more prone to develop the following side effects from phenothiazines:
  Hypotension
  Syncope
  Toxic confusional states
  Extrapyramidal symptoms, especially parkinsonism
  Excessive sedation

Precautions: Temaril (trimeprazine tartrate, SK&F) may significantly affect the actions of other drugs. It may increase, prolong or intensify the sedative action of central nervous system depressants such as anesthetics, barbiturates or alcohol. When 'Temaril' is administered concomitantly the dose of a narcotic or barbiturate should be reduced to ¼ or ½ the usual amount. In the patient with pain, receiving treatment with narcotics, excessive amounts of 'Temaril' may lead to restlessness and motor hyperactivity. 'Temaril' can block and even reverse the usual pressor effect of epinephrine.

'Temaril' should be used cautiously in persons with acute or chronic respiratory impairment, particularly children, as it may suppress the cough reflex.

This drug should be used cautiously in persons with cardiovascular disease, impairment of liver function, or those with a history of ulcer disease. Since 'Temaril' has a slight antiemetic action, it may obscure signs of intestinal obstruction, brain tumor, or overdosage of toxic drugs.

Phenothiazines have been shown to elevate prolactin levels; the elevation persists during chronic administration. Tissue culture experiments indicate that approximately one-third of human breast cancers are prolactin-dependent in vitro, a factor of potential importance if the prescribing of these drugs is contemplated in a patient with a previously detected breast cancer. Although disturbances such as galactorrhea, amenorrhea, gynecomastia, and impotence have been reported, the clinical significance of elevated serum prolactin levels is unknown for most patients. An increase in mammary neoplasms has been found in rodents after chronic administration of neuroleptic drugs. Neither clinical nor epidemiologic studies conducted to date, however, have shown an association between chronic administration of these drugs and mammary tumorigenesis; the available evidence is considered too limited to be conclusive at this time.

Drugs which lower the seizure threshold, including phenothiazine derivatives, should not be used with 'Amipaque'.* As with other phenothiazine derivatives, 'Temaril' should be discontinued at least 48 hours before myelography, should not be resumed for at least 24 hours postprocedure, and should not be used for the control of nausea and vomiting occurring either prior to myelography or postprocedure.

Adverse Reactions: Temaril (trimeprazine tartrate, SK&F) may produce adverse reactions attributable to both phenothiazines and antihistamines.

Note: Not all of the following adverse reactions have been reported with 'Temaril'; however, pharmacological similarities among the phenothiazine derivatives require that each be considered when 'Temaril' is administered. There have been occasional reports of sudden death in patients receiving phenothiazine derivatives chronically.

C.N.S. Effects: Drowsiness is the most common C.N.S. effect of this drug. Extrapyramidal reactions (opisthotonos, dystonia, akathisia, dyskinesia, parkinsonism) occur, particularly with high doses. (See Overdosage section for management of extrapyramidal symptoms). Hyperreflexia has been reported in the newborn when a phenothiazine was used during pregnancy. Other reported reactions include dizziness, headache, lassitude, tinnitus, incoordination, fatigue, blurred vision, euphoria, diplopia, nervousness, insomnia, tremors and grand mal seizures, excitation, catatonic-like states, neuritis and hysteria, oculogyric crises, disturbing dreams/nightmares, pseudoschizophrenia, and intensification and prolongation of the action of C.N.S. depressants (opiates, analgesics, antihistamines, barbiturates, alcohol), atropine, heat, organophosphorus insecticides.

Cardiovascular Effects: Postural hypotension is the most common cardiovascular effect of phenothiazines. Reflex tachycardia may be seen. Bradycardia, faintness, dizziness and cardiac arrest have been reported. ECG changes, including blunting of T waves and prolongation of the Q-T interval, may be seen.

Gastrointestinal: Anorexia, nausea, vomiting, epigastric distress, diarrhea, constipation, and dry mouth may occur. Increased appetite and weight gain have also been reported.

Genitourinary: Urinary frequency and dysuria, urinary retention, early menses, induced lactation, gynecomastia, decreased libido, inhibition of ejaculation and false positive pregnancy tests have been reported.

Respiratory: Thickening of bronchial secretions, tightness of the chest, wheezing and nasal stuffiness may occur.

Allergic Reactions: These include urticaria, dermatitis, asthma, laryngeal edema, angioneurotic edema, photosensitivity, lupus erythematosus-like syndrome and anaphylactoid reactions.

Other Reported Reactions: Leukopenia, agranulocytosis, pancytopenia, hemolytic anemia, elevation of plasma cholesterol levels and thrombocytopenic purpura have been reported. Jaundice of the obstructive type has also been reported; it is usually reversible but chronic jaundice has been reported. Erythema, peripheral edema, and stomatitis have been reported. High or prolonged glucose tolerance curves, glycosuria, elevated spinal fluid proteins and reversed epinephrine effects may also occur.

Rare occurrences of neuroleptic malignant syndrome (NMS) have been reported in patients receiving phenothiazines. This syndrome is comprised of the symptom complex of hyperthermia, altered consciousness, muscular rigidity and autonomic dysfunction and is potentially fatal.

Long-Term Therapy Considerations: After prolonged phenothiazine administration at high dosage, pigmentation of the skin has occurred, chiefly in the exposed areas. Ocular changes consist of the appearance of lenticular and corneal opacities, epithelial keratopathies and pigmentary retinopathy. Vision may be impaired.

Dosage and Administration:
Tablets and Syrup:
Adults: Usual dosage is 2.5 mg. q.i.d.
Children over three years: Usual dosage is 2.5 mg. h.s., or t.i.d. if needed.
Children 6 months to 3 years: Usual dosage is 1.25 mg. ($\frac{1}{2}$ teaspoonful of syrup) h.s., or t.i.d. if needed.
'Spansule' capsules:
Adults: Usual daily dosage is 1 capsule q12h.
Children over 6 years of age: 1 capsule daily.
This product form is not recommended for children under 6 years of age. Use tablets or syrup for their dosage flexibility.

Because some side effects appear to be dose-related, it is important to use the lowest effective dosage.

Drug Interactions: MAO inhibitors and thiazide diuretics prolong and intensify the anticholinergic effects of 'Temaril'. Combined use of MAO inhibitors and phenothiazines may result in hypertension and extrapyramidal reactions.

Narcotics: The C.N.S. depressant and analgesic effects of narcotics are potentiated by phenothiazines.

The following drugs may result in potentiation of phenothiazine effects:
 Oral contraceptives
 Progesterone
 Reserpine
 Nylidrin hydrochloride

Management of Overdosage: Signs and symptoms of 'Temaril' overdosage range from mild depression of the central nervous system and cardiovascular system to profound hypotension, respiratory depression and unconsciousness. Stimulation may be evident, especially in children and geriatric patients. Atropine-like signs and symptoms—dry mouth, fixed, dilated pupils, flushing, etc.—as well as gastrointestinal symptoms may occur. The treatment of overdosage is essentially symptomatic and supportive. Early gastric lavage may be beneficial. **Do not administer emetics or attempt to induce vomiting because a dystonic reaction of the head or neck might result in aspiration of vomitus.** Extrapyramidal symptoms may be treated with anti-parkinsonism drugs, barbiturates, or 'Benadryl'.†

Avoid analeptics, which may cause convulsions. Severe hypotension usually responds to the administration of levarterenol or phenylephrine. EPINEPHRINE SHOULD NOT BE USED, since its use in a patient with partial adrenergic blockade may further lower the blood pressure. Additional measures include oxygen and intravenous fluids. Limited experience with dialysis indicates that it is not helpful.

Special note on 'Spansule' capsules—Since much of the 'Spansule' capsule medication is coated for gradual release, therapy directed at reversing the effects of the ingested drug and at supporting the patient should be continued for as long as overdosage symptoms remain. Saline cathartics are useful for hastening evacuation of pellets that have not already released medication.

How Supplied:
'Temaril' Tablets—2.5 mg. trimeprazine/tablet in bottles of 100 and 1000; Single Unit Packages of 100 (intended for institutional use only).
'Temaril' Syrup—2.5 mg. trimeprazine/5 ml. (teaspoonful) and alcohol 5.7%, in 4 fl. oz. bottles.
'Temaril' Spansule capsules—5 mg. trimeprazine/capsule in bottles of 50; Single Unit Packages of 100 (intended for institutional use only).
Military—Tablets, 2.5 mg., 1000's, 6505-00-935-9826.

*Trademark Reg. U.S. Pat. Off.: 'Amipaque' for metrizamide, Winthrop Laboratories.
†Trademark Reg. U.S. Pat. Off.: 'Benadryl' for diphenhydramine hydrochloride, Parke-Davis.
Shown in Product Identification Section, page 437
TM:L40

THORAZINE®
[thor'ah-zeen]
(brand of chlorpromazine)

Description: Thorazine (chlorpromazine, SK&F) is 10 - (3 - dimethylaminopropyl) -2-chlorphenothiazine, a dimethylamine derivative of phenothiazine. It is present in oral and injectable forms as the hydrochloride salt, and in the suppositories as the base.

Actions: The precise mechanism whereby the therapeutic effects of chlorpromazine are produced is not known. The principal pharmacological actions are psychotropic: It also exerts sedative and antiemetic activity. Chlorpromazine has actions at all levels of the central nervous system—primarily at subcortical levels—as well as on multiple organ systems. Chlorpromazine has strong antiadrenergic and weaker peripheral anticholinergic activity; ganglionic blocking action is relatively slight. It also possesses slight antihistaminic and antiserotonin activity.

Indications: For the management of manifestations of psychotic disorders.
To control nausea and vomiting.
For relief of restlessness and apprehension before surgery.
For acute intermittent porphyria.
As an adjunct in the treatment of tetanus.
To control the manifestations of the manic type of manic-depressive illness.
For relief of intractable hiccups.
For the treatment of severe behavioral problems in children marked by combativeness and/or explosive hyperexcitable behavior (out of proportion to immediate provocations), and in the short-term treatment of hyperactive children who show excessive motor activity with accompanying conduct disorders consisting of some or all of the following symptoms: impulsivity, difficulty sustaining attention, aggressivity, mood lability and poor frustration tolerance.

Thorazine (chlorpromazine, SK&F) is considered possibly effective in the treatment of non-psychotic anxiety. However, 'Thorazine' is not the first drug to be used in therapy for most patients with non-psychotic anxiety because certain risks associated with its use are not shared by common alternative treatments (e.g., benzodiazepines).

When used in the treatment of non-psychotic anxiety, 'Thorazine' should not be administered in doses of more than 100 mg. per day or for longer than 12 weeks because the use of 'Thorazine' at higher doses or for longer intervals may cause persistent tardive dyskinesia that may prove irreversible. (See Warnings section.)

Final classification by the FDA of the non-psychotic anxiety indication requires further investigation.

Contraindications: Comatose states, presence of large amounts of C.N.S. depressants (alcohol, barbiturates, narcotics, etc.) and in the presence of bone marrow depression.

Warnings: The extrapyramidal symptoms which can occur secondary to 'Thorazine' may be confused with the central nervous system signs of an undiagnosed primary disease responsible for the vomiting, e.g., Reye's syndrome or other encephalopathy. The use of 'Thorazine' and other potential hepatotoxins should be avoided in children and adolescents whose signs and symptoms suggest Reye's syndrome.

Patients who have demonstrated a hypersensitivity reaction (e.g., blood dyscrasias, jaundice with a phenothiazine) should not be reexposed to any phenothiazine, including Thorazine (chlorpromazine, SK&F), unless in the judgment of the physician the potential benefits of treatment outweigh the possible hazard.

'Thorazine' may impair mental and/or physical abilities, especially during the first few days of therapy. Therefore, caution patients about activities requiring alertness (e.g., operating vehicles or machinery).

The use of alcohol with this drug should be avoided due to possible additive effects and hypotension. 'Thorazine' may counteract the antihypertensive effect of guanethidine and related compounds.

Persistent Tardive Dyskinesia: Persistent tardive dyskinesia may appear in some patients on long-term therapy with antipsychotic agents or may appear after drug therapy has been discontinued. In some patients the symptoms appear to be irreversible. There is no known effective treatment for tardive dyskinesia. It is suggested that all antipsychotic agents be discontinued if symptoms of this syndrome appear. (See Adverse Reactions section.)

Usage in Pregnancy: Safety for the use of 'Thorazine' during pregnancy has not been established; therefore, it is recommended that the drug be given to pregnant patients only when, in the judgment of the physician, it is essential. The potential benefits should clearly outweigh possible hazards. There are reported instances of jaundice, prolonged extrapyramidal signs or hyperreflexia in newborn infants whose mothers had received 'Thorazine'.

Reproductive studies in rodents have demonstrated a potential for embryotoxicity, increased neonatal mortality and nursing transfer of the drug. Tests in the offspring of the drug-treated rodents demonstrate decreased performance. The possibility of permanent neurological damage cannot be excluded.

Nursing Mothers: There is evidence that chlorpromazine is excreted in the breast milk of nursing mothers.

Precautions: Thorazine (chlorpromazine, SK&F) should be administered cautiously to persons with cardiovascular or liver disease. There is evidence that patients with a history of hepatic encephalopathy due to cirrhosis have increased sensitivity to the C.N.S. effects of 'Thorazine' (i.e., impaired cerebration and abnormal slowing of the EEG).

Because of its C.N.S. depressant effect, 'Thorazine' should be used with caution in patients with chronic respiratory disorders such as severe asthma, emphysema and acute respiratory infections, particularly in children.

Because 'Thorazine' can suppress the cough reflex, aspiration of vomitus is possible.

Thorazine (chlorpromazine, SK&F) prolongs and intensifies the action of C.N.S. depressants such as anesthetics, barbiturates and narcotics. When 'Thorazine' is administered concomitantly, about $\frac{1}{4}$ to $\frac{1}{2}$ the usual dosage of such agents is required. When 'Thorazine' is not being administered to reduce requirements of C.N.S. depressants, it is best to stop such depressants before starting 'Thorazine' treatment. These agents may subsequently be reinstated at low doses and increased as needed.

Continued on next page

Smith Kline & French—Cont.

Note: 'Thorazine' does *not* intensify the anticonvulsant action of barbiturates. Therefore, dosage of anticonvulsants, including barbiturates, should *not* be reduced if 'Thorazine' is started. Instead, start 'Thorazine' at low doses and increase as needed.

Use with caution in persons who will be exposed to extreme heat, organophosphorus insecticides, and in persons receiving atropine or related drugs.

'Thorazine' tablets have recently been reformulated to remove FD&C Yellow #5 (tartrazine). However, until the transition process is complete, some lots of 'Thorazine' tablets containing FD&C Yellow #5 (tartrazine) will still be in stock. FD&C Yellow #5 (tartrazine) may cause allergic-type reactions (including bronchial asthma) in certain susceptible individuals. Although the overall incidence of FD&C Yellow #5 (tartrazine) sensitivity in the general population is low, it is frequently seen in patients who also have aspirin sensitivity. For specific information, contact Smith Kline &French Laboratories (outside Pa., call toll-free: 1-800-523-4835, ext. 4262; in Pa., call collect: 215-751-4262).

Neuroleptic drugs elevate prolactin levels; the elevation persists during chronic administration. Tissue culture experiments indicate that approximately one-third of human breast cancers are prolactin-dependent in vitro, a factor of potential importance if the prescribing of these drugs is contemplated in a patient with a previously detected breast cancer. Although disturbances such as galactorrhea, amenorrhea, gynecomastia and impotence have been reported, the clinical significance of elevated serum prolactin levels is unknown for most patients. An increase in mammary neoplasms has been found in rodents after chronic administration of neuroleptic drugs. Neither clinical nor epidemiologic studies conducted to date, however, have shown an association between chronic administration of these drugs and mammary tumorigenesis; the available evidence is considered too limited to be conclusive at this time.

As with all drugs which exert an anticholinergic effect, and/or cause mydriasis, chlorpromazine should be used with caution in patients with glaucoma.

Chlorpromazine diminishes the effect of oral anticoagulants.

Phenothiazines can produce alpha-adrenergic blockade.

Chlorpromazine may lower the convulsive threshold; dosage adjustments of anticonvulsants may be necessary. Potentiation of anticonvulsant effects does not occur. However, it has been reported that chlorpromazine may interfere with the metabolism of 'Dilantin' * and thus precipitate 'Dilantin' toxicity.

Concomitant administration with propranolol results in increased plasma levels of both drugs. Drugs which lower the seizure threshold, including phenothiazine derivatives, should not be used with 'Amipaque'.† As with other phenothiazine derivatives, 'Thorazine' should be discontinued at least 48 hours before myelography, should not be resumed for at least 24 hours postprocedure, and should not be used for the control of nausea and vomiting occurring either prior to myelography or postprocedure.

Long-Term Therapy: To lessen the likelihood of adverse reactions related to cumulative drug effect, patients with a history of long-term therapy with 'Thorazine' and/or other neuroleptics should be evaluated periodically to decide whether the maintenance dosage could be lowered or drug therapy discontinued.

Antiemetic Effect: The antiemetic action of 'Thorazine' may mask the signs and symptoms of overdosage of other drugs and may obscure the diagnosis and treatment of other conditions such as intestinal obstruction, brain tumor and Reye's syndrome. (See Warnings).

'Thorazine' should be used cautiously with cancer chemotherapy drugs that cause vomiting at toxic levels because vomiting, as a sign of toxicity, may be obscured.

Abrupt Withdrawal: Like other phenothiazines, Thorazine (chlorpromazine, SK&F) is not known to cause psychic dependence and does not produce tolerance or addiction. There may be, however, following abrupt withdrawal of high-dose therapy, some symptoms resembling those of physical dependence such as gastritis, nausea and vomiting, dizziness and tremulousness. These symptoms can usually be avoided or reduced by gradual reduction of the dosage or by continuing concomitant anti-parkinsonism agents for several weeks after 'Thorazine' is withdrawn.

Adverse Reactions:

Drowsiness, usually mild to moderate, may occur, particularly during the first or second week, after which it generally disappears. If troublesome, dosage may be lowered.

Jaundice: Overall incidence has been low, regardless of indication or dosage. Most investigators conclude it is a sensitivity reaction. Most cases occur between the second and fourth weeks of therapy. The clinical picture resembles infectious hepatitis, with laboratory features of obstructive jaundice, rather than those of parenchymal damage. It is usually promptly reversible on withdrawal of the medication; however, chronic jaundice has been reported.

There is no conclusive evidence that preexisting liver disease makes patients more susceptible to jaundice. Alcoholics with cirrhosis have been successfully treated with Thorazine (chlorpromazine, SK&F) without complications. Nevertheless, the medication should be used cautiously in patients with liver disease. Patients who have experienced jaundice with a phenothiazine should not, if possible, be reexposed to 'Thorazine' or other phenothiazines.

If fever with grippe-like symptoms occurs, appropriate liver studies should be conducted. If tests indicate an abnormality, stop treatment.

Liver function tests in jaundice induced by the drug may mimic extrahepatic obstruction; withhold exploratory laparotomy until extrahepatic obstruction is confirmed.

Hematological Disorders, including agranulocytosis, eosinophilia, leukopenia, hemolytic anemia, aplastic anemia, thrombocytopenic purpura and pancytopenia, though rare, have been reported.

Agranulocytosis—Warn patients to report the sudden appearance of sore throat or other signs of infection. If white blood cell and differential counts indicate cellular depression, stop treatment and start antibiotic and other suitable therapy. Most cases have occurred between the 4th and 10th weeks of therapy; patients should be watched closely during that period.

Moderate suppression of white blood cells is not an indication for stopping treatment unless accompanied by the symptoms described above.

Cardiovascular:

Hypotensive Effects—Postural hypotension, simple tachycardia, momentary fainting and dizziness may occur after the first injection; occasionally after subsequent injections; rarely, after the first oral dose. Usually recovery is spontaneous and symptoms disappear within ½ to 2 hours. Occasionally, these effects may be more severe and prolonged, producing a shock-like condition.

To minimize hypotension after initial injection, keep patient lying down and observe for at least ½ hour. To control hypotension, place patient in head-low position with legs raised. If a vasoconstrictor is required, 'Levophed' and 'Neo-Synephrine'‡ are the most suitable. Other pressor agents, including epinephrine, should not be used as they may cause a paradoxical further lowering of blood pressure.

EKG Changes—particularly nonspecific, usually reversible Q and T wave distortions—have been observed in some patients receiving phenothiazine tranquilizers, including Thorazine (chlorpromazine, SK&F). Their relationship to myocardial damage has not been confirmed.

Note: Sudden death, apparently due to cardiac arrest, has been reported, but there is not sufficient evidence to establish a relationship between such deaths and the administration of the drug.

C.N.S. Reactions:

Neuromuscular (Extrapyramidal) Reactions—Neuromuscular reactions include dystonias, motor restlessness, pseudo-parkinsonism and tardive dyskinesia, and appear to be dose-related. They are discussed in the following paragraphs:

Dystonias: Symptoms may include spasm of the neck muscles, sometimes progressing to acute, reversible torticollis; extensor rigidity of back muscles, sometimes progressing to opisthotonos; carpopedal spasm, trismus, swallowing difficulty, oculogyric crisis and protrusion of the tongue.

These usually subside within a few hours, and almost always within 24 to 48 hours after the drug has been discontinued.

In mild cases, reassurance or a barbiturate is often sufficient. *In moderate cases,* barbiturates will usually bring rapid relief. *In more severe adult cases,* the administration of an anti-parkinsonism agent, except levodopa, usually produces rapid reversal of symptoms. *In children,* reassurance and barbiturates will usually control symptoms. (Or, parenteral 'Benadryl'§ may be useful. See 'Benadryl' prescribing information for appropriate children's dosage.) If appropriate treatment with anti-parkinsonism agents or 'Benadryl' fails to reverse the signs and symptoms, the diagnosis should be reevaluated.

Suitable supportive measures such as maintaining a clear airway and adequate hydration should be employed when needed. If therapy is reinstituted, it should be at a lower dosage. Should these symptoms occur in children or pregnant patients, the drug should not be reinstituted.

Motor Restlessness: Symptoms may include agitation or jitteriness and sometimes insomnia. These symptoms often disappear spontaneously. At times these symptoms may be similar to the original neurotic or psychotic symptoms. Dosage should not be increased until these side effects have subsided.

If these symptoms become too troublesome, they can usually be controlled by a reduction of dosage or concomitant administration of a barbiturate.

Pseudo-parkinsonism: Symptoms may include: mask-like facies, drooling, tremors, pillrolling motion, cogwheel rigidity and shuffling gait. In most cases these symptoms are readily controlled when an anti-parkinsonism agent is administered concomitantly. Anti-parkinsonism agents should be used only when required. Generally, therapy of a few weeks to two or three months will suffice. After this time patients should be evaluated to determine their need for continued treatment. (Note: Levodopa has not been found effective in neuroleptic-induced pseudo-parkinsonism.) Occasionally it is necessary to lower the dosage of Thorazine (chlorpromazine, SK&F) or to discontinue the drug.

Persistent Tardive Dyskinesia: As with all antipsychotic agents, tardive dyskinesia may appear in some patients on long-term therapy or may appear after drug therapy has been discontinued. This condition appears in all age groups. However, the risk appears to be greater in elderly patients on high-dose therapy, especially females. The symptoms are persistent and in some patients appear to be irreversible. The syndrome is characterized by rhythmical involuntary movements of the tongue, face, mouth or jaw (e.g., protrusion of tongue, puffing of cheeks, puckering of mouth, chewing movements). Sometimes these may be accompanied by involuntary movements of extremities. In rare instances, these involuntary movements of the extremities are the only manifestations of tardive dyskinesia.

There is no known effective treatment for tardive dyskinesia; anti-parkinsonism agents do not alleviate the symptoms of this syndrome. It is suggested that all antipsychotic agents be discontinued if these symptoms appear. Should it be necessary to reinstitute treatment, or increase the dosage of the agent, or switch to a different antipsychotic agent, the syndrome may be masked.

It has been reported that fine vermicular movements of the tongue may be an early sign of the syndrome and if the medication is stopped at that time the syndrome may not develop.

Adverse Behavioral Effects—Psychotic symptoms and catatonic-like states have been reported rarely.

Other C.N.S. Effects—Cerebral edema has been reported.

Convulsive seizures *(petit mal* and *grand mal)* have been reported, particularly in patients with EEG abnormalities or history of such disorders.

Abnormality of the cerebrospinal fluid proteins has also been reported.

Allergic Reactions of a mild urticarial type or photosensitivity are seen. Avoid undue exposure to sun. More severe reactions, including exfoliative dermatitis, have been reported occasionally.

Contact dermatitis has been reported in nursing personnel; accordingly, the use of rubber gloves when administering 'Thorazine' liquid or injectable is recommended.

Endocrine Disorders: Lactation and moderate breast engorgement may occur in females on large doses. If persistent, lower dosage or withdraw drug. False-positive pregnancy tests have been reported, but are less likely to occur when a serum test is used. Amenorrhea and gynecomastia have also been reported. Hyperglycemia, hypoglycemia and glycosuria have been reported.

Autonomic Reactions: Occasional dry mouth; nasal congestion; constipation; adynamic ileus; urinary retention; priapism; miosis and mydriasis.

Special Considerations in Long-Term Therapy: Skin pigmentation and ocular changes have occurred in some patients taking substantial doses of Thorazine (chlorpromazine, SK&F) for prolonged periods.

Skin Pigmentation—Rare instances of skin pigmentation have been observed in hospitalized mental patients, primarily females who have received the drug usually for three years or more in dosages ranging from 500 mg. to 1500 mg. daily. The pigmentary changes, restricted to exposed areas of the body, range from an almost imperceptible darkening of the skin to a slate gray color, sometimes with a violet hue. Histological examination reveals a pigment, chiefly in the dermis, which is probably a melanin-like complex. The pigmentation may fade following discontinuance of the drug.

Ocular Changes—Ocular changes have occurred more frequently than skin pigmentation and have been observed both in pigmented and nonpigmented patients receiving Thorazine (chlorpromazine, SK&F) usually for two years or more in dosages of 300 mg. daily and higher. Eye changes are characterized by deposition of fine particulate matter in the lens and cornea. In more advanced cases, star-shaped opacities have also been observed in the anterior portion of the lens. The nature of the eye deposits has not yet been determined. A small number of patients with more severe ocular changes have had some visual impairment. In addition to these corneal and lenticular changes, epithelial keratopathy and pigmentary retinopathy have been reported. Reports suggest that the eye lesions may regress after withdrawal of the drug.

Since the occurrence of eye changes seems to be related to dosage levels and/or duration of therapy, it is suggested that long-term patients on moderate to high dosage levels have periodic ocular examinations.

Etiology—The etiology of both of these reactions is not clear, but exposure to light, along with dosage/duration of therapy, appears to be the most significant factor. If either of these reactions is observed, the physician should weigh the benefits of continued therapy against the possible risks and, on the merits of the individual case, determine whether or not to continue present therapy, lower the dosage, or withdraw the drug.

Other Adverse Reactions: Mild fever may occur after large I.M. doses. Hyperpyrexia has been reported. Increases in appetite and weight sometimes occur. Peripheral edema and a systemic lupus erythematosus-like syndrome have been reported.

Rare occurrences of neuroleptic malignant syndrome (NMS) have been reported in patients receiving neuroleptic drugs. This syndrome is comprised of the symptom complex of hyperthermia, altered consciousness, muscular rigidity and autonomic dysfunction and is potentially fatal.

Note: There have been occasional reports of sudden death in patients receiving phenothiazines. In some cases, the cause appeared to be asphyxia due to failure of the cough reflex. In others, the cause could not be determined. There is not sufficient evidence to establish a relationship between such deaths and the administration of phenothiazines.

Dosage and Administration: Adjust dosage to individual and the severity of his condition, recognizing that the milligram for milligram potency relationship among all dosage forms has not been precisely established clinically. It is important to increase dosage until symptoms are controlled. Dosage should be increased more gradually in debilitated or emaciated patients. In continued therapy, gradually reduce dosage to the lowest effective maintenance level, after symptoms have been controlled for a reasonable period.

In general, dosage recommendations for other oral forms of the drug may be applied to Spansule® brand sustained release capsules on the basis of total daily dosage in milligrams.

Increase parenteral dosage only if hypotension has not occurred. Before using I.M., see Important Notes on Injection.

Elderly Patients: In general, dosages in the lower range are sufficient for most elderly patients. Since they appear to be more susceptible to hypotension and neuromuscular reactions, such patients should be observed closely. Dosage should be tailored to the individual, response carefully monitored, and dosage adjusted accordingly. Dosage should be increased more gradually in elderly patients.

General Medicine:
Adults: EXCESSIVE ANXIETY, TENSION AND AGITATION—*Oral:* 10 mg. t.i.d. or q.i.d., or 25 mg. b.i.d. or t.i.d. MORE SEVERE CASES—*Oral:* 25 mg. t.i.d. After 1 or 2 days, daily dosage may be increased by 20 to 50 mg. semiweekly, until patient becomes calm and cooperative. (Maximum improvement may not be seen for weeks or even months.) Continue optimum dosage for 2 weeks; then gradually reduce to maintenance level. Daily dosage of 200 mg. is not unusual. Some patients require higher dosages (e.g., 800 mg. daily is not uncommon in discharged mental patients).
TREATMENT OF NON-PSYCHOTIC ANXIETY—Do not administer in doses of more than 100 mg. per day or for longer than 12 weeks.
PROMPT CONTROL OF SEVERE SYMPTOMS—*I.M.:* 25 mg. (1 ml.). If necessary, repeat in 1 hour. Subsequent doses should be oral, 25 to 50 mg. t.i.d.
NAUSEA AND VOMITING—*Oral:* 10 to 25 mg. q4-6h, p.r.n., increased, if necessary. *I.M.:* 25 mg. (1 ml.). If no hypotension occurs, give 25 to 50 mg. q3-4h, p.r.n., until vomiting stops. Then switch to oral dosage. *Rectal:* One 100 mg. suppository q6-8h, p.r.n. In some patients, half this dose will do.
INTRACTABLE HICCUPS—*Oral:* 25 to 50 mg. t.i.d. or q.i.d. If symptoms persist for 2-3 days, give 25 to 50 mg. (1-2 ml.) I.M. Should symptoms persist, use *slow* I.V. infusion with patient flat in bed: 25 to 50 mg. (1-2 ml.) in 500 to 1,000 ml. of saline. Follow blood pressure closely.
ACUTE INTERMITTENT PORPHYRIA—*Oral:* 25 to 50 mg. t.i.d. or q.i.d. Can usually be discontinued after several weeks, but maintenance therapy may be necessary for some patients. *I.M.:* 25 mg. (1 ml.) t.i.d. or q.i.d. until patient can take oral therapy.
TETANUS—*I.M.:* 25 to 50 mg. (1-2 ml.) given 3 or 4 times daily, usually in conjunction with barbiturates. Total doses and frequency of administration must be determined by the patient's response, starting with low doses and increasing gradually. *I.V.:* 25 to 50 mg. (1-2 ml.). Dilute to at least 1 mg. per ml. and administer at a rate of 1 mg. per minute.
Children: NAUSEA AND VOMITING—Thorazine (chlorpromazine, SK&F) should generally not be used in children under 6 months of age. It should not be used in conditions for which children's dosages have not been established. Dosage and frequency of administration should be adjusted according to the severity of the symptoms and response of the patient. The duration of activity following intramuscular administration may last up to 12 hours. Subsequent doses may be given by the same route if necessary. *Oral:* ¼ mg./lb. body weight q4-6h (e.g., 40 lb. child—10 mg. q4-6h). *Rectal:* ½ mg./lb. body weight q6-8h, p.r.n. (e.g., 20-30 lb. child—half of a 25 mg. suppository q6-8h). *I.M.:* ¼ mg./lb. body weight q6-8h, p.r.n. *Maximum I.M. Dosage:* Children up to 5 yrs. (or 50 lbs.), not over 40 mg./day; 5-12 yrs. (or 50-100 lbs.), not over 75 mg./day except in severe cases. (For mental and emotional disorders, see Psychiatry, below.)
TETANUS—*I.M.* or *I.V.:* ¼ mg./lb. body weight q6-8h. When given I.V., dilute to at least 1 mg./ml. and administer at rate of 1 mg. per 2 minutes. In children up to 50 lbs., do not exceed 40 mg. daily; 50 to 100 lbs., do not exceed 75 mg., except in severe cases.
Surgery:
Adults: PREOPERATIVE—*Oral:* 25 to 50 mg., 2 to 3 hours before the operation. *I.M.:* 12.5 to 25 mg. (0.5-1 ml.), 1 to 2 hours before operation. DURING SURGERY—Administer only to control acute nausea and vomiting. *I.M.:* 12.5 mg. (0.5 ml.). Repeat in ½ hour if necessary and if no hypotension occurs. *I.V.:* 2 mg. per fractional injection, at 2-minute intervals. Do not exceed 25 mg. Dilute to 1 mg./ml., i.e., 1 ml. (25 mg.) mixed with 24 ml. of saline. POSTOPERATIVE—*Oral:* 10 to 25 mg. q4-6h, p.r.n. *I.M.:* 12.5 to 25 mg. (0.5-1 ml.). Repeat in 1 hour if necessary and if no hypotension occurs.
Children: Thorazine (chlorpromazine, SK&F) should generally not be used in children under 6 months of age except where potentially lifesaving. It should not be used in conditions for which specific children's dosages have not been established. PREOPERATIVE—¼ mg./lb. body weight, either *orally* 2 to 3 hours before operation, or *I.M.* 1 to 2 hours before. DURING SURGERY—*I.M.:* ⅛ mg./lb. body weight. Repeat in ½ hour if necessary and if no hypotension occurs. *I.V.:* 1 mg. per fractional injection at 2-minute intervals and not exceeding recommended I.M. dosage. Always dilute to 1 mg./ml., i.e., 1 ml. (25 mg.) mixed with 24 ml. of saline. POSTOPERATIVE—¼ mg./lb. body weight, either *orally* q4-6h, p.r.n., or *I.M.* Repeat in 1 hour if necessary and if no hypotension occurs.
Psychiatry:
Increase dosage gradually until symptoms are controlled. Maximum improvement may not be seen for weeks or even months. Continue optimum dosage for 2 weeks; then gradually reduce dosage to the lowest effective maintenance level.
Adults: OFFICE PATIENTS OR OUTPATIENTS—*Oral:* 10 mg. t.i.d. or q.i.d., or 25 mg. b.i.d. or t.i.d. MORE SEVERE CASES—*Oral:* 25 mg. t.i.d. After 1 or 2 days, daily dosage may be increased by 20-50 mg. at semiweekly intervals until patient becomes calm and cooperative. TREATMENT OF NON-PSYCHOTIC ANXIETY—Do not administer in doses of more than 100 mg. per day or for longer than 12 weeks. PROMPT CONTROL OF SEVERE SYMPTOMS—*I.M.:* 25 mg. (1 ml.). If necessary, repeat in 1 hour. Subsequent doses should be oral, 25-50 mg. t.i.d.
HOSPITALIZED PATIENTS: ACUTELY AGITATED, MANIC, OR DISTURBED—*I.M.:* 25 mg. (1 ml.). If necessary, give additional 25 to 50 mg. injection in 1 hour. Increase subsequent I.M. doses gradually over several days—up to 400 mg. q4-6h in exceptionally severe cases—until patient is controlled. Usually patient becomes quiet and cooperative within 24 to 48 hours and oral doses may be substituted and increased until the patient is calm. 500 mg. a day is generally sufficient. While gradual increases to 2,000 mg. a day or more may be necessary, there is usually little therapeutic gain to be achieved by exceeding 1,000 mg. a

Continued on next page

Smith Kline & French—Cont.

day for extended periods. In general, dosage levels should be lower in the elderly, the emaciated and the debilitated. LESS ACUTELY AGITATED PATIENTS—*Oral:* 25 mg. t.i.d. Increase gradually until effective dose is reached—usually 400 mg. daily.

Children: OFFICE PATIENTS OR OUTPATIENTS—Select route of administration according to severity of patient's condition and increase dosage gradually as required. *Oral:* ¼ mg./lb. body weight q4-6h, p.r.n. (e.g., for 40 lb. child—10 mg. q4-6h). *Rectal:* ½ mg./lb. body weight q6-8h, p.r.n. (e.g., for 20-30 lb. child—half a 25 mg. suppository q6-8h). *I.M.:* ¼ mg./lb. body weight q6-8h, p.r.n.

HOSPITALIZED PATIENTS—As with outpatients, start with low doses and increase dosage gradually. In severe behavior disorders or psychotic conditions, higher dosages (50-100 mg. daily, and in older children, 200 mg. daily or more) may be necessary. There is little evidence that behavior improvement in severely disturbed mentally retarded patients is further enhanced by doses beyond 500 mg. per day. *Maximum I.M. Dosage:* Children up to 5 years (or 50 lbs.), not over 40 mg./day; 5-12 years (or 50-100 lbs.), not over 75 mg./day except in unmanageable cases.

Important Notes on Injection: Inject slowly, deep into upper outer quadrant of buttock.

Because of possible hypotensive effects, reserve parenteral administration for bedfast patients or for acute ambulatory cases, and keep patient lying down for at least ½ hour after injection. If irritation is a problem, dilute Injection with saline or 2% procaine; mixing with other agents in the syringe is not recommended. Subcutaneous injection is not advised. Avoid injecting undiluted Thorazine (chlorpromazine, SK&F) into vein. I.V. route is only for severe hiccups and surgery.

Because of the possibility of contact dermatitis, avoid getting solution on hands or clothing. Protect from light, and discoloration may occur. Slight yellowing will not alter potency. Discard if markedly discolored.

Note on Concentrate: When the Concentrate is to be used, add the desired dosage of Concentrate to 60 ml. (2 fl. oz.) or more of diluent *just prior to administration.* This will insure palatability and stability. Vehicles suggested for dilution are: tomato or fruit juice, milk, simple syrup, orange syrup, carbonated beverages, coffee, tea, or water. Semisolid foods (soups, puddings, etc.) may also be used. The Concentrate is light sensitive; it should be protected from light and dispensed in amber glass bottles. *Refrigeration is not required.*

Overdosage: (See also Adverse Reactions.)
Symptoms—Primarily symptoms of central nervous system depression to the point of somnolence or coma. Hypotension and extrapyramidal symptoms.

Other possible manifestations include agitation and restlessness, convulsions, fever, autonomic reactions such as dry mouth and ileus, EKG changes and cardiac arrhythmias.

Treatment—It is important to determine other medications taken by the patient since multiple dose therapy is common in overdosage situations. Treatment is essentially symptomatic and supportive. Early gastric lavage is helpful. Keep patient under observation and maintain an open airway, since involvement of the extrapyramidal mechanism may produce dysphagia and respiratory difficulty in severe overdosage. **Do not attempt to induce emesis because a dystonic reaction of the head or neck may develop that could result in aspiration of vomitus.** Extrapyramidal symptoms may be treated with anti-parkinsonism drugs, barbiturates, or 'Benadryl'. See prescribing information for these products. Care should be taken to avoid increasing respiratory depression. If administration of a stimulant is desirable, amphetamine, dextroamphetamine, or caffeine with sodium benzoate is recommended. Stimulants that may cause convulsions (e.g., picrotoxin or pentylenetetrazol) should be avoided.

If hypotension occurs, the standard measures for managing circulatory shock should be initiated. If it is desirable to administer a vasoconstrictor, 'Levophed' and 'Neo-Synephrine' are most suitable. Other pressor agents, including epinephrine, are not recommended because phenothiazine derivatives may reverse the usual elevating action of these agents and cause a further lowering of blood pressure.

Limited experience indicates that phenothiazines are *not* dialyzable.

Special note on 'Spansule' capsules—Since much of the 'Spansule' capsule medication is coated for gradual release, therapy directed at reversing the effects of the ingested drug and at supporting the patient should be continued for as long as overdosage symptoms remain. Saline cathartics are useful for hastening evacuation of pellets that have not already released medication.

How Supplied: Tablets—Each tablet contains chlorpromazine hydrochloride, 10 mg., 25 mg. or 50 mg., in bottles of 100 and 1000; in Single Unit Packages of 100 (intended for institutional use only). For use in severe neuropsychiatric conditions, 100 mg. and 200 mg., in bottles of 100 and 1000; in Single Unit Packages of 100 (intended for institutional use only).

Spansule® brand of sustained release capsules—Each 'Spansule' capsule contains chlorpromazine hydrochloride, so prepared that an initial dose is released promptly and the remaining medication is released gradually over a prolonged period. Available as 30 mg., 75 mg., 150 mg. or 200 mg., in bottles of 50 and 500; in Single Unit Packages of 100 (intended for institutional use only). For use in severe neuropsychiatric conditions, 300 mg., in bottles of 50; in Single Unit Packages of 100 (intended for institutional use only).

Ampuls—1 ml. and 2 ml. (25 mg./ml.), in boxes of 10, 100 and 500. Each ml. contains, in aqueous solution, chlorpromazine hydrochloride, 25 mg.; ascorbic acid, 2 mg.; sodium bisulfite, 1 mg.; sodium sulfite, 1 mg.; sodium chloride, 6 mg.

Multiple-dose Vials—10 ml. (25 mg./ml.), in boxes of 1, 20 and 100. Each ml. contains, in aqueous solution, chlorpromazine hydrochloride, 25 mg.; ascorbic acid, 2 mg.; sodium bisulfite, 1 mg.; sodium sulfite, 1 mg.; sodium chloride, 1 mg. Contains benzyl alcohol, 2%, as a preservative.

Syrup—Each 5 ml. (one teaspoonful) contains chlorpromazine hydrochloride, 10 mg., in 4 fl. oz. bottles.

Suppositories—Each suppository contains chlorpromazine, 25 mg. or 100 mg., glycerin, glyceryl monopalmitate, glyceryl monostearate, hydrogenated cocoanut oil fatty acids, hydrogenated palm kernel oil fatty acids, in boxes of 12.

Concentrate (intended for institutional use only)—*30 mg./ml.:* Each ml. contains chlorpromazine hydrochloride, 30 mg., in 4 fl. oz. bottles, in cartons of 36 bottles, and in 1 gallon bottles. *100 mg./ml.:* Each ml. contains chlorpromazine hydrochloride, 100 mg., in 8 fl. oz. bottles, in cartons of 12.

Military—Concentrate 30 mg./ml., 4 fl. oz., 6505-00-660-1664; Injection, 2 ml., 10's, 6505-00-129-6709; Tablets 25 mg., S.U.P. 100's, 6505-00-118-2529, and 1000's, 6505-00-022-1326; Tablets 50 mg., S.U.P. 100's, 6505-00-132-0371, and 1000's, 6505-00-022-1327; Tablets 100 mg., S.U.P. 100's, 6505-00-132-0372, and 1000's, 6505-00-014-1182.

*Trademark Reg. U.S. Pat. Off.: 'Dilantin' for diphenylhydantoin, Parke-Davis.
†Trademark Reg. U.S. Pat. Off.: 'Amipaque' for metrizamide, Winthrop Laboratories.
‡'Levophed' and 'Neo-Synephrine' are the trademarks (Reg. U.S. Pat. Off.) of Winthrop Laboratories for its brands of levarterenol and phenylephrine respectively.
§Trademark Reg. U.S. Pat. Off.: 'Benadryl' for diphenhydramine hydrochloride, Parke-Davis.

Shown in Product Identification Section, page 437
TZ:L63

TUSS-ORNADE® ℞
[*tuss'or-naid'*]
LIQUID

Description: Each 5 ml. (1 teaspoonful) of 'Tuss-Ornade' Liquid contains caramiphen edisylate, 6.7 mg.; phenylpropanolamine hydrochloride, 12.5 mg.; and alcohol, 5.0%, in a preparation that contains no sugar or dyes.

Actions: The 'Tuss-Ornade' formula contains caramiphen edisylate, a synthetic, non-narcotic cough suppressant, and phenylpropanolamine hydrochloride, a vasoconstrictor with decongestant action on nasal and upper respiratory tract mucosal membranes.

> **Indications:**
> For the symptomatic relief of coughs and nasal congestion associated with common colds.
> N.B.: A final determination has not been made on the effectiveness of this drug combination in accordance with efficacy requirements of the 1962 Amendments to the Food, Drug and Cosmetic Act.

Contraindications: Hypersensitivity to either of the components; concurrent MAO inhibitor therapy; severe hypertension; bronchial asthma; coronary artery disease.

Do not use 'Tuss-Ornade' Liquid in children under 15 pounds or in children less than six months of age.

Warnings: Caution patients about activities requiring alertness (e.g., operating vehicles or machinery). Patients should also be warned about the possible additive effects of alcohol and other CNS depressants.

Precautions: Use with caution in patients with cardiovascular disease, glaucoma, prostatic hypertrophy, thyroid disease or diabetes. Use with caution in patients in whom productive cough is desirable to clear excessive secretions from the bronchial tree. Patients taking this medication should be cautioned not to take simultaneously other products containing phenylpropanolamine HCl or amphetamines.

Usage in Pregnancy: Safe use in pregnancy has not been established. This drug should not be used in pregnancy, nursing mothers, or women of childbearing potential unless, in the judgment of the physician, the anticipated benefits outweigh the potential risks.

Adverse Reactions: Adverse effects associated with products containing a centrally acting antitussive or sympathomimetic amine may occur and include: nausea, gastrointestinal upset, diarrhea, constipation, dizziness, drowsiness, nervousness, insomnia, anorexia, weakness, tightness of chest, angina pain, irritability, palpitations, headache, incoordination, tremor, difficulty in urination, dysuria, hypertension, hypotension, visual disturbances.

Dosage and Administration: Adults and children over 12 years—2 teaspoonfuls every 4 hours; do not exceed 12 teaspoonfuls in 24 hours. Children 6 to 12 years—1 teaspoonful every 4 hours; do not exceed 6 teaspoonfuls in 24 hours. Children 2 to 6 years—½ teaspoonful every 4 hours; do not exceed 3 teaspoonfuls in 24 hours. Data are not available on which to base dosage recommendations for children under 2 years of age. **Do not use in children under 15 pounds or less than 6 months old.**

Overdosage: Symptoms—May include dryness of mouth, dysphagia, thirst, blurred vision, dilated pupils, photophobia, fever, rapid pulse and respiration, disorientation, dizziness, nausea, fainting, tachycardia, and either excitation or depression of the central nervous system.

Treatment—Immediate evacuation of the stomach should be induced by emesis and gastric lavage, repeated as necessary.

Respiratory depression should be treated promptly with oxygen and respiratory stimulants. Do not treat respiratory or CNS depression with analeptics that might precipitate convulsions. If

TUSS-ORNADE®
[tuss'or-naid']
SPANSULE® CAPSULES

Description: Each 'Tuss-Ornade' *Spansule* capsule contains 40 mg. of caramiphen edisylate and 75 mg. of phenylpropanolamine hydrochloride, so prepared that an initial dose is released promptly and the remaining medication is released gradually over a prolonged period.

Actions: The 'Tuss-Ornade' formula contains caramiphen edisylate, a synthetic, non-narcotic cough suppressant, and phenylpropanolamine hydrochloride, a vasoconstrictor with decongestant action on nasal and upper respiratory tract mucosal membranes.

Pharmacokinetics: At steady-state conditions, the following peak levels are reached after the oral administration of a 'Spansule' capsule: 24 ng./ml. caramiphen in 4.6 hours; 200 ng./ml. phenylpropanolamine in 5.5 hours; the half-lives are approximately 11 and 8 hours, respectively.

Indications:
For the symptomatic relief of coughs and nasal congestion associated with common colds. N.B.: A final determination has not been made on the effectiveness of this drug combination in accordance with efficacy requirements of the 1962 Amendments to the Food, Drug and Cosmetic Act.

Contraindications: Hypersensitivity to either of the components; concurrent MAO inhibitor therapy; severe hypertension; bronchial asthma; coronary artery disease.
Do not use 'Tuss-Ornade' *Spansule* capsules in children under 12 years of age.

Warnings: Caution patients about activities requiring alertness (e.g., operating vehicles or machinery). Patients should also be warned about the possible additive effects of alcohol and other CNS depressants.

Precautions: Use with caution in persons with cardiovascular disease, glaucoma, prostatic hypertrophy, thyroid disease or diabetes. Use with caution in patients in whom productive cough is desirable to clear excessive secretions from the bronchial tree. Patients taking this medication should be cautioned not to take simultaneously other products containing phenylpropanolamine HCl or amphetamines.

Usage in Pregnancy: Safe use in pregnancy has not been established. This drug should not be used in pregnancy, nursing mothers, or women of childbearing potential unless, in the judgment of the physician, the anticipated benefits outweigh the potential risks.

Adverse Reactions: Adverse effects associated with products containing a centrally acting antitussive or sympathomimetic amine may occur and include: nausea, gastrointestinal upset, diarrhea, constipation, dizziness, drowsiness, nervousness, insomnia, anorexia, weakness, tightness of chest, angina pain, irritability, palpitation, headache, incoordination, tremor, difficulty in urination, dysuria, hypertension, hypotension, visual disturbances.

Dosage and Administration: 'Tuss-Ornade' *Spansule* capsules: Adults and children over 12 years of age—one 'Tuss-Ornade' *Spansule* capsule every 12 hours. **Do not use in children under 12 years of age.**

Overdosage: Symptoms—May include dryness of mouth, dysphagia, thirst, blurred vision, dilated pupils, photophobia, fever, rapid pulse and respiration, disorientation, dizziness, nausea, fainting, tachycardia, and either excitation or depression of the central nervous system. If marked excitement occurs, a short-acting barbiturate or chloral hydrate may be used.

Supplied: 'Tuss-Ornade' Liquid is supplied as a fruit flavored liquid, in 16 fl. oz. bottles.

TOL:L14

Treatment—Immediate evacuation of the stomach should be induced by emesis and gastric lavage, repeated as necessary.
Respiratory depression should be treated promptly with oxygen and respiratory stimulants. Do not treat respiratory or CNS depression with analeptics that might precipitate convulsions. If marked excitement occurs, a short-acting barbiturate or chloral hydrate may be used.
Since much of the 'Spansule' capsule medication is coated for gradual release, saline cathartics should be administered to hasten evacuation of pellets that have not already released medication.

Supplied: 'Tuss-Ornade' *Spansule* capsules: in bottles of 50 and 500 capsules.
Shown in Product Identification Section, page 437

TO:L30

URISPAS®
[yore'eh-spaz]
(brand of flavoxate HCl)
100 mg. tablets
Urinary tract spasmolytic

Description: Urispas (brand of flavoxate HCl) is a synthetic antispasmodic offered specifically for the relief of symptoms associated with various urologic disorders. 'Urispas' exerts its effect directly on the muscle.
Chemically, flavoxate hydrochloride is 2-piperidinoethyl 3-methyl-4-oxo-2-phenyl-4H-1-benzopyran-8-carboxylate hydrochloride. The empirical formula of flavoxate hydrochloride is $C_{24}H_{25}NO_4 \cdot HCl$.

Action: Flavoxate hydrochloride counteracts smooth muscle spasm of the urinary tract.

Indications: Urispas (brand of flavoxate HCl) is indicated for symptomatic relief of dysuria, urgency, nocturia, suprapubic pain, frequency and incontinence as may occur in cystitis, prostatitis, urethritis, urethrocystitis/urethrotrigonitis. 'Urispas' is not indicated for definitive treatment, but is compatible with drugs used for the treatment of urinary tract infections.

Contraindications: Urispas (brand of flavoxate HCl) is contraindicated in patients who have any of the following obstructive conditions: pyloric or duodenal obstruction, obstructive intestinal lesions or ileus, achalasia, gastrointestinal hemorrhage, and obstructive uropathies of the lower urinary tract.

Warnings: Urispas (brand of flavoxate HCl) should be given cautiously in patients with suspected glaucoma.

Usage in Pregnancy—Safety in women who are or may become pregnant has not been established. Therefore, Urispas (brand of flavoxate HCl) should not be given except when the expected benefits outweigh the possible hazards.

Usage in Children—This drug cannot be recommended for infants and children under 12 years of age because safety and efficacy have not been demonstrated in this age group.

Precautions: In the event of drowsiness and blurred vision, the patient should not operate a motor vehicle or machinery or participate in activities where alertness is required.

Adverse Reactions: Adverse reactions reported include nausea and vomiting, dry mouth, nervousness, vertigo, headache, drowsiness, blurred vision, increased ocular tension, disturbance in eye accommodation, urticaria and other dermatoses, mental confusion especially in the elderly patient, dysuria, tachycardia and palpitation, hyperpyrexia, eosinophilia and leukopenia (1 case which was reversible upon discontinuation of the drug).

Dosage and Administration: *Adults and children over twelve years of age:* one or two 100 mg. tablets three or four times a day. With improvement of symptoms, the dose may be reduced. This drug cannot be recommended for infants and children under 12 years of age because safety and efficacy have not been demonstrated in this age group.

How Supplied: 100 mg. tablets, in bottles of 100; in Single Unit Packages of 100 (intended for institutional use only). **Military**—Tablets, 100 mg., 100's, 6505-00-172-3420.
Shown in Product Identification Section, page 437

UR:L9

VONTROL®
[vohn'trole]
(brand of diphenidol)

'Vontrol' may cause hallucinations, disorientation, or confusion. For this reason, its use is limited to patients who are hospitalized or under comparable, continuous, close, professional supervision. Even then, the physician should carefully weigh the benefits against the possible risks and give due consideration to alternate therapeutic measures.

Description: 'Vontrol', α, α-diphenyl-1-piperidinebutanol, is a compound not related to the antihistamines, phenothiazines, barbiturates, or other agents with antivertigo or antiemetic action.

Actions: 'Vontrol' (diphenidol, SK&F) apparently exerts a specific antivertigo effect on the vestibular apparatus to control vertigo and inhibits the chemoreceptor trigger zone to control nausea and vomiting.

Indications (See Warnings):
1) VERTIGO—'Vontrol' is indicated in peripheral (labyrinthine) vertigo and associated nausea and vomiting, as seen in such conditions as: Meniere's disease, middle- and inner-ear surgery (labyrinthitis).
2) NAUSEA AND VOMITING—'Vontrol' is indicated in the control of nausea and vomiting, as seen in such conditions as: postoperative states, malignant neoplasms and labyrinthine disturbances.

Contraindications: Known hypersensitivity to the drug is a contraindication. Anuria is a contraindication. (Since approximately 90% of the drug is excreted in the urine, renal shutdown could cause systemic accumulation.)

Warnings: 'Vontrol' (diphenidol, SK&F) may cause hallucinations, disorientation or confusion. For this reason, its use is limited to patients who are hospitalized or under comparable, continuous, close, professional supervision. Even then, the physician should carefully weigh the benefits against the possible risks and give due consideration to alternate therapeutic measures.
The incidence of auditory and visual hallucinations, disorientation and confusion appears to be less than ½% or approximately one in 350 patients. The reaction has usually occurred within three days of starting the drug in recommended dosage and has subsided spontaneously usually within three days after discontinuation of the drug. Patients on 'Vontrol' should be observed closely and in the event of such a reaction the drug should be stopped.

Usage in Pregnancy: Use of any drug in pregnancy, lactation or in women of childbearing age requires that the potential benefits of the drug be weighed against its possible hazards to the mother and child.
In animal teratogenesis and reproduction studies of 'Vontrol' (diphenidol, SK&F), there were no significant differences between drug-treated groups and untreated control groups, except as noted under animal Reproduction Studies (see "Pharmacology [animal]").
In 936 patients who received 'Vontrol' during pregnancy, the incidences of normal and abnormal birth were comparable to those reported in the literature for the average population of pregnant patients. And in no instance was there any evidence that 'Vontrol' played a part in birth abnormality (see "In Pregnancy").
'Vontrol' is not indicated for use in nausea and vomiting of pregnancy, since the therapeutic value and safety in this indication have not yet been determined.

Precautions: The antiemetic action of 'Vontrol' (diphenidol, SK&F) may mask signs of overdose of drugs (e.g., digitalis) or may obscure diagnosis of

Continued on next page

Smith Kline & French—Cont.

conditions such as intestinal obstruction and brain tumor.

Although there have been no reports of blood dyscrasias with 'Vontrol', patients should be observed regularly for any idiosyncratic reactions.

'Vontrol' has a weak peripheral anticholinergic effect and should be used with care in patients with glaucoma, obstructive lesions of the gastrointestinal and genitourinary tracts, such as stenosing peptic ulcer, prostatic hypertrophy, pyloric and duodenal obstruction, and organic cardiospasm.

Intravenous administration to persons with a history of sinus tachycardia may be undesirable because this procedure may initiate an episode in such patients.

Several patients were reported to have had a transient decrease in systolic and diastolic blood pressure, up to 20 mm. Hg., following parenteral use of 'Vontrol'.

'Vontrol' Tablets contain FD&C Yellow #5 (tartrazine) which may cause allergic-type reactions (including bronchial asthma) in certain susceptible individuals. Although the overall incidence of FD&C Yellow #5 (tartrazine) sensitivity in the general population is low, it is frequently seen in patients who also have aspirin hypersensitivity.

Usage in Children
'Vontrol' is not recommended for use in children under 50 pounds. (See Dosage and Administration—Children.)

Adverse Reactions: Auditory and visual hallucinations, disorientation and confusion have been reported. Drowsiness, overstimulation, depression, sleep disturbance, dry mouth, g.i. irritation (nausea and indigestion), or blurred vision may occur.

Rarely, slight dizziness, skin rash, malaise, headache, or heartburn may occur. Mild jaundice of questionable relationship to the use of 'Vontrol' (diphenidol, SK&F) has been reported. Slight, transient lowering of blood pressure has been reported in a few patients.

(See laboratory studies under "Pharmacology [human]".)

Dosage and Administration (See Warnings)
Adults—for Vertigo or Nausea and Vomiting:
The usual dose is one tablet (25 mg.) every four hours as needed. Some patients may require two tablets (50 mg.).
Children—for Nausea and Vomiting: These recommendations are for nausea and vomiting only. There has been no experience with 'Vontrol' in vertigo in children.

Unit doses in children are best calculated by body weight: usually 0.4 mg./lb.

Children's doses usually should not be given more often than every four hours. However, if symptoms persist after the first dose, administration may be repeated after one hour. Thereafter, doses may be given every four hours as needed.

The total dose in 24 hours should not exceed 2.5 mg./lb.

NOTE: The drug is not recommended for use in children under 50 pounds. The dosage for children 50 to 100 pounds is one tablet (25 mg.).

Overdosage: In the event of overdosage, the patient should be managed according to his symptoms. Treatment is essentially supportive, with maintenance of blood pressure and respiration, plus careful observation. Early gastric lavage may be indicated depending on the amount of overdose and nature of symptoms.

How Supplied: Bottles of 100—Each tablet contains 25 mg. diphenidol as the hydrochloride.

Pharmacology (animal): 'Vontrol' (diphenidol, SK&F) exerts its antiemetic effect primarily by inhibiting the chemoreceptor trigger zone, as evidenced by its activity in blocking emesis induced by apomorphine in dogs. In this regard 'Vontrol', as the hydrochloride salt, has a potency equal to the potent phenothiazine antiemetic, chlorpromazine hydrochloride. In animals 'Vontrol' has only weak parasympatholytic activity and no significant sedative, tranquilizing or antihistaminic action or effects on blood pressure, heart rate, respiration or the electrocardiogram.

Subacute and chronic toxicity studies in rats and dogs, in which large doses of 'Vontrol', as the hydrochloride salt, were administered orally and intramuscularly for periods up to one year, revealed no significant effects on hematology, liver function, kidney function or blood glucose determinations. Histological examination of the animals' tissues did not reveal any significant lesions attributable to administration of 'Vontrol'.

Reproduction Studies: Teratogenesis and reproduction studies were carried out in rats and rabbits. In rats, 'Vontrol' (diphenidol, SK&F), as the hydrochloride salt, was fed daily to male and female animals in doses of 20 mg./kg. and 40 mg./kg. (approximately three and six times the maximum recommended daily dose in adult humans) for 60 days before mating, and during mating, gestation and lactation for each of two litters. There were no significant differences between drug-treated and untreated control groups with regard to conception rate, litter size, live birth or viability in either of the two litters. There was no congenital anomaly among the offspring. In rabbits, 'Vontrol', as the hydrochloride salt, was fed in the diets in doses of 5 mg./kg. or 75 mg./kg. (approximately equal to, and 12 times as much as, the maximum recommended daily dose in adult humans) from the first day of gestation through the 26th or 27th day of gestation, when the young were delivered by Cesarean section. There were no significant differences between drug-treated and control groups with regard to number and weight of fetuses, numbers of resorption sites or viable fetuses. There was also no statistically significant difference between drug-treated and control groups with regard to the total percentage of underdeveloped fetuses. However, when data were calculated on the basis of a ratio between underdeveloped fetuses and number of pregnant does, an adverse dose-related effect was observed in the high-dose test group.

Pharmacology (human): Three double-blind controlled studies comparing 'Vontrol' (diphenidol, SK&F) to placebo were carried out: one in 32 male volunteers over a four-week period; one in 45 volunteers of whom 15 were studied for 12 weeks and 17 for 24 weeks; and one in 48 volunteers of whom 36 were studied for 12 weeks.

In the first study 'Vontrol', as the hydrochloride salt, was given orally in daily doses that were started at 75 mg. during the first week and graduated up to 200 mg. by the fourth week. In the second study, one group received 'Vontrol' orally, as the hydrochloride salt, titrated up to 500 mg. daily, then down to 200 mg. daily; another group received a maximum of 200 mg. daily. In the third study, patients received oral doses of 200 mg. to 300 mg. of 'Vontrol' daily, as the hydrochloride or pamoate salts.

The studies included these laboratory determinations: complete blood counts (including hemoglobin and hematocrit determinations), urinalyses (including microscopic examination), serum alkaline phosphatase, serum bilirubin, and bromsulphalein retention. The studies also included records of weight and blood pressure and, in one, electrocardiograms.

In two of these studies, clinical laboratory changes were seen among volunteers in both treated and control groups. The changes included: extrasystoles, white cells in the urine, increase in prothrombin time, rise in hematocrit, rise in leucocytes, rise in eosinophils, and rise or reduction in neutrophils. At no time in any study did changes in the treated group differ significantly from those in the control group.

'Vontrol', as the hydrochloride salt, was given orally to 17 children (aged five to 15). Total daily doses ranged from 90 to 240 mg. Complete blood counts and, in some patients, urinalyses were done before treatment and after approximately four days of treatment. There was no significant difference between pre- and post-treatment laboratory determinations in any child. No side effects were seen.

Excretion: Following oral administration of 'Vontrol' (diphenidol, SK&F) to dogs, as the hydrochloride or pamoate salts, and to humans, as the hydrochloride salt, peak blood concentration of the drug generally occurs in one and a half to three hours. In dogs and rats, virtually all of an oral dose of C^{14}-labeled 'Vontrol' is excreted in the urine and feces within three to four days, as determined by radioactivity counts. Approximately the same percentage of an administered dose appeared in the urine of dogs following either oral administration of the hydrochloride salt or rectal administration of the free base.

In Pregnancy: Investigators kept follow-up records on 936 patients who had received 'Vontrol' (diphenidol, SK&F) at some time during pregnancy, primarily during the first trimester.

Of the 936 women, 864 (92%) had normal births of normal infants.

Seventy-two (8%) of the women experienced some birth abnormality. Of the 72, six patients had premature but otherwise normal infants, 40 patients aborted, 10 had stillbirths, and 16 had infants with miscellaneous defects. These included hernias, congenital heart defects, hydrocephalus, internal strabismus, anencephalus, enlarged thyroid, and hypospadia.

These incidences of abnormal birth are lower than those generally reported in the literature for the average population of pregnant patients. And in no instance was there any evidence that the administration of 'Vontrol' played a part in birth abnormality.

Shown in Product Identification Section, page 437
VN:L14

EDUCATIONAL MATERIAL

Patient Information on Dyazide® (triamterene and hydrochlorothiazide). Pad (8½″ × 11″) of 50 sheets. Provides basic information about high blood pressure and 'Dyazide', including special considerations about diet, possible drug interactions, and side effects. Free to physicians.

Patient I.D. Card. "I am taking Eskalith®/Eskalith CR® (brand of lithium carbonate)." Packet of 10 wallet-size (2½″ × 3½″) cards. Provides information to emergency room or other medical personnel about the patient and attending physician and about possible drug-related side effects and their management. Free to physicians.

Instruction Sheets for Patients on Parnate® (brand of tranylcypromine sulfate). Pad (4¼″ × 8″) of 24 sheets. Serves as a reminder of principal instructions about 'Parnate' therapy, e.g.: the importance of following dosage instructions exactly; the need for consulting before taking any other drugs; what foods and beverages must be avoided; what symptoms should be reported promptly. A carbon copy is provided for the physician's records. Free to physicians.

10-Page Booklet (3¾″ × 8½″) for Patients Taking Tagamet® (brand of cimetidine): "Some Facts You Should Know About Ulcer Disease." Provides basic information about peptic ulcer disease and 'Tagamet'. Free to physicians.

Patient I.D. Card. "I am taking Stelazine® (brand of trifluoperazine hydrochloride)." Packet of 10 wallet-size (2½″ × 3½″) fold-out cards. Provides information to emergency room or other medical personnel about the patient and attending physician and about possible drug-related side effects and their management. Free to physicians.

Products are cross-indexed by generic and chemical names in the
YELLOW SECTION

Smith Laboratories, Inc.
2215 SANDERS ROAD
NORTHBROOK, IL 60062

CHYMODIACTIN® ℞
[ki″ mō-dī-ac′ tin]
(chymopapain for injection)
with Diluent

WARNINGS

Chymodiactin® should only be used in a hospital setting by physicians experienced and trained in the diagnosis of lumbar disc disease and all acceptable treatment modalities, including surgery. Additionally, these physicians and their support personnel should be competent in the diagnosis and management of all potential complications from the use of Chymodiactin®, including anaphylaxis, which has occurred in about 0.7% of patients (observed rate of 0.4% in patients receiving local anesthesia v. 0.9% in patients receiving general anesthesia) and can be fatal.

Acute transverse myelitis/acute transverse myelopathy has been reported in association with the injection of chymopapain at a rate of about 1 in 18,000. Although cause and effect relationship to the injection of chymopapain itself has not been established, the reported rate is significantly higher than the incidence reported in the medical literature. These patients are characterized clinically by the delayed (2–3 weeks) onset of paraplegia or paraparesis without prior signs or symptoms. Patients receiving injections at two or more disc spaces following discography appear to be at increased risk.

Paraplegia, cerebral hemorrhage and other serious neurological changes have been reported soon after chymopapain injection. Chymopapain is toxic when injected into the subarachnoid space. Some radio-opaque contrast media are neurotoxic. Great care must be taken to assure that the dura is not penetrated and that chymopapain or contrast agents do not enter the subarachnoid space. If there is any question regarding needle tip location within the nucleus of the disc or if the contrast agent extravasates into the subarachnoid space, the procedure should be abandoned, and chymopapain should not be injected.

Description: Chymodiactin® is a proteolytic enzyme in the form of a sterile, nonpyrogenic, lyophilized powder. The unit of chymopapain activity is the picoKatal. The enzyme forms, under the conditions of the assay, 1 picomole of p-nitroaniline per second from DL-benzoyl arginine-p-nitroanilide (BAPNA) substrate. In general, 1 mg of chymopapain contains approximately 500 units.

Chymodiactin® is available in 2 ml and 5 ml vial sizes, and is accompanied by a vial of Sterile Water for Injection, USP, which is to be used as diluent. The 2 ml vial, which is to be reconstituted with 2 ml of diluent, contains 4,000 units of Chymodiactin® and 1.4 mg of sodium L-cysteinate hydrochloride. The 5 ml vial, which is to be reconstituted with 5 ml of diluent, contains 10,000 units of Chymodiactin® and 3.6 mg of sodium L-cysteinate hydrochloride. The concentration of the solution in a reconstituted vial is 2,000 units of active drug per ml. The vial contains no preservatives.

The proteolytic enzyme chymopapain is derived from the crude latex of *Carica papaya*. Sodium L-cysteinate hydrochloride is added as a reducing agent for this sulphur containing enzyme to maintain the sulphur in the sulphydryl form. The pH of the reconstituted drug is 5.5 to 6.5.

Clinical Pharmacology: Chymodiactin® is injected into the herniated nucleus pulposus of the lumbar intervertebral disc resulting in rapid hydrolysis of the noncollagenous polypeptides or proteins that maintain the tertiary structure of the chondromucoprotein of the nucleus pulposus. By causing degradation of the chondromucoprotein, this lessens the intradiscal osmotic activity, thereby decreasing fluid absorption and reducing intradiscal pressure. The foregoing mechanism of action is based on animal *in vitro* and *in vivo* data. Although the mechanism of action in the human has not been established directly, operative findings in patients who have come to surgery following injection have usually revealed the nucleus pulposus to be absent from its former site. A temporary increase in urinary mucopolysaccharide occurs in man following intervertebral injections of chymopapain. After intradiscal injection of chymopapain in humans it appears that the inhibitory activity of the alpha$_2$-macroglobulin prevents expression of any significant proteolytic activity outside the disc.

As Chymodiactin® is injected directly into the herniated lumbar intervertebral disc, absorption, distribution, and metabolism are not necessary for it to achieve its intended purpose. Pharmacological activity has been demonstrated by direct observation both *in vivo* and *in vitro* in animals, *in vitro* in human disc tissue, and pharmacokinetically in the human by observation of increases in urinary excretion of substances known to be in high concentration in the disc.

After injection into the central portion of human lumbar intervertebral discs (*in vivo*) there is an increase in the urinary concentration of glycosaminoglycans of the type known to occur in human intervertebral discs; and chymopapain or its immunologically reactive fragments (CIP) are also detectable by radioimmunoassay in plasma at 30 minutes and are declining at 24 hours. Small amounts of CIP are also detected in the urine. These findings indicate that, after intradiscal injection of chymopapain, CIP diffuses rapidly into plasma. Due to the inhibitory activity of the plasma alpha$_2$-macroglobulin and the low concentration of CIP, it is unlikely that any proteolytic activity is expressed outside the disc.

In a randomized, double-blind comparison of drug and placebo, approximately 75% of patients responded successfully to drug, compared to approximately 45% for placebo, using the randomization code-break as the criterion for efficacy. When the placebo failures were then treated with drug, 90% of them responded with partial or total relief of their symptoms.

Indications and Usage: Chymodiactin® intradiscal injection is indicated for the treatment of patients with documented herniated lumbar intervertebral discs whose symptoms and signs have not responded to an adequate period or periods of conservative therapy. Chymodiactin® has not been studied in the treatment of herniated discs in areas other than the lumbar spine.

Chymodiactin® should only be used by physicians who routinely care for the patients, described above, who are qualified by training and experience to perform laminectomy, discectomy, or other spinal procedures, and who have received specialized training in chemonucleolysis. The appropriate use of Chymodiactin® in chemonucleolysis requires precise diagnosis, and the ability to employ skillfully all appropriate diagnostic and treatment modalities necessary, including surgical intervention other than chemonucleolysis (laminectomy/discectomy) and all aspects of pre and post operative patient management. Proper selection of patients for whom chemonucleolysis is applicable requires extensive training and experience in the diagnosis and management of all spinal disorders, since there are circumstances in which nerve root compression resulting from conditions other than herniated disc can produce similar signs and symptoms.

Chymodiactin® should be used only in hospitals. Supporting personnel, as well as physicians, should be qualified in the diagnosis and management of all potential complications of the use of Chymodiactin® including anaphylaxis.

Females are more likely to develop anaphylactic reactions secondary to Chymodiactin®. (See **Warnings.**)

Contraindications: Chymodiactin® is contraindicated in patients with a known sensitivity to chymopapain, papaya or papaya derivatives. Other contraindications are severe spondylolisthesis; severe, progressing paralysis as indicated by rapidly progressing neurologic dysfunction; and in patients with evidence of spinal cord tumor or a cauda equina lesion.

Use of Chymodiactin® is contraindicated in patients who have previously been injected with any form of chymopapain.

Chymodiactin® has not been studied in regions of the spine other than the lumbar area; therefore, its use is contraindicated in any spinal region other than the lumbar area.

Warnings:

(1) Anaphylaxis of a severe to mild nature has been observed after injection of Chymodiactin® in about 0.7% of patients and may be life threatening if not treated promptly and correctly. *At least one open intravenous line must always be in place to permit rapid and adequate management of such an occurrence.* The reaction can be immediate or delayed up to one hour after injection and can last for minutes to several hours or longer. The patient may present with almost immediate hypotension and/or bronchospasm, the former being more common. These may proceed to laryngeal edema, cardiac arrhythmia, cardiac arrest, coma, and death. Speed in diagnosis and treatment is of the essence since the clinical signs, severity, progression, and duration of an anaphylactic reaction are highly unpredictable. Other signs of allergic response, such as erythema, pilomotor erection, rash, pruritic urticaria, conjunctivitis, vasomotor rhinitis, angioedema, or various gastrointestinal disturbances, must also be watched for.

Post Marketing Surveillance data confirm that females are more likely to develop an anaphylactic reaction secondary to Chymodiactin® (observed rate of 1.2% v. 0.4% in males). These data have also shown a statistically significant difference in the frequency of anaphylaxis in patients receiving local anesthesia v. those receiving general anesthesia (0.4% v. 0.9%, respectively); however, a direct cause and effect relationship has not been established.

Clinical judgement, speed of therapy, and choice of agents all enter into the treatment of anaphylaxis. *Epinephrine is the definitive therapeutic agent in the immediate treatment of anaphylaxis. Substitution of other agents such as steroids should be reserved for cases where epinephrine is not appropriate.*

Chymopapain is a foreign protein and its injection has the potential for generating an immunological response. Therefore, patients who have already received an injection of any form of chymopapain should not be reinjected with Chymodiactin®.

(2) Acute transverse myelitis/acute transverse myelopathy has been reported in association with the injection of chymopapain at a rate of about 1 in 18,000. Although cause and effect relationship to the injection of chymopapain itself has not been established, the reported rate is significantly higher than the incidence reported in the medical literature. These patients are characterized clinically by the delayed (2–3 weeks) onset of paraplegia or paraparesis without prior signs or symptoms. Patients receiving injections at two or more disc spaces following discography appear to be at increased risk.

Paraplegia, cerebral hemorrhage and other serious neurological changes have been reported soon after chymopapain injection in a small number of patients. Causal relationships to the drug when properly injected have not been established. Needle trauma and/or injection of chymopapain and contrast media into the spinal fluid may be causes in some of these reported cases. Other less severe neurologic reactions have included sacral burning, leg pain, hypalgesia, leg weakness, cramping in

Continued on next page

Smith—Cont.

both calves, pain in the opposite leg, paresthesia, tingling in legs, and numbness of legs/toes.
(3) The drug is extremely toxic when injected intrathecally in animals. Therefore, great caution must be exercised in assuring that Chymodiactin® is not injected intrathecally into the dural canal.
(4) Certain radio-opaque contrast media are neurotoxic. The toxicity of these materials may be enhanced by intrathecal bleeding. If Chymodiactin® is then inadvertently administered intrathecally, disruption of the capillaries may occur resulting in intrathecal bleeding.

Precautions:
General: Because of the potential for anaphylaxis resulting from the intradiscal injection of Chymodiactin®, the following precautions should be observed in the use of the drug:
Patient Selection: (1) A careful history should be conducted to determine if the patient has multiple allergies, especially a known allergy to papaya or papaya derivatives or iodine. Absorbable iodine should not be used during myelography or discography in patients allergic to iodine.
(2) The use of Chymodiactin® in a lumbar disc which has previously undergone surgical treatment has not been systematically studied. Therefore, chemonucleolysis at that disc level is not recommended.
(3) Females are more likely to develop an anaphylactic reaction secondary to Chymodiactin®. (See **Warnings.**).
(4) In case of anaphylaxis, beta-blocker therapy may block the action of epinephrine.
Pretreatment: (1) Patients may be pretreated prior to the injection of Chymodiactin® with histamine receptor (H_1 and H_2) antagonists to lessen the severity of an anaphylactic reaction. One regimen that has been widely used is cimetidine 300 mg orally every 6 hours and diphenhydramine 50 mg orally every 6 hours for 24 hours prior to chemonucleolysis.
(2) Because of the abrupt decrease in intravascular volume during anaphylaxis, patients should be well hydrated by oral or intravenous fluids prior to chemonucleolysis.
Procedure: (1) The choice of anesthetic for a specific patient should be made by the attending surgeon and anesthesiologist.
General anesthesia with endotracheal intubation has been employed in about 65% of patients receiving Chymodiactin® injection in post marketing surveillance reports. The advantages of general anesthesia are thought to be: ease of airway management if anaphylaxis should develop; more precise patient positioning for injection; less patient discomfort. A disadvantage of general anesthesia is a higher rate of anaphylaxis (0.9%). If halothane anesthesia is used, it should be noted that if epinephrine HCl is required for treatment of an anaphylactic reaction, there is a potential arrhythmogenic interaction of the two drugs.
Local anesthesia or supplemented local anesthesia has been employed in about 35% of patients receiving Chymodiactin® injection in post marketing surveillance reports. The advantages of local anesthesia are thought to be: a lower anaphylaxis rate (0.4%); possible ease of recognition of impending anaphylaxis because earliest symptoms can be reported by an awake patient; possible correlation of sciatic pain with a specific disc because the patient is awake.
(2) Needle placement for the intradiscal administration of Chymodiactin® should be made by physicians experienced in needle placement via the lateral approach to avoid puncture of the dura mater. Clinical trials have not been conducted using the posterior approach for needle placement and serious neurological toxicity has been reported using a posterior transdural approach, therefore, this method of needle placement is not recommended. Prior to injection of Chymodiactin®, visualization of the needle tip position in the disc must be confirmed using x-ray image intensifier for both the anteroposterior and lateral view. At least 15 minutes should elapse after the administration of radio-opaque contrast media for a discogram, if performed (see **Warnings**) to allow for diffusion and absorption of the media before injection of Chymodiactin® through the same needle after removal of the obturator.
(3) For 3 minutes prior to Chymodiactin® injection, 100% O_2 may be administered to the patient by the anesthesiologist to maximize oxygenation in case of anaphylaxis.
(4) *A test dose injection of 0.2 ml of Chymodiactin® followed by a 10–15 minute wait is recommended prior to the injection of the full therapeutic dose. The purpose of the test dose is to help identify those patients who are most sensitive to chymopapain, and patients who develop signs and/or symptoms of anaphylaxis following the test dose must not receive the therapeutic dose. However, some patients have been reported who failed to react to the test dose, but developed anaphylaxis to the therapeutic dose, suggesting that sensitivity to Chymodiactin® may be dose related.*
Patient Instructions: (1) Patients should be instructed that after injection they may experience back pain or involuntary muscle spasm in the lower area of the back for several days. This is not uncommon nor is a residual stiffness or soreness of the low back which may persist for several months.
(2) Patients should be instructed to anticipate the possibility of any of the following delayed allergic reactions which may occur as late as 15 days after injection: rash of any type, urticaria, or itching. If any of these occur, patients should contact their physician.
Pregnancy: Pregnancy Category C. Animal reproduction studies have not been conducted with Chymodiactin®. It is also not known whether Chymodiactin® can cause fetal harm when administered to a pregnant woman or can affect reproduction capacity. Chymodiactin® should be given to a pregnant woman only if clearly needed.
Pediatric Use: Safety and effectiveness of Chymodiactin® has not been studied in pediatric patients; therefore, the drug should not be used in children.
Adverse Reactions: The most serious adverse reactions encountered with the use of Chymodiactin® have been anaphylactic in nature. Based on post marketing surveillance reports, the overall frequency of anaphylaxis is 0.7% or about 1 in 125 patients. The frequency in females is approximately 1.2%, in males approximately 0.4%. The frequency when general anesthesia is employed is 0.9%, when local anesthesia is employed, 0.4%. These differences are statistically significant.
Several deaths have been reported in association with Chymodiactin® injection. These have been related to complications secondary to anaphylaxis, to staphylococcal meningitis with disc abscess or of unknown etiology. The mortality rate associated with Chymodiactin® is estimated at less than 1 in 3,000 patients (0.03%). For purposes of comparison, mortality associated with laminectomy has been reported to be 0.1%.
Acute transverse myelitis/acute transverse myelopathy has been reported in association with the injection of chymopapain at a rate of about 1 in 18,000. Although cause and effect relationship to the injection of chymopapain itself has not been established, the reported rate is significantly higher than the incidence reported in the medical literature. These patients are characterized clinically by the delayed (2–3 weeks) onset of paraplegia or paraparesis without prior signs or symptoms. Patients receiving injections at two or more disc spaces following discography appear to be at increased risk.
Paraplegia, cerebral hemorrhage and other serious neurological changes have been reported soon after chymopapain injection in a small number of patients. Causal relationships to the drug when properly injected have not been established. Needle trauma and/or injection of chymopapain and contrast media into the spinal fluid may be causes in some of these reported cases. Other less severe neurologic reactions have included sacral burning, leg pain, hypalgesia, leg weakness, cramping in both calves, pain in the opposite leg, paresthesia, tingling in legs, and numbness of legs/toes.
Discitis, both bacterial and aseptic, has been reported in several patients.
Less severe, but more frequent, adverse reactions include back pain/stiffness/soreness in approximately 50% of treated patients and/or back spasm in approximately 30%. Less frequent adverse reactions, occurring in less than 1% of patients studied include rash, itching, urticaria, nausea, paralytic ileus, urinary retention, headache, and dizziness.
Drug Abuse and Dependence: Chymodiactin® injection does not lend itself to drug abuse and dependence.
Overdosage: Overdosage has not occurred in the clinical trials of Chymodiactin®.
Theoretically, the chance of hypersensitivity reaction may be increased as more drug is used. The 5 ml vial of Chymodiactin® contains only 10,000 units of enzyme and when reconstituted and administered as directed (see **Dosage and Administration**) more than 10,000 units cannot be administered to one patient.
Dosage and Administration: Each 2 ml vial of Chymodiactin® contains 4,000 units (picoKatals) of enzyme and should be reconstituted with 2.0 ml Sterile Water for Injection, USP. Each 5 ml vial of Chymodiactin® contains 10,000 units of the enzyme and should be reconstituted with 5.0 ml Sterile Water for Injection, USP. The concentration of solution in the reconstituted vial is 2,000 units of Chymodiactin® per ml. Recommended dosage is 2,000 to 4,000 units per disc, usually 3,000 units per disc, or a volume of injection of 1 to 2 ml, usually 1.5 ml per disc. Maximum dose in a single patient with multiple disc herniation is 8,000 units.
A 5 ml vial of Sterile Water for Injection, USP is supplied with each vial of Chymodiactin®. *This is the only diluent which should be used to reconstitute the drug. Bacteriostatic Water for Injection, USP, must not be used* because it may inactivate the enzyme.
Alcohol should be used to cleanse the vial stopper prior to insertion of needles into the vial. However, since residual alcohol may inactivate the enzyme, it should be allowed to air dry before continuing with the reconstitution process. Parenteral drug products should be visually inspected for particulate matter and discoloration prior to administration. Care should be exercised in the selection of proper size and use of needles inserted into the vials in the reconstitution process to reduce the possibility of coring the stopper. The manufacturing process results in a residual vacuum in the vial; therefore, the use of automatic filling syringes is not recommended.
The drug must be used within two hours of its reconstitution with Sterile Water for Injection, USP. Unused drug must be promptly discarded and not stored for future use.
Each herniated disc should be treated with a single injection of Chymodiactin® after needle tip placement has been verified by image intensifier. If a discogram is performed (see **Warnings**) at least 15 minutes must elapse between discogram and drug administration to allow for dispersion and absorption of the contrast media.
Chymodiactin® is limited to use under the professional supervision of a physician licensed by law to administer it, with the following additional considerations:

The appropriate use of Chymodiactin® in chemonucleolysis, as pointed out in the **Indications and Usage** section of the labeling, requires precise diagnosis, and the ability to skillfully employ all acceptable diagnostic and treatment modalities as necessary, including surgical intervention other than chemonucleolysis, *e.g.*, laminectomy, including all aspects of pre and post operative patient care.

The proper selection of patients for whom chemonucleolysis is applicable is of the utmost importance and requires extensive training and experience in the diagnosis and management of all spinal disorders and diseases, since there are circumstances in which nerve root compression resulting from conditions other than the herniated disc can produce similar signs and symptoms.

The use of Chymodiactin®, therefore, should be limited to physicians who are trained not only in chemonucleolysis but who are qualified by training and experience to routinely care for such patients in other ways.

Chymodiactin® should be used only in a hospital setting with the assistance of trained personnel, and in such a manner as to assure immediate and proper management of all potential complications, especially including anaphylaxis.

How Supplied: Chymodiactin®, chymopapain for injection.

Chymodiactin® is supplied as a sterile, nonpyrogenic, lyophilized powder in vials containing either 4,000 or 10,000 units (picoKatals) of enzymatic activity. Each vial of Chymodiactin® is accompanied by a 5 ml vial of Sterile Water for Injection, USP, which is to be used as diluent. Chymodiactin® is available, with diluent, in single vials.

Although Chymodiactin® is stable at room temperature (77° F) for periods of time up to 9 months without loss of potency, this product should be stored under refrigeration (36° F to 46° F) until it is reconstituted with Sterile Water for Injection, USP, and used.

Animal Pharmacology and Toxicology: Injection of Chymodiactin® into the lumbar intervertebral disc of mature beagle dogs revealed narrowing of the intervertebral space noted on radiographs obtained at 48 hours and at 14 days. In dogs sacrificed at 14 days following injection, cavitation of the nucleus pulposus was observed, but the end plates were unaffected.

Chymopapain has previously been shown to dissolve the nucleus pulposus of dogs and rabbits at doses as low as 50 units/disc and 100 units/disc, respectively. Doses of 3,000 units/disc cause thinning of only the inner portion of the annulus in rabbits but do not penetrate the entire structure, while doses as high as 24,000 units/disc in dogs resulted in no apparent significant change in the peripheral portion of the annulus. *In vitro* studies demonstrated that chymopapain solubilized the mucopolysaccharide protein complex of human nucleus pulposus, but did not attack the collagen of this structure.

When chymopapain is injected into dogs and rabbits, doses up to 100 times greater than that required to remove the nucleus pulposus were well tolerated when injected intravenously, intradiscally, and epidurally. The drug is extremely toxic when injected intrathecally; the approximate LD_{50} is 15 units/kg in rabbits ,150 units/kg in dogs and 200 units/kg in baboons. Therefore, great caution must be exercised in assuring that Chymodiactin® is not injected intrathecally into the dural canal in the human. Method of injection is described in Dosage and Administration.

In baboons the serial injection into the spinal fluid of contrast agents (Renografin®, Conray® or Amipaque®) followed by Chymodiactin® 15 minutes later produced serious neurotoxicity, including weakness, paralysis and death. When administered singly at the same doses, Conray®, Amipaque® and Chymodiactin® were not toxic; Renografin® was less toxic singly than in combination with Chymodiactin®. This information supports the clinical observation that the documented entry of contrast agent and presumed entry of chymopapain into the spinal fluid can produce serious neurotoxicity including paraplegia and cerebral hemorrhage.

July 1984　　　　　　　　　　　　SL-9050
Shown in Product Identification Section, page 437

Springbok Pharmaceuticals, Inc.
12502 SOUTH GARDEN STREET
HOUSTON, TX 77071

E.N.T. Syrup ℞
Sugar-free decongestant

Each 5 ml. (one teaspoonful) orange-colored syrup contains:
Brompheniramine maleate .... 4 mg.
Phenylephrine hydrochloride .... 5 mg.
Phenylpropanolamine hydrochloride .... 5 mg.
Alcohol .... 2.3 %

How Supplied:
Bottles of 16 fluid ounces NDC 50821-376-16
Bottles of one gallon NDC 50821-376-28

E.N.T. Tablets ℞
Adult dose decongestant

Each prolonged-action, scored tablet contains:
Phenylephrine hydrochloride .... 25 mg.
Phenylpropanolamine hydrochloride .... 50 mg.
Chlorpheniramine maleate .... 8 mg.

How Supplied:
Bottles of 100 tablets NDC 50821-378-01
Bottles of 500 tablets NDC 50821-378-05

STOPAYNE CAPSULES ℞ ©
[stō¹pain]
Analgesic

Each blue/white capsule imprinted STOPAYNE/819 contains:
Hydrocodone Bitartrate .... 5 mg.
　(Warning: May be habit-forming)
Acetaminophen .... 500 mg.

How Supplied:
Bottles of 100 capsules　　NDC 50821-919-01
Bottles of 500 capsules　　NDC 50821-919-05
U/D Packs of 100 capsules　NDC 50821-919-03

STOPAYNE SYRUP ℞ ©
[stō¹pain]
Analgesic, antipyretic

Each 5 ml. (one teaspoonful) orange syrup contains:
Acetaminophen .... 120 mg.
Codeine phosphate .... 12 mg.
　(Warning: May be habit-forming)
Alcohol .... 7 percent

How Supplied:
Bottles of 16 fluid ounces　　NDC 50821-920-16

Products are listed alphabetically in the **PINK SECTION.**

Products are cross-indexed by product classifications in the **BLUE SECTION**

Products are cross-indexed by generic and chemical names in the **YELLOW SECTION**

E. R. Squibb & Sons, Inc.
GENERAL OFFICES
P.O. BOX 4000
PRINCETON, NJ 08540

For listing of standard and purified insulins, see Squibb-Novo, Inc.

For a listing of vaccines and biologicals, see Squibb/Connaught, Inc.

UNILOG®
(Tablet and Capsule Identification Code)
NUMERICAL INDEX

Unilog Number	Product
F16	**Principen with Probenecid** (Ampicillin-Probenecid Capsules)
113	**Velosef '250' Capsules** (Cephradine Capsules USP) 250 mg.
114	**Velosef '500' Capsules** (Cephradine Capsules USP) 500 mg.
160	**Ethril '250'** (Erythromycin Stearate Tablets USP) 250 mg.
161	**Ethril '500'** (Erythromycin Stearate Tablets USP) 500 mg.
164	**Pentids Tablets** (Penicillin G Potassium Tablets USP) 200,000 u.
165	**Pentids '400' Tablets** (Penicillin G Potassium Tablets USP) 400,000 u.
168	**Pentids '800' Tablets** (Penicillin G Potassium Tablets USP) 800,000 u.
194	**Vitamin C Tablets** 100 mg.
196	**Vitamin C Tablets** 250 mg.
197	**Vitamin C Tablets** 500 mg.
201	**Aspirin Tablets USP,** 5 gr. (324 mg.)
207	**Corgard** (Nadolol Tablets) 40 mg.
208	**Corgard** (Nadolol Tablets) 120 mg.
230	**Trimox '250' Capsules** (Amoxicillin Capsules USP) 250 mg.
231	**Trimox '500' Capsules** (Amoxicillin Capsules USP) 500 mg.
241	**Corgard** (Nadolol Tablets) 80 mg.
246	**Corgard** (Nadolol Tablets) 160 mg.
283	**Corzide** (Nadolol-Bendroflumethiazide Tablets) 40 mg.-5 mg.
284	**Corzide** (Nadolol-Bendroflumethiazide Tablets) 80 mg.-5 mg.
355	**Valadol Tablets** (Acetaminophen Tablets USP) 325 mg. (5 gr.)
429	**Florinef Acetate** (Fludrocortisone Acetate Tablets USP) 0.1 mg.
431	**Pronestyl Tablets** (Procainamide Hydrochloride Tablets) 250 mg.
434	**Pronestyl Tablets** (Procainamide Hydrochloride Tablets) 375 mg.
438	**Pronestyl Tablets** (Procainamide Hydrochloride Tablets) 500 mg.
452	**Capoten** (Captopril Tablets) 25 mg.
455	**Oragrafin Sodium Capsules** (Ipodate Sodium Capsules USP) 500 mg.
457	**Mycostatin Vaginal Tablets** (Nystatin Vaginal Tablets USP) 100,000 u.
478	**Engran-HP Tablets** (Multi-Vitamin and Multi-Mineral Supplement)
482	**Capoten** (Captopril Tablets) 50 mg.
485	**Capoten** (Captopril Tablets) 100 mg.
512	**Kenacort** (Triamcinolone Tablets USP) 4 mg.
518	**Kenacort**

Continued on next page

Squibb—Cont.

(Triamcinolone Tablets USP) 8 mg.
535 Theragran Hematinic
 (Therapeutic Formula Vitamin Tablets with Hematinics)
537 Niacin Tablets USP, 500 mg.
538 Rautrax-N Modified
 (Powdered Rauwolfia Serpentina 50 mg. and Bendroflumethiazide 2 mg. with Potassium Chloride 400 mg.)
539 Rautrax N
 (Powdered Rauwolfia Serpentina 50 mg. and Bendroflumethiazide 4 mg. with Potassium Choride 400 mg.)
549 Iron and Vitamin C Tablets
573 Ora-Testryl
 (Fluoxymesterone Tablets USP) 5 mg.
580 Mycostatin Oral Tablets
 (Nystatin Tablets USP) 500,000 u.
602 Naturetin c̄K
 (Bendroflumethiazide 2.5 mg. with Potassium Chloride 500 mg.)
603 Sumycin '500' Tablets
 (Tetracycline Hydrochloride Tablets USP) 500 mg.
605 Naturetin-2.5
 (Bendroflumethiazide Tablets USP) 2.5 mg.
606 Naturetin-5
 (Bendroflumethiazide Tablets USP) 5 mg.
608 Naturetin c̄K
 (Bendroflumethiazide 5 mg. with Potassium Chloride 500 mg.)
610 Niacin Tablets USP, 25 mg.
611 Niacin Tablets USP, 50 mg.
612 Niacin Tablets USP, 100 mg.
618 Naturetin-10
 (Bendroflumethiazide Tablets USP) 10 mg.
623 Noctec Capsules
 (Chloral Hydrate Capsules USP) 250 mg. (3¾ grains)
626 Noctec Capsules
 (Chloral Hydrate Capsules USP) 500 mg. (7½ grains)
637 Nydrazid Tablets
 (Isoniazid Tablets USP) 100 mg.
648 Veetids '500' Tablets
 (Penicillin V Potassium Tablets USP) 500 mg. (800,000 u.)
655 Sumycin '250' Capsules
 (Tetracycline Hydrochloride Capsules USP) 250 mg.
663 Sumycin '250' Tablets
 (Tetracycline Hydrochloride Tablets USP) 250 mg.
684 Veetids '250' Tablets
 (Penicillin V Potassium Tablets USP) 250 mg. (400,000 u.)
685 Rautrax
 (Powdered Rauwolfia Serpentina 50 mg. and Flumethiazide 400 mg. with Potassium Chloride 400 mg.)
690 Teslac Tablets
 (Testolactone Tablets USP) 50 mg.
713 Raudixin
 (Rauwolfia Serpentina Tablets USP) 50 mg.
736 Chlordiazepoxide Hydrochloride Capsules USP, 25 mg.
756 Pronestyl Capsules
 (Procainamide Hydrochloride Capsules USP) 375 mg.
757 Pronestyl Capsules
 (Procainamide Hydrochloride Capsules USP) 500 mg.
758 Pronestyl Capsules
 (Procainamide Hydrochloride Capsules USP) 250 mg.
763 Sumycin '500' Capsules
 (Tetracycline Hydrochloride Capsules USP) 500 mg.
769 Rauzide Tablets
 (50 mg. powdered Rauwolfia serpentina with 4 mg. bendroflumethiazide)
775 Pronestyl-SR Tablets
 (Procainamide Hydrochloride Tablets) 500 mg.
776 Raudixin
 (Rauwolfia Serpentina Tablets USP) 100 mg.
779 Mysteclin-F Capsules
 (Tetracycline - Amphotericin B Capsules) 250 mg. c̄ 50 mg.
788 Vitamin B$_{12}$ Capsules 25 mcg.
829 Chlorothiazide Tablets USP, 500 mg.
830 Hydrea Capsules
 (Hydroxyurea Capsules USP) 500 mg.
863 Prolixin Tablets
 (Fluphenazine Hydrochloride Tablets USP) 1 mg.
864 Prolixin Tablets
 (Fluphenazine Hydrochloride Tablets USP) 2.5 mg.
876 Trigesic Tablets
 (Analgesic Compound)
877 Prolixin Tablets
 (Fluphenazine Hydrochloride Tablets USP) 5 mg.
887 Terfonyl Tablets
 (Trisulfapyrimidines Tablets USP) 500 mg.
889 Vitamin E Capsules 100 I.U.
915 Vitamin B$_1$ Tablets 50 mg.
916 Vitamin B$_1$ Tablets 100 mg.
921 Vesprin Tablets
 (Triflupromazine Hydrochloride Tablets USP) 10 mg.
922 Vesprin Tablets
 (Triflupromazine Hydrochloride Tablets USP) 25 mg.
923 Vesprin Tablets
 (Triflupromazine Hydrochloride Tablets USP) 50 mg.
956 Prolixin Tablets
 (Fluphenazine Hydrochloride Tablets USP) 10 mg.
971 Principen '250' Capsules
 (Ampicillin Capsules USP) 250 mg.
974 Principen '500' Capsules
 (Ampicillin Capsules USP) 500 mg.

CAPOTEN® TABLETS R
[kap'o-ten"]
(Captopril Tablets)

Description: CAPOTEN (captopril) is the first of a new class of antihypertensive agents, a specific competitive inhibitor of angiotensin I-converting enzyme (ACE), the enzyme responsible for the conversion of angiotensin I to angiotensin II. Captopril is also effective in the management of heart failure.

CAPOTEN (captopril) is designated chemically as 1-[(2S)-3-mercapto-2-methylpropionyl]-L-proline [MW 217.29].

Captopril is a white to off-white crystalline powder with a slight acid-sulfhydryl odor; it is soluble in water (approx. 160 mg/ml), methanol, and ethanol and sparingly soluble in chloroform and ethyl acetate.

CAPOTEN (captopril) is available as scored tablets for oral administration.

Clinical Pharmacology: Mechanism of Action—The mechanism of action of CAPOTEN (captopril) has not yet been fully elucidated. It appears to act as an antihypertensive and as an adjunct in the therapy of heart failure primarily through suppression of the renin-angiotensin-aldosterone system; however, no consistent correlation has been described between renin levels and response to the drug. Renin, an enzyme synthesized by the kidneys, is released into the circulation where it acts on a plasma globulin substrate to produce angiotensin I, a relatively inactive decapeptide. Angiotensin I is then converted by angiotensin converting enzyme (ACE) to angiotensin II, a potent endogenous vasoconstrictor substance. Angiotensin II also stimulates aldosterone secretion from the adrenal cortex, thereby contributing to sodium and fluid retention.

CAPOTEN (captopril) prevents the conversion of angiotensin I to antiotensin II by inhibition of ACE, a peptidyldipeptide carboxy hydrolase. This inhibition has been demonstrated in both healthy human subjects and in animals by showing that the elevation of blood pressure caused by exogenously administered angiotensin I was attenuated or abolished by captopril. In animal studies, captopril did not alter the pressor responses to a number of other agents, including angiotensin II and norepinephrine, indicating specificity of action.

ACE is identical to "bradykininase," and CAPOTEN (captopril) may also interfere with the degradation of the vasodepressor peptide, bradykinin. However, the effectiveness of captopril in therapeutic doses appears to be unrelated to potentiation of the actions of bradykinin.

Inhibition of ACE results in decreased plasma angiotensin II and increased plasma renin activity (PRA), the latter resulting from loss of negative feedback on renin release caused by reduction in angiotensin II. The reduction of angiotensin II leads to decreased aldosterone secretion, and, as a result, to small increases in serum potassium.

The antihypertensive effects persist for a longer period of time than does demonstrable inhibition of circulating ACE. It is not known whether the ACE present in vascular endothelium is inhibited longer than the ACE in circulating blood.

Pharmacokinetics—After oral administration of therapeutic doses of CAPOTEN (captopril), rapid absorption occurs with peak blood levels at about one hour. The presence of food in the gastrointestinal tract reduces absorption by about 30 to 40 percent; captopril therefore should be given one hour before meals. Based on carbon-14 labeling, average minimal absorption is approximately 75 percent. In a 24-hour period, over 95 percent of the absorbed dose is eliminated in the urine; 40 to 50 percent is unchanged drug; most of the remainder is the disulfide dimer of captopril and captopril-cysteine disulfide.

Approximately 25 to 30 percent of the circulating drug is bound to plasma proteins. The apparent elimination half-life for total radioactivity in blood is probably less than 3 hours. An accurate determination of half-life of unchanged captopril is not, at present, possible, but it is probably less than 2 hours. In patients with renal impairment, however, retention of captopril occurs (see DOSAGE AND ADMINISTRATION).

Pharmacodynamics—Administration of CAPOTEN (captopril) results in a reduction of peripheral arterial resistance in hypertensive patients with either no change, or an increase, in cardiac output. There is an increase in renal blood flow following administration of CAPOTEN (captopril) and glomerular filtration rate is usually unchanged.

Reductions of blood pressure are usually maximal 60 to 90 minutes after oral administration of an individual dose of CAPOTEN (captopril). The duration of effect is dose related. The reduction in blood pressure may be progressive, so to achieve maximal therapeutic effects, several weeks of therapy may be required. The blood pressure lowering effects of captopril and thiazide-type diuretics are additive. In contrast, captopril and beta-blockers have a less than additive effect.

Blood pressure is lowered to about the same extent in both standing and supine positions. Orthostatic effects and tachycardia are infrequent but may occur in volume-depleted patients. Abrupt withdrawal of CAPOTEN (captopril) has not been associated with a rapid increase in blood pressure.

In patients with heart failure, significantly decreased peripheral (systemic vascular) resistance and blood pressure (afterload), reduced pulmonary capillary wedge pressure (preload) and pulmonary vascular resistance, increased cardiac output, and increased exercise tolerance time (ETT) have been demonstrated. These hemodynamic and clinical effects occur after the first dose and appear to persist for the duration of therapy. Placebo controlled studies of 12 weeks duration show no tolerance to beneficial effects on ETT; open studies, with exposure up to 18 months in some cases, also indicate that ETT benefit is maintained. Clinical improvement has been observed in some patients where acute hemodynamic effects were minimal.

Indications and Usage: Hypertension: Because serious adverse effects have been reported (see WARNINGS), CAPOTEN (captopril) is indicated for treatment of hypertensive patients who on multidrug regimens have either failed to respond satisfactorily or developed unacceptable side effects.

Usually, multidrug regimens include combinations of a diuretic, a sympathetic nervous system-active agent (such as a beta-blocker) and a vasodilator.

CAPOTEN is effective alone, but in the population described above, it should usually be used in combination with a thiazide-type diuretic. The blood pressure lowering effects of captopril and thiazides appear to be additive.

Heart Failure: CAPOTEN (captopril) is indicated in patients with heart failure who have not responded adequately to or cannot be controlled by conventional diuretic and digitalis therapy. CAPOTEN is to be used with diuretics and digitalis.

Warnings: Proteinuria—Total urinary proteins greater than 1 g per day were seen in 1.2 percent of patients receiving captopril and the nephrotic syndrome occurred in about one-fourth of these cases. The existence of prior renal disease increased the likelihood of the development of proteinuria. About 60 percent of affected patients had evidence or prior renal disease; the remainder had no known renal dysfunction. In most cases, proteinuria subsided or cleared within six months whether or not captopril was continued, but some patients had persistent proteinuria. Parameters of renal function, such as BUN and creatinine, were seldom altered in the patients with proteinuria. Membranous glomerulopathy was found in nearly all of the proteinuric patients receiving captopril who were biopsied, and may be drug related. This is uncertain, however, since patients were not biopsied prior to treatment and membranous glomerulopathy may be associated with hypertension in the absence of captopril treatment.

Since most cases of proteinuria occurred by the eighth month of therapy with captopril, patients receiving captopril should have urinary protein estimates (dip-stick on first morning urine, or quantitative 24-hour urine) prior to therapy, at approximately monthly intervals for the first nine months of treatment, and periodically thereafter. When proteinuria is persistent and/or at low levels, 24-hour quantitative determinations provide greater precision. For patients who develop proteinuria exceeding 1 g/day, or proteinuria that is increasing, the benefits and risks of continuing captopril should be evaluated.

Neutropenia/Agranulocytosis — Neutropenia ($<300/mm^3$) associated with myeloid hypoplasia (that was probably drug related) was observed in about 0.3 percent of patients treated with captopril. About half of the neutropenic patients developed systemic or oral cavity infections or other features of the syndrome of agranulocytosis. Most of the neutropenic patients had severe hypertension and renal functional impairment, and about half had systemic lupus erythematosus (SLE), or another autoimmune/collagen disorder. Multiple concomitant drug therapy was common, including immunosuppressive therapy in a few cases. Daily doses of captopril in the leukopenic patients were relatively high, particularly in view of their diminished renal function.

The neutropenia appeared 3 to 12 weeks after starting captopril, and it developed relatively slowly, the white count falling to its nadir over 10 to 30 days. Neutrophils returned to normal in about two weeks (other than in two patients who died of sepsis).

Captopril should be used with caution in patients with impaired renal function, serious autoimmune disease (particularly SLE), or who are exposed to other drugs known to affect the white cells or immune response.

In patients at particular risk (as noted above), white blood cell and differential counts should be performed before starting treatment, at approximately two-week intervals for about the first three months of therapy, and periodically thereafter.

The risk of neutropenia in patients who are less seriously ill or who receive lower dosages appears to be smaller, and it is sufficient in these patients to have white blood cell counts every two weeks for the first three months of captopril therapy, and periodically thereafter. Differential counts should be performed when leukocytes are $<4000/mm^3$, or the pretreatment white count is halved.

All patients treated with captopril should be told to report any signs of infection (e.g., sore throat; fever). If infection is suspected, counts should be performed without delay.

Since discontinuation of captopril and other drugs has generally led to prompt return of the white count to normal, upon confirmation of neutropenia (neutrophil count $<1000/mm^3$) the physician should withdraw captopril and closely follow the patient's course.

Hypotension—Excessive hypotension was rarely seen in hypertensive patients but is a possible consequence of captopril use in severely salt/volume depleted persons such as those treated vigorously with diuretics, for example, patients with severe congestive heart failure (see PRECAUTIONS [Drug Interactions]).

In heart failure, where the blood pressure was either normal or low, transient decreases in mean blood pressure greater than 20 percent were recorded in about half of the patients. This transient hypotension may occur after any of the first several doses and is usually well tolerated, producing either no symptoms or brief mild lightheadedness, although in rare instances it has been associated with arrhythmia or conduction defects. Hypotension was the reason for discontinuation of drug in 3.6 percent of patients with heart failure.

BECAUSE OF THE POTENTIAL FALL IN BLOOD PRESSURE IN THESE PATIENTS, THERAPY SHOULD BE STARTED UNDER VERY CLOSE MEDICAL SUPERVISION. A starting dose of 6.25 or 12.5 mg tid may minimize the hypotensive effect. Patients should be followed closely for the first two weeks of treatment and whenever the dose of captopril and/or diuretic is increased.

Hypotension is not *per se* a reason to discontinue captopril. Some decrease of systemic blood pressure is a common and desirable observation upon initiation of CAPOTEN (captopril) treatment in heart failure. The magnitude of the decrease is greatest early in the course of treatment; this effect stabilizes within a week or two, and generally returns to pretreatment levels, without a decrease in therapeutic efficacy, within two months.

Precautions: General—*Impaired Renal Function*—Hypertension—Some patients with renal disease, particularly those with severe renal artery stenosis, have developed increases in BUN and serum creatinine after reduction of blood pressure with captopril. Captopril dosage reduction and/or discontinuation of diuretic may be required. For some of these patients, it may not be possible to normalize blood pressure and maintain adequate renal perfusion.

Heart Failure—About 20 percent of patients develop stable elevations of BUN and serum creatinine greater than 20 percent above normal or baseline upon long-term treatment with captopril. Less than 5 percent of patients generally those with severe preexisting renal disease, required discontinuaton of treatment due to progressively increasing creatinine; subsequent improvement probably depends upon the severity of the underlying renal disease.

See CLINICAL PHARMACOLOGY, DOSAGE AND ADMINISTRATION, ADVERSE REACTIONS [Altered Laboratory Findings].

Valvular Stenosis: There is concern, on theroretical grounds, that patients with aortic stenosis might be at particular risk of decreased coronary perfusion when treated with vasodilators because they do not develop as much afterload reduction as others.

Surgery/Anesthesia: In patients undergoing major surgery or during anesthesia with agents that produce hypotension, captopril will block angiotensin II formation secondary to compensatory renin release. If hypotension occurs and is considered to be due to this mechanism, it can be corrected by volume expansion.

Information for Patients—Patients should be told to report promptly any indication of infection (e.g., sore throat, fever), which may be a sign of neutropenia, or of progressive edema which might be related to proteinuria and nephrotic syndrome.

All patients should be cautioned that excessive perspiration and dehydration may lead to an excessive fall in blood pressure because of reduction in fluid volume. Other causes of volume depletion such as vomiting or diarrhea may also lead to a fall in blood pressure; patients should be advised to consult with the physician.

Patients should be warned against interruption or discontinuation of medication unless instructed by the physician.

Heart failure patients on captopril therapy should be cautioned against rapid increases in physical activity.

Patients should be informed that CAPOTEN (captopril) should be taken one hour before meals (see DOSAGE AND ADMINISTRATION).

Drug Interactions—*Hypotension—Patients on Diuretic Therapy:* Patients on diuretics and especially those in whom diuretic therapy was recently instituted, as well as those on severe dietary salt restriction or dialysis, may occasionally experience a precipitous reduction of blood pressure within the first three hours after receiving the initial dose of captopril.

The possibility of hypotensive effects can be minimized by either discontinuing the diuretic or increasing the salt intake approximately one week prior to initiation of treatment with CAPOTEN (captopril). Alternatively, provide medical supervision for at least three hours after the initial dose. If hypotension occurs, the patient should be placed in a supine position and, if necessary, receive an intravenous infusion of normal saline. This transient hypotensive response is not a contraindication to further doses which can be given without difficulty once the blood pressure has increased after volume expansion.

Agents Having Vasodilator Activity: Data on the effect of concomitant use of other vasodilators in patients receiving CAPOTEN for heart failure are not available; therefore, nitroglycerin or other nitrates (as used for management of angina) or other drugs having vasodilator activity should, if possible, be discontinued before starting CAPOTEN. If resumed during CAPOTEN therapy, such agents should be administered cautiously, and perhaps at lower dosage.

Agents Causing Renin Release: Captopril's effect will be augmented by antihypertensive agents that cause renin release.

Agents Affecting Sympathetic Activity: The sympathetic nervous system may be especially important in supporting blood pressure in patients receiving captopril alone or with diuretics. Therefore, agents affecting sympathetic activity (e.g., ganglionic blocking agents or adrenergic neuron blocking agents) should be used with caution. Beta-adrenergic blocking drugs add some further antihypertensive effect to captopril, but the overall response is less than additive.

Agents Increasing Serum Potassium: Since captopril decreases aldosterone production, elevation of serum potassium may occur. Potassium-sparing diuretics such as spironolactone, triamterene, or amiloride, or potassium supplements should be given only for documented hypokalemia, and then with caution, since they may lead to a significant increase of serum potassium.

Drug/Laboratory Test Interaction—Captopril may cause a false-positive test for acetone.

Carcinogenesis, Mutagenesis and Impairment of Fertility—Two-year studies with doses of 50 to 1350 mg/kg/day in mice and rats failed to show any evidence of carcinogenic potential.

Studies in rats have revealed no impairment of fertility.

Continued on next page

Squibb—Cont.

Animal Toxicology—Chronic oral toxicity studies were conducted in rats (2 years) dogs (47 weeks; 1 year), mice (2 years), and monkeys (1 year). Significant drug-related toxicity included effects on hematopoiesis, renal toxicity, erosion/ulceration of the stomach, and variation of retinal blood vessels. Reductions in hemoglobin and/or hematocrit values were seen in mice, rats, and monkeys at doses 50 to 150 times the maximum recommended human dose (MRHD). Anemia, leukopenia, thrombocytopenia, and bone marrow suppression occurred in dogs at doses 8 to 30 times MRHD. The reductions in hemoglobin and hematocrit values in rats and mice were only significant at 1 year and returned to normal with continued dosing by the end of the study. Marked anemia was seen at all dose levels (8 to 30 times MRHD) in dogs, whereas moderate to marked leukopenia was noted only at 15 to 30 times MRHD and thrombocytopenia at 30 times MRHD. The anemia could be reversed upon discontinuation of dosing. Bone marrow suppression occurred to a varying degree, being associated only with dogs that died or were sacrificed in a moribund condition in the 1-year study. However, in the 47-week study at a dose 30 times MRHD, bone marrow suppression was found to be reversible upon continued drug administration.

Captopril caused hyperplasia of the juxtaglomerular apparatus of the kidneys at doses 7 to 200 times the MRHD in rats and mice, at 20 to 60 times MRHD in monkeys, and at 30 times the MRHD in dogs.

Gastric erosions/ulcerations were increased in incidence at 20 and 200 times MRHD in male rats and at 30 to 65 times MRHD in dogs and monkeys, respectively. Rabbits developed gastric and intestinal ulcers when given oral doses approximately 30 times MRHD for only 5 to 7 days.

In the two-year rat study, irreversible and progressive variations in the caliber of retinal vessels (focal sacculations and constrictions) occurred at all dose levels (7 to 200 times MRHD) in a dose-related fashion. The effect was first observed in the 88th week of dosing, with a progressively increased incidence thereafter, even after cessation of dosing.

Pregnancy: Category C—Captopril was embryocidal in rabbits when given in doses 2 to 70 times (on a mg/kg basis) the maximum recommended human dose. The marked embryocidal effect in rabbits was most probably due to the particularly marked decrease in blood pressure caused by the drug in this species.

Captopril given to pregnant rats at 400 times the recommended human dose continuously during gestation and lactation caused a reduction in neonatal survival.

No teratogenic effects (malformations) have been observed after large doses of captopril in hamsters, rats, and rabbits.

There are no adequate and well-controlled studies in pregnant women. Captopril should be used during pregnancy only if the potential benefit justifies the potential risk to the fetus.

Nursing Mothers—Concentrations of captopril in human milk are approximately one percent of those in maternal blood. The effect of low levels of captopril on the nursing infant has not been determined. Caution should be exercised when captopril is administered to a nursing woman, and, in general, nursing should be interrupted.

Pediatric Use—Safety and effectiveness in children have not been established although there is limited experience with the use of captopril in children from 2 months to 15 years of age with secondary hypertension and varying degrees of renal insufficiency. Dosage, on a weight basis, was comparable to that used in adults. CAPOTEN (captopril) should be used in children only if other measures for controlling blood pressure have not been effective.

Adverse Reactions: Reported incidences are based on clinical trials involving approximately 4000 patients.

Renal—One to two of 100 patients developed proteinuria (see WARNINGS).

Each of the following has been reported in approximately 1 to 2 of 1000 patients and are of uncertain relationship to drug use: renal insufficiency, renal failure, polyuria, oliguria, and urinary frequency.

Hematologic—Neutropenia/agranulocytosis that was probably drug related occurred in about 0.3 percent of patients treated with captopril (see WARNINGS). Two of these patients developed sepsis and died.

Dermatologic—Rash, often with pruritus, and sometimes with fever and eosinophilia, occurred in about 10 of 100 patients, usually during the first four weeks of therapy. It is usually maculopapular, and rarely urticarial. The rash is usually mild and disappears within a few days of dosage reduction, short-term treatment with an antihistaminic agent, and/or discontinuing therapy; remission may occur even if captopril is continued. Pruritus, without rash, occurs in about 2 of 100 patients. Between 7 and 10 percent of patients with skin rash have shown an eosinophilia and/or positive ANA titers. A reversible associated pemphigoid-like lesion, and photosensitivity have also been reported.

Angioedema of the face, mucous membranes of the mouth, or of the extremities has been observed in approximately 1 of 100 patients and is reversible on discontinuation of captopril therapy. One case of laryngeal edema has been reported.

Flushing or pallor has been reported in 2 to 5 of 1000 patients.

Cardiovascular—Hypotension occurred in approximately 2 of 100 patients. See WARNINGS (Hypotension) and PRECAUTIONS (Drug Interactions) for discussion of hypotension on initiation of captopril therapy.

Tachycardia, chest pain, and palpitations have each been observed in approximately 1 of 100 patients.

Angina pectoris, myocardial infarction, Raynaud's syndrome, and congestive heart failure have each occurred in 2 to 3 of 1000 patients.

Dysgeusia—Approximately 7 of 100 patients developed a diminution or loss of taste perception. Taste impairment is reversible and usually self-limited even with continued drug administration (2 to 3 months). Weight loss may be associated with the loss of taste.

The following have been reported in about 0.5 to 2 percent of patients but did not appear at increased frequency compared to placebo or other treatments used in controlled trials; gastric irritation, abdominal pain, nausea, vomiting, diarrhea, anorexia, constipation, aphthous ulcers, peptic ulcer, dizziness, headache, malaise, fatigue, insomnia, dry mouth, dyspnea, paresthesias.

Altered Laboratory Findings—Elevations of liver enzymes have been noted in a few patients but no causal relationship to captopril use has been established. Rare cases of cholestatic jaundice, and of hepatocellular injury with secondary cholestasis, have been reported in association with captopril administration.

A transient elevation of BUN and serum creatinine may occur, especially in patients who are volume-depleted or who have renovascular hypertension. In instances of rapid reduction of long-standing or severely elevated blood pressure, the glomerular filtration rate may decrease transiently, also resulting in transient rises in serum creatinine and BUN.

Small increases in the serum potassium concentration frequently occur, especially in patients with renal impairment (see PRECAUTIONS).

Overdosage: Correction of hypotension would be of primary concern. Volume expansion with an intravenous infusion of normal saline is the treatment of choice for restoration of blood pressure. Captopril may be removed from the general circulation by hemodialysis.

Dosage and Administration: CAPOTEN (captopril) should be taken one hour before meals. Dosage must be individualized.

Hypertension—Initiation of therapy requires consideration of recent antihypertensive drug treatment, the extent of blood pressure elevation, salt restriction, and other clinical circumstances. If possible, discontinue the patient's previous antihypertensive drug regimen for one week before starting CAPOTEN.

The initial dose of CAPOTEN (captopril) is 25 mg bid or tid. If satisfactory reduction of blood pressure has not been achieved after one or two weeks, the dose may be increased to 50 mg bid or tid.

The dose of CAPOTEN in hypertension usually does not exceed 50 mg tid. Therefore, if the blood pressure has not been satisfactorily controlled after one to two weeks at this dose, (and the patient is not already receiving a diuretic), a modest dose of a thiazide-type diuretic (e.g., hydrochlorothiazide, 25 mg daily), should be added. The diuretic dose may be increased at one- to two-week intervals until its highest usual antihypertensive dose is reached.

If further blood pressure reduction is required, the dose of CAPOTEN may be increased to 100 mg bid or tid and then, if necessary, to 150 mg bid or tid (while continuing the diuretic). The usual dose range is 25 to 150 mg bid or tid. A maximum daily dose of 450 mg CAPOTEN should not be exceeded.

For patients with accelerated or malignant hypertension, when temporary discontinuation of current antihypertensive therapy is not practical, or when prompt titration to more normotensive blood pressure levels is indicated, current antihypertensive medication may be stopped and CAPOTEN dosage promptly initiated at 25 mg bid or tid, under close medical supervision. The daily dose of CAPOTEN may be increased every 24 hours until a satisfactory blood pressure response is obtained or the maximum dose of CAPOTEN is reached. In this regimen, addition of a more potent diuretic, e.g., furosemide, may also be indicated. Beta-blockers may also be used in conjunction with CAPOTEN therapy (see PRECAUTIONS [Drug Interactions]), but the effects of the two drugs are less than additive.

Heart Failure—Initiation of therapy requires consideration of recent diuretic therapy and the possibility of severe salt/volume depletion. In patients with either normal or low blood pressure, who have been vigorously treated with diuretics and who may be hyponatremic and/or hypovolemic, a starting dose of 6.25 or 12.5 mg tid may minimize the magnitude or duration of the hypotensive effect (see WARNINGS, [Hypotension]); for these patients, titration to the usual daily dosage can then occur within the next several days.

For most patients the usual initial daily dosage is 25 mg tid. After a dose of 50 mg tid is reached, further increases in dosage should be delayed, where possible, for at least two weeks to determine if a satisfactory response occurs. Most patients studied have had a satisfactory clinical improvement at 50 or 100 mg tid. A maximum daily dose of 450 mg of CAPOTEN (captopril) should not be exceeded.

CAPOTEN is to be used in conjunction with a diuretic and digitalis. CAPOTEN therapy must be initiated under very close medical supervision.

Dosage Adjustment in Renal Impairment—Because CAPOTEN (captopril) is excreted primarily by the kidneys, excretion rates are reduced in patients with impaired renal function. These patients will take longer to reach steady-state captopril levels and will reach higher steady-state levels for a given daily dose than patients with normal renal function. Therefore, these patients may respond to smaller or less frequent doses.

Accordingly, for patients with significant renal impairment, initial daily dosage of CAPOTEN (captopril) should be reduced, and smaller increments utilized for titration, which should be quite slow (one- to two-week intervals). After the desired therapeutic effect has been achieved, the dose should be slowly back-titrated to determine the minimal effective dose. When concomitant diuretic therapy is required, a loop diuretic (e.g., furosemide), rather than a thiazide diuretic, is preferred in patients with severe renal impairment.

How Supplied: CAPOTEN (captopril) is available as white tablets in potencies of 25, 50, and 100 mg in bottles of 100, and in UNIMATIC® single dose packs of 100 tablets. Bottles contain desiccant and charcoal. The 25 mg tablet is a biconvex rounded square with a quadrisect bar; the 50 and 100 mg tablets are biconvex ovals with a bisect bar. Captopril tablets may exhibit a sight sulfurous odor.

Storage—Do not store above 86°F. Keep bottles tightly closed (protect from moisture).

CORGARD® ℞
[kor'gard]
(Nadolol Tablets)

Description: CORGARD (nadolol) is a synthetic nonselective beta-adrenergic receptor blocking agent chemically described as 2, 3-Naphthalenediol, 5- [3- [(1, 1- dimethylethyl) amino] -2- hydroxypropoxy]-1,2,3,4-tetrahydro-, cis-. Nadolol is a white crystalline powder, slightly soluble in water and freely soluble in ethanol.

CORGARD (nadolol) is available as tablets for oral administration.

Clinical Pharmacology: CORGARD (nadolol) is a nonselective beta-adrenergic receptor blocking agent. Clinical pharmacology studies have demonstrated beta-blocking activity by showing (1) reduction in heart rate and cardiac output at rest and on exercise, (2) reduction of systolic and diastolic blood pressure at rest and on exercise, (3) inhibition of isoproterenol-induced tachycardia, and (4) reduction of reflex orthostatic tachycardia. CORGARD (nadolol) specifically competes with beta-adrenergic receptor agonists for available beta receptor sites; it inhibits both the $beta_1$ receptors located chiefly in cardiac muscle and the $beta_2$ receptors located chiefly in the bronchial and vascular musculature, inhibiting the chronotropic, inotropic, and vasodilator responses to beta-adrenergic stimulation proportionately. CORGARD (nadolol) has no intrinsic sympathomimetic activity and, unlike some other beta-adrenergic blocking agents, nadolol has little direct myocardial depressant activity and does not have an anesthetic-like membrane-stabilizing action. Animal and human studies show that CORGARD (nadolol) slows the sinus rate and depresses AV conduction. In dogs, only minimal amounts of nadolol were detected in the brain relative to amounts in blood and other organs and tissues.

In controlled clinical studies, CORGARD (nadolol) at doses of 40 to 320 mg./day has been shown to decrease both standing and supine blood pressure, the effect persisting for approximately 24 hours after dosing.

The mechanism of the antihypertensive effects of beta-adrenergic receptor blocking agents has not been established; however, factors that may be involved include (1) competitive antagonism of catecholamines at peripheral (non-CNS) adrenergic neuron sites (especially cardiac) leading to decreased cardiac output, (2) a central effect leading to reduced tonic-sympathetic nerve outflow to the periphery, and (3) suppression of renin secretion by blockade of the beta-adrenergic receptors responsible for renin release from the kidneys.

By blocking catecholamine-induced increases in heart rate, velocity and extent of myocardial contraction, and blood pressure, CORGARD (nadolol) generally reduces the oxygen requirements of the heart at any given level of effort, making it useful for many patients in the long-term management of angina pectoris. On the other hand, nadolol can increase oxygen requirements by increasing left ventricular fiber length and end diastolic pressure, particularly in patients with heart failure. Although beta-adrenergic receptor blockade is useful in treatment of angina and hypertension, there are also situations in which sympathetic stimulation is vital. For example, in patients with severely damaged hearts, adequate ventricular function may depend on sympathetic drive. Beta-adrenergic blockade may worsen AV block by preventing the necessary facilitating effects of sympathetic activity on conduction. $Beta_2$-adrenergic blockade results in passive bronchial constriction by interfering with endogenous adrenergic bronchodilator activity in patients subject to bronchospasm and may also interfere with exogenous bronchodilators in such patients.

Absorption of nadolol after oral dosing is variable, averaging about 30 percent. Peak serum concentrations of nadolol usually occur in three to four hours after oral administration and the presence of food in the gastrointestinal tract does not affect the rate or extent of nadolol absorption. Approximately 30 percent of the nadolol present in serum is reversibly bound to plasma protein.

Unlike many other beta-adrenergic blocking agents, nadolol is not metabolized and is excreted unchanged, principally by the kidneys.

The half-life of therapeutic doses of nadolol is about 20 to 24 hours, permitting once-daily dosage. Because nadolol is excreted predominantly in the urine, its half-life increases in renal failure (see PRECAUTIONS and DOSAGE AND ADMINISTRATION). Steady-state serum concentrations of nadolol are attained in six to nine days with once-daily dosage in persons with normal renal function. Because of variable absorption and different individual responsiveness, the proper dosage must be determined by titration.

Exacerbation of angina and, in some cases, myocardial infarction and ventricular dysrhythmias have been reported after abrupt discontinuation of therapy with beta-adrenergic blocking agents in patients with coronary artery disease. Abrupt withdrawal of these agents in patients without coronary artery disease has resulted in transient symptoms, including tremulousness, sweating, palpitation, headache, and malaise. Several mechanisms have been proposed to explain these phenomena, among them increased sensitivity to catecholamines because of increased numbers of beta receptors.

Indications and Usage:

Angina Pectoris—CORGARD (nadolol) is indicated for the long-term management of patients with angina pectoris.

Hypertension—CORGARD (nadolol) is indicated in the management of hypertension; it may be used alone or in combination with other antihypertensive agents, especially thiazide-type diuretics.

Contraindications: Nadolol is contraindicated in bronchial asthma, sinus bradycardia and greater than first degree conduction block, cardiogenic shock, and overt cardiac failure (see WARNINGS).

Warnings:

Cardiac Failure—Sympathetic stimulation may be a vital component supporting circulatory function in patients with congestive heart failure, and its inhibition by beta-blockade may precipitate more severe failure. Although beta-blockers should be avoided in overt congestive heart failure, if necessary, they can be used with caution in patients with a history of failure who are well-compensated, usually with digitalis and diuretics. Beta-adrenergic blocking agents do not abolish the inotropic action of digitalis on heart muscle.

IN PATIENTS WITHOUT A HISTORY OF HEART FAILURE, continued use of beta-blockers can, in some cases, lead to cardiac failure. Therefore, at the first sign or symptom of heart failure, the patient should be digitalized and/or treated with diuretics, and the response observed closely, or nadolol should be discontinued (gradually, if possible).

Exacerbation of Ischemic Heart Disease Following Abrupt Withdrawal—Hypersensitivity to catecholamines has been observed in patients withdrawn from beta-blocker therapy; exacerbation of angina and, in some cases, myocardial infarction have occurred after *abrupt* discontinuation of such therapy. When discontinuing chronically administered nadolol, particularly in patients with ischemic heart disease, the dosage should be gradually reduced over a period of one to two weeks and the patient should be carefully monitored. If angina markedly worsens or acute coronary insufficiency develops, nadolol administration should be reinstituted promptly, at least temporarily, and other measures appropriate for the management of

unstable angina should be taken. Patients should be warned against interruption or discontinuation of therapy without the physician's advice. Because coronary artery disease is common and may be unrecognized, it may be prudent not to discontinue nadolol therapy abruptly even in patients treated only for hypertension.

Nonallergic Bronchospasm (e.g., chronic bronchitis, emphysema)—PATIENTS WITH BRONCHOSPASTIC DISEASES SHOULD IN GENERAL NOT RECEIVE BETA-BLOCKERS. Nadolol should be administered with caution since it may block bronchodilation produced by endogenous or exogenous catecholamine stimulation of $beta_2$ receptors.

Major Surgery—Because beta-blockade impairs the ability of the heart to respond to reflex stimuli and may increase the risks of general anesthesia and surgical procedures, resulting in protracted hypotension or low cardiac output, it has generally been suggested that such therapy should be withdrawn several days prior to surgery. Recognition of the increased sensitivity to catecholamines of patients recently withdrawn from beta-blocker therapy, however, has made this recommendation controversial. If possible, beta-blockers should be withdrawn well before surgery takes place. In the event of emergency surgery, the anesthesiologist should be informed that the patient is on beta-blocker therapy. The effects of nadolol can be reversed by administration of beta-receptor agonists such as isoproterenol, dopamine, dobutamine, or levarterenol. Difficulty in restarting and maintaining the heart beat has also been reported with beta-adrenergic receptor blocking agents.

Diabetes and Hypoglycemia—Beta-adrenergic blockade may prevent the appearance of premonitory signs and symptoms (e.g., tachycardia and blood pressure changes) of acute hypoglycemia. This is especially important with labile diabetics. Beta-blockade also reduces the release of insulin in response to hyperglycemia; therefore, it may be necessary to adjust the dose of antidiabetic drugs.

Thyrotoxicosis—Beta-adrenergic blockade may mask certain clinical signs (e.g., tachycardia) of hyperthyroidism. Patients suspected of developing thyrotoxicosis should be managed carefully to avoid abrupt withdrawal of beta-adrenergic blockade which might precipitate a thyroid storm.

Precautions:

Impaired Hepatic or Renal Function—Nadolol should be used with caution in patients with impaired hepatic or renal function (see DOSAGE AND ADMINISTRATION).

Information for Patients—Patients, especially those with evidence of coronary artery insufficiency, should be warned against interruption or discontinuation of nadolol therapy without the physician's advice. Although cardiac failure rarely occurs in properly selected patients, patients being treated with beta-adrenergic blocking agents should be advised to consult the physician at the first sign or symptom of impending failure.

Drug Interactions — Catecholamine-depleting drugs (e.g., reserpine) may have an additive effect when given with beta-blocking agents. Patients treated with nadolol plus a catecholamine-depleting agent should therefore be closely observed for evidence of hypotension and/or excessive bradycardia which may produce vertigo, syncope, or postural hypotension.

Carcinogenesis, Mutagenesis, Impairment of Fertility—In chronic oral toxicologic studies (one to two years) in mice, rats, and dogs, nadolol did not produce any significant toxic effects. In two-year oral carcinogenic studies in rats and mice, nadolol did not produce any neoplastic, preneoplastic, or nonneoplastic pathologic lesions. In fertility and general reproductive performance studies in rats, nadolol caused no adverse effects.

Pregnancy—Teratogenic Effects: Pregnancy Category C. In animal reproduction studies with nadolol, evidence of embryo- and fetotoxicity was found

Continued on next page

Squibb—Cont.

in rabbits, but not in rats or hamsters, at doses 5 to 10 times greater (on a mg./kg. basis) than the maximum indicated human dose. No teratogenic potential was observed in any of these species. There are no adequate and well-controlled studies in pregnant women. Nadolol should be used during pregnancy only if the potential benefit justifies the potential risk to the fetus.

Nursing Mothers—It is not known whether this drug is excreted in human milk. Because many drugs are excreted in human milk, caution should be exercised when nadolol is administered to a nursing woman.

Animal studies showed that nadolol is found in the milk of lactating rats.

Pediatric Use—Safety and effectiveness in children have not been established.

Adverse Reactions: Most adverse effects have been mild and transient and have rarely required withdrawal of therapy.

Cardiovascular—Bradycardia with heart rates of less than 60 beats per minute occurs commonly, and heart rates below 40 beats per minute and/or symptomatic bradycardia were seen in about 2 of 100 patients. Symptoms of peripheral vascular insufficiency, usually of the Raynaud type, have occurred in approximately 2 of 100 patients. Cardiac failure, hypotension, and rhythm/conduction disturbances have each occurred in about 1 of 100 patients. Single instances of first degree and third degree heart block have been reported; intensification of AV block is a known effect of beta-blockers (see also CONTRAINDICATIONS, WARNINGS, and PRECAUTIONS).

Central Nervous System—Dizziness or fatigue have each been reported in approximately 2 of 100 patients; paresthesias, sedation, and change in behavior have each been reported in approximately 6 of 1000 patients.

Respiratory—Bronchospasm has been reported in approximately 1 of 1000 patients (see CONTRAINDICATIONS and WARNINGS).

Gastrointestinal—Nausea, diarrhea, abdominal discomfort, constipation, vomiting, indigestion, anorexia, bloating, and flatulence have been reported in 1 to 5 of 1000 patients.

Miscellaneous—Each of the following has been reported in 1 to 5 of 1000 patients: rash; pruritus; headache; dry mouth, eyes, or skin; impotence or decreased libido; facial swelling; weight gain; slurred speech; cough; nasal stuffiness; sweating; tinnitus; blurred vision.

Sleep disturbances have been reported, but their relationship to drug usage is not clear.

The oculomucocutaneous syndrome associated with the beta-blocker practolol has not been reported with nadolol.

Potential Adverse Effects: In addition, other adverse effects not reported with nadolol have been reported with other beta-adrenergic blocking agents and should be considered potential adverse effects of nadolol.

Central Nervous System—Reversible mental depression progressing to catatonia; visual disturbances; hallucinations; an acute reversible syndrome characterized by disorientation for time and place, short-term memory loss, emotional lability with slightly clouded sensorium, and decreased performance on neuropsychometrics.

Gastrointestinal—Mesenteric arterial thrombosis; ischemic colitis.

Hematologic—Agranulocytosis; thrombocytopenic or nonthrombocytopenic purpura.

Allergic—Fever combined with aching and sore throat; laryngospasm; respiratory distress.

Miscellaneous—Reversible alopecia; Peyronie's disease; erythematous rash.

Overdosage: Nadolol can be removed from the general circulation by hemodialysis.

In addition to gastric lavage, the following measures should be employed, as appropriate. In determining the duration of corrective therapy, note must be taken of the long duration of the effect of nadolol.

Excessive Bradycardia—Administer atropine (0.25 to 1.0 mg.). If there is no response to vagal blockade, administer isoproterenol cautiously.

Cardiac Failure—Administer a digitalis glycoside and diuretic. It has been reported that glucagon may also be useful in this situation.

Hypotension—Administer vasopressors, e.g., epinephrine or levarterenol. (There is evidence that epinephrine may be the drug of choice.)

Bronchospasm—Administer a $beta_2$-stimulating agent and/or a theophylline derivative.

Dosage and Administration: DOSAGE MUST BE INDIVIDUALIZED. CORGARD (NADOLOL) MAY BE ADMINISTERED WITHOUT REGARD TO MEALS.

Angina Pectoris—The usual initial dose is 40 mg. CORGARD (nadolol) once daily. Dosage should be gradually increased in 40 to 80 mg. increments at 3- to 7-day intervals until optimum clinical response is obtained or there is pronounced slowing of the heart rate. The usual maintenance dose range is 80 to 240 mg. administered once daily, with most patients responding to 160 mg. or less daily.

The usefulness and safety in angina pectoris of dosage exceeding 240 mg. per day have not been established. If treatment is to be discontinued, reduce the dosage gradually over a period of one to two weeks (see WARNINGS).

Hypertension—The usual initial dose is 40 mg CORGARD (nadolol) once daily, whether it is used alone or in addition to diuretic therapy. Dosage may be gradually increased in 40 to 80 mg. increments until optimum blood pressure reduction is achieved. The usual maintenance dose is 80 to 320 mg., administered once daily. In rare instances, daily doses up to 640 mg. may be needed.

Dosage Adjustment in Renal Failure—Absorbed nadolol is excreted principally by the kidneys and, although nonrenal elimination does occur, dosage adjustments are necessary in patients with renal impairment. The following dose intervals are recommended:

Creatinine Clearance (ml/min/1.73m^2)	Dosage Interval (hours)
>50	24
31–50	24–36
10–30	24–48
<10	40–60

How Supplied: CORGARD Tablets (Nadolol Tablets) are supplied as scored tablets containing 40, 80, 120, or 160 mg. nadolol per tablet in bottles of 100 and 1000 tablets and in Unimatic® unit-dose packs of 100 tablets. [Military Depot Item: 40 mg, 100's, NSN 6505-01-113-8345; 40 mg, 1000's, NSN 6505-01-114-9384; 80 mg, 1000's, NSN 6505-01-110-1994; 120 mg, 1000's, NSN 6505-01-110-1995.]

Storage: Store at room temperature; avoid excessive heat. Protect from light. Keep bottle tightly closed. Dispense in tight, light-resistant containers.

Shown in Product Identification Section, page 437

CORZIDE® 40/5
CORZIDE® 80/5
[kor'zīd]
Nadolol-Bendroflumethiazide Tablets

Description: CORZIDE (Nadolol-Bendroflumethiazide Tablets) for oral administration combines two antihypertensive agents: CORGARD® (nadolol), a nonselective beta-adrenergic blocking agent, and NATURETIN® (bendroflumethiazide), a thiazide diuretic-antihypertensive. Formulations: 40 mg and 80 mg nadolol per tablet combined with 5 mg bendroflumethiazide.

Nadolol—Nadolol is a white crystalline powder. It is freely soluble in ethanol, soluble in hydrochloric acid, slightly soluble in water and in chloroform, and very slightly soluble in sodium hydroxide.

Nadolol is designated chemically as 1-(tert-butylamino) -3- [5,6,7,8,-tetrahydro-cis-6,7,-dihydroxy-1-naphthyl)oxy]-2-propanol.

Bendroflumethiazide—Bendroflumethiazide is a white crystalline powder. It is soluble in alcohol and in sodium hydroxide, and insoluble in hydrochloric acid, water, and chloroform.

Bendroflumethiazide is designated chemically as 3-benzyl-3,4,-dihydro-6-(trifluoromethyl)-2H-1,2,4-benzothiadiazine-7-sulfonamide 1,1-dioxide.

Clinical Pharmacology: Nadolol—Nadolol is a nonselective beta-adrenergic receptor blocking agent. Clinical pharmacology studies have demonstrated beta-blocking activity by showing (1) reduction in heart rate and cardiac output at rest and on exercise, (2) reduction of systolic and diastolic blood pressure at rest and on exercise, (3) inhibition of isoproterenol-induced tachycardia, and (4) reduction of reflex orthostatic tachycardia. Nadolol specifically competes with beta-adrenergic receptor agonists for available beta receptor sites; it inhibits both the $beta_1$ receptors located chiefly in cardiac muscle and the $beta_2$ receptors located chiefly in the bronchial and vascular musculature, inhibiting the chronotropic, inotropic, and vasodilator responses to beta-adrenergic stimulation proportionately. Nadolol has no intrinsic sympathomimetic activity and, unlike some other beta-adrenergic blocking agents, nadolol has little direct myocardial depressant activity and does not have an anesthetic-like membrane-stabilizing action. Animal and human studies show that nadolol slows the sinus rate and depresses AV conduction. In dogs, only minimal amounts of nadolol were detected in the brain relative to amounts in blood and other organs and tissues.

In controlled clinical studies, nadolol at doses of 40 to 320 mg/day has been shown to decrease both standing and supine blood pressure, the effect persisting for approximately 24 hours after dosing. The mechanism of the antihypertensive effects of beta-adrenergic receptor blocking agents has not been established; however, factors that may be involved include (1) competitive antagonism of catecholamines at peripheral (non-CNS) adrenergic neuron sites (especially cardiac) leading to decreased cardiac output, (2) a central effect leading to reduced tonic-sympathetic nerve outflow to the periphery, and (3) suppression of renin secretion by blockade of the beta-adrenergic receptors responsible for renin release from the kidneys.

By blocking catecholamine-induced increases in heart rate, velocity and extent of myocardial contraction, and blood pressure, nadolol generally reduces the oxygen requirements of the heart at any given level of effort, making it useful for many patients in the long-term management of angina pectoris. On the other hand, nadolol can increase oxygen requirements by increasing left ventricular fiber length and end diastolic pressure, particularly in patients with heart failure.

Although beta-adrenergic receptor blockade is useful in treatment of angina and hypertension, there are also situations in which sympathetic stimulation is vital. For example, in patients with severely damaged hearts, adequate ventricular function may depend on sympathetic drive. Beta-adrenergic blockade may worsen AV block by preventing the necessary facilitating effects of sympathetic activity on conduction. $Beta_2$-adrenergic blockade results in passive bronchial constriction by interfering with endogenous adrenergic bronchodilator activity in patients subject to bronchospasm and may also interfere with exogenous bronchodilators in such patients.

Absorption of nadolol after oral dosing is variable, averaging about 30 percent. Peak serum concentrations of nadolol usually occur in three to four hours after oral administration and the presence of food in the gastrointestinal tract does not affect the rate or extent of nadolol absorption. Approximately 30 percent of the nadolol present in serum is reversibly bound to plasma protein.

Unlike may other beta-adrenergic blocking agents, nadolol is not metabolized and is excreted unchanged, principally by the kidneys.

The half-life of therapeutic doses of nadolol is about 20 to 24 hours, permitting once-daily dosage. Because nadolol is excreted predominantly in the urine, its half-life increases in renal failure (see PRECAUTIONS, *General*, and DOSAGE AND ADMINISTRATION). Steady state serum concentrations of nadolol are attained in six to nine days with once-daily dosage in persons with normal renal function. Because of variable absorption and different individual responsiveness, the proper dosage must be determined by titration.

Exacerbation of angina and, in some cases, myocardial infarction and ventricular dysrhythmias have been reported after abrupt discontinuation of therapy with beta-adrenergic blocking agents in patients with coronary artery disease. Abrupt withdrawal of these agents in patients without coronary artery disease has resulted in transient symptoms, including tremulousness, sweating, palpitation, headache, and malaise. Several mechamisms have been proposed to explain these phenomena, among them increased sensitivity to catecholamines because of increased numbers of beta receptors.

Bendroflumethiazide—The mechanism of action of bendroflumethiazide results in an interference with the renal tubular mechanism of electrolyte reabsorption. At maximal therapeutic dosage all thiazides are approximately equal in their diuretic potency. The mechamism whereby thiazides function in the control of hypertension is unknown.

Indications: CORZIDE (Nadolol-Bendroflumethiazide Tablets) is indicated in the management of hypertension.

This fixed combination drug is not indicated for initial therapy of hypertension. If the fixed combination represents the dose titrated to the individual patient's needs, it may be more convenient than the separate components.

Contraindications: Nadolol—Nadolol is contraindicated in bronchial asthma, sinus bradycardia and greater than first degree conduction block, cardiogenic shock, and overt cardiac failure (see WARNINGS).

Bendroflumethiazide—Bendroflumethiazide is contraindicated in anuria. It is also contraindicated in patients who have previously demonstrated hypersensitivity to bendroflumethiazide or other sulfonamide-derived drugs.

Warnings: Nadolol—**Cardiac Failure**—Sympathetic stimulation may be a vital component supporting circulatory function in patients with congestive heart failure, and its inhibition by beta-blockade may precipitate more severe failure. Although beta-blockers should be avoided in overt congestive heart failure, if necessary, they can be used with caution in patients with a history of failure who are well compensated, usually with digitalis and diuretics. Beta-adrenergic blocking agents do not abolish the inotropic action of digitalis on heart muscle.

IN PATIENTS WITHOUT A HISTORY OF HEART FAILURE, continued use of beta-blockers can, in some cases, lead to cardiac failure. Therefore, at the first sign or symptom of heart failure, the patient should be digitalized and/or treated with diuretics, and the response observed closely, or nadolol should be discontinued (gradually, if possible).

Exacerbation of Ischemic Heart Disease Following Abrupt Withdrawal—Hypersensitivity to catecholamines has been observed in patients withdrawn from beta-blocker therapy; exacerbation of angina and, in some cases, myocardial infarction have occurred after *abrupt* discontinuation of such therapy. When discontinuing chronically administered nadolol, particularly in patients with ischemic heart disease, the dosage should be gradually reduced over a period of one to two weeks and the patient should be carefully monitored. If angina markedly worsens or acute coronary insufficiency develops, nadolol administration should be reinstituted promptly, at least temporarily, and other measures appropriate for the management of unstable angina should be taken. Patients should be warned against interruption or discontinuation of therapy without the physician's advice. Because coronary artery disease is common and may be unrecognized, it may be prudent not to discontinue nadolol therapy abruptly even in patients treated only for hypertension.

Nonallergic Bronchospasm (e.g., chronic bronchitis, emphysema)—PATIENTS WITH BRONCHOSPASTIC DISEASES SHOULD IN GENERAL NOT RECEIVE BETA-BLOCKERS. Nadolol should be administered with caution since it may block bronchodilation produced by endogenous or exogenous catecholamine stimulation of beta$_2$ receptors.

Major Surgery—Because beta blockade impairs the ability of the heart to respond to reflex stimuli and may increase the risks of general anesthesia and surgical procedures, resulting in protracted hypotension or low cardiac output, it has generally been suggested that such therapy should be withdrawn several days prior to surgery. Recognition of the increased sensitivity to catecholamines of patients recently withdrawn from beta-blocker therapy, however, has made this recommendation controversial. If possible, beta-blockers should be withdrawn well before surgery takes place. In the event of emergency surgery, the anesthesiologist should be informed that the patient is on beta-blocker therapy. The effects of nadolol can be reversed by administration of beta-receptor agonists such as isoproterenol, dopamine, dobutamine, or levarterenol. Difficulty in restarting and maintaining the heart beat has also been reported with beta-adrenergic receptor blocking agents.

Diabetes and Hypoglycemia—Beta-adrenergic blockade may prevent the appearance of premonitory signs and syptoms (e.g., tachycardia and blood pressure changes) of acute hypoglycemia. This is especially important with labile diabetics. Beta-blockade also reduces the release of insulin in response to hyperglycemia; therefore, it may be necessary to adjust the dose of antidiabetic drugs.

Thyrotoxicosis—Beta-adrenergic blockage may mask certain clinical signs (e.g., tachycardia) of hyperthyroidism. Patients suspected of developing thyrotoxicosis should be managed carefully to avoid abrupt withdrawal of beta-adrenergic blockade which might precipitate a thyroid storm.

Bendroflumethiazide—Thiazides should be used with caution in severe renal disease. In patients with renal disease, thiazides may precipitate azotemia. Cumulative effects of the drug may develop in patients with impaired renal function.

Thiazides should be used with caution in patients with impaired hepatic function or progressive liver disease, since minor alterations of fluid and electrolyte balance may precipitate hepatic coma. Sensitivity reactions may occur in patients with a history of allergy or bronchial asthma.

The possibility of exacerbation or activation of systemic lupus erythematosus has been reported.

Precautions: General—**Nadolol**—Nadolol should be used with caution in patients with impaired hepatic or renal function (see DOSAGE AND ADMINISTRATION).

Bendroflumethiazide—All patients receiving thiazide therapy should be observed for clinical signs or fluid or electrolyte imbalance, namely, hyponatremia, hypochloremic alkalosis, and hypokalemia. Serum and urine electrolyte determinations are particularly important when the patient is vomiting excessively or receiving parenteral fluids. Medication such as digitalis may also influence serum electrolytes. Warning signs, irrespective of cause, are: dryness of the mouth, thirst, weakness, lethargy, drowsiness, restlessness, muscle pains or cramps, muscular fatigue, hypotension, oliguria, tachycardia, and gastrointestinal disturbances, such as nausea and vomiting.

Hypokalemia may develop with thiazides as with any other potent diuretic, especially with brisk diuresis, when severe cirrhosis is present.

Interference with adequate oral electrolyte intake will also contribute to hypokalemia. Hypokalemia can sensitize or exaggerate the response of the heart to the toxic effects of digitalis (e.g., increased ventricular irritability). Hypokalemia may be avoided or treated by use of potassium supplements such as foods with a high potassium content.

Any chloride deficit is generally mild and usually does not require specific treatment except under extraordinary circumstances (as in liver disease or renal disease). Dilutional hyponatremia may oc-

cur in edematous patients in hot weather; appropriate therapy is water restriction, rather than administration of salt except in rare instances when the hyponatremia is life threatening. In actual salt depletion, appropriate replacement is the therapy of choice.

Hyperuricemia may occur or frank gout may be precipitated in certain patients receiving thiazide therapy.

Latent diabetes mellitus may become manifest during thiazide administration.

The antihypertensive effects of the drug may be enhanced in the post-sympathectomy patient.

If progressive renal impairment becomes evident, as indicated by rising nonprotein nitrogen or blood urea nitrogen, a careful reappraisal of therapy is necessary with consideration given to withholding or discontinuing diuretic therapy.

Thiazides may decrease serum PBI levels without signs of thyroid disturbances.

Calcium excretion is decreased by thiazides. Pathologic changes in the parathyroid gland with hypercalcemia and hypophosphatemia have been observed in a few patients on prolonged thiazide therapy. The common complications of hyperparathyroidism have not been seen.

Information for Patients—Patients, especially those with evidence of coronary artery insufficiency, should be warned against interruption or discontinuation of therapy without the physician's advice. Although cardiac failure rarely occurs in properly selected patients, patients being treated with beta-adrenergic blocking agents should be advised to consult the physician at the first sign or symptom of impending failure.

The patient should also be advised of a proper course in the event of an inadvertent missed dose.

Laboratory Tests—Serum and urine electrolyte levels should be regularly monitored (see WARNINGS, *Bendroflumethiazide,* also PRECAUTIONS, *General, Bendroflumethiazide*).

Drug Interactions—**Nadolol**—When administered concurrently the following drugs may interact with beta-adrenergic blocking agents:

Anesthetics, general—exaggeration of the hypotension induced by general anesthetics (see WARNINGS, *Nadolol, Major Surgery*).

Antidiabetic drugs (oral agents and insulin)—hypoglycemia or hyperglycemia; adjust dosage of antidiabetic drug accordingly (see WARNINGS, *Nadolol, Diabetes and Hypoglycemia*).

Catecholamine-depleting drugs (e.g., reserpine)—additive effect; monitor closely for evidence of hypotension and/or excessive bradycardia (e.g., vertigo, syncope, postural hypotension).

Bendroflumethiazide—When administered concurrently the following drugs may interact with thiazide diuretics:

Alcohol, barbiturates, or narcotics—potentiation of orthostatic hypotension may occur.

Antidiabetic drugs (oral agents and insulin)—hyperglycemia induced by thiazide may require dosage adjustment of antidiabetic drug.

Other antihypertensive drugs—additive effect or potentiation of other antihypertensive drugs.

Corticosteroids, ACTH—intensified electrolyte depletion, particularly hypokalemia.

Ganglionic or peripheral adrenergic blocking drugs—potentiated effect of ganglionic or peripheral adrenergic blocking drugs.

Preanesthetic and anesthetic agents—effects of preanesthetic and anesthetic agents may be potentiated; adjust dosage of these agents accordingly.

Pressor amines (e.g., norepinephrine)—possible decreased response to pressor amines but not sufficient to preclude their use.

Skeletal muscle relaxants, nondepolarizing (e.g., tubocurarine)—possible increased responsiveness to the muscle relaxant.

Drug/Laboratory Test Interactions—Thiazides should be discontinued before carrying out tests for parathyroid function (see PRECAUTIONS, *General, Bendroflumethiazide*).

Carcinogenesis, Mutagenesis, Impairment of Fertility—**Nadolol**—In chronic oral toxicologic studies

Continued on next page

Squibb—Cont.

(one to two years) in mice, rats, and dogs, nadolol did not produce any significant toxic effects. In two-year oral carcinogenicity studies in rats and mice, nadolol did not produce any neoplastic, preneoplastic, or nonneoplastic pathologic lesions. In fertility and general reproductive performance studies in rats, nadolol caused no adverse effect.

Bendroflumethiazide—Long-term studies in animals have not been performed to evaluate carcinogenic potential, mutagenesis, or whether this drug affects fertility in males or females.

Pregnancy—Teratogenic Effects—Nadolol—Category C. In animal reproduction studies with nadolol, evidence of embryo- and fetotoxicity was found in rabbits, but not in rats or hamsters, at doses 5 to 10 times greater (on a mg/kg basis) than the maximum indicated human dose. No teratogenic potential was observed in any of these species.

There are no adequate and well-controlled studies in pregnant women. Nadolol should be used during pregnancy only if the potential benefit justifies the potential risk to the fetus.

Bendroflumethiazide—Category C. Animal reproduction studies have not been conducted with bendroflumethiazide. It is also not known whether this drug can cause fetal harm when administered to a pregnant woman or can affect reproduction capacity. Bendroflumethiazide should be given to a pregnant woman only if clearly needed.

Pregnancy—Nonteratogenic Effects—Thiazides cross the placental barrier and appear in cord blood. The use of thiazides in pregnant women requires that the anticipated benefit be weighed against possible hazards to the fetus. These hazards include fetal or neonatal jaundice, thrombocytopenia, and possibly other adverse reactions which have occurred in the adult.

Nursing Mothers—Both nadolol and bendroflumethiazide are excreted in human milk. Because of the potential for serious adverse reactions in nursing infants from both drugs, a decision should be made whether to discontinue nursing or to discontinue therapy taking into account the importance of CORZIDE (Nadolol-Bendroflumethiazide Tablets) to the mother.

Pediatric Use—Safety and effectiveness in children have not been established.

Adverse Reactions: Nadolol—Most adverse effects have been mild and transient and have rarely required withdrawal of therapy.

Cardiovascular—Bradycardia with heart rates of less than 60 beats per minute occurs commonly, and heart rates below 40 beats per minute and/or symptomatic bradycardia were seen in about 2 of 100 patients. Symptoms of peripheral vascular insufficiency, usually of the Raynaud type, have occurred in approximately 2 of 100 patients. Cardiac failure, hypotension, and rhythm/conduction disturbances have each occurred in about 1 of 100 patients. Single instances of first degree and third degree heart block have been reported; intensification of AV block is a known effect of beta-blockers (see also CONTRAINDICATIONS, WARNINGS, and PRECAUTIONS).

Central Nervous System—Dizziness or fatigue has each been reported in approximately 2 of 100 patients; paresthesias, sedation, and change in behavior have each been reported in approximately 6 of 1000 patients.

Respiratory—Bronchospasm has been reported in approximately 1 of 1000 patients (see CONTRAINDICATIONS and WARNINGS).

Gastrointestinal—Nausea, diarrhea, abdominal discomfort, constipation, vomiting, indigestion, anorexia, bloating, and flatulence have been reported in 1 to 5 of 1000 patients.

Miscellaneous—Each of the following has been reported in 1 to 5 of 1000 patients: rash; pruritus; headache; dry mouth, eyes, or skin; impotence or decreased libido; facial swelling; weight gain; slurred speech; cough; nasal stuffiness; sweating; tinnitus; blurred vision.

Sleep disturbances have been reported, but their relationship to drug usage is not clear.

The oculomucocutaneous syndrome associated with the beta-blocker practolol has not been reported with nadolol.

In addition, the following adverse reactions may occur:

Central Nervous System—Reversible mental depression progressing to catatonia; visual disturbances; hallucinations; an acute reversible syndrome characterized by disorientation for time and place, short-term memory loss, emotional liability with slightly clouded sensorium, and decreased performance on neuropsychometrics.

Gastrointestinal—Mesenteric arterial thrombosis; ischemic colitis.

Hematologic—Agranulocytosis; thrombocytopenic or nonthrombocytopenic purpura.

Allergic—Fever combined with aching and sore throat; laryngospasm; respiratory distress.

Miscellaneous—Reversible alopecia; Peyronie's disease; erythematous rash; arterial insufficiency.

Bendroflumethiazide — Gastrointestinal System—anorexia, gastric irritation, nausea, vomiting, cramping, diarrhea, constipation, jaundice (intrahepatic cholestatic jaundice), and pancreatitis.

Central Nervous System—dizziness, vertigo, paresthesia, headache, and xanthopsia.

Hematologic—leukopenia, agranulocytosis, thrombocytopenia, and aplastic anemia.

Dermatologic-Hypersensitivity — purpura, photosensitivity, rash, urticaria, and necrotizing angiitis (vasculitis, cutaneous vasculitis).

Cardiovascular—Orthostatic hypotension may occur.

Other—hyperglycemia, glycosuria, occasional metabolic acidosis in diabetic patients, hyperuricemia, allergic glomerulonephritis, muscle spasm, weakness, and restlessness.

Whenever adverse reactions are moderate or severe, thiazide dosage should be reduced or therapy withdrawn.

Overdosage: In the event of overdosage, nadolol may cause excessive bradycardia, cardiac failure, hypotension, or bronchospasm.

In addition to the expected diuresis, overdosage of thiazides may produce varying degrees of lethargy which may progress to coma within a few hours, with minimal depression of respiration and cardiovascular function and without evidence of serum electrolyte changes or dehydration. The mechanism of thiazide-induced CNS depression is unknown. Gastrointestinal irritation and hypermotility may occur. Transitory increase in BUN has been reported, and serum electrolyte changes may occur, especially in patients with impaired renal function.

Treatment—Nadolol can be removed from the general circulation by hemodialysis. In determining the duration of corrective therapy, note must be taken of the long duration of the effect of nadolol. In addition to gastric lavage, the following measures should be employed, as appropriate.

Excessive Bradycardia—Administer atropine (0.25 to 1.0 mg). If there is no response to vagal blockade, administer isoproterenol cautiously.

Cardiac Failure—Administer a digitalis glycoside and diuretic. It has been reported that glucagon may also be useful in this situation.

Hypotension—Administer vasopressors, e.g., epinephrine or levarterenol. (There is evidence that epinephrine may be the drug of choice.)

Bronchospasm—Administer a beta$_2$-stimulating agent and/or a theophylline derivative.

Stupor or Coma—Supportive therapy as warranted.

Gastrointestinal Effects—Symptomatic treatment as needed.

BUN and/or Serum Electrolyte Abnormalities—Institute supportive measures as required to maintain hydration, electrolyte balance, respiration, and cardiovascular and renal function.

Dosage and Administration: DOSAGE MUST BE INDIVIDUALIZED (SEE INDICATIONS). CORZIDE (Nadolol-Bendroflumethiazide Tablets) MAY BE ADMINISTERED WITHOUT REGARD TO MEALS.

Bendroflumethiazide is usually given at a dose of 5 mg daily. The usual initial dose of nadolol is 40 mg once daily whether used alone or in combination with a diuretic. Bendroflumethiazide in CORZIDE is 30 percent more bioavailable than that of 5 mg Naturetin (Bendroflumethiazide) tablets. Conversion from 5 mg Naturetin to CORZIDE represents a 30 percent increase in dose of bendroflumethiazide.

The initial dose of CORZIDE (Nadolol-Bendroflumethiazide Tablets) may therefore be the 40 mg/5 mg tablet once daily. When the antihypertensive response is not satisfactory, the dose may be increased by administering the 80 mg/5 mg tablet once daily.

When necessary, another antihypertensive agent may be added gradually beginning with 50 percent of the usual recommended starting dose to avoid an excessive fall in blood pressure.

Dosage Adjustment In Renal Failure—Absorbed nadolol is excreted principally by the kidneys and, although nonrenal elimination does occur, dosage adjustments are necessary in patients with renal impairment. The following dose intervals are recommended:

Creatinine Clearance (ml/min/1.73m^2)	Dosage Interval (hours)
> 50	24
31-50	24-36
10-30	24-48
< 10	40-60

How Supplied: CORZIDE (Nadolol-Bendroflumethiazide Tablets) is available as tablets containing 40 mg nadolol combined with 5 mg bendroflumethiazide and 80 mg nadolol combined with 5 mg bendroflumethiazide in bottles of 100. The round, biconvex tablets are white to bluish white with dark blue specks. Each tablet has a full bisect bar. Tablet identification numbers: 40 mg/5 mg combination, 283; 80 mg/5 mg combination, 284.

Storage: Keep bottle tightly closed. Store at room temperature; avoid excessive heat.

Shown in Product Identification Section, page 437

CRYSTICILLIN® 300 A.S. ℞
CRYSTICILLIN® 600 A.S. ℞
[kris″ ti-sil′ in]
(Sterile Penicillin G Procaine Suspension USP)

Description: Crysticillin 300 A.S. and Crysticillin 600 A.S. are aqueous suspensions providing 300,000 u. per ml. and 600,000 u. per 1.2 ml. (500,000 u./ml.) penicillin G procaine, respectively. The vials providing 300,000 u. per ml. also contain 0.13% methylparaben, 0.02% propylparaben, and 0.25% phenol as preservatives; 0.5% lecithin; 0.5% povidone; 1% sodium citrate; not more than 0.01% sodium formaldehyde sulfoxylate; and 0.075% sodium carboxymethylcellulose. The vials providing 600,000 u. per 1.2 ml. also contain 0.13% methylparaben, 0.02% propylparaben, and 0.18% phenol as preservatives; 0.3% povidone; 1% sodium citrate; 0.05% sodium carboxymethylcellulose; not more than 0.03% sodium formaldehyde sulfoxylate; and 2.3% lecithin.

Clinical Pharmacology: Penicillin G is bactericidal against penicillin-susceptible microorganisms during the stage of active multiplication. It acts by inhibiting biosynthesis of cell-wall mucopeptide. It is not active against the penicillinase-producing bacteria, which include many strains of staphylococci. Penicillin G is highly active *in vitro* against staphylococci (except penicillinase-producing strains), streptococci (groups A, C, G, H, L, and M), and pneumococci. Other organisms susceptible *in vitro* to penicillin G are *Neisseria gonorrhoeae, Corynebacterium diphtheriae, Bacillus anthracis,* Clostridia, *Actinomyces bovis, Streptobacillus moniliformis, Listeria monocytogenes,* and Leptospira; *Treponema pallidum* is extremely susceptible.

Susceptibility plate testing: If the Kirby-Bauer method of disc susceptibility is used, a 10 u. penicillin disc should give a zone greater than 28 mm. when tested against a penicillin-susceptible bacterial strain.

Penicillin G procaine is an equimolar compound of procaine and penicillin G administered intramuscularly as a suspension. It dissolves slowly at the site of injection, giving a plateau type of blood level at about four hours which falls slowly during the next 15 to 20 hours.

Approximately 60 percent of penicillin G is bound to serum protein. The drug is distributed throughout the body tissues in widely varying amounts. Highest levels are found in the kidneys with lesser amounts in the liver, skin, and intestines. Penicillin G penetrates into all other tissues to a lesser degree with a very small level found in the cerebrospinal fluid. The drug is excreted rapidly by tubular excretion in patients with normal kidney function. In neonates and young infants, and in individuals with impaired kidney function, excretion is considerably delayed. Approximately 60 to 90 percent of a dose of parenteral penicillin G is excreted in the urine within 24 to 36 hours.

Indications and Usage: Crysticillin 300 A.S. and Crysticillin 600 A.S. (Sterile Penicillin G Procaine Suspension USP) are indicated in the treatment of moderately severe infections due to penicillin G-susceptible microorganisms. Therapy should be guided by bacteriological studies, including susceptibility tests, and by clinical response. Note: severe pneumonia, empyema, bacteremia, pericarditis, meningitis, peritonitis, and septic arthritis are better treated with aqueous penicillin G during the acute stage; when high, sustained serum levels are required, aqueous penicillin G, either I.M. or I.V. should be used.

The following infections will usually respond to adequate dosage:

Streptococcal infections Group A without bacteremia—Moderately severe to severe infections of the upper respiratory tract, skin and skin structures infections, scarlet fever, and erysipelas. Note: streptococci in groups A, C, G, H, L, and M are very susceptible to penicillin G. Other groups, including group D (enterococcus) are resistant. Aqueous penicillin is recommended for streptococcal infections with bacteremia.

Pneumococcal infections—Moderately severe infections of the respiratory tract.

Staphylococcal infections—penicillin G susceptible—Moderately severe infections of the skin and skin structures. Note: reports indicate an increasing number of strains of staphylococci resistant to penicillin G, emphasizing the need for culture and susceptibility studies in treating suspected staphylococcal infections. Indicated surgical procedures should be performed.

Vincent's gingivitis and pharyngitis (fusospirochetosis)—Moderately severe infections of the oropharynx. Note: necessary dental care should be accomplished in infections involving the gum tissue.

Syphilis (*T. pallidum*)—All stages; **Gonorrheal infections** (acute and chronic—without bacteremia)—With adequate recommended doses; **Treponema**—Yaws, Bejel, Pinta; **Diphtheria**—as an adjunct to antitoxin for the prevention of the carrier state; **Anthrax; Rat-bite fever** (*S. moniliformis* and *S. minus*); **Erysipeloid.**

Subacute bacterial endocarditis (group A streptococcus)—Only in extremely susceptible infections. **Prophylaxis against bacterial endocarditis**—Although no controlled clinical efficacy studies have been conducted, aqueous crystalline penicillin G for injection and penicillin G procaine suspension have been suggested by the American Heart Association and the American Dental Association for use as part of a combined parenteral-oral regimen for prophylaxis against bacterial endocarditis in patients with congenital heart disease or rheumatic or other acquired valvular heart disease when they undergo dental procedures and surgical procedures of the upper respiratory tract.[1] Since it may happen that *alpha* hemolytic streptococci relatively resistant to penicillin may be found when patients are receiving continuous oral penicillin for secondary prevention of rheumatic fever, prophylactic agents other than penicillin may be chosen for these patients and prescribed in addition to their continuous rheumatic fever prophylactic regimen. **NOTE:** When selecting antibiotics for the prevention of bacterial endocarditis, the physician or dentist should read the full joint statement of the American Heart Association and the American Dental Association.[1]

Contraindications: Contraindicated in patients with a history of hypersensitivity to procaine or any penicillin.

Warnings: Serious and occasional fatal hypersensitivity (anaphylactoid) reactions have been reported in patients on penicillin therapy. Although anaphylaxis is more frequent following parenteral administration, it has occurred in patients on oral penicillins. These reactions are more apt to occur in individuals with a history of sensitivity to multiple allergens.

There have been well-documented reports of individuals with a history of penicillin hypersensitivity who have experienced severe hypersensitivity reactions when treated with cephalosporins. Before therapy with a penicillin, careful inquiry should be made concerning previous hypersensitivity reactions to penicillins, cephalosporins, and other allergens. If an allergic reaction occurs, the drug should be discontinued and the patient treated with the usual agents, e.g., pressor amines, antihistamines, and corticosteroids. Serious anaphylactoid reactions are not controlled by antihistamines alone, and require such emergency measures as the immediate use of epinephrine, aminophylline, oxygen, and intravenous corticosteroids.

Immediate toxic reactions to procaine may occur in some individuals, particularly when a large single dose is administered in the treatment of gonorrhea (4.8 million u.). These reactions may be manifested by mental disturbances including anxiety, confusion, agitation, depression, weakness, seizures, hallucinations, combativeness, and expressed "fear of impending death." The reactions noted in carefully controlled studies occurred in approximately one in 500 patients treated for gonorrhea. Reactions are transient, lasting from 15 to 30 minutes.

Precautions: Penicillin should be used with caution in individuals with histories of significant allergies and/or asthma.

A small percentage of patients are sensitive to procaine. If there is a history of sensitivity, make the usual test: inject intradermally 0.1 ml. of a 1 to 2% procaine hydrochloride solution. Development of an erythema, wheal, flare or eruption indicates procaine sensitivity. Sensitivity should be treated by the usual methods, and procaine penicillin preparations should not be used. Antihistamines appear beneficial in the treatment of procaine reactions.

The use of antibiotics may result in overgrowth of nonsusceptible organisms. Constant observation of the patient is essential. If new infections due to bacteria or fungi appear during therapy, the drug should be discontinued and appropriate measures taken. Whenever allergic reactions occur, penicillin should be withdrawn unless, in the opinion of the physician, the condition being treated is life-threatening and amenable only to penicillin therapy.

Care should be taken to avoid accidental intravenous administration.

In prolonged therapy with penicillin, and particularly with high dosage schedules, periodic evaluation of the renal and hematopoietic systems is recommended.

In streptococcal infections, therapy must be sufficient to eliminate the organism (10 days minimum); otherwise the sequelae of streptococcal disease may occur. Cultures should be taken following the completion of treatment to determine whether streptococci have been eradicated.

In suspected staphylococcal infections, proper laboratory studies, including susceptibility tests, should be performed.

When treating gonococcal infections in which primary or secondary syphilis may be suspected, proper diagnostic procedures, including darkfield examinations, should be done. In all cases in which concomitant syphilis is suspected, monthly serological tests should be made for at least four months. All cases of penicillin-treated syphilis should receive clinical and serological examinations every six months for at least two or three years.

Adverse Reactions: Penicillin is a substance of low toxicity, but does possess a significant index of sensitization. The hypersensitivity reactions reported are skin rashes ranging from maculopapular eruptions to exfoliative dermatitis; urticaria; and serum sickness-like reactions including chills, fever, edema, arthralgia, and prostration. Hemolytic anemia, leukopenia, thrombocytopenia, neuropathy, and nephropathy are infrequent reactions and are usually associated with high doses of parenteral penicillin. Severe and often fatal anaphylaxis has been reported; these reactions require emergency measures (see WARNINGS). As with other treatments for syphilis, the Jarisch-Herxheimer reaction has been reported.

Procaine toxicity manifestations have been reported (see WARNINGS). Procaine hypersensitivity reactions have not been reported with this drug.

Dosage and Administration:
For intramuscular use only

The product is ready for immediate injection after vigorous shaking of the vial to insure a uniform suspension.

Injection is made rapidly by the intramuscular route. The preferred site is the upper outer quadrant of the gluteal area. Injections are easier to make and there is less likelihood of needle blockage if a small bore syringe is used; use a 20-gauge needle. Avoid using a syringe with a loosely-fitting plunger as crystals may creep between the walls and cause it to "freeze". Remove the needle and plunger from the syringe soon after injection to prevent "freezing" of the remaining crystals.

The usual dosage recommendation is as follows:
Streptococcal infections (Group A)—moderately severe to severe tonsillitis, erysipelas, scarlet fever, infections of the upper respiratory tract, and skin and skin structures infections: 600,000 to 1,200,000 u. daily for a minimum of 10 days.

Pneumococcal infections (uncomplicated)— moderately severe: 600,000 to 1,200,000 u. daily.

Staphylococcal infections—moderately severe to severe: 600,000 to 1,200,000 u. daily.

Vincent's gingivitis and pharyngitis (fusospirochetosis): 600,000 to 1,200,000 u. daily.

Syphilis—*Primary, secondary and latent* with a negative spinal fluid in adults and children over 12 years of age: 600,000 u. daily for eight days—total 4,800,000 u.; *Late* (tertiary, neurosyphilis and latent syphilis with positive or no spinal fluid examination): 600,000 u. daily for 10 to 15 days—total 6 to 9 million u.; *Congenital* (under 32 kg. [70 lb.] body weight): 10,000 u./kg./day for 10 days.

Gonorrheal infections (uncomplicated): 4.8 million u. divided into at least two doses at one visit for males and females; one gram of oral probenecid is given 30 minutes before the injections. Follow-up cultures should be obtained from the original site(s) of infection 7 to 14 days after therapy. In women, it is also desirable to obtain culture test-of-cure from both the endocervical and anal canals. Note: gonorrheal endocarditis should be treated intensively with aqueous penicillin G.

Yaws, Bejel, and Pinta—treat same as syphilis in corresponding stage of disease.

Diphtheria—*adjunctive therapy with antitoxin:* 300,000 to 600,000 u. daily; **Anthrax**—cutaneous: 600,000 to 1,200,000 u. daily; **Rat-bite fever** (*S. moniliformis* and *S. minus*) and **Erysipeloid:** 600,000 to 1,200,000 u. daily.

Bacterial endocarditis (group A streptococcus) —only in extremely susceptible infections: 600,000 to 1,200,000 u. daily.

Prophylaxis against bacterial endocarditis—For prophylaxis against bacterial endocarditis[1] in patients with congenital heart disease or rheumatic or other acquired valvular heart disease when undergoing dental procedures or surgical procedures of the upper respiratory tract, use a combined parenteral-oral regimen. One million units of aqueous crystalline penicillin G (30,000 u./kg. in children) mixed with 600,000 u. of penicil-

Continued on next page

Squibb—Cont.

lin G procaine (600,000 u. for children) should be given intramuscularly one-half to one hour before the procedure. Oral penicillin V (phenoxymethyl penicillin), 500 mg. for adults or 250 mg. for children less than 60 lb., should be given every six hours for eight doses. Doses for children should not exceed recommendations for adults for a single dose or for a 24-hour period.

How Supplied: Crysticillin 300 A.S. (Sterile Penicillin G Procaine Suspension USP) is available in 10 ml. vials; Crysticillin 600 A.S. is available in 12 ml. vials.

Storage: Store below 15° C. (59° F.); avoid freezing.

Reference: 1. American Heart Association. 1977. Prevention of bacterial endocarditis. Circulation 56:139A-143A.

E.T. THE EXTRA-TERRESTRIAL™
(Children's Chewable Vitamins)

E.T. Vitamins come in the 4 fruity flavors most preferred by children.

Each tablet contains:

		Percent US RDA* ages 4-12
Vitamin A	5,000 IU	100
Vitamin D	400 IU	100
Vitamin E	30 IU	100
Vitamin C	60 mg	100
Folic Acid	0.4 mg	100
Thiamine	1.5 mg	100
Riboflavin	1.7 mg	100
Niacin	20 mg	100
Vitamin B_6	2 mg	100
Vitamin B_{12}	6 mcg	100

*US Recommended Daily Allowances

Usage: For 12 year olds and under—chew one tablet daily.

How Supplied: Bottles of 60.

Storage: Store at room temperature; avoid excessive heat.

KEEP OUT OF THE REACH OF CHILDREN.

Shown in Product Identification Section, page 438

E.T. THE EXTRA-TERRESTRIAL™
Children's Chewable Vitamins
With Iron

E.T. Vitamins come in the 4 fruity flavors most preferred by children.

Each tablet contains:

		Percent US RDA* ages 4-12
Vitamin A	5,000 IU	100
Vitamin D	400 IU	100
Vitamin E	30 IU	100
Vitamin C	60 mg	100
Folic Acid	0.4 mg	100
Thiamine	1.5 mg	100
Riboflavin	1.7 mg	100
Niacin	20 mg	100
Vitamin B_6	2 mg	100
Vitamin B_{12}	6 mcg	100
Iron	18 mg	100

*US Recommended Daily Allowances

Usage: For 12 year olds and under—chew one tablet daily.

How Supplied: Bottles of 60.

Storage: Store at room temperature; avoid excessive heat.

KEEP OUT OF THE REACH OF CHILDREN.

E.T. THE EXTRA-TERRESTRIAL and Likeness are Trademarks of and Licensed by Universal City Studios, Inc.

Copyright © 1982, Universal City Studios, Inc. All rights reserved.

Shown in Product Identification Section, page 438

FUNGIZONE®   ℞
[fun'ji-zōn]
(Amphotericin B)
CREAM/LOTION/OINTMENT

Description: Fungizone Cream (Amphotericin B Cream USP) contains the antifungal antibiotic Amphotericin B USP at a concentration of 3% (30 mg./gram) in a pleasantly tinted aqueous vehicle, which also contains titanium dioxide, thimerosal, propylene glycol, cetearyl alcohol (and) ceteareth-20, white petrolatum, methylparaben, propylparaben, sorbitol solution, glyceryl monostearate, polyethylene glycol monostearate, simethicone, and sorbic acid.

Fungizone Lotion (Amphotericin B Lotion USP) contains the antifungal antibiotic Amphotericin B USP at a concentration of 3% (30 mg./ml.) in a tinted aqueous lotion vehicle, which is pleasantly scented, and also contains thimerosal, titanium dioxide, guar gum, propylene glycol, cetyl alcohol, stearyl alcohol, sorbitan monopalmitate, polysorbate 20, glyceryl monostearate, polyethylene glycol monostearate, simethicone, sorbic acid, methylparaben, and propylparaben.

Fungizone Ointment (Amphotericin B Ointment USP) contains the antifungal antibiotic Amphotericin B USP at a concentration of 3% (30 mg./gram) in a tinted form of Plastibase® (Plasticized Hydrocarbon Gel), a polyethylene and mineral oil gel base with titanium dioxide.

Clinical Pharmacology: Amphotericin B is an antibiotic with antifungal activity which is produced by a strain of *Streptomyces nodosus*. It has been shown to exhibit greater *in vitro* activity than nystatin against *Candida* (Monilia) *albicans*. In clinical studies involving cutaneous and mucocutaneous candidal infections, results with topical preparations of amphotericin B were comparable to those obtained with nystatin in similar formulations.

Although amphotericin B exhibits some *in vitro* activity against the superficial dermatophytes (ringworm organisms), it has not demonstrated an effectiveness *in vivo* on topical application. Amphotericin B has no significant effect either *in vitro* or clinically against gram-positive or gram-negative bacteria, or viruses.

Indications and Usage: Fungizone (Amphotericin B) topical preparations are indicated in the treatment of cutaneous and mucocutaneous mycotic infections caused by Candida (Monilia) species.

Contraindications: The preparations are contraindicated in patients with a history of hypersensitivity to any of their components.

Precautions: Should a reaction of hypersensitivity occur the drug should be immediately withdrawn and appropriate measures taken.

Adverse Reactions: Fungizone Cream (Amphotericin B Cream USP)—No evidence of any systemic toxicity or side effects has been observed during or following the use of the Cream. The preparation is usually well tolerated by all age groups. It is not a primary irritant and apparently has only a slight sensitizing potential. It may have a "drying" effect on some skin, and local irritation characterized by erythema, pruritus, or a burning sensation sometimes occurs, particularly in intertriginous areas.

Fungizone Lotion (Amphotericin B Lotion USP)—No evidence of any systemic toxicity or side effects has been observed during or following even prolonged, intensive and extensive application of the Lotion. The preparation is extremely well tolerated by all age groups, including infants, even when therapy must be continued for many months. It is not a primary irritant and apparently has only a slight sensitizing potential. Local intolerance, which seldom occurs, has included increased pruritus with or without other subjective or objective evidence of local irritation, or exacerbation of preexisting candidal lesions. Allergic contact dermatitis is rare.

Fungizone Ointment (Amphotericin B Ointment USP)—No evidence of any systemic toxicity or side effects has been observed during or following even prolonged, intensive and extensive application of the Ointment. The preparation is usually well tolerated by all age groups. It is not a primary irritant and apparently has only a slight sensitizing potential. However, it is well to remember that any oleaginous ointment vehicle may occasionally irritate when applied to moist, intertriginous areas.

Dosage and Administration: Fungizone (Amphotericin B) Cream, Lotion, or Ointment should be applied liberally to the candidal lesions two to four times daily. Duration of therapy depends on individual patient response. Intertriginous lesions usually respond within a few days, and treatment may be completed in one to three weeks. Similarly, candidiasis of the diaper area, perleche, and glabrous skin lesions usually clear in one to two weeks. Interdigital (erosio) lesions may require two to four weeks of intensive therapy; paronychias also require relatively prolonged therapy, and those onychomycoses which respond may require several months or more of treatment. (Relapses are frequently encountered in the last three clinical conditions.)

NOTE: When rubbed into the lesion, the Cream discolors the skin minimally. The Lotion and Ointment do not stain the skin when thoroughly rubbed into the lesion although nail lesions may be stained. The patient should be informed that any discoloration of fabrics from the Cream may be removed by hand-washing the fabric with soap and warm water, that any discoloration of fabrics from the Lotion is readily removed with soap and warm water, or that any discoloration of fabrics from the Ointment may be removed by applying a standard cleaning fluid.

How Supplied: Fungizone Cream (Amphotericin B Cream USP) is supplied in tubes of 20 grams.

Fungizone Lotion (Amphotericin B Lotion USP) is supplied in 30 ml. plastic squeeze bottles (Military Depot Item, NSN 6505-00-890-1486).

Fungizone Ointment (Amphotericin B Ointment USP) is supplied in tubes of 20 grams.

Storage: Store the Cream and Lotion at room temperature; avoid freezing. Store the Ointment at room temperature.

FUNGIZONE® INTRAVENOUS   ℞
[fun'ji-zōn]
(Amphotericin B for Injection USP)

> **WARNING**
> This drug should be used *primarily* for treatment of patients with progressive and potentially fatal fungal infections; it should not be used to treat the common clinically inapparent forms of fungal disease which show only positive skin or serologic tests.

Description: Fungizone Intravenous (Amphotericin B for Injection USP) is an antifungal antibiotic derived from a strain of *Streptomyces nodosus*. Crystalline amphotericin B is insoluble in water; therefore, the antibiotic is "solubilized" by the addition of sodium desoxycholate to form a mixture which provides a colloidal dispersion for parenteral administration.

Actions:
Microbiology
Amphotericin B shows a high order of *in vitro* activity against many species of fungi. *Histoplasma capsulatum, Coccidiodes immitis, Candida* species, *Blastomyces dermatitidis, Rhodotorula, Cryptococcus neoformans, Sporotrichum schenckii, Mucor mucedo,* and *Aspergillus fumigatus* are all inhibited by concentrations of amphotericin B ranging from 0.03 to 1.0 mcg./ml. *in vitro*. The antibiotic is without effect on bacteria, rickettsiae, and viruses.

Clinical Pharmacology
Amphotericin B is fungistatic or fungicidal depending on the concentration obtained in body fluids and the susceptibility of the fungus. The drug probably acts by binding to sterols in the fungus cell membrane with a resultant change in membrane permeability which allows leakage of a variety of small molecules. Mammalian cell mem-

branes also contain sterols and it has been suggested that the damage to human cells and fungal cells may share common mechanisms.

An initial intravenous infusion of 1 to 5 mg. of amphotericin B per day, gradually increased to 0.65 mg./kg. daily, produces peak plasma concentrations of approximately 2 to 4 mcg./ml. which can persist between doses since the plasma half-life of amphotericin B is about 24 hours. (For recommended dosages, see the DOSAGE AND ADMINISTRATION section.) It has been reported that amphotericin B is highly bound (>90%) to plasma proteins and is poorly dialyzable.

Amphotericin B is excreted very slowly by the kidneys with two to five percent of a given dose being excreted in biologically active form. After treatment is discontinued, the drug can be detected in the urine for at least seven weeks. The cumulative urinary output over a seven-day period amounts to approximately 40 percent of the amount of drug infused.

Details of tissue distribution and possible metabolic pathways are not known.

Indications: Fungizone Intravenous should be administered primarily to patients with progressive, potentially fatal infections. This potent drug should not be used to treat the common inapparent forms of fungal disease which show only positive skin or serologic tests.

Fungizone Intravenous (Amphotericin B for Injection USP) is specifically intended to treat cryptococcosis (torulosis); North American blastomycosis; the disseminated forms of moniliasis, coccidioidomycosis, and histoplasmosis; mucormycosis (phycomycosis) caused by species of the genera *Mucor, Rhizopus, Absidia, Entomophthora,* and *Basidiobolus;* sporotrichosis (*Sporothrix schenckii* [formerly *Sporotrichum schenckii*]); aspergillosis (*Aspergillus fumigatus*).

Amphotericin B may be helpful in the treatment of American mucocutaneous leishmaniasis, but is not the drug of choice in primary therapy.

Contraindications: This product is contraindicated in those patients who have shown hypersensitivity to it unless, in the opinion of the physician, the condition requiring treatment is life-threatening and amenable only to amphotericin B therapy.

Warnings: Amphotericin B is frequently the only effective treatment available for potentially fatal fungal disease. In each case, its possible life-saving benefit must be balanced against its untoward and dangerous side effects.

Usage in Pregnancy: Safety for use in pregnancy has not been established; therefore, it should be used during pregnancy only if the possible benefits to be derived outweigh the potential risks involved.

Precautions: Prolonged therapy with amphotericin B is usually necessary. Unpleasant reactions are quite common when the drug is given parenterally at therapeutic dosage levels. **Some of these reactions are potentially dangerous.** Hence, amphotericin B should be used parenterally only in hospitalized patients or those under close clinical observation by medically trained personnel and should be reserved for those patients in whom a diagnosis of the progressive, potentially fatal forms of susceptible mycotic infections has been firmly established, preferably by positive culture or histologic study.

Corticosteroids should not be administered concomitantly unless they are necessary to control drug reactions. Other nephrotoxic antibiotics and antineoplastic agents such as nitrogen mustard should not be given concomitantly except with great caution.

Laboratory facilities must be available to perform blood urea nitrogen and serum creatinine or endogenous creatinine clearance tests. These determinations should be made at least weekly during therapy. If the BUN exceeds 40 mg. per 100 ml. or the serum creatinine exceeds 3.0 mg. per 100 ml. the drug should be discontinued or the dosage markedly reduced until renal function is improved. Weekly hemograms and serum potassium determinations are also advisable. Low serum magnesium levels have also been noted during treatment with amphotericin B. Therapy should be discontinued if liver function test results (elevated bromsulphalein, alkaline phosphatase and bilirubin) are abnormal.

Whenever medication is interrupted for a period longer than seven days, therapy should be resumed by starting with the lowest dosage level, e.g., 0.25 mg./kg. of body weight, and increased gradually as outlined under DOSAGE AND ADMINISTRATION.

Adverse Reactions: While some few patients may tolerate full intravenous doses of amphotericin B without difficulty, most will exhibit some intolerance, often at less than the full therapeutic dosage. They may be made less severe by giving aspirin, antihistamines, and antiemetics. Administration of the drug on alternate days may decrease anorexia and phlebitis. Intravenous administration of small doses of adrenal corticosteroids just prior to or during the amphotericin B infusion may decrease febrile reactions. The dosage and duration of such corticosteroid therapy should be kept to a minimum. Adding a small amount of heparin to the infusion may lessen the incidence of thrombophlebitis. Extravasation may cause chemical irritation.

The adverse reactions that are most commonly observed are: fever (sometimes with shaking chills); headache; anorexia; weight loss; nausea and vomiting; malaise; dyspepsia; diarrhea; generalized pain including muscle and joint pains, cramping epigastric pain, and local venous pain at the injection site with phlebitis and thrombophlebitis; and normochromic, normocytic anemia. Abnormal renal function including hypokalemia, azotemia, hyposthenuria, renal tubular acidosis and nephrocalcinosis is also commonly observed, and usually improves upon interruption of therapy; however, some permanent impairment often occurs, especially in those patients receiving large amounts (over 5 g.) of amphotericin B. Supplemental alkali medication may decrease renal tubular acidosis complications.

The following adverse reactions occur less frequently or rarely: anuria; oliguria; cardiovascular toxicity including arrhythmias, ventricular fibrillation, cardiac arrest, hypertension, and hypotension; coagulation defects; thrombocytopenia, leukopenia; agranulocytosis; eosinophilia; leukocytosis; melena or hemorrhagic gastroenteritis; maculopapular rash; hearing loss; tinnitus; transient vertigo; blurred vision or diplopia; peripheral neuropathy; convulsions and other neurologic symptoms; pruritus (without rash); anaphylactoid reactions; acute liver failure; and flushing.

Dosage and Administration: Fungizone Intravenous (Amphotericin B for Injection USP) should be administered by *slow* intravenous infusion. Intravenous infusion should be given over a period of approximately six hours observing the usual precautions for intravenous therapy. The recommended concentration for intravenous infusion is 0.1 mg./ml. (1 mg./10 ml.).

Dosage must be adjusted to the specific requirements of each patient since tolerance to amphotericin B varies individually. Therapy is usually instituted with a daily dose of 0.25 mg./kg. of body weight and **gradually** increased as tolerance permits. There are insufficient data presently available to define total dosage requirements and duration of treatment necessary for eradication of mycoses such as phycomycosis. The optimal dose is unknown. Total daily dosage may range up to 1.0 mg./kg. of body weight or alternate day dosages ranging up to 1.5 mg./kg. Several months of therapy are usually necessary; a shorter period of therapy may produce an inadequate response and lead to relapse.

CAUTION: Under no circumstances should a total daily dosage of 1.5 mg./kg. be exceeded. Therapy with intravenous amphotericin B for sporotrichosis has ranged up to nine months. The usual dose per injection is 20 mg.

Aspergillosis has been treated with amphotericin B intravenously for a period up to 11 months with a total dose up to 3.6 g.

Rhinocerebral phycomycosis, a fulminating disease, generally occurs in association with diabetic ketoacidosis. It is, therefore, imperative that rapid restoration of diabetic control be instituted before successful treatment with Fungizone Intravenous (Amphotericin B for Injection USP) can be accomplished. In contradistinction, pulmonary phycomycosis, which is more common in association with hematologic malignancies, is often an incidental finding at autopsy. A cumulative dose of at least 3 g. of amphotericin B is recommended. Although a total dose of 3 to 4 g. will infrequently cause lasting renal impairment, this would seem a reasonable minimum where there is clinical evidence of invasion of the deep tissues; since rhinocerebral phycomycosis usually follows a rapidly fatal course, the therapeutic approach must necessarily be more aggressive than that used in more indolent mycoses.

Preparation of Solutions: Reconstitute as follows: An initial concentrate of 5 mg. amphotericin B per ml. is first prepared by rapidly expressing 10 ml. Sterile Water for Injection USP *without a bacteriostatic agent* directly into the lyophilized cake, using a sterile needle (minimum diameter: 20 gauge) and syringe. Shake the vial immediately until the colloidal solution is clear. The infusion solution, providing 0.1 mg. amphotericin B per ml., is then obtained by further dilution (1:50) with 5% Dextrose Injection USP *of pH above 4.2.* The pH of each container of Dextrose Injection should be ascertained before use. Commercial Dextrose Injection usually has a pH above 4.2; however, if it is below 4.2, then 1 or 2 ml. of buffer should be added to the Dextrose Injection before it is used to dilute the concentrated solution of amphotericin B. The recommended buffer has the following composition:

Dibasic sodium phosphate (anhydrous)	1.59 g.
Monobasic sodium phosphate (anhydrous)	0.96 g.
Water for Injection USP	qs. 100.0 ml.

The buffer should be sterilized before it is added to the Dextrose Injection, either by filtration through a bacterial retentive stone, mat, or membrane, or by autoclaving for 30 minutes at 15 lb. pressure (121°C.).

CAUTION: Aseptic technique must be strictly observed in all handling, since no preservative or bacteriostatic agent is present in the antibiotic or in the materials used to prepare it for administration. **All entries into the vial or into the diluents must be made with a sterile needle. Do not reconstitute with saline solutions. The use of any diluent other than the ones recommended or the presence of a bacteriostatic agent** (e.g., benzyl alcohol) **in the diluent may cause precipitation of the antibiotic. Do not use the initial concentrate or the infusion solution if there is any evidence of precipitation or foreign matter in either one.**

An in-line membrane filter may be used for intravenous infusion of amphotericin B; **however, the mean pore diameter of the filter should not be less than 1.0 micron in order to assure passage of the antibiotic dispersion.**

How Supplied: Fungizone Intravenous is supplied in vials as a sterile lyophilized cake (which may partially reduce to powder following manufacture) providing 50 mg. amphotericin B and 41 mg. sodium desoxycholate with 20.2 mg. sodium phosphates as a buffer. At the time of manufacture, the air in the container is replaced by nitrogen. [Military Depot Item: NSN 6505-01-084-9453.]

Storage: Prior to reconstitution, Fungizone Intravenous (Amphotericin B for injection USP) should be stored in the refrigerator, protected against exposure to light. The concentrate (5 mg. amphotericin B per ml. after reconstitution with 10 ml. Sterile Water for Injection USP) may be stored in the dark, at room temperature for 24 hours, or at refrigerator temperatures for one week with minimal loss of potency and clarity. Any unused material should then be discarded. Solutions prepared for intravenous infusion (0.1 mg. or less amphotericin B per ml.) should be used promptly after prep-

Continued on next page

Squibb—Cont.

aration and should be protected from light during administration.

HALOG®
[hā'log]
(Halcinonide)
CREAM/OINTMENT/SOLUTION/EMOLLIENT BASE

Description: The topical corticosteroids constitute a class of primarily synthetic steroids used as anti-inflammatory and antipruritic agents. The steroids in this class include halcinonide. Halcinonide is designated chemically as 21-Chloro-9-fluoro-11β, 16α, 17-trihydroxypregn-4-ene-3,20-dione cyclic 16,17-acetal with acetone.

Each gram of 0.025% Halog Cream (Halcinonide Cream) contains 0.25 mg. halcinonide in a specially formulated cream base consisting of glyceryl monostearate NF XII, cetyl alcohol, cetyl esters wax, polysorbate 60, propylene glycol, dimethicone 350, and purified water. Each gram of 0.1% Halog Cream (Halcinonide Cream) contains 1 mg. halcinonide in a specially formulated cream base consisting of glyceryl monostearate NF XII, cetyl alcohol, isopropyl palmitate, dimethicone 350, polysorbate 60, titanium dioxide, propylene glycol, and purified water.

Each gram of 0.1% Halog Ointment (Halcinonide Ointment) contains 1 mg. halcinonide in Plastibase® (Plasticized Hydrocarbon Gel), a polyethylene and mineral oil gel base with polyethylene glycol 400, polyethylene glycol 6000 distearate, polyethylene glycol 300, polyethylene glycol 1540, and butylated hydroxytoluene as a preservative.

Each ml. of 0.1% Halog Solution (Halcinonide Solution) contains 1 mg. halcinonide with edetate disodium, polyethylene glycol 300, purified water, and butylated hydroxytoluene as a preservative.

Each gram of 0.1% Halog-E™ Cream (Halcinonide Cream) contains 1 mg halcinonide in a hydrophilic vanishing cream base consisting of propylene glycol, dimethicone 350, castor oil, cetearyl alcohol (and) ceteareth-20, propylene glycol stearate, white petrolatum, and purified water. This formulation is water-washable, greaseless, and nonstaining, with moisturizing and emollient properties.

Clinical Pharmacology: Topical corticosteroids share anti-inflammatory, antipruritic and vasoconstrictive actions.
The mechanism of anti-inflammatory activity of the topical corticosteroids is unclear. Various laboratory methods, including vasoconstrictor assays, are used to compare and predict potencies and/or clinical efficacies of the topical corticosteroids. There is some evidence to suggest that a recognizable correlation exists between vasoconstrictor potency and therapeutic efficacy in man.

Pharmacokinetics: The extent of percutaneous absorption of topical corticosteroids is determined by many factors including the vehicle, the integrity of the epidermal barrier, and the use of occlusive dressings.
Topical corticosteroids can be absorbed from normal intact skin. Inflammation and/or other disease processes in the skin increase percutaneous absorption. Occlusive dressings substantially increase the percutaneous absorption of topical corticosteroids. Thus, occlusive dressings may be a valuable therapeutic adjunct for treatment of resistant dermatoses (see DOSAGE AND ADMINISTRATION).
Once absorbed through the skin, topical corticosteroids are handled through pharmacokinetic pathways similar to systemically administered corticosteroids. Corticosteroids are bound to plasma proteins in varying degrees. Corticosteroids are metabolized primarily in the liver and are then excreted by the kidneys. Some of the topical corticosteroids and their metabolites are also excreted into the bile.

Indications and Usage: Halog (Halcinonide) preparations are indicated for the relief of the inflammatory and pruritic manifestations of corticosteroid-responsive dermatoses.

Contraindications: Topical corticosteroids are contraindicated in those patients with a history of hypersensitivity to any of the components of the preparations.

Precautions: General: Systemic absorption of topical corticosteroids has produced reversible hypothalamic-pituitary-adrenal (HPA) axis suppression, manifestations of Cushing's syndrome, hyperglycemia, and glucosuria in some patients. Conditions which augment systemic absorption include the application of the more potent steroids, use over large surface areas, prolonged use, and the addition of occlusive dressings.
Therefore, patients receiving a large dose of any potent topical steroid applied to a large surface area or under an occlusive dressing should be evaluated periodically for evidence of HPA axis suppression by using the urinary free cortisol and ACTH stimulation tests, and for impairment of thermal homeostasis. If HPA axis suppression or elevation of the body temperature occurs, an attempt should be made to withdraw the drug, to reduce the frequency of application, substitute a less potent steroid, or use a sequential approach when utilizing the occlusive technique.
Recovery of HPA axis function and thermal homeostasis are generally prompt and complete upon discontinuation of the drug. Infrequently, signs and symptoms of steroid withdrawal may occur, requiring supplemental systemic corticosteroids. Occasionally, a patient may develop a sensitivity reaction to a particular occlusive dressing material or adhesive and a substitute material may be necessary.
Children may absorb proportionally larger amounts of topical corticosteroids and thus be more susceptible to systemic toxicity (see PRECAUTIONS, Pediatric Use).
If irritation develops, topical corticosteroids should be discontinued and appropriate therapy instituted.
In the presence of dermatological infections, the use of an appropriate antifungal or antibacterial agent should be instituted. If a favorable response does not occur promptly, the corticosteroid should be discontinued until the infection has been adequately controlled.

Information for the Patient
Patients using topical corticosteroids should receive the following information and instructions:
1. This medication is to be used as directed by the physician. It is for external use only. Avoid contact with the eyes.
2. Patients should be advised not to use this medication for any disorder other than for which it was prescribed.
3. The treated skin area should not be bandaged or otherwise covered or wrapped as to be occlusive unless directed by the physician.
4. Patients should report any signs of local adverse reactions especially under occlusive dressing.
5. Parents of pediatric patients should be advised not to use tight-fitting diapers or plastic pants on a child being treated in the diaper area, as these garments may constitute occlusive dressings.

Laboratory Tests
A urinary free cortisol test and ACTH stimulation test may be helpful in evaluating HPA axis suppression.

Carcinogenesis, Mutagenesis, and Impairment of Fertility
Long-term animal studies have not been performed to evaluate the carcinogenic potential or the effect on fertility of topical corticosteroids. Studies to determine mutagenicity with prednisolone and hydrocortisone showed negative results.

Pregnancy: Teratogenic Effects
Category C. Corticosteroids are generally teratogenic in laboratory animals when administered systemically at relatively low dosage levels. The more potent corticosteroids have been shown to be teratogenic after dermal application in laboratory animals. There are no adequate and well-controlled studies in pregnant women on teratogenic effects from topically applied corticosteroids. Therefore, topical corticosteroids should be used during pregnancy only if the potential benefit justifies the potential risk to the fetus. Drugs of this class should not be used extensively on pregnant patients, in large amounts, or for prolonged periods of time.

Nursing Mothers
It is not known whether topical administration of corticosteroids could result in sufficient systemic absorption to produce detectable quantities in breast milk. Systemically administered corticosteroids are secreted into breast milk in quantities **not** likely to have a deleterious effect on the infant. Nevertheless, caution should be exercised when topical corticosteroids are administered to a nursing woman.

Pediatric Use
Pediatric patients may demonstrate greater susceptibility to topical corticosteroid-induced HPA axis suppression and Cushing's syndrome than mature patients because of a larger skin surface area to body weight ratio.
HPA axis suppression, Cushing's syndrome, and intracranial hypertension have been reported in children receiving topical corticosteroids. Manifestations of adrenal suppression in children include linear growth retardation, delayed weight gain, low plasma cortisol levels, and absence of response to ACTH stimulation. Manifestations of intracranial hypertension include bulging fontanelles, headaches, and bilateral papilledema.
Administration of topical corticosteroids to children should be limited to the least amount compatible with an effective therapeutic regimen. Chronic corticosteroid therapy may interfere with the growth and development of children.

Adverse Reactions: The following local adverse reactions are reported infrequently with topical corticosteroids, but may occur more frequently with the use of occlusive dressings (reactions are listed in an approximate decreasing order of occurrence): burning, itching, irritation, dryness, folliculitis, hypertrichosis, acneiform eruptions, hypopigmentation, perioral dermatitis, allergic contact dermatitis, maceration of the skin, secondary infection, skin atrophy, striae, and miliaria.

Overdosage: Topically applied corticosteroids can be absorbed in sufficient amounts to produce systemic effects (see PRECAUTIONS, General).

Dosage and Administration: Halog Cream (Halcinonide Cream): Apply the 0.025% or the 0.1% Halog Cream (Halcinonide Cream) to the affected area two to three times daily. Rub in gently.
Halog Ointment (Halcinonide Ointment 0.1%): Apply a thin film to the affected area two to three times daily.
Halog Solution (Halcinonide Solution 0.1%): Apply to the affected area two to three times daily.
Halog Cream (Halcinonide Cream) 0.1%: Apply to the affected area one to three times daily. Rub in gently.

Occlusive Dressing Technique
Occlusive dressings may be used for the management of psoriasis or other recalcitrant conditions. Halog Cream (Halcinonide Cream) 0.025% and 0.1% and Halog-E™ Cream (Halcinonide Cream) 0.1%: Gently rub a small amount of the cream into the lesion until it disappears. Reapply the preparation leaving a thin coating on the lesion, cover with a pliable nonporous film, and seal the edges. If needed, additional moisture may be provided by covering the lesion with a dampened clean cotton cloth before the nonporous film is applied or by briefly wetting the affected area with water immediately prior to applying the medication. The frequency of changing dressings is best determined on an individual basis. It may be convenient to apply the cream under an occlusive dressing in the evening and to remove the dressing in the morning (i.e., 12-hour occlusion). When utilizing the 12-hour occlusion regimen, additional cream should be applied, without occlusion, during the day. Reapplication is essential at each dressing change. If an infection develops, the use of occlusive dressings should be discontinued and appropriate antimicrobial therapy instituted.

Halog Ointment (Halcinonide Ointment 0.1%): Apply a thin film of the ointment to the lesion, cover with a pliable nonporous film, and seal the edges. If needed, additional moisture may be provided by covering the lesion with a dampened clean cotton cloth before the nonporous film is applied or by briefly wetting the affected area with water immediately prior to applying the medication. The frequency of changing dressings is best determined on an individual basis. It may be convenient to apply the ointment under an occlusive dressing in the evening and to remove the dressing in the morning (i.e., 12-hour occlusion). When utilizing the 12-hour occlusion regimen, additional ointment should be applied, without occlusion, during the day. Reapplication is essential at each dressing change. If an infection develops, the use of occlusive dressings should be discontinued and appropriate antimicrobial therapy instituted.

Halog Solution (Halcinonide Solution 0.1%): Apply the solution to the lesion, cover with a pliable nonporous film, and seal the edges. If needed, additional moisture may be provided by covering the lesion with a dampened clean cotton cloth before the nonporous film is applied or by briefly wetting the affected area with water immediately prior to applying the medication. The frequency of changing dressings is best determined on an individual basis. It may be convenient to apply the solution under an occlusive dressing in the evening and to remove the dressing in the morning (i.e., 12-hour occlusion). When utilizing the 12-hour occlusion regimen, additional solution should be applied, without occlusion, during the day. Reapplication is essential at each dressing change. If an infection develops, the use of occlusive dressings should be discontinued and appropriate antimicrobial therapy instituted.

How Supplied: 0.025% Cream Tubes of 15 g. and 60 g.; jars of 240 g. (8 oz.).
0.1% Cream Tubes of 15 g., 30 g., and 60 g.; jars of 240 g. (8 oz.).
0.1% Ointment Tubes of 15 g., 30 g., and 60 g.; jars of 240 g. (8 oz.). 0.1% Solution—Plastic squeeze bottles of 20 ml. and 60 ml.
0.1% Cream (emollient base): Tubes of 15 g, 30 g, and 60 g.

Storage: Store the 0.025% and 0.1% Creams at room temperature; avoid excessive heat (104°F). Store the 0.1% Ointment at room temperature; avoid excessive heat (104°F). Store the Solution at room temperature; avoid freezing and temperatures above 104°F. Store the 0.1% Cream (emollient base) at room temperature; avoid freezing and refrigeration.

HYDREA®
[$hī"drē'ah$]
(Hydroxyurea Capsules USP)

Description: Hydrea (Hydroxyurea Capsules USP) is an antineoplastic agent, available for oral use as capsules providing 500 mg. hydroxyurea. Hydroxyurea occurs as an essentially tasteless, white crystalline powder.

Actions: Mechanism of Action
The precise mechanism by which hydroxyurea produces its cytotoxic effects cannot, at present, be described. However, the reports of various studies in tissue culture in rats and man lend support to the hypothesis that hydroxyurea causes an immediate inhibition of DNA synthesis without interfering with the synthesis of ribonucleic acid or of protein. This hypothesis explains why, under certain conditions, hydroxyurea may induce teratogenic effects.

Three mechanisms of action have been postulated for the increased effectiveness of concomitant use of hydroxyurea therapy with irradiation on squamous cell (epidermoid) carcinomas of the head and neck. In vitro studies utilizing Chinese hamster cells suggest that hydroxyurea (1) is lethal to normally radioresistant S-stage cells, and (2) holds other cells of the cell cycle in the G1 or pre-DNA synthesis stage where they are most susceptible to the effects of irradiation. The third mechanism of action has been theorized on the basis of in vitro studies of HeLa cells: it appears that hydroxyurea, by inhibition of DNA synthesis, hinders the normal repair process of cells damaged but not killed by irradiation, thereby decreasing their survival rate; RNA and protein syntheses have shown no alteration.

Absorption, Metabolism, Fate and Excretion
After oral administration in man, hydroxyurea is readily absorbed from the gastrointestinal tract. The drug reaches peak serum concentrations within 2 hours; by 24 hours the concentration in the serum is essentially zero. Approximately 80 percent of an oral or intravenous dose of 7 to 30 mg./kg. may be recovered in the urine within 12 hours.

Animal Pharmacology and Toxicology
The oral LD_{50} of hydroxyurea is 7330 mg./kg. in mice and 5780 mg./kg. in rats, given as a single dose.

In subacute and chronic toxicity studies in the rat, the most consistent pathological findings were an apparent dose-related mild to moderate bone marrow hypoplasia as well as pulmonary congestion and mottling of the lungs. At the highest dosage levels (1260 mg./kg./day for 37 days then 2520 mg./kg./day for 40 days), testicular atrophy with absence of spermatogenesis occurred; in several animals, hepatic cell damage with fatty metamorphosis was noted. In the dog, mild to marked bone marrow depression was a consistent finding except at the lower dosage levels. Additionally, at the higher dose levels (140 to 420 mg. or 140 to 1260 mg./kg./week given 3 or 7 days weekly for 12 weeks), growth retardation, slightly increased blood glucose values, and hemosiderosis of the liver or spleen were found; reversible spermatogenic arrest was noted. In the monkey, bone marrow depression, lymphoid atrophy of the spleen, and degenerative changes in the epithelium of the small and large intestines were found. At the higher, often lethal, doses (400 to 800 mg./kg./day for 7 to 15 days), hemorrhage and congestion were found in the lungs, brain and urinary tract. Cardiovascular effects (changes in heart rate, blood pressure, orthostatic hypotension, EKG changes) and hematological changes (slight hemolysis, slight methemoglobinemia) were observed in some species of laboratory animals at doses exceeding clinical levels.

Indications and Usage: Significant tumor response to Hydrea (Hydroxyurea Capsules USP) has been demonstrated in melanoma, resistant chronic myelocytic leukemia, and recurrent, metastatic, or inoperable carcinoma of the ovary.

Hydrea used concomitantly with irradiation therapy is intended for use in the local control of primary squamous cell (epidermoid) carcinomas of the head and neck, excluding the lip.

Contraindications: Hydroxyurea is contraindicated in patients with marked bone marrow depression, i.e., leukopenia (less than 2500 WBC) or thrombocytopenia (less than 100,000), or severe anemia.

Warnings: Treatment with hydroxyurea should not be initiated if bone marrow function is markedly depressed (—see CONTRAINDICATIONS). Bone marrow suppression may occur, and leukopenia is generally its first and most common manifestation. Thrombocytopenia and anemia occur less often, and are seldom seen without a preceding leukopenia. However, the recovery from myelosuppression is rapid when therapy is interrupted. It should be borne in mind that bone marrow depression is more likely in patients who have previously received radiotherapy or cytotoxic cancer chemotherapeutic agents; hydroxyurea should be used cautiously in such patients.

Patients who have received irradiation therapy in the past may have an exacerbation of postirradiation erythema.

Severe anemia must be corrected with whole blood replacement before initiating therapy with hydroxyurea.

Erythrocytic abnormalities: megaloblastic erythropoiesis, which is self-limiting, is often seen early in the course of hydroxyurea therapy. The morphologic change resembles pernicious anemia, but is not related to vitamin B_{12} or folic acid deficiency. Hydroxyurea may also delay plasma iron clearance and reduce the rate of iron utilization by erythrocytes, but it does not appear to alter the red blood cell survival time.

Hydroxyurea should be used with caution in patients with marked renal dysfunction.

Elderly patients may be more sensitive to the effects of hydroxyurea, and may require a lower dose regimen.

Usage in Pregnancy—Drugs which affect DNA synthesis, such as hydroxyurea, may be potential mutagenic agents. The physician should carefully consider this possibility before administering this drug to male or female patients who may contemplate conception.

Hydrea (Hydroxyurea Capsules USP) is a known teratogenic agent in animals. Therefore, hydroxyurea should not be used in women who are or may become pregnant unless in the judgment of the physician the potential benefits outweigh the possible hazards.

Precautions: Therapy with hydroxyurea requires close supervision. The complete status of the blood, including bone marrow examination, if indicated, as well as kidney function and liver function should be determined prior to, and repeatedly during, treatment. The determination of the hemoglobin level, total leukocyte counts, and platelet counts should be performed at least once a week throughout the course of hydroxyurea therapy. If the white blood cell count decreases to less than 2500/mm^3, or the platelet count to less than 100,000/mm^3, therapy should be interrupted until the values rise significantly toward normal levels. Anemia, if it occurs, should be managed with whole blood replacement, without interrupting hydroxyurea therapy.

Adverse Reactions: Adverse reactions have been primarily bone marrow depression (leukopenia, anemia, and occasionally thrombocytopenia), and less frequently gastrointestinal symptoms (stomatitis, anorexia, nausea, vomiting, diarrhea, and constipation), and dermatological reactions such as maculopapular rash and facial erythema. Dysuria and alopecia occur very rarely. Large doses may produce moderate drowsiness. Neurological disturbances have occurred extremely rarely and were limited to headache, dizziness, disorientation, hallucinations, and convulsions. Hydroxyurea occasionally may cause temporary impairment of renal tubular function accompanied by elevations in serum uric acid, BUN, and creatinine levels. Abnormal BSP retention has been reported. Fever, chills, malaise, and elevation of hepatic enzymes have also been reported. Adverse reactions observed with combined hydroxyurea and irradiation therapy are similar to those reported with the use of hydroxyurea alone. These effects primarily include bone marrow depression (anemia and leukopenia), and gastric irritation. Almost all patients receiving an adequate course of combined hydroxyurea and irradiation therapy will demonstrate concurrent leukopenia. Platelet depression (less than 100,000 cells/mm^3) has occurred rarely and only in the presence of marked leukopenia. Gastric distress has also been reported with irradiation alone and in combination with hydroxyurea therapy.

It should be borne in mind that therapeutic doses of irradiation alone produce the same adverse reactions as hydroxyurea; combined therapy may cause an increase in the incidence and severity of these side effects.

Although inflammation of the mucous membranes at the irradiated site (mucositis) is attributed to irradiation alone, some investigators believe that the more severe cases are due to combination therapy.

Dosage and Administration: Because of the rarity of melanoma, resistant chronic myelocytic leukemia, carcinoma of the ovary, and carcinomas of the head and neck in children, dosage regimens have not been established.

All dosage should be based on the patient's actual or ideal weight, whichever is less.

Continued on next page

Squibb—Cont.

NOTE: If the patient prefers, or is unable to swallow capsules, the contents of the capsules may be emptied into a glass of water and taken immediately. Some inert material used as a vehicle in the capsule may not dissolve, and may float on the surface.

Solid Tumors

Intermittent Therapy: 80 mg./kg. administered orally as *single* dose every *third* day

Continuous Therapy: 20 to 30 mg./kg. administered orally as a *single* dose *daily* The intermittent dosage schedule offers the advantage of reduced toxicity since patients on this dosage regimen have rarely required complete discontinuance of therapy because of toxicity.

Concomitant Therapy with Irradiation (*Carcinoma of the head and neck*)—80 mg./kg. administered orally as a *single* dose every *third* day.

Administration of Hydrea (Hydroxyurea Capsules USP) should be begun at least seven days before initiation of irradiation and continued during radiotherapy as well as indefinitely afterwards provided that the patient may be kept under adequate observation and evidences no unusual or severe reactions.

Irradiation should be given at the maximum dose considered appropriate for the particular therapeutic situation; adjustment of irradiation dosage is not usually necessary when Hydrea is used concomitantly.

Resistant Chronic Myelocytic Leukemia

Until the intermittent therapy regimen has been evaluated, CONTINUOUS therapy (20 to 30 mg./kg. administered orally as a *single* dose *daily*) is recommended.

An adequate trial period for determining the antineoplastic effectiveness of Hydrea is six weeks of therapy. When there is regression in tumor size or arrest in tumor growth, therapy should be continued indefinitely. Therapy should be interrupted if the white blood cell count drops below 2500/mm³, or the platelet count below 100,000/mm³. In these cases, the counts should be rechecked after three days, and therapy resumed when the counts rise significantly toward normal values. Since the hematopoietic rebound is prompt, it is usually necessary to omit only a few doses. If prompt rebound has not occurred during combined hydroxyurea and irradiation therapy, irradiation may also be interrupted. However, the need for postponement of irradiation has been rare; radiotherapy has usually been continued using the recommended dosage and technique. Anemia, if it occurs, should be corrected with whole blood replacement, without interrupting hydroxyurea therapy. Because hematopoiesis may be compromised by extensive irradiation or by other antineoplastic agents, it is recommended that Hydrea be administered cautiously to patients who have recently received extensive radiation therapy or chemotherapy with other cytotoxic drugs.

Pain or discomfort from inflammation of the mucous membranes at the irradiated site (mucositis) is usually controlled by measures such as topical anesthetics and orally administered analgesics. If the reaction is severe, hydroxyurea therapy may be temporarily interrupted; if it is extremely severe, irradiation dosage may, in addition, be temporarily postponed. However, it has rarely been necessary to terminate these therapies.

Severe gastric distress, such as nausea, vomiting, and anorexia resulting from combined therapy may usually be controlled by temporary interruption of Hydrea (Hydroxyurea Capsules USP) administration; rarely has the additional interruption of irradiation been necessary.

How Supplied: Bottles of 100.

Storage: Store at room temperature; avoid excessive heat; keep bottle tightly closed. Dispense in tight containers.

Shown in Product Identification Section, page 438

KENALOG®
[ken'ah-log]
Triamcinolone Acetonide USP
CREAM/LOTION/OINTMENT/SPRAY

Description: The topical corticosteroids constitute a class of primary synthetic steroids used as anti-inflammatory and antipruritic agents. The steroids in this class include triamcinolone acetonide. Triamcinolone acetonide is designated chemically as 9-Fluoro-11β, 16α, 17, 21,-tetrahydroxypregna-1,4-diene-3, 20-dione cyclic 16, 17-acetal with acetone.

Each gram of 0.025%, 0.1%, and 0.5% Kenalog Cream (Triamcinolone Acetonide Cream) provides 0.25 mg, 1 mg, or 5 mg. triancinolone acetonide, respectively, in a vanishing cream base containing propylene glycol, cetearyl alcohol (and) ceteareth-20, white petrolatum, sorbitol solution, glyceryl monostearate, polyethylene glycol monostearate, simethicone, sorbic acid, and purified water.

Each ml of 0.025% and 0.1% Kenalog Lotion (Triamcinolone Acetonide Lotion) provides 0.25 mg. and 1 mg. triamcinolone acetonide, respectively, in a lotion base containing propylene glycol, cetyl alcohol, stearyl alcohol, sorbitan monopalmitate, polysorbate 20, simethicone, and purified water.

Each gram of 0.025%, 0.1%, and 0.5% Kenalog Ointment (Triamcinolone Acetonide Ointment) provides 0.25 mg, 1 mg, or 5 mg. triamcinolone acetonide, respectively, in Plastibase® (Plasticized Hydrocarbon Gel), a polyethylene and mineral oil gel base.

Kenalog Spray (Triamcinolone Acetonide Topical Aerosol) is **for dermatologic use only.** A two-second application, which covers an area approximately the size of the hand, delivers an amount of triamcinolone acetonide not exceeding 0.2 mg. After spraying, the nonvolatile vehicle remaining on the skin contains approximately 0.2% triamcinolone acetonide. Each gram of spray provides 0.147 mg. triamcinolone acetonide in a vehicle of isopropyl palmitate, dehydrated alcolol (10.3%), and isobutane propellant.

Clinical Pharmacology: Topical corticosteroids share anti-inflammatory, antipruritic and vasoconstrictive actions.

The mechanism of anti-inflammatory activity of the topical corticosteroids is unclear. Various laboratory methods, including vasoconstrictor assays, are used to compare and predict potencies and/or clinical efficacies of the topical corticosteroids. There is some evidence to suggest that a recognizable correlation exists between vasoconstrictor potency and therapeutic efficacy in man.

Pharmacokinetics—The extent of percutaneous absorption of topical corticosteroids is determined by many factors including the vehicle, the integrity of the epidermal barrier, and the use of occlusive dressings.

Topical corticosteroids can be absorbed from normal intact skin. Inflammation and/or other disease processes in the skin increase percutaneous absorption. Occlusive dressings substantially increase the percutaneous absorption of topical corticosteroids. Thus, occlusive dressings may be a valuable therapeutic adjunct for treatment of resistant dermatoses (see DOSAGE AND ADMINISTRATION).

Once absorbed through the skin, topical corticosteroids are handled through pharmacokinetic pathways similar to systemically administered corticosteroids. Corticosteroids are bound to plasma proteins in varying degrees. Corticosteroids are metabolized primarily in the liver and are then excreted by the kidneys. Some of the topical corticosteroids and their metabolites are also excreted into the bile.

Indications and Usage: Kenalog (Triamcinolone Acetonide) Creams, Lotions, Ointments, and Spray are indicated for relief of the inflammatory and pruritic manifestations of corticosteroid-responsive dermatoses.

Contraindications: Topical corticosteroids are contraindicated in those patients with a history of hypersensitivity to any of the components of the preparations.

Precautions: General—Systemic absorption of topical corticosteroids has produced reversible hypothalamic-pituitary-adrenal (HPA) axis suppression, manifestations of Cushing's syndrome, hyperglycemia, and glycosuria in some patients. Conditions which augment systemic absorption include the application of the more potent steroids, use over large surface areas, prolonged use, and the addition of occlusive dressings.

Therefore, patients receiving a large dose of any potent topical steroid applied to a large surface area or under an occlusive dressing should be evaluated periodically for evidence of HPA axis suppression by using the urinary free cortisol and ACTH stimulation tests, and for impairment of thermal homeostasis. If HPA axis suppression or elevation of the body temperature occurs, an attempt should be made to withdraw the drug, to reduce the frequency of application, substitute a less potent steroid, or use a sequential approach when utilizing the occlusive technique.

Recovery of HPA axis function and thermal homeostasis are generally prompt and complete upon discontinuation of the drug. Infrequently, signs and symptoms of steroid withdrawal may occur, requiring supplemental systemic corticosteroids. Occasionally, a patient may develop a sensitivity reaction to a particular occlusive dressing material or adhesive and a substitute material may be necessary.

Children may absorb proportionally larger amounts of topical corticosteroids and thus be more susceptible to systemic toxicity (see PRECAUTIONS, Pediatric Use).

If irritation develops, topical corticosteroids should be discontinued and appropriate therapy instituted.

In the presence of dermatological infections, the use of an appropriate antifungal or antibacterial agent should be instituted. If a favorable response does not occur promptly, the corticosteroid should be discontinued until the infection has been adequately controlled.

Information for the Patient: Patients using topical corticosteroids should receive the following information and instructions:

1. This medication is to be used as directed by the physician. It is for external use only. Avoid contact with the eyes.
2. Patients should be advised not to use this medication for any disorder other than for which it was prescribed.
3. The treated skin area should not be bandaged or otherwise covered or wrapped as to be occlusive unless directed by the physician.
4. Patients should report any signs of local adverse reactions especially under occlusive dressing.
5. Parents of pediatric patients should be advised not to use tight-fitting diapers or plastic pants on a child being treated in the diaper area, as these garments may constitute occlusive dressings.

Laboratory Tests—A urinary free cortisol test and ACTH stimulation test may be helpful in evaluating HPA axis suppression.

Carcinogenesis, Mutagenesis, and Impairment of Fertility—Long-term animal studies have not been performed to evaluate the carcinogenic potential or the effect on fertility of topical corticosteroids. Studies to determine mutagenicity with prednisolone and hydrocortisone showed negative results.

Pregnancy: Teratogenic Effects—Category C. Corticosteroids are generally teratogenic in laboratory animals when administered systemically at relatively low dosage levels. The more potent corticosteroids have been shown to be teratogenic after dermal application in laboratory animals. There are no adequate and well-controlled studies in pregnant women on teratogenic effects from topically applied corticosteroids. Therefore, topical corticosteroids should be used during pregnancy only if the potential benefit justifies the potential risk to the fetus. Drugs of this class should not be used extensively on pregnant patients, in large amounts, or for prolonged periods of time.

Nursing Mothers—It is not known whether topical administration of corticosteroids could result in sufficient systemic absorption to produce detectable quantities in breast milk. Systemically administered corticosteroids are secreted into breast milk in quantities **not** likely to have a deleterious effect on the infant. Nevertheless, caution should be exercised when topical corticosteroids are administered to a nursing woman.

Pediatric Use—Pediatric patients may demonstrate greater susceptibility to topical corticosteroid-induced HPA axis suppression and Cushing's syndrome than mature patients because of a larger skin surface area to body weight ratio.

HPA axis suppression, Cushing's syndrome, and intracranial hypertension have been reported in children receiving topical corticosteroids. Manifestations of adrenal suppression in children include linear growth retardation, delayed weight gain, low plasma cortisol levels, and absence of response to ACTH stimulation. Manifestations of intracranial hypertension include bulging fontanelles, headaches, and bilateral papilledema.

Administration of topical corticosteroids to children should be limited to the least amount compatible with an effective therapeutic regimen. Chronic corticosteroid therapy may interfere with the growth and development of children.

Adverse Reactions: The following local adverse reactions are reported infrequently with topical corticosteroids, but may occur more frequently with the use of occlusive dressings (reactions are listed in an approximate decreasing order of occurrence): burning, itching, irritation, dryness, folliculitis, hypertrichosis, acneiform eruptions, hypopigmentation, perioral dermatitis, allergic contact dermatitis, maceration of the skin, secondary infection, skin atrophy, striae, and miliaria.

Overdosage: Topically applied corticosteroids can be absorbed in sufficient amounts to produce systemic effects (see PRECAUTIONS, General).

Dosage and Administration: Kenalog Cream (Triamcinolone Acetonide Cream) 0.025%: Apply to the affected area two to four times daily. Rub in gently.

Kenalog Cream (Triamcinolone Acetonide Cream) 0.1% or 0.5%: Apply, as appropriate, to the affected area two to three times daily. Rub in gently.

Kenalog Lotion (Triamcinolone Acetonide Lotion) 0.025%: Apply to the affected area two to four times daily. Rub in gently.

Kenalog Lotion (Triamcinolone Acetonide Lotion) 0.1%: Apply to the affected area two to three times daily. Rub in gently.

Kenalog Ointment (Triamcinolone Acetonide Ointment) 0.025%: Apply a thin film to the affected area two to four times daily.

Kenalog Ointment (Triamcinolone Acetonide Ointment) 0.1% or 0.5%: Apply a thin film, as appropriate, to the affected area two to three times daily.

Kenalog Spray (Triamcinolone Acetonide Topical Aerosol): Directions for use of the spray can are provided on the label. The preparation may be applied to any area of the body, but when it is sprayed about the face, care should be taken to see that the eyes are covered, and that inhalation of the spray is avoided. Three or four applications daily are generally adequate.

Occlusive Dressing Technique—Kenalog Cream (Triamcinolone Acetonide Cream) 0.025%, 0.1%, and 0.5% and Kenalog Lotion (Triamcinolone Acetonide Lotion) 0.025% and 0.1%: Occlusive dressings may be used for the management of psoriasis or other recalcitrant conditions. Gently rub a small amount of the preparation into the lesion until it disappears. Reapply the preparation leaving a thin coating on the lesion, cover with a pliable nonporous film, and seal the edges. If needed, additional moisture may be provided by covering the lesion with a dampened clean cotton cloth before the nonporous film is applied or by briefly wetting the affected area with water immediately prior to applying the medication. The frequency of changing dressings is best determined on an individual basis. It may be convenient to apply the preparation under an occlusive dressing in the evening and to remove the dressing in the morning (i.e., 12-hour occlusion). When utilizing the 12-hour occlusion regimen, additional preparation should be applied, without occlusion, during the day. Reapplication is essential at each dressing change.

If an infection develops, the use of occlusive dressings should be discontinued and appropriate antimicrobial therapy instituted.

Kenalog Ointment (Triamcinolone Acetonide Ointment) 0.025%, 0.1% and 0.5% and Kenalog Spray (Triamcinolone Acetonide Topical Aerosol): Occlusive dressings may be used for the management of psoriasis or other recalcitrant conditions. Apply a thin coating of the preparation onto the lesion, cover with a pliable nonporous film, and seal the edges. If needed, additional moisture may be provided by covering the lesion with a dampened clean cotton cloth before the nonporous film is applied or by briefly wetting the affected area with water immediately prior to applying the medication. The frequency of changing dressings is best determined on an individual basis. It may be convenient to apply the preparation under an occlusive dressing in the evening and to remove the dressing in the morning (i.e., 12-hour occlusion). When utilizing the 12-hour occlusion regimen, additional preparation should be applied, without occlusion, during the day. Reapplication is essential at each dressing change.

If an infection develops, the use of occlusive dressings should be discontinued and appropriate antimicrobial therapy instituted.

How Supplied: The 0.025% Cream and Ointment are supplied in 15 g., 60 g. and 80 g. tubes, and 240 g. (8 oz.) jars. The 0.1% Cream and Ointment are supplied in 15 g., 60 g., and 80 g. tubes and in 240 g. (8 oz.) jars. The 0.5% Cream and Ointment are supplied in 20 g. tubes. The 0.1% and 0.025% Creams and 0.1% Ointment are also supplied in 5.25 lb. jars. The 0.025% Lotion is supplied in 60 ml. plastic squeeze bottles. The 0.1% Lotion is supplied in 15 ml. and 60 ml. plastic squeeze bottles. [60 ml. bottle, V.A. Depot Item NSN 6505-00-282-5118A]. The Spray is supplied in 23 g. and 63 g. aerosol cans (each can is supplied with a spray tube applicator). [63 g. cans, Military Depot Item, NSN 6505-01-066-1325].

Storage
Store the creams and lotions at room temperature; avoid freezing. Store the ointments at room temperature. Store the spray at room temperature; avoid excessive heat.

KENALOG®-40 INJECTION   ℞
[ken′ah-log″]
(Sterile Triamcinolone Acetonide Suspension USP)
NOT FOR INTRAVENOUS OR INTRADERMAL USE

Description: Kenalog-40 Injection provides a synthetic corticosteroid with marked anti-inflammatory action. Each ml. of the sterile, aqueous suspension provides 40 mg. of triamcinolone acetonide, with sodium chloride for isotonicity, 0.9% (w/v) benzyl alcohol as a preservative, 0.75% sodium carboxymethylcellulose, and 0.04% polysorbate 80. Sodium hydroxide or hydrochloric acid may be present to adjust pH to 5.0 to 7.5. At the time of manufacture, the air in the container is replaced by nitrogen.

Actions: Naturally occurring glucocorticoids (hydrocortisone), which also have salt-retaining properties, are used as replacement therapy in adrenocortical deficiency states. Their synthetic analogs are primarily used for their potent anti-inflammatory effects in disorders of many organ systems.

Glucocorticoids cause profound and varied metabolic effects. In addition, they modify the body's immune responses to diverse stimuli.

Kenalog-40 Injection has an extended duration of effect which may be permanent, or sustained over a period of several weeks. Studies indicate that following a single intramuscular dose of 60 to 100 mg. of triamcinolone acetonide, adrenal suppression occurs within 24 to 48 hours and then gradually returns to normal, usually in 30 to 40 days. This finding correlates closely with the extended duration of therapeutic action achieved with the drug.

Indications:
Intramuscular
Where oral therapy is not feasible or is temporarily undesirable in the judgment of the physician, Kenalog-40 Injection (Sterile Triamcinolone Acetonide Suspension USP) is indicated for intramuscular use as follows:

1. *Endocrine disorders*—Primary or secondary adrenocortical insufficiency (hydrocortisone or cortisone is the drug of choice; synthetic analogs may be used in conjunction with mineralocorticoids where applicable; in infancy, mineralocorticoid supplementation is of particular importance). Acute adrenocortical insufficiency (hydrocortisone or cortisone is the drug of choice; mineralocorticoid supplementation may be necessary, particularly when synthetic analogs are used).
Preoperatively and in the event of serious trauma or illness, in patients with known adrenal insufficiency or when adrenocortical reserve is doubtful. Shock unresponsive to conventional therapy if adrenocortical insufficiency exists or is suspected. Congenital adrenal hyperplasia. Nonsuppurative thyroiditis.

2. *Rheumatic disorders*—As adjunctive therapy for short-term administration (to tide the patient over an acute episode or exacerbation) in: posttraumatic osteoarthritis; synovitis of osteoarthritis; rheumatoid arthritis; acute and subacute bursitis; epicondylitis; acute nonspecific tenosynovitis; acute gouty arthritis; psoriatic arthritis; ankylosing spondylitis; juvenile rheumatoid arthritis.

3. *Collagen diseases*—During an exacerbation or as maintenance therapy in selected cases of: systemic lupus erythematosus; acute rheumatic carditis.

4. *Dermatologic diseases*—Pemphigus; severe erythema multiforme (Stevens-Johnson syndrome); exfoliative dermatitis; bullous dermatitis herpetiformis; severe seborrheic dermatitis; severe psoriasis.

5. *Allergic states*—Control of severe or incapacitating allergic conditions intractable to adequate trials of conventional treatment in: bronchial asthma; contact dermatitis; atopic dermatitis; serum sickness; seasonal or perennial allergic rhinitis; drug hypersensitivity reactions; urticarial transfusion reactions; acute noninfectious laryngeal edema (epinephrine is the drug of first choice).

6. *Ophthalmic diseases*—Severe acute and chronic allergic and inflammatory processes involving the eye, such as: herpes zoster ophthalmicus; iritis; iridocyclitis; chorioretinitis; diffuse posterior uveitis and choroiditis; optic neuritis; sympathetic ophthalmia; anterior segment inflammation.

7. *Gastrointestinal diseases*—To tide the patient over a critical period of disease in: ulcerative colitis (systemic therapy); regional enteritis (systemic therapy).

8. *Respiratory diseases*—Symptomatic sarcoidosis; berylliosis; fulminating or disseminated pulmonary tuberculosis when concurrently accompanied by appropriate antituberculous chemotherapy; aspiration pneumonitis.

9. *Hematologic disorders*—Acquired (autoimmune) hemolytic anemia.

10. *Neoplastic diseases*—For palliative management of: leukemias and lymphomas in adults; acute leukemia of childhood.

11. *Edematous state*—To induce diuresis or remission of proteinuria in the nephrotic syndrome, without uremia, of the idiopathic type or that due to lupus erythematosus.

12. *Miscellaneous*—Tuberculous meningitis with subarachnoid block or impending block when con-

Continued on next page

Squibb—Cont.

currently accompanied by appropriate antituberculous chemotherapy.

Intra-Articular
Kenalog-40 Injection (Sterile Triamcinolone Acetonide Suspension USP) is indicated for intra-articular or intrabursal administration, and for injections into tendon sheaths, as adjunctive therapy for short-term administration (to tide the patient over an acute episode or exacerbation) in: synovitis of osteoarthritis; rheumatoid arthritis; acute and subacute bursitis; acute gouty arthritis; epicondylitis; acute nonspecific tenosynovitis; posttraumatic osteoarthritis.

Contraindications: Corticosteroids are contraindicated in patients with systemic fungal infections. Intramuscular corticosteroid preparations are contraindicated for idiopathic thrombocytopenic purpura.

Warnings: Because it is a suspension, the preparation should **not** be administered intravenously. Strict aseptic technique is mandatory. This preparation is not recommended for children under six years of age.

When patients who are receiving corticosteroid therapy are subjected to unusual stress, increased dosage of rapidly acting corticosteroids is indicated before, during, and after the stressful situation.

Corticosteroids may mask some signs of infection, and new infections may appear during their use. There may be decreased resistance and inability to localize infection when corticosteroids are used. If an infection occurs during corticosteroid therapy, it should be promptly controlled by suitable antimicrobial therapy (see PRECAUTIONS).

Prolonged use of corticosteroids may produce posterior subcapsular cataracts, glaucoma with possible damage to the optic nerves, and may enhance the establishment of secondary ocular infections due to fungi or viruses.

Average and large doses of hydrocortisone or cortisone can cause elevation of blood pressure, salt and water retention, and increased excretion of potassium. These effects are less likely to occur with the synthetic derivatives except when they are used in large doses; dietary salt restriction and potassium supplementation may be necessary (see PRECAUTIONS). All corticosteroids increase calcium excretion.

Patients should not be vaccinated against smallpox while on corticosteroid therapy. Other immunization procedures should not be undertaken in patients who are on corticosteroids, especially on high dose, because of possible hazards of neurological complications and a lack of antibody response. The use of triamcinolone acetonide in patients with active tuberculosis should be restricted to those cases of fulminating or disseminated tuberculosis in which the corticosteroid is used for the management of the disease in conjunction with an appropriate antituberculous regimen. If corticosteroids are indicated in patients with latent tuberculosis or tuberculin reactivity, close observation is necessary since reactivation of the disease may occur. During prolonged corticosteroid therapy, these patients should receive chemoprophylaxis.

Because rare instances of anaphylactoid reactions have occurred in patients receiving parenteral corticosteroid therapy, appropriate precautionary measures should be taken prior to administration, especially when the patient has a history of allergy to any drug.

Unless a **deep** intramuscular injection is given, local atrophy is likely to occur. (For recommendations on injection techniques, see DOSAGE AND ADMINISTRATION.) Due to the significantly higher incidence of local atrophy when the material is injected into the deltoid area, this injection site should be avoided in favor of the gluteal area. Only very unusual circumstances would warrant injection into the deltoid area.

Usage in Pregnancy: Since adequate human reproduction studies have not been done with corticosteroids, the use of these drugs in pregnancy, nursing mothers, or women of child-bearing potential requires that the possible benefits of the drug be weighed against the potential hazards to the mother and the embryo, fetus, or nursing infant. Infants born of mothers who have received substantial doses of corticosteroids during pregnancy should be carefully observed for signs of hypoadrenalism.

Precautions: Drug-induced secondary adrenocortical insufficiency may be minimized by a gradual reduction of dosage. This type of relative insufficiency may persist for months after discontinuation of therapy; therefore, in any situation of stress (such as trauma, surgery, or severe illness) occurring during that period, hormone therapy should be reinstituted. Since mineralocorticoid secretion may be impaired, salt and/or a mineralocorticoid should be administered concurrently.

There is an enhanced corticosteroid effect in patients with hypothyroidism and in those with cirrhosis.

Corticosteroids should be used cautiously in patients with ocular herpes simplex because of possible corneal perforation.

The lowest possible dose of corticosteroid should be used to control the condition being treated. A gradual reduction in dosage should be made when possible.

Psychic derangements may appear when corticosteroids are used. These may range from euphoria, insomnia, mood swings, personality changes and severe depression to frank psychotic manifestations. Existing emotional instability or psychotic tendencies may also be aggravated by corticosteroids.

Aspirin should be used cautiously in conjunction with corticosteroids in patients with hypoprothrombinemia.

Corticosteroids should be used with caution in patients with nonspecific ulcerative colitis if there is a probability of impending perforation, abscess, or other pyogenic infection. Corticosteroids should also be used cautiously in patients with diverticulitis, fresh intestinal anastomoses, active or latent peptic ulcer, renal insufficiency, hypertension, osteoporosis, acute glomerulonephritis, vaccinia, varicella, exanthema, Cushing's syndrome, antibiotic resistant infections, diabetes mellitus, congestive heart failure, chronic nephritis, thromboembolitic tendencies, thrombophlebitis, convulsive disorders, metastatic carcinoma, and myasthenia gravis.

Growth and development of infants and children on prolonged corticosteroid therapy should be carefully observed.

Although therapy with Kenalog-40 Injection (Sterile Triamcinolone Acetonide Suspension USP) will ameliorate symptoms, it is in no sense a cure and the hormone has no effect on the cause of the inflammation. Therefore, this method of treatment does not obviate the need for the conventional measures usually employed.

Intra-articular injection of a corticosteroid may produce systemic as well as local effects. The inadvertent injection of the suspension into the soft tissues surrounding a joint is not harmful, but may lead to the occurrence of systemic effects, and is the most common cause of failure to achieve the desired local results.

Following intra-articular steroid therapy, patients should be specifically warned to avoid overuse of joints in which symptomatic benefit has been obtained. Negligence in this matter may permit an increase in joint deterioration that will more than offset the beneficial effects of the steroid. To detect deterioration, follow-up x-ray examination is suggested in selected cases.

Overdistention of the joint capsule and deposition of steroid along the needle track should be avoided in intra-articular injection since this may lead to subcutaneous atrophy.

Corticosteroids should not be injected into unstable joints. Repeated intra-articular injection may in some cases result in instability of the joint. In selected cases, particularly when repeated injections are given, x-ray follow-up is suggested.

An increase in joint discomfort has seldom occurred. A marked increase in pain accompanied by local swelling, further restriction of joint motion, fever, and malaise are suggestive of a septic arthritis. If these complications should appear, and the diagnosis of septic arthritis is confirmed, administration of triamcinolone acetonide should be stopped, and antimicrobial therapy should be instituted immediately and continued for 7 to 10 days after all evidence of infection has disappeared. Appropriate examination of any joint fluid present is necessary to exclude a septic process.

Local injection of a steroid into a previously infected joint is to be avoided.

Kenalog-40 Injection (Sterile Triamcinolone Acetonide Suspension USP) should be administered only with full knowledge of characteristic activity of, and varied responses to, adrenocortical hormones. Like other potent corticosteroids, triamcinolone acetonide should be used under close clinical supervision. Triamcinolone acetonide can cause elevation of blood pressure, salt and water retention, and increased potassium and calcium excretion necessitating dietary salt restriction and potassium supplementation. Edema may occur in the presence of renal disease with a fixed or decreased glomerular filtration rate.

During prolonged therapy, **a liberal protein intake is essential** for counteracting the tendency to gradual weight loss sometimes associated with negative nitrogen balance, wasting and weakness of skeletal muscles.

When local or systemic microbial infections are present, therapy with triamcinolone acetonide is not recommended, but may be employed with caution and only in conjunction with appropriate antibiotic or chemotherapeutic medication. Triamcinolone acetonide may mask signs of infection and enhance dissemination of the infecting organism. Hence, all patients receiving triamcinolone acetonide should be watched for evidence of intercurrent infection. Should infection occur, vigorous, appropriate anti-infective therapy should be initiated. If possible, abrupt cessation of steroids should be avoided because of the danger of superimposing adrenocortical insufficiency on the infectious process.

Menstrual irregularities may occur, and this possibility should be mentioned to female patients past menarche.

In peptic ulcer, recurrence may be asymptomatic until perforation or hemorrhage occurs. Long-term adrenocorticoid therapy may evoke hyperacidity or peptic ulcer; therefore, as a prophylactic measure, an ulcer regimen and the administration of an antacid are highly recommended. X-rays should be taken in peptic ulcer patients complaining of gastric distress, or when therapy is prolonged. Whether or not changes are observed, an ulcer regimen is recommended.

As with other corticosteroids, the possibility of other severe reactions should be considered. If such reactions should occur, appropriate corrective measures should be instituted and use of the drug discontinued.

Continued supervision of the patient after termination of triamcinolone acetonide therapy is essential, since there may be a sudden reappearance of severe manifestations of the disease for which the patient was treated.

Adverse Reactions: Following Administration by Any Route — Patients should be watched closely for the following adverse reactions which may be associated with any corticosteroid therapy:
Fluid and electrolyte disturbances — sodium retention, fluid retention, congestive heart failure in susceptible patients, potassium loss, cardiac arrhythmias or ECG changes due to potassium deficiency, hypokalemic alkalosis, and hypertension.
Musculoskeletal — muscle weakness, fatigue, steroid myopathy, loss of muscle mass, osteoporosis, vertebral compression fractures, delayed healing of fractures, aseptic necrosis of femoral and humeral heads, pathologic fractures of long bones, and spontaneous fractures.
Gastrointestinal — peptic ulcer with possible subsequent perforation and hemorrhage, pancreati-

tis, abdominal distention, and ulcerative esophagitis.

Dermatologic — impaired wound healing, thin fragile skin, petechiae and ecchymoses, facial erythema, increased sweating, purpura, striae, hirsutism, acneiform eruptions, lupus erythematosus-like lesions and suppressed reactions to skin tests.

Neurological — convulsions, increased intracranial pressure with papilledema (pseudo-tumor cerebri) usually after treatment, vertigo, headache, neuritis or paresthesias, and aggravation of preexisting psychiatric conditions.

Endocrine — menstrual irregularities; development of the cushingoid state; suppression of growth in children; secondary adrenocortical and pituitary unresponsiveness, particularly in times of stress (e.g., trauma, surgery, or illness); decreased carbohydrate tolerance; manifestations of latent diabetes mellitus and increased requirements for insulin or oral hypoglycemic agents in diabetics.

Ophthalmic — posterior subcapsular cataracts, increased intraocular pressure, glaucoma, and exophthalmos.

Metabolic — hyperglycemia, glycosuria, and negative nitrogen balance due to protein catabolism.

Others — necrotizing angiitis, thrombophlebitis, thromboembolism, aggravation or masking of infections, insomnia, syncopal episodes, and anaphylactoid reactions.

Following Intramuscular Administration — Severe pain has been reported in a few cases. Sterile abscess formation, subcutaneous and cutaneous atrophy, hyperpigmentation and hypopigmentation and charcot-like arthropathy have also occurred.

Following Intra-Articular Administration — Undesirable reactions have included postinjection flare, transient pain, occasional irritation at the injection site, sterile abscess formation, hyperpigmentation and hypopigmentation, charcot-like arthropathy and occasional brief increase in joint discomfort.

Dosage and Administration:
General

The initial dose of Kenalog-40 Injection (Sterile Triamcinolone Acetonide Suspension USP) may vary from 2.5 to 60 mg. per day depending on the specific disease entity being treated (see **Dosage** section below). In situations of less severity, lower doses will generally suffice while in selected patients higher initial doses may be required. Usually the parenteral dosage ranges are one-third to one-half the oral dose given every 12 hours. However, in certain overwhelming, acute, life-threatening situations, administration of dosages exceeding the usual dosages may be justified and may be in multiples of the oral dosages.

The initial dosage should be maintained or adjusted until a satisfactory response is noted. If after a reasonable period of time there is a lack of satisfactory clinical response, Kenalog-40 Injection should be discontinued and the patient transferred to other appropriate therapy. **IT SHOULD BE EMPHASIZED THAT DOSAGE REQUIREMENTS ARE VARIABLE AND MUST BE INDIVIDUALIZED ON THE BASIS OF THE DISEASE UNDER TREATMENT AND THE RESPONSE OF THE PATIENT.** After a favorable response is noted, the proper maintenance dosage should be determined by decreasing the initial drug dosage in small increments at appropriate time intervals until the lowest dosage which will maintain an adequate clinical response is reached. It should be kept in mind that constant monitoring is needed in regard to drug dosage. Included in the situations which may make dosage adjustments necessary are changes in clinical status secondary to remissions or exacerbations in the disease process, the patient's individual drug responsiveness, and the effect of patient exposure to stressful situations not directly related to the disease entity under treatment; in this latter situation it may be necessary to increase the dosage of Kenalog-40 Injection for a period of time consistent with the patient's condition. If after long-term therapy the drug is to be stopped, it is recommended that it be withdrawn gradually rather than abruptly.

Dosage
Systemic: Although Kenalog-40 Injection (Sterile Triamcinolone Acetonide Suspension USP) may be administered intramuscularly for initial therapy, most physicians prefer to adjust the dose orally until adequate control is attained. Intramuscular administration provides a sustained or depot action which can be used to supplement or replace initial oral therapy. With intramuscular therapy, greater supervision of the amount of steroid used is made possible in the patient who is inconsistent in following an oral dosage schedule. In maintenance therapy, the patient-to-patient response is not uniform and, therefore, the dose must be individualized for optimal control.

For **adults and children over 12 years of age**, the suggested initial dose is 60 mg., **injected deeply into the gluteal muscle**. Subcutaneous fat atrophy may occur if care is not taken to inject the preparation intramuscularly. Dosage is usually adjusted within the range of 40 to 80 mg., depending upon patient response and duration of relief. However, some patients may be well controlled on dosages as low as 20 mg. or less. Patients with hay fever or pollen asthma who are not responding to pollen administration and other conventional therapy may obtain a remission of symptoms lasting throughout the pollen season after one injection of 40 to 100 mg.

For **children from 6 to 12 years of age**, the suggested initial dose is 40 mg., although dosage depends more on the severity of symptoms than on age or weight. There is insufficient clinical experience with Kenalog-40 Injection to recommend its use in children under six years of age.

Local: For intra-articular or intrabursal administration and for injection into tendon sheaths, the initial dose of Kenalog-40 Injection (Sterile Triamcinolone Acetonide Suspension USP) may vary from 2.5 to 5 mg. for smaller joints and from 5 to 15 mg. for larger joints depending on the specific disease entity being treated. (A more dilute form of Sterile Triamcinolone Acetonide Suspension USP is available—see ALSO AVAILABLE.) For adults, doses up to 10 mg. for smaller areas and up to 40 mg. for larger areas have usually been sufficient to alleviate symptoms. Single injections into several joints for multiple locus involvement, up to a total of 80 mg., have been given without undue reactions. A single local injection of triamcinolone acetonide is frequently sufficient, but several injections may be needed for adequate relief of symptoms. The lower dosages in the initial dosage range of triamcinolone acetonide may produce the desired effect when the corticosteroid is administered to provide a localized concentration. The site of the injection and the volume of the injection should be carefully considered when triamcinolone acetonide is administered for this purpose.

Administration
General: Shake the vial before use to insure a uniform suspension. After withdrawal, inject without delay to prevent settling in the syringe. Careful technique should be employed to avoid the possibility of entering a blood vessel or introducing infection.

Routine laboratory studies, such as urinalysis, two-hour postprandial blood sugar, determination of blood pressure and body weight and a chest x-ray should be made at regular intervals during prolonged therapy. Upper GI x-rays are desirable in patients with an ulcer history or significant dyspepsia.

Systemic: For systemic therapy, injection should be made **deeply into the gluteal muscle** to insure intramuscular delivery (see WARNINGS). For adults, a minimum needle length of 1 ½ inches is recommended. In obese patients, a longer needle may be required. Use alternate sites for subsequent injections.

Local: For treatment of joints, the usual intra-articular injection technique, as described in standard textbooks, should be followed. If an excessive amount of synovial fluid is present in the joint, some, but not all, should be aspirated to aid in the relief of pain and to prevent undue dilution of the corticosteroid.

With intra-articular or intrabursal administration, and with injection of the drug into tendon sheaths, the use of a local anesthetic may often be desirable. When a local anesthetic is used, its package insert should be read with care and all the precautions connected with its use should be observed. It should be injected into the surrounding soft tissues prior to the injection of the corticosteroid. A small amount of the anesthetic solution may be instilled into the joint.

In treating acute nonspecific tenosynovitis, care should be taken to insure that the injection of the corticosteroid is made into the tendon sheath rather than the tendon substance. Epicondylitis (tennis elbow) may be treated by infiltrating the preparation into the area of greatest tenderness.

How Supplied: In vials of 1, 5, and 10 ml. [5 ml. vial—Military Depot Item, NSN 6505-00-885-6216 and V.A. Depot Item, NSN6505-00-885-6216A].

Also Available: Kenalog-10 Injection (Sterile Triamcinolone Acetonide Suspension USP) providing 10 mg. triamcinolone acetonide per ml., with sodium chloride for isotonicity, 0.9% (w/v) benzyl alcohol as a preservative, 0.75% sodium carboxymethylcellulose, and 0.04% polysorbate 80. See package insert for full information.

Storage: Store at room temperature; avoid freezing. Protect from light.

KENALOG® -10 INJECTION ℞
[ken'ah-log"]
(Sterile Triamcinolone Acetonide Suspension USP)
For Intra-articular, Intrabursal or Intradermal Use
NOT FOR INTRAVENOUS OR INTRAMUSCULAR USE

Description: Kenalog-10 Injection (Sterile Triamcinolone Acetonide Suspension USP) provides triamcinolone acetonide, a synthetic corticosteroid with marked anti-inflammatory action, in a sterile aqueous suspension suitable for intradermal, intra-articular, and intrabursal injection and for injection into tendon sheaths. This preparation is NOT suitable for intravenous or intramuscular use. Each ml. of the sterile aqueous suspension provides 10 mg. triamcinolone acetonide, with sodium chloride for isotonicity, 0.9% (w/v) benzyl alcohol as a preservative, 0.75% carboxymethylcellulose sodium, and 0.04% polysorbate 80; sodium hydroxide or hydrochloric acid may have been added to adjust pH between 5.0 and 7.5. At the time of manufacture, the air in the container is replaced by nitrogen.

The chemical name for triamcinolone acetonide is 9-fluoro-11β, 16α, 17, 21-tetrahydroxypregna-1,4-diene-3,20-dione cyclic 16, 17-acetal with acetone.

Clinical Pharmacology: Naturally occurring glucocorticoids (hydrocortisone), which also have salt-retaining properties, are used as replacement therapy in adrenocortical deficiency states. Their synthetic analogs are primarily used for their potent anti-inflammatory effects in disorders of many organ systems.

Glucocorticoids cause profound and varied metabolic effects. In addition, they modify the body's immune responses to diverse stimuli.

Indications and Usage:
Intra-Articular:
Kenalog-10 Injection (Sterile Triamcinolone Acetonide Suspension USP) is indicated for intra-articular or intrabursal administration, and for injections into tendon sheaths, as adjunctive therapy for short-term administration (to tide the patient over an acute episode or exacerbation) in: synovitis of osteoarthritis, rheumatoid arthritis, acute and subacute bursitis, acute gouty arthritis, epicondylitis, acute nonspecific tenosynovitis, and post-traumatic osteoarthritis.

Intradermal:
Intralesional administration of Kenalog-10 Injection is indicated for the treatment of keloids, dis-

Continued on next page

Squibb—Cont.

coid lupus erythematosus, necrobiosis lipoidica diabeticorum, alopecia areata, and localized hypertrophic, infiltrated, inflammatory lesions of: lichen planus, psoriatic plaques, granuloma annulare, and lichen simplex chronicus (neurodermatitis). Kenalog-10 Injection also may be useful in cystic tumors of an aponeurosis or tendon (ganglia).

Contraindications: Corticosteroids are contraindicated in patients with systemic fungal infections.

Warnings: Because it is a suspension, the preparation should *not* be administered intravenously. Strict aseptic technique is mandatory.

When patients who are receiving corticosteroid therapy are subjected to unusual stress, increased dosage of rapidly acting corticosteroids is indicated before, during, and after the stressful situation. Kenalog-10 Injection (Sterile Triamcinolone Acetonide Suspension USP), as a long-acting preparation, is *not* suitable for use in acute stress situations.

Corticosteroids may mask some signs of infection, and new infections may appear during their use. There may be decreased resistance and inability to localize infection when corticosteroids are used. If an infection occurs during corticosteroid therapy, it should be promptly controlled by suitable antimicrobial therapy (see PRECAUTIONS).

Prolonged use of corticosteroids may produce posterior subcapsular cataracts, glaucoma with possible damage to the optic nerves, and may enhance the establishment of secondary ocular infections due to fungi or viruses.

Average and large doses of hydrocortisone or cortisone can cause elevation of blood pressure, salt and water retention, and increased excretion of potassium. These effects are less likely to occur with the synthetic derivatives except when they are used in large doses; dietary salt restriction and potassium supplementation may be necessary (see PRECAUTIONS). All corticosteroids increase calcium excretion.

Patients should not be vaccinated against smallpox while on corticosteroid therapy. Other immunization procedures should not be undertaken in patients who are on corticosteroids, especially on high dose, because of possible hazards of neurological complications and a lack of antibody response. The use of triamcinolone acetonide in patients with active tuberculosis should be restricted to those cases of fulminating or disseminated tuberculosis in which the corticosteroid is used for the management of the disease in conjunction with an appropriate antituberculous regimen. If corticosteroids are indicated in patients with latent tuberculosis or tuberculin reactivity, close observation is necessary since reactivation of the disease may occur. During prolonged corticosteroid therapy these patients should receive chemoprophylaxis.

Because rare instances of anaphylactoid reactions have occurred in patients receiving parenteral corticosteroid therapy, appropriate precautionary measures should be taken prior to administration, especially when the patient has a history of allergy to any drug.

Safety of use of Kenalog-10 Injection (Sterile Triamcinolone Acetonide Suspension USP) by intraturbinal, subconjunctival, subtenons, and retrobulbar injection has not been established.

Usage in Pregnancy — Since adequate human reproduction studies have not been done with corticosteroids, the use of these drugs in pregnancy, nursing mothers, or women of child-bearing potential requires that the possible benefits of the drug be weighed against the potential hazards to the mother and the embryo, fetus, or nursing infant. Infants born of mothers who have received substantial doses of corticosteroids during pregnancy should be carefully observed for signs of hypoadrenalism.

Precautions: Drug-induced secondary adrenocortical insufficiency may be minimized by a gradual reduction of dosage. This type of relative insufficiency may persist for months after discontinuation of therapy; therefore, in any situation of stress (such as trauma, surgery, or severe illness) occurring during that period, hormone therapy should be reinstituted. Since mineralocorticoid secretion may be impaired, salt and/or a mineralocorticoid should be administered concurrently.

There is enhanced corticosteroid effect in patients with hypothyroidism and in those with cirrhosis.

Corticosteroids should be used cautiously in patients with ocular herpes simplex because of possible corneal perforation.

The lowest possible dose of corticosteroid should be used to control the condition being treated. A gradual reduction in dosage should be made when possible.

Psychic derangements may appear when corticosteroids are used. These may range from euphoria, insomnia, mood swings, personality changes, and severe depression, to frank psychotic manifestations. Existing emotional instability or psychotic tendencies may also be aggravated by corticosteroids.

Aspirin should be used cautiously in conjunction with corticosteroids in patients with hypoprothrombinemia.

Corticosteroids should be used with caution in patients with nonspecific ulcerative colitis if there is a probability of impending perforation, abscess, or other pyogenic infection. Corticosteroids should also be used cautiously in patients with diverticulitis, fresh intestinal anastomoses, active or latent peptic ulcer, renal insufficiency, hypertension, osteoporosis, and myasthenia gravis.

Growth and development of infants and children on prolonged corticosteroid therapy should be carefully observed.

Although therapy with Kenalog-10 Injection (Sterile Triamcinolone Acetonide Suspension USP) may ameliorate symptoms, it is in no sense a cure and the hormone has no effect on the cause of the inflammation. Therefore, this method of treatment does not obviate the need for the conventional measures usually employed.

Intra-articular injection of a corticosteroid may produce systemic as well as local effects. The inadvertent injection of the suspension into the soft tissues surrounding a joint is not harmful, but is the most common cause of failure to achieve the desired local results.

Following intra-articular steroid therapy, patients should be specifically warned to avoid overuse of joints in which symptomatic benefit has been obtained. Negligence in this matter may permit an increase in joint deterioration that will more than offset the beneficial effects of the steroid. To detect deterioration follow-up x-ray examination is suggested in selected cases.

Overdistention of the joint capsule and deposition of steroid along the needle track should be avoided in intra-articular injection since this may lead to subcutaneous atrophy.

Corticosteroids should not be injected into unstable joints. Repeated intra-articular injection may in some cases result in instability of the joint. In selected cases, particularly when repeated injections are given, x-ray follow-up is suggested.

An increase in joint discomfort has seldom occurred. A marked increase in pain accompanied by local swelling, further restriction of joint motion, fever, and malaise are suggestive of a septic arthritis. If these complications should appear, and the diagnosis of septic arthritis is confirmed, administration of triamcinolone acetonide should be stopped, and antimicrobial therapy should be instituted immediately and continued for 7 to 10 days after all evidence of infection has disappeared. Appropriate examination of any joint fluid present is necessary to exclude a septic process.

Local injection of a steroid into a previously infected joint is to be avoided.

Kenalog-10 Injection (Sterile Triamcinolone Acetonide Suspension USP) should be administered only with full knowledge of characteristic activity of, and varied responses to, adrenocortical hormones. Like other potent corticosteroids, triamcinolone acetonide should be used under close clinical supervision. Triamcinolone acetonide can cause elevation of blood pressure, salt and water retention, and increased potassium and calcium excretion necessitating dietary salt restriction and potassium supplementation. Edema may occur in the presence of renal disease with a fixed or decreased glomerular filtration rate.

During prolonged therapy, *a liberal protein intake is essential* for counteracting the tendency to gradual weight loss sometimes associated with negative nitrogen balance, wasting and weakness of skeletal muscles.

When local or systemic microbial infections are present, therapy with triamcinolone acetonide is not recommended, but may be employed with caution and only in conjunction with appropriate antibiotic or chemotherapeutic medication. Triamcinolone acetonide may mask signs of infection and enhance dissemination of the infecting organism. Hence, all patients receiving triamcinolone acetonide should be watched for evidence of intercurrent infection. Should infection occur, vigorous, appropriate anti-infective therapy should be initiated. If possible, abrupt cessation of steroids should be avoided because of the danger of superimposing adrenocortical insufficiency on the infectious process.

Menstrual irregularities may occur, and this possibility should be mentioned to female patients past menarche.

In peptic ulcer, recurrence may be asymptomatic until perforation or hemorrhage occurs. X-rays should be taken in peptic ulcer patients complaining of gastric distress, or when therapy is prolonged. Whether or not changes are observed, an ulcer regimen is recommended.

As with other corticosteroids, the possibility of other severe reactions should be considered. If such reactions should occur, appropriate corrective measures should be instituted and use of the drug discontinued.

Continued supervision of the patient after termination of triamcinolone acetonide therapy is essential, since there may be a sudden reappearance of severe manifestations of the disease for which the patient was treated.

Adverse Reactions: Undesirable reactions following intra-articular administration of the preparation have included postinjection flare, transient pain, occasional local irritation at the injection site, sterile abscesses, hyper- and hypopigmentation, charcot-like arthropathy, and occasional brief increase in joint discomfort; following intradermal administration, rare instances of blindness associated with intralesional therapy around the face and head, transient local discomfort, sterile abscesses, hyper- and hypopigmentation, and subcutaneous and cutaneous atrophy (which usually disappears, unless the basic disease process is itself atrophic) have occurred.

Since systemic absorption may occasionally occur with intra-articular or other local administration, patients should be watched closely for the following adverse reactions which may be associated with any corticosteroid therapy:

Fluid and electrolyte disturbances—sodium retention, fluid retention, congestive heart failure in susceptible patients, potassium loss, cardiac arrythmias or ECG changes due to potassium deficiency, hypokalemic alkalosis, and hypertension.

Musculoskeletal—muscle weakness, fatigue, steroid myopathy, loss of muscle mass, osteoporosis, vertebral compression fractures, delayed healing of fractures, aseptic necrosis of femoral and humeral heads, pathologic fractures of long bones, and spontaneous fractures.

Gastrointenstinal—peptic ulcer with possible subsequent perforation and hemorrhage, pancreatitis, abdominal distention, and ulcerative esophagitis.

Dermatologic—impaired wound healing, thin fragile skin, petechiae and ecchymoses, facial erythema, increased sweating, purpura, striae, hirsutism, acneiform eruptions, lupus erythematosus-like lesions and suppressed reactions to skin tests.

Neurological—convulsions, increased intracranial pressure with papilledema (pseudo-tumor cerebri) usually after treatment, vertigo, headache, neuritis or paresthesias, and aggravation of pre-existing psychiatric conditions.

Endocrine—menstrual irregularities; development of the cushingoid state; suppression of growth in children; secondary adrenocortical and pituitary unresponsiveness, particularly in times of stress (e.g., trauma, surgery, or illness); decreased carbohydrate tolerance; manifestations of latent diabetes mellitus; and increased requirements for insulin or oral hypoglycemic agents in diabetics.

Ophthalmic—posterior subcapsular cataracts, increased intraocular pressure, glaucoma, and exophthalmos.

Metabolic—hyperglycemia, glycosuria, and negative nitrogen balance due to protein catabolism.

Others—necrotizing angiitis, thrombophlebitis, thromboembolism, aggravation or masking of infections, insomnia, syncopal episodes, and anaphylactoid reactions.

Dosage and Administration:

Dosage: The initial dose of Kenalog-10 Injection (Sterile Triamcinolone Acetonide Suspension USP) for intra-articular or intrabursal administration and for injection into tendon sheaths may vary from 2.5 mg. to 5 mg. for smaller joints and from 5 to 15 mg. for larger joints depending on the specific disease entity being treated. Single injections into several joints for multiple locus involvement, up to a total of 20 mg. or more, have been given without incident. For intradermal administration, the initial dose of triamcinolone acetonide will vary depending upon the specific disease entity being treated but should be limited to 1.0 mg. (0.1 ml.) per injection site, since larger volumes are more likely to produce cutaneous atrophy. Multiple sites (separated by one centimeter or more) may be so injected, keeping in mind that the greater the *total* volume employed the more corticosteroid becomes available for possible systemic absorption and subsequent corticosteroid effects. Such injections may be repeated, if necessary, at weekly or less frequent intervals.

The lower dosages in the initial dosage range of triamcinolone acetonide may produce the desired effect when the corticosteroid is administered to provide a localized concentration. The site of the injection and the volume of the injection should be carefully considered when triamcinolone acetonide is administered for this purpose. The inital dosage should be maintained or adjusted until a satisfactory response is noted. If after a reasonable period of time there is a lack of satisfactory clinical response, Kenalog-10 Injection should be discontinued and the patient transferred to other appropriate therapy. IT SHOULD BE EMPHASIZED THAT DOSAGE REQUIREMENTS ARE VARIABLE AND MUST BE INDIVIDUALIZED ON THE BASIS OF THE DISEASE UNDER TREATMENT AND THE RESPONSE OF THE PATIENT. After a favorable response is noted, the proper maintenance dosage should be determined by decreasing the initial drug dosage in small increments at appropriate time intervals until the lowest dosage which will maintain an adequate clinical response is reached. It should be kept in mind that constant monitoring is needed in regard to drug dosage. Included in the situations which may make dosage adjustments necessary are changes in clinical status secondary to remissions or exacerbations in the disease process, the patient's individual drug responsiveness, and the effect of patient exposure to stressful situations not directly related to the disease entity under treatment; in this latter situation it may be necessary to increase the dosage of Kenalog-10 Injection (Sterile Triamcinolone Acetonide Suspension USP) for a period of time consistent with the patient's condition. If the drug is to be stopped after long-term therapy, it is recommended that it be withdrawn gradually rather than abruptly.

Administration: Shake the vial before use to insure a uniform suspension. After withdrawal, inject without delay to prevent settling in the syringe. Careful technique should be employed to avoid the possibility of entering a blood vessel or introducing infection.

Routine laboratory studies, such as urinalysis, two-hour post-prandial blood sugar, determination of blood pressure and body weight, and a chest x-ray should be made at regular intervals during prolonged therapy. Upper GI x-rays are desirable in patients with an ulcer history or significant dyspepsia.

For treatment of joints, the usual intra-articular injection technique, as described in standard textbooks, should be followed. If an excessive amount of synovial fluid is present in the joint, some, but not all, should be aspirated to aid in the relief of pain and to prevent undue dilution of the steroid. With intra-articular or intrabursal administration, and with injection of Kenalog-10 Injection into tendon sheaths, the use of a local anesthetic may often be desirable. When a local anesthetic is used, its package insert should be read with care and all the precautions connected with its use should be observed. It should be injected into the surrounding soft tissue prior to the injection of the corticosteroid. A small amount of the anesthetic solution may be instilled into the joint.

In treating acute nonspecific tenosynovitis, care should be taken to insure that the injection of Kenalog-10 Injection is made into the tendon sheath rather than the tendon substance. Epicondylitis (tennis elbow) may be treated by infiltrating the preparation into the area of greatest tenderness.

For treatment of dermal lesions, Kenalog-10 Injection is injected directly into the lesion, i.e., intradermally or sometimes subcutaneously. For accuracy of dosage measurement and ease of administration, it is preferable to employ a tuberculin syringe and a small bore needle (23 to 25 gauge). Ethyl chloride spray may be used to alleviate the discomfort of the injection.

How Supplied: Kenalog-10 Injection (Sterile Triamcinolone Acetonide Suspension USP) is supplied in 5 ml. multiple-dose vials providing 10 mg. triamcinolone acetonide per ml. [Military Depot Item, NSN 6505-00-065-6772].

Storage: Store at room temperature; avoid freezing; protect from light.

KENALOG® IN ORABASE® ℞
[ken'ah-log" in or'a-bās"]
(Triamcinolone Acetonide Dental Paste USP)

Description: Each gram of Kenalog in Orabase provides 1 mg. (0.1%) triamcinolone acetonide in emollient dental paste containing gelatin, pectin, and carboxymethylcellulose sodium in Plastibase® (Plasticized Hydrocarbon Gel), a polyethylene and mineral oil gel base.

Actions: Triamcinolone acetonide is a synthetic corticosteroid which possesses anti-inflammatory, antipruritic, and antiallergic action. The emollient dental paste acts as an adhesive vehicle for applying the active medication to the oral tissues. The vehicle provides a protective covering which may serve to temporarily reduce the pain associated with oral irritation.

Indications: Kenalog in Orabase (Triamcinolone Acetonide Dental Paste USP) is indicated for adjunctive treatment and for the temporary relief of symptoms associated with oral inflammatory lesions and ulcerative lesions resulting from trauma.

Contraindications: This preparation is contraindicated in patients with a history of hypersensitivity to any of its components.

Because it contains a corticosteroid, the preparation is contraindicated in the presence of fungal, viral, or bacterial infections of the mouth or throat.

Warning: Usage in Pregnancy—Safe use of this preparation during pregnancy has not been established with respect to possible adverse reactions upon fetal development; therefore, it should not be used in women of child-bearing potential and particularly during early pregnancy unless, in the judgment of the physician or dentist, the potential benefits outweigh the possible hazards.

Precautions: Patients with tuberculosis, peptic ulcer or diabetes mellitus should not be treated with any corticosteroid preparation without the advice of the patient's physician.

It should be borne in mind that the normal defensive responses of the oral tissues are depressed in patients receiving topical corticosteroid therapy. Virulent strains of oral microorganisms may multiply without producing the usual warning symptoms of oral infections.

The small amount of steroid released when the preparation is used as recommended makes systemic effects very unlikely; however, they are a possibility when topical corticosteroid preparations are used over a long period of time.

If local irritation or sensitization should develop, the preparation should be discontinued and appropriate therapy instituted.

If significant regeneration or repair of oral tissues has not occurred in seven days, additional investigation into the etiology of the oral lesion is advised.

Adverse Reactions: Prolonged administration may elicit the adverse reactions known to occur with systemic steroid preparations; for example, adrenal suppression, alteration of glucose metabolism, protein catabolism, peptic ulcer activations, and others. These are usually reversible and disappear when the hormone is discontinued.

Dosage and Administration: Press a small dab (about one-quarter of an inch) to the lesion until a thin film develops. A larger quantity may be required for coverage of some lesions. For optimal results use only enough to coat the lesion with a thin film. Do not rub in. Attempting to spread this preparation may result in a granular, gritty sensation and cause it to crumble. After application, however, a smooth, slippery film develops.

The preparation should be applied at bedtime to permit steroid contact with the lesion throughout the night. Depending on the severity of symptoms, it may be necessary to apply the preparation two or three times a day, preferably after meals. If significant repair or regeneration has not occurred in seven days, further investigation is advisable.

How Supplied: 5 gram tubes (Military Depot Item, NSN 6505-00-926-8913).

Storage: Store at room temperature; keep tube tightly closed.

MYCOLOG® ℞
[mīk'ō-log"]
(Nystatin, Neomycin Sulfate, Gramicidin, and Triamcinolone Acetonide Cream and Ointment USP)

Description: Mycolog (Nystatin—Neomycin Sulfate—Gramicidin—Triamcinolone Acetonide) is available as a cream in an aqueous vanishing cream base and as an ointment in Plastibase® (Plasticized Hydrocarbon Gel), a polyethylene and mineral oil gel base. Each gram of the cream or ointment provides 100,000 units nystatin, neomycin sulfate equivalent to 2.5 mg. neomycin base, 0.25 mg. gramicidin and 1 mg. triamcinolone acetonide (0.1%). The cream also contains polysorbate 60, alcohol, aluminum hydroxide concentrated wet gel, titanium dioxide, glyceryl monostearate, polyethylene glycol monostearate, simethicone, sorbic acid, propylene glycol, ethylenediamine hydrochloride, white petrolatum, cetearyl alcohol (and) ceteareth-20, methylparaben, propylparaben, and sorbitol solution.

Actions: Triamcinolone acetonide is primarily effective because of its anti-inflammatory, antipruritic, and vasoconstrictive actions. Nystatin provides specific anticandidal activity and the two topical antibiotics, neomycin and gramicidin, provide antibacterial activity.

Indications

Based on a review of these drugs by the National Academy of Sciences—National Research Council and/or other information, FDA has classified the indications as follows:

Continued on next page

Squibb—Cont.

Possibly effective: In
- cutaneous candidiasis
- superficial bacterial infections
- the following conditions when complicated by candidal and/or bacterial infection: atopic, eczematoid, stasis, nummular, contact, or seborrheic dermatitis; neurodermatitis and dermatitis venenata
- infantile eczema
- lichen simplex chronicus
- the Cream is also possibly effective in pruritus ani and pruritus vulvae

Final classification of the less-than-effective indications requires further investigation.

Contraindications: Topical steroids are contraindicated in viral diseases of the skin, such as vaccinia and varicella. The preparations are also contraindicated in fungal lesions of the skin except candidiasis, and in those patients with a history of hypersensitivity to any of their components.

The preparations are not for ophthalmic use nor should they be applied in the external auditory canal of patients with perforated eardrums.

Topical steroids should not be used when circulation is markedly impaired.

Warnings: Because of the potential hazard of nephrotoxicity and ototoxicity, prolonged use or use of large amounts of these products should be avoided in the treatment of skin infections following extensive burns, trophic ulceration, and other conditions where absorption of neomycin is possible.

Usage in Pregnancy: Although topical steroids have not been reported to have an adverse effect on the fetus, the safety of topical steroid preparations during pregnancy has not been absolutely established; therefore, they should not be used extensively on pregnant patients, in large amounts, or for prolonged periods of time.

Precautions: As with any antibiotic preparation, prolonged use may result in overgrowth of nonsusceptible organisms, including fungi other than Candida. Constant observation of the patient is essential. Should superinfection due to nonsusceptible organisms occur, suitable concomitant antimicrobial therapy must be administered. If a favorable response does not occur promptly, application of Mycolog (Nystatin, Neomycin Sulfate, Gramicidin, and Triamcinolone Acetonide Cream and Ointment USP) should be discontinued until the infection is adequately controlled by other anti-infective measures.

If extensive areas are treated or if the occlusive technique is used, the possibility exists of increased systemic absorption of the corticosteroid and suitable precautions should be taken.

If irritation develops, the product should be discontinued and appropriate therapy instituted.

Adverse Reactions: Hypersensitivity to nystatin is extremely uncommon. Sensitivity reactions following the topical use of gramicidin are rarely encountered. Hypersensitivity to neomycin has been reported and articles in the current medical literature indicate an increase in its prevalence.

The following local adverse reactions have been reported with topical corticosteroids either with or without occlusive dressings: burning sensations, itching, irritation, dryness, folliculitis, secondary infection, skin atrophy, striae, miliaria, hypertrichosis, acneform eruptions, maceration of the skin and hypopigmentation. Contact sensitivity to a particular dressing material or adhesive may occur occasionally.

Ototoxicity and nephrotoxicity have been reported.

Dosage and Administration: *Mycolog Cream* (Nystatin, Neomycin Sulfate, Gramicidin,and Triamcinolone Acetonide Cream USP) —Rub the cream into affected areas two to three times daily.
Mycolog Ointment (Nystatin, Neomycin Sulfate, Gramicidin, and Triamcinolone Acetonide Ointment USP)—Apply a thin film of the ointment to the affected areas two to three times daily.

Occlusive Dressing Technique—Cream: Gently rub a small amount of the cream into the lesion until it disappears. Reapply the cream leaving a thin coating on the lesion and cover with a pliable nonporous film. If needed, additional moisture may be provided by covering the lesion with a dampened clean cotton cloth before the plastic film is applied or by briefly soaking the affected area in water. The frequency of changing dressings is best determined on an individual basis. Reapplication is essential at each dressing change.

Ointment: Apply the ointment leaving a thin coating on the lesion and cover with a pliable nonporous film. If needed, additional moisture may be provided by covering the lesion with a dampened clean cotton cloth before the plastic film is applied or by briefly soaking the affected area in water. The frequency of changing dressings is best determined on an individual basis. Reapplication is essential at each dressing change.

How Supplied: Both preparations are available in tubes of 15, 30, and 60 g. They are also available in jars of 120 g. for hospital or institutional use only. [Cream in 15 g. tubes—V.A. Depot Item, NSN6505-00-961-5504A; Cream in 120 g. (4 oz.) jars—V.A. Depot Item, NSN6505-00-772-0245A; Ointment in 15 g. tubes—Military Depot Item, NSN 6505-01-040-5957; V.A. Depot Item, NSN6505-00-040-5957A.]

Storage: Store the cream at room temperature; avoid freezing. Store the ointment at room temperature.

MYCOSTATIN® CREAM ℞
[mĭk'ō-stat"in]
(Nystatin Cream)
MYCOSTATIN OINTMENT ℞
(Nystatin Ointment USP)
MYCOSTATIN TOPICAL POWDER ℞
(Nystatin Topical Powder)

Description: Mycostatin Cream (Nystatin Cream) contains the antifungal antibiotic Nystatin USP at a concentration of 100,000 units per gram in an aqueous, perfumed vanishing cream base containing aluminum hydroxide concentrated wet gel, titanium dioxide, propylene glycol, cetearyl alcohol (and) ceteareth-20, white petrolatum, sorbitol solution, glyceryl monostearate, polyethylene glycol monostearate, sorbic acid and simethicone.

Mycostatin Ointment (Nystatin Ointment USP) provides 100,000 units Nystatin USP per gram in Plastibase® (Plasticized Hydrocarbon Gel), a polyethylene and mineral oil gel base.

Mycostatin Topical Powder (Nystatin Topical Powder) provides, in each gram, 100,000 units Nystatin USP dispersed in Talc USP.

Clinical Pharmacology: Nystatin is an antifungal antibiotic which is both fungistatic and fungicidal *in vitro* against a wide variety of yeasts and yeast-like fungi. It probably acts by binding to sterols in the cell membrane of the fungus with a resultant change in membrane permeability allowing leakage of intracellular components. Nystatin is a polyene antibiotic of undetermined structural formula that is obtained from *Streptomyces noursei*, and is the first well tolerated antifungal antibiotic of dependable efficacy for the treatment of cutaneous, oral and intestinal infections caused by *Candida* (Monilia) *albicans* and other Candida species. It exhibits no appreciable activity against bacteria.

Nystatin provides specific therapy for all localized forms of candidiasis. Symptomatic relief is rapid, often occurring within 24 to 72 hours after the initiation of treatment. Cure is effected both clinically and mycologically in most cases of localized candidiasis.

Indications and Usage: Mycostatin topical preparations are indicated in the treatment of cutaneous or mucocutaneous mycotic infections caused by *Candida* (Monilia) *albicans* and other Candida species.

Contraindications: Mycostatin topical preparations are contraindicated in patients with a history of hypersensitivity to any of their components.

Precautions: Should a reaction of hypersensitivity occur the drug should be immediately withdrawn and appropriate measures taken.

Adverse Reactions: Nystatin is virtually nontoxic and nonsensitizing and is well tolerated by all age groups including debilitated infants, even on prolonged administration. If irritation on topical application should occur, discontinue medication.

Dosage and Administration: The cream and the ointment should be applied liberally to affected areas twice daily or as indicated until healing is complete. The powder should be applied to candidal lesions two or three times daily until lesions have healed. For fungal infection of the feet caused by Candida species, the powder should be dusted freely on the feet as well as in shoes and socks. The cream is usually preferred to the ointment in candidiasis involving intertriginous areas; very moist lesions, however, are best treated with the topical dusting powder.

The preparations do not stain skin or mucous membranes and they provide a simple, convenient means of treatment.

How Supplied: Mycostatin Cream (Nystatin Cream) is supplied in tubes of 15 g. and 30 g.
Mycostatin Ointment (Nystatin Ointment USP) is supplied in tubes of 15 g. and 30 g.
Mycostatin Topical Powder (Nystatin Topical Powder) is supplied in plastic squeeze bottles of 15 g. (½ oz.) [Military Depot Item, NSN 6505-00-890-1218].

Storage: Store the cream at room temperature; avoid freezing. Store the ointment at room temperature. Store the topical powder at room temperature; avoid excessive heat; keep bottle tightly closed.

MYCOSTATIN® ORAL ℞
SUSPENSION
[mĭk'ō-stat"in]
(Nystatin Oral Suspension USP)

Description: Nystatin is an antifungal antibiotic which is both fungistatic and fungicidal *in vitro* against a wide variety of yeasts and yeast-like fungi. It is a polyene antibiotic of undetermined structural formula that is obtained from *Streptomyces noursei*. Mycostatin Oral Suspension is provided for oral administration containing 100,000 units nystatin per ml. in a vehicle containing 50% sucrose; not more than 1% alcohol by volume.

Clinical Pharmacology: Nystatin probably acts by binding to sterols in the cell membrane of the fungus with a resultant change in membrane permeability allowing leakage of intracellular components. It exhibits no appreciable activity against bacteria or trichomonads.

Following oral administration, nystatin is sparingly absorbed with no detectable blood levels when given in the recommended doses. Most of the orally administered nystatin is passed unchanged in the stool.

Indications and Usage: Mycostatin Oral Suspension is indicated for the treatment of candidiasis in the oral cavity.

Contraindication: The preparation is contraindicated in patients with a history of hypersensitivity to any of its components.

Precautions:

Usage in Pregnancy—No adverse effects or complications have been attributed to nystatin in infants born to women treated with nystatin.

Adverse Reactions: Nystatin is virtually nontoxic and nonsensitizing and is well tolerated by all age groups including debilitated infants, even on prolonged administration. Large oral doses have occasionally produced diarrhea, gastrointestinal distress, nausea, and vomiting.

Dosage and Administration: INFANTS—2 ml. (200,000 units nystatin) four times daily (1 ml. in each side of mouth).

NOTE: Limited clinical studies in premature and low birth weight infants indicate that 1 ml. four times daily is effective.

CHILDREN AND ADULTS—4-6 ml. (400,000 to 600,000 units nystatin) four times daily (one-half of dose in each side of mouth). The preparation should be retained in the mouth as long as possible before swallowing.

Continue treatment for at least 48 hours after perioral symptoms have disappeared and cultures returned to normal.

How Supplied: Mycostatin Oral Suspension (Nystatin Oral Suspension USP) is available as a pleasant-tasting, ready-to-use suspension containing 100,000 units nystatin per ml. in 60 ml. bottles (each supplied with a calibrated dropper), 473 ml. bottles, and UNIMATIC® bottles containing a single 5 ml. dose.

Storage: Store at room temperature; avoid freezing.

MYCOSTATIN® ORAL TABLETS ℞
[mĭk'ō-stat" in]
(Nystatin Tablets USP)

Description: Nystatin is an antifungal antibiotic which is both fungistatic and fungicidal *in vitro* against a wide variety of yeasts and yeast-like fungi. It is a polyene antibiotic of undetermined structural formula that is obtained from *Streptomyces noursei*. Mycostatin Oral Tablets are provided for oral administration as coated tablets containing 500,000 units nystatin.

Clinical Pharmacology: Nystatin probably acts by binding to sterols in the cell membrane of the fungus with a resultant change in membrane permeability allowing leakage of intracellular components. It exhibits no appreciable activity against bacteria or trichomonads.

Following oral administration, nystatin is sparingly absorbed with no detectable blood levels when given in the recommended doses. Most of the orally administered nystatin is passed unchanged in the stool.

Indications and Usage: Mycostatin Oral Tablets (Nystatin Tablets USP) are intended for the treatment of intestinal candidiasis.

Contraindications: Mycostatin Oral Tablets are contraindicated in patients with a history of hypersensitivity to any of their components.

Precautions: Usage in Pregnancy—No adverse effects or complications have been attributed to nystatin in infants born to women treated with nystatin.

Adverse Reactions: Nystatin is virtually nontoxic and nonsensitizing and is well tolerated by all age groups including debilitated infants, even on prolonged administration. Large oral doses have occasionally produced diarrhea, gastrointestinal distress, nausea and vomiting.

Dosage and Administration: The usual therapeutic dosage is one to two tablets (500,000 to 1,000,000 units nystatin) three times daily. Treatment should generally be continued for at least 48 hours after clinical cure to prevent relapse.

How Supplied: Mycostatin Oral Tablets (Nystatin Tablets USP) are available for oral administration as FILMLOK® tablets providing 500,000 units nystatin per tablet in bottles of 100 and UNIMATIC® cartons of 100. (Filmlok is a Squibb trademark for veneer-coated tablets.) [Bottles of 100, Military Depot Item, NSN6505-00-118-1949.]

Storage: Store at room temperature; avoid excessive heat. Dispense in tight, light-resistant containers.

Shown in Product Identification Section, page 438

MYCOSTATIN® VAGINAL TABLETS ℞
[mĭk'ō-stat" in]
(Nystatin Vaginal Tablets USP)

Description: Nystatin is an antimycotic polyene antibiotic obtained from *Streptomyces noursei*. Mycostatin Vaginal Tablets (Nystatin Vaginal Tablets USP) are available as diamond-shaped compressed tablets for intravaginal administration, providing 100,000 units of nystatin dispersed in lactose with ethyl cellulose, stearic acid, and starch.

Clinical Pharmacology: Nystatin is both fungistatic and fungicidal *in vitro* against a wide variety of yeasts and yeast-like fungi. Nystatin acts by binding to sterols in the cell membrane of sensitive fungi with a resultant change in membrane permeability allowing leakage of intracellular components. Nystatin exhibits no appreciable activity against bacteria, protozoa, trichomonads, or viruses.

Nystatin is not absorbed from intact skin or mucous membranes.

Indications and Usage: Mycostatin Vaginal Tablets (Nystatin Vaginal Tablets USP) are effective for the local treatment of vulvovaginal candidiasis (moniliasis). The diagnosis should be confirmed, prior to therapy, by KOH smears and/or cultures. Other pathogens commonly associated with vulvovaginitis (Trichomonas and *Haemophilus vaginalis*) do not respond to nystatin and should be ruled out by appropriate laboratory methods.

Contraindications: This preparation is contraindicated in patients with a history of hypersensitivity to any of its components.

Precautions: General: Discontinue treatment if sensitization or irritation is reported during use.

Information for Patients: The patient should be informed of symptoms of sensitization or irritation and told to report them promptly.

The patient should be warned against interruption or discontinuation of medication even during menstruation and even though symptomatic relief may occur within a few days.

The patient should be advised that adjunctive measures such as therapeutic douches are unnecessary and sometimes inadvisable, but cleansing douches may be used by nonpregnant women, if desired, for esthetic purposes.

Laboratory Tests: If there is a lack of response to Mycostatin Vaginal Tablets (Nystatin Vaginal Tablets USP), appropriate microbiological studies should be repeated to confirm the diagnosis and rule out other pathogens, before instituting another course of antimycotic therapy (see INDICATIONS AND USAGE).

Carcinogenesis, Mutagenesis, Impairment of Fertility: Long-term studies in animals have not been performed to evaluate carcinogenic potential, mutagenesis, or whether this medication affects fertility in females.

Pregnancy: Teratogenic Effects: Category A. There have been no reports that use of nystatin vaginal tablets by pregnant women increases the risk of fetal abnormalities or affects later growth, development, and functional maturation of the child. Nevertheless, because the possibility of harm cannot be ruled out, nystatin vaginal tablets should be used during pregnancy only if the physician considers it essential to the welfare of the patient.

Animal reproduction studies have not been conducted with nystatin vaginal tablets.

Pediatric Use: Safety and effectiveness in children have not been established.

Adverse Reactions: Nystatin is virtually nontoxic and nonsensitizing and is well tolerated by all age groups, even on prolonged administration. Rarely, irritation or sensitization may occur (see PRECAUTIONS).

Dosage and Administration: The usual dosage is one tablet (100,000 units nystatin) daily for two weeks. The tablets should be deposited high in the vagina by means of the applicator. "Instructions for the Patient" are enclosed in each package.

How Supplied: Mycostatin Vaginal Tablets (Nystatin Vaginal Tablets USP) are available in packages of 15 and 30 individually foil wrapped tablets with applicator and in UNIMATIC® cartons of 50 unit-dose packs per carton—each cello-protected unit-dose pack contains one individually foil wrapped tablet, one applicator, and one "Instructions for the Patient" leaflet.

Storage: Store in refrigerator below 15° C (59° F).

Shown in Product Identification Section, page 438

MYSTECLIN-F® CAPSULES ℞
[mī-stek' lin-ef]
(Tetracycline and Amphotericin B Capsules USP)
MYSTECLIN-F® SYRUP ℞
(Tetracycline and Amphotericin B Oral Suspension USP)

> Recently, a panel of the National Academy of Sciences—National Research Council has stated that in its informed judgment Mysteclin-F is ineffective as a fixed combination. Further, it stated, "The Panel is not aware of evidence of proved efficacy of this combination in the prevention of disease due to monilial organisms, although suppression of growth of monilia may be accomplished. It should be noted that the apparent reduction of organisms in the feces may be an artifact due to residual antibiotic activity and thus may not reflect the true state in the patient. It is preferable, in the Panel's opinion, to prescribe antifungal drugs when clinically indicated, rather than to use them indiscriminately as 'prophylaxis' against an uncommon clinical entity seen during therapy with tetracyclines and other antibiotics."

Description: Mysteclin-F Capsules (Tetracycline and Amphotericin B Capsules) contain tetracycline equivalent to 250 mg. tetracycline hydrochloride with 50 mg. amphotericin B, and potassium metaphosphate buffer.

Mysteclin-F Syrup (Tetracycline and Amphotericin B Oral Suspension USP) is a fruit-flavored syrup containing, in each 5 ml. teaspoonful, tetracycline equivalent to 125 mg. tetracycline hydrochloride, buffered with potassium metaphosphate, and 25 mg. amphotericin B.

Clinical Pharmacology: Mysteclin-F (Tetracycline—Amphotericin B) Capsules and Syrup have been designed to provide simultaneous antimicrobial therapy and anticandidal prophylaxis, a concept first developed by Squibb.

The preparations, which contain the broad spectrum antibiotic tetracycline, well known for its pronounced antimicrobial effect against a wide range of pathogenic organisms, produce exceptionally high initial tetracycline blood levels as well as excellent diffusion to tissues and body fluids.

Furthermore, these preparations also contain **prophylactic** amounts of the antifungal antibiotic, amphotericin B. This antibiotic, first isolated and described by the Squibb Institute for Medical Research, is substantially more active *in vitro* against *Candida* strains than nystatin, and has been widely used by the intravenous route in the treatment of many deep-seated mycotic infections. Given orally, amphotericin B is extremely well tolerated and is virtually nontoxic in prophylactic doses. Although poorly absorbed from the gut, amphotericin B has a high degree of activity against *Candida* species in the intestinal tract and prevents the overgrowth of these organisms commonly associated with broad spectrum antibiotic therapy (amphotericin B has no antibacterial activity). By suppressing overgrowth of *Candida* in the gastrointestinal tract, thereby minimizing a possible reservoir of this organism, Mysteclin-F (Tetracycline—Amphotericin B) provides added protection for the patient against troublesome, or even serious, candidal superinfections, e.g., intestinal (diarrheal), anogenital, vulvovaginal, mucocutaneous candidiasis.

Note: Microorganisms that have become insensitive to one tetracycline invariably exhibit cross-resistance to other tetracyclines. In addition, gram-negative bacilli made tetracycline resistant may also show cross-resistance to chloramphenicol.

Indications and Usage: Candidal overgrowth occurs in a large number of patients taking broad spectrum antibiotics. Although it is impossible to predict exactly which patient will develop candidal complications and which will not, certain

Continued on next page

Squibb—Cont.

types of patients are known to be particularly susceptible to candidiasis. Among these are elderly or debilitated patients; patients on high or prolonged antibiotic dosage; diabetics; infants; patients on corticoid therapy; patients who have developed candidiasis on previous broad spectrum therapy; women, particularly during pregnancy. Because the danger of candidal complications is greatest in these patients, they are potential candidates for therapy with Mysteclin-F.

Mysteclin-F (Tetracycline and Amphotericin B) Capsules and Syrup are indicated for the many common infections, including those of the respiratory, gastrointestinal and genitourinary systems, which are amenable to tetracycline therapy. Infections caused by gram-positive and gram-negative bacteria, spirochetes, viruses of the lymphogranuloma-psittacosis-trachoma group, rickettsiae and *Endamoeba histolytica* can be expected to respond. Because of the wide range of antimicrobial activity, the preparations are particularly useful in the treatment of mixed infections due to susceptible organisms.

Mysteclin-F (Tetracycline and Amphotericin B) Capsules and Syrup are also a useful part of the armamentarium in the management of chronic cases of acne vulgaris which, in the judgment of the clinician, require long-term treatment. The cystic and pustular forms of this condition respond most satisfactorily to tetracycline therapy; the papular form may also show improvement in some individuals. Because long-term maintenance therapy with tetracycline is involved, the presence of amphotericin B in the product is a particular advantage, helping to guard against the risk of candidal overgrowth.

Note: A number of strains of staphylococci and streptococci have shown resistance to tetracyclines. A few strains of pneumococci, *E. coli* and shigellae also have been reported as resistant. Indicated laboratory studies, including sensitivity tests, should be performed.

Contraindications: These products should not be used in persons with a history of hypersensitivity to any of their components.

Warnings: THE USE OF DRUGS OF THE TETRACYCLINE CLASS DURING TOOTH DEVELOPMENT (LAST HALF OF PREGNANCY, INFANCY, AND CHILDHOOD TO AGE OF EIGHT YEARS) MAY CAUSE PERMANENT DISCOLORATION OF THE TEETH (YELLOW-GRAY-BROWN). This reaction is more common during long-term use of the drugs but has been observed following repeated short-term courses. Enamel hypoplasia has also been reported. TETRACYCLINE DRUGS, THEREFORE, SHOULD NOT BE USED IN THIS AGE GROUP UNLESS OTHER DRUGS ARE NOT LIKELY TO BE EFFECTIVE OR ARE CONTRAINDICATED.

If renal impairment exists, even usual oral or parenteral doses may lead to excessive systemic accumulation of the drug and possible liver toxicity. Under such conditions, lower-than-usual doses are indicated and if therapy is prolonged, tetracycline serum level determinations may be advisable.

Certain hypersensitive individuals may develop a photodynamic reaction precipitated by exposure to direct sunlight during the use of this drug. This reaction is usually of the photoallergic type which may also be produced by other tetracycline derivatives. Individuals with a history of photosensitivity reactions should be instructed to avoid exposure to direct sunlight while under treatment with this or other tetracycline drugs and treatment should be discontinued at first evidence of skin discomfort.

NOTE: Photosensitization reactions have occurred most frequently with demethylchlortetracycline, less with chlortetracycline and very rarely with oxytetracycline and tetracycline.

Precautions: As with any antibiotic preparation, prolonged use may result in overgrowth of nonsusceptible organisms. Constant observation of the patient is essential. Should superinfection occur, the preparation should be discontinued and/or appropriate therapy instituted. *Note:* Superinfection of the bowel by staphylococci may be life threatening.

Tetracycline may form a stable calcium complex in any bone forming tissue with no serious harmful effects reported thus far in humans. However, use of tetracycline during tooth development (i.e., latter half of gestation, neonatal period and early childhood) may cause discoloration of the teeth (i.e., yellow-gray-brownish). This effect occurs mostly during long-term use of the drug but it has also been observed in usual short treatment courses.

During long-term therapy, periodic assessment of organ system function, including renal, hepatic, and hematopoietic systems, should be made.

Increased intracranial pressure with bulging fontanels has been observed in infants taking therapeutic doses of tetracycline. Occurrence has been rare and all signs and symptoms have disappeared rapidly upon cessation of treatment.

Since sensitivity reactions are more likely to occur in persons with a history of allergy, asthma, hay fever, or urticaria, the preparation should be used with caution in such individuals. Cross-sensitization among the various tetracyclines is extremely common.

In the treatment of gonorrhea, patients with a suspected lesion of syphilis should have darkfield examinations before receiving tetracycline and monthly serologic tests for a minimum of three months.

The use of tetracycline in staphylococcal infections does not preclude the need for indicated surgical procedures.

Adverse Reactions: Oral administration of amphotericin B is usually well tolerated.

The following adverse reactions have been reported with tetracycline preparations:

Gastrointestinal irritation (anorexia, epigastric distress, nausea, vomiting) as well as bulky loose stools, and diarrhea may occur. Glossitis, stomatitis, enterocolitis, proctitis, and pruritus ani may occur in some patients. Black hairy tongue, sore throat, dysphagia, and hoarseness have also been reported. However, tetracycline is generally well tolerated, undesirable gastrointestinal side effects occurring significantly less frequently than with the two analogues, oxytetracycline and chlortetracycline.

Tetracyclines may also cause maculopapular and erythematous skin rashes. A rare case of exfoliative dermatitis has been reported. Photosensitivity, manifested by an exaggerated sunburn reaction has been observed in some individuals (see *Warnings*). Onycholysis and discoloration of the nails have been reported rarely.

Rise in BUN has been reported and is apparently dose related. Urinary loss of nitrogen has been observed in some patients receiving tetracyclines and may result in negative nitrogen balance. Increased excretion of sodium has also been reported. The development of peptic ulcers and bleeding has been observed in uremic patients receiving tetracyclines.

Hypersensitivity reactions may include urticaria, serum sickness-like reactions (fever, rash, arthralgia), angioneurotic edema, and anaphylactoid shock. If allergic reactions occur, or if an individual idiosyncrasy appears, tetracycline therapy should be discontinued.

Increased intracranial pressure with bulging fontanels has been reported in infants following full therapeutic doses of tetracycline. This symptom disappears rapidly when administration of tetracycline is discontinued (see *Precautions*).

The use of tetracycline during the mineralization phase of tooth development (latter half of gestation, neonatal period, and early childhood) may cause discoloration of the teeth (yellow-gray-brownish) which may sometimes be accompanied by enamel hypoplasia (see *Warnings*).

Anemia, thrombocytopenic purpura, neutropenia, and eosinophilia have been reported. Tetracyclines may delay blood coagulation.

Hepatic cholestasis has been reported rarely, and is usually associated with high dosage levels of tetracycline.

Dosage and Administration: Dosage should be based on the tetracycline content. **Adults:** For the many common infections amenable to tetracycline therapy, adults should receive a minimum of 250 mg. four times daily. Higher dosages, such as 500 mg. four times daily, may be required for severe infections or for those infections which do not respond to the smaller dose. **For children above eight years of age:** In general, the pediatric dosage should supply 10 to 20 mg. tetracycline per pound of body weight each day, in divided doses, depending on the type and severity of the infection.

Representative pediatric dosages of Mysteclin-F Syrup (Tetracycline and Amphotericin B Oral Suspension USP) are as follows: 20 lbs.: ½ teaspoonful q.i.d.; 40 lbs.: 1 teaspoonful q.i.d.; 60 lbs.: 1½ teaspoonfuls q.i.d.; 80 lbs.: 2 teaspoonfuls q.i.d.

Oral forms of tetracycline should be given one hour before or two hours following meals. Pediatric dosage forms (oral) should not be given with milk formulas or other calcium containing food, and should be given at least one hour prior to feeding.

Treatment of most common infections should continue for 24 to 48 hours after symptoms and fever subside. However, if the capsules or syrup are used in the treatment of streptococcal infections due to susceptible organisms, therapy should be continued for a full 10 days to guard against the risk of rheumatic fever or glomerulonephritis. Higher dosage and even more prolonged therapy is necessary for subacute bacterial endocarditis and may be required in certain staphylococcal infections.

In chronic cases of acne vulgaris which, in the judgment of the clinician, require long-term treatment, the recommended initial dosage of the capsules or syrup is 1 gram daily in divided doses. When improvement is noted, usually within one week, dosage should be gradually reduced to maintenance levels ranging from 125 to 500 mg. daily. In some patients it may be possible to maintain adequate remission of lesions with alternate-day or intermittent therapy. Tetracycline therapy of acne vulgaris should augment the other standard measures known to be of value.

How Supplied: *Mysteclin-F Capsules (Tetracycline and Amphotericin B Capsules USP) are available with the equivalent of 250 mg tetracycline hydrochloride with 50 mg amphotericin B in bottles of 16 and 100 and Unimatic® unit-dose cartons of 100.

Mysteclin-F Syrup (Tetracycline and Amphotericin B Oral Suspension USP) is a fruit-flavored syrup containing, in each 5 ml teaspoonful, tetracycline equivalent to 125 mg tetracycline hydrochloride and 25 mg amphotericin B, available in bottles of 60 ml. and 240 ml.

Storage: Store the capsules at room temperature; avoid excessive heat; keep tightly closed. Dispense in tight containers. Store the syrup below 30°C. (86°F.); protect from light; keep tightly closed. Dispense in tight light-resistant containers.

*Shown in Product Identification Section, page 438

NATURETIN®-2.5 ℞
NATURETIN®-5 ℞
NATURETIN®-10 ℞
[na″chūr-ē′tin]
(Bendroflumethiazide Tablets USP)

Description: Naturetin is a benzothiadiazine derivative containing a benzyl and a trifluoromethyl group. It is a potent oral diuretic and antihypertensive agent available as compressed tablets providing 2.5, 5, or 10 mg. bendroflumethiazide. The tablets contain FD&C Yellow No. 5 (tartrazine).

Clinical Pharmacology: Thiazides affect the renal tubular mechanism of electrolyte reabsorption. At maximal therapeutic dosage all thiazides are approximately equal in their diuretic potency. Thiazides increase excretion of sodium and chloride in approximately equivalent amounts. Natriuresis causes a secondary loss of potassium and bicarbonate.

The mechanism of the antihypertensive effect of thiazides is unknown. Thiazides do not affect normal blood pressure.

Onset of action of thiazides occurs in two hours and the peak effect at about four hours. Duration of action persists for approximately six to 12 hours. Thiazides are eliminated rapidly by the kidney.

Indications and Usage: Naturetin is indicated as adjunctive therapy in edema associated with congestive heart failure, hepatic cirrhosis, and corticosteroid and estrogen therapy.

Naturetin has also been found useful in edema due to various forms of renal dysfunction such as: nephrotic syndrome, acute glomerulonephritis, and chronic renal failure.

Naturetin (Bendroflumethiazide Tablets USP) tablets are indicated in the management of hypertension either as the sole therapeutic agent or to enhance the effectiveness of other antihypertensive drugs in the more severe forms of hypertension.

Usage in Pregnancy—The routine use of diuretics in an otherwise healthy woman is inappropriate and exposes mother and fetus to unnecessary hazard. Diuretics do not prevent development of toxemia of pregnancy, and there is no satisfactory evidence that they are useful in the treatment of developed toxemia.

Edema during pregnancy may arise from pathological causes or from the physiologic and mechanical consequences of pregnancy. Thiazides are indicated in pregnancy when edema is due to pathologic causes, just as they are in the absence of pregnancy (however, see WARNINGS below). Dependent edema in pregnancy, resulting from restriction of venous return by the expanded uterus, is properly treated through elevation of the lower extremities and use of support hose; use of diuretics to lower intravascular volume in this case is illogical and unnecessary. There is hypervolemia during normal pregnancy which is harmful to neither the fetus nor the mother (in the absence of cardiovascular disease), but which is associated with edema, including generalized edema, in the majority of pregnant women. If this edema produces discomfort, increased recumbency will often provide relief. In rare instances, this edema may cause extreme discomfort which is not relieved by rest. In these cases, a short course of diuretics may provide relief and may be appropriate.

Contraindications: Bendroflumethiazide is contraindicated in anuria.

It is also contraindicated in patients who have previously demonstrated hypersensitivity to it or other sulfonamide-derived drugs.

Warnings: Thiazides should be used with caution in severe renal disease. In patients with renal disease, thiazides may precipitate azotemia. Cumulative effects of the drug may develop in patients with impaired renal function.

Thiazides should be used with caution in patients with impaired hepatic function or progressive liver disease, since minor alterations of fluid and electrolyte balance may precipitate hepatic coma.

Thiazides may be additive or may potentiate the action of other antihypertensive drugs. Potentiation occurs with ganglionic or peripheral adrenergic blocking drugs.

Sensitivity reactions may occur in patients with a history of allergy or bronchial asthma.

The possibility of exacerbation or activation of systemic lupus erythematosus has been reported. Lithium generally should not be given with diuretics; diuretic agents reduce the renal clearance of lithium and add a high risk of lithium toxicity. Refer to the package insert for lithium preparations before use of such concomitant therapy.

Usage in Pregnancy—Thiazides cross the placental barrier and appear in cord blood. The use of thiazides in pregnant women requires that the anticipated benefit be weighed against possible hazards to the fetus. These hazards include fetal or neonatal jaundice, thrombocytopenia, and possibly other adverse reactions which have occurred in the adult.

Nursing Mothers—Thiazides appear in breast milk. If use of the drug is deemed essential, the patient should stop nursing.

Precautions: Periodic determination of serum electrolytes to detect possible electrolyte imbalance should be performed at appropriate intervals. All patients receiving thiazide therapy should be observed for clinical signs of fluid or electrolyte imbalance; namely, hyponatremia, hypochloremic alkalosis, and hypokalemia. Serum and urine electrolyte determinations are particularly important when the patient is vomiting excessively or receiving parenteral fluids. Warning signs or symptoms of fluid and electrolyte imbalance include: dryness of the mouth, thirst, weakness, lethargy, drowsiness, restlessness, muscle pains or cramps, muscular fatigue, hypotension, oliguria, tachycardia, and gastrointestinal disturbances such as nausea and vomiting.

Hypokalemia may develop, especially with brisk diuresis, when severe cirrhosis is present, or during concomitant use of corticosteroids, ACTH, or after prolonged thiazide therapy.

Interference with adequate oral electrolyte intake will also contribute to hypokalemia.

Hypokalemia can sensitize or exaggerate the response of the heart to the toxic effects of digitalis (e.g., increased ventricular irritability). Concurrent administration of a potassium-sparing diuretic or potassium supplements may be indicated in these patients.

Any chloride deficit is generally mild and usually does not require specific treatment except under extraordinary circumstances (as in liver disease or renal disease). Dilutional hyponatremia may occur in edematous patients in hot weather; appropriate therapy is water restriction, rather than administration of salt, except in rare instances when the hyponatremia is life threatening. In actual salt depletion, appropriate replacement is the therapy of choice.

Hyperuricemia may occur or frank gout may be precipitated in certain patients receiving thiazide therapy.

Insulin requirements in diabetic patients may be increased, decreased, or unchanged. Latent diabetes mellitus may become manifest during thiazide administration.

Thiazide drugs may increase the responsiveness to tubocurarine.

The antihypertensive effects of the drug may be enhanced in the postsympathectomy patient.

Thiazides may decrease arterial responsiveness to norepinephrine. This diminution is not sufficient to preclude effectiveness of the pressor agent for therapeutic use. If emergency surgery is indicated, preanesthetic and anesthetic agents should be administered in reduced dosage.

If progressive renal impairment becomes evident, as indicated by a rising nonprotein nitrogen or blood urea nitrogen, a careful reappraisal of therapy is necessary with consideration given to withholding or discontinuing diuretic therapy.

Thiazides may decrease serum PBI levels without signs of thyroid disturbance.

Calcium excretion is decreased by thiazides. Pathological changes in the parathyroid gland with hypercalcemia and hypophosphatemia have been observed in a few patients on prolonged thiazide therapy. The common complications of hyperparathyroidism such as renal lithiasis, bone resorption, and peptic ulceration have not been seen. Thiazides should be discontinued before carrying out tests for parathyroid function.

This product contains FD&C Yellow No. 5 (tartrazine) which may cause allergic-type reactions (including bronchial asthma) in certain susceptible individuals. Although the overall incidence of FD&C Yellow No. 5 (tartrazine) sensitivity in the general population is low, it is frequently seen in patients who also have aspirin hypersensitivity.

Adverse Reactions: 1. *Gastrointestinal system*—anorexia; gastric irritation; nausea; vomiting; cramping; diarrhea; constipation; jaundice (intrahepatic cholestatic jaundice); pancreatitis; sialadenitis.

2. *Central nervous system*—dizziness; vertigo; paresthesia; headache; xanthopsia.

3. *Hematologic*-leukopenia; agranulocytosis; aplastic anemia; hemolytic anemia.

4. *Cardiovascular*—orthostatic hypotension (may be aggravated by alcohol, barbiturates, or narcotics)

5. *Hypersensitivity*—purpura; photosensitivity; rash; urticaria; necrotizing angiitis (vasculitis, cutaneous vasculitis); fever; respiratory distress including pneumonitis; anaphylactic reactions.

6. *Other*—hyperglycemia; glycosuria; hyperuricemia; muscle spasm; weakness; restlessness; transient blurred vision.

Whenever adverse reactions are moderate or severe, thiazide dosage should be reduced or therapy withdrawn.

Dosage and Administration: Therapy should be individualized according to patient response and titrated to obtain maximal therapeutic response as well as the lowest dose possible to maintain that therapeutic response and minimize side effects.

Diuretic: The usual dose is 5 mg. once daily, preferably given in the morning. To initiate therapy, doses up to 20 mg. may be given once daily or divided into two doses. A single daily dose of 2.5 to 5 mg. should suffice for maintenance.

Alternatively, intermittent therapy may be advantageous in many patients. By administering the preparation every other day or on a three to five day per week schedule, electrolyte imbalance is less likely to occur; however, the possibility still exists.

In general, the lowest dosage that achieves the therapeutic response should be employed.

Antihypertensive: The suggested initial dosage is 5 to 20 mg. daily. Maintenance dosage may range from 2.5 to 15 mg. per day depending on the individual response of the patient. When the diuretic is used with other antihypertensive agents, lower maintenance doses for each drug are usually sufficient.

How Supplied: 2.5 mg. in bottles of 100; 5 mg. (scored) in bottles of 100 and 1000; 10 mg. (scored) in bottles of 100.

Storage: Store at room temperature; avoid excessive heat. Dispense in tight containers.

Shown in Product Identification Section, page 438

NOCTEC® CAPSULES ℞ ℭ
[nok'tek]
(Chloral Hydrate Capsules USP)
NOCTEC® SYRUP ℞ ℭ
(Chloral Hydrate Syrup USP)

Description: Noctec capsules and syrup contain chloral hydrate, an effective sedative and hypnotic agent for oral administration. Chemically, chloral hydrate is 1,1-Ethanediol,2,2,2-trichloro-Chloral hydrate [MW 165.40]; its graphic formula is $CCl_3CH(OH)_2$.

Chloral hydrate occurs as colorless or white, volatile, hygroscopic crystals very soluble in water and in olive oil and freely soluble in alcohol. It has an aromatic, pungent odor and a slightly bitter, caustic taste.

Clinical Pharmacology: The mechanism of action by which the central nervous system is affected is not known. Chloral hydrate is readily absorbed from the gastrointestinal tract following oral administration; however, significant amounts of chloral hydrate have not been detected in the blood after oral administration. It is generally believed that the central depressant effects are due to the principal pharmacologically active metabolite trichloroethanol, which has a plasma half-life of 8 to 10 hours. A portion of the drug is oxidized to trichloroacetic acid (TCA) in the liver and kidneys; TCA is excreted in the urine and bile along with trichloroethanol in free or conjugated form.

Hypnotic dosage produces mild cerebral depression and quiet, deep sleep with little or no "hangover"; blood pressure and respiration are depressed only slightly more than in normal sleep and reflexes are not significantly depressed, so the patient can be awakened and completely aroused. Chloral hydrate's effect on rapid eye movement (REM) sleep is uncertain.

Chloral hydrate has been detected in cerebrospinal fluid and human milk, and it crosses the placental barrier.

Continued on next page

Squibb—Cont.

Indications and Usage: Noctec (Chloral Hydrate) is indicated for nocturnal sedation in all types of patients and especially for the ill, the young, and the elderly patient.

In candidates for surgery, it is a satisfactory preoperative sedative that allays anxiety and induces sleep without depressing respiration or cough reflex. In postoperative care and control of pain, it is a valuable adjunct to opiates and analgesics.

Contraindications: Chloral hydrate is contraindicated in patients with marked hepatic or renal impairment and in patients with severe cardiac disease. Oral dosage forms of chloral hydrate are contraindicated in the presence of gastritis. Chloral hydrate is also contraindicated in patients who have previously exhibited an idiosyncrasy or hypersensitivity to the drug.

Warnings: Chloral hydrate may be habit-forming. Long-term use of larger than the usual therapeutic doses may result in psychic and physical dependence; therefore, caution must be exercised when administering the drug to patients susceptible to drug abuse. Sudden withdrawal may result in delirium.

Chloral hydrate may increase the rate of metabolism of concomitantly administered coumarin or coumarin-related anticoagulants, thus reducing their effectiveness. Upon withdrawal of chloral hydrate, the rate of metabolism of the anticoagulant drug may decrease with a concomitant rise in plasma levels and with the possibility of a gradual increase of anticoagulant effects (i.e., development of bleeding tendency and hemorrhage). Patients on oral anticoagulant therapy who are also taking chloral hydrate should have close observation of prothrombin times.

Precautions:
General—Chloral hydrate has been reported to precipitate attacks of acute intermittent porphyria and should be used with caution in susceptible patients.

Continued use of therapeutic doses of chloral hydrate has been shown to be without deleterious effect on the heart. Large doses of chloral hydrate, however, should not be used in patients with *severe* cardiac disease (see CONTRAINDICATIONS).

Information for Patients—Chloral hydrate may cause gastrointestinal upset. The capsules should be taken with a full glass of water or fruit juice; capsules should be taken whole, and not chewed. The syrup should be diluted in half a glass of water or fruit juice.

Chloral hydrate may cause drowsiness; therefore, patients should be instructed to use caution when driving, operating dangerous machinery, or performing any hazardous task.

Patients should avoid alcohol and other CNS depressants. They should also be informed that chloral hydrate may be habit-forming.

Noctec (Chloral Hydrate) and all drugs should be kept out of the reach of children.

Patients should be warned against sudden discontinuation of chloral hydrate except under the advice of the physician; they should also be informed of symptoms that would suggest potential adverse effects.

Drug Interactions—Chloral hydrate may cause hypoprothrombinemic effects in patients taking oral anticoagulants (see WARNINGS).

Administration of chloral hydrate followed by intravenous furosemide may result in sweating, hot flashes, and variable blood pressure including hypertension due to a hypermetabolic state caused by displacement of thyroid hormone from its bound state.

Caution is recommended in combining chloral hydrate with other CNS depressants such as alcohol, barbiturates, and tranquilizers. Administration of chloral hydrate should be delayed in patients who have ingested significant amounts of alcohol in the preceding 12 to 24 hours. CNS depressants are additive in effect and the dosage should be reduced when such combinations are given concurrently.

Drug/Laboratory Test Interactions—Chloral hydrate may interfere with copper sulfate tests for glycosuria (suspected glycosuria should be confirmed by a glucose oxidase test when the patient is receiving chloral hydrate), fluorometric tests for urine catecholamines (it is recommended that the medication not be administered for 48 hours preceding the test), or urinary 17-hydroxycorticosteroid determinations (when using the Reddy, Jenkins, and Thorn procedure).

Carcinogenesis, Mutagenesis, Impairment of Fertility—Long-term studies in animals have not been performed.

Pregnancy Category C—Animal reproduction studies have not been conducted with chloral hydrate. Chloral hydrate crosses the placental barrier and chronic use during pregnancy may cause withdrawal symptoms in the neonate. It is not known whether chloral hydrate can affect reproduction capacity. Chloral hydrate should be given to a pregnant woman only if clearly needed.

Nursing Mothers—Chloral hydrate is excreted in human milk; use by nursing mothers may cause sedation in the infant.

Adverse Reactions:
Central Nervous System—Occasionally a patient becomes somnambulistic and he may be disoriented and incoherent and show paranoid behavior. Rarely, excitement, tolerance, addiction, delirium, drowsiness, staggering gait, ataxia, lightheadedness, vertigo, dizziness, nightmares, malaise, mental confusion, and hallucinations have been reported.

Hematological—Leukopenia and eosinophilia have occasionally occurred.

Dermatological—Allergic skin rashes including hives, erythema, eczematoid dermatitis, urticaria, and scarlatiniform exanthems have occasionally been reported.

Gastrointestinal—Some patients experience gastric irritation and occasionally nausea and vomiting, flatulence, diarrhea, and unpleasant taste occur.

Miscellaneous—Rarely, headache, hangover, idiosyncratic syndrome, and ketonuria have been reported.

Drug Abuse and Dependence:
Controlled Substance—Drug Enforcement Administration Schedule ℭ.

Abuse—Chloral hydrate may be habit-forming. Patients known to be addiction-prone and patients who actively solicit hypnotics in increasing doses are potential addicts. Many patients take higher doses of hypnotics than they admit, and slurring of speech, incoordination, tremulousness, and nystagmus should arouse suspicion. Drowsiness, lethargy, and hangover are frequently observed from excessive drug intake.

Dependence—Prolonged use of larger than usual therapeutic doses may result in psychic and physical dependence. Tolerance and psychologic dependence may develop by the second week of continued administration.

Chloral hydrate addicts may take huge doses of the drug, i.e., up to 12 g. nightly has been reported. This abuse is similar to alcohol addiction and sudden withdrawal may result in central nervous excitation, with tremor, anxiety, hallucination, or even delirium which may be fatal. In patients suffering from chronic chloral hydrate intoxication, gastritis is common and skin eruptions may develop. Parenchymatous renal injury may also occur.

Withdrawal should be undertaken in a hospital and supportive treatment similar to that used during barbiturate withdrawal is recommended.

Overdosage: The signs and symptoms of chloral hydrate overdosage resemble those of barbiturate overdosage and especially affect the CNS and cardiovascular system. They may include: hypothermia; pinpoint pupils; blood pressure falls; comatose state; slow or rapid and shallow breathing. Gastric irritation may result in vomiting and even gastric necrosis. If the patient survives, icterus due to hepatic damage and albuminuria from renal irritation may appear.

The toxic oral dose of chloral hydrate for adults is approximately 10 g.; however, death has been reported from a dose of 4 g. and some patients have survived after taking as much as 30 g.

Accidental overdosage should be treated with gastric lavage or by inducing vomiting to empty the stomach. Supportive measures may be used. Hemodialysis is reported to be effective in promoting the clearance of trichloroethanol.

Dosage and Administration: The capsules should be taken with a full glass of liquid. The syrup may be administered in a half glass of water, fruit juice, or ginger ale.

ADULTS: The usual *hypnotic* dose is 500 mg. to 1 g., taken 15 to 30 minutes before bedtime or ½ hour before surgery. The usual *sedative* dose is 250 mg. three times daily after meals. Generally, single doses or daily dosage should not exceed 2 g.

CHILDREN: The usual daily *hypnotic* dosage is 50 mg./kg. of body weight, with a maximum of 1 g. per single dose. Daily dosage may be given in divided doses, if indicated. The *sedative* dosage is half of the hypnotic dosage.

How Supplied: *Noctec Capsules (Chloral Hydrate Capsules USP) are available in potencies of 250 mg. (3¾ grains) in bottles of 100 capsules and 500 mg. (7½ grains) in bottles of 100 and Unimatic® cartons of 25 and 100 capsules.

Noctec (Chloral Hydrate) is also available as an aromatic, flavored syrup supplying 500 mg. (7½ grains) per 5 ml. teaspoonful in 473 ml. (pint) bottles and 3.8 liter (gallon) bottles.

Storage: Store Noctec (Chloral Hydrate) capsules and syrup at room temperature; avoid excessive heat. Dispense only in glass containers. Dispense the syrup in tight, light-resistant containers.

*Shown in Product Identification Section, page 438

O-V STATIN® ℞
[ō-vē-stat′in]
(oral/vaginal therapy pack)

O-V STATIN (oral/vaginal therapy pack) is designed specifically to provide a convenient therapy pack for use in the treatment of coexisting intestinal candidiasis and vulvovaginal candidiasis.

Mycostatin® Oral Tablets
(Nystatin Tablets USP)
Mycostatin® Vaginal Tablets
(Nystatin Vaginal Tablets USP)

Description: Nystatin is an antifungal antibiotic which is both fungistatic and fungicidal *in vitro* against a wide variety of yeasts and yeast-like fungi. It is a polyene antibiotic of undetermined structural formula that is obtained from *Streptomyces noursei*.

MYCOSTATIN ORAL TABLETS (Nystatin Tablets USP) are provided for oral administration as coated tablets containing 500,000 units nystatin.

MYCOSTATIN VAGINAL TABLETS (Nystatin Vaginal Tablets USP) are provided as diamond-shaped, individually foil wrapped, compressed tablets containing 100,000 units nystatin dispersed in lactose with ethyl cellulose, stearic acid and starch.

Clinical Pharmacology: Nystatin probably acts by binding to sterols in the cell membrane of the fungus with a resultant change in membrane permeability allowing leakage of intracellular components. It exhibits no appreciable activity against bacteria or trichomonads.

Following oral administration, nystatin is sparingly absorbed with no detectable blood levels when given in the recommended doses. Most of the orally administered nystatin is passed unchanged in the stool.

Indications and Usage: O-V STATIN oral/vaginal therapy pack [Mycostatin Oral Tablets (Nystatin Tablets USP) and Mycostatin Vaginal Tablets (Nystatin Vaginal Tablets USP)] is indicated for use in the treatment of coexisting intestinal candidiasis and vulvovaginal candidiasis.

MYCOSTATIN VAGINAL TABLETS (Nystatin Vaginal Tablets USP) are effective for the local treatment of vulvovaginal candidiasis (moniliasis). The diagnosis should be confirmed, prior to therapy, by KOH smears and/ or cultures. Other pathogens commonly associated with vulvovaginitis (Trichomonas and *Hemophilus vaginalis*) do not respond to nystatin and should be ruled out by appropriate laboratory methods.

Contraindications: Both preparations are contraindicated in patients with a history of hypersensitivity to any of their components.

Precautions: General—Discontinue treatment if sensitization or irritation is reported during intravaginal use.

Laboratory Tests—If there is a lack of response to MYCOSTATIN VAGINAL TABLETS (Nystatin Vaginal Tablets USP), appropriate microbiological studies should be repeated to confirm the diagnosis and rule out other pathogens before instituting another course of antimycotic therapy.

Usage in Pregnancy: No adverse effects or complications have been attributed to nystatin in infants born to women treated with nystatin oral or vaginal tablets.

Adverse Reactions: Nystatin is virtually nontoxic and nonsensitizing and is well tolerated by all age groups, even on prolonged administration. Large oral doses have occasionally produced diarrhea, gastrointestinal distress, nausea and vomiting. Rarely, irritation or sensitization on intravaginal use may occur (see PRECAUTIONS).

Dosage and Administration: MYCOSTATIN ORAL TABLETS—The usual therapeutic dosage is one to two tablets (500,000 to 1,000,000 units nystatin) three times daily. Treatment should generally be continued for at least 48 hours after clinical cure to prevent relapse.

MYCOSTATIN VAGINAL TABLETS—The usual dosage is one tablet (100,000 units nystatin) daily for two weeks. The tablets should be deposited high in the vagina by means of the applicator. "Instructions for the Patient" are enclosed in each package.

Even though symptomatic relief may occur within a few days, treatment should be continued for the full course.

It is important that therapy be continued during menstruation. Adjunctive measures such as therapeutic douches are unnecessary and sometimes inadvisable. Cleansing douches may be used by nonpregnant women, if desired, for esthetic purposes.

How Supplied: O-V STATIN oral/vaginal therapy pack—containing one bottle of 42 MYCOSTATIN ORAL TABLETS (Nystatin Tablets USP, 500,000 units nystatin each) and 14 individually foil wrapped MYCOSTATIN VAGINAL TABLETS (Nystatin Vaginal Tablets USP, 100,000 units nystatin each) with one plastic applicator and one "Instructions for the Patient" leaflet.

Storage: Store in refrigerator below 15° C (59° F).

PENICILLIN G POTASSIUM FOR INJECTION USP

[pen" i-sil' in-jē]

Description: Penicillin G Potassium for Injection USP is crystalline penicillin G potassium as a sterile powder. The preparation contains approximately 27 mg. citrate buffer (composed of sodium citrate and not more than 0.94 mg. citric acid) with approximately 1.7 mEq. potassium and 0.3 mEq. sodium per million units of penicillin.

Clinical Pharmacology: Penicillin G is bactericidal against penicillin-susceptible microorganisms during the stage of active multiplication. It acts by inhibiting biosynthesis of cell-wall mucopeptide. It is not active against the penicillinase-producing bacteria, which include many strains of staphylococci. Penicillin G is highly active *in vitro* against staphylococci (except penicillinase-producing strains), streptococci (groups A, C, G, H, L, and M) and pneumococci. Other organisms sensitive *in vitro* to penicillin G are *Neisseria gonorrhoeae, Corynebacterium diphtheriae, Bacillus anthracis,* Clostridia, *Actinomyces bovis, Streptobacillus moniliformis, Listeria monocytogenes* and Leptospira; *Treponema pallidum* is extremely susceptible. Some species of gram-negative bacilli are susceptible to moderate to high concentrations of penicillin G obtained with intravenous administration. These include most strains of *Escherichia coli;* all strains of *Proteus mirabilis,* Salmonella, and Shigella; and some strains of *Enterobacter aerogenes* (formerly *Aerobacter aerogenes*) and *Alcaligenes faecalis.*

Susceptibility plate testing: If the Kirby-Bauer method of disc susceptibility is used, a 10 u. penicillin disc should give a zone greater than 28 mm. when tested against a penicillin-susceptible bacterial strain.

Aqueous penicillin G is rapidly absorbed following both intramuscular and subcutaneous injection. Approximately 60 percent of the total dose of 300,000 u. is excreted in the urine within this five-hour period. Therefore, high and frequent doses are required to maintain the elevated serum levels desirable in treating certain severe infections in individuals with normal kidney function. In neonates and young infants, and in individuals with impaired kidney function, excretion is considerably delayed.

Indications and Usage: Penicillin G Potassium for Injection USP is indicated in the treatment of severe infections caused by penicillin G-susceptible microorganisms when rapid and high penicillinemia is required. Therapy should be guided by bacteriological studies, including susceptibility tests, and by clinical response.

The following infections will usually respond to adequate dosage:

Streptococcal infections. Note: streptococci in groups A, C, G, H, L, and M are very susceptible to penicillin G. Some group D organisms are susceptible to the high serum levels obtained with aqueous penicillin G. Aqueous penicillin G potassium is the penicillin dosage form of choice for bacteremia, empyema, severe pneumonia, pericarditis, endocarditis, meningitis and other severe infections caused by susceptible strains of the gram-positive species listed above.

Pneumococcal infections; Staphylococcal infections—penicillin G-susceptible; **Anthrax; Actinomycosis; Clostridial infections** (including tetanus); **Diphtheria** (to prevent the carrier state); **Erysipeloid endocarditis** (Erysipelothrix insidiosa); **Vincent's gingivitis and pharyngitis** (fusospirochetosis)—Severe infections of the oropharynx (Note: necessary dental care should be accomplished in infections involving gum tissue.), and **lower respiratory tract and genital area infections** due to *F. fusiformisans* spirochetes; **Gram-negative bacillary infections** (bacteremias)—*(E. coli, E. aerogenes, A. faecalis,* Salmonella, Shigella and *P. mirabilis);* **Listeria infections** *(L. monocytogenes);* **Meningitis and endocarditis; Pasteurella infections** *(P. multocida):* Bacteremia and *meningitis;* **Rat-bite fever** *(S. minus* or *S. moniliformis);* **Gonorrheal endocarditis and arthritis** *(N. gonorrhoeae);* **Syphilis** *(T. pallidum)* including congenital syphilis; **Meningococcic meningitis.**

Prevention of bacterial endocarditis—Although no controlled clinical efficacy studies have been conducted, aqueous crystalline penicillin G for injection and penicillin G procaine suspension have been suggested by the American Heart Association and the American Dental Association for use as part of a combined parenteral-oral regimen for prophylaxis against bacterial endocarditis in patients with congenital heart disease or rheumatic or other acquired valvular heart disease when they undergo dental procedures and surgical procedures of the upper respiratory tract.[1] Since it may happen that *alpha* hemolytic streptococci relatively resistant to penicillin may be found when patients are receiving continuous oral penicillin for secondary prevention of rheumatic fever, prophylactic agents other than penicillin may be chosen for these patients and prescribed in addition to their continuous rheumatic fever prophylactic regimen. **NOTE: When selecting antibiotics for the prevention of bacterial endocarditis the physician or dentist should read the full joint statement of the American Heart Association and the American Dental Association.**[1]

Contraindications: Contraindicated in patients with a history of hypersensitivity to any penicillin.

Warnings: Serious and occasional fatal hypersensitivity (anaphylactoid) reactions have been reported in patients on penicillin therapy. Although anaphylaxis is more frequent following parenteral administration, it has occurred in patients on oral penicillins. These reactions are more apt to occur in individuals with a history of sensitivity to multiple allergens.

There have been well-documented reports of individuals with a history of penicillin hypersensitivity who have experienced severe hypersensitivity reactions when treated with cephalosporins. Before therapy with a penicillin, careful inquiry should be made concerning previous hypersensitivity reactions to penicillins, cephalosporins, and other allergens. If an allergic reaction occurs, the drug should be discontinued and the patient treated with the usual agents, e.g., pressor amines, antihistamines, and corticosteroids. Serious anaphylactoid reactions are not controlled by antihistamines alone, and require such emergency measures as the immediate use of epinephrine, aminophylline, oxygen, and intravenous corticosteroids.

Precautions: Penicillin should be used with caution in individuals with histories of significant allergies and/or asthma.

In prolonged therapy with penicillin and particularly with high dosage schedules, periodic evaluation of the renal and hematopoietic systems is recommended.

In streptococcal infections, therapy must be sufficient to eliminate the organism (ten days minimum); otherwise the sequelae of streptococcal disease may occur. Cultures should be taken following the completion of treatment to determine whether streptococci have been eradicated.

In high doses (above 10 million u.), intravenous aqueous penicillin G potassium should be administered slowly because of the adverse effects of electrolyte imbalance from the potassium content of the penicillin. The patient's renal, cardiac and vascular status should be evaluated and if impairment of function is suspected or known to exist, a reduction in the total dosage should be considered. Frequent evaluation of electrolyte balance, and renal and hematopoietic function is recommended during therapy when high doses of intravenous aqueous penicillin G potassium are used.

Prolonged use of antibiotics may promote overgrowth of nonsusceptible organisms, including fungi. Should superinfection occur, appropriate measures should be taken. Indwelling intravenous catheters encourage superinfections and should be avoided whenever possible.

Therapy of susceptible infections should be accompanied by any indicated surgical procedures. In suspected staphylococcal infections, proper laboratory studies, including susceptibility tests, should be performed.

When treating gonococcal infections in which primary or secondary syphilis may be suspected, proper diagnostic procedures, including darkfield examinations, should be done. In all cases in which concomitant syphilis is suspected, monthly serological tests should be made for at least four months. All cases of penicillin-treated syphilis should receive clinical and serological examinations every six months for at least two or three years.

Adverse Reactions: Penicillin is a substance of low toxicity but does possess a significant index of sensitization.

The hypersensitivity reactions reported are skin rashes ranging from maculopapular eruptions to exfoliative dermatitis; urticaria; and serum sickness-like reactions including chills, fever, edema, arthralgia and prostration. Severe and occasionally fatal anaphylaxis has occurred (see WARNINGS).

Hemolytic anemia, leukopenia, thrombocytopenia, neuropathy, and nephropathy are rarely observed adverse reactions and are usually associated with high intravenous dosage. Urticaria, other skin rashes, and serum sickness-like reactions may be controlled by antihistamines and, if necessary, corticosteroids. Whenever such reactions occur, penicillin should be discontinued unless, in the opinion of the physician, the condition

Continued on next page

Squibb—Cont.

being treated is life-threatening and amenable only to penicillin therapy. Patients given continuous intravenous therapy with penicillin G potassium in high dosage (10 million to 100 million u. daily) may suffer severe or even fatal potassium poisoning, particularly if renal insufficiency is present. Hyperreflexia, convulsions and coma may be indicative of this syndrome.
The Jarisch-Herxheimer reaction has been reported in patients treated for syphilis.
Dosage and Administration: Penicillin G Potassium for Injection USP may be given intramuscularly or by continuous intravenous drip.
The 10,000,000 and 20,000,000 u. preparations of Penicillin G Potassium for Injection USP should be administered by intravenous infusion only.
The usual dose recommendation is as follows:
Severe infections due to susceptible strains of streptococci, pneumococci, and staphylococci; bacteremia, pneumonia, endocarditis, pericarditis, empyema, meningitis and other severe infections: a minimum of 5 million u. daily.
Anthrax: a minimum of 5 million u./day in divided doses until cure is effected; **Actinomycosis:** 1 to 6 million u./day for cervicofacial cases; 10 to 20 million u./day for thoracic and abdominal disease; **Clostridial infections** (as adjunctive therapy to antitoxin): 20 million u./day; **Diphtheria**—adjunctive therapy to antitoxin for prevention of the carrier state: 300,000 to 400,000 u./day in divided doses for 10 to 12 days; **Erysipeloid:** *Endocarditis:* 2 to 20 million u./day for four to six weeks; **Fusospirochetal infections** (fusospirochetosis)—severe infections of the oropharynx, lower respiratory tract and genital area: 5 to 10 million u./day; **Gram-negative bacillary infections** *(E. coli, E. aerogenes, A. faecalis,* Salmonella, Shigella, and *P. mirabilis); Bacteremia:* 20 to 80 million u./ day; **Listeria infections** *(L. monocytogenes): Neonates:* 500,000 to 1 million u./day; *Adults with meningitis:* 15 to 20 million u./day for two weeks; *Adults with endocarditis:* 15 to 20 million u./ day for four weeks; **Pasteurella infections** *(P. multocida): Bacteremia* and *meningitis:* 4 to 6 million u./day for two weeks; **Rat-bite fever** *(S. minus* or *S. moniliformis):* 12 to 15 million u./day for three to four weeks.
Gonorrheal endocarditis and arthritis: a minimum of 5 million u. daily.
Syphilis—aqueous penicillin G potassium may be used in the treatment of acquired and congenital syphilis but, because of the necessity of frequent dosage, hospitalization is recommended. Dosage and duration of therapy is determined by the age of the patient and the stage of the disease.
Meningococcic meningitis: 1 to 2 million u. I.M. every two hours or continuous I.V. drip of 20 to 30 million u./day.
Prevention of bacterial endocarditis—For prophylaxis against bacterial endocarditis[1] in patients with congenital heart disease or rheumatic or other acquired valvular heart disease when undergoing dental procedures or surgical procedures of the upper respiratory tract, use a combined parenteral-oral regimen. One million units of aqueous crystalline penicillin G (30,000 u./kg. in children) mixed with 600,000 u. penicillin G procaine (600,000 u. for children) should be given intramuscularly one-half to one hour before the procedure. Oral penicillin V (phenoxymethyl penicillin), 500 mg. for adults or 250 mg. for children less than 60 lb., should be given every six hours for eight doses. Doses for children should not exceed recommendations for adults for a single dose or for a 24-hour period.
Preparation of Solutions: Solutions of penicillin should be prepared as follows: Loosen powder. Hold vial horizontally and rotate it while *slowly* directing the stream of diluent against the wall of the vial. Shake vial vigorously after all the diluent has been added. Depending on the route of administration, use Sterile Water for Injection USP, isotonic Sodium Chloride Injection USP, or Dextrose Injection USP. NOTE: Penicillins are rapidly inactivated in the presence of carbohydrate solutions at alkaline pH.
RECONSTITUTION: 1,000,000 u. vial—add 9.6 ml., 4.6 ml., or 3.6 ml. diluent to provide 100,000 u., 200,000 u., or 250,000 u. per ml., respectively: 5,000,000 u. vial—add 23 ml., 18 ml., 8 ml., or 3 ml. diluent to provide 200,000 u., 250,000 u., 500,000 u., or 1,000,000 u. per ml., respectively. *For I.V. infusion only:* 10,000,000 u. vial—add 15.5 ml. or 5.4 ml. diluent to provide 500,000 u. or 1,000,000 u. per ml., respectively: 20,000,000 u. vial—add 31.6 ml. diluent to provide 500,000 u. per ml.
How Supplied: Penicillin G Potassium for Injection USP is available in vials providing 1, 5, 10, and 20 million units of crystalline penicillin G potassium.
Storage: The dry powder is relatively stable and may be stored at room temperature without significant loss of potency. Sterile solutions may be kept in the refrigerator one week without significant loss of potency. Solutions prepared for intravenous infusion are stable at room temperature for at least 24 hours.
Reference: 1. American Heart Association. 1977. Prevention of bacterial endocarditis. Circulation 56:139A-143A.

PENICILLIN G SODIUM FOR INJECTION USP ℞

[*pen" i-sil' in-jē*]

Description: Penicillin G Sodium for Injection USP is crystalline penicillin G sodium as a sterile powder. The preparation contains 28 mg. citrate buffer (composed of sodium citrate, and not more than 0.92 mg. citric acid) and approximately 2.0 mEq. sodium per million units of penicillin.
Clinical Pharmacology: Penicillin G is bactericidal against penicillin-susceptible microorganisms during the stage of active multiplication. It acts by inhibiting biosynthesis of cell-wall mucopeptide. It is not active against the penicillinase-producing bacteria, which include many strains of staphylococci. Penicillin G is highly active *in vitro* against staphylococci (except penicillinase-producing strains), streptococci (groups A, C, G, H, L, and M) and pneumococci. Other organisms susceptible *in vitro* to penicillin G are *Neisseria gonorrhoeae, Corynebacterium diphtheriae, Bacillus anthracis,* Clostridia, *Actinomyces bovis, Streptobacillus moniliformis, Listeria monocytogenes* and Leptospira; *Treponema pallidum* is extremely susceptible. Some species of gram-negative bacilli are susceptible to moderate to high concentrations of penicillin G obtained with intravenous administration. These include most strains of *Escherichia coli;* all strains of *Proteus mirabilis,* Salmonella and Shigella; and some strains of *Enterobacter aerogenes* (formerly *Aerobacter aerogenes*) and *Alcaligenes faecalis.*
Susceptibility plate testing: If the Kirby-Bauer method of disc susceptibility is used, a 10 u. penicillin disc should give a zone greater than 28 mm. when tested against a penicillin-susceptible bacterial strain.
Aqueous penicillin G is rapidly absorbed following both intramuscular and subcutaneous injection. Approximately 60 percent of the total dose of 300,000 u. is excreted in the urine within this five-hour period. Therefore, high and frequent doses are required to maintain the elevated serum levels desirable in treating certain severe infections in individuals with normal kidney function. In neonates and young infants and in individuals with impaired kidney function, excretion is considerably delayed.
Indications and Usage: Penicillin G Sodium for Injection USP is indicated in the treatment of severe infections caused by penicillin G-susceptible microorganisms when rapid and high penicillinemia is required. Therapy should be guided by bacteriological studies, including susceptibility tests, and by clinical response.
The following infections will usually respond to adequate dosage:
Streptococcal infections. Note: streptococci in groups A, C, G, H, L, and M are very susceptible to penicillin G. Some group D organisms are susceptible to the high serum levels obtained with aqueous penicillin G. Aqueous penicillin G sodium is the penicillin dosage form of choice for bacteremia, empyema, severe pneumonia, pericarditis, endocarditis, meningitis and other severe infections caused by susceptible strains of the gram-positive species listed above.
Pneumococcal infections; Staphylococcal infections—penicillin G-susceptible; **Anthrax; Actinomycosis; Clostridial infections** (including tetanus); **Diphtheria** (to prevent the carrier state); **Erysipeloid endocarditis** *(Erysipelothrix insidiosa);* **Vincent's gingivitis and pharyngitis** (fusospirochetosis)—Severe infections of the oropharynx (Note: necessary dental care should be accomplished in infections involving gum tissue.) and **lower respiratory tract and genital area infections** due to *F. fusiformisans* spirochetes; **Gram-negative bacillary infections** (bacteremias)—*(E. coli, E. aerogenes, A. faecalis,* Salmonella, Shigella and *P. mirabilis);* **Listeria infections** *(L. monocytogenes);* **Meningitis and endocarditis; Pasteurella infections** *(P. multocida):* Bacteremia and meningitis; **Rat-bite fever** *(S. minus* or *S. moniliformis);* **Gonorrheal endocarditis and arthritis** *(N. gonorrhoeae);* **Syphilis** *(T. pallidum)* including congenital syphilis; **Meningococcic meningitis.**
Prevention of bacterial endocarditis—Although no controlled clinical efficacy studies have been conducted, aqueous crystalline penicillin G for injection and penicillin G procaine suspension have been suggested by the American Heart Association and the American Dental Association for use as part of a combined parenteral-oral regimen for prophylaxis against bacterial endocarditis in patients with congenital heart disease or rheumatic or other acquired valvular heart disease when they undergo dental procedures and surgical procedures of the upper respiratory tract.[1] Since it may happen that *alpha* hemolytic streptococci relatively resistant to penicillin may be found when patients are receiving continuous oral penicillin for secondary prevention of rheumatic fever, prophylactic agents other than penicillin may be chosen for these patients and prescribed in addition to their continuous rheumatic fever prophylactic regimen. **NOTE: When selecting antibiotics for the prevention of bacterial endocarditis the physician or dentist should read the full joint statement of the American Heart Association and the American Dental Association.[1]**
Contraindications: Contraindicated in patients with a history of hypersensitivity to any penicillin.
Warnings: Serious and occasional fatal hypersensitivity (anaphylactoid) reactions have been reported in patients on penicillin therapy. Although anaphylaxis is more frequent following parenteral administration, it has occurred in patients on oral penicillins. These reactions are more apt to occur in individuals with a history of sensitivity to multiple allergens.
There have been well-documented reports of individuals with a history of penicillin hypersensitivity who have experienced severe hypersensitivity reactions when treated with cephalosporins. Before therapy with a penicillin, careful inquiry should be made concerning previous hypersensitivity reactions to penicillins, cephalosporins, and other allergens. If an allergic reaction occurs, the drug should be discontinued and the patient treated with the usual agents, e.g., pressor amines, antihistamines, and corticosteroids. Serious anaphylactoid reactions are not controlled by antihistamines alone, and require such emergency measures as the immediate use of epinephrine, aminophylline, oxygen, and intravenous corticosteroids.
Precautions: Penicillin should be used with caution in individuals with histories of significant allergies and/or asthma.
In prolonged therapy with penicillin and particularly with high dosage schedules, periodic evaluation of the renal and hematopoietic systems is recommended.
In streptococcal infections, therapy must be sufficient to eliminate the organism (10 days minimum); otherwise the sequelae of streptococcal disease may occur. Cultures should be taken fol-

lowing the completion of treatment to determine whether streptococci have been eradicated.

In high doses (above 10 million u.), intravenous aqueous penicillin G sodium should be administered slowly because of the adverse effects of electrolyte imbalance from the sodium content of the penicillin. The patient's renal, cardiac and vascular status should be evaluated and if impairment of function is suspected or known to exist, a reduction in the total dosage should be considered. Frequent evaluation of electrolyte balance, and renal and hematopoietic function is recommended during therapy when high doses of intravenous aqueous penicillin G sodium are used.

Prolonged use of antibiotics may promote overgrowth of nonsusceptible organisms, including fungi. Should superinfection occur, appropriate measures should be taken. Indwelling intravenous catheters encourage superinfections and should be avoided whenever possible.

Therapy of susceptible infections should be accompanied by any indicated surgical procedures. In suspected staphylococcal infections, proper laboratory studies, including susceptibility tests, should be performed.

When treating gonococcal infections in which primary or secondary syphilis may be suspected, proper diagnostic procedures, including darkfield examinations, should be done. In all cases in which concomitant syphilis is suspected, monthly serological tests should be made for at least four months. All cases of penicillin-treated syphilis should receive clinical and serological examinations every six months for at least two or three years.

Adverse Reactions: Penicillin is a substance of low toxicity but does possess a significant index of sensitization.

The hypersensitivity reactions reported are skin rashes ranging from maculopapular eruptions to exfoliative dermatitis; urticaria; and serum sickness-like reactions including chills, fever, edema, arthralgia and prostration. Severe and occasionally fatal anaphylaxis has occurred (see WARNINGS).

Hemolytic anemia, leukopenia, thrombocytopenia, neuropathy, and nephropathy are rarely observed adverse reactions and are usually associated with high intravenous dosage. Urticaria, other skin rashes, and serum sickness-like reactions may be controlled by antihistamines and, if necessary, corticosteroids. Whenever such reactions occur, penicillin should be discontinued unless, in the opinion of the physician, the condition being treated is life-threatening and amenable only to penicillin therapy. High dosage of penicillin G sodium may result in congestive heart failure due to high sodium intake.

The Jarisch-Herxheimer reaction has been reported in patients treated for syphilis.

Dosage and Administration: Penicillin G Sodium for Injection USP may be given intramuscularly or by continuous intravenous drip.

The usual dosage recommendation is as follows:
Severe infections due to susceptible strains of streptococci, pneumococci, and staphylococci; bacteremia, pneumonia, endocarditis, pericarditis, empyema, meningitis and other severe infections: a minimum of 5 million u. daily.
Anthrax: a minimum of 5 million u./day in divided doses until cure is effected; **Actinomycosis:** 1 to 6 million u./day for cervicofacial cases; 10 to 20 million u./day for thoracic and abdominal disease; **Clostridial infections** (as adjunctive therapy to antitoxin): 300,000 to 400,000 u./day in divided doses for 10 to 12 days; **Diphtheria**—adjunctive therapy to antitoxin for prevention of the carrier state: 300,000 to 400,000 u./day in divided doses for 10 to 12 days; **Erysipeloid:** *Endocarditis:* 2 to 20 million u./day for four to six weeks: **Fusospirochetal infections** (fusospirochetosis)—severe infections of the oropharynx, lower respiratory tract and genital area: 5 to 10 million u./day; **Gram-negative bacillary infections** (*E. coli, E. aerogenes, A. faecalis,* Salmonella, Shigella and *P. mirabilis); Bacteremia:* 20 to 80 million u./day; **Listeria infections** *(L. monocytogenes): Neonates:* 500,000 to 1 million u./day; *Adults with meningitis:* 15 to 20 million u./day for two weeks; *Adults with endocarditis:* 15 to 20 million u./day for four weeks; **Pasteurella infections** *(P. multocida): Bacteremia* and *meningitis:* 4 to 6 million u./day for two weeks; **Rat-bite fever** *(S. minus* or *S. moniliformis):* 12 to 15 million u./day for three to four weeks.
Gonorrheal endocarditis and arthritis: a minimum of 5 million u. daily.
Syphilis—aqueous penicillin G sodium may be used in the treatment of acquired and congenital syphilis but, because of the necessity of frequent dosage, hospitalization is recommended. Dosage and duration of therapy is determined by the age of the patient and the stage of the disease.
Meningococcic meningitis: 1 to 2 million u. I.M. every two hours or continuous I.V. drip of 20 to 30 million u./day.
Prevention of bacterial endocarditis—For prophylaxis against bacterial endocarditis[1] in patients with congenital heart disease or rheumatic or other acquired valvular heart disease when undergoing dental procedures or surgical procedures of the upper respiratory tract, use a combined parenteral-oral regimen. One million units of aqueous crystalline penicillin G (30,000 u./kg. in children) mixed with 600,000 u. penicillin G procaine (600,000 u. for children) should be given intramuscularly one-half to one hour before the procedure. Oral penicillin V (phenoxymethyl penicillin), 500 mg. for adults or 250 mg. for children less than 60 lb., should be given every six hours for eight doses. Doses for children should not exceed recommendations for adults for a single dose or for a 24-hour period.
Preparation of Solutions: Solutions of penicillin should be prepared as follows: Loosen powder. Hold vial horizontally and rotate it while *slowly* directing the stream of diluent against the wall of the vial. Shake vial vigorously after all the diluent has been added. Depending on the route of administration, use Sterile Water for Injection USP, isotonic Sodium Chloride Injection USP, or Dextrose Injection USP. NOTE: Penicillins are rapidly inactivated in the presence of carbohydrate solutions at alkaline pH.
Reconstitute with 23 ml., 18 ml., 8 ml., or 3 ml diluent to provide concentrations of 200,000 u., 250,000 u., 500,000 u., or 1,000,000 u. per ml., respectively.
How Supplied: In vials providing 5 million units of crystalline penicillin G sodium. [Military Depot Item: 10's, NSN 6505-01-145-5216.]
Storage: The dry powder is relatively stable and may be stored at room temperature without significant loss of potency. Sterile solutions may be kept in the refrigerator one week without significant loss of potency. Solutions prepared for intravenous infusion are stable at room temperature for at least 24 hours.
Reference: 1. American Heart Association. 1977. Prevention of bacterial endocarditis. Circulation 56:139A-143A.

PENTIDS® TABLETS ℞
[pen′tidz]
PENTIDS® '400' TABLETS ℞
PENTIDS® '800' TABLETS ℞
(Penicillin G Potassium Tablets USP)
PENTIDS® FOR SYRUP ℞
PENTIDS® '400' FOR SYRUP ℞
(Penicillin G Potassium for Oral Solution USP)

Description: Pentids Tablets, Pentids '400' Tablets and Pentids '800' Tablets (Penicillin G Potassium Tablets USP) are scored, compressed uncoated tablets of crystalline penicillin G potassium. Pentids '800' Tablets contain FD&C Yellow No. 5 (tartrazine).
Pentids for Syrup and Pentids '400' for Syrup (Penicillin G Potassium for Oral Solution USP) provide penicillin G potassium in flavored powder forms for preparation as syrups when liquid oral penicillin therapy is indicated, especially for infants and children. Pentids for Syrup and Pentids '400' for Syrup contain FD&C Yellow No. 5 (tartrazine).
Clinical Pharmacology: Penicillin G is bactericidal against penicillin-susceptible microorganisms during the stage of active multiplication. It acts by inhibiting biosynthesis of cell-wall mucopeptide. It is not active against the penicillinase-producing bacteria, which include many strains of staphylococci.

Penicillin G is highly active *in vitro* against staphylococci (except penicillinase-producing strains), streptococci (groups A, C, G, H, L, and M) and pneumococci. Other organisms susceptible *in vitro* to penicillin G are *Neisseria gonorrhoeae, Corynebacterium diphtheriae, Bacillus anthracis,* Clostridia, *Actinomyces bovis, Streptobacillus moniliformis, Listeria monocytogenes,* and Leptospira; *Treponema pallidum* is extremely susceptible. Some species of gram-negative bacilli are susceptible to moderate to high concentrations of penicillin G obtained with intravenous administration. These include most strains of *Escherichia coli,* all strains of *Proteus mirabilis,* Salmonella and Shigella and some strains of *Enterobacter aerogenes* (formerly *Aerobacter aerogenes)* and *Alcaligenes faecalis.*

Oral preparations of penicillin G are only slightly affected by normal gastric acidity (pH 2.0 to 3.5); however, a pH below 2.0 may partially or totally inactivate penicillin G. Oral penicillin G is absorbed in the upper small intestine, chiefly the duodenum; however, serum level and urinary excretion data indicate that only approximately 30 percent of the dose is absorbed. For this reason four to five times the dose of oral penicillin G must be given to obtain a blood level comparable to that obtained with parenteral penicillin G. Since gastric acidity, stomach emptying time, and other factors affecting absorption may vary considerably, serum levels may be appreciably reduced to nontherapeutic levels in certain individuals.

Approximately 60 percent of penicillin G is bound to serum protein. The drug is distributed throughout the body tissues in widely varying amounts. Highest levels are found in the kidneys with lesser amounts in the liver, skin, and intestines. Penicillin G penetrates into all other tissues to a lesser degree with very limited amounts found in the cerebrospinal fluid. The drug is excreted rapidly by tubular excretion in patients with normal kidney function. In neonates and young infants, and in individuals with impaired kidney function, excretion is considerably delayed. Normally, approximately 20 percent of a dose of oral penicillin G is excreted in the urine.

Indications and Usage: Pentids (Penicillin G Potassium) are indicated in the treatment of mild to moderately severe infections due to penicillin G-susceptible microorganisms. Therapy should be guided by bacteriological studies, including susceptibility tests, and by clinical response. Note: severe pneumonia, empyema, bacteremia, pericarditis, meningitis, and septic arthritis should not be treated with oral penicillin G during the acute stage.

Oral penicillin G is not recommended for short-term prevention of bacterial endocarditis in patients with valvular heart disease undergoing dental or surgical procedures.
Indicated surgical procedures should be performed.
The following infections will usually respond to adequate dosage:
Streptococcal infections Group A without bacteremia—Mild to moderate infections of the upper respiratory tract, skin and skin structures infections, scarlet fever, and mild erysipelas. Note: streptococci in groups A, C, G, H, L, and M are very susceptible to penicillin G. Other groups, including group D (enterococcus) are resistant.
Pneumococcal infections—Mild to moderately severe infections of the respiratory tract.
Staphylococcal infections — penicillin G-susceptible—Mild infections of the skin and skin structures. Note: reports indicate an increasing number of strains of staphylococci resistant to penicillin G, emphasizing the need for culture and susceptibility studies in treating suspected staphylococcal infections.

Continued on next page

Squibb—Cont.

Vincent's gingivitis and pharyngitis (fusospirochetosis)—Mild to moderately severe infections of the oropharynx usually respond to oral penicillin G. Note: necessary dental care should be accomplished in infections involving gum tissue.

Medical conditions in which oral penicillin G therapy is indicated as prophylaxis: (A) *For the prevention of recurrence following rheumatic fever and/or chorea.* Prophylaxis with oral penicillin G on a continuing basis is effective in preventing recurrence of these conditions.

(B) *Prevention of bacteremia following tooth extraction.*

Contraindications: Contraindicated in patients with a history of hypersensitivity to any penicillin.

Warnings: Serious and occasional fatal hypersensitivity (anaphylactoid) reactions have been reported in patients on penicillin therapy. Although anaphylaxis is more frequent following parenteral administration, it has occurred in patients on oral penicillins. These reactions are more apt to occur in individuals with a history of sensitivity to multiple allergens.

There have been well-documented reports of individuals with a history of penicillin hypersensitivity who have experienced severe hypersensitivity reactions when treated with cephalosporins. Before therapy with a penicillin, careful inquiry should be made concerning previous hypersensitivity reactions to penicillins, cephalosporins, and other allergens. If an allergic reaction occurs, the drug should be discontinued and the patient treated with the usual agents, e.g., pressor amines, antihistamines, and corticosteroids. Serious anaphylactoid reactions are not controlled by antihistamines alone, and require such emergency measures as the immediate use of epinephrine, aminophylline, oxygen, and intravenous corticosteroids.

Precautions: Penicillin should be used with caution in individuals with histories of significant allergies and/or asthma.

The oral route of administration should not be relied upon in patients with severe illness, or with nausea, vomiting, gastric dilatation, cardiospasm or intestinal hypermotility.

Occasional patients will not absorb therapeutic amounts of orally administered penicillin.

In streptococcal infections, therapy must be sufficient to eliminate the organism (10 days minimum); otherwise the sequelae of streptococcal disease may occur. Cultures should be taken following completion of treatment to determine whether streptococci have been eradicated.

Prolonged use of antibiotics may promote the overgrowth of nonsusceptible organisms, including fungi. Should superinfection occur, appropriate measures should be taken.

In prolonged therapy with penicillin, and particularly with high dosage schedules, periodic evaluation of the renal and hematopoietic systems is recommended.

Pentids '800' Tablets (Penicillin G Potassium Tablets USP), Pentids for Syrup (Penicillin G Potassium for Oral Solution USP), and Pentids '400' for Syrup contain FD&C Yellow No. 5 (tartrazine) which may cause allergic-type reactions (including bronchial asthma) in certain susceptible individuals. Although the overall incidence of FD&C Yellow No. 5 (tartrazine) sensitivity in the general population is low, it is frequently seen in patients who also have aspirin hypersensitivity.

Adverse Reactions: Although the incidence of reactions to oral penicillins has been reported with much less frequency than following parenteral therapy, it should be remembered that all degrees of hypersensitivity, including fatal anaphylaxis, have been reported with oral penicillin.

The most common reactions to oral penicillins are nausea, vomiting, epigastric distress, diarrhea, and black hairy tongue. The hypersensitivity reactions reported are skin rashes ranging from maculopapular to exfoliative dermatitis; urticaria; serum sickness-like reactions including chills, fever, edema, arthralgia, and prostration; laryngeal edema; and anaphylaxis. Fever and eosinophilia may frequently be the only reactions observed. Hemolytic anemia, leukopenia, thrombocytopenia, neuropathy, and nephropathy are infrequent reactions usually associated with high doses of parenteral penicillin. Urticaria, other skin rashes, and serum sickness-like reactions may be controlled by antihistamines and, if necessary, corticosteroids. Whenever such reactions occur, penicillin should be discontinued unless, in the opinion of the physician, the condition being treated is life-threatening and amenable only to penicillin therapy. Serious anaphylactoid reactions require emergency measures (see WARNINGS).

An occasional patient may complain of sore mouth or tongue, as with any oral penicillin preparation.

Dosage and Administration: The dosage of penicillin G should be determined according to the susceptibility of the causative microorganisms and the severity of infection, and adjusted to the clinical response of the patient.

Therapy for children under 12 years of age is calculated on the basis of body weight. For infants and small children the suggested dose is 15 to 56 mg. (25,000 to 90,000 u.) per kg./day in three to six divided doses.

For maximum absorption of penicillin, dosage should be given on an empty stomach. Thus, a dose of 200,000 units should be administered one-half hour before or at least two hours after meals. The blood concentration with a dose of 400,000 units is sufficiently high to inhibit susceptible bacteria when the antibiotic is given without regard to meals but, as can be expected, the resultant concentration will be higher when it is given before meals.

The usual dosage recommendation for adults and children 12 years and over is as follows:

Streptococcal infections—mild to moderately severe—of the upper respiratory tract and including otitis media, scarlet fever and mild erysipelas: 125 mg. (200,000 u.) t.i.d. or q.i.d. for 10 days for mild infections; 250 mg. (400,000 u.) t.i.d. for 10 days for moderately severe infections; alternatively, 500 mg. (800,000 u.) may be given b.i.d.

Pneumococcal infections—mild to moderately severe—of the respiratory tract, including otitis media: 250 mg. (400,000 u.) q.i.d. until the patient has been afebrile for at least two days.

Staphylococcal infections—mild infections of skin and skin structures (culture and susceptibility tests should be performed): 125 to 250 mg. (200,000 to 400,000 u.) t.i.d. or q.i.d. until infection is cured.

Vincent's gingivitis and pharyngitis (fusospirochetosis)—mild to moderately severe infections of the oropharynx: 250 mg. (400,000 u.) t.i.d. or q.i.d.

For the prevention of recurrence following rheumatic fever and/or chorea: 125 mg. (200,000 u.) twice daily on a continuing basis.

How Supplied: *Pentids, *Pentids '400' and *Pentids '800' Tablets (Penicillin G Potassium Tablets USP) are available for oral administration as scored, uncoated tablets which provide 125 mg. (200,000 units), 250 mg. (400,000 units) and 500 mg. (800,000 units) crystalline penicillin G potassium, respectively, equivalent to 120 mg., 240 mg. and 480 mg. of penicillin G sodium reference standard; the tablets are buffered with calcium carbonate. Pentids Tablets, in bottles of 100; Pentids '400' Tablets in bottles of 16 and 100 and Unimatic® cartons of 100; and Pentids '800' Tablets in bottles of 30 and 100.

Pentids for Syrup and Pentids '400' for Syrup (Penicillin G Potassium for Oral Solution USP) are available for oral administration as powders that, when prepared as directed, provide fruit-flavored syrups respectively containing 125 mg. (200,000 units) and 250 mg. (400,000 units) of penicillin G potassium (equivalent to 120 mg. and 240 mg. penicillin G sodium reference standard) per 5 ml. teaspoonful; both preparations are buffered with sodium phosphates. Pentids for Syrup and Pentids '400' for Syrup in 100 ml. and 200 ml. bottles.

Storage: Penicillin G Potassium Tablets USP—Store at room temperature; avoid excessive heat; keep bottle tightly closed. Dispense in tight containers.

Penicillin G Potassium for Oral Solution USP—Store at room temperature prior to preparation of syrup; store syrup in refrigerator; keep bottle tightly closed; discard unused portion after 14 days. Shake well before using.

Shown in Product Identification Section, page 438

PRINCIPEN® '250' CAPSULES ℞
[prin'si-pen"]
PRINCIPEN® '500' CAPSULES ℞
(Ampicillin Capsules USP)
PRINCIPEN® '125' FOR ORAL SUSPENSION ℞
PRINCIPEN® '250' FOR ORAL SUSPENSION ℞
(Ampicillin for Oral Suspension USP)

Description: Principen (Ampicillin Trihydrate), a semisynthetic penicillin derived from the basic penicillin nucleus, 6-aminopenicillanic acid, is available for oral administration as Principen '250' Capsules and Principen '500' Capsules (Ampicillin Capsules USP) which provide ampicillin trihydrate equivalent to 250 mg. and 500 mg. ampicillin, respectively. It is also available as Principen '125' for Oral Suspension and Principen '250' for Oral Suspension (Ampicillin for Oral Suspension USP) which provide, after mixing, ampicillin trihydrate equivalent to 125 mg. and 250 mg. ampicillin, respectively, per 5 ml. teaspoonful.

Actions: Human Pharmacology: Ampicillin is bactericidal at low concentrations and is clinically effective not only against the gram-positive organisms usually susceptible to penicillin G but also against a variety of gram-negative organisms. It is stable in the presence of gastric acid and is well absorbed from the gastrointestinal tract. It diffuses readily into most body tissues and fluids; however, penetration into the cerebrospinal fluid and brain occurs only with meningeal inflammation. Ampicillin is excreted largely unchanged in the urine; its excretion can be delayed by concurrent administration of probenecid which inhibits the renal tubular secretion of ampicillin. In blood serum, ampicillin is the least bound of all the penicillins; an average of about 20 percent of the drug is bound to the plasma proteins as compared to 60 to 90 percent for the other penicillins. The administration of a 500 mg. dose of ampicillin trihydrate capsules results in an average peak blood serum level of approximately 3.0 mcg./ml.; the average peak serum level for the same dose of ampicillin trihydrate for oral suspension is approximately 3.4 mcg./ml.

Microbiology: The following microorganisms show *in vitro* sensitivity to ampicillin:

GRAM-POSITIVE—strains of alpha- and beta-hemolytic streptococci, *Diplococcus pneumoniae*, those strains of staphylococci which do not produce penicillinase, *Clostridium* sp., *Bacillus anthracis*, *Corynebacterium xerose*, and most strains of enterococci.

GRAM-NEGATIVE—*Hemophilus influenzae; Neisseria gonorrhoeae* and *N. meningitidis; Proteus mirabilis;* and many strains of Salmonella (including *S. typhosa)*, Shigella, and *Escherichia coli.*

NOTE: Ampicillin is inactivated by penicillinase and therefore is ineffective against penicillinase-producing organisms including certain strains of staphylococci, *Pseudomonas aeruginosa, P. vulgaris, Klebsiella pneumoniae, Aerobacter aerogenes,* and some strains of *E. coli.* Ampicillin is not active against Rickettsia, Mycoplasma, and "large viruses" (Miyagawanella).

TESTING FOR SUSCEPTIBILITY: The invading organism should be cultured and its sensitivity demonstrated as a guide to therapy. If the Kirby-Bauer method of disc sensitivity is used, a 10 mcg. ampicillin disc should be used to determine the relative *in vitro* susceptibility.

Indications: Principen Capsules (Ampicillin Capsules USP) and Principen for Oral Suspension (Ampicillin for Oral Suspension USP) are primarily indicated for the treatment of genitourinary, respiratory, and gastrointestinal tract infections caused by susceptible strains of gram-negative bacteria (including Shigella, *S. typhosa* and other Salmonella, *E. coli, H. influenzae, N. gonorrhoeae* and *N. meningitidis,* and *P. mirabilis).* Ampicillin may also be indicated in certain infections due to susceptible gram-positive bacteria: penicillin G-sensitive staphylococci, streptococci, pneumococci, and enterococci.

Bacteriology studies to determine the causative organisms and their sensitivity to ampicillin should be performed. Therapy may be instituted prior to the results of sensitivity testing.

Contraindications: A history of a previous hypersensitivity reaction to any of the penicillins is a contraindication. Ampicillin is also contraindicated in infections caused by penicillinase-producing organisms.

Warnings: Serious and occasional fatal hypersensitivity (anaphylactoid) reactions have been reported in patients on penicillin therapy. Although anaphylaxis is more frequent following parenteral administration, it has occurred in patients on oral penicillins. These reactions are more apt to occur in individuals with a history of sensitivity to multiple allergens.

There have been well-documented reports of individuals with a history of penicillin hypersensitivity who have experienced severe hypersensitivity reactions when treated with cephalosporins. Before therapy with a penicillin, careful inquiry should be made concerning previous hypersensitivity reactions to penicillins, cephalosporins, and other allergens. If an allergic reaction occurs, the drug should be discontinued and the patient treated with the usual agents, e.g., pressor amines, antihistamines, and corticosteroids. **Serious anaphylactoid reactions require immediate emergency treatment with epinephrine. Oxygen, intravenous steroids and airway management, including intubation, should also be administered as indicated.**

Usage in Pregnancy: The safety of this drug for use in pregnancy has not been established.

Precautions: Prolonged use of antibiotics may promote the overgrowth of nonsusceptible organisms, including fungi. Should superinfection occur, appropriate measures should be taken.

Cases of gonococcal infection with a suspected lesion of syphilis should have darkfield examinations ruling out syphilis before receiving ampicillin. Patients who do not have suspected lesions of syphilis and are treated with ampicillin should have a follow-up serologic test for syphilis each month for four months to detect syphilis that may have been masked by treatment for gonorrhea. Patients with gonorrhea who also have syphilis should be given additional appropriate parenteral penicillin treatment.

Treatment with ampicillin does not preclude the need for surgical procedures, particularly in staphylococcal infections.

In prolonged therapy, and particularly with high dosage schedules, periodic evaluation of the renal, hepatic, and hematopoietic systems is recommended.

Adverse Reactions: As with other penicillins, it may be expected that untoward reactions will be essentially limited to sensitivity phenomena. They are more likely to occur in individuals who have previously demonstrated hypersensitivity to penicillin and in those with a history of allergy, asthma, hay fever, or urticaria.

The following adverse reactions have been reported as associated with the use of ampicillin:

Gastrointestinal: glossitis, stomatitis, nausea, vomiting, enterocolitis, pseudomembranous colitis, and diarrhea. These reactions are usually associated with oral dosage forms of the drug.

Hypersensitivity Reactions: an erythematous, mildly pruritic, maculopapular skin rash has been reported fairly frequently. The rash, which usually does not develop within the first week of therapy, may cover the entire body including the soles, palms, and oral mucosa. The eruption usually disappears in 3 to 7 days. Other hypersensitivity reactions that have been reported are: skin rash, pruritus, urticaria, erythema multiforme, and an occasional case of exfoliative dermatitis. Anaphylaxis is the most serious reaction experienced and has usually been associated with the parenteral dosage form of the drug.

NOTE: Urticaria, other skin rashes, and serum sickness-like reactions may be controlled by antihistamines, and, if necessary, systemic corticosteroids. Whenever such reactions occur, ampicillin should be discontinued unless, in the opinion of the physician, the condition being treated is life-threatening and amenable only to ampicillin therapy. Serious anaphylactoid reactions require emergency measures (see WARNINGS).

Liver: moderate elevation in serum glutamic oxaloacetic transaminase (SGOT) has been noted, but the significance of this finding is unknown.

Hemic and Lymphatic Systems: anemia, thrombocytopenia, thrombocytopenic purpura, eosinophilia, leukopenia, and agranulocytosis have been reported during therapy with penicillins. These reactions are usually reversible on discontinuation of therapy and are believed to be hypersensitivity phenomena.

Other adverse reactions that have been reported with the use of ampicillin are laryngeal stridor and high fever. An occasional patient may complain of sore mouth or tongue as with any oral penicillin preparation.

Dosage and Administration: *Adults, and children weighing over 20 kg.:* **For genitourinary or gastrointestinal tract infections other than gonorrhea in men and women,** the usual dose is 500 mg. q.i.d. in equally spaced doses; severe or chronic infections may require larger doses. For the treatment of gonorrhea in both men and women, a single oral dose of 3.5 grams of ampicillin administered simultaneously with 1.0 gram of probenecid is recommended. Physicians are cautioned to use no less than the above recommended dosage for the treatment of gonorrhea. Follow-up cultures should be obtained from the original site(s) of infection 7 to 14 days after therapy. In women, it is also desirable to obtain culture test-of-cure from both the endocervical and anal canals. Prolonged intensive therapy is needed for complications such as prostatitis and epididymitis. For **respiratory tract infections,** the usual dose is 250 mg. q.i.d. in equally spaced doses.

Children weighing 20 kg. or less: For **genitourinary or gastrointestinal tract infections,** the usual dose is 100 mg./kg./day total, q.i.d. in equally divided and spaced doses. For **respiratory infections,** the usual dose is 50 mg./kg./day total, in equally divided and spaced doses 3 to 4 times daily.

All patients, irrespective of age and weight: Larger doses may be required for severe or chronic infections. Although ampicillin is resistant to degradation by gastric acid, like all antibiotics given orally it should be administered at least two hours after or one-half hour before meals for maximal absorption. Except for the single dose regimen for gonorrhea referred to above, therapy should be continued for a minimum of 48 to 72 hours after the patient becomes asymptomatic or evidence of bacterial eradication has been obtained. In infections caused by hemolytic strains of streptococci, a minimum of 10 days' treatment is recommended to guard against the risk of rheumatic fever or glomerulonephritis. In the treatment of chronic urinary or gastrointestinal infections, frequent bacteriologic and clinical appraisal is necessary during therapy and may be necessary for several months afterwards. Stubborn infections may require treatment for several weeks. Smaller doses than those indicated above should not be used. Doses for children should not exceed doses recommended for adults.

How Supplied: Principen is available for oral administration as *Principen '250' Capsules and *Principen '500' Capsules (Ampicillin Capsules USP) which provide ampicillin trihydrate equivalent to 250 mg. and 500 mg. ampicillin, respectively; the 250 mg. potency in bottles of 100 and 500 and Unimatic® Unit-Dose Packs of 100 and 500; the 500 mg. potency in bottles of 16, 100, and 500 and Unimatic Unit-Dose Packs of 100 and 500. It is also available for oral administration as Principen '125' for Oral Suspension and Principen '250' for Oral Suspension (Ampicillin for Oral Suspension USP) which provide, after mixing, pleasantly flavored suspensions containing ampicillin trihydrate equivalent to 125 mg. and 250 mg. ampicillin, respectively, per 5 ml. teaspoonful; both potencies in 80, 100, 150, and 200 ml. bottles, and in Unimatic® cartons of 4×25 bottles (5 ml. each bottle).

Storage: Principen Capsules—Store at room temperature; avoid excessive heat; keep bottle tightly closed. Dispense in tight containers.

Principen for Oral Suspension—Store at room temperature prior to preparation of suspension; after preparation of suspension, store at room temperature and discard unused portion after 7 days or store in refrigerator and discard unused portion after 14 days; keep bottle tightly closed. Shake well before using.

*Shown in Product Identification Section, page 438

PRINCIPEN® with PROBENECID ℞
[prin'si-pen" with pro"ben'e-sid"]
(Ampicillin and Probenecid Capsules USP)

Description: Ampicillin trihydrate is a semisynthetic penicillin derived from the basic penicillin nucleus, 6-aminopenicillanic acid. Probenecid is a uricosuric and renal tubular blocking agent. Principen with Probenecid is provided in single-dose bottles containing nine capsules; each capsule contains ampicillin trihydrate equivalent to 389 mg. ampicillin and 111 mg. probenecid (9 capsules contain ampicillin trihydrate equivalent to 3.5 g. ampicillin and 1 g. probenecid).

Clinical Pharmacology: Ampicillin is stable in the presence of gastric acid and is well absorbed from the gastrointestinal tract. It diffuses readily into most body tissues and fluids; however, penetration into the cerebrospinal fluid and brain occurs only with meningeal inflammation. Ampicillin is excreted largely unchanged in the urine; its excretion is delayed by concurrent administration of probenecid which inhibits the renal tubular secretion of ampicillin. In blood serum, ampicillin is the least bound of all the penicillins; an average of about 20 percent of the drug is bound to the plasma proteins as compared to 60 to 90 percent for the other penicillins. Probenecid inhibits the tubular reabsorption of urate, thus increasing the urinary excretion of uric acid and decreasing serum uric acid levels. It also inhibits the tubular secretion of penicillin and usually increases penicillin plasma levels by any route the antibiotic is given. A two-fold to four-fold elevation has been demonstrated for various penicillins.

Ampicillin is inactivated by penicillinase and therefore is ineffective against penicillinase-producing organisms.

Indications and Usage: Principen with Probenecid (Ampicillin and Probenecid Capsules USP) is indicated for the treatment of uncomplicated infection (urethral, endocervical, or rectal) caused by *Neisseria gonorrhoeae* in men and women.

Urethritis and the presence of gram-negative diplococci in urethral smears is strong presumptive evidence of gonorrhea. Culture or fluorescent antibody studies will confirm the diagnosis.

Susceptibility studies should be performed with recurrent infections or when resistant strains are encountered. Therapy may be instituted prior to obtaining results of susceptibility testing.

Contraindications: A history of a previous hypersensitivity reaction to any of the penicillins or to probenecid is a contraindication.

Probenecid is not recommended in persons with known blood dyscrasias or uric acid kidney stones or during an acute attack of gout. It is not recommended in conjunction with ampicillin in the presence of known renal impairment.

Warnings: Serious and occasional fatal hypersensitivity (anaphylactoid) reactions have been reported in patients on penicillin therapy. Although anaphylaxis is more frequent following parenteral administration, it has occurred in patients on oral penicillins. These reactions are more apt to occur in individuals with a history of sensitivity to multiple allergens.

Continued on next page

Squibb—Cont.

There have been well-documented reports of individuals with a history of penicillin hypersensitivity who have experienced severe hypersensitivity reactions when treated with cephalosporins. Before therapy with a penicillin, careful inquiry should be made concerning previous hypersensitivity reactions to penicillins, cephalosporins, and other allergens. If an allergic reaction occurs, the patient should be treated with the usual agents, e.g., pressor amines, antihistamines, and corticosteroids. Serious anaphylactoid reactions require immediate emergency treatment with epinephrine. Oxygen, intravenous steroids, and airway management, including intubation, should also be administered as indicated.

Usage in Pregnancy: The safety of these drugs for use in pregnancy has not been established.

Precautions: Cases of gonococcal infection with a suspected lesion of syphilis should have darkfield examinations ruling out syphilis before receiving ampicillin. Patients who do not have suspected lesions of syphilis and are treated with ampicillin should have a follow-up serologic test for syphilis each month for four months to detect syphilis that may have been masked by treatment for gonorrhea. Patients with gonorrhea who also have syphilis should be given additional appropriate parenteral penicillin treatment.

Adverse Reactions: Ampicillin—As with other penicillins, it may be expected that untoward reactions will be essentially limited to sensitivity phenomena. They are more likely to occur in individuals who have previously demonstrated hypersensitivity to penicillin and in those with a history of allergy, asthma, hay fever, or urticaria.

The following adverse reactions have been reported as associated with the use of ampicillin:

Gastrointestinal: glossitis, stomatitis, nausea, vomiting, enterocolitis, pseudomembranous colitis, and diarrhea. These reactions are usually associated with oral dosage forms of the drug.

Hypersensitivity Reactions: An erythematous, mildly pruritic, maculopapular skin rash has been reported fairly frequently. The rash, which usually does not develop within the first week of therapy, may cover the entire body including the soles, palms, and oral mucosa. The eruption usually disappears in three to seven days. Other hypersensitivity reactions that have been reported are: skin rash, pruritus, urticaria, erythema multiforme, and an occasional case of exfoliative dermatitis. Anaphylaxis is the most serious reaction experienced and has usually been associated with the parenteral dosage form of the drug.

NOTE: Urticaria, other skin rashes, and serum sickness-like reactions may be controlled by antihistamines, and, if necessary, systemic corticosteroids. Serious anaphylactoid reactions require emergency measures (see WARNINGS).

Liver: Moderate elevation in serum glutamic oxaloacetic transaminase (SGOT) has been noted, but the significance of this finding is unknown.

Hemic and Lymphatic Systems: Anemia, thrombocytopenia, thrombocytopenic purpura, eosinophilia, leukopenia, and agranulocytosis have been reported during therapy with penicillins. These reactions are usually reversible on discontinuation of therapy and are believed to be hypersensitivity phenomena.

Probenecid—The following are the principal adverse reactions which have been reported as associated with the use of probenecid, generally with more prolonged or repeated administration: hypersensitivity reactions (including anaphylaxis), nephrotic syndrome, hepatic necrosis, aplastic anemia; also other anemias, including hemolytic anemia related to genetic deficiency of glucose-6-phosphate dehydrogenase.

Dosage and Administration: For the treatment of gonorrhea in both men and women—3.5 g. ampicillin and 1 g. probenecid (9 capsules) is administered as a single dose.

Physicians are cautioned to use no less than the above recommended dosage.

Follow-up cultures should be obtained from the original site(s) of infection 7 to 14 days after therapy. In women, it is also desirable to obtain culture test-of-cure from both the endocervical and anal canals.

How Supplied: Principen with Probenecid (Ampicillin and Probenecid Capsules USP) is provided in single-dose bottles containing nine capsules; each capsule contains ampicillin trihydrate equivalent to 389 mg. ampicillin and 111 mg. probenecid (9 capsules contain ampicillin trihydrate equivalent to 3.5 g. ampicillin and 1 g. probenecid).

Storage: Store at room temperature; avoid excessive heat.

PROLIXIN® INJECTION ℞
[pro″lik′sin]
(Fluphenazine Hydrochloride Injection USP)

PROLIXIN® TABLETS ℞
(Fluphenazine Hydrochloride Tablets USP)

PROLIXIN® ELIXIR ℞
(Fluphenazine Hydrochloride Elixir USP)

Description: Prolixin is a trifluoromethyl phenothiazine derivative.

Prolixin Injection (Fluphenazine Hydrochloride Injection USP) is available in multiple-dose vials providing 2.5 mg. fluphenazine hydrochloride per ml. FOR INTRAMUSCULAR USE ONLY. The preparation also includes sodium chloride for isotonicity, sodium hydroxide or hydrochloric acid to adjust the pH to 4.8 to 5.2, and 0.1% methylparaben and 0.01% propylparaben as preservatives. At the time of manufacture, the air in the vials is replaced by nitrogen.

Prolixin Tablets (Fluphenazine Hydrochloride Tablets USP) are available for oral administration as tablets providing 1, 2.5, 5, and 10 mg. fluphenazine hydrochloride. Prolixin 2.5, 5, and 10 mg. tablets contain FD&C Yellow No. 5 (tartrazine).

Prolixin Elixir (Fluphenazine Hydrochloride Elixir USP) is available as an elixir for oral administration which provides 0.5 mg. fluphenazine hydrochloride per ml. (2.5 mg. per 5 ml. teaspoonful) and contains 14% alcohol by volume.

Clinical Pharmacology: Prolixin has activity at all levels of the central nervous system as well as on multiple organ systems. The mechanism whereby its therapeutic action is exerted is unknown.

Indications and Usage: Prolixin (Fluphenazine Hydrochloride) Injection, Tablets, and Elixir are indicated in the management of manifestations of psychotic disorders.

Fluphenazine hydrochloride has not been shown effective in the management of behavorial complications in patients with mental retardation.

Contraindications: Phenothiazines are contraindicated in patients with suspected or established subcortical brain damage, in patients receiving large doses of hypnotics, and in comatose or severely depressed states. The presence of blood dyscrasia or liver damage precludes the use of fluphenazine hydrochloride. Prolixin (Fluphenazine Hydrochloride) is contraindicated in patients who have shown hypersensitivity to fluphenazine; cross-sensitivity to phenothiazine derivatives may occur.

Warnings: The use of this drug may impair the mental and physical abilities required for driving a car or operating heavy machinery.

Potentiation of the effects of alcohol may occur with the use of this drug.

Since there is no adequate experience in children who have received this drug, safety and efficacy in children have not been established.

Usage in Pregnancy: The safety for the use of this drug during pregnancy has not been established; therefore, the possible hazards should be weighed against the potential benefits when administering this drug to pregnant patients.

Precautions: Because of the possibility of cross-sensitivity, fluphenazine hydrochloride should be used cautiously in patients who have developed cholestatic jaundice, dermatoses or other allergic reactions to phenothiazine derivatives.

Prolixin Tablets (Fluphenazine Hydrochloride Tablets USP) 2.5, 5, and 10 mg. contain FD&C Yellow No. 5 (tartrazine) which may cause allergic-type reactions (including bronchial asthma) in certain susceptible individuals. Although the overall incidence of FD&C Yellow No. 5 (tartrazine) sensitivity in the general population is low, it is frequently seen in patients who also have aspirin hypersensitivity.

Psychotic patients on large doses of a phenothiazine drug who are undergoing surgery should be watched carefully for possible hypotensive phenomena. Moreover, it should be remembered that reduced amounts of anesthetics or central nervous system depressants may be necessary.

The effects of atropine may be potentiated in some patients receiving fluphenazine because of added anticholinergic effects.

Fluphenazine hydrochloride should be used cautiously in patients exposed to extreme heat or phosphorus insecticides; in patients with a history of convulsive disorders since grand mal convulsions have been known to occur; and in patients with special medical disorders such as mitral insufficiency or other cardiovascular diseases and pheochromocytoma.

The possibility of liver damage, pigmentary retinopathy, lenticular and corneal deposits, and development of irreversible dyskinesia should be remembered when patients are on prolonged therapy.

Neuroleptic drugs elevate prolactin levels; the elevation persists during chronic administration. Tissue culture experiments indicate that approximately one-third of human breast cancers are prolactin dependent *in vitro*, a factor of potential importance if the prescription of these drugs is contemplated in a patient with a previously detected breast cancer. Although disturbances such as galactorrhea, amenorrhea, gynecomastia, and impotence have been reported, the clinical significance of elevated serum prolactin levels is unknown for most patients. An increase in mammary neoplasms has been found in rodents after chronic administration of neuroleptic drugs. Neither clinical studies nor epidemiologic studies conducted to date, however, have shown an association between chronic administration of these drugs and mammary tumorigenesis; the available evidence is considered too limited to be conclusive at this time.

Abrupt Withdrawal: In general, phenothiazines do not produce psychic dependence; however, gastritis, nausea and vomiting, dizziness, and tremulousness have been reported following abrupt cessation of high dose therapy. Reports suggest that these symptoms can be reduced if concomitant antiparkinsonian agents are continued for several weeks after the phenothiazine is withdrawn.

Facilities should be available for periodic checking of hepatic function, renal function and the blood picture. Renal function of patients on long-term therapy should be monitored; if BUN (blood urea nitrogen) becomes abnormal, treatment should be discontinued.

As with any phenothiazine, the physician should be alert to the possible development of "silent pneumonias" in patients under treatment with fluphenazine hydrochloride.

Adverse Reactions: *Central Nervous System*—The side effects most frequently reported with phenothiazine compounds are extrapyramidal symptoms including pseudoparkinsonism, dystonia, dyskinesia, akathisia, oculogyric crises, opisthotonos, and hyperreflexia. Most often these extrapyramidal symptoms are reversible; however, they may be persistent (see below). With any given phenothiazine derivative, the incidence and severity of such reactions depend more on individual patient sensitivity than on other factors, but dosage level and patient age are also determinants. Extrapyramidal reactions may be alarming, and the patient should be forewarned and reassured. These reactions can usually be controlled by administration of antiparkinsonian drugs, such as Benztropine Mesylate or intravenous Caffeine and Sodium Benzoate Injection, and by subsequent reduction in dosage.

Persistent Tardive Dyskinesia: As with all antipsychotic agents, tardive dyskinesia may appear in some patients on long-term therapy or may occur after drug therapy has been discontinued. The risk seems to be greater in elderly patients on high-dose therapy, especially females. The symptoms are persistent and in some patients appear to be irreversible. The syndrome is characterized by rhythmical involuntary movements of the tongue, face, mouth, or jaw (e.g., protrusion of tongue, puffing of cheeks, puckering of mouth, chewing movements). Sometimes these may be accompanied by involuntary movements of the extremities. There is no known effective treatment for tardive dyskinesia; antiparkinsonism agents usually do not alleviate the symptoms of this syndrome. It is suggested that all antipsychotic agents be discontinued if these symptoms appear. Should it be necessary to reinstitute treatment, or increase the dosage of the agent, or switch to a different antipsychotic agent, the syndrome may be masked. It has been reported that fine vermicular movements of the tongue may be an early sign of the syndrome and if the medication is stopped at that time, the syndrome may not develop.

Drowsiness or lethargy, if they occur, may necessitate a reduction in dosage; the induction of a catatonic-like state has been known to occur with dosages of fluphenazine far in excess of the recommended amounts. As with other phenothiazine compounds, reactivation or aggravation of psychotic processes may be encountered.

Phenothiazine derivatives have been known to cause, in some patients, restlessness, excitement, or bizarre dreams.

Autonomic Nervous System—Hypertension and fluctuation in blood pressure have been reported with fluphenazine hydrochloride.

Hypotension has rarely presented a problem with fluphenazine. However, patients with pheochromocytoma, cerebral vascular or renal insufficiency, or a severe cardiac reserve deficiency such as mitral insufficiency appear to be particularly prone to hypotensive reactions with phenothiazine compounds and should therefore be observed closely when the drug is administered. If severe hypotension should occur, supportive measures including the use of intravenous vasopressor drugs should be instituted immediately. Levarterenol Bitartrate Injection is the most suitable drug for this purpose; *epinephrine should not be used* since phenothiazine derivatives have been found to reverse its action, resulting in a further lowering of blood pressure.

Autonomic reactions including nausea and loss of appetite, salivation, polyuria, perspiration, dry mouth, headache, and constipation may occur. Autonomic effects can usually be controlled by reducing or temporarily discontinuing dosage.

In some patients, phenothiazine derivatives have caused blurred vision, glaucoma, bladder paralysis, fecal impaction, paralytic ileus, tachycardia, or nasal congestion.

Metabolic and Endocrine—Weight change, peripheral edema, abnormal lactation, gynecomastia, menstrual irregularities, false results on pregnancy tests, impotency in men and increased libido in women have all been known to occur in some patients on phenothiazine therapy.

Allergic Reactions—Skin disorders such as itching, erythema, urticaria, seborrhea, photosensitivity, eczema and even exfoliative dermatitis have been reported with phenothiazine derivatives. The possibility of anaphylactoid reactions occurring in some patients should be borne in mind.

Hematologic—Routine blood counts are advisable during therapy since blood dyscrasias including leukopenia, agranulocytosis, thrombocytopenic or nonthrombocytopenic purpura, eosinophilia, and pancytopenia have been observed with phenothiazine derivatives. Furthermore, if any soreness of the mouth, gums, or throat, or any symptoms of upper respiratory infection occur and confirmatory leukocyte count indicates cellular depression, therapy should be discontinued and other appropriate measures instituted immediately.

Hepatic—Liver damage as manifested by cholestatic jaundice may be encountered, particularly during the first months of therapy; treatment should be discontinued if this occurs. An increase in cephalin flocculation, sometimes accompanied by alterations in other liver function tests, have been reported in patients receiving fluphenazine hydrochloride who have had no clinical evidence of liver damage.

Others—Sudden, unexpected and unexplained deaths have been reported in hospitalized psychotic patients receiving phenothiazines. Previous brain damage or seizures may be predisposing factors; high doses should be avoided in known seizure patients. Several patients have shown sudden flare-ups of psychotic behavior patterns shortly before death. Autopsy findings have usually revealed acute fulminating pneumonia or pneumonitis, aspiration of gastric contents, or intramyocardial lesions.

Although this is not a general feature of fluphenazine, potentiation of central nervous system depressants (opiates, analgesics, antihistamines, barbiturates, alcohol) may occur.

The following adverse reactions have also occurred with phenothiazine derivatives: systemic lupus erythematosus-like syndrome, hypotension severe enough to cause fatal cardiac arrest, altered electrocardiographic and electroencephalographic tracings, altered cerebrospinal fluid proteins, cerebral edema, asthma, laryngeal edema and angioneurotic edema; with long-term use—skin pigmentation, and lenticular and corneal opacities.

Dosage and Administration: *Prolixin Injection (Fluphenazine Hydrochloride Injection USP)*—The average well-tolerated parenteral starting dose for adult psychotic patients is 1.25 mg. (0.5 ml.) intramuscularly. Depending on the severity and duration of symptoms, initial total daily parenteral dosage may range from 2.5 to 10.0 mg. and should be divided and given at 6- to 8-hour intervals.

The smallest amount that will produce the desired results must be carefully determined for each individual since optimal dosage levels of this potent drug vary from patient to patient. In general, the parenteral dose for fluphenazine has been found to be approximately ⅓ to ½ the oral dose. Treatment may be instituted with a *low initial dosage,* which may be increased, if necessary, until the desired clinical effects are achieved. Dosages exceeding 10.0 mg. intramuscularly daily should be used with caution.

When symptoms are controlled, oral maintenance therapy can generally be instituted, often with single daily doses. Continued treatment, by the oral route if possible, is needed to achieve maximum therapeutic benefits; further adjustments in dosage may be necessary during the course of therapy to meet the patient's requirements.

Prolixin (Fluphenazine Hydrochloride) Tablets and Elixir—Depending on severity and duration of symptoms, total daily oral dosage for *adult* psychotic patients may range initially from 2.5 to 10.0 mg. and should be divided and given at 6- to 8-hour intervals.

The smallest amount that will produce the desired results must be carefully determined for each individual since optimal dosage levels of this potent drug vary from patient to patient. In general, the oral dose has been found to be approximately two to three times the parenteral dose of fluphenazine. Treatment is best instituted with a *low initial dosage,* which may be increased, if necessary, until the desired clinical effects are achieved. Therapeutic effect is often achieved with doses under 20 mg. daily. Patients remaining severely disturbed or inadequately controlled may require upward titration of dosage. Daily doses up to 40 mg. may be necessary; controlled clinical studies have not been performed to demonstrate safety of prolonged administration of such doses.

When symptoms are controlled, dosage can generally be reduced gradually to daily oral maintenance doses of 1.0 or 5.0 mg., often given as a single daily dose. Continued treatment is needed to achieve maximum therapeutic benefits; further adjustments in dosage may be necessary during the course of therapy to meet the patient's requirements.

For psychotic patients who have been stabilized on a fixed daily dosage of Prolixin (Fluphenazine Hydrochloride) Tablets or Elixir, conversion of therapy from oral fluphenazine hydrochloride dosage forms to the long-acting injectable Prolixin Decanoate® may be indicated [see package insert for Prolixin Decanoate (Fluphenazine Decanoate Injection) for conversion information].

For *geriatric* patients, the suggested starting dose is 1.0 to 2.5 mg. orally daily, adjusted according to the response of the patient.

Prolixin Injection (Fluphenazine Hydrochloride Injection USP) is useful when psychotic patients are unable or unwilling to take oral therapy.

How Supplied: Prolixin Injection (Fluphenazine Hydrochloride Injection USP) is available as a sterile, aqueous solution providing 2.5 mg. fluphenazine hydrochloride per ml. in multiple-dose vials of 10 ml.

*Prolixin Tablets (Fluphenazine Hydrochloride Tablets USP) are available for oral administration as sugar-coated tablets providing 1, 2.5, 5, and 10 mg. fluphenazine hydrochloride. — 1 mg. (pink) and 10 mg. (coral) in bottles of 50 and 500; 2.5 mg. (yellow) and 5 mg. (green) in bottles of 50 and 500 and Unimatic® Unit-Dose Packs of 100 [1.0 mg in bottles of 500—Military Depot Item, NSN 6505-00-764-4323; 2.5 mg in bottles of 500—Military Depot Item, NSN 6505-00-764-4322, V.A. Depot Item, NSN6505-00-764-4322A; 5 mg. in bottles of 500—Military Depot Item, NSN 6505-00-951-4750, V.A. Depot Item, NSN6505-00-951-4750A.]

Prolixin Elixir (Fluphenazine Hydrochloride Elixir USP) is available as an elixir for oral administration which provides 0.5 mg. fluphenazine hydrochloride per ml. (2.5 mg. per 5 ml. teaspoonful) —(orange-flavored and colored) in bottles of 473 ml. (1 pint) and in 60 ml. dropper assembly bottles with dropper calibrated at 0.5 ml. (0.25 mg.), 1 ml. (0.5 mg.), 1.5 ml. (0.75 mg.), and 2 ml. (1 mg.). [1 pint bottles—V.A. Depot Item, NSN6505-00-764-5042A.]

Storage: Prolixin Injection should be protected from exposure to light. Parenteral solutions may vary in color from essentially colorless to light amber. If a solution has become any darker than light amber or is discolored in any other way, it should not be used. Store at room temperature; avoid freezing.

Store the tablets and elixir at room temperature; protect from light; keep tightly closed. Tablets: avoid excessive heat. Elixir: avoid freezing.

**Shown in Product Identification Section, page 438*

PROLIXIN DECANOATE® ℞

[pro" lik' sin dek" ah-nō' āt]

(Fluphenazine Decanoate Injection)

Description: Prolixin Decanoate is the decanoate ester of a trifluoromethyl phenothiazine derivative. It is a highly potent behavior modifier with a markedly extended duration of effect. Prolixin Decanoate is available for intramuscular or subcutaneous administration, providing 25 mg. fluphenazine decanoate per ml. in a sesame oil vehicle with 1.2% (w/v) benzyl alcohol as a preservative. At the time of manufacture, the air in the vials is replaced by nitrogen.

Clinical Pharmacology: The basic effects of fluphenazine decanoate appear to be no different from those of fluphenazine hydrochloride, with the exception of duration of action. The esterification of fluphenazine markedly prolongs the drug's duration of effect without unduly attenuating its beneficial action.

Prolixin Decanoate has activity at all levels of the central nervous system as well as on multiple organ systems. The mechanism whereby its therapeutic action is exerted is unknown.

Fluphenazine differs from other phenothiazine derivatives in several respects: it is more potent on a milligram basis, it has less potentiating effect on central nervous system depressants and anesthetics than do some of the phenothiazines and appears to be less sedating, and it is less likely than some of the older phenothiazines to produce hypotension (nevertheless, appropriate cautions should be observed—see sections on PRECAUTIONS and ADVERSE REACTIONS).

Continued on next page

Squibb—Cont.

Indications and Usage: Prolixin Decanoate is a long-acting parenteral antipsychotic drug intended for use in the management of patients requiring prolonged parenteral neuroleptic therapy (e.g., chronic schizophrenics).

Fluphenazine decanoate has not been shown effective in the management of behavioral complications in patients with mental retardation.

Contraindications: Phenothiazines are contraindicated in patients with suspected or established subcortical brain damage.

Phenothiazine compounds should not be used in patients receiving large doses of hypnotics.

Prolixin Decanoate is contraindicated in comatose or severely depressed states.

The presence of blood dyscrasia or liver damage precludes the use of fluphenazine decanoate.

Fluphenazine decanoate is not intended for use in children under 12 years of age.

Prolixin Decanoate (Fluphenazine Decanoate Injection) is contraindicated in patients who have shown hypersensitivity to fluphenazine; cross-sensitivity to phenothiazine derivatives may occur.

Warnings: The use of this drug may impair the mental and physical abilities required for driving a car or operating heavy machinery.

Physicians should be alert to the possibility that severe adverse reactions may occur which require immediate medical attention.

Potentiation of the effects of alcohol may occur with the use of this drug.

Since there is no adequate experience in children who have received this drug, safety and efficacy in children have not been established.

Usage in Pregnancy—The safety for the use of this drug during pregnancy has not been established; therefore, the possible hazards should be weighed against the potential benefits when administering this drug to pregnant patients.

Precautions: Because of the possibility of cross-sensitivity, fluphenazine decanoate should be used cautiously in patients who have developed cholestatic jaundice, dermatoses, or other allergic reactions to phenothiazine derivatives.

Psychotic patients on large doses of a phenothiazine drug who are undergoing surgery should be watched carefully for possible hypotensive phenomena. Moreover, it should be remembered that reduced amounts of anesthetics or central nervous system depressants may be necessary.

The effects of atropine may be potentiated in some patients receiving fluphenazine because of added anticholinergic effects.

Fluphenazine decanoate should be used cautiously in patients exposed to extreme heat or phosphorus insecticides.

The preparation should be used with caution in patients with a history of convulsive disorders since grand mal convulsions have been known to occur.

Use with caution in patients with special medical disorders such as mitral insufficiency or other cardiovascular diseases and pheochromocytoma.

The possibility of liver damage, pigmentary retinopathy, lenticular and corneal deposits, and development of irreversible dyskinesia should be remembered when patients are on prolonged therapy.

Outside state hospitals or other psychiatric institutions, fluphenazine decanoate should be administered under the direction of a physician experienced in the clinical use of psychotropic drugs, particularly phenothiazine derivatives. Furthermore, facilities should be available for periodic checking of hepatic function, renal function, and the blood picture. Renal function of patients on long-term therapy should be monitored; if BUN (blood urea nitrogen) becomes abnormal, treatment should be discontinued.

As with any phenothiazine, the physician should be alert to the possible development of "silent pneumonias" in patients under treatment with fluphenazine decanoate.

Neuroleptic drugs elevate prolactin levels; the elevation persists during chronic administration. Tissue culture experiments indicate that approximately one-third of human breast cancers are prolactin dependent *in vitro*, a factor of potential importance if the prescription of these drugs is contemplated in a patient with a previously detected breast cancer. Although disturbances such as galactorrhea, amenorrhea, gynecomastia, and impotence have been reported, the clinical significance of elevated serum prolactin levels is unknown for most patients. An increase in mammary neoplasms has been found in rodents after chronic administration of neuroleptic drugs. Neither clinical studies nor epidemiologic studies conducted to date, however, have shown an association between chronic administration of these drugs and mammary tumorigenesis; the available evidence is considered too limited to be conclusive at this time.

Adverse Reactions: *Central Nervous System*—The side effects most frequently reported with phenothiazine compounds are extrapyramidal symptoms including pseudoparkinsonism, dystonia, dyskinesia, akathisia, oculogyric crises, opisthotonos, and hyperreflexia. Muscle rigidity sometimes accompanied by hyperthermia has been reported following use of fluphenazine decanoate. Most often these extrapyramidal symptoms are reversible; however, they may be persistent (see below). The frequency of such reactions is related in part to chemical structure: one can expect a higher incidence with fluphenazine decanoate than with less potent piperazine derivatives or with straight-chain phenothiazines such as chlorpromazine. With any given phenothiazine derivative, the incidence and severity of such reactions depend more on individual patient sensitivity than on other factors, but dosage level and patient age are also determinants.

Extrapyramidal reactions may be alarming, and the patient should be forewarned and reassured. These reactions can usually be controlled by administration of antiparkinsonian drugs, such as Benztropine Mesylate or intravenous Caffeine and Sodium Benzoate Injection, and by subsequent reduction in dosage.

Persistent Tardive Dyskinesia: As with all antipsychotic agents, tardive dyskinesia may appear in some patients on long-term therapy or may occur after drug therapy has been discontinued. The risk seems to be greater in elderly patients on high-dose therapy, especially females. The symptoms are persistent and in some patients appear to be irreversible. The syndrome is characterized by rhythmical involuntary movements of the tongue, face, mouth or jaw (e.g., protrusion of tongue, puffing of cheeks, puckering of mouth, chewing movements). Sometimes these may be accompanied by involuntary movements of the extremities. There is no known effective treatment for tardive dyskinesia; antiparkinsonism agents usually do not alleviate the symptoms of this syndrome. It is suggested that all antipsychotic agents be discontinued if these symptoms appear. Should it be necessary to reinstitute treatment, or increase the dosage of the agent, or switch to a different antipsychotic agent, the syndrome may be masked. It has been reported that fine vermicular movements of the tongue may be an early sign of the syndrome and if the medication is stopped at that time, the syndrome may not develop.

Drowsiness or lethargy, if they occur, may necessitate a reduction in dosage; the induction of a catatonic-like state has been known to occur with dosages of fluphenazine far in excess of the recommended amounts. As with other phenothiazine compounds, reactivation or aggravation of psychotic processes may be encountered.

Phenothiazine derivatives have been known to cause, in some patients, restlessness, excitement, or bizarre dreams.

Autonomic Nervous System—Hypertension and fluctuations in blood pressure have been reported with fluphenazine.

Hypotension has rarely presented a problem with fluphenazine. However, patients with pheochromocytoma, cerebral vascular or renal insufficiency, or a severe cardiac reserve deficiency such as mitral insufficiency appear to be particularly prone to hypotensive reactions with phenothiazine compounds, and should therefore be observed closely when the drug is administered. If severe hypotension should occur, supportive measures including the use of intravenous vasopressor drugs should be instituted immediately. Levarterenol Bitartrate Injection is the most suitable drug for this purpose; *epinephrine should not be used* since phenothiazine derivatives have been found to reverse its action, resulting in a further lowering of blood pressure.

Autonomic reactions including nausea and loss of appetite, salivation, polyuria, perspiration, dry mouth, headache, and constipation may occur. Autonomic effects can usually be controlled by reducing or temporarily discontinuing dosage.

In some patients, phenothiazine derivatives have caused blurred vision, glaucoma, bladder paralysis, fecal impaction, paralytic ileus, tachycardia, or nasal congestion.

Metabolic and Endocrine—Weight change, peripheral edema, abnormal lactation, gynecomastia, menstrual irregularities, false results on pregnancy tests, impotency in men and increased libido in women have all been known to occur in some patients on phenothiazine therapy.

Allergic Reactions—Skin disorders such as itching, erythema, urticaria, seborrhea, photosensitivity, eczema and even exfoliative dermatitis have been reported with phenothiazine derivatives. The possibility of anaphylactoid reactions occurring in some patients should be borne in mind.

Hematologic—Routine blood counts are advisable during therapy since blood dyscrasias including leukopenia, agranulocytosis, thrombocytopenic or nonthrombocytopenic purpura, eosinophilia, and pancytopenia have been observed with phenothiazine derivatives. Furthermore, if any soreness of the mouth, gums, or throat, or any symptoms of upper respiratory infection occur and confirmatory leukocyte count indicates cellular depression, therapy should be discontinued and other appropriate measures instituted immediately.

Hepatic—Liver damage as manifested by cholestatic jaundice may be encountered, particularly during the first months of therapy; treatment should be discontinued if this occurs. An increase in cephalin flocculation, sometimes accompanied by alterations in other liver function tests, has been reported in patients receiving the enanthate ester of fluphenazine (a closely related compound) who have had no clinical evidence of liver damage.

Others—Sudden, unexpected and unexplained deaths have been reported in hospitalized psychotic patients receiving phenothiazines. Previous brain damage or seizures may be predisposing factors; high doses should be avoided in known seizure patients. Several patients have shown sudden flare-ups of psychotic behavior patterns shortly before death. Autopsy findings have usually revealed acute fulminating pneumonia or pneumonitis, aspiration of gastric contents, or intramyocardial lesions.

Although this is not a general feature of fluphenazine, potentiation of central nervous system depressants (opiates, analgesics, antihistamines, barbiturates, alcohol) may occur.

The following adverse reactions have also occurred with phenothiazine derivatives: systemic lupus erythematosus-like syndrome, hypotension severe enough to cause fatal cardiac arrest, altered electrocardiographic and electroencephalographic tracings, altered cerebrospinal fluid proteins, cerebral edema, asthma, laryngeal edema, and angioneurotic edema; with long-term use—skin pigmentation and lenticular and corneal opacities.

Injections of fluphenazine decanoate are extremely well tolerated, local tissue reactions occurring only rarely.

Dosage and Administration: Parenteral drug products should be inspected visually for particulate matter and discoloration prior to administration, whenever solution and container permit.

Prolixin Decanoate (Fluphenazine Decanoate Injection) may be given intramuscularly or subcutaneously. A dry syringe and needle of at least 21

gauge should be used. Use of a wet needle or syringe may cause the solution to become cloudy.
To begin therapy with Prolixin Decanoate the following regimens are suggested:
For *most patients*, a dose of 12.5 to 25 mg. (0.5 to 1 ml.) may be given to initiate therapy. The onset of action generally appears between 24 and 72 hours after injection and the effects of the drug on psychotic symptoms becomes significant within 48 to 96 hours. Subsequent injections and the dosage interval are determined in accordance with the patient's response. When administered as maintenance therapy, a single injection may be effective in controlling schizophrenic symptoms up to four weeks or longer. The response to a single dose has been found to last as long as six weeks in a few patients on maintenance therapy.
It may be advisable that patients who have no history of taking phenothiazines should be treated initially with a shorter-acting form of fluphenazine (see HOW SUPPLIED section for the availability of the shorter-acting fluphenazine hydrochloride dosage forms) before administering the decanoate to determine the patient's response to fluphenazine and to establish appropriate dosage. For psychotic patients who have been stabilized on a fixed daily dosage of Prolixin® Tablets (Fluphenazine Hydrochloride Tablets USP) or Prolixin® Elixir (Fluphenazine Hydrochloride Elixir USP), conversion of therapy from these short-acting oral forms to the long-acting injectable Prolixin Decanoate may be indicated.
Appropriate dosage of Prolixin Decanoate should be individualized for each patient and responses carefully monitored. No precise formula can be given to convert to use of Prolixin Decanoate; however, a controlled multicentered study*, in patients receiving oral doses from 5 to 60 mg. fluphenazine hydrochloride daily, showed that 20 mg. fluphenazine hydrochloride daily was equivalent to 25 mg. (1 ml.) Prolixin Decanoate every three weeks. This represents an approximate conversion ratio of 0.5 ml. (12.5 mg.) of decanoate every three weeks for every 10 mg. of fluphenazine hydrochloride daily.
Once conversion to Prolixin Decanoate is made, careful clinical monitoring of the patient and appropriate dosage adjustment should be made at the time of each injection.
Severely agitated patients may be treated with a rapid-acting phenothiazine compound such as Prolixin Injection (Fluphenazine Hydrochloride Injection USP—see package insert accompanying that product for complete information). When acute symptoms have subsided, 25 mg. (1 ml.) of Prolixin Decanoate may be administered; subsequent dosage is adjusted as necessary.
"Poor risk" patients (those with known hypersensitivity to phenothiazines or with disorders that predispose to undue reactions): Therapy may be initiated cautiously with oral or parenteral fluphenazine hydrochloride (see package inserts accompanying these products for complete information). When the pharmacologic effects and an appropriate dosage are apparent, an equivalent dose of Prolixin Decanoate may be administered. Subsequent dosage adjustments are made in accordance with the response of the patient.
The optimal amount of the drug and the frequency of administration must be determined for each patient, since dosage requirements have been found to vary with clinical circumstances as well as with individual response to the drug.
Dosage should not exceed 100 mg. If doses greater than 50 mg. are deemed necessary, the next dose and succeeding doses should be increased cautiously in increments of 12.5 mg.
How Supplied: Prolixin Decanoate (Fluphenazine Decanoate Injection) is available in 1 ml. Unimatic® single dose preassembled syringes, and 5 ml. vials, providing 25 mg. fluphenazine decanoate per ml. [5 ml. vial—Military Depot Item, NSN 6505-01-147-2083, V.A. Depot Item, NSN 6505-00-264-7759A.] Prolixin (fluphenazine) is also available for oral administration as Prolixin Tablets (Fluphenazine Hydrochloride Tablets USP) providing 1, 2.5, 5, and 10 mg. fluphenazine hydrochloride per tablet, and Prolixin Elixir (Fluphenazine Hydrochloride Elixir USP) providing 0.5 mg. fluphenazine hydrochloride per ml. (2.5 mg. per 5 ml. teaspoonful).
Storage: Store at room temperature; avoid freezing and excessive heat. Protect from light.

---

*The Initiation of Long-Term Pharmacotherapy in Schizophrenia: Dosage and Side Effect Comparisons Between Oral and Depot Fluphenazine; N.R. Schooler; Pharmakopsych. 9:159-169, 1976.

PRONESTYL® CAPSULES ℞
[pro″nes′tl]
(Procainamide Hydrochloride Capsules USP)
PRONESTYL® TABLETS ℞
(Procainamide Hydrochloride Tablets)

> The prolonged administration of procainamide often leads to the development of a positive anti-nuclear antibody (ANA) test with or without symptoms of lupus erythematosus-like syndrome. If a positive ANA titer develops, the benefit/risk ratio related to continued procainamide therapy should be assessed. This may necessitate consideration of alternative antiarrhythmic therapy.

Description: Pronestyl is the amide analogue of procaine hydrochloride. It is available for oral administration as capsules and FILMLOK® tablets in potencies of 250 mg., 375 mg., and 500 mg. Pronestyl tablets contain FD&C Yellow No. 5 (tartrazine). (FILMLOK is a Squibb trademark for veneer-coated tablets.)
Actions: Procainamide depresses the excitability of cardiac muscle to electrical stimulation and slows conduction in the atrium, the bundle of His, and the ventricle. The refractory period of the atrium is considerably more prolonged than that of the ventricle. Contractility of the heart is usually not affected, nor is cardiac output decreased to any extent unless myocardial damage exists. In the absence of any arrhythmia, the heart rate may occasionally be accelerated by conventional doses, suggesting that the drug possesses anticholinergic properties. Larger doses can induce atrioventricular block and ventricular extrasystoles which may proceed to ventricular fibrillation. These effects on the myocardium are reflected in the electrocardiogram; a widening of the QRS complex occurs most consistently; less regularly, the P-R and Q-T intervals are prolonged, and the QRS and T waves show some decrease in voltage.
The action of procainamide begins almost immediately after intramuscular or intravenous administration. Plasma levels after intramuscular injection are at their peak in 15 to 60 minutes. Following oral administration, plasma levels of the drug are comparable to those obtained parenterally, and are maximal within an hour; therapeutic levels are usually attained in half that time.
Therapeutic plasma levels have been reported to be 3 to 10 mcg./ml., with those for the majority of patients in the range of 4 to 8 mcg./ml.
Procainamide is less readily hydrolyzed than procaine, and plasma levels decline slowly—about 10% to 20% per hour. The drug is excreted primarily in the urine, about 10% as free and conjugated p-aminobenzoic acid and about 60% in the unchanged form. The fate of the remainder is unknown.
Indications: Pronestyl (Procainamide Hydrochloride) Capsules and Tablets are indicated in the treatment of premature ventricular contractions and ventricular tachycardia, atrial fibrillation, and paroxysmal atrial tachycardia.
Contraindications: It has been suggested that procainamide be contraindicated in patients with myasthenia gravis. Hypersensitivity to the drug is an absolute contraindication; in this connection, cross sensitivity to procaine and related drugs must be borne in mind. Procainamide should not be administered to patients with complete atrioventricular heart block. Procainamide is also contraindicated in cases of second degree and third degree A-V block unless an electrical pacemaker is operative.
Precautions: During administration of the drug, evidence of untoward myocardial responses should be carefully watched for in all patients. In the presence of an abnormal myocardium, procainamide may at times produce untoward responses. In atrial fibrillation or flutter, the ventricular rate may increase suddenly as the atrial rate is slowed. Adequate digitalization reduces but does not abolish this danger. If myocardial damage exists, ventricular tachysystole is particularly hazardous. Correction of atrial fibrillation, with resultant forceful contractions of the atrium, may cause a dislodgment of mural thrombi and produce an embolic episode. However, it has been suggested that in a patient who is already discharging emboli, procainamide is more likely to stop than to aggravate the process.
Attempts to adjust the heart rate in a patient who has developed ventricular tachycardia during an occlusive coronary episode should be carried out with extreme caution. Caution is also required in marked disturbances of atrioventricular conduction such as second degree and third degree A-V block, bundle branch block, or severe digitalis intoxication, where the use of procainamide may result in additional depression of conduction and ventricular asystole or fibrillation.
Since patients with severe organic heart disease and ventricular tachycardia may also have complete heart block which is difficult to diagnose under these circumstances, this complication should always be kept in mind when treating ventricular arrhythmias with procainamide. If the ventricular rate is significantly slowed by procainamide without attainment of regular atrioventricular conduction, the drug should be stopped and the patient re-evaluated as asystole may result under these circumstances.
In patients receiving normal dosage, but who have both liver and kidney disease, symptoms of overdosage (principally ventricular tachycardia and severe hypotension) may occur due to drug accumulation.
Instances of a syndrome resembling lupus erythematosus have been reported in connection with oral maintenance procainamide therapy. The mechanism of this syndrome is uncertain. Polyarthralgia, arthritis, and pleuritic pain are common symptoms; to a lesser extent fever, myalgia, skin lesions, pleural effusion and pericarditis may occur. Rare cases of thrombocytopenia or Coombs positive hemolytic anemia have been reported which may be related to this syndrome. Patients receiving procainamide for extended periods of time or in whom symptoms suggestive of a lupus-like reaction appear should have anti-nuclear antibody titers measured at regular intervals. If there is a rising titer (anti-nuclear antibody) or clinical symptoms of LE appear, the benefit/risk ratio related to continued procainamide therapy should be assessed (see boxed Warning). The LE syndrome may be reversible upon discontinuance of the drug. If discontinuation of the drug does not cause remission of the symptoms, steroid therapy may be effective. If the syndrome develops in a patient with recurrent life-threatening arrhythmias not controllable by other antiarrhythmic agents, steroid suppressive therapy may be used concomitantly with procainamide.
Pronestyl Tablets (Procainamide Hydrochloride Tablets) contain FD&C Yellow No. 5 (tartrazine) which may cause allergic-type reactions (including bronchial asthma) in certain susceptible individuals. Although the overall incidence of FD&C Yellow No. 5 (tartrazine) sensitivity in the general population is low, it is frequently seen in patients who also have aspirin hypersensitivity.
Adverse Reactions: Hypotension following oral administration is rare. Serious disturbances of cardiac rhythm such as ventricular asystole or fibrillation are more common with intravenous administration.

Continued on next page

Squibb—Cont.

Large oral doses of procainamide may sometimes produce anorexia, nausea, urticaria, and/or pruritus.

A syndrome resembling lupus erythematosus has been reported in patients on oral maintenance therapy (see PRECAUTIONS). Reactions consisting of fever and chills have also been reported, including a case with fever and chills plus nausea, vomiting, abdominal pain, acute hepatomegaly, and a rise in serum glutamic oxaloacetic transaminase following single doses of the drug. Bitter taste, diarrhea, weakness, mental depression, giddiness, and psychosis with hallucinations have been reported. The possibility of such untoward effects should be borne in mind.

Hypersensitivity reactions such as angioneurotic edema and maculopapular rash have also occurred.

Agranulocytosis has occasionally followed the repeated use of the drug, and deaths have occurred. Therefore, routine blood counts are advisable during maintenance procainamide therapy. The patients should be instructed to report any soreness of the mouth, throat, or gums, unexplained fever or any symptoms of upper respiratory tract infection. If any of these should occur, and leukocyte counts indicate cellular depression, procainamide therapy should be discontinued and appropriate treatment should be instituted immediately.

Dosage and Administration: Oral administration is preferred for treatment of arrhythmias which do not require immediate suppression, or to continue treatment after control of serious arrhythmias with Pronestyl Injection (Procainamide Hydrochloride Injection USP) or other antiarrhythmic therapy.

Intravenous therapy for the treatment of serious arrhythmias including those following myocardial infarctions should be limited to use in hospitals where monitoring facilities are available (see package insert accompanying Pronestyl Injection [Procainamide Hydrochloride Injection USP] for complete information).

If oral procainamide therapy is continued for appreciable periods, electrocardiograms should be made occasionally to determine the need for the drug.

Oral dose: For ventricular tachycardia, an initial dose of 1 gram orally followed thereafter by a *total daily dose* of 50 mg./kg. of body weight given at 3 hour intervals. The suggested oral dosage for premature ventricular contractions is 50 mg./kg. of body weight daily given in divided doses at 3 hour intervals.

To provide 50 mg./kg./day: give patients weighing less than 120 lbs. 250 mg. q. 3 hours; give patients between 120 and 200 lbs. 375 mg. q. 3 hours; and give patients over 200 lbs. 500 mg. q. 3 hours. This dosage schedule is for use as a guide for treating the average patient but all patients must be considered on an individual basis.

In atrial fibrillation and paroxysmal atrial tachycardia, an initial dose of 1.25 g. may be followed in one hour by 0.75 g. if there have been no electrocardiographic changes. A dose of 0.5 to 1 g. may then be given every 2 hours until arrhythmia is interrupted or the limit of tolerance is reached. Suggested maintenance dosage is 0.5 to 1 g. every 4 to 6 hours.

How Supplied: Pronestyl Capsules (Procainamide Hydrochloride Capsules USP) providing 250 mg. and 500 mg. are available in bottles of 100 and 1000, and UNIMATIC® unit-dose cartons of 100. The capsules which provide 375 mg. are available in bottles of 100 and UNIMATIC unit-dose cartons of 100. Pronestyl Tablets (Procainamide Hydrochloride Tablets) providing 375 mg. are available in bottles of 100 and Unimatic unit-dose cartons of 100; the 250 mg. and 500 mg. tablets are available in bottles of 100 and 1000.

Storage: Store the capsules and tablets at room temperature; avoid excessive heat.

Shown in Product Identification Section, page 438

PRONESTYL® INJECTION ℞
[pro″nes′tl]
(Procainamide Hydrochloride Injection USP)

Description: Procainamide hydrochloride is the amide analogue of procaine hydrochloride. It is available for parenteral use as a sterile, aqueous solution providing 100 mg. or 500 mg. per ml. The 100 mg./ml. potency contains 0.9% (w/v) benzyl alcohol and not more than 0.09% sodium bisulfite as preservatives; pH adjusted to 4.0–6.0 with hydrochloric acid and/or sodium hydroxide; the 500 mg./ml. potency contains 0.1% methylparaben and not more than 0.2% sodium bisulfite as preservatives; pH adjusted to 4.0–6.0 with hydrochloric acid and/or sodium hydroxide. At the time of manufacture, the air in the containers is replaced by nitrogen.

Actions: Procainamide depresses the excitability of cardiac muscle to electrical stimulation and slows conduction in the atrium, the bundle of His, and the ventricle. The refractory period of the atrium is considerably more prolonged than that of the ventricle. Contractility of the heart is usually not affected, nor is cardiac output decreased to any extent unless myocardial damage exists. In the absence of any arrhythmia, the heart rate may occasionally be accelerated by conventional doses, suggesting that the drug possesses anticholinergic properties. Larger doses can induce atrioventricular block and ventricular extrasystoles which may proceed to ventricular fibrillation. These effects on the myocardium are reflected in the electrocardiogram; a widening of the QRS complex occurs most consistently; less regularly, the P-R and Q-T intervals are prolonged, and the QRS and T waves show some decrease in voltage.

The action of procainamide begins almost immediately after intramuscular or intravenous administration. Plasma levels after intramuscular injection are at their peak in 15 to 60 minutes. Following oral administration, plasma levels of the drug are comparable to those obtained parenterally, and are maximal within an hour; therapeutic levels are usually attained in half that time.

Therapeutic plasma levels have been reported to be 3 to 10 mcg./ml., with those for the majority of patients in the range of 4 to 8 mcg./ml.

Procainamide is less readily hydrolyzed than procaine, and plasma levels decline slowly—about 10% to 20% per hour. The drug is excreted primarily in the urine, about 10% as free and conjugated p-aminobenzoic acid and about 60% in the unchanged form. The fate of the remainder is unknown.

Indications: Pronestyl Injection (Procainamide Hydrochloride Injection USP) is indicated in the treatment of ventricular extrasystoles and tachycardia, atrial fibrillation, paroxysmal atrial tachycardia, and cardiac arrythmias associated with anesthesia and surgery.

Contraindications: It has been suggested that procainamide be contraindicated in patients with myasthenia gravis. Hypersensitivity to the drug is an absolute contraindication; in this connection, cross sensitivity to procaine and related drugs must be borne in mind. Procainamide should not be administered to patients with complete atrioventricular heart block. Procainamide is also contraindicated in cases of high-degree A-V block unless an electrical pacemaker is operative.

Precautions: During administration of the drug, evidence of untoward myocardial responses should be carefully watched for in all patients. In the presence of an abnormal myocardium, procainamide may at times produce untoward responses. In atrial fibrillation or flutter, the ventricular rate may increase suddenly as the atrial rate is slowed. Adequate digitalization reduces, but does not abolish this danger. If myocardial damage exists, ventricular tachysystole is particularly hazardous. Correction of atrial fibrillation, with resultant forceful contractions of the atrium, may cause a dislodgment of mural thrombi and produce an embolic episode. However, it has been suggested that in a patient who is already discharging emboli, procainamide is more likely to stop than to aggravate the process.

Attempts to adjust the heart rate in a patient who has developed ventricular tachycardia during an occlusive coronary episode should be carried out with extreme caution. Caution is also required in marked disturbances of atrioventricular conduction such as A-V block, bundle branch block, or severe digitalis intoxication, where the use of procainamide may result in additional depression of conduction and ventricular asystole or fibrillation. Parenteral administration should be monitored electrocardiographically whenever practicable. If electrocardiograms give evidence of impending heart block, parenteral administration should be discontinued at once. Since patients with severe organic heart disease and ventricular tachycardia may also have complete heart block which is difficult to diagnose under these circumstances, this complication should always be kept in mind when treating ventricular arrhythmias with procainamide (especially parenterally). If the ventricular rate is significantly slowed by procainamide without attainment of regular atrioventricular conduction, the drug should be stopped and the patient reevaluated as asystole may result under these circumstances.

In patients receiving normal dosage, but who have both liver and kidney disease, symptoms of overdosage (principally ventricular tachycardia and severe hypotension) may occur due to drug accumulation.

Instances of a syndrome resembling lupus erythematosus have been reported in connection with oral maintenance procainamide therapy. The mechanism of this syndrome is uncertain. Polyarthralgia, arthritis, and pleuritic pain are common symptoms; to a lesser extent fever, myalgia, skin lesions, pleural effusion and pericarditis may occur. Rare cases of thrombocytopenia or Coombs positive hemolytic anemia have been reported which may be related to this syndrome. Patients receiving procainamide for extended periods of time or in whom symptoms suggestive of a lupus-like reaction appear should have anti-nuclear antibody titers measured at regular intervals. The drug should be discontinued if there is a rising titer (anti-nuclear antibody) or clinical symptoms of LE appear. The LE syndrome may be reversible upon discontinuance of the drug. If discontinuation of the drug does not cause remission of the symptoms, steroid therapy may be effective. If the syndrome develops in a patient with recurrent life-threatening arrhythmias not controllable by other antiarrhythmic agents, steroid suppressive therapy may be used concomitantly with procainamide.

Adverse Reactions: Because procainamide is a peripheral vasodilator, intravenous administration may produce transient but at times severe lowering of blood pressure, particularly in conscious patients. Intramuscular injection is less likely to be accompanied by serious falls in blood pressure. Serious disturbances of cardiac rhythm such as ventricular asystole or fibrillation are also more common with intravenous administration. Precautionary measures to be followed during intravenous injection are given in the section on "DOSAGE AND ADMINISTRATION".

A syndrome resembling lupus erythematosus has been reported in patients on oral maintenance therapy (see PRECAUTIONS). Reactions consisting of fever and chills have also been reported, including a case with fever and chills plus nausea, vomiting, abdominal pain, acute hepatomegaly, and a rise in serum glutamic oxaloacetic transaminase following single doses of the drug. Bitter taste, diarrhea, weakness, mental depression, giddiness, and psychosis with hallucinations have been reported. The possibility of such untoward effects should be borne in mind.

Hypersensitivity reactions such as angioneurotic edema and maculopapular rash have also occurred.

Agranulocytosis has occasionally followed the repeated use of the drug, and deaths have occurred. Therefore, routine blood counts are advisable during maintenance procainamide therapy. The patients should be instructed to report any soreness of the mouth, throat, or gums, unexplained fever or any symptoms of upper respiratory tract infection. If any of these should occur, and leukocyte counts indicate cellular depression, procainamide therapy should be discontinued and appropriate treatment should be instituted immediately.

Dosage and Administration: Oral administration is preferred for treatment of arrhythmias which do not require immediate suppression, or to continue treatment after control of serious arrhythmias with Pronestyl Injection (Procainamide Hydrochloride Injection USP) or other antiarrhythmic therapy.

Intravenous therapy for the treatment of serious arrhythmias including those following myocardial infarction should be limited to use in hospitals where monitoring facilities are available.

Both the 100 mg./ml. and 500 mg./ml. concentrations of Pronestyl Injection (Procainamide Hydrochloride Injection USP) should be diluted prior to intravenous use to facilitate control of dosage rate.

Intramuscular dose: Intramuscular administration may be preferable to the oral route in patients with vomiting, in those who are to receive nothing *per os* before surgery, or in those in whom there is reason to believe absorption may be unreliable. A dose of 0.5 to 1 g. may be given intramuscularly, repeated every four to eight hours until oral therapy is possible.

Intravenous dose: CAUTION—Intravenous use of procainamide hydrochloride may be accompanied by a hypotensive response, sometimes marked, if the dose is excessive or administration too rapid. Therefore, to initiate therapy, the intravenous dose should be diluted in 5% Dextrose Injection USP prior to administration to facilitate control of dosage rate; the dose should be administered at a rate not greater than 25 to 50 mg. per minute by either direct intravenous administration or infusion. Slow administration allows for some initial tissue distribution.

Direct Intravenous Administration—To reduce the possibility of a hypotensive response, 100 mg. doses may be administered every five minutes by direct slow intravenous injection, at a rate not exceeding 50 mg. in any one minute, until the arrhythmia is suppressed or the maximum dosage of 1 g. has been administered. Blood pressure must be taken and the electrocardiogram read before each dose. Some effects may be seen after the first 100 or 200 mg., and it is unusual to require more than 500 to 600 mg. to achieve satisfactory antiarrhythmic effects.

To maintain therapeutic levels, an infusion may then be started at a rate of 2 to 6 mg. procainamide per minute (see Table entitled "DILUTIONS AND RATES FOR INTRAVENOUS INFUSIONS") depending on the patient's body weight, circulatory condition and renal function.

Intravenous Infusion—An alternative method of achieving and then maintaining a therapeutic plasma concentration is to infuse 500 to 600 mg. of procainamide at a constant rate over a period of 25 to 30 minutes and then changing to another infusion for maintenance at a rate of 2 to 6 mg./min. (see Table entitled "DILUTIONS AND RATES FOR INTRAVENOUS INFUSIONS").
[See table above].

Intravenous therapy should be terminated as soon as the patient's basic cardiac rhythm appears to be stabilized and, if indicated, the patient should be placed on oral antiarrhythmic maintenance therapy. A period of about three to four hours (one half-life) should elapse after the last intravenous dose of procainamide before administering the first oral dose of procainamide.

Intravenous administration should be monitored electrocardiographically. Excessive widening of the QRS complex or prolongation of the P-R interval suggests the occurrence of myocardial toxicity. Patients should be kept in a supine position and blood pressure should be measured almost continuously during administration. If the fall in blood pressure exceeds 15 mm Hg, administration should be temporarily discontinued. Phenylephrine Hydrochloride Injection USP or Levarterenol Bitartrate Injection USP should be available to counteract severe hypotensive responses.

DILUTIONS AND RATES FOR INTRAVENOUS INFUSIONS*
PRONESTYL INJECTION (Procainamide Hydrochloride Injection USP)

Approximate Final Concentration	Infusion Bottle Size (ml.)	ml. of Pronestyl (100 mg./ml.) to be added	ml. of Pronestyl (500 mg./ml.) to be added	Infusion Rate
0.2% (2 mg./ml.)	500	10	2	1–3 ml./min.
	250	5	1	
0.4% (4 mg./ml.)	500	20	4	0.5–1.5 ml./min.
	250	10	2	

* CAUTION: The flow rate of all intravenous infusion solutions must be closely monitored. These dilutions are calculated to deliver 2 to 6 mg. per minute at the infusion rates listed.

Surgical Use: For cardiac arrhythmias associated with anesthesia and surgery, the suggested parenteral dose is 0.1 to 0.5 g., preferably given intramuscularly.

How Supplied: Pronestyl Injection (Procainamide Hydrochloride Injection USP) is available as sterile, aqueous solutions in 10 ml. vials providing 100 mg. procainamide hydrochloride per ml. or 2 ml. vials providing 500 mg. procainamide hydrochloride per ml.

The solutions, which are colorless initially, may develop a slightly yellow color in time. This does not indicate a change which would prevent its use, but a solution any darker than light amber or discolored in any other way should not be used.

Pronestyl is also available for oral administration as Pronestyl Tablets (Procainamide Hydrochloride Tablets) and Pronestyl Capsules (Procainamide Hydrochloride Capsules USP) providing 250 mg., 375 mg., and 500 mg. procainamide hydrochloride (see package inserts accompanying the products for complete information).

Storage: Store Pronestyl Injection between 50° and 80° F.

PRONESTYL-SR® TABLETS ℞
[pro″nest′tl es-ahr]
(Procainamide Hydrochloride Tablets)

The prolonged administration of procainamide often leads to the development of a positive antinuclear antibody (ANA) test with or without symptoms of lupus erythematosus-like syndrome. If a positive ANA titer develops, the benefit/risk ratio related to continued procainamide therapy should be assessed. This may necessitate consideration of alternative antiarrhythmic therapy.

Description: Procainamide hydrochloride is the amide analogue of procaine hydrochloride. Chemically, procainamide hydrochloride is p-Amino-N-[2-(diethylamino)ethyl] benzamide monohydrochloride.

Pronestyl-SR Tablets (Procainamide Hydrochloride Tablets), containing 500 mg. procainamide hydrochloride, are for oral administration. The tablet matrix is specially designed for the prolonged release of the drug in the gastrointestinal tract.

Clinical Pharmacology: Procainamide depresses the excitability of cardiac muscle to electrical stimulation and slows conduction in the atrium, the bundle of His, and the ventricle. The refractory period of the atrium is considerably more prolonged than that of the ventricle. Contractility of the heart is usually not affected, nor is cardiac output decreased to any extent unless myocardial damage exists. In the absence of any arrhythmia, the heart rate may occasionally be accelerated by conventional doses, suggesting that the drug possesses anticholinergic properties. Larger doses can induce atrioventricular block and ventricular extrasystoles which may proceed to ventricular fibrillation. These effects on the myocardium are reflected in the electrocardiogram; a widening of the QRS complex occurs most consistently; less regularly, the P-R and Q-T intervals are prolonged, and the QRS and T waves show some decrease in voltage.

Following oral administration q6h, the tablets achieve a mean steady state of procainamide (as well as procainamide plus N-acetylprocainamide) serum concentrations approximately equivalent to those from a comparable dose of Pronestyl® Capsules (Procainamide Hydrochloride Capsules USP) q3h. Pronestyl-SR Tablets (Procainamide Hydrochloride Tablets) have a half-life which is significantly longer than that of the capsules.

The specially-formulated tablet coating and core of Pronestyl-SR (Procainamide Hydrochloride Tablets) was designed to provide the biopharmaceutic characteristics of a sustained and relatively constant rate of release and absorption throughout the entire small intestine.

Therapeutic plasma levels have been reported to be 3 to 10 mcg./ml., with those for the majority of patients in the range of 4 to 8 mcg./ml.

Procainamide is less readily hydrolyzed than procaine, and plasma levels decline slowly—about 10 to 20 percent per hour for standard dosage forms of procainamide. The drug is excreted primarily in the urine, with an average of about 60 percent being excreted unchanged; about 10 percent is excreted as free and conjugated p-aminobenzoic acid. The fate of the remainder is unknown.

Indications and Usage: Pronestyl-SR (Procainamide Hydrochloride Tablets) are indicated in the treatment of premature ventricular contractions and ventricular tachycardia, atrial fibrillation, and paroxysmal atrial tachycardia.

Contraindications: It has been suggested that procainamide be contraindicated in patients with myasthenia gravis. Hypersensitivity to the drug is an absolute contraindication; in this connection, cross sensitivity to procaine and related drugs must be borne in mind. Procainamide should not be administered to patients with complete atrioventricular heart block. Procainamide is also contraindicated in cases of second degree and third degree A-V block unless an electrical pacemaker is operative.

Precautions: During administration of the drug, evidence of untoward myocardial responses should be carefully watched for in all patients. In the presence of an abnormal myocardium, procainamide may at times produce untoward responses. In atrial fibrillation or flutter, the ventricular rate may increase suddenly as the atrial rate is slowed. Adequate digitalization reduces, but does not abolish this danger. If myocardial damage exists, ventricular tachysystole is particularly hazardous. Correction of atrial fibrillation, with resultant forceful contractions of the atrium, may cause a dislodgment of mural thrombi and produce an embolic episode. However, it has been suggested that in a patient who is already discharging emboli, procainamide is more likely to stop than to aggravate the process.

Continued on next page

Squibb—Cont.

Attempts to adjust the heart rate in a patient who has developed ventricular tachycardia during an occlusive coronary episode should be carried out with extreme caution. Caution is also required in marked disturbances of atrioventricular conduction such as second degree and third degree A-V block, bundle branch block, or severe digitalis intoxication, where the use of procainamide may result in additional depression of conduction and ventricular asystole or fibrillation.

Since patients with severe heart disease and ventricular tachycardia may also have complete heart block which is difficult to diagnose under these circumstances, this complication should always be kept in mind when treating ventricular arrhythmias with procainamide. If the ventricular rate is significantly slowed by procainamide without attainment of regular atrioventricular conduction, the drug should be stopped and the patient reevaluated as asystole may result under these circumstances.

In patients receiving normal dosage, but who have both liver and kidney disease, symptoms of overdosage (principally ventricular tachycardia and severe hypotension) may occur due to drug accumulation.

Instances of a syndrome resembling lupus erythematosus have been reported in connection with oral maintenance procainamide therapy. The mechanism of this syndrome is uncertain. Polyarthralgia, arthritis, and pleuritic pain are common symptoms; to a lesser extent fever, myalgia, skin lesions, pleural effusion and pericarditis may occur. Rare cases of thrombocytopenia or Coombs positive hemolytic anemia have been reported which may be related to this syndrome. Patients receiving procainamide for extended periods of time or in whom symptoms suggestive of lupuslike reaction appear should have anti-nuclear antibody titers measured at regular intervals. If there is a rising titer (anti-nuclear antibody) or clinical symptoms of LE appear, the drug should be discontinued. The LE syndrome may be reversible upon discontinuance of the drug. If discontinuation of the drug does not cause remission of the symptoms, steroid therapy may be effective. If the syndrome develops in a patient with recurrent life-threatening arrhythmias not controllable by other antiarrhythmic agents, steroid suppressive therapy may be used concomitantly with procainamide.

Adverse Reactions: Hypotension following oral administration is rare. Serious disturbances of cardiac rhythm such as ventricular asystole or fibrillation are more common with intravenous administration.

Large oral doses of procainamide may sometimes produce anorexia, nausea, urticaria, and/or pruritus.

A syndrome resembling lupus erythematosus has been reported in patients on oral maintenance therapy (see PRECAUTIONS). Reactions consisting of fever and chills have also been reported, including a case with fever and chills plus nausea, vomiting, abdominal pain, acute hepatomegaly, and a rise in serum glutamic oxaloacetic transaminase following single doses of the drug. Bitter taste, diarrhea, weakness, mental depression, giddiness, and psychosis with hallucinations have been reported. The possibility of such untoward effects should be borne in mind.

Hypersensitivity reactions such as angioneurotic edema and maculopapular rash have also occurred.

Agranulocytosis has occasionally followed the repeated use of the drug, and deaths have occurred. Therefore, routine blood counts are advisable during maintenance procainamide therapy. The patients should be instructed to report any soreness of the mouth, throat, or gums, unexplained fever or any symptoms of upper respiratory tract infection. If any of these should occur, and leukocyte counts indicate cellular depression, procainamide therapy should be discontinued and appropriate treatment should be instituted immediately.

Dosage and Administration:
Initial Therapy:
Pronestyl-SR Tablets (Procainamide Hydrochloride Tablets) are a sustained-release dosage form not intended for initial therapy. For initial therapy by oral administration, conventional oral formulations of Pronestyl (procainamide hydrochloride) are recommended (see HOW SUPPLIED). The duration of action of procainamide hydrochloride supplied in this sustained release dosage form allows dosing at intervals of every six hours, a schedule which may encourage patient compliance.

For control of arrhythmias requiring immediate suppression, Pronestyl Injection (Procainamide Hydrochloride Injection USP)—see HOW SUPPLIED) or other antiarrhythmic therapy is recommended; following interruption of the arrhythmia, or when the limit of tolerance is reached, Pronestyl-SR is indicated for maintenance.

Maintenance Therapy:
Dosage:
Ventricular Tachycardia and Premature Ventricular Contractions—The suggested maintenance dosage of Pronestyl-SR (Procainamide Hydrochloride Tablets) is 50 mg./kg. of body weight daily given in divided doses at six hour intervals.
To provide approximately 50 mg. per kg. per day: Give patients weighing less than 120 lbs. (less than 55 kg.) 500 mg. q6h; give patients between 120 and 200 lbs. (55 to 91 kg.) 500 mg. or 1 g. q6h; and give patients over 200 lbs. (more than 91 kg.) 1 g. q6h. This dosage schedule is for use as a guide for treating the average patient; however, each patient must be considered on an individual basis.

Atrial Fibrillation and Paroxysmal Atrial Tachycardia—The suggested maintenance dosage for Pronestyl-SR is 1 g. every six hours.

Administration:
Patients should be advised not to break or chew the tablet, as this would interfere with designed dissolution characteristics. The tablet matrix may be seen in the stool since it does not disintegrate following release of procainamide.

How Supplied: Pronestyl-SR Tablets (Procainamide Hydrochloride Tablets) are available as FILMLOK® tablets containing 500 mg. procainamide hydrochloride; these tablets are unscored, biconvex, greenish-yellow elongated ovals and are available in bottles of 100 and Unimatic® cartons of 100. (FILMLOK is a Squibb trademark for veneer-coated tablets.)

Also Available: For initial therapy, available oral dosage forms include Pronestyl Capsules (Procainamide Hydrochloride Capsules USP) and conventionally-formulated capsule-shaped FILMLOK Pronestyl Tablets (Procainamide Hydrochloride Tablets); tablets and capsules are available in potencies of 250 mg., 375 mg., and 500 mg. procainamide hydrochloride. Consult the common package insert provided with these formulations for complete information.

Pronestyl is also available for parenteral use as Pronestyl Injection (Procainamide Hydrochloride Injection USP) as sterile aqueous solutions in 10 ml. vials providing 100 mg. procainamide hydrochloride per ml. or 2 ml. vials providing 500 mg. procainamide hydrochloride per ml. Consult the package insert provided with this product for complete information.

Storage: Store Pronestyl-SR Tablets (Procainamide Hydrochloride Tablets) at room temperature; avoid excessive heat.

Shown in Product Identification Section, page 438

RAUDIXIN® ℞
[raw″dik′sin]
(Rauwolfia Serpentina Tablets USP)
Whole Root—Biologically Standardized

Description: Raudixin contains Powdered Rauwolfia Serpentina USP, a hypotensive agent prepared from the powdered whole root of *Rauwolfia serpentina* Benth. The powdered rauwolfia serpentina in Raudixin contains not less than 0.15 percent and not more than 0.2 percent of reserpine-rescinnamine group alkaloids, calculated as reserpine. This product contains FD&C Yellow No. 5 (tartrazine).

Clinical Pharmacology: Rauwolfia serpentina probably produces its antihypertensive effects through depletion of tissue stores of catecholamines (epinephrine and norepinephrine) from peripheral sites. By contrast, its sedative and tranquilizing properties are thought to be related to depletion of 5-hydroxytryptamine from the brain. Rauwolfia serpentina is characterized by slow onset of action and sustained effect. Both its cardiovascular and central nervous system effects may persist following withdrawal of the drug.

Indications and Usage: Raudixin (Rauwolfia Serpentina Tablets USP) is indicated in the treatment of mild essential hypertension. It is also useful as adjunctive therapy with other antihypertensive agents in the more severe forms of hypertension.

Raudixin is also indicated for the relief of symptoms in agitated psychotic states (e.g., schizophrenia), primarily in those individuals unable to tolerate phenothiazine derivatives or those who also require antihypertensive medication.

Contraindications: The preparation is contraindicated in patients who have previously demonstrated hypersensitivity to rauwolfia. In this regard, it should be remembered that a past history of bronchial asthma or allergy may increase the possibility of drug sensitivity reactions. It is also contraindicated in patients with mental depression (especially with suicidal tendencies), active peptic ulcer, ulcerative colitis, and in patients receiving electroconvulsive therapy.

Warnings: Extreme caution should be exercised in treating patients with a history of mental depression. Discontinue the drug at the first sign of despondency, early morning insomnia, loss of appetite, impotence, or self-deprecation. Drug-induced depression may persist for several months after drug withdrawal and may be severe enough to result in suicide.

Usage in Pregnancy: Usage of rauwolfia preparations in women of childbearing age requires that the potential benefits of the drug be weighed against its possible hazards to the fetus. The hazards of using rauwolfia preparations include increased respiratory secretions, nasal congestion, cyanosis and anorexia in infants born to rauwolfia alkaloid-treated mothers.

Nursing Mothers: Rauwolfia preparations cross the placental barrier and appear in cord blood and breast milk.

Precautions: Because rauwolfia preparations increase gastrointestinal motility and secretion, this drug should be used cautiously in patients with a history of peptic ulcer, ulcerative colitis, or gallstones where biliary colic may be precipitated. Patients on high dosage should be observed carefully at regular intervals to detect possible reactivation of peptic ulcer.

Caution should be exercised when treating hypertensive patients with renal insufficiency since they adjust poorly to lowered blood pressure levels.

Use rauwolfia serpentina cautiously with digitalis and quinidine since cardiac arrhythmias have occurred with rauwolfia preparations.

Preoperative withdrawal of rauwolfia serpentina does not insure that circulatory instability will not occur. It is important that the anesthesiologist be aware of the patient's drug intake and consider this in the overall management since hypotension has occurred in patients receiving rauwolfia preparations. Anticholinergic and/or adrenergic drugs (metaraminol, norepinephrine) have been employed to treat adverse vagocirculatory effects.

This product contains FD&C Yellow No. 5 (tartrazine) which may cause allergic-type reactions (including bronchial asthma) in certain susceptible individuals. Although the overall incidence of FD&C Yellow No. 5 (tartrazine) sensitivity in the general population is low, it is frequently seen in patients who also have aspirin hypersensitivity.

Animal tumorigenicity: rodent studies have shown that reserpine is an animal tumorigen, causing an increased incidence of mammary fibroadenomas in female mice, malignant tumors of the seminal vesicles in male mice, and malignant adrenal medullary tumors in male rats. These findings arose in two year studies in which the drug was administered in the feed at concentrations of 5 and 10 ppm—about 100 to 300 times the usual human dose. The breast neoplasms are thought to be related to reserpine's prolactin-elevating effect. Several other prolactin-elevating drugs have also been associated with an increased incidence of mammary neoplasia in rodents.

The extent to which these findings indicate a risk to humans is uncertain. Tissue culture experiments show that about one-third of human breast tumors are prolactin-dependent *in vitro*, a factor of considerable importance if the use of the drug is contemplated in a patient with previously detected breast cancer. The possibility of an increased risk of breast cancer in reserpine users has been studied extensively; however, no firm conclusion has emerged. Although a few epidemiologic studies have suggested a slightly increased risk (less than twofold in all studies except one) in women who have used reserpine, other studies of generally similar design have not confirmed this. Epidemiologic studies conducted using other drugs (neuroleptic agents) that, like reserpine, increase prolactin levels and therefore would be considered rodent mammary carcinogens, have not shown an association between chronic administration of the drug and human mammary tumorigenesis. While long-term clinical observation has not suggested such an association, the available evidence is considered too limited to be conclusive at this time. An association of reserpine intake with pheochromocytoma or tumors of the seminal vesicles has not been explored.

Adverse Reactions: *Gastrointestinal System*—hypersecretion, nausea, vomiting, anorexia, and diarrhea. *Central Nervous System*—drowsiness, depression, nervousness, paradoxical anxiety, nightmares, rare Parkinsonian syndrome, C.N.S. sensitization manifested by dull sensorium, deafness, glaucoma, uveitis, and optic atrophy. *Cardiovascular*—angina-like symptoms, arrhythmias, particularly when used concurrently with digitalis or quinidine, and bradycardia. *Other*—nasal congestion, pruritus, rash, dryness of mouth, dizziness, headache, dyspnea, purpura, impotence or decreased libido, dysuria, muscular aches, conjunctival injection, weight gain, and extrapyramidal tract symptoms.

These reactions are usually reversible and disappear when the drug is discontinued.

Water retention with edema in patients with hypertensive vascular disease may occur rarely, but the condition generally clears with cessation of therapy, or with the administration of a diuretic agent.

Dosage and Administration: For adults, the average oral dose is 200 to 400 mg. daily, given in divided doses in the morning and evening. Higher doses should be used cautiously because serious mental depression and other side effects may be considerably increased. (Orally, 200 to 300 mg. of powdered whole root is equivalent to 0.5 mg. of reserpine.) Maintenance doses may vary from 50 to 300 mg. per day given as a single dose or as two divided doses.

Concomitant use of rauwolfia serpentina and ganglionic blocking agents, guanethidine, veratrum, hydralazine, methyldopa, chlorthalidone, or thiazides necessitates careful titration of dosage with each agent.

Dosage for adolescents, children and the aged should be proportionately less than the usual adult dosage.

How Supplied: Raudixin (Rauwolfia Serpentina Tablets USP) is available for oral use as 50 and 100 mg. coated tablets, in bottles of 100 and 1000.

Storage: Store at room temperature; avoid excessive heat; keep bottle tightly closed.

Shown in Product Identification Section, page 438

RAUZIDE® ℞
[*raw'zīd*]
(Powdered Rauwolfia Serpentina [50 mg.] with Bendroflumethiazide [4 mg.])

Description: Rauzide is Powdered Rauwolfia Serpentina with Bendroflumethiazide. The Powdered Rauwolfia Serpentina in Rauzide contains not less than 0.15 percent and not more than 0.2 percent of reserpine-rescinnamine group alkaloids, calculated as reserpine. The preparation has been designed specifically to combine the antihypertensive effects of both rauwolfia and bendroflumethiazide for the treatment of hypertension, and may be useful in those patients not adequately benefited by either component alone. This product contains FD&C Yellow No. 5 (tartrazine).

Actions: The mechanism of action of bendroflumethiazide results in an interference with the renal tubular mechanism of electrolyte reabsorption. At maximal therapeutic dosage all thiazides are approximately equal in their diuretic potency. The mechanism whereby thiazides function in the control of hypertension is unknown.

Rauwolfia serpentina probably produces its antihypertensive effects through depletion of tissue stores of catecholamines (epinephrine and norepinephrine) from peripheral sites. By contrast, its sedative and tranquilizing properties are thought to be related to depletion of 5-hydroxytryptamine from the brain.

Rauwolfia serpentina is characterized by slow onset of action and sustained effect. Both its cardiovascular and central nervous system effects may persist following withdrawal of the drug.

Either of the components of Rauzide, when administered alone, may produce a reduction of blood pressure in hypertension. When the two agents are administered simultaneously, the action of the one appears to supplement that of the other so that a hypotensive effect may be produced which is greater than that produced by either agent alone. Thus, hypertension which does not adequately respond to either drug alone may frequently respond to the combination of both drugs.

Indications: Rauzide is indicated for hypertension (see box under WARNINGS).

Contraindications: The preparation is contraindicated in patients who have previously demonstrated hypersensitivity to thiazides or other sulfonamide-derived drugs, or rauwolfia. In this regard, it should be remembered that a past history of bronchial asthma or allergy may increase the possibility of drug sensitivity reactions.

Bendroflumethiazide is contraindicated in anuria. The routine use of diuretics in otherwise healthy pregnant women with or without mild edema is contraindicated and possibly hazardous.

Rauwolfia serpentina is contraindicated in patients with mental depression (especially with suicidal tendencies), active peptic ulcer, ulcerative colitis, and in patients receiving electroconvulsive therapy.

Warnings:

> This fixed combination drug is not indicated for initial therapy of hypertension. Hypertension requires therapy titrated to the individual patient. If the fixed combination represents the dosage so determined, its use may be more convenient in patient management. The treatment of hypertension is not static, but must be reevaluated as conditions in each patient warrant.

Bendroflumethiazide should be used with caution in severe renal disease. In patients with renal disease, thiazides may precipitate azotemia. Cumulative effects of the drug may develop in patients with impaired renal function.

Thiazides should be used with caution in patients with impaired hepatic function or progressive liver disease, since minor alterations of fluid and electrolyte balance may precipitate hepatic coma. Thiazides may be additive or may potentiate the action of other antihypertensive drugs. Potentiation occurs with ganglionic or peripheral adrenergic blocking drugs.

Sensitivity reactions may occur in patients with a history of allergy or bronchial asthma.

The possibility of exacerbation or activation of systemic lupus erythematosus has been reported. When using rauwolfia serpentina, extreme caution should be exercised in treating patients with a history of mental depression. Discontinue the drug at the first sign of despondency, early morning insomnia, loss of appetite, impotence, or self-deprecation. Drug-induced depression may persist for several months after drug withdrawal and may be severe enough to result in suicide.

Usage in Pregnancy—Usage of thiazides and rauwolfia preparations in women of childbearing age requires that the potential benefits of the drug be weighed against its possible hazards to the fetus. The hazards of using thiazides include fetal or neonatal jaundice, thrombocytopenia and possibly other adverse reactions which have occurred in the adult. The hazards of using rauwolfia preparations include increased respiratory secretions, nasal congestion, cyanosis and anorexia in infants born to rauwolfia alkaloid-treated mothers.

Nursing mothers—Thiazides and rauwolfia preparations cross the placental barrier and appear in cord blood and breast milk.

Precautions: This product contains FD&C Yellow No. 5 (tartrazine) which may cause allergic-type reactions (including bronchial asthma) in certain susceptible individuals. Although the overall incidence of FD&C Yellow No. 5 (tartrazine) sensitivity in the general population is low, it is frequently seen in patients who also have aspirin hypersensitivity.

Bendroflumethiazide—Periodic determination of serum electrolytes to detect possible electrolyte imbalance should be performed at appropriate intervals.

All patients receiving thiazide therapy should be observed for clinical signs of fluid or electrolyte imbalance; namely, hyponatremia, hypochloremic alkalosis, and hypokalemia. Serum and urine electrolyte determinations are particularly important when the patient is vomiting excessively or receiving parenteral fluids. Medication such as digitalis may also influence serum electrolytes. Warning signs, irrespective of cause, are: dryness of the mouth, thirst, weakness, lethargy, drowsiness, restlessness, muscle pains or cramps, muscular fatigue, hypotension, oliguria, tachycardia, and gastrointestinal disturbances such as nausea and vomiting.

Hypokalemia may develop with thiazides as with any other potent diuretic, especially with brisk diuresis, when severe cirrhosis is present, or during concomitant use of corticosteroids or ACTH. Interference with adequate oral electrolyte intake will also contribute to hypokalemia. Digitalis therapy may exaggerate metabolic effects of hypokalemia especially with reference to myocardial activity.

Any chloride deficit is generally mild and usually does not require specific treatment except under extraordinary circumstances (as in liver disease or renal disease). Dilutional hyponatremia may occur in edematous patients in hot weather; appropriate therapy is water restriction, rather than administration of salt except in rare instances when the hyponatremia is life threatening. In actual salt depletion appropriate replacement is the therapy of choice.

Hyperuricemia may occur or frank gout may be precipitated in certain patients receiving thiazide therapy.

Insulin requirements in diabetic patients may be increased, decreased, or unchanged. Latent diabetes mellitus may become manifest during thiazide administration.

Thiazide drugs may increase the responsiveness to tubocurarine.

The antihypertensive effects of the drug may be enhanced in the post-sympathectomy patient.

Continued on next page

Squibb—Cont.

Thiazides may decrease arterial responsiveness to norepinephrine. This diminution is not sufficient to preclude effectiveness of the pressor agent for therapeutic use. If emergency surgery is indicated, preanesthetic and anesthetic agents should be administered in reduced dosage.

If progressive renal impairment becomes evident, as indicated by a rising nonprotein nitrogen or blood urea nitrogen, a careful reappraisal of therapy is necessary with consideration given to withholding or discontinuing diuretic therapy.

Thiazides may decrease serum PBI levels without signs of thyroid disturbance.

Rauwolfia serpentina—Because rauwolfia preparations increase gastrointestinal motility and secretion, this drug should be used cautiously in patients with a history of peptic ulcer, ulcerative colitis, or gallstones where biliary colic may be precipitated. Patients on high dosage should be observed carefully at regular intervals to detect possible reactivation of peptic ulcer.

Caution should be exercised when treating hypertensive patients with renal insufficiency since they adjust poorly to lowered blood pressure levels.

Use Rauwolfia serpentina cautiously with digitalis and quinidine since cardiac arrhythmias have occurred with rauwolfia preparations.

Preoperative withdrawal of rauwolfia serpentina does not insure that circulatory instability will not occur. It is important that the anesthesiologist be aware of the patient's drug intake and consider this in the overall management since hypotension has occurred in patients receiving rauwolfia preparations. Anticholinergic and/or adrenergic drugs (metaraminol, norepinephrine) have been employed to treat adverse vagocirculatory effects.

Animal tumorigenicity: rodent studies have shown that reserpine is an animal tumorigen, causing an increased incidence of mammary fibroadenomas in female mice, malignant tumors of the seminal vesicles in male mice, and malignant adrenal medullary tumors in male rats. These findings arose in two year studies in which the drug was administered in the feed at concentrations of 5 and 10 ppm—about 100 to 300 times the usual human dose. The breast neoplasms are thought to be related to reserpine's prolactin-elevating effect. Several other prolactin-elevating drugs have also been associated with an increased incidence of mammary neoplasia in rodents.

The extent to which these findings indicate a risk to humans is uncertain. Tissue culture experiments show that about one-third of human breast tumors are prolactin-dependent *in vitro*, a factor of considerable importance if the use of the drug is contemplated in a patient with previously detected breast cancer. The possibility of an increased risk of breast cancer in reserpine users has been studied extensively; however, no firm conclusion has emerged. Although a few epidemiologic studies have suggested a slightly increased risk (less than twofold in all studies except one) in women who have used reserpine, other studies of generally similar design have not confirmd this. Epidemiologic studies conducted using other drugs (neuroleptic agents) that, like reserpine, increase prolactin levels and therefore would be considered rodent mammary carcinogens, have not shown an association between chronic administration of the drug and human mammary tumorigenesis. While long-term clinical observation has not suggested such an association, the available evidence is considered too limited to be conclusive at this time. An association of reserpine intake with pheochromocytoma or tumors of the seminal vesicles has not been explored.

Adverse Reactions: Bendroflumethiazide: *Gastrointestinal System*—anorexia, gastric irritation, nausea, vomiting, cramping, diarrhea, constipation, jaundice (intrahepatic cholestatic jaundice), and pancreatitis. *Central Nervous System*—dizziness, vertigo, paresthesias, headache, and xanthopsia. *Hematologic*—leukopenia, agranulocytosis, thrombocytopenia, and aplastic anemia. *Dermatologic-Hypersensitivity*—purpura, photosensitivity, rash, urticaria, and necrotizing angiitis (vasculitis, cutaneous vasculitis). *Cardiovascular*—Orthostatic hypotension may occur and may be aggravated by alcohol, barbiturates or narcotics. *Other*—hyperglycemia, glycosuria, occasional metabolic acidosis in diabetic patients, hyperuricemia, allergic glomerulonephritis, muscle spasm, weakness, and restlessness. Whenever adverse reactions are moderate or severe, thiazide dosage should be reduced or therapy withdrawn.

Rauwolfia serpentina: *Gastrointestinal System*—hypersecretion, nausea, vomiting, anorexia, and diarrhea. *Central Nervous System*—drowsiness, depression, nervousness, paradoxical anxiety, nightmares, rare Parkinsonian syndrome, C.N.S. sensitization manifested by dull sensorium, deafness, glaucoma, uveitis, and optic atrophy. *Cardiovascular*—angina-like symptoms, arrhythmias, particularly when used concurrently with digitalis or quinidine, and bradycardia. *Other*—nasal congestion, pruritus, rash, dryness of mouth, dizziness, headache, dyspnea, purpura, impotence or decreased libido, dysuria, muscular aches, conjunctival injection, weight gain, and extrapyramidal tract symptoms.

These reactions are usually reversible and disappear when the drug is discontinued.

Dosage and Administration: As determined by individual titration (see box under WARNINGS). Usual dosage may range from 1 to 4 tablets daily.

How Supplied: Rauzide is available as tablets providing 50 mg. powdered rauwolfia serpentina and 4 mg. bendroflumethiazide. Bottles of 100 and 1000.

Storage: Store at room temperature; avoid excessive heat; keep bottle tightly closed.

Shown in Product Identification Section, page 438

SUMYCIN® '250' TABLETS   ℞
[sū″mī′sin]
SUMYCIN® '500' TABLETS   ℞
(Tetracycline Hydrochloride Tablets USP)
SUMYCIN® '250' CAPSULES   ℞
SUMYCIN® '500' CAPSULES   ℞
(Tetracycline Hydrochloride Capsules USP)
SUMYCIN® SYRUP   ℞
(Tetracycline Oral Suspension USP)

Description: Sumycin '250' and Sumycin '500' Tablets (Tetracycline Hydrochloride Tablets USP) are available for oral administration as FILMLOK® tablets providing 250 mg. and 500 mg. tetracycline hydrochloride, respectively. (FILMLOK is a Squibb trademark for veneer-coated tablets.) Sumycin '250' and Sumycin '500' Capsules (Tetracycline Hydrochloride Capsules USP) contain 250 mg. and 500 mg. crystalline tetracycline hydrochloride, respectively.

Sumycin Syrup (Tetracycline Oral Suspension USP) is a suspension containing, in each 5 ml. teaspoonful, tetracycline equivalent to 125 mg. tetracycline hydrochloride.

Clinical Pharmacology: The tetracyclines are primarily bacteriostatic antibiotics and are thought to exert their antimicrobial effect by the inhibition of protein synthesis. Tetracyclines are active against a wide range of gram-negative and gram-positive organisms.

The drugs in the tetracycline class have closely similar antimicrobial spectra. Microorganisms that have become insensitive to one tetracycline invariably exhibit cross-resistance to other tetracyclines. In addition, gram-negative bacilli made tetracycline-resistant may also show cross-resistance to chloramphenicol. Microorganisms may be considered susceptible if the MIC (minimum inhibitory concentration) is not more than 4 mcg./ml. and intermediate if the MIC is 4 to 12.5 mcg./ml. Susceptibility plate testing: A tetracycline disc may be used to determine microbial susceptibility to drugs in the tetracycline class. If the Kirby-Bauer method of disc sensitivity is used, a 30 mcg. tetracycline disc should give a zone of at least 19 mm. when tested against a tetracycline-susceptible bacterial strain.

Tetracyclines are readily absorbed and are bound to plasma proteins in varying degree. They are concentrated by the liver in the bile and excreted in the urine and feces at high concentrations and in a biologically active form.

Indications and Usage: Tetracycline is indicated in infections caused by the following microorganisms.

Rickettsiae: Rocky mountain spotted fever, typhus fever and the typhus group, Q fever, rickettsialpox, tick fevers, *Mycoplasma pneumoniae* (PPLO, Eaton agent), agents of psittacosis and ornithosis, agents of *Lymphogranuloma venereum* and *Granuloma inguinale*, and the spirochetal agent of relapsing fever *(B. recurrentis)*.

The following gram-negative organisms: *H. ducreyi* (chancroid), *Pasteurella pestis* and *Past. tularensis*, *Bartonella bacilliformis*, Bacteroides, *Vibrio comma* and *V. fetus*, and Brucella organisms (in conjunction with streptomycin).

Because many strains of the following groups of microorganisms have been shown to be resistant to tetracyclines, culture and susceptibility testing are recommended.

The following gram-negative organisms, when bacteriologic testing indicates appropriate susceptibility to the drug: *E. coli*, *Enterobacter aerogenes* (formerly *A. aerogenes*), Shigella, *Mima*, *Herellea*, *H. influenzae* (respiratory infections), and Klebsiella infections (respiratory and urinary).

The following gram-positive organisms when bacteriologic testing indicates appropriate susceptibility to the drug:

1) Streptococcus species: Up to 44 percent of strains of *Streptococcus pyogenes* and 74 percent of *Streptococcus faecalis* have been found to be resistant to tetracycline drugs. Therefore, tetracyclines should not be used for streptococcal disease unless the organism has been demonstrated to be sensitive.

(For upper respiratory infections due to group A beta-hemolytic streptococci, penicillin is the usual drug of choice including prophylaxis of rheumatic fever.)

2) *D. pneumoniae*.

3) *Staphylococcus aureus* (skin and soft tissue infections). Tetracyclines are not the drugs of choice in the treatment of any type of staphylococcal infections.

When penicillin is contraindicated, tetracyclines are alternative drugs in the treatment of infections due to: *N. gonorrhoeae*, *T. pallidum* and *T. pertenue* (syphilis and yaws), *Listeria monocytogenes*, Clostridia, *B. anthracis*, *Fusobacterium fusiforme* (Vincent's infection), and *Actinomyces*.

Tetracycline hydrochloride is indicated for the treatment of uncomplicated urethral, endocervical, or rectal infections in adults caused by *Chlamydia trachomalis*.[1]

In acute intestinal amebiasis, the tetracyclines may be a useful adjunct to amebicides.

In severe acne the tetracyclines may be useful adjunctive therapy.

Tetracyclines are indicated in the treatment of trachoma, although the infectious agent is not always eliminated, as judged by immunofluorescence.

Inclusion conjunctivitis may be treated with oral tetracyclines or with a combination of oral and topical agents.

Contraindications: This drug is contraindicated in persons who have shown hypersensitivity to any of the tetracyclines.

Warnings: THE USE OF DRUGS OF THE TETRACYCLINE CLASS DURING TOOTH DEVELOPMENT (LAST HALF OF PREGNANCY, INFANCY AND CHILDHOOD TO AGE OF EIGHT YEARS) MAY CAUSE PERMANENT DISCOLORATION OF THE TEETH (YELLOW-GRAY-BROWN). This reaction is more common during long-term use of the drugs but has been observed following repeated short-term courses. Enamel hypoplasia has also been reported. TETRACYCLINE DRUGS, THEREFORE, SHOULD NOT BE USED IN THIS AGE GROUP UNLESS OTHER DRUGS ARE NOT LIKELY TO BE EFFECTIVE OR ARE CONTRAINDICATED.

If renal impairment exists, even usual oral or parenteral doses may lead to excessive systemic accumulation of the drug and possible liver toxicity. Under such conditions, lower than usual doses are indicated and, if therapy is prolonged, serum level determinations of the drug may be advisable. The antianabolic action of tetracycline may cause an increase in BUN. While this is not a problem in those with normal renal function, in patients with significantly impaired function, higher serum levels of tetracycline may lead to azotemia, hyperphosphatemia, and acidosis.

Photosensitivity, manifested by an exaggerated sunburn reaction, has been observed in some individuals taking tetracyclines. Patients apt to be exposed to direct sunlight or ultra-violet light should be advised that this reaction can occur with tetracycline drugs, and treatment should be discontinued at the first evidence of skin erythema. NOTE: Photosensitization reactions have occurred most frequently with demeclocycline, less with chlortetracycline, and very rarely with oxytetracycline and tetracycline.

Usage in Pregnancy: (See WARNINGS about use during tooth development.)

Results of animal studies indicate that tetracyclines cross the placenta, are found in fetal tissues and can have toxic effects on the developing fetus (often related to retardation of skeletal development). Evidence of embryotoxicity has also been noted in animals treated early in pregnancy.

Usage in Newborns, Infants, and Children: (See WARNINGS about use during tooth development.)

Tetracyclines form a stable calcium complex in any bone-forming tissue. A decrease in the fibula growth rate has been observed in prematures given oral tetracycline in doses of 25 mg./kg. every six hours. This reaction was shown to be reversible when the drug was discontinued.

Tetracyclines are present in the milk of lactating women who are taking a drug in this class.

Precautions: As with other antibiotics, use of this drug may result in overgrowth of nonsusceptible organisms, including fungi. If superinfection occurs, the antibiotic should be discontinued and appropriate therapy instituted. Note: Superinfection of the bowel by staphylococci may be life-threatening.

In venereal diseases when coexistent syphilis is suspected, patients should have darkfield examinations before treatment is started and the blood serology should be repeated monthly for at least four months.

Because the tetracyclines have been shown to depress plasma prothrombin activity, patients who are on anticoagulant therapy may require downward adjustment of their anticoagulant dosage.

During long-term therapy, periodic laboratory evaluation of organ systems, including hematopoietic, renal and hepatic studies should be performed.

All infections due to group A beta-hemolytic streptococci should be treated for at least 10 days.

Since bacteriostatic drugs may interfere with the bactericidal action of penicillin, it is advisable to avoid giving tetracycline in conjunction with penicillin.

Since sensitivity reactions are more likely to occur in persons with a history of allergy, asthma, hay fever, or urticaria, the preparation should be used with caution in such individuals.

Adverse Reactions: Gastrointestinal: anorexia, epigastric distress, nausea, vomiting, diarrhea, bulky loose stools, stomatitis, sore throat, glossitis, black hairy tongue, dysphagia, hoarseness, enterocolitis, and inflammatory lesions (with candidal overgrowth) in the anogenital region, including proctitis and pruritus ani. These reactions have been caused by both the oral and parenteral administration of tetracyclines but are less frequent after parenteral use.

Skin: maculopapular and erythematous rashes. Exfoliative dermatitis has been reported but is uncommon. Onycholysis and discoloration of the nails have been reported rarely. Photosensitivity has occurred (see WARNINGS).

Renal toxicity: rise in BUN has been reported and is apparently dose-related (see WARNINGS).

Hepatic cholestasis has been reported rarely, and is usually associated with high dosage levels of tetracycline.

Hypersensitivity reactions: urticaria, angioneurotic edema, anaphylaxis, anaphylactoid purpura, pericarditis, exacerbation of systemic lupus erythematosus, and serum sickness-like reactions, as fever, rash, and arthralgia.

When given over prolonged periods, tetracyclines have been reported to produce brown-black microscopic discoloration of thyroid glands. No abnormalities of thyroid function studies are known to occur.

Bulging fontanels have been reported in young infants following full therapeutic dosage. This sign disappeared rapidly when the drug was discontinued.

Blood: anemia, hemolytic anemia, thrombocytopenia, thrombocytopenic purpura, neutropenia and eosinophilia have been reported.

Dizziness and headache have been reported.

Dosage and Administration: Adults: Usual daily dose is 1 to 2 g.; for mild to moderate infections: 500 mg. b.i.d. or 250 mg. q.i.d.; higher dosages such as 500 mg. q.i.d. may be required for severe infections.

For children above eight years of age: Usual daily dose is 10 to 20 mg./lb. (25 to 50 mg./kg.) body weight divided in four equal doses.

Representative pediatric dosages for the syrup on a q.i.d. basis are as follows: 20 lbs.—½ teaspoonful; 40 lbs.—1 teaspoonful; 60 lbs.—1½ teaspoonfuls; and 80 lbs.—2 teaspoonfuls.

Therapy should be continued for at least 24 to 48 hours after symptoms and fever have subsided.

The treatment of brucellosis, 500 mg. tetracycline four times daily for three weeks should be accompanied by streptomycin, 1 g. intramuscularly twice daily the first week and once daily the second week.

For treatment of gonorrhea, the recommended dose is 1.5 g. initially, then 0.5 g. every six hours until a total of 9 g. have been given.

For treatment of syphilis, a total of 30 to 40 g. in equally divided doses over a period of 10 to 15 days should be given. Close followup, including laboratory tests, is recommended.

Uncomplicated urethral, endocervical, or rectal infection in adults caused by *Chlamydia trachomatis*: 500 mg., by mouth, four times a day for at least seven days.[1]

In cases of severe acne which, in the judgment of the clinician, require long-term treatment, the recommended initial dosage is 1 g. daily in divided doses. When improvement is noted, usually within one week, dosage should be gradually reduced to maintenance levels ranging from 125 mg. to 500 mg. daily. In some patients it may be possible to maintain adequate remission of lesions with alternate-day or intermittent therapy. Tetracycline therapy of acne should augment the other standard measures known to be of value.

In patients with renal impairment (see WARNINGS) total dosage should be decreased by reduction of recommended individual doses and/or by extending time intervals between doses.

In the treatment of streptococcal infections, a therapeutic dose of tetracycline should be administered for at least 10 days.

Concomitant therapy: Antacids containing aluminum, calcium, or magnesium impair absorption and should not be given to patients taking oral tetracycline.

Foods and some dairy products also interfere with absorption. Oral forms of tetracycline should be given one hour before or two hours after meals. Pediatric oral dosage forms should not be given with milk formulas and should be given at least one hour prior to feeding.

How Supplied: *Sumycin '250' Tablets (Tetracycline Hydrochloride Tablets USP) are available for oral administration as tablets containing 250 mg. tetracycline hydrochloride in bottles of 100 and 1000. *Sumycin '500' Tablets are available for oral administration as tablets containing 500 mg. tetracycline hydrochloride in bottles of 100 and 500. *Sumycin '250' Capsules (Tetracycline Hydrochloride Capsules USP) are available for oral administration as capsules containing 250 mg. tetracycline hydrochloride in bottles of 100 and 1000 and in Unimatic® Unit-Dose Packs of 100. *Sumycin '500' Capsules are available for oral administration as capsules containing 500 mg. tetracycline hydrochloride in bottles of 100 and 500 and in Unimatic Unit-Dose Packs of 100.

Sumycin Syrup (Tetracycline Oral Suspension USP) is available as a fruit-flavored suspension containing, in each 5 ml. teaspoonful, tetracycline equivalent to 125 mg. tetracycline hydrochloride buffered with potassium metaphosphate in bottles of 60 ml. and 473 ml. (1 pint).

Storage: Store the tablets and capsules at room temperature; avoid excessive heat. Store the syrup below 30° C (86° F); avoid freezing; protect from light; keep bottle tightly closed.

Reference: 1. CDC Sexually Transmitted Diseases Guidelines 1982.

*Shown in Product Identification Section, page 438

TESLAC® TABLETS ℞
[*tez'lak*]
(Testolactone Tablets USP)

Description: Teslac (Testolactone) contains testolactone, which is chemically designated as D-Homo-17a-oxaandrosta-1, 4-diene-3, 17-dione (1-dehydrotestololactone, or Δ^1-testololactone).

Testolactone is a white, odorless, crystalline solid, soluble in ethanol and slightly soluble in water.

Teslac Tablets are available for oral administration as tablets containing 50 mg. testolactone.

Clinical Pharmacology: The precise mechanism by which testolactone produces its clinical antineoplastic effects is unknown at present.

Although the chemical configuration of testolactone is similar to that of certain androgenic hormones, it is devoid of androgenic activity in the doses commonly employed.

Teslac was found to be effective in approximately 15% of patients with advanced or disseminated mammary cancer evaluated according to the following criteria: 1) those with a measurable decrease in size of all demonstrable tumor masses; 2) those in whom more than 50% of non-osseous lesions decreased in size although all bone lesions remained static; and 3) those in whom more than 50% of total lesions improved while the remainder were static.

Indications and Usage: Teslac Tablets (Testolactone Tablets USP) are recommended as adjunctive therapy in the palliative treatment of advanced or disseminated breast cancer in postmenopausal women when hormonal therapy is indicated. It may also be used in women who were diagnosed as having had disseminated breast carcinoma when premenopausal, in whom ovarian function has been subsequently terminated.

Contraindications: Testolactone is contraindicated in the treatment of breast cancer in men.

Warnings: Usage in Pregnancy: Since safe use of testolactone has not been established with respect to adverse effects upon fetal development, and since this preparation is intended for use only in postmenopausal women, testolactone should not be used during pregnancy.

Precautions: Plasma calcium levels should be routinely determined in any patient receiving therapy for mammary cancer, particularly during periods of active remission of bony metastases. If hypercalcemia occurs, appropriate measures should be instituted.

Adverse Reactions: Certain signs and symptoms have been reported in association with the use of this drug but, in these instances, it is often impossible to determine the relationship of the underlying disease and drug administration to the reported reaction. Such reactions include maculopapular erythema, increase in blood pressure, paresthesia, aches and edema of the extremities, glossitis, anorexia, and nausea and vomiting. Alopecia alone and with associated nail growth distur-

Continued on next page

Squibb—Cont.

bance have been reported rarely; these side effects subsided without interruption of treatment.

Dosage and Administration: The recommended oral dose is 250 mg. q.i.d.

In order to evaluate the response, therapy with testolactone should be continued for a minimum of three months unless there is active progression of the disease.

How Supplied: Teslac Tablets are available for oral administration as tablets containing 50 mg. testolactone in bottles of 100.

Storage: Store Teslac Tablets (Testolactone Tablets USP) at room temperature; avoid excessive heat. Keep bottle tightly closed.

THERAGRAN HEMATINIC® R
[ther'ah-gran" hē mah-tin'ik]
(Therapeutic Formula Vitamin Tablets with Hematinics)

Description: Theragran Hematinic is a therapeutic iron-containing multivitamin with minerals tablet for oral administration. The tablets contain FD&C Yellow No. 5 (tartrazine).

Graphic formulas and physical/chemical information for the vitamins may be found in the US Pharmacopeia XX. Theragran Hematinic Tablets supply:

Vitamin A Acetate ....(8,333 IU)	2.5 mg
Vitamin D (Ergocalciferol) .....(133 IU)	3.3 mg
Thiamine Mononitrate	3.3 mg
Riboflavin	3.3 mg
Pyridoxine Hydrochloride	3.3 mg
Niacinamide	33.3 mg
Calcium Pantothenate	11.7 mg
Vitamin E (dl-α-Tocopheryl Acetate) ......(5 IU)	5 mg
Copper (as Sulfate)	0.67 mg
Magnesium (as Carbonate)	41.7 mg
Iron, elemental (as Ferrous Fumarate)	66.7 mg
Vitamin B_{12} (as Cyanocobalamin)	50 mcg
Folic Acid	0.33 mg
Vitamin C (as Sodium Ascorbate)	100 mg

Clinical Pharmacology: Vitamins and dietary minerals are fundamentally involved in vital metabolic processes, where they usually serve as oxidizing and reducing agents and as factors in various enzyme systems. These essential micronutrients are so closely interrelated that the lack of any one may affect the body requirements of others.

Metabolic Functions of Inorganic Ions—*Iron* plays an important role in oxygen and electron transport. Iron may be functional (in hemoglobin, myoglobin, heme enzymes, and cofactor and transport iron) or stored as ferritin and hemosiderin in the liver, spleen, bone marrow, and reticuloendothelial system. The hemoglobin (0.34 percent iron) content of blood is about 14 to 17 g. per 100 ml. in adult males; in adult females it ranges between 12 and 14 g. Following ingestion, ferrous iron forms low molecular chelates with amino acids, ascorbic acid, and sugars which may be solubilized and absorbed before they reach the distal small intestine. Iron is probably absorbed passively into the mucosal layer of the small intestine, then transferred actively to transferrin where it is incorporated into red blood cells in bone marrow or into all body cells. Transferrin iron may also be stored in bone marrow, liver and spleen. Iron is removed from the body in the urine, bile, sweat, feces, and via desquamation of cells.

Copper: an essential enzyme cofactor in the utilization of iron in hemoglobin synthesis.

Magnesium: an enzyme activator—certain peptidases and phosphatases require magnesium for maximal activity as do virtually all reactions involving adenosine triphosphate.

Metabolic Functions of the Vitamins— *Fat Soluble Vitamins*—These tend to be stored in the body; their precise mode of action is largely unknown.

Vitamin A: essential to the production and regeneration of the visual purple of the retina; maintenance of the integrity of epithelial tissue; lysosome stability.

Vitamin D: functions in bone metabolism by regulating the intestinal absorption of calcium and phosphorus.

Vitamin E: intracellular antioxidant, important to the stability of biologic membranes.

Water Soluble Vitamins—except for vitamin B_{12}, these micronutrients are not stored in the body.

B Complex Vitamins (thiamine, riboflavin, pyridoxine, niacinamide, pantothenic acid, vitamin B_{12}, folic acid): these function, either alone or as structural components of more complex molecules, in catalytic systems where they usually function as coenzymes in carbohydrate, protein, or amino acid metabolism, synthesis of DNA and other molecules, maturation of RBCs, nerve cell function, or oxidation-reduction reactions.

Vitamin C: a coenzyme, essential to osteoid tissue; collagen formation; vascular function; tissue respiration and wound healing; facilitates absorption of iron.

Indications and Usage: Theragran Hematinic Tablets are indicated in the treatment of many of the common iron-deficiency anemias, particularly those associated with nutritional deficiency states or when nutritional requirements are high, and tropical and nontropical sprue. These iron-deficiency states include anemias associated with dietary inadequacy, convalescence, those frequently encountered in late childhood, early adolescence and old age, menorrhagia, and the anemias of women from menarche to menopause including macrocytic or microcytic anemia of pregnancy. Iron deficiency may result in fatigue, palpitation, smooth and sore tongue, angular stomatitis, dysphagia, gastritis, enteropathy, and koilonychia, as well as anemia. In young children, depressed growth and impaired mental performance occur.

Contraindications: Hemochromatosis and hemosiderosis are contraindications to iron therapy.

Warnings: Folic acid alone is improper therapy in the treatment of pernicious anemia and other megaloblastic anemias where vitamin B_{12} is deficient.

Precautions:

General—The use of niacin-containing preparations in patients with gastritis, peptic ulcer, or asthma should be undertaken carefully.

Since iron-deficiency anemia may be a manifestation of a basic systemic disturbance such as recurrent blood loss, the underlying cause of the anemia should be determined and corrected if possible.

The ingredients in Theragran Hematinic are not sufficient nor are they intended for the treatment of pernicious anemia. Folic acid in doses above 0.1 mg. daily may obscure pernicious anemia in that hematologic remission can occur while neurological manifestations remain progressive; therefore, the possibility of pernicious anemia should be excluded before treatment with this preparation. Parenteral use of vitamin B_{12} is recommended to assure essential medical supervision of the patient (see WARNINGS).

This product contains FD&C Yellow No. 5 (tartrazine) which may cause allergic-type reactions (including bronchial asthma) in certain susceptible individuals. Although the overall incidence of FD&C Yellow No. 5 (tartrazine) sensitivity in the general population is low, it is frequently seen in patients who also have aspirin hypersensitivity.

Information for the Patient—Keep Theragran Hematinic and all other medication out of the reach of children.

Patients should be informed of symptoms of intolerance to components of this preparation; if any of these symptoms appear the patient should be advised to discontinue dosing, and to notify the physician.

Recommended dosage should not be exceeded unless directed by the physician.

Laboratory Tests—Periodic hematologic studies should be performed.

Drug Interactions—Since oral iron products interfere with absorption of oral tetracyclines, these products should not be taken within two hours of each other.

Mineral oil and bile-acid sequestrants such as cholestyramine and colestipol hydrochloride in long-term therapy have been shown to decrease the absorption of fat-soluble vitamins.

Pyridoxine hydrochloride may act as an antagonist to levodopa.

Hydralazine hydrochloride, penicillamine, isoniazid, and cycloserine may antagonize pyridoxine hydrochloride.

Phenytoin, methotrexate, and pyrimethamine may interfere with folic acid absorption.

Colestipol hydrochloride may decrease the bioavailability of niacin.

Vitamin C may decrease the hypoprothrombinemic effect of oral anticoagulants; prothrombin levels should be monitored.

Neomycin and colchicine may impair cyanocobalamin absorption.

Carcinogenesis, Mutagenesis, Impairment of Fertility—Long-term studies in animals have not been performed.

Pregnancy Category C—Animal reproduction studies have not been conducted with therapeutic formula vitamin tablets with hematinics. Controlled clinical studies have not been performed to determine if therapeutic formula vitamin tablets with hematinics can cause fetal harm when administered to a pregnant woman or can affect reproduction capacity. Theragran Hematinic should be given to a pregnant woman only if clearly needed.

Nursing Mothers—It is not known whether components of this product are excreted in human milk. Because many substances are excreted in human milk, caution should be exercised when Theragran Hematinic is administered to a nursing woman.

Pediatric Use—Safety and effectiveness in children have not been established.

Adverse Reactions: Allergic reactions, skin rashes, and gastrointestinal disturbances, such as nausea, vomiting, diarrhea, or constipation may occur.

A generalized flushing and a feeling of warmth has been reported following niacinamide therapy. Allergic sensitization has been reported following both oral and parenteral administration of folic acid.

Dosage and Administration: The usual adult dose is one Theragran Hematinic Tablet three times daily. When prescribed in late childhood and early adolescence, dosage reduction according to the size and weight of the child should be considered by the physician. Dosage may be adjusted according to the response of the patient. Since ferrous fumarate is not likely to cause gastric upsets, dosage need not be given at mealtime.

How Supplied: Theragran Hematinic is supplied in bottles of 90 tablets.

Storage: Store at room temperature; avoid excessive heat.

Shown in Product Identification Section, page 438

THERAGRAN® LIQUID
[ther'ah-gran"]
(High Potency Vitamin Supplement)

Each 5 ml. teaspoonful contains:

		Percent US RDA*
Vitamin A	10,000 IU	200
Vitamin D	400 IU	100
Vitamin C	200 mg	333
Thiamine	10 mg	667
Riboflavin	10 mg	588
Niacin	100 mg	500
Vitamin B_6	4.1 mg	205
Vitamin B_{12}	5 mcg	83
Pantothenic Acid	21.4 mg	214

*US Recommended Daily Allowance

Usage: For 12 year olds and older—1 teaspoonful daily.

How Supplied: In bottles of 4 fl. oz.

Storage: Store at room temperature; avoid excessive heat.

ADVANCED FORMULA THERAGRAN® TABLETS
[ther'ah-gran"]
(High Potency Multivitamin Formula)

Each tablet contains:

		Percent US RDA*
Vitamin A (as Palmitate)	5,500 IU	110
Vitamin C (Ascorbic Acid)	120 mg	200
Vitamin B_1 (as Thiamine Mononitrate)	3 mg	200
Vitamin B_2 (Riboflavin)	3.4 mg	200
Niacin (as Niacinamide)	30 mg	150
Vitamin B_6 (as Pyridoxine Hydrochloride)	3 mg	150
Vitamin B_{12} (Cyanocobalamin)	9 mcg	150
Vitamin D (Ergocalciferol)	400 IU	100
Vitamin E (dl-α-Tocopheryl Acetate)	30 IU	100
Pantothenic Acid (as Calcium Pantothenate)	10 mg	100
Folic Acid	0.4 mg	100
Biotin	15 mcg	5

*US Recommended Daily Allowance
Usage: For 12 year olds and older—1 tablet daily.
How Supplied: Bottles of 1000; Packs of 30, 100, and 180; and Unimatic® cartons of 100.
Storage: Store at room temperature; avoid excessive heat.
Shown in Product Identification Section, page 438

ADVANCED FORMULA THERAGRAN-M® TABLETS
[ther'ah-gran"em]
(High Potency Multivitamin Formula with Minerals)

Each tablet contains:

VITAMINS		Percent US RDA*
Vitamin A (as Palmitate)	5,500 IU	110
Vitamin C (Ascorbic Acid)	120 mg	200
Vitamin B_1 (as Thiamine Mononitrate)	3 mg	200
Vitamin B_2 (Riboflavin)	3.4 mg	200
Niacin (as Niacinamide)	30 mg	150
Vitamin B_6 (as Pyridoxine Hydrochloride)	3 mg	150
Vitamin B_{12} (Cyanocobalamin)	9 mcg	150
Vitamin D (Ergocalciferol)	400 IU	100
Vitamin E (dl-α-Tocopheryl Acetate)	30 IU	100
Pantothenic Acid (as Calcium Pantothenate)	10 mg	100
Folic Acid	0.4 mg	100
Biotin	15 mcg	5
MINERALS		
Iodine (as Potassium Iodide)	150 mcg	100
Iron (as Ferrous Fumarate)	27 mg	150
Magnesium (as Magnesium Oxide)	100 mg	25
Copper (as Cupric Sulfate)	2 mg	100
Zinc (as Zinc Sulfate)	15 mg	100
Manganese (as Manganese Sulfate)	5 mg	**
Chromium (from Processed Yeast)	15 mcg	**
Selenium (from Processed Yeast)	10 mcg	**
Molybdenum (from Processed Yeast)	15 mcg	**
ELECTROLYTES		
Potassium (as Potassium Salts)	7.5 mg	**
Chloride (as Potassium Chloride)	7.5 mg	**

*US Recommended Daily Allowance
**US RDA not established
Usage: For 12 year olds and older—1 tablet daily.
How Supplied: Bottles of 1000; Packs of 30, 60, 100, and 180; and Unimatic® cartons of 100.
Storage: Store at room temperture; avoid excessive heat.
Shown in Product Identification Section, page 438

THERAGRAN® STRESS FORMULA
(High Potency Multivitamin Formula with Iron and Biotin)

Each FILMLOK® tablet contains:		Percent US RDA*
Vitamin E (dl-α-Tocopheryl Acetate)	30 IU	100
Vitamin C (Ascorbic Acid)	600 mg	1000
B VITAMINS		
Folic Acid	400 mcg	100
Vitamin B_1 (as Thiamine Mononitrate)	15 mg	1000
Vitamin B_2 (Riboflavin)	15 mg	882
Niacin (as Niacinamide)	100 mg	500
Vitamin B_6 (as Pyridoxine Hydrochloride)	25 mg	1250
Vitamin B_{12} (Cyanocobalamin)	12 mcg	200
Biotin	45 mcg	15
Pantothenic Acid (as Calcium Pantothenate)	20 mg	200
Iron (as Ferrous Fumarate)	27 mg	150

*US Recommended Daily Allowance for Adults
Usage: For adults—1 tablet daily or as directed by physician.
How Supplied: Bottles of 75.
Storage: Store at room temperature; avoid excessive heat.
FILMOK is a Squibb trademark for veneer-coated tablets.
Shown in Product Identification Section, page 438

TRIMOX® '250' CAPSULES ℞
[tri'mokz]
TRIMOX® '500' CAPSULES ℞
(Amoxicillin Capsules USP)
TRIMOX® '125' FOR ORAL SUSPENSION ℞
TRIMOX® '250' FOR ORAL SUSPENSION ℞
(Amoxicillin for Oral Suspension USP)

Description: Trimox (amoxicillin) is a semisynthetic antibiotic, an analog of ampicillin, with a broad spectrum of bactericidal activity against many gram-positive and gram-negative microorganisms. Chemically it is D-(-)-alpha-amino-p-hydroxybenzyl penicillin trihydrate.

Clinical Pharmacology: Amoxicillin is stable in the presence of gastric acid and may be given without regard to meals. It is rapidly absorbed after oral administration. It diffuses readily into most body tissues and fluids, with the exception of brain and spinal fluid, except when meninges are inflamed. The half-life of amoxicillin is 61.3 minutes. Most of the amoxicillin is excreted unchanged in the urine; its excretion can be delayed by concurrent administration of probenecid. Amoxicillin is not highly protein-bound. In blood serum, amoxicillin is approximately 20 percent protein-bound as compared to 60 percent for penicillin G.

Orally administered doses of 250 mg. and 500 mg. amoxicillin capsules result in average peak blood levels one to two hours after administration in the range of 3.5 mcg./ml. to 5.0 mcg./ml. and 5.5 mcg./ml. to 7.5 mcg./ml., respectively.

Orally administered doses of amoxicillin suspension 125 mg./5 ml. and 250 mg./5 ml. result in average peak blood levels one to two hours after administration in the range of 1.5 mcg./ml. to 3.0 mcg./ml. and 3.5 mcg./ml. to 5.0 mcg./ml., respectively.

Detectable serum levels are observed up to 8 hours after an orally administered dose of amoxicillin. Following a 1 g. dose and utilizing a special skin window technique to determine levels of the antibiotic, it was noted that therapeutic levels were found in the interstitial fluid. Approximately 60 percent of an orally administered dose of amoxicillin is excreted in the urine within six to eight hours.

Microbiology: Trimox (amoxicillin) is similar to ampicillin in its bactericidal action against susceptible organisms during the stage of active multiplication. It acts through the inhibition of biosynthesis of cell wall mucopeptides. *In vitro* studies have demonstrated the susceptibility of most strains of the following gram-positive bacteria: alpha- and beta-hemolytic streptococci, *Streptococcus pneumoniae* (formerly *Diplococcus pneumoniae*), nonpenicillinase-producing staphylococci, and *Streptococcus faecalis*. It is active *in vitro* against many strains of *Hemophilus influenzae*, *Neisseria gonorrhoeae*, *Escherichia coli* and *Proteus mirabilis*. Because it does not resist destruction by penicillinase, it is *not* effective against penicillinase-producing bacteria, particularly resistant staphylococci. All strains of Pseudomonas and most strains of Klebsiella and Enterobacter are resistant.

Disc Susceptibility Tests: Quantitative methods that require measurement of the diameters of zones of inhibition of microbial growth give the most precise estimates of antibiotic susceptibility. One recommended procedure (21 CFR Sec. 460.1) uses discs for testing susceptibility to ampicillin-class antibiotics. Interpretations correlate diameters of the disc test with MIC values for amoxicillin. With this procedure, a report from the laboratory of "susceptible" indicates that the infecting organism is likely to respond to therapy. A report of "resistant" indicates that the infecting organism is not likely to respond to therapy. A report of "intermediate susceptibility" suggests that the organism would be susceptible if high dosage is used, or if the infection is confined to tissues and fluids (e.g., urine) in which high antibiotic levels are attained.

Indications and Usage: Trimox (amoxicillin) is indicated in the treatment of infections due to susceptible strains of the following:

Gram-negative organisms — *H. influenzae*, *E. coli*, *P. mirabilis* and *N. gonorrhoeae*.

Gram-positive organisms — Streptococci (including *Streptococcus faecalis*), *S. pneumoniae* and nonpenicillinase-producing staphylococci.

Therapy may be instituted prior to obtaining results from bacteriological and susceptibility studies to determine the causative organisms and their susceptibility to amoxicillin.

Indicated surgical procedures should be performed.

Contraindications: The use of this drug is contraindicated in individuals with a history of an allergic reaction to any of the penicillins.

Warnings: Serious and occasionally fatal hypersensitivity (anaphylactoid) reactions have been reported in patients on penicillin therapy. Although anaphylaxis is more frequent following parenteral therapy, it has occurred in patients on oral penicillins. These reactions are more likely to occur in individuals with a history of sensitivity to multiple allergens. There have been reports of individuals with a history of penicillin hypersensitivity who have experienced severe reactions when treated with a cephalosporin. Before therapy with any penicillin, careful inquiry should be made concerning previous hypersensitivity reactions to penicillins, cephalosporins, or other allergens. If an allergic reaction occurs, appropriate therapy should be instituted and discontinuance of amoxicillin therapy considered. **Serious anaphylactoid reactions require immediate emergency treatment with epinephrine. Oxygen, intravenous steroids, and airway management, including intubation, should also be administered as indicated.**

Precautions: As with any potent drug, periodic assessment of renal, hepatic and hematopoietic function should be made during prolonged therapy.

The possibility of superinfections with mycotic or bacterial pathogens should be kept in mind during therapy. If superinfections occur (usually involving Enterobacter, Pseudomonas or Candida), amoxicillin should be discontinued and/or appropriate therapy instituted.

Usage in Pregnancy: Safety for use in pregnancy has not been established.

Adverse Reactions: As with other penicillins, it may be expected that untoward reactions will be essentially limited to sensitivity phenomena. They

Continued on next page

Squibb—Cont.

are more likely to occur in individuals who have previously demonstrated hypersensitivity to penicillins and in those with a history of allergy, asthma, hay fever or urticaria. The following adverse reactions have been reported as associated with the use of the penicillins:

Gastrointestinal: Glossitis, stomatitis, black "hairy" tongue, nausea, vomiting and diarrhea.

Hypersensitivity Reactions: Erythematous maculopapular rashes, urticaria, and a few cases of exfoliative dermatitis and erythema multiforme have been reported. Anaphylaxis is the most serious reaction experienced and has usually been associated with parenteral dosage forms (See WARNINGS).

NOTE: Urticaria, other skin rashes and serum sickness-like reactions may be controlled with antihistamines and, if necessary, systemic corticosteroids. Whenever such reactions occur, amoxicillin should be discontinued unless, in the opinion of the physician, the condition being treated is life-threatening and amenable only to amoxicillin therapy.

Liver: A moderate rise in serum glutamic oxaloacetic transaminase (SGOT) has been noted, but the significance of this finding is unknown.

Hemic and Lymphatic Systems: Anemia, thrombocytopenia, thrombocytopenic purpura, eosinophilia, leukopenia and agranulocytosis have been reported during therapy with the penicillins. These reactions are usually reversible on discontinuation of therapy and are believed to be hypersensitivity phenomena.

Dosage and Administration: Infections of the ear, nose and throat due to streptococci, pneumococci, nonpenicillinase-producing staphylococci and *H. influenzae*; Infections of the genitourinary tract due to *E. coli, P. mirabilis* and *S. faecalis*; Infections of the skin and soft tissues due to streptococci, susceptible staphylococci and *E. coli*:

USUAL DOSAGE:
 Adults: 250 mg. every 8 hours
 Children: 20 mg./kg./day in divided doses every 8 hours
 Children weighing 20 kg. or more should be dosed according to the adult recommendations.

In severe infections or those caused by less susceptible organisms:
 500 mg. every 8 hours for adults and 40 mg./kg./day in divided doses every 8 hours for children may be needed.

Infections of the lower respiratory tract due to streptococci, pneumococci, nonpenicillinase-producing staphylococci and *H. influenzae*:

USUAL DOSAGE:
 Adults: 500 mg. every 8 hours
 Children: 40 mg./kg./day in divided doses every 8 hours
 Children weighing 20 kg. or more should be dosed according to the adult recommendations.

Gonorrhea, acute uncomplicated ano-genital and urethral infections due to *N. gonorrhoeae* (males and females):
 3 grams as a single oral dose
 Cases of gonorrhea with a suspected lesion of syphilis should have darkfield examinations before receiving amoxicillin, and monthly serological tests for a minimum of four months.

General: Larger doses may be required for stubborn or severe infections.

The children's dosage is intended for individuals whose weight will not cause a dosage to be calculated greater than that recommended for adults.

It should be recognized that in the treatment of chronic urinary tract infections frequent bacteriological and clinical appraisals are necessary. Smaller doses than those recommended above should not be used. Even higher doses may be needed at times. In stubborn infections, therapy may be required for several weeks. It may be necessary to continue clinical and/or bacteriological follow-up for several months after cessation of therapy. Except for gonorrhea, treatment should be continued for a minimum of 48 to 72 hours beyond the time that the patient becomes asymptomatic or evidence of bacterial eradication has been obtained. It is recommended that there be at least 10 days' treatment for any infection caused by hemolytic streptococci to prevent the occurrence of acute rheumatic fever or glomerulonephritis.

Preparation and Storage of Oral Suspensions: Prepare the suspension at the time of dispensing. Follow the directions for constitution on the label of the package. Discard any unused suspension after 14 days. The suspension may be kept at room temperature; refrigeration is not required. **Shake well before using.**

How Supplied: Trimox (amoxicillin) is available for oral administration as *Trimox '250' Capsules and *Trimox '500' Capsules (Amoxicillin Capsules USP) which provide amoxicillin trihydrate equivalent to 250 mg. and 500 mg. amoxicillin, respectively. The 250 mg. capsules are available in bottles of 100 and 500 and in Unimatic® cartons of 100. The 500 mg. capsules are available in bottles of 50 and 500 and in Unimatic cartons of 100. Trimox is also available as Trimox '125' for Oral Suspension and Trimox '250' for Oral Suspension (Amoxicillin for Oral Suspension USP) which provide, after preparation, pleasantly flavored suspensions containing amoxicillin trihydrate equivalent to 125 mg. and 250 mg. amoxicillin, respectively, per 5 ml. teaspoonful. Available in bottles of 80, 100, and 150 ml. and Unimatic® cartons of 4 × 25 single-dose bottles, 5 ml. per bottle.

Storage: Store Trimox Capsules (Amoxicillin Capsules USP) and Trimox for Oral Suspension (Amoxicillin for Oral Suspension USP) at room temperature. Dispense the capsules in tight containers.

*Shown in Product Identification Section, page 438

VEETIDS® '250' TABLETS ℞
[vē' tidz]
VEETIDS® '500' TABLETS ℞
(Penicillin V Potassium Tablets USP)
VEETIDS® '125' FOR ORAL SOLUTION ℞
VEETIDS® '250' FOR ORAL SOLUTION ℞
(Penicillin V Potassium for Oral Solution USP)

Description: Veetids (Penicillin V Potassium) is the potassium salt of semisynthetically-produced penicillin V. Veetids '125' for Oral Solution contains FD&C Yellow No. 5 (tartrazine).

Clinical Pharmacology: Penicillin V is bactericidal against penicillin-susceptible microorganisms during the stage of active multiplication. It acts by inhibiting biosynthesis of cell-wall mucopeptide. It is not active against the penicillinase-producing bacteria, which include many strains of staphylococci. Penicillin V is highly active *in vitro* against staphylococci (except penicillinase-producing strains), streptococci (groups A, C, G, H, L, and M) and pneumococci. Other organisms susceptible *in vitro* to penicillin V are *Corynebacterium diphtheriae, Bacillus anthracis*, Clostridia, *Actinomyces bovis, Streptobacillus moniliformis, Listeria monocytogenes*, Leptospira and *Neisseria gonorrhoeae; Treponema pallidum* is extremely susceptible.

Penicillin V is more resistant to inactivation by gastric acid than penicillin G; however, it has the same bacterial spectrum as penicillin G. It may be given with meals; however, blood levels are slightly higher when the drug is given on an empty stomach. Average blood levels are two to five times higher than the levels following the same dose of oral penicillin G and also show much less individual variation.

Once absorbed, penicillin V is about 75 percent bound to serum protein. Highest levels are found in the kidneys, with lesser amounts in the liver, skin, and intestines. Penicillin V penetrates into all other tissues to a lesser degree with a very small level found in the cerebrospinal fluid. The drug is excreted rapidly by tubular excretion in patients with normal kidney function. In neonates and young infants, and in individuals with impaired kidney function, excretion is considerably delayed.

Indications and Usage: Veetids (Penicillin V Potassium) are indicated in the treatment of mild to moderately severe infections due to penicillin-susceptible microorganisms. Therapy should be guided by bacteriological studies, including susceptibility tests, and by clinical response. Note: severe pneumonia, empyema, bacteremia, pericarditis, meningitis, and septic arthritis should not be treated with penicillin V during the acute stage. Indicated surgical procedures should be performed.

The following infections will usually respond to adequate oral dosage:

Streptococcal infections Group A without bacteremia—Mild to moderate infections of the upper respiratory tract (including otitis media), scarlet fever, and mild erysipelas. Note: streptococci in groups A, C, G, H, L, and M are very susceptible to penicillin. Other groups including group D (enterococcus) are resistant.

Pneumococcal infections—Mild to moderately severe infections of the respiratory tract, including otitis media.

Staphylococcal infections — penicillin-susceptible—Mild infections of the skin and skin structures. Note: reports indicate an increasing number of strains of staphylococci resistant to penicillin, emphasizing the need for culture and susceptibility studies in treating suspected staphylococcal infections.

Vincent's gingivitis and pharyngitis (fusospirochetosis)—Mild to moderately severe infections of the oropharynx usually respond to oral penicillin. Note: necessary dental care should be accomplished in infections involving gum tissue.

Medical conditions in which oral penicillin therapy is indicated as prophylaxis: *For the prevention of recurrence following rheumatic fever and/or chorea.* Prophylaxis with oral penicillin on a continuing basis is effective in preventing recurrence of these conditions. *To prevent bacterial endocarditis.* Although no controlled clinical efficacy studies have been conducted penicillin V has been suggested by the American Heart Association and the American Dental Association for use as part of a parenteral-oral regimen and as an alternative oral regimen for prophylaxis against bacterial endocarditis in patients with congenital heart disease or rheumatic or other acquired valvular heart disease when they undergo dental procedures and surgical procedures of the respiratory tract.[1] Since it may happen that *alpha* hemolytic streptococci relatively resistant to penicillin may be found when patients are receiving continuous oral penicillin for secondary prevention of rheumatic fever, prophylactic agents other than penicillin may be chosen for these patients and prescribed in addition to their continuous rheumatic fever prophylactic regimen. Oral penicillin should not be used as adjunctive prophylaxis for genitourinary instrumentation or surgery, lower intestinal tract surgery, sigmoidoscopy, and childbirth. **NOTE: When selecting antibiotics for the prevention of bacterial endocarditis the physician or dentist should read the full joint statement of the American Heart Association and the American Dental Association.**[1]

Contraindications: Contraindicated in patients with a history of hypersensitivity to any penicillin.

Warnings: Serious and occasional fatal hypersensitivity (anaphylactoid) reactions have been reported in patients on penicillin therapy. Although anaphylaxis is more frequent following parenteral administration, it has occurred in patients on oral penicillins. These reactions are more apt to occur in individuals with a history of sensitivity to multiple allergens.

There have been well-documented reports of individuals with a history of penicillin hypersensitivity who have experienced severe hypersensitivity reactions when treated with cephalosporins. Before therapy with a penicillin, careful inquiry should be made concerning previous hypersensitivity reactions to penicillins, cephalosporins, and other allergens. If an allergic reaction occurs, the drug should be discontinued and the patient treated with the usual agents, e.g., pressor amines, antihistamines, and corticosteroids. Serious anaphylactoid reactions are not controlled by antihistamines alone, and require such emergency measures as the immediate use of epinephrine, aminophylline, oxygen, and intravenous corticosteroids.

Concomitant use of oral neomycin therapy should be avoided since malabsorption of penicillin V potassium has been reported.

Precautions: Penicillin should be used with caution in individuals with histories of significant allergies and/or asthma.

The oral route of administration should not be relied upon in patients with severe illness, or with nausea, vomiting, gastric dilatation, cardiospasm or intestinal hypermotility.

Occasional patients will not absorb therapeutic amounts of orally administered penicillin.

In streptococcal infections, therapy must be sufficient to eliminate the organism (10 days minimum); otherwise the sequelae of streptococcal disease may occur. Cultures should be taken following completion of treatment to determine whether streptococci have been eradicated.

Prolonged use of antibiotics may promote the overgrowth of nonsusceptible organisms, including fungi. Should superinfection occur, appropriate measures should be taken.

In prolonged therapy with penicillin, and particularly with high dosage schedules, periodic evaluation of the renal and hematopoietic systems is recommended.

Veetids '125' for Oral Solution (Penicillin V Potassium Oral Solution USP) contains FD&C Yellow No. 5 (tartrazine) which may cause allergic-type reactions (including bronchial asthma) in certain susceptible individuals. Although the overall incidence of FD&C Yellow No. 5 (tartrazine) sensitivity in the general population is low, it is frequently seen in patients who also have aspirin hypersensitivity.

Adverse Reactions: Although the incidence of reactions to oral penicillins has been reported with much less frequency than following parenteral therapy, it should be remembered that all degrees of hypersensitivity, including fatal anaphylaxis, have been reported with oral penicillin.

The most common reactions to oral penicillin are nausea, vomiting, epigastric distress, diarrhea, and black hairy tongue. The hypersensitivity reactions reported are skin rashes ranging from maculopapular to exfoliative dermatitis; urticaria; serum sickness-like reactions including chills, fever, edema, arthralgia, and prostration; laryngeal edema; and anaphylaxis. Fever and eosinophilia may frequently be the only reactions observed. Hemolytic anemia, leukopenia, thrombocytopenia, neuropathy, and nephropathy are infrequent reactions usually associated with high doses of parenteral penicillin. Urticaria, other skin rashes, and serum sickness-like reactions may be controlled by antihistamines and, if necessary, corticosteroids. Whenever such reactions occur, penicillin should be discontinued unless, in the opinion of the physician, the condition being treated is life-threatening and amenable only to penicillin therapy. Serious anaphylactoid reactions require emergency measures (see WARNINGS).

An occasional patient may complain of sore mouth or tongue, as with any oral penicillin preparation.

Dosage and Administration: The dosage of Veetids (Penicillin V Potassium) should be determined according to the susceptibility of the causative microorganism and the severity of the infection, and adjusted to the clinical response of the patient.

For Therapeutic Use

Dosage for *children under 12 years* of age is calculated on the basis of body weight. For *infants and small children* the suggested dose is 15 to 56 mg. (25,000 to 90,000 u.) per kg./day in three to six divided doses.

The usual dosage recommendations for *adults and children 12 years and over* are as follows:

Streptococcal infections—mild to moderately severe—of the upper respiratory tract and including otitis media, scarlet fever and mild erysipelas: 125 mg. (200,000 u.) t.i.d. or q.i.d. for 10 days for mild infections; 250 mg. (400,000 u.) t.i.d. for 10 days for moderately severe infections; for mild to moderately severe streptococcal pharyngitis: 500 mg. (800,000 u.) b.i.d. may be used as an alternative regimen.

Pneumococcal infections—mild to moderately severe—of the respiratory tract, including otitis media: 250 to 500 mg. (400,000 to 800,000 u.) q.i.d. until the patient has been afebrile for at least two days.

Staphylococcal infections—mild infections of skin and skin structures (culture and susceptibility tests should be performed): 250 mg. (400,000 u.) t.i.d. or q.i.d., or 500 mg. (800,000 u.) t.i.d.

Vincent's gingivitis and pharyngitis (fusospirochetosis)—mild to moderately severe infections of the oropharynx: 250 mg. (400,000 u.) t.i.d. or q.i.d., or 500 mg. t.i.d.

For Prophylactic Use

For the prevention of recurrence following rheumatic fever and/or chorea: *Adults*—125 mg. (200,000 u.) b.i.d. on a continuing basis. Dosage for *children under 12 years* of age is calculated on the basis of body weight. For *infants and small children* the suggested dose is 15 to 56 mg. (25,000 to 90,000 u.) per kg./day in three to six divided doses.

To prevent bacterial endocarditis. For prophylaxis against bacterial endocarditis[1] in patients with congenital heart disease or rheumatic or other acquired valvular heart disease when undergoing dental procedures or surgical procedures of the upper respiratory tract, one of two regimens may be selected:

(1) For the oral regimen, give 2 g. of penicillin V (1 g. for children under 60 lb.) one-half to one hour before the procedure, and then 500 mg. (250 mg. for children under 60 lb.) every six hours for eight doses; or

(2) For the combined parenteral-oral regimen give 1,000,000 u. of aqueous crystalline penicillin G (30,000 u./kg. in children) intramuscularly mixed with 600,000 u. procaine penicillin G (600,000 u. for children) one-half to one hour before the procedure, and then oral penicillin V, 500 mg. for adults or 250 mg. for children less than 60 lb., every six hours for eight doses. Doses for children should not exceed recommendations for adults for a single dose or for a 24-hour period.

How Supplied: *Veetids '250' Tablets and *Veetids '500' Tablets (Penicillin V Potassium Tablets USP) are available for oral administration as FILMLOK® tablets providing penicillin V potassium equivalent to 250 mg. (400,000 units) and 500 mg. (800,000 units), respectively, of penicillin V. (Filmlok is a Squibb trademark for veneer-coated tablets.) Bottles of 100 and 1000, and Unimatic® cartons of 100.

Veetids '125' for Oral Solution and Veetids '250' for Oral Solution (Penicillin V Potassium for Oral Solution USP) are available as powders that, when constituted as directed, provide pleasantly flavored solutions containing penicillin V potassium equivalent to 125 mg. (200,000 units) and 250 mg. (400,000 units), respectively, of penicillin V per 5 ml. teaspoonful. Bottles of 100 ml. and 200 ml.

Storage: Store Veetids Tablets at room temperature; avoid excessive heat. Dispense in tight containers. Store Veetids for Oral Solution in dry form at room temperature; after preparation of the solution, store in refrigerator and discard unused portion after 14 days. Shake well before using. Keep tightly closed.

Reference: 1. American Heart Association. 1977. Prevention of bacterial endocarditis. Circulation 56:139A-143A.

*Shown in Product Identification Section, page 438

VELOSEF® '250' CAPSULES ℞
[vel'ō-sef]
VELOSEF® '500' CAPSULES ℞
(Cephradine Capsules USP)
VELOSEF® '125' FOR ORAL SUSPENSION ℞
VELOSEF® '250' FOR ORAL SUSPENSION ℞
(Cephradine for Oral Suspension USP)

Description: Velosef (Cephradine, Squibb) is a semisynthetic cephalosporin antibiotic; oral dosage forms include capsules containing 250 mg. and 500 mg. cephradine, and cephradine for oral suspension containing, after constitution, 125 mg. and 250 mg. per 5 ml. dose. Cephradine is chemically designated as (6R,7R)-7-[(R)-2-amino-2-(1,4-cyclohexadien-1-yl) acetamido]-3- methyl-8-oxo-5-thia-1-azabicylo [4.2.0] oct-2- ene-2-carboxylic acid.

Clinical Pharmacology: Velosef (Cephradine, Squibb) is acid stable. It is rapidly absorbed after oral administration in the fasting state. Following single doses of 250 mg., 500 mg., and 1 g. in normal adult volunteers, average peak serum concentrations within one hour were approximately 9 mcg./ml., 16.5 mcg./ml., and 24.2 mcg./ml., respectively.

In vitro studies by an ultracentrifugation technique show that at therapeutic serum antibiotic concentrations, cephradine is minimally bound (8 to 17 percent) to normal serum protein. Cephradine does not pass across the blood-brain barrier to any appreciable extent. The presence of food in the gastrointestinal tract delays absorption but does not affect the total amount of cephradine absorbed. Over 90 percent of the drug is excreted unchanged in the urine within six hours. Peak urine concentrations are approximately 1600 mcg./ml., 3200 mcg./ml., and 4000 mcg./ml. following single doses of 250 mg., 500 mg., and 1 g., respectively.

Microbiology—*In vitro* tests demonstrate that the cephalosporins are bactericidal because of their inhibition of cell-wall synthesis. Cephradine is active against the following organisms *in vitro*:

Group A beta-hemolytic streptococci
Staphylococci, including coagulase-positive, coagulase-negative, and penicillinase-producing strains
Streptococcus pneumoniae (formerly *Diplococcus pneumoniae*)
Escherichia coli
Proteus mirabilis
Klebsiella species
Hemophilus influenzae

Cephradine is not active against most strains of *Enterobacter* species, *P. morganii*, and *P. vulgaris*. It has no activity against *Pseudomonas* or *Herellea* species. When tested by *in vitro* methods, staphylococci exhibit cross-resistance between cephradine and methicillin-type antibiotics.

Note—Most strains of enterococci (*Streptococcus faecalis*) are resistant to cephradine.

Disc Susceptibility Tests—Quantitative methods that require measurement of zone diameters give the most precise estimates of antibiotic susceptibility. One recommended procedure (21 CFR Sec. 460.1) uses cephalosporin class discs for testing susceptibility; interpretations correlate zone diameters of this disc test with MIC values for cephradine. With this procedure, a report from the laboratory of "resistant" indicates that the infecting organism is not likely to respond to therapy. A report of "intermediate susceptibility" suggests that the organism would be susceptible if the infection is confined to the urinary tract, as high antibiotic levels can be obtained in the urine, or if high dosage is used in other types of infection.

Indications and Usage: Velosef Capsules (Cephradine Capsules USP), and Velosef for Oral Suspension (Cephradine for Oral Suspension USP) are indicated in the treatment of the following infections when caused by susceptible strains of the designated microorganisms:

Continued on next page

Squibb—Cont.

RESPIRATORY TRACT INFECTIONS (e.g., tonsillitis, pharyngitis, and lobar pneumonia) caused by group A beta-hemolytic streptococci and *S. pneumoniae* (formerly *D. pneumoniae*).
[Penicillin is the usual drug of choice in the treatment and prevention of streptococcal infections, including the prophylaxis of rheumatic fever. Velosef is generally effective in the eradication of streptococci from the nasopharynx; substantial data establishing the efficacy of Velosef (Cephradine, Squibb) in the subsequent prevention of rheumatic fever are not available at present.]
OTITIS MEDIA caused by group A beta-hemolytic streptococci, *S. pneumoniae* (formerly *D. pneumoniae*), *H. influenzae*, and staphylococci.
SKIN AND SKIN STRUCTURE INFECTIONS caused by staphylococci (penicillin-susceptible and penicillin-resistant) and beta-hemolytic streptococci.
URINARY TRACT INFECTIONS, including prostatitis, caused by *E. coli*, *P. mirabilis*, *Klebsiella* species, and enterococci (*S. faecalis*). The high concentrations of cephradine achievable in the urinary tract will be effective against many strains of enterococci for which disc susceptibility studies indicate relative resistance. It is to be noted that among beta-lactam antibiotics, ampicillin is the drug of choice for enterococcal urinary tract (*S. faecalis*) infection.
Note—Culture and susceptibility tests should be initiated prior to and during therapy.
Following clinical improvement achieved with parenteral therapy, oral cephradine may be utilized for continuation of treatment of persistent or severe conditions where prolonged therapy is indicated.
Contraindications: Cephradine is contraindicated in patients with known hypersensitivity to the cephalosporin group of antibiotics.
Warnings: *In penicillin-sensitive patients, cephalosporin derivatives should be used with great caution. There is clinical and laboratory evidence of partial cross-allergenicity of the penicillins and the cephalosporins, and there are instances of patients who have had reactions to both drug classes (including anaphylaxis after parenteral use).*
Any patient who has demonstrated some form of allergy, particularly to drugs, should receive antibiotics, including cephradine, cautiously and then only when absolutely necessary.
Pseudomembranous colitis has been reported with the use of cephalosporins (and other broad spectrum antibiotics); therefore, it is important to consider its diagnosis in patients who develop diarrhea in association with antibiotic use. Treatment with broad spectrum antibiotics alters normal flora of the colon and may permit overgrowth of clostridia. Studies indicate a toxin produced by *Clostridium difficile* is one primary cause of antibiotic-associated colitis. Cholestyramine and colestipol resins have been shown to bind the toxin *in vitro*. Mild cases of colitis may respond to drug discontinuance alone. Moderate to severe cases should be managed with fluid, electrolyte and protein supplementation as indicated. When the colitis is not relieved by drug discontinuance or when it is severe, oral vancomycin is the treatment of choice for antibiotic-associated pseudomembranous colitis produced by *C. difficile*. Other causes of colitis should also be considered.
Precautions: *General*—Patients should be followed carefully so that any side effects or unusual manifestations of drug idiosyncrasy may be detected. If a hypersensitivity reaction occurs, the drug should be discontinued and the patient treated with the usual agents, e.g., pressor amines, antihistamines, or corticosteroids.
Administer cephradine with caution in the presence of markedly impaired renal function. In patients with known or suspected renal impairment, careful clinical observation and appropriate laboratory studies should be made prior to and during therapy as cephradine accumulates in the serum and tissues. See DOSAGE AND ADMINISTRATION section for information on treatment of patients with impaired renal function.
Cephradine should be prescribed with caution in individuals with a history of gastrointestinal disease, particularly colitis.
Prolonged use of antibiotics may promote the overgrowth of nonsusceptible organisms. Should superinfection occur during therapy, appropriate measures should be taken.
Indicated surgical procedures should be performed in conjunction with antibiotic therapy.
Information for Patients: Caution diabetic patients that false results may occur with urine glucose tests (see PRECAUTIONS, Drug/Laboratory Test Interactions).
Advise the patient to comply with the full course of therapy even if he begins to feel better and to take a missed dose as soon as possible. Inform the patient that this medication may be taken with food or milk since gastrointestinal upset may be a factor in compliance with the dosage regimen. The patient should report current use of any medicines and should be cautioned not to take other medications unless the physician knows and approves of their use (see PRECAUTIONS, Drug Interactions).
Laboratory Tests: In patients with known or suspected renal impairment, it is advisable to monitor renal function (see DOSAGE AND ADMINISTRATION).
Drug Interactions: When administered concurrently, the following drugs may interact with cephalosporins:
Other antibacterial agents—Bacteriostats may interfere with the bactericidal action of cephalosporins in acute infection; other agents, e.g., aminoglycosides, colistin, polymyxins, vancomycin, may increase the possibility of nephrotoxicity.
Diuretics (potent "loop diuretics," e.g., furosemide and ethacrynic acid)—Enhanced possibility for renal toxicity.
Probenecid—Increased and prolonged blood levels of cephalosporins, resulting in increased risk of nephrotoxicity.
Drug/Laboratory Test Interactions: After treatment with cephradine, a false-positive reaction for glucose in the urine may occur with Benedict's solution, Fehling's solution, or with Clinitest® tablets, but not with enzyme-based tests such as Clinistix® and Tes-Tape®.
False-positive Coombs test results may occur in newborns whose mothers received a cephalosporin prior to delivery.
Cephalosporins have been reported to cause false-positive reactions in tests for urinary proteins which use sulfosalicylic acid, false elevations of urinary 17-ketosteroid values, and prolonged prothrombin times.
Carcinogenesis, Mutagenesis: Long-term studies in animals have not been performed to evaluate carcinogenic potential or mutagenesis.
Pregnancy—Category B: Reproduction studies have been peformed in mice and rats at doses up to four times the maximum indicated human dose and have revealed no evidence of impaired fertility or harm to the fetus due to cephradine. There are, however, no adequate and well-controlled studies in pregnant women. Because animal reproduction studies are not always predictive of human response, this drug should be used during pregnancy only if clearly needed.
Nursing Mothers: Since cephradine is excreted in breast milk during lactation, caution should be exercised when cephradine is administered to a nursing woman.
Pediatric Use: See DOSAGE AND ADMINISTRATION. Adequate information is unavailable on the efficacy of b.i.d. regimens in children under nine months of age.
Adverse Reactions: As with other cephalosporins, untoward reactions are limited essentially to gastrointestinal disturbances and, on occasion, to hypersensitivity phenomena. The latter are more likely to occur in individuals who have previously demonstrated hypersensitivity and those with a history of allergy, asthma, hay fever, or urticaria.
The following adverse reactions have been reported following the use of cephradine:
Gastrointestinal: Symptoms of pseudomembranous colitis can appear during treatment. Nausea and vomiting have been reported rarely.
Skin and Hypersensitivity Reactions: Mild urticaria or skin rash, pruritus, and joint pains were reported by very few patients.
Hematologic: Mild, transient eosinophilia, leukopenia, and neutropenia have been reported.
Liver: Transient mild rise of SGOT, SGPT, and total bilirubin have been observed with no evidence of hepatocellular damage.
Renal: Transitory rises in BUN have been observed in some patients treated with cephalosporins; their frequency increases in patients over 50 years old. In adults for whom serum creatinine determinations were performed, the rise in BUN was not accompanied by a rise in serum creatinine. Other adverse reactions have included dizziness and tightness in the chest and candidal vaginitis.
Dosage and Administration: Velosef (Cephradine, Squibb) may be given without regard to meals.
Adults: *For respiratory tract infections (other than lobar pneumonia) and skin and skin structure infections,* the usual dose is 250 mg. every 6 hours or 500 mg. every 12 hours.
For lobar pneumonia, the usual dose is 500 mg. every 6 hours or 1 g. every 12 hours.
For uncomplicated urinary tract infections, the usual dose is 500 mg. every 12 hours. In more serious urinary tract infections, including prostatitis, 500 mg. every 6 hours or 1 g. every 12 hours may be administered.
Larger doses (up to 1 g. every 6 hours) may be given for severe or chronic infections.
Children: No adequate information is available on the efficacy of b.i.d. regimens in children under nine months of age. The usual dose in children over nine months of age is 25 to 50 mg./kg./day administered in equally divided doses every 6 or 12 hours. For otitis media due to *H. influenzae,* doses are from 75 to 100 mg./kg./day administered in equally divided doses every 6 or 12 hours, but should not exceed 4 g. per day. Dosage for children should not exceed dosage recommended for adults. All patients, regardless of age and weight: Larger doses (up to 1 gram q.i.d.) may be given for severe or chronic infections.
As with antibiotic therapy in general, treatment should be continued for a minimum of 48 to 72 hours after the patient becomes asymptomatic or evidence of bacterial eradication has been obtained. In infections caused by group A beta-hemolytic streptococci, a minimum of 10 days of treatment is recommended to guard against the risk of rheumatic fever or glomerulonephritis. In the treatment of chronic urinary tract infection, frequent bacteriologic and clinical appraisal is necessary during therapy and may be necessary for several months afterwards. Persistent infections may require treatment for several weeks. Prolonged intensive therapy is recommended for prostatitis. Doses smaller than those indicated are not recommended.
Patients With Impaired Renal Function
Not on Dialysis: The following initial dosage schedule is suggested as a guideline based on creatinine clearance. Further modification in the dosage schedule may be required because of individual variations in absorption.

Creatinine Clearance	Dose	Time Interval
> 20 mL/min.	500 mg	6 hours
15–20 mL/min.	250 mg	6 hours
< 5 mL/min.	250 mg	12 hours

On Chronic, Intermittent Hemodialysis:
250 mg Start
250 mg at 12 hours
250 mg 36–48 hours (after start)
Children may require dosage modification proportional to their weight and severity of infection.
How Supplied: Velosef is available as *Velosef '250' Capsules and *Velosef '500' Capsules (Cephradine Capsules USP) providing 250 mg. and 500 mg. cephradine per capsule, respectively. The Capsules are available in bottles of 24 and 100 and Unimatic® cartons of 100. [Military/V.A. Depot

Item: 250 mg capsules, 100's NSN 6505-01-009-9531.]

Velosef is also available as Velosef '125' for Oral Suspension and Velosef '250' for Oral Suspension (Cephradine for Oral Suspension USP) which, after constitution, provide 125 mg. and 250 mg. cephradine, respectively, per 5 ml. teaspoonful in a pleasant fruit-flavored suspension. Bottles of 100 ml. and 200 ml.

Storage: Velosef Capsules—Keep tightly closed. Do not store above 86°F.

Velosef for Oral Suspension— Prior to constitution, store at room temperature; avoid excessive heat. After constitution, when the suspension stored at room temperature, discard unused portion after seven days; when stored in refrigerator, discard unused portion after 14 days. Keep tightly closed.

*Shown in Product Identification Section, page 438

VELOSEF® for INFUSION ℞
[*vel' ō-sef*]
(Sterile Cephradine USP)
Sodium–Free

Description: Velosef (Cephradine, Squibb) is a semisynthetic cephalosporin antibiotic. Cephradine is designated chemically as (6R,7R)-7-[(R)-2-amino-2-(1, 4-cyclochexadien-1-yl) acetamido]-3-methyl-8-oxo-5-thia-1-azabicyclo [4.2.0] oct-2-ene-2- carboxylic acid.

Velosef for Infusion is sterile cephradine, a white powder for constitution and intravenous administration by drip infusion; it is available in infusion bottles containing 2 g. cephradine. At the time of manufacture, the air in the container is replaced by nitrogen.

Clinical Pharmacology: Pharmacokinetic studies with Velosef for Injection (Cephradine for Injection USP) (containing sodium carbonate) and Velosef for Infusion (Sterile Cephradine USP) (sodium-free) performed by drip infusion demonstrate bioequivalence for these formulations. The mean steady-state concentration of cephradine maintained in the sera of nine normal adult volunteers during infusion of either solution was approximately 3 mcg. per ml. for each mg. of cephradine infused per hour per kg. of body weight. Serum half-life, serum clearance, and apparent volume of distribution were equivalent following intravenous infusion of either preparation.

Figure 1 depicts mean serum concentrations after administration of Velosef for Infusion (Sterile Cephradine USP) to nine normal adult volunteers at the average rate of 380 mg. cephradine per hour (5.3 mg./kg./hr.) over a four-hour period; the mean cephradine level rises rapidly and approaches a mean steady-state concentration of 17 mcg./ml. in approximately 1.5 hours. After the infusion is discontinued, the cephradine concentration decreases exponentially, declining to 1.5 mcg./ml. at 6.5 hours.

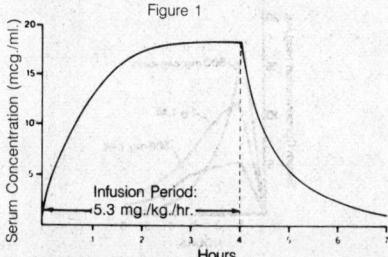

Figure 1

Cephradine is excreted unchanged in the urine. Between 1.5 and 4 hours after the start of the infusion depicted in Figure 1, cephradine is excreted in urine at a mean rate of 312 mg./hr.; a high concentration of cephradine in the urine exists during this period with a mean concentration of 885 mcg./ml. Studies with Velosef for Injection (Cephradine for Injection USP) demonstrate that probenecid slows tubular excretion of cephradine and increases serum concentration.

In vitro studies by an ultracentrifugation technique show that at therapeutic serum antibiotic concentrations, cephradine is minimally bound (8 to 17 percent) to normal human serum protein. Cephradine does not pass across the blood-brain barrier to any appreciable extent.

Assays of bone obtained at surgery have shown that cephradine penetrates bone tissue.

Microbiology: *In vitro* tests demonstrate that the cephalosporins are bactericidal because of their inhibition of cell-wall synthesis. Cephradine is active against the following organisms *in vitro:* group A beta-hemolytic streptococci; staphylococci, including coagulase-positive, coagulase-negative, and penicillinase-producing strains; *Escherichia coli; Streptococcus pneumoniae* (formerly *Diplococcus pneumoniae*); *Proteus mirabilis; Klebsiella* species; and *Hemophilus influenzae.*

It is not active against most strains of *Enterobacter* species, *Proteus morganii,* and *Proteus vulgaris.* It has no activity against *Pseudomonas* or *Herellea* species. When tested by *in vitro* methods, staphylococci exhibit cross-resistance between cephradine and methicillin-type antibiotics.

NOTE—Most strains of enterococci (*Streptococcus faecalis*) are resistant to cephradine.

Disc Susceptibility Tests: Quantitative methods that require measurement of zone diameters give the most precise estimates of antibiotic susceptibility. One recommended procedure (21 CFR Sec. 460.1) uses cephalosporin class discs for testing susceptibility; interpretations correlate zone diameters of this disc test with MIC values for cephradine. With this procedure, a report from the laboratory of "resistant" indicates that the infecting organism is not likely to respond to therapy. A report of "intermediate susceptibility" suggests that the organism would be susceptible if the infection is confined to the urinary tract, as high antibiotic levels can be obtained in the urine, or if high dosage is used in other types of infection.

Indications and Usage: Velosef for Infusion (Sterile Cephradine USP) is indicated in the treatment of the following serious infections when caused by susceptible strains of the designated microorganisms:

RESPIRATORY TRACT INFECTIONS due to *Streptococcus pneumoniae* (formerly *Diplococcus pneumoniae*), *Klebsiella* species, *H. influenzae, Staphylococcus aureus* (penicillin-susceptible and penicillin-resistant), and group A beta-hemolytic streptococci.

[Penicillin is the usual drug of choice in the treatment and prevention of streptococcal infections, including the prophylaxis of rheumatic fever. Velosef (Cephradine, Squibb) is generally effective in the eradication of streptococci from the nasopharynx; substantial data establishing the efficacy of Velosef in the subsequent prevention of rheumatic fever are not available at present.]

URINARY TRACT INFECTIONS due to *E. coli, P. mirabilis,* and *Klebsiella* species.

SKIN AND SKIN STRUCTURES INFECTIONS due to *S. aureus* (penicillin-susceptible and penicillin-resistant) and group A beta-hemolytic streptococci.

BONE INFECTIONS due to *S. aureus* (penicillin-susceptible and penicillin-resistant).

SEPTICEMIA due to *Streptococcus pneumoniae* (formerly *Diplococcus pneumoniae*), *S. aureus* (penicillin-susceptible and penicillin-resistant), *P. mirabilis,* and *E. coli.*

NOTE—Culture and susceptibility tests should be initiated prior to and during therapy.

Contraindications: Cephradine is contraindicated in patients with known hypersensitivity to the cephalosporin group of antibiotics.

Warnings: *In penicillin-sensitive patients, cephalosporin derivatives should be used with great caution. There is clinical and laboratory evidence of partial cross-allergenicity of the penicillins and the cephalosporins, and there are instances of patients who have had reactions to both drug classes (including anaphylaxis after parenteral use).*

Any patient who has demonstrated some form of allergy, particularly to drugs, should receive antibiotics, including cephradine, cautiously and then only when absolutely necessary. Serious anaphy-

lactoid reactions require immediate emergency treatment with epinephrine. Oxygen, intravenous steroids, and airway management, including intubation, should also be administered as indicated.

Pseudomembranous colitis has been reported with the use of cephalosporins (and other broad spectrum antibiotics); therefore, it is important to consider its diagnosis in patients who develop diarrhea in association with antibiotic use. Treatment with broad spectrum antibiotics alters normal flora of the colon and may permit overgrowth of clostridia. Studies indicate a toxin produced by *Clostridium difficile* is one primary cause of antibiotic-associated colitis. Cholestyramine and colestipol resins have been shown to bind the toxin *in vitro.* Mild cases of colitis may respond to drug discontinuance alone. Moderate to severe cases should be managed with fluid, electrolyte and protein supplementation as indicated. When the colitis is not relieved by drug discontinuance or when it is severe, oral vancomycin is the treatment of choice for antibiotic-associated pseudomembranous colitis produced by *C. difficile.* Other causes of colitis should also be considered.

Precautions: *General*—Prolonged use of antibiotics may promote the overgrowth of nonsusceptible organisms. Should superinfection occur during therapy, appropriate measures should be taken.

When cephradine is administered to patients with markedly impaired renal function, lower daily dosage is required. (See DOSAGE AND ADMINISTRATION.) In patients with known or suspected renal impairment, careful clinical observation and appropriate laboratory studies should be conducted because cephradine in the usual recommended dosage will accumulate in the serum and tissues.

Cephradine should be prescribed with caution in individuals with a history of gastrointestinal disease, particularly colitis.

Patients should be followed carefully so that any side effects or unusual manifestations of drug idiosyncrasy may be detected. If a hypersensitivity reaction occurs, the drug should be discontinued and the patient treated with the usual agents, e.g., pressor amines, antihistamines, or corticosteroids. To reduce the risk of phlebitis from intravenous infusion, the injection site should be changed at appropriate intervals during long-term therapy.

Information for Patients: Caution diabetic patients that false test results may occur with urine glucose tests (see PRECAUTIONS, Drug/Laboratory Test Interactions). The patient should report current use of any medicines and should be cautioned not to take other medications unless the physician knows and approves of their use (see PRECAUTIONS, Drug Interactions).

Laboratory Tests: In patients with known or suspected renal impairment, it is advisable to monitor renal function (see DOSAGE AND ADMINISTRATION).

Drug Interactions: When administered concurrently, the following drugs may interact with cephalosporins:

Other antibacterial agents—Bacteriostats may interfere with the bactericidal action of cephalosporins in acute infection; other agents, e.g., aminoglycosides, colistin, polymyxins, vancomycin, may increase the possibility of nephrotoxicity.

Diuretics (potent "loop diuretics," e.g., furosemide and ethacrynic acid)—Enhanced possibility for renal toxicity.

Probenecid—Increased and prolonged blood levels of cephalosporins, resulting in increased risk of nephrotoxicity.

Drug/Laboratory Test Interactions: After treatment with cephradine, a false-positive reaction for glucose in the urine may occur with Benedict's solution, Fehling's solution, or with Clinitest® tablets, but not with enzyme-based tests such as Clinistix® and Tes-Tape®.

False-positive Coombs test results may occur in newborns whose mothers received a cephalosporin prior to delivery.

Continued on next page

Squibb—Cont.

Cephalosporins have been reported to cause false-positive reactions in tests for urinary proteins which use sulfosalicylic acid, false elevations of urinary 17-ketosteroid values, and prolonged prothrombin times.

Carcinogenesis, Mutagenesis: Long-term studies in animals have not been performed to evaluate carcinogenic potential or mutagenesis.

Pregnancy: Teratogenic Effect/Impairment of Fertility: Category B: Reproduction studies have been performed in mice and rats at doses up to four times the maximum indicated human dose and have revealed no evidence of impaired fertility or harm to the fetus due to cephradine. There are, however, no adequate and well-controlled studies in pregnant women. Because animal reproduction studies are not always predictive of human response, this drug should be used during pregnancy only if clearly needed.

Nursing Mothers: Since cephradine is excreted in breast milk during lactation, caution should be exercised when cephradine is administered to a nursing woman.

Pediatric Use: See DOSAGE AND ADMINISTRATION. Cephradine has been effectively used in infants, but all laboratory parameters have not been extensively studied in infants one month to one year of age; therefore, in the treatment of children in this age group, the benefits of the drug to the risk involved must be considered.

Since safety for use in premature infants and in infants under one month of age has not been established, the use of cephradine by injection or infusion should be based on careful consideration of the benefits of the drug against the risk involved.

Adverse Reactions: As with other cephalosporins, untoward reactions are limited essentially to gastrointestinal disturbances and, on occasion, to hypersensitivity phenomena. The latter are more likely to occur in individuals who have previously demonstrated hypersensitivity and those with a history of allergy, asthma, hay fever, or urticaria. The following adverse reactions have been reported following the use of cephradine:

Gastrointestinal: Symptoms of pseudomembranous colitis can appear during antibiotic treatment. Nausea and vomiting have been reported rarely.

Skin and Hypersensitivity Reactions: Mild urticaria or skin rash, edema, erythema, pruritus, joint pains, and drug fever.

Blood: Mild, transient eosinophilia, leukopenia, and neutropenia.

Liver: Instances of elevated SGOT and SGPT of approximately 10 percent and 2 percent of patients, respectively, have been observed; also, a few cases of elevated total bilirubin, alkaline phosphatase and LDH have been observed. In most patients, values tended to return to normal after the end of therapy.

Renal: Mild elevations in BUN have been observed in some patients treated with cephalosporins; their frequency increases in patients over 50 years old and in children under three. In adults for whom serum creatinine determinations were performed, the rise in BUN was not accompanied by a rise in serum creatinine.

Other adverse reactions are headache, dizziness, dyspnea, paresthesia, candidal overgrowth, candidal vaginitis, isolated instances of hepatomegaly, and thrombophlebitis at the site of injection.

Dosage and Administration: Velosef for Infusion (Sterile Cephradine USP) may be administered by continuous or intermittent intravenous infusion. The infusion bottle is designed to be suspended from an I.V. stand and may also be used in any administration procedure where sequential administration of infusion solutions is intended.

Adults: The usual daily dosage of Velosef for Infusion is 2 to 4 g. of cephradine given in equally divided doses four times a day (e.g., 500 mg. to 1 g. q.i.d.). In bone infections the usual dosage is 1 g. q.i.d. A daily dose of 2 g. is adequate in uncomplicated pneumonia, and skin and skin structures infections, and most urinary tract infections. In severe infections, the dosage may be increased.

The maximum daily dose should not exceed 8 g. per day.

Infants and Children: The usual dosage range of Velosef for Infusion is 50 to 100 mg./kg./day (approximately 23 to 45 mg./lb./day) in equally divided doses four times a day and should be determined by age, weight of the patient, and severity of the infection being treated.

All laboratory parameters have not been extensively studied in infants under one year of age; therefore, in the treatment of children in this age group, the benefits of the drug to the risk involved must be considered. In newborn infants, accumulation of other cephalosporin-class antibiotics (with resultant prolongation of drug half-life) has been reported.

The maximum daily pediatric dose should not exceed doses recommended for adults.

PEDIATRIC DOSAGE GUIDE

Weight lbs	kg	50 mg/kg/day Approx. dose mg qid	100 mg/kg/day Approx. dose mg qid
10	4.5	56 mg	112 mg
20	9.1	114 mg	227 mg
30	13.6	170 mg	340 mg
40	18.2	227 mg	455 mg
50	22.7	284 mg	567 mg

As with antibiotic therapy generally: therapy should be continued for a minimum of 48 to 72 hours after the patient becomes asymptomatic or evidence of bacterial eradication has been obtained; in infections caused by group A beta-hemolytic streptococci, a minimum of 10 days of treatment is recommended to guard against the risk of rheumatic fever or glomerulonephritis; in the treatment of chronic urinary tract infection, frequent bacteriologic and clinical appraisal is necessary during therapy and may be necessary for several months afterwards; persistent infections may require treatment for several weeks; doses smaller than those indicated above should not be used.

Parenteral therapy may be followed by oral Velosef (Cephradine, Squibb) either as capsules or as an oral suspension.

Velosef for Infusion (Sterile Cephradine USP) should be administered only by intravenous infusion.

Renal Impairment Dosage: A modified dosage schedule in patients with decreased renal function is necessary. Each patient should be considered individually; the following reduced dosage schedule is recommended as a guideline, based on the creatinine clearance (ml./min./1.73m²).

In adults, the initial loading dose is 750 mg. of Velosef and the maintenance dose is 500 mg. at the time intervals listed below:

Creatinine Clearance	Time Interval
> 20 ml./min.	6 - 12 hours
15 - 19 ml./min.	12 - 24 hours
10 - 14 ml./min.	24 - 40 hours
5 - 9 ml./min.	40 - 50 hours
< 5 ml./min.	50 - 70 hours

Further modification of the dosage schedule may be necessary in children.

Constitution and Storage: The choice of I.V. solution and the volume to be employed are dictated by fluid and electrolyte management. Suitable I.V. solutions are: 5% Dextrose Injection USP, Lactated Ringer's Injection USP, 10% Dextrose Injection USP, Dextrose and Sodium Chloride Injection USP (5% : 0.9% or 5% : 0.45%), 10% Invert Sugar in Water for Injection, Normosol®-R, Ionosol® B with Dextrose 5%, Sodium Chloride Injection USP, or Sodium Lactate Injection USP (M/6 sodium lactate). **Do not use Sterile Water for Injection.** Aseptically add 150 ml. or 200 ml. of the I.V. solution to the infusion bottle for approximate concentrations of 13.3 mg./ml. or 10 mg./ml., respectively. *Note: Complete solution of the preparation requires a minimum of 150 ml. of diluent. Shake well until dissolved.*

Infusion solutions prepared as directed above retain potency for 48 hours at room temperature, or one week under refrigeration (5° C.). Unused solutions must be discarded after these time periods. Constituted solutions may vary in color from nearly colorless to light yellow.

Parenteral drug products should be inspected visually for particulate matter and discoloration prior to administration, whenever solution and container permit.

Store Velosef for Infusion (Sterile Cephradine USP) at room temperature in dry form; avoid excessive heat. Protect the dry form and constituted solutions from concentrated light or direct sunlight.

Extemporaneous mixtures with other antibiotics or drugs are not recommended.

How Supplied: Velosef for Infusion (Sterile Cephradine USP) is available in intravenous infusion bottles (200 ml. size) containing 2 g. cephradine.

VELOSEF® for INJECTION ℞
[*vel' ō-sef*]
(Cephradine for Injection USP)

Description: Velosef (Cephradine, Squibb) is a semisynthetic cephalosporin antibiotic. Cephradine is designated chemically as (6R, 7R)-7-[(R)- 2-amino-2-(1, 4-cyclohexadien-1-yl) acetamido]-3-methyl-8-oxo-5-thia-1-azabicyclo- [4.2.0] oct-2-ene-2-carboxylic acid.

Velosef for Injection is a sterile powder for constitution available in vials containing 250 mg., 500 mg., or 1 g. cephradine; and bottles containing 2 g. or 4 g. cephradine; the preparations also contain 79 mg., 157 mg., 315 mg., 630 mg., or 1.26 g. anhydrous sodium carbonate, respectively. The sodium content is approximately 136 mg. (6 mEq.) per gram of cephradine. At the time of manufacture, the air in the container is replaced by nitrogen.

Clinical Pharmacology: Table I indicates the blood levels following intramuscular administration of a 500 mg. or 1 g. dose to normal adults. [See table on next page].

Figure I depicts representative mean serum concentrations after administration of a 500 mg. and 1 g. I.M. dose, and a 500 mg. oral dose of cephradine. Areas beneath the curves for the 500 mg. oral and I.M. dose are equivalent.

Figure I
VELOSEF FOR INJECTION
(Cephradine for Injection USP)

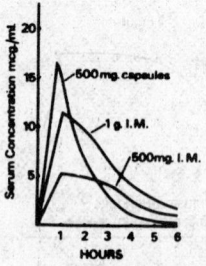

A single intravenous dose of 1 g. cephradine resulted in serum levels of approximately 86 mcg./ml. at 5 minutes, 50 mcg./ml. at 15 minutes, 26 mcg./ml. at 30 minutes, and 12 mcg./ml. at 60 minutes; these levels declined to 1 mcg./ml. at four hours.

In vitro studies by an ultracentrifugation technique show that, at therapeutic serum antibiotic concentrations, cephradine is minimally bound (8 to 17 percent) to normal human serum protein.

Cephradine does not pass across the blood-brain barrier to any appreciable extent.

Velosef (Cephradine, Squibb) is excreted unchanged in the urine. The kidneys excrete 57 to 80 percent of an intramuscular dose in the first six hours; this results in a high urine concentration, e.g., a mean urine concentration of 313 mcg./ml. within a six hour period following a 500 mg. I.M. dose. Probenecid slows tubular excretion and increases serum concentration.

Assays of bone and cardiac tissue (atrial appendage) obtained at surgery have shown that cephradine penetrates these tissues.

Microbiology—In vitro tests demonstrate that the cephalosporins are bactericidal because of their inhibition of cell-wall synthesis. Cephradine is active against the following organisms *in vitro*: group A beta-hemolytic streptococci; staphylococci, including coagulase-positive, coagulase-negative, and penicillinase-producing strains; *Escherichia coli; Streptococcus pneumoniae* (formerly *Diplococcus pneumoniae); Proteus mirabilis; Klebsiella* species; and *Hemophilus influenzae.*

It is not active against most strains of *Enterobacter* species, *Proteus morganii,* and *Proteus vulgaris.* It has no activity against *Pseudomonas* or *Herellea* species. When tested by *in vitro* methods, staphylococci exhibit cross-resistance between cephradine and methicillin-type antibiotics.

NOTE—Most strains of enterococci (*Streptococcus faecalis*) are resistant to cephradine.

Disc Susceptibility Tests—Quantitative methods that require measurement of zone diameters give the most precise estimates of antibiotic susceptibility. One recommended procedure (21 CFR § 460.1) uses cephalosporin class discs for testing susceptibility; interpretations correlate zone diameters of this disc test with MIC values for cephradine. With this procedure, a report from the laboratory of "resistant" indicates that the infecting organism is not likely to respond to therapy. A report of "intermediate susceptibility" suggests that the organism would be susceptible if the infection is confined to the urinary tract, as high antibiotic levels can be obtained in the urine, or if high dosage is used in other types of infection.

Indications and Usage: Treatment—Velosef for Injection (Cephradine for Injection USP) is indicated in the treatment of the following serious infections when caused by susceptible strains of the designated microorganisms:

RESPIRATORY TRACT INFECTIONS due to *Streptococcus pneumoniae* (formerly *Diplococcus pneumoniae*), *Klebsiella* species, *H. influenzae, Staphylococcus aureus* (penicillin-susceptible and penicillin-resistant), and group A beta-hemolytic streptococci.

[Penicillin is the usual drug of choice in the treatment and prevention of streptococcal infections, including the prophylaxis of rheumatic fever. Velosef is generally effective in the eradication of streptococci from the nasopharynx; substantial data establishing the efficacy of Velosef in the subsequent prevention of rheumatic fever are not available at present.]

URINARY TRACT INFECTIONS due to *E. coli, P. mirabilis,* and *Klebsiella* species.

SKIN AND SKIN STRUCTURE INFECTIONS due to *S. aureus* (penicillin-susceptible and penicillin-resistant) and group A beta-hemolytic streptococci.

BONE INFECTIONS due to *S. aureus* (penicillin-susceptible and penicillin-resistant).

SEPTICEMIA due to *Streptococcus pneumoniae* (formerly *Diplococcus pneumoniae), S. aureus* (penicillin-susceptible and penicillin-resistant), *P. mirabilis,* and *E. coli.*

NOTE—Culture and susceptibility tests should be initiated prior to and during therapy.

Prevention: When compared to placebo in randomized controlled studies in patients undergoing vaginal hysterectomy and cesarean section, the prophylactic use of VELOSEF (cephradine) resulted in a significant reduction in the number of postoperative infections.

The prophylactic administration of VELOSEF perioperatively (preoperatively, intraoperatively, and postoperatively) may reduce the incidence of certain postoperative infections in patients undergoing surgical procedures (e.g., vaginal hysterectomy) that are classified as contaminated or potentially contaminated.

In patients undergoing cesarean section, intraoperative (after clamping the umbilical cord) and postoperative use of VELOSEF may reduce the incidence of certain postoperative infections.

Effective perioperative use depends on the time of administration. VELOSEF (Cephradine, Squibb) usually should be given 30 to 90 minutes before surgery, which is sufficient time to achieve effective tissue levels. Prophylactic administration should usually be stopped within 24 hours since continuing administration of any antibiotic increases the possibility of adverse reactions but, in the majority of surgical procedures, does not reduce the incidence of subsequent infection.

If there are signs of infection, specimens for culture should be obtained for identification of the causative organism so that appropriate therapy may be instituted.

Contraindications: Cephradine is contraindicated in patients with known hypersensitivity to the cephalosporin group of antibiotics.

Warnings: *In penicillin-sensitive patients, cephalosporin derivatives should be used with great caution. There is clinical and laboratory evidence of partial cross-allergenicity of the penicillins and the cephalosporins, and there are instances of patients who have had reactions to both drug classes (including fatal anaphylaxis after parenteral use).*

Any patient who has demonstrated some form of allergy, particularly to drugs, should receive antibiotics, including cephradine, cautiously and then only when absolutely necessary. Serious anaphylactoid reactions require immediate emergency treatment with epinephrine. Oxygen, intravenous steroids, and airway management, including intubation, should also be administered as indicated.

Pseudomembranous colitis has been reported with the use of cephalosporins (and other broad spectrum antibiotics); therefore, it is important to consider its diagnosis in patients who develop diarrhea in association with antibiotic use. - Treatment with broad spectrum antibiotics alters normal flora of the colon and may permit overgrowth of clostridia. Studies indicate a toxin produced by *Clostridium difficile* is one primary cause of antibiotic-associated colitis. Cholestyramine and colestipol resins have been shown to bind the toxin *in vitro.* Mild cases of colitis may respond to drug discontinuance alone. Moderate to severe cases should be managed with fluid, electrolyte and protein supplementation as indicated. When the colitis is not relieved by drug discontinuance or when it is severe, oral vancomycin is the treatment of choice for antibiotic-associated pseudomembranous colitis produced by *C. difficile.* Other causes of colitis should also be considered.

Precautions: General—Prolonged use of antibiotics may promote the overgrowth of nonsusceptible organisms. Should superinfection occur during therapy, appropriate measures should be taken.

When cephradine is administered to patients with markedly impaired renal function lower daily dosage is required. (See DOSAGE AND ADMINISTRATION.) In patients with known or suspected renal impairment, careful clinical observation and appropriate laboratory studies should be conducted because cephradine in the usual recommended dosage will accumulate in the serum and tissues.

Cephradine should be prescribed with caution in individuals with a history of gastrointestinal disease, particularly colitis.

Patients should be followed carefully so that any side effects or unusual manifestations of drug idiosyncrasy may be detected. If a hypersensitivity reaction occurs, the drug should be discontinued and the patient treated with the usual agents, e.g., pressor amines, antihistamines, or corticosteroids. Velosef for Injection (Cephradine for Injection USP) is physically compatible with most commonly used intravenous fluids and electrolyte solutions (such as 5% Dextrose Injection or Sodium Chloride Injection or M/6 sodium lactate); however, it is *not* compatible with Lactated Ringer's Injection because of the incompatibility between calcium ions and the sodium carbonate present in Velosef for Injection.

Information for Patients: Caution diabetic patients that false test results may occur with urine glucose tests (see PRECAUTIONS, Drug/Laboratory Test Interactions). The patient should report current use of any medicines and should be cautioned not to take other medications unless the physician knows and approves of their use (see PRECAUTIONS, Drug Interactions).

Laboratory Tests: In patients with known or suspected renal impairment, it is advisable to monitor renal function (see DOSAGE AND ADMINISTRATION).

Drug Interactions: When administered concurrently, the following drugs may interact with cephalosporins:

Other antibacterial agents—Bacteriostats may interfere with the bactericidal action of cephalosporins in acute infection; other agents, e.g., aminoglycosides, colistin, polymyxins, vancomycin, may increase the possibility of nephrotoxicity.

Diuretics (potent "loop diuretics," e.g., furosemide and ethacrynic acid)—Enhanced possibility for renal toxicity.

Probenecid—Increased and prolonged blood levels of cephalosporins, resulting in increased risk of nephrotoxicity.

Drug/Laboratory Test Interactions: After treatment with cephradine, a false-positive reaction for glucose in the urine may occur with Benedict's solution, Fehling's solution, or with Clinitest® tablets, but not with enzyme-based tests such as Clinistix® and Tes-Tape®. False-positive Coombs test results may occur in newborns whose mothers received a cephalosporin prior to delivery.

Cephalosporins have been reported to cause false-positive reactions in tests for urinary proteins which use sulfosalicylic acid, false elevations of urinary 17-ketosteroid values, and prolonged prothrombin times.

Carcinogenesis, Mutagenesis: Long-term studies in animals have not been performed to evaluate carcinogenic potential or mutagenesis.

Pregnancy Category B: Reproduction studies have been performed in mice and rats at doses up to four times the maximum indicated human dose

Continued on next page

TABLE I
VELOSEF FOR INJECTION
(Cephradine for Injection USP)

	MEAN TIME TO PEAK SERUM LEVELS Minutes		MEAN PEAK SERUM CONCENTRATION mcg./ml.		MEAN SERUM CONCENTRATION AT 1 HR. - mcg./ml.	
	500 mg. I.M.	1 g. I.M.	500 mg. I.M.	1 g. I.M.	500 mg. I.M.	1 g. I.M.
MALES	49 (41–59)*	52 (45–61)	6.3 (5.5–7.2)	13.6 (12.2–15.1)	6.2 (5.5–6.9)	12.4 (11.0–14.0)
FEMALES	98 (87–111)	128 (103–157)	5.8 (5.1–6.6)	9.9 (8.7–11.2)	4.3 (3.5–5.2)	6.0 (4.4–8.1)

*Figures in parentheses are 95% confidence limits.

Squibb—Cont.

and have revealed no evidence of impaired fertility or harm to the fetus due to cephradine. There are, however, no adequate and well-controlled studies in pregnant women. Because animal reproduction studies are not always predictive of human response, this drug should be used during pregnancy only if clearly needed.

Nursing Mothers: Since cephradine is excreted in breast milk during lactation, caution should be exercised when cephradine is administered to a nursing woman.

Pediatric Use: See DOSAGE AND ADMINISTRATION. Cephradine has been effectively used in infants, but all laboratory parameters have not been extensively studied in infants one month to one year of age; therefore, in the treatment of children in this age group, the benefits of the drug to the risk involved must be considered.

Since safety for use in premature infants and in infants under one month of age has not been established, the use of cephradine by injection or infusion should be based on careful consideration of the benefits of the drug against the risk involved.

Adverse Reactions: As with other cephalosporins, untoward reactions are limited essentially to gastrointestinal disturbances and, on occasion, to hypersensitivity phenomena. The latter are more likely to occur in individuals who have previously demonstrated hypersensitivity and those with a history of allergy, asthma, hay fever, or urticaria. The following adverse reactions have been reported following the use of cephradine:

Gastrointestinal: Symptoms of pseudomembranous colitis can appear during antibiotic treatment. Nausea and vomiting have been reported rarely.

Skin and Hypersensitivity Reactions: Mild urticaria or skin rash, edema, erythema, pruritus, joint pains and drug fever.

Hematologic: Mild, transient eosinophilia, leukopenia and neutropenia.

Liver: Instances of elevated SGOT and SGPT of approximately 10 percent and 2 percent of patients, respectively, have been observed; also, a few cases of elevated total bilirubin, alkaline phosphatase and LDH have been observed. In most patients, values tended to return to normal after the end of therapy.

Renal: Mild elevations in BUN have been observed in some patients treated with cephalosporins; their frequency increases in patients over 50 years old and in children under three. In adults for whom serum creatinine determinations were performed, the rise in BUN was not accompanied by a rise in serum creatinine.

Other adverse reactions are headache, dizziness, dyspnea, paresthesia, candidal overgrowth, candidal vaginitis, isolated instances of hepatomegaly, and thrombophlebitis at the site of injection. Pain on intramuscular injection has been experienced by some patients. Since sterile abscesses have been reported following accidental subcutaneous injection, the preparation should be administered by deep intramuscular injection.

Dosage and Administration: Adults— Treatment: The usual daily dosage of Velosef for Injection (Cephradine for Injection USP) is 2 to 4 g. of cephradine given in equally divided doses four times a day intramuscularly or intravenously (e.g., 500 mg. to 1 g. q.i.d.). In bone infections the usual dosage is 1 g. q.i.d. administered intravenously. A dosage of 500 mg. q.i.d. is adequate in uncomplicated pneumonia, skin and skin structure and most urinary tract infections. In severe infections, the total daily dose may be increased by using a q. 4 h. dosage regimen or by increasing the dose given q.i.d.; the maximum dose should not exceed 8 g. per day.

Prevention: To prevent postoperative infection in contaminated or potentially contaminated surgery, recommended doses are as follows:
a. 1 g IV or IM administered 30 to 90 minutes prior to start of surgery.
b. 1 g every 4 to 6 hours after the first dose for one or two doses, or for up to 24 hours postoperatively.

Cesarean Section Patients: The first dose of 1 g is administered intravenously as soon as the umbilical cord is clamped. The second and third doses should be given as 1 g intravenously or intramuscularly at 6 and 12 hours after the first dose.

Infants and Children—The usual dosage range of Velosef is 50 to 100 mg./kg./day (approximately 23 to 45 mg./lb./day) in equally divided doses four times a day and should be regulated by age, weight of the patient and severity of the infection being treated.

All laboratory parameters have not been extensively studied in infants under one year of age; therefore, in the treatment of children in this age group, the benefits of the drug to the risk involved must be considered. In newborn infants, accumulation of other cephalosporin-class antibiotics (with resultant prolongation of drug half-life) has been reported.

The maximum daily pediatric dose should not exceed doses recommended for adults.
[See table entitled "Pediatric Dosage Guide".]
[See table below].

As with antibiotic therapy generally: therapy should be continued for a minimum of 48 to 72 hours after the patient becomes asymptomatic or evidence of bacterial eradication has been obtained; in infections caused by group A beta-hemolytic streptococci, a minimum of 10 days of treatment is recommended to guard against the risk of rheumatic fever or glomerulonephritis; in the treatment of chronic urinary tract infection, frequent bacteriologic and clinical appraisal is necessary during therapy and may be necessary for several months afterwards; persistent infections may require treatment for several weeks; doses smaller than those indicated above should not be used. Parenteral therapy may be followed by oral Velosef either as capsules or as an oral suspension.

VELOSEF FOR INJECTION
(Cephradine for Injection USP)

I.M. DILUTION TABLE

Vial Size	Volume of Diluent	Approximate Available Volume	Approximate Available Concentration
250 mg.	1.2 ml.	1.2 ml.	208 mg./ml.
500 mg.	2.0 ml.	2.2 ml.	227 mg./ml.
1 g.	4.0 ml.	4.5 ml.	222 mg./ml.

Velosef for Injection (Cephradine for Injection USP) may be given intravenously or by deep intramuscular injection. To minimize pain and induration, intramuscular injections should be made into a large muscle mass, such as the gluteus or lateral aspect of the thigh.

Patients With Impaired Renal Function
Not on Dialysis: The following initial dosage schedule is suggested as a guideline based on creatinine clearance. Further modification in the dosage schedule may be required because of individual variations in absorption.

Creatinine Clearance	Dose	Time Interval
> 20 mL/min.	500 mg	6 hours
5–20 mL/min.	250 mg	6 hours
< 5 mL/min.	250 mg	12 hours

On Chronic Intermittent Hemodialysis:
250 mg Start
250 mg at 12 hours
250 mg 36–48 hours (after start)

Children may require dosage modification proportional to their weight and severity of infection.

Constitution and Storage:
Parenteral drug products should be inspected visually for particulate matter and discoloration prior to administration, whenever solution and container permit.

For I.M. Use.—Aseptically add Sterile Water for Injection or Bacteriostatic Water for Injection (containing 0.9% [w/v] benzyl alcohol, or 0.12% methylparaben and 0.014% propylparaben) according to the following table [i.e., the table entitled "I.M. Dilution Table"].
[See table above].

Intramuscular solutions should be used within two hours at room temperature; if stored in the refrigerator at 5° C., solutions retain full potency for 24 hours. Constituted solutions may vary in color from light straw to yellow; however, this does not affect the potency.

For I.V. Use—Velosef (Cephradine for Injection USP) may also be administered by direct intravenous injection or by continuous or intermittent infusion. A 3 mcg./ml. serum concentration can be maintained for each mg. of cephradine per kg. body weight per hour of infusion.

For Direct I.V. Administration: Suitable diluents are Sterile Water for Injection, 5% Dextrose Injection, or Sodium Chloride Injection. **Do not use Lactated Ringer's Injection.**

Aseptically add 5 ml. of diluent to the 250 mg. or 500 mg. vials, 10 ml. of diluent to the 1 g. vial, or 20 ml. of diluent to the 2 g. bottle; withdraw entire contents. The solution may be slowly injected directly into a vein over a three to five minute period or may be given as a supplementary injection through the injection site on the administration set when the infusion solution is compatible with cephradine. These Velosef (Cephradine, Squibb) solutions should be used within two hours when held at room temperature; if stored at 5° C., the solutions retain full potency for 24 hours.

For Continuous or Intermittent I.V. Infusion: Suitable intravenous infusion solutions for Velosef are 5% or 10% Dextrose Injection; Sodium Chloride Injection; Sodium Lactate Injection (M/6 sodium lactate); Dextrose and Sodium Chloride Injection (5% : 0.9%) or (5% : 0.45%); 10% Invert Sugar in Water for Injection; Normosol®-R, and Ionosol® B with Dextrose 5%. Sterile Water for Injection may be used as an I.V. infusion solution for Velosef

VELOSEF FOR INJECTION
(Cephradine for Injection USP)

PEDIATRIC DOSAGE GUIDE

Weight lbs.	kg.	50 mg./kg./day Approx. single dose mg. q. 6 h.	Volume needed @ 208 mg./ml. dilution	100 mg./kg./day Approx. single dose mg. q. 6 h.	Volume needed @ 227 mg./ml.
10	4.5	56 mg.	0.27 ml.	112 mg.	0.5 ml.
20	9.1	114 mg.	0.55 ml.	227 mg.	1 ml.
30	13.6	170 mg.	0.82 ml.	340 mg.	1.5 ml.
40	18.2	227 mg.	1.1 ml.	455 mg.	2 ml.
50	22.7	284 mg.	1.4 ml.	567 mg.	2.5 ml.

at a concentration of 30 to 50 mg./ml. (30 mg./ml. is approximately isotonic). **Do not use Lactated Ringer's Injection.**

a) To prepare a Velosef solution for transfer into an I.V. infusion bottle, aseptically add 10 ml., 20 ml., or 40 ml. of Sterile Water for Injection or a suitable infusion solution, respectively, to the 1 g. vial, or 2 g. or 4 g. bottles. Promptly withdraw the entire contents of the resulting solution and aseptically transfer to an I.V. infusion bottle. Intravenous infusion solutions containing Velosef at a concentration of five percent (50 mg./ml.) or less retain potency as noted under (b) below. The choice of I.V. infusion solution and the volume to be employed are dictated by fluid and electrolyte management.

b) Velosef may be infused directly from the 2 g. or 4 g. I.V. bottle. Constitute the 2 g. bottle with 40 ml. and the 4 g. bottle with 80 ml. of a suitable intravenous infusion solution; attach an I.V. administration set directly to the Velosef I.V. infusion bottle. The 2 g. and 4 g. I.V. bottles are designed to be suspended from an I.V. stand.

Intravenous infusion solutions containing Velosef retain full potency for 10 hours at room temperature or 48 hours at 5° C.; infusion solutions of Velosef in Sterile Water for Injection that are frozen immediately after reconstitution in the original container are stable for as long as six weeks when stored at −20° C.

For prolonged infusions, replace the infusion every 10 hours with a freshly prepared solution.

Extemporaneous mixtures of Velosef for Injection (Cephradine for Injection USP) with other antibiotics are not recommmended.

Protect solutions of Velosef from concentrated light or direct sunlight. Velosef for Injection may be stored at room temperature prior to constitution; avoid excessive heat; protect from light.

How Supplied: Velosef for Injection (Cephradine for Injection USP) is available for intramuscular or intravenous use in vials containing 250 mg., 500 mg., or 1 g. cephradine; and for intravenous use in 100 ml. infusion bottles containing 2 g. or 4 g. cephradine.

For information on Squibb products, write to: Squibb Professional Services Department, P.O. Box 4000, Princeton, N.J. 08540.

Squibb/Connaught, Inc.
330 ALEXANDER STREET
PRINCETON, NJ 08540

Distributed in the United States by:
E. R. Squibb & Sons, Inc.
P. O. Box 4000
Princeton, NJ 08540

The following products are manufactured by Connaught Laboratories, Inc., Swiftwater, Pa. Full product and prescribing information is contained in the package insert.

DIPHTHERIA ANTITOXIN, USP ℞
(Purified, Concentrated Globulin—
EQUINE)

Expiration Dating—60 Months
How Supplied: 20,000 unit vial.

DIPHTHERIA AND TETANUS TOXOIDS ADSORBED USP
(For Pediatric Use) (DT)

Expiration dating—24 months
How Supplied: 5 ml vial

DIPHTHERIA AND TETANUS TOXOIDS AND PERTUSSIS VACCINE ADSORBED USP ℞
(For Pediatric Use) (DTP)

Expiration Dating—18 Months
How Supplied: 7.5 ml vial.

FLUZONE® ℞
(Influenza Virus Vaccine USP)
(Zonal Purified, Whole Virion)
and
(Zonal Purified, Subvirion)
(Formula consistent with current USPHS requirements)

Expiration Dating—June 30 of following year.
How Supplied: 5 ml vial (10 doses, 0.5 ml each).

MENOMUNE®-A/C/Y/W-135 ℞
(Meningococcal Polysaccharide Vaccine, Groups A,C,Y and W-135 Combined)
(Freeze-Dried)

Expiration Dating—24 Months
How Supplied: 10 dose vial with 6 ml diluent (needle and syringe administration); 50 dose vial with 27.5 ml diluent (jet injector administration only).

MENOMUNE®- A/C ℞
(Meningococcal Polysaccharide Vaccine, Groups A and C Combined)
(Freeze-Dried)

Expiration Dating—24 Months
How Supplied: 10 dose vial with 6 ml diluent (needle and syringe administration); 50 dose vial with 27.5 ml diluent (jet injector administration only).

TETANUS AND DIPHTHERIA TOXOIDS ADSORBED USP ℞
(For Adult Use) (Td)

Expiration Dating—24 Months
How Supplied: 5 ml vial.

TETANUS TOXOID ADSORBED USP ℞

Expiration Dating—24 Months
How Supplied: 5 ml vial.

TETANUS TOXOID USP ℞
("Fluid" or "Plain")

Expiration Dating—24 Months
How Supplied: 7.5 ml vial

YF-VAX™ (Yellow Fever Vaccine) ℞
(Live, 17D Virus, Avian Leukosis-Free, Stabilized)
(Freeze-Dried)

Expiration Dating—12 Months
How Supplied: 1 dose vial with 0.6 ml diluent; 5 dose vial with 3 ml diluent.

The following products are manufactured by Connaught Laboratories, Ltd., Toronto, Canada. Full product and prescribing information is contained in the package insert.

POLIOMYELITIS VACCINE (PURIFIED) ℞
(For the Prevention of Poliomyelitis [Inactivated, Salk Type])

Expiration Dating—12 Months
How Supplied: 1 ml ampul, package of 5; 10 ml vial.

TUBERSOL® ℞
Tuberculin Purified Protein Derivative
(Mantoux) (PPD)

Expiration Dating—24 Months
How Supplied: 1 U.S. Unit (TU) per test dose (0.1 ml), package of 10 vials; 5 U.S. Units (TU) per test dose (0.1 ml), package of 10 vials and 50 vials; 250 U.S. Units (TU) per test dose (0.1 ml), package of 10 vials.

Squibb-Novo, Inc.
120 ALEXANDER STREET
PRINCETON, NJ 08540

STANDARD INSULIN

REGULAR INSULIN
Insulin Injection
USP (Pork) 100 units/ml

Description: Regular Insulin, Insulin Injection USP, 100 units of insulin per milliliter, is a clear, colorless solution which has a short duration of action. The effect of **Regular Insulin** begins approximately ½ hour after injection. The effect is maximal between 2½ and 5 hours and ends approximately 8 hours after injection. The time course of action of any insulin may vary considerably in different individuals, or at different times in the same individual. Because of this variation, the time periods listed here should be considered as general guidelines only.

SEMILENTE® INSULIN
Prompt Insulin Zinc Suspension
USP (Beef) 100 units/ml

Description: Semilente® Insulin, Prompt Insulin Zinc Suspension USP, 100 units of insulin per milliliter, is a cloudy or milky suspension of amorphous beef insulin. The insulin substance (the cloudy material) settles at the bottom of the vial, therefore, the vial must be gently agitated or rotated so that the contents are uniformly mixed before a dose is withdrawn. The effect of **Semilente® Insulin** begins approximately 1½ hours after injection. The effect is maximal between 5 and 10 hours and ends approximately 16 hours after injection. The time course of action of any insulin may vary considerably in different individuals, or at different times in the same individual. Because of this variation, the time periods listed here should be considered as general guidelines only.

LENTE® INSULIN
Insulin Zinc Suspension
USP (Beef) 100 units/ml

Description: LENTE® Insulin, Insulin Zinc Suspension USP, 100 units of insulin per milliliter, is a cloudy or milky suspension of 70% crystalline and 30% amorphous beef insulin. The Insulin substance (the cloudy material) settles at the bottom of the vial, therefore, the vial must be gently agitated or rotated so that the contents are uniformly mixed before a dose is withdrawn. **Lente® Insulin** has an intermediate duration of action. The effect of **Lente® Insulin** begins approximately 2½ hours after injection. The effect is maximal between 7 and 15 hours and ends approximately 24 hours after injection. The time course of action of any insulin may vary considerably in different individuals, or at different times in the same individual. Because of this variation, the time periods listed here should be considered as general guidelines only.

NPH INSULIN
Isophane Insulin Suspension USP (Beef) 100 units/ml

Description: NPH Insulin, Isophane Insulin Suspension USP, 100 units of insulin per milliliter, is a cloudy or milky suspension of beef insulin with protamine and zinc. The insulin substance (the cloudy material) settles at the bottom of the vial, therefore, the vial must be gently agitated or rotated so that the contents are uniformly mixed before a dose is withdrawn. **NPH Insulin** has an intermediate duration of action. The effect of **NPH Insulin** begins approximately 1½ hours after injection. The effect is maximal between 4 and 12 hours and ends approximately 24 hours after injection. The time course of action of any insulin may vary considerably in different individuals, or at different times in the same individual. Because of this variation, the time periods listed here should be considered as general guidelines only.

Squibb-Novo—Cont.

ULTRALENTE® INSULIN
Extended Insulin Zinc
Suspension USP (Beef) 100 units/ml

Description: Ultralente® Insulin, Extended Insulin Zinc Suspension USP, 100 units of insulin per milliliter, is a cloudy or milky suspension of crystalline beef insulin. The insulin substance (the cloudy material) settles at the bottom of the vial, therefore, the vial must be gently agitated or rotated so that the contents are uniformly mixed before a dose is withdrawn. The effect of Ultralente® Insulin begins approximately 4 hours after injection. The effect is maximal between 10 and 30 hours and ends approximately 36 hours after injection. The time course of action of any insulin may vary considerably in different individuals, or at different times in the same individual. Because of this variation, the time periods listed here should be considered as general guidelines only.

PURIFIED INSULIN
REGULAR PURIFIED PORK INSULIN
INJECTION USP 100 units/ml
(formerly ACTRAPID®)

Description: Regular Purified Pork Insulin Injection, USP, 100 units of insulin per milliliter, is a clear, colorless solution which has a short duration of action. The effect of Regular Purified Insulin begins approximately $\frac{1}{2}$ hour after injection. The effect is maximal between $2\frac{1}{2}$ and 5 hours and ends approximately 8 hours after injection. The time course of action of any insulin may vary considerably in different individuals, or at different times in the same individual. Because of this variation, the time periods listed here should be considered as general guidelines only.

The word "purified" on the label indicates that this insulin differs from standard insulin in that it has undergone additional purification steps (i.e., molecular sieve and ion-exchange chromatography).

SEMILENTE® PURIFIED PORK PROMPT INSULIN ZINC SUSPENSION USP 100 units/ml
(formerly SEMITARD®)

Description: Semilente® Purified Pork Prompt Insulin Zinc Suspension, USP, 100 units of insulin per milliliter, is a cloudy or milky suspension of amorphous purified pork insulin. The insulin substance (the cloudy material) settles at the bottom of the vial, therefore, the vial must be gently agitated or rotated so that the contents are uniformly mixed before a dose is withdrawn. The effect of Semilente® Purified Insulin begins approximately $1\frac{1}{2}$ hours after injection. The effect is maximal between 5 and 10 hours and ends approximately 16 hours after injection. The time course of action of any insulin may vary considerably in different individuals, or at different times in the same individual. Because of this variation, the time periods listed here should be considered as general guidelines only.

The word "purified" on the label indicates that this insulin differs from standard insulin in that it has undergone additional purification steps (i.e., molecular sieve and ion-exchange chromatography).

LENTE® PURIFIED PORK INSULIN ZINC SUSPENSION USP 100 units/ml
(formerly MONOTARD®)

Description: Lente® Purified Pork Insulin Zinc Suspension, USP, 100 units of insulin per milliliter, is a cloudy or milky suspension of 70% crystalline and 30% amorphous purified pork insulin. The insulin substance (the cloudy material) settles at the bottom of the vial, therefore, the vial must be gently agitated or rotated so that the contents are uniformly mixed before a dose is withdrawn. Lente® Purified Insulin has an intermediate duration of action. The effect of Lente® Purified Insulin begins approximately $2\frac{1}{2}$ hours after injection. The effect is maximal between 7 and 15 hours and ends approximately 22 hours after injection. The time course of action of any insulin may vary considerably in different individuals, or at different times in the same individual. Because of this variation, the time periods listed here should be considered as general guidelines only.

The word "purified" on the label indicates that this insulin differs from standard insulin in that it has undergone additional purification steps (i.e., molecular sieve and ion-exchange chromatography).

NPH PURIFIED PORK ISOPHANE INSULIN SUPSENSION USP 100 units/ml
(formerly PROTAPHANE®)

Description: NPH Purified Pork Isophane Insulin Suspension, USP, 100 units of insulin per milliliter, is a cloudy or milky suspension of purified pork insulin with protamine and zinc. The insulin substance (the cloudy material) settles at the bottom of the vial, therefore, the vial must be gently agitated or rotated so that the contents are uniformly mixed before a dose is withdrawn. NPH Purified Insulin has an intermediate duration of action. The effect of NPH Purified Insulin begins approximately $1\frac{1}{2}$ hours after injection. The effect is maximal between 4 and 12 hours and ends approximately 24 hours after injection. The time course of action of any insulin may vary considerably in different individuals, or at different times in the same individual. Because of this variation, the time periods listed here should be considered as general guidelines only.

The word "purified" on the label indicates that this insulin differs from standard insulin in that it has undergone additional purification steps (i.e., molecular sieve and ion-exchange chromatography).

ULTRALENTE® PURIFIED BEEF EXTENDED INSULIN ZINC SUSPENSION USP 100 units/ml
(formerly ULTRATARD®)

Description: Ultralente® Purified Beef Insulin Zinc Suspension, USP, 100 units of insulin per milliliter, is a cloudy or milky suspension of crystalline purified beef insulin. The insulin substance (the cloudy material) settles at the bottom of the vial, therefore, the vial must be gently agitated or rotated so that the contents are uniformly mixed before a dose is withdrawn. The effect of Ultralente® Purified Insulin begins approximately 4 hours after injection. The effect is maximal betwen 10 and 30 hours and ends approximately 36 hours after injection. The time course of action of any insulin may vary considerably in different individuals, or at different times in the same individual. Because of this variation, the time periods listed here should be considered as general guidelines only.

The word "purified" on the label indicates that this insulin differs from standard insulin in that it has undergone additional purification steps (i.e., molecular sieve and ion-exchange chromatography).

HUMAN INSULIN
NOVOLIN™R
Regular Human Insulin Injection (semi-synthetic) USP
100 units/ml
(formerly Actrapid® Human)

NOVOLIN™R is generically known as Regular Human Insulin Injection (semi-synthetic) USP. The concentration of this product is 100 Units per milliliter. It is a clear, colorless solution which has a short duration of action. The effects of NOVOLIN™R begins approximately $\frac{1}{2}$ hour after injection. The effect is maximal between $2\frac{1}{2}$ and 5 hours and ends approximately 8 hours after injection. The time course of action of any insulin may vary considerably in different individuals or a different times in the same individual. Because of this variation, the time periods listed here should be considered as general guidelines only.

This human insulin (semi-synthetic) is structurally identical to the insulin produced by the human pancreas and has undergone a special purification process. A naturally-occurring enzyme is used in a process which converts pork insulin into human insulin. By this enzymatic transpeptidation process the amino acid alanine in pork insulin is selectively substituted by the amino acid threonine thus forming the human insulin molecule.

NOVOLIN™L
Lente® Human Insulin Zinc Suspension
(semi-synthetic) 100 units/ml
(formerly Monotard® Human)

NOVOLIN™L is generically known as Lente® Human Insulin Zinc Suspension (semi-synthetic). The concentration of this product is 100 units of insulin per milliliter. It is a cloudy or milky suspension of 70% crystalline and 30% amorphous human insulin. The insulin substance (the cloudy material) settles at the bottom of the vial, therefore, the vial must be gently agitated or rotated so that the contents are uniformly mixed before a dose is withdrawn. NOVOLIN™L has an intermediate duration of action. The effect of NOVOLIN™L begins approximately $2\frac{1}{2}$ hours after injection. The effect is maximal between 7 and 15 hours and ends approximately 22 hours after injection. The time course of action for any insulin may vary considerably in different individuals or at different times in the same individual. Because of this variation, the periods listed here should be considered as general guidelines only.

This human insulin (semi-synthetic) is structurally identical to the insulin produced by the human pancreas and has undergone a special purification process. A naturally-occurring enzyme is used in a process which converts pork insulin into human insulin. By this enzymatic-transpeptidation process the amino acid alanine in pork insulin is selectively substituted by the amino acid threonine thus forming the human insulin molecule.

NOVOLIN™N
NPH Human Insulin Isophane Suspension
(semi-synthetic) 100 units/ml

NOVOLIN™N is generically known as NPH Human Insulin Isophane Suspension (semi-synthetic). The concentration of this product is 100 units of insulin per milliliter. It is a cloudy or milky suspension of human insulin with protamine and zinc. The insulin substance (the cloudy material) settles at the bottom of the vial, therefore, the vial must be gently agitated or rotated so that the contents are uniformly mixed before a dose is withdrawn. NOVOLIN™N has an intermediate duration of action. The effect of NOVOLIN™N begins approximately $1\frac{1}{2}$ hours after injection. The effect is maximal between 4 and 12 hours. The full duration of action may last up to 24 hours after injection. The time course of action for any insulin may vary considerably in different individuals, or at different times in the same individual. Because of this variation, the periods listed here should be considered as general guidelines only.

This human insulin (semi-synthetic) is structurally identical to the insulin produced by the human pancreas and has undergone a special purification process. A naturally-occurring enzyme is used in a process which converts pork insulin into human insulin. By this enzymatic-transpeptidation process the amino acid alanine in pork insulin is selectively substituted by the amino acid threonine thus forming the human insulin molecule.

Products are cross-indexed by
generic and chemical names
in the
YELLOW SECTION

Standard Process Laboratories, Inc.
2023 WEST WISCONSIN AVENUE
MILWAUKEE, WI 53233

CHLOROPHYLL COMPLEX PERLES

Composition: Crude, natural chlorophyll extracted from Alfalfa and Tillandsia is a steroid rich source of fat soluble natural Vitamin K (6 Perles supply 3.3 mg. of Vitamin K). Vitamin K is indicated to be essential to the normal function of the liver and the formation of prothrombin, one of the normal constituents of the blood.
Action and Uses: Prothrombin is one of the several clotting agents in the blood. (Ref. #1) On the other hand, *water soluble* extracts of chlorophyll, being chemically altered from their natural form, contain no vitamins. Doses of synthetic Vitamin K have produced hemolytic anemia in rats and the toxicity of *synthetic* Vitamin K is attributed to increased breakdown of the red blood cells, (Ref. #2) whereas it is interesting to note, that administering *natural, fat soluble* Vitamin K, causes a prompt response by the body with the formation of prothrombin. The blood returns to its normal composition. (Ref. #3)
Administration: Three to six perles per day or as directed.
How Supplied: CHLOROPHYLL COMPLEX PERLES in bottles of 60 and 350.
Also Available: CHLOROPHYLL, FAT SOLUBLE OINTMENT in 1½-oz. tube.
References: (1) and (3) *Yearbook of Agriculture*, 1959, (U.S. Government Publication) pages 137-138. (2) *Recommended Dietary Allowances*, (Seventh Edition-1968), National Research Council Publication No. 1694, page 30.

ZYPAN TABLETS
An Enzymatic Digestive Supplement for Common Indigestion

Description: Each ZYPAN TABLET contains 1.0 gr. Pancreatin (3x), plus 0.5 gr. of other Pancreas extracts, 1.5 gr. Pepsin (1:3000), 2.75 gr. Betaine Hydrochloride and 0.15 gr. Ammonium Chloride. ZYPAN is a source of digestive enzymes as derived from fresh, frozen beef pancreas (as pancreatin), with betaine hydrochloride as a source of hydrochloric acid, and ammonium chloride as an acidifying agent. Pancreatin is a source of multiple digestive enzymes, notably as follows: (1) Trypsin, which breaks down *protein* into amino acids, (2) Diastase, which converts *starch* to an absorbable form, and (3) Lipase, which assists in the digestion of *fats*.
Indications: When intestinal fermentative processes result in such conditions as flatulence, bloating, and fullness after meals; a lack of digestive enzymes may be present. A long-term inability to absorb foods, because of incomplete digestion, may affect the general health. Deficient protein digestion should be a primary concern, and mere increase of protein in the diet may not correct a deficiency as efficiently as when aided by the proteolytic enzymes.
Administration: One to two tablets with each meal, or as directed.
How Supplied: Bottles of 90 tablets.

Products are listed alphabetically in the **PINK SECTION**.

Star Pharmaceuticals, Inc.
1990 N.W. 44TH STREET
R. R. 2, BOX 904J
POMPANO BEACH, FL 33067-9802

URO–KP–NEUTRAL®   OTC
[ū'ro-kp-nū'tral]
Phosphorous Supplement

Each peach capsule-shaped, film coated tablet contains:
Phosphorous .... 250 mg.
Potassium .... 49.25 mg.
Sodium .... 250 mg.
Derived from Disodium Phosphate Anhydrous, Dipotassium Phosphate Anhydrous, and Sodium Monobasic Anhydrous.
How Supplied: Bottles of 100, 500.
NDC 0076-0109-03 & 04

UROLENE BLUE®   ℞
[ū'ro-lene blue]
Methylene Blue Tablets

Each tablet contains: Methylene blue USP 65 mg.
How Supplied: Bottles of 100 and 1000.
NDC 0076-0501-03 & 04

VIRILON®   ℞
[vir'i-lon]
Methyltestosterone Macro-Beads Capsules
Oral Androgen Macro-Beads

Each capsule contains: Methyltestosterone Macro-Beads USP 10 mg.
How Supplied: Bottles of 100 and 1000.
NDC 0076-0301-03 & 04

Write for complete prescribing information and samples.

Stellar Pharmacal Corp.
1990 N.W. 44TH STREET
R. R. 2, BOX 904J
POMPANO BEACH, FL 33067-9802

STAR-OTIC®
(See PDR For Nonprescription Drugs)

Stiefel Laboratories, Inc.
2801 PONCE DE LEON BLVD.
CORAL GABLES, FL 33134

DUOFILM®   ℞
[dū-ō-film]

Description: Duofilm is a topical preparation containing 16.7% Salicyclic Acid, U.S.P., and 16.7% Lactic Acid, U.S.P., as the active ingredients in a base of Flexible Collodion, U.S.P.
Duofilm's pharmacologic activity is generally attributed to the keratolytic action of Salicyclic Acid and Lactic Acid.
Clinical Pharmacology: The exact mode of action of Salicyclic Acid and Lactic Acid in the treatment of warts is not known. Their activity appears to be associated with keratolytic action which results in mechanical removal of epidermal cells infected with wart viruses.
Indications and Usage: Duofilm is indicated in the treatment of common warts. See Dosage and Administration section for information on frequency and duration of use.
Contraindications: Duofilm should not be used by diabetics or patients with impaired blood circulation. Do not use on moles, birthmarks, or unusual warts with hair growing from them.
Precautions: Duofilm is for external use only. Do not permit Duofilm to contact eyes or mucosal membranes. If spilled in eyes or on mucosal membranes, flush with water, remove precipitated collodion, and flush with water for an additional 15 minutes.
Duofilm should not be allowed to contact normal skin surrounding wart. Treatment should be discontinued if excessive irritation occurs. Duofilm is highly flammable and should be kept away from fire or flame. Keep bottle tightly capped when not in use. Store at controlled room temperature.
Adverse Reactions: A localized irritant reaction will occur if Duofilm is applied to the normal skin surrounding the wart. The irritation will normally be controlled by temporarily discontinuing use of Duofilm, and by applying the medication only to the wart site when treatment is resumed.
Dosage and Administration: Prior to the application of Duofilm, soak affected area in hot water for at least five minutes. Dry thoroughly with a clean towel.
Apply two to four drops of Duofilm directly to wart once a day using the plastic applicator. Each drop should be permitted to dry before the next is added. Duofilm should be applied with care to avoid contact with normal skin surrounding wart. Treated area should be covered by lightly applied Band-Aid.®
Clinically visible improvement will normally occur during the first two to four weeks of therapy. Maximum resolution may be expected after six to twelve weeks of drug use.
How Supplied: Duofilm is supplied in a ½ oz. bottle with plastic applicator, NDC 0145-6788-05. See Precautions section for special handling and storage conditions.

SCABENE® LOTION   ℞
[skā-bēn]
Lindane USP 1%

Description: Active ingredient: lindane USP 1%. Inert ingredients: 99% in a non-greasy, pleasantly scented base, containing purified water, stearic acid, glyceryl stearate laureth-23, carrageenan, triethanolamine, cetyl alcohol, aminomethyl propanol, fragrance, butylparaben, and methylparaben.
Actions: SCABENE LOTION is an ectoparasiticide for Sarcoptes scabiei (scabies), Pediculus capitis (head lice), Phthirus pubis (crab lice), and their ova.
Indications: SCABENE LOTION is indicated for the treatment of Sarcoptes scabiei (scabies), as well as infestations with Pediculus capitis (head lice), Phthirus pubis (crab lice), and their ova.
Contraindications: SCABENE LOTION is contraindicated in individuals with known hypersensitivity to the product or to any of its components.
Warning: SCABENE LOTION SHOULD BE USED WITH CAUTION ESPECIALLY ON INFANTS, CHILDREN AND IN PREGNANCY. LINDANE PENETRATES HUMAN SKIN AND HAS THE POTENTIAL FOR CNS TOXICITY. STUDIES INDICATE THAT POTENTIAL TOXIC EFFECTS OF TOPICALLY APPLIED LINDANE ARE GREATER IN THE YOUNG. Seizures have been reported after the use of lindane but a cause and effect relationship has not been established. Simultaneous application of lotions, ointments or oils may enhance the percutaneous absorption of lindane.
Warning: Do not contaminate water by disposing of waste—DISCARD BOTTLE WHEN EMPTY—DO NOT REUSE.
Precautions: If accidental ingestion occurs, prompt institution of gastric lavage will rid the body of large amounts of the toxicant. However, since oils favor absorption, saline cathartics for intestinal evacuation should be given rather than oil laxatives. If central nervous system manifestations occur, they can be antagonized by the administration of pentobarbital or phenobarbital.
If accidental contact with the eyes occurs, flush with water. If irritation or sensitization occurs, discontinue use and consult a physician.
Adverse Reactions: Eczematous eruptions due to irritation from this product have been reported.

Continued on next page

Stiefel—Cont.

Administration:
CAUTION: USE ONLY AS DIRECTED.
DO NOT EXCEED
RECOMMENDED DOSAGE.
NOTE: PLEASE READ CAREFULLY.

Directions For Use:
Shake well before using.

Pediculosis capitis (head lice)—Apply a quantity sufficient to cover only the affected and adjacent hairy areas.

The lotion should be rubbed into scalp and hair and left in place for 12 hours followed by thorough washing.

Retreatment is usually not necessary. Demonstrable living lice after 7 days is evidence that retreatment is necessary.

Pediculosis pubis (crab lice)—Apply a sufficient quantity only to cover thinly the hair and skin of the pubic area, and if infested, the thighs, trunk, and axillary regions. The material should be rubbed into the skin and hair and left in place for 12 hours followed by a thorough washing.

Retreatment is usually not necessary. Demonstrable living lice after 7 days indicates that retreatment is necessary. Sexual contacts should be treated simultaneously.

Scabies (Sarcoptes scabiei)—The lotion should be applied to dry skin in a thin layer and rubbed in thoroughly. If crusted lesions are present, a warm bath preceding the medication is helpful. If a warm bath is used, allow the skin to dry and cool before applying the lotion. Usually one ounce is sufficient for an adult. A total body application should be made from the neck down. Scabies rarely affects the head of children or adults but may occur in infants. The lotion should be left on for 8-12 hours and should then be removed by thorough washing. ONE APPLICATION IS USUALLY CURATIVE.

Many patients exhibit persistent pruritus after treatment; this is rarely a sign of treatment failure and is not an indication for retreatment unless living mites can be demonstrated.

How Supplied:
Scabene Lotion 2 ounce (59 ml.) bottle NDC 0145-7064-02
Scabene Lotion 16 ounce (472 ml.) bottle NDC 0145-7064-07

SCABENE® SHAMPOO
[skā-bēn]
(Lindane Shampoo, USP, 1%)

Description: Active Ingredient lindane, USP, 10 mg/ml.

Inert Ingredients: 99% in a cosmetically pleasant shampoo base, containing polyoxyethylene sorbitan monostearate, triethanolamine lauryl sulfate, acetone, fragrance, citric acid and purified water.

Actions: SCABENE SHAMPOO is an ectoparasiticide and ovicide toxic to the parasites, Pediculus capitis (head lice), Phthirus pubis (crab lice) and their ova.

Indications: SCABENE SHAMPOO is indicated for the treatment of patients with Pediculus capitis (head lice), Phthirus pubis (crab lice) and their ova.

Contraindications: SCABENE SHAMPOO is contraindicated for individuals with known sensitivity to the product or to any of its components.

Warning: SCABENE SHAMPOO SHOULD BE USED WITH CAUTION, ESPECIALLY ON INFANTS, CHILDREN AND ON PREGNANT WOMEN. LINDANE PENETRATES HUMAN SKIN AND HAS THE POTENTIAL FOR CNS TOXICITY. STUDIES INDICATE THAT POTENTIAL TOXIC EFFECTS OF TOPICALLY APPLIED LINDANE ARE GREATER IN THE YOUNG.

Seizures have been reported after the use of lindane, but a cause and effect relationship has not been established.

Simultaneous application of creams, ointments or oils may enhance the percutaneous absorption of lindane.

Precautions: If accidental ingestion occurs, prompt institution of gastric lavage will rid the body of large amounts of the toxicant. However, since oils favor absorption, saline cathartics for intestinal evacuation should be given rather than oil laxatives. If central nervous system manifestations occur, they can be antagonized by the administration of pentobarbital or phenobarbital.

If accidental contact with the eyes occurs, flush with water. If irritation or sensitization occurs, discontinue use and contact a physician.

Adverse Reactions: Eczematous eruptions due to irritation from this product have been reported.

Administration:
CAUTION: USE ONLY AS DIRECTED. DO NOT EXCEED RECOMMENDED DOSE.
NOTE: PLEASE READ CAREFULLY.

Directions For Use: Pediculosis Capitis (head lice): (1) Apply a sufficient quantity of the shampoo to thoroughly wet the hair and skin of the infested and adjacent hairy areas. (2) When the hair and skin are thoroughly wetted with the shampoo, add small quantities of water at a time working the shampoo into the hair and skin until a good lather forms. (3) Continue shampooing for four minutes. (4) Rinse thoroughly. Towel briskly. When the hair is dry, any remaining nits or nit shells may be removed by fine-tooth combing or with tweezers.

Pediculosis Pubis (crab lice): (1) Apply a sufficient quantity of the shampoo to thoroughly wet the hair and skin of the infested and adjacent hairy areas. (2) When the hair and skin are thoroughly wetted with the shampoo, add small quantities of water at a time working the shampoo into the hair and skin until a good lather forms. (3) Continue shampooing for four minutes. (4) Rinse thoroughly. Towel briskly. (5) Sexual contacts should be examined and treated if necessary.

Retreatment is usually not necessary. Demonstrable living lice after 7 days indicates that retreatment is required.

Note: Scabene Shampoo is intended for head lice and crab lice infestations and should not be used as a routine shampoo. For other ectoparasitic infestations, such as scabies, the use of Scabene Lotion is recommended.

How Supplied:
SCABENE SHAMPOO 2 fl. oz. (59 ml.) bottle NDC 0145-7066-02
SCABENE SHAMPOO 16 fl. oz. (472 ml.) bottle NDC 0145-7066-07

Stuart Pharmaceuticals
Div. of ICI Americas Inc.
WILMINGTON, DE 19897

ALternaGEL®
[all'terna"jel]
Liquid
High-Potency Aluminum Hydroxide Antacid

Composition: ALternaGEL is available as a white, pleasant-tasting, high-potency aluminum hydroxide liquid antacid.

Each 5 ml. teaspoonful contains 600 mg. aluminum hydroxide (equivalent to dried gel, USP) providing 16 milliequivalents (mEq) of acid-neutralizing capacity (ANC), and less than 2.5 mg. (0.109 mEq) of sodium per teaspoonful (5 ml.).

Action and Uses: ALternaGEL is indicated for the symptomatic relief of hyperacidity associated with peptic ulcer, gastritis, peptic esophagitis, gastric hyperacidity, hiatal hernia, and heartburn.

ALternaGEL will be of special value to those patients for whom magnesium-containing antacids are undesirable, such as patients with renal insufficiency, patients requiring control of attendant G.I. complications resulting from steroid or other drug therapy, and patients experiencing the laxation which may result from magnesium or combination antacid regimens.

Dosage and Administration: One or two teaspoonfuls, as needed, between meals and at bedtime, or as directed by a physician. May be followed by a sip of water if desired.

Warnings: As with all medications, ALternaGEL should be kept out of the reach of children.
ALternaGEL may cause constipation.

Except under the advice and supervision of a physician, more than 18 teaspoonfuls should not be taken in a 24-hour period, or the maximum recommended dosage taken for more than two weeks.

Drug Interaction Precaution: ALternaGEL should not be taken concurrently with an antibiotic containing any form of tetracycline.

How Supplied: ALternaGEL is available in bottles of 12 fluid ounces and 5 fluid ounces, and 1 fluid ounce hospital unit doses. NDC 0038-0860.
Shown in Product Identification Section, page 438

BUCLADIN®-S SOFTAB® Tablets
[bu'cla-din]
(buclizine hydrochloride)

Description: Buclizine hydrochloride is 1-(p-tert-Butylbenzyl) -4- (p-chloro- α -phenylbenzyl) piperazine dihydrochloride. Each tablet contains 50 mg. buclizine hydrochloride.

Actions and Uses: BUCLADIN-S (buclizine hydrochloride) acts centrally to suppress nausea and vomiting.

Indications: BUCLADIN-S is effective in the management of nausea, vomiting, and dizziness associated with motion sickness.

Contraindications: Buclizine hydrochloride, when administered to the pregnant rat, induced fetal abnormalities at doses above the human therapeutic range. Clinical data are not adequate to establish nonteratogenicity in early pregnancy. Until such data are available, buclizine hydrochloride is contraindicated for use in early pregnancy. Buclizine hydrochloride is contraindicated in individuals who have shown a previous hypersensitivity to it.

Warnings: Since drowsiness may occur with use of this drug, patients should be warned of this possibility and cautioned against engaging in activities requiring mental alertness, such as driving a car, or operating heavy machinery or appliances. Safe and effective dosage in children has not been established.

Precaution: This product contains FD&C Yellow #5 (tartrazine) which may cause allergic-type reactions (including bronchial asthma) in certain susceptible individuals. Although the overall incidence of FD&C Yellow #5 (tartrazine) sensitivity in the general population is low, it is frequently seen in patients who also have aspirin hypersensitivity.

Adverse Reactions: Occasionally drowsiness, dryness of mouth, headache, and jitteriness are encountered.

Dosage and Administration: BUCLADIN-S (buclizine hydrochloride) SOFTAB Tablets can be taken without swallowing water. Place the SOFTAB tablet in the mouth and allow it to dissolve, or the tablet may be chewed or swallowed whole.

Adults: One tablet usually serves to alleviate nausea. In severe cases, three tablets a day may be taken. The usual maintenance dosage is one tablet twice daily. In the prevention of motion sickness, one tablet taken at least ½ hour before beginning travel usually suffices. For extended travel, a second tablet may be taken after 4 to 6 hours.

How Supplied: Bottles of 100 scored, yellow, SOFTAB Tablets, identified front "STUART", reverse "864". NDC 0038-0864.
Shown in Product Identification Section, page 439

DIALOSE® Capsules
[di'a-lose]
Stool Softener

Composition: Each capsule contains docusate potassium, 100 mg.

Action and Uses: DIALOSE is indicated for treating constipation due to hardness, or lack of moisture in the intestinal contents. DIALOSE is an effective stool softener, whose gentle action will

for possible revisions Product Information 2037

help to restore normal bowel function gradually, without griping or acute discomfort.
Dosage and Administration:
Adults: Initially, one capsule three times a day.
Children, 6 years and over: One capsule at bedtime, or as directed by physician.
Children, under 6 years: As directed by physician.
It is helpful to increase the daily intake of fluids by taking a glass of water with each dose.
When adequate laxation is obtained, the dose may be adjusted to meet individual needs.
Warning: As with any drug, if you are pregnant or nursing a baby, seek the advice of a health professional before using this product. Keep out of the reach of children.
How Supplied: Bottles of 36, 100, and 500 pink capsules, identified "STUART 470". Also available in 100 capsule unit dose boxes (10 strips of 10 capsules each).
NDC 0038-0470.
Shown in Product Identification Section, page 439

DIALOSE® PLUS Capsules
[*di'a-lose Plus*]
Stool Softener
plus **Peristaltic Activator**

Composition: Each capsule contains docusate potassium, 100 mg. and casanthranol, 30 mg.
Action and Uses: DIALOSE PLUS is indicated for the treatment of constipation generally associated with any of the following: hardness, or lack of moisture in the intestinal contents, or decreased intestinal motility.
DIALOSE PLUS combines the advantages of the stool softener, docusate potassium, with the peristaltic activating effect of casanthranol.
Warning: As with any drug, if you are pregnant or nursing a baby, seek the advice of a health professional before using this product. And, as with any laxative, DIALOSE PLUS should not be used when abdominal pain, nausea, or vomiting are present. Frequent or prolonged use may result in dependence on laxatives. Keep out of the reach of children.
Dosage and Administration:
Adults: Initially, one capsule two times a day.
Children: As directed by physician.
When adequate laxation is obtained the dose may be adjusted to meet individual needs.
It is helpful to increase the daily intake of fluids by taking a glass of water with each dose.
How Supplied: Bottles of 36, 100, and 500 yellow capsules, identified "STUART 475". Also available in 100 capsule unit dose boxes (10 strips of 10 capsules each).
NDC 0038-0475.
Shown in Product Identification Section, page 439

EFFERSYLLIUM® Instant Mix
[*ef'fer-sil'lium*]
Natural Fiber Bulking Agent

Composition: Each rounded teaspoonful, or individual packet (7 g.) contains psyllium hydrocolloid, 3 g.
Actions and Uses: EFFERSYLLIUM produces a soft, lubricating bulk which promotes natural elimination.
EFFERSYLLIUM is not a one-dose, fast-acting purgative or cathartic. Administration for several days may be needed to establish regularity.
Effersyllium contains less than 5 mg. sodium per rounded teaspoonful and is considered dietetically sodium free.
Indications: EFFERSYLLIUM is indicated to restore normal bowel habits in chronic constipation, to promote normal elimination in irritable bowel syndrome, and to ease passage of stools in presence of anorectal disorders.
Dosage and Administration:
Adults: One rounded teaspoonful, or one packet, in a glass of water one to three times a day, or as directed by physician.
Children, 6 years and over: One level teaspoonful, or one-half packet (3.5 g.) in one-half glass of water at bedtime, or as directed by physician. *Children, under 6 years:* As directed by physician.

Directions for Mixing: Pour EFFERSYLLIUM into a *dry* glass, add water and stir briskly. Drink immediately. To avoid caking, always use a *dry* spoon to remove EFFERSYLLIUM from its container. Replace cap tightly. Keep in a dry place.
Caution: People sensitive to psyllium powder should avoid inhalation as it may cause an allergic reaction such as wheezing.
Warning: As with all medications, keep out of the reach of children.
How Supplied: Bottles of 9 oz. and 16 oz. of tan, granular powder. Convenient pouch package 7 g. per packet in boxes of 12 or 24.
NDC 0038-0440.

FERANCEE®
[*fer-an-see*]
Chewable Tablets

Composition: Each tablet contains: iron (from 200 mg. ferrous fumarate), 67 mg. and Vitamin C (as ascorbic acid, 49 mg. and sodium ascorbate, 114 mg.), 150 mg. Contains FD&C Yellow #5 (tartrazine) as a color additive.
Action and Uses: A pleasant-tasting hematinic for iron-deficiency anemias, well-tolerated FERANCEE is particularly useful when chronic blood loss, onset of menses, or pregnancy create additional demands for iron supplementation. The peach-cherry flavored chewable tablets dissolve quickly in the mouth and may be either chewed or swallowed.
Dosage and Administration:
Adults: Two tablets daily, or as directed by physician.
Children over 6 years of age: One tablet daily, or as directed by physician.
Children under 6 years of age: As directed by physician.
How Supplied: Bottles of 100 brown and yellow, two-layer tablets identified "STUART 650" on brown layer. A childproof cap is standard on each bottle as a safeguard against accidental ingestion by children.
NDC 0038-0650.
Shown in Product Identification Section, page 439

FERANCEE®-HP Tablets
[*fer-an-see h p*]
High Potency Hematinic

Composition: Each tablet contains: iron (from 330 mg. ferrous fumarate), 110 mg.; Vitamin C (as ascorbic acid, 350 mg. and sodium ascorbate, 281 mg.), 600 mg.
Action and Uses: FERANCEE-HP is a high potency formulation of iron and vitamin C and is intended for use as either:
(1) a maintenance hematinic for those patients needing a daily iron supplement to maintain normal hemoglobin levels, or
(2) intensive therapy for the acute and/or severe iron deficiency anemia where a high intake of elemental iron is required.
The use of well-tolerated ferrous fumarate provides high levels of elemental iron with a low incidence of gastric distress. The inclusion of 600 mg. of Vitamin C per tablet serves to maintain more of the iron in the absorbable ferrous state.
Precautions: Because FERANCEE-HP contains 110 mg. of elemental iron per tablet, it is recommended that its use be limited to adults, i.e. over age 12 years. As with all medication, FERANCEE-HP should be kept out of the reach of children.
Dosage and Administration:
One-tablet-a-day taken after meals should be sufficient to maintain normal hemoglobin levels in most patients with a history of recurring iron deficiency anemia.
For acute and/or severe iron deficiency anemia, two or three tablets per day taken one tablet per dose after meals. (Each tablet provides 110 mg. elemental iron).
How Supplied: FERANCEE-HP is supplied in bottles of 60 red, film coated, oval shaped tablets.

NDC 0038-0863.
Note: A childproof safety cap is standard on each bottle of 60 tablets as a safeguard against accidental ingestion by children.
Shown in Product Identification Section, page 439

HIBICLENS® Antiseptic Antimicrobial
[*hibi-klenz*]
Skin Cleanser
(chlorhexidine gluconate)

Description: HIBICLENS is an antiseptic antimicrobial skin cleanser possessing bactericidal activities. HIBICLENS contains 4% chlorhexidine gluconate, a chemically unique hexamethylenebis biguanide, in a mild, sudsing base adjusted to pH 5.0–6.5 for optimal activity and stability as well as compatability with the normal pH of the skin.
Action: HIBICLENS is bactericidal on contact. It has antiseptic activity and a persistent antimicrobial effect against a wide range of microorganisms, including gram-positive bacteria, and gram-negative bacteria such as *Pseudomonas aeruginosa*. The effectiveness of HIBICLENS is not significantly reduced by the presence of organic matter, such as pus or blood.[1]
In a study[2] simulating surgical use, the immediate bactericidal effect of HIBICLENS after a single six-minute scrub resulted in a 99.9% reduction in resident bacterial flora, with a reduction of 99.98% after the eleventh scrub. Reductions on surgically gloved hands were maintained over the six-hour test period.
HIBICLENS displays persistent antimicrobial action. In one study[2], 93% of a radiolabeled formulation of HIBICLENS remained present on uncovered skin after five hours.
Hibiclens prevents skin infection thereby reducing the risk of cross-infection.
Indications: HIBICLENS is indicated for use as a surgical scrub, as a health-care personnel handwash, for preoperative showering and bathing, as a patient preoperative skin preparation, and as a skin wound cleanser and general skin cleanser.
Safety: The extensive use of chlorhexidine gluconate for over 20 years outside the United States has produced no evidence of absorption of the compound through intact skin. The potential for producing skin reactions is extremely low. HIBICLENS can be used many times a day without causing irritation, dryness, or discomfort. When used for cleaning superficial wounds, HIBICLENS will neither cause additional tissue injury nor delay healing.
Precautions: HIBICLENS is for topical use only. The sudsing formulation may be irritating to the eyes. If HIBICLENS should get into the eyes, rinse out promptly and thoroughly with water. Keep out of ears. Chlorhexidine gluconate, like various other antimicrobial agents, has been reported to cause deafness when instilled in the middle ear. In the presence of a perforated eardrum particular care should be taken to prevent exposure of inner ear tissues to HIBICLENS.
HIBICLENS should not be used by persons with sensitivity to any of its components. Adverse reactions, including dermatitis and photosensitivity, are rare, but if they do occur, discontinue use. Keep this and all other drugs out of the reach of children.
HIBICLENS is nonstaining but hypochlorite bleaches may react with HIBICLENS to cause brown stains in linens or clothing. Soiled fabrics which have come in contact with HIBICLENS should be laundered without bleach or only with an oxidizing bleach such as sodium perborate. An initial flush operation of linen exposed to HIBICLENS will also be helpful in avoiding stains.
Directions for Use:
Skin wound and general skin cleansing
Thoroughly rinse area to be cleansed with water. Apply sufficient HIBICLENS and wash gently. Rinse again thoroughly.
Patient preoperative skin preparation
Apply HIBICLENS liberally to surgical site and swab for at least two minutes. Dry with a sterile

Continued on next page

Stuart—Cont.

towel. Repeat procedure for an additional two minutes and dry with a sterile towel.

Health-care personnel use

SURGICAL HAND SCRUB

Wet hands and forearms with water. Scrub for 3 minutes with about 5 ml. of HIBICLENS and a wet brush, paying particular attention to the nails, cuticles, and interdigital spaces. A separate nail cleaner may be used. Rinse thoroughly. Wash for an additional 3 minutes with 5 ml. of HIBICLENS and rinse under running water. Dry thoroughly.

Directions for use of HIBICLENS™ Sponge/Brush: Open package and remove nail cleaner. Wet hands. Use nail cleaner under fingernails and to clean cuticles. Wet hands and forearms to the elbow with warm water. (Avoid using very cold or very hot water.) Wet sponge side of sponge/brush. Squeeze and pump immediately to work up adequate lather. Apply lather to hands and forearms using *sponge* side of the product. *Start 3 minute scrub* by using the brush side of the product to scrub *only* nails, cuticles, and interdigital areas. Use sponge side for scrubbing hands and forearms. (Avoid using brush on these more sensitive areas.) Rinse thoroughly with warm water. Scrub for an additional 3 minutes *using sponge side* only. To produce additional lather, add a small amount of water and pump the sponge. (While scrubbing, do not use excessive pressure to produce lather—a small amount of lather is all that is required to adequately cleanse skin with HIBICLENS.) Rinse and dry thoroughly, blotting hands and forearms with a soft sterile towel.

HAND WASH

Wet hands with water. Dispense about 5 ml. of HIBICLENS into cupped hands and wash in a vigorous manner for 15 seconds. Rinse and dry thoroughly.

How Supplied: *For general handwashing locations:* pocket-size, 15 ml. foil Packettes; plastic disposable bottles of 4 oz. and 8 oz. with dispenser caps; and 16 oz. filled globes. *For surgical scrub areas:* disposable, unit-of-use 22 ml. impregnated Sponge/Brushes with nail cleaner; plastic disposable bottles of 32 oz. and 1 gal. The 32-oz. bottle is designed for a special foot-operated wall dispenser. A hand-operated wall dispenser is available for the 16-oz. globe. Hand pumps are available for 16 oz., 32 oz., and 1 gal. sizes.   NDC 0038-0575.

References:
1. Lowbury, EJL, and Lilly, HA: The effect of blood on disinfection of surgeons' hands, Brit. J. Surg. 61:19–21 (Jan.) 1974.
2. Peterson RF, Rosenberg A, Alatary SD: Comparative evaluation of surgical scrub preparations, Surg. Gynecol. Obstet. 146:63–65 (Jan.) 1978.

Shown in Product Identification Section, page 439

HIBISTAT®
[hi-bi-stat]
(chlorhexidine gluconate)
Germicidal Hand Rinse

Description: HIBISTAT is a germicidal hand rinse effective against a wide range of microorganisms. HIBISTAT is a clear, colorless liquid containing 0.5% w/w chlorhexidine gluconate in 70% isopropyl alcohol with emollients.

Actions and Uses: HIBISTAT is indicated for health-care personnel use as a germicidal hand rinse. HIBISTAT is for hand hygiene on physically clean hands. It is used in those situations where hands are physically clean, but in need of degerming, when routine handwashing is not convenient or desirable. HIBISTAT provides rapid germicidal action and has a persistent effect.

HIBISTAT should be used in-between patients and procedures where there are no sinks available or continued return to the sink area is inconvenient or time-consuming. HIBISTAT can be used as an alternative to detergent-based products when hands are physically clean. Also, HIBISTAT is an effective germicidal hand rinse following a soap and water handwash.

Cautions: Keep out of eyes and ears. If HIBISTAT should get into eyes or ears, rinse out promptly and thoroughly with water. Chlorhexidine gluconate has been reported to cause deafness when instilled in the middle ear through perforated ear drums. Irritation or other adverse reactions, such as dermatitis or photosensitivity are rare, but if they do occur, discontinue use. Keep this and all other drugs out of the reach of children.

Avoid excessive heat (104°F).

Directions for Use: Dispense about 5 ml. of HIBISTAT into cupped hands and rub vigorously until dry (about 15 seconds), paying particular attention to nails and interdigital spaces. HIBISTAT dries rapidly in use. No water or toweling are necessary.

How Supplied: In plastic disposable bottles of 4 oz. and 8 oz. with flip-top cap.
NDC 0038-0585.

Shown in Product Identification Section, page 439

KASOF® Capsules
[kay'sof]
High Strength Stool Softener

Composition: Each KASOF capsule contains docusate potassium, 240 mg.

Action and Uses: KASOF provides a highly efficient wetting action to restore moisture to the bowel, thus softening the stool to prevent straining. KASOF is especially valuable for the severely constipated, as well as patients with anorectal disorders, such as hemorrhoids and anal fissures. KASOF is ideal for patients with any condition that can be complicated by straining at stool, for example, cardiac patients. The action of KASOF does not interfere with normal peristalsis and generally does not cause griping or extreme sensation of urgency. KASOF is sodium-free, containing a unique potassium formulation, without the problems associated with sodium intake. The simple, one-a-day dosage helps assure patient compliance in maintaining normal bowel function.

Dosage and Administration: Adults: 1 KASOF capsule daily for several days, or until bowel movements are normal and gentle. It is helpful to increase the daily intake of fluids by drinking a glass of water with each dose.

Warning: As with any drug, if you are pregnant or nursing a baby, seek the advice of a health professional before using this product.

How Supplied: KASOF is available in bottles of 30 and 60 brown, gelatin capsules, identified "Stuart 380".
NDC 0038-0380.

Shown in Product Identification Section, page 439

KINESED® Tablets   R
[kin-e-sed]
(belladonna alkaloids and phenobarbital)

Description: Each chewable, fruit-flavored, scored, oval tablet contains:
Phenobarbital..16 mg.
(Warning: May be habit forming)
Hyoscyamine Sulfate...............................0.12 mg.
Atropine Sulfate
Scopolamine Hydrobromide................0.007 mg.

Actions: This drug combination provides natural belladonna alkaloids in a specific, fixed ratio combined with phenobarbital to provide peripheral anticholinergic/antispasmodic action and mild sedation.

Indications: Based on a review of this drug by the National Academy of Sciences—National Research Council, and/or other information, FDA has classified the following indications as "possibly" effective:

For use as adjunctive therapy in the treatment of irritable bowel syndrome (irritable colon, spastic colon, mucous colitis) and acute enterocolitis.

May also be useful as adjunctive therapy in the treatment of duodenal ulcer. IT HAS NOT BEEN SHOWN CONCLUSIVELY WHETHER ANTICHOLINERGIC/ANTISPASMODIC DRUGS AID IN THE HEALING OF A DUODENAL ULCER, DECREASE THE RATE OF RECURRENCES, OR PREVENT COMPLICATIONS.

Contraindications: Glaucoma, obstructive uropathy (for example, bladder neck obstruction due to prostatic hypertrophy); obstructive disease of the gastrointestinal tract (as in achalasia, pyloroduodenal stenosis, etc.); paralytic ileus, intestinal atony of the elderly or debilitated patient; unstable cardiovascular status in acute hemorrhage; severe ulcerative colitis especially if complicated by toxic megacolon; myasthenia gravis; hiatal hernia associated with reflux esophagitis.

KINESED is contraindicated in patients with known hypersensitivity to any of the ingredients. Phenobarbital is contraindicated in acute intermittent porphyria and in those patients in whom phenobarbital produces restlessness and/or excitement.

Warnings: In the presence of a high environmental temperature, heat prostration can occur with belladonna alkaloids (fever and heatstroke due to decreased sweating). Diarrhea may be an early symptom of incomplete intestinal obstruction, especially in patients with ileostomy or colostomy. In this instance treatment with this drug would be inappropriate and possibly harmful.

KINESED may produce drowsiness or blurred vision. The patient should be warned, should these occur, not to engage in activities requiring mental alertness, such as operating a motor vehicle or other machinery, and not to perform hazardous work.

Phenobarbital may decrease the effect of anticoagulants, and necessitate larger doses of the anticoagulant for optimal effect. When the phenobarbital is discontinued, the dose of the anticoagulant may have to be decreased.

Phenobarbital may be habit forming and should not be administered to individuals known to be addiction prone or those with a history of physical and/or psychological dependence upon drugs.

Since barbiturates are metabolized in the liver, they should be used with caution and initial doses should be small in patients with hepatic dysfunction.

Precautions: Use with caution in patients with: autonomic neuropathy, hepatic or renal disease, hyperthyroidism, coronary heart disease, congestive heart failure, cardiac arrhythmias, tachycardia, and hypertension.

Belladonna alkaloids may produce a delay in gastric emptying (antral stasis) which would complicate the management of gastric ulcer. Theoretically, with overdosage, a curare-like action may occur.

Carcinogenesis, mutagenesis. Long-term studies in animals have not been performed to evaluate carcinogenic potential.

Pregnancy Category C. Animal reproduction studies have not been conducted with KINESED. It is not known whether KINESED can cause fetal harm when administered to a pregnant woman or can affect reproduction capacity. KINESED should be given to a pregnant woman only if clearly needed.

Nursing mothers. Because belladonna alkaloids are excreted in human milk, caution should be exercised when KINESED is administered to a nursing mother.

Adverse Reactions: Adverse reactions may include xerostomia; urinary hesitancy and retention; blurred vision; tachycardia; palpitation; mydriasis; cycloplegia; increased ocular tension; loss of taste sense; headache; nervousness; drowsiness; weakness; dizziness; insomnia; nausea; vomiting; impotence; suppression of lactation; constipation; bloated feeling; severe allergic reaction or drug idiosyncrasies, including anaphylaxis, urticaria and other dermal manifestations; and decreased sweating. Elderly patients may react with symptoms of excitement, agitation, drowsiness, and other untoward manifestations to even small doses of the drug.

Phenobarbital may produce excitement in some patients, rather than a sedative effect. In patients habituated to barbiturates, abrupt withdrawal may produce delirium or convulsions.

Dosage and Administration: The dosage of KINESED chewable tablets should be adjusted to the needs of the individual patient to assure symptomatic control with a minimum of adverse effects.
ADULTS: One or two KINESED tablets, three or four times daily, chewed or swallowed with liquids.
CHILDREN, 2 to 12 years: One-half to one KINESED tablet, three or four times daily, chewed or swallowed with liquids.

Overdosage: The signs and symptoms of overdose are headache, nausea, vomiting, blurred vision, dilated pupils, hot and dry skin, dizziness, dryness of the mouth, difficulty in swallowing and CNS stimulation. Treatment should consist of gastric lavage, emetics, and activated charcoal. If indicated, parenteral cholinergic agents such as physostigmine or bethanechol chloride should be added.

How Supplied: Bottles of 100 scored, oval, fruit-flavored, chewable tablets (embossed front "STUART," reverse "220"). Store at room temperature; avoid excess heat. Dispense in well-closed, light-resistant container. NDC 0038-0220.

Shown in Product Identification Section, page 439

MULVIDREN®-F SOFTAB® Tablets ℞
[*mul' vi-dren"*]
(fluoride with multivitamins)

Composition: Each tablet contains: fluoride (as 2.2 mg. sodium fluoride), 1 mg.; Vitamin A (as palmitate), 4,000 USP units; Vitamin D (ergocalciferol), 400 USP units; Vitamin C (as ascorbic acid, and sodium ascorbate), 75 mg.; thiamine mononitrate, 2 mg.; riboflavin, 2 mg.; Vitamin B₆ (as pyridoxine hydrochloride), 1.2 mg.; Vitamin B₁₂ (cyanocobalamin), 3 mcg.; niacinamide, 10 mg.; calcium pantothenate, 3 mg.

Action and Uses: As an aid in promoting the development of caries-resistant teeth, MULVIDREN-F provides a source of daily fluoride supplementation in addition to full nutritional amounts of vitamins. Controlled studies show that a definite decrease in the incidence of dental caries is obtained in children receiving an optimal nutritional supply of fluoride. These studies indicate that in order to achieve maximal anticariogenic effect, fluoride must be provided throughout the stages of tooth formation and calcification. Thus, fluoride should be provided in adequate amounts to the child from birth through the first fifteen years of life. Fluoride should be made available continuously throughout this period by daily dietary supplementation if natural sources are deficient. MULVIDREN-F SOFTAB is a well-accepted and convenient form of administering fluoride for both topical and systemic effects.

Dosage and Administration: It is necessary to know the fluoride content of drinking water in order to adjust the dosage of this product correctly. Where the drinking water is substantially free of fluoride (i.e. less than 3 parts per million) the following dosage schedule is recommended:
Children, three to sixteen years of age: One tablet daily after a meal. Tablets may be chewed or allowed to dissolve in the mouth.
Children, two to three years of age: One-half tablet daily. Tablets may be chewed or crushed and mixed with food.

Important Note: It is recommended that the daily fluoride intake from dietary supplements such as MULVIDREN-F be adjusted according to the amount of fluoride contained in the drinking water. In communities with less than 0.3 ppm of fluoride in the water supply, the recommended dosage is 0.25 mg. of fluoride daily between birth and two years of age, 0.5 mg. between two and three years of age, and 1.0 mg. between 3 and 16 years of age. Where the water supply contains between 0.3 and 0.7 ppm of fluoride the recommendation is for no supplemental fluoride between birth and two years of age, 0.25 mg. between two and three years of age, and 0.5 mg. of fluoride between three and sixteen years of age. If the water supply contains greater than 0.7 ppm of fluoride then no supplemental fluoride is needed. When prescribing MULVIDREN-F, the physician should make sure the child is not receiving significant amounts of fluoride from other medications.

Precautions: Dental fluorosis (mottling) may result from exceeding the recommended dose. In hypersensitive individuals, fluorides occasionally cause skin eruptions such as atopic dermatitis, eczema or urticaria. Gastric distress, headache and weakness have also been reported. These hypersensitivity reactions usually disappear promptly after discontinuation of the fluoride. In rare cases, a delay in the eruption of teeth has been reported.

Warnings: As in the case of all medications, keep out of the reach of children.

How Supplied: On prescription only, in bottles of 100 orange colored, scored SOFTAB tablets, identified front "Stuart", reverse "710". A child-proof safety cap is standard on each 100 tablet bottle as a safeguard against accidental ingestion by children. NDC 0038-710.

Shown in Product Identification Section, page 439

MYLANTA®
[*my' lan" ta*]
Liquid and Tablets
Antacid/Anti-Gas

Composition: Each chewable tablet or each 5 ml. (one teaspoonful) of liquid contains:
Aluminum hydroxide
 (Dried Gel, USP in tablet and equiv.
 to Dried Gel, USP in liquid) .... 200 mg.
Magnesium hydroxide .... 200 mg.
Simethicone .... 20 mg.

Sodium Content: MYLANTA contains an insignificant amount of sodium per daily dose and is considered dietetically sodium free. Typical values are 0.68 mg. (0.03 mEq) sodium per 5 ml. teaspoonful of liquid; 0.77 mg. (0.03 mEq) per tablet.

Sugar Content: 375 mg. dextrose per tablet.

Acid Neutralizing Capacity: Each teaspoonful of MYLANTA liquid will neutralize 12.7 mEq of acid. Each MYLANTA tablet will neutralize 11.5 mEq.

Actions and Uses: MYLANTA, a well-balanced combination of two antacids and simethicone, provides consistently dependable relief of symptoms associated with gastric hyperacidity, and mucus-entrapped air or "gas". These indications include:
 Common heartburn (pyrosis)
 Hiatal hernia
 Peptic esophagitis
 Gastritis
 Peptic ulcer

The exceptionally pleasant tasting liquid and soft, easy-to-chew tablets encourage patients' acceptance, thereby minimizing the skipping of prescribed doses. MYLANTA is appropriate whenever there is a need for effective relief of temporary gastric hyperacidity and mucus-entrapped gas.

Dosage and Administration: One or two teaspoonfuls of liquid or one or two tablets, well-chewed, every two to four hours between meals and at bedtime, or as directed by physician.

Warning: Magnesium hydroxide and other magnesium salts, in the presence of renal insufficiency, may cause central nervous system depression and other symptoms of hypermagnesemia.

Drug Interaction Precaution: Do not use this product for any patient receiving a prescription antibiotic containing any form of tetracycline.

How Supplied: MYLANTA is available as a white, pleasant tasting liquid suspension, and as a two-layer yellow and white chewable tablet, identified on yellow layer "STUART 620". Liquid supplied in bottles of 5 oz. and 12 oz. Tablets supplied in boxes of individually wrapped 40's and 100's, economy size bottles of 180, and consumer convenience packs of 48. Also available for hospital use in liquid unit dose bottles of 1 oz., and bottles of 5 oz.
NDC 0038-0610 (liquid). NDC 0038-0620 (tablets).

Shown in Product Identification Section, page 439

MYLANTA®-II
[*my' lan" ta*]
Liquid and Tablets
Double Strength Antacid/Anti-Gas

Composition: Each chewable tablet or each 5 ml. (one teaspoonful) of liquid contains:
Aluminum hydroxide
 (Dried Gel, USP in tablet and equiv.
 to Dried Gel, USP in liquid)   400 mg.
Magnesium hydroxide   400 mg.
Simethicone   30 mg.

Sodium Content: MYLANTA-II contains an insignificant amount of sodium per daily dose and is considered dietetically sodium free. Typical values are 1.14 mg. (0.05 mEq) sodium per 5 ml. teaspoonful of liquid; 1.3 mg. (0.06 mEq) per tablet.

Sugar Content: 110 mg. sucrose per tablet.

Acid Neutralizing Capacity: Each teaspoonful of MYLANTA-II liquid will neutralize 25.4 mEq of acid. Each MYLANTA-II tablet will neutralize 23.0 mEq.

Actions and Uses: MYLANTA-II is a double strength antacid with an antiflatulent. The exceptionally pleasant tasting liquid and soft, easy-to-chew tablets encourage patient acceptance, thereby minimizing the skipping of prescribed doses. MYLANTA-II provides consistently dependable relief of the symptoms of peptic ulcer and other problems related to acid hypersecretion. The high potency of MYLANTA-II is achieved through its concentration of noncalcium antacid ingredients. Thus MYLANTA-II can produce both rapid and long lasting neutralization without the acid rebound associated with calcium carbonate. The balanced formula of aluminum and magnesium hydroxides minimizes undesirable bowel effects. Simethicone is effective for the relief of concomitant distress caused by mucus-entrapped gas and swallowed air.

Dosage and Administration: One or two teaspoonfuls of liquid, or one or two tablets, well-chewed, between meals and at bedtime, or as directed by physician.
Because patients with peptic ulcer vary greatly in both acid output and gastric emptying time, the amount and schedule of dosages should be varied accordingly.

Warning: Magnesium hydroxide and other magnesium salts, in the presence of renal insufficiency, may cause central nervous system depression and other symptoms of hypermagnesemia.

Drug Interaction Precaution: Do not use this product for any patient receiving a prescription antibiotic containing any form of tetracycline.

How Supplied: MYLANTA-II is available as a white, pleasant tasting liquid suspension, and a two-layer green and white chewable tablet, identified on green layer "STUART 851". Liquid supplied in 5 oz. and 12 oz. bottles. Tablets supplied in boxes of 24 and 60 individually wrapped chewable tablets. Also available for hospital use in liquid unit dose bottles of 1 oz., and bottles of 5 oz.
NDC 0038-0852 (liquid). NDC 0038-0851 (tablets).

Shown in Product Identification Section, page 439

MYLICON® Tablets and Drops
[*my' li-con*]
Antiflatulent

Composition: Each tablet or 0.6 ml. of drops contains simethicone, 40 mg.

Sugar Content: 356 mg. lactose per tablet.

Action and Uses: For relief of the painful symptoms of excess gas in the digestive tract. MYLICON is a valuable adjunct in the treatment of many conditions in which the retention of gas may be a problem, such as: postoperative gaseous distention, air swallowing, functional dyspepsia, peptic ulcer, spastic or irritable colon, diverticulitis. The defoaming action of MYLICON relieves flatulence by dispersing and preventing the formation of mucus-surrounded gas pockets in the gastrointestinal tract. MYLICON acts in the stomach and intestines to change the surface tension of gas bubbles enabling them to coalesce; thus the gas is

Continued on next page

Stuart—Cont.

freed and is eliminated more easily by belching or passing flatus.

Dosage and Administration:
Tablets—One or two tablets four times daily after meals and at bedtime. May also be taken as needed up to 12 tablets daily or as directed by a physician. TABLETS SHOULD BE CHEWED THOROUGHLY.

Drops—0.6 ml. four times daily after meals and at bedtime. May also be taken as needed up to 500 mg. daily or as directed by a physician. Shake well before using.

How Supplied: Bottles of 100 and 500 white, scored, chewable tablets, identified front "STUART", reverse "450," and dropper bottles of 30 ml. (1 fl. oz.) pink, pleasant tasting liquid. Also available in 100 tablet unit dose boxes (10 strips of 10 tablets each).
NDC 0038-0450 (tablets).
NDC 0038-0630 (drops).

Shown in Product Identification Section, page 439

MYLICON®-80 Tablets
[*my'li-con*]
High-Capacity Antiflatulent

Composition: Each tablet contains simethicone, 80 mg.

Sugar Content: 349 mg. lactose per tablet.

Action and Uses: For relief of the painful symptoms of excess gas in the digestive tract. MYLICON-80 is a high capacity antiflatulent for adjunctive treatment of many conditions in which the retention of gas may be a problem, such as the following: air swallowing, functional dyspepsia, postoperative gaseous distention, peptic ulcer, spastic or irritable colon, diverticulitis.

MYLICON-80 has a defoaming action that relieves flatulence by dispersing and preventing the formation of mucus-surrounded gas pockets in the gastrointestinal tract. MYLICON-80 acts in the stomach and intestines to change the surface tension of gas bubbles enabling them to coalesce; thus, the gas is freed and is eliminated more easily by belching or passing flatus.

Dosage and Administration: One tablet four times daily after meals and at bedtime. May also be taken as needed up to 6 tablets daily or as directed by a physician. TABLETS SHOULD BE CHEWED THOROUGHLY.

How Supplied: Economical bottles of 100 and convenience packages of individually wrapped 12 and 48 pink, scored, chewable tablets identified "STUART 858". Also available in 100 tablet unit dose boxes (10 strips of 10 tablets each).
NDC 0038-0858.

Shown in Product Identification Section, page 439

NOLVADEX® 10 mg. Tablets   R
[*nol'va-dex*]
(tamoxifen citrate)

Description: NOLVADEX (tamoxifen citrate) tablets for oral administration contain 15.2 mg. of tamoxifen citrate, which is equivalent to 10 mg. of tamoxifen. It is a nonsteroidal antiestrogen.
Chemically, NOLVADEX is the trans-isomer of a triphenylethylene derivative. The chemical name is (Z)-2-[4-(1,2-diphenyl-1-butenyl) phenoxy]- N, N dimethylethanamine 2-hydroxy-1,2,3-propanetricarboxylate(1:1).

NOLVADEX is intended only for oral administration; the tablets should be protected from heat and light.

Clinical Pharmacology: NOLVADEX is a nonsteroidal agent which has demonstrated potent antiestrogenic properties in animal test systems. The antiestrogenic effects may be related to its ability to compete with estrogen for binding sites in target tissues such as breast. Tamoxifen inhibits the induction of rat mammary carcinoma induced by dimethylbenzanthracene (DMBA), and causes the regression of already established DMBA-induced tumors. In this rat model, tamoxifen appears to exert its antitumor effects by binding to estrogen receptors.

In cytosols derived from human breast adenocarcinomas, tamoxifen competes with estradiol for estrogen receptor protein.

Preliminary pharmacokinetics in women using radio-labeled tamoxifen has shown that most of the radioactivity is slowly excreted in the feces, with only small amounts appearing in urine. The drug is excreted mainly as conjugates, with unchanged drug and hydroxylated metabolites accounting for 30% of the total.

Blood levels of total radioactivity following single oral doses of approximately 0.3 mg./kg. reached peak values of 0.06–0.14 μg/ml. at 4–7 hours after dosing, with only 20–30% of the drug present as tamoxifen. There was an initial half-life of 7–14 hours with secondary peaks four or more days later. The prolongation of blood levels and fecal excretion is believed to be due to enterohepatic circulation.

Indications and Usage: NOLVADEX has proven useful in the palliative treatment of advanced breast cancer in postmenopausal women. Available evidence indicates that patients who have had a recent negative estrogen receptor assay are unlikely to respond to NOLVADEX.

Contraindications: None known.

Warnings: Ocular changes have been reported in a few patients who, as part of a clinical trial, were treated for periods greater than one year with NOLVADEX at doses at least four times the highest recommended daily dose of 40 mg. The ocular changes consist of retinopathy and, in some patients, there are also corneal changes and a decrease in visual acuity.

In addition, a few cases of ocular changes including visual disturbances, corneal changes, and/or retinopathy have been reported in patients treated with NOLVADEX at recommended doses. It is uncertain if these effects are due to NOLVADEX.

As with other additive hormonal therapy (estrogens and androgens), hypercalcemia has been reported in some breast cancer patients with bone metastases within a few weeks of starting treatment with NOLVADEX. If hypercalcemia does occur, appropriate measures should be taken and, if severe, NOLVADEX should be discontinued.

Precautions:
General: NOLVADEX should be used cautiously in patients with existing leukopenia or thrombocytopenia. Observations of leukopenia and thrombocytopenia occasionally have been made, but it is uncertain if these effects are due to NOLVADEX therapy. Transient decreases in platelet counts, usually to 50,000–100,000/ cu. mm., infrequently lower, have been occasionally reported in patients taking NOLVADEX for breast cancer. No hemorrhagic tendency has been recorded and the platelet counts returned to normal levels even though treatment with NOLVADEX continued.

Laboratory Tests: Periodic complete blood counts, including platelet counts, may be appropriate.

Carcinogenesis, Mutagenesis, Impairment of Fertility: Endocrine changes in immature and mature mice were investigated in a 13-month study. Various tumors were found in all treated groups which were related to the estrogenic activity of the compound.

A 14-month chronic study to investigate the effects of low doses in mice was performed. No gonadal tumors were found.

Pregnancy Category C: NOLVADEX has been shown to affect reproductive functions in rats when given at dose levels somewhat higher than the human dose. In reproductive studies in rats, developmental changes of the rib were seen. There are no adequate and well-controlled studies in pregnant women. NOLVADEX should be used during pregnancy only if the potential benefit justifies the potential risk to the fetus.

Nursing Mothers: It is not known whether this drug is excreted in human milk. Because many drugs are excreted in human milk and because of the potential for serious adverse reactions in nursing infants from NOLVADEX, a decision should be made whether to discontinue nursing or to discontinue the drug, taking into account the importance of the drug to the mother.

Adverse Reactions: The most frequent adverse reactions to NOLVADEX are hot flashes, nausea, and vomiting. These may occur in up to one-fourth of patients, but are rarely severe enough to require discontinuation of treatment.

Less frequently reported adverse reactions are vaginal bleeding, vaginal discharge, menstrual irregularities, and skin rash. Usually these have not been of sufficient severity to require dosage reduction or discontinuation of treatment.

Increased bone and tumor pain, and also local disease flare have occurred, which are sometimes associated with a good tumor response. Patients with increased bone pain may require additional analgesics. Patients with soft tissue disease may have sudden increases in the size of preexisting lesions, sometimes associated with marked erythema within and surrounding the lesions, and/or the development of new lesions. When they occur, the bone pain or disease flare are seen shortly after starting NOLVADEX and generally subside rapidly.

Other adverse reactions which are seen infrequently are hypercalcemia, peripheral edema, distaste for food, pruritus vulvae, depression, dizziness, light-headedness, and headache.

If adverse reactions are severe, it is sometimes possible to control them by a simple reduction of dosage without loss of control of the disease.

Overdosage: Acute overdosage in humans has not been reported. Signs observed at the highest doses following studies to determine LD_{50} in animals were respiratory difficulties and convulsions. No specific treatment for overdosage is known; treatment must be symptomatic.

Dosage and Administration: One or two 10 mg. tablets twice a day (morning and evening).

How Supplied: NOLVADEX tablets are white, round, biconvex, uncoated tablets identified with "NOLVADEX 600" debossed on one side and a cameo debossed on the other side. Supplied in bottles of 60 tablets and 250 tablets. Protect from heat and light. NDC0038-0600.

Shown in Product Identification Section, page 439

OREXIN® SOFTAB® Tablets
[*or'ex-in*]

Composition: Each tablet contains: thiamine mononitrate, 10 mg.; Vitamin B_6 (as pyridoxine hydrochloride), 5 mg.; and Vitamin B_{12} (cyanocobalamin), 25 mcg.

Action and Uses: OREXIN is a high-potency vitamin supplement providing thiamine mononitrate and Vitamins B_6 and B_{12}.

OREXIN SOFTAB tablets are specially formulated to dissolve quickly in the mouth. They may be chewed or swallowed. Dissolve tablet in a teaspoonful of water or fruit juice if liquid is preferred.

Dosage and Administration: One tablet daily, or as directed by physician.

How Supplied: Bottles of 100 pale pink SOFTAB tablets, identified "STUART".
NDC 0038-0280.

PROBEC®-T Tablets
[*pro'bek-t*]

Composition: Each tablet contains: Vitamin C (as ascorbic acid, 67 mg. and sodium ascorbate, 600 mg.), 600 mg.; thiamine mononitrate, 15 mg.; riboflavin, 10 mg.; Vitamin B_6 (as pyridoxine hydrochloride), 5 mg.; Vitamin B_{12} (cyanocobalamin), 5 mcg.; niacinamide, 100 mg.; calcium pantothenate, 20 mg.

Action and Uses: PROBEC-T is a high-potency B complex supplement with 600 mg. of Vitamin C in easy to swallow odorless tablets.

Dosage and Administration: One tablet a day with a meal, or as directed by physician.

How Supplied: Bottles of 60, salmon colored, capsule-shaped tablets.
NDC 0038-0840.

Shown in Product Identification Section, page 439

SORBITRATE®
[sorb'i-trate]
(Isosorbide Dinitrate)

Description: SORBITRATE (isosorbide dinitrate), an organic nitrate, is a vasodilator with effects on both arteries and veins.

The chemical name for isosorbide dinitrate is 1,4,3,6-dianhydrosorbitol-2,5-dinitrate.

Isosorbide dinitrate has a molecular weight of 236.14.

Isosorbide dinitrate is a white, crystalline, odorless compound which is stable in air and in solution, has a melting point of 70°C and has an optical rotation of +134° (c = 1.0, alcohol, 20°C). Isosorbide dinitrate is freely soluble in organic solvents such as acetone, alcohol, and ether; but is only sparingly soluble in water.

Clinical Pharmacology: The principal pharmacological action of isosorbide dinitrate is relaxation of vascular smooth muscle, producing a vasodilatory effect on both peripheral arteries and veins, with predominant effects on the latter. Dilation of the post-capillary vessels, including large veins, promotes peripheral pooling of blood and decreases venous return to the heart, thereby reducing left-ventricular end-diastolic pressure (preload). Arteriolar relaxation reduces systemic vascular resistance and arterial pressure (after-load). The mechanism by which isosorbide dinitrate relieves angina pectoris is not fully understood. Myocardial oxygen consumption or demand (as measured by the pressure-rate product, tension-time index, and stroke-work index) is decreased by both the arterial and venous effects of isosorbide dinitrate and, presumably, a more favorable supply-demand ratio is achieved. While the large epicardial coronary arteries are also dilated by isosorbide dinitrate, the extent to which this contributes to relief of exertional angina is unclear.

Therapeutic doses of isosorbide dinitrate may reduce systolic, diastolic, and mean arterial blood pressures, especially in the upright posture. Effective coronary perfusion is usually maintained. The decrease in systemic blood pressure may result in reflex tachycardia, an effect which results in an unfavorable influence on myocardial oxygen demand. Hemodynamic studies indicate that isosorbide dinitrate may reduce the abnormally elevated left ventricular end-diastolic and pulmonary capillary wedge pressures that occur during an acute episode of angina pectoris.

Isosorbide dinitrate is metabolized by enzymatic denitration to the intermediate products isosorbide-2-mononitrate and isosorbide-5-mononitrate. Both metabolites have biological activity, especially the 5-mononitrate which is also the principal metabolite. The liver is a principal site of metabolism and isosorbide dinitrate is subject to a large first-pass effect. The systemic clearance of the drug following intravenous infusion is about 3.4 liters/min. Since the clearance exceeds hepatic blood flow, considerable extrahepatic metabolism must also occur.

The average bioavailability of isosorbide dinitrate is 59 and 22 percent following sublingual and oral administration, respectively. The terminal half-life is about 20 minutes, 60 minutes, and 4 hours following i.v., sublingual, and oral administration, respectively. The dependence of half-life on the route of administration is not understood. Over limited ranges of i.v. dosing, the pharmacokinetics of isosorbide dinitrate appear linear. However, both the 2- and 5-mononitrate metabolites have been shown to decrease the rate of disappearance of the dinitrate from the blood and the half-lives of isosorbide-5-mononitrate and isosorbide-2-mononitrate range from 4.0–5.6 and 1.5–3.1 hours, respectively.

The pharmacokinetics and/or bioavailability of isosorbide dinitrate during multiple dosing have not been well studied. Because the metabolites influence the clearance of isosorbide dinitrate, prediction of blood levels of parent compound or metabolites from single-dose studies is uncertain.

Indications and Usage: SORBITRATE (isosorbide dinitrate) is indicated for the treatment and prevention of angina pectoris. Controlled clinical trials have demonstrated that the sublingual, chewable, immediate release, and controlled release oral dosage forms of isosorbide dinitrate are effective in improving exercise tolerance in patients with angina pectoris. When single sublingual or chewable doses (5 mg) of isosorbide dinitrate were administered prophylactically to patients with angina pectoris in various clinical studies, duration of exercise until chest pain or fatigue was significantly improved for at least 45 minutes (and as long as 2 hours in some studies) following dosing. Similar studies after single oral (15 to 120 mg) and oral controlled-release (40 to 80 mg) doses of isosorbide dinitrate have shown significant improvement in exercise tolerance for up to 8 hours following dosing. The exercise electrocardiographic evidence suggests that improved exercise tolerance with isosorbide dinitrate is not at the expense of greater myocardial ischemia. All dosage forms of isosorbide dinitrate may therefore be used prophylactically to decrease frequency and severity of anginal attacks and can be expected to decrease the need for sublingual nitroglycerin.

The sublingual and chewable forms of the drug are indicated for acute prophylaxis of angina pectoris when taken a few minutes before situations likely to provoke anginal attacks. Because of a slower onset of effect, the oral forms of isosorbide dinitrate are not indicated for acute prophylaxis.

In controlled clinical trials, chewable and sublingual isosorbide dinitrate were effective in relieving an acute attack of angina pectoris. Relief occurred with a mean time of 2.9 and 3.4 minutes (chewable and sublingual respectively) compared to relief of angina with a mean time of 1.9 minutes following sublingual nitroglycerin. Because of the more rapid relief of chest pain with sublingual nitroglycerin, the use of sublingual or chewable isosorbide dinitrate for aborting an acute anginal attack should be limited to patients intolerant or unresponsive to sublingual nitroglycerin.

Contraindications: SORBITRATE is contraindicated in patients who have shown purported hypersensitivity or idiosyncrasy to it or other nitrates or nitrites.

Warnings: The benefits of SORBITRATE during the early days of an acute myocardial infarction have not been established. If one elects to use organic nitrates in early infarction, hemodynamic monitoring and frequent clinical assessment should be used because of the potential deleterious effects of hypotension.

Precautions:

General: Severe hypotensive response, particularly with upright posture, may occur with even small doses of SORBITRATE. The drug should therefore be used with caution in subjects who may have blood volume depletion from diuretic therapy or in subjects who have low systolic blood pressure (e.g., below 90 mmHg). Paradoxical bradycardia and increased angina pectoris may accompany nitrate-induced hypotension.

Nitrate therapy may aggravate the angina caused by hypertrophic cardiomyopathy. Tolerance to this drug and cross-tolerance to other nitrates and nitrites may occur.

Marked symptomatic, orthostatic hypotension has been reported when calcium channel blockers and organic nitrates were used in combination. Dose adjustment of either class of agents may be necessary.

Tolerance to the vascular and antianginal effects of isosorbide dinitrate or nitroglycerin has been demonstrated in clinical trials, experience through occupational exposure, and in isolated tissue experiments in the laboratory. The importance of tolerance to the appropriate use of isosorbide dinitrate in the management of patients with angina pectoris has not been determined. However, one clinical trial using treadmill exercise tolerance (as an endpoint) found an 8-hour duration of action of oral isosorbide dinitrate following the first dose (after a 2-week placebo washout) and only a 2-hour duration of effect of the same dose after 1 week of repetitive dosing at conventional dosing intervals. On the other hand, several trials have been able to differentiate isosorbide dinitrate from placebo after 4 weeks of therapy, and in open trials, an effect seems detectable for as long as several months.

Tolerance clearly occurs in industrial workers continuously exposed to nitroglycerin. Moreover, physical dependence also occurs since chest pain, acute myocardial infarction, and even sudden death have occurred during temporary withdrawal of nitroglycerin from the workers. In clinical trials in angina patients, there are reports of anginal attacks being more easily provoked and of rebound in the hemodynamic effects soon after nitrate withdrawal. The relative importance of these observations to the routine, clinical use of isosorbide dinitrate is not known. However, it seems prudent to gradually withdraw patients from isosorbide dinitrate when the therapy is being terminated, rather than stopping the drug abruptly.

Information for Patients: Headache may occur during initial therapy with SORBITRATE. Headache is usually relieved by the use of standard headache remedies, or by lowering the dose, and tends to disappear after the first week or two of use.

Drug Interactions: Alcohol may enhance any marked sensitivity to the hypotensive effect of nitrates.

Isosorbide dinitrate acts directly on vascular smooth muscle; therefore, any other agent that depends on vascular smooth muscle as the final common path can be expected to have decreased or increased effect depending on the agent.

Carcinogenesis, Mutagenesis, Impairment of Fertility: No long-term studies in animals have been performed to evaluate the carcinogenic potential of this drug. A modified two-litter reproduction study in rats fed isosorbide dinitrate at 25 or 100 mg/kg/day did not reveal any effects on fertility or gestation or any remarkable gross pathology in any parent or offspring fed isosorbide dinitrate as compared with rats fed a basal-controlled diet.

Pregnancy Category C: Isosorbide dinitrate has been shown to cause a dose-related increase in embryotoxicity (increase in mummified pups) in rabbits at oral doses 35 and 150 times the maximum recommended human daily dose. There are no adequate and well-controlled studies in pregnant women. SORBITRATE should be used during pregnancy only if the potential benefit justifies the potential risk to the fetus.

Nursing Mothers: It is not known whether this drug is excreted in human milk. Because many drugs are excreted in human milk, caution should be exercised when SORBITRATE is administered to a nursing woman.

Pediatric Use: The safety and effectiveness of SORBITRATE in children has not been established.

Adverse Reactions: Adverse reactions, particularly headache and hypotension, are dose related. In clinical trials at various doses, the following have been observed.

Headache is the most common (reported incidence varies widely, apparently being dose related, with an average occurrence of about 25%) adverse reaction and may be severe and persistent. Cutaneous vasodilation with flushing may occur. Transient episodes of dizziness and weakness, as well as other signs of cerebral ischemia associated with postural hypotension, may occasionally develop (the incidence of reported symptomatic hypotension ranges from 2% to 36%). An occasional individual will exhibit marked sensitivity to the hypotensive effects of nitrates and severe responses (nausea, vomiting, weakness, restlessness, pallor, perspiration, and collapse) may occur even with the usual therapeutic dose. Drug rash and/or exfoliative dermatitis may occasionally occur. Nausea and vomiting appear to be uncommon.

Overdosage:

Signs and Symptoms: These may include the following: a prompt fall in blood pressure, persistent and throbbing headache, vertigo, palpitation, visual disturbances, flushed and perspiring skin (later becoming cold and cyanotic), nausea and

Continued on next page

Stuart—Cont.

vomiting (possibly with colic and even bloody diarrhea), syncope (especially in the upright position), methemoglobinemia with cyanosis and anoxia, initial hyperpnea, dyspnea and slow breathing, slow pulse (dicrotic and intermittent), heart block, increased intracranial pressure with cerebral symptoms of confusion and moderate fever, paralysis and coma followed by clonic convulsions and possibly death due to circulatory collapse.

It is not known what dose of the drug is associated with symptoms of overdosing or what dose of the drug would be life-threatening. The acute oral LD$_{50}$ of isosorbide dinitrate in rats was found to be approximately 1100 mg/kg of body weight. These animal experiments indicate that approximately 500 times the usual therapeutic dose would be required to produce such toxic symptoms in humans. It is not known whether the drug is dialyzable.

Treatment of Overdose: Prompt removal of the ingested material by gastric lavage is reasonable, but not documented to be useful. Keep the patient recumbent in a shock position and comfortably warm. Passive movements of the extremities may aid venous return. Administer oxygen and artificial respiration if necessary. If methemoglobinemia is present, administer methylene blue (1% solution), 1 to 2 mg/kg intravenously.

Methemoglobin: Case reports of clinically significant methemoglobinemia are rare at conventional doses of organic nitrates. The formation of methemoglobin is dose related and in the case of genetic abnormalities of hemoglobin that favor methemoglobin formulation, even conventional doses of organic nitrate could produce harmful concentrations of methemoglobin.

Warning: Epinephrine is ineffective in reversing the severe hypotensive events associated with overdose. It and related compounds are contraindicated in this situation.

Dosage and Administration: For the treatment of angina pectoris, the usual starting dose for sublingual SORBITRATE is 2.5 to 5 mg; for chewable tablets, 5 mg; for oral (swallowed) tablets, 5 to 20 mg; and for controlled release forms, 40 mg. SORBITRATE should be titrated upward until angina is relieved or side effects limit the dose. In ambulatory patients, the magnitude of the incremental dose increase should be guided by measurements of standing blood pressure.

The initial dosage of sublingual or chewable SORBITRATE for prophylactic therapy in angina pectoris patients is generally 5 or 10 mg every 2 to 3 hours. Adequate, controlled clinical studies demonstrating the effectiveness of chronic maintenance therapy with these dosage forms have not been reported.

SORBITRATE in oral doses of 10 to 40 mg given every 6 hours or in oral controlled release doses of 40 to 80 mg given every 8 to 12 hours is generally recommended. The extent to which development of tolerance should modify the dosage program has not been defined. The oral controlled release forms of isosorbide dinitrate should not be chewed.

How Supplied:
SORBITRATE® Sublingual
2.5 mg Sublingual Tablets. (NDC-0038-0853) White, round tablets (identified front "S", reverse "853") are supplied in bottles of 100, 500, and Unit Dose 100.
Inactive Ingredients: lactose, magnesium stearate, starch.
5 mg Sublingual Tablets. (NDC-0038-0760) Pink, round tablets (identified front "S", reverse "760") are supplied in bottles of 100, 500, and Unit Dose 100.
Inactive Ingredients: FD&C Red #3 aluminum lake, lactose, magnesium stearate, starch.
10 mg Sublingual Tablets. (NDC-0038-0761) Yellow, round tablets (identified front "S", reverse "761") are supplied in bottles of 100 and Unit Dose 100.

Inactive Ingredients: D&C Yellow #10 aluminum lake, FD&C Yellow #6 aluminum lake, lactose, magnesium stearate, starch.
SORBITRATE® Chewable
5 mg Chewable Tablets. (NDC-0038-0810) Green, round, scored tablets (identified front "STUART", reverse "810") are supplied in bottles of 100, 500, and Unit Dose 100.
Inactive Ingredients: confectioner's sugar, D&C Yellow #10 aluminum lake, FD&C Blue #1 aluminum lake, flavor, hydrogenated vegetable oil, magnesium stearate, mannitol, povidone, starch.
10 mg Chewable Tablets. (NDC-0038-0815) Yellow, round, scored tablets (identified front "STUART", reverse "815") are supplied in bottles of 100 and Unit Dose 100.
Inactive Ingredients: confectioner's sugar, D&C Yellow #10 aluminum lake, FD&C Yellow #6 aluminum lake, flavor, hydrogenated vegetable oil, magnesium stearate, mannitol, povidone, starch.
SORBITRATE® Oral
5 mg Oral Tablets. (NDC-0038-0770) Green, oval-shaped, scored tablets (identified front "STUART", reverse "770") are supplied in bottles of 100, 500, and Unit Dose 100.
Inactive Ingredients: D&C Yellow #10 aluminum lake, FD&C Blue #1 aluminum lake, lactose, magnesium stearate, starch.
10 mg Oral Tablets. (NDC-0038-0780) Yellow, oval-shaped, scored tablets (identified front "STUART", reverse "780") are supplied in bottles of 100, 500, and Unit Dose 100.
Inactive Ingredients: D&C Yellow #10 aluminum lake, FD&C Yellow #6 aluminum lake, lactose, magnesium stearate, starch.
20 mg Oral Tablets. (NDC-0038-0820) Blue, oval-shaped, scored tablets (identified front "STUART", reverse "820") are supplied in bottles of 100 and Unit Dose 100.
Inactive Ingredients: FD&C Blue #1 aluminum lake, lactose, magnesium stearate, starch.
30 mg Oral Tablets. (NDC-0038-0773) White, oval-shaped, scored tablets (identified front "STUART", reverse "773") are supplied in bottles of 100 and Unit Dose 100.
Inactive Ingredients: lactose, magnesium stearate, starch.
40 mg Oral Tablets. (NDC-0038-0774) Light blue, oval-shaped, scored tablets (identified front "STUART", reverse "774") are supplied in bottles of 100 and Unit Dose 100.
Inactive Ingredients: D&C Red #30 aluminum lake, FD&C Blue #1 aluminum lake, lactose, magnesium stearate, starch.
SORBITRATE® SA
40 mg Sustained Action Tablets. (NDC-0038-0880) Yellow, round, compression-coated tablets (identified front "STUART", reverse "880") are supplied in bottles of 100 and Unit Dose 100.
Inactive Ingredients: carbomer 934P, D&C Yellow #10 aluminum lake, ethylcellulose, FD&C Yellow #6 aluminum lake, lactose, magnesium stearate, polyethylene glycol.
Store in a dry place at room temperature, avoid excessive heat (over 104°F/40°C).
Shown in Product Identification Section, page 439

THE STUART FORMULA® Tablets

Composition: Each tablet contains:
Vitamins: Vitamin A (as palmitate), 5000 I.U.; Vitamin D (ergocalciferol), 400 I.U.; Vitamin E (as dl-alpha tocopheryl acetate), 15 I.U.; Vitamin C (as ascorbic acid), 60 mg.; folic acid, 0.4 mg.; thiamine (as thiamine mononitrate), 1.5 mg.; riboflavin, 1.7 mg.; niacin (as niacinamide), 20 mg.; Vitamin B$_6$ (as pyridoxine hydrochloride), 2 mg.; Vitamin B$_{12}$ (cyanocobalamin), 6 mcg.
Minerals: calcium 160 mg.; phosphorus, 125 mg.; iodine, 150 mcg.; iron (from 54 mg. ferrous fumarate) 18 mg.; magnesium, 100 mg.
Actions and Uses: The STUART FORMULA tablet provides a well-balanced multivitamin/multimineral formula intended for use as a daily dietary supplement for adults and children over age four.

Dosage and Administration: One tablet daily or as directed by a physician.
How Supplied: Bottles of 100 and 250 white round tablets. Childproof safety caps are standard on both bottles as a safeguard against accidental ingestion by children.
NDC 0038-0866.
Shown in Product Identification Section, page 439

STUART PRENATAL® Tablets

Composition: Each tablet contains:

Vitamins:	% U.S. RDA*	
A (as acetate)	100%	8,000 I.U.
D (ergocalciferol)	100%	400 I.U.
E (as dl-alpha tocopheryl acetate)	100%	30 I.U.
C (ascorbic acid)	100%	60 mg.
Folic Acid	100%	0.8 mg.
Thiamine (as thiamine mononitrate)	100%	1.7 mg.
Riboflavin	100%	2 mg.
Niacin (as niacinamide)	100%	20 mg.
B$_6$ (as pyridoxine hydrochloride)	160%	4 mg.
B$_{12}$ (cyanocobalamin)	100%	8 mcg.
Minerals:		
Calcium (from 679 mg. calcium sulfate anhydrous)	15%	200 mg.
Iodine (from potassium iodide)	100%	150 mcg.
Iron (from 182 mg. ferrous fumarate)	333%	60 mg.
Magnesium (from magnesium oxide)	22%	100 mg.

* Recommended Daily Allowance

Action and Uses: STUART PRENATAL is a non-prescription multivitamin/multimineral supplement for pregnant and lactating women. It provides vitamins equal to 100% or more of the U.S. RDA for pregnant and lactating women, plus essential minerals, including 60 mg. of elemental iron as well-tolerated ferrous fumarate, and 200 mg. of elemental calcium (non-alkalizing and phosphorus-free). Stuart Prenatal also contains .8 mg. folic acid.

Dosage and Administration: During and after pregnancy, one tablet daily after a meal, or as directed by a physician.
How Supplied: Bottles of 100 and 500 pink capsule-shaped tablets. A childproof safety cap is standard on 100 tablet bottles as a safeguard against accidental ingestion by children.
NDC 0038-0270.
Shown in Product Identification Section, page 439

STUARTINIC® Tablets
[stu'ar tin"ik]

Composition: Each tablet contains: iron (from 300 mg. ferrous fumarate), 100 mg.; Vitamin C (as ascorbic acid, 300 mg. and sodium ascorbate, 225 mg.), 500 mg.; Vitamin B$_{12}$ (cyanocobalamin), 25 mcg.; thiamine mononitrate, 6 mg.; riboflavin, 6 mg.; Vitamin B$_6$ (as pyridoxine hydrochloride), 1 mg.; niacinamide, 20 mg.; calcium pantothenate, 10 mg.

Action and Uses: STUARTINIC is a complete hematinic for patients with history of iron deficiency anemia who also lack proper amounts of B-complex vitamins due to inadequate diet.

The use of well-tolerated ferrous fumarate in STUARTINIC provides a high level of elemental iron with a low incidence of gastric distress. The inclusion of 500 mg. of Vitamin C per tablet serves to maintain more of the iron in the absorbable ferrous state. The B-complex vitamins improve nutrition where B-complex deficient diets contribute to the anemia.

Precautions: Because STUARTINIC contains 100 mg. of elemental iron per tablet, use should be confined to adults, i.e. over age 12 years. As with all medications, STUARTINIC should be kept out of the reach of children.

Dosage and Administration: One tablet daily taken after a meal to maintain normal hemoglobin

levels in most patients with chronic iron deficiency anemia resulting from inadequate diet. Higher doses of STUARTINIC can be taken as directed by the physician.
How Supplied: STUARTINIC is supplied in bottles of 60 yellow, film coated, oval shaped tablets. NDC 0038-0862.
Note: A childproof safety cap is standard on each 60 tablet bottle as a safeguard against accidental ingestion by children.
Shown in Product Identification Section, page 439

STUARTNATAL® 1+1 Tablets   R
[stu'art na'tal]

Composition: Each tablet contains:

Vitamins:	% U.S. RDA*	
A (as acetate)	100%	8,000 I.U.
D (ergocalciferol)	100%	400 I.U.
E (as dl-alpha tocopheryl acetate)	100%	30 I.U.
C (ascorbic acid)	150%	90 mg.
Folic Acid	125%	1 mg.
Thiamine (as thiamine mononitrate)	150%	2.55 mg.
Riboflavin	150%	3 mg.
Niacin (as niacinamide)	100%	20 mg.
B_6 (as pyridoxine hydrochloride)	400%	10 mg.
B_{12} (cyanocobalamin)	150%	12 mcg.

Minerals:		
Calcium (from 679 mg. calcium sulfate anhydrous)	15%	200 mg.
Iodine (from potassium iodide)	100%	150 mcg.
Iron (from 197 mg. ferrous fumarate)	361%	65 mg.
Magnesium (from magnesium oxide)	22%	100 mg.

*Recommended Daily Allowance

Action and Uses: STUARTNATAL 1+1 is indicated to provide potent vitamin and mineral supplementation throughout pregnancy and during the postnatal period—for both the lactating and non-lactating mother.
Each tablet provides vitamins equal to 100% or more of U.S. RDA for pregnant and lactating women plus essential minerals, including 1 full grain of elemental iron and 200 mg. of elemental calcium (non-alkalizing and phosphorus-free). STUARTNATAL 1+1 also offers 1 mg. folic acid to aid in the prevention of megaloblastic anemia.
Precaution: Folic acid may partially correct the hematological damage due to Vitamin B_{12} deficiency of pernicious anemia, while the associated neurological damage progresses.
Dosage and Administration: During and after pregnancy, one tablet daily after a meal, or as directed by a physician.
How Supplied: Bottles of 100 and 500 light yellow capsule-shaped tablets identified "Stuart 850". A childproof safety cap is standard on 100 tablet bottles as a safeguard against accidental ingestion by children.
NDC 0038-0850.
Shown in Product Identification Section, page 439

TENORETIC®   R
[ten'or-et ik"]
(atenolol and chlorthalidone)

Description: TENORETIC (atenolol and chlorthalidone) is for the treatment of hypertension. It combines the antihypertensive activity of two agents: a $beta_1$-selective (cardioselective) hydrophilic blocking agent (atenolol, TENORMIN®) and a monosulfonamyl diuretic (chlorthalidone).
Atenolol is Benzeneacetamide,4-[2'-hydroxy-3'-[(1-methylethyl) amino]propoxy]-.
Atenolol (free base) is a relatively polar hydrophilic compound with a water solubility of 26.5 mg/mL at 37°C. It is freely soluble in 1 N HCl (300 mg/mL at 25°C) and less soluble in chloroform (3 mg/mL at 25°C).
Chlorthalidone is 2-Chloro-5-(1-hydroxy-3-oxo-1-isoindolinyl) benzene sulfonamide.

Chlorthalidone has a water solubility of 12 mg/100 mL at 20°C.
Each TENORETIC 50 tablet contains:
   Atenolol (TENORMIN) ....50 mg
   Chlorthalidone ....25 mg
Each TENORETIC 100 tablet contains:
   Atenolol (TENORMIN) ....100 mg
   Chlorthalidone ....25 mg
Clinical Pharmacology: Atenolol and chlorthalidone have been used singly and concomitantly for the treatment of hypertension. The antihypertensive effects of these agents are additive and studies have shown that there is no interference with bioavailability when these agents are given together in the single combination tablet. Therefore, this combination provides a convenient formulation for the concomitant administration of these two entities. In patients with more severe hypertension, TENORETIC may be administered with other antihypertensives such as vasodilators.
Atenolol: A $beta_1$-selective (cardioselective) beta-adrenergic receptor blocking agent without membrane stabilizing or intrinsic sympathomimetic (partial agonist) activities. This preferential effect is not absolute however and, at higher doses, atenolol inhibits $beta_2$-adrenoreceptors, chiefly located in the bronchial and vascular musculature.
Pharmacodynamics: In standard animal or human pharmacological tests, beta-adrenoreceptor blocking activity of atenolol has been demonstrated by: 1) reduction in resting and exercise heart rate and cardiac output, 2) reduction of systolic and diastolic blood pressure at rest and on exercise, 3) inhibition of isoproterenol induced tachycardia, and 4) reduction in reflex orthostatic tachycardia.
A significant beta-blocking effect of atenolol, as measured by reduction of exercise tachycardia, is apparent within 1 hour following oral administration of a single dose. This effect is maximal at about 2 to 4 hours and persists for at least 24 hours. The effect at 24 hours is dose-related and also bears a linear relationship to the logarithm of plasma atenolol concentration. However, as has been shown for all beta-blocking agents, the antihypertensive effect does not appear to be related to plasma level.
In normal subjects, the $beta_1$-selectivity of atenolol has been shown by its reduced ability to reverse the $beta_2$-mediated vasodilating effect of isoproterenol as compared to equivalent beta-blocking doses of propranolol. In asthmatic patients, a dose of atenolol producing a greater effect on resting heart rate than propranolol resulted in much less increase in airway resistance. In a placebo-controlled comparison of approximately equipotent oral doses of several beta blockers, atenolol produced a significantly smaller decrease of FEV_1 than nonselective beta blockers such as propranolol and unlike those agents did not inhibit bronchodilation in response to isoproterenol.
Consistent with its negative chronotropic effect due to beta blockade of the SA node, atenolol increases sinus cycle length and sinus node recovery time. Conduction in the AV node is also prolonged. Atenolol is devoid of membrane stabilizing activity, and increasing the dose well beyond that producing beta blockade does not further depress myocardial contractility. Several studies have demonstrated a moderate (approximately 10%) increase in stroke volume at rest and exercise.
In controlled clinical trials, atenolol given as a single daily dose, was an effective antihypertensive agent providing 24-hour reduction of blood pressure. Atenolol has been studied in combination with thiazide-type diuretics and the blood pressure effects of the combination are approximately additive. Atenolol is also compatible with methyldopa, hydralazine, and prazosin, the combination resulting in a larger fall in blood pressure than with the single agents. The dose range of atenolol is narrow, and increasing the dose beyond 100 mg once daily is not associated with increased antihypertensive effect. The mechanisms of the antihypertensive effects of beta-blocking agents have not been established. Several mechanisms have been proposed and include: 1) competitive

antagonism of catecholamines at peripheral (especially cardiac) adrenergic neuron sites, leading to decreased cardiac output, 2) a central effect leading to reduced sympathetic outflow to the periphery, and 3) suppression of renin activity. The results from long-term studies have not shown any diminution of the antihypertensive efficacy of atenolol with prolonged use.
Pharmacokinetics and Metabolism: In man, absorption of an oral dose is rapid and consistent but incomplete. Approximately 50% of an oral dose is absorbed from the gastrointestinal tract, the remainder being excreted unchanged in the feces. Peak blood levels are reached between 2 and 4 hours after ingestion. Unlike propranolol or metoprolol, but like nadolol, hydrophilic atenolol undergoes little or no metabolism by the liver and the absorbed portion is eliminated primarily by renal excretion. Atenolol also differs from propranolol in that only a small amount (6-16%) is bound to proteins in the plasma. This kinetic profile results in relatively consistent plasma drug levels with about a fourfold interpatient variation. There is no information as to the pharmacokinetic effect of atenolol on chlorthalidone.
The elimination half-life of atenolol is approximately 6 to 7 hours, and there is no alteration of the kinetic profile of the drug by chronic administration. Following doses of 50 mg or 100 mg, both beta-blocking and antihypertensive effects persist for at least 24 hours. When renal function is impaired, elimination of atenolol is closely related to the glomerular filtration rate; but significant accumulation does not occur until the creatinine clearance falls below 35 mL/min/1.73 m^2. (See circular for atenolol [TENORMIN]).
Chlorthalidone: A monosulfonamyl diuretic which differs chemically from thiazide diuretics in that a double ring system is incorporated in its structure. It is an oral diuretic with prolonged action and low toxicity. The diuretic effect of the drug occurs within 2 hours of an oral dose. It produces diuresis with greatly increased excretion of sodium and chloride. At maximal therapeutic dosage, chlorthalidone is approximately equal in its diuretic effect to comparable maximal therapeutic doses of benzothiadiazine diuretics. The site of action appears to be the cortical diluting segment of the ascending limb of Henle's loop of the nephron.
Indications and Usage: TENORETIC is indicated for the treatment of hypertension. This fixed-dose combination drug is not indicated for initial therapy of hypertension. If the fixed-dose combination represents the dose appropriate to the individual patient's needs, it may be more convenient than the separate components.
Contraindications: TENORETIC is contraindicated in patients with: sinus bradycardia, heart block greater than first degree, cardiogenic shock, overt cardiac failure (see WARNINGS), anuria, hypersensitivity to this product or to sulfonamide-derived drugs.
Warnings: Cardiac Failure: Sympathetic stimulation is necessary in supporting circulatory function in congestive heart failure, and beta blockade carries the potential hazard of further depressing myocardial contractility and precipitating more severe failure. In hypertensive patients who have congestive heart failure controlled by digitalis and diuretics, TENORETIC should be administered cautiously. Both digitalis and atenolol slow AV conduction.
IN PATIENTS WITHOUT A HISTORY OF CARDIAC FAILURE, continued depression of the myocardium with beta-blocking agents over a period of time can, in some cases, lead to cardiac failure. At the first sign or symptom of impending cardiac failure, patients receiving TENORETIC should be digitalized and/or be given additional diuretic therapy. Observe the patient closely. If cardiac failure continues despite adequate digitalization and diuretic therapy, TENORETIC therapy should be withdrawn.

Continued on next page

Stuart—Cont.

Renal and Hepatic Disease and Electrolyte Disturbances: Since atenolol is excreted via the kidneys, TENORETIC should be used with caution in patients with impaired renal function.

In patients with renal disease, thiazides may precipitate azotemia. Since cumulative effects may develop in the presence of impaired renal function, if progressive renal impairment becomes evident TENORETIC should be discontinued.

In patients with impaired hepatic function or progressive liver disease, minor alterations in fluid and electrolyte balance may precipitate hepatic coma. TENORETIC should be used with caution in these patients.

Ischemic Heart Disease: Although not yet reported with atenolol following abrupt cessation of therapy with certain beta-blocking agents in patients with coronary artery disease, exacerbations of angina pectoris and, in some cases, myocardial infarction have been reported. Therefore, such patients should be cautioned against interruption of therapy without the physician's advice. Even in the absence of overt angina pectoris, when discontinuation of TENORETIC is planned, the patient should be carefully observed and should be advised to limit physical activity to a minimum. TENORETIC should be reinstated if withdrawal symptoms occur.

Bronchospastic Diseases: PATIENTS WITH BRONCHOSPASTIC DISEASE SHOULD, IN GENERAL, NOT RECEIVE BETA BLOCKERS. Because of its relative beta$_1$-selectivity, however, TENORETIC may be used with caution in patients with bronchospastic disease who do not respond to, or cannot tolerate, other antihypertensive treatment. Since beta$_1$-selectivity is not absolute, the lowest possible dose of TENORETIC should be used and a beta$_2$-stimulating agent (bronchodilator) should be made available. If dosage must be increased, dividing the dose should be considered in order to achieve lower peak blood levels.

Anesthesia and Major Surgery: As with all beta-receptor blocking drugs, it may be decided to withdraw TENORETIC before surgery. In this case, 48 hours should be allowed to elapse between the last dose and anesthesia. If treatment is continued, care should be taken when using anesthetic agents because of the risk of further depression of the myocardium.

Beta blockers are competitive inhibitors of beta-receptor agonists and their effects on the heart can be reversed by administration of such agents; eg, dobutamine or isoproterenol with caution (see section on OVERDOSAGE). Manifestations of excessive vagal tone (eg, profound bradycardia, hypotension) may be corrected with atropine (1-2 mg I.V.).

Metabolic and Endocrine Effects: TENORETIC may be used with caution in diabetic patients. Beta blockers may mask tachycardia occurring with hypoglycemia, but other manifestations such as dizziness and sweating may not be significantly affected. Atenolol does not potentiate insulin-induced hypoglycemia and, unlike nonselective beta blockers, does not delay recovery of blood glucose to normal levels.

Insulin requirements in diabetic patients may be increased, decreased, or unchanged, latent diabetes mellitus may become manifest during chlorthalidone administration.

Beta-adrenergic blockade may mask certain clinical signs (eg, tachycardia) of hyperthyroidism. Abrupt withdrawal of beta blockade might precipitate a thyroid storm; therefore, patients suspected of developing thyrotoxicosis and from whom TENORETIC therapy is to be withdrawn should be monitored closely.

Because calcium excretion is decreased by thiazides, TENORETIC should be discontinued before carrying out tests for parathyroid function. Pathologic changes in the parathyroid glands, with hypercalcemia and hypophosphatemia, have been observed in a few patients on prolonged thiazide therapy; however, the common complications of hyperparathyroidism such as renal lithiasis, bone resorption, and peptic ulceration have not been seen.

Hyperuricemia may occur or acute gout may be precipitated in certain patients receiving thiazide therapy.

Precautions, General—Electrolyte and Fluid Balance Status: Periodic determination of serum electrolytes to detect possible electrolyte imbalance should be performed at appropriate intervals. Patients should be observed for clinical signs of fluid or electrolyte imbalance, ie, hyponatremia, hypochloremic alkalosis, and hypokalemia. Serum and urine electrolyte determinations are particularly important when the patient is vomiting excessively or receiving parenteral fluids. Warning signs or symptoms of fluid and electrolyte imbalance include dryness of the mouth, thirst, weakness, lethargy, drowsiness, restlessness, muscle pains or cramps, muscular fatigue, hypotension, oliguria, tachycardia, and gastrointestinal disturbances such as nausea and vomiting.

Hypokalemia may develop, especially with brisk diuresis, when severe cirrhosis is present, or during concomitant use of corticosteroids or ACTH. Interference with adequate oral electrolyte intake will also contribute to hypokalemia. Hypokalemia can sensitize or exaggerate the response of the heart to the toxic effects of digitalis (eg, increased ventricular irritability). Hypokalemia may be avoided or treated by use of potassium supplements or foods with a high potassium content.

Any chloride deficit during thiazide therapy is generally mild and usually does not require specific treatment except under extraordinary circumstances (as in liver disease or renal disease). Dilutional hyponatremia may occur in edematous patients in hot weather, appropriate therapy is water restriction rather than administration of salt except in rare instances when the hyponatremia is life-threatening. In actual salt depletion, appropriate replacement is the therapy of choice.

Drug Interactions: TENORETIC may potentiate the action of other antihypertensive agents used concomitantly. Patients treated with TENORETIC plus a catecholamine depletor (eg. reserpine) should be closely observed for evidence of hypotension and/or marked bradycardia which may produce vertigo, syncope, or postural hypotension.

Thiazides may decrease arterial responsiveness to norepinephrine. This diminution is not sufficient to preclude the therapeutic effectiveness of norepinephrine. Thiazides may increase the responsiveness to tubocurarine.

Lithium generally should not be given with diuretics because they reduce its renal clearance and add a high risk of lithium toxicity. Read circulars for lithium preparations before use of such preparations with TENORETIC.

Should it be decided to discontinue therapy in patients receiving TENORETIC and clonidine concurrently, the TENORETIC should be discontinued several days before the gradual withdrawal of clonidine.

Other Precautions: In patients receiving thiazides, sensitivity reactions may occur with or without a history of allergy or bronchial asthma. The possible exacerbation or activation of systemic lupus erythematosus has been reported. The antihypertensive effects of thiazides may be enhanced in the postsympathectomy patient.

Carcinogenesis, Mutagenesis, Impairment of Fertility: Two long-term (maximum dosing duration of 18 or 24 months) rat studies and one long-term (maximum dosing duration of 18 months) mouse study with atenolol, each employing dose levels as high as 300 mg/kg/day or 150 times the maximum recommended human dose, did not indicate a carcinogenic potential in rodents.

Atenolol was negative in the mouse dominant lethal test, the Chinese hamster in vivo cytogenetic test and the Salmonella typhimurium back mutation test (Ames test), with or without metabolic activation.

Fertility of male or female rats (evaluated at dose levels as high as 200 mg/kg/day or 100 times the maximum recommended human dose) was unaffected by atenolol administration.

Animal Toxicology: Six month oral studies were conducted in rats and dogs using TENORETIC dosages up to 12.5 mg/kg/day (approximately 5 times the proposed maximum therapeutic dose). There were no functional or morphological abnormalities resulting from dosing either compound alone or together other than minor changes in heart rate, blood pressure, and urine chemistry, which were attributed to the known pharmacologic properties of atenolol and/or chlorthalidone. Chronic studies of atenolol performed in animals have revealed the occurrence of vacuolation of epithelial cells of Brunner's glands in the duodenum of both male and female dogs at all tested dose levels (starting at 15 mg/kg/day or 7.5 times the maximum recommended human dose) and increased incidence of atrial degeneration of hearts of male rats at 300 mg but not 150 mg atenolol/kg/day (150 and 75 times the maximum recommended human dose, respectively).

Use in Pregnancy: Pregnancy Category C. TENORETIC was studied for teratogenic potential in the rat and rabbit. Doses of 10, 100, and 300 mg/kg/day were administered orally to pregnant rats, with no teratologic effects observed. Two studies were conducted in rabbits. In the first study, pregnant rabbits were dosed with 10, 100, or 200 mg/kg/day. No teratologic changes were noted; embryonic resorptions were observed at all dose levels (ranging from approximately 5 times to 100 times the maximum recommended human dose). In a second rabbit study, dosages were 5, 10, and 25 mg/kg/day. No teratogenic or embryotoxic effects were demonstrated. It is concluded that the no-effect level for embryonic resorptions is 25 mg/kg/day (approximately 12.5 times the maximum recommended human dose) or greater. TENORETIC should be used during pregnancy only if the potential benefit justifies the potential risk to the fetus.

Atenolol—Atenolol has been shown to produce a dose-related increase in embryo/fetal resorptions in rats at doses equal to or greater than 50 mg/kg or 25 or more times the maximum recommended human dose. Although similar effects were not seen in rabbits, the compound was not evaluated in rabbits at doses above 25 mg/kg or 12.5 times the maximum recommended human dose. There are no adequate and well-controlled studies in pregnant women.

Chlorthalidone—Thiazides cross the placental barrier and appear in cord blood. The use of chlorthalidone and related drugs in pregnant women requires that the anticipated benefits of the drug be weighed against possible hazards to the fetus. These hazards include fetal or neonatal jaundice, thrombocytopenia, and possibly other adverse reactions which have occurred in the adult.

Nursing Mothers: It is not established to what extent this drug is excreted in human milk. Since most drugs are excreted in human milk, nursing should not be undertaken by mothers receiving TENORETIC.

Pediatric Use: Safety and effectiveness in children have not been established.

Adverse Reactions: TENORETIC is usually well tolerated in properly selected patients. Most adverse effects have been mild and transient. The adverse effects observed for TENORETIC are essentially the same as those seen with the individual components.

Atenolol: The frequency estimates that follow derive from controlled studies in which adverse reactions were either volunteered by the patient (U.S. studies) or elicited, eg, by checklist (foreign studies). The reported frequency of elicited adverse effects was higher for both atenolol and placebo-treated patients than when these reactions were volunteered. Where frequency of adverse effects for atenolol and placebo is similar, causal relationship to atenolol is uncertain.

The data present these estimates in terms of percentages: first from the U.S. studies (volunteered side effects) and then from both U.S. and foreign studies (volunteered and elicited side effects).

U.S. Studies (% Atenolol -% Placebo):
CARDIOVASCULAR: bradycardia (3%-0%), cold extremities (0%-0.5%), postural hypotension (2%-1%), leg pain (0%-0.5%).
CENTRAL NERVOUS SYSTEM/NEUROMUSCULAR: dizziness (4%-1%), vertigo (2%-0.5%), light-headedness (1%-0%), tiredness (0.6%-0.5%), fatigue (3%-1%), lethargy (1%-0%), drowsiness (0.6%-0%), depression (0.6%-0.5%), dreaming (0%-0%).
GASTROINTESTINAL: diarrhea (2%-0%), nausea (4%-1%).
RESPIRATORY (See WARNINGS): wheeziness (0%-0%), dyspnea (0.6%-1%).

Totals U.S. and Foreign Studies:
CARDIOVASCULAR: bradycardia (3%-0%), cold extremities (12%-5%), postural hypotension (4%-5%), leg pain (3%-1%).
CENTRAL NERVOUS SYSTEM/NEUROMUSCULAR: dizziness (13%-6%), vertigo (2%-0.2%), light-headedness (3%-0.7%), tiredness (26%-13%), fatigue (6%-5%), lethargy (3%-0.7%), drowsiness (2%-0.5%), depression (12%-9%), dreaming (3%-1%).
GASTROINTESTINAL: diarrhea (3%-2%), nausea (3%-1%).
RESPIRATORY (see WARNINGS): wheeziness (3%-3%), dyspnea (6%-4%).

Miscellaneous: There have been reports of skin rashes and/or dry eyes associated with the use of beta-adrenergic blocking drugs. The reported incidence is small and, in most cases the symptoms have cleared when treatment was withdrawn. Discontinuance of the drug should be considered if any such reaction is not otherwise explicable. Patients should be closely monitored following cessation of therapy.

Chlorthalidone: Cardiovascular: orthostatic hypotension; Gastrointestinal: anorexia, gastric irritation, vomiting, cramping, constipation, jaundice (intrahepatic cholestatic jaundice), pancreatitis; CNS: vertigo, paresthesias, xanthopsia; Hematologic: leukopenia, agranulocytosis, thrombocytopenia, aplastic anemia; Hypersensitivity: purpura, photosensitivity, rash, urticaria, necrotizing angiitis (vasculitis), (cutaneous vasculitis), Lyell's syndrome (toxic epidermal necrolysis); Miscellaneous: hyperglycemia, glycosuria, hyperuricemia, muscle spasm, weakness, restlessness. Clinical trials of TENORETIC conducted in the United States (69 patients treated with TENORETIC) revealed no new or unexpected adverse effects.

Potential Adverse Effects: In addition, a variety of adverse effects not observed in clinical trials with atenolol but reported with other beta-adrenergic blocking agents, should be considered potential adverse effects of atenolol. Nervous System: reversible mental depression progressing to catatonia, hallucinations, an acute reversible syndrome characterized by disorientation for time and place, short-term memory loss, emotional lability, slightly clouded sensorium, decreased performance on neuropsychometrics; Cardiovascular: intensification of AV block (see CONTRAINDICATIONS); Gastrointestinal: mesenteric arterial thrombosis, ischemic colitis; Hematologic: agranulocytosis, nonthrombocytopenic purpura, thrombocytopenic purpura; Allergic: erythematous rash, fever combined with aching and sore throat, laryngospasm and respiratory distress; Miscellaneous: reversible alopecia, Peyronie's disease.

There have been reports of a syndrome comprising psoriasiform skin rash, conjunctivitis sicca, otitis, and sclerosing serositis attributed to the beta-adrenergic receptor blocking agent, practolol. This syndrome has not been reported with TENORETIC or TENORMIN (atenolol).

Clinical Laboratory Test Findings: Clinically important changes in standard laboratory parameters were rarely associated with the administration of TENORETIC. The changes in laboratory parameters were not progressive and usually were not associated with clinical manifestations. The most common changes were increases in uric acid and decreases in serum potassium.

Overdosage: No specific information is available with regard to overdosage with TENORETIC in humans. Treatment is symptomatic and supportive. Therapy with TENORETIC should be discontinued and the patient observed closely. Suggested measures include induction of emesis and/or gastric lavage, and correction of dehydration, electrolyte imbalance, and hypotension by established procedures.

Atenolol: To date, there is no known case of acute overdosage with atenolol. The most common effects expected with overdosage of a beta-adrenergic blocking agent are bradycardia, congestive heart failure, hypotension, bronchospasm, and hypoglycemia. Atenolol can be removed from the general circulation by hemodialysis. In addition to gastric lavage, the following therapeutic measures are suggested if warranted.
BRADYCARDIA: atropine or another anticholinergic drug.
HEART BLOCK (second or third degree): isoproterenol or transvenous cardiac pacemaker.
CONGESTIVE HEART FAILURE: conventional therapy.
HYPOTENSION (depending on associated factors): epinephrine rather than isoproterenol or norepinephrine may be useful in addition to atropine and digitalis.
BRONCHOSPASM: aminophylline, isoproterenol, or atropine.
HYPOGLYCEMIA: intravenous glucose.
ELECTROLYTE IMBALANCE: supportive treatment; where necessary, intravenous dextrose-saline with potassium, administered with caution.
Chlorthalidone: Symptoms of chlorthalidone overdose include nausea, weakness, dizziness, and disturbances of electrolyte balance.

Dosage and Administration—DOSAGE MUST BE INDIVIDUALIZED (SEE INDICATIONS): Chlorthalidone is usually given at a dose of 25 mg daily; the usual initial dose of atenolol is 50 mg daily. Therefore, the initial dose should be one TENORETIC 50 tablet given once a day. If an optimal response is not achieved, the dosage should be increased to one TENORETIC 100 tablet given once a day.
When necessary, another antihypertensive agent may be added gradually beginning with 50% of the usual recommended starting dose to avoid an excessive fall in blood pressure.
Since atenolol is excreted via the kidneys, dosage should be adjusted in cases of severe impairment of renal function. No significant accumulation of atenolol occurs until creatinine clearance falls below 35 mL/min/1.73 m² (normal range is 100–150 mL/min/1.73 m²), therefore, the following maximum dosages are recommended for patients with renal impairment.

Creatinine Clearance (mL/min/1.73 m²)	Atenolol Elimination Half-life (hrs)	Maximum Dosage
15–35	16–27	50 mg daily
< 15	> 27	50 mg every other day

How Supplied: TENORETIC 50 Tablets (atenolol 50 mg and chlorthalidone 25 mg), NDC 0038-0115 (round, biconvex, uncoated, peach-colored tablets with TENORETIC 50/25 on one side and Stuart 115 on the other side) are supplied in bottles of 100 tablets. TENORETIC 100 Tablets (atenolol 100 mg and chlorthalidone 25 mg), NDC 0038-0117 (round, biconvex, uncoated, light-peach colored tablets with TENORETIC 100/25 on one side and Stuart 117 on the other side) are supplied in bottles of 100 tablets.
Protect from heat, light, and moisture. Dispense in well-closed, light-resistant container.

B/6/84

Shown in Product Identification Section, page 439

TENORMIN® ℞
[ten'or min"]
(atenolol)

Description: TENORMIN (atenolol), a synthetic, beta₁-selective (cardioselective) adrenoceptor blocking agent, may be chemically described as benzeneacetamide, 4-[2'-hydroxy-3'-[(1-methylethyl) amino] propoxy]-.
Atenolol (free base) has a molecular weight of 266. It is a relatively polar hydrophilic compound with a water solubility of 26.5 mg/ml at 37°C and a log partition coefficient (octanol/water) of 0.23. It is freely soluble in 1N HCl (300 mg/ml at 25°C) and less soluble in chloroform (3 mg/ml at 25°C).
TENORMIN is available as 50 mg. and 100 mg. tablets for oral administration.

Clinical Pharmacology: TENORMIN is a beta₁-selective (cardioselective) beta-adrenergic receptor blocking agent without membrane-stabilizing or intrinsic sympathomimetic (partial agonist) activities. This preferential effect is not absolute, however and, at higher doses, TENORMIN inhibits beta₂ adrenoceptors, chiefly located in the bronchial and vascular musculature.

Pharmacokinetics and Metabolism: In man, absorption of an oral dose is rapid and consistent but incomplete. Approximately 50% of an oral dose is absorbed from the gastrointestinal tract, the remainder being excreted unchanged in the feces. Peak blood levels are reached between 2 and 4 hours after ingestion. Unlike propranolol or metoprolol, but like nadolol, TENORMIN undergoes little or no metabolism by the liver and the absorbed portion is eliminated primarily by renal excretion. TENORMIN also differs from propranolol in that only a small amount (6%–16%) is bound to proteins in the plasma. This kinetic profile results in relatively consistent plasma drug levels with about a fourfold interpatient variation.

The elimination half-life of TENORMIN is approximately 6 to 7 hours and there is no alteration of the kinetic profile of the drug by chronic administration. Following doses of 50 mg or 100 mg, both beta-blocking and antihypertensive effects persist for at least 24 hours. When renal function is impaired, elimination of TENORMIN is closely related to the glomerular filtration rate; but, significant accumulation does not occur until the creatinine clearance falls below 35 ml/min/1.73 m² (see DOSAGE AND ADMINISTRATION).

Pharmacodynamics.: In standard animal or human pharmacological tests, beta-adrenoreceptor blocking activity of TENORMIN has been demonstrated by: (1) reduction in resting and exercise heart rate and cardiac output, (2) reduction of systolic and diastolic blood pressure at rest and on exercise, (3) inhibition of isoproterenol-induced tachycardia, and (4) reduction in reflex orthostatic tachycardia.

A significant beta-blocking effect of TENORMIN, as measured by reduction of exercise tachycardia, is apparent within 1 hour following oral administration of a single dose. This effect is maximal at about 2 to 4 hours, and persists for at least 24 hours. The effect at 24 hours is dose-related and also bears a linear relationship to the logarithm of plasma TENORMIN concentration. However, as has been shown for all beta-blocking agents, the antihypertensive effect does not appear to be related to plasma level.

In normal subjects, the beta₁ selectivity of TENORMIN has been shown by its reduced ability to reverse the beta₂-mediated vasodilating effect of isoproterenol as compared to equivalent beta-blocking doses of propranolol. In asthmatic patients, a dose of TENORMIN producing a greater effect on resting heart rate than propranolol resulted in much less increase in airway resistance. In a placebo-controlled comparison of approximately equipotent oral doses of several beta blockers, TENORMIN produced a significantly smaller decrease of FEV₁ than nonselective beta blockers such as propranolol and, unlike those agents, did not inhibit bronchodilation in response to isoproterenol.

Consistent with its negative chronotropic effect due to beta blockade of the SA node, TENORMIN increases sinus cycle length and sinus node recovery time. Conduction in the AV node is also prolonged. TENORMIN is devoid of membrane-stabilizing activity, and increasing the dose well beyond that producing beta blockade does not further depress myocardial contractility. Several studies

Continued on next page

Stuart—Cont.

have demonstrated a moderate (approximately 10%) increase in stroke volume at rest and during exercise.

In controlled clinical trials TENORMIN given as a single daily dose was an effective antihypertensive agent providing 24-hour reduction of blood pressure. TENORMIN has been studied in combination with thiazide-type diuretics and the blood pressure effects of the combination are approximately additive. TENORMIN is also compatible with methyldopa, hydralazine, and prazosin, the combination resulting in a larger fall in blood pressure than with the single agents. The dose range of TENORMIN is narrow and increasing the dose beyond 100 mg. once daily is not associated with increased antihypertensive effect. The mechanisms of the antihypertensive effects of beta-blocking agents have not been established. Several possible mechanisms have been proposed and include: (1) competitive antagonism of catecholamines at peripheral (especially cardiac) adrenergic neuron sites, leading to decreased cardiac output, (2) a central effect leading to reduced sympathetic outflow to the periphery, and (3) suppression of renin activity. The results from long-term studies have not shown any diminution of the antihypertensive efficacy of TENORMIN with prolonged use.

Indications and Usage: TENORMIN is indicated in the management of hypertension. It may be used alone or concomitantly with other antihypertensive agents, particularly with a thiazide-type diuretic.

Contraindications: TENORMIN is contraindicated in sinus bradycardia, heart block greater than first degree, cardiogenic shock, and overt cardiac failure (see WARNINGS).

Warnings: Cardiac Failure: Sympathetic stimulation is necessary in supporting circulatory function in congestive heart failure, and beta blockade carries the potential hazard of further depressing myocardial contractility and precipitating more severe failure. In hypertensive patients who have congestive heart failure controlled by digitalis and diuretics, TENORMIN should be administered cautiously. Both digitalis and atenolol slow AV conduction.

In Patients Without a History of Cardiac Failure: Continued depression of the myocardium with beta-blocking agents over a period of time can, in some cases, lead to cardiac failure. At the first sign or symptom of impending cardiac failure, patients should be fully digitalized and/or be given a diuretic and the response observed closely. If cardiac failure continues, despite adequate digitalization and diuresis, TENORMIN should be withdrawn.

Ischemic Heart Disease: Following abrupt cessation of therapy with certain beta-blocking agents in patients with coronary artery disease, exacerbations of angina pectoris and, in some cases, myocardial infarction have been reported. Therefore, such patients should be cautioned against interruption of therapy without the physician's advice. Even in the absence of overt angina pectoris, when discontinuation of TENORMIN is planned, the patient should be carefully observed and should be advised to limit physical activity to a minimum. TENORMIN should be reinstated if withdrawal symptoms occur.

Bronchospastic Diseases: PATIENTS WITH BRONCHOSPASTIC DISEASE SHOULD IN GENERAL NOT RECEIVE BETA BLOCKERS. Because of its relative beta$_1$ selectivity, however, TENORMIN may be used with caution in patients with bronchospastic disease who do not respond to, or cannot tolerate, other antihypertensive treatment. Since beta$_1$ selectivity is not absolute, the lowest possible dose of TENORMIN should be used with therapy initiated at 50 mg. and a beta$_2$-stimulating agent (bronchodilator) should be made available. If dosage must be increased, dividing the dose should be considered in order to achieve lower peak blood levels.

Anesthesia and Major Surgery: As with all beta-receptor blocking drugs it may be decided to withdraw TENORMIN before surgery. In this case, 48 hours should be allowed to elapse between the last dose and anesthesia. If treatment is continued, care should be taken when using anesthetic agents which depress the myocardium such as ether, cyclopropane, and trichloroethylene.

TENORMIN, like other beta blockers, is a competitive inhibitor of beta-receptor agonists and its effects on the heart can be reversed by administration of such agents (eg, dobutamine or isoproterenol with caution, see section on OVERDOSAGE). Manifestations of excessive vagal tone (eg, profound bradycardia, hypotension) may be corrected with atropine (1–2 mg. IV).

Diabetes and Hypoglycemia: TENORMIN should be used with caution in diabetic patients if a beta-blocking agent is required. Beta blockers may mask tachycardia occurring with hypoglycemia, but other manifestations such as dizziness and sweating may not be significantly affected. TENORMIN does not potentiate insulin-induced hypoglycemia and, unlike nonselective beta blockers, does not delay recovery of blood glucose to normal levels.

Thyrotoxicosis: Beta-adrenergic blockade may mask certain clinical signs (eg, tachycardia) of hyperthyroidism. Abrupt withdrawal of beta blockade might precipitate a thyroid storm; therefore, patients suspected of developing thyrotoxicosis from whom TENORMIN is to be withdrawn should be monitored closely.

Precautions: Impaired Renal Function: The drug should be used with caution in patients with impaired renal function (see DOSAGE AND ADMINISTRATION).

Drug Interactions: Catecholamine-depleting drugs (eg, reserpine) may have an additive effect when given with beta-blocking agents. Patients treated with TENORMIN plus a catecholamine depletor should therefore be closely observed for evidence of hypotension and or marked bradycardia which may produce vertigo, syncope, or postural hypotension.

Should it be decided to discontinue therapy in patients receiving beta blockers and clonidine concurrently, the beta blocker should be discontinued several days before the gradual withdrawal of clonidine.

Carcinogenesis, Mutagenesis, Impairment of Fertility: Two long-term (maximum dosing duration of 18 or 24 months) rat studies and one long-term (maximum dosing duration of 18 months) mouse study, each employing dose levels as high as 300 mg./kg./day or 150 times the maximum recommended human dose, did not indicate a carcinogenic potential in rodents. Results of various mutagenicity studies support this finding.

Fertility of male or female rats (evaluated at dose levels as high as 200 mg./kg./day or 100 times the maximum recommended human dose) was unaffected by atenolol administration.

Animal Toxicology: Chronic studies performed in animals have revealed the occurrence of vacuolation of epithelial cells of Brunner's glands in the duodenum of both male and female dogs at all tested dose levels of atenolol (starting at 15 mg./kg./day or 7.5 times the maximum recommended human dose) and increased incidence of atrial degeneration of hearts of male rats at 300 mg. but not 150 mg. atenolol/kg./day (150 and 75 times the maximum recommended human dose, respectively).

Usage in Pregnancy: Pregnancy Category C. Atenolol has been shown to produce a dose-related increase in embryo/fetal resorptions in rats at doses equal to or greater than 50 mg./kg. or 25 or more times the maximum recommended human dose. Although similar effects were not seen in rabbits, the compound was not evaluated in rabbits at doses above 25 mg./kg. or 12.5 times the maximum recommended human dose. There are no adequate and well-controlled studies in pregnant women. TENORMIN should be used during pregnancy only if the potential benefit justifies the potential risk to the fetus.

Nursing Mothers: It is not established to what extent this drug is excreted in human milk. Since most drugs are excreted in human milk, nursing should not be undertaken by mothers receiving TENORMIN.

Pediatric Use: Safety and effectiveness in children have not been established.

Adverse Reactions: Most adverse effects have been mild and transient. Frequency estimates were derived from controlled studies in which adverse reactions were either volunteered by the patient (U.S. studies) or elicited (eg, by checklist—foreign studies). The reported frequency of elicited adverse effects was higher for both TENORMIN and placebo-treated patients than when these reactions were volunteered. Where frequency of adverse effects for TENORMIN and placebo is similar, causal relationship is uncertain.

The following adverse-reaction data present frequency estimates in terms of percentages: first from the U.S. studies (volunteered side effects) and then from both U.S. and foreign studies (volunteered and elicited side effects):

U.S. STUDIES (% ATENOLOL—% PLACEBO):
CARDIOVASCULAR: bradycardia (3%–0%), cold extremities (0%–0.5%), postural hypotension (2%–1%), leg pain (0%–0.5%)
CENTRAL NERVOUS SYSTEM/NEUROMUSCULAR: dizziness (4%–1%), vertigo (2%–0.5%), light-headedness (1%–0%), tiredness (0.6%–0.5%), fatigue (3%–1%), lethargy (1%–0%), drowsiness (0.6%–0%), depression (0.6%–0.5%), dreaming (0%–0%)
GASTROINTESTINAL: diarrhea (2%–0%), nausea (4%–1%)
RESPIRATORY (See WARNINGS): wheeziness (0%–0%), dyspnea (0.6%–1%)

TOTALS U.S. AND FOREIGN STUDIES:
CARDIOVASCULAR: bradycardia (3%–0%), cold extremities (12%–5%), postural hypotension (4%–5%), leg pain (3%–1%)
CENTRAL NERVOUS SYSTEM/NEUROMUSCULAR: dizziness (13%–6%), vertigo (2%–0.2%), light-headedness (3%–0.7%), tiredness (26%–13%), fatigue (6%–5%), lethargy (3%–0.7%), drowsiness (2%–0.5%), depression (12%–9%), dreaming (3%–1%)
GASTROINTESTINAL: diarrhea (3%–2%), nausea (3%–1%)
RESPIRATORY (see WARNINGS): wheeziness (3%–3%), dyspnea (6%–4%)
MISCELLANEOUS: There have been reports of skin rashes and/or dry eyes associated with the use of beta-adrenergic blocking drugs. The reported incidence is small, and in most cases, the symptoms have cleared when treatment was withdrawn. Discontinuance of the drug should be considered if any such reaction is not otherwise explicable. Patients should be closely monitored following cessation of therapy.

Potential Adverse Effects: In addition, a variety of adverse effects have been reported with other beta-adrenergic blocking agents and may be considered potential adverse effects of TENORMIN.
HEMATOLOGIC: Agranulocytosis, nonthrombocytopenic purpura, thrombocytopenic purpura.
ALLERGIC: Fever, combined with aching and sore throat, laryngospasm, respiratory distress.
CENTRAL NERVOUS SYSTEM: Reversible mental depression progressing to catatonia, visual disturbances, hallucinations, an acute reversible syndrome characterized by disorientation of time and place, short-term memory loss, emotional lability with slightly clouded sensorium, and decreased performance on neuropsychometrics.
GASTROINTESTINAL: Mesenteric arterial thrombosis, ischemic colitis.
OTHER: Reversible alopecia, Peyronie's disease, erythematous rash, Raynaud's phenomenon.
MISCELLANEOUS: The oculomucocutaneous syndrome associated with the beta blocker practolol has not been reported with TENORMIN during investigational use and foreign marketing experience. Furthermore, a number of patients who had previously demonstrated established practolol reactions were transferred to TENORMIN with subsequent resolution or quiescence of the reaction.

Overdosage: To date, there is no known case of acute overdosage, and no specific information on emergency treatment of overdosage is available. The most common effects expected with overdosage of a beta-adrenergic blocking agent are bradycardia, congestive heart failure, hypotension, bronchospasm, and hypoglycemia.

In the case of overdosage, treatment with TENORMIN should be stopped and the patient carefully observed. TENORMIN can be removed from the general circulation by hemodialysis. In addition to gastric lavage, the following therapeutic measures are suggested if warranted:

BRADYCARDIA: Atropine or another anticholinergic drug.
HEART BLOCK (SECOND OR THIRD DEGREE): Isoproterenol or transvenous cardiac pacemaker.
CONGESTIVE HEART FAILURE: Conventional therapy.
HYPOTENSION (DEPENDING ON ASSOCIATED FACTORS): Epinephrine rather than isoproterenol or norepinephrine may be useful in addition to atropine and digitalis.
BRONCHOSPASM: Aminophylline, isoproterenol, or atropine.
HYPOGLYCEMIA: Intravenous glucose.

Dosage and Administration: The initial dose of TENORMIN is 50 mg. given as one tablet a day either alone or added to diuretic therapy. The full effect of this dose will usually be seen within 1 to 2 weeks. If an optimal response is not achieved, the dosage should be increased to TENORMIN 100 mg. given as one tablet a day. Increasing the dosage beyond 100 mg. a day is unlikely to produce any further benefit.

TENORMIN may be used alone or concomitantly with other antihypertensive agents including thiazide-type diuretics, hydralazine, prazosin, and alpha-methyldopa.

Since TENORMIN is excreted via the kidneys, dosage should be adjusted in cases of severe impairment of renal function. No significant accumulation of TENORMIN occurs until creatinine clearance falls below 35 ml./min./1.73 m^2 (normal range is 100–150 ml./min./1.73 m^2); therefore, the following maximum dosages are recommended for patients with renal impairment:
[See table above].

Patients on hemodialysis should be given 50 mg. after each dialysis; this should be done under hospital supervision as marked falls in blood pressure can occur.

How Supplied: Tablets of 50 mg atenolol (round, flat, uncoated, white tablets identified with TENORMIN 50 debossed on one side and NDC number 105 debossed and scored on the other side) are supplied in bottles of 100 tablets and unit-dose packages of 100 tablets. NDC 0038-0105.

Tablets of 100 mg atenolol (round, flat, uncoated, white tablets identified with TENORMIN 100 debossed on one side and NDC number 101 debossed on the other side) are supplied in bottles of 100 tablets and unit-dose packages of 100 tablets. NDC 0038-0101.

Protect from heat, light, and moisture. Store unit-dose packages at controlled room temperature.
Shown in Product Identification Section, page 439

IDENTIFICATION PROBLEM?
Consult PDR's
Product Identification Section
where you'll find over 1200
products pictured actual size
and in full color.

Tenormin

Creatinine Clearance (ml./min./1.73 m^2)	Atenolol Elimination Half-life (hrs.)	Maximum Dosage
15–35	16–27	50 mg. daily
<15	>27	50 mg. every other day

Sween Corporation
SWEEN BUILDING
P.O. BOX 980
LAKE CRYSTAL, MN 56055

FORDUSTIN'®
[fŏr-dŭs'tĭn]
Natural Cornstarch Body Powder

Description: A non-caking natural corn-starch based body powder with Sodium Bicarbonate, Silica, Methylbenzethonium Chloride and Fragrance. National Drug Code (NDC) 11701-005.

Indications and Usage: Lubrication of skin subject to excoriation from friction. Helps absorb perspiration to aid in the protection of the skin from perspiration irritation.

Contraindications: Hypersensitivity to any components of the preparation.

Precautions and Adverse Reactions: Transmission electron microscopy and electron diffraction examinations of Fordustin' powder found the product free of any form of fibrous material (asbestiform minerals included) or inorganic materials. For External Use Only. Avoid contact with eyes. Fordustin' is not considered a primary eye or skin irritant under normal use conditions and is not toxic by oral ingestion.

Dosage and Administration: Apply liberally to areas subject to friction and perspiration irritations.

How Supplied: 3 oz. and 8 oz. containers, 8 oz. refill bags.

GENTLE RAIN™ Shampoo
[gĕntle rāin]
and Skin Cleanser

Description: A shampoo and skin cleanser consisting of Water, Sodium Lauryl Sulfate, Ammonium Lauryl Sulfate, Cocamidopropyl Betaine, Lauramide DEA, Glycol Stearate, Hydrolyzed Animal Protein, Quaternium-33, Ethyl Hexanediol, Citric Acid, Fragrance, Quaternium-15, Tetrasodium EDTA and FD&C Yellow #5.

Indications and Usage: Gentle Rain is a luxurious, non-alkaline formulation designed to condition hair as it cleans, plus cleanse sensitive skin gently and thoroughly. The pH has been carefully adjusted for compatibility with the normal range of hair and skin. The low pH, along with the benefits of the special protein and built-in conditioning ingredients, leave hair extremely manageable and easy to care for. Used as a skin cleanser, this same combination leaves the skin soft and supple. This formulation is safe for color treated hair and gentle enough for daily use.

Contraindications: Hypersensitivity to any components of the preparation.

Precautions and Adverse Reactions: For External Use Only. May cause eye irritation. In case of eye contact, flush eyes with water. Gentle Rain is not toxic by oral ingestion and is not considered a primary skin irritant under normal use conditions.

Dosage and Administration:
Shampooing: Wet hair. Lather, rinse thoroughly and repeat.
Bathing: Apply liberally to a warm washcloth and gently wash skin. Rinse thoroughly and pat dry.

How Supplied: 2 fl.oz., 4 fl. oz. and 16 fl.oz. bottles with flip-top caps, 21 fl. oz. with pump dispenser, in addition to larger bulk sizes.

SWEEN KIND TOUCH™
[swēen kĭnd Tŏuch]
Lotion Skin Cleanser

Description: Sween Kind Touch is a lotion skin cleanser consisting of Water, Sodium C14-16 Olefin Sulfonate, Cocamidopropyl Betaine, Sodium Chloride, Lauramide DEA, Glycerin, Glycol Stearate, Quaternium-33, Ethyl Hexanediol, Citric Acid, Fragrance, Quaternium-15, Tetrasodium EDTA and FD&C Blue #1.

Indications and Usage: Sween Kind Touch is a unique conditioning lotion skin cleanser formulated to incorporate richness, creaminess, quick sudsing action, easy rinsing, and a delightful light fragrance. Gentle enough for repeated daily use for all types of general skin cleansing. The pH has been carefully adjusted for compatibility with the normal range of the skin.

Contraindications: Hypersensitivity to any components of the preparation.

Precautions and Adverse Reactions: For External Use Only. Avoid contact with eyes. If contact should occur, flush eyes with water. Sween Kind Touch is not toxic by oral ingestion and is not considered a primary skin irritant under normal use conditions.

Dosage and Administration: Wet hands with warm water. Dispense a small amount of Sween Kind Touch into palm of hand. Wash thoroughly, rinse and dry.

How Supplied: 2 fl. oz. and 16 fl. oz. with flip top caps; 21 fl. oz. and 32 fl. oz. with pump dispenser; in addition to larger sizes.

METHYLBENZETHONIUM CHLORIDE (MBC)
[mĕth'ĭl-bĕn'zĕ-thō'nē-ŭm-klōr'rĭd]
Microbicide for Compounding Drugs/Cosmetics

Description: A quaternary ammonium compound used in the formulation of products for the control of a wide range of microorganisms including proprietary pharmaceutical products as preservatives or antimicrobial agents for topical applications. Specifically used as the active ingredient in formulations for ammonia dermatitis (urine scald) diaper-type rashes, diarrheal breakdowns and similar superficial skin infections. A 1:1000 dilution immediately controls odors of personal illness or putrefaction on contact without contributing an odor of its own.

MBC was developed approximately 10 years after Benzethonium Chloride as an improvement on that compound because of the desire for one that was more potent in microbicidal action yet less toxic to humans. MBC has 3 times the hard-water ceiling of Benzethonium Chloride and, in addition, has a minimum phenol coefficient of twice that of the older product. MBC has ½ the acute oral toxicity of Benzethonium Chloride. Human patch tests on adult and children demonstrated no primary irritation or sensitization and a 0.1% solution of MBC used repeatedly as an eye wash in humans produced only mild irritation.

Contraindications: Not to be used with oxidizing agents such as calcium hypochlorite, nitric acids, or solid perchlorates because of possible explosions (mixture of organic materials with oxidants). Not compatible with anionic wetting agents, potassium chromate, potassium dichromate, sodium heptaphosphate. Pharmaceutical formulations are subject to the Federal Food, Drug, and Cosmetic Act as amended.

Precautions and Adverse Reactions: Safety and Health Statement. In pure form, Danger, Keep out of Reach of Children. Corrosive. Causes severe eye and skin damage. Do not get in eyes, on skin or on clothing. Wear goggles or face shield

Continued on next page

Sween—Cont.

and rubber gloves when handling. Harmful or fatal if swallowed. Avoid contamination of food. When handling crystals, use an exhaust fan to keep dusts away from operators. In case of contact, immediately flush eyes or skin with plenty of water for at least 15 minutes. For eyes, call a physician. Remove and wash contaminated clothing before reuse. If swallowed, drink promptly a large quantity of milk, egg whites, gelatin solution, or if these are not available, drink large quantities of water. Avoid alcohol. Call a physician immediately. Probable mucosal damage may contraindicate the use of gastric lavage. Measures against circulatory shock as well as oxygen and measures to support breathing manually or mechanically may be needed. If persistent, convulsions may be controlled by the cautious intravenous injection of a short-acting barbiturate drug.

How Supplied: White crystalline powder.

MICRO-GUARD™
[mī′ crō-gūard]
Antimicrobial Skin Cream

Description: Micro-Guard Skin Cream contains the antimicrobial agent Chloroxylenol (PCMX) in a water washable, vanishing cream base. National Drug Code (NDC) 11701-012.

Indications and Usage: Micro-Guard is a soothing antiseptic and antifungal cream. Micro-Guard's antifungal action is effective treatment for conditions such as Athlete's Foot, Jock Itch and Ringworm, while its antiseptic activity helps prevent skin infection. Micro-Guard can be used for adjunctive topical treatment of superficial skin infections when oral antibiotic agents are concurrently being administered.

Contraindications: Micro-Guard is contraindicated in individuals who have shown hypersensitivity to any of its components.

Warnings: Micro-Guard is not for ophthalmic, otic or vaginal use.

Precautions: For External Use Only. Do not use near eyes. If accidental contact occurs, flush eyes immediately with water for 15 minutes and consult a physician. If irritation occurs or if there is no improvement within two weeks, discontinue use and consult a physician.

Adverse Reactions: Micro-Guard is not considered a primary skin irritant or sensitizer, but occasional erythema, stinging and eczematous reactions have occurred following its use. If irritation or sensitivity develops with the use of Micro-Guard, treatment should be discontinued and appropriate therapy instituted.

Dosage and Administration: Gently and thoroughly cleanse affected area and pat dry. Apply a thin layer of Micro-Guard over involved area. Repeat application 2 to 3 times daily or as directed by physician.

How Supplied: ½ oz. tube and 2 oz. jars.

PERI–CARE®
Moisture Barrier Ointment for Perineal Protection

Description: A soft petrolatum based ointment incorporating Petrolatum, Natural Vitamins A & D, Sodium Caseinate, Methylbenzethonium Chloride, Chloroxylenol, BHT, Propylparaben and D & C Green #6. National Drug Code (NDC) 11701-010.

Indications and Usage: Used in the perineal area, Peri-Care acts as a buffer between the skin and proteolytic enzymes present in feces and urine, helping avoid skin breakdown and infection. The petrolatum base offers added protection through its physical barrier properties.

Contraindications: Hypersensitivity to any components of the preparation.

Precautions and Adverse Reactions: For External Use Only. Avoid contact with eyes. Peri-Care ointment is not toxic by oral ingestion and is not considered a primary eye or skin irritant under normal use conditions.

Dosage and Administration: Cleanse and rinse soiled perineal area thoroughly. Pat or air dry. Apply Peri-Care ointment liberally to perineal area to be protected. Repeat cleansing procedure promptly whenever discharge occurs and reapply Peri-Care.

How Supplied: Unit dose packets, ½ oz., 1.75 oz. and 5 oz. tubes, 2-oz. and 8-oz. jars.

PERI-WASH®
[pĕri-wăsh]
Perineal Area Cleanser

Description: A skin cleanser. A feces and urine emulsifier consisting of Water, TEA-Lauryl Sulfate, Cocoamphocarboxypropionate, Sodium Lauryl Sulfate, Propylene Glycol, PPG-12-PEG-65 Lanolin Oil, Citric Acid, Styrene/PVP Copolymer, PEG-8 Laurate, PEG-75 Lanolin, Laureth-23, PEG-4 Oleate, Glycol Stearate, Quaternium-15, Methylbenzethonium Chloride, PEG-90M, FD & C Yellow #5 and Other Ingredients. National Drug Code (NDC) 11701-014.

Indications and Usage: Peri-Wash is used for daily care of the perineal area. It is indicated for cleansing of perineal areas afflicted with dermatitis and ammonia dermatitis associated with diarrhea. Through the process of emulsification, Peri-Wash makes the removal of fecal matter from the skin easier, thereby reducing the irritation and formation of denuded skin around the anus. Peri-Wash reduces or eliminates the ammonia odors from urine or feces. Peri-Wash cleanses peristomal skin. Used in ostomy appliances and urine collecting bags, it controls offensive odors. Additional uses for odor control: Cleaning bed pans, urinals, wheel chairs, soiled linens and garments, and hands.

Contraindications: Hypersensitivity to any components of the preparation.

Precautions and Adverse Reactions: For External Use Only. Peri-Wash is not toxic by oral ingestion and is not considered a primary skin irritant under normal use conditions. Peri-Wash is an eye irritant (Sodium Lauryl Sulfate) and should be rinsed thoroughly from eyes if accidental contact occurs.

Dosage and Administration: Apply liberally to perineal area. Wash and rinse thoroughly with clean warm water in the normal manner.

How Supplied: 2 fl. oz., 4 fl. oz. and 8 fl. oz. bottles with spray fitment, in addition to larger bulk sizes.

PURI-CLENS™
[pūrĭ-clĕns]
(formerly Wound Depurant)
Wound Deodorizer and Cleanser

Description: Puri-Clens contains a safe and effective non-irritating antimicrobial ingredient, Methylbenzethonium Chloride, in a water washable, soothing base. National Drug Code (NDC) 11701-008.

Indications and Usage: Puri-Clens deodorizes wounds and aids in the removal of foreign materials and exudates. Will not delay wound healing.

Contraindications: Hypersensitivity to any components of the preparation.

Precautions and Adverse Reactions: For External Use Only. Do not use on animal bites or puncture wounds. Do not use for more than ten days without consulting physician. Puri-Clens is not toxic by oral ingestion and is not considered a primary eye or skin irritant under normal use conditions.

Dosage and Administration: Apply Puri-Clens liberally to a sterile 4″ × 4″ pad. Gently and throughly cleanse wound and surrounding area. To aid in removing foreign material and exudates, dab wound carefully with clean 4″ × 4″ pad saturated with Puri-Clens. May be rinsed with sterile saline, water or hydrogen peroxide solution.

Deodorization: Apply Puri-Clens directly to wound and cover with a sterile absorbent pad. Do not use solution with occlusive dressing. Repeat one to three times daily as necessary to control odors.

How Supplied: 2 oz. unit dose and 8 fl. oz bottles with flip top caps.

SURGI-KLEEN™
[sŭrgĭ-klēēn]
Skin cleanser and shampoo

Description: A skin cleanser consisting of Water, Sodium Lauryl Sulfate, TEA-Lauryl Sulfate, Cocoamphocarboxypropionate, Propylene Glycol, PPG-12-PEG-65 Lanolin Oil, Citric Acid, Styrene/PVP Copolymer, PEG-8 Laurate, PEG-75 Lanolin, Laureth-23, PEG-4 Oleate, Glycol Stearate, Quaternium-15, Fragrance, Methylbenzethonium Chloride, PEG-90M, FD & C Yellow #5, D & C Red #19 and Other Ingredients. National Drug Code (NDC) 11701-003

Indications and Usage: Surgi-Kleen, a gentle and effective liquid skin cleanser and shampoo replaces the need for all bar soap and shampoos. One container for both tasks! Containing a special refined lanolin, Surgi-Kleen helps retain a soft and supple skin. This easy-to-use, low sudsing liquid rinses free, leaving no residue or film on the skin or hair. The convenient flip-top helps reduce the incidence of cross contamination. Problem head and body odors are controlled when using this one versatile cleanser.

Contraindications: Hypersensitivity to any components of the preparation.

Precautions and Adverse Reactions: For External Use Only. Surgi-Kleen is not toxic by oral ingestion and is not considered a primary skin irritant under normal use conditions. Surgi-Kleen is an eye irritant (Sodium Lauryl Sulfate) and should be rinsed thoroughly from eyes if accidental contact occurs.

Dosage and Administration: Surgi-Kleen may be used full strength or diluted one part to three parts of water.

For Regular Bathing: Apply diluted product to moistened wash cloth and gently wash skin, rinse thoroughly and pat dry.

For Shampooing: Apply diluted or undiluted to moistened hair. Massage hair and scalp until lather develops. Then rinse thoroughly and lather again. A very small quantity of Surgi-Kleen will develop a thick, rich lather when hair is clean.

How Supplied: 2 fl. oz., 8 fl. oz. and 16 fl. oz. bottles with flip-top caps, 21 fl. oz. with pump dispenser, in addition to larger bulk sizes.

SWEEN-A-PEEL™
Wafer Skin Protectant

Description: Sween-A-Peel is a wafer skin protectant containing the following:
1. WA4 hydrophilic polymer—to provide moisture absorption.
2. High molecular weight synthetic rubber polymers—to provide elasticity and strength.
3. Low molecular weight synthetic rubber polymers—to provide adhesion to dry surfaces.
4. Karaya gum powder—to provide adhesion to moist surfaces.

Indications and Usage: Sween-A-Peel wafers applied to the peristomal area in ostomy care or to the area surrounding draining wounds, aids in protecting the skin against contact with exudates. Sween-A-Peel may also be applied to pressure points of immobile patients to help preserve skin integrity and reduce the possible occurrence of decubitus ulcers. Sween-A-Peel has also proven effective when incorporated into a decubitus ulcer treatment procedure.

Contraindications: Hypersensitivity to any components of the preparation.

Precautions: Avoid excess heat and humidity. Store below 77°F (25°C). Reseal container after each use.

Administration: RECOMMENDED SKIN CLEANSING PROCEDURE—Before using Sween-A-Peel: (1) Cleanse entire area with Peri-Wash®, a gentle, odor eliminating cleanser. (2) Apply MINIMAL AMOUNT of Sween Cream® to area. Massage until completely absorbed. Soothes red, irritated skin, maintains healthy skin (will not interfere with adhesives). IMPORTANT: Re-

OSTOMY CARE

1. **IMPORTANT:** Use measuring guide to trace and cut pattern of stoma base. NO AREA SHOULD BE EXPOSED. Transfer pattern to wafer using pencil, then cut. (Precision fit is a must to prevent body wastes from coming in contact with and excoriating unprotected skin).
2. Remove backing paper. Position wafer carefully onto skin. Take care not to touch adhesive surface of Sween-A-Peel prior to fitting, as this may impair effective adhesion.
3. After positioning, APPLY EVEN, BUT GENTLE PRESSURE FOR A FEW SECONDS to wafer with palm of hands, particularly on area immediately surrounding the aperture. The warming effect helps ensure even adhesion to body. "Picture frame" the edges of the wafer with porous (paper) tape.

DRAINING WOUND

Using same procedure as above to protect the area skin from contact with wound exudates. Trace pattern, cut, fit, apply gentle, warming, hand pressure and follow prescribed wound care procedure.

How Supplied: 4″ x 4″ wafer in compacts of 5 and tubs of 20 wafers each; 12″ x 12″ square in packages of 2 and 12 squares.

SWEEN CREAM®
[*Swēen Crēam*]
Protective Cream

Description: A vanishing cream consisting of Water, Lanolin Oil, Cetyl Alcohol, Propylene Glycol, Natural Vitamins A & D, Sodium Lauryl Sulfate, Beeswax, Fragrance, Quaternium-15, Methylbenzethonium Chloride and BHT. National Drug Code (NDC) 11701-002.

Indications and Usage: Sween Cream is used for long-term care of incontinent, geriatric, ostomy, and para/quadraplegic skin. Apply as needed to red, sore, irritated skin such as urine scald, diaper rash, diarrheal breakdowns, rectal itch, psoriasis, minor burns, chaffing and itching. Also apply to folds of skin subject to perspiration irritation, to dry or cracked skin and to pressure sore areas. For ostomy patients, apply a small amount around stoma area before attaching appliance to protect skin, relieve itching, and improve tape adhesion.

Contraindications: Hypersensitivity to any components of the preparation.

Precautions and Adverse Reactions: For External Use Only. Avoid contact with eyes. Sween Cream is not toxic by oral ingestion and is not considered a primary eye or skin irritant under normal use conditions.

Dosage and Administration: Apply liberally as required.

How Supplied: Unit dose packets; ½ oz., 2 oz. and 5 oz. tubes; 2-oz. and 9-oz. jars.

SWEEN PREP™
[*Swēen Prēp*]
Protective Skin Barrier Film

Description: Sween Prep is a medicated skin barrier which contains Chloroxylenol (PCMX), a well known antimicrobial agent, in a protective film forming base.

Indications and Usage: Sween Prep applies to the skin as a liquid, with the aid of the special "Dab-O-Matic" applicator, the non-aerosol sprayer or the single use wipe. It dries rapidly to form a tough film which provides a visable shield on the skin... a barrier between the skin and irritants. This protective film creates a surface other than the skin itself for the application of tapes, cements and doublefaced adhesives.

Contraindications: Hypersensitivity to any components of the preparation.

Precautions and Adverse Reactions: If irritation or pain persists, discontinue use and consult physician. For External Use Only. If accidental ingestion occurs or if it comes into contact with the eyes, seek professional help. Flammable. Do not use near flame or while smoking. Sween Prep is not toxic by oral ingestion and is not considered a primary skin irritant under normal use conditions.

Dosage and Administration: Wash the skin area thoroughly, rinse and pat dry. Apply Sween Prep liberally to the entire area to be protected (slight stinging may be experienced if the skin is excoriated). Allow to dry (approximately 2 minutes) and apply tapes, adhesives, etc., in the normal manner to the Sween Prepped skin. Sween Prep may be removed from the skin with soap and water or for easier removal, with isopropyl alcohol. Removal is, however, not necessary and the skin may be recoated as frequently as required.

How Supplied: Unit dose wipes (NDC 11701-007-20), 2 fl. oz. "Dab-O-Matic" applicator (NDC 11701-007-03) and 4 fl. oz. non-aerosol spray (NDC 11701-006-04).

SWEEN SOFT TOUCH™
[*Swēen Sŏft Tŏuch*]
Medicated, Antimicrobial Lotion Skin Cleanser

Description: Sween Soft Touch is an antimicrobial lotion skin cleanser which contains Chloroxylenol (PCMX), a well known antimicrobial agent, in a mild, densely sudsing, soap-free base, adjusted to pH 5.0–5.5 for optimal activity and maintenance of the "acid-balanced" range for healthy skin. National Drug Code (NDC) 11701-015

Indications and Usage: Sween Soft Touch is recommended for repeated daily use as a health care personnel handwash. It decreases bacteria on the skin, reducing the risk and/or chance of cross-infection.

Contraindications: Hypersensitivity to any components of the preparation.

Precautions and Adverse Reactions: For External Use Only. Avoid contact with eyes. If accidental contact occurs, immediately flush eyes with water for 15 minutes and consult a physician. Sween Soft Touch is not toxic by oral ingestion and is not considered a primary skin irritant under normal use conditions.

Dosage and Administration: Wet skin with warm water. Spread a small amount on hands and forearms. Scrub well and rinse thoroughly with warm water after washing.

How Supplied: 2 fl. oz. and 16 fl. oz. bottles with flip-top caps, 21 fl. oz. and 32 fl. oz. with pump dispenser; in addition to larger bulk sizes.

WHIRL-SOL®
[*whĭrl-sŏl*]
Skin Conditioner

Description: Mineral Oil, Propylene Glycol Dipelargonate, Lanolin Oil, PEG-8 Dioleate, Fragrance, D&C Green #6. National Drug Code (NDC) 11701-001.

Indications and Usage: Whirl-Sol is a completely water dispersible oil easily absorbed by the skin to aid in the relief of dry, pruritic conditions. Whirl-Sol helps soothe and restore skin to a more elastic and pliable condition. It is an effective aid in treating skin problems such as soap dermatitis, pruritus senilis and hiemalis, chronic atopic dermatitis, asteatosis, xerosis, ichthyosis, psoriasis, etc. Whirl-Sol promotes a normal healthy skin with natural-like oils.

Contraindications: Hypersensitivity to any components of the preparation.

Precautions and Adverse Reactions: For External Use Only. Avoid contact with eyes. Whirl-Sol is not toxic by oral ingestion and is not considered a primary eye or skin irritant under normal use conditions. Guard against slipping in tub or shower.

Dosage and Administration: Whirl-Sol is always used with water. It is added, 1 to 2 capfuls to whirlpool bathing systems, regular bath tubs, or wash basins. Apply to washcloth for use in the shower.

How Supplied: 2 fl. oz., 8 fl. oz. and 16 fl. oz. bottles, with flip-top caps, 21 fl. oz. with pump dispenser; in addition to larger bulk sizes.

XTRACARE® II
[*xtrӑ-cӑre*]
Moisturizing Body Lotion

Description: A thick-bodied, high moisturizing cream consisting of Water, Cetyl Alcohol, Propylene Glycol, Lanolin Oil, Beeswax, Sodium Lauryl Sulfate, Quaternium-15, Fragrance and Methylbenzethonium Chloride.
National Drug Code (NDC) 11701-004.

Indications and Usage: Xtracare II is an unusually rich moisturizer which serves as an exceptional massage vehicle for the entire body. Its creamy consistency applies easily and uniformly to soothe and moisturize skin. The special emollient and humectant properties provide long lasting retardation of skin moisture evaporation. This leaves the skin feeling smooth, cool and comfortable without greasiness and tackiness or interference of normal skin respiration. Apply as needed for back rubs, dry skin problems and physical therapy. Especially suited for foot and lower leg care. Liberal application recommended before applying plaster casts.

Contraindications: Hypersensitivity to any components of the preparation.

Precautions and Adverse Reactions: For External Use Only. Avoid contact with eyes. Xtracare II in not toxic by oral ingestion and is not considered a primary eye or skin irritant under normal use conditions.

Dosage and Administration: Apply liberally as often as needed for dry skin management. Use as a massage lubricant for back rubs and for therapeutic muscle massage.

How Supplied: 2 fl. oz., 4 fl. oz. and 8 fl. oz. bottles with dispenser caps, 21 fl. oz. with pump dispenser, in addition to larger bulk sizes.

Syntex (F.P.) Inc.
HUMACAO, PUERTO RICO 00661

Syntex Laboratories, Inc
3401 HILLVIEW AVE.
P.O. BOX 10850
PALO ALTO, CA 94303

Syntex Puerto Rico, Inc.
HUMACAO, PUERTO RICO 00661

ANADROL®-50   B
[*an'ӑ-drawl*]
(oxymetholone)
50 mg. Tablets

A product of Syntex Laboratories, Inc.

Description: Anadrol-50 contains 50 mg. of the steroid, oxymetholone, which has the chemical name 17 β-hydroxy-2-(hydroxymethylene)-17-methyl-5α-androstan-3-one.

Action: Anadrol-50 is a potent anabolic and androgenic drug. It enhances the production and urinary excretion of erythropoietin in patients with anemias due to bone marrow failure and often stimulates erythropoiesis in anemias due to deficient red cell production.

Indications: Anadrol-50 is indicated in the treatment of anemias caused by deficient red cell production. Acquired aplastic anemia, congenital aplastic anemia, myelofibrosis and the hypoplastic anemias due to the administration of myelotoxic drugs often respond. Anadrol-50 should not replace other supportive measures such as transfusion, correction of iron, folic acid, vitamin B_{12} or pyridoxine deficiency, antibacterial therapy and the appropriate use of corticosteroids.

Contraindications: Since anabolic agents are generally contraindicated in the following situations, before instituting therapy, the clinician

Continued on next page

Syntex—Cont.

must weigh the risk involved against the patients' needs.
1. Carcinoma of the prostate or breast in male patients.
2. Pregnancy—primarily because of masculinization of the fetus.
3. Infancy. Since evidence of beneficial effect in prematures and newborns is lacking, and consequences of the use of anabolic steroids in these patients are unknown, their use is not recommended.
4. Nephrosis or the nephrotic phase of nephritis.
5. Hypersensitivity.
6. Hepatic dysfunction.

Warnings: Anabolic steroids do not enhance athletic ability.

Precautions:
1. *Hepatotoxicity*
Hepatotoxic effects, including jaundice, are common with the prescribed dosage. Clinical jaundice may be painless, with or without pruritus. It may also be associated with acute hepatic enlargement and right-upper quadrant pain, which has been mistaken for acute (surgical) obstruction of the bile duct. Drug-induced jaundice is usually reversible when the medication is discontinued. Continued therapy has been associated with hepatic coma and death. Because of the hepatotoxicity associated with Anadrol-50 (oxymetholone) administration, periodic liver function tests are recommended.
Hepatocellular carcinoma and peliosis hepatis,[1] a rare condition of ill-defined etiology consisting of blood-filled cysts in the liver, have been observed in patients with congenital and acquired aplastic anemia treated with oxymetholone and other androgens for prolonged periods. In some cases withdrawal of the drug has been associated with regression of the hepatic lesions.

2. *Virilization*
In the female virilization may occur. Amenorrhea usually occurs in the adult female, even in the presence of thrombocytopenia. Concomitant administration of large doses of progestational agents to control menorrhagia is not recommended.

3. *Iron deficiency*
The development of iron deficiency anemia, manifested by a low serum iron and decreased percent saturation of transferrin, has been observed in some patients treated with Anadrol-50 (oxymetholone). Periodic determination of the serum iron and iron binding capacity is recommended. If iron deficiency is detected, it should be appropriately treated with supplementary iron.

4. Leukemia has been observed in patients with aplastic anemia treated with oxymetholone. The role, if any, of oxymetholone is unclear because malignant transformation has been seen in blood dyscrasias and leukemia has been reported in patients with aplastic anemia who have not been treated with oxymetholone.

5. Caution is required in administering these agents to patients with cardiac, renal, or hepatic disease. Edema, with or without congestive heart failure, may occur occasionally. Concomitant administration with adrenal steroids or ACTH may add to the edema. This is generally controllable with appropriate diuretic and/or digitalis therapy.

6. Hypercalcemia may develop both spontaneously and as a result of hormonal therapy in women with disseminated breast carcinoma. If it develops while on this agent, the drug should be stopped.

7. Anabolic steroids may increase sensitivity to anticoagulants. Dosage of the anticoagulant may have to be decreased in order to maintain the prothrombin time at the desired therapeutic level.

8. Anabolic steroids have been shown to alter glucose tolerance tests. Diabetics should be followed carefully and the insulin or oral hypoglycemic dosage adjusted accordingly.

9. Anabolic steroids should be used with caution in patients with benign prostatic hypertrophy.

10. Serum cholesterol may increase or decrease during therapy. Therefore, caution is required in administering these agents to patients with a history of myocardial infarction or coronary artery disease. Serial determinations of serum cholesterol should be made and therapy adjusted accordingly.

Adverse Reactions:
1. *Hepatotoxicity* is the most serious adverse reaction associated with anabolic steroid therapy. Reversible increase in BSP retention occurs early and appears to be directly related to the dose. Increase in serum bilirubin, with or without an increase in the serum alkaline phosphatase and transaminases (SGOT and SGPT) indicate a higher degree of excretory dysfunction. Clinical jaundice, which is reversible when the drug is discontinued, may occur. The histologic picture is one of intrahepatic cholestasis with little or no cellular damage. Continued therapy may be associated with hepatic coma and death.

2. Virilization is the most common undesirable effect associated with anabolic steroid therapy. Acne occurs frequently in all age groups.
Prepuberal male: The first signs of virilization in the prepuberal male are phallic enlargement and an increase in frequency of erection. Hirsutism and increased skin pigmentation may also occur.
Postpuberal male: Inhibition of testicular function with oligospermia: decrease in seminal volume, alteration in libido, and impotence may occur with prolonged or intensive anabolic therapy. Gynecomastia, and testicular atrophy may occur. Chronic priapism, male-pattern of hair loss, epididymitis and bladder irritability have been reported. In females, hirsutism, hoarseness or deepening of the voice, clitoral enlargement, alteration of libido, and menstrual irregularities and male-pattern baldness may occur. The voice change and clitoral enlargement are usually irreversible even after prompt discontinuance of therapy. The use of estrogens in combination with androgens will not prevent virilization in females.

3. Other adverse reactions associated with anabolic/androgenic therapy include: muscle cramps, nausea, excitation and sleeplessness, chills, bleeding in patients on concomitant anticoagulant therapy, premature closure of epiphyses in children, vomiting and diarrhea.

4. Alterations in these clinical laboratory tests:
 a. The metyrapone test
 b. The FBS and glucose tolerance test
 c. The thyroid function tests: a decrease in the PBI, in thyroxine-binding capacity and radioactive iodine uptake and an increase in T[3] uptake by the rbc's or resin may occur. Free thyroxine is normal. Altered tests usually persist for 2-3 weeks after stopping anabolic therapy.
 d. The electrolytes: retention of sodium, chlorides, water, potassium, phosphates and calcium.
 e. Increased or decreased serum cholesterol.
 f. Suppression of clotting factors II, V, VII, and X.
 g. Increased creatine and creatinine excretion lasting up to two weeks after discontinuing therapy.
 h. Decreased 17-ketosteroid excretion.

5. There have been rare reports of hepatocellular neoplasms and peliosis hepatis in association with long-term androgenic-anabolic steroid therapy.

Dosage and Administration: The recommended daily dose in children and adults, 1-5 mg./kg. body weight per day. The usual effective dose is 1-2 mg./kg./day but higher doses may be required and the dose should be individualized. Response is not often immediate and a minimum trial of three to six months should be given. Following remission, some patients may be maintained without the drug; others may be maintained on an established lower daily dosage. A continued maintenance dose is usually necessary in patients with congenital aplastic anemia.

Availability: Anadrol-50 (oxymetholone) is available in bottles of 100 white scored tablets imprinted with the code "2902" and "Syntex".
Revised 12/79

---

[1]Zak, F. G., Peliosis Hepatis. Am. J. Path. 26:1-15, (Jan.) 1950.
Shown in Product Identification Section, page 440

ANAPROX® ℞
[an'ă-prox]
(naproxen sodium)
Tablets

Manufactured for Syntex Laboratories, Inc. by Syntex Puerto Rico, Inc.

Description: ANAPROX filmcoated tablets for oral administration each contain 275 mg of naproxen sodium, which is equivalent to 250 mg naproxen with 25 mg (about 1 mEq) sodium. It is a member of the arylacetic acid group of nonsteroidal anti-inflammatory drugs.
The chemical name of naproxen sodium is 2-naphthaleneacetic acid, 6-methoxy-α-methyl-, sodium salt, (—).
Naproxen sodium is a white to creamy white, crystalline solid, freely soluble in water.

Clinical Pharmacology: ANAPROX, the sodium salt of naproxen, has been developed as an analgesic because it is more rapidly absorbed. Naproxen is a nonsteroidal anti-inflammatory drug with analgesic and antipyretic properties. Naproxen anion inhibits prostaglandin synthesis but beyond this its mode of action is unknown.
Naproxen sodium is rapidly and completely absorbed from the gastrointestinal tract. After administration of naproxen sodium, peak plasma levels of naproxen anion are attained at 1-2 hours with steady-state conditions normally achieved after 4-5 doses. The mean biological half-life of the anion in humans is approximately 13 hours, and at therapeutic levels it is greater than 99% albumin bound. Approximately 95% of the dose is excreted in the urine, primarily as naproxen, 6-0-desmethyl naproxen or their conjugates. The rate of excretion has been found to coincide closely with the rate of drug disappearance from the plasma. The drug does not induce metabolizing enzymes.
The drug was studied in patients with mild to moderate pain, and pain relief was obtained within 1 hour. It is not a narcotic and is not a CNS-acting drug. Controlled double-blind studies have demonstrated the analgesic properties of the drug in, for example, post-operative, post-partum, orthopedic and uterine contraction pain and dysmenorrhea. In dysmenorrheic patients, the drug reduces the level of prostaglandins in the uterus, which correlates with a reduction in the frequency and severity of uterine contractions. Analgesic action has been shown by such measures as reduction of pain intensity scores, increase in pain relief scores, decrease in number of patients requiring additional analgesic medication, and delay in time for required remedication. The analgesic effect has been found to last for up to 7 hours.
The drug was studied in patients with rheumatoid arthritis, osteoarthritis, ankylosing spondylitis, tendinitis and bursitis, and acute gout. It is not a corticosteroid. Improvement in patients treated for rheumatoid arthritis has been demonstrated by a reduction in joint swelling, a reduction in pain, a reduction in duration of morning stiffness, a reduction in disease activity as assessed by both the investigator and patient, and by increased mobility as demonstrated by a reduction in walking time.
In patients with osteoarthritis, the therapeutic action of the drug has been shown by a reduction in joint pain or tenderness, an increase in range of motion in knee joints, increased mobility as demonstrated by a reduction in walking time, and improvement in capacity to perform activities of daily living impaired by the disease.
In clinical studies in patients with rheumatoid arthritis and osteoarthritis, the drug has been shown to be comparable to aspirin and indomethacin in controlling the aforementioned measures of

disease activity, but the frequency and severity of the milder gastrointestinal adverse effects (nausea, dyspepsia, heartburn) and nervous system adverse effects (tinnitus, dizziness, lightheadedness) were less than in both the aspirin- and indomethacin-treated patients. It is not known whether the drug causes less peptic ulceration than aspirin.

In patients with ankylosing spondylitis, the drug has been shown to decrease night pain, morning stiffness and pain at rest. In double-blind studies the drug was shown to be as effective as aspirin, but with fewer side effects.

In patients with acute gout, a favorable response to the drug was shown by significant clearing of inflammatory changes (e.g., decrease in swelling, heat) within 24–48 hours, as well as by relief of pain and tenderness.

The drug may be used safely in combination with gold salts and/or corticosteroids; however, in controlled clinical trials, when added to the regimen of patients receiving corticosteroids it did not appear to cause greater improvement over that seen with corticosteroids alone. Whether the drug could be used in conjunction with partially effective doses of corticosteroid for a "steroid-sparing" effect has not been adequately studied. When added to the regimen of patients receiving gold salts, the drug did result in greater improvement. Its use in combination with salicylates is not recommended because data are inadequate to demonstrate that the drug produces greater improvement over that achieved with aspirin alone. Further, there is some evidence that aspirin increases the rate of excretion of the drug.

Generally, improvement due to the drug has not been found to be dependent on age, sex, severity or duration of disease.

In ^{51}Cr blood loss and gastroscopy studies with normal volunteers, daily administration of 1100 mg of ANAPROX (naproxen sodium) has been demonstrated to cause statistically significantly less gastric bleeding and erosion than 3250 mg of aspirin.

Indications and Usage: ANAPROX (naproxen sodium) is indicated in the relief of mild to moderate pain and for the treatment of primary dysmenorrhea.

It is also indicated for the treatment of rheumatoid arthritis, osteoarthritis, ankylosing spondylitis, tendinitis and bursitis, and acute gout.

Contraindications: The drug is contraindicated in patients who have had allergic reactions to ANAPROX® (naproxen sodium) or to NAPROSYN® (naproxen). It is also contraindicated in patients in whom aspirin or other nonsteroidal anti-inflammatory/analgesic drugs induce the syndrome of asthma, rhinitis, and nasal polyps. Both types of reactions have the potential of being fatal.

Warnings: Gastrointestinal bleeding, sometimes severe, and occasionally fatal, has been reported in patients receiving the drug. Among 960 patients treated for rheumatoid arthritis or osteoarthritis during the course of clinical trials in the United States (260 treated for more than two years), 16 cases of peptic ulceration were reported. More than half were on concomitant corticosteroid and/or salicylate therapy and about a third had a prior history of peptic ulcer. Gastrointestinal bleeding, including nine potentially serious cases, was also reported in this population. These were not always preceded by premonitory gastrointestinal symptoms. Although most of the patients with serious bleeding were receiving concomitant therapy and had a history of peptic ulcer disease, it should be kept in mind that the drug also has the potential for causing gastrointestinal bleeding on its own. Therefore, it should not be given to patients with active peptic ulcer unless the potential benefit outweighs the potential risk. In such patients, and in other patients with a history of gastrointestinal disease, it should be given under close supervision.

Precautions:
General:
ANAPROX (NAPROXEN SODIUM) SHOULD NOT BE USED CONCOMITANTLY WITH THE RELATED DRUG NAPROSYN (NAPROXEN) SINCE THEY BOTH CIRCULATE IN PLASMA AS THE NAPROXEN ANION.

Anaphylactic reactions to ANAPROX or NAPROSYN, whether of the true allergic type or the pharmacologic idiosyncratic (e.g., aspirin syndrome) type, usually but not always occur in patients with a known history of such reactions. Therefore, careful questioning of patients for such things as asthma, nasal polyps, urticaria, and hypotension associated with nonsteroidal anti-inflammatory drugs before starting therapy is important. In addition, if such symptoms occur during therapy, treatment should be discontinued.

In chronic studies in laboratory animals, the drug has caused nephritis. Glomerular nephritis, interstitial nephritis and nephrotic syndrome have been reported in humans. This drug should therefore be used with great caution in patients with significantly impaired renal function and the monitoring of serum creatinine and/or creatinine clearance is advised in these patients. Caution should be used if the drug is given to patients with creatinine clearance less than 20 ml/minute because accumulation of naproxen metabolites has been seen in such patients.

Certain patients, specifically those where renal blood flow is compromised, such as in extracellular volume depletion, cirrhosis of the liver, sodium restriction, congestive heart failure, and pre-existing renal disease, should have renal function assessed before and during therapy with this drug. Some elderly in whom impaired renal function may be expected could also fall within this category. A reduction in daily dosage should be considered to avoid the possibility of excessive drug accumulation in these patients.

Chronic alcoholic liver disease and probably other forms of cirrhosis reduce the total plasma concentration of naproxen, but the plasma concentration of unbound naproxen is increased. Caution is advised when huge doses are required and some adjustment of dosage may be required in these patients.

One study indicates that although total plasma concentration of naproxen is unchanged, the unbound plasma fraction of naproxen is increased in the elderly. Caution is advised when high doses are required and some adjustment of dosage may be required in elderly patients.

As with other nonsteroidal anti-inflammatory drugs borderline elevations of one or more liver tests may occur in up to 15% of patients. These abnormalities may progress, may remain essentially unchanged, or may be transient with continued therapy. The SGPT (ALT) test is probably the most sensitive indicator of liver dysfunction. Meaningful (3 times the upper limit of normal) elevations of SGPT or SGOT (AST) occurred in controlled clinical trials in less than 1% of patients. A patient with symptoms and/or signs suggesting liver dysfunction, or in whom an abnormal liver test has occurred, should be evaluated for evidence of the development of more severe hepatic reaction while on therapy with this drug. Severe hepatic reactions, including jaundice and cases of fatal hepatitis, have been reported with this drug as with other nonsteroidal anti-inflammatory drugs. Although such reactions are rare, if abnormal liver tests persist or worsen, if clinical signs and symptoms consistent with liver disease develop, or if systemic manifestations occur (e.g. eosinophilia, rash, etc.), this drug should be discontinued.

If steroid dosage is reduced or eliminated during therapy, the steroid dosage should be reduced slowly and the patients must be observed closely for any evidence of adverse effects, including adrenal insufficiency and exacerbation of symptoms of arthritis.

Patients with initial hemoglobin values of 10 grams or less who are to receive long-term therapy should have hemoglobin values determined frequently.

Peripheral edema has been observed in some patients. Since each naproxen sodium tablet contains approximately 25 mg (about 1 mEq) of sodium, this should be considered in patients whose overall intake of sodium must be markedly restricted. For these reasons, the drug should be used with caution in patients with fluid retention, hypertension or heart failure.

The antipyretic and anti-inflammatory activities of the drug may reduce fever and inflammation, thus diminishing their utility as diagnostic signs in detecting complications of presumed non-infectious, non-inflammatory painful conditions.

Because of adverse eye findings in animal studies with drugs of this class it is recommended that ophthalmic studies be carried out within a reasonable period of time after starting therapy and at periodic intervals thereafter if the drug is to be used for an extended period of time.

Information for Patients:
Caution should be exercised by patients whose activities require alertness if they experience drowsiness, dizziness, vertigo or depression during therapy with the drug.

Drug Interactions:
In vitro studies have shown that naproxen anion, because of its affinity for protein, may displace from their binding sites other drugs which are also albumin-bound. Theoretically, the naproxen anion itself could likewise be displaced. Short-term controlled studies failed to show that taking the drug significantly affects prothrombin times when administered to individuals on coumarin-type anticoagulants. Caution is advised nonetheless, since interactions have been seen with other nonsteroidal agents of this class. Similarly, patients receiving the drug and a hydantoin, sulfonamide or sulfonylurea should be observed for signs of toxicity to these drugs.

The natriuretic effect of furosemide has been reported to be inhibited by some drugs of this class. Inhibition of renal lithium clearance leading to increases in plasma lithium concentrations has also been reported.

This and other nonsteroidal anti-inflammatory drugs can reduce the antihypertensive effect of propranolol and other beta-blockers.

Probenecid given concurrently increases naproxen anion plasma levels and extends its plasma half-life significantly.

Caution should be used if this drug is administered concomitantly with methotrexate. Naproxen and other nonsteroidal anti-inflammatory drugs have been reported to reduce the tubular secretion of methotrexate in an animal model, possibly enhancing the toxicity of that drug.

Drug/Laboratory Test Interactions:
The drug may decrease platelet aggregation and prolong bleeding time. This effect should be kept in mind when bleeding times are determined.

The administration of the drug may result in increased urinary values for 17-ketogenic steroids because of an interaction between the drug and/or its metabolites with m-dinitro-benzene used in this assay. Although 17-hydroxy-corticosteroid measurements (Porter-Silber test) do not appear to be artifactually altered, it is suggested that therapy with the drug be temporarily discontinued 72 hours before adrenal function tests are performed. The drug may interfere with some urinary assays of 5-hydroxy indoleacetic acid (5HIAA).

Carcinogenesis:
A two-year study was performed in rats to evaluate the carcinogenic potential of the drug. No evidence of carcinogenicity was found.

Pregnancy:
Teratogenic Effects: Pregnancy Category B. Reproduction studies have been performed in rats, rabbits and mice at doses up to six times the human dose and have revealed no evidence of impaired fertility or harm to the fetus due to the drug. There are, however, no adequate and well-controlled studies in pregnant women. Because animal reproduction studies are not always predictive of human response, the drug should not be used during pregnancy unless clearly needed. Because of the known effect of drugs of this class on the human fetal cardiovascular system (closure of

Continued on next page

Syntex—Cont.

ductus arteriosus), use during late pregnancy should be avoided.

Non-teratogenic Effects: As with other drugs known to inhibit prostaglandin synthesis, an increased incidence of dystocia and delayed parturition occurred in rats.

Nursing Mothers:
The naproxen anion has been found in the milk of lactating women at a concentration of approximately 1% of that found in the plasma. Because of the possible adverse effects of prostaglandin-inhibiting drugs on neonates, use in nursing mothers should be avoided.

Pediatric Use:
Pediatric indications and dosage recommendations have not been established for ANAPROX® (naproxen sodium).

Adverse Reactions: Adverse reactions reported in controlled clinical trials in 960 patients treated for rheumatoid arthritis or osteoarthritis are listed below. In general, these reactions were reported 2 to 10 times more frequently than they were in studies in the 962 patients treated for mild to moderate pain or for dysmenorrhea.

Incidence greater than 1%
Gastrointestinal: The most frequent complaints reported related to the gastrointestinal tract. They were: constipation*, heartburn*, abdominal pain*, nausea*, dyspepsia, diarrhea, stomatitis.
Central Nervous System: Headache*, dizziness*, drowsiness*, lightheadedness, vertigo.
Dermatologic: Itching (pruritus)*, skin eruptions*, ecchymoses*, sweating, purpura.
Special Senses: Tinnitus*, hearing disturbances, visual disturbances.
Cardiovascular: Edema*, dyspnea*, palpitations.
General: Thirst.
*Incidence of reported reaction between 3% and 9%. Those reactions occurring in less than 3% of the patients are unmarked.

Incidence less than 1%
Probable Causal Relationship:
The following adverse reactions were reported less frequently than 1% during controlled clinical trials and through voluntary reports since marketing. The probability of a causal relationship exists between the drug and these adverse reactions.
Gastrointestinal: Abnormal liver function tests, gastrointestinal bleeding, hematemesis, jaundice, melena, peptic ulceration with bleeding and/or perforation, vomiting.
Renal: Glomerular nephritis, hematuria, interstitial nephritis, nephrotic syndrome, renal disease.
Hematologic: Eosinophilia, granulocytopenia, leukopenia, thrombocytopenia.
Central Nervous System: Depression, dream abnormalities, inability to concentrate, insomnia, malaise, myalgia and muscle weakness.
Dermatologic: Alopecia, skin rashes.
Special Senses: Hearing impairment.
Cardiovascular: Congestive heart failure.
General: Anaphylactoid reactions, menstrual disorders, pyrexia (chills and fever).
Causal Relationship Unknown:
Other reactions have been reported in circumstances in which a causal relationship could not be established. However, in these rarely reported events, the possibility cannot be excluded. Therefore these observations are being listed to serve as alerting information to the physicians.
Hematologic: Agranulocytosis, aplastic anemia, hemolytic anemia.
Central Nervous System: Cognitive dysfunction.
Dermatologic: Urticaria.
General: Angioneurotic edema, hyperglycemia, hypoglycemia.
Overdosage: Significant overdosage may be characterized by drowsiness, heartburn, indigestion, nausea or vomiting. Because naproxen sodium may be rapidly absorbed, high and early blood levels should be anticipated. No evidence of toxicity or late sequelae have been reported 5 to 15 months after ingestion for three to seven days of doses equivalent to up to 3,300 mg of naproxen sodium. One patient ingested a single dose equivalent to 27.5 g of naproxen sodium and experienced mild nausea and indigestion. It is not known what dose of the drug would be life threatening. The oral LD_{50} of the drug is 543 mg/kg in rats, 1234 mg/kg in mice, 4110 mg/kg in hamsters and greater than 1000 mg/kg in dogs.

Should a patient ingest a large number of tablets, accidentally or purposefully, the stomach may be emptied and usual supportive measures employed. Animal studies suggest that the prompt administration of 5 grams of activated charcoal would tend to reduce markedly the absorption of the drug. It is not known if the drug is dialyzable.

Dosage and Administration:
For Mild to Moderate Pain, Primary Dysmenorrhea, and Acute Tendinitis and Bursitis:
The recommended starting dose is two 275 mg tablets, followed by one 275 mg tablet every 6 to 8 hours, as required. The total daily dose should not exceed 5 tablets (1,375 mg).
For Rheumatoid Arthritis, Osteoarthritis, and Ankylosing Spondylitis:
The recommended starting dose in adults is one 275 mg tablet twice daily (morning and evening) or one 275 mg tablet in the morning and two 275 mg tablets in the evening. During long-term administration, the dose may be adjusted up or down depending on the clinical response of the patient. A lower daily dose may suffice for long-term administration. Daily doses higher than 1100 mg in these indications have not been studied. The morning and evening doses do not have to be equal in size and the administration of the drug more frequently than twice daily is not necessary. Symptomatic improvement in arthritis usually begins within two weeks. However, if improvement is not seen within this period, a trial for an additional two weeks should be considered.

For Acute Gout:
The recommended starting dose is three 275 mg tablets, followed by one 275 mg tablet every eight hours until the attack has subsided.

How Supplied: ANAPROX® (naproxen sodium) is available in filmcoated tablets of 275 mg (light blue), in bottles of 100 tablets (NDC 18393-274-42) and 500 tablets (NDC 18393-274-62) or in cartons of 100 individually blister packed tablets (NDC 18393-274-53). Store at room temperature in well-closed containers.

CAUTION: Federal law prohibits dispensing without prescription.

Revised May 1984
Shown in Product Identification Section, page 440

BREVICON® Tablets   ℞
[*brev'i-kahn*]
(norethindrone and
  ethinyl estradiol tablets)

NORINYL® 1 + 35 Tablets   ℞
[*nor'i-nil*]
(norethindrone and
  ethinyl estradiol tablets)

NORINYL® 1 + 50 Tablets   ℞
(norethindrone and mestranol tablets)

NORINYL® 1 + 80 Tablets   ℞
(norethindrone and mestranol tablets)

NORINYL® 2 mg. Tablets   ℞
(norethindrone and mestranol tablets)

NOR-Q.D.®   ℞
(norethindrone)
Tablets 0.35 mg.

TRI–NORINYL® Tablets
(norethindrone and
  ethinyl estradiol tablets)
Oral Contraceptives

Products of Syntex (F.P.) Inc.

Description: BREVICON 21-DAY Tablets provide an oral contraceptive regimen consisting of 21 blue tablets containing norethindrone 0.5 mg. with ethinyl estradiol 0.035 mg.

BREVICON 28-DAY Tablets provide a continuous oral contraceptive regimen consisting of 21 blue tablets containing norethindrone 0.5 mg. with ethinyl estradiol 0.035 mg. and 7 orange tablets containing inert ingredients.

NORINYL 1 + 35 21-DAY Tablets provide an oral contraceptive regimen consisting of 21 green tablets containing norethindrone 1 mg. with ethinyl estradiol 0.035 mg.

NORINYL 1 + 35 28-DAY Tablets provide a continuous oral contraceptive regimen consisting of 21 green tablets containing norethindrone 1 mg. with ethinyl estradiol 0.035 mg. and 7 orange tablets containing inert ingredients.

NORINYL 1 + 50 21-DAY Tablets provide an oral contraceptive regimen consisting of 21 white tablets containing norethindrone 1 mg. with mestranol 0.05 mg.

NORINYL 1 + 50 28-DAY Tablets provide a continuous oral contraceptive regimen consisting of 21 white tablets containing norethindrone 1 mg. with mestranol 0.05 mg. and 7 orange tablets containing inert ingredients.

NORINYL 1 + 80 21-DAY Tablets provide an oral contraceptive regimen consisting of 21 yellow tablets containing norethindrone 1 mg. with mestranol 0.08 mg.

NORINYL 1 + 80 28-DAY Tablets provide a continuous oral contraceptive regimen consisting of 21 yellow tablets containing norethindrone 1 mg. with mestranol 0.08 mg. and 7 orange tablets containing inert ingredients.

NORINYL 2 mg. Tablets provide an oral contraceptive regimen consisting of 20 white tablets containing norethindrone 2 mg. with mestranol 0.1 mg.

NOR-Q.D. (norethindrone) Tablets provide a continuous oral contraceptive regimen of one yellow norethindrone 0.35 mg. tablet daily.

TRI-NORINYL 21-DAY Tablets provide an oral contraceptive regimen of 7 blue tablets followed by 9 green tablets and 5 more blue tablets. Each blue tablet contains norethindrone 0.5 mg with ethinyl estradiol 0.035 mg and each green tablet contains norethindrone 1.0 mg with ethinyl estradiol 0.035 mg.

TRI-NORINYL 28-DAY Tablets provide a continuous oral contraceptive regimen of 7 blue tablets, 9 green tablets, 5 more blue tablets, and then 7 orange tablets. Each blue tablet contains norethindrone 0.5 mg with ethinyl estradiol 0.035 mg, each green tablet contains norethindrone 1.0 mg with ethinyl estradiol 0.035 mg, and each orange tablet contains inert ingredients.

Norethindrone is a potent progestational agent with the chemical name 17-hydroxy-19-nor-17α-pregn-4-en-20-yn-3-one. Ethinyl estradiol is an estrogen with the chemical name 19-nor-17α-pregna-1, 3, 5(10)-trien-20-yne-3, 17-diol. Mestranol is an estrogen with the chemical name 3-methoxy-19-nor-17α-pregna-1, 3, 5(10)-trien-20-yn-17-ol.

Clinical Pharmacology: Combination oral contraceptives act primarily through the mechanism of gonadotrophin suppression due to the estrogenic and progestational activity of the ingredients. Although the primary mechanism of action is inhibition of ovulation, alterations in the genital tract including changes in the cervical mucus (which increase the difficulty of sperm penetration) and the endometrium (which reduce the likelihood of implantation) may also contribute to contraceptive effectiveness.

The primary mechanism through which NOR-Q.D. prevents conception is not known, but progestogen-only contraceptives are known to alter the cervical mucus, exert a progestational effect on the endometrium, interfering with implantation, and, in some patients, suppress ovulation.

Indications and Usage: Oral contraceptives are indicated for the prevention of pregnancy in women who elect to use oral contraceptives as a method of contraception. NORINYL 2 mg. is also indicated in the treatment of hypermenorrhea.

Oral contraceptives are highly effective. The pregnancy rate in women using conventional combination oral contraceptives (containing 0.035 mg. or more of ethinyl estradiol or 0.05 mg. or more of mestranol) is generally reported as less than one pregnancy per 100 woman-years of use. Slightly higher rates (somewhat more than 1 pregnancy per 100 woman-years of use) are reported for some combination products containing 0.035 mg. or less of ethinyl estradiol, and rates on the order of 3 pregnancies per 100 woman-years are reported for the progestogen-only oral contraceptives.

These rates are derived from separate studies conducted by different investigators in several population groups and cannot be compared precisely. Furthermore, pregnancy rates tend to be lower as clinical studies are continued, possibly due to selective retention in the longer studies of those patients who accept the treatment regimen and do not discontinue as a result of adverse reactions, pregnancy, or other reasons.

In clinical trials with BREVICON, 1,168 patients completed 16,345 cycles and a total of 3 pregnancies was reported. This represents a pregnancy rate of 0.22 per 100 woman-years.

In clinical trials with NORINYL 1 + 35, 940 patients completed 14,366 cycles and a total of 2 pregnancies was reported. This represents a pregnancy rate of 0.17 per 100 woman-years.

The dropout rate for medical reasons, as observed in the clinical trials conducted with BREVICON and NORINYL 1 + 35, appears to be somewhat higher than observed with higher dose combination products. The dropout rate due to menstrual disorders and irregularities was also somewhat higher, dropouts being equally split between menstrual disorders and irregularities and other medical reasons attributable to the drug.

In clinical trials with NORINYL 1 + 50 21-DAY, 3,852 patients completed 45,937 cycles and a total of 10 pregnancies was reported. This represents a pregnancy rate of 0.26 per 100 woman-years. In clinical trials with NORINYL 1 + 50 28-DAY, 1,590 patients completed 7,330 cycles and a total of 3 pregnancies was reported. This represents a pregnancy rate of 0.5 per 100 woman-years. In clinical trials with NORINYL 1 + 80 21- and 28-DAY, 3,464 patients completed 34,068 cycles and a total of 5 pregnancies was reported. This represents a pregnancy rate of 0.18 per 100 woman-years. In clinical trials with NORINYL 2 mg. 6,097 patients completed 121,233 cycles and a total of 13 pregnancies was reported. This represents a pregnancy rate of 0.13 per 100 woman-years. In clinical trials with NOR-Q.D. (norethindrone) 2,963 patients completed 25,901 cycles of therapy and a total of 55 pregnancies was reported. This represents an average pregnancy rate of 2.54 per 100 woman-years. A higher pregnancy rate of 3.72 is recorded in "fresh" patients (those who had never taken oral contraceptives prior to starting NOR-Q.D. therapy) to a large extent because of incorrect tablet intake. This compares to the lower pregnancy rate of 1.95 recorded in "changeover" patients (those switched from other oral contraceptives). This difference was found to be statistically significant. Furthermore, an even greater statistically significant difference in pregnancy rates between these two groups was found during the first six months of NOR-Q.D. therapy. Therefore, it is especially important for "fresh" patients to strictly adhere to the regimen.

The TRI-NORINYL 21-DAY Tablet regimen is 7 blue tablets, 9 green tablets, and then 5 blue tablets. The TRI-NORINYL 28-DAY Tablet regimen is 7 blue tablets, 9 green tablets, 5 blue tablets, and then 7 orange placebo tablets.

Each blue tablet contains norethindrone 0.5 mg with ethinyl estradiol 0.035 mg. In clinical trials with this formulation, 1,168 patients completed 16,345 cycles and 3 pregnancies were reported. This represents a pregnancy rate of 0.22 per 100 woman-years.

Each green tablet contains norethindrone 1.0 mg with ethinyl estradiol 0.035 mg. In clinical trials with this formulation, 940 patients completed 14,366 cycles and 2 pregnancies were reported. This represents a pregnancy rate of 0.17 per 100 woman-years.

Table 1 gives ranges of pregnancy rates reported in the literature[1] for other means of contraception. The efficacy of these means of contraception (except the IUD) depends upon the degree of adherence to the method.

TABLE 1. *Pregnancies per 100 Woman-Years*
IUD, less than 1–6;
Diaphragm with spermicidal products (creams or jellies), 2–20;
Condom, 3–36;
Aerosol foams, 2–29;
Jellies and creams, 4–36;
Periodic abstinence (rhythm) all types, less than 1–47;
— Calendar method, 14–47;
— Temperature method, 1–20;
— Temperature method—intercourse only in post-ovulatory phase, less than 1–7;
— Mucus method, 1–25;
No contraception, 60–80.

Dose-Related Risk of Thromboembolism From Oral Contraceptives. Studies have shown a positive association between the dose of estrogens in oral contraceptives and the risk of thromboembolism[2,3,81,82]. For this reason, it is prudent and in keeping with good principles of therapeutics to minimize exposure to estrogen. The oral contraceptive product prescribed for any given patient should be that product which contains the least amount of estrogen that is compatible with an acceptable pregnancy rate and patient acceptance. It is recommended that new acceptors of oral contraceptives should be started on preparations containing 0.05 mg or less of estrogen.

Contraindications:
1. Known or suspected pregnancy (see Warning No. 5).
2. Thrombophlebitis or thromboembolic disorders.
3. A past history of deep vein thrombophlebitis or thromboembolic disorders.
4. Undiagnosed abnormal genital bleeding.
5. Oral contraceptives should not be used by women who have or have had any of the following conditions:
   a. Cerebral vascular or coronary artery disease, including myocardial infarction.
   b. Known or suspected carcinoma of the breast.
   c. Known or suspected estrogen dependent neoplasia.
   d. Benign or malignant liver tumor which developed during the use of oral contraceptives or other estrogen containing products.

Warnings:

Cigarette smoking increases the risk of serious cardiovascular side effects from oral contraceptive use. This risk increases with age and with heavy smoking (15 or more cigarettes per day) and is quite marked in women over 35 years of age. Women who use oral contraceptives should be strongly advised not to smoke.

The use of oral contraceptives is associated with increased risk of several serious conditions including thromboembolism, stroke, myocardial infarction, liver tumor, gall bladder disease, visual disturbances, fetal abnormalities, and hypertension. Practitioners prescribing oral contraceptives should be familiar with the following information relating to these risks.

1. *Thromboembolic Disorders and Other Vascular Problems:* An increased risk of thromboembolic and thrombotic disease associated with the use of oral contraceptives is well established. One British study[4] demonstrated an increased relative risk for fatal venous thromboembolism, several British[5,6,11,20,72] and three American[3,7,8,21] studies demonstrated an increased relative risk for non-fatal venous thromboembolism. These studies estimate that users of oral contraceptives are 4 to 11 times more likely than nonusers to develop these diseases without evident cause (Table 2). An analysis of deaths in one British study[73] reported an excess death rate of 40% in oral contraceptive users, most of which resulted from cardiovascular disease. A somewhat similar British study[74] showed a lower death rate in oral contraceptive users than controls; here an increase in cardiovascular deaths was seen although the findings were not statistically significant. A U.S. prospective study[75] failed to disclose increased mortality rates from cardiovascular disorders. However, a selected subset of this study, analyzed as a retrospective, case-control study[76] showed significant increases in venous thromboembolism.

Cerebrovascular Disorders. Two American studies[7,9,10] demonstrated an increased relative risk for stroke, which had not been shown in prior British studies[4–6]. In a collaborative American study[9,10] of cerebrovascular disorders in women with and without predisposing causes, it was estimated that the relative risk of hemorrhagic stroke was 2.0 times greater in users than nonusers and the relative risk of thrombotic stroke was 4 to 9.5 times greater in users than in nonusers (Table 2). A British long-term, follow-up study[11] reported in 1976 a highly significant association between oral contraceptive use and stroke. Another British long-term, follow-up study[12] had suggested such an association in 1974, but the number of cases was too small to estimate the risk. Subarachnoid hemorrhage has been shown to be increased by oral contraceptive use in British[73] and American studies[75,77]. Smoking alone increases the incidence of these accidents and smoking and pill use appear to work together to produce a combined risk greater than either alone.

Myocardial Infarction. An increased relative risk of myocardial infarction associated with the use of oral contraceptives has been reported[13–15], confirming a previously suspected association[4]. One study[14,15] conducted in the United Kingdom found, as expected, that the greater the number of underlying risk factors for coronary artery disease (cigarette smoking, hypertension, hypercholesterolemia, obesity, diabetes, history of preeclamptic toxemia) the higher the risk of developing myocardial infarction, regardless of whether the patient was an oral contraceptive user or not. Oral contraceptives, however, were found to be an additional risk factor.

In terms of relative risk, it has been estimated[16,17] that oral contraceptive users who do not smoke (smoking is considered a major predisposing condition to myocardial infarction) are about twice as likely to have a fatal myocardial infarction as nonusers who do not smoke. Oral contraceptive users who are also smokers have about a 5-fold increased risk of fatal infarction compared to users who do not smoke, and about a 10- to 12-fold increased risk compared to nonusers who do not smoke. Furthermore, the number of cigarettes smoked is also an important factor. In determining the importance of these relative risks, however, the baseline rates for various age groups, as shown in Table 3, must be given serious consideration. (The estimates in Table 3 are based on British vital statistics which show acute myocardial infarction death rates 2- to 3-times less than in the U.S. for women in these age groups; consequently, actual U.S. death rates could be higher than those in Table 3[17].) The importance of other predisposing conditions mentioned above in determining relative and absolute risks has not been quantified; other synergistic actions may exist.

TABLE 2. *Summary of relative risk of thromboembolic disorders and other vascular problems in oral contraceptive users compared to nonusers*

	Relative risk, times greater
Idiopathic thromboembolic disease	4–11
Post surgery thromboembolic complications	4–6
Thrombotic stroke	4–9.5
Hemorrhagic stroke	2

Continued on next page

Syntex—Cont.

Myocardial infarction 2–12
Subarachnoid hemorrhage 6–22

TABLE 3. *Estimated[16] annual mortality rate per 100,000 women from myocardial infarction by use of oral contraceptives, smoking habits, and age (in years)*

Myocardial infarction

Smoking habits	Women aged 30–39 Users	Women aged 30–39 Non-users	Women aged 40–44 Users	Women aged 40–44 Non-users
All smokers	10.2	2.6	62.0	15.9
Heavy*	13.0	5.1	78.7	31.3
Light	4.7	0.9	28.6	5.7
Nonsmokers	1.8	1.2	10.7	7.4
Smokers and nonsmokers	5.4	1.9	32.8	11.7

*Heavy smoker: 15 or more cigarettes per day.

Risk of Dose. In an analysis of data derived from several national adverse reaction reporting systems[2], British investigators concluded that the risk of thromboembolism including coronary thrombosis is directly related to the dose of estrogen used in oral contraceptives. Preparations containing 0.1 mg or more of estrogen were associated with a higher risk of thromboembolism than those containing 0.05–0.08 mg of estrogen. Their analysis did suggest, however, that the quantity of estrogen may not be the sole factor involved. This finding has been supported by a study in the United States[3]. A subsequent study in Great Britain[81] found a positive association between dose of progestogen or estrogen and certain thromboembolic conditions. Swedish authorities[82] noted decreased reporting of thromboembolic episodes when higher estrogen preparations were no longer prescribed. Careful epidemiological studies to determine the degree of thromboembolic risk associated with progestogen-only oral contraceptives have not been performed. Cases of thromboembolic disease have been reported in women using these products, and they should not be presumed to be free of excess risk.

Persistence of Risk: In confirmation of earlier reports,[18,73] two studies have suggested that an increased risk may persist for as long as 6 years after discontinuation of oral contraceptive use for cerebrovascular disease[87] and 9 years for myocardial infarction.[88] In addition, a prospective study suggested the persistence of risk for subarachnoid hemorrhage.[77]

Estimate of Excess Mortality from Circulatory Diseases. A large British prospective study[12,18] estimated[18] the mortality rate per 100,000 women per year from diseases of the circulatory system for users and nonusers of oral contraceptives according to age, smoking habits, and duration of use. The overall excess death rate annually from circulatory diseases for oral contraceptive users was estimated to be 20 per 100,000 (ages 15–34—5/100,000; ages 35–44—33/100,000; ages 45–49—140/100,000). The risk is concentrated in older women, in those with a long duration of use, and in cigarette smokers, and may persist after discontinuation of oral contraceptive use. It was not possible, however, to examine the interrelationships of age, smoking, and duration of use, nor to compare the effects of continuous vs. intermittent use. Although the study showed a 10-fold increase in death due to circulatory diseases in users for 5 or more years, all of these deaths occurred in women 35 or older. An update of this study[73] provided the following rates: ages 15–34—1/6700 for non-smokers and 1/2000 for smokers; ages 45 and over—1/2500 for non-smokers and 1/500 for smokers.

Risk appeared to increase with parity, but not with duration of use. Until larger numbers of women under 35 with continuous use for 5 or more years are available, it is not possible to assess the magnitude of the relative risk for this younger age group.

The available data from a variety of sources have been analyzed[19] to estimate the risk of death associated with various methods of contraception. The estimates of risk of death for each method include the combined risk of the contraceptive method (e.g., thromboembolic and thrombotic disease in the case of oral contraceptives) plus the risk attributable to pregnancy or abortion in the event of method failure. This latter risk varies with the effectiveness of the contraceptive method. The findings of this analysis are shown in Figure 1[19]. The study concluded that the mortality associated with all methods of birth control is low and below that of childbirth, with the exception of oral contraceptives in women over 40 who smoke. (The rates given for pill only/smokers for each age group are for smokers as a class. For "heavy" smokers (more than 15 cigarettes a day), the rates given would be about double; for "light" smokers (less than 15 cigarettes a day), about 50 percent.) The lowest mortality is associated with the condom or diaphragm backed up by early abortion. The study also concluded that oral contraceptive users who smoke, especially those over the age of 30, have a greater mortality risk than oral contraceptive users who do not smoke.

Figure 1. Annual number of deaths associated with control of fertility and no control per 100,000 nonsterile women, by regimen of control and age of woman

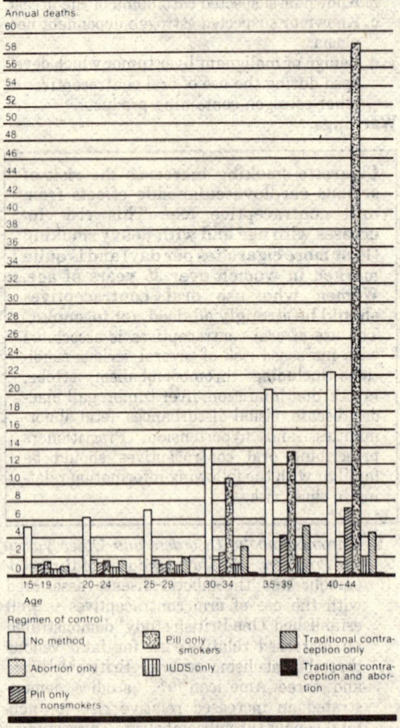

Regimen of control:
- No method
- Abortion only
- Pill only nonsmokers
- Pill only smokers
- IUDS only
- Traditional contraception only
- Traditional contraception and abortion

The risk of thromboembolic and thrombotic disease associated with oral contraceptives increases with age after approximately age 30 and, for myocardial infarction, is further increased by hypertension, hyperlipidemias, obesity, diabetes, or history of preeclamptic toxemia and especially by cigarette smoking[16,17].

Based on the data currently available, the following chart gives a gross estimate of the risk of death from circulatory disorders associated with the use of oral contraceptives: Smoking Habits and Other Predisposing Conditions—Risk Associated with Use of Oral Contraceptives

Age	Below 30	30–39	40+
Heavy smokers	C	B	A
Light smokers	D	C	B
Nonsmokers (no predisposing conditions)	D	C, D	C
Nonsmokers (other predisposing conditions)	C	C, B	B, A

A—Use associated with very high risk.
B—Use associated with high risk.
C—Use associated with moderate risk.
D—Use associated with low risk.

The physician and the patient should be alert to the earliest manifestations of thromboembolic and thrombotic disorders (e.g., thrombophlebitis, pulmonary embolism, cerebrovascular insufficiency, coronary occlusion, retinal thrombosis, and mesenteric thrombosis). Should any of these occur or be suspected, the drug should be discontinued immediately.

A four- to six-fold increased risk of post-surgery thromboembolic complications has been reported in oral contraceptive users[20,21]. If feasible, oral contraceptives should be discontinued at least 4 weeks before surgery of a type associated with an increased risk of thromboembolism or prolonged immobilization. The decision as to when to resume oral contraception following major surgery or bedrest should balance the recognized risks of post-surgery thromboembolic complications with the need to reinstate contraceptive practices.

Data[72] also suggest that the presence of varicose veins substantially increases the risk of superficial venous thrombosis of the leg, the risk depending on the severity of the varicosities.

2. *Ocular Lesions:* There have been reports of neuro-ocular lesions such as optic neuritis or retinal thrombosis associated with the use of oral contraceptives. Discontinue oral contraceptive medication if there is unexplained, sudden or gradual, partial or complete loss of vision; onset of proptosis or diplopia; papilledema; or retinal vascular lesions; and institute appropriate diagnostic and therapeutic measures.

3. *Carcinoma:* Long-term continuous administration of either natural or synthetic estrogen in certain animal species increases the frequency of certain tumors, benign or malignant, such as those of the breast, cervix, vagina, uterus, ovary, pituitary and liver. Certain synthetic progestogens, none currently contained in oral contraceptives, have been noted to increase the incidence of mammary nodules, benign and malignant, in dogs.

Several retrospective case-control studies[22–27] have reported an increased relative risk (3.1 to 13.9 times) associating endometrial carcinoma with the prolonged use of estrogens in postmenopausal women who took estrogen replacement medication to relieve menopausal symptoms. One publication[28] reported on the first 30 cases submitted by physicians to a registry of cases of adenocarcinoma of the endometrium in women under 40 on oral contraceptives. Of the adenocarcinomas found in women without predisposing risk factors for adenocarcinoma of the endometrium (e.g., irregular bleeding at the time oral contraceptives were first given, polycystic ovaries) nearly all occurred in women who had used a sequential oral contraceptive. These products are no longer marketed. No statistical association has been reported suggesting an increased risk of endometrial cancer in users of conventional combination or progestogen-only oral contraceptives, although individual cases have been reported.

Several studies[8,29-33] have shown no increased risk of breast cancer to women taking oral contraceptives or estrogens. In one study[34,35], however, while no overall increased risk of breast cancer was noted in women treated with oral contraceptives, a greater risk was suggested for the subgroups of oral contraceptive users with documented benign breast disease and for long-term (2-4 years) users. In one study, it was found that a history of breast cancer among grandmothers or aunts was significantly more frequent among breast cancer patients who had used an oral contraceptive continuously for one or more years than among non-users with breast cancer[83]. One other study[36] indicated an increasing risk of breast cancer in women taking menopausal estrogens, which increased with duration of follow-up. A reduced occurrence of benign breast tumors in users of oral contraceptives has been well documented[8,11,12,29,34,37,38]. In contrast, one author[79] suggests that extended (over 6 years) use of oral contraceptives prior to the first full term pregnancy was associated with a significant relative risk of breast cancer.

One study[75] reported malignant melanoma more frequently in oral contraceptive users than in controls and suggests an increased incidence of urinary tract cancers and thyroid cancers.

In a prospective study[39] of women with cervical dysplasia, there was an increase in severity and of conversion to cancer *in situ* in oral contraceptive users compared with nonusers. This became statistically significant after 3 to 4 years of use. Nonreversal of dysplasia within the first 6 months of pill use was suggested to be predictive of progression after prolonged exposure. One study[75] disclosed an increased risk of cancer of the cervix (largely carcinoma-*in-situ*) in oral contraceptive users under 40, particularly those who had used these drugs for over four years. There have been other reports of microglandular hyperplasia of the cervix in users of oral contraceptives.

One study reported an association between oral contraceptive use and endocervical adenocarcinoma.[89]

In summary, there is at present no confirmed evidence from human studies of an increased risk of cancer associated with oral contraceptives. Close clinical surveillance of all women taking oral contraceptives is, nevertheless, essential. In all cases of undiagnosed persistent or recurrent abnormal vaginal bleeding, appropriate diagnostic measures should be taken to rule out malignancy. Women with a strong family history of breast cancer or who have breast nodules, fibrocystic disease or abnormal mammograms should be monitored with particular care if they elect to use oral contraceptives instead of other methods of contraception.

4. *Liver Tumors:* Sudden severe abdominal pain or shock may be due to rupture and hemorrhage of a liver tumor. There have been reports associating benign or malignant liver tumors with oral contraceptive use[40-44]. This has been reported in short-term as well as long-term users of oral contraceptives. One study[44] reported that use of oral contraceptives with high hormonal potency and age over 30 years may further increase a woman's risk of hepatocellular adenoma. Two studies[41,44] relate risk with duration of use, the risk being much greater after 4 or more years of use. Long-term users of oral contraceptives have an estimated annual incidence of hepatocellular adenoma of 3-4 per 100,000.[44] Although it is an uncommon lesion, it should be considered in women presenting with an "acute abdomen". The tumor may cause serious or fatal hemorrhage. Patients with liver tumors have demonstrated variable clinical features which may make preoperative diagnosis difficult. Some cases presented because of right upper quadrant masses, while most had signs and symptoms of acute intraperitoneal hemorrhage. Routine radiological and laboratory studies may not be helpful. Liver scans may clearly show a focal defect. Hepatic arteriography may be a useful procedure in diagnosing primary liver neoplasm.

5. *Use in or Immediately Preceding Pregnancy, Birth Defects in Offspring, and Malignancy in Female Offspring:* The use of female sex hormones—both estrogenic and progestational agents—during early pregnancy may seriously damage the offspring. It has been shown that females exposed *in utero* to diethylstilbestrol, a nonsteroidal estrogen, have an increased risk of developing in later life a form of vaginal or cervical cancer that is ordinarily extremely rare[45,46]. This risk has been estimated to be of the order of 1 in 1,000 exposures or less[47,48]. Although there is no evidence at the present time that oral contraceptives further enhance the risk of developing this type of malignancy, such patients should be monitored with particular care if they elect to use oral contraceptives instead of other methods of contraception.

Furthermore, a high percentage of women exposed to diethylstilbestrol (from 30 to 90%) have been found to have epithelial changes of the vagina and cervix[49-53]. Although these changes are histologically benign, it is not known whether this condition is a precursor of vaginal malignancy. Male children so exposed may develop abnormalities of the urogenital tract[54-56]. Although similar data are not available with the use of other estrogens, it cannot be presumed that they would not induce similar changes.

An increased risk of congenital anomalies, including heart defects and limb defects, has been reported following use of sex hormones, including oral contraceptives, in pregnancy[57-61]. In one case-control study[60] it was estimated that there was a 4.7-fold increased relative risk of limb-reduction defects in infants exposed *in utero* to sex hormones (oral contraceptives, hormonal withdrawal tests for pregnancy or attempted treatment for threatened abortion). Some of these exposures were very short and involved only a few days of treatment. The data suggest that the risk of limb-reduction defects in exposed fetuses is somewhat less than 1 in 1,000 live births. In a large prospective study[61], cardiovascular defects in children born to women who received female hormones, including oral contraceptives, during early pregnancy occurred at a rate of 18.2 per 1,000 births, compared to 7.8 per 1,000 for children not so exposed *in utero*. These results are statistically significant. A Welsh study[80] identified a statistically significant excess of neural tube defects among offspring of prior users (within 3 months) of oral contraceptives than among controls. The incidence of twin births may be increased for women who conceive shortly after discontinuing use of the pill[11,60,84,85,86]. In the past, female sex hormones have been used during pregnancy in an attempt to treat threatened or habitual abortion. There is considerable evidence that estrogens are ineffective for these indications, and there is no evidence from well controlled studies that progestogens are effective for these uses.

There is some evidence that triploidy and possibly other types of polyploidy are increased among abortuses from women who become pregnant soon after ceasing oral contraceptives.[62] Embryos with these anomalies are virtually always aborted spontaneously. Whether there is an overall increase in spontaneous abortion of pregnancies conceived soon after stopping oral contraceptives is unknown.

If the patient has not adhered to the prescribed schedule, the possibility of pregnancy should be considered at the time of the first missed period (or after 45 days from the last menstrual period if progestogen-only contraceptives are used) and further use of oral contraceptives should be withheld until pregnancy has been ruled out. It is recommended that for any patient who has missed two consecutive periods, pregnancy should be ruled out before continuing the contraceptive regimen. If pregnancy is confirmed, the patient should be apprised of the potential risks to the fetus and the advisability of continuation of the pregnancy should be discussed in the light of these risks.

It is also recommended that women who discontinue oral contraceptives with the intent of becoming pregnant use an alternate form of contraception for a period of time before attempting to conceive. Many clinicians recommend 3 months; this recommendation is supported by a study suggesting an increased frequency of neural tube defects in women impregnated during the first three months after cessation of pill use[80].

The administration of progestogen-only or progestogen-estrogen combinations to induce withdrawal bleeding should not be used as a test of pregnancy.

6. *Gall Bladder Disease:* Studies[3,8,11,12,31] report an increased risk of gall bladder disease in users of oral contraceptives or estrogens. In one study[12], an increased risk appeared after 2 years of use and doubled after 4 or 5 years of use. In another study[8], an increased risk was apparent between 6 and 12 months of use.

7. *Carbohydrate and Lipid Metabolic Effects:* A decrease in glucose tolerance has been observed in a significant percentage of patients on oral contraceptives. For this reason, prediabetic and diabetic patients should be carefully observed while receiving oral contraceptives.

An increase in triglycerides and total phospholipids has been observed in patients receiving oral contraceptives[63]. The clinical significance of this finding is unknown.

8. *Elevated Blood Pressure:* An increase in blood pressure has been reported[12,64] with oral contraceptive use. In some women, hypertension may occur within a few months of beginning oral contraceptive use. In the first year of use, the prevalence of women with hypertension is low in users and may be no higher than that of a comparable group of nonusers. The prevalence in users increases, however, with longer exposure, and in the fifth year of use is two and a half to three times the reported prevalence in the first year. Age is also strongly correlated with the development of hypertension in oral contraceptive users. Women with a history of elevated blood pressure (hypertension), preexisting renal disease, a history of toxemia or elevated blood pressure during pregnancy, a familial tendency to hypertension or its consequences, or a history of excessive weight gain or fluid retention during the menstrual cycle may be more likely to develop elevation of blood pressure when given oral contraceptives and, therefore, should be monitored closely[65].

Even though elevated blood pressure may remain within the "normal" range, the clinical implications of elevations should not be ignored and close surveillance is indicated, particularly for women with other risk factors for cardiovascular disease or stroke[64]. High blood pressure may or may not persist after discontinuation of the oral contraceptive.

Continued on next page

Syntex—Cont.

9. *Headache:* The onset or exacerbation of migraine or development of headache of a new pattern which is recurrent, persistent, or severe, requires discontinuation of oral contraceptives and evaluation of the cause.
10. *Bleeding Irregularities:* Breakthrough bleeding, spotting, and missed menses are frequent reasons for patients discontinuing oral contraceptives. In breakthrough bleeding, as in all cases of irregular bleeding from the vagina, nonfunctional causes should be borne in mind. In undiagnosed persistent or recurrent abnormal bleeding from the vagina, adequate diagnostic measures are indicated to rule out pregnancy or malignancy. If pathology has been excluded, time or a change to another formulation may solve the problem. Changing to an oral contraceptive with a higher estrogen content, while potentially useful in minimizing menstrual irregularity, should be done only if necessary since this may increase the risk of thromboembolic disease.

    Women with a past history of oligomenorrhea or secondary amenorrhea or young women without regular cycles may have a tendency to remain anovulatory or to become amenorrheic after discontinuation of oral contraceptives. Women with these preexisting problems should be advised of this possibility and encouraged to use other contraceptive methods.

    Post-use anovulation, possibly prolonged, may also occur in women without previous irregularities. A higher incidence of galactorrhea and of pituitary tumors (e.g., adenomas) has been associated with amenorrhea in former users compared with nonusers[66,67]. One study[67] reported a 16-fold increased prevalence of pituitary prolactin-secreting tumors among patients with postpill amenorrhea when galactorrhea was present.
11. *Infertility:* There is evidence of impairment of fertility in women discontinuing oral contraceptives in comparison with those discontinuing other methods of contraception. The impairment appears to be independent of the duration of use of the preparations. While the impairment diminishes with time, there is still an appreciable difference in the results in nulliparous women for the oral contraceptive and non-oral contraceptive groups 30 months after discontinuation of birth control. For parous women the difference is no longer apparent 30 months after cessation of contraception[11].
12. *Ectopic Pregnancy:* Ectopic as well as intrauterine pregnancy may occur in contraceptive failures. However, in progestogen-only oral contraceptive failures, the ratio of ectopic to intrauterine pregnancies is higher than in women who are not receiving oral contraceptives, since the drugs are more effective in preventing intrauterine than ectopic pregnancies.
13. *Breast Feeding:* Oral contraceptives given in the postpartum period may interfere with lactation. There may be a decrease in the quantity and quality of the breast milk. Furthermore, a small fraction of the hormonal agents in oral contraceptives has been identified in the milk of mothers receiving these drugs[68]. The effects, if any, on the breast fed child have not been determined. If feasible, the use of oral contraceptives should be deferred until the infant has been weaned.

Precautions:
General
1. A complete medical and family history should be taken prior to the initiation of oral contraceptives. The pretreatment and periodic physical examinations should include special reference to blood pressure, breasts, abdomen and pelvic organs, including Papanicolaou smear and relevant laboratory tests. As a general rule, oral contraceptives should not be prescribed for longer than 1 year without another physical examination being performed.
2. Under the influence of estrogen-progestogen preparations, preexisting uterine leiomyomata may increase in size.
3. Patients with a history of psychic depression should be carefully observed and the drug discontinued if depression recurs to a serious degree. Patients becoming significantly depressed while taking oral contraceptives should stop the medication and use an alternate method of contraception in an attempt to determine whether the symptom is drug related.
4. Oral contraceptives may cause some degree of fluid retention. They should be prescribed with caution, and only with careful monitoring, in patients with conditions which might be aggravated by fluid retention, such as convulsive disorders, migraine syndrome, asthma or cardiac, hepatic or renal insufficiency.
5. Patients with a past history of jaundice during pregnancy have an increased risk of recurrence of jaundice while receiving oral contraceptive therapy. If jaundice develops in any patient receiving such drugs, the medication should be discontinued.
6. Steroid hormones may be poorly metabolized in patients with impaired liver function and should be administered with caution in such patients.
7. Oral contraceptive users may have disturbances in normal tryptophan metabolism which may result in a relative pyridoxine deficiency. The clinical significance of this is unknown.
8. Serum folate levels may be depressed by oral contraceptive therapy. Since the pregnant woman is predisposed to the development of folate deficiency and the incidence of folate deficiency increases with increasing gestation, it is possible that if a woman becomes pregnant shortly after stopping oral contraceptives, she may have a greater chance of developing folate deficiency and complications attributed to this deficiency.
9. The pathologist should be advised of oral contraceptive therapy when relevant specimens are submitted.
10. Certain endocrine and liver function tests and blood components may be affected by estrogen-containing oral contraceptives. For example:
    a. Increased sulfobromophthalein retention.
    b. Increased prothrombin and factors VII, VIII, IX, and X; decreased antithrombin 3; increased norepinephrine-induced platelet aggregability.
    c. Increased thyroid binding globulin (TBG) leading to increased circulating total thyroid hormone, as measured by protein-bound iodine (PBI), T4 by column, or T4 by radioimmunoassay. Free T3 resin uptake is decreased, reflecting the elevated TBG, free T4 concentration is unaltered.
    d. Decreased pregnanediol excretion.
    e. Reduced response to metyrapone test.
    f. Increased phospholipids and triglycerides.
    g. Temporarily decreased glucose tolerance.
11. Contact lens wearers who develop visual changes or changes in lens tolerance should be assessed by an ophthalmologist and temporary or permanent cessation of wear considered.

DRUG INTERACTIONS
Oral contraceptives may be rendered less effective and an increased incidence of breakthrough bleeding may occur by virtue of drug interaction with rifampin, isoniazid, ampicillin, tetracycline, neomycin, penicillin V, chloramphenicol, sulfonamides, nitrofurantoin, barbiturates, phenytoin, primidone, analgesics, tranquilizers, antimigraine preparations, and antihistamines[66-71,78,90]. Oral contraceptives may alter the effectiveness of other types of drugs, such as oral anticoagulants, anticonvulsants, tricyclic antidepressants, antihypertensive agents (e.g., guanethidine), vitamins, hypoglycemic agents, tranquilizers, hypnotic preparations, and theophylline.[69,91]

INFORMATION FOR THE PATIENT
See detailed patient labeling below.

CARCINOGENESIS
See Warnings section for information on the carcinogenic potential of oral contraceptives.

PREGNANCY
Pregnancy category X. See Contraindications and Warnings.

NURSING MOTHERS
See Warnings.

Adverse Reactions: An increased risk of the following serious adverse reactions has been associated with the use of oral contraceptives (see Warnings):

  Thrombophlebitis, thrombosis
  Pulmonary embolism
  Coronary thrombosis
  Cerebral thrombosis
  Mesenteric thrombosis
  Raynaud's disease
  Arterial thromboembolism
  Liver tumors
  Cerebral hemorrhage
  Hypertension
  Gall bladder disease
  Congenital anomalies
  Neuro-ocular lesions, e.g., retinal thrombosis and optic neuritis

The following adverse reactions have been reported in patients receiving oral contraceptives and are believed to be drug related:

  Bleeding irregularities
    Breakthrough bleeding
    Spotting
    Missed menses during treatment
    Amenorrhea after treatment
  Gastrointestinal symptoms
    Nausea
    Vomiting
    Bloating
    Abdominal cramps
  Dysmenorrhea
  Infertility after discontinuance of treatment
  Edema
  Chloasma or melasma which may persist after drug is discontinued
  Breast changes: tenderness, enlargement, and secretion
  Intolerance to contact lenses
  Change in corneal curvature (steepening)
  Change in weight (increase or decrease)
  Change in cervical erosion and cervical secretion
  Possible diminution in lactation when given immediately postpartum
  Cholestatic jaundice
  Migraine
  Increase in size of uterine leiomyomata
  Rash (allergic)
  Mental depression
  Reduced tolerance to carbohydrates
  Vaginal candidiasis
  Prolaction-secreting pituitary tumors
  Chilblains

The following adverse reactions have been reported in users of oral contraceptives, and the association has been neither confirmed nor refuted:

  Premenstrual-like syndrome
  Cataracts
  Changes in libido
  Chorea
  Changes in appetite
  Cystitis-like syndrome
  Headache
  Nervousness
  Dizziness
  Hirsutism
  Loss of hair
  Erythema multiforme
  Erythema nodosum
  Hemorrhagic eruption
  Vaginitis

Porphyria
Impaired renal function
Malignant nephrosclerosis (hemolytic uremic syndrome)

Acute Overdose: Serious ill effects have not been reported following acute ingestion of large doses of oral contraceptives by young children. Overdosage may cause nausea. Withdrawal bleeding may occur in females.

Dosage and Administration: To achieve maximum contraceptive effectiveness, oral contraceptives must be taken exactly as directed and at intervals not exceeding 24 hours.

Important: The patient should be instructed to use an additional method of protection until after the first week of administration in the initial cycle. The possibility of ovulation and conception prior to initiation of use should be considered.

21-Day Regimen Dosage Schedule for BREVICON, NORINYL 1 & 35, NORINYL 1 & 50, NORINYL 1 & 80: For the initial cycle of therapy the first tablet may be taken on Day 5 of the menstrual cycle, counting the first day of menstrual flow as Day 1 (DAY 5 START), or the first tablet may be taken on the first Sunday after menstrual flow begins (SUNDAY START). For SUNDAY START when menstrual flow begins on Sunday, the first tablet is taken on that day. With either DAY 5 START or SUNDAY START, one tablet is taken each evening at bedtime for 21 days. No tablets are taken for 7 days, then, whether bleeding has stopped or not, a new course is started of one tablet a day for 21 days. This institutes a three weeks on, one week off dosage regimen.

28-Day Regimen Dosage Schedule for BREVICON, NORINYL 1 & 35, NORINYL 1 & 50, NORINYL 1 & 80: For the initial cycle of therapy the first tablet may be taken on Day 5 of the menstrual cycle, counting the first day of menstrual flow as Day 1 (DAY 5 START), or the first tablet may be taken on the first Sunday after menstrual flow begins (SUNDAY START). For SUNDAY START when menstrual flow begins on Sunday, the first tablet is taken on that day. With either DAY 5 START or SUNDAY START, one white, yellow, blue, or green tablet is taken each evening at bedtime for 21 days. Then the orange tablets are taken, one each evening at bedtime for 7 days. After all 28 tablets have been taken, whether bleeding has stopped or not, repeat the same dosage schedule beginning on the following day.

21-Day Regimen Dosage Schedule for TRI-NORINYL: The first blue tablet is taken on the first Sunday after menstrual flow begins. If menstrual flow begins on Sunday, the first blue tablet is taken on that day. One blue tablet is taken each evening at bedtime for 7 days, then one green tablet each evening for 9 days, then one blue tablet each evening for 5 days. No tablets are taken for 7 days; then, whether bleeding has stopped or not, a new sequence of tablets is started for 21 days. This institutes a three weeks on, one week off dosage regimen.

28-Day Regimen Dosage Schedule for TRI-NORINYL: The first blue tablet is taken on the first Sunday after menstrual flow begins. If menstrual flow begins on Sunday, the first blue tablet is taken on that day. One blue tablet is taken each evening at bedtime for 7 days, then one green tablet each evening for 9 days, then one blue tablet each evening for 5 days, then one orange (inert) tablet each evening for 7 days. After all 28 tablets have been taken, whether bleeding has stopped or not, the same dosage schedule is repeated beginning on the following day.

NORINYL 2 mg. Tablets: To prevent conception, one tablet is taken each evening at bedtime for 20 days beginning on DAY 5 of the menstrual cycle, counting the first day of menstrual flow as DAY 1. In the vast majority of women on this schedule menses occur within two to three days following the termination of each 20-day course, but tend to be scantier than normal menses. In those cases where withdrawal bleeding may be delayed until 4, 5 or 6 days after the 20-day course of therapy, the patient should start the next course of medication on the 7th day following completion of the previous 20-day course. For the treatment of hypermenorrhea, one tablet is taken each evening at bedtime from day 5 through day 24 of each menstrual cycle. Following three months of treatment of hypermenorrhea, medication may be discontinued to determine the need for further therapy.

20, 21, 28-Day Schedules for All Products: Even if spotting or breakthrough bleeding should occur, continue the medication according to the schedule. Should spotting or breakthrough bleeding persist, your physician should be notified.

Use of oral contraceptives in the event of a missed menstrual period:

1. If the patient has not adhered to the prescribed dosage regimen, the possibility of pregnancy should be considered after the first missed period and oral contraceptives should be withheld until pregnancy has been ruled out.
2. If the patient has adhered to the prescribed regimen and misses two consecutive periods, pregnancy should be ruled out before continuing the contraceptive regimen.

NOR-Q.D.® (norethindrone) is administered as a continuous daily dosage regimen starting on the first day of menstruation, i.e., one tablet each day, every day of the year. Tablets should be taken at the same time each day and continued daily, without interruption, whether bleeding occurs or not. This is especially important for patients new to progestogen alone oral contraception. The patient should be advised that if prolonged bleeding occurs, she should consult her physician. In the nonnursing mother, NOR-Q.D. may be prescribed in the post-partum period either immediately or at the first post-partum examination whether or not menstruation has resumed.

The risk of pregnancy increases with each tablet missed. If the patient misses one tablet, she should be instructed to take it as soon as she remembers and also to take her next tablet at the regular time which means she will be taking two tablets on that day. If she misses two tablets in a row, she should take one of the missed tablets as soon as she remembers, discard the other missed tablet, and take her regular tablet for that day at the proper time. Furthermore, she should use an additional method of contraception in addition to taking NOR-Q.D. until menses has appeared or pregnancy has been excluded. If more than two tablets in a row have been missed, NOR-Q.D. should be discontinued immediately and an additional method of contraception should be used until menses has appeared or pregnancy has been excluded. Whether or not the patient has adhered to the prescribed schedule, if she does not have a period within 45 days of her last period, she should stop taking NOR-Q.D. and depend upon a method of nonhormonal contraception until pregnancy has been ruled out.

How Supplied:

BREVICON® 21-Day Tablets (norethindrone and ethinyl estradiol tablets) and BREVICON® 28-Day Tablets (norethindrone and ethinyl estradiol tablets) are available in 21-pill or 28-pill blister cards with a WALLETTE™ pill dispenser. Each 28-pill card contains 7 orange inert pills.

NORINYL® 1 + 35 21-Day Tablets (norethindrone and ethinyl estradiol tablets) and NORINYL® 1 + 35 28-Day Tablets (norethindrone and ethinyl estradiol tablets) are available in 21-pill or 28-pill blister cards with a WALLETTE™ pill dispenser. Each 28-pill card contains 7 orange inert pills.

NORINYL® 1 + 50 21-Day Tablets and NORINYL® 1 + 50 28-Day Tablets (norethindrone and mestranol tablets) and NORINYL® 1 + 80 21-Day Tablets and NORINYL® 1 + 80 28-Day Tablets (norethindrone and mestranol tablets) are available in 21-pill or 28-pill blister cards with a WALLETTE™ pill dispenser. Each 28-pill card contains 7 orange inert pills.

NORINYL® 2 mg. Tablets (norethindrone and mestranol tablets) are available in MEMORETTE® Tablet Dispensers, each containing 20 tablets. Also supplied are 20-tablet refills.

NOR-Q.D.® (norethindrone) tablets are available in 42-tablet dispensers.

TRI-NORINYL® 21-DAY Tablets (norethindrone and ethinyl estradiol tablets) and TRI-NORINYL 28-DAY Tablets (northindrone and ethinyl estradiol tablets) are each available in 21-pill or 28-pill blister cards with a WALLETTE pill dispenser. Each 28-pill card contains 7 orange inert pills.

CAUTION: Federal law prohibits dispensing without prescription.

References:

[1]Population Reports, Series H, Number 2, May 1974; Series I, Number 1, June 1974: Series B, Number 2, January 1975; Series H, Number 3, January 1975; Series H, Number 4, January 1976 (published by the Population Information Program, The George Washington University Medical Center, 2001 S St. NW, Washington, D. C.). [2]Inman, W., et al.: *Brit Med J* 2:203–209, 1970. [3]Stolley, P., et al.: *Am J Epidemiol* 102:197–208, 1975. [4]Inman, W., et al.: *Brit Med J* 2:193–199, 1968. [5]Royal College of General Practitioners: *J Coll Gen Pract* 13:267–279, 1967. [6]Vessey, M., et al.: *Brit Med J* 2:651–657, 1969. [7]Sartwell, P., et al.: *Am J Epidemiol* 90:365–380, 1969. [8]Boston Collaborative Drug Surveillance Program: *Lancet* 1:1399–1404, 1973. [9]Collaborative Group for the Study of Stroke in Young Women: *N Engl J Med* 288:871–878, 1973. [10]Collaborative Group for the Study of Stroke in Young Women: *JAMA* 231:718–722, 1975. [11]Vessey, M., et al.: *J Biosoc Sci* 8:373–427, (Oct.) 1976. [12]Royal College of General Practitioners: Oral Contraceptives and Health, London, Pitman, 1974. [13]Mann, J., et al.: *Brit Med J* 2:245–248, 1975. [14]Mann, J., et al.: *Brit Med J* 2:445–447, 1976. [15]Mann, J., et al.: *Brit Med J* 2:241–245, 1975. [16]Jain, A.: *Studies in Family Planning* 8:50–54, 1977. [17]Ory, H.: *JAMA* 237:2619–2622, (June 13) 1977. [18]Beral, V.: *Lancet* 2:727–731, 1977. [19]Tietze, C.: *Family Planning Perspectives* 9:74–76, 1977. [20]Vessey, M., et al.: *Brit Med J* 3:123–126, 1970. [21]Greene, G., et al.: *Am J Pub Health* 62:680–685, 1972. [22]Ziel, H., et al.: *N Engl J Med* 293:1167–1170, 1975. [23]Gordon, J., et al.: *N Engl J Med* 297:570–571, (Sept. 15) 1977. [24]Smith, D., et al.: *N Engl J Med* 293:1164–1167, 1975. [25]Mack, T., et al.: *N Engl J Med* 294:1262–1267, 1976. [26]Gray, L., et al.: *Obstet Gyncecol* 49:385–389, (April) 1977. [27]McDonald, T., et al.: *Am J Obstet Gynecol* 127:572–580, (Mar. 20) 1977. [28]Silverberg, S., et al.: *Cancer* 39:592–598, (Feb.) 1977). [29]Vessey, M., et al.: *Brit Med J* 3:719–724, 1972. [30]Vessey, M., et al.: *Lancet* 1:941–943, 1975. [31]Boston Collaborative Drug Surveillance Program: *N Engl J Med* 290:15–19, 1974. [32]Arthes, F., et al.: *Cancer* 28:1391–1394, 1971. [33]Casagrande, J., et al.: *J Natl Cancer Inst* 56:839–841, (April) 1976). [34]Fasal, E., et al.: *J Natl Cancer Inst* 55:767–773, 1975. [35]Paffenbarger, R., et al.: *Cancer* 49:1887–1891, (April Suppl.) 1977. [36]Hoover, R., et al.: *N Engl J Med* 295:401–405, (Aug. 19) 1976. [37]Kelsey, J., et al.: *Internat J Epidemiol* 3:333–340, 1974. [38]Ory, H., et al.: *N Engl J Med* 294:419–422, 1976. [39]Stern, E., et al.: *Science* 196:1460–1462, (June 24) 1977. [40]Mays, E., et al.: *JAMA* 235:730–732, 1976. [41]Edmondson, H., et al.: *N Engl J Med* 294:470–472, 1976. [42]Murphy, G.: *Am Col of Surg Bull*, (April) 1977. [43]Klatskin, G.: *Gastroent* 73:386–394, (Aug.) 1977. [44]Rooks, et al: *JAMA* 242:644, 1979. [45]Herbst, A., et al.: *N Engl J Med* 284:878–881, 1971. [46]Greenwald, P., et al.: *N Engl J Med* 285:390–392, 1971. [47]Lanier, A., et al.: *Mayo Clin Pro* 48:793–799, 1973. [48]Herbst, A., et al.: *Am J Obstet Gynecol* 128:43–50, 1977. [49]Herbst, A., et al.: *Obstet Gyncecol* 40:287–298, 1972. [50]Herbst, A., et al.: *Am J Obstet Gyncecol* 118:607–615, 1974. [51]Herbst, A., et al.: *N Engl J Med* 292:334–339, 1975. [52]Stafl, A., et al.: *Obstet Gynecol* 43:118–128, 1974. [53]Sherman, A., et al.: *Obstet Gynecol* 44:531–545, 1974. [54]Bibbo, M., et al.: *Jour of Repro Med* 15:29–32, 1975. [55]Gill, W., et al.: *Jour of Repro Med* 16:147–153, 1976. [56]Henderson, B., et al.: *Pediatrics* 58:505–507, 1976. [57]Gal, I., et al.: *Nature* 216:83, 1967. [58]Levy, E., et al.: *Lancet* 1:611, 1973. [59]Nora, J., et al.: *Lancet* 1:941–942, 1973. [60]Janerich, D., et al.: *N Engl J Med* 291:697–700, 1974. [61]Heinonen, O., et al.: *N Engl J Med* 296:67–70, 1977. [62]Carr, D.: *Canad Med Assoc J* 103:343–348, 1970. [63]Wynn, V., et al.: *Lancet*

Continued on next page

Syntex—Cont.

2:720–723, 1966. [64]Fisch, I., et al.: *JAMA* 237:2499–2503, (June 6) 1977. [65]Laragh, J.: *Am J Obstet Gynecol* 126:141–147, (Sept.) 1976. [66]March, C., et al.: *Fertil and Steril* 28:346, (Mar.) 1977. [67]Van Campenhout, J., et al.: *Fertil and Steril* 28:728–732, (July) 1977. [68]Laumas, K., et al.: *Am J Obstet Gynecol* 98:411–413, 1967. [69]Stockley, I.: *Pharm J* 216:140–143, (Feb. 14) 1976. [70]Hempel, E., et al.: *Drugs* 12:442–448, (Dec.) 1976. [71]Bessot, J.-C., et al.: *Nouv Press Med* 6:1568, (Apr. 30) 1977. [72]Royal College of General Practitioners: *J Coll Gen Pract* 28:393–399, 1978. [73]Layde, P. M., et al.: *Lancet* 1:541–546, 1981. [74]Vessey, M. P., et al.: *Lancet* 1:549–550, 1981. [75]Ramcharan, S., et al.: *The Walnut Creek Contraceptive Drug Study*, Volume III, NIH Publication 81-564, 1981. [76]Petitti, D. B., et al.: *Am J Epidemiol* 108:480–485, 1978. [77]Petitti, D. B., et al.: *Lancet* 2:234, 1978. [78]Abernethy, D. R., et al.: *N Engl J Med* 306:791, 1982. [79]Pike, M. C., et al.: *Brit J Cancer* 43:72, 1981. [80]Kasan, P. N., et al.: *Brit J Obstet Gynecol* 87:545, 1980. [81]Meade, T. W., et al.: *Brit Med J* 280:1157, 1980. [82]Bottiger, L. E., et al.: *Lancet* 1:1097, 1980. [83]Black, M. M., et al.: *Cancer* 46:2747, 1980. [84]Rothman, E. J.: *N Engl J Med* 297:468, 1977. [85]Bracken, M. B.: *Am J Obstet Gynecol* 133:432, 1979. [86]Harlap, S., et al.: *Obstet Gynecol* 55:447, 1980. [87]Royal College of General Practitioners: *J Coll Gen Pract* 33:75, 1983. [88]Slone, D., et al.: *N Engl J Med* 305:420, 1981. [89]Dallenbach-Hellweg, G.: *Geburtsh u Fauenheilk* 42:249, 1982. [90]De Sano, C. A., et al.: *Fertil and Steril* 37:853, 1982. [91]Tornatore, K. M., et al.: *Eur J Clin Pharmacol* 23:129, 1982.

Detailed Patient Labeling: Oral contraceptives ("the pill") are the most effective way (except for sterilization) to prevent pregnancy. They are also convenient and, for most women, free of serious or unpleasant side effects. Oral contraceptives must always be taken under the continuous supervision of a physician.

It is important that any woman who considers using an oral contraceptive understand the risks involved. Although the oral contraceptives have important advantages over the other methods of contraception, they have certain risks that no other method has, and some of these risks may continue after you have stopped using the pill. Only you can decide whether the advantages are worth these risks. This leaflet will tell you about the most important risks. It will explain how you can help your doctor prescribe the pill as safely as possible by telling him/her about yourself and being alert for the earliest signs of trouble. And it will tell you how to use the pill properly, so that it will be as effective as possible. There is more detailed information available in the leaflet prepared for doctors. If you need further help, ask your physician or pharmacist.

Who Should Not Use Oral Contraceptives:

A. If you have any of the following conditions you should not use the pill:
  1. Unusual vaginal bleeding that has not yet been diagnosed.
  2. Known or suspected pregnancy.

B. If you have or have had any of the following conditions you should not use the pill:
  1. Heart attack or stroke.
  2. Clots in the legs, lungs, brain, heart or elsewhere.
  3. Chest pain (angina pectoris).
  4. Known or suspected cancer of the breast or sex organs.
  5. Liver tumor associated with the use of the pill or other estrogen containing products.

C. Cigarette smoking increases the risk of serious adverse effects on the heart and blood vessels from oral contraceptive use. This risk increases with age and with heavy smoking (15 or more cigarettes per day) and is quite marked in women over 35 years of age. Women who use oral contraceptives should not smoke.

D. If you have scanty or irregular periods or are a young woman without a regular cycle, you should use another method of contraception because, if you use the pill, you may have difficulty becoming pregnant or may fail to have menstrual periods after discontinuing the pill.

What You Should Know About Oral Contraceptives: This leaflet describes the advantages and risks of oral contraceptives. Except for sterilization, the IUD and abortion, which have their own exclusive risks, the only risks of other methods of contraception are those due to pregnancy should the method fail or not be used conscientiously. Your doctor can answer questions you may have with respect to methods of contraception.

1. What Oral Contraceptives Are and How They Work. Oral contraceptives are of two types. The most common, often simply called "the pill", is a combination of an estrogen and a progestogen, the two kinds of female hormones. The amount of estrogen and progestogen can vary, but the amount of estrogen is most important because both the effectiveness and some of the dangers of oral contraceptives are related to the amount of estrogen. This kind of oral contraceptive works principally by preventing release of an egg from the ovary. When the amount of estrogen is 0.05 milligrams or more, and the pill is taken as directed, oral contraceptives are more than 99% effective (i.e., there would be less than one pregnancy if 100 women used the pill for 1 year). Pills that contain 0.02 to 0.035 milligrams of estrogen vary slightly in effectiveness, ranging from 98% to more than 99% effective.

The second type of oral contraceptive, often called the "mini-pill", contains only a progestogen. It works in part by preventing release of an egg from the ovary but also by keeping sperm from reaching the egg and by making the uterus (womb) less receptive to any fertilized egg that reaches it. The mini-pill is less effective than the combination oral contraceptive, about 97% effective. In addition, the progestogen-only pill has a tendency to cause irregular bleeding which may be quite inconvenient, or cessation of bleeding entirely. The progestogen-only pill is used despite its lower effectiveness in the hope that it will prove not to have some of the serious side effects of the estrogen-containing pill (see below) but it is not yet certain that the mini-pill does in fact have fewer serious side effects. The discussion below, while based mainly on information about the combination pills, should be considered to apply as well to the mini-pill.

2. Other Nonsurgical Ways to Prevent Pregnancy. As this leaflet will explain, oral contraceptives have several serious risks. Some other methods of contraception have lesser risks. They are usually less effective than oral contraceptives, but, used properly, may be effective enough for many women. The following table gives reported pregnancy rates (the number of women out of 100 who would become pregnant in 1 year) for these methods:

Pregnancies per 100 Women per Year
Intrauterine device (IUD), less than 1–6;
Diaphragm with spermicidal products (creams or jellies), 2–20;
Condom (rubber), 3–36;
Aerosol foams, 2–29;
Jellies and creams, 4–36;
Periodic abstinence (rhythm), all types, less than 1–47;
  — Calendar method, 14–47;
  — Temperature method, 1–20;
  — Temperature method—intercourse only in post-ovulatory phase, less than 1–7;
  — Mucus method, 1–25;
No contraception, 60–80.

The figures (except for the IUD) vary widely because people differ in how well they use each method. Very faithful users of the various methods, with the exception of the calendar method of periodic abstinence (rhythm), may achieve lower pregnancy rates than those given above, which are the average results for large groups of women. Except for the IUD, effective use of these methods requires somewhat more effort than simply taking a single pill every evening, but it is an effort that many couples undertake successfully. Your doctor can tell you a great deal more about these methods of contraception.

3. The Dangers of Oral Contraceptives

a. *Circulatory disorders (abnormal blood clots, strokes, and heart attacks).* Blood clots (in various blood vessels of the body) are the most common of the serious side effects of oral contraceptives. A clot can result in a stroke (if the clot is in the brain), a heart attack (if the clot is in a blood vessel of the heart), a pulmonary embolus (a clot which forms in the legs or pelvis, then breaks off and travels to the lungs), or loss of a limb (a clot in a blood vessel in or leading to an arm or leg). Any of these can cause death or disability. Clots also occur rarely in the blood vessels of the eye, resulting in blindness or impairment of vision in that eye. There is evidence that the risk of clotting increases with higher estrogen doses. It is therefore important to keep the dose of estrogen as low as possible, so long as the oral contraceptive used has an acceptable pregnancy rate and doesn't cause unacceptable changes in the menstrual pattern. The risk of abnormal clotting increases with age in both users and nonusers of oral contraceptives, but the increased risk from the contraceptive appears to be present at all ages.

In addition to blood-clotting disorders, it has been estimated that women taking oral contraceptives are twice as likely as nonusers to have a stroke due to rupture of a blood vessel in the brain.

Furthermore, cigarette smoking by oral contraceptive users increases the risk of serious adverse effects on the heart and blood vessels. This risk increases with age and with heavy smoking (15 or more cigarettes per day) and becomes quite marked in women over 35 years of age. For this reason, women who use oral contraceptives should not smoke.

For oral contraceptive users in general, it has been estimated that in women between the ages of 15 and 34 the risk of death due to a circulatory disorder is about 1 in 12,000 per year, whereas for nonusers the rate is about 1 in 50,000 per year. In the age group 35 to 44, the risk is estimated to be about 1 in 2,500 per year for oral contraceptive users and about 1 in 10,000 per year for nonusers. The risk is concentrated in older women, in those with a long duration of use, and in cigarette smokers. The effects on the circulatory system may persist after oral contraceptives are discontinued.

Even without the pill the risk of having a heart attack increases with age and is also increased by such heart attack risk factors as high blood pressure, high cholesterol, obesity, diabetes, and cigarette smoking. Without any risk factors present, the use of oral contraceptives alone may double the risk of heart attack. However, the combination of cigarette smoking, especially heavy smoking, and oral contraceptive use greatly increases the risk of heart attack. Oral contraceptive users who smoke are about 5 times more likely to have a heart attack than users who do not smoke and about 10 times more likely to have a heart attack than nonusers who do not smoke. It has been estimated that users between the ages of 30 and 39 who smoke have about a 1 in 10,000 chance each year of having a fatal heart attack compared to about a 1 in 50,000 chance in users who do not smoke, and about a 1 in 100,000 chance in nonusers who do not smoke.

In the age group 40 to 44, the risk is about 1 in 1,700 per year for users who smoke compared to about 1 in 10,000 for users who do not smoke and to about 1 in 14,000 per year for nonusers who do not smoke. These are average figures for Great Britain; comparable estimates for the U.S. may be higher. Heavy smoking (about 15 cigarettes or more a day) further increases the risk. If you do not smoke and have none of the other heart attack risk factors described above, you will have a smaller risk than listed. If you have several heart attack risk factors, the risk may be considerably greater than listed.

b. *Formation of tumors.* Studies have found that when certain animals are given the female sex hormone estrogen, which is an ingredient of oral contraceptives, continuously for long periods, cancers may develop in the breast, cervix, vagina, uterus, ovary, pituitary and liver.

These findings suggest that oral contraceptives may cause cancer in humans. However, studies to date in women taking currently marketed oral contraceptives have not confirmed that oral contraceptives cause cancer in humans. Several studies have found no increase in breast cancer in users, although one study suggested oral contraceptives might cause an increase in breast cancer in women who already have benign breast disease (e.g., cysts) or who have used oral contraceptives for long periods (2–4 years).

Women with a strong family history of breast cancer or who have breast nodules, fibrocystic disease, or abnormal mammograms or who were exposed to DES (diethylstilbestrol), an estrogen, during their mother's pregnancy must be followed very closely by their doctors if they choose to use oral contraceptives instead of another method of contraception. Many studies have shown that women taking oral contraceptives have less risk of getting benign breast disease than those who have not used oral contraceptives. Strong evidence has emerged that estrogens (one component of oral contraceptives) when given alone (unaccompanied by progestogen) for periods of more than one year to women after the menopause, increase the risk of cancer of the uterus (womb). There is also some evidence that a kind of oral contraceptive which is no longer marketed, the sequential oral contraceptive, may increase the risk of cancer of the uterus. There remains no evidence, however, that the oral contraceptives now available (containing estrogen and progestogen in combination or progestogen alone) increase the risk of this cancer. Cancer of the cervix may develop more readily in long-term (3–4 years) users of the pill who had preexisting abnormal Pap smears. One study reported malignant melanoma (skin cancer), urinary tract cancers, and thyroid cancers more frequently in pill users than in non-users.

Benign or malignant liver tumors have been associated with short-term as well as long-term oral contraceptive use. The benign (non-malignant) tumors do not spread, but they may rupture and produce internal bleeding, which may cause death.

c. *Dangers to a developing child if oral contraceptives are used in or immediately preceding pregnancy.* Oral contraceptives should not be taken by pregnant women because they may damage the developing child. An increased risk of birth defects, including heart defects and limb defects, has been associated with the use of sex hormones, including oral contraceptives, in pregnancy. In addition, the developing female child whose mother has received DES (diethylstilbestrol), an estrogen, during pregnancy has a risk of getting cancer of the vagina or cervix in her teens or young adulthood. This risk is estimated to be about 1 in 1,000 exposures or less. Abnormalities of the urinary and sex organs have been reported in male offspring so exposed. It is possible that other estrogens, such as the estrogens in oral contraceptives, could have the same effect in the child if the mother takes them during pregnancy.

If you stop taking oral contraceptives to become pregnant, your doctor may recommend that you use another method of contraception for a short while. The reason for this is that there is evidence from studies in women who have had "miscarriages" soon after stopping the pill, that the lost fetuses are more likely to be abnormal. Whether there is an overall increase in "miscarriage" in women who become pregnant soon after stopping the pill as compared with women who do not use the pill is not known, but it is possible that there may be. If, however, you do become pregnant soon after stopping oral contraceptives, and do not have a miscarriage, there is no evidence that the baby has an increased risk of being abnormal.

d. *Gallbladder disease.* Women who use oral contraceptives have a greater risk than nonusers of having gallbladder disease requiring surgery. The increased risk may first appear within 1 year of use and may double after 4 to 5 years of use.

e. *Other side effects of oral contraceptives.* Some women using oral contraceptives experience unpleasant side effects that are not dangerous and are not likely to damage their health. Some of these may be temporary. Your breasts may feel tender, nausea and vomiting may occur, you may gain or lose weight, and your ankles may swell. A spotty darkening of the skin, particularly of the face, is possible and may persist. Many of these effects are seen more frequently with combination oral contraceptives containing 0.05 milligrams or more of estrogen. You may notice unexpected vaginal bleeding or changes in your menstrual period. Irregular bleeding is frequently seen when using the mini-pill or combination oral contraceptives containing less than 0.05 milligrams of estrogen. More serious side effects include worsening of migraine, asthma, epilepsy, and kidney or heart disease because of a tendency for water to be retained in the body when oral contraceptives are used. Other side effects are growth of preexisting fibroid tumors of the uterus; mental depression; and liver problems with jaundice (yellowing of the skin). Your doctor may find that levels of sugar and fatty substances in your blood are elevated; the long-term effects of these changes are not known. Some women develop high blood pressure while taking oral contraceptives, which may persist after discontinuation. High blood pressure may lead to serious disease of the kidney and circulatory system. Your physician may wish to check your blood pressure more frequently if you have a history of toxemia of pregnancy, kidney disease or increased blood pressure.

Other reactions have been reported occasionally. These include more frequent urination and some discomfort when urinating, kidney disease, blood cell breakdown with kidney failure, nervousness, dizziness, an increase in or loss of hair, an increase or decrease in sex drive, appetite changes, cataracts, and a need for a change in contact lens prescription or inability to use contact lenses.

After you stop using oral contraceptives, your ability to menstruate or become pregnant may be impaired. This impairment may be greater if you have never been pregnant.

As discussed previously, you should wait a few months after stopping the pill before you try to become pregnant. An increased incidence of twin births has been reported in women who have conceived soon after stopping the pill. During these few months, use another form of contraception. You should consult your physician before resuming use of oral contraceptives after childbirth, especially if you plan to nurse your baby. Drugs in oral contraceptives are known to appear in the milk, and the long-range effect on infants is not known. Furthermore, oral contraceptives may cause a decrease in your milk supply as well as in the quality of the milk.

4. Comparison of the Risks of Oral Contraceptives and Other Contraceptive Methods. The many studies on the risks and effectiveness of oral contraceptives and other methods of contraception have been analyzed to estimate the risk of death associated with various methods of contraception. This risk has two parts: (a) the risk associated with the method itself (e.g., the risk that an oral contraceptive user will die due to abnormal clotting), and (b) the risk associated with failure of the method (death due to pregnancy or abortion). The results of this analysis are shown in the bar graph (Figure 1). The height of the bars is the estimated number of deaths per 100,000 women each year. There are six sets of bars, each set referring to a specific age group of women. Within each set of bars, there are two bars for oral contraceptive users, one referring to users who smoke and one referring to users who do not smoke, and five bars for other contraceptive methods including one bar representing no method of contraception. ("Traditional contraception" means diaphragm or condom.)

This analysis is based on present knowledge and new information could, of course, alter it. The analysis shows that the risk of death from all methods of birth control is low compared to the risks of childbirth, *except for oral contraceptives in women over 40 who smoke.* It shows that the lowest risk of death is associated with the condom or diaphragm (traditional contraception) backed up by early abortion in case of failure of the condom or diaphragm to prevent pregnancy. Also, at any age the risk of death (due to unexpected pregnancy) from use of traditional contraception even without a backup of abortion is generally the same as, or less than, that from use of oral contraceptives.

Careful Use of Oral Contraceptives:
1. Tell Your Doctor About Any Of The Following:
   a. Present or past conditions that mean you should not use oral contraceptives:
   > Clots in the legs, lungs or elsewhere
   > A stroke, heart attack, or chest pain (angina pectoris)
   > Known or suspected cancer of the breast or sex organs
   > Irregular or scanty menstrual periods before starting to take the pill
   > Liver tumor associated with the use of the pill or other estrogen containing products.
   b. Present conditions that mean you should not use oral contraceptives:
   > Unusual vaginal bleeding that has not yet been diagnosed.
   > Known or suspected pregnancy.
   c. Conditions that your doctor will want to watch closely or which might cause him to suggest another method of contraception:
   A family history of breast cancer
   Breast nodules, fibrocystic disease of the breast, or an abnormal mammogram
   Diabetes
   High blood pressure
   High cholesterol
   Cigarette smoking
   Migraine headaches
   Heart or kidney disease
   Epilepsy
   Mental depression
   Tingling of the fingers or toes
   Fibroid tumors of the uterus
   Gallbladder disease
   Asthma
   Problems during a prior pregnancy
   Plans for elective surgery
   History of jaundice or other liver disease
   d. Use of any of the following kinds of drugs, which might interact with the pill: antibiotics, sulfa drugs, drugs for epilepsy or migraine, pain killers, tranquilizers, sedatives or sleeping pills, blood thinning drugs, vitamins, drugs being used for the treatment of depression, high blood pressure, high blood sugar (diabetes), asthma, bronchitis, emphysema, or colds.
   e. Once you are using oral contraceptives, you should be alert for signs of a serious adverse effect and call your doctor if they occur:
   Sharp pain in the chest, coughing blood, or sudden shortness of breath (indicating possible clots in the lungs)
   Pain in the calf (possible clot in the leg)
   Crushing chest pain or heaviness (indicating possible heart attack)
   Sudden severe headache or vomiting, dizziness or fainting, disturbance of vision or speech, or weakness or numbness in an arm or leg (indicating a possible stroke)
   Sudden partial or complete loss of vision (indicating a possible clot in the eye)
   Breast lumps (you should ask your doctor to show you how to examine your own breasts)
   Severe pain or mass in the abdomen (indicating a possible tumor of the liver)
   Severe depression
   Yellowing of the skin (jaundice)
   Unusual swelling.
2. How to Take the Pill So That It is Most Effective
Reduced effectiveness and an increased incidence of breakthrough bleeding have been associated with the use of oral contraceptives with antibiotics such as rifampicin, ampicillin, and tetracycline or with certain other drugs, such as barbiturates, phenylbutazone or phenytoin sodium. You should

Continued on next page

Syntex—Cont.

use an additional means of contraception during any cycle in which any of these drugs are taken. When you first begin to use the pill, you should use an additional method of protection until you have taken your first seven pills.

Your physician has prescribed one of the following dosage schedules. Please follow the instructions appropriate for your schedule.

20-Day Schedule: Counting the onset of flow as day 1, take the first pill on day 5 of the menstrual cycle whether or not the flow has stopped. Take another pill the same time each day, preferably at bedtime, for 20 days. Then wait for 7 days, during which time a menstrual period usually occurs, and begin taking 1 pill every day on the 8th day after you took your last pill, whether or not the menstrual flow has stopped. This cycle is repeated 20 days on pills and 7 days off pills until time for the physician's examination and pill refill. If you are taking NORINYL® 2 mg Tablets for the control of excessive bleeding (hypermenorrhea), your physician may instruct you to stop taking the pills after 3 cycles to determine the need for further treatment. The information contained in this leaflet regarding who should not use the pill, the dangers of the pill and safe use of the pill applies to the use of the pill for hypermenorrhea, as well as for contraception.

21-Day Schedule for BREVICON, NORINYL 1 & 35, NORINYL 1 & 50, NORINYL 1 & 80 Tablets: You may start taking the pill on Day 5 of your menstrual cycle or on Sunday. To start on Day 5, count the first day of menstrual flow as Day 1 and take the first pill on Day 5 of the menstrual cycle whether or not the flow has stopped. To start on Sunday, take the first pill on the first Sunday after your menstrual period begins. If it begins on Sunday, take the first pill that day. Whether you start on Day 5 or on Sunday, take another pill the same time each day, preferably at bedtime, for 21 days. Then wait for 7 days, during which time a menstrual period usually occurs, and begin taking 1 pill every day on the 8th day after you took your last pill, whether or not the menstrual flow has stopped. This cycle is repeated 21 days on pills and 7 days off pills until time for the physician's examination and pill refill.

28-Day Schedule for BREVICON, NORINYL 1 & 35, NORINYL 1 & 50, NORINYL 1 & 80 Tablets: You may start taking the pill on Day 5 of your menstrual cycle or on Sunday. To start on Day 5, count the first day of menstrual flow as Day 1 and take the first white, yellow, green, or blue pill on Day 5 of the menstrual cycle whether or not the flow has stopped. To start on Sunday, take the first white, yellow, green, or blue pill on the first Sunday after your menstrual period begins. If it begins on Sunday, take the first pill that day. Whether you start on Day 5 or on Sunday, follow the sequence around the card and continue taking another pill at the same time each day, preferably at bedtime, for 21 days. Then take an orange pill from the bottom of the card each day for seven days and expect a menstrual period during this week. The orange pills contain no active drug and are included simply for your convenience—to eliminate the need for counting days. After all 28 pills have been taken, whether bleeding has stopped or not, take the first white, yellow, green, or blue pill of the next cycle without any interruption. With the 28-day package, pills are taken every day of the year with no gap between cycles.

21-Day Schedule for TRI-NORINYL Tablets: Take the first blue pill on the first Sunday after menstrual flow begins. If menstrual flow begins on Sunday, take the first blue pill on that day. Take one blue pill the same time each day, preferably at bedtime, for the first 7 days, one green pill daily for the next 9 days, and then one blue pill each day for 5 days. Wait for 7 days, during which time a menstrual period usually occurs, then begin a new cycle of pills on the eighth day after you took your last pill, whether or not the menstrual flow has stopped. This cycle is repeated 21 days on pills and 7 days off pills until time for the physician's examination and pill refill.

28-Day Schedule for TRI-NORINYL Tablets: Take the first blue pill on the first Sunday after menstrual flow begins. If menstrual flow begins on Sunday, take the first blue pill on that day. Take one blue pill the same time each day, preferably at bedtime, for the first 7 days, one green pill daily for the next 9 days and then one blue pill each day for 5 days. Take one orange pill daily for the next 7 days and expect a menstrual period during this week. The orange pills contain no active drug and are included simply for your convenience—to eliminate the need of counting days. After all 28 pills have been taken, whether bleeding has stopped or not, take the first blue pill of the next cycle without any interruption. With the 28-day package, a pill is taken every day of the year with no gap between cycles.

Important Additional Instructions for the 20-Day, 21-Day and 28-Day Schedules

The prescribed dosage schedule must be followed exactly. The chance of becoming pregnant increases with each pill missed. If you miss one pill, you should take it as soon as you remember and also take your next pill at the regular time, which means you will be taking two pills on that day. If you miss two pills in a row, you should take one of the missed pills as soon as you remember, discard the other missed pill, and take your regular pill for that day at the proper time. Furthermore, you should use an additional method of contraception in addition to taking your pills for the remainder of the cycle. If more than 2 pills in a row have been missed, discontinue taking your pills immediately and use an additional method of contraception until you have a period or your doctor determines that you are not pregnant. Missing orange pills in the 28-day schedule does not increase your chances of becoming pregnant.

At times there may be no menstrual period after a cycle of pills. Therefore, if you miss one menstrual period but have taken the pills *exactly as you were supposed to*, continue as usual into the next cycle. If you have not taken the pills correctly, and have missed a menstrual period, *you may be pregnant* and should stop taking oral contraceptives until your doctor determines whether or not you are pregnant. Until you can get to your doctor, use another form of contraception. If two consecutive menstrual periods are missed, you should stop taking pills until it is determined whether you are pregnant. If you do become pregnant while using oral contraceptives, you should discuss the risks to the developing child with your doctor.

Even if spotting or breakthrough bleeding should occur, continue the medication according to the schedule. Should spotting or breakthrough bleeding persist you should notify your physician.
NOR-Q.D.® (norethindrone) Tablets 0.35 mg.

Schedule: Take the first pill on the first day of the menstrual flow, and take another pill each day, every day of the year. The pill should be taken at the same time of day, preferably at bedtime, and *continued daily, without interruption, whether bleeding occurs or not.* If prolonged bleeding occurs, you should consult your physician.
The chance of becoming pregnant increases with each pill missed. If you miss one pill, you should take it as soon as you remember and also take your next pill at the regular time, which means you will be taking two pills on that day. If you miss two pills in a row you should take one of the missed pills as soon as you remember, discard the other missed pill, and take your regular pill for that day at the proper time. Furthermore, you should use an additional method of contraception in addition to taking NOR-Q.D.® until you have a period or your doctor determines you are not pregnant. If more than 2 pills in a row have been missed, NOR-Q.D. should be discontinued immediately and an additional method of contraception should be used until you have a period or your doctor determines that you are not pregnant.

Whether or not you have missed a pill, if you have not had a period within 45 days of your last period, *you may be pregnant.* You should stop taking NOR-Q.D. until your doctor determines whether or not you are pregnant. Until you can get to your doctor, use another form of contraception. If you do become pregnant while using NOR-Q.D., you should discuss the risks to the developing child with your doctor.

3. Periodic Examination

Your doctor will take a complete medical and family history before prescribing oral contraceptives. At that time and about once a year thereafter, he will generally examine your blood pressure, breasts, abdomen, and pelvic organs (including a Papanicolaou smear).

Summary: Oral contraceptives are the most effective method, except sterilization, for preventing pregnancy. Other methods, when used conscientiously, are also very effective and have fewer risks. Although the serious risks of oral contraceptives are uncommon, some of the risks may persist after you stop using the pill. On the other hand, the "pill" is a very convenient method of preventing pregnancy.

If you have certain conditions or have had these conditions in the past, you should not use oral contraceptives because the risk is too great. These conditions are listed in this leaflet. If you do not have these conditions, and decide to use the "pill", please read this leaflet carefully so that you can use the "pill" most safely and effectively.

Based on his or her assessment of your medical needs, your doctor has prescribed this drug for you. Do not give the drug to anyone else.

Revised 7/84
Shown in Product Identification Section, page 440

CARMOL® 10   OTC
[kahr' mawl]
**10% urea lotion
for total body
dry skin care.**

A product of Syntex Laboratories, Inc.

(See PDR For Nonprescription Drugs)

CARMOL® 20   OTC
[kahr' mawl]
**20% Urea Cream
Extra strength for
rough, dry skin**

A product of Syntex Laboratories, Inc.

(See PDR For Nonprescription Drugs)

CARMOL® HC   R
[kahr' mawl]
**(hydrocortisone acetate)
Cream**

Refer to entry under LIDEX® (fluocinonide) Cream 0.05%.

Product Information

LIDEX®
[li'dex]
(fluocinonide)
Cream 0.05%
Gel 0.05%
Ointment 0.05%
Topical Solution 0.05%

LIDEX®-E
(fluocinonide)
Cream 0.05%

CARMOL® HC
(hydrocortisone acetate)
Cream 1%

NEO-SYNALAR® Cream
[ne"o sin'ă-lahr]
[neomycin sulfate 0.5% (0.35% neomycin base), fluocinolone acetonide 0.025%]

SYNACORT®
[sin'ă-cort]
(hydrocortisone)
Cream 1%
Cream 2.5%

SYNALAR®
[sin'ă-lahr]
(fluocinolone acetonide)
Cream 0.025%
Cream 0.01%
Ointment 0.025%
Topical Solution 0.01%

SYNALAR-HP®
(fluocinolone acetonide)
Cream 0.2%

SYNEMOL®
[sin'ĕ-mol]
(fluocinolone acetonide)
Cream 0.025%

Products of Syntex Laboratories, Inc.

Description: These preparations are all intended for topical administration.

LIDEX preparations have as their active component the corticosteroid fluocinonide, which is the 21-acetate ester of fluocinolone acetonide and has the chemical name pregna-1,4-diene-3,20-dione, 21-(acetyloxy)-6, 9-difluoro-11-hydroxy -16,17- ((1-methylethylidene)bis(oxy))-, $(6\alpha, 11\beta, 16\alpha)$-.

LIDEX cream contains fluocinonide 0.5 mg/g in FAPG® cream, a specially formulated cream base consisting of stearyl alcohol, polyethylene glycol 8000, propylene glycol, 1,2,6-hexanetriol and citric acid. This white cream vehicle is greaseless, non-staining, anhydrous and completely water miscible. The base provides emollient and hydrophilic properties. In this formulation the active ingredient is totally in solution.

LIDEX gel contains fluocinonide 0.5 mg/g in a specially formulated gel base consisting of propylene glycol, propyl gallate, edetate disodium, and carbomer 940, with NaOH and/or HCl added to adjust the pH. This clear, colorless thixotropic vehicle is greaseless, non-staining and completely water miscible. In this formulation the active ingredient is totally in solution.

LIDEX ointment contains fluocinonide 0.5 mg/g in a specially formulated ointment base consisting of Amerchol CAB (mixture of sterols and higher alcohols), white petrolatum, propylene carbonate and propylene glycol. It provides the occlusive and emollient effects desirable in an ointment. In this formulation the active ingredient is totally in solution.

LIDEX solution contains fluocinonide 0.5 mg/ml in a solution of propylene glycol, alcohol (35%), diisopropyl adipate, and citric acid. In this formulation the active ingredient is totally in solution.

LIDEX-E cream contains fluocinonide 0.5 mg/g in a water-washable aqueous emollient base of stearyl alcohol, cetyl alcohol, mineral oil, propylene glycol, sorbitan monostearate, polysorbate 60, citric acid and purified water.

CARMOL HC Cream has the corticosteroid hydrocortisone acetate, which has the chemical name pregna-4-ene-3,20-dione,21-(acetyloxy)-11,17-dihydroxy-,(11β)-, as its active component. CARMOL HC contains micronized hydrocortisone acetate, USP, 10 mg/g, in a water-washable vanishing cream containing urea (10%), purified water, stearic acid, isopropyl myristate, PPG-26 oleate, isopropyl palmitate, propylene glycol, trolamine, cetyl alcohol, carbomer 940, sodium bisulfite, sodium laureth sulfate, edetate disodium, xanthan gum; scented with hypoallergenic perfume.

CARMOL HC is non-lipid, non-occlusive and hypoallergenic; it contains no mineral oil, petrolatum, lanolin or parabens.

NEO-SYNALAR cream contains neomycin sulfate 5 mg/g (3.5 mg/g neomycin base) and fluocinolone acetonide 0.25 mg/g in a water-washable aqueous base of stearic acid, propylene glycol, sorbitan monostearate and monooleate, polysorbate 60, purified water, with methylparaben and propylparaben as preservatives.

SYNACORT creams have as their active component the corticosteroid hydrocortisone, which has the chemical name pregn-4-ene-3,20-dione, 11,17,21-trihydroxy-,(11β).

SYNACORT creams contain hydrocortisone, USP, 10 mg/g or 25 mg/g in a cream containing propylene glycol, stearyl alcohol, mineral oil, cetyl alcohol, sorbitan monostearate, polysorbate 60, citric acid and purified water.

SYNALAR preparations, SYNALAR-HP cream, and SYNEMOL cream have as their active component the corticosteroid fluocinolone acetonide, which has the chemical name pregna-1,4-diene-3,20-dione,6,9-difluoro-11,21-dihydroxy-16,17-[(1-methylethylidene)bix(oxy)]-,$(6\alpha, 11\beta, 16\alpha)$-.

SYNALAR creams contains fluocinolone acetonide 0.25 mg/g or 0.1 mg/g in a water-washable aqueous base of stearic acid, propylene glycol, sorbitan monostearate and monooleate, polysorbate 60, purified water and citric acid with methylparaben and propylparaben as preservatives.

SYNALAR ointment contains fluocinolone acetonide 0.25 mg/g in a white petrolatum USP vehicle.

SYNALAR solution contains fluocinolone acetonide 0.1 mg/ml in a water-washable base of propylene glycol with citric acid.

SYNALAR-HP cream contains fluocinolone acetonide 2 mg/g in a water-washable aqueous base of stearyl alcohol, cetyl alcohol, mineral oil, propylene glycol, sorbitan monostearate, polysorbate 60, purified water and citric acid with methylparaben and propylparaben as preservatives.

SYNEMOL cream contains fluocinolone acetonide 0.25 mg/g in a water-washable aqueous emollient base of stearyl alcohol, cetyl alcohol, mineral oil, propylene glycol, sorbitan monostearate, polysorbate 60, purified water and citric acid.

Clinical Pharmacology: Topical corticosteroids share anti-inflammatory, anti-pruritic and vasoconstrictive actions.

The mechanism of anti-inflammatory activity of the topical corticosteroids is unclear. Various laboratory methods including vasoconstrictor assays, are used to compare and predict potencies and/or clinical efficacies of the topical corticosteroids. There is some evidence to suggest that a recognizable correlation exists between vasoconstrictor potency and therapeutic efficacy in man.

Pharmacokinetics: The extent of percutaneous absorption of topical corticosteroids is determined by many factors including the vehicle, the integrity of the epidermal barrier, and the use of occlusive dressings. A significantly greater amount of fluocinonide is absorbed from the solution than from the cream or gel formulations.

Topical corticosteroids can be absorbed from normal intact skin. Inflammation and/or other disease processes in the skin increase percutaneous absorption. Occlusive dressings substantially increase the percutaneous absorption of topical corticosteroids. Thus, occlusive dressings may be a valuable therapeutic adjunct for treatment of resistant dermatoses. (See DOSAGE AND ADMINISTRATION).

Once absorbed through the skin, topical corticosteroids are handled through pharmacokinetic pathways similar to systemically administered corticosteroids. Corticosteroids are bound to plasma proteins in varying degrees. Corticosteroids are metabolized primarily in the liver and are then excreted by the kidneys. Some of the topical corticosteroids and their metabolites are also excreted into the bile.

Indications and Usage: Relief of the inflammatory and pruritic manifestations of corticosteroid-responsive dermatoses.

NEO-SYNALAR is indicated for the treatment of corticosteroid-responsive dermatoses with secondary infection. It has not been demonstrated that this steroid-antibiotic combination provides greater benefit then the steroid component alone after 7 days of treatment (see WARNINGS).

Contraindications: Topical corticosteroids are contraindicated in those patients with a history of hypersensitivity to any of the components of the preparation. NEO-SYNALAR should not be used in the external auditory canal if the eardrum is perforated.

Warnings for NEO-SYNALAR: If local infection should continue or become severe, or in the presence of systemic infection, appropriate systemic antibacterial therapy, based on susceptibility testing, should be considered.

Because of the concern of nephrotoxicity and ototoxicity associated with neomycin, this combination should not be used over a wide area or for extended periods of time.

There are articles in the current medical literature that indicate an increase in the prevalence of persons sensitive to neomycin.

Precautions: General: It is recommended that NEO-SYNALAR not be used under occlusive dressing. Systemic absorption of topical corticosteroids has produced reversible hypothalamic-pituitary-adrenal (HPA) axis suppression, manifestations of Cushing's syndrome, hyperglycemia, and glucosuria in some patients.

Conditions which augment systemic absorption include the application of the more potent steroids, use over large surface areas, prolonged use, and the addition of occlusive dressings and dosage form.

Therefore, patients receiving a large dose of a potent topical steroid applied to a large surface area or under an occlusive dressing should be evaluated periodically for evidence of HPA axis suppression by using the urinary free cortisol and ACTH stimulation tests. If HPA axis suppression is noted, an attempt should be made to withdraw the drug, to reduce the frequency of application, or to substitute a less potent steroid.

Recovery of HPA axis function is generally prompt and complete upon discontinuation of the drug. Infrequently, signs and symptoms of steroid withdrawal may occur, requiring supplemental systemic corticosteroids.

Children may absorb proportionally larger amounts of topical corticosteroids and thus be more susceptible to systemic toxicity. (See PRECAUTIONS—Pediatric Use).

Not for ophthalmic use. Severe irritation is possible if fluocinonide solution contacts the eye. If that should occur, immediate flushing of the eye with a large volume of water is recommended.

If irritation develops, topical corticosteroids should be discontinued and appropriate therapy instituted.

In the presence of dermatological infections, the use of an appropriate antifungal or anti-bacterial agent should be instituted. If a favorable response does not occur promptly, the corticosteroid should be discontinued until the infection has been adequately controlled.

As with all antibiotics, prolonged use of NEO-SYNALAR may result in over-growth of nonsusceptible organisms. If superinfection occurs, appropriate measures should be taken.

SYNALAR-HP cream should not be used for prolonged periods and the quantity per day should not exceed 2 g. of formulated material.

Information for the Patient: Patients using topical corticosteroids should receive the following information and instructions:

Continued on next page

Syntex—Cont.

1. This medication is to be used as directed by the physician. It is for external use only. Avoid contact with the eyes. If there is contact with the eyes and severe irritation occurs, immediately flush with a large volume of water.
2. Patients should be advised not to use this medication for any disorder other than for which is was prescribed.
3. The treated skin area should not be bandaged or otherwise covered or wrapped as to be occlusive unless directed by the physician.
4. Patients should report any signs of local adverse reactions especially under occlusive dressing.
5. Parents of pediatric patients should be advised not to use tight-fitting diapers or plastic pants on a child being treated in the diaper area, as these garments may constitute occlusive dressings.

Laboratory Tests: The following tests may be helpful in evaluating the HPA axis suppression: Urinary free cortisol test and ACTH stimulation test.

Carcinogenesis, Mutagenesis, and Impairment of Fertility: Long-term animal studies have not been performed to evaluate the carcinogenic potential or the effect on fertility of topical corticosteroids. Studies to determine mutagenicity with prednisolone and hydrocortisone have revealed negative results.

Pregnancy Category C: Corticosteroids are generally teratogenic in laboratory animals when administered systemically at relatively low dosage levels. The more potent corticosteroids have been shown to be teratogenic after dermal application in laboratory animals. There are no adequate and well-controlled studies in pregnant women on teratogenic effects from topically applied corticosteroids. Therefore, topical corticosteroids should be used during pregnancy only if the potential benefit justifies the potential risk to the fetus. Drugs of this class should not be used extensively on pregnant patients, in large amounts, or for prolonged periods of time.

Nursing Mothers: It is not known whether topical administration of corticosteroids could result in sufficient systemic absorption to produce detectable quantities in breast milk. Systemically administered corticosteroids are secreted into breast milk in quantities *not* likely to have a deleterious effect on the infant. Nevertheless, caution should be exercised when topical corticosteroids are administered to a nursing mother.

Pediatric Use: SYNALAR-HP® (fluocinolone acetonide) cream 0.2% should not be used on infants up to 2 years of age.

Pediatric patients may demonstrate greater susceptibility to topical corticosteroid-induced HPA axis suppression and Cushing's syndrome than mature patients because of a larger skin surface area to body weight ratio.

Hypothalamic-pituitary-adrenal (HPA) axis suppression, Cushing's syndrome, and intracranial hypertension have been reported in children receiving topical corticosteroids. Manifestations of adrenal suppression in children include linear growth retardation, delayed weight gain, low plasma cortisol levels, and absence of response to ACTH stimulation. Manifestations of intracranial hypertension include bulging fontanelles, headaches, and bilateral papilledema.

Administration of topical corticosteroids to children should be limited to the least amount compatible with an effective therapeutic regimen. Chronic corticosteroid therapy may interfere with the growth and development of children.

Adverse Reactions: The following local adverse reactions are reported infrequently with topical corticosteroids, but may occur more frequently with the use of occlusive dressings. These reactions are listed in an approximate decreasing order of occurrence: burning, itching, irritation, dryness, folliculitis, hypertrichosis, acneiform eruptions, hypopigmentation, perioral dermatitis, allergic contact dermatitis, maceration of the skin, secondary infection, skin atrophy, striae, miliaria. The following reactions have been reported with the topical use of neomycin: ototoxicity and nephrotoxicity.

Overdosage: Topically applied corticosteroids can be absorbed in sufficient amounts to produce systemic effects (See PRECAUTIONS).

Dosage and Administration: Topical corticosteroids are generally applied to the affected area as a thin film from two or four times daily depending on the severity of the condition. In hairy sites, the hair should be parted to allow direct contact with the lesion.

Occlusive dressings may be used for the management of psoriasis or recalcitrant conditions. Some plastic films may be flammable and due care should be exercised in their use. Similarly, caution should be employed when such films are used on children or left in their proximity, to avoid the possibility of accidental suffocation.

If an infection develops, the use of occlusive dressings should be discontinued and appropriate antimicrobial therapy instituted.

How Supplied: LIDEX® (fluocinonide) cream 0.05%—15 g Tube (NDC 0033-2511-13), 30 g Tube (NDC 0033-2511-14), 60 g Tube (NDC 0033-2511-17), and 120 g Tube (NDC 0033-2511-22). Store at room temperature. Avoid excessive heat, above 40°C (104°F).
LIDEX® (fluocinonide) gel 0.05%—15 g Tube (NDC 0033-2507-13), 30 g Tube (NDC 0033-2507-14), 60 g Tube (NDC 0033-2507-17), and 120 g Tube (NDC 0033-2507-22). Store at controlled room temperature, 15–30°C (59–86°F).
LIDEX® (fluocinonide) ointment 0.05%—15 g Tube (NDC 0033-2514-13), 30 g Tube (NDC 0033-2514-14), 60 g Tube (NDC 0033-2514-17), and 120 g Tube (NDC 0033-2514-22). Store at room temperature. Avoid excessive heat, above 40°C (104°F).
LIDEX® (fluocinonide) topical solution 0.05%—Plastic squeeze bottles: 20 cc (NDC 0033-2517-44) and 60 cc (NDC 0033-2517-46). Store at room temperature. Avoid excessive heat, above 40°C (104°F).
LIDEX-E® (fluocinonide) cream 0.05%—15 g Tube (NDC 0033-2513-13), 30 g Tube (NDC 0033-2513-14), 60 g Tube (NDC 0033-2513-17), and 120 g Tube (NDC 0033-2513-22). Store at room temperature. Avoid excessive heat, above 40°C (104°F).
CARMOL® HC (hydrocortisone acetate) cream 1%—1 oz. Tube (NDC 0033-2550-15) and 4 oz. Jar (NDC 0033-2550-11). Avoid excessive heat, above 40°C (104°F).
NEO-SYNALAR cream—15 g Tube (NDC 0033-2505-13), 30 g Tube (NDC 0033-2505-14), 60 g Tube (NDC 0033-2505-17). Store at room temperature. Avoid freezing.
SYNACORT® (hydrocortisone) cream 1%—15 g Tube (NDC 0033-2519-13), 30 g Tube (NDC 0033-2519-14), and 60 g Tube (NDC 0033-2519-17).
SYNACORT® (hydrocortisone) cream 2.5%—30 g Tube (NDC 0033-2520-14). Store at room temperature. Avoid excessive heat, above 40°C (104°F).
SYNALAR® (fluocinolone acetonide) cream 0.025%—15 g Tube (NDC 0033-2501-13), 30 g Tube (NDC 0033-2501-14), 60 g Tube—(NDC 0033-2501-17), 120 g Jar (NDC 0033-2501-21), and 425 g Jar (NDC 0033-2501-23). Store at room temperature. Avoid excessive heat, above 40°C (104°F).
SYNALAR® (fluocinolone acetonide) cream 0.01%—15 g Tube (NDC 0033-2502-13), 45 g Tube (NDC 0033-2502-15), 60 g Tube (NDC 0033-2502-17), 120 g Jar (NDC 0033-2502-21), and 425 g Jar (NDC 0033-2502-23). Store at room temperature. Avoid excessive heat, above 40°C (104°F).
SYNALAR® (fluocinoline acetonide) ointment 0.025%—15 g Tube (NDC 0033-2504-13), 30 g Tube (NDC 0033-2504-14), 60 g Tube (NDC 0033-2504-17), 120 g Tube (NDC 0033-2504-22), and 425 g Jar (NDC 0033-2504-23). Store at room temperature. Avoid excessive heat, above 40°C (104°F).
SYNALAR® (fluocinolone acetonide) topical solution 0.01%—Plastic squeeze bottles: 20 cc (NDC 0033-2506-44) and 60 cc (NDC 0033-2506-46). Store at room temperature. Avoid freezing.
SYNALAR-HP® (fluocinolone acetonide) cream 0.2%—12 g Tube (NDC 0033-2503-12). Store at room temperature. Avoid excessive heat, above 40°C (104°F).
SYNEMOL® (fluocinolone acetonide) cream 0.025%—15 g Tube (NDC 0033-2509-13), 30 g Tube (NDC 0033-2509-14), 60 g Tube (NDC 0033-2509-17), and 120 g Tube (NDC 0033-2509-22). Store at room temperature. Avoid excessive heat, above 40°C (104°F).

CAUTION: Federal law prohibits dispensing without a prescription.

Revised 4/84

NAPROSYN® ℞
[nă'pro-sin]
(naproxen)
Tablets

Manufactured for Syntex Laboratories, Inc. by Syntex Puerto Rico, Inc.

Description: NAPROSYN® (naproxen) tablets for oral administration each contain 250 mg, 375 mg or 500 mg of naproxen. NAPROSYN is a member of the arylacetic acid group of nonsteroidal anti-inflammatory drugs.

The chemical name for naproxen is 2-naphthaleneacetic acid, 6-methoxy-α-methyl-,(+). Naproxen is an odorless, white to off-white crystalline substance. It is lipid soluble, practically insoluble in water at low pH and freely soluble in water at high pH.

Clinical Pharmacology: NAPROSYN (naproxen) is a nonsteroidal anti-inflammatory drug with analgesic and antipyretic properties. Naproxen sodium, the sodium salt of naproxen, has been developed as an analgesic because it is more rapidly absorbed. The naproxen anion inhibits prostaglandin synthesis but beyond this its mode of action is unknown.

Naproxen is rapidly and completely absorbed from the gastrointestinal tract. After administration of naproxen, peak plasma levels of naproxen anion are attained in 2 to 4 hours, with steady-state conditions normally achieved after 4–5 doses. The mean biological half-life of the anion in humans is approximately 13 hours, and at therapeutic levels it is greater than 99% albumin bound. Approximately 95% of the dose is excreted in the urine, primarily as naproxen, 6-0-desmethyl naproxen or their conjugates. The rate of excretion has been found to coincide closely with the rate of drug disappearance from the plasma. The drug does not induce metabolizing enzymes.

The drug was studied in patients with rheumatoid arthritis, osteoarthritis, ankylosing spondylitis, tendinitis and bursitis, and acute gout. It is not a corticosteroid. Improvement in patients treated for rheumatoid arthritis has been demonstrated by a reduction in joint swelling, a reduction in pain, a reduction in duration of morning stiffness, a reduction in disease activity as assessed by both the investigator and patient, and by increased mobility as demonstrated by a reduction in walking time.

In patients with osteoarthritis, the therapeutic action of the drug has been shown by a reduction in joint pain or tenderness, an increase in range of motion in knee joints, increased mobility as demonstrated by a reduction in walking time, and improvement in capacity to perform activities of daily living impaired by the disease.

In clinical studies in patients with rheumatoid arthritis and osteoarthritis, the drug has been shown to be comparable to aspirin and indomethacin in controlling the aforementioned measures of disease activity, but the frequency and severity of the milder gastrointestinal adverse effects (nausea, dyspepsia, heartburn) and nervous system adverse effects (tinnitus, dizziness, lightheadedness) were less than in both the aspirin- and indomethacin-treated patients. It is not known whether the drug causes less peptic ulceration than aspirin.

In patients with ankylosing spondylitis, the drug has been shown to decrease night pain, morning stiffness and pain at rest. In double-blind studies the drug was shown to be as effective as aspirin, but with fewer side effects.

In patients with acute gout, a favorable response to the drug was shown by significant clearing of inflammatory changes (e.g., decrease in swelling, heat) within 24–48 hours, as well as by relief of pain and tenderness.

The drug may be used safely in combination with gold salts and/or corticosteroids; however, in controlled clinical trials, when added to the regimen of patients receiving corticosteroids it did not appear to cause greater improvement over that seen with corticosteroids alone. Whether the drug could be used in conjunction with partially effective doses of corticosteroid for a "steroid-sparing" effect has not been adequately studied. When added to the regimen of patients receiving gold salts the drug did result in greater improvement. Its use in combination with salicylates is not recommended because data are inadequate to demonstrate that the drug produces greater improvement over that achieved with aspirin alone. Further, there is some evidence that aspirin increases the rate of excretion of the drug.

Generally, improvement due to the drug has not been found to be dependent on age, sex, severity or duration of disease.

The drug was studied in patients with mild to moderate pain, and pain relief was obtained within 1 hour. It is not a narcotic and is not a CNS-acting drug. Controlled double-blind studies have demonstrated the analgesic properties of the drug in, for example, post-operative, post-partum, orthopedic and uterine contraction pain and dysmenorrhea. In dysmenorrheic patients, the drug reduces the level of prostaglandins in the uterus, which correlates with a reduction in the frequency and severity of uterine contractions. Analgesic action has been shown by such measures as a reduction of pain intensity scores, increase in pain relief scores, decrease in numbers of patients requiring additional analgesic medication, and delay in time for required remedication. The analgesic effect has been found to last for up to 7 hours.

In ^{51}Cr blood loss and gastroscopy studies with normal volunteers, daily administration of 1000 mg of the drug has been demonstrated to cause statistically significantly less gastric bleeding and erosion than 3250 mg of aspirin.

Indications and Usage: NAPROSYN (naproxen) is indicated for the treatment of rheumatoid arthritis, osteoarthritis, ankylosing spondylitis, tendinitis and bursitis, and acute gout.

It is also indicated in the relief of mild to moderate pain and for the treatment of primary dysmenorrhea.

Contraindications: The drug is contraindicated in patients who have had allergic reactions to NAPROSYN® (naproxen) or to ANAPROX® (naproxen sodium). It is also contraindicated in patients in whom aspirin or other nonsteroidal anti-inflammatory/analgesic drugs induce the syndrome of asthma, rhinitis, and nasal polyps. Both types of reactions have the potential of being fatal.

Warnings: Gastrointestinal bleeding, sometimes severe, and occasionally fatal, has been reported in patients receiving the drug. Among 960 patients treated for rheumatoid arthritis or osteoarthritis during the course of clinical trials in the United States (260 treated for more than two years), 16 cases of peptic ulceration were reported. More than half were on concomitant corticosteroid and/or salicylate therapy and about a third had a prior history of peptic ulcer. Gastrointestinal bleeding, including nine potentially serious cases, was also reported in this population. These were not always preceded by premonitory gastrointestinal symptoms. Although most of the patients with serious bleeding were receiving concomitant therapy and had a history of peptic ulcer disease, it should be kept in mind that the drug also has the potential for causing gastrointestinal bleeding on its own. Therefore, it should not be given to patients with active peptic ulcer unless the potential benefit outweighs the potential risk. In such patients, and in other patients with a history of gastrointestinal disease, it should be given under close supervision.

Precautions:
General:
NAPROSYN (NAPROXEN) SHOULD NOT BE USED CONCOMITANTLY WITH THE RELATED DRUG *ANAPROX* (NAPROXEN SODIUM) SINCE THEY BOTH CIRCULATE IN PLASMA AS THE NAPROXEN ANION.

Anaphylactoid reactions to NAPROSYN or ANAPROX, whether of the true allergic type or the pharmacologic idiosyncratic (e.g., aspirin syndrome) type, usually but not always occur in patients with a known history of such reactions. Therefore, careful questioning of patients for such things as asthma, nasal polyps, urticaria, and hypotension associated with nonsteroidal anti-inflammatory drugs before starting therapy is important. In addition, if such symptoms occur during therapy, treatment should be discontinued.

In chronic studies in laboratory animals, the drug has caused nephritis. Glomerular nephritis, interstitial nephritis and nephrotic syndrome have been reported in humans. Naproxen should therefore be used with great caution in patients with significantly impaired renal function and the monitoring of serum creatinine and/or creatinine clearance is advised in these patients. Caution should be used if the drug is given to patients with creatinine clearance less than 20 ml/minute because accumulation of naproxen metabolites has been seen in such patients.

Certain patients, specifically those where renal blood flow is compromised, such as in extracellular volume depletion, cirrhosis of the liver, sodium restriction, congestive heart failure, and pre-existing renal disease, should have renal function assessed before and during therapy with this drug. Some elderly in whom impaired renal function may be expected could also fall within this category. A reduction in daily dosage should be considered to avoid the possibility of excessive drug accumulation in these patients.

Chronic alcoholic liver disease and probably other forms of cirrhosis reduce the total plasma concentration of naproxen, but the plasma concentration of unbound naproxen is increased. Caution is advised when high doses are required and some adjustment of dosage may be required in these patients.

One study indicates that although total plasma concentration of naproxen is unchanged, the unbound plasma fraction of naproxen is increased in the elderly. Caution is advised when high doses are required and some adjustment of dosage may be required in elderly patients.

As with other nonsteroidal anti-inflammatory drugs borderline elevations of one or more liver tests may occur in up to 15% of patients. These abnormalities may progress, may remain essentially unchanged, or may be transient with continued therapy. The SGPT (ALT) test is probably the most sensitive indicator of liver dysfunction. Meaningful (3 times the upper limit of normal) elevations of SGPT and SGOT (AST) occurred in controlled clinical trials in less than 1% of patients. A patient with symptoms and/or signs suggesting liver dysfunction, or in whom an abnormal liver test has occurred, should be evaluated for evidence of the development of more severe hepatic reaction while on therapy with this drug. Severe hepatic reactions, including jaundice and cases of fatal hepatitis, have been reported with this drug as with other nonsteroidal anti-inflammatory drugs. Although such reactions are rare, if abnormal liver tests persist or worsen, if clinical signs and symptoms consistent with liver disease develop, or if systemic manifestations occur (e.g. eosinophilia, rash, etc.), this drug should be discontinued.

If steroid dosage is reduced or eliminated during therapy, the steroid dosage should be reduced slowly and the patients must be observed closely for any evidence of adverse effects, including adrenal insufficiency and exacerbation of symptoms of arthritis.

Patients with initial hemoglobin values of 10 grams or less who are to receive long-term therapy should have hemoglobin values determined frequently.

Peripheral edema has been observed in some patients. For this reason, the drug should be used with caution in patients with fluid retention, hypertension or heart failure.

The antipyretic and anti-inflammatory activities of the drug may reduce fever and inflammation, thus diminishing their utility as diagnostic signs in detecting complications of presumed non-infectious, non-inflammatory painful conditions.

Because of adverse eye findings in animal studies with drugs of this class it is recommended that ophthalmic studies be carried out within a reasonable period of time after starting therapy and at periodic intervals thereafter if the drug is to be used for an extended period of time.

Information for Patients:
Caution should be exercised by patients whose activities require alertness if they experience drowsiness, dizziness, vertigo or depression during therapy with the drug.

Drug Interactions:
In vitro studies have shown that naproxen anion, because of its affinity for protein, may displace from their binding sites other drugs which are also albumin-bound. Theoretically, the naproxen anion itself could likewise be displaced. Short-term controlled studies failed to show that taking the drug significantly affects prothrombin times when administered to individuals on coumarin-type anticoagulants. Caution is advised nonetheless, since interactions have been seen with other nonsteroidal agents of this class. Similarly, patients receiving the drug and a hydantoin, sulfonamide or sulfonylurea should be observed for signs of toxicity to these drugs.

The natriuretic effect of furosemide has been reported to be inhibited by some drugs of this class. Inhibition of renal lithium clearance leading to increases in plasma lithium concentrations has also been reported.

This and other nonsteroidal anti-inflammatory drugs can reduce the antihypertensive effect of propranolol and other beta-blockers.

Probenecid given concurrently increases naproxen anion plasma levels and extends its plasma half-life significantly.

Caution should be used if this drug is administered concomitantly with methotrexate. Naproxen and other nonsteroidal anti-inflammatory drugs have been reported to reduce the tubular secretion of methotrexate in an animal model, possibly enhancing the toxicity of that drug.

Drug/Laboratory Test Interactions:
The drug may decrease platelet aggregation and prolong bleeding time. This effect should be kept in mind when bleeding times are determined.

The administration of the drug may result in increased urinary values for 17-ketogenic steroids because of an interaction between the drug and/or its metabolites with m-dinitrobenzene used in this assay. Although 17-hydroxy-corticosteroid measurements (Porter-Silber test) do not appear to be artifactually altered, it is suggested that therapy with the drug be temporarily discontinued 72 hours before adrenal function tests are performed. The drug may interfere with some urinary assays of 5-hydroxy indoleacetic acid (5HIAA).

Carcinogenesis:
A two-year study was performed in rats to evaluate the carcinogenic potential of the drug. No evidence of carcinogenicity was found.

Pregnancy:
Teratogenic Effects: Pregnancy Category B. Reproduction studies have been performed in rats, rabbits and mice at doses up to six times the human dose and have revealed no evidence of impaired fertility or harm to the fetus due to the drug. There are, however, no adequate and well-controlled studies in pregnant women. Because animal reproduction studies are not always predictive of human response, the drug should not be used during pregnancy unless clearly needed. Because of the known effect of drugs of this class on the human fetal cardiovascular system (closure of

Continued on next page

Syntex—Cont.

ductus arteriosus), use during late pregnancy should be avoided.

Non-teratogenic Effects: As with other drugs known to inhibit prostaglandin synthesis, an increased incidence of dystocia and delayed parturition occurred in rats.

Nursing Mothers:
The naproxen anion has been found in the milk of lactating women at a concentration of approximately 1% of that found in the plasma. Because of the possible adverse effects of prostaglandin-inhibiting drugs on neonates, use in nursing mothers should be avoided.

Pediatric Use:
Pediatric indications and dosage recommendations have not been established for NAPROSYN® (naproxen).

Adverse Reactions: Adverse reactions reported in controlled clinical trials in 960 patients treated for rheumatoid arthritis or osteoarthritis are listed below. In general, these reactions were reported 2 to 10 times more frequently than they were in studies in the 962 patients treated for mild to moderate pain or for dysmenorrhea.

Incidence greater than 1%
Gastrointestinal: The most frequent complaints reported related to the gastrointestinal tract. They were: constipation*, heartburn*, abdominal pain*, nausea*, dyspepsia, diarrhea, stomatitis.
Central Nervous System: Headache*, dizziness*, drowsiness*, lightheadedness, vertigo.
Dermatologic: Itching (pruritus)*, skin eruptions*, ecchymoses*, sweating, purpura.
Special Senses: Tinnitus*, hearing disturbances, visual disturbances.
Cardiovascular: Edema*, dyspnea*, palpitations.
General: Thirst.

* Incidence of reported reactions between 3% and 9%. Those reactions occurring in less than 3% of the patients are unmarked.

Incidence less than 1%
Probable Causal Relationship:
The following adverse reactions were reported less frequently than 1% during controlled clinical trials and through voluntary reports since marketing. The probability of a causal relationship exists between the drug and these adverse reactions:
Gastrointestinal: Abnormal liver function tests, gastrointestinal bleeding, hematemesis, jaundice, melena, peptic ulceration with bleeding and/or perforation, vomiting.
Renal: Glomerular nephritis, hematuria, interstitial nephritis, nephrotic syndrome, renal disease.
Hematologic: Eosinophilia, granulocytopenia, leukopenia, thrombocytopenia.
Central Nervous System: Depression, dream abnormalities, inability to concentrate, insomnia, malaise, myalgia and muscle weakness.
Dermatologic: Alopecia, skin rashes.
Special Senses: Hearing impairment.
Cardiovascular: Congestive heart failure.
General: Anaphylactoid reactions, menstrual disorders, pyrexia (chills and fever).
Causal Relationship Unknown:
Other reactions have been reported in circumstances in which a causal relationship could not be established. However, in these rarely reported events, the possibility cannot be excluded. Therefore these observations are being listed to serve as alerting information to the physicians:
Hematologic: Agranulocytosis, aplastic anemia, hemolytic anemia.
Central Nervous System: Cognitive dysfunction.
Dermatologic: Urticaria.
General: Angioneurotic edema, hyperglycemia, hypoglycemia.
Overdosage: Significant overdosage may be characterized by drowsiness, heartburn, indigestion, nausea or vomiting. No evidence of toxicity or late sequelae have been reported 5 to 15 months after ingestion for three to seven days of doses up to 3,000 mg of naproxen. One patient ingested a single dose of 25 g of naproxen and experienced mild nausea and indigestion. It is not known what dose of the drug would be life threatening. The oral LD_{50} of the drug is 543 mg/kg in rats, 1234 mg/kg in mice, 4110 mg/kg in hamsters and greater than 1000 mg/kg in dogs.

Should a patient ingest a large number of tablets, accidentally or purposefully, the stomach may be emptied and usual supportive measures employed. Animal studies suggest that the prompt administration of 5 grams of activated charcoal would tend to reduce markedly the absorption of the drug. It is not known if the drug is dialyzable.

Dosage and Administration:
For Rheumatoid Arthritis, Osteoarthritis, and Ankylosing Spondylitis:
The recommended starting dose in adults is one 250 mg tablet or one 375 mg tablet twice daily (morning and evening). During long-term administration, the dose may be adjusted up or down depending on the clinical response of the patient. A lower daily dose may suffice for long-term administration. Daily doses higher than 1000 mg in these indications have not been studied. The morning and evening doses do not have to be equal in size and the administration of the drug more frequently than twice daily is not necessary. Symptomatic improvement in arthritis usually begins within two weeks. However, if improvement is not seen within this period, a trial for an additional two weeks should be considered.

For Acute Gout:
The recommended starting dose is 750 mg, followed by 250 mg every eight hours until the attack has subsided.

For Mild to Moderate Pain, Primary Dysmenorrhea and Acute Tendinitis and Bursitis:
The recommended starting dose is 500 mg, followed by 250 mg every 6 to 8 hours, as required. The total daily dose should not exceed 1,250 mg.

How Supplied: NAPROSYN (naproxen) is available in scored tablets of 250 mg (yellow) in bottles of 100 tablets (NDC 18393-272-42) and 500 tablets (NDC 18393-272-62) or in cartons of 100 individually blister packed tablets (NDC 18393-272-53) and in 375 mg (peach) tablets in bottles of 100 tablets (NDC 18393-273-42) and 500 tablets (NDC 18393-273-62) or in cartons of 100 individually blister packed tablets (NDC 18393-273-53). The 500 mg (yellow) tablets are available in bottles of 100 tablets (NDC 18393-277-42) and 500 tablets (NDC 18393-277-62). Store at room temperature in well-closed containers; dispense in light-resistant containers.

CAUTION: Federal law prohibits dispensing without prescription.

Revised May 1984
Shown in Product Identification Section, page 440

NASALIDE® ℞
[na'ză-lide]
(flunisolide)
Nasal Solution
0.025%
For Nasal Use Only

A product of Syntex Laboratories, Inc.

Description: NASALIDE® (flunisolide) nasal solution is intended for administration as a spray to the nasal mucosa. Flunisolide, the active component of NASALIDE nasal solution, is an anti-inflammatory steroid with the chemical name: 6α-fluoro-11β, 16α, 17,21-tetrahydroxypregna-1,4-diene-3,20-dione cyclic 16,17-acetal with acetone (USAN).

Flunisolide is a white to creamy white crystalline powder with a molecular weight of 434.49. It is soluble in acetone, sparingly soluble in chloroform, slightly soluble in methanol, and practically insoluble in water. It has a melting point of about 245°C.

Each 25 ml spray bottle contains flunisolide 6.25 mg (0.25 mg/ml) in a solution of propylene glycol, polyethylene glycol 3350, citric acid, sodium citrate, butylated hydroxyanisole, edetate disodium, benzalkonium chloride, and purified water, with NaOH and/or HCl added to adjust the pH to approximately 5.3. It contains no fluorocarbons.

After priming the delivery system for NASALIDE, each actuation of the unit delivers a metered droplet spray containing approximately 25 mcg of flunisolide. The size of the droplets produced by the unit is in excess of 8 microns to facilitate deposition on the nasal mucosa. The contents of one nasal spray bottle deliver at least 200 sprays.

Clinical Pharmacology: NASALIDE® (flunisolide) has demonstrated potent glucocorticoid and weak mineralocorticoid activity in classical animal test systems. As a glucocorticoid it is several hundred times more potent that the cortisol standard. Clinical studies with flunisolide have shown therapeutic activity on nasal mucous membranes with minimal evidence of systemic activity at the recommended doses.

Following administration of flunisolide to man, approximately half of the administered dose is recovered in the urine and half in the stool; 65–70% of the dose recovered in urine is the primary metabolite, which has undergone loss of the 6α fluorine and addition of a 6β hydroxy group. Flunisolide is well absorbed but is rapidly converted by the liver to the much less active primary metabolite and to glucuronate and/or sulfate conjugates. Because of first-pass liver metabolism, only 20% of the flunisolide reaches the systemic circulation when it is given orally whereas 50% of the flunisolide administered intranasally reaches the systemic circulation unmetabolized. The plasma half-life of flunisolide is 1–2 hours.

The effects of flunisolide on hypothalamic-pituitary-adrenal (HPA) axis function have been studied in adult volunteers. NASALIDE was administered intranasally as a spray in total doses over 7 times the recommended dose (2200 mcg, equivalent to 88 sprays/day) in 2 subjects for 4 days, about 3 times the recommended dose (800 mcg, equivalent to 32 sprays/day) in 4 subjects for 4 days, and over twice the recommended dose (700 mcg, equivalent to 28 sprays/day) in 6 subjects for 10 days. Early morning plasma cortisol concentrations and 24-hour urinary 17-ketogenic steroids were measured daily. There was evidence of decreased endogenous cortisol production at all three doses.

In controlled studies, NASALIDE was found to be effective in reducing symptoms of stuffy nose, runny nose and sneezing in most patients. These controlled clinical studies have been conducted in 488 adult patients at doses ranging from 8 to 16 sprays (200–400 mcg) per day and 127 children at doses ranging from 6 to 8 sprays (150–200 mcg) per day for periods as long as 3 months. In 170 patients who had cortisol levels evaluated at baseline and after 3 months or more of flunisolide treatment, there was no unequivocal flunisolide-related depression of plasma cortisol levels.

The mechanisms responsible for the anti-inflammatory action of corticosteroids and for the activity of the aerosolized drug on the nasal mucosa are unknown.

Indications: NASALIDE® (flunisolide) is indicated for the relief of the symptoms of seasonal or perennial rhinitis when effectiveness of or tolerance to conventional treatment is unsatisfactory. Clinical studies have shown that improvement is usually apparent within a few days after starting NASALIDE. However, symptomatic relief may not occur in some patients for as long as two weeks. Although systemic effects are minimal at recommended doses, NASALIDE should not be continued beyond 3 weeks in the absence of significant symptomatic improvement.

NASALIDE should not be used in the presence of untreated localized infection involving nasal mucosa.

Contraindications: Hypersensitivity to any of the ingredients.

Warnings: The replacement of a systemic corticosteroid with a topical corticoid can be accompanied by signs of adrenal insufficiency, and in addition some patients may experience symptoms of withdrawal, e.g., joint and/or muscular pain, lassitude and depression. Patients previously treated for prolonged periods with systemic corticosteroids and transferred to NASALIDE® (flunisolide) should be carefully monitored to avoid acute adrenal insufficiency in response to stress.

When transferred to NASALIDE, careful attention must be given to patients previously treated for prolonged periods with systemic corticosteroids. This is particularly important in those patients who have associated asthma or other clinical conditions, where too rapid a decrease in systemic corticosteroids may cause a severe exacerbation of their symptoms.

The use of NASALIDE with alternate-day prednisone systemic treatment could increase the likelihood of HPA suppression compared to a therapeutic dose of either one alone. Therefore, NASALIDE treatment should be used with caution in patients already on alternate-day prednisone regimens for any disease.

Precautions:

General: In clinical studies with flunisolide administered intranasally, the development of localized infections of the nose and pharynx with *Candida albicans* has occurred only rarely. When such an infection develops it may require treatment with appropriate local therapy or discontinuance of treatment with NASALIDE® (flunisolide).

Flunisolide is absorbed into the circulation. Use of excessive doses of NASALIDE may suppress hypothalamic-pituitary-adrenal function.

Flunisolide should be used with caution, if at all, in patients with active or quiescent tuberculosis infections of the respiratory tract or in untreated fungal, bacterial or systemic viral infections or ocular herpes simplex.

Because of the inhibitory effect of corticosteroids on wound healing, in patients who have experienced recent nasal septal ulcers, recurrent epistaxis, nasal surgery or trauma, a nasal corticosteroid should be used with caution until healing has occurred.

Although systemic effects have been minimal with recommended doses, this potential increases with excessive dosages. Therefore, larger than recommended doses should be avoided.

Information for Patients: Patients should use NASALIDE at regular intervals since its effectiveness depends on its regular use. The patient should take the medication as directed. It is not acutely effective and the prescribed dosage should not be increased. Instead, nasal vasoconstrictors or oral antihistamines may be needed until the effects of NASALIDE are fully manifested. One to two weeks may pass before full relief is obtained. The patient should contact the physician if symptoms do not improve, or if the condition worsens, or if sneezing or nasal irritation occurs.

For the proper use of this unit and to attain maximum improvement, the patient should read and follow the accompanying Patient Instructions carefully.

Carcinogenesis: A 22-month study was conducted in Swiss derived mice to evaluate the carcinogenic potential of the drug. While no evidence of carcinogenicity was found, there was a slight increase in the incidence of pulmonary adenomas which was well within the range of spontaneous adenomas previously reported in the literature for untreated or control Swiss derived mice. An additional study is being conducted in a species with a lower incidence of spontaneous pulmonary tumors.

Impairment of fertility: Female rats receiving high doses of flunisolide (200 mcg/kg/day) showed some evidence of impaired fertility. Reproductive performance in the low (8 mcg/kg/day) and mid-dose (40 mcg/kg/day) groups was comparable to controls.

Pregnancy: Teratogenic effects: Pregnancy Category C. As with other corticosteroids, flunisolide has been shown to be teratogenic in rabbits and rats at doses of 40 and 200 mcg/kg/day respectively. It was also fetotoxic in these animal reproductive studies. There are no adequate and well-controlled studies in pregnant women. Flunisolide should be used during pregnancy only if the potential benefit justifies the potential risk to the fetus.

Nursing Mothers: It is not known whether this drug is excreted in human milk. Because other corticosteroids are excreted in human milk, caution should be exercised when flunisolide is administered to nursing women.

Adverse Reactions: Adverse reactions reported in controlled clinical trials and long-term open studies in 595 patients treated with NASALIDE are described below. Of these patients, 409 were treated for 3 months or longer, 323 for 6 months or longer, 259 for 1 year or longer, and 91 for 2 years or longer.

In general, side effects elicited in the clinical studies have been primarily associated with the nasal mucous membranes. The most frequent complaints were those of mild transient nasal burning and stinging, which were reported in approximately 45% of the patients treated with NASALIDE in placebo-controlled and long-term studies. These complaints do not usually interfere with treatment; in only 3% of patients was it necessary to decrease dosage or stop treatment because of these symptoms. Approximately the same incidence of mild transient nasal burning and stinging was reported in patients on placebo as was reported in patients treated with NASALIDE in controlled studies, implying that these complaints may be related to the vehicle or the delivery system. The incidence of complaints of nasal burning and stinging decreased with increasing duration of treatment.

Other side effects reported at a frequency of 5% or less were: nasal congestion, sneezing, epistaxis and/or bloody mucus, nasal irritation, watery eyes, sore throat, nausea and/or vomiting, headaches and loss of sense of smell and taste. In rare instances, nasal septal perforations were observed during the studies but a causal relationship with NASALIDE was not established.

Systemic corticosteroid side effects were not reported during the controlled clinical trials. If recommended doses are exceeded, or if individuals are particularly sensitive, symptoms of hypercorticism, i.e., Cushing's syndrome, could occur.

Overdosage: I.V. flunisolide in animals at doses up to 4 mg/kg showed no effect. One spray bottle contains 6.25 mg of NASALIDE; therefore acute overdosage is unlikely.

Dosage and Administration: The therapeutic effects of corticosteroids, unlike those of decongestants, are not immediate. This should be explained to the patient in advance in order to ensure cooperation and continuation of treatment with the prescribed dosage regimen. Full therapeutic benefit requires regular use, and is usually evident within a few days. However, a longer period of therapy may be required for some patients to achieve maximum benefit (up to 3 weeks). If no improvement is evident by that time, NASALIDE® (flunisolide) should not be continued.

Patients with blocked nasal passages should be encouraged to use a decongestant just before NASALIDE administration to ensure adequate penetration of the spray. Patients should also be advised to clear their nasal passages of secretions prior to use.

Adults: The recommended starting dose of NASALIDE is 2 sprays (50 mcg) in each nostril 2 times a day (total dose 200 mcg/day). If needed, this dose may be increased to 2 sprays in each nostril 3 times a day (total dose 300 mcg/day).

Children 6 to 14 years: The recommended starting dose of NASALIDE is one spray (25 mcg) in each nostril 3 times a day or two sprays (50 mcg) in each nostril 2 times a day (total dose 150-200 mcg/day). NASALIDE is not recommended for use in children less than 6 years of age as safety and efficacy studies, including possible adverse effects on growth, have not been conducted.

Maximum total daily doses should not exceed 8 sprays in each nostril for adults (total dose 400 mcg/day) and 4 sprays in each nostril for children under 14 years of age (total dose 200 mcg/day). Since there is no evidence that exceeding the maximum recommended dosage is more effective and increased systemic absorption would occur, higher doses should be avoided.

After the desired clinical effect is obtained, the maintenance dose should be reduced to the smallest amount necessary to control the symptoms. Approximately 15% of patients with perennial rhinitis may be maintained on as little as 1 spray in each nostril per day.

How Supplied: Each 25 ml NASALIDE® (flunisolide) nasal solution spray bottle (NDC 0033-2906-40) contains 6.25 mg (0.25 mg/ml) of flunisolide and is supplied with a nasal pump unit with dust cover and a patient leaflet of instructions.

Revised 4/83

NORINYL® 1+35 Tablets ℞
(norethindrone and ethinyl estradiol tablets)
NORINYL® 1+50 Tablets ℞
(norethindrone and mestranol tablets)
NORINYL® 1+80 Tablets ℞
(norethindrone and mestranol tablets)
NORINYL® 2 mg. Tablets ℞
(norethindrone and mestranol tablets)

Refer to entry under BREVICON® Tablets (norethindrone and ethinyl estradiol tablets).

NOR—Q.D.® ℞
(norethindrone)
Tablets 0.35 mg.

Refer to entry under BREVICON® Tablets (norethindrone and ethinyl estradiol).

SYNACORT® ℞
(hydrocortisone)
Cream 1%
Cream 2.5%
SYNALAR® ℞
(fluocinolone acetonide)
Cream 0.025%
Cream 0.01%
Ointment 0.025%
Topical Solution 0.01%
SYNALAR-HP® ℞
(fluocinolone acetonide)
Cream 0.2%
SYNEMOL® ℞
(fluocinolone acetonide)
Cream 0.025%

Refer to entry under LIDEX® (fluocinonide) Cream 0.05%.

TOPIC® OTC
Benzyl alcohol gel
Relieves itching

A product of Syntex Laboratories, Inc.

(See PDR For Nonprescription Drugs)

Thompson Medical Company, Inc.
919 THIRD AVENUE
NEW YORK, NY 10022

MAXIMUM STRENGTH
APPEDRINE® OTC
[ăpp-ĕ-drine]
Anorectic for Weight Control

Each tablet contains:
phenylpropanolamine HCl	25 mg
caffeine	100 mg

Each three tablets contain:
Vitamin A	5000 IU
Vitamin D	400 IU
Vitamin E	30 IU
Vitamin C (Ascorbic Acid)	60 mg
Folic Acid	0.4 mg
Vitamin B₁ (Thiamine HCl)	1.5 mg
Vitamin B₂ (Riboflavin)	1.7 mg
Niacinamide	20 mg
Vitamin B₆ (Pyridoxine HCl)	2 mg
Vitamin B₁₂ (Cyanocobalamin)	6 mcg
d-Calcium Pantothenate	10 mg
Iodine (as Potassium Iodide)	150 mcg
Iron (as Ferrous Sulfate)	12 mg

Continued on next page

Thompson—Cont.

Copper (as Cupric Sulfate) 2 mg
Zinc (as Zinc Oxide) 15 mg

Description: Each tablet contains phenylpropanolamine HCl, an anorexiant and one third of the recommended daily adult requirement of major vitamins.

Indications: Maximum Strength APPEDRINE is indicated as adjunctive therapy in a regimen of weight reduction and control based on caloric restriction in the management of simple exogenous obesity.

Caution: READ BEFORE USING. For adult use only. Do not give this product to children under 12 years of age. Persons between the age of 12 and 18 or over 60 are advised to consult their physician or pharmacist before using this or any drug. As with this or any drug, unwanted symptoms such as headaches, nervousness, rapid pulse, dizziness, sleeplessness, palpitations or other symptoms have occasionally been reported. Should any occur, discontinue use and consult your physician.

Warning: DO NOT EXCEED RECOMMENDED DOSAGE. Taking more of this or any other drug than is recommended can cause untoward health complications. It is sensible to check your blood pressure regularly. Do not use if you have high blood pressure, diabetes, heart, thyroid, kidney, or other disease or are being treated for high blood pressure or depression except under the advice and supervision of a physician. As with any drug if you are pregnant or nursing a baby, seek the advice of a health professional before using this product. When you have attained your desired weight loss or are able to control your appetite naturally, use Appedrine only as needed.

Drug Interaction Precaution: Do not take if you are presently taking another medication containing phenylpropanolamine, or any type of nasal decongestant, or a prescription antihypertensive or antidepressant drug containing a monoamine oxidase inhibitor, or any other type of prescription medication except under the advice and supervision of a physician.
KEEP THIS AND ALL MEDICATION OUT OF THE REACH OF CHILDREN. In case of accidental overdose seek professional assistance or contact a poison control center immediately.

Adverse Reactions: Side effects are rare when taken as directed. Nausea or nasal dryness may occasionally occur.

Dosage and Administration: Adults: One tablet 30–60 minutes before each meal three times a day with one or two full glasses of water.

How Supplied: Maximum Strength APPEDRINE® packages of 30 and 60 tablets packaged with 1200 Calorie Extra Strength Appedrine Diet Plan.

Reference: Griboff, Solomon, I., M.D., F.A.C.P. et al., A Double-Blind Clinical Evaluation of a Phenylpropanolamine-Caffeine Combination and a Placebo in the Treatment of Exogenous Obesity, Current Therapeutic Research 17, 6:535, (1975) June.
Silverman, H.I., D.Sc., Kreger, B.E., M.D., Lewis, G.P., M.D., et. al., Lack of Side Effects from Orally Administered Phenylpropanolamine and Phenylpropanolamine with Caffeine: A Controlled Three-Phase Study, Current Therapeutic Research 28, 2:185 (1980) August.
Altschuler, S., Conte, A., Sebok, M., Marlin, R., Winick, C., Three Controlled Trials of Weight Loss with Phenylpropanolamine, International Journal of Obesity (1982) 6, 549–556.

ASPERCREME™
[ăs-per-crēme]
External Analgesic Rub

Description: 10% Trolamine Salicylate in a lotion and odorless creme. ASPERCREME is a clinically proven rub that relieves pain effectively without stomach upset aspirin may cause.

Actions: External analgesic with rapid penetration and absorption.

Indications: An effective salicylate analgesic for temporary relief from minor pains of arthritis, rheumatism and muscular aches.

Contraindications: Do not use in patients allergic to salicylates.

Warnings: Use only as directed. If redness is present or condition worsens, or if pain persists for more than 7 days, discontinue use and consult a physician. Do not use on children under 10 years of age. Do not apply if skin is irritated or if irritation develops. As with any drug, if you are pregnant or nursing a baby, seek the advice of a health professional before using this product. For external use only. Avoid contact with eyes. Keep this and all medicines out of the reach of children.

Precautions: Occasionally where this product has been used extensively, moderate peeling of the skin may occur. This is a normal reaction to salicylates on the skin, and should not warrant discontinuing use of the product.

Dosage and Administration: Apply generously. Massage into painful area until thoroughly absorbed into skin, 3 or 4 times daily, especially before retiring. Relief lasts for hours.

How Supplied: Lotion; 6 oz. plastic bottle. Cream; 3 oz., 5 oz and 1¼ oz. plastic tubes.

References: Golden, Emanuel L., M.D., A Double-Blind Comparison of Orally Ingested Aspirin and a Topically Appled Salicylate Cream in the Relief of Rheumatic Pain, Current Therapeutic Research, 24, 5:524, 1978 (Sept.).
Rabinowitz, J. L., M.D., "Comparative Tissue Absorption of Oral 14C Aspirin and Topical Triethanolamine 14C-Salicylate in Human and Canine Knee Joints," Journal of Clinical Pharmacology 1982, 22:42–48.

CONTROL Capsules   OTC
Maximum Strength
Prolonged action anorectic for weight control containing
phenylpropanolamine HCl 75 mg

Description: Phenylpropanolamine HCl is a sympathomimetic with anorectic action.

Indication: CONTROL is indicated as adjunctive therapy in a regimen of weight reduction based on caloric restriction in the management and control of simple exogenous obesity.

Caution: READ BEFORE USING. For adult use only. Do not give this product to children under 12 years of age. Persons between the age of 12 and 18 or over 60 are advised to consult their physician or pharmacist before using this or any drug. As with this or any drug, unwanted symptoms such as headaches, nervousness, rapid pulse, dizziness, sleeplessness, palpitations or other symptoms have occasionally been reported. Should any occur, discontinue use and consult your physician.

Warning: DO NOT EXCEED RECOMMENDED DOSAGE. Taking more of this or any other drug than is recommended can cause untoward health complications. It is sensible to check your blood pressure regularly. Do not use if you have high blood pressure, diabetes, heart, thyroid, kidney, or other disease or are being treated for high blood pressure or depression except under the advice and supervision of a physician. As with any drug if you are pregnant or nursing a baby, seek the advice of a health professional before using this product. When you have attained your desired weight loss or are able to control your appetite naturally, use Control only as needed.

Drug Interaction Precaution: Do not take if you are presently taking another medication containing phenylpropanolamine, or any type of nasal decongestant, or a prescription antihypertensive or antidepressant drug containing a monoamine oxidase inhibitor, or any other type of prescription medication except under the advice and supervision of a physician.
KEEP THIS AND ALL MEDICATION OUT OF THE REACH OF CHILDREN. In case of accidental overdose seek professional assistance or contact a poison control center immediately.

Adverse Reactions: Side effects are rare when taken as directed. Nausea or nasal dryness may occasionally occur.

Dosage and Administration: One capsule with a full glass of water once a day at mid-morning (10:00 A.M.).

How Supplied: CONTROL Capsules—Packages of 14, 28 and 56 capsules, packaged with 1200 Calorie CONTROL Diet Plan.

Reference: Griboff, Solomon, I., M.D., F.A.C.P. et al., A Double-Blind Clinical Evaluation of a Phenylpropanolamine-Caffeine Combination and a Placebo in the Treatment of Exogenous Obesity, Current Therapeutic Research 17, 6:535, (1975) June.
Silverman, H.I., D.Sc., Kreger, B.E., M.D., Lewis, G.P., M.D., et. al., Lack of Side Effects from Orally Administered Phenylpropanolamine and Phenylpropanolamine with Caffeine: A Controlled Three-Phase Study, Current Therapeutic Research 28, 2:185 (1980) August.
Altschuler, S., Conte, A., Sebok, M., Marlin, R., Winick, C., Three Controlled Trials of Weight Loss with Phenylpropanolamine, International Journal of Obesity (1982), 6, 549–556.

DEXATRIM® Capsules   OTC
[dĕx-a-trĭm]
Prolonged action anorectic for weight control contains
phenylpropanolamine HCl 50 mg

DEXATRIM® Extra Strength   OTC Capsules
phenylpropanolamine HCl 75 mg
Vitamin C 180 mg

Caffeine-Free DEXATRIM®   OTC
Extra Strength Capsules
phenylpropanolamine HCl 75 mg

DEXATRIM® • 15 Caffeine Free   OTC
phenylpropanolamine 75 mg

DEXATRIM® • 15   OTC
phenylpropanolamine HCl 75 mg
Vitamin C 180 mg

DEXATRIM® Extra Strength   OTC
Plus Vitamins
phenylpropanolamine HCl 75 mg
plus multi-vitamins

Description: Phenylpropanolamine hydrochloride is a sympathomimetic with anorectic action.

Indication: DEXATRIM, Extra Strength DEXATRIM, Caffeine-Free DEXATRIM Extra Strength, DEXATRIM • 15 and DEXATRIM Extra Strength Plus Vitamins are indicated as adjunctive therapy in a regimen of weight reduction based on caloric restriction in the management and control of simple exogenous obesity.
In a six week double-blind parallel study comparing phenylpropanolamine HCl to diethylpropion similar weight losses occurred in 62 clinically obese patients. Ninety-six percent of the patients receiving phenylpropanolamine HCl and 87% of the patients receiving diethylpropion lost weight.*

Caution: READ BEFORE USING. For adult use only. Do not give this product to children under 12 years of age. Persons between the age of 12 and 18 or over 60 are advised to consult their physician or pharmacist before using this or any drug. As with this or any drug, unwanted symptoms such as headaches, nervousness, rapid pulse, dizziness, sleeplessness, palpitations or other symptoms have occasionally been reported. Should any occur, discontinue use and consult your physician.

Warning: DO NOT EXCEED RECOMMENDED DOSAGE. Taking more of this or any other drug than is recommended can cause untoward health complications. It is sensible to check your blood pressure regularly. Do not use if you have high blood pressure, diabetes, heart, thyroid, kidney, or other disease or are being treated for high blood pressure or depression except under the advice and supervision of a physician. As with any drug if you are pregnant or nursing a baby, seek the advice of a health professional before using this product. When you have attained your desired weight loss or are able to control your appetite naturally, use Dexatrim only as needed.

Drug Interaction Precaution: Do not take if you are presently taking another medication containing phenylpropanolamine, or any type of nasal

decongestant, or a prescription antihypertensive or antidepressant drug containing a monoamine oxidase inhibitor, or any other type of prescription medication except under the advice and supervision of a physician.
KEEP THIS AND ALL MEDICATION OUT OF THE REACH OF CHILDREN. In case of accidental overdose seek professional assistance or contact a poison control center immediately.
Adverse Reactions: Side effects are rare when taken as directed. Nausea or nasal dryness may occasionally occur.
Dosage and Administration:
DEXATRIM® Capsules: One capsule with a full glass of water mid-morning (10:00 AM)
Extra Strength DEXATRIM® Capsules: One capsule with a full glass of water mid-morning (10:00 AM)
DEXATRIM® ● 15 Capsules: One capsule with a full glass of water in morning (9:00 AM)
How Supplied:
DEXATRIM® Capsules: Packages of 28 and 56 with 1200 calorie DEXATRIM Diet Plan.
Extra Strength DEXATRIM® Capsules: Packages of 10, 20, and 40 with 1200 calorie DEXATRIM Diet Plan.
Caffeine-Free DEXATRIM® Extra Strength: Packages of 10, 20, and 40 capsules with 1200 calorie DEXATRIM Diet Plan.
DEXATRIM® ● 15 Capsules: Packages of 20, and 40 with 1200 calorie Dexatrim Diet Plan.
DEXATRIM Extra Strength Plus Vitamins: Packages of 16 and 32 capsules with 1200 calorie DEXATRIM Diet Plan.
* Report on file, Professional Services, Thompson Medical Company, Inc. 919 Third Avenue, New York, New York 10022.
Reference: Griboff, Solomon, I., M.D., F.A.C.P. et. al., A Double-Blind Clinical Evaluation of a Phenylpropanolamine-Caffeine Combination and a Placebo in the Treatment of Exogenous Obesity, Current Therapeutic Research 17, 6:535, (1975) June.
Silverman, H.I., D.Sc., Kreger, B.E., M.D., Lewis, G.P., M.D., et. al., Lack of Side Effects from Orally Administered Phenylpropanolamine and Phenylpropanolamine with Caffeine: A Controlled Three-Phase Study, Current Therapeutic Research 28, 2:185 (1980) August.
Altschuler, S., Conte, A., Sebok, M., Marlin, R., Winick, C., Three Controlled Trials of Weight Loss with Phenylpropanolamine, International Journal of Obesity (1982) 6, 549–556.

Maximum Strength   OTC
PROLAMINE™ Capsules
[prō-la-mine]
Continous Action Anorectic for Weight Control

Each capsule contains:
phenylpropanolamine HCl   37½ mg
Description: Each capsule contains phenylpropanolamine hydrochloride an anorexiant.
Indication: Maximum Strength PROLAMINE is indicated as adjunctive therapy in the regimen of weight reduction based on caloric restriction in the management and control of simple exogenous obesity.
In a six week double-blind study of 70 obese patients comparing phenylpropanolamine HCl to a placebo, 35% of the subjects taking phenylpropanolamine HCl experienced a weight loss of 8 pounds or more. Only 9% of the subjects taking placebo lost that amount of weight. Results were statistically significant at the 0.05 probability level.[1]
Caution: READ BEFORE USING. For adult use only. Do not give this product to children under 12 years of age. Persons between the age of 12 and 18 or over 60 are advised to consult their physician or pharmacist before using this or any drug. As with this or any drug, unwanted symptoms such as headaches, nervousness, rapid pulse, dizziness, sleeplessness, palpitations or other symptoms have occasionally been reported. Should any occur, discontinue use and consult your physician.

Warning: DO NOT EXCEED RECOMMENDED DOSAGE. Taking more of this or any other drug than is recommended can cause untoward health complications. It is sensible to check your blood pressure regularly. Do not use if you have high blood pressure, diabetes, heart, thyroid, kidney, or other disease or are being treated for high blood pressure or depression except under the advice and supervision of a physician. As with any drug if you are pregnant or nursing a baby, seek the advice of a health professional before using this product. When you have attained your desired weight loss or are able to control your appetite naturally, use Prolamine only as needed.
Drug Interaction Precaution: Do not take if you are presently taking another medication containing phenylpropanolamine, or any type of nasal decongestant, or a prescription antihypertensive or antidepressant drug containing a monoamine oxidase inhibitor, or any other type of prescription medication except under the advice and supervision of a physician.
KEEP THIS AND ALL MEDICATION OUT OF THE REACH OF CHILDREN. In case of accidental overdose seek professional assistance or contact a poison control center immediately.
Adverse Reactions: Side effects are rare when taken as directed. Nausea or nasal dryness may occasionally occur.
Dosage and Administration: One capsule at 10 A.M. and 1 capsule at 4 P.M.
How Supplied: Maximum Strength PROLAMINE™ Capsules: Packages of 20 and 50 packaged with 1200 Calorie PROLAMINE Diet Plan.
1. Report on file, Professional Services, Thompson Medical Company, Inc. 919 Third Avenue, New York, New York 10022
Reference: Griboff, Solomon, I., M.D., F.A.C.P. et. al., A Double-Blind Clinical Evaluation of a Phenylpropanolamine-Caffeine Combination and a Placebo in the Treatment of Exogenous Obesity, Current Therapeutic Research 17, 6:535, (1975) June.
Silverman, H.I., D.Sc., Kreger, B.E., M.D., Lewis, G.P., M.D., et. al., Lack of Side Effects from Orally Administered Phenylpropanolamine and Phenylpropanolamine with Caffeine: A Controlled Three-Phase Study, Current Therapeutic Research 28, 2:185 (1980) August.
Altschuler, S., Conte, A., Sebok, M., Marlin, R., Winick, C., Three Controlled Trials of Weight loss with Phenylpropanolamine, International Journal of Obesity (1982) 6, 549–556.

Trimen Laboratories, Inc.
Pharmaceutical Division
80 TWENTY-SIXTH STREET
PITTSBURGH, PA 15222

AMACODONE™ TABLETS
Acetaminophen/Hydrocodone

Each tablet contains:
Acetaminophen .... 500 mg
Hydrocodone Bitartrate* .... 5 mg
    *(WARNING: May be habit forming)
How Supplied: Bottles of 100's, capsule shaped, scored white tablet with blue specks embossed with TRIMEN.

AMAPHEN® CAPSULES
(Non-Narcotic Analgesic)

Each Capsule contains:
50 mg .... Butalbital
    (WARNING: May be habit forming)
40 mg .... Caffeine
325 mg .... Acetaminophen.
How Supplied: Bottles of 100's; opaque white and opaque pink capsule, imprinted "TRIMEN".

AMAPHEN® with CODEINE #3
Analgesic

Each Amaphen with Codeine Capsule contains: 50 mg butalbital, U.S.P. (Warning: May be habit forming; 325 mg acetaminophen, U.S.P., and 40 mg caffeine, U.S.P.
In addition, Amaphen with Codeine also contains 30 mg of codeine phosphate, U.S.P. (Warning: May be habit forming).
How Supplied: Bottles of 100's, pink and maroon capsules, imprinted TRIMEN.

DYREXAN™-OD
Brand of Phendimetrazine Tartrate
Slow-Release Capsules 105 mg

How Supplied: Bottles of 100's, clear yellow and opaque brown 105 mg capsules imprinted with TRIMEN.

HYDREX® TABLETS
(Benzthiazide 50 mg.) Diuretic-Antihypertensive

How Supplied: Bottles of 100's, white, scored tablet embossed with logo.

KORIGESIC® TABLETS
Analgesic Decongestant

Each Tablet contains: 4 mg. Chlorpheniramine Maleate, 14 mg. Phenylpropanolamine Hydrochloride, 5 mg. Phenylephrine Hydrochloride, 150 mg. Salicylamide, 200 mg. Acetaminophen, 30 mg. Caffeine.
How Supplied: Bottles of 100's, two-layer, scored blue and white tablet, embossed with logo.

NATACOMP-FA® TABLETS
Multivitamin, Multimineral supplement for pregnant or lactating women

How Supplied: Bottles of 100's pink, oval, film coated tablet.

SORATE®
Isosorbide Dinitrate

How Supplied:
Sorate®-5 Chewable as 5 mg orange, round, scored, chewable tablet, embossed with logo.
Sorate®-10 Chewable as 10 mg, white, round, scored, orange flavored chewable tablets, embossed with logo.

VIOPAN-T™ TABLETS
High Potency Vitamin Mineral Formula

How Supplied: Red, film coated tablet, embossed with TRIMEN.

Tyson and Associates, Inc.
1661 LINCOLN
SANTA MONICA, CA 90404

AMINOLETE   OTC

Description: Free form amino acid supplement. Capsules contain 700 mg of 13 free form amino acids without fillers, binders, preservatives or sugars. Contains 102 mg of Nitrogen per capsule.
Composition: L-Glutamine, L-Lysine, L-Methionine, Glycine, L-Leucine, L-Arginine, L-Phenylalanine, L-Valine, L-Isoleucine, L-Threonine, L-Tryptophan, L-Histidine, L-Tyrosine.
Dosage and Administration: Initially it is recommended 2–4 capsules t.i.d. ¼-½ teaspoon t.i.d.
How Supplied: 700 mg capsules. Bottles of 100 capsules. Bottles of 200 grams of free flowing powder.
Literature: Available upon request.

AMINOMINE   OTC

Description: Free form amino acid supplement. Capsules contain 700 mg of 15 amino acids without fillers, binders, preservatives or sugars. Contains 103 mg Nitrogen per capsule.

Continued on next page

Tyson—Cont.

Composition: L-Glutamine, Glycine, L-Alanine, L-Leucine, L-Lysine, L-Valine, L-Isoleucine, L-Arginine, L-Methionine, L-Histidine, L-Threonine, L-Phenylalanine, Proline, L-Tyrosine, L-Tryptophan.
Dosage and Administration: Initially it is recommended 1-2 capsules b.i.d., ¼-½ teaspoon b.i.d.
How Supplied: Bottles of 100 capsules. Bottles of 200 grams of free flowing powder.
Literature: Available upon request.

AMINOPLEX™ OTC

Description: Free form amino acid supplement for adults and children 4 or more years of age. Capsules contain 740 mg of 19 free form amino acids without fillers, binders, preservatives or sugars. Contains 130 mg Nitrogen per capsule. Formula contains sulfur amino acids and neurotransmitter precursors.
Composition: L-Lysine, L-Tryptophan, L-Arginine, L-Isoleucine, L-Leucine, L-Alanine, L-Threonine, L-Histidine, L-Cystine, L-Methionine, L-Glutamine, L-Tyrosine, L-Aspartic Acid, L-Valine, L-Glutamic Acid, L-Phenylalanine, Glycine, L-Serine, L-Cysteine.
Dosage and Administration: Initially it is recommended 2-4 capsules t.i.d. ¼-½ teaspoon t.i.d.
How Supplied: 740 mg capsules. Bottles of 100, 250 & 500 capsules.
370 mg capsules. Bottles of 100, 250 & 500 capsules.
Bottles of 50 & 350 grams of free flowing powder.
Literature: Available upon request.

AMINOSINE OTC

Description: Free form amino acid supplement. Capsules contain 700 mg of 19 amino acids without fillers, binders, preservatives or sugars. Contains 85.5 mg Nitrogen per capsule. Formula does not contain Arginine.
Composition: L-Lysine, L-Tryptophan, L-Threonine, L-Isoleucine, L-Leucine, L-Alanine, L-Histidine, L-Tyrosine, L-Cystine, L-Glutamine, L-Aspartic Acid, L-Valine, L-Methionine, L-Citrulline, L-Glutamic Acid, L-Ornithine, Glycine, L-Serine, L-Phenylalanine.
Dosage and Administration: Initially it is recommended 2-4 capsules t.i.d. ¼-½ teaspoon t.i.d.
How Supplied: 700 mg capsules. Bottles of 100 capsules. Bottles of 200 grams of free flowing powder.
Literature: Available upon request.

AMINOSTASIS™ OTC

Description: Free form amino acid supplement. Capsules contain 700 mg of 12 free form amino acids without fillers, binders, preservatives or sugars. Contains 107 mg of Nitrogen per capsule. Formula rich source of Branched Chain amino acids.
Composition: L-Lysine, Glycine, L-Leucine, L-Methionine, L-Arginine, L-Phenylalanine, L-Valine, L-Isoleucine, L-Histidine, L-Threonine, L-Tyrosine, L-Tryptophan.
Dosage and Administration: Initially it is recommended 2-4 capsules t.i.d. ¼-½ teaspoon t.i.d.
How Supplied: 700 mg capsules: Bottles of 100 capsules. Bottles of 200 and 90 grams of free powder.
Literature: Available upon request.

AMINOTATE® OTC

Description: Free form amino acid supplement for adults and children 4 or more years of age. Capsules contain 700 mg of 15 free form amino acids without fillers, binders, preservatives or sugars. Contains 102 mg Nitrogen per capsule. Formula rich source of glycogenic amino acids.
Composition: Glycine, L-Alanine, L-Leucine, L-Lysine, L-Valine, L-Isoleucine, L-Arginine, L-Methionine, L-Histidine, L-Threonine, L-Phenylalanine, Proline, L-Glutamine, L-Tyrosine, L-Tryptophan.
Dosage and Administration: Initially it is recommended 2-4 capsules b.i.d. in between meals. Powder ¼-½ teaspoon b.i.d.
How Supplied: 700 mg capsule: Bottles of 100 capsules. Bottles of 200 and 90 grams of free powder.
Literature: Available upon request.

DL-CARNITINE OTC

Description: Free form singular amino acid supplement. Capsules containing 600 mg of DL-Carnitine.
How Supplied: 600 mg capsules: Bottles of 60 capsules.
Literature: Available upon request.

L-CARNITINE OTC

Description: Free form singular amino acid supplement. Capsules containing 250 mg of L-Carnitine.
How Supplied: 250 mg capsules: Bottles of 30 capsules.
Literature: Available upon request.

ENDORPHENYL™ OTC
(D-phenylalanine)

Description: Free form singular amino acid capsules containing 200 mg of pure D-Phenylalanine.
How Supplied: 200 mg capsules. Bottles of 50 capsules.
Literature: Available upon request.

ISO-B OTC
(Encapsulated Coenzymatic B Complex)

Description: A nutritional supplement containing several of the active coenzymatic forms of B Complex.
Composition:
CONTENTS PER 2 CAPSULES

Thiamine HCL	50	mg
Riboflavin 5' Phosphate	50	mg
Niacinamide	150	mg
Calcium Pantothenate	250	mg
Pyridoxine HCL	100	mg
Pyridoxal 5' Phosphate	5	mg
Para Amino Benzoic Acid	100	mg
Inositol	100	mg
Choline Bitartrate	250	mg
Biotin	200	mcg
Folic Acid	400	mcg
Vitamin B_{12} (Cyanocobalamin)	200	mcg

Folic Acid, Cyanocobalamin and Biotin are derived from bacterial sources. The other B vitamins are synthesized from the purest yeast free U.S.P. grade materials.
Dosage and Administration: 2 capsules per day as a dietary supplement.
How Supplied: Bottles of 60 capsules.
Lierature: Available upon request.

LYTE-C OTC
(Corn Free Vitamin C with Electrolytes)

Description: Corn free buffered Vitamin C complex. Vitamin C from Sago Palm. Contains 2100 mg Ascorbic Acid; 114 mg Magnesium; 85 mg Calcium; and 80 mg Potassium per every 3 grams.
Dosage and Administration: Initially it is recommended ¼-½ teaspoon t.i.d. as a dietary supplement.
How Supplied: Bottles of 200 grams free flowing powder.
Literature: Available upon request.

MVM OTC
(High Potency Multi-Vitamin/Mineral)

Description: Encapsulated powdered multi-vitamin/mineral. Contains no wheat, liver, corn, soy, yeast, excipients or preservatives (preservative free capsule). Coenzymatic forms of Vitamins B_2 & B_6 as well as a corn free source of Vitamin C.
Composition:
CONTENTS PER 5 CAPSULES

Vitamin A Palmitate	20,000	I.U.
Ascorbic Acid (Corn Free)	250	mg
Thiamine HCL	100	mg
Riboflavin 5' Phosphate	50	mg
Niacin	50	mg
Tryptophan	50	mg
Calcium Pantothenate	500	mg
Pyridoxine HCL	150	mg
Pyridoxal 5' Phosphate	5	mg
Vitamin B_{12} (Cyanocobalamin)	800	mcg
Folic Acid	400	mcg
Biotin	800	mcg
Para Amino Benzoic Acid	100	mg
Vitamin E (d'Alpha Tocopheral Acetate)	300	I.U.
Calcium (DiCalcium Phosphate)	200	mg
Magnesium (Oxide)	125	mg
Potassium (Chloride)	98	mg
Manganese (Sulfate)	15	mg
Zinc (Sulfate)	30	mg
Copper (Sulfate)	1.5	mg
Selenium (Dioxide)	100	mcg
Molybdenum (sodium Molybdate)	150	mcg
Glutamic Acid	100	mg
Chromium (Chloride)	150	mcg
Iron (Ammonium Ferric Citrate)	18	mg
Iodine (Potassium Iodide)	75	mcg

Folic Acid, Cyanocobalamin and Biotin are derived from bacterial sources. The other B vitamins are synthesized from the purest U.S.P. grade materials.
Dosage and Administration: 5 capsules per day in divided doses as a dietary supplement.
How Supplied: Bottles of 150 capsules.
Literature: Available upon request.

MAXOVITE OTC
(Sustained Release Multi-Vitamin/Mineral)

Description: A corn and yeast free multi-vitamin/mineral. Contains lipo and hydro soluble vitamins. Minerals are in amino acid chelated forms for maximum uptake.
Composition
FIVE TABLETS PROVIDE:
VITAMINS
LIPSOLUBLE

Vitamin A (Palmitate) (Water Dispersed)	12,500	I.U.
Vitamin E (d'Alpha Tocopheral)	100	I.U.
Vitamin D_3 (Cholecalciferol)	100	I.U.

HYDROSOLUBLE (Sustained Release)

Folic Acid	200	mcg
Vitamin B_1 (Thiamine HCL)	30	mg
Vitamin B_2 (Riboflavin)	25	mg
Niacinamide	25	mg
Vitamin B_6 (Pyridoxine HCL)	325	mg
Vitamin B_{12} (Cyanocobalamin Concentrate)	65	mcg
Biotin	70	mcg
Pantothenic Acid (d-Calcium Pantothenate)	25	mg
Choline Bitartrate	300	mg
Inositol	25	mg
Para Amino Benzoic Acid	25	mg
Vitamin C (Corn Free)	1,500	mg

Bioflavonoid	250	mg
Rutin	25	mg
MINERALS		
Calcium	125	mg
(Amino Acid Chelate)		
Magnesium	250	mg
(Amino Acid Chelate)		
Iodine	75	mcg
(Potassium Iodide)		
Iron	15	mg
(Amino Acid Chelate)		
Copper	0.5	mg
(Amino Acid Chelate)		
Zinc	30	mg
(Amino Acid Chelate)		
Manganese	10	mg
(Amino Acid Chelate)		
Potassium	49.0	mg
(Amino Acid Complex)		
Selenium	100	mcg
(Amino Acid Complex)		
Chromium	100	mcg
(Amino Acid Complex)		

Dosage and Administration: 5 tablets per day with meals as a dietary supplement.
How Supplied: Bottles of 105 and 210 tablets.
Literature: Available upon request.

NUTROX   OTC
(Encapsulated Anti-Oxidant)

Description: Each capsule of this supplement provides a broad spectrum anti-oxidant complex. Included in this complex are Beta Carotene, Cysteine, DMG, Ascorbic Acid, Zinc and Selenium.
Composition:

	ONE CAPSULE AMOUNT	3 CAPSULE AMOUNT
Vitamin E (d'Alpha Tocopherol Acetate)	150 I.U.	450 I.U.
L-Cysteine HCL	60 mg	180 mg
Ascorbic Acid (Corn Free)	80 mg	240 mg
Niacinamide	50 mg	150 mg
Dimethylglycine	25 mg	75 mg
Glutathione	40 mg	120 mg
Riboflavin 5' Phosphate	25 mg	75 mg
Thiamine HCL	25 mg	75 mg
Calcium Pantothenate	22 mg	66 mg
Zinc Oxide	15 mg	45 mg
Vitamin A (Beta Carotene)	10,000 I.U.	30,000 I.U.
Selenium (Dioxide)	75 mcg	225 mcg

Dosage and Administration: 1–3 capsules per day with meals.
How Supplied: Bottles of 90 capsules.
Literature: Available upon request.

UAD Laboratories, Inc.
6635 HIGHWAY 18 WEST
JACKSON, MS 39209

LORCET®   ℞

Description: Each film coated reddish-orange tablet contains:
Propoxyphene Hydrochloride..........65 mg.
Acetaminophen..........650 mg.
How Supplied: In bottles of 100's—NDC 0785-1111-01.

LORCET-HD®   ℞

Description: Each Lorcet-HD capsule contains 5 mg. of Hydrocodone Bitartrate (WARNING: May be habit forming) and 500 mg. of Acetaminophen.
How Supplied: Lorcet-HD Capsules are opaque maroon capsules and are supplied in bottles of 100 capsules. Each capsule contains Acetaminophen (APAP), 500 mg., and Hydrocodone Bitartrate, 5 mg. (WARNING: May be habit forming). The NDC number for containers of 100 capsules is 0785-1120-01.

ZONE-A LOTION 1%   ℞

Description: Zone-A Lotion is a topical preparation containing Hydrocortisone acetate 1% and Pramoxine HCL 1% in a hydrophylic lotion base containing stearic acid, cetyl alcohol, forlan-L glycerine, Triethanolamine, Myrj-52, Di-isopropyl adipate, polyvinyl-pyrrolidone, silicone, potassium sorbate 0.1% and sorbic acid 0.1% and water. Topical corticosteroids are anti-inflammatory and antipruritic agents.

Clinical Pharmacology: Topical corticosteroids share anti-inflammatory, anti-pruritic and vasoconstrictive actions.

The mechanism of anti-inflammatory activity of the topical corticosteroids is unclear. Various laboratory methods, including vasoconstrictor assays, are used to compare and predict potencies and/or clinical efficacies of the topical corticosteroids. There is some evidence to suggest that a recognizable correlation exists between vasoconstrictor potency and therapeutic efficacy in man.

Pramoxine hydrochloride is a topical anesthetic agent which provides temporary relief from itching and pain. It acts by stabilizing the neuronal membrane of nerve endings with which it comes into contact.

Indications and Usage: Topical corticosteroids are indicated for the relief of the inflammatory and pruritic manifestations of corticosteroid-responsive dermatoses.

Contraindications: Topical corticosteroids are contraindicated in those patients with a history of hypersensitivity to any of the components of the preparation.

Precautions:
General: Systemic absorption of topical corticosteroids has produced reversible hypothalamic-pituitary-adrenal (HPA) axis suppression, manifestations of Cushing's syndrome, hyperglycemia, and glucosuria in some patients.

Conditions which augment systemic absorption include the application of the more potent steroids, use over large surface areas, prolonged use, and the addition of occlusive dressings.

Therefore, patients receiving a large dose of a potent topical steroid applied to a large surface area and under an occlusive dressing should be evaluated periodically for evidence of HPA axis suppression by using the urinary free cortisol and ACTH stimulation tests. If HPA axis suppression is noted, an attempt should be made to withdraw the drug, to reduce the frequency of application, or to substitute a less potent steroid.

Recovery of HPA axis function is generally prompt and complete upon discontinuation of the drug. Infrequently, signs and symptoms of steroid withdrawal may occur, requiring supplemental systemic corticosteroids.

Children may absorb proportionally larger amounts of topical corticosteroids and thus be more susceptible fo systemic toxicity. (See PRECAUTIONS—Pediatric Use).

If irritation develops topical corticosteroids should be discontinued and appropriate therapy instituted.

In the presence of dermatological infections, the use of an appropriate antifngal or antibacterial agent should be instituted. If a favorable response does not occur promptly, the corticosteroid should be discontinued until the infection has been adequately controlled.

Information for the Patient: Patients using topical corticosteroids should receive the following information and instructions:
1. This medication is to be used as directed by the physician. It is for external use only. Avoid contact with the eyes.
2. Patients should be advised not to use this medication for any disorder other than for which it was prescribed.
3. The treated skin area should not be bandaged or otherwise covered or wrapped as to be occlusive unless directed by the physician.
4. Patients should report any signs of local adverse reactions, especially under occlusive dressings.
5. Parents of pediatric patients should be advised not to use tight-fitting diapers or plastic pants on a child being treated in the diaper area, as these garments may constitute occlusive dressings.

Laboratory Tests: The following tests may be helpful in evaluating the HPA axis suppression:
Urinary free cortisol test
ACTH stimulation test

Carcinogenesis, Mutagenesis, and Impairment of Fertility: Long term animal studies have not been performed to evaluate the carcinogenic potential or the effect on fertility of topical corticosteroids. Studies to determine mutagenicity with prednisolone and hydrocortisone have revealed negative results.

Pregnancy Category C: Corticosteroids are generally teratogenic in laboratory animals when administered systemically at relatively low dosage levels. The more potent corticosteroids have been shown to be teratogenic after dermal application in laboratory animals. There are no adequate and well-controlled studies in pregnant women on teratogenic effects from topically applied corticosteroids. Therefore topical corticosteroids should be used during pregnancy only if the potential benefit justifies the potential risk to the fetus. Drugs of this class should not be used extensively on pregnant patients, in large amounts, or for prolonged periods of time.

Nursing Mothers: It is not known whether topical administration of corticosteroids could result in sufficient systemic absorption to produce detectable amounts in breast milk. Systemically administered corticosteroids are secreted into breast milk in quantities NOT likely to have a deleterious effect on the infant. Nevertheless, caution should be exercised when topical corticosteroids are administered to a nursing woman.

Pediatric Use: Pediatric patients may demonstrate greater susceptibility to topical corticosteroid-induced HPA axis suppression and Cushing's syndrome than mature patients because of a larger skin surface area to body weight ratio. Hypothalamic-pituitary-adrenal (HPA) axis suppression, Cushing's syndrome, and intracranial hypertension have been reported in children receiving topical corticosteroids. Manifestations of adrenal suppression in children include linear growth retardation, delayed weight gain, low plasma cortisol levels, and absence of response to ACTH stimulation. Manifestations of intracranial hypertension include bulging fontanelles, headaches, and bilateral papilledema.

Administration of topical corticosteroids to children should be limited to the least amount compatible with an effective therapeutic regimen. Chronic corticosteroids therapy may interfere with the growth and development of children.

Adverse Reactions: The following local adverse reactions are reported infrequently with topical corticosteroids, but may occur more frequently with the use of occlusive dressings. These reactions are listed in an approximate decreasing order of occurence: Burning, Itching, Irritation, Dryness, Folliculitis, Hypertrichosis, Acneiform eruptions, Hypopigmentation, Perioral dermatitis, Allergic contact dermatitis, Maceration of the skin, Secondary infection, Skin Atrophy, Striae and Miliaria.

Overdosage: Topically applied corticosteroids can be absorbed in sufficient amounts to produce systematic effects (See PRECAUTIONS).

Dosage and Administration: Topical corticosteroids are generally applied to the affected area as a thin film three or four times daily depending on the severity of the condition.

Occlusive dressings may be used for the management of psoriasis or recalcitrant conditions.

If an infection develops, the use of occlusive dressings should be discontinued and appropriate antimicrobial therapy instituted.

How Supplied: 2 fl. oz.
Caution: Federal law prohibits dispensing without prescription.

Manufactured for:
UAD LABORATORIES, INC.
Jackson, Mississippi 39209

U.S. Pharmaceutical Corporation
2500 PARK CENTRAL BLVD.
DECATUR, GA 30035

HEMOCYTE Tablets OTC
(ferrous fumarate 324 mg.)

How Supplied:
Bottles of 100 NDC 52747-307-60

HEMOCYTE PLUS™ Tabules ℞
Iron-Vitamin-Mineral Complex

Description: Each tabule contains:

Ferrous Fumarate (anhydrous)	324 mg.
[Equivalent to about 106 mg. of Elemental Iron]	
Sodium Ascorbate (Vit. C)	200 mg.
Vit. B-1—Thiamine Mononitrate	10 mg.
Vit. B-2—Riboflavin	6 mg.
Vit. B-6—Pyridoxine HCl	5 mg.
Vit. B-12—Cyanocobalamin Concentrate	15 mcg.
Folic Acid	1 mg.
Niacinamide	30 mg.
Calcium Pantothenate	10 mg.
Zinc Sulfate	80 mg.
Magnesium Sulfate	70 mg.
Manganese Sulfate	4 mg.
Copper Sulfate	2 mg.

How Supplied:
Bottles of 100 NDC 52747-308-60

HEMOCYTE–F TABLETS ℞

Description: Each tablet contains:

Ferrous Fumarate	324 mg.
Folic Acid	1 mg.

How Supplied:
Bottles of 100 NDC 52747-306-60

MAGSAL™ TABLETS ℞

Description: Each tablet contains:

Magnesium Salicylate	600 mg.
Phenyltoloxamine Citrate	25 mg.

How Supplied:
Bottles of 100
NDC 52747-321-60

ISOVEX® Capsules ℞
(ethaverine hydrochloride 100 mg.)

How Supplied:
Bottles of 100 NDC 52747-204-60
Bottles of 1000 NDC 52747-204-80

MEDIPLEX
Vitamin/Mineral Complex

Description: Each tabule contains:

Vitamin E— dl-alpha Tocopherol Acetate	60 I.U.
Vitamin C—Ascorbic Acid	300 mg.
Vitamin B¹²—Cyanocobalmin Concentrate	25 mcg.
Vitamin B¹—Thiamine	25 mg.
Niacinamide	100 mg.
Vitamin B⁶—Pyridoxine	10 mg.
Vitamin B²—Riboflavin	10 mg.
Calcium Pantothenate	25 mg.
Zinc Sulfate	80 mg.
Magnesium Sulfate	70 mg.
Manganese Sulfate	4 mg.
Copper Sulfate	2 mg.

How Supplied: Bottles of 100 Tabules.
NDC 52747-142-60

Products are cross-indexed by generic and chemical names in the **YELLOW SECTION**

USV Laboratories, Division
USV Pharmaceutical Corp.
TARRYTOWN, NY 10591

USV Laboratories Inc.
MANATI, P.R. 00701

USV (P.R.) Development Corp.
MANATI, P.R. 00701

ARLIDIN® ℞
[ar'lĭ-din"]
(nylidrin HCl)
Vasodilator/Vasorelaxant

Description: Tablets of 6 and 12 mg nylidrin HCl.

Actions: Arlidin acts predominantly by beta-receptor stimulation. Beta stimulation with Arlidin has been demonstrated in a variety of isolated tissues from rabbits, guinea pigs and dogs. It has been shown to dilate arterioles in skeletal muscle and to increase cardiac output in the anesthetized dog and cat and in unanesthetized man.

Indications: Based on a review of this drug by the National Academy of Sciences—National Research Council and/or other information, FDA has classified the indications as follows:

"Possibly" effective whenever an increase in blood supply is desirable in vasospastic disorders such as:

Peripheral vascular disease: arteriosclerosis obliterans, thromboangiitis obliterans, diabetic vascular disease, night leg cramps, Raynaud's phenomenon and disease, ischemic ulcer, frostbite, acrocyanosis, acroparesthesia, thrombophlebitis, cold feet, legs and hands.

Circulatory disturbances of the inner ear: primary cochlear cell ischemia, cochlear stria vascular ischemia, macular or ampullar ischemia and other disturbances due to labyrinthine artery spasm or obstruction.

Final classification of the less-than-effective indications requires further investigation.

Contraindications: Acute myocardial infarction, paroxysmal tachycardia, progressive angina pectoris and thyrotoxicosis.

Warnings: In patients with cardiac disease such as tachyarrhythmias and uncompensated congestive heart failure, the benefit/risk ratio should be weighed prior to therapy and reconsidered at intervals during treatment.

Adverse Reactions: Trembling, nervousness, weakness, dizziness (not associated with labyrinthine artery insufficiency), palpitations, nausea and vomiting may occur. Postural hypotension, while not reported, may also occur.

Dosage: Orally, 3 to 12 mg three or four times a day.

How Supplied: ARLIDIN (nylidrin HCl)—White, scored tablets, 6 mg and 12 mg. Bottles of 100 and 1000. Unit-dose blister packs, boxes of 100 (10 x 10 strips).
NSN 6505-00-685-5435A, V.A. Depots (6 mg., 1000s).
Revised: September, 1976
Shown in Product Identification Section, page 440

AZOLID® ℞
[ă'zōl-id]
phenylbutazone

100 mg tablets, capsules

Important Note: AZOLID (phenylbutazone) cannot be considered a simple analgesic and should never be administered casually. Each patient should be carefully evaluated before treatment is started and should remain constantly under the close supervision of the physician. The following precautions should be observed:

1. Therapy should not be initiated until a careful, detailed history and complete hemogram and urinalysis, etc., of the patient have been made. These examinations should be made at regular, frequent intervals throughout the duration of this drug therapy.
2. Patients should be carefully selected, avoiding those in whom it is contraindicated as well as those who will respond to ordinary therapeutic measures, or those who cannot be observed at frequent intervals.
3. Patients taking AZOLID should be warned not to exceed the recommended dosage because this may lead to toxic effects. Patients should report to the physician immediately any sign of:
   a. fever, sore throat, lesions in the mouth (symptoms of blood dyscrasia);
   b. dyspepsia, epigastric pain, symptoms of anemia, unusual bleeding, unusual bruising, black or tarry stools, or other evidence of intestinal ulceration;
   c. skin reactions;
   d. significant weight gain or edema.
4. A TRIAL PERIOD OF ONE WEEK IS CONSIDERED ADEQUATE TO DETERMINE THE THERAPEUTIC EFFECT OF THE DRUG. IN THE ABSENCE OF A FAVORABLE RESPONSE, THERAPY SHOULD BE DISCONTINUED.
In patients 60 years of age and over, AZOLID should be restricted to a short-term period of no more than seven days.
5. BEFORE PRESCRIBING AZOLID FOR AN INDIVIDUAL PATIENT, READ THOROUGHLY THE INFORMATION CONTAINED UNDER EACH HEADING THAT FOLLOWS:

Description: Chemically, AZOLID is 4-butyl-1,2-diphenyl-3,5-pyrazolidinedione. It is closely related chemically to the pyrazoles.
It is very slightly soluble in water; freely soluble in acetone and in ether; soluble in alcohol.

Clinical Pharmacology: AZOLID is closely related pharmacologically, including toxic effects, to the pyrazole compounds, aminopyrine and antipyrine. It is entirely unrelated to the steroid hormones.
It has analgesic, antipyretic and anti-inflammatory actions as well as mild uricosuric properties resulting in symptomatic relief only. THE DISEASE PROCESS ITSELF IS UNALTERED BY THE DRUG.
The exact mechanism of the anti-inflammatory effects of phenylbutazone has not been elucidated, but clinical pharmacology studies have shown that phenylbutazone inhibits certain factors believed to be involved in the inflammatory process. These processes are (1) prostaglandin synthesis; (2) leucocyte migration; (3) release and/or activity of lysosomal enzymes.
Phenylbutazone is rapidly absorbed after oral administration. Tests conducted in 18 healthy adult male volunteers indicated that a peak plasma concentration of 43.3 ($\pm$3.1) mg/liter was attained within 2.5 ($\pm$1.4) hours after the ingestion of three 100-mg tablets. In these same volunteers, the apparent elimination half-life was 84 ($\pm$23) hours. About 98% of the drug is bound to human serum albumin.
Twenty-one days after oral administration of ^{14}C-labeled drug, 61% was recovered from the urine and 27% from the feces. However, only about 1% of total urinary radioactivity represents unchanged drug. The sum of nonconjugated urinary metabolites (oxyphenbutazone, γ-hydroxyphenylbutazone, p, γ-dihydroxyphenylbutazone), and phenylbutazone itself amounted to only about 10%. About 40% of the total urinary radioactivity was excreted as the C(4)-glucuronide of phenylbutazone and an additional 12% was identified as the C(4)-glucuronide of γ-hydroxyphenylbutazone.
The major metabolite of phenylbutazone in human plasma is oxyphenbutazone; steady-state plasma levels are about 50% of those of phenylbutazone. Less than 2% of the dose of phenylbutazone appears in the urine as oxyphenbutazone.

Indications: The indications for AZOLID (phenylbutazone) are as follows:

Acute gouty arthritis
Acute rheumatoid arthritis
Active ankylosing spondylitis
Short-term treatment of acute attacks of degenerative joint disease of the hips and knees not responsive to other treatment
Painful shoulder (peritendinitis, capsulitis, bursitis, and acute arthritis of that joint).

Contraindications:
AGE: Phenylbutazone is contraindicated in children 14 years of age or younger because controlled clinical trials in patients of this age group have not been conducted.
OTHER MEDICAL CONDITIONS: Phenylbutazone is contraindicated in patients with incipient cardiac failure, blood dyscrasias, pancreatitis, parotitis, stomatitis, polymyalgia rheumatica, temporal arteritis, senility, drug allergy, and in the presence of severe renal, cardiac and hepatic disease, and in patients with a history of peptic ulcer disease, or symptoms of gastrointestinal inflammation or active ulceration because serious adverse reactions or aggravation of existing medical problems can occur.
CONCOMITANT MEDICATIONS: Phenylbutazone should not be used in combination with other drugs that accentuate or share a potential for similar toxicity.
It is also inadvisable to administer phenylbutazone in combination with other potent drugs because of the possibility of increased toxic reactions from phenylbutazone and other agents. (See also PRECAUTIONS: Drug Interactions.)
Phenylbutazone is contraindicated in patients with a history or suggestion of prior toxicity, sensitivity, or idiosyncrasy to phenylbutazone or oxyphenbutazone.

Warnings: Based upon reports of clinical experience with phenylbutazone and related compounds, the following warnings should be considered by the physician prior to prescribing the drug:
GASTROINTESTINAL: Upper G.I. diagnostic tests should be performed in patients with persistent or severe dyspepsia. Peptic ulceration, reactivation of latent peptic ulcer, perforation and gastrointestinal bleeding, sometimes severe, have been reported.
As with other nonsteroidal anti-inflammatory drugs, borderline elevations of one or more liver tests may occur in up to 15% of patients. These abnormalities may progress, may remain essentially unchanged, or may be transient with continued therapy. The SGPT (ALT) test is probably the most sensitive indicator of liver dysfunction. Meaningful (three times the upper limit of normal) elevations of SGPT or SGOT (AST) occurred in controlled clinical trials in less than 1% of patients. A patient with symptoms and/or signs suggesting liver dysfunction, or in whom an abnormal liver test has occurred, should be evaluated for evidence of the development of more severe hepatic reaction while on therapy with phenylbutazone. Severe hepatic reactions, including jaundice and cases of fatal hepatitis, have been reported with phenylbutazone as with other nonsteroidal anti-inflammatory drugs. Although such reactions are rare, if abnormal liver tests persist or worsen, if clinical signs and symptoms consistent with liver disease develop, or if systemic manifestations occur (e.g. eosinophilia, rash, etc.), phenylbutazone should be discontinued.
HEMATOLOGIC: Frequent and regular hematologic evaluations should be performed on patients receiving the drug for periods over one week. Any significant change in the total white count, relative decrease in granulocytes, appearance of immature forms or fall in hematocrit should be a signal for immediate cessation of therapy and a complete hematologic investigation. Serious, sometimes fatal blood dyscrasias, including aplastic anemia have been reported to occur. Hematologic toxicity may occur suddenly or many days or weeks after cessation of treatment as manifested by the appearance of anemia, leukopenia, thrombocytopenia or clinically significant hemorrhagic diathesis. There have been published reports associating phenylbutazone with leukemia. However, the circumstances involved in these reports are such that a cause and effect relationship to the drug has not been established.

Precautions:
GENERAL: Because of potential serious adverse reactions to phenylbutazone, the following precautions should be observed in the use of the drug:
1. A careful diagnostic physical examination and history should be performed on all patients at regular intervals while the patient is receiving the drug.
2. Phenylbutazone is not recommended for chronic use in the elderly.
3. Hematologic evaluation should be performed at frequent and regular intervals and additional laboratory examinations performed as indicated.
4. Patients should be instructed to report immediately the occurrence of high fever, severe sore throat, stomatitis, salivary gland enlargement, tarry stools, unusual bleeding or bruising, sudden weight gain, or edema.
5. The drug reduces iodine uptake by the thyroid and may interfere with laboratory tests of thyroid function. (See ADVERSE REACTIONS: Endocrine-Metabolic.)
6. The patient should be cautioned regarding participation in activities requiring alertness and coordination and that the concomitant ingestion of alcohol with phenylbutazone may further impair psychomotor skills.
DRUG INTERACTIONS: Phenylbutazone is highly bound to serum proteins. If its affinity for protein binding is higher than other concurrently administered drugs, the actions and toxicity of the other drug may be increased.
Phenylbutazone accentuates the prothrombin depression produced by coumarin-type anticoagulants. When administered alone, it does not affect prothrombin activity. The pharmacologic action of insulin, and anti-diabetic and sulfonamide drugs may be potentiated by the simultaneous administration of phenylbutazone.
Concomitant administration of phenylbutazone and phenytoin may result in increased serum levels of phenytoin which could lead to increased phenytoin toxicity.
PREGNANCY CATEGORY C: Reproductive studies in animals, although inconclusive, exhibited evidence of possible embryotoxicity. It is, therefore, recommended that this drug should be used with caution during pregnancy. The benefits should be weighed against the potential risk to the fetus.
NURSING MOTHERS: Caution is also advised in prescribing phenylbutazone in nursing mothers because the drug may appear in cord blood and breast milk.
PEDIATRIC USE: Phenylbutazone is contraindicated in children 14 years of age or younger because controlled clinical trials in patients of this age group have not been conducted.

Adverse Reactions: Based upon reports of clinical experience with phenylbutazone and related compounds, the following adverse reactions have been reported.
TABLE 1: (1)* = Incidence greater than 1%; (2) = Incidence less than 1%.

Gastrointestinal
(1) Nausea*; dyspepsia/including indigestion and heartburn*; abdominal discomfort/distress*.
(2) Vomiting; abdominal distention with flatulence; constipation; diarrhea; esophagitis; gastritis; salivary gland enlargement; stomatitis, sometimes with ulceration; ulceration and perforation of the intestinal tract, including acute and reactivated peptic ulcer with perforation, hemorrhage and hematemesis; anemia due to gastrointestinal bleeding which may be occult; hepatitis, both fatal and nonfatal, sometimes associated with evidence of cholestasis.

Hematological
(1) None.
(2) Anemia; leukopenia; thrombocytopenia with associated purpura, petechiae and hemorrhage; pancytopenia; aplastic anemia; bone marrow depression; agranulocytosis and agranulocytic anginal syndrome; hemolytic anemia.

Hypersensitivity
(1) None.
(2) Urticaria; anaphylactic shock; arthralgia, drug fever; hypersensitivity angiitis (polyarteritis) and vasculitis; Lyell's syndrome; serum sickness; Stevens-Johnson syndrome; activation of systemic lupus erythematosus; aggravation of temporal arteritis in patients with polymyalgia rheumatica.

Dermatologic
(1) Rash*.
(2) Pruritis; erythema nodosum; erythema multiforme; non-thrombocytopenic purpura.

Cardiovascular, Fluid, and Electrolyte
(1) Edema/water retention*.
(2) Sodium and chloride retention; fluid retention and plasma dilution; cardiac decompensation (congestive heart failure) with edema and dyspnea; metabolic acidosis; respiratory alkalosis; hypertension; pericarditis; interstitial myocarditis with muscle necrosis and perivascular granulomata.

Renal
(1) None.
(2) Hematuria; proteinuria; ureteral obstruction with uric acid crystals; anuria; glomerulonephritis; acute tubular necrosis; cortial necrosis; renal stones; nephrotic syndrome; impaired renal function and renal failure associated with azotemia.

Central Nervous System
(1) None
(2) Headache; drowsiness; agitation; confusional states and lethargy; tremors; numbness; weakness.

Endocrine-Metabolic
(1) None.
(2) Hyperglycemia.

Special Senses
(1) Ocular: none; otic: none.
(2) Ocular: none; otic: hearing loss; tinnitus.
Adverse reactions have also been listed in a Group (3)—Causal Relationship Unknown. The reactions in this group have been reported but occurred under circumstances where a causal relationship could not be established. In some patients the reported reactions may have been unrelated to the administration of phenylbutazone. However, in these reported events, the possibility cannot be excluded. Therefore these observations are being listed to serve as alerting information to physicians. Before prescribing this drug for an individual patient, the physician should be familiar with the following:
TABLE 2: (3) = Causal Relationship Unknown —incidence less than 1%.

Hematological
Leukemia. (There have been reports associating phenylbutazone with leukemia. However, the circumstances involved in these reports are such that a cause-and-effect relationship to the drug has not been clearly established.)

Endocrine-Metabolic
Thyroid hyperplasia; goiters associated with hyperthyroidism and hypothyroidism; pancreatitis.

Special Senses
Blurred vision; optic neuritis; toxic amblyopia; scotomata; retinal detachment; retinal hemorrhage; oculomotor palsy.

Overdosage: SIGNS AND SYMPTOMS: Include any of the following: nausea, vomiting, epigastric pain, excessive perspiration, euphoria, psychosis, headaches, giddiness, vertigo, hyperventilation, insomnia, tinnitus, difficulty in hearing, edema (sodium retention), hypertension, cyanosis, respiratory depression, agitation, hallucinations, stupor, convulsions, coma, hematuria, and oliguria. Hepatomegaly, jaundice, and ulceration of the buccal or gastrointestinal mucosa have been reported as late manifestations of massive overdosage.
Reported laboratory abnormalities following overdosage include: respiratory or metabolic acidosis, impaired hepatic or renal function, and abnormalities of formed blood elements.
TREATMENT: In the alert patient, empty the stomach promptly by induced emesis followed by lavage. In the obtunded patient, secure the airway

Continued on next page

USV—Cont.

with a cuffed endotracheal tube before beginning lavage (do not induce emesis). Maintain adequate respiratory exchange; do not use respiratory stimulants. Treat shock with appropriate supportive measures. Control seizures with intravenous diazepam or short-acting barbiturates. Dialysis may be helpful if renal function is impaired.

Dosage and Administration: AZOLID (phenylbutazone) should be used at the smallest effective dosage to afford rapid relief of severe symptoms. It is contraindicated in children under 14 years of age and in senile patients.

If a favorable symptomatic response to treatment is not obtained after one week, the drug should be discontinued. When a favorable therapeutic response has been obtained, the dosage should be reduced and then discontinued as soon as possible. In elderly patients (60 years and over) every effort must be made to discontinue therapy on, or as soon as possible after the seventh day, because of the exceedingly high risk of severe fatal toxic reactions in this age group.

To minimize gastric upset, the drug should be taken with milk or with meals.

In selecting the appropriate dosage in any specific case, consideration should be given to the patient's age, weight, general health, and any other factors that may influence his response to the drug.

Rheumatoid Arthritis, Ankylosing Spondylitis, Acute Attacks of Degenerative Joint Disease, and Painful Shoulder:

Initial Dosage: The daily dose in adult patients is 300 to 600 mg in three or four divided doses. Maximum therapeutic response is usually obtained at a total daily dose of 400 mg. A trial period of one week of therapy is considered adequate to determine the therapeutic effect of the drug. In the absence of a favorable response, therapy should be discontinued.

Maintenance Dosage: When improvement is obtained, dosage should be promptly decreased to the minimum effective level necessary to maintain relief, not exceeding 400 mg daily because of the possibility of cumulative toxicity. A satisfactory clinical response may be obtained with daily doses as low as 100 to 200 mg daily.

Acute Gouty Arthritis:
Satisfactory results are obtained after an initial dose of 400 mg followed by 100 mg every four hours. The articular inflammation usually subsides within four days and treatment should not be continued longer than one week.

How Supplied: AZOLID tablets, 100 mg (yellow, coated), and capsules, 100 mg (yellow and white), bottles of 100 (tablets: NDC 0105-0060-00; capsules: NDC 0105-0112-00) and 1000 (tablets: NDC 0105-0060-99; capsules: NDC 0105-0112-99).
Revised: January, 1984

Bi–K™
potassium supplement ℞

Description: Each 15 ml (one tablespoonful) supplies 20 mEq of potassium ions as a combination of potassium gluconate and potassium citrate in a sorbitol and saccharin solution.

Indications: For use as oral potassium therapy in the prevention or treatment of hypokalemia which may occur as a result of diuretic or corticosteroid administration. It may be used in the treatment of cardiac arrhythmias due to digitalis intoxication.

Contraindications: Severe renal impairment with oliguria or azotemia, untreated Addison's disease, adynamia episodica hereditaria, acute dehydration, heat cramps and hyperkalemia from any cause. This product should not be used in patients receiving aldosterone antagonists or triamterene.

Warnings: Bi-K (potassium gluconate and potassium citrate) is a palatable form of oral potassium replacement. It appears that little if any potassium gluconate-citrate penetrates as far as the jejunum or ileum where enteric coated potassium chloride lesions have been noted. Excessive, undiluted doses of Bi-K may cause a saline laxative effect.

To minimize gastrointestinal irritation, it is recommended that Bi-K be taken with meals or diluted with water or fruit juice. A tablespoonful (15 ml) in 8 ounces of water is approximately isotonic. More than a single tablespoonful should not be taken without prior dilution.

Precautions: Potassium is a major intracellular cation which plays a significant role in body physiology. The serum level of potassium is normally 3.8–5.0 mEq/liter. While the serum or plasma level is a poor indicator of total body stores, a plasma or serum level below 3.5 mEq/liter is considered to be indicative of hypokalemia.

The most common cause of hypokalemia is excessive loss of potassium in the urine. However, hypokalemia can also occur with vomiting, gastric drainage and diarrhea.

Usually a potassium deficiency can be corrected by oral administration of potassium supplements. With normal kidney function it is difficult to produce potassium intoxication by oral administration. However, potassium supplements must be administered with caution since, usually, the exact amount of the deficiency is not accurately known. Checks on the patient's clinical status and periodic E.K.G. and/or serum potassium levels should be made. High serum potassium levels may cause death by cardiac depression, arrhythmias or arrest.

In patients with hypokalemia who also have alkalosis and a chloride deficiency, (hypokalemia hypochloremic alkalosis) there will be a requirement for chloride ions. Bi-K is not recommended for use in these patients.

Adverse Reactions: Symptoms of potassium intoxication include paresthesias of the extremities, flaccid paralysis, listlessness, mental confusion, weakness and heaviness of the legs, fall in blood pressure, cardiac arrhythmias and heart block. Hyperkalemia may exhibit the following electrocardiographic abnormalities: disappearance of the P wave, widening and slurring of the QRS complex, changes of the ST segment and tall peaked T waves.

Bi-K taken on an empty stomach in undiluted doses larger than 30 ml (two tablespoons) can produce gastric irritation with nausea, vomiting, diarrhea and abdominal discomfort.

Overdosage: The administration of oral potassium supplements to persons with normal kidney function rarely causes serious hyperkalemia. However, if the renal excretory function is impaired, potentially fatal hyperkalemia can result. It is important to note that hyperkalemia is usually asymptomatic and may be manifested only by an increased serum potassium concentration with E.K.G. changes.

Treatment measures include:
1. Elimination of potassium containing drugs or foods.
2. Intravenous administration of 300 to 500 ml/hr of a 10% dextrose solution containing 10–20 units of crystalline insulin per 1000 milliliters.
3. Correction of acidosis.
4. Use of exchange resins or peritoneal dialysis.

In treating hyperkalemia, it should be noted that patients stabilized on digitalis can develop digitalis toxicity when the serum potassium concentration is changed too rapidly.

Dosage and Administration: The usual dosage is one tablespoonful (15 ml) in 6–8 fluid ounces of water or fruit juice, two to four times a day. This will supply 40 to 80 mEq of potassium ions. The usual preventive dose of potassium is 20 mEq per day while therapeutic doses range from 30 mEq to 100 mEq per day. Because of the potential for gastrointestinal irritation, undiluted large single doses (30 ml or more) of Bi-K are to be avoided. Deviations from this schedule may be indicated, since no average total daily dose can be defined, but must be governed by close observation for clinical effects.

How Supplied: 1 pint (16 fl. oz.).
Manufactured for USV Laboratories, Division USV Pharmaceutical Corp., Tarrytown, NY 10591 by Boots Pharmaceuticals, Inc., Shreveport, LA 71106.
Revised: November, 1980

CALCIMAR® ℞
[kal'sĭ-mar]
(calcitonin-salmon), USV
SOLUTION

Description: Calcitonin is a polypeptide hormone secreted by the parafollicular cells of the thyroid gland in mammals and by the ultimobranchial gland of birds and fish.

CALCIMAR® (calcitonin-salmon) is a synthetic polypeptide of 32 amino acids in the same linear sequence that is found in calcitonin of salmon origin. This is shown by the following graphic formula:

Cys- Ser- Asn- Leu- Ser- Thr- Cys- Val- Leu- Gly-
 1   2   3   4   5   6   7   8   9   10
Lys- Leu- Ser- Gln- Glu- Leu- His- Lys- Leu- Gln-
11   12   13   14   15   16   17   18   19   20
Thr- Tyr- Pro- Arg- Thr- Asn- Thr- Gly- Ser- Gly-
21   22   23   24   25   26   27   28   29   30
Thr- Pro- NH_2
31   32

It is provided in sterile solution for subcutaneous or intramuscular injection. Each milliliter contains 200 I.U. (MRC) of Calcitonin-Salmon, USV, 5 mg Phenol (as preservative), with Sodium Chloride, Sodium Acetate, Acetic Acid, and Sodium Hydroxide to adjust tonicity and pH.

The activity of CALCIMAR® is stated in International Units (equal to MRC or Medical Research Council units) based on bioassay in comparison with the International Reference Preparation of Calcitonin, Salmon for Bioassay, distributed by the National Institute for Biological Standards and Control, Holly Hill, London.

Clinical Pharmacology: Calcitonin acts primarily on bone, but direct renal effects and actions on the gastrointestinal tract are also recognized. Salmon calcitonin appears to have actions essentially identical to calcitonins of mammalian origin, but its potency per mg is greater and it has a longer duration of action. The actions of calcitonin on bone and its role in normal human bone physiology are still incompletely understood.

Bone—Single injections of calcitonin cause a marked transient inhibition of the ongoing bone resorptive process. With prolonged use, there is a persistent, smaller decrease in the rate of bone resorption. Histologically this is associated with a decreased number of osteoclasts and an apparent decrease in their resorptive activity. Decreased osteocytic resorption may also be involved. There is some evidence that initially bone formation may be augmented by calcitonin through increased osteoblastic activity. However, calcitonin will probably not induce a long-term increase in bone formation.

Animal studies indicate that endogenous calcitonin, primarily through its action on bone, participates with parathyroid hormone in the homeostatic regulation of blood calcium. Thus, high blood calcium levels cause increased secretion of calcitonin which, in turn, inhibits bone resorption. This reduces the transfer of calcium from bone to blood and tends to return blood calcium to the normal level. The importance of this process in humans has not been determined. In normal adults, who have a relatively low rate of bone resorption, the administration of exogenous calcitonin results in only a slight decrease in serum calcium. In normal children and in patients with generalized Paget's disease, bone resorption is more rapid and decreases in serum calcium are more pronounced in response to calcitonin.

Paget's Disease of Bone (osteitis deformans)— Paget's disease is a disorder of uncertain etiology characterized by abnormal and accelerated bone formation and resorption in one or more bones. In most patients only small areas of bone are involved and the disease is not symptomatic. In a small fraction of patients, however, the abnormal bone may lead to bone pain and bone deformity, cranial and spinal nerve entrapment, or spinal cord compression. The increased vascularity of the abnormal bone may lead to high output congestive heart failure.

Active Paget's disease involving a large mass of bone may increase the urinary hydroxyproline excretion (reflecting breakdown of collagen-containing bone matrix) and serum alkaline phosphatase (reflecting increased bone formation).

Salmon calcitonin, presumably by an initial blocking effect on bone resorption, causes a decreased rate of bone turnover with a resultant fall in the serum alkaline phosphatase and urinary hydroxyproline excretion in approximately $2/3$ of patients treated. These biochemical changes appear to correspond to changes toward more normal bone, as evidenced by a small number of documented examples of: 1) radiologic regression of Pagetic lesions, 2) improvement of impaired auditory nerve and other neurologic function, 3) decreases (measured) in abnormally elevated cardiac output. These improvements occur extremely rarely, if ever, spontaneously (elevated cardiac output may disappear over a period of years when the disease slowly enters a sclerotic phase; in the cases treated with calcitonin, however, the decreases were seen in less than one year).

Some patients with Paget's disease who have good biochemical and/or symptomatic responses initially, later relapse. Suggested explanations have included the formation of neutralizing antibodies and the development of secondary hyperparathyroidism, but neither suggestion appears to explain adequately the majority of relapses.

Although the parathyroid hormone levels do appear to rise transiently during each hypocalcemic response to calcitonin, most investigators have been unable to demonstrate persistent hypersecretion of parathyroid hormone in patients treated chronically with calcitonin.

Circulating antibodies to calcitonin after 2–18 months' treatment have been reported in about half of the patients with Paget's disease in whom antibody studies were done, but calcitonin treatment remained effective in many of these cases. Occasionally patients with high antibody titers are found. These patients usually will have suffered a biochemical relapse of Paget's disease and are unresponsive to the acute hypocalcemic effects of calcitonin.

Hypercalcemia—In clinical trials, CALCIMAR® has been shown to lower the elevated serum calcium of patients with carcinoma (with or without demonstrated metastases), multiple myeloma or primary hyperparathyroidism (lesser response). Patients with higher values for serum calcium tend to show greater reduction during CALCIMAR® therapy. The decrease in calcium occurs about 2 hours after the first injection and lasts for about 6–8 hours. CALCIMAR® given every 12 hours maintained a calcium lowering effect for about 5–8 days, the time period evaluated for most patients during the clinical studies. The average reduction of 8-hour post-injection serum calcium during this period was about 9 percent.

Kidney—Calcitonin increases the excretion of filtered phosphate, calcium, and sodium by decreasing their tubular reabsorption. In some patients the inhibition of bone resorption by calcitonin is of such magnitude that the consequent reduction of filtered calcium load more than compensates for the decrease in tubular reabsorption of calcium. The result in these patients is a decrease rather than an increase in urinary calcium. Transient increases in sodium and water excretion may occur after the initial injection of calcitonin. In most patients these changes return to pre-treatment levels with continued therapy.

Gastrointestinal tract—Increasing evidence indicates that calcitonin has significant actions on the gastrointestinal tract. Short-term administration results in marked transient decreases in the volume and acidity of gastric juice and in the volume and the trypsin and amylase content of pancreatic juice. Whether these effects continue to be elicited after each injection of calcitonin during chronic therapy has not been investigated.

Metabolism—The metabolism of salmon calcitonin has not yet been studied clinically. Information from animal studies with salmon calcitonin and from clinical studies with calcitonins of porcine and human origin suggest that salmon calcitonin is rapidly metabolized by conversion to smaller inactive fragments, primarily in the kidneys, but also in the blood and peripheral tissues. A small amount of unchanged hormone and its inactive metabolites are excreted in the urine.

It appears that salmon calcitonin cannot cross the placental barrier and its passage to the cerebrospinal fluid or to breast milk has not been determined.

Indications and Usage: CALCIMAR® (Calcitonin-Salmon) is indicated for the treatment of symptomatic Paget's disease of bone and for the treatment of hypercalcemia.

Paget's Disease—At the present time effectiveness has been demonstrated principally in patients with moderate to severe disease characterized by polyostotic involvement with elevated serum alkaline phosphatase and urinary hydroxyproline excretion.

In these patients, the biochemical abnormalities were substantially improved (more than 30% reduction) in about $2/3$ of patients studied, and bone pain was improved in a similar fraction. A small number of documented instances of reversal of neurologic deficits has occurred, including improvement in the basilar compression syndrome, and improvement of spinal cord and spinal nerve lesions. At present there is too little experience to predict the likelihood of improvement of any given neurologic lesion. Hearing loss, the most common neurologic lesion of Paget's disease is improved infrequently (4 of 29 patients studied audiometrically).

Patients with increased cardiac output due to extensive Paget's disease have had measured decreases in cardiac output while receiving calcitonin. The number of treated patients in this category is still too small to predict how likely such a result will be.

The large majority of patients with localized, especially monostotic disease do not develop symptoms and most patients with mild symptoms can be managed with analgesics. There is no evidence that the prophylactic use of calcitonin is beneficial in asymptomatic patients, although treatment may be considered in exceptional circumstances in which there is extensive involvement of the skull or spinal cord with the possibility of irreversible neurologic damage. In these instances treatment would be based on the demonstrated effect of calcitonin on Pagetic bone, rather than on clinical studies in the patient population in question.

Hypercalcemia—CALCIMAR® (Calcitonin-Salmon) is indicated for early treatment of hypercalcemic emergencies, along with other appropriate agents, when a rapid decrease in serum calcium is required, until more specific treatment of the underlying disease can be accomplished. It may also be added to existing therapeutic regimens for hypercalcemia such as intravenous fluids and furosemide, oral phosphate or corticosteroids, or other agents.

Contraindications: Clinical allergy to synthetic salmon calcitonin.

Warnings:

Allergic Reactions

Because calcitonin is protein in nature, the possibility of a systemic allergic reaction cannot be overlooked. The usual provisions should be made for the emergency treatment of such a reaction should it occur. Patients with a positive skin test to CALCIMAR® were excluded from clinical trials. Skin testing should be considered prior to treatment with calcitonin, particularly for patients with suspected sensitivity to calcitonin. The following procedure is suggested: Prepare a dilution at 10 I.U. (MRC) per ml by withdrawing 1/20 ml (0.05 ml) in a tuberculin syringe and filling it to 1.0 ml with Sodium Chloride Injection, U.S.P. Mix well, discard 0.9 ml and inject intracutaneously 0.1 ml (approximately 1 I.U.) on the inner aspect of the forearm. Observe the injection site 15 minutes after injection. The appearance of more than mild erythema or wheal constitutes a positive response.

The incidence of osteogenic sarcoma is known to be increased in Paget's disease. Pagetic lesions, with or without therapy, may appear by x-ray to progress markedly, possibly with some loss of definition or periosteal margins. Such lesions should be evaluated carefully to differentiate these from osteogenic sarcoma.

Precautions:

1. General

The administration of calcitonin possibly could lead to hypocalcemic tetany under special circumstances although no cases have yet been reported. Provisions for parenteral calcium administration should be available during the first several administrations of calcitonin.

2. Laboratory Tests

Periodic examinations of urine sediment of patients on chronic therapy are recommended.

Coarse granular casts and casts containing renal tubular epithelial cells were reported in young adult volunteers at bed rest who were given salmon calcitonin to study the effect on immobilization osteoporosis. There was no other evidence of renal abnormality and the urine sediment became normal after calcitonin was stopped. Urine sediment abnormalities have not been reported by other investigators.

3. Instructions for the Patient

Careful instruction in sterile injection technique should be given to the patient, and to other persons who may administer CALCIMAR®.

4. Carcinogenesis

No long-term studies have been performed to evaluate carcinogenic potential of salmon calcitonin.

5. Pregnancy

Salmon calcitonin has been shown to cause decrease in fetal birth weights in rabbits when given in doses 14–56 times the dose recommended for human use. Since calcitonin does not cross the placental barrier, this finding may be due to metabolic effects of calcitonin on the pregnant animal. There are no studies in pregnant women. Salmon calcitonin should be used only when clearly needed in women who are or may become pregnant.

6. Nursing Mothers

It is not known whether this drug is excreted in human milk. As a general rule, nursing should not be undertaken while a patient is on this drug since many drugs are excreted in human milk. Calcitonin has been shown to inhibit lactation in animals.

7. Pediatric Use

Disorders of bone in children referred to as juvenile Paget's disease have been reported rarely. The relationship of these disorders to adult Paget's disease has not been established and experience with the use of calcitonin in these disorders is very limited. There are no adequate data to support the use of CALCIMAR® in children.

Adverse Reactions: Nausea with or without vomiting has been noted in about 10% of patients treated with calcitonin. It is most evident when treatment is first initiated and tends to decrease or disappear with continued administration.

Local inflammatory reactions at the site of subcutaneous or intramuscular injection have been reported in about 10% of patients. Flushing of face or hands occurred in about 2 to 5% of patients. Skin rashes have been reported occasionally.

Overdosage: A dose of 1000 I.U. (MRC) subcutaneously may produce nausea and vomiting as the only adverse effects. Doses of 32 units per kg per day for one or two days demonstrate no other adverse effects.

Data on chronic high dose administration are insufficient to judge toxicity.

Dosage and Administration:

Paget's Disease—The recommended starting dose of calcitonin in Paget's disease is 100 I.U. (MRC) (0.5 ml) per day administered subcutaneously (preferred for outpatient self-administration) or intramuscularly. Drug effect should be monitored by periodic measurement of serum alkaline phosphatase and 24-hour urinary hydroxyproline (if available) and evaluation of symptoms. A decrease to-

Continued on next page

USV—Cont.

ward normal of the biochemical abnormalities is usually seen, if it is going to occur, within the first few months. Bone pain may also decrease during that time. Improvement of neurologic lesions, when it occurs, requires a longer period of treatment, often more than one year.

In many patients doses of 50 I.U. (MRC) (0.25 ml) per day or every-other day are sufficient to maintain biochemical and clinical improvement. At the present time, however, there are insufficient data to determine whether this reduced dose will have the same effect as the higher dose on forming more normal bone structure. It appears preferable, therefore, to maintain the higher dose in any patient with serious deformity or neurological involvement.

In any patient with a good response initially who later relapses, either clinically or biochemically, the possibility of antibody formation should be explored. Although specialized tests for antibody titer are not widely available, the patients can be tested for high antibody titer as follows:

After overnight fasting, a sample of the patient's blood is taken for determination of serum calcium and 100 I.U. (MRC) of CALCIMAR® (Calcitonin-Salmon) are injected IM. The patient is then permitted to eat his usual breakfast. At 3 and 6 hours post-injection additional blood samples are drawn and the patient is released. The serum calcium values are then compared. A decrease of 0.5 mg % or more from fasting level at 3 and 6 hours is usually seen in the responsive patient. Decreases of 0.3 mg % or less constitute an inadequate response to calcitonin in the patient with active Paget's disease. If the hypocalcemic action of calcitonin is lost, further therapy with CALCIMAR® will not be effective. Patient compliance should also be assessed in the event of relapse.

In patients who relapse, whether because of antibodies or for unexplained reasons, a dosage increase beyond 100 I.U. (MRC) per day does not usually appear to elicit an improved response.

Hypercalcemia—The recommended starting dose of CALCIMAR® (Calcitonin-Salmon) in hypercalcemia is 4 I.U. (MRC)/kg body weight every 12 hours by subcutaneous or intramuscular injection. If the response to this dose is not satisfactory after one or two days, the dose may be increased to 8 I.U. (MRC)/kg every 12 hours. If the response remains unsatisfactory after two more days, the dose may be further increased to a maximum of 8 I.U. (MRC)/kg every 6 hours.

If the volume of CALCIMAR® (Calcitonin-Salmon) to be injected exceeds 2 ml, intramuscular injection is preferable and multiple sites of injection should be used.

How Supplied: CALCIMAR® Solution (Calcitonin-Salmon), USV is available as a sterile solution in 2 ml vials containing 200 I.U. (MRC) per ml.

STORE IN REFRIGERATOR—Between 2°–8° C (36°–46° F)

Revised: 12/82

Shown in Product Identification Section, page 440

CERESPAN® ℞
[sĕr'ĕs-păn"]
(papaverine HCl)
in sustained-release micro-dialysis cells

Composition: Each capsule provides 150 mg papaverine hydrochloride in micro-dialysis cells, uniquely processed for sustained release of medication to provide prolonged therapeutic effect.

Actions and Uses: The main actions of papaverine are exerted on cardiac and various smooth muscles. It relaxes the smooth musculature of the larger blood vessels, especially coronary, systemic peripheral, cerebral and pulmonary arteries. This relaxation may be prominent if spasm exists. The muscle cell is not paralyzed by papaverine, and still responds to drugs and other stimuli causing contraction. The antispasmodic effect is a direct one, and unrelated to muscle innervation. Papaverine is practically devoid of effects on the central nervous system.

Perhaps by its direct vasodilating action on cerebral blood vessels, papaverine increases cerebral blood flow and decreases cerebral vascular resistance in normal subjects; oxygen consumption is unaltered. These effects may explain the benefit reported from the drug in cerebral vascular encephalopathy.

Like quinidine, papaverine acts directly on heart muscle to depress conduction and prolong the refractory period. These direct actions provide the basis for its clinical trial in abrogating atrial and ventricular premature systoles and ominous ventricular arrhythmias.

The coronary vasodilator action could be an additional factor of therapeutic value when such rhythms are secondary to insufficiency or occlusion of the coronary arteries.

In patients with acute coronary thrombosis, the occurrence of ventricular rhythms is serious and requires measures designed to decrease myocardial irritability. Papaverine may have advantages over quinidine, used for a similar purpose, in that it may be given in an emergency by the intravenous route, does not depress myocardial contraction or cause cinchonism, and produces coronary vasodilation.

Indications: For the relief of cerebral and peripheral ischemia associated with arterial spasm and myocardial ischemia complicated by arrhythmias.

Precautions: Use with caution in patients with glaucoma. Hepatic hypersensitivity has been reported with gastrointestinal symptoms, jaundice, eosinophilia and altered liver function tests. Discontinue drug if these occur.

Side Effects: Although occurring rarely, the reported side effects of papaverine include nausea, abdominal distress, anorexia, constipation or diarrhea, skin rash, malaise, drowsiness, vertigo, sweating, and headache.

Administration and Dosage: One capsule every 12 hours. In difficult cases administration may be increased to one capsule every 8 hours, or two capsules every 12 hours.

How Supplied: Bottles of 100 and 1000.
Revised: June, 1983

DDAVP® ℞
(desmopressin acetate)

Description: DDAVP (desmopressin acetate) is a hormone affecting renal water conservation and a synthetic analogue of 8-arginine vasopressin. It is chemically defined as follows: Mol. wt. 1183.2. 1-(3-mercaptopropionic acid)-8-D-arginine vasopressin monoacetate (salt) trihydrate.

DDAVP (desmopressin acetate) is provided as a sterile, aqueous solution for intranasal use.
Each ml contains:

Desmopressin acetate   0.1 mg
Chlorobutanol   5.0 mg
Sodium chloride   9.0 mg
Hydrochloric acid to adjust pH to approximately 4

Clinical Pharmacology: DDAVP (desmopressin acetate) contains as active substance 1-(3-mercaptopropionic acid)-8-D-arginine vasopressin, which is a synthetic analogue of the natural hormone arginine vasopressin. One ml (0.1 mg) of DDAVP (desmopressin acetate) has an antidiuretic activity of about 400 IU as compared with arginine vasopressin.

1. The biphasic half-lives for DDAVP (desmopressin acetate) were 7.8 and 75.5 minutes for the fast and slow phases, compared with 2.5 and 14.5 minutes for lysine vasopressin. As a result, DDAVP (desmopressin acetate) provides a prompt onset of antidiuretic action with a long duration after each administration.

2. The change in structure of arginine vasopressin to DDAVP (desmopressin acetate) has resulted in a decreased vasopressor action and decreased actions on visceral smooth muscle relative to the enhanced antidiuretic activity, so that clinically effective antidiuretic doses are usually below threshold levels for effects on vascular or visceral smooth muscle.

Indications and Usage: DDAVP (desmopressin acetate) is indicated as replacement therapy in the management of central diabetes insipidus and for management of the temporary polyuria and polydipsia following head trauma or surgery in the pituitary region. It is ineffective for the treatment of nephrogenic diabetes insipidus.

The use of DDAVP (desmopressin acetate) in patients with an established diagnosis will result in a reduction in urinary output with increase in urine osmolality and a decrease in plasma osmolality. This will allow the resumption of a more normal life style with a decrease in urinary frequency and nocturia.

There are reports of an occasional change in response with time, usually greater than 6 months. Some patients may show a decreased responsiveness, others a shortened duration of effect. There is no evidence this effect is due to the development of binding antibodies but may be due to a local inactivation of the peptide.

Patients are selected for therapy by establishing the diagnosis by means of the water deprivation test, the hypertonic saline infusion test, and/or the response to antidiuretic hormone. Continued response to DDAVP (desmopressin acetate) can be monitored by urine volume and osmolality.

Contraindications: Hypersensitivity to DDAVP (desmopressin acetate).

Warnings: 1. For intranasal use only.
2. In very young and elderly patients in particular, fluid intake should be adjusted in order to decrease the potential occurrence of water intoxication and hyponatremia.

Precautions:

General: DDAVP (desmopressin acetate) at high dosage has infrequently produced a slight elevation of blood pressure, which disappeared with a reduction in dosage. The drug should be used with caution in patients with coronary artery insufficiency and/or hypertensive cardiovascular disease.

Since DDAVP (desmopressin acetate) is used intranasally, changes in the nasal mucosa such as scarring, edema, or other disease may cause erratic, unreliable absorption in which case intranasal DDAVP (desmopressin acetate) should not be used.

Laboratory Tests: Laboratory tests for following the patient include urine volume and osmolality. In some cases plasma osmolality may be required.

Drug Interactions: Although the pressor activity of DDAVP (desmopressin acetate) is very low compared to the antidiuretic activity, use of large doses of DDAVP (desmopressin acetate) with other pressor agents should only be done with careful patient monitoring.

Carcinogenesis, Mutagenesis, Impairment of Fertility: Teratology studies in rats have shown no abnormalities. No further information is available.

Pregnancy—Category B: Reproduction studies performed in rats and rabbits with doses up to 12.5 times the human intranasal dose (i.e. about 125 times the total adult human dose given systemically) have revealed no evidence of a harmful action of DDAVP (desmopressin acetate) on the fetus. There are several publications of management of diabetes insipidus in pregnant women with no harm to the fetus reported, however no controlled studies in pregnant women have been carried out. Published reports stress that, as opposed to preparations containing the natural hormones, DDAVP (desmopressin acetate) in antidiuretic doses has no uterotonic action, but the physician will have to weigh possible therapeutic advantages against possible dangers in each individual case.

Nursing Mothers: There have been no controlled studies in nursing mothers. A single study in a post-partum woman demonstrated a marked change in plasma, but little if any change in assayable DDAVP in breast milk following an intranasal dose of 10 mg.

Pediatric Use: DDAVP (desmopressin acetate) has been used in children with diabetes insipidus. The dose must be individually adjusted to the patient with attention in the very young to the danger of an extreme decrease in plasma osmolality with resulting convulsions. Dose should start at 0.05 ml or less.

Adverse Reactions: Infrequently, high dosages have produced transient headache and nausea. Nasal congestion, rhinitis and flushing have also been reported occasionally along with mild abdominal cramps. These symptoms disappeared with reduction in dosage.

Overdosage: See adverse reactions above. In case of overdosage, the dose should be reduced, frequency of administration decreased, or the drug withdrawn according to the severity of the condition.

There is no known specific antidote for DDAVP. If considerable fluid retention is causing concern, a saluretic such as furosemide may induce a diuresis.

An oral LD_{50} has not been established. An intravenous dose of 2 mg/kg in mice demonstrated no effect.

Dosage and Administration: This drug is administered into the nose through a soft, flexible plastic nasal tube which has four graduation marks on it that measure 0.2, 0.15, 0.1 and 0.05 ml. DDAVP (desmopressin acetate) dosage must be determined for each individual patient and adjusted according to the diurnal pattern of response. Response should be estimated by two parameters: adequate duration of sleep and adequate, not excessive, water turnover. Patients with nasal congestion and blockage have often responded well to DDAVP (desmopressin acetate). The usual dose range in adults is 0.1 to 0.4 ml daily, either as a single dose or divided into two or three doses. Most adults require 0.2 ml daily in two divided doses. The morning and evening doses should be separately adjusted for an adequate diurnal rhythm of water turnover. For children aged 3 months to 12 years, the usual dosage range is 0.05 to 0.3 ml daily, either as a single dose or divided into two doses.

About $1/4$ to $1/3$ of patients can be controlled by a single daily dose.

How Supplied: 2.5 ml per vial, packaged with two applicator tubes per carton. Keep refrigerated at about 4°C. When travelling—controlled room temperature (22°C) closed sterile bottles will maintain stability for 3 weeks.

Manufactured for USV Laboratories, Division USV Pharmaceutical Corp., Tarrytown, NY 10591, by Ferring Phatmaceuticals, Malmö, Sweden.

Revised: March, 1983
Shown in Product Identification Section, page 440

DDAVP® INJECTION ℞
(desmopressin acetate)

Description: DDAVP® Injection (desmopressin acetate) is an antidiuretic hormone affecting renal water conservation and is a synthetic analogue of 8-arginine vasopressin. It is chemically defined as follows:

Mol. Wt. 1183.2

Empirical Formula: $C_{48}H_{74}N_{14}O_{17}S_2$

SCH$_2$CH$_2$CO-Tyr-Phe-Gln-Asn-Cys-Pro-D-Arg-

Gly-NH$_2 \cdot C_2H_4O_2 \cdot 3H_2O$

1-(3-mercaptopropionic acid)-8-D-arginine vasopressin mono-acetate (salt) trihydrate.

DDAVP® Injection is provided as a sterile, aqueous solution for injection.

Each ml provides:
Desmopressin acetate   4.0 mcg
Chlorobutanol   5.0 mg
Sodium chloride   9.0 mg
Hydrochloric acid to adjust pH to 3.5.

Clinical Pharmacology: DDAVP® Injection contains as active substance, 1-(3-mercaptopropionic acid)-8-D-arginine vasopressin, a synthetic analogue of the natural hormone arginine vasopressin. One ml (4 mcg) of DDAVP (desmopressin acetate) solution has an antidiuretic activity of about 16 IU; 1 mcg of DDAVP is equivalent to 4 IU. DDAVP has been shown to be more potent than arginine vasopressin in increasing plasma levels of factor VIII activity in patients with hemophilia and von Willebrand's disease Type I.

Dose-response studies were performed in healthy persons, using doses of 0.1 to 0.4 mcg/kg body weight, infused over a 10-minute period. Maximal dose response occurred at 0.3 to 0.4 mcg/kg. The response to DDAVP of factor VIII activity and plasminogen activator is dose-related, with maximal plasma levels of 300 to 400 percent of initial concentrations obtained after infusion of 0.4 mcg/kg body weight. The increase is rapid and evident within 30 minutes, reaching a maximum at a point ranging from 90 minutes to two hours. The factor VIII related antigen and ristocetin cofactor activity were also increased to a smaller degree, but still dose-dependent.

1. The biphasic half-lives of DDAVP were 7.8 and 75.5 minutes for the fast and slow phases, respectively compared with 2.5 and 14.5 minutes for lysine vasopressin, another form of the hormone. As a result, DDAVP (desmopressin acetate) provides a prompt onset of antidiuretic action with a long duration after each administration.
2. The change in structure of arginine vasopressin to DDAVP has resulted in a decreased vasopressor action and decreased actions on visceral smooth muscle relative to the enhanced antidiuretic activity, so that clinically effective antidiuretic doses are usually below threshold levels for effects on vascular or visceral smooth muscle.
3. When administered by injection, DDAVP has an antidiuretic effect about ten times that of an equivalent dose administered intranasally.
4. The bioavailability of the subcutaneous route of administration was determined qualitatively using urine output data. The exact fraction of drug absorbed by that route of administration has not been quantitatively determined.
5. The percentage increase of factor VIII levels in patients with mild hemophilia A and von Willebrand's disease was not significantly different from that observed in normal healthy individuals when treated with 0.3 mcg/kg of DDAVP infused over 10 minutes.
6. Plasminogen activator activity increases rapidly after DDAVP infusion, but there has been no clinically significant fibrinolysis in patients treated with DDAVP.
7. The effect of repeated DDAVP administration when doses were given every 12 to 24 hours has generally shown a gradual diminution of the factor VIII activity increase noted with a single dose. The initial response is reproducible in any particular patient if there are 2 or 3 days between administrations.

Indications and Usage:
Diabetes Insipidus
DDAVP® Injection is indicated as antidiuretic replacement therapy in the management of central (cranial) diabetes insipidus and for the management of the temporary polyuria following head trauma or surgery in the pituitary region. DDAVP is ineffective for the treatment of nephrogenic diabetes insipidus.

DDAVP is also available as an intranasal preparation. However, this means of delivery can be compromised by a variety of factors that can make nasal insufflation ineffective or inappropriate. These include poor intranasal absorption, nasal congestion and blockage, nasal discharge, atrophy of nasal mucosa, and severe atrophic rhinitis. Intranasal delivery may be inappropriate where there is an impaired level of consciousness. In addition, cranial surgical procedures, such as transphenoidal hypophysectomy, create situations where an alternative route of administration is needed as in cases of nasal packing or recovery from surgery.

Hemophilia A
DDAVP® Injection is indicated for patients with hemophilia A with factor VIII coagulant activity levels greater than 5%.
DDAVP will often maintain hemostasis in patients with hemophilia A during surgical procedures and postoperatively when administered 30 minutes prior to scheduled procedure.

DDAVP will also stop bleeding in hemophilia A patients with episodes of spontaneous or trauma-induced injuries such as hemarthroses, intramuscular hematomas or mucosal bleeding.

DDAVP is not indicated for the treatment of hemophilia A with factor VIII coagulant activity levels equal to or less than 5%, or for the treatment of hemophilia B, or in patients who have factor VIII antibodies.

In certain clinical situations, it may be justified to try DDAVP in patients with factor VIII levels between 2–5%; however, these patients should be carefully monitored.

Von Willebrand's Disease (Type I)
DDAVP® Injection is indicated for patients with mild to moderate classic von Willebrand's disease (Type I) with factor VIII levels greater than 5%. DDAVP will often maintain hemostasis in patients with mild to moderate von Willebrand's disease during surgical procedures and postoperatively when administered 30 minutes prior to the scheduled procedure.

DDAVP will usually stop bleeding in mild to moderate von Willebrand's patients with episodes of spontaneous or trauma-induced injuries such as hemarthroses, intramuscular hematomas or mucosal bleeding.

Those von Willebrand's disease patients who are least likely to respond are those with severe homozygous von Willebrand's disease with factor VIII coagulant activity and factor VIII von Willebrand factor antigen levels less than 1%. Other patients may respond in a variable fashion depending on the type of molecular defect they have. Bleeding time and factor VIII coagulant activity, ristocetin cofactor activity, and von Willebrand factor antigen should be checked during administration of DDAVP to ensure that adequate levels are being achieved.

DDAVP is not indicated for the treatment of severe classic von Willebrand's disease (Type I) and when there is evidence of an abnormal molecular form of factor VIII antigen. See WARNING.

Contraindication: Known hypersensitivity to DDAVP.

Warning: Patients who do not have need of antidiuretic hormone for its antidiuretic effect, in particular those who are young or elderly, should be cautioned to ingest only enough fluid to satisfy thirst, in order to decrease the potential occurrence of water intoxication and hyponatremia. DDAVP should not be used to treat patients with Type IIB von Willebrand's disease since platelet aggregation may be induced.

Precautions:
GENERAL: For injection use only.
DDAVP® Injection (desmopressin acetate) has infrequently produced a slight elevation of blood pressure, which disappeared with a reduction in dosage. The drug should be used with caution in patients with coronary artery insufficiency and/or hypertensive cardiovascular disease, because of possible rise in blood pressure.

Severe allergic reactions have not been reported with DDAVP® Injection (desmopressin acetate). It is not known whether antibodies to DDAVP® Injection (desmopressin acetate) are produced after repeated injections.

Diabetes Insipidus
Laboratory tests for monitoring the patient include urine volume and osmolality. In some cases, plasma osmolality may be required.

Hemophilia A
Laboratory tests for assessing patient status include levels of factor VIII coagulant, factor VIII antigen and factor VIII ristocetin cofactor (von Willebrand factor) as well as activated partial thromboplastin time. Factor VIII coagulant activity should be determined before giving DDAVP for hemostasis. If factor VIII coagulant activity is present at less than 5% of normal, DDAVP should not be relied on.

Continued on next page

USV—Cont.

Von Willebrand's Disease
Laboratory tests for assessing patient status include levels of factor VIII coagulant activity, factor VIII ristocetin cofactor activity, and factor VIII von Willebrand factor antigen. The skin bleeding time may be helpful in following these patients.

DRUG INTERACTIONS: Although the pressor activity of DDAVP is very low compared with the antidiuretic activity, use of doses as large as 0.3 mcg/kg of DDAVP with other pressor agents should be done only with careful patient monitoring.

DDAVP has been used with epsilon aminocaproic acid without adverse effects.

CARCINOGENICITY, MUTAGENICITY, IMPAIRMENT OF FERTILITY: Teratology studies in rats have shown no abnormalities. No further data are available.

PREGNANCY CATEGORY B: Reproduction studies performed in rats and rabbits with subcutaneous doses up to 12.5 times the human dose when used for factor VIII stimulation and 125 times the human dose when used in diabetes insipidus have revealed no evidence of harm to the fetus due to DDAVP. There are several publications of management of diabetes insipidus in pregnant women with no harm to the fetus reported; however, there are no adequate and well-controlled studies in pregnant women. Published reports stress that, as opposed to preparations containing the natural hormones, DDAVP in antidiuretic doses has no uterotonic action, but the physician will have to weigh possible therapeutic advantages against possible danger in each case.

NURSING MOTHERS: It is not known whether this drug is excreted in human milk. Because many drugs are excreted in human milk, caution should be exercised when DDAVP is administered to a nursing woman.

PEDIATRIC USE: Use in infants and children will require careful fluid intake restriction to prevent possible hyponatremia and water intoxication. *DDAVP® Injection should not be used in infants younger than three months* in the treatment of hemophilia A or von Willebrand's disease; safety and effectiveness in children under 12 years of age with diabetes insipidus have not been established.

Adverse Reactions: Infrequently, DDAVP has produced transient headache, nausea, mild abdominal cramps and vulval pain. These symptoms disappeared with reduction in dosage. Occasionally, injection of DDAVP has produced local erythema, swelling or burning pain. Occasional facial flushing has been reported with the administration of DDAVP.

DDAVP has infrequently produced a slight elevation of blood pressure, which disappeared with a reduction in dosage.

See WARNING for the possibility of water intoxication and hyponatremia.

Overdosage: See ADVERSE REACTIONS above. In case of overdosage, the dosage should be reduced, frequency of administration decreased, or the drug withdrawn according to the severity of the condition.

There is no known specific antidote for DDAVP. If considerable fluid retention causes concern, a saluretic may induce a diuresis.

An oral LD$_{50}$ has not been established. An intravenous dose of 2 mg/kg in mice demonstrated no effect.

Dosage and Administration:
Diabetes Insipidus
This formulation is administered subcutaneously or by direct intravenous injection. DDAVP® Injection (desmopressin acetate) dosage must be determined for each patient and adjusted according to the pattern of response. Response should be estimated by two parameters: adequate duration of sleep and adequate, not excessive, water turnover.

The usual dosage range in adults is 0.5 ml (2.0 mcg) to 1 ml (4.0 mcg) daily, administered intravenously or subcutaneously, usually in two divided doses. The morning and evening doses should be separately adjusted for an adequate diurnal rhythm of water turnover. For patients who have been controlled on intranasal DDAVP and who must be switched to the injection form, either because of poor intranasal absorption or because of the need for surgery, the comparable antidiuretic dose of the injection is about one-tenth the intranasal dose.

Hemophilia A and von Willebrand's Disease (Type I)
DDAVP® Injection is administered as an intravenous infusion at a dose of 0.3 mcg DDAVP/kg body weight diluted in sterile physiological saline and infused slowly over 15 to 30 minutes. In adults and children weighing more than 10 kg, 50 ml of diluent is used; in children weighing 10 kg or less, 10 ml of diluent is used. Blood pressure and pulse should be monitored during infusion. If DDAVP® Injection is used preoperatively, it should be administered 30 minutes prior to the scheduled procedure.

The necessity for repeat administration of DDAVP or use of any blood products for hemostasis should be determined by laboratory response as well as the clinical condition of the patient. The tendency toward tachyphylaxis (lessening of response) with repeated administration given more frequently than every 48 hours should be considered in treating each patient.

Parenteral drug products should be inspected visually for particulate matter and discoloration prior to administration whenever solution and container permit.

How Supplied: DDAVP® Injection (desmopressin acetate) is available as a sterile solution in cartons of ten 1 ml single-dose ampules (NDC 0075-2451-01) each containing 4.0 mcg DDAVP® per ml. Keep refrigerated at about 4°C.

CAUTION: Federal (USA) law prohibits dispensing without prescription.

Manufactured for USV Laboratories, Division USV Pharmaceutical Corp., Tarrytown, NY 10591, USA By Ferring Pharmaceuticals, Malmö, Sweden

Revised: February, 1984
Shown in Product Identification Section, page 440

DEMI–REGROTON®
[děm″ē-rĕg′rō-tŏn]
Oral antihypertensive

See under Regroton®.

DORIDEN®
[dôr′ĭ-dĭn″]
glutethimide USP

0.5 g tablets
0.25 g tablets

Description: DORIDEN (glutethimide), an oral hypnotic, is a piperidinedione derivative that occurs as a white, crystalline powder and is practically insoluble in water, soluble in alcohol. Its chemical name is 2-ethyl-2-phenylglutarimide.

Clinical Pharmacology: Doriden is erratically absorbed from the gastrointestinal tract. Following single oral doses of 500 mg, wide variations in absorption of the drug were observed, and the peak plasma concentration occurred from one to six hours after administration. The average plasma half-life is 10–12 hours. Glutethimide is a racemate; both isomers are hydroxylated; the d-isomer on the piperidinedione ring and the l-isomer on the phenyl substituent. Both hydroxylates are conjugated with glucuronic acid; the glucuronides pass into the enterohepatic circulation, and thence are excreted in the urine. Less than 2% of a usual dose is excreted in the urine unchanged. About 50% of the drug is bound to plasma proteins.

Glutethimide exhibits pronounced anticholinergic activity, which is manifested by mydriasis, inhibition of salivary secretions, and decreased intestinal motility.

Indications and Usage: Glutethimide has been shown to be effective as a hypnotic for three to seven days. It is not indicated for chronic administration. Should insomnia persist, a drug-free interval of one or more weeks should elapse before retreatment is considered. Attempts should be made to find alternative nondrug therapy in chronic insomnia.

Contraindications: Glutethimide is contraindicated in patients with known hypersensitivity to the drug. It is also contraindicated in patients with porphyria.

Warnings: The concomitant use of alcohol or other CNS depressants may produce additive CNS depressant effects.

Precautions:
Information for Patients: The patient should be warned about the possible additive effects when glutethimide is taken concomitantly with other central nervous system depressants such as alcohol.

The patient on Doriden must be warned against driving a car or operating dangerous machinery while on the drug, since glutethimide may impair the ability to perform hazardous activities requiring mental alertness or physical coordination.

Drug Interactions: Glutethimide induces hepatic microsomal enzymes resulting in increased metabolism of coumarin anticoagulants and decreased anticoagulant response.

Carcinogenesis: No carcinogenicity studies in animals have been performed.

Pregnancy/Teratogenic Effects: *Pregnancy Category C.* Animal reproduction studies have not been conducted with glutethimide. It is also not known *whether glutethimide can cause fetal harm when administered to a pregnant woman or can affect reproduction capacity. Glutethimide should be given to a pregnant woman only if clearly needed.*

Nursing Mothers: Because of the potential for serious adverse reactions in nursing infants from glutethimide, a decision should be made whether to discontinue nursing or to discontinue the drug, taking into account the importance of the drug to the mother.

Pediatric Use: Glutethimide is not recommended for use in children, because its safety and effectiveness in the pediatric age group have not been established by clinical trials.

Adverse Reactions: In clinical studies in more than 796 patients 8.6% exhibited skin rash, 2.7% reported nausea, 1.1% hangover, and 1% reported drowsiness. The following reactions occurred in less than 1% of the patient population: vertigo, headache, depression, dizziness, ataxia, confusion, edema, indigestion, lightheadedness, nocturnal diaphoresis, vomiting, dry mouth, euphoria, impaired memory, slurred speech, and tinnitus. Paradoxical excitation, blurred vision, acute hypersensitivity, porphyria, and blood dyscrasia such as thrombocytopenic purpura, aplastic anemia, and leukopenia are rare.

In cases in which a generalized skin rash occurs, the medication should be withdrawn. This rash usually clears spontaneously within a few days after drug withdrawal.

Drug Abuse and Dependence:
Controlled Substance: This drug is controlled in Schedule III.

Dependence: Both physical and psychological dependence have occurred; therefore patients should be carefully evaluated before prescribing Doriden (glutethimide). Ordinarily, an amount adequate for one week is sufficient. The patient should be reevaluated before represcribing, after an interval of one or more weeks. Withdrawal symptoms include nausea, abdominal discomfort, tremors, convulsions, and delirium. Newborn infants of mothers dependent on glutethimide may also exhibit withdrawal symptoms. In the presence of dependence dosage should be reduced gradually.

Overdosage:
Acute Overdosage: The single acute lethal dose of glutethimide in humans ranges from 10 g to 20 g. Although the majority of fatalities have resulted from single doses in this range, patients have died from single doses as low as 5 g and have recovered from single doses as high as 35 g. A single oral dose of 5 g usually produces severe intoxication. A plasma level of 3 mg/100 ml is indicative

of severe poisoning, but the level may be higher if the patient is tolerant to the drug. However, the level may also be lower because of sequestration of the drug in body fat depots and in the gastrointestinal tract. A lower level does not preclude the possibility of severe poisoning; therefore, the extent of intoxication may not be accurately reflected by single glutethimide plasma level determinations. Serial determinations are mandatory for proper patient evaluation.

Ingestion of acutely excessive dosage of glutethimide can give rise to a life-threatening situation. The effects of glutethimide are exaggerated by concomitant ingestion of other hypnotics or sedatives such as alcohol, barbiturates, etc., and suicidal effects commonly involve multiple drugs of the sedative-hypnotic-tranquilizer types.

Signs and Symptoms: The principal signs and symptoms caused by glutethimide intoxication vary in severity in ratio to the ingested dosage, in general, and are indistinguishable from those caused by barbiturate intoxication. The degree of CNS depression often fluctuates, possibly due to irregular absorption of the drug and/or accumulation of an active toxic metabolite, 4-hydroxy-2-ethyl-2-phenyl-glutarimide (4-HG). They are: CNS depression, including coma *(profound and prolonged in severe intoxication);* hypothermia, which may be followed by fever even without apparent infection; depressed or lost deep tendon reflexes; depression or absence of corneal and pupillary reflexes; dilation of pupils; depressed or absent response to painful stimuli; inadequate ventilation (even with relatively normal respiratory rate), sometimes with cyanosis; sudden apnea, especially with manipulation such as gastric lavage or endotracheal intubation; diminished or absent peristalsis. Severe hypotension unresponsive to volume expansion, tonic muscular spasms, twitching and convulsions may occur.

Treatment: As with all forms of acute intoxication, the sooner adequate treatment is instituted, the better the prognosis. Early and vigorous cardiopulmonary supportive measures should be employed and should include:
1) Maintenance of a patent airway with assisted ventilation if necessary.
2) Monitoring of vital signs and level of consciousness.
3) Continuous electrocardiogram to detect arrhythmias.
4) Maintenance of blood pressure with plasma volume expanders and, if absolutely essential, pressor drugs.

Blood for glutethimide levels and other chemical determinations should be obtained as well as arterial blood for blood gas determinations.

Vomiting should be induced if the patient is fully conscious. Gastric lavage should be done in all cases regardless of elapsed time since drug ingestion, with due caution to prevent aspiration of gastric contents or respiratory arrest during manipulation, including prior insertion of a cuffed endotracheal tube or employment of tracheostomy. Lavage with a 1:1 mixture of castor oil and water is capable of removing larger amounts of glutethimide from the stomach than with aqueous lavage. Fifty ml. of castor oil should be left in the stomach as a cathartic.

Intestinal lavage is used to remove unabsorbed Doriden (glutethimide) from the intestines (100–250 ml of 20–40% sorbitol or mannitol). If emesis or gastric lavage cannot be effected in the fully conscious patient, delay absorption of Doriden by giving one pint of water, milk or fruit juice; flour or cornstarch suspension, or activated charcoal in water. Follow up as soon as possible with production of emesis or gastric lavage.

Adequate respiratory gas exchange must be maintained and may require tracheostomy and mechanical assistance. If coma is prolonged, urine output must be monitored and maintained while preventing overhydration which might contribute to pulmonary or cerebral edema.

In *Severe Intoxication,* in addition to intensive supportive measures and symptomatic care, consideration should be given to dialysis or hemoperfusion in the following circumstances: Grade III or Grade IV coma, but the level of coma per se is not a mandatory indication for the procedure. Hemodialysis may also be required when renal shutdown or impaired renal function are manifest and in life-threatening overdose situations complicated by (a) pulmonary edema, (b) heart failure, (c) circulatory collapse, (d) significant liver disease, (e) major metabolic disturbance, (f) uremia. While aqueous hemodialysis is less effective for glutethimide than for readily water-soluble compounds that are not bound by proteins or sequestered in body fat depots, glutethimide blood levels may decline more rapidly with hemodialysis and the duration of coma may be shortened; efficacy of the procedure, however, is largely controversial. As long as significant amounts of glutethimide remain in fat depots or as an unabsorbed bolus in the intestinal tract, the fall in serum level accelerated by hemodialysis may be followed by increased absorption into the bloodstream on termination of dialysis and may require further dialysis.

Recent clinical data indicate that use of pure food-grade soybean oil as the dialysate enhances removal of glutethimide and some other lipidsoluble substances by means of hemodialysis. Peritoneal dialysis, while able to remove some glutethimide, apparently is of minimal value.

Hemoperfusion appears to be a promising technique for eliminating glutethimide from the body. Charcoal hemoperfusion utilizing acrylic hydrogel microencapsulated of activated charcoal has been reported to be simpler and more effective than hemodialysis. Similarly, a microcapsule artificial kidney has been developed utilizing activated charcoal granules encapsulated with cellulose nitrate and albumin. *Resin* hemoperfusion utilizing a column containing Amerberlite XAD-2 has demonstrated exceptionally high clearance capabilities in glutethimide intoxication and has been reported to be clinically superior to hemodialysis in patients with profound life-threatening coma and potentially lethal blood concentrations of intoxicant drugs.

Drug extraction techniques should be continued for at least two hours after the patient regains consciousness. Glutethimide is highly lipid soluble and therefore, rapidly accumulated in lipid tissue. As the drug is removed from the bloodstream by any technique, it is gradually released from fat storage depots back into the bloodstream. Even after substantial quantities of the drug have been extracted, this blood-level rebound can cause coma to persist or recur.

As in the case of any prolonged coma, appropriate antibiotic therapy is indicated if pulmonary or other infection intervenes.

Chronic Overdosage: Signs and symptoms of chronic glutethimide intoxication (and for all drugs producing barbiturate-alcohol type of dependence in chronic overdosage) include impairment of memory and ability to concentrate, impaired gait, ataxia, tremors, hyporeflexia, and slurring of speech. Abrupt discontinuance of glutethimide after prolonged overdosage will in most cases cause withdrawal reactions ranging from nervousness and anxiety to grand mal seizures, and may include abdominal cramping, chills, numbness of extremities and dysphagia.

Treatment: Chronic glutethimide intoxication may be treated by gradual, stepwise reduction of dosage over a period of days or weeks. Watch patient carefully. If withdrawal reactions occur, they can be controlled by readministration of glutethimide, or substitution of pentobarbital, and subsequent gradual withdrawal.

Dosage and Administration: For use as a hypnotic, dosage should be individualized. The usual adult dosage is 0.25 to 0.5 g at bedtime. For elderly or debilitated patients, the initial daily dosage should not exceed 0.5 g at bedtime, in order to avoid oversedation.

How Supplied: DORIDEN (glutethimide). Tablets, 0.5 g (white, scored); bottles of 100 (NDC 0105-0354-00), 500 (NDC 0105-0354-05), 1000 (NDC 0105-0354-99) and Strip Dispensers of 100 (NDC 0105-0354-61). Tablets, 0.25 g (white, scored); bottles of 100 (NDC 0105-0353-00).

Revised: 5/82

HISTASPAN-D® ℞
[hĭst'ŭ-spăn-dē"]
in sustained-release micro-dialysis cells

Composition: Each Histaspan-D capsule provides 8 mg chlorpheniramine maleate, 20 mg phenylephrine hydrochloride, and 2.5 mg methscopolamine nitrate in sustained-release micro-dialysis cells, uniquely processed for sustained release of medication to provide prolonged therapeutic effect.

Action: Histaspan-D combines the highly effective and widely used antihistamine, chlorpheniramine maleate, with a decongestant, phenylephrine hydrochloride, and a drying agent, methscopolamine nitrate, for relief of rhinorrhea, sneezing, lacrimation, nasal congestion, and other respiratory symptoms accompanying the common cold, sinusitis, hay fever and similar allergic conditions. Prolonged therapeutic effect is obtained by sustained release of medication through the micro-dialysis process.

Indications: One capsule q. 12 h. usually provides relief of rhinorrhea, sneezing, lacrimation, itching of eyes and nose, and nasal congestion accompanying upper respiratory infections such as the common cold and sinusitis; and hay fever and similar allergic conditions.

Contraindications: Hypersensitivity to any component of the drug, glaucoma, paralytic ileus, pyloric obstruction and prostatic hypertrophy.

Precautions: Use with caution in diabetes mellitus, hyperthyroidism, hypertension, cardiovascular disease, debilitated patients with chronic lung disease, in the aged and in children under age 12. Since blurred vision, drowsiness and dizziness may occur, patients should be cautioned about driving or operating machinery.

Adverse Reactions: May include drowsiness, dizziness, blurred vision, and excessive dryness of the nose, throat and mouth. Other possible adverse reactions to individual components, infrequently seen, include photophobia, tachycardia, gastrointestinal symptoms, increased irritability or excitement, flushing, incoordination, headache, nervousness, weakness and urinary disturbances.

Administration and Dosage: Adults and children over age 12, one capsule in the morning and one at night (q. 12 h.).

How Supplied: Bottles of 100 and 1000 capsules.
Issued: 6/83

HISTASPAN®-PLUS ℞
[hĭst'ŭ-spăn-plŭs"]
in sustained-release micro-dialysis cells

Composition: Each Histaspan-Plus capsule provides 8 mg chlorpheniramine maleate and 20 mg phenylephrine hydrochloride in sustained-release micro-dialysis cells, uniquely processed for sustained release of medication to provide prolonged therapeutic effect.

Indications: Antihistaminic and decongestant for relief of nasal congestion and other respiratory symptoms accompanying the common cold, sinusitis, hay fever and similar allergic conditions.

Contraindication: Hypersensitivity to any component of the drug.

Precautions: Use with caution in diabetes mellitus, hyperthyroidism, hypertension and cardiovascular disease. Since blurred vision, drowsiness or dizziness may occur, patients should be cautioned about driving or operating machinery.

Adverse Reactions: May include drowsiness, dizziness, blurred vision, dry mouth, disturbed coordination, G.I. disturbance, tachycardia, headache, nervousness, weakness and urinary disturbances.

Dosage: Adults and children over age 12, one capsule every 12 hours.

How Supplied: Bottles of 100.
7/83

Continued on next page

USV—Cont.

HYGROTON® ℞
[hĭ'grō-tŏn"]
(chlorthalidone USP)
Oral antihypertensive-diuretic

Composition: Each tablet provides 25 mg, 50 mg or 100 mg chlorthalidone.

Description: Hygroton is a monosulfamyl diuretic which differs chemically from thiazide diuretics in that a double-ring system is incorporated in its structure. Chlorthalidone is practically insoluble in water, in ether, and in chloroform; soluble in methanol; slightly soluble in alcohol.

Actions: Hygroton is an oral diuretic with prolonged action (48-72 hours) and low toxicity. The diuretic effect of the drug occurs within two hours of an oral dose and continues for up to 72 hours. It produces copious diuresis with greatly increased excretion of sodium and chloride. At maximal therapeutic dosage, chlorthalidone is approximately equal in its diuretic effect to comparable maximal therapeutic doses of benzothiadiazine diuretics. The site of action appears to be the cortical diluting segment of the ascending limb of Henle's loop of the nephron.

Indications: Diuretics such as Hygroton are indicated in the management of hypertension either as the sole therapeutic agent or to enhance the effect of other antihypertensive drugs in the more severe forms of hypertension.

Hygroton is indicated as adjunctive therapy in edema associated with congestive heart failure, hepatic cirrhosis, and corticosteroid and estrogen therapy.

Hygroton has also been found useful in edema due to various forms of renal dysfunction such as nephrotic syndrome, acute glomerulonephritis, and chronic renal failure.

Usage in Pregnancy: The routine use of diuretics in an otherwise healthy woman is inappropriate and exposes mother and fetus to unnecessary hazard. Diuretics do not prevent development of toxemia of pregnancy, and there is no satisfactory evidence that they are useful in the treatment of developed toxemia.

Edema during pregnancy may arise from pathological causes or from the physiologic and mechanical consequences of pregnancy. Chlorthalidone is indicated in pregnancy when edema is due to pathologic causes, just as it is in the absence of pregnancy (however, see Warnings, below). Dependent edema in pregnancy, resulting from restriction of venous return by the expanded uterus, is properly treated through elevation of the lower extremities and use of support hose; use of diuretics to lower intravascular volume in this case is illogical and unnecessary. There is hypervolemia during normal pregnancy which is harmful to neither the fetus nor the mother (in the absence of cardiovascular disease), but which is associated with edema, including generalized edema, in the majority of pregnant women. If this edema produces discomfort, increased recumbency will often provide relief. In rare instances, this edema may cause extreme discomfort which is not relieved by rest. In these cases, a short course of diuretics may provide relief and may be appropriate.

Contraindications: Anuria. Hypersensitivity to chlorthalidone or other sulfonamide-derived drugs.

Warnings: Should be used with caution in severe renal disease. In patients with renal disease, chlorthalidone or related drugs may precipitate azotemia. Cumulative effects of the drug may develop in patients with impaired renal function.

Chlorthalidone should be used with caution in patients with impaired hepatic function or progressive liver disease, since minor alterations of fluid and electrolyte balance may precipitate hepatic coma.

Chlorthalidone may add to or potentiate the action of other antihypertensive drugs. Potentiation occurs with ganglionic or peripheral adrenergic blocking drugs.

Sensitivity reactions may occur in patients with a history of allergy or bronchial asthma.

The possibility of exacerbation or activation of systemic lupus erythematosus has been reported with thiazide diuretics, which are structurally related to chlorthalidone. However, systemic lupus erythematosus has not been reported following chlorthalidone administration.

USAGE IN PREGNANCY: Reproduction studies in various animal species at multiples of the human dose showed no significant level of teratogenicity; no fetal or congenital abnormalities were observed. Animal data should not be extrapolated for clinical application.

Thiazides cross the placental barrier and appear in cord blood. The use of chlorthalidone and related drugs in pregnant women requires that the anticipated benefits of the drug be weighed against possible hazards to the fetus. These hazards include fetal or neonatal jaundice, thrombocytopenia, and possibly other adverse reactions which have occurred in the adult.

NURSING MOTHERS: Thiazides cross the placental barrier and appear in breast milk. If use of the drug is deemed essential, the patient should stop nursing.

Precautions: Periodic determination of serum electrolytes to detect possible electrolyte imbalance should be performed at appropriate intervals. All patients receiving chlorthalidone should be observed for clinical signs of fluid or electrolyte imbalance; namely, hyponatremia, hypochloremic alkalosis, and hypokalemia. Serum and urine electrolyte determinations are particularly important when the patient is vomiting excessively or receiving parenteral fluids. Medication such as digitalis may also influence serum electrolytes. Warning signs, irrespective of cause, are: Dryness of mouth, thirst, weakness, lethargy, drowsiness, restlessness, muscle pains or cramps, muscular fatigue, hypotension, oliguria, tachycardia, and gastrointestinal disturbances such as nausea and vomiting.

Hypokalemia may develop with chlorthalidone as with any other potent diuretic, especially with brisk diuresis, when severe cirrhosis is present, or during concomitant use of corticosteroids or ACTH.

Interference with adequate oral electrolyte intake will also contribute to hypokalemia. Digitalis therapy may exaggerate metabolic effects of hypokalemia especially with reference to myocardial activity.

Any chloride deficit is generally mild and usually does not require specific treatment except under extraordinary circumstances (as in liver disease or renal disease). Dilutional hyponatremia may occur in edematous patients in hot weather; appropriate therapy is water restriction, rather than administration of salt except in rare instances when the hyponatremia is life threatening. In actual salt depletion, appropriate replacement is the therapy of choice.

Hyperuricemia may occur or frank gout may be precipitated in certain patients receiving chlorthalidone.

Insulin requirements in diabetic patients may be increased, decreased, or unchanged. Latent diabetes mellitus may become manifest during chlorthalidone administration.

Chlorthalidone and related drugs may increase the responsiveness to tubocurarine.

The antihypertensive effects of the drug may be enhanced in the postsympathectomy patient.

Chlorthalidone and related drugs may decrease arterial responsiveness to norepinephrine. This diminution is not sufficient to preclude effectiveness of the pressor agent for therapeutic use.

If progressive renal impairment becomes evident, as indicated by a rising nonprotein nitrogen or blood urea nitrogen, a careful reappraisal of therapy is necessary with consideration given to withholding or discontinuing diuretic therapy.

Chlorthalidone and related drugs may decrease serum PBI levels without signs of thyroid disturbance.

Adverse Reactions: *Gastrointestinal System Reactions:* anorexia, gastric irritation, nausea, vomiting, cramping, diarrhea, constipation, jaundice (intrahepatic cholestatic jaundice), pancreatitis; *Central Nervous System Reactions:* dizziness, vertigo, paresthesias, headache, xanthopsia; *Hematologic Reactions:* leukopenia, agranulocytosis, thrombocytopenia, aplastic anemia; *Dermatologic—Hypersensitivity Reactions:* purpura, photosensitivity, rash, urticaria, necrotizing angiitis (vasculitis) (cutaneous vasculitis), Lyell's syndrome (toxic epidermal necrolysis); *Cardiovascular Reaction:* Orthostatic hypotension may occur and may be aggravated by alcohol, barbiturates or narcotics. *Other Adverse Reactions:* hyperglycemia, glycosuria, hyperuricemia, muscle spasm, weakness, restlessness, impotence.

Whenever adverse reactions are moderate or severe, chlorthalidone dosage should be reduced or therapy withdrawn.

Dosage and Administration: Therapy should be initiated with the lowest possible dose. This dose should be titrated according to individual patient response to gain maximal therapeutic benefit while maintaining the minimal dosage possible. A single dose given in the morning with food is recommended; divided doses are unnecessary.

<u>Hypertension.</u> *Initiation:* Therapy, in most patients should be initiated with a single daily dose of 25 mg. If the response is insufficient after single suitable trial, the dosage may be increased to a single daily dose of 50 mg. If additional control is required, the dosage of Hygroton may be increased to 100 mg once daily or a second antihypertensive drug (step-2 therapy) may be added. Dosage above 100 mg daily usually does not increase effectiveness. Increases in serum uric acid and decreases in serum potassium are dose-related over the 25–100 mg per day range.

Maintenance: Maintenance doses may be lower than initial doses and should be adjusted according to individual patient response. Effectiveness is well sustained during continued use.

<u>Edema.</u> *Initiation:* Adults, initially 50 to 100 mg daily, or 100 mg on alternate days. Some patients may require 150 to 200 mg at these intervals, or up to 200 mg daily. Dosages above this level, however, do not usually produce a greater response.

Maintenance: Maintenance doses may often be lower than initial doses and should be adjusted according to the individual patient. Effectiveness is well sustained during continued use.

Overdosage: Symptoms of overdosage include nausea, weakness, dizziness and disturbances of electrolyte balance. There is no specific antidote, but gastric lavage is recommended, followed by supportive treatment. Where necessary, this may include intravenous dextrose-saline with potassium, administered with caution.

How Supplied: Hygroton (chlorthalidone) is available as 25 mg peach-color tablets in bottles of 100 (NDC 0070-0022-00), 1000 (NDC 0070-0022-99), and unit-dose blister packs, boxes of 100 (10 × 10 strips) (NDC 0070-0022-62); 50 mg aqua tablets in bottles of 100 (NDC 0070-0020-00), 1000 (NDC 0070-0020-99), 5000 (NDC 0070-0020-65), and unit-dose blister packs, boxes of 100 (10 × 10 strips) (NDC 0070-0020-62); 100 mg white, single-scored tablets in bottles of 100 (NDC 0070-0021-00), 1000 (NDC 0070-0021-99), 5000 (NDC 0070-0021-65), and unit-dose blister packs, boxes of 100 (10 × 10 strips) (NDC 0070-0021-62). Store at room temperature; avoid excessive heat. Dispense in tight containers as defined in USP.

Animal Pharmacology: Biochemical studies in animals have suggested reasons for the prolonged effect of chlorthalidone. Absorption from the gastrointestinal tract is slow due to its low solubility. After passage to the liver, some of the drug enters the general circulation, while some is excreted in the bile, to be reabsorbed later. In the general circulation, it is distributed widely to the tissues, but is taken up in highest concentrations by the kidneys, where amounts have been found 72 hours after ingestion, long after it has disappeared from other tissues. The drug is excreted unchanged in the urine.

Revised: January, 1983
Shown in Product Identification Section, page 440

LEVOTHROID®
[lē-vō-throid]
(levothyroxine sodium)
FOR INJECTION

Description: LEVOTHROID® (Levothyroxine Sodium) for Injection is a sterile, lyophilized powder supplied in 6 ml vials containing 200 or 500 mcg of levothyroxine sodium U.S.P. with 15 mg of mannitol.

Clinical Pharmacology: The major thyroid hormones are L-thyroxine (T_4) and L-triiodothyronine (T_3). The amounts of T_4 and T_3 released into the circulation from the normally functioning thyroid gland are regulated by the amount of Thyrotropin (TSH) secreted from the anterior pituitary gland. TSH secretion is in turn regulated by the levels of circulating T_4 and T_3 and by secretion of thyrotropin releasing factor (TRH) from the hypothalamus. Recognition of this complex feedback system is important in the diagnosis and treatment of thyroid dysfunction.

The principal effect of exogenous thyroid hormone is to increase the metabolic rate of body tissues. The thyroid hormones are also concerned with growth and differentiation of tissues. In deficiency states in the young there is a retardation of growth and failure of maturation of the skeletal and other body systems, especially in failure of ossification in the epiphyses and in the growth and development of the brain.

The precise mechanism of action by which thyroid hormones affect thermogenesis and cellular growth and differentiation is not known. It is recognized that these physiologic effects are mediated at the cellular level primarily by T_3, a large part of which is derived from T_4 by deiodination in the peripheral tissues. Thyroxine (T_4) is the major component of normal secretions of the thyroid gland and is thus the primary determinant of normal thyroid function.

More than 99 percent of circulating hormones are bound to serum proteins, including thyroid-binding globulin (TBg), thyroid-binding prealbumin (TBPA), and albumin (TBa), whose capacities and affinities vary for the hormones. L-thyroxine displays greater binding affinity than L-triiodothyronine, both in the circulation and at the cellular level, which explains its longer duration of action. The half-life of T_4 in normal plasma is 6-7 days while that of T_3 is about 1 day. The plasma half-lives of T_4 and T_3 are decreased in hyperthyroidism and increased in hypothyroidism.

Indications and Usage: LEVOTHROID® (Levothyroxine Sodium) for Injection is indicated as replacement or substitution therapy for diminished or absent thyroid function (e.g., cretinism, myxedema, non-toxic goiter or hypothyroidism generally, including the hypothyroid state in children, in pregnancy and in the elderly) resulting from functional deficiency, primary atrophy, from partial or complete absence of the gland or from the effects of surgery, radiation or antithyroid agents. Therapy must be maintained continuously to control the symptoms of hypothyroidism.

It may also be used to suppress the secretion of thyrotropin (TSH), action which may be beneficial in simple nonendemic goiter and in chronic lymphocytic thyroiditis. This may cause a reduction in the goiter size.

Thyroid hormone drugs are indicated as a diagnostic agent in suppression tests to differentiate suspected mild hyperthyroidism or thyroid gland autonomy.

Thyroid hormones may also be used with antithyroid drugs to treat thyrotoxicosis. This combination has been used to prevent goitrogenesis and hypothyroidism. This may be particularly useful in the management of thyrotoxicosis during pregnancy.

Contraindications: LEVOTHROID® for Injection administration is contraindicated in untreated thyrotoxicosis and in acute myocardial infarction. LEVOTHROID® for Injection is contraindicated in the presence of uncorrected adrenal insufficiency because it increases the tissue demands for adrenocortical hormones and may cause an acute adrenal crisis in such patients. (See PRECAUTIONS). LEVOTHROID® for Injection is also contraindicated in cases of hypersensitivity to any of the ingredients.

Warnings

Drugs with thyroid hormone activity, alone or together with other therapeutic agents, have been used for the treatment of obesity. In euthyroid patients, doses within the range of daily hormonal requirements are ineffective for weight reduction. Larger doses may produce serious or even life-threatening manifestations of toxicity, particularly when given in association with sympathomimetic amines such as those used for their anorectic effects.

The use of thyroid hormones in the therapy of obesity, alone or combined with other drugs, is unjustified and has been shown to be ineffective. Neither is their use justified for the treatment of male or female infertility unless this condition is accompanied by hypothyroidism.

Precautions:

General—LEVOTHROID® for Injection should be used with caution in patients with cardiovascular disease, inluding hypertension. The development of chest pain or other aggravation of cardiovascular disease will require a decrease in dosage.

Thyroid hormone therapy in patients with concomitant diabetes mellitus or diabetes insipidus or adrenal cortical insufficiency aggravates the intensity of their symptoms. Appropriate adjustments of the various therapeutic measures directed at these concomitant endocrine diseases are required. The therapy of myxedema coma requires simultaneous administration of glucocorticoids (See DOSAGE AND ADMINISTRATION).

Information for the Patient—Patients on thyroid preparations and parents of children on thyroid therapy should be informed that:

1. Replacement therapy is to be taken essentially for life, with the exception of cases of transient hypothyroidism, usually associated with thyroiditis, and in those patients receiving a therapeutic trial of the drug.
2. They should immediately report during the course of therapy any signs or symptoms of thyroid hormone toxicity, e.g., chest pain, increased pulse rate, palpitations, excessive sweating, heat intolerance, nervousness, or any other unusual event.
3. In case of concomitant diabetes mellitus, the daily dosage of antidiabetic medication may need readjustment as thyroid hormone replacement is achieved. If thyroid medication is stopped, a downward readjustment of the dosage of insulin or oral hypoglycemic agent may be necessary to avoid hypoglycemia. At all times, close monitoring of urinary glucose levels is mandatory in such patients.
4. In case of concomitant oral anticoagulant therapy, the prothrombin time should be measured frequently to determine if the dosage of oral anticoagulants is to be readjusted.
5. Partial loss of hair may be experienced by children in the first few months of thyroid therapy, but this is usually a transient phenomenon and later recovery is usually the rule.

Laboratory Tests—The patient's response to thyroid replacement may be followed by laboratory tests such as serum thyroxine (T_4), serum triiodothyronine (T_3), free thyroxine index and thyroid stimulating hormone (TSH) blood levels.

Drug Interactions—In patients with diabetes mellitus, addition of thyroid hormone therapy may cause an increase in the required dosage of insulin or oral hypoglycemic agents. Conversely, decreasing the dose of thyroid hormone may possibly cause hypoglycemic reactions if the dosage of insulin or oral hypoglycemic agents is not adjusted.

Thyroid replacement may potentiate anticoagulant effects with agents such as warfarin or bishydroxycoumarin and reduction of one-third of anticoagulant dosage should be undertaken upon initiation of LEVOTHROID® for Injection therapy. Subsequent anticoagulant dosage adjustment should be made on the basis of frequent prothrombin determinations. Injection of epinephrine in patients with coronary artery disease may precipitate an episode of coronary insufficiency. This may be enhanced in patients receiving thyroid preparations. Careful observation is required if catecholamines are administered to patients in this category.

Estrogens tend to increase serum thyroxine-binding globulin (TBg). Thus during pregnancy or when using estrogen containing drug products, the total serum thyroxine (T_4) will increase. The ratio of bound to free T_4 will increase but the available free T_4 concentration remains normal. An adjustment in the exogenous dose of T_4 should be made on the basis of free T_4 measurements.

Drug/Laboratory Test Interactions—The following drugs or moieties are known to interfere with laboratory tests performed in patients on thyroid hormone therapy: androgens, corticosteroids, estrogens, oral contraceptives containing estrogens, iodine-containing preparations, and the numerous preparations containing salicylates.

1. Changes in TBg concentration should be taken into consideration in the interpretation of T_4 and T_3 values. In such cases, the unbound (free) hormone should be measured. Pregnancy, estrogens, and estrogen-containing oral contraceptives increase TBg concentrations. TBg may also be increased during infectious hepatitis. Decreases in TBg concentrations are observed in nephrosis, acromegaly, and after androgen or corticosteroid therapy. Familial hyper- or hypo-thyroxine-binding-globulinemias have been described. The incidence of TBg deficiency approximates 1 in 9000. The binding of thyroxine by thyroid-binding prealbumin (TBPA) is inhibited by salicylates.

2. Medical or dietary iodine interferes with all in vivo tests of radio-iodine uptake, producing low uptakes which may not be reflective of a true decrease in hormone synthesis.

3. The persistence of clinical and laboratory evidence of hypothyroidism in spite of adequate dosage replacement indicates either poor patient compliance, poor absorption, excessive fecal loss, or inactivity of the preparation. Intracellular resistance to thyroid hormone is quite rare.

Carcinogenesis, Mutagenesis, and Impairment of Fertility—A reportedly apparent association between prolonged thyroid therapy and breast cancer has not been confirmed and patients on thyroid for established indications should not discontinue therapy. No confirmatory long-term studies in animals have been performed to evaluate carcinogenic potential, mutagenicity, or impairment of fertility in either males or females.

Pregnancy-Category A—Thyroid hormones do not readily cross the placental barrier. The clinical experience to date does not indicate any adverse effect on fetuses when thyroid hormones are administered to pregnant women. On the basis of current knowledge, thyroid replacement therapy to hypothyroid women should not be discontinued during pregnancy.

Nursing Mothers—Minimal amounts of thyroid hormones are excreted in human milk. Thyroid is not associated with serious adverse reactions and does not have a known tumorigenic potential. However, caution should be exercised when thyroid is administered to a nursing woman.

Pediatric Use—The diagnosis and institution of therapy for cretinism should be done as soon after birth as feasible to prevent developmental deficiency. Screening tests for serum T_4 and TSH will identify this group of newborn patients.

Adverse Reactions: Adverse reactions other than those indicative of hyperthyroidism because of therapeutic overdosage, either initially or during the maintenance period, are rare (See OVERDOSAGE).

Overdosage: Excessive dosage of thyroid medication may result in symptoms of hyperthyroidism. Since, however, the effects do not appear at once, the symptoms may not appear for one to three weeks after the dosage regimen is begun. The most common signs and symptoms of overdosage are weight loss, palpitation, nervousness, diar-

Continued on next page

USV—Cont.

rhea or abdominal cramps, sweating, tachycardia, cardiac arrhythmias, angina pectoris, tremors, headache, insomnia, intolerance to heat and fever. If symptoms of overdosage appear, discontinue medication for several days and reinstitute treatment at a lower dosage level.

Laboratory tests such as serum T_4 and serum T_3 and the free thyroxine index will be elevated during the period of overdosage.

Complications as a result of the induced hypermetabolic state may include cardiac failure and death due to arrhythmia or failure.

TREATMENT OF OVERDOSAGE—Dosage should be reduced or therapy temporarily discontinued if signs and symptoms of overdosage appear. Treatment may be reinstituted at a lower dosage. In normal individuals, normal hypothalamic-pituitary-thyroid axis function is restored in 6 to 8 weeks after thyroid suppression.

Treatment of acute massive thyroid hormone overdosage is aimed at counteracting central and peripheral effects, mainly those of increased sympathetic activity. Treatment is symptomatic and supportive. Oxygen may be administered and ventilation maintained. Cardiac glycosides may be indicated if congestive heart failure develops. Measures to control fever, hypoglycemia, or fluid loss shold be instituted if needed. Antiadrenergic agents, particularly propranolol, have been used advantageously in the treatment of increased sympathetic activity. Propranolol may be administered intravenously at a dosage of 1 to 3 mg over a 10 minute period or orally, 80 to 160 mg/day, especially when no contraindications exist for its use.

Dosage and Administration: Myxedema coma is usually precipitated in the hypothyroid patient of long-standing by intercurrent illness or drugs such as sedatives and anesthetics and should be considered a medical emergency. Therapy should be directed at the correction of electrolyte disturbances and possible infection besides the administration of thyroid hormones. Corticosteroids should be administered routinely. T_4 and T_3 may be administered by a nasogastric tube, but the preferred route of administration is intravenous.

LEVOTHROID® (Levothyroxine Sodium) for Injection is given at a starting dose of 200–500 mcg in patients without severe cardiac disease. This initial dose is followed in 24 hours by 100 to 200 mcg given intravenously. Normal T_4 levels may be achieved in 24 hours followed in 3 days by a threefold increase in T_3. Oral therapy with Levothroid® Tablets should be resumed as soon as the clinical situation permits.

In the presence of severe cardiac disease, the risk of a rapid increase in metabolism should be weighed against the danger of prolonging the severe hypothyroid state. This may necessitate a smaller initial I.V. dose of Levothroid® for Injection.

Directions for reconstitution: using aseptic technique add 2 ml, 0.9% Sodium Chloride Injection, U.S.P. to the 200 mcg vial and 5 ml, 0.9% Sodium Chloride Injection, U.S.P. to the 500 mcg vial.

Note: Do not use Bacteriostatic Sodium Chloride Injection, U.S.P. Shake to dissolve the contents of the vial. Use immediately and discard the unused portion.

Parenteral drug products should be inspected visually for particulate matter and discoloration prior to administration whenever solution and container permit.

How Supplied: LEVOTHROID® (Levothyroxine Sodium) for Injection is supplied in 6 ml vials containing 200 or 500 mcg of levothyroxine sodium, U.S.P.

The vials should be stored at controlled room temperature between 15°–30°C (59°–86°F).

Issued: March, 1984

Shown in Product Identification Section, page 440

LEVOTHROID® Tablets ℞
[lēʹ vō-throid]
(levothyroxine sodium tablets, USP)

Description: LEVOTHROID® TABLETS (Levothyroxine Sodium Tablets, USP) provide crystalline sodium levothyroxine (T_4), a potent thyroid hormone, in nine different strengths to permit easy convenient dosage adjustment.

Clinical Pharmacology: The major thyroid hormones are L-thyroxine (T_4) and L-triiodothyronine (T_3). The amounts of T_4 and T_3 released into the circulation from the normally functioning thyroid gland are regulated by the amount of thyrotropin (TSH) secreted from the anterior pituitary gland. TSH secretion is in turn regulated by the levels of circulating T_4 and T_3 and by secretion of thyrotropin releasing factor (TRH) from the hypothalamus. Recognition of this complex feedback system is important in the diagnosis and treatment of thyroid dysfunction.

The principal effect of exogenous thyroid hormones is to increase the metabolic rate of body tissues.

The thyroid hormones are also concerned with growth and differentiation of tissues. In deficiency states in the young there is retardation of growth and failure of maturation of the skeletal and other body systems, especially in failure of ossification in the epiphyses and in the growth and development of the brain.

The precise mechanism of action by which thyroid hormones affect thermogenesis and cellular growth and differentiation is not known. It is recognized that these physiologic effects are mediated at the cellular level primarily by T_3, a large part of which is derived from T_4 by deiodination in the peripheral tissues. Thyroxine (T_4) is the major component of normal secretions of the thyroid gland and is thus the primary determinant of normal thyroid function.

Depending on other factors, absorption has varied from 48 to 79 percent of the administered dose. Fasting increases absorption. Malabsorption syndromes, as well as dietary factors, (children's soybean formula, concomitant use of anionic exchange resins such as cholestyramine) cause excessive fecal loss.

More than 99 percent of circulating hormones are bound to serum proteins, including thyroid-binding globulin (TBg), thyroid-binding prealbumin (TBPA), and albumin (TBa), whose capacities and affinities vary for the hormones. L-thyroxine displays greater binding affinity than L-triiodothyronine, both in the circulation and at the cellular level, which explains its longer duration of action. The half-life of T_4 in normal plasma is 6–7 days while that of T_3 is about 1 day. The plasma half-lives of T_4 and T_3 are decreased in hyperthyroidism and increased in hypothyroidism.

Indications and Usage: LEVOTHROID® Tablets (levothyroxine sodium, USP) are indicated as replacement or substitution therapy for diminished or absent thyroid function (e.g., cretinism, myxedema, non-toxic goiter or hypothyroidism generally, including the hypothyroid state in children, in pregnancy and in the elderly) resulting from functional deficiency, primary atrophy, from partial or complete absence of the gland or from the effects of surgery, radiation or anti-thyroid agents. Therapy must be maintained continuously to control the symptoms of hypothyroidism.

It may also be used to suppress the secretion of thyrotropin (TSH) action which may be beneficial in suppress nonendemic goiter and in chronic lymphocytic thyroiditis. This may cause a reduction in the goiter size.

Thyroid hormone drugs are indicated as a diagnostic agent in suppression tests to differentiate suspected mild hyperthyroidism or thyroid gland autonomy.

Thyroid hormones may also be used with antithyroid drugs to treat thyrotoxicosis. This combination has been used to prevent goitrogenesis and hypothyroidism. This may be particularly useful in the management of thyrotoxicosis during pregnancy.

Contraindications: LEVOTHROID® Tablets administration is contraindicated in untreated thyrotoxicosis and in acute myocardial infarction. LEVOTHROID® Tablets are contraindicated in the presence of uncorrected adrenal insufficiency because they increase the tissue demands for adrenocortical hormones and may cause an acute adrenal crisis in such patients. (See PRECAUTIONS)

Warnings:

> Drugs with thyroid hormone activity, alone or together with other therapeutic agents, have been used for the treatment of obesity. In euthyroid patients, doses within the range of daily hormonal requirements are ineffective for weight reduction. Larger doses may produce serious or even life-threatening manifestations of toxicity, particularly when given in association with sympathomimetic amines such as those used for their anorectic effects.

The use of thryoid hormones in the therapy of obesity, alone or combined with other drugs, is unjustified and has been shown to be ineffective. Neither is their use justified for the treatment of male or female infertility unless this condition is accompanied by hypothyroidism.

Precautions:

General—LEVOTHROID® Tablets should be used with caution in patients with cardiovascular disease, including hypertension. The development of chest pain or other aggravation of cardiovascular disease will require a decrease in dosage.

Thyroid hormone therapy in patients with concomitant diabetes mellitus or insipidus or adrenal cortical insufficiency aggravates the intensity of their symptoms. Appropriate adjustments of the various therapeutic measures directed at these concomitant endocrine diseases are required. The therapy of myxedema coma requires simultaneous administration of glucocorticoids (See DOSAGE AND ADMINISTRATION).

Information for the Patient—Patients on thyroid preparations and parents of children on thyroid therapy should be informed that:

1. Replacement therapy is to be taken essentially for life, with the exception of cases of transient hypothyroidism, usually associated with thyroiditis, and in those patients receiving a therapeutic trial of the drug.

2. They should immediately report during the course of therapy any signs or symptoms of thyroid hormone toxicity, e.g., chest pain, increased pulse rate, palpitations, excessive sweating, heat intolerance, nervousness, or any other unusual event.

3. In case of concomitant diabetes mellitus, the daily dosage of antidiabetic medication may need readjustment as thyroid hormone replacement is achieved. If thyroid medication is stopped, a downward readjustment of the dosage of insulin or oral hypoglycemic agent may be necessary to avoid hypoglycemia. At all times, close monitoring of urinary glucose levels is mandatory in such patients.

4. In case of concomitant oral anticoagulant therapy, the prothrombin time should be measured frequently to determine if the dosage of oral anticoagulants is to be readjusted.

5. Partial loss of hair may be experienced by children in the first few months of thyroid therapy, but this is usually a transient phenomenon and later recovery is usually the rule.

Laboratory Tests—The patient's response to thyroid replacement therapy may be followed by laboratory tests such as serum thyroxine (T_4), serum triiodothyronine (T_3), free thyroxine index and thyroid stimulating hormone (TSH) blood levels.

Drug Interactions—In patients with diabetes mellitus, addition of thyroid hormone therapy may cause an increase in the required dosage of insulin or oral hypoglycemic agents. Conversely, decreasing the dose of thyroid hormone may possibly cause hypoglycemic reactions if the dosage of insulin or oral hypoglycemic agents is not adjusted.

Thyroid replacement may potentiate anticoagulant effects with agents such as warfarin or bishydroxycoumarin and reduction of one-third in anticoagulant dosage should be undertaken upon initiation of **LEVOTHROID® Tablets** therapy. Subsequent anticoagulant dosage adjustment should be made on the basis of frequent prothrombin determinations.

Injection of epinephrine in patients with coronary artery disease may precipitate an episode of coronary insufficiency. This may be enhanced in patients receiving thyroid preparations. Careful observation is required if catecholamines are administered to patients in this category.

Cholestyramine binds both T_4 and T_3 in the intestine, thus impairing absorption of these thyroid hormones. In vitro studies indicate that the binding is not easily removed. Therefore, four to five hours should elapse between administration of cholestyramine and thyroid hormones.

Estrogens tend to increase serum thyroxine-binding globulin (TBg). In a patient with a nonfunctioning thyroid gland who is receiving thyroid replacement therapy, free levothyroxine may be decreased when estrogens are started thus increasing thyroid requirements. However, if the patient's thyroid gland has sufficient function the decreased free thyroxine will result in a compensatory increase in thyroxine output by the thyroid. Therefore, patients without a functioning thyroid gland who are on thyroid replacement therapy may need to increase their thyroid dose if estrogens or estrogen-containing oral contraceptives are given.

Drug/Laboratory Test Interactions—The following drugs or moieties are known to interfere with laboratory tests performed in patients on thyroid hormone therapy: androgens, corticosteroids, estrogens, oral contraceptives containing estrogens, iodine-containing preparations, and the numerous preparations containing salicylates.

1. Changes in TBg concentration should be taken into consideration in the interpretation of T_4 and T_3 values. In such cases, the unbound (free) hormone should be measured. Pregnancy, estrogens, and estrogen-containing oral contraceptives increase TBg concentrations. TBg may also be increased during infectious hepatitis. Decreases in TBg concentrations are observed in nephrosis, acromegaly, and after androgen or corticosteroid therapy. Familial hyper- or hypo-thyroxine-binding globulinemias have been described. The incidence of TBg deficiency approximates 1 in 9000. The binding of thyroxine by thyroxine-binding prealbumin (TBPA) is inhibited by salicylates.

2. Medical or dietary iodine interferes with all in vivo tests of radio-iodine uptake, producing low uptakes which may not be reflective of a true decrease in hormone synthesis.

3. The persistence of clinical and laboratory evidence of hypothyroidism in spite of adequate dosage replacement indicates either poor patient compliance, poor absorption, excessive fecal loss, or inactivity of the preparation. Intracellular resistance to thyroid hormone is quite rare.

Carcinogenesis, Mutagenesis, and Impairment of Fertility—A reportedly apparent association between prolonged thyroid therapy and breast cancer has not been confirmed and patients on thyroid for established indications should not discontinue therapy. No confirmatory long-term studies in animals have been performed to evaluate carcinogenic potential, mutagenicity, or impairment of fertility in either males or females.

Pregnancy-Category A—Thyroid hormones do not readily cross the placental barrier. The clinical experience to date does not indicate any adverse effect on fetuses when thyroid hormones are administered to pregnant women. On the basis of current knowledge, thyroid replacement therapy to hypothyroid women should not be discontinued during pregnancy.

Nursing Mothers—Minimal amounts of thyroid hormones are excreted in human milk. Thyroid is not associated with serious adverse reactions and does not have a known tumorigenic potential. However, caution should be exercised when thyroid is administered to a nursing woman.

Pediatric Use—The diagnosis and institution of therapy for cretinism should be done as soon after birth as feasible to prevent developmental deficiency. Screening tests for serum T_4 and TSH will identify this group of newborn patients.

Adverse Reactions: Patients who are sensitive to lactose may show intolerance to **LEVOTHROID® Tablets** since this substance is used in the manufacture of the product.

Adverse reactions other than those indicative of hyperthyroidism because of therapeutic overdosage, either initially or during the maintenance period, are rare (See OVERDOSAGE).

Overdosage: Excessive dosage of thyroid medication may result in symptoms of hyperthyroidism. Since, however, the effects do not appear at once, the symptoms may not appear for one to three weeks after the dosage regimen is begun. The most common signs and symptoms of overdosage are weight loss, palpitation, nervousness, diarrhea or abdominal cramps, sweating, tachycardia, cardiac arrhythmias, angina pectoris, tremors, headache, insomnia, intolerance to heat and fever. If symptoms of overdosage appear, discontinue medication for several days and reinstitute treatment at a lower dosage level.

Laboratory tests such as serum T_4, serum T_3 and the free thyroxine index will be elevated during the period of overdosage.

Complications as a result of the induced hypermetabolic state may include cardiac failure and death due to arrhythmia or failure.

Treatment of Overdosage—Dosage should be reduced or therapy temporarily discontinued if signs and symptoms of overdosage appear. Treatment may be reinstituted at a lower dosage. In normal individuals, normal hypothalamic-pituitary-thyroid axis function is restored in 6 to 8 weeks after thyroid suppression.

Treatment of acute massive thyroid hormone overdosage is aimed at reducing gastrointestinal absorption of the drugs and counteracting central and peripheral effects, mainly those of increased sympathetic activity. Vomiting may be induced initially if further gastrointestinal absorption can reasonably be prevented and barring contraindications such as coma, convulsions, or loss of the gagging reflex. Treatment is symptomatic and supportive. Oxygen may be administered and ventilation maintained. Cardiac glycosides may be indicated if congestive heart failure develops. Measures to control fever, hypoglycemia, or fluid loss should be instituted if needed. Antiadrenergic agents, particularly propranolol, have been used advantageously in the treatment of increased sympathetic activity. Propranolol may be administered intravenously at a dosage of 1 to 3 mg over a 10 minute period or orally, 80 to 160 mg/day, especially when no contraindications exist for its use.

Dosage and Administration: The goal of therapy should be the restoration of euthyroidism as judged by clinical response and confirmed by appropriate laboratory values. In adults with no complicating endocrine or cardiovascular disease, the predicted full maintenance dose may be achieved immediately with adjustments made as indicated by clinical evaluation. The usual maintenance dose of **LEVOTHROID® Tablets** is 0.1 mg to 0.2 mg daily.

In patients with known complications or in case of doubt, individual dose titration at 2 to 4 week intervals is recommended. The usual starting dose is 0.05 mg with increases of 0.05 mg at 2 to 4 week intervals until the patient is euthyroid or symptoms ensue which preclude further dose increase. In adult myxedema or hypothyroid patients with angina, the starting dose should be 0.025 mg with increases at 2 to 4 week intervals of 0.025 to 0.05 mg as determined by clinical response.

Myxedema coma is usually precipitated in the hypothyroid patient of long-standing by intercurrent illness or drugs such as sedatives and anesthetics and should be considered a medical emergency. Therapy should be directed at the correction of electrolyte disturbances and possible infection besides the administration of thyroid hormones. Corticosteroids should be administered routinely. T_4 and T_3 may be administered via a nasogastric tube but the preferred route of administration of both hormones is intravenous. Sodium levothyroxine (T_4) is given at a starting dose of 400 mcg (100 mcg/ml given rapidly), and is usually well tolerated, even in the elderly. This initial dose is followed by daily supplements of 100 to 200 mcg given IV. Normal T_4 levels are achieved in 24 hours followed in 3 days by threefold elevation of T_3. Oral therapy with **LEVOTHROID® Tablets** should be resumed as soon as the clinical situation has been stabilized and the patient is able to take oral medication.

In cretinism or severe hypothyroidism in children, the initial dosage should be 0.025 to 0.05 mg with increases of 0.05 to 0.01 mg at weekly intervals until the child is clinically euthyroid and laboratory values are in the normal range. In growing children, the usual maintenance dose may be as high as 0.3 to 0.4 mg daily. It is essential in children to reach the euthyroid state as rapidly as possible because of the importance of thyroid in growth and maturation.

How Supplied: **LEVOTHROID® Tablets** (Levothyroxine Sodium Tablets, USP) are available in bottles of 100 and 1000 tablets. The 0.05 mg, 0.1 mg, 0.125 mg, 0.15 mg, 0.175 mg, 0.2 mg, and 0.3 mg potencies are also available in cartons of 100 (10 strips of 10 tablets) packaged in Unit Dose as Armadose®. Each **LEVOTHROID® Tablet** is distinctively colored and bears identifying markings.

Strength (mg)	Tablets Color	Markings
0.025	Orange	¼ LK
0.05	White	½ LL
0.075	Grey	LT
0.1	Yellow	1 LM
0.125	Purple	1¼ LH
0.15	Blue	1½ LN
0.175	Turquoise	1¾ LP
0.2	Pink	2 LR
0.3	Green	3 LS

Tablets should be stored at controlled room temperature—between 15°-30°C (59°-86°F) in capped bottles or unbroken plastic strip packaging.
Revised: April, 1984

Shown in Product Identification Section, page 440

LOZOL® ℞
[lō'zôl]
indapamide
2.5 mg tablets

Description: LOZOL (indapamide) is an oral antihypertensive/diuretic. Its molecule contains both a polar sulfamoyl chlorobenzamide moiety and a lipid-soluble methylindoline moiety. It differs chemically from the thiazides in that it does not possess the thiazide ring system and contains only one sulfonamide group. The chemical name of LOZOL is 1-(4-chloro-3-sulfamoylbenzamido) -2-methylindoline, and its molecular weight is 365.84. The compound is a weak acid, $pK_a = 8.8$, and is soluble in aqueous solutions of strong bases. It is a white to yellow-white crystalline (tetragonal) powder.

Clinical Pharmacology: Indapamide is the first of a new class of antihypertensive/diuretics, the indolines. The oral administration of 5 mg (two 2.5-mg tablets) of indapamide to healthy male subjects produced peak concentrations of approximately 260 ng/ml of the drug in the blood within two hours. A minimum of 70% of a single oral dose is eliminated by the kidneys and an additional 23% by the gastrointestinal tract, probably including the biliary route. The half-life of LOZOL in whole blood is approximately 14 hours.

LOZOL is preferentially and reversibly taken up by the erythrocytes in the peripheral blood. The whole blood/plasma ratio is approximately 6:1 at the time of peak concentration and decreases to 3.5:1 at eight hours. From 71 to 79% of the LOZOL in plasma is reversibly bound to plasma proteins. LOZOL is extensively metabolized, unchanged drug accounting for approximately 7% of the total dose recovered in the urine during the first 48 hours after administration. The urinary elimination of ^{14}C-labeled indapamide and metabolites is biphasic with a terminal half-life of excretion of total radioactivity of 26 hours.

Continued on next page

USV—Cont.

In parallel design, dose-ranging clinical trials in hypertension and edema, daily doses of indapamide between 0.5 and 5.0 mg produced dose-related effects. Generally, doses of 2.5 and 5.0 mg were not distinguishable from each other although each was differentiated from placebo and from 0.5 or 1.0 mg indapamide. At daily doses of 2.5 and 5.0 mg a mean decrease of serum potassium of 0.5 and 0.6 mEq/liter, respectively, was observed and uric acid increased by about 1.0 mg/100 ml.

Thus, at these doses, the effects of indapamide on blood pressure and edema are approximately equal to those obtained with conventional doses of other antihypertensive/diuretics.

In hypertensive patients, daily doses of 2.5 and 5.0 mg of indapamide have no appreciable cardiac inotropic or chronotropic effect. The drug decreases peripheral resistance, with little or no effect on cardiac output, rate or rhythm. Chronic administration of indapamide to hypertensive patients has little or no effect on glomerular filtration rate or renal plasma flow.

LOZOL had an antihypertensive effect in patients with varying degrees of renal impairment, although in general, diuretic effects declined as renal function decreased.

In limited controlled studies adding LOZOL to other antihypertensive drugs such as hydralazine, propranolol, guanethidine, and methyldopa, indapamide appeared to have the additive effect typical of thiazide-type diuretics.

Indications: LOZOL is indicated for the treatment of hypertension, alone or in combination with other antihypertensive drugs.

LOZOL is also indicated for the treatment of salt and fluid retention associated with congestive heart failure.

Usage in Pregnancy: The routine use of diuretics in an otherwise healthy woman is inappropriate and exposes mother and fetus to unnecessary hazard (see PRECAUTIONS below).

Diuretics do not prevent development of toxemia of pregnancy, and there is no satisfactory evidence that they are useful in the treatment of developed toxemia.

Edema during pregnancy may arise from pathological causes or from the physiologic and mechanical consequences of pregnancy. Indapamide is indicated in pregnancy when edema is due to pathologic causes, just as it is in the absence of pregnancy (however, see PRECAUTIONS below). Dependent edema in pregnancy, resulting from restriction of venous return by the expanded uterus, is properly treated through elevation of the lower extremities and use of support hose; use of diuretics to lower intravascular volume in this case is illogical and unnecessary. There is hypervolemia during normal pregnancy which is not harmful to either the fetus or the mother (in the absence of cardiovascular disease), but which is associated with edema, including generalized edema in the majority of pregnant women. If this edema produces discomfort, increased recumbency will often provide relief. In rare instances, this edema may cause extreme discomfort which is not relieved by rest. In these cases, a short course of diuretics may provide relief and may be appropriate.

Contraindications: Anuria. Known hypersensitivity to indapamide or to other sulfonamide-derived drugs.

Warnings: Hypokalemia occurs commonly with diuretics, and electrolyte monitoring is essential, particularly in patients who would be at increased risk from hypokalemia, such as those with cardiac arrhythmias or who are receiving concomitant cardiac glycosides.

In general, diuretics should not be given concomitantly with lithium because they reduce its renal clearance and add a high risk of lithium toxicity. Read prescribing information for lithium preparations before use of such concomitant therapy.

Precautions:
General:
1. *Hypokalemia and Other Fluid and Electrolyte Imbalances:* Periodic determinations of serum electrolytes should be performed at appropriate intervals. In addition, patients should be observed for clinical signs of fluid or electrolyte imbalance, such as hyponatremia, hypochloremic alkalosis, or hypokalemia. Warning signs include dry mouth, thirst, weakness, fatigue, lethargy, drowsiness, restlessness, muscle pains or cramps, hypotension, oliguria, tachycardia and gastrointestinal disturbance. Electrolyte determinations are particularly important in patients who are vomiting excessively or receiving parenteral fluids, in patients subject to electrolyte imbalance (including those with heart failure, kidney disease, and cirrhosis), and in patients on a salt-restricted diet.

The risk of hypokalemia secondary to diuresis and natriuresis is increased when larger doses are used, when the diuresis is brisk, when severe cirrhosis is present and during concomitant use of corticosteroids or ACTH. Interference with adequate oral intake of electrolytes will also contribute to hypokalemia. Hypokalemia can sensitize or exaggerate the response of the heart to the toxic effects of digitalis, such as increased ventricular irritability.

Dilutional hyponatremia may occur in edematous patients; the appropriate treatment is restriction of water rather than administration of salt, except in rare instances when the hyponatremia is life threatening. However, in actual salt depletion, appropriate replacement is the treatment of choice. Any chloride deficit that may occur during treatment is generally mild and usually does not require specific treatment except in extraordinary circumstances as in liver or renal disease.

2. *Hyperuricemia and Gout:* Serum concentrations of uric acid increased by an average of 1.0 mg/100 ml in patients treated with indapamide, and frank gout may be precipitated in certain patients receiving indapamide (see ADVERSE REACTIONS below). Serum concentrations of uric acid should therefore be monitored periodically during treatment.

3. *Renal Impairment:* Indapamide, like the thiazides, should be used with caution in patients with severe renal disease, as reduced plasma volume may exacerbate or precipitate azotemia. If progressive renal impairment is observed in a patient receiving indapamide, withholding or discontinuing diuretic therapy should be considered. Renal function tests should be performed periodically during treatment with indapamide.

4. *Impaired Hepatic Function:* Indapamide, like the thiazides, should be used with caution in patients with impaired hepatic function or progressive liver disease, since minor alterations of fluid and electrolyte balance may precipitate hepatic coma.

5. *Glucose Tolerance:* Latent diabetes may become manifest and insulin requirements in diabetic patients may be altered during thiazide administration. Serum concentrations of glucose should be monitored routinely during treatment with LOZOL.

6. *Calcium Excretion:* Calcium excretion is decreased by diuretics pharmacologically related to indapamide. In long-term studies of hypertensive patients, however, serum concentrations of calcium increased only slightly with indapamide. Prolonged treatment with drugs pharmacologically related to indapamide may in rare instances be associated with hypercalcemia and hypophosphatemia secondary to physiologic changes in the parathyroid gland; however, the common complications of hyperparathyroidism, such as renal lithiasis, bone resorption, and peptic ulcer, have not been seen. Treatment should be discontinued before tests for parathyroid function are performed. Like the thiazides, indapamide may decrease serum PBI levels without signs of thyroid disturbance.

7. *Interaction With Systemic Lupus Erythematosus:* Thiazides have exacerbated or activated systemic lupus erythematosus and this possibility should be considered with indapamide as well.

Drug Interactions:
1. *Other Antihypertensives:* LOZOL may add to or potentiate the action of other antihypertensive drugs. In limited controlled trials that compared the effect of indapamide combined with other antihypertensive drugs with the effect of the other drugs administered alone, there was no notable change in the nature or frequency of adverse reactions associated with the combined therapy.
2. *Lithium:* See WARNINGS.
3. *Post-Sympathectomy Patient:* The antihypertensive effect of the drug may be enhanced in the postsympathectomized patient.
4. *Norepinephrine:* Indapamide, like the thiazides, may decrease arterial responsiveness to norepinephrine, but this diminution is not sufficient to preclude effectiveness of the pressor agent for therapeutic use.

CARCINOGENESIS, MUTAGENESIS, IMPAIRMENT OF FERTILITY: Both mouse and rat lifetime carcinogenicity studies were conducted. There was no significant difference in the incidence of tumors between the indapamide-treated animals and the control groups.

Pregnancy/Teratogenic Effects: Pregnancy Category B. Reproduction studies have been performed in rats, mice, and rabbits at doses up to 6,250 times the therapeutic human dose and have revealed no evidence of impaired fertility or harm to the fetus due to LOZOL (indapamide). Postnatal development in rats and mice was unaffected by pretreatment of parent animals during gestation. There are, however, no adequate and well-controlled studies in pregnant women. Moreover, diuretics are known to cross the placental barrier and appear in cord blood. Because animal reproduction studies are not always predictive of human response, this drug should be used during pregnancy only if clearly needed. There may be hazards associated with this use such as fetal or neonatal jaundice, thrombocytopenia, and possibly other adverse reactions that have occurred in the adult.

Nursing Mothers: It is not known whether this drug is excreted in human milk. Because most drugs are excreted in human milk, if use of this drug is deemed essential, the patient should stop nursing.

Adverse Reactions: Most adverse effects have been mild and transient.

The clinical adverse reactions listed in the following table represent data from Phase II placebo-controlled studies and long-term controlled clinical trials (426 patients given LOZOL 2.5 mg or 5.0 mg). The reactions are arranged into two groups: 1) a cumulative incidence equal to or greater than 5%; and 2) a cumulative incidence less than 5%. Reactions are counted regardless of relation to drug.

Incidence ≥ 5%	Incidence < 5%
CENTRAL NERVOUS SYSTEM/ NEUROMUSCULAR	
Headache	Lightheadedness
Dizziness	Drowsiness
Fatigue, weakness, loss of energy, lethargy, tiredness, or malaise	Vertigo
	Insomnia
	Depression
Muscle cramps or spasm or numbness of the extremities	Blurred Vision
Nervousness, tension, anxiety, irritability, or agitation	
GASTROINTESTINAL SYSTEM	
	Constipation
	Nausea
	Vomiting
	Diarrhea
	Gastric irritation
	Abdominal pain or cramps
	Anorexia
CARDIOVASCULAR SYSTEM	
	Orthostatic hypotension

Premature ventricular contractions
Irregular heart beat
Palpitations
GENITOURINARY SYSTEM
Frequency of urination
Nocturia
Polyuria
DERMATOLOGIC/HYPERSENSITIVITY
Rash
Hives
Pruritus
Vasculitis
OTHER
Impotence or reduced libido
Rhinorrhea
Flushing
Hyperuricemia
Hyperglycemia
Hyponatremia
Hypochloremia
Increase in serum urea nitrogen (BUN) or creatinine
Glycosuria
Weight loss
Dry mouth
Tingling of extremities

Because most of these data are from long-term studies (up to 40 weeks of treatment), it is probable that many of the adverse experiences reported are due to causes other than the drug. Approximately 10% of patients given indapamide discontinued treatment in long-term trials because of reactions either related or unrelated to the drug.

Clinical hypokalemia (i.e., lowered serum potassium concentration with concomitant clinical signs or symptoms) occurred in 3% and 7% of patients given indapamide 2.5 mg and 5.0 mg respectively. In a long-term study of both doses (157 patients given indapamide), potassium supplementation was given to 12% of patients on indapamide 2.5 mg and 27% of patients on indapamide 5.0 mg. As expected in long-term clinical trials, many patients experienced single instances of abnormal clinical laboratory test results. However, over time, the mean changes in selected values are slight, as shown in the table below:
[See table above].

Other adverse reactions reported with antihypertensive/diuretics are jaundice (intrahepatic cholestatic jaundice), sialadenitis, xanthopsia, photosensitivity, purpura, necrotizing angiitis, fever, respiratory distress (including pneumonitis), and anaphylactic reactions; also, agranulocytosis, leukopenia, thrombocytopenia, and aplastic anemia. However, these reactions have not been reported following LOZOL administration.

Overdosage: Symptoms of overdosage include nausea, vomiting, weakness, gastrointestinal disorders and disturbances of electrolyte balance. In severe instances, hypotension and depressed respiration may be observed. If this occurs, support of respiration and cardiac circulation should be instituted. There is no specific antidote. An evacuation of the stomach is recommended by emesis and gastric lavage after which the electrolyte and fluid balance should be evaluated carefully.

Dosage and Administration:
Hypertension and edema of congestive heart failure: The adult starting dose for hypertension or edema of congestive heart failure is 2.5 mg as a *single daily dose* taken in the morning. If the response to 2.5 mg is not satisfactory after one (edema) to four (hypertension) weeks, the daily dose may be increased to 5.0 mg taken once daily.

If the antihypertensive response to indapamide is insufficient, LOZOL may be combined with other antihypertensive drugs, with careful monitoring of blood pressure. It is recommended that the usual dose of other agents be reduced by 50% during initial combination therapy. As the blood pressure response becomes evident, further dosage adjustments may be necessary.

In general, doses of 5.0 mg and larger have not appeared to provide additional effects on blood pressure or heart failure, but are associated with a greater degree of hypokalemia. There is little clinical trial experience in patients with doses greater than 5.0 mg once a day.

How Supplied: LOZOL (indapamide). White, round film-coated tablets of 2.5 mg in bottles of 100 (NDC 0075-0082-00) and 1,000 (NDC 0075-0082-99) and in unit-dose blister packs, boxes of 100 (10 × 10 strips) (NDC 0075-0082-62).
Issued: 10/83
Shown in Product Identification Section, page 440

NICOBID® Tempules® ℞
(niacin, USV)
TIMED–RELEASE NICOTINIC ACID SUPPLEMENT

Description: Each black-and-clear Tempule (timed-release capsule) contains 125 mg niacin (nicotinic acid); each green-and-clear Tempule (timed-release capsule) contains 250 mg niacin (nicotinic acid); and each opaque blue and white Tempule (timed-release capsule) contains 500 mg niacin (nicotinic acid). Nicobid Tempules® provides the full actions of niacin (nicotinic acid). Portions of the pellets contained in the Tempule are released immediately. The remainder is released over several hours.

Uses: Nicobid (niacin, USV) is used in all those conditions in which niacin (nicotinic acid) supplementation is indicated. It has the advantage of a slower release of niacin (nicotinic acid) than conventional tablet dosage forms. This may permit its use by those who do not tolerate the tablets.

Cautions: Nicobid should not be used by persons with a known sensitivity to niacin (nicotinic acid) and by persons with arterial bleeding, glaucoma, severe diabetes, impaired liver function, peptic ulcer, or by pregnant women.

Side Effects: Temporary flushing and feeling of warmth may be expected. These seldom reach levels so as to necessitate discontinuance. If these symptoms persist, discontinue use and consult a physician. Temporary headache, itching and tingling, gastric disturbances, skin rash and allergies may occur.

Dosage: Usual adult dose—one Tempule, 125 mg, 250 mg or 500 mg morning and evening.
KEEP OUT OF THE REACH OF CHILDREN
Revised: 9-83
Shown in Product Identification Section, page 440

NICOLAR® ℞
[nic̄ ō-lär″]
(niacin tablets, USV)

Description: Nicolar® (niacin tablets, USV) is a scored yellow colored tablet containing 500 mg. of niacin (nicotinic acid).

Actions: Niacin functions in the body as a component of two hydrogen transporting coenzymes; Coenzyme I (Nicotinamide Adenine Dinucleotide [NAD], sometimes called Diphosphopyridine Nucleotide [DPN]) and Coenzyme II (Nicotinamide Adenine Dinucleotide Phosphate [NADP], sometimes called Triphosphopyridine Nucleotide [TPN]). Niacin in addition to its functions as a vitamin, exerts several distinctive pharmacologic effects which vary according to the dosage level employed.

Niacin, in large doses, causes a reduction in serum lipids. The exact mechanism of this action is unknown.

Indications: Nicolar® is indicated as adjunctive therapy in patients with significant hyperlipidemia (elevated cholesterol and/or triglycerides) who do not respond adequately to diet and weight loss.

Notice: It has not been established whether the drug-induced lowering of serum cholesterol or triglyceride levels has a beneficial effect, no effect, or a detrimental effect on the morbidity or mortality due to atherosclerosis including coronary heart disease. Investigations now in progress may yield an answer to this question.

Contraindications: Niacin is contraindicated in patients with hepatic dysfunction or in patients with active acute peptic ulcer.

Warnings: Use of this drug in pregnancy, lactation or in women of child-bearing age requires that the potential benefits of the drug be weighed against its possible hazards to the mother and child. Although fetal abnormalities have not been reported with this drug, its use as an antilipidemic agent requires high dosages, and animal reproduction or teratology studies have not been done. There are insufficient studies done for usage in children.

Precautions: Patients with gall bladder disease, or those with a past history of jaundice, liver disease or peptic ulcer should be observed closely while taking this medication.

Frequent monitoring of liver function tests and blood glucose should be performed in the initial stage of therapy until it is ascertained that the drug has no adverse effects on these organ systems.

Diabetic or potential diabetic patients should be observed closely in the event of decreased tolerance. Adjustment of diet and/or hypoglycemic therapy may be necessary.

Patients receiving antihypertensive drugs of the adrenal-blocking type may have an additive vasodilating effect and produce postural hypotension. Elevated uric acid levels have occurred; therefore use with caution in patients predisposed to gout.
This product contains FD&C Yellow No. 5 (tartrazine) which may cause allergic-type reactions (including asthma) in certain susceptible individuals. Although the overall incidence of FD&C Yellow No. 5 (tartrazine) sensitivity in the general population is low, it is frequently seen in patients who also have aspirin hypersensitivity.

Adverse Reactions: Severe generalized flushing
Decreased glucose tolerance
Activation of peptic ulcers
Abnormalities of hepatic functional tests
Jaundice
Gastrointestinal disorders
Dryness of the skin
Keratosis nigricans
Pruritus
Hyperuricemia
Toxic amblyopia
Hypotension
Transient headache

Dosage and Administration: Two to four tablets (1–2 grams) three times a day with or following meals or as directed by physician.
Since flushing, pruritus and gastrointestinal distress appear frequently, begin therapy with small doses and slowly build up dose in gradual increments observing for adverse effects and efficacy. The usual maximum daily dose is 8 grams.
How Supplied: Nicolar® (niacin tablets, USV) is available in bottles of 100 scored tablets, each containing 500 mg. of nicotinic acid (identified by the code NE).
Revised: 12/82
Shown in Product Identification Section, page 440

Continued on next page

	Mean Changes from Baseline after 40 Weeks of Treatment			
	Serum Electrolytes (mEq/l) Potassium Sodium Chloride		Serum Uric Acid (mg/dl)	BUN (mg/dl)
Indapamide 2.5 mg (n=76)	−0.4 −0.6 −3.6		0.7	−0.1
Indapamide 5.0 mg (n=81)	−0.6 −0.7 −5.1		1.1	1.4

USV—Cont.

NITROSPAN®
[nĭ′ trō-span″]
(nitroglycerin)
in sustained-release capsules

Composition: Each capsule provides 2.5 mg or 6.5 mg nitroglycerin in a sustained-release vehicle processed to release medication gradually and continuously for prolonged therapeutic effect.

Actions: The mechanism of action of nitroglycerin in the relief of angina pectoris is not as yet known. However, its main pharmacologic action is to relax smooth muscle, principally in the smaller blood vessels, thus dilating arterioles and capillaries, especially in the coronary circulation. In therapeutic doses, nitroglycerin is thought to increase the blood supply to the myocardium which may in turn relieve myocardial ischemia, the possible functional basis for the pain of angina pectoris.

In Nitrospan the micro-dialysis cells permit smooth, continuous release of nitroglycerin, requiring only the presence of fluid in the gastrointestinal tract.

> **Indications:** Based on a review of this drug by the National Academy of Sciences—National Research Council and/or other information, FDA has classified the indication as follows:
> "Possibly" effective: For the management, prophylaxis, or treatment of anginal attacks. Final classification of the less-than-effective indication requires further investigation.

Contraindications: Acute or recent myocardial infarction, severe anemia, closed-angle glaucoma, postural hypotension, increased intracranial pressure and idiosyncrasy to the drug.

Warnings: Nitrospan Capsules must be swallowed. FOR ORAL, NOT SUBLINGUAL USE. This form of the drug is not intended for immediate relief of anginal attacks.

Precautions: Intraocular pressure may be increased; therefore, caution is required in administering to patients with glaucoma. Tolerance to this drug and cross-tolerance to other organic nitrites and nitrates may occur. If blurring of vision, dryness of mouth or lack of benefit occurs, the drug should be discontinued.

Adverse Reactions: Severe and persistent headaches, cutaneous flushing, dizziness and weakness. Occasionally, drug rash or exfoliative dermatitis, and nausea and vomiting may occur; these responses may disappear with a decrease in dosage. Adverse effects are enhanced by ingestion of alcohol, which appears to increase absorption from the gastrointestinal tract.

Dosage and Administration: Administer the smallest effective dose 2 or 3 times daily at 8- to 12-hour intervals, unless clinical response suggests a different regimen. Discontinue if not effective.

How Supplied: Capsules: 2.5 mg (light green and clear), bottles of 100; 6.5 mg (dark green and clear), bottles of 60.
NSN 6505-00-998-5871A (2.5 mg), V.A. Depots.
Revised: May 1979
Shown in Product Identification Section, page 440

OXALID®
[ŏks′a-lĭd]
oxyphenbutazone

100 mg tablets

Important Note: OXALID (oxyphenbutazone) cannot be considered a simple analgesic and should never be administered casually. Each patient should be carefully evaluated before treatment is started and should remain constantly under the close supervision of the physician. The following cautions should be observed:

1. Therapy should not be initiated until a careful detailed history and complete physical and laboratory examination, including a complete hemogram and urinalysis, etc., of the patient have been made. These examinations should be made at regular, frequent intervals throughout the duration of this drug therapy.
2. Patients should be carefully selected, avoiding those in whom it is contraindicated as well as those who will respond to ordinary therapeutic measures, or those who cannot be observed at frequent intervals.
3. Patients taking this drug should be warned not to exceed the recommended dosage, since this may lead to toxic effects, and should discontinue the drug and report to the physician immediately any sign of:
   a. Fever, sore throat, lesions in the mouth (symptoms of blood dyscrasia).
   b. Dyspepsia, epigastric pain, symptoms of anemia, unusual bleeding, unusual bruising, black or tarry stools or other evidence of intestinal ulceration.
   c. Skin rashes.
   d. Significant weight gain or edema.
4. A trial period of one week of therapy is considered adequate to determine the therapeutic effect of the drug. In the absence of a favorable response, therapy should be discontinued.
In the elderly (sixty years and over) the drug should be restricted to short-term treatment periods only—if possible, *one week* maximum.
5. BEFORE PRESCRIBING OXALID FOR AN INDIVIDUAL PATIENT, READ THOROUGHLY THE INFORMATION CONTAINED UNDER EACH HEADING WHICH FOLLOWS:

Description and Actions: OXALID should not be considered as a simple analgesic that can be prescribed for indiscriminate use.
OXALID is closely related chemically and pharmacologically, including toxic effects, to the well-known pyrazolines (pyrazole compounds) amidopyrine and antipyrine.
Chemically, OXALID is 4-butyl-1-(p-hydroxyphenyl)-2-phenyl-3, 5-pyrazolidinedione monohydrate, the parahydroxy analog of phenylbutazone.
It has anti-inflammatory and antipyretic action as well as analgesic and mild uricosuric properties resulting in symptomatic relief only. THE DISEASE PROCESS ITSELF IS UNALTERED BY THIS DRUG.

Clinical Pharmacology: In man, oxyphenbutazone is completely absorbed after oral administration of OXALID. After ingestion of three 100-mg tablets, peak plasma concentration of oxyphenbutazone has been measured at 34.9 ($\pm$ 5.3) mg/l within six hours. After therapeutic doses, about 98 percent of the drug is bound to human serum albumin. Elimination is mainly by biotransformation in the liver, and the plasma halflife has been measured as 72 ($\pm$ 15 hours). Urinary excretion consists mostly of metabolites.

Indications: The indications for OXALID are:
Acute Gouty Arthritis
Active Rheumatoid Arthritis
Active Ankylosing Spondylitis
Short-term treatment of acute attacks of degenerative joint disease of the hips and knees not responsive to other treatment.
Painful Shoulder (peritendinitis, capsulitis, bursitis, and acute arthritis of that joint)

Contraindications:
1. *Age:* OXALID is contraindicated in children 14 years of age or younger since controlled clinical trials in patients of this age group have not been conducted.
2. *Other Medical Conditions:* OXALID is contraindicated in patients with incipient cardiac failure, blood dyscrasias, pancreatitis, parotitis, stomatitis, polymyalgia rheumatica, temporal arteritis, senility, drug allergy, and in the presence of severe renal, cardiac and hepatic disease, and in patients with a history of peptic ulcer disease, or symptoms of gastrointestinal inflammation or active ulceration because serious adverse reactions or aggravation of existing medical problems can occur.

3. *Concomitant Medications:* OXALID (oxyphenbutazone) should not be used in combination with other drugs which accentuate or share a potential for similar toxicity.
It is also inadvisable to administer OXALID in combination with other potent drugs because of the possibility of increased toxic reactions from OXALID and other agents. (See also *Drug Interactions.*)
OXALID is contraindicated in patients with a history or suggestion of prior toxicity, sensitivity, or idiosyncrasy to phenylbutazone or oxyphenbutazone.

Warnings: Based on reports of clinical experience with oxyphenbutazone and related compounds, the following warnings should be considered by the physician prior to prescribing the drug:
1. *Gastrointestinal:* Upper G.I. diagnostic tests should be performed in patients with persistent or severe dyspepsia. Peptic ulceration, reactivation of latent peptic ulcer, perforation and gastrointestinal bleeding, sometimes severe, have been reported.
As with other nonsteroidal anti-inflammatory drugs, borderline elevations of one or more liver tests may occur in up to 15% of patients. These abnormalities may progress, may remain essentially unchanged, or may be transient with continued therapy. The SGPT (ALT) test is probably the most sensitive indicator of liver dysfunction. Meaningful (three times the upper limit of normal) elevations of SGPT or SGOT (AST) occurred in controlled clinical trials in less than 1% of patients. A patient with symptoms and/or signs suggesting liver dysfunction, or in whom an abnormal liver test has occurred, should be evaluated for evidence of the development of more severe hepatic reaction while on therapy with OXALID. Severe hepatic reactions, including jaundice and cases of fatal hepatitis, have been reported with OXALID as with other nonsteroidal anti-inflammatory drugs. Although such reactions are rare, if abnormal liver tests persist or worsen, if clinical signs and symptoms consistent with liver disease develop, or if systemic manifestations occur (e.g. eosinophilia, rash, etc.), OXALID should be discontinued.
2. *Hematologic: Frequent and regular hematologic evaluations should be performed on patients receiving the drug for periods over one week.* Any significant change in the total white count, relative decrease in granulocytes, appearance of immature forms, or fall in hematocrit should be a signal for immediate cessation of therapy and a complete hematologic investigation. Serious, sometimes fatal blood dyscrasias, including aplastic anemia have been reported to occur. Hematologic toxicity may occur suddenly or many days or weeks after cessation of treatment as manifest by the appearance of anemia, leukopenia, thrombocytopenia or clinically significant hemorrhagic diathesis. There have been published reports associating oxyphenbutazone with leukemia. However, the circumstances involved in these reports are such that a cause-and-effect relationship to the drug has not been clearly established.
3. *Pregnancy:* Reproductive studies in animals, although inconclusive, exhibited evidence of possible embryotoxicity. It is, therefore, recommended that this drug should be used with caution during pregnancy. The benefits should be weighed against the potential risk to the fetus.
4. *Nursing Mothers:* Caution is also advised in prescribing OXALID in nursing mothers since the drug may appear in cord blood and breast milk.
5. Patients reporting visual disturbances while receiving the drug should discontinue treatment and have an ophthalmologic examination because ophthalmologic adverse reactions have been reported (see **Adverse Reactions:** *Special Senses*).
6. In the aging (forty years and over), there appears to be an increase in the possibility of adverse reactions. OXALID should be used with commensurately greater care in the elderly and should be avoided altogether in the senile patient.
7. Like other drugs with prostaglandin synthetase inhibition activity, OXALID (oxyphenbutazone)

for possible revisions   **Product Information**   **2085**

may precipitate acute episodes of asthmatic attacks in patients with asthma.

8. OXALID increases sodium retention. Evidence of fluid retention in patients in whom there is danger of cardiac decompensation is an indication to discontinue the drug.

Precautions: Because of potential serious adverse reactions to OXALID, the following precautions should be observed in the use of the drug:

1. A careful diagnostic physical examination and history should be performed on all patients at regular intervals while the patient is receiving the drug.

2. OXALID is not recommended for chronic use in the elderly.

3. Hematologic evaluation should be performed at frequent and regular intervals and additional laboratory examinations performed as indicated.

4. Patients should be instructed to report immediately the occurrence of high fever, severe sore throat, stomatitis, salivary gland enlargement, tarry stools, unusual bleeding or bruising, sudden weight gain, or edema.

5. The drug reduces iodine uptake by the thyroid and may interfere with laboratory tests of thyroid function (see **Adverse Reactions:** *Endocrine-Metabolic*).

6. The patient should be cautioned regarding participation in activities requiring alertness and coordination, and that the concomitant ingestion of alcohol with OXALID may further impair psychomotor skills.

Drug Interactions: OXALID is highly bound to serum proteins. If its affinity for protein binding is higher than other concurrently administered drugs, the actions and toxicity of the other drug may be increased.

OXALID accentuates the prothrombin depression produced by coumarin-type anticoagulants. When administered alone, it does not affect prothrombin activity.

The pharmacologic action of insulin, anti-diabetic, and sulfonamide drugs may be potentiated by the simultaneous administration of OXALID.

Concomitant administration of oxyphenbutazone and phenytoin may result in increased serum levels of phenytoin which could lead to increased phenytoin toxicity.

Adverse Reactions: Based upon reports of clinical experience with oxyphenbutazone and related compounds, the following adverse reactions have been reported.

The adverse reactions listed in the following table have been arranged into three groups: (1) incidence greater than 1%, (2) incidence less than 1% and (3) causal relationship unknown. The incidence for group (1) was obtained from fifty-seven (57) clinical trials reported in the literature (3713 patients). The incidence for group (2) was based on reports in clinical trials, in the literature, and on voluntary reports. The reactions in group (3) have been reported but occurred under circumstances where a causal relationship could not be established. In some patients the reported reactions may have been unrelated to the administration of the drug. However, in these reported events, the possibility cannot be excluded. Therefore these observations are being listed to serve as alerting information to physicians. Before prescribing this drug for an individual patient, the physician should be familiar with the following:

GASTROINTESTINAL (see **Warnings**)
1. Incidence greater than 1%
gastrointestinal upset
2. Incidence less than 1%
nausea
dyspepsia/including indigestion and heartburn
abdominal and epigastric distress
vomiting
abdominal distention with flatulence
constipation
diarrhea
esophagitis
gastritis
salivary gland enlargement
stomatitis, sometimes with ulceration
ulceration and perforation of the intestinal tract including acute and reactivated peptic ulcer with perforation, hemorrhage and hematemesis
anemia due to gastrointestinal bleeding which may be occult
hepatitis, both fatal and nonfatal, sometimes associated with evidence of cholestasis

HEMATOLOGICAL (see **Warnings**)
1. Incidence greater than 1%
None
2. Incidence less than 1%
anemia
leukopenia
thrombocytopenia with associated purpura, petechiae, and hemorrhage
pancytopenia
aplastic anemia
bone marrow depression
agranulocytosis and agranulocytic anginal syndrome
hemolytic anemia

HYPERSENSITIVITY
1. Incidence greater than 1%
None
2. Incidence less than 1%
urticaria
anaphylactic shock
arthralgia, drug fever
hypersensitivity angiitis (polyarteritis) and vasculitis
Lyell's syndrome
serum sickness
Stevens-Johnson syndrome
activation of systemic lupus erythematosus
aggravation of temporal arteritis in patients with polymyalgia rheumatica

DERMATOLOGIC
1. Incidence greater than 1%
None
2. Incidence less than 1%
pruritus
erythema nodosum
erythema multiforme
nonthrombocytopenic purpura

CARDIOVASCULAR, FLUID AND ELECTROLYTE
1. Incidence greater than 1%
None
2. Incidence less than 1%
sodium and chloride retention
fluid retention and plasma dilution
cardiac decompensation (congestive heart failure) with edema and dyspnea
metabolic acidosis
respiratory alkalosis
hypertension
pericarditis
interstitial myorcarditis with muscle necrosis and perivascular granulomata

RENAL
1. Incidence greater than 1%
None
2. Incidence less than 1%
hematuria
proteinuria
ureteral obstruction with uric acid crystals
anuria
glomerulonephritis
acute tubular necrosis
cortical necrosis
renal stones
nephrotic syndrome
impaired renal function and renal failure associated with azotemia

CENTRAL NERVOUS SYSTEM
1. Incidence greater than 1%
None
2. Incidence less than 1%
headache
drowsiness
agitation
confusional states and lethargy
tremors
numbness
weakness

ENDOCRINE-METABOLIC (see **Precautions**)
1. Incidence greater than 1%
None
2. Incidence less than 1%
None

SPECIAL SENSES (see **Warnings**)
1. Incidence greater than 1%
Ocular: none
Otic: none
2. Incidence less than 1%
Ocular: none
Otic: hearing loss, tinnitus

(3) **Causal relationship unknown—Incidence less than 1%:** *Hematological* (see **Warnings**)—Leukemia (There have been reports associating oxyphenbutazone with leukemia. However, the circumstances involved in these reports are such that a cause-and-effect relationship to the drug has not been clearly established.) *Endocrine-Metabolic* (see **Precautions**)—Thyroid hyperplasia; goiters associated with hyperthyroidism and hypothyroidism; pancreatitis; hyperglycemia. *Special Senses* (see **Warnings**)—Blurred vision; optic neuritis; toxic amblyopia; scotomata; retinal detachment; retinal hemorrhage; oculomotor palsy.

Overdosage:

Signs and Symptoms: Include any of the following: nausea, vomiting, epigastric pain, excessive perspiration, euphoria, psychosis, headaches, giddiness, vertigo, hyperventilation, insomnia, tinnitus, difficulty in hearing, edema (sodium retention), hypertension, cyanosis, respiratory depression, agitation, hallucinations, stupor, convulsions, coma, hematuria, and oliguria. Hepatomegaly, jaundice, and ulceration of the buccal or gastrointestinal mucosa have been reported as late manifestations of massive overdosage.

Reported laboratory abnormalities following overdosage include: respiratory or metabolic acidosis, impaired hepatic or renal function, and abnormalities of formed blood elements.

Treatment: In the alert patient, empty the stomach promptly by induced emesis followed by lavage. In the obtunded patient, secure the airway with a cuffed endotracheal tube before beginning lavage (do not induce emesis). Maintain adequate respiratory exchange, do not use respiratory stimulants. Treat shock with appropriate supportive measures. Control seizures with intravenous diazepam or short-acting barbiturates. Dialysis may be helpful if renal function is impaired.

Dosage and Administration: OXALID (oxyphenbutazone) should be used at the smallest effective dosage to afford rapid relief of severe symptoms. It is contraindicated in children under 14 years of age and in senile patients.

If a favorable symptomatic response to treatment is not obtained after one week, the drug should be discontinued. When a favorable therapeutic response has been obtained, the dosage should be reduced and then discontinued as soon as possible. In elderly patients (sixty years and over) every effort must be made to discontinue therapy on, or as soon as possible after the seventh day, because of the exceedingly high risk of severe fatal toxic reactions in this age group.

To minimize gastric upset, the drug should be taken with milk or with meals.

In selecting the appropriate dosage in any specific case, consideration should be given to the patient's age, weight, general health, and any other factors that may influence his response to the drug.

Rheumatoid Arthritis, Ankylosing Spondylitis, Acute Attacks of Degenerative Joint Disease, and Painful Shoulder. Initial Dosage: The initial daily dose in adult patients is 300 to 600 mg as 3 to 4 divided doses. Maximum therapeutic response is usually obtained at a total daily dose of 400 mg. A trial period of one week of therapy is considered adequate to determine the therapeutic effect of the drug. In the absence of a favorable response, therapy should be discontinued.

Maintenance Dosage: When improvement is obtained, dosage should be promptly decreased to the minimum effective level necessary to maintain relief, not exceeding 400 mg daily because of the

Continued on next page

USV—Cont.

possibility of cumulative toxicity. A satisfactory clinical response may be obtained with daily doses as low as 100 to 200 mg daily.

Acute Gouty Arthritis: Satisfactory results are obtained after an initial dose of 400 mg followed by 100 mg every 4 hours. The articular inflammation usually subsides within 4 days and treatment should not be continued longer than one week.

How Supplied: 100 mg Tablets (white, round, sugar coated), bottles of 100 and 1000.
Revised: 7/82

PENTRITOL® ℞
[pĕn-trĭ-tōl]
(pentaerythritol tetranitrate)

Composition: Each timed-release capsule (Tempules®) USV provides 30 mg or 60 mg pentaerythritol tetranitrate.

Description:
Empirical Formula: $C_5H_8N_4O_{12}$
Molecular Weight: 316.15

The pentaerythritol tetranitrate is in a special timed-release base (Tempules®) designed to give prolonged systemic effect.

Action: The mechanism of action in the relief of angina pectoris is unknown at this time, although the basic pharmacologic action is to relax smooth muscle.

Indication
Based on a review of this drug by the National Academy of Science—National Research Council and/or other information, FDA has classified the indication as follows:
"Possibly" effective for the relief of angina pectoris (pain of coronary artery disease). It is not intended to abort the acute anginal episode, but is widely regarded as useful in the prophylactic treatment of angina pectoris.
Final classification of the less-than-effective indications requires further investigation.

Contraindications: Idiosyncrasy to this drug.

Warning: Data supporting the use of nitrites during the early days of the acute phase of myocardial infarction (the period during which clinical and laboratory findings are unstable) are insufficient to establish safety.

Precautions: Intraocular pressure is increased; therefore, caution is required in administering to patients with glaucoma. Tolerance to this drug, and cross-tolerance to other nitrites and nitrates may occur.

Adverse Reactions: Cutaneous vasodilation with flushing. Headache is common and may be severe and persistent. Transient episodes of dizziness and weakness, as well as other signs of cerebral ischemia associated with postural hypotension, occasionally may develop. This drug can act as a physiological antagonist to norepinephrine, acetylcholine, histamine, and many other agents. An occasional individual exhibits marked sensitivity to the hypotensive effects of nitrite and severe responses (nausea, vomiting, weakness, restlessness, pallor, perspiration, and collapse) can occur, even with the usual therapeutic dose. Alcohol may enhance this effect. Drug rash and/or exfoliative dermatitis may occasionally occur.

Dosage and Administration: One 30 mg or 60 mg oral timed-release capsule (Tempules®) every 12 hours on an empty stomach. (Not recommended for sublingual use.)

Although the onset of effect and the duration of effect of this drug are quite variable, the following are the generally reported ranges for these values:
Onset of effect: estimated to be 30 minutes.
Duration of effect: considered to be up to 12 hours.

How Supplied: Pentritol® 30 mg Tempules® are available in bottles of 100 and 250. Pentritol® 60 mg Tempules® are available in bottles of 60 and 250.

Manufactured by KV PHARMACEUTICAL COMPANY, St. Louis, Missouri 63144

Manufactured for USV LABORATORIES, DIVISION USV PHARMACEUTICAL CORP., Tarrytown, NY 10591
Revised: 12/82

PERTOFRANE® ℞
[pert'ō-frān]
(desipramine hydrochloride USP)

Composition: Each capsule provides 25 mg or 50 mg desipramine hydrochloride.

Description: PERTOFRANE is a metabolite of imipramine hydrochloride. It is a dibenzazepine derivative, representing the desmethyl analog of imipramine hydrochloride. Chemically, it is 10,11-dihydro-5-[3-(methylamino) propyl]-5H-dibenz [b,f] azepine Monohydrochloride, and differs from the parent substance by having only one methyl group on the side chain nitrogen.

Desipramine hydrochloride is a white, crystalline substance with a molecular weight of 302.8. It is soluble to the extent of about 10% w/v in water, and melts within a range of 5° between 208-218°C.

Actions: PERTOFRANE has been found in some studies to have a more rapid onset of action than imipramine; antidepressant efficacy is similar though potency on a weight basis may be less. The earliest manifestations consist mainly of an increase in psychomotor activity. Full treatment benefit is seldom attained before the end of the second week.

PERTOFRANE is not a monoamine oxidase inhibitor and does not act primarily as a central nervous system stimulant. Like all tricyclic antidepressants, PERTOFRANE blocks the reuptake of norepinephrine by adrenergic nerve terminals. Demethylated analogs such as desipramine are more potent in increasing norepinephrine turnover rate than the methylated compounds. However, the exact mechanism of action of tricyclics in depression is still unknown.

A mechanism of action proposed for antidepressant drugs, the biogenic amine theory, postulates that some, if not all, depression is associated with a deficiency or depletion of catecholamines and that some antidepressant drugs increase the amount of amine available at the synaptic receptor.

Desipramine is metabolized in the liver and approximately 70% is excreted in the urine.

Indications: PERTOFRANE is indicated for the relief of mental depression (see Note before How Supplied section for additional information on depressive symptomatologies often responsive to this drug).

Contraindications: The use of PERTOFRANE concomitantly or within two weeks of the administration of MAO inhibitors, is contraindicated. Hyperpyretic crises or severe convulsive seizures may occur in patients receiving such combinations. The potentiation of adverse reactions can be serious, or even fatal. When it is desired to substitute PERTOFRANE in patients receiving a monoamine oxidase inhibitor, as long an interval should elapse as the clinical situation allows, with a minimum of 14 days. Initial dosage should be low and increases should be gradual and cautiously prescribed.

The drug is contraindicated following recent myocardial infarction.

Patients with a known hypersensitivity to tricyclic antidepressants should not be given PERTOFRANE.

Warnings: As with other potent antidepressants, an activation of the psychosis may occasionally be observed in schizophrenic patients.

Due to the drug's atropine-like effects and sympathomimetic potentiation, PERTOFRANE should be used only with the greatest care in patients with narrow-angle glaucoma and with urethral or ureteral spasm.

Likewise, only when patient need outweighs the risk of serious adverse reactions should the drug be used in the presence of any of the following conditions: severe coronary heart disease with EKG abnormalities, progressive heart failure, angina pectoris, paroxysmal tachycardia and active seizure disorder (this agent has been shown to lower the seizure threshold).

In some instances, desipramine and the parent compound, imipramine, have been shown to block the pharmacologic action of the antihypertensive, guanethidine, and related adrenergic neuron-blocking agents.

Hypertensive episodes have been observed during surgery in patients on desipramine hydrochloride therapy.

The concurrent use of other central nervous system drugs or alcohol may potentiate the adverse effects of desipramine hydrochloride. Since many such drugs may be used during surgery, it is recommended that desipramine hydrochloride be discontinued for as long as the clinical situation will allow prior to elective surgery.

In patients who may use alcohol excessively, it should be borne in mind that the potentiation may increase the danger inherent in any suicide attempt or overdosage.

Patients should be cautioned about the possibility of impaired ability to operate a motor vehicle or other dangerous machinery.

Usage in Pregnancy: Although teratogenic studies in mice, rats and rabbits have revealed no adverse effects, safe use of this drug in women who are or may become pregnant has not been definitely established. Therefore, PERTOFRANE (desipramine hydrochloride USP) should be withheld from these women unless the clinical situation warrants the potential risk.

In view of the lack of experience in children, the drug is not recommended for use in patients under twelve years of age.

Elderly and adolescent patients can usually be managed on lower dosage than that recommended for other patients and may not tolerate higher doses as well because of an increased incidence of adverse reactions.

Precautions: It should be kept in mind that the possibility of suicide in seriously depressed patients is inherent in the illness and may persist until remission occurs. These patients require careful supervision and protective measures during therapy.

Anxiety and increased agitation have been reported, particularly where depression is not the primary disorder. A shift to hypomanic or manic excitement may occur during therapy. Such reactions may necessitate discontinuation of the drug. Although the anticholinergic activity of the drug is weak, in susceptible patients and in those receiving anticholinergic drugs (including antiparkinsonism agents), atropine-like effects may be more pronounced (e.g. paralytic ileus).

Caution should be observed in prescribing the drug in hyperthyroid patients and in those receiving thyroid medications. Transient cardiac arrhythmias have occurred in rare instances.

In all patients undergoing extended courses of therapy, periodic blood and liver studies for signs of toxicity should supplement careful clinical observations.

Adverse Reactions: PERTOFRANE is well tolerated by most patients and severe complications or adverse reactions are infrequent. Those most often reported cause little discomfort and seldom require discontinuation of the drug.

Nervous System: Dizziness, drowsiness, insomnia, headache and disturbed visual accommodation have been reported with the drug. In addition, tremor, unsteadiness, tinnitus and paresthesias have been reported. Occasionally, mild extrapyramidal activity, falling, and neuromuscular incoordination have been seen. A confusional state (with such symptoms as hallucinations and disorientation) may be produced, particularly in older patients and at higher dosage, and may require discontinuation of the drug. Changes in EEG patterns have been reported. Epileptiform seizures may occur. The syndrome of inappropriate ADH (antidiuretic hormone) secretion may occur. A reduction in dosage may help control some of these adverse reactions.

Gastrointestinal Tract: Anorexia, dryness of the mouth, nausea, epigastric distress, constipation and diarrhea have been reported in patients receiving PERTOFRANE.

Skin: Skin rashes (including photosensitization), perspiration and flushing sensations have been reported during therapy.

Liver: Transient jaundice, apparently of an obstructive nature, and liver damage have been observed in rare cases. Elevation in transaminase and changes in alkaline phosphatase have occurred and should indicate repeated liver-function profiles. If progressive elevation occurs, the drug should be discontinued.

Blood Elements: Bone-marrow depression, agranulocytosis, thrombocytopenia and purpura have been reported. If these occur, the drug should be discontinued. Transient eosinophilia has been observed in some instances.

Cardiovascular System: Orthostatic hypotension and tachycardia have been observed but seldom require discontinuation of treatment. Patients who require concomitant vasodilating therapy should be carefully supervised, particularly during the initial phases.

Genitourinary System: Urinary frequency or retention and impotence have been reported.

Endocrine System: Occasional hormonal effects, including gynecomastia, galactorrhea and breast enlargement have been reported with PERTOFRANE (desipramine hydrochloride USP). In addition, decreased libido and estrogenic effect have been noted. The exact relationship of these adverse effects to the administration of the drug has not been established.

Sensitivity: Urticaria and rare instances of drug fever and cross-sensitivity with imipramine have been observed.

Withdrawal Symptoms: Abrupt cessation of treatment after prolonged administration may produce nausea, headache, and malaise. These are not indicative of addiction. Rare instances have been reported of mania or hypomania occurring within 2–7 days following cessation of chronic therapy with tricyclic antidepressants.

Dosage and Administration: All Patients Except Geriatric and Adolescent: The usual dosage range is from 75 to 150 mg/day in divided doses or as a single daily dose. Titration to a maintenance dose should be based on clinical response and tolerance by starting in the low dose range and increasing dosage when required. When necessary, dosage may be increased, after initiation of therapy, up to 200 mg daily in divided doses. Continued therapy at the optimal dosage level should be maintained during the active phase of the depression.

It is recommended that a lower maintenance dosage be continued for at least two months after a satisfactory response has been achieved. This, too, may be given on a once-daily schedule for convenience and compliance.

In cases of relapse due to premature withdrawal of the drug, a prompt response may be obtained by immediate resumption of treatment.

Geriatric and Adolescent Patients: Elderly and adolescent patients can usually be managed on lower dosage and may not tolerate higher doses as well as other patients. Therapy in these age groups may be initiated with 25 to 50 mg daily. Dosage may be increased according to response and tolerance to a maximum of 100 mg daily. It is recommended that a lower maintenance dosage be continued for at least two months after a satisfactory response has been achieved. Therapy may be given in divided doses or as a single daily dose.

Overdosage:

Signs and Symptoms: These may vary in severity depending on several factors, including the amount absorbed, age, interval between ingestion and start of treatment, etc. In infants and young children, especially, acute overdosage in any amount must be considered serious and potentially fatal.

CNS abnormalities may include drowsiness, stupor, coma, ataxia, restlessness, agitation, hyperactive reflexes, muscle rigidity, athetoid and choreiform movements, and convulsions.

Cardiac abnormalities may include arrhythmia, tachycardia, ECG evidence of impaired conduction, and signs of congestive failure.

Respiratory depression, cyanosis, hypotension, shock, vomiting, hyperpyrexia, mydriasis, and diaphoresis may also be present.

Treatment: Because CNS involvement, respiratory depression and cardiac arrhythmia can occur suddenly, hospitalization and close observation are necessary, even when the amount ingested is thought to be small or the initial degree of intoxication appears slight or moderate. All patients with ECG abnormalities should have continuous cardiac monitoring for at least 72 hours and be closely observed until well after cardiac status has returned to normal; relapses may occur after apparent recovery.

The *slow* intravenous administration of physostigmine salicylate has been reported to reverse most of the cardiovascular and CNS effects of overdosage with tricyclic antidepressants. In adults, 1 to 3 mg has been reported to be effective. In children, start with 0.5 mg and repeat at 5 minute intervals to determine the minimum effective dose; do not exceed 2 mg. Because of the short duration of action of physostigmine, repeat the effective dose at 30 to 50 minute intervals, as necessary. Avoid rapid injection to reduce the possibility of physostigmine-induced convulsions.

In the alert patient, empty the stomach promptly by induced emesis followed by lavage. In the obtunded patient, secure the airway with a cuffed endotracheal tube before beginning lavage (do not induce emesis). Continue lavage for 24 hours or longer, depending on the apparent severity of intoxication. Use normal or half-normal saline to avoid water intoxication, especially in children. Instillation of activated charcoal slurry may help reduce absorption of desipramine.

Minimize external stimulation to reduce the tendency to convulsions. If anticonvulsants are necessary, diazepam, short-acting barbiturates, paraldehyde or methocarbamol may be useful. Do not use barbiturates if MAO inhibitors have been taken recently.

Maintain adequate respiratory exchange. Do not use respiratory stimulants.

Shock should be treated with supportive measures, such as intravenous fluids, oxygen and corticosteroids. Digitalis may increase conduction abnormalities and further irritate an already sensitized myocardium. If congestive heart failure necessitates rapid digitalization, particular care must be exercised.

Hyperpyrexia should be controlled by whatever external means are available, including ice packs and cooling sponge baths, if necessary.

Hemodialysis, peritoneal dialysis, exchange transfusions and forced diuresis have been generally reported as ineffective because of the rapid fixation of desipramine in tissues. Blood desipramine levels may not correlate with the degree of intoxication, and are unreliable indicators in the clinical management of the patient.

Note: Depressions which are most responsive to PERTOFRANE (desipramine hydrochloride USP) may be described in terms of "target symptoms." These include:

Despondency, sadness and depressed mood
Fatigue
Lack of interest and emotional response
Helplessness, hopelessness, pessimism and despair
Feelings of incapacity and inferiority
Psychomotor retardation and inhibition
Delusions of guilt and unworthiness
Psychosomatic complaints
Insomnia
Anorexia and weight loss
Depression-related anxiety and agitation
Suicidal drive

It should be borne in mind that these "target symptoms" of depression assume their proper significance only after careful history, physical and mental evaluations and other investigative procedures have confirmed a diagnosis of one of the several types of depression.

How Supplied: 25 mg Capsules (pink), bottles of 100 and 1000 (NSN 6505-00-913-0382A—V.A. Depots); 50 mg Capsules (maroon and pink), bottles of 100 and 1000.

Revised: October, 1983
Shown in Product Identification Section, page 440

REGROTON® ℞
[rĕ-grō-tŏn]
DEMI-REGROTON® ℞
Oral antihypertensives

Composition: Each REGROTON tablet provides 50 mg chlorthalidone USP and 0.25 mg reserpine USP. Each DEMI-REGROTON tablet provides 25 mg chlorthalidone USP and 0.125 mg reserpine USP.

Description: REGROTON and DEMI-REGROTON are drug combinations of two well-known antihypertensive agents, chlorthalidone and reserpine.

Chemistry: A monosulfamyl diuretic, chlorthalidone differs from thiazide diuretics in that a double-ring system is incorporated in its structure. Chemically, it is 2-Chloro-5-(1-hydroxy - 3 - oxo - 1-isoindolinyl) benzenesulfonamide.

Reserpine is a pure crystalline alkaloid from the root of Rauwolfia serpentina.

Actions: The pharmacologic effects are those of the constituent drugs. Chlorthalidone produces a saluretic effect in humans, beginning within two hours after an oral dose and continuing for as long as 72 hours. Copious diuresis is produced, with greatly increased excretion of sodium and chloride.

Reserpine, because it reduces arterial blood pressure and exerts a sedative effect, is particularly useful in the therapy of hypertension with related emotional disturbance. Reserpine is characterized by slow onset of action and sustained effect. Both its cardiovascular and central nervous system effects may persist following withdrawal of the drug. (See Precautions.)

Both chlorthalidone and reserpine have prolonged action, and the combination is thus able to exert a smooth and concerted effect over a long period. The two drugs appear to enhance each other, and this gives the combination a high degree of effectiveness. When considered necessary the combination may be prescribed together with other antihypertensive agents, which may then be given in lower dosage with lessened chance of side reactions.

Indication: Treatment of hypertension. (See box warning.)

Contraindications: Mental depression, demonstrated hypersensitivity, and most cases of severe renal or hepatic diseases are the only contraindications.

Warnings:

> These fixed combination drugs are not indicated for initial therapy of hypertension. Hypertension requires therapy titrated to the individual patient. If the fixed combination represents the dosage so determined, its use may be more convenient in patient management. The treatment of hypertension is not static, but must be reevaluated as conditions in each patient warrant.

These drugs should be used with caution in severe renal disease, since products containing chlorthalidone or similar drugs may precipitate azotemia. Cumulative effects of the drug may develop in patients with impaired renal function.

They should be used with caution in patients with impaired hepatic function or progressive liver disease, since minor alterations of fluid and electrolyte balance may precipitate hepatic coma.

REGROTON or DEMI-REGROTON may add to or potentiate the action of other antihypertensive drugs. Potentiation occurs with ganglionic or peripheral adrenergic blocking drugs.

Sensitivity reactions may occur in patients with a history of allergy or bronchial asthma.

Discontinue the drug in patients in whom mental depression develops while on the drug (the possibility of suicide should be kept in mind). In pa-

Continued on next page

USV—Cont.

tients who have had depression, the drug should not be started. Electroshock therapy should not be given to patients taking reserpine, since severe and even fatal reactions have occurred. The drug should be stopped at least seven days before giving electroshock therapy.

In susceptible patients, peptic ulcer may be precipitated or activated, in which case the drug should be discontinued.

Usage in Pregnancy: Reproduction studies with chlorthalidone in various animal species at multiples of the human dose showed no significant level of teratogenicity; no fetal or congenital abnormalities were observed. Animal data should not be extrapolated for clinical application.

Thiazides cross the placental barrier and appear in cord blood. The use of chlorthalidone and related drugs in pregnant women requires that the anticipated benefits of the drug be weighed against possible hazards to the fetus. These hazards include fetal or neonatal jaundice, thrombocytopenia, and possibly other adverse reactions which have occurred in the adult.

NURSING MOTHERS: Thiazides and reserpine cross the placental barrier and appear in cord blood and breast milk. Increased respiratory secretions, nasal congestion, cyanosis and anorexia may occur in infants born to reserpine-treated mothers. If use of the drug is deemed essential, the patient should stop nursing.

Precautions: Antihypertensive therapy with chlorthalidone/reserpine combinations should always be initiated cautiously in postsympathectomy patients and in those receiving ganglionic blocking agents, other potent antihypertensive drugs, or curare. At least a one-half reduction in the usual dosage of such agents may be advisable. Careful and continuous supervision of patients on such multiple-drug regimens is necessary.

Since some patients receiving Rauwolfia preparations have experienced hypotension when undergoing surgery, it may be advisable to discontinue chlorthalidone/reserpine combination drugs therapy about two weeks prior to elective surgical procedures. Emergency surgery may be carried out by using, if necessary, anticholinergic or adrenergic drugs to prevent vagocirculatory responses; other supportive measures may be used as indicated.

Because of the possibility of progression of renal damage, periodic kidney function tests are indicated. In case of a rising BUN, the drug should be stopped.

The drug should be discontinued in cases of aggravated liver dysfunction (hepatic coma may be precipitated).

Periodic determination of serum electrolytes to detect possible electrolyte imbalance should be performed at appropriate intervals.

All patients receiving chlorthalidone should be observed for clinical signs of fluid or electrolyte imbalance; namely, hyponatremia, hypochloremic alkalosis, and hypokalemia. Serum and urine electrolyte determinations are particularly important when the patient is vomiting excessively or receiving parenteral fluids. Medication such as digitalis may also influence serum electrolytes. Warning signs, irrespective of cause, are: Dryness of mouth, thirst, weakness, lethargy, drowsiness, restlessness, muscle pains or cramps, muscular fatigue, hypotension, oliguria, tachycardia, and gastrointestinal disturbances such as nausea and vomiting.

Hypokalemia may develop with chlorthalidone as with any other potent diuretic, especially with brisk diuresis, when severe cirrhosis is present, or during concomitant use of corticosteroids or ACTH.

Interference with adequate oral electrolyte intake will also contribute to hypokalemia. Digitalis therapy may exaggerate metabolic effects of hypokalemia especially with reference to myocardial activity.

Any chloride deficit is generally mild and usually does not require specific treatment except under extraordinary circumstances (as in liver disease or renal disease). Dilutional hyponatremia may occur in edematous patients in hot weather; appropriate therapy is water restriction, rather than administration of salt except in rare instances when the hyponatremia is life threatening. In actual salt depletion, appropriate replacement is the therapy of choice.

Hyperuricemia may occur or frank gout may be precipitated in certain patients receiving chlorthalidone.

Insulin requirements in diabetic patients may be increased, decreased, or unchanged. Latent diabetes mellitus may become manifest during chlorthalidone administration.

Chlorthalidone and related drugs may decrease arterial responsiveness to norepinephrine. This diminution is not sufficient to preclude effectiveness of the pressor agent for therapeutic use.

Chlorthalidone and related drugs may decrease serum PBI levels without signs of thyroid disturbance.

Because reserpine increases gastrointestinal motility and secretion, REGROTON or DEMI-REGROTON should be used cautiously in patients with ulcerative colitis or gallstones, where biliary colic may be precipitated. In susceptible patients, bronchial asthma may occur.

Animal tumorigenicity: rodent studies have shown that reserpine is an animal tumorigen, causing an increased incidence of mammary fibroadenomas in female mice, malignant tumors of the seminal vesicles in male mice, and malignant adrenal medullary tumors in male rats. These findings arose in 2-year studies in which the drug was administered in the feed at concentrations of 5 and 10 ppm—about 100 to 300 times the usual human dose. The breast neoplasms are thought to be related to reserpine's prolactin-elevating effect. Several other prolactin-elevating drugs have also been associated with an increased incidence of mammary neoplasia in rodents.

The extent to which these findings indicate a risk to humans is uncertain. Tissue culture experiments show that about one third of human breast tumors are prolactin dependent in vitro, a factor of considerable importance if the use of the drug is contemplated in a patient with previously detected breast cancer. The possibility of an increased risk of breast cancer in reserpine users has been studied extensively; however, no firm conclusion has emerged. Although a few epidemiologic studies have suggested a slightly increased risk (less than twofold in all studies except one) in women who have used reserpine, other studies of generally similar design have not confirmed this. Epidemiologic studies conducted using other drugs (neuroleptic agents) that, like reserpine, increase prolactin levels and, therefore, would be considered rodent mammary carcinogens, have not shown an association between chronic administration of the drug and human mammary tumorigenesis. While long-term clinical observation has not suggested such an association, the available evidence is considered too limited to be conclusive at this time. An association of reserpine intake with pheochromocytoma or tumors of the seminal vesicles has not been explored.

Adverse Reactions: Clinical trials indicate that the combination of chlorthalidone with reserpine is generally well tolerated. The adverse reactions most frequently seen include anorexia, gastric irritation, nausea, vomiting, diarrhea, constipation, nasal congestion, muscle cramps, dizziness, weakness, headache, drowsiness, and mental depression. Skin rashes, urticaria, and a case of ecchymosis have been reported. (Other dermatologic manifestations may occur—see below.)

A decreased glucose tolerance evidenced by hyperglycemia and glycosuria may develop inconsistently. This condition—usually reversible on discontinuation of therapy—responds to control with antidiabetic treatment. Diabetics and those predisposed should be checked regularly.

Hyperuricemia may be observed on occasion and acute attacks of gout have been precipitated. In cases where prolonged and significant elevation of blood uric acid concentration is considered potentially deleterious, concomitant use of a uricosuric agent is effective in reversing hyperuricemia without loss of diuretic and/or antihypertensive activity.

In addition to the reactions listed above, certain adverse reactions attributable to the drugs' components are shown below. Since REGROTON and DEMI-REGROTON combine chlorthalidone and reserpine in relatively small doses, such reactions may be less than when those drugs are used in full dosage.

Chlorthalidone: Idiosyncratic drug reactions such as aplastic anemia, purpura, thrombocytopenia, leukopenia, agranulocytosis, necrotizing angiitis and Lyell's syndrome (toxic epidermal necrolysis) have occurred, but are rare.

The remote possibility of pancreatitis should be considered when epigastric pain or unexplained gastrointestinal symptoms develop after prolonged administration.

Other reported reactions include restlessness, transient myopia, impotence or dysuria, and orthostatic hypotension, which may be potentiated when chlorthalidone is combined with alcohol, barbiturates or narcotics. Since jaundice, xanthopsia, paresthesia, and photosensitization have been documented in related compounds, the possibility of these reactions should be kept in mind.

Reserpine: The sedative effect of reserpine may lead to drowsiness or lassitude in some patients. Frequently, this effect disappears with continued administration. Nasal stuffiness sometimes occurs. Gastrointestinal reactions include increased gastric secretions, loose stools, or increased bowel frequency.

Symptoms of mental depression may occur in a small percentage of patients, although the recommended dosage of REGROTON contains substantially less reserpine than that usually implicated in such reactions. The same is true of other rare side effects recorded for reserpine, which include bradycardia and ectopic cardiac rhythms (especially when used with digitalis), pruritus, eruptions and/or flushing of skin, angina pectoris, headache, dizziness, paradoxical anxiety, nightmare, dull sensorium, muscular aches, a reversible paralysis agitans-like syndrome, blurred vision, conjunctival injection, uveitis, optic atrophy and glaucoma, increased susceptibility to colds, dyspnea, weight gain, decreased libido or impotence, dryness of the mouth, deafness, and anorexia.

Dosage and Administration:
Selection of drug and dosage should be determined by individual titration. (See box warning.) According to the requirement, the recommended dose of either REGROTON or DEMI-REGROTON is usually *one tablet once a day.* Some patients may require two tablets once a day. Divided doses are unnecessary, and a single dose given in the morning with food is recommended.

Maintenance: Maintenance dosage must be individually adjusted. Mild cases may be adequately controlled with one DEMI-REGROTON tablet daily. Optimal lowering of elevated blood pressure may require two weeks or more in some cases because of the slow onset of action of reserpine.

Combination With Other Drugs: In more severe cases, if the response to a chlorthalidone/reserpine combination alone is inadequate, potent antihypertensives may be added gradually in dosages at least 50% lower than those usually employed. Such patients should be supervised carefully and continuously. As soon as desired blood pressure levels have been attained, the lowest effective maintenance dosage should be followed.

Overdosage: Adverse reactions resulting from accidental acute overdosage may include nausea, weakness, dizziness, syncope, and disturbances of electrolyte balance. There is no specific antidote. However, the following is recommended: gastric lavage followed by supportive treatment, including intravenous dextrose-saline with potassium chloride if necessary, to be given with the usual caution. If marked hypotension results from overdosage, it can be treated with vasopressor drugs.

How Supplied: REGROTON is available as pink, round, single-scored tablets, in bottles of 100 and 1000; DEMI-REGROTON as white, round tablets, bottles of 100 and 1000.

Animal Pharmacology: In animal biochemical studies, chlorthalidone is absorbed slowly from the gastrointestinal tract, due to low solubility. After passage to the liver, some of the drug enters the general circulation, while some is excreted in the bile, to be reabsorbed later. In the general circulation, the drug is distributed widely to the tissues, but is taken up in the highest concentrations in the kidneys, where amounts have been found 72 hours after ingestion, long after it has disappeared from other tissues. The drug is excreted unchanged in the urine. The high renal concentration of chlorthalidone may be causally associated with the prolonged saluretic effect of the drug. Chlorthalidone appears to inhibit sodium and chloride reabsorption in the cortical diluting segment of ascending limb of Henle's loop. The reduction of plasma volume following diuresis is a probable mechanism in the initial antihypertensive action of the drug.

Reserpine probably produces its sedative and hypotensive effects through a depletion in tissue stores of catecholamines. The antihypertensive action of reserpine is probably due to loss of epinephrine and norepinephrine from peripheral sites. By contrast, its sedative and tranquilizing properties are thought to be related to depletion of 5-hydroxytryptamine from the brain.

Revised: April, 1983
Shown in Product Identification Section, page 440

ARMOUR® THYROID Tablets ℞
[thī′roid]

Description: Armour® Thyroid (Thyroid, U.S.P.) Tablets for oral use are derived from porcine thyroid glands. They contain both tetraiodothyronine sodium (T_4 levothyroxine) and triiodothyronine sodium (T_3 liothyronine).

Armour® Thyroid is standardized by the U.S.P. method for iodine content and biologically assayed to assure metabolic potency.

Clinical Pharmacology: The steps in the synthesis of the thyroid hormones are controlled by thyrotropin (Thyroid Stimulating Hormone, THS) secreted by the anterior pituitary. This hormone's secretion is in turn controlled by a feedback mechanism effected by the thyroid hormones themselves and by thyrotropin releasing hormone (THR), a tripeptide of hypothalamic origin. Endogenous thyroid hormone secretion is suppressed when exogenous thyroid hormones are administered to euthyroid individuals in excess of the normal gland's secretion.

The mechanisms by which thyroid hormones exert their physiologic action are not well understood. These hormones enhance oxygen consumption by most tissues of the body, increase the basal metabolic rate, and the metabolism of carbohydrates, lipids, and proteins. Thus, they exert a profound influence on every organ system in the body and are of particular importance in the development of the central nervous system.

The normal thyroid gland contains approximately 200 mcg of levothyroxine (T_4) per gram of gland, and 15 mcg of triiodothyronine (T_3) per gram. The ratio of these two hormones in the circulation does not represent the ratio in the thyroid gland, since about 80 percent of peripheral triiodothyronine comes from monodeiodination of levothyroxine. Peripheral monodeiodination of levothyroxine at the 5 position (inner ring) also results in the formation of reverse triiodothyronine (T_3), which is calorigenically inactive.

Triiodothyronine (T_3) levels are low in the fetus and newborn, in old age, in chronic caloric deprivation, hepatic cirrhosis, renal failure, surgical stress, and chronic illnesses representing what has been called the "low triiodothyronine syndrome."

Pharmacokinetics—Animal studies have shown that T_4 is only partially absorbed from the gastrointestinal tract. The degree of absorption is dependent on the vehicle used for its administration and by the character of the intestinal contents, the intestinal flora, including plasma protein, soluble dietary factors, all of which bind thyroid and thereby make it unavailable for diffusion. Only 41 percent is absorbed when given in a gelatin capsule as opposed to a 74 percent absorption when given with an albumin carrier. Depending on other factors, absorption has varied from 48 to 79 percent of the administered dose. Fasting increases absorption. Malabsorption syndromes, as well as dietary factors, (children's soybean formula, concomitant use of anionic exchange resins such as cholestyramine) cause excessive fecal loss. T_3 is almost totally absorbed, 95 percent in 4 hours. The hormones contained in the natural preparations are absorbed in a manner similar to the synthetic hormones.

More than 99 percent of circulating hormones are bound to serum proteins, including thyroid-binding globulin (TBg), thyroid-binding prealbumin (TBPA), and albumin (TBa), whose capacities and affinities vary for the hormones. The higher affinity of levothyroxine (T_4) for both TBg and TBPA as compared to triiodothyronine (T_3) partially explains the higher serum levels and longer half-life of the former hormone. Both protein-bound hormones exist in reverse equilibrium with minute amounts of free hormone, the latter accounting for the metabolic activity.

Deiodination of levothyroxine (T_4) occurs at a number of sites, including liver, kidney, and other tissues. The conjugated hormone, in the form of glucuronide or sulfate, is found in the bile and gut where it may complete an enterophepatic circulation. Eighty-five percent of levothyroxine (T_4) metabolized daily is deiodinated.

Indications and Usage: Armour® Thyroid (Thyroid U.S.P.) is indicated:

1. As replacement or supplemental therapy in patients with hypothyroidism of any etiology, except transient hypothyroidism during the recovery phase of subacute thyroiditis. This category includes cretinism, myxedema, and ordinary hypothyroidism in patients of any age (children, adults, the elderly), or state (including pregnancy); primary hypothyroidism resulting from functional deficiency, primary atrophy, partial or total absence of thyroid gland, or the effects of surgery, radiation, or drugs, with or without the presence of goiter; and secondary (pituitary), or tertiary (hypothalamic) hypothyroidism (See WARNINGS).
2. As pituitary TSH suppressants, in the treatment or prevention of various types of euthyroid goiters, including thyroid nodules, sub-acute or chronic lymphocytic thyroiditis (Hashimoto's), multinodular goiter, and in the management of thyroid cancer.
3. As diagnostic agents in suppression tests to differentiate suspected mild hyperthyroidism or thyroid gland autonomy.

Contraindications: Thyroid hormone preparations are generally contraindicated in patients with diagnosed but as yet uncorrected adrenal cortical insufficiency, untreated thyrotoxicosis, and apparent hypersensitivity to any of their active or extraneous constituents. There is no well documented evidence from the literature, however, of true allergic or idiosyncratic reactions to thyroid hormone.

WARNINGS

Drugs with thyroid hormone activity, alone or together with other therapeutic agents, have been used for the treatment of obesity. In euthyroid patients, doses within the range of daily hormonal requiremnts are ineffective for weight reduction. Larger doses may produce serious or even life-threatening manifestations of toxicity, particularly when given in association with sympathomimetic amines such as those used for their anorectic effects.

The use of thyroid hormones in the therapy of obesity, alone or combined with other drugs, is unjustified and has been shown to be ineffective. Neither is their use justified for the treatment of male or female infertility unless this condition is accompanied by hypothyroidism.

Precautions:
General—Thyroid hormones should be used with great caution in a number of circumstances where the integrity of the cardiovascular system, particularly the coronary arteries, is suspected. These include patients with angina pectoris or the elderly, in whom there is a greater likelihood of occult cardiac disease. In these patients thyroid therapy should be initiated with low doses, i.e. 15–30 mg Armour® Thyroid. When, in such patients, a euthyroid state can only be reached at the expense of an aggravation of the cardiovascular disease, thyroid hormone dosage should be reduced.

Thyroid hormone therapy in patients with concomitant diabetes mellitus or diabetes insipidus or adrenal cortical insufficiency aggravates the intensity of their symptoms. Appropriate adjustments of the various therapeutic measures directed at these concomitant endocrine diseases are required. The therapy of myxedema coma requires simultaneous administration of glucocorticoids (See DOSAGE AND ADMINISTRATION).

Hypothyroidism decreases and hyperthyroidism increases the sensitivity to oral anticoagulants. Prothrombin time should be closely monitored in thyroid treated patients on oral anticoagulants and dosage of the latter agents adjusted on the basis of frequent prothrombin time determinations. In infants, excessive doses of thyroid hormone preparations may produce craniosynostosis.

Information for the Patient—Patients on thyroid hormone preparations and parents of children on thyroid therapy should be informed that:

1. Replacement therapy is to be taken essentially for life, with the exception of cases of transient hypothyroidism, usually associated with thyroiditis, and in those patients receiving a therapeutic trial of the drug.
2. They should immediately report during the course of therapy any signs or symptoms of thyroid hormone toxicity, e.g., chest pain, increased pulse rate, palpitations, excessive sweating, heat intolerance, nervousness, or any other unusual event.
3. In case of concomitant diabetes mellitus, the daily dosage of antidiabetic medication may need readjustment as thyroid hormone replacement is achieved. If thyroid medication is stopped, a downward readjustment of the dosage of insulin or oral hypoglycemic agent may be necessary to avoid hypoglycemia. At all times, close monitoring of urinary glucose levels is mandatory in such patients.
4. In case of concomitant oral anticoagulant therapy, the prothrombin time should be measured frequently to determine if the dosage of oral anticoagulants is to be readjusted.
5. Partial loss of hair may be experienced by children in the first few months of thyroid therapy, but this is usually a transient phenomenon and later recovery is usually the rule.

Laboratory Tests—Treatment of patients with thyroid hormones requires the periodic assessment of thyroid status by means of appropriate laboratory tests besides the full clinical evaluation. The TSH suppression test can be used to test the effectiveness of any thyroid preparation bearing in mind the relative insensitivity of the infant pituitary to the negative feedback effect of thyroid hormones. Serum T_4 levels can be used to test the effectiveness of all thyroid medications except T_3. When the total serum T_4 is low but TSH is normal, a test specific to assess unbound (free) T_4 levels is warranted. Specific measurements of T_4 and T_3 by competitive protein binding or radioimmunoassay are not influenced by blood levels of organic or inorganic iodine.

Drug Interactions—Oral Anticoagulants—Thyroid hormones appear to increase catabolism of vitamin K-dependent clotting factors. If oral anticoagulants are also being given, compensatory increases in clotting factor synthesis are impaired. Patients stabilized on oral anticoagulants who are

Continued on next page

USV—Cont.

found to require thyroid replacement therapy should be watched very closely when thyroid is started. If a patient is truly hypothyroid, it is likely that a reduction in anticoagulant dosage will be required. No special precautions appear to be necessary when oral anticoagulant therapy is begun in a patient already stabilized on maintenance thyroid replacement therapy.

Insulin or Oral Hypoglycemics—Initiating thyroid replacement therapy may cause increases in insulin or oral hypoglycemic requirements. The effects seen are poorly understood and depend upon a variety of factors such as dose and type of thyroid preparations and endocrine status of the patient. Patients receiving insulin or oral hypoglycemics should be closely watched during initiation of thyroid replacement therapy.

Cholestyramine—Cholestyramine binds both T_4 and T_3 in the intestine, thus impairing absorption of these thyroid hormones. *In vitro* studies indicate that the binding is not easily removed. Therefore, four to five hours should elapse between administration of cholestyramine and thyroid hormones.

Estrogen, Oral Contraceptives—Estrogens tend to increase serum thyroxine-binding globulin (TBg). In a patient with a nonfunctioning thyroid gland who is receiving thyroid replacement therapy, free levothyroxine may be decreased when estrogens are started thus increasing thyroid requirements. However, if the patient's thyroid gland has sufficient function, the decreased free thyroxine will result in a compensatory increase in thyroxine output by the thyroid. Therefore, patients without a functioning thyroid gland who are on thyroid replacement therapy may need to increase their thyroid dose if estrogens or estrogen-containing oral contraceptives are given.

Drug/Laboratory Test Interactions—The following drugs or moieties are known to interfere with laboratory tests performed in patients on thyroid hormone therapy: androgens, corticosteroids, estrogens, oral contraceptives containing estrogens, iodine-containing preparations, and the numerous preparations containing salicylates.

1. Changes in TBg concentration should be taken into consideration in the interpretation of T_4 and T_3 values. In such cases, the unbound (free) hormone should be measured. Pregnancy, estrogens, and estrogen-containing oral contraceptives increase TBg concentrations. TBg may also be increased during infectious hepatitis. Decreases in TBg concentrations are observed in nephrosis, acromegaly, and after androgen or corticosteroid therapy. Familial hyper- or hypothyroxine-binding-globulinemias have been described. The incidence of TBg deficiency approximates 1 in 9,000. The binding of thyroxine by TBPA is inhibited by salicylates.
2. Medicinal or dietary iodine interferes with all *in vivo* tests of radio-iodine uptake, producing low uptakes which may not be relative of a true decrease in hormone synthesis.
3. The persistence of clinical and laboratory evidence of hypothyroidism in spite of adequate dosage replacement indicates either poor patient compliance, poor absorption, excessive fecal loss, or inactivity of the preparation. Intracellular resistance to thyroid hormone is quite rare.

Carcinogenesis, Mutagenesis, and Impairment of Fertility—A reportedly apparent association between prolonged thyroid therapy and breast cancer has not been confirmed and patients on thyroid for established indications should not discontinue therapy. No confirmatory long-term studies in animals have been performed to evaluate carcinogenic potential, mutagenicity, or impairment of fertility in either males or females.

Pregnancy-Category A—Thyroid hormones do not readily cross the placental barrier. The clinical experience to date does not indicate any adverse effect on fetuses when thyroid hormones are administered to pregnant women. On the basis of current knowledge, thyroid replacement therapy to hypothyroid women should not be discontinued during pregnancy.

Nursing Mothers—Minimal amounts of thyroid hormones are excreted in human milk. Thyroid is not associated with serious adverse reactions and does not have a known tumorigenic potential. However, caution should be exercised when thyroid is administered to a nursing woman.

Pediatric Use—Pregnant mothers provide little or no thyroid hormone to the fetus. The incidence of congenital hypothyroidism is relatively high (1:4,000) and the hypothyroid fetus would not derive any benefit from the small amounts of hormone crossing the placental barrier. Routine determinations of serum (T_4) and/or TSH is strongly advised in neonates in view of the deleterious effects of thyroid deficiency on growth and development.

Treatment should be initiated immediately upon diagnosis, and maintained for life, unless transient hypothyroidism is suspected; in which case, therapy may be interrupted for 2 to 8 weeks after the age of 3 years to reassess the condition. Cessation of therapy is justified in patients who have maintained a normal TSH during those 2 to 8 weeks.

Adverse Reactions: Adverse reactions other than those indicative of hyperthyroidism because of therapeutic overdosage, either initially or during the maintenance period, are rare (See OVERDOSAGE).

Overdosage:

Signs and Symptoms—Excessive doses of thyroid result in a hypermetabolic state resembling in every respect the condition of endogenous origin. The condition may be self-induced.

Treatment of Overdosage—Dosage should be reduced or therapy temporarily discontinued if signs and symptoms of overdosage appear.

Treatment may be reinstituted at a lower dosage. In normal individuals, normal hypothalamic-pituitary-thyroid axis function is restored in 6 to 8 weeks after thyroid suppression.

Treatment of acute massive thyroid hormone overdosage is aimed at reducing gastrointestinal absorption of the drugs and counteracting central and peripheral effects, mainly those of increased sympathetic activity. Vomiting may be induced initially if further gastrointestinal absorption can reasonably be prevented and barring contraindications such as coma, convulsions, or loss of the gagging reflex. Treatment is symptomatic and supportive. Oxygen may be administered and ventilation maintained. Cardiac glycosides may be indicated if congestive heart failure develops. Measures to control fever, hypoglycemia, or fluid loss should be instituted if needed. Antiadrenergic agents, particularly propranolol, have been used advantageously in the treatment of increased sympathetic activity. Propranolol may be administered intravenously at a dosage of 1 to 3 mg over a 10 minute period or orally, 80 to 160 mg/day, especially when no contraindications exist for its use.

Dosage and Administration: The dosage of thyroid hormones is determined by the indication and must in every case be individualized according to patient response and laboratory findings.

Thyroid hormones are given orally. In acute, emergency conditions, injectable sodium levothyroxine may be given intravenously when oral administration is not feasible or desirable, as in the treatment of myxedema coma, or during total parenteral nutrition. Intramuscular administration is not advisable because of reported poor absorption.

Hypothyroidism—Therapy is usually instituted using low doses, with increments which depend on the cardiovascular status of the patient. The usual starting dose is 30 mg Armour® Thyroid, with increments of 15 mg every 2 to 3 weeks. A lower starting dosage, 15 mg/day, is recommended in patients with long standing myxedema, particularly if cardiovascular impairment is suspected, in which case extreme caution is recommended. The appearance of angina is an indication for a reduction in dosage. Most patients require 60–120 mg/day. Failure to respond to doses of 180 mg suggests lack of compliance or malabsorption. Maintenance dosages 60–120 mg/day usually result in normal serum levothyroxine (T_4) and triiodothyronine (T_3) levels. Adequate therapy usually results in normal TSH and T_4 levels after 2 to 3 weeks of therapy.

Readjustment of thyroid hormone dosage should be made within the first four weeks of therapy, after proper clinical and laboratory evaluations, including serum levels of T_4, bound and free, and TSH.

T_3 may be used in preference to levothyroxine (T_4) during radio-isotope scanning procedures, since induction of hypothyroidism in those cases is more abrupt and can be of shorter duration. It may also be preferred when impairment of peripheral conversion of T_4 and T_3 is suspected.

Myxedema Coma—Myxedema coma is usually precipitated in the hypothyroid patient of long-standing by intercurrent illness or drugs such as sedatives and anesthetics and should be considered a medical emergency. Therapy should be directed at the correction of electrolyte disturbances and possible infection besides the administration of thyroid hormones. Corticosteroids should be administered routinely. T_4 and T_3 may be administered via a nasogastric tube but the preferred route of administration of both hormones is intravenous. Sodium levothroxine (T_4) is given at a starting dose of 400 mcg (100 mcg/ml) given rapidly, and is usually well tolerated, even in the elderly. This initial dose is followed by daily supplements of 100 to 200 mcg given IV. Normal T_4 levels are achieved in 24 hours followed in 3 days by threefold elevation of T_3. Oral therapy with thyroid hormone would be resumed as soon as the clinical situation has been stabilized and the patient is able to take oral medication.

Thyroid Cancer—Exogenous thyroid hormone may produce regression of metastases from follicular and papillary carcinoma of the thyroid and is used as ancillary therapy of these conditions with radioactive iodine. TSH should be suppressed to low or undetectable levels. Therefore, larger amounts of thyroid hormone than those used for replacement therapy are required. Medullary carcinoma of the thyroid is usually unresponsive to this therapy.

Thyroid Suppression Therapy—Administration of thyroid hormone in doses higher than those produced physiologically by the gland results in suppression of the production of endogenous hormone. This is the basis for the thyroid suppression test and is used as an aid in the diagnosis of patients with signs of mild hyperthyroidism in whom base line laboratory tests appear normal, or to demonstrate thyroid gland autonomy in patients with Grave's ophthalmopathy. [131]I uptake is determined before and after the administration of the exogenous hormone. A fifty percent or greater suppression of uptake indicates a normal thyroid-pituitary axis and thus rules out thyroid gland autonomy.

For adults, the usual suppressive dose of levothyroxine (T_4) 1.56 mg/kg of body weight per day given for 7 to 10 days. These doses usually yield normal serum T_4 and T_3 levels and lack of response to TSH.

Thyroid hormones should be administered cautiously to patients to whom there is strong suspicion of thyroid gland autonomy, in view of the fact that the exogenous hormone effects will be additive to the endogenous source.

Pediatric Dosage—Pediatric dosage should follow the recommendations summarized in Table 1. In infants with congenital hypothyroidism, therapy with full doses should be instituted as soon as the diagnosis has been made.

Recommended Pediatric Dosage for Congenital Hypothyroidism

Armour® Thyroid

Age	Dose per day	Daily dose per kg of body weight
0–6 mos	15–30 mg	4.8–6 mg
6–12 mos	30–45 mg	3.6–4.8 mg
1–5 yrs	45–60 mg	3–3.6 mg

6–12 yrs	60–90 mg	2.4–3 mg
Over 12 yrs	Over 90 mg	1.2–1.8 mg

Table 1

How Supplied: Armour® Thyroid Tablets, U.S.P. are supplied as follows: 30 mg (½ gr) and 60 mg (1 gr) tablets in bottles of 100, 1000, and 5000; 120 mg (2 gr) tablets in bottles of 100, 1000, and 2500; 15 mg (¼ gr) and 180 mg (3 gr) tablets in bottles of 100 and 1000; and 90 mg (1½ gr), 240 mg (4 gr), and 300 mg (5 gr) tablets in bottles of 100. The 15 mg (¼ gr), 30 mg (½ gr), 60 mg (1 gr), 90 mg (1½ gr), 120 mg (2 gr), 180 mg (3 gr), 240 mg (4 gr), and 300 mg (5 gr) potencies are available in special dispensing bottles of 100 tablets designated as Handy 100s® (child-resistant closure with tear-off label). The 30 mg (½ gr), 60 mg (1 gr), and 120 mg (2 gr) potencies are also available in cartons of 100 tablets (10 strips of 10 tablets) packaged in Unit Dose as Armadose.®

Tablets should be stored at controlled room temperature—between 15°–30°C (59°–86°F) in capped bottles or unbroken plastic strip packing.

Revised: March, 1984

THYROLAR® ℞
[thī-rō-lär]
(liotrix, USV)

Description: Thyrolar® tablets provide a combination of the synthetic active thyroid hormones, sodium levothyroxine and sodium liothyronine in a ratio of 4:1 by weight. Thyrolar® is available in five potencies approximately equivalent in therapeutic effect to ¼ gr., ½ gr., 1 gr., 2 gr. and 3 gr. of desiccated thyroid. In Thyrolar®-1 tablets a combination of 50 mcg. of sodium levothyroxine and 12.5 mcg. of sodium liothyronine represent the approximate activity of 1 gr. of desiccated thyroid. The other available potencies are proportional in strength.

Action: Thyrolar® is an effective agent for correcting the hypothyroid state and inducing clinical euthyroidism. The ratio of active hormones present closely simulates the clinical biochemical effects of desiccated thyroid and of the natural endogenous thyroid secretion. Thus, the various thyroid function parameters respond to Thyrolar® as they do to the administration of desiccated thyroid.

The principal effect of thyroid hormones is to increase the metabolic rate of body tissues. Sodium liothyronine is more readily absorbed from the gastrointestinal tract than is sodium levothyroxine. Excretion is rapid so that the action is dissipated more readily than is that of levothyroxine (T_4).

The effects of sodium levothyroxine develop slowly but are more prolonged.

With Thyrolar® the most widely used parameters of thyroid function may be used to aid in the assessment of the response since, when the euthyroid state is achieved, the values may ordinarily be expected to fall within the normal range. This is not true with sodium liothyronine administration alone where subnormal values are present or with sodium levothyroxine alone where abnormally high values are associated with clinical euthyroidism.

Indications: Thyrolar® is indicated in the treatment of hypothyroidism as a source of exogenous thyroid hormone in diminished or absent thyroid function. This may be due to the use of antithyroid agents, radiation therapy, primary atrophy, partial or complete surgical removal of the gland or it may be functional in nature.

Thyrolar® is efficacious in the treatment of hypothyroidism regardless of the etiology. The use of Thyrolar® for suppression therapy in simple (non-toxic) goiter gives prompt results in reducing the size of the gland.

Contraindications: Thyrolar® administration is contraindicated in thyrotoxicosis and in acute myocardial infarction.

Thyrolar® is contraindicated in the presence of uncorrected adrenal insufficiency because it increases the tissue demands for adrenocortical hormones and may cause an acute adrenal crisis in such patients (See Warnings).

Warnings:

> Drugs with thyroid hormone activity, alone or together with other therapeutic agents, have been used for the treatment of obesity. In euthyroid patients, doses within the range of daily hormonal requirements are ineffective for weight reduction. Larger doses may produce serious or even life-threatening manifestations of toxicity, particularly when given in association with sympathomimetic amines such as those used for their anorectic effects.

Thyrolar® should be used with caution in patients with cardiovascular disease, including hypertension. The development of chest pain or other aggravation of cardiovascular disease will require a decrease in dosage.

Injection of epinephrine in patients with coronary artery disease may precipitate an episode of coronary insufficiency. This may be enhanced in patients receiving thyroid preparations. Careful observation is required if catecholamines are administered to patients in this category. Thyrolar® treated patients with concomitant coronary artery disease should be carefully observed during surgery since the possibility of precipitating cardiac arrhythmias may be greater in patients treated with thyroid hormones.

The institution of thyroid replacement therapy may potentiate anticoagulant effects with agents such as warfarin or bishydroxycoumarin and reduction of one-third in anticoagulant dosage should be undertaken upon initiation of Thyrolar® therapy. Subsequent anticoagulant dosage adjustment should be made on the basis of frequent prothrombin determinations.

In patients whose hypothyroidism is secondary to hypopituitarism, adrenal insufficiency will probably also be present. When the adrenal insufficiency and hypothyroidism coexist, the adrenal insufficiency should be corrected by corticosteroids before administering thyroid hormones.

Precautions: Patients with hypothyroidism and especially myxedema are particularly sensitive to thyroid preparations so that treatment should begin with small doses and increments should be gradual. In patients with diabetes mellitus addition of thyroid hormone therapy may cause an increase in the required dosage of insulin or oral hypoglycemic agents. Conversely, decreasing the dose of thyroid hormone may possibly cause hypoglycemic reactions if the dosage of insulin or oral agents is not adjusted.

Adverse Reactions: Excessive dosage of thyroid medication may result in symptoms of hyperthyroidism. Since, however, the effects do not appear at once, the symptoms may not appear for 1 to 3 weeks after the dosage regimen is begun. The most common signs and symptoms of overdosage are weight loss, palpitation, nervousness, diarrhea or abdominal cramps, sweating, tachycardia, cardiac arrhythmias, angina pectoris, tremors, headache, insomnia, intolerance to heat, fever. If symptoms of overdosage appear, discontinue medication for several days and reinstitute treatment at a lower dosage level.

In some individuals who are euthyroid on Thyrolar® headache may appear. Dosage should be decreased. If headache persists or the patient develops signs of hypothyroidism on the lower dosage, another thyroid preparation should be substituted.

Dosage and Administration: As with all thyroid preparations, the dosage of Thyrolar® must be individualized to approximate the deficit in the patient's thyroid secretion. The response of the patient is determined by clinical judgment in conjunction with laboratory findings.

For newly diagnosed or untreated hypothyroidism, therapy may be initiated with one tablet of Thyrolar®-¼ or Thyrolar®-½ daily depending on the patient's status and increased gradually every one or two weeks. In children, increments in dosage should be made every two weeks. For unstabilized hypothyroid patients receiving some form of thyroid therapy direct substitution of Thyrolar® for the current dose of the other product can be made, with gradual increase in dose every one to two weeks.

In patients previously rendered euthyroid with desiccated thyroid, sodium levothyroxine or sodium liothyronine, each Thyrolar®-1 tablet will usually replace 1 grain of desiccated thyroid, 0.1 mg. sodium levothyroxine or 25 mcg. sodium liothyronine. Dosage adjustments, other than those routinely necessary with any thyroid therapy, are seldom necessary.

Thyrolar® is usually given as a single daily dose preferably before breakfast in the morning.

In the normal euthyroid individual, PBI values range from 4 to 8 micrograms/100 ml. and with Thyrolar® values in this range usually correspond to the clinical euthyroid state. Other useful tests include the T_3-resin uptake tests, T_4 by Column and Free thyroxine. In patients rendered euthyroid with Thyrolar®, these tests usually give values within the normal range.

Tablets should be stored at controlled room temperature—between 15°–30°C (59°-86°F) in a light-resistant container.

How Supplied: Thyrolar® is available in five potencies, coded as follows:
[See table above].

Supplied in bottles of 100, two-layered compressed tablets. Thyrolar®-½, Thyrolar®-1, Thyrolar®-2, and Thyrolar®-3 are also supplied in bottles of 1000.

Revised: 12/82

Shown in Product Identification Section, page 440

Name	Composition (T_4/T_3 per Tablet)	Color	Armacode®	Desiccated Thyroid— Approximate Equivalence
Thyrolar®–¼	12.5 mcg./3.1 mcg.	Violet/White	YC	¼ gr.
Thyrolar®–½	25 mcg./6.25 mcg.	Peach/White	YD	½ gr.
Thyrolar®–1	50 mcg./12.5 mcg.	Pink/White	YE	1 gr.
Thyrolar®–2	100 mcg./25 mcg.	Green/White	YF	2 gr.
Thyrolar®–3	150 mcg./37.5 mcg.	Yellow/White	YH	3 gr.

TUSSAR® DM OTC
[tŭs'är]
Cough Syrup
Non-narcotic, Alcohol Free
Antitussive/Decongestant/Antihistaminic

Each 5 ml (one teaspoonful) contains:
Dextromethorphan
 Hydrobromide, U.S.P. ....15 mg
Chlorpheniramine Maleate, U.S.P. ....2 mg
Phenylephrine Hydrochloride, U.S.P. ....5 mg
Methylparaben, N.F. 0.1%

Indications: For relief of cough due to common cold and minor throat and bronchial irritations. TUSSAR DM provides relief of nasal congestion, running nose and watery eyes as may occur in allergic rhinitis (such as hay fever).

Directions For Use: ADULTS—One or two teaspoonfuls (5 or 10 ml) every six to eight hours, not to exceed eight teaspoonfuls in any 24-hour period.

Continued on next page

USV—Cont.

CHILDREN 6–12 YEARS—One teaspoonful (5 ml) every six to eight hours, not to exceed four teaspoonfuls in any 24-hour period.
CHILDREN UNDER 6 YEARS—Not to be administered unless directed by a physician.
Warnings: Do not take this product for persistent cough which may indicate a serious condition except under the supervision of a physician. Do not take this product if you have high blood pressure, heart disease or thyroid disease unless directed by a physician. Do not exceed recommended dosage. As with any drug, if you are pregnant or nursing a baby, seek the advice of a health professional before using this product.
Cautions: If symptoms persist for more than 7 days or are accompanied by a high fever, rash or persistent headache, consult a physician. If drowsiness occurs, do not drive a car or operate machinery.
3/84

TUSSAR®-2
[tŭs-är]
(exempt narcotic cough syrup)

Each 5 ml (one teaspoonful) contains:
Codeine Phosphate, USP ....10 mg
(Warning—may be habit-forming)
Carbetapentane Citrate ....7.5 mg
Chlorpheniramine Maleate, USP ....2.0 mg
Guaifenesin, USP ....50 mg
Sodium Citrate, USP ....130 mg
Citric Acid, USP ....20 mg
Methylparaben, N.F. 0.1%
Alcohol 5%

Indications: For relief of severe coughs due to respiratory conditions such as common cold, bronchitis, and influenza.
Directions for Use: Adults—One teaspoonful 3 to 4 times a day as needed for cough, but no more than 8 teaspoonfuls in any 24-hour period.
Cautions: Persistent cough may indicate the presence of a serious condition. Seek medical advice if there is a high fever or if relief does not occur within 3 days. Persons with a high fever or persistent cough should use only on advice of a physician. Not to be administered to infants or children unless directed by a physician. If drowsiness occurs, do not drive a car or operate machinery.
Warning: As with any drug, if you are pregnant or nursing a baby, seek the advice of a health professional before using this product.
12/82

TUSSAR® SF (Sugar Free)
[tŭs'är]
(exempt narcotic cough syrup)

Formulation identical to Tussar®-2, except Tussar SF contains saccharin-sorbitol base for patients who must limit sugar intake. Alcohol content 12 percent instead of 5 percent.

EDUCATIONAL MATERIAL

For further information, contact your local USV Sales Representative or USV Corporate Headquarters. Your request will be forwarded to the appropriate Sales Representative.

Products are cross-indexed by generic and chemical names in the **YELLOW SECTION**

Ulmer Pharmacal Company
(A Krelitz Industries Company)
2440 FERNBROOK LANE
MINNEAPOLIS, MN 55441

CLINITAR™ CREAM
[klin'i-tar]
(See PDR For Nonprescription Drugs)

CLINITAR™ SHAMPOO
[klin'i-tar]
(See PDR For Nonprescription Drugs)

CLINITAR™ STICK
[klin'i-tar]
(See PDR For Nonprescription Drugs)

LOBANA® BATH OIL
[lō-ban'a]
(See PDR For Nonprescription Drugs)

LOBANA® BODY LOTION
[lō-ban'a]
(See PDR For Nonprescription Drugs)

LOBANA® BODY POWDER
[lō-ban'a]
(See PDR For Nonprescription Drugs)

LOBANA® BODY SHAMPOO
[lō-ban'a]
(See PDR For Nonprescription Drugs)

LOBANA® CONDITIONING SHAMPOO
[lō-ban'a]
(See PDR For Nonprescription Drugs)

LOBANA® DERM-ADE CREAM
[lō-ban'a]
(See PDR For Nonprescription Drugs)

LOBANA® LIQUID HAND SOAP
[lō-ban'a]
(See PDR For Nonprescription Drugs)

LOBANA® PERI-GARD
[lō-ban'a]
(See PDR For Nonprescription Drugs)

LOBANA® PERINEAL CLEANSE
[lō-ban'a]
(See PDR For Nonprescription Drugs)

VERUCID™ GEL
[ver'ū-sid]
(See PDR For Nonprescription Drugs)

VLEMINCKX' Solution
[vlem'inks]
(Topical Acne Treatment and Scabicide)
(See PDR For Nonprescription Drugs)

Products are cross-indexed by product classifications in the **BLUE SECTION**

The Upjohn Company
KALAMAZOO, MI 49001

The Upjohn Manufacturing Company*
BARCELONETA, PUERTO RICO 00617

UPJOHN PRODUCT IDENTIFICATION CODE
Most capsules and tablets manufactured by The Upjohn Company and The Upjohn Manufacturing Company are imprinted with one or a combination of the following: (1) Product trademark (2) Dosage strength (3) "Upjohn" or "U" (4) That portion of the National Drug Code (NDC) number which indicates product and strength.
A complete list of oral solid dosage forms with their assigned NDC numbers is provided below.

Code #	Product	Strength
11	**FEMINONE®** Tablets (ethinyl estradiol tablets, USP)	0.05 mg
12	**CORTEF®** Tablets (hydrocortisone tablets, USP)	5 mg
14	**HALOTESTIN®** Tablets (fluoxymesterone tablets, USP) *See Product Identification Section*	2 mg
15	**CORTISONE ACETATE** Tablets, USP	5 mg
17	**HALCION®** Tablets (triazolam) *See Product Identification Section*	0.25 mg
18	**DIDREX®** Tablets (benzphetamine hydrochloride) *See Product Identification Section*	25 mg
19	**HALOTESTIN®** Tablets (fluoxymesterone tablets, USP) *See Product Identification Section*	5 mg
22	**MEDROL®** Tablets (methylprednisolone tablets, USP) *See Product Identification Section*	8 mg
23	**CORTISONE ACETATE** Tablets, USP	10 mg
24	**DIDREX®** Tablets (benzphetamine hydrochloride) *See Product Identification Section*	50 mg
25	**DELTA-CORTEF®** Tablets (prednisolone tablets, USP)	5 mg
27	**HALCION®** Tablets (triazalam) *See Product Identification Section*	0.5 mg
29	**XANAX®** Tablets (alprazolam) *See Product Identification Section*	0.25 mg
31	**CORTEF®** Tablets (hydrocortisone tablets, USP)	10 mg
32	**DELTASONE®** Tablets (prednisone tablets, USP) *See Product Identification Section*	2.5 mg.
34	**CORTISONE ACETATE** Tablets, USP	25 mg
36	**HALOTESTIN®** Tablets (fluoxymesterone tablets, USP) *See Product Identification Section*	10 mg
38	**HALODRIN®** Tablets (fluoxymesterone and ethinyl estradiol)	
44	**CORTEF®** Tablets (hydrocortisone tablets, USP)	20 mg
45	**DELTASONE®** Tablets (prednisone tablets, USP) *See Product Identification Section*	5 mg
49	**MEDROL®** Tablets (methylprednisolone tablets, USP) *See Product Identification Section*	2 mg
50	**PROVERA®** Tablets (medroxyprogesterone acetate tablets, USP) *See Product Identification Section*	10 mg
55	**XANAX®** Tablets (alprazolam) *See Product Identification Section*	0.5 mg
56	**MEDROL®** Tablets (methylprednisolone tablets, USP) *See Product Identification Section*	4 mg

Product Information

#	Product	Dose
61	**PAMINE®** Tablets (methscopolamine bromide tablets, USP)	2.5 mg
62	**CALDEROL®** Capsules (calcifediol) *See Product Identification Section*	20 mcg
64	**PROVERA®** Tablets (medroxyprogesterone acetate tablets, USP) *See Product Identification Section*	2.5 mg
70	**TOLINASE®** Tablets (tolazamide tablets, USP) *See Product Identification Section*	100 mg
73	**MEDROL®** Tablets (methylprednisolone tablets, USP) *See Product Identification Section*	16 mg
74	**CALDEROL®** Capsules (calcifediol)	50 mcg
81	**ADEFLOR CHEWABLE®** Tablets Fluoride and vitamins *See Product Identification Section*	0.5 mg
90	**XANAX®** Tablets (alprazolam) *See Product Identification Section*	1 mg
92	**ADEFLOR CHEWABLE®** Tablets Fluoride and vitamins *See Product Identification Section*	1 mg
100	**ORINASE®** Tablets (tolbutamide tablets, USP) *See Product Identification Section*	0.5 Gm
101	**ALBAMYCIN®** Capsules (novobiocin sodium)	250 mg
103	**E-MYCIN®** Tablets (erythromycin enteric-coated tablets) *See Product Identification Section*	250 mg
106	**DIOSTATE D®** Tablets Vitamin, calcium and phosphorus supplement	
114	**TOLINASE®** Tablets (tolazamide tablets, USP) *See Product Identification Section*	250 mg
115	**ADEFLOR M®** Tablets Vitamins and minerals with fluoride	
121	**LONITEN®** Tablets (minoxidil) *See Product Identification Section*	2.5 mg
122	**CEBENASE®** Tablets	
131	**MICRONASE®** Tablets (glyburide) *See Product Identification Section*	1.25 mg
137	**LONITEN®** Tablets (minoxidil) *See Product Identification Section*	10 mg
138	**UNICAP®** Capsules Multivitamin Supplement	
141	**MICRONASE®** Tablets (glyburide) *See Product Identification Section*	2.5 mg
149	**UNICAP T®** Tablets Vitamins with minerals	
155	**MEDROL®** Tablets (methylprednisolone tablets, USP) *See Product Identification Section*	24 mg
165	**DELTASONE®** Tablets (prednisone tablets, USP) *See Product Identification Section*	20 mg
171	**MICRONASE®** Tablets (glyburide) *See Product Identification Section*	5.0 mg
176	**MEDROL®** Tablets (methylprednisolone tablets, USP) *See Product Identification Section*	32 mg
193	**DELTASONE®** Tablets (prednisone tablets, USP) *See Product Identification Section*	10 mg
198	**UNICAP CHEWABLE®** Tablets Multivitamin	
225	***CLEOCIN HCl™** Capsules (clindamycin HCl capsules, USP) *See Product Identification Section*	150 mg
243	**ALKETS®** Tablets	
251	**CALCIUM GLUCONATE** Tablets, USP	975 mg
272	**CALCIUM LACTATE** Tablets, USP	650 mg
284	**UNICAP M®** Tablets Vitamins with minerals	
285	**UNICAP PLUS IRON®** Tablets	
299	**UNICAP®** Tablets Multivitamin Supplement	
331	***CLEOCIN HCl™** Capsules (clindamycin HCl capsules, USP) *See Product Identification Section*	75 mg
336	**LINCOCIN®** Pediatric Capsules (lincomycin hydrochloride capsules, USP)	250 mg
348	**UNICAP SENIOR®** Tablets Vitamins with minerals	
363	**ZYMACAP®** Capsules Multivitamins	
388	**DELTASONE®** Tablets (prednisone tablets, USP) *See Product Identification Section*	50 mg
412	**MAOLATE®** Tablets (chlorphenesin carbamate) *See Product Identification Section*	400 mg
461	**SIGTAB®** Tablets High potency vitamin supplement	
477	**TOLINASE®** Tablets (tolazamide tablets, USP) *See Product Identification Section*	500 mg
500	**LINCOCIN®** Capsules (lincomycin hydrochloride capsules, USP)	500 mg
521	**MYCIFRADIN®** Tablets (neomycin sulfate tablets, USP)	0.5 Gm
586	**UTICILLIN VK®** Tablets (penicillin V potassium tablets, USP)	250 mg
671	**UTICILLIN VK®** Tablets (penicillin V potassium tablets, USP)	500 mg
701	**ORINASE®** Tablets (tolbutamide tablets, USP) *See Product Identification Section*	250 mg
730	**PHENOLAX®** Wafers (phenolphthalein)	
733	***MOTRIN®** Tablets (ibuprofen tablets, USP) *See Product Identification Section*	300 mg
742	***MOTRIN®** Tablets (ibuprofen tablets, USP) *See Product Identification Section*	600 mg
750	***MOTRIN®** Tablets (ibuprofen tablets, USP) *See Product Identification Section*	400 mg
782	**PANMYCIN®** Capsules (tetracycline hydrochloride capsules, USP)	250 mg
873	**SUPER D®** Perles (oleovitamins A and D capsules, N.F.)	
949	**URACIL MUSTARD** Capsules	1 mg
3176	**E-MYCIN®** Tablets (erythromycin base enteric-coated tablets) *See Product Identification Section*	333 mg
3212	**PYRROXATE®** Capsules	
3293	**KAOPECTATE®** Tablet Formula	
3300	**P-A-C®** Revised Formula Analgesic Tablets (aspirin and caffeine tablets)	

* Product of The Upjohn Manufacturing Company

Cleocin Pediatric, Cleocin Phosphate, Cleocin T and *Motrin* are registered trademarks of The Upjohn Manufacturing Company.

Cleocin HCl is a trademark of The Upjohn Manufacturing Company.

ADEFLOR CHEWABLE®
brand of fluoride with vitamins tablets

Composition: Each 0.5 mg or 1 mg tablet contains:
Fluoride (as sodium fluoride)..........................0.5 mg
or 1 mg
Vitamin A ....4000 Int. Units
Vitamin D...400 Int. Units
Ascorbic Acid
(as sodium ascorbate) ....75 mg
Thiamine Mononitrate....................................2 mg
Riboflavin ....2 mg
Niacinamide..18 mg
Pyridoxine Hydrochloride ....1 mg
Calcium Pantothenate ....5 mg
Cyanocobalamin ....2 mcg

The palatable cherry-flavored ADEFLOR CHEWABLE Tablets 0.5 mg or raspberry-flavored 1 mg tablets may be chewed, dissolved in the mouth or swallowed whole.

How Supplied:
0.5 mg	Bottles of 100	NDC 0009-0081-01
	Bottles of 500	NDC 0009-0081-02
1 mg	Bottles of 100	NDC 0009-0092-01
	Bottles of 500	NDC 0009-0092-02

Shown in Product Identification Section, page 440

ADEFLOR®
brand of fluoride with vitamins A, C, D and B₆ drops

Composition: Each 0.6 ml contains:
Fluoride (as sodium fluoride)......................0.5 mg
Vitamin A ....2000 Int. Units
Vitamin D...400 Int. Units
Ascorbic Acid (C)..50 mg
Pyridoxine Hydrochloride (B₆)......................1 mg

How Supplied: Aqueous solution in calibrated dropper bottles.
50 ml   NDC 0009-0211-02

BACIGUENT® Antibiotic Ointment
(See PDR For Nonprescription Drugs)

CALDEROL®
brand of calcifediol capsules

Description: CALDEROL Capsules contain calcifediol which is the colorless, crystalline monohydrate of 25-hydroxycholecalciferol prepared by chemical synthesis and is identical to the natural vitamin metabolite. Calcifediol has a calculated molecular weight of 418.67 and is soluble in organic solvents but relatively insoluble in water. Chemically, calcifediol is (5Z,7E)-9,10 - secocholesta - 5,7,10(19) - triene - 3β,25 - diol monohydrate.
The other names frequently used for 25-hydroxycholecalciferol are 25-hydroxyvitamin D_3, 25-HCC, 25-OHCC, and 25-OHD₃.
CALDEROL Capsules (calcifediol) for oral administration are available in two strengths: a white capsule containing 20 mcg calcifediol and an orange capsule containing 50 mcg calcifediol.

Clinical Pharmacology: The natural supply of vitamin D in man mainly depends on the ultraviolet rays of the sun for conversion of 7-dehydrocholesterol to vitamin D_3 (cholecalciferol). It is now known that vitamin D_3 must first be converted to 25-OHD₃ (25-hydroxycholecalciferol) by a vitamin D_3-25-hydroxylase enzyme (25-OHase) present in the liver. 25-Hydroxycholecalciferol is the major transport form of vitamin D_3 and can be readily monitored in the serum. It is further converted to 1,25-dihydroxycholecalciferol (1,25-(OH)₂D₃) and 24,25-dihydroxycholecalciferol (24,25-(OH)₂D₃) in the kidney. 1,25-(OH)₂D₃ stimulates resorption of calcium from bone and increases intestinal calcium absorption. The physiologic role of 24,25-(OH)₂D₃ has not been clearly established. The metabolic activity of calcifediol in clinical use appears to be related not only to its conversion to other metabolites but also due to its intrinsic activity.
When administered orally, calcifediol is rapidly absorbed from the intestine, with peak 25-OHD₃ concentrations in the serum reported after about 4 hours. 25-Hydroxycholecalciferol is known to be transported in blood, bound to a specific plasma protein. The terminal half-life of orally administered calcifediol in the serum is about 16 days.

Continued on next page

Information on these Upjohn products is based on labeling in effect on November 30, 1984. Further information concerning these and other Upjohn products may be obtained from the package insert or by direct inquiry to Medical Information, The Upjohn Company, Kalamazoo, Michigan 49001.

Upjohn—Cont.

Indications and Usage: CALDEROL Capsules (calcifediol) are indicated in the treatment and management of metabolic bone disease or hypocalcemia associated with chronic renal failure in patients undergoing renal dialysis.

In studies to date it has been shown to increase serum calcium levels, to decrease alkaline phosphatase and parathyroid hormone levels in some patients, to decrease subperiosteal bone resorption in some patients, and to decrease histological signs of hyperparathyroid bone disease and mineralization defects in some patients.

Contraindications: CALDEROL Capsules (calcifediol) should not be given to patients with hypercalcemia or evidence of vitamin D toxicity.

Warnings: Since calcifediol is a metabolite of vitamin D, vitamin D and its derivatives should be withheld during treatment.

Aluminum carbonate or hydroxide gels should be used to control serum phosphorus levels in patients undergoing dialysis.

Overdosage of any form of vitamin D is dangerous (see also **OVERDOSAGE**). Progressive hypercalcemia may be so severe as to require emergency attention. Chronic hypercalcemia can lead to generalized vascular calcification, nephrocalcinosis, and other soft-tissue calcification. The serum calcium times phosphorus (Ca × P) product should not be allowed to exceed 70. Radiographic and/or slit lamp evaluation of suspect anatomical regions may be useful in the early detection of this condition.

Precautions:

General: Excessive dosage of CALDEROL Capsules (calcifediol) induces hypercalcemia and in some instances hypercalciuria; therefore, early in treatment during dosage adjustment, serum calcium should be determined frequently (at least weekly). Should hypercalcemia develop, the drug should be discontinued immediately. After achieving normocalcemia, the drug may be readministered at a lower dosage. CALDEROL should be given cautiously to patients receiving digitalis, because hypercalcemia in such patients may precipitate cardiac arrhythmias.

Information for the Patient: The patient and his or her parents or spouse should be informed about compliance with dosage instructions, adherence to instructions about diet, calcium supplementation, phosphate binder usage, and avoidance of non approved prescription drugs. Patients should also be informed about the symptoms of hypercalcemia (see Adverse Reactions).

Essential Laboratory Tests: Serum calcium, phosphorus and alkaline phosphatase and 24-hour urinary calcium and phosphorus should be determined periodically. During the initial phase of the medication, serum calcium should be determined more frequently (at least weekly).

Drug Interactions: Cholestyramine has been reported to reduce absorption of fat-soluble vitamins; as such, it may impair intestinal absorption of calcifediol. The administration of anticonvulsants has been shown to affect the calcifediol requirements in some patients.

Carcinogenesis, Mutagenesis, Impairment of Fertility: Long-term studies in animals have not been completed to evaluate the carcinogenic potential of CALDEROL. No significant effects of calcifediol on fertility and/or general reproductive performances were reported.

Use in Pregnancy: Teratogenic effects: Pregnancy Category C: Calcifediol has been shown to be teratogenic in rabbits when given in doses of 6 to 12 times the human dose. There are no adequate and well-controlled studies in pregnant women. CALDEROL should be used during pregnancy only if the potential benefit justifies potential risk to the fetus.

When calcifediol was given orally to bred rabbits on the 6th through the 18th day of gestation, gross visceral and skeletal examination of pups indicated that the compound was teratogenic at doses of 25 and 50 mcg/kg/day. A dose of 5 mcg/kg/day was not teratogenic. In a similar study in rats, calcifediol was not teratogenic at doses up to and including 60 mcg/kg/day.

Nursing Mothers: It is not known whether this drug is excreted in human milk. Because many drugs are excreted in human milk, caution should be exercised when CALDEROL is administered to a nursing woman.

Pediatric Use: The safety and effectiveness of CALDEROL in children have not been established.

Adverse Reactions: Since calcifediol is an active metabolite of vitamin D, adverse effects are, in general, similar to those encountered with excessive vitamin D intake. The early and late signs and symptoms of vitamin D intoxication associated with hypercalcemia include:

a. *Early:* Weakness, headache, somnolence, nausea, vomiting, dry mouth, constipation, muscle pain, bone pain, and metallic taste.
b. *Late:* Polyuria, polydipsia, anorexia, irritability, weight loss, nocturia, conjunctivitis (calcific), pancreatitis, photophobia, rhinorrhea, pruritus, hyperthermia, decreased libido, elevated BUN, albuminuria, hypercholesterolemia, elevated SGOT and SGPT, ectopic calcification, hypertension, cardiac arrhythmias, and rarely, overt psychosis.

Overdosage: Administration of CALDEROL Capsules (calcifediol) to patients in excess of their daily requirements can cause hypercalcemia, hypercalciuria, and hyperphosphatemia. High intake of calcium and phosphate concomitant with CALDEROL may lead to similar abnormalities.

Treatment of Hypercalcemia and Overdosages: General treatment of hypercalcemia (greater than 1 mg/dl above the upper limit of the normal range) consists of discontinuation of therapy with CALDEROL. Serum calcium measurements should be performed regularly until normocalcemia ensues. Hypercalcemia usually resolves in two to four weeks. When serum calcium levels have returned to within normal limits, therapy with CALDEROL may be reinstituted at a dosage lower than prior therapy. Serum calcium levels should be obtained at least weekly after all dosage changes and subsequent dosage titration. Persistent or markedly elevated calcium levels in dialysis patients may be corrected by dialysis against a calcium-free dialysate.

Treatment of Accidental Overdosage: The treatment of acute accidental overdosage of CALDEROL should consist of general supportive measures. If drug ingestion is discovered within a relatively short time, induction of emesis or gastric lavage may be of benefit in preventing further absorption. If the drug has passed through the stomach, the administration of mineral oil may promote fecal elimination. Serial serum calcium determination, rate of urinary calcium excretion, and an assessment of electrocardiographic abnormalities due to hypercalcemia should be obtained. Such monitoring is critical in patients receiving digitalis. Discontinuation of supplemental calcium and a low calcium diet are also indicated in accidental overdosage. Because the conversion of calcifediol to 1,25-(OH)$_2$D$_3$ is tightly regulated by the body's needs, further measures are probably unnecessary. Should persistent and marked hypercalcemia occur, however, there are a variety of therapeutic measures that may be considered, depending on the patient's underlying condition. These include the use of drugs such as phosphates and corticosteroids as well as measures to induce an appropriate forced diuresis. The use of peritoneal dialysis against a calcium-free dialysate may also be considered.

Dosage and Administration: The optimal daily dose of CALDEROL Capsules (calcifediol) must be carefully determined for each patient. The recommended initial dosage of CALDEROL is based on the assumption that each patient is receiving an adequate daily intake of calcium from dietary sources or from the addition of calcium supplements. The RDA for calcium in adults is 1000 mg. To insure that each patient receives an adequate daily intake of calcium, the physician should either prescribe a calcium supplement or instruct the patients in proper dietary measures.

Chronic Renal Failure—Dialysis Patients: The recommended initial dose of CALDEROL is 300 to 350 mcg of calcifediol weekly, administered on a daily or alternate-day schedule. If a satisfactory response in the biochemical parameters and clinical manifestations of the disease state is not observed, dosage may be increased at four-week intervals. During this titration period serum calcium levels should be obtained at least weekly, and if hypercalcemia is noted, the drug should be discontinued until normocalcemia ensues.

Some patients with normal serum calcium levels may respond to doses of 20 mcg of calcifediol every other day. Most patients respond to doses between 50 and 100 mcg daily or between 100 and 200 mcg on alternate days.

How Supplied: CALDEROL Capsules (calcifediol) are available in the following strengths and package sizes:

Strength	Package Size	NDC Number
20 mcg (white, soft elastic capsules)	Bottles of 60	0009-0062-01
50 mcg (orange, soft elastic capsules)	Bottles of 60	0009-0074-01

Code 811 357 102

CHERACOL D® Cough Formula

(See PDR For Nonprescription Drugs)

CHERACOL PLUS® Head Cold/Cough Formula

(See PDR For Nonprescription Drugs)

CITROCARBONATE® Antacid

(See PDR For Nonprescription Drugs)

CLEOCIN HCl™ ℞
brand of clindamycin hydrochloride capsules, USP

150 mg (100's):
NSN 6505-00-159-4892 (M & VA)

WARNING

Clindamycin therapy has been associated with severe colitis which may end fatally. Therefore, it should be reserved for serious infections where less toxic antimicrobial agents are inappropriate, as described in the Indications section. It should not be used in patients with nonbacterial infections, such as most upper respiratory tract infections. Studies indicate a toxin(s) produced by *Clostridia* is one primary cause of antibiotic associated colitis. Cholestyramine and colestipol resins have been shown to bind the toxin *in vitro*. See WARNINGS section. The colitis is usually characterized by severe, persistent diarrhea and severe abdominal cramps and may be associated with the passage of blood and mucus. Endoscopic examination may reveal pseudomembranous colitis.

When significant diarrhea occurs, the drug should be discontinued or, if necessary, continued only with close observation of the patient. Large bowel endoscopy has been recommended.

Antiperistaltic agents such as opiates and diphenoxylate with atropine (Lomotil) may prolong and/or worsen the condition. Vancomycin has been found to be effective in the treatment of antibiotic associated pseudomembranous colitis produced by *Clostridium difficile*. The usual adult dosage is 500 milligrams to 2 grams of vancomycin orally per day in three to four divided doses administered for 7 to 10 days. Cholestyramine or colestipol resins bind vancomycin *in vitro*. If both a resin and vancomycin are to be administered concurrently, it may be advisable to separate the time of administration of each drug.

Diarrhea, colitis, and pseudomembranous colitis have been observed to begin up to several weeks following cessation of therapy with clindamycin.

Description: CLEOCIN HCL Capsules contain clindamycin hydrochloride, equivalent to 75 mg or 150 mg of clindamycin. Clindamycin hydrochloride is the hydrated hydrochloride salt of clindamycin. Clindamycin is a semisynthetic antibiotic produced by a 7(S)-chloro-substitution of the 7(R)-hydroxyl group of the parent compound lincomycin.

Actions:
Microbiology: Clindamycin has been shown to have *in vitro* activity against isolates of the following organisms:
Aerobic gram-positive cocci, including:
Staphylococcus aureus
Staphylococcus epidermidis
(penicillinase and nonpenicillinase producing strains). When tested by *in vitro* methods some staphylococcal strains originally resistant to erythromycin rapidly develop resistance to clindamycin.
Streptococci (except *Streptococcus faecalis*)
Pneumococci
Anaerobic gram-negative bacilli, including:
Bacteroides species (including *Bacteroides fragilis* group and *Bacteroides melaninogenicus* group)
Fusobacterium species
Anaerobic gram-positive nonsporeforming bacilli, including:
Propionibacterium
Eubacterium
Actinomyces species
Anaerobic and microaerophilic gram-positive cocci, including:
Peptococcus species
Peptostreptococcus species
Microaerophilic streptococci
Clostridia: Clostridia are more resistant than most anaerobes to clindamycin. Most *Clostridium perfringens* are susceptible, but other species, eg, *Clostridium sporogenes* and *Clostridium tertium*, are frequently resistant to clindamycin. Susceptibility testing should be done.
Cross resistance has been demonstrated between clindamycin and lincomycin.
Antagonism has been demonstrated between clindamycin and erythromycin.

Human Pharmacology. Serum level studies with a 150 mg oral dose of clindamycin hydrochloride in 24 normal adult volunteers showed that clindamycin was rapidly absorbed after oral administration. An average peak serum level of 2.50 mcg/ml was reached in 45 minutes; serum levels averaged 1.51 mcg/ml at 3 hours and 0.70 mcg/ml at 6 hours. Absorption of an oral dose is virtually complete (90%), and the concomitant administration of food does not appreciably modify the serum concentrations; serum levels have been uniform and predictable from person to person and dose to dose. Serum level studies following multiple doses of CLEOCIN HCL Capsules (clindamycin hydrochloride) for up to 14 days show no evidence of accumulation or altered metabolism of drug.
Serum half-life of clindamycin is increased slightly in patients with markedly reduced renal function. Hemodialysis and peritoneal dialysis are not effective in removing clindamycin from the serum.
Concentrations of clindamycin in the serum increased linearly with increased dose. Serum levels exceed the MIC (minimum inhibitory concentration) for most indicated organisms for at least six hours following administration of the usually recommended doses. Clindamycin is widely distributed in body fluids and tissues (including bones). The average biological half-life is 2.4 hours. Approximately 10% of the bio-activity is excreted in the urine and 3.6% in the feces; the remainder is excreted as bio-inactive metabolites.
Doses of up to 2 grams of clindamycin per day for 14 days have been well tolerated by healthy volunteers, except that the incidence of gastrointestinal side effects is greater with the higher doses.

No significant levels of clindamycin are attained in the cerebrospinal fluid, even in the presence of inflamed meninges.

Indications: Clindamycin is indicated in the treatment of serious infections caused by susceptible anaerobic bacteria.
Clindamycin is also indicated in the treatment of serious infections due to susceptible strains of streptococci, pneumococci, and staphylococci. Its use should be reserved for penicillin-allergic patients or other patients for whom, in the judgment of the physician, a penicillin is inappropriate. Because of the risk of colitis, as described in the WARNING box, before selecting clindamycin the physician should consider the nature of the infection and the suitability of less toxic alternatives (eg, erythromycin).

Anaerobes: Serious respiratory tract infections such as empyema, anaerobic pneumonitis and lung abscess; serious skin and soft tissue infections; septicemia; intra-abdominal infections such as peritonitis and intra-abdominal abscess (typically resulting from anaerobic organisms resident in the normal gastrointestinal tract); infections of the female pelvis and genital tract such as endometritis, nongonococcal tubo-ovarian abscess, pelvic cellulitis and postsurgical vaginal cuff infection.

Streptococci: Serious respiratory tract infections; serious skin and soft tissue infections.
Staphylococci: Serious respiratory tract infections; serious skin and soft tissue infections.
Pneumococci: Serious respiratory tract infections.

Bacteriologic studies should be performed to determine the causative organisms and their susceptibility to clindamycin.

In Vitro Susceptibility Testing: A standardized disk testing procedure* is recommended for determining susceptibility of aerobic bacteria to clindamycin. A description is contained in the CLEOCIN® Susceptibility Disk (clindamycin) insert. Using this method, the laboratory can designate isolates as resistant, intermediate, or susceptible. Tube or agar dilution methods may be used for both anaerobic and aerobic bacteria. When the directions in the CLEOCIN® Susceptibility Powder insert are followed, an MIC of 1.6 mcg/ml may be considered susceptible; MICs of 1.6 to 4.8 mcg/ml may be considered intermediate and MICs greater than 4.8 mcg/ml may be considered resistant.
CLEOCIN Susceptibility Disks 2 mcg. See package insert for use.
CLEOCIN Susceptibility Powder 20 mg. See package insert for use.
For anaerobic bacteria the minimal inhibitory concentration (MIC) of clindamycin can be determined by agar dilution and broth dilution (including microdilution) techniques. If MICs are not determined routinely, the disk broth method is recommended for routine use. THE KIRBY-BAUER DISK DIFFUSION METHOD AND ITS INTERPRETIVE STANDARDS ARE NOT RECOMMENDED FOR ANAEROBES.
*Bauer, A.W., Kirby, W.M.M., Sherris, J.C., Turck, M.; Antibiotic susceptibility testing by a standardized single disc method, *Am. J. Clin. Path.* 45:493-496, 1966. Standardized Disc Susceptibility Test, *Federal Register* 37:20527-29, 1972.

Contraindications: CLEOCIN HCL Capsules (clindamycin hydrochloride) are contraindicated in individuals with a history of hypersensitivity to preparations containing clindamycin or lincomycin.

Warnings:
See WARNING box. Studies indicate a toxin(s) produced by *Clostridia* is one primary cause of antibiotic associated colitis.[1-5] Cholestyramine and colestipol resins have been shown to bind the toxin *in vitro*. Mild cases of colitis may respond to drug discontinuance alone. Moderate to severe cases should be managed with fluid, electrolyte and protein supplementation as indicated. Vancomycin has been found to be effective in the treatment of antibiotic associated pseudomembranous colitis produced by *Clostridium difficile*. The usual adult dosage is 500 milligrams to 2 grams of vancomycin orally per day in three to four divided doses administered for 7 to 10 days. Cholestyramine or colestipol resins bind vancomycin *in vitro*. If both a resin and vancomycin are to be administered concurrently, it may be advisable to separate the time of administration of each drug. Systemic corticoids and corticoid retention enemas may help relieve the colitis. Other causes of colitis should also be considered.

A careful inquiry should be made concerning previous sensitivities to drugs and other allergens.

Usage in Pregnancy - Safety for use in pregnancy has not been established.

Usage in Newborns and Infants: When CLEOCIN HCL Capsules (clindamycin hydrochloride) are administered to newborns and infants, appropriate monitoring of organ system functions is desirable.

Nursing Mothers—Clindamycin has been reported to appear in breast milk in ranges of 0.7 to 3.8 mcg/ml.

Usage in Meningitis: Since clindamycin does not diffuse adequately into the cerebrospinal fluid, the drug should not be used in the treatment of meningitis.

Antagonism has been demonstrated between clindamycin and erythromycin *in vitro*. Because of possible clinical significance, these two drugs should not be administered concurrently.

1. Bartlett JG, et al: Antibiotic associated Pseudomembranous Colitis Due to Toxin-producing *Clostridia*. *N Engl J Med* 298(10):531-534, 1978.
2. George RH, et al: Identification of *Clostridium difficile* as a cause of Pseudomembranous Colitis. *Br Med J* 6114:669-671, 1978.
3. Larson HE, Price AB: Pseudomembranous Colitis Presence of Clostridial Toxin, *Lancet* 8052/3:1312-1314, 1977.
4. Rifkin GD, Fekety FR, Silva J: Antibiotic-induced Colitis Implication of a Toxin Neutralized by *Clostridium sordellii* Antitoxin. *Lancet* 8048:1103-1106, 1977.
5. Bailey WR, Scott EG: Diagnostic Microbiology. The CV Mosby Company, St. Louis, 1978.

Precautions: Review of experience to date suggests that a subgroup of older patients with associated severe illness may tolerate diarrhea less well. When clindamycin is indicated in these patients, they should be carefully monitored for change in bowel frequency.
CLEOCIN HCL Capsules (clindamycin hydrochloride) should be prescribed with caution in individuals with a history of gastrointestinal disease, particularly colitis.
CLEOCIN HCL should be prescribed with caution in atopic individuals.
During prolonged therapy, periodic liver and kidney function tests and blood counts should be performed.
Indicated surgical procedures should be performed in conjunction with antibiotic therapy.
The use of CLEOCIN HCL occasionally results in overgrowth of nonsusceptible organisms—particularly yeasts. Should superinfections occur, appropriate measures should be taken as indicated by the clinical situation.
Patients with very severe renal disease and/or very severe hepatic disease accompanied by severe metabolic aberrations should be dosed with caution, and serum clindamycin levels monitored during high-dose therapy.
Clindamycin has been shown to have neuromuscular blocking properties that may enhance the action of other neuromuscular blocking agents. Therefore, it should be used with caution in patients receiving such agents.

Continued on next page

Information on these Upjohn products is based on labeling in effect on November 30, 1984. Further information concerning these and other Upjohn products may be obtained from the package insert or by direct inquiry to Medical Information, The Upjohn Company, Kalamazoo, Michigan 49001.

Upjohn—Cont.

This product contains FD&C Yellow No. 5 (tartrazine) which may cause allergic-type reactions (including bronchial asthma) in certain susceptible individuals. Although the overall incidence of FD&C Yellow No. 5 (tartrazine) sensitivity in the general population is low, it is frequently seen in patients who also have aspirin hypersensitivity.

Adverse Reactions: The following reactions have been reported with the use of clindamycin.

Gastrointestinal: Abdominal pain, esophagitis, nausea, vomiting and diarrhea. (See **Warning** Box)

Hypersensitivity Reactions: Maculopapular rash and urticaria have been observed during drug therapy. Generalized mild to moderate morbilliform-like skin rashes are the most frequently reported of all adverse reactions. Rare instances of erythema multiforme, some resembling Stevens-Johnson syndrome, have been associated with clindamycin. A few cases of anaphylactoid reactions have been reported. If a hypersensitivity reaction occurs, the drug should be discontinued. The usual agents (epinephrine, corticosteroids, antihistamines) should be available for emergency treatment of serious reactions.

Liver: Jaundice and abnormalities in liver function tests have been observed during clindamycin therapy.

Hematopoietic: Transient neutropenia (leukopenia) and eosinophilia have been reported. Reports of agranulocytosis and thrombocytopenia have been made. No direct etiologic relationship to concurrent clindamycin therapy could be made in any of the foregoing.

Musculoskeletal: Rare instances of polyarthritis have been reported.

Dosage and Administration:
If significant diarrhea occurs during therapy, this antibiotic should be discontinued. (See **Warning** box).

Adults: *Serious infections*—150 to 300 mg every 6 hours. *More severe infections*—300 to 450 mg every 6 hours.

Children: *Serious infections*—8 to 16 mg/kg/day (4 to 8 mg/lb/day) divided into three or four equal doses. *More severe infections*—16 to 20 mg/kg/day (8 to 10 mg/lb/day) divided into three or four equal doses.

To avoid the possibility of esophageal irritation, CLEOCIN HCL Capsules (clindamycin hydrochloride) should be taken with a full glass of water.
In the treatment of anaerobic infections, CLEOCIN PHOSPHATE® Sterile Solution (clindamycin phosphate injection) should be used initially. This may be followed by oral therapy with CLEOCIN HCL Capsules or CLEOCIN PEDIATRIC® Flavored Granules (clindamycin palmitate HCl) at the discretion of the physician.
In cases of β-hemolytic streptococcal infections, treatment should continue for at least 10 days.

How Supplied: CLEOCIN HCL Capsules (clindamycin hydrochloride) are available as:

75 mg Capsules. Each capsule contains clindamycin hydrochloride equivalent to 75 mg clindamycin.
Bottles of 100   NDC 0009-0331-02

150 mg Capsules. Each capsule contains clindamycin hydrochloride equivalent to 150 mg clindamycin.
Bottles of 16   NDC 0009-0225-01
Bottles of 100   NDC 0009-0225-02
Unit Dose Package
(100)   NDC 0009-0225-03

Toxicology: Animal toxicity studies showed the following:

LD$_{50}$ I.P. Administration—
  Mouse .... 361 mg/kg
LD$_{50}$ I.V. Administration—
  Mouse .... 245 mg/kg
LD$_{50}$ Oral Administration—
  Rat .... 2,618 mg/kg

One year oral toxicity studies in Spartan Sprague-Dawley rats and Beagle dogs at levels of 30, 100 and 300 mg/kg/day (3 grams/day per dog) have shown CLEOCIN HCL to be well tolerated. No appreciable difference in pathological findings has been obtained in CLEOCIN HCL treated groups of animals from comparable control groups. Rats receiving CLEOCIN HCL Capsules (clindamycin hydrochloride) at 600 mg/kg/day for six months tolerated the drug well; however, dogs dosed at this level vomited, would not eat, and lost weight.
Code 810 570 006
Shown in Product Identification Section, page 441
*Product of The Upjohn Manufacturing Company
CLEOCIN HCL is a trademark of The Upjohn Manufacturing Company.
CLEOCIN, CLEOCIN PEDIATRIC and CLEOCIN PHOSPHATE are registered trademarks of The Upjohn Manufacturing Company.
UPJOHN is a trademark registered in the U.S. Patent and Trademark office by The Upjohn Company, Kalamazoo, Michigan, U.S.A.

CLEOCIN PEDIATRIC®
brand of clindamycin palmitate hydrochloride flavored granules*
(clindamycin palmitate HCl for oral solution, USP)
Not for Injection

> **WARNING**
> Clindamycin therapy has been associated with severe colitis which may end fatally. Therefore, it should be reserved for serious infections where less toxic antimicrobial agents are inappropriate, as described in the Indications Section. It should not be used in patients with nonbacterial infections, such as most upper respiratory tract infections. Studies indicate a toxin(s) produced by *Clostridia* is one primary cause of antibiotic associated colitis. Cholestyramine and colestipol resins have been shown to bind the toxin *in vitro*. See WARNINGS section. The colitis is usually characterized by severe, persistent diarrhea and severe abdominal cramps and may be associated with the passage of blood and mucus. Endoscopic examination may reveal pseudomembranous colitis.
> When significant diarrhea occurs, the drug should be discontinued or, if necessary, continued only with close observation of the patient. Large bowel endoscopy has been recommended.
> Antiperistaltic agents such as opiates and diphenoxylate with atropine (Lomotil) may prolong and/or worsen the condition. Vancomycin has been found to be effective in the treatment of antibiotic associated pseudomembranous colitis produced by *Clostridium difficile*. The usual adult dosage is 500 milligrams to 2 grams of vancomycin orally per day in three to four divided doses administered for 7 to 10 days. Cholestyramine or colestipol resins bind vancomycin *in vitro*. If both a resin and vancomycin are to be administered concurrently, it may be advisable to separate the time of administration of each drug.
> Diarrhea, colitis, and pseudomembranous colitis have been observed to begin up to several weeks following cessation of therapy with clindamycin.

Description: CLEOCIN PEDIATRIC Flavored Granules contain clindamycin palmitate hydrochloride for reconstitution. Each 5 ml contains the equivalent of 75 mg clindamycin. Clindamycin palmitate hydrochloride is a water soluble hydrochloride salt of the ester of clindamycin and palmitic acid. Clindamycin is a semisynthetic antibiotic produced by a 7(S)-chloro-substitution of the 7(R)-hydroxyl group of the parent compound lincomycin.

Actions:
Microbiology: Although clindamycin palmitate HCl is inactive *in vitro*, rapid *in vivo* hydrolysis converts this compound to the antibacterially active clindamycin.

Clindamycin has been shown to have *in vitro* activity against isolates of the following organisms:
Aerobic gram positive cocci, including:
  Staphylococcus aureus
  Staphylococcus epidermidis
  (penicillinase and non-penicillinase producing strains). When tested by *in vitro* methods some staphylococcal strains originally resistant to erythromycin rapidly develop resistance to clindamycin.
  Streptococci (except *Streptococcus faecalis*)
  Pneumococci
Anaerobic gram negative bacilli, including:
  Bacteroides species (including *Bacteroides fragilis* group and *Bacteroides melaninogenicus* group)
  Fusobacterium species
Anaerobic gram positive nonsporeforming bacilli, including:
  Propionibacterium
  Eubacterium
  Actinomyces species
Anaerobic and microaerophilic gram positive cocci, including:
  Peptococcus species
  Peptostreptococcus species
  Microaerophilic streptococci

  Clostridia: Clostridia are more resistant than most anaerobes to clindamycin. Most *Clostridium perfringens* are susceptible, but other species, eg, *Clostridium sporogenes* and *Clostridium tertium* are frequently resistant to clindamycin. Susceptibility testing should be done.
Cross resistance has been demonstrated between clindamycin and lincomycin.
Antagonism has been demonstrated between clindamycin and erythromycin.
Human Pharmacology: Blood level studies comparing clindamycin palmitate HCl with clindamycin hydrochloride show that both products reach their peak active serum levels at the same time, indicating a rapid hydrolysis of the palmitate to the clindamycin.
Clindamycin is widely distributed in body fluids and tissues (including bones). Approximately 10% of the biological activity is excreted in the urine. The average biological half-life after doses of clindamycin is approximately two hours in children. Serum half-life of clindamycin is increased slightly in patients with markedly reduced renal function. Hemodialysis and peritoneal dialysis do not appreciably affect the half-life of clindamycin in the serum.
Serum level studies with clindamycin palmitate HCl in normal children weighing 50-100 lbs given 2, 3 or 4 mg/kg every 6 hours (8, 12 or 16 mg/kg/day) demonstrated mean peak clindamycin serum levels of 1.24, 2.25 and 2.44 mcg/ml respectively, one hour after the first dose. By the fifth dose, the 6-hour serum concentration had reached equilibrium. Peak serum concentrations after this time would be about 2.46, 2.98 and 3.79 mcg/ml with doses of 8, 12, 16 mg/kg/day, respectively. Serum levels have been uniform and predictable from person to person and dose to dose. Multiple-dose studies in newborns and infants up to 6 months of age show that the drug does not accumulate in the serum and is excreted rapidly. Serum levels exceed the MICs for most indicated organisms for at least six hours following administration of the usually recommended doses of CLEOCIN PEDIATRIC in adults and children.
No significant levels of clindamycin are attained in the cerebrospinal fluid, even in the presence of inflamed meninges.
Indications: CLEOCIN PEDIATRIC Flavored Granules (clindamycin palmitate HCl) are indicated in the treatment of serious infections caused by susceptible anaerobic bacteria.
Clindamycin is also indicated in the treatment of serious infections due to susceptible strains of streptococci, pneumococci, and staphylococci. Its use should be reserved for penicillin-allergic patients or other patients for whom, in the judgment of the physician, a penicillin is inappropriate. Because of the risk of colitis, as described in the WARNING box, before selecting clindamycin the physician should consider the nature of the infec-

tion and the suitability of less toxic alternatives (eg, erythromycin).

Anaerobes: Serious respiratory tract infections such as empyema, anaerobic pneumonitis and lung abscess; serious skin and soft tissue infections; septicemia; intra-abdominal infections such as peritonitis and intra-abdominal abscess (typically resulting from anaerobic organisms resident in the normal gastrointestinal tract); infections of the female pelvis and genital tract such as endometritis, nongonococcal tubo-ovarian abscess, pelvic cellulitis and postsurgical vaginal cuff infection.

Streptococci: Serious respiratory tract infections; serious skin and soft tissue infections.

Staphylococci: Serious respiratory tract infections; serious skin and soft tissue infections.

Pneumococci: Serious respiratory tract infections.

Bacteriologic studies should be performed to determine the causative organisms and their susceptibility to clindamycin.

In Vitro Susceptibility Testing: A standardized disk testing procedure* is recommended for determining susceptibility of aerobic bacteria to clindamycin. A description is contained in the CLEOCIN® Susceptibility Disk (clindamycin) insert. Using this method, the laboratory can designate isolates as resistant, intermediate, or susceptible. Tube or agar dilution methods may be used for both anaerobic and aerobic bacteria. When the directions in the CLEOCIN Susceptibility Powder insert are followed, an MIC (minimal inhibitory concentration) of 1.6 mcg/ml may be considered susceptible; MICs of 1.6 to 4.8 mcg/ml may be considered intermediate and MICs greater than 4.8 mcg/ml may be considered resistant.

CLEOCIN Susceptibility Disks 2 mcg. See package insert for use.

CLEOCIN Susceptibility Powder 20 mg. See package insert for use.

For anaerobic bacteria the minimal inhibitory concentration (MIC) of clindamycin can be determined by agar dilution and broth dilution (including microdilution) techniques. If MICs are not determined routinely, the disk broth method is recommended for routine use. THE KIRBY-BAUER DISK DIFFUSION METHOD AND ITS INTERPRETIVE STANDARDS ARE NOT RECOMMENDED FOR ANAEROBES.

*Bauer, AW, Kirby, WMM, Sherris, JC, Turck, M.: Antibiotic susceptibility testing by a standardized single disc method, *Am J Clin Path*, **45**:493-496, 1966. Standardized Disc Susceptibility Test, *Federal Register* **37**:20527-29, 1972.

Contraindications: This drug is contraindicated in individuals with a history of hypersensitivity to preparations containing clindamycin or lincomycin.

Warnings:
See WARNING box. Studies indicate a toxin(s) produced by *Clostridia* is one primary cause of antibiotic associated colitis.[1-5] Cholestyramine and colestipol resins have been shown to bind the toxin *in vitro*. Mild cases of colitis may respond to drug discontinuance alone. Moderate to severe cases should be managed promptly with fluid, electrolyte and protein supplementation as indicated. Vancomycin has been found to be effective in the treatment of antibiotic associated pseudomembranous colitis produced by *Clostridium difficile*. The usual adult dosage is 500 milligrams to 2 grams of vancomycin orally per day in three to four divided doses administered for 7 to 10 days. Cholestyramine or colestipol resins bind vancomycin *in vitro*. If both a resin and vancomycin are to be administered concurrently, it may be advisable to separate the time of administration of each drug. Systemic corticoids and corticoid retention enemas may help relieve the colitis. Other causes of colitis should also be considered.

A careful inquiry should be made concerning previous sensitivities to drugs and other allergens.

Usage in Pregnancy—Safety for use in pregnancy has not been established.

Usage in Newborns and Infants: When CLEOCIN PEDIATRIC Flavored Granules (clindamycin palmitate HCl) are administered to newborns and infants, appropriate monitoring of organ system functions is desirable.

Nursing Mothers—Clindamycin has been reported to appear in breast milk in ranges of 0.7 to 3.8 mcg/ml.

Usage in Meningitis: Since clindamycin does not diffuse adequately into the cerebrospinal fluid, the drug should not be used in the treatment of meningitis.

Antagonism has been demonstrated between clindamycin and erythromycin *in vitro*. Because of possible clinical significance, these two drugs should not be administered concurrently.

1. Bartlett JG, et al: Antibiotic associated Pseudomembranous Colitis Due to Toxin-producing *Clostridia. N Engl J Med* 298(10):531-534, 1978.
2. George RH, et al: Identification of *Clostridium difficile* as a cause of Pseudomembranous Colitis. *Br Med J* 6114:669-671, 1978.
3. Larson HE, Price AB: Pseudomembranous Colitis Presence of Clostridial Toxin. *Lancet* 8052/3:1312-1314, 1977.
4. Rifkin GD, Fekety FR, Silva J: Antibiotic-induced Colitis Implication of a Toxin Neutralized by *Clostridium sordellii* Antitoxin. *Lancet* 8048:1103-1106, 1977.
5. Bailey WR, Scott EG: Diagnostic Microbiology. The CV Mosby Company, St. Louis, 1978.

Precautions: Review of experience to date suggests that a subgroup of older patients with associated severe illness may tolerate diarrhea less well. When clindamycin is indicated in these patients, they should be carefully monitored for change in bowel frequency.

CLEOCIN PEDIATRIC Flavored Granules (clindamycin palmitate HCl) should be prescribed with caution in individuals with a history of gastrointestinal disease, particularly colitis.

CLEOCIN PEDIATRIC should be prescribed with caution in atopic individuals.

During prolonged therapy periodic liver and kidney function tests and blood counts should be performed.

Indicated surgical procedures should be performed in conjunction with antibiotic therapy.

The use of CLEOCIN PEDIATRIC may result in overgrowth of nonsusceptible organisms—particularly yeasts. Should superinfections occur, appropriate measures should be taken as indicated by the clinical situation.

Patients with very severe renal disease and/or very severe hepatic disease accompanied by severe metabolic aberrations should be dosed with caution, and serum clindamycin levels monitored during high-dose therapy.

Clindamycin has been shown to have neuromuscular blocking properties that may enhance the action of other neuromuscular blocking agents. Therefore, it should be used with caution in patients receiving such agents.

Adverse Reactions: The following reactions have been reported with the use of clindamycin.

Gastrointestinal: Abdominal pain, nausea, vomiting and diarrhea. (See **Warning** box)

Hypersensitivity Reactions: Maculopapular rash and urticaria have been observed during drug therapy. Generalized mild to moderate morbilliform-like skin rashes are the most frequently reported of all adverse reactions. Rare instances of erythema multiforme, some resembling Stevens-Johnson syndrome, have been associated with clindamycin. A few cases of anaphylactoid reactions have been reported. If a hypersensitivity reaction occurs, the drug should be discontinued. The usual agents (epinephrine, corticosteroids, antihistamines) should be available for emergency treatment of serious reactions.

Liver: Jaundice and abnormalities in liver function tests have been observed during clindamycin therapy.

Hematopoietic: Transient neutropenia (leukopenia) and eosinophilia have been reported. Reports of agranulocytosis and thrombocytopenia have been made. No direct etiologic relationship to concurrent clindamycin therapy could be made in any of the foregoing.

Musculoskeletal: Rare instances of polyarthritis have been reported.

Dosage and Administration: If significant diarrhea occurs during therapy, this antibiotic should be discontinued. (See **Warning** box.) Concomitant administration of food does not adversely affect the absorption of clindamycin palmitate HCl contained in CLEOCIN PEDIATRIC Flavored Granules.

Serious infections: 8-12 mg/kg/day (4-6 mg/lb/day) divided into 3 or 4 equal doses.
Severe infections: 13-16 mg/kg/day (6.5-8 mg/lb/day) divided into 3 or 4 equal doses.
More severe infections: 17-25 mg/kg/day (8.5-12.5 mg/lb/day) divided into 3 or 4 equal doses.

In children weighing 10 kg or less, ½ teaspoon (37.5 mg) three times a day should be considered the minimum recommended dose.

In the treatment of anaerobic infections, CLEOCIN PHOSPHATE ® Sterile Solution (clindamycin phosphate) should be used initially. This may be followed by oral therapy with CLEOCIN PEDIATRIC or CLEOCIN HCl™ Capsules (clindamycin HCl) at the discretion of the physician.

NOTE: In cases of β-hemolytic streptococcal infections, treatment should be continued for at least 10 days.

Reconstitution instructions:
When reconstituted with water as follows, each 5 ml (teaspoon) of solution contains clindamycin palmitate HCl equivalent to 75 mg clindamycin. Reconstitute bottles of 100 ml with **75 ml** of water. Add a large portion of the water and shake vigorously; add the remainder of the water and shake until the solution is uniform.

Storage conditions:
Store unreconstituted product at controlled room temperature 15°-30°C (59°-86°F).

Do **NOT** refrigerate the reconstituted solution; when chilled, the solution may thicken and be difficult to pour. The solution is stable for 2 weeks at room temperature.

How Supplied: CLEOCIN PEDIATRIC Flavored Granules (clindamycin palmitate HCl) for oral solution is available as follows:

100 ml bottles   NDC 0009-0760-04

When reconstituted as directed, each bottle yields a solution containing 75 mg of clindamycin per 5 ml.

Code 810 568 006

*Product of The Upjohn Manufacturing Company
CLEOCIN PEDIATRIC, CLEOCIN PHOSPHATE and CLEOCIN are registered trademarks of The Upjohn Manufacturing Company.
CLEOCIN HCl is a trademark of The Upjohn Manufacturing Company.
UPJOHN is a trademark registered in the U.S. Patent and Trademark office by The Upjohn Company, Kalamazoo, Michigan, U.S.A.

CLEOCIN PHOSPHATE®   ℞
brand of clindamycin phosphate sterile solution *
(clindamycin phosphate injection, USP)
For Intramuscular and Intravenous Use

2 ml ampoule:
NSN 6505-00-138-8474 (M&VA)
4 ml ampoule:
NSN 6505-00-139-1318 (M&VA)
6 ml vial 100's
NSN 6505-01-181-8688 (VA)

WARNING
Clindamycin therapy has been associated with severe colitis which may end fatally. Therefore, it should be reserved for serious infections where less toxic antimicrobial

Continued on next page

Information on these Upjohn products is based on labeling in effect on November 30, 1984. Further information concerning these and other Upjohn products may be obtained from the package insert or by direct inquiry to Medical Information, The Upjohn Company, Kalamazoo, Michigan 49001.

Upjohn—Cont.

agents are inappropriate, as described in the Indications Section. It should not be used in patients with nonbacterial infections, such as most upper respiratory tract infections. Studies indicate a toxin(s) produced by *Clostridia* is one primary cause of antibiotic associated colitis. Cholestyramine and colestipol resins have been shown to bind the toxin *in vitro*. See WARNINGS section. The colitis is usually characterized by severe, persistent diarrhea and severe abdominal cramps and may be associated with the passage of blood and mucus. Endoscopic examination may reveal pseudomembranous colitis.

When significant diarrhea occurs, the drug should be discontinued or, if necessary, continued only with close observation of the patient. Large bowel endoscopy has been recommended.

Antiperistaltic agents such as opiates and diphenoxylate with atropine (Lomotil) may prolong and/or worsen the condition. Vancomycin has been found to be effective in the treatment of antibiotic associated pseudomembranous colitis produced by *Clostridium difficile*. The usual adult dosage is 500 milligrams to 2 grams of vancomycin orally per day in three to four divided doses administered for 7 to 10 days. Cholestyramine or colestipol resins bind vancomycin *in vitro*. If both a resin and vancomycin are to be administered concurrently, it may be advisable to separate the time of administration of each drug.

Diarrhea, colitis, and pseudomembranous colitis have been observed to begin up to several weeks following cessation of therapy with clindamycin.

Description: CLEOCIN PHOSPHATE Sterile Solution contains clindamycin phosphate, a water soluble ester of clindamycin and phosphoric acid. Each ml contains the equivalent of 150 mg clindamycin, 0.5 mg disodium edetate and 9.45 mg benzyl alcohol added as preservative in each ml. Clindamycin is a semisynthetic antibiotic produced by a 7(S)-chloro-substitution of the 7(R)-hydroxyl group of the parent compound lincomycin.

Clinical Pharmacology:
Microbiology: Although clindamycin phosphate is inactive *in vitro*, rapid *in vivo* hydrolysis converts this compound to the antibacterially active clindamycin.

Clindamycin has been shown to have *in vitro* activity against isolates of the following organisms:
Aerobic gram positive cocci, including:
 Staphylococcus aureus
 Staphylococcus epidermidis
 (penicillinase and nonpenicillinase producing strains). When tested by *in vitro* methods some staphylococcal strains originally resistant to erythromycin rapidly develop resistance to clindamycin.

 Streptococci (except *S. faecalis*)
 Pneumococci
Anaerobic gram negative bacilli, including:
 Bacteroides species (including *Bacteroides fragilis* group and *Bacteroides melaninogenicus* group)
 Fusobacterium species
Anaerobic gram positive nonsporeforming bacilli, including:
 Propionibacterium
 Eubacterium
 Actinomyces species
Anaerobic and microaerophilic gram positive cocci, including:
 Peptococcus species
 Peptostreptococcus species
 Microaerophilic streptococci
 Clostridia: Clostridia are more resistant than most anaerobes to clindamycin. Most *Clostridium perfringens* are susceptible, but other species, eg, *Clostridium sporogenes* and *Clostridium Tertium* are frequently resistant to clindamycin. Susceptibility testing should be done.
Cross resistance has been demonstrated between clindamycin and lincomycin.
Antagonism has been demonstrated between clindamycin and erythromycin.

Human Pharmacology:
Biologically inactive clindamycin phosphate is rapidly converted to active clindamycin.
By the end of short-term intravenous infusion, peak serum levels of active clindamycin are reached. Biologically inactive clindamycin phosphate disappears rapidly from the serum; the average disappearance half-life is 6 minutes; however, the serum disappearance half-life of active clindamycin is about 3 hours in adults and 2 ½ hours in children.
After intramuscular injection of clindamycin phosphate, peak levels of active clindamycin are reached within 3 hours in adults and 1 hour in children. Serum level curves may be constructed from IV peak serum levels as given in Table 1 by application of disappearance half-lives listed above.
Serum levels of clindamycin can be maintained above the *in vitro* minimum inhibitory concentrations for most indicated organisms by administration of clindamycin phosphate every 8-12 hours in adults and every 6-8 hours in children, or by continuous intravenous infusion. An equilibrium state is reached by the third dose.
The disappearance half-life of clindamycin is increased slightly in patients with markedly reduced renal or hepatic function. Hemodialysis and peritoneal dialysis are not effective in removing clindamycin from the serum. Dosage schedules need not be modified in the presence of mild or moderate renal or hepatic disease.
No significant levels of clindamycin are attained in the cerebrospinal fluid, even in the presence of inflamed meninges.
Serum assays for active clindamycin require an inhibitor to prevent *in vitro* hydrolysis of clindamycin phosphate.
[See table below].

Indications and Usage: CLEOCIN PHOSPHATE Sterile Solution (clindamycin phosphate) is indicated in the treatment of serious infections caused by susceptible anaerobic bacteria.
CLEOCIN PHOSPHATE is also indicated in the treatment of serious infections due to susceptible strains of streptococci, pneumococci, and staphylococci. Its use should be reserved for penicillin-allergic patients or other patients for whom, in the judgment of the physician, a penicillin is inappropriate. Because of the risk of colitis, as described in the WARNING box, before selecting clindamycin the physician should consider the nature of the infection and the suitability of less toxic alternatives (e.g., erythromycin).

Anaerobes: Serious respiratory tract infections such as empyema, anaerobic pneumonitis and lung abscess; serious skin and soft tissue infections; septicemia; intra-abdominal infections such as peritonitis and intra-abdominal abscess (typically resulting from anaerobic organisms resident in the normal gastrointestinal tract); infections of the female pelvis and genital tract such as endometritis, nongonococcal tubo-ovarian abscess, pelvic cellulitis and postsurgical vaginal cuff infection.

Streptococci: Serious respiratory tract infections; serious skin and soft tissue infections; septicemia.

Staphylococci: Serious respiratory tract infections; serious skin and soft tissue infections; septicemia; acute hematogenous osteomyelitis.

Pneumococci: Serious respiratory tract infections.

Adjunctive Therapy: In the surgical treatment of chronic bone and joint infections due to susceptible organisms.
Indicated surgical procedures should be performed in conjunction with antibiotic therapy.
Bacteriologic studies should be performed to determine the causative organisms and their susceptibility to clindamycin.

In Vitro Susceptibility Testing: A standardized disk testing procedure*** is recommended for determining susceptibility of aerobic bacteria to clindamycin. A description is contained in the CLEOCIN® Susceptibility Disk (clindamycin) insert. Using this method, the laboratory can designate isolates as resistant, intermediate, or susceptible. Tube or agar dilution methods may be used for both anaerobic and aerobic bacteria. When the directions in the CLEOCIN Susceptibility Powder insert are followed, an MIC (minimal inhibitory concentration) of 1.6 mcg/ml may be considered susceptible; MICs of 1.6 to 4.8 mcg/ml may be considered intermediate and MICs greater than 4.8 mcg/ml may be considered resistant.
CLEOCIN Susceptibility Disks 2 mcg. See package insert for use.
CLEOCIN Susceptibility Powder 20 mg. See package insert for use.
For anaerobic bacteria the minimal inhibitory concentration (MIC) of clindamycin can be determined by agar dilution and broth dilution (including microdilution) techniques. If MICs are not determined routinely, the disk broth method is recommended for routine use. The KIRBY-BAUER DISK DIFFUSION METHOD AND ITS INTERPRETIVE STANDARDS ARE NOT RECOMMENDED FOR ANAEROBES.

***Bauer, AW, Kirby, WMM, Sherris, JC, Turck, M: Antibiotic susceptibility testing by a standardized single disc method, *Am J Clin Path*, 45:493-496, 1966. Standardized Disc Susceptibility Test, *Federal Register* 37:20527-29, 1972.

Contraindications: This drug is contraindicated in individuals with a history of hypersensitivity to preparations containing clindamycin or lincomycin.

Warnings:
See WARNING box. Studies indicate a toxin(s) produced by *Clostridia* is one primary cause of antibiotic associated colitis.[1-5] Cholestyramine and colestipol resins have been shown to bind the toxin *in vitro*. Mild cases of colitis may respond to drug discontinuance alone. Moderate to severe cases should be managed promptly with fluid, electrolyte and protein supplementation as indicated.

Table 1. Average Peak Serum Concentrations After Dosing with Clindamycin Phosphate

CLEOCIN PHOSPHATE Dosage Regimen	Clindamycin mcg/ml	Clindamycin Phosphate mcg/ml
Healthy Adult Males (Post equilibrium)		
300 mg IV in 10 min, q8h	7	15
600 mg IV in 20 min, q8h	10	23
900 mg IV in 30 min, q12h	11	29
1200 mg IV in 45 min, q12h	14	49
300 mg IM q8h	6	3
600 mg IM q12h**	9	3
Children (first dose)**		
5-7 mg/kg IV in 1 hr	10	
3-5 mg/kg IM	4	
5-7 mg/kg IM	8	

**Data in this group from patients being treated for infection

Vancomycin has been found to be effective in the treatment of antibiotic associated pseudomembranous colitis produced by *Clostridium difficile.* The usual adult dosage is 500 milligrams to 2 grams of vancomycin orally per day in three to four divided doses administered for 7 to 10 days. Cholestyramine or colestipol resins bind vancomycin *in vitro.* If both a resin and vancomycin are to be administered concurrently, it may be advisable to separate the time of administration of each drug. Systemic corticoids and corticoid retention enemas may help relieve the colitis. Other causes of colitis should also be considered.

A careful inquiry should be made concerning previous sensitivities to drugs and other allergens.

Usage in Pregnancy—Safety for use in pregnancy has not been established.

Usage in Newborns and infants: When CLEOCIN PHOSPHATE Sterile Solution (clindamycin phosphate) is administered to newborns and infants, appropriate monitoring of organ system functions is desirable.

Nursing Mothers—Clindamycin has been reported to appear in breast milk in ranges of 0.7 to 3.8 mcg/ml.

Usage in Meningitis: Since clindamycin does not diffuse adequately into the cerebrospinal fluid, the drug should not be used in the treatment of meningitis.

Antagonism has been demonstrated between clindamycin and erythromycin *in vitro.* Because of possible clinical significance, these two drugs should not be administered concurrently.

SERIOUS ANAPHYLACTOID REACTIONS REQUIRE IMMEDIATE EMERGENCY TREATMENT WITH EPINEPHRINE. OXYGEN AND INTRAVENOUS CORTICOSTEROIDS SHOULD ALSO BE ADMINISTERED AS INDICATED.

1. Bartlett JG, et al: Antibiotic associated Pseudomembranous Colitis Due to Toxin-producing *Clostridia. N Engl J Med* 298(10):531-534, 1978.
2. George RH, et al: Identification of *Clostridium difficile* as a cause of Pseudomembranous Colitis. *Br Med J* 6114:669-671, 1978.
3. Larson HE, Price AB: Pseudomembranous Colitis Presence of Clostridial Toxin. *Lancet* 8052/3:1312-1314, 1977.
4. Rifkin GD, Fekety FR, Silva J: Antibiotic-induced Colitis Implication of a Toxin Neutralized by *Clostridium sordellii* Antitoxin. *Lancet* 8048:1103-1106, 1977.
5. Bailey WR, Scott EG: Diagnostic Microbiology. The CV Mosby Company, St. Louis, 1978.

Precautions: Review of experience to date suggests that a subgroup of older patients with associated severe illness may tolerate diarrhea less well. When clindamycin is indicated in these patients, they should be carefully monitored for change in bowel frequency.

CLEOCIN PHOSPHATE Sterile Solution (clindamycin phosphate) should be prescribed with caution in individuals with a history of gastrointestinal disease, particularly colitis.

CLEOCIN PHOSPHATE should be prescribed with caution in atopic individuals.

During prolonged therapy periodic liver and kidney function tests and blood counts should be performed.

Indicated surgical procedures should be performed in conjunction with antibiotic therapy.

The use of CLEOCIN PHOSPHATE may result in overgrowth of nonsusceptible organisms—particularly yeasts. Should superinfections occur, appropriate measures should be taken as indicated by the clinical situation.

CLEOCIN PHOSPHATE should not be injected intravenously undiluted as a bolus, but should be infused over at least 10-60 minutes as directed in the **Dosage and Administration** Section.

Patients with very severe renal disease and/or very severe hepatic disease accompanied by severe metabolic aberrations should be dosed with caution, and serum clindamycin levels monitored during high-dose therapy.

Clindamycin has been shown to have neuromuscular blocking properties that may enhance the action of other neuromuscular blocking agents.

CLEOCIN PHOSPHATE

To maintain serum clindamycin levels	Rapid infusion rate	Maintenance infusion rate
Above 4 mcg/ml	10 mg/min for 30 min	0.75 mg/min
Above 5 mcg/ml	15 mg/min for 30 min	1.00 mg/min
Above 6 mcg/ml	20 mg/min for 30 min	1.25 mg/min

Therefore, it should be used with caution in patients receiving such agents.

Adverse Reactions: The following reactions have been reported with the use of clindamycin.

Gastrointestinal: Abdominal pain, nausea, vomiting and diarrhea (See **Warning** box).

Hypersensitivity Reactions: Maculopapular rash and urticaria have been observed during drug therapy. Generalized mild to moderate morbilliform-like skin rashes are the most frequently reported of all adverse reactions. Rare instances of erythema multiforme, some resembling Stevens-Johnson syndrome, have been associated with clindamycin. A few cases of anaphylactoid reactions have been reported.

If a hypersensitivity reaction occurs, the drug should be discontinued. The usual agents (epinephrine, corticosteroids, antihistamines) should be available for emergency treatment of serious reactions.

Liver: Jaundice and abnormalities in liver function tests have been observed during clindamycin therapy.

Hematopoietic: Transient neutropenia (leukopenia) and eosinophilia have been reported. Reports of agranulocytosis and thrombocytopenia have been made. No direct etiologic relationship to concurrent clindamycin therapy could be made in any of the foregoing.

Local Reactions: Pain, induration and sterile abscess have been reported after intramuscular injection and thrombophlebitis after intravenous infusion. Reactions can be minimized or avoided by giving deep intramuscular injections and avoiding prolonged use of indwelling intravenous catheters.

Musculoskeletal: Rare instances of polyarthritis have been reported.

Cardiovascular: Rare instances of cardiopulmonary arrest and hypotension have been reported following too rapid intravenous administration. (See Dosage and Administration Section)

Dosage and Administration:

If significant diarrhea occurs during therapy, this antibiotic should be discontinued. (See **Warning** box.)

Adults

Parenteral (IM or IV Administration):
Serious infections due to aerobic gram-positive cocci and the more sensitive anaerobes (NOT generally including *Bacteroides fragilis, Peptococcus* species and *Clostridium* species other than *Clostridium perfringens*):
600–1200 mg/day in 2, 3 or 4 equal doses
More severe infections, particularly those due to proven or suspected *Bacteroides fragilis, Peptococcus* species, or *Clostridium* species other than *Clostridium perfringens:*
1200–2700 mg/day in 2, 3 or 4 equal doses
For more serious infections, these doses may have to be increased. In life threatening situations due to aerobes or anaerobes, these doses may be increased. Doses of as much as 4800 mg daily have been given intravenously to adults. See **Dilution and Infusion Rates** section below.
Single IM injections of greater than 600 mg are not recommended.
Alternatively, drug may be administered in the form of a single rapid infusion of the first dose followed by continuous IV infusion as follows:
[See table above].

Children (over 1 month of age)
Parenteral (IM or IV Administration):
Serious infections:
15–25 mg/kg/day in 3 or 4 equal doses
More severe infections:
25–40 mg/kg/day in 3 or 4 equal doses
As an alternative to dosing on a body weight basis, children may be dosed on the basis of square meters body surface: 350 mg/m^2/day for serious infections and 450 mg/m^2/day for more severe infections.

Neonates (less than 1 month):
15 to 20 mg/kg/day in three to four equal doses. The lower dosage may be adequate for small prematures.
Children (over 1 month):
20 to 40 mg/kg/day in three to four equal doses. An equivalent dosage may be given based on body surface area calculation.

Parenteral therapy may be changed to oral CLEOCIN PEDIATRIC® Flavored Granules (clindamycin palmitate hydrochloride) or CLEOCIN HCl™ Capsules (clindamycin hydrochloride) when the condition warrants and at the discretion of the physician.

In cases of β-hemolytic streptococcal infections, treatment should be continued for at least 10 days.

Dilution and Infusion Rates

Clindamycin phosphate must be diluted prior to IV administration. The concentration of clindamycin in diluent for infusion should not exceed 12 mg per ml and infusion rates should not exceed 30 mg per minute. The usual infusion dilutions and rates are as follows:

Dose	Diluent	Time
300 mg	50 ml	10 min
600 mg	50 ml	20 min
900 mg	100 ml	30 min
1200 mg	100 ml	40 min

Administration of more than 1200 mg in a single 1-hour infusion is not recommended.

Dilution and Compatibility

Physical and biological compatibility studies monitored for 24 hours at room temperature have demonstrated no inactivation or incompatibility with the use of CLEOCIN PHOSPHATE Sterile Solution (clindamycin phosphate) in IV solutions containing NaCl, glucose, calcium or potassium and solutions containing vitamin B complex in concentrations usually used clinically. No incompatibility has been demonstrated with the antibiotics cephalothin, kanamycin, gentamicin, penicillin or carbenicillin.

The following drugs are physically incompatible with CLEOCIN PHOSPHATE: ampicillin, phenytoin sodium, barbiturates, aminophylline, calcium gluconate, and magnesium sulfate.

Physico-Chemical Stability of CLEOCIN PHOSPHATE

Room temperature: 6, 9 and 12 mg/ml (equivalent to clindamycin base) in dextrose 5% in water, sodium chloride 0.9%, or Lactated Ringers in glass bottles or minibags, demonstrated physical and chemical stability for at least 16 days at 25°C.

Refrigeration: 6, 9 and 12 mg/ml (equivalent to clindamycin base) in dextrose 5% in water, sodium chloride 0.9%, or Lactated Ringers in glass bottles or minibags, demonstrated physical and chemical stability for at least 32 days at 4°C.

Frozen: 6,9 and 12 mg/ml (equivalent to clindamycin base) in dextrose 5% in water, sodium chloride 0.9%, or Lactated Ringers in minibags demonstrated physical and chemical stability for at least eight weeks at −10°C.

How Supplied: Each ml of CLEOCIN PHOSPHATE Sterile Solution contains clindamy-

Continued on next page

Information on these Upjohn products is based on labeling in effect on November 30, 1984. Further information concerning these and other Upjohn products may be obtained from the package insert or by direct inquiry to Medical Information, The Upjohn Company, Kalamazoo, Michigan 49001.

Upjohn—Cont.

cin phosphate equivalent to 150 mg clindamycin; 0.5 mg disodium edetate; 9.45 mg benzyl alcohol added as preservative. When necessary, pH is adjusted with sodium hydroxide and/or hydrochloric acid.

The following sizes are available:

25-2 ml ampoules	NDC 0009-0870-17
100-2 ml ampoules	NDC 0009-0870-03
25-4 ml ampoules	NDC 0009-0775-16
100-4 ml ampoules	NDC 0009-0775-03
25-2 ml vials	NDC 0009-0870-21
100-2 ml vials	NDC 0009-0870-22
25-4 ml vials	NDC 0009-0775-20
100-4 ml vials	NDC 0009-0775-21
25-6 ml vials	NDC 0009-0902-11
100-6 ml vials	NDC 0009-0902-12

Code 810 020 14

Shown in Product Identification Section, page 440
*Product of The Upjohn Manufacturing Company
CLEOCIN HCl is a trademark of The Upjohn Manufacturing Company.
CLEOCIN, CLEOCIN PEDIATRIC and CLEOCIN PHOSPHATE are registered trademarks of The Upjohn Manufacturing Company.
UPJOHN is a trademark registered in the US Patent and Trademark Office by The Upjohn Company, Kalamazoo, Michigan 49001, USA.

CLEOCIN T® ℞
brand of clindamycin phosphate topical solution, USP
For External Use
30 ml bottle
NSN 6505-01-140-6450(M)
60 ml bottle
NSN 6505-01-116-5655 (M & VA)

Description: CLEOCIN T Topical Solution contains clindamycin phosphate, USP, at a concentration equivalent to 10 mg clindamycin per milliliter in an isopropyl alcohol and water solution.
Clindamycin phosphate is a water soluble ester of the semi-synthetic antibiotic produced by a 7(S)-chloro-substitution of the 7(R)-hydroxy group of the parent antibiotic lincomycin.
The solution contains isopropyl alcohol 50% v/v, propylene glycol, and water.
The chemical name for clindamycin phosphate is 7(S)-chloro-7-deoxylincomycin-2-phosphate.
Clinical Pharmacology: Although clindamycin phosphate is inactive *in vitro*, rapid *in vivo* hydrolysis converts this compound to the antibacterially active clindamycin.
Clindamycin has been shown to have *in vivo* activity against isolates of *Propionibacterium acnes*. This may account for its usefulness in acne.
Cross resistance has been demonstrated between clindamycin and lincomycin.
Antagonism has been demonstrated between clindamycin and erythromycin.
Studies of penetration into human skin with radiolabelled clindamycin have shown that approximately 10% of the dose is absorbed as indicated by concentration in the stratum corneum. Microbiological assay of urine has shown varying concentrations of clindamycin.
Clindamycin activity has been demonstrated in comedones from acne patients. The mean concentration of antibiotic activity in extracted comedones after application of CLEOCIN T for 4 weeks was 597 mcg/g of comedonal material (range 0–1490). Clindamycin *in vitro* inhibits all *Propionibacterium acnes* cultures tested (MICs 0.4 mcg/ml). Free fatty acids on the skin surface have been decreased from approximately 14% to 2% following application of clindamycin.
Indications and Usage: CLEOCIN T Topical Solution (clindamycin phosphate) is indicated in the treatment of acne vulgaris. In view of the potential for diarrhea, bloody diarrhea and pseudomembranous colitis, the physician should consider whether other agents are more appropriate. (See **Contraindications, Warnings and Adverse Reactions.**)

Contraindications: CLEOCIN T Topical Solution (clindamycin phosphate) is contraindicated in individuals with a history of hypersensitivity to preparations containing clindamycin or lincomycin, a history of regional enteritis or ulcerative colitis, or a history of antibiotic-associated colitis.
Warnings: Orally and parenterally administered clindamycin has been associated with severe colitis which may end fatally. Use of the topical formulation results in absorption of the antibiotic from the skin surface. Diarrhea, bloody diarrhea, and colitis (including pseudomembranous colitis) have been reported with the use of topical and systemic clindamycin. Symptoms can occur after a few days, weeks or months following initiation of clindamycin therapy. They have also been observed to begin up to several weeks after cessation of therapy with clindamycin. Studies indicate a toxin(s) produced by *Clostridium difficile* is one primary cause of antibiotic-associated colitis. The colitis is usually characterized by severe persistent diarrhea and severe abdominal cramps and may be associated with the passage of blood and mucus. Endoscopic examination may reveal pseudomembranous colitis.
When significant diarrhea occurs, the drug should be discontinued. Large bowel endoscopy should be considered in cases of severe diarrhea.
Antiperistaltic agents such as opiates and diphenoxylate with atropine (Lomotil) may prolong and/or worsen the condition. Vancomycin has been found to be effective in the treatment of antibiotic-associated pseudomembranous colitis produced by *Clostridium difficile*. The usual adult dosage is 500 mg to 2 grams of vancomycin orally per day in three to four divided doses administered for 7 to 10 days.
Mild cases of colitis may respond to discontinuance of clindamycin. Moderate to severe cases should be managed promptly with fluid, electrolyte, and protein supplementation as indicated. Cholestyramine and colestipol resins have been shown to bind the toxin *in vitro*. If both a resin and vancomycin are to be administered concurrently, it may be advisable to separate the time of administration of each drug. Systemic corticoids and corticoid retention enemas may help relieve the colitis. Other causes of colitis should also be considered. A careful inquiry should be made concerning previous sensitivities to drugs and other allergens.
Precautions: CLEOCIN T Topical Solution (clindamycin phosphate) contains an alcohol base which will cause burning and irritation of the eye. In the event of accidental contact with sensitive surfaces (eye, abraded skin, mucous membranes), bathe with copious amounts of cool tap water. The solution has an unpleasant taste and caution should be exercised when applying medication around the mouth.
CLEOCIN T Topical Solution should be prescribed with caution in atopic individuals.
Pregnancy Category B
Reproduction studies have been performed in rats and mice using subcutaneous and oral doses of clindamycin ranging from 100 to 600 mg/kg/day and have revealed no evidence of impaired fertility or harm to the fetus due to clindamycin. There are, however, no adequate and well-controlled studies in pregnant women. Because animal reproduction studies are not always predictive of human response, this drug should be used during pregnancy only if clearly needed.
Nursing Mothers
It is not known whether clindamycin is excreted in human milk following use of CLEOCIN T Topical Solution. However, orally and parenterally administered clindamycin has been reported to appear in breast milk. As a general rule, nursing should not be undertaken while a patient is on a drug since many drugs are excreted in human milk.
Adverse Reactions: Skin dryness is the most common adverse reaction.
Clindamycin has been associated with severe colitis which may end fatally (See WARNINGS).
Cases of diarrhea, bloody diarrhea and colitis (including pseudomembranous colitis) have been reported as adverse reactions in patients treated with topical formulations of clindamycin.
Other effects which have been reported in association with the use of topical formulations of clindamycin include:
- Abdominal pain
- Contact dermatitis
- Gastrointestinal disturbances
- Gram-negative folliculitis
- Irritation
- Oily skin
- Sensitization
- Stinging of the eye

Dosage and Administration: Apply a thin film of CLEOCIN T Topical Solution (clindamycin phosphate) twice daily to affected area.
How Supplied: CLEOCIN T Topical Solution (clindamycin phosphate) is available as follows:
30 ml applicator bottle (10 mg/ml) NDC 0009-3116-01
60 ml applicator bottle (10 mg/ml) NDC 0009-3116-02
16 oz (473 ml) bottle—NDC 0009-3116-04
The applicator is designed so that the solution may be applied directly to the involved skin.
Code 811 373 109
Shown in Product Identification Section, page 441
*Product of The Upjohn Manufacturing Company
CLEOCIN T is a registered trademark of The Upjohn Manufacturing Company.
UPJOHN is a trademark registered in U.S. Patent and Trademark Office by The Upjohn Company, Kalamazoo, Michigan 49001, USA.

COLESTID® ℞
brand of colestipol hydrochloride granules

Description: COLESTID Granules consist of colestipol hydrochloride, which is a hyperlipidemia agent for oral use. COLESTID, is an insoluble, high molecular weight basic anion-exchange copolymer of diethylenetriamine and 1-chloro-2,3-epoxypropane, with approximately 1 out of 5 amine nitrogens protonated (chloride form). It is a light yellow resin which is hygroscopic and swells when placed in water or aqueous fluids. COLESTID is tasteless and odorless.
Clinical Pharmacology: Cholesterol is the major, and probably the sole precursor of bile acids. During normal digestion, bile acids are secreted via the bile from the liver and gall bladder into the intestines. Bile acids emulsify the fat and lipid materials present in food, thus facilitating absorption. A major portion of the bile acids secreted is reabsorbed from the intestines and returned via the portal circulation to the liver, thus completing the enterohepatic cycle. Only very small amounts of bile acids are found in normal serum.
COLESTID Granules (colestipol hydrochloride) bind bile acids in the intestine forming a complex that is excreted in the feces. This nonsystemic action results in a partial removal of the bile acids from the enterohepatic circulation, preventing their reabsorption. Since colestipol hydrochloride is an anion exchange resin, the chloride anions of the resin can be replaced by other anions, usually those with a greater affinity for the resin than chloride ion.
Colestipol hydrochloride is hydrophilic, but it is virtually water insoluble (99.75%) and it is not hydrolyzed by digestive enzymes. The high molecular weight polymer in COLESTID apparently is not absorbed. Less than 0.05% of ^{14}C-labeled colestipol hydrochloride is excreted in the urine.
The increased fecal loss of bile acids due to COLESTID administration leads to an increased oxidation of cholesterol to bile acids, a decrease in beta lipoprotein or low density lipoprotein serum levels, and a decrease in serum cholesterol levels. Although COLESTID produces an increase in the hepatic synthesis of cholesterol in man, serum cholesterol levels fall.
There is evidence to show that this fall in cholesterol is secondary to an increased rate of cholesterol rich lipoproteins (beta or low density lipoproteins) from the plasma. Serum triglyceride levels may increase or remain unchanged in colestipol treated patients.

The decline in serum cholesterol levels with treatment with COLESTID is usually evident by one month. When COLESTID is discontinued, serum cholesterol levels usually return to baseline levels within one month. Cholesterol may rise even with continued use of COLESTID, and serum levels should be determined periodically to confirm that a favorable initial response is maintained.

COLESTID is more effective than clofibrate in lowering total serum cholesterol and low density lipoprotein cholesterol in Frederickson type IIa hyperlipoproteinemia (pure hypercholesterolemia without hypertriglyceridemia) without affecting high density lipoprotein cholesterol.

In patients with heterozygous familial hypercholesterolemia who have not obtained an optimal response to colestipol hydrochloride alone in maximal doses, the combination of colestipol hydrochloride and nicotinic acid has been shown to provide effective further lowering of serum cholesterol, triglyceride, and LDL cholesterol values. Simultaneously, HDL cholesterol values increased significantly. In many such patients it is possible to normalize serum lipid values.[1-3]

Indications and Usage: Since no drug is innocuous, strict attention should be paid to the indications and contraindications, particularly when selecting drugs for chronic long-term use.

COLESTID Granules (colestipol hydrochloride) are indicated as adjunctive therapy to diet for the reduction of elevated serum cholesterol in patients with primary hypercholesterolemia (elevated low density lipoproteins). COLESTID has been shown to have no effect on or to increase triglyceride levels.

It has not been established whether the drug-induced lowering of serum colesterol or triglyceride levels has a beneficial effect, no effect, or a detrimental effect on the morbidity or mortality due to atherosclerosis including coronary heart disease. Investigations now in progress may yield an answer to this question.

Contraindications: COLESTID Granules (colestipol hydrochloride) are contraindicated in those individuals who have shown hypersensitivity to any of its components.

Warnings: TO AVOID ACCIDENTAL INHALATION OR ESOPHAGEAL DISTRESS, COLESTID GRANULES (colestipol hydrochloride) SHOULD NOT BE TAKEN IN ITS DRY FORM. ALWAYS MIX COLESTID WITH WATER OR OTHER FLUIDS BEFORE INGESTING.

Precautions: Before instituting therapy with COLESTID Granules (colestipol hydrochloride), a vigorous attempt should be made to control serum cholesterol by an appropriate dietary regimen and weight reduction; any underlying disorder that may contribute to the hypercholesterolemia should be treated.

Because it sequesters bile acids, COLESTID may interfere with normal fat absorption and thus may prevent absorption of fat soluble vitamins such as A, D, and K. If COLESTID resin is to be given for long periods of time, supplemental vitamin A and D should be considered.

Chronic use of COLESTID may be associated with an increased bleeding tendency due to hypoprothrombinemia from vitamin K deficiency. This will usually respond promptly to parenteral vitamin K$_1$ and recurrences can be prevented by oral administration of vitamin K$_1$.

Serum cholesterol and triglyceride levels should be measured periodically to detect significant changes. COLESTID may raise the serum triglycerides in long term use and, in some patients, the cholesterol levels return to baseline or rise above baseline.

COLESTID may produce or severely worsen pre-existing constipation. The dosage should be decreased in these patients since impaction may occur. Particular effort should be made to avoid constipation in patients with symptomatic coronary artery disease. Constipation associated with COLESTID may aggravate hemorrhoids.

While there have been no reports of hypothyroidism induced in individuals with normal thyroid function, the theoretical possibility exists, particularly in patients with limited thyroid reserve.

Use in Pregnancy
The use of COLESTID in pregnancy or lactation or by women of childbearing age requires that the potential benefits of drug therapy be weighed against the possible hazards to the mother and child. The safe use of COLESTID resin by pregnant women has not been established.

Use in Children
Safety and effectiveness in children have not been established.

Drug Interactions: Since colestipol hydrochloride is an anion exchange resin, it may have a strong affinity for anions other than the bile acids. Therefore, colestipol hydrochloride resin may delay or reduce the absorption of concomitant oral medication. The interval between the administration of COLESTID and any other medication should be as long as possible. Patients should take other drugs at least one hour before or four hours after COLESTID to avoid impeding their absorption.

In vitro studies have indicated that COLESTID binds a number of drugs. Studies in humans show that the absorption of chlorothiazide as reflected in urinary excretion is markedly decreased even when administered one hour before COLESTID. The absorption of tetracycline and of penicillin G was significantly decreased when either one was given at the same time as COLESTID; these drugs were not tested to determine the effect of administration one hour before COLESTID.

No depressant effect on blood levels in humans was noted when COLESTID was administered with any of the following drugs: aspirin, clindamycin, clofibrate, methyldopa, tolbutamide or warfarin. Particular caution should be observed with digitalis preparations since there are conflicting results for the effect of COLESTID on the availability of digoxin and digitoxin. The potential for binding of these drugs if given concomitantly is present. Discontinuing COLESTID could pose a hazard to health if a potentially toxic drug that is significantly bound to the resin has been titrated to a maintenance level while the patient was taking COLESTID.

Adverse Reactions:
1. *Gastrointestinal*
The most common adverse reactions are confined to the gastrointestinal tract. Constipation, reported by about one patient in 10, is the major single complaint and at times is severe and occasionally accompanied by fecal impaction. Hemorrhoids may be aggravated. Most instances of constipation are mild, transient, and controlled with standard treatment. Some patients require decreased dosage or discontinuation of therapy. Less frequent gastrointestinal complaints occurring in about one in 30 to one in 100 patients, are abdominal discomfort (abdominal pain and distention), belching, flatulence, nausea, vomiting, and diarrhea. Peptic ulceration, gastrointestinal irritation and bleeding, cholecystitis, and cholelithiasis have been reported by fewer than one in 500 patients and are not necessarily drug related.

2. *Hypersensitivity*
Urticaria and dermatitis were noted in fewer than one in 1,000 patients. Asthma and wheezing were not reported in the COLESTID studies but have been noted during treatment with other cholesterol-lowering agents.

3. *Musculoskeletal*
Muscle and joint pains, and arthritis have had a reported incidence of less than one in 1,000 patients.

4. *Neurologic*
Headache and dizziness were noted in about one in 300 patients; anxiety, vertigo, and drowsiness were reported in fewer than one in 1,000.

5. *Miscellaneous*
Anorexia, fatigue, weakness, and shortness of breath have been seen in 1–3 patients in 1,000. Transient and modest elevations of serum glutamic oxaloacetic transaminase and of alkaline phosphatase were observed in one or more occasions in various patients treated with COLESTID Granules (colestipol hydrochloride). Some patients have shown an increase in serum phosphorus and chloride with a decrease in sodium and potassium.

Overdose: Overdosage of COLESTID Granules (colestipol hydrochloride) has not been reported. Should overdosage occur, however, the chief potential harm would be obstruction of the gastrointestinal tract. The location of such potential obstruction, the degree of obstruction and the presence or absence of normal gut motility would determine treatment.

Dosage and Administration: For adults, COLESTID Granules (colestipol hydrochloride) are recommended in doses of 15–30 grams/day taken in divided doses two to four times daily. To avoid accidental inhalation or esophageal distress, COLESTID should not be taken in its dry form. COLESTID should always be mixed with water or other fluids before ingesting. Patients should take other drugs at least one hour before or four hours after COLESTID to minimize possible interference with their absorption. (See DRUG INTERACTIONS).

Before COLESTID Administration
1. Define the type of hyperlipoproteinemia.
2. Institute a trial of diet and weight reduction.
3. Establish baseline serum cholesterol and triglyceride levels.

During COLESTID Administration
1. The patient should be carefully monitored clinically, including serum cholesterol and triglyceride levels.
2. Failure of cholesterol to fall or significant rise in triglyceride level should be considered as indications to discontinue medication.

Mixing and Administration Guide
COLESTID Granules (colestipol hydrochloride) should always be taken mixed in a liquid such as orange or tomato juice, water, milk, or carbonated beverage. It may also be taken in soups or with cereals or pulpy fruits. COLESTID should never be taken in its dry form.

With beverages
1. Add the prescribed amount of COLESTID to a glassful (three ounces or more) of water, milk, flavored drink, or a favorite juice (orange, tomato, pineapple, or other fruit juice).
2. Stir the mixture until the medication is completely mixed. (COLESTID will not dissolve in the liquid.) COLESTID may also be mixed with carbonated beverages, slowly stirred in a large glass.
Rinse the glass with a small amount of additional beverage to make sure all the medication is taken.

With cereals, soups, and fruits
COLESTID may be taken mixed with milk in hot or regular breakfast cereals, or even mixed in soups that have a high fluid content (tomato or chicken noodle soup). It may also be added to fruits that are pulpy such as crushed pineapple, pears, peaches, or fruit cocktail.

How Supplied: COLESTID Granules (colestipol hydrochloride) are available as follows:
Box of 30–5 gram packets   NDC 0009-0260-01
500 gram bottle   NDC 0009-0260-02
Each packet or each level scoop supplies 5 grams of COLESTID.
Store at controlled room temperature 15°-30°C (59°-86°F).

References:
1. Kane JP, Malloy MJ, Tun P et al: Normalization of low-density-lipoprotein levels in heterozygous familial hypercholesterolemia with a combined drug regimen. *N. Engl J Med* 304:251–258, 1981.
2. Illingworth DR, Phillipson BE, JH Rapp et al: Colestipol plus nicotinic acid in treatment of

Continued on next page

Information on these Upjohn products is based on labeling in effect on November 30, 1984. Further information concerning these and other Upjohn products may be obtained from the package insert or by direct inquiry to Medical Information, The Upjohn Company, Kalamazoo, Michigan 49001.

Upjohn—Cont.

heterozygous familial hypercholesterolemia. *Lancet* 1:296–298, 1981.
3. Kuo PT, Kostis JB, Moreyra AE et al: Familial type II hyperlipoproteinemia with coronary heart disease: Effect of diet-colestipol-nicotinic acid treatment. *Chest* 79:286–291, 1981.

Code 810 307 001

CORTAID® Cream
(See PDR For Nonprescription Drugs)

CORTAID® Lotion
(See PDR For Nonprescription Drugs)

CORTAID® Ointment
(See PDR For Nonprescription Drugs)

CORTAID® Spray
(See PDR For Nonprescription Drugs)

CORTEF® Feminine Itch Cream
(See PDR For Nonprescription Drugs)

CORTEF® Rectal Itch Ointment
(See PDR For Nonprescription Drugs)

CYTOSAR-U® ℞
brand of cytarabine sterile powder
(sterile cytarabine, USP)
(ara-C)

For Intravenous and Subcutaneous Use Only

WARNING

Only physicians experienced in cancer chemotherapy should use CYTOSAR-U Sterile Powder.
For induction therapy patients should be treated in a facility with laboratory and supportive resources sufficient to monitor drug tolerance and protect and maintain a patient compromised by drug toxicity. The main toxic effect of CYTOSAR-U is bone marrow suppression with leukopenia, thrombocytopenia and anemia. Less serious toxicity includes nausea, vomiting, diarrhea and abdominal pain, oral ulceration, and hepatic dysfunction.
The physician must judge possible benefit to the patient against known toxic effects of this drug in considering the advisability of therapy with CYTOSAR-U. Before making this judgment or beginning treatment, the physician should be familiar with the following text.

Description: CYTOSAR-U Sterile Powder contains cytarabine (1-β-D-arabinofuranosylcytosine; β-cytosine arabinoside). Cytarabine is a synthetic nucleoside which differs from the normal nucleosides cytidine and deoxycytidine in that the sugar moiety is arabinose rather than ribose or deoxyribose.
CYTOSAR-U is an antineoplastic agent for parenteral administration. It is available as a sterile freeze-dried preparation in two sizes:
100 mg vials—when prepared as directed, each ml contains:
20 mg cytarabine (Supplied with 5 ml ampoule of Bacteriostatic Water for Injection with Benzyl Alcohol 0.945% w/v added as preservative. **Do not use this diluent for intrathecal use. See WARNINGS).**
500 mg vials—when prepared as directed, each ml contains:
50 mg cytarabine (Supplied with 10 ml ampoule of Bacteriostatic Water for Injection with Benzyl Alcohol 0.945% w/v added as preservative. **Do not use this diluent for intrathecal use. See WARNINGS).**
When necessary, the pH of CYTOSAR-U was adjusted with hydrochloric acid and/or sodium hydroxide.

Pharmacology:
Cell Culture Studies
Cytarabine is cytotoxic to a wide variety of proliferating mammalian cells in culture. It exhibits cell phase specificity, primarily killing cells undergoing DNA synthesis (S-phase) and under certain conditions blocking the progression of cells from the G_1 phase to the S-phase. Although the mechanism of action is not completely understood, it appears that cytarabine acts through the inhibition of DNA polymerase. A limited, but significant, incorporation of cytarabine into both DNA and RNA has also been reported. Extensive chromosomal damage, including chromatoid breaks, have been produced by cytarabine and malignant transformation of rodent cells in culture has been reported. Deoxycytidine prevents or delays (but does not reverse) the cytotoxic activity.
Cell culture studies have shown an antiviral effect.[1] However, efficacy against herpes zoster or smallpox could not be demonstrated in controlled clinical trials.[2–4]

Cellular Resistance and Sensitivity
Cytarabine is metabolized by deoxycytidine kinase and other nucleotide kinases to the nucleotide triphosphate, an effective inhibitor of DNA polymerase; it is inactivated by a pyrimidine nucleoside deaminase which converts it to the nontoxic uracil derivative. It appears that the balance of kinase and deaminase levels may be an important factor in determining sensitivity or resistance of the cell to cytarabine.

Animal Studies
In experimental studies with mouse tumors, cytarabine was most effective in those tumors with a high growth fraction. The effect was dependent on the treatment schedule; optimal effects were achieved when the schedule (multiple closely spaced doses or constant infusion) ensured contact of the drug with the tumor cells when the maximum number of cells were in the susceptible S-phase. The best results were obtained when courses of therapy were separated by intervals sufficient to permit adequate host recovery.

Human Pharmacology
Cytarabine is rapidly metabolized and is not effective orally; less than 20 percent of the orally administered dose is absorbed from the gastrointestinal tract.
Following rapid intravenous injection of cytarabine with tritium, the disappearance from plasma is biphasic. There is an initial distributive phase with a half-life of about 10 minutes, followed by a second elimination phase with a half-life of about 1 to 3 hours. After the distributive phase, over 80 percent of plasma radioactivity can be accounted for by the inactive metabolite 1-β-D-arabinofuranosyluracil (ara-U). Within 24 hours about 80 percent of the administered radioactivity can be recovered in the urine, approximately 90 percent of which is excreted as ara-U.
Relatively constant plasma levels can be achieved by continuous intravenous infusion.
After subcutaneous or intramuscular administration of cytarabine labeled with tritium, peak-plasma levels of radioactivity are achieved about 20 to 60 minutes after injection and are considerably lower than those after intravenous administration.
Cerebrospinal fluid levels of cytarabine are low in comparison to plasma levels after single intravenous injection. However, in one patient in whom cerebrospinal levels were examined after 2 hours of constant intravenous infusion, levels approached 40 percent of the steady state plasma level. With intrathecal administration, levels of cytarabine in the cerebrospinal fluid declined with a first order half-life of about 2 hours. Because cerebrospinal fluid levels of deaminase are low, little conversion to ara-U was observed.

Immunosuppressive Action
CYTOSAR-U Sterile Powder (cytarabine) is capable of obliterating immune responses in man during administration with little or no accompanying toxicity.[5,6] Suppression of antibody responses to E-coli-VI antigen and tetanus toxoid have been demonstrated. This suppression was obtained during both primary and secondary antibody responses.
CYTOSAR-U also suppressed the development of cell-mediated immune responses such as delayed hypersensitivity skin reaction to dinitrochlorobenzene. However, it had no effect on already established delayed hypersensitivity reactions.
Following 5-day courses of intensive therapy with CYTOSAR-U the immune response was suppressed, as indicated by the following parameters: macrophage ingress into skin windows; circulating antibody response following primary antigenic stimulation; lymphocyte blastogenesis with phytohemagglutinin. A few days after termination of therapy there was a rapid return to normal.[7]

Indications and Usage: CYTOSAR-U Sterile Powder (cytarabine) is indicated primarily for induction and maintenance of remission in acute myelocytic leukemia of both adults and children. It has also been found useful in the treatment of other leukemias, such as acute lymphocytic leukemia, chronic myelocytic leukemia (blast phase) and erythroleukemia. CYTOSAR-U may be used alone or in combination with other antineoplastic agents; the best results are often obtained with combination therapy.
CYTOSAR-U has been used experimentally in a variety of neoplastic diseases. In general, few patients with solid tumors have benefited.
Children with non-Hodgkin's lymphoma have benefited from a combination drug program (LSA_2L_2) that includes CYTOSAR-U.[8,9,10]
Remissions induced by CYTOSAR-U not followed by maintenance treatment have been brief. Maintenance therapy has extended these and provided useful and comfortable remissions with relatively little toxicity.

Acute Myelocytic Leukemia
The following tables outline the results of treatment with CYTOSAR-U alone and in combination with other chemotherapeutic agents, in the treatment of acute myelocytic leukemia in adults and children.
The treatment regimens outlined in the tables should not be compared for efficacy. These were independent studies with a number of variables involved, such as patient population, duration of disease, and previous treatment.
[See table on next page].
The responsiveness and course of childhood acute myelocytic leukemia (AML) appears to be different from that in adults.[23–25] Numerous studies show response rates to be higher in children than in adults with similar treatment schedules. Experience indicates that at least with induction and initial drug responsiveness, childhood AML appears to be more similar to childhood acute lymphocytic leukemia (ALL) than to its adult variant.

Acute Lymphocytic Leukemia
CYTOSAR-U has been used in the treatment of acute lymphocytic leukemia in both adults and children. When CYTOSAR-U was used with other antineoplastic agents as part of a total therapy program, results were equal to or better than those reported with such programs which did not include CYTOSAR-U.[26,27] Used singly, or in combination with other agents, CYTOSAR-U has also been effective in treating patients who had relapsed on other therapy. Table III summarizes the results obtained in previously treated patients. Since these are independent studies with such variables as patient population, duration of disease and previous treatment, results shown should not be used for comparing the efficacy of the outlined treatment programs.

Intrathecal Use in Meningeal Leukemia
CYTOSAR-U has been used intrathecally in acute leukemia in doses ranging from 5 mg/m^2 to 75 mg/m^2 of body surface area. The frequency of administration varied from once a day for 4 days to once every 4 days. The most frequently used dose was 30 mg/m^2 every 4 days until cerebrospinal fluid findings were normal, followed by one additional treatment.[36–40] The dosage schedule is usu-

TABLE I
ACUTE MYELOCYTIC LEUKEMIA
REMISSION INDUCTION
ADULTS

Drug-Dosage Schedule*	No. Patients Evaluated	Complete Remissions	Investigator
(CYTOSAR-U) SINGLE-DRUG THERAPY			
(infusion)			
10 mg/m^2/12 hrs/day	12	2 (17%)	Ellison[11] (1968)
30 mg/m^2/12 hrs/day	41	10 (24%)	
10 mg/m^2/24 hrs/day	9	2 (22%)	
30 mg/m^2/24 hrs/day	36	2 (6%)	
(infusion)			
200 mg/m^2/24 hrs/5 days	36	9 (25%)	Bodey[12] (1969)
10 mg/m^2 IV injection initially, then infusions of 30 mg/m^2/12 hrs or 60 mg/m^2/day for 4 days	49	21 (43%)	Goodell[13] (1970)
(infusion therapy)			Southwest Oncology Group[14] (1974)
800 mg/m^2/2 days	53	12 (23%)	
1000 mg/m^2/5 days	60	24 (40%)	
100 mg/m^2/day 1 hr infusion	49	7 (14%)	Carey[15] (1975)
5–12.5 mg/kg/12 hour infusion following IV synchronizing dose**	5	5 (100%)	Lampkin[16] (1976)
COMBINED THERAPY			
CYTOSAR-U, doxorubicin	41	30 (73%)	Preisler[17] (1979)
CYTOSAR-U, thioguanine, daunorubicin	28	22 (79%)	Gale[18] (1977)
CYTOSAR-U, doxorubicin, vincristine, prednisolone	35	23 (66%)	Weinstein[19] (1980)
CYTOSAR-U, daunorubicin, thioguanine, prednisone, vincristine	139	84 (60%)	Glucksberg[20] (1981)
CYTOSAR-U, daunorubicin	21	14 (67%)	Cassileth[21] (1977)

*Unless otherwise stated all doses given until drug effect—modifications then based on hematologic response. See references
**Highly experimental-requires ability to study mitotic indices

ally governed by the type and severity of central nervous system manifestations and the response to previous therapy.
CYTOSAR-U has been used intrathecally with SOLU-CORTEF® Sterile Powder (hydrocortisone sodium succinate) and methotrexate, both as prophylaxis in newly diagnosed children with acute lymphocytic leukemia, as well as in the treatment of meningeal leukemia. Sullivan has reported that prophylactic triple therapy has prevented late CNS disease and given overall cure and survival rates similar to those seen in patients in whom CNS radiation and intrathecal methotrexate were used as initial CNS prophylaxis.[41] The dose of CYTOSAR-U was 30 mg/m^2 of cytarabine, SOLU-CORTEF 15 mg/m^2 of hydrocortisone sodium succinate, and methotrexate 15 mg/m^2. The physician should be familiar with this report before initiation of the regimen.
Prophylactic triple therapy following the successful treatment of the acute meningeal episode may be useful. The physician should familiarize himself with the current literature before instituting such a program.
CYTOSAR-U given intrathecally may cause systemic toxicity and careful monitoring of the hemopoietic system is indicated. Modification of other anti-leukemia therapy may be necessary. Major toxicity is rare. The most frequently reported reactions after intrathecal administration were nausea, vomiting and fever; these reactions are mild and self-limiting. Paraplegia has been reported.[42] Necrotizing leukoencephalopathy occurred in 5 children; these patients had also been treated with intrathecal methotrexate and hydrocortisone, as well as by central nervous system radiation.[43] Isolated neurotoxicity has been reported.[44] Blindness occurred in two patients in remission whose treatment had consisted of combination systemic chemotherapy, prophylactic central nervous system radiation and intrathecal CYTOSAR-U.[45] Focal leukemic involvement of the central nervous system may not respond to intrathecal CYTOSAR-U and may better be treated with radiotherapy.

Non-Hodgkin's Lymphoma in Children
CYTOSAR-U has been used as part of a multi-drug program (LSA$_2$L$_2$) to treat non-Hodgkin's lymphoma in children.[8,9,10]

Contraindications: CYTOSAR-U Sterile Powder (cytarabine) is contraindicated in those patients who are hypersensitive to the drug.

Warnings (See boxed WARNING): CYTOSAR-U Sterile Powder (cytarabine) is a potent bone marrow suppressant. Therapy should be started cautiously in patients with pre-existing drug-induced bone marrow suppression. Patients receiving this drug must be under close medical supervision and, during induction therapy, should have leukocyte and platelet counts performed daily. Bone marrow examinations should be performed frequently after blasts have disappeared from the peripheral blood. Facilities should be available for management of complications, possibly fatal, of bone marrow suppression (infection resulting from granulocytopenia and other impaired body defenses, and hemorrhage secondary to thrombocytopenia). One case of anaphylaxis that resulted in acute cardiopulmonary arrest and required resuscitation has been reported. This occurred immediately after the intravenous administration of CYTOSAR-U.

Severe and at times fatal CNS, GI and pulmonary toxicity (different from that seen with conventional therapy regimens of CYTOSAR-U) has been reported following some experimental CYTOSAR-U dose schedules.[46–49] These reactions include reversible corneal toxicity, and hemorrhagic conjunctivitis, which may be prevented or diminished by prophylaxis with a local corticosteroid eye drop; cerebral and cerebellar dysfunction, including personality changes, somnolence and coma, usually reversible; severe gastrointestinal ulceration, including pneumatosis cystoides intestinalis leading to peritonitis; sepsis and liver abscess; pulmonary edema, liver damage with increased hyperbilirubinemia; bowel necrosis; and necrotizing colitis. Rarely, severe skin rash, leading to desquamation has been reported. Complete alopecia is more commonly seen with experimental high dose therapy than with standard CYTOSAR-U treatment programs. If experimental high dose therapy is used, do not use a diluent containing benzyl alcohol. Benzyl alcohol is contained in the diluent for this product. Benzyl alcohol has been reported to be associated with a fatal "Gasping Syndrome" in premature infants.

Continued on next page

Information on these Upjohn products is based on labeling in effect on November 30, 1984. Further information concerning these and other Upjohn products may be obtained from the package insert or by direct inquiry to Medical Information, The Upjohn Company, Kalamazoo, Michigan 49001.

Upjohn—Cont.

If used intrathecally, do not use a diluent containing benzyl alcohol. Many clinicians reconstitute with preservative-free 0.9% sodium chloride for injection and use immediately.

Use in Pregnancy

Pregnancy Category C. CYTOSAR-U is known to be teratogenic in some animal species. Use of the drug in women who are or who may become pregnant should be undertaken only after due consideration of potential benefit and potential hazard to both mother and child.

A review of the literature has shown 32 reported cases where CYTOSAR-U was given during pregnancy, either alone or in combination with other cytotoxic agents.

Eighteen normal infants were delivered. Four of these had first trimester exposure. Five infants were premature or of low birth weight. Twelve of the 18 normal infants were followed up at ages ranging from six weeks to seven years, and showed no abnormalities. One apparently normal infant died at 90 days of gastroenteritis.

Two cases of congenital abnormalities have been reported, one with upper and lower distal limb defects,[50] and the other with extremity and ear deformities.[51] Both of these cases had first trimester exposure.

There were seven infants with various problems in the neonatal period, including pancytopenia; transient depression of WBC, hematocrit or platelets; electrolyte abnormalities; transient eosinophilia; and one case of increased IgM levels and hyperpyrexia possibly due to sepsis. Six of the seven infants were also premature. The child with pancytopenia died at 21 days of sepsis.

Therapeutic abortions were done in five cases. Four fetuses were grossly normal, but one had an enlarged spleen and another showed Trisomy C chromosome abnormality in the chorionic tissue.

Because of the potential for abnormalities with cytotoxic therapy, particularly during the first trimester, a patient who is or who may become pregnant while on CYTOSAR-U should be apprised of the potential risk to the fetus and the advisability of pregnancy continuation. There is a definite, but considerably reduced risk if therapy is initiated during the second or third trimester. Although normal infants have been delivered to patients treated in all three trimesters of pregnancy, follow-up of such infants would be advisable.

Precautions: Patients receiving CYTOSAR-U Sterile Powder (cytarabine) must be monitored closely. Frequent platelet and leukocyte counts and bone marrow examinations are mandatory. Consider suspending or modifying therapy when drug-induced marrow depression has resulted in a platelet count under 50,000 or a polymorphonuclear granulocyte count under 1000/mm^3. Counts of formed elements in the peripheral blood may continue to fall after the drug is stopped and lowest values after drug-free intervals of 12 to 24 days. When indicated, restart therapy when definite signs of marrow recovery appear (on successive bone marrow studies). Patients whose drug is withheld until "normal" peripheral blood values are attained may escape from control.

When large intravenous doses are given quickly, patients are frequently nauseated and may vomit for several hours postinjection. This problem tends to be less severe when the drug is infused. The human liver apparently detoxifies a substantial fraction of an administered dose. Use the drug with caution and at reduced dose in patients whose liver function is poor.

Periodic checks of bone marrow, liver and kidney functions should be performed in patients receiving CYTOSAR-U.

Like other cytotoxic drugs, CYTOSAR-U may induce hyperuricemia secondary to rapid lysis of neoplastic cells. The clinician should monitor the patient's blood uric acid level and be prepared to use such supportive and pharmacologic measures as might be necessary to control this problem.

Acute pancreatitis has been reported to occur in patients being treated with CYTOSAR-U who have had prior treatment with L-asparaginase.[52]

Adverse Reactions:
Expected Reactions

Because cytarabine is a bone marrow suppressant, anemia, leukopenia, thrombocytopenia, megaloblastosis and reduced reticulocytes can be expected as a result of administration with CYTOSAR-U Sterile Powder. The severity of these reactions are dose and schedule dependent.[53] Cellular changes in the morphology of bone marrow and peripheral smears can be expected.[54]

Following 5-day constant infusions or acute injections of 50 mg/m^2 to 600 mg/m^2, white cell depression follows a biphasic course. Regardless of initial count, dosage level, or schedule, there is an initial fall starting the first 24 hours with a nadir at days 7–9. This is followed by a brief rise which peaks around the twelfth day. A second and deeper fall reaches nadir at days 15–24. Then there is rapid rise to above baseline in the next 10 days. Platelet depression is noticeable at 5 days with a peak depression occurring between days 12–15. Thereupon, a rapid rise to above baseline occurs in the next 10 days.[55]

The Cytarabine (Ara-C) Syndrome

A cytarabine syndrome has been described by Castleberry.[56] It is characterized by fever, myalgia, bone pain, occasionally chest pain, maculopapular rash, conjunctivitis and malaise. It usually occurs 6-12 hours following drug administration. Corticosteroids have been shown to be beneficial in treating or preventing this syndrome. If the symptoms of the syndrome are deemed treatable, corticosteroids should be contemplated as well as continuation of therapy with CYTOSAR-U Sterile Powder (cytarabine).

Most Frequent Adverse Reactions

anorexia
nausea
vomiting
diarrhea
oral and anal inflammation or ulceration
hepatic dysfunction
fever
rash
thrombophlebitis
bleeding (all sites)

Nausea and vomiting are most frequent following rapid intravenous injection.

Less Frequent Adverse Reactions

sepsis
pneumonia
cellulitis at injection site
skin ulceration
urinary retention
renal dysfunction
neuritis
neural toxicity
sore throat
esophageal ulceration
esophagitis
chest pain
bowel necrosis
abdominal pain
freckling
jaundice
conjunctivitis (may occur with rash)
dizziness
alopecia
anaphylaxis (See WARNINGS)
allergic edema
pruritus
shortness of breath
urticaria
headache

Experimental Doses

Severe and at times fatal CNS, GI and pulmonary toxicity (different from that seen with conventional therapy regimens of CYTOSAR-U) has been reported following some experimental dose schedules of CYTOSAR-U.[46-49] These reactions include reversible corneal toxicity and hemorrhagic conjunctivitis, which may be prevented or diminished by prophylaxis with a local corticosteroid eye drop; cerebral and cerebellar dysfunction, including personality changes, somnolence and coma, usually reversible; severe gastrointestinal ulceration, including pneumatosis cystoides intestinalis leading to peritonitis; sepsis and liver abscess; pulmonary edema, liver damage with increased hyperbilirubinemia; bowel necrosis; and necrotizing colitis. Rarely, severe skin rash, leading to desquamation has been reported. Complete alopecia is more commonly seen with experimental high dose therapy than with standard CYTOSAR-U treatment programs. If experimental high dose therapy is used, do not use a diluent containing benzyl alcohol.

Overdosage

There is no antidote for CYTOSAR-U overdosage. Doses of 4.5 g/m^2 by intravenous infusion over 1 hour every 12 hours for 12 doses has caused an unacceptable increase in irreversible CNS toxicity and death.[47]

Dosage and Administration: CYTOSAR-U Sterile Powder (cytarabine) is not active orally. The schedule and method of administration varies with the program of therapy to be used. CYTOSAR-U Sterile Powder may be given by intravenous infusion or injection or subcutaneously. Thrombophlebitis has occurred at the site of drug injection or infusion in some patients, and rarely patients have noted pain and inflammation at subcutaneous injection sites. In most instances, however, the drug has been well tolerated.

Patients can tolerate higher total doses when they receive the drug by rapid intravenous injection as compared with slow infusion. This phenomenon is related to the drug's rapid inactivation and brief exposure of susceptible normal and neoplastic cells to significant levels after rapid injection. Normal and neoplastic cells seem to respond in somewhat parallel fashion to these different modes of administration and no clear-cut clinical advantage has been demonstrated for either.

Clinical experience accumulated to date suggests that success with CYTOSAR-U is dependent more on adeptness in modifying day-to-day dosage to obtain maximum leukemic cell kill with tolerable toxicity than on the basic treatment schedule chosen at the outset of therapy. Toxicity necessitating dosage alteration almost always occurs.

In many chemotherapeutic programs, CYTOSAR-U is used in combination with other cytotoxic drugs. The addition of these cytotoxic drugs has necessitated changes and dose alterations. The dosage schedules for combination therapy outlined below have been reported in the literature (see **References**).

[See table on next page].

Dosage Schedules:

Acute myelocytic leukemia—induction remission, adults

CYTOSAR-U Sterile Powder (cytarabine)—200 mg/m^2 daily by continuous infusion for 5 days (120 hours)—total dose 1000 mg/m^2. This course is repeated approximately every 2 weeks. Modifications must be made and based on hematologic response.

Combined Chemotherapy

Before instituting a program of combined chemotherapy, the physician should be familiar with the literature, adverse reactions, precautions, contraindications, and warnings applicable to all the drugs involved in the program.

CYTOSAR-U, doxorubicin[17]

CYTOSAR-U: 100 mg/m^2/day, continuous IV infusion (Days 1–10)

Doxorubicin: 30 mg/m^2/day, IV infusion of 30 minutes (Days 1–3)

Additional (complete or modified) courses as necessary at 2–4 week intervals if leukemia is persistent.

CYTOSAR-U, thioguanine, daunorubicin[18]

CYTOSAR-U: 100 mg/m^2/day IV infusion over 30 minutes every 12 hours (Days 1–7)

Thioguanine: 100 mg/m^2, orally every 12 hours (Days 1–7)

Daunorubicin: 60 mg/m^2/day, IV infusion (Days 5–7)

Additional (complete or modified) courses as necessary at 2–4 week intervals if leukemia is persistent.

TABLE II
ACUTE MYELOCYTIC LEUKEMIA
REMISSION INDUCTION
CHILDREN (21 and under)

Drug Therapy	No. Patients Evaluated	Complete Remissions	Investigator
CYTOSAR-U, (5–12.5 mg/kg following IV synchronizing dose**)	16	12 (75%)	Lampkin[16] (1976)
CYTOSAR-U, vincristine, doxorubicin, prednisolone	48	35 (73%)	Weinstein[19] (1980)
CYTOSAR-U, thioguanine-doxorubicin	11	8 (72%)	Hagbin[22] (1975)
CYTOSAR-U, thioguanine	47	20 (43%)	Pizzo[23] (1976)
CYTOSAR-U, cyclophosphamide	12	7 (58%)	

**Highly experimental-requires ability to study mitotic indices

CYTOSAR-U, doxorubicin, vincristine, prednisolone[19]
CYTOSAR-U: 100 mg/m²/day, continuous IV infusion (Days 1–7)
Doxorubicin: 30 mg/m²/day, IV infusion (Days 1–3)
Vincristine: 1.5 mg/m²/day, IV infusion (Days 1, 5)
Prednisolone: 40 mg/m²/day, IV infusion every 12 hours (Days 1–5)
Additional (complete or modified) courses as necessary at 2–4 week intervals if leukemia is persistent.

CYTOSAR-U, daunorubicin, thioguanine, prednisone, vincristine[20]
CYTOSAR-U: 100 mg/m²/day, IV every 12 hours (Days 1–7)
Daunorubicin: 70 mg/m²/Day, IV infusion (Days 1–3)
Thioguanine: 100 mg/m², orally every 12 hours (Days 1–7)
Prednisone: 40 mg/m²/day, orally (Days 1–7)
Vincristine: 1 mg/m²/day, IV infusion (Days 1, 7)
Additional (complete or modified) courses as necessary at 2–4 week intervals if leukemia is persistent.

CYTOSAR-U, daunorubicin[21]
CYTOSAR-U: 100 mg/m²/day, continuous infusion (Days 1–7)
Daunorubicin: 45 mg/m²/day, IV push (Days 1–3)
Additional (complete or modified) courses as necessary at 2–4 week intervals if leukemia is persistent.

Acute myelocytic leukemia-maintenance, adults
Maintenance programs are modifications of induction programs and, in general, use similar schedules of drug therapy as were used during induction. Most programs have a greater time spacing between courses of therapy during remission maintenance.

Acute myelocytic leukemia-induction and maintenance in children
Numerous studies have shown that childhood AML responds better than adult AML given similar regimens. Where the adult dosage is stated in terms of body weight or surface area, the children's dosage may be calculated on the same basis. When specified amounts of a drug are indicated for the adult dosage, these should be adjusted for children on the basis of such factors as age, body weight or body surface area.

Acute lymphocytic leukemia
In general, dosage schedules are similar to those used in acute myelocytic leukemia with some modifications. For dosage recommendations see referenced literature in Table III under INDICATIONS AND USAGE.

Dosage Modification—The dosage of CYTOSAR-U must be modified or suspended when signs of serious hematologic depression appear. In general, consider discontinuing the drug if the patient has less than 50,000 platelets or 1000 polymorphonuclear granulocytes/mm³ in his peripheral blood. These guidelines may be modified depending on signs of toxicity in other systems and on the rapidity of fall in formed blood elements. Restart the drug when there are signs of marrow recovery and the above platelet and granulocyte levels have been attained. Withholding therapy until the patient's blood values are normal may result in escape of the patient's disease from control by the drug.

How Supplied: Store unreconstituted product at controlled room temperature: 15°-30°C (59°-86°F). CYTOSAR-U Sterile Powder (cytarabine) is available as a freeze-dried preparation in multidose vials of two sizes:

100 mg* vial—Must be reconstituted with 5 ml of Bacteriostatic Water for Injection with Benzyl Alcohol 0.945% w/v added as preservative, the resulting solution contains 20 mg of cytarabine per ml. (Do not use this diluent for intrathecal use. See WARNINGS.)

500 mg* vial—Must be reconstituted with 10 ml of Bacteriostatic Water for Injection with Benzyl Alcohol 0.945% w/v added as preservative, the resulting solution contains 50 mg of cytarabine per ml. (Do not use this diluent for intrathecal use. See WARNINGS.)

*When necessary, the pH was adjusted with hydrochloric acid and/or sodium hydroxide.

In this form the drug is suitable for intravenous or subcutaneous administration. The pH of the reconstituted solution is about 5. THESE SOLUTIONS MAY BE STORED AT CONTROLLED ROOM TEMPERATURE 15°-30°C (59°-86°F) FOR 48 HOURS. DISCARD ANY SOLUTION IN WHICH A SLIGHT HAZE DEVELOPS.

Chemical Stability in Infusion Solutions
Chemical stability studies were performed by ultraviolet assay on CYTOSAR-U infusion solutions. These studies showed that when the reconstituted CYTOSAR-U Sterile Powder (cytarabine) was added to Water for Injection, 5% Dextrose in Water or Sodium Chloride Injection, 94 to 96 percent of the cytarabine was present after 192 hours storage at room temperature.

References:
1. Zaky DA, Betts RF, Douglas RG, et al: Varicella-Zoster Virus and Subcutaneous Cytarabine: Correlation of In Vitro Sensitivities to Blood Levels, Antimicrob Agents Chemother 7:229–232, 1975
2. Davis CM, VanDarsarl JV, Coltman CA Jr: Failure of Cytarabine in Varicella-Zoster Infections, JAMA 224:122–123, 1973
3. Betts RF, Zaky DA, Douglas RG, et al: Ineffectiveness of Subcutaneous Cytosine Arabinoside in Localized Herpes Zoster, Ann Intern Med 82:778–783, 1975
4. Dennis DT, Doberstyn EB, Awoke S, et al: Failure of Cytosine Arabinoside in Treating Smallpox; A Double-blind Study, Lancet 2:377–379, 1974
5. Gray GD: ARA-C And Derivatives as Examples of Immunosuppressive Nucleoside Analogs, Ann NY Acad Sci 255:372–379, 1975
6. Mitchell MS, Wade ME, DeConti RC, et al: Immunosuppressive Effects of Cytosine Arabinoside and Methotrexate in Man, Ann Intern Med 70:535–547, 1969
7. Frei E, Ho DHW, Bodey GP, et al: Pharmacologic and Cytokinetic Studies of Arabinosyl Cytosine. In Unifying Concepts of Leukemia, Bibl. Hematol. No. 39. Karger, Basel 1973, pp 1085–1097
8. Wollner N, Burchenal JH, Lieberman PH, et al: Non-Hodgkin's Lymphoma in Children—A Comparative Study of Two Modalities of Therapy, Cancer 37:123–134, 1976
9. Wollner N, Exelby PR, Lieberman PH: Non-Hodgkin's Lymphoma in Children—A Progress Report on the Original Patients Treated with the LSA_2-L_2 Protocol, Cancer 44:1990–1999, 1979
10. Sullivan MP, Pullen J, Moore T, et al: Pediatric Oncology Group Trial of LSA_2-L_2 Therapy in Non-Hodgkin's Lymphoma, abstracted, Proc AACR and ASCO 22:C-180, 1981
11. Ellison RR, Holland JF, Weil M, et al: Arabinosyl Cytosine: A Useful Agent in the Treatment of Acute Leukemia in Adults, Blood 32:507–523, 1968
12. Bodey GP, Freireich EJ, Monto RW, et al: Cytosine Arabinoside (NSC-63878) Therapy for Acute Leukemia in Adults, Cancer Chemother Rep 53:59–66, 1969
13. Goodell B, Leventhal B, Henderson E: Cytosine Arabinoside in Acute Granulocytic Leukemia, Clin Pharmacol Ther 12:599–606, 1970
14. Southwest Oncology Group: Cytarabine for Acute Leukemia in Adults, Arch Intern Med 133:251–259, 1974
15. Carey RW, Ribas-Mundo M, Ellison RR, et al: Comparative Study of Cytosine Arabinoside Therapy Alone and Combined with Thioguanine, Mercaptopurine or Daunorubicin in Acute Myelocytic Leukemia, Cancer 36:1560–1566, 1975
16. Lampkin BC, McWilliam NB, Mauer AM, et al: Manipulation of the Mitotic Cycle in the Treatment of Acute Myelogenous Leukemia, Brit J Haematol 32:29–40, 1976
17. Preisler H, Bjornsson S, Henderson ES, et al: Remission Induction in Acute Nonlymphocytic Leukemia—Comparison of a Seven-Day and Ten-Day Infusion of Cytosine Arabinoside in Combination With Adriamycin, Med Pediatr Oncol 7:269–275, 1979
18. Gale RP, Cline MJ: High Remission–Induction Rate in Acute Myeloid Leukemia, Lancet 1:497–499, 1977

Continued on next page

Information on these Upjohn products is based on labeling in effect on November 30, 1984. Further information concerning these and other Upjohn products may be obtained from the package insert or by direct inquiry to Medical Information, The Upjohn Company, Kalamazoo, Michigan 49001.

Upjohn—Cont.

19. Weinstein HJ, Mayer RJ, Rosenthal DS, et al: Treatment of Acute Myelogenous Leukemia In Children and Adults, N Eng J Med 303:473-478, 1980
20. Glucksberg H, Cheever MA, Farewell UT, et al: High-Dose Combination Chemotherapy for Acute Nonlymphoblastic Leukemia in Adults, Cancer 48:1073-1081, 1981
21. Cassileth PA, Katz ME: Chemotherapy for Adult Acute Nonlymphocytic Leukemia with Daunorubicin and Cytosine Arabinoside, Cancer Treat Rep 61:1441-1445, 1977
22. Haghbin M: Acute Non-lymphoblastic Leukemia; Clinical and Morphological Characterization, Mod Prob Pediatr 16:39-58, 1975
23. Pizzo PA, Henderson ES, Leventhal BG: Acute Myelogenous Leukemia in Children: A Preliminary Report of Combination Chemotherapy, J Pediatr 88:125-130, 1976
24. Report of the Medical Research Council's Working Party on Leukaemia in Adults: Treatment of Acute Myeloid Leukaemia with Daunorubicin, Cytosine Arabinoside, Mercaptopurine, L-Asparaginase, Prednisone and Thioguanine: Results of Treatment with Five Multiple-Drug Schedules, Brit J Haematol 27:373-389, 1974
25. Ansari BM, Thompson EN, Whittaker JA: A Comparative Study of Acute Myeloblastic Leukaemia in Children and Adults, Brit J Haematol 31:269-277, 1975
26. Gee TS, Haghbin M, Dowling MD Jr, et al: Acute Lymphoblastic Leukemia in Adults and Children; Differences in Response with Similar Therapeutic Regimens, Cancer 37:1256-1264, 1976
27. Spiers ASD, Roberts PD, Marsh GW, et al: Acute Lymphoblastic Leukaemia: Cyclical Chemotherapy with three Combinations of Four Drugs (COAP-POMP-CART Regimen). Brit Med J 4:614-617, 1975
28. Howard JP, Albo V, Newton WA Jr: Cytosine Arabinoside: Results of a Cooperative Study in Acute Childhood Leukemia, Cancer 21:341-345, 1968
29. McElwain TJ, Hardisty RM: Remission Induction with Cytosine Arabinoside and L-Asparaginase in Acute Lymphoblastic Leukaemia, Brit Med J 4:596-598, 1969
30. Bodey GP, Rodriguez, V, Hart J, et al: Therapy of Acute Leukemia with the Combination of Cytosine Arabinoside (NSC-63878) and Cyclophosphamide (NSC-26271), Cancer Chemother Rep 54:255-262, 1970
31. Nesbit ME Jr, Hammond D: Cytosine Arabinoside (ARAC) and Prednisone Therapy of Previously Treated Acute Lymphoblastic and Undifferentiated Leukemia (ALL-/AUL) of Childhood, Proc Am Assoc Cancer Res 11:59, 1970
32. Wang JJ, Selawry OS, Vietti TJ, et al: Prolonged Infusion of Arabinosyl Cytosine in Childhood Leukemia, Cancer 25:1-6, 1970
33. Klemperer M, Coccia P, Albo V, et al: Reinduction of Remission After First Bone Marrow Relapse in Childhood Acute Lymphoblastic Leukemia, Proc Am Assoc Cancer Res 19:414, 1978
34. Ortega JA, Finklestein JZ, Ertell, et al: Effective Combination Treatment of Advanced Acute Lymphocytic Leukemia with Cytosine Arabinoside (NSC-63878) and L-Asparaginase (NSC-109229), Cancer Chemother Rep 56:363-368, 1972
35. Bryan JH, Henderson ES, Leventhal BG: Cytosine Arabinoside and 6-Thioguanine in Refractory Acute Lymphocytic Leukemia, Cancer 33:539-544, 1974
36. Proceedings of the Chemotherapy Conference on ARA-C: Development and Application (Cytosine Arabinoside Hydrochloride—NSC 63878), Oct. 10, 1969
37. Lay HN, Colebatch JH, Ekert H: Experiences with Cytosine Arabinoside in Childhood Leukaemia and Lymphoma, Med J Aust 2:187-192, 1971
38. Halikowski B, Cyklis R, Armata J, et al: Cytosine Arabinoside Administered Intrathecally in Cerebromeningeal Leukemia, Acta Paediat Scand 59:164-168, 1970
39. Wang JJ, Pratt CB: Intrathecal Arabinosyl Cytosine in Meningeal Leukemia, Cancer 25:531-534, 1970
40. Band PR, Holland JF, Bernard J, et al: Treatment of Central Nervous System Leukemia with Intrathecal Cytosine Arabinoside, Cancer 32:744-748, 1973
41. Sullivan MP, Dyment P, Hvizdala E, et al: Favorable Comparison of All Out #2 with "Total" Therapy in the Treatment of Childhood Leukemia—The Equivalence of Intrathecal Chemotherapy and Radiotherapy as CNS
42. Saiki JH, Thompson S, Smith F, et al: Paraplegia Following Intrathecal Chemotherapy, Cancer 29:370-374, 1972
43. Rubinstein LJ, Herman MM, Long TF, et al: Disseminated Necrotizing Leukoencephalopathy: A Complication of Treated Central System Leukemia and Lymphoma, Cancer 35:291-305, 1975
44. Marmont Am, Damasio EE: Neurotoxicity of Intrathecal Chemotherapy for Leukemia, Brit Med J 4:47, 1973
45. Margileth DA, Poplack DG, Pizzo PA, et al: Blindness During Remission in Two Patients with Acute Lymphoblastic Leukemia, Cancer 39:58-61, 1977
46. Hopen G, Mondino BJ, Johnson BL, et al: Corneal Toxicity with Systemic Cytarabine, Am J Ophthalmol 91:500-504, 1981
47. Lazarus HM, Herzig RH, Herzig GP, et al: Central Nervous System Toxicity of High-Dose Systemic Cytosine Arabinoside, Cancer 48:2577-2582, 1981.
48. Slavin RE, Dias MA, Soral R: Cytosine Arabinoside Induced Gastrointestinal Toxic Alterations in Sequential Chemotherapeutic Protocols—A Clinical Pathologic Study of 33 Patients, Cancer 42:1747-1759, 1978.
49. Haupt HM, Hutchins GM, Moore GW; Ara-C Lung: Noncardiogenic Pulmonary Edema Complicating Cytosine Arabinoside Therapy of Leukemia, Am J Med 70:256-261, 1981.
50. Shafer AI: Teratogenic Effects of Antileukemic Chemotherapy. Arch Intern Med 141:514-515, 1981.
51. Wagner VM, et al: Congenital Abnormalities in Baby Born to Cytarabine Treated Mother, Lancet 2:98-99, 1980.
52. Altman AJ, Dinndorf P, Quinn JJ: Acute Pancreatitis in Association with Cytosine Arabinoside Therapy, Cancer 49:1384-1386, 1982
53. Frei E III, Bickers JN, Hewlett JS, et al: Dose Schedule and Antitumor Studies of Arabinosyl Cytosine (NSC 63878), Cancer Res 29:1325-1332, 1969
54. Bell WR, Whang JJ, Carbone PP, et al: Cytogenetic and Morphologic Abnormalities in Human Bone Marrow Cells during Cytosine Arabinoside Therapy, J. Hematol 27:771-781, 1966
55. Burke PJ, Serpick AA, Carbone PP, et al: A Clinical Evaluation of Dose and Schedule of Administration of Cytosine Arabinoside (NSC 63878), Cancer Res 28:274-279, 1968
56. Castleberry RP, Crist WM, Holbrook T, et al: The Cytosine Arabinoside (Ara-C) Syndrome, Med Pediatr Oncol 9:257-264, 1981.

[See table below]

Animal Toxicology: Toxicity of cytarabine in experimental animals, as well as activity, is markedly influenced by the schedule of administration. For example, in mice the LD_{10} for single intraperitoneal administration is greater than 6000 mg/m². However, when administered in 8 doses, each separated by 3 hours, the LD_{10} is less than 750 mg/m²

TABLE III
ACUTE LYMPHATIC LEUKEMIA
REMISSION INDUCTION
PREVIOUSLY TREATED PATIENTS

ADULTS AND CHILDREN

Drug Therapy	No. of Patients Evaluated	Complete Remissions	Response	Investigator
CYTOSAR-U, 3-5 mg/kg/day (IV injection)	43	2 (5%)	15 (35%)	Howard[28] (1968)
CYTOSAR-U, asparaginase	9	8 (89%)	8 (89%)	McElwain[29] (1969)
CYTOSAR-U, cyclophosphamide	11	7 (64%)	9 (82%)	Bodey[30] (1970)
CYTOSAR-U, prednisone	83		(49%)	Nesbit[31] (1970)
CYTOSAR-U,-150-200 mg/m²/5 days (infusion)	34	1 (3%)	4 (12%)	Wang[32] (1970)
CYTOSAR-U, L-asparaginase, prednisone, vincristine, doxorubicin	91	72 (79%)	—	Klemperer[33] (1978)
CYTOSAR-U, L-asparaginase, prednisone, vincristine, doxorubicin	55	42 (76%)	—	Klemperer[33] (1978)
CYTOSAR-U, asparaginase	22	13 (59%)	15 (68%)	Ortega[34] (1972)
CYTOSAR-U, thioguanine	19	9 (47%)	9 (47%)	Bryan[35] (1974)

total dose. Similarly, although a total dose of 1920 mg/m² administered as 12 injections at 6-hour intervals was lethal to beagle dogs (severe bone marrow hypoplasia with evidence of liver and kidney damage), dogs receiving the same total dose administered as 8 injections (again at 6-hour intervals) over a 48-hour period survived with minimal signs of toxicity. The most consistent observation in surviving dogs was elevated transaminase levels. In all experimental species the primary limiting toxic effect is marrow suppression with leukopenia. In addition, cytarabine causes abnormal cerebellar development in the neonatal hamster and is teratogenic to the rat fetus.
Code 810 126 107

DELTA-CORTEF® ℞
brand of prednisolone tablets, USP

How Supplied: 5 mg scored tablets.
Bottles of 100   NDC 0009-0025-01
Bottles of 500   NDC 0009-0025-02

DELTASONE® ℞
brand of prednisone tablets, USP

How Supplied: Scored tablets in the following strength and sizes:

2.5 mg	Bottles of 100	NDC 0009-0032-01
5 mg	Bottles of 100	NDC 0009-0045-01
	Bottles of 500	NDC 0009-0045-02
	Dosepak™ Unit of use (21)	NDC 0009-0045-04
	Unit Dose Package (100)	NDC 0009-0045-05
10 mg	Bottles of 100	NDC 0009-0193-01
	Bottles of 500	NDC 0009-0193-02
	Unit Dose Packages (100)	NDC 0009-0193-03
20 mg	Bottles of 100	NDC 0009-0165-01
	Bottles of 500	NDC 0009-0165-02
	Unit dose Packages (100)	NDC 0009-0165-03
50 mg	Bottles of 100	NDC 0009-0388-01
	Unit dose Packages (100)	NDC 0009-0388-02

Code 810 342 304
Shown in Product Identification Section, page 441

DEPO–MEDROL® ℞
brand of methylprednisolone acetate sterile aqueous suspension
(sterile methylprednisolone acetate suspension, USP)
Not for Intravenous Use

40 mg/ml (1 ml vial):
NSN 6505-00-952-0267 (M)
40 mg/ml (5 ml vial):
NSN 6505-00-890-1186A (M & VA)

Description: DEPO-MEDROL Sterile Aqueous Suspension contains methylprednisolone acetate which is the 6-methyl derivative of prednisolone. Methylprednisolone acetate is a white or practically white, odorless, crystalline powder which melts at about 215° with some decomposition. It is soluble in dioxane, sparingly soluble in acetone, in alcohol, in chloroform, and in methanol, and slightly soluble in ether. It is practically insoluble in water.
The chemical name for methylprednisolone acetate is pregna-1,4-diene-3,20-dione,21-(acetyloxy)-11, 17-dihydroxy-6-methyl-,(6α, 11β)- and the molecular weight is 416.51.
DEPO-MEDROL Sterile Aqueous Suspension (methylprednisolone acetate) is an anti-inflammatory glucocorticoid in a sterile aqueous suspension for intramuscular, intra-articular, soft tissue or intralesional injection. It is available in three strengths: 20 mg/ml; 40 mg/ml; 80 mg/ml. [See table above].
Actions: Naturally occurring glucocorticoids (hydrocortisone), which also have salt retaining properties, are used in replacement therapy in adrenocortical deficiency states. Their synthetic analogs are used primarily for their potent anti-inflammatory effects in disorders of many organ systems.

DEPO-MEDROL
Each ml of these preparations contains:

	20 mg	40 mg	80 mg
Methylprednisolone Acetate	20 mg	40 mg	80 mg
Polyethylene Glycol 3350	29.6 mg	29 mg	28 mg
Sodium Chloride	8.9 mg	8.7 mg	8.5 mg
Myristyl-gamma-picolinium Chloride added as preservative	0.198 mg	0.195 mg	0.189 mg

When necessary, pH was adjusted with sodium hydroxide and/or hydrochloric acid.
The pH of the finished product remains within the USP specified range; ie, 3.5 to 7.0.

Glucocorticoids cause profound and varied metabolic effects. In addition, they modify the body's immune response to diverse stimuli.
Indications
A. FOR INTRAMUSCULAR ADMINISTRATION
When oral therapy is not feasible and the strength, dosage form, and route of administration of the drug reasonably lend the preparation to the treatment of the condition, the intramuscular use of DEPO-MEDROL Sterile Aqueous Suspension (methylprednisolone acetate) is indicated as follows:
1. **Endocrine Disorders**
   Primary or secondary adrenocortical insufficiency (hydrocortisone or cortisone is the drug of choice; synthetic analogs may be used in conjunction with mineralocorticoids where applicable; in infancy, mineralocorticoid supplementation is of particular importance)
   Acute adrenocortical insufficiency (hydrocortisone or cortisone is the drug of choice; mineralocorticoid supplementation may be necessary, particularly when synthetic analogs are used)
   Preoperatively and in the event of serious trauma or illness, in patients with known adrenal insufficiency or when adrenocortical reserve is doubtful
   Congenital adrenal hyperplasia
   Hypercalcemia associated with cancer
   Nonsuppurative thyroiditis
2. **Rheumatic Disorders**
   As adjunctive therapy for short-term administration (to tide the patient over an acute episode or exacerbation) in:
   Post-traumatic osteoarthritis
   Synovitis of osteoarthritis
   Rheumatoid arthritis, including juvenile rheumatoid arthritis (selected cases may require low-dose maintenance therapy)
   Acute and subacute bursitis
   Epicondylitis
   Acute nonspecific tenosynovitis
   Acute gouty arthritis
   Psoriatic arthritis
   Ankylosing spondylitis
3. **Collagen Diseases**
   During an exacerbation or as maintenance therapy in selected cases of:
   Systemic lupus erythematosus
   Systemic dermatomyositis (polymyositis)
   Acute rheumatic carditis
4. **Dermatologic Diseases**
   Pemphigus
   Severe erythema multiforme (Stevens-Johnson syndrome)
   Exfoliative dermatitis
   Bullous dermatitis herpetiformis
   Severe seborrheic dermatitis
   Severe psoriasis
   Mycosis fungoides
5. **Allergic States**
   Control of severe or incapacitating allergic conditions intractable to adequate trials of conventional treatment in:
   Bronchial asthma
   Contact dermatitis
   Atopic dermatitis
   Serum sickness
   Seasonal or perennial allergic rhinitis
   Drug hypersensitivity reactions
   Urticarial transfusion reactions
   Acute noninfectious laryngeal edema (epinephrine is the drug of first choice)

6. **Ophthalmic Diseases**
   Severe acute and chronic allergic and inflammatory processes involving the eye, such as:
   Herpes zoster ophthalmicus
   Iritis, iridocyclitis
   Chorioretinitis
   Diffuse posterior uveitis and choroiditis
   Optic neuritis
   Sympathetic ophthalmia
   Anterior segment inflammation
   Allergic conjunctivitis
   Allergic corneal marginal ulcers
   Keratitis
7. **Gastrointestinal Diseases**
   To tide the patient over a critical period of the disease in:
   Ulcerative colitis (systemic therapy)
   Regional enteritis (systemic therapy)
8. **Respiratory Diseases**
   Symptomatic sarcoidosis
   Berylliosis
   Fulminating or disseminated pulmonary tuberculosis when used concurrently with appropriate antituberculous chemotherapy
   Loeffler's syndrome not manageable by other means
   Aspiration pneumonitis
9. **Hematologic Disorders**
   Acquired (autoimmune) hemolytic anemia
   Secondary thrombocytopenia in adults
   Erythroblastopenia (RBC anemia)
   Congenital (erythroid) hypoplastic anemia
10. **Neoplastic Diseases**
    For palliative management of:
    Leukemias and lymphomas in adults
    Acute leukemia of childhood
11. **Edematous States**
    To induce diuresis or remission of proteinuria in the nephrotic syndrome, without uremia, of the idiopathic type or that due to lupus erythematosus
12. **Nervous System**
    Acute exacerbations of multiple sclerosis
13. **Miscellaneous**
    Tuberculous meningitis with subarachnoid block or impending block when used concurrently with appropriate antituberculous chemotherapy
    Trichinosis with neurologic or myocardial involvement

B. FOR INTRA-ARTICULAR OR SOFT TISSUE ADMINISTRATION
DEPO-MEDROL is indicated as adjunctive therapy for short-term administration (to tide the patient over an acute episode or exacerbation) in:
Synovitis of osteoarthritis
Rheumatoid arthritis
Acute and subacute bursitis
Acute gouty arthritis
Epicondylitis
Acute nonspecific tenosynovitis
Post-traumatic osteoarthritis
C. FOR INTRALESIONAL ADMINISTRATION
DEPO-MEDROL is indicated for intralesional use in the following conditions:

Continued on next page

Information on these Upjohn products is based on labeling in effect on November 30, 1984. Further information concerning these and other Upjohn products may be obtained from the package insert or by direct inquiry to Medical Information, The Upjohn Company, Kalamazoo, Michigan 49001.

Upjohn—Cont.

Keloids
Localized hypertrophic, infiltrated inflammatory lesions of:
    lichen planus, psoriatic plaques, granuloma annulare, and lichen simplex chronicus (neurodermatitis)
Discoid lupus erythematosus
Necrobiosis lipodica diabeticorum
Alopecia areata
DEPO-MEDROL also may be useful in cystic tumors of an aponeurosis or tendon (ganglia).
Contraindications: Systemic fungal infections.
Warnings:
Multidose Use
Although initially sterile, any multidose use of vials may lead to contamination unless strict aseptic technique is observed. The preservative in DEPO-MEDROL Sterile Aqueous Suspension (methylprednisolone acetate) will prevent growth of most pathogenic organisms, but certain ones (eg *Serratia marcescens*) may remain viable. Particular care, such as use of disposable sterile syringes and needles, should be observed if intrasynovial use is intended.
While crystals of adrenal steroids in the dermis suppress inflammatory reactions, their presence may cause disintegration of the cellular elements and physiochemical changes in the ground substance of the connective tissue. The resultant infrequently occurring dermal and/or subdermal changes may form depressions in the skin at the injection site. The degree to which this reaction occurs will vary with the amount of adrenal steroid injected. Regeneration is usually complete within a few months or after all crystals of the adrenal steroid have been absorbed.
In order to minimize the incidence of dermal and subdermal atrophy, care must be exercised not to exceed recommended doses in injections. Multiple small injections into the area of the lesion should be made whenever possible. The technique of intra-articular and intramuscular injection should include precautions against injection or leakage into the dermis. Injection into the deltoid muscle should be avoided because of a high incidence of subcutaneous atrophy.
DEPO-MEDROL is Not Recommended For Intrathecal Administration.
In patients on corticosteroid therapy subjected to any unusual stress, increased dosage of rapidly acting corticosteroids before, during, and after the stressful situation is indicated.
Corticosteroids may mask some signs of infection, and new infections may appear during their use. There may be decreased resistance and inability to localize infection when corticosteroids are used. Do not use intra-articularly, intrabursally or for intratendinous administration for *local* effect in the presence of acute infection.
Prolonged use of corticosteroids may produce posterior subcapsular cataracts, glaucoma with possible damage to the optic nerves, and may enhance the establishment of secondary ocular infections due to fungi or viruses.
Usage in pregnancy. Since adequate human reproduction studies have not been done with corticosteroids, the use of these drugs in pregnancy, nursing mothers, or women of childbearing potential requires that the possible benefits of the drug be weighed against the potential hazards to the mother and embryo or fetus. Infants born of mothers who have received substantial doses of corticosteroids during pregnancy should be carefully observed for signs of hypoadrenalism.
Average and large doses of cortisone or hydrocortisone can cause elevation of blood pressure, salt and water retention, and increased excretion of potassium. These effects are less likely to occur with the synthetic derivatives except when used in large doses. Dietary salt restriction and potassium supplementation may be necessary. All corticosteroids increase calcium excretion.
While on corticosteroid therapy patients should not be vaccinated against smallpox. Other immunization procedures should not be undertaken in patients who are on corticosteroids, especially in high doses, because of possible hazards of neurological complications and lack of antibody response.
The use of DEPO-MEDROL in active tuberculosis should be restricted to those cases of fulminating or disseminated tuberculosis in which the corticosteroid is used for the management of the disease in conjunction with appropriate antituberculous regimen.
If corticosteroids are indicated in patients with latent tuberculosis or tuberculin reactivity, close observation is necessary as reactivation of the disease may occur. During prolonged corticosteroid therapy, these patients should receive chemoprophylaxis.
Because rare instances of anaphylactoid reactions have occurred in patients receiving parenteral corticosteroid therapy, appropriate precautionary measures should be taken prior to administration especially when the patient has a history of allergy to any drug.
Precautions: Drug-induced secondary adrenocortical insufficiency may be minimized by gradual reduction of dosage. This type of relative insufficiency may persist for months after discontinuation of therapy; therefore, in any situation of stress occurring during that period, hormone therapy should be reinstituted. Since mineralocorticoid secretion may be impaired, salt and/or a mineralocorticoid should be administered concurrently.
When multidose vials are used, special care to prevent contamination of the contents is essential (See WARNINGS).
There is an enhanced effect of corticosteroids in patients with hypothyroidism and in those with cirrhosis.
Corticosteroids should be used cautiously in patients with ocular herpes simplex for fear of corneal perforation.
The lowest possible dose of corticosteroid should be used to control the condition under treatment, and when reduction in dosage is possible, the reduction must be gradual.
Psychic derangements may appear when corticosteroids are used, ranging from euphoria, insomnia, mood swings, personality changes, and severe depression to frank psychotic manifestations. Also, existing emotional instability or psychotic tendencies may be aggravated by corticosteroids.
Aspirin should be used cautiously in conjunction with corticosteroids in hypoprothrombinemia.
Steroids should be used with caution in nonspecific ulcerative colitis, if there is a probability of impending perforation, abscess or other pyogenic infection. Caution must also be used in diverticulitis, fresh intestinal anastomoses, active or latent peptic ulcer, renal insufficiency, hypertension, osteoporosis, and myasthenia gravis, when steroids are used as direct or adjunctive therapy.
Growth and development of infants and children on prolonged corticosteroid therapy should be carefully followed.
The following additional precautions apply for parenteral corticosteroids. Intra-articular injection of a corticosteroid may produce systemic as well as local effects.
Appropriate examination of any joint fluid present is necessary to exclude a septic process.
A marked increase in pain accompanied by local swelling, further restriction of joint motion, fever, and malaise are suggestive of septic arthritis. If this complication occurs and the diagnosis of sepsis is confirmed, appropriate antimicrobial therapy should be instituted.
Local injection of a steroid into a previously infected joint is to be avoided.
Corticosteroids should not be injected into unstable joints.
The slower rate of absorption by intramuscular administration should be recognized.
Although controlled clinical trials have shown corticosteroids to be effective in speeding the resolution of acute exacerbations of multiple sclerosis, they do not show that corticosteroids affect the ultimate outcome or natural history of the disease. The studies do show that relatively high doses of corticosteroids are necessary to demonstrate a significant effect. (See **Dosage And Administration**).
Since complications of treatment with glucocorticoids are dependent on the size of the dose and the duration of treatment, a risk/benefit decision must be made in each individual case as to dose and duration of treatment and as to whether daily or intermittent therapy should be used.
Adverse Reactions:
Fluid and electrolyte disturbances:
  Sodium retention
  Fluid retention
  Congestive heart failure in susceptible patients
  Potassium loss
  Hypokalemic alkalosis
  Hypertension
Musculoskeletal:
  Muscle weakness
  Steroid myopathy
  Loss of muscle mass
  Osteoporosis
  Vertebral compression fractures
  Aseptic necrosis of femoral and humeral heads
  Pathologic fracture of long bones
Gastrointestinal:
  Peptic ulcer with possible subsequent perforation and hemorrhage
  Pancreatitis
  Abdominal distention
  Ulcerative esophagitis
Dermatologic:
  Impaired wound healing
  Thin fragile skin
  Petechiae and ecchymoses
  Facial erythema
  Increased sweating
  May suppress reactions to skin tests
Neurological:
  Convulsions
  Increased intracranial pressure with papilledema (pseudotumor cerebri) usually after treatment
  Vertigo
  Headache
Endocrine:
  Menstrual irregularities
  Development of Cushingoid state
  Suppression of growth in children
  Secondary adrenocortical and pituitary unresponsiveness, particularly in times of stress, as in trauma, surgery or illness
  Decreased carbohydrate tolerance
  Manifestations of latent diabetes mellitus
  Increased requirements for insulin or oral hypoglycemic agents in diabetes
Ophthalmic:
  Posterior subcapsular cataracts
  Increased intraocular pressure
  Glaucoma
  Exophthalmos
Metabolic:
  Negative nitrogen balance due to protein catabolism
The following *additional* adverse reactions are related to parenteral corticosteroid therapy:
  Rare instances of blindness associated with intralesional therapy around the face and head
  Anaphylactic reaction
  Allergic or hypersensitivity reactions
  Urticaria
  Hyperpigmentation or hypopigmentation
  Subcutaneous and cutaneous atrophy
  Sterile abscess
  Injection site infections following non-sterile administration (see WARNINGS)
  Postinjection flare, following intra-articular use
  Charcot-like arthropathy
  Arachnoiditis has been reported following intrathecal administration
Dosage And Administration: Because of possible physical incompatibilities, DEPO-MEDROL Sterile Aqueous Suspension (methylprednisolone acetate) should not be diluted or mixed with other solutions.
A. Administration for Local Effect
Therapy with DEPO-MEDROL does not obviate the need for the conventional measures usually

employed. Although this method of treatment will ameliorate symptoms, it is in no sense a cure and the hormone has no effect on the cause of the inflammation.

1. **Rheumatoid and Osteoarthritis.** The dose for intra-articular administration depends upon the size of the joint and varies with the severity of the condition in the individual patient. In chronic cases, injections may be repeated at intervals ranging from one to five or more weeks depending upon the degree of relief obtained from the initial injection. The doses in the following table are given as a general guide:

Size of Joint	Examples	Range of Dosage
Large	Knees Ankles Shoulders	20 to 80 mg
Medium	Elbows Wrists	10 to 40 mg
Small	Metacarpophalangeal Interphalangeal Sternoclavicular Acromioclavicular	4 to 10 mg

Procedure: It is recommended that the anatomy of the joint involved be reviewed before attempting intra-articular injection. In order to obtain the full anti-inflammatory effect it is important that the injection be made into the synovial space. Employing the same sterile technique as for a lumbar puncture, a sterile 20 to 24 gauge needle (on a dry syringe) is quickly inserted into the synovial cavity. Procaine infiltration is elective. The aspiration of only a few drops of joint fluid proves the joint space has been entered by the needle. *The injection site for each joint is determined by that location where the synovial cavity is most superficial and most free of large vessels and nerves.* With the needle in place, the aspirating syringe is removed and replaced by a second syringe containing the desired amount of DEPO-MEDROL Sterile Aqueous Suspension. The plunger is then pulled outward slightly to aspirate synovial fluid and to make sure the needle is still in the synovial space. After injection, the joint is moved gently a few times to aid mixing of the synovial fluid and the suspension. The site is covered with a small sterile dressing.

Suitable sites for intra-articular injection are the knee, ankle, wrist, elbow, shoulder, phalangeal, and hip joints. Since difficulty is not infrequently encountered in entering the hip joint, precautions should be taken to avoid any large blood vessels in the area. Joints not suitable for injection are those that are anatomically inaccessible such as the spinal joints and those like the sacroiliac joints that are devoid of synovial space. Treatment failures are most frequently the result of failure to enter the joint space. Little or no benefit follows injection into surrounding tissue. If failures occur when injections into the synovial spaces are certain, as determined by aspiration of fluid, repeated injections are usually futile. Local therapy does not alter the underlying disease process, and whenever possible comprehensive therapy including physiotherapy and orthopedic correction should be employed.

Following intra-articular steroid therapy, care should be taken to avoid overuse of joints in which symptomatic benefit has been obtained. Negligence in this matter may permit an increase in joint deterioration that will more than offset the beneficial effects of the steroid.

Unstable joints should not be injected. Repeated intra-articular injection may in some cases result in instability of the joint. X-ray follow-up is suggested in selected cases to detect deterioration.

If a local anesthetic is used prior to injection of DEPO-MEDROL the anesthetic package insert should be read carefully and all the precautions observed.

2. **Bursitis.** The area around the injection site is prepared in a sterile way and a wheal at the site made with 1 percent procaine hydrochloride solution. A 20 to 24 gauge needle attached to a dry syringe is inserted into the bursa and the fluid aspirated. The needle is left in place and the aspirating syringe changed for a small syringe containing the desired dose. After injection, the needle is withdrawn and a small dressing applied.

3. **Miscellaneous: Ganglion, Tendinitis, Epicondylitis.** In the treatment of conditions such as tendinitis or tenosynovitis, care should be taken, following application of a suitable antiseptic to the overlying skin, to inject the suspension into the tendon sheath rather than into the substance of the tendon. The tendon may be readily palpated when placed on a stretch. When treating conditions such as epicondylitis, the area of greatest tenderness should be outlined carefully and the suspension infiltrated into the area. For ganglia of the tendon sheaths, the suspension is injected directly into the cyst. In many cases, a single injection causes a marked decrease in the size of the cystic tumor and may effect disappearance. The usual sterile precautions should be observed, of course, with each injection.

The dose in the treatment of the various conditions of the tendinous or bursal structures listed above varies with the condition being treated and ranges from 4 to 30 mg. In recurrent or chronic conditions, repeated injections may be necessary.

4. **Injections for Local Effect in Dermatologic Conditions.** Following cleansing with an appropriate antiseptic such as 70% alcohol, 20 to 60 mg of the suspension is injected into the lesion. It may be necessary to distribute doses ranging from 20 to 40 mg by repeated local injections in the case of large lesions. Care should be taken to avoid injection of sufficient material to cause blanching since this may be followed by a small slough. One to four injections are usually employed, the intervals between injections varying with the type of lesion being treated and the duration of improvement produced by the initial injection.

When multidose vials are used, special care to prevent contamination of the contents is essential (See WARNINGS).

B. **Administration for Systemic Effect**

The intramuscular dosage will vary with the condition being treated. When employed as a temporary substitute for oral therapy, a single injection during each 24-hour period of a dose of the suspension equal to the total daily oral dose of MEDROL® Tablets (methylprednisolone) is usually sufficient. When a prolonged effect is desired, the weekly dose may be calculated by multiplying the daily oral dose by 7 and given as a single intramuscular injection.

Dosage must be individualized according to the severity of the disease and response of the patient. For infants and children, the recommended dosage will have to be reduced, but dosage should be governed by the severity of the condition rather than by strict adherence to the ratio indicated by age or body weight.

Hormone therapy is an adjunct to, and not a replacement for, conventional therapy. Dosage must be decreased or discontinued gradually when the drug has been administered for more than a few days. The severity, prognosis and expected duration of the disease and the reaction of the patient to medication are primary factors in determining dosage. If a period of spontaneous remission occurs in a chronic condition, treatment should be discontinued. Routine laboratory studies, such as urinalysis, two-hour postprandial blood sugar, determination of blood pressure and body weight, and a chest X-ray should be made at regular intervals during prolonged therapy. Upper GI X-rays are desirable in patients with an ulcer history or significant dyspepsia.

In patients with the **adrenogenital syndrome**, a single intramuscular injection of 40 mg every two weeks may be adequate. For maintenance of patients with **rheumatoid arthritis**, the weekly intramuscular dose will vary from 40 to 120 mg. The usual dosage for patients with **dermatologic lesions** benefited by systemic corticoid therapy is 40 to 120 mg of methylprednisolone acetate administered intramuscularly at weekly intervals for one to four weeks. In acute severe dermatitis due to poison ivy, relief may result within 8 to 12 hours following intramuscular administration of a single dose of 80 to 120 mg. In chronic contact dermatitis repeated injections at 5 to 10 day intervals may be necessary. In seborrheic dermatitis, a weekly dose of 80 mg may be adequate to control the condition. Following intramuscular administration of 80 to 120 mg to asthmatic patients, relief may result within 6 to 48 hours and persist for several days to two weeks. Similarly in patients with allergic rhinitis (hay fever) an intramuscular dose of 80 to 120 mg may be followed by relief of coryzal symptoms within six hours persisting for several days to three weeks.

If signs of stress are associated with the condition being treated, the dosage of the suspension should be increased. If a rapid hormonal effect of maximum intensity is required, the intravenous administration of highly soluble methylprednisolone sodium succinate is indicated.

Multiple Sclerosis

In treatment of acute exacerbations of multiple sclerosis daily doses of 200 mg of prednisolone for a week followed by 80 mg every other day for 1 month have been shown to be effective (4 mg of methylprednisolone is equivalent to 5 mg of prednisolone).

How Supplied: DEPO-MEDROL Sterile Aqueous Suspension (methylprednisolone acetate) is available in the following strengths and sizes:

20 mg/ml	5 ml vial	NDC 0009-0274-01
	25–5 ml vials	NDC 0009-0274-05
40 mg/ml	1 ml vial	NDC 0009-0280-01
	25-1 ml vials	NDC 0009-0280-23
	5 ml vial	NDC 0009-0280-02
	25-5 ml vials	NDC 0009-0280-32
	10 ml vial	NDC 0009-0280-03
	25-10 ml vials	NDC 0009-0280-33
80 mg/ml	1 ml vial	NDC 0009-0306-01
	25-1 ml vials	NDC 0009-0306-09
	1 ml U-Ject® Disposable Syringe	NDC 0009-0306-04
	5 ml vial	NDC 0009-0306-02
	25–5 ml vials	NDC 0009-0306-10

Store at controlled room temperature 15°–30° C (59°–86° F)

Code 810 341 007

Shown in Product Identification Section, page 441

DEPO–PROVERA® ℞
brand of medroxyprogesterone sterile aqueous suspension
(sterile medroxyprogesterone acetate suspension, USP)

400 mg/ml
2.5 ml vial
NSN 6505-01-059-9006 (VA)
10 ml vial
NSN 6505-01-059-9005 (VA)

WARNING

THE USE OF PROGESTATIONAL AGENTS DURING THE FIRST FOUR MONTHS OF PREGNANCY IS NOT RECOMMENDED

Progestational agents have been used beginning with the first trimester of pregnancy in an attempt to prevent habitual abortion or treat threatened abortion. There is no adequate evidence that such use is effective and there is evidence of potential harm to the fetus when such drugs are given during the first four months of pregnancy. Furthermore, in the vast majority of women, the cause of abor-

---

Continued on next page

Information on these Upjohn products is based on labeling in effect on November 30, 1984. Further information concerning these and other Upjohn products may be obtained from the package insert or by direct inquiry to Medical Information, The Upjohn Company, Kalamazoo, Michigan 49001.

Upjohn—Cont.

tion is a defective ovum, which progestational agents could not be expected to influence. In addition, the use of progestational agents, with their uterine-relaxant properties, in patients with fertilized defective ova may cause a delay in spontaneous abortion. Therefore, the use of such drugs during the first four months of pregnancy is not recommended.

Several reports suggest an association between intrauterine exposure to female sex hormones and congenital anomalies, including congenital heart defects and limb reduction defects[1-5]. One study[4] estimated a 4.7-fold increased risk of limb reduction defects in infants exposed in utero to sex hormones (oral contraceptives, hormone withdrawal tests for pregnancy, or attempted treatment for threatened abortion). Some of these exposures were very short and involved only a few days of treatment. The data suggest that the risk of limb reduction defects in exposed fetuses is somewhat less than 1 in 1000.

If the patient is exposed to DEPO-PROVERA Sterile Aqueous Suspension (medroxyprogesterone acetate) during the first four months of pregnancy or if she becomes pregnant while taking this drug, she should be apprised of the potential risks to the fetus.

Description: DEPO-PROVERA Sterile Aqueous Suspension contains medroxyprogesterone acetate which is a derivative of progesterone and is active by the parenteral and oral routes of administration. It is a white to off-white, odorless crystalline powder, stable in air, melting between 200 and 210° C. It is freely soluble in chloroform, soluble in acetone and dioxane, sparingly soluble in alcohol and methanol, slightly soluble in ether and insoluble in water.

The chemical name for medroxyprogesterone acetate is Pregn-4-ene-3,20-dione, 17-(acetyloxy)-6-methyl-, (6α)-.

DEPO-PROVERA for intramuscular injection is available in 2 strengths, 100 mg/ml and 400 mg/ml medroxyprogesterone acetate.

Each ml of the **100 mg/ml** suspension contains:
Medroxyprogesterone Acetate .... 100 mg
Also
Polyethylene Glycol 3350 .... 27.6 mg
Polysorbate 80 .... 1.84 mg
Sodium Chloride .... 8.3 mg
Methylparaben .... 1.75 mg
Propylparaben .... 0.194 mg
added as preservatives

Each ml of the **400 mg/ml** suspension contains:
Medroxyprogesterone Acetate .... 400 mg
Polyethylene Glycol 3350 .... 20.3 mg
Sodium Sulfate Anhydrous .... 11 mg
Myristyl-gamma-picolinium
  Chloride .... 1.69 mg
added as preservative

When necessary, pH was adjusted with sodium hydroxide and/or hydrochloric acid.

Actions: Medroxyprogesterone acetate administered parenterally in the recommended doses to women with adequate endogenous estrogen transforms proliferative endometrium into secretory endometrium.

Medroxyprogesterone acetate inhibits (in the usual dose range) the secretion of pituitary gonadotropin which, in turn, prevents follicular maturation and ovulation.

Because of its prolonged action and the resulting difficulty in predicting the time of withdrawal bleeding following injection, medroxyprogesterone acetate is not recommended in secondary amenorrhea or dysfunctional uterine bleeding. In these conditions oral therapy is recommended.

Indications: Adjunctive therapy and palliative treatment of inoperable, recurrent, and metastatic endometrial carcinoma or renal carcinoma.

Contraindications:
1. Thrombophlebitis, thromboembolic disorders, cerebral apoplexy or patients with a past history of these conditions.
2. Carcinoma of the breast.
3. Undiagnosed vaginal bleeding.
4. Missed abortion.
5. As a diagnostic test for pregnancy.
6. Known sensitivity to DEPO-PROVERA Sterile Aqueous Suspension (medroxyprogesterone acetate).

Warnings:
1. The physician should be alert to the earliest manifestations of thrombotic disorders (thrombophlebitis, cerebrovascular disorders, pulmonary embolism, and retinal thrombosis). Should any of these occur or be suspected, the drug should be discontinued immediately.
2. Long term toxicology studies in the monkey, dog and rat disclose:
   1) Beagle dogs receiving 75 mg/kg and 3 mg/kg every 90 days developed mammary nodules, as did some of the control animals. The nodules appearing in the control animals were intermittent in nature, whereas the nodules in the drug treated animals were larger, more numerous, persistent, and there were two high dose animals that developed breast malignancies.
   2) Two of the monkeys receiving 150 mg/kg every 90 days developed undifferentiated carcinoma of the uterus. No uterine malignancies were found in monkeys receiving 30 mg/kg, 3 mg/kg, or placebo every 90 days. Transient mammary nodules were found during the study in the control, 3 mg/kg and 30 mg/kg groups, but not in the 150 mg/kg group. At sacrifice, the only nodules extant were in three of the monkeys in the 30 mg/kg group. Upon histopathologic examination these nodules have been determined to be hyperplastic.
   3) No uterine or breast abnormalities were revealed in the rat.
   The relevance of any of these findings with respect to humans has not been established.
3. The use of DEPO-PROVERA Sterile Aqueous Suspension (medroxyprogesterone acetate) for contraception is investigational since there are unresolved questions relating to its safety for this indication. Therefore, this is not an approved indication.
4. Discontinue medication pending examination if there is sudden partial or complete loss of vision, or if there is a sudden onset of proptosis, diplopia or migraine. If examination reveals papilledema or retinal vascular lesions, medication should be withdrawn.
5. Usage in pregnancy (See WARNING Box).
6. Retrospective studies of morbidity and mortality in Great Britain and studies of morbidity in the United States have shown a statistically significant association between thrombophlebitis, pulmonary embolism, and cerebral thrombosis and embolism and the use of oral contraceptives.[6-9] The estimate of the relative risk of thromboembolism in the study by Vessey and Doll[8] was about sevenfold, while Sartwell and associates[9] in the United States found a relative risk of 4.4, meaning that the users are several times as likely to undergo thromboembolic disease without evident cause as non-users. The American study also indicated that the risk did not persist after discontinuation of administration, and that it was not enhanced by long continued administration. The American study was not designed to evaluate a difference between products.
7. Following repeated injections, amenorrhea and infertility may persist for periods up to 18 months and occasionally longer.
8. The physician should be alert to the earliest manifestations of impaired liver function.

Precautions:
1. The pretreatment physical examination should include special reference to breast and pelvic organs, as well as Papanicolaou smear.
2. Because progestogens may cause some degree of fluid retention, conditions which might be influenced by this factor, such as epilepsy, migraine, asthma, cardiac or renal dysfunction, require careful observation.
3. In cases of breakthrough bleeding, as in all cases of irregular bleeding per vaginum, nonfunctional causes should be borne in mind. In cases of undiagnosed vaginal bleeding, adequate diagnostic measures are indicated.
4. Patients who have a history of psychic depression should be carefully observed and the drug discontinued if the depression recurs to a serious degree.
5. Any possible influence of prolonged progestin therapy on pituitary, ovarian, adrenal, hepatic or uterine functions awaits further study.
6. A decrease in glucose tolerance has been observed in a small percentage of patients on estrogen-progestin combination drugs. The mechanism of this decrease is obscure. For this reason, diabetic patients should be carefully observed while receiving progestin therapy.
7. The age of the patient constitutes no absolute limiting factor although treatment with progestins may mask the onset of the climacteric.
8. The pathologist should be advised of progestin therapy when relevant specimens are submitted.
9. Because of the occasional occurrence of thrombotic disorders, (thrombophlebitis, pulmonary embolism, retinal thrombosis, and cerebrovascular disorders) in patients taking estrogen-progestin combinations and since the mechanism is obscure, the physician should be alert to the earliest manifestation of these disorders.

Information for the Patient
See Patient Information at the end of the insert.
The patient insert should be given to all premenopausal women, except those in whom childbearing is impossible.

Adverse Reactions: (See WARNING Box for possible adverse effects on the fetus).
In a few instances there have been undesirable sequelae at the site of injection, such as residual lump, change in color of skin or sterile abscess.
The following adverse reactions have been associated with the use of DEPO-PROVERA Sterile Aqueous Suspension (medroxyprogesterone acetate).

Breast—In a few instances, breast tenderness or galactorrhea have occurred.

Psychic—An occasional patient has experienced nervousness, insomnia, somnolence, fatigue or dizziness.

Thromboembolic Phenomena—Thromboembolic phenomena including thrombophlebitis and pulmonary embolism have been reported.

Skin and Mucous Membranes—Sensitivity reactions ranging from pruritus, urticaria, angioneurotic edema to generalized rash and anaphylaxis and/or anaphylactoid reactions have occasionally been reported. Acne, alopecia, or hirsutism have been reported in a few cases.

Gastrointestinal—Rarely, nausea has been reported. Jaundice, including neonatal jaundice, has been noted in a few instances.

Miscellaneous—Rare cases of headache and hyperpyrexia have been reported.

The following adverse reactions have been observed in women taking progestins including DEPO-PROVERA:
breakthrough bleeding
spotting
change in menstrual flow
amenorrhea
edema
change in weight
  (increase or decrease)
changes in cervical erosion and
  cervical secretions
cholestatic jaundice
rash (allergic) with and
  without pruritus

melasma or chloasma
mental depression

A statistically significant association has been demonstrated between use of estrogen-progestin combination drugs and the following serious adverse reactions: thrombophlebitis; pulmonary embolism and cerebral thrombosis and embolism. For this reason patients on progestin therapy should be carefully observed.

Although available evidence is suggestive of an association, such a relationship has been neither confirmed nor refuted for the following serious adverse reactions: neuro-ocular lesions, eg, retinal thrombosis and optic neuritis.

The following adverse reactions have been observed in patients receiving estrogen-progestin combination drugs:
rise in blood pressure in susceptible individuals
premenstrual-like syndrome
changes in libido
changes in appetite
cystitis-like syndrome
headache
nervousness
dizziness
fatigue
backache
hirsutism
loss of scalp hair
erythema multiforme
erythema nodosum
hemorrhagic eruption
itching

In view of these observations, patients on progestin therapy should be carefully observed.

The following laboratory results may be altered by the use of estrogen-progestin combination drugs:
Increased sulfobromophthalein retention and other hepatic function tests.
Coagulation tests: increase in prothrombin factors VII, VIII, IX and X.
Metyrapone test.
Pregnanediol determination.
Thyroid function: increase in PBI, and butanol extractable protein bound iodine and decrease in T^3 uptake values.

Dosage and Administration: The suspension is intended for intramuscular administration only. This product must be vigorously shaken immediately before each use to ensure complete suspension of the drug.

Endometrial or renal carcinoma—doses of 400 mg to 1000 mg of DEPO-PROVERA Sterile Aqueous Suspension (medroxyprogesterone acetate) per week are recommended initially. If improvement is noted within a few weeks or months and the disease appears stabilized, it may be possible to maintain improvement with as little as 400 mg per month. Medroxyprogesterone acetate is not recommended as primary therapy, but as adjunctive and palliative treatment in advanced inoperable cases including those with recurrent or metastatic disease.

How Supplied: DEPO-PROVERA Sterile Aqueous Suspension (medroxyprogesterone acetate) is available in 2 strengths:
100 mg/ml:
  5 ml vials   NDC 0009-0248-02
400 mg/ml:
  1 ml unit dose
    U-JECT® Disposable   NDC 0009-0626-03
    Syringe
  2.5 ml vial   NDC 0009-0626-01
  10 ml vial   NDC 0009-0626-02

References:
1. Gal I, Kirman B, Stern J: Hormonal pregnancy tests and congenital malformation. Nature 216:83, 1967.
2. Levy EP, Cohen A, Fraser FC: Hormone treatment during pregnancy and congenital heart defects. Lancet 1:611, 1973.
3. Nora JJ, Nora AH: Birth defects and oral contraceptives. Lancet 1:941–942, 1973.
4. Janerich DT, Piper JM, Glebatis DM: Oral contraceptives and congenital limb-reduction defects. N Engl J Med 291:697–700, 1974.
5. Heinonen OP, Slone D, Monson RR, et al: Cardiovascular birth defects and antenatal exposure to female sex hormones. N Engl J Med 296:67–70, 1977.
6. Royal College of General Practitioners: Oral contraception and thromboembolic disease. J Coll Gen Pract 13:267–279, 1967.
7. Inman WHW, Vessey MP: Investigation of deaths from pulmonary, coronary, and cerebral thrombosis and embolism in women of child-bearing age. Br Med J 2:193–199, 1968.
8. Vessey MP, Doll R: Investigation of relation between use of oral contraceptives and thromboembolic disease. A further report. Br Med J 2:651–657, 1969.
9. Sartwell PE, Masi AT, Arthes FG, et al: Thromboembolism and oral contraceptives: An epidemiological case-control study. Am J Epidemiol 90:365–380, 1969.

The text of the patient insert for progesterone and progesterone-like drugs is set forth below.

Patient Information: DEPO-PROVERA Sterile Aqueous Suspension contains a progesterone (medroxyprogesterone acetate). The information below is that which the U.S. Food and Drug Administration requires be provided for all patients taking progesterones. The information below relates only to the risk to the unborn child associated with use of progesterone during pregnancy. For further information on the use, side effects and other risks associated with this product, ask your doctor.

WARNING FOR WOMEN

There is an increased risk of birth defects in children whose mothers take this drug during the first four months of pregnancy.

Medroxyprogesterone acetate is similar to the progesterone hormones naturally produced by the body. Progesterone and progesterone-like drugs are used to treat menstrual disorders, to test if the body is producing certain hormones, and to treat some forms of cancer in women.

They have been used as a test for pregnancy but such use is no longer considered safe because of possible damage to a developing baby. Also, more rapid methods for testing for pregnancy are now available.

These drugs have also been used to prevent miscarriage in the first few months of pregnancy. No adequate evidence is available to show that they are effective for this purpose. Furthermore, most cases of early miscarriage are due to causes which could not be helped by these drugs.

There is an increased risk of birth defects, such as heart or limb defects, if progesterone and progesterone-like drugs are taken during the first four months of pregnancy.

The exact risk of taking this drug early in pregnancy and having a baby with a birth defect is not known. However, one study found that babies born to women who had taken sex hormones (such as progesterone-like drugs) during the first three months of pregnancy were 4 to 5 times more likely to have abnormalities of the arms or legs than if their mothers had not taken such drugs. Some of these women had taken these drugs for only a few days. The chance that an infant whose mother had taken this drug will have this type of defect is about 1 in 1,000.

If you take DEPO-PROVERA Sterile Aqueous Suspension and later find you were pregnant when you took it, be sure to discuss this with your doctor as soon as possible.

Code 810 597 004

DEPO®-TESTOSTERONE ℞
brand of testosterone cypionate sterile solution (testosterone cypionate injection, USP)
For Intramuscular Use Only

How Supplied: *Depo*-Testosterone Sterile Solution is available in the following packages:
50 mg per ml. Each ml contains 50 mg testosterone cypionate, also 5.4 mg chlorobutanol anhydrous (chloral deriv.), in 874 mg cottonseed oil.
  10 ml vial   NDC 0009-0303-01
100 mg per ml. Each ml contains 100 mg testosterone cypionate, also 0.1 ml benzyl benzoate, 9.45 mg benzyl alcohol in 736 mg cottonseed oil.
  1 ml vial   NDC 0009-0347-01
  10 ml vial   NDC 0009-0347-02
200 mg per ml. Each ml contains 200 mg testosterone cypionate, also 0.2 ml benzyl benzoate, 9.45 mg benzyl alcohol, in 560 mg cottonseed oil.
  1 ml vial   NDC 0009-0417-01
  10 ml vial   NDC 0009-0417-02

DIDREX® ℞
brand of benzphetamine hydrochloride tablets

Description: DIDREX Tablets contain the anorectic agent benzphetamine hydrochloride. Benzphetamine hydrochloride is a white crystalline powder readily soluble in water and 95% ethanol. The chemical name for benzphetamine hydrochloride is d-N,α-Dimethyl-N-(phenylmethyl)-benzeneethanamine hydrochloride and its molecular weight is 275.82.

Each DIDREX tablet, for oral administration, contains 25 or 50 mg of benzphetamine hydrochloride.

Clinical Pharmacology: Benzphetamine hydrochloride is a sympathomimetic amine with pharmacologic activity similar to the prototype drugs of this class used in obesity, the amphetamines. Actions include central nervous system stimulation and elevation of blood pressure. Tachyphylaxis and tolerance have been demonstrated with all drugs of this class in which these phenomena have been looked for.

Drugs of this class used in obesity are commonly known as "anorectics" or "anorexigenics." It has not been established, however, that the action of such drugs in treating obesity is primarily one of appetite suppression. Other central nervous system actions, or metabolic effects, may be involved. Adult obese subjects instructed in dietary management and treated with "anorectic" drugs, lose more weight on the average than those treated with placebo and diet, as determined in relatively short term clinical trials.

The magnitude of increased weight loss of drug treated patients over placebo treated patients is only a fraction of a pound a week. The rate of weight loss is greatest in the first weeks of therapy for both drug and placebo subjects and tends to decrease in succeeding weeks. The possible origins of the increased weight loss due to the various drug effects are not established. The amount of weight loss associated with the use of an "anorectic" drug varies from trial to trial, and the increased weight loss appears to be related in part to variables other than the drug prescribed, such as the physician-investigator, the population treated, and the diet prescribed. Studies do not permit conclusions as to the relative importance of the drug and nondrug factors on weight loss.

The natural history of obesity is measured in years, whereas the studies cited are restricted to a few weeks duration; thus, the total impact of drug induced weight loss over that of diet alone must be considered to be clinically limited.

Pharmacokinetic data in humans are not available.

Indications and Usage: DIDREX Tablets (benzphetamine hydrochloride) are indicated in the management of exogenous obesity as a short term adjunct (a few weeks) in a regimen of weight reduction based on caloric restriction. The limited usefulness of agents of this class (see **Clinical Pharmacology**) should be weighed against possible risks inherent in their use such as those described above.

Contraindications: DIDREX Tablets (benzphetamine hydrochloride) are contraindicated in patients with advanced arteriosclerosis, symptomatic cardiovascular disease, moderate to severe

Continued on next page

Information on these Upjohn products is based on labeling in effect on November 30, 1984. Further information concerning these and other Upjohn products may be obtained from the package insert or by direct inquiry to Medical Information, The Upjohn Company, Kalamazoo, Michigan 49001.

Upjohn—Cont.

hypertension, hyperthyroidism, known hypersensitivity or idiosyncrasy to sympathomimetic amines, and glaucoma. Benzphetamine should not be given to patients who are in an agitated state or who have a history of drug abuse.

Hypertensive crises have resulted when sympathomimetic amines have been used concomitantly or within 14 days following use of monamine oxidase inhibitors. DIDREX should not be used concomitantly with other CNS stimulants.

DIDREX may cause fetal harm when administered to a pregnant woman. Amphetamines have been shown to be teratogenic and embryotoxic in mammals at high multiples of the human dose. DIDREX is containdicated in women who are or may become pregnant. If this drug is used during pregnancy, or if the patient becomes pregnant while taking this drug, the patient should be apprised of the potential hazard to te fetus.

Warnings: When tolerance to the anorectic effect develops, the recommended dose should not be exceeded in an attempt to increase the effect; rather, the drug should be discontinued.

Precautions: General: Insulin requirements in diabetes mellitus may be altered in association with use of anorexigenic drugs and the concomitant dietary restrictions.

Psychological disturbances have been reported in patients who receive an anorectic agent together with a restrictive dietary regimen.

Caution is to be exercised in prescribing amphetamines for patients with even mild hypertension. The least amount feasible should be prescribed or dispensed at one time in order to minimize the possibility of overdosage.

DIDREX Tablets, 25 mg, contain FD&C Yellow No. 5 (tartrazine) which may cause allergic-type reactions (including bronchial asthma) in certain susceptible individuals. Although the overall incidence of FD&C Yellow No. 5 (tartrazine) sensitivity in the general population is low, it is frequently seen in patients who also have aspirin hypersensitivity.

Information for Patients: Amphetamines may impair the ability of the patient to engage in potentially hazardous activities such as operating machinery or driving a motor vehicle; the patient should therefore be cautioned accordingly.

Drug Interactions: Hypertensive crises have resulted when sympathomimetic amines have been used concomitantly or within 14 days following use of monoamine oxidase inhibitors. DIDREX should not be used concomitantly with other CNS stimulants.

Amphetamines may decrease the hypotensive effect of antihypertensives. Amphetamines may enhance the effects of tricyclic antidepressants.

Urinary alkalinizing agents increase blood levels and decrease excretion of amphetamines. Urinary acidifying agents decrease blood levels and increase excretion of amphetamines.

Carcinogenesis, Mutagenesis, Impairment of Fertility: Animal studies to evaluate the potential for carcinogenesis, mutagenesis or impairment of fertility have not been performed by the Upjohn Company.

Pregnancy: Pregnancy Category X. (See CONTRAINDICATIONS section).

Nursing Mothers: It is not known whether this drug is excreted in human milk. Because many drugs are excreted in human milk and because of the potential for serious adverse reactions from DIDREX in nursing infants, a decision should be made whether to discontinue nursing or to discontinue the drug taking into account the importance of the drug to the mother.

Pediatric Use: Use of benzphetaine hydrochloride is not recommended in children under 12 years of age.

Adverse Reactions: The following have been associated with the use of benzphetamine hydrochloride:

Cardiovascular
Palpitation, tachycardia, elevation of blood pressure.
CNS
Overstimulation, restlessness, dizziness, insomnia, tremor, sweating, headache; rarely, psychotic episodes at recommended doses; depression following withdrawal of the drug.
Gastrointestinal
Dryness of the mouth, unpleasant taste, nausea, diarrhea, other gastrointestinal disturbances.
Allergic
Urticaria and other allergic reactions involving the skin.
Endocrine
Changes in libido.

Drug Abuse and Dependence: Benzphetamine is a controlled substance under the Controlled Substance Act by the Drug Enforcement Administration and has been assigned to Schedule III.

Benzphetamine hydrochloride is related chemically and pharmacologically to the amphetamines. Amphetamines and related stimulant drugs have been extensively abused and the possibility of abuse of DIDREX Tablets should be kept in mind when evaluating the desirability of including a drug as part of a weight reduction program. Abuse of amphetamines and related drugs may be associated with intense psychological dependence and severe social dysfunction. There are reports of patients who have increased the dosage to many times that recommended. Abrupt cessation following prolonged high dosage administration results in extreme fatigue and mental depression; changes are also noted on the sleep EEG. Manifestations of chronic intoxication with anorectic drugs include severe dermatoses, marked insomnia, irritability, hyperactivity, and personality changes. The most severe manifestation of chronic intoxication is psychosis, often clinically indistinguishable from schizophrenia.

Overdosage:

Treatment of Overdosage: (See **Warnings**) Information concerning the effects of overdosage with DIDREX Tablets (benzphetamine hydrochloride) is extremely limited. The following is based on experience with other anorexiants.

Management of acute amphetamine intoxication is largely symptomatic and includes sedation with a barbiturate. If hypertension is marked, the use of a nitrite or rapidly acting alpha receptor blocking agent should be considered. Experience with hemodialysis or peritoneal dialysis is inadequate to permit recommendations in this regard.

The oral LD_{50} is 174 mg/kg in mice and 104 mg/kg in rats. The intraperitoneal LD_{50} in mice is 153 mg/kg.

Dosage and Administration: Dosage should be individualized according to the response of the patient. The suggested dosage ranges from 25 to 50 mg one to three times daily. Treatment should begin with 25 to 50 mg once daily with subsequent increase in individual dose or frequency according to response. A single daily dose is preferably given in mid-morning or mid-afternoon, according to the patient's eating habits. In an occasional patient it may be desirable to avoid late afternoon administration. Use of benzphetamine hydrochloride is not recommended in children under 12 years of age.

How Supplied: DIDREX Tablets (benzphetamine hydrochloride), scored, are available in the following strengths and colors:

25 mg
Bottles of 100   NDC 0009-0018-01
50 mg
Bottles of 100   NDC 0009-0024-01
Bottles of 500   NDC 0009-0024-02
Code 810 735 203

Shown in Product Identification Section, page 441

E-MYCIN® ℞
brand of erythromycin base enteric-coated tablets
Each tablet contains erythromycin as the base

250 mg (40's) Unit of Use
NSN 6505-01-113-4758 (M)
250 mg (100's)
NSN 6505-00-604-1223 (M)

Description: E-MYCIN Tablets contain erythromycin which is produced by a strain of *Streptomyces erythraeus* and belongs to the macrolide group of antibiotics. It is basic and readily forms salts with acids. The base is a white to off-white crystals or powder slightly soluble in water, soluble in alcohol, in chloroform, and in ether. E-MYCIN Tablets (erythromycin) are specially coated to protect the contents from the inactivating effects of gastric acidity and to permit efficient absorption of the antibiotic in the small intestine.

Clinical Pharmacology: The mode of action of erythromycin is inhibition of protein synthesis without affecting nucleic acid synthesis. Resistance to erythromycin of some strains of *Haemophilus influenzae* and staphylococci has been demonstrated. Culture and susceptibility testing should be done. If the Kirby-Bauer method of disk susceptibility is used, a 15 mcg erythromycin disk should give a zone diameter of at least 18 mm when tested against an erythromycin susceptible organism.

Bioavailability data are available from The Upjohn Company.

E-MYCIN Tablets (erythromycin base enteric-coated tablets) are well absorbed and may be given without regard to meals.

After absorption, erythromycin diffuses readily into most body fluids. In the absence of meningeal inflammation, low concentrations are normally achieved in the spinal fluid but passage of the drug across the blood-brain barrier increases in meningitis. In the presence of normal hepatic function, erythromycin is concentrated in the liver and excreted in the bile; the effect of hepatic dysfunction on excretion of erythromycin by the liver into the bile is not known. After oral administration, less than 5 percent of the activity of the administered dose can be recovered in the urine.

Erythromycin crosses the placental barrier but fetal plasma levels are low.

Indications and Usage:
Streptococcus pyogenes (Group A beta hemolytic streptococcus): For upper and lower respiratory tract, skin, and soft tissue infections of mild to moderate severity.

Injectable benzathine penicillin G is considered by the American Heart Association to be the drug of choice in the treatment and prevention of streptococcal pharyngitis and in long-term prophylaxis of rheumatic fever.

When oral medication is preferred for treatment of the above conditions, penicillin G, V, or erythromycin are alternate drugs of choice.

When oral medication is given, the importance of strict adherence by the patient to the prescribed dosage regimen must be stressed. A therapeutic dose should be administered for at least 10 days.

Alpha-hemolytic streptococci (viridans group): Although no controlled clinical efficacy trials have been conducted, oral erythromycin has been suggested by the American Heart Association and American Dental Association for use in a regimen for prophylaxis against bacterial endocarditis in patients hypersensitive to penicillin who have congenital heart disease or rheumatic or other acquired valvular heart disease when they undergo dental procedures and surgical procedures of the upper respiratory tract.[1] Erythromycin is not suitable prior to genitourinary or gastrointestinal tract surgery.

Note: When selecting antibiotics for the prevention of bacterial endocarditis the physician or dentist should read the full joint statement of the American Heart Association and the American Dental Association.[1]

Staphylococcus aureus: For acute infections of skin and soft tissue of mild to moderate severity. Resistant organisms may emerge during treatment.

Streptococcus pneumoniae (Diplococcus pneumoniae): For upper respiratory tract infections (eg, otitis media, pharyngitis) and lower respiratory tract infections (eg, pneumonia) of mild to moderate degree.

Mycoplasma pneumoniae (Eaton agent, PPLO): For respiratory infections due to this organism.

Hemophilus influenzae: For upper respiratory tract infections of mild to moderate severity when used concomitantly with adequate doses of sulfonamides. Not all strains of this organism are susceptible at the erythromycin concentrations ordinarily achieved (see appropriate sulfonamide labeling for prescribing information).

Treponema pallidum: Erythromycin is an alternate choice of treatment for primary syphilis in patients allergic to the penicillins. In treatment of primary syphilis, spinal fluid examinations should be done before treatment and as part of follow-up after therapy.

Corynebacterium diphtheriae and C. minutissimum: As an adjunct to antitoxin, to prevent establishment of carriers, and to eradicate the organism in carriers.

In the treatment of erythrasma.

Entamoeba histolytica: In the treatment of intestinal amebiasis only. Extraenteric amebiasis requires treatment with other agents.

Listeria monocytogenes: Infections due to this organism.

Neisseria gonorrhoeae: Erythromycin lactobionate for injection in conjunction with erythromycin base orally, as an alternative drug in treatment of acute pelvic inflammatory disease caused by *N. gonorrhoeae* in female patients with a history of sensitivity to penicillin. Before treatment of gonorrhea, patients who are suspected of also having syphilis should have a microscopic examination for *T. pallidum* (by immunofluorescence or darkfield) before receiving erythromycin, and monthly serologic tests for a minimum of 4 months.

Chlamydia trachomatis: Erythromycins are indicated for treatment of the following infections caused by *Chlamydia trachomatis:* conjunctivitis of the newborn, pneumonia of infancy, urogenital infections during pregnancy. When tetracyclines are contraindicated or not tolerated, erythromycin is indicated for the treatment of uncomplicated urethral, endocervical, or rectal infections in adults due to *Chlamydia trachomatis.*[2]

Bordetella pertussis: Erythromycin is effective in eliminating the organism from the nasopharynx of infected individuals, rendering them noninfectious. Some clinical studies suggest that erythromycin may be helpful in the prophylaxis of pertussis in exposed susceptible individuals.

Legionnaires Disease: Although no controlled clinical efficacy studies have been conducted, *in vitro* and limited preliminary clinical data suggest that erythromycin can be effective in treating Legionnaires Disease.

Contraindications: Erythromycin is contraindicated in patients with known hypersensitivity to this antibiotic.

Warning: Usage in pregnancy: Safety for use in pregnancy has not been established.

Precautions: Erythromycin is principally excreted by the liver. Caution should be exercised in administering the antibiotic to patients with impaired hepatic function.

There have been reports of hepatic dysfunction, with or without jaundice, occurring in patients receiving oral erythromycin products.

Surgical procedures should be performed when indicated.

Drug Interactions: Recent data from studies of erythromycin reveal that its use in patients who are receiving high doses of theophylline may be associated with an increase of serum theophylline levels and potential theophylline toxicity. In cases of theophylline toxicity and/or elevated serum theophylline levels, the dose of theophylline should be reduced while the patient is receiving concomitant erythromycin therapy.

Erythromycin administration in children receiving carbamazepine has been reported to cause increased blood levels of carbamazepine with subsequent development of signs of carbamazepine toxicity (ataxia, dizziness, vomiting).

Adverse Reactions: The most frequent side effects of erythromycin preparations are gastrointestinal, such as abdominal cramping and discomfort, and are dose related. Nausea, vomiting, and diarrhea occur infrequently with usual oral doses. During prolonged or repeated therapy, there is a possibility of overgrowth of nonsusceptible bacteria or fungi. If such infections occur, the drug should be discontinued and appropriate therapy instituted.

Mild allergic reactions such as urticaria and other skin rashes have occurred. Serious allergic reactions, including anaphylaxis, have been reported. There have been isolated reports of reversible hearing loss occurring chiefly in patients with renal insufficiency and in patients receiving high doses of erythromycin.

Dosage and Administration: E-MYCIN Tablets (erythromycin base enteric-coated tablets) are well absorbed and may be given without regard to meals.

Adults: The usual dose is 250 mg four times daily or 333 mg every 8 hours.

If twice a day dosage is desired, the recommended dose is 500 mg every 12 hours.

Dosage may be increased up to 4 or more grams per day according to the severity of the infection. Twice-a-day dosing is not recommended when doses larger than 1 gram daily are administered.

Children: Age, weight, and severity of the infection are important factors in determining the proper dosage. 30 to 50 mg/kg/day, in divided doses, is the usual dose. For more severe infections, this dose may be doubled.

In the treatment of streptococcal infections, a therapeutic dosage of erythromycin should be administered for at least 10 days. In continuous prophylaxis of streptococcal infections in persons with a history of rheumatic heart disease, the dose is 250 mg twice a day.

For prophylaxis against bacterial endocarditis[1] in patients with rheumatic, congenital, or other acquired valvular heart disease when undergoing dental procedures or surgical procedures of the upper respiratory tract, give 1.0 gram (20 mg/kg for children) orally 1 ½–2 hours before the procedure and then 500 mg (10 mg/kg for children) orally every 6 hours for 8 doses.

For treatment of primary syphilis: 30 to 40 grams given in divided doses over a period of 10 to 15 days.

For treatment of acute pelvic inflammatory disease caused by *N. gonorrhoeae:* After initial treatment with erythromycin lactobionate for injection (500 mg every 6 hours for 3 days), the oral dosage recommendation is 250 mg every 6 hours for 7 days or 333 mg every 8 hours for 7 days.

Urogenital infections during pregnancy due to *Chlamydia trachomatis:* Although the optimal dose and duration of therapy have not been established, the suggested treatment is erythromycin 500 mg, by mouth, four times a day or two 333 mg tablets every eight hours for at least seven days. For women who cannot tolerate this regimen, a decreased dose of 250 mg, by mouth, four times a day or one 333 mg tablet every eight hours should be used for at least 14 days.[2]

For adults with uncomplicated urethral, endocervical, or rectal infections caused by *Chlamydia trachomatis* in whom tetracyclines are contraindicated or not tolerated: 500 mg, by mouth, four times a day or two 333 mg tablets every eight hours for at least seven days.[2]

For dysenteric amebiasis: 250 mg four times daily or 333 mg every 8 hours for 10 to 14 days, for adults; 30 to 50 mg/kg/day in divided doses for 10 to 14 days, for children.

For use in pertussis: Although optimal dosage and duration have not been established, doses of erythromycin utilized in reported clinical studies were 40 to 50 mg/kg/day, given in divided doses for 5 to 14 days.

For treatment of Legionnaires Disease: Although optimal doses have not been established, doses utilized in reported clinical data were those recommended above (1 to 4 grams erythromycin base daily in divided doses).

Treatment of Overdosage: Allergic reactions associated with acute overdosage should be handled in the usual manner—that is, by the administration of adrenalin, corticosteroids, and antihistamines as indicated and the prompt elimination of unabsorbed drug, in addition to all needed supportive measures.

How Supplied: E-MYCIN Tablets (erythromycin base enteric-coated tablets) are available in the following packages:

250 mg Tablets
Bottles of 100	NDC 0009-0103-02
Bottles of 500	NDC 0009-0103-15
Unit dose packages (100)	NDC 0009-0103-03
Bottles of 40, unit of use	NDC 0009-0103-39

333 mg Tablets
Bottles of 100	NDC 0009-3176-01
Unit dose packages (100)	NDC 0009-3176-03
Bottles of 500	NDC 0009-3176-04

[1] American Heart Association 1977. Prevention of bacterial endocarditis. Circulation 56:139A–143A.
[2] CDC Sexually Transmitted Diseases Treatment Guidelines 1982.
Code 810 386 112
Shown in Product Identification Section, page 441

E-MYCIN E® ℞
brand of erythromycin ethylsuccinate liquid
(erythromycin ethylsuccinate oral suspension)

Each 5 ml (one teaspoon) of *E-Mycin E* Liquid contains erythromycin ethylsuccinate equivalent to erythromycin 200 mg or 400 mg in a pleasant tasting oral suspension suitable for oral administration.

How Supplied: *E-Mycin E* Liquid (erythromycin ethylsuccinate oral suspension) is supplied in the following sizes and strengths:

200 mg/5 ml
500 ml bottle — NDC 0009-0939-01
400 mg/5 ml
500 ml bottle — NDC 0009-0940-01

GELFOAM®
brand of absorbable gelatin sterile sponge
(absorbable gelatin sponge, USP)

Size 12-7 mm:
NSN 6510-00-080-2053 (M)
Size 100:
NSN 6510-00-080-2054 (M)
Dental Packs, Size 4:
NSN 6510-00-064-4858 (M)

Description: GELFOAM Sterile Sponge is a sterile, pliable, surgical sponge prepared from specially treated, purified gelatin solution and capable of absorbing and holding within its meshes many times its weight of whole blood. It is used as a hemostatic device.

Actions: When implanted in tissues, GELFOAM Sterile Sponge (absorbable gelatin sponge) is absorbed completely in from four to six weeks without inducing excessive scar tissue. When applied to bleeding areas of nasal, rectal, or vaginal mucosa, it completely liquefies within two to five days.

Indications and Usage:

Hemostasis: GELFOAM Sterile Sponge (absorbable gelatin sponge), dry or saturated with sodium chloride, is indicated in surgical procedures as an adjunct to hemostasis when control of bleeding by ligature or conventional procedures is ineffective or impractical.

Continued on next page

Information on these Upjohn products is based on labeling in effect on November 30, 1984. Further information concerning these and other Upjohn products may be obtained from the package insert or by direct inquiry to Medical Information, The Upjohn Company, Kalamazoo, Michigan 49001.

Upjohn—Cont.

Directions For Use: Pieces of GELFOAM Sterile Sponge (absorbable gelatin sponge), cut to the desired size, may be applied dry or saturated with sodium chloride injection. When applied dry, pieces of GELFOAM should be compressed before application to the bleeding surface and should then be held in place with moderate pressure for 10 to 15 seconds. When used with saline, pieces of GELFOAM should be immersed in the solution, then withdrawn, squeezed between the gloved fingers to remove the air bubbles present in the meshes, replaced in the solution, and left there until needed. The GELFOAM should immediately swell to its original size and shape when dropped into the solution the second time. If it does not swell, it should be removed and kneaded vigorously until all air is expelled and it does expand to its original shape when dropped into the solution. The piece of GELFOAM is then left wet or blotted to dampness on gauze and applied to the bleeding point. It should be held in place for 10 to 15 seconds with a pledget of cotton or small gauze sponge. Removal of the pledget of cotton or gauze is made easier by wetting it with a few drops of water to prevent pulling up the GELFOAM, which now encloses a firm clot. If desired, suction may be applied over the pledget of cotton or gauze to draw blood into the GELFOAM where it promptly clots. However, while suction hastens clotting, it is not essential, since GELFOAM will draw up blood by capillary attraction and cause clotting satisfactorily. Usually the first application of GELFOAM will control bleeding, but if not, additional applications should be made, using fresh pieces of GELFOAM prepared as previously described.

When bleeding is controlled, the pieces of GELFOAM should be left in place; otherwise bleeding may start again. Since GELFOAM causes but little more cellular infiltration than the blood clot, the wound may be closed over it. When applied to bleeding mucosa, GELFOAM will stay in place until it liquefies.

Contraindications: GELFOAM Sterile Sponge (absorbable gelatin sponge) should not be used in the closure of skin incisions as it may interfere with the healing of skin edges.

Warnings: This product should not be resterilized by heat, because heating may change absorption time. Ethylene oxide is not recommended for resterilization since it may be trapped in the interstices of the foam. Although not reported for GELFOAM Sterile Sponge (absorbable gelatin sponge) the gas is toxic to tissue, and in trace amounts may cause burns or irritation.

Precautions: Use of GELFOAM Sterile Sponge (absorbable gelatin sponge) is not recommended in the presence of frank infection. If signs of infection or abscess develop in an area where GELFOAM has been placed, reoperation may be necessary to remove the infected material and allow drainage. GELFOAM should not be employed for controlling postpartum bleeding or menorrhagia.

By absorbing fluid, GELFOAM may expand and impinge on neighboring structures. Therefore, when placed into cavities or closed tissue spaces, minimal preliminary compression is advised and care should be exercised to avoid overpacking.

Adverse Reactions: GELFOAM Sterile Sponge (absorbable gelatin sponge) may form a nidus of infection and abscess formation. Giant cell granuloma has been reported at the site of absorbable gelatin product implantation in the brain, as has compression of the brain and spinal cord as a result of accumulation of sterile fluid. Excessive fibrosis and prolonged fixation of the tendon have been reported when absorbable gelatin products were used about a tendon juncture in repair of severed tendons.

How Supplied: GELFOAM Sterile Sponge (absorbable gelatin sponge) is available in the following sizes:

Size 12—3 mm 20 mm × 60 mm (12 sq cm) × 3 mm [³⁄₄ in × 2³⁄₈ in (1²⁄₄ sq in) × ¹⁄₈ in] in boxes of 4 sponges in individual envelopes.

NDC 0009-0301-01
Size 12—7 mm 20 mm × 60 mm (12 sq cm) × 7 mm [³⁄₄ in × 2³⁄₈ in (1³⁄₄ sq in) × ¹⁄₄ in] in boxes of 12 sponges in individual envelopes, and in jars of 4 sponges.
Box NDC 0009-0315-03
Jar NDC 0009-0315-02
Size 50, 80 mm × 62.5 mm (50 sq cm) × 10 mm [3¹⁄₈ in × 2¹⁄₂ in (7⁷⁄₈ sq in) × ³⁄₈ in] in boxes of 4 sponges in individual envelopes.
NDC 0009-0323-01
Size 100, 80 mm × 125 mm (100 sq cm) × 10 mm [3¹⁄₈ in × 5 in (15⁵⁄₈ sq in) × ³⁄₈ in] in boxes of 6 sponges in individual envelopes.
NDC 0009-0342-01
Size 200, 80 mm × 250 mm (200 sq cm) × 10 mm [3¹⁄₈ in × 10 in (31¹⁄₄ sq in) × ³⁄₈ in] in boxes of 6 sponges in individual envelopes.
NDC 0009-0349-01
Size 2 cm (approximately 40 cm × 2 cm) [15³⁄₄ in × ³⁄₄ in] packaged in individual jars.
NDC 0009-0364-01
Size 6 cm (approximately 40 cm × 6 cm) [15³⁄₄ in × 2³⁄₈ in] packaged in cartons of six sponges in individual envelopes.
NDC 0009-0371-01

Storage and Handling: GELFOAM Sterile Sponge (absorbable gelatin sponge) should be stored under normal conditions. Once the package is opened, contents are subject to contamination. It is recommended that GELFOAM be used as soon as the package is opened and unused contents discarded.

Caution: Federal law restricts this device to sale by or on the order of a physician.
Code 812 250 004
Also available:
Gelfoam Sterile Compressed Sponge (absorbable gelatin sponge, USP) Size 100. For application in dry state. Sponges measure 80 mm × 125 mm and are available in boxes of 6 sponges in individual envelopes.
NDC 0009-0353-01
Gelfoam Sterile Dental Packs (absorbable gelatin sponge, USP), Size 2 or 4. Each measures 10 × 20 × 7 mm or 20 × 20 × 7 mm, respectively; packaged in jars of 15 packs.
Size 2 NDC 0009-0379-01
Size 4 NDC 0009-0396-01
Gelfoam Sterile Prostatectomy Cones, (absorbable gelatin sponge, USP), Size 13 cm or 18 cm (for use with Foley bag catheter). Each cone diameter measures 13 cm or 18 cm, respectively; packaged in boxes of 6 cones in individual envelopes.
Size 13 cm NDC 0009-0449-01
Size 18 cm NDC 0009-0457-01

GELFOAM®
brand of absorbable gelatin sterile powder

How Supplied: GELFOAM Sterile Powder (absorbable gelatin powder) is supplied in jars containing 1 gram.
NDC 0009-0433-01

HALCION®
brand of triazolam tablets

0.25 mg 100's
NSN 6505-01-161-5036 (VA)
0.5 mg 100's
NSN 6505-01-161-5034 (VA)
Description: HALCION Tablets contain triazolam, a triazolobenzodiazepine hypnotic agent. Triazolam is a white crystalline powder, soluble in alcohol and poorly soluble in water. It has a molecular weight of 343.21.
The chemical name for triazolam is 8-chloro- 6- (o-chlorophenyl) -1- methyl-4H-s-triazolo- [4,3-a] [1,4] benzodiazepine.
Each HALCION tablet, for oral administration, contains 0.25 mg or 0.5 mg of triazolam.
Clinical Pharmacology: Triazolam is a hypnotic with a short mean plasma half-life of 2.3 hours, and a range of 1.7–3.0 hours. Following oral administration, triazolam is readily absorbed. The mean peak concentration occurred at 1.3 hours following a single dose of triazolam ^{14}C. The nature of the relationship between dose and bioavailability of triazolam has not yet been established. Triazolam and its metabolites, principally as conjugated glucuronides which are presumably inactive, are excreted primarily in the urine. Only small amounts of unmetabolized triazolam appear in the urine. The two primary metabolites accounted for 79.9% of urinary excretion. Urinary excretion appeared to be biphasic in its time course.

HALCION Tablets (triazolam) 0.5 mg, in two separate studies, did not affect the prothrombin times or plasma warfarin levels in male volunteers administered sodium warfarin orally.

Extremely high concentrations of triazolam do not displace bilirubin bound to human serum albumin in vitro.

Triazolam ^{14}C was administered orally to pregnant mice. Drug-related material appeared uniformly distributed in the fetus with ^{14}C concentrations approximately the same as in the brain of the mother.

In sleep laboratory studies, HALCION Tablets significantly decreased sleep latency, increased the duration of sleep and decreased the number of nocturnal awakenings. After two weeks of consecutive nightly administration, the drug's effect on total wake time is decreased, and the values recorded in the last third of the night approach baseline levels. On the first night after drug discontinuance (first post-drug night), total time asleep, percentage of time spent sleeping, and rapidity of falling asleep frequently were significantly less than on baseline (pre-drug) nights. This effect is often called "rebound" insomnia.

The type and duration of hypnotic effects and the profile of unwanted effects during administration of benzodiazepine drugs may be influenced by the biologic half-life of administered drug and any active metabolites formed. When half-lives are long, drug or metabolites may accumulate during periods of nightly administration and be associated with impairments of congnitive and motor performance during waking hours; the possibility of interaction with other psychoactive drugs or alcohol will be enhanced. In contrast, if half-lives are short, drug and metabolites will be cleared before the next dose is ingested, and carry-over effects related to excessive sedation or CNS depression should be minimal or absent. However, during nightly use for an extended period, pharmacodynamic tolerance or adaptation to some effects of benzodiazepine hypnotics may develop. If the drug has a short half-life of elimination, it is possible that a relative deficiency of the drug or its active metabolites (ie, in relationship to the receptor site) may occur at some point in the interval between each night's use. This sequence of events may account for two clinical findings reported to occur after several weeks of nightly use of rapidly eliminated benzodiazepine hypnotics: 1) increased wakefulness during the last third of the night, and 2) the appearance of increased signs of day-time anxiety reported by one author in a selected group of patients.

Indications and Usage: HALCION Tablets contain triazolam which is a hypnotic agent useful in the short-term management of insomnia characterized by difficulty in falling asleep, frequent nocturnal awakenings, and/or early morning awakenings.

In polysomnographic studies in man of 1 to 42 days duration, triazolam decreased sleep latency, increased duration of sleep, and decreased the number of nocturnal awakenings.

It is recommended that HALCION not be prescribed in quantities exceeding a one-month supply.

Contraindications: HALCION Tablets (triazolam) are contraindicated in patients with known hypersensitivity to this drug or other benzodiazepines.

Benzodiazepines may cause fetal damage when administered during pregnancy. An increased risk of congenital malformations associated with the use of diazepam and chlordiazepoxide during the first trimester of pregnancy has been suggested in several studies. Transplacental distribution has resulted in neonatal CNS depression following the ingestion of therapeutic doses of a benzodiazepine hypnotic during the last weeks of pregnancy. HALCION is contraindicated in pregnant women. If there is a likelihood of the patient becoming pregnant while receiving HALCION she should be warned of the potential risk to the fetus. Patients should be instructed to discontinue the drug prior to becoming pregnant. The possibility that a woman of childbearing potential may be pregnant at the time of institution of therapy should be considered.

Warnings: Overdosage may occur at four times the maximum recommended therapeutic dose (see DOSAGE AND ADMINISTRATION section). Patients should be cautioned *not* to exceed prescribed dosage.

Because of its depressant CNS effects, patients receiving triazolam should be cautioned against engaging in hazardous occupations requiring complete mental alertness such as operating machinery or driving a motor vehicle. For the same reason, patients should be cautioned about the simultaneous ingestion of alcohol and other CNS depressant drugs during treatment with HALCION Tablets (triazolam).

As with some but not all benzodiazepines, anterograde amnesia of varying severity and paradoxical reactions have been reported following therapeutic doses of HALCION.

Precautions:
General: In elderly and/or debilitated patients, it is recommended that treatment with HALCION Tablets (triazolam) be initiated at 0.125 mg to decrease the possibility of development of oversedation, dizziness, or impaired coordination. (See Dosage & Administration Section).

Caution should be exercised if HALCION is prescribed to patients with signs or symptoms of depression which could be intensified by hypnotic drugs. Suicidal tendencies may be present in such patients and protective measures may be required. Intentional overdosage is more common in these patients, and the least amount of drug that is feasible should be available to the patient at any one time.

The usual precautions should be observed in patients with impaired renal or hepatic function and chronic pulmonary insufficiency.

Information for Patients: To assure safe and effective use of HALCION Tablets (triazolam), the following information and instructions should be given to patients:
1. Inform your physician about any alcohol consumption and medicine you are taking now, including drugs you may buy without a prescription. Alcohol should generally not be used during treatment with hypnotics.
2. Inform your physician if you are planning to become pregnant, if you are pregnant, or if you become pregnant while you are taking this medicine.
3. Inform your physician if you are nursing.
4. Until you experience how this medication affects you, do not drive a car or operate potentially dangerous machinery, etc.
5. Do *not* increase prescribed dosage.
6. Patients should also be advised that they may experience an increase in sleep complaints (rebound insomnia) on the first night or two after discontinuing the drug.

Laboratory Tests: Laboratory tests are not ordinarily required in otherwise healthy patients.

Drug Interactions: The benzodiazepines, including triazolam, produce additive CNS depressant effects when co-administered with other psychotropic medications, anticonvulsants, anti-histaminics, ethanol, and other drugs which themselves produce CNS depression.

Pharmacokinetic interactions of benzodiazepines with other drugs have been reported. For example, the co-administration of triazolam and cimetidine in a controlled clinical trial in normal subjects resulted in a reduction of triazolam clearance and an increase in the elimination half-life from 2.2 to 3.7 hours. The plasma concentration of triazolam approximately doubled when co-administered with cimetidine. However, this did not result in any drug accumulation

Carcinogenesis, Mutagenesis, Impairment of Fertility: No evidence of carcinogenic potential was observed in mice during a 24-month study with HALCION in doses up to 4000 times the human dose.

Pregnancy:
1. Teratogenic Effects: Pregnancy Category X. See CONTRAINDICATIONS.
2. Non-Teratogenic Effects: It is to be considered that the child born of a mother who is on benzodiazepines may be at some risk for withdrawal symptoms from the drug, during the postnatal period. Also, neonatal flaccidity has been reported in an infant born of a mother who had been receiving benzodiazepines.

Nursing Mothers: Human studies have not been performed; however, studies in rats have indicated that HALCION and its metabolites are secreted in milk. Therfore, administration of HALCION to nursing mothers is not recommended.

Pediatric Use: Safety and efficacy of HALCION in children below the age of 18 have not been established.

Adverse Reactions: During placebo-controlled clinical studies in which 1003 patients received HALCION Tablets (triazolam), the most troublesome side effects were extensions of the pharmacologic activity of triazolam, eg drowsiness, dizziness, or lightheadedness.

The figures cited below are estimates of untoward clinical event incidence among subjects who participated in the relatively short duration (ie, 1 to 42 days) placebo-controlled clinical trials of HALCION. The figures cannot be used to predict precisely the incidence of untoward events in the course of usual medical practice where patient characteristics and other factors often differ from those in the clinical trials. These figures cannot be compared with those obtained from other clinical studies involving related drug products and placebo as each group of drug trials are conducted under a different set of conditions.

Comparison of the cited figures, however, can provide the prescriber with some basis for estimating the relative contributions of drug and non-drug factors to the untoward event incidence rate in the population studied. Even this use must be approached cautiously, as a drug may relieve a symptom in one patient while inducing it in others. [For example, an anticholinergic, anxiolytic drug may relieve dry mouth (a sign of anxiety) in some subjects but induce it (an untoward event) in others.]

	HALCION	Placebo
Number of Patients	1003	997
% of Patients Reporting:		
Central Nervous System		
Drowsiness	14.0	6.4
Headache	9.7	8.4
Dizziness	7.8	3.1
Nervousness	5.2	4.5
Lightheadedness	4.9	0.9
Coordination Disorders/Ataxia	4.6	0.8
Gastrointestinal		
Nausea/Vomiting	4.6	3.7

In addition to the relatively common (ie, 1% or greater) untoward events enumerated above, the following adverse events have been reported less frequently (ie, 0.9–0.5%): euphoria, tachycardia, tiredness, confusional states/memory impairment, cramps/pain, depression, visual disturbances.

Rare (ie, less than 0.5%) adverse reactions included constipation, taste alterations, diarrhea, dry mouth, dermatitis/allergy, dreaming/nightmares, insomnia, paresthesia, tinnitus, dysesthesia, weakness, congestion, death from hepatic failure in a patient also receiving diuretic drugs.

In addition to these untoward events, the following adverse events have been reported in association with the use of benzodiazepines: dystonia, irritability, anorexia, fatigue, sedation, slurred speech, jaundice, pruritus, dysarthria, changes in libido, menstrual irregularities, incontinence and urinary retention.

As with all benzodiazepines, paradoxical reactions such as stimulation, agitation, increased muscle spasticity, sleep disturbances, hallucinations and other adverse behavioral effects may occur in rare instances and in a random fashion. Should these occur, use of the drug should be discontinued.

Laboratory analyses were performed on all patients participating in the HALCION clinical program. The following incidences of abnormalities were observed in patients receiving HALCION and the corresponding placebo group. None of these changes were considered to be of physiological significance.

[See table above].

When treatment with HALCION is protracted, periodic blood counts, urinalysis and blood chemistry analyses are advisable.

Minor changes in EEG patterns, usually low-voltage fast activity have been observed in patients during therapy with HALCION and are of no known significance.

Drug Abuse and Dependence
Controlled Substance: Triazolam is a controlled substance under the Controlled Substance Act and HALCION Tablets have been assigned to Schedule IV.

Continued on next page

	HALCION		Placebo	
Number of patients	380		361	
% of Patients Reporting:	Low	High	Low	High
Hematology				
Hematocrit	*	*	*	*
Hemoglobin	*	*	*	*
Total WBC Count	1.7	2.1	*	1.3
Neutrophil Count	1.5	1.5	3.3	1.0
Lymphocyte Count	2.3	4.0	3.1	3.8
Monocyte Count	3.6	*	4.4	1.5
Eosinophil Count	10.2	3.2	9.8	3.4
Basophil Count	1.7	2.1	*	1.8
Urinalysis				
Albumin	—	1.1	—	*
Sugar	—	*	—	*
RBC/HPF	—	2.9	—	2.9
WBC/HPF	—	11.7	—	7.9
Blood Chemistry				
Creatinine	2.4	1.9	3.6	1.5
Bilirubin	*	1.5	1.0	*
SGOT	*	5.3	*	4.5
Alkaline Phosphatase	*	2.2	*	2.6

*Less than 1%

Information on these Upjohn products is based on labeling in effect on November 30, 1984. Further information concerning these and other Upjohn products may be obtained from the package insert or by direct inquiry to Medical Information, The Upjohn Company, Kalamazoo, Michigan 49001.

Upjohn—Cont.

Abuse and Dependence: Withdrawal symptoms similar in character to those noted with barbiturates and alcohol have occurred following abrupt discontinuance of benzodiazepine drugs. These can range from mild dysphoria to a major syndrome which may include abdominal and muscle cramps, vomiting, sweating, tremor, and convulsions.
Patients with a history of seizures should not be abruptly withdrawn from any CNS depressant agent, including HALCION. Addiction-prone individuals, such as drug addicts and alcoholics, should be under careful surveillance when receiving triazolam because of the predisposition of such patients to habituation and dependence. As with all hypnotics, repeat prescriptions should be limited to those who are under medical supervision.

Overdosage: Because of the potency of triazolam, overdosage may occur at 2 mg. four times the maximum recommended therapeutic dose (0.5 mg).
Manifestations of overdosage with HALCION Tablets (triazolam) include somnolence, confusion, impaired coordination, slurred speech, and ultimately, coma. As in all cases of drug overdosage, respiration, pulse, and blood pressure should be monitored and supported by general measures when necessary. Immediate gastric lavage should be performed. An adequate airway should be maintained. Intravenous fluids may be administered.
Experiments in animals have indicated that cardiopulmonary collapse can occur with massive intravenous doses of HALCION (over 100 mg/kg, more than 10,000 times the maximum daily human dose). This could be reversed with positive mechanical respiration and the intravenous infusion of levarterenol or metaraminol. Hemodialysis and forced diuresis are probably of little value. As with the management of intentional overdosage with any drug, the physician should bear in mind that multiple agents may have been ingested by the patient.
The oral LD_{50} in mice is greater than 1000 mg/kg and in rats is greater than 5000 mg/kg.

Dosage and Administration: It is important to individualize the dosage of HALCION Tablets (triazolam) for maximum beneficial effect and to help avoid significant adverse effects. The recommended dosage range for adults is 0.25 to 0.5 mg before retiring. In geriatric and/or debilitated patients, the dosage range is 0.125 to 0.25 mg. Therapy should be initiated at 0.125 mg (half of a 0.25 mg scored tablet) until individual response is determined.

How Supplied: HALCION Tablets (triazolam) scored, are available in the following strengths and package sizes:

0.25 mg (powder blue):
  Bottles of 100   NDC 0009-0017-01
  Unit Dose Pkg (100)   NDC 0009-0017-08
  Unit Dose Pkg (100)   NDC 0009-0017-17
0.5 mg (white)
  Bottles of 100   NDC 0009-0027-01
  Unit Dose Pkg (100)   NDC 0009-0027-08
  Unit Dose Pkg (100)   NDC 0009-0027-18

Store at controlled room temperature 15°–30°C (59°–86°F).
Code 812 110 003
Shown in Product Identification Section, page 441

HALOTESTIN®
brand of fluoxymesterone tablets, USP

10 mg-100s
NSN 6505-01-053-8669A (VA)

Description: HALOTESTIN Tablets contain fluoxymesterone, an androgenic hormone.
Fluoxymesterone is a white or practically white odorless, crystalline powder, melting at about 240° C. with some decomposition. It is practically insoluble in water, sparingly soluble in alcohol and slightly soluble in chloroform.
The chemical name for fluoxymesterone is androst-4-en-3-one, 9-fluoro -11, 17- dihydroxy-17-methyl-,(11β,17β)-. The molecular formula is $C_{20}H_{29}FO_3$ and the molecular weight 336.45.
Each HALOTESTIN tablet, for oral administration, contains 2 mg, 5 mg or 10 mg fluoxymesterone.

Clinical Pharmacology: Endogenous androgens are responsible for normal growth and development of the male sex organs and for maintenance of secondary sex characteristics. These effects include growth and maturation of the prostate, seminal vesicles, penis, and scrotum; development of male hair distribution, such as beard, pubic, chest, and axillary hair; laryngeal enlargement, vocal cord thickening, and alterations in body musculature and fat distribution. Drugs in this class also cause retention of nitrogen, sodium, potassium, and phosphorus, and decreased urinary excretion of calcium. Androgens have been reported to increase protein anabolism and decrease protein catabolism. Nitrogen balance is improved only when there is sufficient intake of calories and protein.
Androgens are responsible for the growth spurt of adolescence and for eventual termination of linear growth, brought about by fusion of the epiphyseal growth centers. In children, exogenous androgens accelerate linear growth rates, but may cause disproportionate advancement in bone maturation. Use over long periods may result in fusion of the epiphyseal growth centers and termination of the growth process. Androgens have been reported to stimulate production of red blood cells by enhancing production of erythropoietic stimulation factor.
During exogenous administration of androgens, endogenous testosterone release is inhibited through feedback inhibition of pituitary luteinizing hormone (LH). At large doses of exogenous androgen, spermatogenesis may also be suppressed through feedback inhibition of pituitary follicle stimulating hormone (FSH).
Inactivation of testosterone occurs primarily in the liver.
The half-life of fluoxymesterone after oral administration is approximately 9.2 hours.

Indications and Usage:
In the male—HALOTESTIN Tablets (fluoxymesterone) are indicated for:
1. Replacement therapy in conditions associated with symptoms of deficiency or absence of endogenous testosterone:
   a. Primary hypogonadism (congenital or acquired)—testicular failure due to cryptorchidism, bilateral torsion, orchitis, vanishing testis syndrome; or orchidectomy.
   b. Hypogonadotropic hypogonadism (congenital or acquired)—idiopathic gonadotropin or LHRH deficiency, or pituitary-hypothalamic injury from tumors, trauma, or radiation.
2. Delayed puberty, provided it has been definitely established as such, and is not just a familial trait.

In the female—HALOTESTIN Tablets are indicated for palliation of androgen-responsive recurrent mammary cancer in women who are more than one year but less than five years postmenopausal, or who have been proven to have a hormone-dependent tumor as shown by previous beneficial response to castration.

Contraindications:
1. Known hypersensitivity to the drug
2. Males with carcinoma of the breast
3. Males with known or suspected carcinoma of the prostate gland
4. Women known or suspected to be pregnant
5. Patients with serious cardiac, hepatic or renal disease

Warnings: Hypercalcemia may occur in immobilized patients and in patients with breast cancer. If this occurs, the drug should be discontinued.
Prolonged use of high doses of androgens (principally the 17-α alkyl-androgens) has been associated with development of hepatic adenomas, hepatocellular carcinoma, and peliosis hepatis—all potentially life-threatening complications.
Cholestatic hepatitis and jaundice may occur with 17-α-alkyl-androgens. Should this occur, the drug should be discontinued. This is reversible with discontinuation of the drug.
Geriatric patients treated with androgens may be at an increased risk of developing prostatic hypertrophy and prostatic carcinoma although conclusive evidence to support this concept is lacking.
Edema, with or without congestive heart failure, may be a serious complication in patients with pre-existing cardiac, renal or hepatic disease.
Gynecomastia may develop and occasionally persists in patients being treated for hypogonadism.
Androgen therapy should be used cautiously in males with delayed puberty. Androgens can accelerate bone maturation without producing compensatory gain in linear growth. The effect on bone maturation should be monitored by assessing bone age of the wrist and hand every six months.

Precautions:
General
Women should be observed for signs of virilization which is usual following androgen use at high doses. Discontinuation of drug therapy at the time of evidence of mild virilism is necessary to prevent irreversible virilization. A decision may be made by the patient and the physician that some virilization will be tolerated during treatment for breast carcinoma.
Patients with benign prostatic hypertrophy may develop acute urethral obstruction. Priapism or excessive sexual stimulation may develop. Oligospermia may occur after prolonged administration or excessive dosage. If any of these effects appear, the androgen should be stopped and if restarted, a lower dosage should be utilized.
This product contains FD&C Yellow No. 5 (tartrazine) which may cause allergic-type reactions (including bronchial asthma) in certain susceptible individuals. Although the overall incidence of FD&C Yellow No. 5 (tartrazine) sensitivity in the general population is low, it is frequently seen in patients who also have aspirin hypersensitivity.

Information for patients
Patients should be instructed to report any of the following: nausea, vomiting, changes in skin color, and ankle swelling. Males should be instructed to report too frequent or persistent erections of the penis and females any hoarseness, acne, changes in menstrual periods or increase in facial hair.

Laboratory tests
Women with disseminated breast carcinoma should have frequent determination of urine and serum calcium levels during the course of androgen therapy (See WARNINGS).
Because of the hepatotoxicity associated with the use of 17-alpha-alkylated androgens, liver function tests should be obtained periodically.
Periodic (every six months) x-ray examinations of bone age should be made during treatment of prepubertal males to determine the rate of bone maturation and the effects of androgen therapy on the epiphyseal centers.
Hemoglobin and hematocrit levels (to detect polycythemia) should be checked periodically in patients receiving long-term androgen administration.
Serum cholesterol may increase during androgen therapy.

Drug Interactions
Androgens may increase sensitivity to oral anticoagulants. Dosage of the anticoagulant may require reduction in order to maintain satisfactory therapeutic hypoprothrombinemia.
Concurrent administration of oxyphenbutazone and androgens may result in elevated serum levels of oxyphenbutazone.
In diabetic patients, the metabolic effects of androgens may decrease blood glucose and, therefore, insulin requirements.

Drug/Laboratory test interferences
Androgens may decrease levels of thyroxine-binding globulin, resulting in decreased total T_4 serum levels and increased resin uptake of T_3 and T_4. Free thyroid hormone levels remain unchanged, however, and there is no clinical evidence of thyroid dysfunction.

Carcinogenesis
Animal data: Testosterone has been tested by subcutaneous injection and implantation in mice

and rats. The implant induced cervical-uterine tumors in mice, which metastasized in some cases. There is suggestive evidence that injection of testosterone into some strains of female mice increases their susceptibility to hepatoma. Testosterone is also known to increase the number of tumors and decrease the degree of differentiation of chemically-induced carcinomas of the liver in rats. Human data: There are rare reports of hepatocellular carcinoma in patients receiving long-term therapy with androgens in high doses. Withdrawal of the drugs did not lead to regression of the tumors in all cases.

Geriatric patients treated with androgens may be at an increased risk of developing prostatic hypertrophy and prostatic carcinoma although conclusive evidence to support this concept is lacking.

Pregnancy
Teratogenic effects: Pregnancy Category X. (See CONTRAINDICATIONS).

Nursing mothers
HALOTESTIN Tablets (fluoxymesterone) are not recommended for use in nursing mothers.

Pediatric use
Androgen therapy should be used very cautiously in children and only by specialists aware of the adverse effects on bone maturation. Skeletal maturation must be monitored every six months by an x-ray of the hand and wrist (See WARNINGS).

Adverse Reactions:
Endocrine and urogenital
Female: The most common side effects of androgen therapy are amenorrhea and other menstrual irregularities; inhibition of gonadotropin secretion; and virilization, including deepening of the voice and clitoral enlargement. The latter usually is not reversible after androgens are discontinued. When administered to a pregnant woman, androgens can cause virilization of external genitalia of the female fetus.
Male: Gynecomastia, and excessive frequency and duration of penile erections. Oligospermia may occur at high dosage.
Skin and appendages
Hirsutism, male pattern of baldness, seborrhea, and acne.
Fluid and electrolyte disturbances
Retention of sodium, chloride, water, potassium, calcium, and inorganic phosphates.
Gastrointestinal
Nausea, cholestatic jaundice, alterations in liver function tests, rarely hepatocellular neoplasms and peliosis hepatis (see WARNINGS).
Hematologic
Suppression of clotting factors II, V, VII, and X, bleeding in patients on concomitant anticoagulant therapy, and polycythemia.
Nervous system
Increased or decreased libido, headache, anxiety, depression, and generalized paresthesia.
Allergic
Hypersensitivity, including skin manifestations and anaphylactoid reactions.

Overdosage: There have been no reports of acute overdosage with the androgens.

Dosage and Administration: The dosage will vary depending upon the individual, the condition being treated, and its severity. The total daily oral dose may be administered singly or in divided (three or four) doses.

Male hypogonadism: For complete replacement in the hypogonadal male, a daily dose of 5 to 20 mg will suffice in the majority of patients. It is usually preferable to begin treatment with full therapeutic doses which are later adjusted to individual requirements. Priapism is indicative of excessive dosage and is indication for temporary withdrawal of the drug.

Delayed puberty: Dosage should be carefully titrated utilizing a low dose, appropriate skeletal monitoring, and by limiting the duration of therapy to four to six months.

Inoperable carcinoma of the breast in the female: The recommended total daily dose for palliative therapy in advanced inoperable carcinoma of the breast is 10 to 40 mg. Because of its short action, fluoxymesterone should be administered to patients divided, rather than single, daily doses to ensure more stable blood levels. In general, it appears necessary to continue therapy for at least one month for a satisfactory subjective response, and for two to three months for an objective response.

How Supplied: HALOTESTIN Tablets (fluoxymesterone), scored, are available in the following strengths and colors:
2 mg (peach)
 Bottles of 100   NDC 0009-0014-01
5 mg (light green)
 Bottles of 100   NDC 0009-0019-06
10 mg (green)
 Bottles of 30   NDC 0009-0036-03
 Bottles of 100   NDC 0009-0036-04
Code 810 804 201
Shown in Product Identification Section, page 441

HEPARIN SODIUM INJECTION, USP ℞
Sterile Solution

Description: Heparin Sodium Injection, USP, a mixture of substances having the property of prolonging the clotting time of blood, is usually obtained from the lungs of intestinal mucosa of domestic mammals used for food by man. The potency is determined by biological assay using a USP reference standard based upon units of heparin activity per milligram. The preparations of Heparin Sodium Injection are standardized aqueous solutions of the physiological anticoagulant obtained from beef lung. Slight variations in the color of heparin sodium solutions do not affect the therapeutic efficiency. Each ml of the 1,000 and 5,000 USP Units per ml preparations contains: heparin sodium 1,000 or 5,000 USP Units: 9 mg sodium chloride; 9.45 mg benzyl alcohol added as preservative. Each ml of the 10,000 USP Units per ml preparations contains: heparin sodium 10,000 USP Units; 9.45 mg benzyl alcohol added as preservative.

Actions: Heparin inhibits the clotting of blood and the formation of fibrin clots both *in vitro* and *in vivo*. In combination with a co-factor, it inactivates thrombin thus preventing the conversion of fibrinogen to fibrin. Heparin also prevents the formation of a stable fibrin clot by inhibiting the activation of the fibrin stabilizing factor.
Heparin sodium inhibits reactions which lead to clotting but does not alter the normal components of the blood. Although clotting time is prolonged by therapeutic doses, bleeding time is usually unaffected. Heparin sodium does not have fibrinolytic activity; therefore, it will not lyse existing clots.

Indications: Heparin Sodium Injection is indicated for anticoagulant therapy in prophylaxis and treatment of venous thrombosis and its extension; in low-dose regimen for prevention of postoperative deep venous thrombosis and pulmonary embolism in patients undergoing major abdominothoracic surgery who are at risk of developing thromboembolic disease (see DOSAGE AND ADMINISTRATION); for prophylaxis and treatment of pulmonary embolism; in atrial fibrillation with embolization; for diagnosis and treatment of acute and chronic consumptive coagulopathies (disseminated intravascular coagulation); for prevention of clotting in arterial and cardiac surgery; and for the prevention of cerebral thrombosis in evolving stroke.
Heparin Sodium Injection is indicated as an adjunct in treatment of coronary occlusion with acute myocardial infarction, and in prophylaxis and treatment of peripheral arterial embolism.
Heparin sodium may also be employed as an anticoagulant in blood transfusions, extracorporeal circulation, dialysis procedures, and in blood samples for laboratory purposes.

Contraindications:
Hypersensitivity to heparin.
Inability to perform suitable blood coagulation tests, e.g., the whole blood clotting time, partial thromboplastin time, etc., at required intervals.
Uncontrollable bleeding.

Warnings

> Heparin sodium should be used with extreme caution in disease states where there is increased danger of hemorrhage.

Heparin Sodium Injection, USP when used in therapeutic dosage should be regulated by frequent blood coagulation tests. If these are unduly prolonged or if hemorrhage occurs, heparin sodium should be promptly discontinued. See OVERDOSAGE section.
Some of the conditions in which increased danger of hemorrhage exists are:
Cardiovascular—subacute bacterial endocarditis, arterial sclerosis; increased capillary permeability; during and immediately following (a) spinal tap or spinal anesthesia, (b) major surgery, especially involving the brain, spinal cord, or eye.
Hematologic—conditions associated with increased bleeding tendencies such as hemophilia, some purpuras, and thrombocytopenia.
Gastrointestinal—inaccessible ulcerative lesions; continuous tube drainage of stomach or small intestine.
Heparin sodium may prolong the one-stage prothrombin time. Accordingly, when heparin sodium is given with dicumarol or warfarin sodium, a period of at least 5 hours after the last intravenous dose and 24 hours after the last subcutaneous (intrafat) dose of heparin sodium should elapse before blood is drawn, if a valid prothrombin time is to be obtained.
Drugs (such as acetylsalicylic acid, dextran, phenylbutazone, ibuprofen, indomethacin, dipyridamole and hydroxychloroquine) which interefere with platelet aggregation reactions (the main hemostatic defense of heparinized patients) may induce bleeding and should be used with caution in patients on heparin therapy.
While there is experimental evidence that heparin may antagonize the action of ACTH, insulin or corticoids, this effect has not been clearly defined. There is also evidence in animal experiments that heparin may modify or inhibit allergic reactions. However, the application of these findings to human patients has not been fully defined.
Larger doses of heparin may be necessary in the febrile state.
The use of digitalis, tetracyclines, nicotine, or antihistamines may partially counteract the anticoagulant action of heparin. An increased resistance to heparin is frequently encountered in cases of thrombosis, thrombophlebitis, infections with thrombosing tendency, myocardial infarction, cancer, and in the postoperative patient.
Elevation of the serum transaminases without elevation in bilirubin or alkaline phosphatase may occur in patients on heparin therapy and has been observed in normal volunteers who have received heparin. Caution should be exercised in interpreting this finding as indicative of hepatic or myocardial damage.
Because of the possibility of acute thrombocytopenia occurring when heparin is administered, platelet counts should be monitored before and during heparin therapy. If significant thrombocytopenia occurs, heparin should be immediately terminated, and oral anticoagulation substituted, if necessary. If new evidence of thrombosis appears during heparin therapy, especially in the arterial system, it should be borne in mind that it may be a paradoxical result of the therapy itself, possibly as a result of platelet aggregation. Heparin should be discontinued and oral anticoagulation employed,

Continued on next page

Information on these Upjohn products is based on labeling in effect on November 30, 1984. Further information concerning these and other Upjohn products may be obtained from the package insert or by direct inquiry to Medical Information, The Upjohn Company, Kalamazoo, Michigan 49001.

Upjohn—Cont.

especially if there is associated thrombocytopenia, as noted above.

This product contains benzyl alcohol. Benzyl alcohol has been reported to be associated with a fatal "Gasping Syndrome" in premature infants.

Usage in Pregnancy
Heparin Sodium Injection should be used with caution during pregnancy, especially during the last trimester and in the immediate postpartum period.

There is no adequate information as to whether heparin may affect human fertility or have a teratogenic potential or other adverse effects to the fetus.

Heparin does not cross the placental barrier; it is not excreted in human milk.

Precautions: Because Heparin Sodium Injection is derived from animal tissue, it should be used with caution in patients with a history of allergy. Before a therapeutic dose is given to such a patient, a trial dose of 1,000 units may be advisable.

Heparin sodium should also be used with caution in the presence of mild hepatic or renal disease, hypertension, during menstruation, or in patients with indwelling catheters. A higher incidence of bleeding may be seen in women over 60 years of age.

Caution should be used when administering ACD-converted blood (i.e. blood collected in heparin sodium and later converted to ACD blood), since the anticoagulant activity of its heparin sodium content persists without loss for 22 days. ACD-converted blood may alter the coagulation system of the recipient, especially if it is given in multiple transfusions.

Adverse Reactions: Hemorrhage is the chief complication that may result from heparin therapy. An overly prolonged clotting time or minor bleeding during therapy can usually be controlled by withdrawing the drug. See OVERDOSAGE section.

The occurrence of significant gastrointestinal or urinary tract bleeding during anticoagulant therapy may indicate the presence of an underlying occult lesion.

Adrenal hemorrhage with resultant acute adrenal insufficiency has occurred during anticoagulant therapy. Therefore such treatment should be discontinued in patients who develop signs and symptoms compatible with acute adrenal hemorrhage and insufficiency. Plasma cortisol levels should be measured immediately, and vigorous therapy with intravenous corticosteroids should be instituted promptly. Initiation of therapy should not depend upon laboratory confirmation of the diagnosis, since any delay in an acute situation may result in the patient's death.

Intramuscular injection of heparin sodium frequently causes local irritation, mild pain, hematoma or ulceration, and for these reasons should be avoided. These effects are less frequently seen following deep subcutaneous (intrafat) administration. Histamine-like reactions have also been observed at the site of injection.

Hypersensitivity reactions have been reported with chills, fever, and urticaria as the most usual manifestations. Asthma, rhinitis, lacrimation, headache, nausea and vomiting, and anaphylactoid reactions have also been reported. Vasospastic reactions may develop independent of the origin of heparin, 6 to 10 days after the initiation of therapy and last for 4 to 6 hours. The affected limb is painful, ischemic and cyanosed. An artery to this limb may have been recently catheterized. After repeat injections, the reaction may gradually increase, to include generalized vasospasm, with cyanosis, tachypnea, feeling of oppression, and headache. Protamine sulfate treatment has no marked therapeutic effect. Itching and burning, especially on the plantar side of the feet, is possibly based on a similar allergic vasospastic reaction. Chest pain, elevated blood pressure, arthralgias, and/or headache have also been reported in the absence of definite peripheral vasospasm. Anaphylactic shock has been reported rarely following the intravenous administration of heparin sodium.

Elevations of serum transminases without elevation in bilirubin or alkaline phosphatase occur in a high percentage of patients receiving heparin, by either subcutaneous or intravenous route. This was also observed in normal volunteers who received heparin. Whether this represents toxicity or nonspecific stimulation of the enzymes is not known.

Necrosis of the skin has been reported at the site of subcutaneous injection of heparin, occasionally requiring skin grafting.

During clinical studies, acute reversible thrombocytopenia was reported at frequencies varying from 0 to 31%. This occurred 2 to 20 days (average 5 to 9) following the onset of therapy. In some cases this has been associated with immunologically demonstrable factors in the patients' serum resulting in in vitro platelet aggregation when heparin and platelets are added. In isolated cases, localized or disseminated thromboses have occurred which may have been related to in vivo platelet aggregation. Osteoporosis and suppression of renal function following long-term high-dose administration, suppression of aldosterone synthesis, delayed transient alopecia, priapism, and rebound hyperlipemia following discontinuation of heparin sodium have also been reported.

Dosage and Administration: Heparin sodium is not effective by oral administration and should be given by deep subcutaneous (intrafat, i.e. above iliac crest or into the abdominal fat layer) injection, by intermittent intravenous injection, or intravenous infusion. The intramuscular route of administration should be avoided because of the frequent occurrence of hematoma at the injection site.

The dosage of heparin sodium should be adjusted according to the patient's coagulation test results, which, during the first day of treatment, should be determined just prior to each injection. (There is usually no need to monitor the effect of low-dose heparin in patients with normal coagulation parameters.) Dosage is considered adequate when the whole blood clotting time is elevated approximately 2.5 to 3 times the control value.

When heparin sodium is administered by continuous intravenous infusion, coagulation tests should be performed approximately every four hours during the early stages of therapy. When it is administered intermittently by intravenous, or deep subcutaneous (intrafat) injection, coagulation tests should be performed before each injection during the early stages of treatment and daily thereafter.

When an oral anticoagulant such as warfarin sodium or similar type is administered with heparin sodium, coagulation tests and prothrombin activity should be determined at the start of therapy. For immediate anticoagulant effect, administer heparin sodium in the usual therapeutic dosage. When the results of the initial prothrombin determination are known, administer the first dose of an oral anticoagulant in the usual amount. Thereafter, perform a coagulation test and determine the prothrombin activity at appropriate intervals. A period of at least five hours after the last intravenous dose and 24 hours after the last subcutaneous (intrafat) dose of heparin sodium should elapse before blood is drawn if a valid prothrombin time is to be obtained. When the oral anticoagulant shows full effect and prothrombin activity is in the desired therapeutic range, heparin sodium may be discontinued and therapy continued with the oral anticoagulant.

When heparin is added to an infusion solution for continuous intravenous administration, the container should be inverted at least 6 times to insure adequate mixing and prevent pooling of the heparin in the solution.

Therapeutic anticoagulant effect with full-dose heparin: Although dosage must be adjusted for the individual patient according to the results of suitable laboratory tests, the following dosage schedules may be used as guidelines:
[See table below].

1. **By deep subcutaneous (intrafat) injection.** After an initial I.V. injection of 5,000 units, inject 10,000 to 20,000 units of a concentrated heparin sodium solution subcutaneously, followed by 8,000 to 10,000 units of a concentrated solution subcutaneously every 8 hours, or 15,000 to 20,000 units of a concentrated solution every 12 hours. A different site should be used for each injection to prevent the development of a massive hematoma.

2. **By intermittent intravenous injection.** 10,000 units initially, then 5,000 to 10,000 units every 4 to 6 hours. These amounts may be given either undiluted or diluted with 50 to 100 milliliters of isotonic sodium chloride injection.

3. **By continuous intravenous infusion.** After an initial I.V. injection of 5,000 units of heparin sodium, add 20,000 to 40,000 units to 1,000 milliliters of isotonic sodium chloride solution for infusion. For most patients, the rate of flow should be adjusted to deliver approximately 20,000 to 40,000 units in 24 hours.

Heparin Sodium Inj. Method of Administration	Frequency	Recommended Dose [based on 150 lb (68 kg) patient]
Deep Subcutaneous (Intrafat) Injection	Initial Dose	5,000 units by I.V. injection followed by 10,000–20,000 units of a concentrated solution, subcutaneously
	Every 8 hours	8,000–10,000 units of a concentrated solution
	(or) Every 12 hours	15,000–20,000 units of a concentrated solution
Intermittent Intravenous Injection	Initial Dose	10,000 units, either undiluted or in 50–100 ml isotonic sodium chloride injection
	Every 4 to 6 hours	5,000–10,000 units, either undiluted or in 50–100 ml isotonic sodium chloride injection
Intravenous Infusion	Initial Dose	5,000 units by I.V. injection
	Continuous	20,000–40,000 units in 1,000 ml of isotonic sodium chloride solution for infusion/day

Surgery of the Heart and Blood Vessels: Patients undergoing total body perfusion for open heart surgery should receive an initial dose of not less than 150 units of heparin sodium per kilogram of body weight. Frequently a dose of 300 units of heparin sodium per kilogram of body weight is used for procedures estimated to last less than 60 minutes; or 400 units/kg for those estimated to last longer than 60 minutes.

Low-dose prophylaxis of postoperative thromboembolism: A number of well-controlled clinical trials have demonstrated that low-dose heparin prophylaxis, given just prior to and after surgery, will reduce the incidence of postoperative deep vein thrombosis in the legs, as measured by the I-125 fibrinogen technique and venography, and of clinical pulmonary embolism. The most widely used dosage has been 5,000 units 2 hours before surgery and 5,000 units every 8 to 12 hours thereafter for 7 days or until the patient is fully ambulatory, whichever is longer. The heparin is given by deep subcutaneous injection in the arm or abdomen with a fine needle (25-26 gauge) to minimize tissue trauma. A concentrated solution of heparin sodium is recommended. Such prophylaxis should be reserved for patients over 40 undergoing major surgery. Patients with bleeding disorders, those having neurosurgery, spinal anesthesia, eye surgery, or potentially sanguineous operations should be excluded, as well as patients receiving oral anticoagulants or platelet-active drugs (see WARNINGS). The value of such prophylaxis in hip surgery has not been established. The possibility of increased bleeding during surgery or postoperatively should be borne in mind. If such bleeding occurs, discontinuation of heparin and neutralization with protamine sulfate is advisable. If clinical evidence of thromboembolism develops despite low-dose prophylaxis, full therapeutic doses of anticoagulants should be given unless contraindicated. All patients should be screened prior to heparinization to rule out bleeding disorders, and monitoring should be performed with appropriate coagulation tests just prior to surgery. Coagulation test values should be normal or only slightly elevated. There is usually no need for daily minitoring of the effect of low-dose heparin in patients with normal coagulation parameters.

Extracorporeal Dialysis Use: Follow equipment manufacturer's operating directions carefully.

Blood Transfusion: Addition of 400 to 600 USP Units per 100 ml of whole blood. Usually 7,500 USP heparin sodium units are added to 100 ml of Sterile Sodium Chloride Injection and mixed (or 75,000 USP Units per 1,000 ml of Sodium Chloride Injection) and from this sterile solution, 6 ml to 8 ml are added per 100 ml of whole blood. Leukocyte counts should be performed on heparinized blood within two hours after addition of the heparin. Heparinized blood should not be used for isoagglutinin, complement or erythrocyte fragility tests.

Laboratory Samples: Addition of 70 to 150 units of heparin sodium per 10 to 20 ml sample of whole blood are usually employed to prevent coagulation of the same. See comments above under "Blood Transfusion."

Overdosage: Protamine sulfate (1% solution) by slow infusion will neutralize heparin. No more than 50 mg should be given in any 10 minute period. Decreasing amounts of protamine are required as time from last heparin injection increases. Thirty minutes after a dose of heparin approximately 0.5 mg of protamine is sufficient to neutralize each mg of heparin. Single doses of protamine should not exceed 50 mg. Blood or plasma transfusions may be necessary; these dilute but do not neutralize heparin.

The *in vitro* relationship between protamine sulfate and heparin sodium may be expressed as follows:

heparin derived from beef lung
1 mg of protamine sulfate will neutralize approximately 90 USP Units of heparin sodium of beef lung origin.

heparin derived from porcine intestinal mucosa
1 mg of protamine sulfate will neutralize approximately 115 USP Units of heparin sodium of intestinal mucosa origin.

How Supplied: Heparin Sodium Injection, USP derived **from beef lung** is available in the following strengths and package sizes:

1,000 USP Units per ml
10 ml vials	NDC 0009-0268-01
25-10 ml vials	NDC 0009-0268-07
30 ml vials	NDC 0009-0268-02

5,000 USP Units per ml
1 ml vials	NDC 0009-0291-02
10 ml vials	NDC 0009-0291-01

10,000 USP Units per ml
1 ml vials	NDC 0009-0317-01
25-1 ml vials	NDC 0009-0317-08
4 ml vials	NDC 0009-0317-02
25-4 ml vials	NDC 0009-0317-09

Code 810 670 110

KAOPECTATE® Anti-Diarrhea Medicine
(See PDR For Nonprescription Drugs)

KAOPECTATE CONCENTRATE®
Anti-Diarrhea Medicine
(See PDR For Nonprescription Drugs)

LINCOCIN® ℞
brand of lincomycin hydrochloride capsules and lincomycin hydrochloride sterile solution
(lincomycin hydrochloride, USP)

WARNING

Lincomycin therapy has been associated with severe colitis which may end fatally. Therefore, it should be reserved for serious infections where less toxic antimicrobial agents are inappropriate, as described in the Indications Section. It should not be used in patients with nonbacterial infections, such as most upper respiratory tract infections. Studies indicate a toxin(s) produced by *Clostridia* is one primary cause of antibiotic associated colitis. The colitis is usually characterized by severe, persistent diarrhea and severe abdominal cramps and may be associated with the passage of blood and mucus. Endoscopic examination may reveal pseudomembranous colitis.

When significant diarrhea occurs, the drug should be discontinued or, if necessary, continued only with close observation of the patient. Large bowel endoscopy has been recommended.

Antiperistaltic agents such as opiates and diphenoxylate with atropine (Lomotil) may prolong and/or worsen the condition. Vancomycin has been found to be effective in the treatment of antibiotic associated pseudomembranous colitis produced by *Clostridium difficile*. The usual adult dose is 500 milligrams to 2 grams of vancomycin orally per day in three to four divided doses administered for 7 to 10 days. Cholestyramine or colestipol resins bind vancomycin *in vitro*. If both a resin and vancomycin are to be administered concurrently, it may be advisable to separate the time of administration of each drug.

Diarrhea, colitis, and pseudomembranous colitis have been observed to begin up to several weeks following cessation of therapy with lincomycin.

Description: LINCOCIN preparations contain lincomycin hydrochloride which is the monohydrated salt of lincomycin, a substance produced by the growth of a member of the *lincolnensis* group of *Streptomyces lincolnensis* (Fam. *Streptomycetaceae*). It is a white, or practically white, crystalline powder and is odorless or has a faint odor. Its solutions are acid and are dextrorotatory. Lincomycin hydrochloride is freely soluble in water; soluble in dimethylformamide and very slightly soluble in acetone.

Clinical Pharmacology: Microbiology—Lincomycin has been shown to be effective against most of the common gram-positive pathogens. Depending on the sensitivity of the organism and concentration of the antibiotic, it may be either bactericidal or bacteriostatic. Cross resistance has not been demonstrated with penicillin, chloramphenicol, ampicillin, cephalosporins or the tetracyclines. Despite chemical differences, lincomycin exhibits antibacterial activity similar but not identical to the macrolide antibiotics (e.g. erythromycin). Some cross resistance (with erythromycin) including a phenomenon known as dissociated cross resistance or macrolide effect has been reported. Microorganisms have not developed resistance to lincomycin rapidly when tested by *in vitro* or *in vivo* methods. Staphylococci develop resistance to lincomycin in a slow, step-wise manner based on *in vitro*, serial subculture experiments. This pattern of resistance development is unlike that shown for streptomycin.

Studies indicate that lincomycin does not share antigenicity with penicillin compounds.

Biological Studies—*In vitro* studies indicate that the spectrum of activity includes *Staphylococcus aureus*, *Staphylococcus albus*, β-hemolytic *Streptococcus*, *Streptococcus viridans*, *Diplococcus pneumoniae*, *Clostridium tetani*, *Clostridium perfringens*, *Corynebacterium diphtheriae* and *Corynebacterium acnes*.

NOTE: The drug is not active against most strains of *Streptococcus faecalis*, nor against *Neisseria gonorrhoeae*, *Neisseria meningitidis*, *Hemophilus influenzae*, or other gram-negative organisms or yeasts.

Human Pharmacology—Lincomycin is absorbed rapidly after a 500 mg oral dose, reaching peak levels in 2 to 4 hours. Levels are maintained above the MIC (minimum inhibitory concentration) for most gram-positive organisms for 6 to 8 hours. Urinary recovery of drug in a 24-hour period ranges from 1.0 to 31 percent (mean: 4.0) after a single oral dose of 500 mg of lincomycin. Tissue level studies indicate that bile is an important route of excretion. Significant levels have been demonstrated in the majority of body tissues. Although the drug is not present in significant amounts in the spinal fluid of normal volunteers, it has been demonstrated in the spinal fluid of one patient with pneumococcal meningitis.

Intramuscular administration of a single dose of 600 mg produces a peak serum level at 30 minutes with detectable levels persisting for 24 hours. Urinary excretion after this dose ranges from 1.8 to 24.8 percent (mean: 17.3).

The intravenous infusion over a 2-hour interval of 600 mg of lincomycin hydrochloride in 500 ml of 5 percent glucose in distilled water yields therapeutic levels for 14 hours. Urinary excretion ranges from 4.9 to 30.3 percent (mean: 13.8).

The biological half-life, after oral, intramuscular or intravenous administration is 5.4 ± 1.0 hours. Hemodialysis and peritoneal dialysis do not effectively remove lincomycin from the blood.

Indications and Usage: LINCOCIN preparations (lincomycin) are indicated in the treatment of serious infections due to susceptible strains of streptococci, pneumococci, and staphylococci. Its use should be reserved for penicillin-allergic patients or other patients for whom, in the judgment of the physician, a penicillin is inappropriate. Because of the risk of colitis, as described in the WARNING box, before selecting lincomycin the physician should consider the nature of the infection and the suitability of less toxic alternatives (e.g., erythromycin).

Lincomycin has been demonstrated to be effective in the treatment of staphylococcal infections resistant to other antibiotics and susceptible to lincomycin. Staphylococcal strains resistant to

Continued on next page

Information on these Upjohn products is based on labeling in effect on November 30, 1984. Further information concerning these and other Upjohn products may be obtained from the package insert or by direct inquiry to Medical Information, The Upjohn Company, Kalamazoo, Michigan 49001.

Upjohn—Cont.

LINCOCIN have been recovered; culture and susceptibility studies should be done in conjunction with therapy with LINCOCIN. In the case of macrolides, partial but not complete cross resistance may occur (see **Microbiology**). The drug may be administered concomitantly with other antimicrobial agents when indicated.

Contraindications: This drug is contraindicated in patients previously found to be hypersensitive to lincomycin or clindamycin. It is not indicated in the treatment of minor bacterial infections or viral infections.

WARNINGS:
See WARNING box. Studies indicate a toxin(s) produced by *Clostridia* is one primary cause of antibiotic associated colitis.[1-5] Mild cases of colitis may respond to drug discontinuance alone. Moderate to severe cases should be managed promptly with fluid, electrolyte and protein supplementation as indicated. Vancomycin has been found to be effective in the treatment of antibiotic associated pseudomembranous colitis produced by *Clostridium difficile*. The usual adult dosage is 500 milligrams to 2 grams of vancomycin orally per day in three to four divided doses administered for 7 to 10 days. Cholestyramine or colestipol resins bind vancomycin *in vitro*. If both a resin and vancomycin are to be administered concurrently, it may be advisable to separate the time of administration of each drug. Systemic corticoids and corticoid retention enemas may help relieve the colitis. Other causes of colitis should also be considered. A careful inquiry should be made concerning previous sensitivities to drugs and other allergens.

Usage in Pregnancy—Safety for use in pregnancy has not been established.

Usage in Newborn—Until further clinical experience is obtained, LINCOCIN preparations (lincomycin) are not indicated in the newborn.

Nursing Mothers—LINCOCIN has been reported to appear in breast milk in ranges of 0.5 to 2.4 mcg/ml.

1. Bailey, WR, Scott, EG, *Diagnostic Microbiology* CV Mosby Company, St. Louis, 1978.
2. Bartlett, JG, et al, "Clindamycin-associated Colitis due to a Toxin-producing Species of *Clostridium* in Hamsters", *J. Inf. Dis.* 136(5): 701–705, (November) 1977.
3. Larson, HE, Price, AB, "Pseudomembranous Colitis: Presence of Clostridial Toxin," *Lancet*, 1312–1314 (December) 24 and 31, 1977.
4. Lusk, RH, et al, "Clindamycin-Induced Enterocolitis in Hamsters", *J. Inf. Dis.* 137(4): 464–474 (April) 1978.
5. "Antibiotic-associated Colitis: A Progress Report", *British Med. J.* 1:669–671 (March 18) 1978.

Precautions: Review of experience to date suggests that a subgroup of older patients with associated severe illness may tolerate diarrhea less well. When LINCOCIN preparations (lincomycin) are indicated in these patients, they should be carefully monitored for change in bowel frequency.

LINCOCIN should be prescribed with caution in individuals with a history of gastrointestinal disease, particularly colitis.

LINCOCIN, like any drug, should be used with caution in patients with a history of asthma or significant allergies.

The use of antibiotics occasionally results in overgrowth of nonsusceptible organisms—particularly yeasts. Should superinfections occur, appropriate measures should be taken. When patients with pre-existing monilial infections require therapy with LINCOCIN, concomitant antimonilial treatment should be given.

During prolonged therapy with LINCOCIN, periodic liver function studies and blood counts should be performed.

Since adequate data are not yet available in patients with pre-existing liver disease, its use in such patients is not recommended at this time unless special clinical circumstances so indicate.

Lincomycin has been shown to have neuromuscular blocking properties that may enhance the action of other neuromuscular blocking agents. Therefore, it should be used with caution in patients receiving such agents.

Indicated surgical procedures should be performed in conjunction with antibiotic therapy.

Adverse Reactions:
Gastrointestinal—Glossitis, stomatitis, nausea, vomiting. Persistent diarrhea, enterocolitis and pruritus ani. (See **Warning** box)

Hematopoietic: Neutropenia, leukopenia, agranulocytosis and thrombocytopenic purpura have been reported. There have been rare reports of aplastic anemia and pancytopenia in which LINCOCIN preparations (lincomycin hydrochloride) could not be ruled out as the causative agent.

Hypersensitivity Reactions—Hypersensitivity reactions such as angioneurotic edema, serum sickness and anaphylaxis have been reported, some of these in patients known to be sensitive to penicillin. Rare instances of erythema multiforme, some resembling Stevens-Johnson syndrome, have been associated with LINCOCIN. If an allergic reaction should occur, the drug should be discontinued and the usual agents (epinephrine, corticosteroids, antihistamines) should be available for emergency treatment.

Skin and Mucous Membranes—Skin rashes, urticaria and vaginitis and rare instances of exfoliative and vesiculobullous dermatitis have been reported.

Liver—Although no direct relationship of LINCOCIN to liver dysfunction has been established, jaundice and abnormal liver function tests (particularly elevations of serum transaminase) have been observed in a few instances.

Cardiovascular—After too rapid intravenous administration, rare instances of cardiopulmonary arrest and hypotension have been reported. (See **Dosage and Administration**).

Special Senses—Tinnitus and vertigo have been reported occasionally.

Local Reactions—Patients have demonstrated excellent local tolerance to intramuscularly administered LINCOCIN. Reports of pain following injection have been infrequent. Intravenous administration of LINCOCIN in 250 to 500 ml of 5 percent glucose in distilled water or normal saline produced no local irritation or phlebitis.

Dosage and Administration:
If significant diarrhea occurs during therapy, this antibiotic should be discontinued. (See **Warning** box).

Oral—**Adults:** *Serious infections*—500 mg 3 times per day (500 mg approximately every 8 hours). *More severe infections*—500 mg or more 4 times per day (500 mg or more approximately every 6 hours). **Children over 1 month of age:** *Serious infections*—30 mg/kg/day (15 mg/lb/day) divided into 3 or 4 equal doses. *More severe infections*—60 mg/kg/day (30 mg/lb/day) divided into 3 or 4 equal doses.

With β-hemolytic streptococcal infections, treatment should continue for at least 10 days to diminish the likelihood of subsequent rheumatic fever or glomerulonephritis.

NOTE: For optimal absorption it is recommended that nothing be given by mouth except water for a period of one to two hours before and after oral administration of LINCOCIN preparations (lincomycin).

Intramuscular—**Adults:** *Serious infections*—600 mg (2 ml) intramuscularly every 24 hours. *More severe infections*—600 mg (2 ml) intramuscularly every 12 hours or more often. **Children over 1 month of age:** *Serious infections*—one intramuscular injection of 10 mg/kg (5 mg/lb) every 24 hours. *More severe infections*—one intramuscular injection of 10 mg/kg (5 mg/lb) every 12 hours or more often.

Intravenous—**Adults:** The intravenous dose will be determined by the severity of the infection. For serious infections doses of 600 mg (2 ml of LINCOCIN Sterile Solution) to 1 gram are given every 8-12 hours. For more severe infections these doses may have to be increased. In life-threatening situations daily intravenous doses of as much as 8 grams have been given. Intravenous doses are given on the basis of 1 gram of lincomycin diluted in not less than 100 ml of appropriate solution (see **PHYSICAL COMPATIBILITIES**) and infused over a period of not less than one hour.

Dose	Vol. Diluent	Time
600 mg	100 ml	1 hr
1 gram	100 ml	1 hr
2 grams	200 ml	2 hr
3 grams	300 ml	3 hr
4 grams	400 ml	4 hr

These doses may be repeated as often as required to the limit of the maximum recommended daily dose of 8 grams of lincomycin.

Children over 1 month of age: 10-20 mg/kg/day (5-10 mg/lb/day) depending on the severity of the infection may be infused in divided doses as described above for adults.

NOTE: Severe cardiopulmonary reactions have occurred when this drug has been given at greater than the recommended concentration and rate.

Subconjunctival Injection—0.25 ml (75 mg) injected subconjunctivally will result in ocular fluid levels of antibiotic (lasting for at least 5 hours) with MIC's sufficient for most susceptible pathogens.

Patients with diminished renal function: *When therapy with LINCOCIN is required in individuals with severe impairment of renal function, an appropriate dose is 25 to 30% of that recommended for patients with normally functioning kidneys.*

How Supplied:
LINCOCIN preparations (lincomycin) are available as:

250 mg Pediatric Capsules: Each capsule contains lincomycin hydrochloride equivalent to lincomycin 250 mg.
Bottles of 24   NDC 0009-0336-01

500 mg Capsules: Each capsule contains lincomycin hydrochloride equivalent to lincomycin 500 mg.
Bottles of 24   NDC 0009-0500-01
Bottles of 100   NDC 0009-0500-02

Sterile Solution: Each ml contains lincomycin hydrochloride equivalent to lincomycin 300 mg; also Benzyl Alcohol, 9.45 mg added as preservative—available in single dose 2 ml syringes, in 2 ml and 10 ml vials.

2 ml *U-Ject®*   NDC 0009-0600-01
Disposable Syringe
2 ml vial   NDC 0009-0555-01
10 ml vial   NDC 0009-0555-02

Animal Pharmacology: *In vivo* experimental animal studies demonstrated the effectiveness of LINCOCIN preparations (lincomycin) in protecting animals infected with *Streptococcus viridans*, *β-hemolytic Streptococcus*, *Staphylococcus aureus*, *Diplococcus pneumoniae* and *Leptospira pomona*. It was ineffective in *Klebsiella, Pasteurella, Pseudomonas, Salmonella* and *Shigella* infections.

Clinical Studies: Experience with 345 obstetrical patients receiving this drug revealed no ill effects related to pregnancy.

Physical Compatibilities
[See table on next page].
Code 810 174 204

LONITEN®
brand of minoxidil tablets

10 mg, 100's
NSN 6505-01-088-8120(M & VA)

2.5 mg, 100's
NSN 6505-01-088-8121(VA)

Warnings: LONITEN Tablets contain the powerful antihypertensive agent, minoxidil, which may produce serious adverse effects. It can cause pericardial effusion, occasionally progressing to tamponade, and angina pectoris may be exacerbated. LONITEN should be reserved for hypertensive patients who do not respond adequately to maximum therapeutic doses of a diuretic and two other antihypertensive agents.

In experimental animals, minoxidil caused several kinds of myocardial lesions as well as other adverse cardiac effects (see Cardiac Lesions in Animals).

LONITEN must be administered under close supervision, usually concomitantly with therapeutic doses of a beta-adrenergic blocking agent to prevent tachycardia and increased myocardial workload. It must also usually be given with a diuretic, frequently one acting in the ascending limb of the loop of Henle, to present serious fluid accumulation. Patients with malignant hypertension and those already receiving guanethidine (see Warnings) should be hospitalized when LONITEN is first administered so that they can be monitored to avoid too rapid, or large orthostatic, decreases in blood pressure.

Description: LONITEN Tablets contain minoxidil, an antihypertensive peripheral vasodilator. Minoxidil occurs as a white or off-white, odorless, crystalline solid that is soluble in water to the extent of approximately 2 mg/ml; is readily soluble in propylene glycol or ethanol; and is almost insoluble in acetone, chloroform or ethyl acetate. The chemical name for minoxidil is 2,4-pyrimidinediamine, 6-(1-piperidinyl)-, 3-oxide (mw = 209.25).

LONITEN Tablets for oral administration contain either 2.5 mg or 10 mg of minoxidil.

Clinical Pharmacology:

1. General Pharmacologic Properties

Minoxidil is an orally effective direct acting peripheral vasodilator that reduces elevated systolic and diastolic blood pressure by decreasing peripheral vascular resistance. Microcirculatory blood flow in animals is enhanced or maintained in all systemic vascular beds. In man, forearm and renal vascular resistance decline; forearm blood flow increases while renal blood flow and glomerular filtration rate are preserved.

Because it causes peripheral vasodilation, minoxidil elicits a number of predictable reactions. Reduction of peripheral arteriolar resistance and the associated fall in blood pressure trigger sympathetic, vagal inhibitory, and renal homeostatic mechanisms, including an increase in renin secretion, that lead to increased cardiac rate and output and salt and water retention. These adverse effects can usually be minimized by concomitant administration of a diuretic and a beta-adrenergic blocking agent or other sympathetic nervous system suppressant.

Minoxidil does not interfere with vasomotor reflexes and therefore does not produce orthostatic hypotension. The drug does not enter the central nervous system in experimental animals in significant amounts, and it does not affect CNS function in man.

2. Effects on Blood Pressure and Target Organs

The extent and time-course of blood pressure reduction by minoxidil do not correspond closely to its concentration in plasma. After an effective single oral dose, blood pressure usually starts to decline within one-half hour, reaches a minimum between 2 and 3 hours and recovers at an arithmetically linear rate of about 30%/day. The total duration of effect is approximately 75 hours. When minoxidil is administered chronically, once or twice a day, the time required to achieve maximum effect on blood pressure with a given daily dose is inversely related to the size of the dose. Thus, maximum effect is achieved on 10 mg/day within 7 days, on 20 mg/day within 5 days, and on 40 mg/day within 3 days.

The blood pressure response to minoxidil is linearly related to the logarithm of the dose administered. The slope of this log-linear dose-response relationship is proportional to the degree of hypertension and approaches zero at a supine diastolic blood pressure of approximately 85 mmHg.

When used in severely hypertensive patients resistant to other therapy, frequently with an accompanying diuretic and beta-blocker, LONITEN Tablets (minoxidil) usually decreased the blood pressure and reversed encephalopathy and retinopathy."

LINCOCIN
Physical Compatibilities:

Physically compatible for 24 hours at room temperature unless otherwise indicated.

Infusion Solutions
Dextrose in Water, 5% and 10%
Dextrose in Saline, 5% and 10%
Ringer's Solution
Sodium Lactate 1/6 Molar
Travert 10%—Electrolyte No. 1
Dextran in Saline 6% w/v

Vitamins in Infusion Solutions
B-Complex
B-Complex with Ascorbic Acid

Antibiotics in Infusion Solutions
Penicillin G Sodium (Satisfactory for 4 hours)
Cephalothin
Tetracycline HCl
Cephaloridine
Colistimethate (Satisfactory for 4 hours)
Ampicillin
Methicillin
Chloramphenicol
Polymyxin B Sulfate

Physically Incompatible With:
Novobiocin
Kanamycin

IT SHOULD BE EMPHASIZED THAT THE COMPATIBLE AND INCOMPATIBLE DETERMINATIONS ARE PHYSICAL OBSERVATIONS ONLY, NOT CHEMICAL DETERMINATIONS. ADEQUATE CLINICAL EVALUATION OF THE SAFETY AND EFFICACY OF THESE COMBINATIONS HAS NOT BEEN PERFORMED.

3. Absorption and Metabolism

Minoxidil is at least 90% absorbed from the GI tract in experimental animals and man. Plasma levels of the parent drug reach maximum within the first hour and decline rapidly thereafter. The average plasma half-life in man is 4.2 hours. Approximately 90% of the administered drug is metabolized, predominantly by conjugation with glucuronic acid at the N-oxide position in the pyrimidine ring, but also by conversion to more polar products. Known metabolites exert much less pharmacologic effect than minoxidil itself; all are excreted principally in the urine. Minoxidil does not bind to plasma proteins, and its renal clearance corresponds to the glomerular filtration rate. In the absence of functional renal tissue, minoxidil and its metabolites can be removed by hemodialysis.

4. Cardiac Lesions in Animals

Minoxidil produced two types of cardiac lesions in non-primate species:

(a) *Dog atrial lesion*—
Daily oral doses of 0.5 mg/kg for several days to 1 month or longer produced a grossly visible hemorrhagic lesion of the right atrium of the dog. This lesion has not been seen in other species. Microscopic examination showed replacement of myocardial cells by proliferating fibroblasts and angioblasts; phagocytosis; and hemosiderin accumulation in macrophages.

(b) *Papillary muscle lesion*—
Short term treatment (about 3 days) in several species (dog, rat, minipig) produced necrosis of the papillary muscles and, in some cases subendocardial areas of the left ventricle, lesions similar to those produced by other peripheral dilators and by beta-adrenergic receptor agonists such as isoproterenol and epinephrine. These are thought to result from myocardial ischemia resulting from reflex sympathetic or vagal withdrawal-induced tachycardia in combination with hypotension. These lesions were reduced in incidence and severity by beta-adrenergic receptor blockade.

(c) *Hemorrhagic lesions* were seen in many parts of the heart, mainly in the epicardium, endocardium, and walls of small coronary arteries and arterioles, after acute minoxidil treatment in dogs, and left atrial hemorrhagic lesions were seen in minipigs.

In addition to these lesions, longer term studies in rats, dogs, and monkeys showed cardiac hypertrophy and (in rats) cardiac dilation. In monkeys, hydrochlorothiazide partly reversed the increased heart weight, suggesting it may be related to fluid overload. In a one-year dog study, serosanguineous pericardial fluid was seen.

Autopsies of 79 patients who died from various causes and who had received minoxidil did not reveal right atrial or other hemorrhagic pathology of the kind seen in dogs. Instances of necrotic areas in the papillary muscles were seen, but these occurred in the presence of known pre-existing ischemic heart disease and did not appear different from, or more common than, lesions seen in patients never exposed to minoxidil. Studies to date cannot rule out the possibility that minoxidil can be associated with cardiac damage in humans.

Indications and Usage: Because of the potential for serious adverse effects, LONITEN Tablets (minoxidil) are indicated only in the treatment of hypertension that is symptomatic or associated with target organ damage and is not manageable with maximum therapeutic doses of a diuretic plus two other antihypertensive drugs. At the present time use in milder degrees of hypertension is not recommended because the benefit-risk relationship in such patients has not been defined.

LONITEN reduced supine diastolic blood pressure by 20 mm Hg or to 90 mm Hg or less in approximately 75% of patients, most of whom had hypertension that could not be controlled by other drugs.

Contraindications: LONITEN Tablets (minoxidil) are contraindicated in pheochromocytoma, because it may stimulate secretion of catecholamines from the tumor through its antihypertensive action.

Warnings:

1. Salt and Water Retention; Congestive Heart Failure—concomitant use of an adequate diuretic is required—

LONITEN Tablets (minoxidil) must usually be administered concomitantly with a diuretic adequate to prevent fluid retention and possible congestive heart failure; a high ceiling (loop) diuretic is *almost always* required. Body weight should be monitored closely. If LONITEN is used without a diuretic, retention of several hundred milli-equivalents of salt and corresponding volumes of water can occur within a few days, leading to increased plasma and interstitial fluid volume and local or generalized edema. Diuretic treatment alone, or in combination with restricted salt intake, will usually minimize fluid retention, although reversible edema did develop in approximately 10% of nondialysis patients so treated. Ascites has also been reported. Diuretic effectiveness was limited mostly by disease-related impaired renal function. The condition of patients with preexisting congestive heart failure occasionally deteriorated in association with fluid retention although because of the fall in blood pressure (reduction of afterload), more than twice as many improved than worsened. Rarely, refractory fluid retention may require discontinuation of LONITEN. Provided that the patient is under close medical supervision, it may be possible to resolve refractory salt retention

Continued on next page

Information on these Upjohn products is based on labeling in effect on November 30, 1984. Further information concerning these and other Upjohn products may be obtained from the package insert or by direct inquiry to Medical Information, The Upjohn Company, Kalamazoo, Michigan 49001.

Upjohn—Cont.

by discontinuing LONITEN for 1 or 2 days and then resuming treatment in conjunction with vigorous diuretic therapy.

2. **Concomitant Treatment to Prevent Tachycardia is Usually Required**—LONITEN increases the heart rate. Angina may worsen or appear for the first time during LONITEN treatment, probably because of the increased oxygen demands associated with increased heart rate and cardiac output. The increase in rate and the occurrence of angina generally can be prevented by the concomitant administration of a beta-adrenergic blocking drug or other sympathetic nervous system suppressant. The ability of beta-adrenergic blocking agents to minimize papillary muscle lesions in animals is further reason to utilize such an agent concomitantly. Round-the-clock effectiveness of the sympathetic suppressant should be ensured.

3. **Pericardial Effusion and Tamponade**—Pericardial effusion, occasionally with tamponade, has been observed in about 3% of treated patients not on dialysis, especially those with inadequate or compromised renal function. Although in many cases, the pericardial effusion was associated with a connective tissue disease, the uremic syndrome, congestive heart failure, or marked fluid retention, there have been instances in which these potential causes of effusion were not present. Patients should be observed closely for any suggestion of a pericardial disorder, and echocardiographic studies should be carried out if suspicion arises. More vigorous diuretic therapy, dialysis, pericardiocentesis, or surgery may be required. If the effusion persists, withdrawal of LONITEN should be considered in light of other means of controlling the hypertension and the patient's clinical status.

4. *Interaction with Guanethidine:*
Although minoxidil does not itself cause orthostatic hypotension, its administration to patients already receiving guanethidine can result in profound orthostatic effects. If at all possible, guanethidine should be discontinued well before minoxidil is begun. Where this is not possible, minoxidil therapy should be started in the hospital and the patient should remain institutionalized until severe orthostatic effects are no longer present or the patient has learned to avoid activities that provoke them.

5. *Hazard of Rapid Control of Blood Pressure:*
In patients with very severe blood pressure elevation, too rapid control of blood pressure, especially with intravenous agents, can precipitate syncope, cerebrovascular accidents, myocardial infarction and ischemia of special sense organs with resulting decrease or loss of vision or hearing. Patients with compromised circulation or cryoglobulinemia may also suffer ischemic episodes of the affected organs. Although such events have not been unequivocally associated with minoxidil use, total experience is limited at present.
Any patient with malignant hypertension should have initial treatment with minoxidil carried out in a hospital setting, both to assure that blood pressure is falling and to assure that it is not falling more rapidly than intended.

Precautions:

1. **General Precautions**—(a) **Monitor fluid and electrolyte balance and body weight** (see **Warnings:** Salt and Water Retention).
(b) **Observe patients for signs and symptoms of pericardial effusion** (see **Warnings:** Pericardial Effusion and Tamponade).
(c) **Use after myocardial infarction**—LONITEN Tablets (minoxidil) have not been used in patients who have had a myocardial infarction within the preceding month. It is possible that a reduction of arterial pressure with LONITEN might further limit blood flow to the myocardium, although this might be compensated by decreased oxygen demand because of lower blood pressure.
(d) **Hypersensitivity**—Possible hypersensitivity to LONITEN, manifested as a skin rash, has been seen in less than 1% of patients; whether the drug should be discontinued when this occurs depends on treatment alternatives.
(e) **Renal failure or dialysis patients** may require smaller doses of LONITEN and should have close medical supervision to prevent exacerbation of renal failure or precipitation of cardiac failure.

2. **Information for patient**—The patient should be made fully aware of the importance of continuing all of his antihypertensive medications and of the nature of symptoms that would suggest fluid overload. A patient brochure has been prepared and is included with each LONITEN package. The text of this brochure is reprinted at the end of the insert.

3. **Laboratory tests**
Those laboratory tests which are abnormal at the time of initiation of minoxidil therapy, such as urinalysis, renal function tests, EKG, chest x-ray, echocardiogram, etc., should be repeated at intervals to ascertain whether improvement or deterioration is occuring under minoxidil therapy. Initially, such tests should be performed frequently, eg, 1–3 month intervals; later as stabilization occurs, at intervals of 6–12 months.

4. **Drug Interactions**
See "Interaction with guanethidine" under **WARNINGS**.

5. **Carcinogenesis, Mutagenesis and Impairment of Fertility**—Twenty-two month carcinogenicity studies in rats at doses 15 times the human dose did not provide evidence of tumorigenicity. The drug was not mutagenic in the Salmonella (Ames) test.
Rats receiving up to five times the human dose of minoxidil had a reduction in conception rate, possibly related to drug treatment. There was no evidence of increased fetal resorptions in rats but they did occur in rabbits.

6. **Pregnancy-Teratogenic Effects**—Pregnancy Category C. Minoxidil has been shown to reduce the conception rate in rats and to show evidence of increased fetal absorption in rabbits when administered at five times the human dose. There was no evidence of teratogenic effects in rats and rabbits. There are no adequate and well controlled studies in pregnant women. LONITEN should be used during pregnancy only if the potential benefit justifies the potential risk to the fetus.

7. **Labor and delivery**
The effects on labor and delivery are unknown.

8. **Nursing Mothers**—It is not known whether this drug is secreted in human milk. As a general rule, nursing should not be undertaken while a patient is on LONITEN.

9. **Pediatric Use**—Use in children has been limited to date, particularly in infants. The recommendations under **Dosage and Administration** can be considered only a rough guide at present and careful titration is essential.

Adverse Reactions:

1. **Salt and Water Retention** (see **Warnings:** Concomitant Use of Adequate Diuretic is Required)—Temporary edema developed in 7% of patients who were not edematous at the start of therapy.

2. **Pericardial Effusion and Tamponade** (see **Warnings**).

3. **Dermatologic - Hypertrichosis**—Elongation, thickening, and enhanced pigmentation of fine body hair are seen in about 80% of patients taking LONITEN Tablets (minoxidil). This develops within 3 to 6 weeks after starting therapy. It is usually first noticed on the temples, between the eyebrows, between the hairline and the eyebrows, or in the side-burn area of the upper lateral cheek, later extending to the back, arms, legs, and scalp. Upon discontinuation of LONITEN, new hair growth stops, but 1 to 6 months may be required for restoration to pretreatment appearance. No endocrine abnormalities have been found to explain the abnormal hair growth; thus, it is hypertrichosis without virilism. Hair growth is especially disturbing to children and women and such patients should be thoroughly informed about this effect before therapy with LONITEN is begun.
Allergic—Rashes have been reported, including rare reports of bullous eruptions, and Stevens-Johnson Syndrome.

4. **Hematologic**—Thrombocytopenia and leukopenia (WBC < 3000/mm^3) have rarely been reported.

5. **Gastrointestinal**—Nausea and/or vomiting has been reported. In clinical trials the incidence of nausea and vomiting associated with the underlying disease has shown a decrease from pretrial levels.

6. **Miscellaneous**—Breast tenderness—This developed in less than 1% of patients.

7. **Altered Laboratory Findings**—(a) ECG changes—changes in direction and magnitude of the ECG T-waves occur in approximately 60% of patients treated with LONITEN. In rare instances a large negative amplitude of the T-wave may encroach upon the S-T segment, but the S-T segment is not independently altered. These changes usually disappear with continuance of treatment and revert to the pretreatment state if LONITEN is discontinued. No symptoms have been associated with these changes, nor have there been alterations in blood cell counts or in plasma enzyme concentrations that would suggest myocardial damage. Long-term treatment of patients manifesting such changes has provided no evidence of deteriorating cardiac function. At present the changes appear to be nonspecific and without identifiable clinical significance. (b) Effects of hemodilution—hematocrit, hemoglobin and erythrocyte count usually fall about 7% initially and then recover to pretreatment levels. (c) Other—Alkaline phosphatase increased varyingly without other evidence of liver or bone abnormality. Serum creatinine increased an average of 6% and BUN slightly more, but later declined to pretreatment levels.

Overdosage: There have been only a few instances of deliberate or accidental overdosage with LONITEN Tablets (minoxidil). One patient recovered after taking 50 mg of minoxidil together with 500 mg of a barbiturate. When exaggerated hypotension is encountered, it is most likely to occur in association with residual sympathetic nervous system blockade from previous therapy (guanethidine-like effects or alpha-adrenergic blockage), which prevents the usual compensatory maintenance of blood pressure. Intravenous administration of normal saline will help to maintain blood pressure and facilitate urine formation in these patients. Sympathomimetic drugs such as norepinephrine or epinephrine should be avoided because of their excessive cardiac stimulating action. Phenylephrine, angiotensin II, vasopressin, and dopamine all reverse hypotension due to LONITEN, but should only be used if underperfusion of a vital organ is evident.
Radioimmunoassay can be performed to determine the concentration of minoxidil in the blood. At the maximum adult dosage of 100 mg/day, peak blood levels of 1641 ng/ml and 2441 ng/ml were observed in two patients, respectively. Due to patient-to-patient variation in blood levels, it is difficult to establish an overdosage warning level. In general, a substantial increase above 2000 ng/ml should be regarded as overdosage, unless the physician is aware that the patient has taken no more than the maximum dose.
Oral LD$_{50}$ in rats has ranged from 1321–3492 mg/kg; in mice, 2456-2648 mg/kg.

Dosage and Administration:

Patients over 12 years of age: The recommended initial dosage of LONITEN Tablets (minoxidil) is 5 mg given as a single daily dose. Daily dosage can be increased to 10, 20 and then to 40 mg in single or divided doses if required for optimum blood pressure control. The effective dosage range is usually 10 to 40 mg per day. The maximum recommended dosage is 100 mg per day.

Patients under 12 years of age: The initial dosage is 0.2 mg/kg minoxidil as a single daily dose. The dosage may be increased in 50 to 100% increments until optimum blood pressure control is achieved. The effective dosage range is usually 0.25 to 1.0 mg/kg/day. The maximum recommended dosage is 50 mg daily. (see **9. Pediatric Use** under **Precautions**).

Dose frequency: The magnitude of within-day fluctuation of arterial pressure during therapy with LONITEN is directly proportional to the extent of pressure reduction. If supine diastolic pressure has been reduced less than 30 mmHg, the drug need be administered only once a day; if supine diastolic pressure has been reduced more than 30 mmHg, the daily dosage should be divided into two equal parts.

Frequency of dosage adjustment: Dosage must be titrated carefully according to individual response. Intervals between dosage adjustments normally should be at least 3 days since the full response to a given dose is not obtained for at least that amount of time. **Where a more rapid management of hypertension is required, dose adjustments can be made every 6 hours if the patient is carefully monitored.**

Concomitant therapy: Diuretic and beta-blocker or other sympathetic nervous system supressant.

Diuretics: LONITEN must be used in conjunction with a diuretic in patients relying on renal function for maintaining salt and water balance. Diuretics have been used at the following dosages when starting therapy with LONITEN: hydrochlorothiazide (50 mg, b.i.d.) or other thiazides at equieffective dosage; chlorthalidone (50 to 100 mg, once daily); furosemide (40 mg, b.i.d.). If excessive salt and water retention results in a weight gain of more than 5 pounds, diuretic therapy should be changed to furosemide; if the patient is already taking furosemide, dosage should be increased in accordance with the patient's requirements.

Beta-blocker or other sympathetic nervous system suppressants: When therapy with LONITEN is begun, the dosage of a beta-adrenergic receptor blocking drug should be the equivalent of 80 to 160 mg of propranolol per day in divided doses.

If beta-blockers are contraindicated, methyldopa (250 to 750 mg, b.i.d.) may be used instead. Methyldopa must be given for at least 24 hours before starting therapy with LONITEN because of the delay in the onset of methyldopa's action. Limited clinical experience indicates that clonidine may also be used to prevent tachycardia induced by LONITEN; the usual dosage is 0.1 to 0.2 mg twice daily.

Sympathetic nervous system suppressants may not completely prevent an increase in heart rate due to LONITEN but usually do prevent tachycardia. Typically, patients receiving a beta-blocker prior to initiation of therapy with LONITEN have a bradycardia and can be expected to have an increase in heart rate toward normal when LONITEN is added. When treatment with LONITEN and beta-blocker or other sympathetic nervous system suppressant are begun simultaneously, their opposing cardiac effects usually nullify each other, leading to little change in heart rate.

How Supplied: LONITEN Tablets (minoxidil) are available as round, scored, white tablets. Dosage strengths are imprinted on one convex surface. The following strengths and container sizes are available:

Strength	Container and Size	NDC Number
2.5 mg	Bottles of 100, Unit of Use	0009-0121-01
10 mg	Bottles of 100, Unit of Use	0009-0137-01

Store at controlled room temperature 15°–30°C (59°–86°F).

Patient Information: LONITEN Tablets contain minoxidil, a medicine for the treatment of high blood pressure in the patient who has not been controlled or is experiencing unacceptable side effects with other medications. It must usually be taken with other medicines.

Be absolutely sure to take all of your medicines for high blood pressure according to your doctor's instructions. Do not stop taking LONITEN unless your doctor tells you to. Do not give any of your medicine to other people.

It is important that you look for the warning signals of certain undesired effects of LONITEN. Call your doctor if they occur. Your doctor will want to see you regularly while you are taking LONITEN. Be sure to keep all your appointments or to arrange for new ones if you must miss one.

Do not hesitate to call your doctor if any discomforts or problems occur.

The information here is intended to help you take LONITEN properly. It does not tell you all there is to know about LONITEN. There is a more technical leaflet that you may request from the pharmacist; you may need your doctor's help in understanding parts of that leaflet.

What is LONITEN?
LONITEN Tablets contain minoxidil which is a drug for lowering the blood pressure. It works by relaxing and enlarging certain small blood vessels so that blood flows through them more easily.

Why lower blood pressure?
Your doctor has prescribed LONITEN to lower your blood pressure and protect vital parts of your body. Uncontrolled blood pressure can cause stroke, heart failure, blindness, kidney failure, and heart attacks.

Most people with high blood pressure need to take medicines to treat it for their whole lives.

Who should take LONITEN?
There are many people with high blood pressure, but most of them do not need LONITEN. LONITEN is used ONLY when your doctor decides that:
1. your high blood pressure is severe;
2. your high blood pressure is causing symptoms or damage to vital organs; and
3. other medicines did not work well enough or had very disturbing side effects.

LONITEN should be taken only when a doctor prescribes it. Never give any of your LONITEN Tablets, or any other high blood pressure medicine, to a friend or relative.

Pregnancy: In some cases doctors may prescribe LONITEN for women who are pregnant or who are planning to have children. However, its safe use in pregnancy has not been established. Laboratory animals had a reduced ability to become pregnant and a reduced survival of offspring while taking LONITEN. If you are pregnant or are planning to become pregnant, be sure to tell your doctor.

How to take LONITEN.
Usually, your doctor will prescribe two other medicines along with LONITEN. These will help lower blood pressure and will help prevent undesired effects of LONITEN.

Often, when a medicine like LONITEN lowers blood pressure, your body tries to return the blood pressure to the original, higher level. It does this by holding on to water and salt (so there will be more fluid to pump) and by making your heart beat faster. To prevent this, your doctor will usually prescribe a water tablet to remove the extra salt and water from your body (a diuretic dye-u-RET-tic) and another medicine to slow your heart beat.

You must follow your doctor's instructions exactly, taking all the prescribed medicines, in the right amounts, each day. These medicines will help keep your blood pressure down.

The water tablet and heart beat medicine will help prevent the undesired effects of LONITEN.

LONITEN Tablets come in two strengths (2 ½ milligrams and 10 milligrams) that are marked on each tablet. Pay close attention to the tablet markings to be sure you are taking the correct strength. Your doctor may prescribe half a tablet; the tablets are scored (partly cut on one side) so that you can easily break them.

When you first start taking LONITEN, your doctor may need to see you often in order to adjust your dosage. Take all your medicine according to the schedule prescribed by your doctor. **Do not skip any doses. If you should forget a dose of LONITEN, wait until it is time for your next dose, then continue with your regular schedule. Remember: do not stop taking LONITEN, or any of your other high blood pressure medicines, without checking with your doctor.** Make sure that any doctor treating or examining you knows that you are taking high blood pressure medicines, including LONITEN.

Warning Signals: Even if you take all your medicines correctly, LONITEN Tablets may cause undesired effects. Some of these are serious and you should be on the lookout for them. **If any of the following warning signals occur, you must call your doctor immediately:**

1. **Increase in heart rate**—You should measure your heart rate by counting your pulse rate **while you are resting.** If you have an increase of 20 beats or more a minute over your normal pulse, contact your doctor immediately. If you do not know how to take your pulse rate, ask your doctor. Also ask your doctor how often to check your pulse.
2. **Rapid weight gain of more than 5 pounds**—You should weigh yourself daily. If you quickly gain five or more pounds, or if there is any swelling or puffiness in the face, hands, ankles, or stomach area, this could be a sign that you are retaining body fluids. Your doctor may have to change your drugs or change the dose of your drugs. You may also need to reduce the amount of salt you eat. A smaller weight gain (2 to 3 pounds) often occurs when treatment is started. You may lose this extra weight with continued treatment.
3. **Increased difficulty in breathing**, especially when lying down. This too may be due to an increase of body fluids. It can also happen because your high blood pressure is getting worse. In either case, you might require treatment with other medicines.
4. **New or worsening of pain in the chest, arm, or shoulder or signs of severe indigestion** — These could be signs of serious heart problems.
5. **Dizziness, lightheadedness or fainting** — These can be signs of high blood pressure or they may be side effects from one of the medicines. Your doctor may need to change or adjust the dosage of the medicines you are taking.

Other Undesired Effects: LONITEN Tablets can cause other undesired effects such as nausea and/or vomiting that are annoying but not dangerous. Do not stop taking the drug because of these other undesired effects without talking to your doctor.

Hair growth: About 8 out of every 10 patients who have taken LONITEN noticed that fine **body hair grew darker or longer** on certain parts of the body. This happened about three to six weeks after beginning treatment. The hair may first be noticed on the forehead and temples, between the eyebrows, or on the upper part of the cheeks. Later, hair may grow on the back, arms, legs, or scalp. Although hair growth may not be noticeable to some patients, it often is bothersome in women and children. **Unwanted hair can be controlled with a hair remover or by shaving.** The extra hair is not permanent, it disappears within 1 to 6 months of stopping LONITEN. Nevertheless, **you should not stop taking LONITEN without first talking to your doctor.**

A few patients have developed a rash or breast tenderness while taking LONITEN Tablets (minoxidil), but this is unusual.

Code 810 384 106

Shown in Product Identification Section, page 441

MAOLATE® R
brand of chlorphenesin carbamate tablets

500's
NSN 6505-00-998-7143A (M & VA)
How Supplied: Scored tablets containing 400 mg chlorphenesin carbamate are available in the following packages.

	Bottles of 50	NDC 0009-0412-01
	Bottles of 500	NDC 0009-0412-02
	Unit dose package (100)	NDC 0009-0412-03

Shown in Product Identification Section, page 441

Continued on next page

Information on these Upjohn products is based on labeling in effect on November 30, 1984. Further information concerning these and other Upjohn products may be obtained from the package insert or by direct inquiry to Medical Information, The Upjohn Company, Kalamazoo, Michigan 49001.

Upjohn—Cont.

MEDROL®
brand of methylprednisolone acetate topical
For External Use Only

How Supplied: In two concentrations-2.5 mg (0.25%) or 10 mg (1.0%) methylprednisolone acetate per gram.

0.25%	7.5 gram tubes	NDC 0009-0483-01
	30 gram tubes	NDC 0009-0483-02
1%	7.5 gram tubes	NDC 0009-0505-01
	30 gram tubes	NDC 0009-0505-02

MEDROL®
brand of methylprednisolone tablets, USP
4 mg (500's):
NSN 6505-00-050-3068A (VA)
16 mg (50's):
NSN 6505-00-764-4358A (VA)

Description: MEDROL Tablets contain methylprednisolone which is a glucocorticord. Glucocorticoids are adrenocortical steroids, both naturally occurring and synthetic, which are readily absorbed from the gastrointestinal tract. Methylpredniso- lone occurs as a white to practically white, odorless, crystalline powder. It is sparingly soluble in alcohol, in dioxane, and in methanol, slightly soluble in acetone, and in chloroform, and very slightly soluble in ether. It is practically insoluble in water.

The chemical name for methylprednisolone is pregna-1, 4-diene-3, 20-dione,11, 17, 21-trihydroxy-6-methyl-,(6α, 11β)- and the molecular weight is 374.48.

MEDROL Tablets (methylprednisolone) are available as scored tablets in the following strengths: 2 mg, 4 mg, 8 mg, 16 mg, 24 mg, 32 mg.

Actions: Naturally occurring glucocorticoids (hydrocortisone and cortisone), which also have salt-retaining properties, are used as replacement therapy in adrenocortical deficiency states. Their synthetic analogs are primarily used for their potent anti-inflammatory effects in disorders of many organ systems.

Glucocorticoids cause profound and varied metabolic effects. In addition, they modify the body's immune responses to diverse stimuli.

Indications: MEDROL Tablets (methylprednisolone) are indicated in the following conditions:

1. **Endocrine Disorders**
   Primary or secondary adrenocortical insufficiency (hydrocortisone or cortisone is the first choice; synthetic analogs may be used in conjunction with mineralocorticoids where applicable; in infancy mineralocorticoid supplementation is of particular importance).
   Congenital adrenal hyperplasia
   Nonsuppurative thyroiditis
   Hypercalcemia associated with cancer
2. **Rheumatic Disorders**
   As adjunctive therapy for short-term administration (to tide the patient over an acute episode or exacerbation) in:
   Psoriatic arthritis
   Rheumatoid arthritis, including juvenile rheumatoid arthritis (selected cases may require low-dose maintenance therapy)
   Ankylosing spondylitis
   Acute and subacute bursitis
   Acute nonspecific tenosynovitis
   Acute gouty arthritis
   Post-traumatic osteoarthritis
   Synovitis of osteoarthritis
   Epicondylitis
3. **Collagen Diseases**
   During an exacerbation or as maintenance therapy in selected cases of:
   Systemic lupus erythematosus
   Acute rheumatic carditis
   Systemic dermatomyositis (polymyositis)
4. **Dermatologic Diseases**
   Pemphigus
   Bullous dermatitis herpetiformis
   Severe erythema multiforme (Stevens-Johnson syndrome)
   Exfoliative dermatitis
   Mycosis fungoides
   Severe psoriasis
   Severe seborrheic dermatitis
5. **Allergic States**
   Control of severe or incapacitating allergic conditions intractable to adequate trials of conventional treatment:
   Seasonal or perennial allergic rhinitis
   Serum sickness
   Bronchial asthma
   Drug hypersensitivity reactions
   Contact dermatitis
   Atopic dermatitis
6. **Ophthalmic Diseases**
   Severe acute and chronic allergic and inflammatory processes involving the eye and its adnexa such as:
   Allergic corneal marginal ulcers
   Herpes zoster ophthalmicus
   Anterior segment inflammation
   Diffuse posterior uveitis and choroiditis
   Sympathetic ophthalmia
   Allergic conjunctivitis
   Keratitis
   Chorioretinitis
   Optic neuritis
   Iritis and iridocyclitis
7. **Respiratory Diseases**
   Symptomatic sarcoidosis
   Loeffler's syndrome not manageable by other means
   Berylliosis
   Fulminating or disseminated pulmonary tuberculosis when used concurrently with appropriate antituberculous chemotherapy
   Aspiration pneumonitis
8. **Hematologic Disorders**
   Idiopathic thrombocytopenic purpura in adults
   Secondary thrombocytopenia in adults
   Acquired (autoimmune) hemolytic anemia
   Erythroblastopenia (RBC anemia)
   Congenital (erythroid) hypoplastic anemia
9. **Neoplastic Diseases**
   For palliative management of:
   Leukemias and lymphomas in adults
   Acute leukemia of childhood
10. **Edematous States**
    To induce a diuresis or remission of proteinuria in the nephrotic syndrome, without uremia, of the idiopathic type or that due to lupus erythematosus.
11. **Gastrointestinal diseases**
    To tide the patient over a critical period of the disease in:
    Ulcerative colitis
    Regional enteritis
12. **Nervous System**
    Acute exacerbations of multiple sclerosis
13. **Miscellaneous**
    Tuberculous meningitis with subarachnoid block or impending block when used concurrently with appropriate antituberculous chemotherapy.
    Trichinosis with neurologic or myocardial involvement

Contraindications: Systemic fungal infections.
Warnings: In patients on corticosteroid therapy subjected to unusual stress, increased dosage of rapidly acting corticosteroids before, during, and after the stressful situation is indicated.

Corticosteroids may mask some signs of infection and new infections may appear during their use. There may be decreased resistance and inability to localize infection when corticosteroids are used.
Prolonged use of corticosteroids may produce posterior subcapsular cataracts, glaucoma with possible damage to the optic nerves, and may enhance the establishment of secondary ocular infections due to fungi or viruses.

Usage in pregnancy: Since adequate human reproduction studies have not been done with corticosteroids, the use of these drugs in pregnancy, nursing mothers or women of childbearing potential requires that the possible benefits of the drug be weighed against the potential hazards to the mother and embryo or fetus. Infants born of mothers who have received substantial doses of corticosteroids during pregnancy should be carefully observed for signs of hypoadrenalism.

Average and large doses of hydrocortisone or cortisone can cause elevation of blood pressure, salt and water retention, and increased excretion of potassium. These effects are less likely to occur with the synthetic derivatives except when used in large doses. Dietary salt restriction and potassium supplementation may be necessary. All corticosteroids increase calcium excretion.

While on corticosteroid therapy patients should not be vaccinated against smallpox. Other immunization procedures should not be undertaken in patients who are on corticosteroids, especially on high dose, because of possible hazards of neurological complications and a lack of antibody response.

The use of MEDROL Tablets (methylprednisolone) in active tuberculosis should be restricted to those cases of fulminating or disseminated tuberculosis in which the corticosteroid is used for the management of the disease in conjunction with an appropriate antituberculous regimen.

If corticosteroids are indicated in patients with latent tuberculosis or tuberculin reactivity, close observation is necessary as reactivation of the disease may occur. During prolonged corticosteroid therapy, these patients should receive chemoprophylaxis.

Precautions: Drug-induced secondary adrenocortical insufficiency may be minimized by gradual reduction of dosage. This type of relative insufficiency may persist for months after discontinuation of therapy; therefore, in any situation of stress occurring during that period, hormone therapy should be reinstituted. Since mineralocorticoid secretion may be impaired, salt and/or a mineralocorticoid should be administered concurrently.

There is an enhanced effect of corticosteroids on patients with hypothyroidism and in those with cirrhosis.

Corticosteroids should be used cautiously in patients with ocular herpes simplex because of possible corneal perforation.

The lowest possible dose of corticosteroid should be used to control the condition under treatment, and when reduction in dosage is possible, the reduction should be gradual.

Psychic derangements may appear when corticosteroids are used, ranging from euphoria, insomnia, mood swings, personality changes and severe depression, to frank psychotic manifestations. Also, existing emotional instability or psychotic tendencies may be aggravated by corticosteroids.

Aspirin should be used cautiously in conjunction with corticosteroids in hypoprothrombinemia.

Steroids should be used with caution in nonspecific ulcerative colitis, if there is a probability of impending perforation, abscess or other pyogenic infection; diverticulitis; fresh intestinal anastomoses; active or latent peptic ulcer; renal insufficiency; hypertension; osteoporosis; and myasthenia gravis.

Growth and development of infants and children on prolonged corticosteroid therapy should be carefully observed.

Although controlled clinical trials have shown corticosteroids to be effective in speeding the resolution of acute exacerbations of multiple sclerosis, they do not show that corticosteroids affect the ultimate outcome or natural history of the disease. The studies do show that relatively high doses of corticosteroids are necessary to demonstrate a significant effect. (See **Dosage and Administration**)

Since complications of treatment with glucocorticoids are dependent on the size of the dose and the duration of treatment, a risk/benefit decision must be made in each individual case as to dose and duration of treatment and as to whether daily or intermittent therapy should be used.

The 24 mg tablet contains FD&C Yellow No. 5 (tartrazine) which may cause allergic-type reactions (including bronchial asthma) in certain susceptible individuals. Although the overall incidence of FD&C Yellow No. 5 (tartrazine) sensitivity in the general population is low, it is frequently seen in patients who also have aspirin hypersensitivity.

Adverse Reactions:
Fluid and Electrolyte Disturbances
Sodium retention
Fluid retention
Congestive heart failure in susceptible patients
Potassium loss
Hypokalemic alkalosis
Hypertension

Musculoskeletal
Muscle weakness
Steroid myopathy
Loss of muscle mass
Osteoporosis
Vertebral compression fractures
Aseptic necrosis of femoral and humeral heads
Pathologic fracture of long bones

Gastrointestinal
Peptic ulcer with possible perforation and hemorrhage
Pancreatitis
Abdominal distention
Ulcerative esophagitis

Dermatologic
Impaired wound healing
Thin fragile skin
Petechiae and ecchymoses
Facial erythema
Increased sweating
May suppress reactions to skin tests

Neurological
Increased intracranial pressure with papilledema (pseudo-tumor cerebri) usually after treatment
Convulsions
Vertigo
Headache

Endocrine
Development of Cushingoid state
Suppression of growth in children
Secondary adrenocortical and pituitary unresponsiveness, particularly in times of stress, as in trauma, surgery or illness.
Menstrual irregularities
Decreased carbohydrate tolerance
Manifestations of latent diabetes mellitus
Increased requirements for insulin or oral hypoglycemic agents in diabetics

Ophthalmic
Posterior subcapsular cataracts
Increased intraocular pressure
Glaucoma
Exophthalmos

Metabolic
Negative nitrogen balance due to protein catabolism

The following additional reactions have been reported following oral as well as parenteral therapy: Urticaria and other allergic, anaphylactic or hypersensitivity reactions.

Dosage and Administration:
The initial dosage of MEDROL Tablets (methylprednisolone) may vary from 4 mg to 48 mg per day depending on the specific disease entity being treated. In situations of less severity lower doses will generally suffice while in selected patients higher initial doses may be required. The initial dosage should be maintained or adjusted until a satisfactory response is noted. If after a reasonable period of time there is a lack of satisfactory clinical response, MEDROL should be discontinued and the patient transferred to other appropriate therapy. **IT SHOULD BE EMPHASIZED THAT DOSAGE REQUIREMENTS ARE VARIABLE AND MUST BE INDIVIDUALIZED ON THE BASIS OF THE DISEASE UNDER TREATMENT AND THE RESPONSE OF THE PATIENT.** After a favorable response is noted, the proper maintenance dosage should be determined by decreasing the initial drug dosage in small decrements at appropriate time intervals until the lowest dosage which will maintain an adequate clinical response is reached. It should be kept in mind that constant monitoring is needed in regard to drug dosage. Included in the situations which may make dosage adjustments necessary are changes in clinical status secondary to remissions or exacerbations in the disease process, the patient's individual drug responsiveness, and the effect of patient exposure to stressful situations not directly related to the disease entity under treatment; in this latter situation it may be necessary to increase the dosage of MEDROL for a period of time consistent with the patient's condition. If after long-term therapy the drug is to be stopped, it is recommended that it be withdrawn gradually rather than abruptly.

Multiple Sclerosis
In treatment of acute exacerbations of multiple sclerosis daily doses of 200 mg of prednisolone for a week followed by 80 mg every other day for 1 month have been shown to be effective (4 mg of methylprednisolone is equivalent to 5 mg of prednisolone).

ADT® (Alternate Day Therapy)
Alternate day therapy is a corticosteroid dosing regimen in which twice the usual daily dose of corticoid is administered every other morning. The purpose of this mode of therapy is to provide the patient requiring long-term pharmacologic dose treatment with the beneficial effects of corticoids while minimizing certain undesirable effects, including pituitary-adrenal suppression, the Cushingoid state, corticoid withdrawal symptoms, and growth suppression in children.

The rationale for this treatment schedule is based on two major premises: (a) the anti-inflammatory or therapeutic effect of corticoids persists longer than their physical presence and metabolic effects and (b) administration of the corticosteroid every other morning allows for re-establishment of more nearly normal hypothalamic-pituitary-adrenal (HPA) activity on the off-steroid day.

A brief review of the HPA physiology may be helpful in understanding this rationale. Acting primarily through the hypothalamus a fall in free cortisol stimulates the pituitary gland to produce increasing amounts of corticotropin (ACTH) while a rise in free cortisol inhibits ACTH secretion. Normally the HPA system is characterized by diurnal (circadian) rhythm. Serum levels of ACTH rise from a low point about 10 pm to a peak level about 6 am. Increasing levels of ACTH stimulate adrenal cortical activity resulting in a rise in plasma cortisol with maximal levels occurring between 2 am and 8 am. This rise in cortisol dampens ACTH production and in turn adrenal cortical activity. There is a gradual fall in plasma corticoids during the day with lowest levels occurring about midnight.

The diurnal rhythm of the HPA axis is lost in Cushing's disease, a syndrome of adrenal cortical hyperfunction characterized by obesity with centripetal fat distribution, thinning of the skin with easy bruisability, muscle wasting with weakness, hypertension, latent diabetes, osteoporosis, electrolyte imbalance, etc. The same clinical findings of hyperadrenocorticism may be noted during long-term pharmacologic dose corticoid therapy administered in conventional daily divided doses. It would appear, then, that a disturbance in the diurnal cycle with maintenance of elevated corticoid values during the night may play a significant role in the development of undesirable corticoid effects. Escape from these constantly elevated plasma levels for even short periods of time may be instrumental in protecting against undesirable pharmacologic effects.

During conventional pharmacologic dose corticosteroid therapy, ACTH production is inhibited with subsequent suppression of cortisol production by the adrenal cortex. Recovery time for normal HPA activity is variable depending upon the dose and duration of treatment. During this time the patient is vulnerable to any stressful situation. Although it has been shown that there is considerably less adrenal suppression following a single morning dose of prednisolone (10 mg) as opposed to a quarter of that dose administered every 6 hours, there is evidence that some suppressive effect on adrenal activity may be carried over into the following day when pharmacologic doses are used. Further, it has been shown that a single dose of certain corticosteroids will produce adrenal cortical suppression for two or more days. Other corticoids, including methylprednisolone, hydrocortisone, prednisone, and prednisolone, are considered to be short acting (producing adrenal cortical suppression for $1\frac{1}{4}$ to $1\frac{1}{2}$ days following a single dose) and thus are recommended for alternate day therapy.

The following should be kept in mind when considering alternate day therapy:

1) Basic principles and indications for corticosteroid therapy should apply. The benefits of ADT should not encourage the indiscriminate use of steroids.

2) ADT is a therapeutic technique primarily designed for patients in whom long-term pharmacologic corticoid therapy is anticipated.

3) In less severe disease processes in which corticoid therapy is indicated, it may be possible to initiate treatment with ADT. More severe disease states usually will require daily divided high dose therapy for initial control of the disease process. The initial suppressive dose level should be continued until satisfactory clinical response is obtained, usually four to ten days in the case of many allergic and collagen diseases. It is important to keep the period of initial suppressive dose as brief as possible particularly when subsequent use of alternate day therapy is intended.

Once control has been established, two courses are available: (a) change to ADT and then gradually reduce the amount of corticoid given every other day *or* (b) following control of the disease process reduce the daily dose of corticoid to the lowest effective level as rapidly as possible and then change over to an alternate day schedule. Theoretically, course (a) may be preferable.

4) Because of the advantages of ADT, it may be desirable to try patients on this form of therapy who have been on daily corticoids for long periods of time (eg, patients with rheumatoid arthritis). Since these patients may already have a suppressed HPA axis, establishing them on ADT may be difficult and not always successful. However, it is recommended that regular attempts be made to change them over. It may be helpful to triple or even quadruple the daily maintenance dose and administer this every other day rather than just doubling the daily dose if difficulty is encountered. Once the patient is again controlled, an attempt should be made to reduce this dose to a minimum.

5) As indicated above, certain corticosteroids, because of their prolonged suppressive effect on adrenal activity, are not recommended for alternate day therapy (eg, dexamethasone and betamethasone).

6) The maximal activity of the adrenal cortex is between 2 am and 8 am, and it is minimal between 4 pm and midnight. Exogenous corticosteroids suppress adrenocortical activity the least, when given at the time of maximal activity (am).

7) In using ADT it is important, as in all therapeutic situations, to individualize and tailor the therapy to each patient. Complete control of symptoms will not be possible in all patients. An explanation of the benefits of ADT will help the patient to understand and tolerate the possible flare-up in symptoms which may occur in the latter part of the off-steroid day. Other symptomatic therapy may be added or increased at this time if needed.

8) In the event of an acute flare-up of the disease process, it may be necessary to return to a full suppressive daily divided corticoid dose for control.

Continued on next page

Information on these Upjohn products is based on labeling in effect on November 30, 1984. Further information concerning these and other Upjohn products may be obtained from the package insert or by direct inquiry to Medical Information, The Upjohn Company, Kalamazoo, Michigan 49001.

Upjohn—Cont.

Once control is again established alternate day therapy may be reinstituted.
9) Although many of the undesirable features of corticosteroid therapy can be minimized by ADT, as in any therapeutic situation, the physician must carefully weigh the benefit-risk ratio for each patient in whom corticoid therapy is being considered.

How Supplied:
MEDROL Tablets (methylprednisolone) are available in the following strengths and sizes:

2 mg	Bottles of 100	NDC 0009-0049-02
4 mg	Bottles of 30	NDC 0009-0056-01
	Bottles of 100	NDC 0009-0056-02
	Bottles of 500	NDC 0009-0056-03
	Unit Dose Package (100)	NDC 0009-0056-05
	Dosepak™ Unit of Use (21 tablets)	NDC 0009-0056-04
8 mg	Bottles of 25	NDC 0009-0022-01
16 mg	Bottles of 50	NDC 0009-0073-01
	ADT Pak® (14 tablets) Unit of Use	NDC 0009-0073-02
24 mg	Bottles of 25	NDC 0009-0155-01
32 mg	Bottles of 25	NDC 0009-0176-01

Code 810 487 106
Shown in Product Identification Section, page 441

MICRONASE®
brand of glyburide tablets
1.25, 2.5, and 5.0 mg

℞

Description: MICRONASE Tablets contain glyburide, which is an oral blood-glucose-lowering drug of the sulfonylurea class. Glyburide is a white, crystalline compound, formulated as MICRONASE Tablets of 1.25, 2.5, and 5 mg strengths for oral administration. The chemical name for glyburide is 1-[[p-[2-(5-chloro-o-anisamido) ethyl]phenyl]-sulfonyl]-3-cyclohexylurea and the molecular weight is 493.99.

Clinical Pharmacology:
Actions
Glyburide appears to lower the blood glucose acutely by stimulating the release of insulin from the pancreas, an effect dependent upon functioning beta cells in the pancreatic islets. The mechanism by which glyburide lowers blood glucose during long-term administration has not been clearly established. With chronic administration in Type II diabetic patients, the blood glucose lowering effect persists despite a gradual decline in the insulin secretory response to the drug. Extrapancreatic effects may be involved in the mechanism of action of oral sulfonylurea hypoglycemic drugs. Some patients who are initially responsive to oral hypoglycemic drugs, including MICRONASE Tablets (glyburide), may become unresponsive or poorly responsive over time. Alternatively, MICRONASE may be effective in some patients who have become unresponsive to one or more other sulfonylurea drugs.

In addition to its blood glucose lowering actions, glyburide produces a mild diuresis by enhancement of renal free water clearance. Disulfiram-like reactions have very rarely been reported in patients treated with MICRONASE Tablets.

Pharmacokinetics
Single dose studies with MICRONASE Tablets in normal subjects demonstrate significant absorption of glyburide within one hour, peak drug levels at about four hours, and low but detectable levels at twenty-four hours. Mean serum levels of glyburide, as reflected by areas under the serum concentration-time curve, increase in proportion to corresponding increases in dose. Multiple dose studies with MICRONASE in diabetic patients demonstrate drug level concentration-time curves similar to single dose studies, indicating no buildup of drug in tissue depots. The decrease of glyburide in the serum of normal healthy individuals is biphasic; the terminal half-life is about 10 hours. In single dose studies in fasting normal subjects, the degree and duration of blood glucose lowering is proportional to the dose administered and to the area under the drug level concentration-time curve. The blood glucose lowering effect persists for 24 hours following single morning doses in non-fasting diabetic patients. Under conditions of repeated administration in diabetic patients, however, there is no reliable correlation between blood drug levels and fasting blood glucose levels. A one year study of diabetic patients treated with MICRONASE showed no reliable correlation between administered dose and serum drug level.

The major metabolite of glyburide is the 4-trans-hydroxy derivative. A second metabolite, the 3-cis-hydroxy derivative, also occurs. These metabolites probably contribute no significant hypoglycemic action in humans since they are only weakly active (1/400th and 1/40th as active, respectively, as glyburide) in rabbits.

Glyburide is excreted as metabolites in the bile and urine, approximately 50% by each route. This dual excretory pathway is qualitatively different from that of other sulfonylureas, which are excreted primarily in the urine.

Sulfonylurea drugs are extensively bound to serum proteins. Displacement from protein binding sites by other drugs may lead to enhanced hypoglycemic action. *In vitro*, the protein binding exhibited by glyburide is predominantly non-ionic, whereas that of other sulfonylureas (chlorpropamide, tolbutamide, tolazamide) is predominantly ionic. Acidic drugs such as phenylbutazone, warfarin, and salicylates displace the ionic-binding sulfonylureas from serum proteins to a far greater extent than the non-ionic binding glyburide. It has not been shown that this difference in protein binding will result in fewer drug-drug interactions with MICRONASE Tablets in clinical use.

Indications and Usage: MICRONASE Tablets (glyburide) are indicated as an adjunct to diet to lower the blood glucose in patients with non-insulin-dependent diabetes mellitus (type II) whose hyperglycemia cannot be satisfactorily controlled by diet alone.

In initiating treatment for non-insulin-dependent diabetes, diet should be emphasized as the primary form of treatment. Caloric restriction and weight loss are essential in the obese diabetic patient. Proper dietary management alone may be effective in controlling the blood glucose and symptoms of hyperglycemia. The importance of regular physical activity should also be stressed, and cardiovascular risk factors should be identified and corrective measures taken where possible. If this treatment program fails to reduce symptoms and /or blood glucose, the use of an oral sulfonylurea or insulin should be considered. Use of MICRONASE must be viewed by both the physician and patient as a treatment in addition to diet and not as a substitution or as a convenient mechanism for avoiding dietary restraint. Furthermore, loss of blood glucose control on diet alone may be transient, thus requiring only short-term administration of MICRONASE.

During maintenance programs, MICRONASE should be discontinued if satisfactory lowering of blood glucose is no longer achieved. Judgment should be based on regular clinical and laboratory evaluations.

In considering the use of MICRONASE in asymptomatic patients, it should be recognized that controlling blood glucose in non-insulin-dependent diabetes has not been definitely established to be effective in preventing the long-term cardiovascular or neural complications of diabetes.

Contraindications: MICRONASE Tablets (glyburide) are contraindicated in patients with:
1. Known hypersensitivity or allergy to the drug.
2. Diabetic ketoacidosis, with or without coma. This condition should be treated with insulin.
3. Type I diabetes mellitus, as sole therapy.

Special Warning on Increased Risk of Cardiovascular Mortality: The administration of oral hypoglycemic drugs has been reported to be associated with increased cardiovascular mortality as compared to treatment with diet alone or diet plus insulin. This warning is based on the study conducted by the University Group Diabetes Program (UGDP), a long-term prospective clinical trial designed to evaluate the effectiveness of glucose-lowering drugs in preventing or delaying vascular complications in patients with non-insulin-dependent diabetes. The study involved 823 patients who were randomly assigned to one of four treatment groups (*Diabetes*, 19 (Suppl. 2):747–830, 1970).

UGDP reported that patients treated for 5 to 8 years with diet plus a fixed dose of tolbutamide (1.5 grams per day) had a rate of cardiovascular mortality approximately 2½ times that of patients treated with diet alone. A significant increase in total mortality was not observed, but the use of tolbutamide was discontinued based on the increase in cardiovascular mortality, thus limiting the opportunity for the study to show an increase in overall mortality. Despite controversy regarding the interpretation of these results, the findings of the UGDP study provide an adequate basis for this warning. The patient should be informed of the potential risks and advantages of MICRONASE and of alternative modes of therapy.

Although only one drug in the sulfonylurea class (tolbutamide) was included in this study, it is prudent from a safety standpoint to consider that this warning may also apply to other oral hypoglycemic drugs in this class, in view of their close similarities in mode of action and chemical structure.

Precautions:
General
Hypoglycemia: All sulfonylureas are capable of producing severe hypoglycemia. Proper patient selection and dosage and instructions are important to avoid hypoglycemic episodes. Renal or hepatic insufficiency may cause elevated drug levels of glyburide and the latter may also diminish gluconeogenic capacity, both of which increase the risk of serious hypoglycemic reactions. Elderly, debilitated or malnourished patients, and those with adrenal or pituitary insufficiency, are particularly susceptible to the hypoglycemic action of glucose-lowering drugs. Hypoglycemia may be difficult to recognize in the elderly and in people who are taking beta-adrenergic blocking drugs. Hypoglycemia is more likely to occur when caloric intake is deficient, after severe or prolonged exercise, when alcohol is ingested, or when more than one glucose lowering drug is used.

Loss of Control of Blood Glucose: When a patient stabilized on any diabetic regimen is exposed to stress such as fever, trauma, infection or surgery, a loss of control may occur. At such times it may be necessary to discontinue MICRONASE Tablets (glyburide) and administer insulin.

The effectiveness of any hypoglycemic drug, including MICRONASE, in lowering blood glucose to a desired level decreases in many patients over a period of time which may be due to progression of the severity of diabetes or to diminished responsiveness to the drug. This phenomenon is known as secondary failure, to distinguish it from primary failure in which the drug is ineffective in an individual patient when MICRONASE is first given. Adequate adjustment of dose and adherence to diet should be assessed before classifying a patient as a secondary failure.

Information for Patients: Patients should be informed of the potential risks and advantages of MICRONASE and of alternative modes of therapy. They also should be informed about the importance of adherence to dietary instructions, of a regular exercise program, and of regular testing of urine and/or blood glucose.

The risks of hypoglycemia, its symptoms and treatment, and conditions that predispose to its development should be explained to patients and responsible family members. Primary and secondary failure also should be explained.

Laboratory Tests
Therapeutic response to MICRONASE Tablets should be monitored by frequent urine glucose tests and periodic blood glucose tests. Measurement of glycosylated hemoglobin levels may be helpful in some patients.

Drug Interactions
The hypoglycemic action of sulfonylureas may be potentiated by certain drugs including nonsteroidal anti-inflammatory agents and other drugs that

are highly protein bound, salicylates, sulfonamides, chloramphenicol, probenecid, coumarins, monoamine oxidase inhibitors, and beta adrenergic blocking agents. When such drugs are administered to a patient receiving MICRONASE, the patient should be observed closely for hypoglycemia. When such drugs are withdrawn from a patient receiving MICRONASE, the patient should be observed closely for loss of control.

Certain drugs tend to produce hyperglycemia and may lead to loss of control. These drugs include the thiazides and other diuretics, corticosteroids, phenothiazines, thyroid products, estrogens, oral contraceptives, phenytoin, nicotinic acid, sympathomimetics, calcium channel blocking drugs, and isoniazid. When such drugs are administered to a patient receiving MICRONASE, the patient should be closely observed for loss of control. When such drugs are withdrawn from a patient receiving MICRONASE, the patient should be observed closely for hypoglycemia.

Carcinogenesis, Mutagenesis, and Impairment of Fertility

Studies in rats at doses to 300 mg/kg/day for 18 months showed no carcinogenic effects. Glyburide is non-mutagenic when studied in the Salmonella microsome test (Ames test) and in the DNA damage/alkaline elution assay.

Pregnancy

Teratogenic Effects: Pregnancy Category B Reproduction studies have been performed in rats and rabbits at doses up to 500 times the human dose and have revealed no evidence of impaired fertility or harm to the fetus due to glyburide. There are, however, no adequate and well controlled studies in pregnant women. Because animal reproduction studies are not always predictive of human response, this drug should be used during pregnancy only if clearly needed.

Because recent information suggests that abnormal blood glucose levels during pregnancy are associated with a higher incidence of congenital abnormalities, many experts recommend that insulin be used during pregnancy to maintain blood glucose as close to normal as possible.

Nonteratogenic Effects: Prolonged severe hypoglycemia (4 to 10 days) has been reported in neonates born to mothers who were receiving a sulfonylurea drug at the time of delivery. This has been reported more frequently with the use of agents with prolonged half-lives. If MICRONASE is used during pregnancy, it should be discontinued at least two weeks before the expected delivery date.

Nursing Mothers

Although it is not known whether glyburide is excreted in human milk, some sulfonylurea drugs are known to be excreted in human milk. Because the potential for hypoglycemia in nursing infants may exist, a decision should be made whether to discontinue nursing or to discontinue the drug, taking into account the importance of the drug to the mother. If the drug is discontinued, and if diet alone is inadequate for controlling blood glucose, insulin therapy should be considered.

Pediatric Use

Safety and effectiveness in children have not been established.

Adverse Reactions:

Hypoglycemia: See Precautions and Overdosage Sections.

Gastrointestinal Reactions: Cholestatic jaundice may occur rarely; MICRONASE Tablets (glyburide) should be discontinued if this occurs.

Gastrointestinal disturbances, e.g., nausea, epigastric fullness, and heartburn are the most common reactions, having occurred in 1.8% of treated patients during clinical trials. They tend to be dose related and may disappear when dosage is reduced.

Dermatologic Reactions: Allergic skin reactions, e.g., pruritus, erythema, urticaria, and morbilliform or maculopapular eruptions occurred in 1.5% of treated patients during clinical trials. These may be transient and may disappear despite continued use of MICRONASE; if skin reactions persist, the drug should be discontinued.

Porphyria cutanea tarda and photosensitivity reactions have been reported with sulfonylureas.

Hematologic Reactions: Leukopenia, agranulocytosis, thrombocytopenia, hemolytic anemia, aplastic anemia, and pancytopenia have been reported with sulfonylureas.

Metabolic Reactions: Hepatic porphyria and disulfiram-like reactions have been reported with sulfonylureas; however, hepatic porphyria has not been reported with MICRONASE and disulfiram-like reactions have been reported very rarely.

Overdosage: Overdosage of sulfonylureas, including MICRONASE Tablets (glyburide), can produce hypoglycemia. Mild hypoglycemic symptoms, without loss of consciousness or neurological findings, should be treated aggressively with oral glucose and adjustments in drug dosage and/or meal patterns. Close monitoring should continue until the physician is assured that the patient is out of danger. Severe hypoglycemic reactions with coma, seizure, or other neurological impairment occur infrequently, but constitute medical emergencies requiring immediate hospitalization. If hypoglycemic coma is diagnosed or suspected, the patient should be given a rapid intravenous injection of concentrated (50%) glucose solution. This should be followed by a continuous infusion of a more dilute (10%) glucose solution at a rate which will maintain the blood glucose at a level above 100 mg/dL. Patients should be closely monitored for a minimum of 24 to 48 hours, since hypoglycemia may recur after apparent clinical recovery.

Dosage and Administration: There is no fixed dosage regimen for the management of diabetes mellitus with MICRONASE Tablets (glyburide) or any other hypoglycemic agent. In addition to the usual monitoring of urinary glucose, the patient's blood glucose must also be monitored periodically to determine the minimum effective dose for the patient; to detect primary failure, i.e., inadequate lowering of blood glucose at the maximum recommended dose of medication; and to detect secondary failure, i.e., loss of adequate blood glucose lowering response after an initial period of effectiveness. Glycosylated hemoglobin levels may also be of value in monitoring the patient's response to therapy.

Short-term administration of MICRONASE may be sufficient during periods of transient loss of control in patients usually controlled well on diet.

Usual Starting Dose

The usual starting dose of MICRONASE Tablets is 2.5 to 5.0 mg daily, administered with breakfast or the first main meal. Those patients who may be more sensitive to hypoglycemic drugs should be started at 1.25 mg daily. (See Precautions Sections for patients at increased risk.) Failure to follow an appropriate dosage regimen may precipitate hypoglycemia. Patients who do not adhere to their prescribed dietary and drug regimen are more prone to exhibit unsatisfactory response to therapy.

Transfer From Other Hypoglycemic Therapy

Patients Receiving Other Oral Antidiabetic Therapy: Transfer of patients from other oral antidiabetic regimens to MICRONASE should be done conservatively and the initial daily dose should be 2.5 to 5 mg. When transferring patients from oral hypoglycemic agents other than chlorpropamide to MICRONASE, no transition period and no initial or priming dose are necessary. When transferring patients from chlorpropamide, particular care should be exercised during the first two weeks because the prolonged retention of chlorpropamide in the body and subsequent overlapping drug effects may provoke hypoglycemia.

Patients Receiving Insulin: Some type II diabetic patients being treated with insulin may respond satisfactorily to MICRONASE. If the insulin dose is less than 20 units daily, substitution of MICRONASE Tablets 2.5 to 5.0 mg as a single daily dose may be tried. If the insulin dose is between 20 and 40 units daily, the patient may be placed directly on MICRONASE Tablets 5.0 mg daily as a single dose. If the insulin dose is more than 40 units daily, a transition period is required for conversion to MICRONASE. In these patients, insulin dosage is decreased by 50% and MICRONASE Tablets 5 mg daily is started. Please refer to Titration to Maintenance Dose for further explanation.

Titration to Maintenance Dose

The usual maintenance dose is in the range of 1.25 to 20 mg daily, which may be given as a single dose or in divided doses (See Dosage Interval Section). Dosage increases should be made in increments of no more than 2.5 mg at weekly intervals based upon the patient's blood glucose response.

No exact dosage relationship exists between MICRONASE and the other oral hypoglycemic agents. Although patients may be transferred from the maximum dose of other sulfonylureas, the maximum starting dose of 5.0 mg of MICRONASE Tablets should be observed. A maintenance dose of 5 mg of MICRONASE Tablets provides approximately the same degree of blood glucose control as 250 to 375 mg chlorpropamide, 250 to 375 mg tolazamide, 500 to 750 mg acetohexamide, or 1000 to 1500 mg tolbutamide.

When transferring patients receiving more than 40 units of insulin daily, they may be started on a daily dose of MICRONASE Tablets 5 mg concomitantly with a 50% reduction in insulin dose. Progressive withdrawal of insulin and increase of MICRONASE in increments of 1.25 to 2.5 mg every 2 to 10 days is then carried out. During this conversion period when both insulin and MICRONASE are being used, hypoglycemia may rarely occur. During insulin withdrawal, patients should test their urine for glucose and acetone at least three times daily and report results to their physician. The appearance of persistent acetonuria with glycosuria indicates that the patient is a type I diabetic who requires insulin therapy.

Maximum Dose

Daily doses of more than 20 mg are not recommended.

Dosage Interval

Once-a-day therapy is usually satisfactory. Some patients, particularly those receiving more than 10 mg daily, may have a more satisfactory response with twice-a-day dosage.

Specific Patient Populations

MICRONASE is not recommended for use in pregnancy or for use in children.

In elderly patients, debilitated or malnourished patients, and patients with impaired renal or hepatic function, the initial and maintenance dosing should be conservative to avoid hypoglycemic reactions. (See Precautions Section.)

How Supplied: MICRONASE Tablets (glyburide), scored, are available in the following strengths, colors and sizes:

1.25 mg	White NDC 0009-0131-01	Bottles of 100
2.5 mg	Dark Pink NDC 0009-0141-01	Bottles of 100
5.0 mg	Blue NDC 0009-0171-01	Bottles of 100
5.0 mg	Blue NDC 0009-0171-02	Bottles of 500

Caution: Federal law prohibits dispensing without prescription. Store at controlled room temperature 15°–30° C (59°–86° F). Dispensed in well closed containers with safety closures. Keep container tightly closed.

Code 811 985 000

Shown in Product Identification Section, page 441

Continued on next page

Information on these Upjohn products is based on labeling in effect on November 30, 1984. Further information concerning these and other Upjohn products may be obtained from the package insert or by direct inquiry to Medical Information, The Upjohn Company, Kalamazoo, Michigan 49001.

Upjohn—Cont.

MOTRIN®
brand of ibuprofen tablets, USP
400 mg, Unit Dose, 100's
NSN 6505-01-041-6911A (VA)
600 mg, Unit of Use, 90's
NSN 6505-01-135-9655 (M & VA)
600 mg, 500's
NSN 6505-01-098-0247A (M & VA)

Description: MOTRIN Tablets contain the active ingredient ibuprofen, which is $(\pm)$-2-(p-isobutylphenyl) propionic acid. Ibuprofen is a white powder with a melting point of 74–77°C and is very slightly soluble in water (<1 mg/ml) and readily soluble in organic solvents such as ethanol and acetone.

MOTRIN, a nonsteroidal anti-inflammatory agent, is available in 300, 400 and 600 mg tablets for oral administration.

Clinical Pharmacology: MOTRIN Tablets contain ibuprofen which possesses analgesic and antipyretic activities. Its mode of action, like that of other nonsteroidal anti-inflammatory agents, is not completely understood, but may be related to prostaglandin synthetase inhibition. MOTRIN does not alter the course of the underlying disease.

In patients treated with MOTRIN for rheumatoid arthritis and osteoarthritis, the anti-inflammatory action of ibuprofen has been shown by reduction in joint swelling, reduction in pain, reduction in duration of morning stiffness, reduction in disease activity as assessed by both the investigator and patient; and by improved functional capacity as demonstrated by an increase in grip strength, a delay in the time to onset of fatigue, and a decrease in time to walk 50 feet.

In clinical studies in patients with rheumatoid arthritis and osteoarthritis, MOTRIN has been shown to be comparable to aspirin in controlling the aforementioned signs and symptoms of disease activity and to be associated with a statistically significant reduction in the milder gastrointestinal side effects (see ADVERSE REACTIONS). MOTRIN may be well tolerated in some patients who have had gastrointestinal side effects with aspirin, but these patients when treated with MOTRIN should be carefully followed for signs and symptoms of gastrointestinal ulceration and bleeding. Although it is not definitely known whether MOTRIN causes less peptic ulceration than aspirin, in one study involving 885 patients with rheumatoid arthritis treated for up to one year, there were no reports of gastric ulceration with MOTRIN whereas frank ulceration was reported in 13 patients in the aspirin group (statistically significant $p < .001$).

In clinical studies in patients with rheumatoid arthritis, MOTRIN has been shown to be comparable to indomethacin in controlling the aforementioned signs and symptoms of disease activity and to be associated with a statistically significant reduction of the milder gastrointestinal (see ADVERSE REACTIONS) and CNS side effects.

MOTRIN may be used in combination with gold salts and/or corticosteroids. When MOTRIN and placebo were compared in gold-treated rheumatoid arthritis patients, MOTRIN was consistently more effective in relieving symptoms than was placebo. However, it cannot be inferred that MOTRIN potentiates the effect of gold on the underlying disease. Whether or not MOTRIN can be used in conjunction with partially effective doses of corticosteroid for a "steroid-sparing" effect, and result in greater improvement, has not been adequately studied.

Controlled studies have demonstrated that MOTRIN is a more effective analgesic than propoxyphene for the relief of episiotomy pain, pain following dental extraction procedures, and for the relief of the symptoms of primary dysmenorrhea.

In patients with primary dysmenorrhea, MOTRIN has been shown to reduce elevated levels of prostaglandin activity in the menstrual fluid and to reduce resting and active intrauterine pressure, as well as the frequency of uterine contractions. The probable mechanism of action is to inhibit prostaglandin synthesis rather than simply to provide analgesia.

The ibuprofen in MOTRIN is rapidly absorbed when administered orally. Peak serum ibuprofen levels are generally attained one to two hours after administration. With single doses ranging from 200 mg to 800 mg, a linear dose-response relationship exists between amount of drug administered and the integrated area under the serum drug concentration vs time curve. Above 800 mg, however, the area under the curve increases less than proportional to increases in dose. There is no evidence of drug accumulation or enzyme induction. The administration of MOTRIN Tablets either under fasting conditions or immediately before meals yields quite similar serum ibuprofen concentration-time profiles. When MOTRIN is administered immediately after a meal, there is a reduction in the rate of absorption but no appreciable decrease in the extent of absorption. The bioavailability of the drug is minimally altered by the presence of food.

A bioavailability study has shown that there was no interference with the absorption of ibuprofen when MOTRIN was given in conjunction with an antacid containing both aluminum hydroxide and magnesium hydroxide.

Ibuprofen is rapidly metabolized and eliminated in the urine. The excretion of ibuprofen is virtually complete 24 hours after the last dose. The serum half-life is 1.8 to 2.0 hours.

Studies have shown that following ingestion of the drug, 45% to 79% of the dose was recovered in the urine within 24 hours as metabolite A (25%), (+)-2-[p-(2hydroxymethylpropyl)-phenyl] propionic acid and metabolite B (37%), (+)-2-[p-(2carboxypropyl)-phenyl] propionic acid; the percentages of free and conjugated ibuprofen were approximately 1% and 14%, respectively.

Indications and Usage: MOTRIN Tablets (ibuprofen) are indicated for relief of the signs and symptoms of rheumatoid arthritis and osteoarthritis.

MOTRIN is indicated for relief of mild to moderate pain.

MOTRIN is also indicated for the treatment of primary dysmenorrhea.

Since there have been no controlled clinical trials to demonstrate whether or not there is any beneficial effect or harmful interaction with the use of MOTRIN in conjunction with aspirin, the combination cannot be recommended (see **Drug Interactions**).

Controlled clinical trials to establish the safety and effectiveness of MOTRIN in children have not been conducted.

Contraindications: MOTRIN Tablets (ibuprofen) should not be used in patients who have previously exhibited hypersensitivity to it, or in individuals with the syndrome of nasal polyps, angioedema and bronchospastic reactivity to aspirin or other nonsteroidal anti-inflammatory agents. Anaphylactoid reactions have occurred in such patients.

Warnings: Peptic ulceration and gastrointestinal bleeding, sometimes severe, have been reported in patients receiving MOTRIN Tablets (ibuprofen). Peptic ulceration, perforation, or severe gastrointestinal bleeding can have a fatal outcome, and although a few such reports have been received with MOTRIN, a cause and effect relationship has not been established. MOTRIN should be given under close supervision to patients with a history of upper gastrointestinal tract disease, and only after consulting the ADVERSE REACTIONS section.

In patients with active peptic ulcer and active rheumatoid arthritis, attempts should be made to treat the arthritis with nonulcerogenic drugs, such as gold. If MOTRIN must be given, the patient should be under close supervision for signs of ulcer perforation or gastrointestinal bleeding.

As with other nonsteroidal anti-inflammatory agents, chronic studies in rats and monkeys have shown histologic evidence of mild renal toxicity as demonstrated by papillary edema and papillary necrosis in some animals. Renal papillary necrosis has been rarely reported in humans in association with treatment with MOTRIN.

Precautions: Blurred and/or diminished vision, scotomata, and/or changes in color vision have been reported. If a patient develops such complaints while receiving MOTRIN Tablets (ibuprofen), the drug should be discontinued and the patient should have an ophthalmologic examination which includes central visual fields and color vision testing.

Fluid retention and edema have been reported in association with MOTRIN; therefore, the drug should be used with caution in patients with a history of cardiac decompensation or hypertension. Since ibuprofen is eliminated primarily by the kidneys, patients with significantly impaired renal function should be closely monitored and a reduction in dosage should be anticipated to avoid drug accumulation. Prospective studies on the safety of MOTRIN in patients with chronic renal failure have not been conducted.

MOTRIN, like other nonsteroidal anti-inflammatory agents, can inhibit platelet aggregation but the effect is quantitatively less and of shorter duration than that seen with aspirin. MOTRIN has been shown to prolong bleeding time (but within the normal range) in normal subjects. Because this prolonged bleeding effect may be exaggerated in patients with underlying hemostatic defects, MOTRIN should be used with caution in persons with intrinsic coagulation defects and those on anticoagulant therapy.

Patients on MOTRIN should report to their physicians signs or symptoms of gastrointestinal ulceration or bleeding, blurred vision or other eye symptoms, skin rash, weight gain, or edema.

In order to avoid exacerbation of disease or adrenal insufficiency, patients who have been on prolonged corticosteroid therapy should have their therapy tapered slowly rather than discontinued abruptly when MOTRIN is added to the treatment program.

The antipyretic and anti-inflammatory activity of ibuprofen may reduce fever and inflammation, thus diminishing their utility as diagnostic signs in detecting complications of presumed noninfectious noninflammatory painful conditions.

As with other nonsteroidal anti-inflammatory drugs, borderline elevations of one or more liver tests may occur in up to 15% of patients. These abnormalities may progress, may remain essentially unchanged, or may be transient with continued therapy. The SGPT (ALT) test is probably the most sensitive indicator of liver dysfunction. Meaningful (3 times the upper limit of normal) elevations of SGPT or SGOT (AST) occurred in controlled clinical trials in less than 1% of patients. A patient with symptoms and/or signs suggesting liver dysfunction, or in whom an abnormal liver test has occurred, should be evaluated for evidence of the development of more severe hepatic reaction while on therapy with MOTRIN. Severe hepatic reactions, including jaundice and cases of fatal hepatitis, have been reported with ibuprofen as with other nonsteroidal anti-inflammatory drugs. Although such reactions are rare, if abnormal liver tests persist or worsen, if clinical signs and symptoms consistent with liver disease develop, or if systemic manifestations occur (e.g., eosinophilia, rash, etc.), MOTRIN should be discontinued.

Drug Interactions

Coumarin-type anticoagulants. Several short-term controlled studies failed to show that MOTRIN significantly affected prothrombin times or a variety of other clotting factors when administered to individuals on coumarin-type anticoagulants. However, because bleeding has been reported when MOTRIN and other nonsteroidal anti-inflammatory agents have been administered to patients on coumarin-type anticoagulants, the physician should be cautious when administering MOTRIN to patients on anticoagulants.

Aspirin. Animal studies show that aspirin given with nonsteroidal anti-inflammatory agents, including MOTRIN, yields a net decrease in anti-inflammatory activity with lowered blood levels of the non-aspirin drug. Single dose bioavailability

MOTRIN

Incidence Greater than 1% (but less than 3%) Probable Causal Relationship	Precise Incidence Unknown (but less than 1%) Probable Causal Relationship**	Precise Incidence Unknown (but less than 1%) Causal Relationship Unknown**
GASTROINTESTINAL Nausea*, epigastric pain*, heartburn*, diarrhea, abdominal distress, nausea and vomiting, indigestion, constipation, abdominal cramps or pain, fullness of GI tract (bloating and flatulence)	Gastric or duodenal ulcer with bleeding and/or perforation, gastrointestinal hemorrhage, melena, gastritis, hepatitis, jaundice, abnormal liver function tests	Pancreatitis
CENTRAL NERVOUS SYSTEM Dizziness*, headache, nervousness	Depression, insomnia, confusion, emotional lability, somnolence, aseptic meningitis with fever and coma	Paresthesias, hallucinations, dream abnormalities, pseudotumor cerebri
DERMATOLOGIC Rash* (including maculopapular type), pruritis	Vesiculobullous eruptions, urticaria, erythema multiforme, Stevens-Johnson syndrome, alopecia	Toxic epidermal necrolysis, photoallergic skin reactions
SPECIAL SENSES Tinnitus	Hearing loss, amblyopia (blurred and/or diminished vision, scotomata and/or changes in color vision) (see PRECAUTIONS)	Conjunctivitis, diplopia, optic neuritis, cataracts
HEMATOLOGIC	Neutropenia, agranulocytosis, aplastic anemia, hemolytic anemia (sometimes Coombs positive), thrombocytopenia with or without purpura, eosinophilia, decreases in hemoglobin and hematocrit	Bleeding episodes (eg epistaxis, menorrhagia)
METABOLIC/ENDOCRINE Decreased appetite		Gynecomastia, hypoglycemic reaction, acidosis
CARDIOVASCULAR Edema, fluid retention (generally responds promptly to drug discontinuation; see PRECAUTIONS)	Congestive heart failure in patients with marginal cardiac function, elevated blood pressure, palpitations	Arrhythmias (sinus tachycardia, sinus bradycardia)
ALLERGIC	Syndrome of abdominal pain, fever, chills, nausea and vomiting; anaphylaxis; bronchospasm (see CONTRAINDICATIONS)	Serum sickness, lupus erythematosus syndrome, Henoch-Schönlein vasculitis, angioedema
RENAL	Acute renal failure in patients with pre-existing significantly impaired renal function, decreased creatinine clearance, polyuria, azotemia, cystitis, hematuria	Renal papillary necrosis
MISCELLANEOUS	Dry eyes and mouth, gingival ulcer, rhinitis	

* Reactions occurring in 3% to 9% of patients treated with MOTRIN. (Those reactions occurring in less than 3% of the patients are unmarked).
** Reactions are classified under "*Probable Causal Relationship (PCR)*" if there has been one positive rechallenge or if three or more cases occur which might be causally related. Reactions are classified under "*Causal Relationship Unknown*" if seven or more events have been reported but the criteria for PCR have not been met.

---

studies in normal volunteers have failed to show an effect of aspirin on ibuprofen blood levels. Correlative clinical studies have not been done.

Pregnancy
Reproductive studies conducted in rats and rabbits at doses somewhat less than the maximal clinical dose did not demonstrate evidence of developmental abnormalities. However, animal reproduction studies are not always predictive of human response. As there are no adequate and well-controlled studies in pregnant women, this drug should be used during pregnancy only if clearly needed. Because of the known effects of nonsteroidal anti-inflammatory drugs on the fetal cardiovascular system (closure of ductus arteriosus), use during late pregnancy should be avoided. As with other drugs known to inhibit prostaglandin synthesis, an increased incidence of dystocia and delayed parturition occurred in rats. Administration of MOTRIN is not recommended during pregnancy.

Nursing Mothers
In limited studies, an assay capable of detecting 1 mcg/ml did not demonstrate ibuprofen in the milk of lactating mothers. However, because of the limited nature of the studies, and the possible adverse effects of prostaglandin-inhibiting drugs on neonates, MOTRIN is not recommended for use in nursing mothers.

Adverse Reactions: The most frequent type of adverse reaction occurring with MOTRIN Tablets (ibuprofen) is gastrointestinal. In controlled clinical trials the percentage of patients reporting one or more gastrointestinal complaints ranged from 4% to 16%.

In controlled studies when MOTRIN was compared to aspirin and indomethacin in equally effective doses, the overall incidence of gastrointestinal complaints was about half that seen in either the aspirin- or indomethacin-treated patients.

Adverse reactions observed during controlled clinical trials at an incidence greater than 1% are listed in the following table. Those reactions listed in Column one encompass observations in approximately 3,000 patients. More than 500 of these patients were treated for periods of at least 54 weeks.

Still other reactions occurring less frequently than 1 in 100 were reported in controlled clinical trials and from marketing experience. These reactions have been divided into two categories: Column two of the following table lists reactions with therapy with MOTRIN where the probability of a causal relationship exists: for the reactions in Column three, a causal relationship with MOTRIN has not been established.
[See table above].

Overdosage: Approximately 1½ hours after the reported ingestion of from 7 to 10 MOTRIN Tablets (ibuprofen) (400 mg), a 19-month old child weighing 12 kg was seen in the hospital emergency room, apneic and cyanotic, responding only to painful stimuli. This type of stimulus, however, was sufficient to induce respiration. Oxygen and parenteral fluids were given; a greenish-yellow fluid was aspirated from the stomach with no evidence to indicate the presence of ibuprofen. Two hours after ingestion the child's condition seemed stable; she still responded only to painful stimuli and continued to have periods of apnea lasting from 5 to 10 seconds. She was admitted to intensive care and sodium bicarbonate was administered as well as infusions of dextrose and normal saline. By four hours post-ingestion she could be aroused easily, sit by herself and respond to spoken commands. Blood level of ibuprofen was 102.9 µg/ml approximately 8½ hours after accidental ingestion. At 12 hours she appeared to be completely recovered.

Continued on next page

Information on these Upjohn products is based on labeling in effect on November 30, 1984. Further information concerning these and other Upjohn products may be obtained from the package insert or by direct inquiry to Medical Information, The Upjohn Company, Kalamazoo, Michigan 49001.

Upjohn—Cont.

In two other reported cases where children (each weighing approximately 10 kg) had taken six tablets for an estimated acute intake of approximately 120 mg/kg, there were no signs of acute intoxication or late sequelae. Blood level in one child 90 minutes after ingestion was 700 µg/ml—about 10 times the peak levels seen in absorption-excretion studies.

A 19-year old male who had taken 8,000 mg of ibuprofen over a period of a few hours complained of dizziness, and nystagmus was noted. After hospitalization, parenteral hydration and three days' bed rest, he recovered with no reported sequelae. In cases of acute overdosage, the stomach should be emptied by vomiting or lavage, though little drug will likely be recovered if more than an hour has elapsed since ingestion. Because the drug is acidic and is excreted in the urine, it is theoretically beneficial to administer alkali and induce diuresis.

Dosage and Administration:

Do not exceed 2,400 mg total daily dose. If gastrointestinal complaints occur, administer MOTRIN Tablets (ibuprofen) with meals or milk.

Rheumatoid arthritis and osteoarthritis, including flare-ups of chronic disease:

Suggested Dosage: 300 mg, 400 mg, or 600 mg t.i.d. or q.i.d. The dose should be tailored to each patient, and may be lowered or raised depending on the severity of symptoms either at time of initiating drug therapy or as the patient responds or fails to respond.

In general, patients with rheumatoid arthritis seem to require higher doses of MOTRIN than do patients with osteoarthritis.

The smallest dose of MOTRIN that yields acceptable control should be employed.

In chronic conditions, a therapeutic response to therapy with MOTRIN is sometimes seen in a few days to a week but most often is observed by two weeks. After a satisfactory response has been achieved, the patient's dose should be reviewed and adjusted as required.

Mild to moderate pain:

400 mg every 4 to 6 hours as necessary for relief of pain.

In controlled analgesic clinical trials, doses of MOTRIN greater than 400 mg were no more effective than the 400 mg dose.

Dysmenorrhea:

For the treatment of dysmenorrhea, beginning with the earliest onset of such pain, MOTRIN should be given in a dose of 400 mg every 4 hours as necessary for the relief of pain.

How Supplied:

MOTRIN Tablets (ibuprofen) are supplied as follows:

MOTRIN Tablets, 300 mg (white)
Unit of Use Bottles of 60   NDC 0009-0733-01
Bottles of 500   NDC 0009-0733-02

MOTRIN Tablets, 400 mg (orange)
Bottles of 500   NDC 0009-0750-02
Unit-dose package of 100   NDC 0009-0750-06
Unit of Use bottles of 100 NDC 0009-0750-25

MOTRIN Tablets, 600 mg (peach)
Unit-dose package of 100   NDC 0009-0742-05
Bottles of 500   NDC 0009-0742-02
Unit of Use bottles of 100 NDC 0009-0742-03
Code 810 015 211

* Product of The Upjohn Manufacturing Company.

MOTRIN is registered in the US Patent and Trademark Office by The Upjohn Manufacturing Company.

UPJOHN is registered in the US Patent and Trademark office by The Upjohn Company, Kalamazoo, Michigan, U.S.A.

Shown in Product Identification Section, page 441

MYCIGUENT® Antibiotic Ointment
(See PDR For Nonprescription Drugs)

MYCITRACIN® Antibiotic Ointment
(See PDR For Nonprescription Drugs)

ORINASE® ℞
brand of tolbutamide tablets, USP

Description: ORINASE Tablets contain tolbutamide, an oral blood glucose lowering drug of the sulfonylurea category. Tolbutamide is a pure white crystalline compound practically insoluble in water but forming water-soluble salts with alkalies.

The chemical names for tolbutamide are (1) Benzenesulfonamide, N-[(butylamino) carbonyl]-4-methyl; (2) 1-Butyl-3-(p-tolylsulfonyl)urea and its molecular weight is 270.35.

ORINASE Tablets for oral administration are available as scored, white tablets containing 25 mg or 500 mg tolbutamide.

Clinical Pharmacology:
Actions

Tolbutamide appears to lower blood glucose acutely by stimulating the release of insulin from the pancreas, an effect dependent upon functioning beta cells in the pancreatic islets. The mechanism by which tolbutamide lowers blood glucose during long-term administration has not been clearly established. With chronic administration in Type II diabetic patients, the blood glucose lowering effect persists despite a gradual decline in the insulin secretory response to the drug. Extrapancreatic effects may be involved in the mechanism of action of oral sulfonylurea hypoglycemic drugs.

Some patients who are initially responsive to oral hypoglycemic drugs, including ORINASE, may become unresponsive or poorly responsive over time. Alternatively, ORINASE may be effective in some patients who have become unresponsive to one or more other sulfonylurea drugs.

Pharmacokinetics

When administered orally, the tolbutamide in ORINASE Tablets is readily absorbed from the gastrointestinal tract. Absorption is not impaired and glucose lowering and insulin releasing effects are not altered if the drug is taken with food. Detectable levels are present in the plasma within twenty minutes after oral ingestion of a 500 mg ORINASE Tablet, with peak levels occurring at three to four hours and only small amounts detectable at 24 hours. The half-life of tolbutamide is 4.5 to 6.5 hours. As tolbutamide has no p-amino group, it cannot be acetylated, which is one of the common modes of metabolic degradation for the antibacterial sulfonamides. However, the presence of the p-methyl group renders tolbutamide susceptible to oxidation, and this appears to be the principal manner of its metabolic degradation in man. The p-methyl group is oxidized to form a carboxyl group, converting tolbutamide into the totally inactive metabolite 1-butyl-3-p-carboxy-phenylsulfonylurea, which can be recovered in the urine within 24 hours in amounts accounting for up to 75% of the administered dose.

The major tolbutamide metabolite has been found to have no hypoglycemic or other action when administered orally and IV to both normal and diabetic subjects. This tolbutamide metabolite is highly soluble over the critical acid range of urinary pH values, and its solubility increases with increase in pH. Because of the marked solubility of the tolbutamide metabolite, crystalluria does not occur. A second metabolite, 1-butyl-3-(p-hydroxymethyl) phenyl sulfonylurea also occurs to a limited extent. It is an inactive metabolite.

The administration of 3 grams of tolbutamide to either nondiabetic or tolbutamide-responsive diabetic subjects will, in both instances, occasion a gradual lowering of blood glucose. Increasing the dose to 6 grams does not usually cause a response which is significantly different from that produced by the 3 gram dose. Following the administration of a 3 gram dose of ORINASE solution, nondiabetic fasting adults exhibit a 30% or greater reduction in blood glucose within one hour, following which the blood glucose gradually returns to the fasting level over six to twelve hours. Following the administration of a 3 gram dose of ORINASE solution, tolbutamide responsive diabetic patients show a gradually progressive blood glucose lowering effect, the maximal response being reached between five to eight hours after ingestion of a single 3 gram dose. The blood glucose then rises gradually and by the 24th hour has usually returned to pretest levels. The magnitude of the reduction, when expressed in terms of precent of the protest blood glucose, tends to be similar to the response seen in the nondiabetic subject.

Indications and Usage: ORINASE Tablets (tolbutamide) are indicated as an adjunct to diet to lower the blood glucose in patients with noninsulin-dependent diabetes whose hyperglycemia cannot be satisfactorily controlled by diet alone. In initiating treatment for noninsulin-dependent diabetes, diet should be emphasized as the primary form of treatment. Caloric restriction and weight loss are essential in the obese diabetic patient. Proper dietary management alone may be effective in controlling the blood glucose and symptoms of hyperglycemia. The importance of regular physical activity should also be stressed and cardiovascular risk factors should be identified and corrective measures taken where possible.

If this treatment program fails to reduce symptoms and/or blood glucose, the use of an oral sulfonylurea or insulin should be considered. The use of ORINASE must be viewed by both the physician and patient as a treatment in addition to diet, and not as a substitute for diet or as a convenient mechanism for avoiding dietary restraint. Furthermore, loss of blood glucose control on diet alone may be transient, thus requiring only short-term administration of ORINASE.

During maintenance programs, ORINASE should be discontinued if satisfactory lowering of blood glucose is no longer achieved. Judgments should be based on regular clinical and laboratory evaluations.

In considering the use of ORINASE in asymptomatic patients, it should be recognized that controlling the blood glucose in noninsulin-dependent diabetes has not been definitely established to be effective in preventing the long-term cardiovascular or neural complications of diabetes.

Contraindications: ORINASE Tablets (tolbutamide) are contraindicated in patients with: 1) known hypersensitivity or allergy to ORINASE; 2) diabetic ketoacidosis, with or without coma. This condition should be treated with insulin. 3) Type I diabetes, as sole therapy.

Special Warning on Increased Risk of Cardiovascular Mortality: The administration of oral hypoglycemic drugs has been reported to be associated with increased cardiovascular mortality as compared to treatment with diet alone or diet plus insulin. This warning is based on the study conducted by the University Group Diabetes Program (UGDP), a long-term prospective clinical trial designed to evaluate the effectiveness of glucose-lowering drugs in preventing or delaying vascular complications in patients with noninsulin-dependent diabetes. The study involved 823 patients who were randomly assigned to one of four treatment groups (Diabetes, 19 (supp. 2):747-830, 1970.)

UGDP reported that patients treated for five to eight years with diet plus a fixed dose of tolbutamide (1.5 grams per day) had a rate of cardiovascular mortality approximately 2½ times that of patients with diet alone. A significant increase in total mortality was not observed, but the use of tolbutamide was discontinued based on the increase in cardiovascular mortality, thus limiting the opportunity for the study to show an increase in overall mortality. Despite controversy regarding the interpretation of these results, the findings of the UGDP study provide an adequate basis for this warning. The patient should be informed of the potential risks and advantages of ORINASE and of alternative modes of therapy.

Although only one drug in the sulfonylurea class (tolbutamide) was included in this study, it is prudent from a safety standpoint to consider that this warning may also apply to other oral hypoglycemic drugs in this class, in view of their close similarities in mode of action and chemical structure.

Precautions:

General

Hypoglycemia—All sulfonylurea drugs are capable of producing severe hypoglycemia. Proper patient selection and dosage and instructions are important to avoid hypoglycemic episodes. Renal or hepatic insufficiency may cause elevated blood levels of ORINASE Tablets (tolbutamide) and the latter may also diminish gluconeogenic capacity, both of which increase the risk of serious hypoglycemic reactions. Elderly, debilitated or malnourished patients and those with adrenal or pituitary insufficiency are particularly susceptible to the hypoglycemic action of glucose lowering drugs. Hypoglycemia may be difficult to recognize in the elderly and people who are taking beta-adrenergic blocking drugs. Hypoglycemia is more likely to occur when caloric intake is deficient, after severe or prolonged exercise, or when more than one glucose lowering drug is used.

Loss of Control of Blood Glucose—When a patient stabilized on any diabetic regimen is exposed to stress such as fever, trauma, infection, or surgery, loss of blood glucose control may occur. At such times it may be necessary to discontinue ORINASE and administer insulin.

The effectiveness of any hypoglycemic drug, including ORINASE, in lowering blood glucose to a desired level decreases in patients over a period of time, which may be due to progression of the severity of the diabetes or to diminished responsiveness to the drug. This phenomenon is known as secondary drug failure to distinguish it from primary failure in which the drug is ineffective in an individual patient when first given. Adequate adjustment of dose and adherence to diet should be assessed before classifying a patient as a secondary failure.

Information for Patients

Patients should be informed of the potential risks and advantages of ORINASE Tablets (tolbutamide) and of alternative modes of therapy. They should also be informed about the importance of adherence to dietary instructions, of a regular exercise program, and of regular testing of urine and/or blood glucose.

The risks of hypoglycemia, its symptoms and treatment, and conditions that predispose to its development should be explained to patients and responsible family members. Primary and secondary failure should also be explained.

Laboratory Tests

Blood and urine glucose should be monitored periodically. Measurement of glycosylated hemoglobin may be useful in some patients.

A metabolite of tolbutamide in urine may give a false positive reaction for albumin if measured by the acidification-after-boiling test, which causes the metabolite to precipitate. There is no interference with the sulfosalicylic acid test.

Drug Interactions

The hypoglycemic action of sulfonylureas may be potentiated by certain drugs including nonsteroidal anti-inflammatory agents and other drugs that are highly protein bound, salicylates, sulfonamides, chloramphenicol, probenecid, coumarins, monoamine oxidase inhibitors, and beta adrenergic blocking agents. When such drugs are administered to a patient receiving ORINASE, the patient should be closely observed for hypoglycemia. When such drugs are withdrawn from a patient receiving ORINASE, the patient should be observed closely for loss of control.

Certain drugs tend to produce hyperglycemia and may lead to loss of control. These drugs include the thiazides and other diuretics, corticosteroids, phenothiazines, thyroid products, estrogens, oral contraceptives, phenytoin, nicotinic acid, sympathomimetics, calcium channel blocking drugs and isoniazid. When such drugs are administered to a patient receiving ORINASE, the patient should be closely observed for loss of control of blood glucose. When such drugs are withdrawn from a patient receiving ORINASE, the patient should be observed closely for hypoglycemia.

Carcinogenesis, and Mutagenicity

Bioassay for carcinogenicity was performed in both sexes of rats and mice following ingestion of tolbutamide for 78 weeks. No evidence of carcinogenicity was found.

Tolbutamide has also been demonstrated to be nonmutagenic in the Ames salmonella/mammalian microsome mutagenicity test.

Pregnancy

Teratogenic Effects

Pregnancy Category C. ORINASE has been shown to be teratogenic in rats given in doses 25 to 100 times the human dose. In some studies, pregnant rats given high doses of tolbutamide have shown increased mortality in offspring and ocular and bony abnormalities. Repeat studies in other species (rabbits) have not demonstrated a teratogenic effect. There are no adequate and well controlled studies in pregnant women. ORINASE is not recommended for the treatment of pregnant diabetic patients. Serious consideration should also be given to the possible hazards of the use of ORINASE in women of child-bearing age and in those who might become pregnant while using the drug.

Because recent information suggests that abnormal blood glucose levels during pregnancy are associated with a higher incidence of congenital abnormalities, many experts recommend that insulin be used during pregnancy to maintain blood glucose levels as close to normal as possible.

Nonteratogenic Effects

Prolonged severe hypoglycemia (four to ten days) has been reported in neonates born to mothers who were receiving a sulfonylurea drug at the time of delivery. This has been reported more frequently with the use of agents with prolonged half lives. if ORINASE is used during pregnancy, it should be discontinued at least two weeks before the expected delivery date.

Nursing Mothers

Although it is not known whether tolbutamide is excreted in human milk, some sulfonylurea drugs are known to be excreted in human milk. Because the potential for hypoglycemia in nursing infants may exist, a decision should be made whether to discontinue nursing or to discontinue the drug, taking into account the importance of the drug to the mother. If the drug is discontinued and if diet alone is inadequate for controlling blood glucose, insulin therapy should be considered.

Pediatric Use

Safety and effectiveness in children have not been established.

Adverse Reactions:

Hypoglycemia—See **Precautions** and **Overdosage** sections.

Gastrointestinal Reactions: Cholestatic jaundice may occur rarely; ORINASE Tablets (tolbutamide) should be discontinued if this occurs. Gastrointestinal disturbances, eg, nausea, epigastric fullness, and heartburn, are the most common reactions and occurred in 1.4% of patients treated during clinical trials. They tend to be dose-related and may disappear when dosage is reduced.

Dermatologic Reactions: Allergic skin reactions, eg, pruritus, erythema, urticaria, and morbilliform or maculopapular eruptions, occurred in 1.1% of patients treated during clinical trials. These may be transient and may disappear despite continued use of ORINASE; if skin reactions persist, the drug should be discontinued.

Porphyria cutanea tarda and photosensitivity reactions have been reported with sulfonylureas.

Hematologic Reactions: Leukopenia, agranulocytosis, thrombocytopenia, hemolytic anemia, aplastic anemia, and pancytopenia have been reported with sulfonylureas.

Metabolic Reactions: Hepatic porphria and disulfiram-like reactions have been reported with sulfonylureas.

Miscellaneous Reactions: Headache and taste alterations have occasionally been reported with tolbutamide administration.

Overdosage: Overdosage of sulfonylureas, including ORINASE Tablets, can produce symptoms of hypoglycemia.

Mild hypoglycemic symptoms without loss of consciousness or neurologic findings should be treated aggressively with oral glucose and adjustments in drug dosage and/or meal patterns. Close monitoring should continue until the physician is assured the patient is out of danger. Severe hyoglycemic reactions with coma, seizure, or other neurological impairment occur infrequently but constitute medical emergencies requiring immediate hospitalization. If hypoglycemic coma is suspected or diagnosed, the patient should be given a rapid intravenous injection of concentrated (50%) glucose solution. This should be followed by a continuous infusion of a more dilute (10%) glucose solution at a rate which will maintain the blood glucose level above 100 mg/dl. Patients should be closely monitored for a minimum of 24 to 48 hours, since hypoglycemia may recur after apparent clinical recovery.

Dosage and Administration: There is no fixed dosage regimen for the management of diabetes mellitus with ORINASE Tablets (tolbutamide) or any other hypoglycemic agent. In addition to the usual monitoring of urinary glucose, the patient's blood glucose must also be monitored periodically to determine the minimum effective dose for the patient; to detect primary failure, ie, inadequate lowering of blood glucose at the maximum recommended dose of medication; and to detect secondary failure, ie, loss of adequate blood glucose response after an initial period of effectiveness. Glycosylated hemoglobin levels may also be of value in monitoring the patient's response to therapy.

Short-term administration of ORINASE may be sufficient during periods of transient loss of control in patients usually controlled well on diet.

Usual Starting Dose

The usual starting dose is 1 to 2 grams daily. This may be increased or decreased depending on individual patient response. Failure to follow an appropriate dosage regimen may precipitate hypoglycemia. Patients who do not adhere to their prescribed dietary regimens are more prone to exhibit unsatisfactory response to drug therapy.

Transfer From Other Hypoglycemic Therapy

Patients Receiving Other Oral Antidiabetic Therapy—Transfer of patients from other oral antidiabetes regimens to ORINASE should be done conservatively. When transferring patients from oral hypoglycemic agents other than chlorpropamide to ORINASE, no transition period and no initial or priming doses are necessary. When transferring patients from chlorpropamide, however, particular care should be exercised during the first two weeks because of the prolonged retention of chlorpropamide in the body and the possibility that subsequent overlapping drug effects might provoke hypoglycemia.

Patients Receiving Insulin—Patients requiring 20 units or less of insulin daily may be placed directly on ORINASE and insulin abruptly discontinued. Patients whose insulin requirement is between 20 and 40 units daily may be started on therapy with ORINASE with a concurrent 30 to 50% reduction in insulin dose, with further daily reduction of the insulin when response to tolbutamide is observed. In patients requiring more than 40 units of insulin daily, therapy with ORINASE may be initiated in conjunction with a 20% reduction in insulin dose the first day, with further careful reduction of insulin as response is observed. Occasionally, conversion to ORINASE in the hospital may be advisable in candidates who require more than 40 units of insulin daily. During this conversion period when both insulin and ORINASE are being used, hypoglycemia may rarely occur. During insulin

Continued on next page

Information on these Upjohn products is based on labeling in effect on November 30, 1984. Further information concerning these and other Upjohn products may be obtained from the package insert or by direct inquiry to Medical Information, The Upjohn Company, Kalamazoo, Michigan 49001.

Upjohn—Cont.

withdrawal, patients should test their urine for glucose and acetone at least three times daily and report results to their physician. The appearance of persistent acetonuria with glycosuria indicates that the patient is a type 1 diabetic patient who requires insulin therapy.

Maximum Dose
Daily doses of greater than 3 grams are not recommended.

Usual Maintenance Dose
The maintenance dose is in the range of 0.25 - 3 grams daily. Maintenance doses above 2 grams are seldom required.

Dosage Interval
The total daily dose may be taken either in the morning or in divided doses through the day. While either schedule is usually effective, the divided dose system is preferred by some clinicians from the standpoint of digestive tolerance.
In elderly, debilitated or malnourished patients and patients with impaired renal or hepatic function, the initial and maintenance dosing should be conservative to avoid hypoglycemic reactions (see **Precautions** section).

How Supplied: ORINASE Tablets (tolbutamide) are available in the following strengths and package size:

250 mg (scored, round, white)
Unit-of-Use bottles of 100   NDC 0009-0701-01

0.5 gram (scored, round, white)
Bottles of 200   NDC 0009-0100-02
Bottles of 500   NDC 0009-0100-03
Bottles of 1000   NDC 0009-0100-05
Unit-of-Use bottles of 50   NDC 0009-0100-01
Unit of Use bottles of 100   NDC 0009-0100-11
Unit-Dose package of 100   NDC 0009-0100-06

Store at controlled room temperature 15–30°C (59–86°F).
Code 811 646 001
Shown in Product Identification Section, page 441

PAMINE®
brand of methscopolamine bromide tablets, USP

How Supplied: Each tablet contains 2.5 mg methscopolamine bromide.
Bottles of 100   *NDC 0009-0061-01*
Bottles of 500   *NDC 0009-0061-02*

PROSTIN VR PEDIATRIC®
brand of alprostadil sterile solution
500 micrograms per ml

WARNING
Apnea is experienced by about 10 to 12% of neonates with congenital heart defects treated with PROSTIN VR PEDIATRIC Sterile Solution (alprostadil). Apnea is most often seen in neonates weighing less than 2 kg at birth and usually appears during the first hour of drug infusion. Therefore, respiratory status should be monitored throughout treatment, and PROSTIN VR PEDIATRIC should be used where ventilatory assistance is immediately available.

Description: PROSTIN VR PEDIATRIC Sterile Solution for intravascular infusion contains 500 micrograms alprostadil, more commonly known as prostaglandin E_1, in 1.0 ml dehydrated alcohol. The chemical name for alprostadil is (11α, 13E, 15S)-11,15 dihydroxy-9-oxoprost-13-en-1-oic acid, and the molecular weight is 354.49.
Alprostadil is a white to off-white crystalline powder with a melting point between 110° and 116°C. Its solubility at 35°C is 8000 micrograms per 100 ml double distilled water.

Clinical Pharmacology: Alprostadil (prostaglandin E_1) is one of a family of naturally occurring acidic lipids with various pharmacologic effects. Vasodilation, inhibition of platelet aggregation, and stimulation of intestinal and uterine smooth muscle are among the most notable of these effects. Intravenous doses of 1 to 10 micrograms of alprostadil per kilogram of body weight lower the blood pressure in mammals by decreasing peripheral resistance. Reflex increases in cardiac output and rate accompany the reduction in blood pressure.
Smooth muscle of the ductus arteriosus is especially sensitive to alprostadil, and strips of lamb ductus markedly relax in the presence of the drug. In addition, administration of alprostadil reopened the closing ductus of newborn rats, rabbits, and lambs. These observations led to the investigation of alprostadil in infants who had congenital heart defects which restricted the pulmonary or systemic blood flow and who depended on a patent ductus arteriosus for adequate blood oxygenation and lower body perfusion.
In infants with restricted pulmonary blood flow, about 50% responded to alprostadil infusion with at least a 10 torr increase in blood pO_2 (mean increase about 14 torr and mean increase in oxygen saturation about 23%). In general, patients who responded best had low pretreatment blood pO_2 and were 4 days old or less.
In infants with restricted systemic blood flow, alprostadil often increased pH in those having acidosis, increased systemic blood pressure, and decreased the ratio of pulmonary artery pressure to aortic pressure.
Alprostadil must be infused continuously because it is very rapidly metabolized. As much as 80% of the circulating alprostadil may be metabolized in one pass through the lungs, primarily by β- and ω-oxidation. The metabolites are excreted primarily by the kidney, and excretion is essentially complete within 24 hours after administration. No unchanged alprostadil has been found in the urine, and there is no evidence of tissue retention of alprostadil or its metabolites.

Indications and Usage: PROSTIN VR PEDIATRIC Sterile Solution (alprostadil) is indicated for palliative, not definitive, therapy to temporarily maintain the patency of the ductus arteriosus until corrective or palliative surgery can be performed in neonates who have congenital heart defects and who depend upon the patent ductus for survival. Such congenital heart defects include pulmonary atresia, pulmonary stenosis, tricuspid atresia, tetralogy of Fallot, interruption of the aortic arch, coarctation of the aorta, or transposition of the great vessels with or without other defects.
In infants with restricted pulmonary blood flow, the increase in blood oxygenation is inversely proportional to pretreatment pO_2 values; that is, patients with low pO_2 values respond best, and patients with pO_2 values of 40 torr or more usually have little response.
PROSTIN VR PEDIATRIC should be administered only by trained personnel in facilities that provide pediatric intensive care.

Contraindications: None.
Warnings: See WARNING box.
Note: PROSTIN VR PEDIATRIC Sterile Solution (alprostadil) must be diluted before it is administered. See dilution instructions in DOSAGE AND ADMINISTRATION section.

Precautions:
General Precautions
Cortical proliferation of the long bones, first observed in dogs, has also been observed in infants during long-term infusions of alprostadil. The cortical proliferation in infants regressed after withdrawal of the drug.
PROSTIN VR PEDIATRIC Sterile Solution (alprostadil) should be infused for the shortest time and at the lowest dose that will produce the desired effects. The risks of long-term infusion of PROSTIN VR PEDIATRIC should be weighed against the possible benefits that critically ill infants may derive from its administration.
Because alprostadil inhibits platelet aggregation, use PROSTIN VR PEDIATRIC cautiously in neonates with bleeding tendencies.
PROSTIN VR PEDIATRIC should not be used in neonates with respiratory distress syndrome. A differential diagnosis should be made between respiratory distress syndrome (hyaline membrane disease) and cyanotic heart disease (restricted pulmonary blood flow). If full diagnostic facilities are not immediately available, cyanosis (pO_2 less than 40 torr) and restricted pulmonary blood flow apparent on an X-ray are appropriate indicators of congenital heart defects.

Necessary Monitoring: In all neonates, arterial pressure should be monitored intermittently by umbilical artery catheter, auscultation, or with a Doppler transducer. *Should arterial pressure fall significantly, decrease the rate of infusion immediately.*
In infants with restricted pulmonary blood flow, measure efficacy of PROSTIN VR PEDIATRIC by monitoring improvement in blood oxygenation. In infants with restricted systemic blood flow, measure efficacy by monitoring improvement of systemic blood pressure and blood pH.

Drug Interactions: No drug interactions have been reported between PROSTIN VR PEDIATRIC and the therapy standard in neonates with restricted pulmonary or systemic blood flow. Standard therapy includes antibiotics, such as penicillin and gentamicin; vasopressors, such as dopamine and isoproterenol; cardiac glycosides; and diuretics, such as furosemide.

Carcinogenesis, Mutagenesis, and Impairment of Fertility: Long-term carcinogenicity studies and fertility studies have not been done. The Ames and Alkaline Elution assays reveal no potential for mutagenesis.

Adverse Reactions:
Central Nervous System: *Apnea has been reported in about 12% of the neonates treated.* (See WARNING box.) Other common adverse reactions reported have been fever in about 14% of the patients treated and seizures in about 4%. The following reactions have been reported in less than 1% of the patients: cerebral bleeding, hyperextension of the neck, hyperirritability, hypothermia, jitteriness, lethargy, and stiffness.
Cardiovascular System: The most common adverse reactions reported have been flushing in about 10% of patients (more common after intra-arterial dosing), bradycardia in about 7%, hypotension in about 4%, tachycardia in about 3%, cardiac arrest in about 1%, and edema in about 1%. The following reactions have been reported in less than 1% of the patients: congestive heart failure, hyperemia, second degree heart block, shock, spasm of the right ventricle infundibulum, supraventricular tachycardia, and ventricular fibrillation.
Respiratory System: The following reactions have been reported in less than 1% of the patients: bradypnea, bronchial wheezing, hypercapnia, respiratory depression, respiratory distress, and tachypnea.
Gastrointestinal System: The most common adverse reaction reported has been diarrhea in about 2% of the patients. The following reactions have been reported in less than 1% of the patients; gastric regurgitation, and hyperbilirubinemia.
Hematologic System: The most common hematologic event reported has been disseminated intravascular coagulation in about 1% of the patients. The following events have been reported in less than 1% of the patients: anemia, bleeding, and thrombocytopenia.
Excretory System: Anuria and hematuria have been reported in less than 1% of the patients.
Skeletal System: Cortical proliferation of the long bones has been reported. See PRECAUTIONS.
Miscellaneous: Sepsis has been reported in about 2% of the patients. Peritonitis has been reported in less than 1% of the patients. Hypokalemia has been reported in about 1%, and hypoglycemia and hyperkalemia have been reported in less than 1% of the patients.

Overdosage: Apnea, bradycardia, pyrexia, hypotension, and flushing may be signs of drug overdosage. If apnea or bradycardia occurs, discontinue the infusion, and provide appropriate medical treatment. Caution should be used in restarting the infusion. If pyrexia or hypotension occurs, reduce the infusion rate until these symptoms subside. Flushing is usually a result of incorrect intraarterial catheter placement, and the catheter should be repositioned.

Dosage and Administration: The preferred route of administration for PROSTIN VR PEDIATRIC Sterile Solution (alprostadil) is continuous intravenous infusion into a large vein. Alternatively, PROSTIN VR PEDIATRIC may be administered through an umbilical artery catheter placed at the ductal opening. Increases in blood pO_2 (torr) have been the same in neonates who received the drug by either route of administration.

Begin infusion with 0.1 micrograms alprostadil per kilogram of body weight per minute. After a therapeutic response is achieved (increased pO_2 in infants with restricted pulmonary blood flow or increased systemic blood pressure and blood pH in infants with restricted systemic blood flow), reduce the infusion rate to provide the lowest possible dosage that maintains the response. This may be accomplished by reducing the dosage from 0.1 to 0.05 to 0.025 to 0.01 micrograms per kilogram of body weight per minute. If response to 0.1 micrograms per kilogram of body weight per minute is inadequate, dosage can be increased up to 0.4 micrograms per kilogram of body weight per minute although, in general, higher infusion rates do not produce greater effects.

Dilution instructions: To prepare infusion solutions, dilute 1 ml of PROSTIN VR PEDIATRIC Sterile Solution with Sodium Chloride Injection USP or Dextrose Injection USP. Dilute to volumes appropriate for the pump delivery system available. Prepare fresh infusion solutions every 24 hours. *Discard any solution more than 24 hours old.*

Sample Dilutions and Infusion Rates to Provide a Dosage of 0.1 Micrograms per Kilogram of Body Weight per Minute

Add 1 ampoule (500 micrograms) alprostadil to:	Approximate concentration of resulting solution (micrograms/ml)	Infusion rate (ml/min per kg of body weight)
250 ml	2	0.05
100 ml	5	0.02
50 ml	10	0.01
25 ml	20	0.005

Example: To provide 0.1 micrograms/kilogram of body weight per minute to an infant weighing 2.8 kilograms using a solution of 1 ampoule PROSTIN VR PEDIATRIC in 100 ml of saline or dextrose: INFUSION RATE = 0.02 ml/min per kg × 2.8 kg = 0.056 ml/min or 3.36 ml/hr.

How Supplied: PROSTIN VR PEDIATRIC Sterile Solution (alprostadil) is available in packages of 5—1 ml ampoules (NDC 0009-3169-01). Each ml contains 500 micrograms alprostadil in dehydrated alcohol.

Store PROSTIN VR PEDIATRIC Sterile Solution in a refrigerator at 2°-8°C (36°-46°F).

Code 811 987 001

PROTAMINE SULFATE FOR INJECTION, USP ℞
Sterile Powder
50 mg, 250 mg

Description: Protamines are simple proteins of low molecular weight, rich in arginine and strongly basic. They occur in the sperm of salmon, and certain other species of fish.

Protamine Sulfate for Injection is available as a sterile freeze-dried preparation in two sizes: vials containing **50 mg** of protamine sulfate and 45 mg of sodium chloride and vials containing **250 mg** of protamine sulfate and 225 mg of sodium chloride. When reconstituted as directed, the solution contains 10 mg of protamine sulfate per ml. When necessary pH was adjusted with sodium hydroxide and/or hydrochloric acid to conform to the USP specified range of 6.5 to 7.5.

Actions: The strongly basic nature of protamines accounts for their antiheparin effect. Protamine combines with the strongly acidic heparin to form a stable salt with the loss of anticoagulant activity. Protamine itself has an anticoagulant effect.

Indications: Antidote to heparin overdosage.

Warnings: Hyperheparinemia or bleeding has been reported in experimental animals and in some patients from 30 minutes to 18 hours after cardiac surgery (under cardiopulmonary bypass). The bleeding occurred in spite of complete neutralization of heparin with protamine sulfate after surgery. Therefore, the patient should be kept under close observation after cardiac surgery. If indicated by coagulation studies, eg, the heparin titration test with protamine and the determination of plasma thrombin time, additional doses of protamine sulfate should be given.

When protamine sulfate is administered, it should be given slowly (in 1 to 3 minutes), intravenously, in doses not exceeding 50 mg in any 10-minute period; facilities to treat shock should be available. Reproduction studies have not been performed in animals. There is no adequate information on whether this drug may affect fertility in human males or females or have a teratogenic potential or other adverse effect on the fetus.

If Bacteriostatic Water for Injection with Benzyl Alcohol is used as the diluent, benzyl alcohol has been reported to be associated with a fatal "Gasping Syndrome" in premature infants.

Precautions: Because of the anticoagulant effect of protamine, it is unwise to give more than 100 mg over a short period unless there is certain knowledge of a larger requirement.

Protamine sulfate can be inactivated by blood, and when it is used to neutralize large doses of heparin, a heparin "rebound" may be encountered. This complication is treated by additional protamine injections as needed.

Hypersensitivity reactions have been reported in patients with a history of allergy to fish. However, no definitive relationship has been established between allergic reactions to protamine sulfate and fish allergy.

Adverse Reactions: Intravenous injections of protamine may cause a sudden fall in blood pressure, bradycardia, dyspnea, or transitory flushing and a feeling of warmth. Anaphylaxis resulting in respiratory embarrassment has been reported with protamine (see PRECAUTIONS). Because fatal reactions, often resembling anaphylaxis, have been reported after administration of protamine sulfate, the drug should be given only when resuscitation techniques and treatment of anaphylactoid shock are readily available.

Dosage and Administration: Protamine sulfate is for intravenous administration only. It should be given intravenously **very slowly**—no more than 50 mg in any 10-minute period. Each mg of protamine sulfate neutralizes approximately 90 USP Units of heparin of beef lung origin or 115 USP Units of heparin derived from intestinal mucosa. After the intravenous administration of heparin, the quantity of protamine required decreases rapidly with the time elapsed after heparin injection. Thirty minutes after a dose of heparin, the dose of protamine required for neutralization will be approximately half that required immediately after the heparin injection. Blood or plasma transfusions may also be necessary; these dilute but do not neutralize heparin. The dosage of protamine sulfate should be guided by blood coagulation studies (See Warnings).

Preparation of Solution—To prepare solution, aseptically add 5 ml of Bacteriostatic Water for Injection with Benzyl Alcohol to the vial of Protamine Sulfate for Injection **50 mg** or 25 ml of the same diluent to the vial of Sterile Protamine for Injection **250 mg**. Shake vial vigorously to effect complete solution. Each ml of the prepared solution will contain 10 mg of protamine sulfate. Protamine sulfate should not be mixed with other drugs without knowledge of compatibility, since protamine sulfate has been shown to be incompatible with certain antibiotics, including several of the cephalosporins and penicillins. Solutions of protamine sulfate may be kept for 24 hours if stored in a refrigerator. However, the usual precautions to maintain sterility of prepared solutions should be observed.

Storage Conditions: Store unreconstituted product at controlled room temperature 15°-30° C (59°-86° F). If reconstituted with Sterile Water for Injection, the solution should be used immediately and any unused portion discarded. If reconstituted with Bacteriostatic Water for Injection with Benzyl Alcohol, the solution should be stored at controlled room temperature 15°-30° C (59°-86°F) and used within 72 hours.

How Supplied: Protamine Sulfate for Injection Sterile Powder is available in a dry stable form in rubber-capped vials, each vial containing either **50 mg** protamine sulfate and 45 mg sodium chloride or **250 mg** protamine sulfate and 225 mg sodium chloride. Sodium hydroxide and/or hydrochloric acid were added when necessary to adjust the pH.

Caution: The **250** mg package provides a total dose five times that in the **50** mg size and is intended only for single dose use. It is designed only for antiheparin treatment in certain instances where large doses of heparin have been given during surgery and large doses of protamine sulfate are required for neutralization after the surgical procedure.

50 mg vial   NDC 0009-0811-03
250 mg vial   NDC 0009-0852-01
Code 811 589 003

PROVERA® ℞
brand of medroxyprogesterone acetate tablets, USP
10 mg
10s (unit of use)
NSN 6505-01-071-5605 (VA)
100s (bottle)
NSN 6505-00-890-1355 (M)

> **WARNING:**
> THE USE OF PROGESTATIONAL AGENTS DURING THE FIRST FOUR MONTHS OF PREGNANCY IS NOT RECOMMENDED
>
> Progestational agents have been used beginning with the first trimester of pregnancy in an attempt to prevent habitual abortion or treat threatened abortion. There is no adequate evidence that such use is effective and there is evidence of potential harm to the fetus when such drugs are given during the first four months of pregnancy. Furthermore, in the vast majority of women, the cause of abortion is a defective ovum, which progestational agents could not be expected to influence. In addition, the use of progestational agents with their uterine-relaxant properties, in patients with fertilized defective ova may cause a delay in spontaneous abortion. Therefore, the use of such drugs during the first four months of pregnancy is not recommended.
>
> Several reports suggest an association between intrauterine exposure to female sex hormones and congenital anomalies, including congenital heart defects and limb reduction defects[1-5]. One study[4] estimated a 4.7-fold increased risk of limb reduction defects in infants exposed in utero to sex hormones (oral contraceptives, hormone withdrawal tests for pregnancy, or attempted treatment for

Continued on next page

Information on these Upjohn products is based on labeling in effect on November 30, 1984. Further information concerning these and other Upjohn products may be obtained from the package insert or by direct inquiry to Medical Information, The Upjohn Company, Kalamazoo, Michigan 49001.

Upjohn—Cont.

threatened abortion). Some of these exposures were very short and involved only a few days of treatment. The data suggest that the risk of limb reduction defects in exposed fetuses is somewhat less than 1 in 1,000.

If the patient is exposed to PROVERA Tablets (medroxyprogesterone acetate) during the first four months of pregnancy or if she becomes pregnant while taking this drug, she should be apprised of the potential risks to the fetus.

Description: PROVERA Tablets contain medroxyprogesterone acetate, which is a derivative of progesterone. It is a white to off-white, odorless crystalline powder, stable in air, melting between 200 and 210° C. It is freely soluble in chloroform, soluble in acetone and in dioxane, sparingly soluble in alcohol and in methanol, slightly soluble in ether, and insoluble in water.

The chemical name for medroxyprogesterone acetate is Pregn-4-ene-3,20-dione, 17-(acetyloxy)-6-methyl-, (6α).

PROVERA Tablets are available in two strengths, each tablet containing either 2.5 or 10 mg medroxyprogesterone acetate.

Actions: Medroxyprogesterone acetate, administered orally or parenterally in the recommended doses to women with adequate endogenous estrogen, transforms proliferative into secretory endometrium. Androgenic and anabolic effects have been noted, but the drug is apparently devoid of significant estrogenic activity. While parenterally administered medroxyprogesterone acetate inhibits gonadotropin production, which in turn prevents follicular maturation and ovulation, available data indicate that this does not occur when the usually recommended oral dosage is given as single daily doses.

Indications: Secondary amenorrhea; abnormal uterine bleeding due to hormonal imbalance in the absence of organic pathology, such as fibroids or uterine cancer.

Contraindications:
1. Thrombophlebitis, thromboembolic disorders, cerebral apoplexy or patients with a past history of these conditions.
2. Liver dysfunction or disease.
3. Known or suspected malignancy of breast or genital organs.
4. Undiagnosed vaginal bleeding.
5. Missed abortion.
6. As a diagnostic test for pregnancy.
7. Known sensitivity to PROVERA Tablets (medroxyprogesterone acetate).

Warnings:
1. The physician should be alert to the earliest manifestations of thrombotic disorders (thrombophlebitis, cerebrovascular disorders, pulmonary embolism, and retinal thrombosis). Should any of these occur or be suspected, the drug should be discontinued immediately.
2. Beagle dogs treated with medroxyprogesterone acetate developed mammary nodules some of which were malignant. Although nodules occasionally appeared in control animals, they were intermittent in nature, whereas the nodules in the drug-treated animals were larger, more numerous, persistent, and there were some breast malignancies with metastases. Their significance with respect to humans has not been established.
3. Discontinue medication pending examination if there is sudden partial or complete loss of vision, or if there is a sudden onset of proptosis, diplopia or migraine. If examination reveals papilledema or retinal vascular lesions, medication should be withdrawn.
4. Detectable amounts of progestin have been identified in the milk of mothers receiving the drug. The effect of this on the nursing infant has not been determined.
5. Usage in pregnancy is not recommended (See WARNING Box).
6. Retrospective studies of morbidity and mortality in Great Britain and studies of morbidity in the United States have shown a statistically significant association between thrombophlebitis, pulmonary embolism, and cerebral thrombosis and embolism and the use of oral contraceptives.[6-9] The estimate of the relative risk of thromboembolism in the study by Vessey and Doll[8] was about sevenfold, while Sartwell and associates[9] in the United States found a relative risk of 4.4, meaning that the users are several times as likely to undergo thromboembolic disease without evident cause as nonusers. The American study also indicated that the risk did not persist after discontinuation of administration, and that it was not enhanced by long continued administration. The American study was not designed to evaluate a difference between products.

Precautions:
1. The pretreatment physical examination should include special reference to breast and pelvic organs, as well as Papanicolaou smear.
2. Because progestogens may cause some degree of fluid retention, conditions which might be influenced by this factor, such as epilepsy, migraine, asthma, cardiac or renal dysfunction, require careful observation.
3. In cases of breakthrough bleeding, as in all cases of irregular bleeding per vaginum, nonfunctional causes should be borne in mind. In cases of undiagnosed vaginal bleeding, adequate diagnostic measures are indicated.
4. Patients who have a history of psychic depression should be carefully observed and the drug discontinued if the depression recurs to a serious degree.
5. Any possible influence of prolonged progestin therapy on pituitary, ovarian, adrenal, hepatic or uterine functions awaits further study.
6. A decrease in glucose tolerance has been observed in a small percentage of patients on estrogen-progestin combination drugs. The mechanism of this decrease is obscure. For this reason, diabetic patients should be carefully observed while receiving progestin therapy.
7. The age of the patient constitutes no absolute limiting factor although treatment with progestins may mask the onset of the climacteric.
8. The pathologist should be advised of progestin therapy when relevant specimens are submitted.
9. Because of the occasional occurrence of thrombotic disorders, (thrombophlebitis, pulmonary embolism, retinal thrombosis, and cerebrovascular disorders) in patients taking estrogen-progestin combinations and since the mechanism is obscure, the physician should be alert to the earliest manifestation of these disorders.

Information for the Patient
See Patient Information at the end of insert.

Adverse Reactions:
Pregnancy—(See WARNING Box for possible adverse effects on the fetus)
Breast—Breast tenderness or galactorrhea has been reported rarely.
Skin—Sensitivity reactions consisting of urticaria, pruritus, edema and generalized rash have occurred in an occasional patient. Acne, alopecia and hirsutism have been reported in a few cases.
Thromboembolic Phenomena—Thromboembolic phenomena including thrombophlebitis and pulmonary embolism have been reported.

The following adverse reactions have been observed in women taking progestins including PROVERA Tablets (medroxyprogesterone acetate):

breakthrough bleeding
spotting
change in menstrual flow
amenorrhea
edema
change in weight
 (increase or decrease)
changes in cervical erosion
 and cervical secretions
cholestatic jaundice
anaphylactoid reactions and
 anaphylaxis
rash (allergic) with and
 without pruritus
mental depression
pyrexia
insomnia
nausea
somnolence

A statistically significant association has been demonstrated between use of estrogen-progestin combination drugs and the following serious adverse reactions: thrombophlebitis; pulmonary embolism and cerebral thrombosis and embolism. For this reason patients on progestin therapy should be carefully observed.

Although available evidence is suggestive of an association, such a relationship has been neither confirmed nor refuted for the following serious adverse reactions:

neuro-ocular lesions, eg, retinal thrombosis and optic neuritis.

The following adverse reactions have been observed in patients receiving estrogen-progestin combination drugs:

rise in blood pressure in susceptible individuals
premenstrual-like syndrome
changes in libido
changes in appetite
cystitis-like syndrome
headache
nervousness
dizziness
fatigue
backache
hirsutism
loss of scalp hair
erythema multiforme
erythema nodosum
hemorrhagic eruption
itching

In view of these observations, patients on progestin therapy should be carefully observed.

The following laboratory results may be altered by the use of estrogen-progestin combination drugs:
Increased sulfobromophthalein retention and other hepatic function tests.
Coagulation tests: increase in prothrombin factors VII, VIII, IX and X.
Metyrapone test.
Pregnanediol determination.
Thyroid function: increase in PBI, and butanol extractable protein bound iodine and decrease in T^3 uptake values.

Dosage and Administration:
Secondary Amenorrhea—PROVERA Tablets (medroxyprogesterone acetate) may be given in dosages of 5 to 10 mg daily for from 5 to 10 days. A dose for inducing an optimum secretory transformation of an endometrium that has been adequately primed with either endogenous or exogenous estrogen is 10 mg of PROVERA Tablets daily for 10 days. In cases of secondary amenorrhea, therapy may be started at any time. Progestin withdrawal bleeding usually occurs within three to seven days after discontinuing therapy with PROVERA.

Abnormal Uterine Bleeding Due to Hormonal Imbalance in the Absence of Organic Pathology—Beginning on the calculated 16th or 21st day of the menstrual cycle, 5 to 10 mg of PROVERA Tablets may be given daily for from 5 to 10 days. To produce an optimum secretory transformation of an endometrium that has been adequately primed with either endogenous or exogenous estrogen, 10 mg of PROVERA Tablets daily for 10 days beginning on the 16th day of the cycle is suggested. Progestin withdrawal bleeding usually occurs within three to seven days after discontinuing therapy with PROVERA. Patients with a past history of recurrent episodes of abnormal uterine bleeding may benefit from planned menstrual cycling with PROVERA.

How Supplied: PROVERA Tablets (medroxyprogesterone acetate) are available in two strengths:

2.5 mg—bottles of 25.   NDC 0009-0064-01
10 mg—bottles of 25.   NDC 0009-0050-01
          bottles of 100. NDC 0009-0050-02

Dosepak™ Unit-of-Use of 10   NDC 0009-0050-08

References:
1. Gal I, Kirman B, Stern J: Hormonal pregnancy tests and congenital malformation. Nature 216:83, 1967.
2. Levy EP, Cohen A, Fraser FC: Hormone treatment during pregnancy and congenital heart defects. Lancet 1:611, 1973.
3. Nora JJ, Nora AH: Birth defects and oral contraceptives. Lancet 1:941–942, 1973.
4. Janerich DT, Piper JM, Glebatis DM: Oral contraceptives and congenital limb-reduction defects. N Engl J Med 291:697–700, 1974.
5. Heinonen OP, Slone D, Monson RR, et al: Cardiovascular birth defects and antenatal exposure to female sex hormones. N Engl J Med 296:67–70, 1977.
6. Royal College of General Practitioners: Oral contraception and thromboembolic disease. J Coll Gen Pract 13:267–279, 1967.
7. Inman WHW, Vessey MP: Investigation of deaths from pulmonary, coronary, and cerebral thrombosis and embolism in women of childbearing age. Br Med J 2:193–199, 1968.
8. Vessey MP, Doll R: Investigation of relation between use of oral contraceptives and thromboembolic disease. A further report. Br Med J 2:651–657, 1969.
9. Sartwell PE, Masi AT, Arthes FG, et al: Thromboembolism and oral contraceptives: An epidemiological case-control study. Am J Epidemiol 90:365–380, 1969.

The text of the patient insert for progesterone and progesterone-like drugs is set forth below.

Patient Information: PROVERA Tablets contain medroxyprogesterone acetate, a progesterone. The information below is that which the U.S. Food and Drug Administration requires be provided for all patients taking progesterones. The information below relates only to the risk to the unborn child associated with use of progesterone during pregnancy. For further information on the use, side effects and other risks associated with this product, ask your doctor.

WARNING FOR WOMEN
There is an increased risk of birth defects in children whose mothers take this drug during the first four months of pregnancy.

Medroxyprogesterone acetate is similar to the progesterone hormones naturally produced by the body. Progesterone and progesterone-like drugs are used to treat menstrual disorders, to test if the body is producing certain hormones, and to treat some forms of cancer in women.

They have been used as a test for pregnancy but such use is no longer considered safe because of possible damage to a developing baby. Also, more rapid methods for testing for pregnancy are now available.

These drugs have also been used to prevent miscarriage in the first few months of pregnancy. No adequate evidence is available to show that they are effective for this purpose. Furthermore, most cases of early miscarriage are due to causes which could not be helped by these drugs.

There is an increased risk of birth defects, such as heart or limb defects if progesterone and progesterone-like drugs are taken during the first four months of pregnancy. The exact risk of taking this drug early in pregnancy and having a baby with a birth defect is not known. However, one study found that babies born to women who had taken sex hormones (such as progesterone-like drugs) during the first three months of pregnancy were 4 to 5 times more likely to have abnormalities of the arms or legs than if their mothers had not taken such drugs. Some of these women had taken these drugs for only a few days. The chance that an infant whose mother had taken this drug will have this type of defect is about 1 in 1,000.

If you take PROVERA Tablets and later find you were pregnant when you took it, be sure to discuss this with your doctor as soon as possible.
Code 812 584 000

Shown in Product Identification Section, page 441

SOLU-CORTEF	100 mg MIX-O-VIAL Each 2 ml contains: (when mixed) equiv. to	250 mg MIX-O-VIAL Each 2 ml contains: (when mixed) equiv. to	500 mg MIX-O-VIAL Each 4 ml contains: (when mixed) equiv. to	1000 mg MIX-O-VIAL Each 8 ml contains: (when mixed) equiv. to
Hydrocortisone sodium succinate	100 mg hydrocortisone	250 mg hydrocortisone	500 mg hydrocortisone	1000 mg hydrocortisone
Monobasic sodium phosphate anhydrous	0.8 mg	2 mg	4 mg	8 mg
Diabasic sodium phosphate dried	8.76 mg	21.8 mg	44 mg	88 mg
Benzyl alcohol added as preservative	18.1 mg	16.4 mg	33.4 mg	66.9 mg

When necessary, the pH of each formula was adjusted with sodium hydroxide so that the pH of the reconstituted solution is within the USP specified range of 7 to 8.

PYRROXATE® Capsules
(See PDR For Nonprescription Drugs)

SIGTAB® Tablets
Composition: Each tablet contains:
Vitamin A	5000 IU
Vitamin D	400 IU
Vitamin E	15 IU
Vitamin C	333 mg
Folic Acid	0.4 mg
Thiamine	10.3 mg
Riboflavin	10 mg
Niacin	100 mg
Vitamin B$_6$	6 mg
Vitamin B$_{12}$	18 mcg
Pantothenic Acid	20 mg

How Supplied: Coated compressed tablets in the following sizes:
Bottles of 30   NDC 0009-0461-01
Bottles of 90   NDC 0009-0461-02
Bottles of 500 NDC 0009-0461-03

SOLU–CORTEF®   ℞
brand of hydrocortisone sodium succinate sterile powder
(hydrocortisone sodium succinate for injection, USP)
For Intravenous or Intramuscular Administration

100 mg MIX-O-VIAL®:
NSN 6505-00-753-9609A (M & VA)
250 mg MIX-O-VIAL:
NSN 6505-00-951-5533A (M & VA)
500 mg MIX-O-VIAL:
NSN 6505-00-116-5055A (VA)
1000 mg MIX-O-VIAL:
NSN 6505-00-238-5222A (VA)

Description: SOLU-CORTEF Sterile Powder contains hydrocortisone sodium succinate as the active ingredient. Hydrocortisone sodium succinate is a white or nearly white, odorless, hygroscopic amorphous solid. It is very soluble in water and in alcohol, very slightly soluble in acetone and insoluble in chloroform. The chemical name is pregn-4-ene-3,20-dione,21-(3-carboxy-1-oxopropoxy)-11,17-dihydroxy-, monosodium salt, (11β)-and its molecular weight is 484.52.

Hydrocortisone sodium succinate is an anti-inflammatory adrenocortical steroid. This highly water-soluble sodium succinate ester of hydrocortisone permits the immediate intravenous administration of high doses of hydrocortisone in a small volume of diluent and is particularly useful where high blood levels of hydrocortisone are required rapidly.

SOLU-CORTEF Sterile Powder (hydrocortisone sodium succinate) is available in several packages for intravenous or intramuscular administration.

100 mg Plain—Vials containing hydrocortisone sodium succinate equivalent to 100 mg hydrocortisone, also 0.8 mg sodium biphosphate anhydrous, 8.73 mg dried sodium phosphate. [See table above].

Actions: Hydrocortisone sodium succinate has the same metabolic and anti-inflammatory actions as hydrocortisone. When given parenterally and in equimolar quantities, the two compounds are equivalent in biologic activity. Following the intravenous injection of hydrocortisone sodium succinate, demonstrable effects are evident within one hour and persist for a variable period. Excretion of the administered dose is nearly complete within 12 hours. Thus, if constantly high blood levels are required, injections should be made every 4 to 6 hours. This preparation is also rapidly absorbed when administered intramuscularly and is excreted in a pattern similar to that observed after intravenous injection.

Indications: When oral therapy is not feasible, and the strength, dosage form and route of administration of the drug reasonably lend the preparation to the treatment of the condition, SOLU-CORTEF Sterile Powder (hydrocortisone sodium succinate) is indicated for intravenous or intramuscular use in the following conditions:

1. **Endocrine Disorders**

   Primary or secondary adrenocortical insufficiency (hydrocortisone or cortisone is the drug of choice; synthetic analogs may be used in conjunction with mineralocorticoids where applicable; in infancy, mineralocorticord supplementation is of particular importance)

   Acute adrenocortical insufficiency (hydrocortisone or cortisone is the drug of choice; mineralocorticoid supplementation may be necessary, particularly when synthetic analogs are used)

   Preoperatively and in the event of serious trauma or illness, in patients with known adrenal insufficiency or when adrenocortical reserve is doubtful

   Shock unresponsive to conventional therapy if adrenocortical insufficiency exists or is suspected
   Congenital adrenal hyperplasia
   Hypercalcemia associated with cancer
   Nonsuppurative thyroiditis

2. **Rheumatic Disorders**
   As adjunctive therapy for short-term administration (to tide the patient over an acute episode or exacerbation) in:
   Post-traumatic osteoarthritis
   Synovitis of osteoarthritis
   Rheumatoid arthritis, including juvenile rheumatoid arthritis (selected cases may require low-dose maintenance therapy)
   Acute and subacute bursitis
   Epicondylitis
   Acute nonspecific tenosynovitis
   Acute gouty arthritis
   Psoriatic arthritis

Continued on next page

Information on these Upjohn products is based on labeling in effect on November 30, 1984. Further information concerning these and other Upjohn products may be obtained from the package insert or by direct inquiry to Medical Information, The Upjohn Company, Kalamazoo, Michigan 49001.

Upjohn—Cont.

　　Ankylosing spondylitis
3. **Collagen Diseases**
　　During an exacerbation or as maintenance therapy in selected cases of:
　　Systemic lupus erythematosus
　　Systemic dermatomyositis (polymyositis)
　　Acute rheumatic carditis
4. **Dermatologic Diseases**
　　Pemphigus
　　Severe erythema multiforme (Stevens-Johnson syndrome)
　　Exfoliative dermatitis
　　Bullous dermatitis herpetiformis
　　Severe seborrheic dermatitis
　　Severe psoriasis
　　Mycosis fungoides
5. **Allergic States**
　　Control of severe or incapacitating allergic conditions intractable to adequate trials of conventional treatment in:
　　Bronchial asthma
　　Contact dermatitis
　　Atopic dermatitis
　　Serum sickness
　　Seasonal or perennial allergic rhinitis
　　Drug hypersensitivity reactions
　　Urticarial transfusion reactions
　　Acute noninfectious laryngeal edema (epinephrine is the drug of first choice)
6. **Ophthalmic Diseases**
　　Severe acute and chronic allergic and inflammatory processes involving the eye, such as:
　　Herpes zoster ophthalmicus
　　Iritis, iridocyclitis
　　Chorioretinitis
　　Diffuse posterior uveitis and choroiditis
　　Optic neuritis
　　Sympathetic ophthalmia
　　Anterior segment inflammation
　　Allergic conjunctivitis
　　Allergic corneal marginal ulcers
　　Keratitis
7. **Gastrointestinal Diseases**
　　To tide the patient over a critical period of the disease in:
　　Ulcerative colitis (systemic therapy)
　　Regional enteritis (systemic therapy)
8. **Respiratory Diseases**
　　Symptomatic sarcoidosis
　　Berylliosis
　　Fulminating or disseminated pulmonary tuberculosis when used concurrently with appropriate antituberculous chemotherapy
　　Loeffler's syndrome not manageable by other means
　　Aspiration pneumonitis
9. **Hematologic Disorders**
　　Acquired (autoimmune) hemolytic anemia
　　Idiopathic thrombocytopenic purpura in adults (IV only; IM administration is contraindicated)
　　Secondary thrombocytopenia in adults
　　Erythroblastopenia (RBC anemia)
　　Congenital (erythroid) hypoplastic anemia
10. **Neoplastic Diseases**
　　For palliative mangement of:
　　Leukemias and lymphomas in adults
　　Acute leukemia of childhood
11. **Edematous States**
　　To induce diuresis or remission of proteinuria in the nephrotic syndrome, without uremia, of the idiopathic type or that due to lupus erythematosus
12. **Nervous System**
　　Acute exacerbations of multiple sclerosis
13. **Miscellaneous**
　　Tuberculous meningitis with subarachnoid block or impending block when used concurrently with appropriate antituberculous chemotherapy
　　Trichinosis with neurologic or myocardial involvement

Contraindications: Systemic fungal infections.
Warnings: In patients on corticosteroid therapy subjected to unusual stress, increased dosage of rapidly acting corticosteroids before, during, and after the stressful situation is indicated.
Corticosteroids may mask some signs of infection, and new infections may appear during their use. There may be decreased resistance and inability to localize infection when corticosteroids are used.
Prolonged use of corticosteroids may produce posterior subcapsular cataracts, glaucoma with possible damage to the optic nerves, and may enhance the establishment of secondary ocular infections due to fungi or viruses.
Usage in pregnancy. Since adequate human reproduction studies have not been done with corticosteroids, the use of these drugs in pregnancy, nursing mothers, or women of childbearing potential requires that the possible benefits of the drug be weighed against the potential hazards to the mother and embryo or fetus. Infants born of mothers who have received substantial doses of corticosteroids during pregnancy should be carefully observed for signs of hypoadrenalism.
Average and large doses of hydrocortisone can cause elevation of blood pressure, salt and water retention, and increased excretion of potassium. These effects are less likely to occur with the synthetic derivatives except when used in large doses. Dietary salt restriction and potassium supplementation may be necessary. All corticosteroids increase calcium excretion.
While on corticosteroid therapy patients should not be vaccinated against smallpox. Other immunization procedures should not be undertaken in patients who are on corticosteroids, especially on high dose, because of possible hazards of neurological complications and a lack of antibody response.
The use of SOLU-CORTEF Sterile Powder (hydrocortisone sodium succinate) in active tuberculosis should be restricted to those cases of fulminating or disseminated tuberculosis in which the corticosteroid is used for the management of the disease in conjunction with appropriate antituberculous regimen.
If corticosteroids are indicated in patients with latent tuberculosis or tuberculin reactivity, close observation is necessary as reactivation of the disease may occur. During prolonged corticosteroid therapy, these patients should receive chemoprophylaxis.
Because rare instances of anaphylactoid reactions (eg, bronchospasm) have occurred in patients receiving parenteral corticosteroid therapy, appropriate precautionary measures should be taken prior to administration, especially when the patient has a history of allergy to any drug.
The SOLU-CORTEF 100 mg, 250 mg, 500 mg and 1000 mg MIX-O-VIAL two-compartment vials contain benzyl alcohol. Benzyl alcohol has been reported to be associated with a fatal "Gasping Syndrome" in premature infants.
Precautions: Drug-induced secondary adrenocortical insufficiency may be minimized by gradual reduction of dosage. This type of relative insufficiency may persist for months after discontinuation of therapy; therefore, in any situation of stress occurring during that period, hormone therapy should be reinstituted. Since mineralocorticoid secretion may be impaired, salt and/or a mineralocorticoid should be administered concurrently.
There is an enhanced effect of corticosteroids in patients with hypothyroidism and in those with cirrhosis.
Corticosteroids should be used cautiously in patients with ocular herpes simplex for fear of corneal perforation.
The lowest possible dose of corticosteroid should be used to control the condition under treatment, and when reduction in dosage is possible, the reduction must be gradual.
Psychic derangements may appear when corticosteroids are used, ranging from euphoria, insomnia, mood swings, personality changes, and severe depression to frank psychotic manifestations. Also, existing emotional instability or psychotic tendencies may be aggravated by corticosteroids.
Aspirin should be used cautiously in conjunction with corticosteroids in hypoprothrombinemia.
Steroids should be used with caution in nonspecific ulcerative colitis, if there is a probability of impending perforation, abscess or other pyogenic infection, also in diverticulitis, fresh intestinal anastomoses, active or latent peptic ulcer, renal insufficiency, hypertension, osteoporosis, and myasthenia gravis.
Growth and development of infants and children on prolonged corticosteroid therapy should be carefully followed.
Although controlled clinical trials have shown corticosteroids to be effective in speeding the resolution of acute exacerbations of multiple sclerosis, they do not show that corticosteroids affect the ultimate outcome or natural history of the disease. The studies do show that relatively high doses of corticosteroids are necessary to demonstrate a significant effect. (See **Administration and Dosage**).
Since complications of treatment with glucocorticoides are dependent on the size of the dose and the duration of treatment, a risk/benefit decision must be made in each individual case as to dose and duration of treatment and as to whether daily or intermittent therapy should be used.

Adverse Reactions:
Fluid and Electrolyte Disturbances
　　Sodium retention
　　Fluid retention
　　Congestive heart failure in susceptible patients
　　Potassium loss
　　Hypokalemic alkalosis
　　Hypertension
Musculoskeletal
　　Muscle weakness
　　Steroid myopathy
　　Loss of muscle mass
　　Osteoporosis
　　Vertebral compression fractures
　　Aseptic necrosis of femoral and humeral heads
　　Pathologic fracture of long bones
Gastrointestinal
　　Peptic ulcer with possible perforation and hemorrhage
　　Pancreatitis
　　Abdominal distention
　　Ulcerative esophagitis
Dermatologic
　　Impaired wound healing
　　Thin fragile skin
　　Petechiae and ecchymoses
　　Facial erythema
　　Increased sweating
　　May suppress reactions to skin tests
Neurological
　　Convulsions
　　Increased intracranial pressure with papilledema (pseudotumor cerebri) usually after treatment
　　Vertigo
　　Headache
Endocrine
　　Menstrual irregularities
　　Development of Cushingoid state
　　Suppression of growth in children
　　Secondary adrenocortical and pituitary unresponsiveness, particularly in times of stress, as in trauma, surgery, or illness
　　Decreased carbohydrate tolerance
　　Manifestations of latent diabetes mellitus
　　Increased requirements for insulin or oral hypoglycemic agents in diabetics
Ophthalmic
　　Posterior subcapsular cataracts
　　Increased intraocular pressure
　　Glaucoma
　　Exophthalmos
Metabolic
　　Negative nitrogen balance due to protein catabolism
The following additional reactions are related to parenteral corticosteroid therapy:
　　Allergic, anaphylactic or other hypersensitivity reactions

Hyperpigmentation or hypopigmentation
Subcutaneous and cutaneous atrophy
Sterile abscess

Administration and Dosage: This preparation may be administered by intravenous injection, by intravenous infusion, or by intramuscular injection, the preferred method for initial emergency use being intravenous injection. Following the initial emergency period, consideration should be given to employing a longer acting injectable preparation or an oral preparation.

Therapy is initiated by administering SOLU-CORTEF Sterile Powder (hydrocortisone sodium succinate) intravenously over a period of 30 seconds (eg, 100 mg) to 10 minutes (eg, 500 mg or more). In general, high dose corticosteroid therapy should be continued only until the patient's condition has stabilized—usually not beyond 48 to 72 hours. Although adverse effects associated with high dose, short-term corticoid therapy are uncommon, peptic ulceration may occur. Prophylactic anatacid therapy may be indicated.

When high dose hydrocortisone therapy must be continued beyond 48-72 hours, hypernatremia may occur. Under such circumstances it may be desirable to replace SOLU-CORTEF with a corticoid such as methylprednisolone sodium succinate which causes little or no sodium retention.

The initial dose of SOLU-CORTEF Sterile Powder is 100 mg to 500 mg, depending on the severity of the condition. This dose may be repeated at intervals of 2, 4 or 6 hours as indicated by the patient's response and clinical condition. While the dose may be reduced for infants and children, it is governed more by the severity of the condition and response of the patient than by age or body weight but should not be less than 25 mg daily.

Patients subjected to severe stress following corticosteroid therapy should be observed closely for signs and symptoms of adrenocortical insufficiency.

Corticoid therapy is an adjunct to, and not a replacement for, conventional therapy.

Preparation of Solutions

100 mg Plain—For intravenous or intramuscular injection, prepare solution by aseptically adding **not more than 2 ml** of Bacteriostatic Water for Injection or Bacteriostatic Sodium Chloride Injection to the contents of one vial. **For intravenous infusion**, first prepare solution by adding **not more than 2 ml** of Bacteriostatic Water for Injection to the vial; this solution may then be added to 100 to 1000 ml (but not less than 100 ml) of the following: 5% dextrose in water (or isotonic saline solution or 5% dextrose in isotonic saline solution if patient is not on sodium restriction).

Directions for using MIX-O-VIAL Two-Compartment Vial
1. Remove protective cap, give the plunger-stopper a quarter-turn and press to force diluent into the lower compartment.
2. Gently agitate to effect solution.
3. Sterilize top of plunger-stopper with a suitable germicide.
4. Insert needle **squarely through center** of plunger-stopper until tip is just visible. Invert vial and withdraw dose.

Further dilution is not necessary for intravenous or intramuscular injection. For intravenous infusion, first prepare solution as just described. The **100 mg** solution may then be added to 100 to 1000 ml of 5% dextrose in water (or isotonic saline solution or 5% dextrose in isotonic saline solution if patient is not on sodium restriction). The **250 mg** solution may be added to 250 to 1000 ml, the **500 mg** solution may be added to 500 to 1000 ml and the **1000 mg** solution to 1000 ml of the same diluents. In cases where administration of a small volume of fluid is desirable, 100 mg to 3000 mg of SOLU-CORTEF Sterile Powder may be added to 50 ml of the above diluents. The resulting solutions are stable for at least 4 hours and may be administered either directly or by IV piggyback.

When reconstituted as directed, pH's of the solutions range from 7 to 8 and the tonicities are: 100 mg MIX-O-VIAL, .36 osmolar; 250 mg MIX-O-VIAL, 500 mg MIX-O-VIAL, and the 1000 mg MIX-O-VIAL, .57 osmolar. (Isotonic saline = .28 osmolar.)

How Supplied: SOLU-CORTEF Sterile Powder (hydrocortisone sodium succinate) is available in the following packages:
100 mg Plain—NDC 0009-0825-01
100 mg MIX-O-VIAL
   2 ml—NDC 0009-0900-01
   25-2 ml—NDC 0009-0900-12
250 mg MIX-O-VIAL
   2 ml—NDC 0009-0909-01
   25-2 ml—NDC 0009-0909-07
500 mg MIX-O-VIAL—NDC 0009-0912-01
1000 mg MIX-O-VIAL—NDC 0009-0920-01

Storage Conditions: Store unreconstituted product at controlled room temperature 15°–30°C (59°–86°F).
Store solution at controlled room temperature 15°–30°C (59°–86°F) and protect from light. Use solution only if it is clear. Unused solution should be discarded after 3 days.
Code 810 379 008

SOLU–MEDROL®   B
brand of methylprednisolone sodium succinate sterile powder
(methylprednisolone sodium succinate for injection, USP)
For Intravenous or Intramuscular Administration
40 mg (1 ml MIX-O-VIAL® Two-Compartment Vial):
NSN 6505-00-768-3598A (M & VA)
125 mg (2 ml MIX-O-VIAL):
NSN 6505-00-943-4380A (M & VA)
500 mg:
NSN 6505-00-432-1124A (VA)
1 gram:
NSN 6505-00-104-8069A (VA)

Description: SOLU-MEDROL Sterile Powder contains methylprednisolone sodium succinate as the active ingredient. Methylprednisolone sodium succinate, USP, occurs as a white, or nearly white, odorless hygroscopic, amorphous solid. It is very soluble in water and in alcohol; it is insoluble in chloroform and is very slightly soluble in acetone. The chemical name for methylprednisolone sodium succinate is pregna-1,4-diene-3,20-dione,21-(3-carboxy-1-oxopropoxy)-11,17-dihydroxy-6-methyl-,monosodium salt, (6α, 11β), and the molecular weight is 496.53.

Methylprednisolone sodium succinate is so extremely soluble in water that it may be administered in a small volume of diluent and is especially well suited for intravenous use in situations in which high blood levels of methylprednisolone are required rapidly.

SOLU-MEDROL is available in several strengths and packages for intravenous or intramuscular administration. **40 mg ACT-O-VIAL® System and 40 mg MIX-O-VIAL® Two-Compartment Vial** —Each ml (when mixed) contains methylprednisolone sodium succinate equivalent to 40 mg methylprednisolone; also 1.6 mg monobasic sodium phosphate anhydrous; 17.46 mg dibasic sodium phosphate dried; 25 mg lactose hydrous; 8.8 mg benzyl alcohol added as preservative. **125 mg ACT-O-VIAL System and 125 mg MIX-O-VIAL** Two-Compartment Vial— Each 2 ml (when mixed) contains methylprednisolone sodium succinate equivalent to 125 mg methylprednisolone; also 1.6 mg monobasic sodium biphosphate anhydrous; 17.4 mg dibasic sodium phosphate dried; 17.6 mg benzyl alcohol added as preservative. **500 mg Vial** —Each 8 ml (when mixed as directed) contains methylprednisolone sodium succinate equivalent to 500 mg methylprednisolone; also 6.4 mg monobasic sodium biphosphate anhydrous; 69.6 mg dibasic sodium phosphate dried. **500 mg Vial with Diluent** —Each 8 ml (when mixed as directed) contains methylprednisolone sodium succinate equivalent to 500 mg methylprednisolone; also 6.4 mg monobasic sodium phosphate anhydrous; 69.6 mg dibasic sodium phosphate dried; 70.2 mg benzyl alcohol added as preservative. **1 gram Vial**—Each 16 ml (when mixed as directed) contains methylprednisolone sodium succinate equivalent to 1 gram methylprednisolone; also 12.8 mg monobasic sodium phosphate anhydrous; 139.2 mg dibasic sodium phosphate dried. **1 gram Vial with Diluent** —Each 16 ml (when mixed as directed) contains methylprednisolone sodium succinate equivalent to 1 gram methylprednisolone; also 12.8 mg monobasic sodium phosphate anhydrous; 139.2 mg dibasic sodium phosphate dried; 141 mg benzyl alcohol added as preservative.

When necessary, the pH of each formula was adjusted with sodium hydroxide so that the pH of the reconstituted solution is within the USP specified range of 7 to 8 and the tonicities are, for the 40 mg per ml solution, 0.50 osmolar; for the 125 mg per 2 ml, 500 mg per 8 ml and 1 gram per 16 ml solutions, 0.40 osmolar. (Isotonic saline = 0.28 osmolar).

IMPORTANT—Use only the accompanying diluent or Bacteriostac Water For Injection with Benzyl Alcohol when reconstituting SOLU-MEDROL.

Use within 48 hours after mixing

Actions: Methylprednisolone is a potent anti-inflammatory steroid synthesized in the Research Laboratories of The Upjohn Company. It has a greater anti-inflammatory potency than prednisolone and even less tendency than prednisolone to induce sodium and water retention.

Methylprednisolone sodium succinate has the same metabolic and anti-inflammatory actions as methylprednisolone. When given parenterally and in equimolar quantities, the two compounds are equivalent in biologic activity. The relative potency of SOLU-MEDROL Sterile Powder (methylprednisolone sodium succinate) and hydrocortisone sodium succinate, as indicated by depression of eosinophil count, following intravenous administration, is at least four to one. This is in good agreement with the relative oral potency of methylprednisolone and hydrocortisone.

Indications: When oral therapy is not feasible, and the strength, dosage form and route of administration of the drug reasonably lend the preparation to the treatment of the condition, SOLU-MEDROL Sterile Powder (methylprednisolone sodium succinate) is indicated for intravenous or intramuscular use in the following conditions:

1. **Endocrine Disorders**

   Primary or secondary adrenocortical insufficiency (hydrocortisone or cortisone is the drug of choice; synthetic analogs may be used in conjunction with mineralocorticoids where applicable; in infancy, mineralocorticoid supplementation is of particular importance)

   Acute adrenocortical insufficiency (hydrocortisone or cortisone is the drug of choice; mineralocorticoid supplementation may be necessary, particularly when synthetic analogs are used)

   Preoperatively and in the event of serious trauma or illness, in patients with known adrenal insufficiency or when adrenocortical reserve is doubtful

   Shock unresponsive to conventional therapy if adrenocortical insufficiency exists or is suspected

   Congenital adrenal hyperplasia

   Hypercalcemia associated with cancer

   Nonsuppurative thyroiditis

2. **Rheumatic Disorders**

   As adjunctive therapy for short-term administration (to tide the patient over an acute episode or exacerbation) in:

Continued on next page

Information on these Upjohn products is based on labeling in effect on November 30, 1984. Further information concerning these and other Upjohn products may be obtained from the package insert or by direct inquiry to Medical Information, The Upjohn Company, Kalamazoo, Michigan 49001.

Upjohn—Cont.

Post-traumatic osteoarthritis
Synovitis of osteoarthritis
Rheumatoid arthritis, including juvenile rheumatoid arthritis (selected cases may require low-dose maintenance therapy)
Acute and subacute bursitis
Epicondylitis
Acute nonspecific tenosynovitis
Acute gouty arthritis
Psoriatic arthritis
Ankylosing spondylitis

3. **Collagen Diseases**
During an exacerbation or as maintenance therapy in selected cases of:
Systemic lupus erythematosus
Systemic dermatomyositis (polymyositis)
Acute rheumatic carditis

4. **Dermatologic Diseases**
Pemphigus
Severe erythema multiforme (Stevens-Johnson syndrome)
Exfoliative dermatitis
Bullous dermatitis herpetiformis
Severe seborrheic dermatitis
Severe psoriasis
Mycosis fungoides

5. **Allergic States**
Control of severe or incapacitating allergic conditions intractable to adequate trials of conventional treatment in:
Bronchial asthma
Contact dermatitis
Atopic dermatitis
Serum sickness
Seasonal or perennial allergic rhinitis
Drug hypersensitivity reactions
Urticarial transfusion reactions
Acute noninfectious laryngeal edema (epinephrine is the drug of first choice)

6. **Ophthalmic Diseases**
Severe acute and chronic allergic and inflammatory processes involving the eye, such as:
Herpes zoster ophthalmicus
Iritis, iridocyclitis
Chorioretinitis
Diffuse posterior uveitis and choroiditis
Optic neuritis
Sympathetic ophthalmia
Anterior segment inflammation
Allergic conjunctivitis
Allergic corneal marginal ulcers
Keratitis

7. **Gastrointestinal Diseases**
To tide the patient over a critical period of the disease in:
Ulcerative colitis (systemic therapy)
Regional enteritis (systemic therapy)

8. **Respiratory Diseases**
Symptomatic sarcoidosis
Berylliosis
Fulminating or disseminated pulmonary tuberculosis when used concurrently with appropriate antituberculous chemotherapy
Loeffler's syndrome not manageable by other means
Aspiration pneumonitis

9. **Hematologic Disorders**
Acquired (autoimmune) hemolytic anemia
Idiopathic thrombocytopenic purpura in adults (IV only; IM administration is contraindicated)
Secondary thrombocytopenia in adults
Erythroblastopenia (RBC anemia)
Congenital (erythroid) hypoplastic anemia

10. **Neoplastic Diseases**
For palliative management of:
Leukemias and lymphomas in adults
Acute leukemia of childhood

11. **Edematous States**
To induce diuresis or remission of proteinuria in the nephrotic syndrome, without uremia, of the idiopathic type or that due to lupus erythematosus

12. **Nervous System**
Acute exacerbations of multiple sclerosis

13. **Miscellaneous**
Tuberculous meningitis with subarachnoid block or impending block when used concurrently with appropriate antituberculous chemotherapy
Trichinosis with neurologic or myocardial involvement

Contraindications: Systemic fungal infections.

Warnings: In patients on corticosteroid therapy subjected to any unusual stress, increased dosage of rapidly acting corticosteroids before, during, and after the stressful situation is indicated.

Corticosteroids may mask some signs of infection, and new infections may appear during their use. There may be decreased resistance and inability to localize infection when corticosteroids are used.

Prolonged use of corticosteroids may produce posterior subcapsular cataracts, glaucoma with possible damage to the optic nerves, and may enhance the establishment of secondary ocular infections due to fungi or viruses.

Usage in pregnancy. Since adequate human reproduction studies have not been done with corticosteroids, the use of these drugs in pregnancy, nursing mothers, or women of childbearing potential requires that the possible benefits of the drug be weighed against the potential hazards to the mother and embryo or fetus. Infants born of mothers who have received substantial doses of corticosteroids during pregnancy should be carefully observed for signs of hypoadrenalism.

Average and large doses of cortisone or hydrocortisone can cause elevation of blood pressure, salt and water retention, and increased excretion of potassium. These effects are less likely to occur with the synthetic derivatives except when used in large doses. Dietary salt restriction and potassium supplementation may be necessary. All corticosteroids increase calcium excretion.

While on corticosteroid therapy patients should not be vaccinated against smallpox. Other immunization procedures should not be undertaken in patients who are on corticosteroids, especially on high dose, because of possible hazards of neurological complications and a lack of antibody response.

The use of SOLU-MEDROL Sterile Powder (methylprednisolone sodium succinate) in active tuberculosis should be restricted to those cases of fulminating or disseminated tuberculosis in which the corticosteroid is used for the management of the disease in conjunction with appropriate antituberculous regimen.

If corticosteroids are indicated in patients with latent tuberculosis or tuberculin reactivity, close observation is necessary as reactivation of the disease may occur. During prolonged corticosteroid therapy, these patients should receive chemoprophylaxis.

Because rare instances of anaphylactic (eg, bronchospasm) reactions have occurred in patients receiving parenteral corticosteroid therapy, appropriate precautionary measures should be taken prior to administration, especially when the patient has a history of allergy to any drug.

There are reports of cardiac arrhythmias and/or circulatory collapse and/or cardiac arrest following the rapid administration of large IV doses of SOLU-MEDROL (greater than 0.5 gram administered over a period of less than 10 minutes).

Benzyl alcohol is contained in the 40 mg MIX-O-VIAL, 40 mg ACT-O-VIAL, 125 mg MIX-O-VIAL, and the 125 mg ACT-O-VIAL, and in the accompanying diluent for the 500 mg and 1 gram vials. Benzyl alcohol has been reported to be associated with a fatal "Gasping Syndrome" in premature infants.

Precautions: Drug-induced secondary adrenocortical insufficiency may be minimized by gradual reduction of dosage. This type of relative insufficiency may persist for months after discontinuation of therapy; therefore, in any situation of stress occurring during that period, hormone therapy should be reinstituted. Since mineralocorticoid secretion may be impaired, salt and/or a mineralocorticoid should be administered concurrently.

There is an enhanced effect of corticosteroids on patients with hypothyroidism and in those with cirrhosis.

Corticosteroids should be used cautiously in patients with ocular herpes simplex because of possible corneal perforation.

The lowest possible dose of corticosteroid should be used to control the condition under treatment, and when reduction in dosage is possible, the reduction should be gradual.

Psychic derangements may appear when corticosteroids are used, ranging from euphoria, insomnia, mood swings, personality changes and severe depression, to frank psychotic manifestations. Also, existing emotional instability or psychotic tendencies may be aggravated by corticosteroids.

Aspirin should be used cautiously in conjunction with corticosteroids in hypoprothrombinemia.

Steroids should be used with caution in nonspecific ulcerative colitis, if there is a probability of impending perforation, abscess or other pyogenic infection; diverticulitis; fresh intestinal anastomoses; active or latent peptic ulcer; renal insufficiency; hypertension; osteoporosis; and myasthenia gravis.

Growth and development of infants and children on prolonged corticosteroid therapy should be carefully observed.

Although controlled clinical trials have shown corticosteroids to be effective in speeding the resolution of acute exacerbations of multiple sclerosis, they do not show that corticosteroids affect the ultimate outcome or natural history of the disease. The studies do show that relatively high doses of corticosteroids are necessary to demonstrate a significant effect. (See DOSAGE AND ADMINISTRATION).

Since complications of treatment with glucocorticoids are dependent on the size of the dose and the duration of treatment, a risk/benefit decision must be made in each individual case as to dose and duration of treatment and as to whether daily or intermittent therapy should be used.

Adverse Reactions:

Fluid and Electrolyte Disturbances
Sodium retention
Fluid retention
Congestive heart failure in susceptible patients
Potassium loss
Hypokalemic alkalosis
Hypertension

Musculoskeletal
Muscle weakness
Steroid myopathy
Loss of muscle mass
Severe arthralgia
Vertebral compression fractures
Aseptic necrosis of femoral and humeral heads
Pathologic fracture of long bones
Osteoporosis

Gastrointestinal
Peptic ulcer with possible perforation and hemorrhage
Pancreatitis
Abdominal distention
Ulcerative esophagitis

Dermatologic
Impaired wound healing
Thin fragile skin
Petechiae and ecchymoses
Facial erythema
Increased sweating
May suppress reactions to skin tests

Neurological
Increased intracranial pressure with papilledema (pseudo-tumor cerebri) usually after treatment
Convulsions
Vertigo
Headache

Endocrine
Development of Cushingoid state
Suppression of growth in children
Secondary adrenocortical and pituitary unresponsiveness, particularly in times of stress, as in trauma, surgery or illness

Menstrual irregularities
Decreased carbohydrate tolerance
Manifestations of latent diabetes mellitus
Increased requirements for insulin or oral hypoglycemic agents in diabetics

Ophthalmic
Posterior subcapsular cataracts
Increased intraocular pressure
Glaucoma
Exophthalmos

Metabolic
Negative nitrogen balance due to protein catabolism

The following *additional* adverse reactions are related to parenteral corticosteroid therapy:
Hyperpigmentation or hypopigmentation
Subcutaneous and cutaneous atrophy
Sterile abscess
  Anaphylactic reaction with or without circulatory collapse, cardiac arrest, bronchospasm
Urticaria
Nausea and vomiting
Cardiac arrhythmias; hypotension or hypertension

Dosage and Administration: When high dose therapy is desired, the recommended dose of SOLU-MEDROL Sterile Powder (methylprednisolone sodium succinate) is 30 mg/kg administered intravenously over a 10–20 minute period. This dose may be repeated every 4 to 6 hours for 48 hours.

Therapy is initiated by administering SOLU-MEDROL intravenously over a period of one to several minutes. In general, high dose corticosteroid therapy should be continued only until the patient's condition has stabilized; usually not beyond 48 to 72 hours.

Although adverse effects associated with high dose short-term corticoid therapy are uncommon, peptic ulceration may occur. Prophylactic antacid therapy may be indicated.

In other indications initial dosage will vary from 10 to 40 mg of methylprednisolone depending on the clinical problem being treated. The larger doses may be required for short-term management of severe, acute conditions. The initial dose usually should be given intravenously over a period of one to several minutes. Subsequent doses may be given intravenously or intramuscularly at intervals dictated by the patient's response and clinical condition. Corticoid therapy is an adjunct to, and not replacement for conventional therapy.

Dosage may be reduced for infants and children but should be governed more by the severity of the condition and response of the patient than by age or size. It should not be less than 0.5 mg per kg every 24 hours.

Dosage must be decreased or discontinued gradually when the drug has been administered for more than a few days. If a period of spontaneous remission occurs in a chronic condition, treatment should be discontinued. Routine laboratory studies, such as urinalysis, two-hour postprandial blood sugar, determination of blood pressure and body weight, and a chest X-ray should be made at regular intervals during prolonged therapy. Upper GI X-rays are desirable in patients with an ulcer history or significant dyspepsia.

SOLU-MEDROL may be administered by intravenous or intramuscular injection or by intravenous infusion, the preferred method for initial emergency use being intravenous injection. To administer by intravenous (or intramuscular) injection, prepare solution as directed. The desired dose may be administered intravenously over a period of approximately 60 seconds. Subsequent doses may be withdrawn and administered similarly. If desired, the medication may be administered in diluted solutions by adding Water for Injection or other suitable diluent (see below) to the MIX-O-VIAL and withdrawing the indicated dose.

To prepare solutions for intravenous infusion, first prepare the solution for injection as directed. This solution may then be added to indicated amounts of 5% dextrose in water, isotonic saline solution or 5% dextrose in isotonic saline solution.

Multiple Sclerosis
In treatment of acute exacerbations of multiple sclerosis, daily doses of 200 mg of prednisolone for a week followed by 80 mg every other day for 1 month have been shown to be effective (4 mg of methylprednisolone is equivalent to 5 mg of prednisolone).

Directions for Using the MIX-O-VIAL Two-Compartment Vial
1. Remove protective cap, give the plunger-stopper a quarter turn and press to force diluent into the lower compartment.
2. Gently agitate to effect solution. Use solution within 48 hours.
3. Sterilize top of plunger-stopper with a suitable germicide.
4. Insert needle **squarely through center** of plunger-stopper until tip is just visible. Invert vial and withdraw dose.

Directions for Using the ACT-O-VIAL System
1. Press down on plastic activator to force diluent into the lower compartment.
2. Gently agitate to effect solution.
3. Remove plastic tab covering center of stopper.
4. Sterilize top of stopper with a suitable germicide.
5. Insert needle **squarely through center** of stopper unitl tip is just visible. Invert vial and withdraw dose.

Storage Conditions: Store unreconstituted product at controlled room temperature 15°–30°C (59°–86°F).
Store solution at controlled room temperature 15°–30°C (59°–86°F).
Use solution within 48 hours after mixing.

How Supplied: SOLU-MEDROL Sterile Powder (methylprednisolone sodium succinate) is available in the following packages:
40 mg MIX-O-VIAL Two-Compartment Vial
  1 ml NDC 0009-0113-01
  25-1 ml NDC 0009-0113-11
40 mg ACT-O-VIAL System
  1 ml NDC 0009-0113-12
  25—1 ml NDC 0009-0113-13
125 mg MIX-O-VIAL Two-Compartment Vial
  2 ml NDC 0009-0190-01
  25-2 ml NDC 0009-0190-08
125 mg ACT-O-VIAL System
  2 ml NDC 0009-0190-09
  25—2 ml NDC 0009-0190-100
500 mg Vial NDC 0009-0758-01
500 mg Vial with Diluent
  NDC 0009-0887-01
1 gram Vial NDC 0009-0698-01
1 gram Vial with Diluent
  NDC 0009-0911-01
1 gram Vial with Diluent and IV Administration Set
  NDC 0009-0911-05

Code 810 431 010
Shown in Product Identification Section, page 441

TOLINASE®
brand of tolazamide tablets, USP
  250 mg (30s)
  NSN 6505-01-061-6992 (VA)
  250 mg (100s):
  NSN 6505-00-159-4990A (VA)
  250 mg (1000s):
  NSN 6505-00-105-5842A (M & VA)

Description: TOLINASE Tablets contain tolazamide, an oral blood glucose lowering drug of the sulfonylurea class. Tolazamide is a white or creamy-white powder with a melting point of 165° to 173° C. The solubility of tolazamide at pH 6.0 (mean urinary pH) is 27.8 mg per 100 ml.
The chemical names for tolazamide are (1) Benzenesulfonamide, N-[[hexahydro-1H -azepin-1-yl]amino]-carbonyl]-4-methyl-; (2) 1-(Hexahydro-1H-azepin-1-yl)-3-(p-tolylsulfonyl)urea and its molecular weight is 311.40.
TOLINASE Tablets for oral administration are available as scored, white tablets containing 100 mg, 250 mg or 500 mg tolazamide.

Clinical Pharmacology:
Actions
Tolazamide appears to lower the blood glucose acutely by stimulating the release of insulin from the pancreas, an effect dependent upon functioning beta cells in the pancreatic islets. The mechanism by which tolazamide lowers blood glucose during long-term administration has not been clearly established. With chronic administration in type II diabetic patients, the blood glucose lowering effect persists despite a gradual decline in the insulin secretory response to the drug. Extrapancreatic effects may be involved in the mechanism of action of oral sulfonylurea hypoglycemic drugs.

Some patients who are initially responsive to oral hypoglycemic drugs, including TOLINASE Tablets (tolazamide), may become unresponsive or poorly responsive over time. Alternatively, TOLINASE may be effective in some patients who have become unresponsive to one or more sulfonylurea drugs.

In addition to its blood glucose lowering actions, tolazamide produces a mild diuresis by enhancement of renal free water clearance.

Phrmacokinetics
Tolazamide is rapidly and well absorbed from the gastrointestinal tract. Peak serum concentrations occur at three to four hours following a single oral dose of the drug. The average biological half-life of the drug is seven hours. The drug does not continue to accumulate in the blood after the first four to six doses are administered. A steady or equilibrium state is reached during which the peak and nadir values do not change from day to day after the fourth to sixth doses.

Tolazamide is metabolized to five major metabolites ranging in hypoglycemic activity from 0–70%. They are excreted principally in the urine. Following a single oral dose of tritiated tolazamide, 85% of the dose was excreted in the urine and 7% in the feces over a five-day period. Most of the urinary excretion of the drug occurred within the first 24 hours postadministration.

When normal fasting nondiabetic subjects are given a single 500 mg dose of tolazamide orally, a hypoglycemic effect can be noted within 20 minutes after ingestion with a peak hypoglycemic effect occurring in two to four hours. Following a single oral dose of 500 mg tolazamide, a statistically significant hypoglycemic effect was demonstrated in fasted nondiabetic subjects 20 hours after administration. With fasting diabetic patients, the peak hypoglycemic effect occurs at four to six hours. The duration of maximal hypoglycemic effect in fed diabetic patients is about ten hours, with the onset occurring at four to six hours and with the blood glucose levels beginning to rise at 14 to 16 hours. Single dose potency of tolazamide in normal subjects has been shown to be 6.7 times that of tolbutamide on a milligram basis. Clinical experience in diabetic patients has demonstrated tolazamide to be approximately five times more potent than tolbutamide on a milligram basis, and approximately equivalent in milligram potency to chlorpropamide.

Indications and Usage: TOLINASE Tablets (tolazamide) are indicated as an adjunct to diet to lower the blood glucose in patients with noninsulin dependent diabetes mellitus (type II) whose hyperglycemia cannot be satisfactorily controlled by diet alone.

In initiating treatment for noninsulin-dependent diabetes, diet should be emphasized as the primary form of treatment. Caloric restriction and weight loss are essential in the obese diabetic patient. Proper dietary management alone may be effec-

Continued on next page

Information on these Upjohn products is based on labeling in effect on November 30, 1984. Further information concerning these and other Upjohn products may be obtained from the package insert or by direct inquiry to Medical Information, The Upjohn Company, Kalamazoo, Michigan 49001.

Upjohn—Cont.

tive in controlling the blood glucose and symptoms of hyperglycemia. The importance of regular physical activity should also be stressed and cardiovascular risk factors should be identified and corrective measures taken where possible.

If this treatment program fails to reduce symptoms and/or blood glucose, the use of an oral sulfonylurea or insulin should be considered. Use of TOLINASE must be viewed by both the physician and patient as a treatment in addition to diet and not as a substitute for diet or as a convenient mechanism for avoiding dietary restraint. Furthermore, loss of blood glucose control on diet alone may be transient thus requiring only short-term administration of TOLINASE.

Duing maintenance programs, TOLINASE should be discontinued if satisfactory lowering of blood glucose is no longer achieved. Judgments should be based on regular clinical and laboratory evaluations.

In considering the use of TOLINASE in asymptomatic patients, it should be recognized that controlling the blood glucose in noninsulin-dependent diabetes has not been definitely established to be effective in preventing the long-term cardiovascular or neural complications of diabetes.

Contraindications: TOLINASE Tablets (tolazamide) are contraindicated in patients with: 1) known hypersensitivity or allergy to TOLINASE; 2) diabetic ketoacidosis, with or without coma. This condition should be treated with insulin; 3) Type I diabetes, as sole therapy.

Special Warning on Increased Risk of Cardiovascular Mortality: The administration of oral hypoglycemic drugs has been reported to be associated with increased cardiovascular mortality as compared to treatment with diet alone or diet plus insulin. This warning is based on the study conducted by the University Group Diabetes Program (UGDP), a long-term prospective clinical trial designed to evaluate the effectiveness of glucose-lowering drugs in preventing or delaying vascular complications in patients with noninsulin-dependent diabetes. The study involved 823 patients who were randomly assigned to one of four treatment groups (DIABETES, 19 (supp. 2):747-830, 1970.)

UGDP reported that patients treated for five to eight years with diet plus a fixed dose of tolbutamide (1.5 grams per day) had a rate of cardiovascular mortality approximately 2½ times that of patients with diet alone. A significant increase in total mortality was not observed, but the use of tolbutamide was discontinued based on the increase on cardiovascular mortality, thus limiting the opportunity for the study to show an increase in overall mortality. Despite controversy regarding the interpretation of these results, the findings of the UGDP study provide an adequate basis for this warning. The patient should be informed of the potential risks and advantages of TOLINASE and of alternative modes of therapy.

Although only one drug in the sulfonylurea class (tolbutamide) was included in this study, it is prudent from a safety standpoint to consider that this warning may also apply to other oral hypoglycemic drugs in this class, in view of their close similarities in mode of action and chemical structure.

Precautions:
General
Hypoglycemia—All sulfonylurea drugs are capable of producing severe hypoglycemia. Proper patient selection and dosage and instructions are important to avoid hypoglycemic episodes. Renal or hepatic insufficiency may cause elevated blood levels of TOLINASE Tablets (tolazamide) and the latter may also diminish gluconeogenic capacity, both of which increase the risk of serious hypoglycemic reactions. Elderly, debilitated, or malnourished patients and those with adrenal or pituitary insufficiency are particularly susceptible to the hypoglycemic action of glucose lowering drugs. Hypoglycemia may be difficult to recognize in the elderly and in people who are taking beta-adrenergic blocking drugs. Hypoglycemia is more likely to occur when caloric intake is deficient, after severe or prolonged exercise, when alcohol is ingested, or when more than one glucose-lowering drug is used.

Loss of Control of Blood Glucose—When a patient stabilized on any diabetic regimen is exposed to stress such as fever, trauma, infection, or surgery, loss of control of blood glucose may occur. At such times it may be necessary to discontinue TOLINASE and administer insulin.

The effectiveness of any hypoglycemic drug, including TOLINASE, in lowering blood glucose to a desired level decreases in many patients over a period of time, which may be due to progression of the severity of the diabetes or to diminished responsiveness to the drug. This phenomenon is known as secondary failure to distinguish it from primary failure in which the drug is ineffective in an individual patient when first given. Adequate adjustment of dose and adherence to diet should be assessed before classifying a patient as a secondary failure.

Information for Patients
Patients should be informed of the potential risks and advantages of TOLINASE Tablets (tolazamide) and of alternative modes of therapy. They should also be informed about the importance of adherence to dietary instructions, of a regular exercise program, and of regular testing of urine and/or blood glucose.

The risks of hypoglycemia, its symptoms and treatment, and conditions that predispose to its development should be explained to patients and responsible family members. Primary and secondary failure should also be explained.

Laboratory Tests
Blood and urine glucose should be monitored periodically. Measurement of glycosylated hemoglobin may be useful in some patients.

Drug Interactions
The hypoglycemia action of sulfonylureas may be potentiated by certain drugs including nonsteroidal anti-inflammatory agents and other drugs that are highly protein bound, salicylates, sulfonamides, chloramphenicol, probenecid, coumarins, monoamine oxidase inhibitors, and beta-adrenergic blocking agents. When such drugs are administered to a patient receiving TOLINASE, the patient should be closely observed for hypoglycemia. When such drugs are withdrawn from a patient receiving TOLINASE, the patient should be observed closely for loss of control.

Certain drugs tend to produce hyperglycemia and may lead to loss of control. These drugs include the thiazides and other diuretics, corticosteroids, phenothiazines, thyroid products, estrogens, oral contraceptives, phenytoin, nicotinic acid, sympathomimetics, calcium channel blocking drugs, and isoniazid. When such drugs are administered to a patient receiving TOLINASE, the patient should be closely observed for loss of control. When such drugs are withdrawn from a patient receiving TOLINASE, the patient should be observed closely for hypoglycemia.

Carcinogenicity
In a bioassay for carcinogenicity, rats and mice of both sexes were treated with tolazamide for 103 weeks at low and high doses. No evidence of carcinogenicity was found.

Pregnancy
Teratogenic Effects:
Pregnancy Category C. TOLINASE, administered to pregnant rats at ten times the human dose, decreased litter size but did not produce teratogenic effects in the offspring. In rats treated at a daily dose of 14 mg/kg no reproductive aberrations or drug related fetal anomalies were noted. At an elevated dose of 100 mg/kg per day there was a reduction in the number of pups born and an increased perinatal mortality. There are, however, no adequate and well-controlled studies in pregnant women. Because animal reproduction studies are not always predictive of human response, TOLINASE is not recommended for the treatment of the pregnant diabetic patient. Serious consideration should also be given to the possible hazards of the use of TOLINASE in women of child bearing age and in those who might become pregnant while using the drug.

Because recent information suggests that abnormal blood glucose levels during pregnancy are associated with a higher incidence of congenital abnormalities, many experts recommend that insulin be used during pregnancy to maintain blood glucose levels as close to normal as possible.

Nonteratogenic Effects:
Prolonged severe hypoglycemia (four to ten days) has been reported in neonates born to mothers who were receiving a sulfonylurea drug at the time of delivery. This has been reported more frequently with the use of agents with prolonged half-lives. If TOLINASE is used during pregnancy, it should be discontinued at least two weeks before the expected delivery date.

Nursing Mothers
Altough it is not known whether tolazamide is excreted in human milk, some sulfonylurea drugs are known to be excreted in human milk. Because the potential for hypoglycemia in nursing infants may exist, a decision should be made whether to discontinue nursing or to discontinue the drug, taking into account the importance of the drug to the mother. If the drug is discontinued and if diet alone is inadequate for controlling blood glucose, insulin therapy should be considered.

Pediatric Use
Safety and effectiveness in children have not been established.

Adverse Reactions: TOLINASE Tablets (tolazamide) have generally been well tolerated. In clinical studies in which more than 1,784 diabetic patients were specifically evaluated for incidence of side effects, only 2.1% were discontinued from therapy because of side effects.

Hypoglycemia: See **Precautions** and **Overdosage** sections.

Gastrointestinal Reactions: Cholestatic jaundice may occur rarely; TOLINASE Tablets should be discontinued if this occurs. Gastrointestinal disturbances, eg, nausea, epigastric fullness, and heartburn, are the most common reactions and occurred in 1% of patients treated during clinical trials. They tend to be dose-related and may disappear when dosage is reduced.

Dermatologic Reactions: Allergic skin reactions, eg, pruritus, erythema, urticaria, and morbilliform or maculopapular eruptions, occurred in 0.4% of patients treated during clinical trials. These may be transient and may disappear despite continued use of TOLINASE; if skin reactions persist, the drug should be discontinued.

Porphyria cutanea tarda and photosensitivity reactions have been reported with sulfonylureas.

Hematologic Reactions: Leukopenia, agranulocytosis, thrombocytopenia, hemolytic anemia, aplastic anemia, and pancytopenia have been reported with sulfonylureas.

Metabolic Reactions: Hepatic porphyria and disulfiram-like reactions have been reported with sulfonylureas; however, disulfiram-like reactions with TOLINASE have been reported very rarely.

Miscellaneous: Weakness, fatigue, dizziness, vertigo, malaise and headache were reported infrequently in patients treated during clinical trials. The relationship to therapy with TOLINASE is difficult to assess.

Overdosage: Overdosage of sulfonylureas, including TOLINASE Tablets (tolazamide), can produce hypoglycemia.

Mild hypoglycemic symptoms without loss of consciousness or neurologic findings should be treated aggressively with oral glucose and adjustment in drug dosage and/or meal patterns. Close monitoring should continue until the physician is assured the patient is out of danger. Severe hypoglycemic reactions with coma, seizure, or other neurological impairment occur infrequently, but constitute medical emergencies requiring immediate hospitalization. If hypoglycemic coma is suspected or diagnosed, the patient should be given a rapid intravenous injection of concentrated (50%) glucose solution. This should be followed by a continuous infusion of a more dilute (10%) glucose solution at a rate which will maintain the blood glucose at a level above 100 mg/dl. Patients should be closely monitored for a minimum of 24 to 48 hours since hypoglycemia may recur after apparent clinical recovery.

Dosage and Administration: There is no fixed dosage regimen for the management of diabetes mellitus with TOLINASE Tablets (tolazamide) or any other hypoglycemic agent. In addition to the usual monitoring of urinary glucose, the patient's blood glucose must also be monitored periodically to determine the minimum effective dose for the patient; to detect primary failure, ie, inadequate lowering of blood glucose at the maximum recommended dose of medication; and to detect secondary failure, ie, loss of adequate blood glucose response after an initial period of effectiveness. Glycosylated hemoglobin levels may also be of value in monitoring the patient's response to therapy.

Short-term administration of TOLINASE may be sufficient during periods of transient loss of control in patients usually controlled well on diet.

Usual Starting Dose

The usual starting dose of TOLINASE Tablets for the mild to moderately severe type II diabetic patient is 100–250 mg daily administered with breakfast or the first main meal. Generally, if the fasting blood glucose is less than 200 mg/dl, the starting dose is 100 mg/day as a single daily dose. If the fasting blood glucose value is greater than 200 mg/dl, the starting dose is 250 mg/day as a single dose. If the patient is malnourished, underweight, elderly, or not eating properly, the initial therapy should be 100 mg once a day. Failure to follow an appropriate dosage regimen may precipitate hypoglycemia. Patients who do not adhere to their prescribed dietary regimen are more prone to exhibit unsatisfactory response to drug therapy.

Transfer From Other Hypoglycemic Therapy

Patients Receiving Other Oral Antidiabetic Therapy—Transfer of patients from other oral antidiabetes regimens to TOLINASE should be done conservatively. When transferring patients from oral hypoglycemic agents other than chlorpropamide to TOLINASE, no transition period or initial or priming dose is necessary. When transferring from chlorpropamide, particular care should be exercised to avoid hypoglycemia.

Tolbutamide: If receiving less than 1 gm/day, begin at 100 mg of tolazamide per day. If receiving 1 gm or more per day, initiate at 250 mg of tolazamide per day as a single dose.

Chlorpropamide: 250 mg of chlorpropamide may be considered to provide approximately the same degree of blood glucose control as 250 mg of tolazamide. The patient should be observed carefully for hypoglycemia during the transition period from chlorpropamide to TOLINASE (one to two weeks) due to the prolonged retention of chlorpropamide in the body and the possibility of a subsequent overlapping drug effect.

Acetohexamide: 100 mg of tolazamide may be considered to provide approximately the same degree of blood glucose control as 250 mg of acetohexamide.

Patients Receiving Insulin—Some type II diabetic patients who have been treated only with insulin may respond satisfactorily to therapy with TOLINASE. If the patient's previous insulin dosage has been less than 20 units, substitutioin of 100 mg of tolazamide per day as a single daily dose may be tried. If the previous insulin dosage was less than 40 units, but more than 20 units, the patient should be placed directly on 250 mg of tolazamide per day as a single dose. If the previous insulin dosage was greater than 40 units, the insulin dosage should be decreased by 50% and 250 mg of tolazamide per day started. The dosage of TOLINASE should be adjusted weekly (or more often in the group previously requiring more than 40 units of insulin). During this conversion period when both insulin and TOLINASE are being used, hypoglycemia may rarely occur. During insulin withdrawal, patients should test their urine for glucose and acetone at least three times daily and report results to their physician. The appearance of persistent acetonuria with glycosuria indicates that the patient is a type I diabetic who requires insulin therapy.

Maximum Dose

Daily doses of greater than 1000 mg are not recommended. Patients will generally have no further response to doses larger than this.

Usual Maintenance Dose

The usual maintenance dose is in the range of 100–1000 mg/day with the average maintenance dose being 250–500 mg/day. Following initiation of therapy, dosage adjustment is made in increments of 100 mg to 250 mg at weekly intervals based on the patient's blood glucose response.

Dosage Interval

Once a day therapy is usually satisfactory. Doses up to 500 mg/day should be given as a single dose in the morning. 500 mg once daily is as effective as 250 mg twice daily. When a dose of more than 500 mg/day is required, the dose may be divided and given twice daily.

In elderly patients, debilitated or malnourished patients, and patients with impaired renal or hepatic function, the initial and maintenance dosing should be conservative to avoid hypoglycemic reactions (see **PRECAUTIONS** section).

How Supplied: TOLINASE Tablets (tolazamide) are available in the following strengths and package sizes:

100 mg (scored, round, white)
   Unit-of-Use bottles of 100   NDC 0009-0070-02
250 mg (scored, round, white)
   Bottles of 200   NDC 0009-0114-04
   Bottles of 1000   NDC 0009-0114-02
   Unit-of-Use bottles of 100   NDC 0009-0114-05
   Unit-Dose package of 100   NDC 0009-0114-06
500 mg (scored, round, white)
   Unit-of-Use bottles of 100   NDC 0009-0477-06

Store at controlled room temperature 15–30° C (59–86° F).
Code 811 417 103
Shown in Product Identification Section, page 441

TROBICIN® ℞
brand of spectinomycin hydrochloride sterile powder
(sterile spectinomycin hydrochloride, USP)
For Intramuscular Injection

2 Gm vial
NSN 6505-00-079-7611 (M)
4 Gm vial
NSN 6505-00-079-7643 (M)

Description: TROBICIN Sterile Powder contains spectinomycin hydrochloride which is an aminocyclitol antibiotic produced by a species of soil microorganism designated as *Streptomyces spectabilis*. Sterile spectinomycin hydrochloride is the pentahydrated dihydrochloride salt of spectinomycin. Spectinomycin hydrochloride is isolated as a white to pale buff crystalline dihydrochloride pentahydrate powder, molecular weight 495, and is stable in the dry state for 36 months.

Actions: Spectinomycin hydrochloride is an inhibitor of protein synthesis in the bacterial cell; the site of action is the 30S ribosomal subunit.

In vitro studies have shown spectinomycin hydrochloride to be active against most strains of *Neisseria gonorrhoeae* (minimum inhibitory concentration < 7.5 to 20 mcg/ml).

Definitive *in vitro* studies have shown no cross-resistance of *N. gonorrhoeae* between streptinomycin hydrochloride and penicillin. The antibiotic is not significantly bound to plasma protein.

Indications: TROBICIN Sterile Powder (spectinomycin hydrochloride) is indicated in the treatment of acute gonorrheal urethritis and proctitis in the male and acute gonorrheal cervicitis and proctitis in the female when due to susceptible strains of *Neisseria gonorrhoeae*. Men and women with known recent exposure to gonorrhea should be treated as those known to have gonorrhea.

The *in vitro* susceptibility of *Neisseria gonorrhoeae* to spectinomycin hydrochloride can be tested by agar dilution methods. TROBICIN Susceptibility Powder is available for this purpose, and its package insert should be consulted for details.

Contraindications: The use of TROBICIN Sterile Powder (spectinomycin hydrochloride) is contraindicated in patients previously found hypersensitive to it.

Warnings: Spectinomycin hydrochloride is not effective in the treatment of syphilis. Antibiotics used in high doses for short periods of time to treat gonorrhea may mask or delay the symptoms of incubating syphilis. Since the treatment of syphilis demands prolonged therapy with any effective antibiotic, patients being treated for gonorrhea should be closely observed clinically. All patients with gonorrhea should have a serologic test for syphilis at the time of diagnosis. Patients treated with spectinomycin hydrochloride should have a follow-up serologic test for syphilis after three months.

Usage in pregnancy: Safety for use in pregnancy has not been established.

Usage in infants and children: Safety for use in infants and children has not been established.

Precautions: The usual precautions should be observed with atopic individuals.

The clinical effectiveness of TROBICIN Sterile Powder (spectinomycin hydrochloride) should be monitored to detect evidence of development of resistance by *Neisseria gonorrhoeae*.

Adverse Reactions: The following reactions were observed during the single dose clinical trials: soreness at the injection site, urticaria, dizziness, nausea, chills, fever and insomnia.

During multiple dose subchronic tolerance studies in normal human volunteers, the following were noted: a decrease in hemoglobin, hematocrit and creatinine clearance; elevation of alkaline phosphatase, BUN and SGPT. In single and multiple dose studies in normal volunteers, a reduction in urine output was noted. Extensive renal function studies demonstrated no consistent changes indicative of renal toxicity.

Although no clearly defined case of anaphylaxis has been reported with TROBICIN Sterile Powder, the possibility of such reactions should be considered particularly when using antibiotics.

Dosage and Administration:
Preparation of Drug for Intramuscular Injection
TROBICIN Sterile Powder, 2 gram (spectinomycin hydrochloride): reconstitute with 3.2 ml of the accompanying diluent.*
TROBICIN Sterile Powder 4 gram: reconstitute with 6.2 ml of the accompanying diluent.*
*Bacteriostatic Water for Injection with Benzyl Alcohol 0.945% w/v added as preservative.
Shake vials vigorously immediately after adding diluent and before withdrawing dose. It is recommended that disposable syringes and needles be used to avoid contamination with penicillin residue, especially when treating patients known to be highly sensitive to penicillin. **Use of 20 gauge needle is recommended.**

Dosage
Intramuscular injections should be made deep into the upper outer quadrant of the gluteal muscle.

Adults (Men and Women)—Inject 5 ml intramuscularly for a 2 gram dose. This is also the recommended dose for patients being treated after failure of previous antibiotic therapy.

In geographic areas where antibiotic resistance is known to be prevalent, initial treatment with 4 grams (10 ml) intramuscularly is preferred. The 10 ml injection may be divided between two gluteal injection sites.

Storage Conditions: Store unreconstituted product at controlled room temperature 15°–30°C (59°–86°F). Store prepared suspension at controlled room temperature 15°–30°C (59°–86°F) and use within 24 hours.

Continued on next page

Information on these Upjohn products is based on labeling in effect on November 30, 1984. Further information concerning these and other Upjohn products may be obtained from the package insert or by direct inquiry to Medical Information, The Upjohn Company, Kalamazoo, Michigan 49001.

Upjohn—Cont.

How Supplied: TROBICIN Sterile Powder (spectinomycin hydrochloride) is available as:

TROBICIN Sterile Powder, 2 gram vial—with one ampoule of Bacteriostatic Water for Injection with Benzyl Alcohol 0.945% w/v added as preservative. When reconstituted with 3.2 ml of the accompanying diluent, each vial yields a sufficient quantity for withdrawal of 5 ml of a suspension containing 400 mg spectinomycin per ml (as the hydrochloride). 5 ml provides 2 grams spectinomycin. For intramuscular use only.

NDC 0009-0566-01

TROBICIN Sterile Powder 4 gram vial—with one ampoule of Bacteriostatic Water for Injection with Benzyl Alcohol 0.945% w/v added as preservative. When reconstituted with 6.2 ml of the accompanying diluent, each vial yields a sufficient quantity for withdrawal of 10 ml of a suspension containing spectinomycin hydrochloride equivalent to 400 mg spectinomycin per ml. 10 ml provides 4 grams spectinomycin. For intramuscular use only.

NDC 0009-0592-01

TROBICIN Susceptibility Powder—100 mg. See package insert for *in vitro* testing procedure.

Human Pharmacology: TROBICIN Sterile Powder (spectinomycin hydrochloride) is rapidly absorbed after intramuscular injection. A single, two gram injection produces peak serum concentrations averaging about 100 mcg/ml at one hour; a single, four gram injection produces peak serum concentrations averaging 160 mcg/ml at two hours. Average serum concentrations of 15 mcg/ml for the two gram dose and 31 mcg/ml for the four gram dose were present eight hours after dosing.

Code 810 130 004

UNICAP® Capsules/Tablets
(See PDR For Nonprescription Drugs)

UNICAP CHEWABLE® Tablets
(See PDR For Nonprescription Drugs)

UNICAP M® Tablets
(See PDR For Nonprescription Drugs)

UNICAP PLUS IRON® Tablets
(See PDR For Nonprescription Drugs)

UNICAP SENIOR® Tablets
(See PDR For Nonprescription Drugs)

UNICAP T® Tablets
(See PDR For Nonprescription Drugs)

XANAX®
brand of alprazolam tablets
0.25 mg, 100's
NSN 6505-01-143-9269 (M and VA)
0.5 mg, 100's
NSN 6505-01-140-3199 (M and VA)
1 mg, 100's
NSN 6505-01-140-3200 (M and VA)

Description: XANAX Tablets contain alprazolam which is a triazolo analog of the 1,4 benzodiazepine class of central nervous system-active compounds.

The chemical name of alprazolam is 8-Chloro-1-methyl-6-phenyl-4H-s-triazolo[4,3-α] [1,4]benzodiazepine.

Alprazolam is a white crystalline powder, soluble in methanol or ethanol but with no appreciable solublity in water at physiological pH.

Each XANAX tablet, for oral administration, contains, 0.25, 0.5 or 1.0 mg of alprazolam.

Clinical Pharmacology: CNS agents of the 1,4 benzodiazepine class presumably exert their effects by binding at stereo specific receptors at several sites within the central nervous system. Their exact mechanism of action is unknown. Clinically, all benzodiazepines cause a dose-related central nervous system depressant activity varying from mild impairment of task performance to hypnosis.

Following oral administration, alprazolam is readily absorbed. Peak concentrations in the plasma occur in one to two hours following administration. Plasma levels are proportionate to the dose given; over the dose range of 0.5 to 3.0 mg, peak levels of 8.0 to 37 ng/ml were observed. The mean elimination half-life of alprazolam is 12–15 hours. The predominant metabolites are α-hydroxy-alprazolam and a benzophenone derived from alprazolam. The biological activity of α-hydroxy-alprazolam is approximately one-half that of alprazolam. The benzophenone metabolite is essentially inactive. Plasma levels of these metabolites are extremely low, thus precluding precise pharmacokinetic description. However, their half-lives appear to be of the same order of magnitude as alprazolam. Alprazolam and its metabolites are excreted primarily in the urine.

The ability of alprazolam to induce human hepatic enzyme systems has not yet been determined. However, this is not a property of benzodiazepines in general. Further, alprazolam did not affect the prothrombin or plasma warfarin levels in male volunteers administered sodium warfarin orally.

In vitro, alprazolam is bound (80 percent) to human serum protein.

Changes in the absorption, distribution, metabolism and excretion of benzodiazepines have been reported in a variety of disease states including alcoholism, impaired hepatic function and impaired renal function. Changes have also been demonstrated in geriatric patients. It has not yet been determined if similar changes occur in the pharmacokinetics of alprazolam.

Because of its similarity to other benzodiazepines, it is assumed that alprazolam undergoes transplacental passage and is excreted in human milk.

Indications and Usage: XANAX Tablets (alprazolam) are indicated for the management of anxiety disorders or the short-term relief of the symptoms of anxiety. Anxiety or tension associated with the stress of everyday life usually does not require treatment with an anxiolytic.

Anxiety associated with depression is also responsive to XANAX.

The effectiveness of XANAX for long-term use, that is, more than four months, has not been established by systematic clinical trials. The physician should periodically reassess the usefulness of the drug for the individual patient.

Contraindications: XANAX Tablets (alprazolam) are contraindicated in patients with known sensitivity to this drug or other benzodiazepines. XANAX may be used in patients with open angle glaucoma who are receiving appropriate therapy, but is contraindicated in acute narrow angle glaucoma.

Warnings: XANAX Tablets (alprazolam) are not of value in the treatment of psychotic patients and should not be employed in lieu of appropriate treatment for psychosis. Because of its depressant CNS effects, patients receiving XANAX should be cautioned against engaging in hazardous occupations requiring complete mental alertness such as operating machinery or driving a motor vehicle. For the same reason, patients should be cautioned about the simultaneous ingestion of alcohol and other CNS depressant drugs during treatment with XANAX.

Benzodiazepines can potentially cause fetal harm when administered to pregnant women. If XANAX is used during pregnancy, or if the patient becomes pregnant while taking this drug, the patient should be appraised of the potential hazard to the fetus. Because of experience with other members of the benzodiazepine class, XANAX is assumed to be capable of causing an increased risk of congenital abnormalities when administered to a pregnant woman during the first trimester. Because use of these drugs is rarely a matter of urgency, their use during the first trimester should almost always be avoided. The possibility that a woman of childbearing potential may be pregnant at the time of institution of therapy should be considered. Patients should be advised that if they become pregnant during therapy or intend to become pregnant they should communicate with their physicians about the desirability of discontinuing the drug.

Precautions

General: In some patients receiving recommended (or higher) doses of XANAX Tablets (alprazolam) for relatively brief periods of time (eg, one week to four months), withdrawal seizures have been reported upon rapid decrease of dosage or abrupt discontinuation. Therefore, the dosage of XANAX should be reduced or withdrawn gradually (see DOSAGE AND ADMINISTRATION.)

If XANAX Tablets are to be combined with other psychotropic agents or anticonvulsant drugs, careful consideration should be given to the pharmacology of the agents to be employed—particularly with compounds which might potentiate the action of benzodiazepines (See Drug Interaction Section).

As with other psychotropic medications, the usual precautions with respect to administration of the drug and size of the prescription are indicated for severely depressed patients or those in whom there is reason to expect concealed suicidal ideation or plans.

In elderly and debilitated patients, it is recommended that the dosage be limited to the smallest effective amount to preclude the development of ataxia or oversedation (See Dosage and Administration Section). The usual precautions in treating patients with impaired renal or hepatic function should be observed.

Information for Patients: To assure safe and effective use of benzodiazepines, the following information and instructions should be given to patients:

1) Inform your physician about any alcohol consumption and medicine you are taking now, including drugs you may buy without a prescription. Alcohol should generally not be used during treatment with benzodiazepines.

2) Inform your physician if you are planning to become pregnant, if you are pregnant, or if you become pregnant while you are taking this medication.

3) Inform your physician if you are nursing.

4) Until you experience how this medication affects you, do not drive a car or operate potentially dangerous machinery, etc.

5) If benzodiazepines are used in large doses and/or for extended periods of time, they may produce habituation and emotional and physical dependence. Therefore, do not increase the dose even if you think the drug "does not work anymore."

6) Do not stop taking the drug abruptly without consulting your physician, since withdrawal symptoms can occur.

Laboratory Tests: Laboratory tests are not ordinarily required in otherwise healthy patients.

Drug interactions: The benzodiazepines, including alprazolam, produce additive CNS depressant effects when co-administered with other psychotropic medications, anticonvulsants, anti-histaminics, ethanol and other drugs which themselves produce CNS depression.

Pharmacokinetic interactions of benzodiazepines with other drugs have been reported. For example, the clearance of alprazolam and certain other benzodiazepines can be delayed by the co-administration of cimetidine. The clinical significance of this is unclear.

Drug/Laboratory Test Interactions: Although interactions between benzodiazepines and commonly employed clinical laboratory tests have occasionally been reported, there is no consistent pattern for a specific drug or specific test.

Carcinogenesis, Mutagenesis, Impairment of Fertility: No evidence of carcinogenic potential was observed in rats during a 24-month study with alprazolam in doses up to 375 times the human dose.

Alprazolam was not mutagenic in the rat micronucleus test at doses up to 1250 times the human dose.

Product Information

Alprazolam produced no impairment of fertility in rats at doses up to 62.5 times the human dose.

Pregnancy: Teratogenic Effects: Pregnancy Category D: (See Warnings Section)

Nonteratogenic Effects: It is to be considered that the child born of a mother who is on benzodiazepines may be at some risk for withdrawal symptoms from the drug during the postnatal period. Also, neonatal flaccidity has been reported in children born of a mother who has been receiving benzodiazepines.

Labor and Delivery: XANAX has no established use in labor or delivery.

Nursing Mothers: Benzodiazepines are known to be excreted in human milk. It is to be assumed that alprazolam is as well. Chronic administration of diazepam to nursing mothers has been reported to cause their infants to become lethargic and lose weight. As a general rule, nursing should not be undertaken by mothers who must use XANAX.

Pediatric Use: Safety and effectiveness in children below the age of 18 have not been established.

Adverse Reactions: Side effects to XANAX Tablets (alprazolam), if they occur are generally observed at the beginning of therapy and usually disappear upon continued medication. In the usual patient, the most frequent side effects are likely to be an extension of the pharmacological activity of alprazolam, eg, drowsiness or lightheadedness.

The figures cited below are estimates of untoward clinical event incidence among subjects who participated in the relatively short duration (ie, four weeks) placebo-controlled clinical trials of XANAX. The figures cannot be used to predict precisely the incidence of untoward events in the course of usual medical practice where patient characteristics, and other factors often differ from those which obtained in the clinical trials. These figures cannot be compared with those obtained from other clinical studies involving related drug products and placebo as each group of drug trials are conducted under a different set of conditions. Comparison of the cited figures, however, can provide the prescriber with some basis for estimating the relative contributions of drug and non-drug factors to the untoward event incidence rate in the population studied. Even this use must be approached cautiously, as a drug may relieve a symptom in one patient while inducing it in others. [For example, an anxiolytic drug may relieve dry mouth (a symptom of anxiety) in some subjects but induces (an untoward event) in others.]

Additionally, the cited figures can provide the prescriber with an indication as to the frequency with which physician intervention (eg increased surveillance, decreased dosage or discontinuation of drug therapy) may be necessary because of the untoward clinical event.

[See table above].

There have also been reports of withdrawal seizures upon rapid decrease or abrupt discontinuation of XANAX TAblets (See PRECAUTIONS—General).

In addition to the relatively common (i.e., greater than 1%) untoward events enumerated above, the following adverse events have been reported in association with the use of anxiolytic benzodiazepines: dystonia, irritability, concentration difficulties, anorexia, loss of coordination, fatigue, sedation, slurred speech, jaundice, musculoskeletal weakness, pruritus, diplopia, dysarthria, changes in libido, menstrual irregularities, incontinence and urinary retention.

As with all benzodiazepines, paradoxical reactions such as stimulation, agitation, increased muscle spasticity, sleep disturbances, hallucinations and other adverse behavioral effects may occur in rare instances and in a random fashion. Should these occur, use of the drug should be discontinued.

Laboratory analyses were performed on all patients participating in the XANAX clinical program. The following incidences of abnormalities were observed in patients receiving XANAX and the corresponding placebo group. None of these changes were considered to be of physiological significance.

XANAX	Treatment Symptom XANAX	Emergent Incidence Placebo	Incidence of Intervention Because of Symptoms XANAX
Number of Patients	565	505	565
% of Patients Reporting:			
Central Nervous System			
Drowsiness	41.0	21.6	15.1
Light-headedness	20.8	19.3	1.2
Depression	13.9	18.1	2.4
Headache	12.9	19.6	1.1
Confusion	9.9	10.0	0.9
Insomnia	8.9	18.4	1.3
Nervousness	4.1	10.3	1.1
Syncope	3.1	4.0	*
Dizziness	1.8	0.8	2.5
Akathisia	1.6	1.2	*
Tiredness/Sleepiness	*	*	1.8
Gastrointestinal			
Dry Mouth	14.7	13.3	0.7
Constipation	10.4	11.4	0.9
Diarrhea	10.1	10.3	1.2
Nausea/Vomiting	9.6	12.8	1.7
Increased Salivation	4.2	2.4	*
Cardiovascular			
Tachycardia/Palpitations	7.7	15.6	0.4
Hypotension	4.7	2.2	*
Sensory			
Blurred Vision	6.2	6.2	0.4
Musculoskeletal			
Rigidity	4.2	5.3	*
Tremor	4.0	8.8	0.4
Cutaneous			
Dermatitis/Allergy	3.8	3.1	0.6
Other			
Nasal Congestion	7.3	9.3	*
Weight Gain	2.7	2.7	*
Weight Loss	2.3	3.0	*

* None reported

	XANAX Low	XANAX High	Placebo Low	Placebo High
Hematology				
Hematocrit	*	*	*	*
Hemoglobin	*	*	*	*
Total WBC Count	1.4	2.3	1.0	2.0
Neutrophil Count	2.3	3.0	4.2	1.7
Lymphocyte Count	5.5	7.4	5.4	9.5
Monocyte Count	5.3	2.8	6.4	*
Eosinophil Count	3.2	9.5	3.3	7.2
Basophil Count	*	*	*	*
Urinalysis				
Albumin	—	*	—	*
Sugar	—	*	—	*
RBC/HPF	—	3.4	—	5.0
WBC/HPF	—	25.7	—	25.9
Blood Chemistry				
Creatinine	2.2	1.9	3.5	1.0
Bilirubin	*	1.6	*	*
SGOT	*	3.2	1.0	1.8
Alkaline Phosphatase	*	1.7	*	1.8

* Less than 1%

When treatment with XANAX is protracted, periodic blood counts, urinalysis and blood chemistry analyses are advisable.

Minor changes in EEG patterns, usually low-voltage fast activity have been observed in patients during therapy with XANAX and are of no known significance.

Drug Abuse and Dependence

Physical and Psychological Dependence: Withdrawal symptoms (similar in character to those noted with barbiturates and alcohol) have occurred following abrupt discontinuance of benzodiazepines. (These can range from mild dysphoria and insomnia to a major syndrome which may include abdominal and muscle cramps, vomiting, sweating, tremor and convulsions). In addition, withdrawal seizures have occurred upon rapid decrease or abrupt discontinuation of therapy with XANAX Tablets (See PRECAUTIONS—General). It is recommended that all patients on XANAX who require a dosage reduction be gradually tapered under close supervision (See DOSAGE AND ADMINISTRATION).

Patients with a history of seizures or epilepsy, regardless of their concomitant anti-seizure drug therapy, should not be abruptly withdrawn from any CNS depressant agent, including XANAX Tablets (alprazolam). Addiction-prone individuals (such as drug addicts or alcoholics) should be under careful surveillance when receiving alprazolam or other psychotropic agents because of the predisposition of such patients to habituation and dependence.

Controlled Substance Class:

XANAX is a controlled substance under the Controlled Substance Act by the Drug Enforcement

Continued on next page

Information on these Upjohn products is based on labeling in effect on November 30, 1984. Further information concerning these and other Upjohn products may be obtained from the package insert or by direct inquiry to Medical Information, The Upjohn Company, Kalamazoo, Michigan 49001.

Upjohn—Cont.

Administration and has been assigned to Schedule IV.

Overdosage: Manifestations of alprazolam overdosage include somnolence, confusion, impaired coordination, diminished reflexes and coma.

No delayed reactions (eg, organ toxicity) or clinical laboratory abnormalities have been reported.

The acute oral LD_{50} in rats is 331–2171 mg/kg. Other experiments in animals have indicated that cardiopulmonary collapse can occur following massive intravenous doses of alprazolam (over 195 mg/kg; 2000 times the maximum usual daily human dose). Animals could be resuscitated with positive mechanical ventilation and the intravenous infusion of levarterenol.

Animal experiments have suggested that forced diuresis or hemodialysis are probably of little value in treating overdosage.

General Treatment of Overdose: Overdosage reports with XANAX are limited. Respiration, pulse, and blood pressure should be monitored, as in all cases of drug overdosage. General supportive measures should be employed, along with immediate gastric lavage. Intravenous fluids should be administered and an adequate airway maintained. Hypotension may be combated by the use of Levophed (levarterenol) or Aramine (metaraminol). Dialysis is of limited value. As with the management of intentional overdosing with any drug, it should be borne in mind that multiple agents may have been ingested.

Dosage and Administration: Dosage should be individualized for maximum beneficial effect. While the usual daily dosages given below will meet the needs of most patients, there will be some who require higher doses. In such cases, dosage should be increased cautiously to avoid adverse effects. Dosage should be reduced gradually when terminating therapy or decreasing the daily dose. Although clinical studies have not been conducted to determine a tapering regimen, it is suggested that dosage be decreased no more than one milligram every three days.

Daily Dosage Schedule: The usual starting dose is 0.25 to 0.5 mg, given three times daily. This may be titrated according to the needs of the patient to a maximum total daily dose of 4 mg, given in divided doses.

In the elderly, or in the presence of debilitating disease, the usual starting dose is 0.25 mg, given two or three times daily. This may be gradually increased if needed and tolerated.

If side effects occur with the starting dose, the dose should be lowered.

How Supplied:
XANAX Tablets (alprazolam), ovoid-shaped and scored, are available as follows:
  0.25 mg (white)
    Bottles of 100 **NDC** 0009-0029-01
    Unit-Dose Pkg (100) **NDC** 0009-0029-09
    Bottles of 500 **NDC** 0009-0029-02
  0.5 mg (peach)
    Bottles of 100 **NDC** 0009-0055-01
    Unit-Dose Pkg (100) **NDC** 0009-0055-02
    Bottles of 500 **NDC** 0009-0055-03
  1 mg (lavender)
    Bottles of 100 **NDC** 0009-0090-01
    Unit-Dose Pkg (100) **NDC** 0009-0090-02
    Bottles of 500 **NDC** 0009-0090-04

Store at controlled room temperature 15°–30°C (59°–86°F).

Caution: Federal law prohibits dispensing without prescription.

Animal Studies: When rats were treated with alprazolam at 3, 10, and 30 mg/kg/day (37.5 to 375 times the maximum recommended human dose) orally for 2 years, a tendency for a dose related increase in the number of cataracts was observed in females and a tendency for a dose related increase in corneal vascularization was observed in males. These lesions did not appear until after 11 months of treatment.

Clinical Studies: XANAX Tablets (alprazolam) were compared to placebo in double blind clinical trials in patients with a diagnosis of anxiety or anxiety with associated depressive symptomatology. XANAX was significantly better than placebo at each of the evaluation periods of these four week studies as judged by the psychometric instruments: Physician's Global Impressions, Hamilton Anxiety Rating Scale Target Symptoms, Patient's Global Impressions and Self-Rating Symptom Scale.

Code 811 557 206

Shown in Product Identification Section, page 441

Upsher-Smith Laboratories, Inc.
14905 23RD AVE., NORTH MINNEAPOLIS, MN 55441

ACETAMINOPHEN UNISERTS® OTC
Rectal Suppositories

Description: Acetaminophen Uniserts suppositories are supplied in 120 mg. (pediatric), 325 mg. and 650 mg. strengths. Acetaminophen Uniserts are foil strip-wrapped and unit dose labeled.

Indications: For the temporary relief of fever, minor aches, pains and headaches.

Dosage: Adults—One 650 mg. suppository every 4 to 6 hours. No more than a total of 6 suppositories in any 24-hour period.
Children (over 6)—One 325 mg. suppository every 4 to 6 hours. No more than a total of 8 suppositories in any 24-hour period.
Children (3 to 6)—One 120 mg. (pediatric) suppository every 4 to 6 hours. No more than a total of 6 suppositories in any 24-hour period. Children (under 3)—Consult a physician.

Warning: Severe or recurrent pain or high or continued fever may be indicative of serious illness. Under these conditions, consult a physician. Do not use consistently for more than 2 days except on the advice of a physician.

How Supplied: 120 mg., boxes of 12. 325 mg., boxes of 12 and 50. 650 mg., boxes of 12, 50 and 500.

KLOR-10%™ ℞
(potassium chloride oral solution, USP 10%)

How Supplied: 4 fl. oz., pints and gallons.

KLOR–CON® 20% ℞
(potassium chloride oral solution, USP 20%)

How Supplied: 4 fl. oz., pints and gallons.

KLOR–CON® Powder ℞
(Potassium Chloride for Oral Solution, U.S.P.) 20 mEq. (1.5g) per packet

Description: Each packet contains 1.5g potassium chloride providing potassium 20 mEq and chloride 20 mEq. Fruit-flavored with artificial color and sweetener (saccharin) added.

Indications: Treatment of potassium deficiency which may occur with long-term diuretic therapy, corticosteroid therapy, digitalis intoxication, low dietary intake of potassium or loss of potassium due to vomiting and diarrhea.

Contraindications: Renal impairment, untreated Addison's disease, dehydration, heat cramps and hyperkalemia. Potassium chloride should not be employed in patients receiving potassium-sparing agents such as aldosterone antagonists and triamterene.

Precautions: Potassium chloride must be administered with caution since the degree of potassium deficiency and the corresponding daily dosage is often not accurately known. Excessive or even therapeutic dosages may result in potassium intoxication. The patient should be checked frequently and periodic ECG and/or plasma potassium levels made. High plasma concentrations of potassium ion may cause cardiac depression, arrhythmias or arrest. Use with caution in the presence of cardiac disease. Patients should be cautioned to adhere to dilution instructions.

Adverse Reactions: Vomiting, diarrhea, nausea and abdominal discomfort may occur. Symptoms and signs of potassium intoxication include mental confusion, listlessness, paresthesias of the extremities, flaccid paralysis, weakness of the legs, fall in blood pressure, cardiac arrhythmias and heart block. Hyperkalemia, when detected, must be treated promptly.

Dosage and Administration: The usual adult dose is 20 to 80 mEq of potassium per day (1 packet 1 to 4 times daily after meals.) The contents of 1 packet should be dissolved in at least 4 oz cold water or fruit juice. This preparation, like other potassium supplements, must be properly diluted to avoid the possibility of gastrointestinal irritation.

How Supplied: KLOR-CON Powder 20 mEq (1.5g) (Potassium Chloride). In cartons of 30 and 100 packets.

KLOR-CON®/25 Powder ℞
(Potassium Chloride for Oral Solution, U.S.P.) 25 mEq. per packet

How Supplied: Cartons of 30, 100 and 250 packets.

LUBRIN™ Vaginal Lubricating Inserts

(See PDR For Nonprescription Drugs)

RMS™ Suppositories © ℞
(Rectal Morphine Sulfate)

WARNING—MAY BE HABIT FORMING

Description: Suppositories contain 5, 10 or 20 mg of morphine sulfate. Morphine sulfate occurs as white, feathery, silky crystals, cubical masses of crystals, or white, crystalline powder. The chemical name of morphine sulfate is 7,8-didehydro-4,5α-epoxy-17 methylmorphinan-3, 6α-diol sulfate (2:1) (salt) pentahydrate. The empirical formula is $(C_{17}H_{19}NO_3)_2 \cdot H_2SO_4 \cdot 5H_2O$. Morphine sulfate suppositories are for rectal administration.

Clinical Pharmacology: Morphine sulfate is a potent analgesic, with major effects on the central nervous system and the bowel. Opioids act as agonists, interacting with stereospecific and saturable binding sites on receptors in the brain and other tissues. Morphine sulfate given as a rectal suppository can produce analgesic effects and duration similar to that of oral administration at similar dose levels. Analgesic effects are commonly seen 20 to 60 minutes after administration.

Indications and Usage: Morphine is a potent analgesic used for the relief of severe pain. It has also been used preoperatively to sedate the patient and allay apprehension, facilitate induction of anesthesia, and reduce anesthesia dosage.

Contraindications: Hypersensitivity to morphine; respiratory insufficiency or depression; severe CNS depression; attack of bronchial asthma; heart failure secondary to chronic lung disease; cardiac arrhythmias; increased intracranial or cerebrospinal pressure; head injuries, brain tumor; acute alcoholism; delerium tremens; convulsive disorders; after biliary tract surgery; suspected surgical abdomen; surgical anastomosis; concomitantly with MAO inhibitors or within 14 days of such treatment.

Warnings: Morphine can cause tolerance, psychological and physical dependence. Withdrawal will occur on abrupt discontinuation or administration of a narcotic antagonist. *Interaction with Other Central-Nervous System Depressants*—Morphine should be used with caution and in reduced dosage in patients who are concurrently receiving other narcotic analgesics, general anesthetics, phenothiazines, other tranquilizers, sedative-hypnotics, tricyclic antidepressants, and other CNS depressants (including alcohol). Respiratory depression, hypotension, and profound sedation or coma may result.

Precautions: *Acute Abdominal Condition*—The administration of morphine or other narcotics may obscure the diagnosis or clinical course in patients with acute abdominal conditions. *Special Risk Patients*—Morphine should be given with caution to certain patients, such as the elderly or debilitated and those with severe impairment of hepatic or renal function, hypothyroidism, Addison's disease, and prostatic hypertrophy or urethral stricture. Morphine sulfate should be used with extreme caution in patients with disorders characterized by hypoxia, since even usual therapeutic doses of narcotics may decrease respiratory drive to the point of apnea while simultaneously increasing airway resistance. *Hypotensive Effect*—The administration of morphine sulfate may result in severe hypotension in the postoperative patient or any individual whose ability to maintain blood pressure has been compromised by a depleted blood volume or the administration of such drugs as the phenothiazines or certain anesthetics. *Supraventricular Tachycardias*—Because of possible vagolytic action that may produce a significant increase in the ventricular response rate, morphine sulfate should be used with caution in patients with atrial flutter and other supraventricular tachycardias. *Convulsions*—Morphine sulfate may aggravate preexisting convulsions in patients with convulsive disorders. If dosage is escalated substantially above recommended levels because of tolerance development, convulsions may occur in individuals without a history of convulsive disorders. *Kidney or Liver Dysfunction*—Morphine sulfate may have a prolonged duration and cumulative effect in patients with kidney or liver dysfunction. *Information for Patients*—Morphine may impair the mental and/or physical abilities required for the performance of potentially hazardous tasks, such as driving a car or operating machinery. Morphine in combination with other narcotic analgesics, phenothiazines, sedative/hypnotics, and alcohol has additive depressant effects. The patient should be cautioned accordingly. *Drug Interactions*—Morphine in combination with other narcotic analgesics, general anesthetics, phenothiazines, tranquilizers, sedative/hypnotics, or other CNS depressants (including alcohol) has additive depressant effects. When such combination therapy is contemplated, the dosage of one or both agents should be reduced. *Carcinogenesis, Mutagenesis, Impairment of Fertility*—Morphine has no known carcinogenic or mutagenic potential. However, no long-term animal studies are available to support this observation. *Usage in Pregnancy—Pregnancy Category C*—Animal reproduction studies have not been conducted with morphine sulfate. It is not known whether morphine sulfate can cause fetal harm when administered to a pregnant woman or can affect reproduction capacity. On the basis of the historical use of morphine sulfate during all stages of pregnancy, there is no known risk of fetal abnormality. Morphine sulfate should be given to a pregnant woman only if clearly needed. *Labor and Delivery*—The use of morphine sulfate in obstetrics may prolong labor. It passes the placental barrier and may produce depression of respiration in the newborn. Resuscitation and in severe depression, the administration of a narcotic antagonist such as naloxone or nalorphine may be required. *Nursing Mothers*—Morphine sulfate appears in the milk of nursing mothers. Caution should be exercised when it is administered to a nursing mother.

Adverse Reactions: The major hazards of morphine as of other narcotic analgesics, are respiratory depression and, to a lesser degree, circulatory depression, respiratory arrest, shock, and cardiac arrest have occurred. The most frequently observed adverse reactions include lightheadedness, dizziness, sedation, nausea, vomiting, and sweating. These effects seem to be more prominent in ambulatory patients and in those who are not suffering severe pain. In such individuals, lower doses are advisable. Some adverse reactions may be alleviated in the ambulatory patient if he lies down. Other adverse reactions include the following: *Central Nervous System*—Euphoria, dysphoria, weakness, headache, insomnia, agitation, disorientation, and visual disturbances. *Gastrointestinal*—Dry mouth, anorexia, constipation, and biliary tract spasms. *Cardiovascular*—Flushing of the face, bradycardia, palpitation, faintness, and syncope. *Genitourinary*—Urinary retention or hesitancy, anti-diuretic effect and reduced libido and/or potency. *Allergic*—Pruritus, urticaria, other skin rashes, edema, and rarely hemorrhagic urticaria.

Drug Abuse and Dependence: *Controlled Substance*—Morphine sulfate is a Schedule II narcotic. *Dependence*—Morphine can produce drug dependence and therefore, has the potential for being abused. Patients receiving therapeutic dosage regimens of 10 mg every 4 hours for 1 to 2 weeks have exhibited mild withdrawal symptoms. Development of the dependent state is recognizable by an increased tolerance to the analgesic effect and the appearance of purposive phenomena (complaints, pleas, demands, or manipulative actions) shortly before the time of the next scheduled dose. A patient in withdrawal should be treated in a hospital environment. Usually, it is necessary only to provide supportive care with administration of a tranquilizer to suppress anxiety. Severe symptoms of withdrawal may require administration of a replacement narcotic.

Overdosage: *Signs and Symptoms*—Serious overdosage of morphine is characterized by respiratory depression (a decrease in respiratory rate and/or tidal volume, Cheyne-Stokes respiration, cyanosis), extreme somnolence progressing to stupor or coma, skeletal-muscle flaccidity, cold and clammy skin, and, sometimes, bradycardia and hypotension. In severe overdosage, apnea, circulatory collapse, cardiac arrest, and death may occur. *Treatment*—Primary attention should be given to the re-establishment of adequate respiratory exchange through provision of a patient's airway and institution of assisted or controlled ventilation. The narcotic antagonists—naloxone, nalorphine, and levallorphan—are specific antidotes against the respiratory depression that may result from overdosage or unusual sensitivity to narcotics. Therefore, an appropriate dose of one of these antagonists should be administered, preferably by the intravenous route, simultaneously with efforts at respiratory resuscitation. Since the duration of action of morphine may exceed that of the antagonist, the patient should be kept under continued surveillance, and repeated doses of the antagonist should be administered as needed to maintain adequate respiration. Oxygen, intravenous fluids, vasopressors, and other supportive measures should be employed as indicated.

Dosage and Administration: Dosage should be adjusted according to the severity of the pain and the response of the patient. RMS™ suppositories are to be administered rectally. *For Analgesia*—Usual Adult Dose: 10 to 20 mg every 4 hours or as directed by physician. Dosage is a patient dependent variable, and increased dosage may be required for adequate analgesia.

Morphine Dosage Reduction: During the first two to three days of effective pain relief, the patient may sleep for many hours. This can be misinterpreted as the effect of excessive analgesic dosing rather than the first sign of relief in a pain exhausted patient. The dose, therefore, should be maintained for at least three days before reduction, if respiratory activity and other vital signs are adequate. Following successful relief of severe pain, periodic attempts to reduce the narcotic dose should be made. Smaller doses or complete discontinuation of the narcotic analgesic may become feasible due to a physiologic change or the improved mental state of the patient.

How Supplied: RMS™ suppositories are individually sealed and color-coded to aid in identification. 5 mg suppositories: NDC 0245-0160-12: 12 suppositories per carton. 10 mg suppositories: NDC 0245-0161-12: 12 suppositories per carton. 20 mg suppositories: NDC 0245-0162-12: 12 suppositories per carton.

DEA Order Form Required: Caution: Federal law prohibits dispensing without prescription.

SSKI® ℞
(potassium iodide oral solution, U.S.P.)

Composition: Each 0.3ml. contains potassium iodide 300 mg.

Action and Uses: An expectorant in the symptomatic treatment of chronic pulmonary diseases where tenacious mucus complicates the problem, including bronchial asthma, bronchitis and pulmonary emphysema.

Contraindications: Contraindicated in patients with hyperthyroidism or known sensitivity to iodides.

Adverse Reactions: May include gastrointestinal upset, metallic taste, minor skin eruptions, nausea, vomiting and epigastric pain. If these symptoms develop, discontinue use.

Precautions: Caution is recommended in patients during pregnancy. In some patients prolonged use of iodides can lead to hypothyroidism.

Administration and Dosage: Adults, 0.3ml. or 0.6ml. diluted in one glassful of water 3 or 4 times daily.

How Supplied: In bottles of 1 oz. (calibrated dropper, marked to deliver 0.3ml. and 0.6ml.) and 8 oz.

TROFAN®
L-Tryptophan Tablets, 0.5 Gm.

Composition: Each capsule shaped tablet contains L-Tryptophan, 0.5 Gm.
How Supplied: Trofan tablets 0.5 Gm. in bottles of 30 and 100.

The Vale Chemical Co., Inc.
1201 LIBERTY ST.
ALLENTOWN, PA 18102

GLYCOTUSS
[gli'cō-tuss]
(Guaifenesin)

(See PDR For Nonprescription Drugs)

Verex Laboratories, Inc.
8925 EAST NICHOLS AVENUE
ENGLEWOOD, CO 80112

HELP® Tablets OTC
(Constant Ordered Release Phenylpropanolamine HCl)

Description: Each tablet contains 75 mg of phenylpropanolamine, uniquely formulated to control the release of the drug after ingestion. Phenylpropanolamine is a stimulant, related to ephedrine, but has less stimulant effect on the nervous system than amphetamine like diet capsules. Constant release rate means that the tablet will release the drug slowly, at a constant rate as it dissolves in the gastrointestinal tract.

Indications and Usage: This product is indicated as a temporary diet aid for those people who wish to lose weight. The tablet is designed to be used once daily, in the morning, along with a program of dietary management and caloric restrictions. HELP has no value in causing weight reduction other than controlling appetite. Taken alone without a proper program of dietary restriction, HELP will not cause weight loss.

Warning: Use in Pregnancy: This drug should not be used during pregnancy or by mothers who are breast feeding their baby.

Precautions: This product is intended for use only by adults. Do not exceed the recommended dose of one tablet daily.

If nervousness, dizziness, sleeplessness, rapid pulse or other symptoms of stimulation occur, stop taking the drug and notify your family doctor. People with high blood pressure, heart disease, or thyroid disorders should not take this medication except under the supervision of their physician.

Continued on next page

Verex—Cont.

You should not use HELP if you are taking medication for high blood pressure. Some drugs used to treat mental depression will react in an unfavorable manner with HELP. Therefore if you are being treated with medication for depression, you should talk with your doctor before starting a diet program with this drug.

Side Effects: Side effects may occur with this product which are generally a result of the stimulant effects of the drug. Reported side effects are nausea, dry nose, shaking of the hands and general irritability.

Drug Overdose: In case of accidental or intentional drug overdose, call your doctor, or contact a poison control center immediately.

Adult Dosage: One HELP tablet daily in the morning with a full glass of water or fruit juice. It is recommended that a person not take this medication longer than 60 days or as a continuous form of diet control. This product should not be used by children under 12 years of age.

How Supplied: HELP®, 75 mg. orange capsule shaped tablets embossed with the word HELP. Available in boxes of 30. (NDC 51296-003-03)

Shown in Product Identification Section, page 442

VERIN® 650 mg. TABLETS
Aspirin (Constant Release Rate Aspirin)

Description: Each tablet contains 650 mg (10 grs) of aspirin, specially formulated to control the release rate of aspirin after ingestion. Constant release rate, means, that the tablet will release the aspirin slowly, at a constant rate, into the blood stream as it dissolves in the gastrointestinal tract.

Indications and Usage: VERIN is indicated for the treatment of osteoarthritis, rheumatoid arthritis, bursitis, tendinitis and menstrual cramps when used under the supervision of a physician. VERIN may be used by the patient for the temporary relief of pain associated with arthritis, tendinitis, bursitis or menstrual cramps. However, this drug should not be used longer than 10 days, unless the product is being used as directed by a physician. Because VERIN works slowly over a period of time, it is not recommended as a treatment for headache, muscle pains or feverish conditions.

Contraindications: This drug should not be taken by persons known to be allergic to salicylates or individuals with advanced kidney disease.

Warnings: Use in Pregnancy: VERIN, or other aspirin containing products should not be used by a woman when pregnant, except as directed by her physician.

Precautions: Many non-prescription items contain aspirin, salicylates or other aspirin like products. Precaution should be used when taking VERIN with any other non prescription drug. If you are taking VERIN, make sure you tell your doctor. People who have a recent history of gastritis or peptic ulcer should use this drug with caution. This product should not be used if you have a bleeding tendency or are taking anticoagulant drugs.

Side Effects:
Blood

Aspirin may interfere with blood clotting. Patients with a history of blood coagulation problems or individuals receiving anticoagulant drugs should avoid VERIN. Aspirin used chronically may cause an iron deficiency anemia.

Stomach

Aspirin may irritate peptic ulcers and cause heartburn. In some people, aspirin can cause a large amount of bleeding due to erosions and ulcers in the stomach and small intestine. VERIN is released slowly, and the greatest amount of active drug is released in the small intestine over a period of time, subsequently there are less gastrointestinal side effects with this form of constant release rate aspirin. For this reason, individuals who have had gastrointestinal related side effects with other aspirin preparations may tolerate VERIN.

Allergic

Allergic reactions have been noted with aspirin products. People with known sensitivity to aspirin or salicylate type drugs should not take VERIN.

Ears-Hearing

Aspirin when given in high doses may produce ringing or a buzzing noise in the ears.

Drug Interactions

Aspirin may interfere with some anticoagulant or antidiabetic drugs. Drugs to lower uric acid in patients with gout are blocked by the simultaneous use of aspirin. Some anti-arthritic drugs may produce irritation of the stomach, this effect is aggravated by aspirin. Alcohol and aspirin do not mix! Together, alcohol and aspirin may cause irritation, erosion and/or gastrointestinal bleeding.

Drug Overdose: In case of an accidental or intentional drug overdosage, call your doctor, or contact a poison control center immediately.

Dosage and Administration: In order to achieve a constant release rate, VERIN tablets should be swallowed whole. Breaking the tablets will alter the release profile of the drug.

Adult Dosage: For mild to moderate pain associated with rheumatoid arthritis, osteoarthritis, tendinitis, bursitis as well as menstrual cramps, the initial dose of VERIN is 1300 mg (two 650 mg tablets) taken twice a day, in the morning and evening. Because VERIN releases the drug into the blood stream over 12–14 hours, the tablets need only be taken twice a day. Dosage may be increased or decreased depending upon the severity of the pain. However, you should not take more than 6 tablets in any 24 hour period. Do not continue the drug for more than 10 days unless your doctor has advised you to do so.

Dosage for Children: This drug is not intended for use in children below the age of 12 years, except at the specific direction of a physician

How Supplied: VERIN®, 650 mg white capsule shaped tablets embossed with the word VERIN. Available in bottles of 100. (NDC 51296-001-01)

Shown in Product Identification Section, page 442

Vicks Health Care Division
RICHARDSON-VICKS INC.
TEN WESTPORT ROAD
WILTON, CT 06897

DAYCARE® LIQUID
DAYCARE® CAPSULES
Multi-Symptom Colds Medicine

(See PDR For Nonprescription Drugs)

FORMULA 44® COUGH CONTROL DISCS
(See PDR For Nonprescription Drugs)

FORMULA 44® COUGH MIXTURE
(See PDR For Nonprescription Drugs)

FORMULA 44D®
DECONGESTANT COUGH MIXTURE
(See PDR For Nonprescription Drugs)

HEADWAY® CAPSULES
HEADWAY® TABLETS
For colds, sinus, allergy.

(See PDR For Nonprescription Drugs)

NYQUIL®
[nī′ quĭl]
Nighttime Colds Medicine
in oral liquid form.

(See PDR For Nonprescription Drugs)

ORACIN COOLING THROAT LOZENGES
[ō′ rǎ″ sĭn]
ORACIN CHERRY FLAVOR COOLING THROAT LOZENGES

(See PDR For Nonprescription Drugs)

SINEX™
[sī′ něx]
Decongestant Nasal Spray

(See PDR For Nonprescription Drugs)

SINEX™ LONG-ACTING
[sī′ něx]
Decongestant Nasal Spray

(See PDR For Nonprescription Drugs)

TEMPO®
[těm′ pō]
Antacid with Antigas Action

(See PDR For Nonprescription Drugs)

VAPOSTEAM®
[vā′ pō″ stēm]
Liquid Medication for
Hot Steam Vaporizers.

(See PDR For Nonprescription Drugs)

VATRONOL®
[vā′ trō″ nŏl]
Nose Drops

(See PDR For Nonprescription Drugs)

VICKS® COUGH SILENCERS
Cough Drops

(See PDR For Nonprescription Drugs)

VICKS® COUGH SYRUP
Expectorant, Antitussive Cough Syrup

(See PDR For Nonprescription Drugs)

VICKS® INHALER
with decongestant action

(See PDR For Nonprescription Drugs)

VICKS® THROAT LOZENGES
(See PDR For Nonprescription Drugs)

VICKS® VAPORUB®
Decongestant Vaporizing Ointment

(See PDR For Nonprescription Drugs)

Vicks Pharmacy Products Division
RICHARDSON-VICKS INC.
TEN WESTPORT ROAD
WILTON, CT 06897

CREMACOAT™ 1
[krěm′ à kōte]
Throat Coating Cough Medicine

Active Ingredients: Each 15 ml (3 teaspoonfuls) contains:
Dextromethorpan Hydrobromide .... 30 mg.
In a red, cherry-flavored, creamy liquid. Also contains Alcohol 10%.

Indications: CREMACOAT 1 calms, quiets coughs due to colds.

Actions: CREMACOAT 1 is a nonnarcotic antitussive and demulcent formulation. Dextromethorphan acts centrally to calm coughs while the thick and creamy demulcent formula of CREMACOAT 1 soothes cough-irritated throats and shields sensitive cough receptors in the mucosa of the oropharynx and hypopharynx where coughs due to colds frequently begin.

Warning: Do not exceed recommended dosage. Do not administer to children under 2 years of age unless directed by a physician. Persistent cough may indicate the presence of a serious condition. Persons with a high fever or persistent cough should not use this preparation unless directed by a physician. In case of accidental overdose, seek professional assistance or contact a Poison Control Center immediately. As with any drug, if pregnant or nursing a baby, seek the advice of a health professional before using this product. Keep this and all drugs out of the reach of children.

Symptoms and Treatment of Overdosage: These symptoms are based on medical judgment, not on actual experience, since no incidents of overdosage in clinical or consumer experience have been brought to our attention. Ingestion of large amounts might be anticipated to cause nausea, vomiting, dizziness, or CNS depression. Treatment is symptomatic, with bedrest and observation.

Dosage:
ADULTS
(12 years and older) .... 3 teaspoonfuls
CHILDREN
(6 to 12 years) .... 1½ teaspoonfuls
CHILDREN (2 to 6 years) .... ¾ teaspoonfuls
Repeat every 6 hours as needed. No more than 4 doses per day.

How Supplied: Available in 3 fl. oz. and 6 fl. oz. bottles.

Shown in Product Identification Section, page 442

CREMACOAT™ 2
[krĕm¹ a kōte]
Throat Coating Cough Medicine

Active Ingredient: Each 15 ml (3 teaspoonfuls) contains:
Guaifenesin (Glyceryl Guaiacolate)...........200 mg.
In a orange-colored, orange-flavored creamy liquid. Also contains Alcohol 10%.

Indications: CREMACOAT 2 relieves coughs due to colds.

Actions: CREMACOAT 2 is an expectorant and demulcent formulation. Guaifenesin loosens phlegm in upper chest and makes coughs due to colds more productive. In addition, the thick, creamy formulation soothes cough-irritated throats and shields sensitive cough receptors in the mucosa of the oropharynx and hypopharynx where coughs frequently begin.

Warning: Do not exceed recommended dosage. Do not administer to children under 2 years of age unless directed by a physician. Persistent cough may indicate the presence of a serious condition. Persons with a high fever or cough which persists for more than 1 week should not use this preparation unless directed by a physician. In case of accidental overdose, seek professional assistance or contact a Poison Control Center immediately. As with any drug, if pregnant or nursing a baby, seek the advice of a health professional before using this product. Keep this and all drugs out of the reach of children.

Symptoms and Treatment of Overdosage: These symptoms are based on medical judgment, not on actual experience, since no incidents of overdosage have been brought to our attention in clinical or consumer experience. Ingestion of large amounts might be anticipated to case nausea and vomiting. Treatment is symptomatic, with bedrest and observation.

Dosage:
ADULTS
(12 years and older) .... 3 teaspoonfuls
CHILDREN
(6 to 12 years) .... 1½ teaspoonfuls
CHILDREN (2 to 6 years) .... ¾ teaspoonful
Repeat every 4 hours as needed. No more than 6 doses per day.

How Supplied: Available in 3 fl. oz. and 6 fl. oz. bottles.

Shown in Product Identification Section, page 442

CREMACOAT™ 3
[krĕm¹ a kōte]
Throat Coating Cough Medicine

Active Ingredients: Each 15 ml (3 teaspoonfuls) contains:
Dextromethorphan Hydrobromide..............20 mg.
Phenylpropanolamine
Hydrochloride..37.5 mg.
Guaifenesin (Glyceryl Guaiacolate)...........200 mg.
In a bluish-red, raspberry-flavored creamy liquid. Also contains Alcohol 10%.

Indications: CREMACOAT 3 calms, quiets coughs, loosens phlegm and mucus in upper chest, and relieves nasal congestion due to colds.

Actions: CREMACOAT 3 is a nonnarcotic antitussive, nasal decongestant, expectorant, and demulcent formulation. Guaifenesin loosens phlegm and mucus in upper chest. Phenylpropanolamine hydrochloride relieves nasal congestion. Dextromethorphan acts centrally to calm coughs, while the thick, creamy formulation soothes cough-irritated throats and shields sensitive cough receptors in the mucosa of the oropharynx and hypopharynx where coughs due to colds frequently begin.

Warning: Do not exceed recommended dosage. Do not administer to children under 2 years of age unless directed by a physician. Persistent cough may indicate the presence of a serious condition. Persons with a high fever or persistent cough or with high blood pressure, diabetes, heart or thyroid disease should not use this preparation unless directed by a physician. In case of accidental overdose, seek professional assistance or contact a Poison Control Center immediately. As with any drug, if pregnant or nursing a baby, seek the advice of a health professional before using this product. Keep this and all drugs out of the reach of children.

Symptoms and Treatment of Overdose: These symptoms are based on medical judgment, not on actual experience, since no incidents of overdosage in clinical or consumer experience have been brought to our attention. Ingestion of large amounts may cause restlessness, anxiety, sweating, tremor, rapid pulse, hypertension, extrasystoles, confusion, delirium, nausea and vomiting. Treatment is symptomatic, with bedrest and observation.

Dosage:
ADULTS
(12 years and older) .... 3 teaspoonfuls
CHILDREN
(6 to 12 years) .... 1½ teaspoonfuls
CHILDREN (2 to 6 years) .... ¾ teaspoonfuls
Repeat every 4 hours as needed. No more than 4 doses per day.

How Supplied: Available in 3 fl. oz. and 6 fl. oz. bottles.

Shown in Product Identification Section, page 442

CREMACOAT™ 4
[krĕm¹ a kōte]
Throat Coating Cough Medicine

Active Ingredients: Each 15 ml (3 teaspoonfuls) contain:
Dextromethorphan Hydrobromide .... 20 mg.
Phenylpropanolamine
Hydrochloride .... 37.5 mg.
Doxylamine Succinate .... 7.5 mg.
In a pink, black cherry-flavored creamy liquid. Also contains Alcohol 10%.

Indications: CREMACOAT 4 quiets coughs, relieves nasal congestion, dries nasal drip due to colds.

Actions: CREMACOAT 4 is a nonnarcotic antitussive, nasal decongestant, antihistamine and demulcent formulation. Phenylpropanolamine hydrochloride relieves nasal congestion. Doxylamine succinate relieves sneezing and dries nasal drip. The dextromethorphan hydrobromide acts centrally to calm coughs, while the thick, creamy formulation soothes cough-irritated throats and shields sensitive cough receptors in the mucosa of the oropharynx and hypopharynx where coughs due to colds frequently begin.

Warning: Do not exceed recommended dosage. Do not administer to children under 6 years of age unless directed by a physician. Persistent cough may indicate the presence of a serious condition. Persons with a high fever or cough or with high blood pressure, diabetes, heart or thyroid disease should not use this preparation unless directed by a physician. This preparation may cause drowsiness. Do not drive or operate machinery while taking this medication. If relief does not occur within 3 days, discontinue use and see a physician. In case of accidental overdose, seek professional assistance or call a Poison Control Center immediately. As with any drug, if pregnant or nursing a baby, seek the advice of a health professional before using this product. Keep this and all drugs out of the reach of children.

Symptoms and Treatment of Overdosage: These symptoms are based on medical judgment, not on actual experience, since no incidents of overdosage in clinical or consumer experience have been brought to our attention. Ingestion of very large amounts may cause nausea and vomiting, restlessness, anxiety, sweating, tremor, rapid pulse, hypertension, extrasystoles, confusion, delirium and drowsiness. Treatment is symptomatic, with bedrest and observation.

Dosage:
ADULT (12 years and older)...........3 teaspoonfuls
CHILDREN
(6 to 12 years).............................1½ teaspoonfuls
Repeat every 4 hours as needed. No more than 4 doses per day.

How Supplied: Available in 3 fl. oz. and 6 fl. oz. bottles.

Shown in Product Identification Section, page 442

PERCOGESIC®
[pĕr kō-gē′sĭk]
Analgesic Tablets

Description: Each tablet contains:
Acetaminophen ....325 mg
Phenyltoloxamine citrate ....30 mg

Indications: For relief of pain and discomfort due to headache, for temporary relief of pain associated with muscle and joint soreness, neuralgia, sinusitis, minor menstrual cramps, the common cold, toothache, and minor aches and pains of rheumatism and arthritis.

Warning: If arthritic or rheumatic pain persists for more than 10 days; in the presence of redness or swelling; or in arthritic or rheumatic conditions affecting children under 12 years of age, consult a physician immediately. When used for temporary, symptomatic relief of colds, do not use for more than 3 days, except as directed by a physician. This preparation may cause drowsiness. Do not drive or operate machinery while taking this medication. Do not administer to children under 6 years of age or exceed recommended dosage unless directed by a physician. Keep this and all drugs out of the reach of children. In case of overdosage, seek professional assistance or contact a poison control center immediately. As with any drug, if you are pregnant or nursing a baby, seek the advice of a health professional before using this product.

Dosage and Administration:
ADULTS (12 years and over)—1 or 2 tablets every four hours. Maximum daily dose—8 tablets
CHILDREN (6-12 years)—one-half adult dose. Maximum daily dose—4 tablets
Do not use for more than 10 days unless directed by a physician.

How Supplied: Child-resistant sealed packets of 24 tablets and bottles of 50 and 90 tablets.

Shown in Product Identification Section, page 442

Products are cross-indexed by generic and chemical names in the **YELLOW SECTION**

Vitaline Formulas
P.O. BOX 6757
INCLINE VILLAGE, NV 89450

ENVIRO-STRESS™ with ZINC and SELENIUM
High Potency
Stress Formula with Vitamins and Minerals

Each slow release ENVIRO-STRESS tablet provides:

600 mg	Vitamin C	
132 mg	Zinc Sulfate, buffered	
	(equal to 30 mg zinc)	
100 mg	Magnesium	
	(equal to 60 mg magnesium)	
25 mcg	Selenium	
	(organically bound)	
50 mg	Vitamin B1	
	(thiamine mononitrate)	
50 mg	Vitamin B2	
	(riboflavin)	
50 mg	Vitamin B6	
	(pyridoxine HCL)	
25 mcg	Vitamin B12	
100 mg	Niacinamide	
50 mg	Pantothenic Acid	
400 mcg	Folic Acid	
5 mg	Para-Amino Benzoic Acid	
30 I.U.	Vitamin E	

ENVIRO-STRESS Tablets contain no sugar, yeast, wheat, corn, soya, salicylates, phenol, preservatives or artificial coloring agents.
Recommended Intake: Adults, 1 tablet daily or as directed by the physician.
How Supplied: Bottles of 90 and 1000 tablets.
Literature Available: Complete literature available upon request by physician.

PANCREATIN 2400 mg. N.F.
(High Lipase)

Description: Vitaline's Pancreatin 2400 mg. N.F. is an **uncoated** compressed tablet, specially buffered to prevent the destruction of unknown amounts of pancreatin by gastric pepsin. No agents have been added to the tablet formulation to mask possible undesirable attributes of odor or taste imparted by the enzymes of pancreatin. Each tablet contains no less than:

Lipase .... 12,000 N.F. Units
Amylase .... 60,000 N.F. Units
Protease .... 60,000 N.F. Units

Indications and Usage: Pancreatin 2400 mg. N.F. is indicated for patients with exocrine pancreatic enzyme deficiency as in:
*chronic pancreatitis
*pancreatectomy or gastrectomy
*cystic fibrosis

Precautions: Use with caution in patients known to be allergic to pork protein.
Vitaline's Pancreatin 2400 mg. N.F. tablets contain no sugar, corn, wheat, soya, yeast, phenol, salicylates, preservatives or artificial coloring agents.
Dosage and Administration: Usual dosage: One or two tablets during each meal and one tablet with snacks. Occasionally a third tablet with meals may be required depending upon individual requirements for control of steatorrhea.
How Supplied: Uncoated tablets in bottles of 90, 500 and 1000 tablets.
Literature Available: Complete literature available upon request by physician.

SELENIUM 200 MCG

Description: Each tablet contains: Selenium 200 mcg (organically bound in kelp)
Advantages of Kelp Bound Selenium Source
- Free of yeast protein allergens
- High bioavailability
- Uniformly distributed selenium
- Non toxic—not extractable
- Organic selenium—selenium is contained in a colloidal polymannuronate complex
- High trace element content

Action and Uses: A convenient source of selenium for patients deficient in this essential element.
Administration and Dosage: As a dietary supplement, adults—1 tablet daily, or as directed by physician.
Side Effects: None reported.
How Supplied: Bottles of 90 and 1000.
Literature and Samples: On request by physician.

TOTAL FORMULA®
(High Potency Multivitamin/Multimineral Supplement with micro-trace elements; Chromium, Selenium and Molybdenum)

Description: TOTAL FORMULA utilizes a unique technique of microspheres within the tablet to protect the delicate nutrients from moisture, air and the incompatibilities of certain minerals. Vitaline's microsphere technique also protects those nutrients that are suspectible to acid hydrolysis.

Each tablet provides:

Vitamins		RDA %
A (Water Soluble, Palmitate)	10,000 I.U.	200%
D-3	400 I.U.	100%
E (d-alpha tocopherol succinate) Water Soluble)	30 I.U.	100%
K (Water Soluble)	70 mcg	70%
C (Ascorbic Acid, from Sago Palm)	100 mg	166%
B-1 (Thiamine)	15 mg	1000%
B-2 (Riboflavin)	15 mg	882%
B-3 (Niacinamide)	25 mg	400%
B-5 (Pantothenic Acid)	25 mg	250%
B-6 (Pyridoxine HCL)	25 mg	1250%
B-12 (on ion exchange resin)	25 mcg	416%
Folic Acid	400 mcg	100%
Biotin	300 mcg	100%
Choline (Bitartrate)	10 mg	**
Hesperidin Complex	10 mg	***
Citrus Bioflavinoids	10 mg	***
Rutin	10 mg	***
Inositol	10 mg	***
PABA (para amino benzoic acid)	8 mg	***
Minerals		
Calcium (oyster shell)	100 mg	10%
Magnesium (chelate)	100 mg	25%
Phosphorus	52 mg	5%
Potassium (chelate)	25 mg	**
Iron (Fumarate)	20 mg	111%
Zinc (Gluconate)	30 mg	200%
Copper (Gluconate)	2 mg	100%
Manganese (Gluconate)	6 mg	**
Iodine (kelp)	100 mcg	66%
Chromium (GTF factor)	500 mcg	**
Selenium (organically bound chelate)	10 mcg	**
Molybdenum (chelate)	100 mcg	**
Silicon (kelp)	2.4 mg	**
Vanadium (chelate)	25 mcg	**

Chlorophyll coloring in coating. *RDA—recommended daily allowance. **Need in human nutrition established, RDA not determined. ***Need in human nutrition not determined.
TOTAL FORMULA contains no yeast, corn, wheat, soya, sugar, phenol, preservatives, dairy products, artificial colors, or added salicylates.
Directions: Adults, 1 tablet daily as a dietary supplement . . . children, as directed by physician.
How Supplied: Bottles of 90 and 1000.
Literature and Samples: On request by physician.

Products are
listed alphabetically
in the
PINK SECTION.

Walker, Corp & Co., Inc.
P.O. BOX 1320
EASTHAMPTON PL. &
N. COLLINGWOOD AVE.
SYRACUSE, NY 13201

EVAC–U–GEN®

Description: Evac-U-Gen® is available as purple scored tablets, each containing 97.2 mg. of yellow phenolphthalein.
Action and Uses: For temporary relief of occasional constipation and to help restore a normal pattern of evacuation. A mild, non-griping, stimulant laxative in chewable, anise-flavored form, Evac-U-Gen provides softening of the feces through selective action on the intramural nerve plexus of intestinal smooth muscle, and increases the propulsive peristaltic activity of the colon. It is frequently helpful in preparing the bowel for diagnostic procedures.
Indications: Because of its gentle action and non-toxic nature, Evac-U-Gen is suitable in pregnancy, in the presence of hemorrhoids, for children and the elderly. Safe for nursing mothers, it dose not affect the infant. It may be especially useful when straining at the stool is a hazard, as in hernia, cardiac or hypertensive patients.
Contraindications: Contraindicated in patients with a history of sensitivity to phenolphthalein. Evac-U-Gen should not be used when abdominal pain, nausea, vomiting, or other symptoms of appendicitis are present.
Side Effects: If skin rash appears, use of Evac-U-Gen or other preparations containing phenolphthalein should be discontinued. May cause coloration of feces or urine if such are sufficiently alkaline.
Warning: Frequent or prolonged use may result in dependence on laxatives. Keep this and all medication out of reach of children.
Administration and Dosage: Adults: chew one or two tablets night or morning. **Children:** 3 to 10 years, chew ½ tablet daily. Intensity of action is proportional to dosage, but individually effective doses vary. Evac-U-Gen is usually active 6 to 8 hours after administration, but residual action may last 3 to 4 days.
How Supplied: Evac-U-Gen is available in bottles of 35, 100, 500, 1000 and 6000 tablets.

Walker Pharmacal Company
4200 LACLEDE AVENUE
ST. LOUIS, MO 63108

SUCCUS CINERARIA MARITIMA   R
[suk′us si-ne′ra″ria mar′ i-te″ma]
(Senecio Cineraria Compound Solution)
Sterile—Ophthalmic

Description: Succus Cineraria Maritima is an aqueous and glycerin solution of the total extractives of the fresh Senecio Cineraria USPH 8th (Senecio Compositae) with extract of Hamamelis V. (Witch Hazel) and boric acid USP. The Alkaloids included in the total extract include Senecine and Senecionine. Total nonvolatiles is approximately 20%. The pH is adjusted to 4.1 pH; osmotic pressure is 5.5 osmols.
Actions and Uses: Succus Cineraria Maritima applied locally to the eyes acts as a safe lymphagogue, increasing circulation in the intraocular tissues, also stimulating collateral circulation and normal metabolism, functions so necessary from the standpoint of the physiology of the eye. Clinical observation indicates the definite value of local applications of Succus Cineraria Maritima in checking, or even aborting existing opacities. The benefits attained are obviously more satisfactory when treatment is instituted in the early stage of Cataract. In cases of well advanced opacity, and where pathological changes caused by the deterioration of the Metabolic functions have occurred, as

is characteristic in senility, less favorable results can be expected.

The use of Succus Cineraria Maritima, however, is justified in certain cases well past the incipient stage, particularly when an operation is not contemplated or is contraindicated. It gives comfort to the patient to know that something potentially beneficial is being done. Clinical studies of advanced stages of cataract treated with Succus Cineraria Maritima indicated that in 22.5% of these cases beneficial results were obtained. In many of the cases which did not show improvement the process of the opacity was retarded or checked. In certain cases Succus Cineraria Maritima only gives temporary relief or serves to postpone the surgical removal.

Indications: Succus Cineraria Maritima is indicated in the treatment of various cases of optic opacity caused by cataract.

Contraindications: A history of a previous hypersensitivity reaction to any of the Senecio Alkaloids or the Hamamelis V. is a contraindication.

Warning: The possibility of sensitivity reactions should be considered in patients with a history of allergy. If excessive irritation occurs it may be advisable to dilute the dosage, or discontinue treatment. (pH of 4.1 may cause minor irritation). For topical ophthalmic use only. If excessive irritation should develop, patient should consult the prescribing physician.

Caution: Federal Law prohibits dispensing without prescription.

Caution: Not intended for use in Glaucoma.

Dosage and Administration: Succus Cineraria Maritima should be instilled in the affected eye, two drops morning and evening, or as directed by physician. Do not touch dropper tip to any surface, since this may contaminate the solution.

Supplied: In sterile 1/4 oz. dropper vial (7 cc). NDC 619-4021-38.

EDUCATIONAL MATERIAL

Booklet: "Cataract—Is Surgery the Only Way?" Free to physicians, pharmacists and patients. Call (314) 533-9600 for your copy.

Wallace Laboratories
P.O. BOX 1
CRANBURY, NJ 08512

AQUATENSEN® ℞
(methyclothiazide, USP 5 mg)
Tablets

Description: AQUATENSEN (methyclothiazide) is a member of the benzothiadiazine (thiazide) family of drugs. It is an analogue of hydrochlorothiazide.

Clinically, AQUATENSEN is an oral diuretic-antihypertensive agent.

Actions: The diuretic and saluretic effects of AQUATENSEN result from a drug-induced inhibition of the renal tubular reabsorption of electrolytes. The excretion of sodium and chloride is greatly enhanced. Potassium excretion is also enhanced to a variable degree, as it is with the other thiazides. Although urinary excretion of bicarbonate is increased slightly, there is usually no significant change in urinary pH. Methyclothiazide has a per mg natriuretic activity approximately 100 times that of the prototype thiazide, chlorothiazide. At maximal therapeutic dosages, all thiazides are approximately equal in their diuretic/natriuretic effects.

There is significant natriuresis and diuresis within two hours after administration of a single dose of methyclothiazide. These effects reach a peak in about six hours and persist for 24 hours following oral administration of a single dose.

Like other benzothiadiazines, AQUATENSEN also has antihypertensive properties, and may be used for this purpose either alone or to enhance the antihypertensive action of other drugs. The mechanism by which the benzothiadiazines, including methyclothiazide, produce a reduction of elevated blood pressure is not known. However, sodium depletion appears to be involved.

AQUATENSEN is readily absorbed from the gastrointestinal tract and is excreted unchanged by the kidneys.

Indications: AQUATENSEN is indicated in the management of hypertension either as the sole therapeutic agent or to enhance the effect of other antihypertensive drugs in the more severe forms of hypertension.

AQUATENSEN is indicated as adjunctive therapy in edema associated with congestive heart failure, hepatic cirrhosis, and corticosteroid and estrogen therapy.

AQUATENSEN has also been found useful in edema due to various forms of renal dysfunction such as the nephrotic syndrome, acute glomerulonephritis and chronic renal failure.

Usage in pregnancy: The routine use of diuretics in an otherwise healthy woman is inappropriate and exposes the mother and fetus to unnecessary hazard. Diuretics do not prevent development of toxemia of pregnancy, and there is no satisfactory evidence that they are useful in the treatment of developed toxemia.

Edema during pregnancy may arise from pathological causes or from the physiological and mechanical consequences of pregnancy. Thiazides are indicated in pregnancy when edema is due to pathologic causes, just as they are in the absence of pregnancy (however, see Warnings, below). Dependent edema in pregnancy, resulting from restriction of venous return by the expanded uterus, is properly treated through elevation of the lower extremities and use of support hose; use of diuretics to lower intravascular volume in this case is illogical and unnecessary. There is hypervolemia during normal pregnancy which is harmful to neither the fetus nor the mother (in the absence of cardiovascular disease), but which is associated with edema, including generalized edema, in the majority of pregnant women. If this edema produces discomfort, increased recumbency will often provide relief. In rare instances, this edema may cause extreme discomfort which is not relieved by rest. In these cases, a short course of diuretics may provide relief and may be appropriate.

Contraindications: Renal decompensation. Hypersensitivity to this or other sulfonamide derived drugs.

Warnings: Methyclothiazide shares with other thiazides the propensity to deplete potassium reserves to an unpredictable degree.

Thiazides should be used with caution in patients with renal disease or significant impairment of renal function, since azotemia may be precipitated and cumulative drug effects may occur.

Thiazides should be used with caution in patients with impaired hepatic function or progressive liver disease, since minor alterations of fluid and electrolyte balance may precipitate hepatic coma.

Thiazides may be additive or potentiative of the action of other antihypertensive drugs. Potentiation occurs with ganglionic or pheripheral adrenergic blocking drugs.

Sensitivity reactions may occur in patients with a history of allergy or bronchial asthma.

The possibility of exacerbation or activation of systemic lupus erythematosus has been reported.

Usage in pregnancy: Thiazides cross the placental barrier and appear in cord blood. The use of thiazides in pregnant women requires that the anticipated benefit be weighed against possible hazards to the fetus. These hazards include fetal or neonatal jaundice, thrombocytopenia, and possibly other adverse reactions, that have occurred in the adult.

Nursing mothers: Thiazides appear in breast milk. If use of the drug is deemed essential, the patient should stop nursing.

Precautions: Periodic determination of serum electrolytes should be performed at appropriate intervals for the purpose of detecting possible electrolyte imbalances such as hyponatremia, hypochloremic alkalosis, and hypokalemia. Serum and urine electrolyte determinations are particularly important when a patient is vomiting excessively or receiving parenteral fluids. All patients should be observed for other clinical signs of electrolyte imbalances such as dryness of mouth, thirst, weakness, lethargy, drowsiness, restlessness, muscle pains or cramps, muscular fatigue, hypotension, oliguria, tachycardia, and gastrointestinal disturbances such as nausea and vomiting.

Hypokalemia may develop with thiazides as with any other potent diuretic, especially when brisk diuresis occurs, severe cirrhosis is present, or when corticosteroids or ACTH are given concomitantly. Interference with the adequate oral intake of electrolytes will also contribute to the possible development of hypokalemia. Potassium depletion, even of a mild degree, resulting from thiazide use, may sensitize a patient to the effects of cardiac glycosides such as digitalis.

Any chloride deficit is generally mild and usually does not require specific treatment except under extraordinary circumstances (as in liver disease or renal disease). Dilutional hyponatremia may occur in edematous patients in hot weather; appropriate therapy is water restriction, rather than administration of salt except in rare instances when the hyponatremia is life threatening.

In actual salt depletion, appropriate replacement is the therapy of choice.

Hyperuricemia may occur or frank gout may be precipitated in certain patients receiving thiazide therapy.

Insulin requirements in diabetic patients may be increased, decreased, or unchanged. Latent diabetes mellitus may become manifest during thiazide administration.

Thiazide drugs may increase the responsiveness to tubocurarine.

The antihypertensive effects of the drug may be enhanced in the postsympathectomy patient.

Thiazides may decrease arterial responsiveness to norepinephrine. This diminution is not sufficient to preclude effectiveness of the pressor agent for therapeutic use.

If progressive renal impairment becomes evident as indicated by a rising nonprotein nitrogen or blood urea nitrogen, a careful reappraisal of therapy is necessary with consideration given to withholding or discontinuing diuretic therapy.

Thiazides may decrease serum PBI levels without signs of thyroid disturbance.

Thiazides have been reported, on rare occasions, to have elevated serum calcium to hypercalcemic levels. The serum calcium levels have returned to normal when the medication has been stopped. This phenomenon may be related to the ability of the thiazide diuretics to lower the amount of calcium excreted in the urine.

Adverse Reactions:

Gastrointestinal system reactions: Anorexia, gastric irritation, nausea, vomiting, cramping, diarrhea, constipation, jaundice (intrahepatic cholestatic jaundice), pancreatitis.

Central nervous system reactions: Dizziness, vertigo, paresthesia, headache, xanthopsia.

Hematologic reactions: Leukopenia, agranulocytosis, thrombocytopenia, aplastic anemia.

Dermatologic-hypersensitivity reactions: Purpura, photosensitivity, rash, urticaria, necrotizing angiitis (vasculitis) (cutaneous vasculitis).

Cardiovascular reactions: Orthostatic hypotension may occur and may be aggravated by alcohol, barbiturates, or narcotics.

Other: Hyperglycemia, glycosuria, hypercalcemia, hyperuricemia, muscle spasm, weakness, restlessness.

There have been isolated reports that certain nonedematous individuals developed severe fluid and electrolyte derangements after only brief exposure to normal doses of thiazide and non-thiazide diuretics. The condition is usually manifested as severe dilutional hyponatremia, hypokalemia, and hypochloremia. It has been reported to be due to inappropriately increased ADH secretion and appears to be idiosyncratic. Potassium replace-

Continued on next page

Wallace—Cont.

ment is apparently the most important therapy in the treatment of this syndrome along with removal of the offending drug.
Whenever adverse reactions are severe, treatment should be discontinued.

Dosage and Administration: AQUATENSEN (methyclothiazide) is administered orally. The usual adult dose ranges from 2.5 to 10 mg once daily.
Therapy should be individualized according to patient response. This therapy should be titrated to gain maximal therapeutic response as well as the minimal dose possible to maintain that therapeutic response.
To maintain an edema-free state or as an adjunct in the management of hypertension, 2.5 to 5.0 mg once daily is often adequate.
Maximum effective single dose is 10 mg; larger single doses do not accomplish greater diuresis, and are not recommended.
In the treatment of hypertension, methyclothiazide may be either employed alone or concurrently with other antihypertensive drugs. Combined therapy may provide adequate control of hypertension with lower dosage of the component drugs and fewer or less severe side effects.
For treatment of moderately severe or severe hypertension, supplemental use of other more potent antihypertensive agents may be indicated.
When other antihypertensive agents are to be added to the regimen, this should be accomplished gradually. Ganglionic blocking agents should be given at only half the usual dose since their effect is potentiated by pretreatment with AQUATENSEN.

Overdosage: Symptoms of overdosage include electrolyte imbalance and signs of potassium deficiency such as confusion, dizziness, muscular weakness, and gastrointestinal disturbances. General supportive measures including replacement of fluids and electrolytes may be indicated in treatment of overdosage.

How Supplied: AQUATENSEN (methyclothiazide) is supplied as a 5 mg, peach-colored, monogrammed, grooved, rectangular-shaped tablet.

NDC 0037-0153-92, bottle of 100.
NDC 0037-0153-96, bottle of 500.

CAUTION: Federal law prohibits dispensing without prescription.

Rev. 4/83
Shown in Product Identification Section, page 442

BUTISOL SODIUM®
(butabarbital sodium)
Tablets and Elixir

Description: BUTISOL SODIUM (butabarbital sodium) is a nonselective central nervous system depressant which is used as a sedative or hypnotic (WARNING: May be habit-forming). It is available for oral administration as *Tablets* containing 15 mg, 30 mg, 50 mg or 100 mg butabarbital sodium; and as *Elixir* containing 30 mg/5 ml, with alcohol (by volume) 7%. Butabarbital sodium occurs as a white, bitter powder which is freely soluble in water and alcohol, but practically insoluble in benzene and ether.

Clinical Pharmacology: BUTISOL SODIUM (butabarbital sodium), like other barbiturates, is capable of producing all levels of CNS mood alteration from excitation to mild sedation, to hypnosis, and deep coma. Overdosage can produce death. Barbiturates depress the sensory cortex, decrease motor activity, alter cerebellar function, and produce drowsiness, sedation, and hypnosis.
Barbiturate-induced sleep differs from physiological sleep. Sleep laboratory studies have demonstrated that barbiturates reduce the amount of time spent in the rapid eye movement (REM) phase of sleep or dreaming stage. Also, Stages III and IV sleep are decreased. Following abrupt cessation of barbiturates used regularly, patients may experience markedly increased dreaming, nightmares, and/or insomnia. Therefore, withdrawal of a single therapeutic dose over 5 or 6 days has been recommended to lessen the REM rebound and disturbed sleep which contribute to drug withdrawal syndrome (for example, decrease the dose from 3 to 2 doses a day for 1 week).
In studies, secobarbital sodium and pentobarbital sodium have been found to lose most of their effectiveness for both inducing and maintaining sleep by the end of 2 weeks of continued drug administration even with the use of multple doses. As with secobarbital sodium and pentobarbital sodium, other barbiturates might be expected to lose their effectiveness for inducing and maintaining sleep after about 2 weeks. The short-, intermediate-, and, to a lesser degree, long-acting barbiturates have been widely prescribed for treating insomnia. Although the clinical literature abounds with claims that the short-acting barbiturates are superior for producing sleep while the intermediate-acting compounds are more effective in maintaining sleep, controlled studies have failed to demonstrate these differential effects. Therefore, as sleep medications, the barbiturates are of limited value beyond the short-term use.
Barbiturates are respiratory depressants. The degree of respiratory depression is dependent upon dose. With hypnotic doses, respiratory depression produced by barbiturates is similar to that which occurs during physiologic sleep with slight decrease in blood pressure and heart rate.
Barbiturates do not impair noraml hepatic function, but have been shown to induce liver microsomal enzymes, thus increasing and/or altering the metabolism of barbiturates and other drugs (see PRECAUTIONS—Drug interactions).

Pharmacokinetics: BUTISOL SODIUM (butabarbital sodium) is the sodium salt of a weak acid. Barbiturates are weak acids that are absorbed and rapidly distributed to all tissues and fluids with high concentrations in the brain, liver, and kidneys. Barbiturates are bound to plasma and tissue proteins. The rate of absorption is increased if it is ingested as a dilute solution or taken on an empty stomach.
Barbiturates are metabolized primarily by the hepatic microsomal enzyme system, and most metabolic products are excreted in the urine. The excretion of unchanged butabarbital in the urine is negligible. BUTISOL SODIUM (butabarbital sodium) is classified as an intermediate-acting barbiturate. The average plasma half-life for butabarbital is 100 hours in the adult.
Although variable from patient to patient, butabarbital has an onset of action of about ¾ to 1 hour, and a duration of action of about 6 to 8 hours.

Indications and Usage: BUTISOL SODIUM (butabarbital sodium) is indicated for use as a sedative or hypnotic.
Since barbiturates appear to lose their effectiveness for sleep induction and sleep maintenance after 2 weeks, use of BUTISOL SODIUM in treating insomnia should be limited to this time (see CLINICAL PHARMACOLOGY above).

Contraindications: Barbiturates are contraindicated in patients with known barbiturate sensitivity. Barbiturates are also contraindicated in patients with a history of manifest or latent porphyria.

Warnings: Habit-forming: Barbiturates may be habit-forming. Tolerance, psychological and physical dependence may occur with continued use (see DRUG ABUSE AND DEPENDENCE below). Patients who have psychological dependence on barbiturates may increase the dosage or decrease the dosage interval without consulting a physician and may subsequently develop a physical dependence on barbiturates. To minimize the possibility of overdosage or the development of dependence, the prescribing and dispensing of sedative-hypnotic barbiturates should be limited to the amount required for the interval until the next appointment. Abrupt cessation after prolonged use in the dependent person may result in withdrawal symptoms, including delirium, convulsions, and possibly death. Barbiturates should be withdrawn gradually from any patient known to be taking excessive dosage over long periods of time. (See DRUG ABUSE AND DEPENDENCE below.)

Acute or chronic pain: Caution should be exercised when barbiturates are administered to patients with acute or chronic pain, because paradoxical excitement could be induced, or important symptoms could be masked. However, the use of barbiturates as sedatives in the postoperative surgical period, and as adjuncts to cancer chemotherapy, is well established.

Use in pregnancy: Barbiturates may cause fetal damage when administered to a pregnant woman. Retrospective, case-controlled studies have suggested a connection between the maternal consumption of barbiturates and a higher than expected incidence of fetal abnormalities. Following oral administration, barbiturates readily cross the placental barrier and are distributed throughout fetal tissues with highest concentrations found in the placenta, fetal liver, and brain.
Withdrawal symptoms occur in infants born to mothers who receive barbiturates throughout the last trimester of pregnancy (see DRUG ABUSE AND DEPENDENCE). If this drug is used during pregnancy, or if the patient becomes pregnant while taking this drug, the patient should be apprised of the potential hazard to the fetus.

Precautions: General: Barbiturates should be administered with caution, if at all, to patients who are mentally depressed, have suicidal tendencies, or a history of drug abuse.
Elderly or debilitated patients may react to barbiturates with marked excitement, depression, and confusion. In some persons, barbiturates repeatedly produce excitement rather than depression.
In patients with hepatic damage, barbiturates should be administered with caution and initially in reduced doses. Barbiturates should not be administered to patients showing the premonitory signs of hepatic coma.
BUTISOL SODIUM (butabarbital sodium) Tablets, 30 mg and 50 mg, and Elixir contain FD&C Yellow No. 5 (tartrazine) which may cause allergic-type reactions (including bronchial asthma) in certain susceptible individuals. Although the overall incidence of FD&C Yellow No. 5 (tartrazine) sensitivity in the general population is low, it is frequently seen in patients who also have aspirin hypersensitivity.

Information for Patients: Practitioners should give the following information and instructions to patients receiving barbiturates.
The use of barbiturates carries with it an associated risk of psychological and/or physical dependence. The patient should be warned against increasing the dose of the drug without consulting a physician.
Barbiturates may impair mental and/or physical abilities required for the performance of potentially hazardous tasks, such as driving or operating machinery.
Alcohol should not be consumed while taking barbiturates. Concurrent use of the barbiturates with other CNS depressants, including other sedatives or hypnotics, alcohol, narcotics, tranquilizers, and antihistamines, may result in additional CNS depressant effects.

Laboratory Tests: Prolonged therapy with barbiturates should be accompanied by periodic laboratory evaluation of organ systems, including hematopoietic, renal, and hepatic systems (see PRECAUTIONS—General and ADVERSE REACTIONS).

Drug interactions: Most reports of clinically significant drug interactions occurring with the barbiturates have involved phenobarbital. However, the application of these data to other barbiturates appears valid and warrants serial blood level determinations of the relevant drugs when there are multiple therapies.

1. *Anticoagulants.* Phenobarbital lowers the plasma levels of dicumarol and causes a decrease in anticoagulant activity as measured by the prothrombin time. Barbiturates can induce hepatic microsomal enzymes resulting in increased metabolism and decreased anticoagulant response of oral anticoagulants (e.g., warfarin, acenocoumarol, dicumarol, and phenprocoumon). Patients stabilized on anticoagulant therapy may require

dosage adjustments if barbiturates are added to or withdrawn from their dosage regimen.

2. *Corticosteroids.* Barbiturates appear to enhance the metabolism of exogenous corticosteroids probably through the induction of hepatic microsomal enzymes. Patients stabilized on corticosteroid therapy may require dosage adjustments if barbiturates are added to or withdrawn from their dosage regimen.

3. *Griseofulvin.* Phenobarbital appears to interfere with the absorption of orally administered griseofulvin, thus decreasing its blood level. The effect of the resultant decreased blood levels of griseofulvin on therapeutic response has not been established. However, it would be preferable to avoid concomitant administration of these drugs.

4. *Doxycycline.* Phenobarbital has been shown to shorten the half-life of doxycycline for as long as 2 weeks after barbiturate therapy is discontinued. The mechanism is probably through the induction of hepatic microsomal exzymes that metabolize the antibiotic. If phenobarbital and doxycycline are administered concurrently, the clinical response to doxycycline should be monitered closely.

5. *Phenytoin, sodium valproate, valproic acid.* The effect of barbiturates on the metabolism of phenytoin appears to be variable. Some investigators report an accelerating effect, while others report no effect. Because the effect of barbiturates on the metabolism of phenytoin is not predictable, phenytoin and barbiturate blood levels should be monitored more frequently if these drugs are given concurrently. Sodium valproate and valproic acid appear to decrease barbiturate metabolism; therefore, barbiturate blood levels should be monitored and appropriate adjustments made as indicated.

6. *Central nervous system.* The concomitant use of other central nervous system depressants, including other sedatives or hypnotics, antihistamines, tranquilizers, or alcohol, may produce additive depressant effects.

7. *Monoamine oxidase inhibitors (MAOI).* MAOI prolong the effects of barbiturates probably because metabolism of the barbiturate is inhibited.

8. *Estradiol, estrone, progesterone and other steroid hormones.* Pretreatment with or concurrent administration of phenobarbital may decrease the effect of estradiol by increasing its metabolism. There have been reports of patients treated with antiepileptic drugs (e.g. phenobarbital) who become pregnant while taking oral contraceptives. An alternate contraceptive method might be suggested to women taking phenobarbital.

Carcinogenesis, mutagenesis, impairment of fertility: No long-term studies in animals have been performed with butabarbital sodium to determine carcinogenic and mutagenic potential, or effects on fertility.

Pregnancy: Teratogenic effects—Pregnancy Category D (See WARNINGS—**Use in pregnancy** above).

Nonteratogenic effects—Infants suffering from long-term barbiturate exposure *in utero* may have an acute withdrawal syndrome of seizures and hyperirritability from birth to a delayed onset of up to 14 days (see DRUG ABUSE AND DEPENDENCE).

Labor and delivery: Hypnotic doses of barbiturates do not appear to significantly impair uterine activity during labor. Administration of sedative-hypnotic barbiturates to the mother during labor may result in respiratory depression in the newborn. Premature infants are particularly susceptible to the depressant effects of barbiturates. If barbiturates are used during labor and delivery, resuscitation equipment should be available.

Nursing mothers: Caution should be exercised when a barbiturate is administered to a nursing woman since small amounts of some barbiturates are excreted in the milk.

Adverse Reactions: The following adverse reactions have been observed with the use of barbiturates in hospitalized patients. Because such patients may be less aware of certain of the milder adverse effects of barbiturates, the incidence of these reactions may be somewhat higher in fully ambulatory patients.

More than 1 in 100 patients. The most common adverse reaction, somnolence, is estimated to occur at a rate of 1 to 3 patients per 100.

Less than 1 in 100 patients. The most common adverse reactions estimated to occur at a rate of less than 1 in 100 patients listed below, grouped by organ system, and by decreasing order of occurrence are:

Central nervous system/psychiatric: Agitation, confusion, hyperkinesia, ataxia, CNS depression, nightmares, nervousness, psychiatric disturbance, hallucinations, insomnia, anxiety, dizziness, thinking abnormality.

Respiratory: Hypoventilation, apnea.

Cardiovascular: Bradycardia, hypotension, syncope.

Gastrointestinal: Nausea, vomiting, constipation.

Other reported reactions: Headache, hypersensitivity (angioedema, skin rashes, exfoliative dermatitis), fever, liver damage.

Drug Abuse and Dependence: Controlled substance: Schedule III.

Abuse and dependence: Barbiturates may be habit-forming. Tolerance, psychological dependence, and physical dependence may occur especially following prolonged use of high doses of barbiturates. Daily administration in excess of 400 milligrams (mg) of pentobarbital or secobarbital for approximately 90 days is likely to produce some degree of physical dependence. A dosage of from 600 to 800 mg taken for at least 35 days is sufficient to produce withdrawal seizures. The average daily dose for the barbiturate addict is usually about 1.5 grams. As tolerance to barbiturates develops, the amount needed to maintain the same level of intoxication increases; tolerance to a fatal dosage, however, does not increase more than two-fold. As this occurs, the margin between an intoxicating dosage and fatal dosage becomes smaller.

Symptoms of acute intoxication with barbiturates include unsteady gait, slurred speech, and sustained nystagmus. Mental signs of chronic intoxication include confusion, poor judgment, irritability, insomnia, and somatic complaints. Symptoms of barbiturate dependence are similar to those of chronic alcoholism.

If an individual appears to be intoxicated with alcohol to a degree that is radically disproportionate to the amount of alcohol in his or her blood, the use of barbiturates should be suspected. The lethal dose of a barbiturate is far less if alcohol is also ingested.

The symptoms of barbiturate withdrawal can be severe and may cause death. Minor withdrawal symptoms may appear 8 to 12 hours after the last dose of a barbiturate. These symptoms usually appear in the following order: anxiety, muscle twitching, tremor of hands and fingers, progressive weakness, dizziness, distortion in visual perception, nausea, vomiting, insomnia, and orthostatic hypotension. Major withdrawal symptoms (convulsions and delirium) may occur within 16 hours and last up to 5 days after abrupt cessation of these drugs. Intensity of withdrawal symptoms gradually declines over a period of approximately 15 days.

Drug dependence to barbiturates arises from repeated administration of a barbiturate or agent with barbiturate-like effect on a continuous basis, generally in amounts exceeding the therapeutic dose levels. The characteristics of drug dependence to barbiturates include: (a) a strong desire or need to continue taking the drug; (b) a tendency to increase the dose; (c) a psychic dependence on the effects of the drug related to subjective and individual appreciation for those effects; and (d) a physical dependence on the effects of the drug requiring its presence for maintenance of homeostasis and resulting in a definite, characteristic, and self-limited abstinence syndrome when the drug is withdrawn.

Treatment of barbiturate dependence consists of cautious and gradual withdrawal of the drug. Barbiturate-dependent patients can be withdrawn by using a number of different withdrawal regimens. In all cases, withdrawal takes an extended period of time. One method involves initiating treatment at the patient's regular dosage level, in 3 to 4 divided doses, and decreasing the daily dose by 10 percent if tolerated by the patient.

Infants physically dependent on barbiturates may be given phenobarbital 3 to 10 mg/kg/day. After withdrawal symptoms (hyperactivity, disturbed sleep, tremors, hyperreflexia) are relieved, the dosage of phenobarbital should be gradually decreased and completely withdrawn over a 2-week period.

Overdosage: Signs and symptoms: The toxic dose of barbiturates varies considerably. In general, an oral dose of 1 gram of most barbiturates produces serious poisoning in an adult. Death commonly occurs after 2 to 10 grams of ingested barbiturate. Symptoms of acute intoxication with barbiturates include unsteady gait, slurred speech, and sustained nystagmus. Mental signs of chronic intoxication include confusion, poor judgment, irritability, insomnia, and somatic complaints. Barbiturate intoxication may be confused with alcoholism, bromide intoxication, and with various neurological disorders.

Acute overdosage with barbiturates is manifested by CNS and respiratory depression which may progress to Cheyne-Stokes respiration, areflexia, constriction of the pupils to a slight degree (though in severe poisoning they may show paralytic dilation), oliguria, tachycardia, hypotension, lowered body temperature, and coma. Typical shock syndrome (apnea, circulatory collapse, respiratory arrest, and death) may occur.

In extreme overdose, all electrical activity in the brain may cease, in which case a "flat" EEG normally equated with clinical death cannot be accepted. This effect is fully reversible unless hypoxic damage occurs. Consideration should be given to the possibility of barbiturate intoxication even in situations that appear to involve trauma.

Complications: Pneumonia, pulmonary edema, cardiac arrhythmias, congestive heart failure, and renal failure may occur. Uremia may increase CNS sensitivity to barbiturates if renal function is impaired. Differential diagnosis should include hypoglycemia, head trauma, cerebrovascular accidents, convulsive states, and diabetic coma.

Treatment: Treatment of overdosage is mainly supportive and consists of the following:

1. Maintenance of an adequate airway, with assisted respiration and oxygen administration as necessary.
2. Monitoring of vital signs and fluid balance.
3. If the patient is conscious and has not lost the gag reflex, emesis may be induced with ipecac. Care should be taken to prevent pulmonary aspiration of vomitus. After completion of vomiting, 30 grams activated charcoal in a glass of water may be administered.
4. If emesis is contraindicated, gastric lavage may be performed with a cuffed endotracheal tube in place with the patient in the face down position. Activated charcoal may be left in the emptied stomach and a saline cathartic administered.
5. Fluid therapy and other standard treatment for shock, if needed.
6. If renal function is normal, forced diuresis may aid in the elimination of the barbiturate.
7. Although not recommended as a routine procedure, hemodialysis may be used in severe barbiturate intoxications or if the patient is anuric or in shock.
8. Appropriate nursing care, including rolling patients from side-to-side every 30 minutes, to prevent hypostatic pneumonia, decubiti, aspiration, and other complications of patients with altered states of consciousness.
9. Antibiotics should be given if pneumonia is expected.

Dosage and Administration:

Usual adult dosage:

Daytime sedative—15 to 30 mg, 3 or 4 times daily.

Bedtime hypnotic—50 to 100 mg.

Preoperative sedative—50 to 100 mg, 60 to 90 minutes before surgery.

Continued on next page

Wallace—Cont.

Usual pediatric dosage:
Preoperative sedative—2 to 6 mg/kg maximum 100 mg.

Special patient population:
Dosage should be reduced in the elderly or debilitated because these patients may be more sensitive to barbiturates. Dosage should be reduced for patients with impaired renal function or hepatic disease (see PRECAUTIONS).

How Supplied: BUTISOL SODIUM® (butabarbital sodium) Tablets:

15 mg—colored lavender, scored, imprinted "BUTISOL SODIUM" and $37/_{112}$ in bottles of 100 (NDC 0037-0112-60) and 1000 (NDC 0037-0112-80).

30 mg*—colored green, scored, imprinted "BUTISOL SODIUM" and $37/_{113}$ in bottles of 100 (NDC 0037-0113-60) and 1000 (NDC 0037-0113-80).

50 mg*—colored orange, scored, imprinted "BUTISOL SODIUM" and $37/_{114}$ in bottles of 100 (NDC 0037-0114-60).

100 mg—colored pink, scored, imprinted "BUTISOL SODIUM" and $37/_{115}$ in bottles of 100 (NDC 0037-0115-60).

BUTISOL SODIUM® (butabarbital sodium) Elixir*: 30 mg/5 ml, alcohol (by volume) 7%—colored green in bottles of one pint (NDC 0037-0110-16) and one gallon (NDC 0037-0110-28).

*Contains FD&C Yellow No. 5 (see PRECAUTIONS).

Storage: Tablets and Elixir—Store at room temperature. Keep bottle tightly closed.

Rev. 11/83

Shown in Product Identification Section, page 442

DEPEN® ℞
(Penicillamine, Wallace)
Titratable Tablets

> Physicians planning to use penicillamine should thoroughly familiarize themselves with its toxicity, special dosage considerations, and therapeutic benefits. Penicillamine should never be used casually. Each patient should remain constantly under the close supervision of the physician. Patients should be warned to report promptly any symptoms suggesting toxicity.

Description: Penicillamine is 3-mercapto-D-valine. It is a white or practically white, crystalline powder, freely soluble in water, slightly soluble in alcohol, and insoluble in chloroform and ether. Although its configuration is D, it is levoratatory as usually measured:

25°
[α] D = −62.5° ± 2° (C = 0.05%, 1N NaOH)

The empirical formula is $C_5H_{11}NO_2S$, giving it a molecular weight of 149.21.

It reacts readily with formaldehyde or acetone to form a thiazolidine-carboxylic acid.

Clinical Pharmacology: Penicillamine is a chelating agent recommended for the removal of excess copper in patients with Wilson's disease. From *in vitro* studies which indicate that one atom of copper combines with two molecules of penicillamine, it would appear that one gram of penicillamine should be followed by the excretion of about 200 milligrams of copper; however, the actual amount excreted is about one percent of this.

Penicillamine also reduces excess cystine excretion in cystinuria. This is done, at least in part, by disulfide interchange between penicillamine and cystine, resulting in formation of penicillamine-cysteine disulfide, a substance that is much more soluble than cystine and is excreted readily.

Penicillamine interferes with the formation of cross-links between tropocollagen molecules and cleaves them when newly formed. The mechanism of action of penicillamine in rheumatoid arthritis is unknown, although it appears to suppress disease activity. Unlike cytotoxic immunosuppressants, penicillamine markedly lowers IgM rheumatoid factor but produces no significant depression in absolute levels of serum immunoglobulins. Also unlike cytotoxic immunosuppressants, which act on both, penicillamine *in vitro* depresses T-cell activity but not B-cell activity. *In vitro*, penicillamine dissociates macroglobulins (rheumatoid factor) although the relationship of the activity to its effect in rheumatoid arthritis is not known.

In rheumatoid arthritis, the onset of therapeutic response to DEPEN (Penicillamine, Wallace) may not be seen for two or three months. In those patients who respond, however, the first evidence of suppression of symptoms such as pain, tenderness, and swelling usually is apparent within three months. The optimum duration of therapy has not been determined. If remissions occur, they may last from months to years but usually require continued treatment (see DOSAGE AND ADMINISTRATION).

In patients with rheumatoid arthritis, it is important that DEPEN be given on an empty stomach, at least one hour before meals and at least one hour apart from any other drug, food or milk. This permits maximum absorption and reduces the likelihood of metal binding.

Methodology for determining the bioavailability of penicillamine is not available; however, penicillamine is known to be a very soluble substance.

Indications: DEPEN is indicated in the treatment of Wilson's disease, cystinuria, and in patients with severe, active rheumatoid arthritis who have failed to respond to an adequate trial of conventional therapy. Available evidence suggests that DEPEN is not of value in ankylosing spondylitis.

Wilson's Disease—Wilson's disease (hepatolenticular degeneration) results from the interaction of an inherited defect and an abnormality in copper metabolism. The metabolic defect, which is the consequence of the autosomal inheritance of one abnormal gene from each parent, manifests itself in a greater positive copper balance than normal. As a result, copper is deposited in several organs and appears eventually to produce pathologic effects most prominently seen in the brain, where degeneration is widespread; in the liver, where fatty infiltration, inflammation, and hepatocellular damage progress to postnecrotic cirrhosis; in the kidney, where tubular and glomerular dysfunction results; and in the eye, where characteristic corneal copper deposits are known as Kayser-Fleischer rings.

Two types of patients require treatment for Wilson's disease: (1) the symptomatic, and (2) the asymptomatic in whom it can be assumed the disease will develop in the future if the patient is not treated.

Diagnosis, suspected on the basis of family or individual history, physical examination, or a low serum concentration of ceruloplasmin*, is confirmed by the demonstration of Kayser-Fleischer rings or, particularly in the asymptomatic patient, by the quantitative demonstration in a liver biopsy specimen of a concentration of copper in excess of 250 mcg/g dry weight.

---
*For quantitative test for serum ceruloplasmin see: Morell, A. G.; Windsor, J.; Sternlieb, I.; Scheinberg, I. H.: Measurement of the concentration of ceruloplasmin in serum by determination of its oxidase activity, in "Laboratory Diagnosis of Liver Disease," F. W. Sunderman; F. W Sunderman, Jr. (eds.), St. Louis, Warren H. Green, Inc., 1968, pp. 193–195.

Treatment has two objectives:
(1) to minimize dietary intake and absorption of copper.
(2) to promote excretion of copper deposited in tissues.

The first objective is attained by a daily diet that contains no more than one or two milligrams of copper. Such a diet should exclude, most importantly, chocolate, nuts, shellfish, mushrooms, liver, molasses, broccoli, and cereals enriched with copper, and be composed to as great an extent as possible of foods with a low copper content. Distilled or demineralized water should be used if the patient's drinking water contains more than 0.1 mg of copper per liter.

For the second objective, a copper chelating agent is used. Penicillamine is the only one of these agents that is orally effective.

In symptomatic patients, this treatment usually produces marked neurologic improvement, fading of Kayser-Fleischer rings, and gradual amelioration of hepatic dysfunction and psychic disturbances.

Clinical experience to date suggests that life is prolonged with the above regimen.

Noticeable improvement may not occur for one to three months. Occasionally, neurologic symptoms become worse during initiation of therapy with DEPEN. Despite this, the drug should not be discontinued permanently, although temporary interruption may result in clinical improvement of the neurological symptoms but it carries an increased risk of developing a sensitivity reaction upon resumption of therapy (See WARNINGS).

Treatment of asymptomatic patients has been carried out for over ten years. Symptoms and signs of the disease appear to be prevented indefinitely if daily treatment with DEPEN can be continued.

Cystinuria—Cystinuria is characterized by excessive urinary excretion of the dibasic amino acids, arginine, lysine, ornithine, and cystine, and the mixed disulfide of cysteine and homocysteine. The metabolic defect that leads to cystinuria is inherited as an autosomal, recessive trait. Metabolism of the affected amino acids is influenced by at least two abnormal factors: (1) defective gastrointestinal absorption and (2) renal tubular dysfunction.

Arginine, lysine, ornithine, and cysteine are soluble substances, readily excreted. There is no apparent pathology connected with their excretion in excessive quantities.

Cystine, however, is so slightly soluble at the usual range of urinary pH that it is not excreted readily, and so crystallizes and forms stones in the urinary tract. Stone formation is the only known pathology in cystinuria.

Normal daily output of cystine is 40 to 80 mg. In cystinuria, output is greatly increased and may exceed 1 g/day. At 500 to 600 mg/day, stone formation is almost certain. When it is more than 300 mg/day, treatment is indicated. Conventional treatment is directed at keeping urinary cystine diluted enough to prevent stone formation, keeping the urine alkaline enough to dissolve as much cystine as possible, and minimizing cystine production by a diet low in methionine (the major dietary precursor of cystine). Patients must drink enough fluid to keep urine specific gravity below 1.010, take enough alkali to keep urinary pH at 7.5 to 8, and maintain a diet low in methionine. This diet is not recommended in growing children and probably is contraindicated in pregnancy because of its low protein content (see PRECAUTIONS).

When these measures are inadequate to control recurrent stone formation, DEPEN may be used as additional therapy. When patients refuse to adhere to conventional treatment, DEPEN may be a useful substitute. It is capable of keeping cystine excretion to near normal values, thereby hindering stone formation and the serious consequences of pyelonephritis and impaired renal function that develop in some patients.

Bartter and colleagues depict the process by which penicillamine interacts with cystine to form penicillamine-cysteine mixed disulfide as:

CSSC + PS′ ⇌ CS′ + CSSP
PSSP + CS′ ⇌ PS′ + CSSP
CSSC + PSSP ⇌ 2 CSSP

CSSC = cystine
CS′ = deprotonated cysteine
PSSP = penicillamine
PS′ = deprotonated penicillamine sulfhydryl
CSSP = penicillamine-cysteine mixed disulfide

In this process, it is assumed that the deprotonated form of penicillamine, PS′, is the active factor in bringing about the disulfide interchange.

Rheumatoid Arthritis—Because DEPEN can cause severe adverse reactions, its use in rheumatoid arthritis should be restricted to patients who have severe, active disease and who have failed to respond to an adequate trial of conventional therapy. Even then, benefit-to-risk ratio should be carefully considered. Other measures, such as rest, physiotherapy, salicylates and corticosteroids should be used, when indicated, in conjunction with DEPEN (see PRECAUTIONS).

Contraindications—Penicillamine should not be administered to patients with rheumatoid arthritis who are pregnant (see PRECAUTIONS). Patients with a history of penicillamine-related aplastic anemia or agranulocytosis should not be restarted on penicillamine (see WARNINGS and ADVERSE REACTIONS).

Because of its potential for causing renal damage, penicillamine should not be administered to rheumatoid arthritis patients with a history or other evidence of renal insufficiency.

Warnings: The use of penicillamine has been associated with fatalities due to certain diseases, such as aplastic anemia, agranulocytosis, thrombocytopenia, Goodpasture's syndrome, and myasthenia gravis.

Because of the potential for serious hematological and renal adverse reactions, routine urinalysis, white and differential blood cell count, hemoglobin determination, and direct platelet count must be done every two weeks for the first six months of penicillamine therapy and monthly thereafter. Patients should be instructed to report promptly signs and symptoms of granulocytopenia and/or thrombocytopenia such as fever, sore throat, chills, bruising or bleeding and the above laboratory studies should be promptly repeated.

Leukopenia and thrombocytopenia have been reported to occur in up to 5% of patients during penicillamine therapy. Leukopenia is of the granulocytic series and may or may not be associated with an increase in eosinophils. A confirmed reduction in WBC below 3500 mandates discontinuance of penicillamine therapy. Thrombocytopenia may be on an idiosyncratic basis with decreased or absent megakaryocytes in the marrow, when it is part of an aplastic anemia. In other cases the thrombocytopenia is presumably on an immune basis since the number of megakaryocytes in the marrow has been reported to be normal or sometimes increased. The development of a platelet count below 100,000, even in the absence of clinical bleeding, requires at least temporary cessation of penicillamine therapy. A progressive fall in either platelet count or WBC in three successive determinations, even though values are still within the normal range, likewise requires at least temporary cessation.

Proteinuria and/or hematuria may develop during therapy and may be warning signs of membranous glomerulopathy which can progress to a nephrotic syndrome. Close observation of these patients is essential. In some patients the proteinuria disappears with continued therapy; in others penicillamine must be discontinued. When a patient develops proteinuria or hematuria the physician must ascertain whether it is a sign of drug-induced glomerulopathy or is unrelated to penicillamine.

Rheumatoid arthritis patients who develop moderate degrees of proteinuria may be continued cautiously on penicillamine therapy, provided that quantitative 24-hour urinary protein determinations are obtained at intervals of one to two weeks. Penicillamine dosage should not be increased under these circumstances. Proteinuria which exceeds 1 g/24 hours, or proteinuria which is progressively increasing requires either discontinuance of the drug or a reduction in the dosage. In some patients, proteinuria has been reported to clear following reduction in dosage.

In rheumatoid arthritis patients, penicillamine should be discontinued if unexplained gross hematuria or presistent microscopic hematuria develops.

In patients with Wilson's disease or cystinuria the risks of continued penicillamine therapy in patients manifesting potentially serious urinary abnormalities must be weighed against the expected therapeutic benefits.

When penicillamine is used in cystinuria, an annual x-ray for renal stones is advised. Cystine stones form rapidly, sometimes in six months. Up to one year or more may be required for any urinary abnormalities to disappear after penicillamine has been discontinued.

Because of rare reports of intrahepatic cholestasis and toxic hepatitis, liver function tests are recommended every six months during therapy.

Goodpasture's syndrome has occurred rarely. The development of abnormal urinary findings associated with hemoptysis and pulmonary infiltrates on x-ray requires immediate cessation of penicillamine.

Myasthenic syndrome sometimes progressing to myasthenia gravis has been reported. In the majority of cases, symptoms of myasthenia have receded after withdrawal of penicillamine.

Pemphigoid-type reactions characterized by bullous lesions clinically indistinguishable from pemphigus have occurred and have required discontinuation of penicillamine and treatment with corticosteroids.

Once instituted for Wilson's disease or cystinuria, treatment with penicillamine should, as a rule, be continued on a daily basis. Interruptions for even a few days have been followed by sensitivity reactions after reinstitution of therapy.

Precautions: Some patients may experience drug fever, a marked febrile response to penicillamine, usually in the second or third week following initiation of therapy. Drug fever may sometimes be accompanied by a macular cutaneous eruption.

In the case of drug fever in patients with Wilson's disease or cystinuria, because no alternative treatment is available, penicillamine should be temporarily discontinued until the reaction subsides. Then penicillamine should be reinstituted with a small dose that is gradually increased until the desired dosage is attained. Systemic steroid therapy may be necessary, and is usually helpful, in such patients in whom toxic reactions develop a second or third time.

In the case of drug fever in rheumatoid arthritis patients, because other treatments are available, penicillamine should be discontinued and another therapeutic alternative tried, since experience indicates that the febrile reaction will recur in a very high percentage of patients upon readministration of penicillamine.

The skin and mucous membranes should be observed for allergic reactions. Early and late rashes have occurred. Early rash occurs during the first few months of treatment and is more common. It is usually a generalized pruritic, erythematous, maculopapular or morbilliform rash and resembles the allergic rash seen with other drugs. Early rash usually disappears within days after stopping penicillamine and seldom recurs when the drug is restarted at a lower dosage. Pruritus and early rash may often be controlled by the concomitant administration of antihistamines. Less commonly, a late rash may be seen, usually after six months or more of treatment, and requires discontinuation of penicillamine. It is usually on the trunk, is accompanied by intense pruritus, and is usually unresponsive to topical corticosteroid therapy. Late rash may take weeks to disappear after penicillamine is stopped and usually recurs if the drug is restarted.

The appearance of drug eruption accompanied by fever, arthralgia, lymphadenopathy or other allergic manifestations usually requires discontinuation of penicillamine.

Certain patients will develop a positive antinuclear antibody (ANA) test and some of these may show a lupus erythematosus-like syndrome similar to drug-induced lupus associated with other drugs. The lupus erythematosus-like syndrome is not associated with hypocomplementemia and may be present without nephropathy. The development of a positive ANA test does not mandate discontinuance of the drug; however, the physician should be alerted to the possibility that a lupus erythematosus-like syndrome may develop in the future.

Some patients may develop oral ulcerations which in some cases have the appearance of aphthous stomatitis. The stomatitis usually recurs on rechallenge but often clears on a lower dosage. Although rare, cheilosis, glossitis and gingivostomatitis have also been reported. These oral lesions are frequently dose-related and may preclude further increase in penicillamine dosage or require discontinuation of the drug.

Hypogeusia (a blunting or diminution in taste perception) has occurred in some patients. This may last two to three months or more and may develop into a total loss of taste; however, it is usually self-limited, despite continued penicillamine treatment. Such taste impairment is rare in patients with Wilson's disease.

Penicillamine should not be used in patients who are receiving concurrent gold therapy, antimalarial or cytotoxic drugs, oxyphenbutazone or phenylbutazone because these drugs are also associated with similar serious hematologic and/or renal adverse reactions. Patients who have had gold salt therapy discontinued due to a major toxic reaction may be at greater risk of serious side effects with penicillamine, but not necessarily of the same type. Patients who are allergic to penicillin may theoretically have cross-sensitivity to penicillamine. The possibility of reactions from contamination of penicillamine by trace amounts of penicillin has been precluded now that penicillamine is being produced synthetically rather than as a degradation product of penicillin.

Because of their dietary restrictions, patients with Wilson's disease and cystinuria should be given 25 mg/day of pyridoxine during therapy, since penicillamine increases the requirement for this vitamin. Patients also may receive benefit from a multivitamin preparation, although there is no evidence that deficiency of any vitamin other than pyridoxine is associated with penicillamine. In Wilson's disease, multivitamin preparations must be copper-free.

Rheumatoid arthritis patients whose nutrition is impaired should also be given a daily supplement of pyridoxine. Mineral supplements should not be given, since they may block the response to penicillamine.

Iron deficiency may develop, especially in children and in menstruating women. In Wilson's disease, this may be a result of adding the effects of the low copper diet, which is probably also low in iron, and the penicillamine to the effects of blood loss or growth. In cystinuria, a low methionine diet may contribute to iron deficiency, since it is necessarily low in protein. If necessary, iron may be given in short courses, but a period of two hours should elapse between administration of penicillamine and iron, since orally administered iron has been shown to reduce the effects of penicillamine.

Penicillamine causes an increase in the amount of soluble collagen. In the rat this results in inhibition of normal healing and also a decrease in tensile strength of intact skin. In man this may be the cause of increased skin friability at sites especially subject to pressure or trauma, such as shoulders, elbows, knees, toes, and buttocks. Extravasations of blood may occur and may appear as purpuric areas, with external bleeding if the skin is broken, or as vesicles containing dark blood. Neither type is progressive. There is no apparent association with bleeding elsewhere in the body and no associated coagulation defect has been found. Therapy with penicillamine may be continued in the presence of these lesions. They may disappear if dosage is reduced. Other reported effects probably due to the action of penicillamine on collagen are excessive wrinkling of the skin and development of small, white papules at venipuncture and surgical sites.

The effects of penicillamine on collagen and elastin make it advisable to consider a reduction in dosage to 250 mg/day when surgery is contemplated. Reinstitution of full therapy should be delayed until wound healing is complete.

Caution patients to report immediately any abrupt onset of pulmonary symptoms, such as exertional dyspnea, wheezing, or cough and have appropriate pulmonary function studies done to rule out obstructive bronchiolitis.

Continued on next page

Wallace—Cont.

Carcinogenesis—Long-term animal carcinogenicity studies have not been done with penicillamine. There is a report that 5 of 10 autoimmune disease-prone NZB Hybrid mice developed lymphocytic leukemia after 6 months' intraperitoneal treatment with a dose of 400 mg/kg penicillamine 5 days per week.

Usage in Pregnancy—Penicillamine has been shown to be teratogenic in rats when given in doses several times higher than the highest dose recommended for human use. Skeletal defects, cleft palates and fetal toxicity (resorptions) have been reported.

Wilson's disease—There are no controlled studies in pregnant women with Wilson's disease, but experience does not include any positive evidence of adverse effects to the fetus. Reported experience* shows that continued treatment with penicillamine throughout pregnancy protects the mother against relapse of the Wilson's disease, and that discontinuation of penicillamine has deleterious effects on the mother. It indicates that the drug does not increase the risk of fetal abnormalities, but it does not exclude the possibility of infrequent or subtle damage to the fetus.

*Scheinberg, I. H., Sternlieb, I.: *N Engl J Med* 293: 1300–1302, Dec. 18, 1975.

If penicillamine is administered during pregnancy to patients with Wilson's disease, it is recommended that the daily dosage be limited to 1 g. If Caesarean section is planned, the daily dosage should be limited to 250 mg during the last six weeks of pregnancy and postoperatively until wound healing is complete.

Cystinuria—If possible, penicillamine should not be given during pregnancy to women with cystinuria. There is a report of a woman with cystinuria treated with 2 g/day of penicillamine during pregnancy who gave birth to a child with a generalized connective tissue defect that may have been caused by penicillamine. If stones continue to form in these patients, the benefits of therapy to the mother must be evaluated against the risk to the fetus.

Rheumatoid Arthritis—Penicillamine should not be administered to rheumatoid arthritis patients who are pregnant (see CONTRAINDICATIONS) and should be discontinued promptly in patients in whom pregnancy is suspected or diagnosed. Penicillamine should be used in women of childbearing potential only when the expected benefits outweigh possible hazards. Women of childbearing potential should be informed of the possible hazards of penicillamine to the developing fetus and should be advised to report promptly any missed menstrual periods or other indications of possible pregnancy.

There is a report that a woman with rheumatoid arthritis treated with less than 1 g/day of penicillamine during pregnancy gave birth (Caesarean delivery) to an infant with growth retardation, flattened face with broad nasal bridge, low set ears, short neck with loose skin folds, and unusually lax body skin.

Usage in Children—The efficacy of DEPEN in juvenile rheumatoid arthritis has not been established.

Adverse Reactions: Penicillamine is a drug with a high incidence of untoward reactions, some of which are potentially fatal. Therefore, it is mandatory that patients receiving penicillamine therapy remain under close medical supervision throughout the period of drug administration (see WARNINGS and PRECAUTIONS).

Reported incidences (%) for the most commonly occurring adverse reactions in rheumatoid arthritis patients are noted, based on 17 representative clinical trials reported in the literature (1270 patients).

Allergic—Generalized pruritus, early and late rashes (5%), pemphigoid-type reactions and drug eruptions which may be accompanied by fever, arthralgia or lymphadenopathy have occurred (see WARNINGS and PRECAUTIONS). Some patients may show a lupus erythematosus-like syndrome similar to drug induced lupus produced by other pharmacological agents (see PRECAUTIONS).

Urticaria and exfoliative dermatitis have occurred.

Thyroiditis has been reported but is extremely rare.

Some patients may develop a migratory polyarthralgia, often with objective synovitis (see DOSAGE AND ADMINISTRATION).

Gastrointestinal—Anorexia, epigastric pain, nausea, vomiting or occasional diarrhea may occur (17%).

Isolated cases of reactivated peptic ulcer have occurred, as have hepatic dysfunction, cholestatic jaundice and pancreatitis. There have been a few reports of increased serum alkaline phosphatase, lactic dehydrogenase, and positive cephalin flocculation and thymol turbidity tests.

Some patients may report a blunting, diminution or total loss of taste perception (12%) or may develop oral ulcerations. Although rare, cheilosis, glossitis and gingivostomatitis have been reported (see PRECAUTIONS).

Gastrointestinal side effects are usually reversible following cessation of therapy.

Hematological—Penicillamine can cause bone marrow depression (see WARNINGS). Leukopenia (2%) and thrombocytopenia (4%) have occurred. Fatalities have been reported as a result of thrombocytopenia, agranulocytosis and aplastic anemia. Thrombotic thrombocytopenic purpura, hemolytic anemia, red cell aplasia, monocytosis, leukocytosis, eosinophilia and thrombocytosis have also been reported.

Renal—Patients on penicillamine therapy may develop proteinuria (6%) and/or hematuria which, in some, may progress to the development of the nephrotic syndrome as a result of an immune complex membranous glomerulopathy (see WARNINGS)

Central Nervous System—Tinnitus has been reported. Reversible optic neuritis has been reported with the administration of penicillamine and may be related to pyridoxine deficiency.

Neuromuscular—Myasthenia gravis (see WARNINGS).

Other—Adverse reactions that have been reported rarely include thrombophlebitis; hyperpyrexia (see PRECAUTIONS); falling hair or alopecia; polymyositis; dermatomyositis; mammary hyperplasia; elastosis perforans serpiginosa; toxic epidermal necrolysis; anetoderma (cutaneous macular atrophy); Goodpasture's syndrome, a severe and ultimately fatal glomerulonephritis associated with intra-alveolar hemorrhage (see WARNINGS); and fatal renal vasculitis. Allergic alveolitis and obliterative bronchiolitis have been reported in patients with severe rheumatoid arthritis, some of whom were receiving penicillamine (see PRECAUTIONS).

Increased skin friability, excessive wrinkling of skin, and development of small, white papules at venipuncture and surgical sites have been reported (See PRECAUTIONS).

The chelating action of the drug may cause increased excretion of other heavy metals such as zinc, mercury and lead.

There have been reports associating penicillamine with leukemia. However, circumstances involved in these reports are such that a cause and effect relationship to the drug has not been established.

Dosage and Administration:

Wilson's Disease—DEPEN tablets should be given on an empty stomach, four times a day; one-half to one hour before meals and at bedtime—at least two hours after the evening meal.

Optimal dosage can be determined only by measurement of urinary copper excretion. The urine must be collected in copper-free glassware, and should be quantitatively analyzed for copper before and soon after initiation of therapy with DEPEN. Continued therapy should be monitored by doing a 24-hour urinary copper analysis every three months or so for the duration of therapy. Since a low copper diet should keep copper absorption down to less than one milligram a day, the patient probably will be in negative copper balance if 0.5 to one milligram of copper is present in a 24-hour collection of urine.

To achieve this, the suggested initial dosage of DEPEN in the treatment of Wilson's disease is 1 g/day for children or adults. This may be increased, as indicated by the urinary copper analyses, but it is seldom necessary to exceed a dosage of 2 g/day.

In patients who cannot tolerate as much as 1 g/day initially, initiating dosage with 250 mg/day, and increasing gradually to the requisite amount, gives closer control of the effects of the drug and may help to reduce the incidence of adverse reactions.

Cystinuria—It is recommended that DEPEN be used along with conventional therapy. By reducing urinary cystine, it decreases crystalluria and stone formation. In some instances, it has been reported to decrease the size of, and even to dissolve, stones already formed.

The usual dosage of DEPEN in the treatment of cystinuria is 2 g/day for adults; with a range of 1 to 4 g/day. For children, dosage can be based on 30 mg/kg/day. The total daily amount should be divided into four doses. If four equal doses are not feasible, give the larger portion at bedtime. If adverse reactions necessitate a reduction in dosage, it is important to retain the bedtime dose.

Initiating dosage with 250 mg/day, and increasing gradually to the requisite amount, gives closer control of the effects of the drug and may help to reduce the incidence of adverse reactions.

In addition to taking DEPEN, patients should drink copiously. It is especially important to drink about a pint of fluid at bedtime and another pint once during the night when urine is more concentrated and more acid than during the day. The greater the fluid intake, the lower the required dosage of DEPEN.

Dosage must be individualized to an amount that limits cystine excretion to 100–200 mg/day in those with no history of stones, and below 100 mg/day in those who have had stone formation and/or pain. Thus, in determining dosage, the inherent tubular defect, the patient's size, age, and rate of growth, and his diet and water intake all must be taken into consideration.

The standard nitroprusside cyanide test has been reported useful as a qualitative measure of the effective dose*: Add 2 ml of freshly prepared 5 percent sodium cyanide to 5 ml of a 24-hour aliquot of protein-free urine and let stand ten minutes. Add 5 drops of freshly prepared 5 percent sodium nitroprusside and mix. Cystine will turn the mixture magenta. If the result is negative, it can be assumed that cystine excretion is less than 100 mg/g creatinine.

*Lotz, M., Potts, J. T. and Bartter, F. C.: *Brit Med J* 2:521, Aug. 28, 1965 (in Medical Memoranda).

Although penicillamine is rarely excreted unchanged, it also will turn the mixture magenta. If there is any question as to which substance is causing the reaction, a ferric chloride test can be done to eliminate doubt: Add 3 percent ferric chloride dropwise to the urine. Penicillamine will turn the urine an immediate and quickly fading blue. Cystine will not produce any change in appearance.

Rheumatoid Arthritis—The principal rule of treatment with DEPEN in rheumatoid arthritis is patience. The onset of therapeutic response is typically delayed. Two or three months may be required before the first evidence of a clinical response is noted (see CLINICAL PHARMACOLOGY).

When treatment with DEPEN has been interrupted because of adverse reactions or other reasons, the drug should be reintroduced cautiously by starting with a lower dosage and increasing slowly.

Initial Therapy—

The currently recommended dosage regimen in rheumatoid arthritis begins with a single daily dose of 125 mg or 250 mg which is thereafter increased at one to three month intervals, by 125 mg or 250 mg/day, as patient response and tolerance indicate. If a satisfactory remission of symptoms is achieved, the dose associated with the remission should be continued (see **Maintenance Therapy**). If there is no improvement and there are no signs of potentially serious toxicity after two to three months of treatment with doses of 500–750 mg/day, increases of 250 mg/day at two to three month intervals may be continued until a satisfactory remission occurs (see **Maintenance Therapy**) or signs of toxicity develop (see **WARNINGS** and **PRECAUTIONS**). If there is no discernible improvement after three to four months of treatment with 1000 to 1500 mg penicillamine/day, it may be assumed the patient will not respond and DEPEN should be discontinued.

It is important that DEPEN be given on an empty stomach at least one hour before meals and at least one hour apart from any other drug, food or milk (see **CLINICAL PHARMACOLOGY**).

Maintenance Therapy—
The maintenance dosage of DEPEN must be individualized, and may require adjustment during the course of treatment. Many patients respond satisfactorily to a dosage within the 500–750 mg/day range. Some need less.

Changes in maintenance dosage levels may not be reflected clinically or in the erythrocyte sedimentation rate for two to three months after each dosage adjustment.

Some patients will subsequently require an increase in the maintenance dosage to achieve maximal disease suppression. In those patients who do respond, but who evidence incomplete suppression of their disease after the first six to nine months of treatment, the daily dosage of DEPEN may be increased by 125 mg or 250 mg/day at three-month intervals. It is unusual in current practice to employ a dosage in excess of 1 g/day, but up to 1.5 g/day has sometimes been required.

Management of Exacerbations—
During the course of treatment some patients may experience an exacerbation of disease activity following an initial good response. These may be self-limited and can subside within twelve weeks. They are usually controlled by the addition of non-steroidal anti-inflammatory drugs, and only if the patient has demonstrated a true "escape" phenomenon (as evidenced by failure of the flare to subside within this time period) should an increase in the maintenance dose ordinarily be considered.

In the rheumatoid patient, migratory polyarthralgia due to penicillamine is extremely difficult to differentiate from an exacerbation of the rheumatoid arthritis. Discontinuance or a substantial reduction in the dosage of DEPEN for up to several weeks will usually determine which of these processes is responsible for the arthralgia.

Duration of Therapy—
The optimum duration of DEPEN therapy in rheumatoid arthritis has not been determined. If the patient has been in remission for six months or more, a gradual, stepwise dosage reduction in decrements of 125 mg or 250 mg/day at approximately three month intervals may be attempted.

Concomitant Drug Therapy—
DEPEN should not be used in patients who are receiving gold therapy, antimalarial or cytotoxic drugs, oxyphenbutazone or phenylbutazone (see **PRECAUTIONS**). Other measures, such as salicylates, other nonsteroidal anti-inflammatory drugs or systemic corticosteroids may be continued when DEPEN is initiated. After improvement commences, analgesic and anti-inflammatory drugs may be slowly discontinued as symptoms permit. Steroid withdrawal must be done gradually, and many months of DEPEN treatment may be required before steroids can be completely eliminated.

Dosage Frequency—
Based on clinical experience, dosages up to 500 mg/day can be given as a single daily dose. Dosages in excess of 500 mg/day should be administered in divided doses.

How Supplied: DEPEN® Titratable Tablets: 250 mg scored, oval, white tablets imprinted in red with 37-4401; available in bottles of 100 (NDC 0037-4401-01).

Manufactured under license from HOMBURG (Degussa), West Germany.

Rev. 7/83

DEPROL® ℞ ©
(meprobamate 400 mg + benactyzine hydrochloride 1 mg)

Description: 'Deprol' is available as light pink, scored tablets, each containing meprobamate, U.S.P., 400 mg and benactyzine hydrochloride 1 mg.

Actions: 'Deprol' (meprobamate + benactyzine hydrochloride) combines the tranquilizing action of meprobamate with the antidepressant action of benactyzine hydrochloride.

Benactyzine hydrochloride
Benactyzine hydrochloride is a mild antidepressant and anticholinergic agent which in animals has been shown to reduce the autonomic response to emotion-provoking stress.

Meprobamate
Meprobamate is a carbamate derivative which has been shown in animal studies to have effects at multiple sites in the central nervous system, including the thalamus and limbic system.

Indications: Based on a review of this drug by the National Academy of Sciences—National Research Council and/or other information, FDA has classified the indication as follows:

"Possibly" effective: in the management of depression, both acute (reactive) and chronic. It is particularly useful in the less severe depressions and where the depression is accompanied by anxiety, insomnia, agitation, or rumination. It is also useful for management of depression and associated anxiety accompanying or related to organic illnesses.

Final classification of this indication requires further investigation.

Contraindications:
Benactyzine hydrochloride
Glaucoma and allergic or idiosyncratic reactions to benactyzine hydrochloride or related compounds.
Meprobamate
Acute intermittent porphyria as well as allergic or idiosyncratic reactions to meprobamate or related compounds such as carisoprodol, mebutamate, tybamate, or carbromal.

Warnings: The following information on meprobamate pertains to 'Deprol' (meprobamate + benactyzine hydrochloride):
Meprobamate
Drug Dependence—Physical dependence, psychological dependence, and abuse have occurred. When chronic intoxication from prolonged use occurs, it usually involves ingestion of greater than recommended doses and is manifested by ataxia, slurred speech, and vertigo. Therefore, careful supervision of dose and amounts prescribed is advised, as well as avoidance of prolonged administration, especially for alcoholics and other patients with a known propensity for taking excessive quantities of drugs.

Sudden withdrawal of the drug after prolonged and excessive use may precipitate recurrence of pre-existing symptoms, such as anxiety, anorexia, or insomnia, or withdrawal reactions, such as vomiting, ataxia, tremors, muscle twitching, confusional states, hallucinosis, and, rarely, convulsive seizures. Such seizures are more likely to occur in persons with central nervous system damage or pre-existent or latent convulsive disorders. Onset of withdrawal symptoms occurs usually within 12 to 48 hours after discontinuation of meprobamate; symptoms usually cease within the next 12 to 48 hours.

When excessive dosage has continued for weeks or months, dosage should be reduced gradually over a period of one or two weeks rather than abruptly stopped. Alternatively, a short-acting barbiturate may be substituted, then gradually withdrawn.

Potentially Hazardous Tasks—Patients should be warned that this drug may impair the mental and/or physical abilities required for the performance of potentially hazardous tasks such as driving a motor vehicle or operating machinery.

Additive Effects—Since the effects of meprobamate and alcohol or meprobamate and other CNS depressants or psychotropic drugs may be additive, appropriate caution should be exercised with patients who take more than one of these agents simultaneously.

Usage in Pregnancy and Lactation
An increased risk of congenital malformations associated with the use of minor tranquilizers (meprobamate, chlordiazepoxide, and diazepam) during the first trimester of pregnancy has been suggested in several studies. Because use of these drugs is rarely a matter of urgency, their use during this period should almost always be avoided. The possibility that a woman of childbearing potential may be pregnant at the time of institution of therapy should be considered. Patients should be advised that if they become pregnant during therapy or intend to become pregnant they should communicate with their physicians about the desirability of discontinuing the drug.

Meprobamate passes the placental barrier. It is present both in umbilical cord blood at or near maternal plasma levels and in breast milk of lactating mothers at concentrations two to four times that of maternal plasma. When use of meprobamate is contemplated in breast-feeding patients, the drug's higher concentrations in breast milk as compared to maternal plasma levels should be considered.

Usage in Children—This combination is not intended for use in children.

Precautions: This product contains FD&C Yellow No. 5 (tartrazine) which may cause allergic-type reactions (including bronchial asthma) in certain susceptible individuals. Although the overall incidence of FD&C Yellow No. 5 (tartrazine) sensitivity in the general population is low, it is frequently seen in patients who also have aspirin hypersensitivity.

Meprobamate
The lowest effective dose should be administered, particularly to elderly and/or debilitated patients, in order to preclude oversedation.

The possibility of suicide attempts should be considered and the least amount of drug feasible should be dispensed at any one time.

Meprobamate is metabolized in the liver and excreted by the kidney; to avoid its excess accumulation, caution should be exercised in administration to patients with compromised liver or kidney function.

Meprobamate occasionally may precipitate seizures in epileptic patients.

Adverse Reactions: Side effects have included nausea, dryness of mouth, and other gastrointestinal symptoms; syncope; and one case each of severe nervousness and loss of power of concentration.

The following side effects, which have occurred after administration of its components alone, have either occurred or might occur when the combination is taken.

Benactyzine hydrochloride
Benactyzine hydrochloride alone, particularly in high dosage, may produce dizziness, thought-blocking, a sense of depersonalization, aggravation of anxiety, or disturbance of sleep patterns, and a subjective feeling of muscle relaxation. There may also be anticholinergic effects such as blurred vision, dryness of mouth, or failure of visual accommodation. Other reported side effects have included gastric distress, allergic response, ataxia, and euphoria.

Meprobamate
Central Nervous System—Drowsiness, ataxia, dizziness, slurred speech, headache, vertigo, weakness, paresthesias, impairment of visual accommodation, euphoria, overstimulation, paradoxical excitement, fast EEG activity.

Continued on next page

Wallace—Cont.

Gastrointestinal—Nausea, vomiting, diarrhea.
Cardiovascular—Palpitations, tachycardia, various forms of arrhythmia, transient ECG changes, syncope; also, hypotensive crises (including one fatal case).
Allergic or Idiosyncratic—Allergic or idiosyncratic reactions are usually seen within the period of the first to fourth dose in patients having had no previous contact with the drug. Milder reactions are characterized by an itchy, urticarial, or erythematous maculopapular rash which may be generalized or confined to the groin. Other reactions have included leukopenia, acute nonthrombocytopenic purpura, petechiae, ecchymoses, eosinophilia, peripheral edema, adenopathy, fever, fixed drug eruption with cross reaction to carisoprodol, and cross sensitivity between meprobamate/mebutamate and meprobamate/carbromal.
More severe hypersensitivity reactions, rarely reported, include hyperpyrexia, chills, angioneurotic edema, bronchospasm, oliguria, and anuria. Also, anaphylaxis, erythema multiforme, exfoliative dermatitis, stomatitis, proctitis, Stevens-Johnson syndrome, and bullous dermatitis, including one fatal case of the latter following administration of meprobamate in combination with prednisolone.
In case of allergic or idiosyncratic reactions to meprobamate, discontinue the drug and initiate appropriate symptomatic therapy, which may include epinephrine, antihistamines, and in severe cases corticosteroids. In evaluating possible allergic reactions, also consider allergy to excipients (information on excipients is available to physicians on request).
Hematologic (See also **Allergic or Idiosyncratic**.)—Agranulocytosis and aplastic anemia have been reported, although no causal relationship has been established. These cases rarely were fatal. Rare cases of thrombocytopenic purpura have been reported.
Other—Exacerbation of porphyric symptoms.
Dosage and Administration: The usual adult starting dosage of 'Deprol' (meprobamate +benactyzine hydrochloride) is one tablet three or four times daily, which may be increased gradually to six tablets daily and gradually reduced to maintenance levels upon establishment of relief. Doses above six tablets daily are not recommended, even though higher doses have been used by some clinicians to control depression, and in chronic psychotic patients.
Overdosage: Overdosage of 'Deprol' (meprobamate +benactyzine hydrochloride) has not differed substantially from meprobamate overdosage:
Meprobamate
Suicidal attempts with meprobamate have resulted in drowsiness, lethargy, stupor, ataxia, coma, shock, vasomotor and respiratory collapse. Some suicidal attempts have been fatal.
The following data on meprobamate tablets have been reported in the literature and from other sources. These data are not expected to correlate with each case (considering factors such as individual susceptibility and length of time from ingestion to treatment), but represent the *usual ranges* reported.
Acute simple overdose (meprobamate alone): Death has been reported with ingestion of as little as 12 gm meprobamate and survival with as much as 40 gm.
Blood Levels:
0.5–2.0 mg% represents the usual blood level range of meprobamate after therapeutic doses. The level may occasionally be as high as 3.0 mg%.
3 —10 mg% usually corresponds to findings of mild to moderate symptoms of overdosage, such as stupor or light coma.
10 —20 mg% usually corresponds to deeper coma, requiring more intensive treatment. Some fatalities occur.
At levels greater than 20 mg%, more fatalities than survivals can be expected.

Acute combined overdose (meprobamate with alcohol or other CNS depressants or psychotropic drugs): Since effects can be additive, a history of ingestion of a low dose of meprobamate plus any of these compounds (or of a relatively low blood or tissue level) cannot be used as a prognostic indicator.
In cases where excessive doses have been taken, sleep ensues rapidly and blood pressure, pulse, and respiratory rates are reduced to basal levels. Any drug remaining in the stomach should be removed and symptomatic therapy given. Should respiration or blood pressure become compromised, respiratory assistance, central nervous system stimulants, and pressor agents should be administered cautiously as indicated. Meprobamate is metabolized in the liver and excreted by the kidney. Diuresis, osmotic (mannitol) diuresis, peritoneal dialysis, and hemodialysis have been used successfully. Careful monitoring of urinary output is necessary and caution should be taken to avoid overhydration. Relapse and death, after initial recovery, have been attributed to incomplete gastric emptying and delayed absorption. Meprobamate can be measured in biological fluids by two methods: colorimetric (Hoffman, A.J. and Ludwig, B.J.: *J Amer Pharm Assn* **48**: 740, 1959) and gas chromatographic (Douglas, J.F. et al: *Anal Chem* **39**: 956, 1967).
How Supplied: Bottles of 100 (NDC 0037-3001-01). Bottles of 500 (NDC 0037-3001-03). Unit Dose: 500 (NDC 0037-3001-05). Unit Dose: 1000 (NDC 0037-3001-04).
Rev. 7/79

DIUTENSEN® Tablets
R

Description: DIUTENSEN® is a round, white-blue mottled tablet. Each tablet contains:
Cryptenamine .... 2 mg †
(as tannate salts)
Methyclothiazide .... 2.5 mg
† Equivalent to 260 Carotid Sinus Reflex Units.
Actions: Cryptenamine is an alkaloidal fraction obtained from *Veratrum viride* by a nonaqueous extraction procedure. The antihypertensive response to cryptenamine is widely documented. The principal mechanism of action of the drug in reducing the blood pressure involves widespread arteriolar dilatation mediated centrally, without peripheral adrenergic or ganglionic blockade. The major cardiovascular effects are reflex in nature and are mainly due to stimulation of afferent pressor receptors predominantly in the heart and carotid sinus area. These receptors initiate an increase in impulses which are interpreted by areas in the brain stem as denoting a pressure higher than that actually present. As a result, the mechanism concerned with blood pressure homeostasis is activated, sympathetic tone is decreased, vagal tone is increased, and the blood pressure is therefore reduced. Both systolic and diastolic pressure are decreased and the heart is slowed. Atropine abolishes the bradycrotic effect but only partially reverses the hypotensive effect.
Methyclothiazide is a synthetic saluretic-antihypertensive agent. It is a potent analogue of hydrochlorothiazide, being about 20 times as active, by weight, as the latter compound. The renal mechanism involved in the diuretic action of methyclothiazide is indistinguishable from that elicited by chlorothiazide or hydrochlorothiazide, but the duration of action of methyclothiazide is longer than that of either of these compounds. The principal mechanism of action of methyclothiazide is the production of diuresis by inhibition of renal tubular reabsorption of electrolytes, resulting in a marked increase in the urinary excretion of sodium, chloride, and water, and moderate increase in the excretion of potassium and bicarbonate.

Indications:
Based on a review of this drug by the National Academy of Sciences—National Research Council and/or other information, FDA has classified the indications as follows:

Lacking substantial evidence of effectiveness as a fixed combination for use in basic hypertensive therapy and for essential hypertension of all grades of severity. (See box warning.)
Final classification of the less-than-effective indications requires further investigation.

Contraindications: DIUTENSEN is contraindicated for patients with known idiosyncrasy to *Veratrum viride* or thiazide compounds and for those who have recently experienced either coronary artery occlusion or cerebral thrombosis. Treatment with thiazide diuretics (including methyclothiazide) is also contraindicated for patients with severe renal or hepatic disease.

> **WARNING:** THIS FIXED COMBINATION DRUG IS NOT INDICATED FOR INITIAL THERAPY OF HYPERTENSION. HYPERTENSION REQUIRES THERAPY TITRATED TO THE INDIVIDUAL PATIENT. IF THE FIXED COMBINATION REPRESENTS THE DOSAGE SO DETERMINED, ITS USE MAY BE MORE CONVENIENT IN PATIENT MANAGEMENT. THE TREATMENT OF HYPERTENSION IS NOT STATIC, BUT MUST BE RE-EVALUATED AS CONDITIONS IN EACH PATIENT WARRANT.

Warnings: There have been several reports, published and unpublished, concerning non-specific small bowel lesions consisting of stenosis with or without ulceration, associated with the administration of enteric-coated thiazides with potassium salts. These lesions may occur with enteric-coated potassium tablets alone or when they are used with non-enteric-coated thiazides, or certain other oral diuretics. These small bowel lesions have caused obstruction, hemorrhage, and perforation. Surgery was frequently required and deaths have occurred. Available information tends to implicate enteric-coated potassium salts although lesions of this type also occur spontaneously. Therefore, coated potassium-containing formulations should be administered only when indicated, and should be discontinued immediately if abdominal pain, distention, nausea, vomiting, or gastrointestinal bleeding occur. Coated potassium tablets should be used only when adequate dietary supplementation is not practical.
USE IN PREGNANCY: USE OF ANY DRUG IN PREGNANCY, LACTATION, OR IN WOMEN OF CHILDBEARING AGE REQUIRES THAT THE POTENTIAL BENEFITS OF THE DRUG SHOULD BE WEIGHED AGAINST THE POSSIBLE HAZARDS TO THE MOTHER AND CHILD. DIUTENSEN SHOULD BE USED WITH CARE IN PREGNANT AND NURSING MOTHERS SINCE THIAZIDES CROSS THE PLACENTAL BARRIER AND APPEAR IN CORD BLOOD AND BREAST MILK. THIAZIDES MAY RESULT IN FETAL OR NEONATAL JAUNDICE, THROMBOCYTOPENIA, AND POSSIBLY OTHER ADVERSE REACTIONS WHICH HAVE OCCURRED IN THE ADULT.
Thiazides potentiate the action of other antihypertensive drugs. Therefore the dosage of these agents, especially the ganglion blockers, must be reduced by at least 50 percent as soon as thiazides are added to the regimen.
Exacerbation or activation of systemic lupus erythematosus has been reported with sulfonamide derived drugs, including thiazides.
Precautions: Cryptenamine is a potent hypotensive and occasionally bradycrotic drug. Overdosage may produce nausea and vomiting, excessive hypotension and prostration and, rarely, bronchoconstriction. If necessary, atropine sulfate (0.5 to 1.0 mg) may be administered to reverse the bradycrotic effect. In the event of excessive fall in blood pressure, administer vasopressor drugs, such as ephedrine sulfate (30 to 50 mg) or phenylephrine hydrochloride (5 mg) subcutaneously. If

left untended, the reaction will gradually disappear within 60 to 90 minutes.

Particular caution is warranted when treating patients with angina pectoris, coronary thrombosis, or cerebrovascular disease. Caution should also be exercised when treating hypertensive patients with chronic renal disease, since they adjust poorly to lowered blood pressure.

Special caution is warranted when treating patients with histories of bronchial asthma who may respond adversely to the cholinergic effect of cryptenamine.

The bradycrotic effect of veratrum alkaloids is additive to, but not synergistic with, that produced by morphine and related drugs.

Methyclothiazide is a potent saluretic drug. After initiation of therapy, the patient should be seen regularly to determine his individual response to therapy. Ordinarily, a total daily dose of 10 mg (4 DIUTENSEN tablets daily), or less, is not accompanied by significant untoward reactions. However, certain patients may be unusually responsive to the saluretic effect of methyclothiazide and they may experience disturbances in electrolyte balance with subsequent development of hypokalemia. Serum electrolytes should be checked periodically during treatment, particularly in patients receiving relatively large doses of the drug. Patients who are receiving simultaneous treatment either with DIUTENSEN and digitalis or DIUTENSEN and potassium-depleting corticosteroids and those with impending hepatic coma should be carefully watched for signs and symptoms of disturbances in serum electrolyte balance. In the event evidence of electrolyte imbalance with hypokalemia is seen, it may be necessary to give supplemental potassium therapy in the form of fruit juices or direct potassium supplements of one gram, two to four times daily. In severe cases not responding to supplemental potassium therapy, it may be necessary to withdraw the drug.

Hypochloremic alkalosis occurs infrequently with methyclothiazide. Nevertheless, it is a possibility and if this condition develops, it may be treated by the addition of ammonium chloride to the dosage schedule. However, ammonium chloride should not be administered concurrently with a thiazide compound to patients with liver disease because each may cause an elevation in serum ammonia and precipitate onset of coma.

Some elevation of the blood urea nitrogen has been noted occasionally in patients receiving methyclothiazide. This reaction occurs more frequently in patients with decreased renal function. If serum nitrogen (BUN, NPN, creatinine) increases progressively, thiazide therapy should be discontinued.

As with other thiazide diuretics, hyperglycemia has been noted during treatment with methyclothiazide. If a significant elevation in blood sugar is noted, the drug should be withdrawn.

As with thiazides in general, serum uric acid has been observed to rise in a few patients treated with methyclothiazide, with overt symptoms of gout appearing in some of these. Symptoms of gout are readily controlled by treatment with colchicine.

Because some patients receiving veratrum alkaloids have experienced marked hypotension when undergoing surgical procedures, it may be advisable to discontinue treatment with DIUTENSEN for a period of approximately two weeks prior to elective surgery. Thiazide drugs may increase the responsiveness of patients to tubocurarine. Thiazides may decrease arterial responsiveness to norepinephrine and therefore should be withdrawn 48 hours before elective surgery. If emergency surgery is indicated, preanesthetic and anesthetic agents should be administered in reduced dosage. Emergency surgery may be carried out with the use, if necessary, of anticholinergic or adrenergic drugs to prevent vagal circulatory responses and of other supportive measures, as indicated.

Thiazides may decrease serum protein bound iodine levels without signs of thyroid disturbance. The antihypertensive effects of these drugs may be enhanced in the post-sympathectomy patient.

The concurrent use of DIUTENSEN with digitalis may increase the possibility of digitalis intoxication (due chiefly to the saluretic effects of methyclothiazide and perhaps to the vagotonic effects of cryptenamine). If there is evidence of myocardial irritability (extrasystoles, bigeminy, or AV block) dosage of DIUTENSEN should be reduced or discontinued.

Adverse Reactions: *Thiazides*—Varied reactions have been noted in patients treated with thiazides as follows:
Gastrointestinal: Anorexia, gastric irritation, nausea, vomiting, cramping, diarrhea, constipation, jaundice (intrahepatic cholestatic) and pancreatitis.
Central nervous system: Vertigo, paresthesia, headache and xanthopsia.
Dermatologic-hypersensitivity: Skin rash, photosensitivity, urticaria and cutaneous vasculitis.
Hematologic: Purpura, thrombocytopenia, leukopenia, agranulocytosis and aplastic anemia.
In addition, orthostatic hypotension (aggravated when thiazides were administered in combination with either alcohol, barbiturates or narcotics), hyperglycemia, glycosuria, muscle cramps, dizziness, weakness, and restlessness have been reported.
Cryptenamine—Patients treated with cryptenamine have experienced a variety of reactions as follows: excessive hypotension, prostration, anorexia, nausea and vomiting, epigastric and substernal burning, which may be mistaken for angina pectoris, unpleasant taste, salivation, sweating, hiccough, blurring of vision, mental confusion, cardiac arrhythmias, bradycardia, and, with excessive doses, bronchiolar constriction and respiratory depression.
When adverse reactions occur during treatment with DIUTENSEN, they are usually reversible and disappear when treatment is discontinued.

Dosage and Administration: As determined by individual titration (see box warning). The usual adult dosage of DIUTENSEN is one to four tablets a day depending on the individual patient response.

How Supplied: NDC 0037-0272-92, bottle of 100. NDC 0037-0272-96, bottle of 500.

CAUTION: Federal law prohibits dispensing without prescription.

Rev. 1/84

WALLACE LABORATORIES
Division of
CARTER-WALLACE, Inc.
Cranbury, New Jersey 08512

DIUTENSEN®-R ℞
Tablets

Warning: THIS FIXED COMBINATION DRUG IS NOT INDICATED FOR INITIAL THERAPY OF HYPERTENSION. HYPERTENSION REQUIRES THERAPY TITRATED TO THE INDIVIDUAL PATIENT. IF THE FIXED COMBINATION REPRESENTS THE DOSAGE SO DETERMINED, ITS USE MAY BE MORE CONVENIENT IN PATIENT MANAGEMENT. THE TREATMENT OF HYPERTENSION IS NOT STATIC, BUT MUST BE RE-EVALUATED AS CONDITIONS IN EACH PATIENT WARRANT.

Description: DIUTENSEN®-R is a two-component system of active ingredients containing 2.5 mg. methyclothiazide and 0.1 mg. reserpine per tablet. DIUTENSEN-R thus provides for easier titration of hypertensive patients than does a three-component system. DIUTENSEN-R tablets are round, white, pink-mottled tablets.
NOTE: DIUTENSEN-R previously contained cryptenamine tannate as a third antihypertensive agent.

Actions: Methyclothiazide—The predominant effects of methyclothiazide are diuresis, natriuresis, and chloruresis. The mechanism of action results in an interference with the renal tubular mechanism of electrolyte reabsorption. There is significant natriuresis and diuresis within two hours after administration of a single dose of methyclothiazide. These effects reach a peak in about six hours and persist for 24 hours following oral administration of a single dose.

In nonedematous patients the "peak" (maximum effective) natriuretic single dose of methyclothiazide is 10 mg., whereas the peak kaliuretic dose is 5 mg. Thus, doubling a daily dose of 5 mg. results in an increase of sodium output without significantly increasing potassium excretion.
Like other benzothiadiazines, methyclothiazide also has antihypertensive properties. It also may be used to enhance the antihypertensive action of other drugs. The mechanism by which benzothiadiazines, including methyclothiazide, produce a reduction of elevated blood pressure has not been definitely established. Sodium depletion, however, appears to be of primary importance.
Methyclothiazide is readily absorbed from the gastrointestinal tract and is excreted unchanged by the kidneys.
Reserpine—Reserpine is a pure crystalline alkaloid from the root of *Rauwolfia serpentina*. The drug has mild antihypertensive and bradycrotic effects in addition to sedative and tranquilizing properties.
Reserpine probably produces its antihypertensive effects through depletion of tissue stores of catecholamines (epinephrine and norepinephrine) from peripheral sites. By contrast, its sedative and tranquilizing properties are thought to be due to a depletion of 5-hydroxytryptamine from the brain. Reserpine is characterized by slow onset of action and sustained effect. Both its cardiovascular and central nervous system effects may persist following withdrawal of the drug.

Indications: Hypertension (see box warning).

Contraindications: Methyclothiazide—This compound should not be used in anuric patients or those who exhibit a hypersensitivity to this or other sulfonamide derived drugs.
Reserpine—Reserpine is contraindicated in patients with known hypersensitivity, mental depression, especially with suicidal tendencies, active peptic ulcer, and ulcerative colitis. It is also contraindicated in patients receiving electroconvulsive therapy.

Warnings: Methyclothiazide—Thiazides should be used with caution in severe renal disease. In patients with renal disease, thiazides may precipitate azotemia. Cumulative effects of the drug may develop in patients with impaired renal function. Thiazides should be used with caution in patients with impaired hepatic function or progressive liver disease, since minor alterations of fluid and electrolyte balance may precipitate hepatic coma. Thiazides may be additive or potentiate the action of other antihypertensive drugs. Potentiation occurs with ganglionic or peripheral adrenergic blocking drugs.
Sensitivity reactions may occur in patients with a history of allergy or bronchial asthma. The possibility of exacerbation or activation of systemic lupus erythematosus has been reported.
Reserpine—Extreme caution should be exercised in treating patients with a history of mental depression. Discontinue the drug at the first sign of despondency, early morning insomnia, loss of appetite, impotence, or self-deprecation. Drug-induced depression may persist for several months after drug withdrawal and may be severe enough to result in suicide.
Electroshock therapy should not be given to patients under treatment with reserpine since severe and even fatal reactions to such therapy have been reported in patients receiving reserpine. Reserpine should be discontinued for two weeks before electroshock therapy is given.
USE IN PREGNANCY: USE OF ANY DRUG IN PREGNANCY, LACTATION, OR IN WOMEN OF CHILDBEARING AGE REQUIRES THAT THE POTENTIAL BENEFITS OF THE DRUG SHOULD BE WEIGHED AGAINST THE POSSIBLE HAZARDS TO THE MOTHER AND CHILD. DIUTENSEN-R SHOULD BE USED WITH CARE IN PREGNANT AND NURSING MOTHERS SINCE METHYCLOTHIAZIDE AND RESERPINE CROSS THE PLACENTAL BARRIER AND APPEAR IN CORD BLOOD AND BREAST MILK.

Continued on next page

Wallace—Cont.

THE SAFETY OF RESERPINE FOR USE DURING PREGNANCY OR LACTATION HAS NOT BEEN ESTABLISHED. INCREASED RESPIRATORY SECRETIONS, NASAL CONGESTION, CYANOSIS, AND ANOREXIA MAY OCCUR IN INFANTS BORN TO RESERPINE-TREATED MOTHERS.

THIAZIDES MAY RESULT IN FETAL OR NEONATAL JAUNDICE, THROMBOCYTOPENIA, AND POSSIBLE OTHER ADVERSE REACTIONS WHICH HAVE OCCURRED IN THE ADULT.

Precautions: Methyclothiazide—Periodic determinations of serum electrolytes to detect possible electrolyte imbalance should be performed at appropriate intervals.

All patients receiving thiazide therapy should be observed for clinical signs of fluid or electrolyte imbalance; namely, hyponatremia, hypochloremic alkalosis, and hypokalemia. Serum and urine electrolyte determinations are particularly important when the patient is vomiting excessively or receiving parenteral fluids. Medication such as digitalis may also influence serum electrolytes. Warning signs, irrespective of cause, are: Dryness of mouth, thirst, weakness, lethargy, drowsiness, restlessness, muscle pains or cramps, muscular fatigue, hypotension, oliguria, tachycardia, and gastrointestinal disturbances such as nausea and vomiting.

Hypokalemia may develop with thiazides as with any other potent diuretic, especially with brisk diuresis, when severe cirrhosis is present, or during concomitant use of corticosteroids or ACTH. Interference with adequate oral electrolyte intake will also contribute to hypokalemia. Digitalis therapy may exaggerate metabolic effects of hypokalemia especially with reference to myocardial activity.

Any chloride deficit is generally mild and usually does not require specific treatment except under extraordinary circumstances (as in liver disease or renal disease). Dilutional hyponatremia may occur in edematous patients in hot weather; appropriate therapy is water restriction, rather than administration of salt except in rare instances when the hyponatremia is life threatening. In actual salt depletion, appropriate replacement is the therapy of choice.

Hyperuricemia may occur or frank gout may be precipitated in certain patients receiving thiazide therapy.

Insulin requirements in diabetic patients may be increased, decreased, or unchanged. Latent diabetes mellitus may become manifest during thiazide administration.

Thiazide drugs may increase the responsiveness of tubocurarine.

The antihypertensive effects of the drug may be enhanced in the postsympathectomy patient.

Thiazides may decrease arterial responsiveness to norepinephrine. This diminution is not sufficient to preclude effectiveness of the pressor agent for therapeutic use.

If progressive renal impairment becomes evident, as indicated by a rising non-protein nitrogen or blood urea nitrogen, a careful reappraisal of therapy is necessary with consideration given to withholding or discontinuing diuretic therapy.

Thiazides may decrease serum PBI levels without signs of thyroid disturbance.

Reserpine—Because reserpine preparations increase gastrointestinal motility and secretion, this drug should be used cautiously in patients with a history of peptic ulcer, ulcerative colitis, or gallstones, where biliary colic may be precipitated.

Caution should be exercised when treating hypertensive patients with renal insufficiency since they adjust poorly to lowered blood pressure levels.

Use reserpine cautiously with digitalis and quinidine since cardiac arrhythmias have occurred with the concurrent use of rauwolfia preparations.

Preoperative withdrawal of reserpine does not assure that circulatory instability will not occur. It is important that the anesthesiologist be aware of the patient's drug intake and consider this in the overall management, since hypotension has occurred in patients receiving rauwolfia preparations. Anticholinergic and/or adrenergic drugs (metaraminol, norepinephrine) have been employed to treat adverse vagocirculatory effects.

Animal tumorigenicity: Rodent studies have shown that reserpine is an animal turmorigen, causing an increased incidence of mammary fibroadenomas in female mice, malignant tumors of the seminal vesicles in male mice, and malignant adrenal medullary tumors in male rats. These findings arose in 2 year studies in which the drug was administered in the feed at concentrations of 5 and 10 ppm—about 100 to 300 times the usual human dose. The breast neoplasms are thought to be related to reserpine's prolactin-elevating effect. Several other prolactin-elevating drugs have also been associated with an increased incidence of mammary neoplasia in rodents.

The extent to which these findings indicate a risk to humans is uncertain. Tissue culture experiments show that about one-third of human breast tumors are prolactin-dependent in vitro, a factor of considerable importance if the use of the drug is contemplated in a patient with previously detected breast cancer. The possibility of an increased risk of breast cancer in reserpine users has been studied extensively; however, no firm conclusion has emerged. Although a few epidemiologic studies have suggested a slightly increased risk (less than twofold in all studies except one) in women who have used reserpine, other studies of generally similar design have not confirmed this. Epidemiologic studies conducted using other drugs (neuroleptic agents) that, like reserpine, increase prolactin levels and therefore would be considered rodent mammary carcinogens, have not shown an association between chronic administration of the drug and human mammary tumorigenesis. While long-term clinical observation has not suggested such an association, the available evidence is considered too limited to be conclusive at this time. An association of reserpine intake with pheochromocytoma or tumors of the seminal vesicles has not been explored.

Adverse Reactions: Methyclothiazide—The following adverse reactions have been associated with the use of thiazide diuretics.

Gastrointestinal: Anorexia, gastric irritation, nausea, vomiting, cramping, diarrhea, constipation, jaundice (intrahepatic cholestatic jaundice), pancreatitis.

Central nervous system: Dizziness, vertigo, paresthesia, headache, xanthopsia.

Dermatologic-Hypersensitivity: Purpura, photosensitivity, rash, urticaria, necrotizing angiitis (vasculitis) (cutaneous vasculitis).

Hematologic: Leukopenia, agranulocytosis, thrombocytopenia, aplastic anemia.

Cardiovascular: Orthostatic hypotension may occur and may be aggravated by alcohol, barbiturates or narcotics.

Miscellaneous: Hyperglycemia, glycosuria, hyperuricemia, muscle spasm, weakness, restlessness.

Reserpine—Reserpine preparations have caused gastrointestinal reactions including hypersecretion, nausea and vomiting, anorexia, and diarrhea; cardiovascular reactions including angina-like symptoms, arrhythmias particularly when used concurrently with digitalis or quinidine, and bradycardia; and central nervous system reactions including drowsiness, depression, nervousness, paradoxical anxiety, nightmares, rare parkinsonian syndrome, CNS sensitization manifested by dull sensorium, deafness, glaucoma, uveitis, and optic atrophy. Nasal congestion is a frequent complaint, and pruritus, rash, dryness of mouth, dizziness, headache, dyspnea, purpura, impotence or decreased libido, dysuria, muscular aches, conjunctival injection, and weight gain have been reported. Extrapyramidal tract symptoms have also occurred. These reactions are usually reversible and disappear when the drug is discontinued.

Whenever DIUTENSEN-R therapy results in adverse reactions which are moderate or severe, dosage should be reduced or therapy withdrawn.

Dosage and Administration: As determined by individual titration (see box warning). The usual adult dosage of DIUTENSEN-R is 1 to 4 tablets a day depending on the individual patient response.

How Supplied:
NDC 0037-0274-92, bottle of 100
NDC 0037-0274-96, bottle of 500

Caution: Federal law prohibits dispensing without prescription.

Rev. 5/83
Shown in Product Identification Section, page 442

LUFYLLIN® ℞
(dyphylline)
Elixir

Description: LUFYLLIN (dyphylline) Elixir is a bronchodilator available for oral administration as a clear red liquid. Each 15 ml (one tablespoonful) contains dyphylline, 100 mg, and alcohol, 20% (by volume).

Chemically, dyphylline is 7-(2,3-dihydroxypropyl)-theophylline, a white, extremely bitter, amorphous powder that is freely soluble in water and soluble in alcohol to the extent of 2 g/100 ml. Dyphylline forms a neutral solution that is stable in gastrointestinal fluids over a wide range of pH. The molecular formula for dyphylline is $C_{10}H_{14}N_4O_4$ with a molecular weight of 254.25.

Clinical Pharmacology: Dyphylline is a xanthine derivative with pharmacologic actions similar to theophylline and other members of this class of drugs. Its primary action is that of bronchodilation, but it also exhibits peripheral vasodilatory and other smooth muscle relaxant activity to a lesser degree. The bronchodilatory action of dyphylline, as with other xanthines, is thought to be mediated through competitive inhibition of phosphodiesterase with a resulting increase in cyclic AMP producing relaxation of bronchial smooth muscle.

Dyphylline is well tolerated and produces less nausea than aminophylline and other alkaline theophylline compounds when administered orally. Unlike the hydrolyzable salts of theophylline, dyphylline is not converted to free theophylline *in vivo*. It is absorbed rapidly in therapeutically active form and in healthy volunteers reaches a mean peak plasma concentration of 17.1 mcg/ml in approximately 45 minutes following a single oral dose of 1000 mg.

Dyphylline exerts its bronchodilatory effects directly and, unlike theophylline, is excreted unchanged by the kidneys without being metabolized by the liver. Because of this, dyphylline pharmacokinetics and plasma levels are not influenced by various factors that affect liver function and hepatic enzyme activity, such as smoking, age, congestive heart failure or concomitant use of drugs which effect liver function.

The elimination half-life of dyphylline is approximately two hours (1.8–2.1 hr) and approximately 88% of a single oral dose can be recovered from the urine unchanged. The renal clearance would be correspondingly reduced in patients with impaired renal function. In anuric patients, the half-life may be increased 3 to 4 times normal.

Dyphylline plasma levels are dose-related and generally predictable. The range of plasma levels within which dyphylline can be expected to produce effective bronchodilation has not been determined.

Dyphylline plasma concentrations can be accurately determined using high pressure liquid chromatography (HPLC)* or gas-liquid chromatography (GLC).

* *See Valia, et al, J Chromatogr 221:170 (1980). Small quantities of pure dyphylline powder may be obtained from Wallace Laboratories, Cranbury, N.J. The internal standard, β-hydroxyethyltheophylline may be obtained from companies supplying analytic chemicals.*

Indications and Usage: For relief of acute bronchial asthma and for reversible bronchospasm

associated with chronic bronchitis and emphysema.
Contraindications: Hypersensitivity to dyphylline or related xanthine compounds.
Warnings: LUFYLLIN Elixir is not indicated in the management of status asthmaticus which is a serious medical emergency.
Although the relationship between plasma levels of dyphylline and appearance of toxicity is unknown, excessive doses may be expected to be associated with an increased risk of adverse effects.
Precautions:
General: Use LUFYLLIN Elixir with caution in patients with severe cardiac disease, hypertension, hyperthyroidism, or acute myocardial injury or peptic ulcer.
Drug interactions: Synergism betwen xanthine bronchodilators (e.g., theophylline), ephedrine and other sympathomimetic bronchodilators has been reported. This should be considered whenever these agents are prescribed concomitantly.
Concurrent administration of dyphylline and probenecid, which competes for tubular secretion, has been shown to increase the plasma half-life of dyphylline (see CLINICAL PHARMACOLOGY).
Carcinogenesis, mutagenesis, impairment of fertility: No long-term animal studies have been performed with LUFYLLIN Elixir.
Pregnancy: Teratogenic effects—Pregnancy category C. Animal reproduction studies have not been conducted with LUFYLLIN Elixir. It is also not known if 'Lufyllin' Elixir can cause fetal harm when administered to a pregnant woman or can affect reproduction capacity. LUFYLLIN Elixir should be given to a pregnant woman only if clearly needed.
Nursing mothers: Dyphylline is present in human milk at approximately twice the maternal plasma concentration. Caution should be exercised when 'Lufyllin' Elixir is administered to a nursing woman.
Pediatric use: Safety and effectiveness in children have not been established.
Adverse Reactions: Adverse reactions with the use of LUFYLLIN Elixir have been infrequent, relatively mild, and rarely required reduction in dosage or withdrawal of therapy.
The following adverse reactions which have been reported with other xanthine bronchodilators, and which have most often been related to excessive drug plasma levels, should be considered as potential adverse effects when dyphylline is administered:
Gastrointestinal: nausea, vomiting, epigastric pain, hematemesis, diarrhea.
Central nervous system: headache, irritability, restlessness, insomnia, hyperexcitability, agitation, muscle twitching, generalized clonic and tonic convulsions.
Cardiovascular: palpitation, tachycardia, extrasystoles, flushing, hypotension, circulatory failure, ventricular arrhythmias.
Respiratory: tachypnea.
Renal: albuminuria, gross and microscopic hematuria, diuresis.
Others: hyperglycemia, inappropriate ADH syndrome.
Overdosage: There have been no reports, in the literature, of overdosage with LUFYLLIN Elixir. However, the following information based on reports of theophylline overdosage are considered typical of the xanthine class of drugs and should be kept in mind.
Signs and symptoms: Restlessness, anorexia, nausea, vomiting, diarrhea, insomnia, irritability, and headache. Marked overdosage with resulting severe toxicity has produced agitation, severe vomiting, dehydration, excessive thirst, tinnitus, cardiac arrhythmias, hyperthermia, diaphoresis, and generalized clonic and tonic convulsions. Cardiovascular collapse has also occurred, with some fatalities. Seizures have occured in some cases associated with very high theophylline plasma concentrations, without any premonitory symptoms of toxicity.
Treatment: There is no specific antidote for overdosage with drugs of the xanthine class. Symptomatic treatment and general supportive measures should be instituted with careful monitoring and maintenance of vital signs, fluids and electrolytes. The stomach should be emptied by inducing emesis if the patient is conscious and responsive, or by gastric lavage, taking care to protect against aspiration, especially in stuporous or comatose patients. Maintenance of an adequate airway is essential in case oxygen or assisted respiration is needed. Symptomatic agents should be avoided but sedatives such as short-acting barbiturates may be useful.
Dyphylline is dialyzable and, although not recommended as a routine procedure in overdosage cases, hemodialysis may be of some benefit when severe intoxication is present or when the patient has not responded to general supportive and symptomatic treatment.
Dosage and Administration: Dosage should be individually titrated according to the severity of the condition and the response of the patient.
Usual adult dosage: 2 to 4 tablespoonfuls every six hours.
Appropriate dosage adjustments should be made in patients with impaired renal function (see CLINICAL PHARMACOLOGY).
How Supplied:
LUFYLLIN Elixir:
 NDC 0037-0515-68, pint bottle.
 NDC 0037-0515-69, gallon bottle.
Storage: Store below 30°C (86°F).
CAUTION: Federal law prohibits dispensing without prescription.
Rev. 4/83

LUFYLLIN® ℞
(dyphylline)
Injection
FOR INTRAMUSCULAR USE ONLY

Description: Chemically, dyphylline is 7-(2,3-dihydroxypropyl)-theophylline, a white, extremely bitter, amorphous powder that is freely soluble in water and alcohol to the extent of 2 g/100 ml.
LUFYLLIN Injection is a clear, colorless, sterile solution of dyphylline, a xanthine derivative available as a bronchodilator *for intramuscular use only*.
Each ml of LUFYLLIN Injection contains 250 mg of dyphylline (pH adjusted with sodium hydroxide and/or hydrochloric acid).
The molecular formula for dyphylline is $C_{10}H_{14}N_4O_4$ with a molecular weight of 254.25.
Clinical Pharmacology: Dyphylline is a xanthine derivative with pharmacologic actions similar to theophylline and other members of this class of drugs. Its primary action is that of bronchodilation, but it also exhibits peripheral vasodilatory and other smooth muscle relaxant activity to a lesser degree. The bronchodilatory action of dyphylline, as with other xanthines, is thought to be mediated through competitive inhibition of phosphodiesterase with a resulting increase in cyclic AMP producing relaxation of bronchial smooth muscle.
LUFYLLIN Injection is well tolerated and causes little or no discomfort, by the intramuscular route, and produces less nausea than aminophylline and other alkaline theophylline compounds. Unlike the hydrolyzable salts of theophylline, dyphylline is not converted to free theophylline *in vivo*. It is absorbed rapidly in therapeutically active form and in healthy volunteers reaches a mean peak plasma concentration comparable to that achieved with equivalent oral doses in approximately 45 minutes (17.1 mg following a single oral dose of 1000 mg).
Dyphylline exerts it bronchodilatory effects directly and, unlike theophylline, is excreted unchanged by the kidneys without being metabolized by the liver. Because of this, dyphylline pharmacokinetics and plasma levels are not influenced by various factors that affect liver function and hepatic enzyme activity, such as smoking, age, congestive heart failure or concomitant use of drugs which effect liver function. The renal clearance would be correspondingly reduced in patients with impaired renal function. In anuric patients, the half-life may be increased 3 to 4 times normal.
The range of plasma levels within which dyphylline can be expected to produce effective bronchodilation has not been determined.
Dyphylline plasma concentrations can be accurately determined using high pressure liquid chromatography (HPLC)* or gas-liquid chromatography (GLC).
* *See Valia, et al: J. Chromatogr.* **221**:170 (1980). Small quantities of pure dyphylline powder may be obtained from Wallace Laboratories, Cranbury, N.J. The internal standard, β-hydroxyethyltheophylline, may be obtained from companies supplying analytical chemicals.
Indications and Usage: For relief of acute bronchial asthma and for reversible bronchospasm associated with chronic bronchitis and emphysema.
Contraindications: Hypersensitivity to dyphylline or related xanthine compounds.
Warnings: LUFYLLIN Injection is not indicated in the management of status asthmaticus or apnea in the newborn, which are serious medical emergencies.
Although the relationship between plasma levels of dyphylline and appearance of toxicity is unknown, excessive doses may be expected to be associated with an increased risk of adverse effects.
Precautions: General: Use LUFYLLIN Injection with caution in patients with severe cardiac disease, hypertension, hyperthyroidism, acute myocardial injury or peptic ulcer.
Drug interactions: Synergism between xanthine bronchodilators (e.g., theophylline), ephedrine and other sympathomimetic bronchodilators has been reported. This should be considered whenever these agents are prescribed concomitantly.
Concurrent administration of dyphylline and probenecid, which competes for tubular secretion, has been shown to increase the plasma half-life of dyphylline (see CLINICAL PHARMACOLOGY).
Carcinogenesis, mutagenesis, impairment of fertility: No long-term animal studies have been performed with LUFYLLIN Injection.
Pregnancy: Teratogenic effects—Pregnancy Category C. Animal reproduction studies have not been conducted with LUFYLLIN Injection. It is also not known if LUFYLLIN Injection can cause fetal harm when administered to a pregnant woman or can affect reproduction capacity. LUFYLLIN Injection should be given to a pregnant woman only if clearly needed.
Nursing mothers: Dyphylline is present in human milk at approximately twice the maternal plasma concentration. Caution should be exercised when LUFYLLIN Injection is administered to a nursing woman.
Pediatric use: Safety and effectiveness in children have not been established.
Adverse Reactions: Adverse reactions with the use of LUFYLLIN Injection have been infrequent, relatively mild, and rarely required reduction in dosage or withdrawal of therapy.
The following adverse reactions which have been reported with other xanthine bronchodilators, and which have most often been related to excessive drug plasma levels, should be considered as potential adverse effects when dyphylline is administered:
Gastrointestinal: nausea, vomiting, epigastric pain, hematemesis, diarrhea.
Central nervous system: headache, irritability, restlessness, insomnia, hyperexcitability, agitation, muscle twitching, generalized clonic and tonic convulsions.
Cardiovascular: palpitation, tachycardia, extrasystoles, flushing, hypotension, circulatory failure, ventricular arrhythmias.
Respiratory: tachypnea.
Renal: albuminuria, gross and microscopic hematuria, diuresis.
Other: hyperglycemia, inappropriate ADH syndrome.

Continued on next page

Wallace—Cont.

Overdosage: There have been no reports, in the literature, of overdosage with LUFYLLIN Injection. However, the following information based on reports of theophylline overdosage are considered typical of the xanthine class of drugs and should be kept in mind.

Signs and symptoms: Restlessness, anorexia, nausea, vomiting, diarrhea, insomnia, irritability, and headache. Marked overdosage with resulting severe toxicity has produced agitation, severe vomiting, dehydration, excessive thirst, tinnitus, cardiac arrhythmias, hyperthermia, diaphoresis, and generalized clonic and tonic convulsions. Cardiovascular collapse has also occurred, with some fatalities. Seizures have occurred, in some cases associated with very high theophylline plasma concentrations, without any premonitory symptoms of toxicity.

Treatment: There is no specific antidote for overdosage with drugs of the xanthine class. Symptomatic treatment and general supportive measures should be instituted with careful monitoring and maintenance of vital signs, fluids and electrolytes. The stomach should be emptied by inducing emesis if the patient is conscious and responsive, or by gastric lavage, taking care to protect against aspiration, especially in stuporous or comatose patients. Maintenance of an adequate airway is essential in case oxygen or assisted respiration is needed. Sympathomimetic agents should be avoided but sedatives such as short-acting barbiturates may be useful.

Dyphylline is dialyzable and, although not recommended as a routine procedure in overdosage cases, hemodialysis may be of some benefit when severe intoxication is present or when the patient has not responded to general supportive and symptomatic treatment.

Dosage and Administration: LUFYLLIN Injection is *for intramuscular use only.*

Usual adult dosage: 500 mg (2 ml) I.M. initially, followed by 250-500 mg (1 to 2 ml) every two to six hours, as indicated by the patient's response. Do not exceed total dosage of 15 mg/kg every six hours.

How Supplied: Box of 25 × 2 ml ampuls (NDC 0037-0537-01).

Storage: Store below 40°C (104°F), preferably between 15° and 30°C (59° to 86°F). Excessive cold may cause formation of a precipitate. DO NOT USE if preciptiate is present.

CAUTION: Federal law prohibits dispensing without prescription.

Distributed by
WALLACE LABORATORIES
Division of
CARTER-WALLACE, INC.
Cranbury, New Jersey 08512

Manufactured by:
Taylor Pharmacal Co.
Decatur, Illinois 62526

Rev. 4/83

Shown in Product Identification Section, page 442

LUFYLLIN® R
LUFYLLIN®-400 R
(dyphylline)
Tablets

Description: LUFYLLIN (dyphylline), a xanthine derivative, is a bronchodilator available for oral administration as tablets containing 200 mg and 400 mg of dyphylline.

Chemically, dyphylline is 7-(2,3-dihydroxypropyl)-theophylline, a white, extremely bitter, amorphous powder that is freely soluble in water and soluble in alcohol to the extent of 2 g/100 ml. Dyphylline forms a neutral solution that is stable in gastrointestinal fluids over a wide range of pH. The molecular formula for dyphylline is $C_{10}H_{14}N_4O_4$ with a molecular weight of 254.25.

Clinical Pharmacology: Dyphylline is a xanthine derivative with pharmacologic actions similar to theophylline and other members of this class of drugs. Its primary action is that of bronchodilation, but it also exhibits peripheral vasodilatory and other smooth muscle relaxant activity to a lesser degree. The bronchodilatory action of dyphylline, as with other xanthines, is thought to be mediated through competitive inhibition of phosphodiesterase with a resulting increase in cyclic AMP producing relaxation of bronchial smooth muscle.

LUFYLLIN is well tolerated and produces less nausea than aminophylline and other alkaline theophylline compounds when administered orally. Unlike the hydrolyzable salts of theophylline, dyphylline is not converted to free theophylline *in vivo.* It is absorbed rapidly in therapeutically active form and in healthy volunteers reaches a mean peak plasma concentration of 17.1 mcg/ml in approximately 45 minutes following a single oral dose of 1000 mg of LUFYLLIN.

Dyphylline exerts its bronchodilatory effects directly and, unlike theophylline, is excreted unchanged by the kidneys without being metabolized by the liver. Because of this, dyphylline pharmacokinetics and plasma levels are not influenced by various factors that affect liver function and hepatic enzyme activity, such as smoking, age, congestive heart failure or concomitant use of drugs which affect liver function.

The elimination half-life of dyphylline is approximately two hours (1.8-2.1 hr) and approximately 88% of a single oral dose can be recovered from the urine unchanged. The renal clearance would be correspondingly reduced in patients with impaired renal function. In anuric patients, the half-life may be increased 3 to 4 times normal.

Dyphylline plasma levels are dose-related and generally predictable. The range of plasma levels within which dyphylline can be expected to produce effective bronchodilation has not been determined.

Dyphylline plasma concentrations can be accurately determined using high pressure liquid chromatography (HPLC)* or gas-liquid chromatography (GLC).

* *See* Valia, et al, *J. Chromatogr.* **221**:170 (1980). Small quantities of pure dyphylline powder may be obtained from Wallace Laboratories, Cranbury, N.J. The internal standard, β-hydroxyethyltheophylline, may be obtained from companies supplying analytical chemicals.

Indications and Usage: For relief of acute bronchial asthma and for reversible bronchospasm associated with chronic bronchitits and emphysema.

Contraindications: Hypersensitivity to dyphylline or related xanthine compounds.

Warnings: LUFYLLIN is not indicated in the management of status asthmaticus, which is a serious medical emergency.

Although the relationship between plasma levels of dyphylline and appearance of toxicity is unknown, excessive doses may be expected to be associated with an increased risk of adverse effects.

Precautions: General: Use LUFYLLIN with caution in patients with severe cardiac disease, hypertension, hyperthyroidism, acute myocardial injury or peptic ulcer.

Drug interactions: Synergism between xanthine bronchodilators (e.g., theophylline), ephedrine and other sympathomimetic bronchodilators has been reported. This should be considered whenever these agents are prescribed concomitantly.

Concurrent administration of dyphylline and probenecid, which competes for tubular secretion, has been shown to increase the plasma half-life of dyphylline (see CLINICAL PHARMACOLOGY).

Carcinogenesis, mutagenesis, impairment of fertility: No long-term animal studies have been performed with LUFYLLIN.

Pregnancy: Teratogenic effects—Pregnancy Category C. Animal reproduction studies have not been conducted with LUFYLLIN. It is also not known if LUFYLLIN can cause fetal harm when administered to a pregnant woman or can affect reproduction capacity. LUFYLLIN should be given to a pregnant woman only if clearly needed.

Nursing mothers: Dyphylline is present in human milk at approximately twice the maternal plasma concentration. Caution should be exercised when LUFYLLIN is administered to a nursing woman.

Pediatric use: Safety and effectiveness in children have not been established.

Adverse Reactions: Adverse reactions with the use of LUFYLLIN have been infrequent, relatively mild, and rarely required reduction in dosage or withdrawal of therapy.

The following adverse reactions which have been reported with other xanthine bronchodilators, and which have most often been related to excessive drug plasma levels, should be considered as potential adverse effects when dyphylline is administered:

Gastrointestinal: nausea, vomiting, epigastric pain, hematemesis, diarrhea.

Central nervous system: headache, irritability, restlessness, insomnia, hyperexcitability, agitation, muscle twitching, generalized clonic and tonic convulsions.

Cardiovascular: palpitation, tachycardia, extrasystoles, flushing, hypotension, circulatory failure, ventricular arrhythmias.

Respiratory: tachypnea.

Renal: albuminuria, gross and microscopic hematuria, diuresis.

Other: hyperglycemia, inappropriate ADH syndrome.

Overdosage: There have been no reports, in the literature, of overdosage with LUFYLLIN. However, the following information based on reports of theophylline overdosage are considered typical of the xanthine class of drugs and should be kept in mind.

Signs and symptoms: Restlessness, anorexia, nausea, vomiting, diarrhea, insomnia, irritability, and headache. Marked overdosage with resulting severe toxicity has produced agitation, severe vomiting, dehydration, excessive thirst, tinnitus, cardiac arrhythmias, hyperthermia, diaphoresis, and generalized clonic and tonic convulsions. Cardiovascular collapse has also occcurred, with some fatalities. Seizures have occurred in some cases associated with very high theophylline plasma concentrations, without any premonitory symptoms of toxicity.

Treatment: There is no specific antidote for overdosage with drugs of the xanthine class. Symptomatic treatment and general supportive measures should be instituted with careful monitoring and maintenance of vital signs, fluid and electrolytes. The stomach should be emptied by inducing emesis if the patient is conscious and responsive, or by gastric lavage, taking care to protect against aspiration, especially in stuporous or comatose patients. Maintenance of an adequate airway is essential in case oxygen or assisted respiration is needed. Sympathomimetic agents should be avoided but sedatives such as short-acting barbiturates may be useful.

Dyphylline is dialyzable and, although not recommended as a routine procedure in overdosage cases, hemodialysis may be of some benefit when severe intoxication is present or when the patient has not responded to general supportive and symptomatic treatment.

Dosage and Administration: Dosage should be individually titrated according to the severity of the condition and the response of the patient.

Usual adult dosage: Up to 15 mg/kg every six hours.

Appropriate dosage adjustments should be made in patients with impaired renal function (see CLINICAL PHARMACOLOGY).

How Supplied:

LUFYLLIN Tablets: Available as white, rectangular, monogrammed tablets containing 200 mg dyphylline in bottles of 100 (NDC 0037-0521-92) and 1000 (NDC 0037-0521-97), and individually film-sealed tablets in unit-dose boxes of 100 (NDC 0037-0521-85).

LUFYLLIN-400 Tablets: Available as white, capsule-shaped, monogrammed tablets containing 400 mg dyphylline in bottles of 100 (NDC 0037-0731-92) and 1000 (NDC 0037-0731-97), and individually film-sealed tablets in unit-dose boxes of 100 (NDC 0037-0731-85).

LUFYLLIN®–GG
Tablets and Elixir

Description: LUFYLLIN®-GG is a bronchodilator/expectorant combination available for oral administration as *Tablets* and *Elixir*.
Each Tablet contains:
Dyphylline .... 200 mg
Guaifenesin .... 200 mg
Each 15 ml (one tablespoonful) of Elixir contains:
Dyphylline .... 100 mg
Guaifenesin .... 100 mg
Alcohol (by volume) 17%
Dyphylline is 7-(2,3-dihydroxypropyl)-theophylline, a white, extremely bitter, amorphous powder that is fully soluble in water and soluble in alcohol to the extent of 2 g/100 ml. Dyphylline forms a neutral solution that is stable in gastrointestinal fluids over a wide range of pH.

Clinical Pharmacology: Dyphylline is a xanthine derivative with pharmacologic actions similar to theophylline and other members of this class of drugs. Its primary action is that of bronchodilation, but it also exhibits peripheral vasodilatory and other smooth muscle relaxant activity to a lesser degree. The bronchodilatory action of dyphylline, as well as other xanthines, is thought to be mediated through competitive inhibition of phosphodiesterase with a resulting increase in cyclic AMP producing relaxation of bronchial smooth muscle.
Dyphylline in LUFYLLIN-GG is well tolerated and produces less nausea than aminophylline and other alkaline theophylline compounds when administered orally. Unlike the hydrolyzable salts of theophylline, dyphylline is not converted to free theophylline *in vivo*. It is absorbed rapidly in therapeutically active form and in healthy volunteers reaches a mean peak plasma concentration of 17.1 mcg/ml in approximately 45 minutes following a single oral dose of 1000 mg of dyphylline.
Dyphylline exerts its bronchodilatory effects directly and, unlike theophylline, is excreted unchanged by the kidneys without being metabolized by the liver. Because of this, dyphylline pharmacokinetics and plasma levels are not influenced by various factors that affect liver function and hepatic enzyme activity, such as smoking, age, or concomitant use of drugs which affect liver function.
The elimination half-life of dyphylline is approximately two hours (1.8–2.1 hr) and approximately 88% of a single oral dose can be recovered from the urine unchanged. The renal clearance would be correspondingly reduced in patients with impaired renal function. In anuric patients, the half-life may be increased 3 to 4 times normal.
Dyphylline plasma levels are dose-related and generally predictable. The therapeutic range of plasma levels within which dyphylline can be expected to produce effective bronchodilation has not been determined.
Dyphylline plasma concentrations can be accurately determined using high pressure liquid chromatography (HPLC)* or gas-liquid chromatography (GLC).
Guaifenesin is an expectorant whose action helps increase the output of thin respiratory tract fluid to facilitate mucociliary clearance and removal of inspissated mucus.

* *See Valia, et al, J Chromatogr 221:170 (1980). Small quantities of pure dyphylline powder may be obtained from Wallace Laboratories, Cranbury, N.J. The internal standard, β-hydroxyethyltheophylline, may be obtained from companies supplying analytical chemicals.*

Indications and Usage: For relief of acute bronchial asthma and for reversible bronchospasm associated with chronic bronchitis and emphysema.

Contraindications: Hypersensitivity to any of the ingredients or related compounds.

Warnings: LUFYLLIN-GG is not indicated in the management of status asthmaticus, which is a serious medical emergency.
Although the relationship between plasma levels of dyphylline and appearance of toxicity is unknown, excessive doses may be expected to be associated with an increased risk of adverse effects.

Precautions:
General: Use LUFYLLIN-GG with caution in patients with severe cardiac disease, hypertension, hyperthyroidism, acute myocardial injury or peptic ulcer.
Drug interactions: Synergism between xanthine bronchodilators (e.g., theophylline), ephedrine and other sympathomimetic bronchodilators has been reported. This should be considered whenever these agents are prescribed concomitantly.
Concurrent administration of dyphylline and probenecid, which competes for tubular secretion, has been shown to increase plasma half-life of dyphylline (see Clinical Pharmacology).
Carcinogenesis, mutagenesis, impairment of fertility: No long-term animal studies have been performed with 'Lufyllin'-GG.
Pregnancy: Teratogenic effects — Pregnancy Category C. Animal reproduction studies have not been conducted with LUFYLLIN-GG. It is also not known whether the product can cause fetal harm when administered to a pregnant woman or can affect reproduction capacity. LUFYLLIN-GG should be given to a pregnant woman only if clearly needed.
Nursing mothers: Dyphylline is present in human milk at approximately twice the maternal plasma concentration. Caution should be exercised when LUFYLLIN-GG is administered to a nursing woman.
Pediatric use: Safety and effectiveness in children below the age of six have not been established. Use caution when administering to children six years of age or older.
Adverse Reactions: LUFYLLIN-GG may cause nausea, headache, cardiac palpitation and CNS stimulation. Postprandial administration may help avoid gastric discomfort.
The following adverse reactions which have been reported with other xanthine bronchodilators, and which have most often been related to excessive drug plasma levels, should be considered as potential adverse effects when dyphylline is administered:
Gastrointestinal: nausea, vomiting, epigastric pain, hematemesis, diarrhea.
Central nervous system: headache, irritability, restlessness, insomnia, hyperexcitability, agitation, muscle twitching, generalized clonic and tonic convulsions.
Cardiovascular: palpitation, tachycardia, extrasystoles, flushing, hypotension, circulatory failure, ventricular arrhythmias.
Respiratory: tachypnea.
Renal: albuminuria, gross and microscopic hematuria, diuresis.
Other: hyperglycemia, inappropriate ADH syndrome.
Overdosage: There have been no reports, in the literature, of overdosage with LUFYLLIN-GG. However, the following information based on reports of theophylline overdosage are considered typical of the xanthine class of drugs and should be kept in mind.
Signs and symptoms: Restlessness, anorexia, nausea, vomiting, diarrhea, insomnia, irritability, and headache. Marked overdosage with resulting severe toxicity has produced agitation, severe vomiting, dehydration, excessive thirst, tinnitus, cardiac arrhythmias, hyperthermia, diaphoresis, and generalized clonic and tonic convulsions. Cardiovascular collapse has also occured, with some fatalities. Seizures have occured in some cases associated with very high theophylline plasma concentrations, without any premonitory symptoms of toxicity.
Treatment: There is no specific antidote for overdosage with drugs of the xanthine class. Symptomatic treatment and general supportive measures should be instituted with careful monitoring and maintenance of vital signs, fluids and electrolytes. The stomach should be emptied by inducing emesis if the patient is conscious and responsive, or by gastric lavage, taking care to protect against aspiration, especially in stuporous or comatose patients. Maintenance of an adequate airway is essential in case oxygen or assisted respiration is needed. Sympathomimetic agents should be avoided but sedatives such as short-acting barbiturates may be useful.
Dyphylline is dialyzable and, although not recommended as a routine procedure in overdosage cases, hemodialysis may be of some benefit when severe intoxication is present or when the patient has not responded to general supportive and symptomatic treatment.

Dosage and Administration: Dosage should be individually titrated according to the severity of the condition and the response of the patient.
Usual adult dosage: 1 tablet or 30 ml (2 tablespoonfuls) Elixir, four times daily.
Children above age six: ½ to 1 tablet or 15 to 30 ml (1 to 2 tablespoonfuls) Elixir, 3 or 4 times daily.
Not recommended for use in children below age 6 (see Precautions).

How Supplied: LUFYLLIN-GG Tablets: round, light yellow, monogrammed tablets, scored on one side, in bottles of 100 (NDC 0037-0541-92) and 1000 (NDC 0037-0541-97) and boxes of 100 unit-dose, individually film-sealed tablets (NDC 0037-0541-85).
LUFYLLIN-GG Elixir: clear, light yellow-orange liquid with a mild wine-like odor and taste, in bottles of one pint (NDC 0037-0545-68) and one gallon (NDC 0037-0545-69).

Storage:
Tablets—Avoid excessive heat; above 40°C (104°F).
Elixir—Store below 30°C (86°F).
CAUTION: Federal law prohibits dispensing without prescription.

WALLACE LABORATORIES
Division of
CARTER-WALLACE, INC.
Cranbury, New Jersey 08512
Issued 12/83
Shown in Product Identification Section, page 442

MALTSUPEX®   OTC
(malt soup extract)
Powder, Liquid, Tablets
(See PDR for Nonprescription Drugs)

MEPROSPAN®
(meprobamate, sustained-release capsules)

Description: Meprobamate is a white powder with a characteristic odor and a bitter taste. It is slightly soluble in water, freely soluble in acetone and alcohol, and sparingly soluble in ether.

Actions: Meprobamate is a carbamate derivative which has been shown in animal studies to have effects at multiple sites in the central nervous system, including the thalamus and limbic system.

Indications: 'Meprospan' (meprobamate) is indicated for the management of anxiety disorders or for the short-term relief of the symptoms of anxiety. Anxiety or tension associated with the stress of everyday life usually do not require treatment with an anxiolytic.
The effectiveness of 'Meprospan' in long-term use, that is, more than 4 months, has not been assessed by systematic clinical studies. The physician should periodically reassess the usefulness of the drug for the individual patient.

Contraindications: Acute intermittent porphyria as well as allergic or idiosyncratic reactions to meprobamate or related compounds such as carisoprodol, mebutamate, tybamate, or carbromal.

Continued on next page

Storage: Avoid excessive heat—above 40°C (104°F).
CAUTION: Federal law prohibits dispensing without prescription.
Rev. 3/83
Shown in Product Identification Section, page 442

Wallace—Cont.

Warnings
Drug Dependence
Physical dependence, psychological dependence, and abuse have occurred. When chronic intoxication from prolonged use occurs, it usually involves ingestion of greater than recommended doses and is manifested by ataxia, slurred speech, and vertigo. Therefore, careful supervision of dose and amounts prescribed is advised, as well as avoidance of prolonged administration, especially for alcoholics and other patients with a known propensity for taking excessive quantities of drugs. Sudden withdrawal of the drug after prolonged and excessive use may precipitate recurrence of pre-existing symptoms, such as anxiety, anorexia, or insomnia, or withdrawal reactions, such as vomiting, ataxia, tremors, muscle twitching, confusional states, hallucinosis, and, rarely, convulsive seizures. Such seizures are more likely to occur in persons with central nervous system damage or pre-existent or latent convulsive disorders. Onset of withdrawal symptoms occurs usually within 12 to 48 hours after discontinuation of meprobamate; symptoms usually cease within the next 12 to 48 hours.

When excessive dosage has continued for weeks or months, dosage should be reduced gradually over a period of one or two weeks rather than abruptly stopped. Alternatively, a short-acting barbiturate may be substituted, then gradually withdrawn.

Potentially Hazardous Tasks
Patients should be warned that this drug may impair the mental and/or physical abilities required for the performance of potentially hazardous tasks such as driving a motor vehicle or operating machinery.

Additive Effects
Since the effects of meprobamate and alcohol or meprobamate and other CNS depressants or psychotropic drugs may be additive, appropriate caution should be exercised with patients who take more than one of these agents simultaneously.

USAGE IN PREGNANCY AND LACTATION
An increased risk of congenital malformations associated with the use of minor tranquilizers (meprobamate, chlordiazepoxide, and diazepam) during the first trimester of pregnancy has been suggested in several studies. Because use of these drugs is rarely a matter of urgency, their use during this period should almost always be avoided. The possibility that a woman of childbearing potential may be pregnant at the time of institution of therapy should be considered.

Patients should be advised that if they become pregnant during therapy or intend to become pregnant they should communicate with their physicians about the desirability of discontinuing the drug.

Meprobamate passes the placental barrier. It is present both in umbilical cord blood at or near maternal plasma levels and in breast milk of lactating mothers at concentrations two or four times that of maternal plasma. When use of meprobamate is contemplated in breast-feeding patients, the drug's higher concentration in breast milk as compared to maternal plasma levels should be considered.

Usage in Children
Meprobamate should not be administered to children under age six, since there is a lack of documented evidence for safety and effectiveness in this age group.

Precautions: The lowest effective dose should be administered, particularly to elderly and/or debilitated patients, in order to preclude oversedation. The possibility of suicide attempts should be considered and the least amount of drug feasible should be dispensed at any one time.

Meprobamate is metabolized in the liver and excreted by the kidney; to avoid its excess accumulation, caution should be exercised in administration to patients with compromised liver or kidney function.

Meprobamate occasionally may precipitate seizures in epileptic patients.

Adverse Reactions
Central Nervous System
Drowsiness, ataxia, dizziness, slurred speech, headache, vertigo, weakness, paresthesias, impairment of visual accommodation, euphoria, overstimulation, paradoxical excitement, fast EEG activity.

Gastrointestinal
Nausea, vomiting, diarrhea.

Cardiovascular
Palpitations, tachycardia, various forms of arrhythmia, transient ECG changes, syncope; also, hypotensive crises (including one fatal case).

Allergic or Idiosyncratic
Allergic or idiosyncratic reactions are usually seen within the period of the first to fourth dose in patients having had no previous contact with the drug. Milder reactions are characterized by an itchy, urticarial, or erythematous maculopapular rash which may be generalized or confined to the groin. Other reactions have included leukopenia, acute nonthrombocytopenic purpura, petechiae, ecchymoses, eosinophilia, peripheral edema, adenopathy, fever, fixed drug eruption with cross reaction to carisoprodol, and cross sensitivity between meprobamate/mebutamate and meprobamate/carbromal.

More severe hypersensitivity reactions, rarely reported, include hyperpyrexia, chills, angioneurotic edema, bronchospasm, oliguria, and anuria. Also, anaphylaxis, erythema multiforme, exfoliative dermatitis, stomatitis, proctitis, Stevens-Johnson syndrome, and bullous dermatitis, including one fatal case of the latter following administration of meprobamate in combination with prednisolone.

In case of allergic or idiosyncratic reactions to meprobamate, discontinue the drug and initiate appropriate symptomatic therapy, which may include epinephrine, antihistamines, and in severe cases corticosteroids. In evaluating possible allergic reactions, also consider allergy to excipients (information on excipients is available to physicians on request).

Hematologic
(See also **Allergic or Idiosyncratic.**) Agranulocytosis and aplastic anemia have been reported, although no causal relationship has been established. These cases rarely were fatal. Rare cases of thrombocytopenic purpura have been reported.

Other
Exacerbation of porphyric symptoms.

Dosage and Administration: The usual adult dosage of 'Meprospan' (meprobamate, sustained-release capsules) is one to two 400 mg capsules in the morning and again at bedtime; doses above 2400 mg daily are not recommended. The usual dosage for children ages six to twelve is one 200 mg capsule in the morning and again at bedtime. Meprobamate is not recommended for children under age six.

Overdosage: Suicidal attempts with meprobamate have resulted in drowsiness, lethargy, stupor, ataxia, coma, shock, vasomotor and respiratory collapse. Some suicidal attempts have been fatal. Overdosage experience with 'Meprospan' (meprobamate, sustained-release capsules) is limited. However, the following data on meprobamate tablets have been reported in the literature and from other sources. These data are not expected to correlate with each case (considering factors such as individual susceptibility and length of time from ingestion to treatment), but represent the *usual ranges* reported.

Acute simple overdose (meprobamate alone): Death has been reported with ingestion of as little as 12 gm meprobamate and survival with as much as 40 gm.

Blood Levels:
0.5 —2.0 mg% represents the usual blood level range of meprobamate after therapeutic doses. The level may occasionally be as high as 3.0 mg%.

3 —10 mg% usually corresonds to findings of mild to moderate symptoms of overdosage, such as stupor or light coma.

10 —20 mg% usually corresponds to deeper coma, requiring more intensive treatment. Some fatalities occur.

At levels greater than 20 mg%, more fatalities than survivals can be expected.

Acute combined overdose (meprobamate with alcohol or other CNS depressants or psychotropic drugs): Since effects can be additive, a history of ingestion of a low dose of meprobamate plus any of these compounds (or of a relatively low blood or tissue level) cannot be used as a prognostic indicator.

In cases where excessive doses have been taken, sleep ensues rapidly and blood pressure, pulse, and respiratory rates are reduced to basal levels. Any drug remaining in the stomach should be removed and symptomatic therapy given. Should respiration or blood pressure become compromised, respiratory assistance, central nervous system stimulants, and pressor agents should be administered cautiously as indicated. Meprobamate is metabolized in the liver and excreted by the kidney. Diuresis, osmotic (mannitol) diuresis, peritoneal dialysis, and hemodialysis have been used successfully. Careful monitoring of urinary output is necessary and caution should be taken to avoid overhydration. Relapse and death, after initial recovery, have been attributed to incomplete gastric emptying and delayed absorption. Meprobamate can be measured in biological fluids by two methods: colorimetric (Hoffman, A.J. and Ludwig, B.J.: *J Amer Pharm Assn 48:* 740, 1959) and gas chromatographic (Douglas, J.F. et al: *Anal Chem 39:* 956, 1967).

How Supplied: 'Meprospan' 400: Each sustained-release, blue-topped capsule contains meprobamate, U.S.P., 400 mg in bottles of 100 (NDC 0037-1301-01).

'Meprospan' 200: Each sustained-release, yellow-topped capsule contains meprobamate, U.S.P., 200 mg in bottles of 100 (NDC 0037-1401-01).

Distributed by
WALLACE LABORATORIES
Division of
CARTER-WALLACE, INC.
Cranbury, New Jersey 08512
Manufactured by KV Pharmacal, St. Louis, Mo. 63144

Rev. 10/80

MILTOWN® Tablets ℞ ℭ
(meprobamate)
MILTOWN® 600 Tablets ℞ ℭ
(meprobamate 600 mg)

Description: Meprobamate is a white powder with a characteristic odor and a bitter taste. It is slightly soluble in water, freely soluble in acetone and alcohol, and sparingly soluble in ether.

Actions: Meprobamate is a carbamate derivative which has been shown in animal studies to have effects at multiple sites in the central nervous system, including the thalamus and limbic system.

Indications: 'Miltown' (meprobamate) is indicated for the management of anxiety disorders or for the short-term relief of the symptoms of anxiety. Anxiety or tension associated with the stress of everyday life usually do not require treatment with an anxiolytic.

The effectiveness of 'Miltown' in long-term use, that is, more than 4 months, has not been assessed by systematic clinical studies. The physician should periodically reassess the usefulness of the drug for the individual patient.

Contraindications: Acute intermittent porphyria as well as allergic or idiosyncratic reactions to meprobamate or related compounds such as carisoprodol, mebutamate, tybamate, or carbromal.

Warnings:
Drug Dependence
Physical dependence, psychological dependence, and abuse have occurred. When chronic intoxication from prolonged use occurs, it usually involves ingestion of greater than recommended doses and is manifested by ataxia, slurred speech, and vertigo. Therefore, careful supervision of dose and

amounts prescribed is advised, as well as avoidance of prolonged administration, especially for alcoholics and other patients with a known propensity for taking excessive quantities of drugs.
Sudden withdrawal of the drug after prolonged and excessive use may precipitate recurrence of pre-existing symptoms, such as anxiety, anorexia, or insomnia, or withdrawal reactions, such as vomiting, ataxia, tremors, muscle twitching, confusional states, hallucinosis, and, rarely, convulsive seizures. Such seizures are more likely to occur in persons with central nervous system damage or pre-existent or latent convulsive disorders. Onset of withdrawal symptoms occurs usually within 12 to 48 hours after discontinuation of meprobamate; symptoms usually cease within the next 12 to 48 hours.
When excessive dosage has continued for weeks or months, dosage should be reduced gradually over a period of one or two weeks rather than abruptly stopped. Alternatively, a short-acting barbiturate may be substituted, then gradually withdrawn.

Potentially Hazardous Tasks
Patients should be warned that this drug may impair the mental and/or physical abilities required for the performance of potentially hazardous tasks such as driving a motor vehicle or operating machinery.

Additive Effects
Since the effects of meprobamate and alcohol or meprobamate and other CNS depressants or psychotropic drugs may be additive, appropriate caution should be exercised with patients who take more than one of these agents simultaneously.

Usage in Pregnancy and Lactation
An increased risk of congenital malformations associated with the use of minor tranquilizers (meprobamate, chlordiazepoxide, and diazepam) during the first trimester of pregnancy has been suggested in several studies. Because use of these drugs is rarely a matter of urgency, their use during this period should almost always be avoided. The possibility that a woman of childbearing potential may be pregnant at the time of institution of therapy should be considered. Patients should be advised that if they become pregnant during therapy or intend to become pregnant they should communicate with their physicians about the desirability of discontinuing the drug.
Meprobamate passes the placental barrier. It is present both in umbilical cord blood at or near maternal plasma levels and in breast milk of lactating mothers at concentrations two to four times that of maternal plasma. When use of meprobamate is contemplated in breast-feeding patients, the drug's higher concentration in breast milk as compared to maternal plasma levels should be considered.

Usage in Children
'Miltown' (meprobamate)—Meprobamate should not be administered to children under age six, since there is a lack of documented evidence for safety and effectiveness in this age group.
'Miltown' 600 (meprobamate 600 mg)—This dosage form is not intended for use in children.
Precautions: The lowest effective dose should be administered, particularly to elderly and/or debilitated patients, in order to preclude oversedation.
The possibility of suicide attempts should be considered and the least amount of drug feasible should be dispensed at any one time.
Meprobamate is metabolized in the liver and excreted by the kidney; to avoid its excess accumulation, caution should be exercised in administration to patients with compromised liver or kidney function.
Meprobamate occasionally may precipitate seizures in epileptic patients.

Adverse Reactions:
Central Nervous System
Drowsiness, ataxia, dizziness, slurred speech, headache, vertigo, weakness, paresthesias, impairment of visual accommodation, euphoria, overstimulation, paradoxical excitement, fast EEG activity.

Gastrointestinal
Nausea, vomiting, diarrhea.
Cardiovascular
Palpitations, tachycardia, various forms of arrhythmia, transient ECG changes, syncope; also, hypotensive crises (including one fatal case).
Allergic or Idiosyncratic
Allergic or idiosyncratic reactions are usually seen within the period of the first to fourth dose in patients having had no previous contact with the drug. Milder reactions are characterized by an itchy, urticarial, or erythematous maculopapular rash which may be generalized or confined to the groin. Other reactions have included leukopenia, acute nonthrombocytopenic purpura, petechiae, ecchymoses, eosinophilia, peripheral edema, adenopathy, fever, fixed drug eruption with cross reaction to carisoprodol, and cross sensitivity between meprobamate/mebutamate and meprobamate/carbromal.
More severe hypersensitivity reactions, rarely reported, include hyperpyrexia, chills, angioneurotic edema, bronchospasm, oliguria, and anuria. Also, anaphylaxis, erythema multiforme, exfoliative dermatitis, stomatitis, proctitis, Stevens-Johnson syndrome, and bullous dermatitis, including one fatal case of the latter following administration of meprobamate in combination with prednisolone.
In case of allergic or idiosyncratic reactions to meprobamate, discontinue the drug and initiate appropriate symptomatic therapy, which may include epinephrine, antihistamines, and in severe cases corticosteroids. In evaluating possible allergic reactions, also consider allergy to excipients (information on excipients is available to physicians on request).
Hematologic
(See also **Allergic or Idiosyncratic**.) Agranulocytosis and aplastic anemia have been reported, although no causal relationship has been established. These cases rarely were fatal. Rare cases of thrombocytopenic purpura have been reported.
Other
Exacerbation of porphyric symptoms.
Dosage and Administration:
Doses of meprobamate above 2400 mg daily are not recommended.
'Miltown' (meprobamate)—**Adults:** the usual dosage is 1200 to 1600 mg daily, in three or four divided doses. **Children:** the usual dosage for children ages six to twelve is 100 to 200 mg two or three times daily. Meprobamate is not recommended for children under six.
'Miltown' 600 (meprobamate 600 mg)—**Adults:** the recommended dosage is one tablet twice a day. **Children:** not intended for use in children.
Overdosage: Suicidal attempts with meprobamate have resulted in drowsiness, lethargy, stupor, ataxia, coma, shock, vasomotor and respiratory collapse. Some suicidal attempts have been fatal. The following data on meprobamate tablets have been reported in the literature and from other sources. These data are not expected to correlate with each case (considering factors such as individual susceptibility and length of time from ingestion to treatment), but represent the **usual ranges** reported.
Acute simple overdose (meprobamate alone): Death has been reported with ingestion of as little as 12 gm meprobamate and survival with as much as 40 gm.
Blood levels:
0.5 - 2.0 mg% represents the usual blood level range of meprobamate after therapeutic doses. The level may occasionally be as high as 3.0 mg%.
3 - 10 mg% usually corresponds to findings of mild to moderate symptoms of overdosage, such as stupor or light coma.
10 - 20 mg% usually corresponds to deeper coma, requiring more intensive treatment. Some fatalities occur.
At levels greater than 20 mg%, more fatalities than survivals can be expected.
Acute combined overdose (meprobamate with alcohol or other CNS depressants or psychotropic drugs): Since effects can be additive, a history of

ingestion of a low dose of meprobamate plus any of these compounds (or of a relatively low blood or tissue level) cannot be used as a prognostic indicator.
In cases where excessive doses have been taken, sleep ensues rapidly and blood pressure, pulse, and respiratory rates are reduced to basal levels. Any drug remaining in the stomach should be removed and symptomatic therapy given. Should respiration or blood pressure become compromised, respiratory assistance, central nervous system stimulants, and pressor agents should be administered cautiously as indicated. Meprobamate is metabolized in the liver and excreted by the kidney. Diuresis, osmotic (mannitol) diuresis, peritoneal dialysis, and hemodialysis have been used successfully. Careful monitoring of urinary output is necessary and caution should be taken to avoid overhydration. Relapse and death, after initial recovery, have been attributed to incomplete gastric emptying and delayed absorption. Meprobamate can be measured in biological fluids by two methods: colorimetric (Hoffman, A.J. and Ludwig, B.J.: *J Amer Pharm Assn 48:* 740, 1959) and gas chromatographic (Douglas, J.F. et al: *Anal Chem 39:* 956, 1967).
How Supplied: 'Miltown' (meprobamate, U.S.P.) is available as 400 mg white, scored tablets in bottles of:
100 (NDC 0037-1001-01)
500 (NDC 0037-1001-03)
1000 (NDC 0037-1001-02)
and 200 mg white, sugar-coated tablets in bottles of 100 (NDC 0037-1101-01).
'Miltown' 600 is available as white, capsule-shaped tablets, each containing 600 mg meprobamate, U.S.P., in bottles of 100 (NDC 0037-1601-01).
WALLACE LABORATORIES
Division of CARTER-WALLACE, INC.
Cranbury, New Jersey 08512
Rev. 10/80
Shown in Product Identification Section, page 442

ORGANIDIN® ℞
(iodinated glycerol)
Solution, Tablets, Elixir

Description: Organidin® (iodinated glycerol), a mucolytic-expectorant, is an isomeric mixture formed by the interaction of iodine and glycerol, whose active ingredient is thought to be iodopropylidene glycerol but whose structural and chemical formulas have not been precisely established. Iodinated glycerol is a viscous, amber liquid stable in acid media, including gastric juice, which contains virtually no inorganic iodide and no free iodine. ORGANIDIN is available for oral administration as: *Solution*—5%, containing 50 mg ORGANIDIN (25 mg organically bound iodine) per mL; *Tablets*—Each containing 30 mg ORGANIDIN (15 mg organically bound iodine); and *Elixir*—1.2%, containing 60 mg ORGANIDIN (30 mg organically bound iodine) per 5 mL (teaspoonful); and alcohol, 21.75% by volume.
Clinical Pharmacology: ORGANIDIN increases the output of thin respiratory tract fluid and helps liquefy tenacious mucus in the bronchial tree. Iodines are readily absorbed from the gastrointestinal tract and concentrated primarily in the secretions of the respiratory tract, but their mechanism of action as mucolytic-expectorants is not clear.
Indications and Usage: ORGANIDIN is indicated for adjunctive treatment as a mucolytic-expectorant in respiratory tract conditions such as bronchitis, bronchial asthma, pulmonary emphysema, cystic fibrosis, chronic sinusitis, or after surgery to help prevent atelectasis.
Contraindications: History of marked sensitivity to inorganic iodides; hypersensitivity to any of the ingredients or related compounds; pregnancy; newborns; and nursing mothers.
The human fetal thyroid begins to concentrate iodine in the 12th to 14th week of gestation and the use of inorganic iodides in pregnant women during this period and thereafter has rarely been re-

Continued on next page

Wallace—Cont.

ported to induce fetal goiter (with or without hypothyroidism) with the potential for airway obstruction. If the patient becomes pregnant while taking ORGANIDIN, the drug should be discontinued and the patient should be apprised of the potential risk to the fetus.

Warnings: Discontinue use if rash or other evidence of hypersensitivity appears. Use with caution or avoid use in patients with history or evidence of thyroid disease.

Precautions: *General*—Iodides have been reported to cause a flare-up of adolescent acne. Children with cystic fibrosis appear to have an exaggerated susceptibility to the goitrogenic effect of iodides.

Dermatitis and other reversible manifestations of iodism have been reported with chronic use of inorganic iodides. Although these have not been reported to be a problem clinically with ORGANIDIN, they should be kept in mind in patients receiving these preparations for prolonged periods.

Drug Interactions: Iodides may potentiate the hypothyroid effect of lithium and other antithyroid drugs.

Carcinogenesis, Mutagenesis, impairment of fertility: No long-term animal studies have been performed with ORGANIDIN.

Pregnancy Teratogenic Effects: Pregnancy Category X (see CONTRAINDICATIONS).

Nursing Mothers: ORGANIDIN should not be administered to a nursing woman.

Adverse Reactions: Reports of gastrointestinal irritation, rash, hypersensitivity, thyroid gland enlargement, and acute parotitis have been rare.

Overdosage: Acute overdosage experience with ORGANIDIN has been rare and there have been no reports of any serious problems.

Dosage and Administration: *Note:* Add *Solution* to fruit juice or other liquid. One drop *Solution* equals approximately 3 mg ORGANIDIN.
Adults: Solution—20 drops 4 times a day.
Tablets—2 tablets 4 times a day, with liquid.
Elixir— 1 teaspoonful 4 times a day.
Children: Up to one-half the adult dosage based on the child's weight.

How Supplied: ORGANIDIN is available as—
- **Solution:** 5%—clear amber liquid, in 30 ml dropper bottles (NDC 0037-4211-10).
- **Tablets:** 30 mg—round, scored, rose-colored tablets, in bottles of 100 (NDC 0037-4224-40).
- **Elixir:** 1.2%—clear amber liquid, in bottles of one pint (NDC 0037-4213-30) and one gallon (NDC 0037-4213-40).

Storage: Store at room temperature; avoid excessive heat. Keep bottle tightly closed.

ORGANIDIN *Solution* and *Elixir* are distributed by
WALLACE LABORATORIES
Division of
CARTER-WALLACE, Inc.
Cranbury, New Jersey 08512
Manufactured by
DENVER CHEMICAL (Puerto Rico), Inc.
Humacao, Puerto Rico 00661
ORGANIDIN *Tablets* are manufactured by
WALLACE LABORATORIES
Division of
CARTER-WALLACE, Inc.
Cranbury, New Jersey 08512
Rev. 3/84
Shown in Product Identification Section, page 442

RONDOMYCIN®
(methacycline HCl)

Description: 'Rondomycin' (methacycline HCl) is a broad-spectrum antibiotic synthetically derived from oxytetracycline. Chemical dehydration at the 6-position yields a structural homologue which is a light-yellow crystalline powder with a chemical designation of 6-methylene-5-oxytetracycline.

Actions: The tetracyclines are primarily bacteriostatic and are thought to exert their antimicrobial effect by the inhibition of protein synthesis. Tetracyclines are active against a wide range of gram-negative and gram-positive organisms.

The drugs in the tetracycline class have closely similar antimicrobial spectra, and cross-resistance among them is common. Micro-organisms may be considered susceptible if the MIC (minimum inhibitory concentration) is not more than 4.0 mcg/ml and intermediate if the MIC is 4.0 to 12.5 mcg/ml.
Susceptibility plate testing: A tetracycline disc may be used to determine microbial susceptibility to drugs in the tetracycline class. If the kirby-Bauer method of disc susceptibility testing is used, a 30 mcg tetracycline disc should give a zone of at least 19 mm when tested against a tetracycline-susceptible bacterial strain.

Tetracyclines are readily absorbed and are bound to plasma proteins in varying degree. They are concentrated by the liver in the bile and excreted in the urine and feces at high concentrations and in a biologically active form.

Indications: 'Rondomycin' (methacycline HCl) is indicated in infections caused by the following micro-organisms:
Rickettsiae (Rocky Mountain spotted fever, typhus fever and the typhus group, Q fever, rickettsialpox and tick fevers),
Mycoplasma pneumoniae (PPLO, Eaton Agent),
Agents of psittacosis and ornithosis,
Agents of lymphogranuloma venereum and granuloma inguinale,
The spirochetal agent of relapsing fever (*Borrelia recurrentis*).
The following gram-negative micro-organisms:
Haemophilus ducreyi (chancroid),
Pasteurella pestis and *Pasteurella tularensis*,
Bartonella bacilliformis,
Bacteroides species,
Vibrio comma and *Vibrio fetus*,
Brucella species (in conjunction with streptomycin).

Because many strains of the following groups of micro-organisms have been shown to be resistant to tetracyclines, culture and susceptibility testing are recommended.

'Rondomycin' (methacycline HCl) is indicated for treatment of infections caused by the following gram-negative micro-organisms, when bacteriologic testing indicates appropriate susceptibility to the drug:
Escherichia coli,
Enterobacter aerogenes (formerly *Aerobacter aerogenes*),
Shigella species,
Mima species and *Herellea* species,
Haemophilus influenzae (respiratory infections),
Klebsiella species (respiratory and urinary infections).

'Rondomycin' (methacycline HCl) is indicated for treatment of infections caused by the following gram-positive micro-organisms when bacteriologic testing indicates appropriate susceptibility to the drug:
Streptococcus species: Up to 44 percent of strains of *streptococcus pyogenes* and 74 percent of *streptococcus faecalis* have been found to be resistant to tetracycline drugs. Therefore, tetracyclines should not be used for streptococcal disease unless the organism has been demonstrated to be sensitive.

For upper respiratory infections due to group A beta-hemolytic streptococci, penicillin is the usual drug of choice, including prophylaxis of rheumatic fever.
Diplococcus pneumoniae,
Staphylococcus aureus, skin and soft tissue infections. Tetracyclines are not the drugs of choice in the treatment of any type of staphylococcal infections.

When penicillin is contraindicated, tetracyclines are alternative drugs in the treatment of infections due to:
Neisseria gonorrhoeae,
Treponema pallidum and *Treponema pertenue* (syphilis and yaws),
Listeria monocytogenes,
Clostridium species,
Bacillus anthracis,
Fusobacterium fusiforme (Vincent's infection),
Actinomyces species.

In acute intestinal amebiasis, the tetracyclines may be a useful adjunct to amebicides.

In severe acne, the tetracyclines may be useful adjunctive therapy.

Tetracyclines are indicated in the treatment of trachoma, although the infectious agent is not always eliminated, as judged by immunofluorescence.

Inclusion conjunctivitis may be treated with oral tetracyclines or with a combination of oral and topical agents.

Contraindications: This drug is contraindicated in persons who have shown hypersensitivity to any of the tetracyclines.

Warnings: THE USE OF DRUGS OF THE TETRACYCLINE CLASS DURING TOOTH DEVELOPMENT (LAST HALF OF PREGNANCY, INFANCY, AND CHILDHOOD TO THE AGE OF 8 YEARS) MAY CAUSE PERMANENT DISCOLORATION OF THE TEETH (YELLOW-GRAY-BROWN). This adverse reaction is more common during long-term use of the drugs but has been observed following repeated short-term courses. Enamel hypoplasia has also been reported. TETRACYCLINE DRUGS, THEREFORE, SHOULD NOT BE USED IN THIS AGE GROUP UNLESS OTHER DRUGS ARE NOT LIKELY TO BE EFFECTIVE OR ARE CONTRAINDICATED.

If renal impairment exists, even usual oral or parenteral doses may lead to excessive systemic accumulation of the drug and possible liver toxicity. Under such conditions, lower than usual total doses are indicated, and, if therapy is prolonged, serum level determinations of the drug may be advisable.

Photosensitivity manifested by an exaggerated sunburn reaction has been observed in some individuals taking tetracyclines. Patients apt to be exposed to direct sunlight or ultraviolet light should be advised that this reaction can occur with tetracycline drugs, and treatment should be discontinued at the first evidence of skin erythema.
The anti-anabolic action of the tetracyclines may cause an increase in BUN. While this is not a problem in those with normal renal function, in patients with significantly impaired function, higher serum levels of tetracyclines may lead to azotemia, hyperphosphatemia, and acidosis.

Usage in pregnancy. (See above "Warnings" about use during tooth development.)

Results of animal studies indicate that tetracyclines cross the placenta, are found in fetal tissues and can have toxic effects on the developing fetus (often related to retardation of skeletal development). Evidence of embryotoxicity has also been noted in animals treated early in pregnancy.

Usage in newborns, infants, and children. (See above "Warnings" about use during tooth development.)

All tetracyclines form a stable calcium complex in any bone-forming tissue. A decrease in the fibula growth rate has been observed in prematures given oral tetracycline in doses of 25 mg/kg every 6 hours. This reaction was shown to be reversible when the drug was discontinued.

Tetracyclines are present in the milk of lactating women who are taking a drug in this class.

Precautions: As with other antibiotic preparations, use of this drug may result in overgrowth of nonsusceptible organisms, including fungi. If superinfection occurs, the antibiotic should be discontinued and appropriate therapy instituted.

In venereal diseases when coexistent syphilis is suspected, darkfield examination should be done before treatment is started and the blood serology repeated monthly for at least 4 months.

Because tetracyclines have been shown to depress plasma prothrombin activity, patients who are on anticoagulant therapy may require downward adjustment of their anticoagulant dosage.

In long-term therapy, periodic laboratory evaluation of organ systems, including hematopoietic, renal and hepatic studies should be performed.

All infections due to Group A beta-hemolytic streptococci should be treated for at least 10 days.

Since bacteriostatic drugs may interfere with the bactericidal action of penicillin, it is advisable to avoid giving tetracycline in conjunction with penicillin.

Adverse Reactions:
Gastrointestinal: Anorexia, nausea, vomiting, diarrhea, glossitis, dysphagia, enterocolitis, and inflammatory lesions (with monilial overgrowth) in the anogenital region. These reactions have been caused by both the oral and parenteral administration of tetracyclines.
Skin: Maculopapular and erythematous rashes. Exfoliative dermatitis has been reported but is uncommon. Photosensitivity is discussed above. (See "Warnings".)
Renal toxicity: Rise in BUN has been reported and is apparently dose related. (See "Warnings".)
Hypersensitivity reactions: Urticaria, angioneurotic edema, anaphylaxis, anaphylactoid purpura, pericarditis and exacerbation of systemic lupus erythematosus.
Bulging fontanels in infants and benign intracranial hypertension in adults have been reported in individuals receiving full therapeutic dosages. These conditions disappeared rapidly when the drug was discontinued.
Blood: Hemolytic anemia, thrombocytopenia, neutropenia and eosinophilia have been reported. When given over prolonged periods, tetracyclines have been reported to produce brown-black microscopic discoloration of thyroid glands. No abnormalities of thyroid function studies are known to occur.
Dosage and Administration: The usual adult dosage of 'Rondomycin' (methacycline HCl) is 600 mg daily. This may be given in four divided doses of 150 mg each or two divided doses of 300 mg each. An initial dose of 300 mg followed by 150 mg every six hours or 300 mg every 12 hours may be used in the management of more severe infections.
In uncomplicated gonorrhea, when penicillin is contraindicated, 'Rondomycin' (methacycline HCl) may be used for treating both males and females in the following clinical dosage schedule: 900 mg initially, followed by 300 mg q.i.d. for a total of 5.4 grams.
For treatment of syphilis, when penicillin is contraindicated, a total of 18 to 24 grams of 'Rondomycin' (methacycline HCl) in equally divided doses over a period of 10–15 days should be given. Close follow-up, including laboratory tests, is recommended.
In Eaton Agent pneumonia, the usual adult dosage is 900 mg daily for 6 days.
The recommended dosage schedule for children above eight years of age is 3 to 6 mg/lb of body weight per day divided into two or four equally spaced doses.
Therapy should be continued for at least 24–48 hours after symptoms and fever have subsided. It should be noted, however, that antibacterial serum levels may usually be present from 24 to 36 hours following the discontinuation of 'Rondomycin' (methacycline HCl).
Concomitant therapy: Antacids containing aluminum, calcium, or magnesium impair absorption and should no be given to patients taking oral tetracyclines.
Food and some dairy products also interfere with absorption. Oral forms of tetracycline should be given 1 hour before or 2 hours after meals. Pediatric oral dosage forms should not be given with milk formulas and should be given at least 1 hour prior to feeding.
In patients with renal impairment (see "Warnings"): Total dosage should be decreased by reduction of recommended individual doses and/or by extending time intervals between doses.
In the treatment of streptococcal infections, a therapeutic dose of tetracycline should be administered for at least 10 days.
How Supplied: 'Rondomycin'-300 is available as blue and white capsules, each containing 300 mg methacycline HCl equivalent to 280 mg methacycline base, supplied in bottles of 50 (NDC 0037-4101-06).
'Rondomycin'-150 is available as blue and white capsules, each containing 150 mg methacycline HCl equivalent to 140 mg methacycline base, supplied in bottles of 100 (NDC 0037-4001-01).

Rev. 6/81

WALLACE LABORATORIES
Division of
CARTER-WALLACE, INC.
Cranbury, New Jersey 08512
Shown in Product Identification Section, page 442

RYNA™(Liquid)
RYNA–C® ℭ
(Liquid)
RYNA–CX® ℭ
(Liquid)

(See PDR for Nonprescription Drugs)

RYNATAN® ℞
Tablets
Pediatric Suspension

Description: Rynatan® is an antihistaminic/decongestant combination available for oral administration as **Tablets** and as **Pediatric Suspension.** Each tablet contains:
Phenylephrine Tannate ....25 mg
Chlorpheniramine Tannate ....8 mg
Pyrilamine Tannate ....25 mg
Each 5 ml (teaspoonful) of the Pediatric Suspension contains:
Phenylephrine Tannate ....5 mg
Chlorpheniramine Tannate ....2 mg
Pyrilamine Tannate ....12.5 mg
Clinical Pharmacology: Rynatan combines the sympathomimetic decongestant effect of phenylephrine with the antihistaminic actions of chlorpheniramine and pyrilamine.
Indications and Usage: Rynatan is indicated for symptomatic relief of the coryza and nasal congestion associated with the common cold, sinusitis, allergic rhinitis and other upper respiratory tract conditions. Appropriate therapy should be provided for the primary disease.
Contraindications: Rynatan is contraindicated for newborns, nursing mothers and patients sensitive to any of the ingredients or related compounds.
Warnings: Use with caution in patients with hypertension, cardiovascular disease, hyperthyroidism, diabetes, narrow angle glaucoma or prostatic hypertrophy. Use with caution or avoid use in patients taking monoamine oxidase (MAO) inhibitors. This product contains antihistamines which may cause drowsiness and may have additive central nervous system (CNS) effects with alcohol or other CNS depressants (e.g., hypnotics, sedatives, tranquilizers).
Precautions: General: Antihistamines are more likely to cause dizziness, sedation and hypotension in elderly patients. Antihistamines may cause excitation, particularly in children, but their combination with sympathomimetics may cause either mild stimulation or mild sedation.
Information for Patients: Caution patients against drinking alcoholic beverages or engaging in potentially hazardous activities requiring alertness, such as driving a car or operating machinery, while using this product.
Drug Interactions: MAO inhibitors may prolong and intensify the anticholinergic effects of antihistamines and the overall effects of sympathomimetic agents.
Carcinogenesis, Mutagenesis, Impairment of Fertility: No long-term animal studies have been performed with Rynatan.
Pregnancy: Teratogenic Effects: Pregnancy Category C. Animal reproduction studies have not been conducted with Rynatan. It is also not known whether Rynatan can cause fetal harm when administered to a pregnant woman or can affect reproduction capacity. Rynatan should be given to a pregnant woman only if clearly needed.
Nursing Mothers: Rynatan should not be administered to a nursing woman.
Adverse Reactions: Adverse effects associated with Rynatan at recommended doses have been minimal. The most common have been drowsiness, sedation, dryness of mucous membranes, and gastrointestinal effects. Serious side effects with oral antihistimines or sympathomimetics have been rare.
Overdosage: Signs & Symptoms—may vary from CNS depression to stimulation (restlessness to convulsions). Antihistamine overdosage in young children may lead to convulsions and death. Atropine-like signs and symptoms may be prominent.
Treatment—Induce vomiting if it has not occurred spontaneously. Precautions must be taken against aspiration especially in infants, children and comatose patients. If gastric lavage is indicated, isotonic or half-isotonic saline solution is preferred. Stimulants should not be used. If hypotension is a problem, vasopressor agents may be considered.
Dosage and Administration: Administer the recommended dose every 12 hours.
Rynatan Tablets: Adults—1 or 2 tablets.
Rynatan Pediatric Suspension: Children over six years of age—5 to 10 ml (1 to 2 teaspoonfuls); **Children two to six years of age**—2.5 to 5 ml (½ to 1 teaspoonful); **Children under two years of age**—Titrate dose individually.
How Supplied: Rynatan® Tablets: buff, capsule-shaped, compressed tablets in bottles of 100 (NDC 0037-0713-92) and bottles of 500 (NDC 0037-0713-96)
Rynatan® Pediatric Suspension: dark-pink with strawberry-currant flavor, in pint bottles (NDC-0037-0715-68)
Storage: Rynatan Tablets—Store at room temperature; avoid excessive heat—(above 40°C/104°F).
Rynatan Pediatric Suspension—Store at controlled room temperature—between 15°C-30°C (59°F-86°F); protect from freezing.

Rev. 2/80
Shown in Product Identification Section, page 442

RYNATUSS® ℞
Tablets
Pediatric Suspension

Description: RYNATUSS® is an antitussive/antihistaminic/decongestant/bronchodilator combination available for oral administration as *Tablets* and as *Pediatric Suspension.*
Each tablet contains:
Carbetapentane Tannate ....60 mg
Chlorpheniramine Tannate ....5 mg
Ephedrine Tannate ....10 mg
Phenylephrine Tannate ....10 mg
Each 5 ml (one teaspoonful) of the Pediatric Suspension contains:
Carbetapentane Tannate ....30 mg
Chlorpheniramine Tannate ....4 mg
Ephedrine Tannate ....5 mg
Phenylephrine Tannate ....5 mg
Clinical Pharmacology: RYNATUSS combines the antitussive action of carbetapentane, the sympathomimetic decongestant effect of phenylephrine, the antihistaminic action of chlorpheniramine, and the bronchodilator action of ephedrine.
Indications and Usage: RYNATUSS is indicated for the symptomatic relief of cough associated with respiratory tract conditions such as the common cold, bronchial asthma, acute and chronic bronchitis. Appropriate therapy should be provided for the primary disease.
Contraindications: RYNATUSS is contraindicated for newborns, nursing mothers and patients who are sensitive to any of the ingredients or related compounds.
Warnings: Use with caution in patients with hypertension, cardiovascular disease, hyperthyroidism, diabetes, narrow angle glaucoma or prostatic hypertrophy. Use with caution or avoid use in patients taking monoamine oxidase (MAO) Inhibitors.
This product contains antihistamines which may cause drowsiness and may have additive central nervous system (CNS) effects with alcohol or other CNS depressants (e.g., hypnotics, sedatives, tranquilizers).
Precautions: *For RYNATUSS Pediatric Suspension only:* This product contains FD&C Yellow No. 5 (tartrazine) which may cause allergic-type reac-

Continued on next page

Wallace—Cont.

tions (including bronchial asthma) in certain susceptible individuals. Although the overall incidence of FD&C Yellow No. 5 (tartrazine) sensitivity in the general population is low, it is frequently seen in patients who also have aspirin hypersensitivity.

General: Antihistamines are more likely to cause dizziness, sedation and hypotension in elderly patients. Antihistamines may cause excitation, particularly in children, but their combination with sympathomimetics may cause either mild stimulation or mild sedation.

Information for patients: Caution patients against drinking alcoholic beverages or engaging in potentially hazardous activities requiring alertness, such as driving a car or operating machinery, while using this product.

Drug interactions: MAO inhibitors may prolong and intensify the anticholinergic effects of antihistamines and the overall effects of sympathomimetic agents.

Carcinogenesis, mutagenesis, impairment of fertility: No long term animal studies have been performed with RYNATUSS.

Pregnancy: Teratogenic Effects: Pregnancy Category C. Animal reproduction studies have not been conducted with RYNATUSS. It is also not known whether RYNATUSS can cause fetal harm when administered to a pregnant woman or can affect reproduction capacity. RYNATUSS should be given to a pregnant woman only if clearly needed.

Nursing mothers: RYNATUSS should not be administered to a nursing woman.

Adverse Reactions: Adverse effects associated with RYNATUSS at recommended doses have been minimal. The most common have been drowsiness, sedation, dryness of mucous membranes, and gastrointestinal effects. Serious side effects with oral antihistamines or sympathomimetics have been rare.

Overdosage: *Signs and Symptoms:* May vary from CNS depression to stimulation (restlessness to convulsions). Antihistamine overdosage in young children may lead to convulsions and death. Atropine-like signs and symptoms may be prominent.

Treatment: Induce vomiting if it has not occurred spontaneously. Precautions must be taken against aspiration especially in infants, children and comatose patients. If gastric lavage is indicated, isotonic or half-isotonic saline solution is preferred. Stimulants should not be used. If hypotension is a problem, vasopressor agents may be considered.

Dosage and Administration: Administer the recommended dose every 12 hours.

RYNATUSS Tablets: Adults—1 to 2 tablets.

RYNATUSS Pediatric Suspension: Children over six years of age—5 to 10 mL (1 to 2 teaspoonfuls); Children two to six years of age—2.5 to 5 mL (½ to 1 teaspoonful); Children under two years of age—Titrate dose individually.

How Supplied:

RYNATUSS® Tablets: mauve, capsule-shaped, compressed tablets in bottles of 100 (NDC 0037-0717-92) and bottles of 500 (NDC 0037-0717-96).

RYNATUSS® Pediatric Suspension: pink with strawberry-currant flavor, in bottles of 8 fl oz (NDC 0037-0718-67) and one pint (NDC 0037-0718-68).

Storage: RYNATUSS Tablets: Store at room temperature; avoid excessive heat—above 40°C (104°F).

RYNATUSS Pediatric Suspension: Store at controlled room temperature—between 15°C-30°C (59°F-86°F); protect from freezing. Rev. 8/83

WALLACE LABORATORIES
Division of
CARTER-WALLACE, Inc.
Cranbury, New Jersey 08512

Shown in Product Identification Section, page 442

SOMA® ℞
(carisoprodol)

Description: 'Soma' (carisoprodol) is available as 350 mg white tablets. Carisoprodol is N-isopropyl-2-methyl-2-propyl-1,3-propanediol dicarbamate.

Actions: Carisoprodol produces muscle relaxation in animals by blocking interneuronal activity in the descending reticular formation and spinal cord. The onset of action is rapid and effects last four to six hours.

Indications: Carisoprodol is indicated as an adjunct to rest, physical therapy, and other measures for the relief of discomfort associated with acute, painful musculoskeletal conditions. The mode of action of this drug has not been clearly identified, but may be related to its sedative properties. Carisoprodol does not directly relax tense skeletal muscles in man.

Contraindications: Acute intermittent porphyria as well as allergic or idiosyncratic reactions to carisoprodol or related compounds such as meprobamate, mebutamate, or tybamate.

Warnings:

Idiosyncratic Reactions—On very rare occasions, the first dose of carisoprodol has been followed by idiosyncratic symptoms appearing within minutes or hours. Symptoms reported include: extreme weakness, transient quadriplegia, dizziness, ataxia, temporary loss of vision, diplopia, mydriasis, dysarthria, agitation, euphoria, confusion, and disorientation. Symptoms usually subside over the course of the next several hours. Supportive and symptomatic therapy, including hospitalization, may be necessary.

Usage in Pregnancy and Lactation—Safe usage of this drug in pregnancy or lactation has not been established. Therefore, use of this drug in pregnancy, in nursing mothers, or in women of childbearing potential requires that the potential benefits of the drug be weighed against the potential hazards to mother and child. Carisoprodol is present in breast milk of lactating mothers at concentrations two to four times that of maternal plasma. This factor should be taken into account when use of the drug is contemplated in breast-feeding patients.

Usage in Children—Because of limited clinical experience, 'Soma' is not recommended for use in patients under 12 years of age.

Potentially Hazardous Tasks—Patients should be warned that this drug may impair the mental and/or physical abilities required for the performance of potentially hazardous tasks such as driving a motor vehicle or operating machinery.

Additive Effects—Since the effects of carisoprodol and alcohol or carisoprodol and other CNS depressants or psychotropic drugs may be additive, appropriate caution should be exercised with patients who take more than one of these agents simultaneously.

Drug Dependence—In dogs, no withdrawal symptoms occurred after abrupt cessation of carisoprodol from dosages as high as 1 gm/kg/day. In a study in man, abrupt cessation of 100 mg/kg/day (about five times the recommended daily adult dosage) was followed in some subjects by mild withdrawal symptoms such as abdominal cramps, insomnia, chilliness, headache, and nausea. Delirium and convulsions did not occur. In clinical use, psychological dependence and abuse have been rare, and there have been no reports of significant abstinence signs. Nevertheless, the drug should be used with caution in addiction-prone individuals.

Precautions: Carisoprodol is metabolized in the liver and excreted by the kidney; to avoid its excess accumulation, caution should be exercised in administration to patients with compromised liver or kidney function.

Adverse Reactions: Central Nervous System—Drowsiness and other CNS effects may require dosage reduction. Also observed: dizziness, vertigo, ataxia, tremor, agitation, irritability, headache, depressive reactions, syncope, and insomnia. (See also Idiosyncratic Reactions under "Warnings".)

Allergic or Idiosyncratic—Allergic or idiosyncratic reactions occasionally develop. They are usually seen within the period of the first to fourth dose in patients having had no previous contact with the drug. Skin rash, erythema multiforme, pruritus, eosinophilia, and fixed drug eruption with cross reaction to meprobamate have been reported with carisoprodol. Severe reactions have been manifested by asthmatic episodes, fever, weakness, dizziness, angioneurotic edema, smarting eyes, hypotension, and anaphylactoid shock. (See also Idiosyncratic Reactions under "Warnings".)

In case of allergic or idiosyncratic reactions to carisoprodol, discontinue the drug and initiate appropriate symptomatic therapy, which may include epinephrine, antihistamines, and in severe cases corticosteroids. In evaluating possible allergic reactions, also consider allergy to excipients (information on excipients is available to physicians on request).

Cardiovascular—Tachycardia, postural hypotension, and facial flushing.

Gastrointestinal—Nausea, vomiting, hiccup, and epigastric distress.

Hematologic—Leukopenia, in which other drugs or viral infection may have been responsible, and pancytopenia, attributed to phenylbutazone, have been reported. No serious blood dyscrasias have been attributed to carisoprodol.

Dosage and Administration: The usual adult dosage of 'Soma' (carisoprodol) is one 350 mg tablet, three times daily and at bedtime. Usage in patients under age 12 is not recommended.

Overdosage: Overdosage of carisoprodol has produced stupor, coma, shock, respiratory depression, and, very rarely, death. The effects of an overdosage of carisoprodol and alcohol or other CNS depressants or psychotropic agents can be additive even when one of the drugs has been taken in the usual recommended dosage. Any drug remaining in the stomach should be removed and symptomatic therapy given. Should respiration or blood pressure become compromised, respiratory assistance, central nervous system stimulants, and pressor agents should be administered cautiously as indicated. Carisoprodol is metabolized in the liver and excreted by the kidney. Although carisoprodol overdosage experience is limited, the following types of treatment have been used successfully with the related drug meprobamate: diuresis, osmotic (mannitol) diuresis, peritoneal dialysis, and hemodialysis (carisoprodol is dialyzable). Careful monitoring of urinary output is necessary and caution should be taken to avoid overhydration. Observe for possible relapse due to incomplete gastric emptying and delayed absorption. Carisoprodol can be measured in biological fluids by gas chromatography (Douglas, J.F. et al: *J Pharm Sci* 58: 145, 1969).

How Supplied: 'Soma' 350: Bottles of 100 (NDC 0037-2001-01) and 500 (NDC 0037-2001-03).

Rev. 8/74

Shown in Product Identification Section, page 442

SOMA® ℞
COMPOUND TABLETS
(carisoprodol 200 mg + aspirin 325 mg)

Description: 'Soma' Compound is a combination product containing carisoprodol, a centrally-acting muscle relaxant, plus aspirin, an analgesic with antipyretic and anti-inflammatory properties. It is available as a two-layered, white and orange, round tablet for oral administration. Each tablet contains carisoprodol 200 mg and aspirin 325 mg. Chemically, carisoprodol is N-isopropyl-2-methyl-2-propyl-1,3-propanediol dicarbamate. Its empirical formula is $C_{12}H_{24}N_2O_4$, with a molecular weight of 260.33. The structural formula is:

$$H_2NCOOCH_2CCH_2OOCNHCH(CH_3)_2$$
with side chains $CH_2CH_2CH_3$ and CH_3

Clinical Pharmacology—*Carisprodol:* Carisprodol is a centrally-acting muscle relaxant that does not directly relax tense skeletal muscles in man. The mode of action of carisoprodol in relieving acute muscle spasm of local origin has not been clearly identified, but may be related to its sedative properties. In animals, carisoprodol has been shown to produce muscle relaxation by blocking interneuronal activity and depressing transmission of polysynaptic neurons in the spinal cord and in the descending reticular formation of the brain. The onset of action is rapid and lasts four to six hours.

Carisoprodol is metabolized in the liver and is excreted by the kidneys. It is dialyzable by peritoneal and hemodialysis.

Aspirin: Aspirin is a non-narcotic analgesic with anti-inflammatory and antipyretic activity. Inhibition of prostaglandin biosynthesis appears to account for most of its anti-inflammatory and for at least part of its analgesic and antipyretic properties.

Aspirin is rapidly absorbed and almost totally hydrolyzed to salicylic acid following oral administration. Although aspirin has a half-life of only about 15 minutes, the apparent biologic half-life of salicylic acid in the therapeutic plasma concentration range is between 6 and 12 hours. Salicylic acid is eliminated by renal excretion and by biotransformation to inactive metabolites. Clearance of salicylic acid in the high-dose range is sensitive to urinary pH (see *Drug Interactions*) and is reduced by renal dysfunction.

Indications and Usage: 'Soma' Compound is indicated as an adjunct to rest, physical therapy, and other measures for the relief of pain, muscle spasm, and limited mobility associated with acute, painful musculoskeletal conditions.

Contraindications: Acute intermittent porphyria; bleeding disorders, allergic or idiosyncratic reactions to carisoprodol, aspirin or related compounds.

Warnings: On very rare occasions, the first dose of carisoprodol has been followed by an idiosyncratic reaction with symptoms appearing within minutes or hours. These may include extreme weakness, transient quadriplegia, dizziness, ataxia, temporary loss of vision, diplopia, mydriasis, dysarthria, agitation, euphoria, confusion, and disorientation. Although symptoms usually subside over the course of the next several hours, discontinue 'Soma' Compound and initiate appropriate supportive and symptomatic therapy, which may include epinephrine and/or antihistamines. In severe cases, corticosteroids may be necessary. Severe reactions have been manifested by asthmatic episodes, fever, weakness, dizziness, angioneurotic edema, smarting eyes, hypotension, and anaphylactoid shock.

The effects of carisoprodol with agents such as alcohol, other CNS depressants, or psychotropic drugs may be additive. Appropriate caution should be exercised with patients who may take one or more of these agents simultaneously with 'Soma' Compound.

Precautions—*General:* To avoid excessive accumulation of carisoprodol, aspirin, or their metabolites, use 'Soma' Compound with caution in patients with compromised liver or kidney function, or in elderly or debilitated patients (see CLINICAL PHARMACOLOGY).

Use with caution in patients with history of gastritis or peptic ulcer, in patients on anticoagulant therapy, and in addiction-prone individuals.

Information for Patients: Caution patients that this drug may impair the mental and/or physical abilities required for the performance of potentially hazardous tasks such as driving a motor vehicle or operating machinery.

Caution patients with a predisposition for gastrointestinal bleeding that concomitant use of aspirin and alcohol may have an addictive effect in this regard.

Caution patients that dosage of medications used for gout, arthritis, or diabetes may have to be adjusted when aspirin is administered or discontinued (see *Drug Interactions*).

Drug Interactions: Clinically important interactions may occur when certain drugs are administered concomitantly with aspirin or aspirin-containing drugs.

1. *Oral Anticoagulants*—By interfering with platelet function or decreasing plasma prothrombin concentration, aspirin enhances the potential for bleeding in patients on anticoagulants.
2. *Methotrexate*—aspirin enhances the toxic effects of this drug.
3. *Probenecid and Sulfinpyrazone*—large doses of aspirin reduce the uricosuric effect of both drugs. Renal excretion of salicylate may also be reduced.
4. *Oral Antidiabetic Drugs*—enhancement of hypoglycemia may occur.
5. *Antacids*—to the extent that they raise urinary pH, antacids may substantially decrease plasma salicylate concentrations; conversely, their withdrawal can result in a substantial increase.
6. *Ammonium Chloride*—this and other drugs that acidify a relatively alkaline urine can elevate plasma salicylate concentrations.
7. *Ethyl Alcohol*—enhanced aspirin-induced fecal blood loss has been reported.
8. *Corticosteroids*—salicylate plasma levels may be decreased when adrenal corticosteroids are given, and may be increased substantially when they are discontinued.

Carcinogenesis, Mutagenesis, Impairment of Fertility: No long-term studies have been done with 'Soma' Compound.

Pregnancy—Teratogenic Effects: Pregnancy Category C. Adequate animal reproduction studies have not been conducted with 'Soma' Compound. It is also not known whether 'Soma' Compound can cause fetal harm when administered to a pregnant woman or can affect reproduction capacity. 'Soma' Compound should be given to a pregnant woman only if clearly needed.

Studies in rodents have shown salicylates to be teratogenic when given in early gestation, and embryocidal when given in later gestation in doses considerably greater than usual therapeutic doses in humans. Studies in women who took aspirin during pregnancy have not demonstrated an increased incidence of congenital abnormalities in the offspring.

Labor and Delivery: Ingestion of aspirin near term or prior to delivery may prolong delivery or lead to bleeding in mother, fetus, or neonate.

Nursing Mothers: Carisoprodol is excreted in human milk in concentrations two-to-four times that in maternal plasma. Aspirin is excreted in human milk in moderate amounts and can produce a bleeding tendency in nursing infants. Because of the potential for serious adverse reactions in nursing infants, a decision should be made whether to discontinue nursing or the drug, taking into account the importance of the drug to the mother.

Pediatric Use: Safety and effectiveness in children below the age of twelve have not been established.

Adverse Reactions: If severe reactions occur, discontinue 'Soma' Compound and initiate appropriate symptomatic and supportive therapy.

The following side effects which have occurred with the administration of the individual ingredients alone may also occur with the combination.

Carisoprodol: *Central Nervous System*—Drowsiness is the most frequent complaint and along with other CNS effects may require dosage reduction. Observed less frequently are dizziness, vertigo and ataxia. Tremor, agitation, irritability, headache, depressive reactions, syncope, and insomnia have been infrequent or rare.

Idiosyncratic—Idiosyncratic reactions are very rare. They are usually seen within the period of the first to fourth dose in patients having had no previous contact with the drug (see WARNINGS).

Allergic—Skin rash, erythema multiforme, pruritus, eosinophilia, and fixed drug eruptions with cross-reaction to meprobamate have been reported. If allergic reactions occur, discontinue 'Soma' Compound and treat symptomatically. In evaluating possible allergic reactions, also consider allergy to excipients (information on excipients is available to physicians on request).

Cardiovascular—Tachycardia, postural hypotension, and facial flushing.

Gastrointestinal—Nausea, vomiting, epigastric distress and hiccup.

Hematologic—No serious blood dyscrasias have been attributed to carisoprodol alone. Leukopenia and pancytopenia have been reported, very rarely, in situations in which other drugs or viral infections may have been responsible.

Aspirin: The most common adverse reactions associated with the use of aspirin have been gastrointestinal, including nausea, vomiting, gastritis, occult bleeding, constipation and diarrhea. Gastric erosion, angioedema, asthma, rash, pruritus and urticaria have been reported less commonly. Tinnitus is a sign of high serum salicylate levels (see OVERDOSAGE).

Aspirin Intolerance—Allergic type reactions in aspirin-sensitive individuals may involve the respiratory tract or the skin. Symptoms of the former range from rhinorrhea and shortness of breath to severe asthma, and the latter may consist of urticaria, edema, rash, or angioedema (giant hives). These may occur independently or in combination.

Drug Abuse and Dependence—
Abuse: In clinical use, abuse has been rare.
Dependence: In clinical use, dependence with 'Soma' Compound has been rare and there have been no reports of significant abstinence signs. Nevertheless, the following information on the individual ingredients should be kept in mind.

Carisoprodol—In dogs, no withdrawal symptoms occurred after abrupt cessation of carisoprodol from dosages as high as 1 gm/kg/day. In a study in man, abrupt cessation of 100 mg/kg/day (about five times the recommended daily adult dosage) was followed in some subjects by mild withdrawal symptoms such as abdominal cramps, insomnia, chills, headache, and nausea. Delirium and convulsions did not occur (see PRECAUTIONS).

Overdosage—*Signs and Symptoms:* Any of the following which have been reported with the individual ingredients may occur and may be modified to a varying degree by the effects of the other ingredients present in 'Soma' Compound.

Carisoprodol—Stupor, coma, shock, respiratory depression and, very rarely, death. Overdosage with carisoprodol in combination with alcohol, other CNS depressants, or psychotropic agents can have additive effects, even when one of the agents has been taken in the usually recommended dosage.

Aspirin—Headache, tinnitus, hearing difficulty, dim vision, dizziness, lassitude, hyperpnea, rapid breathing, thirst, nausea, vomiting, sweating and occasionally diarrhea are characteristic of mild to moderate salicylate poisoning. Salicylate poisoning should be considered in children with symptoms of vomiting, hyperpnea, and hyperthermia. Hyperpnea is an early sign of salicylate poisoning, but dyspnea supervenes at plasma levels above 50 mg/dl. These respiratory changes eventually lead to serious acid-base disturbances. Metabolic acidosis is a constant finding in infants but occurs in older children only with severe poisoning; adults usually exhibit respiratory alkalosis initially and acidosis terminally.

Other symptoms of severe salicylate poisoning include hyperthermia, dehydration, delirium, and mental disturbances. Skin eruptions, GI hemorrhage, or pulmonary edema are less common. Early CNS stimulation is replaced by increasing depression, stupor, and coma. Death is usually due to respiratory failure or cardiovascular collapse.

Treatment—*General:* Provide symptomatic and supportive treatment, as indicated. Any drug remaining in the stomach should be removed using appropriate procedures and caution to protect the airway and prevent aspiration, especially in the stuporous or comatose patient. Incomplete gastric emptying with delayed absorption of carisoprodol has been reported as a cause for relapse. Should respiration or blood pressure become compromised, respiratory assistance, central nervous system stimulants, and pressor agents should be administered cautiously, as indicated.

Carisoprodol: The following have been used successfully in overdosage with the related drug meprobamate: diuretics, osmotic (mannitol) diuresis, peritoneal dialysis, and hemodialysis (see CLINICAL PHARMACOLOGY). Careful monitoring of urinary output is necessary and caution should be taken to avoid overhydration. Carisoprodol can be measured in biological fluid by gas chromatography (Douglas, J.F., et al: *J Pharm Sci* 58: 145, 1969).

Aspirin—Since there are no specific antidotes for salicylate poisoning, the aim of treatment is to enhance elimination of salicylate and prevent or

Continued on page 2169

Memorandum

Wallace—Cont.

reduce further absorption; to correct any fluid electrolyte or metabolic imbalance; and to provide general and cardiorespiratory support. If acidosis is present, intravenous sodium bicarbonate must be given, along with adequate hydration, until salicylate levels decrease to within the therapeutic range. To enhance elimination, forced diuresis and alkalinization of the urine may be beneficial. The need for hemoperfusion or hemodialysis is rare and should be used only when other measures have failed.

Dosage and Administration—*Usual Adult Dosage:* 1 or 2 tablets, four times daily.
Not recommended for use in children under age twelve (see PRECAUTIONS).

How Supplied: 'Soma' Compound Tablets: In bottles of 100 (NDC 0037-2103-01) and 500 (NDC 0037-2103-03) and Unit dose packages of 100 (NDC 0037-2103-85).

Storage: Store at room temperature. Keep bottle
Rev.12/83

WALLACE LABORATORIES
Division of
CARTER-WALLACE, INC.
Cranbury, New Jersey 08512

Shown in Product Identification Section, page 442

SOMA® COMPOUND with CODEINE
(carisoprodol 200 mg + aspirin 325 mg + codeine phosphate 16 mg—
Warning: May be habit-forming)
Tablets

Description: 'Soma' Compound with Codeine is a combination product containing carisprodol, a centrally-acting muscle relaxant, plus aspirin, an analgesic with antipyretic and anti-inflammatory properties and codeine phosphate, a centrally-acting narcotic analgesic. It is available as a two-layered, white and yellow, oval shaped tablet for oral administration. Each tablet contains carisoprodol 200 mg, aspirin 325 mg, and codeine phosphate 16 mg. Chemically, carisoprodol is N-isopropyl-2-methyl-2-propyl-1,3-propanediol dicarbamate. Its empirical formula is $C_{12}H_{24}N_2O_4$ with a molecular weight of 260.33

Clinical Pharmacology:

Carisoprodol: Carisoprodol is a centrally-acting muscle relaxant that does not directly relax tense skeletal muscles in man. The mode of action of carisoprodol in relieving acute muscle spasm of local origin has not been clearly identified, but may be related to its sedative properties. In animals, carisoprodol has been shown to produce muscle relaxation by blocking interneuronal activity and depressing transmission of polysynaptic neurons in the spinal cord and in the descending reticular formation of the brain. The onset of action is rapid and lasts four to six hours.

Carisoprodol is metabolized in the liver and is excreted by the kidneys. It is dialyzable by peritoneal and hemodialysis.

Aspirin: Aspirin is a non-narcotic analgesic with anti-inflammatory and antipyretic activity. Inhibition of prostaglandin biosynthesis appears to account for most of its anti-inflammatory and for at least part of this analgesic and antipyretic properties.

Aspirin is rapidly absorbed and almost totally hydrolyzed to salicylic acid following oral administration. Although aspirin has a half-life of only about 15 minutes, the apparent biologic half-life of salicylic acid in the therapeutic plasma concentration range is between 6 and 12 hours. Salicylic acid is eliminated by renal excretion and by biotransformation to inactive metabolite. Clearance of salicylic acid in the high-dose range is sensitive to urinary pH (see **Drug Interactions**) and is reduced by renal dysfunction.

Codeine Phosphate: Codeine phosphate is a centrally-acting narcotic-analgesic. Its actions are qualitatively similar to morphine, but its potency is substantially less.

Clinical studies have shown that combining aspirin and codeine produces a significant additive effect in analgesic efficacy.

Indications and Usage: 'Soma' Compound with Codeine is indicated as an adjunct to rest, physical therapy, and other measures for relief of pain, muscle spasm, and limited mobility associated with acute, painful musculoskeletal conditions when the additional action of codeine is desired.

Contraindications: Acute intermittent porphyria; bleeding disorders; allergic or idiosyncratic reactions to carisoprodol, aspirin, codeine, or related compounds.

Warnings: On very rare occasions, the first dose of carisoprodol has been followed by idiosyncratic reactions with symptoms appearing within minutes or hours. These may include extreme weakness, transient quadriplegia, dizziness, ataxia, temporary loss of vision, diplopia, mydriasis, agitation, euphoria, confusion, and disorientation. Although symptoms usually subside over the course of the next several hours, discontinue 'Soma' Compound with Codeine and initiate appropriate supportive and symptomatic therapy, which may include epinephrine and/or antihistamines. In severe cases, corticosteroids may be necessary. Severe reactions have been manifested by asthmatic episodes, fever, weakness, dizziness, angioneurotic edema, smarting eyes, hypotension, and anaphylactoid shock.

The effects of carisoprodol with agents such as alcohol, other CNS depressants, or psychotropic drugs may be additive. Appropriate caution should be exercised with patients who take one or more of these agents simultaneously with 'Soma' Compound with Codeine.

Precautions:

General: To avoid excessive accumulation of carisoprodol, aspirin, or their metabolites, use 'Soma' Compound with Codeine with caution in patients with compromised liver or kidney function, or in elderly or debilitated patients (see CLINICAL PHARMACOLOGY.)

Use with caution in patients with history of gastritis or peptic ulcer, in patients on anticoagulant therapy, and in addiction-prone individuals.

Information for Patients: Caution patients that this drug may impair the mental and/or physical abilities required for the performance of potentially hazardous tasks such as driving a motor vehicle or operating machinery.

Caution patients with a predisposition for gastrointestinal bleeding that concomitant use of aspirin and alcohol may have an additive effect in this regard.

Caution patients that dosage of medications used for gout, arthritis, or diabetes may have to be adjusted when aspirin is administered or discontinued (see **Drug Interactions**).

Drug Interactions: Clinically important interactions may occur when certain drugs are administered concomitantly with aspirin or aspirin-containing drugs.

1. *Oral anticoagulants*—By interfering with platelet function or decreasing plasma prothrombin concentration, aspirin enhances the potential for bleeding in patients on anticoagulants.
2. *Methotrexate*—aspirin enhances the toxic effects of this drug.
3. *Probenecid and Sulfinpyrazone*—large doses of aspirin reduce the uricosuric effect of both drugs. Renal excretion of salicylate may also be reduced.
4. *Oral Antidiabetic Drugs*—enhancement of hypoglycemia may occur.
5. *Antacids*—to the extent that they raise urinary pH, antacids may substantially decrease plasma salicylate concentrations; conversely, their withdrawal can result in a substantial increase.
6. *Ammonium Chloride*—this and other drugs that acidify a relatively alkaline urine can elevate plasma salicylate concentrations.
7. *Ethyl Alcohol*—enhanced aspirin-induced fecal blood loss has been reported.
8. *Corticosteroids*—salicylate plasma levels may be decreased when adrenal corticosteroids are given, and may be increased substantially when they are discontinued.

Carcinogenesis, Mutagenesis, Impairment of Fertility: No long-term studies have been done with 'Soma' Compound with Codeine.

Pregnancy—Teratogenic Effects: Pregnancy Category C. Adequate animal reproduction studies have not been conducted with 'Soma' Compound with Codeine. It is also not known whether 'Soma' Compound with Codeine can cause fetal harm when administered to a pregnant woman or can affect reproduction capacity. 'Soma' Compound with Codeine should be given to a pregnant woman only if clearly needed.

Studies in rodents have shown salicylates to be teratogenic when given in early gestation, and embryocidal when given in later gestation in doses considerably greater than usual therapeutic doses in humans. Studies in women who took aspirin during pregnancy have not demonstrated an increased incidence of congenital abnormalities in the offspring.

Labor and Delivery: Ingestion of aspirin near term or prior to delivery may prolong delivery or lead to bleeding in mother, fetus, or neonate.

Nursing Mothers: Carisoprodol is excreted in human milk in concentrations two-to-four times that in maternal plasma. Aspirin is excreted in human milk in moderate amounts and can produce a bleeding tendency in nursing infants. Because of the potential for serious adverse reactions in nursing infants, a decision should be made whether to discontinue nursing or the drug, taking into account the importance of the drug to the mother.

Pediatric Use: Safety and effectiveness in children below the age of twelve have not been established.

Adverse Reactions: If severe reactions occur, discontinue 'Soma' Compound with Codeine and initiate appropriate symptomatic and supportive therapy.

The following side effects which have occurred with the administration of the individual ingredients alone may also occur with the combination.

Carisoprodol: Central Nervous System—Drowsiness is the most frequent complaint and along with other CNS effects may require dosage reduction. Observed less frequently are dizziness, vertigo and ataxia. Tremor, agitation, irritability, headache, depressive reactions, syncope, and insomina have been infrequent or rare.

Idiosyncratic—Idiosyncratic reactions are very rare. They are usually seen within the period of the first to fourth dose in patients having had no previous contact with the drug (see WARNINGS).

Allergic—Skin rash, erythema multiforme, pruritus, eosinophilia, and fixed drug eruptions with cross-reaction to meprobamate have been reported. If allergic reactions occur, discontinue 'Soma' Compound with Codeine and treat symptomatically. In evaluating possible allergic rections, also consider allergy to excipients (information on excipients is available to physicians on request).

Cardiovascular—Tachycardia, postural hypotension, and facial flushing.

Gastrointestinal—nausea, vomiting, epigastric distress and hiccup.

Hematological—No serious blood dyscrasias have been attributed to carisoprodol alone. Leukopenia and pancytopenia have been reported, very rarely, in situations in which other drugs or viral infections may have been responsible.

Aspirin: The most common adverse reactions associated with the use of aspirin have been gastrointestinal, including nausea, vomiting, gastritis, occult bleeding, constipation and diarrhea. Gastric erosion, angioedema, asthma, rash, pruritus and urticaria have been reported less commonly. Tinnitus is a sign of high serum salicylate levels (see OVERDOSAGE).

Aspirin Intolerance—Allergic type reactions in aspirin-sensitive indiviuals may involve the respiratory tract or the skin. Symptoms of the former range from rhinorrhea and shortness of breath to severe asthma, and the latter may consist of urticaria, edema, rash, or angioedema (giant hives). These may occur independently or in combination.

Codeine Phosphate: Nausea, vomiting, constipation, miosis, sedation, and dizziness have been reported.

Drug Abuse and Dependence:

Controlled Substance: Schedule C-III (see PRECAUTIONS).

Wallace—Cont.

Abuse: In clincal use, abuse has been rare.
Dependence: In clinical use, dependence with 'Soma' Compound with Codeine has been rare and there have been no reports of significant abstinence signs. Nevertheless, the following information on the indiviual ingredients should be kept in mind.
Carisoprodol—In dogs, no withdrawal symptoms occurred after abrupt cessation of carisoprodol from dosages as high as 1 gm/kg/day. In a study in man, abrupt cessation of 100 mg/kg/day (about five times the recommended daily adult dosage) was followed in some subjects by mild withdrawal symptoms such as abdominal cramps, insomnia, chills, headache, and nausea. Delirium and convulsions did not occur (see PRECAUTIONS).
Codeine Phosphate—Drug dependence of the morphine type may result.

Overdosage:
Signs and Symptoms: Any of the following which have been reported with the individual ingredients may occur and may be modified to a varying degree by the effects of the other ingredients present in 'Soma' Compound with Codeine.
Carisoprodol—Stupor, coma, shock, respiratory depression and, very rarely, death. Overdosage with carisoprodol in combination with alcohol, other CNS depressants, or psychotropic agents can have additive effects, even when one of the agents has been taken in the usually recommended dosage.
Aspirin—headache, tinnitus, hearing difficulty, dim vision, dizziness, lassitude, hyperpnea, rapid breathing, thirst, nausea, vomiting, sweating and occasionally diarrhea are characteristic of mild to moderate salicylate poisoning. Salicylate poisoning should be considered in children with symptoms of vomiting, hyperpnea, and hyperthermia. Hyperpnea is an early sign of salicylate poisoning, but dyspnea supervenes at plasma levels above 50 mg/dl. These respiratory changes eventually lead to serious acid-base disturbances. Metabolic acidosis is a constant finding in infants but occurs in older children only with severe poisoning; adults usually exhibit respiratory alkalosis initially and acidosis terminally.
Other symptoms of severe salicylate poisoning include hyperthermia, dehydration, delirium, and mental disturbances. Skin eruptions, GI hemorrhage, or pulmonary edema are less common. Early CNS stimulation is replaced by increasing depression, stupor, and coma. Death is usually due to respiratory failure or cardiovascular collapse.
Codeine Phosphate—pinpoint pupils, CNS depression, coma, respiratory depression, and shock.
Treatment: General:—Provide symptomatic and supportive treatment, as indicated. Any drug remaining in the stomach should be removed using appropriate procedures and caution to protect the airway and prevent aspiration, especially in the stuporous or comatose patient. Incomplete gastric emptying with delayed absorption of carisoprodol has been reported as a cause for relapse. Should respiration or blood pressure become compromised, respiratory assistance, central nervous system stimulants, and pressor agents should be administered cautiously, as indicated.
Carisoprodol—The following have been used successfully in overdosage with the related drug meprobamate: diuretics, osmotic (mannitol) diuresis, peritoneal dialysis, and hemodialysis (see CLINICAL PHARMACOLOGY). Careful monitoring of urinary output is necessary and caution should be taken to avoid overhydration. Carisoprodol can be measured in biological fluid by gas chromatography (Douglas, J.F., et al: *J Pharm Sci* 58:145, 1969).
Aspirin—Since there are no specific antidotes for salicylate poisoning, the aim of treatment is to enhance elimination of salicylate and prevent or reduce further absorption; to correct any fluid electrolyte and metabolic imbalance; and to provide general and cardiorespiratory support. If acidosis is present, intravenous sodium bicarbonate must be given, along with adequate hydration, until salicylate levels decrease to within the therapeutic range. To enhance elimination, forced diuresis and alkalinization of the urine may be beneficial. The need for hemoperfusion or hemodialysis is rare and should be used only when other measures have failed.
Codeine Phosphate—Narcotic antagonists, such as nalorphine and levallorphan, may be indicated.
Dosage and Administration:
Usual Adult Dosage: 1 or 2 tablets, four times daily.
Not recommended for use in children under age twelve.
How Supplied: 'Soma' Compound with Codeine Tablets: In bottles of 100 (NDC 0037-2403-01).
Storage: Store at room temperature; avoid excessive heat and prolonged light exposure. Keep bottle tightly closed.

Rev. 10/83
Shown in Product Identification Section, page 442

THEO–ORGANIDIN®
Elixir

Description: Theo-Organidin is a bronchodilator/mucolytic-expectorant combination available for oral administration as an *Elixir*. Each 15 ml (tablespoonful) contains theophylline (anhydrous), 120 mg; Organidin® (iodinated glycerol), 30 mg (15 mg organically bound iodine); and alcohol, 15% by volume.
Clinical Pharmacology: Theo-Organidin combines the bronchodilator effects of theophylline, a xanthine derivative, and the mucolytic-expectorant action of Organidin. Therapeutic blood levels of theophylline are reached in approximately 15 minutes and peak blood levels in one hour.
Indications and Usage: Theo-Organidin is indicated for symptomatic treatment in bronchial asthma and other bronchospastic conditions such as bronchitis, bronchiolitis, and pulmonary emphysema; for the relief of wheezing and respiratory distress due to reversible bronchospasm and tenacious mucous secretions; and for daily maintenance therapy of patients with bronchial asthma and other chronic bronchospastic pulmonary disorders.
Contraindications: History of marked sensitivity to inorganic iodides; hypersensitivity to any of the ingredients or related compounds; pregnancy; newborns; and nursing mothers.
The human fetal thyroid begins to concentrate iodine in the 12th to 14th week of gestation and the use of inorganic iodides in pregnant women during this period and thereafter has rarely been reported to induce fetal goiter (with or without hypothyroidism) with the potential for airway obstruction. If the patient becomes pregnant while taking Theo-Organidin, the drug should be discontinued and the patient should be apprised of the potential risk to the fetus.
Warnings: Discontinue use if rash or other evidence of hypersensitivity appears. Use with caution or avoid use in patients with history or evidence of thyroid disease. Do not exceed recommended dosage. Do not administer more often than every 6 hours or within 12 hours after rectal administration of any preparation containing theophylline or aminophylline. Use with caution or avoid use with other xanthine derivatives or CNS stimulants.
Precautions:
General—Children have been know to exhibit marked sensitivity to the CNS stimulant action of the xanthines. Toxic synergism (i.e., CNS stimulation) may occur with other sympathomimetic bronchodilator agents, particularly in children. Iodides have been reported to cause a flare-up of adolescent acne. Children with cystic fibrosis appear to have an exaggerated susceptibility to the goitrogenic effects of iodides.
Dermatitis and other reversible manifestations of iodism have been reported with chronic use of inorganic iodides. Although these have not been reported to be a problem clinically with Organidin formulations, they should be kept in mind in patients receiving these preparations for prolonged periods.
Drug Interactions—Iodides may potentiate the hypothyroid effect of lithium and other antithyroid drugs.
Carcinogenesis, Mutagenesis, Impairment of Fertility—No long-term animal studies have been performed with Theo-Organidin.
Pregnancy—Teratogenic Effects: Pregnancy Category X (see CONTRAINDICATIONS).
Nursing Mothers—Theo-Organidin should not be administered to a nursing woman.
Adverse Reactions: Side effects sometimes seen with individual ingredients may occur and may be modified as a result of their combination. *Theophylline*—Gastric irritation, nausea, and vomiting may occur; these can be minimized by taking Theo-Organidin after meals. Palpitations and mild central nervous system stimulation (e.g., restlessness, sleeplessness) have been reported, particularly in children. *Organidin*—Reports of gastrointestinal irritation, rash, hypersensitivity, thyroid enlargement, and acute parotitis have been rare.
Overdosage: There have been no reports of any serious problems from overdosage with Theo-Organidin. However, overdosage with theophylline has been reported and the following may be expected if overdosage with Theo-Organidin should occur:
Signs and Symptoms—Toxic overdosage with theophylline may produce severe gastrointestinal adverse effects including nausea, vomiting, epigastric pain, hematemesis and diarrhea; CNS effects including insomnia, headache, irritability, restlessness, severe agitation and convulsions; cardiovascular effects including hypotension, circulatory failure, and life-threatening arrhythmias; renal effects including diuresis and hypokalemia; and respiratory arrest. Serious toxicity leading to seizures and death can occur with serum concentrations of 40 mcg/ml or more.
Treatment—There is no specific antidote for theophylline toxicity. Discontinue drug immediately. Avoid sympathomimetic agents. Emetics and gastric lavage may be of value. Provide general supportive measures to prevent hypotension, overcome hydration, and maintain adequate ventilation. Hemodialysis with the use of resin or charcoal hemoperfusion may be helpful in reducing theophylline serum levels.
Dosage and Administration: Do not exceed recommended dosage. Acute attacks of asthma can usually be terminated fairly rapidly with the recommended dosage of Theo-Organidin; but in severe attacks, or when initiating treatment, the dose may be increased by $\frac{1}{2}$ for up to 24 hours. The need for intravenous aminophylline and/or other regimens should also be considered in the management of severe episodes.
Usual Adult Dosage: For maintenance therapy: 1–2 tablespoonfuls 3 times a day (every 6–8 hours). *For the acute asthmatic attack:* 3 tablespoonfuls initially, then reduce to maintenance dosage.
Children: 1 teaspoonful per 20 lbs. (9 kg) body weight, 2–3 times daily. Children over 99 lbs (45 kg) may require adult dosage.
How Supplied: *Theo-Organidin Elixir*—clear amber liquid, in bottles of one pint (NDC 0037-4611-10) and one gallon (NDC 0037-4611-20).
Storage: Store at room temperature; avoid excessive heat; protect from freezing. Keep bottle tightly closed.

Distributed by
WALLACE LABORATORIES
Division of CARTER-WALLACE, INC.
Cranbury, New Jersey 08512
Manufactured by
Denver Chemical (Puerto Rico), Inc.
Humacao, Puerto Rico 00661

Rev. 2/80
Shown in Product Identification Section, page 442

TUSSI-ORGANIDIN® ℞
C-V/TUSSI-ORGANIDIN® DM
Liquid

Description: *Tussi-Organidin* and *Tussi-Organidin DM* are antitussive/mucolytic-expectorant combinations available for oral administration as a *Liquid*. *Tussi-Organidin*—Each 5 ml (teaspoonful) contains: Organidin® (iodinated glycerol), 30 mg (15 mg organically bound iodine); and codeine phosphate (*Warning:* May be habit-forming), 10 mg.

Tussi-Organidin DM—Each 5 ml (teaspoonful) contains: Organidin (iodinated glycerol), 30 mg (15 mg organically bound iodine); dextromethorphan hydrobromide, 10 mg.

Clinical Pharmacology: *Tussi-Organidin* combines the antitussive action of codeine with the mucolytic-expectorant action of Organidin.

Tussi-Organidin DM combines the non-narcotic antitussive action of dextromethorphan with the mucolytic-expectorant action of Organidin.

Indications and Usage: *Tussi-Organidin* and *Tussi-Organidin DM* are indicated for the symptomatic relief of irritating, nonproductive cough associated with respiratory tract conditions such as chronic bronchitis, bronchial asthma, tracheobronchitis, and the common cold; also for the symptomatic relief of cough accompanying other respiratory tract conditions such as laryngitis, pharyngitis, croup, pertussis and emphysema. Appropriate therapy should be provided for the primary disease.

Contraindications: History of marked sensitivity to inorganic iodides; hypersensitivity to any of the ingredients or related compounds; pregnancy; newborns; and nursing mothers.

The human fetal thyroid begins to concentrate iodine in the 12th to 14th week of gestation and the use of inorganic iodides in pregnant women during this period and thereafter has rarely been reported to induce fetal goiter (with or without hypothyroidism) with the potential for airway obstruction. If the patient becomes pregnant while taking any of these products, the drug should be discontinued and the patient should be apprised of the potential risk to the fetus.

Warnings: Discontinue use if rash or other evidence of hypersensitivity appears. Use with caution or avoid use in patients with history or evidence of thyroid disease.

Precautions: *General*—Iodides have been reported to cause a flare-up of adolescent acne. Children with cystic fibrosis appear to have an exaggerated susceptibility to the goitrogenic effects of iodides.

Dermatitis and other reversible manifestations of iodism have been reported with chronic use of inorganic iodides. Although these have not been a problem clinically with Organidin formulations, they should be kept in mind in patients receiving these preparations for prolonged periods.

Drug Interactions—Iodides may potentiate the hypothyroid effect of lithium and other antithyroid drugs.

Carcinogenesis, Mutagenesis, Impairment of Fertility—No long-term animal studies have been performed with Tussi-Organidin or Tussi-Organidin DM.

Pregnancy—Teratogenic effects: Pregnancy Category X (see CONTRAINDICATIONS).

Nursing Mothers—Tussi-Organidin or Tussi-Organidin DM should not be administered to a nursing woman.

Adverse Reactions: Side effects with Tussi-Organidin and Tussi-Organidin DM have been rare, including those which may occur with the individual ingredients and which may be modified as a result of their combination:

Organidin—Rare side effects include gastrointestinal irritation, rash, hypersensitivity, thyroid gland enlargement, and acute parotitis.

Codeine—(Tussi-Organidin only): Nausea, vomiting, constipation, drowsiness, dizziness, and miosis have been reported.

Dextromethorphan—(Tussi-Organidin DM only): Rarely produces drowsiness or gastrointestinal disturbances.

Drug Abuse and Dependence (*Tussi-Organidin only*):
Controlled Substance—Schedule V.
Dependence—Codeine may be habit-forming.

Overdosage: There have been no reports of any serious problems from overdosage with Tussi-Organidin nor Tussi-Organidin DM.

Dosage and Administration:
Adults: 1 to 2 teaspoonfuls every 4 hours.
Children: ½ to 1 teaspoonful every 4 hours.

How Supplied: *Tussi-Organidin Liquid*—clear red liquid, in bottles of one pint (NDC 0037-4811-10) and one gallon (NDC 0037-4811-20).

Tussi-Organidin DM Liquid—clear yellow liquid, in bottles of one pint (NDC 0037-4712-10) and one gallon (NDC 0037-4712-20).

Storage: Store at room temperature; avoid excessive heat. Keep bottle tightly closed.

Distributed by
WALLACE LABORATORIES
Division of
CARTER-WALLACE, INC.
Cranbury, New Jersey 08512
Manufactured by
Denver Chemical (Puerto Rico) Inc.
Humacao, Puerto Rico 00661
Rev. 4/84
Shown in Product Identification Section, page 442

VōSoL® Otic Solution ℞
(acetic acid-nonaqueous 2%)

VōSoL® HC Otic Solution ℞
(hydrocortisone 1%, acetic acid–nonaqueous 2%)

Description: VōSoL is a nonaqueous solution of acetic acid (2%), in a propylene glycol vehicle containing propylene glycol diacetate (3%), benzethonium chloride (0.02%), and sodium acetate (0.015%).

VōSoL HC also contains hydrocortisone (1%) and citric acid (0.2%).

Actions: VōSoL is antibacterial, antifungal, and hydrophilic; it has an acid pH and a low surface tension.

VōSoL HC is, in addition, anti-inflammatory and anti-pruritic.

Indications: VōSoL: For the treatment of superficial infections of the external auditory canal caused by organisms susceptible to the action of the antimicrobial.

VōSol HC: For the treatment of superficial infections of the external auditory canal caused by organisms susceptible to the action of the antimicrobial, complicated by inflammation.

Contraindications: These products are contraindicated in those individuals who have shown hypersensitivity to any of their components; perforated tympanic membranes are frequently considered a contraindication to the use of external ear canal medication. VōSoL HC is contraindicated in vaccinia and varicella.

Precautions: VōSol and VōSol HC: If sensitization or irritation occurs, medication should be discontinued promptly.

VōSoL HC : As safety of topical steroids during pregnancy has not been confirmed, they should not be used for an extended period during pregnancy. Systemic side effects may occur with extensive use of topical steroids.

Dosage and Administration: Carefully remove all cerumen and debris to allow VōSoL (or VōSoL HC) to contact infected surfaces immediately. To promote continuous contact, insert a VōSoL (or VōSoL HC) saturated cotton wick in the ear with instructions to the patient to keep wick moist for the next 24 hours by occasionally adding a few drops on the wick. Remove wick after first 24 hours and continue to instill 5 drops of VōSoL (or VōSoL HC) three or four times daily thereafter.

How Supplied: VōSoL Otic Solution, in 15 ml (NDC 0037-3611-10) and 30 ml (NDC 0037-3611-30) measured-drop, safety-tip plastic bottles.

VōSoL HC Otic Solution, in 10 ml measured-drop, safety-tip plastic bottle (NDC 0037-3811-12).

Distributed by
WALLACE LABORATORIES
Division of
CARTER-WALLACE, INC.
Cranbury, New Jersey 08512
Manufactured by
Denver Chemical (Puerto Rico), Inc.
Humacao, Puerto Rico 00661
Rev. 2/83
Shown in Product Identification Section, page 442

Webcon Pharmaceuticals
Division of
ALCON (Puerto Rico) INC.
P.O. BOX 1629
FORT WORTH, TX 76101

SUPPRETTES®, Webcon's identifying trademark for suppository medication in the NEOCERA® BASE, a unique blend of water-soluble Carbowaxes* that release drugs by hydrophilic action.
*TM Union Carbide.

ANESTACON® ℞
[*ăne'stăcon*]
(2% lidocaine hydrochloride viscous solution for topical use)

Description: A sterile anesthetic for endo-urethral use. Each ml contains: Active: Lidocaine Hydrochloride 20 mg (2%). Vehicle: Hydroxypropyl Methylcellulose 10 mg (1%). Preservative: Benzalkonium Chloride 0.1 mg (0.01%). Inactive: Sodium Chloride, Hydrochloric Acid and/or Sodium Hydroxide (to adjust pH), Purified Water.

Clinical Pharmacology: Lidocaine HCl acts on surface mucous membranes of the urethra to produce local anesthesia by altering the permeability of the nerve cell membrane to sodium and potassium ions, resulting in an increased threshold for electrical excitability and a decreased conduction of impulses whereby depolarization and ion exchanges are inhibited. The anesthetic effect usually begins within two to five minutes and lasts for at least 30 minutes.

Lidocaine is metabolized mainly in the liver and excreted via the kidneys. Approximately 90% of lidocaine administered is excreted in the form of various metabolites, while less than 10% is excreted unchanged.

Indications and Usage: For prevention and control of pain in procedures involving the male and female urethra and for topical treatment of painful urethritis.

Contraindications: Contraindicated in patients with a known sensitivity (allergy) to lidocaine or other drugs of a similar chemical nature, or to other components of the formulation.

Warnings: RESUSCITATIVE EQUIPMENT AND DRUGS SHOULD BE IMMEDIATELY AVAILABLE WHEN ANY LOCAL ANESTHETIC IS USED. Lidocaine should be used with extreme caution on traumatized mucosa or in a region of sepsis.

NOTE: After initial use of the 15 ml single dose container, the remaining contents of the container should be discarded. The 240 ml container should be used for only an individual patient. See CAUTION under DOSAGE AND ADMINISTRATION.

Precautions: The smallest volume that will produce effective anesthesia is recommended, and caution should be exercised to avoid overdosage. The safety and effectiveness are dependent on proper dosage, correct technique, adequate precautions, and readiness for emergencies. The debilitated, elderly, acutely ill, and children should be given reduced doses commensurate with their age and physical condition. Use cautiously in persons with known drug sensitivities or allergies.

PREGNANCY CATEGORY C: Animal reproduction studies have not been conducted with Anestacon®. It is also not known whether Anestacon can

Continued on next page

Webcon—Cont.

cause fetal harm when administered to a pregnant woman or can affect reproduction capacity. Anestacon should be administered to a pregnant woman only if clearly needed.

NURSING MOTHERS: It is not known whether this drug is excreted in human milk. Because many drugs are excreted in human milk, caution should be exercised when Anestacon is administered to a nursing mother.

Adverse Reactions: Adverse reactions result from high plasma levels due to excessive dosage, rapid absorption, or inadvertent intravascular injection. Hypersensitivity, idiosyncrasy, or diminished tolerance may also be the cause of reactions. Reactions due to overdosage (high plasma levels) are systemic and involve the central nervous system and the cardiovascular system.

Reactions involving the central nervous system are characterized by excitation and/or depression. Nervousness, dizziness, blurred vision or tremors may occur, followed by convulsions, unconsciousness, drowsiness, and possible respiratory arrest. Excitement may be transient or absent, and the first manifestations may be drowsiness, merging into unconsciousness and respiratory arrest.

Reactions involving the cardiovascular system include depression of the myocardium, hypotension, bradycardia, and even cardiac arrest. Treatment of a patient with toxic manifestations consists of maintaining an airway, and supporting ventilation using oxygen and assisted or controlled respiration as required. Supportive treatment of the cardiovascular system consists of using vasopressors, preferably those that stimulate the myocardium (e.g. ephedrine, metaraminol, etc.) and intravenous fluids. Convulsions may be controlled by the intravenous administration in small increments of an ultra-short-acting barbiturate (i.e. thiopental, thiamylal) or a short-acting muscle relaxant (succinylcholine), together with oxygen. Muscle relaxants and intravenous barbiturates should only be used by those familiar with their use.

Allergic reactions are characterized by cutaneous lesions of delayed onset, urticaria, edema, or other manifestations of allergy. The detection of sensitivity by skin testing is of doubtful value.

Dosage and Administration: Dosage varies and depends upon the area to be anesthetized, vascularity of the tissues, individual tolerance, and the technique of anesthesia. The least volume of the drug needed to provide effective anesthesia should be administered. For specific techniques and procedures refer to standard texts. THE USUAL DOSE SHOULD NOT EXCEED 600 mg or 30 ml IN ANY TWELVE HOUR PERIOD.

15 ML SINGLE-DOSE CONTAINER: ADULT MALES: Immediately before use, remove the label and cap and firmly insert the sterile tip into the urethral orifice. Slowly instill 5 ml to 15 ml by exerting pressure on opposite sides of the container - the full dose should be administered in a single action without removing the tip. While waiting two to five minutes for induction of anesthesia, the urethra should be occluded with a penile clamp or by manual compression. ADULT FEMALES: The sterile tip may be used to insert about 1 ml.

240 ml CONTAINER: Note: This is for use for an individual patient only. CAUTION: Care should be taken to prevent contamination of bottle contents (e.g., aspiration of urethral contents into the container when using insertion tip).

ADULT MALES: Instill slowly into the urethra 5 ml to 15 ml and allow two to five minutes for induction of anesthesia. The medication is retained in the urethra by means of a penile clamp or by manual compression of the distal urethra. ADULT FEMALES: Apply liberal amount of medication on a cotton swab and insert into urethra for two to five minutes, or a dropper may be employed to insert about 1 ml.

How Supplied: In 15 ml (NDC 0998-0300-10) and 240 ml multiple-dose (NDC 0998-0300-20) disposable containers for single patient use.

B & O SUPPRETTES®
No. 15A and No. 16A
(belladonna and opium rectal suppositories)

Description: Each B & O Suprette® contains (in water-soluble Neocera® Suppository Base for rectal administration):
B & O No. 15A: powdered opium* 30 mg (½ gr.) and powdered belladonna extract 16.2 mg (equivalent to 0.21 mg or 0.0035 gr. alkaloid of belladonna).
B & O No. 16A: powdered opium* 60 mg (1 gr.) and powdered belladonna extract 16.2 mg (equivalent to 0.21 mg or 0.0035 gr. alkaloid of belladonna).
Neocera® Base is a blend of polyethylene glycol 400, 1450, 8000 and Polysorbate 60. This drug falls into the pharmacological/therapeutic class of narcotic analgesic/antispasmodic agents.

The pharmacologically active principles present in the belladonna extract component of B & O Suprettes are Atropine and Scopolamine.

Opium contains more than a score of alkaloids, the principal ones being morphine (10%), narcotine (6%), papaverine (1%) and codeine (0.5%). The major pharmacologically active principle of the powdered opium component of B & O Suprettes, however, is morphine.

Clinical Pharmacology: Through its parasympatholytic action, atropine relaxes smooth muscle resulting from parasympathetic stimulation. It is the dl isomer of l-hyoscyamine and therefore exhibits the same clinical effects. It is, however, approximately one-half as active peripherally as l-hyoscyamine, the latter being the major active plant principle. The dl isomer atropine is formed during the process of isolation of the belladonna extract.[1]

Morphine, the major active principle of powdered opium, is responsible for the action of powdered opium although the other alkaloids present also contribute to it. The sedative and analgesic action of morphine, the effect desired by inclusion in B & O Suprettes of powdered opium, are thought to be due to its depressant effect on the cerebral cortex, hypothalamus and medullary centers. In large doses the opiates and their analogs also inhibit synaptic conduction in the spinothalamic tracts, depress the function of the reticular formation, the lemniscus and the thalamic relays, and inhibit spinal synaptic reflexes; but these inhibitor actions are not elicited with therapeutic doses of the drug. Moderate doses of powder opium do not alter the electroencephalogram.

The action of morphine consists mainly of a descending depression of the central nervous system. It exerts its analgesic action by increasing the pain threshold or the magnitude of stimulus required to evoke pain and by dulling the sensibility or reaction to pain. In addition to its action in abolishing pain, morphine induces a sense of well being (euphoria) facilitating certain mental processes while retarding others. Upon absorption of morphine, oxidative dealkylation to produce nor-compounds appears to be the first step in the reaction sequence which imparts analgesia. Morphine is conjugated in the liver to form the 3-glucuronide which passes into the bile and is reabsorbed and excreted in the urine.

The atropine effect of the belladonna extract serves to eliminate morphine induced smooth muscle spasm without affecting the sedative analgesic action of powdered opium.[2]

Indications and Usage: B & O Suprettes are used for the relief of moderate to severe pain associated with ureteral spasm not responsive to non-narcotic analgesics and to space intervals between injections of opiates.

Contraindications: Do not use B & O Suprettes in patients suffering from glaucoma, severe hepatic or renal disease, bronchial asthma, narcotic idiosyncrasies, respiratory depression, convulsive disorders, acute alcoholism, delirium tremens and premature labor.

*Warnings: True addiction may result from opium usage. These preparations are not recommended for use in children.

Precautions: Administer with caution to persons with a known idiosyncrasy to atropine or atropine-like compounds; to persons known to be sensitive to or addicted to morphine or morphine-like drugs; to persons with cardiac disease, incipient glaucoma or prostatic hypertrophy. Caution should be used in the administration of this drug to old and debilitated patients and patients with increased intracranial pressure, toxic psychosis and myxedema.

Pregnancy Category C. Animal studies have not been conducted with B & O Suprettes 15A and 16A. It is also not known whether B & O Suprettes 15A and 16A can affect reproduction capacity. The active principles of B & O Suprettes, atropine and morphine, are known to enter the fetal circulation. B & O Suprettes 15A and 16A therefore should be used by a pregnant woman with caution and only when clearly indicated.

Nursing Mothers: It is not known whether this drug is excreted in human milk. Because many drugs are excreted in human milk, caution should be exercised when B & O Suprettes are administered to a nursing woman.

Adverse Reactions: Belladonna may cause drowsiness, dry mouth, urinary retention, photophobia, rapid pulse, dizziness and blurred vision. Opium usage may result in constipation, nausea, vomiting. Pruritis and urticaria may occasionally occur.

Drug Abuse and Dependence: Because of their content of opium, B & O Suprettes 15A and 16A are considered as Schedule II drugs by the Drug Enforcement Agency. No data exists on chronic abuse effects or dependence characteristics of B & O Suprettes 15A and 16A.

Overdosage: As with morphine and related narcotics, overdosage is characterized by respiratory depression, pinpoint pupils and coma. Respiratory depression may be reversed by intravenous administration of naloxone hydrochloride or levallorphan tartrate. In addition, supportive measures such as oxygenation, intravenous fluids and vasopressors should be used as indicated.

Dosage and Administration: Adults: One B & O No. 15A or No. 16A Suprette rectally once or twice daily, or as recommended by the physician. Moisten finger and Suprette with water before inserting. Not recommended for use in children.

How Supplied: In strip packaged units of 12 (scored for ½ dosage). DEA order required (Schedule II).
B & O No. 15A NDC 0998-5015-75.
B & O No. 16A NDC 0998-5016-75.

References:
1. Grollman, A., and Grollman, E. F., Pharmacology and Therapeutics, 7th Edition, Lea and Febiger, Philadelphia, 1970, pp. 338 to 346.
2. Ibid., pp. 96 to 107.

CYSTOSPAZ®
(Hyoscyamine Tablets)
CYSTOSPAZ-M®
(Hyoscyamine Sulfate)

Description: CYSTOSPAZ® is a pale blue uncoated compressed tablet for oral administration. It contains the parasympatholytic agent hyoscyamine as the free base. Each tablet contains hyoscyamine 0.15 mg.
CYSTOSPAZ-M® is a light blue timed-release capsule containing hyoscyamine sulfate 0.375 mg.

Clinical Pharmacology: Through its parasympatholytic action, hyoscyamine relaxes smooth muscle spasm resulting from parasympathetic stimulation. It is the λ-isomer of atropine and therefore exhibits the same clinical effects as atropine. It is, however, approximately twice as active peripherally as atropine, since the latter is the racemic (dλ) form of hyoscyamine and d-hyoscyamine possesses only a very weak anticholinergic action. Since only one-half the atropine dose is required for λ-hyoscyamine it has only one-half the unwanted central effects of atropine.[1]

Indications and Usage: In the management of disorders of the lower urinary tract associated with hypermotility. Although specific therapy is often required to remove the underlying cause of spasm, Cystospaz and Cystospaz-M are offered as antispasmodic agent dosage forms which may be combined with other forms of therapy where indicated.

Contraindications: Glaucoma, urinary bladder neck or pyloric obstruction, duodenal obstruction and cardiospasm. Hypersensitivity to any of the ingredients.

Precautions: Administer with caution to persons with known idiosyncrasy to atropine-like compounds and to patients suffering cardiac disease.

Pregnancy Category C. Animal Reproduction studies have not been conducted with Cystospaz or Cystospaz-M. It is also not known whether Cystospaz or Cystospaz-M can cause fetal harm when administered to a pregnant woman or can affect reproduction capacity. Cystospaz and Cystospaz-M should be taken by a pregnant woman only if clearly needed.

Nursing Mothers: It is not known whether this drug is excreted in human milk. Because many drugs are excreted in human milk, caution should be exercised when Cystospaz or Cystospaz-M is administered to a nursing woman.

Adverse Reactions: Though rarely a problem, the side effects encountered with this class of antispasmodic-antisecretory agents (drowsiness, dryness of mouth, photophobia, constipation, urinary retention) may also be seen with this drug. If rapid pulse, dizziness or blurring of vision occurs, discontinue use immediately. Acute urinary retention may be precipitated in prostatic hypertrophy.

Note: Slight dryness of mouth is an indication that parasympathetic blockage is effective. The patient should be warned that this may occur.

Drug Abuse and Dependence: A dependence on the use of Cystospaz or Cystospaz-M has not been reported and due to the nature of its ingredients abuse of Cystospaz or Cystospaz-M is not expected.

Overdosage: Symptoms of overdosage include severe dryness of mouth and throat, dryness of skin, difficulty or inability to swallow, difficult speech, dilated pupils until iris almost disappears, restlessness and garrulity indicating an irritability of the brain, marked tremors, convulsions, respiratory failure, death.[2] In adults, symptoms of overdosage may be in the range of ingestion of 0.6 to 1 mg with doses exceeding 1–2 mg eliciting more profound toxicity.

Dosage and Administration:
Adults: Cystospaz®—One or two tablets four times daily or fewer if needed.
Cystospaz-M®—One capsule every twelve hours.
Older Children: Reduce dosage in proportion to age and weight.

How Supplied: Cystospaz — Bottles of 100 light blue tablets NDC 0998-2225-10. Tablets are imprinted with a "W 2225". Cystospaz-M—Bottles of 100 light blue timed-release capsules NDC 0998-2260-10. Capsules are identified with "W-2260" printed in black.

References:
1. Grollman, A. and Grollman, E. F.: *Pharmacology and Therapeutics*, 7th Edition, p. 346.
2. Ibid., p. 347.

URISED®

Description: URISED® is a purple, round, sugar coated tablet for oral administration. It is a combination of antiseptics (Methenamine, Methylene Blue, Phenyl Salicylate, Benzoic Acid) and parasympatholytics (Atropine Sulfate, Hyoscyamine).

Each tablet contains: Methenamine 40.8 mg, Phenyl Salicylate 18.1 mg, Methylene Blue 5.4 mg, Benzoic Acid 4.5 mg, Atropine Sulfate 0.03 mg and Hyoscyamine 0.03 mg.

Clinical Pharmacology: Methenamine itself does not have antiseptic, irritant, or toxic properties in the urine. Methenamine, in an acid urine (pH 6 or below) hydrolyzes into formaldehyde within the urinary tract providing mild antiseptic activity[1]. When given as directed and the daily urine volume is 1000 to 1500 ml, a daily dose of 2 grams will yield a urinary concentration of 18–60 mcg/ml of free formaldehyde in the urine. This is more than the minimal inhibitory dose of formaldehyde which must be available for most urinary tract pathogens. Methenamine is readily absorbed from the gastrointestinal tract and is rapidly excreted almost entirely in the urine. Methylene Blue and Benzoic Acid are mild but effective antiseptics which contribute to the antiseptic properties of Methenamine. Phenyl Salicylate is a mild analgesic and antipyretic with weak antiseptic activity. All of these compounds are readily absorbed from the gastrointestinal tract and excreted in the urine. Through parasympatholytic action, atropine and hyoscyamine relax smooth muscle spasm resulting from parasympathetic stimulation.[2]

Indications and Usage: URISED is indicated for the relief of discomfort of the lower urinary tract caused by hypermotility resulting from inflammation or diagnostic procedures and in the treatment of cystitis, urethritis, and trigonitis when caused by organisms which maintain or produce an acid urine and are susceptible to formaldehyde.

Contraindications: Glaucoma, urinary bladder neck obstruction, pyloric or duodenal obstruction, or cardiospasm. Hypersensitivity to any of the ingredients.

Warnings: Do not exceed recommended dose. Methenamine may combine with sulfonamides in the urine to give mutual antagonism and should not be used with sulfonamides.

Precautions: Administer with caution to persons with known idiosyncrasy to atropine-like compounds and to patients suffering from cardiac disease. Bacteriological studies of the urine may be helpful in following the patient response. Methylene Blue interferes with the analysis for some urinary components such as free formaldehyde. Drugs and/or foods which produce an alkaline urine should be restricted.[3]

Patient should be advised that the urine may become blue to blue-green and the feces may be discolored as a result of excretion of Methylene Blue. Methenamine preparations should not be given to patients taking sulfonamides since insoluble precipitates may form with formaldehyde in the urine. No known long-term animal studies have been performed to evaluate carcinogenic potential.

Pregnancy Category C. Animal reproduction studies have not been conducted with URISED® tablets. It is also not known whether URISED tablets can cause fetal harm when administered to a pregnant woman or can affect reproduction capacity. URISED tablets should be given to a pregnant woman only if clearly needed.

Nursing Mothers: It is not known whether this drug is excreted in human milk. Because many drugs are excreted in human milk, caution should be exercised when URISED tablets are administered to a nursing woman.

Adverse Reactions: If pronounced dryness of the mouth, flushing, or difficulty in initiating micturition occurs, decrease dosage. If rapid pulse, dizziness or blurring of vision occurs, discontinue use immediately. Acute urinary retention may be precipitated in prostatic hypertrophy.

Drug Abuse and Dependence: A dependence on the use of URISED has not been reported and due to the nature of its ingredients, abuse of URISED is not expected.

Overdosage: By exceeding the recommended dosage of URISED, symptomology related to the overdose of its individual active ingredients may be expected as follows:
Atropine Sulfate, Hyoscyamine: Symptoms associated with an overdose of URISED will most probably be manifested in the symptoms related to overdosage of the alkaloids Atropine Sulfate and Hyoscyamine. Such symptoms as dryness of mucous membranes; dilatation of pupils, hot, dry, flushed skin; hyperpyrexia, tachycardia palpatations; elevated blood pressure; coma; circulatory collapse and death from respiratory failure can occur due to overdosage of these alkaloids.
Methenamine: If large amounts of the drug (2-8 gm daily) are used over extended periods, (3-4 weeks), bladder and gastrointestinal irritation, painful and frequent micturition, albuminuria and gross hematuria may be expected.
Methylene Blue: Symptoms of Methylene Blue overdosage associated with the overdosage of URISED are not expected to be discernible from those associated with the other active ingredients in URISED.
Benzoic Acid: Symptoms of Benzoic Acid overdosage associated with the overdosage of URISED are not expected to be discernible from those associated with the other active ingredients in URISED.
Phenyl Salicylate: Symptoms of Phenyl Salicylate overdosage include burning pain in throat and mouth, white necrotic lesions in the mouth, abdominal pain, vomiting, bloody diarrhea, pallor, sweating, weakness, headache, dizziness and tinnitus. The symptoms, however, are not expected to be discernible from those associated with the other active ingredients in URISED.

Dosage and Administration: Adults: Two tablets four times daily.

Children (12 years and older): Reduce dosage in proportion to age and weight.

How Supplied: Bottles of 100 (NDC 0998-2183-10), 500 (NDC 0998-2183-20) and 1000 (NDC 0998-2183-30) tablets. Tablets are imprinted with a "W 2183".

References:
1. Stamey, T. A., *Urinary Infections*. Williams & Wilkins Co., Baltimore 1972.
2. Goodman, L. S. and Gilman, G., *The Pharmacological Basis of Therapeutics*, Sixth Edition, Macmillan Pub. Co. 121, 971, 1119 (1980).
3. *AMA Drug Evaluation*, Fifth Edition, 1745 (1983).

WANS®
(pyrilamine maleate and pentobarbital sodium)
ANTI-NAUSEA SUPPRETTES®

Description: WANS® is a combination of an antihistamine (Pyrilamine Maleate) and a sedative (Pentobarbital Sodium) in suppository form for rectal administration. Each WANS® SUPPRETTE® contains (in water-soluble Neocera® Base):

WANS® Children (blue): pyrilamine maleate 25 mg and pentobarbital sodium* 30 mg; scored for ½ dosage.

WANS® No. 1 (pink): pyrilamine maleate 50 mg and pentobarbital sodium* 50 mg; scored for ½ dosage.

WANS® No. 2 (yellow): pyrilamine maleate 50 mg and pentobarbital sodium* 100 mg; scored for ½ dosage.

*Warning: May be habit forming.

The Neocera Base is a blend of Polyethylene Glycol 400, 1450 and 8000, Polysorbate 60 and color additives including FD&C Yellow No. 5 (Tartrazine) in WANS No. 2.

Clinical Pharmacology: Pyrilamine maleate is an antihistamine of the ethylenediamine family, which exhibits recognized antiemetic activity. Pyrilamine maleate may exhibit a noticeable stimulating effect on the central nervous system (CNS) and, on occasion, a weak CNS-depressant effect. Pentobarbital sodium is an effective, short-acting barbiturate which acts as a general CNS-depressant. Pentobarbital sodium suppresses the vomiting center itself, and at the same time, provides sedation.

Indications and Usage: WANS® is indicated in the symptomatic treatment of nausea and vomiting. The suppository dosage form is a particularly useful method of drug administration in patients with nausea and vomiting who are unable to retain oral medication.

Continued on next page

Webcon—Cont.

Contraindications: Acute intermittent porphyria, known hypersensitivity to barbiturates or antihistamines, known barbiturate addiction, in senility, severe hepatic impairment, and in the presence of uncontrolled pain, acute head injury associated with vomiting or other signs of CNS injury. Not for use in infants under 6 months of age since they are more sensitive to the central nervous system stimulating effects of pyrilamine maleate than adults. Pyrilamine maleate may cause convulsions in infants, particularly in excessive dosage.

Warnings:

> Caution should be exercised when administering WANS® to children for the treatment of vomiting. Antiemetics are not recommended for treatment of uncomplicated vomiting in children and their use should be limited to prolonged vomiting of known etiology. There are three principal reasons for caution:
> 1. There have been some recent reports of toxic encephalopathy, characterized by a depressed level of consciousness, marked irritability and ataxia in infants and children following administration of higher-than-recommended doses of pyrilamine maleate and pentobarbital sodium combination products such as WANS®. **The recommended dosage should therefore not be exceeded.**
> 2. There has been some suspicion that centrally acting antiemetics may contribute, in combination with viral illnesses (a possible cause of vomiting in children), to development of Reye's syndrome, a potentially fatal acute childhood encephalopathy with visceral fatty degeneration, especially involving the liver. Although there is no confirmation of this suspicion, caution is nevertheless recommended.
> 3. It should also be noted that salicylates and acetaminophen are hepatotoxic at large doses. Although it is not known that at usual doses they would represent a hazard in patients with the underlying hepatic disorder of Reye's syndrome, these drugs should be avoided in children whose signs and symptoms could represent Reye's syndrome, unless alternative methods of controlling fever are not successful.

Barbiturates may be habit forming. Administration in the presence of pre-existing psychological disturbances may result in confusion, delirium, and accentuation of symptoms. Idiosyncratic reactions may occur and include lassitude, vertigo, nausea, vomiting, and diarrhea. Acquired sensitivity to barbiturates may result in allergic reactions including urticaria, dermatitis, and rarely, exfoliative dermatitis and degenerative changes in the liver and kidney.

Pentobarbital sodium may cause fetal harm when administered to a pregnant woman. Pentobarbital sodium can cross the placental barrier and may depress the fetal central nervous system so that respiration is not adequately established at birth. If this drug is used during pregnancy, or if the patient becomes pregnant while taking this drug, the patient should be apprised of the potential hazard to the fetus.

Precautions: General: WANS® should be administered with caution to patients with a history of drug dependence or suicidal tendencies. Caution should be exercised when the drug is used concurrently with other sedative, hypnotic, or narcotic agents. This drug should be given with caution to patients with known acute or chronic hepatic disease, fever, hyperthyroidism, diabetes mellitus, severe anemia, and congestive heart failure.

WANS® No. 2 contains FD&C Yellow No. 5 (tartrazine) which may cause allergic-type reactions (including bronchial asthma) in certain susceptible individuals. Although the overall incidence of sensitivity to FD&C Yellow No. 5 (tartrazine) in the general population is low, it is frequently seen in patients who also have aspirin hypersensitivity.

Information for Patients: Do not take alcoholic beverages or other CNS depressants while taking this product. This product may cause drowsiness. Do not drive, operate machinery, or otherwise engage in activities where impairment of alertness and coordination could result in accidents or injury.

Drug Interactions: Alcohol and other CNS depressants taken in conjunction with this product produce an additive depressant effect on the central nervous system. Patients taking other CNS depressants concomitantly with this product should be observed more frequently, especially during the initiation of therapy. Also, barbiturates and antihistamines must be used with caution in patients receiving monoamine oxidase inhibitors since these drugs may potentiate the depressant effect of the barbiturate or augment the anticholinergic effect of the antihistamine.

Carcinogenesis, Mutagenesis, Impairment of Fertility: Long-term studies in animals to evaluate the carcinogenic potential of this drug have not been performed. There is no evidence in the published literature that the ingredients of this product are carcinogenic, mutagenic, or impair fertility.

Pregnancy:
Teratogenic Effects: Pregnancy Category D. See "Warnings" section.
Non-Teratogenic Effects: Dependence of the mother on pentobarbital sodium may result in withdrawal symptoms (e.g., hyperirritability, vomiting, shrill cry) in the baby after delivery.

Nursing Mothers: Antihistamines may inhibit lactation and may be excreted in breast milk. Since the risk of adverse reactions is higher in infants, use of antihistamines is not recommended in nursing mothers. Barbiturates may also be excreted in breast milk. The effects of barbiturates in the nursing infant may include sedation and induction of hepatic metabolizing enzymes. Therefore, because of the potential for serious adverse reactions in nursing infants from the use of this product, a decision should be made whether to discontinue nursing or to discontinue the drug, taking into account the importance of the drug to the mother.

Pediatric Use: See "Contraindications" and "Warnings" sections for information regarding the use of this product in infants and children.

Adverse Reactions: Antihistamine side effects include drowsiness, potentiation of the sedative effect of barbiturates, fatigue, vertigo, incoordination, tremor, muscle weakness, dryness of the nose, mouth and throat, tinnitus, pupillary dilation and blurred vision, urinary retention, impotence, epigastric and intestinal pain, anorexia, nausea, vomiting, diarrhea, excitation, euphoria, insomnia, nervousness, palpitation, tachycardia, hypotension, hypersensitivity reactions such as allergic dermatitis, and rarely, blood dyscrasias. Side effects associated with barbiturates include drowsiness, lethargy, sedation, paradoxic restlessness or excitement in susceptible persons, respiratory depression, coma, and delirium.

Drug Abuse and Dependence:
Controlled Substance: WANS® is a Schedule III controlled drug.
Dependence: As with other CNS-depressants, the use of pentobarbital sodium may induce a psychological dependence in some patients. Prolonged, uninterrupted use of barbiturates, even in therapeutic doses, may result in physical and psychological dependence. The symptoms of chronic intoxication are similar to those of alcohol intoxication (e.g., disorientation, ataxia, euphoria). In such cases, abrupt discontinuance may precipitate typical withdrawal symptoms, including convulsions. Therefore, the drug should be withdrawn gradually.
Abuse: Those persons who develop a psychological dependence on pentobarbital sodium may increase the dosage without consulting a physician and may subsequently develop a physical dependence on the drug.

Overdosage: Antihistamine overdosage, particularly in children, may result in hallucination, excitement, ataxia, incoordination, athetosis, convulsions and death. Mechanical ventilation and supportive care are important, and drugs likely to potentiate the effects of the antihistamine should not be given.

Overdosage of pentobarbital sodium is manifested by drowsiness, lethargy, sedation, paradoxic restlessness or excitement in susceptible persons, respiratory depression, delirium, hypothermia, latent fever, sluggishness or absence of reflexes, coma, gradual appearance of circulatory collapse, pulmonary edema and death. Supportive care is of primary importance in the treatment of barbiturate overdosage.

1. Maintain and assist respiration as indicated.
2. Support circulation with vasopressors and intravenous fluids as required.
3. Aspirate stomach contents, taking care to avoid pulmonary aspiration.
4. Use osmotic diuretic and measure intake and output of fluids.

In severe overdosage, hemodialysis may be lifesaving, especially if a vigorous diuresis cannot be maintained.

Dosage and Administration:
Children: For children 2 to 12 years of age (over 15 kg bodyweight) the usual dose is one WANS® Children, rectally, every 6 to 8 hours as required. Do not exceed three doses in 24 hours. Children 6 months to 2 years of age (less than 15 kg bodyweight) should use not more than $\frac{1}{2}$ the above dosage. **Do not use in infants below the age of 6 months.** In determining the optimum dosage in infants and children, consideration should be given in each case to the age and weight of the patient, the etiology and severity of the condition being treated and the clinical response. **The above recommended dosages should not be exceeded (see "Warnings").**

Adults: Rectally, one WANS® No. 1 to inhibit mild nausea and/or vomiting or one WANS® No. 2 to control pernicious vomiting. Repeat doses for adults should be 4 to 6 hours apart; do not exceed four doses in 24 hours. The optimum dosage must be determined in each case by the clinical response. Moisten finger and SUPPRETTE® with water before inserting.

How Supplied: In foil strip packaged units of 12 (scored for $\frac{1}{2}$ dosage).
WANS® CHILDREN (blue): NDC 0998-1000-75
WANS® No. 1 (pink): NDC 0998-1001-75
WANS® No. 2 (yellow): NDC 0998-1002-75
Storage: Store at room temperature. Do not refrigerate.

Westwood Pharmaceuticals Inc.
100 FOREST AVENUE
BUFFALO, NY 14213

ALPHA KERI®
Therapeutic Shower and Bath Oil

Composition: Contains mineral oil, Hydroloc™ brand of Westwood's PEG-4 dilaurate, lanolin oil, fragrance, benzophenone-3, D&C green 6.

Action and Uses: ALPHA KERI is a water-dispersible, antipruritic oil for the care of dry skin. ALPHA KERI effectively deposits a thin, uniform, emulsified film of oil over the skin. This film helps relieve itching, lubricates and softens the skin. ALPHA KERI Shower and Bath Oil is an all-over skin moisturizer. Only Alpha Keri contains Hydroloc™ — the unique emulsifier that provides a more uniform distribution of the therapeutic oils to moisturize dry skin. ALPHA KERI is valuable as an aid in the treatment of dry, pruritic skin and mild skin irritations such as chronic atopic dermatitis; pruritus senilis and hiemalis; contact dermatitis; "bath-itch"; xerosis or asteatosis; ichthyosis; soap dermatitis; psoriasis.

Administration and Dosage: ALPHA KERI *should always be used with water, either added to water or rubbed on to wet skin.* Because of its inher-

ent cleansing properties it is not necessary to use soap when ALPHA KERI is being used.
For exact dosage, label directions should be followed.
BATH: Added as directed to bathtub of water. For optimum relief: 10 to 20 minute soak.
SHOWER: Dispense a small amount into hand and rub on to wet skin. Rinse as desired and pat dry.
SPONGE BATH: Added as directed to a basin of warm water then rubbed over entire body with washcloth.
SITZ BATH: Added as directed to tub water. Soak should last for 10 to 20 minutes.
INFANT BATH: Added as directed to basin or bathinette of water.
SKIN CLEANSING OTHER THAN BATH OR SHOWER: A small amount is rubbed on to wet skin. Rinse. Pat dry.
Precaution: The patient should be warned to guard against slipping in tub or shower.
How Supplied: 4 fl. oz. (NDC 0072-3600-04), 8 fl. oz. (NDC 0072-3600-08; NSN 6505-00-890-2027) and 16 fl. oz. (NDC 0072-3600-16) plastic bottles. Also available for patients who prefer to shower —ALPHA KERI SPRAY—5 oz. (NDC 0072-3600-05) aerosol container.

ALPHA KERI® SOAP
Non-detergent Soap

Composition: Sodium tallowate, sodium cocoate, water, mineral oil, fragrance, PEG-75, glycerin, titanium dioxide, lanolin oil, sodium chloride, BHT, EDTA, D&C Green 5, D&C Yellow 10.
Action and Uses: ALPHA KERI SOAP, rich in emollient oils, thoroughly cleanses as it soothes and softens the skin.
Indications: Adjunctive use in dry skin care.
Administration and Dosage: To be used as any other soap.
How Supplied: 4 oz. (NDC 0072-3500-04) bar.

BALNETAR®
Water-dispersible Emollient Tar

Composition: Contains WESTWOOD® TAR (equivalent to 2.5% Coal Tar USP).
Action and Uses: For temporary relief of itching and scaling due to psoriasis, eczema, and other tar-responsive dermatoses. Tar ingredient is chemically and biologically standardized to insure uniform therapeutic activity. BALNETAR exerts keratoplastic, antieczematous, antipruritic, and emollient actions. It deposits microfine particles of tar over the skin in a lubricant-moisturizing film that helps soften and remove scales and crusts, making the skin smoother and more supple. BALNETAR is an important adjunct in a wide range of dermatoses, including: atopic dermatitis; chronic eczematoid dermatitis; seborrheic dermatitis.
Contraindications: Not indicated when acute inflammation is present.
Administration and Dosage: BALNETAR *should always be used with water... either added to water or rubbed onto wet skin.* For exact dosage label directions are to be followed.
IN THE TUB—Add as directed to a bathtub of water. Soap is not used. The patient soaks for 10 to 20 minutes and then pats dry.
FOR DIRECT APPLICATION—A small amount is rubbed onto the wet skin. Excess is wiped off with tissue to help prevent staining of clothes or linens.
FOR SCALP APPLICATION —A small amount is rubbed onto the wet scalp with fingertips.
Caution: If irritation persists, discontinue use. May temporarily discolor blond, bleached or tinted hair. In rare cases BALNETAR may cause allergic sensitization attributable to coal tar.
Precaution: After use of BALNETAR, patient should avoid exposure to direct sunlight unless sunlight is being used therapeutically in a supervised, modified Goeckerman regimen. Contact with the eyes should be avoided. Patient should be cautioned against slipping when BALNETAR is used in bathtub. Also advise patient that use in a plastic or fiberglass tub may cause staining of the tub.

How Supplied: 8 fl. oz. (NDC 0072-4200-08; NSN 6505-00-928-5890) plastic shatterproof bottle.

CAPITROL®
(chloroxine 2%)
Cream Shampoo

Description: Capitrol is an antibacterial cream shampoo containing 2% chloroxine (each gram contains 20 mg chloroxine) suspended in a base of sodium octoxynol-3 sulfonate, PEG-6 lauramide, dextrin, stearyl alcohol/ceteareth-20, sodium lauryl sulfoacetate, dioctyl sodium sulfosuccinate, magnesium aluminum silicate, PEG-14M, EDTA, citric acid, water, color, fragrance and 1% benzyl alcohol. The pH of the shampoo is 7.0.
Chloroxine is a synthetic antibacterial compound that is effective in the treatment of dandruff and seborrheic dermatitis when incorporated in a shampoo.
The chemical name of chloroxine 5,7-dichloro-8-hydroxyquinoline. The chemical structure of chloroxine is:

Clinical Pharmacology: Well controlled studies demonstrate Capitrol effectively reduces the excess scaling in patients with dandruff or seborrheic dermatitis. Though the cause of dandruff is not known it is thought to be the result of accelerated mitotic activity in the epidermis. The presumed mechanism of action to reduce scaling would be to slow down the mitotic activity.
The role of microbes in seborrheic dermatitis is not known; however, *Staphylococcus aureus* and *Pityrosporon* species are often present in increased numbers during the course of the disease. Chloroxine is antibacterial, inhibiting the growth of Grampositive as well as some Gram-negative organisms. Antifungal activity against some dermatophytes and yeasts also has been shown.
The absorption, metabolism and pharmacokinetics of Capitrol in humans have not been studied.
Indications and Usage: Capitrol is indicated in the treatment of dandruff and mild-to-moderately severe seborrheic dermatitis of the scalp. Clinical studies indicate that improvement may be observed after 14 days of therapy.
Contraindications: Capitrol is contraindicated in those patients with a history of hypersensitivity to any of the listed ingredients.
Warnings: Capitrol should not be used on acutely inflamed (exudative) lesions of the scalp.
Precautions:
Information for patients: Exercise care to prevent Capitrol from entering the eyes. If contact occurs, the patient should flush eyes with cool water. Discoloration of light-colored hair (e.g. blond, gray or bleached) may follow use of this preparation.
Irritation and a burning sensation on the scalp and adjacent areas have been reported.
Drug/Laboratory Test Interactions: There is no known interference of Capitrol with laboratory tests.
Carcinogenesis, Mutagenesis: No long term studies in animals have been performed to evaluate the carcinogenic potential of Capitrol.
Results of the *in vitro* Ames Salmonella/Microsome Plate test show that Capitrol does not demonstrate genetic activity and is considered non-mutagenic.
Teratogenic Effects
Pregnancy Category C: Animal reproduction studies have not been conducted with Capitrol. It is also not known whether Capitrol can cause fetal harm when administered to a pregnant woman or can affect reproduction capacity. Capitrol should be given to a pregnant woman only if clearly needed.
Nursing Mothers: It is not known whether this drug is excreted in human milk. Because many drugs are excreted in human milk, caution should be exercised when Capitrol is administered to a nursing woman.
Pediatric Use: Specific studies to demonstrate the safety and effectiveness for use of Capitrol in children have not been conducted.
Adverse Reaction: One patient out of 225 in clinical studies was reported to have contact dermatitis.
Overdosage: The acute oral LD_{50} in mice was found to be 200 mg/kg and in rats 450 mg/kg. On the basis of these animal studies, Capitrol may be considered practically non-toxic.
Dosage and Administration: Capitrol should be massaged thoroughly onto the wet scalp, avoiding contact with the eyes. Lather should remain on the scalp for approximately three minutes, then rinsed. The application should be repeated and the scalp rinsed thoroughly. Two treatments per week are usually sufficient.
How Supplied: Capitrol shampoo contains 2% chloroxine (20 mg chloroxine per gram) and is supplied in 85 g plastic tubes, (NDC 0072-6800-02).

DESQUAM-X$^{2.5}$® Gel
2.5% Benzoyl Peroxide, 6% Laureth-4

DESQUAM-X^5® Gel
5% Benzoyl Peroxide, 6% Laureth-4

DESQUAM-X^{10}® Gel
10% Benzoyl Peroxide, 6% Laureth-4

Caution: Federal law prohibits dispensing without prescription.
Description: DESQUAM-X2.5, DESQUAM-X5 and DESQUAM-X10 brand topical anti-acne gels contain benzoyl peroxide (2.5, 5 and 10%) and laureth-4 (6%), in a water-base vehicle of carbomer 940, diisopropanolamine and disodium edetate.

Clinical Pharmacology: The effectiveness of benzoyl peroxide in the treatment of acne vulgaris is primarily attributable to its antibacterial activity, especially with respect to *Propionibacterium acnes*, the predominant organism in sebaceous follicles and comedones. The antibacterial activity of this compound is presumably due to the release of active or free-radical oxygen capable of oxidizing bacterial proteins. In acne patients treated topically with benzoyl peroxide, resolution of the acne usually coincides with reduction in the levels of *P. acnes* and free fatty acids (FFA). Mild desquamation is another observed action of topically applied benzoyl peroxide and may also play a role in the drug's effectiveness in acne. Studies also indicate that topical benzoyl peroxide may exert a sebostatic effect with a resultant reduction of skin surface lipids.
Benzoyl peroxide has been shown to be absorbed by the skin, where it is metabolized to benzoic acid and then excreted as benzoate in the urine. Laureth-4 is a non-toxic surfactant which exerts its action through cleansing and mild desquamation. The result of these actions is a drying and degreasing of the skin.
Indications and Usage: DESQUAM-X (2.5, 5 or 10) GEL is indicated for the topical treatment of mild to moderate acne vulgaris and as an adjunct in therapeutic regimens including antibiotics, retinoic acid products and sulfur/salicylic acid-containing preparations. DESQUAM-X GEL has been shown effective in the treatment of the following acne lesion types: papules, pustules, open and closed comedones. Clinical studies have demonstrated therapeutic response after two to three weeks. DESQUAM-X GEL may also be used as adjunctive treatment for nodulo-cystic acne (acne

Continued on next page

Westwood—Cont.

conglobata), although its effectiveness for this condition has not been proven.

Contraindications: This product should not be used in patients known to be hypersensitive to benzoyl peroxide or any of the other listed ingredients.

Precautions: *General:* Avoid contact with eyes and other mucous membranes. For external use only. In patients known to be sensitive to the following substances, there is a possibility of cross-sensitization: benzoic acid derivatives (including certain topical anesthetics) and cinnamon.

Information for Patients: This product may bleach colored fabric or hair. Concurrent use with PABA-containing sunscreens may result in transient discoloration of the skin.

Carcinogenesis, Mutagenesis, Impairment of Fertility: Based upon considerable evidence, benzoyl peroxide is not considered to be a carcinogen. However, in one study, using mice known to be highly susceptible to cancer, there was evidence for benzoyl peroxide as a tumor promoter. Benzoyl peroxide has been found to be inactive as a mutagen in the *Ames Salmonella* and other assays, including the mouse dominant lethal assay. This assay is frequently used to assess the effect of substances on spermatogenesis.

Pregnancy (Category C): Animal reproduction studies have not been conducted with benzoyl peroxide (DESQUAM-X GEL). It is also not known whether benzoyl peroxide (DESQUAM-X GEL) can cause fetal harm when administered to a pregnant woman or can affect reproductive capacity. Benzoyl peroxide (DESQUAM-X GEL) should be given to a pregnant woman only if clearly needed.

Nursing Mothers: It is not known whether this drug is excreted in human milk. Caution should be exercised when benzoyl peroxide is administered to a nursing woman.

Pediatric Use: Safety and effectiveness in children below the age of 12 have not been established.

Adverse Reactions: Adverse reactions which may be encountered with topical benzoyl peroxide include excessive drying (manifested by marked peeling, erythema and possibly edema), and allergic contact sensitization.

Excessive dryness appears to occur in approximately 2 patients in 50.

Pertinent literature seems to indicate that allergic sensitization to benzoyl peroxide may occur in 10 to 25 patients in 1,000. There is one reference that reports an occurrence of sensitization in 5 of 100 patients.

Overdosage: In the event that excessive scaling, erythema or edema occur, the use of this preparation should be discontinued. If the reaction is judged to be due to excessive use and not allergenicity, after symptoms and signs subside, a reduced dosage schedule may be cautiously tried. To hasten resolution of the adverse effects, emollients, cool compresses and/or topical corticosteroid preparations may be used.

Dosage and Administration: DESQUAM-X GEL should be gently rubbed into all affected areas once or twice daily. Suitable cleansing of the affected area should precede application. In fair-skinned individuals or under excessively drying conditions, it is suggested that therapy be initiated with one application daily. The degree of drying or peeling may be controlled by modification of dose frequency or drug concentration. The use of DESQUAM-X GEL may be continued as long as deemed necessary.

How Supplied:

DESQUAM-X 2.5 GEL
1.5 oz. (42.5 g)   Plastic Tubes
NDC 0072-6300-01

DESQUAM-X 5 GEL
1.5 oz. (42.5 g)   Plastic Tubes
NDC 0072-6621-01
NSN 6505-01-036-8629
3 oz. (85 g)   Plastic Tubes
NDC 0072-6621-03

DESQUAM-X 10 GEL
1.5 oz. (42.5 g)   Plastic Tubes
NDC 0072-6721-01
NSN 6505-01-036-8628
3 oz. (85 g)   Plastic Tubes
NDC 0072-6721-03
Store at controlled room temperature (59°–86° F).

WATER BASE
DESQUAM-X® 5 WASH   ℞
(5% benzoyl peroxide)
WATER BASE
DESQUAM-X® 10 WASH   ℞
(10% benzoyl peroxide)

Caution: Federal law prohibits dispensing without prescription.

Description: DESQUAM-X^5 and DESQUAM-X^{10} brand topical therapeutic anti-acne cleansers contain benzoyl peroxide (5% and 10%) in a lathering water base of sodium octoxynol-3 sulfonate, dioctyl sodium sulfosuccinate, magnesium aluminum silicate, methylcellulose and EDTA.

benzoyl peroxide

Clinical Pharmacology: The effectiveness of benzoyl peroxide in the treatment of acne vulgaris is primarily attributable to its antibacterial activity, especially with respect to *Propionibacterium acnes*, the predominant organism in sebaceous follicles and comedones. The antibacterial activity of this compound is presumably due to the release of active or free-radical oxygen capable of oxidizing bacterial proteins. In acne patients treated topically with benzoyl peroxide, resolution of the acne usually coincides with reduction in the levels of *P. acnes* and free fatty acids (FFA). Mild desquamation is another observed action of topically applied benzoyl peroxide and may also play a role in the drug's effectiveness in acne. Studies also indicate that topical benzoyl peroxide may exert a sebostatic effect with a resultant reduction of skin surface lipids.

Benzoyl peroxide has been shown to be absorbed by the skin, where it is metabolized to benzoic acid and then excreted as benzoate in the urine.

Indications and Usage: DESQUAM-X (5 or 10) WASH is indicated for the topical treatment of mild to moderate acne. In more severe cases, it may be used as an adjunct in therapeutic regimens including benzoyl peroxide gels, antibiotics, retinoic acid products and sulfur/salicylic acid-containing preparations. The improvement of the treated condition is dependent on the degree and type of acne, the frequency of use of DESQUAM-X WASH and the nature of other therapies employed.

Contraindications: This product should not be used in patients known to be sensitive to benzoyl peroxide or any other of the listed ingredients.

Precautions: *General:* Avoid contact with eyes and other mucous membranes. For external use only. In patients known to be sensitive to the following substances, there is a possibility of cross-sensitization: benzoic acid derivatives (including certain topical anesthetics) and cinnamon.

Information for Patients: This product may bleach colored fabric or hair. Concurrent use with PABA-containing sunscreens may result in transient discoloration of the skin.

Carcinogenesis, Mutagenesis, Impairment of Fertility: Based upon considerable evidence, benzoyl peroxide is not considered to be a carcinogen. However, in one study, using mice known to be highly susceptible to cancer, there was evidence for benzoyl peroxide as a tumor promoter. Benzoyl peroxide has been found to be inactive as a mutagen in the *Ames Salmonella* and other assays, including the mouse dominant lethal assay. This assay is frequently used to assess the effect of substances on spermatogenesis.

Pregnancy (Category C): Animal reproduction studies have not been conducted with benzoyl peroxide (DESQUAM-X WASH). It is also not known whether benzoyl peroxide can cause fetal harm when administered to a pregnant woman or can affect reproductive capacity. Benzoyl peroxide should be given to a pregnant woman only if clearly needed.

Nursing Mothers: It is not known whether this drug is excreted in human milk. Caution should be exercised when benzoyl peroxide is administered to a nursing woman.

Pediatric Use: Safety and effectiveness in children below the age of 12 have not been established.

Adverse Reactions: Adverse reactions which may be encountered with topical benzoyl peroxide include excessive drying (manifested by marked peeling, erythema and possible edema), and allergic contact sensitization.

Excessive dryness would appear to occur in approximately 2 patients in 50.

Pertinent literature would seem to indicate that allergic sensitization to benzoyl peroxide may occur in 10 to 25 patients in 1,000. There is one reference that reports an occurrence of sensitization in 5 of 100 patients.

Overdosage: In the event that excessive scaling, erythema or edema occur, the use of this preparation should be discontinued. If the reaction is judged to be due to excessive use and not allergenicity, after symptoms and signs subside, a reduced dosage schedule may be cautiously tried. To hasten resolution of the adverse effects, emollients, cool compresses and/or topical corticosteroid preparations may be used.

Dosage and Administration: Shake well before use. Wash affected areas once or twice daily, avoiding contact with eyes or mucous membranes. Wet skin areas to be treated prior to administration; apply DESQUAM-X WASH, work to a full lather, rinse thoroughly and pat dry. The amount of drying or peeling may be controlled by modification of dose frequency or drug concentration.

How Supplied:
Desquam-X Wash (5%):   5 oz. plastic bottle, NDC 0072-6905-05.
Desquam-X Wash (10%):   5 oz. plastic bottle, NDC 0072-7000-05.
Store at controlled room temperature (59°-86°F; 15°-30°C).

ESTAR®
Therapeutic Tar Gel

Composition: Westwood® Tar (biologically equivalent to 5% Coal Tar USP) in a hydro-alcoholic gel (13.8% alcohol).

Actions and Uses: A therapeutic aid in the treatment of eczema, psoriasis, and other tar-responsive dermatoses such as atopic dermatitis, lichen simplex chronicus, and nummular eczema. ESTAR exerts keratoplastic, antieczematous, and antipruritic actions. It is equivalent in its photodynamic activity to 5% crude coal tar in either hydrophilic ointment or petrolatum. ESTAR provides the characteristic benefits of tar therapy in a form that is readily accepted by patients and nursing staff, due to its negligible tar odor and staining potential, and the superior cosmetic qualities of its gel base. ESTAR is suitable for use in a modified Goeckerman regimen, either in the hospital or on an outpatient basis; it also can be used in follow-up treatment to help maintain remissions. Substantivity to the skin can be demonstrated by examination with a Wood's light, which shows residual microfine particles of tar on the skin several days after application.

Contraindications: ESTAR should not be applied to acutely inflamed skin or used by individuals who are known to be sensitive to coal tar.

Administration and Dosage:

Psoriasis: ESTAR can be applied at bedtime in the following manner: the patient should massage ESTAR into affected areas, allowing the gel to remain for five minutes, and then remove excess by patting with tissues. This procedure minimizes staining of skin and clothing, leaving behind an almost invisible layer of the active tar. If any staining of fabric should occur, it can be removed easily by standard laundry procedures.

The same technique of application may be used the following morning. If dryness occurs, an emollient may be applied one hour after ESTAR.

Because of ESTAR's superior substantivity and cosmetic qualities, patients who might otherwise be hospitalized for tar/UV therapy can now be treated as outpatients. The patient can easily apply ESTAR at bedtime and the following morning, then report for UV treatment that day. Laboratory tests and clinical experience to date suggest that it may be advisable to carefully regulate the length of UV exposure.

Chronic atopic dermatitis, lichen simplex chronicus, nummular eczema, and seborrheic dermatitis: One or two applications per day, as described above, are suggested. If dryness occurs, an emollient may be applied one hour after ESTAR and between applications as needed.

Caution: PROTECT TREATED AREAS FROM DIRECT SUNLIGHT, FOR AT LEAST 24 HOURS AFTER APPLICATION, UNLESS DIRECTED BY A PHYSICIAN. AVOID USE ON INFECTED, HIGHLY INFLAMED OR BROKEN SKIN. DO NOT APPLY TO GENITAL AREA. If used on the scalp, temporary discoloration of blond, bleached, or tinted hair may occur. If undue irritation develops or increases, the usage schedule should be changed or ESTAR discontinued. Contact with the eyes should be avoided. In case of contact, flush eyes with water.

Slight staining of clothing may occur. Standard laundry procedures will usually remove stains. For external use only.

How Supplied: 3 oz. (NDC 0072-7603-03; NSN 6505-01-056-2916) plastic tube.

EURAX®
(crotamiton USP)
Lotion/Cream
Scabicide/Antipruritic

Description: Eurax, crotamiton USP, is a scabicidal and antipruritic agent available as a cream or lotion for topical use only. Eurax provides 10% of the synthetic, crotamiton USP, in a vanishing-cream or emollient-lotion base containing: glyceryl monostearate, anhydrous lanolin, PEG 6-32, glycerin, polysorbate 80, water, benzyl alcohol, quaternium-15 and fragrance. In addition, the cream contains mineral oil and white wax; the lotion, light mineral oil, carboxymethylcellulose sodium and simethicone. Crotamiton is N-ethyl-N-(o-methylphenyl)-2-butenamide and its structural formula is:

$CH_3 CH = CHCONCH_2CH_3$ / CH_3

Crotamiton USP is a colorless to slightly yellowish oil, having a faint amine-like odor. It is miscible with alcohol and with methanol. The Crotamiton in Eurax is a mixture of the *cis* and *trans* isomers. Its molecular weight is 203.28.

Clinical Pharmacology: Eurax has scabicidal and antipruritic actions. The mechanisms of these actions are not known.

Indications and Usage: For eradication of scabies (*Sarcoptes scabiei*) and for symptomatic treatment of pruritic skin.

Contraindications: Eurax should not be applied topically to patients who develop a sensitivity or are allergic to it or who manifest a primary irritation response to topical medications.

Warnings: If severe irritation or sensitization develops, treatment with this product should be discontinued and appropriate therapy instituted.

Precautions: *General:* Eurax should not be applied in the eyes or mouth because it may cause irritation. It should not be applied to acutely inflamed skin or raw or weeping surfaces until the acute inflammation has subsided.

Information for Patients: See "Directions for patients with scabies".

Drug Interactions: None known.

Carcinogenesis, Mutagenesis, Impairment of Fertility: Long-term carcinogenicity studies in animals have not been conducted.

Pregnancy (Category C): Animal reproduction studies have not been conducted with Eurax. It is also not known whether Eurax can cause fetal harm when applied topically to a pregnant woman or can affect reproduction capacity. Eurax should be given to a pregnant woman only if clearly needed.

Pediatric Use: Safety and effectiveness in children have not been established.

Adverse Reactions: Allergic sensitivity or primary irritation reactions may occur in some patients.

Overdosage: There is no specific information on the effect of overtreatment with repeated topical applications in humans. Acute toxicity (after accidental oral administration in children): No deaths have occurred. Highest known doses ingested: Cream: small children—2g (age 1½ years): Lotion: small children—2.8g (age 2 years).

Oral LD_{50} in animals (mg/kg): rats, 2212; mice, 2011.

Signs and symptoms (of oral ingestion): Burning sensation in the mouth, irritation of the buccal, esophageal and gastric mucosa, nausea, vomiting, abdominal pain.

Treatment: There is no specific antidote if taken orally. General measures to eliminate the drug and reduce its absorption, combined with symptomatic treatment, are recommended.

Dosage and Administration: LOTION Shake well before using—*In Scabies:* Thoroughly massage into the skin of the whole body from the chin down, paying particular attention to all folds and creases. A second application is advisable 24 hours later.

Clothing and bed linen should be changed the next morning. A cleansing bath should be taken 48 hours after the last application.

In Pruritus: Massage gently into affected areas until medication is completely absorbed. Repeat as needed.

Directions for Patients with Scabies:
1. Take a routine bath or shower. Thoroughly massage Eurax cream or lotion into the skin from the chin to the toes including folds and creases.
2. A second application is advisable 24 hours later.
3. This 60 gram tube or bottle is sufficient for two applications.
4. Clothing and bed linen should be changed the next day. Contaminated clothing and bed linen may be dry-cleaned, or washed in the hot cycle of the washing machine.
5. A cleansing bath should be taken 48 hours after the last application.

How Supplied:
Cream: 60 g tubes (NDC 0072-2100-60; NSN 6505-00-116-0200).
Lotion: 60 g (2 oz.) bottles (NDC 0072-2200-60). 454 g (16 oz.) bottles (NDC 0072-2200-16).

FOSTEX® MEDICATED CLEANSING BAR
Acne Skin Cleanser

Composition: Contains 2% sulfur, 2% salicylic acid, plus a combination of soapless cleansers and wetting agents.

Action and Uses: FOSTEX MEDICATED CLEANSING BAR is a surface-active, penetrating anti-seborrheic cleanser for therapeutic washing of the skin in the local treatment of acne and other skin conditions characterized by excessive oiliness. Degreases, dries and mildly desquamates.

Administration and Dosage: Use FOSTEX MEDICATED CLEANSING BAR instead of soap. Wash entire affected area 2 or 3 times daily, or as physician directs. Rinse well. The desired degree of dryness and peeling may be obtained by regulating frequency of use.

Caution: Avoid contact with eyes. In case of contact, flush with water. If undue skin irritation develops or increases, discontinue use and consult physician. For external use only.

How Supplied: 3¾ oz. (NDC 0072-3000-01; NSN 6505-00-116-1315) bar.

FOSTEX® MEDICATED CLEANSING CREAM
Acne Skin Cleanser and Dandruff Shampoo

Composition: Contains 2% sulfur, 2% salicylic acid, plus a combination of soapless cleansers and wetting agents.

Action and Uses: A penetrating antiseborrheic cleanser for the local treatment of acne, dandruff and other seborrheic skin conditions, characterized by excessive oiliness. Degreases, dries and mildly desquamates.

Administration and Dosage: AS A WASH: Wet skin; wash entire affected area with FOSTEX MEDICATED CLEANSING CREAM instead of soap. Rinse thoroughly. Use 2 or 3 times daily or as physician directs. The desired degree of dryness and peeling may be obtained by regulating frequency of use.

AS A SHAMPOO: Use liberal amount on wet scalp and hair. Shampoo thoroughly, rinse, and repeat shampoo. Rinse thoroughly. No other shampoos are required. To help keep scalp free from excessive oiliness or scaling, use FOSTEX MEDICATED CLEANSING CREAM as often as necessary or as physician directs.

Caution: Avoid contact with eyes. In case of contact, flush with water. If undue skin irritation develops or increases, discontinue use and consult physician. For external use only.

How Supplied: FOSTEX CREAM in 4 oz. (NDC 0072-3200-01; NSN 6505-01-030-9067) tube.

FOSTEX® 5% BENZOYL PEROXIDE GEL
Antibacterial Acne Gel

Composition: Contains 5% benzoyl peroxide.

Action and Uses: FOSTEX 5% BENZOYL PEROXIDE GEL is a penetrating, disappearing gel which helps kill bacteria that can cause acne. Helps prevent new pimples before they appear. Drying action promotes gentle peeling to help clear acne skin.

Indications: A topical aid for the control of acne vulgarica.

Administration and Dosage: After washing, rub FOSTEX 5% BPO into affected areas twice daily. In fair-skinned individuals or in excessively dry climates start with only one application daily. The desired degree of dryness and peeling may be obtained by regulating frequency of use.

Caution: Avoid contact with eyes, lips and mucous membranes. In case of contact, flush with water. Persons with very sensitive skin or a known allergy to benzoyl peroxide should not use this medication. If itching, redness, burning or swelling occurs, discontinue use. For external use only. May bleach dyed fabrics. Keep this and all drugs out of the reach of children. Store at controlled room temperature (59°-86°F).

How Supplied: 1.5 oz (NDC 0072-3300-02) plastic tube.

FOSTEX 10% BENZOYL PEROXIDE CLEANSING BAR
Antibacterial Acne Cleanser

Composition: 10% Benzoyl peroxide.

Action and Uses: FOSTEX 10% BENZOYL PEROXIDE CLEANSING BAR helps kill bacteria that can cause acne. Helps prevent new pimples before they appear. Drying action promotes gentle peeling to help clear your skin.

Indications: A topical aid for the control of acne vulgaris.

Administration and Dosage: Use FOSTEX 10% BENZOYL PEROXIDE CLEANSING BAR instead of soap. For best results, wash entire affected area gently with fingertips for 1 to 2 minutes, 2 to 3 times daily, or as physician directs. Rinse well. The desired degree of dryness and peeling may be obtained by regulating frequency of use.

Caution: Avoid contact with eyes, lips and mucous membranes. In case of contact, flush with water. Persons with very sensitive skin or a known allergy to benzoyl peroxide should not use this

Continued on next page

Westwood—Cont.

medication. If itching, redness, burning or swelling occurs, discontinue use. If symptoms persist, consult a physician. For external use only. May bleach hair and dyed fabrics. Store at controlled room temperature (59°-86°F).
How Supplied: 3 3/4 oz. (NDC 0072-2900-03) bar.

FOSTEX® 10% BENZOYL PEROXIDE GEL
Antibacterial Acne Gel

Composition: Contains 10% benzoyl peroxide.
Action and Uses: FOSTEX 10% BENZOYL PEROXIDE GEL provides super strong protection against acne with 10% benzoyl peroxide... the strongest concentration of the most effective acne fighter you can buy without a prescription. Penetrates to kill bacteria that can cause acne. Helps prevent new pimples before they appear. Drying action promotes peeling to help clear skin. Wear day and night for invisible acne treatment.
Administration and Dosage: Before applying Fostex 10% Benzoyl Peroxide Gel, start fresh with a Fostex cleanser—to clean skin effectively. After washing, rub Fostex 10% Benzoyl Peroxide Gel into entire affected area twice daily, or as physician directs. In fair-skinned individuals or in excessively dry climates, start with only one application daily. The desired degree of dryness and peeling may be obtained by regulating frequency of use.
Caution: Avoid contact with eyes, lips and mucous membranes. In case of contact, flush with water. Persons with very sensitive skin or a known allergy to benzoyl peroxide should not use this medication. If itching, redness, burning or swelling occurs, discontinue use. If symptoms persist, consult a physician. For external use only. May bleach dyed fabrics. Keep this and all drugs out of the reach of children.
How Supplied: 1.5 oz. (NDC 0072-4300-01) plastic tube.

FOSTEX 10% BENZOYL PEROXIDE TINTED CREAM
Antibacterial Acne Cream

Composition: 10% Benzoyl Peroxide
Action and Uses: Fostex 10% Benzoyl Peroxide Tinted Cream provides super-strong protection against acne with 10% benzoyl peroxide... the strongest concentration of the most effective acne fighter you can buy without a prescription. Conceals as it helps heal. Helps prevent new pimples. Drying action promotes peeling to help clear skin. Wear this skin-tone acne medication day and night.
Administration and Dosage: Start fresh with a Fostex cleanser to clean skin effectively. After washing, rub Fostex 10% Benzoyl Peroxide Tinted Cream to entire affected area twice daily, or as a physician directs. In fair-skinned individuals or in excessively dry climates, start with only one application daily. The desired degree of dryness and peeling may be obtained by regulating frequency of use.
Caution: Avoid contact with eyes, lips and mucous membranes. In case of contact, flush with water. Persons with very sensitive skin or a known allergy to benzoyl peroxide should not use this medication. If itching, redness, burning or swelling occurs, discontinue use. If symptoms persist consult a physician. For external use only. May bleach dyed fabrics. Keep this and all drugs out of reach of children. Store at controlled room temperature (59–86°F).
How Supplied: 1 1/2 oz. (NDC 0072-4002-01).

FOSTEX 10% BENZOYL PEROXIDE WASH
Antibacterial Acne Wash

Composition: 10% Benzoyl peroxide.
Action and Uses: FOSTEX 10% BENZOYL PEROXIDE WASH helps kill bacteria that can cause acne. Helps prevent new pimples before they appear. Drying action promotes gentle peeling to help clear your acne.
Indications: A topical aid for the control of acne vulgaris.
Administration and Dosage: Shake well. Wet skin; wash entire affected are with FOSTEX 10% BENZOYL PEROXIDE WASH instead of soap. Wash gently for 1 to 2 minutes, 2 to 3 times daily, or as physician directs. The desired degree of dryness and peeling may be obtained by regulating frequency of use.
Caution: Avoid contact with eyes, lips and mucous membranes. In case of contact, flush with water. Persons with very sensitive skin or a known allergy to benzoyl peroxide should not use this medication. If itching, redness, burning or swelling occurs, discontinue use. If symptoms persist, consult a physician. May bleach dyed fabrics. Store at controlled room temperature (59°-86°F).
How Supplied: 5 oz. (NDC 0072-3100-05) plastic bottles.

FOSTRIL®
Drying Lotion for Acne

Composition: Contains 2% sulfur, in a greaseless base with laureth-4.
Action and Uses: Promotes drying and peeling of the skin in the treatment of acne. Daily use of FOSTRIL should result in a desirable degree of dryness and peeling in about 7 days. FOSTRIL removes excess oil and follicular obstruction, helping to remove comedones. It also helps prevent epithelial closure of pores and formation of new lesions.
Administration and Dosage: A thin film is applied to affected areas once or twice daily, or as directed.
Caution: If undue skin irritation develops or increases, adjust usage schedule or discontinue use. Anti-inflammatory measures may be used if necessary. For external use only. Contact with eyes should be avoided. In case of contact, flush eyes thoroughly with water.
How Supplied: 1 oz. (NDC 0072-3800-01; NSN 6505-00-116-1159) tube.

HALOTEX®
(Haloprogin)
Cream 1%, Solution 1%
Antifungal Agent for Topical Use
℞

Description: HALOTEX (brand of haloprogin) Cream/Solution for topical use. Each gram of the cream contains 10 mg haloprogin in a water-dispersible base composed of polyethylene glycol 400, polyethylene glycol 4000, diethyl sebacate and polyvinylpyrrolidone.
Each ml of the solution contains 10 mg haloprogin in a clear, colorless vehicle composed of 75% alcohol and diethyl sebacate.
These preparations are effective topical antifungal agents. The chemical name for haloprogin is: 1,2,4-trichloro-5[(3-iodo-2-propynyl)oxy]benzene. The structure is:

Clinical Pharmacology: The mechanism of antifungal activity for haloprogin in yeast cells is believed to be inhibition of respiration and disruption of the yeast cell membrane. The mechanism of antifungal activity in dermatophytes is unknown.
Dermal penetration studies utilizing single applications of ^{14}C ring-labeled haloprogin formulated as creams, or dissolved in acetone or alcoholic solutions, were performed in 18 male subjects. Urinary recovery from 3 subjects ranged from 9.47% (0.25% cream) to 14.89% (1% cream) over 5 days. The 0.25% and 1% alcoholic solutions were associated with lesser recoveries of 3% and 6%, respectively. Subtotal inunction studies have been conducted with both the cream and the solution. Fifteen grams of HALOTEX Cream (n=8) and 15 ml of HALOTEX Solution (n=14) were administered to the entire body for 10 consecutive days. Physical examinations and clinical laboratory tests conducted throughout the study showed no abnormalities. Repeat patch testing for contact sensitization and photosensitivity also were negative.
The following *in-vitro* data on haloprogin are available, but their clinical significance is not known.

Organism (# Strains Tested)	MIC[1] (µg/ml) Range Found
Microsporum audouini (2)	< 0.0470 – 0.390
M. canis (2)	< 0.0470 – 0.390
M. gypseum (2)	0.0950 – 0.190
Other *Microsporum* spp (3)	0.0030 – 0.190
Trichophyton mentagrophytes (5)	0.0950 – 0.780
T. rubrum (4)	0.0120 – 0.780
Other *Trichophyton* spp (9)	0.0015 – 0.095
Candida albicans (3)	0.0500 – 0.400
Other *Candida* spp (2)	0.4000 – 0.800
Other Yeasts/yeast-like fungi (8)	0.0500 – 0.400
Staphylococcus aureus (5)	1.5600 – 3.120
Streptococcus pyrogenes (3)	0.7800 –50.000
Other gram pos. organisms (6)	25.00 – > 100.000
Gram neg. organisms	> 100

[1] Minimal Inhibitory Concentration

Indications and Usage: HALOTEX Cream and Solution are indicated for the treatment of superficial mycotic infections including tinea pedis, tinea cruris, tinea corporis and tinea manuum due to infection with *Tricophyton rubrum*, *T. tonsurans*, *T. mentaprophytes*, *Microsporum canis* and *Epidermophyton floccosum*. HALOTEX also is indicated for the treatment of tinea versicolor caused by *Malassezia furfur*.
Contraindications: HALOTEX Cream and Solution should not be used by patients known to have hypersensitivity to any of the listed ingredients.
Warnings: See Contraindications and Precautions.
Precautions:
General: Treatment with HALOTEX Cream or Solution should be discontinued in case of sensitization or persistent irritation and appropriate therapy instituted. The diagnosis in patients showing no improvement after four weeks of treatment with HALOTEX should be reconsidered.
In mixed infections, where bacteria or nonsusceptible fungi are present, supplementary antiinfective therapy may be indicated.
Information for Patients: HALOTEX is for topical use only.
Contact of this drug with the eyes should be avoided.
Use of HALOTEX should be discontinued and a physician contacted in the event of increased irritation.
In order to minimize the risk of recurrence, use the prescribed medication for the full duration even if symptoms have abated.
Laboratory Tests: KOH preparations of the afflicted areas may be useful to verify the diagnosis of fungal infection prior to treatment. Periodic repeat KOH preparations at 2-week intervals during treatment and at 2–4 weeks after treatment will document the beneficial response to treatment. Cultures for bacteria or fungi of specimens from affected area, not responding to treatment may help to elucidate the lack of response.
In the event of a suspected irritation or sensitization, patch testing with components of the formulation used may help verify the reaction and identify its cause.
Carcinogenesis, Mutagenesis, Impairment of Fertility: The carcinogenic potential of haloprogin in laboratory animals has not been evaluated. HALOTEX was shown to be non-mutagenic in The Ames-Salmonella/Microsome Plate Assay.
Pregnancy: Pregnancy Category B: Reproduction studies have been performed in rats and rabbits, each group being given 10 daily topical applications, representing up to 3 times the estimated total human dose needed for a 30-day course of therapy. No evidence of impaired fertility or harm to the fetus due to haloprogin was revealed. There are, however, no adequate and well-controlled studies in pregnant women. Because animal repro-

duction studies are not always predictive of human response, this drug should be used during pregnancy only if clearly needed.
Nursing Mothers: It is not known whether this drug is excreted in huma milk. Because many drugs are excreted in human milk, caution should be exercised when HALOTEX formulations are applied to a nursing mother.
Pediatric Use: Safety and efficacy studies in children have not been performed.
Adverse Reactions: In clinical studies with the cream and the solution 26 adverse reactions were noted out of a total 1796 patients treated. These reactions are tabulated below for each formulation.

REACTION	FORMULATION Cream (n=977)	Solution (n=819)
Burning and/or irritation on application	8	14
Erythema and Scaling	1	—
Erythema and Itching	1	—
Folliculitis	1	—
Pruritus and Vesicle Formation	—	1

Reactions noted did not always require interruption of treatment.
Overdosage: The oral LD_{50} of haloprogin is >3000 mg/kg in mice, rats, dogs and rabbits. The maximum haloprogin in any single package is 300 mg total. There is no experience to allow extrapolation of acute toxicity and expected symptoms in man.
Dosage and Administration: HALOTEX Cream and Solution should be applied liberally to the affected areas twice daily for 2–3 weeks. Intertriginous areas may require 4 weeks of treatment.
How Supplied: HALOTEX (haloprogin) Cream 1% is supplied in 15 g (NDC 0072-7130-15) and 30 g (NDC 0072-7130-02) NSN 6505-00-118-2318 tubes. Store below 45°C (113°F). HALOTEX (haloprogin) Solution 1% is supplied in 10 ml (NDC 0072-7200-10) NSN 6505-00-118-2211 and 30 ml (NDC 0072-7200-30) NSN 6505-00-118-2308 bottles with controlled drop tip.

KERALYT® GEL
Salicylic Acid

Description: KERALYT is a gel for topical administration containing 6% salicylic acid in a vehicle composed of propylene glycol, alcohol (19.4%), hydroxypropylcellulose and water. Salicylic acid is the 2-hydroxy derivative of benzoic acid.
Clinical Pharmacology: Salicylic acid has been shown to produce desquamation of the horny layer of skin while not effecting qualitative or quantitative changes in the structure of the viable epidermis. The mechanism of action has been attributed to a dissolution of intracellular cement substance. In a study of the percutaneous absorption of salicylic acid from KERALYT GEL in four patients with extensive active psoriasis, Taylor and Halprin showed that the peak serum salicylate levels never exceeded 5 mg/100 ml even though more than 60% of the applied salicylic acid was absorbed. Systemic toxic reactions are usually associated with much higher serum levels (30 to 40 mg/100 ml). Peak serum levels occurred within 5 hours of the topical application under occlusion. The sites were occluded for 10 hours over the entire body surface below the neck. Since salicylates are distributed in the extracellular space, patients with a contracted extracellular space due to dehydration or diuretics have higher salicylate levels than those with a normal extracellular space. (See PRECAUTIONS.)
The major metabolites identified in the urine after topical administration are salicyluric acid (52%), salicylate glucuronides (42%) and free salicylic acid (6%). The urinary metabolites after percutaneous administration differ from those after oral salicylate administration; those derived from percutaneous absorption contain more salicylate glucuronides and less salicyluric and salicylic acid. Almost 95% of a single dose of salicylate is excreted within 24 hours of its entrance into the extracellular space.

Fifty to eighty percent of salicylate is protein bound to albumin. Salicylates compete with the binding of several drugs and can modify the action of these drugs; by similar competitive mechanisms other drugs can influence the serum levels of salicylate. (See PRECAUTIONS.)
Indications and Usage: For Dermatologic Use: KERALYT GEL is a topical aid in the removal of excessive keratin in hyperkeratotic skin disorders, including verrucae, and the various ichthyoses (vulgaris, sex-linked and lamellar), keratosis palmaris and plantaris, keratosis pilaris, pityriasis rubra pilaris, psoriasis (including body, scalp, palms and soles).
For Podiatric Use: KERALYT GEL is a topical aid in the removal of excessive keratin on dorsal and plantar hyperkeratotic lesions. KERALYT has been reported to be useful adjunctive therapy for verrucae plantares.
Contraindications: KERALYT GEL should not be used in any patient known to be sensitive to salicylic acid or any other listed ingredients. KERALYT should not be used in children under 2 years of age.
Warnings: Prolonged use over large areas, especially in children and those patients with significant renal or hepatic impairment, could result in salicylism. Concomitant use of other drugs which may contribute to elevated serum salicylate levels should be avoided where the potential for toxicity is present. In children under 12 years of age and those patients with renal or hepatic impairment, the area to be treated should be limited and the patient monitored closely for signs of salicylate toxicity: nausea, vomiting, dizziness, loss of hearing, tinnitus, lethargy, hyperpnea, diarrhea, psychic disturbances.
In the event of salicylic acid toxicity, the use of KERALYT GEL should be discontinued. Fluids should be administered to promote urinary excretion. Treatment with sodium bicarbonate (oral or intravenous) should be instituted as appropriate.
Precautions: For external use only. Avoid contact with eyes and other mucous membranes.
Drug Interactions: (The following interactions are from a published review and include reports concerning both oral and topical salicylate administration. The relationship of these interactions to the use of KERALYT GEL is not known.)

I. Due to the competition of salicylate with other drugs for binding to serum albumin the following drug interactions may occur:

DRUG	DESCRIPTION OF INTERACTION
Tolbutamide	Hypoglycemia potentiated.
Methotrexate	Decreases tubular reabsorption; clinical toxicity from methotrexate can result.

II. Drugs changing salicylate levels by altering renal tubular reabsorption:

DRUG	DESCRIPTION
Corticosteroids	Decreases plasma salicylate level; tapering doses of steroids may promote salicylism
Ammonium Sulfate	Increases plasma salicylate level.

III. Drugs with Complicated Interactions with Salicylates

DRUG	DESCRIPTION
Heparin	Salicylate decreases platelet adhesiveness and interferes with hemostasis in heparin-treated patients.
Pyrazinamide	Inhibits pyrazinamide-induced hyperuricemia.
Uricosuric Agents	Effect of probenemide, sulfinpyrazone and phenylbutazone inhibited.

The following alterations of laboratory tests have been reported during salicylate therapy.

LABORATORY TESTS	EFFECT OF SALICYLATES
Thyroid Function	Decreased PBI; increased T_3 uptake.
Urinary Sugar	False negative with glucose oxidase; false positive with Clinitest with high-dose salicylate therapy (2-5g q.d.).
5-Hydroxyindole acetic acid	False negative with fluorometric test.
Acetone, ketone bodies	False positive $FeCl_3$ in Gerhardt reaction; red color persists with boiling.
17-OH corticosteroids	False reduced values with >4.8g q.d. salicylate.
Vanilmandelic acid	False reduced values.
Uric acid	May increase or decrease depending on dose.
Prothrombin	Decreased levels; slightly increased prothrombin time.

Pregnancy (Category C): Salicylic acid has been shown to be teratogenic in rats and monkeys. It is difficult to extrapolate from oral doses of acetylsalicylic acid used in these studies to topical administration as the oral dose to monkeys may represent 6 times the maximal daily human dose of salicylic acid (as supplied in one tube, 28 g, of Keralyt) when applied topically over a large body surface. There are no adequate and well-controlled studies in pregnant women. KERALYT GEL should be used during pregnancy only if the potential benefit justifies the potential risk to the fetus.
Nursing Mothers: Because of the potential for serious adverse reactions in nursing infants from the mother's use of KERALYT GEL, a decision should be made whether to discontinue nursing or to discontinue the drug, taking into account the importance of the drug to the mother.
Carcinogenesis, Mutagenesis, Impairment of Fertility: No data are available concerning potential carcinogenic or reproductive effects of KERALYT GEL. It has been shown to lack mutagenic potential in the Ames Salmonella test.
Adverse Reactions: Excessive erythema and scaling conceivably could result from use on open skin lesions.
Overdosage: See Warnings.
Dosage and Administraton: The preferable method of use is to apply KERALYT GEL thoroughly to the affected area and occlude the area at night. Preferably, the skin should be hydrated for at least five minutes prior to application. The medication is washed off in the morning and if excessive drying and/or irritation is observed a bland cream or lotion may be applied. Once clearing is apparent, the occasional use of KERALYT GEL will usually maintain the remission. In those areas where occlusion is difficult or impossible, application may be made more frequently; hydration by wet packs or baths prior to application apparently enhances the effect. Unless hands are being treated, hands should be rinsed thoroughly after application.
How Supplied: 1 oz. (28.4g) (NDC 0072-6500-01; NSN 6505-01-546-7319) plastic tube.

KERI® CREME
Concentrated Moisturizer—Nongreasy Emollient

Composition: Contains water, mineral oil, talc, sorbitol, ceresin, lanolin alcohol/mineral oil, magnesium stearate, glyceryl oleate/propylene glycol, isopropyl myristate, methylparaben, propylparaben, fragrance, quaternium-15.
Actions and Uses: KERI CREME is a concentrated moisturizer and nongreasy emollient for problem dry skin—hands, face, elbows, feet, legs. KERI CREME helps retain moisture that makes skin feel soft, smooth, supple. Helps resist the drying effects of soaps, detergents and chemicals.
Administration and Dosage: A small amount is rubbed into dry skin areas as needed.

Continued on next page

Westwood—Cont.

How Supplied: 2.25 oz. (NDC 0072-5800-01) tube.

KERI® FACIAL SOAP
Non-detergent Facial Soap

Composition: KERI LOTION® concentrate in a gentle, non-detergent soap containing: sodium tallowate, sodium cocoate, water, mineral oil, octyl hydroxystearate, fragrance, glycerin, titanium dioxide, PEG-75, lanolin oil, dioctyl sodium sulfosuccinate, PEG-4 dilaurate, propylparaben, PEG-40 stearate, glyceryl monostrearate, PEG-100 stearate, sodium chloride, BHT, EDTA.
Action and Uses: KERI FACIAL SOAP helps keep skin soft while thoroughly cleansing.
Administration and Dosage: To be used as facial soap.
How Supplied: 3.25 oz. (NDC 0072-4900-03) bar.

KERI® LOTION
Skin Lubricant—Moisturizer

Composition: Contains mineral oil in a base of water, propylene glycol, glyceryl stearate/ PEG-100 stearate, PEG-40 stearate, PEG-4 dilaurate, laureth-4, lanolin oil, methylparaben, propylparaben, fragrance, carbomer-934, triethanolamine, dioctyl sodium sulfosuccinate, quaternium-15. Freshly-scented: FD&C blue 1, D&C yellow 10.
Action and Uses: KERI LOTION lubricates and helps hydrate the skin, making it soft and smooth. It relieves itching, helps maintain a normal moisture balance and supplements the protective action of skin lipids. Indicated for generalized dryness and itching; detergent hands; chapped or chafed skin; sunburn; "winter-itch"; aging, dry skin; diaper rash; heat rash.
Administration and Dosage: Apply as often as needed. Use particularly after bathing and exposure to sun, water, soaps and detergents.
How Supplied: 6½ oz. (NDC 0072-4600-56; NSN 6505-01-009-2897), 13 oz. (NDC 0072-4600-63) and 20 oz. (NDC 0072-4600-70) plastic bottles. Also available as KERI LOTION FRESHLY SCENTED—6½ oz. (NDC 0072-4500-56), 13 oz. (NDC 0072-4500-63), and 20 oz. (NDC 0072-4500-70) plastic bottles.

LOWILA® CAKE
Soap-free Skin Cleanser

Composition: Contains dextrin, sodium α olefin (C_{14}-C_{16}) sulfonate, water, boric acid, urea, sorbitol, mineral oil, PEG-14 M, lactic acid, dioctyl sodium sulfosuccinate, cellulose gum, fragrance.
Action and Uses: LOWILA CAKE is indicated when soap should not be used, for cleansing skin that is sensitive or irritated, or in dermatitic and eczematous conditions. Used for general bathing, infant bathing, routine washing of hands and face and shampooing. The pH of LOWILA CAKE helps protect the skin's normal acid mantle and create an environment favorable to therapy and healing.
Administration and Dosage: LOWILA CAKE is used in place of soap. Lathers well in both hard and soft water.
How Supplied: 3¾ oz. (NDC 0072-2304-01) bar.

MOISTUREL™
Skin Lubricant—Moisturizer

Composition: Water, petrolatum, glycerin, dimethicone, steareth-2, cetyl alcohol, benzyl alcohol, laureth-23, carbomer-934, Mg Al silicate, quaternium-15, sodium hydroxide.
Action and Uses: Moisturel is a non-greasy formula that leaves the skin feeling smooth and soft. Clinically proven to relieve dry skin. Free of parabens and fragrances that can sensitize or irritate skin. Indicated for generalized dry skin, chapped or chafed skin, diaper rash, sunburn, heat rash, itching and dryness associated with eczema.
Administration and Dosages: Apply as often as needed.

How Supplied: 8 oz. (NDC 0072-9100-08) plastic bottle.

PERNOX®
Medicated Lathering Scrub Cleanser for Acne

Composition: Contains 2% Sulfur, 1.5% salicylic acid, plus a combination of soapless cleansers and wetting agents and abradant polyethylene granules.
Actions and Uses: A lathering scrub cleanser for acne, oily skin. PERNOX provides microfine, uniform-size scrub particles with a rounded surface area to enable patients to achieve effective and gentle desquamation as they wash their skin. PERNOX helps loosen and remove comedones, dries, peels and degreases acne skin. It lathers abundantly and leaves the skin feeling smooth.
Contraindications: Not indicated when acute inflammation is present or in nodular or cystic acne.
Administration and Dosage: After wetting the skin, PERNOX is applied with the fingertips and massaged onto the skin for about one-half to one minute. The skin is then thoroughly rinsed. May be used instead of soap one to two times daily, or as directed.
Caution: If undue skin irritation develops or increases, adjust usage schedule or discontinue use. If necessary, anti-inflammatory measures may be used after discontinuance. For external use only. Contact with eyes should be avoided. In case of contact, flush eyes thoroughly with water.
How Supplied: 2 oz. (NDC 0072-5200-02; NSN 6505-01-035-1719), and 4 oz. (NDC 0072-5200-04) tubes; lemon scented: 2 oz. (NDC 0072-5300-02), and 4 oz. (NDC 0072-5300-04) tubes.

PERNOX® LOTION
Lathering Scrub Cleanser for Acne

Composition: Contains 2% Sulfur, 1.5% salicylic acid, plus a combination of soapless cleansers and wetting agents and abradant polyethylene granules.
Actions and Uses: PERNOX LOTION is a therapeutic scrub cleanser in lotion form that is to be used routinely instead of soap. It gently desquamates or peels acne or oily skin. PERNOX LOTION also removes excessive oil from the skin surface and will produce mild drying of the affected skin areas when used regularly. It helps skin feel fresher and smoother with each wash.
Contraindications: Not indicated when acute inflammation is present or in nodular or cystic acne.
Administration and Dosage: To be shaken well before using. PERNOX may be used instead of soap one or two times daily or as directed. The skin should be wet first and PERNOX applied with the fingertips. The lather should be massaged into skin for one-half to one minute. The patient then rinses thoroughly and pats dry.
Caution: If undue skin irritation develops or increases, adjust usage schedule or discontinue use. For external use only. Contact with eyes should be avoided. In case of contact, flush eyes with water.
How Supplied: 5 oz. (NDC 0072-7900-05) plastic bottle.

PERNOX® SHAMPOO
For Oily Hair

Composition: A blend of biodegradable cleansers and hair conditioners, containing: sodium laureth sulfate, water, lauramide DEA, quaternium 22, PEG-75 lanolin/hydrolyzed animal protein, sodium chloride, fragrance, lactic acid, sorbic acid, disodium EDTA, FD&C yellow 6, FD&C blue 1.
Actions and Uses: A gentle but thorough shampoo especially formulated to cleanse, control and condition oily hair. Especially suitable for adjunctive use with acne patients. PERNOX SHAMPOO works into a rich, pleasant lather, leaves the hair lustrous and manageable. Its special conditioners help prevent tangles and fly away hair. Gentle enough to be used every day. It contains a refreshing natural scent.
Administration and Dosage: A liberal amount is massaged into wet hair and scalp. A good lather is worked up, massaging thoroughly. This is followed by a rinse and repeat application. A final rinse is used. No other shampoos or hair conditioners are necessary. May be used as needed.
Caution: For external use only. Contact with the eyes should be avoided. In case of contact, flush eyes with water.
How Supplied: 8 fl. oz. (NDC 0072-5500-08) shatterproof plastic bottle.

PRESUN® 4 CREAMY SUNSCREEN
Moderate Sunscreen Protection

Composition: Contains 1.4% Padimate O (Octyl dimethyl PABA).
Action and Uses: PRESUN 4 CREAMY, a water-resistant, non-staining moisturizing formula, provides 4 times an individual's natural protection. Liberal and regular use may reduce the chance of premature aging of the skin and skin cancer from overexposure to the sun. PRESUN 4 CREAMY provides moderate protection, permits limited tanning while reducing the chance of sunburn. PRESUN 4 CREAMY maintains its degree of sunburn protection even after 40 minutes in the water.
Administration and Dosage: Shake well. Gently smooth liberal amount evenly onto dry skin before sun exposure. Do not rub in. Reapply to dry skin after prolonged swimming or excessive perspiration, or after towel drying. Repeated applications during prolonged sun exposure are recommended.
If used, cosmetics or emollients may be applied after PRESUN.
Warnings: For external use only. Do not use if sensitive to p-aminobenzoic acid (PABA), or related compounds (such as benzocaine, sulfonamides, aniline dyes, or PABA esters). Discontinue use if irritation or rash appears. Avoid contact with eyes. In case of contact, flush eyes with water. Keep out of the reach of children.
How Supplied: 4 oz. (NDC 0072-5904-04) plastic bottle.

PRESUN® 8; LOTION, CREAMY AND GEL
Maximal Sunscreen Protection

Composition: Lotion: 7.3% (w/w) Padimate O (Octyl dimethyl PABA), 2.3% (w/w) oxybenzone, 60% (w/w) SD alcohol 40. Creamy Lotion: Contains: 5% Padimate 0 (Octyl dimethyl PABA), 2% oxybenzone. Gel: contains: PABA, 55% SD alcohol 40.
Action and Uses: PreSun 8 provides 8 times an individual's natural protection. Liberal and regular use may reduce the chance of premature aging of the skin and skin cancer . PreSun 8 permits limited tanning and reduces the chance of sunburn. It gives maximum protection in the erythemogenic range, screening out the burning rays of the sun. Creamy: a water resistant, non-staining moisturizing formula which maintains its degree of sunburn protection even after 40 minutes in the water. Lotion: a non- staining formula which permits limited tanning while reducing the chance of sunburn.
Warnings: For external use only. Do not use if sensitive to p-aminobenzoic acid (PABA), or related compounds (such as benzocaine, sulfonamides, aniline dyes, or PABA esters). Discontinue use if irritation or rash appears. Avoid contact with eyes. In case of contact, flush eyes with water. Keep out of the reach of children. Lotion: Avoid flame. Gel: Avoid flame. Avoid contact with fabric or other materials as staining may result.
Administration and Dosage: Apply liberally and evenly to dry skin, let dry before dressing. Reapply after swimming or excessive perspiration, or after towel drying. Repeated applications during prolonged sun expo sure are recommended. Creamy: Do not rub in. Gel: apply liberally and evenly one hour before exposure. Let dry before dressing.

How Supplied: Lotion: 4 fl. oz. (NDC 0072-5403-04; NSN 6505-01-037-8636) and 7 fl. oz. (NDC 0072-5400-07) plastic bottles. Creamy Lotion: 4 oz. (NDC 0072-8404-04) plastic bottle. Gel: 3 oz. (NDC 0072-7700-03) plastic tube.

PRESUN® 15 SUNSCREEN LOTION
Ultra Sunscreen Protection

Composition: 5% Aminobenzoic acid (PABA), 5% Padimate O (octyl dimethyl PABA) 3% oxybenzone, 58% SD alcohol 40.

Actions and Uses: PRESUN 15, a clear PABA formula, provides 15 times an individual's natural protection. Liberal and regular use may reduce the chance of premature aging of the skin and skin cancer from overexposure to the sun. PRESUN 15 provides the highest degree of sunburn protection.

Administration and Dosage: Shake well. Apply liberally and evenly to **dry skin** before exposure; let dry before dressing. Reapply to dry skin after swimming or excessive perspiration, or after towel drying. Repeated applications during prolonged exposure ae recommended. If used, cosmetics or emollients may be applied after PRESUN.

Warnings: For external use only. Do not use if sensitive to p-aminobenzoic acid (PABA), or related compounds (such as benzocaine, sulfonamides, aniline dyes or PABA esters). Discontinue use if irritation or rash appars. Transient facial stinging may occur in hot, humid weather. Avoid contact with eyes. In case of contact, flush eyes with water. Avoid flame. Avoid contact with fabric or other materials as staining may result. Keep out of the reach of children.

How Supplied: 4 oz. (NDC 0072-8800-04) plastic bottle, NSN 6505-01-121-2335.

PRESUN® 15 CREAMY SUNSCREEN
Ultra Sunscreen Protection

Composition: 8% Padimate O (Octyl dimethyl PABA), 3% oxybenzone.

Action and Uses: PRESUN 15 CREAMY, a water-resistant, non-staining moisturizing formula, provides 15 times an individual's natural protection. Liberal and regular use may help reduce the chance of premature aging of the skin and skin cancer from overexposure to the sun. PRESUN 15 CREAMY permits limited tanning while reducing the chance of sunburn. PRESUN 15 CREAMY maintains its degree of protection even after 40 minutes in the water.

Administration and Dosage: Shake well. Gently smooth liberal amount evenly onto **dry skin** before sun exposure. Do not rub in. Reapply to dry skin after prolonged swimming or excessive perspiration, or after towel drying. Repeated applications during prolonged sun exposure are recommended.

Warnings: For external use only. Do not use if sensitive to p-aminobenzoic acid (PABA), or related compounds (such as benzocaine, sulfonamides, aniline dyes, or PABA esters). Discontinue use if irritation or rash appears. Avoid contact with eyes. In case of contact, flush eyes with water. Keep out of the reach of children.

How Supplied: 4 oz. (NDC 0072-8904-04) plastic bottle, NSN 6505-01-121-2336.

SEBUCARE®
Antiseborrheic Scalp Lotion

Contains: 1.8% Salicylic acid, 61% alcohol, water, PPG-40 butyl ether, laureth-4, dihydroabietyl alcohol, fragrance.

Action and Uses: An aid in the treatment of dandruff, seborrhea capitis and other scaling conditions of the scalp. SEBUCARE helps control scaling, oiliness and itching. The unique base helps soften brittle hair and grooms the hair, thus eliminating the need for hair dressing which often impedes antiseborrheic treatment. SEBUCARE should be used every day in conjunction with therapeutic shampoos such as SEBULEX® or FOSTEX® CREAM.

Administration and Dosage: SEBUCARE is applied directly to scalp and massaged thoroughly with fingertips. Comb or brush as usual. Grooms as it medicates. Use once or twice daily or as directed..

Precaution: Volatile—Avoid flame. For external use only. Keep this and all drugs out of reach of children. Avoid contact with eyes. In case of contact, flush eyes with water.

How Supplied: 4 fl. oz. (NDC 0072-4800-04) plastic bottle.

SEBULEX® and SEBULEX® CREAM
Antiseborrheic Treatment Shampoo

Composition: Contains 2% sulfur and 2% salicylic acid in SEBULYTIC® brand of surface-active cleansers and wetting agents.

Action and Uses: A penetrating therapeutic shampoo for the temporary relief of itchy scalp and the scaling of dandruff, SEBULEX helps relieve itching, remove dandruff, excess oil. It penetrates and softens the crusty, matted layers of scales adhering to the scalp, and leaves the hair soft and manageable.

Administration and Dosage: SEBULEX liquid should be shaken before being used. SEBULEX or SEBULEX CREAM is massaged into wet scalp. Lather should be allowed to remain on scalp for about 5 minutes and then rinsed. Application is repeated, followed by a thorough rinse. Initially, SEBULEX or SEBULEX CREAM can be used daily, or every other day, or as directed, depending on the condition. Once symptoms are under control, one or two treatments a week usually will maintain control of itching, oiliness and scaling.

Caution: If undue skin irritation develops or increases, discontinue use. For external use only. Contact with eyes should be avoided. In case of contact, flush eyes thoroughly with water.

How Supplied: SEBULEX in 4 oz. (NDC 0072-2700-04), NSN 6508-00-116-1362 and 8 oz. (NDC 0072-2700-08) plastic bottles. SEBULEX CREAM in 4 oz. (NDC 0072-2800-04) plastic tube.

SEBULEX® SHAMPOO WITH CONDITIONERS
Antiseborrheic Treatment and Conditioning Shampoo

Composition: Contains 2% sulfur, 2% salicylic acid, water, sodium octoxynol-3 sulfonate, sodium lauryl sulfate, lauramide DEA, acetamide MEA, amphoteric-2, hydrolyzed animal protein, magnesium aluminum silicate, pro- pylene glycol, methylcellulose, PEG-14 M, fragrance, disodium EDTA, dioctyl sodium sulfosuccinate, FD & C blue 1, D & C yellow 10.

Action and Uses: SEBULEX SHAMPOO WITH CONDITIONERS provides effective temporary control of the scaling and itching of dandruff and seborrheic dermatitis, while adding protein to the hair shaft to increase its manageability.

Administration and Dosage: SEBULEX SHAMPOO WITH CONDITIONERS should be shaken well before use. Shampoo five minutes. For optimum dandruff control and conditioning leave lather on scalp for the full five minutes. Rinse. Repeat. Use two to three times weekly to maintain control, although daily use may be continued. Consult physician for severe or unresponsive scalp conditions.

Caution: If undue skin irritation develops or increases, use should be discontinued. Contact with eyes should be avoided. In cases of contact, eyes should be flushed thoroughly with water.

How Supplied: 4 oz. (NDC 0072-2600-04) and 8 oz. (NDC 0072-2600-08) plastic bottles.

SEBULON® DANDRUFF SHAMPOO
Antiseborrheic Treatment and Conditioning Shampoo

Composition: 2% Zinc pyrithione. Also contains: Water, TEA-lauryl sulfate, disodium oleamido PEG-2 sulfosuccinate, cocamide DEA, acetamide MEA, magnesium aluminum silicate, dydroxpropyl guar, fragrance, FD & D green 3 and D & C green 5.

Action and Uses: Sebulon Shampoo—specially formulated to relieve the itching and flaking of dandruff and seborrheic dermatitis. Leaves hair clean and manageable.

Administration and Dosage: Shake well before using. For best results use at least twice a week. Can be used daily, if desired. Wet hair, apply to scalp and massage vigorously. Rinse and repeat.

Caution: For external use only. If condition worsens or does not improve after regular use of this product as directed, discontinue use. Avoid contact with the eyes—if this occurs, flush thoroughly with water.

How Supplied: 4 oz. (0072-2500-04) and 8 oz. (0072-2500-08) plastic bottles.

SEBUTONE® and SEBUTONE® CREAM
Antiseborrheic Tar Shampoo

Composition: WESTWOOD® TAR (equivalent to 0.5% Coal Tar USP), 2% sulfur and 2% salicylic acid in SEBULYTIC® brand of surface-active cleansers and wetting agents.

Action and Uses: A surface-active, penetrating therapeutic shampoo for the temporary relief of itchy scalp and the scaling of stubborn dandruff and psoriasis. Provides prompt and prolonged relief of itching, helps control oiliness and rid the scalp of scales and crust. Tar ingredient is chemically and biologically standardized to produce uniform therapeutic activity. Wood's light demonstrates residual microfine particles of tar on the scalp several days after a course of SEBUTONE shampoo. In addition to its antipruritic and antiseborrheic actions, SEBUTONE also helps offset excessive scalp dryness with a special moisturizing emollient.

Administration and Dosage: SEBUTONE liquid should be shaken before being used. A liberal amount of SEBUTONE or SEBUTONE CREAM is massaged into the wet scalp for 5 minutes and the scalp is then rinsed. Application is repeated, followed by a thorough rinse. Use as often as necessary to keep the scalp free from itching and scaling or as directed. No other shampoo or soap washings are required.

Caution: If undue skin irritation develops or increases, discontinue use. In rare instances, temporary discoloration of white, blond, bleached or tinted hair may occur. Contact with the eyes is to be avoided. In case of contact flush eyes with water.

How Supplied: SEBUTONE in 4 oz. (NDC 0072-5000-04) NSN 6508-00-116-1367 and 8 oz. (NDC 0072-5000-08) plastic bottles.
SEBUTONE CREAM in 4 oz. (NDC 0072-5100-01) tubes.

STATICIN®/T-STAT™ R
(erythromycin)
15% Topical Solution, 20% Topical Solution

Description: STATICIN (erythromycin) 1.5% Topical Solution contains 15 mg/ml erythromycin base in a clear solution vehicle of 55% alcohol, propylene glycol, laureth-4 and fragrance.
T-STAT (erythromycin) 2.0% Topical Solution is a clear liquid antibiotic preparation formulated for the topical treatment of acne. It contains 20 mg of erythromycin per milliliter in a solution of alcohol 71.2%, propylene glycol, fragrance, and citric acid. Erythromycin is a member of the macrolide class of antibiotics and is produced by the actinomycete *Streptomyces erythaeus*.

Actions: Although the mechanism by which STATICIN & T-STAT act in reducing inflammatory lesions of acne vulgaris is unknown, it is presumably due to its antibiotic action.

Indications: STATICIN & T-STAT are indicated for the topical control of acne vulgaris.

Contraindications: STATICIN & T-STAT are contraindicated in persons who have shown hypersensitivity to erythromycin or any of the other listed ingredients.

Continued on next page

Westwood—Cont.

Warnings: The safe use of STATICIN or T-STAT during pregnancy or lactation has not been established.

Precautions: STATICIN & T-STAT are recommended for external use only and should be kept away from the eyes, nose, mouth and other mucous membranes. Concomitant topical acne therapy should be used with caution because a cumulative irritancy effect may occur, especially with the use of peeling, desquamating or abrasive agents.

The use of antibiotic agents may be associated with the overgrowth of antibiotic-resistant organisms. If this occurs, administration of this drug should be discontinued and appropriate measures taken.

Adverse Reactions: STATCIN—Adverse conditions experienced include erythema, desquamation, tenderness, dryness, pruritius and oiliness. Of a total of 193 patients exposed to the drug during clinical effectiveness trials, 155 experienced some type of adverse effect, with approximately half of the patients treated experiencing local drying of the treated areas. There was one case of a generalized urticarial reaction, possibly related to the drug, which required the use of systemic steroid therapy.

Adverse Reactions: T-STAT—Adverse reactions associated with the use of topical erythromycin include dryness, erythema, pruritus, desquamation and burning.

Dosage and Administration: STATICIN & T-STAT should be applied each morning and evening to affected areas. These areas first should be washed, rinsed well, and patted dry. STATICIN & T-STAT should be applied with applicator top, using a dabbing motion. If fingertips are used, wash hands after application. Drying and peeling may be controlled by reducing the frequency of application.

How Supplied: STATICIN solution, 60 ml plastic bottle with optional applicator, NDC 0072-8000-60, NSN 6505-01-118-6098.

T-STAT solution, 60 ml plastic bottle with optional applicator, NDC 0072-8300-60.

Store at controlled room temperature 15°–30°C (59°–86°F).

TACARYL Tablets and Syrup ℞
(Methdilazine HCl)
TACARYL Chewable Tablets ℞
(Methdilazine)

Description: TACARYL, available as methdilazine or methdilazine HCl, a phenothiazine derivative, is 10-(1-methyl-3-pyrrolidinyl) methyl phenothiazine.

Actions: TACARYL and TACARYL HCl are phenothiazine derivatives, possessing antipruritic and antihistaminic properties with anticholinergic (drying) and sedative side effects.

Indication: TACARYL and TACARYL HCl are indicated for the symptomatic relief of pruritic symptoms in urticaria.

Contraindications: TACARYL is contraindicated in comatose states, in patients who have received large amounts of central nervous system depressants (alcohol, barbiturates, narcotics, etc.). It is contraindicated in patients who have bone marrow depression, jaundice, or in those who have demonstrated an idiosyncrasy or hypersensitivity to TACARYL or other phenothiazines. This drug is contraindicated in newborn or premature infants. Further, it should not be used in children acutely ill and dehydrated, as there may be an increased susceptibility to dystonias. Because of the higher risk of drugs of this type for infants generally and prematures in particular, TACARYL is contraindicated in nursing mothers.

Warnings: TACARYL may impair the mental and/or physical ability required for the performance of potentially hazardous tasks, such as driving a vehicle or operating machinery. Similarly, it may impair mental alertness in children. The concomitant use of alcohol or other central nervous system depressants may have an additive effect. Patients should be warned accordingly. TACARYL should be used with extreme caution in patients with: asthmatic attack, narrow-angle glaucoma, prostatic hypertrophy, stenosing peptic ulcer, pyloroduodenal obstruction, bladder neck obstruction, as well as in patients receiving monoamine oxidase inhibitors.

Usage in Pregnancy: The safe use of TACARYL has not been established with respect to the possible adverse effects upon fetal development. Therefore, it is recommended that this medication be given to pregnant patients, or women of child-bearing potential, only when in the judgment of the physician the potential benefits outweigh the possible hazards. There are reports of jaundice and prolonged extrapyramidal symptoms in infants whose mothers received phenothiazines during pregnancy.

Use in Children: TACARYL should be used with caution, as administration in the young child may result in excitation. Overdosage may produce hallucinations, convulsions, and sudden death.

Use in the Elderly (60 Years or Older): The elderly are more prone to develop the following side effects from phenothiazines: hypotension; syncope; toxic confusional states; excessive sedation; extrapyramidal signs, especially parkinsonism; akathisia; persistent dyskinesia.

Precautions: TACARYL may significantly affect the actions of other drugs. It may increase, prolong or intensify the sedative action of central nervous system depressants such as anesthetics, barbiturates or alcohol. The dose of a narcotic or barbiturate may be reduced to ¼ or ½ the usual amount when TACARYL is administered concomitantly. Excessive amounts of TACARYL, relative to a narcotic, may lead to restlessness and motor hyperactivity in the patient with pain.

Phenothiazines may block and even reverse some of the actions of epinephrine.

TACARYL should be used cautiously in persons with acute or chronic respiratory impairment, particularly children. The cough reflex can be suppressed.

TACARYL should be used cautiously in persons with cardiovascular disease, impairment of liver function or those with a history of ulcer disease.

Adverse Reactions: This drug may produce adverse reactions common to both phenothiazines and antihistamines.

Note: Not all of the following adverse reactions have been reported with this specific drug; however, pharmacological similarities among the phenothiazine derivatives require that each be considered when TACARYL is administered. There have been occasional reports of sudden death in patients receiving phenothiazine derivatives chronically.

CNS: Drowsiness is the most prominent CNS effect of this drug. Extrapyramidal reactions occur, particularly with high doses. Hyper-reflexia has been reported in the newborn when a phenothiazine was used during pregnancy. Other reported reactions include dizziness, lassitude, tinnitus, incoordination, fatigue, blurred vision, euphoria, diplopia, nervousness, insomnia, tremors and grand mal seizures; excitation, catatonic-like states, neuritis and hysteria.

Cardiovascular: Postural hypotension is the most common cardiovascular effect of the phenothiazines. Reflex tachycardia may be seen. Bradycardia, faintness, dizziness and cardiac arrest have been reported. ECG changes, including blunting of T waves and prolongation of the Q-T interval, may be seen.

Gastrointestinal: Anorexia, nausea, vomiting, epigastric distress, constipation and dry mouth may occur. Diarrhea has also been reported as well as increased appetite and weight gain.

Genitourinary: Urinary frequency and dysuria, urinary retention, early menses, induced lactation, gynecomastia, decreased libido, inhibition of ejaculation and false pregnancy tests have been reported.

Respiratory: Thickening of bronchial secretions, tightness of the chest, wheezing and nasal stuffiness may occur.

Allergic Reactions: These include urticaria, dermatitis, asthma, laryngeal edema, photosensitivity, lupus erythematosus-like syndrome and anaphylactoid reactions.

Other Reported Reactions: Leukopenia, agranulocytosis, elevation of plasma cholesterol levels, thrombocytopenic purpura and jaundice of the obstructive type have been reported. The jaundice is usually reversible, but chronic jaundice has been reported. High or prolonged glucose tolerance curves, glycosuria, elevated spinal fluid proteins may also occur.

Long-Term Therapy Considerations: After prolonged administration at high dosage, pigmentation of the skin has occurred, chiefly in the exposed areas. Ocular changes consist of the appearance of lenticular and corneal opacities, epithelial keratopathies and pigmentary retinopathy. Vision may be impaired.

Dosage and Administration:
TACARYL® Hydrochloride Tablets (methdilazine HCl)
  Adults: 1 tablet (8 mg.) 2 to 4 times daily.
  Children over 3 years: ½ tablet (4 mg.) 2 to 4 times daily.
TACARYL® Hydrochloride Syrup (methdilazine HCl)
  Adults: 2 teaspoons (8 mg.) 2 to 4 times daily.
  Children over 3 years: 1 teaspoon (4 mg.) 2 to 4 times daily.
TACARYL® Chewable Tablets (methdilazine)
  Adults: 2 tablets (7.2 mg.) 2 to 4 times daily.
  Children over 3 years: 1 tablet (3.6 mg.) 2 to 4 times daily.
  This product form should be chewed and swallowed promptly.

The above doses should be considered maximal daily doses and every effort should be made to minimize side-effects and adverse reactions, through the use of the minimal effective dosage.

Drug Interactions: MAO inhibitors and thiazide diuretics prolong and intensify the anticholinergic effects of the phenothiazines. Combined use of MAO inhibitors and phenothiazines may result in hypotension and extrapyramidal reactions.

Narcotics: The CNS depressant and analgesic effects of narcotics are potentiated by phenothiazines.

The following drugs result in potentiation of phenothiazine effect: oral contraceptives, progesterone, reserpine, nylidrin hydrochloride.

Management of Overdosage: Signs and symptoms of overdosage range from mild depression of the central nervous system and cardiovascular system, to profound hypotension, respiratory depression and unconsciousness. Stimulation may be evident, especially in children and geriatric patients. Atropine-like signs and symptoms—dry mouth; fixed, dilated pupils; flushing; etc.—as well as gastrointestinal symptoms may occur. The treatment of overdosage is essentially symptomatic and supportive. Early gastric lavage may be beneficial. Centrally acting emetics are of little use.

Avoid analeptics, which may cause convulsions. Severe hypotension usually responds to the administration of levarterenol or phenylephrine. EPINEPHRINE SHOULD NOT BE USED, since its use in the patient with partial adrenergic blockade may further lower the blood pressure. Additional measures include oxygen and intravenous fluids. Limited experience with dialysis indicates that it is not helpful.

How Supplied:
TACARYL® Hydrochloride (methdilazine HCl) Tablets 8 mg. each, scored, peach colored tablet (w logo):
  NDC 0072-7400-01   Bottles of 100 (with child-resistant closures)
TACARYL® Hydrochloride (methdilazine HCl) Syrup 4 mg./5 ml:
  NDC 0072-7500-01   Bottles of 16 fl. oz. (1 pint) (with child-resistant closures)
TACARYL® (methdilazine) Chewable Tablets 3.6 mg. each (equivalent to 4 mg. methdilazine HCl), pink, unscored tablet (w logo):

NDC 0072-7300-01 Bottles of 100 (with child-resistant closures)
Shown in Product Identification Section, page 442

TRANSACT®
Transparent Medicated Acne Gel

Composition: Contains 2% Sulfur and 37% alcohol in a greaseless gel base with laureth-4.

Action and Uses: TRANSACT is a transparent, nonstaining and greaseless gel, which leaves a fresh, clean fragrance on the skin. It dries, peels and degreases the skin of acne patients. Its effect is controlled by frequency of application and climatic conditions.

Administration and Dosage: After washing acne skin thoroughly, a thin film is applied to affected areas once daily or as directed. A brief tingling sensation may be expected upon application. Patient should anticipate beneficial drying and peeling in 5 to 7 days. Since TRANSACT is a highly active drying agent it should be used sparingly when initiating therapy, particularly for patients with sensitive skin. 1. Patients with tender skin may best be started on one application every other day. 2. Most other patients can be started on one daily application. 3. When patients develop tolerance, applications may be increased to two and then three times daily to maintain an adequate therapeutic effect. 4. TRANSACT is also for use on the shoulders and back. In dry or cold climates skin is more reactive to TRANSACT and frequency of use should be reduced. During warm, humid months, frequency of use may be increased.

Caution: If undue skin irritation develops, usage schedule should be adjusted or TRANSACT discontinued. For external use only. Avoid contact with eyes. In case of contact, flush eyes with water.

How Supplied: 1 oz. (NDC 0072-5600-01) plastic tube.

WESTCORT®
(hydrocortisone valerate)
Cream/Ointment, 0.2%

Caution: Federal law prohibits dispensing without a prescription.

Description: WESTCORT is a topical formulation containing hydrocortisone valerate, a nonfluorinated steroid. It has the chemical name Pregn-4-ene-3, 20-dione, 11, 21-dihydroxy-17-[(1-oxopentyl) oxy]-, (11β)-; the empirical formula is: $C_{26}H_{38}O_6$; the molecular weight is 446.58, and the CAS registry number is: 57524-89-7. The structural formula is:

Each gram of WESTCORT CREAM contains 2.0 mg hydrocortisone valerate in a hydrophilic base composed of white petrolatum, stearyl alcohol, propylene glycol, amphoteric-9, carbomer 940, sodium phosphate, sodium lauryl sulfate, sorbic acid and water.

Each gram of Westcort Ointment contains 2.0 mg hydrocortisone valerate in a hydrophilic base composed of white petrolatum, stearyl alcohol, propylene glycol, sorbic acid, sodium lauryl sulfate, carbomer 934, sodium phosphate, mineral oil, steareth-2, steareth-100, and water.

Clinical Pharmacology: Topical corticosteroids share anti-inflammatory, anti-pruritic and vasoconstrictive actions.

The mechanism of anti-inflammatory activity of the topical corticosteroids is unclear. Various laboratory methods, including vasoconstrictor assays, are used to compare and predict potencies and/or clinical efficacies of the topical corticosteroids. There is some evidence to suggest that a recognizable correlation exists between vasoconstrictor potency and therapeutic efficacy in man.

Pharmacokinetics: The extent of percutaneous absorption of topical corticosteroids is determined by many factors including the vehicle, the integrity of the epidermal barrier, and the use of occlusive dressings.

Topical corticosteroids can be absorbed from normal intact skin. Inflammation and/or other disease processes in the skin increase percutaneous absorption. Occlusive dressings substantially increase the percutaneous absorption of topical corticosteroids. Thus, occlusive dressings may be a valuable therapeutic adjunct for treatment of resistant dermatoses (see DOSAGE AND ADMINISTRATION).

Once absorbed through the skin, topical corticosteroids are handled through pharmacokinetic pathways similar to systemically administered corticosteroids. Corticosteroids are bound to plasma proteins in varying degrees. Corticosteroids are metabolized primarily in the liver and are then excreted by the kidneys. Some of the topical corticosteroids and their metabolites are also excreted into the bile.

Indications and Usage: WESTCORT is indicated for the relief of the inflammatory and pruritic manifestations of the corticosteroid-responsive dermatoses.

Contraindications: Topical corticosteroids are contraindicated in those patients with a history of hypersensitivity to any of the components of the preparation.

Precautions: *General:* Systemic absorption of topical corticosteroids has produced reversible hypothalamic-pituitary-adrenal (HPA) axis suppression, manifestations of Cushing's syndrome, hyperglycemia, and glucosuria in some patients. Conditions which augment systemic absorption include the application of the more potent steroids, use over large surface areas, prolonged use, and the addition of occlusive dressings.

Therefore, patients receiving a large dose of a potent topical steroid applied to a large surface area or under an occlusive dressing should be evaluated periodically for evidence of HPA axis suppression by using the urinary free cortisol and ACTH stimulation tests. If HPA axis suppression is noted, an attempt should be made to withdraw the drug, to reduce the frequency of application, or to substitute a less potent steroid.

Recovery of HPA axis function is generally prompt and complete upon discontinuation of the drug. Infrequently, signs and symptoms of steroid withdrawal may occur, requiring supplemental systemic corticosteroids.

Children may absorb proportionally larger amounts of topical corticosteroids and thus be more susceptible to systemic toxicity (see PRECAUTIONS—Pediatric Use).

If irritation develops, topical corticosteroids should be discontinued and appropriate therapy instituted.

In the presence of dermatological infections, the use of an appropriate antifungal or antibacterial agent should be instituted. If a favorable response does not occur promptly, the corticosteroids should be discontinued until the infection has been adequately controlled.

Information for the Patient: Patients using topical corticosteroids should receive the following information and instructions:
1. This medication is to be used as directed by the physician. It is for external use only. Avoid contact with the eyes.
2. Patients should be advised not to use this medication for any disorder other than for which it was prescribed.
3. The treated skin area should not be bandaged or otherwise covered or wrapped as to be occlusive unless directed by the physician.
4. Patients should report any signs of local adverse reactions especially under occlusive dressing.
5. Parents of pediatric patients should be advised not to use tight-fitting diapers or plastic pants on a child being treated in the diaper area, as these garments may constitute occlusive dressing.

Laboratory Tests: The following tests may be helpful in evaluating the HPA axis suppression:
Urinary free cortisol test
ACTH stimulation test

Carcinogenesis, Mutagenesis, and Impairment of Fertility: Long-term animal studies have not been performed to evaluate the carcinogenic potential or the effect on fertility of topical corticosteroids.

Studies to determine mutagenicity with prednisolone and hydrocortisone have revealed negative results.

Pregnancy Category C: Corticosteroids are generally teratogenic in laboratory animals when administered systemically at relatively low dosage levels. The more potent corticosteroids have been shown to be teratogenic after dermal application in laboratory animals. There are no adequate and well-controlled studies in pregnant women on teratogenic effects from topically applied corticosteroids. Therefore, topical corticosteroids should be used during pregnancy only if the potential benefit justifies the potential risk to the fetus. Drugs of this class should not be used extensively on pregnant patients, in large amounts, or for prolonged periods of time.

Nursing Mothers: It is not known whether topical administration of corticosteroids could result in sufficient systemic absorption to produce detectable quantities in breast milk. Systemically administered corticosteroids are secreted into breast milk in quantities *not* likely to have a deleterious effect on the infant. Nevertheless, caution should be exercised when topical corticosteroids are administered to a nursing woman.

Pediatric Use: Pediatric patients may demonstrate greater susceptibility to topical corticosteroid-induced HPA axis suppression and Cushing's syndrome than mature patients because of a larger skin surface area to body weight ratio.

Hypothalamic-pituitary-adrenal (HPA) axis suppression, Cushing's syndrome, and intracranial hypertension have been reported in children receiving topical corticosteroids. Manifestations of adrenal suppression in children include linear growth retardation, delayed weight gain, low plasma cortisol levels, and absence of response to ACTH stimulation. Manifestations of intracranial hypertension include bulging fontanelles, headaches, and bilateral papilledema.

Administration of topical corticosteroids to children should be limited to the least amount compatible with an effective therapeutic regimen. Chronic corticosteroid therapy may interfere with the growth and development of children.

Adverse Reactions: The following local adverse reactions are reported infrequently with topical corticosteroids, but may occur more frequently with the use of occlusive dressings. These reactions are listed in an approximate decreasing order of occurrence: burning; itching; irritation; dryness; folliculitis; hypertrichosis; acneiform eruptions; hypopigmentation; perioral dermatitis; allergic contact dermatitis; maceration of the skin; secondary infection; skin atrophy; striae; miliaria.

Overdosage: Topically applied corticosteroids can be absorbed in sufficient amounts to produce systemic effects (see PRECAUTIONS).

Dosage and Administration: WESTCORT should be applied to the affected area as a thin film two or three times daily depending on the severity of the condition.

Occlusive dressings may be used for the management of psoriasis or recalcitrant conditions.

If an infection develops, the use of occlusive dressings should be discontinued and appropriate antimicrobial therapy instituted.

How Supplied: WESTCORT CREAM, 0.2% is supplied in the following tube sizes:
15 g NDC 0072-8100-15; NSN 6505-01-093-9901
45 g NDC 0072-8100-45; NSN 6505-01-083-9395
60 g NDC 0072-8100-60; NSN 6505-01-121-0118
120 g NDC 0072-8100-12

WESTCORT OINTMENT, 0.2% is supplied in the following tube sizes:

Continued on next page

Westwood—Cont.

15 g NDC 0072-7800-15
45 g NDC 0072-7800-45
60 g NDC 0072-7800-60
Store below 78°F (26°C).

Wharton Laboratories, Inc.
37-02 FORTY-EIGHTH AVE.
LONG ISLAND CITY, NY 11101

ECLABRON® ℞
(Guaiacolglycerylether-theophyllinate)

Description: Each tablespoon (15 ml) contains 240 mg. guaiacolglycerylether-theophyllinate equivalent to 150 mg of theophylline (anhydrous) and 90 mg of guaifenesin.
How Supplied: 120 ml bottles—(NDC 0195-0017-53).

NITRONG® OINTMENT ℞
(Nitroglycerin 2%)

Description: NITRONG® Ointment contains 2% nitroglycerin in a special absorptive lanolin-white petrolatum base for topical administration, to provide a controlled-release of the active ingredient. Each inch, as squeezed from the tube, contains approx. 15 mg nitroglycerin.
How Supplied:
30 gram tube (NDC 0195-280-50)
60 gram tube (NDC 0195-280-51)
Unit Dose (1″ Equivalent) (NDC 0195-280-77)

NITRONG® 2.6 mg. Tablets ℞
(nitroglycerin, oral, controlled-release)

Description: Each NITRONG 2.6 mg. tablet for oral administration contains 2.6 mg. nitroglycerin in controlled-release form with light green granules, identified by the U.S. Ethicals trademark. (NDC 0195-0021-20)

NITRONG® 6.5 mg. Tablets ℞
(nitroglycerin, oral, controlled-release)

Description: Each NITRONG 6.5 mg. tablets for oral administration contains 6.5 mg. nitroglycerin in controlled-release form with light orange granules, identified by the U.S. Ethicals trademark. (NDC 0195-0274-20)

NITRONG® 9 mg. Tablets ℞
(nitroglycerin, oral, controlled-release)

Description: Each NITRONG 9.0 mg. tablet for oral administration contains 9.0 mg. nitroglycerin in controlled-release form with blue granules identified by the U.S. Ethicals trademark. (NDC 0195-0300-17)

How Supplied: NITRONG 2.6 mg. and 6.5 mg. are available in bottles of 100 tablets. NITRONG 9.0 mg. is available in bottles of 60 tablets. The tablets are scored and have a mottled appearance.

Important Notice
Before prescribing or administering any product described in PHYSICIANS' DESK REFERENCE always consult the PDR Supplement for possible new or revised information

---

Whitehall Laboratories Inc.
Division of American Home Products Corporation
685 THIRD AVENUE
NEW YORK, NY 10017

ADVIL™
Ibuprofen Tablets, USP
Pain Reliever/Fever Reducer

Warning: ASPIRIN SENSITIVE PATIENTS. Do not take this product if you have had a severe allergic reaction to aspirin, e.g.—asthma, swelling, shock or hives, because even though this product contains no aspirin or salicylates cross-reactions may occur in patients allergic to aspirin.
Active Ingredient: Each tablet contains ibuprofen 200 mg.
Indications: For the temporary relief of minor aches and pains associated with the common cold, headache, toothache, muscular aches, backache, for the minor pain of arthritis, for the pain of menstrual cramps, and for reduction of fever.
Dosage and Administration: Adults: Take one tablet every 4 to 6 hours while symptoms persist. If pain or fever does not respond to one tablet, two tablets may be used but do not exceed six tablets in 24 hours unless directed by a doctor. The smallest effective dose should be used. Take with food or milk if occasional and mild heartburn, upset stomach, or stomach pain occurs with use. Consult a doctor if these symptoms are more than mild or if they persist. Children: Do not give this product to children under 12 except under the advice and supervision of a doctor. Keep this and all drugs out of the reach of children. In case of accidental overdose, seek professional assistance or contact a poison control center immediately.
Warnings: Do not take for pain for more than 10 days or for fever for more than 3 days unless directed by a doctor. If pain or fever persists or gets worse, if new symptoms occur, or if the painful area is red or swollen, consult a doctor. These could be signs of serious illness. If you are under a doctor's care for any serious condition, consult a doctor before taking this product. As with aspirin and acetaminophen, if you have any condition which requires you to take prescription drugs or if you have had any problems or serious side effects from taking any non-prescription pain reliever, do not take this product without first discussing it with your doctor. If you experience any symptoms which are unusual or seem unrelated to the condition for which you took ibuprofen, consult a doctor before taking any more of it. Although ibuprofen is indicated for the same conditions as aspirin and acetaminophen, it should not be taken with them except under a doctor's direction. Before using any drug, including this product, you should seek the advice of a health professional if you are pregnant or nursing a baby. IT IS ESPECIALLY IMPORTANT NOT TO USE IBUPROFEN DURING THE LAST 3 MONTHS OF PREGNANCY UNLESS SPECIFICALLY DIRECTED TO DO SO BY A DOCTOR BECAUSE IT MAY CAUSE PROBLEMS IN THE UNBORN CHILD OR COMPLICATIONS DURING DELIVERY.
Professional Labeling: Same as stated under Indications.
How Supplied: Coated tablets in bottles of 8, 24, 50, and 100.
Storage: Store at room temperature; avoid excessive heat (40°C, 104°F).
Shown in Product Identification Section, page 443

ANACIN®
[an'a-sin]
Analgesic Tablets and Capsules

Active Ingredients: Each tablet or capsule contains: Aspirin 400 mg., Caffeine 32 mg.
Indications and Actions: Anacin relieves pain of headaches, neuralgia, neuritis, sprains, muscular aches, discomforts and fever of colds, pain caused by tooth extraction and toothache, menstrual discomfort. Anacin also temporarily relieves the minor aches and pains of arthritis and rheumatism.
Warnings: As with any drug, if you are pregnant or nursing a baby, seek the advice of a health professional before using this product. Keep this and all medicines out of children's reach. In case of accidental overdose, contact a physician immediately.
Precautions: If pain persists for more than 10 days, or redness is present, or in arthritic or rheumatic conditions affecting children under 12 years of age, consult a physician immediately.
Dosage: Two tablets or capsules with water every 4 hours, as needed. Do not exceed 10 tablets or 10 capsules daily. For children 6–12, half the adult dosage.
Professional Labeling: Same as those outlined under Indications.
How Supplied: Tablets: In tins of 12's and bottles of 30's, 50's, 100's, 200's and 300's. Capsules: In bottles of 20's, 40's, 75's and 125's. Professional Samples: Available upon request. Write Whitehall Laboratories, PDR Dept., New York, N.Y. 10017.
Shown in Product Identification Section, page 443

Children's
ANACIN-3®
[an'a-sin thre]
Acetaminophen
Chewable Tablets, Elixir, Drops

Description: Each Children's Anacin-3 Chewable Tablet contains 80 mg. acetaminophen in a cherry flavored tablet. Children's Anacin-3 acetaminophen Elixir is stable, cherry flavored, red in color and contains 7% alcohol. Infants' Anacin-3 Drops are stable, fruit flavored, red in color and contain 7% alcohol.
Children's Anacin-3 Elixir: Each 5 ml. contains 160 mg. acetaminophen.
Infants' Anacin-3 Drops: Each 0.8 ml. (one calibrated dropperful) contains 80 mg. acetaminophen.
Indications and Actions: Children's Anacin-3 Chewable Tablets, Elixir and Infants' Anacin-3 drops are safe and effective 100% aspirin free products designed for treatment of infants and children with conditions requiring reduction of fever or relief of pain—such as mild upper respiratory infections (tonsillitis, common cold, "grippe"), headache, myalgia, post-immunization reactions, post-tonsillectomy discomfort and gastroenteritis. In conjunction with antibiotics or sulfanomides, Anacin-3 acetaminophen is useful as an analgesic and antipyretic in many bacterial or viral infections, such as bronchitis, pharyngitis, tracheobronchitis, sinusitis, pneumonia, otitis media, and cervical adenitis.
Caution: If fever persists for more than 3 days or recurs, or if pain continues for more than 5 days, consult your physician immediately.
Phenylketonurics: tablets contain Phenylalanine.
Warnings: Keep this and all medicines out of the reach of children. In case of accidental overdose contact a physician immediately.
Dosage: All dosages may be repeated every 4 hours. Do not exceed 5 dosages in any 24 hour period.
Children's Anacin-3 Chewable Tablets: 1–2 years, 18 to 23 lbs: one and one half tablets. 2–3 years, 24 to 35 lbs: two tablets. 4–5 years, 36 to 47 lbs: three tablets. 6–8 years, 48–59 lbs: four tablets. 9–10 years, 60 to 71 lbs: five tablets. 11–12 years, 72 to 95 lbs: six tablets.
Children's Anacin-3 Elixir: (Special cup for measuring dosage is provided) 4–11 months, 12 to 17 lbs: one-half teaspoon. 12–23 months, 18 to 23 lbs: three-quarters teaspoon. 2–3 years, 24 to 35 lbs: one teaspoon. 4–5 years, 36 to 47 lbs: one and one-half teaspoons. 6–8 years, 48 to 59 lbs: two teaspoons. 9–10 years, 60 to 71 lbs: two and one-half teaspoons. 11–12 years, 72 to 95 lbs: three teaspoons.
Infants' Anacin-3 Drops: 0–3 months, 6 to 11 lbs: one-half dropperful. 4–11 months, 12 to 17 lbs: one dropperful. 12–23 months, 18 to 23 lbs: one and one-half dropperful. 2–3 years, 24 to 35 lbs: 2 droppersful. 4–5 years, 36 to 47 lbs: 3 dropperful.

Overdosage: Acetaminophen in massive overdosage may cause hepatic toxicity in some patients. In all cases of suspected overdose, immediately call your regional poison center for assistance in diagnosis and for directions in the use of N-acetylcysteine as an antidote. Adverse effects are rare when acetaminophen is used as recommended.

How Supplied: Chewable Tablets (colored pink, scored, imprinted "CHILDREN A-3")—Bottles of 30. Elixir (colored red)—bottles of 2 and 4 fl. oz. Drops (colored red)—bottles of ½ oz. (15 ml.) with calibrated plastic dropper.

All packages listed above have child-resistant safety caps and tamper resistant packaging.

Shown in Product Identification Section, page 443

Maximum Strength
ANACIN-3®
[an'a-sin thre]
Acetaminophen Tablets and Capsules
Regular Strength
ANACIN-3®
Acetaminophen Tablets

Active Ingredients: Maximum Strength—Each tablet or capsule contains acetaminophen 500 mg. Regular strength—Each tablet contains acetaminophen 325 mg.

Indications and Actions: Anacin-3 is a safe and effective 100% aspirin-free analgesic product that acts fast to provide temporary relief from pain of headache, colds or "flu", sinusitis, muscle aches, bursitis, sprains, overexertion, backache, menstrual discomfort, minor arthritis pain, toothaches and to reduce fever.

Warnings: Keep this and all medicines out of reach of children. In case of accidental overdose, contact a physician immediately. As with any drug, if you are pregnant or nursing a baby, seek the advice of a health professional before using this product.

Caution: If pain persists for more than 10 days or redness is present or in arthritic or rheumatic conditions affecting children under 12, consult a physician immediately.

Dosage and Administration: Maximum Strength—Adults: Two tablets or capsules 3 or 4 times a day. Do not exceed 8 tablets or capsules in any 24-hour period. Regular Strength—Adults: 2 or 3 tablets every 4 hours not to exceed 12 tablets in a 24-hour period. Children (6-12): ½ to 1 tablet 3 to 4 times daily. Consult a physician for use by children under 6 or for use longer than 10 days.

Overdosage: Acetaminophen in massive overdosage may cause hepatic toxicity in some patients. In all cases of suspected overdose, immediately call your regional poison center for assistance in diagnosis and for directions in the use of N-acetylcysteine as an antidote. Adverse effects are rare when acetaminophen is used as recommended.

Professional Labeling: Same as those outlined under Indications.

How Supplied: Maximum Strength—Tablets (colored white, imprinted "A-3" and "500")—tins of 12 and bottles of 30, 60, and 100; Capsules (colored blue and white, imprinted "Anacin-3")—bottles of 20, 40, and 72. Regular Strength—Tablets (colored white, scored, imprinted "A-3") in bottles of 24, 50, and 100.

Shown in Product Identification Section, page 443

ANBESOL® Gel and Liquid
[an'ba-sol'']
Antiseptic Anesthetic

Description: Anbesol is a safe and effective antiseptic-anesthetic that can be used by all family members for the temporary relief of minor mouth pain such as toothache, teething, sore gums and denture irritation. Anbesol also soothes, relieves the pain and helps dry cold sores and fever blisters. Anbesol is also an excellent first-aid measure that provides fast, temporary pain relief and helps prevent infection from minor cuts, scrapes and burns.

Active Ingredients: Gel: Benzocaine (6.3% w/v), Phenol (0.5% w/v), Alcohol (70%). Liquid: Benzocaine (6.3% w/v), Phenol (0.5% w/v), Povidone-Iodine (Yields 0.04% Iodine), Alcohol (70%).

Indications: For fast temporary pain relief of toothache, teething, denture irritation, minor mouth irritations, cold sores, fever blisters, minor cuts, scrapes, and burns.

Actions: Temporarily deadens sensations of nerve endings to provide relief of pain and discomfort; reduces oral bacterial flora temporarily as an aid in oral hygiene.

Warnings: Flammable. Keep away from fire or flame. Avoid smoking during application and until product has dried. Do not use near eyes. Keep this and all medicines out of the reach of children.

Precautions: Not for prolonged use. If the condition persists or irritation develops, discontinue use and consult your physician or dentist. Not for use under dental work.

Dosage and Administration: Apply topically to the affected area on or around the lips, or within the mouth. FOR DENTURE IRRITATION: Apply thin layer to affected area and do not reinsert dental work until irritation/pain is relieved. Rinse mouth before reinserting. If irritation/pain persists, contact your physician.

Professional Labeling: Same as outlined under Indications.

How Supplied: Gel in .25 oz. (7.2 gram) tube. Liquid in two sizes—.31 fl. oz. (9 ml.) and .74 fl. oz. (22 ml.) bottles.

Shown in Product Identification Section, page 443

BABY ANBESOL®
[an'ba-sol'']
Anesthetic Gel

Description: Baby Anbesol Gel is a safe and effective anesthetic developed to soothe the sore gums of an infant by providing temporary relief from pain due to teething.

Active Ingredient: Benzocaine (7.5%) in a special base, flavored with clove oil.

Indications: For fast, temporary relief from the pain and irritation associated with teething.

Actions: A topical anesthetic that temporarily inhibits the conduction of nerve impulses from sensory nerves in the gums to provide relief of pain and discomfort.

Warning: Avoid getting into eyes. Keep this and all medicines out of the reach of children.

Precautions: For persistent or excessive teething pain, consult your pediatrician.

Dosage and Administration: Apply a small amount of Baby Anbesol on the infant's irritated gums with cotton swab or finger tip.

Professional Labeling: Baby Anbesol has been specially formulated to soothe your baby's sore gums and relieve teething pain on contact.

How Supplied: Clear gel in .25 oz. (7.2 grams) tube.

Shown in roduct Identification Section, page 443

ARTHRITIS PAIN FORMULA
[är' thrīt-ıs' pān' for-mye-la]
By the Makers of Anacin® Analgesic Tablets

Active Ingredients: Each tablet contains 7½ grains microfined aspirin. Also contains two buffers, 20 mg. dried Aluminum Hydroxide Gel and 60 mg. Magnesium Hydroxide.

Indications: Fast, temporary relief from minor aches and pain of arthritis and rheumatism and low back pain. Also relieves the pain of headache, neuralgia, neuritis, sprains, muscular aches, discomforts and fever of colds, pain caused by tooth extraction and toothache, and menstrual discomfort.

Actions: Arthritis Pain Formula contains 50% more pain relief medicine than ordinary aspirin or regular buffered aspirin. Arthritis Pain Formula also provides extra stomach protection because, in addition to containing two buffers, the pain reliever is microfined. This means the pain relieving particles are so fine they dissolve rapidly and so are less apt to cause stomach upset.

Warnings: Keep this and all medications out of children's reach. In case of accidental overdose, contact a physician immediately.

Caution: In arthritic or rheumatic conditions, if pain persists for more than 10 days, or redness is present, consult a physician immediately. As with any drug, if you are pregnant or nursing a baby, seek the advice of a health professional before using this product.

Dosage and Administration: Adult Dosage: 2 tablets, 3 or 4 times a day. Do not exceed 8 tablets in any 24 hour period. For children under 12, consult your physician.

Professional Labeling: Same as stated under "Indications".

How Supplied: In plastic bottles of 40, 100 and 175 tablets.

Shown in Product Identification Section, page 443

SAFETY COATED APF®
[sāf-tē kōt-ed APF]
ARTHRITIS PAIN FORMULA™
By the makers of Anacin® Analgesic Tablets

Active Ingredients: Each tablet contains 500 mg. aspirin with a special enteric safety coating.

Indications: Safety Coated APF provides hours of temporary relief from minor aches and pains of arthritis and rheumatism. It also helps relieve low back pain and the pain of neuralgia, neuritis and muscular aches.

Actions: Safety Coated APF contains 500 mg. aspirin and is maximum strength. Its special safety coating is designed to dissolve in the small intestine, not in the stomach, for maximum stomach protection.

Warning: Discontinue use if ringing in the ears or other symptoms occur. Keep this and all medications out of children's reach. In case of accidental overdose, consult a physician immediately. As with any drug, if you are pregnant or nursing a baby, seek the advice of a health professional before using this product.

Caution: In arthritic or rheumatic conditions, if pain persists for more than 10 days or redness is present, consult a physician immediately.

Dosage and Administration: Adult Dosage: 2 tablets every 6 hours with water. Do not exceed 8 tablets in any 24 hour period. In children under 12, consult your physician.

Professional Labeling: Same as those outlined under Indications.

How Supplied: In plastic bottles of 24, 60 and 125 tablets.

Shown in Product Identification Section, page 443

DENOREX®
[děn' ō-reks]
Medicated Shampoo
DENOREX®
Mountain Fresh Herbal Scent
Medicated Shampoo
DENOREX®
Medicated Shampoo and Conditioner

Active Ingredients:
Lotion: Coal Tar Solution 9.0%, Menthol 1.5%, Alcohol 7.5%. Also contains TEA-Lauryl Sulfate, Water, Lauramide DEA, Stearic Acid, Chloroxylenol.
Shampoo and Conditioner: Coal Tar Solution 9.0%, Menthol 1.5%, Alcohol 7.5%. Also contains TEA-Lauryl Sulfate, Water, Lauramide DEA, PEG-27 Lanolin, Quaterium 23, Fragrance, Chloroxylenol Hydroxypropyl Methylcellulose, Citric Acid.
Gel: Coal Tar Solution 9.0%, Menthol 1.5%, Alcohol 7.5%. Also contains TEA-Lauryl Sulfate, Water, Hydroxypropyl Methylcellulose, Chloroxylenol.

Indications: Relieves scaling—itching—flaking of dandruff, seborrhea and psoriasis. Regular use promotes cleaner, healthier hair and scalp.

Actions: Denorex Shampoo is antiseborrheic and antipruritic. Loosens and softens scales and crusts. Coal tar helps correct abnormalities of ke-

Continued on next page

Whitehall—Cont.

ratinization by decreasing epidermal proliferation and dermal infiltration. Denorex also contains the antipruritic agent, menthol, which is "one of the most widely used antipruritics in dermatologic therapy of various diseases accompanied by itching". (The United States Dispensatory—26th Edition).

Warnings: For external use only. Discontinue treatment if irritation develops. Avoid contact with eyes. Keep this and all medicines out of children's reach.

Directions: For best results, shampoo every other day. For severe scalp problems use daily. Wet hair thoroughly and briskly massage until a rich lather is obtained. Rinse thoroughly and repeat. Scalp may tingle slightly during treatment.

Professional Labeling: Same as stated under Indications.

How Supplied:

Lotion: 4 oz. and 8 oz. and 12 oz. bottles in Regular Scent, Mountain Fresh Herbal Scent, and Shampoo and Conditioner.

Gel: 2 oz. Tube and 4 oz. Tube in Regular Scent

Shown in Product Identification Section, page 443

DRISTAN®
[drĭs'tăn]
Nasal Spray
DRISTAN®
Menthol Nasal Spray

Active Ingredients: Phenylephrine HCl 0.5%, Pheniramine Maleate 0.2%.

Other Ingredients: Dristan Nasal Spray: Benzalkonium Chloride 1:5000 in buffered isotonic aqueous solution, Thimerosal preservative 0.002% (loss is unavoidable), Alcohol 0.4%.

Dristan Menthol Nasal Spray: Benzalkonium Chloride 1:5000 in buffered isotonic aqueous solution, Thimerosal preservative 0.002% (loss is unavoidable) with aromatics (Menthol, Eucalyptol, Camphor, Methyl Salicylate).

Indications: For prompt temporary relief of nasal congestion due to the common cold, sinusitis, hay fever or other upper respiratory allergies.

Actions: Phenylephrine HCl is a sympathomimetic agent that constricts the smaller arterioles of the nasal passages producing a gentle and predictable decongesting effect. Pheniramine Maleate is an antihistamine that controls rhinorrhea, sneezing, and lacrimation associated with elevated histamine levels in disorders of the respiratory tract.

Warnings: Do not exceed recommended dosage because symptoms may occur such as burning, stinging, sneezing, or increase of nasal discharge. Do not use this product for more than 3 days. If symptoms persist, consult a physician. As with any drug, if you are pregnant or nursing a baby, seek the advice of a health professional before using this product. The use of this dispenser by more than one person may spread infection. For adult use only. Do not give this product to children under 12 years except under the advice and supervision of a physician. Keep these and all medicines out of the reach of children. In case of accidental ingestion, seek professional assistance or contact a poison control center immediately.

Dosage and Administration: With head upright, insert nozzle in nostril. Spray quickly, firmly and sniff deeply. Adults: Spray 2 or 3 times into each nostril. Repeat every 4 hours as needed. Children under 12 years: As directed by a physician.

Professional Labeling: Same as those outlined under Indications.

How Supplied: 15 ml. and 30 ml. plastic squeeze bottles.

Shown in Product Identification Section, page 443

DRISTAN®
[drĭs'tăn]
Long Lasting Nasal Spray
DRISTAN®
Long Lasting Menthol Nasal Spray

Active Ingredient: Oxymetazoline HCl 0.05%.
Other Ingredients: Dristan Long Lasting Nasal Spray: Benzalkonium Chloride 1:5000 in buffered isotonic aqueous solution, Thimerosal preservative 0.002% (loss is unavoidable).

Dristan Long Lasting Menthol Nasal Spray: Benzalkonium Chloride 1:5000 in buffered isotonic aqueous solution with aromatics (Menthol, Eucalyptol, Camphor), Thimerosal preservative 0.002% (loss is unavoidable).

Indications: Dristan Long Lasting Nasal Spray and Dristan Long Lasting Menthol Nasal Spray are indicated for prompt temporary relief of nasal congestion due to the common cold, sinusitis, hay fever, or other upper respiratory allergies for up to 12 hours.

Actions: The sympathomimetic action of Dristan Long Lasting Nasal Spray and Dristan Long Lasting Menthol Nasal Spray constricts the smaller arterioles of the nasal passages, producing a prolonged, up to 12 hours, gentle and predictable decongesting effect.

Warnings: Do not exceed recommended dosage because symptoms may occur, such as burning, stinging, sneezing, or an increase of nasal discharge. Do not use this product for more than 3 days. If symptoms persist, consult a physician. As with any drug, if you are pregnant or nursing a baby, seek the advice of a health professional before using this product. The use of the dispenser by more than one person may spread infection. Keep these and all medicines out of the reach of children. In case of accidental ingestion, seek professional assistance or contact a poison control center immediately.

Dosage and Administration: With head upright, insert nozzle in nostril. Spray quickly, firmly and sniff deeply. Adults and children 6 years of age and over, spray 2 or 3 times into each nostril. Repeat twice daily—morning and evening. Not recommended for children under six.

Professional labeling: Same as those outlined under Indications.

How Supplied: Dristan Long Lasting Nasal Spray: 15 ml. and 30 ml. plastic squeeze bottles. Dristan Long Lasting Menthol Nasal Spray: 15 ml. plastic squeeze bottle.

Shown in Product Identification Section, page 443

Advanced Formula
DRISTAN®
[drĭs'tăn]
Decongestant/Antihistamine/Analgesic
Tablets and Capsules

Active Ingredients: Each Dristan Tablet or Capsule contains: Phenylephrine HCl 5 mg., Chlorpheniramine Maleate 2 mg., Acetaminophen 325 mg.

Indications: For hours of effective multi-symptom relief of colds/flu, sinusitis, hay fever, or other upper respiratory allergies: nasal congestion, sneezing, runny nose, fever, headache and minor aches and pains.

Actions: Acetaminophen is both analgesic and antipyretic. Therapeutic doses of acetaminophen will effectively reduce an elevated body temperature. Also, acetaminophen is effective in reducing the discomfort of pain associated with headache. Phenylephrine HCl is an oral nasal decongestant (Sympathomimetic Amine), effective as a vasoconstrictor to help reduce nasal/sinus congestion. Chlorpheniramine Maleate is an antihistamine effective in the control of rhinorrhea, sneezing and lacrimation associated with elevated histamine levels in disorders of the respiratory tract.

Dosage and Administration: Adults: Two tablets or capsules every four hours, not to exceed 12 tablets or capsules in 24 hours. Children 6–12: One tablet or capsule every four hours, not to exceed six tablets or capsules in 24 hours.

Warnings: Avoid alcoholic beverages and driving a motor vehicle or operating heavy machinery while taking this product. May cause drowsiness or excitability, especially in children. Persons with asthma, glaucoma, high blood pressure, diabetes, heart or thyroid disease, difficulty in urination due to enlarged prostate gland or taking an antidepressant drug, should use only as directed by a physician. Do not exceed recommended dosage because at higher doses nervousness, dizziness, or sleeplessness may occur. If symptoms do not improve within 7 days or are accompanied by a high fever, discontinue use and see a physician. As with any drug, if you are pregnant or nursing a baby, seek the advice of a health professional before using this product.

Do not give to children under 6. Keep this and all medication out of children's reach. In case of accidental overdose contact a physician immediately.

Professional Labeling: Same as those outlined under Indications.

How Supplied: Yellow/White uncoated tablets in tins of 12's and bottles of 24's, 50's, and 100's, and physician dispensers of 100 2-tablet patient sample pouches. Red/White capsules in bottles of 20 and 40.

Shown in Product Identification Section, page 443

PREPARATION H®
[prep-e'rā-shen āch]
Hemorrhoidal Ointment
PREPARATION H®
Hemorrhoidal Suppositories

Active Ingredients: Live Yeast Cell Derivative, supplying 2,000 units skin respiratory factor per ounce of ointment or suppository base. Shark liver oil 3.0%; in a specially prepared base with Phenylmercuric Nitrate 1:10,000 (as a preservative).

Indications: To help shrink swelling of hemorrhoidal tissues caused by inflammation, and to give prompt, temporary relief in many cases from pain and itch in tissues.

Actions: Live Yeast Cell Derivative acts to: A) Increase the oxygen utilization of dermal tissue. B) Increases collagen formation. C) Increases the rate of wound healing. Shark liver oil has been incorporated to act as a protectant which softens and soothes the tissue. Preparation H also lubricates inflamed, irritated surfaces to help make bowel movements less painful.

Precaution: In case of bleeding, or if your condition persists, a physician should be consulted.

Dosage and Administration: Ointment: Apply freely, night, morning, after each bowel movement and whenever symptoms occur. Lubricate applicator before each application and thoroughly cleanse after use.

Suppository: Remove wrapper and insert one suppository night, morning, after each bowel movement and whenever symptoms occur. Store at controlled room temperature in cool place but not over 80° F.

Professional Labeling: Same as those outlined under Indications.

How Supplied: Ointment: Net wt. 1 oz. and 2 oz. Suppository: 12's, 24's and 48's.

Shown in Product Identification Section, page 443

PRIMATENE®
[prīm'a-tēn]
Mist
(Epinephrine)

Active Ingredients: Each spray delivers approximately 0.2 mg. Epinephrine. A 0.5% w/w (= 5.5 mg./cc.) solution of U.S.P. Epinephrine containing Absorbic Acid as a preservative in an inert propellant. Alcohol 34%.

Indications: Provides temporary relief from acute paroxysms of bronchial asthma.

Warnings: For INHALATION ONLY. Contents under pressure. Do not puncture or throw container into incinerator.

Using or storing near open flame or heating above 120° F may cause bursting.

Do not use unless a diagnosis of asthma has been established by a physician. Reduce dosage if bronchial irritation, nervousness, restlessness or sleeplessness occurs. Overdose may cause nervousness and rapid heartbeat. Use only on the advice of a physician if heart disease, high blood pressure, diabetes, or thyroid disease is present. If difficulty in breathing persists, or if relief does not occur within 20 minutes of inhalation, discontinue use and seek medical assistance immediately. As with any drug, if you are pregnant or nursing a baby, seek the advice of a health professional before using this product. Children under 6 years of age should use Primatene Mist only on the advice of a physician. KEEP THIS AND ALL MEDICINES OUT OF REACH OF CHILDREN.

Directions:
1. Take plastic cap off mouthpiece. (For refills, use mouthpiece from previous purchase).
2. Take plastic mouthpiece off bottle.
3. Place other end of mouthpiece on bottle.
4. Turn bottle upside down. Place thumb on bottom of mouthpiece over the circular button and forefinger on top of vial. Empty the lungs as completely as possible by exhaling.
5. Place mouthpiece in mouth with lips closed around opening. Inhale deeply while squeezing mouthpiece and bottle together. Release immediately and remove unit from mouth, then complete taking the deep breath, drawing medication into your lungs, holding breath as long as comfortable.
6. Then exhale slowly keeping lips nearly closed. This distributes the medication in the lungs.

Dosage: Start with one inhalation by squeezing mouthpiece and bottle together. Release immediately and remove unit from mouth. Then wait at least one minute. If not relieved, use Primatene Mist once more; do not repeat treatment for at least 4 hours.

Professional Labeling: Same as stated under Indications.

How Supplied: ½ fl. oz (15 cc) with mouthpiece.
½ fl. oz. (15 cc) refill
¾ fl. oz. (22.5 cc) refill

Shown in Product Identification Section, page 443

PRIMATENE®
[prīm′a-tēn]
**Mist Suspension
(Epinephrine Bitartrate)**

Active Ingredients: Each spray delivers 0.3 mg. Epinephrine Bitartrate equivalent to 0.16 mg. Epinephrine base. Contains Epinephrine Bitartrate 7.0 mg. per cc. in an inert propellant.

Indications: Provides temporary relief from acute paroxysms of bronchial asthma.

Warnings: For INHALATION ONLY. Contents under pressure. Do not puncture or throw container into incinerator. Using or storing near open flame or heating above 120°F may cause bursting. Do not use unless a diagnosis of asthma has been established by a physician. Reduce dosage if bronchial irritation, nervousness, restlessness or sleeplessness occurs. Overdose may cause nervousness and rapid heartbeat. Use only on the advice of a physician if heart disease, high blood pressure, diabetes, or thyroid disease is present. If difficulty in breathing persists, or if relief does not occur within 20 minutes of inhalation, discontinue use and seek medical assistance immediately. As with any drug, if you are pregnant or nursing a baby, seek the advice of a health professional before using this product. Children under 6 years of age should use Primatene Mist only on the advice of a physician. KEEP THIS AND ALL MEDICINES OUT OF REACH OF CHILDREN.

Administration: Directions: 1. Shake well. 2. Hold inhaler with nozzle down while using. Empty the lungs as completely as possible by exhaling. 3. Purse the lips as in saying "o" and hold the nozzle up to the lips, keeping the tongue flat. As you start to take a deep breath, squeeze nozzle and can together, releasing one one full application. Complete taking deep breath, drawing medication into your lungs. 4. Hold breath for as long as comfortable. This distributes the medication in the lungs. Then exhale slowly, keeping the lips nearly closed.

5. Rinse nozzle daily with soap and hot water after removing from vial. Dry with clean cloth.

Dosage: Start with one inhalation—then wait at least one minute; if not relieved, use Primatene Mist Suspension once more; do not repeat treatment for at least 4 hours.

Professional Labeling: Same as stated under Indications.

How Supplied: ⅓ fl. oz. (10 cc.) pocket-size aerosol inhaler.

PRIMATENE®
[prīm′a-tēn]
Tablets

Available in two formulas, "M" or "P", depending on state. See details below in section on "How Supplied".

Active Ingredients: Theophylline 130 mg., Ephedrine Hydrochloride 24 mg., Phenobarbital 8 mg. (⅛ gr.) per tablet. In those states where Phenobarbital is ℞ only, Pyrilamine Maleate 16.6 mg. is substituted for the Phenobarbital.

Indications: For relief and control of attacks of bronchial asthma and associated hay fever.

Actions: Theophylline and ephedrine both produce bronchodilation through relaxation of bronchial muscle spasm, as occurs in attacks of bronchial asthma. Because theophylline is a methylxanthine and ephedrine is a sympathomimetic, they are believed to have different mechanisms of action.

Warnings: If symptoms persist, consult your physician. Some people are sensitive to ephedrine and, in such cases, temporary sleeplessness and nervousness may occur. These reactions will disappear if the use of the medication is discontinued. Do not exceed recommended dosage.
People who have heart disease, high blood pressure, diabetes or thyroid trouble should take this preparation only on the advice of a physician. "M" Formula, may cause drowsiness. People taking the "M" Formula should not drive or operate machinery. "P" Formula may be habit forming.

Caution: As with any drug, if you are pregnant or nursing a baby, seek the advice of a health professional before using this product. Keep all medicines out of reach of children.

Dosage and Administration: Adults: 1 or 2 tablets initially and then one every 4 hours, as needed, not to exceed 6 tablets in 24 hours. Children (6–12): One half adult dose. For children under 6, consult a physician.

Professional Labeling: Same as stated under Indications.

How Supplied: Available in two forms coded "M" or "P". "M" formula, containing pyrilamine maleate, is available in those states where phenobarbital is ℞ only. "P" formula, containing phenobarbital, is available in all other states. Both "M" and "P" formulas are supplied in glass bottles of 24 and 60 tablets.

Shown in Product Identification Section, page 443

SEMICID®
[sĕm′ē-sĭd]
Vaginal Contraceptive Suppositories

Description: Semicid is a safe, effective, vaginal contraceptive in suppository form.
Convenient, Individually Wrapped, No Hormones, odorless, non-messy.

Active Ingredient: Each suppository contains nonoxynol-9, 100 mg.

Indication: For the prevention of pregnancy.

Actions: Semicid dissolves in the vagina and blends with natural vaginal secretions to provide double birth control protection: a physical barrier, plus an effective sperm killing barrier that covers the cervical opening and adjoining vaginal walls. Each Semicid suppository contains the maximum allowable amount of nonoxynol-9, the most widely used nonprescription spermicide.
Semicid requires no applicator and has no unpleasant taste or odor. Semicid is not messy and it does not drip or run like foams, creams and jellies. And it's not awkward to use like the diaphragm. As with all spermicides, some Semicid users experience irritation in using the product, but for years most women have used Semicid safely and effectively with full satisfaction. Also, Semicid does not effervesce like some suppositories, so it is not as likely to cause a burning feeling.
Semicid is approximately as effective as vaginal foam contraceptives in actual use, but is not as effective as the Pill or IUD.
Semicid provides effective contraceptive protection when used properly. However, no contraceptive method or product can provide an absolute guarantee against becoming pregnant.

Dosage and Administration: To use, just unwrap one suppository and insert it deeply into the vagina. It is essential that Semicid be inserted at least 15 minutes before intercourse, however Semicid is also effective when inserted up to 1 hour before intercourse. If intercourse is delayed for more than 1 hour after Semicid is inserted, or if intercourse is repeated, then another suppository must be inserted. Semicid can be used as frequently as needed.

Warnings: Do not insert in urinary opening. Do not take orally. If irritation occurs, discontinue use. If irritation persists, consult your physician. Keep this and all contraceptives out of the reach of children.

How to Store: Keep Semicid at room temperature (not over 86°F or 30°C).

Precautions: If douching is desired, one should wait at least six hours after intercourse before douching. If either partner experiences irritation, discontinue use. If irritation persists, consult a physician.
If your doctor has told you that you should not become pregnant, ask your doctor if you can use Semicid.
If menstrual period is missed, a physician should be consulted.

How Supplied: Strip packaging of 3's, 10's and 20's.

Shown in Product Identification Section, page 443

Willen Drug Company
**18 NORTH HIGH STREET
BALTIMORE, MD 21202**

BICITRA®—Sugar-Free   ℞
[bye″sit-rah]
**(Brand of Sodium Citrate & Citric
Acid Oral Solution USP)**

Description: BICITRA is a stable and pleasant tasting oral systemic alkalizer and neutralizing buffer composed of Sodium Citrate and Citric Acid in a sugar-free base. BICITRA is the USP formula for SHOHL'S Solution.

Composition: BICITRA contains in each teaspoonful (5 ml): Sodium Citrate Dihydrate 500mg (0.34 Molar) and Citric Acid Monohydrate 334mg (0.32 Molar). Each ml contains 1 mEq Sodium ion and is equivalent to 1 mEq. Bicarbonate (HCO_3).

Actions: Sodium Citrate is absorbed and metabolized to sodium bicarbonate, thus acting as a systemic alkalizer. The effects are essentially those of chlorides before absorption and those of bicarbonates subsequently. BICITRA is useful for effectively buffering and neutralizing gastric acid, especially in preanesthesia medication.

Indications and Advantages: BICITRA is an effective oral alkalizing agent and a non-particulate acid neutralizing buffer. BICITRA offers the advantage over particulate antacids by being absorbed and metabolized, since it is a systemic alkalizer. It is useful in those conditions where long term maintenance of an alkaline urine is desirable, and is of value in the alleviation of chronic metabolic acidosis such as results from chronic renal insufficiency or the syndrome of renal tubular acidosis, especially when the administration of potassium salts is undesirable or contraindicated. BICITRA is fast-acting and useful in raising the pH value of gastric acid. In vitro tests have shown that 15ml BICITRA plus 15ml water will neutral-

Continued on next page

Willen—Cont.

ize and buffer 117ml of 0.1N HCl to a pH value of 2.5, with no alteration or changes in pH value after 2 hours elapsed time. BICITRA is concentrated, and when administered after meals and before bedtime, allows one to maintain an alkaline urine pH around the clock, usually without the necessity of a 2 A.M. dose. BICITRA alkalinizes the urine without producing a systemic alkalosis in the recommended dosage. BICITRA is pleasant tasting and tolerable, even when administered for long periods, and offers these advantages over SHOHL'S Solution, while supplying the equivalent sodium content. BICITRA is sugar-free.
Contraindications: Patients on sodium-restricted diet or with severe renal impairment. In certain situations, Potassium Citrate, as contained in Syrup POLYCITRA-K may be preferable.
Precautions: Should be used with caution by patients with low urinary output unless under the supervision of a physician. Patients should be directed to dilute adequately with water and preferably, to take each dose after meals to avoid saline laxative effect. Sodium salts should be used cautiously in patients with cardiac failure, hypertension, impaired renal function, peripheral and pulmonary edema and toxemia of pregnancy. Periodic examinations and determinations of serum electrolytes, particularly serum bicarbonate level, should be carried out in those patients with renal disease in order to avoid these complications.
Adverse Reactions: BICITRA is generally well tolerated without any unpleasant side effects when given in recommended doses to patients with normal renal function and urinary output. However, as with any alkalinizing agent, caution must be used in certain patients with abnormal renal mechanisms to avoid development of alkalosis, especially in the presence of hypocalcemia.
Dosage and Administration: BICITRA should be taken diluted in water followed by additional water, if desired.
For Systemic Alkalization:
Usual Adult Dose: 10 to 30ml diluted in 1 to 3 ounces of water after meals and at bedtime, or as directed by physician.
As a Neutralizing Buffer: 15ml diluted with 15ml water, taken as a single dose, or as directed by physician.
Overdosage: Overdosage with sodium salts may cause diarrhea, nausea and vomiting, hypernoea, and convulsions.
How Supplied: BICITRA—16 fl oz. (473ml) (NDC 11414-207-01); 1 gallon (NDC 11414-207-08); 4 fl oz (120ml) (NDC 11414-207-04); 15ml Unit-Dose (NDC 11414-207-15).
Literature Available: Yes

NEUTRA-PHOS® Powder & Capsules
NEUTRA-PHOS®-K Powder & Capsules
[new" trah foss']
Oral Phosphorus Dietary Supplement

NEUTRA-PHOS and NEUTRA-PHOS-K supply the physiologically important element—PHOSPHORUS—as inorganic orthophosphate, in a well tolerated oral compound. Each contains a chemically balanced combination of readily soluble inorganic phosphates, affording a very high source of elemental Phosphorus. Both products supply equal concentration of elemental Phosphorus.
Composition: NEUTRA-PHOS is a stable powder combination of monobasic and dibasic Sodium and Potassium Phosphates. NEUTRA-PHOS-K is a stable sodium-free powder combination of monobasic and dibasic Potassium Phosphates intended for oral use in low sodium diets. Both products form an oral solution by reconstitution with water and are neutral (pH 7.3), isotonic, pleasant tasting sources of Phosphorus. There is less than 1 calorie per average dose.
Indications: NEUTRA-PHOS and NEUTRA-PHOS-K are recommended as oral Phosphorus supplements, particularly if the diet is low in mineral intake or if needs are increased.

Advantages: NEUTRA-PHOS and NEUTRA-PHOS-K, reconstituted to an oral liquid, provide rapid absorption and utilization from the alimentary tract. This is very advantageous compared to the use of coated or uncoated tablet dosage forms. (The patient ingests a liquid rather than a slowly dissolving tablet which may cause localized irritation or inflamation in sensitive individuals.) Both products are highly concentrated and thus economically provide inorganic Phosphate. They are especially useful for long term maintenance requirements. NEUTRA-PHOS also supplies Sodium and Potassium in equimolar proportions—a decided advantage over products which supply a high amount of sodium and a low amount of potassium per dose. NEUTRA-PHOS-K supplies only Potassium and is recommended when a low sodium diet is indicated.
Electrolytes Supplied: 2-½ fluid ounces (75 ml) of the reconstituted solution or contents of 1 capsule* supplies:

Electrolyte	NEUTRA-PHOS mg.	mEq
Phosphorus	250	14.25
Phosphate (PO$_4$)	765	—
Sodium	164	7.125
Potassium	278	7.125

Electrolyte	NEUTRA-PHOS-K mg.	mEq
Phosphorus	250	14.25
Phosphate (PO$_4$)	765	—
Sodium	none	none
Potassium	556	14.25

(*reconstituted in water as per label directions. Refer to Capsules description.)
Average Directions for Adults and Children: 4 or more years of age: 2-½ fl. oz. (75 ml) of the oral solution, or contents of 1 capsule, equivalent to 250 mg Phosphorus, taken 4 times a day. (See Capsules description.)
Pediatric Dose: Infants and children under 4 years of age: 2 fl. oz. (60 ml) of the oral solution, equivalent to 200 mg of Phosphorus, taken 4 times a day.
Usual Dose Range: 2-½ fl. oz. to 20 fl. oz. (75 ml to 600 ml) of the oral solution, or contents of 1 to 8 capsules (equivalent from 250 mg to 2 grams of Phosphorus) taken daily in divided doses, after meals and at bedtime.
2-½ fl. oz. (75 ml) or 1 capsule, 4 times a day supplies 1 gm. Phosphorus. 5 fl. oz. (150 ml) or 2 capsules, 3 times a day supplies 1.5 gm. Phosphorus. 5 fl. oz. (150 ml) or 2 capsules, 4 times a day supplies 2 gm. Phosphorus. (See Capsules description).
Precautions and Side Effects: Reconstitute powder and contents of capsules as directed before taking. Occasionally some individuals may experience a mild laxative effect for the first day or two when beginning to use NEUTRA-PHOS. If this persists to an unpleasant degree, reduce the daily intake until this effect subsides or, if necessary, discontinue its use.
How Supplied: Both products are supplied as powder concentrates, to be reconstituted with water by the patient, and are available in multiple dose or single dose capsule sizes.
Multiple Dose Powder Concentrate: For patient convenience, these powder concentrates are packaged in a size sufficient to make 1 gallon (3.785 Liters) and are intended for use while at home. This economical dosage form is prepared by the patient who is instructed to dissolve the entire contents of 1 bottle in sufficient water to make 1 gallon of solution. This solution is not to be diluted and can be stored for 60 days. It can be chilled if desired, to increase palatability. 2-½ fl. oz. (75 ml) of this solution supplies 250 mg Phosphorus (refer to electrolyte chart).
Capsules: These products are also supplied in pre-measured capsules which are intended for use if the above multiple dose form precludes transportation of liquid. The contents of 1 capsule makes 2-½ fl. oz. (75 ml) of an oral suspension equal to the oral solution prepared above. To use, empty the contents of 1 capsule into ⅓ glass water (approx. 2-½ fl. oz.) and stir well and take promptly. Each capsule supplies 250 mg Phosphorus (refer to electrolyte chart).
NEUTRA-PHOS Powder Concentrate—2-¼ oz. (64 gm) bottle. Reconstitutes to 1 gallon Stock No. 201-01.
NEUTRA-PHOS Capsules—1.25 gm powder concentrate per capsule, 48 capsules per bottle Stock No. 202-01.
NEUTRA-PHOS-K Powder Concentrate—2-½ oz. (71 gm) bottle. Reconstitutes to 1 gallon Stock No. 203-01.
NEUTRA-PHOS-K Capsules—1.45 gm powder concentrate per capsule, 48 capsules per bottle Stock No. 204-01.
Is this product O.T.C.: Yes.
Literature Available: Yes.

POLYCITRA® Syrup
POLYCITRA®-LC-Sugar-Free
[polly"sit-rah]
(Brand of Tricitrates Oral Solution U.S.P.)

Description: Syrup POLYCITRA and POLYCITRA-LC are stable and pleasant-tasting oral systemic alkalizers containing Potassium Citrate, Sodium Citrate and Citric Acid. Syrup POLYCITRA is a sugar-base preparation. POLYCITRA-LC is a sugar-free solution, to be used by patients who desire a low-carbohydrate diet. Both products are non-alcoholic and contain identical amounts of active ingredients.
Composition: Syrup POLYCITRA and POLYCITRA-LC contains in each teaspoonful (5 ml): Potassium Citrate Monohydrate 550 mg (0.34 Molar), Sodium Citrate Dihydrate 500 mg (0.34 Molar), and Citric Acid Monohydrate 334 mg (0.32 Molar). Each ml contains 1 mEq. Potassium ion and 1 mEq. Sodium ion and is equivalent to 2 mEq. Bicarbonate (HCO$_3$).
Actions: Potassium Citrate and Sodium Citrate are absorbed and metabolized to potassium bicarbonate and sodium bicarbonate, thus acting as systemic alkalizers. The effects are essentially those of chlorides before absorption and those of bicarbonates subsequently.
Indications and Advantages: Syrup POLYCITRA and POLYCITRA-LC are effective alkalinizing agents useful in those conditions where long term maintenance of an alkaline urine is desirable, such as in patients with uric acid and cystine calculi of the urinary tract. In addition, they are valuable adjuvants when administered with uricosuric agents in gout therapy, since urates tend to crystallize out of an acid urine. They are also effective in correcting the acidosis of certain renal tubular disorders. Syrup POLYCITRA and POLYCITRA-LC are highly concentrated, and when administered after meals and before bedtime, allows one to maintain an alkaline urine pH around the clock, usually without the necessity of a 2 AM dose. Syrup POLYCITRA and POLYCITRA-LC alkalinize the urine without producing a systemic alkalosis in recommended dosage. They are highly palatable, pleasant tasting and tolerable, even when administered for long periods. POLYCITRA-LC is a fast-acting and effective non-particulate neutralizing buffer, useful in raising the pH value of gastric acid. In vitro tests have shown that 15 ml POLYCITRA-LC plus 15 ml water will neutralize and buffer 234 ml of 0.1N HCl to a pH value of 2.9, with no alteration or changes in pH value after 2 hours elapsed time.
Contraindications: Severe renal impairment with oliguria or azotemia, untreated Addison's disease or severe myocardial damage. In certain situations, when patients are on a sodium-restricted diet, the use of Potassium Citrate, as contained in Syrup POLYCITRA-K, may be preferable; or when patients are on a potassium-restricted diet, the use of Sodium Citrate, as contained in BICITRA, may be preferable.
Precautions and Warnings: Should be used with caution by patients with low urinary output unless under the supervision of a physician. Pa-

tients should be directed to dilute adequately with water and preferably, to take each dose after meals, to minimize the possibility of gastrointestinal injury associated with oral ingestion of potassium salt preparations and to avoid saline laxative effect. Sodium salts should be used cautiously in patients with cardiac failure, hypertension, peripheral and pulmonary edema and toxemia of pregnancy. Concurrent administration of potassium-containing medication, potassium-sparing diuretics, or cardiac glycosides may lead to toxicity. Periodic examination and determinations of serum electrolytes, particularly serum bicarbonate level, should be carried out in those patients with renal disease in order to avoid these complications.
Adverse Reactions: Syrup POLYCITRA and POLYCITRA-LC are generally well tolerated without any unpleasant side effects when given in recommended doses to patients with normal renal function and urinary output. However, as with any alkalinizing agent, caution must be used in certain patients with abnormal renal mechanisms to avoid development of hyperkalemia or alkalosis, especially in the presence of hypocalcemia. Potassium intoxication causes listlessness, weakness, mental confusion and tingling of extremities.
Dosage and Administration: Syrup POLYCITRA and POLYCITRA-LC should be taken diluted in water, followed by additional water if desired. Palatability is enhanced if chilled before taking.
Usual Dosage: Adults: 15 to 30 ml diluted in water, four times a day after meals and at bedtime, or as directed by physician. Children: 5 to 15 ml diluted in water, four times a day after meals and at bedtime or as directed by physician.
Usual Dosage Range: 10 to 15 ml diluted with water, taken four times a day, will usually maintain a urine pH of 6.5–7.4. 15 to 20 ml diluted with water, taken four times a day, will usually maintain a urine pH of 7.0–7.6 throughout most of the 24 hours without unpleasant side effects.
As a Neutralizing Buffer: 15 ml diluted with 15 ml water, taken as a single dose, or as directed by physician.
Overdosage: Overdosage with sodium salts may cause diarrhea, nausea and vomiting, hypernoea, and convulsions. Overdosage with potassium salts may cause hyperkalemia and alkalosis, especially in the presence of renal disease.
How Supplied: Syrup POLYCITRA—16 fl oz (473 ml) (NDC 11414-205-01) and 4 fl oz (120 ml) hospital size (NDC 11414-205-04).
POLYCITRA-LC—16 fl oz (473 ml) (NDC 11414-208-01) and 4 fl oz (120 ml) hospital size (NDC 11414-208-04)
Literature Available: Yes.

POLYCITRA-K Syrup ℞
[polly"sit-rah-ka'y]
(Brand of Potassium Citrate and Citric Acid Oral Solution USP)

Description: Syrup POLYCITRA-K is a stable and pleasant tasting oral systemic alkalizer containing Potassium Citrate and Citric Acid in a non-alcoholic syrup base.
Composition: Syrup POLYCITRA-K contains in each teaspoonful (5ml): Potassium Citrate Monohydrate 1100mg (0.68 Molar) and Citric Acid Monohydrate 334mg (0.32 Molar). Each ml contains 2 mEq. Potassium ion and is equivalent to 2 mEq. Bicarbonate (HCO$_3$).
Actions: Potassium Citrate is absorbed and metabolized to potassium bicarbonate, thus acting as a systemic alkalizer. The effects are essentially those of chlorides before absorption and those of bicarbonates subsequently.
Indications and Advantages: Syrup POLYCITRA-K is an effective alkalinizing agent useful in those conditions where long term maintenance of an alkaline urine is desireable, such as patients with uric acid and cystine calculi of the urinary tract, especially when the administration of sodium salts is undesirable or contraindicated. In addition, it is a valuable adjuvant when administered with uricosuric agents in gout therapy, since urates tend to crystallize out of an acid urine. It is also effective in correcting the acidosis of certain renal tubular disorders where the administration of Potassium Citrate may be preferable. Syrup POLYCITRA-K is highly concentrated, and when administered after meals and before bedtime allows one to maintain an alkaline urine pH around the clock, usually without the necessity of a 2 A.M. dose. Syrup POLYCITRA-K alkalinizes the urine without producing a systemic alkalosis in recommended dosage. It is highly palatable, pleasant tasting and tolerable even when administered for long periods.
Contraindications: Severe renal impairment with oliguria or azotemia, untreated Addison's disease, adynamia episodica hereditaria, acute dehydration, heat cramps, anuria, severe myocardial damage, and hyperkalemia from any cause.
Warning: Large doses may cause hyperkalemia and alkalosis, especially in the presence of renal disease. Concurrent administration of potassium-containing medication, potassium-sparing diuretics, or cardiac glycosides may lead to toxicity.
Precautions: Should be used with caution by patients with low urinary output unless under the supervision of a physician. As with all liquids containing a high concentration of potassium, patients should be directed to dilute adequately with water to minimize the possibility of gastrointestinal injury associated with the oral ingestion of concentrated potassium salt preparations; and preferably, to take each dose after meals to avoid saline laxative effect.
Adverse Reactions: Syrup POLYCITRA-K is generally well tolerated without any unpleasant side effects when given in recommended doses to patients with normal renal function and urinary output. However, as with any alkalinizing agent, caution must be used in certain patients with abnormal renal mechanisms to avoid development of hyperkalemia or alkalosis. Potassium intoxication causes listlessness, weakness, mental confusion, tingling of extremities, and other symptoms associated with a high concentration of potassium in the serum. Periodic determinations of serum electrolytes should be carried out in those patients with renal disease in order to avoid these complications. Hyperkalemia may exhibit the following electrocardiographic abnormalities; Disappearance of the P wave, widening and slurring of QRS complex, changes of the S-T segment, tall peaked T waves, etc.
Dosage and Administration: Syrup POLYCITRA-K should be taken diluted in water according to directions, followed by additional water if desired.
Usual Adult Dose: 3 to 6 teaspoonfuls (15 to 30ml), diluted with 1 glass of water, after meals and at bedtime, or as directed by physician.
Usual Pediatric Dose: 1 to 3 teaspoonfuls (5 to 15ml), diluted with ½ glass of water, after meals and at bedtime or as directed by physician.
Usual Dosage Range: 10 to 15ml diluted with a glassful of water, taken four times a day, will usually maintain a urine pH of 6.5–7.4. 15 to 20ml diluted with a glassful of water, taken four times a day will usually maintain a urine pH of 7.0–7.6 throughout most of the 24 hours without unpleasant side effects.
Overdosage: The administration of oral potassium salts to persons with normal excretory mechanisms for potassium rarely causes serious hyperkalemia. However, if excretory mechanisms are impaired, hyperkalemia can result (see Contraindications and Warnings). Hyperkalemia, when detected, must be treated immediately because lethal levels can be reached in a few hours.
Treatment of Hyperkalemia: Should hyperkalemia occur, treatment measures include the following: (1) elimination of foods or medications containing potassium. (2) The intravenous administration of 300 to 500 ml/hr of dextrose solution (10 to 25%) containing 10 units of insulin/20gm dextrose. (3) The use of exchange resins, hemodialysis, or peritoneal dialysis. In treating hyperkalemia, it should be recalled that in patients who have been stabilized on digitalis, too rapid a lowering of the plasma potassium concentration can produce digitalis toxicity.
How Supplied: Syrup POLYCITRA-K—16 fl oz (473ml) (NDC 11414-206-01) and 4 fl oz (120ml hospital size) (NDC 11414-206-04)
Literature Available: Yes.

Winthrop-Breon Laboratories
90 PARK AVENUE
NEW YORK, NY 10016

AMIPAQUE® ℞
brand of metrizamide
(See Diagnostic Section.)

ARALEN® Hydrochloride ℞
brand of chloroquine hydrochloride
injection, USP

For Malaria and Extraintestinal Amebiasis

WARNING: PHYSICIANS SHOULD COMPLETELY FAMILIARIZE THEMSELVES WITH THE COMPLETE CONTENTS OF THIS LEAFLET BEFORE PRESCRIBING ARALEN.

Description: Parenteral solution, each ml containing 50 mg of the dihydrochloride salt equivalent to 40 mg of chloroquine base. ARALEN hydrochloride, a 4-aminoquinoline compound, is chemically 7-(chloro-4-[[4-diethylamino)-1-methylbutyl] amino]-quinoline dihydrochloride, a white, crystalline substance, freely soluble in water.
Actions: The compound is a highly active antimalarial and amebicidal agent.
ARALEN hydrochloride has been found to be highly active against the erythrocytic forms of *Plasmodium vivax* and *malariae* and most strains of *Plasmodium falciparum* (but not the gametocytes of *P. falciparum*). The precise mechanism of action of the drug is not known.
ARALEN hydrochloride does not prevent relapses in patients with vivax or malariae malaria because it is not effective against exoerythrocytic forms of the parasite, nor will it prevent vivax or malariae infection when administered as a prophylactic. It is highly effective as a suppressive agent in patients with vivax or malariae malaria, in terminating acute attacks, and significantly lengthening the interval between treatment and relapse. In patients with falciparum malaria it abolishes the acute attack and effects complete cure of the infection, unless due to a resistant strain of *P. falciparum*.
Indications: ARALEN hydrochloride is indicated for the treatment of extraintestinal amebiasis and for treatment of acute attacks of malaria due to *P. vivax, P. malariae, P. ovale,* and susceptible strains of *P. falciparum* when oral therapy is not feasible.
Contraindications: Use of this drug is contraindicated in the presence of retinal or visual field changes either attributable to 4-aminoquinoline compounds or to any other etiology, and in patients with known hypersensitivity to 4-aminoquinoline compounds. However, in the

Continued on next page

This product information was effective as of December 3, 1984. On these and other products of Winthrop-Breon Laboratories, detailed information may be obtained on a current basis by direct inquiry to the Professional Services Department, 90 Park Avenue, New York, NY 10016 (212) 907-2525.

Winthrop-Breon—Cont.

treatment of acute attacks of malaria caused by susceptible strains of plasmodia, the physician may elect to use this drug after carefully weighing the possible benefits and risks to the patient.

Warnings: *Children and infants are extremely susceptible to adverse effects from an overdose of parenteral ARALEN and sudden deaths have been recorded after such administration. In no instance should the single dose of parenteral ARALEN administered to infants or children exceed 5 mg base per kg.*

In recent years it has been found that certain strains of *P. falciparum* have become resistant to 4-aminoquinoline compounds (including chloroquine and hydroxychloroquine) as shown by the fact that normally adequate doses have failed to prevent or cure clinical malaria or parasitemia. Treatment with quinine or other specific forms of therapy is therefore advised for patients infected with a resistant strain of parasites.

Use of ARALEN should be avoided in patients with psoriasis, for it may precipitate a severe attack of psoriasis. Some authors consider the use of 4-aminoquinoline compounds contraindicated in patients with porphyria since the condition may be exacerbated.

Irreversible retinal damage has been observed in some patients who had received long-term or high-dosage 4-aminoquinoline therapy. Retinopathy has been reported to be dose related.

If there is any indication (past or present) of abnormality in the visual acuity, visual field, or retinal macular areas (such as pigmentary changes, loss of foveal reflex), or any visual symptoms (such as light flashes and streaks) which are not fully explainable by difficulties of accommodation or corneal opacities, the drug should be discontinued immediately and the patient closely observed for possible progression. Retinal changes (and visual disturbances) may progress even after cessation of therapy.

Usage in Pregnancy. Usage of this drug during pregnancy should be avoided except in the suppression or treatment of malaria when in the judgment of the physician the benefit outweighs the possible hazard. It should be noted that radioactively tagged chloroquine administered intravenously to pregnant pigmented CBA mice passed rapidly across the placenta, accumulated selectively in the melanin structures of the fetal eyes and was retained in the ocular tissues for five months after the drug had been eliminated from the rest of the body.[1]

Precautions: Since the drug is known to concentrate in the liver, it should be used with caution in patients with hepatic disease or alcoholism or in conjunction with known hepatotoxic drugs.

The drug should be administered with caution to patients having G-6-PD (glucose-6- phosphate dehydrogenase) deficiency.

Adverse Reactions: Respiratory depression, cardiovascular collapse, shock, convulsions, and death have been reported with overdoses of ARALEN hydrochloride, brand of chloroquine hydrochloride injection, especially in infants and children.

Any of the adverse reactions associated with short-term oral administration of chloroquine phosphate must be considered a possibility with chloroquine hydrochloride. Cardiovascular effects, such as hypotension and electrocardiographic changes (particularly inversion or depression of the T-wave, widening of the QRS complex), have rarely been noted in patients receiving usual antimalarial doses of the drug. Mild and transient headache, pruritus, psychic stimulation, visual disturbances (blurring of vision and difficulty of focusing or accommodation), pleomorphic skin eruptions, and gastrointestinal complaints (anorexia, nausea, vomiting, diarrhea, abdominal cramps) have been observed.

Instances of convulsive seizures associated with oral chloroquine therapy in patients with extraintestinal amebiasis have been reported.

A few cases of a nerve type of deafness have been reported after prolonged therapy, usually in high doses. Tinnitus and reduced hearing have been reported, in a patient with preexistent auditory damage, after administration of only 500 mg once a week for a few months. Since neuromyopathy, blood dyscrasias, lichen planus-like eruptions, and skin and mucosal pigmentary changes have been noted during prolonged oral therapy, their occurrence with this dosage form is possible.

Patients with retinal changes may be asymptomatic, especially in early cases, or may complain of nyctalopia and scotomatous vision with field defects of paracentral, pericentral ring types, and typically temporal scotomas, e.g., difficulty in reading with words tending to disappear, seeing only half an object, misty vision, and fog before the eyes. Rarely scotomatous vision may occur without observable retinal changes.

Dosage and Administration: *Malaria—*
Adult Dose. An initial dose of 4 mL or 5 mL (160 mg to 200 mg chloroquine base) may be injected intramuscularly and repeated in 6 hours if necessary. The total parenteral dosage in the first 24 hours should not exceed 800 mg chloroquine base. Treatment by mouth should be started as soon as practicable and continued until a course of approximately 1.5 g of base in 3 days is completed.

Pediatric Dose. Infants and children are extremely susceptible to overdosage of parenteral ARALEN. Severe reactions and deaths have occurred. In the pediatric age range, parenteral ARALEN dosage should be calculated in proportion to the adult dose based upon body weight. The recommended single dose in infants and children is 5 mg base per kg. This dose may be repeated in 6 hours; however, the total dose in any 24 hour period should not exceed 10 mg base per kg of body weight. Parenteral administration should be terminated and oral therapy instituted as soon as possible.

*Extraintestinal Amebiasis—*In adult patients not able to tolerate oral therapy, from 4 mL to 5 mL (160 mg to 200 mg chloroquine base) may be injected daily for 10 to 12 days. Oral administration should be substituted or resumed as soon as possible.

Overdosage: Inadvertent toxic doses may produce respiratory depression or shock with hypotension. Respiratory depression is treated by artificial respiration and administration of oxygen. In shock with hypotension, a potent vasopressor, such as NEO-SYNEPHRINE® hydrochloride, brand of phenylephrine hydrochloride, USP, should be given intramuscularly in doses of 2 mg to 5 mg.

How Supplied: Ampuls of 5 mL, box of 5 (NDC 0024-0074-01)

Reference: Ullberg S, Lindquist N G, Sjostrand S E: Accumulation of chorio-retinotoxic drugs in the foetal eye, *Nature* 1970; 227:1257.

AW-100-G

ARALEN® Phosphate ℞
brand of chloroquine phosphate tablets, USP

For Malaria and
Extraintestinal Amebiasis

WARNING: PHYSICIANS SHOULD COMPLETELY FAMILIARIZE THEMSELVES WITH THE COMPLETE CONTENTS OF THIS LEAFLET BEFORE PRESCRIBING ARALEN.

Description: ARALEN phosphate, a 4-aminoquinoline compound, is chemically 7-Chloro-4-[[4- (diethylamino) -1-methylbutyl]amino]-quinoline phosphate (1:2), a white, crystalline substance, freely soluble in water.

Actions: ARALEN phosphate has been found to be highly active against the erythrocytic forms of *Plasmodium vivax* and *malariae* and most strains of *Plasmodium falciparum* (but not the gametocytes of *P. falciparum*). The precise mechanism of action of the drug is not known.

ARALEN phosphate does not prevent relapses in patients with vivax or malariae malaria because it is not effective against exo-erythrocytic forms of the parasite, nor will it prevent vivax or malariae infection when administered as a prophylactic. It is highly effective as a suppressive agent in patients with vivax or malariae malaria, in terminating acute attacks, and significantly lengthening the interval between treatment and relapse. In patients with falciparum malaria it abolishes the acute attack and effects complete cure of the infection, unless due to a resistant strain of *P. falciparum*.

In vitro studies with trophozoites of *Entamoeba histolytica* have demonstrated that ARALEN phosphate also possesses amebicidal activity comparable to that of emetine.

Indications: ARALEN phosphate is indicated for the suppressive treatment and for acute attacks of malaria due to *P. vivax, P. malariae, P. ovale,* and susceptible strains of *P. falciparum.* The drug is also indicated for treatment of extraintestinal amebiasis.

Contraindications: Use of this drug is contraindicated in the presence of retinal or visual field changes either attributable to 4- aminoquinoline compounds or to any other etiology, and in patients with known hypersensitivity to 4-aminoquinoline compounds. However, in the treatment of acute attacks of malaria caused by susceptible strains of plasmodia, the physician may elect to use this drug after carefully weighing the possible benefits and risks to the patient.

Warnings: In recent years it has been found that certain strains of *P. falciparum* have become resistant to 4-aminoquinoline compounds (including chloroquine and hydroxychloroquine) as shown by the fact that normally adequate doses have failed to prevent or cure clinical malaria or parasitemia. Treatment with quinine or other specific forms of therapy is therefore advised for patients infected with a resistant strain of parasites.

Irreversible retinal damage has been observed in some patients who had received long-term or high-dosage 4-aminoquinoline therapy. Retinopathy has been reported to be dose related.

When prolonged therapy with any antimalarial compound is contemplated, initial (base line) and periodic ophthalmologic examinations (including visual acuity, expert slit-lamp, funduscopic, and visual field tests) should be performed.

If there is any indication (past or present) of abnormality in the visual acuity, visual field, or retinal macular areas (such as pigmentary changes, loss of foveal reflex), or any visual symptoms (such as light flashes and streaks) which are not fully explainable by difficulties of accommodation or corneal opacities, the drug should be discontinued immediately and the patient closely observed for possible progression. Retinal changes (and visual disturbances) may progress even after cessation of therapy.

All patients on long-term therapy with this preparation should be questioned and examined periodically, including testing knee and ankle reflexes, to detect any evidence of muscular weakness. If weakness occurs, discontinue the drug.

A number of fatalities have been reported following the accidental ingestion of chloroquine, sometimes in relatively small doses (0.75 or 1 g chloroquine phosphate in one 3-year-old child). Patients should be strongly warned to keep this drug out of the reach of children because they are especially sensitive to the 4- aminoquinoline compounds.

Use of ARALEN phosphate, brand of chloroquine phosphate tablets, in patients with psoriasis may precipitate a severe attack of psoriasis. When used in patients with porphyria the condition may be exacerbated. The drug should not be used in these conditions unless in the judgment of the physician the benefit to the patient outweighs the possible hazard.

Usage in Pregnancy. Usage of this drug during pregnancy should be avoided except in the suppression or treatment of malaria when in the judgment of the physician the benefit outweighs the

for possible revisions

possible hazard. It should be noted that radioactively tagged chloroquine administered intravenously to pregnant pigmented CBA mice passed rapidly across the placenta, accumulated selectively in the melanin structures of the fetal eyes and was retained in the ocular tissues for five months after the drug had been eliminated from the rest of the body.[1]

Precautions: Since the drug is known to concentrate in the liver, it should be used with caution in patients with hepatic disease or alcoholism or in conjunction with known hepatotoxic drugs.

Complete blood cell counts should be made periodically if patients are given prolonged therapy. If any severe blood disorder appears which is not attributable to the disease under treatment, discontinuance of the drug should be considered. The drug should be administered with caution to patients having G-6-PD (glucose-6-phosphate dehydrogenase) deficiency.

Adverse Reactions: Following the administration of ARALEN phosphate in doses adequate for the treatment of an acute malarial attack or extraintestinal amebiasis, mild and transient headache, pruritus, gastrointestinal complaints (anorexia, nausea, vomiting, diarrhea, abdominal cramps), psychic stimulation, and rarely psychotic episodes or convulsions have been observed. Cardiovascular effects, such as hypotension and electrocardiographic changes (particularly inversion or depression of the T-wave, widening of the QRS complex), have rarely been noted in patients receiving usual antimalarial doses of the drug. A few cases of a nerve type of deafness have been reported after prolonged therapy, usually in high doses. Tinnitus and reduced hearing have been reported, in a patient with preexistent auditory damage, after administration of only 500 mg once a week for a few months. Neuromyopathy, blood dyscrasias, lichen planus-like eruptions, and skin and mucosal pigmentary changes have also been noted during prolonged therapy.

When employed for the indications (malaria and extraintestinal amebiasis) and in the dosages recommended in this leaflet, visual disturbances, consisting of blurring of vision or difficulty in focusing or accommodation, occasionally may be noted; they are reversible and disappear on discontinuation of therapy. Other types of visual disturbances and ocular complications have been reported during the use of chloroquine for long-term therapy usually in daily doses exceeding 250 mg of chloroquine phosphate. These consisted of (1) reversible corneal changes (transient edema or opaque deposits in the epithelium) which may be asymptomatic or cause visual halos, focusing difficulties, or blurred vision and (2) generally irreversible, sometimes progressive, or, rarely delayed, retinal changes, such as narrowing of the arterioles, macular lesions (loss of foveal reflex, areas of edema, atrophy, and abnormal pigmentation), pallor of the optic disc, optic atrophy, and patchy retinal pigmentation.

Patients with retinal changes may be asymptomatic, especially in early cases, or may complain of nyctalopia and scotomatous vision with field defects of paracentral, pericentral ring types, and typically temporal scotomas, eg, difficulty in reading with words tending to disappear, seeing only half an object, misty vision, and fog before the eyes. Rarely scotomatous vision may occur without observable retinal changes.

Dosage and Administration: The dosage of chloroquine phosphate is often expressed or calculated as the base. Each 500 mg tablet of ARALEN phosphate, brand of chloroquine phosphate tablets, is equivalent to 300 mg base. In infants and children the dosage is preferably calculated on the body weight.

Malaria: Suppression — In adults, 500 mg (= 300 mg base) on exactly the same day of each week. **In infants and children** the weekly suppressive dosage is 5 mg, calculated as base, per kg of body weight, but should not exceed the adult dose regardless of weight.

If circumstances permit, suppressive therapy should begin two weeks prior to exposure. However, failing this in adults, an initial double (loading) dose of 1 g (= 600 mg base), or in children 10 mg base/kg may be taken in two divided doses, six hours apart. The suppressive therapy should be continued for eight weeks after leaving the endemic area.

Treatment of the acute attack—**In adults,** an initial dose of 1 g (= 600 mg base) followed by an additional 500 mg (= 300 mg base) after six to eight hours and a single dose of 500 mg (= 300 mg base) on each of two consecutive days. This represents a total dose of 2.5 g chloroquine phosphate or 1.5 g base in three days.

The dosage for adults may also be calculated on the basis of body weight; this method is preferred for infants and children. A total dose representing 25 mg of base per kg of body weight is administered in three days, as follows:

First dose: 10 mg base per kg (but not exceeding a single dose of 600 mg base).

Second dose: 5 mg base per kg (but not exceeding a single dose of 300 mg base) 6 hours after first dose.

Third dose: 5 mg base per kg 18 hours after second dose.

Fourth dose: 5 mg base per kg 24 hours after third dose.

For radical cure of *vivax* and *malariae* malaria concomitant therapy with an 8- aminoquinoline compound is necessary.

Extraintestinal Amebiasis: Adults, 1 g (600 mg base) daily for two days, followed by 500 mg (300 mg base) daily for at least two to three weeks. Treatment is usually combined with an effective intestinal amebicide.

Overdosage: Chloroquine is very rapidly and completely absorbed after ingestion, and in accidental overdosage, or rarely with lower doses in hypersensitive patients, toxic symptoms may occur within thirty minutes. These consist of headache, drowsiness, visual disturbances, cardiovascular collapse, and convulsions followed by sudden and early respiratory and cardiac arrest. The electrocardiogram may reveal atrial standstill, nodal rhythm, prolonged intraventricular conduction time, and progressive bradycardia leading to ventricular fibrillation and/or arrest. Treatment is symptomatic and must be prompt with immediate evacuation of the stomach by emesis (at home, before transportation to the hospital) or gastric lavage until the stomach is completely emptied. If finely powdered, activated charcoal is introduced by stomach tube, after lavage, and within 30 minutes after ingestion of the antimalarial, it may inhibit further intestinal absorption of the drug. To be effective, the dose of activated charcoal should be at least five times the estimated dose of chloroquine ingested.

Convulsions, if present, should be controlled before attempting gastric lavage. If due to cerebral stimulation, cautious administration of an ultrashort-acting barbiturate may be tried but, if due to anoxia, it should be corrected by oxygen administration, artificial respiration or, in shock with hypotension, by vasopressor therapy. Because of the importance of supporting respiration, tracheal intubation or tracheostomy, followed by gastric lavage, may also be necessary. Peritoneal dialysis and exchange transfusions have also been suggested to reduce the level of the drug in the blood. A patient who survives the acute phase and is asymptomatic should be closely observed for at least six hours. Fluids may be forced, and sufficient ammonium chloride (8 g daily in divided doses for adults) may be administered for a few days to acidify the urine to help promote urinary excretion in cases of both overdosage or sensitivity.

How Supplied: Tablets of 500 mg (= 300 mg base), bottle of 25 (NDC 0024-0077-01)

Reference: 1. Ullberg S, Lindquist N G, Sjostrand S E: Accumulation of chorio-retinotoxic drugs in the foetal eye. *Nature* 1970; 227:1257.

Shown in Product Identification Section, page 443

AW-123 E

ARALEN® Phosphate
brand of chloroquine phosphate, USP
with
PRIMAQUINE Phosphate, USP

℞

For Malaria Prophylaxis Only

WARNING: PHYSICIANS SHOULD COMPLETELY FAMILIARIZE THEMSELVES WITH THE COMPLETE CONTENTS OF THIS LEAFLET BEFORE PRESCRIBING ARALEN PHOSPHATE WITH PRIMAQUINE PHOSPHATE.

Description: Each tablet contains ARALEN phosphate, brand of chloroquine phosphate, USP, 500 mg (equivalent to 300 mg base) and primaquine phosphate 79 mg (equivalent to 45 mg base).

Actions: ARALEN is a 4-aminoquinoline compound which is highly active against the erythrocytic forms of *Plasmodium vivax* and most strains of *Plasmodium falciparum* (but not the gametocytes of *P. falciparum*).

Primaquine is an 8-aminoquinoline compound which eliminates tissue (exo-erythrocytic) infection. Thereby, it prevents the development of the blood (erythrocytic) forms of the parasite which are responsible for relapses in vivax malaria. Primaquine phosphate is active against gametocytes of *P. falciparum*.

ARALEN phosphate with primaquine phosphate demonstrates antimalarial activity against all stages of human-malaria parasites, except for certain strains of *P. falciparum* resistant to chloroquine.

Indication: ARALEN phosphate with primaquine phosphate is intended solely for use in the prophylaxis of malaria, regardless of species, in all areas where this disease is endemic.

Contraindications: The drug is contraindicated in acutely ill patients suffering from systemic disease manifested by tendency to granulocytopenia, such as rheumatoid arthritis and lupus erythematosus. The drug is also contraindicated in those patients receiving concurrently other potentially hemolytic drugs or depressants of myeloid elements of the bone marrow.

Primaquine should not be administered to patients who have received quinacrine recently, as toxicity is increased.

Warnings: Children are especially sensitive to 4-aminoquinoline compounds. A number of fatalities have been reported following the accidental ingestion of chloroquine, sometimes in relatively small doses (0.75 or 1 g in one 3- year-old child). Patients should be strongly warned to keep these drugs out of the reach of children.

Hemolytic reactions (moderate to severe) may occur after even a weekly dose of this preparation in glucose-6-phosphate dehydrogenase (G-6-PD) deficient Caucasians (particularly, in Sardinians and in individuals with a family or personal history of favism).

Usage in Pregnancy. Safe usage of this preparation in pregnancy has not been established. Therefore, use of it during pregnancy should be avoided except when in the judgment of the physician the benefit outweighs the possible hazard. It should be noted that radioactively tagged chloroquine administered intravenously to pregnant pigmented CBA mice passed rapidly across the placenta, accumulated selectively in the melanin structures of the fetal eyes and was retained in the ocular tis-

Continued on next page

This product information was effective as of December 3, 1984. On these and other products of Winthrop-Breon Laboratories, detailed information may be obtained on a current basis by direct inquiry to the Professional Services Department, 90 Park Avenue, New York, NY 10016 (212) 907-2525.

Winthrop-Breon—Cont.

sues for five months after the drug had been eliminated from the rest of the body.[1]

Precautions: ARALEN phosphate, brand of chloroquine phosphate, with primaquine phosphate is intended for malaria prophylaxis only; it should not be used for the treatment of clinical malaria. The recommended dosage (one tablet weekly, on the same day each week) should not be exceeded. The drug should not be taken more often than once every seven days to minimize danger of toxicity. If the combination is prescribed for (1) an individual who has shown a previous idiosyncrasy to either chloroquine or primaquine (as manifested by dermatitis, hemolytic anemia, methemoglobinemia, or leukopenia), (2) an individual with a family or personal history of favism, or (3) an individual with erythrocytic glucose-6-phosphate dehydrogenase (G-6-PD) deficiency or nicotinamide adenine dinucleotide (NADH) methemoglobin reductase deficiency, the person should be observed closely for tolerance. The drug should be discontinued immediately if marked darkening of the urine, sudden decrease in hemoglobin concentration or leukocyte count, or severe skin reaction occurs.

In areas with endemic falciparum malaria due to strains that are resistant to the 4-aminoquinolines (chloroquine, amodiaquine, hydroxychloroquine), chemoprophylaxis with this combination alone may not be effective.

Adverse Reactions: *Gastrointestinal reactions:* anorexia, nausea, vomiting, epigastric distress, and abdominal cramps. *Hematologic reactions:* leukopenia, hemolytic anemia in glucose-6-phosphate dehydrogenase (G-6-PD) deficient individuals, methemoglobinemia in nicotinamide adenine dinucleotide (NADH) methemoglobin reductase deficient individuals.

Cardiovascular effects, such as hypotension and electrocardiographic changes (particularly inversion or depression of the T wave, widening of the QRS complex), have rarely been noted in patients receiving usual antimalarial doses of the drug.

Visual disturbances, consisting of blurring of vision or difficulty in focusing or accommodation, have occasionally been noted when chloroquine has been employed for malaria. These symptoms are reversible and disappear on discontinuation of therapy. Other types of visual disturbances (reversible corneal changes) and ocular complications including retinal changes (narrowing of the arterioles, macular lesions, pallor of the optic disc, optic atrophy, and patchy retinal pigmentation) have been reported during the use of chloroquine for long-term therapy usually in daily doses exceeding 250 mg of chloroquine phosphate. These changes have not been reported with the use of ARALEN phosphate, brand of chloroquine phosphate, with primaquine phosphate for malaria prophylaxis.

Auditory disturbances: tinnitus and reduced hearing have been reported, in a patient with preexistent auditory damage, after administration of only 500 mg of ARALEN phosphate, brand of chloroquine phosphate, once a week for a few months.

Dosage and Administration:
Adults—Starting at least one day before entering the malarious area, one tablet weekly, taken on the same day each week. This schedule (one tablet weekly) should be continued for eight weeks after leaving the endemic area.

Children—The following dosage, based on body weight, is suggested.

Weight (lb)	ARALEN base (mg)	Primaquine base (mg)	Dose* (mL)
10-15	20	3	2.5
16-25	40	6	5.0
26-35	60	9	7.5
36-45	80	12	10.0
46-55	100	15	12.5
56-100	150	22.5	½ tab
100+	300	45	1 tab

*Dose based on liquid containing approximately 40 mg of chloroquine base and 6 mg of primaquine base per 5 mL (1 teaspoon) prepared from ARALEN phosphate, brand of chloroquine phosphate, with primaquine phosphate tablets. Chocolate syrup could be used to prepare a suspension (one tablet crushed and suspended in 40 mL of liquid). Shake well before use.

Overdosage: Symptoms of overdosage are due to the two drug components.

Chloroquine is very rapidly and completely absorbed after ingestion, and in accidental overdosage, or rarely with lower doses in hypersensitive patients, toxic symptoms may occur within thirty minutes. These consist of headache, drowsiness, visual disturbances, cardiovascular collapse, and convulsions followed by sudden and early respiratory and cardiac arrest. The electrocardiogram may reveal atrial standstill, nodal rhythm, prolonged intraventricular conduction time, and progressive bradycardia leading to ventricular fibrillation and/or arrest.

Symptoms of overdosage of primaquine are similar to those seen after overdosage of pamaquine. They include abdominal cramps, vomiting, burning epigastric distress, central nervous system and cardiovascular disturbances, cyanosis, methemoglobinemia, moderate leukocytosis or leukopenia, and anemia. The most striking symptoms are granulocytopenia and acute hemolytic anemia in sensitive persons. Acute hemolysis occurs, but patients recover completely if the dosage is discontinued.

Treatment is symptomatic and must be prompt with immediate evacuation of the stomach by emesis (at home, before transportation to the hospital) or gastric lavage until the stomach is completely emptied. Finely powdered, activated charcoal in a dose not less than five times the estimated dose of chloroquine ingested, if introduced by the stomach tube after lavage within thirty minutes after ingestion of the antimalarial, may inhibit further intestinal absorption of the drug.

Convulsions, if present, should be controlled before attempting gastric lavage. If due to cerebral stimulation, cautious administration of an ultra-short-acting barbiturate may be tried but, if due to anoxia, it should be corrected by oxygen administration, artificial respiration or, in shock with hypotension, by vasopressor therapy. Because of the importance of supporting respiration, tracheal intubation or tracheostomy, followed by gastric lavage, may also be necessary. Exchange transfusions have also been suggested to reduce the level of the drug in the blood.

The patient should be kept in bed and warm. If methemoglobinemia and cyanosis occur, oxygen may be administered and use of methylene blue may be considered. If collapse and hypotension or shock occur, vasopressors may be used. The patient should be observed for the possible development of leukopenia or hemolytic anemia.

A patient who survives the acute stage and is asymptomatic should be closely observed for at least six hours. Fluids may be forced, and sufficient ammonium chloride (8 g daily in divided doses for adults) may be administered for a few days to acidify the urine to help promote urinary excretion in cases of both overdosage or sensitivity.

How Supplied: Tablets, bottle of 100 (NDC 0024-0079-04)

Clinical Studies: On the basis of carefully controlled preliminary clinical trials, Alving and his associates[2] found that the weekly administration of 300 mg chloroquine base and 45 mg primaquine base (administered as the phosphate salts) proved highly effective as a prophylactic against severe *P. vivax* infections with the Chesson strain and did not produce clinical hemolysis even among primaquine-sensitive American Negro adult volunteers. A weekly dose of primaquine phosphate equivalent to 45 mg primaquine base cured 90 percent of infections.

The studies of these workers indicate that the toxicity of primaquine phosphate, as regards the production of hemolysis, is markedly diminished when administered in weekly doses. When administered with standard suppressive doses of chloroquine phosphate, its therapeutic effectiveness in the radical cure of Chesson vivax malaria is increased. Thus, a weekly dose equivalent to 60 mg of primaquine base is less toxic than 15 mg base administered daily; and a dose equivalent to 45 mg base administered weekly was found to be practically without demonstrable toxicity. A dose equivalent to 45 mg base weekly for 8 weeks was more effective in the radical cure of infections than 15 mg base daily for 14 days.

Wittmer[3] conducted a double-blind study in 24 Caucasian male adults who received ARALEN phosphate, brand of chloroquine phosphate, with primaquine phosphate once each week (Friday) for 15 weeks to determine its safety and suitability for use in Armed Forces flying personnel. The author concluded that there appear to be no contraindications to the long-term use of the combination in flying personnel since there was no effect on vision, time of useful consciousness, or psychomotor performance. No deleterious synergistic effect of the two drugs was demonstrated. Charles[4] investigated the effects of 5 weekly doses of primaquine phosphate (1 mg to 1.5 mg base per kg body weight) in combination with a 4-aminoquinoline antimalarial agent on the parasitemia and blood picture of 100 Ghanaian children from 2½ to 8 years old. Although the enzyme-deficiency trait (glucose-6-phosphate dehydrogenase deficiency) for primaquine sensitivity occurred in approximately 25 percent of the group, no general evidence of hemolysis was observed. Eight of the treated subjects were positive for the glucose-6-phosphate dehydrogenase deficiency test but maintained their pre-treatment hemoglobin values.

However, Ziai and his associates[5] noted that serious hematologic reactions can occur in persons with a glucose-6-phosphate dehydrogenase (G-6-PD) deficiency with the small weekly doses of chloroquine-primaquine used for malaria suppressive therapy. This has been reported primarily in patients with a family history and/or personal history of favism.

Methemoglobinemia has been discovered in individuals with nicotinamide adenine dinucleotide methemoglobin reductase deficiency.[6]

The susceptibility of primaquine-sensitive children to hemolysis by primaquine phosphate is considered to be of the same order of magnitude as that of adults on an equal drug/body weight basis.

References:
1. Ullberg S, Lindquist N G, Sjostrand S E: Accumulation of chorio-retinotoxic drugs in the foetal eye. *Nature* 1970; 227:1257.
2. Alving A S. et al: Mitigation of the haemolytic effect of primaquine and enhancement of its action against exo-erythrocytic forms of the Chesson strain of *Plasmodium vivax* by intermittent regimens of drug administration. *Bull. WHO* 1960; 22:621.
3. Wittmer J F: Aeromedical aspects of malaria prophylaxis with chloroquine-primaquine. *Aerospace Med* 1963; 34:944.
4. Charles L J: Observations on the haemolytic effect of primaquine in 100 Ghanaian children. *Ann Trop Med* 1960; 54:460.
5. Ziai M, et al.: Malaria prophylaxis and treatment in G-6-PD deficiency. *Clin Pediat* 1967; 6:242.
6. Cohen R, et al: Methemoglobinemia provoked by malarial chemoprophylaxis in Vietnam. *New Eng J Med* 1968; 279:1127-1131.

AW-109 H

ATABRINE® Hydrochloride ℞
brand of quinacrine hydrochloride tablets, USP

Each tablet contains 100 mg of quinacrine hydrochloride, a bright yellow, odorless, bitter crystalline powder that is water soluble (1:35), and bears identifying number A 82.

How Supplied: Tablets of 100 mg (bright yellow, shellac-coated), bottle of 100 (NDC 0024-0082-04)

For complete prescribing information contact Winthrop-Breon Professional Services Department.
AW-91-I

BILOPAQUE® SODIUM
brand of tyropanoate sodium, USP

(See Diagnostic Section.)

BREONESIN®
brand of guaifenesin capsules, USP

Description: Each red, oval-shaped BREONESIN capsule contains 200 mg of guaifenesin in an easy-to-swallow, soft gelatin capsule. BREONESIN contains no sugar or alcohol.
Indications: BREONESIN is indicated for the temporary relief of coughs. BREONESIN is an expectorant which helps to loosen phlegm (sputum) and bronchial secretions, and acts to thin mucus. Coughs due to minor throat and bronchial irritation that occur with the common cold are temporarily relieved.
Warnings: Persistent cough may indicate a serious condition. Consult your physician if cough persists for more than 1 week, recurs, or is accompanied by high fever, rash, or persistent headache. Do not take this product for persistent coughs due to smoking, asthma, or emphysema, or coughs accompanied by excessive secretions, except under the advice and supervision of your physician. As with any drug, if you are pregnant or nursing a baby, seek the advice of a health professional before using this product.
Dosage: *Adults and Children 12 years of age and over:* 1 or 2 capsules every 4 hours, not to exceed 12 capsules in a 24-hour period. *Children under 12 years:* as directed by your physician.
Store at controlled room temperature, between 15°C and 30°C (59°F and 86°F).
How Supplied: Capsules of 200 mg (red), bottle of 100 (NDC 0024-1050-10)
Marketed by
Winthrop-Breon Laboratories
New York, NY 10016
Mfg. by R.P. Scherer Corp.
Clearwater, Florida 33518

BRONKAID® Mist — OTC
(See PDR For Nonprescription Drugs)

BRONKAID® Mist Suspension — OTC
(See PDR For Nonprescription Drugs)

BRONKAID® Tablets — OTC
(See PDR For Nonprescription Drugs)

BRONKEPHRINE®
(ethylnorepinephrine hydrochloride injection, USP)
IN AQUEOUS SOLUTION

Description: BRONKEPHRINE is ethylnorepinephrine hydrochloride injection, USP. Each mL contains 2 mg ethylnorepinephrine HCl in a sterile isotonic solution of 0.7% sodium chloride with sodium acetone bisulfite 0.2% as preservative. The pH is adjusted to 2.9–4.5 with NaOH or HCl. BRONKEPHRINE is a synthetic sympathomimetic amine intended for subcutaneous or intramuscular injection. The chemical name is 1-(3,4-dihydroxyphenyl)-2-amino-1-butanol hydrochloride.
Clinical Pharmacology: BRONKEPHRINE is primarily a beta-adrenergic agonist. Its actions are similar to those of isoproterenol, although it is less potent. Its bronchodilating properties closely simulate those of epinephrine but without significant pressor effects. It thus may be safer than epinephrine for hypertensive patients and severely ill patients in whom such effects are undesirable. It is particularly adapted for use in children because of its relative lack of adverse effects, especially central nervous system excitation. It also may be of value in diabetic asthmatics due to its lack of glycogenolytic activity.
Metabolic and pharmacokinetic data are unavailable.
Indications and Usage: BRONKEPHRINE is indicated for use as a bronchodilator for bronchial asthma and for reversible bronchospasm that may occur in association with bronchitis and emphysema.
Contraindications: BRONKEPHRINE is contraindicated in patients who are hypersensitive to any of its ingredients or with idiosyncrasy to sympathomimetic drugs.
Warnings: BRONKEPHRINE should not be administered along with epinephrine or other sympathomimetic amines because these drugs are direct cardiac stimulants and may cause excessive tachycardia.
Precautions: BRONKEPHRINE should be used with caution in persons with cardiovascular disease, a history of stroke or coronary artery disease. It is a potent drug and may cause toxic symptoms through idiosyncratic response or overdosage.
Care should be taken in anatomical selection of injection sites to avoid inadvertent intraneural or intravascular injection.
Carcinogenesis, mutagenesis, impairment of fertility: Long-term animal studies of BRONKEPHRINE to evaluate carcinogenic potential and reproduction studies in animals have not been performed. There is no evidence from human data that BRONKEPHRINE may be carcinogenic or mutagenic or that it impairs fertility.
Pregnancy Category C: Animal reproduction studies have not been conducted with BRONKEPHRINE. It is not known whether BRONKEPHRINE can cause fetal harm when administered to a pregnant woman or can affect reproduction capacity. BRONKEPHRINE should be given to a pregnant woman only if clearly needed and the potential benefits outweigh the risk.
Nursing mothers: It is not known whether BRONKEPHRINE is excreted in human milk; however, because many drugs are excreted in human milk, caution should be exercised when BRONKEPHRINE is administered to a nursing woman.
Adverse Reactions: BRONKEPHRINE (ethylnorepinephrine) is generally well tolerated. It may, however, produce changes in blood pressure (elevation or depression) or pulse rate (elevation), palpitation, headache, dizziness or nausea; as with other sympathomimetic amines.
Overdosage: The signs and symptoms of overdosage with BRONKEPHRINE are those typical of any sympathomimetic amine. Treatment should be symptomatic.
Dosage and Administration: The usual adult dose by subcutaneous or intramuscular injection is 0.5 mL–1.0 mL. Depending on severity of the asthmatic attack, smaller doses (0.3 mL–0.5 mL) may suffice. Dosage in children varies according to age and weight; usually 0.1 mL to 0.5 mL is sufficient.
How Supplied:
1 mL sterile single-dose ampuls, UNI-NEST™ PAK of 25. (NDC 0024-1001-25)
PROTECT AMPULS FROM LIGHT.
BW-96

BRONKODYL®
brand of theophylline anhydrous capsules
100 mg and 200 mg

How Supplied:
BRONKODYL 100 mg NDC 0024-1036-10 brown and white capsules in bottle of 100
BRONKODYL 200 mg NDC 0024-1037-10 green and white capsules in bottle of 100
Marketed by
Winthrop-Breon Laboratories
Manufactured by
KV Pharmaceutical Co.
St. Louis, Missouri 63144

BRONKOLIXIR®

Composition: Each 5 mL teaspoonful contains:
Ephedrine sulfate, USP .... 12 mg
Guaifenesin, USP .... 50 mg
Theophylline, USP .... 15 mg
Phenobarbital, USP .... 4 mg
(Warning: May be habit forming.)
in a cherry-flavored solution containing alcohol, USP, 19% (v/v).
How Supplied: Bottle of 16 fl oz

BRONKOSOL®
brand of isoetharine inhalation solution, USP, 1.0%
BRONCHODILATOR SOLUTION FOR ORAL INHALATION

Description:
Isoetharine HCl, USP 1.0%
in an aqueous-glycerin solution containing sodium chloride, citric acid, and sodium hydroxide, with methylparaben, propylparaben, and acetone sodium bisulfite.

BRONKOMETER®
brand of isoetharine mesylate inhalation aerosol, USP

Description: BRONKOMETER is a complete pocket nebulizer containing isoetharine mesylate 0.61% (w/w) with saccharin, menthol, alcohol 30% (w/w), and fluorochlorohydrocarbons as gaseous propellants. Preserved with ascorbic acid 0.1% (w/w).
Isoetharine is 1-(3,4 dihydroxyphenyl)-2-isopropylamino-1-butanol. The BRONKOMETER unit delivers approximately 20 metered doses per mL of solution. Each average 56 mg delivery contains 340 mcg isoetharine.
Action: Isoetharine is a sympathomimetic amine with preferential affinity for Beta$_2$ adrenergic receptor sites of bronchial and certain arteriolar musculature, and a lower order of affinity for Beta$_1$ adrenergic receptors. Its activity in symptomatic relief of bronchospasm is rapid and of relatively long duration. By relieving bronchospasm, BRONKOSOL and BRONKOMETER help give prompt relief and significantly increase vital capacity.
Indications: BRONKOSOL and BRONKOMETER are indicated for use as bronchodilators for bronchial asthma and for reversible bronchospasm that may occur in association with bronchitis and emphysema.
Contraindication: BRONKOSOL and BRONKOMETER should not be administered to patients who are hypersensitive to any of their ingredients.
Warnings: Excessive use of an adrenergic aerosol should be discouraged as it may lose its effectiveness. Occasional patients have been reported to develop severe paradoxical airway resistance with repeated excessive use of an aerosol adrenergic inhalation preparation. The cause of this refractory state is unknown. It is advisable that in such instances the use of the aerosol adrenergic be discontinued immediately and alternative therapy instituted, since in the reported cases the patients did not respond to other forms of therapy until the drug was withdrawn. Cardiac arrest has been noted in several instances.
BRONKOSOL and BRONKOMETER should not be administered along with epinephrine or other sympathomimetic amines, since these drugs are direct cardiac stimulants and may cause excessive tachycardia. They may, however, be alternated if desired.

Continued on next page

This product information was effective as of December 3, 1984. On these and other products of Winthrop-Breon Laboratories, detailed information may be obtained on a current basis by direct inquiry to the Professional Services Department, 90 Park Avenue, New York, NY 10016 (212) 907-2525.

Winthrop-Breon—Cont.

Usage in Pregnancy: Although there has been no evidence of teratogenic effects with this drug, use of any drug in pregnancy, lactation, or in women of childbearing potential requires that the potential benefit of the drug be weighed against its possible hazard to the mother or child.

Precautions: Dosage must be carefully adjusted in patients with hyperthyroidism, hypertension, acute coronary disease, cardiac asthma, limited cardiac reserve, and in individuals sensitive to sympathomimetic amines, since overdosage may result in tachycardia, palpitation, nausea, headache, or epinephrine-like side effects.

Adverse Reactions: Although BRONKOSOL and BRONKOMETER are relatively free of toxic side effects, too frequent use may cause tachycardia, palpitation, nausea, headache, changes in blood pressure, anxiety, tension, restlessness, insomnia, tremor, weakness, dizziness, and excitement, as is the case with other sympathomimetic amines.

Dosage and Administration: BRONKOSOL can be administered by hand nebulizer, oxygen aerosolization, or intermittent positive pressure breathing (IPPB). Usually treatment need not be repeated more often than every four hours, although in severe cases more frequent administration may be necessary.

Method of Administration	Usual Dose	Usual Range	Usual Dilution
Hand nebulizer	4 inhalations	3-7 inhalations	undiluted
Oxygen aerosolization*	½ mL	¼-½ mL	1:3 with saline or other diluent
IPPB†	½ mL	¼-1 mL	1:3 with saline or other diluent

* Administered with oxygen flow adjusted to 4 to 6 liters/minute over a period of 15 to 20 minutes.
† Usually an inspiratory flow rate of 15 liters/minute at a cycling pressure of 15 cm H_2O is recommended. It may be necessary, according to patient and type of IPPB apparatus, to adjust flow rate to 6 to 30 liters per minute, cycling pressure to 10-15 cm H_2O, and further dilution according to needs of patient.

BRONKOMETER®

Ced Administration: The average adult dose is one or two inhalations. Occasionally, more may be required. It is important, however, to wait one full minute after the initial one or two inhalations in order to be certain whether another is necessary. In most cases, inhalations need not be repeated more often than every four hours, although more frequent administration may be necessary in severe cases.

How Supplied: BRONKOSOL, brand of isoetharine inhalation solution, for inhalation—

Vial of 1% 10 mL   NDC 0024-1071-10
Vial of 1% 30 mL   NDC 0024-1072-30
BRONKOMETER, brand of isoetharine mesylate inhalation aerosol
Vial of 10 mL with Oral Nebulizer
Vial of 10 mL, with oral nebulizer (NDC 0024-1040-01)
Refill only, 10 mL (NDC 0024-1041-01)
Vial of 15 mL, with oral nebulizer (NDC 0024-1040-03)
Refill only, 15 mL (NDC 0024-1041-03)
Vial of 20 mL, with oral nebulizer (NDC 0024-1040-02)
Refill only, 20 mL (NDC 0024-1041-02)

BW-105

Marketed by Winthrop-Breon Laboratories
Division of Sterling Drug Inc
New York, NY 10016
Manufactured by
Sterling Pharmaceuticals Inc
Barceloneta, Puerto Rico 00617

BRONKOTABS®

Composition: Each tablet contains ephedrine sulfate, USP, 24 mg; guaifenesin, USP, 100 mg; theophylline, USP, 100 mg; phenobarbital, USP, 8 mg. (Warning: May be habit forming.)
How Supplied: Bottle of 100 (NDC 0024-1006-10)
Bottle of 1000 (NDC 0024-1006-00)

CAMPHO–PHENIQUE®   OTC
Liquid and Gel

(See PDR For Nonprescription Drugs)

CARBOCAINE® Hydrochloride   R
brand of mepivacaine hydrochloride injection, USP

THESE SOLUTIONS ARE NOT INTENDED FOR SPINAL ANESTHESIA OR DENTAL USE.

Description: Mepivacaine hydrochloride is 1-methyl-2′, 6′-pipecoloxylidide monohydrochloride. It is a white crystalline, odorless powder, soluble in water, but very resistant to both acid and alkaline hydrolysis. Solutions may be stored for extended periods of time without decomposition and if without vasoconstrictors may be reautoclaved when necessary.
[See table below].

Actions: Mepivacaine stabilizes the neuronal membrane and prevents the initiation and transmission of nerve impulses, thereby effecting local anesthesia.
Onset of anesthesia is rapid, the time of onset for sensory block ranging from about 3 to 20 minutes depending upon such factors as the anesthetic technique, the type of block, the concentration of the solution, and the individual patient. The degree of motor blockade produced is dependent on the concentration of the solution. A 0.5 percent solution will be effective in small superficial nerve blocks while the 1 percent concentration will block sensory and sympathetic conduction without loss of motor function. The 1.5 percent solution will provide extensive and often complete motor block and the 2 percent concentration of CARBOCAINE will produce complete sensory and motor block of any nerve group.

The duration of anesthesia also varies depending upon the technique and type of block, the concentration, and the individual. Mepivacaine will normally provide anesthesia which is adequate for 2 to 2½ hours of surgery. It has been reported that vasoconstrictors do not significantly prolong anesthesia with mepivacaine but epinephrine (1:200,000) may be added to the mepivacaine solution to promote local hemostasis and to delay systemic absorption of the anesthetic.

Mepivacaine, because of its amide structure, is not detoxified by the circulating plasma esterases. It is rapidly metabolized, with only a small percentage of the anesthetic (5 to 10 percent) being excreted unchanged in the urine. The liver is the principal site of metabolism, with over 50 percent of the administered dose being excreted into the bile as metabolites. Most of the metabolized mepivacaine is probably resorbed in the intestine and then excreted into the urine since only a small percentage is found in the feces. The principal route of excretion is via the kidney. Most of the anesthetic and its metabolites are eliminated within 30 hours. It has been shown that hydroxylation and N-demethylation, which are detoxification reactions, play important roles in the metabolism of the anesthetic. Three metabolites of mepivacaine have been identified from adult humans: two phenols, which are excreted almost exclusively as their glucuronide conjugates, and the N-demethylated compound (2′, 6′-pipecoloxylidide).

Mepivacaine does not ordinarily produce irritation or tissue damage.

Indications: CARBOCAINE is indicated for the production of local anesthesia by infiltration injection, peripheral nerve block, and central neural blocks by the lumbar or caudal epidural route.

Contraindication: Mepivacaine is contraindicated in patients with known hypersensitivity to the amide-type local anesthetics or to methylparaben, which is added to the multiple-dose vials.

Warnings: RESUSCITATIVE EQUIPMENT AND DRUGS SHOULD BE IMMEDIATELY AVAILABLE WHENEVER ANY LOCAL ANESTHETIC DRUG IS USED.

Large doses of local anesthetics should not be used in patients with heart block.

Reactions resulting in fatality have occurred on rare occasions with the use of local anesthetics, even in the absence of a history of hypersensitivity.

Solutions which contain a vasoconstrictor should be used with extreme caution in patients receiving drugs known to produce alterations in blood pressure (ie, monoamine oxidase (MAO) inhibitors, tricyclic antidepressants, phenothiazines, etc) as either severe sustained hypertension or hypotension may occur.

Usage in Children. Great care must be exercised in adhering to safe concentrations and dosages for pediatric administration (see Dosage and Administration).

Usage in Pregnancy. Safe use of mepivacaine has not been established with respect to adverse effects on fetal development. Careful consideration should be given to this fact before administering this drug to women of childbearing potential, particularly during early pregnancy. This does not exclude the use of the drug at term for obstetrical analgesia. Vasopressor agents (administered for the treatment of hypotension related to caudal or other epidural blocks) should be used with extreme caution in the presence of oxytocic drugs as they are known to interact and may produce severe, persistent hypertension and/or rupture of cerebral blood vessels. CARBOCAINE, brand of mepivacaine hydrochloride, has been used for obstetrical analgesia by the peridural and paracervical routes without evidence of adverse effects on the fetus when no more than the maximum safe dosages are used and strict adherence to technique is followed.

Local anesthetic procedures should be used with caution when there is inflammation and/or sepsis in the region of the proposed injection.

Composition of Available Solutions

Each mL contains	Single-dose 1% vial	Multiple-dose 1% vial	Single-dose 1.5% vial	Single-dose 2% vial	Multiple-dose 2% vial
Mepivacaine hydrochloride	10 mg	10 mg	15 mg	20 mg	20 mg
Sodium chloride	6.6 mg	7 mg	5.6 mg	4.6 mg	5 mg
Potassium chloride	0.3 mg	—	0.3 mg	0.3 mg	—
Calcium chloride	0.33 mg	—	0.33 mg	0.33 mg	—
Methylparaben	—	1 mg	—	—	1 mg
Water for injection	30 mL	50 mL	30 mL	20 mL	50 mL

The pH of the solutions is adjusted between 4.5 and 6.8 with sodium hydroxide or hydrochloric acid.

Precautions: Standard textbooks should be consulted for specific techniques and precautions for various regional anesthetic procedures.

The safety and effectiveness of a local anesthetic drug depend upon proper dosage, correct technique, adequate precautions, and readiness for emergencies.

The lowest dosage that results in effective anesthesia should be used to avoid high plasma levels and possible adverse effects. Injection of repeated doses of mepivacaine may cause significant increase in blood levels with each repeated dose due to slow accumulation of the drug or its metabolites or due to slower metabolic degradation than normal.

Tolerance varies with the status of the patient. Debilitated, elderly patients, or acutely ill patients should be given reduced doses commensurate with their weight and physical status.

Mepivacaine should be used with caution in patients with severe disturbances of cardiac rhythm, shock or heart block.

INJECTION SHOULD ALWAYS BE MADE SLOWLY AND WITH FREQUENT ASPIRATIONS TO AVOID INADVERTENT RAPID INTRAVASCULAR ADMINISTRATION WHICH CAN PRODUCE SYSTEMIC TOXICITY.

Fetal bradycardia which frequently follows paracervical block may be indicative of high fetal blood concentrations of CARBOCAINE with resultant fetal acidosis. Fetal heart rate should be monitored prior to and during paracervical block. Added risk appears to be present in prematurity, toxemia of pregnancy, and fetal distress. The physician should weigh the benefits against the risks in considering paracervical block in these conditions. Careful adherence to recommended dosage is of the utmost importance in paracervical block. Failure to achieve adequate analgesia with these doses should arouse suspicion of intravascular or fetal injection.

Case reports of maternal convulsions and cardiovascular collapse following use of mepivacaine for paracervical block in early pregnancy (as anesthesia for elective abortion) suggest that systemic absorption under these circumstances may be rapid. Therefore the recommended maximum dose of 100 mg per side should not be exceeded. Injection should be made slowly and with frequent aspiration. Allow a 5-minute interval between sides.

Vasoconstrictors. Solutions containing a vasoconstrictor should be used cautiously. The decision whether or not to use a vasoconstrictor with local anesthesia depends on the physician's appraisal of the benefits as opposed to the risk, eg, in injection of solutions containing a vasoconstrictor into areas where the blood supply is limited (eg, ears, nose, digits) or when peripheral vascular disease is present. Furthermore, serious cardiac arrhythmias may occur if preparations containing a vasoconstrictor are employed in patients during or immediately following the administration of halothane, cyclopropane, trichloroethylene, or other related agents.

MEPIVACAINE SHOULD BE USED WITH CAUTION IN PATIENTS WITH KNOWN DRUG ALLERGIES AND SENSITIVITIES. A thorough history of the patient's prior experience with CARBOCAINE or other local anesthetics as well as concomitant or recent drug use should be taken (see Contraindications). Patients allergic to methylparaben or para-aminobenzoic acid derivatives (procaine, tetracaine, benzocaine, etc) have not shown cross-sensitivity to agents of the amide-type such as mepivacaine. Since mepivacaine is metabolized in the liver and excreted by the kidneys, it should be used cautiously in patients with liver and renal disease.

Adverse Reactions: Systemic adverse reactions involving the central nervous system and the cardiovascular system usually result from high plasma levels due to excessive dosage, rapid absorption, or inadvertent intravascular injection. A small number of reactions may result from hypersensitivity, idiosyncrasy, or diminished tolerance to normal dosage.

Excitatory CNS effects commonly represent the initial signs of local anesthetic systemic toxicity. However, these reactions may be very brief or absent in some patients in which case the first manifestation of toxicity may be drowsiness merging into unconsciousness and respiratory arrest.

Cardiovascular system reactions include depression of the myocardium, hypotension (or sometimes hypertension), bradycardia, and even cardiac arrest. In obstetrics, cases of fetal bradycardia have occurred (see Precautions).

Allergic reactions are characterized by cutaneous lesions of delayed onset, or urticaria, edema, and other manifestations of allergy. The detection of sensitivity by skin testing is of limited value. As with other local anesthetics, hypersensitivity, idiosyncrasy, and anaphylactoid reactions to CARBOCAINE, brand of mepivacaine hydrochloride, have occurred rarely. The reaction may be abrupt and severe, and is not usually dose related. Sensitivity to methylparaben, a preservative added to multiple-dose vials, has been reported. Single-dose vials without methylparaben are also available.

Reactions following epidural or caudal anesthesia also may include: high or total spinal block; urinary retention; fecal incontinence; loss of perineal sensation and sexual function; persistent analgesia, paresthesia, and paralysis of the lower extremities; headache and backache; and slowing of labor and consequent increased incidence of forceps delivery.

Treatment of Reactions. Toxic effects of local anesthetics require symptomatic treatment; there is no specific cure. The physician should be prepared to maintain an airway and to support ventilation with oxygen and assisted or controlled respiration as required. Supportive treatment of the cardiovascular system includes intravenous fluids and, when appropriate, vasopressors (preferably those that stimulate the myocardium, such as ephedrine). *Convulsions* may be controlled with oxygen and by the intravenous administration of diazepam or short or ultrashort-acting barbiturates. Intravenous anticonvulsant agents should only be administered by those familiar with their use and only when ventilation and oxygenation are assured. In epidural anesthesia, sympathetic blockade also occurs as a pharmacological reaction, resulting in peripheral vasodilation and often *hypotension.* The extent of the hypotension will usually depend on the number of dermatomes blocked. The blood pressure should therefore be monitored in the early phases of anesthesia. If hypotension occurs, it is readily controlled by vasoconstrictors administered either by the intramuscular or the intravenous route, the dosage of which would depend on the severity of the hypotension and the response to treatment.

Dosage and Administration: As with all local anesthetics, the dose varies and depends upon the area to be anesthetized, the vascularity of the tissues, the number of neuronal segments to be blocked, individual tolerance, and the technique of anesthesia. The lowest dose needed to provide effective anesthesia should be administered. For specific techniques and procedures, refer to standard textbooks.

The recommended single adult dose (or the total of a series of doses given in one procedure) of CARBOCAINE, brand of mepivacaine hydrochloride,for unsedated, healthy, normal-sized individuals should not usually exceed 400 mg. The recommended dosage is based on requirements for the average adult and should be reduced for elderly or debilitated patients.

While maximum doses of 7 mg/kg (550 mg) have been administered without adverse effect, these are not recommended, except in exceptional circumstances and under no circumstances should the administration be repeated at intervals of less than 1½ hours. The total dose for any 24-hour period should not exceed 1000 mg because of a slow accumulation of the anesthetic or its derivatives or slower than normal metabolic degradation or detoxification with repeat administration (see Actions and Precautions).

Children tolerate the local anesthetic as well as adults. However, the pediatric dose should be carefully measured as a percentage of the total adult dose based on weight, and should not exceed 5 to 6 mg/kg (2.5 to 3 mg/lb) in children, especially those weighing less than 30 lbs. In children under 3 years of age or weighing less than 30 lbs. concentrations less than 2 percent (eg, 0.5 to 1.5 percent) should be employed.

[See table on next page].

How Supplied:
These solutions are not intended for spinal anesthesia or dental use.
1% single-dose vials of 30 mL (NDC 0024-0231-01)
1% multiple-dose vials of 50 mL (NDC 0024-0232-01)
1.5% single-dose vials of 30 mL (NDC 0024-0234-01)
2% single-dose vials of 20 mL (NDC 0024-0236-01)
2 multiple-dose vials of 50 mL
(NDC 0024-0237-01)

> For full prescribing information on the dental use of CARBOCAINE see Cook-Waite Laboratories, Inc. product listing in this publication.

CW-60-Q

DANOCRINE®
brand of danazol capsules, USP

Description: DANOCRINE, brand of danazol, is a synthetic androgen derived from ethisterone. Chemically, danazol is 17α-pregna-2,4-dien-20-yno[2,3-d]-isoxazol-17-ol.

Clinical Pharmacology: DANOCRINE suppresses the pituitary-ovarian axis by inhibiting the output of gonadotropins from the pituitary gland. The only other demonstrable hormonal effect is weak androgenic activity which is dose related. Studies have established that the drug is neither estrogenic nor progestational. DANOCRINE depresses the output of both follicle-stimulating hormone (FSH) and luteinizing hormone (LH).

Recent evidence suggests a direct inhibitory effect at gonadal sites and a binding of DANOCRINE to receptors of gonadal steroids at target organs. Bioavailability studies indicate that blood levels do not increase proportionally with increases in the administered dose. When the dose of DANOCRINE is doubled the increase in plasma levels is only about 35% to 40%.

In the treatment of endometriosis, DANOCRINE alters the normal and ectopic endometrial tissue so that it becomes inactive and atrophic. Complete resolution of endometrial lesions occurs in the majority of cases.

Changes in vaginal cytology and cervical mucus reflect the suppressive effect of DANOCRINE on the pituitary-ovarian axis.

In the treatment of fibrocystic breast disease, DANOCRINE usually produces partial to complete disappearance of nodularity and complete relief of pain and tenderness. Changes in the menstrual pattern may occur.

Generally the pituitary-suppressive action of DANOCRINE is reversible. Ovulation and cyclic bleeding usually return within 60 to 90 days when DANOCRINE therapy is discontinued.

In the treatment of hereditary angioedema, DANOCRINE at effective doses prevents attacks of the disease characterized by episodic edema of the abdominal viscera, extremities, face, and airway which may be disabling and, if the airway is involved, fatal. In addition, DANOCRINE corrects partially or completely the primary biochemical abnormality of hereditary angioedema by increasing the levels of the deficient C1 esterase inhibitor (C1EI). As a result of this action the serum levels of

Continued on next page

This product information was effective as of December 3, 1984. On these and other products of Winthrop-Breon Laboratories, detailed information may be obtained on a current basis by direct inquiry to the Professional Services Department, 90 Park Avenue, New York, NY 10016 (212) 907-2525.

Winthrop-Breon—Cont.

the C4 component of the complement system are also increased.

Indications and Usage: *Endometriosis.* DANOCRINE is indicated for the treatment of endometriosis amenable to hormonal management.

Fibrocystic Breast Disease. Most cases of symptomatic fibrocystic breast disease may be treated by simple measures (eg, padded brassieres and analgesics).

In infrequent patients, symptoms of pain and tenderness may be severe enough to warrant treatment by suppression of ovarian function. DANOCRINE is usually effective in decreasing nodularity, pain, and tenderness. It should be stressed to the patient that this treatment is not innocuous in that it involves considerable alterations of hormone levels and that recurrence of symptoms is very common after cessation of therapy.

Hereditary Angioedema. DANOCRINE is indicated for the prevention of attacks of angioedema of all types (cutaneous, abdominal, laryngeal) in males and females.

Contraindications: DANOCRINE should not be administered to patients with:
1. Undiagnosed abnormal genital bleeding.
2. Markedly impaired hepatic, renal, or cardiac function.
3. Pregnancy.
4. Breast feeding.

Warnings: Safe use of the drug in pregnancy has not been established clinically. Therefore, a nonhormonal method of contraception should be recommended. If a patient becomes pregnant during treatment, administration of the drug should be discontinued. Continuing treatment may result in an androgenic effect on the fetus, which to date has been limited to clitoral hypertrophy and labial fusion of the external genitalia in the female fetus. If the patient becomes pregnant while taking DANOCRINE, she should be apprised of the potential risk to the fetus.

Before initiating therapy of fibrocystic breast disease with DANOCRINE, carcinoma of the breast should be excluded. However, nodularity, pain, tenderness due to fibrocystic breast disease may prevent recognition of underlying carcinoma before treatment is begun. Therefore, if any nodule persists or enlarges during treatment, carcinoma should be considered and ruled out.

Long-term experience with danazol is limited. Long-term therapy with other steroids alkylated at the 17 position has been associated with serious toxicity (cholestatic jaundice, peliosis hepatis). The physician therefore should be alert to the possibility that similar toxicity may develop after long-term therapy with danazol. Attempts should be made to determine the lowest dose that will provide adequate protection. If the drug was begun at a time of exacerbation of angioneurotic edema due to trauma, stress or other cause, periodic attempts to decrease or withdraw therapy should be considered.

Patients should be watched closely for signs of virilization. Some androgenic effects may not be reversible even when drug administration is stopped.

Precautions: Because DANOCRINE may cause some degree of fluid retention, conditions that might be influenced by this factor, such as epilepsy, migraine, or cardiac or renal dysfunction, require careful observation.

Since hepatic dysfunction has been reported in patients treated with DANOCRINE, periodic liver function tests should be performed (see ADVERSE REACTIONS section).

Check semen for volume, viscosity, sperm count and motility every 3 to 4 months, especially in adolescents.

Adverse Reactions: The following androgenic effects have occurred in patients receiving DANOCRINE: acne, edema, mild hirsutism, decrease in breast size, deepening of the voice, oiliness of the skin or hair, weight gain, and rarely, clitoral hypertrophy, or testicular atrophy.

Also hypoestrogenic manifestations such as flushing, sweating, vaginitis including itching, dryness, burning and vaginal bleeding, nervousness, and emotional lability have been reported.

Hepatic dysfunction, as evidenced by elevated serum enzymes and/or jaundice, has been reported in patients receiving a daily dosage of DANOCRINE of 400 mg or more. It is recommended that patients receiving DANOCRINE, brand of danazol capsules, be monitored for hepatic dysfunction by laboratory tests and clinical observation. Prolongation of prothrombin time in patients stabilized on warfarin has also been reported.

Although the following reactions have also been reported, a causal relationship to the administration of DANOCRINE has neither been confirmed nor refuted: *allergic:* skin rashes and rarely, nasal congestion; *CNS effects:* dizziness, headache, sleep disorders, fatigue, tremor, and rarely, paresthesia in extremities, visual disturbances, anxiety, depression, changes in appetite, and chills; *gastrointestinal:* gastroenteritis, and rarely, nausea, vomiting, constipation; *musculoskeletal:* muscle cramps or spasms, joint lock-up, joint swelling, and pain in back, neck, or legs; *genitourinary:* rarely, hematuria; *other:* abnormal glucose tolerance test and increased insulin requirements in diabetic patients, loss of hair, changes in libido, elevation in blood pressure, and rarely, pelvic pain.

Dosage and Administration: *Endometriosis.* In moderate to severe disease, or in patients infertile due to endometriosis, a starting dose of 800 mg given in two divided doses is recommended. Amenorrhea and a rapid response to painful symptoms is best achieved at this dosage level. Gradual downward titration to a dose sufficient to maintain amenorrhea may be considered depending upon patient response. For mild cases, an initial daily dose of 200 mg to 400 mg given in two divided doses is recommended and may be adjusted depending on patient response. Therapy should begin during menstruation. Otherwise, appropriate tests should be performed to ensure that the patient is not pregnant while on DANOCRINE therapy. (See WARNINGS.) It is essential that therapy continue uninterrupted for 3 to 6 months but may be extended to 9 months if necessary. After termination of therapy, if symptoms recur, treatment can be reinstituted.

Fibrocystic Breast Disease. The total daily dosage of DANOCRINE for fibrocystic breast disease ranges from 100 mg to 400 mg given in two divided doses depending upon patient response. Therapy should begin during menstruation. Otherwise, appropriate tests should be performed to ensure that the patient is not pregnant while on DANOCRINE therapy. A nonhormonal method of contraception is recommended when DANOCRINE is administered at this dose, since ovulation may not be suppressed.

In most instances, breast pain and tenderness are significantly relieved by the first month and eliminated in 2 to 3 months. Usually elimination of nodularity requires 4 to 6 months of uninterrupted therapy. Regular menstrual patterns, irregular menstrual patterns, and amenorrhea each occur in approximately one-third of patients treated with 100 mg of DANOCRINE, brand of danazol capsules. Irregular menstrual patterns and amenorrhea are observed more frequently with higher doses. Clinical studies have demonstrated that 50% of patients may show evidence of recurrence of symptoms within one year. In this event, treatment may be reinstated.

Hereditary Angioedema. The dosage requirements for continuous treatment of hereditary angioedema with DANOCRINE should be individualized on the basis of the clinical response of the patient. It is recommended that the patient be started on 200 mg, two or three times a day. After a favorable initial response is obtained in terms of prevention of episodes of edematous attacks, the proper continuing dosage should be determined by decreasing the dosage by 50% or less at intervals of one to three months or longer if frequency of attacks prior to treatment dictates. If an attack occurs the daily dosage may be increased by up to 200 mg. During the dose adjusting phase, close monitoring of the patient's response is indicated,

Recommended Concentrations and Doses of CARBOCAINE

Procedure	Concentration	Total Dose mL	Total Dose mg	Comments
Cervical, brachial, intercostal, pudendal nerve block	1%	5–40	50–400	Pudendal block; one half of total dose injected each side.
	2%	5–20	100–400	
Transvaginal block (paracervical plus pudendal)	1%	up to 30 (both sides)	up to 300 (both sides)	One half of total dose injected each side. See Precautions.
Paracervical block	1%	up to 20 (both sides)	up to 200 (both sides)	One half of total dose injected each side. This is maximum recommended dose per 90 minute period in obstetrical and non-obstetrical patients. Inject slowly, 5 minutes between sides. See Precautions.
Caudal and Epidural block	1%	15–30	150–300	Use only single dose vials which do not contain a preservative.
	1.5%	10–25	150–375	
	2%	10–20	200–400	
Infiltration	1%	up to 40	up to 400	An equivalent amount of a 0.5% solution (prepared by diluting the 1% solution with Sodium Chloride Injection, USP) may be used for large areas.
Therapeutic block	1%	1–5	10–50	
	2%	1–5	20–50	

Unused portions of solutions not containing preservatives should be discarded.

particularly if the patient has a history of airway involvement.

How Supplied: Capsules of 200 mg (orange), bottles of 100 (NDC 0024-0305-06).
Capsules of 100 mg (yellow), bottles of 100 (NDC 0024-0304-06).
Capsules of 50 mg (orange and white), bottles of 100 (NDC 0024-0303-06).

Distributed by Winthrop-Breon Laboratories
Division of Sterling Drug Inc.
New York, NY 10016
Manufactured by
Sterling Pharmaceuticals Inc.
Barceloneta, Puerto Rico 00617

Shown in Product Identification Section, page 443

DW-254 M(O)

DEMEROL® Hydrochloride
brand of meperidine hydrochloride, USP

Description: Meperidine hydrochloride is ethyl 1-methyl-4-phenylisonipecotate hydrochloride, a white crystalline substance with a melting point of 186° C to 189° C. It is readily soluble in water and has a neutral reaction and a slightly bitter taste. The solution is not decomposed by a short period of boiling.

The syrup is a pleasant-tasting, nonalcoholic, banana-flavored solution containing 50 mg of DEMEROL hydrochloride, brand of meperidine hydrochloride, per 5 mL teaspoon (25 drops contain 13 mg of DEMEROL hydrochloride). The tablets contain 50 mg or 100 mg of the analgesic.

DEMEROL hydrochloride, brand of meperidine hydrochloride, 5 percent solution has a specific gravity of 1.0086 at 20°C and 10 percent solution, a specific gravity of 1.0165 at 20°C.

Clinical Pharmacology: Meperidine hydrochloride is a narcotic analgesic with multiple actions qualitatively similar to those of morphine; the most prominent of these involve the central nervous system and organs composed of smooth muscle. The principal actions of therapeutic value are analgesia and sedation.

There is some evidence which suggests that meperidine may produce less smooth muscle spasm, constipation, and depression of the cough reflex than equianalgesic doses of morphine. Meperidine, in 60 mg to 80 mg parenteral doses, is approximately equivalent in analgesic effect to 10 mg of morphine. The onset of action is slightly more rapid than with morphine, and the duration of action is slightly shorter. Meperidine is significantly less effective by the oral than by the parenteral route, but the exact ratio of oral to parenteral effectiveness is unknown.

Indications and Usage:
For the relief of moderate to severe pain (parenteral and oral forms)
For preoperative medication (parenteral form only)
For support of anesthesia (parenteral form only)
For obstetrical analgesia (parenteral form only)

Contraindications:
Hypersensitivity to meperidine.
Meperidine is contraindicated in patients who are receiving monoamine oxidase (MAO) inhibitors or those who have recently received such agents. Therapeutic doses of meperidine have occasionally precipitated unpredictable, severe, and occasionally fatal reactions in patients who have received such agents within 14 days. The mechanism of these reactions is unclear, but may be related to a preexisting hyperphenylalaninemia. Some have been characterized by coma, severe respiratory depression, cyanosis, and hypotension, and have resembled the syndrome of acute narcotic overdose. In other reactions the predominant manifestations have been hyperexcitability, convulsions, tachycardia, hyperpyrexia, and hypertension. Although it is not known that other narcotics are free of the risk of such reactions, virtually all of the reported reactions have occurred with meperidine. If a narcotic is needed in such patients, a sensitivity test should be performed in which repeated, small, incremental doses of morphine are administered over the course of several hours while the patient's condition and vital signs are under careful observation. (Intravenous hydrocortisone or prednisolone have been used to treat severe reactions, with the addition of intravenous chlorpromazine in those cases exhibiting hypertension and hyperpyrexia. The usefulness and safety of narcotic antagonists in the treatment of these reactions is unknown.)

Solutions of DEMEROL and barbiturates are chemically incompatible.

Warnings: *Drug Dependence.* Meperidine can produce drug dependence of the morphine type and therefore has the potential for being abused. Psychic dependence, physical dependence, and tolerance may develop upon repeated administration of meperidine, and it should be prescribed and administered with the same degree of caution appropriate to the use of morphine. Like other narcotics, meperidine is subject to the provisions of the Federal narcotic laws.

Interaction with Other Central Nervous System Depressants. Meperidine should be used with great caution and in reduced dosage in patients who are concurrently receiving other narcotic analgesics, general anesthetics, phenothiazines, other tranquilizers (see Dosage and Administration), sedative-hypnotics (including barbiturates), tricyclic antidepressants, and other CNS depressants (including alcohol). Respiratory depression, hypotension, and profound sedation or coma may result.

Head Injury and Increased Intracranial Pressure. The respiratory depressant effects of meperidine and its capacity to elevate cerebrospinal fluid pressure may be markedly exaggerated in the presence of head injury, other intracranial lesions, or a preexisting increase in intracranial pressure. Furthermore, narcotics produce adverse reactions which may obscure the clinical course of patients with head injuries. In such patients, meperidine must be used with extreme caution and only if its use is deemed essential.

Intravenous Use. If necessary, meperidine may be given intravenously, but the injection should be given very slowly, preferably in the form of a diluted solution. Rapid intravenous injection of narcotic analgesics, including meperidine, increases the incidence of adverse reactions; severe respiratory depression, apnea, hypotension, peripheral circulatory collapse, and cardiac arrest have occurred. Meperidine should not be administered intravenously unless a narcotic antagonist and the facilities for assisted or controlled respiration are immediately available. When meperidine is given parenterally, especially intravenously, the patient should be lying down.

Asthma and Other Respiratory Conditions. Meperidine should be used with extreme caution in patients having an acute asthmatic attack, patients with chronic obstructive pulmonary disease or cor pulmonale, patients having a substantially decreased respiratory reserve, and patients with preexisting respiratory depression, hypoxia, or hypercapnia. In such patients, even usual therapeutic doses of narcotics may decrease respiratory drive while simultaneously increasing airway resistance to the point of apnea.

Hypotensive Effect. The administration of meperidine may result in severe hypotension in the postoperative patient or any individual whose ability to maintain blood pressure has been compromised by a depleted blood volume or the administration of drugs such as the phenothiazines or certain anesthetics.

Usage in Ambulatory Patients. Meperidine may impair the mental and/or physical abilities required for the performance of potentially hazardous tasks such as driving a car or operating machinery. The patient should be cautioned accordingly.

Meperidine, like other narcotics, may produce orthostatic hypotension in ambulatory patients.

Usage in Pregnancy and Lactation. Meperidine should not be used in pregnant women prior to the labor period, unless in the judgment of the physician the potential benefits outweigh the possible hazards, because safe use in pregnancy prior to labor has not been established relative to possible adverse effects on fetal development.

When used as an obstetrical analgesic, meperidine crosses the placental barrier and can produce depression of respiration and psychophysiologic functions in the newborn. Resuscitation may be required (see section on Overdosage).

Meperidine appears in the milk of nursing mothers receiving the drug.

Precautions: *Supraventricular Tachycardias.* Meperidine should be used with caution in patients with atrial flutter and other supraventricular tachycardias because of a possible vagolytic action which may produce a significant increase in the ventricular response rate.

Convulsions. Meperidine may aggravate preexisting convulsions in patients with convulsive disorders. If dosage is escalated substantially above recommended levels because of tolerance development, convulsions may occur in individuals without a history of convulsive disorders.

Acute Abdominal Conditions. The administration of meperidine or other narcotics may obscure the diagnosis or clinical course in patients with acute abdominal conditions.

Special Risk Patients. Meperidine should be given with caution and the initial dose should be reduced in certain patients such as the elderly or debilitated, and those with severe impairment of hepatic or renal function, hypothyroidism, Addison's disease, and prostatic hypertrophy or urethral stricture.

Adverse Reactions: The major hazards of meperidine, as with other narcotic analgesics, are respiratory depression and, to a lesser degree, circulatory depression; respiratory arrest, shock, and cardiac arrest have occurred.

The most frequently observed adverse reactions include lightheadedness, dizziness, sedation, nausea, vomiting, and sweating. These effects seem to be more prominent in ambulatory patients and in those who are not experiencing severe pain. In such individuals, lower doses are advisable. Some adverse reactions in ambulatory patients may be alleviated if the patient lies down.

Other adverse reactions include:
Nervous System. Euphoria, dysphoria, weakness, headache, agitation, tremor, uncoordinated muscle movements, transient hallucinations and disorientation, visual disturbances. Inadvertent injection about a nerve trunk may result in sensorimotor paralysis which is usually, though not always, transitory.

Gastrointestinal. Dry mouth, constipation, biliary tract spasm.

Cardiovascular. Flushing of the face, tachycardia, bradycardia, palpitation, hypotension (see Warnings), syncope, phlebitis following intravenous injection.

Genitourinary. Urinary retention.

Allergic. Pruritus, urticaria, other skin rashes, wheal and flare over the vein with intravenous injection.

Other. Pain at injection site; local tissue irritation and induration following subcutaneous injection, particularly when repeated; antidiuretic effect.

Dosage and Administration:
For Relief of Pain
Dosage should be adjusted according to the severity of the pain and the response of the patient. While subcutaneous administration is suitable for occasional use, intramuscular administration is preferred when repeated doses are required. If intravenous administration is required, dosage should be decreased and the injection made very slowly, preferably utilizing a diluted solution. Meperidine is less effective orally than on parenteral administration. The dose of DEMEROL should be

Continued on next page

This product information was effective as of December 3, 1984. On these and other products of Winthrop-Breon Laboratories, detailed information may be obtained on a current basis by direct inquiry to the Professional Services Department, 90 Park Avenue, New York, NY 10016 (212) 907-2525.

Winthrop-Breon—Cont.

proportionately reduced (usually by 25 to 50 percent) when administered concomitantly with phenothiazines and many other tranquilizers since they potentiate the action of DEMEROL, brand of meperidine.

Adults. The usual dosage is 50 mg to 150 mg intramuscularly, subcutaneously, or orally, every 3 or 4 hours as necessary.

Children. The usual dosage is 0.5 mg/lb to 0.8 mg/lb intramuscularly, subcutaneously, or orally up to the adult dose, every 3 or 4 hours as necessary.

Each dose of the syrup should be taken in one-half glass of water, since if taken undiluted, it may exert a slight topical anesthetic effect on mucous membranes.

For Preoperative Medication

Adults. The usual dosage is 50 mg to 100 mg intramuscularly or subcutaneously, 30 to 90 minutes before the beginning of anesthesia.

Children. The usual dosage is 0.5 mg/lb to 1 mg/lb intramuscularly or subcutaneously up to the adult dose, 30 to 90 minutes before the beginning of anesthesia.

For Support of Anesthesia

Repeated slow intravenous injections of fractional doses (eg, 10 mg/mL) or continuous intravenous infusion of a more dilute solution (eg, 1 mg/mL) should be used. The dose should be titrated to the needs of the patient and will depend on the premedication and type of anesthesia being employed, the characteristics of the particular patient, and the nature and duration of the operative procedure.

For Obstetrical Analgesia

The usual dosage is 50 mg to 100 mg intramuscularly or subcutaneously when pain becomes regular, and may be repeated at 1- to 3-hour intervals.

Overdosage: *Symptoms.* Serious overdosage with meperidine is characterized by respiratory depression (a decrease in respiratory rate and/or tidal volume, Cheyne-Stokes respiration, cyanosis), extreme somnolence progressing to stupor or coma, skeletal muscle flaccidity, cold and clammy skin, and sometimes bradycardia and hypotension. In severe overdosage, particularly by the intravenous route, apnea, circulatory collapse, cardiac arrest, and death may occur.

Treatment. Primary attention should be given to the reestablishment of adequate respiratory exchange through provision of a patent airway and institution of assisted or controlled ventilation. The narcotic antagonist, naloxone hydrochloride, is a specific antidote against respiratory depression which may result from overdosage or unusual sensitivity to narcotics, including meperidine. Therefore, an appropriate dose of this antagonist should be administered, preferably by the intravenous route, simultaneously with efforts at respiratory resuscitation.

An antagonist should not be administered in the absence of clinically significant respiratory or cardiovascular depression.

Oxygen, intravenous fluids, vasopressors, and other supportive measures should be employed as indicated.

In cases of overdosage with DEMEROL, brand of meperidine, tablets, the stomach should be evacuated by emesis or gastric lavage.

NOTE: In an individual physically dependent on narcotics, the administration of the usual dose of a narcotic antagonist will precipitate an acute withdrawal syndrome. The severity of this syndrome will depend on the degree of physical dependence and the dose of antagonist administered. The use of narcotic antagonists in such individuals should be avoided if possible. If a narcotic antagonist must be used to treat serious respiratory depression in the physically dependent patient, the antagonist should be administered with extreme care and only one-fifth to one-tenth the usual initial dose administered.

How Supplied:
For Parenteral Use
Detecto-Seal® — *Carpuject®* **Sterile Cartridge-Needle Units**—*2.5 percent* (25 mg per 1 mL) NDC 0024-0324-02, *5 percent* (50 mg per 1 mL) NDC 0024-0325-02, *7.5 percent* (75 mg per 1 mL) NDC 0024-0326-02; and *10 percent* (100 mg per 1 mL) NDC 0024-0328-02 all in boxes of 10.

Each cartridge is only partially-filled based upon product volume to permit mixture with other sterile materials in accordance with the best judgment of the physician.

Uni-Amp—*5 percent solution;* ampuls of 0.5 mL (25 mg) NDC 0024-0361-04, 1 mL (50 mg) NDC 0024-0362-04, 1½ mL (75 mg) NDC 0024-0363-04, and 2 mL (100 mg) NDC 0024-0364-04 all in boxes of 25; and *10 percent solution,* ampuls of 1 mL (100 mg) NDC 0024-0365-04 in boxes of 25.

Uni-Nest™—*5 percent solution;* ampuls of 0.5 mL (25 mg) NDC 0024-0371-04, 1 mL (50 mg) NDC 0024-0372-04, 1½ mL (75 mg) NDC 0024-0373-04, and 2 mL (100 mg) NDC 0024-0374-04 all in boxes of 25; and *10 percent solution,* ampuls of 1 mL (100 mg) NDC 0024-0375-04 in boxes of 25.

Vials—*5 percent* multiple-dose vials of 30 mL NDC 0024-0329-01, and *10 percent* multiple-dose vials of 20 mL NDC 0024-0331-01 all in boxes of 1.

Note: The pH of DEMEROL solutions is adjusted between 3.5 and 6.0 with sodium hydroxide or hydrochloric acid. Multiple-dose vials contain metacresol 0.1 percent as preservative. No preservatives are added to the ampuls or CARPUJECT Sterile Cartridge-Needle Units.

For Oral Use
Tablets of 50 mg, bottles of 100 (NDC 0024-0335-04) and 500 (NDC 0024-0335-06); Hospital Blister Pak of 25 (NDC 0024-0335-02); 100 mg, bottles of 100 (NDC 0024-0337-04) and 500 (NDC 0024-0337-06); Hospital Blister Pak of 25 (NDC 0024-0337-02).

Syrup, nonalcoholic, banana-flavored 50 mg per 5 mL teaspoon, bottles of 16 fl oz (NDC 0024-0332-06).

Shown in Product Identification Section, page 443

DW-55-DD(R)

FERGON® CAPSULES
FERGON®
brand of ferrous gluconate
FERGON® ELIXIR

Composition: FERGON (ferrous gluconate) is stabilized to maintain a minimum of ferric ions. It contains not less than 11.5 percent iron. Each FERGON Capsule contains 435 mg of ferrous gluconate, yielding 50 mg of elemental iron. Each FERGON tablet contains 320 mg. FERGON Elixir 6% contains 300 mg per teaspoon.

Action and Uses: FERGON preparations produce rapid hemoglobin regeneration in patients with iron deficiency anemias. FERGON is better utilized and better tolerated than other forms of iron because of its low ionization constant and solubility in the entire pH range of the gastrointestinal tract. It does not precipitate proteins or have the astringency of more ionizable forms of iron, does not interfere with proteolytic or diastatic activities of the digestive system, and will not produce nausea, abdominal cramps, constipation or diarrhea in the great majority of patients. The pellets of ferrous gluconate contained in FERGON Capsules are coated to permit maximum availability of iron in the upper small bowel, the site of maximum absorption.

FERGON preparations are indicated in anemias amenable to iron therapy (1) hypochromic anemia of infancy and childhood; (2) idiopathic hypochromic anemia; (3) hypochromic anemia of pregnancy; and (4) anemia associated with chronic blood loss.

Dosage and Administration: *Adults*—1 FERGON Capsule daily for mild to moderate iron deficiency anemia. For more severe anemia the dosage may be increased. One to two FERGON tablets or one to two teaspoons of FERGON Elixir daily. *For children and infants,* consult physician.

How Supplied: FERGON Capsules, bottle of 30 (NDC 0024-1016-03). FERGON, tablets of 320 mg (5 grains), bottles of 100 (NDC 0024-1015-10), 500 (NDC 0024-1015-50), and 1,000 (NDC 0024-1015-00). FERGON Elixir 6% (5 grains per teaspoon), bottle of 1 pint (NDC 0024-1019-16).

Shown in Product Identification Section, page 443

FERGON® PLUS
FOR IRON DEFICIENCY AND MACROCYTIC ANEMIAS

℞

Description:
Ferrous gluconate, USP .... 500 mg
Vitamin B_{12} with Intrinsic Factor
Concentrate NF·XI .... 1/2 unit (oral)
Ascorbic Acid, USP .... 75 mg
  contained in each pink-colored, sugar-coated caplet

Ferrous gluconate contains 12% metallic iron. Intrinsic Factor is a glycoprotein with a molecular weight in the range of 60,000.

Clinical Pharmacology: Vitamin B_{12} with Intrinsic Factor Concentrate as contained in 2 FERGON PLUS Caplets® represents 1 NF XI oral unit of anti-anemia activity, that is, the amount of material which, when administered daily by mouth, produces a satisfactory hematologic and symptomatic response in patients in relapse with pernicious anemia.

Vitamin B_{12} is the principal active anti-pernicious anemia factor of liver extract and is believed to be essentially extrinsic factor. Its anti-pernicious anemia activity is approximately the same as that produced by liver extract and, like the latter, it is more effective by injection than by mouth. However, its activity on oral administration is increased by the concomitant ingestion of Intrinsic Factor Concentrate which facilitates absorption of vitamin B_{12} from the alimentary tract.

Ferrous gluconate is better utilized and better tolerated than other forms of iron and produces rapid hemoglobin regeneration when iron deficiency is present. Ascorbic acid appears to play a role in the absorption of iron. Its deficiency leads to depression of bone marrow activity.

Indications and Usage: Dietary Supplement: FERGON PLUS is useful as a dietary supplement and as a maintenance source of vitamin B_{12}, vitamin C, and iron. However, it should be remembered that the development of the classic symptoms of pernicious anemia may in some cases be delayed by oral ingestion of Intrinsic Factor.

Therapy: FERGON PLUS is indicated for all anemias amenable to iron therapy including (1) hypochromic anemia of infancy and childhood; (2) idiopathic hypochromic anemia; (3) hypochromic anemia of pregnancy; and (4) anemia associated with chronic blood loss.

FERGON PLUS is also indicated for patients with anemias responding to oral Vitamin B_{12} therapy, viz, those in whom the bone marrow is in a state of megaloblastic arrest reflected in the blood stream by macrocytosis, anisocytosis and poikilocytosis, including macrocytic anemia of tropical and nontropical sprue, megaloblastic anemias of pregnancy and infancy, and pernicious anemia amenable to oral B_{12} therapy. Similarly, FERGON PLUS may be given orally to patients with pernicious anemia to supplement parenterally administered vitamin B_{12} therapy.

Contraindications: FERGON PLUS is contraindicated in patients with known hypersensitivity to any of its ingredients.

Warnings: The treatment of any anemic condition should be under the advice and supervision of a physician.

Precautions: All patients with pernicious anemia should be given periodic examinations and laboratory studies should be performed. Recommended laboratory tests include hemoglobin, hematocrit and reticulocyte count. Some patients may not respond to orally ingested vitamin B_{12} with Intrinsic Factor Concentrate. There is no known way to predict which patients may cease to respond.

Drug Interactions: Antacids reduce the absorption of iron if given concurrently. Absorption of FERGON® PLUS is optimal when the ferrous salt is taken by the patient when fasting. Food variably reduces the availability of an iron salt, depending on the composition of the diet.

Carcinogenesis, Mutagenesis, Impairment of Fertility: Long-term animal studies have not been done to evaluate the potential of FERGON PLUS in these areas.

Pregnancy Category C: Animal reproduction studies have not been conducted with FERGON PLUS. On the basis of the high prevalence of iron deficiency in the population of pregnant females, iron balance studies, and therapeutic trials, the FDA's Panel on OTC Vitamin, Mineral, and Hematinic Drug Products, recommends a daily dose of 30 mg to 60 mg iron be made available to pregnant females to maintain iron stores and prevent iron deficiency.

Nursing Mothers: The FDA's Panel on OTC Vitamin, Mineral, and Hematinic Drug Products recommends a daily dose of 10 mg to 30 mg of exogenous iron be made available to nursing mothers to compensate for iron loss through lactation.

Adverse Reactions: Intolerance to oral preparations of iron is primarily a function of the amount of soluble iron in the upper gastrointestinal tract and of psychological factors. Symptoms include heartburn, nausea, upper gastric discomfort, constipation, and diarrhea.

Overdosage: Signs and symptoms of severe iron poisoning may occur within 30 minutes or may be delayed for several hours after ingestion. Overdosage may lead to cyanosis, pallor, acidosis, and cardiovascular collapse. In overdosages, efforts should be made to hasten the elimination of the CAPLETS. An emetic should be administered as soon as possible followed by gastric lavage. Following emesis a saline cathartic should be administered to hasten passage through the gastrointestinal system. X-rays should be taken to evaluate the number of CAPLETS remaining in the small bowel.

Dosage and Administration: As a dietary supplement: 1 caplet daily.

Therapeutic dose: 1 caplet twice daily (before the morning and evening meals). When the condition is severe, the initial dose should be increased to 2 CAPLETS twice daily for one or two weeks, or specific parenteral therapy should be employed.

How Supplied: Bottle of 100 (NDC 0024-1017-10)

CAUTION: Federal law prohibits dispensing without prescription.

FW-36-A

HALEY'S M-O®   OTC

(See PDR For Nonprescription Drugs)

HYPAQUE® SODIUM   ℞
brand of diatrizoate sodium, USP
ORAL POWDER

(See Diagnostic Section.)

HYPAQUE® SODIUM   ℞
ORAL SOLUTION
brand of diatrizoate sodium solution, USP

(See Diagnostic Section.)

HYPAQUE® SODIUM 20%   ℞
brand of diatrizoate sodium injection, USP
Sterile Aqueous Solution

(See Diagnostic Section.)

HYPAQUE® SODIUM 25%   ℞
brand of diatrizoate sodium injection, USP
Sterile Aqueous Solution

(See Diagnostic Section.)

HYPAQUE-CYSTO®   ℞
brand of diatrizoate meglumine injection, USP
Sterile Aqueous Solution

(See Diagnostic Section.)

HYPAQUE® MEGLUMINE 30%   ℞
brand of diatrizoate meglumine injection, USP
Sterile Aqueous Solution

(See Diagnostic Section.)

HYPAQUE® SODIUM 50%   ℞
brand of diatrizoate sodium injection, USP
Sterile Aqueous Injection

(See Diagnostic Section.)

HYPAQUE® MEGLUMINE 60%   ℞
brand of diatrizoate meglumine injection, USP
Sterile Aqueous Injection

(See Diagnostic Section.)

HYPAQUE®-M, 75%   ℞
brand of diatrizoate meglumine and diatrizoate sodium injection, USP
Sterile Aqueous Injection

(See Diagnostic Section.)

HYPAQUE®-76   ℞
brand of diatrizoate meglumine and diatrizoate sodium injection, USP
Sterile Aqueous Injection

(See Diagnostic Section.)

HYPAQUE®-M, 90%   ℞
brand of diatrizoate meglumine and diatrizoate sodium injection, USP
Sterile Aqueous Injection

(See Diagnostic Section.)

INOCOR® LACTATE INJECTION   ℞
brand of amrinone lactate
Sterile Intravenous Solution

Description: INOCOR lactate injection, brand of amrinone lactate, represents a new class of cardiac inotropic agents distinct from digitalis glycosides or catecholamines. Amrinone lactate is designated chemically as 5-Amino[3,4'-bipyridin]-6(1H)-one lactate.

Amrinone is a pale yellow crystalline compound with a molecular weight of 187.2 and an empirical formula of $C_{10}H_9N_3O$. Each mole of lactic acid has a molecular weight of 90.08 and an empirical formula of $C_3H_6O_3$. The solubilities of amrinone at pH's 4.1, 6.0, and 8.0 are 25, 0.9, and 0.7 mg/mL, respectively.

INOCOR lactate injection is available as a sterile solution in 20 mL ampuls for intravenous administration. Each mL contains INOCOR lactate equivalent to 5 mg of base and 0.25 mg of sodium metabisulfite added as a preservative in Water for Injection. All dosages expressed in the package insert are expressed in terms of the base, amrinone. The pH is adjusted to between 3.2 to 4.0 with lactic acid or sodium hydroxide. The total concentration of lactic acid can vary between 5.0 mg/mL and 7.5 mg/mL.

Clinical Pharmacology: INOCOR lactate injection is a positive inotropic agent with vasodilator activity, different in structure and mode of action from either digitalis glycosides or catecholamines.

The mechanism of its inotropic and vasodilator effects has not been fully elucidated.

With respect to its inotropic effect, experimental evidence indicates that it is not a beta-adrenergic agonist. It inhibits myocardial cyclic adenosine monophosphate phosphodiesterase (c-AMP) activity and increases cellular levels of c-AMP. Unlike digitalis, it does not inhibit sodium-potassium adenosine triphosphatase activity.

With respect to its vasodilatory activity, INOCOR reduces afterload and preload by its direct relaxant effect on vascular smooth muscle.

Pharmacokinetics

Following intravenous bolus (1 to 2 minutes) injection of 0.68 mg/kg to 1.2 mg/kg to normal volunteers, INOCOR had a volume of distribution of 1.2 liters/kg, and following a distributive phase half-life of about 4.6 minutes in plasma, had a mean apparent first-order terminal elimination half-life of about 3.6 hours. In patients with congestive heart failure receiving infusions of INOCOR the mean apparent first-order terminal elimination half-life was about 5.8 hours.

Amrinone has been shown in one study to be 10% to 22% bound to human plasma protein by ultrafiltration in vitro, and in another study 35% to 49% bound by either ultrafiltration or equilibrium dialysis.

The primary route of excretion in man is *via* the urine as both amrinone and several metabolites (N-glycolyl, N-acetate, O-glucuronide and N-glucuronide). In normal volunteers, approximately 63% of an oral dose of ^{14}C-labelled amrinone was excreted in the urine over a 96-hour period. In the first 8 hours, 51% of the radioactivity in the urine was amrinone with 5% as the N-acetate, 8% as the N-glycolate, and less than 5% for each glucuronide. Approximately 18% of the administered dose was excreted in the feces in 72 hours.

In a 24-hour nonradioactive intravenous study, 10% to 40% of the dose was excreted in urine as unchanged amrinone with the N-acetyl metabolite representing less than 2% of the dose.

In congestive heart failure patients, after a loading bolus dose, steady-state plasma levels of about 2.4 µg/mL were able to be maintained by an infusion of 5 µg/kg/min to 10 µg/kg/min. In some congestive heart failure patients, with associated compromised renal and hepatic perfusion, it is possible that plasma levels of amrinone may rise during the infusion period; therefore, in these patients, it may be necessary to monitor the hemodynamic response and/or drug level. The principal measures of patient response include cardiac index, pulmonary capillary wedge pressure, central venous pressure, and their relationship to plasma concentrations. Additionally, measures of blood pressure, urine output, and body weight may prove useful, as may such clinical symptoms as orthopnea, dyspnea, and fatigue.

Pharmacodynamics

In patients with depressed myocardial function, INOCOR lactate injection produces a prompt increase in cardiac output due to its inotropic and vasodilator actions.

Following a single intravenous bolus dose of INOCOR of 0.75 mg/kg to 3 mg/kg in patients with congestive heart failure, dose-related maximum increases in cardiac output occur (of about 28% on 0.75 mg/kg to about 61% at 3 mg/kg). The peak effect occurs within 10 minutes at all doses. The duration of effect depends upon dose, lasting about ½ hour at 0.75 mg/kg and approximately 2 hours at 3 mg/kg.

Over the same range of doses, pulmonary capillary wedge pressure and total peripheral resistance show dose-related decreases (mean maximum decreases of 29% in pulmonary capillary wedge pressure and 33% in systemic vascular resistance). At doses up to 3.0 mg/kg dose-related decreases in diastolic pressure (up to 13%) have been observed. Mean arterial pressure decreases (9.7%) at a dose of 3.0 mg/kg. The heart rate is generally unchanged.

The changes in hemodynamic parameters are maintained during continuous intravenous infusion and for several hours thereafter.

INOCOR lactate injection, brand of amrinone lactate, is effective in fully digitalized patients without causing signs of cardiac glycoside toxicity. Its inotropic effects are additive to those of digitalis. In cases of atrial flutter/fibrillation, it is possi-

Continued on next page

This product information was effective as of December 3, 1984. On these and other products of Winthrop-Breon Laboratories, detailed information may be obtained on a current basis by direct inquiry to the Professional Services Department, 90 Park Avenue, New York, NY 10016 (212) 907-2525.

Winthrop-Breon—Cont.

ble that INOCOR may increase ventricular response rate because of its slight enhancement of A/V conduction. In these cases, prior treatment with digitalis is recommended.

Improvement in left ventricular function and relief of congestive heart failure in patients with ischemic heart disease have been observed. The improvement has occurred without inducing symptoms or electrocardiographic signs of myocardial ischemia.

At constant heart rate and blood pressure, increases in cardiac output occur without measurable increases in myocardial oxygen consumption or changes in arterio-venous oxygen difference.

Inotropic activity is maintained following repeated intravenous doses of INOCOR. INOCOR administration produces hemodynamic and symptomatic benefits to patients not satisfactorily controlled by conventional therapy with diuretics and cardiac glycosides.

Indications and Usage: INOCOR lactate injection is indicated for the short-term management of congestive heart failure. Because of limited experience and potential for serious adverse effects (see ADVERSE REACTIONS), INOCOR should be used only in patients who can be closely monitored and who have not responded adequately to digitalis, diuretics, and/or vasodilators. Although most patients have been studied hemodynamically for periods only up to 24 hours, some patients were studied for longer periods and demonstrated consistent hemodynamic and clinical effects. The duration of therapy should depend on patient responsiveness.

Contraindications: INOCOR lactate injection is contraindicated in patients who are hypersensitive to it.

It is also contraindicated in those patients known to be hypersensitive to bisulfites.

Precautions: General: INOCOR lactate injection should not be used in patients with severe aortic or pulmonic valvular disease in lieu of surgical relief of the obstruction. Like other inotropic agents, it may aggravate outflow tract obstruction in hypertrophic subaortic stenosis.

During intravenous therapy with INOCOR lactate injection, blood pressure and heart rate should be monitored and the rate of infusion slowed or stopped in patients showing excessive decreases in blood pressure.

Patients who have received vigorous diuretic therapy may have insufficient cardiac filling pressure to respond adequately to INOCOR lactate injection, in which case cautious liberalization of fluid and electrolyte intake may be indicated.

Supraventricular and ventricular arrhythmias have been observed in the very high-risk population treated. While amrinone per se has not been shown to be arrhythmogenic, the potential for arrhythmia, present in congestive heart failure itself, may be increased by any drug or combination of drugs.

Thrombocytopenia and hepatotoxicity have been noted (see ADVERSE REACTIONS).

USE IN ACUTE MYOCARDIAL INFARCTION: No clinical trials have been carried out in patients in the acute phase of postmyocardial infarction. Therefore, INOCOR lactate injection, brand of amrinone lactate, is not recommended in these cases.

Laboratory Tests

Fluid and Electrolytes: Fluid and electrolyte changes and renal function should be carefully monitored during amrinone lactate therapy. Improvement in cardiac output with resultant diuresis may necessitate a reduction in the dose of diuretic. Potassium loss due to excessive diuresis may predispose digitalized patients to arrhythmias. Therefore, hypokalemia should be corrected by potassium supplementation in advance of or during amrinone use.

Drug Interactions

In a relatively limited experience, no untoward clinical manifestations have been observed in patients in which INOCOR lactate injection was used concurrently with the following drugs: digitalis glycosides; lidocaine, quinidine; metoprolol, propranolol; hydralazine, prazosin; isosorbide dinitrate, nitroglycerine; chlorthalidone, ethacrynic acid, furosemide, hydrochlorothiazide, spironolactone; captopril; heparin, warfarin; potassium supplements; insulin; diazepam.

One case report of excessive hypotension has been reported when amrinone was used concurrently with disopyramide.

Until additional experience is available, concurrent administration with NORPACE® (disopyramide) should be undertaken with caution.

Carcinogenesis, Mutagenesis, Impairment of Fertility

The 1-year interim evaluation of the 2-year oral carcinogenicity study on F344 rats indicated no tumor induction at that time.

The mouse micronucleus test (at 7.5 to 10 times the maximum human dose) and the Chinese hamster ovary chromosome aberration assay were positive indicating both clastogenic potential and suppression of the number of polychromatic erythrocytes. However, the Ames Salmonella assay, mouse lymphoma study, and cultured human lymphocyte metaphase analysis were all negative. The clastogenic effects are in contrast to negative results obtained in the rat male and female fertility studies, and a three-generation study in rats, both with oral dosing.

Slight prolongation of the rat gestation period was seen in these studies at dose levels of 50 mg/kg/day and 100 mg/kg/day. Dystocia occurred in dams receiving 100 mg/kg/day resulting in increased numbers of stillbirths, decreased litter size, and poor pup survival.

Pregnancy Category C

In New Zealand white rabbits, amrinone has been shown to produce fetal skeletal and gross external malformations at oral doses of 16 mg/kg and 50 mg/kg which were toxic for the rabbit. Studies in French Hy/Cr rabbits using oral doses up to 32 mg/kg/day did not confirm this finding. No malformations were seen in rats receiving amrinone intravenously at the maximum dose used, 15 mg/kg/day (approximately the recommended daily intravenous dose for patients with congestive heart failure). There are no adequate and well-controlled studies in pregnant women. Amrinone should be used during pregnancy only if the potential benefit justifies the potential risk to the fetus.

Nursing Mothers

Caution should be exercised when amrinone is administered to nursing women, since it is not known whether it is excreted in human milk.

Pediatric Use

Safety and effectiveness in children have not been established.

Adverse Reactions: *Thrombocytopenia:* Intravenous INOCOR lactate injection, brand of amrinone lactate, resulted in platelet count reductions to below 100,000/mm³ or normal limits in 2.4 percent of the patients.

It is more common in patients receiving prolonged therapy. To date, in closely-monitored clinical trials, in patients whose platelet counts were not allowed to remain depressed, no bleeding phenomena have been observed.

Platelet reduction is dose dependent and appears due to a decrease in platelet survival time. Several patients who developed thrombocytopenia while receiving amrinone had bone marrow examinations which were normal. There is no evidence relating platelet reduction to immune response or to a platelet activating factor.

Gastrointestinal Effects: Gastrointestinal adverse reactions reported with INOCOR lactate injection during clinical use included nausea (1.7%), vomiting (0.9%), abdominal pain (0.4%), and anorexia (0.4%).

Cardiovascular Effects: Cardiovascular adverse reactions reported with INOCOR lactate injection include arrhythmia (3%) and hypotension (1.3%).

Hepatic Toxicity: In dogs, at IV doses between 9 mg/kg/day and 32 mg/kg/day, amrinone showed dose-related hepatotoxicity manifested either as enzyme elevation or hepatic cell necrosis or both. Hepatotoxicity has been observed in man following long-term oral dosing and has been observed, in a limited experience (0.2%), following intravenous administration of amrinone.

Hypersensitivity: There have been reports of several apparent hypersensitivity reactions in patients treated with oral amrinone for about two weeks. Signs and symptoms were variable but included pericarditis, pleuritis and ascites (1 case), myositis with interstitial shadowing on chest x-ray and elevated sedimentation rate (1 case) and vasculitis with nodular pulmonary densities, hypoxemia, and jaundice (1 case). The first patient died, not necessarily of the possible reaction, while the last two resolved with discontinuation of therapy. None of the cases were rechallenged so that attribution to amrinone is not certain, but possible hypersensitivity reactions should be considered in any patient maintained for a prolonged period on amrinone.

General: Additional adverse reactions observed in intravenous amrinone clinical studies include fever (0.9%), chest pain (0.2%), and burning at the site of injection (0.2%).

Management of Adverse Reactions

Platelet Count Reductions: Asymptomatic platelet count reduction (to < 150,000/mm³) may be reversed within one week of a decrease in drug dosage. Further, with no change in drug dosage, the count may stabilize at lower than pre-drug levels without any clinical sequelae. Pre-drug platelet counts and frequent platelet counts during therapy are recommended to assist in decisions regarding dosage modifications.

Should a platelet count less than 150,000/mm³ occur, the following actions may be considered:
- Maintain total daily dose unchanged, since in some cases counts have either stabilized or returned to pretreatment levels.
- Decrease total daily dose.
- Discontinue amrinone if, in the clinical judgment of the physician, risk exceeds the potential benefit.

Gastrointestinal Side Effects: While gastrointestinal side effects were seen infrequently with intravenous therapy, should severe or debilitating ones occur, the physician may wish to reduce dosage or discontinue the drug based on the usual benefit-to-risk considerations.

Hepatic Toxicity: In clinical experience to date with intravenous administration, hepatotoxicity has been observed rarely. If acute marked alterations in liver enzymes occur together with clinical symptoms suggesting an idiosyncratic hypersensitivity reaction, amrinone therapy should be promptly discontinued.

If less than marked enzyme alterations occur without clinical symptoms, these nonspecific changes should be evaluated on an individual basis. The clinician may wish to continue amrinone, reduce dosage, or discontinue the drug based on the usual benefit/risk considerations.

Overdosage: Doses of INOCOR lactate injection may produce hypotension because of its vasodilator effect. If this occurs, amrinone administration should be reduced or discontinued. No specific antidote is known, but general measures for circulatory support should be taken.

In rats, the LD_{50} of amrinone, as the lactate salt, was 102 mg/kg or 130 mg/kg intravenously in two different studies and 132 mg/kg orally (intragastrically); as a suspension in aqueous gum tragacanth the oral LD_{50} was 239 mg/kg.

Dosage and Administration: INOCOR lactate injection may be administered as supplied or diluted in normal, or half normal saline solution to a concentration of 1 mg/mL to 3 mg/mL. Diluted solutions should be used within 24 hours.

INOCOR lactate injection, brand of amrinone lactate, may be injected into running dextrose (glucose) infusions through a Y-Connector or directly into the tubing where preferable.

A chemical interaction occurs slowly over a 24-hour period when the intravenous solution of INOCOR lactate injection is mixed directly with dextrose (glucose)-containing solutions. THEREFORE, INOCOR LACTATE INJECTION SHOULD NOT BE DILUTED WITH SOLUTIONS THAT CON-

for possible revisions

TAIN DEXTROSE (GLUCOSE) PRIOR TO INJECTION.
The following procedure is recommended for the administration of INOCOR lactate injection:
1. Initiate therapy with a 0.75 mg/kg bolus given slowly over 2 to 3 minutes.
2. Continue therapy with a maintenance infusion between 5 µg/kg/min and 10 µg/kg/min.
3. Based on clinical response, an additional bolus injection of 0.75 mg/kg may be given 30 minutes after the initiation of therapy.
4. The rate of infusion usually ranges from 5 µg/kg/min to 10 µg/kg/min such that the recommended total daily dose (including boluses) does not exceed 10 mg/kg. A limited number of patients studied at higher doses support a dosage regimen up to 18 mg/kg/day for shortened durations of therapy.
5. The rate of administration and the duration of therapy should be adjusted according to the response of the patient. The physician may wish to reduce or titrate the infusion downward based on clinical responsiveness or untoward effects.

The above dosing regimens can be expected to place most patient's plasma concentration of amrinone at approximately 3 µg/mL. Increases in cardiac index show a linear relationship to plasma concentration of a range of 0.5 µg/mL to 7 µg/mL. No observations have been made at greater plasma concentrations.

Patient improvement may be reflected by increases in cardiac output, reduction in pulmonary capillary wedge pressure, and such clinical responses as a lessening of dyspnea and an improvement in other symptoms of heart failure, such as orthopnea and fatigue.

Monitoring central venous pressure (CVP) may be valuable in the assessment of hypotension and fluid balance management. Prior correction or adjustment of fluid/electrolytes is essential to obtain satisfactory response with amrinone.

Parenteral drug products should be inspected visually and should not be used if particulate matter or discoloration is observed.

How Supplied: Ampuls of 20 mL sterile, clear yellow solution containing INOCOR 5 mg/mL, box of 5 (NDC 0024-0888-20). Each 1 mL contains INOCOR lactate equivalent to 5 mg base and 0.25 mg sodium metabisulfite in Water for Injection. The pH of INOCOR lactate injection, brand of amrinone lactate, is adjusted to a range of 3.2 to 4.0 with lactic acid or sodium hydroxide.
Protect INOCOR lactate ampuls from light. Ampul packaging is light resistant for protection during storage.
Store at room temperature.
NOTE: Parenteral drug products should be inspected visually and should not be used if particulate matter or discoloration is observed.

NORPACE, trademark, G. D. Searle & Co.
IW-161 B
FOR INOCOR MEDICAL INFORMATION CALL TOLL FREE 1-800-4-INOCOR

ISUPREL® Hydrochloride ℞
brand of isoproterenol hydrochloride injection, USP
Sterile Injection 1:5000
Description: ISUPREL hydrochloride, brand of isoproterenol hydrochloride, is 3,4-dihydroxy-α-[(isopropylamino) methyl] benzyl alcohol hydrochloride, a synthetic sympathomimetic amine that is structurally related to epinephrine but acts almost exclusively on beta receptors.
Each milliliter of the sterile 1:5000 solution contains 0.2 mg ISUPREL hydrochloride, brand of isoproterenol hydrochloride, 0.12 mg lactic acid, 1.8 mg sodium lactate, 7 mg sodium chloride, and not more than 1 mg sodium bisulfite as preservative. The pH is adjusted with hydrochloric acid. The air in the ampuls has been displaced by nitrogen gas.

Action: The primary actions of ISUPREL are on the heart and on smooth muscle of bronchi, skeletal muscle vasculature, and alimentary tract. The positive inotropic and chronotropic actions of the drug increase cardiac output. There is also an increase in venous return to the heart. With usual therapeutic doses, the increase in cardiac output is generally sufficient to maintain or increase systolic blood pressure. ISUPREL also lowers peripheral vascular resistance; the diastolic pressure, therefore, may be expected to fall in normal individuals. Thus, the mean pressure may be reduced. The rate of discharge of cardiac pacemakers is increased with isoproterenol.
ISUPREL relaxes most smooth muscle, the most pronounced effect being on bronchial and gastrointestinal smooth muscle. It produces marked relaxation in the smaller bronchi and may even dilate the trachea and main bronchi past the resting diameter.
The acute toxicity of ISUPREL in animals is much less than that of epinephrine. Excessive doses in animals or man can cause a striking drop in blood pressure, and repeated large doses in animals may result in cardiac enlargement and focal myocarditis.
Indications: Parenteral isoproterenol hydrochloride is indicated as an adjunct in the management of shock (hypoperfusion syndrome) and in the treatment of cardiac standstill or arrest; carotid sinus hypersensitivity; Adams-Stokes syndrome; and ventricular tachycardia and ventricular arrhythmias that require increased inotropic cardiac activity for therapy. It may also be used in the management of bronchospasm during anesthesia.

SHOCK (HYPOPERFUSION SYNDROME)

Shock is a complex clinical syndrome characterized by inadequate tissue perfusion, which results from one or more of the following mechanisms: loss of effective blood volume, cardiac failure, peripheral vascular failure. Rational therapy must be aimed at correcting this perfusion deficit.
Since shock is often, but by no means always, associated with lowered blood pressure, administration of vasoactive drugs that increase blood pressure without increasing blood flow may not be in the best interests of the patient. However, in cases of shock characterized chiefly by peripheral vasodilatation and in shock following acute myocardial infarction, according to one group of investigators, a vasopressor such as norepinephrine bitartrate injection, USP, may be indicated.[1,2]
In addition to the routine monitoring of systemic blood pressure, heart rate, urine flow, and the use of the electrocardiogram, the shock state and the response to therapy should be monitored by frequent determinations of the central venous pressure, blood pH, and blood pCO_2 (or bicarbonate). Determinations of cardiac output and circulation time may also be helpful.
Adequate filling of the intravascular compartment by suitable volume expanders is of primary importance in most cases of shock, and should precede the administration of vasoactive drugs. Determination of central venous pressure is a reliable guide during volume replacement. If evidence of hypoperfusion persists after adequate volume replacement, ISUPREL may be given.
ISUPREL increases cardiac output by increasing the strength of cardiac contraction and, to a limited extent, the rate of contraction. ISUPREL also increases venous return to the heart by mobilizing blood from vascular reservoirs.[3] In addition, the peripheral and coronary vasodilating effects of the drug may aid tissue perfusion. ISUPREL may be given to patients who are fully digitalized;[4,5] in fact, ISUPREL may be particularly useful when cardiac competence cannot be restored by digitalization.
Appropriate measures should be taken to ensure adequate ventilation. Careful attention should be paid to acid-base balance and to the correction of electrolyte disturbance. In cases of shock associated with bacteremia, suitable antimicrobial therapy is, of course, imperative.
In a group of 10 patients with elevated central venous pressures who were in shock from cardiac failure, isoproterenol produced increases in cardiac output of 0.33 to 4.34 liters per minute in nine of the ten.[6] Similarly, in a series of 12 patients with shock due to gram-negative bacteremia, Kardos[7] found isoproterenol to be useful in correcting the hemodynamic alterations.
Although the ultimate effect of ISUPREL on patient survival has not yet been documented, experimental studies in rats have shown that the fatal course of shock caused by transient hemorrhage was reversed by treatment with isoproterenol after replacement of blood volume.[3] In addition, clinical studies[5-15] have indicated that in a majority of patients in shock, administration of ISUPREL tends to correct the hemodynamic abnormalities.
Contraindication: Administration of ISUPREL is contraindicated in patients with tachycardia caused by digitalis intoxication.
Warning: Isoproterenol infusions may produce an increase in myocardial work and oxygen consumption. These effects may be detrimental to myocardial metabolism and functioning in patients who are in cardiogenic shock secondary to coronary artery occlusion and myocardial infarction.
Precautions: ISUPREL and epinephrine should not be administered simultaneously, since both drugs are direct cardiac stimulants and their combined effects may induce serious arrhythmia. The drugs may, however, be administered alternately provided a proper interval has elapsed between doses.
Dosage of ISUPREL should be carefully adjusted particularly in patients with coronary insufficiency, diabetes, or hyperthyroidism, and in patients sensitive to sympathomimetic amines.
Hypovolemia should be corrected by suitable volume expanders before treatment with ISUPREL. Patients in shock should be closely observed during isoproterenol administration. If the heart rate exceeds 110 beats per minute, it may be advisable to decrease the infusion rate or temporarily discontinue the infusion. Doses of ISUPREL sufficient to increase the heart rate to more than 130 beats per minute may induce ventricular arrhythmia.
There has been no clinical evidence of teratogenic effects attributable to ISUPREL in more than 20 years' use of the drug. However, before administration of any drug to pregnant women or women of childbearing potential, the expected benefit of the drug should be carefully weighed against the possible risk to the mother or child.
Dosage and Administration: ISUPREL hydrochloride Solution 1:5000 should be diluted in 5 percent Dextrose Injection, USP, before it is administered to patients in shock.
- A convenient dilution is 1 mg ISUPREL (5 mL) in 500 mL diluent (final concentration, 1:500,000).
- Concentrations up to 10 times greater have been used.[6] This may be important in patients in whom limitation of volume is essential.
- Infusion rates of 0.5 µg to 5 µg per minute (0.25 mL to 2.5 mL diluted solution 1:500,000) have been recommended.
- Rates over 30 µg per minute have been used in advanced stages of shock.

The speed of infusion should be adjusted on the basis of heart rate, central venous pressure, sys-

Continued on next page

This product information was effective as of December 3, 1984. On these and other products of Winthrop-Breon Laboratories, detailed information may be obtained on a current basis by direct inquiry to the Professional Services Department, 90 Park Avenue, New York, NY 10016 (212) 907-2525.

Winthrop-Breon—Cont.

temic blood pressure, and urine flow. If the heart rate exceeds 110 beats per minute, it may be advisable to decrease the infusion rate or temporarily discontinue the infusion.

CARDIAC STANDSTILL AND CARDIAC ARRHYTHMIAS

Because it has potent inotropic cardiac stimulant action with little or no pressor activity, ISUPREL hydrochloride, brand of isoproterenol hydrochloride, has been effective for the treatment of the following:
1. Adams-Stokes syndrome—atrioventricular heart block
2. Cardiac standstill (arrest)
3. Carotid sinus hypersensitivity
4. Ventricular arrhythmias, especially certain types of ventricular tachycardia and fibrillation occurring during the course of atrioventricular block.

It should be noted that in symptomatic heart block, electrical pacing is the preferred method of treatment for maintenance of an adequate ventricular rate. Moreover, in ventricular arrhythmias, especially certain types of ventricular tachycardia and fibrillation, electroshock may have to be used, and is usually the treatment of choice.

If, however, therapy with ISUPREL is elected in these conditions, intravenous administration, with constant monitoring, is preferred.

In patients with heart block and episodic ventricular tachycardia or fibrillation, ISUPREL stimulates the higher centers or nodal tissue without exciting the lower ventricular foci. In so doing, the normal idioventricular pacemaker function may take over, thereby abolishing ventricular acceleration. Epinephrine is contraindicated in patients with ventricular fibrillation because it may precipitate or prolong fibrillation by stimulation of multiple higher and lower foci. It also may further embarrass the cardiovascular system by its hypertensive action.

Intravenous administration of ISUPREL has been recommended for the management of patients with complete heart block following closure of ventricular septal defects. A 1:50,000 solution may be administered intravenously in doses ranging from 0.5 mL to 1.5 mL for infants and from 2 mL to 3 mL for adults. With such doses the heart rate accelerates and the effect often lasts for 15 or 20 minutes. Sinus rhythm sometimes occurs and persists for a variable period but often relapses again into complete block. In other cases, ISUPREL merely maintains an acceptable heart rate somewhere above 90 to 100 beats per minute. The patient must be monitored constantly by electrocardiography.

Contraindications: Use of isoproterenol in patients with preexisting cardiac arrhythmias associated with tachycardia is generally considered contraindicated because the chronotropic effect of the drug on the heart may aggravate such disorders. Exceptions consist only of those ventricular tachycardias and ventricular arrhythmias which require increased inotropic cardiac activity for therapy.

Administration of ISUPREL is contraindicated in patients with tachycardia caused by digitalis intoxication.

Precautions: ISUPREL and epinephrine should not be administered simultaneously, since both drugs are direct cardiac stimulants and their combined effects may induce serious arrhythmia. The drugs may, however, be administered alternately provided a proper interval has elapsed between doses.

Dosage of ISUPREL should be carefully adjusted in patients with coronary insufficiency, diabetes, or hyperthyroidism, and in patients sensitive to sympathomimetic amines.

If the cardiac rate increases sharply, patients with angina pectoris may experience anginal pain until the cardiac rate decreases.

There has been no clinical evidence of teratogenic effects attributable to ISUPREL in more than 20 years' use of the drug. However, before administration of any drug to pregnant women or women of childbearing potential, the expected benefit of the drug should be carefully weighed against the possible risk to the mother or child.

Adverse Reactions: Serious reactions to ISUPREL are infrequent. The following reactions, however, have been reported: flushing of the face, sweating, mild tremors, nervousness, headache, and tachycardia with palpitation manifested as a sensation of pounding in the chest. These reactions disappear quickly and usually do not require discontinuation of treatment with ISUPREL. No cumulative effects have been reported. Pulmonary edema has been reported in a patient extremely intolerant to all sympathomimetic drugs.[16]

In a few patients, presumably with organic disease of the A-V node and its branches, ISUPREL has been reported, paradoxically, to precipitate Adams-Stokes seizures during normal sinus rhythm or transient heart block.[16]

Dosage and Administration: In the treatment and prevention of cardiac standstill and cardiac arrhythmias, parenteral ISUPREL may be administered by intravenous injection, infusion, intramuscular and subcutaneous injection, and *in extremis*, by intracardiac injection.

The following table summarizes the dosage regimen suggested for various routes of administration in adults. Children may be given half the initial adult dose. In all patients, subsequent dosage and method of administration depend on the response of the ventricular rate and the rapidity with which the cardiac pacemaker can take over when the drug is gradually withdrawn.

The usual route of administration in emergency treatment of patients threatened with cardiac standstill or arrhythmia is by intravenous injection or infusion. Dosage must be regulated by monitoring of the electrocardiogram. If time is not of utmost importance, initial therapy by intramuscular or subcutaneous injection is preferred.
[See table below].

BRONCHOSPASM DURING ANESTHESIA

Parenteral ISUPREL hydrochloride, brand of isoproterenol hydrochloride, has been shown under experimental and clinical conditions to be a potent bronchodilating agent. However, when given in dosages to achieve this effect, it may also have a stimulating effect on the cardiovascular system. Like epinephrine, it may produce arrhythmias in patients anesthetized with cyclopropane, and should be used with caution. ISUPREL can be used for the management of bronchospasm by helping the patient to maintain adequate ventilation and a normally functioning circulatory system.

Precautions and Adverse Reactions: See corresponding sections under "Cardiac Standstill and Cardiac Arrhythmias."

Dosage and Administration: For the management of bronchospasm during anesthesia, 1 mL of ISUPREL Solution 1:5000 is diluted to 10 mL with Sodium Chloride Injection, USP, or 5 percent Dextrose Injection, USP. An initial dose of 0.01 mg to 0.02 mg (0.5 mL to 1 mL of the diluted solution, 1:50,000) is administered intravenously, and may be repeated when necessary.

How Supplied:
Ampuls of 1 mL (0.2 mg)
UNI-NEST™ PAK of 25   NDC-0024-0866-25
Ampuls of 5 mL (1 mg) box of 10
NDC-0024-0866-02

Keep in a cool place. Protect from light—keep in opaque container until used.

Bibliography:
1. Gunnar, R.M., Loeb, H.S., Pietras, R.J., and Tobin, J.R., Jr.: *J.A.M.A. 202*:1124, Dec. 25, 1967.
2. Loeb, H.S., Pietras, R.J., Tobin, J.R., Jr., and Gunnar, R. M.: *Clin. Res. 15*:213, April 1967.
3. Weil, M. H. and Bradley, E.C.: *Bull. N.Y. Acad. Med. 42*:1023, Nov. 1966.
4. Cohn, J. N.: *GP 34*:78, Aug. 1966.
5. du Toit, H. J., du Plessis, J. M. E., Dommisse, J., Rorke, M. J., Theron, M. S., and de Villiers, V. P.: *Lancet 2*:143, July 16, 1966.
6. MacLean, L. D., Duff, J. H., Scott, H. M., and Peretz, D. I.: *Surg. Gynec. Obstet. 120*:1, Jan. 1965.
7. Kardos, G. G.: *New Eng. J. Med. 274*:868, April 21, 1966.
8. Duff, J. H., Scott, H. M., Peretz, D. I., Mulligan, G. W., and MacLean, L. D.: *J. Trauma 6*:145, March 1966.
9. Duff, J. H., McLean, A. P. H., Mulligan, G. W., and MacLean, L. D.: *Acad. Med. New Jersey Bull. 12*:193, Sept. 1966.
10. Duff, J. H., Peretz, D. I., Scott, H. M., Wigmore, R. A., and MacLean, L. D.: *J. Okla. Med. Ass. 59*:437, Aug. 1966.
11. Brown, R. S., Carey, J. S., Mohr, Patricia A., Monson, D. O., and Shoemaker, W. C.: *Circulation 34*:260, Aug. 1966.
12. Brown, R. S., Carey, J. S., Woodward, N. W., Mohr, Patricia A., and Shoemaker, W. C.: *Surg. Gynec. Obstet. 122*:303, Feb. 1966.
13. Wilson, J. N.: *Arch. Surg. 91*:92, July 1965.
14. Loeb, H. S., Stavrakos, C., Pietras, R. J., Tobin, J. R., Jr., and Gunnar, R. M.: *Circulation 34*:III, Oct., Suppl. 3, 1966. (abstr.)
15. Torpey, D. J.: *J.A.M.A. 202*:955, Dec. 4, 1967.
16. Schwartz, S. P. and Schwartz, L. S.: *Amer. Heart J. 57*:849, June 1959.

IW-33-R

Dosage of ISUPREL for Cardiac Standstill and Cardiac Arrhythmias in Adults

Route of Administration	Preparation of Dilution	Initial Dose	Subsequent Dose Range
Intravenous	Dilute 1 mL of Solution 1:5000 (0.2 mg) to 10 mL with Sodium Chloride Injection, USP, or 5% Dextrose Injection, USP.	0.02 to 0.06 mg (1 to 3 mL of diluted solution 1:50,000)	0.01 to 0.2 mg (0.5 to 10 mL of diluted solution)
Intravenous infusion	Dilute 10 mL of Solution 1:5000 (2 mg) in 500 mL of 5% Dextrose Injection, USP.	5 µg/min (1.25 mL of diluted solution 1:250,000 per minute)	
Intramuscular	Use Solution 1:5000 undiluted	0.2 mg (1 mL)	0.02 to 1 mg (0.1 to 5 mL)
Subcutaneous	Use Solution 1:5000 undiluted	0.2 mg (1 mL)	0.15 to 0.2 mg (0.75 to 1 mL)
Intracardiac	Use Solution 1:5000 undiluted	0.02 mg (0.1 mL)	

ISUPREL® Hydrochloride ℞
brand of isoproterenol hydrochloride, USP
MISTOMETER®

Potent Bronchodilator

Description: ISUPREL MISTOMETER is a complete nebulizing unit consisting of a plastic-coated vial of aerosol solution, detachable plastic mouthpiece with built-in nebulizer, and protective cap. The vial contains isoproterenol hydrochloride in inert propellants (dichlorodifluoromethane and dichlorotetrafluoroethane) with alcohol 33 percent (w/w) and ascorbic acid. The contents permit the delivery of not less than 200 actuations from the 11.2 g (10 mL) vial, not less than 300 actuations from the 16.8 g (15 mL) vial, or not less than 450 actuations from the 25.2 g (22.5 mL) vial. The MISTOMETER unit delivers a measured dose of 131 µg of the bronchodilator in a fine, even mist for inhalation.

Action: ISUPREL relaxes bronchial spasm and facilitates expectoration of pulmonary secretions. It is frequently effective when epinephrine and other drugs fail, and it has a wide margin of safety. In dogs the toxic dose is 1000 times the therapeutic dose. Converted to the amount used clinically in man, this would be about 2500 times the therapeutic dose.

Indications: ISUPREL is indicated for the treatment of bronchospasm associated with acute and chronic bronchial asthma, pulmonary emphysema, bronchitis, and bronchiectasis.

Contraindication: Use of isoproterenol in patients with preexisting cardiac arrhythmias associated with tachycardia is generally considered contraindicated because the cardiac stimulant effect of the drug may aggravate such disorders.

Warnings: Excessive use of an adrenergic aerosol should be discouraged as it may lose its effectiveness.

In patients with status asthmaticus and abnormal blood gas tensions, improvement in vital capacity and in blood gas tensions may not accompany apparent relief of bronchospasm. Facilities for administering oxygen mixtures and ventilatory assistance are necessary for such patients.

Occasional patients have been reported to develop severe paradoxical airway resistance with repeated, excessive use of isoproterenol inhalation preparations. The cause of this refractory state is unknown. It is advisable that in such instances the use of this preparation be discontinued immediately and alternative therapy instituted, since in the reported cases the patients did not respond to other forms of therapy until the drug was withdrawn.

Deaths have been reported following excessive use of isoproterenol inhalation preparations and the exact cause is unknown. Cardiac arrest was noted in several instances.

Precautions: Epinephrine should not be administered concomitantly with ISUPREL, as both drugs are direct cardiac stimulants and their combined effects may induce serious arrhythmia. If desired they may, however, be alternated, provided an interval of at least four hours has elapsed. Isoproterenol should be used with caution in patients with cardiovascular disorders including coronary insufficiency, diabetes, or hyperthyroidism, and in persons sensitive to sympathomimetic amines.

A single treatment with the ISUPREL MISTOMETER unit is usually sufficient for controlling isolated attacks of asthma. Any patient who requires more than three aerosol treatments within a 24-hour period should be under the close supervision of a physician. Further therapy with the bronchodilator aerosol alone is inadvisable when three to five treatments within six to twelve hours produce minimal or no relief.

During the course of over 30 years of use of ISUPREL (isoproterenol), there has been no clinical evidence of teratogenic effects. However, use of any drug in pregnancy, lactation, or in women of childbearing age requires that the potential benefit of the drug be weighed against its possible hazards to the mother or child.

Adverse Reactions: The mist from the ISUPREL MISTOMETER unit contains alcohol but is generally very well tolerated. An occasional patient may experience some transient throat irritation which has been attributed to the alcohol content.

Tachycardia, palpitation, nervousness, nausea, and vomiting may occur from overdosage. Rarely do headache, flushing of the skin, tremor, dizziness, weakness, sweating, precordial distress, or anginal-type pain occur. The inhalation route is usually accompanied by a minimum of side effects. These untoward reactions disappear quickly and do not, as a rule, inconvenience the patient to the extent that the drug must be discontinued. No cumulative effects have been reported.

Dosage and Administration:
Acute Bronchial Asthma: Hold the MISTOMETER unit in an inverted position. Close lips and teeth around open end of mouthpiece. Breathe out, expelling as much air from the lungs as possible; then inhale deeply while pressing down on the bottle to activate spray mechanism. Try to hold breath for a few seconds before exhaling. Wait one full minute in order to determine the effect before considering a second inhalation. A treatment may be repeated up to 5 times daily if necessary. (See Precautions.) If carefully instructed, children quickly learn to keep the stream of mist clear of the teeth and tongue, thereby assuring inhalation into the lungs. Occlusion of the nares of very young children may be advisable to make inhalation certain.

Warm water should be run through the mouthpiece once daily to wash it and prevent clogging. The mouthpiece may also be sanitized by immersion in alcohol.

Bronchospasm in Chronic Obstructive Lung Disease: The MISTOMETER unit provides a convenient aerosol method for delivering ISUPREL (isoproterenol). The treatment described for Acute Bronchial Asthma may be repeated at not less than 3 to 4 hour intervals as part of a programmed regimen of treatment of obstructive lung disease complicated by a reversible bronchospastic component. One application from the MISTOMETER unit may be regarded as equivalent in effectiveness to 5 to 7 operations of a hand-bulb nebulizer using a 1:100 solution.

Children's Dosage. In general, the technique of ISUPREL MISTOMETER administration to children is similar to that of adults, since children's smaller ventilatory exchange capacity automatically provides proportionally smaller aerosol intake.

How Supplied:
Vial of 11.2 g (10 mL) with oral nebulizer (NDC 0024-0878-05)
Vial of 16.8 g (15 mL) with oral nebulizer (NDC 0024-0878-01)
Refill only, 16.8 g (15 mL) (NDC 0024-0879-01)
Vial of 25.2 g (22.5 mL) with oral nebulizer (NDC 0024-0878-02)
Refill only, 25.2 g (22.5 mL) (NDC 0024-0879-02)

IW-67-X

ISUPREL® Hydrochloride ℞
brand of isoproterenol hydrochloride
inhalation, USP
SOLUTION 1:200
SOLUTION 1:100

Potent Bronchodilator

Description: ISUPREL hydrochloride, brand of isoproterenol hydrochloride, is available as:
Solution 1:200 in a buffered aqueous vehicle containing sodium chloride, citric acid, and glycerin with chlorobutanol 0.5 percent and sodium bisulfite 0.3 percent as preservatives.
Solution 1:100 in a buffered aqueous vehicle containing sodium chloride, sodium citrate, citric acid, and saccharin with chlorobutanol 0.5 percent and sodium bisulfite 0.3 per cent as preservatives.
The air in the bottles has been displaced by nitrogen gas.

Do not use the solutions if a precipitate or discoloration is observed. Although solutions of ISUPREL left in nebulizers will remain clear and potent for many days, for sanitary reasons it is recommended that they be changed daily.

Action: ISUPREL relaxes bronchial spasm and facilitates expectoration of pulmonary secretions. It is frequently effective when epinephrine and other drugs fail, and it has a wide margin of safety. In dogs the toxic dose is 1000 times the therapeutic dose. Converted to the amount used clinically in man, this would be about 2500 times the therapeutic dose.

Indications: ISUPREL is indicated for the treatment of bronchospasm associated with acute and chronic bronchial asthma, pulmonary emphysema, bronchitis, and bronchiectasis.

Contraindication: Use of isoproterenol in patients with preexisting cardiac arrhythmias associated with tachycardia is generally considered contraindicated because the cardiac stimulant effect of the drug may aggravate such disorders.

Warnings: Excessive use of an adrenergic aerosol should be discouraged as it may lose its effectiveness.

In patients with status asthmaticus and abnormal blood gas tensions, improvement in vital capacity and in blood gas tensions may not accompany apparent relief of bronchospasm. Facilities for administering oxygen mixtures and ventilatory assistance are necessary for such patients.

Occasional patients have been reported to develop severe paradoxical airway resistance with repeated, excessive use of isoproterenol inhalation preparations. The cause of this refractory state is unknown. It is advisable that in such instances the use of this preparation be discontinued immediately and alternative therapy instituted, since in the reported cases the patients did not respond to other forms of therapy until the drug was withdrawn.

Deaths have been reported following excessive use of isoproterenol inhalation preparations and the exact cause is unknown. Cardiac arrest was noted in several instances.

Precautions: Epinephrine should not be administered concomitantly with ISUPREL, as both drugs are direct cardiac stimulants and their combined effects may induce serious arrhythmia. If desired they may, however, be alternated, provided an interval of at least four hours has elapsed.

Isoproterenol should be used with caution in patients with cardiovascular disorders including coronary insufficiency, diabetes, or hyperthyroidism, and in persons sensitive to sympathomimetic amines.

Any patient who requires more than three aerosol treatments within a 24-hour period should be under the close supervision of his physician. Further therapy with the bronchodilator aerosol alone is inadvisable when three to five treatments within six to twelve hours produce minimal or no relief. During the course of over 25 years of use of ISUPREL (isoproterenol) there has been no clinical evidence of teratogenic effects. However, use of any drug in pregnancy, lactation, or in women of childbearing age requires that the potential benefit of the drug be weighed against its possible hazards to the mother or child.

When compressed oxygen is employed as the aerosol propellant, the percentage of oxygen used should be determined by the patient's individual requirements to avoid depression of respiratory drive.

Continued on next page

This product information was effective as of December 3, 1984. On these and other products of Winthrop-Breon Laboratories, detailed information may be obtained on a current basis by direct inquiry to the Professional Services Department, 90 Park Avenue, New York, NY 10016 (212) 907-2525.

Winthrop-Breon—Cont.

Adverse Reactions: Tachycardia, palpitation, nervousness, nausea, and vomiting may occur from overdosage. Rarely do headache, flushing of the skin, tremor, dizziness, weakness, sweating, precordial distress, or anginal-type pain occur. The inhalation route is usually accompanied by a minimum of side effects. These untoward reactions disappear quickly and do not, as a rule, inconvenience the patient to the extent that the drug must be discontinued. No cumulative effects have been reported.

Dosage and Administration: ISUPREL hydrochloride solutions can be administered as an aerosol mist by hand-bulb nebulizer, compressed air or oxygen operated nebulizer, or by intermittent positive pressure breathing (IPPB) devices. The method of delivery, and the treatment regimen employed in the management of the reversible bronchospastic element accompanying bronchial asthma, chronic bronchitis, and chronic obstructive lung diseases, will depend on such factors as the severity of the bronchospasm, patient age, tolerance to the medication, complicating cardiopulmonary conditions, and whether therapy is for an intermittent acute attack of bronchospasm or is part of a programmed treatment regimen for constant bronchospasm.

Acute Bronchial Asthma. *Hand-Bulb Nebulizer*—Depending on the frequency of treatment and the type of nebulizer used, a volume of solution of ISUPREL, sufficient for not more than one day's treatment, should be placed in the nebulizer using the dropper provided. In time, the patient can learn to adjust the volume required. For adults and children, the 1:200 solution is administered by hand-bulb nebulization in a dosage of 5 to 15 deep inhalations (using an all glass or plastic nebulizer). In adults, the 1:100 solution may be used if a stronger solution seems to be indicated. The dose is 3 to 7 deep inhalations. If after about 5 to 10 minutes inadequate relief is observed, these doses may be repeated one more time. If the acute attack recurs, treatments may be repeated up to 5 times daily if necessary. (See Precautions.)

Bronchospasm in Chronic Obstructive Lung Disease. *Hand-Bulb Nebulizer*—ISUPREL 1:200 or 1:100 solution may be administered daily at not less than 3 to 4 hour intervals for subacute bronchospastic attacks or as part of a programmed treatment regimen in patients with chronic obstructive lung disease with a reversible bronchospastic component. An adequate dose is usually 5 to 15 deep inhalations, using the 1:200 solution. Some patients with severe attacks of bronchospasm may require 3 to 7 deep inhalations using the ISUPREL 1:100 solution.
Nebulization by Compressed Air or Oxygen—A method often used in patients with severe chronic obstructive lung disease is to deliver the ISUPREL (isoproterenol) mist *in more dilute form over a longer period of time*. The purpose is, not so much to increase the dose supplied, as to achieve progressively deeper bronchodilatation and thus insure that the mist achieves maximum penetration of the finer bronchioles. In this method, 0.5 mL of an ISUPREL 1:200 solution is diluted to 2 mL to 2.5 mL with water or isotonic saline to achieve a use concentration of 1:800 to 1:1000. If desired, 0.25 mL of the 1:100 solution may be similarly diluted to achieve the same use concentration. The diluted solution is placed in a nebulizer (eg, DeVilbiss #640 unit) connected to either a source of compressed air or oxygen. The flow rate is regulated to suit the particular nebulizer so that the diluted solution of ISUPREL will be delivered over approximately 10 to 20 minutes. A treatment may be repeated up to 5 times daily if necessary. Although the total delivered dose of ISUPREL is somewhat higher than with the treatment regimen employing the hand-bulb nebulizer, patients usually tolerate it well because of the greater dilution and longer application-time factors.

Intermittent Positive Pressure Breathing (IPPB)—Diluted solutions of ISUPREL 1:200 or 1:100 are used in a programmed regimen for the treatment of reversible bronchospasm in patients with chronic obstructive lung disease who require intermittent positive pressure breathing therapy. These devices generally have a small nebulizer, usually of 3 mL to 5 mL capacity, on a patient-operated side arm. The effectiveness of IPPB therapy is greatly enhanced by the simultaneous use of aerosolized bronchodilators. As with compressed air or oxygen operated nebulizers, the usual regimen is to place 0.5 mL of ISUPREL 1:200 solution diluted to 2 mL to 2.5 mL with water or isotonic saline in the nebulizer cup and follow the IPPB manufacturer's operating instructions. IPPB-bronchodilator treatments are usually administered over 15 to 20 minutes, up to 5 times daily if necessary.

Children's Dosage: In general, the technique of ISUPREL hydrochloride solution administration to children is similar to that of adults, since children's smaller ventilatory exchange capacity automatically provides proportionally smaller aerosol intake. However, it is generally recommended that the 1:200 solution (rather than the 1:100) be used for an acute attack of bronchospasm, and no more than 0.25 mL of the 1:200 solution should be used for each 10 to 15 minute programmed treatment in chronic bronchospastic disease.

How Supplied:
Solution 1:100
  bottle of 10 mL   (**NDC** 0024-0873-01)
Solution 1:200
  bottle of 10 mL   (**NDC** 0024 0871-01)
  bottle of 60 mL   (**NDC** 0024-0871-03)

IW-154-A

ISUPREL® Hydrochloride ℞
brand of isoproterenol hydrochloride tablets, USP
GLOSSETS®

Each tablet contains 10 mg or 15 mg isoproterenol hydrochloride in a rapidly disintegrating base consisting of starch, lactose, sodium saccharin, and talcum with sodium bisulfite 2 mg per tablet as antioxidant.

How Supplied:
ISUPREL GLOSSETS   10 mg, bottle of 50
(NDC 0024-0875-02)
ISUPREL GLOSSETS   15 mg, bottle of 50
(NDC 0024-0877-02)
Shown in Product Identification Section, page 443

IW-121-D

KAYEXALATE® ℞
brand of sodium polystyrene sulfonate, USP

Cation-Exchange Resin

Description: The drug is a light brown to brown, finely ground, powdered form of sodium polystyrene sulfonate, a cation-exchange resin prepared in the sodium phase with an *in vitro* exchange capacity of approximately 3.1 mEq (*in vivo* approximately 1 mEq) of potassium per gram. The sodium content is approximately 100 mg (4.1 mEq) per gram of the drug.

Action: As the resin passes along the intestine or is retained in the colon after administration by enema, the sodium ions are partially released and are replaced by potassium ions. For the most part, this action occurs in the large intestine, which excretes potassium ions to a greater degree than does the small intestine. The efficiency of this process is limited and unpredictably variable. It commonly approximates the order of 33 percent but the range is so large that definitive indices of electrolyte balance must be clearly monitored.

Indication: KAYEXALATE is indicated for the treatment of hyperkalemia.

Warnings: Since effective lowering of serum potassium with KAYEXALATE may take hours to days, treatment with this drug alone may be insufficient to rapidly correct severe hyperkalemia associated with states of rapid tissue breakdown (eg, burns and renal failure) or hyperkalemia so marked as to constitute a medical emergency. Therefore, other definitive measures, including dialysis, should always be considered and may be imperative.
Serious potassium deficiency can occur from KAYEXALATE therapy. The effect must be carefully controlled by frequent serum potassium determinations within each 24-hour period. Since intracellular potassium deficiency is not always reflected by serum potassium levels, the level at which treatment with KAYEXALATE should be discontinued must be determined individually for each patient. Important aids in making this determination are the patient's clinical condition and electrocardiogram. Early clinical signs of severe hypokalemia include a pattern of irritable confusion and delayed thought processes. Electrocardiographically, severe hypokalemia is often associated with a lengthened Q-T interval, widening, flattening, or inversion of the T wave, and prominent U waves. Also, cardiac arrhythmias may occur, such as premature atrial, nodal, and ventricular contractions, and supraventricular and ventricular tachycardias. The toxic effects of digitalis are likely to be exaggerated. Marked hypokalemia can also be manifested by severe muscle weakness, at times extending into frank paralysis. Like all cation-exchange resins, KAYEXALATE is not totally selective (for potassium) in its actions, and small amounts of other cations such as magnesium and calcium can also be lost during treatment. Accordingly, patients receiving KAYEXALATE should be monitored for all applicable electrolyte disturbances. Systemic alkalosis has been reported after cation-exchange resins were administered orally in combination with nonabsorbable cation-donating antacids and laxatives such as magnesium hydroxide and aluminum carbonate. Magnesium hydroxide should not be administered with KAYEXALATE. One case of grand mal seizure has been reported in a patient with chronic hypocalcemia of renal failure who was given KAYEXALATE with magnesium hydroxide as laxative. Also, the simultaneous oral administration of KAYEXALATE with nonabsorbable cation-donating antacids and laxatives may reduce the resin's potassium exchange capability.

Precautions: Caution is advised when KAYEXALATE is administered to patients who cannot tolerate even a small increase in sodium loads (ie, severe congestive heart failure, severe hypertension, or marked edema). In such instances compensatory restriction of sodium intake from other sources may be indicated.
If constipation occurs, patients should be treated with sorbitol (from 10 to 20 mL of 70 percent syrup every two hours or as needed to produce one or two watery stools daily), a measure which also reduces any tendency to fecal impaction.

Adverse Reactions: KAYEXALATE may cause some degree of gastric irritation. Anorexia, nausea, vomiting, and constipation may occur especially if high doses are given. Also, hypokalemia, hypocalcemia, and significant sodium retention may occur. Occasionally diarrhea develops. Large doses in elderly individuals may cause fecal impaction (see Precautions). This effect may be obviated through usage of the resin in enemas as described under Dosage and Administration. Intestinal obstruction due to concretions of aluminum hydroxide, when used in combination with KAYEXALATE, has been reported.

Dosage and Administration: Suspension of this drug should be freshly prepared and not stored beyond 24 hours.

The average daily adult dose of the resin is 15 g to 60 g. This is best provided by administering 15 g (approximately 4 *level* teaspoons) of KAYEXALATE, one to four times daily. One gram of KAYEXALATE contains 4.1 mEq of sodium; one level teaspoon contains approximately 3.5 g of KAYEXALATE and 15 mEq of sodium. (A heaping teaspoon may contain as much as 10 g to 12 g of KAYEXALATE, brand of sodium polystyrene sulfonate.) Since the *in vivo* efficiency of sodium-potassium exchange resins is approximately 33 percent, about one third of the resin's actual sodium content is being delivered to the body.

In smaller children and infants lower doses should be employed by using as a guide a rate of 1 mEq of potassium per gram of resin as the basis for calculation.

Each dose should be given as a suspension in a small quantity of water or, for greater palatability, in syrup. The amount of fluid usually ranges from 20 mL to 100 mL, depending on the dose, or may be simply determined by allowing 3 mL to 4 mL per gram of resin. Sorbitol may be administered in order to combat constipation.

The resin may be introduced into the stomach through a plastic tube and, if desired, mixed with a diet appropriate for a patient in renal failure.

The resin may also be given, although with less effective results, in an enema consisting (for adults) of 30 g to 50 g every six hours. Each dose is administered as a warm emulsion (at body temperature) in 100 mL of aqueous vehicle, such as sorbitol. The emulsion should be agitated gently during administration. The enema should be retained as long as possible and followed by a cleansing enema.

After an initial cleansing enema, a soft, large size (French 28) rubber tube is inserted into the rectum for a distance of about 20 cm, with the tip well into the sigmoid colon, and taped in place. The resin is then suspended in the appropriate amount of aqueous vehicle at body temperature and introduced by gravity, while the particles are kept in suspension by stirring. The suspension is flushed with 50 mL or 100 mL of fluid, following which the tube is clamped and left in place. If back leakage occurs, the hips are elevated on pillows or a knee-chest position is taken temporarily. A somewhat thicker suspension may be used, but care should be taken that no paste is formed, because the latter has a greatly reduced exchange surface and will be particularly ineffective if deposited in the rectal ampulla. The suspension is kept in the sigmoid colon for several hours, if possible. Then, the colon is irrigated with nonsodium containing solution at body temperature in order to remove the resin. Two quarts of flushing solution may be necessary. The returns are drained constantly through a Y tube connection.

The intensity and duration of therapy depend upon the severity and resistance of hyperkalemia. KAYEXALATE, brand of sodium polystyrene sulfonate, should not be heated for to do so may alter the exchange properties of the resin.

How Supplied: Jars of 1 pound (453.6 g)
NDC 0024-1075-01

KW 2-L

LEVOPHED® Bitartrate
brand of norepinephrine bitartrate injection, USP

R

Description: Levarterenol (sometimes referred to as *l-arterenolor* or as *l-norepinephrine*) is a primary amine which differs from epinephrine by the absence of a methyl group on the nitrogen atom. LEVOPHED is supplied in sterile aqueous solution in the form of the bitartrate. Each 1 mL of LEVOPHED solution contains 1 mg of LEVOPHED base, sodium chloride for isotonicity, and not more than 2 mg of sodium bisulfite as preservative. The air in the ampuls has been displaced by nitrogen gas.

Actions: LEVOPHED functions as a powerful peripheral vasoconstrictor (alpha-adrenergic action) and as a potent inotropic stimulator of the heart and dilator of coronary arteries (beta-adrenergic action). Both of these actions result in an increase in systemic blood pressure and coronary artery blood flow. Cardiac output will vary reflexly in response to systemic hypertension but is usually increased in hypotensive man when the blood pressure is raised to an optimal level. In myocardial infarction accompanied by hypotension, LEVOPHED usually increases aortic blood pressure, coronary artery blood flow, and myocardial oxygenation, thereby helping to limit the area of myocardial ischemia and infarction. Venous return is increased and the heart tends to resume a more normal rate and rhythm than in the hypotensive state.

In hypotension that persists after correction of blood volume deficits, LEVOPHED helps raise the blood pressure to an optimal level and establish a more adequate circulation.

Indications: For the restoration of blood pressure in controlling certain acute hypotensive states (eg, pheochromocytomectomy, sympathectomy, poliomyelitis, spinal anesthesia, myocardial infarction, septicemia, blood transfusion, and drug reactions).

As an adjunct in the treatment of cardiac arrest and profound hypotension.

Contraindications: LEVOPHED should not be given to patients who are hypotensive from blood volume deficits except as an emergency measure to maintain coronary and cerebral artery perfusion until blood volume replacement therapy can be completed. If LEVOPHED is continuously administered to maintain blood pressure in the absence of blood volume replacement, the following may occur: severe peripheral and visceral vasoconstriction, decreased renal perfusion and urine output, poor systemic blood flow despite "normal" blood pressure, tissue hypoxia, and lactate acidosis.

LEVOPHED should also not be given to patients with mesenteric or peripheral vascular thrombosis (because of the risk of increasing ischemia and extending the area of infarction) unless, in the opinion of the attending physician, the administration of LEVOPHED is necessary as a life-saving procedure.

Cyclopropane and halothane anesthetics increase cardiac autonomic irritability and therefore seem to sensitize the myocardium to the action of intravenously administered epinephrine or levarterenol. Hence, the use of LEVOPHED during cyclopropane and halothane anesthesia is generally considered contraindicated because of the risk of producing ventricular tachycardia or fibrillation. The same type of cardiac arrhythmias may result from the use of LEVOPHED in patients with profound hypoxia or hypercarbia.

Warning: LEVOPHED should be used with extreme caution in patients receiving monoamine oxidase (MAO) inhibitors or antidepressants of the triptyline or imipramine types, because severe, prolonged hypertension may result.

Precautions: Avoid Hypertension: Because of the potency of LEVOPHED and because of varying response to pressor substances, the possibility always exists that dangerously high blood pressure may be produced with overdoses of this pressor agent. It is desirable, therefore, to record the blood pressure every two minutes from the time administration is started until the desired blood pressure is obtained, then every five minutes if administration is to be continued. The rate of flow must be watched constantly, and the patient should never be left unattended while receiving LEVOPHED. Headache may be a symptom of hypertension due to overdosage.

Site of Infusion: Whenever possible, LEVOPHED should be given into a large vein, particularly an antecubital vein because, when administered into this vein, the risk of necrosis of the overlying skin from prolonged vasoconstriction is apparently very slight. Some authors have indicated that the femoral vein is also an acceptable route of administration. A catheter tie-in technique should be avoided, if possible, since the obstruction to blood flow around the tubing may cause stasis and increased local concentration of the drug. Occlusive vascular diseases (for example, atherosclerosis, arteriosclerosis, diabetic endarteritis, Buerger's disease) are more likely to occur in the lower than in the upper extremity. Therefore, one should avoid the veins of the leg in elderly patients or in those suffering from such disorders. Gangrene has been reported in a lower extremity when LEVOPHED was given in an ankle vein.

Extravasation: The infusion site should be checked frequently for free flow. Care should be taken to avoid extravasation of LEVOPHED (norepinephrine) into the tissues, as local necrosis might ensue due to the vasoconstrictive action of the drug. Blanching along the course of the infused vein, sometimes without obvious extravasation, has been attributed to vasa vasorum constriction with increased permeability of the vein wall, permitting some leakage. This also may progress on rare occasions to superficial slough, particularly during infusion into leg veins in elderly patients or in those suffering from obliterative vascular disease. Hence, if blanching occurs, consideration should be given to the advisability of changing the infusion site at intervals to allow the effects of local vasoconstriction to subside.

IMPORTANT—Antidote for Extravasation Ischemia: To prevent sloughing and necrosis in areas in which extravasation has taken place, the area should be infiltrated as soon as possible with 10 mL to 15 mL of saline solution containing from 5 mg to 10 mg of **Regitine®** (brand of phentolamine), an adrenergic blocking agent. A syringe with a fine hypodermic needle is used, and the solution is infiltrated liberally throughout the area, which is easily identified by its cold, hard, and pallid appearance. Sympathetic blockade with phentolamine causes immediate and conspicuous local hyperemic changes if the area is infiltrated within 12 hours. Therefore, phentolamine should be given as soon as possible after the extravasation is noted.

Some investigators[1] add phentolamine (5 mg to 10 mg) directly to the infusion flask because it is believed that the drug used in this manner is an effective antidote against sloughing should extravasation occur, whereas the systemic vasopressor activity of the LEVOPHED is not impaired.

Two investigators[2] stated that, in the treatment of patients with severe hypotension following *myocardial infarction*, thrombosis in the infused vein and perivenous reactions and necrosis may usually be prevented if 10 mg of heparin are added to each 500 mL of infusion fluid (5 percent dextrose) containing LEVOPHED.

Sympathetic nerve block has also been suggested.

Adverse Reactions: When used as directed, LEVOPHED is more certain in action and better tolerated systemically than other pressor amines. Its therapeutic index is four times that of epinephrine. Bradycardia sometimes occurs, probably as a reflex result of a rise in blood pressure. Headache may indicate overdosage and extreme hypertension.

Overdosage with LEVOPHED may also result in severe hypertension, reflex bradycardia, marked increase in peripheral resistance, and decreased cardiac output.

Prolonged administration of any potent vasopressor may result in plasma volume depletion which

Continued on next page

This product information was effective as of December 3, 1984. On these and other products of Winthrop-Breon Laboratories, detailed information may be obtained on a current basis by direct inquiry to the Professional Services Department, 90 Park Avenue, New York, NY 10016 (212) 907-2525.

Winthrop-Breon—Cont.

should be continuously corrected by appropriate fluid and electrolyte replacement therapy. If plasma volumes are not corrected, hypotension may recur when LEVOPHED is discontinued, or blood pressure may be maintained at the risk of severe peripheral vasoconstriction with diminution in blood flow and tissue perfusion.

Dosage and Administration:
Restoration of Blood Pressure in Acute Hypotensive States
Blood volume depletion should always be corrected as fully as possible before any vasopressor is administered. When, as an emergency measure, intraaortic pressures must be maintained to prevent cerebral or coronary artery ischemia, LEVOPHED bitartrate, brand of norepinephrine bitartrate injection, can be administered before and concurrently with blood volume replacement.
Diluent: Norepinephrine solution should be administered in 5 percent dextrose solution in distilled water or 5 percent dextrose in saline solution. These fluids containing dextrose are protection against significant loss of potency due to oxidation. Administration in saline solution alone is not recommended. Whole blood or plasma, if indicated to increase blood volume, should be administered separately (for example, by use of a Y-tube and individual flasks if given simultaneously).
Average Dosage: Add 4 mL of norepinephrine solution to 1000 mL of 5 percent dextrose solution. Each 1 mL of this dilution contains 4 μg of LEVOPHED base. Give this dilution intravenously. Insert a plastic intravenous catheter through a suitable bore needle well advanced centrally into the vein and securely fixed with adhesive tape, avoiding, if possible, a catheter tie-in technique as this promotes stasis. A drip bulb is necessary to permit an accurate estimation of the rate of flow in drops per minute. After observing the response to an initial dose of 2 mL to 3 mL (from 8 μg to 12 μg of base) per minute, adjust the rate of flow to establish and maintain a low normal blood pressure (usually 80 to 100 mm Hg systolic) sufficient to maintain the circulation to vital organs. In previously hypertensive patients, it is recommended that the blood pressure should be raised no higher than 40 mm Hg below the preexisting systolic pressure. The average maintenance dose ranges from 0.5 mL to 1 mL per minute (from 2 μg to 4 μg of base).
High Dosage: Great individual variation occurs in the dose required to attain and maintain an adequate blood pressure. In all cases, dosage of LEVOPHED should be titrated according to the response of the patient. Occasionally much larger or even enormous daily doses (as high as 68 mg base or 17 ampuls) may be necessary if the patient remains hypotensive, but occult blood volume depletion should always be suspected and corrected when present. Central venous pressure monitoring is usually helpful in detecting and treating this situation.
Fluid Intake: The degree of dilution depends on clinical fluid volume requirements. If large volumes of fluid (dextrose) are needed at a flow rate that would involve an excessive dose of the pressor agent per unit of time, a more dilute solution than 4 μg per mL should be used. On the other hand, when large volumes of fluid are clinically undesirable, a concentration greater than 4 μg per mL may be used.
Duration of Therapy: The infusion should be continued until adequate blood pressure and tissue perfusion are maintained without therapy. Norepinephrine infusion should be reduced gradually, avoiding abrupt withdrawal. In some of the reported cases of vascular collapse due to acute myocardial infarction, treatment was required for up to six days.

Adjunctive Treatment in Cardiac Arrest
LEVOPHED is usually administered intravenously during cardiac resuscitation to restore and maintain an adequate blood pressure after an effective heartbeat and ventilation have been established by other means. [The powerful beta-adrenergic stimulating action of LEVOPHED is also thought to increase the strength and effectiveness of systolic contractions once they occur.]
Average Dosage: To maintain systemic blood pressure during the management of cardiac arrest, LEVOPHED bitartrate, brand of norepinephrine bitartrate injection, is used in the same manner as described under Restoration of Blood Pressure in Acute Hypotensive States.
How Supplied: Ampuls of 4 mL containing 4 mg LEVOPHED base, box of 10 NDC 0024-1123-02
References:
1. Zucker, G. *et al.*: *Circulation* 22:935, Nov. 1960.
2. Sampson, J. and Griffith, G.: *Geriatrics* 11:60, Feb. 1956.

Regitine, trademark, CIBA Pharmaceutical Company.

LW-34-PP

LOTUSATE® Caplets®
brand of talbutal tablets, USP

Each caplet contains 120 mg of 5-Allyl-5-*sec*-butyl-barbituric acid, is lavender in color, and bears identifying number L 53.
How Supplied: CAPLETS of 120 mg, bottle of 100 (NDC 0024-1153-04)
For complete prescribing information contact Winthrop-Breon Laboratories Professional Services Department.

LW-87-Q

MARCAINE® HYDROCHLORIDE
bupivacaine hydrochloride injection, USP

MARCAINE® HYDROCHLORIDE WITH EPINEPHRINE 1:200,000 (AS BITARTRATE)
bupivacaine hydrochloride and epinephrine injection, USP

Description: Bupivacaine hydrochloride is 2-Piperidinecarboxamide, 1-butyl-*N*-(2,6-dimethylphenyl)-, monohydrochloride, a white crystalline powder that is freely soluble in 95 percent ethanol, soluble in water, and slightly soluble in chloroform or acetone.
Epinephrine is (-)-3, 4-Dihydroxy-α-[(methylamino)methyl] benzyl alcohol.
MARCAINE hydrochloride is available in sterile isotonic solutions with and without epinephrine (as bitartrate) 1:200,000 for injection via local infiltration, peripheral nerve block, and caudal and lumbar epidural blocks. Solutions of MARCAINE may be autoclaved if they do not contain epinephrine.
Bupivacaine is related chemically and pharmacologically to the aminoacyl local anesthetics. It is a homologue of mepivacaine and is chemically related to lidocaine. All three of these anesthetics contain an amide linkage between the aromatic nucleus and the amino, or piperidine group. They differ in this respect from the procaine-type local anesthetics, which have an ester linkage.
MARCAINE hydrochloride —Sterile isotonic solutions containing sodium chloride. In multiple-dose vials, each 1 mL also contains 1 mg methylparaben as antiseptic preservative. The pH of these solutions is adjusted to between 4.0 and 6.5 with sodium hydroxide or hydrochloric acid.
MARCAINE hydrochloride with epinephrine 1:200,000 (as bitartrate)—Sterile isotonic solutions containing sodium chloride. Each 1 mL contains bupivacaine hydrochloride and 0.0091 mg epinephrine bitartrate, with 0.5 mg sodium bisulfite, 0.001 mL monothioglycerol, and 2 mg ascorbic acid as antioxidants, 0.0017 mL 60% sodium lactate buffer, and 0.1 mg edetate calcium disodium as stabilizer. In multiple-dose vials, each 1 mL also contains 1 mg methylparaben as antiseptic preservative. The pH of these solutions is adjusted to between 3.4 and 4.5 with sodium hydroxide or hydrochloric acid. The specific gravity of MARCAINE 0.5% with epinephrine 1:200,000 (as bitartrate) at 25°C is 1.008 and at 37°C is 1.008.

Clinical Pharmacology: Local anesthetics block the generation and the conduction of nerve impulses, presumably by increasing the threshold for electrical excitation in the nerve, by slowing the propagation of the nerve impulse, and by reducing the rate of rise of the action potential. In general, the progression of anesthesia is related to the diameter, myelination, and conduction velocity of affected nerve fibers. Clinically, the order of loss of nerve function is as follows: (1) pain, (2) temperature, (3) touch, (4) proprioception, and (5) skeletal muscle tone.
Systemic absorption of local anesthetics produces effects on the cardiovascular and central nervous systems (CNS). At blood concentrations achieved with normal therapeutic doses, changes in cardiac conduction, excitability, refractoriness, contractility, and peripheral vascular resistance are minimal. However, toxic blood concentrations depress cardiac conduction and excitability, which may lead to atrioventricular block, ventricular arrhythmias, and cardiac arrest, sometimes resulting in fatalities. In addition, myocardial contractility is depressed and peripheral vasodilation occurs, leading to decreased cardiac output and arterial blood pressure. Recent clinical reports and animal research suggest that these cardiovascular changes are more likely to occur after unintended intravascular injection of bupivacaine. Therefore, incremental dosing is necessary.
Following systemic absorption, local anesthetics can produce central nervous system stimulation, depression, or both. Apparent central stimulation is manifested as restlessness, tremors and shivering progressing to convulsions, followed by depression and coma progressing ultimately to respiratory arrest. However, the local anesthetics have a primary depressant effect on the medulla and on higher centers. The depressed stage may occur without a prior excited state.
Pharmacokinetics: The rate of systemic absorption of local anesthetics is dependent upon the total dose and concentration of drug administered, the route of administration, the vascularity of the administration site, and the presence or absence of epinephrine in the anesthetic solution. A dilute concentration of epinephrine (1:200,000 or 5 mcg/mL) usually reduces the rate of absorption and peak plasma concentration of MARCAINE, permitting the use of moderately larger total doses and sometimes prolonging the duration of action. The onset of action with MARCAINE is rapid and anesthesia is long-lasting. The duration of anesthesia is significantly longer with MARCAINE than with any other commonly used local anesthetic. It has also been noted that there is a period of analgesia that persists after the return of sensation, during which time the need for strong analgesics is reduced.
The onset of action following dental injections is usually 2 to 10 minutes and anesthesia may last two or three times longer than lidocaine and mepivacaine for dental use, in many patients up to 7 hours. The duration of anesthetic effect is prolonged by the addition of epinephrine 1:200,000.
Local anesthetics are bound to plasma proteins in varying degrees. Generally, the lower the plasma concentration of drug the higher the percentage of drug bound to plasma proteins.
Local anesthetics appear to cross the placenta by passive diffusion. The rate and degree of diffusion is governed by (1) the degree of plasma protein binding, (2) the degree of ionization, and (3) the degree of lipid solubility. Fetal/maternal ratios of local anesthetics appear to be inversely related to the degree of plasma protein binding, because only the free, unbound drug is available for placental transfer. MARCAINE with a high protein binding capacity (95%) has a low fetal/maternal ratio (0.2 to 0.4). The extent of placental transfer is also determined by the degree of ionization and lipid solubility of the drug. Lipid soluble, nonionized drugs readily enter the fetal blood from the maternal circulation.
Depending upon the route of administration, local anesthetics are distributed to some extent to all body tissues, with high concentrations found in

highly perfused organs such as the liver, lungs, heart, and brain.

Pharmacokinetic studies on the plasma profile of MARCAINE after direct intravenous injection suggest a three-compartment open model. The first compartment is represented by the rapid intravascular distribution of the drug. The second compartment represents the equilibration of the drug throughout the highly perfused organs such as the brain, myocardium, lungs, kidneys, and liver. The third compartment represents an equilibration of the drug with poorly perfused tissues, such as muscle and fat. The elimination of drug from tissue distribution depends largely upon the ability of binding sites in the circulation to carry it to the liver where it is metabolized.

After injection of MARCAINE for caudal, epidural, or peripheral nerve block in man, peak levels of bupivacaine in the blood are reached in 30 to 45 minutes, followed by a decline to insignificant levels during the next three to six hours.

Various pharmacokinetic parameters of the local anesthetics can be significantly altered by the presence of hepatic or renal disease, addition of epinephrine, factors affecting urinary pH, renal blood flow, the route of drug administration, and the age of the patient. The half-life of MARCAINE (bupivacaine) in adults is 2.7 hours and in neonates 8.1 hours.

Amide-type local anesthetics such as MARCAINE are metabolized primarily in the liver via conjugation with glucuronic acid. Patients with hepatic disease, especially those with severe hepatic disease, may be more susceptible to the potential toxicities of the amide-type local anesthetics. Pipecolylxylidine is the major metabolite of MARCAINE.

The kidney is the main excretory organ for most local anesthetics and their metabolites. Urinary excretion is affected by urinary perfusion and factors affecting urinary pH. Only 6% of bupivacaine is excreted unchanged in the urine.

When administered in recommended doses and concentrations, MARCAINE does not ordinarily produce irritation or tissue damage and does not cause methemoglobinemia.

Indications and Usage: MARCAINE is indicated for the production of local or regional anesthesia or analgesia for surgery, dental and oral surgery procedures, diagnostic and therapeutic procedures, and for diagnostic procedures. Only the 0.25% and 0.5% concentrations are indicated for obstetrical anesthesia. (See WARNINGS.)

Experience with nonobstetrical surgical procedures in pregnant patients is not sufficient to recommend use of 0.75% concentration of MARCAINE in these patients.

MARCAINE is not recommended for intravenous regional anesthesia (Bier Block). See WARNINGS. The routes of administration and indicated MARCAINE concentrations are:

- local infiltration   0.25%
- peripheral nerve block 0.25% and 0.5%
- retrobulbar block   0.75%
- sympathetic block   0.25%
- lumbar epidural   0.25%, 0.5%, and 0.75% (0.75% not for obstetrical anesthesia)
- caudal   0.25% and 0.5%
- epidural test dose   0.5% with epinephrine 1:200,000
- dental blocks   0.5% with epinephrine 1:200,000

(See DOSAGE AND ADMINISTRATION for additional information.)

Standard textbooks should be consulted to determine the accepted procedures and techniques for the administration of MARCAINE.

Contraindications: MARCAINE is contraindicated in obstetrical paracervical block anesthesia. Its use in this technique has resulted in fetal bradycardia and death.

MARCAINE (bupivacaine) is contraindicated in patients with a known hypersensitivity to it or to any local anesthetic agent of the amide type or to other components of MARCAINE solutions.

Warnings:

THE 0.75% CONCENTRATION OF MARCAINE IS NOT RECOMMENDED FOR OBSTETRICAL ANESTHESIA. THERE HAVE BEEN REPORTS OF CARDIAC ARREST WITH DIFFICULT RESUSCITATION OR DEATH DURING USE OF MARCAINE FOR EPIDURAL ANESTHESIA IN OBSTETRICAL PATIENTS. IN MOST CASES, THIS HAS FOLLOWED USE OF THE 0.75% CONCENTRATION. RESUSCITATION HAS BEEN DIFFICULT OR IMPOSSIBLE DESPITE APPARENTLY ADEQUATE PREPARATION AND APPROPRIATE MANAGEMENT. CARDIAC ARREST HAS OCCURRED AFTER CONVULSIONS RESULTING FROM SYSTEMIC TOXICITY, PRESUMABLY FOLLOWING UNINTENTIONAL INTRAVASCULAR INJECTION. THE 0.75% CONCENTRATION SHOULD BE RESERVED FOR SURGICAL PROCEDURES WHERE A HIGH DEGREE OF MUSCLE RELAXATION AND PROLONGED EFFECT ARE NECESSARY.

LOCAL ANESTHETICS SHOULD ONLY BE EMPLOYED BY CLINICIANS WHO ARE WELL VERSED IN DIAGNOSIS AND MANAGEMENT OF DOSE-RELATED TOXICITY AND OTHER ACUTE EMERGENCIES WHICH MIGHT ARISE FROM THE BLOCK TO BE EMPLOYED, AND THEN ONLY AFTER INSURING THE *IMMEDIATE* AVAILABILITY OF OXYGEN, OTHER RESUSCITATIVE DRUGS, CARDIOPULMONARY RESUSCITATIVE EQUIPMENT, AND THE PERSONNEL RESOURCES NEEDED FOR PROPER MANAGEMENT OF TOXIC REACTIONS AND RELATED EMERGENCIES. (See also ADVERSE REACTIONS, PRECAUTIONS, and OVERDOSAGE.) DELAY IN PROPER MANAGEMENT OF DOSE-RELATED TOXICITY, UNDERVENTILATION FROM ANY CAUSE, AND/OR ALTERED SENSITIVITY MAY LEAD TO THE DEVELOPMENT OF ACIDOSIS, CARDIAC ARREST, AND POSSIBLY, DEATH.

Local anesthetic solutions containing antimicrobial preservatives, ie, those supplied in multiple-dose vials, should not be used for epidural or caudal anesthesia because safety has not been established with regard to intrathecal injection, either intentionally or unintentionally, of such preservatives.

It is essential that aspiration for blood or cerebrospinal fluid (where applicable) be done prior to injecting any local anesthetic, both the original dose and all subsequent doses, to avoid intravascular or subarachnoid injection. However, a negative aspiration does *not* ensure against an intravascular or subarachnoid injection.

MARCAINE with epinephrine 1:200,000 or other vasopressors should not be used concomitantly with ergot-type oxytocic drugs, because a severe persistent hypertension may occur. Likewise, solutions of MARCAINE containing a vasoconstrictor, such as epinephrine, should be used with extreme caution in patients receiving monoamine oxidase inhibitors (MAOI) or antidepressants of the triptyline or imipramine types, because severe prolonged hypertension may result.

Until further experience is gained in children younger than 12 years, administration of MARCAINE in this age group is not recommended.

Mixing or the prior or intercurrent use of any other local anesthetic with MARCAINE cannot be recommended because of insufficient data on the clinical use of such mixtures.

There have been reports of cardiac arrest and death during the use of MARCAINE for intravenous regional anesthesia (Bier Block). Information on safe dosages and techniques of administration of MARCAINE in this procedure is lacking. Therefore, MARCAINE is not recommended for use in this technique.

Precautions:

General: The safety and effectiveness of local anesthetics depend on proper dosage, correct technique, adequate precautions, and readiness for emergencies. Resuscitative equipment, oxygen, and other resuscitative drugs should be available for immediate use. (See WARNINGS, ADVERSE REACTIONS and OVERDOSAGE.) During major regional nerve blocks, the patient should have IV fluids running via an indwelling catheter to assure a functioning intravenous pathway. The lowest dosage of local anesthetic that results in effective anesthesia should be used to avoid high plasma levels and serious adverse effects. The rapid injection of a large volume of local anesthetic solution should be avoided and fractional (incremental) doses should be used when feasible.

Epidural Anesthesia: During epidural administration of MARCAINE, 0.5% and 0.75% solutions should be administered in incremental doses of 3 mL to 5 mL with sufficient time between doses to detect toxic manifestations of unintentional intravascular or intrathecal injection. Injections should be made slowly, with frequent aspirations before and during the injection to avoid intravascular injection. Syringe aspirations should also be performed before and during each supplemental injection in continuous (intermittent) catheter techniques. An intravascular injection is still possible even if aspirations for blood are negative.

During the administration of epidural anesthesia, it is recommended that a test dose be administered initially and the effects monitored before the full dose is given. When using a "continuous" catheter technique, test doses should be given prior to both the original and all reinforcing doses, because plastic tubing in the epidural space can migrate into a blood vessel or through the dura. When clinical conditions permit, the test dose should contain epinephrine (10 mcg to 15 mcg have been suggested) to serve as a warning of unintended intravascular injection. If injected into a blood vessel, this amount of epinephrine is likely to produce a transient "epinephrine response" within 45 seconds, consisting of an increase in heart rate and/or systolic blood pressure, circumoral pallor, palpitations, and nervousness in the unsedated patient. The sedated patient may exhibit only a pulse rate increase of 20 or more beats per minute for 15 or more seconds. Therefore, following the test dose, the heart rate should be monitored for a heart rate increase. Patients on beta-blockers may not manifest changes in heart rate, but blood pressure monitoring can detect a transient rise in systolic blood pressure. The test dose should also contain 10 mg to 15 mg of MARCAINE or an equivalent amount of another local anesthetic to detect an unintended intrathecal administration. This will be evidenced within a few minutes by signs of spinal block (eg, decreased sensation of the buttocks, paresis of the legs, or, in the sedated patient, absent knee jerk). The MARCAINE Test Dose formulation contains 15 mg of bupivacaine and 15 mcg of epinephrine in a volume of 3 mL. An intravascular or subarachnoid injection is still possible even if results of the test dose are negative. The test dose itself may produce a systemic toxic reaction, high spinal or epinephrine-induced cardiovascular effects.

Injection of repeated doses of local anesthetics may cause significant increases in plasma levels with each repeated dose due to slow accumulation of the drug or its metabolites, or to slow metabolic degradation. Tolerance to elevated blood levels varies with the status of the patient. Debilitated, elderly patients and acutely ill patients should be given reduced doses commensurate with their age and physical status. Local anesthetics should also be used with caution in patients with hypotension or heart block.

Continued on next page

This product information was effective as of December 3, 1984. On these and other products of Winthrop-Breon Laboratories, detailed information may be obtained on a current basis by direct inquiry to the Professional Services Department, 90 Park Avenue, New York, NY 10016 (212) 907-2525.

Winthrop-Breon—Cont.

Careful and constant monitoring of cardiovascular and respiratory (adequacy of ventilation) vital signs and the patient's state of consciousness should be performed after each local anesthetic injection. It should be kept in mind at such times that restlessness, anxiety, incoherent speech, lightheadedness, numbness and tingling of the mouth and lips, metallic taste, tinnitus, dizziness, blurred vision, tremors, twitching, depression, or drowsiness may be early warning signs of central nervous system toxicity.

Local anesthetic solutions containing a vasoconstrictor should be used cautiously and in carefully restricted quantities in areas of the body supplied by end arteries or having otherwise compromised blood supply such as digits, nose, external ear, or penis. Patients with hypertensive vascular disease may exhibit exaggerated vasoconstrictor response. Ischemic injury or necrosis may result.

Because amide-type local anesthetics such as MARCAINE (bupivacaine) are metabolized by the liver, these drugs, especially repeat doses, should be used cautiously in patients with hepatic disease. Patients with severe hepatic disease, because of their inability to metabolize local anesthetics normally, are at a greater risk of developing toxic plasma concentrations. Local anesthetics should also be used with caution in patients with impaired cardiovascular function because they may be less able to compensate for functional changes associated with the prolongation of A-V conduction produced by these drugs.

Serious dose-related cardiac arrhythmias may occur if preparations containing a vasoconstrictor such as epinephrine are employed in patients during or following the administration of potent inhalation anesthetics. In deciding whether to use these products concurrently in the same patient, the combined action of both agents upon the myocardium, the concentration and volume of vasoconstrictor used, and the time since injection, when applicable, should be taken into account.

Many drugs used during the conduct of anesthesia are considered potential triggering agents for familial malignant hyperthermia. Because it is not known whether amide-type local anesthetics may trigger this reaction and because the need for supplemental general anesthesia cannot be predicted in advance, it is suggested that a standard protocol for management should be available. Early unexplained signs of tachycardia, tachypnea, labile blood pressure and metabolic acidosis may precede temperature elevation. Successful outcome is dependent on early diagnosis, prompt discontinuance of the suspect triggering agent(s) and prompt institution of treatment, including oxygen therapy, indicated supportive measures and dantrolene. (Consult dantrolene sodium intravenous package insert before using.)

Use in Head and Neck Area: Small doses of local anesthetics injected into the head and neck area, including retrobulbar, dental, and stellate ganglion blocks, may produce adverse reactions similar to systemic toxicity seen with unintentional intravascular injections of larger doses. Confusion, convulsions, respiratory depression and/or respiratory arrest, and cardiovascular stimulation or depression have been reported. These reactions may be due to intra-arterial injection of the local anesthetic with retrograde flow to the cerebral circulation. Patients receiving these blocks should have their circulation and respiration monitored and be constantly observed. Resuscitative equipment and personnel for treating adverse reactions should be immediately available. Dosage recommendations should not be exceeded. (See DOSAGE AND ADMINISTRATION.)

Use in Ophthalmic Surgery: When MARCAINE 0.75% is used for retrobulbar block, complete corneal anesthesia usually precedes onset of clinically acceptable external ocular muscle akinesia. Therefore, presence of akinesia rather than anesthesia alone should determine readiness of the patient for surgery.

Use in Dentistry: Because of the long duration of anesthesia, when MARCAINE 0.5% with epinephrine is used for dental injections, patients should be cautioned about the possibility of inadvertent trauma to tongue, lips, and buccal mucosa and advised not to chew solid foods or test the anesthetized area by biting or probing.

Information for Patients: When appropriate, patients should be informed in advance that they may experience temporary loss of sensation and motor activity, usually in the lower half of the body, following proper administration of caudal or epidural anesthesia. Also, when appropriate, the physician should discuss other information including adverse reactions in the MARCAINE package insert.

Patients receiving dental injections of MARCAINE should be cautioned not to chew solid foods or test the anesthetized area by biting or probing until anesthesia has worn off (up to 7 hours).

Clinically Significant Drug Interactions: The administration of local anesthetic solutions containing epinephrine or norepinephrine to patients receiving monoamine oxidase inhibitors or tricyclic antidepressants may produce severe, prolonged hypertension. Concurrent use of these agents should generally be avoided. In situations when concurrent therapy is necessary, careful patient monitoring is essential.

Concurrent administration of vasopressor drugs and of ergot-type oxytocic drugs may cause severe, persistent hypertension or cerebrovascular accidents.

Phenothiazines and butyrophenones may reduce or reverse the pressor effect of epinephrine.

Carcinogenesis, Mutagenesis, Impairment of Fertility: Long-term studies in animals of most local anesthetics including bupivacaine to evaluate the carcinogenic potential have not been conducted. Mutagenic potential or the effect on fertility has not been determined. There is no evidence from human data that MARCAINE may be carcinogenic or mutagenic or that it impairs fertility.

Pregnancy Category C: Decreased pup survival in rats and an embryocidal effect in rabbits have been observed when bupivacaine hydrochloride was administered to these species in doses comparable to nine and five times respectively the maximum recommended daily human dose (400 mg). There are no adequate and well-controlled studies in pregnant women of the effect of bupivacaine on the developing fetus. Bupivacaine hydrochloride should be used during pregnancy only if the potential benefit justifies the potential risk to the fetus. This does not exclude the use of MARCAINE at term for obstetrical anesthesia or analgesia. (See *Labor and Delivery.*)

Labor and Delivery: SEE BOXED WARNING REGARDING OBSTETRICAL USE OF 0.75% MARCAINE.

MARCAINE is contraindicated for obstetrical paracervical block anesthesia.

Local anesthetics rapidly cross the placenta, and when used for epidural, caudal, or pudendal block anesthesia, can cause varying degrees of maternal, fetal and neonatal toxicity. (See *Pharmacokinetics* in **CLINICAL PHARMACOLOGY.**) The incidence and degree of toxicity depend upon the procedure performed, the type, and amount of drug used, and the technique of drug administration. Adverse reactions in the parturient, fetus, and neonate involve alterations of the central nervous system, peripheral vascular tone, and cardiac function.

Maternal hypotension has resulted from regional anesthesia. Local anesthetics produce vasodilation by blocking sympathetic nerves. Elevating the patient's legs and positioning her on her left side will help prevent decreases in blood pressure. The fetal heart rate also should be monitored continuously and electronic fetal monitoring is highly advisable.

Epidural, caudal, or pudendal anesthesia may alter the forces of parturition through changes in uterine contractility or maternal expulsive efforts. Epidural anesthesia has been reported to prolong the second stage of labor by removing the parturient's reflex urge to bear down or by interfering with motor function. The use of obstetrical anesthesia may increase the need for forceps assistance.

The use of some local anesthetic drug products during labor and delivery may be followed by diminished muscle strength and tone for the first day or two of life. This has not been reported with bupivacaine.

It is extremely important to avoid aortocaval compression by the gravid uterus during administration of regional block to parturients. To do this, the patient must be maintained in the left lateral decubitus position or a blanket roll or sandbag may be placed beneath the right hip and the gravid uterus displaced to the left.

Nursing Mothers: It is not known whether local anesthetic drugs are excreted in human milk. Because many drugs are excreted in human milk, caution should be exercised when local anesthetics are administered to a nursing woman.

Pediatric Use: Until further experience is gained in children younger than 12 years, administration of MARCAINE in this age group is not recommended.

Adverse Reactions: Reactions to MARCAINE (bupivacaine) are characteristic of those associated with other amide-type local anesthetics. A major cause of adverse reactions to this group of drugs is excessive plasma levels, which may be due to overdosage, unintentional intravascular injection, or slow metabolic degradation.

The most commonly encountered acute adverse experiences which demand immediate countermeasures are related to the central nervous system and the cardiovascular system. These adverse experiences are generally dose related and due to high plasma levels which may result from overdosage, rapid absorption from the injection site, diminished tolerance, or from unintentional intravascular injection of the local anesthetic solution. In addition to systemic dose-related toxicity, unintentional subarachnoid injection of drug during the intended performance of caudal or lumbar epidural block or nerve blocks near the vertebral column (especially in the head and neck region) may result in underventilation or apnea ("Total or High Spinal"). Also, hypotension due to loss of sympathetic tone and respiratory paralysis or underventilation due to cephalad extension of the motor level of anesthesia may occur. This may lead to secondary cardiac arrest if untreated. Factors influencing plasma protein binding, such as acidosis, systemic diseases which alter protein production, or competition of other drugs for protein binding sites, may diminish individual tolerance.

Central Nervous System Reactions: These are characterized by excitation and/or depression. Restlessness, anxiety, dizziness, tinnitus, blurred vision or tremors may occur, possibly proceeding to convulsions. However, excitement may be transient or absent, with depression being the first manifestation of an adverse reaction. This may quickly be followed by drowsiness merging into unconsciousness and respiratory arrest. Other central nervous system effects may be nausea, vomiting, chills, and constriction of the pupils.

The incidence of convulsions associated with the use of local anesthetics varies with the procedure used and the total dose administered. In a survey of studies of epidural anesthesia, over toxicity progressing to convulsions occurred in approximately 0.1 % of local anesthetic administrations.

Cardiovascular System Reactions: High doses or unintentional intravascular injection may lead to high plasma levels and related depression of the myocardium, decreased cardiac output, heart block, hypotension, bradycardia, ventricular arrhythmias, including ventricular tachycardia and ventricular fibrillation, and cardiac arrest. (See WARNINGS, PRECAUTIONS, and OVERDOSAGE sections.)

Allergic: Allergic-type reactions are rare and may occur as a result of sensitivity to the local anesthetic or to other formulation ingredients, such as the antimicrobial preservative methylparaben contained in multiple-dose vials or sulfites in epinephrine-containing solutions. These reactions are characterized by signs such as urticaria, pruritus, erythema, angioneurotic edema (including laryngeal edema), tachycardia, sneezing, nausea, vomiting, dizziness, syncope, excessive sweating, elevated temperature, and, possibly, anaphylactoid-like symptomatology (including severe hypotension). Cross sensitivity among members of the amide-type local anesthetic group has been reported. The usefulness of screening for sensitivity has not been definitely established.

Neurologic: The incidences of adverse neurologic reactions associated with the use of local anesthetics may be related to the total dose of local anesthetic administered and are also dependent upon the particular drug used, the route of administration, and the physical status of the patient. Many of these effects may be related to local anesthetic techniques, with or without a contribution from the drug.

In the practice of caudal or lumbar epidural block, occasional unintentional penetration of the subarachnoid space by the catheter or needle may occur. Subsequent adverse effects may depend partially on the amount of drug administered intrathecally and the physiological and physical effects of a dural puncture. A high spinal is characterized by paralysis of the legs, loss of consciousness, respiratory paralysis, and bradycardia.

Neurologic effects following epidural or caudal anesthesia may include spinal block of varying magnitude (including high or total spinal block); hypotension secondary to spinal block; urinary retention; fecal and urinary incontinence; loss of perineal sensation and sexual function; persistent anesthesia, paresthesia, weakness, paralysis of the lower extremities and loss of sphincter control all of which may have slow, incomplete, or no recovery; headache; backache; septic meningitis; meningismus; slowing of labor; increased incidence of forceps delivery; and cranial nerve palsies due to traction on nerves from loss of cerebrospinal fluid.

Overdosage: Acute emergencies from local anesthetics are generally related to high plasma levels encountered during therapeutic use of local anesthetics or to unintended subarachnoid injection of local anesthetic solution. (See ADVERSE REACTIONS, WARNINGS, and PRECAUTIONS.)

Management of Local Anesthetic Emergencies: The first consideration is prevention, best accomplished by careful and constant monitoring of cardiovascular and respiratory vital signs and the patient's state of consciousness after each local anesthetic injection. At the first sign of change, oxygen should be administered.

*The first step in the management of systemic toxic reactions, as well as underventilation or apnea due to unintentional subarachnoid injection of drug solution, consists of **immediate** attention to the establishment and maintenance of a patent airway and effective assisted or controlled ventilation with 100% oxygen with a delivery system capable of permitting immediate positive airway pressure by mask.* This may prevent convulsions if they have not already occurred.

If necessary, use drugs to control the convulsions. A 50 mg to 100 mg bolus IV injection of succinylcholine will paralyze the patient without depressing the central nervous or cardiovascular systems and facilitate ventilation. A bolus IV dose of 5 mg to 10 mg of diazepam or 50 mg to 100 mg of thiopental will permit ventilation and counteract central nervous system stimulation, but these drugs also depress central nervous system, respiratory, and cardiac function, add to postictal depression and may result in apnea. Intravenous barbiturates, anticonvulsant agents, or muscle relaxants should only be administered by those familiar with their use. Immediately after the institution of these ventilatory measures, the adequacy of the circulation should be evaluated. Supportive treatment of circulatory depression may require administration of intravenous fluids, and, when appropriate, a vasopressor dictated by the clinical situation (such as ephedrine or epinephrine to enhance myocardial contractile force).

Endotracheal intubation, employing drugs and techniques familiar to the clinician, may be indicated after initial administration of oxygen by mask if difficulty is encountered in the maintenance of a patent airway, or if prolonged ventilatory support (assisted or controlled) is indicated.

Recent clinical data from patients experiencing local anesthetic-induced convulsions demonstrated rapid development of hypoxia, hypercarbia, and acidosis with bupivacaine within a minute of the onset of convulsions. These observations suggest that oxygen consumption and carbon dioxide production are greatly increased during local anesthetic convulsions and emphasize the importance of immediate and effective ventilation with oxygen which may avoid cardiac arrest.

If not treated immediately, convulsions with simultaneous hypoxia, hypercarbia, and acidosis plus myocardial depression from the direct effects of the local anesthetic may result in cardiac arrhythmias, bradycardia, asystole, ventricular fibrillation, or cardiac arrest. Respiratory abnormalities, including apnea, may occur. Underventilation or apnea due to unintentional subarachnoid injection of local anesthetic solution may produce these same signs and also lead to cardiac arrest if ventilatory support is not instituted. *If cardiac arrest should occur, successful outcome may require prolonged resuscitative efforts.*

The supine position is dangerous in pregnant women at term because of aortocaval compression by the gravid uterus. Therefore during treatment of systemic toxicity, maternal hypotension or fetal bradycardia following regional block, the parturient should be maintained in the left lateral decubitus position if possible, or manual displacement of the uterus off the great vessels be accomplished.

The mean seizure dosage of bupivacaine in rhesus monkeys was found to be 4.4 mg/kg with mean arterial plasma concentration of 4.5 mcg/mL. The intravenous and subcutaneous LD_{50} in mice is 6 mg/kg to 8 mg/kg and 38 mg/kg to 54 mg/kg respectively.

Dosage and Administration: The dose of any local anesthetic administered varies with the anesthetic procedure, the area to be anesthetized, the vascularity of the tissues, the number of neuronal segments to be blocked, the depth of anesthesia and degree of muscle relaxation required, the duration of anesthesia desired, individual tolerance, and the physical condition of the patient. The smallest dose and concentration required to produce the desired result should be administered. Dosages of MARCAINE should be reduced for elderly and debilitated patients and patients with cardiac and/or liver disease. The rapid injection of a large volume of local anesthetic solution should be avoided and fractional (incremental) doses should be used when feasible.

For specific techniques and procedures, refer to standard textbooks.

In recommended doses, MARCAINE produces complete sensory block, but the effect on motor function differs among the three concentrations.

0.25%—when used for caudal, epidural, or peripheral nerve block, produces incomplete motor block. Should be used for operations in which muscle relaxation is not important, or when another means of providing muscle relaxation is used concurrently. Onset of action may be slower than with the 0.5% or 0.75% solutions.

0.5%—provides motor blockade for caudal, epidural, or nerve block, but muscle relaxation may be inadequate for operations in which complete muscle relaxation is essential.

0.75%—produces complete motor block. Most useful for epidural block in abdominal operations requiring complete muscle relaxation, and for retrobulbar anesthesia. Not for obstetrical anesthesia.

The duration of anesthesia with MARCAINE is such that for most indications, a single dose is sufficient.

Maximum dosage limit must be individualized in each case after evaluating the size and physical status of the patient, as well as the usual rate of systemic absorption from a particular injection site. Most experience to date is with single doses of MARCAINE up to 225 mg with epinephrine 1:200,000 and 175 mg without epinephrine; more or less drug may be used depending on individualization of each case.

These doses may be repeated up to once every three hours. In clinical studies to date, total daily doses have been up to 400 mg. Until further experience is gained, this dose should not be exceeded in 24 hours. The duration of anesthetic effect may be prolonged by the addition of epinephrine.

The dosages in Table 1 have generally proved satisfactory and are recommended as a guide for use in the average adult. These dosages should be reduced for elderly or debilitated patients. Until further experience is gained, MARCAINE (bupivacaine) is not recommended for children younger than 12 years. MARCAINE is contraindicated for obstetrical paracervical blocks, and is not recommended for intravenous regional anesthesia (Bier Block).

Use in Epidural Anesthesia: During epidural administration of MARCAINE, 0.5% and 0.75% solutions should be administered in incremental doses of 3 mL to 5 mL with sufficient time between doses to detect toxic manifestatons of unintentional intravascular or intrathecal injection. In obstetrics, only the 0.5% and 0.25% concentrations should be used; incremental doses of 3 mL to 5 mL of the 0.5% solution not exceeding 50 mg to 100 mg at any dosing interval are recommended. Repeat doses should be preceded by a test dose containing epinephrine if not contraindicated. Use only the single-dose ampuls and single-dose vials for caudal or epidural anesthesia; the multiple-dose vials contain a preservative and therefore should not be used for these procedures.

Test Dose for Caudal and Lumbar Epidural Blocks: MARCAINE Test Dose (0.5% bupivacaine with 1:200,000 epinephrine in a 3 mL ampul) is recommended for use as a test dose when clinical conditions permit prior to caudal and lumbar epidural blocks. This may serve as a warning of unintended intravascular or subarachnoid injection. (See PRECAUTIONS.) The pulse rate and other signs should be monitored carefully immediately following each test dose administration to detect possible intravascular injection, and adequate time for onset of spinal block should be allotted to detect possible intrathecal injection. An intravascular or subarachnoid injection is still possible even if results of the test dose are negative. The test dose itself may produce a systemic toxic reaction, high spinal or cardiovascular effects from the epinephrine. (See WARNINGS and OVERDOSAGE.)

Use in Dentistry: The 0.5% concentration with epinephrine is recommended for infiltration and block injection in the maxillary and mandibular area when a longer duration of local anesthetic action is desired, such as for oral surgical procedures generally associated with significant postoperative pain. The average dose of 1.8 mL (9 mg) per injection site will usually suffice; an occasional second dose of 1.8 mL (9 mg) may be used if necessary to produce adequate anesthesia after making allowance for 2 to 10 minutes onset time. (See CLINICAL PHARMACOLOGY.) The lowest effective dose should be employed and time should be allowed between injections; it is recommended that the total dose for all injection sites, *spread out* over a single dental sitting, should not ordinarily exceed 90 mg for a healthy adult patient (ten 1.8 mL injections of 0.5% MARCAINE with epinephrine, bupivacaine and epinephrine). Injections should be made slowly and with frequent aspirations. Until further experience is gained, MARCAINE in dentistry is not recommended for children younger than 12 years.

Unused portions of solutions not containing preservatives, ie, those supplied in single-dose ampuls

Continued on next page

This product information was effective as of December 3, 1984. On these and other products of Winthrop-Breon Laboratories, detailed information may be obtained on a current basis by direct inquiry to the Professional Services Department, 90 Park Avenue, New York, NY 10016 (212) 907-2525.

Winthrop-Breon—Cont.

and single-dose vials, should be discarded following initial use.
This product should be inspected visually for particulate matter and discoloration prior to administration whenever solution and container permit. Solutions which are discolored or which contain particulate matter should not be administered. [See table below].

How Supplied:
These solutions are not for spinal anesthesia.
Store at controlled room temperature, between 15°C and 30°C (59°F and 86°F).

MARCAINE hydrochloride— Solutions of MARCAINE (bupivacaine) that do not contain epinephrine may be autoclaved. Autoclave at 15-pound pressure, 121°C (250°F) for 15 minutes.

0.25%—Contains 2.5 mg bupivacaine hydrochloride per mL.
   Single-dose ampuls of 50 mL, box of 5
      NDC 0024-1212-02
   Single-dose vials of 10 mL, box of 10
      NDC 0024-1212-10
   Single-dose vials of 30 mL, box of 10
      NDC 0024-1212-30
   Multiple-dose vials of 50 mL, box of 1
      NDC 0024-1217-01

0.5%—Contains 5 mg bupivacaine hydrochloride per mL.
   Single-dose ampuls of 30 mL, box of 5
      NDC 0024-1213-02
   Single-dose vials of 10 mL, box of 10
      NDC 0024-1213-10
   Single-dose vials of 30 mL, box of 10
      NDC 0024-1213-30
   Multiple-dose vials of 50 mL, box of 1
      NDC 0024-1218-01

0.75%—Contains 7.5 mg bupivacaine hydrochloride per mL.
   Single-dose ampuls of 30 mL, box of 5
      NDC 0024-1214-02
   Single-dose vials of 10 mL, box of 10
      NDC 0024-1214-10
   Single-dose vials of 30 mL, box of 10
      NDC 0024-1214-30

MARCAINE hydrochloride with epinephrine 1:200,000 (as bitartrate).—Solutions of MARCAINE that contain epinephrine should not be autoclaved and should be protected from light. Do not use if solution is discolored or contains a precipitate.

0.25%—with epinephrine 1:200,000
Contains 2.5 mg bupivacaine hydrochloride per mL.
   Single-dose ampuls of 50 mL, box of 5
      NDC 0024-1222-02
   Single-dose vials of 10 mL, box of 10
      NDC 0024-1222-10
   Single-dose vials of 30 mL, box of 10
      NDC 0024-1222-30
   Multiple-dose vials of 50 mL, box of 1
      NDC 0024-1227-01

0.5%—with epinephrine 1:200,000
Contains 5 mg bupivacaine hydrochloride per mL.
   Single-dose ampuls of 3 mL, box of 10
      NDC 0024-1223-03
   Single-dose ampuls of 30 mL, box of 5
      NDC 0024-1223-02
   Single-dose vials of 10 mL, box of 10
      NDC 0024-1223-10
   Single-dose vials of 30 mL, box of 10
      NDC 0024-1223-30
   Multiple-dose vials of 50 mL, box of 1
      NDC 0024-1228-01

0.75%—with epinephrine 1:200,000
Contains 7.5 mg bupivacaine hydrochloride per mL.
   Single-dose ampuls of 30 mL, box of 5
      NDC 0024-1224-02
      MW-126-G

MARCAINE® Spinal   ℞
brand of bupivacaine HCl, USP, 0.75% with dextrose, USP,
8.25% injection
STERILE HYPERBARIC SOLUTION FOR SPINAL ANESTHESIA

Description: Bupivacaine hydrochloride is 2-Piperidinecarboxamide, 1-butyl-N-(2,6-dimethylphenyl)-, monohydrochloride, a white crystalline powder that is freely soluble in 95 percent ethanol, soluble in water, and slightly soluble in chloroform or acetone.
Dextrose is D-glucopyranose monohydrate.
MARCAINE Spinal is available in sterile hyperbaric solution for subarachnoid injection (spinal block).
Bupivacaine hydrochloride is related chemically and pharmacologically to the aminoacyl local anesthetics. It is a homologue of mepivacaine and is chemically related to lidocaine. All three of these anesthetics contain an amide linkage between the aromatic nucleus and the amino or piperidine group. They differ in this respect from the procaine-type local anesthetics, which have an ester linkage.
Each 1 mL of MARCAINE Spinal contains 7.5 mg bupivacaine hydrochloride and 82.5 mg dextrose. The pH of this solution is adjusted to between 4.0 and 6.5 with sodium hydroxide or hydrochloric acid.
The specific gravity of MARCAINE Spinal is between 1.030 and 1.035 at 25°C and 1.03 at 37°C.
MARCAINE Spinal does not contain any preservatives.

Clinical Pharmacology: Local anesthetics block the generation and the conduction of nerve impulses, presumably by increasing the threshold for electrical excitation in the nerve, by slowing the propagation of the nerve impulse, and by reducing the rate of rise of the acton potential. In general, the progression of anesthesia is related to the diameter, myelination, and conduction velocity of affected nerve fibers. Clinically, the order of loss of nerve function is as follows: (1) pain, (2) temperature, (3) touch, (4) proprioception, and (5) skeletal muscle tone.
Systemic absorption of local anesthetics produces effects on the cardiovascular and central nervous systems (CNS). At blood concentrations achieved with normal therapeutic doses, changes in cardiac conduction, excitability, refractoriness, contractility, and peripheral vascular resistance are minimal. However, toxic blood concentrations depress cardiac conduction and excitability, which may lead to atrioventricular block, ventricular arrhythmias, and cardiac arrest, sometimes resulting in fatalities. In addition, myocardial contractility is depressed and peripheral vasodilation occurs, leading to decreased cardiac output and arterial blood pressure. Recent clinical reports and animal research suggest that these cardiovascular changes are more likely to occur after unintended direct intravascular injection of bupivacaine. Therefore, when epidural anesthesia with bupivacaine is considered, incremental dosing is necessary.
Following systemic absorption, local anesthetics can produce central nervous system stimulation, depression, or both. Apparent central stimulation is manifested as restlessness, tremors and shivering, progressing to convulsions, followed by depression and coma progressing ultimately to respiratory arrest. However, the local anesthetics have a primary depressant effect on the medulla and on higher centers. The depressed stage may occur without a prior excited stage.

Pharmacokinetics: The rate of systemic absorption of local anesthetics is dependent upon the total dose and concentration of drug administered, the route of administration, the vascularity of the administraton site, and the presence or absence of epinephrine in the anesthetic solution. A dilute concentration of epinephrine (1:200,000 or 5 mcg/mL) usually reduces the rate of absorption and peak plasma concentration of MARCAINE, permitting the use of moderately larger total doses and sometimes prolonging the duration of action. The onset of action with MARCAINE is rapid and anesthesia is long lasting. The duration of anesthesia is significantly longer with MARCAINE than with any other commonly used local anesthetic. It has also been noted that there is a period of analgesia that persists after the return of sensation, during which time the need for strong analgesics is reduced.
The onset of sensory blockade following spinal block with MARCAINE Spinal is very rapid (within one minute); maximum motor blockade and maximum dermatome level are achieved within 15 minutes in most cases. Duration of sensory blockade (time to return of complete sensation in the operative site or regression of two dermatomes) following a 12 mg dose averages 2 hours with or without 0.2 mg epinephrine. The time to return of complete motor ability with 12 mg MARCAINE Spinal averages 3½ hours without the addition of epinephrine and 4½ hours if 0.2 mg epinephrine is added. When compared to equal milligram doses of hyperbaric tetracaine, the duration of sensory blockade was the same but the time to complete motor recovery was significantly

Table 1. Recommended Concentrations and Doses of MARCAINE

Type of Block	Conc.	Each Dose (mL)	Each Dose (mg)	Motor Block[1]
Local Infiltration	0.25%[4]	up to max.	up to max.	—
Epidural	0.75%[2,4]	10–20	75–150	complete
	0.5%[4]	10–20	50–100	moderate to complete
	0.25%[4]	10–20	25–50	partial to moderate
Caudal	0.5%[4]	15–30	75–150	moderate to complete
	0.25%[4]	15–30	37.5–75	moderate
Peripheral nerves	0.5%[4]	5 to max.	25 to max.	moderate to complete
	0.25%[4]	5 to max.	12.5 to max.	moderate to complete
Retrobulbar[3]	0.75%[4]	2–4	15–30	complete
Sympathetic	0.25%	20–50	50–125	—
Dental[3]	0.5% w/epi	1.8–3.6 per site	9–18 per site	—
Epidural[3] Test Dose	0.5% w/epi	2–3	10–15 (10–15 micrograms epinephrine)	—

[1] With continuous (intermittent) techniques, repeat doses increase the degree of motor block. The first repeat dose of 0.5% may produce complete motor block. Intercostal nerve block with 0.25% may also produce complete motor block for intraabdominal surgery.
[2] For single dose use, not for intermittent (catheter) epidural technique. Not for obstetrical anesthesia.
[3] See PRECAUTIONS.
[4] Solutions with or without epinephrine.

longer for tetracaine. Addition of 0.2 mg epinephrine significantly prolongs the motor blockade and time to first postoperative narcotic with MARCAINE Spinal.

Local anesthetics appear to cross the placenta by passive diffusion. The rate and degree of diffusion is governed by (1) the degree of plasma protein binding, (2) the degree of ionization, and (3) the degree of lipid solubility. Fetal/maternal ratios of local anesthetics appear to be inversely related to the degree of plasma protein binding, because only the free, unbound drug is available for placental transfer. MARCAINE with a high protein binding capacity (95%) has a low fetal/maternal ratio (0.2 to 0.4). The extent of placental transfer is also determined by the degree of ionization and lipid solubility of the drug. Lipid soluble, nonionized drugs readily enter the fetal blood from the maternal circulation.

Depending upon the route of administration, local anesthetics are distributed to some extent to all body tissues, with high concentrations found in highly perfused organs such as the liver, lungs, heart, and brain.

Pharmacokinetic studies on the plasma profiles of MARCAINE after direct intravenous injection suggest a three-compartment open model. The first compartment is represented by the rapid intravascular distribution of the drug. The second compartment represents the equilibration of the drug throughout the highly perfused organs such as the brain, myocardium, lungs, kidneys, and liver. The third compartment represents an equilibration of the drug with poorly perfused tissues, such as muscle and fat. The elimination of drug from tissue distribution depends largely upon the ability of binding sites in the circulation to carry it to the liver where it is metabolized.

Various pharmacokinetic parameters of the local anesthetics can be significantly altered by the presence of hepatic or renal disease, addition of epinephrine, factors affecting urinary pH, renal blood flow, the route of drug administration, and the age of the patient. The half-life of MARCAINE in adults is 2.7 hours and in neonates 8.1 hours. Amide-type local anesthetics such as MARCAINE are metabolized primarily in the liver via conjugation with glucuronic acid. Patients with hepatic disease, especially those with severe hepatic disease, may be more susceptible to the potential toxicities of the amide-type local anesthetics. Pipecolylxylidine is the major metabolite of MARCAINE

The kidney is the main excretory organ for most local anesthetics and their metabolites. Urinary excretion is affected by urinary perfusion and factors affecting urinary pH. Only 6% of bupivacaine is excreted unchanged in the urine.

When administered in recommended doses and concentrations, MARCAINE does not ordinarily produce irritation or tissue damage and does not cause methemoglobinemia.

Indications and Usage: MARCAINE Spinal, brand of bupivacaine HCl, 0.75% with dextrose, 8.25% injection, is indicated for the production of subarachnoid block (spinal anesthesia).

Standard textbooks should be consulted to determine the accepted procedures and techniques for the administration of spinal anesthesia.

Contraindications: MARCAINE Spinal is contraindicated in patients with a known hypersensitivity to it or to any local anesthetic agent of the amide-type.

The following conditions preclude the use of spinal anesthesia:
1. Severe hemorrhage, severe hypotension or shock and arrhythmias, such as complete heart block, which severely restrict cardiac output.
2. Local infection at the site of proposed lumbar puncture.
3. Septicemia.

Warnings: LOCAL ANESTHETICS SHOULD ONLY BE EMPLOYED BY CLINICIANS WHO ARE WELL VERSED IN DIAGNOSIS AND MANAGEMENT OF DOSE-RELATED TOXICITY AND OTHER ACUTE EMERGENCIES WHICH MIGHT ARISE FROM THE BLOCK TO BE EMPLOYED, AND THEN ONLY AFTER IN- SURING THE **IMMEDIATE** AVAILABILITY OF OXYGEN, OTHER RESUSCITATIVE DRUGS, CARDIOPULMONARY RESUSCITATIVE EQUIPMENT, AND THE PERSONNEL RESOURCES NEEDED FOR PROPER MANAGEMENT OF TOXIC REACTIONS AND RELATED EMERGENCIES. (See also ADVERSE REACTIONS and PRECAUTIONS.) DELAY IN PROPER MANAGEMENT OF DOSE-RELATED TOXICITY, UNDERVENTILATION FROM ANY CAUSE AND/OR ALTERED SENSITIVITY MAY LEAD TO THE DEVELOPMENT OF ACIDOSIS, CARDIAC ARREST, AND, POSSIBLY, DEATH.

Spinal anesthetics should not be injected during uterine contractions, because spinal fluid current may carry the drug further cephalad than desired.

A free flow of cerebrospinal fluid during the performance of spinal anesthesia is indicative of entry into the subarachnoid space. However, aspiration should be performed before the anesthetic solution is injected to confirm entry into the subarachnoid space and to avoid intravascular injection.

MARCAINE solutions containing epinephrine or other vasopressors should not be used concomitantly with ergot-type oxytocic drugs, because a severe persistent hypertension may occur. Likewise, solutions of MARCAINE containing a vasoconstrictor, such as epinephrine, should be used with extreme caution in patients receiving monoamine oxidase inhibitors (MAOI) or antidepressants of the triptyline or imipramine types, because severe prolonged hypertension may result.

Until further experience is gained in patients younger than 18 years, administration of MARCAINE in this age group is not recommended.

Mixing or the prior or intercurrent use of any other local anesthetic with MARCAINE cannot be recommended because of insufficient data on the clinical use of such mixtures.

Precautions: *General:* The safety and effectiveness of spinal anesthetics depend on proper dosage, correct technique, adequate precautions, and readiness for emergencies. Resuscitative equipment, oxygen, and other resuscitative drugs should be available for immediate use. (See WARNINGS and ADVERSE REACTONS.) The patient should have IV fluids running via an indwelling catheter to assure a functioning intravenous pathway. The lowest dosage of local anesthetic that results in effective anesthesia should be used. Aspiration for blood should be performed before injection and injection should be made slowly. Tolerance varies with the status of the patient. Elderly patients and acutely ill patients may require reduced doses. Reduced doses may also be indicated in patients with increased intra-abdominal pressure (including obstetrical patients), if otherwise suitable for spinal anesthesia.

There should be careful and constant monitoring of cardiovascular and respiratory (adequacy of ventilation) vital signs and the patient's state of consciousness after local anesthetic injection. Restlessness, anxiety, incoherent speech, lightheadedness, numbness and tingling of the mouth and lips, metallic taste, tinnitus, dizziness, blurred vision, tremors, depression, or drowsiness may be early warning signs of central nervous system toxicity.

Spinal anesthetics should be used with caution in patients with severe disturbances of cardiac rhythm, shock, or heart block.

Sympathetic blockade occurring during spinal anesthesia may result in peripheral vasodilation and hypotension, the extent depending on the number of dermatomes blocked. Blood pressure should, therefore, be carefully monitored especially in the early phases of anesthesia. Hypotension may be controlled by vasoconstrictors in dosages depending on the severity of hypotension and response of treatment. The level of anesthesia should be carefully monitored because it is not always controllable in spinal techniques.

Because amide-type local anesthetics such as MARCAINE are metabolized by the liver, these drugs, especially repeat doses, should be used cautiously in patients with hepatic disease. Patients with severe hepatic disease, because of their in- ability to metabolize local anesthetics normally, are at a greater risk of developing toxic plasma concentrations. Local anesthetics should also be used with caution in patients with impaired cardiovascular function because they may be less able to compensate for functional changes associated with the prolongation of A-V conduction produced by these drugs. However, dosage recommendations for spinal anesthesia are much lower than dosage recommendations for other major blocks and most experience regarding hepatic and cardiovascular disease dose-related toxicity is derived from these other major blocks.

Serious dose-related cardiac arrhythmias may occur if preparations containing a vasoconstrictor such as epinephrine are employed in patients during or following the administration of potent inhalation agents. In deciding whether to use these products concurrently in the same patient, the combined action of both agents upon the myocardium, the concentration and volume of vasoconstrictor used, and the time since injection, when applicable, should be taken into account.

Many drugs used during the conduct of anesthesia are considered potential triggering agents for familial malignant hyperthermia. Because it is not known whether amide-type local anesthetics may trigger this reaction and because the need for supplemental general anesthesia cannot be predicted in advance, it is suggested that a standard protocol for management should be available. Early unexplained signs of tachycardia, tachypnea, labile blood pressure, and metabolic acidosis may precede temperature elevation. Successful outcome is dependent on early diagnosis, prompt discontinuance of the suspect triggering agent(s) and institution of treatment, including oxygen therapy, indicated supportive measures, and dantrolene. (Consult dantrolene sodium intravenous package insert before using.)

The following conditions may preclude the use of spinal anesthesia, depending upon the physician's evaluation of the situation and ability to deal with the complications or complaints which may occur:
- Preexisting diseases of the central nervous system, such as those attributable to pernicious anemia, poliomyelitis, syphilis, or tumor.
- Hematological disorders predisposing to coagulopathies or patients on anticoagulant therapy. Trauma to a blood vessel during the conduct of spinal anesthesia may, in some instances, result in uncontrollable central nervous system hemorrhage or soft tissue hemorrhage.
- Chronic backache and preoperative headache.
- Hypotension and hypertension.
- Technical problems (persistent paresthesias, persistent bloody tap).
- Arthritis or spinal deformity.
- Extremes of age.
- Psychosis or other causes of poor cooperation by the patient.

Information for Patients: When appropriate, patients should be informed in advance that they may experience temporary loss of sensation and motor activity, usually in the lower half of the body, following proper administration of spinal anesthesia. Also, when appropriate, the physician should discuss other information including adverse reactions in the MARCAINE Spinal package insert.

Clinically Significant Drug Interactions: The administration of local anesthetic solutions containing epinephrine or norepinephrine to patients receiving monoamine oxidase inhibitors or tricyclic antidepressants may produce severe, pro-

Continued on next page

This product information was effective as of December 3, 1984. On these and other products of Winthrop-Breon Laboratories, detailed information may be obtained on a current basis by direct inquiry to the Professional Services Department, 90 Park Avenue, New York, NY 10016 (212) 907-2525.

Winthrop-Breon—Cont.

longed hypertension. Concurrent use of these agents should generally be avoided. In situations when concurrent theapy is necessary, careful patient monitoring is essential.

Concurrent administration of vasopressor drugs and of ergot-type oxytocic drugs may cause severe persistent hypertension or cerebrovascular accidents.

Phenothiazines and butyrophenones may reduce or reverse the pressor effect of epinephrine.

Carcinogenesis, Mutagenesis, Impairment of Fertility: Long-term studies in animals of most local anesthetics including bupivacaine to evaluate the carcinogenic potential have not been conducted. Mutagenic potential or the effect on fertility have not been determined. There is no evidence from human data that MARCAINE Spinal, brand of bupivacaine HCl, 0.75% with dextrose, 8.25% injection, may be carcinogenic or mutagenic or that it impairs fertility.

Pregnancy Category C: Decreased pup survival in rats and an embryocidal effect in rabbits have been observed when bupivacaine hydrochloride was administered to these species in doses comparable to 230 and 130 times respectively the maximum recommended human spinal dose. There are no adequate and well-controlled studies in pregnant women of the effect of bupivacaine on the developing fetus. Bupivacaine hydrochloride should be used during pregnancy only if the potential benefit justifies the potential risk to the fetus. This does not exclude the use of MARCAINE Spinal at term for obstetrical anesthesia. (See **Labor and Delivery.**)

Labor and Delivery: Spinal anesthesia has a recognized use during labor and delivery. Bupivacaine hydrochloride, when administered properly, via the epidural route in doses 10 to 12 times the amount used in spinal anesthesia has been used for obstetrical analgesia and anesthesia without evidence of adverse effects on the fetus.

Maternal hypotension has resulted from regional anesthesia. Local anesthetics produce vasodilation by blocking sympathetic nerves. Elevating the patient's legs and positioning her on her left side will help prevent decreases in blood pressure. The fetal heart rate also should be monitored continuously and electronic fetal monitoring is highly advisable.

It is extremely important to avoid aortocaval compression by the gravid uterus during administrations of regional block to parturients. To do this, the patient must be maintained in the left lateral decubitus position or a blanket roll or sandbag may be placed beneath the right hip and the gravid uterus displaced to the left.

Spinal anesthesia may alter the forces of parturition through changes in uterine contractility or maternal expulsive efforts. Spinal anesthesia has also been reported to prolong the second stage of labor by removing the parturient's reflex urge to bear down or by interfering with motor function. The use of obstetrical anesthesia may increase the need for forceps assistance.

The use of some local anesthetic drug products during labor and delivery may be followed by diminished muscle strength and tone for the first day or two of life. This has not been reported with bupivacaine.

There have been reports of cardiac arrest during use of MARCAINE 0.75% solution for epidural anesthesia in obstetrical patients. The package insert for MARCAINE hydrochloride for epidural, nerve block, etc, has a more complete discussion of preparation for, and management of, this problem. These cases are compatible with systemic toxicity following unintended intravascular injection of the much larger doses recommended for epidural anesthesia and have not occurred within the dose range of bupivacaine hydrochloride 0.75% recommended for spinal anesthesia in obstetrics. The 0.75% concentration of MARCAINE is therefore not recommended for obstetrical epidural anesthesia. MARCAINE Spinal (bupivacaine HCl 0.75% with dextrose 8.25%) is recommended for spinal anesthesia in obstetrics.

Nursing Mothers: It is not known whether local anesthetic drugs are excreted in human milk. Because many drugs are excreted in human milk, caution should be exercised when local anesthetics are administered to a nursing woman.

Pediatric Use: Until further experience is gained in patients younger than 18 years, administration of MARCAINE Spinal in this age group is not recommended.

Adverse Reactions: Reactions to bupivacaine are characteristic of those associated with other amide-type local anesthetics.

The most commonly encountered acute adverse experiences which demand immediate countermeasures following the administration of spinal anesthesia are hypotension due to loss of sympathetic tone and respiratory paralysis or underventilation due to cephalad extension of the motor level of anesthesia. These may lead to cardiac arrest if untreated. In addition, dose-related convulsions and cardiovascular collapse may result from diminished tolerance, rapid absorption from the injection site, or from unintentional intravascular injection of a local anesthetic solution. Factors influencing plasma protein binding, such as acidosis, systemic diseases which alter protein production, or competition of other drugs for protein binding sites, may diminish individual tolerance.

Respiratory System: Respiratory paralysis or underventilation may be noted as a result of upward extension of the level of spinal anesthesia and may lead to secondary hypoxic cardiac arrest if untreated. Preanesthetic medication, intraoperative analgesics and sedatives, as well as surgical manipulation, may contribute to underventilation. This will usually be noted within minutes of the injection of spinal anesthetic solution, but because of differing maximal onset times, differing intercurrent drug usage and differing surgical manipulation, it may occur at any time during surgery or the immediate recovery period.

Cardiovascular System: Hypertension due to loss of sympathetic tone is a commonly encountered extension of the clinical pharmacology of spinal anesthesia. This is more commonly observed in patients with shrunken blood volume, shrunken interstitial fluid volume, cephalad spread of the local anesthetic, and/or mechanical obstruction of venous return. Nausea and vomiting are frequently associated with hypotensive episodes following the administration of spinal anesthesia. High doses, or inadvertent intravascular injection, may lead to high plasma levels and related depression of the myocardium, decreased cardiac output, bradycardia, heart block, ventricular arrhythmias, and, possibly, cardiac arrest. (See **WARNINGS, PRECAUTIONS,** and **OVERDOSAGE** sections.)

Central Nervous System: Respiratory paralysis or underventilation secondary to cephalad spread of the level of spinal anesthesia (See *Respiratory System*) and hypotension for the same reason (see *Cardiovascular System*) are the two most commonly encountered central nervous system-related adverse observations which demand immediate countermeasures.

High doses or inadvertent intravascular injection may lead to high plasma levels and related central nervous sytem toxicity characterized by excitement and/or depression. Restlessness, anxiety, dizziness, tinnitus, blurred vision, or tremors may occur, possibly proceeding to convulsions. However, excitement may be transient or absent, with depression being the first manifestation of an adverse reaction. This may quickly be followed by drowsiness merging into unconsciousness and respiratory arrest.

Neurologic: The incidences of adverse neurologic reactions associated with the use of local anesthetics may be related to the total dose of local anesthetic administered and are also dependent upon the particular drug used, the route of administration, and the physical status of the patient. Many of these effects may be related to local anesthetic techniques, with or without a contribution from the drug.

Neurologic effects following spinal anesthesia may include loss of perineal sensation and sexual function; persistent anesthesia, paresthesia, weakness and paralysis of the lower extremities, and loss of sphincter control all of which may have slow, incomplete, or no recovery; hypotension; high or total spinal block; urinary retention; headache; backache; septic meningitis; meningismus; arachnoiditis; slowing of labor; increased incidence of forceps delivery; shivering; cranial nerve palsies due to traction on nerves from loss of cerebrospinal fluid; and fecal and urinary incontinence.

Allergic: Allergic-type reactions are rare and may occur as a result of sensitivity to the local anesthetic. These reactions are characterized by signs such as urticaria, pruritus, erythema, angioneurotic edema (including laryngeal edema), tachycardia, sneezing, nausea, vomiting, dizziness, syncope, excessive sweating, elevated temperature, and, possibly, anaphylactoid-like symptomatology (including severe hpotension). Cross sensitivity among members of the amide-type local anesthetic group has been reported. The usefulness of screening for sensitivity has not been definitely established.

Other: Nausea and vomiting may occur during spinal anesthesia.

Overdosage: Acute emergencies from local anesthetics are generally related to high plasma levels encountered during therapeutic use or to underventilation (and perhaps apnea) secondary to upward extension of spinal anesthesia. Hypotension is commonly encountered during the conduct of spinal anesthesia due to relaxation of sympathetic tone, and sometimes, contributory mechanical obstruction of venous return.

Management of Local Anesthetic Emergencies: - The first consideration is prevention, best accomplished by careful and constant monitoring of cardiovascular and respiratory vital signs and the patient's state of consciousness after each local anesthetic injection. At the first sign of change, oxygen should be administered.

*The first step in the management of systemic toxic reactions, as well as underventilation or apnea due to a high or total spinal, consists of **immediate** attention to the establishment and maintenance of a patent airway and effective assisted or controlled ventilation with 100% oxygen with a delivery system capable of permitting immediate positive airway pressure by mask. This may prevent convulsions if they have not already occurred.*

If necessary, use drugs to control the convulsions. A 50 mg to 100 mg bolus IV injection of succinylcholine will paralyze the patient without depressing the central nervous or cardiovascular systems and facilitate ventilation. A bolus IV dose of 5 mg to 10 mg of diazepam or 50 mg to 100 mg of thiopental will permit ventilation and counteract central nervous system stimulation, but these drugs also depress central nervous system, respiratory and cardiac function, add to postictal depression and may result in apnea. Intravenous barbiturates, anticonvulsant agents, or muscle relaxants should only be administered by those familiar with their use. Immediately after the institution of these ventilatory measures, the adequacy of the circulation should be evaluated. Supportive treatment of circulatory depression may require administration of intravenous fluids, and, when appropriate, a vasopressor dictated by the clinical situation (such as ephedrine or epinephrine to enhance myocardial contractile force).

Hypotension due to sympathetic relaxation may be managed by giving intravenous fluids (such as isotonic saline or lactated Ringer's solution), in an attempt to relieve mechanical obstruction of venous return, or by using vasopressors (such as ephedrine which increases the force of myocardial contractions) and, if indicated, by giving plasma expanders or whole blood.

Endotracheal intubation, employing drugs and techniques familiar to the clinician, may be indicated after initial administration of oxygen by mask if difficulty is encountered in the maintenance of a patent airway, or if prolonged ventilatory support (assisted or controlled) is indicated.

Recent clinical data from patients experiencing local anesthetic-induced convulsions demonstrated rapid development of hypoxia, hypercarbia, and acidosis with bupivacaine within a minute of the onset of convulsions. These observations suggest that oxygen consumption and carbon dioxide production are greatly increased during local anesthetic convulsions and emphasize the importance of immediate and effective ventilation with oxygen which may avoid cardiac arrest.

If not treated immediately, convulsions with simultaneous hypoxia, hypercarbia, and acidosis plus myocardial depression from the direct effects of the local anesthetic may result in cardiac arrhythmias, bradycardia, asystole, ventricular fibrillation, or cardiac arrest. Respiratory abnormalities, including apnea, may occur. Underventilation or apnea due to a high or total spinal may produce these same signs and also lead to cardiac arrest if ventilatory support is not instituted. If cardiac arrest should occur, standard cardiopulmonary resuscitative measures should be instituted and maintained for a prolonged period if necessary. Recovery has been reported after prolonged resuscitative efforts.

The supine position is dangerous in pregnant women at term because of aortocaval compression by the gravid uterus. Therefore during treatment of systemic toxicity, maternal hypotension, or fetal bradycardia following regional block, the parturient should be maintained in the left lateral decubitus position if possible, or manual displacement of the uterus off the great vessels be accomplished.

The mean seizure dosage of bupivacaine in rhesus monkeys was found to be 4.4 mg/kg with mean arterial plasma concentration of 4.5 mcg/mL. The intravenous and subcutaneous LD_{50} in mice is 6 mg/kg to 8 mg/kg and 38 mg/kg to 54 mg/kg respectively.

Dosage and Administration: The dose of any local anesthetic administered varies with the anesthetic procedure, the area to be anesthetized, the vascularity of the tissues, the number of neuronal segments to be blocked, the depth of anesthesia and degree of muscle relaxation required, the duration of anesthesia desired, individual tolerance, and the physical condition of the patient. The smallest dose and concentration required to produce the desired result should be administered. Dosages of MARCAINE Spinal, brand of bupivacaine HCl, 0.75% with dextrose, 8.25% injection, should be reduced for elderly and debilitated patients and patients with cardiac and/or liver disease.

For specific techniques and procedures, refer to standard textbooks.

The extent and degree of spinal anesthesia depend upon several factors including dosage, specific gravity of the anesthetic solution, volume of solution used, force of injection, level of puncture, and position of the patient during and immediately after injection.

Seven and one-half mg (7.5 mg or 1.0 mL) MARCAINE Spinal has generally proven satisfactory for spinal anesthesia for lower extremity and perineal procedures including TURP and vaginal hysterectomy. Twelve mg (12.0 mg or 1.6 mL) has been used for lower abdominal procedures such as abdominal hysterectomy, tubal ligation, and appendectomy. These doses are recommended as a guide for use in the average adult and may be reduced for the elderly or debilitated patients. Because experience with MARCAINE Spinal is limited in patients below the age of 18 years, dosage recommendations in this age group cannot be made.

Obstetrical Use: Doses as low as 6 mg bupivacaine hydrochloride have been used for vaginal delivery under spinal anesthesia. The dose range of 7.5 mg to 10.5 mg (1 mL to 1.4 mL) bupivacaine hydrochloride has been used for Cesarean section under spinal anesthesia.

In recommended doses, MARCAINE Spinal produces complete motor and sensory block.

Unused portions of solutions should be discarded following initial use.

MARCAINE Spinal should be inspected visually for discoloration and particulate matter prior to administration; solutions which are discolored or which contain particulate matter should not be administered.

How Supplied: Single-dose ampuls of 2 mL (15 mg bupivacaine hydrochloride with 165 mg dextrose), in Uni-Nest™ Unit Dose Pak of 10 (NDC 0024-1229-10)

Store at controlled room temperature, between 15°C and 30°C (59°F and 86°F).

MARCAINE Spinal solution may be autoclaved once at 15 pound pressure, 121°C (250°F) for 15 minutes. Do not administer any solution which is discolored or contains particulate matter.

MW-246

MEBARAL®
(brand of mephobarbital tablets)

Description: Mephobarbital, 5-Ethyl-1-methyl-5-phenylbarbituric acid, is a barbiturate with sedative, hypnotic, and anticonvulsant properties. It occurs as a white, nearly odorless, tasteless powder and is slightly soluble in water and in alcohol. MEBARAL is available as tablets for oral administration.

Clinical Pharmacology: Barbiturates are capable of producing all levels of CNS mood alteration from excitation to mild sedation, to hypnosis, and deep coma. Overdosage can produce death. In high enough therapeutic doses, barbiturates induce anesthesia.

Barbiturates depress the sensory cortex, decrease motor activity, alter cerebellar function, and produce drowsiness, sedation, and hypnosis.

Barbiturates are respiratory depressants. The degree of respiratory depression is dependent upon dose. With hypnotic doses, respiratory depression produced by barbiturates is similar to that which occurs during physiologic sleep with slight decrease in blood pressure and heart rate.

Studies in laboratory animals have shown that barbiturates cause reduction in the tone and contractility of the uterus, ureters, and urinary bladder. However, concentrations of the drugs required to produce this effect in humans are not reached with sedative-hypnotic doses.

Barbiturates do not impair normal hepatic function, but have been shown to induce liver microsomal enzymes, thus increasing and/or altering the metabolism of barbiturates and other drugs. (See PRECAUTIONS—DRUG INTERACTIONS.)

MEBARAL exerts a strong sedative and anticonvulsant action but has a relatively mild hypnotic effect. It reduces the incidence of epileptic seizures in grand mal and petit mal. MEBARAL usually causes little or no drowsiness or lassitude. Hence, when it is used as a sedative or anticonvulsant, patients usually become more calm, more cheerful, and better adjusted to their surroundings without clouding of mental faculties. MEBARAL is reported to produce less sedation than does phenobarbital.

Barbiturates are weak acids that are absorbed and rapidly distributed to all tissues and fluids with high concentrations in the brain, liver, and kidneys. Lipid solubility of the barbiturates is the dominant factor in their distribution within the body. Barbiturates are bound to plasma and tissue proteins to a varying degree with the degree of binding increasing directly as a function of lipid solubility.

Approximately 50% of an oral dose of mephobarbital is absorbed from the gastrointestinal tract. Therapeutic plasma concentrations for mephobarbital have not been established nor has the half-life been determined. Following oral administration, the onset of action of the drug is 30 to 60 minutes and the duration of action is 10 to 16 hours. The primary route of mephobarbital metabolism is N-demethylation by the microsomal enzymes of the liver to form phenobarbital. Phenobarbital may be excreted in the urine unchanged or further metabolized to *p*-hydroxyphenobarbital and excreted in the urine as glucuronide or sulfate conjugates. About 75% of a single oral dose of mephobarbital is converted to phenobarbital in 24 hours. Therefore, chronic administration of mephobarbital may lead to an accumulation of phenobarbital (not mephobarbital) in plasma. It has not been determined whether mephobarbital or phenobarbital is the active agent during long-time mephobarbital therapy.

Indications and Usage: MEBARAL is indicated for use as a sedative for the relief of anxiety, tension and apprehension, and as an anticonvulsant for the treatment of grand mal and petit mal epilepsy.

Contraindications: Hypersensitivity to any barbiturate. Manifest or latent porphyria.

Warnings: 1. *Habit forming.* Barbiturates may be habit forming. Tolerance, psychological and physical dependence may occur with continued use. (See DRUG ABUSE AND DEPENDENCE and CLINICAL PHARMACOLOGY.) Patients who have psychological dependence on barbiturates may increase the dosage or decrease the dosage interval without consulting a physician and may subsequently develop a physical dependence on barbiturates. To minimize the possibility of overdosage or the development of dependence, the prescribing and dispensing of sedative-hypnotic barbiturates should be limited to the amount required for the interval until the next appointment. Abrupt cessation after prolonged use in the dependent person may result in withdrawal symptoms, including delirium, convulsions, and possibly death. Barbiturates should be withdrawn gradually from any patient known to be taking excessive dosage over long periods of time. (See DRUG ABUSE AND DEPENDENCE.)

2. *Acute or chronic pain.* Caution should be exercised when barbiturates are administered to patients with acute or chronic pain, because paradoxical excitement could be induced or important symptoms could be masked. However, the use of barbiturates as sedatives in the postoperative surgical period and as adjuncts to cancer chemotherapy is well established.

3. *Use in pregnancy.* Barbiturates can cause fetal damage when administered to a pregnant woman. Retrospective, case-controlled studies have suggested a connection between the maternal consumption of barbiturates and a higher than expected incidence of fetal abnormalities. Following oral or parenteral administration, barbiturates readily cross the placental barrier and are distributed throughout fetal tissues with highest concentrations found in the placenta, fetal liver, and brain. Fetal blood levels approach maternal blood levels following parenteral administration.

Withdrawal symptoms occur in infants born to mothers who receive barbiturates throughout the last trimester of pregnancy. (See DRUG ABUSE AND DEPENDENCE.) If this drug is used during pregnancy, or if the patient becomes pregnant while taking this drug, the patient should be apprised of the potential hazard to the fetus.

4. *Synergistic effects.* The concomitant use of alcohol or other CNS depressants may produce additive CNS depressant effects.

Precautions: *General.* Barbiturates may be habit forming. Tolerance and psychological and physical dependence may occur with continuing use. (See DRUG ABUSE AND DEPENDENCE.) Barbiturates should be administered with caution, if at all, to patients who are mentally depressed, have suicidal tendencies, or a history of drug abuse.

Elderly or debilitated patients may react to barbiturates with marked excitement, depression, and confusion. In some persons, barbiturates repeatedly produce excitement rather than depression.

Continued on next page

This product information was effective as of December 3, 1984. On these and other products of Winthrop-Breon Laboratories, detailed information may be obtained on a current basis by direct inquiry to the Professional Services Department, 90 Park Avenue, New York, NY 10016 (212) 907-2525.

Winthrop-Breon—Cont.

In patients with hepatic damage, barbiturates should be administered with caution and initially in reduced doses. Barbiturates should not be administered to patients showing the premonitory signs of hepatic coma.

Status epilepticus may result from the abrupt discontinuation of MEBARAL, even when administered in small daily doses in the treatment of epilepsy.

Caution and careful adjustment of dosage are required when MEBARAL, brand of mephobarbital tablets, is used in patients with impaired renal, cardiac, or respiratory function and in patients with myasthenia gravis and myxedema. The least quantity feasible should be prescribed or dispensed at any one time in order to minimize the possibility of acute or chronic overdosage.

Vitamin D Deficiency: MEBARAL may increase vitamin D requirements, possibly by increasing vitamin D metabolism via enzyme induction. Rarely, rickets and osteomalacia have been reported following prolonged use of barbiturates.

Vitamin K: Bleeding in the early neonatal period due to coagulation defects may follow exposure to anticonvulsant drugs *in utero;* therefore, vitamin K should be given to the mother before delivery or to the child at birth.

Information for the patient: Practitioners should give the following information and instructions to patients receiving barbiturates.
1. The use of barbiturates carries with it an associated risk of psychological and/or physical dependence. The patient should be warned against increasing the dose of the drug without consulting a physician.
2. Barbiturates may impair mental and/or physical abilities required for the performance of potentially hazardous tasks (eg, driving, operating machinery, etc).
3. Alcohol should not be consumed while taking barbiturates. Concurrent use of the barbiturates with other CNS depressants (eg, alcohol, narcotics, tranquilizers, and antihistamines) may result in additional CNS depressant effects.

Laboratory tests. Prolonged therapy with barbiturates should be accompanied by periodic laboratory evaluation or organ systems, including hematopoietic, renal, and hepatic systems. (See PRECAUTIONS [*General*] and ADVERSE REACTIONS.)

Drug interactions. Most reports of clinically significant drug interactions occurring with the barbiturates have involved phenobarbital. However, the application of these data to other barbiturates appears valid and warrants serial blood level determinations of the relevant drugs when there are multiple therapies.

1. *Anticoagulants.* Phenobarbital lowers the plasma levels of dicumarol (name previously used: bishydroxycoumarin) and causes a decrease in anticoagulant activity as measured by the prothrombin time. Barbiturates can induce hepatic microsomal enzymes resulting in increased metabolism and decreased anticoagulant response of oral anticoagulants (eg, warfarin, acenocoumarol, dicumarol, and phenprocoumon). Patients stablized on anticoagulant therapy may require dosage adjustments if barbiturates are added to or withdrawn from their dosage regimen.

2. *Corticosteroids.* Barbiturates appear to enhance the metabolism of exogenous corticosteroids probably through the induction of hepatic microsomal enzymes. Patients stabilized on corticosteroid therapy may require dosage adjustments if barbiturates are added to or withdrawn from their dosage regimen.

3. *Griseofulvin.* Phenobarbital appears to interfere with the absorption of orally administered griseofulvin, thus decreasing its blood level. The effect of the resultant decreased blood levels of griseofulvin on therapeutic response has not been established. However, it would be preferable to avoid concomitant administration of these drugs.

4. *Doxycycline.* Phenobarbital has been shown to shorten the half-life of doxycycline for as long as 2 weeks after barbiturate therapy is discontinued. This mechanism is probably through the induction of hepatic microsomal enzymes that metabolize the antibiotic. If phenobarbital and doxycycline are administered concurrently, the clinical response to doxycycline should be monitored closely.

5. *Phenytoin, sodium valproate, valproic acid.* The effect of barbiturates on the metabolism of phenytoin appears to be variable. Some investigators report an accelerating effect, while others report no effect. Because the effect of barbiturates on the metabolism of phenytoin is not predictable, phenytoin and barbiturate blood levels should be monitored more frequently if these drugs are given concurrently. Sodium valproate and valproic acid appear to decrease barbiturate metabolism; therefore, barbiturate blood levels should be monitored and appropriate dosage adjustments made as indicated.

6. *Central nervous system depressants.* The concomitant use of other central nervous system depressants, including other sedatives or hypnotics, antihistamines, tranquilizers, or alcohol, may produce additive depressant effects.

7. *Monoamine oxidase inhibitors (MAOI).* MAOI prolong the effects of barbiturates probably because metabolism of the barbiturate is inhibited.

8. *Estradiol, estone, progesterone and other steroidal hormones.* Pretreatment with or concurrent administration of phenobarbital may decrease the effect of estradiol by increasing its metabolism. There have been reports of patients treated with antiepileptic drugs (eg, phenobarbital) who become pregnant while taking oral contraceptives. An alternate contraceptive method might be suggested to women taking phenobarbital.

Carcinogenesis
1. *Animal data.* Phenobarbital sodium is carcinogenic in mice and rats after lifetime administration. In mice, it produced benign and malignant liver cell tumors. In rats, benign liver cell tumors were observed very late in life. Phenobarbital is the major metabolite of MEBARAL.
2. *Human data.* In a 29-year epidemiological study of 9136 patients who were treated on an anticonvulsant protocol which included phenobarbital, results indicated a higher than normal incidence of hepatic carcinoma. Previously, some of these patients were treated with thorotrast, a drug which is known to produce hepatic carcinomas. Thus, this study did not provide sufficient evidence that phenobarbital sodium is carcinogenic in humans. Phenobarbital is the major metabolite of MEBARAL, brand of mephobarbital tablets.

A retrospective study of 84 children with brain tumors matched to 73 normal controls and 78 cancer controls (malignant disease other than brain tumors) suggested an association between exposure to barbiturates prenatally and an increased incidence of brain tumors.

Pregnancy
1. *Teratogenic effects.* Pregnancy Category D—See WARNINGS—Use in Pregnancy above.
2. *Nonteratogenic effects.* Reports of infants suffering from long-term barbiturate exposure *in utero* included the acute withdrawal syndrome of seizures and hyperirritability from birth to a delayed onset of up to 14 days. (See DRUG ABUSE AND DEPENDENCE.)

Labor and delivery. Hypnotic doses of these barbiturates do not appear to significantly impair uterine activity during labor. Full anesthetic doses of barbiturates decrease the force and frequency of uterine contractions. Administration of sedative-hypnotic barbiturates to the mother during labor may result in respiratory depression in the newborn. Premature infants are particularly susceptible to the depressant effects of barbiturates. If barbiturates are used during labor and delivery, resuscitation equipment should be available.

Data are currently not available to evaluate the effect of these barbiturates when forceps delivery or other intervention is necessary. Also, data are not available to determine the effect of these barbiturates on the later growth, development, and functional maturation of the child.

Nursing Mothers. Caution should be exercised when a barbiturate is administered to a nursing woman since small amounts of barbiturates are excreted in the milk.

Adverse Reactions: The following adverse reactions and their incidence were compiled from surveillance of thousands of hospitalized patients. Because such patients may be less aware of certain of the milder adverse effects of barbiturates, the incidence of these reactions may be somewhat higher in fully ambulatory patients.

More than 1 in 100 patients. The most common adverse reactions estimated to occur at a rate of 1 to 3 patients per 100 is:
Nervous system: Somnolence.

Less than 1 in 100 patients. Adverse reactions estimated to occur at a rate of less than 1 in 100 patients listed below, grouped by organ system, and by decreasing order of occurrence are:
Nervous system: Agitation, confusion, hyperkinesia, ataxia, CNS depression, nightmares, nervousness, psychiatric disturbance, hallucinations, insomnia, anxiety, dizziness, thinking abnormality.
Respiratory system: Hypoventilation, apnea.
Cardiovascular system: Bradycardia, hypotension, syncope.
Digestive system: Nausea, vomiting, constipation.
Other reported reactions: Headache, hypersensitivity reactions (angioedema, skin rashes, exfoliative dermatitis), fever, liver damage, megaloblastic anemia following chronic phenobarbital use.

Drug Abuse and Dependence: Mephobarbital is a controlled substance in Narcotic Schedule IV. Barbiturates may be habit forming. Tolerance, psychological dependence, and physical dependence may occur especially following prolonged use of high doses of barbiturates. As tolerance to barbiturates develops, the amount needed to maintain the same level of intoxication increases; tolerance to a fatal dosage, however, does not increase more than two-fold. As this occurs, the margin between an intoxicating dosage and fatal dosage becomes smaller.

Symptoms of acute intoxication with barbiturates include unsteady gait, slurred speech, and sustained nystagmus. Mental signs of chronic intoxication include confusion, poor judgment, irritability, insomnia, and somatic complaints.

Symptoms of barbiturate dependence are similar to those of chronic alcoholism. If an individual appears to be intoxicated with alcohol to a degree that is radically disproportionate to the amount of alcohol in his or her blood the use of barbiturates should be suspected. The lethal dose of a barbiturate is far less if alcohol is also ingested.

The symptoms of barbiturate withdrawal can be severe and may cause death. Minor withdrawal symptoms may appear 8 to 12 hours after the last dose of a barbiturate. These symptoms usually appear in the following order: anxiety, muscle twitching, tremor of hands and fingers, progressive weakness, dizziness, distortion in visual perception, nausea, vomiting, insomnia, and orthostatic hypotension. Major withdrawal symptoms (convulsions and delirium) may occur within 16 hours and last up to 5 days after abrupt cessation of these drugs. Intensity of withdrawal symptoms gradually declines over a period of approximately 15 days. Individuals susceptible to a barbiturate abuse and dependence include alcoholics and opiate abusers, as well as other sedative-hypnotic and amphetamine abusers.

Drug dependence to barbiturates arises from repeated administration of a barbiturate or agent with barbiturate-like effect on a continuous basis, generally in amounts exceeding therapeutic dose levels. The characteristics of drug dependence to barbiturates include: (a) a strong desire or need to continue taking the drug; (b) a tendency to increase the dose; (c) a psychic dependence on the effects of the drug related to subjective and individual appreciation of those effects; and (d) a physical dependence on the effects of the drug requiring its presence for maintenance of homeostasis and resulting in a definite, characteristic, and self-limited abstinence syndrome when the drug is withdrawn.

Treatment of barbiturate dependence consists of cautious and gradual withdrawal of the drug. Barbiturate-dependent patients can be withdrawn by using a number of different withdrawal regimens. In all cases withdrawal takes an extended period of time. One method involves substituting a 30 mg dose of phenobarbital for each 100 mg to 200 mg dose of barbiturate that the patient has been taking. The total daily amount of phenobarbital is then administered in 3 to 4 divided doses, not to exceed 600 mg daily. Should signs of withdrawal occur on the first day of treatment, a loading dose of 100 mg to 200 mg of phenobarbital may be administered IM in addition to the oral dose. After stablization on phenobarbital, the total daily dose is decreased by 30 mg a day as long as withdrawal is proceeding smoothly. A modification of this regimen involves initiating treatment at the patient's regular dosage level and decreasing the daily dosage by 10% if tolerated by the patient.

Infants physically dependent on barbiturates may be given phenobarbital 3 mg/kg/day to 10 mg/kg/day. After withdrawal symptoms (hyperactivity, disturbed sleep, tremors, hyperreflexia) are relieved, the dosage of phenobarbital should be gradually decreased and completely withdrawn over a 2-week period.

Overdosage: The toxic dose of barbiturates varies considerably. In general, an oral dose of 1 gram of most barbiturates produces serious poisoning in an adult. Death commonly occurs after 2 to 10 grams of ingested barbiturate. Barbiturate intoxication may be confused with alcoholism, bromide intoxication, and with various neurological disorders.

Acute overdosage with barbiturates is manifested by CNS and respiratory depression which may progress to Cheyne-Stokes respiration, areflexia, constriction of the pupils to a slight degree (though in severe poisoning they may show paralytic dilation), oliguria, tachycardia, hypotension, lowered body temperature, and coma. Typical shock syndrome (apnea, circulatory collapse, respiratory arrest, and death) may occur.

In extreme overdose, all electrical activity in the brain may cease, in which case a "flat" EEG normally equated with clinical death cannot be accepted. This effect is fully reversible unless hypoxic damage occurs. Consideration should be given to the possibility of barbiturate intoxication even in situations that appear to involve trauma.

Complications such as pneumonia, pulmonary edema, cardiac arrhythmias, congestive heart failure, and renal failure may occur. Uremia may increase CNS sensitivity to barbiturates if renal function is impaired. Differential diagnosis should include hypoglycemia, head trauma, cerebrovascular accidents, convulsive states, and diabetic coma.

Treatment of overdosage is mainly supportive and consists of the following:
1. Maintenance of an adequate airway, with assisted respiration and oxygen administration as necessary.
2. Monitoring of vital signs and fluid balance.
3. If the patient is conscious and has not lost the gag reflex, emesis may be induced with ipecac. Care should be taken to prevent pulmonary aspiration of vomitus. After completion of vomiting, 30 grams activated charcoal in a glass of water may be administered.
4. If emesis is contraindicated, gastric lavage may be performed with a cuffed endotracheal tube in place with the patient in the face down position. Activated charcoal may be left in the emptied stomach and a saline cathartic administered.
5. Fluid therapy and other standard treatment for shock, if needed.
6. If renal function is normal, forced diuresis may aid in the elimination of the barbiturate. Alkalinization of the urine increases renal excretion of some barbiturates, including mephobarbital (which is metabolized to phenobarbital).
7. Although not recommended as a routine procedure, hemodialysis may be used in severe barbiturate intoxications or if the patient is anuric or in shock.
8. Patient should be rolled from side to side every 30 minutes.
9. Antibiotics should be given if pneumonia is suspected.
10. Appropriate nursing care to prevent hypostatic pneumonia, decubiti aspiration, and other complications of patients with altered states of consciousness.

Dosage and Administration: Epilepsy: Average dose for adults: 400 mg to 600 mg (6 grains to 9 grains) daily; children under 5 years: 16 mg to 32 mg ($\frac{1}{4}$ grain to $\frac{1}{2}$ grain) three or four times daily; children over 5 years: 32 mg to 64 mg ($\frac{1}{2}$ grain to 1 grain) three or four times daily. MEBARAL is best taken at bedtime if seizures generally occur at night, and during the day if attacks are diurnal. Treatment should be started with a small dose which is gradually increased over four or five days until the optimum dosage is determined. If the patient has been taking some other antiepileptic drug, it should be tapered off as the doses of MEBARAL are increased, to guard against the temporary marked attacks that may occur when any treatment for epilepsy is changed abruptly. Similarly, when the dose is to be lowered to a maintenance level or to be discontinued, the amount should be reduced gradually over four or five days.

Special patient population. Dosage should be reduced in the elderly or debilitated because these patients may be more sensitive to barbiturates. Dosage should be reduced for patients with impaired renal function or hepatic disease.

Combination with Other Drugs: MEBARAL may be used in combination with phenobarbital, either in the form of alternating courses or concurrently. When the two drugs are used at the same time, the dose should be about one-half the amount of each used alone. The average daily dose for an adult is from 50 mg to 100 mg ($\frac{3}{4}$ grain to $1\frac{1}{2}$ grains) of phenobarbital and from 200 mg to 300 mg (3 grains to $4\frac{1}{2}$ grains) of MEBARAL, brand of mephobarbital tablets.

MEBARAL may also be used with phenytoin sodium; in some cases, combined therapy appears to give better results than either agent used alone, since phenytoin sodium is particularly effective for the psychomotor types of seizure but relatively ineffective for petit mal. When the drugs are employed concurrently, a reduced dose of phenytoin sodium is advisable, but the full dose of MEBARAL may be given. Satisfactory results have been obtained with an average daily dose of 230 mg ($3\frac{1}{2}$ grains) of phenytoin sodium plus about 600 mg (9 grains) of MEBARAL.

Sedation: Adults: 32 mg to 100 mg ($\frac{1}{2}$ grain to $1\frac{1}{2}$ grains)—optimum dose, 50 mg ($\frac{3}{4}$ grain)—three or four times daily. Children: 16 mg to 32 mg ($\frac{1}{4}$ grain to $\frac{1}{2}$ grain) three or four times daily.

How Supplied: Tablets:
32 mg ($\frac{1}{2}$ grain)—bottles of 250
(NDC 0024-1231-05)
32 mg ($\frac{1}{2}$ grain)—bottles of 1000
(NDC 0024-1231-08)
50 mg ($\frac{3}{4}$ grain)—bottles of 250
(NDC 0024-1232-05)
100 mg ($1\frac{1}{2}$ grains)—bottles of 250
(NDC 0024-1233-05)

Shown in Product Identification Section, page 444
MW-86-S

NegGram® Caplets® ℞
brand of nalidixic acid tablets, USP
NegGram® Suspension ℞
brand of nalidixic acid oral suspension, USP

Description: Nalidixic acid, an oral antibacterial agent, is 1-Ethyl-1,4-dihydro-7-methyl-4-oxo-1,8-naphthyridin-3-carboxylic acid. It is a pale yellow, crystalline substance and a very weak organic acid.

Clinical Pharmacology: NegGram has marked antibacterial activity against gram-negative bacteria including *Proteus mirabilis*, *P. morganii*, *P. vulgaris*, and *P. rettgeri*; *Escherichia coli*; Enterobacter (Aerobacter), and Klebsiella. Pseudomonas strains are generally resistant to the drug. NegGram is bactericidal and is effective over the entire urinary pH range. Conventional chromosomal resistance to NegGram taken in full dosage has been reported to emerge in approximately 2 to 14 percent of patients during treatment; however, bacterial resistance to NegGram has not been shown to be transferable via R factor.

Indications and Usage: NegGram is indicated for the treatment of urinary tract infections caused by susceptible gram-negative microorganisms, including the majority of Proteus strains, Klebsiella, Enterobacter (Aerobacter), and *E. coli*. Disc susceptibility testing with the 30 μg disc should be performed prior to administration of the drug, and during treatment if clinical response warrants.

Contraindications: NegGram is contraindicated in patients with known hypersensitivity to nalidixic acid and in patients with a history of convulsive disorders.

Warnings: CNS effects including brief convulsions, increased intracranial pressure, and toxic psychosis have been reported rarely. These have occurred in infants and children or in geriatric patients, usually from overdosage or in patients with predisposing factors, and have been completely and rapidly reversible upon discontinuation of the drug. If these reactions occur, NegGram should be discontinued and appropriate therapeutic measures instituted; only if rapid disappearance of CNS symptoms does not occur within 48 hours should diagnostic procedures involving risk to the patient be undertaken. (See Adverse Reactions and Overdosage.)

Precautions: Blood counts and renal and liver function tests should be performed periodically if treatment is continued for more than two weeks. NegGram should be used with caution in patients with liver disease, epilepsy, or severe cerebral arteriosclerosis. While caution should be used in patients with severe renal failure, therapeutic concentrations of NegGram in the urine, without increased toxicity due to drug accumulation in the blood, have been observed in patients on full dosage with creatinine clearances as low as 2 mL/minute to 8 mL/minute.

Patients should be cautioned to avoid undue exposure to direct sunlight while receiving NegGram. Therapy should be discontinued if photosensitivity occurs.

If bacterial resistance to NegGram emerges during treatment, it usually does so within 48 hours, permitting rapid change to another antimicrobial. Therefore, if the clinical response is unsatisfactory or if relapse occurs, cultures and sensitivity tests should be repeated. Underdosage with NegGram during initial treatment (with less than 4 g per day for adults) may predispose to emergence of bacterial resistance. (See Dosage and Administration.) Cross resistance between NegGram and other antimicrobials has been observed only with oxolinic acid.

Nalidixic acid may enhance the effects of oral anticoagulants, warfarin or bishydroxycoumarin, by displacing significant amounts from serum albumin binding sites.

When Benedict's or Fehling's solutions or Clinitest® Reagent Tablets are used to test the urine of

Continued on next page

This product information was effective as of December 3, 1984. On these and other products of Winthrop-Breon Laboratories, detailed information may be obtained on a current basis by direct inquiry to the Professional Services Department, 90 Park Avenue, New York, NY 10016 (212) 907-2525.

Winthrop-Breon—Cont.

patients taking NegGram, a false-positive reaction for glucose may be obtained, due to the liberation of glucuronic acid from the metabolites excreted. However, a colorimetric test for glucose based on an enzyme reaction (eg, with Clinistix® Reagent Strips or Tes-Tape®) does not give a false-positive reaction to the liberated glucuronic acid.

Incorrect values may be obtained for urinary 17-keto and ketogenic steroids in patients receiving NegGram, brand of nalidixic acid, because of an interaction between the drug and the m-dinitrobenzene used in the usual assay method. In such cases, the Porter-Silber test for 17-hydroxycorticoids may be used.

Usage in Prepubertal Children. Recent toxicological studies have shown that nalidixic acid and related drugs can produce erosions of the cartilage in weight-bearing joints and other signs of arthropathy in immature animals of most species tested. No such joint lesions have been reported in man to date. Nevertheless, until the significance of this finding is clarified, care should be exercised when prescribing this product for prepubertal children.

Usage in Pregnancy. Safe use of NegGram during the first trimester of pregnancy has not been established. However, the drug has been used during the last two trimesters without producing apparent ill effects in mother or child.

Adverse Reactions: Reactions reported after oral administration of NegGram include *CNS effects:* drowsiness, weakness, headache, and dizziness and vertigo. Reversible subjective visual disturbances without objective findings have occurred infrequently (generally with each dose during the first few days of treatment). These reactions include overbrightness of lights, change in color perception, difficulty in focusing, decrease in visual acuity, and double vision. They usually disappeared promptly when dosage was reduced or therapy was discontinued. Toxic psychosis or brief convulsions have been reported rarely, usually following excessive doses. In general, the convulsions have occurred in patients with predisposing factors such as epilepsy or cerebral arteriosclerosis. In infants and children receiving therapeutic doses of NegGram, increased intracranial pressure with bulging anterior fontanel, papilledema, and headache has occasionally been observed. A few cases of 6th cranial nerve palsy have been reported. Although the mechanisms of these reactions are unknown, the signs and symptoms usually disappeared rapidly with no sequelae when treatment was discontinued. *Gastrointestinal:* abdominal pain, nausea, vomiting, and diarrhea. *Allergic:* rash, pruritus, urticaria, angioedema, eosinophilia, arthralgia with joint stiffness and swelling, and rarely, anaphylactoid reaction. Photosensitivity reactions consisting of erythema and bullae on exposed skin surfaces usually resolve completely in 2 weeks to 2 months after NegGram is discontinued; however, bullae may continue to appear with successive exposures to sunlight or with mild skin trauma for up to 3 months after discontinuation of drug. (See Precautions.) *Other:* rarely, cholestasis, paresthesia, metabolic acidosis, thrombocytopenia, leukopenia, or hemolytic anemia, sometimes associated with glucose-6-phosphate dehydrogenase deficiency.

Dosage and Administration: *Adults.* The recommended dosage for initial therapy in adults is 1 g administered four times daily for one or two weeks (total daily dose, 4 g). For prolonged therapy, the total daily dose may be reduced to 2 g after the initial treatment period. Underdosage during initial treatment may predispose to emergence of bacterial resistance.

Children. Until further experience is gained, NegGram should not be administered to infants younger than three months. Dosage in children 12 years of age and under should be calculated on the basis of body weight. The recommended total daily dosage for initial therapy is 25 mg/lb/day (55 mg/kg/day), administered in four equally divided doses. For prolonged therapy, the total daily dose may be reduced to 15 mg/lb/day (33 mg/kg/day). NegGram Suspension or NegGram CAPLETS of 250 mg may be used. One 250 mg tablet is equivalent to one teaspoon (5 mL) of the Suspension.

Overdosage: *Manifestations:* Toxic psychosis, convulsions, increased intracranial pressure, or metabolic acidosis may occur in patients taking more than the recommended dosage. Vomiting, nausea, and lethargy may also occur following overdosage.

Treatment: Reactions are short-lived (two to three hours) because the drug is rapidly excreted. If overdosage is noted early, gastric lavage is indicated. If absorption has occurred, increased fluid administration is advisable and supportive measures such as oxygen and means of artificial respiration should be available. Although anticonvulsant therapy has not been used in the few instances of overdosage reported, it may be indicated in a severe case.

How Supplied:
Suspension (250 mg/5 mL tsp), raspberry flavored, bottles of 1 pint (NDC 0024-1318-06)
CAPLETS of 1 g, scored, bottles of 100 (NDC 0024-1323-04)
Unit Dose Pack of 100 (NDC 0024-1323-14)—10 strips of ten—1 g CAPLETS each
CAPLETS of 500 mg, scored, bottles of 56 (NDC 0024-1322-03), 500 (NDC 0024-1322-06), and 1000 (NDC 0024-1322-08)
Unit Dose Pack of 100 (NDC 0024-1322-14)–10 strips of ten-500 mg CAPLETS each
CAPLETS of 250 mg, scored, bottles of 56 (NDC 0024-1321-03)

Pharmacology: Following oral administration, NegGram, brand of nalidixic acid, is rapidly absorbed from the gastrointestinal tract, partially metabolized in the liver, and rapidly excreted through the kidneys. Unchanged nalidixic acid appears in the urine along with an active metabolite, hydroxynalidixic acid, which has antibacterial activity similar to that of nalidixic acid. Other metabolites include glucuronic acid conjugates of nalidixic acid and hydroxynalidixic acid, and the dicarboxylic acid derivative. The hydroxy metabolite represents 30 percent of the biologically active drug in the blood and 85 percent in the urine. Peak serum levels of active drug average approximately 20 µg to 40 µg per mL (90 percent protein bound), one to two hours after administration of a 1 g dose to a fasting normal individual, with a half-life of about 90 minutes. Peak urine levels of active drug average approximately 150 µg to 200 µg per mL, three to four hours after administration, with a half-life of about six hours. Approximately four percent of NegGram is excreted in the feces. Traces of nalidixic acid were found in blood and urine of an infant whose mother had received the drug during the last trimester of pregnancy.

Animal Pharmacology: NegGram (nalidixic acid) and related drugs have been shown to cause arthropathy in juvenile animals of most species tested. (See PRECAUTIONS.)

Hydroxynalidixic acid, the principal metabolite of NegGram, did not produce any oculotoxic effects at any dosage level in seven species of animals including three primate species. However, oral administration of this metabolite in high doses has been shown to have oculotoxic potential, namely in dogs and cats where it produced retinal degeneration upon prolonged administration leading, in some cases, to blindness.

In experiments with NegGram itself, little if any such activity could be elicited in either dogs or cats. Sensitivity to CNS side effects in these species limited the doses of NegGram that could be used; this factor, together with a low conversion rate to the hydroxy metabolite in these species, may explain the absence of these effects.

Shown in Product Identification Section, page 444

NW-375- I(O)

NEO—SYNEPHRINE®   OTC
oxymetazoline hydrochloride
12 HOUR

(See PDR For Nonprescription Drugs)

Long Acting
NEO–SYNEPHRINE® II   OTC
xylometazoline hydrochloride

(See PDR For Nonprescription Drugs)

NEO-SYNEPHRINE® Hydrochloride   ℞
brand of phenylephrine hydrochloride
injection, USP
1% INJECTION

Well-Tolerated Vasoconstrictor and Pressor

> **WARNING:** PHYSICIANS SHOULD COMPLETELY FAMILIARIZE THEMSELVES WITH THE COMPLETE CONTENTS OF THIS LEAFLET BEFORE PRESCRIBING NEO-SYNEPHRINE.

Description: NEO-SYNEPHRINE hydrochloride, brand of phenylephrine hydrochloride injection, is a vasoconstrictor and pressor drug chemically related to epinephrine and ephedrine.

NEO-SYNEPHRINE hydrochloride is a synthetic sympathomimetic agent in sterile form for parenteral injection. Chemically, phenylephrine hydrochloride is (−)-m-Hydroxy-α-[(methylamino)methyl] benzyl alcohol hydrochloride.

Clinical Pharmacology: NEO-SYNEPHRINE hydrochloride produces vasoconstriction that lasts longer than that of epinephrine and ephedrine. Responses are more sustained than those to epinephrine, lasting 20 minutes after intravenous and as long as 50 minutes after subcutaneous injection. Its action on the heart contrasts sharply with that of epinephrine and ephedrine, in that it slows the heart rate and increases the stroke output, producing no disturbance in the rhythm of the pulse.

Phenylephrine is a powerful postsynaptic alpha-receptor stimulant with little effect on the beta receptors of the heart. In therapeutic doses, it produces little if any stimulation of either the spinal cord or cerebrum. A singular advantage of this drug is the fact that repeated injections produce comparable effects.

The predominant actions of phenylephrine are on the cardiovascular system. Parenteral administration causes a rise in systolic and diastolic pressures in man and other species. Accompanying the pressor response to phenylephrine is a marked reflex bradycardia that can be blocked by atropine; after atropine, large doses of the drug increase the heart rate only slightly. In man, cardiac output is slightly decreased and peripheral resistance is considerably increased. Circulation time is slightly prolonged, and venous pressure is slightly increased; venous constriction is not marked. Most vascular beds are constricted; renal splanchnic, cutaneous, and limb blood flows are reduced but coronary blood flow is increased. Pulmonary vessels are constricted, and pulmonary arterial pressure is raised.

The drug is a powerful vasoconstrictor, with properties very similar to those of norepinephrine but almost completely lacking the chronotropic and inotropic actions on the heart. Cardiac irregularities are seen only very rarely even with large doses.

Indications and Usage: NEO-SYNEPHRINE is intended for the maintenance of an adequate level of blood pressure during spinal and inhalation anesthesia and for the treatment of vascular failure in shock, shocklike states, and drug-induced hypotension, or hypersensitivity. It is also employed to overcome paroxysmal supraventricular tachycardia, to prolong spinal anesthesia, and as a vasoconstrictor in regional analgesia.

Contraindications: NEO-SYNEPHRINE hydrochloride should not be used in patients with severe hypertension, ventricular tachycardia, or in patients who are hypersensitive to it.

Warnings: If used in conjunction with oxytocic drugs, the pressor effect of sympathomimetic pressor amines is potentiated (see Drug Interaction). The obstetrician should be warned that some oxytocic drugs may cause severe persistent hyperten-

sion and that even a rupture of a cerebral blood vessel may occur during the postpartum period.
Precautions: NEO-SYNEPHRINE hydrochloride should be employed only with extreme caution in elderly patients or in patients with hyperthyroidism, bradycardia, partial heart block, myocardial disease, or severe arteriosclerosis.
Drug Interactions—Vasopressors, particularly metaraminol, may cause serious cardiac arrhythmias during halothane anesthesia and therefore should be used only with great caution or not at all.
MAO Inhibitors—The pressor effect of sympathomimetic pressor amines is markedly potentiated in patients receiving monoamine oxidase inhibitors (MAOI). Therefore, when initiating pressor therapy in these patients, the initial dose should be small and used with due caution. The pressor response of adrenergic agents may also be potentiated by tricyclic antidepressants.
Carcinogenesis, Mutagenesis, Impairment of Fertility—No long-term animal studies have been done to evaluate the potential of NEO-SYNEPHRINE in these areas.
Pregnancy Category C—Animal reproduction studies have not been conducted with NEO-SYNEPHRINE. It is also not known whether NEO-SYNEPHRINE can cause fetal harm when administered to a pregnant woman or can affect reproduction capacity. NEO-SYNEPHRINE should be given to a pregnant woman only if clearly needed.
Labor and Delivery—If vasopressor drugs are either used to correct hypotension or added to the local anesthetic solution, the obstetrician should be cautioned that some oxytocic drugs may cause severe persistent hypertension and that even a rupture of a cerebral blood vessel may occur during the postpartum period (see WARNINGS).
Nursing Mother—It is not known whether this drug is excreted in human milk. Because many are excreted in human milk, caution should be exercised when NEO-SYNEPHRINE hydrochloride, brand of phenylephrine hydrochloride injection, is administered to a nursing woman.
Pediatric Use—To combat hypotension during spinal anesthesia in children, a dose of 0.5 mg to 1 mg per 25 pounds of body weight, administered subcutaneously or intramuscularly, is recommended.
Adverse Reactions: Headache, reflex bradycardia, excitability, restlessness, and rarely arrhythmias.
Overdosage: Overdosage may induce ventricular extrasystoles and short paroxysms of ventricular tachycardia, a sensation of fullness in the head and tingling of the extremities.
Should an excessive elevation of blood pressure occur, it may be immediately relieved by an α-adrenergic blocking agent, eg, phentolamine.
The oral LD_{50} in the rat is 350 mg/kg, in the mouse 120 mg/kg.
Dosage and Administration:
NEO-SYNEPHRINE is generally injected subcutaneously, intramuscularly, slowly intravenously, or in dilute solution as a continuous intravenous infusion. In patients with paroxysmal supraventricular tachycardia and, if indicated, in case of emergency, NEO-SYNEPHRINE is administered directly intravenously. The dose should be adjusted according to the pressor response.

Dosage Calculations

Dose Required	Use NEO-SYNEPHRINE 1%
10 mg	1 mL
5 mg	0.5 mL
1 mg	0.1 mL

For convenience in intermittent intravenous administration, dilute 1 mL NEO-SYNEPHRINE 1% with 9 mL Sterile Water for Injection, USP, to yield 0.1% NEO-SYNEPHRINE.

Dose Required	Use Diluted NEO-SYNEPHRINE (0.1%)
0.1 mg	0.1 mL
0.2 mg	0.2 mL
0.5 mg	0.5 mL

Mild or Moderate Hypotension
Subcutaneously or Intramuscularly: Usual dose, from 2 mg to 5 mg. Range, from 1 mg to 10 mg. Initial dose should not exceed 5 mg.
Intravenously: Usual dose, 0.2 mg. Range, from 0.1 mg to 0.5 mg. Initial dose should not exceed 0.5 mg.
Injections should not be repeated more often than every 10 to 15 minutes. A 5 mg intramuscular dose should raise blood pressure for one to two hours. A 0.5 mg intravenous dose should elevate the pressure for about 15 minutes.
Severe Hypotension and Shock—Including Drug-Related Hypotension
Blood volume depletion should always be corrected as fully as possible before any vasopressor is administered. When, as an emergency measure, intraaortic pressures must be maintained to prevent cerebral or coronary artery ischemia, NEO-SYNEPHRINE hydrochloride, brand of phenylephrine hydrochloride injection, can be administered before and concurrently with blood volume replacement.
Hypotension and occasionally severe shock may result from overdosage or idiosyncrasy following the administration of certain drugs, especially adrenergic and ganglionic blocking agents, rauwolfia and veratrum alkaloids, and phenothiazine tranquilizers. Patients who receive a phenothiazine derivative as preoperative medication are especially susceptible to these reactions. As an adjunct in the management of such episodes, NEO-SYNEPHRINE hydrochloride is a suitable agent for restoring blood pressure.
Higher initial and maintenance doses of NEO-SYNEPHRINE are required in patients with persistent or untreated severe hypotension or shock. Hypotension produced by powerful peripheral adrenergic blocking agents, chlorpromazine, or pheochromocytomectomy may also require more intensive therapy.
Continuous Infusion—Add 10 mg of the drug (1 mL of 1 percent solution) to 500 mL of Dextrose Injection, USP, or Sodium Chloride Injection, USP (providing a 1:50,000 solution). To raise the blood pressure rapidly, start the infusion at about 100 μg to 180 μg per minute (based on 20 drops per mL this would be 100 to 180 drops per minute). When the blood pressure is stabilized (at a low normal level for the individual), a maintenance rate of 40 μg to 60 μg per minute usually suffices (based on 20 drops per mL this would be 40 to 60 drops per minute). If the drop size of the infusion system varies from the 20 drops per mL, the dose must be adjusted accordingly.
If a prompt initial pressor response is not obtained, additional increments of NEO-SYNEPHRINE (10 mg or more) are added to the infusion bottle. The rate of flow is then adjusted until the desired blood pressure level is obtained. (In some cases, a more potent vasopressor, such as norepinephrine bitartrate, may be required.) Hypertension should be avoided. The blood pressure should be checked frequently. Headache and/or bradycardia may indicate hypertension. Arrhythmias are rare.
Spinal Anesthesia—Hypotension
Routine parenteral use of NEO-SYNEPHRINE has been recommended for the prophylaxis and treatment of hypotension during spinal anesthesia. It is best administered subcutaneously or intramuscularly three or four minutes before injection of the spinal anesthetic. The total requirement for high anesthetic levels is usually 3 mg, and for lower levels, 2 mg. For hypotensive emergencies during spinal anesthesia, NEO-SYNEPHRINE may be injected intravenously, using an initial dose of 0.2 mg. Any subsequent dose should not exceed the previous dose by more than 0.1 mg to 0.2 mg and no more than 0.5 mg should be administered in a single dose. To combat hypotension during spinal anesthesia in children, a dose of 0.5 mg to 1 mg per 25 pounds body weight, administered subcutaneously or intramuscularly, is recommended.
Prolongation of Spinal Anesthesia
The addition of 2 mg to 5 mg of NEO-SYNEPHRINE hydrochloride to the anesthetic solution increases the duration of motor block by as much as approximately 50 percent without any increase in the incidence of complications such as nausea, vomiting, or blood pressure disturbances.
Vasoconstrictor for Regional Analgesia
Concentrations about ten times those employed when epinephrine is used as a vasoconstrictor are recommended. The optimum strength is 1:20,000 (made by adding 1 mg of NEO-SYNEPHRINE hydrochloride to every 20 mL of local anesthetic solution). Some pressor responses can be expected when 2 mg or more are injected.
Paroxysmal Supraventricular Tachycardia
Rapid intravenous injection (within 20 to 30 seconds) is recommended; the initial dose should not exceed 0.5 mg, and subsequent doses, which are determined by the initial blood pressure response, should not exceed the preceding dose by more than 0.1 mg to 0.2 mg, and should never exceed 1 mg.
How Supplied:
Solution 1 percent
Each 1 mL contains 10 mg of NEO-SYNEPHRINE hydrochloride, 3.5 mg of sodium chloride, 4 mg of sodium citrate, 1 mg of citric acid monohydrate, and not more than 2 mg of sodium bisulfite.
Uni-Nest™ ampuls of mL , box of 25 (NDC 0024-1342-04).
CARPUJECT® Sterile Cartridge-Needle Units, 10 mg/mL (1 mL fill in 2 mL cartridge), 22-gauge, 1¼ inch needle, dispensing bins of 50 (NDC 0024-1340-02).
The air in all ampuls and Cartridge-Needle Units has been displaced by nitrogen gas.
Protect from light if removed from carton or dispensing bin.

NW-64-BB

NEO-SYNEPHRINE® Hydrochloride ℞
brand of phenylephrine hydrochloride
ophthalmic solution, USP
Vasoconstrictor and Mydriatic
SOLUTIONS 2.5% AND 10%
VISCOUS SOLUTION 10%

For Use in Ophthalmology

> WARNING: PHYSICIANS SHOULD COMPLETELY FAMILIARIZE THEMSELVES WITH THE COMPLETE CONTENTS OF THIS LEAFLET BEFORE PRESCRIBING NEO-SYNEPHRINE.

Description: NEO-SYNEPHRINE hydrochloride, brand of phenylephrine hydrochloride ophthalmic solution, is a sterile solution used as a vasoconstrictor and mydriatic for use in ophthalmology.
NEO-SYNEPHRINE hydrochloride is a synthetic sympathomimetic compound structurally similar to epinephrine and ephedrine.
Phenylephrine hydrochloride is (−)-m-Hydroxy-α-[(methylamino)methyl] benzyl alcohol hydrochloride.
Clinical Pharmacology:
NEO-SYNEPHRINE possesses predominantly α-adrenergic effects. In the eye, phenylephrine acts locally as a potent vasoconstrictor and mydriatic, by constricting ophthalmic blood vessels and the radial muscle of the iris.

Continued on next page

This product information was effective as of December 3, 1984. On these and other products of Winthrop-Breon Laboratories, detailed information may be obtained on a current basis by direct inquiry to the Professional Services Department, 90 Park Avenue, New York, NY 10016 (212) 907-2525.

Winthrop-Breon—Cont.

The ophthalmologic usefulness of NEO-SYNEPHRINE hydrochloride is due to its rapid effect and moderately prolonged action, as well as to the fact that it produces no compensatory vasodilatation.

The action of different concentrations of ophthalmic solutions of NEO-SYNEPHRINE hydrochloride is shown in the following table:

Strength of solution (%)	Mydriasis Maximal (minutes)	Recovery time (hours)	Paralysis of accommodation
2.5	15-60	3	trace
10	10-60	6	slight

Although rare, systemic absorption of sufficient quantities of phenylephrine may lead to systemic α-adrenergic effects, such as rise in blood pressure which may be accompanied by a reflex atropine-sensitive bradycardia.

Indications and Usage: NEO-SYNEPHRINE hydrochloride is recommended for use as a decongestant and vasoconstrictor and for pupil dilatation in uveitis (posterior synechiae), wide angle glaucoma, prior to surgery, refraction, ophthalmoscopic examination, and diagnostic procedures.

Contraindications: Ophthalmic solutions of NEO-SYNEPHRINE hydrochloride are contraindicated in persons with narrow angle glaucoma (and in those individuals who are hypersensitive to NEO-SYNEPHRINE). NEO-SYNEPHRINE hydrochloride 10 percent ophthalmic solutions are contraindicated in infants and in patients with aneurysms.

Warnings: There have been rare reports associating the use of NEO-SYNEPHRINE 10 percent ophthalmic solutions with the development of serious cardiovascular reactions, including ventricular arrhythmias and myocardial infarctions. These episodes, some ending fatally, have usually occurred in elderly patients with preexisting cardiovascular diseases.

Precautions: Exceeding recommended dosages or applying NEO-SYNEPHRINE hydrochloride ophthalmic solutions to the instrumented, traumatized, diseased or postsurgical eye or adnexa, or to patients with suppressed lacrimation, as during anesthesia, may result in the absorption of sufficient quantities of phenylephrine to produce a systemic vasopressor response.

A significant elevation in blood pressure is rare but has been reported following conjunctival instillation of recommended doses of NEO-SYNEPHRINE 10 percent ophthalmic solutions. Caution, therefore, should be exercised in administering the 10 percent solutions to children of low body weight, the elderly, and patients with insulin-dependent diabetes, hypertension, hyperthyroidism, generalized arteriosclerosis, or cardiovascular disease. The posttreatment blood pressure of these patients, and any patients who develop symptoms, should be carefully monitored.

Ordinarily, any mydriatic, including NEO-SYNEPHRINE hydrochloride, brand of phenylephrine hydrochloride ophthalmic solution, is contraindicated in patients with glaucoma, since it may occasionally raise intraocular pressure. However, when temporary dilatation of the pupil may free adhesions or when vasoconstriction of intrinsic vessels may lower intraocular tension, these advantages may temporarily outweigh the danger from coincident dilatation of the pupil.

Rebound miosis has been reported in older persons one day after receiving NEO-SYNEPHRINE hydrochloride ophthalmic solutions, and reinstillation of the drug produced a reduction in mydriasis. This may be of clinical importance in dilating the pupils of older subjects prior to retinal detachment or cataract surgery.

Due to a strong action of the drug on the dilator muscle, older individuals may also develop transient pigment floaters in the aqueous humor 30 to 45 minutes following the administration of NEO-SYNEPHRINE hydrochloride ophthalmic solutions. The appearance may be similar to anterior uveitis or to a microscopic hyphema.

To prevent pain, a drop of suitable topical anesthetic may be applied before using the 10 percent ophthalmic solution.

Drug Interaction: As with all other adrenergic drugs, when NEO-SYNEPHRINE 10 percent ophthalmic solutions or 2.5 percent ophthalmic solution is administered simultaneously with, or up to 21 days after, administration of monoamine oxidase (MAO) inhibitors, careful supervision and adjustment of dosages are required since exaggerated adrenergic effects may occur. The pressor response of adrenergic agents may also be potentiated by tricyclic antidepressants, propranolol, reserpine, guanethidine, methyldopa, and atropine-like drugs.

It has been reported that the concomitant use of NEO-SYNEPHRINE 10 percent ophthalmic solutions and systemic beta blockers has caused acute hypertension and, in one case, the rupture of a congenital cerebral aneurysm.

Carcinogenesis, Mutagenesis, Impairment of Fertility: No long-term animal studies have been done to evaluate the potential of NEO-SYNEPHRINE in these areas.

Pregnancy Category C: Animal reproduction studies have not been conducted with NEO-SYNEPHRINE. It is also not known whether NEO-SYNEPHRINE can cause fetal harm when administered to a pregnant woman or can affect reproduction capacity. NEO-SYNEPHRINE should be given to a pregnant woman only if clearly needed.

Nursing Mothers: It is not known whether this drug is excreted in milk; many are. Caution should be exercised when NEO-SYNEPHRINE hydrochloride ophthalmic solution is administered to a nursing woman.

Pediatric Use: NEO-SYNEPHRINE hydrochloride 10 percent ophthalmic solutions are contraindicated in infants. (See CONTRAINDICATIONS.) For use in older children see DOSAGE AND ADMINISTRATION.

Exceeding recommended dosages or applying NEO-SYNEPHRINE hydrochloride ophthalmic solutions to the instrumented, traumatized, diseased or postsurgical eye or adnexa, or to patients with suppressed lacrimation, as during anesthesia, may result in the absorption of sufficient quantities of phenylephrine to produce a systemic vasopressor response.

The hypertensive effects of phenylephrine may be treated with an alpha-adrenergic blocking agent such as phentolamine mesylate, 5 mg to 10 mg intravenously, repeated as necessary.

The oral LD_{50} of phenylephrine in the rat: 350 mg/kg, in the mouse: 120 mg/kg.

Dosage and Administration: Prolonged exposure to air or strong light may cause oxidation and discoloration. Do not use if solution is brown or contains a precipitate.

Vasoconstriction and Pupil Dilatation
NEO-SYNEPHRINE hydrochloride 10 percent ophthalmic solutions is especially useful when rapid and powerful dilatation of the pupil and reduction of congestion in the capillary bed are desired. A drop of a suitable topical anesthetic may be applied, followed in a few minutes by 1 drop of the NEO-SYNEPHRINE hydrochloride 10 percent ophthalmic solution on the upper limbus. The anesthetic prevents stinging and consequent dilution of the solution by lacrimation. It may occasionally be necessary to repeat the instillation after one hour, again preceded by the use of the topical anesthetic.

Uveitis: Posterior Synechiae
NEO-SYNEPHRINE hydrochloride 10 percent ophthalmic solutions may be used in patients with uveitis when synechiae are present or may develop. The formation of synechiae may be prevented by the use of the 10 percent ophthalmic solutions and atropine to produce wide dilatation of the pupil. It should be emphasized, however, that the vasoconstrictor effect of NEO-SYNEPHRINE hydrochloride may be antagonistic to the increase of local blood flow in uveal infection.

To free recently formed posterior synechiae, 1 drop of the 10 percent ophthalmic solutions may be applied to the upper surface of the cornea. On the following day, treatment may be continued if necessary. In the interim, hot compresses should be applied for five or ten minutes three times a day, with 1 drop of a 1 or 2 percent solution of atropine sulfate before and after each series of compresses.

Glaucoma
In certain patients with glaucoma, temporary reduction of intraocular tension may be attained by producing vasoconstriction of the intraocular vessels; this may be accomplished by placing 1 drop of the 10 percent ophthalmic solutions on the upper surface of the cornea. This treatment may be repeated as often as necessary.

NEO-SYNEPHRINE hydrochloride, brand of phenylephrine hydrochloride ophthalmic solution, may be used with miotics in patients with wide angle glaucoma. It reduces the difficulties experienced by the patient because of the small field produced by miosis, and still it permits and often supports the effect of the miotic in lowering the intraocular pressure. Hence, there may be marked improvement in visual acuity after using NEO-SYNEPHRINE hydrochloride in conjunction with miotic drugs.

Surgery
When a short-acting mydriatic is needed for wide dilatation of the pupil before intraocular surgery, the 10 percent ophthalmic solutions or 2.5 percent ophthalmic solution may be applied topically from 30 to 60 minutes before the operation.

Refraction
Prior to determination of refractive errors, NEO-SYNEPHRINE hydrochloride 2.5 percent ophthalmic solution may be used effectively with homatropine hydrobromide, atropine sulfate, or a combination of homatropine and cocaine hydrochloride.

For *adults*, a drop of the preferred cycloplegic is placed in each eye, followed in five minutes by 1 drop of NEO-SYNEPHRINE hydrochloride 2.5 percent ophthalmic solution and in ten minutes by another drop of the cycloplegic. In 50 to 60 minutes, the eyes are ready for refraction.

For *children*, a drop of atropine sulfate 1 percent is placed in each eye, followed in 10 to 15 minutes by 1 drop of NEO-SYNEPHRINE hydrochloride 2.5 percent ophthalmic solution and in five to ten minutes by a second drop of atropine sulfate 1 percent. In one to two hours, the eyes are ready for refraction.

For a "one application method," NEO-SYNEPHRINE hydrochloride 2.5 percent ophthalmic solution may be combined with a cycloplegic to elicit synergistic action. The additive effect varies depending on the patient. Therefore, when using a "one application method," it may be desirable to increase the concentration of the cycloplegic.

Ophthalmoscopic Examination
One drop of NEO-SYNEPHRINE hydrochloride 2.5 percent ophthalmic solution is placed in each eye. Sufficient mydriasis to permit examination is produced in 15 to 30 minutes. Dilatation lasts from one to three hours.

Diagnostic Procedures
Provocative Test for Angle Block in Patients with Glaucoma: The 2.5 percent ophthalmic solution may be used as a provocative test when latent increased intraocular pressure is suspected. Tension is measured before application of NEO-SYNEPHRINE hydrochloride and again after dilatation. A 3 to 5 mm of mercury rise in pressure suggests the presence of angle block in patients with glaucoma; however, failure to obtain such a rise does not preclude the presence of glaucoma from other causes.

Shadow Test (Retinoscopy): When dilatation of the pupil without cycloplegic action is desired for the

shadow test, the 2.5 percent ophthalmic solution may be used alone.
Blanching Test: One or 2 drops of the 2.5 percent ophthalmic solution should be applied to the injected eye. After five minutes, examine for perilimbal blanching. If blanching occurs, the congestion is superficial and probably does not indicate iritis.

How Supplied: *In Mono-Drop® (plastic dropper) bottle:*
Low surface tension solutions
  2.5 percent ophthalmic solution — NEO-SYNEPHRINE hydrochloride, brand of phenylephrine hydrochloride ophthalmic solution, 2.5 percent in a sterile, isotonic, buffered, low surface tension vehicle with sodium phosphate, sodium biphosphate, boric acid, and, as antiseptic preservative, benzalkonium chloride, NF, 1:7500. The pH is adjusted with phosphoric acid or sodium hydroxide.
  Bottles of 15 mL (NDC 0024-1358-01)
  10 percent ophthalmic solution — NEO-SYNEPHRINE hydrochloride
  10 percent in a sterile, buffered, low surface tension vehicle with sodium phosphate, sodium biphosphate, and, as antiseptic preservative, benzalkonium chloride 1:10,000. The pH is adjusted with phosphoric acid or sodium hydroxide.
  Bottles of 5 mL (NDC 0024-1359-01)
Viscous solution
  10 percent ophthalmic solution — NEO-SYNEPHRINE hydrochloride
  10 percent in a sterile, buffered, viscous vehicle with sodium phosphate, sodium biphosphate, methylcellulose, and, as antiseptic preservative, benzalkonium chloride 1:10,000. The pH is adjusted with phosphoric acid or sodium hydroxide.
  Bottles of 5 mL (NDC 0024-1362-01)

NW-147-AA

NEO—SYNEPHRINE®   OTC
phenylephrine hydrochloride
(See PDR For Nonprescription Drugs)

Long Acting
NTZ®   OTC
oxymetazoline hydrochloride
(See PDR For Nonprescription Drugs)

NOVOCAIN®   ℞
brand of procaine hydrochloride
injection, USP
Local Anesthetic
for Major and Minor Surgery
THESE SOLUTIONS ARE NOT INTENDED FOR SPINAL OR EPIDURAL ANESTHESIA OR DENTAL USE

Description: Procaine hydrochloride, is benzoic acid, 4-amino-, 2-(diethylamino)ethyl ester, monohydrochloride, the ester of diethylaminoethanol and para-aminobenzoic acid.
It is a white crystalline, odorless powder that is freely soluble in water, but less soluble in alcohol.
Composition of Available Solutions.
[See table above].
The solutions are made isotonic with sodium chloride and the pH is adjusted between 3.0 and 5.5 with sodium hydroxide and hydrochloric acid. DO NOT USE SOLUTIONS IF CRYSTALS, CLOUDINESS, OR DISCOLORATION IS OBSERVED. EXAMINE SOLUTIONS CAREFULLY BEFORE USE. REAUTOCLAVING INCREASES LIKELIHOOD OF CRYSTAL FORMATION.
Clinical Pharmacology: NOVOCAIN stabilizes the neuronal membrane and prevents the initiation and transmission of nerve impulses, thereby effecting local anesthesia. NOVOCAIN lacks surface anesthetic activity. The onset of action is rapid (2 to 5 minutes) and the duration of action is relatively short (average 1 hour), depending upon the anesthetic technique, the type of block, the concentration, and the individual patient.

NOVOCAIN is readily absorbed following parenteral administration and is rapidly hydrolyzed by plasma cholinesterase to para-aminobenzoic acid and diethylaminoethanol.
A vasoconstrictor may be added to the NOVOCAIN solution to promote local hemostasis, delay systemic absorption, and increase duration of anesthesia.

Indications and Usage: NOVOCAIN is indicated for the production of local anesthesia by infiltration injection, nerve block, and other peripheral blocks.

Contraindication: NOVOCAIN is contraindicated in patients with a known hypersensitivity to the drug, drugs of a similar chemical configuration, or para-aminobenzoic acid or its derivatives.

Warnings: RESUSCITATIVE EQUIPMENT AND DRUGS SHOULD BE IMMEDIATELY AVAILABLE WHENEVER ANY LOCAL ANESTHETIC DRUG IS USED.
Large doses of local anesthetics should not be used in patients with heart block.
Reactions resulting in fatality have occurred on rare occasions with the use of local anesthetics, even in the absence of a history of hypersensitivity.
Solutions which contain a vasoconstrictor should be used with extreme caution in patients receiving drugs known to produce alterations in blood pressure (ie , monoamine oxidase (MAO) inhibitors, tricyclic antidepressants, phenothiazines, etc) as either severe or sustained hypertension or hypotension or disturbances of cardiac rhythm may occur.

Usage in Pregnancy. Safe use of NOVOCAIN has not been established with respect to adverse effects on fetal development. Careful consideration should be given to this fact before administering this drug to women of childbearing potential particularly during early pregnancy. This does not exclude the use of the drug at term for obstetrical analgesia. Vasopressor agents (administered for the treatment of hypotension or added to the anesthetic solution for vasoconstriction) should be used with extreme caution in the presence of oxytocic drugs as they may produce severe, persistent hypertension with possible rupture of a cerebral blood vessel.
Local anesthetic procedures should be used with caution when there is inflammation and/or sepsis in the region of the proposed injection.

Precautions: Standard textbooks should be consulted for specific techniques and precautions for various regional anesthetic procedures.
The safety and effectiveness of a local anesthetic drug depend upon proper dosage, correct technique, adequate precautions, and readiness for emergencies.
Tolerance varies with the status of the patient. Debilitated, elderly patients, or acutely ill patients should be given reduced doses commensurate with their weight and physical status.
NOVOCAIN, brand of procaine hydrochloride injection, should be used with caution in patients with severe disturbances of cardiac rhythm, shock, or heart block.
INJECTION SHOULD ALWAYS BE MADE SLOWLY AND WITH FREQUENT ASPIRATIONS TO AVOID INADVERTENT RAPID INTRAVASCULAR ADMINISTRATION WHICH CAN PRODUCE SYSTEMIC TOXICITY.
Fetal bradycardia which frequently follows paracervical block may be indicative of high fetal blood concentrations of NOVOCAIN with resultant fetal acidosis. Fetal heart rate should be monitored

NOVOCAIN

Each mL contains	1% ampul	1% vial	2% vial
Procaine hydrochloride	10 mg	10 mg	20 mg
Acetone sodium bisulfite	≤ 1 mg	≤ 2 mg	≤ 2 mg
Chlorobutanol	—	≤ 2.5 mg	≤ 2.5 mg

[Acetone sodium bisulfite is added as antioxidant and chlorobutanol as antimalarial preservative for the multiple-dose vials.]

prior to and during paracervical block. Added risk appears to be present in prematurity, toxemia of pregnancy, and fetal distress. The physician should weigh the benefits against the risks in considering paracervical block in these conditions. Careful adherence to recommended dosage is of the utmost importance in paracervical block. Failure to achieve adequate analgesia with these doses should arouse suspicion of intravascular or fetal injection.
VASOCONSTRICTORS. Solutions containing a vasoconstrictor should be used cautiously. The decision whether or not to use a vasoconstrictor with local anesthesia depends on the physician's appraisal of the benefits as opposed to the risk, eg, in injection of solutions containing a vasoconstrictor into areas where the blood supply is limited (eg, ears, nose, digits) or when peripheral vascular disease is present. Furthermore, serious cardiac arrhythmias may occur if preparations containing a vasoconstrictor are employed in patients during or immediately following the administration of halothane, cyclopropane, trichloroethylene, or other related agents.
NOVOCAIN SHOULD BE USED WITH CAUTION IN PATIENTS WITH KNOWN DRUG ALLERGIES AND SENSITIVITIES. A thorough history of the patient's prior experience with NOVOCAIN or other local anesthetics as well as concomitant or recent drug use should be taken (see Contraindications). NOVOCAIN should not be used in any conditions in which a sulfonamide drug is being employed since para-aminobenzoic acid inhibits the action of the sulfonamides.

Adverse Reactions: Systemic adverse reactions involving the central nervous system and the cardiovascular system usually result from high plasma levels due to excessive dosage, rapid absorption, or inadvertent intravascular injection.
A small number of reactions may result from hypersensitivity, idiosyncrasy, or diminished tolerance to normal dosage.
Excitatory CNS effects (nervousness, dizziness, blurred vision, tremors) commonly represent the initial signs of local anesthetic systemic toxicity. However, these reactions may be very brief or absent in some patients in which case the first manifestation of toxicity may be drowsiness or convulsions merging into unconsciousness and respiratory arrest.
Cardiovascular system reactions include depression of the myocardium, hypotension (or sometimes hypertension), bradycardia, and even cardiac arrest. In obstetrics, cases of fetal bradycardia have occurred (see Precautions).
Allergic reactions are characterized by cutaneous lesions of delayed onset, or urticaria, edema, and other manifestations of allergy. The detection of sensitivity by skin testing is of limited value. As with other local anesthetics, hypersensitivity, idiosyncrasy and anaphylactoid reactions have occurred rarely. The reaction may be abrupt and severe and is not usually dose related.
Treatment of Reactions. Treatment of a patient with toxic manifestations consists of assuring and maintaining a patent airway and supporting ven-

Continued on next page

This product information was effective as of December 3, 1984. On these and other products of Winthrop-Breon Laboratories, detailed information may be obtained on a current basis by direct inquiry to the Professional Services Department, 90 Park Avenue, New York, NY 10016 (212) 907-2525.

Winthrop-Breon—Cont.

tilation with oxygen and assisted or controlled ventilation (respiration) as required. This usually will be sufficient in the management of most reactions. Should a convulsion persist despite ventilatory therapy, small increments of anticonvulsive agents may be given intravenously, such as benzodiazepine (eg, diazepam), or ultrashort-acting barbiturates (eg, thiopental or thiamylal) or a short-acting barbiturate (eg, pentobarbital or secobarbital). Cardiovascular depression may require circulatory assistance with intravenous fluids and/or vasopressors (eg, ephedrine) as dictated by the clinical situation. Allergic reactions are rare and may occur as a result of sensitivity to the local anesthetic or methylparaben used as a preservative and are characterized by cutaneous lesions, urticaria, edema, and anaphylactoid-type symptomatology. These allergic reactions should be managed by conventional means. The detection of potential sensitivity by skin testing is of limited value.

Dosage and Administration: As with all local anesthetics, the dose of NOVOCAIN varies and depends upon the area to be anesthetized, the vascularity of the tissues, the number of neuronal segments to be blocked, individual tolerance, and the technique of anesthesia. The lowest dose needed to provide effective anesthesia should be administered. For specific techniques and procedures, refer to standard textbooks.

For infiltration anesthesia, 0.25 or 0.5 percent solution; 350 mg to 600 mg is generally considered to be a single safe total dose. To prepare 60 mL of a 0.5 percent solution (5 mg/mL), dilute 30 mL of the 1 percent solution with 30 mL sterile distilled water. To prepare 60 mL of a 0.25 percent solution (2.5 mg/mL), dilute 15 mL of the 1 percent solution with 45 mL sterile distilled water. 0.5 to 1 mL of epinephrine 1:1000 per 100 mL anesthetic solution may be added for vasoconstrictive effect (1:200,000 to 1:100,000) (see Warnings and Precautions).

For peripheral nerve block, 0.5 percent solution (up to 200 mL), 1 percent solution (up to 100 mL) or 2 percent solution (up to 50 mL). The use of the 2 percent solution should usually be limited to cases requiring a small volume of anesthetic solution (10 mL to 25 mL). 0.5 to 1 mL of epinephrine 1:1000 per 100 mL anesthetic solution may be added for vasoconstrictive effect (1:200,000 to 1:100,000) (see Warnings and Precautions).

THE USUAL INITIAL DOSE SHOULD NOT EXCEED 1000 MG.

Sterilization: Disinfecting agents containing heavy metals, which cause release of respective ions (mercury, zinc, copper, etc) should not be used for skin or mucous membrane disinfection as they have been related to incidence of swelling and edema.

When chemical disinfection of multiple-dose vials is desired, either pure undiluted isopropyl alcohol (91%) or 70% ethyl alcohol USP is recommended. Many commercially available brands of rubbing alcohol, as well as solutions of ethyl alcohol not of USP grade, contain denaturants which are injurious to rubber and, therefore, are not to be used. It is recommended that chemical disinfection be accomplished, by wiping the vial or ampul thoroughly with cotton or gauze that has been moistened with the recommended alcohol just prior to use.

The drug in intact ampuls and vials is sterile. The preferred method of destroying bacteria on the exterior before opening is heat sterilization (autoclaving). Immersion in antiseptic solution is not recommended.

Autoclave at 15-pound pressure, at 121°C (250°F), for 15 minutes.

How Supplied:
NOVOCAIN, brand of procaine hydrochloride injection, Solution 1 percent
Ampuls of 2 mL UNI-NEST™ PAK of 25
(NDC 0024-1381-25)
Ampuls of 6 mL, box of 50 (NDC 0024-1382-05)
Vials of 30 mL, box of 100 (NDC 0024-1385-01)
NOVOCAIN Solution 2 percent
Vials of 30 mL, box of 100 (NDC 0024-1386-01)
Protect solutions from light.
The air in all ampuls and vials has been displaced by nitrogen gas.

NW 63-S

NOVOCAIN® ℞
brand of procaine hydrochloride injection, USP
10% Solution for Spinal Anesthesia

Description: NOVOCAIN, brand of procaine hydrochloride, is benzoic acid, 4-amino-, 2-(diethylamino) ethyl ester, monohydrochloride, the ester of diethylaminoethanol and para-aminobenzoic acid.

It is a white crystalline, odorless powder that is freely soluble in water, but less soluble in alcohol. Each mL in the ampuls contains 100 mg procaine hydrochloride and 8 mg acetone sodium bisulfite as antioxidant. DO NOT USE SOLUTIONS IF CRYSTALS, CLOUDINESS, OR DISCOLORATION IS OBSERVED. EXAMINE SOLUTIONS CAREFULLY BEFORE USE. REAUTOCLAVING INCREASES LIKELIHOOD OF CRYSTAL FORMATION.

Clinical Pharmacology: NOVOCAIN stabilizes the neuronal membrane and prevents the initiation and transmission of nerve impulses, thereby effecting local anesthesia. NOVOCAIN lacks surface anesthetic activity. The onset of action is rapid (2 to 5 minutes) and the duration of action is relatively short (average 1 to 1½ hours), depending upon the anesthetic technique, the type of block, the concentration, and the individual patient.

NOVOCAIN is readily absorbed following parenteral administration and is rapidly hydrolyzed by plasma cholinesterase to para-aminobenzoic acid and diethylaminoethanol.

A vasoconstrictor may be added to the NOVOCAIN solution to promote local hemostasis, delay systemic absorption, and increase duration of anesthesia.

Indications and Usage: NOVOCAIN is indicated for spinal anesthesia.

Contraindications: Spinal anesthesia with NOVOCAIN is contraindicated in patients with generalized septicemia; sepsis at the proposed injection site; certain diseases of the cerebrospinal system, eg, meningitis, syphilis; and a known hypersensitivity to the drug, drugs of a similar chemical configuration, or para-aminobenzoic acid or its derivatives.

The decision as to whether or not spinal anesthesia should be used in an individual case should be made by the physician after weighing the advantages with the risks and possible complications.

Warnings: RESUSCITATIVE EQUIPMENT AND DRUGS SHOULD BE IMMEDIATELY AVAILABLE WHENEVER ANY LOCAL ANESTHETIC DRUG IS USED. Spinal anesthesia should only be administered by those qualified to do so.

Large doses of local anesthetics should not be used in patients with heart block.

Reactions resulting in fatality have occurred on rare occasions with the use of local anesthetics, even in the absence of a history of hypersensitivity.

Usage in Pregnancy. Safe use of NOVOCAIN has not been established with respect to adverse effects on fetal development. Careful consideration should be given to this fact before administering this drug to women of childbearing potential particularly during early pregnancy. This does not exclude the use of the drug at term for obstetrical analgesia. Vasopressor agents (administered for the treatment of hypotension or added to the anesthetic solution for vasoconstriction) should be used with extreme caution in the presence of oxytocic drugs as they may produce severe, persistent hypertension with possible rupture of a cerebral blood vessel.

Solutions which contain a vasoconstrictor should be used with extreme caution in patients receiving drugs known to produce alterations in blood pressure (ie, monoamine oxidase (MAO) inhibitors, tricyclic antidepressants, phenothiazines, etc) as either severe sustained hypertension or hypotension may occur.

Local anesthetic procedures should be used with caution when there is inflammation and/or sepsis in the region of the proposed injection.

Precautions: Standard textbooks should be consulted for specific techniques and precautions for various spinal anesthetic procedures.

The safety and effectiveness of a spinal anesthetic depend upon proper dosage, correct technique, adequate precautions, and readiness for emergencies. The lowest dosage that results in effective anesthesia should be used to avoid high plasma levels and possible adverse effects. Tolerance varies with the status of the patient. Debilitated, elderly patients, or acutely ill patients should be given reduced doses commensurate with their weight and physical status. Reduced dosages are also indicated for obstetric delivery and patients with increased intraabdominal pressure.

The decision whether or not to use spinal anesthesia in the following disease states depends on the physician's appraisal of the advantages as opposed to the risk: cardiovascular disease (ie, shock, hypertension, anemia, etc), pulmonary disease, renal impairment, metabolic or endocrine disorders, gastrointestinal disorders (ie, intestinal obstruction, peritonitis, etc), or complicated obstetrical deliveries.

NOVOCAIN SHOULD BE USED WITH CAUTION IN PATIENTS WITH KNOWN DRUG ALLERGIES AND SENSITIVITIES. A thorough history of the patient's prior experience with NOVOCAIN or other local anesthetics as well as concomitant or recent drug use should be taken (see Contraindications). NOVOCAIN should not be used in any condition in which a sulfonamide drug is being employed since para-aminobenzoic acid inhibits the action of sulfonamides.

Solutions containing a vasopressor should be used with caution in the presence of diseases which may adversely affect the cardiovascular system.

NOVOCAIN, brand of procaine hydrochloride injection, should be used with caution in patients with severe disturbances of cardiac rhythm, shock or heart block.

Adverse Reactions: Systemic adverse reactions involving the central nervous system and the cardiovascular system usually result from high plasma levels due to excessive dosage, rapid absorption, or inadvertent intravascular injection. In addition, use of inappropriate doses or techniques may result in extensive spinal blockade leading to hypotension and respiratory arrest.

A small number of reactions may result from hypersensitivity, idiosyncrasy, or diminished tolerance to normal dosage.

Excitatory CNS effects (nervousness, dizziness, blurred vision, tremors) commonly represent the initial signs of local anesthetic systemic toxicity. However, these reactions may be very brief or absent in some patients in which case the first manifestation of toxicity may be drowsiness or convulsions merging into unconsciousness and respiratory arrest.

Cardiovascular system reactions include depression of the myocardium, hypotension (or sometimes hypertension), bradycardia, and even cardiac arrest.

Allergic reactions are characterized by cutaneous lesions of delayed onset, or urticaria, edema, and other manifestations of allergy. The detection of sensitivity by skin testing is of limited value. As with other local anesthetics, hypersensitivity, idiosyncrasy and anaphylactoid reactions have occurred rarely. The reaction may be abrupt and severe and is not usually dose related.

The following adverse reactions may occur with spinal anesthesia: *Central Nervous System:* postspinal headache, meningismus, arachnoiditis, palsies, or spinal nerve paralysis. *Cardiovascular:* hypotension due to vasomotor paralysis and pooling of the blood in the venous bed. *Respiratory:* respiratory impairment or paralysis due to the level of anesthesia extending to the upper thoracic and cervical segments. *Gastrointestinal:* nausea and vomiting.

Treatment of Reactions. Toxic effects of local anesthetics require symptomatic treatment: there is no specific cure. The physician should be prepared to maintain an airway and to support ventilation with oxygen and assisted or controlled respiration as required. Supportive treatment of the cardiovascular system includes intravenous fluids and, when appropriate, vasopressors (preferably those that stimulate the myocardium, such as ephedrine). Convulsions may be controlled with oxygen and by the intravenous administration of diazepam or ultrashort-acting barbiturates or a short-acting muscle relaxant (succinylcholine). Intravenous anticonvulsant agents and muscle relaxants should only be administered by those familiar with their use and only when ventilation and oxygenation are assured. In spinal and epidural anesthesia, sympathetic blockade also occurs as a pharmacological reaction, resulting in peripheral vasodilation and often *hypotension*. The extent of the hypotension will usually depend on the number of dermatomes blocked. The blood pressure should therefore be monitored in the early phases of anesthesia. If hypotension occurs, it is readily controlled by vasoconstrictors administered either by the intramuscular or the intravenous route, the dosage of which would depend on the severity of the hypotension and the response to treatment.

Dosage and Administration: As with all local anesthetics, the dose of NOVOCAIN, brand of procaine hydrochloride injection, varies and depends upon the area to be anesthetized, the vascularity of the tissues, the number of neuronal segments to be blocked, individual tolerance, and the technique of anesthesia. The lowest dose needed to provide effective anesthesia should be administered. For specific techniques and procedures, refer to standard textbooks.

[See table above].

The diluent may be sterile normal saline, sterile distilled water, spinal fluid; and for hyperbaric technique, sterile dextrose solution.

The usual rate of injection is 1 mL per 5 seconds. Full anesthesia and fixation usually occur in 5 minutes.

Sterilization: The drug in intact ampuls is sterile. The preferred method of destroying bacteria on the exterior of ampuls before opening is heat sterilization (autoclaving). Immersion in antiseptic solution is not recommended.

Autoclave at 15-pound pressure, at 121°C (250°F), for 15 minutes. The diluent dextrose may show some brown discoloration due to caramelization.

How Supplied: NOVOCAIN Solution 10 percent, ampuls of 2 mL (200 mg) UNI-NEST PAK of 25 (NDC 0024-1384-25).

Protect solutions from light.

The air in the ampuls has been displaced by nitrogen gas.

NW 62-M

PEDIACOF®   C R

Decongestant and Soothing Cough Syrup for Children

Description: Each teaspoon (5 mL) contains:
Codeine phosphate, USP .... 5.0 mg
(Warning: May be habit forming.)
Phenylephrine hydrochloride, USP .... 2.5 mg
Chlorpheniramine maleate, USP .... 0.75 mg
Potassium iodide, USP .... 75.0 mg
with sodium benzoate 0.2% as preservative and alcohol 5%.

PEDIACOF is a pleasant-tasting, raspberry-flavored cough syrup. It contains four active ingredients in proper proportion for children. Codeine phosphate is a white crystalline, odorless powder which is freely soluble in water. It is a narcotic analgesic.

Codeine phosphate is 7,8-Didehydro-4,5α-epoxy-3-methoxy-17 methylmorphinan-6α-ol phosphate.

Phenylephrine hydrochloride is a vasoconstrictor and pressor drug chemically related to epinephrine and ephedrine. It is a synthetic sympathomimetic agent. Chemically, phenylephrine hydrochloride is (−)-m-Hydroxy-α-[(methylamino)methyl] benzyl alcohol hydrochloride.

Chlorpheniramine maleate is an alkylamine H_1-blocking agent (antihistamine) which is chemically 2-pyridinepropanamine γ-(4-chlorophenyl)-N, N-dimethyl-, (Z)-2-butenedioate.

Potassium iodide is an expectorant.

Clinical Pharmacology: Codeine phosphate is an antitussive that is well recognized not only because of its efficiency and rapidity of action but also because of its relative safety in clinical use. Thus, irritating, nonproductive cough is suppressed by codeine. The codeine content of PEDIACOF is reduced to the proportion that is most suitable for children. When codeine is combined with the expectorant potassium iodide, which tends to increase bronchial secretion, coughing, although minimized, is more productive when it does occur. The continuous fatiguing effect of useless coughing is thereby avoided. Codeine is a narcotic analgesic and antitussive which resembles morphine pharmacologically. Codeine is metabolized by the liver and excreted chiefly in the urine, largely in inactive forms. A small fraction (10%) of administered codeine is demethylated to form morphine, and both free and conjugated morphine can be found in the urine after therapeutic doses of codeine. When administered subcutaneously, 120 mg of codeine is approximately equivalent to 10 mg of morphine. The abuse liability of codeine is generally considered to be much lower than that of morphine.

The half-life of codeine in plasma is 2.5 to 3.0 hours.

Codeine has diverse additional actions. It depresses the respiratory center, stimulates the vomiting center, depresses the cough reflex, constricts the pupils, increases the tone of the gastrointestinal and genitourinary tracts, and produces mild vasodilation.

Neo-Synephrine® hydrochloride, brand of phenylephrine hydrochloride produces effective decongestion of the mucous membranes of the respiratory tract via its powerful postsynaptic α-receptor stimulant action. It has little effect on cardiac β-receptors. Most of its effects are due to direct action on receptors and only a small part is due to norepinephrine release. Central stimulant activity is minimal.

Chlorpheniramine maleate helps control allergic coughs and mucosal congestion. The mild anticholinergic action of chlorpheniramine maleate may aid in reducing rhinorrhea, and its mild sedative action may also be beneficial to patients whose excessive coughing has caused them to lose sleep. Clinical experience with PEDIACOF has shown it to be a dependable medication for the relief of cough and the reduction of nasal congestion in children.

Indications and Usage: Coughs due to colds as well as coughs and congestive symptoms associated with upper respiratory tract infections such as tracheobronchitis or laryngobronchitis, croup, pharyngitis, allergic bronchitis, and infectious bronchitis, when accompanied by disturbing and fatiguing cough, have been treated successfully with PEDIACOF in children.

Contraindications: PEDIACOF is contraindicated in patients who are hypersensitive to any of its ingredients. Due to the component phenylephrine, PEDIACOF is contraindicated in patients with ventricular tachycardia or severe hypertension.

Warnings:

Respiratory Depression: Codeine produces dose-related respiratory depression by acting directly on brain stem respiratory centers. Codeine also affects centers that control respiratory rhythm and may produce irregular and periodic breathing. If significant respiratory depression occurs, it may be antagonized by the use of naloxone hydrochloride. (See OVERDOSAGE.)

Head Injury and Increased Intracranial Pressure: The respiratory depressant effects of narcotics and their capacity to elevate cerebrospinal fluid pressure may be markedly exaggerated in the presence of head injury, other intracranial lesions, or a preexisting increase in intracranial pressure. Furthermore, narcotics can produce adverse reactions which may obscure the clinical course of patients with head injuries.

Acute Abdominal Conditions: The administration of narcotics may obscure the diagnosis or clinical course of patients with acute abdominal conditions.

Precautions: Caution should be exercised if PEDIACOF is administered to patients with cardiac disorders other than ventricular tachycardia which is contraindicated, mild hypertension and hyperthyroidism.

Special Risk Patients:

Codeine should be used with caution in patients with impaired renal or hepatic function, hypothyroidism, Addison's disease, or urethral stricture. In asthma, the indiscriminate use of codeine may, due to its drying action upon the mucosa of the respiratory tract, precipitate severe respiratory insufficiency resulting from increased viscosity of the bronchial secretions and suppression of the cough reflex. As with any narcotic analgesic agent, the usual precautions should be observed and the possibility of respiratory depression should be kept in mind.

Phenylephrine hydrochloride should be employed only with extreme caution in patients with hyperthyroidism, bradycardia, partial heart block, or myocardial disease.

Chlorpheniramine maleate should be used with considerable caution in patients with narrow angle glaucoma, pyloroduodenal obstruction, and bladder neck obstruction. Chlorpheniramine maleate has an atropine-like action and therefore should be used with caution in patients with a history of bronchial asthma, increased intraocular pressure, hyperthyroidism; cardiovascular disease, and hypertension.

Drug Interactions: Patients receiving other narcotic analgesics, general anesthetics, phenothiazines, tranquilizers, sedative-hypnotics, MAO in-

Continued on next page

This product information was effective as of December 3, 1984. On these and other products of Winthrop-Breon Laboratories, detailed information may be obtained on a current basis by direct inquiry to the Professional Services Department, 90 Park Avenue, New York, NY 10016 (212) 907-2525.

RECOMMENDED DOSAGE FOR SPINAL ANESTHESIA

Extent of anesthesia	NOVOCAIN 10% Solution Volume of 10% Solution (mL)	Volume of Diluent (mL)	Total Dose (mg)	Site of Injection (lumbar interspace)
Perineum	0.5	0.5	50	4th
Perineum and lower extremities	1	1	100	3rd or 4th
Up to costal margin	2	1	200	2nd, 3rd or 4th

THE USUAL INITIAL DOSE SHOULD NOT EXCEED 1000 MG.

Winthrop-Breon—Cont.

hibitors, tricyclic antidepressants, or other CNS depressants (including alcohol) concomitantly with codeine may exhibit an additive CNS depression. When such combined therapy is contemplated, the dose of one or both agents should be reduced.

Carcinogenesis, Mutagenesis, Impairment of Fertility: No long-term animal studies have been performed to evaluate the potential of PEDIACOF in these areas.

Nonteratogenic Effects: Dependence has been reported in newborns whose mothers received opiates regularly during pregnancy. Withdrawal signs include irritability, excessive crying, tremors, hyperreflexia, fever, vomiting, and diarrhea. Signs usually appear during the first few days of life.

Adverse Reactions: The only significant untoward effects that have occurred are mild anorexia and an occasional tendency to constipation. However, discontinuance of PEDIACOF has seldom been required. Mild drowsiness occurs in some patients but, when cough is relieved, the quieting effect of PEDIACOF is considered beneficial in many instances. Because of its iodine content, PEDIACOF may cause elevation of the protein-bound iodine. Adverse reactions to codeine include: *Central Nervous System:* Sedation, drowsiness, mental clouding, dizziness, lethargy, impairment of mental and physical performance, anxiety, convulsions, fear, miosis, dysphoria, psychic dependence, mood changes, and respiratory depression. *Gastrointestinal System:* Nausea, vomiting, increased pressure in the biliary tract, and constipation. *Cardiovascular System:* Orthostatic hypotension, fainting, and tachycardia. *Genitourinary System:* Ureteral spasm, spasm of vesical sphincters and urinary retention have been reported. *Other:* Flushing, sweating, pruritus, allergic reactions; and suppressed cough reflex. Adverse reactions to phenylephrine hydrochloride include headache, reflex bradycardia, excitability, restlessness, and, rarely, arrhythmias.

Adverse reactions to chlorpheniramine maleate include: slight to moderate drowsiness. Other possible side effects common to antihistamines in general include: *General:* urticaria, drug rash, anaphylactic shock, photosensitivity, excessive perspiration, chills, dryness of mouth, nose, and throat. *Cardiovascular System:* hypotension, headache, palpitations, tachycardia, and extrasystoles. *Hematologic System:* hemolytic anemia, thrombocytopenia, and agranulocytosis. *Nervous System:* sedation, dizziness, disturbed coordination, fatigue, confusion, restlessness, excitation, nervousness, tremor, irritability, insomnia, euphoria, paresthesias, blurred vision, diplopia, vertigo, tinnitus, acute labyrinthitis, hysteria, neuritis, and convulsions. *Gastrointestinal System:* epigastric distress, anorexia, nausea, vomiting, diarrhea, and constipation. *Genitourinary System:* urinary frequency, difficult urination, urinary retention, and early menses. *Respiratory System:* thickening of bronchial secretions, tightness of chest and wheezing, and nasal stuffiness.

Overdosage:
Codeine:
Signs and Symptoms: Overdosage with codeine is characterized by respiratory depression (a decrease in respiratory rate and/or tidal volume, Cheyne-Stokes respiration, cyanosis), pinpoint pupils, extreme somnolence progressing to stupor or coma, skeletal muscle flaccidity, cold and clammy skin, and sometimes bradycardia and hypotension. In severe overdosage, particularly by the intravenous route, apnea, circulatory collapse, cardiac arrest, and death may occur.

Treatment: Primary attention should be given to the reestablishment of adequate respiratory exchange through provision of a patent airway and institution of assisted or controlled ventilation. Naloxone hydrochloride is a specific and effective antagonist for respiratory depression which may result from overdosage. If the desired degree of counteraction and improvement in respiratory function is not obtained immediately following IV administration, it may be repeated intravenously at 2 to 3 minute intervals. Failure to obtain significant improvement after 2 or 3 doses suggests that the condition may be due partly or completely to other disease processes or nonopioid drugs. The usual initial pediatric dose is 0.01 mg/kg body weight given IV, IM, or SC. If necessary, naloxone can be diluted with Sterile Water for Injection, USP, Oxygen, intravenous fluids, vasopressors, and other supportive measures should be employed as indicated.

Oral LD$_{50}$ in the mouse is 693 mg/kg. Codeine is not dialyzable.

Phenylephrine hydrochloride:
Signs and Symptoms: Overdosage may induce ventricular extrasystoles and short paroxysms of ventricular tachycardia, a sensation of fullness in the head, and tingling of the extremities.

Treatment: Should an excessive elevation of blood pressure occur, it may be immediately relieved by an α-adrenergic blocking agent, eg, phentolamine. The oral LD$_{50}$ in the rat: 350 mg/kg; mouse: 120 mg/kg.

Chlorpheniramine maleate:
Signs and Symptoms: Antihistamine overdosage may vary from central nervous system depression (sedation, apnea, and cardiovascular collapse) to stimulation (insomnia, hallucinations, tremors or convulsions). Other signs and symptoms may be dizziness, tinnitus, ataxia, blurred vision, and hypotension. Stimulation and atropine-like signs and symptoms (dry mouth; fixed, dilated pupils; flushing; hyperthermia, and gastrointestinal symptoms) are particularly likely in children.

Treatment: Emergency treatment should be started immediately. Vomiting should be induced, even if it has occurred spontaneously. Vomiting by the administration of ipecac syrup is preferred. Vomiting should *not* be induced in patients with impaired consciousness. The action of ipecac is facilitated by physical activity and by the administration of eight to twelve fluid ounces of water. If emesis does not occur within fifteen minutes, the dose of ipecac should be repeated. Precautions against aspiration must be taken, especially in infants and children. Following emesis, any drug remaining in the stomach may be absorbed by activated charcoal administered as a slurry with water. If vomiting is unsuccessful or contraindicated, gastric lavage should be performed. Isotonic and one-half isotonic saline are the lavage solutions of choice. Saline cathartics, such as milk of magnesia, draw water into the bowel by osmosis and, therefore, may be valuable for their action in rapid dilution of bowel content. After emergency treatment the patient should continue to be medically monitored. Treatment of the signs and symptoms of overdosage is symptomatic and supportive. Stimulants (analeptic agents) should *not* be used. Vasopressors may be used to treat hypotension. Short-acting barbiturates, diazepam, or paraldehyde may be administered to control seizures. Hyperpyrexia, especially in children, may require treatment with tepid water sponge baths or a hypothermic blanket. Apnea is treated with ventilatory support.

Dosage and Administration:
PEDIACOF should be given in accordance with the needs and age of the patient. Frequency of administration may be adjusted as cough is brought under control. The following doses, to be given at 4 to 6 hour intervals, are suggested for patients under 12 years of age: **from 6 months to 1 year,** $\frac{1}{4}$ teaspoon; **from 1 to 3 years,** $\frac{1}{2}$ teaspoon; **from 3 to 6 years,** 1 to 2 teaspoons; and **from 6 to 12 years,** 2 teaspoons.

How Supplied:
Bottle of 16 fl oz (**NDC** 0024-1509-06)
Available on prescription only.

PW-295-J

pHisoDerm®   OTC
(See PDR For Nonprescription Drugs)

pHisoHex®   ℞
brand of hexachlorophene detergent cleanser
sudsing antibacterial soapless skin cleanser

Description: pHisoHex is an antibacterial sudsing emulsion. It contains a colloidal dispersion of hexachlorophene 3% (w/w) in a stable emulsion consisting of entsufon sodium, petrolatum, lanolin cholesterols, methylcellulose, polyethylene glycol, polyethylene glycol monostearate, lauryl myristyl diethanolamide, sodium benzoate, and water. pH is adjusted with hydrochloric acid. Entsufon sodium is a synthetic detergent.

Clinical Pharmacology: pHisoHex is a bacteriostatic cleansing agent. It cleanses the skin thoroughly and has bacteriostatic action against staphylococci and other gram-positive bacteria. Cumulative antibacterial action develops with repeated use. This antibacterial residue is resistant to removal by many solvents, soaps, and detergents for several days.

pHisoHex has the same slight acidity as normal skin (pH value 5.0 to 6.0).

Indications and Usage: pHisoHex is indicated for use as a surgical scrub and a bacteriostatic skin cleanser. It may also be used to control an outbreak of gram-positive infection where other infection control procedures have been unsuccessful. Use only as long as necessary for infection control.

Contraindications: pHisoHex should not be used on burned or denuded skin.

It should not be used as an occlusive dressing, wet pack, or lotion.

It should not be used routinely for prophylactic total body bathing.

It should not be used as a vaginal pack or tampon, or on any mucous membranes.

pHisoHex should not be used on persons with sensitivity to any of its components. It should not be used on persons who have demonstrated primary light sensitivity to halogenated phenol derivatives because of the possibility of cross-sensitivity to hexachlorophene.

Warnings: RINSE THOROUGHLY AFTER ALL USES, especially from sensitive areas such as the scrotum and perineum.

Rapid absorption of hexachlorophene may occur with resultant toxic blood levels when preparations containing hexachlorophene are applied to skin lesions such as ichthyosis congenita, the dermatitis of Letterer-Siwe's syndrome, or other generalized dermatological conditions. Application to burns has also produced neurotoxicity and death.
PHISOHEX SHOULD BE DISCONTINUED PROMPTLY IF SIGNS OR SYMPTOMS OF CEREBRAL IRRITABILITY OCCUR.
Infants, especially premature infants or those with dermatoses, are particularly susceptible to hexachlorophene absorption. Systemic toxicity may be manifested by signs of stimulation (irritation) of the central nervous system, sometimes with convulsions.

Infants have developed dermatitis, irritability, generalized clonic muscular contractions and decerebrate rigidity following application of a 6 percent hexachlorophene powder. Examination of brainstems of those infants revealed vacuolization like that which can be produced in newborn experimental animals following repeated topical application of 3 percent hexachlorophene. Moreover, a study of histologic sections of premature infants who died of unrelated causes has shown a positive correlation between hexachlorophene baths and lesions in white matter of brains.

ORAL TOXICITY: pHisoHex is intended for *external use only.* If swallowed, pHisoHex is harmful, especially to infants and children. **pHisoHex, brand of hexachlorophene detergent cleanser, should not be poured into measuring cups, medicine bottles, or similar containers since it may be mistaken for baby formula or other medications. (See TREATMENT OF ACCIDENTAL INGESTION.)**
KEEP OUT OF THE REACH OF CHILDREN.
Precaution: pHisoHex suds that get into the eyes accidentally during washing should be rinsed out promptly and thoroughly with water.

Adverse Reactions: Adverse reactions to pHisoHex may include dermatitis and photosensitivity. Sensitivity to hexachlorophene is rare; however, persons who have developed photoallergy to similar compounds also may become sensitive to hexachlorophene.

In persons with highly sensitive skin, the use of pHisoHex may at times produce a reaction characterized by redness and/or mild scaling or dryness, especially when it is combined with such mechanical factors as excessive rubbing or exposure to heat or cold.

Directions for Use:
Surgical Hand Scrub—
1. Wet hands and forearms with water. Apply approximately 5 mL of pHisoHex over the hands and rub into a copious lather by adding small amounts of water. Spread suds over hands and forearms and scrub well with a wet brush for 3 minutes. Pay particular attention to the nails and interdigital spaces. A separate nail cleaner may be used. *Rinse thoroughly* under running water.
2. Apply 5 mL of pHisoHex to hands again and scrub as above for another 3 minutes. *Rinse thoroughly* with running water and dry.
3. For repeat surgical scrubs during the day, scrub thoroughly with the same amount of pHisoHex for 3 minutes only. *Rinse thoroughly* with water and dry.

Bacteriostatic Cleansing—
Wet hands with water. Dispense approximately 5 mL of pHisoHex into the palm, work up a lather with water and apply to area to be cleansed. *Rinse thoroughly after each washing.*
INFANT CARE: pHisoHex should not be used routinely for bathing infants. See **WARNINGS.**
PREMATURE INFANTS: See **WARNINGS.**
Use of baby skin products containing alcohol may decrease the antibacterial action of pHisoHex, brand of hexachlorophene detergent cleanser.
Treatment of Accidental Ingestion: The accidental ingestion of pHisoHex in amounts from 1 to 4 oz has caused anorexia, vomiting, abdominal cramps, diarrhea, dehydration, convulsions, hypotension and shock, and in several reported instances, fatalities.
If patients are seen early, the stomach should be evacuated by emesis or gastric lavage. Olive oil or vegetable oil (60 mL or 2 fl oz) may then be given to delay absorption of hexachlorophene, followed by a saline cathartic to hasten removal. Treatment is symptomatic and supportive; intravenous fluids (5 per cent dextrose in physiologic saline solution) may be given for dehydration. Any other electrolyte derangement should be corrected. If marked hypotension occurs, vasopressor therapy is indicated. Use of opiates may be considered if gastrointestinal symptoms (cramping, diarrhea) are severe. Scheduled medical or surgical procedures should be postponed for a few days and until the patient's condition has been evaluated and stabilized.
How Supplied: pHisoHex is available in plastic squeeze bottles of 5 ounces (NDC 0024-1535-02) and 1 pint (NDC 0024-1535-06); in plastic bottles of 1 gallon (NDC 0024-1535-08) and $\frac{1}{4}$ oz (8 mL) unit packets, boxes of 50 (NDC 0024-1535-05).
The following, specially constructed, refillable dispensers made with metals and plastics compatible with pHisoHex can also be supplied: 16 oz hand operated wall dispensers; 30 oz pedal operated wall dispensers; 30 oz pedal operated wall dispenser with stand; portable stand with two 30 oz pedal operated dispensers.
Prolonged direct exposure of pHisoHex to strong light may cause brownish surface discoloration but does not affect its antibacterial or detergent properties. Shaking will disperse the color. If pHisoHex is spilled or splashed on porous surfaces, rinse off to avoid discoloration.
pHisoHex should not be dispensed from, or stored in, containers with ordinary metal parts. A special type of stainless steel must be used or undesirable discoloration of the product or oxidation of metal may occur. Specially designed dispensers for hospital or office use may be obtained through your local dealer.

Directions for Cleaning Dispensers: Before initial installation and use, run an antiseptic, such as an aqueous solution of benzalkonium chloride, NF, 1:500 to 1:750, or alcohol, through the working parts; rinse with sterile water. At weekly intervals thereafter, remove dispenser and pour off remainder of pHisoHex emulsion. Rinse empty dispenser with water. Run water through the working parts by operating the dispenser. Sanitize as described above. Rinse thoroughly with sterile water.

PW-61-AA

PLAQUENIL® Sulfate ℞
brand of hydroxychloroquine sulfate tablets, USP

WARNING
PHYSICIANS SHOULD COMPLETELY FAMILIARIZE THEMSELVES WITH THE COMPLETE CONTENTS OF THIS LEAFLET BEFORE PRESCRIBING HYDROXYCHLOROQUINE.

Description: The compound is a colorless crystalline solid, soluble in water to at least 20 percent; chemically the drug is 2-[[4-[(7-Chloro-4-quinolyl)amino] pentyl] ethylamino] ethanol sulfate (1:1).
Actions: The drug possesses antimalarial actions and also exerts a beneficial effect in lupus erythematosus (chronic discoid or systemic) and acute or chronic rheumatoid arthritis. The precise mechanism of action is not known.
Indications: PLAQUENIL is indicated for the suppressive treatment and treatment of acute attacks of malaria due to *Plasmodium vivax, P. malariae, P. ovale*, and susceptible strains of *P. falciparum*. It is also indicated for the treatment of discoid and systemic lupus erythematosus, and rheumatoid arthritis.
Contraindications: Use of this drug is contraindicated (1) in the presence of retinal or visual field changes attributable to any 4-aminoquinoline compound, (2) in patients with known hypersensitivity to 4-aminoquinoline compounds and (3) for long-term therapy in children.
Warnings, General: PLAQUENIL is not effective against chloroquine-resistant strains of *P. falciparum.*
Children are especially sensitive to the 4-aminoquinoline compounds. A number of fatalities have been reported following the accidental ingestion of chloroquine, sometimes in relatively small doses (0.75 g or 1 g in one 3- year-old child). Patients should be strongly warned to keep these drugs out of the reach of children.
Use of PLAQUENIL in patients with psoriasis may precipitate a severe attack of psoriasis. When used in patients with porphyria the condition may be exacerbated. The preparation should not be used in these conditions unless in the judgment of the physician the benefit to the patient outweighs the possible hazard.
Usage in Pregnancy—Usage of this drug during pregnancy should be avoided except in the suppression or treatment of malaria when in the judgment of the physician the benefit outweighs the possible hazard. It should be noted that radioactively-tagged chloroquine administered intravenously to pregnant, pigmented CBA mice passed rapidly across the placenta. It accumulated selectively in the melanin structures of the fetal eyes and was retained in the ocular tissues for five months after the drug had been eliminated from the rest of the body.
Precautions, General: Antimalarial compounds should be used with caution in patients with hepatic disease or alcoholism or in conjunction with known hepatotoxic drugs.
Periodic blood cell counts should be made if patients are given prolonged therapy. If any severe blood disorder appears which is not attributable to the disease under treatment, discontinuation of the drug should be considered. The drug should be administered with caution in patients having G-6-PD (glucose-6-phosphate dehydrogenase) deficiency.
Overdosage: The 4-aminoquinoline compounds are very rapidly and completely absorbed after ingestion, and in accidental overdosage, or rarely with lower doses in hypersensitive patients, toxic symptoms may occur within 30 minutes. These consist of headache, drowsiness, visual disturbances, cardiovascular collapse, and convulsions, followed by sudden and early respiratory and cardiac arrest. The electrocardiogram may reveal atrial standstill, nodal rhythm, prolonged intraventricular conduction time, and progressive bradycardia leading to ventricular fibrillation and/or arrest. Treatment is symptomatic and must be prompt with immediate evacuation of the stomach by emesis (at home, before transportation to the hospital) or gastric lavage until the stomach is completely emptied. If finely powdered, activated charcoal is introduced by the stomach tube, after lavage, and within 30 minutes after ingestion of the tablets, it may inhibit further intestinal absorption of the drug. To be effective, the dose of activated charcoal should be at least five times the estimated dose of hydroxychloroquine ingested. Convulsions, if present, should be controlled before attempting gastric lavage. If due to cerebral stimulation, cautious administration of an ultrashort-acting barbiturate may be tried but, if due to anoxia, it should be corrected by oxygen administration, artificial respiration or, in shock with hypotension, by vasopressor therapy. Because of the importance of supporting respiration, tracheal intubation or tracheostomy, followed by gastric lavage, may also be necessary. Exchange transfusions have been used to reduce the level of 4-aminoquinoline drug in the blood.
A patient who survives the acute phase and is asymptomatic should be closely observed for at least six hours. Fluids may be forced, and sufficient ammonium chloride (8 g daily in divided doses for adults) may be administered for a few days to acidify the urine to help promote urinary excretion in cases of both overdosage and sensitivity.

MALARIA

Actions: Like chloroquine phosphate, USP, PLAQUENIL sulfate is highly active against the erythrocytic forms of *P. vivax* and *malariae* and most strains of *P. falciparum* (but not the gametocytes of *P. falciparum*).
PLAQUENIL sulfate does not prevent relapses in patients with *vivax* or *malariae* malaria because it is not effective against exo-erythrocytic forms of the parasite, nor will it prevent *vivax* or *malariae* infection when administered as a prophylactic. It is highly effective as a suppressive agent in patients with *vivax* or *malariae* malaria, in terminating acute attacks, and significantly lengthening the interval between treatment and relapse. In patients with *falciparum* malaria, it abolishes the acute attack and effects complete cure of the infection, unless due to a resistant strain of *P. falciparum.*
Indications: PLAQUENIL sulfate, brand of hydroxychloroquine sulfate tablets, is indicated for the treatment of acute attacks and suppression of malaria.
Warning: In recent years, it has been found that certain strains of *P. falciparum* have become resistant to 4-aminoquinoline compounds (including hydroxychloroquine) as shown by the fact that normally adequate doses have failed to prevent or cure clinical malaria or parasitemia. Treatment

Continued on next page

This product information was effective as of December 3, 1984. On these and other products of Winthrop-Breon Laboratories, detailed information may be obtained on a current basis by direct inquiry to the Professional Services Department, 90 Park Avenue, New York, NY 10016 (212) 907-2525.

Winthrop-Breon—Cont.

with quinine or other specific forms of therapy is therefore advised for patients infected with a resistant strain of parasites.

Adverse Reactions: Following the administration in doses adequate for the treatment of an acute malarial attack, mild and transient headache, dizziness, and gastrointestinal complaints (diarrhea, anorexia, nausea, abdominal cramps and, on rare occasions, vomiting) may occur.

Dosage and Administration: One tablet of 200 mg of hydroxychloroquine sulfate is equivalent to 155 mg base.

Malaria: Suppression—*In adults,* 400 mg (=310 mg base) on exactly the same day of each week. *In infants and children,* the weekly suppressive dosage is 5 mg, calculated as base, per kg of body weight, but should not exceed the adult dose regardless of weight.

If circumstances permit, suppressive therapy should begin two weeks prior to exposure. However, failing this, in adults an initial double (loading) dose of 800 mg (= 620 mg base), or in children 10 mg base/kg may be taken in two divided doses, six hours apart. The suppressive therapy should be continued for eight weeks after leaving the endemic area.

Treatment of the acute attack—*In adults,* an initial dose of 800 mg (= 620 mg base) followed by 400 mg (= 310 mg base) in six to eight hours and 400 mg (310 mg base) on each of two consecutive days (total 2 g hydroxychloroquine sulfate or 1.55 g base). An alternative method, employing a single dose of 800 mg (= 620 mg base), has also proved effective.

The dosage for adults may also be calculated on the basis of body weight; this method is preferred for infants and children. A total dose representing 25 mg of base per kg of body weight is administered in three days, as follows:

First dose: 10 mg base per kg (but not exceeding a single dose of 620 mg base).

Second dose: 5 mg base per kg (but not exceeding a single dose of 310 mg base) 6 hours after first dose.

Third dose: 5 mg base per kg 18 hours after second dose.

Fourth dose: 5 mg base per kg 24 hours after third dose.

For radical cure of *vivax* and *malariae* malaria concomitant therapy with an 8-aminoquinoline compound is necessary.

LUPUS ERYTHEMATOSUS AND RHEUMATOID ARTHRITIS

Indications: PLAQUENIL is useful in patients with the following disorders who have not responded satisfactorily to drugs with less potential for serious side effects: lupus erythematosus (chronic discoid and systemic) and acute or chronic rheumatoid arthritis.

Warnings: PHYSICIANS SHOULD COMPLETELY FAMILIARIZE THEMSELVES WITH THE COMPLETE CONTENTS OF THIS LEAFLET BEFORE PRESCRIBING PLAQUENIL.

Irreversible retinal damage has been observed in some patients who had received long-term or high-dosage 4-aminoquinoline therapy for discoid and systemic lupus erythematosus, or rheumatoid arthritis. Retinopathy has been reported to be dose related.

When prolonged therapy with any antimalarial compound is contemplated, initial (base line) and periodic (every three months) ophthalmologic examinations (including visual acuity, expert slit-lamp, funduscopic, and visual field tests) should be performed.

If there is any indication of abnormality in the visual acuity, visual field, or retinal macular areas (such as pigmentary changes, loss of foveal reflex), or any visual symptoms (such as light flashes and streaks) which are not fully explainable by difficulties of accommodation or corneal opacities, the drug should be discontinued immediately and the patient closely observed for possible progression. Retinal changes (and visual disturbances) may progress even after cessation of therapy.

All patients on long-term therapy with this preparation should be questioned and examined periodically, including the testing of knee and ankle reflexes, to detect any evidence of muscular weakness. If weakness occurs, discontinue the drug.

In the treatment of rheumatoid arthritis, if objective improvement (such as reduced joint swelling, increased mobility) does not occur within six months, the drug should be discontinued. Safe use of the drug in the treatment of juvenile arthritis has not been established.

Precautions: Dermatologic reactions to PLAQUENIL sulfate, brand of hydroxychloroquine sulfate tablets, may occur and, therefore, proper care should be exercised when it is administered to any patient receiving a drug with a significant tendency to produce dermatitis.

The methods recommended for early diagnosis of "chloroquine retinopathy" consist of (1) funduscopic examination of the macula for fine pigmentary disturbances or loss of the foveal reflex and (2) examination of the central visual field with a small red test object for pericentral or paracentral scotoma or determination of retinal thresholds to red. Any unexplained visual symptoms, such as light flashes or streaks should also be regarded with suspicion as possible manifestations of retinopathy.

If serious toxic symptoms occur from overdosage or sensitivity, it has been suggested that ammonium chloride (8 g daily in divided doses for adults) be administered orally three or four days a week for several months after therapy has been stopped, as acidification of the urine increases renal excretion of the 4-aminoquinoline compounds by 20 to 90 percent. However, caution must be exercised in patients with impaired renal function and/or metabolic acidosis.

Adverse Reactions: Not all of the following reactions have been observed with every 4-aminoquinoline compound during long-term therapy, but they have been reported with one or more and should be borne in mind when drugs of this class are administered. Adverse effects with different compounds vary in type and frequency.

CNS Reactions: irritability, nervousness, emotional changes, nightmares, psychosis, headache, dizziness, vertigo, tinnitus, nystagmus, nerve deafness, convulsions, ataxia.

Neuromuscular Reactions: extraocular muscle palsies, skeletal muscle weakness, absent or hypoactive deep tendon reflexes.

Ocular Reactions:

A. *Ciliary body:* disturbance of accommodation with symptoms of blurred vision. This reaction is dose related and reversible with cessation of therapy.

B. *Cornea:* transient edema, punctate to lineal opacities, decreased corneal sensitivity. The corneal changes, with or without accompanying symptoms (blurred vision, halos around lights, photophobia), are fairly common, but reversible. Corneal deposits may appear as early as three weeks following initiation of therapy.

The incidence of corneal changes and visual side effects appears to be considerably lower with hydroxychloroquine than with chloroquine.

C. *Retina:*

Macula: Edema, atrophy, abnormal pigmentation (mild pigment stippling to a "bull's-eye" appearance), loss of foveal reflex, increased macular recovery time following exposure to a bright light (photo-stress test), elevated retinal threshold to red light in macular, paramacular and peripheral retinal areas.

Other fundus changes include optic disc pallor and atrophy, attenuation of retinal arterioles, fine granular pigmentary disturbances in the peripheral retina and prominent choroidal patterns in advanced stage.

D. *Visual field defects:* pericentral or paracentral scotoma, central scotoma with decreased visual acuity, rarely field constriction.

The most common visual symptoms attributed to the retinopathy are: reading and seeing difficulties (words, letters, or parts of objects missing), photophobia, blurred distance vision, missing or blacked out areas in the central or peripheral visual field, light flashes and streaks.

Retinopathy appears to be dose related and has occurred within several months (rarely) to several years of daily therapy; a small number of cases have been reported several years after antimalarial drug therapy was discontinued. It has not been noted during prolonged use of weekly doses of the 4-aminoquinoline compounds for suppression of malaria.

Patients with retinal changes may have visual symptoms or may be asymptomatic (with or without visual field changes). Rarely scotomatous vision or field defects may occur without obvious retinal change.

Retinopathy may progress even after the drug is discontinued. In a number of patients, early retinopathy (macular pigmentation sometimes with central field defects) diminished or regressed completely after therapy was discontinued. Paracentral scotoma to red targets (sometimes called "premaculopathy") is indicative of early retinal dysfunction which is usually reversible with cessation of therapy.

A small number of cases of retinal changes have been reported as occurring in patients who received only hydroxychloroquine. These usually consisted of alteration in retinal pigmentation which was detected on periodic ophthalmologic examination; visual field defects were also present in some instances. A case of delayed retinopathy has been reported with loss of vision starting one year after administration of hydroxychloroquine had been discontinued.

Dermatologic Reactions: Bleaching of hair, alopecia, pruritus, skin and mucosal pigmentation, skin eruptions (urticarial, morbilliform, lichenoid, maculopapular, purpuric, erythema annulare centrifugum and exfoliative dermatitis).

Hematologic Reactions: Various blood dyscrasias such as aplastic anemia, agranulocytosis, leukopenia, thrombocytopenia (hemolysis in individuals with glucose-6-phosphate dehydrogenase (G-6-PD) deficiency).

Gastrointestinal Reactions: Anorexia, nausea, vomiting, diarrhea, and abdominal cramps.

Miscellaneous Reactions: Weight loss, lassitude, exacerbation or precipitation of porphyria and nonlight-sensitive psoriasis.

Dosage and Administration: One tablet of hydroxychloroquine sulfate, 200 mg, is equivalent to 155 mg base.

Lupus erythematosus—Initially, the average *adult* dose is 400 mg (=310 mg base) once or twice daily. This may be continued for several weeks or months, depending on the response of the patient. For prolonged maintenance therapy, a smaller dose, from 200 mg to 400 mg (=155 mg to 310 mg base) daily will frequently suffice.

The incidence of retinopathy has been reported to be higher when this maintenance dose is exceeded.

Rheumatoid arthritis—The compound is cumulative in action and will require several weeks to exert its beneficial therapeutic effects, whereas minor side effects may occur relatively early. Several months of therapy may be required before maximum effects can be obtained. If objective improvement (such as reduced joint swelling, increased mobility) does not occur within six months, the drug should be discontinued. Safe use of the drug in the treatment of juvenile rheumatoid arthritis has not been established.

Initial dosage—In *adults,* from 400 mg to 600 mg (=310 mg to 465 mg base) daily, each dose to be taken with a meal or a glass of milk. In a small percentage of patients, troublesome side effects may require temporary reduction of the initial dosage. Later (usually from five to ten days), the dose may gradually be increased to the optimum response level, often without return of side effects.

Maintenance dosage—When a good response is obtained (usually in four to twelve weeks), the dosage is reduced by 50 percent and continued at a usual maintenance level of 200 mg to 400 mg (=155 mg to 310 mg base) daily, each dose to be taken with a meal or a glass of milk. The incidence

of retinopathy has been reported to be higher when this maintenance dose is exceeded.
Should a relapse occur after medication is withdrawn, therapy may be resumed or continued on an intermittent schedule if there are no ocular contraindications.

Corticosteroids and salicylates may be used in conjunction with this compound, and they can generally be decreased gradually in dosage or eliminated after the drug has been used for several weeks. When gradual reduction of steroid dosage is indicated, it may be done by reducing every four to five days the dose of cortisone by no more than from 5 mg to 15 mg; of hydrocortisone from 5 mg to 10 mg; of prednisolone and prednisone from 1 mg to 2.5 mg; of methylprednisolone and triamcinolone from 1 mg to 2 mg; and of dexamethasone from 0.25 mg to 0.5 mg.

How Supplied: Tablets of 200 mg (equivalent to 155 mg of base), bottles of 100.

Shown in Product Identification Section, page 444
PW-306-M

PONTOCAINE® Hydrochloride R
brand of tetracaine hydrochloride, USP

Prolonged Spinal Anesthesia

Description: Tetracaine hydrochloride is 2-(dimethylamino) ethyl *p*-(butylamino) benzoate monohydrochloride. It is a white crystalline, odorless powder that is readily soluble in water, physiologic saline solution, and dextrose solution.
Tetracaine hydrochloride is a local anesthetic of the ester-linkage type, related to procaine.
PONTOCAINE hydrochloride is supplied in two forms for prolonged spinal anesthesia: NIPHANOID® and 1% solution.
Niphanoid: A sterile, instantly soluble form consisting of a network of extremely fine, highly purified particles, resembling snow.
1% solution: A sterile, isotonic, isobaric solution, each 1 mL containing 10 mg tetracaine hydrochloride, 6.7 mg sodium chloride, and not more than 2 mg acetone sodium bisulfite. The air in the ampuls has been displaced by nitrogen gas. The pH is 3.2 to 6.0.
These formulations do not contain preservatives.
Clinical Pharmacology: Parenteral administration of PONTOCAINE stabilizes the neuronal membrane and prevents initiation transmission of nerve impulses thereby effecting local anesthesia.
The onset of action is rapid, and the duration prolonged (up to two or three hours or longer of surgical anesthesia).
PONTOCAINE is detoxified by plasma esterases to para-aminobenzoic acid and diethylaminoethanol.
Indications and Usage: PONTOCAINE is indicated for the production of spinal anesthesia for procedures requiring two to three hours.
Contraindications: Spinal anesthesia with PONTOCAINE is contraindicated in patients with known hypersensitivity to tetracaine hydrochloride or to drugs of a similar chemical configuration (ester-type local anesthetics), or para-aminobenzoic acid or its derivatives; and in patients for whom spinal anesthesia as a technique is contraindicated.
The decision as to whether or not spinal anesthesia should be used for an individual patient should be made by the physician after weighing the advantages with the risks and possible complications. Contraindications to spinal anesthesia as a technique can be found in standard reference texts, and usually include generalized septicemia, infection at the site of injection, certain diseases of the cerebrospinal system, uncontrolled hypotension, etc.
Warnings: RESUSCITATIVE EQUIPMENT AND DRUGS SHOULD BE IMMEDIATELY AVAILABLE WHENEVER ANY LOCAL ANESTHETIC DRUG IS USED.
Large doses of local anesthetics should not be used in patients with heart block.

Reactions resulting in fatality have occurred on rare occasions with the use of local anesthetics, even in the absence of a history of hypersensitivity.
Precautions: The safety and effectiveness of any spinal anesthetic depend upon proper dosage, correct technique, adequate precautions, and readiness for emergencies. The lowest dosage that results in effective anesthesia should be used to avoid high plasma levels and serious systemic side effects. Tolerance varies with the status of the patient; debilitated, elderly patients or acutely ill patients should be given reduced doses commensurate with their weight, age, and physical status. Reduced doses are also indicated for obstetric patients and those with increased intraabdominal pressure.
Caution should be used in administering PONTOCAINE to patients with abnormal or reduced levels of plasma esterases.
Blood pressure should be frequently monitored during spinal anesthesia and hypotension immediately corrected.
Spinal anesthetics should be used with caution in patients with severe disturbances of cardiac rhythm, shock or heart block.
Drug Interactions: PONTOCAINE should not be used if the patient is being treated with a sulfonamide because para-aminobenzoic acid inhibits the action of sulfonamides.
Carcinogenesis, mutagenesis, impairment of fertility: Long-term animal studies to evaluate carcinogenic potential and reproduction studies in animals have not been performed. There is no evidence from human data that PONTOCAINE may be carcinogenic or that it impairs fertility.
Pregnancy Category C: Animal reproduction studies have not been conducted with PONTOCAINE. It is not known whether PONTOCAINE can cause fetal harm when administered to a pregnant woman or can affect reproduction capacity. PONTOCAINE should be given to a pregnant woman only if clearly needed and the potential benefits outweigh the risk.
Labor and delivery: Vasopressor agents administered for the treatment of hypotension resulting from spinal anesthesia may result in severe persistent hypertension and/or rupture of cerebral blood vessels if oxytocic drugs have also been administered; therefore, vasopressors should be used with extreme caution in the presence of oxytocic drugs.
PONTOCAINE has a recognized use during labor and delivery; the effect of the drug on duration of labor, incidence of forceps delivery, status of the newborn, and later growth and development of the child have not been studied.
Nursing mothers: It is not known whether PONTOCAINE is excreted in human milk; however it is rapidly metabolized following absorption into the plasma. Because many drugs are excreted in human milk, caution should be exercised when PONTOCAINE, brand of tetracaine hydrochloride, is administered to a nursing woman.
Pediatric use: Safety and effectiveness of PONTOCAINE in children have not been established.
Adverse Reactions: Systemic adverse reactions to PONTOCAINE are characteristic of those associated with other local anesthetics and can involve the central nervous system and the cardiovascular system. Systemic reactions usually result from high plasma levels due to excessive dosage, rapid absorption, or inadvertent intravascular injection.
A small number of reactions to PONTOCAINE may result from hypersensitivity, idiosyncrasy or diminished tolerance to normal dosage.
Central nervous system effects are characterized by excitation or depression. The first manifestation may be nervousness, dizziness, blurred vision, or tremors, followed by drowsiness, convulsions, unconsciousness and possibly respiratory and cardiac arrest. Since excitement may be transient or absent, the first manifestation may be drowsiness, sometimes merging into unconsciousness and respiratory and cardiac arrest. Other central nervous system effects may be nausea, vomiting, chills, constriction of the pupils, or tinnitus.

Cardiovascular system reactions include depression of the myocardium, blood pressure changes (usually hypotension), and cardiac arrest.
Allergic reactions, which may be due to hypersensitivity, idiosyncrasy or diminished tolerance, are characterized by cutaneous lesions (urticaria), edema, and other manifestations of allergy. Detection of sensitivity by skin testing is of limited value. Severe allergic reactions including anaphylaxis have occurred rarely and are not usually dose-related.
Reactions associated with spinal anesthesia techniques: Central nervous system: postspinal headache, meningismus, arachnoiditis, palsies, or spinal nerve paralysis. Cardiovascular: hypotension due to vasomotor paralysis and pooling of the blood in the venous bed. Respiratory: respiratory impairment or paralysis due to the level of anesthesia extending to the upper thoracic and cervical segments. Gastrointestinal: nausea and vomiting.
Treatment of reactions: Toxic effects of local anesthetics require symptomatic treatment; there is no specific cure. **The most important measure is oxygenation of the patient by maintaining an airway and supporting ventilation.** Supportive treatment of the cardiovascular system includes intravenous fluids and, when appropriate, vasopressors (preferably those that stimulate the myocardium). Convulsions are usually controlled with adequate oxygenation alone but intravenous administration in small increments of a barbiturate (preferably an ultrashort-acting barbiturate such as thiopental and thiamylal) or diazepam can be utilized. Intravenous barbiturates or anticonvulsant agents should only be administered by those familiar with their use and only if ventilation and oxygenation have first been assured. In spinal anesthesia, sympathetic blockade also occurs as a pharmacological action, resulting in peripheral vasodilation and often hypotension. The extent of the hypotension will usually depend on the number of dermatomes blocked. The blood pressure should therefore be monitored in the early phases of anesthesia. If hypotension occurs, it is readily controlled by vasoconstrictors administered either by the intramuscular or the intravenous route, the dosage of which would depend on the severity of the hypotension and the response to treatment.
Dosage and Administration: As with all anesthetics, the dosage varies and depends upon the area to be anesthetized, the number of neuronal segments to be blocked, individual tolerance, and the technique of anesthesia. The lowest dosage needed to provide effective anesthesia should be administered. For specific techniques and procedures, refer to standard textbooks.
[See table on next page].
The extent and degree of spinal anesthesia depend upon dosage, specific gravity of the anesthetic solution, volume of solution used, force of the injection, level of puncture, position of the patient during and immediately after injection, etc.
When spinal fluid is added to either the NIPHANOID or solution, some turbidity results, the degree depending on the pH of the spinal fluid, the temperature of the solution during mixing, as well as the amount of drug and diluent employed. This cloudiness is due to the release of the *base* from the hydrochloride. Liberation of base (which is completed within the spinal canal) is held to be essential for satisfactory results with any spinal anesthetic.
The specific gravity of spinal fluid at 25°/25°C varies under normal conditions from 1.0063 to 1.0075. A solution of the instantly soluble form (NIPHANOID) in spinal fluid has only a slightly

Continued on next page

This product information was effective as of December 3, 1984. On these and other products of Winthrop-Breon Laboratories, detailed information may be obtained on a current basis by direct inquiry to the Professional Services Department, 90 Park Avenue, New York, NY 10016 (212) 907-2525.

Winthrop-Breon—Cont.

greater specific gravity. The 1% concentration in saline solution has a specific gravity of 1.0060 to 1.0074 at 25°/25°C.

A hyperbaric solution may be prepared by mixing equal volumes of the 1% solution and Dextrose Solution 10% (which is available in ampuls of 3 mL).

If the NIPHANOID form is preferred, it is first dissolved in Dextrose Solution 10% in a ratio of 1 mL dextrose to 10 mg of the anesthetic. Further dilution is made with an equal volume of spinal fluid. The resulting solution now contains 5% dextrose with 5 mg of anesthetic agent per milliliter.

A hypobaric solution may be prepared by dissolving the NIPHANOID in Sterile Water for Injection, USP (1 mg per milliliter). The specific gravity of this solution is essentially the same as that of water, 1.000 at 25°/25°C.

Examine ampuls carefully before use. Do not use solution if crystals, cloudiness, or discoloration is observed.

These formulations of tetracaine hydrochloride do not contain preservatives; therefore, unused portions should be discarded and the reconstituted NIPHANOID should be used immediately.

Sterilization of Ampuls: The drug in intact ampuls is sterile. The preferred method of destroying bacteria on the exterior of ampuls before opening is heat sterilization (autoclaving). Immersion in antiseptic solution is not recommended.

Autoclave at 15-pound pressure, at 121°C (250°F) for 15 minutes. The NIPHANOID form may also be autoclaved in the same way but may lose its snowlike appearance and tend to adhere to the sides of the ampul. This may slightly decrease the rate at which the drug dissolves but does not interfere with its anesthetic potency.

Autoclaving increases likelihood of crystal formation. Unused autoclaved ampuls should be discarded. In no case should unused autoclaved ampuls be placed back in stock for later use.

How Supplied:
Protect ampuls from light and store solution under refrigeration.
NIPHANOID (instantly soluble): ampuls of 20mg, box of 100 (NDC 0024-1577-06)
1% isotonic isobaric solution: ampuls of 2 mL, UNI-NEST™ PAK of 25 (NDC 0024-1574-25)

PW-56-W

SULFAMYLON® Cream ℞
brand of mafenide acetate cream, USP

Topical Antibacterial Agent for Adjunctive Therapy in Second- and Third-Degree Burns

Description: SULFAMYLON Cream is a soft, white, nonstaining, water-miscible, anti-infective cream for topical administration to burn wounds. SULFAMYLON Cream spreads easily, and can be washed off readily with water. It has a slight acetic odor. Each gram of SULFAMYLON Cream contains mafenide acetate equivalent to 85 mg of the base. The cream vehicle consists of cetyl alcohol, stearyl alcohol, cetyl esters wax, polyoxyl 40 stearate, polyoxyl 8 stearate, glycerin, and water, with methylparaben, propylparaben, sodium bisulfite, and edetate disodium as preservatives.

Chemically, mafenide acetate is α-Amino-p-toluenesulfonamide monoacetate.

Clinical Pharmacology: SULFAMYLON Cream, applied topically, produces a marked reduction in the bacterial population present in the avascular tissues of second- and third-degree burns. Reduction in bacterial growth after application of SULFAMYLON Cream has also been reported to permit spontaneous healing of deep partial-thickness burns, and thus prevent conversion of burn wounds from partial thickness to full thickness. It should be noted, however, that delayed eschar separation has occurred in some cases.

Absorption and Metabolism. Applied topically, SULFAMYLON Cream diffuses through devascularized areas, is absorbed, and rapidly converted to a metabolite (p-carboxybenzenesulfonamide) which is cleared through the kidneys. SULFAMYLON is active in the presence of pus and serum, and its activity is not altered by changes in the acidity of the environment.

Antibacterial Activity. SULFAMYLON exerts bacteriostatic action against many gram-negative and gram-positive organisms, including *Pseudomonas aeruginosa* and certain strains of anaerobes.

Indications and Usage: SULFAMYLON Cream is a topical agent indicated for adjunctive therapy of patients with second- and third-degree burns.

Contraindications: SULFAMYLON is contraindicated in patients who are hypersensitive to it. It is not known whether there is cross sensitivity to other sulfonamides.

Warnings: Fatal hemolytic anemia with disseminated intravascular coagulation, presumably related to a glucose-6-phosphate dehydrogenase deficiency, has been reported following SULFAMYLON Cream therapy.

Precautions: SULFAMYLON and its metabolite, p-carboxybenzenesulfonamide, inhibit carbonic anhydrase, which may result in metabolic acidosis, usually compensated by hyperventilation. In the presence of impaired renal function, high blood levels of SULFAMYLON and its metabolite may exaggerate the carbonic anhydrase inhibition. Therefore, close monitoring of acid-base balance is necessary, particularly in patients with extensive second-degree or partial thickness burns and in those with pulmonary or renal dysfunction. Some burn patients treated with SULFAMYLON Cream have also been reported to manifest all unexplained syndrome of marked hyperventilation with resulting respiratory alkalosis (slightly alkaline blood pH, low arterial pCO_2, and decreased total CO_2); change in arterial pO_2 is variable. The etiology and significance of these findings are unknown.

Mafenide acetate cream should be used with caution in burn patients with acute renal failure.

SULFAMYLON Cream should be administered with caution to patients with history of hypersensitivity to mafenide. It is not known whether there is cross sensitivity to other sulfonamides.

Fungal colonization in and below the eschar may occur concomitantly with reduction of bacterial growth in the burn wound. However, fungal dissemination through the infected burn wound is rare.

Carcinogenesis, Mutagenesis, Impairment of Fertility. No long-term animal studies have been performed to evaluate the drug's potential in these areas.

Pregnancy Category C. Animal reproduction studies have not been conducted with SULFAMYLON. It is also not known whether SULFAMYLON can cause fetal harm when administered to a pregnant woman or can affect reproduction capacity. Therefore, the preparation is not recommended for the treatment of women of childbearing potential, unless the burned area covers more than 20% of the total body surface, or the need for the therapeutic benefit of SULFAMYLON Cream is, in the physician's judgment, greater than the possible risk to the fetus.

Nursing Mothers. It is not known whether mafenide acetate is excreted in human milk. Because many drugs are excreted in human milk and because of the potential for serious adverse reaction in nursing infants from SULFAMYLON, a decision should be made whether to discontinue nursing or to discontinue the drug, taking into account the importance of the drug to the mother.

Pediatric Use. Same as for adults. (See DOSAGE AND ADMINISTRATION.)

Adverse Reactions: It is frequently difficult to distinguish between an adverse reaction to SULFAMYLON Cream and the effect of a severe burn. A single case of bone marrow depression and a single case of an acute attack of porphyria have been reported following SULFAMYLON Cream therapy. Fatal hemolytic anemia with disseminated intravascular coagulation, presumably related to a glucose-6-phosphate dehydrogenase deficiency, has been reported following SULFAMYLON Cream therapy.

Dermatologic: The most frequently reported reaction was pain on application or a burning sensation. Rare occurrences are excoriation of new skin, and bleeding of skin.

Allergic: Rash, itching, facial edema, swelling, hives, blisters, erythema, and eosinophilia.

Respiratory: Tachypnea or hyperventilation, decrease in arterial pCO_2.

Metabolic: Acidosis, increase in serum chloride. Accidental ingestion of SULFAMYLON Cream has been reported to cause diarrhea.

Administration: Prompt institution of appropriate measures for controlling shock and pain is of prime importance. The burn wounds are then cleansed and debrided, and SULFAMYLON Cream, brand of mafenide acetate cream, is applied with a sterile gloved hand. Satisfactory results can be achieved with application of the cream once or twice daily, to a thickness of approximately 1/16 inch; thicker application is not recommended. The burned areas should be covered with

---

PONTOCAINE — SUGGESTED DOSAGE FOR SPINAL ANESTHESIA

Extent of anesthesia	Using NIPHANOID			Using 1% solution		
	Dose of NIPHANOID (mg)	Volume of spinal fluid (mL)		Dose of solution (mL)	Volume of spinal fluid (mL)	Site of injection (lumbar interspace)
Perineum	5*	1		0.5 (=5 mg)*	0.5	4th
Perineum and lower extremities	10	2		1.0 (=10 mg)	1.0	3d or 4th
Up to costal margin	15 to 20†	3		1.5 to 2.0 (=15 mg to 20 mg)†	1.5 to 2.0	2d, 3d, or 4th

*For vaginal delivery (saddle block), from 2 mg to 5 mg in dextrose.

† Doses exceeding 15 mg are rarely required and should be used only in exceptional cases. Inject solution at rate of about 1 mL per 5 seconds.

SULFAMYLON Cream at all times. Therefore, whenever necessary, the cream should be reapplied to any areas from which it has been removed (eg, by patient activity). The routine of administration can be accomplished in minimal time, since dressings usually are not required. If individual patient demands make them necessary, however, only a thin layer of dressing should be used.

When feasible, the patient should be bathed daily, to aid in debridement. A whirlpool bath is particularly helpful, but the patient may be bathed in bed or in a shower.

The duration of therapy with SULFAMYLON Cream depends on each patient's requirements. Treatment is usually continued until healing is progressing well or until the burn site is ready for grafting. *SULFAMYLON Cream should not be withdrawn from the therapeutic regimen while there is the possibility of infection.* However, if allergic manifestations occur during treatment with SULFAMYLON Cream, discontinuation of treatment should be considered.

If acidosis occurs and becomes difficult to control, particularly in patients with pulmonary dysfunction, discontinuing SULFAMYLON Cream therapy for 24 to 48 hours while continuing fluid therapy may aid in restoring acid-base balance.

How Supplied:
Cans of 14.5 ounces (411 g)—NDC 0024-1884-09
Collapsible tubes of 4 ounces (113.4 g) NDC 0024-1884-02
Collapsible tubes of 2 ounces (56.7 g) NDC 0024-1884-01

SW-89-I

TALACEN®
Pentazocine hydrochloride, USP, equivalent to 25 mg base and acetaminophen, USP, 650 mg.

Description: TALACEN is a combination of pentazocine hydrochloride, USP, equivalent to 25 mg base and acetaminophen, USP, 650 mg. Pentazocine is a member of the benzazocine series (also known as the benzomorphan series). Chemically, pentazocine is 1,2,3,4,5,6-Hexahydro-6,11-dimethyl-3-(3-methyl-2-butenyl)-2,6-methano-3-benzazocin-8-ol, a white, crystalline substance soluble in acidic aqueous solutions.

Chemically, acetaminophen is Acetamide, *N*-(4-hydroxy-phenyl).

Pentazocine is an analgesic and acetaminophen is an analgesic and antipyretic.

TALACEN is a pale blue, scored caplet for oral administration.

Clinical Pharmacology: TALACEN is an analgesic possessing antipyretic actions.

Pentazocine is an analgesic with agonist/antagonist action which when administered orally is approximately equivalent on a mg for mg basis in analgesic effect to codeine.

Acetaminophen is an analgesic and antipyretic. Onset of significant analgesia with pentazocine usually occurs between 15 and 30 minutes after oral administration, and duration of action is usually three hours or longer. Onset and duration of action and the degree of pain relief are related both to dose and the severity of pretreatment pain. Pentazocine weakly antagonizes the analgesic effects of morphine, meperidine, and phenazocine; in addition, it produces incomplete reversal of cardiovascular, respiratory, and behavioral depression induced by morphine and meperidine. Pentazocine has about 1/50 the antagonistic activity of nalorphine. It also has sedative activity.

Pentazocine is well absorbed from the gastrointestinal tract. Plasma levels closely correspond to the onset, duration, and intensity of analgesia. The mean peak concentration in 24 normal volunteers was 1.7 hours (range 0.5 to 4.0 hours) after oral administration and the mean plasma elimination half-life was 3.6 hours (range 1.5 to 10 hours).

The action of pentazocine is terminated for the most part by biotransformation in the liver with some free pentazocine excreted in the urine. The products of the oxidation of the terminal methyl groups and glucuronide conjugates are excreted by the kidney. Elimination of approximately 60% of the total dose occurs within 24 hours. Pentazocine passes the placental barrier.

Onset of significant analgesic and antipyretic activity of acetaminophen when administered orally occurs within 30 minutes and is maximal at approximately 2½ hours. The pharmacological mode of action of acetaminophen is unknown at this time.

Acetaminophen is rapidly and almost completely absorbed from the gastrointestinal tract. In 24 normal volunteers the mean peak plasma concentration was 1 hour (range 0.25 to 3 hours) after oral administration and the mean plasma elimination half-life was 2.8 hours (range 2 to 4 hours).

The effect of pentazocine on acetaminophen plasma protein binding or vice versa has not been established. For acetaminophen there is little or no plasma protein binding at normal therapeutic doses. When toxic doses of acetaminophen are ingested and drug plasma levels exceed 90 mcg/mL, plasma binding may vary from 8% to 43%.

Acetaminophen is conjugated in the liver with glucuronic acid and to a lesser extent with sulfuric acid. Approximately 80% of acetaminophen is excreted in the urine after conjugation and about 3% is excreted unchanged. The drug is also conjugated to a lesser extent with cysteine and additionally metabolized by hydroxylation.

If TALACEN is taken every 4 hours over an extended period of time, accumulation of pentazocine and to a lesser extent, acetaminophen, may occur.

Indications and Usage: TALACEN is indicated for the relief of mild to moderate pain.

Contraindications: TALACEN should not be administered to patients who are hypersensitive to either pentazocine or acetaminophen.

Warnings: *Head Injury and Increased Intracranial Pressure.* As in the case of other potent analgesics, the potential of pentazocine for elevating cerebrospinal fluid pressure may be attributed to CO_2 retention due to the respiratory depressant effects of the drug. These effects may be markedly exaggerated in the presence of head injury, other intracranial lesions, or a preexisting increase in intracranial pressure. Furthermore, pentazocine can produce effects which may obscure the clinical course of patients with head injuries. In such patients, TALACEN must be used with extreme caution and only if its use is deemed essential.

Acute CNS Manifestations. Patients receiving pentazocine in doses of 50 mg or more have experienced, in rare instances, hallucinations (usually visual), disorientation, and confusion which have cleared spontaneously within a period of hours. The mechanism of this reaction is not known. Such patients should be very closely observed and vital signs checked. If the drug is reinstituted, it should be done with caution since the acute CNS manifestations may recur.

There have been instances of psychological and physical dependence on parenteral pentazocine in patients with a history of drug abuse, and rarely, in patients without such a history. (See DRUG ABUSE AND DEPENDENCE.)

Due to the potential for increased CNS depressant effects, alcohol should be used with caution in patients who are currently receiving pentazocine.

Pentazocine may precipitate opioid abstinence symptoms in patients receiving courses of opiates for pain relief.

Precautions: *In prescribing TALACEN for chronic use, the physician should take precautions to avoid increases in dose by the patient.*

Myocardial Infarction. As with all drugs, TALACEN should be used with caution in patients with myocardial infarction who have nausea or vomiting.

Certain Respiratory Conditions. Although respiratory depression has rarely been reported after oral administration of pentazocine, the drug should be administered with caution to patients with respiratory depression from any cause, severely limited respiratory reserve, severe bronchial asthma and other obstructive respiratory conditions, or cyanosis.

Impaired Renal or Hepatic Function. Decreased metabolism of the drug by the liver in extensive liver disease may predispose to accentuation of side effects. Although laboratory tests have not indicated that pentazocine causes or increases renal or hepatic impairment, the drug should be administered with caution to patients with such impairment.

Since acetaminophen is metabolized by the liver, the question of the safety of its use in the presence of liver disease should be considered.

Biliary Surgery. Narcotic drug products are generally considered to elevate biliary tract pressure for varying periods following their administration. Some evidence suggests that pentazocine may differ from other marketed narcotics in this respect (ie, it causes little or no elevation in biliary tract pressures). The clinical significance of these findings, however, is not yet known.

CNS Effect. Caution should be used when TALACEN is administered to patients prone to seizures; seizures have occurred in a few such patients in association with the use of pentazocine although no cause and effect relationship has been established.

Information for Patients: Since sedation, dizziness, and occasional euphoria have been noted, ambulatory patients should be warned not to operate machinery, drive cars, or unnecessarily expose themselves to hazards. Pentazocine may cause physical and psychological dependence when taken alone and may have additive CNS depressant properties when taken in combination with alcohol or other CNS depressants.

Drug Interactions. Pentazocine is a mild narcotic antagonist. Some patients previously given narcotics, including methadone for the daily treatment of narcotic dependence, have experienced withdrawal symptoms after receiving pentazocine.

Carcinogenesis, Mutagenesis, Impairment of Fertility. Carcinogenesis, mutagenesis, and impairment of fertility studies have not been done with this combination product.

Pentazocine, when administered orally or parenterally, had no adverse effect on either the reproductive capabilities or the course of pregnancy in rabbits and rats. Embryotoxic effects on the fetuses were not shown.

The daily administration of 4 mg/kg to 20 mg/kg pentazocine subcutaneously to female rats during a 14 day pre-mating period and until the 13th day of pregnancy did not have any adverse effects on the fertility rate.

There is no evidence in long-term animal studies to demonstrate that pentazocine is carcinogenic.

Pregnancy Category C. Animal reproduction studies have not been conducted with TALACEN. It is also not known whether TALACEN can cause fetal harm when administered to pregnant women or can effect reproduction capacity. TALACEN should be given to pregnant women only if clearly needed. However, animal reproduction studies with pentazocine have not demonstrated teratogenic embryotoxic effects.

Nonteratogenic Effects. There has been no experience in this regard with the combination pentazocine and acetaminophen. However, there have been rare reports of possible abstinence syndromes in newborns after prolonged use of pentazocine during pregnancy.

Labor and Delivery. Patients receiving pentazocine during labor have experienced no adverse effects other than those that occur with commonly used analgesics. TALACEN should be used with caution in women delivering premature infants. The effect of TALACEN on the mother and fetus,

Continued on next page

This product information was effective as of December 3, 1984. On these and other products of Winthrop-Breon Laboratories, detailed information may be obtained on a current basis by direct inquiry to the Professional Services Department, 90 Park Avenue, New York, NY 10016 (212) 907-2525.

Winthrop-Breon—Cont.

the duration of labor or delivery, the possibility that forceps delivery or other intervention or resuscitation of the newborn may be necessary, or the effect of TALACEN, on the later growth, development, and functional maturation of the child are unknown at the present time.

Nursing Mothers. It is not known whether this drug is excreted in human milk. Because many drugs are excreted in human milk, caution should be exercised when TALACEN is administered to a nursing woman.

Pediatric Use. Safety and effectiveness in children below the age of 12 have not been established.

Adverse Reactions: Clinical experience with TALACEN has been insufficient to define all possible adverse reactions with this combination. However, reactions reported after oral administration of pentazocine hydrochloride in 50 mg dosage include *gastrointestinal:* nausea, vomiting, infrequently constipation; and rarely abdominal distress, anorexia, diarrhea. *CNS effects:* dizziness, lightheadedness, sedation, euphoria, headache; infrequently weakness, disturbed dreams, insomnia, syncope, visual blurring and focusing difficulty, hallucinations (see *Acute CNS Manifestations* under WARNINGS); and rarely tremor, irritability, excitement, tinnitus. *Autonomic:* sweating; infrequently flushing; and rarely chills. *Allergic:* infrequently rash; and rarely urticaria, edema of the face. *Cardiovascular:* infrequently decrease in blood pressure, tachycardia. *Hematologic:* rarely depression of white blood cells (especially granulocytes), which is usually reversible, moderate transient eosinophilia. *Other:* rarely respiratory depression, urinary retention, paresthesia, toxic epidermal necrolysis.

Numerous clinical studies have shown that acetaminophen, when taken in recommended doses, is relatively free of adverse effects in most age groups, even in the presence of a variety of disease states.

A few cases of hypersensitivity to acetaminophen have been reported, as manifested by skin rashes, thrombocytopenic purpura, rarely hemolytic anemia and agranulocytosis. Occasional individuals respond to ordinary doses with nausea and vomiting or diarrhea.

Drug Abuse and Dependence: *Controlled Substance.* TALACEN is a Schedule IV controlled substance.

Abuse and Dependence. There have been some reports of dependence and of withdrawal symptoms with orally administered pentazocine. There have been recorded instances of psychological and physical dependence in patients using parenteral pentazocine. Abrupt discontinuance following the extended use of parenteral pentazocine has resulted in withdrawal symptoms. Patients with a history of drug dependence should be under close supervision while receiving TALACEN. There have been rare reports of possible abstinence syndromes in newborns after prolonged use of pentazocine during pregnancy.

Some tolerance to the analgesic and subjective effects of pentazocine develops with frequent and repeated use.

Drug addicts who are given closely spaced doses of pentazocine (eg, 60 mg to 90 mg every 4 hours) develop physical dependence which is demonstrated by abrupt withdrawal or by administration of naloxone. The withdrawal symptoms exhibited after chronic doses of more than 500 mg of pentazocine per day have similar characteristics, but to a lesser degree, of opioid withdrawal and may be associated with drug seeking behavior.

Overdosage: *Manifestations.* Clinical experience with TALACEN has been insufficient to define the signs of overdosage with this product. It may be assumed that signs and symptoms of TALACEN overdose would be a combination of those observed with pentazocine overdose and acetaminophen overdose.

For pentazocine alone in single doses above 60 mg there have been reports of the occurrence of nalorphine-like psychotomimetic effects such as anxiety, nightmares, strange thoughts, and hallucinations. Marked respiratory depression associated with increased blood pressure and tachycardia have also resulted from excessive doses as have dizziness, nausea, vomiting, lethargy, and paresthesias. The respiratory depression is antagonized by naloxone (see *Treatment*).

In acute acetaminophen overdosage, dose-dependent, potentially fatal hepatic necrosis is the most serious adverse effect. Renal tubular necrosis, hypoglycemic coma, and thrombocytopenia may also occur.

In adults, a single dose of 10 g to 15 g (200 mg/kg to 250 mg/kg) of acetaminophen may cause hepatotoxicity. A dose of 25 g or more is potentially fatal. The potential seriousness of the intoxication may not be evident during the first two days of acute acetaminophen poisoning. During the first 24 hours, nausea, vomiting, anorexia, and abdominal pain occur. These may persist for a week or more. Liver injury may become evident the second day, initial signs being elevation of serum transaminase and lactic dehydrogenase activity, increased serum bilirubin concentration, and prolongation of prothrombin time. Serum albumin concentration and alkaline phosphatase activity may remain normal. The hepatotoxicity may lead to encephalopathy, coma, and death. Transient azotemia is evident in a majority of patients and acute renal failure occurs in some.

There have been reports of glycosuria and impaired glucose tolerance, but hypoglycemia may also occur. Metabolic acidosis and metabolic alkalosis have been reported. Cerebral edema and nonspecific myocardial depression have also been noted. Biopsy reveals centrolobular necrosis with sparing of the periportal area. The hepatic lesions are reversible over a period of weeks or months in nonfatal cases.

The severity of the liver injury can be determined by measurement of the plasma half-time of acetaminophen during the first day of acute poisoning. If the half-time exceeds 4 hours, hepatic necrosis is likely and if the half-time is greater than 12 hours, hepatic coma will probably occur. Only minimal liver damage has developed when the serum concentration was below 120 µg/mL at 12 hours after ingestion of the drug. If serum bilirubin concentration is greater than 4 mg/100 mL during the first 5 days, encephalopathy may occur.

The seven day oral LD$_{50}$ value for TALACEN in mice is 3,570 mg/kg.

Treatment. Oxygen, intravenous fluids, vasopressors, and other supportive measures should be employed as indicated. Assisted or controlled ventilation should also be considered. For respiratory depression due to overdosage or unusual sensitivity to TALACEN, parenteral naloxone is a specific and effective antagonist.

The toxic effects of acetaminophen may be prevented or minimized by antidotal therapy with N-acetylcysteine. In order to obtain the best possible results, N-acetylcysteine should be administered within approximately 16 hours of ingestion of the overdose.

The use of N-acetylcysteine as an antidote is currently restricted to investigational use. For information and directions for use, contact the Rocky Mountain Poison Center (800-525-6115).

Vigorous supportive therapy is required in severe intoxication. Procedures to limit the continuing absorption of the drug must be readily performed since the hepatic injury is dose dependent and occurs early in the course of intoxication. Induction of vomiting or gastric lavage, followed by oral administration of activated charcoal should be done in all cases.

If hemodialysis can be initiated within the first 12 hours, it is advocated for patients with a plasma acetaminophen concentration exceeding 120 µg/mL at 4 hours after ingestion of the drug.

Dosage and Administration: *Adult.* The usual adult dose is 1 tablet every 4 hours as needed for pain relief, up to a maximum of 6 tablets per day. The usual duration of therapy is dependent upon the condition being treated but in any case should be reviewed regularly by the physician. The effect of meals on the rate and extent of bioavailability of both pentazocine and acetaminophen has not been documented.

How Supplied: Caplets®, pale blue, scored, each containing pentazocine hydrochloride equivalent to 25 mg base and acetaminophen 650 mg. Bottles of 100 (NDC 0024-1937-04).

Unit Dose Dispenser Package of 250 (NDC 0024-1937-14), 10 sleeves of 25 CAPLETS each.

Distributed by
Winthrop-Breon Laboratories
Division of Sterling Drug Inc
New York, NY 10016
Manufactured by
Sterling Pharmaceuticals Inc
Barceloneta, Puerto Rico 00617

Shown in Product Identification Section, page 444

TW-262-D

TALWIN® Injection © ℞
brand of pentazocine lactate injection, USP

Analgesic for Parenteral Use

Description: TALWIN injection, brand of pentazocine lactate injection, is a member of the benzazocine series (also known as the benzomorphan series). Chemically, pentazocine lactate is 1, 2, 3, 4, 5, 6- Hexahydro-6, 11-dimethyl-3-(3-methyl-2-butenyl) -2,6-methano-3- benzazocin-8-ol lactate, a white, crystalline substance soluble in acidic aqueous solutions.

Actions: TALWIN is a potent analgesic and 30 mg is usually as effective an analgesic as morphine 10 mg or meperidine 75 mg to 100 mg; however, a few studies suggest the TALWIN to morphine ratio may range from 20 mg to 40 mg TALWIN to 10 mg morphine. The duration of analgesia may sometimes be less than that of morphine. Analgesia usually occurs within 15 to 20 minutes after intramuscular or subcutaneous injection and within 2 to 3 minutes after intravenous injection. TALWIN weakly antagonizes the analgesic effects of morphine, meperidine, and phenazocine; in addition, it produces incomplete reversal of cardiovascular, respiratory, and behavioral depression induced by morphine and meperidine. TALWIN has about 1/50 the antagonistic activity of nalorphine. It also has sedative activity.

Indications: For the relief of moderate to severe pain. TALWIN may also be used for preoperative or preanesthetic medication and as a supplement to surgical anesthesia.

Contraindication: TALWIN should not be administered to patients who are hypersensitive to it.

Warnings: Drug Dependence. *Special care should be exercised in prescribing pentazocine for emotionally unstable patients and for those with a history of drug misuse. Such patients should be closely supervised when greater than 4 or 5 days of therapy is contemplated. There have been instances of psychological and physical dependence on TALWIN in patients with such a history and, rarely, in patients without such a history. Extended use of parenteral TALWIN may lead to physical or psychological dependence in some patients. When TALWIN is abruptly discontinued, withdrawal symptoms such as abdominal cramps, elevated temperature, rhinorrhea, restlessness, anxiety, and lacrimation may occur. However, even when these have occurred, discontinuance has been accomplished with minimal difficulty. In the rare patient in whom more than minor difficulty has been encountered, reinstitution of parenteral TALWIN with gradual withdrawal has ameliorated the patient's symptoms. Substituting methadone or other narcotics for TALWIN in the treatment of the pentazocine abstinence syndrome should be avoided. There have been rare reports of possible abstinence syndromes in newborns after prolonged use of TALWIN during pregnancy.*

In prescribing parenteral TALWIN for chronic use, particularly if the drug is to be self-administered, the physician should take precautions to avoid increases in dose and frequency of injection by the patient.

Just as with all medication, the oral form of TALWIN is preferable for chronic administration.

Tissue Damage at Injection Sites. Severe sclerosis of the skin, subcutaneous tissues, and underlying muscle have occurred at the injection sites of patients who have received multiple doses of pentazocine lactate. Constant rotation of injection sites is, therefore, essential. In addition, animal studies have demonstrated that TALWIN is tolerated less well subcutaneously than intramuscularly. (See DOSAGE AND ADMINISTRATION.)

Head Injury and Increased Intracranial Pressure. As in the case of other potent analgesics, the potential of TALWIN injection for elevating cerebrospinal fluid pressure may be attributed to CO_2 retention due to the respiratory depressant effects of the drug. These effects may be markedly exaggerated in the presence of head injury, other intracranial lesions, or a preexisting increase in intracranial pressure. Furthermore, TALWIN can produce effects which may obscure the clinical course of patients with head injuries. In such patients, TALWIN must be used with extreme caution and only if its use is deemed essential.

Usage in Pregnancy. Safe use of TALWIN during pregnancy (other than labor) has not been established. Animal reproduction studies have not demonstrated teratogenic or embryotoxic effects. However, TALWIN should be administered to pregnant patients (other than labor) only when, in the judgment of the physician, the potential benefits outweigh the possible hazards. Patients receiving TALWIN during labor have experienced no adverse effects other than those that occur with commonly used analgesics. TALWIN should be used with caution in women delivering premature infants.

Acute CNS Manifestations. Patients receiving therapeutic doses of TALWIN have experienced, in rare instances, hallucinations (usually visual), disorientation, and confusion which have cleared spontaneously within a period of hours. The mechanism of this reaction is not known. Such patients should be very closely observed and vital signs checked. If the drug is reinstituted, it should be done with caution since the acute CNS manifestations may recur.

Due to the potential for increased CNS depressant effects, alcohol should be used with caution in patients who are currently receiving pentazocine.

Usage in Children. Because clinical experience in children under twelve years of age is limited, the use of TALWIN in this age group is not recommended.

Ambulatory Patients. Since sedation, dizziness, and occasional euphoria have been noted, ambulatory patients should be warned not to operate machinery, drive cars, or unnecessarily expose themselves to hazards.

Myocardial Infarction. Caution should be exercised in the intravenous use of pentazocine for patients with acute myocardial infarction accompanied by hypertension or left ventricular failure. Data suggest that intravenous administration of pentazocine increases systemic and pulmonary arterial pressure and systemic vascular resistance in patients with acute myocardial infarction.

Precautions: Certain Respiratory Conditions. The possibility that TALWIN may cause respiratory depression should be considered in treatment of patients with bronchial asthma. TALWIN injection, brand of pentazocine lactate injection, should be administered only with caution and in low dosage to patients with respiratory depression (eg, from other medication, uremia, or severe infection), severely limited respiratory reserve, obstructive respiratory conditions, or cyanosis.

Impaired Renal or Hepatic Function. Although laboratory tests have not indicated that TALWIN causes or increases renal or hepatic impairment, the drug should be administered with caution to patients with such impairment. Extensive liver disease appears to predispose to greater side effects (eg, marked apprehension, anxiety, dizziness, sleepiness) from the usual clinical dose, and may be the result of decreased metabolism of the drug by the liver.

Biliary Surgery. Narcotic drug products are generally considered to elevate biliary tract pressure for varying periods following their administration. Some evidence suggests that pentazocine may differ from other marketed narcotics in this respect (ie, it causes little or no elevation in biliary tract pressures). The clinical significance of these findings, however, is not yet known.

Patients Receiving Narcotics. TALWIN is a mild narcotic antagonist. Some patients previously given narcotics, including methadone for the daily treatment of narcotic dependence, have experienced withdrawal symptoms after receiving TALWIN.

CNS Effect. Caution should be used when TALWIN is administered to patients prone to seizures; seizures have occurred in a few such patients in association with the use of TALWIN although no cause and effect relationship has been established.

Use in Anesthesia. Concomitant use of CNS depressants with parenteral TALWIN, brand of pentazocine lactate injection, may produce additive CNS depression. Adequate equipment and facilities should be available to identify and treat systemic emergencies should they occur.

Adverse Reactions: The most commonly occurring reactions are: nausea, dizziness or lightheadedness, vomiting, euphoria.

Dermatologic Reactions: Soft tissue induration, nodules, and cutaneous depression can occur at injection sites. Ulceration (sloughing) and severe sclerosis of the skin and subcutaneous tissues (and, rarely, underlying muscle) have been reported after multiple doses.

Infrequently occurring reactions are—*respiratory:* respiratory depression, dyspnea, transient apnea in a small number of newborn infants whose mothers received TALWIN during labor; *cardiovascular:* circulatory depression, shock, hypertension; *CNS effects:* sedation, alteration of mood (nervousness, apprehension, depression, floating feeling), dreams; *gastrointestinal:* constipation, dry mouth; *dermatologic including local:* diaphoresis, sting on injection, flushed skin including plethora, dermatitis including pruritus; *other:* urinary retention, headache, paresthesia, alterations in rate or strength of uterine contractions during labor.

Rarely reported reactions include—*neuromuscular and psychiatric:* muscle tremor, insomnia, disorientation, hallucinations; *gastrointestinal:* taste alteration, diarrhea and cramps; *ophthalmic:* blurred vision, nystagmus, diplopia, miosis; *hematologic:* depression of white blood cells (especially granulocytes), which is usually reversible, moderate transient eosinophilia; *other:* tachycardia, weakness or faintness, chills, allergic reactions including edema of the face, toxic epidermal necrolysis.

See **Acute CNS Manifestations** and **Drug Dependence** under **WARNINGS**.

Dosage and Administration: Adults, Excluding Patients in Labor. The recommended single parenteral dose is 30 mg by intramuscular, subcutaneous, or intravenous route. This may be repeated every 3 to 4 hours. Doses in excess of 30 mg intravenously or 60 mg intramuscularly or subcutaneously are not recommended. Total daily dosage should not exceed 360 mg.

The subcutaneous route of administration should be used only when necessary because of possible severe tissue damage at injection sites (see WARNINGS). When frequent injections are needed, the drug should be administered intramuscularly. In addition, constant rotation of injection sites (eg, the upper outer quadrants of the buttocks, mid-lateral aspects of the thighs, and the deltoid areas) is essential.

Patients in Labor. A single, intramuscular 30 mg dose has been most commonly administered. An intravenous 20 mg dose has given adequate pain relief to some patients in labor when contractions become regular, and this dose may be given two or three times at two-to three-hour intervals, as needed.

Children Under 12 Years of Age. Since clinical experience in children under twelve years of age is limited, the use of TALWIN in this age group is not recommended.

CAUTION. TALWIN should not be mixed in the same syringe with soluble barbiturates because precipitation will occur.

Overdosage: Manifestations: Clinical experience with TALWIN overdosage has been insufficient to define the signs of this condition.

Treatment: Oxygen, intravenous fluids, vasopressors, and other supportive measures should be employed as indicated. Assisted or controlled ventilation should also be considered. For respiratory depression due to overdosage or unusual sensitivity to TALWIN, parenteral naloxone is a specific and effective antagonist.

How Supplied: *Uni-Amp®—Individual unit dose ampuls of 1 mL (30 mg)* NDC 0024-1924-04, *1.5 mL (45 mg)* NDC 0024-1925-04, *and 2 mL (60 mg)* NDC 0024-1926-04 in box of 25.
Uni-Nest™ ampuls of 1 mL (30 mg) NDC 0024-1924-14 *and 2 mL (60 mg)* NDC 0024-1926-14 in box of 25.
Each 1 mL contains pentazocine lactate equivalent to 30 mg base and 2.8 mg sodium chloride, in Water for Injection.
*Carpuject® **Sterile Cartridge-Needle Units**, 1 mL (30 mg)* NDC 0024-1917-02, *1.5 mL (45 mg)* NDC 0024-1918-02, *and 2 mL (60 mg)* NDC 0024-1919-02, all in 2 mL cartridges, box of 10. Each 1 mL contains pentazocine lactate equivalent to 30 mg base, 1 mg acetone sodium bisulfite, and 2.2 mg sodium chloride, in Water for Injection.
Multiple-dose vials of 10 mL NDC 0024-1916-01, box of 1. Each 1 mL contains pentazocine lactate equivalent to 30 mg base, 2 mg acetone sodium bisulfite, 1.5 mg sodium chloride, and 1 mg methylparaben as preservative, in Water for Injection. The pH of TALWIN solutions is adjusted between 4 and 5 with lactic acid or sodium hydroxide. The air in the ampuls, vials, and Cartridge-Needle Units has been displaced by nitrogen gas.

TW-109-DD

TALWIN® Compound © ℞
brand of pentazocine hydrochloride and aspirin tablets, USP

Description: TALWIN Compound is a combination of pentazocine hydrochloride equivalent to 12.5 mg base and aspirin 325 mg.
Pentazocine is a member of the benzazocine series (also known as the benzomorphan series). Chemically, pentazocine is 1, 2, 3, 4, 5, 6-Hexahydro-6, 11-dimethyl-3-(3-methyl-2-butenyl)-2, 6-methano-3-benzazocin-8-ol, a white, crystalline substance soluble in acidic aqueous solutions.

Clinical Pharmacology: Pentazocine is a potent analgesic which when administered orally is approximately equivalent, on a mg for mg basis, in analgesic effect to codeine. Two Caplets® of TALWIN Compound when administered orally have the additive analgesic effect equivalent to 25 mg of TALWIN plus 650 mg of aspirin. TALWIN Compound provides the analgesic effects of pentazocine and the analgesic, anti-inflammatory, and antipyretic actions of aspirin.
Onset of significant analgesia usually occurs between 15 and 30 minutes after oral administration, and duration of action is usually three hours or longer. Onset and duration of action and the degree of pain relief are related both to dose and the severity of pretreatment pain. Pentazocine weakly antagonizes the analgesic effects of morphine, meperidine, and phenazocine; in addition, it produces incomplete reversal of cardiovascular, respiratory, and behavioral depression induced by morphine and meperidine. Pentazocine has about

Continued on next page

This product information was effective as of December 3, 1984. On these and other products of Winthrop-Breon Laboratories, detailed information may be obtained on a current basis by direct inquiry to the Professional Services Department, 90 Park Avenue, New York, NY 10016 (212) 907-2525.

Winthrop-Breon—Cont.

1/50 the antagonistic activity of nalorphine. It also has sedative activity.

Indication and Usage: For the relief of moderate pain

Contraindications: TALWIN Compound should not be administered to patients who are hypersensitive to either pentazocine or salicylates, or in any situation where aspirin is contraindicated.

Warnings: *Drug Dependence.* There have been instances of psychological and physical dependence on parenteral pentazocine in patients with a history of drug abuse, and rarely, in patients without such a history. Abrupt discontinuance following the extended use of parenteral pentazocine has resulted in withdrawal symptoms. There have been a few reports of dependence and of withdrawal symptoms with orally administered pentazocine. Patients with a history of drug dependence should be under close supervision while receiving TALWIN Compound orally. There have been rare reports of possible abstinence syndromes in newborns after prolonged use of pentazocine during pregnancy.
In prescribing TALWIN Compound for chronic use, the physician should take precautions to avoid increases in dose by the patient and to prevent the use of the drug in anticipation of pain rather than for the relief of pain.
Head Injury and Increased Intracranial Pressure. The respiratory depressant effects of pentazocine and its potential for elevating cerebrospinal fluid pressure may be markedly exaggerated in the presence of head injury, other intracranial lesions, or a preexisting increase in intracranial pressure. Furthermore, pentazocine can produce effects which may obscure the clinical course of patients with head injuries. In such patients, TALWIN Compound must be used with extreme caution and only if its use is deemed essential.
Usage in Pregnancy. Safe use of pentazocine during pregnancy (other than labor) has not been established. Animal reproduction studies have not demonstrated teratogenic or embryotoxic effects. However, TALWIN Compound should be administered to pregnant patients (other than labor) only when, in the judgment of the physician, the potential benefits outweigh the possible hazards. Patients receiving pentazocine during labor have experienced no adverse effects other than those that occur with commonly used analgesics. TALWIN Compound should be used with caution in women delivering premature infants.
Acute CNS Manifestations. Patients receiving therapeutic doses of pentazocine have experienced, in rare instances, hallucinations (usually visual), disorientation, and confusion which have cleared spontaneously within a period of hours. The mechanism of this reaction is not known. Such patients should be very closely observed and vital signs checked. If the drug is reinstituted it should be done with caution since the acute CNS manifestations may recur.
Due to the potential for increased CNS depressant effects, alcohol should be used with caution in patients who are currently receiving pentazocine.
Usage in Children. Because clinical experience in children under 12 years of age is limited, administration of TALWIN Compound in this age group is not recommended.
Ambulatory Patients. Since sedation, dizziness, and occasional euphoria have been noted, ambulatory patients should be warned not to operate machinery, drive cars, or unnecessarily expose themselves to hazards.
Other. Because of its aspirin content, TALWIN Compound should be used with caution in the presence of peptic ulcer, in conjunction with anticoagulant therapy, or in any situation where the effects of aspirin may be deleterious.
Precautions: *Certain Respiratory Conditions.* Although respiratory depression has rarely been reported after oral administration of pentazocine, TALWIN Compound should be administered with caution to patients with respiratory depression from any cause, severely limited respiratory reserve, severe bronchial asthma and other obstructive respiratory conditions, or cyanosis.
Impaired Renal or Hepatic Function. Decreased metabolism of the drug by the liver in extensive liver disease may predispose to accentuation of side effects. Although laboratory tests have not indicated that pentazocine causes or increases renal or hepatic impairment, TALWIN Compound should be administered with caution to patients with such impairment.
Myocardial Infarction. As with all drugs, TALWIN Compound should be used with caution in patients with myocardial infarction who have nausea or vomiting.
Biliary Surgery. Narcotic drug products are generally considered to elevate biliary tract pressure for varying periods following their administration. Some evidence suggests that pentazocine may differ from other marketed narcotics in this respect (ie, it causes little or no elevation in biliary tract pressure). The clinical significance of these findings, however, is not yet known.
Patients Receiving Narcotics. Pentazocine is a mild narcotic antagonist. Some patients previously given narcotics, including methadone for the daily treatment of narcotic dependence, have experienced withdrawal symptoms after receiving pentazocine.
CNS Effect. Caution should be used when pentazocine is administered to patients prone to seizures. Seizures have occurred in a few such patients in association with the use of pentazocine although no cause and effect relationship has been established.

Adverse Reactions: Reactions reported after oral administration of pentazocine or TALWIN Compound include *gastrointestinal:* nausea, vomiting; infrequently constipation; and rarely abdominal distress, anorexia, diarrhea. *CNS Effects:* dizziness, lightheadedness, sedation, euphoria, headache; infrequently weakness, disturbed dreams, insomnia, syncope, visual blurring and focusing difficulty, depression, hallucinations (see *Acute CNS Manifestations* under **WARNINGS**); and rarely confusion, tremor, irritability, excitement, tinnitus. *Autonomic:* sweating; infrequently flushing; and rarely chills. *Allergic:* infrequently rash; and rarely urticaria, edema of the face. *Cardiovascular:* infrequently decrease in blood pressure, tachycardia. *Hematologic:* rarely depression of white blood cells (especially granulocytes), which is usually reversible, moderate transient eosinophilia. *Other:* rarely respiratory depression, urinary retention, paresthesia, toxic epidermal necrolysis.

Dosage and Administration: *Adults.* The usual adult dose is 2 CAPLETS three or four times a day.
Children Under 12 Years of Age. Since clinical experience in children under 12 years of age is limited, administration of TALWIN Compound in this age group is not recommended.
Duration of Therapy. Patients with chronic pain who receive pentazocine orally for prolonged periods have only rarely been reported to experience withdrawal symptoms when administration was abruptly discontinued (see WARNINGS). Tolerance to the analgesic effect of pentazocine has also been reported only rarely. Significant abnormalities of liver and kidney function tests have not been reported, even after prolonged administration of pentazocine.
Overdosage: *Manifestations:* Clinical experience with pentazocine overdosage has been insufficient to define the signs of this condition. Signs of salicylate overdosage include headache, dizziness, confusion, tinnitus, diaphoresis, thirst, nausea, vomiting, diarrhea, tachycardia, tachypnea, Kussmaul breathing, convulsions, and coma. Death is usually from respiratory failure.
Treatment: Treatment for overdosage of TALWIN Compound should include treatment for salicylate poisoning as outlined in standard references.
Oxygen, intravenous fluids, vasopressors, and other supportive measures should be employed as indicated. Assisted or controlled ventilation should also be considered. For respiratory depression due to overdosage or unusual sensitivity to pentazocine, parenteral naloxone is a specific and effective antagonist.
How Supplied: CAPLETS, white, each containing pentazocine hydrochloride equivalent to 12.5 mg base and aspirin 325 mg. Bottles of 100 (NDC 0024-1927-04).
Distributed by Winthrop-Breon Laboratories Division of Sterling Drug Inc., New York, NY 10016. Manufactured by Sterling Pharmaceuticals Inc., Barceloneta, Puerto Rico 00617

TW-225-I(O)

TALWIN® Nx © ℞
Pentazocine hydrochloride, USP, equivalent to 50 mg base and naloxone hydrochloride, USP, equivalent to 0.5 mg base

Analgesic for Oral Use Only

> TALWIN® Nx is intended for oral use only. Severe, potentially lethal, reactions may result from misuse of TALWIN® Nx by injection either alone or in combination with other substances. (See **DRUG ABUSE AND DEPENDENCE** section.)

Description: TALWIN Nx contains pentazocine hydrochloride, USP, equivalent to 50 mg base and is a member of the benzazocine series (also known as the benzomorphan series), and naloxone hydrochloride, USP, equivalent to 0.5 mg base.
TALWIN Nx is an analgesic for oral administration.
Chemically, pentazocine hydrochloride is 1,2,3,4,5,6-Hexahydro-6,11-dimethyl-3-(3-methyl-2-butenyl)-2, 6-methano-3-benzazocin-8-ol hydrochloride, a white, crystalline substance soluble in acidic aqueous solutions.
Chemically, naloxone hydrochloride is Morphinan-6-one, 4, 5-epoxy-3, 14-dihydroxy-17-(2-propenyl)-, hydrochloride, (5α)-. It is a slightly off-white powder, and is soluble in water and dilute acids.
Clinical Pharmacology: Pentazocine is a potent analgesic which when administered orally in a 50 mg dose appears equivalent in analgesic effect to 60 mg (1 grain) of codeine. Onset of significant analgesia usually occurs between 15 and 30 minutes after oral administration, and duration of action is usually three hours or longer. Onset and duration of action and the degree of pain relief are related both to dose and the severity of pretreatment pain. Pentazocine weakly antagonizes the analgesic effects of morphine and meperidine; in addition, it produces incomplete reversal of cardiovascular, respiratory, and behavioral depression induced by morphine and meperidine. Pentazocine has about 1/50 the antagonistic activity of nalorphine. It also has sedative activity.
Pentazocine is well absorbed from the gastrointestinal tract. Concentrations in plasma coincide closely with the onset, duration, and intensity of analgesia; peak values occur 1 to 3 hours after oral administration. The half-life in plasma is 2 to 3 hours.
Pentazocine is metabolized in the liver and excreted primarily in the urine. Pentazocine passes into the fetal circulation.
Naloxone when administered orally at 0.5 mg has no pharmacologic activity. Naloxone hydrochloride administered parenterally at the same dose is an effective antagonist to pentazocine and a pure antagonist to narcotic analgesics.
TALWIN Nx is a potent analgesic when administered orally. However, the presence of naloxone in TALWIN Nx will prevent the effect of pentazocine if the product is misused by injection.
Studies in animals indicate that the presence of naloxone does not effect pentazocine analgesia when the combination is given orally. If the combination is given by injection the action of pentazocine is neutralized.
Indications and Usage:

> TALWIN® Nx is intended for oral use only. Severe, potentially lethal, reactions may result from misuse of TALWIN® Nx by injec-

tion either alone or in combination with other substances. (See **DRUG ABUSE AND DEPENDENCE** section.)

TALWIN Nx is indicated for the relief of moderate to severe pain.
TALWIN Nx is indicated for oral use only.
Contraindications: TALWIN Nx should not be administered to patients who are hypersensitive to either pentazocine or naloxone.

Warnings:

> TALWIN® Nx is intended for oral use only. Severe, potentially lethal, reactions may result from misuse of TALWIN® Nx by injection either alone or in combination with other substances. (See **DRUG ABUSE AND DEPENDENCE** section.)

Drug Dependence. Pentazocine can cause a physical and psychological dependence. (See **DRUG ABUSE AND DEPENDENCE**.)
Head Injury and Increased Intracranial Pressure. As in the case of other potent analgesics, the potential of pentazocine for elevating cerebrospinal fluid pressure may be attributed to CO_2 retention due to the respiratory depressant effects of the drug. These effects may be markedly exaggerated in the presence of head injury, other intracranial lesions, or a preexisting increase in intracranial pressure. Furthermore, pentazocine can produce effects which may obscure the clinical course of patients with head injuries. In such patients, pentazocine must be used with extreme caution and only if its use is deemed essential.
Usage with Alcohol. Due to the potential for increased CNS depressant effects, alcohol should be used with caution in patients who are currently receiving pentazocine.
Patients Receiving Narcotics. Pentazocine is a mild narcotic antagonist. Some patients previously given narcotics, including methadone for the daily treatment of narcotic dependence, have experienced withdrawal symptoms after receiving pentazocine.
Certain Respiratory Conditions. Although respiratory depression has rarely been reported after oral administration of pentazocine, the drug should be administered with caution to patients with respiratory depression from any cause, severely limited respiratory reserve, severe bronchial asthma, and other obstructive respiratory conditions, or cyanosis.
Precautions: *CNS Effect.* Caution should be used when pentazocine is administered to patients prone to seizures; seizures have occurred in a few such patients in association with the use of pentazocine though no cause and effect relationship has been established.
Patients receiving therapeutic doses of pentazocine have experienced, in rare instances, hallucinations (usually visual), disorientation, and confusion which have cleared spontaneously within a period of hours. The mechanism of this reaction is not known. Such patients should be very closely observed and vital signs checked. If the drug is reinstituted, it should be done with caution since the acute CNS manifestations may recur.
Impaired Renal or Hepatic Function. Decreased metabolism of pentazocine by the liver in extensive liver disease may predispose to accentuation of side effects. Although laboratory tests have not indicated that pentazocine causes or increases renal or hepatic impairment, the drug should be administered with caution to patients with such impairment.
In prescribing pentazocine for long-term use, the physician should take precautions to avoid increases in dose by the patient.
Biliary Surgery. Narcotic drug products are generally considered to elevate biliary tract pressure for varying periods following their administration. Some evidence suggests that pentazocine may differ from other marketed narcotics in this respect (ie, it causes little or no elevation in biliary tract pressures). The clinical significance of these findings, however, is not yet known.
Information for Patients. Since sedation, dizziness, and occasional euphoria have been noted, ambulatory patients should be warned not to operate machinery, drive cars, or unnecessarily expose themselves to hazards. Pentazocine may cause physical and psychological dependence when taken alone and may have additive CNS depressant properties when taken in combination with alcohol or other CNS depressants.
Myocardial Infarction. As with all drugs, pentazocine should be used with caution in patients with myocardial infarction who have nausea or vomiting.
Drug Interactions. Usage with Alcohol: See Warnings.
Carcinogenesis, Mutagenesis, Impairment of Fertility. No long-term studies in animals to test for carcinogenesis have been performed with the components of TALWIN Nx.
Pregnancy Category C. Animal reproduction studies have not been conducted with TALWIN Nx. It is also not known whether TALWIN Nx can cause fetal harm when administered to pregnant women or can affect reproduction capacity. TALWIN Nx should be given to pregnant women only if clearly needed. However, animal reproduction studies with pentazocine have not demonstrated teratogenic embryotoxic effects.
Labor and Delivery. Patients receiving pentazocine during labor have experienced no adverse effects other than those that occur with commonly used analgesics. TALWIN Nx should be used with caution in women delivering premature infants. The effect of TALWIN Nx on the mother and fetus, the duration of labor or delivery, the possibility that forceps delivery or other intervention or resusitation of the newborn may be necessary, or the effect of TALWIN Nx on the later growth, development, and functional maturation of the child are unknown at the present time.
Nursing Mothers. It is not known whether this drug is excreted in human milk. Because many drugs are excreted in human milk, caution should be exercised when TALWIN Nx is administered to a nursing woman.
Pediatric Use. Safety and effectiveness in children below the age of 12 years have not been established.
Adverse Reactions: *Cardiovascular:* Hypotension, tachycardia, syncope.
Respiratory: Rarely, respiratory depression.
CNS. Acute CNS Manifestations: Patients receiving therapeutic doses of pentazocine have experienced, in rare instances, hallucinations (usually visual), disorientation, and confusion which have cleared spontaneously within a period of hours. The mechanism of this reaction is not known and may recur if the drug is reinstituted.
Other CNS Effects: Dizziness, lightheadedness, sedation, euphoria, disturbed dreams, hallucinations, irritability, excitement, tinnitus, tremor.
Gastrointestinal: Nausea, vomiting, constipation, diarrhea, anorexia, rarely abdominal distress.
Allergic: Edema of the face; dermatitis, including pruritus; flushed skin, including plethora.
Ophthalmic: Visual blurring and focusing difficulty.
Hematologic: Depression of white blood cells (especially granulocytes), which is usually reversible, moderate transient eosinophilia.
Other: Headache, chills, insomnia, weakness, urinary retention.
Drug Abuse and Dependence: *Controlled Substance.* TALWIN Nx is a Schedule IV controlled substance.
There have been some reports of dependence and of withdrawal symptoms wth orally administered pentazocine. Patients with a history of drug dependence should be under close supervision while receiving pentazocine orally. There have been rare reports of possible abstinence syndromes in newborns after prolonged use of pentazocine during pregnancy.
There have been instances of psychological and physical dependence on parenteral pentazocine in patients with a history of drug abuse and, rarely, in patients without such a history. Abrupt discontinuance following the extended use of parenteral pentazocine has resulted in withdrawal symptoms. In prescribing pentazocine for chronic use, the physician should take precautions to avoid increases in dose by the patient.
The amount of naloxone present in TALWIN Nx (0.5 mg per tablet) has no action when taken orally and will not interfere with the pharmacologic action of pentazocine. However, this amount of naloxone given by injection has profound antagonistic action to narcotic analgesics.
Severe, even lethal, consequences may result from misuse of tablets by injection either alone or in combination with other substances, such as pulmonary emboli, vascular occlusion, ulceration and abscesses, and withdrawal symptoms in narcotic dependent individuals.
TALWIN Nx contains an opioid antagonist, naloxone (0.5 mg). Naloxone is inactive when administered orally at this dose, and its inclusion in TALWIN Nx is intended to curb a form of misuse of oral pentazocine. Parenterally, naloxone is an active narcotic antagonist. Thus, TALWIN Nx has a lower potential for parenteral misuse than the previous oral pentazocine formulation TALWIN® 50 (pentazocine hydrochloride tablets, USP). However, it is still subject to patient misuse and abuse by the oral route.
Overdosage: *Manifestations.* Clinical experience of overdosage with this oral medication has been insufficient to define the signs of this condition.
Treatment. Oxygen, intravenous fluids, vasopressors, and other supportive measures should be employed as indicated. Assisted or controlled ventilation should also be considered. For respiratory depression due to overdosage or unusual sensitivity to pentazocine, parenteral naloxone is a specific and effective antagonist.

Dosage and Administration:

> TALWIN® Nx is intended for oral use only. Severe, potentially lethal, reactions may result from misuse of TALWIN® Nx by injection either alone or in combination with other substances. (See **DRUG ABUSE AND DEPENDENCE** section.)

Adults: The usual initial adult dose is 1 tablet every three or four hours. This may be increased to 2 tablets when needed. Total daily dosage should not exceed 12 tablets.
When anti-inflammatory or antipyretic effects are desired in addition to analgesia, aspirin can be administered concomitantly with this product.
Children Under 12 Years of Age. Since clinical experience in children under 12 years of age is limited, administration of this product in this age group is not recommended.
Duration of Therapy. Patients with chronic pain who receive TALWIN Nx orally for prolonged periods have only rarely been reported to experience withdrawal symptoms when administration was abruptly discontinued (see Warnings). Tolerance to the analgesic effect of pentazocine has also been reported only rarely. However, there is no long-term experience with the oral administration of TALWIN Nx.
How Supplied: Tablets (oblong), yellow, scored, each containing pentazocine hydrochloride equivalent to 50 mg base and naloxone hydrochloride equivalent to 0.5 mg base.

Continued on next page

This product information was effective as of December 3, 1984. On these and other products of Winthrop-Breon Laboratories, detailed information may be obtained on a current basis by direct inquiry to the Professional Services Department, 90 Park Avenue, New York, NY 10016 (212) 907-2525.

Winthrop-Breon—Cont.

Bottles of 100 (NDC 0024-1951-04).
Unit Dose Dispenser Package of 250 (NDC 0024-1951-24), 10 sleeves of 25 tablets each.
Distributed by
Winthrop-Breon Laboratories
Division of Sterling Drug Inc.
New York, NY 10016
Manufactured by
Sterling Pharmaceuticals Inc.
Barceloneta, Puerto Rico 00617
Shown in Product Identification Section, page 444
TW-267-D

TELEPAQUE®
brand of iopanoic acid tablets, USP

(See Diagnostic Section.)

TRANCOPAL®
brand of chlormezanone
Nonhypnotic Antianxiety Agent

Description: Trancopal (brand of chlormezanone) is [2-(p-chlorophenyl)-tetrahydro-3-methyl-4H-1, 3-thiazin-4-one 1, 1-dioxide], a white, virtually tasteless, crystalline powder with a solubility of less than 0.25 percent w/v in water.
Clinical Pharmacology: TRANCOPAL improves the emotional state by allaying mild anxiety, usually without impairing clarity of consciousness.
The relief of symptoms is often apparent in fifteen to thirty minutes after administration and may last up to six hours or longer.
Indications and Usage: TRANCOPAL is indicated for the treatment of mild anxiety and tension states.
The effectiveness of chlormezanone in long-term use, that is, more than 4 months, has not been assessed by systematic clinical studies. The physician should periodically reassess the usefulness of the drug for the individual patient.
Contraindication: Contraindicated in patients with a history of a previous hypersensitivity reaction to chlormezanone.
Warnings: Should drowsiness occur, the dose should be reduced. As with other CNS-acting drugs, patients receiving chlormezanone should be warned against performing potentially hazardous tasks which require complete mental alertness, such as operating a motor vehicle or dangerous machinery. Patients should also be warned of the possible additive effects which may occur when the drug is taken with alcohol or other CNS-acting drugs.
Usage in Pregnancy. Safe use of this preparation in pregnancy or lactation has not been established, as no animal reproduction studies have been performed; therefore, use of the drug in pregnancy, lactation, or in women of childbearing age requires that the potential benefit of the drug be weighed against its possible hazards to the mother and fetus.
Adverse Reactions: Adverse effects reported to occur with TRANCOPAL include drowsiness, drug rash, dizziness, flushing, nausea, depression, edema, inability to void, weakness, excitement, tremor, confusion, and headache. Medication should be discontinued or modified as the case demands.
Jaundice, apparently of the cholestatic type, has been reported as occurring rarely during the use of chlormezanone, but was reversible on discontinuance of therapy.
Dosage and Administration: The usual **adult** dosage is 200 mg orally three or four times daily but in some patients 100 mg may suffice. The dosage for **children from 5 to 12 years** is 50 mg to 100 mg three or four times daily. Since the effect of CNS-acting drugs varies, treatment, particularly in children, should begin with the lowest dosage which may be increased as needed.
How Supplied:
100 mg (peach colored, scored Caplets®)
bottle of 100 (NDC 0024-1973-04)
200 mg (green colored, scored CAPLETS)
bottle of 100 (NDC 0024-1974-04)
bottle of 1000 (NDC 0024-1974-08)
Shown in Product Identification Section, page 444
TW 72-K

WinGel®   OTC
(See PDR For Nonprescription Drugs)

WINSTROL®
brand of stanozolol tablets, USP
For Oral Administration

Description: WINSTROL, brand of stanozolol tablets, is an anabolic steroid, a synthetic derivative of testosterone. Each tablet contains 2 mg of stanozolol. It is designated chemically as 17-methyl-2′ H-5α-androst-2-eno[3,2-c]pyrazol-17β-ol.
Clinical Pharmacology: Anabolic steroids are synthetic derivatives of testosterone.
Certain clinical effects and adverse reactions demonstrate the androgenic properties of this class of drugs. Complete dissociation of anabolic and androgenic effects has not been achieved. The actions of anabolic steroids are therefore similar to those of male sex hormones with the possibility of causing serious disturbances of growth and sexual development if given to young children. They suppress the gonadotropic functions of the pituitary and may exert a direct effect upon the testes.
WINSTROL has been found to increase low-density lipoproteins and decrease high-density lipoproteins. These changes are not associated with any increase in total cholesterol or triglyceride levels and revert to normal on discontinuation of treatment.
Hereditary angioedema (HAE) is an autosomal dominant disorder caused by a deficient or non-functional C1 esterase inhibitor (C1 INH) and clinically characterized by episodes of swelling of the face, extremities, genitalia, bowel wall, and upper respiratory tract.
In small scale clinical studies, stanozolol was effective in controlling the frequency and severity of attacks of angioedema and in increasing serum levels of C1 INH and C4. WINSTROL is not effective in stopping HAE attacks while they are under way. The effect of WINSTROL on increasing serum levels of C1 INH and C4 may be related to an increase in protein anabolism.
Indications and Usage:
Hereditary Angioedema. WINSTROL is indicated prophylactically to decrease the frequency and severity of attacks of angioedema.
Contraindications: The use of WINSTROL is contraindicated in the following:
1. Carcinoma of the prostate or breast in male patients.
2. Carcinoma of the breast in some females.
3. Nephrosis or the nephrotic phase of nephritis.
4. WINSTROL can cause fetal harm when administered to a pregnant woman.
WINSTROL is contraindicated in women who are or may become pregnant. If this drug is used during pregnancy, or if the patient becomes pregnant while taking this drug, the patient should be apprised of the potential hazard to the fetus.
Warnings:

Peliosis hepatis, a condition in which liver and sometimes splenic tissue is replaced with blood-filled cysts, has been reported in patients receiving androgenic anabolic steroid therapy. These cysts are sometimes present with minimal hepatic dysfunction, but at other times they have been associated with liver failure. They are often not recognized until life-threatening liver failure or intra-abdominal hemorrhage develops. Withdrawal of drug usually results in complete disappearance of lesions.
Liver cell tumors are also reported. Most often these tumors are benign and androgen-dependent, but fatal malignant tumors have been reported. Withdrawal of drug often results in regression or cessation of progression of the tumor. However, hepatic tumors associated with androgens or anabolic steroids are much more vascular than other hepatic tumors and may be silent until life-threatening intra-abdominal hemorrhage develops.
Blood lipid changes that are known to be associated with increased risk of atherosclerosis are seen in patients treated with androgens and anabolic steroids. These changes include decreased high-density lipoprotein and sometimes increased low-density lipoprotein. The changes may be very marked and could have a serious impact on the risk of atherosclerosis and coronary artery disease.

Cholestatic hepatitis and jaundice occur with 17-alpha-alkylated androgens at relatively low doses. If cholestatic hepatitis with jaundice appears, the anabolic steroid should be discontinued. If liver function tests become abnormal, the patient should be monitored closely and the etiology determined. Generally, the anabolic steroid should be discontinued although in cases of mild abnormalities, the physician may elect to follow the patient carefully at a reduced drug dosage.
In patients with breast cancer, anabolic steroid therapy may cause hypercalcemia by stimulating osteolysis. In this case, the drug should be discontinued.
Edema with or without congestive heart failure may be a serious complication in patients with preexisting cardiac, renal, or hepatic disease.
Geriatric male patients treated with androgenic anabolic steroids may be at an increased risk for the development of prostatic hypertrophy and prostatic carcinoma.
Anabolic steroids have not been clearly shown to enhance athletic ability.
Precautions:
General. Women should be observed for signs of virilization (deepening of the voice, hirsutism, acne, and clitoromegaly). To prevent irreversible change, drug therapy must be discontinued, or the dosage significantly reduced when mild virilism is first detected. Such virilization is usual following androgenic anabolic steroid use at high doses. Some virilizing changes in women are irreversible even after prompt discontinuance of therapy and are not prevented by concomitant use of estrogens. Menstrual irregularities may also occur.
The insulin or oral hypoglycemic dosage may need adjustment in diabetic patients who receive anabolic steroids.
Information for the Patient. The physician should instruct patients to report any of the following side effects of androgens:
Adult or Adolescent Males. Too frequent or persistent erections of the penis, appearance or aggravation of acne.
Women. Hoarseness, acne, changes in menstrual periods, or more hair on the face.
All Patients. Any nausea, vomiting, changes in skin color, or ankle swelling.
Laboratory Tests. Women with disseminated breast carcinoma should have frequent determination of urine and serum calcium levels during the course of androgenic anabolic steroid therapy (see WARNINGS).
Because of the hepatotoxicity associated with the use of 17-alpha-alkylated androgens, liver function tests should be obtained periodically.
Periodic (every 6 months) x-ray examinations of bone age should be made during treatment of prepubertal patients to determine the rate of bone maturation and the effects of androgenic anabolic steroid therapy on the epiphyseal centers.
In common with other anabolic steroids, WINSTROL, brand of stanozolol tablets, has been reported to lower the level of high-density lipoproteins and raise the level of low-density lipoproteins. These changes usually revert to normal on discontinuation of treatment. Increased low-density lipoproteins and decreased high-density lipoproteins are considered cardiovascular risk factors. Serum lipids and high-density lipoprotein cholesterol should be determined periodically.

Drug Interaction. Anabolic steroids may increase sensitivity to anticoagulants; therefore, dosage of an anticoagulant may have to be decreased in order to maintain the prothrombin time at the desired therapeutic level.

Drug/Laboratory Test Interferences. Therapy with androgenic anabolic steroids may decrease levels of thyroxine-binding globulin resulting in decreased total T_4 serum levels and increase resin uptake of T_3 and T_4. Free thyroid hormone levels remain unchanged and there is no clinical evidence of thyroid dysfunction.

Anabolic steroids may cause an increase in prothrombin time.

Carcinogenesis, Mutagenesis, Impairment of Fertility. WINSTROL has not been tested in laboratory animals for carcinogenic or mutagenic effects. No tumorigenic or cancer-inducing properties of WINSTROL, tablets, were seen in one-year toxicity studies in rats.

WINSTROL administered orally (intragastrically) to pregnant rats at dosages of 2.5 mg/kg/day to 20 mg/kg/day increased the ano-genital distance in rat fetuses, indicative of a masculinizing effect. WINSTROL prevented pregnancy when given orally to rats from the 1st to the 21st day of gestation.

No teratogenic effects or congenital malformation were observed in offspring of rabbits given 0.5 mg/day, 1.0 mg/day, or 5.0 mg/day of WINSTROL from the 8th through the 16th day of pregnancy, nor were there any adverse effects on the course of pregnancy at these dose levels.

Pregnancy Category X. See CONTRAINDICATIONS section.

Nursing Mothers. It is not known whether anabolic steroids are excreted in human milk. Many drugs are excreted in human milk and because of the potential for adverse reactions in nursing infants from WINSTROL, a decision should be made whether to discontinue nursing or discontinue the drug, taking into account the importance of the drug to the mother.

Pediatric Use. Anabolic agents may accelerate epiphyseal maturation more rapidly than linear growth in children, and the effect may continue for 6 months after the drug has been stopped. Therefore, therapy should be monitored by x-ray studies at 6 month intervals in order to avoid the risk of compromising the adult height. The safety and efficacy of WINSTROL in children with hereditary angioedema have not been established.

Adverse Reactions: *Hepatic:* Cholestatic jaundice with, rarely, hepatic necrosis and death. Hepatocellular neoplasms and peliosis hepatis have been reported in association with long-term androgenic-anabolic steroid therapy (see WARNINGS). Reversible changes in liver function tests also occur including increased bromsulphalein (BSP) retention and increases in serum bilirubin, glutamic oxaloacetic transaminase (SGOT), and alkaline phosphatase.

Genitourinary System: *In men. Prepubertal:* Phallic enlargement and increased frequency of erections.

Postpubertal: Inhibition of testicular function, testicular atrophy and oligospermia, impotence, chronic priapism, epididymitis and bladder irritability.

In women: Clitoral enlargement, menstrual irregularities.

In both sexes: Increased or decreased libido.

CNS: Habituation, excitation, insomnia, depression.

Gastrointestinal: Nausea, vomiting, diarrhea.

Hematologic: Bleeding in patients on concomitant anticoagulant therapy.

Breast: Gynecomastia.

Larynx: Deepening of the voice in women.

Hair: Hirsutism and male pattern baldness in women.

Skin: Acne (especially in women and prepubertal boys).

Skeletal: Premature closure of epiphyses in children (see PRECAUTIONS, **Pediatric Use**).

Fluid and Electrolytes: Edema, retention of serum electrolytes (sodium, chloride, potassium, phosphate, calcium).

Metabolic/Endocrine: Decreased glucose tolerance (see PRECAUTIONS), increased serum levels of low-density lipoproteins and decreased levels of high-density lipoproteins (see PRECAUTIONS, **Laboratory Tests**), increased creatine and creatinine excretion, increased serum levels of creatinine phosphokinase (CPK).

Some virilizing changes in women are irreversible even after prompt discontinuance of therapy and are not prevented by concomitant use of estrogens (see PRECAUTIONS).

Dosage and Administration: The use of anabolic steroids may be associated with serious adverse reactions, many of which are dose related; therefore, patients should be placed on the lowest possible effective dose.

Hereditary Angioedema. The dosage requirements for continuous treatment of hereditary angioedema with WINSTROL should be individualized on the basis of the clinical response of the patient. It is recommended that the patient be started on 2 mg, three times a day. After a favorable initial response is obtained in terms of prevention of episodes of edematous attacks, the proper continuing dosage should be determined by decreasing the dosage at intervals of one to three months to a maintenance dosage of 2 mg a day. Some patients may be successfully managed on a 2 mg alternate day schedule. During the dose adjusting phase, close monitoring of the patient's response is indicated, particularly if the patient has a history of airway involvement.

The prophylactic dose of WINSTROL, brand of stanozolol tablets, to be used prior to dental extraction, or other traumatic or stressful situations has not been established and may be substantially larger.

Attacks of hereditary angioedema are generally infrequent in childhood and the risks from stanozolol administration are substantially increased. Therefore, long-term prophylactic therapy with this drug is generally not recommended in children, and should only be undertaken with due consideration of the benefits and risks involved (see PRECAUTIONS, **Pediatric Use**).

How Supplied: Tablets of 2 mg, scored, bottles of 100 (NDC 0024-2253-04)

Distributed by Winthrop-Breon Laboratories
Division of Sterling Drug Inc New York, NY 10016
Manufactured by Sterling Pharmaceuticals Inc
Barceloneta, Puerto Rico 00617

Shown in Product Identification Section, page 444

WW 5-U

ZEPHIRAN® CHLORIDE   OTC
brand of benzalkonium chloride

ANTISEPTIC

AQUEOUS SOLUTION 1:750
TINTED TINCTURE 1:750
SPRAY—TINTED TINCTURE 1:750

Description: ZEPHIRAN Chloride, brand of benzalkonium chloride, NF, a mixture of alkylbenzyldimethylammonium chlorides, is a cationic quaternary ammonium surface-acting agent. It is very soluble in water, alcohol, and acetone. Aqueous solutions of ZEPHIRAN Chloride are neutral to slightly alkaline, generally colorless, and nonstaining. They have a bitter taste, aromatic odor, and foam when shaken. ZEPHIRAN Chloride Tinted Tincture 1:750 contains alcohol 50 percent and acetone 10 percent by volume. ZEPHIRAN Chloride Spray—Tinted Tincture 1:750 contains alcohol 92 percent. The Tinted Tincture and Spray also contain an orange-red coloring agent.

Clinical Pharmacology: ZEPHIRAN Chloride solutions are rapidly acting antiinfective agents with a moderately long duration of action. They are active against bacteria and some viruses, fungi, and protozoa. Bacterial spores are considered to be resistant. Solutions are bacteriostatic or bactericidal according to their concentration. The exact mechanism of bactericidal action is unknown but it is thought to be due to enzyme inactivation. Activity generally increases with increasing temperature and pH. Gram-positive bacteria are more susceptible than gram-negative bacteria (TABLE 1).

TABLE 1
Highest Dilution of ZEPHIRAN
Chloride Aqueous Solution
Destroying the Organism in
10 but not in 5 Minutes

Organisms	20°C
Streptococcus pyogenes	1:75,000
Staphylococcus aureus	1:52,500
Salmonella typhosa	1:37,500
Escherichia coli	1:10,500

Pseudomonas is the most resistant gram-negative genus. Using the AOAC Use-Dilution Confirmation Method, no growth was obtained when *Staphylococcus aureus*, *Salmonella choleraesuis*, and *Pseudomonas aeruginosa* (strain PRD-10) were exposed for ten minutes at 20°C to ZEPHIRAN Chloride Aqueous Solution 1:750 and Tinted Tincture 1:750.

ZEPHIRAN Chloride Aqueous Solution 1:750 has been shown to retain its bactericidal activity following autoclaving for 30 minutes at 15 lb pressure, freezing, and then thawing.

The tubercle bacillus may be resistant to aqueous ZEPHIRAN Chloride solutions but is susceptible to the 1:750 tincture (AOAC Method, 10 minutes at 20°C).

ZEPHIRAN Chloride solutions also demonstrate deodorant, wetting, detergent, keratolytic, and emulsifying activity.

Indications and Usage: ZEPHIRAN Chloride aqueous solutions in appropriate dilutions (see Recommended Dilutions) are indicated for the antisepsis of skin, mucous membranes, and wounds. They are used for preoperative preparation of the skin, surgeons' hand and arm soaks, treatment of wounds, preservation of ophthalmic solutions, irrigations of the eye, body cavities, bladder, urethra, and vaginal douching.

ZEPHIRAN Chloride Tinted Tincture 1:750 and Spray are indicated for preoperative preparation of the skin and for treatment of minor skin wounds and abrasions.

Contraindication: The use of ZEPHIRAN Chloride solutions in occlusive dressings, casts, and anal or vaginal packs is inadvisable, as they may produce irritation or chemical burns.

Warnings: Sterile Water for Injection, USP, should be used as diluent in preparing diluted aqueous solutions intended for use on deep wounds or for irrigation of body cavities. Otherwise, freshly distilled water should be used. Tap water, containing metallic ions and organic matter, may reduce antibacterial potency. Resin deionized water should not be used since it may contain pathogenic bacteria.

Organic, inorganic, and synthetic materials and surfaces may adsorb sufficient quantities of ZEPHIRAN Chloride to significantly reduce its antibacterial potency in solutions. This has resulted in serious contamination of solutions of ZEPHIRAN Chloride with viable pathogenic bacteria. Solutions should not be stored in bottles stoppered with cork closures, but rather in those equipped with appropriate screw-caps. Cotton, wool, rayon, and other materials should not be stored in ZEPHIRAN Chloride solutions. Gauze sponges and fiber pledgets used to apply solutions of ZEPHIRAN Chloride to the skin should be sterilized and stored in separate containers. Only immediately prior to application should they be immersed in ZEPHIRAN Chloride solutions.

Continued on next page

This product information was effective as of December 3, 1984. On these and other products of Winthrop-Breon Laboratories, detailed information may be obtained on a current basis by direct inquiry to the Professional Services Department, 90 Park Avenue, New York, NY 10016 (212) 907-2525.

Winthrop-Breon—Cont.

Since ZEPHIRAN Chloride solutions are inactivated by soaps and anionic detergents, thorough rinsing is necessary if these agents are employed prior to their use.

Antiseptics such as ZEPHIRAN Chloride solutions must not be relied upon to achieve complete sterilization, because they do not destroy bacterial spores and certain viruses, including the etiologic agent of infectious hepatitis, and may not destroy *Mycobacterium tuberculosis* and other rare bacterial strains.

ZEPHIRAN Chloride Tinted Tincture 1:750 and Spray contain flammable organic solvents and should not be used near an open flame or cautery. If solutions stronger than 1:3000 enter the eyes, irrigate immediately and repeatedly with water. Prompt medical attention should then be obtained. Concentrations greater than 1:5000 should not be used on mucous membranes, with the exception of the vaginal mucosa (see Recommended Dilutions).

Precautions: In preoperative antisepsis of the skin, ZEPHIRAN Chloride solutions should not be permitted to remain in prolonged contact with the patient's skin. Avoid pooling of the solution on the operating table.

ZEPHIRAN Chloride solutions that are used on inflamed or irritated tissues must be more dilute than those used on normal tissues (see Recommended Dilutions). ZEPHIRAN Chloride Tinted Tincture 1:750 and Spray, which contain irritating organic solvents, should be kept away from the eyes or other mucous membranes.

Adverse Reactions: ZEPHIRAN Chloride solutions in normally used concentrations have low systemic and local toxicity and are generally well tolerated, although a rare individual may exhibit hypersensitivity.

Directions for Use:

General: For most surgical applications, the recommended concentration of ZEPHIRAN Chloride Aqueous Solution or ZEPHIRAN Chloride Tinted Tincture is 1:750 (0.13 percent). Liberal use of the solution is recommended to compensate for any adsorption of ZEPHIRAN Chloride by cotton or other materials.

To use ZEPHIRAN Chloride Spray—Tinted Tincture 1:750, remove protective cap, hold in an UPRIGHT position several inches away from the surgical field or injured area, and apply by spraying freely.

Preoperative preparation of skin: ZEPHIRAN Chloride solutions 1:750 are recommended as an antiseptic for use on unbroken skin in the preoperative preparation of the surgical field. Detergents and soaps should be thoroughly rinsed from the skin before applying ZEPHIRAN Chloride solutions. The detergent action of ZEPHIRAN Chloride solutions, particularly when used alternately with alcohol, leaves the skin smooth and clean. When ZEPHIRAN Chloride solutions are applied by friction (using several changes of sponges), dirt, skin fats, desquamating epithelium, and superficial bacteria are effectively removed, thus exposing the underlying skin to the antiseptic activity of the solutions.

The following procedure has been found satisfactory for preparation of the surgical field. On the day prior to surgery, the operative site is shaved and then scrubbed thoroughly with ZEPHIRAN Chloride Aqueous Solution 1:750. Immediately before surgery, ZEPHIRAN Chloride Tinted Tincture 1:750 or Spray is applied to the site in the usual manner (see Precautions). If the red tinted solution turns yellow during the preparation of patient's skin for surgery, it usually indicates the presence of soap (alkali) residue which is incompatible with ZEPHIRAN solutions. Therefore, rinse thoroughly and reapply the antiseptic. Because ZEPHIRAN Chloride Tinted Tincture 1:750 contains alcohol and acetone, its cleansing action on the skin is particularly effective and it dries more rapidly than the aqueous solution. The Tinted Tincture is recommended when it is desirable to outline the operative site.

Recommended Dilutions: For specific directions, see TABLES 2 and 3.

Surgery
Preoperative preparation of skin: Aqueous solution 1:750 and Tinted Tincture 1:750 or Spray
Surgeons' hand and arm soaks: Aqueous solution 1:750
Treatment of minor wounds and lacerations: Tinted Tincture 1:750 or Spray
Irrigation of deep infected wounds: Aqueous solution 1:3000 to 1:20,000
Denuded skin and mucous membranes: Aqueous solution 1:5000 to 1:10,000

Obstetrics and Gynecology
Preoperative preparation of skin: Aqueous solution 1:750 and Tinted Tincture 1:750 or Spray
Vaginal douche and irrigation: Aqueous solution 1:2000 to 1:5000
Postepisiotomy care: Aqueous solution 1:5000 to 1:10,000
Breast and nipple hygiene: Aqueous solution 1:1000 to 1:2000

Urology
Bladder and urethral irrigation: Aqueous solution 1:5000 to 1:20,000
Bladder retention lavage: Aqueous solution 1:20,000 to 1:40,000

Dermatology
Oozing and open infections: Aqueous solution 1:2000 to 1:5000

TABLE 2
Correct Use of ZEPHIRAN Chloride

ZEPHIRAN Chloride solutions must be prepared, stored, and used correctly to achieve and maintain their antiseptic action. Serious inactivation and contamination of ZEPHIRAN Chloride solutions may occur with misuse.

CORRECT DILUENTS	INCOMPATIBILITIES	PREFERRED FORM
Sterile Water for Injection is recommended for irrigation of body cavities.	Anionic detergents and soaps should be thoroughly rinsed from the skin or other areas prior to use of ZEPHIRAN Chloride solutions because they reduce the antibacterial activity of the solutions.	ZEPHIRAN Chloride Tinted Tincture 1:750 is recommended for preoperative skin preparation because it contains alcohol and acetone which enhance its cleansing action and promote rapid drying.
Sterile distilled water is recommended for irrigating traumatized tissue and in the eye.		
Freshly distilled water is recommended for skin antisepsis.	Serum and protein material also decrease the activity of ZEPHIRAN Chloride solutions.	ZEPHIRAN Chloride Tinted Tincture 1:750, containing acetone, is recommended when it is desirable to outline the operative site. (Aqueous solutions of ZEPHIRAN Chloride used in skin preparation have a tendency to "run off" the skin.)
Resin deionized water should not be used because the deionizing resins can carry pathogens (especially gram-negative bacteria); they also inactivate quaternary ammonium compounds.	Corks should not be used to stopper bottles containing ZEPHIRAN Chloride solutions.	

Stored water is not recommended since it may contain many organisms.	Fibers or fabrics when stored in ZEPHIRAN Chloride solutions adsorb ZEPHIRAN from the surrounding liquid. Examples are:
	
	    Cotton Gauze sponges
	    Wool Rayon
	    Rubber materials
		Caution: Because of the flammable organic solvents in ZEPHIRAN Chloride Tinted Tincture 1:750 and Spray, these products should be kept away from open flame or cautery.

Saline should not be used since it may decrease the antibacterial potency of ZEPHIRAN Chloride solutions.	Applicators or sponges, intended for a skin prep, should be stored separately and dipped in ZEPHIRAN Chloride solutions immediately before use.	

	Under certain circumstances the following commonly encountered substances are incompatible with ZEPHIRAN Chloride solutions:
	
	    Iodine Aluminum
	    Silver nitrate Caramel
	    Fluorescein Kaolin
	    Nitrates Pine oil
	    Peroxide Zinc sulfate
	    Lanolin Zinc oxide
	    Potassium permanganate Yellow oxide of mercury	

Product Information

Wet dressings by irrigation or open dressing (Use in occlusive dressings is inadvisable.): Aqueous solution 1:5000 or less

Ophthalmology

Eye irrigation: Aqueous solution 1:5000 to 1:10,000

Preservation of ophthalmic solutions: Aqueous solution 1:5000 to 1:7500
[See table on preceding page].

TABLE 3
Dilutions of ZEPHIRAN Chloride
Aqueous Solution 1:750

Final Dilution	ZEPHIRAN Chloride Aqueous Solution 1:750 (parts)	Distilled Water (parts)
1:1000	3	1
1:2000	3	5
1:2500	3	7
1:3000	3	9
1:4000	3	13
1:5000	3	17
1:10,000	3	37
1:20,000	3	77
1:40,000	3	157

Accidental Ingestion: If ZEPHIRAN Chloride solution, particularly a concentrated solution, is ingested, marked local irritation of the gastrointestinal tract, manifested by nausea and vomiting, may occur. Signs of systemic toxicity include restlessness, apprehension, weakness, confusion, dyspnea, cyanosis, collapse, convulsions, and coma. Death occurs as a result of paralysis of the respiratory muscles.

Treatment: Immediate administration of several glasses of a mild soap solution, milk, or egg whites beaten in water is recommended. This may be followed by gastric lavage with a mild soap solution. Alcohol should be avoided as it promotes absorption.

To support respiration, the airway should be clear and oxygen should be administered, employing artificial respiration if necessary. If convulsions occur, a short-acting barbiturate may be given parenterally with caution.

How Supplied:
ZEPHIRAN Chloride Aqueous Solution 1:750
Bottles of 8 fl oz (NDC 0024-2521-04) and 1 gallon (NDC 0024-2521-08)
ZEPHIRAN Chloride Tinted Tincture 1:750 (*flammable*)
Bottles of 1 gallon (NDC 0024-2523-08)
ZEPHIRAN Chloride Spray—Tinted Tincture 1:750
(*flammable*)
Bottles of
1 fl oz (NDC 0024-2527-01) and
6 fl oz (NDC 0024-2527-03)

ZW-83 G

Wyeth Laboratories
Division of American Home Products Corporation
P.O. BOX 8299
PHILADELPHIA, PA 19101

Product Identification Codes

The process of imprinting all oral solid dosage forms manufactured by Wyeth with their respective National Drug Code (NDC) numbers is at present incomplete. In the future that portion of the number indicating product and strength will appear on each tablet and capsule, together with the name Wyeth.

The following is a numerical list of NDC code numbers with their corresponding product names.

Numerical Listing

Product Ident. Code	Product
1	Equanil® (meprobamate) Tablet 400 mg.
2	Equanil® (meprobamate) Tablet 200 mg.
6	Serax® (oxazepam) Capsule 15 mg.
7	Equagesic® (meprobamate with aspirin) Tablet
13	Amphojel® (dried aluminum hydroxide gel) Tablet 0.6 Gm. (10 gr.)
16	Purodigin® (crystalline digitoxin) Tablet 0.1 mg.
19	Phenergan® (promethazine HCl) Tablet 12.5 mg.
22	Aludrox® (alumina and magnesia) Tablet
27	Phenergan® (promethazine HCl) Tablet 25 mg.
28	Sparine® (promazine HCl) Tablet 50 mg.
29	Sparine® (promazine HCl) Tablet 25 mg.
33	Equanil® (meprobamate) Tablet Wyseals® 400 mg.
51	Serax® (oxazepam) Capsule 10 mg.
52	Serax® (oxazepam) Capsule 30 mg.
53	Omnipen® (ampicillin) Capsule 250 mg.
56	Ovral® (each tablet contains 0.5 mg. norgestrel with 0.05 mg. ethinyl estradiol) Tablet, white
57	Unipen® [(nafcillin sodium) as the monohydrate] Capsule 250 mg.
58	Pen•Vee® K (penicillin V potassium) Tablet 125 mg.
59	Pen•Vee® K (penicillin V potassium) Tablet 250 mg.
62	Ovrette® (norgestrel) Tablet
64	Ativan® (lorazepam) Tablet 1 mg.
65	Ativan® (lorazepam) Tablet 2 mg.
71	Mazanor® (mazindol) Tablet 1 mg.
73	Wytensin® (guanabenz acetate) Tablet 4 mg.
74	Wytensin® (guanabenz acetate) Tablet 8 mg.
75	Nordette-21® (each tablet contains 0.15 mg. levonorgestrel with 0.03 mg. ethinyl estradiol) Tablet
78	Lo/Ovral® (each tablet contains 0.3 mg. norgestrel with 0.03 mg. ethinyl estradiol) Tablet, white
81	Ativan® (lorazepam) Tablet 0.5 mg.
85	Wygesic® (each tablet contains 65 mg. propoxyphene HCl, U.S.P., and 650 mg. acetaminophen, U.S.P.) Tablet
114	Purodigin® (crystalline digitoxin) Tablet 0.2 mg.
119	Amphojel® (dried aluminum hydroxide gel) Tablet 0.3 Gm. (5 gr.)
165	Bicillin® (penicillin G benzathine) Tablet 200,000 units
200	Sparine® (promazine HCl) Tablet 100 mg.
202	Sparine® (promazine HCl) Tablet 10 mg.
227	Phenergan® (promethazine HCl) Tablet 50 mg.
261	Mepergan® Fortis (meperidine HCl and promethazine HCl) Capsule
267	Phenobarbital Tablet 15 mg.
268	Phenobarbital Tablet 30 mg.
269	Phenobarbital Tablet 100 mg.
272	Penicillin G Potassium Tablet 400,000 units (250 mg)
308	Meperidine HCl Tablet 50 mg.
309	Omnipen® (ampicillin) Capsule 500 mg.
313	Aspirin Tablet 300 mg. (5 gr.)
317	Serax® (oxazepam) Tablet 15 mg.
320	Phenobarbital Tablet 60 mg.
322	Chloral Hydrate Capsule 500 mg.
325	Codeine Sulfate Tablet 15 mg.
326	Codeine Sulfate Tablet 30 mg.
327	Codeine Sulfate Tablet 60 mg.
360	Pathocil® (dicloxacillin sodium monohydrate) Capsule 250 mg.
389	Tetracycline HCl Capsule 250 mg.
390	Pen•Vee® K (penicillin V potassium) Tablet 500 mg.
434	Phenergan®-D (promethazine HCl with pseudoephedrine HCl) Tablet
445	Ovral®-28 pink inert tablet
464	Unipen® [(nafcillin sodium) as the monohydrate] 500 mg. Tablet
471	Tetracycline HCl Capsule 500 mg.
472	Basaljel® (dried basic aluminum carbonate gel) Capsule
473	Basaljel® (dried basic aluminum carbonate gel) Swallow Tablet
486	Nordette®-28, Lo/Ovral®-28 pink inert tablet
559	Wymox® (amoxicillin) 250 mg. Capsule
560	Wymox® (amoxicillin) 500 mg. Capsule
576	Wyamycin®S (erythromycin stearate) Tablet 250 mg.
578	Wyamycin®S (erythromycin stearate) Tablet 500 mg.
593	Pathocil® (dicloxacillin sodium monohydrate) Capsule 500 mg
607	Polymagma® Plain Tablet (each tablet contains Claysorb® [activated attapulgite] 500 mg., pectin 45 mg.
614	Cyclapen-W® (cyclacillin) Tablet 250 mg.
615	Cyclapen-W® (cyclacillin) Tablet 500 mg.
2511	Ovral®-28 Pilpak® (21 white tablets each containing 0.5 mg. norgestrel with 0.05 mg. ethinyl estradiol and 7 pink inert tablets)
2514	Lo/Ovral®-28 Pilpak® (21 white tablets each containing 0.3 mg. norgestrel with 0.03 mg. ethinyl estradiol and 7 pink inert tablets)
2533	Nordette®-28 Pilpak® (21 light-orange tablets each containing 0.15 mg. levonorgestrel with 0.03 mg ethinyl estradiol and 7 pink inert tablets)

ALUDROX® OTC
[al'u-drox]
(alumina and magnesia)
ORAL SUSPENSION • TABLETS

Composition: Nonconstipating, noncathartic, effective and palatable antacid containing, in each 5 ml. teaspoonful of suspension, 307 mg. of aluminum hydroxide as a gel, and 103 mg. of magnesium hydroxide. Each tablet contains 233 mg. aluminum hydroxide as a dried gel and 83 mg. magnesium hydroxide. Sodium content is 0.07 mEq per tablet and 0.05 mEq per 5 ml suspension.

Indications: For the symptomatic relief of hyperacidity associated with the diagnosis of peptic ulcer, gastritis, peptic esophagitis, gastric hyperacidity, and hiatal hernia.

Dosage and Administration: Two tablets or 2 teaspoonfuls (10 ml.) of suspension every four hours, or as required. Suspension may be followed by a sip of water if desired. Tablets are designed to be chewed with or without water.

Two ALUDROX tablets have the capacity to neutralize 23 mEq of acid; 10 ml. of ALUDROX suspension have the capacity to neutralize 28 mEq of acid.

Warnings: Patients are advised not to take more than 12 teaspoonfuls (60 ml) or 16 tablets in a 24-hour period or use this maximum dosage for more than two weeks except under the advice and supervision of a physician.

Drug Interaction Precautions: This product must not be taken if the patient is presently taking a prescription antibiotic drug containing any form of tetracycline.

How Supplied: *Oral Suspension,* bottles of 12 fluidounces.

Tablets, boxes of 100; each tablet is safety sealed in cellophane so that a day's supply can be conveniently carried.

Continued on next page

Wyeth—Cont.

AMPHOJEL® OTC
[am'fo-jel]
(aluminum hydroxide gel)
SUSPENSION • TABLETS

Composition: *Suspension*—Each 5 ml. teaspoonful contains 320 mg. of aluminum hydroxide as a gel, and not more than 0.3 mEq of sodium. *Tablets* contain a dried gel. The 0.3 Gm. (5 grain) strength is equivalent to about 1 teaspoonful of the suspension and the 0.6 Gm (10 grain) strength is equivalent to about 2 teaspoonfuls.
Indications: For the symptomatic relief of hyperacidity associated with the diagnosis of peptic ulcer, gastritis, peptic esophagitis, gastric hyperacidity, and hiatal hernia.
Dosage: *Suspension*—two teaspoonfuls followed by a sip of water if desired, five or six times daily, between meals and at bedtime. 2 teaspoonfuls have the capacity to neutralize 13 mEq of acid.
Tablets—Two tablets of the 0.3 Gm. strength, or one tablet of the 0.6 Gm. strength, five or six times daily between meals and at bedtime. 2 tablets have the capacity to neutralize 18 mEq of acid.
Warnings: Patients are advised not to take more than 12 teaspoonfuls (60 ml) or 6 tablets in a 24-hour period or use this maximum dosage for more than two weeks except under the advice and supervision of a physician.
Precaution: May cause constipation.
Drug Interaction Precautions: This product must not be taken if the patient is presently taking a prescription antibiotic drug containing any form of tetracycline.
How Supplied: *Suspension*—Peppermint flavored; without flavor—bottles of 12 fluidounces. *Tablets*—a convenient auxiliary dosage form—0.3 Gm. (5 gr.), bottles of 100; 0.6 Gm. (10 gr.), boxes of 100.

ATIVAN® ℞
[at'i-van]
(lorazepam)

Description: Ativan (lorazepam), an antianxiety agent, has the chemical formula, 7-chloro-5-(o-chlorophenyl)-1,3-dihydro-3-hydroxy-2H-1,4-benzodiazepin-2-one.
It is a nearly white powder almost insoluble in water. Each Ativan (lorazepam) tablet, to be taken orally, contains 0.5 mg, 1 mg or 2 mg of lorazepam.
Clinical Pharmacology: Studies in healthy volunteers show that in single high doses Ativan (lorazepam) has a tranquilizing action on the central nervous system with no appreciable effect on the respiratory or cardiovascular systems.
Ativan (lorazepam) is readily absorbed with an absolute bioavailability of 90 percent. Peak concentrations in plasma occur approximately 2 hours following administration. The peak plasma level of lorazepam from a 2 mg dose is approximately 20 ng/ml.
The mean half-life of unconjugated lorazepam in human plasma is about 12 hours and for its major metabolite, lorazepam glucuronide, about 18 hours. At clinically relevant concentrations, lorazepam is approximately 85% bound to plasma proteins. Ativan (lorazepam) is rapidly conjugated at its 3-hydroxy group into lorazepam glucuronide which is then excreted in the urine. Lorazepam glucuronide has no demonstrable CNS activity in animals.
The plasma levels of lorazepam are proportional to the dose given. There is no evidence of accumulation of lorazepam on administration up to six months.
Studies comparing young and elderly subjects have shown that the pharmacokinetics of lorazepam remain unaltered with advancing age.
Indications and Usage: Ativan (lorazepam) is indicated for the management of anxiety disorders or for the short-term relief of the symptoms of anxiety or anxiety associated with depressive symptoms. Anxiety or tension associated with the stress of everyday life usually does not require treatment with an anxiolytic.
The effectiveness of Ativan (lorazepam) in long-term use, that is, more than 4 months, has not been assessed by systematic clinical studies. The physician should periodically reassess the usefulness of the drug for the individual patient.
Contraindications: Ativan (lorazepam) is contraindicated in patients with known sensitivity to the benzodiazepines or with acute narrow-angle glaucoma.
Warnings: Ativan (lorazepam) is not recommended for use in patients with a primary depressive disorder or psychosis. As with all patients on CNS-acting drugs, patients receiving lorazepam should be warned not to operate dangerous machinery or motor vehicles and that their tolerance for alcohol and other CNS depressants will be diminished.
PHYSICAL AND PSYCHOLOGICAL DEPENDENCE: Withdrawal symptoms similar in character to those noted with barbiturates and alcohol have occurred following abrupt discontinuance of benzodiazepine drugs. These symptoms include convulsions, tremor, abdominal and muscle cramps, vomiting and sweating. Addiction-prone individuals, such as drug addicts and alcoholics, should be under careful surveillance when receiving benzodiazepines because of the predisposition of such patients to habituation and dependence. Withdrawal symptoms have also been reported following abrupt discontinuance of benzodiazepines taken continuously at therapeutic levels for several months.
Precautions: In patients with depression accompanying anxiety, a possibility for suicide should be borne in mind.
For elderly or debilitated patients, the initial daily dosage should not exceed 2 mg in order to avoid oversedation.
Ativan® (lorazepam) dosage should be terminated gradually, since abrupt withdrawal of any anti-anxiety agent may result in symptoms similar to those for which patients are being treated: anxiety, agitation, irritability, tension, insomnia, and occasional convulsions.
The usual precautions for treating patients with impaired renal or hepatic function should be observed.
In patients where gastrointestinal or cardiovascular disorders coexist with anxiety, it should be noted that lorazepam has not been shown to be of significant benefit in treating the gastrointestinal or cardiovascular component.
Esophageal dilation occurred in rats treated with lorazepam for more than one year at 6 mg/kg/day. The no-effect dose was 1.25 mg/kg/day (approximately 6 times the maximum human therapeutic dose of 10 mg per day). The effect was reversible only when the treatment was withdrawn within two months of first observation of the phenomenon. The clinical significance of this is unknown. However, use of lorazepam for prolonged periods and in geriatric patients requires caution, and there should be frequent monitoring for symptoms of upper G.I. disease.
Safety and effectiveness of Ativan (lorazepam) in children of less than 12 years have not been established.
ESSENTIAL LABORATORY TESTS: Some patients on Ativan (lorazepam) have developed leukopenia, and some have had elevations of LDH. As with other benzodiazepines, periodic blood counts and liver-function tests are recommended for patients on long-term therapy.
CLINICALLY SIGNIFICANT DRUG INTERACTIONS: The benzodiazepines, including Ativan (lorazepam), produce CNS depressant effects when administered with such medications as barbiturates or alcohol.
CARCINOGENESIS AND MUTAGENESIS: No evidence of carcinogenic potential emerged in rats during an 18-month study with Ativan (lorazepam). No studies regarding mutagenesis have been performed.
PREGNANCY: Reproductive studies in animals were performed in mice, rats, and two strains of rabbits. Occasional anomalies (reduction of tarsals, tibia, metatarsals, malrotated limbs, gastroschisis, malformed skull, and microphthalmia) were seen in drug-treated rabbits without relationship to dosage. Although all of these anomalies were not present in the concurrent control group, they have been reported to occur randomly in historical controls. At doses of 40 mg/kg and higher, there was evidence of fetal resorption and increased fetal loss in rabbits which was not seen at lower doses.
The clinical significance of the above findings is not known. However, an increased risk of congenital malformations associated with the use of minor tranquilizers (chlordiazepoxide, diazepam, and meprobamate) during the first trimester of pregnancy has been suggested in several studies. Because the use of these drugs is rarely a matter of urgency, the use of lorazepam during this period should almost always be avoided. The possibility that a woman of childbearing potential may be pregnant at the time of institution of therapy should be considered. Patients should be advised that if they become pregnant, they should communicate with their physician about the desirability of discontinuing the drug.
In humans, blood levels obtained from umbilical cord blood indicate placental transfer of lorazepam and lorazepam glucuronide.
NURSING MOTHERS: It is not known whether oral lorazepam is excreted in human milk like the other benzodiazepine tranquilizers. As a general rule, nursing should not be undertaken while a patient is on a drug, since many drugs are excreted in human milk.
Adverse Reactions: Adverse reactions, if they occur, are usually observed at the beginning of therapy and generally disappear on continued medication or upon decreasing the dose. In a sample of about 3,500 anxious patients, the most frequent adverse reaction to Ativan® (lorazepam) is sedation (15.9%), followed by dizziness (6.9%), weakness (4.2%), and unsteadiness (3.4%). Less frequent adverse reactions are disorientation, depression, nausea, change in appetite, headache, sleep disturbance, agitation, dermatological symptoms, eye function disturbance, together with various gastrointestinal symptoms and autonomic manifestations. The incidence of sedation and unsteadiness increased with age.
Small decreases in blood pressure have been noted but are not clinically significant, probably being related to the relief of anxiety produced by Ativan (lorazepam).
Transient amnesia or memory impairment has been reported in association with the use of benzodiazepines.
Overdosage: In the management of overdosage with any drug, it should be borne in mind that multiple agents may have been taken.
Manifestations of Ativan (lorazepam) overdosage include somnolence, confusion, and coma. Induced vomiting and/or gastric lavage should be undertaken, followed by general supportive care, monitoring of vital signs, and close observation of the patient. Hypotension, though unlikely, usually may be controlled with Levarterenol Bitartrate Injection, USP. The usefulness of dialysis has not been determined.
Dosage and Administration: Ativan® (lorazepam) is administered orally. For optimal results, dose, frequency of administration, and duration of therapy should be individualized according to patient response. To facilitate this, 0.5 mg, 1 mg and 2 mg tablets are available.
The usual range is 2 to 6 mg/day given in divided doses, the largest dose being taken before bedtime, but the daily dosage may vary from 1 to 10 mg/day.
For anxiety, most patients require an initial dose of 2 to 3 mg/day given b.i.d. or t.i.d.
For insomnia due to anxiety or transient situational stress, a single daily dose of 2 to 4 mg may be given, usually at bedtime.
For elderly or debilitated patients, an initial dosage of 1 to 2 mg/day in divided doses is recommended, to be adjusted as needed and tolerated.
The dosage of Ativan (lorazepam) should be increased gradually when needed to help avoid ad-

verse effects. When higher dosage is indicated, the evening dose should be increased before the daytime doses.

How Supplied: Ativan® (lorazepam) Tablets, Wyeth®, are available in the following dosage strengths:

0.5 mg, NDC 0008-0081, white, five-sided tablet with a raised "A" on one side and "WYETH" and "81" on reverse side, in bottles of 100 and 500 tablets, and in Redipak® Strip Pack, boxes of 25

1 mg, NDC 0008-0064, white, five-sided tablet with a raised "A" on one side and "WYETH" and "64" on scored reverse side, in bottles of 100, 500, and 1000 tablets, and in Redipak® Strip Pack, boxes of 25.

2 mg, NDC 0008-0065, white, five-sided tablet with a raised "A" on one side and "WYETH" and "65" on scored reverse side, in bottles of 100, 500, and 1000 tablets, and in Redipak® Strip Pack, boxes of 25.

Store at controlled room temperature.
Keep bottles tightly closed.
Dispense in tight container.

The appearance of ATIVAN tablets is a registered trademark of Wyeth Laboratories.
Shown in Product Identification Section, page 444

ATIVAN®
[at'i-van]
(lorazepam)
Injection

Description: Ativan (lorazepam) Injection, a benzodiazepine with anti-anxiety and sedative effects, is intended for intramuscular or intravenous route of administration. It has the chemical formula: 7-chloro-5-(o-chlorophenyl)-1,3-dihydro-3-hydroxy-2 H-1, 4-benzodiazepin-2-one. The molecular weight is 321.2 and the C.A.S. No. is [846-49-1].

Lorazepam is a nearly white powder almost insoluble in water. Each ml of sterile injection contains either 2.0 or 4.0 mg of lorazepam, 0.18 ml polyethylene glycol 400 in propylene glycol with 2.0% benzyl alcohol as preservative.

Clinical Pharmacology: Intravenous or intramuscular administration of the recommended dose of 2–4 mg of Ativan (lorazepam) Injection to adult patients is followed by dose related effects of sedation (sleepiness or drowsiness), relief of preoperative anxiety and lack of recall of events related to the day of surgery in the majority of patients. The clinical sedation (sleepiness or drowsiness), thus noted is such that the majority of patients are able to respond to simple instructions whether they give the appearance of being awake or asleep. The lack of recall is relative rather than absolute, as determined under conditions of careful patient questioning and testing using props designed to enhance recall. The majority of patients under these reinforced conditions had difficulty recalling peri-operative events, or recognizing props from before surgery. The lack of recall and recognition was optimum within 2 hours following intramuscular administration and 15–20 minutes after intravenous injection.

The intended effects of the recommended adult dose of lorazepam injection usually last 6–8 hours. In rare instances and where patients received greater than the recommended dose, excessive sleepiness and prolonged lack of recall were noted. As with other benzodiazepines, unsteadiness, enhanced sensitivity to CNS depressant effects of ethyl alcohol and other drugs were noted in isolated and rare cases for greater than 24 hours.

Studies in healthy adult volunteers reveal that intravenous lorazepam in doses up to 3.5 mg/70 kg does not alter sensitivity to the respiratory stimulating effect of carbon dioxide and does not enhance the respiratory depressant effects of doses of meperidine up to 100 mg/70 kg (also determined by carbon dioxide challenge) as long as patients remain sufficiently awake to undergo testing. Upper airway obstruction has been observed in rare instances where the patient received greater than the recommended dose, and was excessively sleepy and difficult to arouse. (See WARNINGS and ADVERSE REACTIONS.)

Clinically employed doses of lorazepam injectable do not greatly affect the circulatory system in the supine position or employing a 70 degree tilt test. Doses of 8–10 mg of intravenous lorazepam (2 to 2½ times the maximum recommended dosage) will produce loss of lid reflexes within 15 minutes. Studies in six (6) healthy young adults who received lorazepam injection and no other drugs revealed that visual tracking (the ability to keep a moving line centered) was impaired for a mean of eight (8) hours following administration of 4 mg of intramuscular lorazepam and four (4) hours following administration of 2 mg intramuscularly with considerable subject variation. Similar findings were noted with pentobarbital 150 and 75 mg. Although this study showed that both lorazepam and pentobarbital interfered with eye-hand coordination, the data are insufficient to predict when it would be safe to operate a motor vehicle or engage in a hazardous occupation or sport.

PHARMACOKINETICS

Injectable Ativan (lorazepam) is readily absorbed when given intramuscularly. Peak plasma concentrations occur approximately 60–90 minutes following administration and appear to be dose related, e.g. a 2.0 mg dose provides a level of approximately 20 ng/ml and a 4.0 mg dose aproximately 40 ng/ml in plasma. The mean half-life of lorazepam is about 16 hours when given intravenously or intramuscularly. Ativan (lorazepam) is rapidly conjugated at the 3-hydroxyl group into its major metabolite, lorazepam glucuronide, which is then excreted in the urine. Lorazepam glucuronide has no demonstrable CNS activity in animals. When 5 mg of intravenous lorazepam was administered to volunteers once a day for four consecutive days, a steady state of free lorazepam was achieved by the second day (approximately 52 ng/ml of plasma three hours after the first dose and approximately 62 ng/ml three hours after each subsequent dose, one day apart). At clinically relevant concentrations, lorazepam is bound 85% to plasma proteins.

Indications and Usage: Ativan (lorazepam) Injection is indicated in adult patients for preanesthetic medication, producing sedation (sleepiness or drowsiness), relief of anxiety, and a decreased ability to recall events related to the day of surgery. It is most useful in those patients who are anxious about their surgical procedure and who would prefer to have diminished recall of the events of the day of surgery. (see Information for Patients)

Contraindications: Ativan (lorazepam) Injection is contraindicated in patients with a known sensitivity to benzodiazepines or its vehicle (polyethylene glycol, propylene glycol, and benzyl alcohol) and in patients with acute narrow angle glaucoma. The use of Ativan (lorazepam) Injection intra-arterially is contraindicated because, as with other injectable benzodiazepines, inadvertent intra-arterial injection may produce arteriospasm resulting in gangrene which may require amputation. (see Warnings)

Warnings: PRIOR TO INTRAVENOUS USE, ATIVAN INJECTION MUST BE DILUTED WITH AN EQUAL AMOUNT OF COMPATIBLE DILUENT (SEE DOSAGE AND ADMINISTRATION). INTRAVENOUS INJECTION SHOULD BE MADE SLOWLY AND WITH REPEATED ASPIRATION. CARE SHOULD BE TAKEN TO DETERMINE THAT ANY INJECTION WILL NOT BE INTRA-ARTERIAL AND THAT PERIVASCULAR EXTRAVASATION WILL NOT TAKE PLACE.
PARTIAL AIRWAY OBSTRUCTION MAY OCCUR IN HEAVILY SEDATED PATIENTS. INTRAVENOUS LORAZEPAM, WHEN GIVEN ALONE IN GREATER THAN THE RECOMMENDED DOSE, OR AT THE RECOMMENDED DOSE AND ACCOMPANIED BY OTHER DRUGS USED DURING THE ADMINISTRATION OF ANESTHESIA, MAY PRODUCE HEAVY SEDATION, THEREFORE EQUIPMENT NECESSARY TO MAINTAIN A PATENT AIRWAY AND TO SUPPORT RESPIRATION/VENTILATION SHOULD BE AVAILABLE.
There is no evidence to support the use of lorazepam injection in coma, shock or acute alcohol intoxication at this time. Since the liver is the most likely site of conjugation of lorazepam and since excretion of conjugated lorazepam (glucuronide) is a renal function, this drug is not recommended for use in patients with hepatic and/or renal *failure*. This does not preclude use of the drug in patients with mild to moderate hepatic or renal disease. When injectable lorazepam is selected for use in patients with mild to moderate hepatic or renal disease, the lowest effective dose should be considered since drug effect may be prolonged. Experience with other benzodiazepines and limited experience with parenteral lorazepam has demonstrated that tolerance to alcoholic beverages, and other central nervous system depressants is diminished when used concomitantly.

As is true of similar CNS-acting drugs, patients receiving injectable lorazepam should not operate machinery or engage in a hazardous occupations or drive a motor vehicle for a period of 24–48 hours. Impairment of performance may persist for greater intervals because of extremes of age, concomitant use of other drugs, stress of surgery or the general condition of the patient.

Clinical trials have shown that patients over the age of 50 years may have a more profound and prolonged sedation with intravenous lorazepam. Ordinarily an initial dose of 2 mg may be adequate, unless a greater degree of lack of recall is desired.

As with all central nervous system depressant drugs, care should be exercised in patients given injectable lorazepam that premature ambulation may result in injury from falling.

There is no added beneficial effect to the addition of scopolamine to injectable lorazepam and their combined effect may result in an increased incidence of sedation, hallucination and irrational behavior.

PREGNANCY

ATIVAN® (LORAZEPAM) MAY CAUSE FETAL DAMAGE WHEN ADMINISTERED TO PREGNANT WOMEN. An increased risk of congenital malformations associated with the use of minor tranquilizers (chlordiazepoxide, diazepam and meprobamate) during the first trimester of pregnancy has been suggested in several studies. In humans, blood levels obtained from umbilical cord blood indicate placental transfer of lorazepam and lorazepam glucuronide.

Ativan Injection should not be used during pregnancy. There are insufficient data regarding obstetrical safety of parenteral lorazepam, including use in cesarean section. Such use, therefore, is not recommended.

Reproductive studies in animals were performed in mice, rats, and two strains of rabbits. Occasional anomalies (reduction of tarsals, tibia, metatarsals, malrotated limbs, gastroschisis, malformed skull and microphthalmia) were seen in drug-treated rabbits without relationship to dosage. Although all of these anomalies were not present in the concurrent control group, they have been reported to occur randomly in historical controls. At doses of 40 mg/kg orally or 4 mg/kg intravenously and higher, there was evidence of fetal resorption and increased fetal loss in rabbits which was not seen at lower doses.

ENDOSCOPIC PROCEDURES

There are insufficient data to support the use of Ativan (lorazepam) Injection for outpatient endoscopic procedures. Inpatient endoscopic procedures require adequate recovery room observations.

Pharyngeal reflexes are not impaired when Ativan Injection is used for per-oral endoscopic procedures; therefore adequate topical or regional anesthesia is recommended to minimize reflex activity associated with such procedures.

Precautions:
GENERAL

The additive central nervous system effects of other drugs such as phenothiazines, narcotic analgesics, barbiturates, anti-depressants, scopolamine and monoamine oxidase inhibitors should be

Continued on next page

Wyeth—Cont.

borne in mind when these other drugs are used concomitantly with or during the period of recovery from Ativan (lorazepam) Injection. (See CLINICAL PHARMACOLOGY and WARNINGS).

Extreme care must be used in administering Ativan Injection to elderly patients, very ill patients, and to patients with limited pulmonary reserve, because of the possibility that underventilation and/or hypoxic cardiac arrest may occur. Resuscitative equipment for ventilatory support should be readily available. (See WARNINGS and DOSAGE and ADMINISTRATION).

When lorazepam injection is used IV as the premedicant prior to regional or local anesthesia, the possibility of excessive sleepiness or drowsiness may interfere with patient cooperation to determine levels of anesthesia. This is most likely to occur when greater than 0.05 mg/kg is given and when narcotic analgesics are used concomitantly with the recommended dose. (See ADVERSE REACTIONS).

INFORMATION FOR PATIENTS

As appropriate, the patient should be informed of the pharmacological effects of the drug such as sedation, relief of anxiety and lack of recall and the duration of these effects (about 8 hours) so that they may adequately perceive the risks as well as the benefits to be derived from its use.

Patients who receive Ativan Injection as a premedicant should be cautioned that driving an automobile or operating hazardous machinery, or engaging in a hazardous sport should be delayed for 24–48 hours following the injection. Sedatives, tranquilizers, and narcotic analgesics may produce a more prolonged and profound effect when administered along with injectable Ativan. This effect may take the form of excessive sleepiness or drowsiness, and on rare occasions, interfere with recall and recognition of events of the day of surgery and the day after.

Getting out of bed unassisted may result in falling and injury if undertaken within 8 hours of receiving lorazepam injection. Alcoholic beverages should not be consumed for at least 24–48 hours after receiving lorazepam injectable due to the additive effects on central nervous system depression seen with benzodiazepines in general. Elderly patients should be told that Ativan (lorazepam) Injection may make them very sleepy for a period longer than six (6) to eight (8) hours following surgery.

LABORATORY TESTS

In clinical trials no laboratory test abnormalities were identified with either single or multiple doses of Ativan (lorazepam) Injection. These tests included: CBC, urinalysis, SGOT, SGPT, bilirubin, alkaline phosphatase, LDH, cholesterol, uric acid, BUN, glucose, calcium, phosphorus and total proteins.

DRUG INTERACTIONS

Ativan (lorazepam) Injection, like other injectable benzodiazepines, produces depression of the central nervous system when administered with ethyl alcohol, phenothiazines, barbiturates, MAO inhibitors and other antidepressants. When scopolamine is used concomitantly with injectable lorazepam an increased incidence of sedation, hallucinations and irrational behavior has been observed.

DRUG/LABORATORY TEST INTERACTIONS

No laboratory test abnormalities were identified when lorazepam was given alone or concomitantly with another drug, such as narcotic analgesics, inhalation anesthetics, scopolamine, atropine, and a variety of tranquilizing agents.

CARCINOGENESIS, MUTAGENESIS, IMPAIRMENT OF FERTILITY

No evidence of carcinogenic potential emerged in rats and mice during an 18-month study with oral lorazepam. No studies regarding mutagenesis have been performed. Pre-implantation study in rats was performed with oral lorazepam at a 20 mg/kg dose and showed no impairment of fertility.

PREGNANCY

Pregnancy Category D. See WARNINGS.

LABOR AND DELIVERY

There are insufficient data to support the use of Ativan® (lorazepam) injection during labor and delivery, including cesarean section; therefore its use in this situation is not recommended.

NURSING MOTHERS

Injectable lorazepam should not be administered to nursing mothers, because like other benzodiazepines, the possibility exists that lorazepam may be excreted in human milk and sedate the infant.

PEDIATRIC USE

There are insufficient data to support efficacy or make dosage recommendations for injectable lorazepam in patients less than 18 years of age; therefore, such use is not recommended.

Adverse Reactions:

CENTRAL NERVOUS SYSTEM

The most frequent adverse effects seen with injectable lorazepam are an extension of the central nervous system depressant effects of the drug. The incidence varied from one study to another, depending on the dosage, route of administration, use of other central nervous system depressants, and the investigator's opinion concerning the degree and duration of desired sedation. Excessive sleepiness and drowsiness were the main side effects. This interfered with patient cooperation in approximately 6% (25/446) of patients undergoing regional anesthesia in that they were unable to assess levels of anesthesia in regional blocks or with caudal anesthesia. Patients over 50 years of age had a higher incidence of excessive sleepiness or drowsiness when compared with those under 50 (21/106 vs 24/245) when lorazepam was given intravenously. (see DOSAGE and ADMINISTRATION). On rare occasion (3/1580) the patient was unable to give personal identification in the operating room on arrival, and one patient fell when attempting premature ambulation in the postoperative period.

Symptoms such as restlessness, confusion, depression, crying, sobbing, and delirium occurred in about 1.3% (20/1580). One patient injured himself by picking at his incision during the immediate postoperative period.

Hallucinations were present in about 1% (14/1580) of patients, and were visual and self-limiting.

An occasional patient complained of dizziness, diplopia and/or blurred vision. Depressed hearing was infrequently reported during the peak effect period.

An occasional patient had a prolonged recovery room stay, either because of excessive sleepiness or because of some form of inappropriate behavior. The latter was seen most commonly when scopolamine was given concomitantly as a premedicant. Limited information derived from patients who were discharged the day after receiving injectable lorazepam showed one patient complained of some unsteadiness of gait and a reduced ability to perform complex mental functions. Enhanced sensitivity to alcoholic beverages has been reported more than 24 hours after receiving injectable lorazepam, similar to experience with other benzodiazepines.

LOCAL EFFECTS

Intramuscular injection of lorazepam has resulted in pain at the injection site, a sensation of burning, or observed redness in the same area in a very variable incidence from one study to another. The overall incidence of pain and burning was about 17% (146/859) in the immediate post-injection period and about 1.4% (12/859) at the 24-hour observation time. Reactions at the injection site (redness) occurred in approximately 2% (17/859) in the immediate post-injection period, and were present 24 hours later in about 0.8% (7/859).

Intravenous administration of lorazepam resulted in painful responses in 13/771 patients or approximately 1.6% in the immediate post-injection period and 24 hours later 4/771 patients or about 0.5% still complained of pain. Redness did not occur immediately following intravenous injection, but was noted in 19/771 patients at the 24-hour observation period. This incidence is similar to that observed with an intravenous infusion before lorazepam is given.

CARDIOVASCULAR SYSTEM

Hypertension (0.1%) and hypotension (0.1%) have occasionally been observed after patients have received injectable lorazepam.

RESPIRATORY SYSTEM

Five patients (5/446) who underwent regional anesthesia were observed to have partial airway obstruction. This was believed due to excessive sleepiness at the time of the procedure, and resulted in temporary underventilation. Immediate attention to the airway, employing the usual countermeasures, will usually suffice to manage this condition (see also CLINICAL PHARMACOLOGY, WARNINGS and PRECAUTIONS).

OTHER ADVERSE EXPERIENCES

Skin rash, nausea, and vomiting have occasionally been noted in patients who have received injectable lorazepam combined with other drugs during anesthesia and surgery.

Drug Abuse and Dependence: As with other benzodiazepines, Ativan (lorazepam) Injection has a low potential for abuse and may lead to limited dependence. Although there are no clinical data available for injectable lorazepam in this respect, physicians should be aware that repeated doses over a prolonged period of time may result in limited physical and psychological dependence.

Overdosage: Overdosage of benzodiazepines is usually manifested by varying degrees of central nervous system depression ranging from drowsiness to coma. In mild cases symptoms include drowsiness, mental confusion and lethargy. In more serious examples, symptoms may include ataxia, hypotonia, hypotension, hypnosis, stages one (1) to three (3) coma, and very rarely death. Treatment of overdosage is mainly supportive until the drug is eliminated from the body. Vital signs and fluid balance should be carefully monitored. An adequate airway should be maintained and assisted respiration used as needed. With normally functioning kidneys, forced diuresis with intravenous fluids and electrolytes may accelerate elimination of benzodiazepines from the body. In addition, osmotic diuretics such as mannitol may be effective as adjunctive measures. In more critical situations, renal dialysis and exchange blood transfusions may be indicated. Published reports indicate that intravenous infusion of 0.5 to 4 mg of physostigmine at the rate of 1 mg/minute may reverse symptoms and signs suggestive of central anticholinergic overdose (confusion, memory disturbance, visual disturbances, hallucinations, delirium); however, hazards associated with the use of physostigmine (i.e. induction of seizures) should be weighed against its possible clinical benefit.

Dosage and Administration:
INTRAMUSCULAR INJECTION

For the designated indications as a premedicant, the usual recommended dose of lorazepam for intramuscular injection is 0.05 mg/kg up to a maximum of 4 mg. As with all premedicant drugs, the dose should be individualized. (See also CLINICAL PHARMACOLOGY, WARNINGS, PRECAUTIONS, and ADVERSE REACTIONS). Doses of other central nervous system depressant drugs should be ordinarily reduced (See PRECAUTIONS). *For optimum effect, measured as lack of recall, intramuscular lorazepam should be administered at least 2 hours before the anticipated operative procedure.* Narcotic analgesics should be administered at their usual pre-operative time. There are insufficient data to support efficacy to make dosage recommendations for intramuscular lorazepam in patients less than 18 years of age; therefore such use is not recommended.

INTRAVENOUS INJECTION

For the primary purpose of sedation and relief of anxiety, the usual recommended initial dose of lorazepam for intravenous injection is 2 mg total, or 0.02 mg/lb (0.044 mg/kg) whichever is smaller. This dose will suffice for sedating most adult patients, and should not ordinarily be exceeded in patients over 50 years of age. In those patients in whom a greater likelihood of lack of recall for perioperative events would be beneficial, larger doses

as high as 0.05 mg/kg up to a total of 4 mg may be administered. (See CLINICAL PHARMACOLOGY, WARNINGS, PRECAUTIONS, and ADVERSE REACTIONS). Doses of other injectable central nervous system depressant drugs should ordinarily be reduced. (See PRECAUTIONS). *For optimum effect, measured as lack of recall, intravenous lorazepam should be administered 15–20 minutes before the anticipated operative procedure.*
EQUIPMENT NECESSARY TO MAINTAIN A PATENT AIRWAY SHOULD BE IMMEDIATELY AVAILABLE PRIOR TO INTRAVENOUS ADMINISTRATION OF LORAZEPAM (See WARNINGS).
There are insufficient data to support efficacy or make dosage recommendations for intravenous lorazepam in patients less than 18 years of age; therefore, such use is not recommended.
ADMINISTRATION
When given intramuscularly, Ativan® Injection, undiluted, should be injected deep in the muscle mass.
Injectable Ativan (lorazepam) can be used with atropine sulfate, narcotic analgesics, other parenterally used analgesics, commonly used anesthetics, and muscle relaxants.
Immediately prior to intravenous use, Ativan (lorazepam) Injection must be diluted with an equal volume of compatible solution. When properly diluted the drug may be injected directly into a vein or into the tubing of an existing intravenous infusion. The rate of injection should not exceed 2.0 mg per minute.
Parenteral drug products should be inspected visually for particulate matter and discoloration prior to administration whenever solution and container permit. Do not use if solution is discolored or contains a precipitate.
Ativan (lorazepam) Injection is compatible for dilution purposes with the following solutions:
Sterile Water for Injection, USP
Sodium Chloride Injection, USP
5% Dextrose Injection, USP
How Supplied: Ativan® (lorazepam) Injection, Wyeth®, is available in the following dosage strengths in single-dose and in multiple-dose vials and in TUBEX® Sterile Cartridge-Needle Units, packaged in boxes of 10 TUBEX:
2 mg per ml, NDC 0008-0581; 1 ml and 10 ml vials and 1 ml fill in 2 ml TUBEX.
4 mg per ml, NDC 0008-0570; 1 ml and 10 ml vials and 1 ml fill in 2 ml TUBEX.
For IM or IV injection.
Protect from light.
Keep in a refrigerator.
Directions for Dilution for IV Use: To dilute, adhere to the following procedure:
For TUBEX—
1. Extrude the entire amount of air in the half-filled TUBEX.
2. Slowly aspirate the desired volume of diluent.
3. Pull back slightly on the plunger to provide additional mixing space.
4. Immediately mix contents thoroughly by gently inverting TUBEX repeatedly until a homogenous solution results. Do not shake vigorously, as this will result in air entrapment.
For Vial—
Aspirate the desired amount of Ativan Injection into the syringe. Then proceed as described under TUBEX.

BASALJEL®   OTC
[bā′sel-jel]
(basic aluminum carbonate gel)
SUSPENSION ●CAPSULES ●SWALLOW TABLETS

Composition: Suspension—each 5 ml teaspoonful contains basic aluminum carbonate gel equivalent to 400 mg aluminum hydroxide. Extra Strength Suspension—each 5 ml teaspoonful contains basic aluminum carbonate gel equivalent to 1000 mg aluminum hydroxide. Capsule contains dried basic aluminum carbonate gel equivalent to 608 mg of dried aluminum hydroxide gel or 500 mg aluminum hydroxide. Tablet contains dried basic aluminum carbonate gel equivalent to 608 mg of dried aluminum hydroxide gel or 500 mg aluminum hydroxide.
Indications: For the symptomatic relief of hyperacidity associated with the diagnosis of peptic ulcer, gastritis, peptic esophagitis, gastric hyperacidity and hiatal hernia.
Warnings: No more than 24 tablets/capsules/teaspoonfuls of BASALJEL, and no more than 12 teaspoonfuls of BASALJEL Extra Strength Suspension should be taken in a 24-hour period. Dosage should be carefully supervised since continued overdosage, in conjunction with restriction of dietary phosphorous and calcium, may produce a persistently lowered serum phosphate and a mildly elevated alkaline phosphatase. A usually transient hypercalciuria of mild degree may be associated with the early weeks of therapy.
Dosage and Administration: Suspension—two teaspoonfuls (10 ml) in water or fruit juice taken as often as every two hours up to twelve times daily. Two teaspoonfuls have the capacity to neutralize 28 mEq of acid. Extra Strength Suspension—one teaspoonful (5 ml) as often as every two hours up to twelve times daily. One teaspoonful is equivalent to two capsules or tablets and has the capacity to neutralize 22 mEq of acid. Capsules—two capsules as often as every two hours up to twelve times daily. Two capsules have the capacity to neutralize 26 mEq of acid. Swallow Tablets—two tablets as often as every two hours up to twelve times daily. Two tablets have the capacity to neutralize 28 mEq of acid. The sodium content of each dosage form is as follows: 0.1 mEq/5 ml for the suspension, 1.0 mEq/5 ml for the extra strength suspension, 0.12 mEq per capsule, and 0.09 mEq per tablet.
Precautions: May cause constipation. Adequate fluid intake should be maintained in addition to the specific medical or surgical management indicated by the patient's condition.
Drug Interaction Precautions: Alumina-containing antacids should not be used concomitantly with any form of tetracycline therapy.
How Supplied: Suspension—bottles of 12 fluidounces.
Extra Strength Suspension—bottles of 12 fluidounces.
Capsules—bottles of 100 and 500.
Swallow Tablets (scored)—bottles of 100.

BICILLIN® C-R   ℞
[bĭ-sĭl′ in]
(penicillin G benzathine and
penicillin G procaine suspension)
INJECTION

FOR DEEP INTRAMUSCULAR INJECTION ONLY

Description: Multiple-dose vials of 300,000 units per ml contain in each ml 150,000 units penicillin G benzathine and 150,000 units penicillin G procaine in a stabilized aqueous suspension with sodium citrate buffer, approximately 6 mg lecithin, 3 mg povidone, 1 mg carboxymethylcellulose, 0.5 mg sorbitan monopalmitate, 0.5 mg polyoxyethylene sorbitan monopalmitate, 1.2 mg methylparaben and 0.14 mg propylparaben.
Each TUBEX® cartridge (1 ml size) contains 600,000 units of penicillin comprising: 300,000 units penicillin G benzathine and 300,000 units penicillin G procaine in a stabilized aqueous suspension with sodium citrate buffer; and as w/v, approximately 0.5% lecithin, 0.55% carboxymethylcellulose, 0.55% povidone, 0.1% methylparaben, and 0.01% propylparaben.
Each TUBEX cartridge (2 ml size) contains 1,200,000 units of penicillin comprising: 600,000 units penicillin G benzathine and 600,000 units penicillin G procaine in a stabilized aqueous suspension with sodium citrate buffer; and as w/v, approximately 0.5% lecithin, 0.55% carboxymethylcellulose, 0.55% povidone, 0.1% methylparaben, and 0.01% propylparaben.
Each disposable syringe (2 ml size) contains 1,200,000 units of penicillin comprising: 600,000 units penicillin G benzathine and 600,000 units penicillin G procaine in a stabilized aqueous suspension with sodium citrate buffer; and as w/v, approximately 0.5% lecithin, 0.55% carboxymethylcellulose, 0.55% povidone, 0.1% methylparaben, and 0.01% propylparaben.
Each disposable syringe (4 ml size) contains 2,400,000 units of penicillin comprising: 1,200,000 units penicillin G benzathine and 1,200,000 units penicillin G procaine in a stabilized aqueous suspension with sodium citrate buffer; and as w/v, approximately 0.5% lecithin, 0.55% carboxymethylcellulose, 0.55% povidone, 0.1% methylparaben, and 0.01% propylparaben.
Bicillin C-R suspension in the multiple-dose vial, TUBEX, and disposable syringe formulations is viscous and opaque. Read "Contraindications," "Warnings," "Precautions," and "Dosage and Administration" sections prior to use.
Actions and Pharmacology: Penicillin G exerts a bactericidal action against penicillin-sensitive microorganisms during the stage of active multiplication. It acts through the inhibition of biosynthesis of cell-wall mucopeptide. It is not active against the penicillinase-producing bacteria, which include many strains of staphylococci.
Penicillin G exerts high *in vitro* activity against staphylococci (except penicillinase-producing strains) streptococci (Groups A, C, G, H, L, and M), and pneumococci. Other organisms sensitive to penicillin G are *Neisseria gonorrhoeae*, *Corynebacterium diphtheriae*, *Bacillus anthracis*, Clostridia, *Actinomyces bovis*, *Streptobacillus moniliformis*, *Listeria monocytogenes*, and Leptospira. *Treponema pallidum* is extremely sensitive to the bactericidal action for penicillin G.
Sensitivity plate testing: If the Kirby-Bauer method of disc sensitivity is used, a 10-unit penicillin disc should give a zone greater than 28 mm when tested against a penicillin-sensitive bacterial strain.
Intramuscular penicillin G benzathine is absorbed very slowly into the bloodstream from the intramuscular site and converted by hydrolysis to penicillin G. This combination of hydrolysis and slow absorption results in blood serum levels much lower but much more prolonged than other parenteral penicillins.
Penicillin G procaine is an equimolecular compound of procaine and penicillin G, administered intramuscularly as a suspension. It dissolves slowly at the site of injection, giving a plateau type of blood level at about 4 hours which falls slowly over a period of the next 15-20 hours.
Approximately 60% of penicillin G is bound to serum protein. The drug is distributed throughout the body tissues in widely varying amounts. Highest levels are found in the kidneys with lesser amounts in the liver, skin, and intestines. Penicillin G penetrates into all other tissues and the spinal fluid to a lesser degree. With normal kidney function the drug is excreted rapidly by tubular excretion. In neonates and young infants and in individuals with impaired kidney function, excretion is considerably delayed.
Indications: This drug is indicated in the treatment of moderately severe infections due to penicillin-G-susceptible microorganisms which are susceptible to serum levels common to this particular dosage form. Therapy should be guided by bacteriological studies (including susceptibility testing) and by clinical response. NOTE: When high, sustained serum levels are required, penicillin G sodium or potassium, either IM or IV, should be used. This drug should *not* be used in the treatment of venereal diseases, including syphilis, gonorrhea, yaws, bejel, and pinta.
The following infections will usually respond to adequate dosages of this drug:
Streptococcal infections Group A (without bacteremia). Moderately severe to severe infections of the upper respiratory tract, skin and soft-tissue infections, scarlet fever, and erysipelas.
NOTE: Streptococci in Groups A, C, G, H, L, and M are very sensitive to penicillin G. Other groups, including Group D (enterococci), are resistant.

Continued on next page

Wyeth—Cont.

Penicillin G sodium or potassium is recommended for streptococcal infections with bacteremia.

Pneumococcal infections. Moderately severe pneumonia and otitis media.

NOTE: Severe pneumonia, empyema, bacteremia, pericarditis, meningitis, peritonitis, and arthritis of pneumococcal etiology are better treated with penicillin G sodium or potassium during the acute stage.

Contraindications: A previous hypersensitivity reaction to any penicillin or to procaine is a contraindication.

Do not inject into or near an artery or nerve.

Warnings: Serious and occasionally fatal hypersensitivity (anaphylactoid) reactions have been reported in patients on penicillin therapy. Although anaphylaxis is more frequent following parenteral therapy, it has occurred in patients on oral penicillins. These reactions are more apt to occur in individuals with a history of sensitivity to multiple allergens.

There have been well-documented reports of individuals with a history of penicillin hypersensitivity reactions who have experienced severe hypersensitivity reactions when treated with a cephalosporin. Before therapy with a penicillin, careful inquiry should be made concerning previous hypersensitivity reactions to penicillins, cephalosporins, and other allergens. If an allergic reaction occurs, the drug should be discontinued and the patient treated with the usual agents, e.g., pressor amines, antihistamines, and corticosteroids.

Inadvertent intravascular administration, including inadvertent direct intraarterial injection or injection immediately adjacent to arteries, of Bicillin C-R and other penicillin preparations has resulted in severe neurovascular damage, including transverse myelitis with permanent paralysis, gangrene requiring amputation of digits and more proximal portions of extremities, and necrosis and sloughing at and surrounding the injection site. Such severe effects have been reported following injections into the buttock, thigh, and deltoid areas. Other serious complications of suspected intravascular administration which have been reported include immediate pallor, mottling or cyanosis of the extremity both distal and proximal to the injection site followed by bleb formation; severe edema requiring anterior and/or posterior compartment fasciotomy in the lower extremity. The above-described severe effects and complications have most often occurred in infants and small children. Prompt consultation with an appropriate specialist is indicated if any evidence of compromise of the blood supply occurs at, proximal to, or distal to the site of injection.[1-9] See "Contraindications," "Precautions," and "Dosage and Administration."

Quadriceps femoris fibrosis and atrophy have been reported following repeated intramuscular injections of penicillin preparations into the anterolateral thigh.

Injection into or near a nerve may result in permanent neurological damage.

Precautions: Penicillin should be used with caution in individuals with histories of significant allergies and/or asthma.

Care should be taken to avoid intravenous or intraarterial administration, or injection into or near major peripheral nerves or blood vessels, since such injections may produce neurovascular damage. See "Contraindications," "Warnings," and "Dosage and Administration."

In streptococcal infections, therapy must be sufficient to eliminate the organism; otherwise the sequelae of streptococcal disease may occur. Cultures should be taken following completion of treatment to determine whether streptococci have been eradicated.

A small percentage of patients are sensitive to procaine. If there is a history of sensitivity make the usual test: Inject intradermally 0.1 ml of a 1 to 2 percent procaine solution. Development of an erythema, wheal, flare, or eruption indicates procaine sensitivity. Sensitivity should be treated by the usual methods, including barbiturates, and procaine penicillin preparations should not be used. Antihistaminics appear beneficial in treatment of procaine reactions.

The use of antibiotics may result in overgrowth of nonsusceptible organisms. Constant observation of the patient is essential. If new infections due to bacteria or fungi appear during therapy, the drug should be discontinued and appropriate measures taken.

Whenever allergic reactions occur, penicillin should be withdrawn unless, in the opinion of the physician, the condition being treated is life-threatening and amenable only to penicillin therapy.

In prolonged therapy with penicillin, and particularly with high-dosage schedules, periodic evaluation of the renal and hematopoietic systems is recommended.

Adverse Reactions: Penicillin is a substance of low toxicity but does possess a significant index of sensitization. The following hypersensitivity reactions associated with use of penicillin have been reported: Skin rashes, ranging from maculopapular eruptions to exfoliative dermatitis; urticaria; serum-sickness-like reactions, including chills, fever, edema, arthralgia, and prostration. Severe and often fatal anaphylaxis has been reported (see "Warnings").

Dosage and Administration: Shake multiple-dose vial vigorously before withdrawing the desired dose.

Administer by DEEP, INTRAMUSCULAR INJECTION in the upper, outer quadrant of the buttock. In infants and small children, the midlateral aspect of the thigh may be preferable. When doses are repeated, vary the injection site.

When using the multiple-dose vial:

After selection of the proper site and insertion of the needle into the selected muscle, aspirate by pulling back on the plunger. While maintaining negative pressure for 2–3 seconds, carefully observe the neck of the syringe immediately proximal to the needle hub for appearance of blood or any discoloration. Blood or "typical blood color" may *not* be seen if a blood vessel has been entered —only a mixture of blood and Bicillin C-R. The appearance of any discoloration is reason to withdraw the needle and discard the syringe. If it is elected to inject at another site, a new syringe and needle should be used. If no blood or discoloration appears, inject the contents of the syringe slowly. Discontinue delivery of the dose if the subject complains of severe immediate pain at the injection site or if in infants and young children symptoms or signs occur suggesting onset of severe pain.

When using the TUBEX cartridge:

The Wyeth Tubex® cartridge for this product incorporates several features that are designed to facilitate the visualization of blood on aspiration if a blood vessel is inadvertently entered.

The design of this cartridge is such that blood which enters its needle will be quickly visualized as a red or dark-colored "spot." This "spot" will appear on the barrel of the glass cartridge immediately proximal to the blue hub. Prior to injection, in order to determine where this "spot" can be seen, the operator should first insert and secure the cartridge in the Tubex syringe in the usual fashion. The needle cover should then be removed and the cartridge and syringe held in one hand with the needle pointing away from the operator. If the 2 ml metal syringe is used the glass cartridge should then be rotated by turning the plunger of the syringe clockwise until the flat bevel at the tip of the needle is pointing upward and is horizontal when viewed directly from above. An imaginary straight line then drawn from the middle of the flat bevel to the back edge of the blue hub where it joins the glass will point to the area on the glass cartridge where the "spot" can be visualized. If the 1 ml metal syringe is used it will not be possible to continue to rotate the glass cartridge clockwise once it is properly engaged and fully threaded; it can, however, then be rotated counterclockwise as far as necessary to properly orient the bevel of the needle and locate the observation area. (In this same area in some cartridges a dark spot may sometimes be visualized prior to injection. This is the proximal end of the needle and does not represent a foreign body in, or other abnormality of, the suspension.)

Thus, before the needle is inserted into the selected muscle, it is important for the operator to orient the flat bevel of the needle so that any blood which might enter after its insertion and during aspiration can be visualized in the area of the cartridge where it will appear and not be obscured by the metal syringe or other obstructions.

After selection of the proper site and insertion of the needle into the selected muscle, aspirate by pulling back on the plunger. While maintaining negative pressure for 2-3 seconds, carefully observe the barrel of the cartridge in the area previously identified (see above) for the appearance of a red or dark-colored "spot."

Blood or "typical blood color" may *not* be seen if a blood vessel has been entered—only a mixture of blood and Bicillin C-R. The appearance of any discoloration is reason to withdraw the needle and discard the glass Tubex cartridge. If it is elected to inject at another site, a new cartridge should be used. If no blood or discoloration appears, inject the contents of the cartridge slowly. Discontinue delivery of the dose if the subject complains of severe immediate pain at the injection site or if, especially in infants and young children, symptoms or signs occur suggesting onset of severe pain.

Some TUBEX cartridges may contain a small air bubble which may be disregarded since it does not affect administration of the product. Because of the high concentration of suspended material in this product, the needle may be blocked if the injection is not made at a slow, steady rate.

When using the disposable syringe:

The Wyeth disposable syringe for this product incorporates several new features that are designed to facilitate its use.

A single small indentation, or "dot," has been punched into the metal ring that surrounds the neck of the syringe near the base of the needle. It is important that this "dot" be placed in a position so that it can be easily visualized by the operator following the intramuscular insertion of the syringe needle.

After selection of the proper site and insertion of the needle into the selected muscle, aspirate by pulling back on the plunger. While maintaining negative pressure for 2-3 seconds, carefully observe the barrel of the syringe immediately proximal to the location of the "dot" for appearance of blood or any discoloration. Blood or "typical blood color" may *not* be seen if a blood vessel has been entered—only a mixture of blood and Bicillin C-R. The appearance of any discoloration is reason to withdraw the needle and discard the syringe. If it is elected to inject at another site, a new syringe should be used. If no blood or discoloration appears, inject the contents of the syringe slowly. Discontinue delivery of the dose if the subject complains of severe immediate pain at the injection site or if in infants and young children symptoms or signs occur suggesting onset of severe pain.

Streptococcal infections Group A—Infections of the upper-respiratory tract, skin and soft-tissue infections, scarlet fever, and erysipelas.

The following doses are recommended:

Adults and children over 60 lbs. in weight: 2,400,000 units. Children from 30–60 lbs.: 900,000 units to 1,200,000 units. Infants and children under 30 lbs.: 600,000 units.

NOTE: Treatment with the recommended dosage is usually given at a single session using multiple IM sites when indicated. An alternative dosage schedule may be used, giving one-half (½) the total dose on day 1 and one-half (½) on day 3. This will also insure the penicillinemia required over a 10-day period; however, this alternate schedule should be used only when the physician can be assured of the patient's cooperation.

Pneumococcal infections (except pneumococcal meningitis): 600,000 units in children and 1,200,000 units in adults, repeated every 2 or 3 days until the temperature is normal for 48 hours.

Other forms of penicillin may be necessary for severe cases.

How Supplied: 300,000 units per ml—multiple-dose vials of 10 ml. 600,000 units per ml—1 ml Tubex® Sterile Cartridge-Needle Units, packages of 10 and 50; 2 ml Tubex Sterile Cartridge-Needle Units (1,200,000 units per Tubex), packages of 10 and 50; 2 ml single-dose (1,200,000 units) disposable syringes, packages of 10; 4 ml single-dose (2,400,000 units) disposable syringes, packages of 10.

References:
1. SHAW, E.: Transverse myelitis from injection of penicillin, Am. J. Dis. Child., 111:548, 1966.
2. KNOWLES, J.: Accidental intra-arterial injection of penicillin. Am. J. Dis. Child., 111:552, 1966.
3. DARBY, C., et al: Ischemia following an intragluteal injection of benzathine-procaine penicillin G mixture in a one-year-old boy. Clin. Pediatrics, 12:485, 1973.
4. BROWN, L. & NELSON, A.: Postinfectious intravascular thrombosis with gangrene. Arch. Surg., 94:652, 1967.
5. BORENSTINE, J.: Transverse myelitis and penicillin (Correspondence). Am. J. Dis. Child., 112:166, 1966.
6. ATKINSON, J.: Transverse myelopathy secondary to penicillin injection. J. Pediatrics, 75:867, 1969.
7. TALBERT, J. et al: Gangrene of the foot following intramuscular injection in the lateral thigh: A case report with recommendations for prevention. J. Pediatrics, 70:110, 1967.
8. FISHER, T.: Medicolegal affairs. Canad. Med. Assoc. J., 112:395, 1975.
9. SCHANZER, H. et al: Accidental intra-arterial injection of penicillin G. JAMA, 242:1289, 1979.

BICILLIN® C-R 900/300 ℞
[bī-sil' in]
(penicillin G benzathine and penicillin G procaine suspension)
INJECTION

FOR DEEP INTRAMUSCULAR INJECTION ONLY

Description: Each TUBEX® cartridge (2 ml size) contains 1,200,000 units of penicillin comprising: 900,000 units penicillin G benzathine and 300,000 units penicillin G procaine in a stabilized aqueous suspension with sodium citrate buffer; and as w/v, approximately 0.5% lecithin, 0.55% carboxymethylcellulose, 0.55% povidone, 0.1% methylparaben, and 0.01% propylparaben.
Bicillin C-R 900/300 suspension in the TUBEX formulation is viscous and opaque. Read "Contraindications," "Warnings," "Precautions," and "Dosage and Administration" sections prior to use.

Actions and Pharmacology: Penicillin G exerts a bactericidal action against penicillin-sensitive microorganisms during the stage of active multiplication. It acts through the inhibition of biosynthesis of cell-wall mucopeptide. It is not active against the penicillinase-producing bacteria, which include many strains of staphylococci. Penicillin G exerts high in vitro activity against staphylococci (except penicillinase-producing strains), streptococci (groups A, C, G, H, L, and M), and pneumococci.
Other organisms sensitive to penicillin G are Neisseria gonorrhoeae, Corynebacterium diphtheriae, Bacillus anthracis, Clostridia, Actinomyces bovis, Streptobacillus moniliformis, Listeria monocytogenes, and Leptospira. Treponema pallidum is extremely sensitive to the bactericidal action of penicillin G.
Sensitivity plate testing: If the Kirby-Bauer method of disc sensitivity is used, a 10-unit penicillin disc should give a zone greater than 28 mm when tested against a penicillin-sensitive bacterial strain.
Intramuscular penicillin G benzathine is absorbed very slowly into the bloodstream from the intramuscular site and converted by hydrolysis to penicillin G. This combination of hydrolysis and slow absorption results in blood serum levels much lower but much more prolonged than other parenteral penicillins.
Penicillin G procaine is an equimolecular compound of procaine and penicillin G, administered intramuscularly as a suspension. It dissolves slowly at the site of injection, giving a plateau type of blood level at about 4 hours which falls slowly over a period of the next 15-20 hours.
Approximately 60% of penicillin G is bound to serum protein. The drug is distributed throughout the body tissues in widely varying amounts. Highest levels are found in the kidneys with lesser amounts in the liver, skin, and intestines. Penicillin G penetrates into all other tissues and the spinal fluid to a lesser degree. With normal kidney function, the drug is excreted rapidly by tubular excretion. In neonates and young infants and in individuals with impaired kidney function, excretion is considerably delayed.

Indications: This drug is indicated for use in children of all ages in the treatment of moderately severe infections due to penicillin-G-susceptible microorganisms that are susceptible to serum levels common to this particular dosage form. Therapy should be guided by bacteriological studies (including susceptibility testing) and by clinical response.
NOTE: When high, sustained serum levels are required, penicillin G sodium or potassium, either IM or IV, should be used. This drug should *not* be used in the treatment of venereal diseases, including syphilis, gonorrhea, yaws, bejel, and pinta.
The following infections will usually respond to adequate dosages of this drug:
Streptococcal infections Group A (without bacteremia). Moderately severe to severe infections of the upper respiratory tract, skin and soft-tissue infections, scarlet fever, and erysipelas.
NOTE: Streptococci in groups A, C, G, H, L, and M are very sensitive to penicillin G. Other groups, including group D (enterococci), are resistant. Penicillin G sodium or potassium is recommended for streptococcal infections with bacteremia.
Pneumococcal infections. Moderately severe pneumonia and otitis media.
NOTE: Severe pneumonia, empyema, bacteremia, pericarditis, meningitis, peritonitis, and arthritis of pneumococcal etiology are better treated with penicillin G sodium or potassium during the acute stage.

Contraindications: A previous hypersensitivity reaction to any penicillin or to procaine is a contraindication.
Do not inject into or near an artery or nerve.

Warnings: Serious and occasionally fatal hypersensitivity (anaphylactoid) reactions have been reported in patients on penicillin therapy. Although anaphylaxis is more frequent following parenteral therapy, it has occurred in patients on oral penicillins. These reactions are more apt to occur in individuals with a history of sensitivity to multiple allergens.
There have been well-documented reports of individuals with a history of penicillin hypersensitivity reactions who have experienced severe hypersensitivity reactions when treated with a cephalosporin. Before therapy with a penicillin, careful inquiry should be made concerning previous hypersensitivity reactions to penicillins, cephalosporins, and other allergens. If an allergic reaction occurs, the drug should be discontinued and the patient treated with the usual agents, e.g., pressor amines, antihistamines, and corticosteroids.
Inadvertent intravascular administration, including inadvertent direct intraarterial injection or injection immediately adjacent to arteries, of Bicillin C-R 900/300 and other penicillin preparations has resulted in severe neurovascular damage, including transverse myelitis with permanent paralysis, gangrene requiring amputation of digits and more proximal portions of extremities, and necrosis and sloughing at and surrounding the injection site. Such severe effects have been reported following injections into the buttock, thigh, and deltoid areas. Other serious complications of suspected intravascular administration which have been reported include immediate pallor, mottling or cyanosis of the extremity both distal and proximal to the injection site followed by bleb formation; severe edema requiring anterior and/or posterior compartment fasciotomy in the lower extremity. The above-described severe effects and complications have most often occurred in infants and small children. Prompt consultation with an appropriate specialist is indicated if any evidence of compromise of the blood supply occurs at, proximal to, or distal to the site of injection.[1-9] See "Contraindications," "Precautions," and "Dosage and Administration."
Quadriceps, femoris fibrosis and atrophy have been reported following repeated intramuscular injections of penicillin preparations into the anterolateral thigh.
Injection into or near a nerve may result in permanent neurological damage.

Precautions: Penicillin should be used with caution in individuals with histories of significant allergies and/or asthma.
Care should be taken to avoid intravenous or intraarterial administration, or injection into or near major peripheral nerves or blood vessels, since such injections may produce neurovascular damage. See "Contraindications," "Warnings," and "Dosage and Administration."
In streptococcal infections, therapy must be sufficient to eliminate the organism; otherwise the sequelae of streptococcal disease may occur. Cultures should be taken following completion of treatment to determine whether streptococci have been eradicated.
A small percentage of patients are sensitive to procaine. If there is a history of sensitivity make the usual test: Inject intradermally 0.1 ml of a 1 to 2 percent procaine solution. Development of an erythema, wheal, flare, or eruption indicates procaine sensitivity. Sensitivity should be treated by the usual methods, including barbiturates, and procaine penicillin preparations should not be used. Antihistaminics appear beneficial in treatment of procaine reactions.
The use of antibiotics may result in overgrowth of nonsusceptible organisms. Constant observation of the patient is essential. If new infections due to bacteria or fungi appear during therapy, the drug should be discontinued and appropriate measures taken.
Whenever allergic reactions occur, penicillin should be withdrawn unless, in the opinion of the physician, the condition being treated is life-threatening and amenable only to penicillin therapy.
In prolonged therapy with penicillin, and particularly with high-dosage schedules, periodic evaluation of the renal and hematopoietic systems is recommended.

Adverse Reactions: Penicillin is a substance of low toxicity but does possess a significant index of sensitization. The following hypersensitivity reactions associated with use of penicillin have been reported: skin rashes, ranging from maculopapular eruptions to exfoliative dermatitis; urticaria; serum-sicknesslike reactions, including chills, fever, edema, arthralgia, and prostration. Severe and often fatal anaphylaxis has been reported (see "Warnings").

Dosage and Administration: Administer by DEEP, INTRAMUSCULAR INJECTION in the upper, outer quadrant of the buttock. In infants and small children, the midlateral aspect of the thigh may be preferable. When doses are repeated, vary the injection site.
The Wyeth Tubex® cartridge for this product incorporates several features that are designed to facilitate the visualization of blood on aspiration if a blood vessel is inadvertently entered.
The design of this cartridge is such that blood which enters its needle will be quickly visualized as a red or dark-colored "spot." This "spot" will appear on the barrel of the glass cartridge immediately proximal to the blue hub. Prior to injection, in order to determine where this "spot" can be seen, the operator should first insert and secure the cartridge in the Tubex syringe in the usual

Continued on next page

Wyeth—Cont.

fashion. The needle cover should then be removed and the cartridge and syringe held in one hand with the needle pointing away from the operator. If the 2 ml metal syringe is used the glass cartridge should then be rotated by turning the plunger of the syringe clockwise until the flat bevel at the tip of the needle is pointing upward and is horizontal when viewed directly from above. An imaginary straight line then drawn from the middle of the flat bevel to the back edge of the blue hub where it joins the glass will point to the area on the glass cartridge where the "spot" can be visualized. If the 1 ml metal syringe is used it will not be possible to continue to rotate the glass cartridge clockwise once it is properly engaged and fully threaded; it can, however, then be rotated counterclockwise as far as necessary to properly orient the bevel of the needle and locate the observation area. (In this same area in some cartridges a dark spot may sometimes be visualized prior to injection. This is the proximal end of the needle and does not represent a foreign body in, or other abnormality of, the suspension.)

Thus, before the needle is inserted into the selected muscle, it is important for the operator to orient the flat bevel of the needle so that any blood which might enter after its insertion and during aspiration can be visualized in the area of the cartridge where it will appear and not be obscured by the metal syringe or other obstructions.

After selection of the proper site and insertion of the needle into the selected muscle, aspirate by pulling back on the plunger. While maintaining negative pressure for 2–3 seconds, carefully observe the barrel of the cartridge in the area previously identified (see above) for the appearance of a red or dark-colored "spot."

Blood or "typical blood color" may *not* be seen if a blood vessel has been entered—only a mixture of blood and Bicillin C-R 900/300. The appearance of *any* discoloration is reason to withdraw the needle and discard the glass Tubex cartridge. If it is elected to inject at another site, a new cartridge should be used. If no blood or discoloration appears, inject the contents of the cartridge slowly. Discontinue delivery of the dose if the subject complains of severe immediate pain at the injection site or if, especially in infants and young children, symptoms or signs occur suggesting onset of severe pain.

Some TUBEX cartridges may contain a small air bubble which may be disregarded since it does not affect administration of the product. Because of the high concentration of suspended material in this product, the needle may be blocked if the injection is not made at a slow, steady rate.

Streptococcal infections Group A—Infections of the upper respiratory tract, skin and soft-tissue infections, scarlet fever, and erysipelas.
A single injection of Bicillin C-R 900/300 is usually sufficient for the treatment of Group A streptococcal infections in children of all ages.

Pneumococcal infections (except pneumococcal meningitis): One TUBEX Bicillin C-R 900/300 repeated at 2- or 3-day intervals until the temperature is normal for 48 hours. Other forms of penicillin may be necessary for severe cases.

How Supplied: Bicillin® C-R 900/300 is supplied in 2 ml TUBEX® (Sterile Cartridge-Needle Unit) in packages of 10.

References:
1. SHAW, E.: Transverse myelitis from injection of penicillin. *Am. J. Dis. Child.*, 111:548, 1966.
2. KNOWLES, J.: Accidental intra-arterial injection of penicillin. *Am. J. Dis. Child.*, 111:552, 1966.
3. DARBY, C., et al: Ischemia following an intragluteal injection of benzathine-procaine penicillin G mixture in a one-year-old boy. *Clin. Pediatrics,* 12:485, 1973.
4. BROWN, L. & NELSON, A.: Postinfectious intravascular thrombosis with gangrene. *Arch. Surg.,* 94:652, 1967.
5. BORENSTINE, J.: Transverse myelitis and penicillin (Correspondence). *Am. J. Dis. Child.,* 112:166, 1966.
6. ATKINSON, J.: Transverse myelopathy secondary to penicillin injection. *J. Pediatrics,* 75:867, 1969.
7. TALBERT, J. et al: Gangrene of the foot following intramuscular injection in the lateral thigh: A case report with recommendations for prevention. *J. Pediatrics,* 70:110, 1967.
8. FISHER, T.: Medicolegal affairs. *Canad. Med. Assoc. J.,* 112:395, 1975.
9. SCHANZER, H. et al: Accidental intra-arterial injection of penicillin G. *JAMA,* 242:1289, 1979.

BICILLIN® L-A
[bī-sil'in L-A] ℞
(sterile penicillin G benzathine suspension)
INJECTION
FOR DEEP INTRAMUSCULAR INJECTION ONLY

Description: Each Tubex® Sterile Cartridge-Needle Unit or disposable syringe contains penicillin G benzathine in aqueous suspension with sodium citrate buffer; and as w/v, approximately 0.5% lecithin, 0.6% carboxymethylcellulose, 0.6% povidone, 0.1% methylparaben, and 0.01% propylparaben.

Each multiple-dose vial contains in each milliliter 300,000 units penicillin G benzathine with sodium citrate buffer and approx. 6 mg lecithin, 3 mg povidone, 1 mg carboxymethylcellulose, 0.5 mg sorbitan monopalmitate, 0.5 mg polyoxyethylene sorbitan monopalmitate, 1.2 mg methylparaben, and 0.14 mg propylparaben.

Bicillin L-A suspension in the multiple-dose vial, TUBEX, and disposable syringe formulations is viscous and opaque. Read "Contraindications," "Warnings," "Precautions," and "Dosage and Administration" sections prior to use.

Actions and Pharmacology: Penicillin G exerts a bactericidal action against penicillin-sensitive microorganisms during the stage of active multiplication. It acts through the inhibition of biosynthesis of cell-wall mucopeptide. It is not active against the penicillinase-producing bacteria, which include many strains of staphylococci. Penicillin G exerts high *in vitro* activity against staphylococci (except penicillinase-producing strains), streptococci (Groups A, C, G, H, L, and M), and pneumococci. Other organisms sensitive to penicillin G are: *Neisseria gonorrhoeae, Corynebacterium diphtheriae, Bacillus anthracis,* Clostridia, *Actinomyces bovis, Streptobacillus moniliformis,* Listeria monocytogenes, and Leptospira. *Treponema pallidum* is extremely sensitive to the bactericidal action of penicillin G.

Intramuscular penicillin G benzathine is absorbed very slowly into the bloodstream from the intramuscular site and converted by hydrolysis to penicillin G. This combination of hydrolysis and slow absorption results in blood serum levels much lower but much more prolonged than other parenteral penicillins.

Approximately 60% of penicillin G is bound to serum protein. The drug is distributed throughout the body tissues in widely varying amounts. Highest levels are found in the kidneys with lesser amounts in the liver, skin, and intestines. Penicillin G penetrates into all other tissues and the spinal fluid to a lesser degree. With normal kidney function the drug is excreted rapidly by tubular excretion. In neonates and young infants and in individuals with impaired kidney function, excretion is considerably delayed.

Indications: Intramuscular penicillin G benzathine is indicated in the treatment of infections due to penicillin-G-sensitive microorganisms that are susceptible to the low and very prolonged serum levels common to this particular dosage form. Therapy should be guided by bacteriological studies (including sensitivity tests) and by clinical response.

The following infections will usually respond to adequate dosage of intramuscular penicillin G benzathine:

Streptococcal infections (Group A—without bacteremia). Mild-to-moderate infections of the upper respiratory tract (e.g., pharyngitis).

Venereal infections—Syphilis, yaws, bejel, and pinta.

Medical Conditions in Which Penicillin G Benzathine Therapy Is Indicated as Prophylaxis: Rheumatic fever and/or chorea—Prophylaxis with penicillin G benzathine has proven effective in preventing recurrence of these conditions. It has also been used as follow-up prophylactic therapy for rheumatic heart disease and acute glomerulonephritis.

Contraindications: A history of a previous hypersensitivity reaction to any of the penicillins is a contraindication.

Do not inject into or near an artery or nerve.

Warnings: Serious and occasionally fatal hypersensitivity (anaphylactoid) reactions have been reported in patients on penicillin therapy. Although anaphylaxis is more frequent following parenteral therapy, it has occurred in patients on oral penicillins. These reactions are more apt to occur in individuals with a history of sensitivity to multiple allergens.

There have been well-documented reports of individuals with a history of penicillin hypersensitivity reactions who have experienced severe hypersensitivity reactions when treated with a cephalosporin. Before therapy with a penicillin, careful inquiry should be made concerning previous hypersensitivity reactions to penicillins, cephalosporins, and other allergens. If an allergic reaction occurs, the drug should be discontinued and the patient treated with the usual agents, e.g., pressor amines, antihistamines, and corticosteroids.

Inadvertent intravascular administration, including inadvertent direct intraarterial injection or injection immediately adjacent to arteries, of Bicillin L-A and other penicillin preparations has resulted in severe neurovascular damage, including transverse myelitis with permanent paralysis, gangrene requiring amputation of digits and more proximal portions of extremities, and necrosis and sloughing at and surrounding the injection site. Such severe effects have been reported following injections into the buttock, thigh, and deltoid areas. Other serious complications of suspected intravascular administration which have been reported include immediate pallor, mottling or cyanosis of the extremity both distal and proximal to the injection site followed by bleb formation; severe edema requiring anterior and/or posterior compartment fasciotomy in the lower extremity. The above-described severe effects and complications have most often occurred in infants and small children. Prompt consultation with an appropriate specialist is indicated if any evidence of compromise of the blood supply occurs at, proximal to, or distal to the site of injection.[1-9] See "Contraindications," "Precautions," and "Dosage and Administration" Sections.

Quadriceps femoris fibrosis and atrophy have been reported following repeated intramuscular injections of penicillin preparations into the anterolateral thigh.

Injection into or near a nerve may result in permanent neurological damage.

Precautions: Penicillin should be used with caution in individuals with histories of significant allergies and/or asthma.

Care should be taken to avoid intravenous or intra-arterial administration, or injection into or near major peripheral nerves or blood vessels, since such injection may produce neurovascular damage. See "Contraindications," "Warnings," and "Dosage and Administration" Sections.

In streptococcal infections therapy must be sufficient to eliminate the organism; otherwise, the sequelae of streptococcal disease may occur. Cultures should be taken following completion of treatment to determine whether streptococci have been eradicated.

Prolonged use of antibiotics may promote the overgrowth of nonsusceptible organisms, including fungi. Should superinfection occur, appropriate measures should be taken.

Adverse Reactions: The hypersensitivity reactions reported are skin eruptions (maculopapular to exfoliative dermatitis), urticaria and other serum-sicknesslike reactions, laryngeal edema, and anaphylaxis. Fever and eosinophilia may frequently be the only reaction observed. Hemolytic anemia, leukopenia, thrombocytopenia, neuropathy, and nephropathy are infrequent reactions and usually associated with high doses of parenteral penicillin. As with other treatments for syphilis, the Jarisch-Herxheimer reaction has been reported.

Dosage and Administration: Shake multiple-dose vial vigorously before withdrawing the desired dose.

Administer by DEEP INTRAMUSCULAR INJECTION in the upper, outer quadrant of the buttock. In infants and small children, the midlateral aspect of the thigh may be preferable. When doses are repeated, vary the injection site.

When using the multiple-dose vial:
After selection of the proper site and insertion of the needle into the selected muscle, aspirate by pulling back on the plunger. While maintaining negative pressure for 2-3 seconds, carefully observe the neck of the syringe immediately proximal to the needle hub for appearance of blood or any discoloration. Blood or "typical blood color" may *not* be seen if a blood vessel has been entered—only a mixture of blood and Bicillin L-A. The appearance of any discoloration is reason to withdraw the needle and discard the syringe. If it is elected to inject at another site, a new syringe and needle should be used. If no blood or discoloration appears, inject the contents of the syringe slowly. Discontinue delivery of the dose if the subject complains of severe immediate pain at the injection site or if in infants and young children symptoms or signs occur suggesting onset of severe pain.

When using the TUBEX cartridge:
The Wyeth Tubex® cartridge for this product incorporates several features that are designed to facilitate the visualization of blood on aspiration if a blood vessel is inadvertently entered.

The design of this cartridge is such that blood which enters its needle will be quickly visualized as a red or dark-colored "spot." This "spot" will appear on the barrel of the glass cartridge immediately proximal to the blue hub. Prior to injection, in order to determine where this "spot" can be seen, the operator should first insert and secure the cartridge in the Tubex syringe in the usual fashion. The needle cover should then be removed and the cartridge and syringe held in one hand with the needle pointing away from the operator. If the 2 ml metal syringe is used the glass cartridge should then be rotated by turning the plunger of the syringe clockwise until the flat bevel at the tip of the needle is pointing upward and is horizontal when viewed directly from above. An imaginary straight line, then drawn from the middle of the flat bevel to the back edge of the blue hub where it joins the glass, will point to the area on the glass cartridge where the "spot" can be visualized. If the 1 ml metal syringe is used it will not be possible to continue to rotate the glass cartridge clockwise once it is properly engaged and fully threaded; it can, however, then be rotated counterclockwise as far as necessary to properly orient the bevel of the needle and locate the observation area. (In this same area in some cartridges a dark spot may sometimes be visualized prior to injection. This is the proximal end of the needle and does not represent a foreign body in, or other abnormality of, the suspension.)

Thus, before the needle is inserted into the selected muscle, it is important for the operator to orient the flat bevel of the needle so that any blood which might enter after its insertion and during aspiration can be visualized in the area of the cartridge where it will appear and not be obscured by the metal syringe or other obstructions.

After selection of the proper site and insertion of the needle into the selected muscle, aspirate by pulling back on the plunger. While maintaining negative pressure for 2-3 seconds, carefully observe the barrel of the cartridge in the area previously identified (see above) for the appearance of a red or dark-colored "spot."

Blood or "typical blood color" may *not* be seen if a blood vessel has been entered—only a mixture of blood and Bicillin L-A. The appearance of *any* discoloration is reason to withdraw the needle and discard the glass Tubex cartridge. If it is elected to inject at another site, a new cartridge should be used. If no blood or discoloration appears, inject the contents of the cartridge slowly. Discontinue delivery of the dose if the subject complains of severe immediate pain at the injection site or if, especially in infants and young children, symptoms or signs occur suggesting onset of severe pain.

Some TUBEX cartridges may contain a small air bubble which may be disregarded since it does not affect administration of the product. Because of the high concentration of suspended material in this product, the needle may be blocked if the injection is not made at a slow, steady rate.

When using the disposable syringe:
The Wyeth disposable syringe for this product incorporates several new features that are designed to facilitate its use.

A single small indentation, or "dot", has been punched into the metal ring that surrounds the neck of the syringe near the base of the needle. It is important that this "dot" be placed in a position so that it can be easily visualized by the operator following the intramuscular insertion of the syringe needle.

After selection of the proper site and insertion of the needle into the selected muscle, aspirate by pulling back on the plunger. While maintaining negative pressure for 2-3 seconds, carefully observe the barrel of the syringe immediately proximal to the location of the "dot" for appearance of blood or any discoloration. Blood or "typical blood color" may *not* be seen if a blood vessel has been entered—only a mixture of blood and Bicillin L-A. The appearance of any discoloration is reason to withdraw the needle and discard the syringe. If it is elected to inject at another site, a new syringe should be used. If no blood or discoloration appears, inject the contents of the syringe slowly. Discontinue delivery of the dose if the subject complains of severe immediate pain at the injection site or if in infants and young children symptoms or signs occur suggesting onset of severe pain.

Some disposable syringes may contain a small air bubble which may be disregarded since it does not affect administration of the product. Because of the high concentration of suspended material in this product, the needle may be blocked if the injection is not made at a slow, steady rate.

Streptococcal (Group A) upper respiratory infections (for example, pharyngitis).

A single injection of 1,200,000 units for adults.

A single injection of 900,000 units for older children.

A single injection of 300,000 to 600,000 units for infants and for children under 60 pounds.

Venereal infections—
Syphilis—Primary, secondary, and latent—2.4 million units (1 dose). Late (tertiary and neurosyphilis)—2.4 million units at 7-day intervals for three doses.

Congenital—under 2 years of age: 50,000 units/kg/body weight; ages 2–12 years: adjust dosage based on adult dosage schedule.

Yaws, Bejel, and Pinta—1.2 million units (1 injection).

Prophylaxis—for rheumatic fever and glomerulonephritis.

Following an acute attack, penicillin G benzathine (parenteral) may be given in doses of 1,200,000 units once a month or 600,000 units every 2 weeks.

How Supplied: BICILLIN® L-A (sterile penicillin G benzathine suspension) Injection: *300,000 units per ml*—vials of 10 ml; *600,000 units per 1 ml* TUBEX® sterile cartridge-needle unit, packages of 10; *900,000 units per* TUBEX—1.5 ml fill in 2 ml size, packages of 10; *1,200,000 units per 2 ml* disposable syringe or TUBEX, packages of 10; *2,400,000 units per 4 ml* disposable syringe, packages of 10.

References:
1. SHAW, E.: Transverse myelitis from injection of penicillin. *Am. J. Dis. Child.*, 111:548, 1966.
2. KNOWLES, J.: Accidental intra-arterial injection of penicillin. *Am. J. Dis. Child.*, 111:552, 1966.
3. DARBY, C., et al: Ischemia following an intragluteal injection of benzathine-procaine penicillin G mixture in a one-year-old boy. *Clin. Pediatrics*, 12:485, 1973.
4. BROWN, L. & NELSON, A.: Postinfectious intravascular thrombosis with gangrene. *Arch. Surg.*, 94:652, 1967.
5. BORENSTINE, J.: Transverse myelitis and penicillin (Correspondence). *Am. J. Dis. Child.*, 112:166, 1966.
6. ATKINSON, J.: Transverse myelopathy secondary to penicillin injection. *J. Pediatrics*, 75:867, 1969.
7. TALBERT, J. et al: Gangrene of the foot following intramuscular injection in the lateral thigh: A case report with recommendations for prevention. *J. Pediatrics*, 70:110, 1967.
8. FISHER, T.: Medicolegal affairs. *Canad. Med. Assoc. J.*, 112:395, 1975.
9. SCHANZER, H. et al: Accidental intra-arterial injection of penicillin G. *JAMA*, 242:1289, 1979.

BIOLOGICALS

For prescribing information on products listed—and for which full prescribing information is not provided—write to Professional Service, Wyeth Laboratories, Box 8299, Philadelphia, PA, 19101, or contact your local Wyeth representative.

ANTIVENIN (CROTALIDAE) ℞
[an"te ven'in]
POLYVALENT
(equine origin)

Important: Pit viper bites may cause severe tissue damage or fatal envenomation, or both. The physician responsible for treatment of an envenomated patient should be familiar with the contents of this brochure and the pertinent medical literature concerning current concepts of first-aid and general supportive therapy as presented in the references listed at the end of this pamphlet.

Composition: Antivenin (Crotalidae) Polyvalent, Wyeth, is a refined and concentrated preparation of serum globulins obtained by fractionating blood from healthy horses immunized with the following venoms: *Crotalus adamanteus* (eastern diamond rattlesnake), *C. atrox* (western diamond rattlesnake), *C. durissus terrificus* (tropical rattlesnake, Cascabel), and Bothrops atrox ("Fer-de-lance"). Phenol, 0.25%, and thimerosal, 0.005%, are added as preservatives. The product is standardized by its ability to neutralize the lethal action of standard venoms by intravenous injection in mice.[1] Dried from the frozen state, the lyophilized serum has a moisture content of less than 1% and is soluble on addition of the diluent contained in each package (Bacteriostatic Water for Injection, USP, with preservative: 0.001% phenylmercuric nitrate).

Antivenin (Crotalidae) Polyvalent, Wyeth (hereinafter referred to as Antivenin) contains protective substances capable of neutralizing the toxic effects of venoms of crotalids (pit vipers) native to North, Central, and South America, including rattlesnakes *(Crotalus, Sistrurus);* copperhead and cottonmouth moccasins *(Agkistrodon),* including *A. halys* of Korea and Japan; the Fer-de-lance and other species of *Bothrops;* the tropical rattler *(Crotalus durissus* and similar species); the Cantil *(A. bilineatus);* and bushmaster *(Lachesis mutus)* of South and Central America.

Indication: Antivenin is indicated only for the treatment of envenomation caused by bites of those crotalids (pit vipers) specified in the immediately preceding paragraph.

Pit Viper Bites and Envenomation: The symptoms, signs, and severity of snake-venom poisoning resulting from pit viper bites depend on many factors, including, but not limited to, the following

Continued on next page

Wyeth—Cont.

variables: species, age, and size of the biting snake; the number and location of bite(s); the depth of venom deposit by the snake's fangs; the condition of the snake's fangs and venom glands; the length of time the snake "hangs on"; the age, general health, and size of the victim; the type and efficacy of any first-aid treatment rendered in an attempt to remove venom and how soon such treatment was applied. In any venomous snake bite, the actual amount of venom introduced into the victim is always an unknown. Even the type of clothing or leg-footwear through which the snake's fangs pass may affect the amount of venom delivered by the bite. Although most North American pit vipers tend to bite and introduce venom superficially, their fangs may get hung-up in the subcutaneous tissues during the biting act and can penetrate deeper tissues during the attempt to release the bitten part. In some bites the fangs may penetrate into muscle. In such cases, the usual local superficial manifestations of envenomation may not appear early in the course of poisoning. In bites by some species, systemic evidence of envenomation may be present in the absence of significant local manifestations. It may be difficult to determine the severity of envenomation during the first several hours after a pit viper bite and estimates of severity may need to be revised as poisoning progresses. It must be remembered, too, that not all pit viper bites result in envenomation. In approximately 20% of rattlesnake bites, the snake may not inject any venom. The local and systemic symptoms and signs of envenomation include the following:

LOCAL:
Fang puncture(s).
Swelling—edema is usually seen around the site of bite within five minutes. It may progress rapidly and involve the entire extremity within an hour. More than 95% of all snakebites are inflicted on extremities.[2] Generally, however, edema spreads more slowly, usually over a period of 8 or more hours. Swelling is usually most severe following envenomation by the eastern diamondback; less severe after bites by the western diamondback, prairie, timber, red, Pacific, Mojave, and black-tailed rattlers, the sidewinder and cottonmouth moccasins; least severe after bites by copperheads, massasaugas, and pygmy rattlers.
Ecchymosis and discoloration of the skin —often appear in the area of the bite within a few hours. Vesicles may form within a few hours and are usually present at 24 hours. Hemorrhagic blebs and petechiae are common. Necrosis may develop, necessitating amputation of an extremity or a portion thereof.
Pain—frequently a complaint of the victim beginning shortly after the bite by most pit vipers. Pain may be absent after bites by Mojave rattlers.

SYSTEMIC:
Weakness; faintness; nausea; sweating; numbness or tingling around the mouth, tongue, scalp, fingers, toes, site of bite; muscle fasciculations; hypotension; prolongation of bleeding and clotting times; hemoconcentration, early followed by a decrease in erythrocytes; thrombocytopenia; hematuria; proteinuria; vomiting, including hematemesis; melena; hemoptysis; epistaxis. In fatal poisoning, a frequent cause of death is associated with destruction of erythrocytes and changes in capillary permeability, especially of the pulmonary vascular system, leading to pulmonary edema; hemoconcentration usually occurs early, probably as a result of plasma loss secondary to vascular permeability; the hemoglobin may fall, and bleeding may occur throughout the body as early as 6 hours after the bite. Renal involvement is not uncommon. Mojave rattler venom may cause neuromuscular changes leading to respiratory failure.
An estimate of the severity of envenomation should be made as soon as possible and before any Antivenin is administered. The amount (volume) of the first dose of Antivenin is determined on this estimate of severity. Every symptom, sign, laboratory-test result, and any other pertinent information should be considered in estimating severity— local manifestations; systemic manifestations, including abnormal laboratory findings; species and size of the biting snake, if known; number and location of bites(s); size and health of the patient; type of first-aid treatment rendered; and interval between bite and arrival for treatment. Russell et al,[3] and Wingert and Wainschel[4] grade severity as follows:
No envenomation—no local or systemic manifestations.
Minimal envenomation—local swelling and other local changes; no systemic manifestations; normal laboratory findings.
Moderate envenomation—swelling progressing beyond the site of bite and one or more systemic manifestations; abnormal laboratory findings, for example, a fall in hematocrit or platelets.
Severe envenomation—marked local response, severe systemic manifestations and significant alteration in laboratory findings.
Parrish and Hayes,[5] McCollough and Gennaro,[6] and Watt and Gennaro[7] have used a Grade 0 (no envenomation) through Grade IV (very severe) classification of severity which was developed for the most part in treatment of envenomation by the eastern diamondback and timber rattlers. This classification is more dependent on local manifestations, or the absence thereof, as the venoms of these species seem to be more consistent in inducing local tissue damage.
Any suspected envenomation should be treated as a medical emergency, and until careful observation provides clear evidence that envenomation has not occurred or is minimal, the following procedures are recommended:
Monitor vital signs at frequent intervals: Blood pressure, pulse, respiration.
Draw sufficient blood as soon as possible for baseline laboratory studies, including type and cross-match, CBC, hematocrit, platelet count, prothrombin time, clot retraction, bleeding and coagulation times, BUN, electrolytes, bilirubin. Some of these studies may need to be repeated at daily intervals, or less, depending on the severity of envenomation and the response to treatment. During the first 4 or 5 days of severe envenomations, hemoglobin, hematocrit, and platelet counts should be carried out several times a day.
Obtain urine samples at frequent intervals for analysis, with special attention to microscopic examination for presence of erythrocytes.
Chart fluid intake and urine output.
Measure and record the circumference of the bitten extremity just proximal to the bite and at one or more additional points each several inches closer to the trunk. Repeat measurements every 15-30 minutes to obtain information about progression of edema.
Have available and ready for immediate use:
Oxygen, resuscitation equipment including airway, tourniquet, epinephrine, injectable antihistaminic agents, and corticosteroids.
Start an intravenous infusion in one or two extremities: one line to be used for supportive therapy, if needed, such as whole blood, plasma, packed red cells, specific clotting factors, platelet transfusion, plasma expanders; the other line to be used for administration of Antivenin and electrolytes.
Carry out and interpret a skin test for horse-serum sensitivity. (See Precautions section below.)
Dosage and Administration: Before administration, read Precautions and Systemic Reactions sections below. Since the possibility of a severe immediate reaction (anaphylaxis) exists whenever a horse-serum-containing product is administered, appropriate therapeutic agents, including a tourniquet, airway, oxygen, epinephrine, an injectable pressor amine, and corticosteroid, must be available and ready for immediate use. Constant attendance and observation of the patient for untoward reactions are mandatory when Antivenin is administered. Should any systemic reaction occur, administration should be discontinued immediately and appropriate treatment initiated.

The intravenous route of administration is preferred, and probably should always be used for moderate or severe envenomation. Intravenous administration is mandatory if venom-induced shock is present. To be most effective, Antivenin should be administered within 4 hours of the bite; it is less effective when given after 8 hours and may be of questionable value after 12 hours. However, it is recommended that Antivenin therapy be given in severe poisonings, even if 24 hours have elapsed since the time of the bite. It should be kept in mind that maximum blood levels of Antivenin may not be obtained for 8 or more hours after intramuscular administration.
For intravenous-drip use, prepare a 1:1 to 1:10 dilution of reconstituted Antivenin in Sodium Chloride Injection, USP, or 5% Dextrose Injection, USP. To avoid foaming, mix by gently swirling rather than shaking. Allow the initial 5 to 10 ml to infuse over a 3- to 5-minute period, with careful observation of the patient for evidence of untoward reaction. If no symptoms or signs of an immediate systemic reaction appear, continue the infusion with delivery at the maximum safe rate for intravenous fluid administration. The dilution of Antivenin to be used, the type of electrolyte solution used for dilution, and the rate of intravenous delivery of the diluted Antivenin must take into consideration the age, weight, and cardiac status of the patient; the severity of envenomation; the total amount and type of parenteral fluids it is anticipated will be given or are needed; and the interval between bite and initiation of specific therapy.
It is important to give as soon as possible the entire initial dose of Antivenin as based on the best estimate of the severity of envenomation at the time treatment is begun. The following initial doses are recommended:[3,4,8]
no envenomation—none
minimal envenomation—20-40 ml (contents of 2-4 vials)
moderate envenomation—50-90 ml (contents of 5-9 vials)
severe envenomation—100-150 ml or more (contents of 10-15 or more vials)
These recommended initial-dosage volumes are in general accord with those of others.[5-7,9]
The need for additional Antivenin must be based on the clinical response to the initial dose and continuing assessment of the severity of poisoning. If swelling continues to progress or if systemic symptoms or signs of envenomation increase in severity or if new manifestations appear, for example, fall in hematocrit or hypotension, administer an additional 10-50 ml (contents of 1-5 vials) intravenously.
Envenomation by large snakes in children or small adults requires larger doses of Antivenin. The amount administered to a child is not based on weight.
If Antivenin is given intramuscularly, it should be given into a large muscle mass, preferably the gluteal area, with care to avoid nerve trunks. Antivenin should never be injected into a finger or toe. The effectiveness of corticosteroids in treatment of envenomation per se or venom shock is not resolved. Russell[3] and others[9,10] believe corticosteroids may mask the seriousness of hypovolemia in moderate or severe poisoning and have little, if any, effect on the local-tissue response to rattler venoms. Corticosteroids should not be given simultaneously with Antivenin on a routine basis or during the acute stage of envenomation; however, their use may be necessary to treat immediate allergic reactions to Antivenin, and corticosteroids are the agents of choice for treating serious delayed reactions to Antivenin.
Snakes' mouths do not harbor *Clostridium tetani*. However, appropriate tetanus prophylaxis is indicated, since tetanus spores may be carried into the fang puncture wounds by dirt present on skin at time of bite or by nonsterile first-aid procedures. A broad-spectrum antibiotic in adequate dosage is indicated if local tissue damage is evident.
Shock following envenomation is treated like shock resulting from hypovolemia from any cause,

including administration of whole blood, plasma, albumin, or other plasma expanders, as indicated. Aspirin or codeine is usually adequate for relieving pain. Sedation with phenobarbital or mild tranquilizers may be used if indicated, but not in the presence of respiratory failure.

The bitten extremity should not be packed in ice, and so-called "cryotherapy" is contraindicated. Compartment syndromes may complicate pit viper envenomations, especially those caused by bites on the lower extremities. Prompt surgical consultation is indicated whenever a closed-compartment syndrome is suspected.[3,12]

Defibrination and disseminated intravascular coagulation (DIC) syndromes have been associated with envenomation caused by some pit vipers native to the United States, and appropriate therapy may be indicated.[3,9,10,13-17]

Technic for Reconstituting the Dried Antivenin: Pry off the small metal disc in the cap over the diaphragms of the vials of Antivenin and diluent. Swab the exposed surface of the rubber diaphragms of both vials with an appropriate germicide. With a sterile 10 ml syringe and needle, withdraw the diluent (Bacteriostatic Water for Injection, USP, containing phenylmercuric nitrate 1:100,000) from the vial of diluent and inject it into the vial of antivenin. Gentle agitation will hasten complete dissolution of the lyophilized Antivenin.

Precautions: Before administration of any product prepared from horse serum, appropriate measures must be taken in an effort to detect the presence of dangerous sensitivity: (1) A careful review of the patient's history, including any report of (a) asthma, hay fever, urticaria, or other allergic manifestations; (b) allergic reactions upon exposure to horses; and (c) prior injections of horse serum. (2) A suitable test for detection of sensitivity. A skin test should be performed in every patient prior to administration, regardless of clinical history.

Skin test—Inject intracutaneously 0.02 to 0.03 ml of a 1:10 dilution of Normal Horse Serum or Antivenin. A control test on the opposite extremity, using Sodium Chloride Injection, USP, facilitates interpretation. Use of larger amounts for the skin-test dose increases the likelihood of false-positive reactions, and in the exquisitely sensitive patient, increases the risk of a systemic reaction from the skin-test dose. A 1:100 or greater dilution should be used for preliminary skin testing if the history suggests sensitivity. A positive reaction to a skin test occurs within five to thirty minutes and is manifested by a wheal with or without pseudopodia and surrounding erythema. In general, the shorter the interval between injection and the beginning of the skin reaction, the greater the sensitivity.

If the history is negative for allergy and the result of a skin test is negative, proceed with administration of Antivenin as outlined above. If the history is positive and a skin test is strongly positive, administration may be dangerous, especially if the positive sensitivity test is accompanied by systemic allergic manifestations. In such instances, the risk of administering Antivenin must be weighed against the risk of withholding it, keeping in mind that severe envenomation can be fatal. (See last paragraph of this section.)

A negative allergic history and absence of reaction to a properly applied skin test do not rule out the possibility of an immediate reaction. Also, a negative skin test has no bearing on whether or not delayed serum reactions (serum sickness) will occur after administration of the full dose.

If the history is negative, and the skin test is mildly or questionably positive, administer as follows to reduce the risk of a severe immediate systemic reaction: (a) Prepare, in separate sterile vials or syringes, 1:100 and 1:10 dilutions of Antivenin. (b) Allow at least 15 minutes between injections and proceed with the next dose if no reaction follows the previous dose. (c) Inject subcutaneously, using a tuberculin-type syringe, 0.1, 0.2, and 0.5 ml of the 1:100 dilution at 15-minute intervals; repeat with the 1:10 dilution, and finally undiluted Antivenin. (d) If a systemic reaction occurs after any injection, place a tourniquet proximal to the site of injections and administer an appropriate dose of epinephrine, 1:1000, proximal to the tourniquet or into another extremity. Wait at least 30 minutes before injecting another dose. The amount of the next dose should be the same as the last that did not evoke a reaction. (e) If no reaction occurs after 0.5 ml of undiluted Antivenin has been administered, switch to the intramuscular route and continue doubling the dose at 15-minute intervals until the entire dose has been injected intramuscularly or proceed to the intravenous route as described above under Dosage and Administration.

Obviously, if the just-described schedule is used, 3 to 5 or more hours would be required to administer the initial dose suggested for a moderate or severe envenomation, and time is an important factor in neutralization of venom in a critically ill patient. Wingert and Wainschel[4] have described a procedure based on the experience of their group which they have used in some severely envenomated patients who have positive sensitivity tests: 50 to 100 mg of diphenhydramine hydrochloride is given intravenously, followed by slow intravenous infusion of diluted Antivenin for 15 to 20 minutes while carefully observing the patient for symptoms and signs of anaphylaxis; if anaphylaxis does not occur, Antivenin is continued maintaining close observation of the patient. Patients who require Antivenin but develop signs of impending anaphylaxis in spite of this or the procedure described earlier present a difficult problem, and consultation should be sought.

Systemic Reactions: A. The immediate reaction (shock, anaphylaxis) usually occurs within 30 minutes. Symptoms and signs may develop before the needle is withdrawn and may include apprehension, flushing, itching, urticaria; edema of the face, tongue, and throat; cough, dyspnea, cyanosis, vomiting, and collapse.

B. Serum sickness usually occurs 5 to 24 days after administration. The incubation period may be less than 5 days, especially in those who have received horse-serum-containing preparations in the past. The usual symptoms and signs are malaise, fever, urticaria, lymphadenopathy, edema, arthralgia, nausea, and vomiting. Occasionally, neurological manifestations develop, such as meningismus or peripheral neuritis. Peripheral neuritis usually involves the shoulders and arms. Pain and muscle weakness are frequently present, and permanent atrophy may develop.

References:
1. GINGRICH, W. & HOHENADEL, J.: Standardization of polyvalent antivenin. "Venoms", edited by E. Buckley and N. Porges. Publication No. 44, Amer. Assoc. for the Advancement of Science, Washington, D.C., 1956, Pages 337–80.
2. PARRISH, H.: Incidence of treated snakebite in the United States. Pub. Hlth. Rep. 81:269, 1966.
3. RUSSELL, F., et al.: Snake venom poisoning in the United States. Experiences with 550 cases. JAMA 233:341, 1975. RUSSELL, F.: Venomous Bites and stings: Poisonous snakes. In The Merck Manual of Diagnosis and Therapy, pp. 1982–1987, 13th Ed., 1977.
4. WINGERT, W. and WAINSCHEL, J.: Diagnosis and management of envenomation by poisonous snakes. South. Med. J. 68:1015, 1975.
5. PARRISH, H. & HAYES, R.: Hospital management of pit viper venenations. Clinical Toxicol. 3:501, 1970.
6. McCOLLOUGH, N. & GENNARO, J.: Diagnosis, symptoms, treatment and sequelae of envenomation by *Crotalus adamanteus* and Genus *Agkistrodon.* J. Florida Med. Assoc. 55:327, 1968.
7. WATT, C. & GENNARO, J.: Pit viper bites in South Georgia and North Florida. Tr. South. Surg. Assoc. 77:378, 1966.
8. MINTON, S.: Venom Diseases: Snakebite. In Textbook of Medicine, P. Beeson and W. McDermott (Eds.), pp. 88–92; Saunders, Philadelphia, 1975.
9. VAN MIEROP, L.: Snakebite symposium. J. Florida Med. Assoc. 63:101, 1976.
10. ARNOLD, R.: Treatment of snakebite. JAMA 236:1843, 1976.
11. Poisonous Snakes of the World. U.S. Government Printing Office, Washington, D.C., NAVMED, 1965.
12. GARFIN, S. et al.: Rattlesnake bites: Current concepts. Clin. Orthop. 140:50, 1979; Role of surgical decompression in treatment of rattlesnake bites. Surg. Forum 30:502, 1979.
13. VAN MIEROP, L. & KITCHENS, C.: Defibrination syndrome following bites by the eastern diamondback rattlesnake, J. Florida Med. Assoc. 67:21, 1980.
14. HASIBA, U. et al.: DIC-like syndrome after envenomation by the snake, *Crotalus horridus horridus.* New Eng. J. Med. 292:505, 1975.
15. WEISS, H. et al.: Afibrinogenemia in man following the bite of a rattlesnake *(Crotalus adamanteus)*. Am. J. Med. 47:625, 1969.
16. SIVAPRASAD, R. & CANTINI, E.: Western diamondback rattlesnake *(Crotalus atrox)* poisoning. Postgrad. Med. 71:223, 1982.
17. SABBACK, M. et al.: A study of the treatment of pit viper envenomization in 45 patients. J. Trauma 17:569, 1977.

How Supplied: Each combination package contains one vacuum vial to yield 10 ml of serum—to be used immediately after reconstitution—(with preservatives: phenol 0.25% and thimerosal [mercury derivative] 0.005%). One vial containing 10 ml of Bacteriostatic Water for Injection, USP (with preservative: phenylmercuric nitrate 0.001%). One 1 ml vial of normal horse serum (diluted 1:10) as sensitivity testing material with preservatives: thimerosal (mercury derivative) 0.005% and phenol 0.35%. Not returnable.

ANTIVENIN (Micrurus fulvius) ℞
[an″te ven′in]
(equine origin)
North American Coral Snake Antivenin

Composition: Each combination package contains one vial of lyophilized Antivenin (Micrurus fulvius) with 0.25% phenol and 0.005% thimerosal (mercury derivative) as preservatives (before lyophilization); one vial of diluent containing 10 ml of Bacteriostatic Water for Injection, U.S.P., with phenylmercuric nitrate (1:100,000) as preservative.

How Supplied: Combination packages as described (not returnable).

CHOLERA VACCINE, U.S.P. ℞
[kol′er-ah vak′sēn]

Description: Each ml. contains 8 units each serotype antigen (Ogawa and Inaba). The preservative is 0.5% phenol.

How Supplied: Vials of 1.5 ml. and 20 ml.

DIPHTHERIA AND TETANUS TOXOIDS ℞
[dif-the′re-ah and tet′ah-nus tok′soids]
ADSORBED (PEDIATRIC)
aluminum phosphate adsorbed,
ULTRAFINED®

Description: Antigens adsorbed on aluminum phosphate. Preservative is 0.01% thimerosal (mercury derivative).

How Supplied: Vials of 5 ml.; and 0.5-ml. TUBEX® Sterile Cartridge-Needle Units, packages of 10.

IMMUNE SERUM GLOBULIN ℞
[ĭ-mūn′se′rum glob′u-lin]
(human), U.S.P.

Description: Immune Serum Globulin (Human)[ISG] is a sterile solution of immunoglobulin, primarily immunoglobulin G (IgG), containing 16.5± 1.5% protein. It is prepared by cold alcohol fractionation of pooled plasma. All plasma units have been tested and found nonreactive for hepatitis B surface antigen (HBsAg). ISG contains the mercurial preservative, sodium ethylmercurithiosalicylate (thimerosal), at a concentration of 100

Continued on next page

Wyeth—Cont.

mg per liter and 0.3 M glycine. The solution has been adjusted to a physiological pH of 6.8± 0.4 with the aid of sodium carbonate, sodium bicarbonate and/or sodium acetate—acetic acid buffer.
How Supplied: Vials of 10 ml; and 2 ml Tubex® Sterile Cartridge-Needle Units, packages of 1.

INFLUENZA VIRUS VACCINE, SUBVIRION TYPE
[in"flu-en'zah vi'rus vak'sēn sub vir'ēon]

The formulation of influenza virus vaccine for use during each season is established by the office of Biologics Research and Review, Food and Drug Administration. For current information about formulation, dosage and recommended use, consult product direction circular which can be obtained by writing Professional Service, Wyeth Laboratories, P.O. Box 8299, Philadelphia, PA, 19101, or through your local Wyeth representative.

RABIES VACCINE
[rā'bēz vak'sēn]
(Human Diploid-Cell Strain)
Subvirion Antigen

(See WYVAC® [Rabies Vaccine])

TETANUS AND DIPHTHERIA TOXOIDS ADSORBED
[tet'ah-nus and dif-the're-ah tok'soids]
(for adult use)
aluminum phosphate adsorbed
ULTRAFINED®

Description: A combination of refined tetanus and diphtheria toxoids for adult use, in which the fully potent antigens are adsorbed on aluminum phosphate. The preservative is 0.01% thimerosal (mercury derivative). Each dose contains no more than 2 Lf of purified diphtheria toxoid.
How Supplied: Vials of 5 ml.; and 0.5-ml. TUBEX® Sterile Cartridge-Needle Units, packages of 10.

TETANUS IMMUNE GLOBULIN
[tet'ah-nus ĭ-mūn' glob'u-lin]
(human)

Description: Tetanus Immune Globulin (Human) (TIG) is a sterile 10- to 18-percent solution of human immunoglobulin prepared by the cold ethanol fractionation method from the plasma of persons who have been hyperimmunized with tetanus toxoid. The final product contains 0.3 molar glycine as a stabilizer and 0.01 percent thimerosal (mercury derivative) as preservative. This product was prepared from plasma that was nonreactive when tested with licensed third generation reagents for hepatitis B surface antigen (HBsAg).
How Supplied: 1 ml TUBEX® Sterile Cartridge-Needle Unit, packages of 10.

TETANUS TOXOID ADSORBED
[tet'ah-nus tok'soid]
aluminum phosphate adsorbed,
ULTRAFINED®

Description: A refined toxoid, in which the antigen is adsorbed on aluminum phosphate. The preservative is 0.01% thimerosal (mercury derivative).
How Supplied: Vials of 5 ml.; and 0.5-ml. TUBEX® Sterile Cartridge-Needle Units, packages of 10.

TETANUS TOXOID,
[tet'ahnus tok'soid]
fluid purified, ULTRAFINED®

Description: A refined tetanus toxoid. The preservative is 0.01% thimerosal (mercury derivative).
How Supplied: Vials of 7.5 ml.; and 0.5-ml. TUBEX® Sterile Cartridge-Needle Units, packages of 10.

TYPHOID VACCINE, U.S.P.
[ti'foid vak'sēn]

Description: Each ml. contains not more than 1000 million Salmonella typhosa (Ty-2 strain) organisms, killed and suspended in buffered sodium chloride injection. The preservative is 0.5% phenol. Contains 8 units per ml.
How Supplied: Vials of 5 ml., 10 ml., and 20 ml.

Rabies Vaccine
(Human Diploid-Cell Strain)
Subvirion Antigen
WYVAC®
[wi'vak]

Description: Rabies Vaccine, Wyeth (WYVAC), is a sterile, stable, cell-culture rabies virus vaccine for human use by intramuscular injection. It is prepared with the Pasteur-derived Pitman-Moore virus strain adapted from material grown in rabbit brain—as used in the production of Semple-type vaccine—to cultivation in the Human Diploid-Cell Strain (HDCS), WI-38.[1] Seed stocks and vaccine lots have been prepared with cell-free virus harvests from infected cultures after 63 or more consecutive HDCS passages. The virus is propagated in these cells, in a chemically defined nutrient medium with normal serum albumin (human) with the following antibiotics added: neomycin sulfate, amphotericin B, and gentamicin sulfate.
The virus harvest is freed of debris by membrane filtration and then concentrated to a standard antigen content by aseptic ultrafiltration. The virus particles in the concentrate are disrupted into smaller antigenic units by the addition of tri(n)butylphosphate (0.1%) and Polysorbate 80, USP (0.1%); and inactivation is completed by further treatment with beta propiolactone (0.025%). The vaccine is preserved with thimerosal (mercury derivative), added to the ultra-filtrate to a final concentration of 0.01% (1:10,000). The vaccine is stabilized by lyophilization. Each 1 ml dose of vaccine, which is colorless to faintly pink after reconstitution because of a phenol red indicator, contains approximately 2.5% normal human serum albumin and not more than 50 mcg neomycin, 2.5 mcg amphotericin, 50 mcg gentamicin, 0.01% tri(n)butylphosphate (as determined by assay), 0.1% Polysorbate 80, USP, and 0.01% thimerosal (mercury derivative).
The potency of the vaccine is equal to or greater than 2.5 International Units (IU) of rabies antigen per dose, which is established by tests in parallel with the Standard Rabies Vaccine in the NIH mouse potency test as required by the Office of Biologics Research and Review, Food and Drug Administration.
Clinical Pharmacology: The administration of the inactivated rabies vaccine stimulates rapid production of specific antibodies.
In *preexposure trials* involving more than 2,000 volunteers, after three injections of vaccine over a four-week period, at least 99% of recipients developed antibodies. Geometric mean titers for various groups 35 days after the start of immunization were approximately ten IU, with only a few vaccinees falling below one IU. The definition of a minimally acceptable antibody titer varies among laboratories and is influenced by the type of test conducted. CDC currently specifies a 1:5 titer by the rapid fluorescent-focus inhibition test (RFFIT) as acceptable. The World Health Organization (WHO) specifies a titer of 0.5 IU.
In ongoing *postexposure* clinical trials utilizing a five- or six-dose regimen in conjunction with Rabies Immune Globulin, Human RIG(H), over 500 adults and children have been successfully treated. Treatment groups consisting of subjects allergic to Duck Embryo Vaccine (DEV), nonresponders to DEV, and subjects receiving primary postexposure therapy have been successfully immunized in 100% of cases. No cases of human rabies have occurred in these patients who have had varying degrees of exposure to confirmed or suspected rabid animals.[2,3,4,5]

A group of ten children, ranging in age from 2–16 years, has also been successfully treated on the same regimen.[6] All developed significant rabies antibody titers within 14 days, with a geometric mean titer (GMT) of 3.7 IU/ml at 14 days, 8.7 IU/ml at 28 days, and 20.1 IU/ml at 42 days after beginning treatment, as determined by the RFFIT. As a result of exposure to two cases of human rabies, seventy individuals with histories of contact up to two months prior to receiving vaccine all developed protective responses. The GMTs ranged from 0.9 IU at 14 days to 14.6 IU at 42 days after a five-dose regimen, and RIG(H).
Data on persistence of antibody demonstrated that in 546 subjects who received preexposure inoculations, sera obtained at 9–12 months after primary immunization with a three-dose regimen demonstrated antibody levels of 0.5 to 8.4 IU/ml in nearly 93% of vaccinees. Single booster doses of 1.0 ml given to several different groups, immunized previously with 3 or 4 doses of WYVAC or a routine course of DEV, induced four-fold increases in titer in 99% of vaccinees. The GMT was 4.7 IU/ml by RFFIT 14–35 days after receipt of the booster dose. A small group of these individuals tested one year later still had a range of titers of 1.0–2.0 IU/ml.[7]
Indications and Usage[3]**:**
1. RATIONALE OF TREATMENT
In the United States and Canada, the following factors should be considered before specific antirabies treatment is indicated:

A. *Species of Biting Animal*
Carnivorous wild animals (especially skunks, raccoons, foxes, coyotes, and bobcats) and bats are the animals most commonly infected with rabies and have caused most of the indigenous cases of human rabies in the United States since 1960. Unless an animal is tested and shown not to be rabid, postexposure prophylaxis should be initiated upon bite or nonbite exposure to the animals. (See definition in "Type of Exposure" below.) If treatment has been initiated and subsequent testing in a competent laboratory shows the exposing animal is not rabid, treatment can be discontinued.
The likelihood that a domestic dog or cat is infected with rabies varies from region to region; hence, the need for postexposure prophylaxis also varies.
Rodents (such as squirrels, hamsters, guinea pigs, gerbils, chipmunks, rats, and mice) and lagomorphs (including rabbits and hares) are rarely found to be infected with rabies and have not been known to cause human rabies in the United States. In these cases, the state or local health department should be consulted before a decision is made to initiate postexposure antirabies prophylaxis.

B. *Circumstances of Biting Incident*
An UNPROVOKED attack is more likely than a provoked attack to indicate that the animal is rabid. Bites inflicted on a person attempting to feed or handle an apparently healthy animal should generally be regarded as PROVOKED.

C. *Type of Exposure*
Rabies is commonly transmitted by inoculation with infectious saliva. The likelihood that rabies infection will result from exposure to a rabid animal varies with the nature and extent of the exposure. Two categories of exposure should be considered:
Bite: Any penetration of the skin by teeth.
Nonbite: Scratches, abrasions, open wounds or mucous membranes contaminated with saliva or other potentially infectious material, such as the brain from a rabid animal. In addition, there have been two instances of airborne rabies acquired in the laboratory and two probable airborne rabies cases acquired in one bat-infested cave (Frio Cave, Texas).
Casual contact with a rabid animal, such as petting the animal (without a bite or nonbite exposure as described above), does not constitute an exposure and is not an indication for prophylaxis.
The only documented cases of rabies due to human-to-human transmission occurred in patients who received corneal transplants from persons

who died of rabies undiagnosed at the time of death.

Each exposure to possible rabies infection must be individually evaluated.

Local or state public health officials should be consulted if questions arise about the need for rabies prophylaxis.

II. PRE- AND POSTEXPOSURE TREATMENT OF RABIES

A. *Preexposure* (See Table 1)

Preexposure immunization may be offered to persons in high-risk groups, such as veterinarians, animal handlers, certain laboratory workers, and persons spending time (e.g., 1 month or more) in foreign countries where rabies is a constant threat. Persons whose vocational or avocational pursuits bring them into contact with potentially rabid dogs, cats, foxes, skunks, bats, or other species at risk of having rabies should also be considered for preexposure prophylaxis.

Immunization is recommended for children living in or visiting countries where exposure to rabid animals is a constant threat. Worldwide statistics indicate that children are more at risk than adults.

Preexposure prophylaxis is given for several reasons. First, it may provide protection to persons with inapparent exposures to rabies. Second, it may protect persons whose postexposure therapy might be expected to be delayed. Finally, although it does not eliminate the need for additional therapy after a rabies exposure, it simplifies therapy by eliminating the need for globulin and decreasing the number of doses of vaccine needed. This is of particular importance for persons at high risk of being exposed in countries where the available rabies immunizing products may carry a higher risk of adverse reactions.

Preexposure immunization does not eliminate the need for prompt postexposure prophylaxis following an exposure; it only reduces the postexposure regimen.

TABLE 1
PREEXPOSURE IMMUNIZATION. Preexposure immunization consists of three doses of HDCV, 1.0 ml, IM (i.e., deltoid area), one each on days 0, 7, and 28. Administration of routine booster doses of vaccine depends on exposure risk category as noted below. Preexposure immunization of immunosuppressed persons is not recommended. [See table above].

B. *Postexposure*

1. Local Treatment of Wounds: Immediate and thorough local treatment of all bite wounds and scratches is perhaps the most effective preventive measure. The wound should be thoroughly cleansed immediately with soap and water.

Tetanus prophylaxis and measures to control bacterial infection should be given as indicated.

2. Specific Treatment: Postexposure antirabies treatment should always include both passive [preferably Rabies Immune Globulin of human origin—RIG(H)] and active (Rabies Vaccine) immunization, with one exception: persons who have been previously immunized with the recommended preexposure or postexposure regimen with HDCV or who have been immunized with other types of vaccines and have a history of documented adequate rabies antibody titer should receive only vaccine. Antirabies serum of horse origin (ARS) should only be used where human immune globulin is unavailable. The combination of globulin and vaccine is recommended for both bite exposures and nonbite exposures (as described under "Rationale of Treatment") and regardless of the interval between exposure and treatment. The sooner treatment is begun after exposure, the better.

POSTEXPOSURE RABIES TREATMENT GUIDE (Table 2)

The following recommendations are only a guide. They should be applied in conjunction with knowledge of the animal species involved, circumstances of the bite or other exposure, vaccination status of the animal, and presence of rabies in the region. Local and state public health officials should be

Criteria for Preexposure Immunization

Risk category	Nature of risk	Typical populations	Preexposure regimen
Continuous	Virus present continuously, often in high concentrations. Aerosol, mucous membrane, bite, or nonbite exposure possible. Specific exposures may go unrecognized.	Rabies research lab workers.* Rabies biologics production workers.	Primary preexposure immunization course. Serology every 6 months. Booster immunization when antibody titer falls below acceptable level.*
Frequent	Exposure usually episodic, with source recognized, but exposure may also be unrecognized. Aerosol, mucous membrane, bite, or nonbite exposure.	Rabies diagnostic lab workers,* spelunkers, veterinarians, and animal control and wildlife workers in rabies-epizootic areas.	Primary preexposure immunization course. Booster immunization or serology every 2 years.†
Infrequent (greater than population-at-large)	Exposure nearly always episodic with source recognized. Mucous membrane, bite, or nonbite exposure.	Veterinarians and animal control and wildlife workers in areas of low rabies endemicity. Certain travelers to foreign rabies-epizootic areas. Veterinary students.	Primary preexposure immunization course. No routine booster immunization or serology.
Rare (population-at-large)	Exposure always episodic, mucous membrane, or bite with source recognized.	U.S. population-at-large, including individuals in rabies-epizootic areas.	No preexposure immunization.

*Judgment of relative risk and extra monitoring of immunization status of laboratory workers is the responsibility of the laboratory supervisor (see U.S. Department of Health and Human Services' *Biosafety in Microbiological and Biomedical Laboratories*, 1984).

†Preexposure booster immunization consists of one dose of HDCV, 1.0 ml/dose, IM (deltoid area). Acceptable antibody level is 1:5 titer (complete inhibition in RFFIT at 1:5 dilution). (See "Clinical Pharmacology.") Boost if titer falls below 1:5.

consulted if questions arise about the need for rabies prophylaxis.
[See table on next page].

Contraindications: For postexposure treatment there are no known specific contraindications for the use of this vaccine. In cases of preexposure immunization, there are no known specific contraindications other than situations such as developing febrile illness.

Warnings: In both preexposure and postexposure immunization, the full 1.0 ml dose should be given intramuscularly. There are no data to establish the efficacy of using either reduced volumes of vaccine or of that injected intradermally.

Systemic allergic reactions to HDCV have been reported (11 per 10,000 vaccinees).[8] Few patients required hospitalization, and no deaths secondary to the reactions were reported. Such reports have included cases of presumed Type I immediate hypersensitivity, presumed Type III hypersensitivity, and cases of allergic reactions of indeterminate type. Type I reactions refer to immediate hypersensitivity, such as atopy or anaphylaxis. Type III reactions were primarily observed following booster immunization and occurred 2 to 21 days after HDCV administration. Patients presented with a generalized or pruritic rash or urticaria, sometimes accompanied by arthralgias, angioedema, fever, nausea, vomiting, and malaise. Preliminary data suggest this "immune complex-like" illness may occur in up to 6% of persons receiving booster vaccines and much less frequently in persons receiving primary immunization. Individuals with histories of presumed Type III hypersensitivity to HDCV may be at higher risk of subsequent hypersensitivity reactions, and vaccine should be administered under appropriate medical supervision.

Neurological events reported following receipt of HDCS rabies vaccine include two cases of acute polyradiculoneuropathy (Guillain-Barré Syndrome)[9], a transient neuroparalytic illness that completely resolved within 12 weeks[10], and a focal subacute CNS disorder. While these have been temporally associated with vaccine administration, no causal relationship has been established. Should a neurological complication develop, advice and assistance on managing the patient as well as making a decision about discontinuing vaccine treatment is available from state health departments or the Centers for Disease Control (CDC). Any serious reactions should be immediately reported to the state health department or the Viral Disease Division, Bureau of Epidemiology, CDC, Atlanta, Georgia (telephone 404-329-3095 during working hours or 404-329-2888 at other times).

Precautions:

GENERAL

While the concentration of antibiotics in each dose of vaccine is extremely small, persons with known hypersensitivity to any of these agents could manifest an allergic reaction. While the risk is small, it should be weighed in light of the potential risk of contracting rabies. Epinephrine injection (1:1000) must be immediately available should an acute anaphylactic reaction occur due to any component of the vaccine.

DRUG INTERACTIONS

Corticosteroids and immunosuppressive agents may interfere with the development of active immunity and predispose the patient to developing rabies. They should not be administered during postexposure therapy unless essential for the treatment of other serious conditions. If rabies postexposure therapy is administered to persons receiving steroids or immunosuppressive therapy, it is especially important that serum be tested for rabies antibody to ensure that an adequate response has developed.

USAGE IN PREGNANCY—PREGNANCY CATEGORY C

Continued on next page

Wyeth—Cont.

Animal reproductive studies have not been conducted with WYVAC. It is also not known whether WYVAC can cause fetal harm when administered to a pregnant woman or can affect reproduction capacity. Pregnancy is not a contraindication to rabies postexposure therapy. Based on limited data, there have been no fetal abnormalities associated with rabies vaccination. If there is substantial risk of rabies exposure, preexposure treatment may also be indicated during pregnancy.

PEDIATRIC USE: Both safety and efficacy in children have been established.

Adverse Reactions: Once initiated, rabies prophylaxis should not be interrupted or discontinued because of local, or mild systemic, adverse reactions to rabies vaccine. Usually such reactions can be successfully managed with antiinflammatory and antipyretic agents (aspirin, for example).

Reactions after vaccination with HDCV are less common than with previously available vaccines. In a study using five doses of HDCV, local reactions, such as pain, erythema, and swelling or itching at the injection site, were reported in about 25% of recipients of HDCV, and mild systemic reactions, such as headache, nausea, abdominal pain, muscle aches, and dizziness, were reported in about 20% of recipients. Two cases of neurologic illness, resembling Guillain-Barré syndrome that resolved without sequelae in 12 weeks and a focal subacute central nervous system disorder temporally associated with HDCV vaccine, have been reported.

Systemic allergic reactions have included reports of Type I hypersensitivity (atopy and anaphylaxis); Type III hypersensitivity (generalized or pruritic rash or urticaria, arthralgias, angioedema, fever, nausea, vomiting, and malaise); and reactions of indeterminate type (see "Warnings").[8]

Constitutional reactions and symptoms may arise in patients faced with a life-threatening situation and may not be caused by the vaccine. However, the development of fever, malaise, fatigue, nausea, and arthralgia merits careful observation.

The occurrence of neuroparalytic reactions, such as transverse myelitis, encephalomyelitis, Guillain-Barré Syndrome, and other cranial or peripheral neuropathies with resultant permanent neurological sequelae and/or death, have been reported in recipients of inactivated rabies vaccines of nervous-tissue and duck embryo origin. The possibility of the occurrence of such neuroparalytic or other major neurologic reactions following the use of inactivated rabies vaccines of human-diploid-cell origin should be kept in mind. Also see "Warnings" section.

Serious systemic, anaphylactic, or neuroparalytic reactions, occurring during the administration of rabies vaccines, pose a serious dilemma for the attending physician. A patient's risk of developing rabies must be carefully considered before deciding to discontinue vaccination or to choose an alternate vaccine. Moreover, the use of corticosteroids to treat life-threatening neuroparalytic reactions carries the risk of inhibiting the development of active immunity to rabies. It is especially important in these cases that the serum of the patient be tested for rabies antibodies. Advice and assistance on the management of serious adverse reactions in persons receiving rabies vaccines may be sought from the state health department or the CDC.

Dosage and Administration[3]:
Parenteral drug products should be inspected visually for particulate matter and discoloration prior to administration, whenever solution and container permit.

DIRECTIONS FOR USE
Using a sterile syringe, inject 1.0 ml of Sterile Water for Injection, USP, into the vial of vaccine. Shake vial gently until vaccine is completely dissolved. The reconstituted vaccine should be used immediately.

Withdraw entire dose and inject intramuscularly, preferably into the deltoid muscle or upper, outer quadrant of the buttock. In infants and small children, the midlateral aspect of the thigh may be preferable. Care should be taken to avoid injection into or near blood vessels and nerves. After aspiration, if blood or any suspicious discoloration appears in the syringe, do not inject but instead, discard its contents and repeat procedure using fresh vaccine with new needle and syringe at a different site.

A. PREEXPOSURE IMMUNIZATION
Three 1-ml injections of WYVAC should be given intramuscularly (for example, in the deltoid area), 1 on each of days 0, 7, and 28.

Booster doses of vaccine: Persons who work with live rabies virus in research laboratories or vaccine production facilities and are at risk of inapparent exposure should have the rabies antibody titer of their serum determined every 6 months. Booster doses of vaccine should be given, as needed, to maintain an adequate titer. (For definition of adequate titer, see "Clinical Pharmacology.") Other laboratory workers, such as those doing rabies diagnostic tests, spelunkers, and those veterinarians, animal control and wildlife officers in areas where animal rabies is epizootic, should have boosters every 2 years or have their serum tested for rabies antibody every 2 years and, if the titer is inadequate, have a booster dose. Veterinarians and animal control and wildlife officers, if working in areas of low rabies endemicity, do not require routine booster doses of HDCV after completion of primary preexposure immunization (Table 2).

Persons who have experienced Type III hypersensitivity reactions should receive no further doses of HDCV unless: 1) they are exposed to rabies (see below) or 2) they are truly likely to be inapparently and/or unavoidably exposed to rabies virus and have unsatisfactory antibody titers. The routine use of booster immunization in persons without histories of hypersensitivity reactions is clearly indicated only in those subjected to inapparent and/or unavoidable exposure to rabies virus.

B. POSTEXPOSURE IMMUNIZATION
Postexposure antirabies immunization should always include both passively administered antibody [preferably RIG(H)] and vaccine with 1 exception: persons who have been previously immunized with the recommended preexposure or postexposure regimen with HDCV or who have been immunized with other types of rabies vaccine and have a documented adequate rabies antibody titer should receive only vaccine. The combination of globulin and vaccine is recommended for both bite exposures and nonbite exposures (as described under "Rationale of Treatment") and regardless of the interval between exposure and treatment. RIG(H) is administered only once, at the beginning of postexposure therapy, as described below. The sooner treatment is begun after exposure, the better. However, there have been instances in which the decision to begin treatment was indicated as late as 6 months and longer after the exposure.

In 1977 the World Health Organization (WHO) established a recommendation for 6 intramuscular doses of HDCV based on studies in Germany and Iran of a regimen of RIG(H) or ARS and 6 doses of HDCV. Used in this way the vaccine was found to be effective in protecting 76 persons bitten by proven rabid animals and induced an excellent antibody response in all recipients. Since 1977, studies conducted by the CDC in the United States have shown that a regimen of 1 dose of RIG(H) and 5 doses of WYVAC induced an excellent antibody response in all recipients. Of 77 persons bitten by proven rabid animals and so treated, none developed rabies.

Five 1-ml doses of WYVAC should be given intramuscularly (for example, in the deltoid regions). Other routes of administration, such as the intradermal route, have not been tested for postexposure prophylaxis and should not be used. The first dose should be given as soon as possible after the exposure and be administered in conjunction with RIG(H); an additional dose should be given on each of days 3, 7, 14, and 28 after the first dose. (WHO currently recommends a sixth dose 90 days after the first dose.)

C. POSTEXPOSURE THERAPY OF PREVIOUSLY IMMUNIZED PERSONS
When an immunized person who received the recommended preexposure or postexposure regimen with HDCV or who has been immunized with any other type of rabies vaccine and has previously demonstrated rabies antibody is exposed to rabies, that person should receive 2 doses (1 ml each) of WYVAC, 1 immediately and 1 three days

TABLE 2 WYVAC

Animal Species	Condition of Animal at Time of Attack	Treatment of Exposed Person (1). All bites and wounds should immediately be thoroughly cleansed with soap and water (see preceding text).
Domestic: Dog & Cat	Healthy and available for 10 days of observation	None, unless animal develops rabies (2).
	Rabid or suspected rabid	Rabies Immune Globulin (3) AND Rabies Vaccine (4).
	Unknown (escaped)	Consultation with public health officials. If treatment is indicated, give Rabies Immune Globulin (3) AND Rabies Vaccine (4).
Wild: Skunk, bat, fox, coyote, raccoon, bobcat, and other carnivores	Regard as rabid unless proven negative by laboratory test (5)	Rabies Immune Globulin (3) AND Rabies Vaccine (4).
Other: Livestock, rodents, rabbits, and hares		Consider Individually: provoked bites of squirrels, hamsters, guinea pigs, gerbils, chipmunks, rats, mice and other rodents or rabbits and hares almost never call for antirabies prophylaxis. Local or state public health officials should be consulted about questions that arise about the need for rabies prophylaxis.

(1) If antirabies treatment is indicated, both Rabies Immune Globulin and Rabies Vaccine should be given as soon as possible, *regardless* of the interval from exposure.
(2) Begin treatment with Rabies Immune Globulin and Rabies Vaccine at first sign of rabies in biting domestic animals during the usual holding period of 10 days. The symptomatic animal should be killed immediately and tested.
(3) If Rabies Immune Globulin is not available, use antirabies serum of equine origin. Do not use more than the recommended dosage.
(4) Discontinue vaccine if fluorescent antibody tests of animal are negative.
(5) The animal should be killed and tested as soon as possible. Holding for observation is not recommended.

later. Passive immunization should not be given in these cases. If the immune status of a person immunized previously with a non-HDCV vaccine is not known, full primary postexposure antirabies treatment [RIG(H) plus 5 doses of WYVAC] may be necessary. In such cases, if antibody can be demonstrated in a serum sample collected before vaccine is given, treatment can be discontinued after at least 2 doses of WYVAC.

SEROLOGIC TESTING
The Immunization Practices Advisory Committee (ACIP) does not recommend routine serologic testing of persons who receive the recommended preexposure or postexposure treatment regimen of HDCV except as indicated in Table 1. Serologic testing is still recommended for persons whose immune responses might be diminished by drug therapy or for other reasons.[11] If the need arises to determine the antibody status of a patient, the CDC or state health department should be contacted.

How Supplied: Rabies Vaccine (HDCS WI-38) Subvirion Antigen, WYVAC®, is supplied as a single-dose vial of lyophilized vaccine with one ampule of diluent (Sterile Water for Injection).

Storage: DO NOT FREEZE. Keep between 2°C and 8°C (35°F and 46°F).

References:
1. WIKTOR TJ, FERNANDES MV, KOPROWSKI H: Cultivation of Rabies Virus in Human Diploid Cell Strain WI-38. J Immunol 93:353, 1964.
2. Human Diploid Cell Strain Rabies Vaccine. Centers for Disease Control. Morbidity and Mortality Weekly Rep 27:333-339, 1978.
3. Recommendations of the Public Health Service Advisory Committee on Immunization Practices—Rabies Prevention—United States, 1984. Centers for Disease Control. Morbidity and Mortality Weekly Rep 33:393-408, 1984.
4. ANDERSON LJ, SIKES RK, LANGKOP CW, MANN JW, SMITH JS, WINKLER WG, DEITCH MW: Post-Exposure Trial with 5 Doses of HDCS Rabies Vaccine. J Inf Dis 142:133-138, 1980.
5. ANDERSON LJ, WINKLER WG, HAFKIN B, KEENLYSIDE RA, D'ANGELO LJ, DEITCH MW: Clinical Experience with a Human Diploid Cell Rabies Vaccine. JAMA 244:781-784, 1980.
6. SIEBER O, ROSANOFF E, DEITCH M, GOLDEN F, TENNICAN P: Post-exposure Rabies Treatment with Wyeth Rabies Human Diploid Cell Vaccine. Proceedings of 19th Interscience Conf. on Antimicrobial Agents & Chemotherapy, October 1979.
7. ROSANOFF E, DEITCH M, PLOTKIN S, WIKTOR T, SWANGO L: Clinical Trial of Human Diploid Cell Strain (HDCS) Rabies Vaccine. Proceedings of 19th Interscience Conf. on Antimicrobial Agents & Chemotherapy, October 1979.
8. Systemic allergic reactions following immunization with human diploid cell rabies vaccine. Morbidity and Mortality Weekly Rep 33:185-187, 1984.
9. BOE E, NYLAND H: Guillain-Barré Syndrome after Vaccination with Human Diploid Cell Rabies Vaccine. Scand J Infect Dis 12:231-232, 1980.
10. BERNARD, KW (Personal Communication).
11. Recommendations of the Immunization Practices Advisory Committee (ACIP). Morbidity and Mortality Weekly Rep 30:535, 1981.

COLLYRIUM   OTC
[ko-lir'e-um]
a neutral borate solution
SOOTHING EYE LOTION

Description: A neutral borate solution containing boric acid and sodium borate as buffers, not more than 0.002% thimerosal as a preservative, and water.

Indications: For flushing or irrigating the eye to remove loose foreign material, air pollutants, or chlorinated water.

Dosage and Administration: Patients are advised to rinse cup clean before each use and to avoid contamination of rim and inside surfaces of cup. The half-filled cup should be applied to the affected eye and pressed tightly to the eye to prevent the escape of the liquid, and the head tilted backward. Eyelids should be opened wide and the eyeball rotated to ensure thorough bathing with the wash or lotion. The cup should be rinsed with clean water after each use. After every use, the bottle can be reclosed by placing the threaded eyecup on the bottle which replaces the disposable top after opening.

Warnings: Patients are advised of the following. To avoid contamination of this product, do not touch tip of container to any other surface. Replace cap after using. Not for use in open wounds in or near the eyes. Consult a doctor if you experience eye pain, changes in vision, continued redness or irritation of the eye, or if the condition worsens or persists.

This product contains thimerosal as a preservative. Do not use this product if you are sensitive to mercury. Do not use if solution changes color or becomes cloudy, or with a wetting solution for contact lens or other eye lotions containing polyvinyl alcohol. Container should be kept tightly closed at room temperature, approx. 77°F (25°C).

How Supplied: Bottles of 6 fl. oz. with eyecup.

COLLYRIUM 2™   OTC
[ko-lir'e-um]
eye drops with tetrahydrozoline

Description: Collyrium 2™ Eye Drops contain tetrahydrozoline hydrochloride (0.05%), zinc sulfate (0.25%), and glycerin (1.0%), with boric acid and sodium borate as buffering agents, and benzalkonium chloride (0.01%) and edetate disodium (0.1%) as preservatives.

Indications: For the relief of redness of the eye due to minor irritations, temporary relief of burning and irritation due to dryness of the eye and/or discomfort due to minor irritations of the eye or to exposure to wind and sun.

Dosage and Administration: One to two drops in the affected eye(s). Procedure may be repeated up to four times daily.

Warnings: Patients are advised of the following: To avoid contamination of this product, do not touch tip of container to any other surface. Replace cap after using.

If you experience eye pain, changes in vision, continued redness or irritation of the eye, or if the condition worsens or persists for more than 72 hours, discontinue use and consult a doctor.

If you have glaucoma, do not use this product except under the advice and supervision of a doctor. Overuse of this product may produce increased redness of the eye.

Do not use if solution changes color or becomes cloudy, or with povidone-containing contact lens wetting solutions. Container should be kept tightly closed and stored at room temperature, approx. 77°F (25°C).

How Supplied: Bottles of ½ fl. oz. with built-in eye dropper.

CYCLAPEN-W®   R
[si'klah-pen-w]
(cyclacillin)
Tablets and Oral Suspension

Description: Cyclapen-W (cyclacillin, Wyeth) is a semisynthetic penicillin of the ampicillin class chemically designated as a 6-(1-amino-cyclohexanecarboxamido) penicillanic acid. It differs from ampicillin in having an aminocyclohexanecarboxamido substitution on the penicillin nucleus in place of the aminophenylacetamido substitution contained in ampicillin. It is available for oral administration as 250 mg and 500 mg Tablets and for Oral Suspension, bottles providing 125 mg or 250 mg Cyclapen-W per 5 ml teaspoonful when reconstituted. Cyclacillin is a white, crystalline, anhydrous powder sparingly soluble in water.

Actions: HUMAN PHARMACOLOGY
Cyclacillin is acid stable and is rapidly and well absorbed from the gastrointestinal tract and rapidly excreted in the urine after oral administration in the fasting state (Graphs I and II).
Peak serum concentration is attained within 40-60 minutes after oral administration in the fasting state. Following oral doses of 250 mg and 500 mg in normal adult human subjects, the average peak serum levels (C max) were approximately 6-7 mcg/ml and 11-12 mcg/ml respectively. Measurable serum levels were present up to 4 hours. Mean serum concentrations over time are shown in the graphs below:

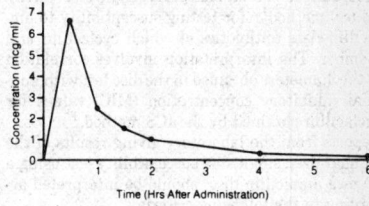

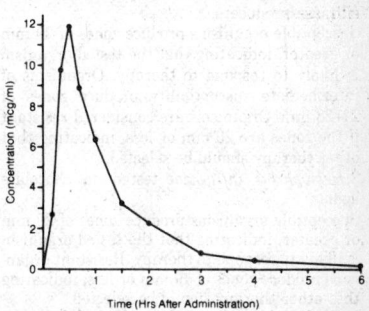

In blood, cyclacillin is one of the least-bound penicillins; an average of about 20% of the drug is bound to plasma proteins.

The biological half-life of the drug in normal adult subjects is about 30-40 minutes with renal clearance accounting for approximately 80 percent. Within 6 hours following administration, 65-70 percent of the cyclacillin dose is excreted unchanged in the urine. Additionally, approximately 15-17 percent of the dose is excreted in the urine in the form of the principal metabolite, 6-(1-aminocyclohexanecarboxamido) penicilloic acid.

Patients with Renal Failure
Cyclacillin may be safely administered to patients with reduced renal function. Normal adult subjects achieve a renal clearance of approximately 450-500 ml/min for cyclacillin. In patients with renal insufficiency (creatinine clearance less than 30 ml/min but greater than 6 ml/min), the mean renal clearance for cyclacillin was about 70 ml/min and the total body clearance was 184 ml/min, resulting in a mean biological half-life of 3.5 hours (210 min). In such patients this renal clearance accounts for approximately 38 percent of the total body clearance. In patients receiving hemodialysis the total body clearance was about 90 ml/min, resulting in a biological half-life of 8 hours (480 minutes). Due to this prolonged serum half-life of cyclacillin, patients with various degrees of renal impairment may require a change in dosage level. (See DOSAGE AND ADMINISTRATION.)

MICROBIOLOGY
Cyclacillin is an orally active, bactericidal semisynthetic penicillin for oral administration. *In vitro* studies have shown that cyclacillin is usually active against the following bacteria:
Group A beta-hemolytic streptococci
Streptococcus pneumoniae (formerly *D. pneumoniae*)
Staphylococci, non-penicillinase producers
Hemophilus influenzae
Escherichia coli
Proteus mirabilis
All strains of *Pseudomonas* and most strains of *Klebsiella* and *Enterobacter* are resistant; some

Continued on next page

Wyeth—Cont.

strains of *Escherichia coli* and *Hemophilus influenzae* may be resistant.

DISC SUSCEPTIBILITY TESTS
Quantitative methods that require measurement of zone diameters give the most precise estimates of antibiotic susceptibility. The recommended procedure is the standardized single-disc (Kirby-Bauer) method[1,2] for testing susceptibility to ampicillin-class antibiotics of which cyclacillin is a member. The interpretation involves correlation of the diameters obtained in the disc test with minimal inhibitory concentration (MIC) values for cyclacillin obtained by the ICS method.[3]

Reports from the laboratory giving results of the standardized single-disc susceptibility test using a 10 mcg ampicillin disc[1] should be interpreted according to the following criteria:

1. Group A beta-hemolytic streptococci, *Streptococcus pneumoniae*, and staphylococci, non-penicillinase producers.
Susceptible organisms produce zones of 29 mm or greater, indicating that the tested organism is likely to respond to therapy. Organisms of intermediate susceptibility produce zones of 21–28 mm. Organisms are considered resistant if the zones are 20 mm or less, indicating that other therapy should be selected.

2. *Hemophilus influenzae* tested on chocolate agar.
Susceptible organisms produce zones of 20 mm or greater, indicating that the tested organism is likely to respond to therapy. Resistant organisms produce zones of 19 mm or less, indicating that other therapy should be selected.

3. *Escherichia coli* and *Proteus mirabilis*.
(The following information applies only to urinary tract infections caused by these gram-negative organisms.)

If the standardized single-disc method of susceptibility testing is used, a disc containing 10 mcg of ampicillin should give a zone diameter of at least 14 mm when tested against a cyclacillin-susceptible strain of *Escherichia coli*, or *Proteus mirabilis*, a zone of 12–13 mm for a strain of intermediate susceptibility and a zone of 11 mm or less for a cyclacillin-resistant strain. Strains may be considered susceptible if the minimal inhibitory concentration (MIC) in Mueller-Hinton broth is not more than 125 mcg of cyclacillin per ml. Strains may be considered resistant if the MIC in Mueller-Hinton broth is greater than 250 mcg of cyclacillin per ml. The MIC value of ampicillin and cyclacillin can be affected by the method of assay and components and pH of the assay medium.

Indications: Cyclapen-W® (cyclacillin) has less in vitro activity than other drugs in the ampicillin class of antibiotics, and its use should be confined to the indications listed below.

Cyclapen-W is indicated for the treatment of the following infections:

RESPIRATORY TRACT
Tonsillitis and pharyngitis caused by Group A beta-hemolytic streptococci.
Bronchitis and pneumonia caused by *S. pneumoniae* (formerly *D. pneumoniae*).
Otitis Media caused by *S. pneumoniae* (formerly *D. pneumoniae*), *H. influenzae*, and Group A beta-hemolytic streptococci.
Acute exacerbation of chronic bronchitis caused by *H. influenzae*.*
*Though clinical improvement has been shown, bacteriologic cures cannot be expected in all patients with chronic respiratory disease due to *H. influenzae*.

SKIN AND SKIN STRUCTURES (integumentary) infections caused by Group A beta-hemolytic streptococci and staphylococci, non-penicillinase producers.

URINARY TRACT INFECTIONS caused by *E. coli* and *P. mirabilis*. (This drug should not be used in any infections caused by *E. coli* and *P. mirabilis* other than urinary tract infections.)

NOTE: Cultures and susceptibility tests should be performed initially and during treatment to monitor the effectiveness of therapy and the susceptibility of bacteria. Therapy may be instituted prior to the results of sensitivity testing.

Contraindications: The use of this drug is contraindicated in individuals with a history of an allergic reaction to penicillins.

Warnings: CYCLACILLIN SHOULD ONLY BE PRESCRIBED FOR THE INDICATIONS LISTED IN THIS INSERT.
CYCLACILLIN HAS LESS *IN VITRO* ACTIVITY THAN OTHER DRUGS OF THE AMPICILLIN-CLASS ANTIBIOTICS. HOWEVER, CLINICAL TRIALS HAVE DEMONSTRATED THAT IT IS EFFICACIOUS FOR THE RECOMMENDED INDICATIONS.
SERIOUS AND OCCASIONAL FATAL HYPERSENSITIVITY (ANAPHALOID) REACTIONS HAVE BEEN REPORTED IN PATIENTS RECEIVING PENICILLIN. ALTHOUGH ANAPHYLAXIS IS MORE FREQUENT FOLLOWING PARENTERAL ADMINISTRATION, IT HAS OCCURRED IN PATIENTS ON ORAL PENICILLINS. THESE REACTIONS ARE MORE APT TO OCCUR IN INDIVIDUALS WITH A HISTORY OF SENSITIVITY TO MULTIPLE ALLERGENS. THERE ARE REPORTS OF PATIENTS WITH A HISTORY OF PENICILLIN HYPERSENSITIVITY REACTIONS WHO EXPERIENCED SEVERE HYPERSENSITIVITY REACTIONS WHEN TREATED WITH A CEPHALOSPORIN. BEFORE THERAPY WITH A PENICILLIN, CAREFUL INQUIRY SHOULD BE MADE ABOUT PREVIOUS HYPERSENSITIVITY REACTIONS TO PENICILLINS, CEPHALOSPORINS, AND OTHER ALLERGENS. IF AN ALLERGIC REACTION OCCURS, THE DRUG SHOULD BE DISCONTINUED AND APPROPRIATE THERAPY SHOULD BE INITIATED. SERIOUS ANAPHYLACTOID REACTIONS REQUIRE IMMEDIATE EMERGENCY TREATMENT WITH EPINEPHRINE. OXYGEN, INTRAVENOUS STEROIDS, AIRWAY MANAGEMENT, INCLUDING INTUBATION, SHOULD ALSO BE ADMINISTERED AS INDICATED.

Precautions: Prolonged use of antibiotics may promote the overgrowth of nonsusceptible organisms. If superinfection occurs during therapy, appropriate measures should be taken.

PREGNANCY: Pregnancy Category B. Reproduction studies have been performed in mice and rats at doses up to ten times the human dose and have revealed no evidence of impaired fertility or harm to the fetus due to cyclacillin. There are, however, no adequate and well-controlled studies in pregnant women. Because animal reproduction studies are not always predictive of human response, this drug should be used during pregnancy only if clearly needed.

NURSING MOTHERS: It is not known whether this drug is excreted in human milk. Because many drugs are excreted in human milk, caution should be exercised when cyclacillin is administered to a nursing woman.

Adverse Reactions: The oral administration of cyclacillin is generally well-tolerated.
As with other penicillins, untoward reactions of the sensitivity phenomena are likely to occur, particularly in individuals who have previously demonstrated hypersensitivity to penicillins or in those with a history of allergy, asthma, hay fever, or urticaria.

The following adverse reactions have been reported with the use of cyclacillin: diarrhea (in approximately 1 out of 20 patients treated), nausea and vomiting (in approximately 1 in 50), and skin rash (in approximately 1 in 60). Isolated instances of headache, dizziness, abdominal pain, vaginitis, and urticaria have been reported. (See WARNINGS)

Other less-frequent adverse reactions which may occur and that have been reported during therapy with other penicillins are: anemia, thrombocytopenia, thrombocytopenic purpura, leukopenia, neutropenia, and eosinophilia. These reactions are usually reversible on discontinuation of therapy.

As with other semisynthetic penicillins, SGOT elevations have been reported.

Dosage and Administration:
[See table on next page]
Patients with Renal Failure
Based on a dosage of 500 mg q.i.d., the following adjustment in dosage interval is recommended:
Patients with a creatinine clearance of > 50 ml/min need no dosage interval adjustment.
Patients with a creatinine clearance of 30–50 ml/min should receive full doses every 12 hours.
Patients with a creatinine clearance of between 15–30 ml/min should receive full doses every 18 hours.
Patients with a creatinine clearance of between 10–15 ml/min should receive full doses every 24 hours.
In patients with a creatinine clearance of ≤ 10 ml/min or serum creatinine values of ≥ 10 mg%, serum cyclacillin levels are recommended to determine both subsequent dosage and frequency.

How Supplied: Cyclapen-W® (cyclacillin) tablets are available in the following strengths:
250 mg, NDC 0008-0614, yellow capsule-shaped scored tablet embossed with "WYETH" and "614", supplied in bottles of 100 tablets.
500 mg, NDC 0008-0615, yellow capsule-shaped scored tablet embossed with "WYETH" and "615", supplied in bottles of 100 tablets.

Keep bottles tightly closed.
Dispense in tight containers.
Cyclapen-W (cyclacillin) for oral suspension is available in the following strengths:
125 mg per 5 ml, NDC 0008-0599, white to pinkish-white powder supplied in bottles to make 100, 150, and 200 ml of suspension.
250 mg per 5 ml, NDC 0008-0600, white to pinkish-white powder supplied in bottles to make 100, 150, and 200 ml of suspension.

After reconstituting, as directed on the package label, store under refrigeration.
Discard any unused portion after 14 days.

References:
1. BAUER, A.W., KIRBY, W.M.M., SHERRIS, J.C. and TURCK, M.; Antibiotic Testing by a Standardized Single Disc Method, Am. J. Clin. Pathol. 45:493, 1966. Standardized Disc Susceptibility Test, FEDERAL REGISTER 37:20527-29, 1972.
2. National Committee for Laboratory Standards; Approved Standard-2; Performance Standards for Antimicrobial Disc Susceptibility Tests, 1976.
3. ERICSON, H. M., and SHERRIS, J.C.; Antibiotic Sensitivity Testing Report of an International Collaborative Study, ACTA, Pathol. Microbiol. Scand., Section B:217, 1971.

Shown in Product Identification Section, page 444

EQUAGESIC® ℰ ℬ
[ek″ wa-je′ zik]
(meprobamate with aspirin)

Description: Each tablet of Equagesic contains 200 mg meprobamate and 325 mg aspirin.

Actions: Meprobamate is a carbamate derivative which has been shown (in animal and/or human studies) to have effects at multiple sites in the central nervous system, including the thalamus and limbic system.
Aspirin, acetylsalicylic acid, is a nonnarcotic analgesic with antipyretic and anti-inflammatory properties.

Indications: As an adjunct in the short-term treatment of pain accompanied by tension and/or anxiety in patients with musculoskeletal disease. Clinical trials have demonstrated that in these situations relief of pain is somewhat greater than with aspirin alone.
The effectiveness of Equagesic in long-term use, that is, more than 4 months, has not been assessed by systematic clinical studies. The physician should periodically reassess the usefulness of the drug for the individual patient.

Contraindications:
ASPIRIN:
Allergic or idiosyncratic reactions to aspirin or related compounds.

Product Information

MEPROBAMATE:
Acute intermittent porphyria and allergic or idiosyncratic reactions to meprobamate or related compounds, such as carisoprodol, mebutamate, or carbromal.

Warnings:
ASPIRIN:
Salicylates should be used with extreme caution in patients with peptic ulcer, asthma, coagulation abnormalities, hypoprothrombinemia, vitamin K deficiency, or in those on anticoagulant therapy. In rare instances, the use of aspirin in persons allergic to salicylates may result in life-threatening allergic episodes.

MEPROBAMATE:
DRUG DEPENDENCE: Physical dependence, psychological dependence, and abuse have occurred. Chronic intoxication from prolonged ingestion of, usually, greater-than-recommended doses is manifested by ataxia, slurred speech and vertigo. Therefore, careful supervision of dose and amounts prescribed is advised, as well as avoidance of prolonged administration, especially for alcoholics and other patients with a known propensity for taking excessive quantities of drugs. Sudden withdrawal of the drug after prolonged and excessive use may precipitate recurrence of preexisting symptoms such as anxiety, anorexia, or insomnia, or withdrawal reactions such as vomiting, ataxia, tremors, muscle twitching, confusional states, hallucinosis, and, rarely, convulsive seizures. Such seizures are more likely to occur in persons with central-nervous-system damage or preexistent or latent convulsive disorders. Onset of withdrawal symptoms occurs usually within 12 to 48 hours after discontinuation of meprobamate; symptoms usually cease within the next 12- to 48-hour period.
When excessive dosage has continued for weeks or months, dosage should be reduced gradually over a period of 1 to 2 weeks rather than abruptly stopped. Alternatively, a short-acting barbiturate may be substituted, then gradually withdrawn.
POTENTIALLY HAZARDOUS TASKS: Patients should be warned that meprobamate may impair the mental or physical abilities required for performance of potentially hazardous tasks, such as driving or operating machinery.
ADDITIVE EFFECTS: Since CNS-suppressant effects of meprobamate and alcohol or meprobamate and other psychotropic drugs may be additive, appropriate caution should be exercised with patients who take more than one of these agents simultaneously.

USAGE IN PREGNANCY AND LACTATION
An increased risk of congenital malformations associated with the use of minor tranquilizers (meprobamate, chlordiazepoxide, and diazepam) during the first trimester of pregnancy has been suggested in several studies. Because use of these drugs is rarely a matter of urgency, their use during this period should almost always be avoided. The possibility that a woman of childbearing potential may be pregnant at the time of institution of therapy should be considered. Patients should be advised that if they become pregnant during therapy or intend to become pregnant they should communicate with their physicians about the desirability of discontinuing the drug.
Meprobamate passes the placental barrier. It is present both in umbilical-cord blood at or near maternal plasma levels and in breast milk of lactating mothers at concentrations two to four times that of maternal plasma. When use of meprobamate is contemplated in breast-feeding patients, the drug's higher concentrations in breast milk as compared to maternal plasma levels should be considered.
USAGE IN CHILDREN: Preparations containing aspirin should be kept out of the reach of children. Equagesic (meprobamate with aspirin) is not recommended for patients 12 years of age and under.

Precautions:
ASPIRIN:
Salicylates antagonize the uricosuric activity of probenecid and sulfinpyrazone. Salicylates are reported to enhance the hypoglycemic effect of the sulfonylurea antidiabetic drugs.

MEPROBAMATE:
The lowest effective dose should be administered, particularly to elderly and/or debilitated patients, in order to preclude oversedation.
Meprobamate is metabolized in the liver and excreted by the kidney; to avoid its excess accumulation, caution should be exercised in the administration to patients with compromised liver or kidney function.
Meprobamate occasionally may precipitate seizures in epileptic patients.
The drug should be prescribed cautiously and in small quantities to patients with suicidal tendencies.

Adverse Reactions:
ASPIRIN:
Aspirin may cause epigastric discomfort, nausea, and vomiting. Hypersensitivity reactions, including urticaria, angioneurotic edema, purpura, asthma, and anaphylaxis, may rarely occur.
Patients receiving large doses of salicylates may develop tinnitus.

MEPROBAMATE:
CENTRAL NERVOUS SYSTEM: Drowsiness, ataxia, dizziness, slurred speech, headache, vertigo, weakness, paresthesias, impairment of visual accommodation, euphoria, overstimulation, paradoxical excitement, fast EEG activity.
GASTROINTESTINAL: Nausea, vomiting, diarrhea.
CARDIOVASCULAR: Palpitation, tachycardia, various forms of arrhythmia, transient ECG changes, syncope, hypotensive crisis.
ALLERGIC OR IDIOSYNCRATIC: Milder reactions are characterized by an itchy, urticarial, or erythematous maculopapular rash which may be generalized or confined to the groin. Other reactions have included leukopenia, acute nonthrombocytopenic purpura, petechiae, ecchymoses, eosinophilia, peripheral edema, adenopathy, fever, fixed drug eruption with cross-reaction to carisoprodol, and cross-sensitivity between meprobamate/mebutamate and meprobamate/carbromal.
More severe hypersensitivity reactions, rarely reported, include hyperpyrexia, chills, angioneurotic edema, bronchospasm, oliguria, and anuria. Also, anaphylaxis, exfoliative dermatitis, stomatitis and proctitis, Stevens-Johnson syndrome and bullous dermatitis have occurred.
HEMATOLOGIC (SEE ALSO "ALLERGIC OR IDIOSYNCRATIC"): Agranulocytosis, aplastic anemia have been reported, although no causal relationship has been established, and thrombocytopenic purpura.
OTHER: Exacerbation of porphyric symptoms.
Dosage and Administration: The usual dosage of Equagesic (meprobamate with aspirin) is one or two tablets, each tablet containing meprobamate, 200 mg, and aspirin, 325 mg, orally 3 to 4 times daily as needed for the relief of pain when tension or anxiety is present.
Equagesic is not recommended for patients 12 years of age and under.
Overdosage: Treatment of overdose with Equagesic is essentially symptomatic and supportive. Any drug remaining in the stomach should be removed. Induction of vomiting or gastric lavage may be indicated. Activated charcoal may reduce absorption of both aspirin and meprobamate.
Overdosage with aspirin produces the usual symptoms and signs of salicylate intoxication. Observation and treatment should include management of hyperthermia, specific parenteral electrolyte therapy for ketoacidosis and dehydration, watching for

Continued on next page

Cyclapen-W

INFECTION*	ADULTS	CHILDREN
		Dosage should not result in a dose higher than that for adults.
Respiratory Tract Tonsillitis & Pharyngitis**	250 mg q.i.d. in equally spaced doses	body weight < 20 kg (44 lbs) 125 mg t.i.d. in equally spaced doses body weight > 20 kg (44 lbs) 250 mg t.i.d. in equally spaced doses
Bronchitis and Pneumonia Mild or Moderate Infections	250 mg q.i.d. in equally spaced doses	50 mg/kg/day q.i.d. in equally spaced doses
Chronic Infections	500 mg q.i.d. in equally spaced doses	100 mg/kg/day q.i.d. in equally spaced doses
Otitis Media	250 mg to 500 mg q.i.d. in equally spaced doses depending on severity	50 to 100 mg/kg/day t.i.d. in equally spaced doses depending on severity
Skin & Skin Structures	250 mg to 500 mg q.i.d. in equally spaced doses depending on severity	50 to 100 mg/kg/day in equally spaced doses depending on severity
Urinary Tract	500 mg q.i.d. in equally spaced doses	100 mg/kg/day in equally spaced doses

*As with antibiotic therapy generally, treatment should be continued for a minimum of 48 to 72 hours after the patient becomes asymptomatic or until evidence of bacterial eradication has been obtained.
**In infections caused by Group A beta-hemolytic streptococci, a minimum of 10 days of treatment is recommended to guard against the risk of rheumatic fever or glomerulonephritis.
In the treatment of chronic urinary tract infection, frequent bacteriologic and clinical appraisal is necessary during therapy and may be required for several months afterwards.
Persistent infection may require treatment for several weeks.
Cyclacillin is not indicated in children under 2 months of age.

Wyeth—Cont.

evidence of hemorrhagic manifestations due to hypoprothrombinemia which, if it occurs, usually requires whole-blood transfusions.

Suicidal attempts with meprobamate have resulted in drowsiness, lethargy, stupor, ataxia, coma, shock, vasomotor and respiratory collapse. Some suicidal attempts have been fatal.

The following data have been reported in the literature and from other sources. These data are not expected to correlate with each case (considering factors such as individual susceptibility and length of time from ingestion to treatment), but represent the usual ranges reported.

Acute simple overdose (meprobamate alone): Death has been reported with ingestion of as little as 12 grams meprobamate and survival with as much as 40 grams.

BLOOD LEVELS:

0.5–2.0 mg percent represents the usual blood-level range of meprobamate after therapeutic doses. The level may occasionally be as high as 3.0 mg percent.

3–10 mg percent usually corresponds to findings of mild-to-moderate symptoms of overdosage, such as stupor or light coma.

10–20 mg percent usually corresponds to deeper coma, requiring more intensive treatment. Some fatalities occur.

At levels greater than 20 mg percent, more fatalities than survivals can be expected.

Acute combined overdose (meprobamate with other psychotropic drugs or alcohol): Since effects can be additive, a history of ingestion of a low dose of meprobamate plus any of these compounds (or of a relatively low blood or tissue level) cannot be used as a prognostic indicator.

In cases where excessive doses have been taken, sleep ensues rapidly and blood pressure, pulse, and respiratory rates are reduced to basal levels. Any drug remaining in the stomach should be removed and symptomatic treatment given. Should respiration or blood pressure become compromised, respiratory assistance, central-nervous-system stimulants, and pressor agents should be administered cautiously as indicated. Diuresis, osmotic (mannitol) diuresis, peritoneal dialysis, and hemodialysis have been used successfully in removing both aspirin and meprobamate. Alkalinization of the urine increases the excretion of salicylates. Careful monitoring of urinary output is necessary, and caution should be taken to avoid overhydration. Relapse and death, after initial recovery, have been attributed to incomplete gastric emptying and delayed absorption.

How Supplied: Equagesic® (meprobamate with aspirin) scored tablets are available in bottles of 100 tablets, in Redipak® strip packs of 25 tablets, and in Redipak unit-dose cartons of 100 individually wrapped tablets.

The appearance of EQUAGESIC tablets is a registered trademark of Wyeth Laboratories.

Shown in Product Identification Section, page 444

EQUANIL®
[ek'wah-nil]
(meprobamate)
Tablets

How Supplied: Tablets (white, scored)—200 mg and 400 mg, bottles of 50, 100, 500, 1000, and REDIPAK® (Strip Pack), boxes of 25; REDIPAK® (Unit Dose Medication), boxes of 100 (individually wrapped). WYSEALS® EQUANIL (meprobamate), especially coated for easy swallowing, sealed yellow tablets—400 mg, bottles of 50.

For prescribing information write to Professional Service, Wyeth Laboratories,
Box 8299, Philadelphia, PA, 19101,
or contact your local Wyeth representative.

Shown in Product Identification Section, page 444

FUROSEMIDE
[fu-roh'sa-mide]
Injection, USP

> **Warning**
> Furosemide is a potent diuretic which, if given in excessive amounts, can lead to a profound diuresis with water and electrolyte depletion. Therefore, careful medical supervision is required, and the individual dose and the dosage schedule have to be adjusted to each patient's needs. (See under "Dosage and Administration.")

Description: Furosemide is an anthranilic acid derivative, chemically known as 4-chloro-N-furfuryl-5-sulfamoyl-anthranilic acid.

Furosemide is a white to slightly yellow, odorless, crystalline powder. It is practically insoluble in water and acid; freely soluble in acetone, in dimethylformamide, and in solutions of base; soluble in methanol; sparingly soluble in alcohol; slightly soluble in ether; very slightly soluble in chloroform.

Furosemide Injection, USP, is a sterile solution of furosemide in water for injection prepared with the aid of sodium hydroxide to make the solution slightly alkaline. Each ml contains furosemide, 10 mg, and sodium chloride for isotonicity. The preparation contains no antimicrobial preservatives and is intended for single use only. Any portion of the solution remaining after injection must be discarded.

Clinical Pharmacology: Furosemide has been demonstrated to act primarily by inhibiting the reabsorption of sodium in the loop of Henle as well as in the proximal and distal tubules. Its high degree of efficacy is attributed to its principal site of action. The action on the distal tubule is independent of any inhibitory effect on carbonic anhydrase and aldosterone.

Diuresis commences within five minutes following an intravenous injection and somewhat later after intramuscular injection. The diuresis reaches its peak within the first half hour and lasts for approximately two hours.

Furosemide is often effective in patients with markedly reduced glomerular filtration rates in whom other diuretics usually fail. This is because furosemide inhibits the reabsorption of a very high percentage of the filtered sodium.

Indications: For the treatment of the edema associated with congestive heart failure, cirrhosis of the liver, and renal disease, including the nephrotic syndrome. Furosemide is particularly useful when an agent with greater diuretic potential than that of the more commonly used agents is desired. Furosemide is indicated as adjunctive therapy in acute pulmonary edema.

Intravenous administration is indicated when a rapid onset of diuresis is desired, e.g., acute pulmonary edema. The intramuscular or intravenous route is indicated if gastrointestinal absorption is impaired or oral medication is not practical for any reason. Oral furosemide should be substituted for parenteral as soon as possible.

NOTE: Parenteral administration should be reserved for patients for whom oral medication is not practical or for emergency clinical situations.

Contraindications: Furosemide is contraindicated in anuria. If increasing azotemia and oliguria occur during treatment of severe progressive renal disease, the drug should be discontinued. In hepatic coma and in states of electrolyte depletion, furosemide therapy should not be instituted until the basic condition is improved or corrected. Furosemide is also contraindicated in patients with a history of hypersensitivity to this compound.

Because animal-reproductive studies have shown that furosemide may cause fetal abnormalities and maternal death, the drug is contraindicated in women of childbearing potential. An exception exists in life-threatening situations where the use of a diuretic, such as furosemide by injection, is considered of paramount importance over the use of alternative drugs and where the physician has considered the efficacy potential against the risks. (See "Precautions"—"Teratogenic Effects.")

Furosemide should not be used concomitantly with cephaloridine, since diuretics, such as furosemide, are reported to enhance the nephrotoxicity of cephaloridine.

Warnings: Excessive diuresis may result in dehydration and reduction in blood volume, with circulatory collapse and the possibility of vascular thrombosis and embolism, particularly in elderly patients.

Excessive loss of potassium in patients receiving digitalis glycosides may precipitate digitalis toxicity. Care should also be exercised in patients receiving potassium-depleting steroids because of the added potassium loss due to furosemide.

Frequent serum electrolyte, CO_2, and BUN determinations should be performed during the first few months of therapy and periodically thereafter, and abnormalities corrected or the drug temporarily withdrawn.

In patients with hepatic cirrhosis and ascites, initiation of therapy with furosemide is best carried out in the hospital. Sudden alteration of fluid and electrolyte balance in patients with cirrhosis may precipitate hepatic coma; therefore, strict observation is necessary during the period of diuresis. Supplemental potassium chloride and, if required, an aldosterone antagonist are helpful in preventing hypokalemia and metabolic alkalosis.

Patients with known sulfonamide sensitivity may show allergic reactions to furosemide.

Cases of tinnitus and reversible hearing impairment have been reported. There have also been some reports of cases in which irreversible hearing impairment occurred. Usually, ototoxicity has been reported when furosemide was injected rapidly in patients with severe impairment of renal function at doses exceeding several times the usual recommended dose and to whom other drugs known to be ototoxic were also given.

If the physician elects to use high-dose parenteral therapy in patients with severely impaired renal function, controlled intravenous infusion is advisable (for adults, it has been reported that an infusion rate not exceeding 4 mg furosemide per minute has been used). (See "Dosage and Administration.")

Parenterally administered furosemide may increase the ototoxic potential of aminoglycoside antibiotics. Especially in the presence of impaired renal function, the use of parenterally administered furosemide in patients to whom aminoglycoside antibiotics are also being given should be avoided except in life-threatening situations.

The possibility exists of exacerbation or activation of systemic lupus erythematosus.

Furosemide appears in breast milk. If use of the drug is deemed essential, the patient should stop nursing.

Precautions: As with any effective diuretic, electrolyte depletion may occur during therapy with furosemide, especially in patients receiving higher doses and on a restricted salt intake.

All patients receiving furosemide therapy should have laboratory determinations of serum electrolytes at appropriate intervals to detect fluid or electrolyte imbalance, namely, hyponatremia, hypochloremic alkalosis, or hypokalemia. Serum and urine electrolyte determinations are particularly important when the patient is vomiting excessively or receiving parenteral fluids. Hypokalemia may develop with furosemide as with any other potent diuretic, especially with brisk diuresis, when cirrhosis is present, or during concomitant use of corticosteroids or ACTH. Interference with adequate oral electrolyte intake will also contribute to hypokalemia. Medication, such as digitalis, may also influence serum electrolytes. Warning signs of fluid or electrolyte imbalance, irrespective of cause, are: dryness of mouth, thirst, weakness, mental confusion, lethargy, drowsiness, restlessness, muscle pains or cramps, muscular fatigue, hypotension, oliguria, tachycardia, arrhythmia, and gastrointestinal disturbances, such as nausea and vomiting.

Furosemide may lower serum calcium levels, and rare cases of tetany have been reported. Accordingly, periodic serum calcium levels should be obtained.

Asymptomatic hyperuricemia can occur, and gout may rarely be precipitated. Reversible elevations of BUN may be seen. These have been observed in association with dehydration which should be avoided, particularly in patients with renal insufficiency.

As with many other drugs, patients should be observed regularly for the possible occurrence of blood dyscrasias, liver damage, or other idiosyncratic reactions.

In patients being treated with antihypertensive agents, care should be taken to reduce the dose of these drugs when furosemide is administered, since furosemide potentiates the hypotensive effect of antihypertensive medications.

Periodic checks on urine and blood glucose should be made in diabetics and even those suspected of latent diabetes when receiving furosemide. Increases in blood glucose and alterations in glucose tolerance tests, with abnormalities of the fasting and two-hour postprandial sugar, have been observed; rare cases of precipitation of diabetes mellitus have been reported.

Patients receiving high doses of salicylates, as in rheumatic diseases, in conjunction with furosemide may experience salicylate toxicity at lower doses because of competitive renal excretory sites.

Sulfonamide diuretics have been reported to decrease arterial responsiveness to pressor amines and to enhance the effect of tubocurarine. Therefore, great caution should be exercised in administering curare or its derivatives to patients undergoing therapy with furosemide, and it is advisable to discontinue furosemide two days prior to any elective surgery.

It has been reported in the literature that coadministration of indomethacin may reduce the natriuretic and antihypertensive effects of furosemide in some patients. This effect has been attributed to inhibition of prostaglandin synthesis by indomethacin. Indomethacin may also affect plasma renin levels and aldosterone excretion; this should be borne in mind when a renin profile is evaluated in hypertensive patients. Patients receiving both indomethacin and furosemide should be observed closely to determine if the desired diuretic and/or antihypertensive effect of furosemide is achieved.

Lithium generally should not be given with diuretics, because they reduce its renal clearance and add a high risk of lithium toxicity.

TERATOGENIC EFFECTS—PREGNANCY CATEGORY C

Furosemide has been shown to cause unexplained maternal deaths and abortions in rabbits at 2, 4 and 8 times the human dose. There are no adequate and well-controlled studies in pregnant women. Furosemide should be used during pregnancy only if the potential benefit justifies the potential risk to the fetus and mother. (See "Contraindications.")

The effects of furosemide on the embryonic and fetal development and on pregnant dams were studied in mice, rats, and rabbits.

Furosemide caused unexplained maternal deaths and abortions in the rabbit when 50 mg/kg (4 times the maximal recommended human dose of 600 mg per day) was administered between days 12 and 17 of gestation. In a previous study the lowest dose of only 25 mg/kg (2 times the maximal recommended human dose of 600 mg per day) caused maternal deaths and abortions. In a third study, none of the pregnant rabbits survived a dose of 100 mg/kg. Data from the above studies indicate fetal lethality which can precede maternal deaths.

The results of the mouse study and one of the three rabbit studies also showed an increased incidence of hydronephrosis (distention of the renal pelvis and, in some cases, of the ureters) in fetuses derived from treated dams as compared to the incidence in fetuses from the control group.

Adverse Reactions:
GASTROINTESTINAL: anorexia, nausea, vomiting, cramping, diarrhea, and constipation.

CENTRAL NERVOUS SYSTEM: dizziness, vertigo, paresthesias, headache, xanthopsia, blurred vision, and tinnitus and hearing loss.
HEMATOLOGIC: anemia, leukopenia, agranulocytosis (rare), thrombocytopenia (with purpura), and aplastic anemia (rare).
DERMATOLOGIC-HYPERSENSITIVITY: photosensitivity, rash, urticaria, necrotizing angiitis (vasculitis, cutaneous vasculitis), exfoliative dermatitis, erythema multiforme, and pruritus.
CARDIOVASCULAR: Orthostatic hypotension may occur and be aggravated by alcohol, barbiturates, or narcotics.
OTHER: hyperglycemia, glycosuria, hyperuricemia and gout, muscle spasm, weakness, restlessness, urinary bladder spasm, thrombophlebitis, and transient pain at the injection site following intramuscular injection.

In addition the following rare adverse reactions have been reported; however, relationship to the drug has not been established with certainty: sweet taste, oral and gastric burning, paradoxical swelling, headache, intrahepatic cholestatic jaundice, and acute pancreatitis.

In children, complaints of mild-to-moderate abdominal pain and cramping have been reported after intravenous furosemide.

Whenever adverse reactions are moderate or severe, furosemide dosage should be reduced or therapy withdrawn.

Dosage and Administration: Parenteral drug products should be inspected visually for particulate matter and discoloration prior to administration whenever solution and container permit.

Do not use if solution is discolored or contains a precipitate.

ADULTS

Parenteral therapy should be reserved for patients for whom oral medication is not practical or in emergency situations where prompt diuresis is desired. Parenteral therapy should be replaced by oral therapy as soon as this is practical for continued mobilization of edema.

Edema

The usual initial dose of furosemide is 20 to 40 mg given as a single dose, injected intramuscularly or intravenously. The intravenous injection should be given slowly (1 to 2 minutes).

Ordinarily, a prompt diuresis ensues. Depending on the patient's response, a second dose can be administered 2 hours after the first dose or later. If the diuretic response with a single dose of 20 to 40 mg is not satisfactory, increase this dose by increments of 20 mg not sooner than 2 hours after the previous dose until the desired diuretic effect has been obtained. This individually determined single dose should then be given once or twice daily.

Therapy should be individualized according to patient response. This therapy should be titrated to gain maximal therapeutic response as well as the minimal dose possible to maintain that therapeutic response. Close medical supervision is necessary.

If the physician elects to use high-dose parenteral therapy, it should be administered as a controlled infusion at a rate not exceeding 4 mg/min. Furosemide injection is a mildly buffered alkaline solution which should not be mixed with acidic solutions of pH below 5.5. To prepare infusion solutions, isotonic saline and lactated Ringer's injection and 5% dextrose injection have been used after pH has been adjusted when necessary.

Before diluting with any other intravenous solution or combining with any medication, consult specialized literature. Do not use if there is any indication of precipitation or other signs of incompatibility.

Acute Pulmonary Edema

The usual initial dose of furosemide is 40 mg, injected intravenously. The injection should be given slowly (1 to 2 minutes). If 40 mg furosemide does not produce a satisfactory response within one hour, the dose may be increased to 80 mg, given intravenously (over 1 to 2 minutes).

If deemed necessary, additional therapy (e.g., digitalis, oxygen) can be administered concomitantly

with caution (see "Warnings" regarding digitalis toxicity).
INFANTS AND CHILDREN
Parenteral therapy should be reserved for patients for whom oral medication is not practical or in emergency situations where prompt diuresis is desired. Parenteral therapy should be replaced by oral therapy as soon as this is practical for continued mobilization of edema.

The usual initial dose of furosemide injection (intravenously or intramuscularly) in infants and children is 1 mg/kg body weight and should be given slowly under close medical supervision. If the diuretic response after the initial dose is not satisfactory, dosage may be increased by 1 mg/kg, not sooner than 2 hours after the previous dose, until the desired diuretic effect has been obtained. Doses greater than 6 mg/kg body weight are not recommended.

How Supplied: Furosemide Injection, USP, Wyeth®, is available in the following dosage strength in packages of 25 ampuls and in TUBEX® Sterile Cartridge-Needle Units, packaged in boxes of 10 TUBEX.

10 mg per ml, NDC 0008-0628; 2 ml, 4 ml, and 10 ml ampuls and 2 ml TUBEX.

Store at Controlled Room Temperature, 15°–30° C (59°–86° F).

Protect TUBEX from light.

HEPARIN ℞
[hep'ah-rin]
Lock Flush Solution, USP
anticoagulant for clearing
intermittent infusion sets

Description: Wyeth's TUBEX® Heparin Lock Flush Solution, USP, is a sterile solution. Each ml contains either 10 or 100 USP units heparin sodium derived from porcine intestinal mucosa (standardized for use as an anticoagulant) in normal saline solution, and not more than 10 mg benzyl alcohol as a preservative.

The potency is determined by biological assay, using a USP reference standard based upon units of heparin activity per milligram.

Actions: See Heparin Sodium Injection, USP.
Indications: See Heparin Sodium Injection, USP.
Contraindications: See Heparin Sodium Injection, USP.
Warnings: See Heparin Sodium Injection, USP.
Precautions: See Heparin Sodium Injection, USP.
Adverse Reactions: See Heparin Sodium Injection, USP.
Dosage and Administration: See Heparin Sodium Injection, USP.
CLEARING INTERMITTENT INFUSION (HEPARIN LOCK) SETS

To prevent clot formation in a heparin lock set following its proper insertion, dilute heparin solution is injected via the injection hub in a quantity sufficient to fill the entire set to the needle tip. This solution should be replaced each time the heparin lock is used. Aspirate before administering any solution via the lock in order to confirm patency and location of needle or catheter tip. If the drug to be administered is incompatible with heparin, the entire heparin lock set should be flushed with sterile water or normal saline before and after the medication is administered; following the second flush, the dilute heparin solution may be reinstilled into the set. The set manufacturer's instructions should be consulted for specifics concerning the heparin lock set in use at a given time.

NOTE: Since repeated injections of small doses of heparin can alter tests for activated partial thromboplastin time (APTT), a baseline value for APTT should be obtained prior to insertion of a heparin lock set.

Overdosage: See Heparin Sodium Injection, USP.

How Supplied: Heparin Lock Flush Solution, USP, anticoagulant for clearing intermittent infu-

Continued on next page

Wyeth—Cont.

sion sets, is available as 1 ml and 2.5 ml TUBEX® Sterile Cartridge-Needle Units, each ml containing 10 USP units or 100 USP units of Heparin Sodium, in packages of 50 TUBEX.

HEPARIN ℞
[*hep'ah-rin*]
Sodium Injection, USP

Description: Wyeth's TUBEX® Heparin Sodium Injection, USP, is a sterile solution. Each ml contains 1,000, 2,500, 5,000, 7,500, 10,000, 15,000, or 20,000 USP units heparin sodium, derived from porcine intestinal mucosa (standardized for use as an anticoagulant), in water for injection, and not more than 10 mg benzyl alcohol as a preservative. The potency is determined by biological assay, using a USP reference standard based upon units of heparin activity per milligram.

Actions: Heparin inhibits reactions which lead to the clotting of blood and the formation of fibrin clots both *in vitro* and *in vivo*. Heparin acts at multiple sites in the normal coagulation system. Small amounts of heparin in combination with antithrombin III (heparin cofactor) can prevent the development of a hypercoagulable state by inactivating activated Factor X, preventing the conversion of prothrombin to thrombin. Once a hypercoagulable state exists, larger amounts of heparin in combination with antithrombin III can inhibit the coagulation process by inactivating thrombin and earlier clotting intermediates, thus preventing the conversion of fibrinogen to fibrin. Heparin also prevents the formation of a stable fibrin clot by inhibiting the activation of the fibrin stabilizing factor.

Bleeding time is usually unaffected by heparin. Clotting time is prolonged by full therapeutic doses of heparin; in most cases it is not measurably affected by low doses of heparin.

Heparin does not have fibrinolytic activity; therefore, it will not lyse existing clots.

Indications: Heparin sodium injection is indicated for anticoagulant therapy in prophylaxis and treatment of venous thrombosis and its extension; in low-dose regimen for prevention of postoperative deep venous thrombosis and pulmonary embolism in patients undergoing major abdominothoracic surgery who are at risk of developing thromboembolic disease (see "Dosage and Administration"); for prophylaxis and treatment of pulmonary embolism; in atrial fibrillation with embolization; for diagnosis and treatment of acute and chronic consumptive coagulopathies (disseminated intravascular coagulation); for prevention of clotting in arterial and cardiac surgery; and for prevention of cerebral thrombosis in evolving stroke.

Heparin is indicated as an adjunct in treatment of coronary occlusion with acute myocardial infarction, and in prophylaxis and treatment of peripheral arterial embolism.

Heparin may also be employed as an anticoagulant in blood transfusions, extracorporeal circulation, dialysis procedures, and in blood samples for laboratory purposes.

Contraindications: Hypersensitivity to heparin.
Inability to perform suitable blood-coagulation tests, e.g., the whole-blood clotting time, partial thromboplastin time, etc., at required intervals. There is usually no need to monitor the effect of low-dose heparin in patients with normal coagulation parameters.
Uncontrollable bleeding.

Warnings:

> Heparin sodium should be used with extreme caution in disease states in which there is an increased danger of hemorrhage.

Administration of Heparin Sodium Injection, USP, when used in therapeutic dosage, should be regulated by frequent blood-coagulation tests. If these are unduly prolonged or if hemorrhage occurs, heparin sodium should be promptly discontinued. See "Overdosage."

Some of the conditions in which increased danger of hemorrhage exists are:

CARDIOVASCULAR—subacute bacterial endocarditis; arteriosclerosis; dissecting aneurysm; severe hypertension; capillary permeability; during and immediately following a) spinal tap or spinal anesthesia, b) major surgery, especially involving the brain, spinal cord, or eye.

HEMATOLOGIC—conditions associated with increased bleeding tendencies, such as hemophilia, some purpuras, and thrombocytopenia.

GASTROINTESTINAL—diverticulitis, ulcerative colitis, inaccessible ulcerative lesions, and continuous tube drainage of the stomach or small intestine.

Also in the presence of severe hepatic, renal, or biliary disease and threatened abortion.

Heparin sodium may prolong the one-stage prothrombin time. Accordingly, when heparin sodium is given with dicumarol or warfarin sodium, a period of at least 5 hours after the last intravenous dose and 24 hours after the last subcutaneous (intrafat) dose of heparin sodium should elapse before blood is drawn, if a valid prothrombin time is to be obtained.

Drugs (such as aspirin, dextran, phenylbutazone, ibuprofen, indomethacin, dipyridamole, and hydroxychloroquine) which interfere with platelet aggregation reactions (the main hemostatic defense of heparinized patients) may induce bleeding and should be used with caution in patients on heparin therapy.

While there is experimental evidence that heparin may antagonize the action of ACTH, insulin, or corticoids, this effect has not been clearly defined. There is also evidence in animal experiments that heparin may modify or inhibit allergic reactions. However, the application of these findings to human patients has not been fully defined.

Larger doses of heparin may be necessary in the febrile state.

The use of digitalis, tetracyclines, nicotine, or antihistamines may partially counteract the anticoagulant action of heparin. An increased resistance to heparin is frequently encountered in cases of thrombosis, thrombophlebitis, infections with thrombosing tendency, myocardial infarction, cancer, and in the postoperative patient.

Because of the possibility of acute thrombocytopenia occurring when heparin is administered, platelet counts should be monitored before and during heparin therapy. If significant thrombocytopenia occurs, heparin should be immediately terminated, and oral anticoagulation substituted, if necessary. If new evidence of thrombosis appears during heparin therapy, especially in the arterial system, it should be borne in mind that it may be a paradoxical result of the therapy itself, possibly as a result of platelet aggregation. Heparin should be discontinued and oral anticoagulation employed, especially if there is associated thrombocytopenia, as noted above.

USAGE IN PREGNANCY

Heparin sodium injection should be used with caution during pregnancy, especially during the last trimester and in the immediate postpartum period.

There is no adequate information as to whether heparin may affect human fertility, or have a teratogenic potential or other adverse effects to the fetus.

Heparin does not cross the placental barrier; it is not excreted in human milk.

Precautions

Because heparin sodium injection is derived from animal tissue, it should be used with caution in patients with a history of allergy. Before a therapeutic dose is given to such a patient, a trial dose of 1,000 units may be advisable.

Heparin sodium should also be used with caution in the presence of hepatic or renal disease, hypertension, during menstruation, or in patients with indwelling catheters.

A higher incidence of bleeding may be seen in women over 60 years of age.

Caution should be exercised when administering ACD-converted blood (i.e., blood collected in heparin sodium and later converted to ACD blood), since the anticoagulant activity of its heparin sodium content persists without loss for 22 days. ACD-converted blood may alter the coagulation system of the recipient, especially if it is given in multiple transfusions.

Adverse Reactions

Hemorrhage is the chief complication that may result from heparin therapy. An overly prolonged clotting time or minor bleeding during therapy can usually be controlled by withdrawing the drug. See "Overdosage."

The occurrence of significant gastrointestinal or urinary-tract bleeding during anticoagulant therapy may indicate the presence of an underlying occult lesion.

Adrenal hemorrhage with resultant acute adrenal insufficiency has occurred during anticoagulant therapy. Therefore, such treatment should be discontinued in patients who develop signs and symptoms compatible with acute adrenal hemorrhage and insufficiency. Plasma cortisol levels should be measured immediately, and vigorous therapy with intravenous corticosteroids should be instituted promptly. Initiation of therapy should not depend upon laboratory confirmation of the diagnosis, since any delay in an acute situation may result in the patient's death.

Intramuscular injection of heparin sodium frequently causes local irritation, mild pain, or hematoma, and for these reasons should be avoided. These effects are less often seen following deep, subcutaneous (intrafat) injection. Histaminelike reactions have also been observed at the site of injection.

Hypersensitivity reactions have been reported with chills, fever, and urticaria as the most usual manifestations. Asthma, rhinitis, lacrimation, and anaphylactoid reactions have also been reported. Vasospastic reactions may develop independent of the origin of heparin, 6 to 10 days after the initiation of therapy and last for 4 to 6 hours. The affected limb is painful, ischemic, and cyanosed. An artery to this limb may have been recently catheterized. After repeat injections, the reaction may gradually increase, to include generalized vasospasms, with cyanosis, tachypnea, feeling of oppression, and headache. Protamine sulfate treatment has no marked therapeutic effect. Itching and burning, especially on the plantar surface of the feet, is possibly based on a similar allergic vasospastic reaction. Chest pain, elevated blood pressure, arthralgias, and/or headache have also been reported in the absence of definite peripheral vasospasm. Anaphylactic shock has been reported rarely following the intravenous administration of heparin sodium.

During clinical studies, acute reversible thrombocytopenia was reported at frequencies varying from 0 to 31%. This occurred 2 to 20 days (average 5 to 9) following the onset of therapy. In some cases this has been associated with immunologically demonstrable factors in the patients' serum resulting in *in vitro* platelet aggregation when heparin and platelets are added. In isolated cases, localized or disseminated thromboses have occurred which may have been related to *in vivo* platelet aggregation. Osteoporosis and suppression of renal function following long-term, high-dose administration, suppression of aldosterone synthesis, delayed transient alopecia, priapism, and rebound hyperlipemia following discontinuation of heparin sodium have also been reported.

Dosage and Administration

Heparin sodium is not effective by oral administration and should be given by deep, subcutaneous (intrafat, i.e., above iliac crest or into the abdominal fat layer) injection, by intermittent intravenous injection, or intravenous infusion. The intramuscular route of administration should be avoided because of the frequent occurrence of hematoma at the injection site.

The dosage of heparin sodium should be adjusted according to the patient's coagulation-test results, which during the first day of treatment should be determined just prior to each injection. Dosage is considered adequate when the whole-blood clotting time is elevated approximately 2.5 to 3 times the control value. (There is usually no need for daily monitoring of the effect of low-dose prophylactic heparin in patients with normal coagulation parameters.)

When heparin sodium is administered by continuous intravenous infusion, coagulation tests should be performed approximately every 4 hours during the early stages of therapy. When it is administered intermittently by intravenous or deep, subcutaneous (intrafat) injection, coagulation tests should be performed before each injection during the early stages of treatment, and daily thereafter. When an oral anticoagulant of the coumarin derivatives, or similar type, is administered with heparin sodium, coagulation tests and prothrombin activity should be determined at the start of therapy. For immediate anticoagulant effect, administer heparin sodium in the usual therapeutic dosage. When the results of the initial prothrombin determination are known, administer the first dose of an oral anticoagulant in the usual initial amount. Thereafter, perform a coagulation test and determine the prothrombin activity at appropriate intervals. A period of at least 5 hours after the last intravenous dose and 24 hours after the last subcutaneous (intrafat) dose of heparin sodium should elapse before blood is drawn if a valid prothrombin time is to be obtained. When the oral anticoagulant shows full effect and prothrombin activity is in the desired therapeutic range, heparin sodium may be discontinued and therapy continued with the oral anticoagulant.

THERAPEUTIC ANTICOAGULANT EFFECT WITH FULL-DOSE HEPARIN

Although dosage must be adjusted for the individual patient according to the results of suitable laboratory tests, the following dosage schedules may be used as guidelines:

[See table above]:

1. *By Deep, Subcutaneous (Intrafat) Injection:* After an initial IV injection of 5,000 units, inject 10,000 to 20,000 units of a concentrated heparin sodium solution subcutaneously, followed by 8,000 to 10,000 units of a concentrated solution subcutaneously every eight hours, or 15,000 to 20,000 units of a concentrated solution every twelve hours. A different site should be used for each injection to prevent the development of a massive hematoma.

2. *By Intermittent Intravenous Injection:* 10,000 units initially, then 5,000 to 10,000 units every four to six hours. These amounts may be given either undiluted or diluted with 50 to 100 ml of isotonic sodium chloride injection.

3. *By Continuous Intravenous Infusion:* After an initial IV injection of 5,000 units of heparin sodium, add 20,000 to 40,000 units to 1,000 ml of isotonic sodium chloride solution for infusion. For most patients, the rate of flow should be adjusted to deliver approximately 20,000 to 40,000 units in 24 hours.

SURGERY OF THE HEART AND BLOOD VESSELS

Patients undergoing total body perfusion for open-heart surgery should receive an initial dose of not less than 150 units of heparin sodium per kilogram of body weight. Frequently, a dose of 300 units of heparin sodium per kilogram of body weight is used for procedures estimated to last less than 60 minutes; or 400 units per kilogram for those estimated to last longer than 60 minutes.

LOW-DOSE PROPHYLAXIS OF POSTOPERATIVE THROMBOEMBOLISM

A number of well-controlled clinical trials have demonstrated that low-dose heparin prophylaxis, given just prior to and after surgery, will reduce the incidence of postoperative deep-vein thrombosis in the legs, as measured by the l-125 fibrinogen technique and venography, and of clinical pulmonary embolism. The most widely used dosage has been 5,000 units 2 hours before surgery and 5,000 units every 8 to 12 hours thereafter for 7 days or until the patient is fully ambulatory, whichever is longer. The heparin is given by deep, subcutaneous injection in the arm or abdomen with a fine needle (25–26 gauge) to minimize tissue trauma. A con-

Method of Administration	Frequency	Recommended Dose [based on 150 lb (68 kg) patient]
Deep, Subcutaneous (Intrafat) Injection	Initial Dose	5,000 units by IV injection followed by 10,000–20,000 units of a concentrated solution, subcutaneously
	Every 8 hours	8,000–10,000 units of a concentrated solution
	(or) Every 12 hours	15,000–20,000 units of a concentrated solution
Intermittent, Intravenous Injection	Initial Dose	10,000 units, either undiluted or in 50–100 ml isotonic sodium chloride injection
	Every 4 to 6 hours	5,000–10,000 units, either undiluted or in 50–100 ml isotonic sodium chloride injection
Intravenous Infusion	Initial Dose	5,000 units by IV injection
	Continuous	20,000–40,000 units in 1,000 ml of isotonic sodium-chloride solution for infusion/day

centrated solution of heparin sodium is recommended. Such prophylaxis should be reserved for patients over 40 undergoing major surgery. Patients with bleeding disorders, those having neurosurgery, spinal anesthesia, eye surgery, or potentially sanguineous operations should be excluded, as well as patients receiving oral anticoagulants or platelet-active drugs (see "Warnings"). The value of such prophylaxis in hip surgery has not been established. The possibility of increased bleeding during surgery or postoperatively should be borne in mind. If such bleeding occurs, discontinuance of heparin and neutralization with protamine sulfate is advisable. If clinical evidence of thromboembolism develops despite low-dose prophylaxis, full therapeutic doses of anticoagulants should be given unless contraindicated. All patients should be screened prior to heparinization to rule out bleeding disorders, and monitoring should be performed with appropriate coagulation tests just prior to surgery. Coagulation-test values should be normal or only slightly elevated. There is usually no need for daily monitoring of the effect of low-dose heparin in patients with normal coagulation parameters.

EXTRACORPOREAL DIALYSIS USE

Follow equipment manufacturer's operating directions carefully.

BLOOD TRANSFUSION

Addition of 400 to 600 USP units per 100 ml of whole blood. Usually, 7,500 USP units of heparin sodium are added to 100 ml of Sterile Sodium Chloride Injection (or 75,000 USP units per 1,000 ml of Sterile Sodium Chloride Injection) and mixed, and from this sterile solution, 6 to 8 ml is added per 100 ml of whole blood. Leukocyte counts should be performed on heparinized blood within two hours after addition of the heparin. Heparinized blood should not be used for isoagglutinin, complement, erythrocyte fragility tests, or platelet counts.

LABORATORY SAMPLES

Addition of 70 to 150 units of heparin sodium per 10 to 20 ml sample of whole blood is usually employed to prevent coagulation of the sample. See comments under "Blood Transfusion."

Overdosage: Protamine sulfate (1% solution) by slow infusion will neutralize heparin. No more than 50 mg should be given, very slowly, in any 10-minute period. Each mg of protamine sulfate neutralizes approximately 100 USP units of heparin (or 1.0 to 1.5 mg neutralizes approximately 1.0 mg of heparin). Heparins derived from various animal sources require different amounts of protamine sulfate for neutralization. This fact is of most importance during procedures of regional heparinization, including dialysis.

Decreasing amounts of protamine are required as time from last heparin injection increases. Thirty minutes after a dose of heparin, approximately 0.5 mg of protamine sulfate is sufficient to neutralize each 100 units of administered heparin. Blood or plasma transfusions may be necessary; these dilute but do not neutralize heparin.

How Supplied: Heparin Sodium Injection, USP, is supplied as follows in TUBEX® Sterile Cartridge-Needle Units:

Each 1 ml size TUBEX contains one of the following concentrations of heparin sodium, in packages of ten TUBEX:

1,000 USP Units per ml (22 gauge × 1-1/4 inch needle)

2,500 USP Units per ml (25 gauge × 5/8 inch needle)

5,000 USP Units per 0.5 ml (10,000 USP Units per ml) (25 gauge × 5/8 inch needle)

5,000 USP Units per ml (22 gauge × 1-1/4 inch needle)

5,000 USP Units per ml (25 gauge × 5/8 inch needle)

7,500 USP Units per ml (25 gauge × 5/8 inch needle)

10,000 USP Units per ml (25 gauge × 5/8 inch needle)

15,000 USP Units per ml (25 gauge × 5/8 inch needle)

20,000 USP Units per ml (25 gauge × 5/8 inch needle)

Each 2.5 ml size contains the following concentration of heparin sodium, in packages of 50 TUBEX:

2,500 USP Units per TUBEX or 1,000 USP Units per ml (25 gauge × 5/8 inch needle)

LO/OVRAL®   ℞

[lōh-ōh'vral]

Tablets

(norgestrel and ethinyl estradiol tablets)

Description: Each LO/OVRAL® tablet contains 0.3 mg of norgestrel (dl-13-beta-ethyl-17-alpha-ethinyl-17-beta-hydroxygon- 4-en-3-one), a totally synthetic progestogen, and 0.03 mg of ethinyl estradiol (19-nor-17α-pregna-1,3,5 (10)-trien-20-yne-3,17-diol).

Clinical Pharmacology: Combination oral contraceptives act primarily through the mechanism of gonadotropin suppression due to the estrogenic and progestational activity of the ingredients. Although the primary mechanism of action is inhibition of ovulation, alterations in the genital tract, including changes in the cervical mucus (which increase the difficulty of sperm penetration) and the endometrium (which reduce the likelihood of implantation), may also contribute to contraceptive effectiveness.

Indications and Usage: LO/OVRAL® is indicated for the prevention of pregnancy in women who elect to use oral contraceptives as a method of contraception.

Oral contraceptives are highly effective. The pregnancy rate in women using conventional combination oral contraceptives (containing 35 mcg or

Continued on next page

Wyeth—Cont.

more of ethinyl estradiol or 50 mcg or more of mestranol) is generally reported as less than one pregnancy per 100 woman-years of use. Slightly higher rates (somewhat more than 1 pregnancy per 100 woman-years of use) are reported for some combination products containing 35 mcg or less of ethinyl estradiol, and rates on the order of 3 pregnancies per 100 woman-years are reported for the progestogen-only oral contraceptives.

These rates are derived from separate studies conducted by different investigators in several population groups and cannot be compared precisely. Furthermore, pregnancy rates tend to be lower as clinical studies are continued, possibly due to selective retention in the longer studies of those patients who accept the treatment regimen and do not discontinue as a result of adverse reactions, pregnancy, or other reasons.

In clinical trials with LO/OVRAL®, 1,700 patients completed 22,489 cycles, and a total of two pregnancies were reported. This represents a pregnancy rate of 0.12 per 100 woman-years.

Table 1 gives ranges of pregnancy rates reported in the literature[1] for other means of contraception. The efficacy of these means of contraception (except the IUD) depends upon the degree of adherence to the method.

TABLE 1
PREGNANCIES PER 100 WOMAN-YEARS

IUD, less than 1–6; Diaphragm with spermicidal products (creams or jellies), 2–20; Condom, 3–36; Aerosol foams, 2–29; Jellies and creams, 4–36; Periodic abstinence (rhythm) all types, less than 1–47;
 1. Calendar method, 14–47;
 2. Temperature method, 1–20;
 3. Temperature method—intercourse only in postovulatory phase, less than 1–7;
 4. Mucus method, 1–25;

No contraception, 60–80.

Dose-Related Risk of Thromboembolism from Oral Contraceptives: Two studies have shown a positive association between the dose of estrogens in oral contraceptives and the risk of thromboembolism.[2,3] For this reason, it is prudent and in keeping with good principles of therapeutics to minimize exposure to estrogen. The oral-contraceptive product prescribed for any given patient should be that product which contains the least amount of estrogen that is compatible with an acceptable pregnancy rate and patient acceptance. It is recommended that new acceptors of oral contraceptives be started on preparations containing 0.05 mg or less of estrogen.

Contraindications: Oral contraceptives should not be used in women with any of the following conditions:
1. Thrombophlebitis or thromboembolic disorders.
2. A past history of deep-vein thrombophlebitis or thromboembolic disorders.
3. Cerebral-vascular or coronary-artery disease.
4. Known or suspected carcinoma of the breast.
5. Known or suspected estrogen-dependent neoplasia.
6. Undiagnosed abnormal genital bleeding.
7. Known or suspected pregnancy (see Warning No. 5).
8. Benign or malignant liver tumor which developed during the use of oral contraceptives or other estrogen-containing products.

Warnings:

> Cigarette smoking increases the risk of serious cardiovascular side effects from oral-contraceptive use. This risk increases with age and with heavy smoking (15 or more cigarettes per day) and is quite marked in women over 35 years of age. Women who use oral contraceptives should be strongly advised not to smoke.

The use of oral contraceptives is associated with increased risk of several serious conditions, including thromboembolism, stroke, myocardial infarction, hepatic adenoma, gallbladder disease, hypertension. Practitioners prescribing oral contraceptives should be familiar with the following information relating to these risks.

1. *Thromboembolic Disorders and Other Vascular Problems:* An increased risk of thromboembolic and thrombotic disease associated with the use of oral contraceptives is well-established. Three principal studies in Great Britain[4–6] and three in the United States[7–10] have demonstrated an increased risk of fatal and nonfatal venous thromboembolism and stroke, both hemorrhagic and thrombotic.

These studies estimate that users of oral contraceptives are 4 to 11 times more likely than nonusers to develop these diseases without evident cause (Table 2).

CEREBROVASCULAR DISORDERS

In a collaborative American study[9,10] of cerebrovascular disorders in women with and without predisposing causes, it was estimated that the risk of hemorrhagic stroke was 2.0 times greater in users than nonusers and the risk of thrombotic stroke was 4 to 9.5 times greater in users than in nonusers (Table 2).

TABLE 2
SUMMARY OF RELATIVE RISK OF THROMBOEMBOLIC DISORDERS AND OTHER VASCULAR PROBLEMS IN ORAL-CONTRACEPTIVE USERS COMPARED TO NONUSERS

	Relative risk, times greater
Idiopathic thromboembolic disease	4–11
Postsurgery thromboembolic complications	4–6
Thrombotic stroke	4–9.5
Hemorrhagic stroke	2
Myocardial infarction	2–12

MYOCARDIAL INFARCTION

An increased risk of myocardial infarction associated with the use of oral contraceptives has been reported,[11,12,13] confirming a previously suspected association. These studies, conducted in the United Kingdom, found, as expected, that the greater the number of underlying risk factors for coronary-artery disease (cigarette smoking, hypertension, hypercholesterolemia, obesity, diabetes, history of pre-eclamptic toxemia) the higher the risk of developing myocardial infarction, regardless of whether the patient was an oral-contraceptive user or not. Oral contraceptives, however, were found to be a clear additional risk factor.

In terms of relative risk, it has been estimated[52] that oral-contraceptive users who do not smoke (smoking is considered a major predisposing condition to myocardial infarction) are about twice as likely to have a fatal myocardial infarction as nonusers who do not smoke. Oral-contraceptive users who are also smokers have about a 5-fold increased risk of fatal infarction compared to users who do not smoke, but about a 10- to 12-fold increased risk compared to non-users who do not smoke. Furthermore, the amount of smoking is also an important factor. In determining the importance of these relative risks, however, the baseline rates for various age groups, as shown in Table 3, must be given serious consideration. The importance of other predisposing conditions mentioned above in determining relative and absolute risks has not as yet been quantified; it is quite likely that the same synergistic action exists, but perhaps to a lesser extent.

TABLE 3
Estimated annual mortality rate per 100,000 women from myocardial infarction by use of oral contraceptives, smoking habits, and age (in years):

	Myocardial infarction			
	Women aged 30–39		Women aged 40–44	
Smoking habits	Users	Non-users	Users	Non-users
All smokers	10.2	2.6	62.0	15.9
Heavy*	13.0	5.1	78.7	31.3
Light	4.7	0.9	28.6	5.7
Nonsmokers	1.8	1.2	10.7	7.4
Smokers and nonsmokers	5.4	1.9	32.8	11.7

*Heavy smoker: 15 or more cigarettes per day. From JAIN, A.K., *Studies in Family Planning*, 8:50, 1977

RISK OF DOSE

In an analysis of data derived from several national adverse-reaction reporting systems,[2] British investigators concluded that the risk of thromboembolism, including coronary thrombosis, is directly related to the dose of estrogen used in oral contraceptives. Preparations containing 100 mcg or more of estrogen were associated with a higher risk of thromboembolism than those containing 50–80 mcg of estrogen. Their analysis did suggest, however, that the quantity of estrogen may not be the sole factor involved. This finding has been confirmed in the United States.[3] Careful epidemiological studies to determine the degree of thromboembolic risk associated with progestogen-only oral contraceptives have not been performed.

Cases of thromboembolic disease have been reported in women using these products, and they should not be presumed to be free of excess risk.

ESTIMATE OF EXCESS MORTALITY FROM CIRCULATORY DISEASES

A large prospective study[53] carried out in the U.K. estimated the mortality rate per 100,000 women per year from diseases of the circulatory system for users and nonusers of oral contraceptives according to age, smoking habits, and duration of use. The overall excess death rate annually from circulatory diseases for oral-contraceptive users was estimated to be 20 per 100,000 (ages 15–34—5/100,000; ages 35–44—33/100,000; ages 45–49—140/100,000), the risk being concentrated in older women, in those with a long duration of use, and in cigarette smokers. It was not possible, however, to examine the interrelationships of age, smoking, and duration of use, nor to compare the effects of continuous vs. intermittent use. Although the study showed a 10-fold increase in death due to circulatory diseases in users for 5 or more years, all of these deaths occurred in women 35 or older. Until larger numbers of women under 35 with continuous use for 5 or more years are available, it is not possible to assess the magnitude of the relative risk for this younger age group.

The available data from a variety of sources have been analyzed[14] to estimate the risk of death associated with various methods of contraception. The estimates of risk of death for each method include the combined risk of the contraceptive method (e.g., thromboembolic and thrombotic disease in the case of oral contraceptives) plus the risk attributable to pregnancy or abortion in the event of method failure. This latter risk varies with the effectiveness of the contraceptive method. The findings of this analysis are shown in Figure 1 below.[14] The study concluded that the mortality associated with all methods of birth control is low and below that associated with childbirth, with the exception of oral contraceptives in women over 40 who smoke. (The rates given for Pill only/smokers for each age group are for smokers as a class. For "heavy" smokers (more than 15 cigarettes a day), the rates given would be about double; for "light" smokers (less than 15 cigarettes a day), about 50 percent. The lowest mortality is associated with the condom or diaphragm backed up by early abortion. The risk of thromboembolic and thrombotic disease associated with oral contraceptives increases with age after approximately age 30 and, for myocardial infarction, is further increased by hypertension, hypercholesterolemia, obesity, diabetes, or history of preeclamptic toxemia and especially by cigarette smoking.

Based on the data currently available, the following chart gives a gross estimate of the risk of death from circulatory disorders associated with the use of oral contraceptives:

SMOKING HABITS AND OTHER PREDISPOSING CONDITIONS—

RISK ASSOCIATED WITH USE OF ORAL CONTRACEPTIVES

Age	Below 30	30-39	40+
Heavy smokers	C	B	A
Light smokers	D	C	B
Nonsmokers (no predisposing conditions)	D	C,D	C
Nonsmokers (other predisposing conditions)	C	C,B	B,A

A—Use associated with very high risk.
B—Use associated with high risk.
C—Use associated with moderate risk.
D—Use associated with low risk.

The physician and the patient should be alert to the earliest manifestations of thromboembolic and thrombotic disorders (e.g., thrombophlebitis, pulmonary embolism, cerebrovascular insufficiency, coronary occlusion, retinal thrombosis, and mesenteric thrombosis). Should any of these occur or be suspected, the drug should be discontinued immediately.

A four- to six-fold increased risk of postsurgery thromboembolic complications has been reported in oral-contraceptive users.[15,16]

If feasible, oral contraceptives should be discontinued at least 4 weeks before surgery of a type associated with an increased risk of thromboembolism or prolonged immobilization.

PERSISTENCE OF RISK OF VASCULAR DISORDERS

Findings from one study in Great Britain involving cerebrovascular disease[54] and another study in the United States concerning myocardial infarction[55] suggest that an increased risk of these conditions in users of oral contraceptives persists after discontinuation of the oral contraceptive. In the British study, the risk of cerebrovascular disease remained elevated in former oral-contraceptive users for at least six years after discontinuation. In the U.S. study, an increased risk of myocardial infarction persisted for at least 9 years in women 40- to 49-years-old who had used oral contraceptives for five or more years. The findings in both these studies require confirmation since they are inconsistent with other published information.[9,11,13,56-60]

2. *Ocular Lesions:*
There have been reports of neuro-ocular lesions such as optic neuritis or retinal thrombosis associated with the use of oral contraceptives. Discontinue oral-contraceptive medication if there is unexplained, sudden or gradual, partial or complete loss of vision; onset of proptosis or diplopia; papilledema; or retinal-vascular lesions, and institute appropriate diagnostic and therapeutic measures.

3. *Carcinoma:*
Long-term continuous administration of either natural or synthetic estrogen in certain animal species increases the frequency of carcinoma of the breast, cervix, vagina, and liver. Certain synthetic progestogens, none currently contained in oral contraceptives, have been noted to increase the incidence of mammary nodules, benign and malignant, in dogs.

In humans, three case-control studies have reported an increased risk of endometrial carcinoma associated with the prolonged use of exogenous estrogen in postmenopausal women.[17,18,19] One publication[20] reported on the first 21 cases submitted by physicians to a registry of cases of adenocarcinoma of the endometrium in women under 40 on oral contraceptives. Of the cases found in women without predisposing risk factors for adenocarcinoma of the endometrium (e.g., irregular bleeding at the time oral contraceptives were first given, polycystic ovaries), nearly all occurred in women who had used a sequential oral contraceptive. These products are no longer marketed. No evidence has been reported suggesting an increased risk of endometrial cancer in users of conventional combination or progestogen-only oral contraceptives.

Several studies[8,21-24] have found no increase in breast cancer in women taking oral contraceptives or estrogen. One study,[25] however, while also noting no overall increased risk of breast cancer in women treated with oral contraceptives, found an excess risk in the subgroups of oral-contraceptive users with documented benign breast disease. A reduced occurrence of benign breast tumors in users of oral contraceptives has been well-documented.[8,21,25,26,27]

In summary, there is at present no confirmed evidence from human studies of an increased risk of cancer associated with oral contraceptives. Close clinical surveillance of all women taking oral contraceptives is, nevertheless, essential. In all cases of undiagnosed persistent or recurrent abnormal vaginal bleeding, appropriate diagnostic measures should be taken to rule out malignancy. Women with a strong family history of breast cancer or who have breast nodules, fibrocystic disease, or abnormal mammograms should be monitored with particular care if they elect to use oral contraceptives instead of other methods of contraception.

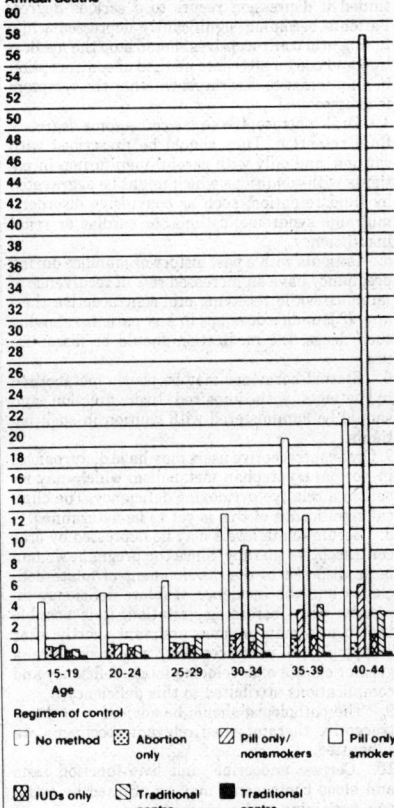

Figure 1. Estimated annual number of deaths associated with control of fertility and no control per 100,000 nonsterile women, by regimen of control and age of woman.

4. *Hepatic Tumors:*
Benign hepatic adenomas have been found to be associated with the use of oral contraceptives.[28,29,30,46] One study[46] showed that oral contraceptive formulations with high hormonal potency were associated with a higher risk than lower potency formulations. Although benign, hepatic adenomas may rupture and may cause death through intra-abdominal hemorrhage. This has been reported in short-term as well as long-term users of oral contraceptives. Two studies relate risk with duration of use of the contraceptive, the risk being much greater after 4 or more years of oral-contraceptive use.[30,46] While hepatic adenoma is a rare lesion, it should be considered in women presenting abdominal pain and tenderness, abdominal mass or shock. A few cases of hepatocellular carcinoma have been reported in women taking oral contraceptives. The relationship of these drugs to this type of malignancy is not known at this time.

5. *Use in or Immediately Preceding Pregnancy, Birth Defects in Offspring, and Malignancy in Female Offspring:*
The use of female sex hormones—both estrogenic and progestational agents—during early pregnancy may seriously damage the offspring. It has been shown that females exposed in utero to diethylstilbestrol, a nonsteroidal estrogen, have an increased risk of developing in later life a form of vaginal or cervical cancer that is ordinarily extremely rare.[31,32] This risk has been estimated to be of the order of 1 in 1,000 exposures or less.[33,47] Although there is no evidence at the present time that oral contraceptives further enhance the risk of developing this type of malignancy, such patients should be monitored with particular care if they elect to use oral contraceptives instead of other methods of contraception. Furthermore, a high percentage of such exposed women (from 30 to 90%) have been found to have epithelial changes of the vagina and cervix.[34-38] Although these changes are histologically benign, it is not known whether this condition is a precursor of vaginal malignancy. Male children so exposed may develop abnormalities of the urogenital tract.[48,49,50] Although similar data are not available with the use of other estrogens, it cannot be presumed that they would not induce similar changes.

An increased risk of congenital anomalies, including heart defects and limb defects, has been reported with the use of sex hormones, including oral contraceptives, in pregnancy.[39-42,51] One case-control study[42] has estimated a 4.7-fold increase in risk of limb-reduction defects in infants exposed in utero to sex hormones (oral contraceptives, hormonal withdrawal tests for pregnancy, or attempted treatment for threatened abortion). Some of these exposures were very short and involved only a few days of treatment. The data suggest that the risk of limb-reduction defects in exposed fetuses is somewhat less than one in 1,000 live births.

In the past, female sex hormones have been used during pregnancy in an attempt to treat threatened or habitual abortion. There is considerable evidence that estrogens are ineffective for these indications, and there is no evidence from well-controlled studies that progestogens are effective for these uses.

There is some evidence that triploidy and possibly other types of polyploidy are increased among abortuses from women who become pregnant soon after ceasing oral contraceptives.[43] Embryos with these anomalies are virtually always aborted spontaneously. Whether there is an overall increase in spontaneous abortion of pregnancies conceived soon after stopping oral contraceptives is unknown.

It is recommended that, for any patient who has missed two consecutive periods, pregnancy should be ruled out before continuing the contraceptive regimen. If the patient has not adhered to the prescribed schedule, the possibility of pregnancy should be considered at the time of the first missed period (or after 45 days from the last menstrual period if the progestogen-only oral contraceptives are used), and further use of oral contraceptives should be withheld until pregnancy has been ruled out. If pregnancy is confirmed, the patient should be apprised of the potential risks to the fetus, and the advisability of continuation of the pregnancy should be discussed in the light of these risks.

It is also recommended that women who discontinue oral contraceptives with the intent of becoming pregnant use an alternate form of contracep-

Continued on next page

Wyeth—Cont.

tion for a period of time before attempting to conceive.

Many clinicians recommend 3 months, although no precise information is available on which to base this recommendation.

The administration of progestogen-only or progestogen-estrogen combinations to induce withdrawal bleeding should not be used as a test of pregnancy.

6. *Gallbladder Disease:*
Studies [8,23,26] report an increased risk of surgically confirmed gallbladder disease in users of oral contraceptives and estrogens. In one study, an increased risk appeared after 2 years of use and doubled after 4 or 5 years of use. In one of the other studies, an increased risk was apparent between 6 and 12 months of use.

7. *Carbohydrate and Lipid Metabolic Effects:*
A decrease in glucose tolerance has been observed in a significant percentage of patients on oral contraceptives. For this reason, prediabetic and diabetic patients should be carefully observed while receiving oral contraceptives.

An increase in triglycerides and total phospholipids has been observed in patients receiving oral contraceptives.[44] The clinical significance of this finding remains to be defined.

8. *Elevated Blood Pressure:*
An increase in blood pressure has been reported in patients receiving oral contraceptives.[26] In some women, hypertension may occur within a few months of beginning oral-contraceptive use. In the first year of use, the prevalence of women with hypertension is low in users and may be no higher than that of a comparable group of nonusers. The prevalence in users increases, however, with longer exposure, and in the fifth year of use is two-and-a-half to three times the reported prevalence in the first year. Age is also strongly correlated with the development of hypertension in oral-contraceptive users. Women who previously have had hypertension during pregnancy may be more likely to develop elevation of blood pressure when given oral contraceptives. Hypertension that develops as a result of taking oral contraceptives usually returns to normal after discontinuing the drug.

9. *Headache:*
The onset or exacerbation of migraine or development of headache of a new pattern which is recurrent, persistent, or severe, requires discontinuation of oral contraceptives and evaluation of the cause.

10. *Bleeding Irregularities:*
Breakthrough bleeding, spotting, and amenorrhea are frequent reasons for patients discontinuing oral contraceptives. In breakthrough bleeding, as in all cases of irregular bleeding from the vagina, nonfunctional causes should be borne in mind. In undiagnosed persistent or recurrent abnormal bleeding from the vagina, adequate diagnostic measures are indicated to rule out pregnancy or malignancy. If pathology has been excluded, time or a change to another formulation may solve the problem. Changing to an oral contraceptive with a higher estrogen content, while potentially useful in minimizing menstrual irregularity, should be done only if necessary, since this may increase the risk of thromboembolic disease.

Women with a past history of oligomenorrhea or secondary amenorrhea or young women without regular cycles may have a tendency to remain anovulatory or to become amenorrheic after discontinuation of oral contraceptives. Women with these preexisting problems should be advised of this possibility and encouraged to use other contraceptive methods. Post-use anovulation, possibly prolonged, may also occur in women without previous irregularities.

11. *Ectopic Pregnancy:*
Ectopic as well as intrauterine pregnancy may occur in contraceptive failures. However, in progestogen-only oral contraceptive failures, the ratio of ectopic to intrauterine pregnancies is higher than in women who are not receiving oral contraceptives, since the drugs are more effective in preventing intrauterine than ectopic pregnancies.

12. *Breast-feeding:*
Oral contraceptives given in the postpartum period may interfere with lactation. There may be a decrease in the quantity and quality of the breast milk. Furthermore, a small fraction of the hormonal agents in oral contraceptives has been identified in the milk of mothers receiving these drugs.[45] The effects, if any, on the breast-fed child have not been determined. If feasible, the use of oral contraceptives should be deferred until the infant has been weaned.

Precautions:
GENERAL
1. A complete medical and family history should be taken prior to initiation of oral contraceptives. The pretreatment and periodic physical examinations should include special reference to blood pressure, breasts, abdomen and pelvic organs, including Papanicolaou smear and relevant laboratory tests. As a general rule, oral contraceptives should not be prescribed for longer than 1 year without another physical examination being performed.

2. Under the influence of estrogen-progestogen preparations, pre-existing uterine leiomyomata may increase in size.

3. Patients with a history of psychic depression should be carefully observed and the drug discontinued if depression recurs to a serious degree. Patients becoming significantly depressed while taking oral contraceptives should stop the medication and use an alternate method of contraception in an attempt to determine whether the symptom is drug-related.

4. Oral contraceptives may cause some degree of fluid retention. They should be prescribed with caution, and only with careful monitoring, in patients with conditions which might be aggravated by fluid retention, such as convulsive disorders, migraine syndrome, asthma, or cardiac or renal insufficiency.

5. Patients with a past history of jaundice during pregnancy have an increased risk of recurrence of jaundice while receiving oral-contraceptive therapy. If jaundice develops in any patient receiving such drugs, the medication should be discontinued.

6. Steroid hormones may be poorly metabolized in patients with impaired liver function and should be administered with caution in such patients.

7. Oral-contraceptive users may have disturbances in normal tryptophan metabolism which may result in a relative pyridoxine deficiency. The clinical significance of this is yet to be determined.

8. Serum folate levels may be depressed by oral-contraceptive therapy. Since the pregnant woman is predisposed to the development of folate deficiency and the incidence of folate deficiency increases with increasing gestation, it is possible that if a woman becomes pregnant shortly after stopping oral contraceptives, she may have a greater chance of developing folate deficiency and complications attributed to this deficiency.

9. The pathologist should be advised of oral-contraceptive therapy when relevant specimens are submitted.

10. Certain endocrine- and liver-function tests and blood components may be affected by estrogen-containing oral contraceptives:
a. Increased sulfobromophthalein retention.
b. Increased prothrombin and factors VII, VIII, IX, and X; decreased antithrombin 3; increased norepinephrine-induced platelet aggregability.
c. Increased thyroid-binding globulin (TBG) leading to increased circulating total-thyroid hormone, as measured by protein-bound iodine (PBI), T4 by column, or T4 by radioimmunoassay. Free T3 resin uptake is decreased, reflecting the elevated TBG; free T4 concentration is unaltered.
d. Decreased pregnanediol excretion.
e. Reduced response to metyrapone test.

Information for the Patient: (See Patient Labeling Printed Below.)

Drug Interactions: Reduced efficacy and increased incidence of breakthrough bleeding have been associated with concomitant use of rifampin. A similar association has been suggested with barbiturates, phenylbutazone, phenytoin sodium, ampicillin, and tetracycline.

Carcinogenesis: See Warnings section for information on the carcinogenic potential of oral contraceptives.

Pregnancy: Pregnancy category X. See Contraindications and Warnings.

Nursing Mothers: See Warnings.

Adverse Reactions: An increased risk of the following serious adverse reactions has been associated with the use of oral contraceptives (see Warnings):

Thrombophlebitis.
Pulmonary embolism.
Coronary thrombosis.
Cerebral thrombosis.
Cerebral hemorrhage.
Hypertension.
Gallbladder disease.
Benign hepatomas.
Congenital anomalies.

There is evidence of an association between the following conditions and the use of oral contraceptives, although additional confirmatory studies are needed:

Mesenteric thrombosis.
Neuro-ocular lesions, e.g., retinal thrombosis and optic neuritis.

The following adverse reactions have been reported in patients receiving oral contraceptives and are believed to be drug-related:

Nausea and/or vomiting, usually the most common adverse reactions, occur in approximately 10% or less of patients during the first cycle. Other reactions, as a general rule, are seen much less frequently or only occasionally.
Gastrointestinal symptoms (such as abdominal cramps and bloating).
Breakthrough bleeding.
Spotting.
Change in menstrual flow.
Dysmenorrhea.
Amenorrhea during and after treatment.
Temporary infertility after discontinuance of treatment.
Edema.
Chloasma or melasma which may persist.
Breast changes: tenderness, enlargement, and secretion.
Change in weight (increase or decrease).
Change in cervical erosion and cervical secretion.
Possible diminution in lactation when given immediately post-partum.
Cholestatic jaundice.
Migraine.
Increase in size of uterine leiomyomata.
Rash (allergic).
Mental depression.
Reduced tolerance to carbohydrates.
Vaginal candidiasis.
Change in corneal curvature (steepening).
Intolerance to contact lenses.

The following adverse reactions have been reported in users of oral contraceptives, and the association has been neither confirmed nor refuted:

Premenstrual-like syndrome.
Cataracts.
Changes in libido.
Chorea.
Changes in appetite.
Cystitis-like syndrome.
Headache.
Nervousness.
Dizziness.
Hirsutism.
Loss of scalp hair.
Erythema multiforme.
Erythema nodosum.
Hemorrhagic eruption.
Vaginitis.
Porphyria.

Acute Overdose: Serious ill effects have not been reported following acute ingestion of large doses of oral contraceptives by young children.

Overdosage may cause nausea, and withdrawal bleeding may occur in females.

Dosage and Administration: To achieve maximum contraceptive effectiveness, LO/OVRAL® must be taken exactly as directed and at intervals not exceeding 24 hours. The dosage of LO/OVRAL® is one tablet daily for 21 consecutive days per menstrual cycle according to prescribed schedule. Tablets are then discontinued for 7 days (three weeks on, one week off).

It is recommended that LO/OVRAL® tablets be taken at the same time each day, preferably after the evening meal or at bedtime.

During the first cycle of medication, the patient is instructed to take one LO/OVRAL® tablet daily for twenty-one consecutive days beginning on day five of her menstrual cycle. (The first day of menstruation is day one.) The tablets are then discontinued for one week (7 days). Withdrawal bleeding should usually occur within three days following discontinuation of LO/OVRAL®.

(If LO/OVRAL® is first taken later than the fifth day of the first menstrual cycle of medication or postpartum, contraceptive reliance should not be placed on LO/OVRAL® until after the first seven consecutive days of administration. The possibility of ovulation and conception prior to initiation of medication should be considered.)

The patient begins her next and all subsequent 21-day courses of LO/OVRAL® tablets on the same day of the week that she began her first course, following the same schedule: 21 days on—7 days off. She begins taking her tablets on the 8th day after discontinuance regardless of whether or not a menstrual period has occurred or is still in progress. Any time a new cycle of LO/OVRAL® is started later than the 8th day the patient should be protected by another means of contraception until she has taken a tablet daily for seven consecutive days.

If spotting or breakthrough bleeding occurs, the patient is instructed to continue on the same regimen. This type of bleeding is usually transient and without significance; however, if the bleeding is persistent or prolonged the patient is advised to consult her physician.

Although the occurrence of pregnancy is highly unlikely if LO/OVRAL® is taken according to directions, if withdrawal bleeding does not occur, the possibility of pregnancy must be considered. If the patient has not adhered to the prescribed schedule (missed one or more tablets or started taking them on a day later than she should have) the probability of pregnancy should be considered at the time of the first missed period and appropriate diagnostic measures taken before the medication is resumed. If the patient has adhered to the prescribed regimen and misses two consecutive periods, pregnancy should be ruled out before continuing the contraceptive regimen.

The patient should be instructed to take a missed tablet as soon as it is remembered. If two consecutive tablets are missed they should both be taken as soon as remembered. The next tablet should be taken at the usual time.

Any time the patient misses one or two tablets she should also use another method of contraception until she has taken a tablet daily for seven consecutive days. If breakthrough bleeding occurs following missed tablets it will usually be transient and of no consequence.

While there is little likelihood of ovulation occurring if only one or two tablets are missed, the possibility of ovulation increases with each successive day that scheduled tablets are missed. If three consecutive tablets are missed, all medication should be discontinued and the remainder of the package discarded. A new tablet cycle should be started on the 8th day after the last tablet was taken, and an alternate means of contraception should be prescribed during the seven days without tablets and until the patient has taken a tablet daily for seven consecutive days. In the nonlactating mother LO/OVRAL® may be prescribed in the postpartum period either immediately or at the first postpartum examination whether or not menstruation has resumed.

How Supplied: LO/OVRAL® tablets (0.3 mg norgestrel and 0.03 mg ethinyl estradiol), Wyeth®, are available in packages of 6 PILPAK® dispensers with 21 tablets each and in 3-PAK packages containing 63 tablets each as follows: NDC 0008-0078, white, round tablet marked "WYETH" and "78".

Also Available: LO/OVRAL®-28 tablets in containers of 28 tablets, consisting of 21 white LO/OVRAL® tablets (0.3 mg norgestrel + 0.03 mg ethinyl estradiol) and 7 pink inert tablets.

References:
1. "Population Reports," Series H, Number 2, May 1974; Series I, Number 1, June 1974; Series B, Number 2, January 1975; Series H, Number 3, 1975; Series H, Number 4, January 1976 (published by the Population Information Program, The George Washington University Medical Center, 2001 S St. NW., Washington, D.C.).
2. Inman, W. H. W., Vessey, M. P., Westerholm, B., and Engelund, A., "Thromboembolic disease and the steroidal content of oral contraceptives. A report to the Committee on Safety of Drugs," Brit Med J 2:203–209, 1970.
3. Stolley, P. D., Tonascia, J. A., Tockman, M. S., Sartwell, P. E., Rutledge, A. H., and Jacobs, M. P., "Thrombosis with low-estrogen oral contraceptives," Am J Epidemiol 102:197–208, 1975.
4. Royal College of General Practitioners, "Oral contraception and thromboembolic disease," J Coll Gen Pract 13:267–279, 1967.
5. Inman, W. H. W., and Vessey, M. P., "Investigation of deaths from pulmonary, coronary and cerebral thrombosis and embolism in women of childbearing age," Brit Med J 2:193–199, 1968.
6. Vessey, M. P., and Doll, R., "Investigation of relation between use of oral contraceptives and thromboembolic disease. A further report," Brit Med J 2:651–657, 1969.
7. Sartwell, P. E., Masi, A. T., Arthes, F. G., Greene, G. R., and Smith, H. E., "Thromboembolism and oral contraceptives: an epidemiological case control study," Am J Epidemiol 90:365–380, 1969.
8. Boston Collaborative Drug Surveillance Program, "Oral contraceptives and venous thromboembolic disease, surgically confirmed gallbladder disease and breast tumors," Lancet 1:1399–1404, 1973.
9. Collaborative Group for the Study of Stroke in Young Women, "Oral contraception and increased risk of cerebral ischemia or thrombosis," N Engl J Med 288:871–878, 1973.
10. Collaborative Group for the Study of Stroke in Young Women, "Oral contraceptives and stroke in young women: associated risk factors," JAMA 231:718–722, 1975.
11. Mann, J. I., and Inman, W. H. W., "Oral contraceptives and death from myocardial infarction," Brit Med J 2:245–248, 1975.
12. Mann, J. I., Inman, W. H. W., and Thorogood, M., "Oral contraceptive use in older women and fatal myocardial infarction," Brit Med J 2:445–447, 1976.
13. Mann, J. I., Vessey, M. P., Thorogood, M., and Doll, R., "Myocardial infarction in young women with special reference to oral contraceptive practice," Brit Med J 2:241–245, 1975.
14. Tietze, C., "New Estimates of Mortality Associated with Fertility Control," Family Planning Perspectives, 9:74–76, 1977.
15. Vessey, M. P., Doll, R., Fairbairn, A. S., and Glober, G., "Post-operative thromboembolism and the use of oral contraceptives," Brit Med J 3:123–126, 1970.
16. Greene, G. R., Sartwell, P. E., "Oral contraceptive use in patients with thromboembolism following surgery, trauma, or infection," Am J Pub Health 62:680–685, 1972.
17. Smith, D. C., Prentice, R., Thompson, D. J., and Herrmann, W. L., "Association of exogenous estrogen and endometrial carcinoma," N Engl J Med 293:1164–1167, 1975.
18. Ziel, H. K., and Finkle, W. D., "Increased risk of endometrial carcinoma among users of conjugated estrogens," N Engl J Med 293:1167–1170, 1975.
19. Mack, T. N., Pike, M. C., Henderson, B. E., Pfeffer, R. I., Gerkins, V. R., Arthur, M., and Brown, S. E., "Estrogens and endometrial cancer in a retirement community," N Engl J Med 294:1262–1267, 1976.
20. Silverberg, S. G., and Makowski, E. L., "Endometrial carcinoma in young women taking oral contraceptive agents," Obstet Gynecol 46:503–506, 1975.
21. Vessey, M. P., Doll, R., and Sutton, P. M., "Oral contraceptives and breast neoplasia: a retrospective study," Brit Med J 3:719–724, 1972.
22. Vessey, M. P., Doll, R., and Jones K., "Oral contraceptives and breast cancer. Progress report of an epidemiological study," Lancet 1:941–943, 1975.
23. Boston Collaborative Drug Surveillance Program, "Surgically confirmed gallbladder disease, venous thromboembolism and breast tumors in relation to postmenopausal estrogen therapy," N Engl J Med 290:15–19, 1974.
24. Arthes, F. G., Sartwell, P. E., and Lewison, E. F., "The pill, estrogens, and the breast. Epidemiologic aspects," Cancer 28:1391–1394, 1971.
25. Fasal, E., and Paffenbarger, R. S., "Oral contraceptives as related to cancer and benign lesions of the breast," J Natl Cancer Inst 55:767–773, 1975.
26. Royal College of General Practitioners, "Oral Contraceptives and Health," London, Pitman, 1974.
27. Ory, H., Cole P., MacMahon, B., and Hoover, R., "Oral contraceptives and reduced risk of benign breast diseases," N Engl J Med 294:419–422, 1976.
28. Baum, J., Holtz, F., Bookstein, J. J., and Klein, E. W., "Possible association between benign hepatomas and oral contraceptives," Lancet 2:926–928, 1973.
29. Mays, E. T., Christopherson, W. M., Mahr, M. M., and Williams, H. C., "Hepatic changes in young women ingesting contraceptive steroids. Hepatic hemorrhage and primary hepatic tumors," JAMA 235:730–732, 1976.
30. Edmondson, H. A., Henderson, B., and Benton, B., "Liver-cell adenomas associated with use of oral contraceptives," N Engl J Med 294:470–472, 1976.
31. Herbst, A. L., Ulfedler, H., and Poskanzer, D. C., "Adenocarcinoma of the vagina," N Engl J Med 284:878–881, 1971.
32. Greenwald, P., Barlow, J. J., Nasca, P. C., and Burnett, W., "Vaginal cancer after maternal treatment with synthetic estrogens," N Engl J Med 285:390–392, 1971.
33. Lanier, A. P., Noller, K. L., Decker, D. G., Elveback, L., and Kurland, L. T., "Cancer and stilbestrol. A follow-up of 1719 persons exposed to estrogens in utero and born 1943–1959," Mayo Clin Pro 48:793–799, 1973.
34. Herbst, A. L., Kurman, R. J., and Scully, R. E., "Vaginal and cervical abnormalities after exposure to stilbestrol in utero," Obstet Gynecol 40:287–298, 1972.
35. Herbst, A. L., Robboy, S. J., Macdonald, G. J., and Scully, R. E., "The effects of local progesterone on stilbestrol-associated vaginal adenosis," Am J Obstet Gynecol 118:607–615, 1974.
36. Herbst, A. L., Poskanzer, D. C., Robboy, S. J., Friedlander, L., and Scully, R. E., "Prenatal exposure to stilbestrol: a prospective comparison of exposed female offspring with unexposed controls," N Engl J Med 292:334–339, 1975.
37. Stafl, A., Mattingly, R. F., Foley, D. V., Fetherston, W., "Clinical diagnosis of vaginal adenosis," Obstet Gynecol 43:118–128, 1974.
38. Sherman, A. I., Goldrath, M., Berlin, A., Vakhariya, V., Banooni, F., Michaels, W., Goodman, P., and Brown, S., "Cervical-vaginal adenosis after in utero exposure to synthetic estrogens," Obstet Gynecol 44:531–545, 1974.
39. Gal, I., Kirman, B., and Stern, J., "Hormone pregnancy tests and congenital malformation," Nature 216:83, 1967.
40. Levy, E. P., Cohen, A., and Fraser, F. C., "Hormone treatment during pregnancy and congenital heart defects," Lancet 1:611, 1973.

Continued on next page

Wyeth—Cont.

41. Nora, J. J., and Nora, A. H., "Birth defects and oral contraceptives," Lancet *1*:941-942, 1973.
42. Janerich, D. T., Piper, J. M., and Glebatis, D. M., "Oral contraceptives and congenital limb-reduction defects," N Engl J Med *291*:697-700, 1974.
43. Carr, D. H., "Chromosome studies in selected spontaneous abortions: I. Conception after oral contraceptives," Canad Med Assoc J *103*:343-348, 1970.
44. Wynn, V., Doar, J. W. H., and Mills, G. L., "Some effects of oral contraceptives on serum-lipid and lipoprotein levels," Lancet *2*:720-723, 1966.
45. Laumas, K. R., Malkani, P. K., Bhatnagar, S., and Laumas, V., "Radioactivity in the breast milk of lactating women after oral administration of 3 H-norethynodrel," Amer J Obstet Gynecol *98*:411-413, 1967.
46. Center for Disease Control, "Increased Risk of Hepatocellular Adenoma in Women with Long-term use of Oral Contraceptives," Morbidity and Mortality Weekly Report, *26*:293-294, 1977.
47. Herbst, A. L., Cole, P., Colton, T., Robboy, S. J., Scully, R. E., "Age-incidence and Risk of Diethylstilbestrol-related Clear Cell Adenocarcinoma of the Vagina and Cervix," Am. J. Obstet. Gynecol., *128*:43-50, 1977.
48. Bibbo, M., Al-Naqeeb, M., Baccarini, I., Gill, W., Newton, M., Sleeper, K. M., Sonek, M., Wied, G. L., "Follow-up Study of Male and Female Offspring of DES-treated Mothers. A Preliminary Report," Jour. of Repro. Med., *15*:29-32, 1975.
49. Gill, W. B., Schumacher, G. F. B., Bibbo, M., "Structural and Functional Abnormalities in the Sex Organs of Male Offspring of Mothers Treated with Diethylstilbestrol (DES)," Jour. of Repro. Med., *16*:147-153, 1976.
50. Henderson, B. E., Senton, B., Cosgrove, M., Baptista, J., Aldrich, J., Townsend, D., Hart, W., Mack, T., "Urogenital Tract Abnormalities in Sons of Women Treated with Diethylstilbestrol," Pediatrics, *58*:505-507, 1976.
51. Heinonen, O. P., Slone, D., Nonson, R. R., Hook, E. B., Shapiro, S., "Cardiovascular Birth Defects and Antenatal Exposure to Female Sex Hormones," N. Engl. J. Med., *296*:67-70, 1977.
52. Jain, A. K., "Mortality Risk Associated with the Use of Oral Contraceptives," Studies in Family Planning, *8*:50-54, 1977.
53. Beral, V., "Mortality Among Oral Contraceptive Users," Lancet, *2*:727-731, 1977.
54. Royal College of General Practitioners' Oral contraception study, "Incidence of arterial disease among oral contraceptive users," J Royal Col Gen Pract *33*:75-82, 1983.
55. Slone, D., Shapiro, S., Kaufman, D. W., Rosenberg, L., Miettinen, O., and Stolley, P., "Risk of myocardial infarction in relation to current and discontinued use of oral contraceptives," N Engl J Med *305*:420-424, 1981.
56. Inman, W.H.W., "Oral contraceptives and fatal subarachnoid haemorrhage," Brit Med J *2*:1468-1470, 1979.
57. Petitti, D. B., and Wingerd, J., "Use of oral contraceptives, cigarette smoking and risk of subarachnoid haemorrhage," Lancet *2*:234-236, 1978.
58. Thorogood, M., Adam, S. A., and Mann, J. I., "Fatal subarachnoid haemorrhage in young women: role of oral contraceptives," Brit Med J *283*:762, 1981.
59. Rosenberg, L., Hennekens, C.H., Rosner, B., Belanger, C., Rothman, K. J., and Speizer, F. E., "Oral contraceptive use in relation to nonfatal myocardial infarction," Am J Epidemiol *111*:59-66, 1980.
60. Adam, S. A., Thorogood, M., and Mann, J. I., "Oral contraception and myocardial infarction revisited: the effects of new preparations and prescribing patterns," Brit J Obstet Gynaecol *88*:838-845, 1981.

The patient labeling for oral-contraceptive drug products is set forth below:

Brief Summary Patient Package Insert

> **Cigarette smoking increases the risk of serious adverse effects on the heart and blood vessels from oral-contraceptive use. This risk increases with age and with heavy smoking (15 or more cigarettes per day) and is quite marked in women over 35 years of age. Women who use oral contraceptives should not smoke.**

Oral contraceptives taken as directed are about 99% effective in preventing pregnancy. (The mini-pill, however, is somewhat less effective.) Forgetting to take your pills increases the chance of pregnancy. Women who have or have had clotting disorders, cancer of the breast or sex organs, unexplained vaginal bleeding, a stroke, heart attack, angina pectoris, or who suspect they may be pregnant should not use oral contraceptives. Various drugs, such as some antibiotics, may also decrease the effectiveness of oral contraceptives.

Most side effects of the pill are not serious. The most common side effects are nausea, vomiting, bleeding between menstrual periods, weight gain, and breast tenderness. However, proper use of oral contraceptives requires that they be taken under your doctor's continuous supervision, because they can be associated with serious side effects which may be fatal. Fortunately, these occur very infrequently. The serious side effects are:

1. Blood clots in the legs, lungs, brain, heart, or other organs, and hemorrhage into the brain due to bursting of a blood vessel. Certain of these effects may occur after pill use has been stopped.
2. Liver tumors, which may rupture and cause severe bleeding.
3. Birth defects if the pill is taken while you are pregnant.
4. High blood pressure.
5. Gallbladder disease.

The symptoms associated with these serious side effects are discussed in the detailed leaflet given you with your supply of pills. Notify your doctor if you notice any unusual physical disturbance while taking the pill.

The estrogen in oral contraceptives has been found to cause breast cancer and other cancers in certain animals. These findings suggest that oral contraceptives may also cause cancer in humans. However, studies to date in women taking currently marketed oral contraceptives have not confirmed that oral contraceptives cause cancer in humans.

The detailed leaflet describes more completely the benefits and risks of oral contraceptives. It also provides information on other forms of contraception. Read it carefully. If you have any questions, consult your doctor.

Caution: Oral contraceptives are of no value in the prevention or treatment of venereal disease.

DETAILED PATIENT LABELING

WHAT YOU SHOULD KNOW ABOUT ORAL CONTRACEPTIVES

Oral contraceptives ("the pill") are the most effective way (except for sterilization) to prevent pregnancy. They are also convenient and, for most women, free of serious or unpleasant side effects. Oral contraceptives must always be taken under the continuous supervision of a physician.

It is important that any woman who considers using an oral contraceptive understand the risks involved. Although the oral contraceptives have important advantages over other methods of contraception, they have certain risks that no other method has. Only you can decide whether the advantages are worth these risks. This leaflet will tell you about the most important risks. It will explain how you can help your doctor prescribe the pill as safely as possible by telling him about yourself and being alert for the earliest signs of trouble. And it will tell you how to use the pill properly, so that it will be as effective as possible. There is more detailed information available in the leaflet prepared for doctors. Your pharmacist can show you a copy; you may need your doctor's help in understanding parts of it.

WHO SHOULD NOT USE ORAL CONTRACEPTIVES

A. If you have any of the following conditions, you should not use the pill:
 1. Clots in the legs or lungs.
 2. Angina pectoris.
 3. Known or suspected cancer of the breast or sex organs.
 4. Unusual vaginal bleeding that has not yet been diagnosed.
 5. Known or suspected pregnancy.

B. If you have had any of the following conditions, you should not use the pill:
 1. Heart attack or stroke.
 2. Clots in the legs or lungs.

> **C. Cigarette smoking increases the risk of serious adverse effects on the heart and blood vessels from oral-contraceptive use. This risk increases with age and with heavy smoking (15 or more cigarettes per day) and is quite marked in women over 35 years of age. Women who use oral contraceptives should not smoke.**

D. If you have scanty or irregular periods or are a young woman without a regular cycle, you should use another method of contraception because, if you use the pill, you may have difficulty becoming pregnant or may fail to have menstrual periods after discontinuing the pill.

DECIDING TO USE ORAL CONTRACEPTIVES

If you do not have any of the conditions listed above and are thinking about using oral contraceptives, to help you decide, you need information about the advantages and risks of oral contraceptives and of other contraceptive methods as well. This leaflet describes the advantages and risks of oral contraceptives. Except for sterilization, the IUD, and abortion, which have their own inherent risks, the only risks of other methods of contraception are those due to pregnancy should the method fail. Your doctor can answer questions you may have with respect to other methods of contraception. He can also answer any questions you may have after reading this leaflet on oral contraceptives.

1. What Oral Contraceptives Are and How They Work. Oral contraceptives are of two types. The most common, often simply called "the pill," is a combination of an estrogen and a progestogen, the two kinds of female hormones. The amount of estrogen and progestogen can vary, but the amount of estrogen is most important because both the effectiveness and some of the dangers of oral contraceptives are related to the amount of estrogen. This kind of oral contraceptive works principally by preventing release of an egg from the ovary. When the amount of estrogen is 50 micrograms or more, and the pill is taken as directed, oral contraceptives are more than 99% effective (i.e., there would be less than 1 pregnancy if 100 women used the pill for 1 year). Pills that contain 20 to 35 micrograms of estrogen vary slightly in effectiveness, ranging from 98% to more than 99% effective. The second type of oral contraceptive, often called the "mini-pill", contains only a progestogen. It works in part by preventing release of an egg from the ovary but also by keeping sperm from reaching the egg and by making the uterus (womb) less receptive to any fertilized egg that reaches it. The mini-pill is less effective than the combination oral contraceptive, about 97% effective. In addition, the progestogen-only pill has a tendency to cause irregular bleeding which may be quite inconvenient, or cessation of bleeding entirely. The progestogen-only pill is used despite its lower effectiveness in the hope that it will prove not to have some of the serious side effects of the estrogen-containing pill (see below), but it is not yet certain that the mini-pill does in fact have fewer serious side effects. The discussion below, while based mainly on information about the combination pills, should be considered to apply as well to the mini-pill.

2. Other Nonsurgical Ways to Prevent Pregnancy. As this leaflet will explain, oral contraceptives have several serious risks. Other methods of con-

traception have lesser risks or none at all. They are also less effective than oral contraceptives, but, used properly, may be effective enough for many women.

The following table gives reported pregnancy rates (the number of women out of 100 who would become pregnant in 1 year) for these methods.

PREGNANCIES PER 100 WOMEN PER YEAR
Intrauterine device (IUD), less than 1-6; Diaphragm with spermicidal products (creams or jellies), 2-20; Condom (rubber), 3-36; Aerosol foams, 2-29; Jellies and creams, 4-36; Periodic abstinence (rhythm) all types, less than 1-47:
1. Calendar method, 14-47;
2. Temperature method, 1-20;
3. Temperature method—intercourse only in postovulatory phase, less than 1-7;
4. Mucus method, 1-25;
No contraception, 60-80.

The figures (except for the IUD) vary widely because people differ in how well they use each method. Very faithful users of the various methods obtain very good results, except for users of the calendar method of periodic abstinence (rhythm). Except for the IUD, effective use of these methods requires somewhat more effort than simply taking a single pill every day, but it is an effort that many couples undertake successfully. Your doctor can tell you a great deal more about these methods of contraception.

3. The Dangers of Oral Contraceptives.
a. *Circulatory disorders (abnormal blood clotting and stroke due to hemorrhage).*
Blood clots (in various blood vessels of the body) are the most common of the serious side effects of oral contraceptives. A clot can result in a stroke (if the clot is in the brain), a heart attack (if the clot is in a blood vessel of the heart), or a pulmonary embolus (a clot which forms in the legs or pelvis, then breaks off and travels to the lungs). Any of these can be fatal. Clots also occur rarely in the blood vessels of the eye, resulting in blindness or impairment of vision in that eye. There is evidence that the risk of clotting increases with higher estrogen doses. It is therefore important to keep the dose of estrogen as low as possible, so long as the oral contraceptive used has an acceptable pregnancy rate and doesn't cause unacceptable changes in the menstrual pattern. Furthermore, cigarette smoking by oral-contraceptive users increases the risk of serious adverse effects on the heart and blood vessels. This risk increases with age and with heavy smoking (15 or more cigarettes per day) and begins to become quite marked in women over 35 years of age. For this reason, women who use oral contraceptives should not smoke. The risk of abnormal clotting increases with age in both users and nonusers of oral contraceptives, but the increased risk from the contraceptive appears to be present at all ages. For oral-contraceptive users in general, it has been estimated that in women between the ages of 15 and 34 the risk of death due to a circulatory disorder is about 1 in 12,000 per year, whereas for nonusers the risk is about 1 in 50,000 per year. In the age group 35 to 44, the risk is estimated to be about 1 in 2,500 per year for oral-contraceptive users and about 1 in 10,000 per year for nonusers. (See chart next column.)

Even without the pill the risk of having a heart attack increases with age and is also increased by such heart attack risk factors as high blood pressure, high cholesterol, obesity, diabetes, and cigarette smoking. Without any risk factors present, the use of oral contraceptives alone may double the risk of heart attack. However, the combination of cigarette smoking, especially heavy smoking, and oral contraceptive use greatly increases the risk of heart attack. Oral-contraceptive users who smoke are about 5 times more likely to have a heart attack than users who do not smoke and about 10 times more likely to have a heart attack than nonusers who do not smoke. It has been estimated that users between the ages of 30 and 39 who smoke have about a 1 in 10,000 chance each year of having a fatal heart attack compared to about a 1 in 50,000 chance in users who do not smoke, and about 1 in 100,000 chance in nonus-

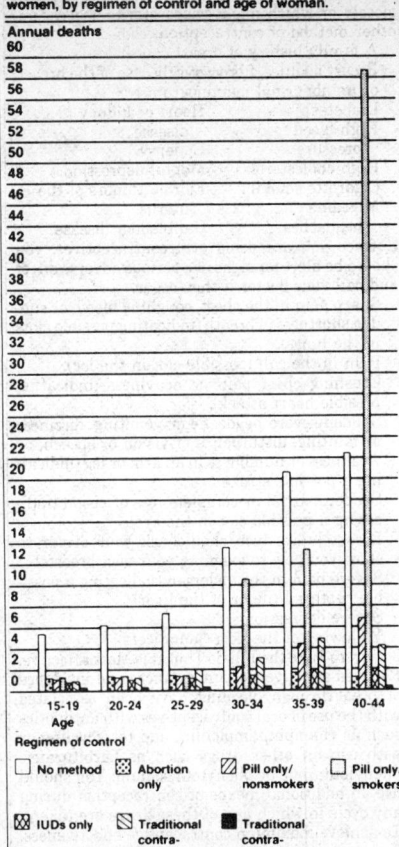

Figure 1. Estimated annual number of deaths associated with control of fertility and no control per 100,000 nonsterile women, by regimen of control and age of woman.

ers who do not smoke. In the age group 40 to 44, the risk is about 1 in 1,700 per year for users who smoke compared to about 1 in 10,000 for users who do not smoke and to about 1 in 14,000 per year for nonusers who do not smoke. Heavy smoking (about 15 cigarettes or more a day) further increases the risk. If you do not smoke and have none of the other heart attack risk factors described above, you will have a smaller risk than listed. If you have several heart attack risk factors, the risk may be considerably greater than listed.

In addition to blood-clotting disorders, it has been estimated that women taking oral contraceptives are twice as likely as nonusers to have a stroke due to rupture of a blood vessel in the brain. There is evidence that patients who stop taking oral contraceptives after using them continuously for five or more years may continue to have an increased risk of stroke or heart attack for at least six to nine years after discontinuation.

b. *Formation of tumors.* Studies have found that when certain animals are given the female sex hormone, estrogen, which is an ingredient of oral contraceptives, continuously for long periods, cancers may develop in the breast, cervix, vagina, and liver.

These findings suggest that oral contraceptives may cause cancer in humans. However, studies to date in women taking currently marketed oral contraceptives have not confirmed that oral contraceptives cause cancer in humans. Several studies have found no increase in breast cancer in users, although one study suggested oral contraceptives might cause an increase in breast cancer in women who already have benign breast disease (e.g., cysts).

Women with a strong family history of breast cancer or who have breast nodules, fibrocystic disease, or abnormal mammograms or who were exposed to DES (Diethylstilbestrol), an estrogen, during their mother's pregnancy must be followed very closely by their doctors if they choose to use oral contraceptives instead of another method of contraception. Many studies have shown that women taking oral contraceptives have less risk of getting benign breast disease than those who have not used oral contraceptives. Recently, strong evidence has emerged that estrogens (one component of oral contraceptives), when given for periods of more than one year to women after the menopause, increase the risk of cancer of the uterus (womb). There is also some evidence that a kind of oral contraceptive which is no longer marketed, the sequential oral contraceptive, may increase the risk of cancer of the uterus. There remains no evidence, however, that the oral contraceptives now available increase the risk of this cancer. Oral contraceptives do cause, although rarely, a benign (nonmalignant) tumor of the liver. These tumors do not spread, but they may rupture and cause internal bleeding, which may be fatal. A few cases of cancer of the liver have been reported in women using oral contraceptives, but it is not yet known whether the drug caused them.

c. *Dangers to a developing child if oral contraceptives are used in or immediately preceding pregnancy.* Oral contraceptives should not be taken by pregnant women because they may damage the developing child. An increased risk of birth defects, including heart defects and limb defects, has been associated with the use of sex hormones, including oral contraceptives, in pregnancy. In addition, the developing female child whose mother has received DES (diethylstilbestrol), an estrogen, during pregnancy has a risk of getting cancer of the vagina or cervix in her teens or young adulthood. This risk is estimated to be about 1 in 1,000 exposures or less. Abnormalities of the urinary and sex organs have been reported in male offspring so exposed. It is possible that other estrogens, such as the estrogens in oral contraceptives, could have the same effect in the child if the mother takes them during pregnancy.

If you stop taking oral contraceptives to become pregnant, your doctor may recommend that you use another method of contraception for a short while. The reason for this is that there is evidence from studies in women who have had "miscarriages" soon after stopping the pill, that the lost fetuses are more likely to be abnormal. Whether there is an overall increase in "miscarriage" in women who become pregnant soon after stopping the pill as compared with women who do not use the pill is not known, but it is possible that there may be. If, however, you do become pregnant soon after stopping oral contraceptives, and do not have a miscarriage, there is no evidence that the baby has an increased risk of being abnormal.

d. *Gallbladder disease.* Women who use oral contraceptives have a greater risk than nonusers of having gallbladder disease requiring surgery. The increased risk may first appear within 1 year of use and may double after 4 or 5 years of use.

e. *Other side effects of oral contraceptives.* Some women using oral contraceptives experience unpleasant side effects that are not dangerous and are not likely to damage their health. Some of these may be temporary. Your breasts may feel tender, nausea and vomiting may occur, you may gain or lose weight, and your ankles may swell. A spotty darkening of the skin, particularly of the face, is possible and may persist. You may notice unexpected vaginal bleeding or changes in your menstrual period. Irregular bleeding is frequently seen when using the mini-pill or combination oral contraceptives containing less than 50 micrograms of estrogen.

More serious side effects include worsening of migraine, asthma, epilepsy, and kidney or heart disease because of a tendency for water to be retained in the body when oral contraceptives are used. Other side effects are growth of preexisting fibroid tumors of the uterus; mental depression, and liver problems with jaundice (yellowing of the skin). Your doctor may find that levels of sugar and fatty substances in your blood are elevated; the long-

Continued on next page

Wyeth—Cont.

term effects of these changes are not known. Some women develop high blood pressure while taking oral contraceptives, which ordinarily returns to the original levels when the oral contraceptive is stopped.

Other reactions, although not proved to be caused by oral contraceptives, are occasionally reported. These include more frequent urination and some discomfort when urinating, nervousness, dizziness, some loss of scalp hair, an increase in body hair, an increase or decrease in sex drive, appetite changes, cataracts, and a need for a change in contact lens prescription, or inability to use contact lenses.

After you stop using oral contraceptives, there may be a delay before you are able to become pregnant or before you resume having menstrual periods. This is especially true of women who had irregular menstrual cycles prior to the use of oral contraceptives. As discussed previously, your doctor may recommend that you wait a short while after stopping the pill before you try to become pregnant. During this time, use another form of contraception. You should consult your physician before resuming use of oral contraceptives after childbirth, especially if you plan to nurse your baby. Drugs in oral contraceptives are known to appear in the milk, and the long-range effect on infants is not known at this time. Furthermore, oral contraceptives may cause a decrease in your milk supply as well as in the quality of the milk.

4. Comparison of the Risks of Oral Contraceptives and Other Contraceptive Methods. The many studies on the risks and effectiveness of oral contraceptives and other methods of contraception have been analyzed to estimate the risk of death associated with various methods of contraception. This risk has two parts: (a) the risk of the method itself (e.g., the risk that oral contraceptives will cause death due to abnormal clotting), and (b) the risk of death due to pregnancy or abortion in the event the method fails. The results of this analysis are shown in the bar graph (Figure 1). The height of the bars is the number of deaths per 100,000 women each year. There are six sets of bars, each set referring to a specific age group of women. Within each set of bars, there is a single bar for each of the different contraceptive methods. For oral contraceptives, there are two bars—one for smokers and the other for nonsmokers. The analysis is based on present knowledge, and new information could, of course, alter it. The analysis shows that the risk of death from all methods of birth control is low and below that associated with childbirth, except for oral contraceptives in women over 40 who smoke. It shows that the lowest risk of death is associated with the condom or diaphragm (traditional contraception) backed up by early abortion in case of failure of the condom or diaphragm to prevent pregnancy. Also, at any age the risk of death (due to unexpected pregnancy) from the use of traditional contraception, even without a backup of abortion, is generally the same as or less than that from use of oral contraceptives.

HOW TO USE ORAL CONTRACEPTIVES AS SAFELY AND EFFECTIVELY AS POSSIBLE, ONCE YOU HAVE DECIDED TO USE THEM

1. What to Tell your Doctor.

You can make use of the pill as safely as possible by telling your doctor if you have any of the following:

a. Conditions that mean you should not use oral contraceptives.
  Clots in the legs or lungs.
  Clots in the legs or lungs in the past.
  A stroke, heart attack, or angina pectoris.
  Known or suspected cancer of the breast or sex organs.
  Unusual vaginal bleeding that has not yet been diagnosed.
  Known or suspected pregnancy.

b. Conditions that your doctor will want to watch closely or which might cause him to suggest another method of contraception:
  A family history of breast cancer.
  Breast nodules, fibrocystic disease of the breast, or an abnormal mammogram.
  Diabetes.
  High blood pressure.
  High cholesterol.
  Cigarette smoking.
  Migraine headaches.
  Heart or kidney disease.
  Epilepsy.
  Mental depression.
  Fibroid tumors of the uterus.
  Gallbladder disease.

c. Once you are using oral contraceptives, you should be alert for signs of a serious adverse effect and call your doctor if they occur.
  Sharp pain in the chest, coughing blood, or sudden shortness of breath (indicating possible clots in the lungs).
  Pain in the calf (possible clot in the leg).
  Crushing chest pain or heaviness (indicating possible heart attack).
  Sudden severe headache or vomiting, dizziness or fainting, disturbance of vision or speech, or weakness or numbness in an arm or leg (indicating a possible stroke).
  Sudden partial or complete loss of vision (indicating a possible clot in the eye).
  Breast lumps (you should ask your doctor to show you how to examine your own breasts).
  Severe pain in the abdomen (indicating a possible ruptured tumor of the liver).
  Severe depression.
  Yellowing of the skin (jaundice).

2. How to Take the Pill So That It is Most Effective.
Reduced effectiveness and an increased incidence of breakthrough bleeding have been associated with the use of oral contraceptives with antibiotics such as rifampin, ampicillin, and tetracycline or with certain other drugs such as barbiturates, phenylbutazone or phenytoin sodium. You should use an additional means of contraception during any cycle in which any of these drugs are taken. To achieve maximum contraceptive effectiveness, oral contraceptives must be taken exactly as directed and at intervals not exceeding 24 hours. It is recommended that tablets be taken at the same time each day, preferably after the evening meal or at bedtime. Taking them on a definite schedule will decrease the chance of forgetting a tablet and also help keep the proper amount of medication in your system. See detailed instructions below for Nordette-21, Ovral® and Lo/Ovral®, Nordette-28, Ovral®-28 and Lo/Ovral®-28, and for Ovrette®.

NORDETTE®-21, OVRAL®, LO/OVRAL®
The dosage of Nordette-21, Ovral® and Lo/Ovral® is one tablet daily for 21 days in a row per menstrual cycle. Tablets are then discontinued for 7 days.
The basic schedule is 21 days on—7 days off.
During the first month, you should begin taking Nordette-21, Ovral® or Lo/Ovral® on Day 5 of your menstrual cycle whether or not you still have your period. (Day 1 is the first day of menstruation, even if it is almost midnight when you start.) Note: During your first month on Nordette-21, Ovral® or Lo/Ovral®, if you start taking tablets later than Day 5 of your menstrual cycle, you should protect yourself by also using another method of birth control until you have taken a tablet daily for seven consecutive days. Thereafter, if you follow directions carefully you will obtain the full contraceptive benefit. If you begin taking tablets later than the proper day, the possibility of ovulation and pregnancy occurring before beginning medication should be considered.
Take one tablet every day until you finish all 21 tablets. No tablets are then taken for one week (7 days). Your period will usually begin about three days after you take the last tablet. Don't be alarmed if the amount of bleeding is not the same as before. On the 8th day, start a new Pilpak®, even if you still have your period. If, for example, you took Nordette-21, Ovral® or Lo/Ovral® for the first time on a Tuesday, the 8th day will also be a Tuesday. Thus, you will always begin a new cycle on the same day of the week as long as you do not interrupt your original schedule. If you start taking tablets later than the 8th day, you should protect yourself by also using another method of birth control until you have taken a tablet daily for seven days in a row.

NORDETTE®-28, OVRAL®-28, LO/OVRAL®-28
The dosage of Nordette-28, Ovral®-28 and Lo/Ovral®-28 is one white or light-orange active tablet daily for 21 consecutive days followed by one pink inactive tablet daily for 7 consecutive days. The basic schedule is 21 days on white or light-orange active tablets—7 days on pink inactive tablets. Always take all 21 white or light-orange tablets in each Pilpak® before taking the pink tablets.
You should begin taking Nordette-28, Ovral®-28 or Lo/Ovral®-28 on the first Sunday after your menstrual period begins, whether or not you are still bleeding. If your period begins on a Sunday, take your first tablet that very same day. Your first white or light-orange tablet is marked with a large arrow and the word "Start". Note: During your first month on Nordette-28, Ovral®-28 or Lo/Ovral®-28, you should protect yourself by also using another method of birth control until you have taken a white or light-orange tablet daily for seven consecutive days. Thereafter, if you follow directions carefully, you will obtain the full contraceptive benefit. If you begin taking tablets later than the proper day, the possibility of ovulation and pregnancy occurring before beginning medication should be considered.
Take one tablet every day until you finish all 21 white or light-orange tablets in a Pilpak®, followed by all seven pink tablets. Your period will usually begin about three days after you take the last white or light-orange tablet, which will be during the time you are taking the pink tablets. Don't be alarmed if the amount of bleeding is not the same as before. The day after you have taken your last pink tablet, begin a new Pilpak® of tablets (taking all 21 white or light-orange tablets first, just as you did before) so that you will take a tablet every day without interruption. The starting day for each new Pilpak® will always be Sunday. If in any cycle you start tablets later than the proper day, you should also use another method of birth control until you have taken a white or light-orange tablet daily for 7 days in a row.

Spotting or Breakthrough Bleeding:
Spotting is slight staining between menstrual periods which may not even require a pad. Breakthrough bleeding is a flow much like a regular period, requiring sanitary protection. Spotting is more common than breakthrough bleeding, and both occur more often in the first few cycles than in later cycles. These types of bleeding are usually temporary and without significance. It is important to continue taking your pills on schedule. If the bleeding persists for more than a few days, consult your doctor.

Forgotten Pills:
Nordette-21, Ovral® and Lo/Ovral® each contain 21 active white or light-orange tablets per Pilpak®. Nordette-28, Ovral®-28 and Lo/Ovral®-28 each contain 21 active white or light-orange tablets plus 7 pink inactive tablets per Pilpak®.
The chance of becoming pregnant is probably quite small if you miss only one white or light-orange tablet in a cycle. Of course, with each additional one you skip, the chance increases. If you miss one or more pink tablets (Nordette-28, Ovral®-28, Lo/Ovral®-28) you are still protected against pregnancy as long as you begin taking your next white or light-orange tablet on the proper day. It is important to take a missed white or light-orange tablet as soon as it is remembered. If two consecutive white or light-orange tablets are missed they should both be taken as soon as remembered. The next tablet should then be taken at the usual time. Any time you miss one or two white or light-orange tablets, or begin a new Pilpak® after the proper starting day, you should also use another method of birth control until you have taken a white or light-orange tablet daily for seven consecutive days. If breakthrough bleeding occurs follow-

ing missed tablets, it will usually be temporary and of no consequence. While there is little likelihood of pregnancy occurring if only one or two white or light-orange tablets are missed, the possibility of pregnancy increases with each successive day that scheduled white or light-orange tablets are missed.

If you are taking Nordette-21, Ovral® or Lo/Ovral® and forget to take three white or light-orange tablets in a row, do not take them when you remember. Wait four more days— which makes a whole week without tablets. Then begin a new Pilpak® on the 8th day after the last tablet was taken. During the seven days without tablets, and until you have taken a white or light-orange tablet daily for seven consecutive days, you should protect yourself from pregnancy by also using another method of birth control.

If you are taking Nordette-28, Ovral®-28 or Lo/Ovral®-28 and forget to take three white or light-orange tablets in a row, do not take them when you remember. Stop taking all medication until the first Sunday following the last missed tablet. Then, whether or not you have had your period, and even if you are still bleeding, start a new Pilpak®. During the days without tablets, and until you have taken a white or light-orange tablet daily for seven consecutive days, you should protect yourself from pregnancy by also using another method of birth control.

OVRETTE®

Ovrette® is administered on a continuous daily dosage schedule, one tablet each day, every day of the year. Take the first tablet on the first day of your menstrual period. Tablets should be taken at the same time every day, without interruption, whether bleeding occurs or not. If bleeding is prolonged (more than 8 days) or unusually heavy, you should contact your doctor.

Forgotten Pills:

The risk of pregnancy increases with each tablet missed. Therefore, it is very important that you take one tablet daily as directed. If you miss one tablet, take it as soon as you remember and also take your next tablet at the regular time. If you miss two tablets, take one of the missed tablets as soon as you remember, as well as your regular tablet for that day at the proper time. Furthermore, you should use another method of birth control in addition to taking Ovrette® until you have taken fourteen days (2 weeks) of medication.

If more than two tablets have been missed, Ovrette® should be discontinued and another method of birth control used until the start of your next menstrual period. Then you may resume taking Ovrette®.

At times there may be no menstrual period after a cycle of pills.

Therefore, if you miss one menstrual period but have taken the pills *exactly as you were supposed to,* continue as usual into the next cycle. If you have not taken the pills correctly and miss a menstrual period, or if you are taking mini-pills and it is 45 days or more from the start of your last menstrual period, you may be pregnant and should stop taking oral contraceptives until your doctor determines whether or not you are pregnant. Until you can get to your doctor, use another form of contraception. If two consecutive menstrual periods are missed, you should stop taking pills until it is determined whether you are pregnant. If you do become pregnant while using oral contraceptives, you should discuss the risks to the developing child with your doctor.

3. Periodic Examination.

Your doctor will take a complete medical and family history before prescribing oral contraceptives. At that time and about once a year thereafter, he will generally examine your blood pressure, breasts, abdomen, and pelvic organs (including a Papanicolaou smear, i.e., test for cancer).

SUMMARY

Oral contraceptives are the most effective method, except sterilization, for preventing pregnancy. Other methods when used conscientiously, are also very effective and have fewer risks. The serious risks of oral contraceptives are uncommon, and the "pill" is a very convenient method of preventing pregnancy.

If you have certain conditions or have had these conditions in the past, you should not use oral contraceptives, because the risk is too great. These conditions are listed in the leaflet. If you do not have these conditions, and decide to use the "pill", please read the leaflet carefully so that you can use the "pill" most safely and effectively.

Based on his or her assessment of your medical needs, your doctor has prescribed this drug for you. Do not give the drug to anyone else.

Shown in Product Identification Section, page 444

LO/OVRAL®-28
[lŏh-oh'vral-28]
Tablets
(norgestrel and ethinyl estradiol tablets)

Description: 21 white LO/OVRAL® tablets, each containing 0.3 mg of norgestrel (*dl*-13-beta-ethyl-17-alpha-ethinyl-17-beta-hydroxygon-4-en-3-one), a totally synthetic progestogen, and 0.03 mg of ethinyl estradiol (19-nor-17α-pregna-1,3,5(10)-trien-20-yne-3,17-diol), and 7 pink inert tablets.

Clinical Pharmacology: See Lo/Ovral®.
Indications and Usage: See Lo/Ovral.
Dose-Related Risk of Thromboembolism from Oral Contraceptives: See Lo/Ovral.
Contraindications: See Lo/Ovral.
Warnings: See Lo/Ovral.
Precautions: See Lo/Ovral.
Information for the Patient: See Lo/Ovral.
Drug Interactions: See Lo/Ovral.
Carcinogenesis: See Lo/Ovral.
Pregnancy: See Lo/Ovral.
Nursing Mothers: See Lo/Ovral.
Adverse Reactions: See Lo/Ovral.
Acute Overdosage: See Lo/Ovral.
Dosage and Administration: To achieve maximum contraceptive effectiveness, LO/OVRAL®-28 must be taken exactly as directed and at intervals not exceeding 24 hours.

The dosage of LO/OVRAL®-28 is one white tablet daily for 21 consecutive days followed by one pink inert tablet daily for 7 consecutive days according to prescribed schedule. It is recommended that tablets be taken at the same time each day, preferably after the evening meal or at bedtime.

During the first cycle of medication, the patient is instructed to begin taking LO/OVRAL®-28 on the first Sunday after the onset of menstruation. If menstruation begins on a Sunday, the first tablet (white) is taken that day. One white tablet should be taken daily for 21 consecutive days followed by one pink inert tablet daily for 7 consecutive days. Withdrawal bleeding should usually occur within three days following discontinuation of white tablets.

During the first cycle, contraceptive reliance should not be placed on LO/OVRAL®-28 until a white tablet has been taken daily for 7 consecutive days. The possibility of ovulation and conception prior to initiation of medication should be considered.

The patient begins her next and all subsequent 28-day courses of tablets on the same day of the week (Sunday) on which she began her first course, following the same schedule: 21 days on white tablets—7 days on pink inert tablets. If in any cycle the patient starts tablets later than the proper day, she should protect herself by using another method of birth control until she has taken a white tablet daily for 7 consecutive days.

If spotting or breakthrough bleeding occurs, the patient is instructed to continue on the same regimen. This type of bleeding is usually transient and without significance; however, if the bleeding is persistent or prolonged the patient is advised to consult her physician. Although the occurrence of pregnancy is highly unlikely if LO/OVRAL®-28 is taken according to directions, if withdrawal bleeding does not occur, the possibility of pregnancy must be considered. If the patient has not adhered to the prescribed schedule (missed one or more tablets or started taking them on a day later than she should have) the probability of pregnancy should be considered at the time of the first missed period and appropriate diagnostic measures taken before the medication is resumed. If the patient has adhered to the prescribed regimen and misses two consecutive periods, pregnancy should be ruled out before continuing the contraceptive regimen.

The patient should be instructed to take a missed white tablet as soon as it is remembered. If two consecutive white tablets are missed they should both be taken as soon as remembered. The next tablet should be taken at the usual time. Any time the patient misses one or two white tablets she should also use another method of contraception until she has taken a white tablet daily for seven consecutive days. If the patient misses one or more pink tablets she is still protected against pregnancy *provided* she begins taking white tablets again on the proper day.

If breakthrough bleeding occurs following missed white tablets it will usually be transient and of no consequence. While there is little likelihood of ovulation occurring if only one or two white tablets are missed the possibility of ovulation increases with each successive day that scheduled white tablets are missed. (If three consecutive days white LO/OVRAL® tablets are missed, all medication should be discontinued and the remainder of the 28-day package discarded. A new tablet cycle should be started on the first Sunday following the last missed tablet, and an alternate means of contraception should be prescribed during the days without tablets and until the patient has taken a white tablet daily for 7 consecutive days.)

In the nonlactating mother LO/OVRAL® may be prescribed in the postpartum period either immediately or at the first postpartum examination whether or not menstruation has resumed.

How Supplied: LO/OVRAL®-28 Tablets (0.3 mg norgestrel and 0.03 mg ethinyl estradiol), Wyeth®, are available in packages of 6 PILPAK® dispensers, each containing 28 tablets as follows: 21 active tablets, NDC 0008-0078, white, round tablet marked "WYETH" and "78".

7 inert tablets, NDC 0008-0486, pink, round tablet marked "WYETH" and "486".

References: See Lo/Ovral.
Brief Summary Patient Package Insert: See Lo/Ovral.
DETAILED PATIENT LABELING: See Lo/Ovral.
Shown in Product Identification Section, page 444

MAZANOR®
[maz'a-nor]
(mazindol)

Description: Mazanor (mazindol) is an imidazoisoindole anorectic agent. It is chemically designated as 5-p-chloro-phenyl-5-hydroxy-2,3-dihydro-5H-imidazo (2,1-a)isoindole, a tautomeric form of 2-[2'-(p-chlorobenzoyl)phenyl]-2-imidazoline.

Actions: Mazanor (mazindol), although an isoindole, has pharmacologic activity similar in many ways to the prototype drugs used in obesity, the amphetamines. Actions include central-nervous-system stimulation in humans and animals, as well as such amphetamine-like effects in animals as the production of stereotyped behavior. Animal experiments also suggest certain differences from phenethylamine anorectic drugs, e.g., amphetamine, with respect to site and mechanism of action; for example, mazindol appears to exert its primary effects on the limbic system. The significance of these differences for humans is uncertain. It does not cause brain norepinephrine depletion in animals; on the other hand, it does appear to inhibit storage-site uptake of norepinephrine as is suggested by its marked potentiation of the effect of exogenous norepinephrine on blood pressure in dogs (see "Warnings") and on smooth-muscle contraction *in vitro.*

Tolerance has been demonstrated with all drugs of this class in which this phenomenon has been studied.

Drugs used in obesity are commonly known as "anorectics" or "anorexigenics." It has not been

Continued on next page

Wyeth—Cont.

established, however, that the action of such drugs in treating obesity is exclusively one of appetite suppression. Other central-nervous-system actions or metabolic effects may be involved as well.

Adult obese subjects, instructed in dietary management and treated with anorectic drugs, lose more weight on the average than those treated with placebo and diet, as determined in relatively short-term clinical trials.

The average magnitude of increased weight loss of drug-treated patients over placebo-treated patients in studies of anorectics in general is ordinarily only a fraction of a pound a week. The rate of weight loss is greatest in the first weeks of therapy for both drug and placebo subjects and tends to decrease in succeeding weeks.

The amount of weight loss associated with the use of Mazanor (mazindol), as with other anorectic drugs, varies from trial to trial, and the increased weight loss appears to be related in part to variables other than the drugs prescribed, such as the interaction between physician-investigator and the patient, the population treated, and the diet prescribed. The importance of non-drug factors in such weight loss has not been elucidated.

The natural history of obesity is measured in years, whereas, most studies cited are restricted to a few weeks duration; thus, the total impact of drug-induced weight loss over that of diet alone must be considered clinically limited.

Indication: Mazanor (mazindol) is indicated in the management of exogenous obesity as a short-term (a few weeks) adjunct in a regimen of weight reduction based on caloric restriction. The limited usefulness of agents of this class (see "Actions") should be measured against possible risk factors inherent in their use, such as those described below.

Contraindications: Glaucoma, hypersensitivity or idiosyncrasy to Mazanor (mazindol). Agitated states.

Patients with a history of drug abuse.

During or within 14 days following the administration of monoamine oxidase inhibitors (hypertensive crises may result).

Warnings: Tolerance to the effect of many anorectic drugs may develop within a few weeks; if this occurs, the recommended dose should not be exceeded in an attempt to increase the effect; rather, the drug should be discontinued.

Mazanor (mazindol) may impair the ability of the patient to engage in potentially hazardous activities, such as operating machinery or driving a motor vehicle; the patient should therefore be cautioned accordingly.

DRUG INTERACTIONS

Mazanor (mazindol) may decrease the hypotensive effect of guanethidine; patients should be monitored accordingly.

Mazanor (mazindol) may markedly potentiate the pressor effect of exogenous catecholamines. If it should be necessary to give a pressor amine agent (e.g., levarterenol or isoproterenol) to a patient in shock (e.g., from a myocardial infarction) who has recently been taking Mazanor (mazindol), extreme care should be taken in monitoring blood pressure at frequent intervals and initiating pressor therapy with a low initial dose and careful titration.

DRUG DEPENDENCE

Mazanor (mazindol) shares important pharmacologic properties with amphetamines. Amphetamines and related stimulant drugs have been extensively abused and can produce tolerance and severe psychologic dependence. In this regard, the manifestations of chronic overdosage or withdrawal of Mazanor (mazindol) have not been determined in humans. Abstinence effects have been observed in dogs after abrupt cessation for prolonged periods. There was some self-administration of the drug in monkeys. EEG studies and "liking" scores in human studies yielded equivocal results. While the abuse potential of Mazanor (mazindol) has not been further defined, the possibility of dependence should be kept in mind when evaluating the desirability of including Mazanor (mazindol) as part of a weight-reduction program.

USAGE IN PREGNANCY

Mazanor (mazindol) was studied in reproduction experiments in rats and rabbits, and an increase in neonatal mortality and a possible increased incidence of rib anomalies in rats were observed at relatively high doses. Although these studies have not indicated important adverse effects, use of mazindol by women who are or may become pregnant requires that the potential benefit be weighed against the possible hazard to mother and fetus.

USAGE IN CHILDREN

Mazanor (mazindol) is not recommended for use in children under 12 years of age.

Precautions: Insulin requirements in diabetes mellitus may be altered in association with the use of mazindol and the concomitant dietary regimen. The least amount feasible should be prescribed or dispensed at one time in order to minimize the possibility of overdosage.

Use only with caution in hypertension with monitoring of blood pressure, since evidence is insufficient to rule out a possible adverse effect on blood pressure in some hypertensive patients. The drug is not recommended in severely hypertensive patients. The drug is not recommended for patients with symptomatic cardiovascular disease including arrhythmias.

Adverse Reactions: The most common adverse effects of Mazanor (mazindol) are: dry mouth, tachycardia, constipation, nervousness, and insomnia.

Cardiovascular: Palpitation, tachycardia.

Central Nervous System: Overstimulation, restlessness, dizziness, insomnia, dysphoria, tremor, headache, depression, drowsiness, weakness.

Gastrointestinal: Dryness of the mouth, unpleasant taste, diarrhea, constipation, nausea, other gastrointestinal disturbances.

Skin: Rash, excessive sweating, clamminess.

Endocrine: Impotence, changes in libido have rarely been observed with Mazanor (mazindol).

Eye: Treatment of dogs with high doses of Mazanor (mazindol) for long periods resulted in some corneal opacities, reversible on cessation of medication. No such effect has been observed in humans.

Dosage and Administration: Usual dosage is 1 mg three times daily, one hour before meals, or 2 mg once daily, one hour before lunch. The lowest effective dose should be used. To determine the lowest effective dose, therapy with Mazanor may be initiated at 1 mg once a day, and adjusted to the need and response of the patient. Should G.I. discomfort occur, Mazanor may be taken with meals.

Overdosage: There are no data as yet on acute overdosage with Mazanor (mazindol) in humans. Manifestations of acute overdosage with amphetamines and related substances include restlessness, tremor, rapid respiration, dizziness. Fatigue and depression may follow the stimulatory phase of overdosage. Cardiovascular effects include tachycardia, hypertension, and circulatory collapse. Gastrointestinal symptoms include nausea, vomiting, and abdominal cramps. While similar manifestations of overdosage may be seen with Mazanor (mazindol), their exact nature has yet to be determined. The management of acute intoxication is largely symptomatic. Data are not available on the treatment of acute intoxication with Mazanor (mazindol) by hemodialysis or peritoneal dialysis, but the substance is poorly soluble except at very acid pH.

How Supplied: Mazanor® (mazindol) Tablets, Wyeth®, are available in the following dosage strength in bottles of 30 tablets:

1 mg, NDC 0008-0071, white, round, scored tablet marked "WYETH" and "71".

Keep bottles tightly closed.

Store below 25° C (77° F).

Dispense in tight containers.

Shown in Product Identification Section, page 444

MEPERGAN®

[mep′er-gan]
(meperidine HCl and promethazine HCl)
Injection

Description: This product is available in concentration providing 25 mg each of meperidine hydrochloride and promethazine hydrochloride per ml with 0.1 mg edetate disodium, 0.04 mg calcium chloride, and not more than 0.75 mg sodium formaldehyde sulfoxylate, 0.25 mg sodium metabisulfite, and 5 mg phenol with sodium acetate buffer.

Actions: Meperidine hydrochloride is a narcotic analgesic with multiple actions qualitatively similar to those of morphine. Phenergan® (promethazine HCl) is a phenothiazine derivative that has several different pharmacologic properties including antihistaminic, sedative, and antiemetic actions.

Indications: As a preanesthetic medication when analgesia and sedation are indicated. As an adjunct to local and general anesthesia.

Contraindications: Hypersensitivity to meperidine or promethazine.

Under no circumstances should Mepergan be given by intra-arterial injection, due to the likelihood of severe arteriospasm and the possibility of resultant gangrene (see Warnings).

Mepergan should not be given by the subcutaneous route; evidence of chemical irritation has been noted and necrotic lesions have resulted on rare occasions following subcutaneous injection. The preferred parenteral route of administration is by deep intramuscular injection.

Meperidine is contraindicated in patients who are receiving monoamine oxidase inhibitors (MAOI) or those who have received such agents within 14 days.

Therapeutic doses of meperidine have inconsistently precipitated unpredictable, severe, and occasionally fatal reactions in patients who have received such agents within 14 days. The mechanism of these reactions is unclear. Some have been characterized by coma, severe respiratory depression, cyanosis, and hypotension, and have resembled the syndrome of acute narcotic overdose. In other reactions the predominant manifestations have been hyperexcitability, convulsions, tachycardia, hyperpyrexia, and hypertension. Although it is not known that other narcotics are free of the risk of such reactions, virtually all of the reported reactions have occurred with meperidine. If a narcotic is needed in such patients, a sensitivity test should be performed in which repeated, small, incremental doses of morphine are administered over the course of several hours while the patient's condition and vital signs are under careful observation.

(Intravenous hydrocortisone or prednisolone have been used to treat severe reactions, with the addition of intravenous chlorpromazine in those cases exhibiting hypertension and hyperpyrexia. The usefulness and safety of narcotic antagonists in the treatment of these reactions is unknown.)

Warnings: Tolerance and Addiction Liability
Warning—may be habit forming

DRUG DEPENDENCE: Meperidine can produce drug dependence of the morphine type and therefore has the potential for being abused. Psychic dependence, physical dependence, and tolerance may develop upon repeated administration of meperidine, and it should be prescribed and administered with the same degree of caution appropriate to the use of morphine. Like other narcotics, meperidine is subject to the provisions of the Federal narcotic laws.

INTERACTION WITH OTHER CENTRAL-NERVOUS-SYSTEM DEPRESSANTS: Meperidine should be used with great caution and in reduced dosage in patients who are concurrently receiving other narcotic analgesics, general anesthetics, phenothiazines, other tranquilizers, sedative-hypnotics, tricyclic antidepressants, and other CNS depressants (including alcohol). Respiratory depression, hypotension, and profound sedation or coma may result.

The sedative action of promethazine hydrochloride is additive to the sedative effects of central-nervous-system depressants; therefore, agents such as alcohol, barbiturates, and narcotic analgesics should either be eliminated or given in reduced dosage in the presence of promethazine hydrochloride. When given concomitantly with promethazine hydrochloride the dose of barbiturates should be reduced by at least one-half and the dose of analgesic depressants, such as morphine or meperidine, should be reduced by one-quarter to one-half.

HEAD INJURY AND INCREASED INTRACRANIAL PRESSURE: The respiratory depressant effects of meperidine and its capacity to elevate cerebrospinal-fluid pressure may be markedly exaggerated in the presence of head injury, other intracranial lesions, or a preexisting increase in intracranial pressure. Furthermore, narcotics produce adverse reactions which may obscure the clinical course of patients with head injuries. In such patients, meperidine must be used with extreme caution and only if its use is deemed essential.

INADVERTENT INTRA-ARTERIAL INJECTION: Due to the close proximity of arteries and veins in the areas most commonly used for intravenous injection, extreme care should be exercised to avoid perivascular extravasation or inadvertent intra-arterial injection of Mepergan. Reports compatible with inadvertent intra-arterial injection suggest that pain, severe chemical irritation, severe spasm of distal vessels, and resultant gangrene requiring amputation is likely under such circumstances. Intravenous injection was intended in all the cases reported, but perivascular extravasation or arterial placement of the needle is now suspect. There is no proven successful management of this condition after it occurs, although sympathetic block and heparinization are commonly employed during the acute management because of the results of animal experiments with other known arteriolar irritants. Aspiration of dark blood does not preclude intra-arterial needle placement, because blood is discolored upon contact with promethazine. Use of syringes with rigid plungers or of small bore needles might obscure typical arterial backflow if this is relied upon alone.

INTRAVENOUS USE: If necessary, meperidine may be given intravenously, but the injection should be given very slowly, preferably in the form of a diluted solution. Rapid intravenous injection of narcotic analgesics, including meperidine, increases the incidence of adverse reactions; severe respiratory depression, apnea, hypotension, peripheral circulatory collapse, and cardiac arrest have occurred. Meperidine should not be administered intravenously unless a narcotic antagonist and the facilities for assisted or controlled respiration are immediately available. When meperidine is given parenterally, especially intravenously, the patient should be lying down.

When used intravenously, Mepergan® (meperidine hydrochloride and promethazine hydrochloride) should be given at a rate not to exceed 1 ml (25 mg of each component) per minute. When administering any irritant drug intravenously it is usually preferable to inject it through the tubing of an intravenous infusion set that is known to be functioning satisfactorily. In the event that a patient complains of pain during intended intravenous injection of Mepergan, the injection should immediately be stopped to provide for evaluation of possible arterial placement or perivascular extravasation.

ASTHMA AND OTHER RESPIRATORY CONDITIONS: Meperidine should be used with extreme caution in patients having an acute asthmatic attack, patients with chronic obstructive pulmonary disease or cor pulmonale, patients having a substantially decreased respiratory reserve, and patients with preexisting respiratory depression, hypoxia, or hypercapnia. In such patients, even usual therapeutic doses of narcotics may decrease respiratory drive while simultaneously increasing airway resistance to the point of apnea.

HYPOTENSIVE EFFECT: The administration of meperidine may result in severe hypotension in an individual whose ability to maintain his blood pressure has already been compromised by a depleted blood volume or concurrent administration of drugs such as the phenothiazines or certain anesthetics.

USAGE IN AMBULATORY PATIENTS: Meperidine may impair the mental and/or physical abilities required for the performance of potentially hazardous tasks such as driving a car or operating machinery. The patient should be cautioned accordingly.

Meperidine, like other narcotics, may produce orthostatic hypotension in ambulatory patients.

USAGE IN PREGNANCY AND LACTATION: Meperidine should not be used in pregnant women prior to the labor period, unless in the judgment of the physician the potential benefits outweigh the possible hazards, because safe use in pregnancy prior to labor has not been established relative to possible adverse effects on fetal development.

When used as an obstetrical analgesic, meperidine crosses the placental barrier and can produce respiratory depression in the newborn; resuscitation may be required (see section on Overdosage).

Meperidine appears in the milk of nursing mothers receiving the drug.

Precautions: SUPRAVENTRICULAR TACHYCARDIAS: Meperidine should be used with caution in patients with atrial flutter and other supraventricular tachycardias because of a possible vagolytic action which may produce a significant increase in the ventricular response rate.

CONVULSIONS: Meperidine may aggravate preexisting convulsions in patients with convulsive disorders. If dosage is escalated substantially above recommended levels because of tolerance development, convulsions may occur in individuals without a history of convulsive disorders.

ACUTE ABDOMINAL CONDITIONS: The administration of meperidine or other narcotics may obscure the diagnosis or clinical course in patients with acute abdominal conditions.

SPECIAL-RISK PATIENTS: Meperidine should be given with caution and the initial dose should be reduced in certain patients such as the elderly or debilitated, and those with severe impairment of hepatic or renal function, hypothyroidism, Addison's disease, and prostatic hypertrophy or urethral stricture. Antiemetics may mask the symptoms of an unrecognized disease and thereby interfere with diagnosis.

Patients in pain who have received inadequate or no analgesia have been noted to develop "athetoid-like" movements of the upper extremities following the parenteral administration of promethazine. These symptoms usually disappear upon adequate control of the pain.

Ambulatory patients should be cautioned against driving automobiles or operating dangerous machinery until it is known that they do not become drowsy or dizzy from promethazine hydrochloride therapy.

Adverse Reactions: The major hazards of meperidine, as with other narcotic analgesics, are respiratory depression and, to a lesser degree, circulatory depression; respiratory arrest, shock, and cardiac arrest have occurred.

The most frequently observed adverse reactions include light-headedness, dizziness, sedation, nausea, vomiting, and sweating. These effects seem to be more prominent in ambulatory patients and in those who are not experiencing severe pain. In such individuals, lower doses are advisable. Some adverse reactions in ambulatory patients may be alleviated if the patient lies down.

Other adverse reactions include:

CENTRAL NERVOUS SYSTEM: Euphoria, dysphoria, weakness, headache, agitation, tremor, uncoordinated muscle movements, transient hallucinations and disorientation, visual disturbances and, rarely, extrapyramidal reactions.

GASTROINTESTINAL: Dry mouth, constipation, biliary-tract spasm.

CARDIOVASCULAR: Flushing of the face, tachycardia, bradycardia, palpitation, faintness, syncope.

Cardiovascular effects from promethazine have been rare. Minor increases in blood pressure and occasional mild hypotension have been reported. Venous thrombosis at the injection site has been reported. Intra-arterial injection of Mepergan may result in gangrene of the affected extremity (see Warnings).

GENITOURINARY: Urinary retention.

ALLERGIC: Pruritus, urticaria, other skin rashes, wheal and flare over the vein with IV injection. Photosensitivity, although extremely rare, has been reported. Occurrence of photosensitivity may be a contraindication to further treatment with promethazine or related drugs.

OTHER: Pain at injection site; local tissue irritation and induration following subcutaneous injection, particularly when repeated; antidiuretic effect.

Patients may occasionally complain of autonomic reactions such as dryness of the mouth, blurring of vision and, rarely, dizziness following the use of promethazine.

Very rare cases have been reported where patients receiving promethazine have developed leukopenia. In one instance agranulocytosis has been reported. In nearly every instance reported, other toxic agents known to have caused these conditions have been associated with the administration of promethazine.

Dosage and Administration: WARNING—BARBITURATES ARE NOT CHEMICALLY COMPATIBLE IN SOLUTION WITH MEPERGAN® (MEPERIDINE HYDROCHLORIDE AND PROMETHAZINE HYDROCHLORIDE), AND SHOULD NOT BE MIXED IN THE SAME SYRINGE.

The TUBEX® (Sterile Cartridge-Needle Unit) is designed for single-dose use. VIALS should be used when required doses are fractions of a milliliter, as indicated below.

Mepergan® is usually administered intramuscularly. However, in certain specific situations, the intravenous route may be employed. INADVERTENT INTRA-ARTERIAL INJECTION CAN RESULT IN GANGRENE OF THE AFFECTED EXTREMITY (see Warnings). SUBCUTANEOUS ADMINISTRATION IS CONTRAINDICATED, AS IT MAY RESULT IN TISSUE NECROSIS (see Contraindications). INJECTION INTO OR NEAR PERIPHERAL NERVES MAY RESULT IN PERMANENT NEUROLOGICAL DEFICIT.

When used intravenously, the rate should not be greater than 1 ml of Mepergan (25 mg of each component) per minute; it is preferable to inject through the tubing of an intravenous infusion set that is known to be functioning satisfactorily.

ADULT DOSE: 1-2 ml (25-50 mg of each component) per single injection, which can be repeated every 3 to 4 hours.

CHILDREN 12 YEARS OF AGE AND UNDER: 0.5 mg of each component per pound of body weight. The dosage may be repeated every 3 to 4 hours as necessary. For preanesthetic medication the usual adult dose is 2 ml (50 mg of each component) intramuscularly with or without appropriate atropine-like drug. Atropine sulfate 0.3 to 0.4 mg or scopolamine hydrobromide 0.25 to 0.4 mg in sterile solution may be mixed in the same syringe with Mepergan. Repeat doses of 50 mg or less of both promethazine and meperidine may be administered by either route at 3- to 4-hour intervals, as necessary. As an adjunct to local or general anesthesia the usual dose is 2 ml (50 mg each of meperidine and promethazine).

Overdosage: SYMPTOMS: Serious overdose with meperidine is characterized by respiratory depression (a decrease in respiratory rate and/or tidal volume, Cheyne-Stokes respiration, cyanosis), extreme somnolence progressing to stupor or coma, skeletal muscle flaccidity, cold and clammy skin, and sometimes bradycardia and hypotension. In severe overdosage, particularly by the intravenous route, apnea, circulatory collapse, cardiac arrest, and death may occur.

Continued on next page

Wyeth—Cont.

TREATMENT: Primary attention should be given to the reestablishment of adequate respiratory exchange through provision of a patent airway and institution of assisted or controlled ventilation. The narcotic antagonists, naloxone hydrochloride, nalorphine hydrochloride, and levallorphan tartrate, are specific antidotes against respiratory depression which may result from overdosage or unusual sensitivity to narcotics, including meperidine. Therefore, an appropriate dose of one of these antagonists should be administered, preferably by the intravenous route, simultaneously with efforts at respiratory resuscitation.

An antagonist should not be administered in absence of clinically significant respiratory or cardiovascular depression.

Oxygen, intravenous fluids, vasopressors, and other supportive measures should be employed as indicated.

NOTE: In an individual physically dependent on narcotics, the administration of the usual dose of a narcotic antagonist will precipitate an acute withdrawal syndrome. The severity of this syndrome will depend on the degree of physical dependence and the dose of antagonist administered. The use of narcotic antagonists in such individuals should be avoided if possible. If a narcotic antagonist must be used to treat serious respiratory depression in the physically dependent patient, the antagonist should be administered with extreme care and only one-fifth to one-tenth the usual initial dose administered.

Attempted suicides with promethazine have resulted in deep sedation, coma, rarely convulsions and cardiorespiratory symptoms compatible with the depth of sedation present. Extrapyramidal reactions may be treated with anticholinergic antiparkinson agents, diphenhydramine, or barbiturates.

If severe hypotension occurs, levarterenol or phenylephrine may be indicated. Epinephrine is probably best avoided, since it has been suggested that promethazine overdosage could produce a partial alpha-adrenergic blockade.

A paradoxical reaction, characterized by hyperexcitability and nightmares, has been reported in children receiving large single doses of promethazine.

How Supplied: Mepergan® (meperidine hydrochloride and promethazine hydrochloride) is supplied in 10 ml vials and TUBEX® Sterile Cartridge-Needle Units.

Subject to Regulations of Federal Bureau Narcotics and Dangerous Drugs.

NORDETTE®-21
[nor-det¹-21]
TABLETS
(levonorgestrel and ethinyl estradiol tablets)

Description:
ORAL CONTRACEPTIVE
Each Nordette® tablet contains 0.15 mg of levonorgestrel (d(-)-13 beta-ethyl-17-alpha-ethinyl-17-beta-hydroxygon-4-en-3-one), a totally synthetic progestogen, and 0.03 mg of ethinyl estradiol (19-nor-17α-pregna-1,3,5 (10)-trien-20-yne-3,17-diol).

Clinical Pharmacology: Combination oral contraceptives act primarily through the mechanism of gonadotropin suppression due to the estrogenic and progestational activity of the ingredients. Although the primary mechanism of action is inhibition of ovulation, alterations in the genital tract, including changes in the cervical mucus (which increase the difficulty of sperm penetration) and the endometrium (which reduce the likelihood of implantation), may also contribute to contraceptive effectiveness.

Indications and Usage: Nordette® is indicated for the prevention of pregnancy in women who elect to use oral contraceptives as a method of contraception.

Oral contraceptives are highly effective. The pregnancy rate in women using conventional combination oral contraceptives (containing 35 mcg or more of ethinyl estradiol or 50 mcg or more of mestranol) is generally reported as less than one pregnancy per 100 woman-years of use. Slightly higher rates (somewhat more than 1 pregnancy per 100 woman-years of use) are reported for some combination products containing 35 mcg or less of ethinyl estradiol, and rates on the order of 3 pregnancies per 100 woman-years are reported for the progestogen-only oral contraceptives.

These rates are derived from separate studies conducted by different investigators in several population groups and cannot be compared precisely. Furthermore, pregnancy rates tend to be lower as clinical studies are continued, possibly due to selective retention in the longer studies of those patients who accept the treatment regimen and do not discontinue as a result of adverse reactions, pregnancy, or other reasons.

In clinical trials with Nordette®, 1,084 patients completed 8,186 cycles, and a total of three pregnancies were reported. This represents a pregnancy rate of 0.48 per 100 woman-years.

Table 1 gives ranges of pregnancy rates reported in the literature[1] for other means of contraception. The efficacy of these means of contraception (except the IUD) depends upon the degree of adherence to the method.

TABLE 1
PREGNANCIES PER 100 WOMAN-YEARS
IUD, less than 1-6; Diaphragm with spermicidal products (creams or jellies), 2-20; Condom, 3-36; Aerosol foams, 2-29; Jellies and creams, 4-36; Periodic abstinence (rhythm) all types, less than 1-47:
1. Calendar method, 14-47;
2. Temperature method, 1-20;
3. Temperature method—intercourse only in postovulatory phase, less than 1-7;
4. Mucus method, 1-25;

No contraception, 60-80.

Dose-Related Risk of Thromboembolism from Oral Contraceptives: Two studies have shown a positive association between the dose of estrogens in oral contraceptives and the risk of thromboembolism.[2,3] For this reason, it is prudent and in keeping with good principles of therapeutics to minimize exposure to estrogen. The oral-contraceptive product prescribed for any given patient should be that product which contains the least amount of estrogen that is compatible with an acceptable pregnancy rate and patient acceptance. It is recommended that new acceptors of oral contraceptives be started on preparations containing 0.05 mg or less of estrogen.

Contraindications: Oral contraceptives should not be used in women with any of the following conditions:
1. Thrombophlebitis or thromboembolic disorders.
2. A past history of deep-vein thrombophlebitis or thromboembolic disorders.
3. Cerebral-vascular or coronary-artery disease.
4. Known or suspected carcinoma of the breast.
5. Known or suspected estrogen-dependent neoplasia.
6. Undiagnosed abnormal genital bleeding.
7. Known or suspected pregnancy (see Warning No. 5).
8. Benign or malignant liver tumor which developed during the use of oral contraceptives or other estrogen-containing products.

Warnings:

Cigarette smoking increases the risk of serious cardiovascular side effects from oral-contraceptive use. This risk increases with age and with heavy smoking (15 or more cigarettes per day) and is quite marked in women over 35 years of age. Women who use oral contraceptives should be strongly advised not to smoke.

The use of oral contraceptives is associated with increased risk of several serious conditions, including thromboembolism, stroke, myocardial infarction, hepatic adenoma, gallbladder disease, hypertension. Practitioners prescribing oral contraceptives should be familiar with the following information relating to these risks.

1. *Thromboembolic Disorders and Other Vascular Problems:* An increased risk of thromboembolic and thrombotic disease associated with the use of oral contraceptives is well-established. Three principal studies in Great Britain[4-6] and three in the United States[7-10] have demonstrated an increased risk of fatal and nonfatal venous thromboembolism and stroke, both hemorrhagic and thrombotic. These studies estimate that users of oral contraceptives are 4 to 11 times more likely than nonusers to develop these diseases without evident cause (Table 2).

CEREBROVASCULAR DISORDERS
In a collaborative American study[9,10] of cerebrovascular disorders in women with and without predisposing causes, it was estimated that the risk of hemorrhagic stroke was 2.0 times greater in users than nonusers and the risk of thrombotic stroke was 4 to 9.5 times greater in users than in nonusers (Table 2).

TABLE 2
SUMMARY OF RELATIVE RISK OF THROMBOEMBOLIC DISORDERS AND OTHER VASCULAR PROBLEMS IN ORAL-CONTRACEPTIVE USERS COMPARED TO NONUSERS

	Relative risk, times greater
Idiopathic thromboembolic disease	4-11
Postsurgery thromboembolic complications	4-6
Thrombotic stroke	4-9.5
Hemorrhagic stroke	2
Myocardial infarction	2-12

MYOCARDIAL INFARCTION
An increased risk of myocardial infarction associated with the use of oral contraceptives has been reported,[11,12,13] confirming a previously suspected association. These studies, conducted in the United Kingdom, found, as expected, that the greater the number of underlying risk factors for coronary-artery disease (cigarette smoking, hypertension, hypercholesterolemia, obesity, diabetes, history of preeclamptic toxemia) the higher the risk of developing myocardial infarction, regardless of whether the patient was an oral-contraceptive user or not. Oral contraceptives, however, were found to be a clear additional risk factor.

In terms of relative risk, it has been estimated[52] that oral-contraceptive users who do not smoke (smoking is considered a major predisposing condition to myocardial infarction) are about twice as likely to have a fatal myocardial infarction as nonusers who do not smoke. Oral-contraceptive users who are also smokers have about a 5-fold increased risk of fatal infarction compared to users who do not smoke, but about a 10- to 12-fold increased risk compared to nonusers who do not smoke. Furthermore, the amount of smoking is also an important factor. In determining the importance of these relative risks, however, the baseline rates for various age groups, as shown in Table 3, must be given serious consideration. The importance of other predisposing conditions mentioned above in determining relative and absolute risks has not as yet been quantified; it is quite likely that the same synergistic action exists, but perhaps to a lesser extent.

TABLE 3
Estimated annual mortality rate per 100,000 women from myocardial infarction by use of oral contraceptives, smoking habits, and age (in years): [See table on next page].

RISK OF DOSE
In an analysis of data derived from several national adverse-reaction reporting systems,[2] British investigators concluded that the risk of thromboembolism, including coronary thrombosis, is directly related to the dose of estrogen used in oral contraceptives. Preparations containing 100 mcg or more of estrogen were associated with a higher risk of thromboembolism than those containing 50-80 mcg of estrogen. Their analysis did suggest, however, that the quantity of estrogen may not be the sole factor involved. This finding has been confirmed in the United States.[3] Careful epidemiolog-

ical studies to determine the degree of thromboembolic risk associated with progestogen-only oral contraceptives have not been performed. Cases of thromboembolic disease have been reported in women using these products, and they should not be presumed to be free of excess risk.

ESTIMATE OF EXCESS MORTALITY FROM CIRCULATORY DISEASES

A large prospective study[53] carried out in the U.K. estimated the mortality rate per 100,000 women per year from diseases of the circulatory system for users and nonusers of oral contraceptives according to age, smoking habits, and duration of use. The overall excess death rate annually from circulatory diseases for oral-contraceptive users was estimated to be 20 per 100,000 (ages 15-34—5/100,000; ages 35-44—33/100,000; ages 45-49—140/100,000), the risk being concentrated in older women, in those with a long duration of use, and in cigarette smokers. It was not possible, however, to examine the interrelationships of age, smoking, and duration of use, nor to compare the effects of continuous vs. intermittent use. Although the study showed a 10-fold increase in death due to circulatory diseases in users for 5 or more years, all of these deaths occurred in women 35 or older. Until larger numbers of women under 35 with continuous use for 5 or more years are available, it is not possible to assess the magnitude of the relative risk for this younger age group.

The available data from a variety of sources have been analyzed[14] to estimate the risk of death associated with various methods of contraception. The estimates of risk of death for each method include the combined risk of the contraceptive method (e.g., thromboembolic and thrombotic disease in the case of oral contraceptives) plus the risk attributable to pregnancy or abortion in the event of method failure. This latter risk varies with the effectiveness of the contraceptive method. The findings of this analysis are shown in Figure 1 below.[14] The study concluded that the mortality associated with all methods of birth control is low and below that associated with childbirth, with the exception of oral contraceptives in women over 40 who smoke. (The rates given for Pill only/smokers for each age group are for smokers as a class. For "heavy" smokers (more than 15 cigarettes a day), the rates given would be about double; for "light" smokers (less than 15 cigarettes a day), about 50 percent. The lowest mortality is associated with the condom or diaphragm backed up by early abortion. The risk of thromboembolic and thrombotic disease associated with oral contraceptives increases with age after approximately age 30 and, for myocardial infarction, is further increased by hypertension, hypercholesterolemia, obesity, diabetes, or history of preeclamptic toxemia and especially by cigarette smoking.

Based on the data currently available, the following chart gives a gross estimate of the risk of death from circulatory disorders associated with the use of oral contraceptives:

SMOKING HABITS AND OTHER PREDISPOSING CONDITIONS—RISK ASSOCIATED WITH USE OF ORAL CONTRACEPTIVES

Age	Below 30	30-39	40+
Heavy smokers	C	B	A
Light smokers	D	C	B
Nonsmokers (no predisposing conditions)	D	C,D	C
Nonsmokers (other predisposing conditions)	C	C,B	B,A

A—Use associated with very high risk.
B—Use associated with high risk.
C—Use associated with moderate risk.
D—Use associated with low risk.

The physician and the patient should be alert to the earliest manifestations of thromboembolic and thrombotic disorders (e.g., thrombophlebitis, pulmonary embolism, cerebrovascular insufficiency, coronary occlusion, retinal thrombosis, and mes-

	Myocardial infarction			
	Women aged 30-39		Women aged 40-44	
Smoking habits	Users	Nonusers	Users	Nonusers
All smokers	10.2	2.6	62.0	15.9
Heavy*	13.0	5.1	78.7	31.3
Light	4.7	0.9	28.6	5.7
Nonsmokers	1.8	1.2	10.7	7.4
Smokers and nonsmokers	5.4	1.9	32.8	11.7

* Heavy smoker: 15 or more cigarettes per day.
From JAIN, A.K., *Studies in Family Planning*, 8:50, 1977

enteric thrombosis). Should any of these occur or be suspected, the drug should be discontinued immediately.

A four- to six-fold increased risk of postsurgery thromboembolic complications has been reported in oral-contraceptive users.[15,16] If feasible, oral contraceptives should be discontinued at least 4 weeks before surgery of a type associated with an increased risk of thromboembolism or prolonged immobilization.

PERSISTENCE OF RISK OF VASCULAR DISORDERS

Findings from one study in Great Britain involving cerebrovascular disease[56] and another study in the United States concerning myocardial infarction[57] suggest that an increased risk of these conditions in users of oral contraceptives persists after discontinuation of the oral contraceptive. In the British study, the risk of cerebrovascular disease remained elevated in former oral-contraceptive users for at least six years after discontinuation. In the U. S. study, an increased risk of myocardial infarction persisted for at least 9 years in women 40- to 49-years-old who had used oral contraceptives for five or more years. The findings in both these studies require confirmation since they are inconsistent with other published information.[9,11,13,58-62]

2. *Ocular Lesions:*
There have been reports of neuro-ocular lesions such as optic neuritis or retinal thrombosis associated with the use of oral contraceptives. Discontinue oral-contraceptive medication if there is unexplained, sudden or gradual, partial or complete loss of vision; onset of proptosis or diplopia; papilledema; or retinal-vascular lesions, and institute appropriate diagnostic and therapeutic measures.

3. *Carcinoma:*
Long-term continuous administration of either natural or synthetic estrogen in certain animal species increases the frequency of carcinoma of the breast, cervix, vagina, and liver. Certain synthetic progestogens, none currently contained in oral contraceptives, have been noted to increase the incidence of mammary nodules, benign and malignant, in dogs.

In humans, three case-control studies have reported an increased risk of endometrial carcinoma associated with the prolonged use of exogenous estrogen in postmenopausal women.[17,18,19] One publication[20] reported on the first 21 cases submitted by physicians to a registry of cases of adenocarcinoma of the endometrium in women under 40 on oral contraceptives. Of the cases found in women without predisposing risk factors for adenocarcinoma of the endometrium (e.g., irregular bleeding at the time oral contraceptives were first given, polycystic ovaries), nearly all occurred in women who had used a sequential oral contraceptive. These products are no longer marketed. No evidence has been reported suggesting an increased risk of endometrial cancer in users of conventional combination or progestogen-only oral contraceptives.

Several studies[8,21-24] have found no increase in breast cancer in women taking oral contraceptives or estrogens. One study,[25] however, while also noting no overall increased risk of breast cancer in women treated with oral contraceptives, found an excess risk in the subgroups of oral-contraceptive users with documented benign breast disease. A reduced occurrence of benign breast tumors in users of oral contraceptives has been well-documented.[8,21,25,26,27]

In summary, there is at present no confirmed evidence from human studies of an increased risk of cancer associated with oral contraceptives. Close clinical surveillance of all women taking oral contraceptives is, nevertheless, essential. In all cases of undiagnosed persistent or recurrent abnormal vaginal bleeding, appropriate diagnostic measures should be taken to rule out malignancy. Women with a strong family history of breast cancer or who have breast nodules, fibrocystic disease, or abnormal mammograms should be monitored with particular care if they elect to use oral contraceptives instead of other methods of contraception.

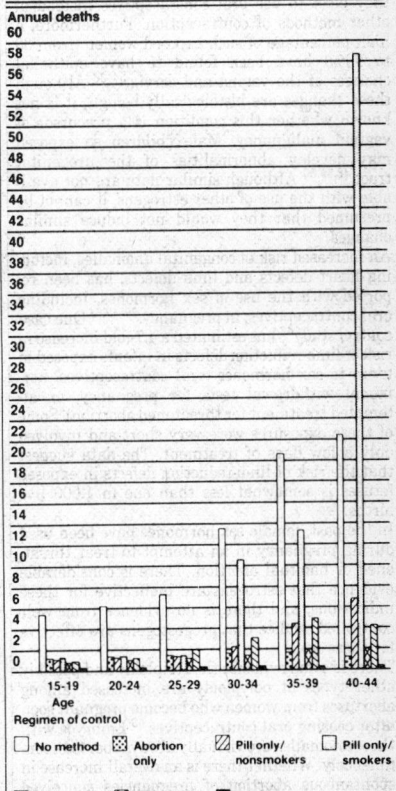

Figure 1. Estimated annual number of deaths associated with control of fertility and no control per 100,000 nonsterile women, by regimen of control and age of woman.

4. *Hepatic Tumors:*
Benign hepatic adenomas have been found to be associated with the use of oral contraceptives.[28,29,30,46] One study[46] showed that oral contraceptive formulations with high hormonal po-

Continued on next page

Wyeth—Cont.

tency were associated with a higher risk than lower potency formulations. Although benign, hepatic adenomas may rupture and may cause death through intra-abdominal hemorrhage. This has been reported in short-term as well as long-term users of oral contraceptives. Two studies relate risk with duration of use of the contraceptive, the risk being much greater after 4 or more years of oral-contraceptive use.[30,46] While hepatic adenoma is a rare lesion, it should be considered in women presenting abdominal pain and tenderness, abdominal mass or shock. A few cases of hepatocellular carcinoma have been reported in women taking oral contraceptives. The relationship of these drugs to this type of malignancy is not known at this time.

5. *Use in or Immediately Preceding Pregnancy, Birth Defects in Offspring, and Malignancy in Female Offspring:*

The use of female sex hormones—both estrogenic and progestational agents—during early pregnancy may seriously damage the offspring. It has been shown that females exposed in utero to diethylstilbestrol, a nonsteroidal estrogen, have an increased risk of developing in later life a form of vaginal or cervical cancer that is ordinarily extremely rare.[31,32] This risk has been estimated to be of the order of 1 in 1,000 exposures or less.[33,47] Although there is no evidence at the present time that oral contraceptives further enhance the risk of developing this type of malignancy, such patients should be monitored with particular care if they elect to use oral contraceptives instead of other methods of contraception. Furthermore, a high percentage of such exposed women (from 30 to 90%) have been found to have epithelial changes of the vagina and cervix.[34–38] Although these changes are histologically benign, it is not known whether this condition is a precursor of vaginal malignancy. Male children so exposed may develop abnormalities of the urogenital tract.[48,49,50] Although similar data are not available with the use of other estrogens, it cannot be presumed that they would not induce similar changes.

An increased risk of congenital anomalies, including heart defects and limb defects, has been reported with the use of sex hormones, including oral contraceptives, in pregnancy.[39–42,51] One case-control study[42] has estimated a 4.7-fold increase in risk of limb-reduction defects in infants exposed in utero to sex hormones (oral contraceptives, hormonal withdrawal tests for pregnancy, or attempted treatment for threatened abortion). Some of these exposures were very short and involved only a few days of treatment. The data suggest that the risk of limb-reduction defects in exposed fetuses is somewhat less than one in 1,000 live births.

In the past, female sex hormones have been used during pregnancy in an attempt to treat threatened or habitual abortion. There is considerable evidence that estrogens are ineffective for these indications, and there is no evidence from well-controlled studies that progestogens are effective for these uses.

There is some evidence that triploidy and possibly other types of polyploidy are increased among abortuses from women who become pregnant soon after ceasing oral contraceptives.[43] Embryos with these anomalies are virtually always aborted spontaneously. Whether there is an overall increase in spontaneous abortion of pregnancies conceived soon after stopping oral contraceptives is unknown. It is recommended that, for any patient who has missed two consecutive periods, pregnancy should be ruled out before continuing the contraceptive regimen. If the patient has not adhered to the prescribed schedule, the possibility of pregnancy should be considered at the time of the first missed period (or after 45 days from the last menstrual period if the progestogen-only oral contraceptives are used), and further use of oral contraceptives should be withheld until pregnancy has been ruled out. If pregnancy is confirmed, the patient should be apprised of the potential risks to the fetus, and the advisability of continuation of the pregnancy should be discussed in the light of these risks.

It is also recommended that women who discontinue oral contraceptives with the intent of becoming pregnant use an alternate form of contraception for a period of time before attempting to conceive. Many clinicians recommend 3 months, although no precise information is available on which to base this recommendation.

The administration of progestogen-only or progestogen-estrogen combinations to induce withdrawal bleeding should not be used as a test of pregnancy.

6. *Gallbladder Disease:*

Studies[8,23,26] report an increased risk of surgically confirmed gallbladder disease in users of oral contraceptives and estrogens. In one study, an increased risk appeared after 2 years of use and doubled after 4 or 5 years of use. In one of the other studies, an increased risk was apparent between 6 and 12 months of use.

7. *Carbohydrate and Lipid Metabolic Effects:*

A decrease in glucose tolerance has been observed in a significant percentage of patients on oral contraceptives. For this reason, prediabetic and diabetic patients should be carefully observed while receiving oral contraceptives.

An increase in triglycerides and total phospholipids has been observed in patients receiving oral contraceptives.[44] The clinical significance of this finding remains to be defined.

8. *Elevated Blood Pressure:*

An increase in blood pressure has been reported in patients receiving oral contraceptives.[26] In some women, hypertension may occur within a few months of beginning oral-contraceptive use. In the first year of use, the prevalence of women with hypertension is low in users and may be no higher than that of a comparable group of nonusers. The prevalence in users increases, however, with longer exposure, and in the fifth year of use is two-and-a-half to three times the reported prevalence in the first year. Age is also strongly correlated with the development of hypertension in oral-contraceptive users. Women who previously have had hypertension during pregnancy may be more likely to develop elevation of blood pressure when given oral contraceptives. Hypertension that develops as a result of taking oral contraceptives usually returns to normal after discontinuing the drug.

9. *Headache:*

The onset or exacerbation of migraine or development of headache of a new pattern which is recurrent, persistent, or severe, requires discontinuation of oral contraceptives and evaluation of the cause.

10. *Bleeding Irregularities:*

Breakthrough bleeding, spotting, and amenorrhea are frequent reasons for patients discontinuing oral contraceptives. In breakthrough bleeding, as in all cases of irregular bleeding from the vagina, nonfunctional causes should be borne in mind. In undiagnosed persistent or recurrent abnormal bleeding from the vagina, adequate diagnostic measures are indicated to rule out pregnancy or malignancy. If pathology has been excluded, time or a change to another formulation may solve the problem. Changing to an oral contraceptive with a higher estrogen content, while potentially useful in minimizing menstrual irregularity, should be done only if necessary, since this may increase the risk of thromboembolic disease.

Women with a past history of oligomenorrhea or secondary amenorrhea or young women without regular cycles may have a tendency to remain anovulatory or to become amenorrheic after discontinuation of oral contraceptives. Women with these preexisting problems should be advised of this possibility and encouraged to use other contraceptive methods. Post-use anovulation, possibly prolonged, may also occur in women without previous irregularities.

11. *Ectopic Pregnancy:*

Ectopic as well as intrauterine pregnancy may occur in contraceptive failures. However, in progestogen-only oral contraceptive failures, the ratio of ectopic to intrauterine pregnancies is higher than in women who are not receiving oral contraceptives, since the drugs are more effective in preventing intrauterine than ectopic pregnancies.

12. *Breast-feeding:*

Oral contraceptives given in the postpartum period may interfere with lactation. There may be a decrease in the quantity and quality of the breast milk. Furthermore, a small fraction of the hormonal agents in oral contraceptives has been identified in the milk of mothers receiving these drugs.[45,54,55] The effects, if any, on the breast-fed child have not been determined. If feasible, the use of oral contraceptives should be deferred until the infant has been weaned.

Precautions:

GENERAL

1. A complete medical and family history should be taken prior to initiation of oral contraceptives. The pretreatment and periodic physical examinations should include special reference to blood pressure, breasts, abdomen and pelvic organs, including Papanicolaou smear and relevant laboratory tests. As a general rule, oral contraceptives should not be prescribed for longer than 1 year without another physical examination being performed.

2. Under the influence of estrogen-progestogen preparations, preexisting uterine leiomyomata may increase in size.

3. Patients with a history of psychic depression should be carefully observed and the drug discontinued if depression recurs to a serious degree. Patients becoming significantly depressed while taking oral contraceptives should stop the medication and use an alternate method of contraception in an attempt to determine whether the symptom is drug-related.

4. Oral contraceptives may cause some degree of fluid retention. They should be prescribed with caution, and only with careful monitoring, in patients with conditions which might be aggravated by fluid retention, such as convulsive disorders, migraine syndrome, asthma, or cardiac or renal insufficiency.

5. Patients with a past history of jaundice during pregnancy have an increased risk of recurrence of jaundice while receiving oral-contraceptive therapy. If jaundice develops in any patient receiving such drugs, the medication should be discontinued.

6. Steroid hormones may be poorly metabolized in patients with impaired liver function and should be administered with caution in such patients.

7. Oral-contraceptive users may have disturbances in normal tryptophan metabolism which may result in a relative pyridoxine deficiency. The clinical significance of this is yet to be determined.

8. Serum folate levels may be depressed by oral-contraceptive therapy. Since the pregnant woman is predisposed to the development of folate deficiency and the incidence of folate deficiency increases with increasing gestation, it is possible that if a woman becomes pregnant shortly after stopping oral contraceptives, she may have a greater chance of developing folate deficiency and complications attributed to this deficiency.

INFORMATION FOR THE PATIENT
(See Patient Labeling Printed Below.)

LABORATORY TESTS

1. The pathologist should be advised of oral-contraceptive therapy when relevant specimens are submitted.

2. Certain endocrine- and liver-function tests and blood components may be affected by estrogen-containing oral contraceptives:

a. Increased sulfobromophthalein retention.

b. Increased prothrombin and factors VII, VIII, IX, and X; decreased antithrombin 3; increased norepinephrine-induced platelet aggregability.

c. Increased thyroid-binding globulin (TBG) leading to increased circulating total-thyroid hormone, as measured by protein-bound iodine (PBI), T4 by column, or T4 by radioimmunoassay. Free T3 resin uptake is decreased, reflecting the elevated TBG; free T4 concentration is unaltered.

d. Decreased pregnanediol excretion.
e. Reduced response to metyrapone test.

DRUG INTERACTIONS

Reduced efficacy and increased incidence of breakthrough bleeding have been associated with concomitant use of rifampin. A similar association has been suggested with barbiturates, phenylbutazone, phenytoin sodium, ampicillin, and tetracycline.

CARCINOGENESIS, MUTAGENESIS, IMPAIRMENT OF FERTILITY

See WARNINGS section #3, 4, and 5 for information on carcinogenesis, mutagenesis, and impairment of fertility.

PREGNANCY

Pregnancy category X. See Contraindications and Warnings.

NURSING MOTHERS

See WARNINGS. Because of the potential for adverse reactions in nursing infants from oral-contraceptive tablets, a decision should be made whether to discontinue the drug, taking into account the importance of the drug to the mother.

Adverse Reactions: An increased risk of the following serious adverse reactions has been associated with the use of oral contraceptives (see Warnings):

Thrombophlebitis
Pulmonary embolism.
Coronary thrombosis.
Cerebral thrombosis.
Cerebral hemorrhage.
Hypertension.
Gallbladder disease.
Benign hepatomas.
Congenital anomalies.

There is evidence of an association between the following conditions and the use of oral contraceptives, although additional confirmatory studies are needed:

Mesenteric thrombosis.
Neuro-ocular lesions, e.g., retinal thrombosis and optic neuritis.

The following adverse reactions have been reported in patients receiving oral contraceptives and are believed to be drug-related:

Nausea and/or vomiting, usually the most common adverse reactions, occur in approximately 10 percent or less of patients during the first cycle. Other reactions, as a general rule, are seen much less frequently or only occasionally.
Gastrointestinal symptoms (such as abdominal cramps and bloating).
Breakthrough bleeding.
Spotting.
Change in menstrual flow.
Dysmenorrhea.
Amenorrhea during and after treatment.
Temporary infertility after discontinuance of treatment.
Edema.
Chloasma or melasma which may persist.
Breast changes: tenderness, enlargement, and secretion.
Change in weight (increase or decrease).
Change in cervical erosion and cervical secretion.
Possible diminution in lactation when given immediately postpartum.
Cholestatic jaundice.
Migraine.
Increase in size of uterine leiomyomata.
Rash (allergic).
Mental depression.
Reduced tolerance to carbohydrates.
Vaginal candidiasis.
Change in corneal curvature (steepening).
Intolerance to contact lenses.

The following adverse reactions have been reported in users of oral contraceptives, and the association has been neither confirmed nor refuted:

Premenstrual-like syndrome.
Cataracts.
Changes in libido.
Chorea.
Changes in appetite.
Cystitis-like syndrome.
Headache.
Nervousness
Dizziness.
Hirsutism.
Loss of scalp hair.
Erythema multiforme.
Erythema nodosum.
Hemorrhagic eruption.
Vaginitis.
Porphyria.

Acute Overdose: Serious ill effects have not been reported following acute ingestion of large doses of oral contraceptives by young children. Overdosage may cause nausea, and withdrawal bleeding may occur in females.

Dosage and Administration: To achieve maximum contraceptive effectiveness, Nordette®-21 must be taken exactly as directed and at intervals not exceeding 24 hours. The dosage of Nordette®-21 is one tablet daily for 21 consecutive days per menstrual cycle according to prescribed schedule. Tablets are then discontinued for 7 days (three weeks on, one week off). It is recommended that Nordette®-21 tablets be taken at the same time each day, preferably after the evening meal or at bedtime.

During the first cycle of medication, the patient is instructed to take one Nordette®-21 tablet daily for twenty-one consecutive days beginning on day five of her menstrual cycle. (The first day of menstruation is day one.) The tablets are then discontinued for one week (7 days). Withdrawal bleeding should usually occur within three days following discontinuation of Nordette®-21.

(If Nordette®-21 is first taken later than the fifth day of the first menstrual cycle of medication or postpartum, contraceptive reliance should not be placed on Nordette®-21 until after the first seven consecutive days of administration. The possibility of ovulation and conception prior to initiation of medication should be considered.)

The patient begins her next and all subsequent 21-day courses of Nordette®-21 tablets on the same day of the week that she began her first course, following the same schedule: 21 days on—7 days off.

She begins taking her tablets on the 8th day after discontinuance regardless of whether or not a menstrual period has occurred or is still in progress. Any time a new cycle of Nordette®-21 is started later than the 8th day the patient should be protected by another means of contraception until she has taken a tablet daily for seven consecutive days.

If spotting or breakthrough bleeding occurs, the patient is instructed to continue on the same regimen. This type of bleeding is usually transient and without significance; however, if the bleeding is persistent or prolonged the patient is advised to consult her physician. Although the occurrence of pregnancy is highly unlikely if Nordette®-21 is taken according to directions, if withdrawal bleeding does not occur, the possibility of pregnancy must be considered. If the patient has not adhered to the prescribed schedule (missed one or more tablets or started taking them on a day later than she should have) the probability of pregnancy should be considered at the time of the first missed period and appropriate diagnostic measures taken before the medication is resumed. If the patient has adhered to the prescribed regimen and misses two consecutive periods, pregnancy should be ruled out before continuing the contraceptive regimen.

The patient should be instructed to take a missed tablet as soon as it is remembered. If two consecutive tablets are missed they should both be taken as soon as remembered. The next tablet should be taken at the usual time.

Any time the patient misses one or two tablets she should also use another method of contraception until she has taken a tablet daily for seven consecutive days. If breakthrough bleeding occurs following missed tablets it will usually be transient and of no consequence. While there is little likelihood of ovulation occurring if only one or two tablets are missed, the possibility of ovulation increases with each successive day that scheduled tablets are missed. If three consecutive tablets are missed, all medication should be discontinued and the remainder of the package discarded. A new tablet cycle should be started on the 8th day after the last tablet was taken, and an alternate means of contraception should be prescribed during the seven days without tablets and until the patient has taken a tablet daily for seven consecutive days. In the nonlactating mother Nordette® may be prescribed in the postpartum period either immediately or at the first postpartum examination whether or not menstruation has resumed.

How Supplied: Nordette®-21 Tablets (0.15 mg levonorgestrel + 0.03 mg ethinyl estradiol tablets), Wyeth®, are available in 6 Pilpak® dispensers of 21 tablets: NDC 0008-0075, light-orange, round tablet marked "WYETH" and "75".

References:

1. "Population Reports," Series H, Number 2, May 1974; Series I, Number 1, June 1974; Series B, Number 2, January 1975; Series H, Number 3, 1975; Series H, Number 4, January 1976 (published by the Population Information Program, The George Washington University Medical Center, 2001 S St. NW., Washington, D.C.).
2. Inman, W. H. W., Vessey, M. P., Westerholm, B., and Engelund, A., "Thromboembolic disease and the steroidal content of oral contraceptives. A report to the Committee on Safety of Drugs," Brit Med J 2:203-209, 1970.
3. Stolley, P. D., Tonascia, J. A., Tockman, M. S., Sartwell, P. E., Rutledge, A. H., and Jacobs, M. P., "Thrombosis with low-estrogen oral contraceptives," Am J Epidemiol 102:197-208, 1975.
4. Royal College of General Practitioners, "Oral contraception and thromboembolic disease," J Coll Gen Pract 13:267-279, 1967.
5. Inman, W. H. W., and Vessey, M. P., "Investigation of deaths from pulmonary, coronary and cerebral thrombosis and embolism in women of childbearing age," Brit Med J 2:193-199, 1968.
6. Vessey, M. P., and Doll, R., "Investigation of relation between use of oral contraceptives and thromboembolic disease. A further report," Brit Med J 2:651-657, 1969.
7. Sartwell, P. E., Masi, A. T., Arthes, F. G., Greene, G. R., and Smith, H. E., "Thromboembolism and oral contraceptives: an epidemiological case control study," Am J Epidemiol 90:365-380, 1969.
8. Boston Collaborative Drug Surveillance Program, "Oral contraceptives and venous thromboembolic disease, surgically confirmed gallbladder disease and breast tumors," Lancet 1:1399-1404, 1973.
9. Collaborative Group for the Study of Stroke in Young Women, "Oral contraception and increased risk of cerebral ischemia or thrombosis," N Engl J Med 288:871-878, 1973.
10. Collaborative Group for the Study of Stroke in Young Women, "Oral contraceptives and stroke in young women: associated risk factors," JAMA 231:718-722, 1975.
11. Mann, J. I., and Inman, W. H. W., "Oral contraceptives and death from myocardial infarction," Brit Med J 2:245-248, 1975.
12. Mann, J. I., Inman, W. H. W., and Thorogood, M., "Oral contraceptive use in older women and fatal myocardial infarction," Brit Med J 2:445-447, 1976.
13. Mann, J. I., Vessey, M. P., Thorogood, M., and Doll, R., "Myocardial infarction in young women with special reference to oral contraceptive practice," Brit Med J 2:241-245, 1975.
14. Tietze, C., "New Estimates of Mortality Associated with Fertility Control," Family Planning Perspectives, 9:74-76, 1977.
15. Vessey, M. P., Doll, R., Fairbairn, A. S., and Glober, G., "Post-operative thromboembolism and the use of oral contraceptives," Brit Med J 3:123-126, 1970.
16. Greene, G. R., Sartwell, P. E., "Oral contraceptive use in patients with thromboembolism following surgery, trauma, or infection," Am J Pub Health 62:680-685, 1972.

Continued on next page

Wyeth—Cont.

17. Smith, D. C., Prentice, R., Thompson, D. J., and Herrmann, W. L., "Association of exogenous estrogen and endometrial carcinoma," N Engl J Med 293:1164-1167, 1975.
18. Ziel, H. K., and Finkle, W. D., "Increased risk of endometrial carcinoma among users of conjugated estrogens," N Engl J Med 293:1167-1170, 1975.
19. Mack, T. N., Pike, M. C., Henderson, B. E., Pfeffer, R. I., Gerkins, V. R., Arthur, M., and Brown, S. E., "Estrogens and endometrial cancer in a retirement community," N Engl J Med 294:1262-1267, 1976.
20. Silverberg, S. G., and Makowski, E. L., "Endometrial carcinoma in young women taking oral contraceptive agents," Obstet Gynecol 46:503-506, 1975.
21. Vessey, M. P., Doll, R., and Sutton, P. M., "Oral contraceptives and breast neoplasia: a retrospective study," Brit Med J 3:719-724, 1972.
22. Vessey, M. P., Doll, R., and Jones K., "Oral contraceptives and breast cancer. Progress report of an epidemiological study," Lancet 1:941-943, 1975.
23. Boston Collaborative Drug Surveillance Program, "Surgically confirmed gallbladder disease, venous thromboembolism and breast tumors in relation to postmenopausal estrogen therapy," N Engl J Med 290:15-19, 1974.
24. Arthes, F. G., Sartwell, P. E., and Lewison, E. F., "The pill, estrogens, and the breast. Epidemiologic aspects," Cancer 28:1391-1394, 1971.
25. Fasal, E., and Paffenbarger, R. S., "Oral contraceptives as related to cancer and benign lesions of the breast," J Natl Cancer Inst 55:767-773, 1975.
26. Royal College of General Practitioners, "Oral Contraceptives and Health," London, Pitman, 1974.
27. Ory, H., Cole, P., MacMahon, B., and Hoover, R., "Oral contraceptives and reduced risk of benign breast diseases," N Engl J Med 294:419-422, 1976.
28. Baum, J., Holtz, F., Bookstein, J. J., and Klein, E. W., "Possible association between benign hepatomas and oral contraceptives," Lancet 2:926-928, 1973.
29. Mays, E. T., Christopherson, W. M., Mahr, M. M., and Williams, H. C., "Hepatic changes in young women ingesting contraceptive steroids. Hepatic hemorrhage and primary hepatic tumors," JAMA 235:730-732, 1976.
30. Edmondson, H. A., Henderson, B., and Benton, B., "Liver-cell adenomas associated with use of oral contraceptives," N Engl J Med 294:470-472, 1976.
31. Herbst, A. L., Ulfedler, H., and Poskanzer, D. C., "Adenocarcinoma of the vagina," N Engl J Med 284:878-881, 1971.
32. Greenwald, P., Barlow, J. J., Nasca, P. C., and Burnett, W., "Vaginal cancer after maternal treatment with synthetic estrogens," N Engl J Med 285:390-392, 1971.
33. Lanier, A. P., Noller, K. L., Decker, D. G., Elveback, L., and Kurland, L. T., "Cancer and stilbestrol. A follow-up of 1719 persons exposed to estrogens in utero and born 1943-1959," Mayo Clin Pro 48:793-799, 1973.
34. Herbst, A. L., Kurman, R., and Scully, R. E., "Vaginal and cervical abnormalities after exposure to stilbestrol in utero," Obstet Gynecol 40:287-298, 1972.
35. Herbst, A. L. Robboy, S. J., Macdonald, G. J., and Scully, R. E., "The effects of local progesterone on stilbestrol-associated vaginal adenosis," Am J Obstet Gynecol 118:607:615, 1974.
36. Herbst, A. L., Poskanzer, D. C., Robboy, S. J., Friedlander, L., and Scully, R. E., "Prenatal exposure to stilbestrol: a prospective comparison of exposed female offspring with unexposed controls," N Engl J Med 292:334-339, 1975.
37. Stafl, A., Mattingly, R. F., Foley, D. V., Fetherston, W., "Clinical diagnosis of vaginal adenosis," Obstet Gynecol 43:118-128, 1974.
38. Sherman, A. I., Goldrath, M., Berlin, A., Vakhariya, V., Banooni, F., Michaels, W., Goodman, P., and Brown S., "Cervical-vaginal adenosis after in utero exposure to synthetic estrogens," Obstet Gynecol 44:531-545, 1974.
39. Gal, I., Kirman, B., and Stern, J., "Hormone pregnancy tests and congenital malformation," Nature 216:83, 1967.
40. Levy, E. P., Cohen, A., and Fraser, F. C., "Hormone treatment during pregnancy and congenital heart defects," Lancet 1:611, 1973.
41. Nora, J. J., and Nora, A. H., "Birth defects and oral contraceptives," Lancet 1:941-942, 1973.
42. Janerich, D. T., Piper, J. M., and Glebatis, D. M., "Oral contraceptives and congenital limb-reduction defects," N Engl J Med 291:697-700, 1974.
43. Carr, D. H., "Chromosome studies in selected spontaneous abortions: I. Conception after oral contraceptives," Canad Med Assoc J 103:343-348, 1970.
44. Wynn, V., Doar, J. W. H., and Mills, G. L., "Some effects of oral contraceptives on serum-lipid and lipoprotein levels," Lancet 2:720-723, 1966.
45. Laumas, K. R., Malkani, P. K., Bhatnagar, S., and Laumas, V., "Radioactivity in the breast milk of lactating women after oral administration of 3 H-norethynodrel," Amer J Obstet Gynecol 98:411-413, 1967.
46. Center for Disease Control, "Increased Risk of Hepatocellular Adenoma in Women with Long-term use of Oral Contraceptives," Morbidity and Mortality Weekly Report, 26:293-294, 1977.
47. Herbst, A. L., Cole, P., Colton, T., Robboy, S. J., Scully, R. E., "Age-incidence and Risk of Diethylstilbestrol-related Clear Cell Adenocarcinoma of the Vagina and Cervix," Am J Obstet Gynecol, 128:43-50, 1977.
48. Bibbo, M., Al-Naqeeb, M., Baccarini, I., Gill, W., Newton, M., Sleeper, K. M., Sonek, M., Wied, G. L., "Follow-up Study of Male and Female Offspring of DES-treated Mothers. A Preliminary Report," Jour of Repro Med, 15:29-32, 1975.
49. Gill, W. B., Schumacher, G. F. B., Bibbo, M., "Structural and Functional Abnormalities in the Sex Organs of Male Offspring of Mothers Treated with Diethylstilbestrol (DES)," Jour of Repro Med, 16:147-153, 1976.
50. Henderson, B. E., Senton, B., Cosgrove, M., Baptista, J., Aldrich, J., Townsend, D., Hart, W., Mack, T., "Urogenital Tract Abnormalities in Sons of Women Treated with Diethylstilbestrol," Pediatrics, 58:505-507, 1976.
51. Heinonen, O. P., Slone, D., Nonson, R. R., Hook, E. B., Shapiro, S., "Cardiovascular Birth Defects and Antenatal Exposure to Female Sex Hormones," N Engl J Med 296:67-70, 1977.
52. Jain, A. K., "Mortality Risk Associated with the Use of Oral Contraceptives," Studies in Family Planning, 8:50-54, 1977.
53. Beral, V., "Mortality Among Oral Contraceptive Users," Lancet, 2:727-731, 1977.
54. Nilsson, S., Nygren, K., and Johansson, E., "Ethinyl Estradiol in Human Milk and Plasma after Oral Administration," Contraception 17:131-139, 1978.
55. Nilsson, S., Nygren, K., and Johansson, E., "d-Norgestrel Concentrations in Maternal Plasma, Milk and Child Plasma During Administration of Oral Contraceptives to Nursing Women," Am J Obstet Gynecol, 129:178, 1977.
56. Royal College of General Practioners' Oral contraception study, "Incidence of arterial disease among oral contraceptive users," J Royal Col Gen Pract 33:75-82, 1983.
57. Slone, D., Shapiro, S., Kaufman, D. W., Rosenberg, L., Miettinen, O., and Stolley, P., "Risk of myocardial infarction in relation to current and discontinued use of oral contraceptives," N Engl J Med 305:420-424, 1981.
58. Inman, W.H.W., "Oral contraceptives and fatal subarachnoid haemorrhage," Brit Med J 2:1468-1470, 1979.
59. Petitti, D. B., and Wingerd, J., "Use of oral contraceptives, cigarette smoking and risk of subarachnoid haemorrhage," Lancet 2:234-236, 1978.
60. Thorogood, M., Adam, S. A., and Mann, J. I., "Fatal subarachnoid haemorrhage in young women: role of oral contraceptives," Brit Med J 283:762, 1981.
61. Rosenberg, L., Hennekens, C. H., Rosner, B., Belanger, C., Rothman, K. J., and Speizer, F. E., "Oral contraceptive use in relation to nonfatal myocardial infarction," Am J Epidemiol 111:59-66, 1980.
62. Adam, S. A., Thorogood, M., and Mann, J. I., "Oral contraception and myocardial infarction revisited: the effects of new preparations and prescribing patterns," Brit J Obstet Gynaecol 88:838-845, 1981.

Brief Summary Patient Package Insert: See Lo/Ovral

DETAILED PATIENT LABELING: See Lo/Ovral Shown in Product Identification Section, page 444

NORDETTE®-28 ℞
[nor-det'-28]
TABLETS
(levonorgestrel and ethinyl estradiol tablets)

Description:
ORAL CONTRACEPTIVE

21 light-orange Nordette® tablets, each containing 0.15 mg of levonorgestrel (d(-)-13 beta-ethyl-17-alpha-ethinyl-17-beta-hydroxygon-4-en-3-one), a totally synthetic progestogen, and 0.03 mg of ethinyl estradiol (19-nor-17α-pregna-1,3,5 (10)-trien-20-yne-3,17-diol), and 7 pink inert tablets.

Clinical Pharmacology: See NORDETTE®-21
Indications and Usage: See NORDETTE®-21
Dose-Related Risk of Thromboembolism from Oral Contraceptives: See NORDETTE®-21
Contraindications: See NORDETTE®-21
Warnings: See NORDETTE®-21
Precautions: See NORDETTE®-21
Adverse Reactions: See NORDETTE®-21
Acute Overdosage: See NORDETTE®-21
Dosage and Administration: To achieve maximum contraceptive effectiveness, Nordette®-28 must be taken exactly as directed and at intervals not exceeding 24 hours. The dosage of Nordette®-28 is one light-orange tablet daily for 21 consecutive days followed by one pink inert tablet daily for 7 consecutive days according to prescribed schedule. It is recommended that tablets be taken at the same time each day, preferably after the evening meal or at bedtime.

During the first cycle of medication, the patient is instructed to begin taking Nordette®-28 on the first Sunday after the onset of menstruation. If menstruation begins on a Sunday, the first tablet (light-orange) is taken that day. One light-orange tablet should be taken daily for 21 consecutive days followed by one pink inert tablet daily for 7 consecutive days. Withdrawal bleeding should usually occur within three days following discontinuation of light-orange tablets.

During the first cycle, contraceptive reliance should not be placed on Nordette®-28 until a light-orange tablet has been taken daily for 7 consecutive days. The possibility of ovulation and conception prior to initiation of medication should be considered.

The patient begins her next and all subsequent 28-day courses of tablets on the same day of the week (Sunday) on which she began her first course, following the same schedule: 21 days on light-orange tablets—7 days on pink inert tablets. If in any cycle the patient starts tablets later than the proper day, she should protect herself by using another method of birth control until she has taken a light-orange tablet daily for 7 consecutive days.

If spotting or breakthrough bleeding occurs, the patient is instructed to continue on the same regimen. This type of bleeding is usually transient and without significance; however, if the bleeding is persistent or prolonged, the patient is advised to consult her physician. Although the occurrence of pregnancy is highly unlikely if Nordette®-28 is taken according to directions, if withdrawal bleeding does not occur, the possibility of pregnancy must be considered. If the patient has not adhered to the prescribed schedule (missed one or more tablets or started taking them on a day later than she should have), the probability of pregnancy should be considered at the time of the first missed period and appropriate diagnostic measures taken before the medication is resumed. If the patient has adhered to the prescribed regimen and misses two consecutive periods, pregnancy should be ruled out before continuing the contraceptive regimen. The patient should be instructed to take a missed light-orange tablet as soon as it is remembered. If two consecutive light-orange tablets are missed, they should both be taken as soon as remembered. The next tablet should be taken at the usual time. Any time the patient misses one or two light-orange tablets she should also use another method of contraception until she has taken a light-orange tablet daily for seven consecutive days. If the patient misses one or more pink tablets, she is still protected against pregnancy *provided* she begins taking light-orange tablets again on the proper day.

If breakthrough bleeding occurs following missed light-orange tablets, it will usually be transient and of no consequence. While there is little likelihood of ovulation occurring if only one or two light-orange tablets are missed, the possibility of ovulation increases with each successive day that scheduled light-orange tablets are missed. (If three consecutive light-orange Nordette® tablets are missed, all medication should be discontinued and the remainder of the 28-day package discarded. A new tablet cycle should be started on the first Sunday following the last missed tablet, and an alternate means of contraception should be prescribed during the days without tablets and until the patient has taken a light-orange tablet daily for 7 consecutive days.) In the nonlactating mother, Nordette® may be prescribed in the postpartum period either immediately or at the first postpartum examination whether or not menstruation has resumed.

How Supplied: Nordette®-28 Tablets (0.15 mg levonorgestrel + 0.03 mg ethinyl estradiol tablets), Wyeth®, NDC 0008-2533, are available in 6 Pilpak® dispensers of 28 tablets, consisting of 21 light-orange, round, active tablets marked "WYETH" and "75" and 7 pink, round, inert tablets marked "WYETH" and "486".

References: See NORDETTE®-21

Brief Summary Patient Package Insert: See LO/OVRAL

DETAILED PATIENT LABELING: See LO/OVRAL

Shown in Product Identification Section, page 444

NURSOY®
[nur-soy]
Soy protein formula
READY-TO-FEED
CONCENTRATED LIQUID

Nursoy® milk free formula is intended to meet the nutritional needs of infants and children who are not breast feeding and are allergic to cow's milk protein or intolerant to lactose. It contains no corn syrup solids. Professional advice should be followed.

Ingredients: (in normal dilution supplying 20 calories per fluidounce): 87% water; 6.7% sucrose; 3.4% oleo, coconut, oleic (safflower) and soybean oils; 2.3% soy protein isolate; 0.10% potassium citrate; 0.09% monobasic sodium phosphate; 0.04% calcium carbonate; 0.04% dibasic calcium phosphate; 0.03% magnesium chloride; 0.03% calcium chloride; 0.03% soy lecithin; 0.03% calcium carrageenan; 0.03% calcium hydroxide; 0.03% l-methionine; 0.01% sodium chloride; 0.01% potassium bicarbonate; ferrous, zinc and cupric sulfates; (68ppb) potassium iodide; ascorbic acid; choline chloride; alpha tocopheryl acetate; niacinamide; calcium pantothenate; riboflavin; vitamin A palmitate; thiamine hydrochloride; pyridoxine hydrochloride; beta-carotene; phytonadione; folic acid; biotin; activated 7-dehydrocholesterol; cyanocobalamin.

PROXIMATE ANALYSIS
at 20 calories per fluidounce

READY-TO-FEED and CONCENTRATED LIQUID:

	(W/V)
Protein	2.1%
Fat	3.6%
Carbohydrate	6.9%
Ash	0.35%
Water	87.0%
Crude fiber	not more than 0.01%
Calories/fl. oz.	20

Vitamins, Minerals: In normal dilution, each quart contains:

A	2,500	IU
D_3	400	IU
E	9	IU
K_1	0.1	mg
C (ascorbic acid)	55	mg
B_1 (thiamine)	0.67	mg
B_2 (riboflavin)	1	mg
B_6	0.4	mg
B_{12}	2	mcg
Niacin mg equivalents	9.5	
Pantothenic acid	3	mg
Folic acid	50	mcg
Choline	85	mg
Inositol	26	mg
Biotin	35	mcg
Calcium	600	mg
Phosphorus	420	mg
Sodium	190	mg
Potassium	700	mg
Chloride	355	mg
Magnesium	65	mg
Manganese	0.2	mg
Iron	12	mg
Copper	0.45	mg
Zinc	3.5	mg
Iodine	65	mcg

Preparation: *Ready-to-Feed* (32 fl. oz. cans of 20 calories per fluidounce formula)—shake can, open and pour into previously sterilized nursing bottle; attach nipple and feed. Cover opened can and immediately store in refrigerator. Use contents of can within 48 hours of opening.
Concentrated Liquid—For normal dilution supplying 20 calories per fluidounce, use equal amounts of Nursoy® liquid and cooled, previously boiled water. *Note: Prepared formula should be used within 24 hours.*

How Supplied: *Ready-to-Feed*—presterilized and premixed, 32 fluidounce (1 quart) cans, cases of 6; *Concentrated Liquid*—13 fluidounce cans, cases of 24.

Also available to hospitals only:
Ready-to-Feed 4 oz. disposable bottles (48 bottles/case) as part of the Wyeth Hospital Infant Feeding System.

OMNIPEN® ℞
[om'nĭ-pen]
(ampicillin)
CAPSULES

How Supplied: Omnipen® (ampicillin) Capsules—250 mg ampicillin anhydrous, bottles of 100 and 500 capsules; 500 mg, bottles of 100 and 500 capsules. Redipak® Unit Dose Medication, 250 mg and 500 mg, boxes of 100 capsules (individually wrapped).

For prescribing information write to Professional Service, Wyeth Laboratories, Box 8299, Philadelphia, PA, 19101, or contact your local Wyeth representative.

Shown in Product Identification Section, page 444

OMNIPEN® ℞
[om'nĭ-pen]
(ampicillin)
ORAL SUSPENSION

How Supplied: Omnipen® (ampicillin) for Oral Suspension in bottles of powder for reconstitution. When reconstituted with water they will make a palatable suspension containing 125 mg, 250 mg, or 500 mg ampicillin per 5 ml.

For prescribing information write to Professional Service, Wyeth Laboratories, Box 8299, Philadelphia, PA, 19101, or contact your local Wyeth representative.

OMNIPEN® Pediatric Drops ℞
[om'nĭ-pen]
(ampicillin)
ORAL SUSPENSION

How Supplied: One bottle of powder for reconstitution with water to make 20 ml suspension. When reconstituted according to instructions on label, each ml contains 100 mg of ampicillin.
For prescribing information write to Professional Service, Wyeth Laboratories, Box 8299, Philadelphia, PA, 19101, or contact your local Wyeth representative.

OMNIPEN®-N ℞
[om'nĭ-pen-N]
(ampicillin sodium)
INJECTION

How Supplied: Omnipen®-N (ampicillin sodium) for Injection: Ampicillin sodium equivalent to 125 mg, 250 mg, 500 mg, 1 gram, or 2 gram ampicillin per standard vial; 10 gram per pharmacy bulk vial. Piggyback Units: Supplied in single units equivalent to 500 mg, 1 gram or 2 gram ampicillin per unit, packed in 10 vials per package.
For prescribing information write to Professional Service, Wyeth Laboratories, Box 8299, Philadelphia, PA, 19101, or contact your local Wyeth representative.

OVRAL® TABLETS ℞
[oh'vral]
(norgestrel and ethinyl estradiol tablets)

Description: Each Ovral® tablet contains 0.5 mg of norgestrel (dl-13-beta-ethyl-17-alpha-ethinyl-17-beta-hydroxygon-4-en-3-one), a totally synthetic progestogen, and 0.05 mg of ethinyl estradiol (19-nor-17α-pregna-1,3,5(10)-trien-20-yne-3, 17-diol).

Clinical Pharmacology: See LO/OVRAL®.

Indications and Usage: Ovral® is indicated for the prevention of pregnancy in women who elect to use oral contraceptives as a method of contraception.
Oral contraceptives are highly effective. The pregnancy rate in women using conventional combination oral contraceptives (containing 35 mcg or more of ethinyl estradiol or 50 mcg or more of mestranol) is generally reported as less than one pregnancy per 100 woman-years of use. Slightly higher rates (somewhat more than 1 pregnancy per 100 woman-years of use) are reported for some combination products containing 35 mcg or less of ethinyl estradiol, and rates on the order of 3 pregnancies per 100 woman-years are reported for the progestogen-only oral contraceptives.
These rates are derived from separate studies conducted by different investigators in several population groups and cannot be compared precisely. Furthermore, pregnancy rates tend to be lower as clinical studies are continued possibly due to selective retention in the longer studies of those patients who accept the treatment regimen and do not discontinue as a result of adverse reactions, pregnancy, or other reasons.
In clinical trials with Ovral®, 6,806 patients completed 127,872 cycles, and a total of 19 pregnancies were reported. This represents a pregnancy rate of 0.19 per 100 woman-years. All of the pregnancies reported in these trials were the result of patient failure.
Table 1 gives ranges of pregnancy rates reported in the literature[1] for other means of contraception. The efficacy of these means of contraception (except the IUD) depends upon the degree of adherence to the method.

TABLE 1
PREGNANCIES PER 100 WOMAN-YEARS
IUD, less than 1-6; Diaphragm with spermicidal products (creams or jellies), 2-20; Condom, 3-36; Aerosol foams, 2-29; Jellies and creams, 4-36; Periodic abstinence (rhythm) all types, less than 1-47;

Continued on next page

Wyeth—Cont.

1. Calendar method, 14–47;
2. Temperature method, 1–20;
3. Temperature method—intercourse only in postovulatory phase, less than 1–7;
4. Mucus method, 1–25;

No contraception, 60–80.

Dose-Related Risk of Thromboembolism from Oral Contraceptives: See LO/OVRAL.
Contraindications: See LO/OVRAL.
Warnings: See LO/OVRAL.
Precautions: See LO/OVRAL.
Information for the Patient: See LO/OVRAL.
Drug Interactions: See LO/OVRAL.
Carcinogenesis: See LO/OVRAL.
Pregnancy: See LO/OVRAL.
Nursing Mothers: See LO/OVRAL.
Adverse Reactions: See LO/OVRAL.
Acute Overdose: See LO/OVRAL.
Dosage and Administration: To achieve maximum contraceptive effectiveness, Ovral® must be taken exactly as directed and at intervals not exceeding 24 hours. The dosage of Ovral® is one tablet daily for 21 consecutive days per menstrual cycle according to prescribed schedule. Tablets are then discontinued for 7 days (three weeks on, one week off).

It is recommended that Ovral® tablets be taken at the same time each day, preferably after the evening meal or at bedtime.

During the first cycle of medication, the patient is instructed to take one Ovral® tablet daily for twenty-one consecutive days beginning on day five of her menstrual cycle. (The first day of menstruation is day one.) The tablets are then discontinued for one week (7 days). Withdrawal bleeding should usually occur within three days following discontinuation of Ovral®. (If Ovral® is first taken later than the fifth day of the first menstrual cycle of medication or postpartum, contraceptive reliance should not be placed on Ovral® until after the first seven consecutive days of administration. The possibility of ovulation and conception prior to initiation of medication should be considered.) The patient begins her next and all subsequent 21-day courses of Ovral® tablets on the same day of the week that she began her first course, following the same schedule: 21 days on—7 days off.

She begins taking her tablets on the 8th day after discontinuance regardless of whether or not a menstrual period has occurred or is still in progress. Any time a new cycle of Ovral® is started later than the 8th day the patient should be protected by another means of contraception until she has taken a tablet daily for seven consecutive days. If spotting or breakthrough bleeding occurs, the patient is instructed to continue on the same regimen. This type of bleeding is usually transient and without significance; however, if the bleeding is persistent or prolonged the patient is advised to consult her physician. Although the occurrence of pregnancy is highly unlikely if Ovral® is taken according to directions, if withdrawal bleeding does not occur, the possibility of pregnancy must be considered. If the patient has not adhered to the prescribed schedule (missed one or more tablets or started taking them on a day later than she should have) the probability of pregnancy should be considered at the time of the first missed period and appropriate diagnostic measures taken before the medication is resumed. If the patient has adhered to the prescribed regimen and misses two consecutive periods, pregnancy should be ruled out before continuing the contraceptive regimen.

The patient should be instructed to take a missed tablet as soon as it is remembered. If two consecutive tablets are missed they should both be taken as soon as remembered. The next tablet should be taken at the usual time.

Any time the patient misses one or two tablets she should also use another method of contraception until she has taken a tablet daily for seven consecutive days. If breakthrough bleeding occurs following missed tablets it will usually be transient and of no consequence. While there is little likelihood of ovulation occurring if only one or two tablets are missed, the possibility of ovulation increases with each successive day that scheduled tablets are missed. If three consecutive tablets are missed, all medication should be discontinued and the remainder of the package discarded. A new tablet cycle should be started on the 8th day after the last tablet was taken, and an alternate means of contraception should be prescribed during the seven days without tablets and until the patient has taken a tablet daily for seven consecutive days. In the nonlactating mother Ovral® may be prescribed in the postpartum period either immediately or at the first postpartum examination whether or not menstruation has resumed.

How Supplied: Ovral® Tablets (0.5 mg norgestrel and 0.05 mg ethinyl estradiol), Wyeth®, are available in packages of 6 PILPAK® dispensers with 21 tablets each and in 3-PAK packages containing 63 tablets each as follows: NDC 0008-0056, white, round tablet marked "WYETH" and "56".

References: See LO/OVRAL®.

Brief Summary Patient Package Insert: See LO/OVRAL.

DETAILED PATIENT LABELING: See LO/OVRAL®.

Shown in Product Identification Section, page 444

OVRAL®-28 ℞
[oh′vral-28]
Tablets
(norgestrel and ethinyl estradiol tablets)

Description: 21 white Ovral® tablets, each containing 0.5 mg of norgestrel (dl-13-beta-ethyl-17-alpha-ethinyl-17-beta-hydroxygon-4-en-3-one), a totally synthetic progestogen, and 0.05 mg of ethinyl estradiol (19-nor-17α-pregna-1,3,5 (10)-trien-20-yne-3,17-diol), and 7 pink inert tablets.

Clinical Pharmacology: See LO/OVRAL®.
Indications and Usage: See OVRAL®.
Dose-Related Risk of Thromboembolism from Oral Contraceptives: See LO/OVRAL.
Contraindications: See LO/OVRAL.
Warnings: See LO/OVRAL.
Precautions: See LO/OVRAL.
Information for the Patient: See LO/OVRAL.
Drug Interactions: See LO/OVRAL.
Carcinogenesis: See LO/OVRAL.
Pregnancy: See LO/OVRAL.
Nursing Mothers: See LO/OVRAL.
Adverse Reactions: See LO/OVRAL.
Acute Overdosage: See LO/OVRAL.
Dosage and Administration: To achieve maximum contraceptive effectiveness, Ovral®-28 must be taken exactly as directed and at intervals not exceeding 24 hours. The dosage of Ovral®-28 is one white tablet daily for 21 consecutive days followed by one pink inert tablet for 7 consecutive days according to prescribed schedule. It is recommended that tablets be taken at the same time each day, preferably after the evening meal or at bedtime. During the first cycle of medication, the patient is instructed to begin taking Ovral®-28 on the first Sunday after the onset of menstruation. If menstruation begins on a Sunday, the first tablet (white) is taken that day. One white tablet should be taken daily for 21 consecutive days followed by one pink inert tablet daily for 7 consecutive days. Withdrawal bleeding should usually occur within three days following discontinuation of white tablets.

During the first cycle, contraceptive reliance should not be placed on Ovral®-28 until a white tablet has been taken daily for 7 consecutive days. The possibility of ovulation and conception prior to initiation of medication should be considered.

The patient begins her next and all subsequent 28-day courses of tablets on the same day of the week (Sunday) on which she began her first course, following the same schedule: 21 days on white tablets—7 days on pink inert tablets. If in any cycle the patient starts tablets later than the proper day, she should protect herself by using another method of birth control until she has taken a white tablet daily for 7 consecutive days.

If spotting or breakthrough bleeding occurs, the patient is instructed to continue on the same regimen. This type of bleeding is usually transient and without significance; however, if the bleeding is persistent or prolonged the patient is advised to consult her physician. Although the occurrence of pregnancy is highly unlikely if Ovral®-28 is taken according to directions, if withdrawal bleeding does not occur, the possibility of pregnancy must be considered. If the patient has not adhered to the prescribed schedule (missed one or more tablets or started taking them on a day later than she should have) the probability of pregnancy should be considered at the time of the first missed period and appropriate diagnostic measures taken before the medication is resumed. If the patient has adhered to the prescribed regimen and misses two consecutive periods, pregnancy should be ruled out before continuing the contraceptive regimen. The patient should be instructed to take a missed white tablet as soon as it is remembered. If two consecutive white tablets are missed they should both be taken as soon as remembered. The next tablet should be taken at the usual time. Any time the patient misses one or two white tablets she should also use another method of contraception until she has taken a white tablet daily for seven consecutive days. If the patient misses one or more pink tablets she is still protected against pregnancy *provided* she begins taking white tablets again on the proper day.

If breakthrough bleeding occurs following missed white tablets it will usually be transient and of no consequence. While there is little likelihood of ovulation occurring if only one or two white tablets are missed the possibility of ovulation increases with each successive day that scheduled white tablets are missed. If three consecutive white Ovral® tablets are missed, all medication should be discontinued and the remainder of the 28-day package discarded. A new tablet cycle should be started on the first Sunday following the last missed tablet, and an alternate means of contraception should be prescribed during the days without tablets and until the patient has taken a white tablet daily for 7 consecutive days. In the nonlactating mother Ovral®-28 may be prescribed in the postpartum period either immediately or at the first postpartum examination whether or not menstruation has resumed.

How Supplied: Ovral®-28 Tablets (0.5 mg norgestrel and 0.05 mg ethinyl estradiol), Wyeth®, are available in packages of 6 PILPAK® dispensers, each containing 28 tablets as follows: 21 active tablets, NDC 0008-0056, white, round tablet marked "WYETH" and "56".
7 inert tablets, NDC 0008-0445, pink, round tablet marked "WYETH" and "445".

References: See LO/OVRAL®.

Brief Summary Patient Package Insert: See LO/OVRAL.

DETAILED PATIENT LABELING: See LO/OVRAL.

Shown in Product Identification Section, page 444

OVRETTE® TABLETS ℞
[oh-vret′]
(norgestrel tablets)

Each OVRETTE® tablet contains 0.075 mg of norgestrel (dl-13-beta-ethyl-17-alpha-ethinyl-17-beta-hydroxygon-4-en-3-one).

Description: Each OVRETTE® tablet contains 0.075 mg of a single active steroid ingredient, norgestrel, a totally synthetic progestogen. The available data suggest that the d-enantiomeric form of norgestrel is the biologically active portion. This form amounts to 0.0375 mg per OVRETTE® tablet.

Clinical Pharmacology: The primary mechanism through which OVRETTE® prevents conception is not known, but progestogen-only contraceptives are known to alter the cervical mucus, exert a progestational effect on the endometrium, interfering with implantation, and, in some patients, suppress ovulation.

Indications and Usage: OVRETTE® is indicated for the prevention of pregnancy in women who elect to use oral contraceptives as a method of contraception. Oral contraceptives are highly effective. The pregnancy rate in women using conventional combination oral contraceptives (containing 35 mcg or more of ethinyl estradiol or 50 mcg or more of mestranol) is generally reported as less than one pregnancy per 100 woman-years of use. Slightly higher rates (somewhat more than 1 pregnancy per 100 woman-years of use) are reported for some combination products containing 35 mcg or less of ethinyl estradiol, and rates on the order of 3 pregnancies per 100 woman-years are reported for the progestogen-only oral contraceptives.

These rates are derived from separate studies conducted by different investigators in several population groups and cannot be compared precisely. Furthermore, pregnancy rates tend to be lower as clinical studies are continued, possibly due to selective retention in the longer studies of those patients who accept the treatment regimen and do not discontinue as a result of adverse reactions, pregnancy, or other reasons.

In clinical trials with OVRETTE®, 2,752 patients completed 38,245 cycles, and a total of 78 pregnancies were reported. This represents a pregnancy rate of 2.45 per 100 woman-years. Approximately one-half of the pregnancies reported in these trials were due to method failure, and the other half were due to patient failure.

Table 1 gives ranges of pregnancy rates reported in the literature[1] for other means of contraception. The efficacy of these means of contraception (except the IUD) depends upon the degree of adherence to the method.

TABLE 1
PREGNANCIES PER 100 WOMAN-YEARS
IUD, less than 1-6; Diaphragm with spermicidal products (creams or jellies), 2-20; Condom, 3-36; Aerosol foams, 2-29; Jellies and creams, 4-36; Periodic abstinence (rhythm) all types, less than 1-47:

1. Calendar method, 14-47;
2. Temperature method, 1-20;
3. Temperature method—intercourse only in postovulatory phase, less than 1-7;
4. Mucus method, 1-25;

No contraception, 60-80.

Dose-Related Risk of Thromboembolism from Oral Contraceptives: See LO/OVRAL.
Contraindications: See LO/OVRAL.
Warnings: See LO/OVRAL.
Precautions: See LO/OVRAL.
Information for the Patient: See LO/OVRAL®.
Drug Interactions: See LO/OVRAL.
Carcinogenesis: See LO/OVRAL.
Pregnancy: See LO/OVRAL.
Nursing Mothers: See LO/OVRAL.
Adverse Reactions: See LO/OVRAL.
Acute Overdose: See LO/OVRAL.
Dosage and Administration: To achieve maximum contraceptive effectiveness, OVRETTE® (norgestrel) must be taken exactly as directed and at intervals not exceeding 24 hours. OVRETTE® is administered on a continuous daily dosage regimen starting on the first day of menstruation, i.e., one tablet each day, every day of the year.
Tablets should be taken at the same time each day and continued daily, without interruption, whether bleeding occurs or not. The patient should be advised that, if prolonged bleeding occurs, she should consult her physician. In the non-nursing mother, OVRETTE® may be prescribed in the postpartum period either immediately or at the first postpartum examination whether or not menstruation has resumed.
The risk of pregnancy increases with each tablet missed. If the patient misses one tablet, she should be instructed to take it as soon as she remembers and to also take her next tablet at the regular time. If she misses two tablets, she should take one of the missed tablets as soon as she remembers, as well as taking her regular tablet for that day at the proper time. Furthermore, she should use a method of non-hormonal contraception in addition to taking OVRETTE® until fourteen tablets have been taken. If more than 2 tablets have been missed, OVRETTE® should be discontinued immediately and a method of nonhormonal contraception should be used until menses has appeared or pregnancy has been excluded. If menses does not appear within 45 days from the last period, a method of nonhormonal contraception should be substituted until the start of the next menstrual period or an appropriate diagnostic procedure is performed to rule out pregnancy.

How Supplied: OVRETTE® (as yellow, round tablets) is available in 28-tablet dispensers.
References: See LO/OVRAL.
Brief Summary Patient Package Insert: See LO/OVRAL®
DETAILED PATIENT LABELING: See LO/OVRAL®.

OXYTOCIN ℞
[ok″se-to′sin]
Injection, USP
(synthetic)

Description: TUBEX® Injection Oxytocin is a sterile aqueous solution containing in each ml an oxytocic activity equivalent to 10 USP Posterior Pituitary Units. The solution contains 0.5% chlorobutanol (a chloroform derivative) as preservative, and acetic acid to adjust pH.

Clinical Pharmacology: The pharmacologic and clinical properties of oxytocin are identical with those of the naturally occurring oxytocin principle of the posterior lobe of the pituitary. Oxytocin exerts a selective action on the smooth musculature of the uterus, particularly toward the end of pregnancy, during labor, and immediately following delivery. Oxytocin stimulates rhythmic contractions of the uterus, increases the frequency of existing contractions, and raises the tone of the uterine musculature.

When given in appropriate doses during pregnancy, oxytocin is capable of eliciting graded increases in uterine motility from a moderate increase in the rate and force of spontaneous motor activity to sustained tetanic contraction. The sensitivity of the uterus to oxytocic activity increases progressively throughout pregnancy until term when it is maximal.

Oxytocin is distributed throughout the extracellular fluid. Small amounts of this drug probably reach the fetal circulation. Oxytocin has a plasma half-life of about 3 to 5 minutes. Following parenteral administration, uterine response occurs within 3 to 5 minutes and persists for 2 to 3 hours. Its rapid removal from plasma is accomplished largely by the kidney and the liver. Only small amounts of oxytocin are excreted in the urine unchanged.

Indications and Usage:

> **IMPORTANT NOTICE**
> Oxytocin is indicated for the medical rather than the elective induction of labor. Available data and information are inadequate to define the benefits-to-risks considerations in the use of the drug product for elective induction. Elective induction of labor is defined as the initiation of labor for convenience in an individual with a term pregnancy who is free of medical indications.

ANTEPARTUM: Oxytocin is indicated for the initiation or improvement of uterine contractions, where this is desirable and considered suitable for reasons of fetal or maternal concern, in order to achieve early vaginal delivery. It is indicated for (1) induction of labor in patients with a medical indication for the initiation of labor, such as Rh problems, maternal diabetes, preeclampsia at or near term, when delivery is in the best interest of mother and fetus or when membranes are prematurely ruptured and delivery is indicated; (2) stimulation or reinforcement of labor, as in selected cases of uterine inertia; (3) as adjunctive therapy in the management of incomplete or inevitable abortion. In the first trimester curettage is generally considered primary therapy. In second trimester abortion, oxytocin infusion will often be successful in emptying the uterus. Other means of therapy, however, may be required in such cases.
POSTPARTUM: Oxytocin is indicated to produce uterine contractions during the third stage of labor and to control postpartum bleeding or hemorrhage.

Contraindications: Oxytocin is contraindicated in any of the following conditions:
significant cephalopelvic disproportion;
unfavorable fetal positions or presentations which are undeliverable without conversion prior to delivery, e.g., transverse lies;
in obstetrical emergencies where the benefit-to-risk ratio for either the fetus or the mother favors surgical intervention;
in cases of fetal distress where delivery is not imminent;
hypertonic uterine patterns;
hypersensitivity to the drug.
Prolonged use in uterine inertia or severe toxemia is contraindicated.
Oxytocin should not be used in cases where vaginal delivery is not indicated, such as cord presentation or prolapse, total placenta previa, and vasa previa.

Warnings: Oxytocin, when given for induction or stimulation of labor, must be administered only by intravenous infusion (drip method) and with adequate medical supervision in a hospital.

Precautions
GENERAL:
1. All patients receiving intravenous infusions of oxytocin must be under continuous observation by trained personnel with a thorough knowledge of the drug and qualified to identify complications. A physician qualified to manage any complications should be immediately available.
2. When properly administered, oxytocin should stimulate uterine contractions similar to those seen in normal labor. Overstimulation of the uterus by improper administration can be hazardous to both mother and fetus. Even with proper administration and adequate supervision, hypertonic contractions can occur in patients whose uteri are hypersensitive to oxytocin.
3. Except in unusual circumstances, oxytocin should not be administered in the following conditions: prematurity, borderline cephalopelvic disproportion, previous major surgery on the cervix or uterus, including cesarean section, overdistention of the uterus, grand multiparity, or invasive cervical carcinoma. Because of the variability of the combinations of factors which may be present in the conditions listed above, the definition of "unusual circumstances" must be left to the judgment of the physician. The decision can only be made by carefully weighing the potential benefits which oxytocin can provide in a given case against the rare occurrence of hypertonicity or tetanic spasm with this drug.
4. Maternal deaths due to hypertensive episodes, subarachnoid hemorrhage, rupture of the uterus, fetal deaths and permanent CNS or brain damage of the infant due to various causes have been reported to be associated with the use of parenteral oxytocic drugs for induction of labor or for augmentation in the first and second stages of labor.
5. Oxytocin has been shown to have an intrinsic antidiuretic effect, acting to increase water reabsorption from the glomerular filtrate. Consideration should, therefore, be given to the possibility of water intoxication, particularly when oxytocin is administered continuously by infusion and the patient is receiving fluids by mouth.
6. Oxytocin should be considered for use only in patients who have been carefully selected. Pelvic adequacy must be considered and maternal and fetal conditions thoroughly evaluated before use of the drug.

DRUG INTERACTIONS
Severe hypertension has been reported when oxytocin was given 3 to 4 hours following prophylactic administration of a vasoconstrictor in conjunction with caudal block anesthesia. Cyclopropane anesthesia may modify oxytocin's cardiovascular ef-

Continued on next page

Wyeth—Cont.

fects, so as to produce unexpected results such as hypotension. Maternal sinus bradycardia with abnormal atrioventricular rhythms has also been noted when oxytocin was used concomitantly with cyclopropane anesthesia.

CARCINOGENESIS, MUTAGENESIS, IMPAIRMENT OF FERTILITY
There are no animal or human studies on the carcinogenicity and mutagenicity of this drug, nor is there any information on its effect on fertility.

PREGNANCY
See "Indications and Usage."
Nonteratogenic Effects.
See "Adverse Reactions" in the fetus or infant.

LABOR AND DELIVERY
See "Indications and Usage."

Adverse Reactions: The following adverse reactions have been reported in the mother:
anaphylactic reaction
postpartum hemorrhage
cardiac arrhythmia
fatal afibrinogenemia
nausea
vomiting
premature ventricular contractions
pelvic hematoma

Excessive dosage or hypersensitivity to the drug may result in uterine hypertonicity, spasm, tetanic contraction, or rupture of the uterus.
The possibility of increased blood loss and afibrinogenemia should be kept in mind when administering the drug.
Severe water intoxication with convulsions and coma has occurred, associated with a slow oxytocin infusion over a 24-hour period. Maternal death due to oxytocin-induced water intoxication has been reported.
The following adverse reactions have been reported in the fetus or infant: (Due to induced uterine motility)
Bradycardia
Premature ventricular contractions and other arrhythmias
Permanent CNS or brain damage
Fetal death
(Due to use of oxytocin in the mother)
Low Apgar scores at five minutes
Neonatal jaundice

Overdosage: Overdosage with oxytocin depends essentially on uterine hyperactivity whether or not due to hypersensitivity to this agent. Hyperstimulation with strong (hypertonic) or prolonged (tetanic) contractions, or a resting tone of 15 to 20 mmH$_2$O or more between contractions can lead to tumultuous labor, uterine rupture, cervical and vaginal lacerations, postpartum hemorrhage, utero-placental hypoperfusion, and variable deceleration of fetal heart, fetal hypoxia, hypercapnia or death. Water intoxication with convulsions, which is caused by the inherent antidiuretic effect of oxytocin, is a serious complication that may occur if large doses (40 to 50 milliunits/minute) are infused for long periods. Management consists of immediate discontinuation of oxytocin, and symptomatic and supportive therapy.

Dosage and Administration: Parenteral drug products should be inspected visually for particulate matter and discoloration prior to administration, whenever solution and container permit.
Dosage of oxytocin is determined by uterine response. The following dosage information is based upon the various regimens and indications in general use.

A. INDUCTION OR STIMULATION OF LABOR
Intravenous infusion (drip method) is the only acceptable method of administration for the induction or stimulation of labor.
Accurate control of the rate of infusion flow is essential. An infusion pump or other such device and frequent monitoring of strength of contractions and fetal heart rate are necessary for the safe administration of oxytocin for the induction or stimulation of labor. If uterine contractions become too powerful, the infusion can be abruptly stopped, and oxytocic stimulation of the uterine musculature will soon wane.

1. An intravenous infusion of non-oxytocin-containing solution should be started. Physiologic electrolyte solution should be used except under unusual circumstances.
2. To prepare the usual solution for infusion, the contents of one 1-ml TUBEX® (10 units) is combined aseptically with 1,000 ml of nonhydrating diluent (physiologic electrolyte solution). The combined solution, rotated in the infusion bottle to insure thorough mixing, contains 10 mU/ml. Add the container with dilute oxytocic solution to the system through use of a constant infusion pump or other such device, to control accurately the rate of infusion.
3. The initial dose should be no more than 1–2 mU/min. The dose may be gradually increased in increments of no more than 1 to 2 mU/min. until a contraction pattern has been established which is similar to normal labor.
4. The fetal heart rate, resting uterine tone, and the frequency, duration, and force of contractions should be monitored.
5. The oxytocin infusion should be discontinued immediately in the event of uterine hyperactivity or fetal distress. Oxygen should be administered to the mother. The mother and the fetus must be evaluated by the responsible physician.

B. CONTROL OF POSTPARTUM UTERINE BLEEDING
1. Intravenous infusion (Drip Method)
To control postpartum bleeding, 10 to 40 units of oxytocin may be added to 1,000 ml of a nonhydrating diluent (physiologic electrolyte solution) and run at a rate necessary to control uterine atony.
2. Intramuscular Administration
1 ml (10 units) of oxytocin can be given after delivery of the placenta.

C. TREATMENT OF INCOMPLETE OR INEVITABLE ABORTION
Intravenous infusion with physiologic saline solution, 500 ml, or 5% dextrose in physiologic saline solution to which 10 units of oxytocin have been added should be infused at a rate of 20 to 40 drops per minute.

How Supplied: Oxytocin Injection, USP (synthetic), 10 USP units in 1 ml TUBEX® (Sterile Cartridge-Needle Units) supplied in packages of 10 TUBEX®.
Keep in a refrigerator, do not freeze.
When stored out of refrigeration at temperatures of up to 26° C (79° F), this product has exhibited acceptable data for a period not exceeding three (3) months.

PATHOCIL® ℞
[path′o-sil]
(dicloxacillin sodium monohydrate)
CAPSULES • ORAL SUSPENSION

Description: Dicloxacillin sodium monohydrate is an isoxazolyl penicillin which resists destruction by the enzyme penicillinase (beta-lactamase). It is the monohydrate sodium salt of 6-[3-(2,6-Dichlorophenyl)-5-methyl-4-isoxazolecarboxamido]-3,3-dimethyl-7-oxo-4-thia-1-azabicyclo [3.2.0] heptane-2-carboxylic acid.

Actions:
Pharmacology
Dicloxacillin sodium monohydrate is resistant to destruction by acid and is exceptionally well absorbed from the gastrointestinal tract. Oral administration of dicloxacillin sodium monohydrate gives blood levels considerably higher than those obtained with equivalent doses of any other presently available oral penicillin.

Microbiology
In vitro dicloxacillin is active against certain gram-positive cocci, including most strains of beta-hemolytic streptococci, pneumococci, penicillin G-sensitive staphylococci and, because of its resistance to penicillinase, penicillin G-resistant staphylococci. Dicloxacillin has less intrinsic antibacterial activity and a narrower spectrum than penicillin G.

DISC SUSCEPTIBILITY TESTS
Quantitative methods that require measurement of zone diameters give the most precise estimates of antibiotic susceptibility. One such procedure* has been recommended for use with discs for testing susceptibility to penicillinase-resistant penicillin-class antibiotics. Interpretations correlate diameters on the disc test with MIC values for penicillinase-resistant penicillins. With this procedure, a report from the laboratory of "susceptible" indicates that the infecting organism is likely to respond to therapy. A report of "resistant" indicates that the infecting organism is not likely to respond to therapy. A report of "intermediate susceptibility" suggests that the organism would be susceptible if high dosage is used, or if the infection is confined to tissues and fluids (e.g., urine), in which high antibiotic levels are attained.

Indications: Although the principal indication for dicloxacillin is in the treatment of infections due to penicillinase-producing staphylococci, it may be used to initiate therapy in such patients in whom a staphylococcal infection is suspected. (See Important Note.)
Bacteriologic studies to determine the causative organisms and their sensitivity to dicloxacillin should be performed.
In serious, life-threatening infections, oral preparations of the penicillinase-resistant penicillins should not be relied on for initial therapy.

Important Note: When it is judged necessary that treatment be initiated before definitive culture and sensitivity results are known, the choice of dicloxacillin should take into consideration the fact that it has been shown to be effective only in the treatment of infections caused by pneumococci, Group A beta-hemolytic streptococci, and penicillin G-resistant and penicillin G-sensitive staphylococci. If the bacteriology report later indicates the infection is due to an organism other than a penicillin G-resistant staphylococcus sensitive to dicloxacillin, the physician is advised to continue therapy with a drug other than dicloxacillin or any other penicillinase-resistant penicillin.
Recent studies have reported that the percentage of staphylococcal isolates resistant to penicillin G outside the hospital is increasing, approximating the high percentage of resistant staphylococcal isolates found in the hospital. For this reason, it is recommended that a penicillinase-resistant penicillin be used as initial therapy for any suspected staphylococcal infection until culture and sensitivity results are known.
Dicloxacillin acts through a mechanism similar to that of methicillin against penicillin G-resistant staphylococci. Strains of staphylococci resistant to methicillin have existed in nature and it is known that the number of these strains reported has been increasing. Such strains of staphylococci have been capable of producing serious disease, in some instances resulting in fatality. Because of this, there is concern that widespread use of the penicillinase-resistant penicillins may result in the appearance of an increasing number of staphylococcal strains which are resistant to these penicillins. Methicillin-resistant strains are almost always resistant to all other penicillinase-resistant penicillins (cross-resistance with cephalosporin derivatives also occurs frequently). Resistance to any penicillinase-resistant penicillin should be interpreted as evidence of clinical resistance to all in spite of the fact that minor variations in *in vitro* sensitivity may be encountered when more than one penicillinase-resistant penicillin is tested against the same strain of staphylococcus.

Contraindications: A history of a previous hypersensitivity reaction to any of the penicillins is a contraindication.

Warnings: Serious and occasionally fatal hypersensitivity (anaphylactoid) reactions have been reported in patients on penicillin therapy. Although anaphylaxis is more frequent following parenteral therapy, it has occurred in patients on oral penicillins. These reactions are more apt to occur in individuals with a history of sensitivity to multiple allergens.

There have been reports of individuals with a history of penicillin hypersensitivity reactions who experienced severe hypersensitivity reactions when treated with cephalosporins. Before therapy with a penicillin, careful inquiry should be made concerning previous hypersensitivity reactions to penicillins, cephalosporins, and other allergens. If an allergic reaction occurs, appropriate therapy should be instituted and discontinuance of dicloxacillin therapy considered. The usual agents (antihistamines, pressor amines, corticosteroids) should be readily available.

Usage in pregnancy
Safety for use in pregnancy has not been established.

Precautions: As with any potent drug, periodic assessment of organ-system function, including renal, hepatic, and hematopoietic, should be made during prolonged therapy.

The possibility of bacterial and fungal superinfection should be kept in mind during long-term therapy. If overgrowth of resistant organisms occurs, appropriate measures should be taken.

This oral preparation should not be relied upon in patients with severe illness or with nausea, vomiting, gastric dilatation, cardiospasm or intestinal hypermotility.

Since experience in neonates is limited, a dose for the newborn is not recommended at this time.

Adverse Reactions: Gastrointestinal disturbances such as nausea, vomiting, epigastric discomfort, flatulence, and loose stools have been noted in some patients receiving dicloxacillin. As with other penicillins, pruritus, urticaria, skin rashes, eosinophilia, anaphylactic reactions, and other allergic symptoms have been occasionally encountered.

Minor changes in the results of liver-function tests such as transient elevation of SGOT and changes in cephalin flocculation tests have been reported. The clinical significance of these changes is unknown.

Dosage and Administration: For mild-to-moderate upper-respiratory and localized skin and soft-tissue infections due to sensitive organisms:
Adults and children weighing 40 kg (88 lbs.) or more: 125 mg q. 6h.
Children weighing less than 40 kg (88 lbs.): 12.5 mg/kg/day in equally divided doses q. 6h.
For more severe infections such as those of the lower-respiratory tract or disseminated infections:
Adults and children weighing 40 kg (88 lbs.) or more: 250 mg q. 6h or higher.
Children weighing less than 40 kg (88 lbs.): 25 mg/kg/day or higher in equally divided doses q. 6h.
Since experience in neonates is limited, a dose for the newborn is not recommended at this time.
Dicloxacillin sodium monohydrate is best absorbed when taken on an empty stomach, preferably one to two hours before meals.
N.B.: INFECTIONS CAUSED BY GROUP A BETA-HEMOLYTIC STREPTOCOCCI SHOULD BE TREATED FOR AT LEAST 10 DAYS TO HELP PREVENT THE OCCURRENCE OF ACUTE RHEUMATIC FEVER OR ACUTE GLOMERULONEPHRITIS.
How Supplied: Pathocil® (dicloxacillin sodium monohydrate) is supplied in capsules equivalent to 250 mg (bottles of 100) and 500 mg (bottles of 50) of dicloxacillin and as a powder to be reconstituted for oral suspension containing dicloxacillin sodium monohydrate equivalent to 62.5 mg dicloxacillin per 5 ml (bottles to yield 100 ml).

*Bauer, A.W., Kirby, W.M.M., Sherris, J.C., and Turck, M.: Antibiotic Testing by a Standardized Single Discs Method, Am. J. Clin. Pathol., 45:493, 1966; Standardized Disc Susceptibility Test, FEDERAL REGISTER 37:20527-29, 1972.

Shown in Product Identification Section, page 444

PEN•VEE® K ℞
[pen-vee-kay]
(penicillin V potassium)
TABLETS • FOR ORAL SOLUTION

How Supplied: Pen·Vee® K (penicillin V potassium) is supplied in tablets containing 125 mg (200,000 units), 250 mg (400,000 units), and 500 mg (800,000 units); and as powders for reconstitution which provide oral solutions containing 125 mg (200,000 units) or 250 mg (400,000 units) per 5 ml.
For prescribing information write to Professional Service, Wyeth Laboratories, Box 8299, Philadelphia, PA, 19101, or contact your local Wyeth representative.
Shown in Product Identification Section, page 444

PHENERGAN® ℞
[fen'er-gan]
(promethazine hydrochloride)
INJECTION

Description: Promethazine HCl (10H-phenothiazine-10-ethanamine, N,N,α-trimethyl-, monohydrochloride). Each ml of TUBEX® (Sterile Cartridge-Needle Unit) contains either 25 or 50 mg promethazine hydrochloride with 0.1 mg edetate disodium, 0.04 mg calcium chloride, not more than 5 mg monothioglycerol and 5 mg phenol with sodium acetate-acetic acid buffer. Each Ampul of injection contains either 25 mg or 50 mg promethazine hydrochloride with 0.1 mg edetate disodium, 0.04 mg calcium chloride, not more than 0.25 mg sodium metabisulfite and 5 mg phenol with sodium acetate-acetic acid buffer.

Actions: Promethazine hydrochloride, a phenothiazine derivative, possesses antihistaminic, sedative, antimotion-sickness, antiemetic, and anticholinergic effects. The duration of action is generally from four to six hours. The major side reaction of this drug is sedation. As an antihistamine it acts by competitive antagonism, but does not block the release of histamine. It antagonizes in varying degrees most but not all of the pharmacological effects of histamine.

Indications: The injectable form of promethazine hydrochloride is indicated for the following conditions:
1. Amelioration of allergic reactions to blood or plasma.
2. In anaphylaxis as an adjunct to epinephrine and other standard measures after the acute symptoms have been controlled.
3. For other uncomplicated allergic conditions of the immediate type when oral therapy is impossible or contraindicated.
4. Active treatment of motion sickness.
5. Preoperative, postoperative, and obstetric (during labor) sedation.
6. Prevention and control of nausea and vomiting associated with certain types of anesthesia and surgery.
7. As an adjunct to analgesics for the control of postoperative pain.
8. For sedation and relief of apprehension and to produce light sleep from which the patient can be easily aroused.
9. Intravenously in special surgical situations, such as repeated bronchoscopy, ophthalmic surgery, and poor-risk patients, with reduced amounts of meperidine or other narcotic analgesic as an adjunct to anesthesia and analgesia.

Contraindications: Promethazine is contraindicated in comatose states, in patients who have received large amounts of central-nervous-system depressants (alcohol, sedative hypnotics, including barbiturates, general anesthetics, narcotics, narcotic analgesics, tranquilizers, etc.), and in patients who have demonstrated an idiosyncrasy or hypersensitivity to promethazine.

Under no circumstances should promethazine be given by intra-arterial injection due to the likelihood of severe arteriospasm and the possibility of resultant gangrene (see Warnings).

Phenergan injection should not be given by the subcutaneous route; evidence of chemical irritation has been noted and necrotic lesions have resulted on rare occasions following subcutaneous injection. The preferred parenteral route of administration is by deep intramuscular injection.

Warnings: Promethazine may impair the mental and/or physical abilities required for the performance of potentially hazardous tasks, such as driving a vehicle or operating machinery. The concomitant use of alcohol, sedative hypnotics (including barbiturates), general anesthetics, narcotics, narcotic analgesics, tranquilizers or other central-nervous-system depressants may have an additive sedative effect. Patients should be warned accordingly.

USAGE IN PREGNANCY: The safe use of promethazine has not been established with respect to the possible adverse effects upon fetal development. Therefore, the need for the use of this drug during pregnancy should be weighed against the possible but unknown hazards to the developing fetus.

USE IN CHILDREN: Excessively large dosages of antihistamines, including promethazine, in children may cause hallucinations, convulsions, and sudden death. In children who are acutely ill associated with dehydration, there is an increased susceptibility to dystonias with the use of promethazine hydrochloride injection.

CAUTION SHOULD BE EXERCISED WHEN ADMINISTERING PHENERGAN TO CHILDREN. ANTIEMETICS ARE NOT RECOMMENDED FOR TREATMENT OF UNCOMPLICATED VOMITING IN CHILDREN, AND THEIR USE SHOULD BE LIMITED TO PROLONGED VOMITING OF KNOWN ETIOLOGY. THE EXTRAPYRAMIDAL SYMPTOMS WHICH CAN OCCUR SECONDARY TO PHENERGAN® ADMINISTRATION MAY BE CONFUSED WITH THE CNS SIGNS OF UNDIAGNOSED PRIMARY DISEASE, e.g., ENCEPHALOPATHY OR REYE'S SYNDROME. THE USE OF PHENERGAN SHOULD BE AVOIDED IN CHILDREN WHOSE SIGNS AND SYMPTOMS MAY SUGGEST REYE'S SYNDROME, OR OTHER HEPATIC DISEASES.

USE IN THE ELDERLY (APPROXIMATELY 60 YEARS OR OLDER): Since therapeutic requirements for sedative drugs tend to be less in elderly patients, the dosage of Phenergan should be reduced for these patients.

OTHER CONSIDERATIONS: Drugs having anticholinergic properties should be used with caution in patients with asthmatic attack, narrow-angle glaucoma, prostatic hypertrophy, stenosing peptic ulcer, pyloroduodenal obstruction, and bladder-neck obstruction.

Phenergan should be used with caution in patients with bone-marrow depression. Leukopenia and agranulocytosis have been reported, usually when Phenergan has been used in association with other known toxic agents.

INADVERTENT INTRA-ARTERIAL INJECTION: Due to the close proximity of arteries and veins in the areas most commonly used for intravenous injection, extreme care should be exercised to avoid perivascular extravasation or inadvertent intra-arterial injection. Reports compatible with inadvertent intra-arterial injection of promethazine, usually in conjunction with other drugs intended for intravenous use, suggest that pain, severe chemical irritation, severe spasm of distal vessels, and resultant gangrene requiring amputation are likely under such circumstances. Intravenous injection was intended in all the cases reported but perivascular extravasation or arterial placement of the needle is now suspect. There is no proven successful management of this condition after it occurs, although sympathetic block and heparinization are commonly employed during the acute management because of the results of animal experiments with other known arteriolar irritants. Aspiration of dark blood does not preclude intra-arterial needle placement, because blood is discolored upon contact with promethazine. Use of syringes with rigid plungers or of small bore needles might obscure typical arterial backflow if this is relied upon alone.

Continued on next page

Wyeth—Cont.

When used intravenously promethazine hydrochloride should be given in a concentration no greater than 25 mg per ml and at a rate not to exceed 25 mg per minute. When administering any irritant drug intravenously it is usually preferable to inject it through the tubing of an intravenous infusion set that is known to be functioning satisfactorily. In the event that a patient complains of pain during intended intravenous injection of promethazine, the injection should immediately be stopped to provide for evaluation of possible arterial placement or perivascular extravasation.

Precautions: Promethazine may significantly affect the actions of other drugs. It may increase, prolong, or intensify the sedative action of central-nervous-system depressants, such as alcohol, sedative hypnotics (including barbiturates), general anesthetics, narcotics, narcotic analgesics, tranquilizers, etc. When given concomitantly with promethazine hydrochloride, the dose of barbiturates should be reduced by at least one-half, and the dose of narcotics should be reduced by one-quarter to one-half. Dosage must be individualized. Excessive amounts of promethazine relative to a narcotic may lead to restlessness and motor hyperactivity in the patient with pain; these symptoms usually disappear with adequate control of the pain. Promethazine should be used cautiously in persons with cardiovascular disease or impairment of liver funtion.

Although reversal of the vasopressor effect of epinephrine has not been reported with promethazine, the possibility should be considered in case of promethazine overdose.

Adverse Reactions: CNS EFFECTS: Drowsiness is the most prominent CNS effect of this drug. Extrapyramidal reactions may occur with high doses; this is almost always responsive to a reduction in dosage. Other reported reactions include dizziness, lassitude, tinnitus, incoordination, fatigue, blurred vision, euphoria, diplopia, nervousness, insomnia, tremors, convulsive seizures, oculogyric crises, excitation, catatonic-like states, and hysteria.

CARDIOVASCULAR EFFECTS: Tachycardia, bradycardia, faintness, dizziness, and increases and decreases in blood pressure have been reported following the use of promethazine hydrochloride injection. Venous thrombosis at the injection site has been reported. INTRA-ARTERIAL INJECTION MAY RESULT IN GANGRENE OF THE AFFECTED EXTREMITY (see Warnings).

GASTROINTESTINAL: Nausea and vomiting have been reported, usually in association with surgical procedures and combination drug therapy.

ALLERGIC REACTIONS: These include urticaria, dermatitis, asthma, and photosensitivity. Angioneurotic edema has been reported.

OTHER REPORTED REACTIONS: Leukopenia and agranulocytosis, usually when Phenergan® has been used in association with other known toxic agents, have been reported. Thrombocytopenic purpura and jaundice of the obstructive type have been associated with the use of promethazine. The jaundice is usually reversible on discontinuation of the drug. Subcutaneous injection has resulted in tissue necrosis. Nasal stuffiness may occur. Dry mouth has been reported.

LABORATORY TESTS: The following laboratory tests may be affected in patients who are receiving therapy with promethazine hydrochloride: Pregnancy Tests—Diagnostic pregnancy tests based on immunological reactions between HCG and anti-HCG may result in false-negative or false-positive interpretations.

Glucose Tolerance Test—An increase in glucose tolerance has been reported in patients receiving promethazine hydrochloride.

PARADOXICAL REACTIONS (OVERDOSAGE): Hyperexcitability and abnormal movements which have been reported in children following a single administration of promethazine may be manifestations of relative overdosage, in which case, consideration should be given to the discontinuation of the promethazine and to the use of other drugs. Respiratory depression, nightmares, delirium, and agitated behavior have also been reported in some of these patients.

Drug Interactions: NARCOTICS AND BARBITURATES: The CNS-depressant effects of narcotics and barbiturates are additive with promethazine hydrochloride.

MAO INHIBITORS: Drug interactions, including an increased incidence of extra-pyramidal effects, have been reported when some MAO inhibitors and phenothiazines are used concomitantly. Although such a reaction has not been reported with promethazine, the possibility should be considered.

Dosage and Administration: The preferred parenteral route of administration for promethazine hydrochloride is by deep, intramuscular injection. The proper intravenous administration of this product is well tolerated, but use of this route is not without some hazard.

INADVERTENT INTRA-ARTERIAL INJECTION CAN RESULT IN GANGRENE OF THE AFFECTED EXTREMITY (see Warnings). SUBCUTANEOUS INJECTION IS CONTRAINDICATED AS IT MAY RESULT IN TISSUE NECROSIS (see Contraindications). When used intravenously, promethazine hydrochloride should be given in concentration no more than 25 mg/ml at a rate not to exceed 25 mg per minute; it is preferable to inject through the tubing of an intravenous infusion set that is known to be functioning satisfactorily.

ALLERGIC CONDITIONS: The average adult dose is 25 mg. This dose may be repeated within two hours if necessary, but continued therapy, if indicated, should be via the oral route as soon as existing circumstances permit. After initiation of treatment, dosage should be adjusted to the smallest amount adequate to relieve symptoms. The average adult dose for amelioration of allergic reactions to blood or plasma is 25 mg.

SEDATION: In hospitalized adult patients, nighttime sedation may be achieved by a dose of 25 to 50 mg of promethazine hydrochloride.

PRE- AND POST-OPERATIVE USE:
As an adjunct to pre- or post-operative medication, 25 to 50 mg of promethazine hydrochloride in adults may be combined with appropriately reduced doses of analgesics and atropine-like drugs as desired. Dosage of concomitant analgesic or hypnotic medication should be reduced accordingly.

NAUSEA AND VOMITING: For control of nausea and vomiting the usual adult dose is 12.5 to 25 mg, not to be repeated more frequently than every four hours. When used for control of post-operative nausea and vomiting, the medication may be administered either intramuscularly or intravenously and dosage of analgesics and barbiturates reduced accordingly.

OBSTETRICS: Phenergan® (promethazine hydrochloride) in doses of 50 mg will provide sedation and relieve apprehension in the early stages of labor. When labor is definitely established, 25 to 75 mg (average dose, 50 mg) promethazine hydrochloride may be given intramuscularly or intravenously with an appropriately reduced dose of any desired narcotic. Amnesic agents may be administered as necesssary. If necessary, Phenergan with a reduced dose of analgesic may be repeated once or twice at four-hour intervals in the course of a normal labor. A maximum total dose of 100 mg of Phenergan may be administered during a 24-hour period to patients in labor.

CHILDREN: In children under the age of 12 years the dosage should not exceed half that of the suggested adult dose. As an adjunct to premedication the suggested dose is 0.5 mg per lb. of body weight in combination with an equal dose of narcotic or barbiturate and the appropriate dose of an atropine-like drug. Antiemetics should not be used in vomiting of unknown etiology in children.

Management of Overdosage: Signs and symptoms of overdosage range from mild depression of the central nervous system and cardiovascular system, to profound hypotension, respiratory depression, and unconsciousness. Stimulation may be evident, especially in children and geriatric patients. Atropine-like signs and symptoms—dry mouth, fixed, dilated pupils, flushing, etc., as well as gastrointestinal symptoms, may occur. The treatment of overdosage is essentially symptomatic and supportive. Early gastric lavage may be beneficial if promethazine has been taken orally. Centrally acting emetics are of little use.

Avoid analeptics, which may cause convulsions. Severe hypotension usually responds to the administration of levarterenol or phenylephrine. EPINEPHRINE SHOULD NOT BE USED, since its use in a patient with partial adrenergic blockade may further lower the blood pressure. Extrapyramidal reactions may be treated with anticholinergic antiparkinson agents, diphenhydramine, or barbiturates. Additional measures include oxygen and intravenous fluids. Limited experience with dialysis indicates that it is not helpful.

How Supplied: Phenergan® (promethazine hydrochloride) Injection as TUBEX® (Sterile Cartridge-Needle Unit), either 25 or 50 mg per ml, in packages of 10 TUBEX, and Ampuls of 1 ml, either 25 or 50 mg per ml, in packages of 5 and 25 Ampuls.

PHENERGAN® ℞
[fen′er-gan]
Syrup Plain and
PHENERGAN® ℞
Syrup Fortis
(promethazine HCl)

Description: Each teaspoon (5 ml) of Phenergan Syrup Plain contains 6.25 mg promethazine hydrochloride in a flavored syrup base with a pH between 4.7 and 5.2.
Alcohol 7%.

Each teaspoon (5 ml) of Phenergan Syrup Fortis contains 25 mg promethazine hydrochloride in a flavored syrup with a pH between 5.0 and 5.5.
Alcohol 1.5%.

Promethazine hydrochloride, a phenothiazine derivative, is designated chemically as N,N,α-trimethyl-10H-phenothiazine-10-ethanamine monohydrochloride with the following structural formula:

$$CH_2CH(CH_3)N(CH_3)_2 \cdot HCl$$

Promethazine hydrochloride occurs as a white to faint yellow, practically odorless, crystalline powder which slowly oxidizes and turns blue on prolonged exposure to air. It is soluble in water and freely soluble in alcohol.

Clinical Pharmacology: Promethazine is a phenothiazine derivative which differs structurally from the antipsychotic phenothiazines by the presence of a branched side chain and no ring substitution. It is thought that this configuration is responsible for its relative lack (1/10 that of chlorpromazine) of dopaminergic (CNS) action.

Promethazine is an H_1 receptor blocking agent. In addition to its antihistaminic action, it provides clinically useful sedative and antiemetic effects. In therapeutic dosage, promethazine produces no significant effects on the cardiovascular system. Promethazine is well absorbed from the gastrointestinal tract. Clinical effects are apparent within 20 minutes after oral administration and generally last four to six hours, although they may persist as long as 12 hours. Promethazine is metabolized by the liver to a variety of compounds; the sulfoxides of promethazine and N-demethylpromethazine are the predominant metabolites appearing in the urine.

Indications and Usage: Phenergan is useful for:

Perennial and seasonal allergic rhinitis.
Vasomotor rhinitis.
Allergic conjunctivitis due to inhalant allergens and foods.

Mild, uncomplicated allergic skin manifestations of urticaria and angioedema.

Amelioration of allergic reactions to blood or plasma.

Dermographism.

Anaphylactic reactions, as adjunctive therapy to epinephrine and other standard measures, after the acute manifestations have been controlled.

Preoperative, postoperative, or obstetric sedation.

Prevention and control of nausea and vomiting associated with certain types of anesthesia and surgery.

Therapy adjunctive to meperidine or other analgesics for control of postoperative pain.

Sedation in both children and adults, as well as relief of apprehension and production of light sleep from which the patient can be easily aroused.

Active and prophylactic treatment of motion sickness.

Antiemetic therapy in postoperative patients.

Contraindications: Promethazine is contraindicated in individuals known to be hypersensitive or to have had an idiosyncratic reaction to promethazine or to other phenothiazines.

Antihistamines are contraindicated for use in the treatment of lower respiratory tract symptoms including asthma.

Warnings: Promethazine may cause marked drowsiness. Ambulatory patients should be cautioned against such activities as driving or operating dangerous machinery until it is known that they do not become drowsy or dizzy from promethazine therapy.

The sedative action of promethazine hydrochloride is additive to the sedative effects of central nervous system depressants; therefore, agents such as alcohol, narcotic analgesics, sedatives, hypnotics, and tranquilizers should either be eliminated or given in reduced dosage in the presence of promethazine hydrochloride. When given concomitantly with promethazine hydrochloride, the dose of barbiturates should be reduced at least one-half, and the dose of analgesic depressants, such as morphine or meperidine, should be reduced by one-quarter to one-half.

Promethazine may lower seizure threshold. This should be taken into consideration when administering to persons with known seizure disorders or when giving in combination with narcotics or local anesthetics which may also affect seizure threshold.

Sedative drugs or CNS depressants should be avoided in patients with a history of sleep apnea.

Antihistamines should be used with caution in patients with narrow-angle glaucoma, stenosing peptic ulcer, pyloroduodenal obstruction, and urinary bladder obstruction due to symptomatic prostatic hypertrophy and narrowing of the bladder neck.

Administration of promethazine has been associated with reported cholestatic jaundice.

Precautions:
GENERAL

Promethazine should be used cautiously in persons with cardiovascular disease or with impairment of liver function.

INFORMATION FOR PATIENTS

Phenergan may cause marked drowsiness or impair the mental and/or physical abilities required for the performance of potentially hazardous tasks, such as driving a vehicle or operating machinery. Ambulatory patients should be told to avoid engaging in such activities until it is known that they do not become drowsy or dizzy from Phenergan therapy. Children should be supervised to avoid potential harm in bike riding or in other hazardous activities.

The concomitant use of alcohol or other central nervous system depressants, including narcotic analgesics, sedatives, hypnotics, and tranquilizers, may have an additive effect and should be avoided or their dosage reduced.

Patients should be advised to report any involuntry muscle movements or unusual sensitivity to sunlight.

DRUG INTERACTIONS

The sedative action of promethazine is additive to the sedative effects of other central nervous system depressants, including alcohol, narcotic analgesics, sedatives, hypnotics, tricyclic antidepressants, and tranquilizers; therefore, these agents should be avoided or administered in reduced dosage to patients receiving promethazine.

DRUG/LABORATORY TEST INTERACTIONS

The following laboratory tests may be affected in patients who are receiving therapy with promethazine hydrochloride:

Pregnancy Tests

Diagnostic pregnancy tests based on immunological reactions between HCG and anti-HCG may result in false-negative or false-positive interpretations.

Glucose Tolerance Test

An increase in blood glucose has been reported in patients receiving promethazine.

CARCINOGENESIS, MUTAGENESIS, IMPAIRMENT OF FERTILITY

Long-term animal studies have not been performed to assess the carcinogenic potential of promethazine, nor are there other animal or human data concerning carcinogenicity, mutagenicity, or impairment of fertility with this drug. Promethazine was nonmutagenic in the *Salmonella* test system of Ames.

PREGNANCY

Teratogenic Effects—Pregnancy Category C

Teratogenic effects have not been demonstrated in rat-feeding studies at doses of 6.25 and 12.5 mg/kg of promethazine. These doses are from approximately 6 to 16.7 times the maximum recommended total daily dose of promethazine for a 50-kg subject, depending upon the indication for which the drug is prescribed. Specific studies to test the action of the drug on parturition, lactation, and development of the animal neonate were not done, but a general preliminary study in rats indicated no effect on these parameters. Although antihistamines, including promethazine, have been found to produce fetal mortality in rodents, the pharmacological effects of histamine in the rodent do not parallel those in man. There are no adequate and well-controlled studies of promethazine in pregnant women. Phenergan should be used during pregnancy only if the potential benefit justifies the potential risk to the fetus.

Nonteratogenic Effects

Promethazine taken within two weeks of delivery my inhibit platelet aggregation in the newborn.

LABOR AND DELIVERY

Phenergan, in appropriate dosage form, may be used alone or an an adjunct to narcotic analgesics during labor and delivery. (See "Indications and Usage" and "Dosage and Administration.") See also "Nonteratogenic Effects."

NURSING MOTHERS

It is not known whether promethazine is excreted in human milk. Caution should be exercised when promethazine is administered to a nursing woman.

PEDIATRIC USE

This product should not be used in children under 2 years of age because safety for such use has not been established.

Adverse Reactions:

Nervous System—Sedation, sleepiness, occasional blurred vision, dryness of mouth, dizziness; rarely confusion, disorientation, and extrapyramidal symptoms such as oculogyric crisis, torticollis, and tongue protrusion (usually in association with parenteral injection or excessive dosage).

Cardiovascular—Increased or decreased blood pressure.

Dermatologic—Rash, rarely photosensitivity.

Hematologic—Rarely leukopenia, thrombocytopenia; agranulocytosis (1 case).

Gastrointestinal—Nausea and vomiting.

Overdosage: Signs and symptoms of overdosage with promethazine range from mild depression of the central nervous system and cardiovascular system to profound hypotension, respiratory depression, and unconsciousness.

Stimulation may be evident, especially in children and geriatric patients. Convulsions may rarely occur. A paradoxical reaction has been reported in children receiving single doses of 75 mg to 125 mg orally, characterized by hyperexcitability and nightmares.

Atropine-like signs and symptoms—dry mouth, fixed, dilated pupils, flushing, as well as gastrointestinal symptoms, may occur.

TREATMENT

Treatment of overdosage is essentially symptomatic and supportive. Only in cases of extreme overdosage or individual sensitivity do vital signs including respiration, pulse, blood pressure, temperature, and EKG need to be monitored. Activated charcoal orally or by lavage may be given, or sodium or magnesium sulfate orally as a cathartic. Attention should be given to the reestablishment of adequate respiratory exchange through provision of a patent airway and institution of assisted or controlled ventilation. Diazepam may be used to control convulsions. Acidosis and electrolyte losses should be corrected. Note that any depressant effects of promethazine are not reversed by naloxone. Avoid analeptics which may cause convulsions.

Severe hypotension usually responds to the administration of norepinephrine or phenylephrine. EPINEPHRINE SHOULD NOT BE USED, since its use in patients with partial adrenergic blockade may further lower the blood pressure.

Limited experience with dialysis indicates that it is not helpful.

Dosage and Administration:
ALLERGY

The average oral dose is 25 mg taken before retiring; however, 12.5 mg may be taken before meals and on retiring, if necessary. Children tolerate this product well. Single 25-mg doses at bedtime or 6.25 to 12.5 mg taken three times daily will usually suffice. After initiation of treatment in children or adults, dosage should be adjusted to the smallest amount adequate to relieve symptoms. The administration of promethazine hydrochloride in 25-mg doses will control minor transfusion reactions of an allergic nature.

MOTION SICKNESS

The average adult dose is 25 mg taken twice daily. The initial dose should be taken one-half to one hour before anticipated travel and be repeated 8 to 12 hours later, if necessary. On succeeding days of travel, it is recommended that 25 mg be given on arising and again before the evening meal. For children, Phenergan Tablets, Syrup, or Rectal Suppositories, 12.5 to 25 mg, twice daily, may be administered.

NAUSEA AND VOMITING

The average effective dose of Phenergan for the active therapy of nausea and vomiting in children or adults is 25 mg. When oral medication cannot be tolerated, the dose should be given parenterally (cf. Phenergan Injection) or by rectal suppository. 12.5 to 25-mg doses may be repeated, as necessary, at 4- to 6-hour intervals.

For nausea and vomiting in children, the usual dose is 0.5 mg per pound of body weight, and the dose should be adjusted to the age and weight of the patient and the severity of the condition being treated.

For prophylaxis of nausea and vomiting, as during surgery and the postoperative period, the average dose is 25 mg repeated at 4- to 6-hour intervals, as necessary.

SEDATION

This product relieves apprehension and induces a quiet sleep from which the patient can be easily aroused. Administration of 12.5 to 25 mg Phenergan by the oral route or by rectal suppository at bedtime will provide sedation in children. Adults usually require 25 to 50 mg for nighttime, presurgical, or obsterical sedation.

PRE- AND POSTOPERATIVE USE

Phenergan in 12.5- to 25-mg doses for children and 50-mg doses for adults the night before surgery relieves apprehension and produces a quiet sleep.

For preoperative medication children require doses of 0.5 mg per pound of body weight in combination with an equal dose of meperidine and the appropriate dose of an atropine-like drug.

Continued on next page

Wyeth—Cont.

Usual adult dosage is 50 mg Phenergan with an equal amount of meperidine and the required amount of a belladonna alkaloid.

Postoperative sedation and adjunctive use with analgesics may be obtained by the administration of 12.5 to 25 mg in children and 25- to 50-mg doses in adults.

Phenergan Syrup Plain and Phenergan Syrup Fortis are not recommended for children under 2 years of age.

How Supplied: Phenergan® (promethazine HCl) Syrup Plain, Wyeth®, is a clear, green solution supplied as follows:
NDC 0008-0549-02, case of 24 bottles of 4 fl. oz.
NDC 0008-0549-06, case of 16 bottles of 6 fl. oz.
NDC 0008-0549-08, case of 12 bottles of 8 fl. oz.
NDC 0008-0549-03, bottle of 1 pint.
NDC 0008-0549-04, bottle of 1 gallon.

Phenergan® (promethazine HCl) Syrup Fortis, Wyeth®, is a clear, light straw-colored solution supplied as follows:
NDC 0008-0231-01, bottle of 1 pint.

Keep bottles tightly closed at Room Temperature, Approx. 25°C (77°F).
Protect from light.
Dispense in light-resistant, glass, tight containers.

PHENERGAN® ℞
[fen´er-gan]
(promethazine hydrochloride)
TABLETS •
RECTAL SUPPOSITORIES

Description: Each tablet contains 12.5 mg., 25 mg., or 50 mg. promethazine hydrochloride; each rectal suppository contains 12.5 mg., 25 mg. or 50 mg. promethazine hydrochloride with ascorbyl palmitate, silicon dioxide, white wax and cocoa butter.

Actions: Phenergan® is a phenothiazine derivative that has several different types of pharmacologic properties. In addition to its antihistaminic action, which is of marked potency and prolonged duration, it also provides antiemetic as well as sedative actions, so that it is useful in a variety of clinical situations.

Indications: Phenergan, either orally or by suppository, is useful in the management of the following conditions:
Perennial and seasonal allergic rhinitis.
Vasomotor rhinitis.
Allergic conjunctivitis due to inhalant allergens and foods.
Mild, uncomplicated allergic skin manifestations of urticaria and angioedema.
Amelioration of allergic reactions to blood or plasma.
Dermographism.
As therapy for anaphylactic reactions adjunctive to epinephrine and other standard measures after the acute manifestations have been controlled.
Preoperative, postoperative, or obstetric sedation.
Prevention and control of nausea and vomiting associated with certain types of anesthesia and surgery.
Therapy adjunctive to meperidine or other analgesics for control of postoperative pain.
Sedation in both children and adults as well as relief of apprehension and production of light sleep from which the patient can be easily aroused.
Active and prophylactic treatment of motion sickness.
Antiemetic effect in postoperative patients.

Contraindications: Phenergan is contraindicated in individuals with a known hypersensitivity to the drug.

Warnings: The sedative action of promethazine hydrochloride is additive to the sedative effects of central-nervous-system depressants; therefore, agents such as alcohol, barbiturates and narcotic analgesics should either be eliminated or given in reduced dosage in the presence of promethazine hydrochloride. When given concomitantly with promethazine hydrochloride the dose of barbiturates should be reduced by at least one-half and the dose of analgesic depressants, such as morphine or meperidine, should be reduced by one-quarter to one-half.

Precautions: Ambulatory patients should be cautioned against driving automobiles or operating dangerous machinery until it is known that they do not become drowsy or dizzy from promethazine hydrochloride therapy.

Antiemetics may mask the symptoms of an unrecognized disease and thereby interfere with diagnosis.

Adverse Reactions: Patients may occasionally complain of autonomic reactions such as dryness of the mouth, blurring of vision and, rarely, dizziness.

Very rare cases have been reported where patients receiving promethazine have developed leukopenia. In one instance agranulocytosis has been reported. In nearly every instance reported, other toxic agents known to have caused these conditions have been associated with the administration of promethazine.

Cardiovascular by-effects from promethazine have been rare. Minor increases in blood pressure and occasional mild hypotension have been reported.

Photosensitivity, although extremely rare, has been reported. Occurrence of photosensitivity may be a contraindication to further treatment with promethazine or related drugs. In the presence of abraded or denuded rectal lesions the patient may experience initial local discomfort following administration of promethazine hydrochloride suppositories.

Attempted suicides with promethazine have resulted in deep sedation, coma, rarely convulsions and cardiorespiratory symptoms compatible with the depth of sedation present. A paradoxical reaction has been reported in children receiving single doses of 75 mg. to 125 mg. orally, characterized by hyperexcitability and nightmares.

Dosage and Administration: Allergy: The average oral dose is 25 mg. taken before retiring; however, 12.5 mg. may be taken before meals and on retiring, if necessary. Children tolerate this product well. Single 25 mg. doses at bedtime or 6.25 to 12.5 mg. taken three times daily will usually suffice. After initiation of treatment, in children or adults, dosage should be adjusted to the smallest amount adequate to relieve symptoms. When the oral route is not feasible, Phenergan HCl Rectal Suppositories in 25 mg. doses may be used.

The dose may be repeated within two hours if necessary, but oral therapy should be resumed if indicated and existing circumstances permit.

The administration of promethazine hydrochloride in 25 mg. doses will control minor transfusion reactions of an allergic nature.

Motion Sickness: The average adult dose is 25 mg. taken twice daily. The initial dose should be taken one-half to one hour before anticipated travel and be repeated eight to twelve hours later if necessary. On succeeding days of travel, it is recommended that 25 mg. be given on arising and again before the evening meal. For children, Phenergan Tablets, or Rectal Suppositories, 12.5 to 25 mg., twice daily, may be administered.

Nausea and Vomiting: The average effective dose of Phenergan (promethazine hydrochloride) for the active therapy of nausea and vomiting in children or adults is 25 mg. When oral medication cannot be tolerated, the dose should be given parenterally (cf. Phenergan Injection) or by rectal suppository. 12.5 to 25 mg. doses may be repeated as necessary at four- to six-hour intervals.

For nausea and vomiting in children the dose should be adjusted to the age and weight of the patient and the severity of the condition being treated.

For prophylaxis of nausea and vomiting, as during surgery and the postoperative period, the average dose is 25 mg. repeated at four- to six-hour intervals as necessary.

Sedation: This product relieves apprehension and induces a quiet sleep from which the patient can be easily aroused. Administration of 12.5 to 25 mg. Phenergan by the oral route or by rectal suppository at bedtime will provide sedation in children.

Adults usually require 25 to 50 mg. for nighttime, presurgical or obstetrical sedation.

Pre- and Postoperative Use: Phenergan in 12.5 to 25 mg. doses for children and 50 mg. doses for adults the night before surgery relieves apprehension and produces a quiet sleep.

For preoperative medication, children require doses of 0.5 mg. per pound of body weight in combination with an equal dose of meperidine and the appropriate dose of an atropine-like drug. Phenergan Suppositories, 25 mg., in children up to three years, and 50 mg. suppositories in older children, may be used in lieu of oral or parenteral medication.

Usual adult dosage is 50 mg. Phenergan with an equal amount of meperidine and the required amount of a belladonna alkaloid.

Postoperative sedation and adjunctive use with analgesics may be obtained by the administration of 12.5 to 25 mg. in children and 25 to 50 mg. doses in adults.

How Supplied: Phenergan® (promethazine HCl) Tablets and Suppositories, Wyeth®, are available as follows:
TABLETS
12.5 mg, NDC 0008-0019, orange tablet with "WYETH" on one side and "19" on the scored reverse side, in bottles of 100 and 1000 tablets and in Redipak® cartons of 100 individually wrapped tablets.
25 mg, NDC 0008-0027, white tablet with "WYETH" and "27" on one side and scored on the reverse side, in bottles of 100 and 1000 tablets, in Redipak cartons of 100 individually wrapped tablets, and in Strip Pack rolls of 25 tablets.
50 mg, NDC 0008-0227, pink tablet with "WYETH" on one side and "227" on the other side, in bottles of 100 tablets.
SUPPOSITORIES
12.5 mg, NDC 0008-0498, ivory, cone-shaped suppository wrapped in copper-colored foil, in cartons of 12 suppositories.
25 mg, NDC 0008-0212, ivory, cone-shaped suppository wrapped in light-green foil, in cartons of 12 suppositories and in Redipak Unit of Use Suppository Pack cartons of 25 suppositories.
50 mg, NDC 0008-0229, ivory, torpedo-shaped suppository wrapped in light-green foil, in cartons of 12 suppositories and in Redipak Unit of Use Suppository Pack cartons of 25 suppositories.

Shown in Product Identification Section, page 444

PHENERGAN® Ⓒ ℞
[fen´er-gan]
with codeine

Description: Each teaspoon (5 ml) of Phenergan with codeine contains 10 mg (1/6 grain) codeine phosphate (Warning—may be habit-forming) and 6.25 mg promethazine hydrochloride in a flavored syrup base with pH between 4.7 and 5.2. Alcohol 7%.

Codeine is one of the naturally occurring phenanthrene alkaloids of opium derived from the opium poppy; it is classified pharmacologically as a narcotic analgesic. Codeine phosphate may be chemically named as $(5\alpha,6\alpha)$-7,8-didehydro-4,5-epoxy-3-methoxy-17-methylmorphinan-6-ol phosphate (1:1) (salt) hemihydrate with the following structural formula:

$$ \cdot H_3PO_4 \cdot \frac{1}{2}H_2O $$

The phosphate salt of codeine occurs as white, needle-shaped crystals or white crystalline powder. Codeine phosphate is freely soluble in water and slightly soluble in alcohol.

Promethazine hydrochloride, a phenothiazine derivative, is designated chemically as N,N,α-trimethyl-10H-phenothiazine-10-ethanamine monohydrochloride with the following structural formula:

Promethazine hydrochloride occurs as a white to faint yellow, practically odorless, crystalline powder which slowly oxidizes and turns blue on prolonged exposure to air. It is soluble in water and freely soluble in alcohol.

Clinical Pharmacology:
CODEINE
Narcotic analgesics, including codeine, exert their primary effects on the central nervous system and gastrointestinal tract. The analgesic effects of codeine are due to its central action; however, the precise sites of action have not been determined, and the mechanisms involved appear to be quite complex. Codeine resembles morphine both structurally and pharmacologically, but its actions at the doses of codeine used therapeutically are milder, with less sedation, respiratory depression, and gastrointestinal, urinary, and pupillary effects. Codeine produces an increase in biliary tract pressure, but less than morphine or meperidine. Codeine is less constipating than morphine.
Codeine has good antitussive activity, although less than that of morphine at equal doses. It is used in preference to morphine, because side effects are infrequent at the usual antitussive dose of codeine. Codeine in oral therapeutic dosage does not usually exert major effects on the cardiovascular system.
Narcotic analgesics may cause nausea and vomiting by stimulating the chemoreceptor trigger zone (CTZ); however, they also depress the vomiting center, so that subsequent doses are unlikely to produce vomiting. Nausea is minimal after usual oral doses of codeine.
Narcotic analgesics cause histamine release, which appears to be responsible for wheals or urticaria sometimes seen at the site of injection on parenteral administration. Histamine release may also produce dilation of cutaneous blood vessels, with resultant flushing of the face and neck, pruritus, and sweating.
Codeine and its salts are well absorbed following both oral and parenteral administration. Codeine is about 2/3 as effective orally as parenterally. Codeine is metabolized primarily in the liver by enzymes of the endoplasmic reticulum, where it undergoes O-demethylation, N-demethylation, and partial conjugation with glucuronic acid. The drug is excreted primarily in the urine, largely as inactive metabolites and small amounts of free and conjugated morphine. Negligible amounts of codeine and its metabolites are found in the feces. Following oral or subcutaneous administration of codeine, the onset of analgesia occurs within 15 to 30 minutes and lasts for four to six hours.
The cough-depressing action, in animal studies, was observed to occur 15 minutes after oral administration of codeine, peak action at 45 to 60 minutes after ingestion. The duration of action, which is dose-dependent, usually did not exceed 3 hours.
PROMETHAZINE
Promethazine is a phenothiazine derivative which differs structurally from the antipsychotic phenothiazines by the presence of a branched side chain and no ring substitution. It is thought that this configuration is responsible for its lack (1/10 that of chlorpromazine) of dopaminergic (CNS) action. Promethazine is an H_1 receptor blocking agent. In addition to its antihistaminic action, it provides clinically useful sedative and antiemetic effects. In therapeutic dosages, promethazine produces no significant effects on the cardiovascular system.
Promethazine is well absorbed from the gastrointestinal tract. Clinical effects are apparent within 20 minutes after oral administration and generally last four to six hours, although they may persist as long as 12 hours. Promethazine is metabolized by the liver to a variety of compounds; the sulfoxides of promethazine and N-demethylpromethazine are the predominant metabolites appearing in the urine.

Indications and Usage: Phenergan with codeine is indicated for the temporary relief of coughs and upper respiratory symptoms associated with allergy or the common cold.

Contraindications: Codeine is contraindicated in patients with a known hypersensitivity to the drug.
Promethazine is contraindicated in individuals known to be hypersensitive or to have had an idiosyncratic reaction to promethazine or to other phenothiazines.
Antihistamines and codeine are both contraindicated for use in the treatment of lower respiratory tract symptoms, including asthma.

Warnings:
CODEINE
Dosage of codeine SHOULD NOT BE INCREASED if cough fails to respond; an unresponsive cough should be reevaluated in 5 days or sooner for possible underlying pathology, such as foreign body or lower respiratory tract disease.
Codeine may cause or aggravate constipation.
Respiratory depression leading to arrest, coma, and death has occurred with the use of codeine antitussives in young children, particularly in the under-one-year infants whose ability to deactivate the drug is not fully developed.
Administration of codeine may be accompanied by histamine release and should be used with caution in atopic children.
Head Injury and Increased Intracranial Pressure
The respiratory-depressant effects of narcotic analgesics and their capacity to elevate cerebrospinal fluid pressure may be markedly exaggerated in the presence of head injury, intracranial lesions, or a preexisting increase in intracranial pressure. Narcotics may produce adverse reactions which may obscure the clinical course of patients with head injuries.
Asthma and Other Respiratory Conditions
Narcotic analgesics or cough suppressants, including codeine, should not be used in asthmatic patients (see "Contraindications"). Nor should they be used in acute febrile illness associated with productive cough or in chronic respiratory disease where interference with ability to clear the tracheobronchial tree of secretions would have a deleterious effect on the patient's respiratory function.
Hypotensive Effect
Codeine may produce orthostatic hypotension in ambulatory patients.
PROMETHAZINE
Promethazine may cause marked drowsiness. Ambulatory patients should be cautioned against such activities as driving or operating dangerous machinery until it is known that they do not become drowsy or dizzy from promethazine therapy.
The sedative action of promethazine hydrochloride is additive to the sedative effects of central nervous system depressants; therefore, agents such as alcohol, narcotic analgesics, sedatives, hypnotics, and tranquilizers should either be eliminated or given in reduced dosage in the presence of promethazine hydrochloride. When given concomitantly with promethazine hydrochloride, the dose of barbiturates should be reduced by at least one-half, and the dose of analgesic depressants, such as morphine or meperidine, should be reduced by one-quarter to one-half.
Promethazine may lower seizure threshold. This should be taken into consideration when administering to persons with known seizure disorders or when giving in combination with narcotics or local anesthetics which may also affect seizure threshold.
Sedative drugs or CNS depressants should be avoided in patients with a history of sleep apnea.
Antihistamines should be used with caution in patients with narrow-angle glaucoma, stenosing peptic ulcer, pyloroduodenal obstruction, and urinary bladder obstruction due to symptomatic prostatic hypertrophy and narrowing of the bladder neck.
Administration of promethazine has been associated with reported cholestatic jaundice.

Precautions: Animal reproduction studies have not been conducted with the drug combination—promethazine and codeine. It is not known whether this drug combination can cause fetal harm when administered to a pregnant woman or can affect reproduction capacity. Phenergan with codeine should be given to a pregnant woman only if clearly needed.

GENERAL
Narcotic analgesics, including codeine, should be administered with caution and the initial dose reduced in patients with acute abdominal conditions, convulsive disorders, significant hepatic or renal impairment, fever, hypothyroidism, Addison's disease, ulcerative colitis, prostatic hypertrophy, in patients with recent gastrointestinal or urinary tract surgery, and in the very young or elderly or debilitated patients.
Promethazine should be used cautiously in persons with cardiovascular disease or with impairment of liver function.
INFORMATION FOR PATIENTS
Phenergan with codeine may cause marked drowsiness or may impair the mental and/or physical abilities required for the performance of potentially hazardous tasks, such as driving a vehicle or operating machinery. Ambulatory patients should be told to avoid engaging in such activities until it is known that they do not become drowsy or dizzy from Phenergan with codeine therapy. Children should be supervised to avoid potential harm in bike riding or in other hazardous activities.
The concomitant use of alcohol or other central nervous system depressants, including narcotic analgesics, sedatives, hypnotics, and tranquilizers, may have an additive effect and should be avoided or their dosage reduced.
Patients should be advised to report any involuntary muscle movements or unusual sensitivity to sunlight.
Codeine, like other narcotic analgesics, may produce orthostatic hypotension in some ambulatory patients. Patients should be cautioned accordingly.
DRUG INTERACTIONS
CODEINE
In patients receiving MAO inhibitors, an initial small test dose is advisable to allow observation of any excessive narcotic effects or MAOI interaction.
PROMETHAZINE
The sedative action of promethazine is additive to the effects of other central nervous system depressants, including alcohol, narcotic analgesics, sedatives, hypnotics, tricyclic antidepressants, and tranquilizers; therefore, these agents should be avoided or administered in reduced dosage to patients receiving promethazine.
DRUG/LABORATORY TEST INTERACTIONS
Because narcotic analgesics may increase biliary tract pressure, with resultant increases in plasma amylase or lipase levels, determination of these enzyme levels may be unreliable for 24 hours after a narcotic analgesic has been given.
The following laboratory tests may be affected in patients who are receiving therapy with promethazine hydrochloride:
Pregnancy Tests
Diagnostic pregnancy tests based on immunological reactions between HCG and anti-HCG may result in false-negative or false-positive interpretations.
Glucose Tolerance Test
An increase in blood glucose has been reported in patients receiving promethazine.
CARCINOGENESIS, MUTAGENESIS, IMPAIRMENT OF FERTILITY
Long-term animal studies have not been performed to assess the carcinogenic potential of codeine or of promethazine, nor are there other animal or human data concerning carcinogenicity, mutagenicity, or impairment of fertility with these agents. Codeine has been reported to show

Continued on next page

Wyeth—Cont.

no evidence of carcinogenicity or mutagenicity in a variety of test systems, including the micronucleus and sperm abnormality assays and the *Salmonella* assay. Promethazine was nonmutagenic in the *Salmonella* test system of Ames.

PREGNANCY
Teratogenic Effects—Pregnancy Category C
CODEINE
A study in rats and rabbits reported no teratogenic effect of codeine administered during the period of organogenesis in doses ranging from 5 to 120 mg/kg. In the rat, doses at the 120-mg/kg level, in the toxic range for the adult animal, were associated with an increase in embryo resorption at the time of implantation. In another study a single 100-mg/kg dose of codeine administered to pregnant mice reportedly resulted in delayed ossification in the offspring.
There are no studies in humans, and the significance of these findings to humans, if any, is not known.
PROMETHAZINE
Teratogenic effects have not been demonstrated in rat-feeding studies at doses of 6.25 and 12.5 mg/kg of promethazine. These doses are 8.3 and 16.7 times the maximum recommended total daily dose of promethazine for a 50-kg subject. Specific studies to test the action of the drug on parturition, lactation, and development of the animal neonate were not done, but a general preliminary study in rats indicated no effect on these parameters. Although antihistamines, including promethazine, have been found to produce fetal mortality in rodents, the pharmacological effects of histamine in the rodent do not parallel those in man. There are no adequate and well-controlled studies of promethazine in pregnant women.
Phenergan with codeine should be used during pregnancy only if the potential benefit justifies the potential risk to the fetus.
Nonteratogenic Effects
Dependence has been reported in newborns whose mothers took opiates regularly during pregnancy. Withdrawal signs include irritability, excessive crying, tremors, hyperreflexia, fever, vomiting, and diarrhea. Signs usually appear during the first few days of life.
Promethazine taken within two weeks of delivery may inhibit platelet aggregation in the newborn.
LABOR AND DELIVERY
Narcotic analgesics cross the placental barrier. The closer to delivery and the larger the dose used, the greater the possibility of respiratory depression in the newborn. Narcotic analgesics should be avoided during labor if delivery of a premature infant is anticipated. If the mother has received narcotic analgesics during labor, newborn infants should be observed closely for signs of respiratory depression. Resuscitation may be required (see "Overdosage"). The effect of codeine, if any, on the later growth, development, and functional maturation of the child is unknown.
See also "Nonteratogenic Effects."
NURSING MOTHERS
Some studies, but not others, have reported detectable amounts of codeine in breast milk. The levels are probably not clinically significant after usual therapeutic dosage. The possibility of clinically important amounts being excreted in breast milk in individuals abusing codeine should be considered.
It is not known whether promethazine is excreted in human milk.
Caution should be exercised when Phenergan with codeine is administered to a nursing woman.
PEDIATRIC USE
This product should not be used in children under 2 years of age because safety for such use has not been established.

Adverse Reactions:
CODEINE
Nervous System—CNS depression, particularly respiratory depression, and to a lesser extent circulatory depression; light-headedness, dizziness, sedation, euphoria, dysphoria, headache, transient hallucination, disorientation, visual disturbances, and convulsions.
Cardiovascular—Tachycardia, bradycardia, palpitation, faintness, syncope, orthostatic hypotension (common to narcotic analgesics).
Gastrointestinal—Nausea, vomiting, constipation, and biliary tract spasm. Patients with chronic ulcerative colitis may experience increased colonic motility; in patients with acute ulcerative colitis, toxic dilation has been reported.
Genitourinary—Oliguria, urinary retention; antidiuretic effect has been reported (common to narcotic analgesics).
Allergic—Infrequent pruritus, giant urticaria, angioneurotic edema, and laryngeal edema.
Other—Flushing of the face, sweating and pruritus (due to opiate-induced histamine release); weakness.
PROMETHAZINE
Nervous System—Sedation, sleepiness, occasional blurred vision, dryness of mouth, dizziness; rarely confusion, disorientation, and extrapyramidal symptoms such as oculogyric crisis, torticollis, and tongue protrusion (usually in association with parenteral injection or excessive dosage).
Cardiovascular—Increased or decreased blood pressure.
Dermatologic—Rash, rarely photosensitivity.
Hematologic—Rarely leukopenia, thrombocytopenia; agranulocytosis (1 case).
Gastrointestinal—Nausea and vomiting.

Drug Abuse and Dependence:
CONTROLLED SUBSTANCE
Phenergan with codeine is a Schedule V Controlled Substance.
ABUSE
Codeine is known to be subject to abuse; however, the abuse potential of oral codeine appears to be quite low. Even parenteral codeine does not appear to offer the psychic effects sought by addicts to the same degree as heroin or morphine. However, codeine must be administered only under close supervision to patients with a history of drug abuse or dependence.
DEPENDENCE
Psychological dependence, physical dependence, and tolerance are known to occur with codeine.

Overdosage:
CODEINE
Serious overdose with codeine is characterized by respiratory depression (a decrease in respiratory rate and/or tidal volume, Cheyne-Stokes respiration, cyanosis), extreme somnolence progressing to stupor or coma, skeletal muscle flaccidity, cold and clammy skin, and sometimes bradycardia and hypotension. The triad of coma, pinpoint pupils, and respiratory depression is strongly suggestive of opiate poisoning. In severe overdosage, particularly by the intravenous route, apnea, circulatory collapse, cardiac arrest, and death may occur. Promethazine is additive to the depressant effects of codeine.
It is difficult to determine what constitutes a standard toxic or lethal dose. However, the lethal oral dose of codeine in an adult is reported to be in the range of 0.5 to 1.0 gram. Infants and children are believed to be relatively more sensitive to opiates on a bodyweight basis. Elderly patients are also comparatively intolerant to opiates.
PROMETHAZINE
Signs and symptoms of overdosage with promethazine range from mild depression of the central nervous system and cardiovascular system to profound hypotension, respiratory depression, and unconsciousness.
Stimulation may be evident, especially in children and geriatric patients. Convulsions may rarely occur. A paradoxical reaction has been reported in children receiving single doses of 75 mg to 125 mg orally, characterized by hyperexcitability and nightmares.
Atropine-like signs and symptoms—dry mouth, fixed, dilated pupils, flushing, as well as gastrointestinal symptoms, may occur.
TREATMENT
The treatment of overdosage with Phenergan with codeine is essentially symptomatic and supportive. Only in cases of extreme overdosage or individual sensitivity do vital signs including respiration, pulse, blood pressure, temperature, and EKG need to be monitored. Activated charcoal orally or by lavage may be given, or sodium or magnesium sulfate orally as a carthartic. Attention should be given to the reestablishment of adequate respiratory exchange through provision of a patent airway and institution of assisted or controlled ventilation. The narcotic antagonist, naloxone hydrochloride, may be administered when significant respiratory depression occurs with Phenergan with codeine; any depressant effects of promethazine are not reversed with naloxone. Diazepam may be used to control convulsions. Avoid analeptics, which may cause convulsions. Acidosis and electrolyte losses should be corrected. A rise in temperature or pulmonary complications may signal the need for institution of antibiotic therapy.
Severe hypotension usually responds to the administration of norepinephrine or phenylephrine. EPINEPHRINE SHOULD NOT BE USED, since its use in a patient with partial adrenergic blockade may further lower the blood pressure.
Limited experience with dialysis indicates that it is not helpful.

Dosage and Administration: The average effective dose is given in the following table:
[See table below].
How Supplied: Phenergan® with codeine, Wyeth®, is a clear, purple solution supplied as follows:
NDC 0008-0550-02, case of 24 bottles of 4 fl. oz.
NDC 0008-0550-06, case of 16 bottles of 6 fl. oz.
NDC 0008-0550-08, case of 12 bottles of 8 fl. oz.
NDC 0008-0550-03, bottle of 1 pint.
NDC 0008-0550-04, bottle of 1 gallon.
Keep bottles tightly closed at Room Temperature, Approx. 25° C (77° F).
Protect from light.
Dispense in light-resistant, glass, tight containers.

PHENERGAN® R
[fen'er-gan]
with dextromethorphan

Description: Each teaspoon (5 ml) of Phenergan with dextromethorphan contains 6.25 mg promethazine hydrochloride and 15 mg dextromethorphan hydrobromide in a flavored syrup base with a pH between 4.7 and 5.2. Alcohol 7%.
Promethazine hydrochloride, a phenothiazine derivative, is designated chemically as N,N, α-trimethyl-10H-phenothiazine-10-ethanamine monohydrochloride with the following structural formula:

Adults	1 teaspoon (5 ml) every 4 to 6 hours, not to exceed 30.0 ml in 24 hours.	
Children 6 years to under 12 years	½ to 1 teaspoon (2.5 to 5 ml) every 4 to 6 hours, not to exceed 30.0 ml in 24 hours.	
Children under 6 years (weight: 18 kg or 40 lbs)	¼ to ½ teaspoon (1.25 to 2.5 ml) every 4 to 6 hours, not to exceed 9.0 ml in 24 hours.	
Children under 6 years (weight: 16 kg or 35 lbs)	¼ to ½ teaspoon (1.25 to 2.5 ml) every 4 to 6 hours, not to exceed 8.0 ml in 24 hours.	
Children under 6 years (weight: 14 kg or 30 lbs)	¼ to ½ teaspoon (1.25 to 2.5 ml) every 4 to 6 hours, not to exceed 7.0 ml in 24 hours.	
Children under 6 years (weight: 12 kg or 25 lbs)	¼ to ½ teaspoon (1.25 to 2.5 ml) every 4 to 6 hours, 4 not to exceed 6.0 ml in 24 hours.	

Phenergan with codeine is not recommended for children under 2 years of age.

Promethazine hydrochloride occurs as a white to faint yellow, practically odorless, crystalline powder which slowly oxidizes and turns blue on prolonged exposure to air. It is soluble in water and freely soluble in alcohol.

Dextromethorphan hydrobromide is a salt of the methyl ether of the dextrorotatory isomer of levorphanol, a narcotic analgesic. It is chemically named as 3-methoxy-17-methyl-9α, 13α, 14α-morphinan hydrobromide monohydrate with the following structural formula:

Dextromethorphan hydrobromide occurs as white crystals sparingly soluble in water and freely soluble in alcohol.

Clinical Pharmacology:
PROMETHAZINE
Promethazine is a phenothiazine derivative which differs structurally from the antipsychotic phenothiazines by the presence of a branched side chain and no ring substitution. It is thought that this configuration is responsible for its relative lack (1/10 that of cholrpromazine) of dopaminergic (CNS) action.

Promethazine is an H_1 receptor blocking agent. In addition to its antihistaminic action, it provides clinically useful sedative and antiemetic effects. In therapeutic dosages, promethazine produces no significant effects on the cardiovascular system.

Promethazine is well absorbed from the gastrointestinal tract. Clinical effects are apparent within 20 minutes after oral administration and generally last four to six hours, although they may persist as long as 12 hours. Promethazine is metabolized by the liver to a variety of compounds; the sulfoxides of promethazine and N-demethylpromethazine are the predominant metabolites appearing in the urine.

DEXTROMETHORPHAN
Dextromethorphan is an antitussive agent and, unlike the isomeric levorphanol, it has no analgesic or addictive properties.

The drug acts centrally and elevates the threshold for coughing. It is about equal to codeine in depressing the cough reflex. In therapeutic dosage dextromethorphan does not inhibit ciliary activity.

Dextromethorphan is rapidly absorbed from the gastrointestinal tract and exerts its effect in 15 to 30 minutes. The duration of action after oral administration is approximately three to six hours. Dextromethorphan is metabolized primarily by liver enzymes undergoing O-demethylation, N-demethylation, and partial conjugation with glucuronic acid and sulfate. In humans, (+)-3-hydroxy-N-methylmorphinan, (+)-3-hydroxymorphinan, and traces of unmetabolized drug were found in urine after oral administration.

Indications and Usage: Phenergan with dextromethorphan is indicated for the temporary relief of coughs and upper respiratory symptoms associated with allergy or the common cold.

Contraindications: Promethazine is contraindicated in individuals known to be hypersensitive or to have had an idiosyncratic reaction to promethazine or to other phenothiazines.

Antihistamines are contraindicated for use in the treatment of lower respiratory tract symptoms, including asthma.

Dextromethorphan should not be used in patients receiving a monoamine oxidase inhibitor (MAOI).

Warnings:
PROMETHAZINE
Promethazine may cause marked drowsiness. Ambulatory patients should be cautioned against such activities as driving or operating dangerous machinery until it is known that they do not become drowsy or dizzy from promethazine therapy.

The sedative action of promethazine hydrochloride is additive to the sedative effects of central nervous system depressants; therefore, agents such as alcohol, narcotic analgesics, sedatives, hypnotics, and tranquilizers should either be eliminated or given in reduced dosage in the presence of promethazine hydrochloride. When given concomitantly with promethazine hydrochloride, the dose of barbiturates should be reduced by at least one-half, and the dose of analgesic depressants, such as morphine or meperidine, should be reduced by one-quarter to one-half.

Promethazine may lower seizure threshold. This should be taken into consideration when administering to persons with known seizure disorders or when giving in combination with narcotics or local anesthetics which may also affect seizure threshold.

Sedative drugs or CNS depressants should be avoided in patients with a history of sleep apnea. Antihistamines should be used with caution in patients with narrow-angle glaucoma, stenosing peptic ulcer, pyloroduodenal obstruction, and urinary bladder obstruction due to symptomatic prostatic hypertrophy and narrowing of the bladder neck.

Administration of promethazine has been associated with reported cholestatic jaundice.

DEXTROMETHORPHAN
Administration of dextromethorphan may be accompanied by histamine release and should be used with caution in atopic children.

Precautions: Animal reproduction studies have not been conducted with the drug combination—promethazine and dextromethorphan. It is not known whether this drug combination can cause fetal harm when administered to a pregnant woman or can affect reproduction capacity. Phenergan with dextromethorphan should be given to a pregnant woman only if clearly needed.

GENERAL
Promethazine should be used cautiously in persons with cardiovascular disease or with impairment of liver function.

Dextromethorphan should be used with caution in sedated patients, in the debilitated, and in patients confined to the supine position.

INFORMATION FOR PATIENTS
Phenergan with dextromethorphan may cause marked drowsiness or impair the mental and/or physical abilities required for the performance of potentially hazardous tasks, such as driving a vehicle or operating machinery. Ambulatory patients should be told to avoid engaging in such activities until it is known that they do not become drowsy or dizzy from Phenergan with dextromethorphan therapy. Children should be supervised to avoid potential harm in bike riding or in other hazardous activities.

The concomitant use of alcohol or other central nervous system depressants, including narcotic analgesics, sedatives, hypnotics, and tranquilizers, may have an additive effect and should be avoided or their dosage reduced.

Patients should be advised to report any involuntary muscle movements or unusual sensitivity to sunlight.

DRUG INTERACTIONS
The sedative action of promethazine is additive to the sedative effects of other central nervous system depressants, including alcohol, narcotic analgesics, sedatives, hypnotics, tricyclic antidepressants, and tranquilizers; therefore, these agents should be avoided or administered in reduced dosage to patients receiving promethazine.

DRUG/LABORATORY TEST INTERACTIONS
The following laboratory tests may be affected in patients who are receiving therapy with promethazine hydrochloride:

Pregnancy Tests
Diagnostic pregnancy tests based on immunological reactions between HCG and anti-HCG may result in false-negative or false-positive interpretations.

Glucose Tolerance Test
An increase in blood glucose has been reported in patients receiving promethazine.

CARCINOGENESIS, MUTAGENESIS, IMPAIRMENT OF FERTILITY
Long-term animal studies have not been performed to assess the carcinogenic potential of promethazine or of dextromethorphan. There are no animal or human data concerning the carcinogenicity, mutagenicity, or impairment of fertility with these drugs. Promethazine was nonmutagenic in the *Salmonella* test system of Ames.

PREGNANCY
Teratogenic Effects—Pregnancy Category C
Teratogenic effects have not been demonstrated in rat-feeding studies at doses of 6.25 and 12.5 mg/kg of promethazine. These doses are 8.3 and 16.7 times the maximum recommended total daily dose for a 50-kg subject. Specific studies to test the action of the drug on parturition, lactation, and development of the animal neonate were not done, but a general preliminary study in rats indicated no effect on these parameters. Although antihistamines, including promethazine, have been found to produce fetal mortality in rodents, the pharmacological effects of histamine in the rodent do not parallel those in man. There are no adequate and well-controlled studies of promethazine in pregnant women.

Phenergan with dextromethorphan should be used during pregnancy only if the potential benefit justifies the potential risk to the fetus.

Nonteratogenic Effects
Promethazine taken within two weeks of delivery may inhibit platelet aggregation in the newborn.

LABOR AND DELIVERY
See "Nonteratogenic Effects.

NURSING MOTHERS
It is not known whether promethazine or dextromethorphan is excreted in human milk. Caution should be exercised when Phenergan with dextromethorphan is administered to a nursing woman.

PEDIATRIC USE
This product should not be used in children under 2 years of age because safety for that use has not been established.

Adverse Reactions:
PROMETHAZINE
Nervous System—Sedation, sleepiness, occasional blurred vision, dryness of mouth, dizziness; rarely confusion, disorientation, and extrapyramidal symptoms such as oculogyric crisis, torticollis, and tongue protrusion (usually in association with parenteral injection or excessive dosage).

Cardiovascular—Increased or decreased blood pressure.

Dermatologic—Rash, rarely photosensitivity.

Hematologic—Rarely leukopenia, thrombocytopenia; agranulocytosis (1 case).

Gastrointestinal—Nausea and vomiting.

DEXTROMETHORPHAN
Dextromethorphan hydrobromide occasionally causes slight drowsiness, dizziness, and gastrointestinal disturbances.

Drug Abuse and Dependence: According to the WHO Expert Committee on Drug Dependence, dextromethorphan could produce very slight psychic dependence but no physical dependence.

Overdosage:
PROMETHAZINE
Signs and symptoms of overdosage with promethazine range from mild depression of the central nervous system and cardiovascular system to profound hypotension, respiratory depression, and unconsciousness.

Stimulation may be evident, especially in children and geriatric patients. Convulsions may rarely occur. A paradoxical reaction has been reported in children receiving single doses of 75 mg to 125 mg

Continued on next page

Wyeth—Cont.

orally, characterized by hyperexcitability and nightmares.

Atropine-like signs and symptoms—dry mouth, fixed, dilated pupils, flushing, as well as gastrointestinal symptoms, may occur.

DEXTROMETHORPHAN

Dextromethorphan may produce central excitement and mental confusion. Very high doses may produce respiratory depression. One case of toxic psychosis (hyperactivity, marked visual and auditory hallucinations) after ingestion of a single dose of 20 tables (300 mg) of dextromethorphan has been reported.

TREATMENT

Treatment of overdosage with Phenergan with dextromethorphan is essentially symptomatic and supportive. Only in cases of extreme overdosage or individual sensitivity do vital signs including respiration, pulse, blood pressure, temperature, and EKG need to be monitored. Activated charcoal orally or by lavage may be given, or sodium or magnesium sulfate orally as a cathartic. Attention should be given to the reestablishment of adequate respiratory exchange through provision of a patent airway and institution of assisted or controlled ventilation. Diazepam may be used to control convulsions. Acidosis and electrolyte losses should be corrected. The antidotal efficacy of narcotic antagonists to dextromethorphan has not been established; note that any of the depressant effects of promethazine are not reversed by naloxone. Avoid analeptics, which may cause convulsions.

Severe hypotension usually responds to the administration of norepinephrine or phenylephrine. EPINEPHRINE SHOULD NOT BE USED, since its use in a patient with partial adrenergic blockade may further lower the blood pressure.

Limited experience with dialysis indicates that it is not helpful.

Dosage and Administration: The average effective dose for adults is one teaspoon (5 ml) every 4 to 6 hours, not to exceed 30.0 ml in 24 hours. For children 6 years to under 12 years of age, the dose is one-half to one teaspoon (2.5 to 5.0 ml) every 4 to 6 hours, not to exceed 20.0 ml in 24 hours. For children 2 years to under 6 years of age, the dose is one-quarter to one-half teaspoon (1.25 to 2.5 ml) every 4 to 6 hours, not to exceed 10.0 ml in 24 hours.

Phenergan with dextromethorphan is not recommended for children under 2 years of age.

How Supplied: Phenergan® with dextromethorphan, Wyeth®, is a clear, yellow solution supplied as follows:

NDC 0008-0548-02, case of 24 bottles of 4 fl. oz.
NDC 0008-0548-06, case of 16 bottles of 6 fl. oz.
NDC 0008-0548-03, bottle of 1 pint.
NDC 0008-0548-04, bottle of 1 gallon.

Keep bottles tightly closed at Room Temperature, Approx. 25° C (77° F).
Protect from light.
Dispense in light-resistant, glass, tight containers.

PHENERGAN® VC ℞
[fen′er-gan]

Description: Each teaspoon (5 ml) of Phenergan VC contains 6.25 mg promethazine hydrochloride and 5 mg phenylephrine hydrochloride in a flavored syrup base with a pH between 4.7 and 5.2. Alcohol 7%.

Promethazine hydrochloride, a phenothiazine derivative, is designated chemically as N,N,α-trimethyl-10H-phenothiazine-10-ethanamine monohydrochloride with the following structural formula:

Promethazine hydrochloride occurs as white to faint yellow, practically odorless, crystalline powder which slowly oxidizes and turns blue on prolonged exposure to air. It is soluble in water and freely soluble in alcohol.

Phenylephrine hydrochloride is a sympathomimetic amine salt. It may be chemically named as 3-hydroxy-α-[(methyl-amino)methyl]-benzenemethanol hydrochloride and has the following chemical formula:

Phenylephrine hydrochloride occurs as white or nearly white crystals, having a bitter taste. It is freely soluble in water and alcohol. Phenylephrine hydrochloride is subject to oxidation and must be protected from light and air.

Clinical Pharmacology

PROMETHAZINE

Promethazine is a phenothiazine derivative which differs structurally from the antipsychotic phenothiazines by the presence of a branched side chain and no ring substitution. It is thought that this configuration is responsible for its relative lack (1/10 that of chlorpromazine) of dopaminergic (CNS) action.

Promethazine is an H_1 receptor blocking agent. In addition to its antihistaminic action, it provides clinically useful sedative and antiemetic effects. In therapeutic dosages, promethazine produces no significant effects on the cardiovascular system. Promethazine is well absorbed from the gastrointestinal tract. Clinical effects are apparent within 20 minutes after oral administration and generally last four to six hours, although they may persist as long as 12 hours. Promethazine is metabolized by the liver to a variety of compounds; the sulfoxides of promethazine and N-demethylpromethazine are the predominant metabolites appearing in the urine.

PHENYLEPHRINE

Phenylephrine is a potent postsynaptic α-receptor agonist with little effect on β receptors of the heart. Phenylephrine has no effect on β-adrenergic receptors of the bronchi or peripheral blood vessels. A direct action at receptors accounts for the greater part of its effects, only a small part being due to its ability to release norepinephrine. Therapeutic doses of phenylephrine mainly cause vasoconstriction. Phenylephrine increases resistance and, to a lesser extent, decreases capacitance of blood vessels. Total peripheral resistance is increased, resulting in increased systolic and diastolic blood pressure. Pulmonary arterial pressure is usually increased, and renal blood flow is usually decreased. Local vasoconstriction and hemostasis occur following topical application or infiltration of phenylephrine into tissues.

The main effect of phenylephrine on the heart is bradycardia; it produces a positive inotropic effect on the myocardium in doses greater than those usually used therapeutically. Rarely, the drug may increase the irritability of the heart, causing arrhythmias. Cardiac output is decreased slightly. Phenylephrine increases the work of the heart by increasing peripheral arterial resistance.

Phenylephrine has a mild central stimulant effect. Following oral administration or topical application of phenylephrine to the mucosa, constriction of blood vessels in the nasal mucosa relieves nasal congestion associated with allergy or head colds. Following oral administration, nasal decongestion may occur within 15 or 20 minutes and may persist for up to 4 hours.

Phenylephrine is irregularly absorbed from and readily metabolized in the gastrointestinal tract. Phenylephrine is metabolized in the liver and intestine by monoamine oxidase. The metabolites and their route and rate of excretion have not been identified. The pharmacologic action of phenylephrine is terminated at least partially by uptake of the drug into tissues.

Indications and Usage: Phenergan VC is indicated for the temporary relief of upper respiratory symptoms, including nasal congestion, associated with allergy or the common cold.

Contraindications: Promethazine is contraindicated in individuals known to be hypersensitive or to have had an idiosyncratic reaction to promethazine or to other phenothiazines.

Antihistamines are contraindicated for use in the treatment of lower respiratory tract symptoms or asthma.

Phenylephrine is contraindicated in patients with hypertension or with peripheral vascular insufficiency (ischemia may result with risk of gangrene or thrombosis of compromised vascular beds). Phenylephrine should not be used in patients known to be hypersensitive to the drug or in those receiving a monoamine oxidase inhibitor (MAOI).

Warnings:

PROMETHAZINE

Promethazine may cause marked drowsiness. Ambulatory patients should be cautioned against such activities as driving or operating dangerous machinery until it is known that they do not become drowsy or dizzy from promethazine therapy.

The sedative action of promethazine hydrochloride is additive to the sedative effects of central nervous system depressants; therefore, agents such as alcohol, narcotic analgesics, sedatives, hypnotics, and tranquilizers should either be eliminated or given in reduced dosage in the presence of promethazine hydrochloride. When given concomitantly with promethazine hydrochloride, the dose of barbiturates should be reduced by at least one-half, and the dose of analgesic depressants, such as morphine or meperidine, should be reduced by one-quarter to one-half.

Promethazine may lower seizure threshold. This should be taken into consideration when administering to persons with known seizure disorders or when giving in combination with narcotics or local anesthetics which may also affect seizure threshold.

Sedative drugs or CNS depressants should be avoided in patients with a history of sleep apnea. Antihistamines should be used with caution in patients with narrow-angle glaucoma, stenosing peptic ulcer, pyloroduodenal obstruction, and urinary bladder obstruction due to symptomatic prostatic hypertrophy and narrowing of the bladder neck.

Administration of promethazine has been associated with reported cholestatic jaundice.

PHENYLEPHRINE

Because phenylephrine is an adrenergic agent, it should be given with caution to patients with thyroid diseases, diabetes mellitus, and heart diseases or those receiving tricyclic antidepressants.

Men with symptomatic, benign prostatic hypertrophy can experience urinary retention when given oral nasal decongestants.

Phenylephrine can cause a decrease in cardiac output, and extreme caution should be used when administering the drug, parenterally or orally, to patients with arteriosclerosis, to elderly individuals, and/or to patients with initially poor cerebral or coronary circulation.

Phenylephrine should be used with caution in patients taking diet preparations, such as amphetamines or phenylpropanolamine, because synergistic adrenergic effects could result in serious hypertensive response and possible stroke.

Precautions: Animal reproduction studies have not been conducted with the drug combination—promethazine and phenylephrine. It is not known whether this drug combination can cause fetal harm when administered to a pregnant woman or can affect reproduction capacity. Phenergan VC should be given to a pregnant woman only if clearly needed.

GENERAL

Promethazine should be used cautiously in persons with cardiovascular disease or impairment of liver function.

Phenylephrine should be used with caution in patients with cardiovascular disease, particularly hypertension.

INFORMATION FOR PATIENTS
Phenergan VC may cause marked drowsiness or impair the mental and/or physical abilities required for the performance of potentially hazardous tasks, such as driving a vehicle or operating machinery. Ambulatory patients should be told to avoid engaging is such activities until it is known that they do not become drowsy or dizzy from Phenergan VC therapy. Children should be supervised to avoid potential harm in bike riding or other hazardous acitvities.

The concomitant use of alcohol or other central nervous system depressants, including narcotic analgesics, sedatives, hypnotics, and tranquilizers, may have an additive effect and should be avoided or their dosage reduced.

Patients should be advised to report any involuntary muscle movements or unusual sensitivity to sunlight.

DRUG INTERACTIONS
PROMETHAZINE
The sedative action of promethazine is additive to the sedative effects of other central nervous system depressants, including alcohol, narcotic analgesics, sedatives, hypnotics, tricyclic antidepressants, and tranquilizers; therefore, these agents should be avoided or administered in reduced dosage to patients receiving promethazine.
[See table above].

PHENYLEPHRINE

Drug	Effect
Phenylephrine with prior administration of monoamine oxidase inhibitors (MAOI).	Cardiac pressor response potentiated. May cause acute hypertensive crisis.
Phenylephrine with tricyclic antidepressants.	Pressor response increased.
Phenylephrine with ergot alkaloids.	Excessive rise in blood pressure.
Phenylephrine with bronchodilator sympathomimetic agents and with epinephrine or other sympathomimetics.	Tachycardia or other arrhythmias may occur.
Phenylephrine with prior administration of propranolol or other β-adrenergic blockers.	Cardiostimulating effects blocked.
Phenylephrine with atropine sulfate.	Reflex bradycardia blocked; pressor response enhanced.
Phenylephrine with prior administration of phentolamine or other α-adrenergic blockers.	Pressor response decreased.
Phenylephrine with diet preparations, such as amphetamines or phenylpropanolamine.	Synergistic adrenergic response.

DRUG/LABORATORY TEST INTERACTIONS
The following laboratory tests may be affected in patients who are receiving therapy with promethazine hydrochloride:
Pregnancy Tests
Diagnostic pregnancy tests based on immunological reactions between HCG and anti-HCG may result in false-negative or false-positive interpretations.
Glucose Tolerance Test
An increase in blood glucose has been reported in patients receiving promethazine.

CARCINOGENESIS, MUTAGENESIS, IMPAIRMENT OF FERTILITY
PROMETHAZINE
Long-term animal studies have not been performed to assess the carcinogenic potential of promethazine, nor are there other animal or human data concerning carcinogenicity, mutagenicity, or impairment of fertility with this drug. Promethazine was nonmutagenic in the *Salmonella* test system of Ames.

PHENYLEPHRINE
A study which followed the develpment of cancer in 143,574 patients over a four-year period indicated that in 11,981 patients who received phenylephrine (systemic or topical), there was no statistically significant association between the drug and cancer at any or all sites.

Long-term animal studies have not been performed to assess the carcinogenic potential of phenylephrine, nor are there other animal or human data concerning mutagenicity.

A study of the effects of adrenergic drugs on ovum transport in rabbits indicated that treatment with phenylephrine did not alter incidence of pregnancy; the number of implantations was significantly reduced when high doses of the drug were used.

PREGNANCY
Teratogenic Effects—Pregnancy Category C
PROMETHAZINE
Teratogenic effects have not been demonstrated in rat-feeding studies at doses of 6.25 and 12.5 mg/kg of promethazine. These doses are 8.3 and 16.7 times the maximum recommended total daily dose of promethazine for a 50-kg subject. Specific studies to test the action of the drug on parturition, lactation, and development of the animal neonate were not done, but a general preliminary study in rats indicated no effect on these parameters. Although antihistamines, including promethazine, have been found to produce fetal mortality in rodents, the pharmacological effects of histamine in the rodent do not parallel those in man. There are no adequate and well-controlled studies of promethazine in pregnant women.

PHENYLEPHRINE
A study in rabbits indicated that continued moderate overexposure to phenylephrine (3 mg/day) during the second half of pregnancy (22nd day of gestation to delivery) may contribute to perinatal wastage, prematurity, premature labor, and possibly fetal anomalies; when phenylephrine (3 mg/day) was given to rabbits during the first half of pregnancy (3rd day after mating for seven days), a significant number gave birth to litters of low birth weight. Another study showed that phenylephrine was associated with anomalies of aortic arch and with ventricular septal defect in the chick embryo.

Phenergan VC should be used during pregnancy only if the potential benefit justifies the potential risk to the fetus.

Nonteratogenic Effects
Promethazine taken within two weeks of delivery may inhibit platelet aggregation in the newborn.

LABOR AND DELIVERY
Administration of phenylephrine to patients in late pregnancy or labor may cause fetal anoxia or bradycardia by increasing contractility of the uterus and decreasing uterine blood flow.
See also "Nonteratogenic Effects."

NURSING MOTHERS
It is not known whether promethazine or phenylephrine are excreted in human milk. Caution should be exercised when Phenergan VC is administered to a nursing woman.

PEDIATRIC USE
This product should not be used in children under 2 years of age because safety for such use has not been established.

Adverse Reactions
PROMETHAZINE
Nervous System—Sedation, sleepiness, occasional blurred vision, dryness of mouth, dizziness; rarely confusion, disorientation, and extrapyramidal symptoms such as oculogyric crisis, torticollis, and tongue protrusion (usually in association with parenteral injection or excessive dosage).
Cardiovascular—Increased or decreased blood pressure.
Dermatologic—Rash, rarely photosensitivity.
Hematologic—Rarely leukopenia, thrombocytopenia; agranulocytosis (1 case).
Gastrointestinal—Nausea and vomiting.

PHENYLEPHRINE
Nervous System—Restlessness, anxiety, nervousness, and dizziness.
Cardiovascular—Hypertension (see "Warnings").
Other—Precordial pain, respiratory distress, tremor, and weakness.

Overdosage
PROMETHAZINE
Signs and symptoms of overdosage with promethazine range from mild depression of the central nervous system and cardiovascular system to profound hypotension, respiratory depression, and unconsciousness.
Stimulation may be evident, especially in children and geriatric patients. Convulsions may rarely occur. A paradoxical reaction has been reported in children receiving single doses of 75 mg to 125 mg orally, characterized by hyperexcitability and nightmares.
Atropine-like signs and symptoms—dry mouth, fixed, dilated pupils, flushing, as well as gastrointestinal symptoms, may occur.

PHENYLEPHRINE
Signs and symptoms of overdosage with phenylephrine include hypertension, headache, convulsions, cerebral hemorrhage, and vomiting. Ventricular premature beats and short paroxysms of ventricular tachycardia may also occur. Headache may be a symptom of hypertension. Bradycardia may also be seen early in phenylephrine overdosage through stimulation of baroreceptors.

TREATMENT
Treatment of overdosage with Phenergan VC is essentially symptomatic and supportive. Only in cases of extreme overdosage or individual sensitivity do vital signs including respiration, pulse, blood pressure, temperature, and EKG need to be monitored. Activated charcoal orally or by lavage may be given, or sodium or magnesium sulfate orally as a cathartic. Attention should be given to the reestablishment of adequate respiratory exchange through provision of a patent airway and institution of assisted or controlled ventilation. Diazepam may be used to control convulsions. Acidosis and electrolyte losses should be corrected. Note that any depressant effects of promethazine are not reversed by naloxone. Avoid analeptics which may cause convulsions.
Severe hypotension usually responds to the administration of norepinephrine or phenylephrine. EPINEPHRINE SHOULD NOT BE USED, since its use in patients with partial adrenergic blockade may further lower the blood pressure.
Limited experience with dialysis indicates that it is not helpful.

Dosage and Administration: The recommended adult dose is one teaspoon (5 ml) every 4 to 6 hours, not to exceed 30.0 ml in 24 hours. For children 6 years to under 12 years of age, the dose is one-half to one teaspoon (2.5 to 5.0 ml) repeated at 4- to 6-hour intervals, not to exceed 30.0 ml in 24 hours. For children 2 years to under 6 years of age, the dose is one-quarter to one-half teaspoon (1.25 to 2.5 ml) every 4 to 6 hours.
Phenergan VC is not recommended for children under 2 years of age.

How Supplied: Phenergan® VC, Wyeth®, is a clear, orange-yellow solution supplied as follows:
NDC 0008-0551-02, case of 24 bottles of 4 fl. oz.
NDC 0008-0551-06, case of 16 bottles of 6 fl. oz.
NDC 0008-0551-08, case of 12 bottles of 8 fl. oz.
NDC 0008-0551-03, bottle of 1 pint.
NDC 0008-0551-04, bottle of 1 gallon.
Keep bottles tightly closed below 25°C (77°F).
Protect from light.
Dispense in light-resistant, glass, tight containers.

Continued on next page

Wyeth—Cont.

PHENERGAN® VC
[fen'er-gan]
with codeine

Description: Each teaspoon (5 ml) of Phenergan VC with codeine contains 10 mg ($\frac{1}{6}$ grain) codeine phosphate (Warning—may be habit-forming), 6.25 mg promethazine hydrochloride, and 5 mg phenylephrine hydrochloride in a flavored syrup base with a pH between 4.7 and 5.2. Alcohol 7%. Codeine is one of the naturally occurring phenanthrene alkaloids of opium derived from the opium poppy; it is classified pharmacologically as a narcotic analgesic. Codeine phosphate may be chemically named as ($5\alpha,6\alpha$)-7,8-didehydro-4,5-epoxy-3-methoxy-17-methylmorphinan-6-ol phosphate (1:1) (salt) hemihydrate with the following structural formula:

The phosphate salt of codeine occurs as white, needle-shaped crystals or white crystalline powder. Codeine phosphate is freely soluble in water and slightly soluble in alcohol.

Promethazine hydrochloride, a phenothiazine derivative, is designated chemically as N,N,α-trimethyl-10H-phenothiazine-10-ethanamine monohydrochloride with the following structural formula:

Promethazine hydrochloride occurs as a white to faint yellow, practically odorless, crystalline powder which slowly oxidizes and turns blue on prolonged exposure to air. It is soluble in water and freely soluble in alcohol. Phenylephrine hydrochloride is a sympathomimetic amine salt. It may be chemically named as 3-hydroxy-α-[(methylamino)methyl]-benzenemethanol hydrochloride and has the following chemical formula:

Phenylephrine hydrochloride occurs as white or nearly white crystals, having a bitter taste. It is freely soluble in water and alcohol. Phenylephrine hydrochloride is subject to oxidation and must be protected from light and air.

Clinical Pharmacology: CODEINE: Narcotic analgesics, including codeine, exert their primary effects on the central nervous system and gastrointestinal tract. The analgesic effects of codeine are due to its central action; however, the precise sites of action have not been determined, and the mechanisms involved appear to be quite complex. Codeine resembles morphine both structurally and pharmacologically, but its actions at the doses of codeine used therapeutically are milder, with less sedation, respiratory depression, and gastrointestinal, urinary, and pupillary effects. Codeine produces an increase in biliary tract pressure, but less than morphine or meperidine. Codeine is less constipating than morphine.

Codeine has good antitussive activity, although less than that of morphine at equal doses. It is used in preference to morphine, because side effects are infrequent at the usual antitussive dose of codeine. Codeine in oral therapeutic dosage does not usually exert major effects on the cardiovascular system. Narcotic analgesics may cause nausea and vomiting by stimulating the chemoreceptor trigger zone (CTZ); however, they also depress the vomiting center, so that subsequent doses are unlikely to produce vomiting. Nausea is minimal after usual oral doses of codeine.

Narcotic analgesics cause histamine release, which appears to be responsible for wheals or urticaria sometimes seen at the site of injection on parenteral administration. Histamine release may also produce dilation of cutaneous blood vessels, with resultant flushing of the face and neck, pruritus, and sweating.

Codeine and its salts are well absorbed following both oral and parenteral administration. Codeine is about $\frac{2}{3}$ as effective orally as parenterally. Codeine is metabolized primarily in the liver by enzymes of the endoplasmic reticulum, where it undergoes O-demethylation, N-demethylation, and partial conjugation with glucuronic acid. The drug is excreted primarily in the urine, largely as inactive metabolites and small amounts of free and conjugated morphine. Negligible amounts of codeine and its metabolites are found in the feces. Following oral or subcutaneous administration of codeine, the onset of analgesia occurs within 15 to 30 minutes and lasts for four to six hours.

The cough-depressing action, in animal studies, was observed to occur 15 minutes after oral administration of codeine, peak action at 45 to 60 minutes after ingestion. The duration of action, which is dose-dependent, usually did not exceed 3 hours.

PROMETHAZINE: Promethazine is a phenothiazine derivative which differs structurally from the antipsychotic phenothiazines by the presence of a branched side chain and no ring substitution. It is thought that this configuration is responsible for its relative lack ($\frac{1}{10}$ that of chlorpromazine) of dopaminergic (CNS) action.

Promethazine is an H_1 receptor blocking agent. In addition to its antihistaminic action, it provides clinically useful sedative and antiemetic effects. In therapeutic dosages, promethazine produces no significant effects on the cardiovascular system. Promethazine is well absorbed from the gastrointestinal tract. Clinical effects are apparent within 20 minutes after oral adminstration and generally last four to six hours, although they may persist as long as 12 hours. Promethazine is metabolized by the liver to a variety of compounds; the sulfoxides of promethazine and N-demethylpromethazine are the predominant metabolites appearing in the urine.

PHENYLEPHRINE: Phenylephrine is a potent postsynaptic α-receptor agonist with little effect on β receptors of the heart. Phenylephrine has no effect on β-adrenergic receptors of the bronchi or peripheral blood vessels. A direct action at receptors accounts for the greater part of its effects, only a small part being due to its ability to release norepinephrine.

Therapeutic doses of phenylephrine mainly cause vasoconstriction. Phenylephrine increases resistance and, to a lesser extent, decreases capacitance of blood vessels. Total peripheral resistance is increased, resulting in increased systolic and diastolic blood pressure. Pulmonary arterial pressure is usually increased, and renal blood flow is usually decreased. Local vasoconstriction and hemostasis occur following topical application or infiltration of phenylephrine into tissues.

The main effect of phenylephrine on the heart is bradycardia; it produces a positive inotropic effect on the myocardium in doses greater than those usually used therapeutically. Rarely, the drug may increase the irritability of the heart, causing arrhythmias. Cardiac output is decreased slightly. Phenylephrine increases the work of the heart by increasing peripheral arterial resistance. Phenylephrine has a mild central stimulant effect.

Following oral administration or topical application of phenylephrine to the mucosa, constriction of blood vessels in the nasal mucosa relieves nasal congestion associated with allergy or head colds. Following oral administration, nasal decongestion may occur within 15 or 20 minutes and may persist for up to 4 hours.

Phenylephrine is irregularly absorbed from and readily metabolized in the gastrointestinal tract. Phenylephrine is metabolized in the liver and intestine by monoamine oxidase. The metabolites and their route and rate of excretion have not been identified. The pharmacologic action of phenylephrine is terminated at least partially by uptake of the drug into tissues.

Indications and Usage: Phenergan VC with codeine is indicated for the temporary relief of coughs and upper respiratory symptoms, including nasal congestion, associated with allergy or the common cold.

Contraindications: Codeine is contraindicated in patients with a known hypersensitivity to the drug.

Promethazine is contraindicated in individuals known to be hypersensitive or to have had an idiosyncratic reaction to promethazine or to other phenothiazines.

Phenylephrine is contraindicated in patients with hypertension or with peripheral vascular insufficiency (ischemia may result wtih risk of gangrene or thrombosis of compromised vascular beds). Phenylephrine should not be used in patients known to be hypersensitive to the drug or in those receiving a monoamine oxidase inhibitor (MAOI). Antihistamines and codeine are both contraindicated for use in the treatment of lower respiratory tract symptoms, including asthma.

Warings: CODEINE: Dosage of codeine SHOULD NOT BE INCREASED if cough fails to respond; an unresponsive cough should be reevaluated in 5 days or sooner for possible underlying pathology, such as foreign body or lower respiratory tract disease.

Codeine may cause or aggravate constipation.
Respiratory depression leading to arrest, coma, and death has occurred with the use of codeine antitussives in young children, particularly in the under-one-year infants whose ability to deactivate the drug is not fully developed.

Administration of codeine may be accompanied by histamine release and should be used with caution in atopic children.

Head Injury and Increased Intracranial Pressure
The respiratory-depressant effects of narcotic analgesics and their capacity to elevate cerebrospinal fluid pressure may be markedly exaggerated in the presence of head injury, intracranial lesions, or a preexisting increase in intracranial pressure. Narcotics may produce adverse reactions which may obscure the clinical course of patients with head injuries.

Asthma and Other Respiratory Conditions
Narcotic analgesics or cough suppressants, including codeine, should not be used in asthmatic patients (see "Contraindications"). Nor should they be used in acute febrile illness associated with productive cough or in chronic respiratory disease where interference with ability to clear the tracheobronchial tree of secretions would have a deleterious effect on the patient's respiratory function.

Hypotensive Effect
Codeine may produce orthostatic hypotension in ambulatory patients.

PROMETHAZINE: Promethazine may cause marked drowsiness. Ambulatory patients should be cautioned against such activities as driving or operating dangerous machinery until it is known that they do not become drowsy or dizzy from promethazine therapy.

The sedative action of promethazine hydrochloride is additive to the sedative effects of central nervous system depressants; therefore, agents such as alcohol, narcotic analgesics, sedatives, hypnotics, and tranquilizers should either be eliminated or given in reduced dosage in the presence of promethazine hydrochloride. When given concomitantly with promethazine hydrochloride, the dose of barbiturates should be reduced by at least one-half, and the dose of analgesic depressants, such as morphine or meperidine, should be reduced by one-quarter to one-half.

Promethazine may lower seizure threshold. This should be taken into consideration when administering to persons with known seizure disorders or when giving in combination with narcotics or local anesthetics which may also affect seizure threshold.

Sedative drugs or CNS depressants should be avoided in patients with a history of sleep apnea. Antihistamines should be used with caution in patients with narrow-angle glaucoma, stenosing peptic ulcer, pyloroduodenal obstruction, and urinary bladder obstruction due to symptomatic prostatic hypertrophy and narrowing of the bladder neck.

Administration of promethazine has been associated with reported cholestatic jaundice.

PHENYLEPHRINE: Because phenlephrine is an adrenergic agent, it should be given with caution to patients with thyroid diseases, diabetes mellitus, and heart diseases or those receiving tricyclic antidepressants.

Men with symptomatic, benign prostatic hypertrophy can experience urinary retention when given oral nasal decongestants.

Phenylephrine can cause a decrease in cardiac output, and extreme caution should be used when administering the drug, parenterally or orally, to patients with arteriosclerosis, to elderly individuals, and/or to patients with initially poor cerebral or coronary circulation.

Phenylephrine should be used with caution in patients taking diet preparations, such as amphetamines or phenylpropanolamine, because synergistic adrenergic effects could result in serious hypertensive response and possible stroke.

Precautions: Animal reproduction studies have not been conducted with the drug combination—promethazine, phenylephrine, and codeine. It is not known whether this drug combination can cause fetal harm when administered to a pregnant woman or can affect reproduction capacity. Phenergan VC with codeine should be given to a pregnant woman only if clearly needed.

GENERAL

Narcotic analgesics, including codeine, should be administered with caution and the initial dose reduced in patients with acute abdominal conditions, convulsive disorders, significant hepatic or renal impairment, fever, hypothyroidism, Addison's disease, ulcerative colitis, prostatic hypertrophy, in patients with recent gastrointestinal or urinary tract surgery, and in the very young or elderly or debilitated patients.

Promethazine should be used cautiously in persons with cardiovascular disease or with impairment of liver function.

Phenylephrine should be used with caution in patients with cardiovascular disease, particularly hypertension.

INFORMATION FOR PATIENTS

Phenergan VC with codeine may cause marked drowsiness or impair the mental and/or physical abilities required for the performance of potentially hazardous tasks, such as driving a vehicle or operating machinery. Ambulatory patients should be told to avoid engaging in such activities until it is known that they do not become drowsy or dizzy from Phenergan VC with codeine therapy. Children should be supervised to avoid potential harm in bike riding or in other hazardous activities. The concomitant use of alcohol or other central nervous system depressants, including narcotic analgesics, sedatives, hypnotics, and tranquilizers, may have an additive effect and should be avoided or their dosage reduced.

Patients should be advised to report any involuntary muscle movements or unusual sensitivity to sunlight.

Codeine, like other narcotic analgesics, may produce orthostatic hypotension is some ambulatory patients. Patients should be cautioned accordingly.

DRUG INTERACTIONS

CODEINE: In patients receiving MAO inhibitors, an initial small test dose is advisable to allow observation of any excessive narcotic effects of MAOI interaction.

PROMETHAZINE: The sedative action of promethazine is additive to the effects of other central nervous system depressants, including alcohol, narcotic analgesics, sedatives, hypnotics, tricyclic antidepressants, and tranquilizers; therefore, these agents should be avoided or administered in reduced dosage to patients receiving promethazine.

[See table above].

DRUG/LABORATORY TEST INTERACTIONS

Because narcotic analgesics may increase biliary tract pressure, with resultant increases in plasma amylase or lipase levels, determination of these enzyme levels may be unreliable for 24 hours after a narcotic analgesic has been given.

The following laboratory tests may be affected in patients who are receiving therapy with promethazine hydrochloride:

Pregnancy Tests

Diagnostic pregnancy tests based on immunological reactions between HCG and anti-HCG may result in false-negative or false-positive interpretations.

Glucose Tolerance Test

An increase in blood glucose has been reported in patients receiving promethazine.

CARCINOGENESIS, MUTAGENESIS, IMPAIRMENT OF FERTILITY

CODEINE AND PROMETHAZINE

Long-term animal studies have not been performed to assess the carcinogenic potential of codeine or of promethazine, nor are there other animal or human data concerning carcinogenicity, mutagenicity, or impairment of fertility with these agents. Codeine has been reported to show no evidence of carcinogencity or mutagenicity in a variety of test systems, including the micronucleus and sperm abnormality assays and the *Salmonella* assay. Promethazine was nonmutagenic in the *Salmonella* test system of Ames.

PHENYLEPHRINE

A study which followed the development of cancer in 143,574 patients over a four-year period indicated that in 11,981 patients who received phenylephrine (systemic or topical), there was no statistically significant association between the drug and cancer at any or all sites.

Long-term animal studies have not been performed to assess the carcinogenic potential of phenylephrine, nor are there other animal or human data concerning mutagenicity.

A study of the effects of adrenergic drugs on ovum transport in rabbits indicated that treatment with phenylephrine did not alter incidence of pregnancy; the number of implantations was significantly reduced when high doses of the drug were used.

PREGNANCY

Teratogenic Effects—Pregnancy Category C

CODEINE: A study in rats and rabbits reported no teratogenic effect of codeine administered during the period of organogenesis in doses ranging from 5 to 120 mg/kg. In the rat, doses at the 120-mg/kg level, in the toxic range for the adult animal, were associated with an increase in embryo resorption at the time of implantation. In another study a single 100-mg/kg dose of codeine administered to pregnant mice reportedly resulted in delayed ossification in the offspring.

There are no studies in humans, and the significance of these findings to humans, if any, is not known.

PROMETHAZINE: Teratogenic effects have not been demonstrated in rat-feeding studies at doses of 6.25 and 12.5 mg/kg of promethazine. These doses are 8.3 and 16.7 times the maximum recommended total daily dose for a 50-kg subject. Specific studies to test the action of the drug on parturition, lactation, and development of the aimal neonate were not done, but a general preliminary study in rats indicated no effect on these parameters. Although antihistamines, including promethazine, have been found to produce fetal mortality in rodents, the pharmacological effects of histamine in the rodent do not parallel those in man. There are no adequate and well-controlled studies of promethazine in pregnant women.

PHENYLEPHRINE: A study in rabbits indicated that continued moderate overexposure to phenylephrine (3 mg/day) during the second half of pregnancy (22nd day of gestation to delivery) may contribute to perinatal wastage, prematurity, premature labor, and possibly fetal anomalies; when phenylephrine (3 mg/day) was given to rabbits during the first half of pregnancy (3rd day after mating for seven days), a significant number gave birth to litters of low birth weight. Another study showed that phenylephrine was associated with anomalies of aortic arch and with ventricular septal defect in the chick embryo.

Phenergan VC with codeine should be used during pregnancy only if the potential benefit justifies the potential risk to the fetus.

Nonteratogenic Effects

Dependence has been reported in newborns whose mothers took opiates regularly during pregnancy. Withdrawal signs include irritability, excessive crying, tremors, hyperreflexia, fever, vomiting, and diarrhea. Signs usually appear during the first few days of life.

Promethazine taken within two weeks of delivery may inhibit platelet aggregation in the newborn.

LABOR AND DELIVERY

Narcotic analgesics cross the placental barrier. The closer to delivery and the larger the dose used, the greater the possibility of respiratory depression in the newborn. Narcotic analgesics should be avoided during labor if delivery of a premature infant is anticipated. If the mother has received narcotic analgesics during labor, newborn infants should be observed closely for signs of respiratory depression. Resuscitation may be required (see

Continued on next page

PHENYLEPHRINE

Drug	Effect
Phenylephrine with prior administration of monoamine oxidase inhibitors (MAOI)	Cardiac pressor response potentiated. May cause acute hypertensive crisis.
Phenylephrine with tricyclic antidepressants.	Pressor response increased.
Phenylephrine with ergot alkaloids.	Excessive rise in blood pressure.
Phenylephrine with bronchodilator sympathomimetic agents and with epinephrine or other sympathomimetics.	Tachycardia or other arrhythmias may occur.
Phenylephrine with prior administration of propranolol or other β-adrenergic blockers.	Cardiostimulating effects blocked.
Phenylephrine with atropine sulfate.	Reflex bradycardia blocked; pressor response enhanced.
Phenylephrine with prior administration of phentolamine or other α-adrenergic blockers.	Pressor response decreased.
Phenylephrine with diet preparations, such as amphetamines or phenylpropanolamine.	Synergistic adrenergic response.

Wyeth—Cont.

"Overdosage"). The effect of codeine, if any, on the later growth, development, and functional maturation of the child is unknown.

Administration of phenylephrine to patients in late pregnancy or labor may cause fetal anoxia or bradycardia by increasing contractility of the uterus and decreasing uterine blood flow.

See also "Nonteratogenic Effects."

NURSING MOTHERS

Some studies, but not others, have reported detectable amounts of codeine in breast milk. The levels are probably not clinically significant after usual therapeutic dosage. The possibility of clinically important amounts being excreted in breast milk in individuals abusing codeine should be considered.

It is not known whether either phenylephrine or promethazine is excreted in human milk.

Caution should be exercised when Phenergan VC with codeine is administered to a nursing woman.

PEDIATRIC USE

This product should not be used in children under 2 years of age because safety for such use has not been established.

Adverse Reactions:
CODEINE

Nervous System—CNS depression, particularly respiratory depression, and to a lesser extent circulatory depression; light-headedness, dizziness, sedation, euphoria, dysphoria, headache, transient hallucination, disorientation, visual disturbances, and convulsions.

Cardiovascular—Tachycardia, bradycardia, palpitation, faintness, syncope, orthostatic hypotension (common to narcotic analgesics).

Gastrointestinal—Nausea, vomiting, constipation, and biliary tract spasm. Patients with chronic ulcerative colitis may experience increased colonic motility; in patients with acute ulcerative colitis, toxic dilation has been reported.

Genitourinary—Oliguria, urinary retention; antidiuretic effect has been reported (common to narcotic analgesics).

Allergic—Infrequent pruritus, giant urticaria, angioneurotic edema, and laryngeal edema.

Other—Flushing of the face, sweating and pruritus (due to opiate-induced histamine release); weakness.

PROMETHAZINE

Nervous System—Sedation, sleepiness, occasional blurred vision, dryness of mouth, dizziness; rarely confusion, disorientation, and extrapyramidal symptoms such as oculogyric crisis, torticollis, and tongue protrusion (usually in association with parenteral injection or excessive dosage).

Cardiovascular—Increased or decreased blood pressure.

Dermatologic—Rash, rarely photosensitivity.

Hematologic—Rarely leukopenia, thrombocytopenia; agranulocytosis (1 case).

Gastrointestinal—Nausea and vomiting.

PHENYLEPHRINE

Nervous System—Restlessness, anxiety, nervousness, and dizziness.

Cardiovascular—Hypertension (see "Warnings").

Other—Precordial pain, respiratory distress, tremor, and weakness.

Drug Abuse and Dependence:
CONTROLLED SUBSTANCE

Phenergan VC with codeine is a Schedule V Controlled Substance.

ABUSE

Codeine is known to be subject to abuse; however, the abuse potential of oral codeine appears to be quite low. Even parenteral codeine does not appear to offer the psychic effects sought by addicts to the same degree as heroin or morphine. However, codeine must be administered only under close supervision to patients with a history of drug abuse or dependence.

DEPENDENCE

Psychological dependence, physical dependence, and tolerance are known to occur with codeine.

Overdosage: CODEINE: Serious overdose with codeine is characterized by respiratory depression (a decrease in respiratory rate and/or tidal volume, Cheyne-Stokes respiration, cyanosis), extreme somnolence progressing to stupor or coma, skeletal muscle flaccidity, cold and clammy skin, and sometimes bradycardia and hypotension. The triad of coma, pinpoint pupils, and respiratory depression is strongly suggestive of opiate poisoning. In severe overdosage, particularly by the intravenous route, apnea, circulatory collapse, cardiac arrest, and death may occur. Promethazine is additive to the depressant effects of codeine.

It is difficult to determine what constitutes a standard toxic or lethal dose. However, the lethal oral dose of codeine in an adult is reported to be in the range of 0.5 to 1.0 gram. Infants and children are believed to be relatively more sensitive to opiates on a body-weight basis. Elderly patients are also comparatively intolerant to opiates.

PROMETHAZINE: Signs and symptoms of overdosage with promethazine range from mild depression of the central nervous system and cariovascular system to profound hypotension, respiratory depression, and unconsciousness.

Stimulation may be evident, especially in children and geriatric patients. Convulsions may rarely occur. A paradoxical reaction has been reported in children receiving single doses of 75 mg to 125 mg orally, characterized by hyperexcitability and nightmares.

Atropine-like signs and symptoms—dry mouth, fixed, dilated pupils, flushing, as well as gastrointestinal symptoms, may occur.

PHENYLEPHRINE: Signs and symptoms of overdosage with phenylephrine include hypertension, headache, convulsions, cerebral hemorrhage, and vomiting. Ventricular premature beats and short paroxysms of ventricular tachycardia may also occur. Headache may be a symptom of hypertension. Bradycardia may also be seen early in phenylephrine overdosage through stimulation of baroreceptors.

TREATMENT

Treatment of overdosage with Phenergan VC with codeine is essentially symptomatic and supportive. Only in cases of extreme overdosage or individual sensitivity do vital signs including respiration, pulse, blood pressure, temperature, and EKG need to be monitored. Activated charcoal orally or by lavage may be given, or sodium or magnesium sulfate orally as a cathartic. Attention should be given to the reestablishment of adequate respiratory exchange through provision of a patent airway and institution of assisted or controlled ventilation. The narcotic antagonist, naloxone hydrochloride, may be administered when significant respiratory depression occurs with Phenergan VC with codeine; any depressant effects of promethazine are not reversed by naloxone. Diazepam may be used to control convulsions. Avoid analeptics, which may cause convulsions. Acidosis and electrolyte losses should be corrected. A rise in temperature of pulmonary complications may signal the need for institution of antibiotic therapy.

Severe hypotension usually responds to the administration of norepinephrine or phenylephrine. EPINEPHRINE SHOULD NOT BE USED, since its use in a patient with partial adrenergic blockade may further lower the blood pressure.

Limited experience with dialysis indicates that is not helpful.

Dosage and Administration: The average effective dose is given in the following table:
[See table below].

How Supplied: Phenergan ® VC with codeine, Wyeth®, is a clear, reddish-orange solution supplied as follows:

NDC 0008-0552-02, case of 24 bottles of 4 fl. oz.
NDC 0008-0552-06, case of 16 bottles of 6 fl. oz.
NDC 0008-0552-08, case of 12 bottles of 8 fl. oz.
NDC 0008-0552-03, bottle of 1 pint.
NDC 0008-0552-04, bottle of 1 gallon.

Keep bottles tightly closed below 25°C (77°F).
Protect from light.
Dispense in light-resistance, glass, tight containers.

SMA®
[ess-em-ay]
Iron fortified
infant formula
READY-TO-FEED
CONCENTRATED LIQUID
POWDER

Breast milk is the preferred feeding for newborns. Infant formula is intended to replace or supplement breast milk when breast feeding is not possible or is insufficient, or when mothers elect not to breast feed.

Good maternal nutrition is important for the preparation and maintenance of breast feeding. Extensive or prolonged use of partial bottle feeding, before breast feeding has been well established, could make breast feeding difficult to maintain. A decision not to breast feed could be difficult to reverse.

Professional advice should be followed on all matters of infant feeding. Infant formula should always be prepared and used as directed. Unnecessary or improper use of infant formula could present a health hazard. Social and financial implications should be considered when selecting the method of infant feeding.

SMA® is unique among prepared formulas for its fat blend, whey-dominated protein composition, amino acid pattern and mineral content.

SMA®, utilizing a hybridized safflower (oleic) oil, became the first infant formula offering fat and calcium absorption equal to that of human milk, with a physiologic level of linoleic acid. Thus, the fat blend in SMA® provides a ready source of energy, helps protect infants against neonatal tetany and produces a ratio of Vitamin E to polyunsaturated fatty acids (linoleic acid) more than adequate to prevent hemolytic anemia.

By combining reduced minerals whey with skimmed cow's milk, SMA® adjusts the protein content to within the range of human milk, reverses the whey-protein to casein ratio of cow's milk so that it is like that of human milk, and reduces the mineral content to a physiologic level. The resultant 60:40 whey-protein to casein ratio provides protein nutrition superior to a casein-dominated formula. In addition, the essential amino acids, including cystine, are present in amounts close to those of human milk. So the protein in SMA® is of high biologic value.

The physiologic mineral content makes possible a low renal solute load which helps protect the functionally immature infant kidney, increases expendable water reserves and helps protect against dehydration.

Adults	1 teaspoon (5 ml) every 4 to 6 hours,	not to exceed 30.0 ml in 24 hours.
Children 6 years to under 12 years	½ to 1 teaspoon (2.5 to 5 ml) every 4 to 6 hours,	not to exceed 30.0 ml in 24 hours.
Children under 6 years (weight: 18 kg or 40 lbs)	¼ to ½ teaspoon (1.25 to 2.5 ml) every 4 to 6 hours,	not to exceed 9.0 ml in 24 hours.
Children under 6 years (weight: 16 kg or 35 lbs)	¼ to ½ teaspoon (1.25 to 2.5 ml) every 4 to 6 hours,	not to exceed 8.0 ml in 24 hours.
Children under 6 years (weight: 14 kg or 30 lbs)	¼ to ½ teaspoon (1.25 to 2.5 ml) every 4 to 6 hours,	not to exceed 7.0 ml in 24 hours.
Children under 6 years (weight: 12 kg or 25 lbs)	¼ to ½ teaspoon (1.25 to 2.5 ml) every 4 to 6 hours,	not to exceed 6.0 ml in 24 hours.

Phenergan VC with codeine is not recommended for children under 2 years of age.

Use of lactose as the carbohydrate results in a physiologic stool flora and a low stool pH, decreasing the incidence of perianal dermatitis.

Ingredients: SMA® Concentrated Liquid or Ready-to-Feed. Water; nonfat milk; reduced minerals whey; lactose; oleo, coconut, oleic (safflower), and soybean oils; soy lecithin; calcium carrageenan. *Minerals:* Potassium bicarbonate; calcium chloride and citrate; potassium chloride; sodium citrate; ferrous sulfate; sodium bicarbonate; zinc, cupric, and manganese sulfates. *Vitamins:* Ascorbic acid, alpha tocopheryl acetate, niacinamide, vitamin A palmitate, calcium pantothenate, thiamine hydrochloride, riboflavin, pyridoxine hydrochloride, beta-carotene, folic acid, phytonadione, activated 7-dehydrocholesterol, biotin, cyanocobalamin.

SMA® Powder. Nonfat milk; reduced minerals whey; lactose; oleo, coconut, oleic (safflower), and soybean oils; soy lecithin.
Minerals: Calcium chloride; sodium bicarbonate; calcium hydroxide; ferrous sulfate; potassium hydroxide and bicarbonate; potassium chloride; zinc, cupric, and manganese sulfates.
Vitamins: Ascorbic acid, alpha tocopheryl acetate, niacinamide, vitamin A palmitate, calcium pantothenate, thiamine hydrochloride, riboflavin, pyridoxine hydrochloride, beta-carotene, folic acid, phytonadione, activated 7-dehydrocholesterol, biotin, cyanocobalamin.

PROXIMATE ANALYSIS
at 20 calories per fluidounce
READY-TO-FEED, POWDER, and CONCENTRATED LIQUID:

	(w/v)
Fat	3.6%
Carbohydrate	7.2%
Protein	1.5%
60% Lactalbumin (whey protein)	0.9%
40% Casein	0.6%
Ash	0.25%
Crude Fiber	None
Total Solids	12.6%
Calories/fl. oz.	20

Vitamins, Minerals: In normal dilution, each quart contains 2500 IU vitamin A, 400 IU vitamin D_3, 9 IU vitamin E, 55 mcg vitamin K_1, 0.67 mg vitamin B_1 (thiamine), 1 mg vitamin B_2 (riboflavin), 55 mg vitamin C (ascorbic acid), 0.4 mg vitamin B_6 (pyridoxine hydrochloride), 1 mcg vitamin B_{12}, 9.5 mg equivalents niacin, 2 mg pantothenic acid, 50 mcg folic acid, 14 mcg biotin, 100 mg choline, 420 mg calcium, 312 mg phosphorus, 50 mg magnesium, 142 mg sodium, 530 mg potassium, 355 mg chloride, 12 mg iron, 0.45 mg copper, 3.5 mg zinc, 150 mcg manganese, 65 mcg iodine.

Preparation: *Ready-to-Feed* (8 and 32 fl. oz. cans of 20 calories per fluidounce formula)— shake can, open and pour into previously sterilized nursing bottle; attach nipple and feed. Cover opened can and immediately store in refrigerator. Use contents of can within 48 hours of opening.
Powder—(1 pound can)—For normal dilution supplying 20 calories per fluidounce, use 1 scoop (or 1 standard tablespoonful) of powder, packed and leveled, to 2 fluidounces of cooled, previously boiled water. For larger amount of formula, use ¼ standard measuring cup of powder, packed and leveled, to 8 fluidounces (1 cup) of water. Three of these portions make 26 fluidounces of formula.
Concentrated Liquid—For normal dilution supplying 20 calories per fluidounce, use equal amounts of SMA® liquid and cooled, previously boiled water.
Note: Prepared formula should be used within 24 hours.
How Supplied: *Ready-to-Feed*—presterilized and premixed, 32 fluidounce (1 quart) cans, cases of 6; 8 fluidounce cans, cases of 24 (4 carriers of 6 cans). *Powder*—1 pound cans with measuring scoop, cases of 12. *Concentrated Liquid*— 13 fluidounce cans, cases of 24.
For Hospital Nursery Use—an infant feeding system which provides premixed, presterilized, ready-to-feed items, thus saving space, time and equipment. It eliminates washing, measuring, mixing, sterilizing, refrigerating and heating.

The system is offered in a choice of two forms:
1. Prefilled and presterilized 4 oz. glass bottles for which sterile nipple assemblies are available, to be attached before feeding. These units may be used again after resterilizing or may be discarded, as desired.
2. The E-Z NURSER® (single unit nurser), also prefilled and presterilized, consists of a 4 oz. glass bottle with sterile nipple already attached; the entire unit is designed to be discarded after use.

The following items are supplied in both the forms described above:

SMA® Ready-to-Feed
13 calories/oz.	48 bottles of 4 fl. oz.
20 calories/oz.	48 bottles of 4 fl. oz.
24 calories/oz.	48 bottles of 4 fl. oz.
27 calories/oz.	48 bottles of 4 fl. oz.

SMA® lo-iron Ready-to-Feed
13 calories/oz.	48 bottles of 4 fl. oz.
20 calories/oz.	48 bottles of 4 fl. oz.
24 calories/oz.	48 bottles of 4 fl. oz.

"preemie" SMA® Ready-to-Feed
24 calories/oz.	48 bottles of 4 fl. oz.

(Not available in the E-Z NURSER®)
Distilled Water	48 bottles of 4 fl. oz.
Glucose, 5% in Distilled Water, 6 calories/oz.	48 bottles of 4 fl. oz.
Glucose, 10% in Distilled Water, 12 calories/oz.	48 bottles of 4 fl. oz.

NURSOY® (soy protein formula)
20 calories/oz.	48 bottles of 4 fl. oz.

(Not available in the E-Z NURSER®)
Supplied in 8 oz. bottles, to which sterile nipple assemblies must be attached before feeding, are the following:

SMA® Ready-to-Feed
20 calories/oz.	24 bottles of 8 fl. oz.
Oral Electrolyte Solution	24 bottles of 8 fl. oz.
Distilled Water	24 bottles of 8 fl. oz.

NIPPLE ASSEMBLIES—presterilized, for both premature and term infants, single-hole and cross-cut, suitable for use with all ready-to-feed products requiring them, cartons of 288 nipple units. Single-hole, cross cut and orthodontic nipples.
ACCUFEED™, Wyeth Graduated Nursers—presterilized, disposable nursers (60 ml capacity) for accurately measured feedings, packages of 200.
Also Available: SMA® lo-iron. For those who appreciate the particular advantages of SMA®, the infant formula closest in composition nutritionally to mother's milk, but who sometimes need or wish to recommend a formula that does not contain a high level of iron, now there is SMA® lo-iron with all the benefits of regular SMA® but with a reduced level of iron of 1.4 mg per quart. Infants should receive supplemental dietary iron from an outside source to meet daily requirements.
Concentrated Liquid, 13 fl. oz. cans, cases of 24. Powder, 1 pound cans with measuring scoop, cases of 12. Ready-to-Feed, 32 fl. oz. cans, cases of 6.
Preparation of the standard 20 calories per fluidounce formula of SMA® lo-iron is the same as SMA® iron fortified given above.

SERAX®
[ser′aks]
(oxazepam)
CAPSULES • TABLETS

Description: A therapeutic agent providing versatility and flexibility in control of common emotional disturbances, this product exerts prompt action in a wide variety of disorders associated with anxiety, tension, agitation and irritability, and anxiety associated with depression. In tolerance and toxicity studies on several animal species, this product reveals significantly greater safety factors than related compounds (chlordiazepoxide and diazepam) and manifests a wide separation of effective doses and doses inducing side effects.
Serax is 7 chloro-1,3-dihydro-3-hydroxy-5- phenyl-2H-1,4-benzodiazepin-2-one, a white crystalline powder with a molecular weight of 286.7.
Animal Pharmacology and Toxicology: In mice, SERAX exerts an anticonvulsant (anti-Metrazol®) activity at 50 percent effective doses of about 0.6 mg/kg orally. (Such anticonvulsant activity of benzodiazepines correlates with their tranquilizing properties.) To produce ataxia (rotabar test) and sedation (abolition of spontaneous motor activity), the 50 percent effective doses of this product are greater than 5 mg/kg orally. Thus about ten times the therapeutic (anticonvulsant) dose must be given before ataxia ensues, indicating a wide separation of effective doses and doses inducing side effects.
In evaluation of antianxiety activity of compounds, conflict behavioral tests in rats differentiate continuous response for food in the presence of anxiety-provoking stress (shock) from drug-induced motor incoordination. This product shows significant separation of doses required to relieve anxiety and doses producing sedation or ataxia. Ataxia-producing doses exceed those of related CNS-acting drugs.
Acute oral LD_{50} in mice is greater than 5000 mg/kg, compared to 800 mg/kg for a related compound (chlordiazepoxide).
Subacute toxicity studies in dogs for four weeks at 480 mg/kg daily showed no specific changes; at 960 mg/kg two out of eight died with evidence of circulatory collapse. This wide margin of safety is significant compared to chlordiazepoxide HCl, which showed nonspecific changes in six dogs at 80 mg/kg. On chlordiazepoxide, two out of six died with evidence of circulatory collapse at 127 mg/kg, and six out of six died at 200 mg/kg daily. Chronic toxicity studies of Serax in dogs at 120 mg/kg/day for 52 weeks produced no toxic manifestation.
Fatty metamorphosis of the liver has been noted in six-week toxicity studies in rats given this product at 0.5% of the diet. Such accumulations of fat are considered reversible as there is no liver necrosis or fibrosis.
Breeding studies in rats through two successive litters did not produce fetal abnormality.
This product has a single major metabolite in man, a glucuronide excreted in the urine.
Indications: SERAX (oxazepam) is indicated for the management of anxiety disorders or for the short-term relief of the symptoms of anxiety. Anxiety or tension associated with the stress of everyday life usually does not require treatment with an anxiolytic.
Anxiety associated with depression is also responsive to SERAX (oxazepam) therapy.
This product has been found particularly useful in the management of anxiety, tension, agitation and irritability in older patients.
Alcoholics with acute tremulousness, inebriation, or with anxiety associated with alcohol withdrawal are responsive to therapy.
The effectiveness of SERAX in long-term use, that is, more than 4 months, has not been assessed by systematic clinical studies. The physician should reassess periodically the usefulness of the drug for the individual patient.
Contraindications: History of previous hypersensitivity reaction to oxazepam. Oxazepam is not indicated in psychoses.
Warnings: As with other CNS-acting drugs, patients should be cautioned against driving automobiles or operating dangerous machinery until it is known that they do not become drowsy or dizzy on oxazepam therapy.
Patients should be warned that the effects of alcohol or other CNS-depressant drugs may be additive to those of Serax, possibly requiring adjustment of dosage or elimination of such agents.

USE IN PREGNANCY
An increased risk of congenital malformations associated with the use of minor tranquilizers (chlordiazepoxide, diazepam, and meprobamate) during the first trimester of pregnancy has been suggested in several studies. Serax, a benzodiazepine derivative, has not been studied adequately to determine whether it, too, may be associated with an increased risk of fetal abnormality. Because use of these drugs is rarely a matter of urgency, their use during this period should almost always be avoided. The possibility that a woman of

Continued on next page

Wyeth—Cont.

childbearing potential may be pregnant at the time of institution of therapy should be considered. Patients should be advised that if they become pregnant during therapy or intend to become pregnant they should communicate with their physician about the desirability of discontinuing the drug.

Precautions: Although hypotension has occurred only rarely, oxazepam should be administered with caution to patients in whom a drop in blood pressure might lead to cardiac complications. This is particularly true in the elderly patient.

In some patients exhibiting drug dependency through chronic overdose with SERAX (oxazepam) withdrawal symptoms have been noted on discontinuance of drug administration. Withdrawal symptoms have also been reported following abrupt discontinuance of benzodiazepines taken continuously at therapeutic levels for several months. Careful supervision of dose and amounts prescribed for patients is advised, especially with those patients with a known propensity for taking excessive quantities of drugs. Excessive and prolonged use in susceptible persons, for example, alcoholics, former addicts, and others, may result in dependence on or habituation to the drug. Where excessive dosage is continued for weeks or months, dosage should be reduced gradually rather than abruptly stopped. Abrupt discontinuance of doses in excess of the recommended dose may result in some cases in the occurrence of epileptiform seizures. Withdrawal symptoms following abrupt discontinuance are similar to those seen with barbiturates.

SERAX 15 mg tablets, *but none of the other available dosage forms of this product,* contain FD&C Yellow No. 5 (tartrazine) which may cause allergic-type reactions (including bronchial asthma) in certain susceptible individuals. Although the overall incidence of FD&C Yellow No. 5 (tartrazine) sensitivity in the general population is low, it is frequently seen in patients who also have aspirin hypersensitivity.

Adverse Reactions: The necessity for discontinuation of therapy due to undesirable effects has been rare. Transient mild drowsiness is commonly seen in the first few days of therapy. If it persists, the dosage should be reduced. In few instances, dizziness, vertigo, headache and rarely syncope have occurred either alone or together with drowsiness. Mild paradoxical reactions, i.e., excitement, stimulation of affect, have been reported in psychiatric patients; these reactions may be secondary to relief of anxiety and usually appear in the first two weeks of therapy.

Other side effects occurring during oxazepam therapy include rare instances of minor diffuse skin rashes—morbilliform, urticarial and maculopapular—nausea, lethargy, edema, slurred speech, tremor and altered libido. Such side effects have been infrequent and are generally controlled with reduction of dosage.

Although rare, leukopenia and hepatic dysfunction including jaundice have been reported during therapy. Periodic blood counts and liver-function tests are advisable.

Ataxia with oxazepam has been reported in rare instances and does not appear to be specifically related to dose or age.

Although the following side reactions have not as yet been reported with oxazepam, they have occurred with related compounds (chlordiazepoxide and diazepam): paradoxical excitation with severe rage reactions, hallucinations, menstrual irregularities, change in EEG pattern, blood dyscrasias including agranulocytosis, blurred vision, diplopia, incontinence, stupor, disorientation, fever and euphoria.

Transient amnesia or memory impairment has been reported in association with the use of benzodiazepines.

Dosage and Administration: Because of the flexibility of this product and the range of emotional disturbances responsive to it, dosage should be individualized for maximum beneficial effects. [See table below].

This product is not indicated in children under 6 years of age. Absolute dosage for children 6–12 years of age is not established.

How Supplied: Serax® (oxazepam) Capsules and Tablets, Wyeth® are available in the following dosage strengths:

10 mg, NDC 0008-0051, white and pink capsule banded with Wyeth logo and marked "SERAX", "10", and "51", in bottles of 100 and 500 capsules and in Redipak® Strip Pack in cartons of 25 capsules.

15 mg, NDC 0008-0006, white and red capsule banded with Wyeth logo and marked "SERAX", "15", and "6", in bottles of 100 and 500 capsules, in Redipak® Strip Pack in cartons of 25 capsules, and in Redipak® individually wrapped capsules in cartons of 100.

30 mg, NDC 0008-0052, white and maroon capsule banded with Wyeth logo and marked "SERAX", "30", and "52", in bottles of 100 and 500 capsules, in Redipak® Strip Pack in cartons of 25 capsules, and in Redipak® individually wrapped capsules in cartons of 100.

15 mg, NDC 0008-0317, yellow, five-sided tablet with a raised "S" and a "15" on one side and "WYETH" and "317" on reverse side, in bottles of 100 tablets.

The appearance of SERAX capsules and tablets is a trademark of Wyeth Laboratories.

Keep bottles tightly closed.
Dispense in tight containers.

Shown in Product Identification Section, page 445

SIMECO®   OTC
[sim'e-ko]
(aluminum hydroxide gel, magnesium hydroxide, simethicone)
SUSPENSION

Composition: Each teaspoonful (5 ml) contains aluminum hydroxide gel equivalent to 365 mg of dried gel, USP, 300 mg of magnesium hydroxide and 30 mg of simethicone. Sodium content is 0.3 mEq-0.6 mEq per teaspoonful. High potency and low dose are provided by high concentration of antacid per teaspoonful.

Indications: For the symptomatic relief of hyperacidity associated with the diagnosis of peptic ulcer, gastritis, peptic esophagitis, gastric hyperacidity and hiatal hernia. To relieve the symptoms of gas.

Dosage and Administration: Usually: 1 or 2 teaspoonfuls undiluted or with a little water to be taken 3 or 4 times daily between meals and at bedtime. 5 ml SIMECO suspension neutralizes 22 mEq of acid.

Warnings: Patients are advised not to take more than 8 teaspoonfuls (40 ml) in a 24-hour period or use the maximum dosage for more than two weeks except under the advice and supervision of a physician. Not to be used except under the advice and supervision of a physician if patient has kidney disease.

Drug Interaction Precautions: Alumina-containing antacids should not be used concomitantly with any form of tetracycline therapy.

How Supplied: Suspension—Cool mint flavor available in 12 fl. oz. plastic bottles.

TUBEX® Closed Injection System
[tū' beks]

The TUBEX® closed injection system delivers injectable medication in accurately machine-measured doses with each sterile, prefilled cartridge-needle unit permanently identified up to the moment of injection. Precisely calibrated single-use cartridge-needle units eliminate cross contamination and minimize dosage errors. Super-sharp, siliconized needles minimize penetration pressure. Medication is easily delivered via the sturdy, stainless TUBEX® hypodermic syringe.

TUBEX sterile cartridge-needle units are ready for instant use, fit easily into the physician's bag, and are readily stored and inventoried in the office.

TAMP-R-TEL® (tamper resistant package) — a clear, sturdy plastic package for all TUBEX narcotics and barbiturates — adds a new dimension to the handling and record keeping of these controlled drugs. In TAMP-R-TEL, each TUBEX® sterile cartridge-needle unit is locked into an individual slot within the package by its own end-lock tab, which is easily broken to release the unit for use. Once the end-lock tab is broken, it is almost impossible to replace it. TAMP-R-TEL thus enhances package integrity, discourages pilferage and facilitates "at a glance" drug count.

The following products are currently available in TUBEX® closed injection system. *For prescribing information on products listed write to Professional Service, Wyeth Laboratories, P.O. Box 8299, Philadelphia, PA, 19101, or contact your local Wyeth representative.*

Product and Needle Size Units Per Pkg	NDC 0008-
NARCOTICS in TAMP-R-TEL® (tamper resistant package)	
CODEINE PHOSPHATE, USP@●	
30 mg (½ gr.) (25 G × ⅝") 10—1 ml	0608-01
60 mg (1 gr.) (25 G × ⅝") 10—1 ml	0609-01
HYDROMORPHONE HYDROCHLORIDE, USP @●	
1 mg (1/60 gr.) (25 G × ⅝") 10—1 ml fill in 2 ml	0387-01
1 mg (1/60 gr.) (22 G × 1¼") 10—1 ml fill in 2 ml	0387-03
2 mg (1/30 gr.) (25 G × ⅝") 10—1 ml fill in 2 ml	0295-02
2 mg (1/30 gr.) (22 G × 1¼") 10—1 ml fill in 2 ml	0295-01
3 mg (1/20 gr.) (25 G × ⅝") 10—1 ml fill in 2 ml	0388-01
4 mg (1/15 gr.) (25 G × ⅝") 10—1 ml fill in 2 ml	0296-02

SERAX (oxazepam)

	Usual Dose
Mild-to moderate-anxiety, with associated tension, irritability, agitation or related symptoms of functional origin or secondary to organic disease.	10 to 15 mg, 3 or 4 times daily
Severe anxiety syndromes, agitation, or anxiety associated with depression.	15 to 30 mg, 3 or 4 times daily
Older patients with anxiety, tension, irritability and agitation.	Initial dosage: 10 mg, 3 times daily. If necessary, increase cautiously to 15 mg, 3 or 4 times daily
Alcoholics with acute inebriation, tremulousness, or anxiety on withdrawal.	15 to 30 mg, 3 or 4 times daily

for possible revisions · Product Information · 2289

4 mg (1/15 gr.) (22 G × 1¼″)
10—1 ml fill in 2 ml — 0296-01

MEPERGAN® (Meperidine HCl and Promethazine HCl) 25 mg each/ml ⓒ●
(22 G × 1¼″)
10—2 ml — 0235-01

MEPERIDINE HYDROCHLORIDE, USP ⓒ●
25 mg (25 G × ⅝″)
10—1 ml fill in 2 ml — 0601-03

25 mg (22 G × 1¼″)
10—1 ml fill in 2 ml — 0601-02

50 mg (25 G × ⅝″)
10—1 ml fill in 2 ml — 0602-03

50 mg (22 G × 1¼″)
10—1 ml fill in 2 ml — 0602-02

75 mg (25 G × ⅝″)
10—1 ml fill in 2 ml — 0605-03

75 mg (22 G × 1¼″)
10—1 ml fill in 2 ml — 0605-02

100 mg (25 G × ⅝″)
10—1 ml fill in 2 ml — 0613-03

100 mg (22 G × 1¼″)
10—1 ml fill in 2 ml — 0613-02

MORPHINE SULFATE, USP ⓒ●
2 mg (1/30 gr.) (25 G × ⅝″)
10—1 ml — 0649-01

4 mg (1/15 gr.) (25 G × ⅝″)
10—1 ml — 0653-01

8 mg (1/8 gr.) (25 G × ⅝″)
10—1 ml — 0655-02

8 mg (1/8 gr.) (25 G × ⅝″)
10—1 ml fill in 2 ml — 0655-01

8 mg (1/8 gr.) (22 G × 1¼″)
10—1 ml fill in 2 ml — 0655-03

10 mg (1/6 gr.) (25 G × ⅝″)
10—1 ml — 0656-03

10 mg (1/6 gr.) (25 G × ⅝″)
10—1 ml fill in 2 ml — 0656-02

10 mg (1/6 gr.) (22 G × 1¼″)
10—1 ml fill in 2 ml — 0656-01

15 mg (¼ gr.) (25 G × ⅝″)
10—1 ml — 0657-03

15 mg (¼ gr.) (25 G × ⅝″)
10—1 ml fill in 2 ml — 0657-02

15 mg (¼ gr.) (22 G × 1¼″)
10—1 ml fill in 2 ml — 0657-01

BARBITURATES in TAMP-R-TEL®
PENTOBARBITAL SODIUM, USP ⓒ●
50 mg (¾ gr.) (22 G × 1¼″)
10—1 ml — 0303-01

100 mg (1½ gr.) (22 G × 1¼″)
10—2 ml — 0303-02

PHENOBARBITAL SODIUM, USP ⓒ
30 mg (½ gr.) (22 G × 1¼″)
10—1 ml — 0499-01

60 mg (1 gr.) (22 G × 1¼″)
10—1 ml — 0457-01

130 mg (2 gr.) (22 G × 1¼″)
10—1 ml — 0304-01

SECOBARBITAL SODIUM, USP ⓒ●
50 mg (¾ gr.) (22 G × 1¼″)

10—1 ml — 0305-01

100 mg (1½ gr.) (22 G × 1¼″)
10—2 ml — 0305-02

● Narcotic order blank required.

ANTIBIOTICS
BICILLIN® C-R (Penicillin G Benzathine and Penicillin G Procaine Suspension) 300,000 U each/ml
600,000 U (20 G × 1¼″)
10—1 ml — 0026-17

600,000 U (20 G × 1¼″)
50—1 ml — 0026-13

600,000 U (20 G × 1″)
10—1 ml — 0026-18

1,200,000 U (20 G × 1¼″)
10—2 ml — 0026-16

1,200,000 U (20 G × 1¼″)
50—2 ml — 0026-14

1,200,00 U (20 G × 1″)
10—2 ml — 0026-19

1,200,000 U (20 G × 1¼″)
10—2 ml — 0026-21
(disposable syringe)

2,400,000 U (18 G × 2″)
10—4 ml — 0026-22
(disposable syringe)

BiCILLIN C-R 900/300
(900,000 units Penicillin G Benzathine and 300,000 units Penicillin G Procaine in suspension)
1,200,000 U (20 G × 1¼″)
10—2 ml — 0079-01

BICILLIN LONG-ACTING (Sterile Penicillin G Benzathine Suspension)
600,000 U (20 G × 1¼″)
10—1 ml — 0021-08

900,000 U (20 G × 1¼″)
10—1.5 ml fill in 2 ml — 0021-13

1,200,000 U (20 G × 1¼″)
10—2 ml — 0021-07

1,200,000 U (20 G × 1¼″)
10—2 ml — 0021-11
(disposable syringe)

2,400,000 U (18 G × 2″)
10—4 ml — 0021-12
(disposable syringe)

WYCILLIN® (Sterile Penicillin G Procaine Suspension)
600,000 U (20 G × 1¼″)
10—1 ml — 0018-10

600,000 U (20 G × 1¼″)
50—1 ml — 0018-07

1,200,000 U (20 G × 1¼″)
10—2 ml — 0018-08

2,400,000 U (18 G × 2″)
10—4 ml — 0018-12
(disposable syringe)

WYCILLIN Injection and PROBENECID Tablets
(Sterile Penicillin G Procaine Suspension and Probenecid Tablets)
2,400,000 U (18 G × 2″)
2—4 ml — 2517-01
(package contains two disposable syringes and two 0.5 gram Probenecid tablets)

BIOLOGICALS
DIPHTHERIA and TETANUS TOXOIDS ADSORBED (PEDIATRIC)

(25 G × ⅝″)
10—0.5 ml — 0338-01

IMMUNE SERUM GLOBULIN (HUMAN), USP
(20 G × 1¼″)
1—2 ml — 0437-02

INFLUENZA VIRUS VACCINE
(purified subvirion)
1984-1985 Formula
(25 G × ⅝″)
10—0.5 ml

TETANUS and DIPHTHERIA TOXOIDS ADSORBED (ADULT)
(25 G × ⅝″)
10—0.5 ml — 0341-01

TETANUS IMMUNE GLOBULIN (HUMAN)
250 U (20 G × 1¼″)
10—1 ml — 0408-03

TETANUS TOXOID ADSORBED
(25 G × ⅝″)
10—0.5 ml — 0339-01

TETANUS TOXOID FLUID
(25 G × ⅝″)
10—0.5 ml — 0340-01

VITAMINS
CYANOCOBALAMIN, USP
100 mcg (22 G × 1¼″)
10—1 ml — 0265-01

1,000 mcg (25 G × ⅝″)
10—1 ml — 0264-03

1,000 mcg (22 G × 1¼″)
10—1 ml — 0264-01

1,000 mcg (22 G × 1¼″)
10—1 ml fill in 2 ml — 0264-02

THIAMINE HYDROCHLORIDE, USP
100 mg (22 G × 1¼″)
10—1 ml fill in 2 ml — 0302-01

CARDIOVASCULAR AGENTS
DIGOXIN, USP
0.25 mg (22 G × 1¼″)
10—1 ml — 0480-02

0.5 mg (22 G × 1¼″)
10—2 ml — 0480-01

EPINEPHRINE, USP (1:1000)
(25 G × ⅝″)
10—1 ml — 0263-01

FUROSEMIDE, USP
20 mg (22 G × 1¼″)
10—2 ml — 0628-04

HEPARIN SODIUM, USP
1,000 USP units (22 G × 1¼″)
10—1 ml — 0275-01

2,500 USP units (25 G × ⅝″)
50—2.5 ml — 0275-02

2,500 USP units (25 G × ⅝″)
10—1 ml — 0482-01

5,000 USP units (25 G × ⅝″)
10—0.5 ml — 0277-02

5,000 USP units (25 G × ⅝″)
10—1 ml — 0278-02

5,000 USP units (22 G × 1¼″)
10—1 ml — 0278-01

7,500 USP units (25 G × ⅝″)
10—1 ml — 0293-01

Continued on next page

Wyeth—Cont.

10,000 USP units (25 G × ⅝") 10—1 ml	0277-01
15,000 USP units (25 G × ⅝") 10—1 ml	0279-01
20,000 USP units (25 G × ⅝") 10—1 ml	0276-01

WYAMINE® SULFATE (Mephentermine Sulfate)

30 mg (22 G × 1¼") 10—1 ml	0239-01

SPECIAL AGENTS

ATIVAN® (Lorazepam)℃

2 mg/ml (22 G × 1¼") 10—1 ml fill in 2 ml	0581-02
4 mg/ml (22 G × 1¼") 10—1 ml fill in 2 ml	0570-02

CHLORPROMAZINE HYDROCHLORIDE, USP

25 mg (22 G × 1¼") 10—1 ml	0435-01
50 mg (22 G × 1¼") 10—2 ml	0435-03

DEXAMETHASONE SODIUM PHOSPHATE, USP

4 mg (22 G × 1¼") 10—1 ml	0546-01

DIMENHYDRINATE, USP

50 mg (22 G × 1¼") 10—1 ml	0485-01

DIPHENHYDRAMINE HYDROCHLORIDE, USP

50 mg (22 G × 1¼") 10—1 ml	0384-01

HEPARIN FLUSH KITS
10 USP units
(25 G × ⅝")
50 Kits   2528-01

Each Unit of Use Kit contains:
One 1 ml size (25 G × ⅝") TUBEX Heparin Lock Flush Solution, USP, 10 USP units per ml and two 2.5 ml size (25 G × ⅝") TUBEX Bacteriostatic Sodium Chloride Injection, USP.

100 USP units
(25 G × ⅝")
50 Kits   2529-01

Each Unit of Use Kit contains:
One 1 ml size (25 G × ⅝") TUBEX Heparin Lock Flush Solution, USP, 100 USP units per ml and two 2.5 ml size (25 G × ⅝") TUBEX Bacteriostatic Sodium Chloride Injection, USP.

HEPARIN LOCK FLUSH Solution, USP

10 USP units per ml (25 G × ⅝") 50—1 ml	0523-01
100 USP units per ml (25 G × ⅝") 50—1 ml	0487-01
10 USP units per ml—25 USP units (25 G × ⅝") 50—2.5 ml	0523-02
100 USP units per ml—250 USP units (25 G × ⅝") 50—2.5 ml	0487-03

HYDROXYZINE HCl, USP

25 mg (22 G × 1¼") 10—1 ml	0540-01
50 mg (22 G × 1¼") 10—1 ml	0541-01
100 mg (22 G × 1¼") 10—2 ml	0541-02

LARGON® (Propiomazine HCl) (1678CB)

20 mg (22 G × 1¼") 10—1 ml	0260-01

LIDOCAINE HYDROCHLORIDE, USP

2% 20 mg/ml (25 G × ⅝") 10—2.5 ml	0460-01

OXYTOCIN, USP (Synthetic)

10 USP units (22 G × 1¼") 10—1 ml	0406-01

PHENERGAN® (Promethazine HCl)

25 mg (22 G × 1¼") 10—1 ml	0416-01
50 mg (22 G × 1¼") 10—1 ml	0417-01

PROCHLORPERAZINE EDISYLATE, USP

5 mg (22 G × 1¼") 10—1 ml	0542-01
10 mg (22 G × 1¼") 10—2 ml	0542-02

SODIUM CHLORIDE, USP (Bacteriostatic)

(22 G × 1¼") 50—2.5 ml	0333-05
(25 G × ⅝") 50—2.5 ml	0333-02

SPARINE® (Promazine HCl)

25 mg (22 G × 1¼") 10—1 ml	0232-01
50 mg (22 G × 1¼") 10—1 ml	0236-01
100 mg (22 G × 1¼") 10—2 ml	0236-02

TUBEX, EMPTY, STERILE CARTRIDGE-NEEDLE UNITS

(25 G × ⅝") 50—1 ml	9103-02
(22 G × 1¼") 50—1 ml	9103-01
(25 G × ⅝") 50—2 ml	9103-04
(22 G × 1¼") 50—2 ml	9103-03

Shown in Product Identification Section, page 445

UNIPEN®   ℞
[ū'ni-pen]
(nafcillin sodium) as the monohydrate
INJECTION • CAPSULES • POWDER
FOR ORAL SOLUTION • TABLETS

Description: UNIPEN (nafcillin sodium) is a semisynthetic penicillin developed by Wyeth research. Although primarily designed as an antistaphylococcal penicillin, in limited clinical trials it has been shown to be effective in the treatment of infections caused by pneumococci and Group A beta-hemolytic streptococci. Because of this wide gram-positive spectrum, this product is particularly suitable for *Initial Therapy* in severe or potentially severe infections before definitive culture results are known and in which staphylococci are suspected.

This product is readily soluble and can be conveniently administered in both oral and parenteral dosage forms. It is resistant to inactivation by staphylococcal penicillinase. Following intramuscular administration in humans, it rapidly appears in the plasma, penetrates body tissues in high concentration, and diffuses well into pleural, pericardial, and synovial fluids.

NOTE: Unipen contains 2.9 milliequivalents of sodium per gram of nafcillin as the sodium salt.

Microbiology: UNIPEN is a bactericidal penicillin which has shown activity *in vitro* against both penicillin G-sensitive and penicillin G-resistant strains of *Staphylococcus aureus* as well as against pneumococcus, beta-hemolytic streptococcus, and alpha streptococcus (viridans).

In experimental mouse infections induced with pneumococci, beta-hemolytic streptococci, and both penicillin G-susceptible and penicillin G-resistant strains of *Staph. aureus*, nafcillin sodium was compared with methicillin and oxacillin. Regardless of the route of drug administration (intramuscular or oral), nafcillin sodium was consistently and significantly more effective than the other two penicillins.

The fate of a penicillin G-resistant strain of *Staph. aureus* was determined in the kidneys of mice treated with penicillin G, methicillin, and nafcillin sodium. Animals injected with the nafcillin sodium showed negative cultures after the fourteenth day, whereas positive kidney cultures were obtained during the entire 28-day period from mice treated with penicillin G and methicillin.

Pharmacology: UNIPEN is relatively nontoxic for animals. The acute LD_{50} of this product by oral administration in rats and mice was greater than 5 g/kg; by intramuscular administration in rats, 2800 mg/kg; by intraperitoneal administration in rats, 1240 mg/kg; and by intravenous administration in mice, 1140 mg/kg. The intraperitoneal LD_{50} in dogs is 600 mg/kg. Animal studies indicated that local tissue responses following intramuscular administration of 25% solutions were minimal and resembled those of penicillin G rather than methicillin.

Animal studies indicate that antibacterial amounts are concentrated in the bile, kidney, lung, heart, spleen, and liver. Eighty-four percent of an intravenously administered dose can be recovered by biliary cannulation and 13 percent by renal excretion in 24 hours. High and prolonged tissue levels can be demonstrated by both biological activity assays and C^{14} distribution patterns. At comparable dosage, intramuscular absorption of this product is nearly equivalent to that of intramuscular methicillin, and oral absorption to that of oral oxacillin. Blood concentrations may be tripled by the concurrent use of probenecid. Clinical studies with nafcillin sodium monohydrate in infants under three days of age and prematures have revealed higher blood levels and slower rates of urinary excretion than in older children and adults.

Studies of the effect of this product on reproduction in rats and rabbits have been completed and reveal no fetal or maternal abnormalities. These studies include the observation of the effects of administration of the drug before conception and continuously through weaning (one generation).

Disc Susceptibility Tests: Quantitative methods that require measurement of zone diameters give the most precise estimates of antibiotic susceptibility. One such procedure* has been recommended for use with discs for testing susceptibility to penicillinase-resistant penicillin-class antibiotics. Interpretations correlate diameters on the disc test with MIC values for penicillinase-resistant penicillins. With this procedure, a report from the laboratory of "susceptible" indicates that the infecting organism is likely to respond to therapy. A report of "resistant" indicates that the infecting organism is not likely to respond to therapy. A report of "intermediate susceptibility" suggests that the organism would be susceptible if high dosage is used, or if the infection is confined to tissues and fluids (e.g., urine) in which high antibiotic levels are attained.

*Bauer, A.W., Kirby, W.M.M., Sherris, J.C., and Turck, M.: Antibiotic Testing by a Standardized Single-Discs Method, Am. J. Clin. Pathol., 45:493, 1966; Standardized Disc Susceptibility Test, FEDERAL REGISTER 37:20527-29, 1972.

Indications: Although the principal indication for nafcillin sodium is in the treatment of infections due to penicillinase-producing staphylococci, it may be used to initiate therapy in such patients in whom a staphylococcal infection is suspected. (See Important Note below.)

Bacteriologic studies to determine the causative organisms and their sensitivity to nafcillin sodium should be performed.

In serious, life-threatening infections, oral preparations of the penicillinase-resistant penicillins should not be relied on for initial therapy.

Important Note: When it is judged necessary that treatment be initiated before definitive culture and sensitivity results are known, the choice of nafcillin sodium should take into consideration the fact that it has been shown to be effective only in the treatment of infections caused by pneumococci, Group A beta-hemolytic streptococci, and penicillin G-resistant and penicillin G-sensitive staphylococci. If the bacteriology report later indicates the infection is due to an organism other than a penicillin G-resistant staphylococcus sensitive to nafcillin sodium, the physician is advised to continue therapy with a drug other than nafcillin sodium or any other penicillinase-resistant, semisynthetic penicillin.

Recent studies have reported that the percentage of staphylococcal isolates resistant to penicillin G outside the hospital is increasing, approximating the high percentage of resistant staphylococcal isolates found in the hospital. For this reason, it is recommended that a penicillinase-resistant penicillin be used as initial therapy for any suspected staphylococcal infection until culture and sensitivity results are known.

Methicillin is a compound that acts through a mechanism similar to that of nafcillin sodium against penicillin G-resistant staphylococci. Strains of staphylococci resistant to methicillin have existed in nature, and it is known that the number of these strains reported has been increasing. Such strains of staphylococci have been capable of producing serious disease, in some instances resulting in fatality. Because of this there is concern that widespread use of the penicillinase-resistant penicillins may result in the appearance of an increasing number of staphylococcal strains which are resistant to these penicillins.

Methicillin-resistant strains are almost always resistant to all other penicillinase-resistant penicillins (cross-resistance with cephalosporin derivatives also occurs frequently). Resistance to any penicillinase-resistant penicillin should be interpreted as evidence of clinical resistance to all, in spite of the fact that minor variations in *in vitro* sensitivity may be encountered when more than one penicillinase-resistant penicillin is tested against the same strain of staphylococcus.

Contraindications: A history of allergic reaction to any of the penicillins is a contraindication.

Warnings: Serious and occasionally fatal hypersensitivity (anaphylactoid) reactions have been reported in patients on penicillin therapy. Although anaphylaxis is more frequent following parenteral therapy, it has occurred in patients on oral penicillins. These reactions are more apt to occur in individuals with a history of sensitivity to multiple allergens.

There have been reports of individuals with a history of penicillin hypersensitivity reactions who have experienced severe hypersensitivity reactions when treated with a cephalosporin. Before therapy with a penicillin, careful inquiry should be made concerning previous hypersensitivity reactions to penicillins, cephalosporins, and other allergens. If an allergic reaction occurs, appropriate therapy should be instituted, and discontinuation of nafcillin therapy considered. The usual agents (antihistamines, pressor amines, corticosteroids) should be readily available.

Precautions: As with any potent drug, periodic assessment of organ-system function, including renal, hepatic and hematopoietic, should be made during prolonged therapy.

The possibility of bacterial and fungal overgrowth should be kept in mind during long-term therapy.

If overgrowth of resistant organisms occurs, appropriate measures should be taken.

The oral route of administration should not be relied upon in patients with severe illness, or with nausea, vomiting, gastric dilatation, cardiospasm, or intestinal hypermotility.

Safety for use in pregnancy has not been established.

Particular care should be taken with intravenous administration because of the possibility of thrombophlebitis.

Adverse Reactions: Reactions to nafcillin sodium have been infrequent and mild in nature. As with other penicillins, the possibility of an anaphylactic reaction or serum-sickness-like reactions should be considered. A careful history should be taken. Patients with histories of hay fever, asthma, urticaria, or previous sensitivity to penicillin are more likely to react adversely.

Transient leukopenia, neutropenia with evidence of granulocytopenia or thrombocytopenia are infrequent and usually associated with prolonged therapy with high doses of penicillin. These alterations have been noted to return to normal after cessation of therapy.

The few reactions associated with the intramuscular use of nafcillin sodium have been skin rash, pruritus, and possible drug fever. As with other penicillins, reactions from oral use of the drug have included nausea, vomiting, diarrhea, urticaria, and pruritus.

Dosage and Administration: It is recommended that parenteral therapy be used initially in severe infections. The patient should be placed on oral therapy with this product as soon as the clinical condition warrants. Very severe infections may require very high doses.

Intravenous Route: 500 mg every 4 hours in adults; double the dose if necessary in very severe infections.

The required amount of drug should be diluted in 15 to 30 ml of Sterile Water for Injection, U.S.P., or Sodium Chloride Injection, U.S.P., and injected over a 5- to 10-minute period. This may be accomplished through the tubing of an intravenous infusion if desirable.

To add nafcillin sodium to an intravenous solution, reconstitute the vials as directed under "How Supplied"—"For Parenteral Administration." Add the reconstituted vial contents immediately to the intravenous solution or within 8 hours following reconstitution if the vials are kept at room temperature (25° C) or within 48 hours following reconstitution if the vials are kept at refrigeration (2°-8° C).

Stability studies on nafcillin sodium at concentrations of 2 mg/ml to 40 mg/ml in the following intravenous solutions indicate the drug will lose less than 10% activity at room temperature (70°F.) or, if kept under refrigeration, during the time period stipulated:

STABILITY OF	ROOM TEMPERATURE	REFRIGERATED
Sterile Water for Injection	24 hours	96 hours
Isotonic sodium chloride	24 hours	96 hours
5% dextrose in water	24 hours	96 hours
5% dextrose in 0.4% sodium chloride solution	24 hours	96 hours
Ringer's solution	24 hours	96 hours
M/6 sodium lactate solution	24 hours	96 hours

Discard any unused portions of intravenous solutions after 24 hours if kept at room temperature or after 96 hours if kept under refrigeration.

Only those solutions listed above should be used for the intravenous infusion of UNIPEN (nafcillin sodium). The concentration of the antibiotic should fall within the range of 2 to 40 mg/ml. The drug concentrate and the rate and volume of the infusion should be adjusted so that the total dose of nafcillin is administered before the drug loses its stability in the solution in use.

There is no clinical experience available on the use of this agent in neonates or infants for this route of administration.

This route of administration should be used for relatively short-term therapy (24-48 hours) because of the occasional occurrence of thrombophlebitis, particularly in elderly patients.

PIGGYBACK UNITS (for Intravenous Drip Use)—

As diluents, use the following solutions: Sterile Water for Injection, Isotonic Sodium Chloride, 5% dextrose in water, 5% dextrose in 0.4% sodium chloride solution, Ringer's solution, or M/6 sodium lactate solution.

1-GRAM BOTTLE:
Add a minimum of 49 ml diluent and shake well. If lower concentrations are desired, the solution could be further diluted with up to a total of 99 ml of diluent.

Amount of Diluent	Concentration of Solution
49 ml	20 mg/ml
99 ml	10 mg/ml

1.5-GRAM BOTTLE:
Add a minimum of 49 ml diluent and shake well. If lower concentrations are desired, the solution could be further diluted with up to a total of 99 ml of diluent.

Amount of Diluent	Concentration of Solution
49 ml	30 mg/ml
99 ml	15 mg/ml

2-GRAM BOTTLE:
Add a minimum of 49 ml diluent and shake well. If lower concentrations are desired, the solution could be further diluted with up to a total of 99 ml of diluent.

Amount of Diluent	Concentration of Solution
49 ml	40 mg/ml
99 ml	20 mg/ml

4-GRAM BOTTLE:
Add 97 ml diluent and shake well. The resulting solution will contain 40 mg/ml.

The resulting solutions may then be administered alone or with the intravenous solutions listed above. Discard unused solution after 24 hours at room temperature (70°F) or 96 hours if kept under refrigeration. Administer piggyback through an IV tubing very slowly (at least 30–60 minutes) to avoid vein irritation.

At times it may be desired to use the contents of the piggyback bottles for addition to large-volume IV fluids. In this case the entire vial contents should be dissolved in not less than 25 ml of Sterile Water for Injection. Use the resulting concentration within 24 hours when kept at room temperature or within 96 hours when kept under refrigeration.

Intramuscular Route: 500 mg every 6 hours in adults; decrease the interval to 4 hours if necessary in severe infections. In infants and children a dose of 25 mg/kg (about 12 mg per pound) twice daily is usually adequate.

For neonates 10 mg/kg is recommended twice daily.

To reconstitute see directions and table below.

The clear solution should be administered by deep intragluteal injection immediately after reconstitution. After reconstitution, keep refrigerated (2°-8° C) and use within 7 days, keep at room temperature (25° C) and use within 3 days, or keep frozen (−20° C) for up to 3 months.

Oral Route: In adults a dose of 250 to 500 mg every 4 to 6 hours is sufficient for mild-to-moderate infections. In severe infections 1 gram every 4 to 6 hours may be necessary.

In children, streptococcal pharyngitis cases have responded to a dosage of 250 mg t.i.d. Beta-hemolytic streptococcal infections should be treated for at least ten days to prevent development of acute rheumatic fever or glomerulonephritis.

Continued on next page

Wyeth—Cont.

Children and infants with scarlet fever and pneumonia should receive 25 mg/kg/day in four divided doses. For staphylococcal infections, 50 mg/kg/day in four divided doses is recommended. For neonates, 10 mg/kg three to four times daily is recommended. If inadequate, resort to parenteral UNIPEN® (nafcillin sodium) Wyeth.
To reconstitute the powder for oral solution, add the water in two separate portions. Shake well after each addition. After reconstitution the solution must be refrigerated. Discard any unused portion after seven days.

How Supplied:
FOR ORAL ADMINISTRATION—
CAPSULES: containing nafcillin sodium, as the monohydrate, equivalent to 250 mg. nafcillin buffered with calcium carbonate, bottles of 100, and REDIPAK® Unit Dose Medication boxes of 100 (individually wrapped).
TABLETS (film-coated): containing nafcillin sodium, as the monohydrate, equivalent to 500 mg. nafcillin buffered with calcium carbonate, bottles of 50.
The appearance of UNIPEN capsules and tablets is a trademark of Wyeth Laboratories.
ORAL SOLUTION: Supplied as a powder for oral solution. When reconstituted with water each 5 ml will contain nafcillin sodium equivalent to 250 mg nafcillin, bottle to make 100 ml.
FOR PARENTERAL ADMINISTRATION—(intravenous or intramuscular)
VIALS: Supplied in vial sizes of 500 mg, 1 gram, and 2 gram nafcillin sodium as the monohydrate, buffered. When reconstituted as recommended (see table below) with Sterile Water for Injection, USP, Sodium Chloride Injection, USP, Bacteriostatic Water for Injection, USP (Tubex®), or Bacteriostatic Water for Injection, USP, with parabens or with benzyl alcohol, each vial contains, respectively, 2, 4, or 8 ml of solution. Each ml contains nafcillin sodium equivalent to 250 mg nafcillin buffered with 10 mg sodium citrate.

Vial Size	Amount of Diluent	Nafcillin Sodium Solution
500 mg	1.7 ml	2 ml
1 gram	3.4 ml	4 ml
2 gram	6.8 ml	8 ml

Also Available: 10 gram pharmacy bulk vial.
FOR INTRAVENOUS USE ONLY—
PIGGYBACK UNITS: Supplied in single units equivalent to 1, 1.5, 2, or 4 gram nafcillin per unit buffered with 40 mg sodium citrate per gram.
Shown in Product Identification Section, page 445

WYAMYCIN® E
[wi-a-mi'sin]
Liquid
(erythromycin ethylsuccinate oral suspension)

Description: Erythromycin is produced by a strain of Streptomyces erythraeus and belongs to the macrolide group of antibiotics. It is basic and readily forms salts with acids. The base, the stearate salt, and the esters are poorly soluble in water. Erythromycin ethylsuccinate is an ester of erythromycin suitable for oral administration.
The pleasant-tasting, fruit-flavored liquids are supplied ready for oral administration.
The ready-made suspensions are intended primarily for pediatric use but can also be used in adults.
Actions: The mode of action of erythromycin is by inhibition of protein synthesis without affecting nucleic acid synthesis. Resistance to erythromycin of some strains of Hemophilus influenzae and staphylococci has been demonstrated. Culture and susceptibility testing should be done. If the Kirby-Bauer method of disc susceptibility is used, a 15 mcg erythromycin disc should give a zone diameter of at least 18 mm when tested against an erythromycin-susceptible organism.
Orally administered erythromycin ethylsuccinate suspensions are readily and reliably absorbed. Serum levels are comparable when the drug is administered in either the fasting or nonfasting state.

After absorption, erythromycin diffuses readily into most body fluids. In the absence of meningeal inflammation, low concentrations are normally achieved in the spinal fluid, but passage of the drug across the blood-brain barrier increases in meningitis. In the presence of normal hepatic function, erythromycin is concentrated in the liver and excreted in the bile; the effect of hepatic dysfunction on excretion of erythromycin by the liver into the bile is not known. After oral administration, less than 5 percent of the activity of the administered dose can be recovered in the urine.
Erythromycin crosses the placental barrier, but fetal plasma levels are generally low.
Indications: Streptococcus Pyogenes (Group A beta-hemolytic streptococcus):
Upper- and lower-respiratory-tract, skin, and soft tissue infections of mild-to-moderate severity.
Injectable penicillin G benzathine is considered by the American Heart Association to be the drug of choice in the treatment and prevention of streptococcal pharyngitis and in long-term prophylaxis of rheumatic fever.
When oral medication is preferred for treatment of the above conditions, penicillin G, V, or erythromycin are alternate drugs of choice.
When oral medication is given, the importance of strict adherence by the patient to the prescribed dosage regimen must be stressed. A therapeutic dose should be administered for at least 10 days.
Although no controlled clinical efficacy trials have been conducted, oral erythromycin has been suggested by the American Heart Association and American Dental Association for use in a regimen for prophylaxis against bacterial endocarditis in patients hypersensitive to penicillin who have congenital heart disease or rheumatic or other acquired valvular heart disease when they undergo dental procedures and surgical procedures of the upper respiratory tract.[1] Erythromycin is not suitable prior to genitourinary or gastrointestinal tract surgery.
NOTE: When selecting antibiotics for the prevention of bacterial endocarditis the physician or dentist should read the full joint statement of the American Heart Association and the American Dental Association.[1]
Staphylococcus Aureus: Acute infections of skin and soft tissue of mild-to-moderate severity. Resistant organisms may emerge during treatment.
Streptococcus Pneumoniae (Diplococcus pneumoniae): Upper-respiratory-tract infections (e.g., otitis media, pharyngitis) and lower-respiratory-tract infections (e.g., pneumonia) of mild-to-moderate degree.
Mycoplasma Pneumoniae (Eaton agent, PPLO): For respiratory infections due to this organism.
Hemophilus Influenzae: For upper-respiratory-tract infections of mild-to-moderate severity when used concomitantly with adequate doses of sulfonamides. Not all strains of this organism are susceptible at the erythromycin concentrations ordinarily achieved (see appropriate sulfonamide labeling for prescribing information).
Treponema Pallidum: Erythromycin is an alternate choice of treatment for primary syphilis in patients allergic to the penicillins. In treatment of primary syphilis, spinal-fluid examinations should be done before treatment and as part of follow-up after therapy.
Corynebacterium Diphtheriae and C. Minutissimum: As an adjunct to antitoxin, to prevent establishment of carriers, and to eradicate the organism in carriers.
In the treatment of erythrasma.
Entamoeba Histolytica: In the treatment of intestinal amebiasis only. Extra-enteric amebiasis requires treatment with other agents.
Listeria Monocytogenes: Infections due to this organism.
Legionnaires' Disease: Although no controlled clinical efficacy studies have been conducted, in vitro and limited preliminary clinical data suggest that erythromycin may be effective in treating Legionnaires' Disease.
Erythromycins are indicated for treatment of the following infections caused by Chlamydia trachomatis: conjunctivitis of the newborn, pneumonia of infancy, urogenital infections during pregnancy. When tetracyclines are contraindicated or not tolerated, erythromycin is indicated for the treatment of uncomplicated urethral, endocervical, or rectal infections in adults due to Chlamydia trachomatis.
Contraindications: Erythromycin is contraindicated in patients with known hypersensitivity to this antibiotic.
Warnings: USAGE IN PREGNANCY: Safety for use in pregnancy has not been established.
Precautions: Erythromycin is principally excreted by the liver. Caution should be exercised in administering the antibiotic to patients with impaired hepatic function. There have been reports of hepatic dysfunction, with or without jaundice, occurring in patients receiving oral erythromycin products.
Recent data from studies of erythromycin reveal that its use in patients who are receiving high doses of theophylline may be associated with an increase of serum theophylline levels and potential theophylline toxicity. In case of theophylline toxicity and/or elevated serum theophylline levels, the dose of theophylline should be reduced while the patient is receiving concomitant erythromycin therapy.
Surgical procedures should be performed when indicated.
Adverse Reactions: The most frequent side effects of erythromycin preparations are gastrointestinal, such as abdominal cramping and discomfort, and are dose-related. Nausea, vomiting, and diarrhea occur infrequently with usual oral doses. During prolonged or repeated therapy, there is a possibility of overgrowth of nonsusceptible bacteria or fungi. If such infections occur, the drug should be discontinued and appropriate therapy instituted.
Mild allergic reactions such as urticaria and other skin rashes have occurred. Serious allergic reactions, including anaphylaxis, have been reported.
There have been isolated reports of reversible hearing loss occurring chiefly in patients with renal insufficiency and in patients receiving high doses of erythromycin.
Dosage and Administration: Erythromycin ethylsuccinate suspensions may be administered without regard to meals.
Children: Age, weight, and severity of the infection are important factors in determining the proper dosage. In mild-to-moderate infections the usual dosage of erythromycin ethylsuccinate for children is 30 to 50 mg/kg/day in divided doses. For more severe infections this dosage may be doubled.
The following dosage schedule is suggested for mild-to-moderate infections:

Body Weight	Total Daily Dose
Under 10 lbs.	30-50 mg/kg/day 15-25 mg/lb/day
10 to 15 lbs.	200 mg
16 to 25 lbs.	400 mg
26 to 50 lbs.	800 mg
51 to 100 lbs.	1200 mg
over 100 lbs.	1600 mg

The total daily dosage must be administered in divided doses.
Adults: 400 mg erythromycin ethylsuccinate every 6 hours is the usual dose. Dosage may be increased up to 4 gram per day according to the severity of the infection.
If twice-a-day dosage is desired in either adults or children, one-half of the total daily dose may be given every 12 hours.
The oral administration of 400 mg of erythromycin ethylsuccinate provides blood levels of erythromycin base (activity) similar to those provided by 250 mg of erythromycin stearate, erythromycin base, or erythromycin estolate (measured in terms of free base levels).

In the treatment of streptococcal infections, a therapeutic dosage of erythromycin ethylsuccinate should be administered for at least 10 days. In continuous prophylaxis against recurrences of streptococcal infections in persons with a history of rheumatic heart disease, the usual dosage is 400 mg twice a day.

For prophylaxis against bacterial endocarditis[1] in patients with congenital heart disease or rheumatic or other acquired valvular heart disease when undergoing dental procedures or surgical procedures of the upper respiratory tract, give 1.0 gm (20 mg/kg for children) orally 1-½ to 2 hours before the procedure, and then 500 mg (10 mg/kg for children) orally every 6 hours for 8 doses.
For Treatment of Primary Syphilis:
Adults—48 to 64 gram, given in divided doses over a period of 10 to 15 days.
For Intestinal Amebiasis:
Adults—400 mg four times daily for 10 to 14 days.
Children—30 to 50 mg/kg/day in divided doses for 10 to 14 days.
For Treatment of Legionnaires' Disease:
Although optimal doses have not been established, doses utilized in reported clinical data were those recommended above, 1.6 to 4 gram daily in divided doses.
Conjunctivitis of the newborn caused by *Chlamydia trachomatis:* Oral erythromycin syrup 50 mg/kg/day in 4 divided doses for at least 2 weeks.[2]
Pneumonia of infancy caused by *Chlamydia trachomatis:* Although the optimal duration of therapy has not been established, the recommended therapy is oral erythromycin syrup 50 mg/kg/day in 4 divided doses for at least 3 weeks.[2]
Urogenital infections during pregnancy due to *Chlamydia trachomatis:* Although the optimal dose and duration of therapy have not been established, the suggested treatment is erythromycin 500 mg. by mouth, 4 times a day on an empty stomach for at least 7 days. For women who cannot tolerate this regimen, a decreased dose of 250 mg, by mouth, 4 times a day should be used for at least 14 days.[2]
For adults with uncomplicated urethral, endocervical, or rectal infections caused by *Chlamydia trachomatis* in whom tetracyclines are contraindicated or not tolerated: 500 mg, by mouth, 4 times a day for at least 7 days.[2]
How Supplied: Wyamycin® E 200 (erythromycin ethylsuccinate oral suspension) is supplied in 1-pint bottles. Each 5 ml teaspoonful of fruit-flavored suspension contains activity equivalent to 200 mg of erythromycin.
Wyamycin® E 400 (erythromycin ethylsuccinate oral suspension) is supplied in 1-pint bottles. Each 5 ml teaspoonful of fruit-flavored suspension contains activity equivalent to 400 mg of erythromycin.
Also Available: Wyamycin® S (erythromycin stearate) tablets, containing the equivalent of 250 mg erythromycin, are available in bottles of 100 and 500 film-coated tablets. Wyamycin® S (erythromycin stearate) tablets, containing the equivalent of 500 mg erythromycin, are available in bottles of 100 film-coated tablets.
References:
1. American Heart Association. 1977. Prevention of bacterial endocarditis. Circulation. 56:139A-143A.
2. CDC Sexually Transmitted Disease Treatment Guidelines, 1982.
Shown in Product Identification Section, page 445

WYANOIDS® OTC
[wi'a-noids]
Hemorrhoidal Suppositories
Description: Each suppository contains 15 mg extract belladonna (0.19 mg equiv. total alkaloids), 3 mg ephedrine sulfate, zinc oxide, boric acid, bismuth oxyiodide, bismuth subcarbonate, and peruvian balsam in cocoa butter and beeswax. Wyeth Wyanoids have an unusual "torpedo" design which facilitates insertion and insures retention.
Indications: For the temporary relief of pain and itching of hemorrhoidal tissue in many cases.

Warning: Not to be used by persons having glaucoma or excessive pressure within the eye, by elderly persons (where undiagnosed glaucoma or excessive pressure within the eye occurs most frequently), or by children under 6 years of age, unless directed by a physician. Discontinue use if blurring of vision, rapid pulse, or dizziness occurs. Do not exceed recommended dosage. Not for frequent or prolonged use. If dryness of the mouth occurs, decrease dosage. If eye pain occurs, discontinue use and see your physician immediately as this may indicate undiagnosed glaucoma. In case of rectal bleeding, consult physician promptly.
Usual Dosage: One suppository twice daily for six days.
Directions: Remove wrapper of suppository and insert suppository rectally with gentle pressure, pointed end first. Use preferably upon arising and at bedtime.
How Supplied: Boxes of 12.
Shown in Product Identification Section, page 445

WYCILLIN® R
[wi-sil' in]
(sterile penicillin G procaine suspension)
INJECTION
FOR DEEP INTRAMUSCULAR INJECTION ONLY
Description: This product is designed to provide a stable aqueous suspension of sterile penicillin G procaine, ready for immediate use. This eliminates the necessity for addition of any diluent, required for the usual dry formulation of injectable penicillin.
Each TUBEX® (Sterile Cartridge-Needle Unit, Wyeth), 1,200,000 units (2 ml size) or 600,000 units (1 ml size) or disposable syringe 2,400,000 units (4 ml size) contains penicillin G procaine in a stabilized aqueous suspension with sodium citrate buffer; and as w/v, approximately 0.5% lecithin, 0.5% carboxymethylcellulose, 0.5% povidone, 0.1% methylparaben and 0.01% propylparaben.
Each TUBEX, 300,000 units (1 ml size), contains penicillin G procaine in a stabilized aqueous suspension with sodium citrate buffer; and as w/v, approximately 0.3% lecithin, 0.9% carboxymethylcellulose, 0.9% povidone, 0.14% methylparaben, and 0.015% propylparaben.
Wycillin (sterile penicillin G procaine suspension) must be stored in a refrigerator. Keep from freezing. This will prevent deterioration and assure that no significant loss of potency occurs within the expiration date.
Wycillin suspension in the TUBEX and disposable syringe formulations is viscous and opaque. Read "Contraindications," "Warnings," "Precautions," and "Dosage and Administration" sections prior to use.
Actions and Pharmacology: Penicillin G exerts a bactericidal action against penicillin-sensitive microorganisms during the stage of active multiplication. It acts through the inhibition of biosynthesis of cell-wall mucopeptide. It is not active against the penicillinase-producing bacteria, which include many strains of staphylococci. Penicillin G exerts high *in vitro* activity against staphylococci (except penicillinase-producing strains), streptococci (Groups A, C, G, H, L, and M), and pneumococci. Other organisms sensitive to penicillin G are *Neisseria gonorrhoeae, Corynebacterium diphtheriae, Bacillus anthracis,* Clostridia, *Actinomyces bovis, Streptobacillus moniliformis, Listeria monocytogenes,* and *Leptospira. Treponema pallidum* is extremely sensitive to the bactericidal action of penicillin G.
Sensitivity plate testing: If the Kirby-Bauer method of disc sensitivity is used, a 10-unit penicillin disc should give a zone greater than 28 mm when tested against a penicillin-sensitive bacterial strain.
Penicillin G procaine is an equimolecular compound of procaine and penicillin G, administered intramuscularly as a suspension. It dissolves slowly at the site of injection, giving a plateau type of blood level at about 4 hours which falls slowly over a period of the next 15–20 hours.

Approximately 60% of penicillin G is bound to serum protein. The drug is distributed throughout the body tissues in widely varying amounts. Highest levels are found in the kidneys with lesser amounts in the liver, skin, and intestines. Penicillin G penetrates into all other tissues to a lesser degree with a very small level found in the cerebrospinal fluid. With normal kidney function the drug is excreted rapidly by tubular excretion. In neonates and young infants and in individuals with impaired kidney functions, excretion is considerably delayed. Approximately 60–90 percent of a dose of parenteral penicillin G is excreted in the urine within 24–36 hours.
Indications: Penicillin G procaine is indicated in the treatment of moderately severe infections due to penicillin-G-sensitive microorganisms that are sensitive to the low and persistent serum levels common to this particular dosage form. Therapy should be guided by bacteriological studies (including sensitivity tests) and by clinical response.
NOTE: When high, sustained serum levels are required, aqueous penicillin G, either IM or IV, should be used.
The following infections will usually respond to adequate dosages of intramuscular penicillin G procaine:
Streptococcal infections (Group A—without bacteremia). Moderately severe to severe infections of the upper respiratory tract, skin and soft-tissue infections, scarlet fever, and erysipelas.
NOTE: Streptococci in Groups A, C, G, H, L, and M are very sensitive to penicillin G. Other groups, including Group D (enterococcus), are resistant. Aqueous penicillin is recommended for streptococcal infections with bacteremia.
Pneumococcal infections. Moderately severe infections of the respiratory tract.
NOTE: Severe pneumonia, empyema, bacteremia, pericarditis, meningitis, peritonitis, and arthritis of pneumococcal etiology are better treated with aqueous penicillin G during the acute stage.
Staphylococcal infections—penicillin-G-sensitive. Moderately severe infections of the skin and soft tissues.
NOTE: Reports indicate an increasing number of strains of staphylococci resistant to penicillin G, emphasizing the need for culture and sensitivity studies in treating suspected staphylococcal infections.
Indicated surgical procedures should be performed.
Fusospirochetosis (Vincent's gingivitis and pharyngitis). Moderately severe infections of the oropharynx respond to therapy with penicillin G procaine.
NOTE: Necessary dental care should be accomplished in infections involving the gum tissue.
Treponema pallidum (syphilis); all stages.
N. gonorrhoeae; acute and chronic (without bacteremia).
Yaws, Bejel, Pinta.
C. diphtheriae—penicillin G procaine as an adjunct to antitoxin for prevention of the carrier stage.
Anthrax.
Streptobacillus moniliformis and *Spirillum minus* infections (rat-bite fever).
Erysipeloid.
Subacute bacterial endocarditis (Group A streptococcus), only in extremely sensitive infections.
Although no controlled clinical efficacy studies have been conducted, aqueous crystalline penicillin G for injection and penicillin G procaine suspension have been suggested by the American Heart Association and the American Dental Association for use as part of a combined parenteral-oral regimen for prophylaxis against bacterial endocarditis in patients who have congenital heart disease or rheumatic or other acquired valvular heart disease when they undergo dental procedures and surgical procedures of the upper respiratory tract.[1]
Since it may happen that *alpha*-hemolytic streptococci relatively resistant to penicillin may be

Continued on next page

Wyeth—Cont.

found when patients are receiving continuous oral penicillin for secondary prevention of rheumatic fever, prophylactic agents other than penicillin may be chosen for these patients and prescribed in addition to their continuous rheumatic fever prophylactic regimen.

NOTE: When selecting antibiotics for the prevention of bacterial endocarditis, the physician or dentist should read the full joint statement of the American Heart Association and the American Dental Association.[1]

Contraindications: A previous hypersensitivity reaction to any penicillin is a contraindication.

Do not inject into or near an artery or nerve.

Warnings: Serious and occasionally fatal hypersensitivity (anaphylactoid) reactions have been reported in patients on penicillin therapy.

Serious anaphylactoid reactions require immediate emergency treatment with epinephrine. Oxygen and intravenous corticosteroids should also be administered as indicated.

Although anaphylaxis is more frequent following parenteral therapy, it has occurred in patients on oral penicillins. These reactions are more apt to occur in individuals with a history of sensitivity to multiple allergens.

There have been well-documented reports of individuals with a history of penicillin hypersensitivity reactions who have experienced severe hypersensitivity reactions when treated with a cephalosporin. Before therapy with a penicillin, careful inquiry should be made concerning previous hypersensitivity reactions to penicillins, cephalosporins, and other allergens. If an allergic reaction occurs, the drug should be discontinued and the patient treated with the usual agents, e.g., pressor amines, antihistamines, and corticosteroids.

Immediate toxic reactions to procaine may occur in some individuals, particularly when a large single dose is administered in the treatment of gonorrhea (4.8 million units). These reactions may be manifested by mental disturbances, including anxiety, confusion, agitation, depression, weakness, seizures, hallucinations, combativeness, and expressed "fear of impending death." The reactions noted in carefully controlled studies occurred in approximately one in 500 patients treated for gonorrhea. Reactions are transient, lasting from 15–30 minutes.

Inadvertent intravascular administration, including inadvertent direct intraarterial injection or injection immediately adjacent to arteries, of Wycillin (sterile penicillin G procaine suspension) and other penicillin preparations has resulted in severe neurovascular damage, including transverse myelitis with permanent paralysis, gangrene requiring amputation of digits and more proximal portions of extremities, and necrosis and sloughing at and surrounding the injection site. Such severe effects have been reported following injections into the buttock, thigh, and deltoid areas. Other serious complications of suspected intravascular administration which have been reported include immediate pallor, mottling or cyanosis of the extremity both distal and proximal to the injection site followed by bleb formation; severe edema requiring anterior and/or posterior compartment fasciotomy in the lower extremity. The above described severe effects and complications have most often occurred in infants and small children. Prompt consultation with an appropriate specialist is indicated if any evidence of compromise of the blood supply occurs at, proximal to, or distal to the site of injection.[2-10] See "Contraindications," "Precautions," and "Dosage and Administration" sections.

Quadriceps femoris fibrosis and atrophy have been reported following repeated intramuscular injections of penicillin preparations into the anterolateral thigh.

Injection into or near a nerve may result in permanent neurological damage.

Precautions: Penicillin should be used with caution in individuals with histories of significant allergies and/or asthma.

Care should be taken to avoid intravenous or intraarterial administration, or injection into or near major peripheral nerves or blood vessels, since such injections may produce neurovascular damage. See "Contraindications," "Warnings," and "Dosage and Administration" sections.

In suspected staphylococcal infections, proper laboratory studies, including sensitivity tests, should be performed.

A small percentage of patients are sensitive to procaine. If there is a history of sensitivity make the usual test: Inject intradermally 0.1 ml of a 1 to 2 percent procaine solution. Development of an erythema, wheal, flare, or eruption indicates procaine sensitivity. Sensitivity should be treated by the usual methods, including barbiturates, and procaine penicillin preparations should not be used. Antihistaminics appear beneficial in treatment of procaine reactions.

The use of antibiotics may result in overgrowth of nonsusceptible organisms. Constant observation of the patient is essential. If new infections due to bacteria or fungi appear during therapy, the drug should be discontinued and appropriate measures taken.

Whenever allergic reactions occur, penicillin should be withdrawn unless, in the opinion of the physician, the condition being treated is life-threatening and amenable only to penicillin therapy.

In prolonged therapy with penicillin, and particularly with high-dosage schedules, periodic evaluation of the renal and hematopoietic systems is recommended.

When treating gonococcal infections in which primary or secondary syphillis may be suspected, proper diagnostic procedures, including dark-field examinations, should be done. In all cases in which concomitant syphilis is suspected, monthly serological tests should be made for at least four months.

Adverse Reactions: Penicillin is a substance of low toxicity but does possess a significant index of sensitization. The following hypersensitivity reactions associated with use of penicillin have been reported: Skin rashes, ranging from maculopapular eruptions to exfoliative dermatitis; urticaria; serum-sickness-like reactions, including chills, fever, edema, arthralgia, and prostration. Severe and often fatal anaphylaxis has been reported (see "Warnings"). As with other treatments for syphilis, the Jarisch-Herxheimer reaction has been reported.

Procaine toxicity manifestations have been reported (see "Warnings"). Although procaine hypersensitivity reactions have not been reported with this drug, there are patients who are sensitive to procaine (see "Precautions").

Dosage and Administration:

Penicillin G procaine (aqueous) is for intramuscular injection only.

Administer by DEEP, INTRAMUSCULAR INJECTION in the upper, outer quadrant of the buttock. In infants and small children, the midlateral aspect of the thigh may be preferable. When doses are repeated, vary the injection site.

When using the TUBEX cartridge:

The Wyeth Tubex® cartridge for this product incorporates several features that are designed to facilitate the visualization of blood on aspiration if a blood vessel is inadvertently entered.

The design of this cartridge is such that blood which enters its needle will be quickly visualized as a red or dark-colored "spot." This "spot" will appear on the barrel of the glass cartridge immediately proximal to the blue hub. Prior to injection, in order to determine where this "spot" can be seen, the operator should first insert and secure the cartridge in the Tubex syringe in the usual fashion. The needle cover should then be removed and the cartridge and syringe held in one hand with the needle pointing away from the operator. If the 2 ml metal syringe is used the glass cartridge should then be rotated by turning the plunger of the syringe clockwise until the flat bevel at the tip of the needle is pointing upward and is horizontal when viewed directly from above. An imaginary straight line then drawn from the middle of the flat bevel to the back edge of the blue hub where it joins the glass will point to the area on the glass cartridge where the "spot" can be visualized. If the 1 ml metal syringe is used it will not be possible to continue to rotate the glass cartridge clockwise once it is properly engaged and fully threaded; it can, however, then be rotated counterclockwise as far as necessary to properly orient the bevel of the needle and locate the observation area. (In this same area in some cartridges a dark spot may sometimes be visualized prior to injection. This is the proximal end of the needle and does not represent a foreign body in, or other abnormality of, the suspension.)

Thus, before the needle is inserted into the selected muscle, it is important for the operator to orient the flat bevel of the needle so that any blood which might enter after its insertion and during aspiration can be visualized in the area of the cartridge where it will appear and not be obscured by the metal syringe or other obstructions.

After selection of the proper site and insertion of the needle into the selected muscle, aspirate by pulling back on the plunger. While maintaining negative pressure for 2–3 seconds, carefully observe the barrel of the cartridge in the area previously identified (see above) for the appearance of a red or dark-colored "spot."

Blood or "typical blood color" may not be seen if a blood vessel has been entered—only a mixture of blood and Wycillin. The appearance of *any* discoloration is reason to withdraw the needle and discard the glass Tubex cartridge. If it is elected to inject at another site, a new cartridge should be used. If no blood or discoloration appears, inject the contents of the cartridge slowly. Discontinue delivery of the dose if the subject complains of severe immediate pain at the injection site or if, especially in infants and young children, symptoms or signs occur suggesting onset of severe pain.

Some Tubex cartridges may contain a small air bubble which may be disregarded, since it does not affect administration of the product.

Because of the high concentration of suspended material in this product, the needle may be blocked if the injection is not made at a slow, steady rate.

When using the disposable syringe:

The Wyeth disposable syringe for this product incorporates several new features that are designed to facilitate its use.

A single small indentation, or "dot," has been punched into the metal ring that surrounds the neck of the syringe near the base of the needle. It is important that this "dot" be placed in a position so that it can be easily visualized by the operator following the intramuscular insertion of the syringe needle.

After selection of the proper site and insertion of the needle into the selected muscle, aspirate by pulling back on the plunger. While maintaining negative pressure for 2–3 seconds, carefully observe the barrel of the syringe immediately proximal to the location of the "dot" for appearance of blood or any discoloration. Blood or "typical blood color" may *not* be seen if a blood vessel has been entered—only a mixture of blood and Wycillin. The appearance of any discoloration is reason to withdraw the needle and discard the syringe. If it is elected to inject at another site, a new syringe should be used. If no blood or discoloration appears, inject the contents of the syringe slowly. Discontinue delivery of the dose if the subject complains of severe immediate pain at the injection site or if in infants and young children symptoms or signs occur suggesting onset of severe pain.

Pneumonia (pneumococcal), moderately severe (uncomplicated): 600,000–1,000,000 units daily.

Streptococcal infections (Group A), moderately severe to severe tonsillitis, erysipelas, scarlet fever, upper respiratory tract, skin and soft tissue: 600,000–1,000,000 units daily for 10-day minimum.

Staphylococcal infections, moderately severe to severe: 600,000–1,000,000 units daily.

In pneumonia, streptococcal (Group A) and staphylococcal infections in children under 60 pounds: 300,000 units daily.

Bacterial endocarditis (Group A streptococci) only in extremely sensitive infections: 600,000–1,000,000 units daily.

For prophylaxis against bacterial endocarditis[1] in patients with congenital heart disease or rheumatic or other acquired valvular heart disease when undergoing dental procedures or surgical procedures of the upper respiratory tract, use a combined parenteral-oral regimen. One million units of aqueous crystalline penicillin G (30,000 units/kg in children) intramuscularly mixed with 600,000 units penicillin G procaine (600,000 units for children) should be given one-half to one hour before the procedure. Oral penicillin V (phenoxymethyl penicillin), 500 mg for adults or 250 mg for children less than 60 lbs., should be given every 6 hours for 8 doses. Doses for children should not exceed recommendations for adults for a single dose or for a 24-hour period.

Syphilis—
Primary, secondary, and latent with a negative spinal fluid in adults and children over 12 years of age: 600,000 units daily for 8 days—total 4,800,000 units.

Late (tertiary, neurosyphilis, and latent syphilis with positive spinal-fluid examination or no spinal-fluid examination): 600,000 units daily for 10–15 days—total 6–9 million units.

Congenital syphilis under 70-lb. body weight: 10,000 units/kg/day for 10 days.

Yaws, Bejel, and Pinta: Treatment as syphilis in corresponding stage of disease.

Although some isolates of *Neisseria gonorrhoeae* have decreased susceptibility to penicillin, this inherent resistance is relative, not absolute, and penicillin in large doses remains the drug of choice for these strains. Strains producing penicillinase, however, are resistant to penicillin G, and a drug other than penicillin G should be used. Physicians are cautioned not to use less than the recommended doses.

Gonorrheal infections (uncomplicated)—Men or Women: Aqueous penicillin G procaine, 4.8 million units intramuscularly, divided into at least two doses and injected at different sites at one visit, together with 1 gram of oral probenecid, preferably given just before the injection.

NOTE: Treatment of severe complications of gonorrhea should be individualized, using large amounts of short-acting penicillin.

Gonorrheal endocarditis should be treated intensively with aqueous penicillin G. Prophylactic or epidemiologic treatment for gonorrhea (male and female) is accomplished with the same treatment schedules as for the uncomplicated gonorrhea.

Retreatment
The National Center for Disease Control, Venereal Disease Branch, U.S. Department of Health and Human Services, Atlanta, Georgia, recommends: Test of cure procedures at approximately 7–14 days after therapy. In the male, a gram-stained smear is adequate if positive; otherwise, a culture specimen should be obtained from the anterior urethra. In the female, culture specimens should be obtained from both the endocervical and anal canal sites.

Retreatment in the male is indicated if the urethral discharge persists for three or more days following initial therapy and the smear or culture remains positive. Follow-up treatment consists of 4,800,000 units of aqueous penicillin G procaine intramuscularly, divided in two injection sites at a single visit.

In uncomplicated gonorrhea in the female, retreatment is indicated if follow-up cervical or rectal cultures remain positive for *N. gonorrhoeae*. Follow-up treatment consists of 4,800,000 units of aqueous penicillin G daily on two successive days.

Syphilis: All gonorrheal patients should have a serologic test for syphilis at the time of diagnosis. Patients with gonorrhea who also have syphilis should be given additional treatment appropriate to the stage of syphilis.

Diphtheria—adjunctive therapy with antitoxin: 300,000–600,000 units daily.

Diphtheria carrier state: 300,000 units daily for 10 days.

Anthrax-cutaneous: 600,000–1,000,000 units/day.
Vincent's infection (fusospirochetosis): 600,000–1,000,000 units/day.
Erysipeloid: 600,000–1,000,000 units/day.
Streptobacillus moniliformis and *Spirillum minus* (rat-bite fever): 600,000–1,000,000 units/day.

How Supplied: *600,000 units per ml*—1 ml TUBEX sterile cartridge-needle unit, packages of 10 and 50; *1,200,000 units in 2 ml* TUBEX, packages of 10; *2,400,000 units in 4 ml* single-dose disposable syringe, packages of 10.

References:
1. American Heart Association: Prevention of bacterial endocarditis. *Circulation*, 56:139A–143A, 1977.
2. SHAW, E.: Transverse myelitis from injection of penicillin. *Am. J. Dis. Child.*, 11:548, 1966.
3. KNOWLES, J.: Accidental intra-arterial injection of penicillin. *Am. J. Dis. Child.*, 111:552, 1966.
4. DARBY, C., et al: Ischemia following an intragluteal injection of benzathine-procaine penicillin G mixture in a one-year-old boy. *Clin. Pediatrics*, 12:485, 1973.
5. BROWN, L. & NELSON, A.: Postinfectious intravascular thrombosis with gangrene. *Arch. Surg.*, 94:652, 1967.
6. BORENSTINE, J.: Transverse myelitis and penicillin (Correspondence). *Am. J. Dis. Child.*, 112:166, 1966.
7. ATKINSON, J.: Transverse myelopathy secondary to penicillin injection. *J. Pediatrics*, 75:867, 1969.
8. TALBERT, J. et al: Gangrene of the foot following intramuscular injection in the lateral thigh: A case report with recommendations for prevention. *J. Pediatrics*, 79:110, 1967.
9. FISHER, T.: Medicolegal affairs. *Canad. Med. Assoc. J.*, 112:395, 1975.
10. SCHANZER, H. et al: Accidental intraarterial injection of penicillin G. *JAMA*, 242:1289, 1979.

WYCILLIN® and PROBENECID ℞
[wi-sil'in and pro-ben'is-id]
(sterile penicillin G procaine suspension and probenecid tablets)
Disposable Syringe and Tablets
Wycillin is for deep IM injection only.

Description: The Wycillin disposable syringe is designed to provide a stable aqueous suspension of sterile penicillin G procaine, ready for immediate use. This eliminates the necessity for addition of any diluent, required for the usual dry formulation of injectable penicillin.

Each syringe, 2,400,000 units (4 ml size), contains penicillin G procaine in a stabilized aqueous suspension with sodium citrate buffer; and as w/v, approximately 0.5% lecithin, 0.5% carboxymethylcellulose, 0.5% povidone, 0.1% methylparaben, and 0.01% propylparaben.

Wycillin must be stored in a refrigerator. Keep from freezing. This will prevent deterioration and assure that no significant loss of potency occurs within the expiration date.

Probenecid is a uricosuric and renal tubular-blocking agent.

Wycillin suspension in the disposable syringe formulation is viscous and opaque. Read "Contraindications," "Warnings," "Precautions," and "Dosage and Administration" sections prior to use.

Actions and Pharmacology: Penicillin G exerts a bactericidal action against penicillin-sensitive microorganisms during the stage of active multiplication. It acts through the inhibition of biosynthesis of cell-wall mucopeptide. It is not active against the penicillinase-producing bacteria, which include many strains of staphylococci. Neisseria gonorrhoeae are included among the various organisms which are sensitive to penicillin G. Penicillin G procaine is an equimolecular salt of procaine and penicillin G, administered intramuscularly as a suspension. It dissolves slowly at the site of injection, giving a plateau type of blood level at about 4 hours which falls slowly over a period of the next 15–20 hours. Approximately 60% to 90% of a dose of penicillin G is excreted in the urine within 24 to 36 hours.

Approximately 60% of penicillin G is bound to serum protein. The drug is distributed throughout the body tissues in widely varying amounts, with highest levels found in the kidneys and lesser amounts in the liver, skin, and intestines. Penicillin G penetrates into all other tissues to a lesser degree, with a very small level found in the cerebrospinal fluid. With normal kidney function the drug is excreted rapidly by tubular excretion. In neonates and young infants and in individuals with impaired kidney function, excretion is considerably delayed.

Probenecid inhibits the tubular reabsorption of urate, thus increasing the urinary excretion of uric acid and decreasing serum uric acid levels. It also inhibits the tubular excretion of penicillin and usually increases penicillin plasma levels, regardless of the route by which the antibiotic is given. A 2-fold to 4-fold elevation has been demonstrated for various penicillins. Probenecid does not influence plasma concentrations of salicylates, nor the excretion of streptomycin, chloramphenicol, chlortetracycline, oxytetracycline, or neomycin.

Indications: Wycillin and Probenecid is indicated for the single-dose treatment of uncomplicated (without bacteremia) urethral, cervical, rectal, or pharyngeal infections caused by *Neisseria gonorrhoeae* (gonorrhea) in men and women.

Susceptibility studies should be performed when recurrent infections or resistant strains are encountered. Urethritis and the presence of gram-negative diplococci in urethral smears are strong presumptive evidence of gonorrhea. Culture or fluorescent antibody studies will confirm the diagnosis. Therapy may be instituted prior to obtaining results of susceptibility testing.

Contraindications: A history of a previous hypersensitivity reaction to any of the penicillins or to Probenecid is a contraindication.

Probenecid is not recommended in persons with known blood dyscrasias or uric kidney stones or during an acute attack of gout. It is not recommended in conjunction with penicillin G procaine suspension in the presence of known renal impairment.

Do not inject into or near an artery or nerve.

Warnings: PENICILLIN G PROCAINE: Serious and occasionally fatal hypersensitivity (anaphylactoid) reactions have been reported in patients on penicillin therapy. Serious anaphylactoid reactions require immediate emergency treatment with epinephrine. Oxygen and intravenous corticosteroids should also be administered as indicated. Although anaphylaxis is more frequent following parenteral therapy, it has occurred in patients on oral penicillins. These reactions are more apt to occur in individuals with a history of sensitivity to multiple allergens.

There have been well-documented reports of individuals with a history of penicillin-hypersensitivity reactions who have experienced severe hypersensitivity reactions when treated with a cephalosporin. Before therapy with a penicillin, careful inquiry should be made concerning previous hypersensitivity reactions to penicillins, cephalosporins, and other allergens. If an allergic reaction occurs, the drug should be discontinued and the patient treated with the usual agents, e.g., pressor amines, antihistamines, and corticosteroids.

Immediate toxic reactions to procaine may occur in some individuals, particularly when a large single dose is administered in the treatment of gonorrhea (4.8 million units). These reactions may be manifested by mental disturbances, including anxiety, confusion, agitation, depression, weakness, seizures, hallucinations, combativeness, and expressed "fear of impending death." The reactions noted in carefully controlled studies occurred in approximately one in 500 patients

Continued on next page

Wyeth—Cont.

treated for gonorrhea. Reactions are transient, lasting from 15-30 minutes.

Inadvertent intravascular administration, including inadvertent direct intraarterial injection or injection immediately adjacent to arteries, of Wycillin (sterile penicillin G procaine suspension) and other penicillin preparations has resulted in severe neurovascular damage, including transverse myelitis with permanent paralysis, gangrene requiring amputation of digits and more proximal portions of extremities, and necrosis and sloughing at and surrounding the injection site. Such severe effects have been reported following injections into the buttock, thigh, and deltoid areas. Other serious complications of suspected intravascular administration which have been reported include immediate pallor, mottling or cyanosis of the extremity both distal and proximal to the injection site followed by bleb formation; severe edema requiring anterior and/ or posterior compartment fasciotomy in the lower extremity. The above-described severe effects and complications have most often occurred in infants and small children. Prompt consultation with an appropriate specialist is indicated if any evidence of compromise of the blood supply occurs at, proximal to, or distal to the site of injection.[1-9] See "Contraindications," "Precautions," and "Dosage and Administration" sections.

Quadriceps femoris fibrosis and atrophy have been reported following repeated intramuscular injections of penicillin preparations into the anterolateral thigh.

Injection into or near a nerve may result in permanent neurological damage.

PROBENECID: Exacerbation of gout following therapy with Probenecid may occur; in such cases colchicine therapy is advisable.

In patients on Probenecid, the use of salicylates in either small or large doses is not recommended because it antagonizes the uricosuric action of Probenecid. Patients on Probenecid who require a mild analgesic agent should receive acetaminophen rather than salicylates, even in small doses.

USAGE IN PREGNANCY: The safety of these drugs for use in pregnancy has not been established.

Precautions: PENICILLIN G PROCAINE: When treating gonococcal infections in which primary or secondary syphilis may be suspected, proper diagnostic procedures, including dark-field examinations, should be done. In all cases in which concomitant syphilis is suspected, monthly serological tests should be made for at least four months. Patients with gonorrhea, who also have syphilis, should be given additional appropriate parenteral penicillin treatment.

Penicillin should be used with caution in individuals with histories of significant allergies and/or asthma. When administering Wycillin, care should be taken to avoid intravenous or intraarterial administration, or injection into or near major peripheral nerves or blood vessels, since such injections may produce neurovascular damage. See "Contraindications," "Warnings," and "Dosage and Administration" sections.

A small percentage of patients are sensitive to procaine. If there is a history of sensitivity, make the usual test: Inject intradermally 0.1 ml of a 1- to 2-percent procaine solution. Development of an erythema, wheal, flare, or eruption indicates procaine sensitivity. Sensitivity should be treated by the usual methods, including barbiturates, and procaine penicillin preparations should not be used. Antihistaminics appear beneficial in treatment of procaine reactions.

PROBENECID: Use Probenecid with caution in patients with a history of peptic ulcer. A reducing substance may appear in the urine of patients receiving Probenecid. Although this disappears with discontinuance of therapy, a false diagnosis of glycosuria may be made because of a false-positive Benedict's test.

Adverse Reactions: WYCILLIN: Penicillin is a substance of low toxicity but does possess a significant index of sensitization. The following hypersensitivity reactions associated with use of penicillin have been reported: Skin rashes, ranging from maculopapular eruptions to exfoliative dermatitis; urticaria; serum-sickness-like reactions, including chills, fever, edema, arthralgia, and prostration. Severe and often fatal anaphylaxis has been reported (see "Warnings"). As with other treatments for syphilis, the Jarisch-Herxheimer reaction has been reported.

Procaine toxicity manifestations have been reported (see "Warnings"). Although procaine hypersensitivity reactions have not been reported with this drug, there are patients who are sensitive to procaine (see "Precautions").

PROBENECID: The following are the principal adverse reactions which have been reported as associated with the use of Probenecid, generally with more prolonged or repeated administration: Hypersensitivity reactions (including anaphylaxis), nephrotic syndrome, hepatic necrosis, aplastic anemia; also other anemias, including hemolytic anemia related to genetic deficiency of glucose-6-phosphate dehydrogenase.

Dosage and Administration:

Penicillin G procaine (aqueous) is for intramuscular injection only.

Administer by DEEP INTRAMUSCULAR INJECTION in the upper, outer quadrant of the buttock. When doses are repeated, vary the injection site. The Wyeth disposable syringe for this product incorporates several new features that are designed to facilitate its use.

A single small indentation, or "dot", has been punched into the metal ring that surrounds the neck of the syringe near the base of the needle. It is important that this "dot" be placed in a position so that it can be easily visualized by the operator following the intramuscular insertion of the syringe needle.

After selection of the proper site and insertion of the needle into the selected muscle, aspirate by pulling back on the plunger. While maintaining negative pressure for 2-3 seconds, carefully observe the barrel of the syringe immediately proximal to the location of the "dot" for appearance of blood or any discoloration. Blood or "typical blood color" may *not* be seen if a blood vessel has been entered—only a mixture of blood and Wycillin. The appearance of any discoloration is reason to withdraw the needle and discard the syringe. If it is elected to inject at another site, a new syringe should be used. If no blood or discoloration appears, inject the contents of the syringe slowly. Discontinue delivery of the dose if the subject complains of severe immediate pain at the injection site or if in infants and young children symptoms or signs occur suggesting onset of severe pain.

Although some isolates of *Neisseria gonorrhoeae* have decreased susceptibility to penicillin, this inherent resistance is relative, not absolute, and penicillin in large doses remains the drug of choice for these strains. Strains producing penicillinase, however, are resistant to penicillin G, and a drug other than penicillin G should be used.

GONORRHEAL INFECTIONS (UNCOMPLICATED) MEN OR WOMEN: Aqueous penicillin G procaine, 4.8 million units intramuscularly, divided into at least two doses and injected at different sites at one visit, together with 1 gram (2 tablets, 0.5 gram each) of Probenecid orally, given just before the injections. Physicians are cautioned to use no less than the recommended dosages.

NOTE: Treatment of severe complications of gonorrhea should be individualized, using large amounts of short-acting penicillin. Gonorrheal endocarditis should be treated intensively with aqueous penicillin G. Prophylactic or epidemiologic treatment for gonorrhea (male and female) is accomplished with the same treatment schedules as for the uncomplicated gonorrhea.

RETREATMENT: The National Center for Disease Control, Venereal Disease Branch, U.S. Department of Health and Human Services, Atlanta, Georgia, recommends:

Test of cure procedures at approximately 7-14 days after therapy. In the male, a gram-stained smear is adequate if positive; otherwise, a culture specimen should be obtained from the anterior urethra. In the female, culture specimens should be obtained from both the endocervical and anal canal sites.

Retreatment in the male is indicated if the urethral discharge persists for three or more days following initial therapy and the smear or culture remains positive. Follow-up treatment consists of 4,800,000 units of aqueous penicillin G procaine, intramuscular, divided in two injection sites at a single visit.

In uncomplicated gonorrhea in the female, retreatment is indicated if follow-up cervical or rectal cultures remain positive for *N. gonorrhoeae.* Follow-up treatment consists of 4,800,000 units of aqueous penicillin G procaine daily on two successive days.

Syphilis: All gonorrhea patients should have a serologic test for syphilis at the time of diagnosis. Patients with gonorrhea who also have syphilis should be given additional treatment appropriate to the stage of syphilis.

How Supplied: Supplied as a combination package containing two disposable syringes of Wycillin® (sterile penicillin G procaine suspension) (2,400,000 units each) and two tablets Probenecid, Benemid® (0.5 gram each).

Wycillin® Disposable Syringes manufactured by **Wyeth Laboratories Inc.**, Philadelphia, PA 19101

Probenecid Tablets (Benemid®) manufactured by **Merck, Sharp and Dohme,** Division of Merck & Co., West Point, PA 19486

References:

1. SHAW, E.: Transverse myelitis from injection of penicillin, *Am. J. Dis. Child., 111:* 548, 1966.
2. KNOWLES, J.: Accidental intra-arterial injection of penicillin. *Am. J. Dis. Child., 111:* 552, 1966.
3. DARBY, C., et al: Ischemia following an intragluteal injection of benzathine-procaine penicillin G mixture in a one-year-old boy. *Clin. Pediatrics, 12:* 485, 1973.
4. BROWN, L. & NELSON, A.: Postinfectious intravascular thrombosis with gangrene, *Arch. Surg., 94:* 652, 1967.
5. BORENSTINE, J.: Transverse myelitis and penicillin (Correspondence), *Am. J. Dis. Child., 112:* 166, 1966.
6. ATKINSON, J.: Transverse myelopathy secondary to penicillin injection. *J. Pediatrics, 75:* 867, 1969.
7. TALBERT, J. et al: Gangrene of the foot following intramuscular injection in the lateral thigh: A case report with recommendations for prevention. *J. Pediatrics, 70:* 110, 1967.
8. FISHER, T.: Medicolegal affairs, *Canad. Med. Assoc. J., 112:* 395, 1975.
9. SCHANZER, H. et al: Accidental intraarterial injection of penicillin G. *JAMA, 242:* 1289, 1979.

WYDASE®   B
[wi-dās]
(hyaluronidase)
INJECTION

Description: This product, a preparation of highly purified bovine testicular hyaluronidase, is available in two dosage forms, as follows: WYDASE LYOPHILIZED: Hyaluronidase, dehydrated in the frozen state under high vacuum, with lactose and thimerosal (mercury derivative).

Reconstitute with Sodium Chloride Injection, USP, before use, usually in the proportion of one milliliter per 150 USP units of hyaluronidase (WYDASE LYOPHILIZED).

Each vial of 1500 USP units contains 1.0 mg thimerosal (mercury derivative), added as a preservative, and 13.3 mg lactose. Each vial of 150 USP units contains 0.075 mg thimerosal (mercury derivative), added as a preservative, and 2.66 mg lactose.

WYDASE SOLUTION (Stabilized): An injection solution ready for use, containing 150 USP units of hyaluronidase per milliliter with 8.5 mg. sodium chloride, 1 mg. edetate disodium, 0.4 mg. calcium chloride, monobasic sodium phosphate buffer, and not more than 0.1 mg. thimerosal (mercury derivative).

The USP hyaluronidase unit is equivalent to the turbidity-reducing (TR) unit and the International Unit.

Action: The enzymatic action of hyaluronidase hydrolyzes hyaluronic acid, a viscous polysaccharide found in the interstices of the tissues, where it normally obstructs diffusion of invasive substances. Thus hyaluronidase promotes diffusion and consequently absorption of fluids in the tissues, and has the action of the spreading factor of Duran-Reynals. When no spreading factor is present, material injected subcutaneously spreads very slowly; but hyaluronidase causes rapid spreading, provided local interstitial pressure is adequate to furnish the necessary mechanical impulse. Such an impulse is normally initiated by injected solutions. The rate of diffusion is proportionate to the amount of enzyme, and the extent is proportionate to the volume of solution.

Intravenous administration of even 75,000 USP units (500 times the maximal therapeutic dose) of hyaluronidase in animals causes no significant change in blood pressure, respiration, body temperature, or kidney function, and no histological changes in the tissues. Results from an experimental study on the influence of hyaluronidase in bone repair supports the conclusion that this enzyme alone, in the usual clinical dosage, does not deter bone healing. Hyaluronidase has no effect on the spread of localized infection provided it is not injected into the infected area, and seems to have no deleterious effect on bacterial or viral infections. But when crude testicular extracts which contained tissue irritants as well as "spreading factor" were used, an increase in area and virulence of the infection was observed.

Indications: This drug is indicated as an adjuvant to increase the absorption and dispersion of other injected drugs, for hypodermoclysis, and as an adjunct in subcutaneous urography for improving resorption of radiopaque agents.

Contraindications: Do not inject hyaluronidase into acutely inflamed or cancerous areas.

Precautions: Discontinue hyaluronidase if sensitization occurs. Sensitivity to hyaluronidase occurs infrequently. A preliminary test for sensitivity should be conducted. The skin test is made by an intradermal injection of approximately 0.02 ml. of the solution. A positive reaction consists of a wheal with pseudopods appearing within five minutes and persisting for 20 to 30 minutes and accompanied by localized itching. Transient vasodilation at the site of the test, i.e., erythema, is not a positive reaction.

When epinephrine is injected along with hyaluronidase the usual precautions for the use of epinephrine in cardiovascular disease, thyroid disease, diabetes, digital nerve block, ischemia of the fingers and toes, etc., should be observed.

Dosage and Administration: WYDASE® (hyaluronidase) should be administered only as discussed below, since its effects relative to the absorption and dispersion of other drugs are not produced when it is administered intravenously.

ABSORPTION AND DISPERSION OF INJECTED DRUGS. Absorption and dispersion of other injected drugs may be enhanced by adding 150 units hyaluronidase to the menstruum containing the other medication.

HYPODERMOCLYSIS. Insert needle with aseptic precautions. With tip lying free and movable between skin and muscle, begin clysis; fluid should start in readily without pain or lump. Then inject Solution Wydase into rubber tubing close to needle. An alternate method is to inject Wydase under skin prior to clysis. 150 units will facilitate absorption of 1000 ml. or more of solution. As with all parenteral fluid therapy, observe effect closely, with same precautions for restoring fluid and electrolyte balance as in intravenous injections. The dose, the rate of injection, and the type of solution (saline, glucose, Ringer's, etc.) must be adjusted carefully to the individual patient. When solutions devoid of inorganic electrolytes are given by hypodermoclysis, hypovolemia may occur. This may be prevented by using solutions containing adequate amounts of inorganic electrolytes and/or controlling the volume and speed of administration. Hyaluronidase may be added to small volumes of solution (up to 200 ml.), such as a small clysis for infants or solutions of drugs for subcutaneous injection. **For children less than 3 years old the volume of a single clysis should be limited to 200 ml.; and in premature infants or during the neonatal period, the daily dosage should not exceed 25 ml. per kilogram of body weight; the rate of administration should not be greater than 2 ml. per minute. For older patients the rate and volume of administration should not exceed those employed for intravenous infusion.**

SUBCUTANEOUS UROGRAPHY. The subcutaneous route of administration of urographic contrast media is indicated when intravenous administration cannot be successfully accomplished, particularly in infants and small children. With the patient prone, 75 units of Wydase® (hyaluronidase) Wyeth is injected subcutaneously over each scapula, followed by injection of the contrast medium at the same sites.

How Supplied:
WYDASE® LYOPHILIZED:
150 USP (TR) units, vials of 1 ml.;
1500 USP (TR) units, vials of 10 ml.
WYDASE® SOLUTION (Stabilized):
150 USP (TR) units per ml., vials of 1 ml. and 10 ml.

WYGESIC®
[wi-je'zik]

Each tablet contains:
65 mg propoxyphene HCl
and 650 mg acetaminophen.

Description: Propoxyphene hydrochloride is an odorless white crystalline powder with a bitter taste. It is freely soluble in water. Chemically, it is alpha-(+)-4-(Dimethylamino)-3-methyl-1,2-diphenyl-2-butanol Propionate Hydrochloride.

Acetaminophen is a white, crystalline powder, possessing a slightly bitter taste. It is soluble in boiling water and freely soluble in alcohol. Chemically, it is N-Acetyl-p-aminophenol.

Clinical Pharmacology: Propoxyphene is a centrally acting narcotic analgesic agent.

Repeated doses of propoxyphene at 6-hour intervals lead to increasing plasma concentrations, with a plateau after the ninth dose at 48 hours. Propoxyphene is metabolized in the liver to yield norpropoxyphene. Propoxyphene has a half-life of 6 to 12 hours, whereas that of norpropoxyphene is 30 to 36 hours.

Norpropoxyphene has substantially less central-nervous-system-depressant effect than propoxyphene, but a greater local anesthetic effect, which is similar to that of amitriptyline and antiarrhythmic agents, such as lidocaine and quinidine.

In animal studies in which propoxyphene and norpropoxyphene were continuously infused in large amounts, intracardiac conduction time (P-R and QRS intervals) was prolonged. Any intracardiac conduction delay attributable to high concentrations of norpropoxyphene may be of relatively long duration.

Actions: Propoxyphene is a mild narcotic analgesic structurally related to methadone.

The combination of propoxyphene and acetaminophen produces greater analgesia than that produced by either propoxyphene or acetaminophen administered alone.

Indications: These products are indicated for the relief of mild-to-moderate pain, either when pain is present alone or when it is accompanied by fever.

Contraindications: Hypersensitivity to propoxyphene or to acetaminophen.

Warnings

Do not prescribe propoxyphene for patients who are suicidal or addiction-prone.
Prescribe propoxyphene with caution for patients taking tranquilizers or antidepressant drugs and patients who use alcohol in excess.
Tell your patients not to exceed the recommended dose and to limit their intake of alcohol.

Propoxyphene products in excessive doses, either alone or in combination with other CNS depressants, including alcohol, are a major cause of drug-related deaths. Fatalities within the first hour of overdosage are not uncommon. In a survey of deaths due to overdosage conducted in 1975, in approximately 20% of the fatal cases, death occurred within the first hour (5% occurred within 15 minutes). Propoxyphene should not be taken in doses higher than those recommended by the physician. The judicious prescribing of propoxyphene is essential to the safe use of this drug. With patients who are depressed or suicidal, consideration should be given to the use of nonnarcotic analgesics. Patients should be cautioned about the concomitant use of propoxyphene products and alcohol because of potentially serious CNS-additive effects of these agents. Because of its added depressant effects, propoxyphene should be prescribed with caution for those patients whose medical condition requires the concomitant administration of sedatives, tranquilizers, muscle relaxants, antidepressants, or other CNS-depressant drugs. Patients should be advised of the additive depressant effects of these combinations.

Many of the propoxyphene-related deaths have occurred in patients with previous histories of emotional disturbances or suicidal ideation or attempts as well as histories of misuse of tranquilizers, alcohol, and other CNS-active drugs. Some deaths have occurred as a consequence of the accidental ingestion of excessive quantities of propoxyphene alone or in combination with other drugs. Patients taking propoxyphene should be warned not to exceed the dosage recommended by the physician.

DRUG DEPENDENCE: Propoxyphene, when taken in higher-than-recommended doses over long periods of time, can produce drug dependence characterized by psychic dependence and, less frequently, physical dependence and tolerance. Propoxyphene will only partially suppress the withdrawal syndrome in individuals physically dependent on morphine or other narcotics. The abuse liability of propoxyphene is qualitatively similar to that of codeine although quantitatively less, and propoxyphene should be prescribed with the same degree of caution appropriate to the use of codeine.

USAGE IN AMBULATORY PATIENTS: - Propoxyphene may impair the mental and/or physical abilities required for the performance of potentially hazardous tasks, such as driving a car or operating machinery. The patient should be cautioned accordingly.

Precautions

DRUG INTERACTIONS: The CNS-depressant effect of propoxyphene is additive with that of other CNS depressants, including alcohol.

USAGE IN PREGNANCY: Safe use in pregnancy has not been established relative to possible adverse effects on fetal development. Instances of withdrawal symptoms in the neonate have been reported following usage during pregnancy. Therefore, propoxyphene should not be used in pregnant women unless, in the judgment of the physician, the potential benefits outweigh the possible hazards.

USAGE IN NURSING MOTHERS: Low levels of propoxyphene have been detected in human milk. In postpartum studies involving nursing mothers who were given propoxyphene, no adverse effects were noted in infants receiving mother's milk.

USAGE IN CHILDREN: Propoxyphene is not recommended for use in children, because documented clinical experience has been insufficient to

Continued on next page

Wyeth—Cont.

establish safety and a suitable dosage regimen in the pediatric age group.

Adverse Reactions: In a survey conducted in hospitalized patients, less than 1% of patients taking propoxyphene hydrochloride at recommended doses experienced side effects. The most frequently reported have been dizziness, sedation, nausea, and vomiting. Some of these adverse reactions may be alleviated if the patient lies down.

Other adverse reactions include constipation, abdominal pain, skin rashes, light-headedness, headache, weakness, euphoria, dysphoria, and minor visual disturbances.

Cases of liver dysfunction have been reported.

Dosage and Administration: This product is given orally. The usual dose is 65 mg propoxyphene HCl and 650 mg acetaminophen every 4 hours as needed for pain. The maximum recommended dose of propoxyphene HCl is 390 mg per day.

Management of Overdosage: Initial consideration should be given to the management of the CNS effects of propoxyphene overdosage. Resuscitative measures should be initiated promptly.

SYMPTOMS OF PROPOXYPHENE OVERDOSAGE: The manifestations of acute overdosage with propoxyphene are those of narcotic overdosage. The patient is usually somnolent, but may be stuporous or comatose and convulsing. Respiratory depression is characteristic. The ventilatory rate and/or tidal volume is decreased, which results in cyanosis and hypoxia. Pupils, initially pinpoint, may become dilated as hypoxia increases. Cheyne-Stokes respiration and apnea may occur. Blood pressure and heart rate are usually normal initially, but blood pressure falls and cardiac performance deteriorates, which ultimately results in pulmonary edema and circulatory collapse unless the respiratory depression is corrected and adequate ventilation is restored promptly. Cardiac arrhythmias and conduction delay may be present. A combined respiratory-metabolic acidosis occurs, owing to retained CO_2 (hypercapnea) and to lactic acid formed during anaerobic glycolysis. Acidosis may be severe if large amounts of salicylates have also been ingested. Death may occur.

TREATMENT OF PROPOXYPHENE OVERDOSAGE: Attention should be directed first to establishing a patent airway and to restoring ventilation. Mechanically assisted ventilation, with or without oxygen, may be required, and positive-pressure respiration may be desirable if pulmonary edema is present. The narcotic antagonist naloxone will markedly reduce the degree of respiratory depression and should be administered promptly, preferably intravenously, 0.4 to 0.8 mg, and carefully repeated as necessary at 20- to 30-minute intervals.

The duration of action of the antagonist may be brief. If no response is observed after 10 mg of naloxone have been administered, the diagnosis of propoxyphene toxicity should be questioned. (Nalorphine and levallorphan may be used if naloxone is not available, but these agents are not as satisfactory as naloxone.)

Blood gases, pH, and electrolytes should be monitored in order that acidosis and any electrolyte disturbance present may be corrected promptly. Acidosis, hypoxia, and generalized CNS depression predispose to the development of cardiac arrhythmias. Ventricular fibrillation or cardiac arrest may occur and necessitate the full complement of cardiopulmonary resuscitation (CPR) measures. Respiratory acidosis rapidly subsides as ventilation is restored and hypercapnea eliminated, but lactic acidosis may require intravenous bicarbonate for prompt correction.

Electrocardiographic monitoring is essential. Prompt correction of hypoxia, acidosis, and electrolyte disturbance (when present) will help prevent these cardiac complications and will increase the effectiveness of agents administered to restore normal cardiac function.

In addition to the use of a narcotic antagonist, the patient may require careful titration with an anticonvulsant to control convulsions. Analeptic drugs (for example, caffeine or amphetamine) should not be used because of their tendency to precipitate convulsions.

General supportive measures, in addition to oxygen, include, when necessary, intravenous fluids, vasopressor-inotropic compounds, and, when infection is likely, anti-infective agents.

Gastric lavage may be useful, and activated charcoal can adsorb a significant amount of ingested propoxyphene. Dialysis is of little value in poisoning due to propoxyphene. Efforts should be made to determine whether other agents, such as alcohol, barbiturates, tranquilizers, or other CNS depressants, were also ingested, since these increase CNS depression as well as cause specific toxic effects.

SYMPTOMS OF ACETAMINOPHEN OVERDOSAGE: Symptoms of massive overdosage with acetaminophen may include nausea, vomiting, anorexia, and abdominal pain, beginning shortly after ingestion and lasting for a period of 12 to 24 hours.

Evidence of liver damage is usually delayed, appearing during the next 24 to 48 hours. However, early recognition may be difficult since early symptoms may be mild and nonspecific. After the initial symptoms, the patient may feel less ill; however, laboratory determinations are likely to show a rapid rise in liver enzymes including serum transaminase and lactic dehydrogenase and bilirubin. In case of serious hepatotoxicity, jaundice, coagulation defects, hypoglycemia, encephalopathy, and coma may follow.

Death from hepatic failure may result 3 to 7 days after overdosage.

TREATMENT OF ACETAMINOPHEN OVERDOSAGE: Acetaminophen is rapidly absorbed, and efforts to remove the drug from the body should not be delayed. Subject to primary consideration of the CNS-depressant effects of propoxyphene, gastric lavage should be instituted.

Activated charcoal is probably ineffective unless administered almost immediately after acetaminophen ingestion.

Neither forced diuresis nor hemodialysis appear to be effective in removing acetaminophen. Since acetaminophen in overdose may have an antidiuretic effect and may produce renal damage, administration of fluids should be carefully monitored to avoid overload.

It has been reported that mercaptamine (cysteamine) or other thiol compounds may protect against liver damage if given soon after overdosage (8-10 hours). N-acetyl-cysteine is under investigation as a less toxic alternative to mercaptamine, which may cause anorexia, nausea, vomiting, and drowsiness. A Poison Control Center should be consulted for the latest antidote information.

Clinical and laboratory evidence of hepatotoxicity may be delayed up to one week. Acetaminophen plasma levels and half-life may be useful in assessing the likelihood of hepatotoxicity. Serial hepatic enzyme determinations are also recommended.

How Supplied: Wygesic® tablets, containing 65 mg propoxyphene hydrochloride and 650 mg acetaminophen per scored tablet, are supplied in bottles of 100 and 500 tablets and in Redipak® Strip Pack, Wyeth®, boxes of 100 (10 strips of 10).

PATIENT INFORMATION
YOUR PRESCRIPTION FOR A PROPOXYPHENE PRODUCT

Your doctor has chosen to prescribe a medicine containing propoxyphene. Propoxyphene is used for the relief of pain.

It is important that you read and understand the information in this leaflet. If you have any questions, ask your doctor or pharmacist.

GENERAL CAUTIONS

OTHER DRUGS: Combinations of excessive doses of propoxyphene, alcohol, and tranquilizers may be dangerous. Make sure your doctor knows that you are taking tranquilizers, sleep aids, antidepressant drugs, antihistamines, or any other drugs that make you sleepy. The use of these drugs with propoxyphene increases their sedative effects and may lead to overdosage symptoms, including death (see "Overdosage" below).

ALCOHOL: Heavy use of alcohol with propoxyphene is hazardous and may lead to overdosage symptoms (see "Overdosage" below). THEREFORE, LIMIT YOUR INTAKE OF ALCOHOL WHILE TAKING PROPOXYPHENE.

REGULAR ACTIVITIES: Propoxyphene may cause drowsiness or impair your mental and/or physical abilities; therefore, use caution when driving a vehicle or operating dangerous machinery. DO NOT perform any hazardous task until you have seen your response to this drug.

PREGNANCY: Do not take propoxyphene or other drugs during pregnancy unless your doctor knows you are pregnant and specifically recommends their use.

CHILDREN: Propoxyphene is not recommended for use in children under 12 years of age.

ALLERGY: Do not take propoxyphene if you have had an allergic reaction to any drug containing propoxyphene.

DEPENDENCE: Propoxyphene, when taken in higher-than-recommended doses over a long period of time, has produced physical and psychologic dependence (a craving for the drug or an inability to function normally without the drug).

Side Effects: When propoxyphene is taken as directed, side effects are infrequent. Among those reported are drowsiness, dizziness, nausea, and vomiting. If these effects occur, some of them may go away if you lie down.

Less frequently reported side effects include constipation, abdominal pain, skin rashes, light-headedness, headache, weakness, minor visual disturbances, and feelings of elation or discomfort.

If one of these side effects occurs and becomes severe, contact your physician.

Dosage: Your prescription should be taken as directed by your doctor. Do not exceed the maximum daily dose shown below. Always follow dosage recommendations carefully—do *not* increase the dosage without your doctor's approval. If you miss a dose of the drug, do *not* take twice as much the next time.

Propoxyphene HCl with Acetaminophen
65 mg   650 mg
MAXIMUM DAILY DOSE
6

Overdosage: An overdosage of propoxyphene, alone or in combination with other drugs, including alcohol, may cause weakness, difficulty in breathing, confusion, anxiety, and more severe drowsiness and dizziness. Extreme overdosage may lead to unconsciousness and death.

In *any* suspected overdosage situation, GET EMERGENCY HELP IMMEDIATELY.

Other Information: This medication was prescribed specifically for you. It should not be given to anyone else even if his/her condition appears to be similar to yours. If you want more information or have any questions about propoxyphene, ask your doctor or pharmacist. There is a more detailed leaflet available from them. You may need their help in understanding parts of the detailed leaflet.

Keep this and all other drugs out of the reach of children.

Shown in Product Identification Section, page 445

WYMOX®   R
[wi'moks]
(amoxicillin)
Capsules and Oral Suspension

How Supplied: Capsules contain 250 mg or 500 mg amoxicillin as the trihydrate, and are supplied in bottles of 100 and 500 for the 250 mg capsules and bottles of 50 and 500 for the 500 mg capsules. WYMOX Oral Suspension is supplied in bottles of powder for reconstitution. When reconstituted with water, it will make a palatable suspension containing amoxicillin trihydrate equivalent to 125 mg or 250 mg amoxicillin per 5 ml.

For prescribing information write to Professional Service, Wyeth Laboratories, Box 8299,

WYTENSIN®
[wi-ten'sin]
(guanabenz acetate)

Description: Wytensin (guanabenz acetate), an antihypertensive agent for oral administration, is an aminoguanidine derivative, 2,6-dichlorobenzylideneaminoguanidine acetate.
It is an odorless, white to off-white, crystalline substance, sparingly soluble in water and soluble in alcohol, with a molecular weight of 291.14. Each tablet of Wytensin is equivalent to 4 mg or 8 mg of free guanabenz base.
Wytensin is available as 4 or 8 mg tablets for oral administration.

Clinical Pharmacology: Wytensin is an orally active central alpha-2 adrenergic agonist. Its antihypertensive action appears to be mediated via stimulation of central alpha adrenergic receptors, resulting in a decrease of sympathetic outflow from the brain at the bulbar level to the peripheral circulatory sytem.

PHARMACOKINETICS
In human studies, about 75% of an orally administered dose of Wytensin is absorbed and metabolized with less than 1% of unchanged drug recovered from the urine. Peak plasma concentrations of unchanged drug occur between two and four hours after a single oral dose. The average half-life for Wytensin is about 6 hours. The site or sites of metabolism of Wytensin and the consequences of renal or hepatic insufficiency on excretion of Wytensin or its metabolites have not been determined. The effect of meals on the absorption of Wytensin has not been studied.

PHARMACODYNAMICS
The onset of the antihypertensive action of Wytensin begins within 60 minutes after a single oral dose and reaches a peak effect within two to four hours. The effect of an acute single dose is reduced appreciably six to eight hours after administration, and blood pressure approaches baseline values within 12 hours of administration.
The acute antihypertensive effect of Wytensin occurs without major changes in peripheral resistance, but its chronic effect appears to be a decrease in peripheral resistance. A decrease in blood pressure is seen in both the supine and standing positions without alterations of normal postural mechanisms, so that postural hypotension has not been observed. Wytensin decreases pulse rate by about 5 beats per minute. Cardiac output and left ventricular ejection fraction are unchanged during long-term therapy.
With effective control of blood pressure in hypertensive patients, Wytensin has not demonstrated any significant effect on glomerular filtration rate, renal blood flow, renal sodium or potassium excretion, renal concentrating ability, body fluid volume, or body weight. In clinical trials of six to thirty months, hypertensive patients whose blood pressure was controlled with Wytensin lost one to four pounds of body weight. The mechanism of this weight loss has not been established. Tolerance to the antihypertensive effect of Wytensin has not been observed.
During long-term administration of Wytensin, there is a small decrease in serum cholesterol and total triglycerides without any change in the high-density lipoprotein fraction. Plasma norepinephrine, serum dopamine beta-hydroxylase and plasma renin activity are decreased during chronic administration of Wytensin. No changes in serum electrolytes, uric acid, blood-urea nitrogen, calcium, or glucose have been observed.
Wytensin and hydrochlorothiazide have been shown to have at least partially additive effects in patients not responding adequately to either drug alone.

Indications and Usage: Wytensin (guanabenz acetate) is indicated in the treatment of hypertension. It may be employed alone or in combination with a thiazide diuretic.

Contraindication: Wytensin is contraindicated in patients with a known sensitivity to the drug.

Precautions:
1. Sedation: Wytensin causes sedation or drowsiness in a large fraction of patients. When Wytensin is used with centrally active depressants, such as phenothiazines, barbiturates, and benzodiazepines, the potential for additive sedative effects should be considered.
2. Patients with vascular insufficiency: Wytensin, like other antihypertensive agents, should be used with caution in patients with severe coronary insufficiency, recent myocardial infarction, cerebrovascular disease, or severe hepatic or renal failure.
3. Rebound: Sudden cessation of therapy with central alpha agonists like Wytensin may rarely result in "overshoot" hypertension and more commonly produces an increase in serum catecholamines and subjective symptomatology.

INFORMATION FOR PATIENTS
Patients who receive Wytensin should be advised to exercise caution when operating dangerous machinery or driving motor vehicles until it is determined that they do not become drowsy or dizzy from the medication. Patients should be warned that their tolerance for alcohol and other CNS depressants may be diminished. Patients should be advised not to discontinue therapy abruptly.

LABORATORY TESTS
In clinical trials, no clinically significant laboratory test abnormalities were identified during either acute or chronic therapy with Wytensin. Tests carried out included CBC, urinalysis, electrolytes, SGOT, bilirubin, alkaline phosphatase, uric acid, BUN, creatinine, glucose, calcium, phosphorus, total protein, and Coombs' test. During long-term administration of Wytensin, there was a small decrease in serum cholesterol and total triglycerides without any change in the high-density lipoprotein fraction. In rare instances an occasional nonprogressive increase in liver enzymes has been observed. However, no clinical evidence of hepatic disease has been found.

DRUG INTERACTIONS
Wytensin has not been demonstrated to cause any drug interactions when administered with other drugs, such as digitalis, diuretics, analgesics, anxiolytics, and antiinflammatory or antiinfective agents, in clinical trials. However, the potential for increased sedation when Wytensin is administered concomitantly with CNS depressant drugs should be noted.

DRUG/LABORATORY TEST INTERACTIONS
No laboratory test abnormalities were identified with the use of Wytensin.

CARCINOGENESIS, MUTAGENESIS, IMPAIRMENT OF FERTILITY
No evidence of carcinogenic potential emerged in rats during a two-year oral study with Wytensin at doses up to 9.5 mg/kg/day, i.e., about 10 times the maximum recommended human dose. In the Salmonella microsome mutagenicity (Ames) test system, Wytensin at 200-500 mcg per plate or at 30-50 mcg/ml in suspension gave dose-related increases in the number of mutants in one (TA 1537) of five *Salmonella typhimurium* strains with or without inclusion of rat liver microsomes. No mutagenic activity was seen at doses up to those which inhibit growth in the eukaryotic microorganism, *Schizosaccharomyces pombe*, or in Chinese hamster ovary cells at doses up to those which were lethal to the cells in culture. In another eukaryotic system, *Saccharomyces cerevisiae*, Wytensin produced no activity in an assay measuring induction of repairable DNA damage. Reproductive studies showed a decreased pregnancy rate in rats administered high oral doses (9.6 mg/kg) of Wytensin, suggesting an impairment of fertility. The fertility of treated males (9.6 mg/kg) may also have been affected, as suggested by the decreased pregnancy rate of their mates, even though the females received Wytensin only during the last third of pregnancy.

PREGNANCY
Pregnancy Category C
WYTENSIN MAY HAVE ADVERSE EFFECTS ON THE FETUS WHEN ADMINISTERED TO PREGNANT WOMEN. A teratology study in mice has indicated a possible increase in skeletal abnormalities when Wytensin is given orally at doses of 3 to 6 times the maximum recommended human dose of 1.0 mg/kg. These abnormalities, principally costal and vertebral, were not noted in similar studies in rats and rabbits. However, increased fetal loss has been observed after oral Wytensin administration to pregnant rats (14 mg/kg) and rabbits (20 mg/kg). Reproductive studies of Wytensin in rats have shown slightly decreased live-birth indices, decreased fetal survival rate, and decreased pup body weight at oral doses of 6.4 and 9.6 mg/kg. There are no adequate, well-controlled studies in pregnant women. Wytensin should be used during pregnancy only if the potential benefit justifies the potential risk to the fetus.

NURSING MOTHERS
Because no information is available on the excretion of Wytensin in human milk, it should not be administered to nursing mothers.

PEDIATRIC USE
The safety and effectiveness of Wytensin in children less than 12 years of age have not been demonstrated. Therefore, its use in this age group cannot be recommended at this time.

Adverse Reactions: The incidence of adverse effects has been ascertained from controlled clinical studies conducted in the United States and is based on data from 859 patients who received Wytensin for up to 3 years. There is some evidence that the side effects are dose-related.
The following table shows the incidence of adverse effects occurring in at least 5% of patients in a study comparing Wytensin (guanabenz acetate) to placebo, at a starting dose of 8 mg b.i.d.

Adverse Effect	Placebo (%) n=102	Wytensin (%) n=109
Dry mouth	7	28
Drowsiness or sedation	12	39
Dizziness	7	17
Weakness	7	10
Headache	6	5

In other controlled clinical trials at the starting dose of 16 mg/day in 476 patients, the incidence of dry mouth was slightly higher (38%) and that of dizziness was slightly lower (12%), but the incidence of the most frequent adverse effects was similar to the placebo-controlled trial. Although these side effects were not serious, they led to discontinuation of treatment about 15% of the time. In more recent studies using an initial dose of 8 mg/day in 274 patients, the incidence of drowsiness or sedation was lower, about 20%.
Other adverse effects were reported during clinical trials with Wytensin but are not clearly distinguished from placebo effects and occurred with a frequency of 3% or less:
Cardiovascular—chest pain, edema, arrhythmias, palpitations.
Gastrointestinal—nausea, epigastric pain, diarrhea, vomiting, constipation, abdominal discomfort.
Central nervous system—anxiety, ataxia, depression, sleep disturbances.
ENT disorders—nasal congestion.
Eye disorders—blurring of vision.
Musculoskeletal—aches in extremities, muscle aches.
Respiratory—dyspnea.
Dermatologic—rash, pruritus.
Urogenital—urinary frequency, disturbances of sexual function.
Other—gynecomastia, taste disorders.

Drug Abuse and Dependence: No reported dependence or abuse has been associated with the administration of Wytensin.

Continued on next page

Wyeth—Cont.

Overdosage: Accidental ingestion of Wytensin caused hypotension, somnolence, lethargy, irritability, miosis, and bradycardia in two children aged one and three years. Gastric lavage and administration of pressor substances, fluids, and oral activated charcoal resulted in complete and uneventful recovery within 12 hours in both patients. Since experience with accidental overdosage is limited, the suggested treatment is mainly supportive while the drug is being eliminated from the body and until the patient is no longer symptomatic. Vital signs and fluid balance should be carefully monitored. An adequate airway should be maintained and, if indicated, assisted respiration instituted. There are no data available on the dialyzability of Wytensin.

Dosage and Administration: Dosage with Wytensin should be individualized. A starting dose of 4 mg twice a day is recommended, whether Wytensin is used alone or with a thiazide diuretic. Dosage may be increased in increments of 4 to 8 mg per day every one to two weeks, depending on the patient's response. The maximum dose studied to date has been 32 mg twice daily, but doses as high as this are rarely needed.

How Supplied: Wytensin® (guanabenz acetate) Tablets, Wyeth®, are available in the following dosage strengths:

4 mg, NDC 0008-0073, white, five-sided tablet with a raised "W" and a "4" under the "W" on one side and "WYETH 73" on reverse side, in bottles of 100 and 500 tablets.

8 mg, NDC 0008-0074, white, five-sided tablet with a raised "W" and an "8" under the "W" on one side and "WYETH 74" on scored reverse side, in bottles of 100 tablets.

The appearance of these tablets is a trademark of Wyeth Laboratories.

Keep bottles of Wytensin Tablets tightly closed.
Dispense in tight containers.
Protect from light.

Shown in Product Identification Section, page 445

EDUCATIONAL MATERIAL

Films—Slides—Videos
The Wyeth Film and Audiovisual Catalog, listing films, audiovisual and slide programs available through the Wyeth Film Library or on loan through the local Wyeth representative, can be obtained by writing Professional Service, Wyeth Laboratories. Box 8299, Philadelphia, PA 19101.

Products are cross-indexed by

generic and chemical names

in the

YELLOW SECTION

Important Notice

Before prescribing or administering

any product described in

PHYSICIANS' DESK REFERENCE

always consult the PDR Supplement for

possible new or revised information

Youngs Drug Products Corp.
P.O. Box 385
865 CENTENNIAL AVENUE
PISCATAWAY, NJ 08854

Sole Distributors for products manufactured by
HOLLAND-RANTOS COMPANY, INC.

KORO-FLEX®
ARCING SPRING DIAPHRAGM

Composition: Improved contouring spring; natural latex diaphragm.

Action and Uses: Half-moon shape when compressed, facilitates introduction along vaginal floor beyond cervix for easy, correct placement.

Administration and Dosage: As directed.

How Supplied: Available as a kit containing trial sizes of KOROMEX CRYSTAL CLEAR GEL and KOROMEX CONTRACEPTIVE CREAM (Stock #136). Also available in a set (Plastic Compact Bag) containing regular size KOROMEX CRYSTAL CLEAR GEL, trial size KOROMEX CONTRACEPTIVE CREAM. AND Jelly/Cream Applicator (stock #536). Sizes 60 mm.–95 mm. at gradations of 5 mm.

KOROMEX® COIL SPRING DIAPHRAGM

Action and Uses: The KOROMEX COIL SPRING DIAPHRAGM is made of pure latex rubber. The cadmium plated coil spring is tension-adjusted. The diaphragm is used with KOROMEX II CONTRACEPTIVE JELLY or KOROMEX II CONTRACEPTIVE CREAM for conception control.

How Supplied: Available as a kit containing trial sizes of KOROMEX CRYSTAL CLEAR GEL and KOROMEX CONTRACEPTIVE CREAM (Stock #131). Also available in a set (plastic compact bag) containing an INTRODUCER, regular size KOROMEX CRYSTAL CLEAR GEL, trial size KOROMEX CONTRACEPTIVE CREAM and Jelly/Cream Applicator (Stock #541). Sizes 50 mm.–95 mm. at gradations of 5 mm.

KOROMEX
CONTRACEPTIVE CREAM   OTC

(See PDR For Nonprescription Drugs)

KOROMEX® CONTRACEPTIVE   OTC
CRYSTAL CLEAR GEL

(See PDR For Nonprescription Drugs)

KOROMEX® CONTRACEPTIVE   OTC
FOAM

(See PDR For Nonprescription Drugs)

KOROMEX   OTC
CONTRACEPTIVE JELLY

(See PDR For Nonprescription Drugs)

KOROSTATIN VAGINAL TABLETS
[koro-stat' in]
(nystatin vaginal tablets)
Nystatin

Description: KOROSTATIN nystatin Vaginal Tablets U.S.P. is an oblong shaped vaginal tablet, each containing 100,000 units Nystatin, U.S.P. Nystatin is a polyene antibiotic of undetermined structural formula that is obtained from Streptomyces noursei.

Clinical Pharmacology: Nystatin is an antifungal antibiotic which is both fungistatic and fungicidal in vitro against a wide variety of yeasts and yeast-like fungi. It probably acts by binding to sterols in the cell membrane of the fungus with a resultant change in membrane permeability allowing leakage of intracellular components. It exhibits no appreciable activity against bacteria or trichomonads.

No detectable blood levels are obtained following topical or vaginal application.

Indications and Usage: Nystatin Vaginal Tablets are effective for the local treatment of vulvovaginal candidiasis (moniliasis). The diagnosis should be confirmed, prior to therapy by KOH smears and/or cultures. Other pathogens commonly associated with vulvovaginitis (Trichomonas and Haemophilus vaginalis) do not respond to nystatin and should be ruled out by appropriate laboratory methods.

Contraindications: This preparation is contraindicated in patients with a history of hypersensitivity to any of its components.

Precautions:
General
Discontinue treatment if sensitization or irritation is reported during use.

Laboratory Tests
If there is a lack of response to Nystatin Vaginal Tablets, appropriate microbiological studies should be repeated to confirm the diagnosis and rule out other pathogens, before instituting another course of antimycotic therapy.

Usage in Pregnancy
No adverse effects or complications have been attributed to nystatin in infants born to women treated with nystatin vaginal tablets.

Adverse Reactions: Nystatin U.S.P. is virtually nontoxic and nonsensitizing and is well tolerated by all age groups, even on prolonged administration. Rarely, irritation or sensitization may occur (see PRECAUTIONS).

Dosage and Administration: The usual dosage is one tablet (100,000 units nystatin) daily for two weeks. The tablets should be deposited high in the vagina by means of the applicator. "Instructions for the Patient" are printed on each package.

Even though symptomatic relief may occur within a few days, treatment should be continued for the full course.

It is important that therapy be continued during menstruation. Adjunctive measures such as therapeutic douches are unnecessary and sometimes inadvisable. Cleansing douches may be used by nonpregnant women, if desired, for esthetic purposes.

How Supplied: In packages of 15 and 30 individual foil wrapped tablets with applicator. Refrigeration is not required for these tablets. KOROSTATIN Vaginal Tablets should be stored below 30°C. (86°F.).

NYLMERATE II® DOUCHE   OTC
[nil' mer-rate]
CONCENTRATE

(See PDR For Nonprescription Drugs)

TRIPLE X

(See PDR For Nonprescription Drugs)

Products are

listed alphabetically

in the

PINK SECTION.

SECTION 7
Diagnostic Product Information

This section is intended to reflect the increased use of diagnostic products in the practice of medicine. It is intended for the use of all practitioners and is included in this format to make it easier for the physician to find the information which he seeks about these products.

Products described in PHYSICIANS' DESK REFERENCE® which have official package circulars must be in full compliance with Food & Drug Administration regulations pertaining to labeling for prescription drugs. These regulations require that for PDR copy, "indications and usage, dosages, routes, methods, and frequency and duration of administration, description, clinical pharmacology and supply and any relevant warnings, hazards, contraindications, adverse reactions, potential for drug abuse and dependence, overdosage and precautions" must be the *"same in language and emphasis"* as the approved labeling for the product. FDA regards the words *"same in language and emphasis"* as requiring VERBATIM use of the approved labeling providing such information. Furthermore, the information in the approved labeling that is emphasized by the use of type set in a box or in capitals, bold face, or italics must be given the same emphasis in PDR. For products which do not have official package circulars, the Publisher emphasized to manufacturers the necessity of describing such products comprehensively so that physicians would have access to all information essential for intelligent and informed prescribing. In organizing and presenting the material in PHYSICIANS' DESK REFERENCE, the Publisher is providing all the information made available to PDR by manufacturers.

This edition of PHYSICIANS' DESK REFERENCE contains the latest product information available at press-time. During the year, however, new and revised information about the products described herein may be furnished us. This information will be published in the PDR Supplement. Therefore, before prescribing or administering any product described in the following pages, you should first consult the PDR Supplement.

In presenting the following material to the medical profession, the Publisher is not necessarily advocating the use of any product listed.

Abbott Laboratories
DIAGNOSTICS DIVISION
ABBOTT PARK 6C4, DEPT. 49B
ABBOTT PARK, IL 60064

THYPINONE® Injection
[thī′ pĭ-nōn]
(Protirelin)

Description: Chemically, Thypinone (protirelin) is identified as 5-oxo-L-prolyl-L-histidyl-L-proline amide. It is a synthetic tripeptide which is believed to be structurally identical with the naturally-occurring thyrotropin-releasing hormone produced by the hypothalamus.

Thypinone (protirelin) is supplied as 1 ml ampules. Each ampule contains 500 mcg protirelin in a sterile non-pyrogenic isotonic saline solution having a pH of 5.5 to 7.5. In addition, each ampule contains sodium chloride, 9.0 mg, water for injection, and hydrochloric acid as needed to adjust pH. Thypinone (protirelin) is intended for intravenous administration.

Clinical Pharmacology: Pharmacologically, Thypinone increases the release of the thyroid stimulating hormone (TSH) from the anterior pituitary. Prolactin release is also increased. It has recently been observed that approximately 65% of acromegalic patients tested with a rise in circulating growth hormone levels; the clinical significance is as yet not clear. Following intravenous administration, the mean plasma half-life of protirelin in normal subjects is approximately five minutes. TSH levels rise rapidly and reach a peak at 20 to 30 minutes. The decline in TSH levels takes place more slowly, approaching baseline levels after approximately three hours.

Indications and Usage: Thypinone (protirelin) is indicated as an adjunctive agent in the diagnostic assessment of thyroid function. As an adjunct to other diagnostic procedures, testing with Thypinone may yield useful information in patients with pituitary or hypothalamic dysfunction.

Thypinone (protirelin) is indicated as an adjunct to evaluate the effectiveness of thyrotropin suppression with a particular dose of T4 in patients with nodular or diffuse goiter. A normal TSH baseline value and a minimal difference between the 30 minute and baseline response to Thypinone (protirelin) injection would indicate adequate suppression of the pituitary secretion of TSH.

Thypinone (protirelin) may be used, adjunctively, for adjustment of thyroid hormone dosage given to patients with primary hypothyroidism. A normal or slightly blunted TSH response, thirty minutes following Thypinone (protirelin) injection, would indicate adequate replacement therapy.

Warnings: Transient changes in blood pressure, either increases or decreases, frequently occur immediately following administration of Thypinone (protirelin). BLOOD PRESSURE SHOULD THEREFORE BE MEASURED BEFORE THYPINONE (PROTIRELIN) IS ADMINISTERED AND AT FREQUENT INTERVALS DURING THE FIRST 15 MINUTES AFTER ITS ADMINISTRATION.

Increases in systolic pressure (usually less than 30 mm Hg) and/or increases in diastolic pressure (usually less than 20 mm Hg) have been observed more frequently than decreases in pressure. These changes have not ordinarily persisted for more than 15 minutes nor have they required therapy. MORE SEVERE DEGREES OF HYPERTENSION OR HYPOTENSION WITH OR WITHOUT SYNCOPE, HAVE BEEN REPORTED IN A FEW PATIENTS.

To minimize the incidence and/or severity of hypotension, THE PATIENT SHOULD BE SUPINE BEFORE, DURING AND AFTER THYPINONE (PROTIRELIN) ADMINISTRATION. IF A CLINICALLY IMPORTANT CHANGE IN BLOOD PRESSURE OCCURS, MONITORING OF BLOOD PRESSURE SHOULD BE CONTINUED UNTIL IT RETURNS TO BASELINE LEVELS. THYPINONE (PROTIRELIN) SHOULD NOT BE ADMINISTERED TO PATIENTS IN WHOM MARKED RAPID CHANGES IN BLOOD PRESSURE WOULD BE DANGEROUS UNLESS THE POTENTIAL BENEFIT CLEARLY OUTWEIGHS THE POTENTIAL RISK.

Precautions: Thyroid hormones reduce the TSH response to Thypinone (protirelin). Accordingly, patients in whom Thypinone is to be used diagnostically should be taken off liothyronine (T3) approximately seven days prior to testing and should be taken off thyroid medications containing levothyroxine (T4), e.g., desiccated thyroid, thyroglobulin, or liotrix, at least 14 days before testing. Hormone therapy is NOT to be discontinued when the test is used to evaluate the effectiveness of thyroid suppression with a particular dose of T4 in patients with nodular or diffuse goiter, or for adjustment of thyroid hormone dosage given to patients with primary hypothyroidism.

Chronic administration of levodopa has been reported to inhibit the TSH response to Thypinone. It is not advisable to withdraw maintenance doses of adrenocortical drugs used in the therapy of known hypopituitarism. Several published reports have shown that prolonged treatment with glucocorticoids at physiologic doses has no significant effect on the TSH response to thyrotropin releasing hormone, but that the administration of pharmacologic doses of steroids reduces the TSH response.

Therapeutic doses of acetylsalicylic acid (2 to 3.6 g/day) have been reported to inhibit the TSH response to protirelin. The ingestion of acetylsalicylic acid caused the peak level of TSH to decrease approximately 30% as compared to values obtained without acetylsalicylic acid administration. In both cases, the TSH peak occurred 30 minutes post-administration of protirelin.

Pregnancy
Reproduction studies have been performed in rats and rabbits. At doses 1-½ and 6 times the human dose, there was an increase in the number of resorption sites in the pregnant rabbit. There are no studies in pregnant women which bear on the safety of Thypinone for the human fetus. Thypinone should be used in pregnant women only when clearly needed.

Adverse Reactions: Side effects have been reported in about 50% of the patients tested with Thypinone (protirelin). Generally, the side effects were minor, have occurred promptly, and have persisted for only a few minutes following injection.

Cardiovascular Reactions
MARKED CHANGES IN BLOOD PRESSURE INCLUDING BOTH HYPERTENSION AND HYPOTENSION WITH OR WITHOUT SYNCOPE, HAVE BEEN REPORTED IN A SMALL NUMBER OF PATIENTS.

Endocrine Reaction
Breast enlargement and leakage in lactating women for up to two or three days.

Other Reactions
Headaches, sometimes severe, and transient amaurosis in patients with pituitary tumors; nausea; urge to urinate; flushed sensation; lightheadedness; bad taste; abdominal discomfort; headache; and dry mouth. Less frequently reported were: anxiety; sweating; tightness in the throat; pressure in the chest; tingling sensation; and drowsiness.

Dosage and Administration: Thypinone (protirelin) is intended for intravenous administration with the patient in the supine position. The drug is administered as a bolus over a period of 15 to 30 seconds, with the patient remaining supine for an additional 15 minutes during which time the blood pressure is monitored.

Dosage
Adults: 500 mcg. Doses between 200 and 500 mcg have been used. 500 mcg is considered the optimum dose to give the maximum response in the greatest number of patients. Doses greater than 500 mcg are unlikely to elicit a greater TSH response.

Children age 6 to 16 years: 7 mcg/kg body weight up to 500 mcg.

Infants and children up to 6 years: Experience is limited in this age group; doses of 7 mcg/kg have been administered.

One blood sample for TSH assay should be drawn immediately prior to the injection of Thypinone, and a second sample should be obtained 30 minutes after injection.

The TSH response to Thypinone (protirelin) is reduced by repetitive administration of the drug. Accordingly, if the Thypinone test is repeated, an interval of seven days before testing is recommended.

Elevated serum lipids may interfere with the TSH assay. Thus, fasting (except in patients with hypopituitarism) or a low-fat meal is recommended prior to the test.

Interpretation of Test Results: Interpretation of the TSH response to Thypinone (protirelin) requires an understanding of thyroid-pituitary-hypothalamic physiology and knowledge of the clinical status of the individual patient.

Because the TSH test results may vary with the laboratory, the physician should be familiar with the TSH assay method used and the normal range for the laboratory performing the assay.

TSH response 30 minutes after Thypinone administration in normal subjects and in patients with hyperthyroidism and hypothyroidism are presented in Figure 1. The diagnoses were established prior to the administration of Thypinone on the basis of the clinical history, physical examination, and the results of other thyroid and/or pituitary function tests. (See below)

Among the normal euthyroid subjects, women and children were found to have higher levels of TSH at 30 minutes than men. Among the patients with hyperthyroidism or primary (thyroidal), secondary (pituitary) or tertiary (hypothalamic) hypothyroidism, no significant differences in TSH levels by age or sex were found.

Normal: Baseline TSH levels of less than 10 microunits/ml (μU/ml) were observed in 97% of euthyroid normal subjects tested. Thirty minutes after Thypinone (protirelin), the serum TSH increased by 2.0 μU/ml or more in 95% of euthyroid subjects.

Hyperthyroidism: All hyperthyroid patients tested had baseline TSH levels of less than 10 μU/ml and a rise of less than 2 μU/ml 30 minutes after Thypinone.

Primary (thyroidal) hypothyroidism: The diagnosis of primary hypothyroidism is frequently supported by finding clearly elevated baseline TSH levels; 93% of patients tested had levels above 10

Figure 1
Mean ± One Standard Deviation of TSH levels Observed at Baseline and 30 Minutes After Thypinone (μU/ml)

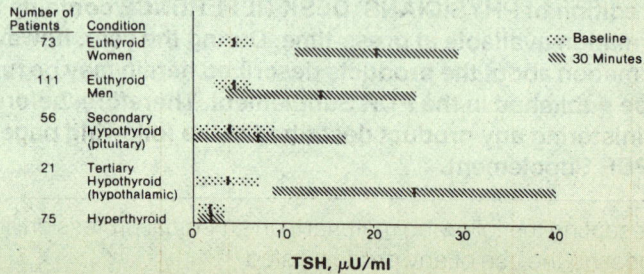

Number of Patients	Condition
73	Euthyroid Women
111	Euthyroid Men
56	Secondary Hypothyroid (pituitary)
21	Tertiary Hypothyroid (hypothalamic)
75	Hyperthyroid

TSH, μU/ml

μU/ml. Thypinone (protirelin) administration to these patients generally would not be expected to yield additional useful information. Ninety-four percent of patients with primary hypothyroidism given Thypinone in clinical trials responded with a rise in TSH of 2.0 μU/ml or greater; since this response is also found in normal subjects, Thypinone testing does not differentiate primary hypothyroidism from normal.

Secondary (pituitary) and tertiary (hypothalamic) hypothyroidism: In the presence of clinical and other laboratory evidence of hypothyroidism, the finding of a baseline TSH level less than 10 μU/ml should suggest secondary or tertiary hypothyroidism. In this situation, a response to Thypinone of less than 2 μU/ml suggests secondary hypothyroidism since this response was observed in about 60% of patients with secondary hypothyroidism and only approximately 5% of patients with tertiary hypothyroidism. A TSH response to Thypinone greater than 2 μU/ml is not helpful in differentiating between secondary and tertiary hypothyroidism since this response was noted in about 40% of the former and about 95% of the latter. Establishing the diagnosis of secondary or tertiary hypothyroidism requires a careful history and physical examination along with appropriate tests of anterior pituitary and or target gland function. The Thypinone test should not be used as the only laboratory determinant for establishing these diagnoses.
[See table above].

How Supplied: As 1 ml ampules—boxes of 5 (NDC 0074-8971-05). Each ml contains Thypinone (protirelin) 0.50 mg (500 mcg), sodium chloride 9.0 mg for isotonicity, and pH adjusted with hydrochloric acid.

Adria Laboratories Inc.
5000 POST ROAD
DUBLIN, OH 43017

CHYMEX®
[kī' mĕx]
(bentiromide)

Description: CHYMEX® (bentiromide) is a peptide which carries the marker PABA (para-aminobenzoic acid). CHYMEX is formulated as a 7.5 ml solution containing 500 mg bentiromide in a 40% propylene glycol solution. CHYMEX is a screening test for the assessment of exocrine pancreatic insufficiency. The chemical names of CHYMEX are benzoic acid, 4-[[2-(benzoylamino)-3-(4-hydroxyphenyl)-1-oxopropyl] amino]-,(S)-; or (S)-p-(α-Benzamido-p-hydroxyhydrocinnamamido) benzoic acid, or N-benzoyl-L-tyrosyl-p-aminobenzoic acid. Bentiromide is practically insoluble in water, dilute acid and ether; sparingly soluble in ethanol; and freely soluble in dilute alkali. The pKa is 5.4. The empirical formula of bentiromide is $C_{23}H_{20}N_2O_5$, the molecular weight is 404.4 and the structural formula is as follows:

Clinical Pharmacology: Following oral administration of CHYMEX, the agent is selectively cleaved by pancreatic chymotrypsin with the liberation of PABA (para-aminobenzoic acid). PABA is readily absorbed through the intestinal mucosa under normal conditions of absorption, conjugated primarily by the liver and rapidly excreted in the urine. PABA is detected in the urine using the Smith modification of the Bratton-Marshall method of analysis for arylamines (see References). This method is suitable for detecting both conjugated and unconjugated arylamines. It is not known whether CHYMEX or PABA crosses either the placental barrier or the blood brain barrier. Under conditions of normal exocrine pancreatic function, normal gastric emptying, normal gut function and normal kidney function, over 50% of the PABA contained in CHYMEX (500 mg of CHYMEX contains 170 mg of PABA) appears in the urine within six hours following administration of this agent.

Indications and Usage: CHYMEX is indicated as a screening test for pancreatic exocrine insufficiency.
CHYMEX may also be used to monitor the adequacy of supplemental pancreatic therapy.

Contraindications: CHYMEX is contraindicated in individuals who have previously shown hypersensitivity to the product.

Precautions:
General—Proper use of CHYMEX requires (1) close attention to the technical details of drug administration and of urine collection, handling and assay for arylamine levels, (2) awareness that "false positive" and "false negative" results can occur (see Interpretation of Results).
Repeat dosings of this agent, if needed, should be scheduled at intervals of seven days or more to assure complete metabolism and excretion of prior doses of the drug.
In testing of diabetic patients, suitable adjustments in insulin may need to be made in order to accommodate the fasting patient.
Hypersensitivity—A single case of hypersensitivity to bentiromide has been reported (see Adverse Reactions). It is not yet possible to determine the frequency of sensitization, but no other cases have been reported in more than 6000 cases reported in the literature, in about 1000 patients studied in clinical trials, or in Japanese post-marketing experience. Following administration of bentiromide, patients should remain in a medical setting and be observed.
Information for Patients—The full text of patient information is reprinted at the end of the labeling.
Laboratory Tests—Because it has not been established whether concurrent gastrointestinal diagnostic testing interferes with the results of this test, all such testing should be conducted at least 24 hours before or after dosing with bentiromide.
Drug Interactions—PABA may compete for binding sites with methotrexate.
Assay Interactions—Drugs that are metabolized to primary arylamines may cause interference in the assay and yield a false elevation of test results. These drugs include the following: acetaminophen, phenacetin, benzocaine, chloramphenicol, lidocaine, procaine, procainamide, sulfonamides and thiazide diuretics. PABA-containing drugs such as sunscreens or certain multiple vitamin preparations may also falsely elevate test results. Drugs such as those listed above should be discontinued three days prior to the administration of bentiromide. In adults, oral pancreatic enzyme supplements should be discontinued five days prior to the administration of bentiromide. In cystic fibrotic children the time interval is reduced to one day.
Carcinogenesis, Mutagenesis, Impairment of Fertility—Long-term studies of carcinogenicity have not been performed. No effects on fertility, embryogenesis and delivery were observed in rats dosed at daily levels as high as 1000 mg/kg (100 times the human dose) during pregnancy. In rabbits this dose level was associated with a high frequency of fetal death and resorption, probably due to maternal emaciation. No maternal or embryo-fetal-toxicity occurred in rabbits treated with 500 mg/kg (50 times the human dose).
Usage in Pregnancy—Pregnancy Category B. Reproduction studies performed in rats and rabbits have revealed no evidence of impaired fertility or harm to the fetus due to CHYMEX at doses up to 100 and 50 times the human dose, respectively. There are, however, no adequate and well-controlled studies in pregnant women. Because animal reproduction studies are not always predictive of human response, this drug should be used during pregnancy only if clearly needed.
Nursing mothers—It is not known whether this drug is excreted in human milk. Because many drugs are excreted in human milk, caution should be exercised when CHYMEX is administered to a nursing woman. In rats dosed with CHYMEX at levels up to 1000 mg/kg during the perinatal period and during lactation, no effect was seen on the functional development, morphological characteristics of the offspring at weaning, behavior, sexual maturation or reproductive function of the offspring.
Pediatric Use—Safety and effectiveness in children below the age of 6 years have not been established.

Adverse Reactions: The most frequent adverse reactions are diarrhea and headache. These occur in less than one in 50 patients. Flatulence, nausea, vomiting and weakness occur rarely, in approximately 1 out of 160 patients. These side effects are transient in nature and rarely require symptomatic therapy. Acute respiratory distress and stridor, requiring symptomatic therapy, has been reported in one patient following a second dose of CHYMEX; the patient had developed coughing and choking after his first dose (see Contraindications).
Other adverse reactions reported for which a causal relationship to CHYMEX has not been established include abdominal pain, drowsiness, lightheadedness, heartburn and transient elevations of liver function tests.

Overdosage: This product is packaged in unit dose bottles and overdose is unlikely. If overdosage occurs treatment should be symptomatic.

Dosage and Administration:
Administration—CHYMEX is administered following an overnight fast. The urine is to be voided prior to administration of the drug. The drug is administered in a single 500 mg dose, followed immediately by 250 ml of water. In patients less

Continued on next page

Table 1
Characterization Based on Serum TSH Levels at Baseline and 30 Minutes after Thypinone

	Baseline Serum TSH (μU/ml)	Change of Serum TSH (μU/ml) at 30 Minutes
Euthyroidism (normal thyroid function)	10 or less (usually 6 or less; 20% have < 1.5 μU/ml)	2 or more (usually 6 to 30)
Hyperthyroidism	10 or less (usually 4 or less)	less than 2
Primary Hypothyroidism (thyroidal)	more than 10 (usually 15 to 200)	2 or more (usually 20 or more)
Secondary Hypothyroidism (pituitary)	10 or less (usually 6 or less)	less than 2 (59%) 2 to 50 (41%)
Tertiary Hypothyroidism (hypothalamic)	10 or less (often less than 2)	2 or more

Adria—Cont.

than 12 years of age, the dose should be calculated on the basis of 14 mg/kg body weight. The patient is then given another 250 ml of water at post-dosing hour 2 and should receive up to an additional 500 ml of water during the post-dosing hours 2 through 6. Drinking of water is encouraged in order to promote diuresis. A total collection of urine is obtained during 0–6 hours post-dosing. The volume of the collection is measured and a 10 ml sample is retained for analysis. The fast is broken following completion of urine collection. Should retesting with CHYMEX become necessary, subsequent administrations should be separated by intervals of at least 7 days to avoid interference of test results by prior CHYMEX dosings. In the testing of diabetic patients, suitable adjustment of insulin may need to be made in order to accommodate the fasting procedure.

Analysis of Urine—Arylamines are assayed in the urine using the Smith modification of the Bratton-Marshall test.

The analysis for urinary arylamines consists of hydrolysis of PABA conjugates to free PABA with hydrochloric acid, formation of the diazonium salt of PABA with sodium nitrite and the condensation of PABA with N- (1-naphthyl) ethylenediamine dihydrochloride (NEDA) to form a colored compound which is assayed colorimetrically (see References below).

Interpretation of Results—PABA recovery in the urine following administration of 500 mg of CHYMEX is dependent upon the chymotrypsin present in the gut. Total 6 hour post-dosing urinary arylamine recovery levels obtained in a study of healthy subjects and in patients with well-established exocrine pancreatic insufficiency are displayed in the graph below.

The distribution of PABA recovery shows that all healthy subjects with normal pancreatic function had a recovery of 50% or more; only in patients with pancreatic disease were PABA recoveries below 50%. At the same time, some of the patients with documented pancreatic insufficiency had recoveries indistinguishable from normal subjects.

The overlap of recoveries in normal and abnormal persons precludes designation of any specific value as diagnostic of abnormal pancreatic exocrine function. The smaller the urinary arylamine recovery, the greater the likelihood that the patient has diminished exocrine pancreatic function. The CHYMEX test result can be affected by gastric retention, impaired gut mucosal function, severe hepatic insufficiency, or chronic renal insufficiency. In these instances, an abnormally low recovery of urinary arylamines can be expected.

Concurrent use of drugs that result in the urinary excretion of arylamines or the concurrent use of pancreatic enzyme supplements can result in a false elevation of test values (see Assay Interactions).

A negative CHYMEX test in the face of a clinical history or other findings suggesting pancreatic exocrine insufficiency should not lead to termination of the search for a pancreatic etiology of maldigestion or other pancreatic disease. A good response to an oral pancreatic enzyme supplement would be confirmatory of a positive CHYMEX test.

How Supplied: Single dose bottles of 500 mg (NDC 0013-1803-41). The total volume per dose is 7.5 ml.

Store at room temperature.

References:
1. Bratton, A. C. and Marshall, K. A new coupling component for sulfanilamide determination. J. Biol. Chem. 1939; **128**:537–550.
2. Smith, H. Y., et al. The renal clearances of substituted hippuric acid derivatives and other aromatic acids in dog and man. J. Clin. Invest. 1945; **24**:388–404.

Information for Patients
How this Test Works:
After CHYMEX is swallowed, it is broken down by the pancreas, similarly to the way the pancreas breaks down food. After CHYMEX is broken down, a part of it goes into the urine.

CHYMEX is used to test how well your pancreas is working. Your doctor will do this by testing your urine after you take the drug. The urine is collected during a six hour period, starting with when you took the drug. Your doctor will need your help to make this an accurate test.

FOLLOW THESE INSTRUCTIONS CAREFULLY. If you don't follow instructions exactly, the test might have to be done over again.

Instructions
1. Don't eat any food after midnight before taking this test. If you have eaten anything since last night, it might change the test results.
2. Urinate before taking the drug. You should have an empty bladder. If you have already urinated this morning, this is O.K.
3. Drink the drug first, then drink a large glass of water (8 oz). You'll also be asked to drink at least one more glass of water during the six hours after dosing. This is to make sure there is plenty of urine to test.
4. Collect ALL the urine you pass for exactly six hours after taking the drug. You will be given a container for collecting the urine.

Other Drugs
If you are taking any of the following drugs they may ruin this test:
1. acetaminophen or phenacetin (these are found in aspirin substitutes that you can buy without a prescription).
2. sulfa drugs
3. "water pills" (diuretics)
4. local anesthetics, such as benzocaine and lidocaine.
5. Sunscreens and multiple vitamin preparations containing PABA (para-aminobenzoic acid) or PABA alone.

Let your doctor know which drugs you are taking, or have taken recently. These include drugs prescribed by the doctor or ones purchased without a prescription.

If you take pancreatic supplements you should have discontinued these at least five days ago in order for this test to produce useful results.

Side Effects
Some side effects such as diarrhea, headaches, nausea and vomiting have been reported with this drug. Flatulence (gas) and weakness have been reported but these are rare. If you experience *any* discomfort or unusual change let your physician know about it at once.

Products are cross-indexed by generic and chemical names in the **YELLOW SECTION**

Ames Division
Miles Laboratories, Inc.
P.O. BOX 70
ELKHART, IN 46515

[See table on next page].

N-MULTISTIX® SG
Reagent Strips

N-MULTISTIX® SG is a firm plastic strip to which are affixed nine separate reagent areas which test for specific gravity, pH, protein, glucose, ketone (acetoacetic acid), bilirubin, blood, nitrite, and urobilinogen in urine. Test results may provide information regarding the status of carbohydrate metabolism, kidney and liver function, acid-base balance and bacteriuria.

No. 2740—N-MULTISTIX® SG Reagent Strips, bottles of 100
No. 2741—MULTISTIX® SG Reagent Strips, bottles of 100

CHEK-STIX®
Urinalysis Control Strips

CHEK-STIX® Urinalysis Control Strips are Reactive Controls for Specific Gravity, pH, Protein, Glucose, Ketone (Acetoacetic Acid), Bilirubin, Blood, Nitrite and Urobilinogen for Use with Ames Visual Reagent Strips.

Each CHEK-STIX® Urinalysis Control Strip is a firm plastic strip to which are affixed six separate analyte areas. These each contain one or more natural or synthetic ingredients which, when dissolved out of the analyte areas in a measured quantity of distilled or deionized water, provide positive or defined results with Ames Visual Reagent Strips used in urinalysis.

No. 1360K—CHEK-STIX bottles of 25

DIASTIX®
Reagent Strips
KETO-DIASTIX®
Reagent Strips

DIASTIX is a clear, flexible plastic strip to which is affixed a reagent area for the quantitative, 30-second determination of glucose in urine. KETO-DIASTIX is designed for the determination of ketone and glucose in urine. Results are read by comparison with color chart (on containers): ketone in 15 seconds, glucose in 30 seconds.

No. 2806—DIASTIX Reagent Strips, plastic vials of 50.
No. 2803—DIASTIX Reagent Strips, bottles of 100.
No. 2882—KETO-DIASTIX Reagent Strips, bottles of 100.
No. 2883—KETO-DIASTIX Reagent Strips, bottles of 50.

AMES TDA®
Therapeutic Drug Assays
Fluorescent Immunoassays for the Quantitative Determination of Therapeutic Drugs in Serum

Ames TDA Tests are used to monitor patient serum drug levels. The data provided assists in establishing and maintaining serum drug levels in the therapeutic range.

Description: Ames TDA®/Therapeutic Drug Assays are a convenient series of nonradioisotopic assays for the quantitative determination of specific therapeutic drugs in serum or plasma. The series utilize a unique homogeneous substrate-labeled fluorescent immunoassay which is both easy to perform and requires no separation steps. Results can be read in any standard fluorometer. Ames TDA/Therapeutic Drug Assays are available in kits of 100 tests each.

No. 3775—Ames TDA Monoclonal Theophylline
No. 3756—Ames TDA Amikacin
No. 3770—Ames TDA Monoclonal Gentamicin
No. 3847—Ames TDA Kanamycin
No. 3849—Ames TDA Monoclonal Netilmicin
No. 3848—Ames TDA Monoclonal Sisomicin

Diagnostic Product Information

for possible revisions

No. 3771—Ames TDA Tobramycin
No. 3776—Ames TDA Carbamazepine
No. 3841—Ames TDA Ethosuximide
No. 3773—Ames TDA Phenobarbital
No. 3772—Ames TDA Phenytoin
No. 3777—Ames TDA Primidone
No. 3842—Ames TDA Valproic Acid
No. 3846—Ames TDA Disopyramide
No. 3844—Ames TDA N-acetylprocainamide
No. 3843—Ames TDA Procainamide
No. 3798—Ames TDA Quinidine

DEXTROSTIX®
Reagent Strips

Descriptions: DEXTROSTIX is a firm plastic strip with an impregnated paper area that provides a reagent system for determination of blood glucose levels with the use of one drop of fingertip or venous blood. DEXTROSTIX is a convenient 60-second test which can be read semiquantitatively against a comparison color chart on bottle label or quantitatively with the EYETONE® Reflectance Colorimeter, DEXTROMETER™ Reflectance Colorimeter, and GLUCOMETER® Reflectance Photometer.

No. 2888—DEXTROSTIX Reagent Strips, bottles of 25.
No. 2893—DEXTROSTIX Reagent Strips, individually foil-wrapped, package of 10.
No. 2895—DEXTROSTIX Reagent Strips, bottles of 100.

Product Descriptions

#5537 DEXTRO-CHEK Calibrator—For use with Ames DEXTROSTIX® Reagent Strips to calibrate either the EYETONE® Reflectance Colorimeter or the DEXTROMETER® Reflectance Colorimeter. The vial cap of this calibrator is color-coded white and each product contains two 5 mL vials of solution.

#5593 DEXTRO-CHEK® Calibrators for GLU-COMETER® Reflectance Photometer—For use in calibrating GLUCOMETER using DEXTROSTIX. Since GLUCOMETER incorporates a two point calibration procedure, this product package contains one 5 mL vial each of Low Calibrator and High Calibrator solution. The vial caps are color-coded blue (Low) and red (High).

#5591 DEXTRO-CHEK® NORMAL Control—For use with all Ames blood glucose instruments/reagent strip systems and for Ames blood glucose reagent strips read visually. The vial cap is color-coded brown and each package contains two 5 mL vials of NORMAL Control Solution. The package insert gives complete directions for use and expected ranges of the test results using the various meters and reagent strips. The ranges of test results have been individually established for each reagent strip/instrument system. This product is for use by those individuals wanting to run a control test in the euglycemic (normal) range of blood glucose values.

#5538 DEXTRO-CHEK HIGH Control—For use with all Ames reagent strip/instrument systems. For visual reading, a range of test results is only given for DEXTROSTIX. The vial cap is color-coded orange and each package contains two 5 mL vials of HIGH Control Solution. The package insert gives complete directions for use and expected ranges of test results. The ranges of test results have been individually established for each reagent strip/instrument system. This product is for use by those individuals wanting to run a control test in the hyperglycemic (elevated) range of blood glucose values.

#5589 DEXTRO-CHEK® LOW Control—For use with the DEXTROMETER/DEXTROSTIX System and the GLUCOMETER/DEXTROSTIX System. The vial cap is color-coded light green and each package contains two 5 mL vials of LOW Control Solution. The package insert gives complete directions for use and expected ranges of test results. The ranges of test results have been individually established for each reagent strip/instrument system. This product is for use by those individuals wanting to run a control test in the hypoglycemic (low) range of blood glucose values.

OTHER AVAILABLE REAGENT STRIPS AND/OR TABLETS

	Glucose	Protein	pH	Blood	Ketones	Bilirubin	Urobilinogen	Phenylketones (PKU)	Nitrite	Specific Gravity
CLINISTIX®	X									
*CLINITEST®	X									
DIASTIX®	X									
URISTIX®	X	X								
ALBUSTIX®		X								
BUMINTEST®		X								
COMBISTIX®	X	X	X							
HEMA-COMBISTIX®	X	X	X	X						
HEMASTIX®				X						
LABSTIX®	X	X	X	X	X					
KETO-DIASTIX®	X				X					
KETOSTIX®					X					
ACETEST®					X					
BILI-LABSTIX®	X	X	X	X	X	X				
BILI-LABSTIX® SG	X	X	X	X	X	X				X
ICTOTEST®						X				
MULTISTIX®	X	X	X	X	X	X	X			
MULTISTIX® SG	X	X	X	X	X	X	X			X
N-MULTISTIX®	X	X	X	X	X	X	X		X	
N-MULTISTIX® SG	X	X	X	X	X	X	X		X	X
UROBILISTIX®							X			
PHENISTIX®								X		
N-URISTIX®	X	X							X	
MICROSTIX®-NITRITE (test for Nitrite)									X	

*Available as 5-drop or 2-drop methods.

system. This product is for use by those individuals wanting to run a control test in the hypoglycemic (low) range of blood glucose values.

HEMA-CHEK®
Slide Test for the Qualitative Determination of Fecal Occult Blood with Control

HEMA-CHEK™ is a slide test for the qualitative determination of occult blood in feces. When a specimen containing occult blood is placed on the HEMA-CHEK impregnated paper, hemoglobin will come in contact with the guaiac reagent. When HEMA-CHEK Developer is added, the presence of hemoglobin is indicated by a blue color. HEMA-CHEK is a simple, convenient and economical test by which results can be obtained within thirty seconds.

No. 2592—HEMA-CHEK Slide Test, 100 Tests, 1 × 25 mL Developer and Applicators
No. 2593—HEMA-CHEK Patient Dispensing Pak, 300 Tests, 3 × 25 mL Developer, Applicators, and 100 Patient Envelopes
No. 2594—HEMA-CHEK, 1000 Tests, 10 × 25 mL Developer, and Applicators

MICROCULT®-GC
Miniaturized Culture Test for the Detection of Neisseria gonorrhoeae

MICROCULT-GC test system consists of a plastic Culture Slide containing two dry culture areas, a bottle of Rehydration Fluid, a CO_2-Generating Tablet to provide the proper environment during incubation, and Cytochrome Oxidase Detection Strips to visualize growth locations after culture. MICROCULT-GC culture tests are available in kits of 25 culture slides (#3026). Also available Ames MICROSTIX® Incubator (#3056).

MICROSTIX®-3
Reagent Strips

Description:

Test for Nitrite, total bacteria and gram negative bacteria in urine

A firm, plastic strip containing 3 separate areas—a chemical test area for immediate recognition of nitrite in urine, and two culture areas for semiquantitation of bacterial growth after 18 hours. One culture area supports total bacterial growth (both gram-positive and gram-negative) the other, only gram negative organisms. The dry-reagent microbiologic technology provides a

Continued on next page

Ames—Cont.

unique culture medium which does not require refrigeration and is more stable than agar plates. A compact MICROSTIX Incubator is available.

No. 3009 — Box of 25 foil-wrapped MICROSTIX-3 Reagent Strips, with 25 incubation pouches and 25 labels.

MICROSTIX®–CANDIDA
Miniaturized Culture Test for the Detection of Candida Species in Vaginal Specimens

MICROSTIX®-CANDIDA is a culture test which contains a selective growth medium for *Candida* species and is intended as an aid to diagnosis of *Candida*.

The MICROSTIX-CANDIDA test system consists of a firm, plastic strip to which is affixed a dry culture area, a bottle of water for rehydration, and a plastic pouch which provides a suitable environment for the strip during incubation. The test area uses a modified Nickerson's medium which contains a support nutrient along with agents to inhibit bacterial growth, and is a selective isolation medium for *Candida* species. The dry-reagent microbiological technology provides a unique culture vehicle which does not require refrigeration, and possesses much longer stability than conventional agar plates or slide tests.

No. 3004—MICROSTIX-CANDIDA culture tests are available in kits of 25 strips.

No. 3056—MICROSTIX Incubator.

N-URISTIX®
Reagent Strips
Dip-and Read Test for Nitrite, Glucose and Protein in Urine

N-URISTIX® is a firm, plastic strip to which three separate reagent areas are affixed for testing for nitrite, glucose and protein in urine. When considered along with other clinical and biochemical tests, N-URISTIX results may provide clinically meaningful information on the status of a number of metabolic and physiological states, such as kidney function, carbohydrate metabolism and urinary tract infection.

No. 2854-N-URISTIX Reagent Strips, bottles of 100 strips.

VISIDEX® II Reagent Strips
Visual Test for Glucose in Whole Blood

VISIDEX Reagent Strips are disposable plastic strips with two reagent pads for determining the concentration of glucose in whole blood. A semipermeable membrane serves as a barrier to blood cell migration into the reagent area. The reagent strip is for visual interpretation only.

No. 2660—VISIDEX II bottles of 25
No. 2661—VISIDEX II bottles of 100

AMES INSTRUMENTS

DEXTROMETER®
Reflectance Colorimeter with Digital Display

Description: DEXTROMETER quantitatively measures whole blood glucose when it is used with DEXTROSTIX® Reagent Strips. It is compact and portable for on-site glucose screening, testing, and monitoring. Operation is simple—a one-step calibration procedure is all that is necessary for routine testing. DEXTRO-CHEK™ Standard and Controls are also available to assure the user of the system's reliability.

No. 5570—DEXTROMETER Reflectance Colorimeter.

No. 5576—DEXTROMETER Rechargeable Battery Pack, (optional—must be ordered separately).

FLUOROSTAT®
Filter Fluorometer

The Ames FLUOROSTAT (Product Code No. 3799A) is a semiautomated, split-beam, ratio-recording filter fluorometer, with microprocessor-based keyboard control. The instrument can perform 10 fluoroimmunoassays (see Listings under Ames TDA® Therapeutic Drug Assays), data analysis, storage, and recording. Alpha-numeric display panel and printer are integrated with the system.

FLUOROSTAT Accessories:

Product Code No.	Description
3779	Pipettor/Diluter
3720	Plastic Cuvettes—500/Case
3721	Printer Paper—4 Rolls
3796	Ames TDM Control Sera and Diluent—12 × 5 ml
3880	Ames Netilmicin Control Serum—3 × 1 ml
3881	Ames Sisomicin Control Serum—3 × 1 ml
3882	Ames Kanamycin Control Serum—3 × 1 ml
3774	Ames Amikacin Control Serum—3 × 1 ml

FLUOROSTAT Test Capabilities USING Ames TDA® Therapeutic Drug Assays

Product Code No.		Description
		Antiasthmatics
No.	3775	Monoclonal Theophylline
		Antibiotics
No.	3756	Amikacin
No.	3770	Monoclonal Gentamicin
No.	3847	Kanamycin
No.	3849	Monoclonal Netilmicin
No.	3848	Monoclonal Sisomicin
No.	3771	Tobramycin
		Anticonvulsants
	3776	Carbamazepine
	3841	Ethosuximide
	3773	Phenobarbital
	3772	Phenytoin
	3777	Primidone
	3842	Valproic Acid
		Antiarrhythmics
	3846	Disopyramide
	3844	N-acetylprocainamide
	3843	Procainamide
	3798	Quinidine

GLUCOMETER®
Battery-Powered Reflectance Photometer with Digital Display and Built-In Timer

GLUCOMETER® quantitatively measures whole blood glucose when it is used with DEXTROSTIX® Reagent Strips. Battery-operated and with a built-in timer, it is compact and portable for on-site glucose testing and monitoring. Operation is simple, with easy calibration procedures using either the DEXTRO-CHEK® Calibrators or Calibration Chips.

No. 5580—GLUCOMETER Reflectance Photometer (4 1.5 V AA Alkaline Batteries; Operating Manual; one pkg. Calibration Chips, one Wash Bottle; Leatherette Carrying Case)

OPTIMATE™ Alpha
Automated Fluorometer/Photometer

The Ames OPTIMATE Alpha system (Product Code No. 6700) is a fully automated, microprocessor-based bench-top analyzer consisting of a single cabinet. This single-unit system is preprogrammed to perform immunoassays in the fluorescence, absorbance, and turbidimetric modes for quantitating serum levels of therapeutic and addictive drugs, enzymes, metabolites, specific proteins, and hormones, as well as blood chemistry values. In addition, the OPTIMATE Alpha system can be operator programmed for performing user-selected assays.

OPTIMATE Alpha Test Capabilities
Preprogrammed Ames TDA substrate-labeled fluorescence immunoassays:

Product Code No.	Description
6718	Monoclonal Theophylline
6712	Amikacin
6710	Monoclonal Gentamicin
6734	Kanamycin
6736	Monoclonal Netilmicin
6735	Monoclonal Sisomicin
6711	Tobramycin
6716	Carbamazepine
6722	Ethosuximide
6715	Phenobarbital
6713	Phenytoin
6714	Primidone
6723	Valproic Acid
6733	Disopyramide
6724	N-acetylprocainamide
6725	Procainamide
6717	Quinidine
6726	IgA
6727	IgG
6729	IgM

Preprogrammed absorbance mode assays:
Description
Acetaminophen*
Amphetamine*
Barbiturate (serum)*
Barbiturate (urine)*
Benzodiazepine (serum)*
Benzodiazepine Metabolite (urine)*
Cannabinoid*
Cocaine Metabolite*
Methadone*
Methaqualone*
Opiates*
Phencyclidine
Propoxyphene*
Tricyclic Antidepressants*
Plus 23 routine blood chemistries
*Manufactured by Syva Company

Preprogrammed turbidimetric assays:
C-reactive protein

Operator-programmable absorbance mode assays:
Lidocaine
Propranolol
Methotrexate

SERALYZER®
Reflectance Photometer and Solid Phase Reagent Strips

The SERALYZER® System for blood chemistries and serum theophilline determinations consists of a Reflectance Photometer, a series of solid-phase Reagent Strips and Test Modules, plus an Accessory Kit for specimen preparation.

No. 5110—SERALYZER Instrument Package: (includes No. 5186 below) SERALYZER Reflectance Photometer, Voltage Regulator, Workstation, Power Cord, Hex Wrenches (2), Strip Guide Clamps (2), Spare Fuses (2), and Operating Manual

No. 5186—SERALYZER Accessory Kit: DipStat™ Diluter, PIP-DIL Pipette Tips (200), MLA® Pipette, MLA Pipette Tips (1,000), Module Rack, and Foot Switch

Reagent Strips

2701	Seralyzer Glucose Reagent Strips—bottles of 25
2711	Seralyzer BUN Reagent Strips—bottles of 25
2712	Seralyzer Uric Acid Reagent Strips—bottles of 25
2713	Seralyzer LDH Reagent Strips—bottles of 25
2729	Seralyzer T. Bilirubin Reagent Strips—bottles of 25
2715	Seralyzer Cholesterol Reagent Strips—bottles of 25
2719	Seralyzer Creatinine Reagent Strips—bottles of 25
2721	Seralyzer CK Reagent Strips—bottles of 25
2718	Seralyzer Hemoglobin Reagent Strips—bottles of 50
2716	Seralyzer Triglycerides Reagent Strips—bottles of 25
2714	Seralyzer AST/SGOT Reagent Strips—bottles of 25
2723	Seralyzer ALT/SGPT Reagent Strips—bottles of 25
2728	Seralyzer Theophylline Reagent Strips—bottles of 25
2730	Seralyzer Theophylline Reagent Strips—bottles of 25 Test Pack (1 vial Hi Calibrator, 1 Vial Lo Calibrator, 1 vial Control, 1 pad Report Forms)

Ayerst Laboratories
Division of American Home Products Corporation
685 THIRD AVE.
NEW YORK, NY 10017

FACTREL®
[făc′ trel]
(gonadorelin hydrochloride)
Synthetic Luteinizing Hormone Releasing Hormone (LH-RH)
DIAGNOSTIC USE ONLY

Caution: Federal law prohibits dispensing without prescription.

Description: An agent for use in evaluating hypothalamic-pituitary gonadotropic function. FACTREL (gonadorelin hydrochloride) injectable is available as a sterile lyophilized powder for reconstitution and administration by subcutaneous or intravenous routes.

Chemical Name: 5-oxo-L-prolyl-L-histidyl-L-tryptophyl -L- seryl -L- tyrosyl-glycyl -L- leucyl-L-arginyl-L-prolyl glycinamide hydrochloride [See formula above].

FACTREL is $C_{55}H_{75}N_{17}O_{13}$·HCl, as the mono- or dihydrochloride, or their mixture. The gonadorelin base has a molecular weight of 1182.33. It is a white powder, soluble in alcohol and water, hygroscopic and moisture-sensitive, and stable at room temperature. The synthetic decapeptide, FACTREL, has a chemical composition and structure identical to the natural hormone, identified from porcine or ovine hypothalami.

Each vial of FACTREL contains 100 or 500 mcg gonadorelin as the hydrochloride, with 100 mg lactose, U.S.P. Each ampul of sterile diluent contains 2% benzyl alcohol and Water for Injection, U.S.P.

Clinical Pharmacology: FACTREL has been shown to have gonadotropin-releasing effects upon the anterior pituitary. The range for normal baseline LH levels, as determined from the literature, is 5–25 mIU/ml in postpubertal males, and postpubertal and premenopausal females. The standard used is the Second International Reference Preparation—HMC. This range may not correspond in each laboratory performing the assay since the concentration of LH in normal individuals varies with different assay methods. The normal responses to FACTREL analyzed from the results of clinical studies included:
(1) LH peak mIU/ml
   (highest LH value post-FACTREL administration)
(2) Maximum LH increase (mIU/ml)
   (peak LH value—LH baseline value)
(3) LH percent response
   $\frac{\text{peak LH—baseline LH}}{\text{baseline LH}} \times 100\%$
(4) Time to peak (minutes)
   (time required to reach LH peak value)

Normal adult subjects were shown to have these LH responses following FACTREL administration by subcutaneous or intravenous routes.

I. MALE ADULTS:
 A) Subcutaneous Administration
  The results are based on 18 tests in males between the ages of 18–42 years, inclusive:
  (1) LH peak: mean 60.3 ± 26.2 mIU/ml
   100% ≥ 24.0 mIU/ml
   90% ≥ 32.8 mIU/ml
  (2) Maximum LH increase: mean 46.7 ± 20.8 mIU/ml
   100% ≥ 12.3 mIU/ml
   90% ≥ 20.9 mIU/ml
  (3) LH percent response: mean 437 ± 243%
   range: 66–1853%
   90% ≥ 188%
  (4) Time to peak: mean 34 ± 13 min.
 B) Intravenous Administration
  The results are based on 26 tests in males between the ages of 19–58 years, inclusive:
  (1) LH peak: mean 63.8 ± 40.3 mIU/ml
   100% ≥ 12.6 mIU/ml
   90% ≥ 26.0 mIU/ml
  (2) Maximum LH increase: mean 51.3 ± 35.2 mIU/ml
   100% ≥ 7.4 mIU/ml
   90% ≥ 14.8 mIU/ml
  (3) LH percent response: mean 481 ± 184%
   range: 67–2139%
   90% ≥ 142%
  (4) Time to peak: mean 27 ± 14 min.

In males older than 50 years, the LH baseline and peak levels tend to be higher; however, the maximum LH increases do not differ in regard to age.

II. FEMALE ADULTS:
 A) Subcutaneous Administration
  The results are based on 38 tests in females between the ages of 19–36 years, inclusive:
  (1) LH peak: mean 67.9 ± 27.5 mIU/ml
   100% ≥ 12.5 mIU/ml
   90% ≥ 39.0 mIU/ml
  (2) Maximum LH increase: mean 52.8 ± 26.4 mIU/ml
   100% ≥ 7.5 mIU/ml
   90% ≥ 23.8 mIU/ml
  (3) LH percent response: mean 374 ± 221%
   range: 108–981%
   90% ≥ 185%
  (4) Time to peak: mean 71.5 ± 49.6 min.
 B) Intravenous Administration
  The results are based on 31 tests in females between the ages of 20–35 years inclusive:
  (1) LH peak: mean 57.6 ± 36.7 mIU/ml
   100% ≥ 20.0 mIU/ml
   90% ≥ 24.6 mIU/ml
  (2) Maximum LH increase: mean 44.5 ± 31.8 mIU/ml
   100% ≥ 7.5 mIU/ml
   90% ≥ 16.2 mIU/ml
  (3) LH percent response: mean 356 ± 282%
   range: 60–1300%
   90% ≥ 142%
  (4) Time to peak: mean 36 ± 24 min.

The FACTREL (gonadorelin hydrochloride) tests on which the normal female responses are based were performed in the early follicular phase of the menstrual cycle (Days 1–7).

In menopausal and postmenopausal females, the baseline LH levels are elevated and the maximum LH increases are exaggerated when compared with the premenopausal levels.

Patients with clinically diagnosed or suspected pituitary and/or hypothalamic dysfunction were often shown to have subnormal or no LH responses following FACTREL administration. For example, in clinical tests of 6 patients with known postpubertal panhypopituitarism, and 11 patients with Prader-Willi Syndrome, 100% showed subnormal responses or no rise in LH. Subnormal responses to the FACTREL test also were observed in 21 (95%) of 22 patients with prepubertal panhypopituitarism. In 19 patients with Sheehan Syndrome, 16 (84%) had a subnormal response. In the FACTREL test in 44 patients with Kallmann Syndrome, 33 (77%) had subnormal LH responses.

Indications and Usage: FACTREL as a single injection is indicated for evaluating the functional capacity and response of the gonadotropes of the anterior pituitary. This single injection test does not measure pituitary gonadotropic reserve for which more prolonged or repeated administration may be required. The LH response is useful in testing patients with suspected gonadotropin deficiency, whether due to the hypothalamus alone or in combination with anterior pituitary failure. FACTREL is also indicated for evaluating residual gonadotropic function of the pituitary following removal of a pituitary tumor by surgery and/or irradiation. In clinical studies to date, however, the single injection test has not been useful in differentiating pituitary disorders from hypothalamic disorders. The FACTREL test can be performed concomitantly with other post-treatment evaluations.

The results of the FACTREL test complement the clinical examination and other laboratory tests used to confirm or substantiate hypogonadotropic hypogonadism.

In cases where there is a normal response, it indicates the presence of functional pituitary gonadotropes. The single injection test does not measure pituitary gonadotropic reserve.

Contraindications: Hypersensitivity to gonadorelin hydrochloride or any of the components.

Precautions: Although allergic and hypersensitivity reactions have been observed with other polypeptide hormones, to date no such reactions have been encountered following the administration of a single 100 mcg dose of FACTREL. Antibody formation has been rarely reported after chronic administration of large doses of FACTREL.

The FACTREL test should be conducted in the absence of other drugs which directly affect the pituitary secretion of the gonadotropins. These would include a variety of preparations which contain androgens, estrogens, progestins, or glucocorticoids. The gonadotropin levels may be transiently elevated by spironolactone, minimally elevated by levodopa, and suppressed by oral contraceptives and digoxin. The response to FACTREL may be blunted by phenothiazines and dopamine antagonists which cause a rise in prolactin.

Pregnancy Category B. Reproduction studies have been performed in mice, rats, and rabbits at doses up to 50 times the human dose, and have revealed no evidence of harm to the fetus due to FACTREL. There are, however, no adequate and well-controlled studies in pregnant women. Because animal reproduction studies are not always predictive of human response, this drug should be used during pregnancy only if clearly needed.

Appropriate precautions should be taken because the effects of LH-RH on the fetus and developing offspring have not been adequately evaluated. Repetitive, high doses of FACTREL may cause luteolysis and inhibition of spermatogenesis.

Adverse Reactions: Systemic complaints such as headaches, nausea, lightheadedness, abdominal discomfort and flushing have been reported rarely following administration of 100 mcg of FACTREL (gonadorelin hydrochloride). Local swelling, occasionally with pain and pruritus, at the injection

Continued on next page

Ayerst—Cont.

site may occur if FACTREL is administered subcutaneously. Local and generalized skin rash have been noted after chronic subcutaneous administration.

Overdosage: FACTREL has been administered parenterally in doses up to 3 mg BID for 28 days without any signs or symptoms of overdosage. In case of overdosage or idiosyncrasy, symptomatic treatment should be administered as required.

Dosage and Administration: Adults: 100 mcg dose, subcutaneously or intravenously. In females for whom the phase of the menstrual cycle can be established, the test should be performed in the early follicular phase (Days 1–7).

Test Methodology: To determine the status of the gonadotropin secretory capacity of the anterior pituitary, a test procedure requiring seven venous blood samples for LH is recommended.

PROCEDURE:
1. Venous blood samples should be drawn at -15 minutes and immediately prior to FACTREL administration. The LH baseline is obtained by averaging the LH values of the two samples.
2. Administer a bolus of 100 mcg of FACTREL subcutaneously or intravenously.
3. Draw venous blood samples at 15, 30, 45, 60, and 120 minutes after administration.
4. Blood samples should be handled as recommended by the laboratory that will determine the LH content. It must be emphasized that the reliability of the test is directly related to the inter-assay and intra-assay reliability of the laboratory performing the assay.

Interpretation of Test Results: Interpretation of the LH response to FACTREL requires an understanding of the hypothalamic-pituitary physiology, knowledge of the clinical status of the individual patient, and familiarity with the normal ranges and the standards used in the laboratory performing the LH assays.

Figures 1 through 4 represent the LH response curves after FACTREL administration in normal subjects. The normal LH response curves were established between the 10th percentile (B line) and 90th percentile (A line) of all LH responses in normal subjects analyzed from the results of clinical studies. LH values are reported in units of mIU/ml and time is displayed in minutes. Individual patient responses should be plotted on the appropriate curve. A subnormal response in patients is defined as three or more LH values which fall below the B line of the normal LH response curve. In cases where there is a blunted or borderline response, the FACTREL (gonadorelin hydrochloride) test should be repeated.

The FACTREL (gonadorelin hydrochloride) test complements the clinical assessment of patients with a variety of endocrine disorders involving the hypothalamic-pituitary axis. In cases where there is a normal response, it indicates the presence of functional pituitary gonadotropes. The single injection test does not determine the pathophysiological cause for the subnormal response and does not measure pituitary gonadotropic reserve.

How Supplied: LYOPHILIZED POWDER—in single-dose vials containing 100 mcg (NDC 0046-0507-05) and 500 mcg (NDC 0046-0509-05) gonadorelin as the hydrochloride with 100 mg lactose, U.S.P. Each vial is accompanied by one ampul containing 2 ml sterile diluent of 2% benzyl alcohol in Water for Injection, U.S.P.

Directions: Store at room temperature (approximately 25°C).
Reconstitute 100 mcg vial with 1.0 ml of the accompanying sterile diluent.
Reconstitute 500 mcg vial with 2.0 ml of the accompanying sterile diluent.
Prepare solution immediately before use.
After reconstitution, store at room temperature and use within 1 day.
Discard unused reconstituted solution and diluent.
Diagnostic Method of Use Patent 3,947,569
Shown in Product Identification Section, page 404

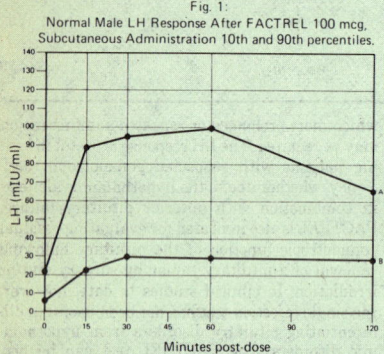

Fig. 1:
Normal Male LH Response After FACTREL 100 mcg, Subcutaneous Administration 10th and 90th percentiles.

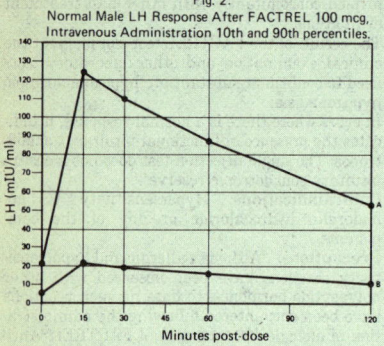

Fig. 2:
Normal Male LH Response After FACTREL 100 mcg, Intravenous Administration 10th and 90th percentiles.

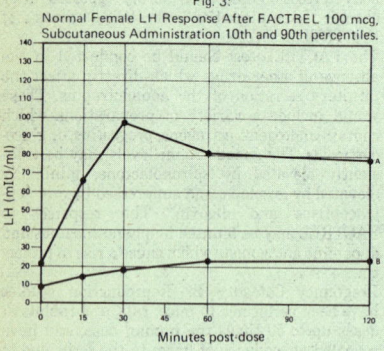

Fig. 3:
Normal Female LH Response After FACTREL 100 mcg, Subcutaneous Administration 10th and 90th percentiles.

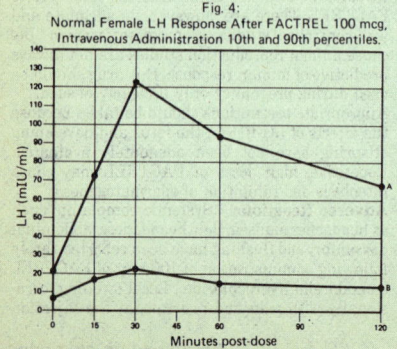

Fig. 4:
Normal Female LH Response After FACTREL 100 mcg, Intravenous Administration 10th and 90th percentiles.

PEPTAVLON®
[pĕp-tăv'lon]
Brand of pentagastrin
A diagnostic agent for evaluation of gastric acid secretory function.

CAUTION: Federal law prohibits dispensing without prescription.

Description:
Chemical name: N-t-butyloxycarbonyl-B-alanyl-L-tryptophyl-L-methionyl-L-aspartyl-L-phenylalanyl amide.

Structural formula:

[Structural formula of pentagastrin]

Pentagastrin is a synthetic pentapeptide containing the carboxyl terminal tetrapeptide, the active portion found in all natural gastrins. Pentagastrin is a colorless crystalline solid. It is soluble in dimethylformamide and dimethylsulfoxide; it is almost insoluble in water, ethanol, ether, benzene, chloroform, and ethyl acetate.

Actions: PEPTAVLON (pentagastrin) contains the C-terminal tetrapeptide responsible for the actions of the natural gastrins and, therefore, acts as a physiologic gastric acid secretagogue. The recommended dose of 6 mcg/kg subcutaneously produces a peak acid output which is reproducible when used in the same individual.

PEPTAVLON stimulates gastric acid secretion approximately ten minutes after subcutaneous injection, with peak responses occurring in most cases twenty to thirty minutes after administration. Duration of activity is usually between sixty and eighty minutes.

Indications: PEPTAVLON (pentagastrin) is used as a diagnostic agent to evaluate gastric acid secretory function. It is useful in testing for:

Anacidity:—as a diagnostic aid in patients with suspected pernicious anemia, atrophic gastritis, or gastric carcinoma.

Hypersecretion:—as a diagnostic aid in patients with suspected duodenal ulcer or postoperative stomal ulcer, and for the diagnosis of Zollinger-Ellison tumor.

PEPTAVLON (pentagastrin) is also useful in determining the adequacy of acid-reducing operations for peptic ulcer.

Contraindications: Hypersensitivity or idiosyncrasy to pentagastrin.

Warnings: *Use in Pregnancy*—The use of pentagastrin in pregnancy has NOT been studied, and the benefit of administration of the drug must be weighed against any possible risk to the mother and/or fetus.

Use in Children—There are insufficient data to recommend the use of, or establish a dosage, in children.

****

In amounts in excess of the recommended dose, pentagastrin may cause inhibition of gastric acid secretion.

Precautions: Use with caution in patients with pancreatic, hepatic, or biliary disease. Like gastrin, pentagastrin could, in some cases, have the physiologic effect of stimulating pancreatic enzyme and bicarbonate secretion, as well as biliary flow.

Adverse Reactions: Pentagastrin causes fewer and less severe cardiovascular and other adverse reactions than histamine or betazole. The majority of reactions to pentagastrin are related to the gastrointestinal tract.

The following reactions associated with the use of pentagastrin have been reported.

Gastrointestinal: abdominal pain, desire to defecate, nausea, vomiting, borborygmi, blood-tinged mucus

Cardiovascular: flushing, tachycardia

Central Nervous System: dizziness, faintness or lightheadedness, drowsiness, sinking feeling, transient blurring of vision, tiredness, headache

Allergic and Hypersensitivity Reactions: May occur in some patients.

Miscellaneous: shortness of breath, heavy sensation in arms and legs, tingling in fingers, chills, sweating, generalized burning sensation, warmth, pain at site of injection, bile in collected specimens

Dosage and Administration: Adults: 6

mcg/kg subcutaneously. Effect begins in about ten minutes; peak response usually occurs in twenty to thirty minutes. (For discussion of the test and explicit directions, consult Baron, J.H.: Gastric Function Tests, in Wastell, C.: Chronic Duodenal Ulcer, New York, Appleton-Century-Crofts, 1972, pp. 82-114.)

Note: Data are inadequate to recommend the use of, or establish a dosage, in children.

Overdosage: In case of overdosage or idiosyncrasy, symptomatic treatment should be administered as required.

How Supplied: PEPTAVLON—In 2 ml ampuls. Each ml contains 0.25 mg (250 mcg) pentagastrin. Also contains 0.88% sodium chloride, and Water for Injection U.S.P. The pH is adjusted with ammonium hydroxide and/or hydrochloric acid. Cartons of 10 (NDC 0046-3290-10).

Clinical Studies:

Gastric Acid Secretion: Peak gastric output in mEq/hr caused by subcutaneous injection of 6 mcg/kg pentagastrin does not differ significantly from that caused by the standard subcutaneous injection of the histamine acid phosphate dose used in the augmented histamine test (40 mcg/kg). For example, in 25 normal volunteers, pentagastrin produced an average peak acid output of 28.4 mEq/hr compared with 24.7 mEq/hr by histamine. In 45 patients with duodenal ulcer, or suspected duodenal ulcer, pentagastrin produced an average peak gastric acid output of 39.7 mEq/hr compared with 33.7 mEq/hr by histamine. In 18 patients with gastric ulcer, or suspected gastric ulcer, pentagastrin produced an average peak acid output of 17.4 mEq/hr compared with 19.4 mEq/hr by histamine. The overall mean for peak acid secretion by pentagastrin was 24.8 mEq/hr compared with 22.6 mEq/hr by histamine. No biochemical abnormality which might indicate specific organ toxicity has been encountered following the administration of pentagastrin.

Boehringer Mannheim Diagnostics, Inc.
Bio-Dynamics Division
9115 HAGUE ROAD
INDIANAPOLIS, IN 46250

CHEMSTRIP bG®
[*kim' strip bee-jee'*]
BLOOD GLUCOSE TEST
Test Strips for Semi-Quantitative Determination of Glucose in Whole Blood

Summary and Explanation: CHEMSTRIP bG is a sensitive and specific test strip which facilitates accurate semi-quantitative determination of blood glucose within 2 minutes.

CHEMSTRIP bG is a glucose test strip with 2 separate test zones whose different reagent concentrations optimize sensitivity and colorimetric accuracy of semi-quantitative values from 20 mg/dl to 800 mg/dl. A wide range of test values permits wide use of CHEMSTRIP bG—for *stat* semi-quantitative assays of hypo- and hyperglycemia in neonatal, surgical, and cardiac care, as well as in emergency diagnosis of coma, mass screening of metabolic status, monitoring of diabetes mellitus and in home blood glucose monitoring programs.

Specimen Collection and Preparation: CHEMSTRIP bG is free from interference when used with fresh capillary blood. It is specific for D-glucose in whole blood and nonreactive to fructose, lactose, galactose, and pentose sugars. Hematocrit values between 30–70% have no significant effect, and neither physiologic concentrations of uric or ascorbic acid, nor therapy with heparin, EDTA or the usual plasma expanders, affect test results with CHEMSTRIP bG.

Procedure for *In Vitro* Diagnostic Use: Two-minute test procedure with CHEMSTRIP bG requires only 3 steps: (1) Place a large enough drop of whole blood on the reagent area to cover both test zones completely. (2) After 60 seconds, wipe off the blood with a dry cotton ball and then rewipe the strip 2 more times. **Do not use water**; unlike other strips, CHEMSTRIP bG needs no washing. (3) After another 60 seconds, read test results by comparing test-zone colors with the vial label's color values for 20, 40, 80, 120, 180, and 240 mg/dl. (For colors **darker** than those for 240 mg/dl, wait an extra minute before reading 400 or 800 mg/dl.) The 8 distinct, precalibrated color values facilitate reproducible reading and permit practical estimation of intermediate values.

How Supplied: Nonbreakable aluminum vials of 25 test strips, moisture-protected by drying agent in vial cap. Cat. No. 00501. Vial of 50 test strips with calibration strip included, may be read visually or may be used with Accu-chek bG blood glucose meter. Cat. No. 00503.

Complete self-testing system also available. Kit includes 25 test strips, lancets, cotton balls, alcohol wipes, illustrated "How-to-Use" card and diabetic information guide. Cat. No. 00505.

Ordering/Pricing/Technical Information: Call (317) 845-2000 or toll-free (800) 428-4674.

CHEMSTRIP®
[*kim' strip*]
URINE TESTING SYSTEM
Dip-and-Read Test Strips for Nitrite-pH-Protein-Glucose-Ketones-Urobilinogen-Bilirubin-Blood-Leukocytes in Urine

Summary and Explanation: CHEMSTRIP is a uniquely constructed test strip of inert plastic to which a nylon mesh bonds, without glue, 1 to 9 reagent papers to determine nitrite, pH, protein, glucose, ketones, urobilinogen, bilirubin, blood and leukocytes in urine. The nylon mesh holds each reagent paper in place, protects it and promotes rapid and even urine-diffusion in each complete test area. To prevent the "run-over" phenomenon, certain test papers also have an inert absorbent paper between the reagent paper and the plastic strip.

[See table above].

CHEMSTRIPS are packaged in an aluminum vial with a tight-fitting cap which contains a drying agent. Each CHEMSTRIP is stable and ready for use when removed from the vial. No additional equipment or instrumentation is required.

Specimen Collection and Preparation: CHEMSTRIPS may be used on any freshly voided urine specimen or on urines collected under special conditions, such as first-morning specimens and postprandial urines. The urine must be collected in a clean container and should be tested as soon as possible after collection (do not centrifuge). It is of particular importance to use fresh urine to obtain the best results with the test for urine bilirubin because this compound is very unstable when exposed to room temperature and daylight. If testing cannot be performed within an hour after collection, the specimen should be refrigerated immediately at 2 to 8° C and returned to room temperature before testing. Mix thoroughly before use.

Procedure for *In Vitro* Diagnostic Use. For convenience, all values on the strip may be read at 60 seconds (during the second minute) after immersion in the urine. Color changes occurring more than 2 minutes after strip immersion are not

Chemstrip Test Parameters

	Nitrite	pH	Protein	Glucose	Ketones	Urobilinogen	Bilirubin	Blood	Leukocytes	Catalog No.	Strips Per Vial
CHEMSTRIP® 9	X	X	X	X	X	X	X	X	X	417109	100
CHEMSTRIP® 7L		X	X	X	X	X	X	X	X	417117	100
CHEMSTRIP® 6L		X	X	X	X			X	X	417126	100
CHEMSTRIP® 5L		X	X	X				X	X	417135	100
CHEMSTRIP® GP			X	X						200743	100
CHEMSTRIP® uGK				X	X					00513 or 00514	100 or 50
CHEMSTRIP® K					X					00515 or 00516	100 or 25
CHEMSTRIP® uG				X						00511	100
CHEMSTRIP® LN	X								X	417152	100

of diagnostic value. (Semi-quantitative assay of abnormally high glucose concentrations may require 4-5 minutes, however.) Color changes that occur only along the edge of the test area should be ignored. Careful removal of excess urine should eliminate this effect.

Calibration of the CHEMSTRIP during use is not required. Color blocks on vial label are previously calibrated by use of precise standards during the manufacturing process.

Ordering / Pricing / Technical Information: Call (317) 845-2000 or toll free (800) 428-4674.

C. B. Fleet Co., Inc.
4615 MURRAY PL.
LYNCHBURG, VA. 24502-2235

FLEET DETECATEST®   OTC
Home use test for determination of presence of fecal occult blood.

Fleet Detecatest contains all the necessary materials to test for occult blood at home. Included are: complete instructions regarding diet, medications, preparation of specimens, development, and reading results; three guaiac impregnated paper slides for two samples from each of three consecutive stools with Control Dots to indicate proper activity of paper and developer; Fleet Detecatest Developing Solution 2 ml.; three stool collection applicator sticks.

When a small stool sample that has blood in it is placed on the Detecatest paper, hemoglobin will come in contact with the guaiac. The addition of Fleet Detecatest Developing Solution causes oxidation of the guaiac resulting in a blue color. Reading the instructions thoroughly before beginning the test is important in performing the test and reading the results.

Important: **This test is not intended to replace a physician's diagnosis:** If a patient reports a positive test, he should be questioned concerning diet, medication intake, and testing procedures. The person should then be tested under physician's supervision.

How Supplied: One dozen test kits per case.
Is This Product OTC: Yes.
Literature Available: Yes.

IDENTIFICATION PROBLEM?
Consult PDR's
Product Identifcation Section
where you'll find over 1200
products pictured actual size
and in full color.

Helena Laboratories
1530 LINDBERGH
P.O. BOX 752
BEAUMONT, TX 77704

COLOSCREEN/VPI™
Fecal Occult Blood Test

Description: ColoScreen/VPI™ (Vegetable Peroxidase Inactivator) is a guaiac paper slide test for the detection of occult blood in stool. Positive results may be indicative of a variety of conditions, including diverticulitis, bleeding gums, ulcers, or hemorrhoids, polyps, or colorectal cancer. Dietary restrictions of certain fruits and vegetables are not required for use of the test, since it contains a vegetable peroxidase inactivator to eliminate the false positive reaction caused by these food sources. Other dietary restrictions, such as red meat and vitamin C, should be avoided during the testing period, as they may interfere with test results.

All ColoScreen/VPI™ slides contain positive and negative controls, and monitors for VPI and color development reagents.
Cat. No. 5085 Office Pack—100 patient kits with envelopes
Cat. No. 5088 Lab Pack—100 triple unit slides
Cat. No. 5089 Bulk Pack—carton of 1000 slides
Cat. No. 5086 Lab Pack—100 single slides
Cat. No. 5087 Bulk Pack—carton of 1000 single slides
Ordering/Pricing Information: (800) 231-5663

Lederle Laboratories
A Division of American Cyanamid Co.
ONE CYANAMID PLAZA
WAYNE, NJ 07470

TUBERCULIN, OLD, TINE TEST® ℞
[to-ber-cu-lĭn]

Description: The Tuberculin, Old, TINE TEST® is a sterile, simple, multiple-puncture, disposable intradermal test device for the detection of tuberculin reactivity. These convenient devices are especially useful in mass tuberculosis screening programs.

Each test unit consists of a stainless steel disc attached to a plastic handle. Projecting from the disk are four triangular-shaped prongs (tines) which are 2 mm long and approximately 4 mm apart. The tines have been mechanically dipped in a solution of Old Tuberculin, containing 7% Acacia (Gum Arabic) and 8.5% lactose as stabilizers, and then dried. The entire unit has been sterilized by Colbalt 60 irradiation. No preservative has been added. The unit is disposable and there is no need for syringes, needles, and other equipment necessary for the standard intradermal tests.

Tuberculin, Old, TINE TEST® UNITS have been standardized by clinical evaluation in human subjects to give reactions equivalent to or more potent than 5 T.U.* of standard old tuberculin administered intradermally in the Mantoux test. However, all multiple puncture-type devices must be regarded as screening tools and other appropriate diagnostic procedures such as the Mantoux test should be utilized for retesting reactors.
*U.S. (International) tuberculin units.

Clinical Pharmacology: Tuberculin deposited in the skin of tuberculin reactive individuals reacts with sensitized lymphocytes to effect the release of mediators of cellular hypersensitivity. Some of these indicators (e.g., skin reactive factor) induce an inflammatory response in the skin causing the edema and erythema characteristic of "positive" reactions.[1,2]

Indications and Usage: Tuberculin, Old, TINE TEST® is indicated to detect tuberculin-sensitive individuals. TINE TEST units are also useful in programs to determine priorities for additional testing (i.e., chest x-rays) and in epidemiological surveys to identify those areas having high levels of infection.

In clinical studies covering various geographical areas of the U.S. and all age groups, with a total of 30,588 test subjects, there were 911 (4%) false positive reactors among 26,236 subjects who were Mantoux negative, and 342 (8%) false negative reactors among 4,352 subjects who were Mantoux positive.

The frequency of repeated tuberculin tests depends on the risk of exposure of the child and on the prevalence of tuberculosis in the population group. For the pediatrician's office or outpatient clinic, an annual or biennial tuberculin test, unless local circumstances clearly indicate otherwise, is appropriate. The initial test should be done at the time of, or preceding, the measles immunization.[3] The repeated testing of uninfected individuals does not sensitize to tuberculin. Among individuals with waning sensitivity to homologous or heterologous mycobacterial antigens, however, the stimulus of a tuberculin test may "boost" or increase the size of the reaction to a second test, even causing an apparent development of sensitivity in some cases.[4]

Tuberculin testing should be done with caution in individuals with active tuberculosis. (See PRECAUTIONS).

Contraindications: There are no known contraindications for use of Tuberculin, Old, TINE TEST®. See PRECAUTIONS section for information regarding special care to be exercised for safe and effective use.

Warning: There are no known serious adverse reactions or potential safety hazards associated with the use of Tuberculin, Old, TINE TEST®. However, as with the use of any biological product, the possibility of anaphylactic reaction should be considered. See PRECAUTION section for information regarding special care to be exercised for safe and effective use.

Precautions: Tuberculin testing should be done with caution in individuals with active tuberculosis. Although activation of quiescent lesions is rare, if a patient has a history of occurrence of vesiculation and necrosis with a previous tuberculin test by any method, tuberculin testing should be avoided.

Although clinical allergy to acacia is very rare, this product contains some acacia as stabilizer and should be used with caution in patients with known allergy to this component. In this instance remedial measures for anaphylactoid reactions, including epinephrine injection (1:1000), must be available for immediate use.

Reactivity to the test may be suppressed in patients who are receiving corticosteroids or immunosuppressive agents, or those who have recently been vaccinated with live virus vaccines such as measles, mumps, rubella, polio, etc.

With a positive reaction further diagnostic procedures must be considered. These may include x-ray of the chest, microbiologic examinations of sputa and other specimens, and confirmation of the positive TINE TEST reaction (except vesiculation reactions) using the Mantoux method. In general, the TINE TEST does not need to be repeated.

Antituberculous chemotherapy should not be instituted solely on the basis of a single positive TINE TEST

When vesiculation occurs, the reaction is to be interpreted as strongly positive and a repeat test by the Mantoux method must not be attempted. Similar or more severe vesiculation with or without necrosis is likely to occur.

Pregnancy Category C. Animal reproduction studies have not been conducted with Tuberculin, Old, TINE TEST®. It is also not known whether Tuberculin, Old, TINE TEST can cause fetal harm when administered to a pregnant woman or can affect reproduction capacity. Tuberculin, Old, TINE TEST should be given to a pregnant woman only if clearly needed.

During pregnancy, known positive reactors may demonstrate a negative response to a Tuberculin TINE TEST.

Tuberculin, Old, TINE TEST® units must never be reused.

Adverse Reactions: Vesiculation (positive reaction), ulceration, or necrosis may occur at the test site in highly sensitive persons. Pain, pruritus, and discomfort at the test site may be relieved by cold packs or by topical glucocorticoid ointment or cream. Transient bleeding may be observed at a puncture site and is of no significance.

Dosage and Administration: Tuberculin, Old, TINE TEST® UNITS have been standardized by clinical evaluation in human subjects to give reactions equivalent to or more potent than 5 T.U.* of standard old tuberculin administered intradermally in the Mantoux test. However, all multiple puncture-type devices must be regarded as screening tools and other appropriate diagnostic procedures such as the Mantoux test should be utilized for retesting reactors.

The volar surface of the upper one-third of the forearm, over a muscle belly, is the preferred site. Hairy areas, and areas without adequate subcutaneous tissue, e.g., concavities over a tendon or bone should be avoided.
*U.S. (International) tuberculin units.

Alcohol, acetone, ether, or soap and water may be used to cleanse the skin. The area must be clean and thoroughly dry before application of the Tuberculin, Old, TINE TEST®.

Expose the four coated tines by removing the protective cap while holding the plastic handle. Grasp the patient's forearm firmly, since the sharp momentary sting may cause the patient to jerk his or her arm, resulting in scratching. Stretch the skin of the forearm tightly and apply the disc with the other hand. **Hold at least one second.** Release tension grip on forearm. Withdraw tine unit.

Sufficient pressure should be exerted so that the four puncture sites, and circular depression of the skin from the plastic base are visible.

Local care of the skin is not necessary.

Tuberculin, Old, TINE TEST® Unit must never be reused.

Reading Reactions. Tests should be read at 48–72 hours. Vesiculation or the extent of induration are the determining factors; erythema without induration is of no significance. Readings should be made in good light with the forearm slightly flexed. The size of the induration in millimeters should be determined by inspection, measuring, and palpation with gentle finger stroking. Identification of the application site is usually easy because of the distinct four-point pattern. The diameter of the largest single reaction around one of the puncture sites should be measured. With pronounced reactions, the areas of induration around the puncture sites may coalesce.

Interpretation:
Positive Reactions

A. Vesiculation. If vesiculation is present, the test may be interpreted as positive, in which case the management of the patient is the same as that for one classified as positive to the Mantoux test.[5]

B. Induration, 2mm or greater. The test may be interpreted as positive but further diagnostic procedures must be considered. These may include x-ray of the chest, microbiologic examination of sputa and other specimens, and confirmation of the positive TINE TEST reaction using the Mantoux Method.

Negative Reaction. Induration less than 2mm. With a negative reaction there is no need for retesting unless the person is a contact of a patient with tuberculosis or there is clinical evidence suggestive of the disease.[5]

Descriptive literature illustrating typical reactions is available upon request.

How Supplied: Tuberculin, Old, TINE TEST® is supplied as follows:
NDC 0005-2722-25 25 individual tests in a jar
NDC 0005-2722-28 100 individual tests
NDC 0005-2722-34 250 individual tests

Storage: Tuberculin, Old, TINE TEST® UNITS should be stored unrefrigerated below 30°C (86°F).

References:
1. Comstock, C.W., et al, The Tuberculin Skin Test, *Amer. Rev. Respiratory Disease* 124:356–363, 1981.
2. Burrows W., *Immunity and Hypersensitivity: Textbook of Microbiology*, 369–424, 1979.
3. Report on the Committee on the Control of Infectious Diseases. American Academy of Pediatrics, 1977.

4. Comstock, G.W., et al, The Tuberculin Skin Test, *Amer. Rev. Respiratory Disease* 104:769–775, No. 5 (Nov) 1971.
5. Committee on Diagnostic Skin Testing of the American Thoracic Society, The Tuberculin Test (Revised 1974). New York, American Lung Association, 1974.

LEDERLE LABORATORIES DIVISION
American Cyanamid Company, Pearl River, N.Y. 10965
Military Depot: NSN 6505-00-890-1534

Tine Test® PPD
[*tīne tĕst*] ℞
Tuberculin, Purified Protein Derivative

Description: THE TUBERCULIN, PURIFIED PROTEIN DERIVATIVE (PPD) TINE TEST® is a sterile, simple, multiple-puncture, disposable intradermal test device for the detection of tuberculin reactivity. These convenient devices are especially useful in mass tuberculosis screening programs.
Each test unit consists of a stainless steel disc attached to a light blue plastic handle. Projecting from the disc are four triangular-shaped prongs (tines) which are 2 mm long and approximately 4 mm apart. The tines have been mechanically dipped into a concentrated solution of PPD. The PPD concentrate is prepared by the Seibert Process[1,2] and is stabilized with seven percent acacia (gum Arabic), thirty percent dextrose and five percent glycerol. The glycerol also acts as a humectant preventing the film on the tines from becoming brittle-dry. The final PPD concentrate is standardized against U.S. Standard PPD. The tines are dipped into concentrated PPD, capped and sterilized with ethylene oxide. No preservative has been added. The TINE TEST (PPD) unit is disposable, and there is no need for syringes, needles, and other equipment necessary for the standard intradermal tests.
The Tine Test (PPD) units have been standardized by clinical evaluation in human subjects to give reactions equivalent to or more potent than 5 T.U.* of standard PPD administered intradermally in the Mantoux test. However, all multiple puncture-type devices must be regarded as screening tools and other appropriate diagnostic procedures such as the Mantoux test should be utilized for retesting reactors.
*U.S. (International) tuberculin units.
Clinical Pharmacology: Tuberculin deposited in the skin of tuberculin reactive individuals reacts with sensitized lymphocytes to effect the release of mediators of cellular hypersensitivity. Some of these indicators (e.g., skin reactive factor) induce an inflammatory response in the skin causing the edema and erythema characteristic of a "positive" reactions.[3,4]
Indications and Usage: TUBERCULIN, PURIFIED PROTEIN DERIVATIVE TINE TEST® PPD is indicated to detect tuberculin-sensitive individuals. Tine Test units are also useful in programs to determine priorities for additional testing (i.e., chest X-rays) and in epidemiological surveys to identify those areas having high levels of infection.
Data obtained from clinical studies with a total of 3,062 volunteer subjects (males and females), ranging in age from 4 to 96 years, of which 47.5% (1,443) were Mantoux positive, clearly demonstrates that TINE TEST PPD, when used as a screening test to determine tuberculin reactivity is associated with very little, if any, adverse reactivity. Other than the skin test reaction itself, slight vesication and slight ulceration were the only adverse experiences reported. The slight to mild vesication was equally divided between the two tests (TINE TEST, 54/3062, 1.78%, and PPD-T Mantoux, 55/3062, 1.81%). The slight ulceration observed with one subject at 72 hours was associated with the TINE TEST site. Of the subjects classified as positive or intermediate by PPD-T Mantoux, 93.8% were classified similarly with the TINE TEST. The results of the clinical trials revealed a 72-hour false positive rate of 10.9% and a false negative rate of 6.2%.

In clinical studies of more than 1,800 PPD-S Mantoux positive subjects only 6.3% gave negative TINE TEST PPD reactions at 72 hours; of more than 1,900 TINE TEST PPD positive tests, less than 11% gave negative Mantoux results.
The frequency of repeated tuberculin tests depends on risk of exposure of the child and on the prevalence of tuberculosis in the population group. For the pediatrician's office or outpatient clinic, an annual or biennial tuberculin test, unless local circumstances clearly indicate otherwise, is appropriate. The initial test should be done at the time of, or preceding, the measles immunization.[5] The repeated testing of uninfected individuals does not sensitize to tuberculin. Among individuals with waning sensitivity to homologous or heterologous mycobacterial antigens, however, the stimulus of a tuberculin test may "boost" or increase the size of the reaction to a second test, even causing an apparent development of sensitivity in some cases.[6] Tuberculin testing should be done with caution in individuals with active tuberculosis. (See PRECAUTIONS).
Contraindications: There are no known contraindications for use of Tuberculin, Purified Protein Derivative (PPD) TINE TEST®. See PRECAUTIONS section for information regarding special care to be exercised for safe and effective use.
Warnings: There are no known serious adverse reactions or potential safety hazards associated with the use of Tuberculin, Purified, Protein Derivative (PPD) TINE TEST®. However, as with the use of any biological product, the possibility of anaphylactic reaction should be considered. See PRECAUTION section for information regarding special care to be exercised for safe and effective use.
Precautions: Tuberculin testing should be done with caution in individuals with active tuberculosis. However, activation of quiescent lesions is rare. If a patient has a history of occurrence of vesication and necrosis with a previous tuberculin test by any method, tuberculin testing should be avoided.
Although clinical allergy to acacia is very rare, this product contains some acacia as stabilizer and should be used with caution in patients with known allergy to this component. In these instances remedial measures for anaphylactoid reactions, including epinephrine injection (1:1000), must be available for immediate use.
Reactivity to the test may be suppressed in patients who are receiving corticosteroids or immunosuppressive agents, or those who have recently been vaccinated with live virus vaccines such as measles, mumps, rubella, polio, etc.
With a positive reaction further diagnostic procedures must be considered. These may include X-ray of the chest, microbiologic examinations of sputa and other specimens, and confirmation of the positive TINE TEST reaction (except vesication reactions) using the Mantoux method. In general, the TINE TEST does not need to be repeated. Antituberculous chemotherapy should not be instituted solely on the basis of a single positive TINE TEST.
When vesication occurs, the reaction is to be interpreted as strongly positive and a repeat test by the Mantoux method must not be attempted. Similar or more severe vesication with or without necrosis is likely to occur.
Pregnancy Category C. Animal reproduction studies have not been conducted with Tuberculin, Purified Protein Derivative (PPD) TINE TEST®. It is also not known whether Tuberculin, Purified Protein Derivative (PPD) Tine Test can cause fetal harm when administered to a pregnant woman or can affect reproduction capacity. Tuberculin, Purified Protein Derivative (PPD) TINE TEST should be given to a pregnant woman only if clearly needed.
During pregnancy, known positive reactors may demonstrate a negative response to a Tuberculin (PPD) TINE TEST.
Tuberculin, Purified Protein Derivative TINE TEST® PPD units must never be reused.
Adverse Reactions: Vesication (positive reaction), ulceration, or necrosis may occur at the test site in highly sensitive persons. Pain, pruritus, and discomfort at the test site may be relieved by cold packs or by topical glucocorticoid ointment or cream. Transient bleeding may be observed at a puncture site and is of no significance.
Dosage and Administration: TUBERCULIN, OLD, TINE TEST® UNITS have been standardized by clinical evaluation in human subjects to give reactions equivalent to or more potent than 5 T.U.* of standard PPD administered intradermally in the Mantoux test. However, all multiple puncture-type devices must be regarded as screening tools and other appropriate diagnostic procedures such as the Mantoux test should be utilized for retesting reactors.
The volar surface of the upper one-third of the forearm, over a muscle belly, is the preferred site. Hairy areas, and areas without adequate subcutaneous tissue, e.g., concavities over a tendon or bone should be avoided.
*U.S. (International) tuberculin units.
Alcohol, acetone, ether, or soap and water may be used to cleanse the skin. The area must be clean and thoroughly dry before application of the TINE TEST PPD.
Expose the four coated tines by removing the protective cap while holding the plastic handle. Grasp the patient's forearm firmly, since the sharp momentary sting may cause the patient to jerk his or her arm, resulting in scratching. Stretch the skin of the forearm tightly and apply the disc with the other hand. **Hold at least one second.** Release tension grip on forearm. Withdraw tine unit. **Sufficient pressure should be exerted so that the four puncture sites, and circular depression of the skin from the plastic base are visible.**
Local care of the skin is not necessary.
TUBERCULIN, PURIFIED PROTEIN DERIVATIVE TINE TEST® PPD Unit *Must never be reused.*
Reading Reactions: Tests should be read at 48–72 hours. Vesication or the extent of induration are the determining factors; erythema without induration is of no significance. Readings should be made in good light with the forearm slightly flexed. The size of the induration in millimeters should be determined by inspection, measuring, and palpation with gentle finger stroking. Identification of the application site is usually easy because of the distinct four-point pattern. The diameter of the largest single reaction around one of the puncture sites should be measured. With pronounced reactions, the areas of induration around the puncture sites may coalesce.
Interpretation:
Positive Reactions
A. **Vesiculation.** If vesiculation is present, the test may be interpreted as positive, in which case the management of the patient is the same as that for one classified as positive to the Mantoux Test.[7]
B. **Induration, 2mm or Greater.** The test may be interpreted as positive but further diagnostic procedures must be considered. These may include X-ray of the chest, microbiologic examination of sputa and other specimens, and confirmation of the positive TINE TEST reaction using the Mantoux Method.

Negative Reaction
Induration Less Than 2mm. With a negative reaction there is no need for retesting unless the person is a contact of a patient with tuberculosis or there is clinical evidence suggestive of the disease.[7]
Descriptive literature illustrating typical reactions is available upon request.

Continued on next page

The information on each product appearing here is based on labelling effective in August, 1984 and is either the entire official brochure or an accurate condensation thereform. Information concerning all Lederle products may be obtained from the Professional Services Department, Lederle Laboratories Pearl River, New York, 10965.

Lederle—Cont.

How Supplied: TUBERCULIN, PURIFIED PROTEIN DERIVATIVE TINE TEST® PPD is supplied as follows:
2720-25 25 individual tests in a jar
2720-28 100 individual tests
Storage: Tine Test PPD Units should be stored unrefrigerated below 30° C (86° F.).

References:
1. Seibert, F.B. "Isolation and Properties of Purified Protein Derivative of Tuberculin." *Am. Rev. Tuberc.*, 30 (1934) 713.
2. Seibert, F.B., and Glenn, J.F. "Tuberculin Purified Protein Derivative—Preparation and Analysis of a Large Quantity for Standard." *Amer. Rev. Tuberc.*, 44 (1941) 9.
3. Comstock, C.W., et al, The Tuberculin Skin Test, Amer. Rev. Respiratory Disease 124:356-363, 1981.
4. Burrows, W., Immunity and Hypersensitivity: Textbook of Microbiology, 369-424, 1979.
5. Report of the Committee on the Control of Infectious Diseases. American Academy of Pediatrics, 1977.
6. Comstock, G.W., et al, The Tuberculin Skin Test, Amer. Rev. Respiratory Disease 104:769-775, No. 5 (Nov) 1971.
7. Committee on Diagnostic Skin Testing of the American Thoracic Society, The Tuberculin Test (Revised 1974). New York, American Lung Association, 1974.

Eli Lilly and Company
307 E. McCARTY ST.
INDIANAPOLIS, IN 46285

HISTAMINE PHOSPHATE ℞
[hĭs' tă-mēn fŏs' făt]
Injection, USP
For Gastric Histamine Test

Description: Histamine is a basic substance which may be obtained by decarboxylation of the amino acid histidine. It is usually administered as the stable, water-soluble acid phosphate. Two molecules of phosphoric acid are attached to each molecule of histamine.
Since the molecular weight of histamine phosphate is 307.15 and that of histamine itself is 111.15, 2.75 mg of the salt are required to obtain 1 mg of the active principle.
Actions: Histamine acts on the vascular system, smooth muscle, and exocrine glands. Histamine increases the volume and acidity of the gastric juice.
Indication: Histamine phosphate solution is intended for subcutaneous administration to test the ability of the gastric mucosa to produce hydrochloric acid.
Contraindications: The gastric histamine test is contraindicated in patients with a history of hypersensitivity to histamine products. It is contraindicated in patients with hypotension, severe hypertension, vasomotor instability, bronchial asthma (past or present), urticaria (past or present), or severe cardiac, pulmonary, or renal disease.
Warnings: Attacks of severe asthma or other serious allergic conditions may be precipitated by the administration of histamine phosphate. The possible benefit that may be derived from the gastric histamine test should be carefully weighed against the serious untoward reactions that may develop in patients with allergic diseases. Small doses by any route of administration may precipitate asthma in patients with bronchial disease. The utmost caution is advised in using histamine in such patients.
When histamine phosphate is administered, pull back on the syringe plunger before the injection is made to be sure the end of the needle is not in a blood vessel. Care should be taken to avoid accidental introduction into a vein or artery. Epinephrine, 1:1000, *should be immediately available to counteract the effects of histamine.*
Usage in Pregnancy—The safety of this agent for use during pregnancy or lactation has not been established; therefore, the benefits must be weighed against its possible hazards to the mother and child.
The physician must carefully weigh the risk/benefit ratio when considering the use of the gastric histamine test in patients with pheochromocytoma.
Precautions: Average or large doses of histamine may cause flushing, dizziness, headache, nervousness, local or generalized allergic manifestations, marked hypertension or hypotension, tachycardia, and abdominal cramps. These reactions may be alarming and are potentially dangerous. Local reactions at the site of injection may include erythema and edema. Histamine increases the acid of the gastric juice and may cause symptoms of peptic ulcer.
A large subcutaneous dose of histamine may cause severe occipital headache, blurred vision, anginal pain, a rapid drop in blood pressure, and cyanosis of the face. Overdosage may cause severe symptoms, including circulatory collapse, shock, and even death. The blood pressure and pulse should be carefully monitored during injection of histamine.
Use with caution in patients with any cardiac abnormality.
Adverse Reactions: Following the injection of an average or large dose of histamine, side effects may include such local reactions as erythema and edema and/or such systemic reactions as flushing, dizziness, headache, bronchial constriction, dyspnea, visual disturbances, faintness, syncope, urticaria, asthma, marked hypertension or hypotension, weakness, palpitation, tachycardia, nervousness, abdominal cramps, diarrhea, nausea, vomiting, metallic taste, local or generalized allergic manifestations, or collapse with convulsions.
Dosage and Administration—Gastric Histamine Test: *Histamine Test*—After the basal gastric secretion has been collected, histamine phosphate is given subcutaneously. The dose is 0.0275 mg of histamine phosphate (or 0.01 mg of the histamine base) per kg of body weight. The gastric contents are then collected in four 15-minute specimens for one hour and analyzed for volume, acidity, pH, and acid output.
Augmented Histamine Test—Initially, a suitable dose of antihistamine is administered intramuscularly, e.g., 10 mg chlorpheniramine maleate, 50 mg pyrilamine maleate, or 50 mg diphenhydramine hydrochloride.
After the conclusion of the basal secretion study, histamine phosphate is given subcutaneously in a dose of 0.04 mg/kg of body weight.
Before undertaking these procedures, the physician should thoroughly familiarize himself with the technique or methodology of performing the gastric histamine test or the augmented histamine test and with the interpretation of the results from standard reference texts.
Overdosage: Overdosage of Histamine Phosphate Injection may cause severe symptoms, including circulatory collapse, shock, and even death (see Warnings, Precautions, and Adverse Reactions). If accidental overdosage is discovered early, temporary application of a tourniquet proximally to the injection site may be tried to slow down the absorption of the drug.
Antidotes to histamine are the following:
Epinephrine hydrochloride, 0.1-0.5 ml of a 1:1000 aqueous solution, given subcutaneously in case of emergency due to severe reactions.
An antihistamine preparation may be given intramuscularly to prevent or ameliorate systemic reactions to the drug.
How Supplied: (℞) *Histamine Phosphate Injection, USP:* Vials No. 328, 2.75 mg (equivalent to 1 mg histamine base) in 5 ml, 5 ml, rubber-stoppered, in singles (10/carton) (NDC 0002-1635-01); 1 ml contains 0.55 mg histamine phosphate (equivalent to 0.2 mg histamine base), with 16 mg glycerin and 2 mg phenol. Phosphoric acid may have been added to adjust the pH. Ampoules No. 269, 2.75 mg (equivalent to 1 mg histamine base), 1 ml, in packages of 6 (NDC 0002-1622-16) and 100 (NDC 0002-1622-02).

[032482]

HISTAMINE PHOSPHATE ℞
[hĭs' tă-mēn fŏs' făt]
Injection, USP
Histamine Test for Pheochromocytoma

Description: Histamine is a basic substance which may be obtained by decarboxylation of the amino acid histidine. It is usually administered as the stable, water-soluble acid phosphate. Two molecules of phosphoric acid are attached to each molecule of histamine.
Since the molecular weight of histamine phosphate is 307.15 and that of histamine itself is 111.15, 2.75 mg of the salt are required to obtain 1 mg of the active principle.
Each ml of Ampoules No. 338, Histamine Phosphate Injection, USP (histamine test for pheochromocytoma), contains 0.275 mg histamine phosphate (equivalent to 0.1 mg histamine) and 9 mg sodium chloride.
Indication: Histamine Phosphate Injection may be used intravenously for the presumptive diagnosis of pheochromocytoma.
Contraindications: The histamine test for pheochromocytoma is contraindicated in the elderly or in the presence of severe hypertension.
Warnings: Attacks of severe asthma or other serious allergic conditions may be precipitated by the administration of histamine phosphate. The possible benefit that may be derived from the histamine test for pheochromocytoma should be carefully weighed against the serious untoward reactions that may develop in patients with severe allergic diseases.
Precautions: Average or large doses of histamine may cause flushing, dizziness, headache, nervousness, local or generalized allergic manifestations, marked hypertension or hypotension, tachycardia, and abdominal cramps. These reactions may be alarming and are potentially dangerous. Histamine increases the acid of the gastric juice and may cause symptoms of peptic ulcer. Small doses by any route of administration may precipitate asthma in patients with bronchial disease. The utmost caution is advised in using histamine in such patients and in those with a history of bronchial asthma.
Frequent checks of the blood pressure and pulse should be made during intravenous injections of histamine. If there is a dangerous fall in blood pressure, a prompt injection of epinephrine should be given.
A large dose of histamine may cause severe occipital headache, blurred vision, anginal pain, a rapid drop in blood pressure, and cyanosis of the face. Overdosage by the intravenous route may cause severe symptoms, including vasomotor collapse, shock, and even death.
Adverse Reactions: Following the injection of an average or large dose of histamine, side effects may include such systemic reactions as flushing, dizziness, headache, bronchial constriction, dyspnea, visual disturbances, faintness, syncope, urticaria, asthma, marked hypertension or hypotension, palpitation, tachycardia, nervousness, abdominal cramps, diarrhea, vomiting, metallic taste, local or generalized allergic manifestations, or collapse with convulsions.
Dosage and Administration—Histamine Test for Pheochromocytoma: Antihypertensive drugs, sympathomimetic agents, sedatives, and narcotics should be withheld from the patient for at least 24 hours, preferably 72 hours, before the histamine test is performed. *Food should not be withheld.*
The histamine test for pheochromocytoma is a provocative test and, therefore, is indicated only for the occasional patient who has paroxysmal signs of excessive catecholamine secretion and who has normal urinary values for assays of catecholamines and metabolites during periods when he is asymptomatic.

A well-conducted test provides information on the symptomatic and physiologic responses and changes in urinary catecholamine levels.

This test is to be used only in patients in whom resting blood pressure does not exceed 150/110. Epinephrine should be available in case a severe hypotensive response is produced. Phentolamine should be on hand to depress any alarming increase in blood pressure.

The patient rests in bed while a slow intravenous infusion of either 5% dextrose or isotonic saline solution is established. The blood pressure is recorded until it is stable. At that time, a two-hour period of urine collection for catecholamine assay is started. At the end of this period, histamine is rapidly administered through the infusion, and another two-hour urine collection is started.

The first dose of histamine should be 0.01 mg, or 10 mcg. This dose is provided in 0.1 ml of Ampoules No. 338 (0.275 mg histamine phosphate, or 0.1 mg histamine, in 1 ml of solution). If no response is observed within five minutes, a dose of 0.05 mg (50 mcg) should be administered. The blood pressure and pulse are to be recorded every 30 seconds for 15 minutes. The expected responses in both positive and negative tests are headache, flushing, and a decrease in blood pressure followed within two minutes by an increase.

Positive tests have been defined as—
1. An increase in blood pressure of at least 20/10 mm Hg greater than that obtained with the cold pressor test.
2. An increase in blood pressure of at least 60/40 mm Hg above the base line and greater than that with the cold pressor test.

An increase in urinary catecholamine levels from normal during the pretest control period to abnormally high during the test lessens the possibility of false-positive tests.

How Supplied: (℞) *Ampoules No. 338, Histamine Phosphate Injection, USP,* 0.275 mg (equivalent to 0.1 mg histamine), 1 ml, in packages of 6 (NDC 0002-1639-16). [051082]

TES-TAPE®   OTC
[těs' tāp]
(glucose enzymatic test strip)
USP

For In Vitro Diagnostic Use in Testing for the Presence and Semiquantitative Measurement of Glucose in Human Urine

Tes-Tape has been used since 1956, when Dr. A. S. Keston described the novel idea of using two enzymes simultaneously to test for glucose and Dr. J. P. Comer published data on the specificity and accuracy of Tes-Tape for the semiquantitative analysis of urine glucose.

During the development and testing of this urine test method, Tes-Tape was found to be an accurate and reliable semiquantitative method for determining urine glucose. To date, relatively few instances of faulty results have occurred with the use of Tes-Tape. Problems associated with the product are usually due to improper techniques or exposure of the tape to adverse conditions or due to drugs which have an inhibitory effect on the enzyme reaction. Considerable data may be found in the published scientific documents.

Tes-Tape is impregnated with the enzymes glucose oxidase and peroxidase and an oxidizable substrate, orthotolidine. When the tape is dipped into urine containing glucose, the glucose oxidase catalyzes the reaction of glucose in the urine with oxygen from the air to form gluconic acid and hydrogen peroxide. The enzyme peroxidase (from horseradish) then catalyzes the reaction of hydrogen peroxide and orthotolidine to form a blue color. With the addition of a yellow dye (FDC Yellow No. 5) to the paper, the possible color range of the test is extended from yellow to light green to deep blue. If no glucose is present, the tape maintains its yellow color.

Reactive Ingredient	Approximate Amount per 1.5 Inches of Tape
Glucose oxidase	3.78 units
Horseradish peroxidase	2.82 PZ units
O-tolidine	0.136 mg

Nonreactive ingredients include filter paper, FDC Yellow No. 5 coloring, buffers, stabilizers, and wetting agents.

For in vitro diagnostic use. Store below 86°F (30°C). Protect from high humidity and light.

Do not use if the tape becomes dark yellow or yellowish-brown or if a 2 percent reading is not obtained when the reliability is tested, as described under the heading **Important.**

The urine should be collected in a container free of chemicals and glucose.

If the freshly voided specimen is not to be tested within four hours, it should be refrigerated.

Drugs that are known to have an inhibitory effect on the enzyme reactions include ascorbic acid (vitamin C), dipyrone, gentisic acid (a metabolite of aspirin), homogentisic acid (present in alkaptonuria), levodopa, meralluride injection, and methyldopa. The inhibiting effect is notable on the dipped part of the tape, but accurate readings may be obtained by observing the narrow band of color at the junction of the dry and wet portions. A separation of glucose from the inhibitory substances occurs as the urine travels along the dry portion of the tape. Ingestion of more than 1.5 g of ascorbic acid may produce urine with inhibitory action on Tes-Tape. Specimens for storage or shipment should be refrigerated or preserved with up to 0.37 percent formaldehyde.

All materials are provided for the test and include dispenser, tape, and color chart.

Results on the color chart are expressed in percent of glucose (urine sugar) and by a corresponding arbitrary system of 0, +, ++, +++, ++++, representing 0, $\frac{1}{10}$, $\frac{1}{4}$, $\frac{1}{2}$, 2 (or more) percent of glucose respectively.

When testing, do not place the tape on the lavatory or on paper or allow moistened portion to contact fingers. Contamination of the tape by glucose from other sources (e.g., perspiration, tears, and saliva) or with a residue of chlorine from lavatory cleansing agents can cause false-positive results.

Patients who are receiving high doses of ascorbic acid or whose urine contains dipyrone, meralluride, homogentisic acid, gentisic acid, levodopa, or methyldopa should read only the very narrow band of color in the moist portion of the tape above the level to which it was dipped into the specimen. Very high doses of ascorbic acid may cause a false-negative test even with the above precaution. (Urinary levels of ascorbic acid in excess of 0.1 percent are necessary to block the test completely. This concentration is most likely to appear within three to seven hours after a single dose of 1.5 g or more.)

Normal urine should test 0 percent with Tes-Tape. Persons using Tes-Tape for a screening test should report all values above 0 percent to their physician. Diabetic urine values in the range of the color chart should also be recorded and reported to the patient's physician. Measured values of 2 percent should be reported as 2 percent or more.

The overall semiquantitative accuracy of Tes-Tape originally reported in 1956 on 1000 determinations was 96 percent. This was confirmed in 1973 on 14,000 determinations over a two-year period. These data were obtained on urine samples containing concentrations of glucose at each increment shown to be measurable on the color chart. The color chart provided is based on the average color perception of many observers. Patients who have difficulty in differentiating color should seek the advice of their physician before using Tes-Tape.

Numerous other clinical and laboratory studies have shown that Tes-Tape is accurate in qualitative and semiquantitative determination of urine sugar. Tes-Tape is specific for glucose in urine sugar testing. Except for instances involving contamination of the tape or urine receptacle with glucose from other sources (e.g., perspiration, tears, and saliva) or with a residue of chlorine from cleansing agents, there is no known clinical situation in which a false-positive test for glucose occurs with Tes-Tape. The sensitivity of Tes-Tape is such that it will react with concentrations of 0.05 percent glucose or more. Trace reactions shown by the development of a very light yellow-green color may be observed with less than this amount of glucose.

After opening plastic wrapper, use tape within four months. It must be used prior to expiration date.

Important: The reliability of a roll of Tes-Tape may easily be checked by dipping a piece into a properly prepared glucose solution.* The tape should be removed immediately, as one would when testing a urine specimen. After two minutes have elapsed, the reading obtained when the tape is compared with the color chart should be approximately + + + + (2 percent). If such a reading is not obtained, the tape has apparently deteriorated and should not be used.

Measurements for the amount of glucose present (semiquantitative) should not be made after two minutes because the colors gradually change as the tape dries. Screening tests for the presence of glucose (qualitative) in urine may be made for several hours after the tape has dried. The patient should consult the package insert in regard to Procedure, What to Do If Tape Breaks, and a record chart for urine sugar tests with Tes-Tape.

---
*If a properly prepared glucose solution is not available, any nationally known *sugar (glucose)-containing* beverage from a freshly opened bottle or can is satisfactory. (Diet cola beverages would not be satisfactory.)

How Supplied: *M-73, Tes-Tape®* *(Glucose Enzymatic Test Strip, USP),* dispenser package, approximately 100 tests, in single packages.
(NDC 0002-2344-41)   [080583]
    M-73—100 tests—6505-00-559-6859

Merieux Institute, Inc.
P. O. BOX 52-3980
MIAMI, FL 33152

MULTITEST® CMI™   ℞
[mul' tĭ-test]
(Skin Test Antigens for Cellular Hypersensitivity)
NDC 50361-780001

Description: Skin Test Antigens for Cellular Hypersensitivity, MULTITEST® CMI™ is a disposable, plastic applicator consisting of eight sterile test heads preloaded with the following seven delayed hypersensitivity skin test antigens and glycerin negative control for precutaneous administration: Tetanus Toxoid Antigen, Diphtheria Toxoid Antigen, Streptococcus Antigen, Old Tuberculin, Candida Antigen, Trichophyton Antigen, and Proteus Antigen.

MULTITEST® CMI™ provides a quick, convenient and uniform procedure for delayed cutaneous hypersensitivity testing.

Supplied in box of 10 individual cartons containing one preloaded MULTITEST® CMI™ per carton.

TUBERCULIN, MONO-VACC®   ℞
TEST (O.T.)
[tu-ber' ku-lin]
(old tuberculin)
Multiple Puncture Device

NDC 50361-772425   25 tests per box
Supplied in plastic tamper proof box of 25 tests per box; test reading cards in English or Spanish also available.

Products are
listed alphabetically in the
pink SECTION

Parke-Davis
DIVISION OF WARNER-LAMBERT COMPANY
201 TABOR ROAD
MORRIS PLAINS, NEW JERSEY
07950

APLISOL®
[ă′plĭ-sōl″]
(Tuberculin Purified Protein Derivative, Diluted [Stabilized Solution])

Description: Aplisol (tuberculin PPD, diluted) is a sterile aqueous solution of a purified protein fraction for intradermal administration as an aid in the diagnosis of tuberculosis. The solution is stabilized with polysorbate (Tween) 80, buffered with potassium and sodium phosphates and contains approximately 0.35% phenol as a preservative.

The product is clinically equivalent in potency to the standard PPD-S* (5 TU** per 0.1 ml) of the U.S. Public Health Service, National Center for Disease Control, and is ready for immediate use without further dilution. This product meets all applicable standards.

Clinical Pharmacology: The purified protein fraction is isolated from culture filtrates of human type strains of *Mycobacterium tuberculosis* by the method of F.B. Seibert.[1,2] This product is made from a single master lot (No. 924994) to eliminate lot to lot variation inherent in manufacturing.

The 5 TU dose of Tuberculin PPD intradermally (Mantoux) is recommended as the standard tuberculin test, and Tuberculin PPD is recommended by the American Lung Association as an aid in the detection of infection with *Mycobacterium tuberculosis*.

Reactions to the Mantoux test are interpreted on the basis of a quantitative measurement of the response to a specific dose (5 TU PPD-S or equivalent) of Tuberculin PPD. Other dosages are regarded as having no demonstrable usefulness in ordinary practice.[3] Accordingly, Aplisol is available in only one potency (5 TU equivalent) and the use of this potency only is recommended. The selection of 5 TU as the test dose is based upon data indicating that (1) the 5 TU dose gives measurable reactions in over 95 percent of the known tuberculous infected; (2) doses larger than 5 TU might elicit reactions not caused by tuberculosis infection; and (3) nonreactors to doses considerably less than 5 TU are not accepted as negative but are retested with a stronger dose.[3]

Indications and Usage: Tuberculin PPD is recommended by the American Lung Association as an aid in the detection of infection with *Mycobacterium tuberculosis*. The standard tuberculin test recommended employs the intradermal (Mantoux) test using a 5 TU dose of tuberculin PPD.[3] The 0.1 ml test dose of Aplisol (tuberculin PPD, diluted) is equivalent to the 5 TU dose recommended as clinically established and standardized with PPD-S.

Contraindications: None known.

Warnings: Tuberculin should not be administered to known tuberculin-positive reactors because of the severity of reactions (e.g., vesiculation, ulceration or necrosis) that may occur at the test site in very highly sensitive individuals.

Avoid injecting tuberculin subcutaneously. If this occurs, no local reaction develops, but a general febrile reaction and/or acute inflammation around old tuberculous lesions may occur in highly sensitive individuals.

Precautions:
General
A separate heat sterilized syringe and needle, or a sterile disposable unit, should be used for each individual patient to prevent possible transmission of homologous serum hepatitis virus and other infectious agents from one person to another.
Syringes that have previously been used with histoplasmin, blastomycin and other antigens should not be used for tuberculin.

As with any biological product, epinephrine should be immediately available in case an anaphylactoid or acute hypersensitivity reaction occurs.

Pregnancy
Teratogenic effects: Pregnancy Category C. Animal reproduction studies have not been conducted with Aplisol. It is also not known whether Aplisol can cause fetal harm when administered to a pregnant woman or can affect the reproduction capacity. Aplisol should be given to a pregnant woman only if clearly needed.

However, the risk of unrecognized tuberculosis and the close postpartum contact between a mother with active disease and an infant leaves the infant in grave danger of tuberculosis and complications such as tuberculous meningitis. Although there have been not been reported any adverse effects upon the fetus recognized as being due to tuberculosis skin testing, the prescribing physician will want to consider if the potential benefits outweigh the possible risks for performing the tuberculin test on a pregnant woman or woman of childbearing age, particularly in certain high risk populations.

Adverse Reactions: In highly sensitive individuals, strongly positive reactions including vesiculation, ulceration or necrosis may occur at the test site. Cold packs or topical steroid preparations may be employed for symptomatic relief of the associated pain, pruritus, and discomfort.
Strongly positive test reactions may result in scarring at the test site.

Dosage and Administration:
Standard Method (Mantoux Test)
The Mantoux test is performed by intradermally injecting with a syringe and needle exactly 0.1 ml of tuberculin PPD, diluted. The result is read 48 to 72 hours later and induration only is considered in interpreting the test. The standard test is performed as follows:
1. The site of the test is usually the flexor or dorsal surface of the forearm about 4″ below the elbow. Other skin sites may be used, but the flexor surface of the forearm is preferred.
2. The skin at the injection site is cleansed with 70% alcohol and allowed to dry.
3. The test material is administered with a tuberculin syringe (0.5 or 1.0 ml) fitted with a short (½″) 26 or 27 gauge needle.
4. The syringe and needle should be of a sterile disposable, single use type or should have been sterilized by autoclaving, boiling or by the use of dry heat. A separate sterile unit should be used for each person tested.
5. The diaphragm of the vial-stopper should be wiped with 70% alcohol.
6. The needle is inserted through the stopper diaphragm of the inverted vial. Exactly 0.1 ml is filled into the syringe, with care being taken to exclude air bubbles and to maintain the lumen of the needle filled.
7. The point of the needle is inserted into the most superficial layers of the skin with the needle bevel pointing upward. As the tuberculin solution is injected, a pale bleb 6 to 10 mm in size (⅜″) will rise over the point of the needle. This is quickly absorbed and no dressing is required.
In the event the injection is delivered subcutaneously (ie, no bleb will form), or if a significant part of the dose leaks from the injection site, the test should be repeated immediately at another site at least 5 cm (2″) removed.
Aplisol vials should be inspected visually for particulate matter and discoloration prior to administration.
The Mantoux test is the standard of comparison for all other tuberculin tests.
Aplisol is a stabilized solution of Tuberculin PPD. Data indicate that Aplisol is stable when prefilled into syringes and stored in a refrigerator for up to 30 days.
However, the practice of storing such prefilled syringes is not recommended as good practice because of the increased potential for contamination.

Interpretation of Tuberculin Reaction
Readings of Mantoux reactions should be made during the period from 48 to 72 hours after the injection. Induration only should be considered in interpreting the test. The diameter of induration should be measured transversely to the long axis of the forearm and recorded in millimeters. Erythema of less than 10 mm should be disregarded. If the area of erythema is greater than 10 mm and induration is absent the injection may have been made too deeply and retesting is indicated.

Reactions should be interpreted as follows:
Positive—Induration measuring 10 mm or more. This indicates hypersensitivity to tuberculoprotein and should be interpreted as positive for past or present infection with *M. tuberculosis*.

Doubtful—Induration measuring 5 to 9 mm. Retesting is indicated using a different site of injection. Evaluation to rule out cross-reaction from other mycobacterial infection should be considered.

Negative—Induration of less than 5 mm. This indicates a lack of hypersensitivity to tuberculoprotein and tuberculous infection is highly unlikely.

It should be noted that reactivity to tuberculin may be depressed or suppressed for as long as four weeks by viral infections, live virus vaccines (i.e., measles, smallpox, polio, rubella and mumps), or by the administration of corticosteroids. Malnutrition may also have a similar effect. When of diagnostic importance, a negative test should be accepted as proof that hypersensitivity is absent only after normal reactivity to nonspecific irritants has been demonstrated. A primary injection of tuberculin may possibly have a boosting effect on subsequent tuberculin reactions.

A child who is known to have been exposed to a tuberculous adult must not be adjudged free of infection until he has a negative tuberculin reaction at least ten weeks after contact with the tuberculous person has ceased.[4]

A positive tuberculin reaction does not necessarily signify the presence of active disease. Further diagnostic procedures should be carried out before a diagnosis of tuberculosis is made. A small percentage of responders may not have been infected with *M. tuberculosis* but by some other mycobacterium.

How Supplied:
N 0071-4525-03 (Bio. 1525)
1 ml (10 tests)—rubber-diaphragm-capped vial
N 0071-4525-08 (Bio. 1607)
5 ml (50 tests)—rubber-diaphragm-capped vial
This product should be stored at 2° to 8°C (36° to 46°F), and protected from light.

References:
1. Seibert, F.B.: Am. Rev. Tuberc. 30:713, 1934.
2. Seibert, F.B., and Glenn, J.T.: Am. Rev. Tuberc. 44:9, 1941.
3. Diagnostic Standards and Classification of Tuberculosis and Other Mycobacterial Diseases, American Lung Association, New York, 1974.
4. Sewell, E.M., O'Hare, D., and Kendig, E.L., Jr.: The Tuberculin Test, Pediatrics, Vol. 54, No. 5, Nov. 1974.

---
* PPD-S (No. 49608) World Health Organization International PPD-Tuberculin Standard (PPD-S is a dried powder from which WHO and U.S. Standard tuberculin solutions are made.)
** U.S. Tuberculin Unit

4525G032

APLITEST®
[ă′plĭ-tĕst″]
Tuberculin Purified Protein Derivative
Multiple-Puncture Device

Description: Aplitest (tuberculin PPD) is a sterile, single-use, multiple-puncture type device for percutaneous administration for use in determining the tuberculin sensitivity status of individuals. Aplitest, a diagnostic aid, has been clinically compared with 5 US Tuberculin Units of PPD-S administered intradermally.

These disposable devices are useful in mass tuberculosis screening programs. The product packaging facilitates the use of Aplitest units for testing of individual patients in office, ward, or clinic settings.

Each Aplitest unit consists of a cylindrical plastic holder bearing four equally spaced stainless steel tines at one end. The tines have been coated by dipping in a solution of tuberculin PPD and dried. The tuberculin solution applied to the tines is buffered with potassium and sodium phosphates and contains approximately 0.5% phenol as a preservative. The narrow (tine-bearing) end of each unit fits into a protective cap to protect the tines and maintain their sterility.

The purified tuberculin protein fraction is isolated from culture filtrates of human-type strains of *Mycobacterium tuberculosis* by the method of F.B. Seibert.[1,2] Purified tuberculin protein solution is prepared from a single master lot (No. 975302) to eliminate lot to lot variation.

Clinical Pharmacology: Tuberculin deposited in the skin of tuberculin-reactive individuals reacts with sensitized lymphocytes to effect the release of mediators of cellular hypersensitivity. Some of these mediators, eg, skin reactive factor, induce an inflammatory response to the skin, causing the induration characteristic of a "positive" or "significant" reaction.

Aplitest has been standardized by clinical studies in human subjects against 5 TU* of PPD-S administered intradermally by the Mantoux test, and guidelines relating response to the two treatments have been formulated. (See "Interpretation of Response" section.)

Indications and Usage: Aplitest is indicated to detect tuberculin-sensitive individuals. Aplitest units are also useful in programs to establish priorities for additional testing (ie, chest x-rays) and in epidemiological surveys to identify areas with high levels of infection.

All multiple-puncture type devices should be regarded as screening tools, and appropriate diagnostic procedures (eg, Mantoux test with tuberculin PPD diluted, Aplisol®) should be employed for retesting "doubtful" reactors.

Regular periodic (annual or biennial)[3] testing of tuberculin-negative persons is recommended and is especially valuable because the conversion of an individual from negative to positive is highly indicative of recent tuberculosis infection. Repeated testing of the uninfected individual does not sensitize to tuberculin. In persons with waning sensitivity to homologous or heterologous mycobacterial antigens, however, the stimulus of a tuberculin test may "boost" or increase the size of reaction to a second test, even causing an apparent development of sensitivity in some instances.

Contraindications: None known.

Warnings: Tuberculin should not be administered to known tuberculin-positive reactors because of the severity of reactions (eg, vesiculation, ulceration or necrosis) that may occur at the test site in very highly sensitive individuals.

As with any biological product, epinephrine should be immediately available in case an anaphylactoid or acute hypersensitivity reaction occurs.

Precautions:

General: A separate, sterile unit must be used for each individual patient and disposed of after use. Sensitivity may decrease or disappear temporarily during or immediately following severe febrile illness, measles, and other exanthemas, live virus vaccination, sarcoidosis, overwhelming miliary or pulmonary tuberculosis, and the administration of corticosteroids or immunosuppressive drugs. Severe malnutrition may also have a similar effect. A positive tuberculin reaction does not necessarily signify the presence of active disease. Further diagnostic procedures should be carried out before a diagnosis of tuberculosis is made.

Simultaneous application of two or more multiple-puncture devices is not recommended. The response of an individual to a single multiple-puncture device may be altered by the simultaneous administration of additional tuberculin tests (multiple-puncture or Mantoux).[4]

Pregnancy: Teratogenic effects: Pregnancy Category C. Animal reproduction studies have not been conducted with Aplitest. It is also not known whether Aplitest can cause fetal harm when administered to a pregnant woman or can affect reproduction capacity. Aplitest should be given to a pregnant woman only if clearly needed.

However, the risk of unrecognized tuberculosis and the close postpartum contact between a mother with active disease and an infant leaves the infant in grave danger of tuberculosis and complications such as tuberculous meningitis. Although there have not been reported any adverse effects upon the fetus recognized as being due to tuberculosis skin testing, the prescribing physician will want to consider if the potential benefits outweigh the possible risks for performing the tuberculin test on a pregnant woman or a woman of childbearing age, particularly in certain high risk populations.

Adverse Reactions: In highly sensitive individuals, strongly positive reactions, including vesiculation, ulceration or necrosis, may occur at the test site. Cold packs or topical steroid preparations may be employed for symptomatic relief of the associated pain, pruritus and discomfort.

Strongly positive test reactions may result in scarring at the test site.

Minimal bleeding may be experienced at a puncture site. This occurs infrequently and does not affect the interpretation of the test.

Dosage and Administration: Each Aplitest unit provides for the intradermal administration of one test-dose of tuberculin PPD.

Method of Application

1. The preferred site of the test is the flexor surface of the forearm about 4 inches below the elbow. Other suitable skin sites, such as the dorsal surface of the forearm, may be used. Areas without adequate subcutaneous tissue, such as over a tendon, should be avoided.
2. The skin at the test site should be cleaned with 70% alcohol, or other suitable agent, and allowed to dry thoroughly.
3. To expose the four impregnated tines, grasp the device and twist to break the perforated label seal.
4. Grasp the patient's forearm firmly to stretch the skin taut at the test site and to prevent any jerking motion of the arm that could cause scratching with the tines.
5. Apply the Aplitest unit firmly and without twisting to the test area for approximately one second. Sufficient pressure should be exerted to assure that all four tines have penetrated the skin of the test area.
6. Dispose of used units in a manner to avoid accidents. Do not reuse.

Interpretation of Response

Selection of the appropriate criteria for interpretation of response to the tuberculin PPD Aplitest should be made in accordance with the objectives of the specific testing program and with consideration of the history and clinical status of the individuals.

Reading of reactions should be made during the period from 48 to 72 hours after application of Aplitest and should be conducted under good lighting conditions. Induration only should be considered in interpreting the test. Erythema should be disregarded. The diameter of the induration of the greatest response at any of the four puncture points should be determined by visual inspection and palpation. If there is coalescence of reaction, the largest diameter of coalescent induration should be measured and recorded.

The American Thoracic Society recommends that all multiple-puncture tuberculin skin test devices be interpreted as follows: If vesiculation is present, the test may be interpreted as positive. If vesiculation is not present, induration of 2 mm or more is considered as a doubtful reaction and a Mantoux test for diagnostic evaluation should be given. Decisions concerning management should be based on the reaction to the Mantoux test and relevant diagnostic criteria. Induration of less than 2 mm and/or erythema of any size is a negative test and there is no need for retesting.[5]

In clinical studies with Aplitest, it has been determined that coalescence of the induration around two or more puncture sites corresponds more than 90% of the time to 10 mm or more of induration in the same individual tested by Mantoux test at the 5 TU level with PPD-S.†

Thus, the following criteria of interpretation have been established.

1. Vesiculation—Positive Reaction

The test should be interpreted as positive and the management of the subject is the same as that for one classified as positive by Mantoux test.

2. Coalescence of induration from two or more puncture points—Doubtful Reaction

A subject with a coalescent reaction may be considered for Mantoux retest. However, more than 90% of the time this reaction was equivalent to a reaction of 10 mm or more of induration with PPD-S (5 TU) administered by Mantoux test.[6] Other criteria, such as contact with tuberculosis patients and case history, should be considered to determine the likelihood that such a reaction is considered positive.

3. 2 mm or more of induration without coalescence—Doubtful Reaction

Reactions of this size range reflect sensitivity that can result from infection with either atypical mycobacteria or *M tuberculosis*; hence, they are classified as doubtful.

A standard Mantoux test should be done on all subjects in this group. Management should be based on the reaction to the Mantoux test, as well as other clinical considerations.

4. Less than 2 mm of induration—Negative Reaction

There is no need for retesting unless the individual is in contact with a case of tuberculosis or there is clinical evidence suggestive of the disease.

How Supplied:

N 0071-4589-13 (Bio. 1590) 25-test package. Twenty-five individually capped Aplitest units in a dispensing package.

Aplitest (tuberculin PPD, multiple-puncture device) units should be stored at no warmer than 30°C (86°F).

References:

1. Seibert, F.B.: Am. Rev. Tuberc. 30:713, 1934.
2. Seibert, F.B., and Glenn J.T.: Am. Rev. Tuberc. 44:9, 1941.
3. Report of the Committee on Infectious Diseases, American Academy of Pediatrics, 1982.
4. Rosenthal, S.R., and Libby, J.E.P.: Bull. Wld. Hlth. Org. 23:689, 1960.
5. Diagnostic Standards and Classification of Tuberculosis and Other Mycobacterial Diseases, American Lung Association, 1974.
6. Unpublished data from Warner-Lambert Co. available upon request.

*U.S. (International) tuberculin units.

†Purified Protein Derivative (Seibert). Lot No. 49608, the standard adopted by the World Health Organization in 1952 as International PPD Tuberculin and used to prepare the official U.S. Public Health Service 5 TU solution of tuberculin for skin testing known as PPD-S.

4589G022

This product information was prepared in August, 1984. On these and other Parke-Davis Products, information may be obtained by addressing PARKE-DAVIS, Division of Warner-Lambert Company, Morris Plains, New Jersey 07950.

Roche Laboratories
Division of Hoffmann-La Roche Inc.
NUTLEY, NJ 07110

TENSILON® ℞
[*ten'sill-on*]
(edrophonium chloride/Roche)
Injectable Solution
ampuls • vials

The following text is complete prescribing information based on official labeling in effect August 1, 1984.

Description: Tensilon is a short and rapid-acting cholinergic drug. Chemically, edrophonium chloride is ethyl (*m*-hydroxyphenyl)-dimethylammonium chloride.

10-ml vials: Each ml contains, in a sterile solution, 10 mg edrophonium chloride/Roche compounded with 0.45% phenol and 0.2% sodium sulfite as preservatives, buffered with sodium citrate

Continued on next page

Roche—Cont.

and citric acid, and pH adjusted to approximately 5.4.

1-ml ampuls: Each ml contains, in a sterile solution, 10 mg edrophonium chloride/Roche compounded with 0.2% sodium sulfite, buffered with sodium citrate and citric acid, and pH adjusted to approximately 5.4.

Actions: Tensilon is an anticholinesterase drug. Its pharmacological action is due primarily to the inhibition or inactivation of acetylcholinesterase at sites of cholinergic transmission. Its effect is manifest within 30 to 60 seconds after injection and lasts an average of 10 minutes.

Indications: Tensilon is recommended for the differential diagnosis of myasthenia gravis and as an adjunct in the evaluation of treatment requirements in this disease. It may also be used for evaluating emergency treatment in myasthenic crises. Because of its brief duration of action, it is not recommended for maintenance therapy in myasthenia gravis.

Tensilon is also useful whenever a curare antagonist is needed to reverse the neuromuscular block produced by curare, tubocurarine, gallamine triethiodide or dimethyl-tubocurarine. It is *not* effective against decamethonium bromide and succinylcholine chloride. It may be used adjunctively in the treatment of respiratory depression caused by curare overdosage.

Contraindications: Known hypersensitivity to anticholinesterase agents; intestinal and urinary obstructions of mechanical type.

Warnings: Whenever anticholinesterase drugs are used for testing, a syringe containing 1 mg of atropine sulfate should be immediately available to be given in aliquots intravenously to counteract severe cholinergic reactions which may occur in the hypersensitive individual, whether he is normal or myasthenic. Tensilon should be used with caution in patients with bronchial asthma or cardiac dysrhythmias. The transient bradycardia which sometimes occurs can be relieved by atropine sulfate. Isolated instances of cardiac and respiratory arrest following administration of Tensilon have been reported. It is postulated that these are vagotonic effects.

Usage in Pregnancy: The safety of Tensilon during pregnancy or lactation in humans has not been established. Therefore, use of Tensilon in women who may become pregnant requires weighing the drug's potential benefits against its possible hazards to mother and child.

Precautions: Patients may develop "anticholinesterase insensitivity" for brief or prolonged periods. During these periods the patients should be carefully monitored and may need respiratory assistance. Dosages of anticholinesterase drugs should be reduced or withheld until patients again become sensitive to them.

Adverse Reactions: Careful observation should be made for severe cholinergic reactions in the hyperreactive individual. The myasthenic patient in crisis who is being tested with Tensilon should be observed for bradycardia or cardiac standstill and cholinergic reactions if an overdose is given. The following reactions common to anticholinesterase agents may occur, although not all of these reactions have been reported with the administration of Tensilon, probably because of its short duration of action and limited indications: **Eye:** Increased lacrimation, pupillary constriction, spasm of accommodation, diplopia, conjunctival hyperemia. **CNS:** Convulsions, dysarthria, dysphonia, dysphagia. **Respiratory:** Increased tracheobronchial secretions, laryngospasm, bronchiolar constriction, paralysis of muscles of respiration, central respiratory paralysis. **Cardiac:** Arrhythmias (especially bradycardia), fall in cardiac output leading to hypotension. **G.I.:** Increased salivary, gastric and intestinal secretion, nausea, vomiting, increased peristalsis, diarrhea, abdominal cramps. **Skeletal Muscle:** Weakness, fasciculations. **Miscellaneous:** Increased urinary frequency and incontinence, diaphoresis.

Dosage and Administration: *Tensilon Test in the Differential Diagnosis of Myasthenia Gravis:*[1-8] *Intravenous Dosage (Adults):* A tuberculin syringe containing 1 ml (10 mg) of Tensilon is prepared with an intravenous needle, and 0.2 ml (2 mg) is injected intravenously within 15 to 30 seconds. The needle is left *in situ. Only* if no reaction occurs after 45 seconds is the remaining 0.8 ml (8 mg) injected. If a cholinergic reaction (muscarinic side effects, skeletal muscle fasciculations and increased muscle weakness) occurs after injection of 0.2 ml (2 mg), the test is discontinued and atropine sulfate 0.4 mg to 0.5 mg is administered intravenously. After one-half hour the test may be repeated.

Intramuscular Dosage (Adults): In adults with inaccessible veins, dosage for intramuscular injection is 1 ml (10 mg) of Tensilon. Subjects who demonstrate hyperreactivity to this injection (cholinergic reaction), should be retested after one-half hour with 0.2 ml (2 mg) of Tensilon intramuscularly to rule out false-negative reactions.

Dosage (Children): The intravenous testing dose of Tensilon in children weighing up to 75 lbs is 0.1 ml (1 mg); above this weight, the dose is 0.2 ml (2 mg). If there is no response after 45 seconds, it may be titrated up to 0.5 ml (5 mg) in children under 75 lbs, given in increments of 0.1 ml (1 mg) every 30 to 45 seconds and up to 1 ml (10 mg) in heavier children. In infants, the recommended dose is 0.05 ml (0.5 mg). Because of technical difficulty with intravenous injection in children, the intramuscular route may be used. In children weighing up to 75 lbs, 0.2 ml (2 mg) is injected intramuscularly. In children weighing more than 75 lbs, 0.5 ml (5 mg) is injected intramuscularly. All signs which would appear with the intravenous test appear with the intramuscular test except that there is a delay of two to ten minutes before a reaction is noted.

Tensilon Test for Evaluation of Treatment Requirements in Myasthenia Gravis: The recommended dose is 0.1 ml to 0.2 ml (1 mg to 2 mg) of Tensilon, administered intravenously one hour after oral intake of the drug being used in treatment.[1-5] Response will be myasthenic in the undertreated patient, adequate in the controlled patient, and cholinergic in the overtreated patient. Responses to Tensilon in myasthenic and nonmyasthenic individuals are summarized in the accompanying chart.[2]

[See table below].

Tensilon Test in Crisis: The term *crisis* is applied to the myasthenic whenever severe respiratory distress with objective ventilatory inadequacy occurs and the response to medication is not predictable. This state may be secondary to a sudden increase in severity of myasthenia gravis (myasthenic crisis), or to overtreatment with anticholinesterase drugs (cholinergic crisis).

When a patient is apneic, controlled ventilation must be secured immediately in order to avoid cardiac arrest and irreversible central nervous system damage. No attempt is made to test with Tensilon until respiratory exchange is adequate. *Dosage used at this time is most important:* If the patient is cholinergic, Tensilon will cause increased oropharyngeal secretions and further weakness in the muscles of respiration. If the crisis is myasthenic, the test clearly improves respiration and the patient can be treated with longer-acting intravenous anticholinesterase medication. When the test is performed, there should not be more than 0.2 ml (2 mg) Tensilon in the syringe. An intravenous dose of 0.1 ml (1 mg) is given initially. The patient's heart action is carefully observed. If, after an interval of one minute, this dose does not further impair the patient, the remaining 0.1 ml (1 mg) can be injected. If no clear improvement of respiration occurs after 0.2 ml (2 mg) dose, it is usually wisest to discontinue all anticholinesterase drug therapy and secure controlled ventilation by tracheostomy with assisted respiration.[5]

For Use as a Curare Antagonist: Tensilon should be administered by intravenous injection in 1 ml (10 mg) doses given slowly over a period of 30 to 45 seconds so that the onset of cholinergic reaction can be detected. This dosage may be repeated whenever necessary. The maximal dose for any one patient should be 4 ml (40 mg). Because of its brief effect, Tensilon should not be given prior to the administration of curare, tubocurarine, gallamine triethiodide or dimethyl-tubocurarine; it should be used at the time when its effect is needed. When given to counteract curare overdosage, the effect of each dose on the respiration should be carefully observed before it is repeated, and assisted ventilation should always be employed.

Drug Interactions: Care should be given when administering this drug to patients with symptoms of myasthenic weakness who are also on anticholinesterase drugs. Since symptoms of anticholinesterase overdose (cholinergic crisis) may mimic underdosage (myasthenic weakness), their condition may be worsened by the use of this drug. (See OVERDOSAGE section for treatment.)

Overdosage: With drugs of this type, muscarine-like symptoms (nausea, vomiting, diarrhea, sweating, increased bronchial and salivary secretions and bradycardia) often appear with overdosage (cholinergic crisis). An important complication that can arise is obstruction of the airway by bronchial secretions. These may be managed with suction (especially if tracheostomy has been performed) and by the use of atropine. Many experts have advocated a wide range of dosages of atropine *(for Tensilon, see atropine dosage below),* but if there are copious secretions, up to 1.2 mg intravenously may be given initially and repeated every 20 minutes until secretions are controlled. Signs of atropine overdosage such as dry mouth, flush and tachycardia should be avoided as tenacious secretions and bronchial plugs may form. A total dose of atropine of 5 to 10 mg or even more may be required. The following steps should be taken in the management of overdosage of Tensilon:

1. Adequate respiratory exchange should be maintained by assuring an open airway, and the use of assisted respiration augmented by oxygen.
2. Cardiac function should be monitored until complete stabilization has been achieved.

Responses to Tensilon in Myasthenic and Nonmyasthenic Individuals

	Myasthenic*	Adequate**	Cholinergic***
Muscle Strength ... (ptosis, diplopia, dysphonia, dysphagia, dysarthria, respiration, limb strength)	Increased	No change	Decreased
Fasciculations ... (orbicularis oculi, facial muscles, limb muscles)	Absent	Present or absent	Present or absent
Side reactions ... (lacrimation, diaphoresis, salivation, abdominal cramps, nausea, vomiting, diarrhea)	Absent	Minimal	Severe

*Myasthenic Response—occurs in untreated myasthenics and may serve to establish diagnosis; in patients under treatment, indicates that therapy is inadequate.

**Adequate Response—observed in treated patients when therapy is stabilized; a typical response in normal individuals. In addition to this response in nonmyasthenics, the phenomenon of forced lid closure is often observed in psychoneurotics.[1]

***Cholinergic Response—seen in myasthenics who have been overtreated with anticholinesterase drugs.

3. Atropine sulfate in doses of 0.4 to 0.5 mg should be administered intravenously. This may be repeated every 3 to 10 minutes. Because of the short duration of action of Tensilon the total dose required will seldom exceed 2 mg.
4. Pralidoxime chloride (a cholinesterase reactivator) may be given intravenously at the rate of 50 to 100 mg per minute; usually the total dose does not exceed 1000 mg. Extreme caution should be exercised in the use of pralidoxime chloride when the cholinergic symptoms are induced by double-bond phosphorous anticholinesterase drugs.[9]
5. If convulsions or shock is present, appropriate measures should be instituted.

How Supplied: *Multiple Dose Vials,* 10 ml. *Ampuls,* 1 ml, boxes of 10.

References:
1. Osserman, K.E. and Kaplan, L.I., *J.A.M.A., 150:*265, 1952.
2. Osserman, K.E., Kaplan, L.I. and Besson, G., *J. Mt. Sinai Hosp., 20:*165, 1953.
3. Osserman, K.E. and Kaplan, L.I., *Arch. Neurol. & Psychiat., 70:*385, 1953.
4. Osserman, K.E. and Teng, P., *J.A.M.A., 160:*153, 1956.
5. Osserman, K.E. and Genkins, G., *Ann. N.Y. Acad. Sci., 135:*312, 1966.
6. Tether, J.E., Second International Symposium Proceedings, Myasthenia Gravis, 1961, p. 444.
7. Tether, J.E., in H.F. Conn: *Current Therapy 1960,* Philadelphia, W. B. Saunders Company, p. 551.
8. Tether, J.E., in H.F. Conn: *Current Therapy 1965,* Philadelphia, W. B. Saunders Company, p. 556.
9. Grob, D. and Johns, R.J., *J.A.M.A., 166:*1855, 1958.

Sclavo Inc.
5 MANSARD COURT
WAYNE, NJ 07470

SclavoTest®-PPD   ℞
Tuberculin Purified Protein Derivative (PPD) Multiple Puncture Device

Composition/Description: SclavoTest-PPD is a sterile multiple-puncture device containing a tuberculin PPD used for the identification of individuals who have a delayed hypersensitivity to tuberculin. SclavoTest-PPD is an easy-to-use, self-contained, unit-dose disposable system which minimizes waste and can be stored at room temperature. No needles, syringes, or vials are needed. The SclavoTest-PPD device is composed of a plastic handle with four sharp stainless steel points to which has been affixed and dried a tuberculin PPD solution. The retracted points are projected, after the device is placed upon the skin, by gentle pressure applied through a spring inside the handle. SclavoTest-PPD is stored at room temperature until the moment of use in a hermetically sealed unit-dose blister pack, which is designed to impede the passage of moisture and maintain sterility.

Adverse Reactions: Vesication, occasionally necrosis, ulceration.

How Supplied: 1, 20 or 250 units individually blister-sealed in strips of 1.

Products are cross-indexed
by product classifications
in the
BLUE SECTION

SmithKline Diagnostics, Inc.
A SmithKline Beckman Company
POST OFFICE BOX 61947
SUNNYVALE, CA 94086

GASTROCCULT™
[*gas' tro-cult*]
Test for Gastric Occult Blood and pH

To meet the need for a reliable test for detecting occult blood in gastric samples (both aspirates and vomitus), SKD has developed Gastroccult™, the only test specifically designed for this purpose. The test is as easy to run as Hemoccult®, but is not affected by the low pH frequently encountered in gastric samples. Also, it is not affected by oral cimetidine (Tagamet®). Further, it also features a convenient test for pH right on the slide.
Gastroccult™ slides are available from leading distributors in economical boxes of 40 slides, SKD product number 66000.

HEMOCCULT®
[*hē' mō-cult*]

Intended Uses: The Hemoccult® test is a rapid, convenient, and virtually odorless method for detecting the presence of fecal occult blood, as an aid to diagnosis of various gastrointestinal conditions:
• during routine physical examinations
• in newly admitted hospital patients
• in postoperative patients
• in newborn infants
• in screening programs for colorectal cancer

Because Hemoccult® tests require only a small stool specimen, offensive odors are minimized and storage or transport of large stool specimens is unnecessary.
Hemoccult® Single Slides are convenient for use when single stool specimens are to be tested.
Hemoccult II® Slides, in cards of three tests, are designed so your patient can collect serial specimens at home over the course of three bowel movements. After the patient collects the specimens, the Hemoccult II® test may be returned to a laboratory, a hospital, or a medical office for developing and evaluation. Serial fecal specimen analysis is recommended when screening asymptomatic patients.[1]
Hemoccult® Tape is designed to complement Hemoccult® slides and is best suited for "on-the-spot" testing for occult blood during rectal or sigmoidoscopic examinations.
The Hemoccult® test and other unmodified guaiac tests are not recommended for use with gastric specimens.[2]

Summary and Explanation of the Test: The Hemoccult® test is a simplified, standardized variation of the guaiac test for occult blood. It contains specially prepared guaiac-impregnated paper and is ready for use without additional preparation.
When a small stool specimen containing occult blood is applied to Hemoccult® test paper, the hemoglobin comes in contact with the guaiac. Application of Hemoccult® Developer (a stabilized hydrogen peroxide solution) creates a guaiac/peroxidase-like reaction which turn the test paper blue within 60 seconds if occult blood is present. The test reacts with hemoglobin released from lysed cells. When blood is present, hemolysis is promoted by substances in the stool, primarily water and salts. As with any occult blood test, results with the Hemoccult® test cannot be considered conclusive evidence of the presence or absence of gastrointestinal bleeding or pathology. Hemoccult® tests are designed for preliminary screening as a diagnostic aid and are not intended to replace other diagnostic procedures such as proctosigmoidoscopic examination, barium enema, or other x-ray studies. (See LIMITATIONS OF PROCEDURE).

Reagents: Natural guaiac resin impregnated into standardized, high-quality filter paper.
A developing solution containing a stabilized dilute mixture of hydrogen peroxide (less than 6%) and 75% denatured ethyl alcohol in aqueous solution.

Performance Monitors®: The function and stability of the slides and Developer can be tested using the on-slide Performance Monitors®. Both a positive and negative Performance Monitor® are located under the flap and below the specimen windows on the back of the Hemoccult II® and Hemoccult® single slides.
The positive Performance Monitor® contains a hemoglobin-derived catalyst which, upon application of Developer, will turn blue within 30 seconds. The negative Performance Monitor® contains no such catalyst and should not turn blue upon application of Developer.
The Performance Monitors® provide additional assurance that the guaiac-impregnated paper and Developer are functional.
In the unlikely event that the Performance Monitors® do not react as expected after application of Developer, the test results should be regarded as invalid. The Product Support Department at SmithKline Diagnostics will provide further assistance should this occur.

Precautions:
Slides and Tape
For *In Vitro* Diagnostic Use. Do not use after expiration date which appears on each Slide or Tape Dispenser.
Prolonged exposure to some air pollutants and light may cause slides to turn blue. This does not affect the performance of the test and results can be read in the usual manner.

Developer
Hemoccult® Developer should be protected from heat and the bottle kept tightly capped when not in use. It is flammable and subject to evaporation.
Hemoccult® Developer is an irritant. Avoid contact with the skin.
Do Not Use in Eyes. Should such contact occur, solution should be rinsed out promptly with water. Do not use after expiration date on bottle.

Storage and Stability: Do not refrigerate. Store at controlled room temperature 15°–30°C (59°–86°F) in original packaging. Protect from heat. Do not store with volatile chemicals (eg. iodine, chlorine, bromine or ammonia). The Hemoccult® test, stored as recommended, will maintain its sensitivity until the expiration date on the slide. The expiration date appears on each slide and tape dispenser.
Hemoccult® Developer, stored as recommended, will remain stable until the expiration date on the bottle. The expiration date appears on each bottle.

Specimen Collection: Only a very small stool sample, about the size of a matchhead, thinly applied is necessary in preparing either slide or tape. When specimen is to be collected from toilet bowl, the patient should flush the toilet before defecating. The slides may be prepared and developed immediately or prepared and stored for up to 12 days.[3]
Patients with bleeding from other conditions which may affect test results (e.g., hemorrhoids, menstrual bleeding, hematuria) are not appropriate test subjects while such bleeding is active.
Since bleeding from gastrointestinal lesions may be intermittent, it is recommended that stool smears for testing be collected from three consecutive bowel movements. To increase the probability of detecting occult blood, Greegor recommends that samples be taken from two different sections of each stool.[4,5]

Patient Preparation: Whenever practicable, patients should be placed on a meat-free, high residue diet[4,5] starting two days before and continuing through the test period. Such a diet may increase the accuracy of the test and at the same time provide roughage to help uncover "silent" lesions which may bleed only intermittently.
An alternative procedure is to omit the special diet initially. Then if a patient has one or more positive tests in the initial three-slide series, he should be placed on the special diet and retested for three days.[6]

Continued on next page

SmithKline Diagnostics—Cont.

Interfering Substances: Some oral medications (e.g. aspirin, indomethacin, phenylbutazone, corticosteroids, reserpine, etc.) can cause g.i. irritation and occult bleeding in some patients.[7,8] These substances should be discontinued two days prior to and during testing.

Ascorbic acid (Vitamin C) in excess of 250 mg/day may cause false-negaltive results[9] and should also be eliminated before testing.

Therapeutic dosages of iron can yield false-positive fecal occult blood test reactions. Use of iron preparations should be suspended before and during testing for fecal occult blood.[10]

Satisfactory Limits of Performance; Expected Results: Results with the Hemoccult® test are visually determined. The Hemoccult® guaiac test paper should be observed for color change within 60 seconds after Developer has been applied. This reading time is important, because the color reaction may fade after two to four minutes.

If any trace of blue on or at the edge of the smear is seen, the test is positive for occult blood.

Note: Because this test is visually read and requires color differentiation, it should not be read by the visually impaired.

The function and stability of the Hemoccult® slides and Developer can be tested using the on-slide Performance Monitors®. The Hemoccult® Tape may be tested by applying a drop of diluted whole blood (1:5,000 in distilled water) to an unused portion of the tape. Add Developer to opposite side. If any blue appears, the guaiac impregnated paper and Developer are functional.

Limitations of Procedure: As with any occult blood test, results with the Hemoccult® test cannot be considered conclusive evidence of the presence or absence of gastrointestinal bleeding or pathology. Hemoccult® tests are designed for preliminary screening as an aid to diagnosis and are not intended to replace other diagnostic procedures such as proctosigmoidoscopic examination, barium enema, or other x-ray studies. Hemoccult® tests are designed to detect fecal blood which normally contains enough water and salts to hemolyze the blood cells so that they will release hemoglobin.

Hemoccult®, as well as other fecal occult blood tests, should not be used to test gastric specimens. Summary of the Hemoccult® test's performance based on reported experience to date:
1. The positive rate in screening situations has been approximately 3% to 5%.
2. False-positive rate in patients receiving adequate preparation has been between 1% and 2%.

A bibliography on the Hemoccult® test is available on request from the Product Support Department, SmithKline Diagnostics, Inc.

HEMOCCULT® TEST ORDERING INFORMATION

(Please order by product number)
Hemoccult® guaiac paper tests for fecal occult blood are available as follows:

Product / Product Number

HEMOCCULT II® DISPENSAPAK®
with on-slide Performance Monitors®
- 100 Patients Kits 61100
  (Each kit contains 3 Hemoccult II® slides, applicators, envelope, diet and test instructions. Six 15 ml. bottles of Developer also included.)

HEMOCCULT® 2-Hole Single Slides
with on-slide Performance Monitors®
- Boxes of 100 60151
  (100 single slides, two 15 ml. bottles of Developer and applicators)
- Cartons of 1000
  (10 boxes, each containing 100 single slides, twenty 15 ml. bottles of Developer and applicators)

HEMOCCULT II® Two-Specimen Units of Three with on-slide Performance Monitors®
- Boxes of 100 61200
  (34 units of 3 slides, two 15 ml. bottles of Developer and applicators)
- Cartons of 1000
  (10 boxes, each containing 34 units of 3 slides, twenty 15 ml. bottles of Developer and applicators)

HEMOCCULT® TAPE
- 2 Tape Kits 63202
  (Each kit contains one plastic tape dispenser with 100-test capacity and one 15 ml. bottle of Developer)

HEMOCCULT® DEVELOPER
- Twenty 15 ml. bottles 62115

References:
[1] Winawer, S.L. et al: "Screening for Colon Cancer," Gastroenterology 70:783 (May) 1976
[2] Layne, E.A., et al.: "Insensitivity of Guaiac Slide Tests for Detection of Blood in Gastric Juice," Annals of Int. Med. 94:774–776, 1981
[3] Data on file, SmithKline Diagnostics, Inc.
[4] Greegor, D.H.: "Detection of Silent Colon Cancer in Routine Examination," Ca 19:330, 1969
[5] Greegor, D.H.: "Occult Blood Testing for Detection of Asymptomatic Colon Cancer," Cancer 28:131, 1971
[6] Ross, T.H. and Johnson, J.C.M.: "Preliminary Report of a Cancer Screening Program by Physicians in Maricopa County (Ariz.) Arizona Med. 33:445 (June) 1976.
[7] Ostrow, J.D., Mulvaney, C.A., Hansell, J.R. and Rhodes, R.S.: "Sensitivity and Reproducibility of Chemical Tests for Fecal Occult Blood with an Emphasis on False-Positive Reactions," Am. J. Digest Dis. 18:930–40 (Nov.) 1973
[8] Grossman, M.I.; Matsumoto, K.K., and Lichter, R.J.: "Fecal Blood Loss Produced by Oral and Intravenous Administration of Various Salicylates," Gastroenterology 40:383–388 1961
[9] Jaffe, R.M. et al.: "False-Negative Stool Occult Blood Tests Caused by Ingestion of Ascorbic Acid (Vitamin C)," Ann. Int. Med. 83:824 (Dec.) 1975
[10] Lifton, L.J., Kreiser, J.: "False-Positive Stool Occult Blood Tests Caused by Iron Preparations," Gastroenterology 83:860–3 1982.
[11] Herzog; Holtemuller, K.H.: "Oral Cimetidine Does Not Cause False Positive Test for Blood in Stool," NEJM, Sept. 10, 1981

ISOCULT®
[ī'sō-cult]

The Isocult® Diagnostic Culturing System is a fast, accurate, cost-effective way to culture certain medically important organisms as an aid to diagnosis. Clinical studies show Isocult® results are equivalent or superior to standard laboratory procedures. All Isocult® tests are ready to use. Media are contained on the culture paddle (or in the bottom of the culture tube for the *T. vaginalis* test) and are specially formulated to encourage the growth of specific micro-organisms and, when necessary, to suppress or inhibit others. Media are usually modified to enhance the visibility of colonies or to increase the contrast between colonies and the surrounding medium.

A color-coded plastic collar identifies each Isocult® test. Patented tines in the collar streak the specimen along the medium to separate the organisms and isolate colonies when the paddle is inserted through the collar into the tube.

CO_2 generating tablets are supplied with some tests to supply an optimal growth environment. The Isocult® prodecure includes three simple steps:

Inoculate Collect specimens, inoculate, and insert paddle into tube.
Incubate Incubate Isocult® culture test at 35–37° C for the time recommended in each test's product instructions.
Interpret Interpret results by comparing appearance of Isocult® culture test with color photographs on the Organism Identification Chart.

Isocult® culture tests are available for:
Throat Streptococci
Bacteriuria
Neisseria gonorrhoeae
Candida
N. gonorrhoeae / Candida combination
Trichomonas vaginalis
T. vaginalis / Candida combination
Pseudomonas aeruginosa
Staphylococcus aureus

EDUCATIONAL MATERIAL

Patient Education Information and Poster Display
Questions & Answers about Colorectal Cancer/Fecal Occult Blood Testing
Reprint Folder
Selected Articles on Colorectal Cancer and Fecal Occult Blood Testing

---

Winthrop-Breon Laboratories
90 PARK AVENUE
NEW YORK, NY 10016

AMIPAQUE® ℞
brand of metrizamide
SECTION I. Intrathecal Use
SECTION II. Intravascular Use

Description: Metrizamide, 2-[3-Acetamido-2, 4, 6- triiodo -5- (*N*-methylacetamido) benzamido]-2-deoxy-D-glucopyranose, is a compound derived from metrizoic acid and glucosamine. It is a nonionic water-soluble contrast medium with a molecular weight of 789 (iodine content: 48.25%).

The viscosity in centipoise of the "use" concentration ranges from 2.9 at 170 mgI/mL to 12.7 at 300 mgI/mL at room temperature (20°C) and from 1.8 to 6.2 at body temperature (37°C) respectively. Osmolality in mosm/kg at 37°C ranges from 300 at 170 mgI/mL concentration to 484 at 300 mgI/mL. CSF is approximately 301. Specific gravity ranges from 1.184 at 170 mgI/mL to 1.329 at 300 mgI/mL. (CSF normal range is 1.005 to 1.009.) The pH of the solution reconstituted from the diluent is approximately 7.4.

AMIPAQUE is provided as a sterile, white lyophilized powder under vacuum. Each 2.5 g/20 mL vial contains 2.5 g metrizamide (1.21 g organically bound iodine) and 0.8 mg edetate calcium disodium. Each 3.75 g/20 mL vial contains 3.75 g metrizamide (1.81 g organically bound iodine) and 1.2 mg edetate calcium disodium. Each 6.75 g/50 mL vial contains 6.75 g metrizamide (3.26 g organically bound iodine) and 2.16 mg edetate calcium disodium. Each 13.5 g/100 mL vial contains 13.5 g metrizamide (6.51 g organically bound iodine) and 4.32 mg edetate calcium disodium.

Each 20 mL vial and 40 mL vial of sterile aqueous diluent contains 0.05 mg/mL sodium bicarbonate in water for injection. pH is adjusted with Carbon Dioxide, USP, if necessary.

AMIPAQUE solution and powder is sensitive to heat or light and, therefore, should be protected from exposure.

SECTION I
Clinical Pharmacology — Intrathecal:
AMIPAQUE is absorbed from cerebrospinal fluid into the bloodstream in adults. Approximately 60 percent of the administered dose is excreted unchanged through the kidneys within 48 hours.

The initial concentration and volume of the medium, in conjunction with appropriate patient manipulation, will determine the extent of the diagnostic contrast that can be achieved. This can be monitored by fluoroscopy.

Following subarachnoid injection conventional radiography will continue to provide good diagnostic contrast for at least 30 minutes. At about 1 hour diagnostic degree of contrast will not usually be available. However, sufficient contrast for CT myelography will be available for several hours. CT myelography, following conventional myelography, should be deferred for at least 4 hours to reduce the degree of contrast.

In a multi-centered study, AMIPAQUE was used in 502 pediatric patients for a variety of procedures. The results and effects of the medium were similar to that in adults.

Following subarachnoid placement, irrespective of the position in which the patient is later maintained, slow upward diffusion of AMIPAQUE takes place through the CSF. After introduction into the lumbar subarachnoid space, without special positioning of the patient, computerized tomography (CT) shows CSF contrast enhancement in the thoracic region in about 1 hour, in the cervical region in about 2 hours, and in the basal cisterns in 3 to 4 hours.

When low doses (4 mL to 6 mL of 170 mgI/mL to 190 mgI/mL) of AMIPAQUE are introduced into the lumbar CSF and moved cephalad under gravity control and examined by CT scanning, they will provide immediate CSF contrast in the basal cisterns. Depending on the specific technique used, the lateral, third, and fourth ventricles may also be visualized. The contrast in this area will markedly diminish at 6 hours and disappear by 24 hours. CSF enhancement will be evident at the cortical sulci and interhemispheric fissures at 6 hours.

Between 12 and 24 hours the surfaces of the cerebrum and cerebellum, in contact with the subarachnoid spaces, will develop a "blush" effect on the scan which will normally disappear in 36 to 48 hours. The rate, time, extent of diffusion, and the disappearance or stasis of AMIPAQUE as demonstrated with CT scanning, can be used to detect or infer the presence of CNS or CSF circulation abnormalities.

Indications and Usage — Intrathecal: AMIPAQUE is indicated in adults and pediatric patients for lumbar, thoracic, cervical, and total columnar myelography and for use in computerized tomography of the intracranial subarachnoid spaces following spinal subarachnoid injection.

In pediatric patients, AMIPAQUE is also indicated for cisternography and ventriculography by direct injection using standard radiologic techniques.

Contraindications — Intrathecal: AMIPAQUE should not be administered to patients with a known hypersensitivity to metrizamide.

Intrathecal administration of corticosteroids with AMIPAQUE, brand of metrizamide, is contraindicated.

Immediate repeat myelography, in the event of technical failure, is contraindicated because of overdosage considerations. (See interval recommendation under DOSAGE AND ADMINISTRATION.)

Lumbar puncture should not be performed in the presence of significant local or systemic infection where bacteremia is likely.

Warnings—Intrathecal: If grossly bloody CSF is encountered, the possible benefits of a myelographic procedure should be considered in terms of the risk to the patient.

Fatal reactions have been associated with the administration of water-soluble contrast media. Therefore, it is of utmost importance that a course of action be carefully planned in advance for the immediate treatment of serious reactions, and that adequate and appropriate facilities and personnel be readily available in case of a severe reaction.

Caution is advised in patients with a history of epilepsy, severe cardiovascular disease, chronic alcoholism or multiple sclerosis.

Elderly patients may present a greater risk following myelography. The need for the procedure in these patients should be evaluated carefully. Special attention must be paid to dose and concentration of the medium, hydration, and technique used.

Patients who are receiving anticonvulsants should be maintained on this therapy. Should a seizure occur, intravenous diazepam or phenobarbital sodium is recommended. In patients with a history of seizure activity who are not on anticonvulsant therapy, premedication with barbiturates or phenytoin should be considered.

Prophylactic anticonvulsant treatment with barbiturates should be considered in patients with evidence of inadvertent intracranial entry of a large or concentrated bolus of the contrast medium since there is an increased risk of seizures in such cases.

Drugs which lower the seizure threshold, especially phenothiazine derivatives, including those used for their antihistamine properties should not be used with AMIPAQUE. Others include MAO inhibitors, tricyclic antidepressants, CNS stimulants, psychoactive drugs described as analeptics, major tranquilizers, or antipsychotic drugs. Such medication should be discontinued at least 48 hours before myelography, should not be used for the control of nausea and vomiting, and should not be resumed for at least 24 hours postprocedure. Care is required in patient management to prevent inadvertent intracranial entry of a large dose or concentrated bolus of the medium. Also, effort should be directed to avoid rapid dispersion of the medium causing inadvertent rise to intracranial levels (eg, by active patient movement). Direct intracisternal or ventricular administration for standard radiography (not CT) is not recommended.

In most reported cases of major motor seizures one or more of the following factors were present. Therefore avoid:
- Deviations from recommended procedure or in myelographic management.
- Use in patients with a history of epilepsy.
- Inadvertent overdosage.
- Intracranial entry of a bolus or premature diffusion of a high concentration of the medium.
- Medication with neuroleptic drugs or phenothiazine antinauseants.
- Failure to maintain elevation of the head during the procedure, on the stretcher, or in bed.
- Excessive and particularly active patient movement or straining.

At concentrations of 200 mgI/mL or less, these seizures have been noted only very rarely.

Treatment with intravenous diazepam or administration of phenobarbital sodium has provided rapid control of seizures. (See PATIENT MANAGEMENT.)

Precautions—Intrathecal: Before a contrast medium is injected, the patient should be questioned for a history of allergy. Although a history of allergy, including asthma, may imply a greater than usual risk, it does not arbitrarily contraindicate the use of the medium. No conclusive relationship between severe reactions and antigen-antibody reactions or other manifestations of allergy has been established.

In patients with severe renal insufficiency or failure, the drug is excreted by the liver into the bile at a much slower rate. Patients with hepatorenal insufficiency should not be examined unless the possibility of benefit clearly outweighs the additional risk.

For Repeat Procedure see DOSAGE AND ADMINISTRATION.

If nondisposable equipment is used, scrupulous care should be taken to prevent residual contamination with traces of cleansing agents.

Pregnancy Category B. Reproduction studies have been performed in rats and rabbits up to 70 times the human dose and have revealed no evidence of impaired fertility or harm to the fetus due to AMIPAQUE, brand of metrizamide. There are, however, no adequate and well controlled studies in pregnant women. Because animal reproduction studies are not always predictive of human response, this drug should be used during pregnancy only if clearly needed.

Nursing Mothers. Caution should be exercised when AMIPAQUE is administered to a nursing woman. AMIPAQUE is excreted in milk to the extent of 1 mg of the injected myelographic dose over 2 days.

Adverse Reactions—Intrathecal: The most frequently occurring adverse reactions are headache, nausea, and vomiting. These reactions occur 3 to 8 hours postinjection, almost all occurring within 24 hours. They are usually mild to moderate in degree lasting for a few hours and usually disappearing within 24 hours. Rarely, headaches may be severe or persist for days. The reported incidence of headaches varies from 20 to over 60 percent and they are often accompanied by nausea and vomiting. Headaches tend to be more frequent and persistent in patients not optimally hydrated. (See PATIENT MANAGEMENT.)

Backache, neck stiffness, numbness and paresthesias, leg or sciatic-type pain occurred less frequently, often in the form of a transient exacerbation of preexisting symptomatology. Temperature elevations constitute the fourth most common reaction in individuals under 18 years of age. Dizziness has also been reported.

The incidence and nature of adverse reactions in pediatric patients is similar to adult patients except for the occurrence of a higher incidence of fever (19%) and occasional incidence of croup, breast feeding problems, and crying spells. Of the 42 percent of pediatric patients who received general anesthesia, the incidence of nausea and vomiting was generally higher.

Cardiovascular: Chest pain, tachycardia, bradycardia and other arrhythmias, hypertension or hypotension, cardiac arrest, vasculitis, hemorrhage, collapse, and shock have also been reported. Transient alterations in vital signs may occur. Their significance must be assessed on an individual basis.

Other rarely occurring adverse reactions include the following:

Major motor seizures: Focal or generalized grand mal seizures have occurred with an incidence reported between 0.1 and 0.3 percent. They have usually occurred 4 to 12 hours following injection, and have consisted of one or two episodes 1 or more hours apart, which have responded promptly to the intravenous injection of diazepam. For prolonged prophylaxis barbiturates have been recommended.

Early onset of seizures (less than 2 hours) is indicative of early substantial intracranial entry.

Transitory EEG changes are frequent and usually take the form of slow wave activity, although sharp activity and paroxysmal activity have been reported up to 24 hours after the procedure, the incidence of EEG changes may be as high as 30 percent.

An **aseptic meningitis** syndrome, has been reported rarely (less than 0.1%). It was usually preceded by pronounced headaches, nausea and vomiting. Onset usually occurred about 12 to 18 hours postprocedure. Prominent features were meningismus, fever, sometimes with oculomotor signs and mental confusion. Lumbar puncture revealed a high white cell count, high protein content often with a low glucose level and with absence of organisms. The condition usually started to clear spontaneously about 10 hours after onset, with complete recovery over 2 to 3 days.

Allergy or idiosyncrasy: Chills, fever, profuse diaphoresis, pruritus, urticaria, nasal congestion, dyspnea, and a case of Guillain-Barre syndrome.

CNS irritation: Mild and transitory perceptual aberrations such as hallucinations, depersonalization, amnesia, hostility, amblyopia, diplopia, photophobia, psychosis, insomnia, anxiety, depression, hyperesthesia, visual, auditory or speech disturbances, confusion and disorientation. In addition, malaise, weakness, EEG changes, menin-

Continued on next page

This product information was effective as of December 3, 1984. On these and other products of Winthrop-Breon Laboratories, detailed information may be obtained on a current basis by direct inquiry to the Professional Services Department, 90 Park Avenue, New York, NY 10016 (212) 907-2525.

Winthrop-Breon—Cont.

gismus, hyperreflexia or areflexia, hypertonia or flaccidity, hemiplegia, paralysis, quadriplegia, restlessness, tremor, echoacousia, echolalia, asterixis or dysphasia have occurred.

Profound mental disturbances have also rarely been reported. They have usually consisted of various forms and degrees of aphasia, mental confusion or disorientation. The onset is usually at 8 to 10 hours and lasts for about 24 hours, without aftereffects. However, occasionally they have been manifest as apprehension, agitation, or progressive withdrawal in several instances to the point of somnolence, stupor and coma. In a few cases these have been accompanied by transitory hearing loss or other auditory symptoms and visual disturbances (believed subjective or delusional), including unilateral or bilateral loss of vision which may last for hours. In one case persistent cortical loss of vision has been reported in association with convulsions. Ventricular block has been reported in two cases, amnesia of varying degrees may be present for the reaction event.

Rarely, persistent though transitory weakness in the leg or ocular muscles has been reported.

Peripheral neuropathies have been rare and transitory. They include sensory and/or motor or nerve root disturbances, myelitis, persistent leg muscle pain or weakness, or 6th nerve palsy, or cauda equina syndrome. Muscle cramps, fasciculation or myoclonia, spinal convulsion, or spasticity are unusual and have responded promptly to a small intravenous dose of diazepam.

Respiratory: Apnea and pulmonary edema have been reported.

Body-General: Asthenia, cellulitis, hyponatremia, hemolytic anemia, generalized angioedema with marked dyspnea and stridor, and deaths have been reported.

Urogenital: Renal failure, polyuria, hematuria, and urinary retention have been reported.

Overdosage—Intrathecal: There is clinical evidence that reactions, particularly seizures and mental aberrations, following the administration of myelographic doses in excess of those recommended tend to be dose related. Even use of a recommended dose can produce effects tantamount to overdosage, if incorrect management of the patient during or immediately following the procedure permits inadvertent early intracranial entry of a large portion of the medium.

Treatment: See ADVERSE REACTIONS—Major motor seizures.

The subarachnoid LD_{50} in mice is greater than 1,500 mgI/kg.

Dosage and Administration—Intrathecal:
See also PATIENT MANAGEMENT

The dosage and concentration of AMIPAQUE will depend on the degree and extent of contrast required in the area(s) under examination and on the equipment and technique employed. Concentrations which are approximately isotonic (170 mgI/mL to 190 mgI/mL) are recommended for examination in the lumbar region. For movement of the medium to distant target areas, higher concentrations are recommended to compensate for dilution of AMIPAQUE with CSF.

A total dose of 3000 mg iodine or a concentration of 300 mgI/mL should not be exceeded. As in all diagnostic procedures, the least amount to produce adequate visualization should be used. Most procedures do not require either maximum dose or concentration. The incidence of serious adverse reactions is considerably less with concentrations of 200 mgI/mL or less. The dose and concentration used in the spinal area influence ultimate intracranial concentrations.

Anesthesia is not necessary. Premedication sedatives or tranquilizers are usually not needed (see PRECAUTIONS). Patients should be well hydrated. Epileptic patients should be maintained on their anticonvulsant medication.

As with any lumbar puncture, sterile technique must be employed. The lumbar puncture is usually made between L3 and L4, but if pathology is suspected at this level the interspace immediately above or below may be selected. A lateral cervical puncture may also be used.

Rate of Injection: To avoid excessive mixing with CSF and consequent loss of contrast as well as premature dispersion upward, injection must be made slowly over 1 to 2 minutes.

The lumbar puncture needle is removed immediately following injection since it is not necessary to remove AMIPAQUE after injection into subarachnoid spaces.

Repeat Procedure: An interval of at least 48 hours should be allowed before repeat examination; however, whenever possible 5 to 7 days is recommended.

The recommended usual and maximum doses of AMIPAQUE, brand of metrizamide, are summarized in the following tables:
[See table below].

The pediatric doses, intended as guidelines, are based on age range rather than weight because brain or CSF capacity is independent of weight. Variations will depend on such factors as height, nature of pathology, condition of the patient, technique used, etc (eg, whether for CSF contrast for CT scan or for standard radiography, or whether movement of the medium is to be directed to an area distal to the site of injection). Direct intracranial placement will require particular care in planning to maintain total dose and concentration as low as practical to avoid convulsive response. Whenever possible (eg, for CT scan) the use of the isotonic concentration (170 mgI/mL) is preferable. In children, loss of contrast due to mixing on movement of the medium is less apt to occur because of their shorter spinal cord. Therefore, the use of relatively lower dosages may be feasible.
[See table on next page].

The medium disperses in about 60 minutes following direct ventricular placement.

Young children may require general anesthesia for technical reasons.

Convulsions occurred in a few patients, only one attributable to the medium, at these dosage schedules.

Prophylactic barbiturates are suggested for inadvertent overdosage. Parenteral diazepam or barbiturates is suggested for treatment of seizures and barbiturates and/or phenytoin for continued suppression.

Preparation of the Solution—Intrathecal:
1. Select the correct iodine concentration recommended for the procedure in the DOSAGE TABLES.
2. The volume of diluent required to obtain that iodine concentration can be obtained from the DILUTION TABLE.
3. Using a sterile technique with a small gauge transfer needle (approximately 22 gauge to help prevent coring), withdraw the required amount of diluent.
4. Insert this volume of diluent into the lyophil vial also using the fine needle. Contents under vacuum. Use only if vacuum is present as evidenced by diluent being drawn into vial when stopper is punctured. Leave syringe and needle in place.
5. Gently swirl the vial (without shaking) until its contents are dissolved (approximately 3 to 10 minutes) to insure complete dissolution of the lyophil. The resulting solution should be clear and colorless to slightly yellow. Do not use if undissolved particulate matter or bubbles are present.
6. Withdraw the volume of AMIPAQUE, brand of metrizamide, recommended for the procedure in the DOSAGE TABLES.
7. Detach syringe and attach to myelographic injection unit. Use immediately after reconstitution. Discard any unused portion.
[See table on page 3022].

Patient Management—Intrathecal:
Suggestions for Usual Patient Management

Preprocedure
- Discontinue neuroleptic drugs (including phenothiazines, eg, chlorpromazine, prochlorperazine, and promethazine) 48 hours beforehand.
- Maintain normal diet up to 2 hours before.
- Ensure hydration—fluids up to procedure.

During Procedure
- Use minimum dose and concentration required for satisfactory contrast. (See DOSAGE AND ADMINISTRATION.)
- In all positioning techniques keep the patient's head elevated above highest level of spine.
- Do not lower head of table more than 15° during thoraco-cervical procedures.
- In patients with excessive lordosis consider lateral position for injection and movement of the medium cephalad.
- Avoid intracranial entry of a bolus.
- Avoid early and high cephalad dispersion of the medium.
- Inject slowly over 1 to 2 minutes to avoid excessive mixing.
- Abrupt or active patient movement causes excessive mixing with CSF. Instruct patient to remain passive. Move patient slowly and only as necessary.
- To maintain as a bolus, move medium to distal area very slowly under fluoroscopic control.
- At completion of direct cervical or lumbo-cervical procedures, raise head of table steeply (45°) for about 2 minutes to restore medium to lower levels.

Postprocedure
- Raise head of stretcher to at least 15° before moving patient onto it.
- Movement onto stretcher, and off the stretcher to bed, should be done slowly with patient completely passive, maintaining head up position.
- Before moving patient onto bed, raise head of bed 15° to 30°.
- Advise patient to remain still in bed, in head up position, especially in first few hours.
- Maintain close observation for at least 12 hours after myelogram.
- After 8 hours, patient may be lowered to a horizontal position for further 16 hours.
- Obtain visitors' cooperation in keeping the patient quiet and in head up position, especially in first few hours.

ADULT DOSAGE TABLE—Iodine Content

Procedure	Conc. of Solution (mgI/mL)	Usual Recommended Dose* (mL)	Max. Dose Total (mgI)
Lumbar myelogram	170–190	10–15	2850
Thoracic myelogram	220	12	2640
Cervical myelogram (lumbar injection)	250–300	10	3000
Cervical myelogram (lateral cervical injection)	220	10	2200
Total columnar myelography	250–280	10	2800
CT cisternography (lumbar injection)	170–190	4–6	1140

* Refer to DILUTION TABLE FOR INTRATHECAL USE for preparation of Solution

- Encourage oral fluids and diet as tolerated.
- If nausea or vomiting occurs, do not use phenothiazine antinauseants. Persistent nausea and vomiting will result in dehydration. Therefore, prompt consideration of replacement by intravenous fluids is recommended.

Alternative Postprocedure Method
- Recent evidence suggests that maintaining the patient postmyelography in an upright position (via wheelchair or ambulation) may help minimize adverse effects. The upright position may help to delay upward dispersion of the medium and to maximize the spinal arachnoid absorption.

SECTION II

Clinical Pharmacology—Intravascular: Intravascular injection of a radiopaque diagnostic agent opacifies those vessels in the path of flow of the contrast medium permitting radiographic visualization of the internal structures of the human body until significant hemodilution occurs. The pharmacokinetics of the intravenously administered radiopaque contrast media are usually best described by a two compartment model with a rapid alpha phase for drug distribution and a slow beta phase for drug elimination. In patients with renal and kidney functional impairment, the elimination half-life for the beta phase may be prolonged for up to several days.

Following intravenous injection, AMIPAQUE is distributed and excreted in a manner similar to the diatrizoates, ie, following initial high serum levels, the level falls rapidly as the medium becomes distributed throughout the extravascular compartment. Thereafter, it is excreted unchanged principally by glomerular filtration. It is not metabolized. About 94% of the medium is excreted in this manner in 24 hours and a further 5% by hepatobiliary excretion via the bowel.

Indications and Usage — Intravascular: AMIPAQUE is indicated for intravenous digital arteriography for head and neck, adult peripheral arteriography, and pediatric angiocardiography.

Contraindications—Intravascular: Known hypersensitivity to AMIPAQUE, brand of metrizamide.

Warnings—Intravascular: In patients with myelomatosis the effects of nonionic media on renal function is unknown. If a decision to use AMIPAQUE is made, the patient should be well hydrated beforehand, a minimal diagnostic dose used, and renal function and extent of urinary precipitation of the myeloma protein checked for a few days afterwards.

Contrast media may promote sickling in individuals who are homozygous for sickle cell disease when the material is injected intravenously or intra-arterially.

Administration of radiopaque materials to patients known or suspected of having pheochromocytoma should be performed with extreme caution. If, in the opinion of the physician, the possible benefits of such procedures outweigh the considered risks, the procedures may be performed; however, the amount of radiopaque medium injected should be kept to an absolute minimum. The blood pressure should be assessed throughout the procedure and measures for treatment of a hypertensive crisis should be available.

Recent reports of thyroid storm occurring following the intravascular use of iodinated radiopaque diagnostic agents in patients with hyperthyroidism or with an autonomously functioning thyroid nodule suggest that this additional risk be evaluated in such patients before use of these drugs.

Arteriography should be performed with caution in patients with severely impaired renal function and patients with combined renal and hepatic disease.

Precautions—Intravascular: Diagnostic procedures which involve the use of radiopaque diagnostic agents should be carried out under the direction of personnel with the prerequisite training and with a thorough knowledge of the particular procedure to be performed. Appropriate facilities should be available for coping with any complication of the procedure, as well as for emergency treatment of severe reactions to the contrast agent itself. After parenteral administration of a radiopaque agent, competent personnel and emergency facilities should be available for at least 30 to 60 minutes since severe delayed reactions have occurred (see ADVERSE REACTIONS).

Since allergic response can occur with the nonionic media, similar preparations to those recommended for ionic media should be planned to handle severe or potentially fatal complications. These measures are to ensure the ready availability of appropriate resuscitative drugs, equipment, and personnel.

A history of allergy to the intravascular use of metrizamide, or other contrast agents, may indicate a greater likelihood of allergic response. However, such history is not a contraindication but calls for caution in use.

The possibility of an idiosyncratic reaction in susceptible patients should always be considered (see ADVERSE REACTIONS). The susceptible population includes patients with a history of a previous reaction to a contrast media, patients with a known sensitivity to iodine per se, and patients with a known clinical hypersensitivity: bronchial asthma, hay fever and food allergies.

The occurrence of severe idiosyncratic reactions has prompted the use of several pretesting methods. However, pretesting cannot be relied upon to predict severe reactions and may itself be hazardous for the patient. It is suggested that a thorough medical history with emphasis on allergy and hypersensitivity, prior to the injection of any contrast media, may be more accurate than pretesting in predicting potential adverse reactions.

A positive history of allergies or hypersensitivity does not arbitrarily contraindicate the use of a contrast agent, where a diagnostic procedure is thought essential, but caution should be exercised (see ADVERSE REACTIONS). Premedication with antihistamines or corticosteroids to avoid or minimize possible allergic reactions in such patients should be considered. Recent reports indicate that such pretreatment does not prevent serious life-threatening reactions, but may reduce both their incidence and severity.

Continued on next page

PEDIATRIC DOSAGE TABLE—Iodine Content

Conventional Radiography

Procedure	Age	Conc. of Solution (mgI/mL)	Usual Recommended Dose* (mL)
Lumbar, thoracic myelography (lumbar injection)	Less than 2 months	170–190	2–3
	2 months to 2 years	170–190	2–4
	3 to 7 years	170–190	4–8
	8 to 12 years	170–190	7–9
	13 to 18 years	170–190	8–10
Cervical myelography (lumbar injection)	Less than 2 months	170–210	2–3
	2 months to 2 years	170–200	2–4
	3 to 7 years	170–210	4–8
	8 to 12 years	170–230	7–9
	13 to 18 years	170–230	8–10
Cervical myelography (lateral cervical injection)	8 to 18 years	200–220	3–5
Cisternography (direct injection)	Less than 2 months	170–220	2–3
	8 to 18 years	170–220	2–5
Cisternography (lumbar injection)	2 months to 2 years	170–220	2–3
	3 to 7 years	170–190	3–5
	8 to 12 years	170–190	5–6
Ventriculography (direct injection)	Less than 2 months	170–220	2–3
	2 months to 2 years	170–220	2–3
	3 to 12 years	170–220	2–4
	13 to 18 years	190–220	2–5
Ventriculography (lumbar injection)	2 months to 2 years	170–220	2–3

CT Radiography

Procedure	Age	Conc. of Solution (mgI/mL)	Usual Recommended Dose* (mL)
CT cisternography (lumbar injection)	3 to 7 years	170–190	3–5
	8 to 12 years	180–190	3–5
	13 to 18 years	170–190	3–5
CT ventriculography (direct injection)	Less than 2 months	170–220	2
	2 months to 2 years	170–220	2
	3 to 7 years	170–220	3
CT ventriculography (lumbar injection)	3 to 7 years	170–220	3

* Refer to DILUTION TABLE FOR INTRATHECAL USE for preparation of Solution

---

This product information was effective as of December 3, 1984. On these and other products of Winthrop-Breon Laboratories, detailed information may be obtained on a current basis by direct inquiry to the Professional Services Department, 90 Park Avenue, New York, NY 10016 (212) 907-2525.

Winthrop-Breon—Cont.

Azotemia is not a contraindication. Care should be taken regarding dosage and hydration status and the patient's renal status should be monitored for days afterwards.

Acute renal failure has been reported in diabetic patients with diabetic nephropathy and in susceptible nondiabetic patients (often elderly with preexisting renal disease) following intravascular use of contrast media. Therefore, careful consideration of the potential risks should be given before performing this radiographic procedure in these patients.

Preparatory dehydration is dangerous and may contribute to acute renal failure in infants, young children, elderly, patients with preexisting renal insufficiency, and patients with advanced vascular disease. Dehydration in these patients seems to be enhanced by the osmotic diuretic action of contrast agents. It is believed that overnight fluid restriction prior to angiography does not provide better visualization in normal patients. Therefore, preparatory dehydration is unnecessary, and is usually contraindicated, in association with the angiographic use of AMIPAQUE, brand of metrizamide.

Angiography should be avoided whenever possible in patients with homocystinuria, because of the risk of inducing thrombosis and embolism.

Drug/Laboratory Test Interactions
It is expected that the results of thyroid function tests, which depend on iodine estimations, will not reflect true function for about 16 days. Tests which directly determine thyroxine levels should not be affected.

Pregnancy Category B. See Intrathecal Uses. Precautions.

Nursing Mothers. Caution should be exercised when AMIPAQUE is administered to a nursing woman. AMIPAQUE is excreted in milk to the extent of 1 mg of the injected myelographic dose over 2 days.

The nature of the adverse effects which occur following intravascular administration of AMIPAQUE is similar to that following corresponding ionic media although their incidence and severity may be less.

The following is based on general vascular experience with both ionic and nonionic media.

Adverse Reactions—Intravascular: Reactions which have been observed are similar in nature to those following the use of ionic media.

Cardiovascular: Various arrhythmias, bradycardia being the most frequent, as well as peripheral vasodilation with brief hypotension have occurred.

Hemodynamic: A feeling of heat, usually mild but which may be moderate in degree, may be evident particularly following selective arterial procedures. Frank pain is very unusual.

Renal: Mild diuresis and transitory mild increase in urine osmolarity.

Allergic: Dermal urticaria or erythemata have occurred. Therefore, other allergic manifestations such as rigors, broncho or laryngospastic attacks with serious cardiopulmonary complications resulting in fatality must be considered a possibility.

Respiratory: Pulmonary or laryngeal edema, dyspnea.

Nervous System: Restlessness, tremors.

Technical Factors: Hematoma, ecchymosis, extravasation of the medium particularly on mechanical high pressure injection, venous rupture or hemorrhage from arterial injection sites (observe areas for at least 24 hours).

Individual Indications and Usage—Intravascular:

INTRAVENOUS DIGITAL ARTERIOGRAPHY FOR THE HEAD AND NECK
AMIPAQUE solution can be injected intravenously as a rapid bolus to provide arterial visualization using digital subtraction radiography. Preprocedural medications are not considered necessary. AMIPAQUE will provide diagnostic arterial radiographs in about 90% of patients. In almost all cases in which poor arterial visualization occurs (10%), it can be attributed to patient movement. AMIPAQUE is very well tolerated in the vascular system. There is very little subjective or objective evidence of patient discomfort (general sensation of heat) following the injection as compared with ionic media. Very few of the reactions are moderate to severe in degree. In about 87% of patients discomfort is either absent or is mild. Some patients exhibit mild nausea which does not appear to be dose related.

Precautions: Since the dose is usually administered mechanically under high pressure, rupture of smaller peripheral veins has occurred. It has been suggested that this can be avoided by using an intravenous catheter threaded proximally beyond larger tributaries or in the case of the antecubital vein, into the superior vena cava. Sometimes the femoral vein is used.

Dosage and Administration: The maximum total dose administered to the patient should not exceed 87.5 g of iodine. See DESCRIPTION section for iodine content.

AMIPAQUE is administered intravenously as a bolus injection in a concentration of 370 mgI/mL.

The usual individual volume is about 40 mL (range 30 mL to 60 mL).

Frequently three injections may be required, up to a total volume of about 120 mL (range 40 mL to 165 mL).

The patient is urged not to move during, or immediately after, the injection. In the case of carotid-cerebral arteriography, the patient is also asked not to swallow during this period. AMIPAQUE is usually administered via 16-18 gauge catheter by mechanical injection at a rate of about 12 mL/sec. A dextrose solution may be layered over the contrast medium in the injector with the purpose of pushing the remnant of the bolus forward into the main circulation, and to flush out the vein.

ADULT PERIPHERAL ARTERIOGRAPHY
AMIPAQUE, brand of metrizamide, solution in a concentration of 370 mgI/mL is recommended for arteriography of the lower limbs. The injection is usually through a catheter introduced into the femoral artery with the tip placed as to achieve lower aortic or aorto-iliac runoff or visualization of individual femoral artery or its distribution throughout the lower limb. When necessary, the catheter tip may be advanced to the level of the renal artery. Pressure injection is usually employed. Visualization is similar to that achieved with ionic media of similar dose and concentration. Sedative premedication may be employed with AMIPAQUE, however, anesthesia is usually not considered necessary.

Adverse Reactions: Very brief (seconds to minutes) nausea immediately following the injection or mild urticaria starting within minutes and of a few hours duration, has been reported in about 3% of patients; these reactions have not interfered with the procedure. Patient discomfort during and immediately following the injection is substantially less than the discomfort which follows injection of ionic media of similar volume and concentrations. Severe discomfort is very unusual.

Dosage and Administration: The maximum total dose administered to the patient should not exceed 87.5 g of iodine. See DESCRIPTION section for iodine content.

The volume required will depend on the size, flow rate and disease status of the injected artery, and on the size and condition of the patient as well as the imaging technique used. The usual individual volume is about 50 mL (range 25 mL to 65 mL). Two injections are usually required, sometimes three, and rarely up to five.

PEDIATRIC ANGIOCARDIOGRAPHY
AMIPAQUE at a maximum concentration of 370 mgI/mL may be used for angiocardiography in infants and young children.

Dosage and Administration: The recommended single dose of AMIPAQUE in 370 mgI/mL concentration is about 1.5 mL/kg (range 1 mL/kg to 2 mL/kg). In addition, small test volumes of about 2 mL may be used for catheter placement. The usual total dose of AMIPAQUE per procedure, which includes diagnostic and test doses, is about 4 mL/kg (range 1.5 mL/kg to 6 mL/kg).

Analgesics and/or sedative tranquilizers may be required in these young patients.

Preparation of the Solution—Intravascular Use: 1. Determine the concentration required for the vascular procedure.

2. The volume of diluent required to obtain that iodine concentration can be obtained from the DILUTION TABLE.

3. Using a sterile technique with a small gauge transfer needle (approximately 22 gauge to help prevent coring), withdraw the required amount of diluent.

4. Insert this volume of diluent into the lyophil vial also using the fine needle. Contents under vacuum. Use only if vacuum is present as evidenced by diluent being drawn into vial when stopper is punctured. Leave syringe and needle in place.

5. Gently swirl the vial (without shaking) until its contents are dissolved (approximately 3 to 10 minutes) to insure complete dissolution of the lyophil. The resulting solution should be clear and colorless to slightly yellow. Do not use if undissolved particulate matter or bubbles are present.

DILUTION TABLE FOR INTRATHECAL USE

Conc. of Solution (mgI/mL)	Volume of Diluent to be Added		
	2.5 g vial (mL)	3.75 g vial (mL)	6.75 g vial (mL)
170	6.0	8.9	16.1
180	5.6	8.3	15.0
190	5.3	7.8	14.0
200	4.9	7.3	13.2
210	4.7	6.9	12.4
220	4.4	6.5	11.7
230	4.2	6.1	11.1
240	3.9	5.8	10.5
250	3.7	5.5	10.0
260	3.6	5.2	9.4
270	3.4	5.0	9.0
280	3.2	4.7	8.5
290	3.1	4.5	8.1
300	2.9	4.3	7.8

The volume of the final solution will equal the volume of the diluent + 1.1 mL

The volume of the final solution will equal the volume of the diluent + 1.7 mL

The volume of the final solution will equal the volume of the diluent + 3.1 mL

The volume of the final solution will exceed the amount required to achieve the recommended dosage. For volume for injection refer to DOSAGE TABLES.

6. Withdraw the volume of AMIPAQUE, brand of metrizamide, required.
[See table above].

How Supplied:
Kits, each containing
  One 3.75 g/20 mL single-dose vial of AMIPAQUE with 1 (20 mL) vial of diluent (NDC 0024-0044-01); or
  One 6.75 g/50 mL single-dose vial of AMIPAQUE with 1 (20 mL) vial of diluent (NDC 0024-0046-01).
Combination packs, each containing
  Five 2.5 g/20 mL single-dose vials of AMIPAQUE with 5 (20 mL) vials of diluent (NDC 0024-0047-12); or
  Five 3.75 g/20 mL single-dose vials of AMIPAQUE with 5 (20 mL) vials of diluent (NDC 0024-0044-12); or
  Five 6.75 g/50 mL single-dose vials of AMIPAQUE with 5 (20 mL) vials of diluent (NDC 0024-0046-12); or
  Five 13.5 g/100 mL single-dose vials of AMIPAQUE with 5 (40 mL) vials of diluent (NDC 0024-0049-12).
Protect vials of AMIPAQUE from light or excessive heat 40°C (104°F).

AW-144 L

DILUTION TABLE FOR INTRAVASCULAR USE

Conc. of Solution (mgI/mL)	Volume of Diluent to be Added	
	6.75 g vial (mL)	13.5 g vial (mL)
300	7.8	15.5
310	7.4	14.8
320	7.1	14.1
330	6.8	13.5
340	6.5	12.9
350	6.2	12.4
360	6.0	11.9
370	5.7	11.4

The volume of the final solution will equal the volume of the diluent + 3.1 mL

The volume of the final solution will equal the volume of the diluent + 6.2 mL

The volume of the final solution will exceed the amount required to achieve the recommended dosage. For volume for injection refer to individual Dosage and Administration sections.

BILOPAQUE® SODIUM ℞
brand of tyropanoate sodium, USP

ORAL CHOLECYSTOGRAPHIC MEDIUM

Description: BILOPAQUE sodium, brand of tyropanoate sodium, is a diagnostic enteral cholecystographic radiopaque agent used for radiographic visualization of the gallbladder and biliary tract. Each 750 mg capsule contains 57.4 percent organically bound iodine.

BILOPAQUE sodium is an off-white, odorless, hygroscopic solid which is soluble in water to 14.7 percent. Sodium content per 3 g dose is 100 mg. The molecular weight is 663.1.

BILOPAQUE sodium is a substituted, triiodinated, benzoic acid derivative. BILOPAQUE is sodium 3-butyramido-α-ethyl-2,4,6-triiodohydrocinnamate.

Clinical Pharmacology: The most important characteristic of contrast media is the iodine content. The relatively high atomic weight of iodine contributes sufficient radiodensity for radiographic contrast with surrounding tissues.

Diagnostic enteral radiopaque agents have few known pharmacological effects. They are moderately uricosuric. Tyropanoate sodium when absorbed systemically may produce iodine-mediated thyrotropic effects described under PRECAUTIONS.

Pharmacokinetics
Tyropanoate sodium is absorbed by passive diffusion across the gastrointestinal mucosa. Absorption of the agent can be improved by increasing the gastrointestinal pH, drug solubility, and availability of bile salts.

Controversy exists regarding the effects of food on the absorption and clinical efficacy of the cholecystographic agents. In one study, the number of satisfactory cholecystograms obtained with the agent administered with a high-fat meal was greater than with a nonfat meal. However, the fat content of the meal had no significant effect on the number of satisfactory cholecystograms obtained with tyropanoate sodium. Therefore, recommendations regarding the size or content of the evening meal on the day prior to oral cholecystography are made at the discretion of the physician.

Once absorbed, tyropanoate sodium enters the systemic circulation via the portal venous system. It is then transported to the liver and bound to plasma albumin. The affinity for albumin may determine the primary route of elimination, biliary or renal, with the more extensively bound agents primarily excreted by the hepatobiliary system.

In the liver, BILOPAQUE is metabolized to glucuronide esters which are then actively excreted into the hepatic ducts and concentrated by the gallbladder. The time of peak opacification of the gallbladder is approximately 4 to 10 hours for BILOPAQUE. However, diagnostically adequate visualization of gallbladder may occur within 5 to 6 hours.

BILOPAQUE is removed from the body by two pathways: excretion into the duodenum via the common bile duct and renal elimination. The ratio of renal to fecal elimination for BILOPAQUE is 50:50 respectively in normal subjects. It appears that the bulk of an administered dose is eliminated from the body within a week. However, effects on thyroid function tests may persist for longer periods.

Oral cholecystographic agents are excreted in breast milk. (See PRECAUTIONS—**Nursing Mothers.**)

Oral cholecystographic agents may produce changes in thyroid studies attributable to changes in circulating iodide. Thyroid function tests may not accurately reflect thyroid status for up to 1 year following cholecystography. Additionally, oral cholecystographic agents tend to elevate BSP (sulfobromophthalein) determinations. (See PRECAUTIONS—**Drug/Laboratory Test Interactions.**)

Indication and Usage: BILOPAQUE sodium is indicated for use in oral cholecystography.

Contraindications: BILOPAQUE should not be administered to patients with advanced hepatorenal disease, severe impairment of renal function, or severe gastrointestinal disorders that prevent absorption.

Higher than recommended or double doses of BILOPAQUE (tyropanoate sodium) to force visualization is contraindicated, especially in elderly patients or in those with vascular disease.

Precautions:
General—Severe, advanced liver disease may interfere with the metabolism of oral cholecystographic agents, and therefore, a greater amount of unchanged drug will be diverted for renal excretion, increasing the load on the kidneys. Acute renal insufficiency has followed the use of oral cholecystographic agents. Most reported cases were attributed to the use of large doses or multiple agents, preexisting dehydration, or hepatic disease.

Renal function, especially in patients with liver disease should be assessed before cholecystography, and urinary output, serum BUN and creatinine, and hepatic function should be observed for a few days after the procedure. Patients with preexisting renal disease should not receive large doses of cholecystographic agents. All patients, especially those with preexisting renal or hepatic diseases should be adequately hydrated prior to oral cholecystography. Liberal fluid intake should be encouraged after ingesting the diagnostic agents. Because oral cholecystographic agents are moderately uricosuric, patients with hyperuricemia may be susceptible to the development of uric acid stones and decreased renal function. Therefore, patients with hyperuricemia receiving oral cholecystographic agents should be well hydrated to maintain adequate urinary output and the possibility of uric acid crystal formation should be kept in mind.

Various factors may result in nonvisualization of the hepatic and biliary ducts and the gallbladder. These include gastrointestinal disorders which interfere with absorption, liver disorders which interfere with glucuronide conjugation and excretion, and obstruction of the hepatic or cystic duct which blocks the flow of the contrast medium to the gallbladder.

Cases of hyperthyroidism have been reported with the use of oral contrast media. Some of these patients reportedly had multinodular goiters which may have been responsible for the increased hormone synthesis in response to excess iodine. Administration of an intravascular iodinated radiopaque diagnostic agent to a hyperthyroid patient precipitated thyroid storm. A similar situation could follow administration of oral preparations of iodides. Therefore, caution should be exercised when administering cholecystographic agents to hyperthyroid and euthyroid goiterous patients.

Information for the Patient—Patients receiving oral cholecystographic agents should be given the following information and instructions.

This drug has been prescribed to perform an x-ray study of the gallbladder. All the medication must be taken with water following dinner the evening prior to the test. Thereafter, nothing except water should be taken until the test has been completed. Patients should be questioned regarding medicine, including nonprescription drugs currently being used. Allergies to iodine, any foods, or x-ray dyes should also be disclosed.

Patients should inform the physician of any liver or kidney disease or pregnancy before taking this drug.

Patients should consult the physician if, at some future date, any thyroid tests are planned. The iodine in this agent may interfere with later thyroid tests.

This drug may cause abdominal cramping, nausea, vomiting, diarrhea, skin rashes, itching, heartburn, dizziness or headache in some patients. Most reactions are mild and pass quickly.

Drug Interactions—Concurrent administration of cholestyramine and cholecystographic agents reportedly resulted in abnormal cholecystography. In vitro studies indicate that cholestyramine

Continued on next page

This product information was effective as of December 3, 1984. On these and other products of Winthrop-Breon Laboratories, detailed information may be obtained on a current basis by direct inquiry to the Professional Services Department, 90 Park Avenue, New York, NY 10016 (212) 907-2525.

Winthrop-Breon—Cont.

has an apparent high affinity for the agents. To avoid nonvisualization or poor visualization, oral cholecystography should be performed after cholestyramine has been discontinued long enough for complete evacuation from at least the small bowel.

The administration of both oral cholecystographic agents and intravenous iodipamide meglumine within 24 hours is not recommended. The prior administration of an oral cholecystographic agent seems to block the hepatic excretion of the intravenously administered iodipamide meglumine.

Renal toxicity has been reported in a few patients with liver dysfunction who were given oral cholecystographic agents followed by urographic agents. Administration of urographic agents should therefore be postponed in any patient with a known or suspected hepatic or biliary disorder who has recently taken a cholecystographic contrast agent.

Drug/Laboratory Test Interactions

Thyroid Function Tests: The results of protein bound iodine (PBI) and radioactive iodine uptake studies will not reliably reflect thyroid function for six months, and possibly as long as one year following the administration of diagnostic enteral radiopaque media.

Thyroid function tests, if indicated, generally should be performed prior to the administration of any iodinated agent. However, thyroid function can be evaluated after use of these agents by using T_3 resin uptake or free thyroxine assays.

Liver Function Tests: Because increases in sulfobromophthalein (BSP) retention may occur after oral cholecystography, the BSP test is not reliable and should not be performed for at least two days following that procedure. Elevated serum bilirubin may render the examination worthless due to no or poor visualization.

Pseudoalbuminuria may be present for three days following oral cholecystography if determined by certain chemical protein precipitation tests. Post cholecystographic pseudoalbuminuria should be verified by the heat and acetic acid or colorimetric dip-strip methods.

Oral cholecystography may lower blood levels and raise urinary excretion of uric acid for a few days.

Carcinogenesis, Mutagenesis, Impairment of Fertility—No long-term studies have been reported.

Pregnancy Category C—Teratogenic effects of tyropanoate sodium are not known at the present time. Therefore, this agent should be used during pregnancy only if clearly needed.

Nursing Mothers—BILOPAQUE sodium is excreted in breast milk. Caution should be exercised when BILOPAQUE sodium, brand of tyropanoate sodium, is administered to a nursing woman.

Pediatric Use—The safety and effectiveness of BILOPAQUE sodium in children under 12 years have not been established.

Adverse Reactions: *Gastrointestinal.* The side effects most frequently encountered during BILOPAQUE cholecystography are related to gastrointestinal response, the upper tract being most frequently affected; mild to moderate nausea 10%, with vomiting 2%, and loose stool or diarrhea in about 5% of patients. Severe or persisting nausea and vomiting, diarrhea with abdominal discomfort or cramps are unusual >1%.

Dermal and allergic reactions are unusual (1% or less) and have been manifest as disseminated pleomorphic rashes, dysphagia, swollen tongue, laryngotracheal or epiglottic edema, periorbital edema, conjunctivitis, wheezing, dyspnea, sneezing, urticaria, or pruritus.

Miscellaneous: Fever, chills, malaise, pain or cramps in limbs, headaches, perspiration, fatigue, and vertigo each occurring >1%.

Cardiovascular: Hypotension, tachycardia, and rarely, syncope or shock, and chest pain.

Renal: Dysuria occurs occasionally. Rarely transitory renal failure.

The nature, incidence or severity of side effects are not materially different with a repeat examination.

Overdosage: There have been no reports on the effect of large overdosage with BILOPAQUE. However, the potential for serious adverse effects with gross overdosage of water-soluble media such as tyropanoate sodium would be expected to be much greater than with poorly soluble iopanoic acid since these media are rapidly absorbed, creating early high serum levels with particular potential for hepatorenal or cardiovascular dysfunction. Therefore, the following empirical measures are suggested:

- Lavage the stomach and administer enemas to remove remaining potentially absorbable contrast material.
- Force fluids to avoid concentration and possible precipitation or crystallization of the contrast material or uric acid in the kidneys.
- Alkalinize the urine to increase the solubility of the drug-glucuronide complex and of uric acid. Administer cholestyramine to chelate and reduce absorption of the drug.
- Monitor blood pressure.

The normal serum levels of iodine following a single 3 g dose achieved between one and four hours is approximately 100 mcgI/mL to 150 mcgI/mL of tyropanoate sodium.

The acute oral LD_{50} of tyropanoate sodium in the mouse is 4.8 ± 1.45 to 16.3 ± 1.83 g/kg $\pm$ Standard Error.

Dosage and Administration: A single dose of 3 g (4 capsules) is recommended for adults. The optimal time interval between administration of BILOPAQUE and cholecystography is 10 to 12 hours, although satisfactory results have been reported as early as 4 to 6 hours.

If no visualizaton occurs after administration of BILOPAQUE, repeat examination with a 3 g dose is recommended on the following day. *Increasing the amount of the repeat dose is not recommended.* Cholestasis is a common cause of nonvisualization in patients who have been on almost completely fat-free diets. To reduce the incidence of false-negative nonvisualization, such patients should eat a diet containing some fat for one or two days before cholecystographic examination. Fat is a long-acting cholecystagogue, and will stimulate emptying of the gallbladder and prepare it to receive the radiopaque medium. *The meal immediately before ingestion of the BILOPAQUE capsules should be fat free.*

Preparatory dehydration is unnecessary and undesirable, especially in elderly patients. After the fat-free evening meal, the patient should swallow 4 BILOPAQUE capsules (3 g) with water. Between ingestion of BILOPAQUE and cholecystographic examination, the patient should take nothing by mouth except water, and should not smoke or chew gum.

Many physicians believe that the quality of gallbladder visualization is enhanced when the intestine is relatively free of residue. This may be achieved with an enema the morning of the examination, or a laxative the day before.

For observation of gallbladder contractility, the patient may be given a fatty meal or a cholecystagogue after the initial x-ray examination. Additional exposures may be made 5 to 30 minutes later.

Nonvisualization

Nonvisualization in routine cholecystography with BILOPAQUE (tyropanoate sodium) usually implies substantial loss of gallbladder function. However, nonvisualization may also result on occasion from other factors not related to disease of the biliary tract.

Repeat Examination

When adequate visualization is not obtained initially, repeat cholecystography with the recommended dose of 3 g helps reduce the possibility of diagnostic error. A larger dose is not recommended. Disease may be inferred with reasonable certainty if the gallbladder does not visualize on repeat examination.

How Supplied: Capsules of 750 mg—Envelopes of 4 capsules (3 g, the recommended dose), box of 25 (NDC 0024-0134-03).

BW-68 H
Shown in Product Identification Section, page 443

HYPAQUE® SODIUM
brand of diatrizoate sodium, USP
ORAL POWDER

For Radiographic Visualization of the Gastrointestinal Tract

Description: HYPAQUE sodium, brand of diatrizoate sodium, is a powder for the preparation of solutions for oral administration for radiographic visualization of the gastrointestinal tract. It is a substituted, triiodinated, benzoic acid derivative, containing 59.87 percent iodine. It thus provides about 600 mg organically bound iodine per gram of powder and contains caramel as a coloring agent. Chemical name: Monosodium 3,5-diacetamido-2,4,6-triiiodobenzoate. Empirical formula: $C_{11}H_8I_3N_2NaO_4$. Molecular weight: 635.90. Chemical Abstract Service: -737-31-5.

Clinical Pharmacology: The most important characteristic of contrast media is the iodine content. The relatively high atomic weight of iodine contributes sufficient radiodensity for radiographic contrast with surrounding tissues.

HYPAQUE solution has few known pharmacological effects other than a laxative action attributable to its high osmolarity.

HYPAQUE solution is sparingly absorbed from the *intact* gastrointestinal tract. It therefore permits gastrointestinal opacification after oral or rectal administration. Oral administration is used for radiographic evaluation of the esophagus, stomach, and proximal small intestine. Rectal administration is used for examination of the colon; however, visualization of the distal small bowel is generally unsatisfactory, since the hypertonicity of the agents causes intraluminal diffusion of water with subsequent dilution of the agent. Enough absorption (0.5% to 2%) from the gastrointestinal tract is sometimes sufficient to provide faint renal tract visualization; this should also be considered when thyroid testing is being contemplated. Also, systemic absorption may have iodine-mediated thyrotropic effects described under PRECAUTIONS.

Indications and Usage: HYPAQUE solutions are indicated for radiographic examination of segments of the gastrointestinal tract, ie, esophagus, stomach, proximal small intestine, and colon.

Contraindications: None known.

Warnings: Solutions of HYPAQUE employed clinically (ie, from 15% to 40%) are hypertonic and may lead to intraluminal movement of fluid with resulting hypovolemia. In young or debilitated children and in elderly cachectic persons, the loss of plasma fluid may be sufficient to cause a shock-like state, which if untreated, could be dangerous to the patient. Lower concentrations (achieved by further dilution) must be used for infants and young children (under 10 kg) and for dehydrated or debilitated patients. *Electrolyte disturbances must be corrected before using these hypertonic solutions.* In debilitated patients and in patients with electrolyte imbalances, postprocedural monitoring of hydration, serum osmolarity, electrolytes and clinical status is essential. In pediatric or severely debilitated patients, the maintenance of an open intravenous fluid line for rehydration may be advisable should hypotension or shock supervene.

Bronchial entry of HYPAQUE (diatrizoate) solution causes a copious osmotic effusion. Therefore, pulmonary entry by aspiration and use in patients with esophogotracheal fistula should be avoided.

Precautions:
General

Cases of hyperthyroidism have been reported with the use of oral contrast media. Some of these patients reportedly had multinodular goiters which may have been responsible for the increased hormone synthesis in response to excess iodine. Injection of an iodinated radiopaque diagnostic agent to a hyperthyroid patient has precipitated thyroid storm. A similar situation could follow administration of oral preparations of iodides.

Diagnostic Product Information

Caution is advised in patients with severe renal or hepatic disease.

In patients with known hypersensitivity to diatrizoic acid compounds, the benefit to risk ratio should be considered.

Information for the Patient

Patients receiving diagnostic agents for gastrointestinal radiography should be given the following information:

1. This drug has been prescribed to perform an x-ray study of the gastrointestinal tract.
2. Patients should be questioned regarding pregnancy or a history of allergy to iodine, any foods, or x-ray dyes.
3. Patients should consult the physician if, at some future date, any thyroid tests are planned. The iodine in this agent may interfere with later thyroid tests.
4. This drug may cause abdominal cramping, nausea, vomiting, diarrhea, skin rashes, itching, heartburn, dizziness or headache in some patients, but most reactions are mild and pass quickly.

Drug/Laboratory Test Interactions

Thyroid Function Tests

The results of protein bound iodine (PBI) and radioactive iodine uptake studies will not reliably reflect thyroid function for six months, and possibly as long as one year, following the administration of diagnostic enteral radiopaque media.

Thyroid function tests, if indicated, generally should be performed prior to the administration of any iodinated agent. However, thyroid function can be evaluated after use of these agents by using T_3 resin uptake or free thyroxine assays.

Pancreatic Test

Small quantities of HYPAQUE solution in the intestinal tract may cause falsely low spectrophotometrically determined trypsin values. Therefore, duodenal instillation of HYPAQUE should not precede pancreatic function tests involving spectrophotometric trypsin assays.

Pregnancy Category B

HYPAQUE solutions when administered intravenously cross the placenta and are evenly distributed in fetal tissues. No teratogenic effects attributable to HYPAQUE have been observed in teratology studies performed in animals. There are, however, no adequate and well-controlled studies in pregnant women. Because small amounts of these agents may be absorbed and animal teratology studies are not always predictive of human response, these agents should be used during pregnancy only if clearly needed.

Nursing Mothers

HYPAQUE administered intravascularly has been found to be excreted in breast milk.

Because small amounts may be absorbed from oral administration, caution should be exercised when HYPAQUE solutions are administered to a nursing woman.

Pediatric Use

Solutions of HYPAQUE employed clinically are hypertonic, which may lead to intraluminal movement of fluid and may lead to hypovolemia. In infants and young children (under 10 kg), the loss of plasma fluid may be sufficient to cause a shock-like state; therefore, low concentrations (achieved by further dilution) must be used (see WARNINGS).

Diatrizoate sodium may be preferred over the diatrizoate meglumine/diatrizoate sodium combination, since the wetting agent (T ween 80) in the latter preparation may be injurious to the colonic mucosa.

Adverse Reactions: Most adverse reactions to HYPAQUE sodium solutions are mild and transitory. Nausea, vomiting and/or diarrhea have occurred particularly when high concentrations or large volumes of solutions are administered. Severe changes in serum osmolarity and electrolyte concentrations may produce shock-like states (see WARNINGS).

In the event of serious or anaphylactoid reactions, it should be kept in mind that the reactions known to occur with intravenous administration of radiopaque contrast materials are theoretically possible.

Directions for Making Solutions from Powder (Approximate Values)

% HYPAQUE Solution Required	Measuring spoonfuls* 10 g each powder in can (per 100 mL of Diluent)	10 g Packets or bottles of Powder (per 100 mL of Diluent)**	25 g Packets of Powder (per 250 mL of Diluent)**	Iodine Content (approx) (mgI/mL)
10	1	1	1	62
15	1½	1½	1½	93
20	2	2	2	125
25	2½	2½	2½	155
40	4	4	4	250

Overdosage: Solutions of HYPAQUE sodium, brand of diatrizoate sodium, employed clinically (ie, from 15% to 40%) are hypertonic and may lead to intraluminal movement of fluid with resulting hypovolemia. In young or debilitated children and in elderly cachectic persons, the loss of plasma fluid may be sufficient to cause a shock-like state. Lower concentrations (achieved by further dilution) must be used for infants and young children (under 10 kg) and for dehydrated or debilitated patients (see WARNINGS).

Dosage and Administration:

Adults: Oral, from 90 mL to 180 mL of a 25 to 40 percent solution.

Enema, from 500 mL to 1000 mL of a 15 to 25 percent solution.

Infants and Children: Oral, from 30 mL to 75 mL of a 20 to 40 percent solution.

Enema, from 100 mL to 500 mL of a 10 to 15 percent solution, depending on weight of patient.

Warning: The powder is not to be used for the preparation of solutions for parenteral injection. [See table above].

*10 g measuring spoon supplied in cans of HYPAQUE Powder.

Dilutions may also be made on the basis that: 1 g Oral Powder to 100 mL = 1% HYPAQUE (6 mgI/mL).

**Solutions may be sweetened or flavored (eg, with vanilla, lemon, chocolate); the diluent may be water, milk, or a carbonated drink. Carbonated diluents should be avoided when gas artifacts are undesirable.

How Supplied:

HYPAQUE Oral powder—Cans of 250 g each with measuring spoon (approximately 10 g capacity), NDC 0024-0769-01.

Bottles of 10 g each, box of 10 (NDC 0024-0769-10)

Foil Packets 10 g each, box of 10 (NDC 0024-0769-45)

Foil Packets 25 g each, box of 10 (NDC 0024-0769-25)

For HYPAQUE Oral Solution, see separate circular.

HW-195 C

HYPAQUE® SODIUM ORAL SOLUTION   B

brand of diatrizoate sodium solution, USP

For Radiographic Visualization of the Gastrointestinal Tract

Description: HYPAQUE sodium, brand of diatrizoate sodium, is an orally administered liquid for radiographic visualization of the gastrointestinal tract. It is a substituted, triiodinated, benzoic acid derivative, which in pure form contains 59.87 percent iodine. The 41.66 percent oral solution as supplied is a thin, slightly viscous, colorless to light brown solution of diatrizoate sodium in water. Each mL contains 416.6 mg of diatrizoate sodium or 249 mg of organically bound iodine.

Chemical name: Monosodium 3,5-diacetamido-2,4,6-triiodobenzoate

Empirical formula: $C_{11}H_8I_3N_2NaO_4$

Molecular weight: 635.90

Chemical Abstract Service: -737-31-5

Clinical Pharmacology: The most important characteristic of contrast media is the iodine content. The relatively high atomic weight of iodine contributes sufficient radiodensity for radiographic contrast with surrounding tissues.

HYPAQUE solution has few known pharmacological effects other than a laxative action attributable to its high osmolarity.

HYPAQUE solution is sparingly absorbed from the *intact* gastrointestinal tract. It therefore permits gastrointestinal opacification after oral or rectal administration. Oral administration is used for radiographic evaluation of the esophagus, stomach, and proximal small intestine. Rectal administration is used for examination of the colon; however, visualization of the distal small bowel is generally unsatisfactory, since the hypertonicity of the agents causes intraluminal diffusion of water with subsequent dilution of the agent. Enough absorption (0.5% to 2%) from the gastrointestinal tract is sometimes sufficient to provide faint renal tract visualization; this should also be considered when thyroid testing is being contemplated. Also, systemic absorption may have iodine-mediated thyrotropic effects described under PRECAUTIONS.

Indications and Usage: HYPAQUE solutions are indicated for radiographic examination of segments of the gastrointestinal tract, ie, esophagus, stomach, proximal small intestine, and colon.

Contraindications: None known.

Warnings: Solutions of HYPAQUE (diatrizoate) employed clinically (ie, from 15% to 40%) are hypertonic and may lead to intraluminal movement of fluid with resulting hypovolemia. In young or debilitated children and in elderly cachectic persons, the loss of plasma fluid may be sufficient to cause a shock-like state, which if untreated, could be dangerous to the patient. Lower concentrations (achieved by further dilution) must be used for infants and young children (under 10 kg) and for dehydrated or debilitated patients. *Electrolyte disturbances must be corrected before using these hypertonic solutions.* In debilitated patients and in patients with electrolyte imbalances, postprocedural monitoring of hydration, serum osmolarity, electrolytes and clinical status is essential. In pediatric or severely debilitated patients, the maintenance of an open intravenous fluid line for rehydration may be advisable should hypotension or shock supervene.

Bronchial entry of HYPAQUE solution causes a copious osmotic effusion. Therefore, pulmonary entry by aspiration and use in patients with esophagotracheal fistula should be avoided.

Precautions:

General

Cases of hyperthyroidism have been reported with the use of oral contrast media. Some of these patients reportedly had multinodular goiters which may have been responsible for the increased hormone synthesis in response to excess iodine. Injection of an iodinated radiopaque diagnostic agent to a hyperthyroid patient has precipitated thyroid storm. A similar situation could follow administration of oral preparations of iodides.

Continued on next page

This product information was effective as of December 3, 1984. On these and other products of Winthrop-Breon Laboratories, detailed information may be obtained on a current basis by direct inquiry to the Professional Services Department, 90 Park Avenue, New York, NY 10016 (212) 907-2525.

Winthrop-Breon—Cont.

Caution is advised in patients with severe renal or hepatic disease.

In patients with known hypersensitivity to diatrizoic acid compounds, the benefit to risk ratio should be considered.

Information for the Patient
Patients receiving diagnostic agents for gastrointestinal radiography should be given the following information:
1. This drug has been prescribed to perform an x-ray study of the gastrointestinal tract.
2. Patients should be questioned regarding pregnancy or a history of allergy to iodine, any foods, or x-ray dyes.
3. Patients should consult the physician if, at some future date, any thyroid tests are planned. The iodine in this agent may interfere with later thyroid tests.
4. This drug may cause abdominal cramping, nausea, vomiting, diarrhea, skin rashes, itching, heartburn, dizziness or headache in some patients, but most reactions are mild and pass quickly.

Drug/Laboratory Test Interactions
Thyroid Function Tests
The results of protein bound iodine (PBI) and radioactive iodine uptake studies will not reliably reflect thyroid function for six months, and possibly as long as one year, following the administration of diagnostic enteral radiopaque media.

Thyroid function tests, if indicated, generally should be performed prior to the administration of any iodinated agent. However, thyroid function can be evaluated after use of these agents by using T_3 resin uptake or free thyroxine assays.

Pancreatic Test
Small quantities of HYPAQUE solution in the intestinal tract may cause falsely low spectrophotometrically determined trypsin values. Therefore, duodenal instillation of HYPAQUE should not precede pancreatic function tests involving spectrophotometric trypsin assays.

Pregnancy Category B
HYPAQUE solutions when administered intravenously cross the placenta and are evenly distributed in fetal tissues. No teratogenic effects attributable to HYPAQUE have been observed in teratology studies performed in animals. There are, however, no adequate and well-controlled studies in pregnant women. Because small amounts of these agents may be absorbed and animal teratology studies are not always predictive of human response, these agents should be used during pregnancy only if clearly needed.

Nursing Mothers
HYPAQUE administered intravascularly has been found to be excreted in breast milk.
Because small amounts may be absorbed from oral administration, caution should be exercised when HYPAQUE solutions are administered to a nursing woman.

Pediatric Use
Solutions of HYPAQUE employed clinically are hypertonic, which may lead to intraluminal movement of fluid and may lead to hypovolemia. In infants and young children (under 10 kg), the loss of plasma fluid may be sufficient to cause a shock-like state; therefore, low concentrations (achieved by further dilution) must be used (see WARNINGS).

Diatrizoate sodium may be preferred over the diatrizoate meglumine/diatrizoate sodium combination, since the wetting agent (Tween 80) in the latter preparation may be injurious to the colonic mucosa.

Adverse Reactions: Most adverse reactions to HYPAQUE sodium, brand of diatrizoate sodium, solutions are mild and transitory. Nausea, vomiting and/or diarrhea have occurred particularly when high concentrations or large volumes of solutions are administered. Severe changes in serum osmolarity and electrolyte concentrations may produce shock-like states (see WARNINGS).

In the event of serious or anaphylactoid reactions, it should be kept in mind that the reactions known to occur with intravenous administration of radiopaque contrast materials are theoretically possible.

Overdosage: Solutions of HYPAQUE sodium employed clinically (ie, from 15% to 40%) are hypertonic and may lead to intraluminal movement of fluid with resulting hypovolemia. In young or debilitated children and in elderly cachectic persons, the loss of plasma fluid may be sufficient to cause a shock-like state. Lower concentrations (achieved by further dilution) must be used for infants and young children (under 10 kg) and for dehydrated or debilitated patients (see WARNINGS).

Dosage and Administration:
Adults: *Oral,* from 90 mL to 180 mL of a 25 to 40 percent solution.
Enema, from 500 mL to 1000 mL of a 15 to 25 percent solution.
Infants and Children: *Oral,* from 30 mL to 75 mL of a 20 to 40 percent solution.
Enema, from 100 mL to 500 mL of a 10 to 15 percent solution, depending on weight of patient.
Warning: The oral liquid is not to be used for the preparation of solutions for parenteral injection. [See table below].
How Supplied: HYPAQUE Oral Solution—Bottles of 120 mL each (50 g of diatrizoate sodium), NDC 0024-0768-01
For HYPAQUE Oral Powder, see separate circular.

HW-48-T

HYPAQUE® sodium 20% ℞
brand of diatrizoate sodium injection, USP
Sterile Aqueous Solution
For Retrograde Pyelography

Description: HYPAQUE sodium, brand of diatrizoate sodium, is a radiopaque diagnostic, water-soluble organic contrast medium. It is a triiodinated benzoic acid derivative. In pure form, it contains 59.87 percent iodine. Each 1 mL of the 20 percent solution contains 120 mg organically bound iodine.

The 20 percent (w/v) solution contains edetate calcium disodium 0.01 percent as stabilizer. Sodium hydroxide or hydrochloric acid has been added to adjust pH between 6.5 and 7.7. The pKa is 3.4 for diatrizoic acid. The sterile aqueous solution is clear, colorless or nearly colorless. The medium can be sterilized by heat in the customary manner without decomposition. It contains benzyl alcohol 1 percent as antiseptic preservative.

It is the sodium salt of 3,5-diacetamido-2,4,6-triiodobenzoate.

Clinical Pharmacology: Retrograde introduction of HYPAQUE sodium 20 percent solution provides radiopacity of the structures of the renal pelvis and ureter.

HYPAQUE sodium 20 percent is not absorbed from the ureteropelvic tract, however, some venous entry by pyelorenal back flow can occur. Therefore, effects similar to direct intravascular injection are possible.

At physiologic pH, the water-soluble contrast media are completely dissociated into a radiopaque anion and a solubilizing cation.

EXCRETION
HYPAQUE sodium is not metabolized but excreted unchanged in the urine, each diatrizoate molecule remaining "obligated" to its sodium moiety.

Diatrizoate solutions may be excreted either through the kidneys or the liver. These two excretory pathways are not mutually exclusive, but the main route of excretion seems to be governed by the affinity of the contrast medium for serum albumin. From 0% to 10% of diatrizoate sodium is bound to serum protein.

Diatrizoate salts are excreted unchanged predominantly through the kidneys by glomerular filtration. The amount excreted during any period of time is determined by the filtered load; ie, the product of plasma contrast media concentration and glomerular filtration rate.

The liver and small intestine provide the major alternate route of excretion for diatrizoate. In patients free of severe renal disease, the fecal recovery is less than 2 percent. In patients with severe renal impairment the excretion of these contrast media through the gallbladder and into the small intestine sharply increases; up to 20 percent in the feces in 48 hours.

Saliva is a minor secretory pathway for injectable radiopaque diagnostic agents. In patients with normal renal function, minimal amounts of contrast media are secreted unchanged.

PREGNANCY AND LACTATION
Diatrizoate sodium crosses the human placental barrier by simple diffusion and appears to enter fetal tissues passively. No apparent harm to the fetus occurs. Procedures including radiation involve a certan risk related to the exposure of the fetus. (See **Pregnancy Category C**.)

Diatrizoate solutions are excreted unchanged in human milk. (See **Nursing Mothers**.)

Indications and Usage: HYPAQUE sodium 20 percent is indicated for retrograde pyelography in adult and pediatric patients.

Contraindication: HYPAQUE sodium 20 percent has no absolute contraindications in its recommended use.

Warnings: Serious or fatal reactions have been associated with vascular entry of radiopaque media. It is important that a course of action be carefully planned in advance for the treatment of possible serious reactions.

Precautions:
General
Diagnostic procedures which involve the use of radiopaque diagnostic agents should be carried out under the direction of personnel with the prerequisite training and with a thorough knowledge of the particular procedure to be performed. Appropriate facilities should be available for the management of any complication of the procedure, as well as for emergency treatment of severe reactions to the contrast agent itself. Competent personnel and emergency facilities should be available for at least 30 to 60 minutes since severe delayed reactions have occurred (see ADVERSE REACTIONS).

ALLERGIC HISTORY
Before injecting a contrast medium, the patient should be questioned for a history of allergy. A positive history does not arbitarily contraindicate the use of a contrast agent where a diagnostic procedure is considered essential, but caution should be exercised (see ADVERSE REACTIONS).

The possibility of an idiosyncratic reaction in susceptible patients should always be considered (see ADVERSE REACTIONS). The susceptible population includes patients with a history of a previous reaction to a contrast media, patients with a known sensitivity to iodine per se, and patients with known clinical hypersensitivity (ie, bronchial asthma, hay fever, and food allergies).

Premedication with antihistamines or corticosteroids to avoid or minimize possible allergic reactions in such patients should be considered. Recent

---

Directions for Measurement and Dilution of HYPAQUE Liquid
(Approximate Values)

HYPAQUE Solution Required	Dilution Required	Iodine Content of Diluted Solution (mgI/mL)
40	Use undiluted	250
25	Dilute each 60 mL to 100 mL	155
20	Dilute each 50 mL to 100 mL	125
15	Dilute each 40 mL to 100 mL	93
10	Dilute each 25 mL to 100 mL	62

reports indicate that such pretreatment does not prevent serious life-threatening reactions, but may reduce both their incidence and severity.

TEST DOSE
The occurrence of severe idiosyncratic reactions has prompted the use of several pretesting methods. However, pretesting cannot be relied upon to predict severe reactions and may itself be hazardous for the patient. It is suggested that a thorough medical history with emphasis on allergy and hypersensitivity, prior to the injection of any contrast media, may be more accurate than pretesting in predicting potential adverse reactions.

Information for Patients
Patients receiving injectable radiopaque diagnostic agents should be instructed to:
- Inform the physician if they are pregnant (see CLINICAL PHARMACOLOGY).
- Inform the physician if they are allergic to any drugs, food, or if they have had any reactions to previous injections of dyes used for x-ray procedures (see PRECAUTIONS).

Drug/Laboratory Test Interactions
Although interference with these laboratory tests have not been reported following the occurrence of renal back flow during retrograde pyelography, they have occurred following direct intravenous injection. Therefore, if any of these studies, which might be affected by contrast media are indicated, it is recommended that they be performed prior to administration of the contrast medium or two or more days afterwards.

Diatrizoate salts interfere with several laboratory urine and blood tests.

Blood Tests
Coagulation: Diatrizoate salts significantly inhibit all stages of coagulation. The fibrinogen concentration, Factors V, VII, and VIII are decreased. Prothrombin time and thromboplastin time are increased.
Platelet aggregation: High levels of plasma and diatrizoates inhibit platelet aggregation.
Serum calcium: Diatrizoate salts may decrease serum calcium levels. However, this depletion of serum calcium may also be the result of the addition of chelating agents (edetate disodium) in the preparation of certain contrast media.
Red cell counts: Transitory decreases in red cell counts. Technetium-99m—RBC labeling interference.
Leukocyte counts: Decrease.
Urea nitrogen (BUN): Transitory increase (see CLINICAL PHARMACOLOGY).
Serum creatinine: Transitory increase.

Urine Tests
Urine osmolarity and specific gravity.
Urine cultures. Diatrizoate in urine cultures may inhibit bacterial growth.

Thyroid Function Tests
Protein-bound iodine (PBI) and total serum organic iodine: Transient increase of both tests following retrograde pyelography have been noticed. The results of PBI and radioactive iodine uptake studies which depend on iodine estimations will not accurately reflect thyroid function for up to 16 days following administration of iodinated media. However, thyroid function tests not depending on iodine estimations, eg, T_3 resin uptake or free thyroxine assays are not affected.

Carcinogenesis, Mutagenesis, Impairment of Fertility
Long-term studies in animals have not been performed in order to evaluate carcinogenic potential, mutagenesis, or whether HYPAQUE sodium, brand of diatrizoate sodium injection, 20 percent can affect fertility in males or females.

Pregnancy Category C
Animal reproduction studies have not been conducted with HYPAQUE sodium. It is also not known whether it can cause fetal harm when administered to a pregnant woman or can affect reproduction capacity. Therefore, HYPAQUE sodium should be given to a pregnant woman only if clearly needed. (See **PREGNANCY AND LACTATION**.)

Labor and Delivery
It is not known whether use of these contrast agents during labor or delivery has immediate or delayed adverse effects on the fetus, prolongs the duration of labor or increases the likelihood that forceps delivery or other obstetrical intervention or resuscitation of the newborn will be necessary.

Nursing Mothers
Diatrizoate salts are excreted unchanged in human milk. Because of the potential adverse reactions, although it has not been established that serious adverse reactions occur in nursing infants, caution should be exercised when these contrast media are administered to a nursing woman.

Adverse Reactions:
Inadvertent entry of HYPAQUE sodium 20 percent into the vascular system is possible if pyeloreenal back flow occurs during retrograde pyelography. Therefore, the occurrence of systemic adverse effects is possible. However, the relative incidence and severity of the following reactions refer only to experience with direct intravascular injection.

Approximately 95 percent of adverse reactions accompanying the intravascular use of diatrizoate salts are of mild to moderate severity. However, life-threatening reactions and fatalities, mostly of cardiovascular origin, have occurred.

Adverse reactions to injectable contrast media fall into two categories: chemotoxic reactions and idiosyncratic reactions.

Chemotoxic reactions result from the physicochemical properties of the contrast media, the dose, and the speed of injection. All hemodynamic disturbances and injuries to organs or vessels perfused by the contrast medium are included in this category.

Idiosyncratic reactions include all other reactions. They occur more frequently in patients 20 to 40 years old. Idiosyncratic reactions may or may not be dependent on the amount of dose injected, the speed of injection, the mode of injection, and the radiographic procedure. Idiosyncratic reactions are subdivided into minor, intermediate, and severe. The minor reactions are self-limited and of short duration; the severe reactions are life-threatening and treatment is urgent and mandatory.

The reported incidence of adverse reactions to contrast media in patients with a history of allergy are twice that of the general population. Patients with a history of previous reactions to a contrast medium are three times more susceptible than other patients. However, sensitivity to contrast media does not appear to increase with repeated examinations.

Most adverse reactions to injectable contrast media appear within one to three minutes after the start of injection, but delayed reactions may occur. Adverse reactions are grouped by organ system and listed below by decreasing order of occurrence and with an approximate incidence of occurrence. Significantly more severe reactions are listed before the other reactions regardless of frequency.

Greater Than 1 in 100 Patients
Body as a Whole: Reported incidences of death range from 6.6 per 1 million (0.00066 percent) to 1 in 10,000 patients (0.01 percent). Most deaths occur during injection or 5 to 10 minutes later, the main feature being cardiac arrest with cardiovascular disease as the main aggravating factor.
Isolated reports of hypotensive collapse and shock following urography are found in the literature. The incidence of shock is estimated to occur in 1 out of 20,000 (0.005 percent) patients.
Cardiovascular System: The most frequent adverse reaction to diatrizoate salts is vasodilation (feeling of warmth). The estimated incidence is 49 percent.
Digestive System: Nausea 6 percent, vomiting 3 percent.
Nervous System: Paresthesia 6 percent, dizziness 5 percent.
Respiratory System: Rhinitis 1 percent, increased cough 2 percent.
Skin and Appendages: Urticaria 1 percent.
Pain at the injection site is estimated to occur in about 12 percent of the patients undergoing urography. Pain is usually due to extravasation.
Painful hot erythematous swelling above the venipuncture site was estimated to occur in more than one percent of the patients undergoing phlebography.

Special Senses: Perversion of taste 11 percent.
Urogenital System: Osmotic nephrosis of the proximal tubular cells is estimated to occur in 23 percent of patients following excretory urography.

Less Than 1 in 100 Patients
Other infrequently reported reactions without accompanying incidence rates are listed below, grouped by organ system.
Body as a Whole: Malaria relapse, uremia, high creatinine and BUN (see PRECAUTIONS—Drug/Laboratory Test Interactions), thrombocytopenia, leukopenia and anemia.
Cardiovascular System: Cerebral hematomas, hemodynamic disturbances, sinus bradycardia, transient electrocardiographic abnormalities, ventricular fibrillation, and petechiae.
Digestive System: Severe unilateral or bilateral swelling of the parotid and submaxillary glands.
Nervous System: Convulsions, paralysis, and coma.
Respiratory System: Asthma, dyspnea, laryngeal edema, pulmonary edema, and bronchospasm.
Skin and Appendages: Skin necrosis.
Special Senses: Bilateral ocular irritation, lacrimation, itching, conjunctival chemosis, infection, and conjunctivitis.
Urogenital: Renal failure, pain.

Overdosage: Signs of overdosage due to the instillation of *excess volume* are those of pyelorenal distention, ie, abdominal discomfort, back pain, renal colic, or shock. (See DOSAGE AND ADMINISTRATION for normal adult and pediatric pelvic capacities.)

Dosage and Administration: Considerable variations in renal pelvic capacity account for differences in the quantities of radiopaque medium suggested for retrograde pyelography. The solution is introduced slowly, avoiding force, and is immediately stopped at the first evidence of renal or abdominal discomfort to avoid overdistention or injury. The procedure is not carried out unless the patient is conscious enough to react to pain. Introduction of the medium by gravity from an elevated buret is considered the best procedure, but injection by syringe is suitable, particularly in small children.

The renal pelvis is relatively nondistensible. The usual volumes of the 20 percent solution suggested for unilateral introduction are:

Infant under 1 year	Less than 1.5 mL
Children 5 years of age and under	1.5 mL to 3.0 mL
Children over 5 years of age	4.0 mL to 50.0 mL
Adults	6.0 mL to 10.0 mL

The volume needed will vary according to the individual and the disorder under examination. Twenty milliliters or more may be necessary for diagnostic pyelograms in patients with hydronephrosis.

When the diagnostic information required warrants a bilateral examination in one procedure, a double volume of the "use" solution is required. The bilateral procedure may be employed, usually without untoward effects. (See PRECAUTIONS.)

Intravascular administration is not recommended since the multiple-dose vials contain an antiseptic preservative.

Dilution and withdrawal of the contrast agents should be accomplished under aseptic conditions with sterile syringes. The solution should be inspected visually for particulate matter and discoloration prior to administration.

How Supplied: Multiple-dose vials of 100 mL, rubber stoppered; contain an antiseptic preservative. Box of 10 (NDC 0024-0754-10).

Continued on next page

This product information was effective as of December 3, 1984. On these and other products of Winthrop-Breon Laboratories, detailed information may be obtained on a current basis by direct inquiry to the Professional Services Department, 90 Park Avenue, New York, NY 10016 (212) 907-2525.

Winthrop-Breon—Cont.

The solution should be protected from strong light.

HW 39-O

HYPAQUE® sodium 25% ℞
brand of diatrizoate sodium injection, USP
Sterile Aqueous Solution

INTRAVENOUS INFUSION FOR UROGRAPHY CONTRAST ENHANCEMENT OF COMPUTED TOMOGRAPHIC HEAD IMAGING

Description: HYPAQUE sodium, brand of diatrizoate sodium, is a radiopaque diagnostic agent, water-soluble organic iodide contrast medium. In pure form, it contains 59.87 percent organically bound iodine.

The 25 percent solution (w/v) contains 150 mg iodine per mL and 0.4 mEq (9.05 mg) sodium per mL. It has an osmolarity of approximately 657 mosm per liter (0.657 mosm per mL) at 25°C and is, therefore, hypertonic. The viscosity (cp) is about 1.59 at 25°C and 1.19 at 37°C. Sodium carbonate or hydrochloric acid has been added to adjust pH between 6.5 and 7.7. The pKa is 3.4 for diatrizoic acid. The sterile, aqueous solution is clear and nearly colorless. It is relatively thermostable and may be autoclaved once. It does not contain an antibacterial preservative. The 25 percent solution contains edetate calcium disodium 1:10,000 as a sequestering stabilizing agent.

Diatrizoate sodium is a triiodinated benzoic acid derivative, the sodium salt of 3,5-diacetamido-2,4,6-triiodobenzoate.

Clinical Pharmacology:
DISTRIBUTION

Intravascular injection of a radiopaque diagnostic agent opacifies those vessels in the path of the flow of the contrast medium, permitting radiographic visualization of the internal structures of the human body until significant hemodilution occurs. During use of HYPAQUE sodium 25 percent for infusion urography high serum levels of diatrizoate sodium are achieved and maintained.

At physiologic pH, the water-soluble contrast media are completely dissociated into a radiopaque anion and a solubilizing cation.

Following intravenous injection, HYPAQUE sodium 25 percent is immediately diluted in the circulating plasma. Equilibrium is reached with the extracellular compartment at about 10 minutes. Hence, the plasma concentration at 10 minutes is closely related to the dose corrected to body size. The pharmacokinetics of the intravenously administered radiopaque contrast media are usually best described by a two compartment model with a rapid alpha phase for drug distribution and a slow beta phase for drug elimination. In patients with normal renal function, the alpha and beta half-lives were respectively 30 and 120 minutes for diatrizoate sodium. However, in patients with renal and kidney functional impairment, the elimination half-life for the beta phase can be prolonged up to several days.

EXCRETION

HYPAQUE sodium 25 percent is not metabolized but excreted unchanged in the urine, each diatrizoate molecule remaining "obligated" to its sodium moiety. Excretion is accompanied by a dose-related osmotic diuresis which is less with the sodium than with the meglumine salt. Fluid deprivation may increase urinary iodine concentration; however, fluid restriction is usually not considered necessary with the higher dose infusion technique. Diatrizoate solutions may be excreted either through the kidneys or the liver. These two excretory pathways are not mutually exclusive, but the main route of excretion seems to be governed by the affinity of the contrast medium for serum albumin. From 0% to 10% of diatrizoate sodium is bound to serum protein.

Diatrizoate salts are excreted predominantly unchanged through the kidneys by glomerular filtration. The amount excreted during any period of time is determined by the filtered load; ie, the product of plasma contrast media concentration and glomerular filtration rate. The plasma concentration is dependent upon the dose administered and the body size. The glomerular filtration rate varies with the body size, sex, age, circulatory dynamics, diuretic effect of the drug, and renal function. In patients with normal renal function the maximum urinary concentration of diatrizoate sodium occurs within 10 minutes with 12 percent of the administered dose being excreted. The mean values of cumulative urinary excretion for diatrizoate sodium expressed as percentage of administered dose are 38 percent at 60 minutes, 45 percent at 3 hours, and 94 to 100 percent at 24 hours.

Urinary excretion of contrast media is delayed in infants younger than 1 month and in patients with urinary tract obstruction. The urinary concentration is higher with the sodium salt of diatrizoic acid than with the meglumine salt.

The liver and small intestine provide the major alternate route of excretion for diatrizoate. In patients free of severe renal disease, the fecal recovery is less than 2 percent of the administered dose. In patients with severe renal impairment the excretion of these contrast media through the gallbladder and into the small intestine sharply increases; up to 20 percent of the administered dose has been recovered in the feces in 48 hours.

Saliva is a minor secretory pathway for injectable radiopaque diagnostic agents. In patients with normal renal function, minimal amounts of contrast media are secreted unchanged. However, in uremic patients small amounts of free iodides resulting from deiodination prior to administration or in vivo, have been detected in the saliva.

PREGNANCY AND LACTATION

Injectable radiopaque diagnostic agents cross the human placental barrier by simple diffusion and appear to enter fetal tissues passively. No apparent harm to the fetus was observed when diatrizoate sodium and diatrizoate meglumine were injected intravenously 24 hours prior to delivery. However, abnormal neonatal opacification of the small intestine and colon were detected 4 to 6 days after delivery. Procedures including radiation involve a certain risk related to the exposure of the fetus.

Diatrizoate solutions are excreted unchanged in human milk.

CT ENHANCEMENT

Intravenous injection of HYPAQUE sodium 25 percent results in increased brain tissue contrast differentials. Initially, this may represent increased local vascular density. Later, however, in certain brain lesions which disrupt the function of the blood-brain barrier, tissue contrast distribution represents accumulated extravascular penetration of the medium.

Indications and Usage:
Urography

Diatrizoate salts are used in small, medium, and large dose urography (See DOSAGE AND ADMINISTRATION). Visualization of the urinary tract can be achieved by either direct intravenous bolus injection or intravenous drip infusion. Visualization of the urinary tract is delayed in infants less than 1 month old, and in patients with urinary tract obstruction (see CLINICAL PHARMACOLOGY).

Contrast Enhancement of Computed Tomographic Head Imaging

Injectable radiopaque contrast media may be used to refine diagnostic precision in areas of the brain which may not otherwise have been satisfactorily visualized.

Tumors. Radiopaque diagnostic agents may be useful to investigate the presence and extent of certain malignancies such as: gliomas including malignant gliomas, glioblastomas, astrocytomas, oligodendrogliomas and gangliomas, ependymomas, medulloblastomas, meningiomas, neuromas, pinealomas, pituitary adenomas, craniopharyngiomas, germinomas, and metastatic lesions.

The usefulness of contrast enhancement for the investigation of the retrobulbar space and in cases of low grade or infiltrative glioma has not been demonstrated.

In calcified lesions or cysts, there is less likelihood of enhancement. Following therapy, tumors may show decreased or no enhancement.

The opacification of the inferior vermis following contrast media administration has resulted in false-positive diagnosis in a number of normal studies.

Non-Neoplastic Conditions. The use of injectable radiopaque diagnostic agents may be beneficial in the image enhancement of non-neoplastic lesions. Cerebral infarctions of recent onset may be better visualized with contrast enhancement in about 60 percent of cerebral infarctions studied from one to four weeks from the onset of symptoms.

Sites of active infection may also be enhanced following contrast media administration.

Arteriovenous malformations and aneurysms will show contrast enhancement. For these vascular lesions, the enhancement is probably dependent on the iodine content of the circulating blood pool. Hematomas and intraparenchymal bleeders seldom demonstrate any contrast enhancement. However, in cases of intraparenchymal clot, for which there is no obvious clinical explanation, contrast media administration may be helpful in ruling out the possibility of associated arteriovenous malformation.

Contraindications: HYPAQUE sodium, brand of diatrizoate sodium injection, 25 percent has no absolute contraindications in its recommended use (see WARNINGS and PRECAUTIONS).

Warnings:
MYELOMATOSIS

Excretory urography is potentially hazardous in patients with multiple myeloma. In some of those patients, therapeutically resistant anuria resulting in progressive uremia, renal failure and eventually death has followed this procedure. Although neither the contrast agent nor dehydration has been proved separately to be the cause of anuria in myelomatous patients, it has been speculated that the combination of both may be causative. The risk of excretory urography in myelomatous patients is not a contraindication to the procedure; however, they require special precautions. Partial dehydration in the preparation of these patients for the examination is not recommended since this may predispose to the precipitation of myeloma protein in the renal tubules. Myeloma, which occurs most commonly in persons over age 40, should be considered before instituting urographic procedures.

SICKLE CELL

Contrast media may promote sickling in individuals who are homozygous for sickle cell disease when the material is injected intravenously or intra-arterially.

PHEOCHROMOCYTOMA

Administration of radiopaque materials to patients known or suspected of having pheochromocytoma should be performed with extreme caution. If, in the opinion of the physician, the possible benefits of such procedures outweigh the considered risks, the procedures may be performed; however, the amount of radiopaque medium injected should be kept to an absolute minimum. The blood pressure should be assessed throughout the procedure and measures for treatment of a hypertensive crisis should be available.

HYPERTHYROIDISM

Recent reports of thyroid storm occurring following the intravascular use of iodinated radiopaque diagnostic agents in patients with hyperthyroidism or with an autonomously functioning thyroid nodule suggest that this additional risk be evaluated in such patients before use of HYPAQUE sodium.

RENAL AND HEPATIC DISEASE

Urography should be performed with caution in patients with severely impaired renal function and patients with combined renal and hepatic disease.

Precautions
General

Diagnostic procedures which involve the use of radiopaque diagnostic agents should be carried out under the direction of personnel with the prerequisite training and with a thorough knowledge of the particular procedure to be performed. Appropriate facilities should be available for the management of any complication of the procedure, as well as for emergency treatment of severe reactions to the contrast agent itself. Competent personnel and emergency facilities should be available for at least 30 to 60 minutes since severe delayed reactions have occurred (see ADVERSE REACTIONS).

ALLERGIC HISTORY

Before injecting a contrast medium, the patient should be questioned for a history of allergy. A positive history does not arbitrarily contraindicate the use of a contrast agent where a diagnostic procedure is considered essential, but caution should be exercised (see ADVERSE REACTIONS).

The possibility of an idiosyncratic reaction in susceptible patients should always be considered (see ADVERSE REACTIONS). The susceptible population includes patients with a history of a previous reaction to a contrast media, patients with a known sensitivity to iodine per se, and patients with known clinical hypersensitivity (ie, bronchial asthma, hay fever, and food allergies).

Premedication with antihistamines or corticosteroids to avoid or minimize possible allergic reactions in such patients should be considered. Recent reports indicate that such pretreatment does not prevent serious life-threatening reactions, but may reduce both their incidence and severity.

TEST DOSE

The occurrence of severe idiosyncratic reactions has prompted the use of several pretesting methods. However, pretesting cannot be relied upon to predict severe reactions and may itself be hazardous for the patient. It is suggested that a thorough medical history with emphasis on allergy and hypersensitivity, prior to the injection of any contrast media, may be more accurate than pretesting in predicting potential adverse reactions.

PREPARATORY DEHYDRATION

Preparatory dehydration is dangerous and may contribute to acute renal failure in infants, young children, the elderly, patients with preexisting renal insufficiency, patients with advanced vascular disease especially in diabetic patients. Dehydration in these patients seems to be enhanced by the osmotic diuretic action of urographic agents. Routine overnight fluid restriction may be undesirable and is considered unnecessary when using the relatively large dose infusion urography technique. In CT enhancement studies, fluid restriction is unnecessary and undesirable.

DIABETES AND NEPHROPATHIES

Acute renal failure has been reported in diabetic patients with diabetic nephropathy and in susceptible nondiabetic patients (often elderly with preexisting renal disease) following excretory urography. Therefore, careful consideration of the potential risks should be given before performing this radiographic procedure in these patients.

RENAL TRANSPLANT

Immediately following surgery, excretory urography should be used with caution in renal transplant recipients.

EFFECTS OF OSMOTIC LOAD

Immediate adverse reactions to infusion urography have not been reported to occur at a higher frequency or greater severity than with routine excretory urography. However, sequelae of this procedure are possible some hours after the examination. The infusion imposes not only a sudden osmotic load, but may also present as much as 160 mEq of sodium (3.7 g) to patients with established, decreased glomerular filtration and renal tubular damage. In addition, these patients may also have coexisting or associated cardiovascular disease. Therefore, the possibility of the development of congestive heart failure hours after the procedure should be considered. Such patients should be observed for several hours following the procedure to detect delayed hemodynamic disturbances.

Information for Patients

Patients receiving injectable radiopaque diagnostic agents should be instructed to:

1. Inform the physician if they are pregnant (see CLINICAL PHARMACOLOGY).
2. Inform the physician if they are diabetic or if they have multiple myeloma, pheochromocytoma, homozygous sickle cell disease or known thyroid disorder (see WARNINGS).
3. Inform the physician if they are allergic to any drugs, food, or if they have had any reactions to previous injections of dyes used for x-ray procedures (see PRECAUTIONS).
4. Inform the physician about any other medications they are currently taking, including nonprescription drugs, before they are administered this drug.

Drug Interactions

Renal toxicity has been reported in a few patients with liver dysfunction who were given oral cholecystographic agents followed by urographic agents. Administration of intravascular urographic agents should therefore be postponed in any patient with a known or suspected hepatic or biliary disorder who has recently received a cholecystographic contrast agent.

Drug/Laboratory Test Interactions

If any of these studies, which might be affected by contrast media are indicated, it is recommended that they be performed prior to administration of the contrast medium or two or more days afterwards.

Diatrizoate salts interfere with several laboratory urine and blood tests.

Blood Tests

Coagulation: Diatrizoate salts significantly inhibit all stages of coagulation. The fibrinogen concentration, Factors V, VII, and VIII are decreased. Prothrombin time and thromboplastin time are increased.

Platelet aggregation: High levels of plasma and diatrizoate meglumine inhibit platelet aggregation.

Serum calcium: Diatrizoate salts may decrease serum calcium levels. However, this depletion of serum calcium may also be the result of the addition of chelating agents (edetate disodium) in the preparation of certain contrast media.

Red cell counts: Transitory decreases in red cell counts. Technetium-99m–RBC labeling interference.

Leukocyte counts: Decrease following injection.

Urea nitrogen (BUN): Transitory increase (see CLINICAL PHARMACOLOGY).

Serum creatinine: Transitory increase.

Urine Tests

Urine osmolarity and specific gravity. Decreased due to induced diuresis.

Urine cultures. Diatrizoate in urine cultures may inhibit bacterial growth.

Thyroid Function Tests

Protein-bound iodine (PBI) and total serum organic iodine: Transient increase of both tests following urography have been noticed. The results of PBI and radioactive iodine uptake studies which depend on iodine estimations will not accurately reflect thyroid function for up to 16 days following administration of iodinated urographic media. However, thyroid function tests not depending on iodine estimations, eg, T_3 resin uptake or free thyroxine assays are not affected.

Carcinogenesis, Mutagenesis, Impairment of Fertility

Long-term studies in animals have not been performed in order to evaluate carcinogenic potential, mutagenesis, or whether HYPAQUE sodium can affect fertility in males or females.

Pregnancy Category C

Animal reproduction studies have not been conducted with HYPAQUE sodium 25 percent. It is also not known whether HYPAQUE sodium, brand of diatrizoate sodium injection, 25 percent can cause fetal harm when administered to a pregnant woman or can affect reproduction capacity. HYPAQUE sodium 25 percent should be given to a pregnant woman only if clearly needed.

Labor and Delivery

It is not known whether use of these contrast agents during labor or delivery has immediate or delayed adverse effects on the fetus, prolongs the duration of labor or increases the likelihood that forceps delivery or other obstetrical intervention or resuscitation of the newborn will be necessary.

Nursing Mothers

Diatrizoate salts are excreted unchanged in human milk. Because of the potential adverse reactions, although it has not been established that serious adverse reactions occur in nursing infants, caution should be exercised when these intravascular contrast media are administered to a nursing woman.

Pediatric Use

Infants and small children should not have fluid restriction prior to injection. Full hydration should be assured. (See PRECAUTIONS.)

Adverse Reactions: Approximately 95 percent of adverse reactions accompanying the intravascular use of diatrizoate salts are of mild to moderate severity. However, life-threatening reactions and fatalities, mostly of cardiovascular origin, have occurred.

Adverse reactions to injectable contrast media fall into two categories: chemotoxic reactions and idiosyncratic reactions.

Chemotoxic reactions result from the physicochemical properties of the contrast media, the dose, and the speed of injection. All hemodynamic disturbances and injuries to organs or vessels perfused by the contrast medium are included in this category.

Idiosyncratic reactions include all other reactions. They occur more frequently in patients 20 to 40 years old. Idiosyncratic reactions may or may not be dependent on the amount of dose injected, the speed of injection, the mode of injection, and the radiographic procedure. Idiosyncratic reactions are subdivided into minor, intermediate, and severe. The minor reactions are self-limited and of short duration; the severe reactions are life-threatening and treatment is urgent and mandatory.

The reported incidence of adverse reactions to contrast media in patients with a history of allergy are twice that of the general population. Patients with a history of previous reactions to a contrast medium are three times more susceptible than other patients. However, sensitivity to contrast media does not appear to increase with repeated examinations.

Most adverse reactions to injectable contrast media appear within one to three minutes after the start of injection, but delayed reactions may occur. Adverse reactions are grouped by organ system and listed below by decreasing order of occurrence and with an approximate incidence of occurrence. Significantly more severe reactions are listed before the other reactions regardless of frequency.

Greater Than 1 in 100 Patients

Body as a Whole: Reported incidences of death range from 6.6 per 1 million (0.00066 percent) to 1 in 10,000 patients (0.01 percent). Most deaths occur during injection or 5 to 10 minutes later, the main feature being cardiac arrest with cardiovascular disease as the main aggravating factor.

Isolated reports of hypotensive collapse and shock following urography are found in the literature. The incidence of shock is estimated to occur in 1 out of 20,000 (0.005 percent) patients.

Cardiovascular System: The most frequent adverse reaction to diatrizoate salts is vasodilation (feeling of warmth). The estimated incidence is 49 percent.

Digestive System: Nausea 6 percent, vomiting 3 percent.

Nervous System: Paresthesia 6 percent, dizziness 5 percent.

Respiratory System: Rhinitis 1 percent, increased cough 2 percent.

Continued on next page

This product information was effective as of December 3, 1984. On these and other products of Winthrop-Breon Laboratories, detailed information may be obtained on a current basis by direct inquiry to the Professional Services Department, 90 Park Avenue, New York, NY 10016 (212) 907-2525.

Winthrop-Breon—Cont.

Skin and Appendages: Urticaria 1 percent.
Pain at the injection site is estimated to occur in about 12 percent of the patients undergoing urography. Pain is usually due to extravasation.
Painful hot erythematous swelling above the venipuncture site was estimated to occur in more than one percent of the patients undergoing phlebography.
Special Senses: Perversion of taste 11 percent.
Urogenital System: Osmotic nephrosis of the proximal tubular cells is estimated to occur in 23 percent of patients following excretory urography.

Less Than 1 in 100 Patients
Other infrequently reported reactions without accompanying incidence rates are listed below, grouped by organ system.
Body as a Whole: Malaria relapse, uremia, high creatinine and BUN (see PRECAUTIONS—Drug/Laboratory Test Interactions), thrombocytopenia, leukopenia and anemia.
Cardiovascular System: Cerebral hematomas, hemodynamic disturbances, sinus bradycardia, transient electrocardiographic abnormalities, ventricular fibrillation, and petechiae.
Digestive System: Severe unilateral or bilateral swelling of the parotid and submaxillary glands.
Nervous System: Convulsions, paralysis, and coma.
Respiratory System: Asthma, dyspnea, laryngeal edema, pulmonary edema, and bronchospasm.
Skin and Appendages: Skin necrosis.
Special Senses: Bilateral ocular irritation, lacrimation, itching, conjunctival chemosis, infection, and conjunctivitis.

Overdosage: At dosage levels of diatrizoate sodium above a level containing 45 g of iodine, the incidence of unpleasant side effects increases. At total dosage equivalent to 80 gI or 90 gI administered over a short period of time (eg, 30 minutes), clinical signs of systemic intolerance appear (mostly related to hyperosmolar effects) and are manifest as tremors, irritability, and tachycardia. Above these maximal tolerated dosage levels in otherwise healthy adults, an increasing incidence and severity of dyspnea and pulmonary edema should be expected.
The acute intravenous LD_{50} of diatrizoate sodium in mice is equivalent in iodine content of 5.3 gI/kg to 8.0 gI/kg and seem to be directly proportional to the rate of injection.
Diatrizoate sodium is dialyzable.

Dosage and Administration:
Preparation of the patient will vary with preference of the radiologist and the type of radiological procedure performed. Specific radiographic procedures used will depend on the state of the patient and the diagnostic indications. Therefore, individual doses should be tailored according to age, conditions, body size, and indication for the examination.
Solutions of radiopaque diagnostic agents for intravascular use should be at body temperature when injected and may need to be warmed before use. In the event that crystallization occurs, the solution may be clarified by placing the vial in a water bath at 40 °C to 50 °C and shaking gently for two to three minutes or until the solids redissolve. If particles still persist, do not use this vial but discard it. The solution should be protected from strong light and any unused portion remaining in the container should be discarded.
Dilution and withdrawal of the contrast agents should be accomplished under aseptic conditions with sterile syringes.
Parenteral drug products should be inspected visually for particulate matter and discoloration prior to administration, whenever solution and container permit.

Infusion Urography
The recommended dose is calculated on the basis of 2 mL of HYPAQUE sodium, brand of diatrizoate sodium injection, 25 percent per pound of body weight. The average dose of the solution for adults is 300 mL; for optimum results, a minimum dose of 250 mL should be used. A maximum dose of 400 mL is generally sufficient for the largest of subjects.
The solution is administered intravenously through an 18-gauge needle over a period of three to ten minutes. Pyelographic films are taken at 10, 20, and 30 minutes from the beginning of the infusion. Early 2, 3, 4, and 5 minute films are obtained when indicated for the evaluation of hypertension. Nephrotomographic sections are best taken just at the end of the infusion, and voiding cystourethrograms when desired are usually made at 30 minutes.

Contrast Enhancement of Computed Tomographic Head Imaging
The dose and administration will depend on the technique and equipment used. The usual dose in adults is 300 mL of HYPAQUE sodium 25 percent, infused over 10 to 20 minutes.

Drug Incompatibilities
Diatrizoate salts are incompatible in vitro with some antihistamines and many other drugs. It is believed that one of the chief causes of in vitro incompatibility is an alteration of pH. Turbidity of solutions of intravascular contrast medium occurs between pH 2.5 and 4.1. Another cause is chemical interaction; therefore, other pharmaceuticals should not be mixed with contrast agents in the same syringe.

How Supplied: Cartons of 10 calibrated bottles of 300 mL (NDC 0024-0758-10). Cartons of 10 calibrated bottles of 300 mL with 10 intravenous infusion sets (NDC 0024-0758-20).
The solution should be protected from strong light. *Contains no preservatives, therefore, discard any unused portion remaining in the container.*
HW-81 L

HYPAQUE-CYSTO® ℞
brand of diatrizoate meglumine injection, USP
Sterile Aqueous Solution
For Retrograde Cystourethrography

Description: HYPAQUE-CYSTO, brand of diatrizoate meglumine, is a water-soluble, radiopaque diagnostic medium. It is a triiodinated benzoic acid derivative. It is constituted as a radiopaque iodinated anion (diatrizoate) and a radiolucent cation (meglumine). It is a colorless, microcrystalline solid which is readily soluble in water.
HYPAQUE-CYSTO is a sterile aqueous solution containing 30 g (w/v) of the meglumine salt of diatrizoic acid per 100 mL aqueous solution. The sterile solution is clear and colorless to pale yellow. The pH is adjusted between 6.5 and 7.7 with hydrochloric acid, or diatrizoic acid, or meglumine. It does not contain an antibacterial preservative. It is relatively thermostable and may be autoclaved. Edetate calcium disodium 1:10,000 has been added as a sequestering stabilizing agent. Each 1 mL contains approximately 141 mg of organically bound iodine.
The viscosity of the solution is 1.94 cp at 25°C and 1.42 cp at 37°C.
HYPAQUE-CYSTO is a 30 percent solution of 1-Deoxy-1-(methylamino)-D-glucitol 3,5-diacet amido-2,4,6-triiodobenzoate ($C_{11}H_9I_3N_2O_4 \cdot C_7H_{17}NO_5$) with a molecular weight of 809.13

Clinical Pharmacology: Retrograde introduction of HYPAQUE-CYSTO solution provides radiopacity of the contents of the urinary bladder. When used during micturation as a function test, it also opacifies the bladder neck and lower urinary tract. Continuous fluoroscopic and monitoring of urinary bladder contractions will demonstrate cystoureteric reflux and its extent, if present.
HYPAQUE-CYSTO is not absorbed from the urinary tract to any extent (<2%), therefore, systemic effects are rare. However, pyelorenal intravasation (especially in patients with ureteric reflux) can occur. Therefore, the potential for adverse effects, such as occur with intravascular use, are possible.
At physiologic pH, the water-soluble contrast media are completely dissociated into a radiopaque anion and a solubilizing cation.

EXCRETION
HYPAQUE-CYSTO which gains inadvertent intravascular entry is not metabolized but excreted unchanged in the urine, each diatrizoate molecule remaining "obligated" to its cation moiety.
Diatrizoate solutions may be excreted either through the kidneys or the liver. These two excretory pathways are not mutually exclusive, but the main route of excretion seems to be governed by the affinity of the contrast medium for serum albumin. From 0% to 10% of diatrizoate meglumine is bound to serum protein.
Diatrizoate salts are excreted unchanged predominantly through the kidneys by glomerular filtration. The amount excreted during any period of time is determined by the filtered load; ie, the product of plasma contrast media concentration and glomerular filtration rate.
The liver and small intestine provide the major alternate route of excretion for diatrizoate. In patients free of severe renal disease, the fecal recovery is less than 2 percent. In patients with severe renal impairment the excretion of these contrast media through the gallbladder and into the small intestine sharply increases; up to 20 percent in the feces in 48 hours.
Saliva is a minor secretory pathway for injectable radiopaque diagnostic agents. In patients with normal renal function, minimal amounts of contrast media are secreted unchanged.

PREGNANCY AND LACTATION
Diatrizoate meglumine crosses the human placental barrier by simple diffusion and appears to enter fetal tissues passively. No apparent harm to the fetus occurs. Procedures including radiation involve a certain risk related to the exposure of the fetus.
Diatrizoate solutions are excreted unchanged in human milk.

Indications and Usage: HYPAQUE-CYSTO, brand of diatrizoate meglumine injection, is indicated for retrograde cystourethrography in adult and pediatric patients.

Contraindication: HYPAQUE-CYSTO has no absolute contraindications in its recommended use.

Warnings: Serious or fatal reactions have been associated with the vascular entry of radiopaque media. It is important that a course of action be carefully planned in advance for the treatment of possible serious reactions.

Precautions
General
Diagnostic procedures which involve the use of radiopaque diagnostic agents should be carried out under the direction of personnel with the prerequisite training and with a thorough knowledge of the particular procedure to be performed. Appropriate facilities should be available for the management of any complication of the procedure, as well as for emergency treatment of severe reactions to the contrast agent itself. Competent personnel and emergency facilities should be available for at least 30 to 60 minutes since severe delayed reactions have occurred (see ADVERSE REACTIONS).

ALLERGIC HISTORY
Before injecting a contrast medium, the patient should be questioned for a history of allergy. A positive history does not arbitrarily contraindicate the use of a contrast agent where a diagnostic procedure is considered essential, but caution should be exercised (see ADVERSE REACTIONS).
The possibility of an idiosyncratic reaction in susceptible patients should always be considered (see ADVERSE REACTIONS). The susceptible population includes patients with a history of a previous reaction to a contrast media, patients with a known sensitivity to iodine per se, and patients with known clinical hypersensitivity (ie, bronchial asthma, hay fever, and food allergies).
Premedication with antihistamines or corticosteroids to avoid or minimize possible allergic reactions in such patients should be considered. Recent reports indicate that such pretreatment does not prevent serious life-threatening reactions, but may reduce both their incidence and severity.

TEST DOSE

The occurrence of severe idiosyncratic reactions has prompted the use of several pretesting methods. However, pretesting cannot be relied upon to predict severe reactions and may itself be hazardous for the patient. It is suggested that a thorough medical history with emphasis on allergy and hypersensitivity, prior to the injection of any contrast media, may be more accurate than pretesting in predicting potential adverse reactions.

Information for Patients
Patients receiving injectable radiopaque diagnostic agents should be instructed to:
- Inform the physician if they are pregnant (see CLINICAL PHARMACOLOGY).
- Inform the physician if they are allergic to any drugs, food, or if they have had any reactions to previous injections of dyes used for x-ray procedures (see PRECAUTIONS).

Drug/Laboratory Test Interactions
Although interference with these laboratory tests have not been reported following cystography absorption (from the bladder or by pyelorenal back flow), they have occurred following direct intravenous injection. Therefore, **if any of these studies, which might be affected by contrast media are indicated, it is recommended that they be performed prior to administration of the contrast medium or two or more days afterwards.**

Diatrizoate salts interfere with several laboratory urine and blood tests.

Blood Tests
Coagulation: Diatrizoate salts significantly inhibit all stages of coagulation. The fibrinogen concentration, Factors V, VII, and VIII are decreased. Prothrombin time and thromboplastin time are increased.

Platelet aggregation: High levels of plasma and diatrizoate meglumine inhibit platelet aggregation.

Serum calcium: Diatrizoate salts may decrease serum calcium levels. However, this depletion of serum calcium may also be the result of the addition of chelating agents (edetate disodium) in the preparation of certain contrast media.

Red cell counts: Transitory decreases in red cell counts. Technetium-99m—RBC labeling interference.

Leukocyte counts: Decrease.

Urea nitrogen (BUN): Transitory increase (see CLINICAL PHARMACOLOGY).

Serum creatinine: Transitory increase.

Urine Tests
Urine osmolarity and specific gravity. Decreased due to induced diuresis.

Urine cultures. Diatrizoate in urine cultures may inhibit bacterial growth.

Thyroid Function Tests
Protein-bound iodine (PBI) and total serum organic iodine: Transient increase of both tests following cystography and retrograde pyelography have been noticed. The results of PBI and radioactive iodine uptake studies which depend on iodine estimations will not accurately reflect thyroid function for up to 16 days following administration of iodinated media. However, thyroid function tests not depending on iodine estimations, eg, T_3 resin uptake or free thyroxine assays are not affected.

Carcinogenesis, Mutagenesis, Impairment of Fertility
Long-term studies in animals have not been performed in order to evaluate carcinogenic potential, mutagenesis, or whether HYPAQUE-CYSTO can affect fertility in males or females.

Pregnancy Category C
Animal reproduction studies have not been conducted with diatrizoate meglumine. It is also not known whether it can cause fetal harm when administered to a pregnant woman or can affect reproduction capacity. Therefore, diatrizoate meglumine should be given to a pregnant woman only if clearly needed.

Labor and Delivery
It is not known whether use of these contrast agents during labor or delivery has immediate or delayed adverse effects on the fetus, prolongs the duration of labor or increases the likelihood that forceps delivery or other obstetrical intervention or resuscitation of the newborn will be necessary.

Nursing Mothers
Diatrizoate salts are excreted unchanged in human milk. Because of the potential adverse reactions, although it has not been established that serious adverse reactions occur in nursing infants, caution should be exercised when these contrast media are administered to a nursing woman.

Adverse Reactions: Because inadvertent intravascular entry of HYPAQUE-CYSTO, brand of diatrizoate meglumine injection, is possible during urethrocystography (bladder absorption or pyelorenal back flow), the occurrence of systemic adverse effects is possible. However, the relative incidence and severity of the following reactions refer only to experience with direct intravascular injection.

Approximately 95 percent of adverse reactions accompanying the intravascular use of diatrizoate salts are of mild to moderate severity. However, life-threatening reactions and fatalities, mostly of cardiovascular origin, have occurred.

Adverse reactions to injectable contrast media fall into two categories: chemotoxic reactions and idiosyncratic reactions.

Chemotoxic reactions result from the physicochemical properties of the contrast media, the dose, and the speed of injection. All hemodynamic disturbances and injuries to organs or vessels perfused by the contrast medium are included in this category.

Idiosyncratic reactions include all other reactions. They occur more frequently in patients 20 to 40 years old. Idiosyncratic reactions may or may not be dependent on the amount of dose injected, the speed of injection, the mode of injection, and the radiographic procedure. Idiosyncratic reactions are subdivided into minor, intermediate, and severe. The minor reactions are self-limited and of short duration; the severe reactions are life-threatening and treatment is urgent and mandatory.

The reported incidence of adverse reactions to contrast media in patients with a history of allergy are twice that of the general population. Patients with a history of previous reactions to a contrast medium are three times more susceptible than other patients. However, sensitivity to contrast media does not appear to increase with repeated examinations.

Most adverse reactions to injectable contrast media appear within one to three minutes after the start of injection, but delayed reactions may occur. Adverse reactions are grouped by organ system and listed below by decreasing order of occurrence and with an approximate incidence of occurrence. Significantly more severe reactions are listed before the other reactions regardless of frequency.

Greater Than 1 in 100 Patients
Body as a Whole: Reported incidences of death range from 6.6 per 1 million (0.00066 percent) to 1 in 10,000 patients (0.01 percent). Most deaths occur during injection or 5 to 10 minutes later, the main feature being cardiac arrest with cardiovascular disease as the main aggravating factor.

Isolated reports of hypotensive collapse and shock following urography are found in the literature. The incidence of shock is estimated to occur in 1 out of 20,000 (0.005 percent) patients.

Cardiovascular System: The most frequent adverse reaction to diatrizoate salts is vasodilation (feeling of warmth). The estimated incidence is 49 percent.

Digestive System: Nausea 6 percent, vomiting 3 percent.

Nervous System: Paresthesia 6 percent, dizziness 5 percent.

Respiratory System: Rhinitis 1 percent, increased cough 2 percent.

Skin and Appendages: Urticaria 1 percent.

Pain at the injection site is estimated to occur in about 12 percent of the patients undergoing urography. Pain is usually due to extravasation.

Painful hot erythematous swelling above the venipuncture site was estimated to occur in more than 1 percent of the patients undergoing phlebography.

Special Senses: Perversion of taste 11 percent.

Urogenital System: Osmotic nephrosis of the proximal tubular cells is estimated to occur in 23 percent of patients following excretory urography.

Less Than 1 in 100 Patients
Other infrequently reported reactions without accompanying incidence rates are listed below, grouped by organ system.

Body as a Whole: Malaria relapse, uremia, high creatinine and BUN (see PRECAUTIONS—Drug/Laboratory Test Interactions), thrombocytopenia, leukopenia, and anemia.

Cardiovascular System: Cerebral hematomas, hemodynamic disturbances, sinus bradycardia, transient electrocardiographic abnormalities, ventricular fibrillation, and petechiae.

Digestive System: Severe unilateral or bilateral swelling of the parotid and submaxillary glands.

Nervous System: Convulsions, paralysis, and coma.

Respiratory System: Asthma, dyspnea, laryngeal edema, pulmonary edema, and bronchospasm.

Skin and Appendages: Skin necrosis.

Special Senses: Bilateral ocular irritation, lacrimation, itching, conjunctival chemosis, infection, and conjunctivitis.

Urogenital: Renal failure, pain.

Dosage and Administration: After the bladder is emptied, HYPAQUE-CYSTO, brand of diatrizoate meglumine injection, is gently instilled without force, often beyond the first desire to micturate, but not beyond the point of urgency or mild discomfort. The volume required to fill the bladder to slightly less than capacity may vary from patient to patient.

Bladder capacity in normal adults is generally 200 mL to 300 mL, and rarely, up to 600 mL. Capacity at birth is 20 mL to 50 mL, and increases about 400 percent in the first year. In children 3 to 5 years old, bladder capacity is 150 mL to 180 mL. In children older than 8 years, it is in the low adult range. In disease, bladder capacity in adults may vary from 50 mL in a hypertonic reflex bladder to over 1000 mL in an atonic or sensory paralytic bladder or chronic lower urinary tract obstruction.

Repeat examination may be required to detect reflux, or in function studies.

The concentration varies with technique and equipment used. HYPAQUE-CYSTO may be diluted with sterile water or 5 percent dextrose solution, as indicated in the following tables. A 10 percent solution is isotonic.

STANDARD PACKAGE
(250 mL of HYPAQUE-CYSTO in 500 mL bottle) [See table on next page].

Dilution and withdrawal of the contrast agents should be accomplished under aseptic conditions with sterile syringes. The solution should be inspected visually for particulate matter and discoloration prior to administration.

How Supplied
STANDARD PACKAGE—Calibrated 500 mL dilution bottles containing 250 mL HYPAQUE-CYSTO, brand of diatrizoate meglumine injection; rubber stoppered, with hangers, inner removable seal and screw neck. Box of 10 (NDC 0024-0734-01)

PEDIATRIC PACKAGE—Calibrated 300 mL dilution bottles containing 100 mL HYPAQUE-CYSTO; rubber stoppered, with hangers, inner removable seal and screw neck. Box of 10 (NDC 0024-0735-10)

The solution should be protected from strong light. *Contains no preservatives, therefore, discard any unused portion remaining in the container.*

HW-143-G

Continued on next page

This product information was effective as of December 3, 1984. On these and other products of Winthrop-Breon Laboratories, detailed information may be obtained on a current basis by direct inquiry to the Professional Services Department, 90 Park Avenue, New York, NY 10016 (212) 907-2525.

Winthrop-Breon—Cont.

HYPAQUE® meglumine 30% ℞
brand of diatrizoate meglumine injection, USP
Sterile Aqueous Solution

INTRAVENOUS INFUSION FOR UROGRAPHY CONTRAST ENHANCEMENT OF COMPUTED TOMOGRAPHIC HEAD IMAGING

Description: HYPAQUE meglumine, brand of diatrizoate meglumine, is a water-soluble, radiopaque diagnostic medium. It is a triiodinated benzoic acid derivative. It is constituted as an iodinated anion (diatrizoate) and a radiolucent cation (meglumine). It is a colorless, microcrystalline solid which is readily soluble in water.

HYPAQUE meglumine 30 percent is a sterile aqueous solution containing 30 g (w/v) of the meglumine salt of diatrizoic acid per 100 mL of solution. The sterile aqueous solution is clear and colorless to pale yellow. The pH is adjusted between 6.5 and 7.7 with hydrochloric acid, or diatrizoic acid, or meglumine. It is relatively thermostable and may be autoclaved once. It does not contain an antibacterial preservative. Edetate calcium disodium 1:10,000 has been added as a sequestering stabilizing agent. Each 1 mL contains approximately 141 mg of organically bound iodine.

The viscosity of the solution is 1.94 cp at 25°C and 1.42 cp at 37°C.

HYPAQUE meglumine 30 percent is a solution of 1-Deoxy-1(methylamino)-D-glucitol 3,5-diacetamido-2, 4, 6-triiodobenzoate $C_{11}H_9I_3N_2O_4 \cdot C_7H_{17}NO_5$) with a molecular weight of 809.13.

Clinical Pharmacology:
DISTRIBUTION

Intravascular injection of a radiopaque diagnostic agent opacifies those vessels in the path of the flow of the contrast medium, permitting radiographic visualization of the internal structures of the human body until significant hemodilution occurs. During use of HYPAQUE meglumine 30 percent for infusion urography high serum levels of diatrizoate meglumine are achieved and maintained. At physiologic pH, HYPAQUE meglumine is completely dissociated into a radiopaque anion and a solubilizing cation.

Following intravenous injection, HYPAQUE meglumine 30 percent is immediately diluted in the circulating plasma. Equilibrium is reached with the extracellular compartment at about 10 minutes. Hence, the plasma concentration at 10 minutes is closely related to the dose corrected to body size.

The pharmacokinetics of the intravenously administered radiopaque contrast media are usually best described by a two compartment model with a rapid alpha phase for drug distribution and a slow beta phase for drug elimination. In patients with normal renal function, the alpha and beta half-lives were respectively 30 and 120 minutes for diatrizoate. However, in patients with renal and kidney functional impairment, the elimination half-life for the beta phase can be prolonged up to several days.

EXCRETION

HYPAQUE meglumine 30 percent is not metabolized but excreted unchanged in the urine, each diatrizoate molecule remaining "obligated" to its meglumine moiety. Excretion is accompanied by a dose-related osmotic diuresis which is less with the sodium than with the meglumine salt. Fluid deprivation may increase urinary iodine concentration; however, fluid restriction is usually not considered necessary with the higher dose infusion technique. Diatrizoate solutions may be excreted either through the kidneys or the liver. These two excretory pathways are not mutually exclusive, but the main route of excretion seems to be governed by the affinity of the contrast medium for serum albumin. From 0% to 10% of diatrizoate meglumine is bound to serum protein.

Diatrizoate salts are excreted unchanged predominately through the kidneys by glomerular filtration. The amount excreted during any period of time is determined by the filtered load; ie, the product of plasma contrast media concentration and glomerular filtration rate. The plasma concentration is dependent upon the dose administered and the body size. The glomerular filtration rate varies with the body size, sex, age, circulatory dynamics, diuretic effect of the drug, and renal function. In patients with normal renal function the maximum urinary concentration of diatrizoate occurs within 10 minutes with 12 percent of the administered dose being excreted. The mean values of cumulative urinary excretion for diatrizoate expressed as percentage of administered dose are 38 percent at 60 minutes, 45 percent at 3 hours, and 94 to 100 percent at 24 hours.

Urinary excretion of contrast media is delayed in infants younger than 1 month and in patients with urinary tract obstruction. The urinary concentration is higher with the sodium salt of diatrizoic acid than with the meglumine salt.

The liver and small intestine provide the major alternate route of excretion for diatrizoate. In patients free of severe renal disease, the fecal recovery is less than 2 percent of the administered dose. In patients with severe renal impairment the excretion of these contrast media through the gallbladder and into the small intestine sharply increases; up to 20 percent of the administered dose has been recovered in the feces in 48 hours.

Saliva is a minor secretory pathway for injectable radiopaque diagnostic agents. In patients with normal renal function, minimal amounts of contrast media are secreted unchanged. However, in uremic patients small amounts of free iodides resulting from deiodination prior to administration or in vivo, have been detected in the saliva.

PREGNANCY AND LACTATION

Injectable radiopaque diagnostic agents cross the human placental barrier by simple diffusion and appear to enter fetal tissues passively. No apparent harm to the fetus was observed when diatrizoate sodium and diatrizoate meglumine were injected intravenously 24 hours prior to delivery. However, abnormal neonatal opacification of the small intestine and colon were detected 4 to 6 days after delivery. Procedures including radiation involve a certain risk related to the exposure of the fetus.

Diatrizoate solutions are excreted unchanged in human milk.

CT ENCHANCEMENT

Intravenous injection of HYPAQUE meglumine, brand of diatrizoate meglumine injection, 30 percent results in increased brain tissue contrast differentials. Initially, this may represent increased local vascular density. Later, however, in certain brain lesions which disrupt the function of the blood-brain barrier, tissue contrast distribution represents accumulated extravascular penetration of the medium.

Indications and Usage:
Urography

Diatrizoate salts are used in small, medium, and large dose urography (see DOSAGE AND ADMINISTRATION). Visualization of the urinary tract can be achieved by either direct intravenous injection or intravenous drip infusion. Visualization of the urinary tract is delayed in infants less than 1 month old, and in patients with urinary tract obstruction (see CLINICAL PHARMACOLOGY).

Contrast Enhancement of Computed Tomographic Head Imaging

Injectable radiopaque contrast media may be used to refine diagnostic precision in areas of the brain which may not otherwise have been satisfactorily visualized.

Tumors. Radiopaque diagnostic agents may be useful to investigate the presence and extent of certain malignancies such as: gliomas including malignant gliomas, glioblastomas, astrocytomas, oligodendrogliomas and gangliomas, ependymomas, medulloblastomas, meningiomas, neuromas, pinealomas, pituitary adenomas, craniopharyngiomas, germinomas, and metastatic lesions.

The usefulness of contrast enhancement for the investigation of the retrobulbar space and in cases of low grade or infiltrative glioma has not been demonstrated.

In calcified lesions, there is less likelihood of enhancement. Following therapy, tumors may show decreased or no enhancement.

The opacification of the inferior vermis following contrast media administration has resulted in false-positive diagnosis in a number of normal studies.

Non-Neoplastic Conditions: The use of injectable radiopaque diagnostic agents may be beneficial in the image enhancement of non-neoplastic lesions. Cerebral infarctions of recent onset may be better visualized with contrast enhancement, while some infarctions are obscured if contrast media are used. The use of iodinated contrast media results in contrast enhancement in about 60 percent of cerebral infarctions studied from one to four weeks from the onset of symptoms.

Sites of active infection may also be enhanced following contrast media administration.

Arteriovenous malformations and aneurysms will show contrast enhancement. For these vascular lesions, the enhancement is probably dependent on the iodine content of the circulating blood pool. Hematomas and intraparenchymal bleeders seldom demonstrate any contrast enhancement. However, in cases of intraparenchymal clot, for which there is no obvious clinical explanation, contrast media administration may be helpful in

Final conc.	TO MAKE Final volume	ADD Sterile water or 5% dextrose solution	FINAL SOLUTION CONTAINS Iodine
30 %	250 mL	—	141 mg/mL
25 %	300 mL	50 mL	118 mg/mL
21.4%	350 mL	100 mL	101 mg/mL
20 %	375 mL	125 mL	94 mg/mL
18.8%	400 mL	150 mL	88 mg/mL
16.7%	450 mL	200 mL	78 mg/mL
15 %	500 mL	250 mL	71 mg/mL

PEDIATRIC PACKAGE
(100 mL of HYPAQUE-CYSTO in 300 mL bottle)

Final conc.	TO MAKE Final volume	ADD Sterile water or 5% dextrose solution	FINAL SOLUTION CONTAINS Iodine
30%	100 mL	—	141 mg/mL
24%	125 mL	25 mL	113 mg/mL
20%	150 mL	50 mL	94 mg/mL
15%	200 mL	100 mL	71 mg/mL
12%	250 mL	150 mL	56 mg/mL
10%	300 mL	200 mL	47 mg/mL

for possible revisions

ruling out the possibility of associated arteriovenous malformation.

Contraindications: HYPAQUE meglumine 30 percent has no absolute contraindications in its recommended uses (see WARNINGS and PRECAUTIONS).

Warnings:

MYELOMATOSIS

Excretory urography is potentially hazardous in patients with multiple myeloma. In some of those patients, therapeutically resistant anuria resulting in progressive uremia, renal failure and eventually death has followed this procedure. Although neither the contrast agent nor dehydration has been proved separately to be the cause of anuria in myelomatous patients, it has been speculated that the combination of both may be causative. The risk of excretory urography in myelomatous patients is not a contraindication to the procedure; however, they require special precautions. Partial dehydration in the preparation of these patients for the examination is not recommended since this may predispose to the precipitation of myeloma protein in the renal tubules. Myeloma, which occurs most commonly in persons over age 40, should be considered before instituting urographic procedures.

SICKLE CELL

Contrast media may promote sickling in individuals who are homozygous for sickle cell disease when the material is injected intravenously or intra-arterially.

PHEOCHROMOCYTOMA

Administration of radiopaque materials to patients known or suspected of having pheochromocytoma should be performed with extreme caution. If, in the opinion of the physician, the possible benefits of such procedures outweigh the considered risks, the procedures may be performed; however, the amount of radiopaque medium injected should be kept to an absolute minimum. The blood pressure should be assessed throughout the procedure and measures for treatment of a hypertensive crisis should be available.

HYPERTHYROIDISM

Recent reports of thyroid storm occurring following the intravascular use of iodinated radiopaque diagnostic agents in patients with hyperthyroidism or with an autonomously functioning thyroid nodule suggest that this additional risk be evaluated in such patients before use of HYPAQUE meglumine, brand of diatrizoate meglumine injection.

RENAL AND HEPATIC DISEASE

Urography should be performed with caution in patients with severely impaired renal function and patients with combined renal and hepatic disease.

Precautions:

General

Diagnostic procedures which involve the use of radiopaque diagnostic agents should be carried out under the direction of personnel with the prerequisite training and with a thorough knowledge of the particular procedure to be performed. Appropriate facilities should be available for the management of any complication of the procedure, as well as for emergency treatment of severe reactions to the contrast agent itself. Competent personnel and emergency facilities should be available for at least 30 to 60 minutes since severe delayed reactions have occurred (see ADVERSE REACTIONS).

ALLERGIC HISTORY

Before injecting a contrast medium, the patient should be questioned for a history of allergy. A positive history does not arbitrarily contraindicate the use of a contrast agent where a diagnostic procedure is considered essential, but caution should be exercised (see ADVERSE REACTIONS).

The possibility of an idiosyncratic reaction in susceptible patients should always be considered (see ADVERSE REACTIONS). The susceptible population includes patients with a history of a previous reaction to a contrast media, patients with a known sensitivity to iodine per se, and patients with known clinical hypersensitivity (ie, bronchial asthma, hay fever, and food allergies).

Premedication with antihistamines or corticosteroids to avoid or minimize possible allergic reactions in such patients should be considered. Recent reports indicate that such pretreatment does not prevent serious life-threatening reactions, but may reduce both their incidence and severity.

TEST DOSE

The occurrence of severe idiosyncratic reactions has prompted the use of several pretesting methods. However, pretesting cannot be relied upon to predict severe reactions and may itself be hazardous for the patient. It is suggested that a thorough medical history with emphasis on allergy and hypersensitivity, prior to the injection of any contrast media, may be more accurate than pretesting in predicting potential adverse reactions.

PREPARATORY DEHYDRATION

Preparatory dehydration is dangerous and may contribute to acute renal failure in infants, young children, the elderly, patients with preexisting renal insufficiency, patients with advanced vascular disease especially in diabetic patients. Dehydration in these patients seems to be enhanced by the osmotic diuretic action of urographic agents. Routine overnight fluid restriction may be undesirable and is considered unnecessary when using the relatively large dose infusion urography technique. In CT enhancement studies, fluid restriction is unnecessary and undesirable.

DIABETES AND NEPHROPATHIES

Acute renal failure has been reported in diabetic patients with diabetic nephropathy and in susceptible nondiabetic patients (often elderly with preexisting renal disease) following excretory urography. Therefore, careful consideration of the potential risks should be given before performing this radiographic procedure in these patients.

RENAL TRANSPLANT

Immediately following surgery, excretory urography should be used with caution in renal transplant recipients.

EFFECTS OF OSMOTIC LOAD

Immediate adverse reactions to infusion urography have not been reported to occur at a higher frequency or greater severity than with routine excretory urography. However, sequelae of this procedure are possible some hours after the examination. The infusion imposes not only a sudden osmotic load, but may also present as much as 160 mEq of sodium (3.7 g) to patients with established, decreased glomerular filtration and renal tubular damage. In addition, these patients may also have coexisting or associated cardiovascular disease. Therefore, the possibility of the development of congestive heart failure hours after the procedure should be considered. Such patients should be observed for several hours following the procedure to detect delayed hemodynamic disturbances.

Information for Patients

Patients receiving injectable radiopaque diagnostic agents should be instructed to:

1. Inform the physician if they are pregnant (see CLINICAL PHARMACOLOGY).
2. Inform the physician if they are diabetic or if they have multiple myeloma, pheochromocytoma, homozygous sickle cell disease or known thyroid disorder (see WARNINGS).
3. Inform the physician if they are allergic to any drugs, food, or if they have had any reactions to previous injections of dyes used for x-ray procedures (see PRECAUTIONS).
4. Inform the physician about any other medications they are currently taking, including nonprescription drugs, before they are administered this drug.

Drug Interactions

Renal toxicity has been reported in a few patients with liver dysfunction who were given oral cholecystographic agents followed by urographic agents. Administration of intravascular urographic agents should therefore be postponed in any patient with a known or suspected hepatic or biliary disorder who has recently received a cholecystographic contrast agent.

Drug/Laboratory Test Interactions

If any of these studies, which might be affected by contrast media are indicated, it is recommended that they be performed prior to administration of the contrast medium or two or more days afterwards.

Diatrizoate salts interfere with several laboratory urine and blood tests.

Blood Tests

Coagulation: Diatrizoate salts significantly inhibit all stages of coagulation. The fibrinogen concentration, Factors V, VII, and VIII are decreased. Prothrombin time and thromboplastin time are increased.

Platelet aggregation: High levels of plasma and diatrizoate meglumine inhibit platelet aggregation.

Serum calcium: Diatrizoate salts may decrease serum calcium levels. However, this depletion of serum calcium may also be the result of the addition of chelating agents (edetate disodium) in the preparation of certain contrast media.

Red cell counts: Transitory decreases in red cell counts. Technetium-99m—RBC labeling interference.

Leukocyte counts: Decrease.

Urea nitrogen (BUN): Transitory increase (see CLINICAL PHARMACOLOGY).

Serum creatinine: Transitory increase.

Urine Tests

Urine osmolarity and specific gravity. Decreased due to induced diuresis.

Urine cultures. Diatrizoate in urine cultures may inhibit bacterial growth.

Thyroid Function Tests

Protein-bound iodine (PBI) and total serum organic iodine: Transient increase of both tests following urography have been noticed. The results of PBI and radioactive iodine uptake studies which depend on iodine estimations will not accurately reflect thyroid function for up to 16 days following administration of iodinated urographic media. However, thyroid function tests not depending on iodine estimations, eg, T_3 resin uptake or free thyroxine assays are not affected.

Carcinogenesis, Mutagenesis, Impairment of Fertility

Long-term studies in animals have not been performed in order to evaluate carcinogenic potential, mutagenesis, or whether HYPAQUE meglumine, brand of diatrizoate meglumine injection 30 percent can affect fertility in males or females.

Pregnancy Category C

Animal reproduction studies have not been conducted with HYPAQUE meglumine, brand of diatrizoate meglumine injection, 30 percent. It is also not known whether HYPAQUE meglumine 30 percent can cause fetal harm when administered to a pregnant woman or can affect reproduction capacity. HYPAQUE meglumine 30 percent should be given to a pregnant woman only if clearly needed.

Labor and Delivery

It is not known whether use of these contrast agents during labor or delivery has immediate or delayed adverse effects on the fetus, prolongs the duration of labor or increases the likelihood that forceps delivery or other obstetrical intervention or resuscitation of the newborn will be necessary.

Nursing Mothers

Diatrizoate salts are excreted unchanged in human milk. Because of the potential adverse reactions, although it has not been established that serious adverse reactions occur in nursing infants, caution should be exercised when these intravascular contrast media are administered to a nursing woman.

Pediatric Use

Infants and small children should not have fluid restriction prior to injection. Full hydration should be assured. (See PRECAUTIONS.)

Continued on next page

This product information was effective as of December 3, 1984. On these and other products of Winthrop-Breon Laboratories, detailed information may be obtained on a current basis by direct inquiry to the Professional Services Department, 90 Park Avenue, New York, NY 10016 (212) 907-2525.

Winthrop-Breon—Cont.

Adverse Reactions: Approximately 95 percent of adverse reactions accompanying the intravascular use of diatrizoate salts are of mild to moderate severity. However, life-threatening reactions and fatalities, mostly of cardiovascular origin, have occurred.

Adverse reactions to injectable contrast media fall into two categories: chemotoxic reactions and idiosyncratic reactions.

Chemotoxic reactions result from the physiochemical properties of the contrast media, the dose, and the speed of injection. All hemodynamic disturbances and injuries to organs or vessels perfused by the contrast medium are included in this category. Idiosyncratic reactions include all other reactions. They occur more frequently in patients 20 to 40 years old. Idiosyncratic reactions may or may not be dependent on the amount of dose injected, the speed of injection, the mode of injection, and the radiographic procedure. Idiosyncratic reactions are subdivided into minor, intermediate, and severe. The minor reactions are self-limited and of short duration; the severe reactions are life-threatening and treatment is urgent and mandatory.

The reported incidence of adverse reactions to contrast media in patients with a history of allergy are twice that of the general population. Patients with a history of previous reactions to a contrast medium are three times more susceptible than other patients. However, sensitivity to contrast media does not appear to increase with repeated examinations.

Most adverse reactions to injectable contrast media appear within one to three minutes after the start of injection, but delayed reactions may occur. Adverse reactions are grouped by organ system and listed below by decreasing order of occurrence and with an approximate incidence of occurrence. Significantly more severe reactions are listed before the other reactions regardless of frequency.

Greater Than 1 in 100 Patients
Body as a Whole: Reported incidences of death range from 6.6 per 1 million (0.00066 percent) to 1 in 10,000 patients (0.01 percent). Most deaths occur during injection or 5 to 10 minutes later, the main feature being cardiac arrest with cardiovascular disease as the main aggravating factor.
Isolated reports of hypotensive collapse and shock following urography are found in the literature. The incidence of shock is estimated to occur in 1 out of 20,000 (0.005 percent) patients.
Cardiovascular System: The most frequent adverse reaction to diatrizoate salts is vasodilation (feeling of warmth). The estimated incidence is 49 percent.
Digestive System: Nausea 6 percent, vomiting 3 percent.
Nervous System: Paresthesia 6 percent, dizziness 5 percent.
Respiratory System: Rhinitis 1 percent, increased cough 2 percent.
Skin and Appendages: Urticaria 1 percent.
Pain at the injection site is estimated to occur in about 12 percent of the patients undergoing urography. Pain is usually due to extravasation.
Painful hot erythematous swelling above the venipuncture site was estimated to occur in more than one percent of the patients undergoing phlebography.
Special Senses: Perversion of taste 11 percent.
Urogenital System: Osmotic nephrosis of the proximal tubular cells is estimated to occur in 23 percent of patients following excretory urography.

Less Than 1 in 100 Patients
Other infrequently reported reactions without accompanying incidence rates are listed below, grouped by organ system.
Body as a Whole: Malaria relapse, uremia, high creatinine and BUN (see PRECAUTIONS—**Drug/ Laboratory Test Interactions**), thrombocytopenia, leukopenia and anemia.
Cardiovascular System: Cerebral hematomas, hemodynamic disturbances, sinus bradycardia, transient electrocardiographic abnormalities, ventricular fibrillation, and petechiae.
Digestive System: Severe unilateral or bilateral swelling of the parotid and submaxillary glands.
Nervous System: Convulsions, paralysis, and coma.
Respiratory System: Asthma, dyspnea, laryngeal edema, pulmonary edema, and bronchospasm.
Skin and Appendages: Skin necrosis.
Special Senses: Bilateral ocular irritation, lacrimation, itching, conjunctival chemosis, infection, and conjunctivitis.
Urogenital: Renal failure, pain.

Overdosage: At dosage levels of diatrizoate salts above a level containing 45 g of iodine, the incidence of unpleasant side effects increases. At total dosage equivalent to 80 gI or 90 gI administered over a short period of time (eg, 30 minutes), clinical signs of systemic intolerance appear (mostly related to hyperosmolar effects) and are manifest as tremors, irritability, and tachycardia. Above these maximal tolerated dosage levels in otherwise healthy adults, an increasing incidence and severity of dyspnea and pulmonary edema should be expected.

The acute intravenous LD_{50} of HYPAQUE meglumine in the rat at 24 hours when administered as a 30 to 60 percent solution is $20,500 \pm 1,300$ $(= 12 \text{ gI}_2)$ mg/kg.

Diatrizoate salts are dialyzable.

Dosage and Administration: Preparation of the patient will vary with preference of the radiologist and the type of radiological procedure performed. Specific radiographic procedures used will depend on the state of the patient and the diagnostic indications. Therefore, individual doses should be tailored according to age, conditions, body size, and indication for the examination.

Parenteral drug products should be inspected visually for particulate matter and discoloration prior to administration, whenever solution and container permit.

Solutions of radiopaque diagnostic agents for intravascular use should be at body temperature when injected and may need to be warmed before use. In the event that crystallization occurs, the solution may be clarified by placing the vial in a water bath at 40°C to 50°C and shaking gently for two to three minutes or until the solids redissolve. If particles still persist, do not use this vial but discard it. The solution should be protected from strong light and any unused portion remaining in the container should be discarded.

Dilution and withdrawal of the contrast agents should be accomplished under aseptic conditions with sterile syringes.

Infusion Urography
The recommended dose is calculated on the basis of 2 mL of HYPAQUE meglumine, brand of diatrizoate meglumine injection, 30 percent per pound of body weight. The average dose of the solution for adults is 300 mL; for optimum results, a minimum dose of 250 mL should be used. A maximum dose of 400 mL is generally sufficient for the largest of subjects.

The solution is administered intravenously through an 18-gauge needle over a period of three to ten minutes. Pyelographic films are taken at 10, 20, and 30 minutes from the beginning of the infusion. Early 2, 3, 4, and 5 minute films are obtained when indicated for the evaluation of hypertension. Nephrotomographic sections are best taken just at the end of the infusion, and voiding cystourethrograms, when desired, are usually made at 30 minutes.

Contrast Enhancement of Computed Tomographic Head Imaging
The dose and administration will depend on the technique and equipment used. The usual dose in adults is 300 mL of HYPAQUE meglumine, brand of diatrizoate meglumine injection, 30 percent, infused over 10 to 20 minutes.

Drug Incompatibilities
Diatrizoate salts are incompatible in vitro with some antihistamines and many other drugs. It is believed that one of the chief causes of in vitro compatibility is an alteration of pH. Turbidity of solutions of intravascular contrast medium occurs between pH 2.5 and 4.1. Another cause is chemical interaction; therefore, other pharmaceuticals should not be mixed with contrast agents in the same syringe.

How Supplied: Calibrated bottles of 300 mL, rubber stoppered, with hangers, box of 10 (NDC 0024-0739-10).
Calibrated bottles of 300 mL, rubber stoppered, with hangers, with 10 intravenous infusion sets, box of 10 (NDC 0024-0739-20).
Vials of 100 mL, rubber stoppered, box of 10 (NDC 0024-0740-20).

The solution should be protected from strong light. *Contains no preservatives, therefore, discard any unused portion remaining in the container.*

HW-142-J

HYPAQUE® sodium 50% B
brand of diatrizoate sodium injection, USP
Sterile Aqueous Solution

For Excretory Urography
Cerebral Angiography
Peripheral Angiography
Aortography
Intraosseous Venography
Direct Cholangiography
Hysterosalpingography
Splenoportography

Description: HYPAQUE sodium, brand of diatrizoate sodium, is a radiopaque diagnostic agent, water-soluble organic iodide contrast medium. In pure form, it contains 59.87 percent organically bound iodine.

The 50 percent (w/v) solution contains 300 mg iodine per mL and 0.8 mEq (18.1 mg) sodium per mL. It has an osmolarity of approximately 1270 mosm per liter (1.27 mosm per mL) and is hypertonic. The viscosity (cp) is about 3.25 at 25°C and 2.34 at 37°C. Sodium carbonate, or sodium hydroxide, or hydrochloric acid has been added to adjust pH between 6.5 and 7.7. The pKa is 3.4 for diatrizoic acid. If a solution of this medium is chilled, crystals may form but readily dissolve if the vial is placed in moderately hot water before use; cool to body temperature before injecting.

The sterile aqueous solution is clear and nearly colorless. It is relatively thermostable and may be autoclaved without harmful effects, although it should be protected from strong light. The 50 percent solution contains edetate calcium disodium 1:10,000 as a sequestering stabilizing agent.

Diatrizoate sodium is a triiodinated benzoic acid derivative, the sodium salt of 3,5-diacetamido-2,4,6-triiodobenzoate wth a molecular weight of 635.90.

Clinical Pharmacology: Intravascular injection of a radiopaque diagnostic agent opacifies those vessels in the path of the flow of the contrast medium, permitting radiographic visualization of the internal structures of the human body until significant hemodilution occurs.

At physiologic pH, the water-soluble contrast media are completely dissociated into a radiopaque anion and a solubilizing cation.

Following intravenous injection, the radiopaque diagnostic agents are immediately diluted in the circulating plasma. Equilibrium is reached with the extracellular compartment at about 10 minutes. Hence, the plasma concentration at 10 minutes is closely related to the dose corrected to body size.

The pharmacokinetics of the intravenously administered radiopaque contrast media are usually best described by a two compartment model with a rapid alpha phase for drug distribution and a slow beta phase for drug elimination. In patients with normal renal function, the alpha and beta half-lives were respectively 30 minutes and 120 minutes for diatrizoate. But in patients with renal and kidney functional impairment, the elimination half-life for the beta phase can be prolonged up to several days.

Injectable radiopaque diagnostic agents are excreted either through the liver or through the kidneys. These two excretory pathways are not mutually exclusive, but the main route of excretion seems to be governed by the affinity of the contrast medium for serum albumin. From 0% to 10% of diatrizoate sodium is bound to serum protein. Diatrizoate salts are excreted predominantly unchanged through the kidneys by glomerular filtration. The amount excreted by the kidney during any period of time is determined by the filtered load; ie, the product of plasma contrast media concentration and glomerular filtration rate. The plasma concentration is dependent upon the dose administered and the body size. The glomerular filtration rate varies with the body size, sex, age, circulatory dynamics, diuretic effect of the drug, and renal funtion. In patients with normal renal function the maximum urinary concentration of diatrizoate sodium occurs within 10 minutes with 12 percent of the administered dose being excreted. The mean values of cumulative urinary excretion for diatrizoate sodium expressed as percentage of administered dose are 38 percent at 60 minutes, 45 percent at 3 hours, and 94 to 100 percent at 24 hours.

Urinary excretion of contrast media is delayed in infants younger than 1 month and in patients with urinary tract obstruction. The urinary concentration is higher with the sodium salt of diatrizoic acid than with the meglumine salt.

The liver and small intestine provide the major alternate route of excretion for diatrizoate. In patients free of severe renal disease, the fecal recovery is less than 2 percent of the administered dose. In patients with severe renal impairment the excretion of these contrast media through the gallbladder and into the small intestine sharply increases; up to 20 percent of the administered dose has been recovered in the feces in 48 hours.

Saliva is a minor secretory pathway for injectable radiopaque diagnostic agents. In patients with normal renal function, minimal amounts of contrast media are secreted unchanged. However, in uremic patients small amounts of free iodides resulting from deiodination prior to administration or in vivo, have been detected in the saliva.

Diatrizoate sodium crosses the placental barrier in humans by simple diffusion and appears to enter fetal tissue passively. No apparent harm to the fetus was observed when diatrizoate sodium and diatrizoate meglumine were injected intravenously 24 hours prior to delivery. However, abnormal neonatal opacification of the small intestine and colon were detected 4 to 6 days after delivery. Procedures including radiation involve a certain risk related to the exposure of the fetus. (See PRECAUTIONS—**General, Pregnancy Category C.**)

Injectable radiopaque diagnostic agents are excreted unchanged in human milk. (See PRECAUTIONS—**General, Nursing Mothers**).

Computerized tomography. HYPAQUE sodium 50 percent can be administered as an intravenous bolus for brain tissue enhancement using computerized tomography. Increased tissue contrast differential for the scan is achieved either because of increased vascular (arterial, venous, or capillary bed) contrast or by blood brain barrier penetration of the medium (or its absence) in certain localized areas of disrupted vascular permeability. The degree of tissue enhancement caused by increased blood contrast is directly related to blood iodine content. However, the degree of enhancement due to extravascular accumulation of iodine resulting from blood brain barrier disruption will depend on the extent of disruption, the blood level of iodine, and the time delay prior to scanning. The nature of the pathology will determine whether an immediate or delayed scan is optimal.

Effects of steroid therapy. The anti-inflammatory and antiedema effects in patients receiving steroid therapy have interfered with the expected distribution of CT tissue enhancement on the scan in certain diseases.

Indications and Usage: HYPAQUE sodium 50 percent is indicated for excretory urography, cerebral and peripheral angiography, aortography, intraosseous venography, direct cholangiography, hysterosalpingography, splenoportography, and contrast enhancement of computed tomographic head imaging.

Urography
Diatrizoate salts are used in small, medium, and large dose urography (see Dosage and Administration—**EXCRETORY UROGRAPHY**). Visualization of the urinary tract can be achieved by either direct intravenous bolus injection, intravenous drip infusion, or sometimes by intramuscular or subcutaneous injections, or incidentally following intra-arterial procedures. Visualization of urinary tract is delayed in infants less than 1 month old, and in patients with urinary tract obstruction (see CLINICAL PHARMACOLOGY).

Contrast Enchancement of Computed Tomographic Head Imaging
Injectable radiopaque contrast media may be used to refine diagnostic precision in areas of the brain which may not otherwise have been satisfactorily visualized.

Tumors. Radiopaque diagnostic agents may be useful to investigate the presence and extent of certain malignancies such as: gliomas including malignant gliomas, glioblastomas, astrocytomas, oligodendrogliomas and gangliomas, ependymonas, medulloblastomas, meningiomas, neuromas, pinealomas, pituitary adenomas, craniopharyngiomas, germinomas, and metastatic lesions.

The usefulness of contrast enhancement for the investigation of the retrobulbar space and in cases of low grade or infiltrative glioma has not been demonstrated.

In calcified lesions, there is less likelihood of enhancement. Following therapy, tumors may show decreased or no enhancement.

The opacification of the inferior vermis following contrast media administration has resulted in false-positive diagnosis in a number of normal studies.

Nonneoplastic Conditions. The use of injectable radiopaque diagnostic agents may be beneficial in the image enhancement of nonneoplastic lesions. Cerebral infarctions of recent onset may be better visualized with contrast enhancement, while some infarctions are obscured if contrast media are used. The use of iodinated contrast media results in contrast enhancement in about 60 percent of cerebral infarctions studied from one to four weeks from the onset of symptoms.

Sites of active infection may also be enhanced following contrast media administration.

Arteriovenous malformations and aneurysms will show contrast enhancement. For these vascular lesions, the enhancement is probably dependent on the iodine content of the circulating blood pool. Hematomas and intraparenchymal bleeders seldom demonstrate any contrast enhancement. However, in cases of intraparenchymal clot, for which there is no obvious clinical explanation, contrast media administration may be helpful in ruling out the possibility of associated arteriovenous malformation.

Angiography
Diatrizoate salts are used for radiographic studies throughout the cardiovascular system.

Intravascular radiopaque diagnostic agents of high viscosity are not recommended for cerebral angiography (see CONTRAINDICATONS—General), and contrast agents with the lowest compatible viscosity and higher concentration of iodine (310 mg/mL to 480 mg/mL of bound iodine) must be used for angiocardiography. Contrast media approaching serum ionic content and osmolarity have less potential for deleterious effects on the myocardium (see PRECAUTIONS—**Drug Interactions**).

Addition of chelating agents may contribute to toxicity in coronary angiography, and the sodium content of angiographic agents used in coronary arteriography is of crucial importance.

In addition to the following general CONTRAINDICATIONS, WARNINGS, PRECAUTIONS, and ADVERSE REACTIONS, there are additional listings in these categories under the particular procedures.

Contraindications:
General
HYPAQUE sodium 50 percent has no absolute contraindications in its recommended uses (see general WARNINGS and PRECAUTIONS).

Do not use HYPAQUE sodium 50 percent for myelography or for examination of dorsal cysts or sinuses which might communicate with the subarachnoid space. Even a small amount of the medium in the subarachnoid space may produce convulsions and result in fatality. Epidural injection is also contraindicated.

Warnings:
General
Excretory urography is potentially hazardous in patients with multiple myeloma. In some of those patients, therapeutically resistant anuria resulting in progressive uremia, renal failure, and eventually death has followed this procedure. Although neither the contrast agent nor dehydration has been proved separately to be the cause of anuria in myelomatous patients, it has been speculated that the combination of both may be causative. The risk of excretory urography in myelomatous patients is not a contraindication to the procedure; however, they require special precautions. Partial dehydration in the preparation of these patients for the examination is not recommended since this may predispose to the precipitation of myeloma protein in the renal tubules. Myeloma, which occurs most commonly in persons over age 40, should be considered before instituting urographic procedures.

Contrast media may promote sickling in individuals who are homozygous for sickle cell disease when the material is injected intravenously or intra-arterially.

Administration of radiopaque materials to patients known or suspected of having pheochromocytoma should be performed with extreme caution. If, in the opinion of the physician, the possible benefits of such procedures outweigh the considered risks, the procedures may be performed; however, the amount of radiopaque medium injected should be kept to an absolute minimum. The blood pressure should be assessed throughout the procedure and measures for treatment of a hypertensive crisis should be available.

Recent reports of thyroid storm occurring following the intravascular use of iodinated radiopaque diagnostic agents in patients with hyperthyroidism or with an autonomously functioning thyroid nodule suggest that this additional risk be evaluated in such patients before use of HYPAQUE sodium.

Contrast media administered for cardiac catheterization and angiocardiography may cause cellular injury to circulating lymphocytes. Chromosomal damage in humans includes inhibition of mitosis, increases in the number of micronuclei, and chromosome aberrations. The damages appear to be related to the contrast medium itself rather than to the x-ray radiation. It is to be noted that those agents have not been adequately tested in animal or laboratory systems.

Urography should be performed with caution in patients with severely impaired renal function and patients with combined renal and hepatic disease.

Selective spinal arteriography or arteriography of trunks providing spinal branches can cause mild to severe muscle spasm. However, serious neurologic sequelae, including permanent paralysis, have occasionally been reported. (See also ANGIOGRAPHY, Precaution.)

Continued on next page

This product information was effective as of December 3, 1984. On these and other products of Winthrop-Breon Laboratories, detailed information may be obtained on a current basis by direct inquiry to the Professional Services Department, 90 Park Avenue, New York, NY 10016 (212) 907-2525.

Winthrop-Breon—Cont.

Precautions:
General

Diagnostic procedures which involve the use of radiopaque diagnostic agents should be carried out under the direction of personnel with the prerequisite training and with a thorough knowledge of the particular procedure to be performed. Appropriate facilities should be available for coping with any complication of the procedure, as well as for emergency treatment of severe reactions to the contrast agent itself. After parenteral administration of a radiopaque agent, competent personnel and emergency facilities should be available for at least 30 to 60 minutes since severe delayed reactions have occurred (see ADVERSE REACTIONS—General).

Preparatory dehydration is dangerous and may contribute to acute renal failure in infants, young children, the elderly, patients with preexisting renal insufficiency, patients with advanced vascular disease, and diabetic patients. Dehydration in these patients seems to be enhanced by the osmotic diuretic action of urographic agents. It is believed that overnight fluid restriction prior to excretory urography generally does not provide better visualization in normal patients.

Acute renal failure has been reported in diabetic patients with diabetic nephropathy and in susceptible nondiabetic patients (often elderly with preexisting renal disease) following excretory urography. Therefore, careful consideration of the potential risks should be given before performing this radiographic procedure in these patients.

Immediately following surgery, excretory urography should be used with caution in renal transplant recipients.

The possibility of an idiosyncratic reaction in susceptible patients should always be considered (see ADVERSE REACTIONS—General). The susceptible population includes patients with a history of a previous reaction to a contrast media, patients with a known sensitivity to iodine per se, and patients with a known clinical hypersensitivity: bronchial asthma, hay fever, and food allergies.

The occurrence of severe idiosyncratic reactions has prompted the use of several pretesting methods. However, pretesting cannot be relied upon to predict severe reactions and may itself be hazardous for the patient. It is suggested that a thorough medical history with emphasis on allergy and hypersensitivity, prior to injection of any contrast media, may be more accurate than pretesting in predicting potential adverse reactions.

A positive history of allergies or hypersensitivity does not arbitrarily contraindicate the use of a contrast agent, where a diagnostic procedure is thought essential, but caution should be exercised (see ADVERSE REACTIONS—General). Premedication with antihistamines or corticosteroids to avoid or minimize possible allergic reactions in such patients should be considered. Recent reports indicate that such pretreatment does not prevent serious life-threatening reactions, but may reduce both their incidence and severity.

Due to the transitory increase in the circulatory osmotic load, injections of urographic agents should be used with caution in patients with congestive heart failure. Such patients should be observed for several hours following the procedure to detect delayed hemodynamic disturbances.

General anesthesia may be indicated in the performance of some procedures in young or uncooperative children and in selected adult patients; however, a higher incidence of adverse reactions has been reported in these patients, and may be attributable to the inability of the patient to identify untoward symptoms, or to the hypotensive effect of anesthesia which can reduce cardiac output and increase the duration of exposure to the contrast agent.

In addition to the general precautions already described, excretory urography, cholangiography, and other uses also have hazards associated with particular techniques employed.

Information for Patients

Patients receiving injectable radiopaque diagnostic agents should be instructed to:
1. Inform the physician if they are pregnant (see CLINICAL PHARMACOLOGY).
2. Inform the physician if they are diabetic or if they have multiple myeloma, pheochromocytoma, homozygous sickle cell disease or known thyroid disorder (see WARNINGS—General).
3. Inform the physician if they are allergic to any drugs, food, or if they have had any reactions to previous injections of dyes used for x-ray procedures (see PRECAUTIONS—General).
4. Inform the physician about any other medications they are currently taking, including nonprescription drugs, before they are administered this drug.

Drug Interactions

Renal toxicity has been reported in a few patients with liver dysfunction who were given oral cholecystographic agents followed by urographic agents. Administration of intravascular urographic agents should therefore be postponed in any patient with a known or suspected hepatic or biliary disorder who has recently received a cholecystographic contrast agent.

Addition of an inotropic agent to contrast agents may produce a paradoxical depressant response which can be deleterious to the ischemic myocardium.

Drug/Laboratory Test Interactions

If any of these studies, which might be affected by contrast media are indicated, it is recommended that they be performed prior to administration of the contrast medium or two or more days afterwards.

Diatrizoate salts interfere with several laboratory urine and blood tests.

Blood Tests

Coagulation: Diatrizoate salts significantly inhibit all stages of coagulation. The fibrinogen concentration, Factors V, VII, and VII are decreased. Prothrombin time and thromboplastin time are increased.

Platelet aggregation: High levels of plasma and diatrizoates inhibit platelet aggregation.

Serum calcium: Diatrizoate salts may decrease serum calcium levels. However, this depletion of serum calcium may also be the result of the addition of chelating agents (edetate disodium) in the preparation of certain contrast media.

Red cell counts: Transitory decreases in red cell counts. Technetium-99m—RBC labeling interference.

Leukocyte counts: Decrease.

Urea nitrogen (BUN): Transitory increase (see CLINICAL PHARMACOLOGY).

Serum creatinine: Transitory increase.

Urine Tests

Contrast media which are excreted in the urine, may interfere with some laboratory determinations eg, proteinuria, specific gravity, osmolarity, or bacterial cultures.

Thyroid Function Tests

Protein-bound iodine (PBI) and total serum organic iodine: Transient increase of both tests following urography have been noticed. The results of PBI and radioactive iodine uptake studies which depend on iodine estimations will not accurately reflect thyroid function for up to 16 days following administration of iodinated urographic media. However, thyroid function tests not depending on iodine estimations, eg, T_3 resin uptake or free thyroxine assays are not affected.

Carcinogenesis, Mutagenesis, Impairment of Fertility

Long-term studies in animals have not been performed in order to evaluate carcinogenic potential, mutagenesis, or whether HYPAQUE sodium 50 percent can affect fertility in males or females.

Pregnancy Category C

Animal reproduction studies have not been conducted with HYPAQUE sodium 50 percent. It is also not known whether HYPAQUE sodium 50 percent can cause fetal harm when administered to a pregnant woman or can affect reproduction capacity. HYPAQUE sodium 50 percent should be given to a pregnant woman only if clearly needed.

Labor and Delivery

It is not known whether use of these contrast agents during labor or delivery has immediate or delayed adverse effects on the fetus, prolongs the duration of labor or increases the likelihood that forceps delivery or other obstetrical intervention or resuscitation of the newborn will be necessary.

Nursing Mothers

Diatrizoate salts are excreted unchanged in human milk. Because of the potential adverse reactions, although it has not been established that serious adverse reactions occur in nursing infants, caution should be exercised when these contrast media are administered to a nursing woman.

Pediatric Use

Infants and small children should not have any fluid restriction prior to excretory urography or any other procedures (see PRECAUTIONS—General). Guidelines for pediatric dosages are presented in DOSAGE AND ADMINISTRATION—General.

Adverse Reactions:
General

Approximately 95 percent of adverse reactions accompanying the intravascular use of diatrizoate salts are of mild to moderate severity. However, life-threatening reactions and fatalities, mostly of cardiovascular origin, have occurred.

Adverse reactions to injectable contrast media fall into two categories: chemotoxic reactions and idiosyncratic reactions.

Chemotoxic reactions result from the physicochemical properties of the contrast media, the dose, and the speed of injection. All hemodynamic disturbances and injuries to organs or vessels perfused by the contrast medium are included in this category.

Idiosyncratic reactions include all other reactions. They occur more frequently in patients 20 to 40 years old. Idiosyncratic reactions may or may not be dependent on the amount of dose injected, the speed of injection, the mode of injection, and the radiographic procedure. Idiosyncratic reactions are subdivided into minor, intermediate, and severe. The minor reactions are self-limited and of short duration; the severe reactions are life-threatening and treatment is urgent and mandatory.

The reported incidence of adverse reactions to contrast media in patients with a history of allergy are twice that of the general population. Patients with a history of previous reactions to a contrast medium are 3 times more susceptible than other patients. However, sensitivity to contrast media does not appear to increase with repeated examinations.

Most adverse reactions to injectable contrast media appear within one to three minutes after the start of injection, but delayed reactions may occur. Adverse reactions are grouped by organ system and listed below by decreasing order of occurrence and with an approximate incidence of occurrence. Significantly more severe reactions are listed before the other reactions regardless of frequency.

Greater Than 1 in 100 Patients

Body as a Whole: Reported incidences of death range from 6.6 per 1 million (0.00066 percent) to 1 in 10,000 patients (0.01 percent). Most deaths occur during injection or 5 to 10 minutes later, the main feature being cardiac arrest with cardiovascular disease as the main aggravating factor. Isolated reports of hypotensive collapse and shock following urography are found in the literature. The incidence of shock is estimated to occur in 1 out of 20,000 (0.005 percent) patients.

Cardiovascular System: The most frequent adverse reaction to diatrizoate salts is vasodilation (feeling of warmth). The estimated incidence is 49 percent.

Digestive System: Nausea 6 percent, vomiting 3 percent.

Nervous System: Paresthesia 6 percent, dizziness 5 percent.

Respiratory System: Rhinitis 1 percent, increased cough 2 percent.

Skin and Appendages: Urticaria 1 percent.

Pain at the injection site is estimated to occur in about 12 percent of the patients undergoing urography. Pain is usually due to extravasation.

Painful hot erythematous swelling above the venipuncture site was estimated to occur in more than one percent of the patients undergoing phlebography.
Special Senses: Perversion of taste 11 percent.
Urogenital System: Osmotic nephrosis of the proximal tubular cells is estimated to occur in 23 percent of patients following excretory urography.

Less Than 1 in 100 Patients
Other infrequently reported reactions without accompanying incidence rates are listed below, grouped by organ system.
Body as a Whole: Malaria relapse, uremia, high creatinine and BUN (see PRECAUTIONS—**Drug/Laboratory Test Interactions**), thrombocytopenia, leukopenia, and anemia.
Cardiovascular System: Cerebral hematomas, hemodynamic disturbances, sinus bradycardia, transient electrocardiographic abnormalities, ventricular fibrillation, and petechiae.
Digestive System: Severe unilateral or bilateral swelling of the parotid and submaxillary glands.
Nervous System: Convulsions, paralysis, and coma.
Respiratory System: Asthma, dyspnea, laryngeal edema, pulmonary edema, and bronchospasm.
Skin and Appendages: Skin necrosis.
Special Senses: Bilateral ocular irritation, lacrimation, itching, conjunctival chemosis, infection, and conjunctivitis.
Urogenital: Renal failure, pain.
Overdosage: At dosage levels of diatrizoate sodium above a level containing 45 g of iodine, the incidence of unpleasant side effects increases. At total dosage equivalent to 80 gI or 90 gI administered over a short period of time (eg, 30 minutes), clinical signs of systemic intolerance appear (mostly related to hyperosmolar effects) and are manifest as tremors, irritability, and tachycardia. Above these maximal tolerated dosage levels in otherwise healthy adults, an increasing incidence and severity of dyspnea and pulmonary edema should be expected.
Four cases of overdosage in infants, during urography, are reported. Three of the infants died within 19 hours of the injection. The overdose ranged from slightly above the recommended pediatric dosage to a dose exceeding 19 g/kg. The symptoms of overdosage appeared between 10 minutes to several hours after injection of the contrast medium. Adverse effects were life-threatening, affecting mainly the pulmonary and cardiovascular systems. The symptoms included: cyanosis, bradycardia, acidosis, pulmonary hemorrhage, convulsions, coma, and cardiac arrest. All infants showed a poor visualization of the kidneys and a diffuse opacification of all the tissues and vasculature. Autopsy findings showed acute pulmonary damage and/or edema of subcutaneous tissues. Treatment of an overdose of injectable radiopaque contrast media is directed toward the support of all vital functions, and prompt institution of symptomatic therapy.
The acute intravenous LD_{50} of diatrizoate sodium in mice is equivalent in iodine content of 5.3 gI/kg to 8.0 gI/kg and seem to be directly proportional to the rate of injection.
Diatrizoate sodium is dialyzable.

Dosage and Administration: General
Preparation of the patient will vary with preference of the radiologist and the type of radiological procedure performed. Specific radiographic procedures used will depend on the state of the patient and the diagnostic indications. Individual doses should be tailored according to age, body size, and indication for examination. (See INDIVIDUAL INDICATIONS AND USAGE section for specific Dosage and Administration.)
Solutions of radiopaque diagnostic agents for intravascular use should be at body temperature when injected and may need to be warmed before use. In the event that crystallization occurs, the solution may be clarified by placing the vial in a water bath at 40°C to 50°C and shaking gently for two to three minutes or until the solids redissolve. If particles still persist, do not use this vial but discard it. The solution should be protected from light and any unused portion remaining in the container should be discarded.
Dilution and withdrawal of the contrast agents should be accomplished under aseptic conditions with sterile syringes.
Parenteral drug products should be inspected visually for particulate matter and discoloration prior to administration. Avoid contaminating catheters, syringes, needles, and contrast media with glove powder or cotton fibers.

Pediatric Dosage
Pediatric doses of injectable radiopaque diagnostic agents are generally determined on a weight basis and should be calculated for each patient individually. (See INDIVIDUAL INDICATIONS AND USAGE sections.)

Drug Incompatibilities
Diatrizoate salts are incompatible in vitro with some antihistamines and many other drugs. It is believed that one of the chief causes of in vitro incompatibility is an alteration of pH. Turbidity of solutions of intravascular contrast medium occurs between pH 2.5 and 4.1. Another cause is chemical interaction; therefore, other pharmaceuticals should not be mixed with contrast agents in the same syringe.

Individual Indications and Usage:
THE FOLLOWING SECTIONS FOR INDIVIDUAL INDICATIONS AND USAGE CONTAIN CONTRAINDICATIONS, WARNINGS, PRECAUTIONS, ADVERSE REACTIONS, AND DOSAGE AND ADMINISTRATION SECTIONS RELATED TO THE SPECIFIC PROCEDURES. HOWEVER, IT SHOULD BE UNDERSTOOD THAT THE INFORMATION IN THE GENERAL SECTIONS IS ALSO LIKELY TO APPLY TO ALL OF THESE SPECIFIC USES.
Hydration—With the possible exception of urography, patients should be fully hydrated prior to the following procedures.

Excretory Urography
Dehydration (fluid deprivation for 12 to 15 hours) improves urographic contrast especially at lower dosage level (see PRECAUTIONS). A preparatory laxative at bedtime to reduce gas and feces is often employed.
Diatrizoate salts are used in small, medium, and large dose urography (See Dosage and Administration—**EXCRETORY UROGRAPHY**). Visualization of the urinary tract can be achieved by either direct intravenous bolus injection, intravenous drip infusion, or sometimes by intramuscular or subcutaneous injections, or incidently following intraarterial procedure.
In infants less than 1 month only visualization of the urinary tract is delayed, therefore the number of roentgen exposures during the early part of the examination should be limited.
In patients with substantially impaired renal function and in patients with urinary tract obstruction, optimal visualization may be delayed for as long as 60 minutes or more. In such patients large doses may be required for adequate urograms.
For distribution and excretion of diatrizoates, see CLINICAL PHARMACOLOGY.

PRECAUTIONS
See PRECAUTIONS—General. Some clinicians consider multiple myeloma a contraindication to excretory urography because of the great possibility of producing transient to fatal renal failure. Others believe that the risk of causing anuria is definite but small. If excretory urography is performed in the presence of multiple myeloma, dehydration should be avoided since it favors protein precipitation in renal tubules.
Preparatory dehydration may be dangerous in infants, young children, the elderly, and azotemic patients (especially those with polyuria, oliguria, diabetes, advanced vascular disease, or preexisting dehydration) . The undesirable dehydration in these patients may be accentuated by the osmotic diuretic action of the medium.

ADVERSE REACTIONS
See ADVERSE REACTIONS—General.

DOSAGE AND ADMINISTRATION
Intravenous Dosage
Adults. A dose of 30 mL of the 50 percent solution administered intravenously with or without compression produces diagnostic shadows in the majority of adults subjected to partial dehydration and to effective purgation. If the administration of 30 mL does not provide satisfactory visualization, this dose may be repeated in 15 to 30 minutes. In persons of slight build 20 mL may produce adequate shadows.
Larger doses ranging from 50 mL to 60 mL of the 50 percent solution may be used for routine excretory urography in adults. The increased dosage offers better and more complete visualization of the urinary tract. This technique requires neither compression nor dehydration and is more effective in obese patients. Adverse reactions to the larger dose are similar to those encountered with lower doses without an increase in incidence, severity, or type of reactions. Voiding cystourethrograms may be obtained when desired. For the best results and minimal side effects, it is advisable to inject the total amount of solution intravenously in one to three minutes.
Children. The dosage of the 50 percent solution for children under 6 months of age is 5 ml; for children 6 to 12 months of age, 6 mL to 8 mL; for children 1 to 2 years of age, 8 mL to 10 mL; for children 2 to 5 years of age, 10 mL to 12 mL; for children 5 to 7 years of age, 12 mL to 15 mL; for children 7 to 11 years of age, 15 mL to 18 mL, and for children 11 to 15 years of age, 18 mL to 20 mL.

Subcutaneous or Intramuscular Urography
HYPAQUE sodium 50 percent may be used for excretory urography via subcutaneous injection, undiluted or diluted; or subcutaneously diluted with equal quantities of sterile water for injection. The intramuscular injection site generally used is the gluteal muscles in two separate, equal doses. Used subcutaneously the medium is generally injected in divided equal doses over each scapula. In both locations the contrast medium is rapidly absorbed providing urograms beginning variously 5 to 10 minutes following intramuscular injection; subsequent exposures being made according to degree of pyelographic contrast.
Radiographs with subcutaneous injection are usually exposed at 10, 20, and 30 minutes. The urograms achieved with either methods will be almost equal to that following intravenous injection.
The usual intramuscular or subcutaneous (diluted) dose of HYPAQUE sodium 50 percent in adults and older children is about 20 mL to 30 mL. For infants and young children, the dose ranges from 5 mL to 16 mL.

Roentgenography
A plain film is often made prior to IVP. A nephrogram effect is available in 30 to 60 seconds. Its duration is dose dependent.
Urograms may be available as early as two minutes. However, urograms of optimal density are usually made at 5, 10, or 15 minutes following injection.
Ureteric films are usually made between 10 and 20 minutes, and cystograms at 30 minutes. In impaired renal function, delayed films may be required.

ANGIOGRAPHY
Angiography should be avoided whenever possible in patients with homocystinuria, because of the risk of inducing thrombosis and embolism.

Continued on next page

This product information was effective as of December 3, 1984. On these and other products of Winthrop-Breon Laboratories, detailed information may be obtained on a current basis by direct inquiry to the Professional Services Department, 90 Park Avenue, New York, NY 10016 (212) 907-2525.

Winthrop-Breon—Cont.

CEREBRAL ANGIOGRAPHY
HYPAQUE sodium 50 percent may be administered for visualization of the cerebral vessels. Inasmuch as cerebral angiography is a highly specialized procedure requiring the use of special techniques, it is recommended that HYPAQUE sodium 50 percent be used for this purpose only by persons skilled and experienced in carrying out the procedure.

Contraindication
Carotid angiography during the progressive period of a stroke should be avoided, particularly on the left side because of the increased risk of cerebral complications.

Precautions
See PRECAUTIONS—General. Patients in whom cerebral angiography is to be performed should be selected with care.
Although cerebral angiography has been considered contraindicated in patients who have recently experienced cerebral embolism or thrombosis (stroke syndrome), many experts now believe that the diagnostic value of the procedure, when employed early as an aid in locating lesions amenable to operation, outweighs any added risk to the patient. Furthermore, a small number of post-angiographic fatalities have been reported, including progressive thrombosis already clinically evident before angiography, in which the procedure did not appear to play any direct role. Patients with severe cerebrovascular disease should be examined primarily by indirect methods of angiography.
In cerebral angiography, every precaution must be taken to prevent untoward reactions. Reactions may vary directly with the concentration of the substance, the amount used, the speed and frequency of injections, and the interval between injections.
In subarachnoid hemorrhage, angiography is expected to be hazardous. In migraine, the procedure can be hazardous because of ischemic complications, particularly if performed during or soon after an attack.

Adverse Reactions
See ADVERSE REACTIONS—General. With any contrast medium introduced into the cerebral vasculature, neurologic complications, including neuromuscular disorders, seizures, loss of consciousness, hemiplegia, unilateral dysesthesias, visual field defects, language disorders (aphasia), amnesia, and respiratory difficulties may occur, particularly when the extent of the intrinsic lesion is unknown. Such untoward reactions are for the most part temporary, although permanent visual field defects have been reported. Some investigators who are experienced in angiographic procedure emphasize the fact that they tend to occur after repeated injections or higher doses of the contrast medium. Other clinicians find that they occur most frequently in elderly patients. Inasmuch as the procedure itself is attended by technical difficulties regardless of the risk the patient presents (eg, mechanical catheter obstruction of the vertebral artery can cause transient blindness), the more experienced the radiologic team, the fewer the complications of any degree that are apt to arise.

Dosage and Administration
A dose of 8 mL to 12 mL injected at a rate not exceeding the normal flow in the carotid artery (about 5 mL per second) is suggested. The dose may be repeated as indicated; however, an increased risk attends each repeat injection. In the retrograde brachial or catheter method (aortic arch), a single injection of 35 mL to 50 mL is generally used. Children require a smaller dose in proportion to weight. Light anesthesia may be required in these procedures.

PERIPHERAL ANGIOGRAPHY
HYPAQUE sodium 50 percent may be administered for peripheral arteriography and for venography.

Precautions
See PRECAUTIONS—General. Extreme caution is advised in considering peripheral arteriography in patients suspected of having thromboangiitis obliterans (Buerger's disease) since any procedure (even insertion of a needle or catheter) may induce a severe arterial or venous spasm. Caution is also advisable in patients with severe ischemia associated with ascending infection.

Adverse Reactions
See ADVERSE REACTIONS—General. Soreness in extremities has also been reported.
Adverse reactions observed during peripheral arteriography may sometimes be due to arterial trauma during the procedure (ie, insertion of needle or catheter, subintimal injection, perforation) as well as to the hypertonicity or effect of the medium. Reported adverse reactions include transient arterial spasm, extravasation, hemorrhage, hematoma formation with tamponode, injury to nerves in close proximity to artery, thrombosis, dissecting aneurysm, arteriovenous fistula (eg, with accidental perforation of femoral artery and vein during the needling), and transient leg pain from contraction of calf muscles in femoral arteriography. Transient hypotension has been reported after intra-arterial (brachial) injection of the medium. Also, brachial plexus injury has been reported with axillary artery injections.
During venography in the presence of venous stasis, inflammatory changes and thrombosis may occur. Thrombosis is rare if the vein is irrigated following the injection.

Dosage and Administration
Diagnostic arteriograms may be obtained with 25 mL to 35 mL of HYPAQUE sodium 50 percent introduced into the larger peripheral arteries by percutaneous or operative methods. Visualization of veins in the extremities may be accomplished with 15 mL to 40 mL.

Aortography
HYPAQUE sodium 50 percent may be administered intravenously or intra-arterially by accepted techniques to visualize the aorta and its major branches.

Warnings
Pheochromocytoma. Administration of angiographic media to patients known or suspected to have pheochromocytoma can cause dangerous changes in blood pressure. A minimum dose should be injected. The blood pressure should be carefully monitored and measures for controlling major fluctuations should be available.
During aortography by the translumbar technique, extreme care is advised to avoid inadvertent intrathecal injection since the injection of even small amounts (5 mL to 7 mL) of the contrast medium may cause convulsions, permanent sequelae, or fatality. Should the accident occur, the patient should be placed upright to confine the hyperbaric solution to a low level, anesthesia may be required to control convulsions, and if there is evidence of a large dose having been administered, a careful cerebrospinal fluid exchange-washout should be considered.

Precautions
The presence of a vigorous pulsatile flow should be established before using a catheter or pressure injection technique. A small "pilot" dose (about 2 mL) sould be administered to locate the exact site of needle or catheter tip to help prevent injection of the main dose into a branch of the aorta or intramurally. In the translumbar technique, severe pain during injection may indicate intramural placement and abdominal or back pain afterwards may indicate hemorrhage from the injection site. Following catheter procedures, gentle pressure hemostasis for 5 to 10 minutes is advised, followed by observation for 30 to 60 minutes and immobilization of the limb for several hours to prevent hemorrhage from the site of arterial puncture.
The care and experience with which the procedure is performed, the amount and type of medium used, the age and condition of the patient, and the premedication and anesthesia employed, influence the incidence and severity of reactions or complications that may be encountered. Since aortography is not without some danger, it should be employed only by persons experienced in the technique.
Repeated injections of the solution during a single study should be avoided whenever possible.
Under conditions of *slowed aortic circulation* there is an increased likelihood of aortography causing muscle spasm. Occasional serious neurologic complications, including paraplegia, have also been reported in patients with aortic-iliac or even femoral artery bed obstruction, abdominal compression, hypotension, hypertension, spinal anesthesia, injection of vasopressors to increase contrast, and low injection sites (L2-3). In these patients the concentration, dose, and number of repeat injections of the medium should be maintained at a minimum with appropriate intervals between injections. The position of the patient and catheter tip should be carefully evaluated.
Aortic Branches. Since serious neurologic complications, including quadriplegia, have occasionally been reported following spinal arteriography or selective injection of arterial trunks providing spinal artery branches (usually the thyrocervical, costocervical, subclavian, vertebral, bronchial, intercostal), great care is necessary to avoid entry of a large concentrated bolus of the medium. Thus, a "pilot" dose may establish correct position of the catheter tip. The concentration of the medium should not be over 50 percent. The carefully individualized dose is usually under 5 mL but preferably 3 mL to 4 mL and the number of repeat injections held to a minimum with appropriate intervals between injections. Pain or muscle spasm during the injection may require reevaluation of the procedure.

Adverse Reactions
The most common reaction to the medium is a mild burning sensation on injection. In addition to the reactions described in the general section, the following have been reported: mesenteric and intestinal necrosis, acute pancreatitis, renal shutdown (usually transitory), and neurologic complications following inadvertent injection of a large part of the aortic dose into a branch of the aorta. Entry of the large aortic dose into the renal artery can cause, even in the absence of symptoms, albuminuria, cylindruria, and hematuria, and an elevated BUN. Rapid and complete return of function usually follows. Also reported are coronary occlusion, hemorrhage from puncture site, arterial perforation by catheter or needle, thrombosis, embolism, and subintimal injection with aortic dissection by the medium.

Dosage and Administration
The amount of each individual dose is a more important consideration than the total dosage used. Sufficient time should elapse between each injection to allow for subsidence of hemodynamic disturbances.
Retrograde (catheter) aortography—For **adults** and **children**, 0.5 mL to 1 mL per kg of body weight.
Intravenous aortography—For **adults** and **children**, 1 mL per kg of body weight.
Translumbar aortography—For **adults**, 10 mL to 30 mL. For **children** under 12 years, the dose is proportionate to age.
Selective renal arteriography—For **adults** and **children** over 14 years of age, 5 mL to 8 mL with repeat injections as indicated. For **younger children**, the dose is proportionate to age.

Intraosseous Venography
The 50 percent solution may be injected directly into the bone marrow in the study of venous circulation of the bone and extraosseous tissue in the immediate drainage area.
A general anesthetic is sometimes necessary since the method is painful. Occasionally, extravasation of the contrast medium from the needle into the soft tissue may occur.

Dosage and Administration
After aspiration of 4 mL of marrow, 10 mL to 20 mL of the medium are injected.
To visualize the pterygoid venous plexus, 5 mL to 8 mL of the contrast medium are injected into the medullary cavity of the mandible.

Direct Cholangiography
Precaution
In the presence of acute pancreatitis, direct cholangiography, if necessary, should be employed with caution, injecting no more than 5 mL to 10 mL without undue pressure.

Adverse Reactions
Adverse reactions may often be attributed to injection pressure or excessive volume of the medium, resulting in overdistention. Such pressure may produce a sensation of epigastric fullness, followed by moderate pain in the back or right upper abdominal quadrant, which will subside when injection is stopped.
Some of the medium may enter the pancreatic duct and cause a transient serum amylase elevation 6 to 18 hours later, without apparent ill effects. Occasionally, nausea, vomiting, fever, and tachycardia have been observed. Pancholangitis resulting in liver abscess or septicemia has been reported.

Dosage and Administration
The solution should be warmed to body temperature before administration. The injection is made slowly without undue pressure, taking great care to avoid introducing bubbles.
Operative—If no resistance is encountered, from 10 mL to 15 mL of a 25 to 50 percent solution is injected or instilled into the cystic duct or common bile duct, as indicated. In patients with obstructive jaundice, 40 mL to 50 mL of the medium may be injected directly into the gallbladder after aspiration of its contents.
Postexploratory or completion T tube cholangiography may also be performed after exploration of the common bile duct.
Postoperative—Delayed cholangiograms are usually made from the fifth to the tenth postoperative day prior to removal of the T tube.
In case of a dilated ductal tract, a larger volume (up to 100 mL) of radiopaque medium may be required for complete filling and visualization.

PERCUTANEOUS TRANSHEPATIC CHOLANGIOGRAPHY
Percutaneous transhepatic cholangiography is recommended for carefully selected patients for the differential diagnosis of jaundice due to extrahepatic biliary obstruction or parenchymal disease. The procedure is only employed where oral or intravenous cholangiography and other procedures have failed to provide the necessary information. In obstructive cases, percutaneous transhepatic cholangiography is used to determine the cause and site of the obstruction to help plan surgery. The technique may also be of value in avoiding laparotomy in poor risk jaundice patients since failure to enter a duct suggest hepatocellular disease. Careful attention to technique is essential for the success and safety of the procedure. The procedure is usually performed under local anesthesia following analgesic premedication (eg, 100 mg meperidine intramuscularly).

Contraindications
Percutaneous transhepatic cholangiography is contraindicated in patients with coagulation defects and prolonged prothrombin times until normal, or near normal, coagulation is achieved, eg, with vitamin K.

Precautions
Percutaneous transhepatic cholangiography should only be attempted when compatible blood for potential transfusions is in readiness and emergency surgical measures are available. The patient should be carefully monitored for at least 24 hours to insure prompt detection of bile leakage and hemorrhage. Cholespastic premedication, as with morphine, should be avoided. Respiratory movements should be controlled during introduction of the needle.

Adverse Reactions
In percutaneous transhepatic cholangiography, some discomfort is common, but severe pain is unusual. Complications of the procedure are often serious and have been reported in four to six percent of patients. These reactions have included bile leakage and peritonitis, which are more likely to occur in patients with obstructions that cause unrelieved high biliary pressure. Bleeding (sometimes massive with exsanguination) may occur, especially in patients with clotting abnormalities. Blood-bile fistula, manifested by an early urogram (within 2 minutes), has been reported. Hypotension with fever and chills, as manifestations of septicemia, have occurred. Tension pneumothorax, cholangitis, and bacteremia have been reported.

Dosage and Administration
As the needle is advanced or withdrawn, a bile duct may be located by frequent aspiration for bile or mucus into a syringe filled with normal saline. As much bile as possible is aspirated. The usual dose of HYPAQUE sodium 50 percent is 20 mL to 40 mL but the range can be from 10 mL to 60 mL depending on degree of biliary dilatation present. The injection may be repeated for exposures in different planes. If a duct is not readily located by aspiration, entry may be established by injection of successive small doses of 1 mL to 2 mL of the medium under x-ray observation as the needle is withdrawn. If a duct is not located after three or four attempts, the procedure should be abandoned. Inability to enter a duct strongly suggests hepatocellular disease.

Hysterosalpingography
Hysterosalpingography may be performed with either the 50 percent solution, or if a somewhat more viscous solution is preferred, diatrizoate meglumine and diatrizoate sodium, 90 percent.

Contraindications
The procedure should not be performed during the menstrual period or when menstrual flow is imminent, nor should it be performed when infection is present in any portion of the genital tract, including the external genitalia. The procedure is also contraindicated for pregnant women or for those in whom pregnancy is suspected. Its use is not advised for six months after termination of pregnancy, or 30 days after conization or curettage.

Precaution
In patients with carcinoma or in those in whom the condition is suspected, caution should be exercised to avoid possible spread of the lesion by the procedure.

Adverse Reactions
Cramping may occur during the injection and sometimes mild lower abdominal pain may be present for an hour or two afterwards. Even when the medium gains entrance into venous or lymphatic channels, systemic effects are rare. Generalized urticaria or slight transient hyperpyrexia, however, has been reported.

Dosage and Administration
Preparation of the Patients
It is preferable to perform the procedure approximately 10 days after the patient's menstrual period. The patient should empty the bladder before the examination. An enema and vaginal douche are not essential but may be given one hour before the study. Premedication is not necessary.
Approximately 4 mL will suffice to fill a normal uterine cavity, with an additional 3 mL or 4 mL for the fallopian tubes. These amounts may vary depending on the nature of the disease.

Splenoportography
Indication
Splenoportography is usually performed under mild preoperative sedation and under local anesthesia.

Contraindications
Splenoportography should not be performed on any patient for whom splenectomy is contraindicated, since complications of the procedure at times make splenectomy necessary. Other contraindications include prolonged prothrombin time or other coagulation defects, significant thrombocytopenia, and any condition which may increase the possibility of rupture of the spleen.

Precautions
Prior gastrointestinal x-ray examination should include particular attention to the lower esophageal area. A hematologic survey, including prothrombin time and platelet count, should be performed. To minimize risk of bleeding, manipulation during or after entry of the needle should be avoided. Caution is advised in patients whose spleen has recently become tender and palpable. Following splenoportography, the patient should lie on his left side for several hours and should be closely observed for 24 hours for signs of internal bleeding.

Adverse Reactions
Internal bleeding is the most common serious complication of splenoportography. Although leakage of up to 300 mL of blood is apparently not uncommon, sometimes blood transfusions and rarely, splenectomy, may be required to control hemorrhage. Peritoneal extravasation may cause transient diaphragmatic irritation or mild to moderate transient pain which may sometimes be referred to the shoulder, the periumbilical region, or other areas. Because of the proximity of the pleural cavity, accidental pneumothorax has been known to occur. Inadvertent injection of the medium into other nearby structures is not likely to cause untoward consequences.

Dosage and Administration
A preliminary small "pilot" dose is injected to confirm splenic entry, followed usually by rapid injection of 20 mL to 25 mL of HYPAQUE sodium 50 percent. Rapid serial exposures are started with the injection of the dose and continued until contrast is observed in the entire portal system.

Contrast Enhancement of Computed Tomographic Head Imaging
Precautions
Metastatic Brain Lesions. Large doses of contrast media should be avoided in patients with suspected metastatic brain lesions. Intravenous administration of large doses to these patients is more likely to result in convulsions; however, these occurrences are rare. This has been attributed to tissue accumulation of the medium in the presence of blood brain barrier disruption caused by disease. Appropriate measures for seizure management should be immediately available.

Dosage and Administration
Bolus intravenous injection of 50 mL to 100 mL, or up to 150 mL by infusion. The rate of injection and the timing of scans will depend principally on the expected nature of the pathology. Dosage in children is proportional to adults, based on weight.

How Supplied: Vials of 20 mL, rubber stoppered, box of 25 (NDC 0024-0764-04)
Vials of 30 mL, rubber stoppered, box of 25 (NDC 0024-0765-04).
Vials of 50 mL, rubber stoppered, box of 25 (NDC 0024-0766-04).
Box of 10 calibrated 200 mL dilution bottles with hangers containing 150 mL HYPAQUE sodium 50%; rubber stoppered, with 10 intravenous infusion sets (NDC 0024-0770-10)
Box of 10 calibrated 200 mL bottles with hangers containing 200 mL HYPAQUE sodium 50%; rubber stoppered (NDC 0024-0771-10)

HW-10-HH

HYPAQUE® meglumine 60% ℞
brand of diatrizoate meglumine injection, USP
Sterile Aqueous Injection

For Excretory Urography
Cerebral Angiography
Peripheral Arteriography
Venography
Direct Cholangiography
Splenoportography
Arthrography
Discography

Contrast Enhancement of Computed Tomographic Head Imaging:
Description: HYPAQUE meglumine, brand of diatrizoate meglumine, is a water-soluble, radiopaque diagnostic medium. It is a triiodinated benzoic acid derivative containing 47.06 percent

Continued on next page

This product information was effective as of December 3, 1984. On these and other products of Winthrop-Breon Laboratories, detailed information may be obtained on a current basis by direct inquiry to the Professional Services Department, 90 Park Avenue, New York, NY 10016 (212) 907-2525.

Winthrop-Breon—Cont.

organically bound iodine. It is constituted as an iodinated anion (diatrizoate) and a radiolucent cation (mgl).
HYPAQUE meglumine 60 percent (w/v) is a sterile aqueous solution containing 60 g of the meglumine salt of diatrizoic acid per 100 mL of solution. The solution is a clear, colorless to pale yellow liquid, and the pH is adjusted between 6.5 and 7.7 with diatrizoic acid or meglumine solution. It is a relatively thermostable solution and may be autoclaved without harmful effects, although it should be protected from strong light. The 60 percent solution contains edetate calcium disodium 1:10,000 as a sequestering stabilizing agent. Each 1 mL contains approximately 282 mg of organically bound iodine. The viscosity of the solution is 6.17 cp at 25°C and 4.12 cp at 37°C.
It is hypertonic to blood with an osmolality of 1270 mosm/L.
It is a colorless, microcrystalline solid which is readily soluble in water.
It is meglumine 3,5-diacetamido- 2,4,6-tri- iodobenzoate ($C_{11}H_9I_3N_2O_4 \cdot C_7H_{17}NO_5$) with a molecular weight of 809.13.
Clinical Pharmacology: Intravascular injection of a radiopaque diagnostic agent opacifies those vessels in the path of the flow of the contrast medium, permitting radiographic visualization of the internal structures of the human body until significant hemodilution occurs.
At physiologic pH, the water soluble contrast media are completely dissociated into a radiopaque anion and a solubilizing cation.
Following intravenous injection, the radiopaque diagnostic agents are immediately diluted in the circulating plasma. Equilibrium is reached with the extracellular compartment at about 10 minutes. Hence, the plasma concentration at 10 minutes is closely related to the dose corrected to body size.
The pharmacokinetics of the intravenously administered radiopaque contrast media are usually best described by a two compartment model with a rapid alpha phase for drug distribution and a slow beta phase for drug elimination. In patients with normal renal function, the alpha and beta half-lives were respectively 30 minutes and 120 minutes for diatrizoate. But in patients with renal and kidney functional impairment, the elimination half-life for the beta phase can be prolonged up to several days.
Injectable radiopaque diagnostic agents are excreted either through the liver or through the kidneys. These two excretory pathways are not mutually exclusive, but the main route of excretion seems to be governed by the affinity of the contrast medium for serum albumin. From 0% to 10% of diatrizoate sodium is bound to serum protein.
Diatrizoate salts are excreted predominantly unchanged through the kidneys by glomerular filtration. The amount excreted by the kidney during any period of time is determined by the filtered load; ie, the product of plasma contrast media concentration and glomerular filtration rate. The plasma concentration is dependent upon the dose administered and the body size. The glomerular filtration rate varies with the body size, sex, age, circulatory dynamics, diuretic effect of the drug, and renal function. In patients with normal renal function the maximum urinary concentration of diatrizoate meglumine occurs within 10 minutes with 12 percent of the administered dose being excreted. The mean values of cumulative urinary excretion for diatrizoate meglumine expressed as percentage of administered dose are 38 percent at 60 minutes, 45 percent at 3 hours, and 94 to 100 percent at 24 hours.

Urinary excretion of contrast media is delayed in infants younger than 1 month and in patients with urinary tract obstruction. The urinary iodine concentration is higher with the sodium salt of diatrizoic acid than with the meglumine salt.
Diatrizoate meglumine is excreted mainly unchanged through the kidneys.

The liver and small intestine provide the major alternate route of excretion for diatrizoate. In patients free of severe renal disease, the fecal recovery is less than 2 percent of the administered dose. In patients with severe renal impairment the excretion of these contrast media through the gallbladder and into the small intestine sharply increases; up to 20 percent of the administered dose has been recovered in the feces in 48 hours.
Saliva is a minor secretory pathway for injectable radiopaque diagnostic agents. In patients with normal renal function, minimal amounts of contrast media are secreted unchanged. However, in uremic patients small amounts of free iodides resulting from deiodination prior to adminstration or in vivo, have been detected in the saliva.
Diatrizoate meglumine crosses the placental barrier in humans by simple diffusion and appears to enter fetal tissue passively. No apparent harm to the fetus was observed when diatrizoate sodium and diatrizoate meglumine were injected intravenously 24 hours prior to delivery. However, abnormal neonatal opacification of the small intestine and colon were detected 4 to 6 days after delivery. Procedures including radiation involve a certain risk related to the exposure of the fetus.
Injectable radiopaque diagnostic agents are excreted unchanged in human milk.
Computerized tomography. HYPAQUE meglumine, brand of diatrizoate meglumine injection, 60 percent can be administered as an intravenous bolus for brain tissue enhancement using computerized tomography. Increased tissue contrast differential for the scan is achieved either because of increased vascular (arterial, venous, or capillary bed) contrast or by blood brain barrier penetration of the medium (or its absence) in certain localized areas of disrupted vascular permeability. The degree of tissue enhancement caused by increased blood contrast is directly related to blood iodine content. However, the degree of enhancement due to extravascular accumulation of iodine resulting from blood brain barrier disruption will depend on the extent of disruption, the blood level of iodine, and the time delay prior to scanning. The nature of the pathology will determine whether an immediate or delayed scan is optimal.
Effects of steroid therapy. The anti-inflammatory and anti-edema effects in patients receiving steroid therapy have interfered with the expected distribution of CT tissue enhancement on the scan in certain diseases.
Indications and Usage: HYPAQUE meglumine 60 percent is indicated for excretory urography; cerebral angiography; peripheral arteriography; venography; operative, T-tube, or percutaneous transhepatic cholangiography; splenoportography; arthrography; discography; and contrast enhancement of computed tomographic head imaging.
Urography
Diatrizoate salts are used in small, medium, and large dose urography (see Dosage and Administration—EXCRETORY UROGRAPHY). Visualization of the urinary tract can be achieved by either direct intravenous injection, intravenous drip infusion, or sometimes by intramuscular or subcutaneous injections, or incidentally following intra-arterial procedure. Visualization of the urinary tract is delayed in infants less than 1 month old, and in patients with urinary tract obstruction (see CLINICAL PHARMACOLOGY).

Contrast Enhancement of Computed Tomographic Head Imaging
Injectable radiopaque contrast media may be used to refine diagnostic precision in areas of the brain which may not otherwise have been satisfactorily visualized.
Tumors. Radiopaque diagnostic agents may be useful to investigate the presence and extent of certain malignancies such as: gliomas including malignant gliomas, glioblastomas, astrocytomas, oligodendrogliomas and gangliomas, ependymomas, medulloblastomas, meningiomas, neuromas, pinealomas, pituitary adenomas, craniopharynigiomas, germinomas, and metastatic lesions.

The usefulness of contrast enhancement for the investigation of the retrobulbar space and in cases of low grade or infiltrative glioma has not been demonstrated.
In calcified lesions, there is less likelihood of enhancement. Following therapy, tumors may show decreased or no enhancement.
The opacification of the inferior vermis following contrast media administration has resulted in false-positive diagnosis in a number of normal studies.
Nonneoplastic Conditions. The use of injectable radiopaque diagnostic agents may be beneficial in the image enhancement of nonneoplastic lesions. Cerebral infarctions of recent onset may be better visualized with contrast enhancement, while some infarctions are obscured if contrast media are used. The use of iodinated contrast media results in contrast enhancement in about 60 percent of cerebral infarctions studied from one to four weeks from the onset of symptoms.
Sites of active infection may also be enhanced following contrast media administration.
Arteriovenous malformations and aneurysms will show contrast enhancement. For these vascular lesions, the enhancement is probably dependent on the iodine content of the circulating blood pool. Hematomas and intraparenchymal bleeders seldom demonstrate any contrast enhancement. However, in cases of intraparenchymal clot, for which there is no obvious clinical explanation, contrast media administration may be helpful in ruling out the possibility of associated arteriovenous malformation.
Angiography
Diatrizoate salts are used for radiographic studies throughout the cardiovascular system.
Intravascular radiopaque diagnostic agents of high viscosity are not recommended for cerebral angiography (see CONTRAINDICATIONS—General), and contrast agents with the lowest compatible viscosity and higher concentration of iodine (310 mg/mL to 480 mg/mL of bound iodine) must be used for angiocardiography. Contrast media approaching serum ionic content and osmolarity have less potential for deleterious effects on the myocardium (see PRECAUTIONS—Drug Interactions).
Addition of chelating agents may contribute to toxicity in coronary angiography, and the sodium content of angiographic agents used in coronary arteriography is of crucial importance.
In addition to the following general CONTRAINDICATIONS, WARNINGS, PRECAUTIONS, and ADVERSE REACTIONS, there are additional listings in these categories under the particular procedures.
Contraindications:
General: HYPAQUE meglumine 60 percent has no absolute contraindications in its recommended uses (see general WARNINGS and PRECAUTIONS).
Do not use HYPAQUE meglumine, brand of diatrizoate meglumine injection, 60 percent solution for myelography or for examination of dorsal cysts or sinuses which might communicate with the subarachnoid space. Injection of even a small amount into the subarachnoid space may produce convulsions and result in fatality. Epidural injection is also contraindicated.
Warnings:
General: Excretory urography is potentially hazardous in patients with multiple myeloma. In some of those patients, therapeutically resistant anuria resulting in progressive uremia, renal failure, and eventually death has followed this procedure. Although neither the contrast agent nor dehydration has been proved separately to be the cause of anuria in myelomatous patients, it has been speculated that the combination of both may be causative. The risk of excretory urography in myelomatous patients is not a contraindication to the procedure; however, they require special precautions. Partial dehydration in the preparation of these patients for the examination is not recommended since this may predispose to the precipitation of myeloma protein in the renal tubules. Myeloma, which occurs most commonly in persons

over age 40, should be considered before instituting urographic procedures.

Contrast media may promote sickling in individuals who are homozygous for sickle cell disease when the material is injected intravenously or intra-arterially.

Administration of radiopaque materials to patients known or suspected of having pheochromocytoma should be performed with extreme caution. If, in the opinion of the physician, the possible benefits of such procedures outweigh the considered risks, the procedures may be performed; however, the amount of radiopaque medium injected should be kept to an absolute minimum. The blood pressure should be assessed throughout the procedure and measures for treatment of a hypertensive crisis should be available.

Recent reports of thyroid storm occurring following the intravascular use of iodinated radiopaque diagnostic agents in patients with hyperthyroidism or with an autonomously functioning thyroid nodule suggest that this additional risk be evaluated in such patients before use of HYPAQUE meglumine.

Contrast media administered for cardiac catheterization and angiocardiography may cause cellular injury to circulating lymphocytes. Chromosomal damage in humans includes inhibition of mitosis, increases in the number of micronuclei, and chromosome aberrations. The damages appear to be related to the contrast medium itself rather than to the x-ray radiation. It is to be noted that those agents have not been adequately tested in animal or laboratory systems.

Urography should be performed with caution in patients with severly impaired renal function and patients with combined renal and hepatic disease.

Selective spinal arteriography or arteriography of trunks providing spinal branches can cause mild to severe muscle spasm. However, serious neurologic sequelae, including permanent paraylsis, have occasionally been reported. (See also Precaution, ANGIOGRAPHY).

Precautions:

General: Diagnostic procedures which involve the use of radiopaque diagnostic agents should be carried out under the direction of personnel with the prerequisite training and with a thorough knowledge of the particular procedure to be performed. Appropriate facilities should be available for coping with any complication of the procedure, as well as for emergency treatment of severe reactions to the contrast agent itself. After parenteral administration of a radiopaque agent, competent personnel and emergency facilities should be available for at least 30 to 60 minutes since severe delayed reactions have occurred (see ADVERSE REACTIONS—General).

Preparatory dehydration is dangerous and may contribute to acute renal failure in infants, young children, the elderly, patients with preexisting renal insufficiency, patients with advanced vascular disease, and diabetic patients. Dehydration in these patients seems to be enhanced by the osmotic diuretic action of urographic agents and by the decreased water clearance and uricosuria induced by cholangiographic agents. It is believed that overnight fluid restriction prior to excretory urography generally does not provide better visualization in normal patients.

Acute renal failure has been reported in diabetic patients with diabetic nephropathy and in susceptible nondiabetic patients (often elderly with preexisting renal disease) following excretory urography. Therefore, careful consideration of the potential risks should be given before performing this radiographic procedure in these patients.

Immediately following surgery, excretory urography should be used with caution in renal transplant recipients.

The possibility of an idiosyncratic reaction in susceptible patients should always be considered (see ADVERSE REACTIONS—General). The susceptible population includes patients with a history of a previous reaction to a contrast medium, patients with a known sensitivity to iodine per se, and patients with a known clinical hypersensitivity: bronchial asthma, hay fever, and food allergies.

The occurrence of severe idiosyncratic reactions has prompted the use of several pretesting methods. However, pretesting cannot be relied upon to predict severe reactions and may itself be hazardous for the patient. It is suggested that a thorough medical history with emphasis on allergy and hypersensitivity, prior to injection of any contrast media, may be more accurate than pretesting in predicting potential adverse reactions.

A positive history of allergies or hypersensitivity does not arbitrarily contraindicate the use of a contrast agent, where a diagnostic procedure is thought essential, but caution should be exercised (see ADVERSE REACTIONS—General). Premedication with antihistamines or corticosteroids to avoid or minimize possible allergic reactions in such patients should be considered. Recent reports indicate that such pretreatment does not prevent serious life-threatening reactions, but may reduce both their incidence and severity.

Due to the transitory increase in the circulatory osmotic load, injections of urographic agents should be used with caution in patients with congestive heart failure. Such patients should be observed for several hours following the procedure to detect delayed hemodynamic disturbances.

General anesthesia may be indicated in the performance of some procedures in young or uncooperative children and in selected adult patients; however, a higher incidence of adverse reactions has been reported in these patients, and may be attributable to the inability of the patient to identify untoward symptoms, or to the hypotensive effect of anesthesia which can reduce cardiac output and increase the duration of exposure to the contrast agent.

In addition to the general precautions already described, excretory urography, cholangiography, and other uses also have hazards associated with the particular techniques employed.

Information for Patients

Patients receiving injectable radiopaque diagnostic agents should be instructed to:
1. Inform the physician if they are pregnant (see CLINICAL PHARMACOLOGY).
2. Inform the physician if they are diabetic or if they have multiple myeloma, pheochromocytoma, homozygous sickle cell disease, or known thyroid disorder (see WARNINGS—General).
3. Inform the physician if they are allergic to any drugs, food, or if they have had any reactions to previous injections of dyes used for x-ray procedures (see PRECAUTIONS—General).
4. Inform the physician about any other medication they are currently taking, including nonprescription drugs, before they are administered this drug.

Drug Interactions

Renal toxicity has been reported in a few patients with liver dysfunction who were given oral cholecystographic agents followed by urographic agents. Administration of intravascular urographic agents should therefore be postponed in any patient with a known or suspected hepatic or biliary disorder who has recently received a cholecystographic contrast agent.

Addition of an inotropic agent to contrast agents may produce a paradoxical depressant response which can be deleterious to the ischemic myocardium.

Drug/Laboratory Test Interactions

If any of these studies, which might be affected by contrast media are indicated, it is recommended that they be performed prior to administration of the contrast medium or two or more days afterwards.

Diatrizoate salts interfere with several laboratory urine and blood tests.

Blood Tests

Coagulation: Diatrizoate salts significantly inhibit all stages of coagulation. The fibrinogen concentration, Factors V, VII, and VIII are decreased. Prothrombin time and thromboplastin time are increased.

Platelet aggregation: High levels of plasma and diatrizoate meglumine inhibit platelet aggregation.

Serum calcium: Diatrizoate salts may decrease serum calcium levels. However, this depletion of serum calcium may also be the result of the addition of chelating agents (edetate disodium) in the preparation of certain contrast media.

Red cell counts: Transitory decreases in red cell counts. Technetium-99m–RBC labeling interference.

Leukocyte counts: Decrease following injection of diatrizoate.

Urea nitrogen (BUN): Transitory increase (see CLINICAL PHARMACOLOGY).

Serum creatinine: Transitory increase.

Urine Tests

Contrast media which are excreted in the urine, may interfere with some laboratory determinations eg, proteinuria, specific gravity, osmolarity, or bacterial cultures.

Thyroid Function Tests

Protein-bound iodine (PBI) and total serum organic iodine: Transient increase of both tests following urography have been noticed. The results of PBI and radioactive iodine uptake studies which depend on iodine estimations will not accurately reflect thyroid function for up to 16 days following administration of iodinated urographic media. However, thyroid function tests not depending on iodine estimations, eg, T_3 resin uptake or free thyroxine assays are not affected.

Carcinogenesis, Mutagenesis, Impairment of Fertility. No long-term animal studies have been performed to evaluate the potential of diatrizoate salts in these areas.

Pregnancy Category C. Animal reproduction studies have not been conducted with HYPAQUE meglumine, brand of diatrizoate meglumine injection, 60 percent. It is also not known whether HYPAQUE meglumine 60 percent can cause fetal harm when administered to a pregnant woman or can affect reproduction capacity. HYPAQUE meglumine 60 percent should be given to a pregnant woman only if clearly needed. Doses up to 2500 mg/kg in rats, given IV daily, administered during gestation days 6 to 15 revealed no teratogenic abnormalities.

Labor and Delivery. It is not known whether use of these contrast agents during labor or delivery has immediate or delayed adverse effects on the fetus, prolongs the duration of labor or increases the likelihood that forceps delivery or other obstetrical intervention or resuscitation of the newborn will be necessary.

Nursing Mothers. Diatrizoate salts are excreted unchanged in human milk. Because of the potential adverse reactions, although it has not been established that serious adverse reactions occur in nursing infants, caution should be exercised when these intravascular contrast media are administered to a nursing woman.

Pediatric Use. Infants and small children should not have any fluid restriction prior to excretory urography or any other procedures (see PRECAUTIONS—General). Guidelines for pediatric dosages are presented in DOSAGE AND ADMINISTRATION—General).

Adverse Reactions:

General: Approximately 95 percent of adverse reactions accompanying the intravascular use of diatrizoate salts are of mild to moderate severity. However, life-threatening reactions and fatalities, mostly of cardiovascular origin, have occurred.

Adverse reactions to injectable contrast media fall into two categories; chemotoxic reactions and idiosyncratic reactions.

Chemotoxic reactions result from the physicochemical properties of the contrast media, the dose, and the speed of injection. All hemodynamic

Continued on next page

This product information was effective as of December 3, 1984. On these and other products of Winthrop-Breon Laboratories, detailed information may be obtained on a current basis by direct inquiry to the Professional Services Department, 90 Park Avenue, New York, NY 10016 (212) 907-2525.

Winthrop-Breon—Cont.

disturbances and injuries to organs or vessels perfused by the contrast medium are included in this category.

Idiosyncratic reactions include all other reactions. They occur more frequently in patients 20 to 40 years old. Idiosyncratic reactions may or may not be dependent on the amount of dose injected, the speed of injection, the mode of injection, and the radiographic procedure. Idiosyncratic reactions are subdivided into minor, intermediate, and severe. The minor reactions are self-limited and of short duration; the severe reactions are life-threatening and treatment is urgent and mandatory.

The reported incidence of adverse reactions to contrast media in patients with a history of allergy are twice that of the general population. Patients with a history of previous reactions to a contrast medium are 3 times more susceptible than other patients. However, sensitivity to contrast media does not appear to increase with repeated examinations.

Most adverse reactions to injectable contrast media appear within one to three minutes after the start of injection, but delayed reactions may occur. Adverse reactions are grouped by organ system and listed below by decreasing order of occurrence and with an approximate incidence of occurrence. Significantly more severe reactions are listed before the other reactions regardless of frequency.

Greater Than 1 in 100 Patients

Body as a Whole: Reported incidences of death range from 6.6 per 1 million (0.00066 percent) to 1 in 10,000 patients (0.01 percent). Most deaths occur during injection or 5 to 10 minutes later, the main feature being cardiac arrest with cardiovascular disease as the main aggravating factor.

Isolated reports of hypotensive collapse and shock following urography are found in the literature. The incidence of shock is estimated to occur in 1 out of 20,000 (0.005 percent) patients.

Cardiovascular System: The most frequent adverse reaction to diatrizoate salts is vasodilation (feeling of warmth). The estimated incidence is 49 percent.

Digestive System: Nausea 6 percent, vomiting 3 percent.

Nervous System: Paresthesia 6 percent, dizziness 5 percent.

Respiratory System: Rhinitis 1 percent, increased cough 2 percent.

Skin and Appendages: Urticaria 1 percent.

Pain at the injection site is estimated to occur in about 12 percent of the patients undergoing urography. Pain is usually due to extravasation. Painful hot erythematous swelling above the venipuncture site was estimated to occur in more than one percent of the patients undergoing phlebography.

Special Senses: Perverson of taste 11 percent.

Urogenital System: Osmotic nephrosis of the proximal tubular cells is estimated to occur in 23 percent of patients following excretory urography.

Less Than 1 in 100 Patients

Other infrequently reported reactions without accompanying incidence rates are listed below, grouped by organ system.

Body as a Whole: Malaria relapse, uremia, high creatinine and BUN (see PRECAUTIONS—Drug/Laboratory Test Interactions), thrombocytopenia, leukopenia, and anemia.

Cardiovascular System: Cerebral hematomas, hemodynamic disturbances, sinus bradycardia, transient electrocardiographic abnormalities, ventricular fibrillation, and petechiae.

Digestive System: Severe unilateral or bilateral swelling of the parotid and submaxillary glands.

Nervous System: Convulsions, paralysis, and coma.

Respiratory System: Asthma, dyspnea, laryngeal edema, pulmonary edema, and bronchospasm.

Skin and Appendages: Skin necrosis.

Special Senses: Bilateral ocular irritation, lacrimation, itching, conjunctival chemosis, infection, and conjunctivitis.

Urogenital: Renal failure, pain.

Overdosage: At dosage levels of 1 mL/lb, the incidence of unpleasant side effects increases. At total dosage of 2 mL/lb, administered over a short period of time (eg, 30 minutes), clinical signs of systemic intolerance appear (mostly related to hyperosmolar effects) and are manifest as tremors, irritability, and tachycardia. Above these maximal tolerated dosage levels in otherwise healthy adults, an increasing incidence and severity of dyspnea and pulmonary edema should be expected.

Four cases of overdosage in infants, during urography, are reported. Three of the infants died within 19 hours of the injection. the overdose ranged from slightly above the recommended pediatric dosage to a dose exceeding 19 g/kg. The symptoms of overdosage appeared between 10 minutes to several hours after injection of the contrast medium. Adverse effects were life-threatening, affecting mainly the pulmonary and cardiovascular systems. The symptoms included: cyanosis, bradycardia, acidosis, pulmonary hemorrhage, convulsions, coma, and cardiac arrest. All infants showed a poor visualization of the kidneys and a diffuse opacification of all the tissues and vasculature. Autopsy findings showed acute pulmonary damage and/or edema of subcutaneous tissues. Treatment of an overdose of injectable radiopaque contrast media is directed toward the support of all vital functions, and prompt institution of symptomatic therapy.

The acute intravenous LD_{50} of diatrizoate meglumine in mice is equivalent in iodine content of 5.3 gI/kg to 8.0 gI/kg and seem to be directly proportional to the rate of injection.

Diatrizoate meglumine is dialyzable.

Dosage and Administration:

General: Preparation of the patient will vary with preference of the radiologist and the type of radiological procedure performed. Specific radiographic procedures used will depend on the state of the patient and the diagnostic indications. (See INDIVIDUAL INDICATIONS AND USAGE section for specific Dosage and Administration.)

Solutions of radiopaque diagnostic agents for intravascular use should be at body temperature when injected and may need to be warmed before use. In the event that crystallization occurs, the solution may be clarified by placing the vial in a water bath at 40°C to 50°C and shaking gently for two to three minutes or until the solids redissolve. If particles still persist, do not use this vial but discard it. The solution should be protected from light and any unused portion remaining in the container should be discarded.

Dilution and withdrawal of the contrast agents should be accomplished under aseptic conditions with sterile syringes.

Parenteral drug products should be inspected visually for particulate matter and discoloration prior to administration, whenever solution and container permit.

Pediatric Dosage

Pediatric doses of injectable radiopaque diagnostic agents are generally determined on a weight basis and should be calculated for each patient individually. (See INDIVIDUAL INDICATIONS AND USAGE sections.)

Drug Incompatibilities

Diatrizoate salts are incompatible in vitro with some antihistamines and many other drugs. It is believed that one of the chief causes of in vitro incompatibility is an alteration of pH. Turbidity of solutions of intravascular contrast medium occurs between pH 2.5 and 4.1. Another cause is chemical interaction; therefore, other pharmaceuticals should not be mixed with contrast agents in the same syringe.

Individual Indications and Usage

Excretory Urography

Indications

Diatrizoate salts are used in small, medium, and large dose urography (see Dosage and Administration—EXCRETORY UROGRAPHY). Visualization of the urinary tract can be achieved by either direct intravenous injection, intravenous drip infusion, or sometimes by intramuscular or subcutaneous injections, or incidentally following intraarterial procedure. Visualization of the urinary tract is delayed in infants less than 1 month old, and in patients with urinary tract obstruction (see CLINICAL PHARMACOLOGY).

Precautions

See PRECAUTIONS—General. Some clinicians consider multiple myeloma a contraindication to excretory urography because of the great possibility of producing transient to fatal renal failure. Others believe that the risk of causing anuria is definite but small. If excretory urography is performed in the presence of mulitple myeloma, dehydration should be avoided since it favors protein precipitation in renal tubules.

Because of the possibility of temporary suppression of urine, it is wise to allow an interval of at least 48 hours before excretory urography is repeated in patients with unilateral or bilateral reduction of normal renal function.

Preparatory dehydration may be dangerous in infants, young children, the elderly, and azotemic patients (especially those with polyuria, oliguria, diabetes, advanced vascular disease, or preexisting dehydration). The undesirable dehydration in these patients may be accentuated by the osmotic diuretic action of the medium.

Adverse Reactions

See ADVERSE REACTIONS—General.

Dosage and Administration

Intravenous Dosage

Adults. A dose of 30 mL to 60 mL produces excellent shadows in the majority of adults subjected to partial dehydration and effective purgation. In persons of slight build, 20 mL produces adequate shadows. For best results and minimal reactions, the total 30 mL to 60 mL should be injected in one to three minutes and compression may be used. A small intravenous test dose may be administered as a possible aid in determining sensitivity to the medium. (See PRECAUTIONS-General.)

Children. The suggested dosage for children up to 12 years old is presented in the table below. Children older than 12 years may be given an adult dose.

[See table below].

Preliminary Preparation of Patient

Although clear shadows are often seen in patients who have had no preliminary preparation for urography, the largest percentage of satisfactory films is obtained in patients who abstain from fluids for 12 to 15 hours before the intravenous injection so that partial dehydration results. (See PRECAUTIONS—General concerning dehydration.) Unless contraindicated, a laxative may be taken at bedtime to eliminate gas from the intestine.

Roentgenographic Technique

A preliminary scout film may be obtained before the intravenous injection. Excellent shadows can often be obtained immediately after administration of the radiopaque medium (within a five-minute period). If preliminary preparation has been carried out, the urinary organs are usually best visualized on films exposed 5, 10, or 15 minutes after intravenous injection. If a film of the bladder is required, it is generally taken 25 or 35 minutes after injection.

Pediatric Dosage for Excretory Urography

Age	Body Weight	Dosage
Under 2 years	up to 10 lb	5 mL to 10 mL
	10 to 30 lb	10 mL to 15 mL
2 to 12 years	30 to 60 lb	15 mL to 30 mL
	over 60 lb	30 mL

In patients with impaired renal function, the best shadows may not be obtainable until later (30 minutes or more) because of delayed excretion, and additional film may have to be exposed.

Most urologists and roentgenologists believe that compression immediately above the symphysis (obtained by application of a small hollow rubber ball about the size of a grapefruit or by the rolled bed sheet technique) assures adequate filling of the pelves and ureters, and hence is of great value. Although compression undoubtedly improves the urogram, it also seems to increase the possibility of pyelorenal backflow or reflux by raising the pressure within the urinary tract.

Angiography
Precaution

Since serious neurologic complications, including quadriplegia, have occasionally been reported following spinal arteriography or selective injection of arterial trunks providing spinal artery branches (usually the thyrocervical, costocervical, subclavian, vertebral, bronchial, intercostal), great care is necessary to avoid entry of a large concentrated bolus of the medium. Thus, a "pilot" dose may establish correct position of the catheter tip. The concentration of the medium should not be over 60 percent. The carefully individualized dose is usually under 5 mL but preferably 3 mL to 4 mL and the number of repeat injections held to a minimum with appropriate intervals between injections. Pain or muscle spasm during the injection may require reevaluation of the procedure. Angiography should be avoided whenever possible in patients with homocystinuria, because of the risk of inducing thrombosis and embolism.

Cerebral Angiography
Indication

HYPAQUE meglumine, brand of diatrizoate meglumine injection, 60 percent may be administered for visualization of the cerebral vessels. Inasmuch as cerebral angiography is a highly specialized procedure requiring the use of special techniques, it is recommended that HYPAQUE meglumine 60 percent be used for this purpose only by persons skilled and experienced in carrying out the procedure.

Carotid angiography during the progressive period of a stroke should be avoided, particularly on the left side because of the increased risk of cerebral complications.

Precautions

See PRECAUTIONS—General. Patients in whom cerebral angiography is to be performed should be selected with care.

Although cerebral angiography has been considered contraindicated in patients who have recently experienced cerebral embolism or thrombosis (stroke syndrome), many experts now believe that the diagnostic value of the procedure, when employed early as an aid in locating lesions amenable to operation, outweighs any added risk to the patient. Furthermore, a small number of postangiographic fatalities have been reported, including progressive thrombosis already clinically evident before angiography, in which the procedure did not appear to play any direct role. Patients with severe cerebrovascular disease should be examined primarily by indirect methods of angiography.

In cerebral angiography, every precaution must be taken to prevent untoward reactions. Reactions may vary directly with the concentration of the substance, the amount used, the speed and frequency of injections, and the interval between injections.

In subarachnoid hemorrhage, angiography is expected to be hazardous. In migraine, the procedure can be hazardous because of ischemic complications, particularly if performed during or soon after an attack.

Adverse Reactions

See ADVERSE REACTIONS—General. With any contrast medium introduced into the cerebral vasculature, neurologic complications, including neuromuscular disorders, seizures, loss of consciousness, hemiplegia, unilateral dysesthesias, visual field defects, language disorders (aphasia), amnesia, and respiratory difficulties may occur, particularly when the extent of the intrinsic lesion is unknown. Such untoward reactions are for the most part temporary, although permanent visual field defects have been reported. Some investigators who are experienced in angiographic procedure emphasize the fact that they tend to occur after repeated injections or higher doses of the contrast medium. Other clinicians find that they occur most frequently in elderly patients. Inasmuch as the procedure itself is attended by technical difficulties regardless of the risk the patient presents (eg, mechanical catheter obstruction of the vertebral artery can cause transient blindness), the more experienced the radiologic team, the fewer the complications of any degree that are apt to arise.

Dosage and Administration

A dose of 8 mL to 12 mL injected at a rate not exceeding the normal flow in the carotid artery (about 5 mL per second) is suggested. The dose may be repeated as indicated; however, an increased risk attends each repeat injection. Children require a smaller dose in proportion to weight. Light anesthesia may be required in these procedures.

Peripheral Arteriography and Venography
Indications

HYPAQUE meglumine, brand of diatrizoate meglumine injection, 60 percent may be administered for peripheral arteriography and for venography.

Precautions

See PRECAUTIONS—General. Extreme caution is advised in considering peripheral arteriography in patients suspected of having thromboangiitis obliterans (Buerger's disease) since any procedure (even insertion of a needle or catheter) may induce a severe arterial or venous spasm. Caution is also advisable in patients with severe ischemia associated with ascending infection.

Adverse Reactions

See ADVERSE REACTIONS—General. Soreness in extremities has also been reported.

Adverse reactions observed during peripheral arteriography may sometimes be due to arterial trauma during the procedure (ie, insertion of needle or catheter, subintimal injection, perforation, etc) as well as to the hypertonicity or effect of the medium. Reported adverse reactions include transient arterial spasm, extravasation, hemorrhage, hematoma formation with tamponade, injury to nerves in close proximity to artery, thrombosis, dissecting aneurysm, arteriovenous fistula (eg, with accidental perforation of femoral artery and vein during the needling), and transient leg pain from contraction of calf muscles in femoral arteriography. Transient hypotension has been reported after intra-arterial (brachial) injection of the medium. Also, brachial plexus injury has been reported with axillary artery injections.

During venography in the presence of venous stasis, inflammatory changes and thrombosis may occur. Thrombosis is rare if the vein is irrigated following the injection.

Dosage and Administration

Diagnostic arteriograms may be obtained with 20 mL to 40 mL of HYPAQUE meglumine 60 percent introduced into the larger peripheral arteries by percutaneous or operative methods. Visualization of veins in the extremities may be accomplished with 10 mL to 20 mL.

Direct Cholangiography
Contraindication

Percutaneous transhepatic cholangiography is contraindicated in patients with coagulation defects and prolonged prothrombin times until normal, or near normal, coagulation is achieved (eg, with vitamin K).

Precautions

In the presence of acute pancreatitis, direct cholangiography, if necessary, should be employed with caution, injecting no more than 5 mL to 10 mL without undue pressure.

Percutaneous transhepatic cholangiography should only be attempted when compatible blood for potential transfusions is in readiness and emergency surgical measures are available. The patient should be carefully monitored for at least 24 hours to insure prompt detection of bile leakage and hemorrhage. Cholespastic premedication, as with morphine, should be avoided. Respiratory movements should be controlled during introduction of the needle.

Adverse Reactions

Adverse reactions may often be attributed to injection pressure or excessive volume of the medium, resulting in overdistention. Such pressure may produce a sensation of epigastric fullness, followed by moderate pain in the back or right upper abdominal quadrant, which will subside when injection is stopped.

Some of the medium may enter the pancreatic duct and cause a transient serum amylase elevation 6 to 18 hours later, without apparent ill effects. Occasionally, nausea, vomiting, fever, and tachycardia have been observed. Pancholangitis resulting in liver abscess or septicemia has been reported.

In percutaneous transhepatic cholangiography, some discomfort is common, but severe pain is unusual. Complications of the procedure are often serious and have been reported in four to six per cent of patients. These reactions have included bile leakage and peritonitis, which are more likely to occur in patients with obstructions that cause unrelieved high biliary pressure. Bleeding (sometimes massive with exsanguination) may occur, especially in patients with clotting abnormalities. Blood-bile fistula, manifested by an early urogram (within 2 minutes) has been reported. Hypotension with fever and chills, as manifestations of septicemia, have occurred. Tension pneumothorax, cholangitis, and bacteremia have been reported.

Dosage and Administration

The solution should be warmed to body temperature before administration. The injection is made slowly without undue pressure, taking great care to avoid introducing bubbles.

Operative—If no resistance is encountered, from 10 mL to 15 mL (sometimes up to 25 mL) of a 30 to 60 percent solution is injected or instilled into the cystic duct or common bile duct, as indicated. In patients with obstructive jaundice, 40 mL to 50 mL of the medium may be injected directly into the gallbladder after aspiration of its contents.

Postexploratory or completion T-tube cholangiography may also be performed after exploration of the common bile duct.

Postoperative—Delayed cholangiograms are usually made from the fifth to the tenth postoperative day prior to removal of the T-tube.

Percutaneous transhepatic cholangiography is recommended for carefully selected patients for the differential diagnosis of jaundice due to extrahepatic biliary obstruction or parenchymal disease. The procedure is only employed where oral or intravenous cholangiography and other procedures have failed to provide the necessary information. In obstructive cases, percutaneous transhepatic cholangiography is used to determine the cause and site of the obstruction to help plan surgery. The technique may also be of value in avoiding laparotomy in poor risk jaundice patients since failure to enter a duct suggests hepatocellular disease. Careful attention to technique is essential for the success and safety of the procedure. The procedure is usually performed under local anesthesia following analgesic premedication (eg, 100 mg meperidine intramuscularly).

As the needle is advanced or withdrawn, a bile duct may be located by frequent aspiration for bile or mucus into a syringe filled with normal saline. As much bile as possible is aspirated. The usual dose of HYPAQUE meglumine, brand of diatrizoate meglumine injection, 60 percent is 20 mL to 40 mL but the range can be from 10 mL to 60 mL depending on degree of biliary dilatation present.

Continued on next page

This product information was effective as of December 3, 1984. On these and other products of Winthrop-Breon Laboratories, detailed information may be obtained on a current basis by direct inquiry to the Professional Services Department, 90 Park Avenue, New York, NY 10016 (212) 907-2525.

Winthrop-Breon—Cont.

The injection may be repeated for exposures in different planes. If a duct is not readily located by aspiration, entry may be established by the injection of successive small doses of 1 mL or 2 mL of the medium under x-ray observation as the needle is withdrawn. If a duct is not located after three or four attempts, the procedure should be abandoned. Inability to enter a duct strongly suggests hepatocellular disease.

Splenoportography
Indication
Splenoportography is usually performed under mild preoperative sedation and under local anesthesia.
Contraindications
Splenoportography should not be performed on any patient for whom splenectomy is contraindicated, since complications of the procedure at times make splenectomy necessary. Other contraindications include prolonged prothrombin time or other coagulation defects, significant thrombocytopenia, and any condition which may increase the possibility of rupture of the spleen.
Precautions
Prior gastrointestinal x-ray examination should include particular attention to the lower esophageal area. A hematologic survey, including prothrombin time and platelet count, should be performed. To minimize risk of bleeding, manipulation during or after entry of the needle should be avoided. Caution is advised in patients whose spleen has recently become tender and palpable. Following splenoportography, the patient should lie on his left side for several hours and should be closely observed for 24 hours for signs of internal bleeding.
Adverse Reactions
Internal bleeding is the most common serious complication of splenoportography. Although leakage of up to 300 mL of blood is apparently not uncommon, sometimes blood transfusions and, rarely, splenectomy, may be required to control hemorrhage. Peritoneal extravasation may cause transient diaphragmatic irritation or mild to moderate transient pain which may sometimes be referred to the shoulder, the periumbilical region, or other areas. Because of the proximity of the pleural cavity, accidental pneumothorax has been known to occur. Inadvertent injection of the medium into other nearby structures is not likely to cause untoward consequences.
Dosage and Administration
A preliminary small "pilot" dose is injected to confirm splenic entry, followed usually by rapid injection of 20 mL to 25 mL of HYPAQUE meglumine, brand of diatrozate meglumine injection, 60 percent. Rapid serial exposures are started with the injection of the dose and continued until contrast is observed in the entire portal system.

Arthrography
Indications
Arthrography may be helpful in the diagnosis of posttraumatic or degenerative joint diseases, synovial rupture, the visualization of communicating bursae or cysts, and in meniscography. However, the technique is of little value unless the arthrograms are interpreted by well-trained personnel.
Contraindication
Arthrography is contraindicated when there is infection in or near the joint.
Precautions
See PRECAUTIONS—General. A strict, aseptic technique is required to avoid introducing infection.
Adverse Reactions
See ADVERSE REACTIONS—General. Injection of HYPAQUE meglumine 60 percent into the joint usually causes immediate but transient discomfort. However, delayed, severe, or persistent pain may occur occasionally. Severe pain often results from undue use of pressure or the injection of large volumes. Joint swelling after injection is rare. Effusion, occasionally requiring aspiration, can occur in patients with rheumatoid arthritis.
Dosage and Administration
The procedure is usually performed with analgesic premedication and under local anesthesia. The amount of HYPAQUE meglumine 60 percent injected depends solely on the capacity of the joint. The damaged joint may require doses greatly exceeding those for normal joints. As much fluid as possible should first be aspirated from the joint; then, the medium should be injected gently to avoid overdistention of the joint capsule. Passive manipulation is sometimes used to disperse the medium in the joint. Sometimes, a 1 mL or 2 mL test dose is injected; immediate pain may indicate extravasation or extracapsular injection which, if confirmed by x-ray, requires relocation of the needle.

A single injection is usually adequate for multiple exposures. Contrast is good during the first 10 minutes after injection, adequate at 10 to 15 minutes, and begins to fade at 15 to 25 minutes.

The following approximate volumes have been used in normal adult joints:
  Knee, shoulder, hip—5 mL to 15 mL
  Temporomandibular—0.5 mL
  Other—1 rL to 4 mL

"Double contrast arthrography," using a mixture of the medium and air or a dilution of HYPAQUE meglumine, brand of diatrozate meglumine injection, 60 percent to a 30 percent concentration, has been employed.

Discography
Indications
Cervical discography is a more hazardous procedure than lumbar discography, and the interpretation of the cervical discograms is more difficult. The injected medium gradually diffuses throughout the disc and is absorbed rapidly. In a normal disc, good contrast is evident for 10 to 15 minutes. In a ruptured disc, the medium is absorbed more rapidly. Aspiration of the medium on completion of discography is considered unnecessary.
Contraindication
Discography is contraindicated when there is infection or open injury near the region to be examined.
Warning
Inadvertent subarachnoid injection must be avoided since even the small dose of the medium used in discography might result in convulsions and death. The onset of signs of pain, cramps, or convulsions (requiring anesthesia) may occur within minutes to an hour.
Precautions
A strict, aseptic technique is required to avoid introducing infection. The examination should be postponed if local or systemic infection is present. In cervical discography, care should be taken to avoid contamination of the disc by inadvertent puncture of the esophagus. Laceration of the disc by use of a needle that has become barbed by forceful impingement on a vertebra, should be avoided. The patient should be cautioned not to move during introduction of the needle.
Adverse Reactions
In the normal disc, only minor discomfort will occur during injection. More discomfort will result if excessive pressure or volume is used. Pain is unusual and may indicate extravasation.
In the damaged disc, however, the injection can cause pain, sometimes severe, which mimics the symptoms. Transient backache or headache, as in lumbar puncture, often occurs. Extravasation from the disc into the lateral recesses and extradurally into the spinal canal or local soft tissue does not usually cause adverse effects.
Dosage and Administration
Discography is usually performed with parenteral analgesia or sedation, and under local anesthesia. To minimize disc and tissue trauma, a two-needle technique is usually employed. An 18 to 20 gauge needle is used to penetrate to the disc and then a very fine (25 or 26 gauge) lumbar puncture-type needle is inserted through the needle to penetrate the disc.
Because of the resistance encountered, it is difficult to inject more than 0.2 mL to 0.3 mL of HYPAQUE meglumine 60 percent into a normal disc. Occasionally, however, a cervical disc can accept up to 0.5 mL and a lumbar disc, 1 mL (rarely, 2 mL) before resistance is encountered. Mild discomfort with little or no frank pain may indicate a normal disc.
In ruptured and some abnormal discs, 1 mL to 2 mL or more can be introduced without resistance; and, particularly if only one disc has pathology, the patient usually experiences pain, sometimes severe, with distribution characteristic of his symptoms. To minimize the amount of HYPAQUE extravasated, no more than 2 mL is injected in any one disc.
The procedure should be planned so that the duration of the discogram allows multiple exposures with a single dose. It has been recommended for diagnostic reasons that the procedure (injection and discogram) be performed on one disc at a time. Injection of a number of discs under suspicion, however, may be performed as part of one procedure.

Contrast Enhancement of Computed Tomographic Head Imaging
Precautions
Metastatic Brain Lesions. Large doses of contrast media should be avoided in patients with suspected metastatic brain lesions. Intravenous administration of large doses to these patients is more likely to result in convulsions; however, these occurrences are rare. This has been attributed to tissue accumulation of the medium in the presence of blood brain barrier disruption caused by disease. Appropriate measures for seizure management should be immediately available.
Dosage and Administration
Bolus intravenous injection by 50 mL to 100 mL, or up to 150 mL by infusion. The rate of injection and the timing of scans will depend principally on the expected nature of the pathology. Dosage in children is proportional to adults, based on weight.
How Supplied:
Vials of 20 mL, rubber stoppered, box of 25 (NDC 0024-0744-04).
Vials of 30 mL, rubber stoppered, box of 25 (NDC 0024-0745-04).
Vials of 50 mL, rubber stoppered, box of 25 (NDC 0024-0746-04).
Vials of 100 mL, rubber stoppered, box of 10 (NDC 0024-0747-02).
Box of 10 calibrated 200 mL dilution bottles with hanger containing 100 mL HYPAQUE meglumine, brand of diatrozate meglumine injection, 60%; rubber stoppered, with 10 intravenous infusion sets (NDC 0024-0748-10).
Box of 10 calibrated 200 mL dilution bottles with hanger containing 150 mL HYPAQUE meglumine 60%; rubber stoppered, with 10 intravenous infusion sets (NDC 0024-0749-10).
Box of 10 calibrated 200 mL dilution bottles with hanger containing 200 mL HYPAQUE meglumine 60%; rubber stoppered (NDC 0024-0750-10).

HW-87 T

HYPAQUE®-M, 75% ℞
brand of diatrizoate meglumine and diatrizoate sodium injection, USP
Sterile Aqueous Injection

For Angiocardiography, Aortography, Angiography, Urography

Description: HYPAQUE-M, 75 percent, brand of diatrizoate meglumine and diatrizoate sodium, is a water-soluble radiopaque diagnostic medium. It is supplied as a 75 percent sterile aqueous solution providing 50 percent (w/v) diatrizoate meglumine and 25 percent (w/v) diatrizoate sodium. It is a triiodonated benzoic acid derivative containing 38.5 percent (w/v) organically bound iodine. Each mL contains 385 mg iodine and 9 mg (0.39 mEq) sodium. It is constituted as a radiopaque iodinated anion (diatrizoate) and the radiolucent cations (meglumine and sodium). It is the organically bound iodine of the anion which opacifies internal structures for x-ray visualization and fluoroscopy. The solution is hypertonic and has a viscosity of approximately 8.3 cp at 37° C. The pH is adjusted between 6.5 and 7.7 with sodium hydroxide, or hydrochloric acid, or sodium carbonate. The pKa is 3.4 for diatrizoic acid. Edetate calcium disodium

1:10,000 has been added as a sequestering stabilizing agent. At body temperature the solution is clear and colorless to pale straw color. The solution may be autoclaved once. Discard any unused portion remaining in the container. The solution should be stored at room temperature and protected from strong light. Crystals may form in the solution on cooling; they are readily redissolved on warming; the solution, however, should be administered at body temperature.

Diatrizoate meglumine is 1-deoxy-1-(methylamino)-D-glucitol 3,5-diacetamido-2,4,6-triiodobenzoate (salt).

Diatrizoate sodium is monosodium 3,5-diacetamido-2,4,6-triiodobenzoate.

Clinical Pharmacology: Intravascular injection of a radiopaque diagnostic agent opacifies those vessels in the path of the flow of the contrast medium, permitting radiographic visualization of the internal structures of the human body until significant hemodilution occurs.

At physiologic pH, the water-soluble contrast media are completely dissociated into a radiopaque anion and a solubilizing cation. While circulating in tissue fluids, the compound remains ionized. However, it is not metabolized but excreted unchanged in the urine, each diatrizoate molecule remaining "obligated" to its sodium or meglumine moiety.

Following intravenous injection, the radiopaque diagnostic agents are immediately diluted in the circulating plasma. Equilibrium is reached with the extracellular compartment at about 10 minutes. Hence, the plasma concentration at 10 minutes is closely related to the dose corrected for body size.

The pharmacokinetics of the intravenously administered radiopaque contrast media are usually best described by a two compartment model with a rapid alpha phase for drug distribution and a slow beta phase for drug elimination. In patients with normal renal function, the alpha and beta half-lives were respectively 30 minutes and 120 minutes for diatrizoate. But in patients with renal and kidney functional impairment, the elimination half-life for the beta phase can be prolonged up to several days.

Injectable radiopaque diagnostic agents are excreted either through the liver or through the kidneys. These two excretory pathways are not mutually exclusive, but the main route of excretion seems to be governed by the affinity of the contrast medium for serum albumin. From 0% to 10% of diatrizoate sodium is bound to serum protein.

Diatrizoate salts are excreted unchanged predominantly through the kidneys by glomerular filtration. The amount excreted by the kidney during any period of time is determined by the filtered load; ie, the product of plasma contrast media concentration and glomerular filtration rate. The plasma concentration is dependent upon the dose administered and the body size. The glomerular filtration rate varies with the body size, sex, age, circulatory dynamics, diuretic effect of the drug, and renal function. In patients with normal renal function the maximum urinary concentration of diatrizoate meglumine occurs within 10 minutes with 12 percent of the administered dose being excreted. The mean values of cumulative urinary excretion for diatrizoate sodium expressed as percentage of administered dose are 38 percent at 60 minutes, 45 percent of 3 hours, and 94 to 100 percent at 24 hours.

Urinary excretion of contrast media is delayed in infants younger than 1 month and in patients with urinary tract obstruction. The urinary iodine concentration is higher with the sodium salt of diatrizoic acid than with the meglumine salt.

The liver and small intestine provide the major alternate route of excretion for diatrizoate. In patients free of severe renal disease, the fecal recovery is less than 2 percent of the administered dose. In patients with severe renal impairment the excretion of these contrast media through the gallbladder and into the small intestine sharply increases; up to 20 percent of the administered dose has been recovered in the feces in 48 hours.

Saliva is a minor secretory pathway for injectable radiopaque diagnostic agents. In patients with normal renal function, minimal amounts of contrast media are secreted unchanged. However, in uremic patients small amounts of free iodides resulting from deiodination prior to administration or in vivo, have been detected in the saliva.

Diatrizoate salts cross the placental barrier in humans by simple diffusion and appear to enter fetal tissue passively. No apparent harm to the fetus was observed when diatrizoate sodium and diatrizoate meglumine were injected intravenously 24 hours prior to delivery. However, abnormal neonatal opacification of the small intestine and colon were detected 4 to 6 days after delivery. Procedures including radiation involve a certain risk related to the exposure of the fetus.

Injectable radiopaque diagnostic agents are excreted unchanged in human milk.

Computerized Tomography. HYPAQUE-M, 75 percent can be administered as an intravenous bolus for brain tissue enhancement using computerized tomography. Increased tissue contrast differential for the scan is achieved either because of increased vascular (arterial, venous, or capillary bed) contrast or by blood brain barrier penetration of the medium (or its absence) in certain localized areas of disrupted vascular permeability. The degree of tissue enhancement caused by increased blood contrast is directly related to blood iodine content. However, the degree of enhancement due to extravascular accumulation of iodine resulting from blood brain barrier disruption will depend on the extent of disruption, the blood level of iodine, and the time delay prior to scanning. The nature of the pathology will determine whether an immediate or delayed scan is optimal.

Effects of Steroid Therapy. The anti-inflammatory and antiedema effects in patients receiving steroid therapy have interfered with the expected distribution of CT tissue enhancement on the scan in certain diseases.

Indications and Usage: HYPAQUE-M, brand of diatrizoate meglumine and diatrizoate sodium injection, 75 percent is indicated for angiocardiography, aortography, angiography, and urography.

Urography
Diatrizoate salts are used in small, medium, and large dose urography (see Dosage and Administration—**EXCRETORY UROGRAPHY**). Visualization of the urinary tract can be achieved by either direct intravenous bolus injection, intravenous drip infusion, or incidentally following intra-arterial procedures. Visualization of the urinary tract is delayed in infants less than 1 month old, and in patients with urinary tract obstruction (see CLINICAL PHARMACOLOGY).

Contrast Enhancement of Computed Tomographic Head Imaging
Injectable radiopaque contrast media may be used to refine diagnostic precision in areas of the brain which may not otherwise have been satisfactorily visualized.

Tumors. Radiopaque diagnostic agents may be useful to investigate the presence and extent of certain malignancies such as: gliomas including malignant gliomas, glioblastomas, astrocytomas, oligodendrogliomas and gangliomas, ependymomas, medulloblastomas, meningiomas, neuromas, pinealomas, pituitary adenomas, craniopharyngiomas, germinomas, and metastatic lesions.

The usefulness of contrast enhancement for the investigation of the retrobulbar space and in cases of low grade or infiltrative glioma has not been demonstrated.

In calcified lesions, there is less likelihood of enhancement. Following therapy, tumors may show decreased or no enhancement.

The opacification of the inferior vermis following contrast media administration has resulted in false-positive diagnosis in a number of normal studies.

Nonneoplastic Conditions. The use of injectable radiopaque diagnostic agents may be beneficial in the image enhancement of nonneoplastic lesions. Cerebral infarctions of recent onset may be better visualized with contrast enhancement, while some infarcations are obscured if contrast media are used. The use of iodinated contrast media results in contrast enhancement in about 60 percent of cerebral infarctions studied from one to four weeks from the onset of symptoms.

Sites of active infection may also be enhanced following contrast media administration.

Arteriovenous malformations and aneurysms will show contrast enhancement. For these vascular lesions, the enhancement is probably dependent on the iodine content of the circulating blood pool. Hematomas and intraparenchymal bleeders seldom demonstrate any contrast enhancement. However, in cases of intraparenchymal clot, for which there is no obvious clinical explanation, contrast media administration may be helpful in ruling out the possibility of associated arteriovenous malformation.

Angiography
Diatrizoate salts are used for radiographic studies throughout the cardiovascular system.

Intravascular radiopaque diagnostic agents of high concentration are not recommended for cerebral or spinal angiography (see CONTRAINDICATIONS—General), and contrast agents with the lowest compatible viscosity and higher concentration of iodine (310 mg/mL to 480 mg/mL of bound iodine) must be used for angiocardiography. Contrast media approaching serum ionic content and osmolarity have less potential for deleterious effects on the myocardium (see PRECAUTIONS—General, **Drug Interactions**).

Addition of chelating agents may contribute to toxicity in coronary angiography, and the sodium content of angiographic agents used in coronary arteriography is of crucial importance.

In addition to the following general CONTRAINDICATIONS, WARNINGS, PRECAUTIONS, and ADVERSE REACTIONS, there are additional listings in these categories under the particular procedures.

Contraindications—General: HYPAQUE-M, 75 percent has no absolute contraindications in its recommended uses (see general WARNINGS and PRECAUTIONS).

Do not use HYPAQUE-M, 75 percent for myelography or for examination of dorsal cysts or sinuses which might communicate with the subarachnoid space. Even a small amount in the subarachnoid space may produce convulsions and result in fatality. (See also **ABDOMINAL AORTOGRAPHY,** Warnings.) Epidural injection is also contraindicated.

HYPAQUE-M, 75 percent should not be injected directly into the carotid, vertebral, or spinal arteries.

HYPAQUE-M, brand of diatrizoate meglumine and diatrizoate sodium injection, 75 percent is contraindicated in patients with a hypersensitivity to salts of diatrizoic acid. Urography is contraindicated in patients with anuria.

Warnings—General: Excretory urography is potentially hazardous in patients with multiple myeloma. In some of those patients, therapeutically resistant anuria resulting in progressive uremia, renal failure, and eventually death has followed this procedure. Although neither the contrast agent nor dehydration has been proved separately to be the cause of anuria in myelomatous patients, it has been speculated that the combination of both may be causative. The risk of excretory urography in myelomatous patients is not a contraindication to the procedure; however, they require special precautions. Partial dehydration in the preparation of these patients for the examination is not recommended since this may predispose to the precipitation of myeloma protein in the renal tubules. Myeloma, which occurs most com-

Continued on next page

This product information was effective as of December 3, 1984. On these and other products of Winthrop-Breon Laboratories, detailed information may be obtained on a current basis by direct inquiry to the Professional Services Department, 90 Park Avenue, New York, NY 10016 (212) 907-2525.

Winthrop-Breon—Cont.

monly in persons over age 40, should be considered before instituting urographic procedures.

Contrast media may promote sickling in individuals who are homozygous for sickel cell disease when the material is injected intravenously or intra-arterially.

Administration of radiopaque materials to patients known or suscepted of having pheochromocytoma should be performed with extreme caution. If, in the opinion of the physician, the possible benefits of such procedures outweigh the considered risks, the procedures may be performed; however, the amount of radiopaque medium injected should be kept to an absolute minimum. The blood pressure should be assessed throughout the procedure and measures for treatment of a hypertensive crisis should be available.

Recent reports of thyroid storm occurring following the intravascular use of iodinated radiopaque diagnostic agents in patients with hyperthyroidism or with an autonomously functioning thyroid nodule suggest that this additional risk be evaluated in such patients before use of diatrizoate salts.

Contrast media administered for cardiac catheterization and angiocardiography may cause cellular injury to circulating lymphocytes. Chromosomal damage in humans includes inhibition of mitosis, increases in the number of micronuclei, and chromosome aberrations. The damages appear to be related to the contrast medium itself rather than to the x-ray radiation. It is to be noted that those agents have not been adequately tested in animal or laboratory systems.

Urography should be performed with caution in patients with severely impaired renal function and patients with combined renal and hepatic disease.

Selective spinal arteriography or arteriography of trunks providing spinal branches can cause mild to severe muscle spasm. However, serious neurologic sequelae, including permanent paralysis, could occur with even small doses of the 75 percent concentration. (See also ANGIOGRAPHY, Precaution.)

Precautions—General: Diagnostic procedures which involve the use of radiopaque diagnostic agents should be carried out under the direction of personnel with the prerequisite training and with a thorough knowledge of the particular procedure to be performed. Appropriate facilities should be available for coping with any complication of the procedure, as well as for emergency treatment of severe reactions to the contrast agent itself. After parenteral administration of a radiopaque agent, competent personnel and emergency facilities should be available for at last 30 to 60 minutes since severe delayed reactions have occurred (see ADVERSE REACTIONS—General).

The possibility of an idiosyncratic reaction in susceptible patients should always be considered (see ADVERSE REACTIONS—General). The susceptible population includes patients with a history of a previous reaction to a contrast media, patients with a known sensitivity to iodine per se, and patients with a known clinical hypersensitivy: bronchial asthma, hay fever, and food allergies.

The occurrence of severe idiosyncratic reactions has prompted the use of several pretesting methods. However, pretesting cannot be relied upon to predict severe reactions and may itself be hazardous for the patient. It is suggested that a thorough medical history with emphasis on allergy and hypersensitivity, prior to the injection of any contrast media, may be more accurate than pretesting in predicting potential adverse reactions.

A positive history of allergies or hypersensitivity does not arbitrarily contraindicate the use of a contrast agent, where a diagnostic procedure is thought essential, but caution should be exercised (see ADVERSE REACTIONS—General). Premedication with antihistamines or corticosteroids to avoid or minimize possible allergic reactions in such patients should be considered. Recent reports indicate that such pretreatment does not prevent serious life-threatening reactions, but may reduce both their incidence and severity.

Preparatory dehydration for angiography and CT procedures is unnecessary and may be dangerous, contributing to acute renal failure in infants, young children, the elderly, patients with preexisting renal insufficiency, patients with advanced vascular disease, and diabetic patients. Dehydration in these patients seems to be enhanced by the osmotic diuretic action of urographic agents. Overnight fluid restriction for urography may be undesirable and is considered unnecessary when using this relatively high (75%) concentration.

Although azotemia is not a contraindication, the medium should be used with great care in patients with advanced renal destruction associated with severe uremia. (See also **EXCRETORY UROGRAPHY**, Precautions.)

Acute renal failure has been reported in diabetic patients with diabetic nephropathy and in susceptible nondiabetic patients (often elderly with preexisting renal disease) following excretory urography. Therefore, careful consideration of the potential risks should be given before performing this radiographic procedure in these patients. (See also **EXCRETORY UROGRAPHY**, Precautions—*Preparatory Dehydration.*)

Immediately following surgery, excretory urography should be used with caution in renal transplant recipients.

Due to the transitory increase in the circulatory osmotic load, injections of urographic agents should be used with caution in patients with congestive heart failure. Such patients should be observed for several hours following the procedure to detect delayed hemodynamic disturbances.

General anesthesia may be indicated in the performance of some procedures, in young or uncooperative children and in selected adult patients; however, a high incidence of adverse reactions has been reported in these patients, and may be attributable to the inability of the patient to identify untoward symptoms, or to the hypotensive effect of anesthesia which can reduce cardiac output and increase the duration of exposure to the contrast agent.

In addition to the general precautions already described, excretory urography, angiography, and other uses also have hazards associated with the particular techniques employed. (See INDIVIDUAL INDICATIONS AND USAGE section.)

Information for Patients

Patients receiving injectable radiopaque diagnostic agents should be instructed to:

1. Inform the physician if they are pregnant (see CLINICAL PHARMACOLOGY).
2. Inform the physician if they are diabetic or if they have multiple myeloma, pheochromocytoma, homozygous sickle cell disease or known thyroid disorder (see WARNINGS—General).
3. Inform the physician if they are allergic to any drugs, food, or if they have had any reactions to previous injections of dyes used for x-ray procedures (see PRECAUTIONS—General).
4. Inform the physician about any other medications they are currently taking, including nonprescription drugs, before they are administered this drug.

Drug Interactions

Renal toxicity has been reported in a few patients with liver dysfunction who were given oral cholecystographic agents followed by urographic agents. Administration of intravascular urographic agents should therefore be postponed in any patient with a known or suspected hepatic or biliary disorder who has recently received a cholecystographic contrast agent.

Addition of an inotropic agent to contrast agents may produce a paradoxical depressant response which can be deleterious to the ischemic myocardium.

Benadryl®, brand of diphenhydramine hydrochloride, may cause precipitation when mixed in the same syringe with HYPAQUE-M, 75 percent.

Drug/Laboratory Test Interactions

If any of these studies, which might be affected by contrast media are indicated, it is recommended that they be performed prior to administration of the contrast medium or two or more days afterwards.

Diatrizoate salts interfere with several laboratory urine and blood tests.

Blood Tests

Coagulation: Diatrizoate salts significantly inhibit all stages of coagulation. The fibrinogen concentration, Factors V, VII, and VIII are decreased. Prothrombin time and thromboplastin time are increased.

Platelet aggregation: High levels of plasma and diatrizoates inhibit platelet aggregation.

Serum calcium: Diatrizoate salts may decrease serum calcium levels. However, this depletion of serum calcium may also be the result of the addition of chelating agents (edetate disodium) in the preparation of certain contrast media.

Red cell counts: Transitory decreases in red cell counts. Technetium-99m— RBC labeling interference.

Leukocyte counts: Decrease.

Urea nitrogen (BUN): Transitory increase (see CLINICAL PHARMACOLOGY).

Serum creatinine: Transitory increase.

Urine Tests

Contrast media which are excreted in the urine, may interfere with some laboratory determinations eg, proteinuria, specific gravity, osmolarity, or bacterial cultures.

Thyroid Function Tests

Protein-bound iodine (PBI) and total serum organic iodine: Transient increase of both tests following urography have been noticed. The results of PBI and radioactive iodine uptake studies which depend on iodine estimations will not accurately reflect thyroid function for up to 16 days following administration of iodinated urographic media. However, thyroid function tests not depending on iodine estimations, eg , T_3 resin uptake or free thyroxine assays are not affected.

Carcinogenesis, Mutagenesis, Impairment of Fertility

Long-term studies in animals have not been performed in order to evaluate carcinogenic potential, mutagenesis, or whether HYPAQUE-M, 75 percent can affect fertility in males or females.

Pregnancy Category C

Animal reproduction studies have not been conducted with HYPAQUE-M, 75 percent. It is also not known whether HYPAQUE-M, 75 percent can cause fetal harm when administered to a pregnant woman or can affect reproduction capacity. HYPAQUE-M, brand of diatrizoate meglumine and diatrizoate sodium injection, 75 percent should be given to a pregnant woman only if clearly needed.

Labor and Delivery

It is not known whether use of these contrast agents during labor or delivery has immediate or delayed adverse effects on the fetus, prolongs the duration of labor or increases the likelihood that forceps delivery of other obstetrical intervention or resuscitation of the newborn will be necessary.

Nursing Mothers

Diatrizoate salts are excreted unchanged in human milk. Because of the potential adverse reactions, although it has not been established that serious adverse reactions occur in nursing infants, caution should be exercised when these contrast media are administered to a nursing woman.

Pediatric Use

Infants and small children should not have any fluid restriction prior to excretory urography or any other procedures (see PRECAUTIONS—General). Guidelines for pediatric dosages are presented in DOSAGE AND ADMINISTRATION—General.

Adverse Reactions—General: Approximately 95 percent of adverse reactions accompanying the intravascular use of diatrizoate salts are of mild to moderate severity. However, life-threatening reactions and fatalities, mostly of cardiovascular origin, have occurred.

Adverse reactions to injectable contrast media fall into two categories: chemotoxic reactions and idiosyncratic reactions.

Chemotoxic reactions result from the physicochemical properties of the contrast media, the dose, and the speed of injection. All hemodynamic disturbances and injuries to organs or vessels perfused by the contrast medium are included in this category.

Idiosyncratic reactions include all other reactions. They occur more frequently in patients 20 to 40 years old. Idiosyncratic reactions may or may not be dependent on the amount of dose injected, the speed of injection, the mode of injection, and the radiographic procedure. Idiosyncratic reactions are subdivided into minor, intermediate, and severe. The minor reactions are self-limited and of short duration; the severe reactions are life-threatening and treatment is urgent and mandatory.

The reported incidence of adverse reactions to contrast media in patients with a history of allergy are twice that of the general population. Patients with a history of previous reactions to a contrast medium are three times more susceptible than other patients. However, sensitivity to contrast media does not appear to increase with repeated examinations.

Most adverse reactions to injectable contrast media appear within one to three minutes after the start of injection, but delayed reactions may occur. Adverse reactions are grouped by organ system and listed below by decreasing order of occurrence and with an approximate incidence of occurrence. Significantly more severe reactions are listed before the other reactions regardless of frequency.

Greater Than 1 in 100 Patients
Body as a Whole: Reported incidences of death range from 6.6 per 1 million (0.00066 percent) to 1 in 10,000 patients (0.01 percent). Most deaths occur during injection or 5 to 10 minutes later, the main feature being cardiac arrest with cardiovascular disease as the main aggravating factor.
Isolated reports of hypotensive collapse and shock following urography are found in the literature. The incidence of shock is estimated to occur in 1 out of 20,000 (0.005 percent) patients.
Cardiovascular System: The most frequent adverse reaction to diatrizoate salts is vasodilation (feeling of warmth). The estimated incidence is 49 percent.
Digestive System: Nausea 6 percent, vomiting 3 percent.
Nervous System: Paresthesia 6 percent, dizziness 5 percent.
Respiratory System: Rhinitis 1 percent, increased cough 2 percent.
Skin and Appendages: Urticaria 1 percent.
Pain at the injection site is estimated to occur in about 12 percent of the patients undergoing urography. Pain is usually due to extravasation.
Painful hot erythematous swelling above the veinipuncture site was estimated to occur in more than one percent of the patients undergoing phlebography.
Special Senses: Perversion of taste 11 percent.
Urogenital System: Osmotic nephrosis of the proximal tubular cells is estimated to occur in 23 percent of patients following excretory urography.

Less Than 1 in 100 Patients
Other infrequently reported reactions without accompanying incidence rates are listed below, grouped by organ system.
Body as a Whole: Malaria relapse, uremia, high creatinine and BUN (see PRECAUTIONS—General, **Drug/Laboratory Test Interactions**), thrombocytopenia, leukopenia, and anemia.
Cardiovascular System: Cerebral hematomas, hemodynamic disturbances, sinus bradycardia, transient electrocardiographic abnormalities, ventricular fibrillation, and petechiae.
Digestive System: Severe unilateral or bilateral swelling of the parotid and submaxillary glands.
Nervous System: Convulsions, paralysis, and coma.
Respiratory System: Asthma, dyspnea, laryngeal edema, pulmonary edema, and bronchospasm.
Skin and Appendages: Skin necrosis.
Special Senses: Bilateral ocular irritation, lacrimation, itching, conjunctival chemosis, infection, and conjunctivitis.
Urogenital: Renal failure, pain.
Overdosage: At dosage levels of diatrizoate sodium above a level containing 45 g of iodine, the incidence of unpleasant side effects increases. At total dosage equivalent to 80 gI or 90 gI administered over a short period of time (eg, 30 minutes), clinical signs of systemic intolerance appear (mostly related to hyperosmolar effects) and are manifest as tremors, irritability, and tachycardia. Above these maximal tolerated dosage levels in otherwise healthy adults, an increasing incidence and severity of dyspnea and pulmonary edema should be expected.

Four cases of overdosage in infants, during urography, are reported. Three of the infants died within 19 hours of the injection. The overdose ranged from slightly above the recommended pediatric dosage to a dose exceeding 19 g/kg. The symptoms of overdosage appeared between 10 minutes to several hours after injection of the contrast medium. Adverse effects were life-threatening, affecting mainly the pulmonary and cardiovascular systems. The symptoms included: cyanosis, bradycardia, acidosis, pulmonary hemorrhage, convulsions, coma, and cardiac arrest. All infants showed a poor visualization of the kidneys and a diffuse opacification of all the tissues and vasculature. Autopsy findings showed acute pulmonary damage and/or edema of subcutaneous tissues. Treatment of an overdose of injectable radiopaque contrast media is directed toward the support of all vital functions, and prompt institution of symptomatic therapy.

The acute intravenous LD_{50} of diatrizoate salts in mice is equivalent in iodine content of 5.3 gI/kg to 8.0 gI/kg and seem to be directly proportional to the rate of injection.

Diatrizoate salts are dialyzable.

Dosage and Administration—General: Preparation of the patient will vary with preference of the radiologist and the type of radiological procedure performed. Specific radiographic procedures used will depend on the state of the patient and the diagnostic indications. Individual dose should be tailored according to age, body size, and indication for examination. (See INDIVIDUAL INDICATIONS AND USAGE section for specific Dosage and Administration.)

Solutions of radiopaque diagnostic agents for intravascular use should be at body temperature when injected and may need to be warmed before use. In the event that crystallization occurs, the solution may be clarified by placing the vial in a water bath at 40° C to 50°C and shaking it gently for two to three minutes or until the solids redissolve. If the particles still persist, do not use this vial but discard it. The solution should be protected from light and any unused portion remaining in the container should be discarded.

Dilution and withdrawal of the contrast agents should be accomplished under aseptic conditions with sterile syringes.

Parenteral drug products should be inspected visually for particulate matter and discoloration prior to administration. Avoid contaminating catheters, syringes, needles, and contrast media with glove powder or cotton fibers.

Pediatric Dosage
Pediatric doses of injectable radiopaque diagnostic agents are generally determined on a weight basis and should be calculated for each patient individually. (See INDIVIDUAL INDICATIONS AND USAGE section.)

Drug Incompatibilities
Diatrizoate salts are incompatible in vitro with some antihistamines and many other drugs. It is believed that one of the chief causes of in vitro incompatibility is an alteration of pH. Turbidity of solutions of intravascular contrast medium occurs between pH 2.5 and 4.1. Another cause is chemical interaction; therefore, other pharmaceuticals should not be mixed with contrast agents in the same syringe.

Individual Indications and Usage
THE FOLLOWING SECTIONS FOR INDIVIDUAL INDICATIONS AND USAGE CONTAIN CONTRAINDICATIONS, WARNINGS, PRECAUTIONS, ADVERSE REACTIONS, AND DOSAGE AND ADMINISTRATION SECTIONS RELATED TO THE SPECIFIC PROCEDURES, HOWEVER, IT SHOULD BE UNDERSTOOD THAT THE INFORMATION IN THE GENERAL SECTIONS IS ALSO LIKELY TO APPLY TO ALL OF THESE SPECIFIC USES.

Hydration—With the possible exception of urography, patients should be fully hydrated prior to the following procedures.

Angiocardiography
Pharmacology—Hemodynamic Changes
Due to its physical characteristics (chiefly tonicity and viscosity) and the volume administered, HYPAQUE-M, 75 percent may cause a number of transitory hemodynamic changes. When the medium is ejected from the left ventricle or introduced at the root of the ascending aorta, a brief (three seconds) hypertensive response is usually induced, followed immediately by a decrease in aortic and peripheral blood pressures below normal levels, lasting for at least two minutes. This hypotensive phase may be followed by a 15-to 20-minute period of fluctuating blood pressure.

Clinical doses (up to 1 mL per kg) injected into the vena cava or right heart outflow tract usually cause an irregular rise in right ventricular blood pressure, a slight increase in pulmonary artery blood pressure, and delayed signs of peripheral hypotension.

Other changes reported clinically include an increase in cardiac output and atrial pressure, a decrease in myocardial contractile force, and at the peak of postinjection hypotension, a marked rise in aortic and carotid blood flow, and elevation of central venous pressure. At dosage levels used in angiocardiography, the hematocrit and hemoglobin level may fall about 10 to 15 percent and serum osmolality may rise 10 to 12 percent. Blood carbon dioxide, pH, and BUN levels may fall. These changes commence immediately after injection, reach a maximum in two to five minutes, and return to normal values in 10 to 15 minutes. However, after the initial rise, plasma volume may decrease and continue to fall below control levels, even beyond 30 minutes, probably due to diuresis. If repeat injections are made in rapid succession, these changes are likely to be more pronounced. (See Dosage and Administration.) HYPAQUE-M, brand of diatrizoate meglumine and diatrizoate sodium injection, 75 percent is not metabolized. It is eliminated unchanged, rapidly and completely, in the urine by glomerular filtration.

Precautions
During administration of large doses of HYPAQUE-M, 75 percent, continuous monitoring of vital signs is desirable. Caution is advised in the administration of large doses to patients with incipient heart failure because of the possibility of aggravation of the preexisting condition. Hypotension should be corrected promptly since it may induce serious arrhythmias.

Because of the hemodynamic changes which may occur on injection into the right heart outflow tract, special care, especially regarding dosage, should be observed in patients with right ventricular failure, pulmonary hypertension, or obliterated pulmonary vascular beds.

Precautions in Infants
Apnea, bradycardia and other arrhythmias, cerebral effects (lethargy and depression), and a tendency to acidosis are more likely to occur in cyanotic infants. It is desirable that vital signs be monitored on an intensive care basis afterwards to detect delayed adverse effects (arrhythmia, electrolyte and hemodynamic disturbances). Infants are more likely than adults to respond with convulsions, particularly after repeated injections. Unlike in the adult, the amount of the total dosage in young infants is of particular importance. (See Dosage and Administration.)

Continued on next page

This product information was effective as of December 3, 1984. On these and other products of Winthrop-Breon Laboratories, detailed information may be obtained on a current basis by direct inquiry to the Professional Services Department, 90 Park Avenue, New York, NY 10016 (212) 907-2525.

Winthrop-Breon—Cont.

Adverse Reactions
See Adverse Reactions, General.
Dosage and Administration
The individual dose is determined by the size of the structure to be visualized, the anticipated degree of hemodilution, and valvular competence. Weight is a minor consideration in adults. The size of each individual dose is a more important consideration than the total dosage used. When large individual doses are administered, as for contrast in the cardiac chambers and thoracic aorta, it has been suggested that 20 minutes be permitted to elapse between each injection to allow for subsidence of hemodynamic disturbances.
Adult Dosage: Adult dose of HYPAQUE-M, 75 percent is usually 35 mL to 50 mL into either left or right chamber, outflow tracts, or aorta. The individual dose for intravenous angiocardiography ranges from 70 mL to 100 mL often injected simultaneously bilaterally by pressure injection, half of the dose into each antecubital vein.
Pediatric Dosage: The usual dose is 0.5 mL to 1 mL per kg for a subject with heart of normal size and intact valves and septum. For patients with stenotic lesions, 0.5 mL per kg is recommended. Doses up to 1.5 mL per kg may be required in cardiomegaly, large volume shunts, or where right cardiac injection is also intended to opacify left chambers.
Young Infant Dosage: The individual dose is similar to that described under Pediatric Dosage. It has been suggested, however, that the total dosage administered should be maintained below 3 mL per kg in infants under two months of age in any one procedure.
Arteriography
Coronary Arteriography
Coronary arteriography should only be used in carefully selected patients when the value of the anticipated information outweighs the risk involved.
Contraindication
Routine coronary arteriography should be deferred for four weeks in patients with clinically apparent myocardial infarction.
Precaution
Continuous EKG monitoring for early detection of arrhythmias is desirable.
Adverse Reactions
Transitory EKG changes occur almost inevitably with good filling. Transient arrhythmia may occur. (See ADVERSE REACTIONS—General.) Serum enzymes may be elevated for 24 hours.
Dosage and Administration
The usual dose for adults is 50 mL of HYPAQUE-M, 75 percent delivered into the **root of the aorta** for simultaneous bilateral angiograms. For injection at the **sinus of Valsalva,** the usual dose is 15 mL to 25 mL on either side. For **selective coronary procedures,** as by the Sones technique, the individual dose recommended is 3 mL to 5 mL into either artery. This dose may be injected alternately into the right and left coronary artery, and repeated.
Abdominal Aortography
HYPAQUE-M, brand of diatrizoate meglumine and diatrizoate sodium injection, 75 percent solution may be injected by commonly accepted techniques, such as translumbar, retrograde catheter, retrograde pressure injection (by cannula) or by antegrade (brachial) catheter for examination of the aorta and its major branches.
Warnings
During aortography by the translumbar technique, extreme care is advised to avoid inadvertent intrathecal injection since the injection of even small amounts (5 mL to 7 mL) of the contrast medium may cause convulsions, permanent sequelae, or fatality. Should the accident occur, the patient should be placed upright to confine the hyperbaric solution to a low level, anesthesia may be required to control convulsions, and if there is evidence of a large dose having been administered, a careful cerebrospinal fluid exchange-washout should be considered.

Pheochromocytoma: Administration of angiographic media to patients known or suspected to have pheochromocytoma can cause dangerous changes in blood pressure. A minimum dose should be injected. The blood pressure should be carefully monitored and measures for controlling major fluctuations should be available.
Precautions
The presence of a vigorous pulsatile flow should be established before using a catheter or pressure injection technique. A small "pilot" dose (about 2 mL) should be administered to locate the exact site of needle or catheter tip to help prevent injection of the main dose into a branch of the aorta or intramurally. In the translumbar technique, severe pain during injection may indicate intramural placement and abdominal or back pain afterwards may indicate hemorrhage from the injection site. Following catheter procedures, gentle pressure hemostasis for 5 to 10 minutes is advised, followed by observation for 30 to 60 minutes and immobilization of the limb for several hours to prevent hemorrhage from the site of arterial puncture.
Under conditions of slowed aortic circulation there is an increased likelihood of aortography causing muscle spasm. Occasional serious neurologic complications, including paraplegia, have also been reported in patients with aortic-iliac or even femoral artery bed obstruction, abdominal compression, hypotension, hypertension, spinal anesthesia, injection of vasopressors to increase contrast, and low injection sites (L2-3). In these patients the concentration, dose, and number of repeat injections of the medium should be maintained at a minimum with appropriate intervals between injections. The position of the patient and catheter tip should be carefully evaluated.
Adverse Reactions
The only adverse reaction expected is a mild burning sensation on injection. Unusual reactions can occur, as in angiocardiography. An abrupt hypertensive episode can occur following entry of the medium into the renal artery in patients with pheochromocytoma. Mesenteric necrosis, acute pancreatitis, and renal shutdown (usually transitory) and neurologic complications have been reported following inadvertent injection of a large part of the aortic dose into a branch of the aorta. Entry of the large aortic dose into the renal artery can cause, even in the absence of symptoms, albuminuria, cylindruria, and hematuria, and an elevated BUN. Rapid and complete return of function usually follows.
Dosage and Administration
The average adult dose range of HYPAQUE-M, 75 percent is 10 mL to 15 mL by translumbar technique and by retrograde catheter, 15 mL to 25 mL. In infants and children and thin adults, the use of a less concentrated medium for aortography, such as diatrizoate sodium 50 percent, is advised in doses of 0.5 mL per kg. For retrograde pressure injection (cannula) the usual adult dose is 35 mL to 40 mL of HYPAQUE-M, 75 percent solution.
Renal Arteriography
Renal arteriography by aortography or by selective catheterization of the renal artery may be used to establish renal vascular status in the diagnosis of renal and immediate extrarenal pathology.
Precaution
In the selective renal procedure, inadvertent entry into a lumbar artery can be avoided by using a test dose.
Adverse Reactions
Transitory increase in resistance of the renovascular bed can occur with a slight disturbance in function. Renal damage is rare even in azotemic patients. Inadvertent entry of a large dose (as in aortography) into the renal artery can cause, even in the absence of symptoms, albuminuria, cylindruria, and hematuria, and an elevated BUN. Rapid and complete return of function usually follows.
Dosage and Administration
By aortography, 10 mL to 25 mL. By selected renal arteriography, 5 mL to 8 mL. The dose may be repeated as indicated.

Peripheral Arteriography
The use of HYPAQUE-M, brand of diatrizoate meglumine and diatrizoate sodium injection, 75 percent is sometimes preferred over less concentrated media in selected cases for femoral and brachio-axillary arteriography in adults.
Precautions
Pulsation should be present in the artery to be injected. In thromboangiitis obliterans, or ascending infection associated with severe ischemia, angiography should be performed with extreme caution, if at all.
Adverse Reactions
Pain or a burning sensation with some spasm may occur, and is more marked in patients with arterial insufficiency. Therefore, the procedure is more satisfactorily performed under general or, for the lower extremity, spinal anesthesia.
Arterial thrombosis, displacement of arterial plaques, and ipsilateral venous thrombosis are very rare complications.
Dosage and Administration
The usual dose of HYPAQUE-M, 75 percent is 10 mL to 25 mL, which may be repeated. Appropriate dosage in infants and children of a less concentrated medium, such as diatrizoate sodium 50 percent, will usually provide adequate contrast.
Urography
Nephrotomography and "Adequate" or High Dose Urography
HYPAQUE-M, 75 percent solution may be used for excretory urography in selected patients. It may be used when prior urography has failed to provide diagnostic contrast and for preliminary excretory tract study to detect obstruction in azotemic patients or to avoid retrograde instrumentation. It may also be used as a high dosage medium to intensify and prolong the nephrographic effect when the prime purpose is examination of the renal parenchyma, especially with tomography. When combined with a urea "washout" technique, HYPAQUE-M, 75 percent provides the necessary increased pyelographic contrast and diuresis required for screening or special examination of patients with suspected renal hypertension.
Contraindication
Urography is contraindicated in patients with anuria.
Precautions
Although azotemia is not considered a contraindication, care is required in patients with advanced renal failure. The usual preparatory dehydration should be omitted, and urinary output should be observed for one to two days in these patients.
When HYPAQUE-M, 75 percent is used with a urea "washout" procedure, the patient should also be observed for a few hours to detect signs of undue dehydration caused by increased diuresis induced by both the medium and the urea. Ingestion of water may be required for rehydration.
In myelomatosis, urography should only be performed with caution. If a weak protein-binding agent such as a diatrizoate is used for the procedure, it is essential to omit preparatory dehydration, administer fluids, and attempt to alkalinize the urine.
Preparatory Dehydration: Preparatory dehydration is dangerous in infants, young children, the elderly, and azotemic patients (especially those with polyuria, oliguria, diabetes, advanced vascular disease, or preexisting dehydration). The undesirable dehydration in these patients may be accentuated by the osmotic diuretic action of the medium.
Adverse Reactions
Side effects following this relatively high dose urography are usually mild and transitory and do not appear to occur more frequently or severely than those induced by "standard dose" urography. Nausea, facial flushing, and emesis are not uncommon reactions. (See ADVERSE REACTIONS—General.)
Dosage and Administration
In adults, the single dose of HYPAQUE-M, 75 percent is usually 50 mL. The dose in infants and children is 0.5 mL to 1 mL/kg (not to exceed 50 mL). It is injected rapidly intravenously.
How Supplied: Vials of 20 mL, rubber stoppered, box of 25 (NDC 0024-0785-04)

Vials of 50 mL, rubber stoppered, box of 25 (NDC 0024-0786-04)

HW-51-R

HYPAQUE®-76 ℞
brand of diatrizoate meglumine and diatrizoate sodium injection, USP
Sterile Aqueous Injection

For Excretory Urography, Aortography, Angiocardiography, (Ventriculography, Pulmonary Angiography, Selective Coronary Arteriography), Peripheral Angiography (Peripheral Arteriography and Peripheral Venography), Intravenous Digital Arteriography, Contrast Enhancement of Computed Tomographic Head Imaging, Contrast Enhancement of Computed Tomographic Body Imaging, Selective Renal Arteriography, Selective Visceral Arteriography, Central Venography, Renal Venography

Description: HYPAQUE-76, brand of diatrizoate meglumine and diatrizoate sodium, is a water-soluble, radiopaque diagnostic medium. It is supplied as a 76 percent sterile aqueous solution providing 66 percent (w/v) diatrizoate meglumine and 10 percent (w/v) diatrizoate sodium. It is a triiodinated benzoic acid derivative containing 37 percent (w/v) organically bound iodine. Each mL contains 370 mg iodine and 3.68 mg (0.16 mEq) sodium. It is constituted as a radiopaque iodinated anion, diatrizoate and the radiolucent cations, meglumine and sodium. It is the organically bound iodine of the anion which opacifies internal structures for x-ray visualization and fluoroscopy.

The solution is hypertonic and has a viscosity of approximately 9 cp at 37°C. The pH is adjusted between 7.0 and 7.6 with Na_2CO_3 and HCl or NaOH. The pKa is 3.4 for diatrizoic acid. Edetate calcium disodium 0.01 percent has been added as a sequestering stabilizing agent. The solution is clear and colorless to pale straw color. The solution may be autoclaved once. Discard any unused portion remaining in the container. The solution should be stored at room temperature and protected from strong light. Crystals may form in the solution on cooling; they are readily redissolved on warming; the solution, however, should be administered at body temperature.

Diatrizoate meglumine is 1-deoxy-1- (methylamino)-D-glucitol 3,5-diacetamido 2,4,6-triiodobenzoate (salt).

Diatrizoate sodium is monosodium 3,5-diacetamido-2,4,6-triiodobenzoate.

Clinical Pharmacology: Intravascular injection of a radiopaque diagnostic agent opacifies those vessels in the path of the flow of the contrast medium, permitting radiographic visualization of the internal structures of the human body until significant hemodilution occurs.

At physiologic pH, the water-soluble contrast media are completely dissociated into a radiopaque anion and a solubilizing cation. While circulating in tissue fluids, the compound remains ionized. However, it is not metabolized but excreted unchanged in the urine, each diatrizoate molecule remaining "obligated" to its sodium or meglumine moiety.

Following intravenous injection, the radiopaque diagnostic agents are immediately diluted in the circulating plasma. Equilibrium is reached with the extracellular compartment at about 10 minutes. Hence, the plasma concentration at 10 minutes is closely related to the dose corrected to body size.

The pharmacokinetics of the intravenously administered radiopaque contrast media are usually best described by a two compartment model with a rapid alpha phase for drug distribution and a slow beta phase for drug elimination. In patients with normal renal function, the alpha and beta half-lives were respectively 30 minutes and 120 minutes for diatrizoate. But in patients with renal and kidney functional impairment, the elimination half-life for the beta phase can be prolonged up to several days.

Injectable radiopaque diagnostic agents are excreted either through the liver or through the kidneys. These two excretory pathways are not mutually exclusive, but the main route of excretion seems to be governed by the affinity of the contrast medium for serum albumin. From 0% to 10% of diatrizoate sodium is bound to serum protein.

Diatrizoate salts are excreted unchanged predominantly through the kidneys by glomerular filtration. The amount excreted by the kidney during any period of time is determined by the filtered load; ie, the product of plasma contrast media concentration and glomerular filtration rate. The plasma concentration is dependent upon the dose administered and the body size. The glomerular filtration rate varies with the body size, sex, age, circulatory dynamics, diuretic effect of the drug, and renal function. In patients with normal renal function the maximum urinary concentration of diatrizoate meglumine occurs within 10 minutes with 12 percent of the administered dose being excreted. The mean values of cumulative urinary excretion for diatrizoate sodium expressed as percentage of administered dose are 38 percent at 60 minutes, 45 percent at 3 hours, and 94 to 100 percent at 24 hours.

Urinary excretion of contrast media is delayed in infants younger than 1 month and in patients with urinary tract obstruction. The urinary iodine concentration is higher with the sodium salt of diatrizoic acid than with the meglumine salt.

The liver and small intestine provide the major alternate route of excretion for diatrizoate. In patients free of severe renal disease, the fecal recovery is less than 2 percent of the administered dose. In patients with severe renal impairment the excretion of these contrast media through the gallbladder and into the small intestine sharply increases; up to 20 percent of the administered dose has been recovered in the feces in 48 hours.

Saliva is a minor secretory pathway for injectable radiopaque diagnostic agents. In patients with normal renal function, minimal amounts of contrast media are secreted unchanged. However, in uremic patients small amounts of free iodides resulting from deiodination prior to administration or in vivo, have been detected in the saliva.

Diatrizoate salts cross the placental barrier in humans by simple diffusion and appears to enter fetal tissue passively. No apparent harm to the fetus was observed when diatrizoate sodium and diatrizoate meglumine were injected intravenously 24 hours prior to delivery. However, abnormal neonatal opacification of the small intestine and colon were detected 4 to 6 days after delivery. Procedures including radiation involve a certain risk related to the exposure of the fetus.

Injectable radiopaque diagnostic agents are excreted unchanged in human milk.

Computerized Tomography. HYPAQUE-76 can be administered as an intravenous bolus for brain tissue enhancement using computerized tomography. Increased tissue contrast differential for the scan is achieved either because of increased vascular (arterial, venous, or capillary bed) contrast or by blood brain barrier penetration of the medium (or its absence) in certain localized areas of disrupted vascular permeability. The degree of tissue enhancement caused by increased blood contrast is directly related to blood iodine content. However, the degree of enhancement due to extravascular accumulation of iodine resulting from blood brain barrier disruption will depend on the extent of disruption, the blood level of iodine, and the time delay prior to scanning. The nature of the pathology will determine whether an immediate or delayed scan is optimal.

Effects of Steroid Therapy. The anti-inflammatory and antiedema effects in patients receiving steroid therapy have interfered with the expected distribution of CT tissue enhancement on the scan in certain diseases.

Indications and Usage: HYPAQUE-76, brand of diatrizoate meglumine and diatrizoate sodium injection, is indicated for excretory urography, aortography, angiocardiography (ventriculography, pulmonary angiography, selective coronary arteriography), peripheral angiography (peripheral arteriography and peripheral venography), intravenous digital arteriography, contrast enhancement of computed tomographic head imaging, contrast enhancement of computed tomographic body imaging, selective renal arteriography, selective visceral arteriography, central venography, and renal venography.

Urography
Diatrizoate salts are used in small, medium, and large dose urography (see Dosage and Administration—**EXCRETORY UROGRAPHY**). Visualization of the urinary tract can be achieved by either direct intravenous bolus injection, intravenous drip infusion, or incidentally following intra-arterial procedures. Visualization of the urinary tract is delayed in infants less than 1 month old, and in patients with urinary tract obstruction (see CLINICAL PHARMACOLOGY).

Contrast Enhancement of Computed Tomographic Head Imaging
Injectable radiopaque contrast media may be used to refine diagnostic precision in areas of the brain which may not otherwise have been satisfactorily visualized.

Tumors. Radiopaque diagnostic agents may be useful to investigate the presence and extent of certain malignancies such as: gliomas including malignant gliomas, gliobastomas, astrocytomas, oligodendrogliomas and gangliomas, ependymomas, medulloblastomas, meningiomas, neuromas, pinealomas, pituitary adenomas, craniopharyngiomas, germinomas, and metastatic lesions.

The usefulness of contrast enhancement for the investigation of the retrobulbar space and in cases of low grade or infiltrative glioma has not been demonstrated.

In calcified lesions, there is less likelihood of enhancement. Following therapy, tumors may show decreased or no enhancement.

The opacification of the inferior vermis following contrast media administration has resulted in false positive diagnosis in a number of normal studies.

Nonneoplastic Conditions. The use of injectable radiopaque diagnostic agents may be beneficial in the image enhancement of nonneoplastic lesions. Cerebral infarctions of recent onset may be better visualized with contrast enhancement, while some infarctions are obscured if contrast media are used. The use of iodinated contrast media results in contrast enhancement in about 60 percent of cerebral infarctions studied from one to four weeks from the onset of symptoms.

Sites of active infection may also be enhanced following contrast media administration.

Arteriovenous malformations and aneurysms will show contrast enhancement. For these vascular lesions, the enhancement is probably dependent on the iodine content of the circulating blood pool. Hematomas and intraparenchymal bleeders seldom demonstrate any contrast enhancement. However, in cases of intraparenchymal clot, for which there is no obvious clinical explanation, contrast media administration may be helpful in ruling out the possibility of associated arteriovenous malformation.

Angiography
Diatrizoate salts are used for radiographic studies throughout the cardiovascular system.

Intravascular radiopaque diagnostic agents of high concentration are not recommended for cerebral or spinal angiography (see CONTRAINDICATIONS—General), and contrast agents with the lowest compatible viscosity and higher concentration of iodine (310 mg/mL to 480 mg/mL of bound

Continued on next page

This product information was effective as of December 3, 1984. On these and other products of Winthrop-Breon Laboratories, detailed information may be obtained on a current basis by direct inquiry to the Professional Services Department, 90 Park Avenue, New York, NY 10016 (212) 907-2525.

Winthrop-Breon—Cont.

iodine) must be used for angiocardiography. Contrast media approaching serum ionic content and osmolarity have less potential for deleterious effects on the myocardium (see PRECAUTIONS—General, **Drug Interactions**).
Addition of chelating agents may contribute to toxicity in coronary angiography, and the sodium content of angiographic agents used in coronary arteriography is of crucial importance.

In addition to the following general CONTRAINDICATIONS, WARNINGS, PRECAUTIONS, and ADVERSE REACTIONS, there are additional listings in these categories under the particular procedures.

Contraindications—General: HYPAQUE-76, brand of diatrizoate meglumine and diatrizoate sodium injection, has no absolute contraindications in its recommended uses (see general WARNINGS and PRECAUTIONS).
Do not use HYPAQUE-76 for myelography or for examination of dorsal cysts or sinuses which might communicate with the subarachnoid space. Even a small amount in the subarachnoid space may produce convulsions and result in fatality. (See also **AORTOGRAPHY**, Warnings.) Epidural injection is also contraindicated.
HYPAQUE-76 should not be injected directly into the carotid, vertebral, or spinal arteries.
HYPAQUE-76, brand of diatrizoate meglumine and diatrizoate sodium injection, is contraindicated in patients with a hypersensitivity to salts of diatrizoic acid.
Urography is contraindicated in patients with anuria.

Warnings—General: Excretory urography is potentially hazardous in patients with multiple myeloma. In some of those patients, therapeutically resistant anuria resulting in progressive uremia, renal failure, and eventually death has followed this procedure. Although neither the contrast agent nor dehydration has been proved separately to be the cause of anuria in myelomatous patients, it has been speculated that the combination of both may be causative. The risk of excretory urography in myelomatous patients is not a contraindication to the procedure; however, they require special precautions. Partial dehydration in the preparation of these patients for the examination is not recommended since this may predispose to the precipitation of myeloma protein in the renal tubules. Myeloma, which occurs most commonly in persons over age 40, should be considered before instituting urographic procedures.
Contrast media may promote sickling in individuals who are homozygous for sickle cell disease when the material is injected intravenously or intra-arterially.
Administration of radiopaque materials to patients known or suspected of having pheochromocytoma should be performed with extreme caution. If, in the opinion of the physician, the possible benefits of such procedures outweigh the considered risks, the procedures may be performed; however, the amount of radiopaque medium injected should be kept to an absolute minimum. The blood pressure should be assessed throughout the procedure and measures for treatment of a hypertensive crisis should be available.
Recent reports of thyroid storm occurring following the intravascular use of iodinated radiopaque diagnostic agents in patients with hyperthyroidism or with an autonomously functioning thyroid nodule suggest that this additional risk be evaluated in such patients before use of diatrizoate salts.
Contrast media administered for cardiac catheterization and angiocardiography may cause cellular injury to circulating lymphocytes. Chromosomal damage in humans includes inhibition of mitosis, increases in the number of micronuclei, and chromosome aberrations. The damages appear to be related to the contrast medium itself rather than to the x-ray radiation. It is to be noted that those agents have not been adequately tested in animal or laboratory systems.
Urography should be performed with caution in patients with severely impaired renal function and patients with combined renal and hepatic disease.
Selective spinal arteriography or arteriography of trunks providing spinal branches can cause mild to severe muscle spasm. However, serious neurologic sequelae, including permanent paralysis, could occur with even small doses of the 76 percent concentration.

Precautions—General: Diagnostic procedures which involve the use of radiopaque diagnostic agents should be carried out under the direction of personnel with the prerequisite training and with a thorough knowledge of the particular procedure to be performed. Appropriate facilities should be available for coping with any complication of the procedure, as well as for emergency treatment of severe reactions to the contrast agent itself. After parenteral administration of a radiopaque agent, competent personnel and emergency facilities should be available for at least 30 to 60 minutes since severe delayed reactions have occurred (see ADVERSE REACTIONS—General).
The possibility of an idiosyncratic reaction in susceptible patients should always be considered (see ADVERSE REACTIONS—General). The susceptible population includes patients with a history of a previous reaction to a contrast media, patients with a known sensitivity to iodine per se, and patients with a known clinical hypersensitivity: bronchial asthma, hay fever, and food allergies.
The occurrence of severe idiosyncratic reactions has prompted the use of several pretesting methods. However, pretesting cannot be relied upon to predict severe reactions and may itself be hazardous for the patient. It is suggested that a thorough medical history with emphasis on allergy and hypersensitivity, prior to the injection of any contrast media, may be more accurate than pretesting in predicting potential adverse reactions.
A positive history of allergies or hypersensitivity does not arbitrarily contraindicate the use of a contrast agent, where a diagnostic procedure is thought essential, but caution should be exercised (see ADVERSE REACTIONS—General). Premedication with antihistamines or corticosteroids to avoid or minimize possible allergic reactions in such patients should be considered. Recent reports indicate that such pretreatment does not prevent serious life-threatening reactions, but may reduce both their incidence and severity.
Preparatory dehydration for angiography and CT procedures is unnecessary and may be dangerous, contributing to acute renal failure in infants, young children, the elderly, patients with preexisting renal insufficiency, patients with advanced vascular disease, and diabetic patients. Dehydration in these patients seems to be enhanced by the osmotic diuretic action of urographic agents. Overnight fluid restriction for urography may be undesirable and is considered unnecessary when using this relatively high (76%) concentration.
Although azotemia is not a contraindication, the medium should be used with great care in patients with advanced renal destruction associated with severe uremia. (See also **EXCRETORY UROGRAHY**, Precautions.)
Acute renal failure has been reported in diabetic patients with diabetic nephropathy and in susceptible nondiabetic patients (often elderly with preexisting renal disease) following excretory urograhy. Therefore, careful consideration of the potential risks should be given before performing this radiographic procedure in these patients. (See also **EXCRETORY UROGRAPHY**, Precautions—*Preparatory Dehydration.*)
Immediately following surgery, excretory urography should be used with caution in renal transplant recipients.
Due to the transitory increase in the circulatory osmotic load, injections of urographic agents should be used with caution in patients with congestive heart failure. Such patients should be observed for several hours following the procedure to detect delayed hemodynamic disturbances.
General anesthesia may be indicated in the performance of some procedures, in young or uncooperative children and in selected adult patients; however, a higher incidence of adverse reactions has been reported in these patients, and may be attributable to the inability of the patient to identify untoward symptoms, or to the hypotensive effect of anesthesia which can reduce cardiac output and increase the duration of exposure to the contrast agent.
In addition to the general precautions already described, excretory urography, angiography, and other uses also have hazards associated with the particular techniques employed. (See INDIVIDUAL INDICATIONS AND USAGE section.)

Information for Patients
Patients receiving injectable radiopaque diagnostic agents should be instructed to:
1. Inform the physician if they are pregnant (see CLINICAL PHARMACOLOGY).
2. Inform the physician if they are diabetic or if they have multiple myeloma, pheochromocytoma, homozygous sickle cell disease or known thyroid disorder (see WARNINGS—General).
3. Inform the physician if they are allergic to any drugs, food, or if they have had any reactions to previous injections of dyes used for x-ray procedures (see PRECAUTIONS—General).
4. Inform the physician about any other medications they are currently taking, including nonprescription drugs, before they are administered this drug.

Drug Interactions
Renal toxicity has been reported in a few patients with liver dysfunction who were given oral cholecystographic agents followed by urographic agents. Administration of intravascular urographic agents should therefore be postponed in any patient with a known or suspected hepatic or biliary disorder who has recently received a cholecystographic contrast agent.
Addition of an inotropic agent to contrast agents may produce a paradoxical depressant response which can be deleterious to the ischemic myocardium.
Benadryl®, brand of diphenhydramine hydrochloride, may cause precipitation when mixed in the same syringe with HYPAQUE-76.

Drug/Laboratory Test Interactions
If any of these studies, which might be affected by contrast media are indicated, it is recommended that they be performed prior to administration of the contrast medium or two or more days afterwards.
Diatrizoate salts interfere with several laboratory urine and blood tests.

Blood Tests
Coagulation: Diatrizoate salts significantly inhibit all stages of coagulation. The fibrinogen concentration, Factors V, VII, and VIII are decreased. Prothrombin time and thromboplastin time are increased.
Platelet aggregation: High levels of plasma and diatrizoates inhibit platelet aggregation.
Serum calcium: Diatrizoate salts may decrease serum calcium levels. However, this depletion of serum calcium may also be the result of the addition of chelating agents (edetate disodium) in the preparation of certain contrast media.
Red cell counts: Transitory decreases in red cell counts. Technetium-99m-RBC labeling interference.
Leukocyte counts: Decrease.
Urea nitrogen (BUN): Transitory increase (see CLINICAL PHARMACOLOGY).
Serum creatinine: Transitory increase.

Urine Tests
Contrast media which are excreted in the urine, may interfere with some laboratory determinations eg, proteinuria, specific gravity, osmolarity, or bacterial cultures.

Thyroid Function Tests
Protein-bound iodine (PBI) and total serum organic iodine: Transient increase of both tests following urography have been noticed. The results of PBI and radioactive iodine uptake studies which depend on iodine estimations will not accurately reflect thyroid function for up to 16 days following administration of iodinated urographic media. However, thyroid function tests not depending on iodine estimations, eg, T_3 resin uptake or free thyroxine assays are not affected.

Diagnostic Product Information

Carcinogenesis, Mutagenesis, Impairment of Fertility
Long-term studies in animals have not been performed in order to evaluate carcinogenic potential, mutagenesis, or whether HYPAQUE-76, brand of diatrizoate meglumine and diatrizoate sodium injection, can affect fertility in males or females.

Pregnancy Category C
Animal reproduction studies have not been conducted with HYPAQUE-76. It is also not known whether HYPAQUE-76 can cause fetal harm when administered to a pregnant woman or can affect reproduction capacity. HYPAQUE-76 should be given to a pregnant woman only if clearly needed.

Labor and Delivery
It is not known whether use of these contrast agents during labor or delivery has immediate or delayed adverse effects on the fetus, prolongs the duration of labor or increases the likelihood that forceps delivery or other obstetrical intervention or resuscitation of the newborn will be necessary.

Nursing Mothers
Diatrizoate salts are excreted unchanged in human milk. Because of the potential adverse reactions, although it has not been established that serious adverse reactions occur in nursing infants, caution should be exercised when these contrast media are administered to a nursing woman.

Pediatric Use
Infants and small children should not have any fluid restriction prior to excretory urography or any other procedures (see PRECAUTIONS—General). Guidelines for pediatric dosages are presented in DOSAGE AND ADMINISTRATION—General.

Adverse Reactions—General: Approximately 95 percent of adverse reactions accompanying the intravascular use of diatrizoate salts are of mild to moderate severity. However, life-threatening reactions and fatalities, mostly of cardiovascular origin, have occurred.

Adverse reactions to injectable contrast media fall into two categories: chemotoxic reactions and idiosyncratic reactions.

Chemotoxic reactions result from the physicochemical properties of the contrast media, the dose, and the speed of injection. All hemodynamic disturbances and injuries to organs or vessels perfused by the contrast medium are included in this category.

Idiosyncratic reactions include all other reactions. They occur more frequently in patients 20 to 40 years old. Idiosyncratic reactions may or may not be dependent on the amount of dose injected, the speed of injection, the mode of injection, and the radiographic procedure. Idiosyncratic reactions are subdivided into minor, intermediate, and severe. The minor reactions are self-limited and of short duration; the severe reactions are life-threatening and treatment is urgent and mandatory.

The reported incidence of adverse reactions to contrast media in patients with a history of allergy are twice that of the general population. Patients with a history of previous reactions to a contrast medium are three times more susceptible than other patients. However, sensitivity to contrast media does not appear to increase with repeated examinations.

Most adverse reactions to injectable contrast media appear within one to three minutes after the start of injection, but delayed reactions may occur. Adverse reactions are grouped by organ system and listed below by decreasing order of occurrence and with an approximate incidence of occurrence. Significantly more severe reactions are listed before the other reactions regardless of frequency.

Greater Than 1 in 100 Patients
Body as a Whole: Reported incidences of death range from 6.6 per 1 million (0.00066 percent) to 1 in 10,000 patients (0.01 percent). Most deaths occur during injection or 5 to 10 minutes later, the main feature being cardiac arrest with cardiovascular disease as the main aggravating factor. Isolated reports of hypotensive collapse and shock following urography are found in the literature. The incidence of shock is estimated to occur in 1 out of 20,000 (0.005 percent) patients.

Cardiovascular System: The most frequent adverse reaction to diatrizoate salts is vasodilation (feeling of warmth). The estimated incidence is 49 percent.
Digestive System: Nausea 6 percent, vomiting 3 percent.
Nervous System: Paresthesia 6 percent, dizziness 5 percent.
Respiratory System: Rhinitis 1 percent, increased cough 2 percent.
Skin and Appendages: Urticaria 1 percent.
Pain at the injection site is estimated to occur in about 12 percent of the patients undergoing urography. Pain is usually due to extravasation.
Painful hot erythematous swelling above the venipuncture site was estimated to occur in more than one percent of the patients undergoing phlebography.
Special Senses: Perversion of taste 11 percent.
Urogenital System: Osmotic nephrosis of the proximal tubular cells is estimated to occur in 23 percent of patients following excretory urography.

Less Than 1 in 100 Patients
Other infrequently reported reactions without accompanying incidence rates are listed below, grouped by organ system.
Body as a Whole: Malaria relapse, uremia, high creatinine and BUN (see PRECAUTIONS—General, **Drug/Laboratory Test Interactions**), thrombocytopenia, leukopenia, and anemia.
Cardiovascular System: Cerebral hematomas, hemodynamic disturbances, sinus bradycardia, transient electrocardiographic abnormalities, ventricular fibrillation, and petechiae.
Digestive System: Severe unilateral or bilateral swelling of the parotid and submaxillary glands.
Nervous System: Convulsions, paralysis, and coma.
Respiratory System: Asthma, dyspnea, laryngeal edema, pulmonary edema, and bronchospasm.
Skin and Appendages: Skin necrosis.
Special Senses: Bilateral ocular irritation, lacrimation, itching, conjunctival chemosis, infection, and conjunctivitis.
Urogenital: Renal failure, pain.

Overdosage:
At dosage levels of diatrizoate sodium above a level containing 45 g of iodine, the incidence of unpleasant side effects increases. At total dosage equivalent to 80 gI or 90 gI administered over a short period of time (eg, 30 minutes), clinical signs of systemic intolerance appear (mostly related to hyperosmolar effects) and are manifest as tremors, irritability, and tachycardia. Above these maximal tolerated dosage levels in otherwise healthy adults, an increasing incidence and severity of dyspnea and pulmonary edema should be expected.

Four cases of overdosage in infants, during urography, are reported. Three of the infants died within 19 hours of the injection. The overdose ranged from slightly above the recommended pediatric dosage to a dose exceeding 19 g/kg. The symptoms of overdosage appeared between 10 minutes to several hours after injection of the contrast medium. Adverse effects were life-theatening, affecting mainly the pulmonary and cardiovascular systems. The symptoms included: cyanosis, bradycardia, acidosis, pulmonary hemorrhage, convulsions, coma, and cardiac arrest. All infants showed a poor visualization of the kidneys and a diffuse opacification of all the tissues and vasculature. Autopsy findings showed acute pulmonary damage and/or edema of subcutaneous tissues. Treatment of an overdose of injectable radiopaque contrast media is directed toward the support of all vital functions, and prompt institution of symptomatic therapy.

The acute intravenous LD_{50} of diatrizoate salts in mice is equivalent in iodine content of 5.3 gI/kg to 8.0 gI/kg and seem to be directly proportional to the rate of injection.

Diatrizoate salts are dialyzable.

Dosage and Administration—General:
Preparation of the patient will vary with preference of the radiologist and the type of radiological procedure performed. Specific radiographic procedures used will depend on the state of the patient and the diagnostic indications. Individual dose should be tailored according to age, body size, and indication for examination. (See INDIVIDUAL INDICATIONS AND USAGE section for specific Dosage and Administration.)

Solutions of radiopaque diagnostic agents for intravascular use should be at body temperature when injected and may need to be warmed before use. In the event that crystallization occurs, the solution may be clarified by placing the vial in a water bath at 40°C to 50°C and shaking it gently for two to three minutes or until the solids redissolve. If the particles still persist, do not use this vial but discard it. The solution should be protected from light and any unused portion remaining in the container should be discarded.

Dilution and withdrawal of the contrast agents should be accomplished under aseptic conditions with sterile syringes.

Parenteral drug products should be inspected visually for particulate matter and discoloration prior to administration. Avoid contaminating catheters, syringes, needles, and contrast media with glove powder or cotton fibers.

Pediatric Dosage
Pediatric doses of injectable radiopaque diagnostic agents are generally determined on a weight basis and should be calculated for each patient individually. (See INDIVIDUAL INDICATIONS AND USAGE section.)

Drug Incompatibilities
Diatrizoate salts are incompatible in vitro with some antihistamines and many other drugs. It is believed that one of the chief causes of in vitro incompatibility is an alteration of pH. Turbidity of solutions of intravascular contrast medium occurs between pH 2.5 and 4.1. Another cause is chemical interaction; therefore, other pharmaceuticals should not be mixed with contrast agents in the same syringe.

Individual Indications and Usage
THE FOLLOWING SECTIONS FOR INDIVIDUAL INDICATIONS AND USAGE CONTAIN CONTRAINDICATIONS, WARNINGS, PRECAUTIONS, ADVERSE REACTIONS, AND DOSAGE AND ADMINISTRATION SECTIONS RELATED TO THE SPECIFIC PROCEDURES. HOWEVER, IT SHOULD BE UNDERSTOOD THAT THE INFORMATION IN THE GENERAL SECTIONS IS ALSO LIKELY TO APPLY TO ALL OF THESE SPECIFIC USES.

Hydration—With the possible exception of urography, patients should be fully hydrated prior to the following procedures.

Excretory Urography
Nephrotomography and "Adequate" or High Dose Urography
HYPAQUE-76 solution may be used for excretory urography in selected patients. It may be used when prior urography has failed to provide diagnostic contrast and for preliminary excretory tract study to detect obstruction in azotemic patients or to avoid retrograde instrumentation. It may also be used as a high dosage medium to intensify and prolong the nephrographic effect when the prime purpose is examination of the renal parenchyma, especially with tomography. When combined with the urea "washout" technique, HYPAQUE-76, brand of diatrizoate meglumine and diatrizoate sodium injection, provides the necessary increased pyelographic contrast and diuresis required for screening or special examination of patients with suspected renal hypertension.

Contraindication
Urography is contraindicated in patients with anuria.

Continued on next page

This product information was effective as of December 3, 1984. On these and other products of Winthrop-Breon Laboratories, detailed information may be obtained on a current basis by direct inquiry to the Professional Services Department, 90 Park Avenue, New York, NY 10016 (212) 907-2525.

Winthrop-Breon—Cont.

Precautions
Although azotemia is not considered a contraindication, care is required in patients with advanced renal failure. The usual preparatory dehydration should be omitted, and urinary output should be observed for one to two days in these patients. Adequate visualization may be difficult or impossible to attain in patients with severely impaired renal and/or hepatic function. Use with extreme caution in patients with concomitant hepatorenal disease.

When HYPAQUE-76 is used with a urea "wash-out" procedure, the patient should also be observed for a few hours to detect signs of undue dehydration caused by increased diuresis induced by both the medium and the urea. Ingestion of water may be required for rehydration.

In myelomatosis, urography should only be performed with caution. If a weak protein-binding agent such as a diatrizoate is used for the procedure, it is essential to omit preparatory dehydration, administer fluids, and attempt to alkalinize the urine.

Preparatory Dehydration: Preparatory dehydration is dangerous in infants, young children, the elderly, and azotemic patients (especially those with polyuria, oliguria, diabetes, advanced vascular disease, or preexisting dehydration). The undesirable dehydration in these patients may be accentuated by the osmotic diuretic action of the medium.

Adverse Reactions
Side effects following this relatively high dose urography are usually mild and transitory and do not appear to occur more frequently or severely than those induced by "standard dose" urography. Nausea, facial flushing, and emesis are not uncommon reactions. (See also Adverse Reactions—General.)

Dosage and Administration
The usual intravenous dose for adults is 50 mL, with a range of 40 mL to 100 mL. Children require less in proportion to weight: Under 6 months of age—4mL; 6 to 12 months—6 mL; 1 to 2 years—8 mL; 2 to 5 years—10 mL; 5 to 7 years—12 mL; 8 to 10 years—14 mL; 11 to 15 years—16 mL.

Aortography
HYPAQUE-76, brand of diatrizoate meglumine and diatrizoate sodium injection, solution may be injected by commonly accepted techniques, such as translumbar, retrograde catheter, retrograde pressure injection (by cannula) or by antegrade (brachial) catheter for examination of the aorta and its major branches.

Warnings
During aortography by the translumbar technique, extreme care is advised to avoid inadvertent intrathecal injection since the injection of even small amounts (5 mL to 7 mL) of the contrast medium may cause convulsions, permanent sequelae, or fatality. Should the accident occur, the patient should be placed upright to confine the hyperbaric solution to a low level, anesthesia may be required to control convulsions, and if there is evidence of a large dose having been administered, a careful cerebrospinal fluid exchange-washout should be considered.

Pheochromocytoma: Administration of angiographic media to patients known or suspected to have pheochromocytoma can cause dangerous changes in blood pressure. A minimum dose should be injected. The blood pressure should be carefully monitored and measures for controlling major fluctuations should be available.

Precautions
The presence of a vigorous pulsatile flow should be established before using a cathether or pressure injection technique. A small "pilot" dose (about 2 mL) should be administered to locate the exact site of needle or catheter tip to help prevent injection of the main dose into a branch of the aorta or intramurally. In the translumbar technique, severe pain during injection may indicate intramural placement and abdominal or back pain afterwards may indicate hemorrhage from the injection site. Following catheter procedures, gentle pressure hemostasis for 5 to 10 minutes is advised, followed by observation for 30 to 60 minutes and immobilization of the limb for several hours to prevent hemorrhage from the site of arterial puncture.

Under conditions of slowed aortic circulation there is an increased likelihood of aortography causing muscle spasm. Occasional serious neurologic complications, including paraplegia, have also been reported in patients with aortic-iliac or even femoral artery bed obstruction, abdominal compression, hypotension, hypertension, spinal anesthesia, injection of vasopressors to increase contrast, and low injection sites (L2–3). In these patients the concentration, dose, and number of repeat injections of the medium should be maintained at a minimum with appropriate intervals between injections. The position of the patient and catheter tip should be carefully evaluated.

Adverse Reactions
The only adverse reaction expected is a mild burning or painful sensation on injection. Unusual reactions can occur, as in angiocardiography. An abrupt hypertensive episode can occur following entry of the medium into the renal artery in patients with pheochromocytoma. Mesenteric necrosis, acute pancreatitis, renal shutdown (usually transitory), and neurologic complications have been reported following inadvertent injection of a large part of the aortic dose into a branch of the aorta. Entry of the large aortic dose into the renal artery can cause, even in the absence of symptoms, albuminuria, cylindruria, hematuria, and an elevated BUN. Rapid and complete return of function usually follows.

Additional procedural reactions include injury to the aorta and neighboring organs, pleural puncture, renal damage including infarction and acute tubular necrosis with oliguria and anuria, accidental selective filling of the right renal artery during the translumbar procedure in the presence of preexistent renal disease, retroperitoneal hemorrhage from the translumbar approach.

Dosage and Administration
Adult: The usual adult dose as a single injection is 40 mL to 50 mL, repeated if indicated, to a total of 160 mL.
Pediatric: The usual single pediatric dose ranges from 0.3 mL/kg to 0.9 mL/kg. The total dose should not exceed 1 mL/kg.

Angiocardiography
Pharmacology-Hemodynamic Changes
Due to its physical characteristics (chiefly tonicity and viscosity) and the volume administered, HYPAQUE-76, brand of diatrizoate meglumine and diatrizoate sodium injection, may cause a number of transitory hemodynamic changes. When the medium is ejected from the left ventricle or introduced at the root of the ascending aorta, a brief (three seconds) hypertensive response is usually induced, followed immediately by a decrease in aortic and peripheral blood pressures below normal levels, lasting for at least two minutes. This hypotensive phase may be followed by a 15- to 20-minute period of fluctuating blood pressure.

Clinical doses (up to 1 mL per kg) injected into the vena cava or right heart outflow tract usually cause an irregular rise in right ventricular blood pressure, a slight increase in pulmonary artery blood pressure, and delayed signs of peripheral hypotension.

Other changes reported clinically include an increase in cardiac output and atrial pressure, a decrease in myocardial contractile force, and at the peak of postinjection hypotension, a marked rise in aortic and carotid blood flow, and elevation of central venous pressure. At dosage levels used in angiocardiography, the hematocrit and hemoglobin level may fall about 10 to 15 percent and serum osmolality may rise 10 to 12 percent. Blood carbon dioxide, pH, and BUN levels may fall. These changes commence immediately after injection, reach a maximum in two to five minutes, and return to normal values in 10 to 15 minutes. However, after the initial rise, plasma volume may decrease and continue to fall below control levels, even beyond 30 minutes, probably due to diuresis. If repeat injections are made in rapid succession these changes are likely to be more pronounced. (See also Dosage and Administration.) HYPAQUE-76 is not metabolized. It is eliminated unchanged, rapidly and completely in the urine by glomerular filtration.

Precautions
During administration of large doses of HYPAQUE-76 continuous monitoring of vital signs is desirable. Caution is advised in the administration of large doses to patients with incipient heart failure because of the possibility of aggravation of the preexisting condition. Hypotension should be corrected promptly since it may induce serious arrhythmias.

Because of the hemodynamic changes which may occur on injection into the right heart outflow tract, special care especially regarding dosage, should be observed in patients with right ventricular failure, pulmonary hypertension, or obliterated pulmonary vascular beds.

Precautions in Infants
Apnea, bradycardia and other arrhythmias, cerebral effects (lethargy and depression), and a tendency to acidosis are more likely to occur in cyanotic infants. It is desirable that vital signs be monitored on an intensive care basis afterwards to detect delayed adverse effects (arrhythmia, electrolyte and hemodynamic disturbances). Infants are more likely than adults to respond with convulsions, particularly after repeated injections. Unlike in the adult, the amount of the total dosage in young infants is of particular importance. (See Dosage and Administration.)

Adverse Reactions
See Adverse Reactions, General

Dosage and Administration
The individual dose is determined by the size of the structure to be visualized, the anticipated degree of hemodilution, and valvular competence. Weight is a minor consideration in adults. The size of each individual dose is a more important consideration than the total dosage used. When large individual doses are administered, as for contrast in the cardiac chambers and thoracic aorta, it has been suggested that 20 minutes be permitted to elapse between each injection to allow for subsidence of hemodynamic disturbances.

Ventriculography
Adult: The usual adult dose in a single injection is 45 mL, with a range of 40 mL to 50 mL. This may be repeated as necessary. However, when combined with selective coronary arteriography, the total dose should not exceed 225 mL.
Pediatric: The usual single pediatric dose is 0.2 mL/kg to 0.3 mL/kg. The total dose should not exceed 50 mL.

Pulmonary Angiography or Arch Study Used Alone
Adult: The usual single adult dose is 30 mL, with a range of 10 mL to 56 mL.
Pediatric: The pediatric dose ranges from 0.3 mL/kg to 0.9 mL/kg. The total dose should not exceed 1 mL/kg.

Combined Angiocardiographic Procedures
Multiple Procedures
With continuing advances in radiologic techniques and the development of more sophisticated equipment as well as more versatile and reliable radiopaque media, it is possible to examine multiple vascular systems and target organs during a single radiographic examination of the patient.

Multiple procedures of selective angiography require multiple injections of the contrast medium into several specific target organs and result in a greater dosage. Large doses of HYPAQUE-76 were well tolerated in multiple injections and multiple procedures of angiography.

See general sections for Contraindications, Warnings, Precautions, Adverse Reactions, and Dosage and Administration recommendations as well as those sections pertinent to the specific procedures.
Adult: The maximum total dose for multiple procedures in adult use, should not exceed 225 mL.
Pediatric: When multiple procedures are required in pediatric use, the total dose administered should be maintained below 4 mL/kg, or especially in young infants below 3 mL/kg.

Selective Coronary Arteriography
Adult: The usual single adult dose for right or left coronary arteriography is mL (range 4 mL to 10 mL) repeated as required up to a total dose of 120 mL for coronary arteriography alone.

Peripheral Angiography
The use of HYPAQUE-76, brand of diatrizoate meglumine and diatrizote sodium injection, is sometimes preferred over less concentrated media in selected cases for femoral and brachio-axillary arteriography in adults.

Precautions
Pulsation should be present in the artery to be injected. In thromboangiitis obliterans, or ascending infection associated with severe ischemia, angiography should be performed with extreme caution, if at all.

Adverse Reactions
Pain or a burning sensation with some spasm may occur, and is more marked in patients with arterial insufficiency. Therefore, the procedure is more satisfactorily performed under general or, for the lower extremity, spinal anesthesia.

Technical complications have included hemorrhage from the puncture site, and brachial plexus palsy following axillary artery injections.

Arterial thrombosis, displacement of arterial plaques, and ipsilateral venous thrombosis are very rare complications.

Dosage and Administration
Arteriography (aorto-iliac runoff and peripheral)
Adult: The single adult dose for femoral arteriography varies from 20 mL to 60 mL, depending on the site of placement, ie, aort iliac runoff, iliofemoral, femoral. For the upper limb, 20 mL to 40 mL is usually sufficient. These doses may be repeated up to three times.

Venography
Dosage and Administration
Central Venography
Adult: For central venography (inferior or superior vena cava), the total adult dose is 40 mL to 50 mL, repeated up to two times.

Renal Venography
Adult: The usual single adult dose is 20 mL to 40 mL.

Peripheral Venography
Adult: The usual single adult dose is 40 mL, with a range of 40 mL to 60 mL.

Selective Renal Arteriography
Dosage and Administration
Adult: The usual single adult dose is 8 mL, repeated up to three times. The dose ranges from 5 mL to 10 mL.

Selective Visceral Arteriography
Dosage and Administration
Celiac Axis: The usual adult dose ranges from 30 mL to 40 mL with subselective arteriography of its branches, eg, hepatic, usual dose of 25 mL with a range of 15 mL to 30 mL; mesenteric, usual dose of 30 mL with a range of 20 mL to 40 mL; splenic, usual dose of 20 mL with a range of 20 mL to 50 mL.

Superior Mesenteric: The usual single adult dose is 30 mL with a range of 20 mL to 40 mL.

The maximum total dose should not exceed 175 mL.

Intravenous Digital Arteriography
Arteriograms of diagnostic quality can be obtained following the intravenous administration of HYPAQUE-76, brand of diatrizoate meglumine and diatrizoate sodium injection, employing digital subtraction and computer imaging enhancement equipment. The intravenous route of administration using these techniques has the advantage of being less invasive than the corresponding selective catheter placement of the medium. The dose is administered into a peripheral vein usually by mechanical injection although sometimes by rapid manual injection. The technique has been used most frequently to visualize the ventricles, the aorta and most of its larger branches including carotid, cerebral, vertebral, renal, celiac, mesenterics, and the major peripheral vessels of the limbs.

Precautions
Since the dose is usually administered mechanically under high pressure, rupture of smaller peripheral veins has occurred. It has been suggested that this can be avoided by using an intravenous catheter threaded proximally beyond larger tributaries or in the case of the antecubital vein, into the superior vena cava. Sometimes the femoral vein is used.

Dosage and Administration
The usual dose of HYPAQUE-76 per injection by the intravenous digital technique is 30 mL to 60 mL with a range of 0.5 mL/kg to 1 mL/kg administered as a bolus 7.5 mL/second to 30 mL/second using a pressure injector. The dose and rate of injection will depend primarily on the type of equipment and technique used, with first exposures made on calculated circulation time.

Contrast Enhancement of Computed Tomographic Head Imaging
Injectable radiopaque contrast media may be used to refine diagnostic precision in areas of the brain which may not otherwise have been satisfactorily visualized.

Tumors. Radiopaque diagnostic agents may be useful to investigate the presence and extent of certain malignancies such as: gliomas including malignant gliomas, glioblastomas, astrocytomas, oligodendrogliomas and gangliomas, ependymomas, medulloblastomas, meningiomas, neuromas, pinealomas, pituitary adenomas, craniopharyngiomas, germinomas, and metastatic lesions. The usefulness of contrast enhancement for the investigation of the retrobulbar space and in cases of low grade or infiltrative glioma has not been demonstrated.

In calcified lesions, there is less likelihood of enhancement. Following therapy, tumors may show decreased or no enhancement.

The opacification of the inferior vermis following contrast media administration has resulted in false positive diagnosis in a number of normal studies.

Nonneoplastic Conditions. The use of injectable radiopaque diagnostic agents may be beneficial in the image enhancement of nonneoplastic lesions. Cerebral infarctions of recent onset may be better visualized with contrast enhancement, while some infarctions are obscured if contrast media are used. The use of iodinated contrast media results in contrast enhancement in about 60 percent of cerebral infarctions studied from one to four weeks from the onset of symptoms.

Sites of active infection may also be enhanced following contrast media administration.

Arteriovenous malformations and aneurysms will show contrast enhancement. For these vascular lesions, the enhancement is probably dependent on the iodine content of the circulating blood pool. Hematomas and intraparenchymal bleeders seldom demonstrate any contrast enhancement. However, in cases of intraparenchymal clot, for which there is no obvious clinical explanation, contrast media administration may be helpful in ruling out the possibility of associated arteriovenous malformation.

Dosage and Administration
The suggested dose is 50 mL to 125 mL by intravenous administration; scanning may be performed immediately after completion of administration. Doses for children should be proportionately less, depending on age and weight.

Contrast Enhancement of Computed Tomographic Body Imaging
Injectable radiopaque contrast media may be used to refine diagnostic precision in areas of the body which may not otherwise have been satisfactorily visualized.

When HYPAQUE-76, brand of diatrizoate meglumine and diatrizoate sodium injection, is injected by a rapid bolus technique, slight density differences between dissimilar tissues and structures can be observed radiologically using computed tomography. This phenomenon reflects vascularity and corresponds to the capillary phase of angiography.

The pharmacokinetics of these radiographic or attenuation differences can best be described by the two compartment open model. This model considers the body to consist of a central and peripheral compartment. The central compartment consists of the plasma and extracellular space of highly perfused tissues and organs. The peripheral compartment is less well perfused, and therefore, the contrast agents do not reach it so rapidly.

Following the intravenous injection of HYPAQUE-76, there is immediate dilution in the circulating plasma. Equilibrium is reached in the extracellular compartment in about ten minutes. During the first few minutes after contrast injection, tissue-dependent temporal changes in contrast distribution may affect the relative enhancement of neighboring tissues and organs. Therefore, in order to achieve maximum enhancement in a given tissue, it is necessary to perform the scan at the appropriate time after contrast injection.

Generally, because of the rapid attainment of equilibrium between the circulation and the extravascular space, maximum enhancement is usually obtained in the first few minutes following the bolus injection. Scans usually appear isodense after the first five minutes.

Because of the nature of the time-density curves, it is suggested that a high-concentration, bolus injection, early continuous dynamic scanning technique be employed in enhanced computed tomographic body imaging.

Since contrast enhancement appears to be greatest soon after administration of the contrast agent, a series of consecutive 2 to 3 second CT scans beginning 15 to 30 seconds after contrast injection would best assess the enhancement. This technique would be suitable for the evaluation of neoplastic and nonneoplastic lesions of both the abdomen and thorax.

Dosage and Administration
The suggested dose is 50 mL to 125 mL by rapid intravenous bolus administration; scanning may be performed immediately after completion of administration. Doses for children should be proportionately less, depending on age and weight.

How Supplied:
Vials of 30 mL, rubber stoppered, box of 25 (NDC 0024-0775-04)
Vials of 50 mL, rubber stoppered, box of 25 (NDC 0024-0776-04)
Vials of 100 mL, rubber stoppered, box of 10 0024-0777-02)
Calibrated bottles of 200 mL, rubber stoppered, with hangers, box of 10 (NDC 0024-0778-02)
Calibrated 200 mL dilution bottles containing 100 mL HYPAQUE-76; rubber-stoppered, with hangers, box of 10 (NDC 0024-0779-02)
Calibrated 200 mL dilution bottles containing 150 mL HYPAQUE-76, brand of diatrizoate meglumine and diatrizoate sodium injection; rubber-stoppered, with hangers, box of 10 (NDC 0024-0778-03)

HW-196-J

HYPAQUE®-M, 90% ℞
brand of diatrizoate meglumine and diatrizoate sodium injection, USP
Sterile Aqueous Injection

For Angiocardiography, Aortography, Angiography, Urography, Hysterosalpingography

Description: HYPAQUE-M, 90 percent, brand of diatrizoate meglumine and diatrizoate sodium, is a water-soluble radiopaque diagnostic medium. It is supplied as a 90 percent sterile aqueous solution providing 60 percent (w/v) diatrizoate meglumine and 30 percent (w/v) diatrizoate sodium. It is a triiodinated benzoic acid derivative containing 46.2 percent (w/v) organically bound iodine. Each mL contains 462 mg iodine and 10.9 mg (0.47 mEq) sodium. It is constituted as a radiopaque iodinated anion (diatrizoate) and the radiolucent cations (meglumine and sodium). It is the organically bound iodine of the anion which opacifies internal structures for x-ray visualization and fluoroscopy.

This product information was effective as of December 3, 1984. On these and other products of Winthrop-Breon Laboratories, detailed information may be obtained on a current basis by direct inquiry to the Professional Services Department, 90 Park Avenue, New York, NY 10016 (212) 907-2525.

Continued on next page

Winthrop-Breon—Cont.

The solution is hypertonic and has a viscosity of approximately 18.7 cp at 37°C. The pH is adjusted between 6.5 and 7.7 with sodium hydroxide, or hydrochloric acid, or sodium carbonate. The pKa is 3.4 for diatrizoic acid. Edetate calcium disodium 1:10,000 has been added as a sequestering stabilizing agent. At body temperature the solution is clear and colorless to pale straw color. The solution may be autoclaved once. Discard any unused portion remaining in the container. The solution should be stored at room temperature and protected from strong light. Crystals may form in the solution on cooling; they are readily redissolved on warming; the solution, however, should be administered at body temperature.

Diatrizoate meglumine is 1-deoxy-1 (methylamino)-D-glucitol 3,5-diacetamido - 2,4,6-triiodobenzoate (salt).

Diatrizoate sodium is monosodium 3,5-diacetamido-2,4,6-triiodobenzoate.

Clinical Pharmacology: Intravascular injection of a radiopaque diagnostic agent opacifies those vessels in the path of the flow of the contrast medium, permitting radiographic visualization of the internal structures of the human body until significant hemodilution occurs.

At physiologic pH, the water-soluble contrast media are completely dissociated into a radiopaque anion and a solubilizing cation. While circulating in tissue fluids, the compound remains ionized. However, it is not metabolized but excreted unchanged in the urine, each diatrizoate molecule remaining "obligated" to its sodium or meglumine moiety.

Following intravenous injection, the radiopaque diagnostic agents are immediately diluted in the circulating plasma. Equilibrium is reached with the extracellular compartment at about 10 minutes. Hence, the plasma concentration at 10 minutes is closely related to the dose corrected to body size.

The pharmacokinetics of the intravenously administered radiopaque contrast media are usually best described by a two compartment model with a rapid alpha phase for drug distribution and a slow beta phase for drug elimination. In patients with normal renal function, the alpha and beta half-lives were respectively 30 minutes and 120 minutes for diatrizoate. But in patients with renal and kidney functional impairment, the elimination half-life for the beta phase can be prolonged up to several days.

Injectable radiopaque diagnostic agents are excreted either through the liver or through the kidneys. These two excretory pathways are not mutually exclusive, but the main route of excretion seems to be governed by the affinity of the contrast medium for serum albumin. From 0% to 10% of diatrizoate sodium is bound to serum protein.

Diatrizoate salts are excreted unchanged predominantly through the kidneys by glomerular filtration. The amount excreted by the kidney during any period of time is determined by the filtered load; ie, the product of plasma contrast media concentration and glomerular filtration rate. The plasma concentration is dependent upon the dose administered and the body size. The glomerular filtration rate varies with the body size, sex, age, circulatory dynamics, diuretic effect of the drug, and renal function. In patients with normal renal function the maximum urinary concentration of diatrizoate meglumine occurs within 10 minutes with 12 percent of the administered dose being excreted. The mean values of cumulative urinary excretion for diatrizoate sodium expressed as percentage of administered dose are 38 percent at 60 minutes, 45 percent at 3 hours, and 94 to 100 percent at 24 hours.

Urinary excretion of contrast media is delayed in infants younger than 1 month and in patients with urinary tract obstruction. The urinary iodine concentration is higher with the sodium salt of diatrizoic acid than with the meglumine salt.

The liver and small intestine provide the major alternate route of excretion for diatrizoate. In patients free of severe renal disease, the fecal recovery is less than 2 percent of the administered dose. In patients with severe renal impairment the excretion of these contrast media through the gallbladder and into the small intestine sharply increases; up to 20 percent of the administered dose has been recovered in the feces in 48 hours.

Saliva is a minor secretory pathway for injectable radiopaque diagnostic agents. In patients with normal renal function, minimal amounts of contrast media are secreted unchanged. However, in uremic patients small amounts of free iodides resulting from deiodination prior to administration or in vivo, have been detected in the saliva.

Diatrizoate salts cross the placental barrier in humans by simple diffusion and appear to enter fetal tissue passively. No apparent harm to the fetus was observed when diatrizoate sodium and diatrizoate meglumine were injected intravenously 24 hours prior to delivery. However, abnormal neonatal opacification of the small intestine and colon were detected 4 to 6 days after delivery. Procedures including radiation involve a certain risk related to the exposure of the fetus.

Injectable radiopaque diagnostic agents are excreted unchanged in human milk.

Computerized Tomography: HYPAQUE-M, 90 percent can be administered as an intravenous bolus for brain tissue enhancement using computerized tomography. Increased tissue contrast differential for the scan is achieved either because of increased vascular (arterial, venous, or capillary bed) contrast or by blood brain barrier penetration of the medium (or its absence) in certain localized areas of disrupted vascular permeability. The degree of tissue enhancement caused by increased blood contrast is directly related to blood iodine content. However, the degree of enhancement due to extravascular accumulation of iodine resulting from blood brain barrier disruption will depend on the extent of disruption, the blood level of iodine, and the time delay prior to scanning. The nature of the pathology will determine whether an immediate or delayed scan is optimal.

Effects of Steroid Therapy: The anti-inflammatory and antiedema effects in patients receiving steroid therapy have interfered with the expected distribution of CT tissue enhancement on the scan in certain diseases.

Indications and Usage: HYPAQUE-M, brand of diatrizoate meglumine and diatrizoate sodium injection, 90 percent is indicated for angiocardiography, aortography, angiography, urography, and hysterosalpingography.

Urography

Diatrizoate salts are used in small, medium, and large dose urography (see Dosage and Administration—**EXCRETORY UROGRAPHY**). Visualization of the urinary tract can be achieved by either direct intravenous bolus injection, intravenous drip infusion, or incidentally following intra-arterial procedures. Visualization of the urinary tract is delayed in infants less than 1 month old, and in patients with urinary tract obstruction (see CLINICAL PHARMACOLOGY).

Contrast Enhancement of Computed Tomographic Head Imaging

Injectable radiopaque contrast media may be used to refine diagnostic precision in areas of the brain which may not otherwise have been satisfactorily visualized.

Tumors. Radiopaque diagnostic agents may be useful to investigate the presence and extent of certain malignancies such as: gliomas including malignant gliomas, glioblastomas, astrocytomas, oligodendrogliomas and gangliomas, ependymomas, medulloblastomas, meningiomas, neuromas, pinealomas, pituitary adenomas, craniopharyngiomas, germinomas, and metastatic lesions.

The usefulness of contrast enhancement for the investigation of the retrobulbar space and in cases of low grade or infiltrative glioma has not been demonstrated.

In calcified lesions, there is less likelihood of enhancement. Following therapy, tumors may show decreased or no enhancement.

The opacification of the inferior vermis following contrast media administration has resulted in false-positive diagnosis in a number of normal studies.

Nonneoplastic Conditions. The use of injectable radiopaque diagnostic agents may be beneficial in the image enhancement of nonneoplastic lesions. Cerebral infarctions of recent onset may be better visualized with contrast enhancement, while some infarctions are obscured if contrast media are used. The use of iodinated contrast media results in contrast enhancement in about 60 percent of cerebral infarctions studied from one to four weeks from the onset of symptoms.

Sites of active infection may also be enhanced following contrast media administration.

Arteriovenous malformations and aneurysms will show contrast enhancement. For these vascular lesions, the enhancement is probably dependent on the iodine content of the circulating blood pool. Hematomas and intraparenchymal bleeders seldom demonstrate any contrast enhancement. However, in cases of intraparenchymal clot, for which there is no obvious clinical explanation, contrast media administration may be helpful in ruling out the possibility of associated arteriovenous malformation.

Angiography

Diatrizoate salts are used for radiographic studies throughout the cardiovascular system.

Intravascular radiopaque diagnostic agents of high concentration are not recommended for cerebral or spinal angiography (see CONTRAINDICATIONS—General), and contrast agents with the lowest compatible viscosity and higher concentration of iodine (310 mg/mL to 480 mg/mL of bound iodine) must be used for angiocardiography. Contrast media approaching serum ionic content and osmolarity have less potential for deleterious effects on the myocardium (see PRECAUTIONS—General, **Drug Interactions**).

Addition of chelating agents may contribute to toxicity in coronary angiography, and the sodium content of angiographic agents used in coronary arteriography is of crucial importance.

In addition to the following general CONTRAINDICATIONS, WARNINGS, PRECAUTIONS, and ADVERSE REACTIONS, there are additional listings in these categories under the particular procedures.

Contraindications—General: HYPAQUE-M, 90 percent has no absolute contraindications in its recommended uses (see general WARNINGS and PRECAUTIONS).

Do not use HYPAQUE-M, 90 percent for myelography or for examination of dorsal cysts or sinuses which might communicate with the subarachnoid space. Even a small amount in the subarachnoid space may produce convulsions and result in fatality. (See also **ABDOMINAL AORTOGRAPHY**, Warnings.) Epidural injection is also contraindicated.

HYPAQUE-M, brand of diatrizoate meglumine and diatrizoate sodium injection, 90 percent should not be injected directly into the carotid, vertebral, or spinal arteries.

HYPAQUE-M, 90 percent is contraindicated in patients with a hypersensitivity to salts of diatrizoic acid. Urography is contraindicated in patients with anuria.

Warnings—General: Excretory urography is potentially hazardous in patients with multiple myeloma. In some of those patients, therapeutically resistant anuria resulting in progressive uremia, renal failure, and eventually death has followed this procedure. Although neither the contrast agent nor dehydration has been proved separately to be the cause of anuria in myelomatous patients, it has been speculated that the combination of both may be causative. The risk of excretory urography in myelomatous patients is not a contraindication to the procedure; however, they require special precautions. Partial dehydration in the preparation of these patients for the examination is not recommended since this may predispose to the precipitation of myeloma protein in the renal tubules. Myeloma, which occurs most commonly in persons over age 40, should be considered before instituting urographic procedures.

Contrast media may promote sickling in individuals who are homozygous for sickle cell disease when the material is injected intravenously or intra-arterially.

Administration of radiopaque materials to patients known or suspected of having pheochromocytoma should be performed with extreme caution. If, in the opinion of the physician, the possible benefits of such procedures outweigh the considered risks, the procedures may be performed; however, the amount of radiopaque medium injected should be kept to an absolute minimum. The blood pressure should be assessed throughout the procedure and measures for treatment of a hypertensive crisis should be available.

Recent reports of thyroid storm occurring following the intravascular use of iodinated radiopaque diagnostic agents in patients with hyperthyroidism or with an autonomously functioning thyroid nodule suggest that this additional risk be evaluated in such patients before use of diatrizoate salts.

Contrast media administered for cardiac catheterization and angiocardiography may cause cellular injury to circulating lymphocytes. Chromosomal damage in humans includes inhibition of mitosis, increases in the number of micronuclei, and chromosome aberrations. The damages appear to be related to the contrast medium itself rather than to the x-ray radiation. It is to be noted that those agents have not been adequately tested in animal or laboratory systems.

Urography should be performed with caution in patients with severely impaired renal function and patients with combined renal and hepatic disease.

Selective spinal arteriography or arteriography of trunks providing spinal branches can cause mild to severe muscle spasm. However, serious neurologic sequelae, including permanent paralysis, could occur with even small doses of the 90 percent concentration. (See also ANGIOGRAPHY, Precaution.)

Precautions—General: Diagnostic procedures which involve the use of radiopaque diagnostic agents should be carried out under the direction of personnel with the prerequisite training and with a thorough knowledge of the particular procedure to be performed. Appropriate facilities should be available for coping with any complication of the procedure, as well as, for emergency treatment of severe reactions to the contrast agent itself. After parenteral administration of a radiopaque agent, competent personnel and emergency facilities should be available for at least 30 to 60 minutes since severe delayed reactions have occurred (see ADVERSE REACTIONS—General).

The possibility of an idiosyncratic reaction in susceptible patients should always be considered (see ADVERSE REACTIONS—General). The susceptible population includes patients with a history of a previous reaction to a contrast media, patients with a known sensitivity to iodine per se, and patients with a known clinical hypersensitivity: bronchial asthma, hay fever, and food allergies.

The occurrence of severe idiosyncratic reactions has prompted the use of several pretesting methods. However, pretesting cannot be relied upon to predict severe reactions and may itself be hazardous for the patient. It is suggested that a thorough medical history with emphasis on allergy and hypersensitivity, prior to the injection of any contrast media, may be more accurate than pretesting in predicting potential adverse reactions.

A positive history of allergies or hypersensitivity does not arbitrarily contraindicate the use of a contrast agent, where a diagnostic procedure is thought essential, but caution should be exercised (see ADVERSE REACTIONS—General). Premedication with antihistamines or corticosteroids to avoid or minimize possible allergic reactions in such patients should be considered. Recent reports indicate that such pretreatment does not prevent serious life-threatening reactions, but may reduce both their incidence and severity.

Preparatory dehydration for angiography and CT procedures is unnecessary and may be dangerous, contributing to acute renal failure in infants, young children, the elderly, patients with preexisting renal insufficiency, patients with advanced vascular disease, and diabetic patients. Dehydration in these patients seems to be enhanced by the osmotic diuretic action of urographic agents. Overnight fluid restriction for urography may be undesirable and is considered unnecessary when using this relatively high (90%) concentration.

Although azotemia is not a contraindication, the medium should be used with great care in patients with advanced renal destruction associated with severe uremia. (See also **EXCRETORY UROGRAPHY,** Precautions.)

Acute renal failure has been reported in diabetic patients with diabetic nephropathy and in susceptible nondiabetic patients (often elderly with preexisting renal disease) following excretory urography. Therefore, careful consideration of the potential risks should be given before performing this radiographic procedure in these patients. (See also **EXCRETORY UROGRAPHY,** Precautions—*Preparatory Dehydration*.)

Immediately following surgery, excretory urography should be used with caution in renal transplant recipients.

Due to the transitory increase in the circulatory osmotic load, injections of urographic agents should be used with caution in patients with congestive heart failure. Such patients should be observed for several hours following the procedure to detect delayed hemodynamic disturbances.

General anesthesia may be indicated in the performance of some procedures, in young or uncooperative children and in selected adult patients; however, a higher incidence of adverse reactions has been reported in these patients, and may be attributable to the inability of the patient to identify untoward symptoms, or to the hypotensive effect of anesthesia which can reduce cardiac output and increase the duration of exposure to the contrast agent.

In addition to the general precautions already described, excretory urography, angiography, and other uses also have hazards associated with the particular techniques employed. (See INDIVIDUAL INDICATIONS AND USAGE section.)

Information for Patients
Patients receiving injectable radiopaque diagnostic agents should be instructed to:
1. Inform the physician if they are pregnant (see CLINICAL PHARMACOLOGY).
2. Inform the physician if they are diabetic or if they have multiple myeloma, pheochromocytoma, homozygous sickle cell disease or known thyroid disorder (see WARNINGS—General).
3. Inform the physician if they are allergic to any drugs, food, or if they have had any reactions to previous injections of dyes used for x-ray procedures (see PRECAUTIONS—General).
4. Inform the physician about any other medications they are currently taking, including nonprescription drugs, before they are administered this drug.

Drug Interactions
Renal toxicity has been reported in a few patients with liver dysfunction who were given oral cholecystographic agents followed by urographic agents. Administration of intravascular urographic agents should therefore be postponed in any patient with a known or suspected hepatic or biliary disorder who has recently received a cholecystographic contrast agent.

Addition of an inotropic agent to contrast agents may produce a paradoxical depressant response which can be deleterious to the ischemic myocardium.

Benadryl®, brand of diphenhydramine hydrochloride, may cause precipitation when mixed in the same syringe with HYPAQUE-M, 90 percent.

Drug/Laboratory Test Interactions
If any of these studies, which might be affected by contrast media are indicated, it is recommended that they be performed prior to administration of the contrast medium or two or more days afterwards.

Diatrizoate salts interfere with several laboratory urine and blood tests.

Blood Tests
Coagulation: Diatrizoate salts significantly inhibit all stages of coagulation. The fibrinogen concentration, Factors V, VII, and VIII are decreased. Prothrombin time and thromboplastin time are increased.

Platelet aggregation: High levels of plasma and diatrizoates inhibit platelet aggregation.

Serum calcium: Diatrizoate salts may decrease serum calcium levels. However, this depletion of serum calcium may also be the result of the addition of chelating agents (edetate disodium) in the preparation of certain contrast media.

Red cell counts: Transitory decreases in red cell counts. Technetium-99m—RBC labeling interference.

Leukocyte counts: Decrease.

Urea nitrogen (BUN): Transitory increase (see CLINICAL PHARMACOLOGY).

Serum creatinine: Transitory increase.

Urine Tests
Contrast media which are excreted in the urine, may interfere with some laboratory determinations eg, proteinuria, specific gravity, osmolarity, or bacterial cultures.

Thyroid Function Tests
Protein-bound iodine (PBI) and total serum organic iodine: Transient increase of both tests following urography have been noticed. The results of PBI and radioactive iodine uptake studies which depend on iodine estimations will not accurately reflect thyroid function for up to 16 days following administration of iodinated urographic media. However, thyroid function tests not depending on iodine estimations, eg, T_3 resin uptake or free thyroxine assays are not affected.

Carcinogenesis, Mutagenesis, Impairment of Fertility
Long-term studies in animals have not been performed in order to evaluate carcinogenic potential, mutagenesis, or whether HYPAQUE-M, 90 percent can affect fertility in males or females.

Pregnancy Category C
Animal reproduction studies have not been conducted with HYPAQUE-M, 90 percent. It is also not known whether HYPAQUE-M, 90 percent can cause fetal harm when administered to a pregnant woman or can affect reproduction capacity. HYPAQUE-M, brand of diatrizoate meglumine and diatrizoate sodium injection, 90 percent should be given to a pregnant woman only if clearly needed.

Labor and Delivery
It is not known whether use of these contrast agents during labor or delivery has immediate or delayed adverse effects on the fetus, prolongs the duration of labor or increases the likelihood that forceps delivery or other obstetrical intervention or resuscitation of the newborn will be necessary.

Nursing Mothers
Diatrizoate salts are excreted unchanged in human milk. Because of the potential adverse reactions, although it has not been established that serious adverse reactions occur in nursing infants, caution should be exercised when these contrast media are administered to a nursing woman.

Pediatric Use
Infants and small children should not have any fluid restriction prior to excretory urography or any other procedures (see PRECAUTIONS—General). Guidelines for pediatric dosages are presented in DOSAGE AND ADMINISTRATION—General.

Adverse Reactions—General: Approximately 95 percent of adverse reactions accompanying the intravascular use of diatrizoate salts are of mild to

---

This product information was effective as of December 3, 1984. On these and other products of Winthrop-Breon Laboratories, detailed information may be obtained on a current basis by direct inquiry to the Professional Services Department, 90 Park Avenue, New York, NY 10016 (212) 907-2525.

Continued on next page

Winthrop-Breon—Cont.

moderate severity. However, life-threatening reactions and fatalities, mostly of cardiovascular origin, have occurred.

Adverse reactions to injectable contrast media fall into two categories: chemotoxic reactions and idiosyncratic reactions.

Chemotoxic reactions result from the physicochemical properties of the contrast media, the dose, and the speed of injection. All hemodynamic disturbances and injuries to organs or vessels perfused by the contrast medium are included in this category.

Idiosyncratic reactions include all other reactions. They occur more frequently in patients 20 to 40 years old. Idiosyncratic reactions may or may not be dependent on the amount of dose injected, the speed of injection, the mode of injection, and the radiographic procedure. Idiosyncratic reactions are subdivided into minor, intermediate, and severe. The minor reactions are self-limited and of short duration; the severe reactions are life-threatening and treatment is urgent and mandatory.

The reported incidence of adverse reactions to contrast media in patients with a history of allergy are twice that of the general population. Patients with a history of previous reactions to a contrast medium are three times more susceptible than other patients. However, sensitivity to contrast media does not appear to increase with repeated examinations.

Most adverse reactions to injectable contrast media appear within one to three minutes after the start of injection, but delayed reactions may occur. Adverse reactions are grouped by organ system and listed below by decreasing order of occurrence and with an approximate incidence of occurrence. Significantly more severe reactions are listed before the other reactions regardless of frequency.

Greater Than 1 in 100 Patients

Body as a Whole: Reported incidences of death range from 6.6 per 1 million (0.00066 percent) to 1 in 10,000 patients (0.01 percent). Most deaths occur during injection or 5 to 10 minutes later, the main feature being cardiac arrest with cardiovascular disease as the main aggravating factor.

Isolated reports of hypotensive collapse and shock following urography are found in the literature. The incidence of shock is estimated to occur in 1 out of 20,000 (0.005 percent) patients.

Cardiovascular System: The most frequent adverse reaction to diatrizoate salts is vasodilation (feeling of warmth). The estimated incidence is 49 percent.

Digestive System: Nausea 6 percent, vomiting 3 percent.

Nervous System: Paresthesia 6 percent, dizziness 5 percent.

Respiratory System: Rhinitis 1 percent, increased cough 2 percent.

Skin and Appendages: Urticaria 1 percent.

Pain at the injection site is estimated to occur in about 12 percent of the patients undergoing urography. Pain is usually due to extravasation.

Painful hot erythematous swelling above the venipuncture site was estimated to occur in more than one percent of the patients undergoing phlebography.

Special Senses: Perversion of taste 11 percent.

Urogenital System: Osmotic nephrosis of the proximal tubular cells is estimated to occur in 23 percent of patients following excretory urography.

Less Than 1 in 100 Patients

Other infrequently reported reactions without accompanying incidence rates are listed below, grouped by organ system.

Body as a Whole: Malaria relapse, uremia, high creatinine and BUN (see PRECAUTIONS—General, **Drug/Laboraotory Test Interactions**), thrombocytopenia, leukopenia, and anemia.

Cardiovascular System: Cerebral hematomas, hemodynamic disturbances, sinus bradycardia, transient electrocardiographic abnormalities, ventricular fibrillation, and petechiae.

Digestive System: Severe unilateral or bilateral swelling of the parotid and submaxillary glands.

Nervous System: Convulsions, paralysis, and coma.

Respiratory System: Asthma, dyspnea, laryngeal edema, pulmonary edema, and bronchospasm.

Skin and Appendages: Skin necrosis.

Special Senses: Bilateral ocular irritation, lacrimation, itching, conjunctival chemosis, infection, and conjunctivitis.

Urogenital: Renal failure, pain.

Overdosage: At dosage levels of diatrizoate sodium above a level containing 45 g of iodine, the incidence of unpleasant side effects increases. At total dosage equivalent to 80 gI or 90 gI administered over a short period of time (eg, 30 minutes), clinical signs of systemic intolerance appear (mostly related to hyperosmolar effects) and are manifest as temors, irritability, and tachycardia. Above these maximal tolerated dosage levels in otherwise healthy adults, an increasing incidence and severity of dyspnea and pulmonary edema should be expected.

Four cases of overdosage in infants, during urography, are reported. Three of the infants died within 19 hours of the injection. The overdose ranged from slightly above the recommended pediatric dosage to a dose exceeding 19 g/kg. The symptoms of overdosage appeared between 10 minutes to several hours after injection of the contrast medium. Adverse effects were life-threatening, affecting mainly the pulmonary and cardiovascular systems. The symptoms included: cyanosis, bradycardia, acidosis, pulmonary hemorrhage, convulsions, coma, and cardiac arrest. All infants showed a poor visualization of the kidneys and a diffuse opacification of all the tissues and vasculature. Autopsy findings showed acute pulmonary damage and/or edema of subcutaneous tissues. Treatment of an overdose of injectable radiopaque contrast media is directed toward the support of all vital functions, and prompt institution of symptomatic therapy.

The acute intravenous LD_{50} of diatrizoate salts in mice is equivalent in iodine content of 5.3 gI/kg to 8.0 gI/kg and seem to be directly proportional to the rate of injection.

Diatrizoate salts are dialyzable.

Dosage and Administration—General: Preparation of the patient will vary with preference of the radiologist and the type of radiological procedure performed. Specific radiographic procedures used will depend on the state of the patient and the diagnostic indications. Individual dose should be tailored according to age, body size, and indication for examination. (See INDIVIDUAL INDICATIONS AND USAGE section for specific Dosage and Administration.)

Solutions of radiopaque diagnostic agents for intravascular use should be at body temperature when injected and may need to be warmed before use. In the event that crystallization occurs, the solution may be clarified by placing the vial in a water bath at 40°C to 50°C and shaking it gently for two to three minutes or until the solids redissolve. If the particles still persist, do not use this vial but discard it. The solution should be protected from light and any unused portion remaining in the container should be discarded.

Dilution and withdrawal of the contrast agents should be accomplished under aseptic conditions with sterile syringes.

Parenteral drug products should be inspected visually for particulate matter and discoloration prior to administration. Avoid contaminating catheters, syringes, needles, and contrast media with glove powder or cotton fibers.

Pediatric Dosage

Pediatric doses of injectable radiopaque diagnostic agents are generally determined on a weight basis and should be calculated for each patient individually. (See INDIVIDUAL INDICATIONS AND USAGE section.)

Drug Incompatibilities

Diatrizoate salts are incompatible in vitro with some antihistamines and many other drugs. It is believed that one of the chief causes of in vitro incompatibility is an alteration of pH. Turbidity of solutions of intravascular contrast medium occurs between pH 2.5 and 4.1. Another cause is chemical interaction; therefore, other pharmaceuticals should not be mixed with contrast agents in the same syringe.

Individual Indications and Usage

THE FOLLOWING SECTIONS FOR INDIVIDUAL INDICATIONS AND USAGE CONTAIN CONTRAINDICATIONS, WARNINGS, PRECAUTIONS, ADVERSE REACTIONS, AND DOSAGE AND ADMINISTRATION SECTIONS RELATED TO THE SPECIFIC PROCEDURES. HOWEVER, IT SHOULD BE UNDERSTOOD THAT THE INFORMATION IN THE GENERAL SECTIONS IS ALSO LIKELY TO APPLY TO ALL OF THESE SPECIFIC USES.

Hydration—With the possible exception of urography, patients should be fully hydrated prior to the following procedures.

Angiocardiography

Pharmacology—Hemodynamic Changes

Due to its physical characteristics (chiefly tonicity and viscosity) and the volume administered, HYPAQUE-M, 90 percent may cause a number of transitory hemodynamic changes. When the medium is ejected from the left ventricle or introduced at the root of the ascending aorta, a brief (three seconds) hypertensive response is usually induced, followed immediately by a decrease in aortic and peripheral blood pressures below normal levels, lasting for at least two minutes. This hypotensive phase may be followed by a 15- to 20-minute period of fluctuating blood pressure.

Clinical doses (up to 1 mL per kg) injected into the vena cava or right heart outflow tract usually cause an irregular rise in right ventricular blood pressure, a slight increase in pulmonary artery blood pressure, and delayed signs of peripheral hypotension.

Other changes reported clinically include an increase in cardiac output and atrial pressure, a decrease in myocardial contractile force, and at the peak of postinjection hypotension, a marked rise in aortic and carotid blood flow, and elevation of central venous pressure. At dosage levels used in angiocardiography, the hematocrit and hemoglobin level may fall about 10 to 15 percent and serum osmolality may rise 10 to 12 percent. Blood carbon dioxide, pH, and BUN levels may fall. These changes commence immediately after injection, reach a maximum in two to five minutes, and return to normal values in 10 to 15 minutes. However, after the initial rise, plasma volume may decrease and continue to fall below control levels, even beyond 30 minutes, probably due to diuresis. If repeat injections are made in rapid succesion, these changes are likely to be more pronounced. (See Dosage and Administration.) HYPAQUE-M, brand of diatrizoate meglumine and diatrizoate sodium injection 90 percent is not metabolized. It is eliminated unchanged, rapidly and completely, in the urine by glomerular filtration.

Precautions

During administration of large doses of HYPAQUE-M, 90 percent, continuous monitoring of vital signs is desirable. Caution is advised in the administration of large doses to patients with incipient heart failure because of the possibility of aggravation of the preexisting condition. Hypotension should be corrected promptly since it may induce serious arrhythmias.

Because of the hemodynamic changes which may occur on injection into the right heart outflow tract, special care, especially regarding dosage, should be observed in patients with right ventricular failure, pulmonary hypertension, or obliterated pulmonary vascular beds.

Precautions in Infants

Apnea, bradycardia and other arrhythmias, cerebral effects (lethargy and depression), and a tendency to acidosis are more likely to occur in cyanotic infants. It is desirable that vital signs be monitored on an intensive care basis afterwards to detect delayed adverse effects (arrhythmia, electrolyte and hemodynamic disturbances). Infants are more likely than adults to respond with convulsions, particularly after repeated injections. Unlike in the adult, the amount of the total dosage in young infants is of particular importance. (See Dosage and Administration.)

Adverse Reactions
See Adverse Reactions, General.

Dosage and Administration
The individual dose is determined by the size of the structure to be visualized, the anticipated degree of hemodilution, and valvular competence. Weight is a minor consideration in adults. The size of each individual dose is a more important consideration than the total dosage used. When large individual doses are administered, as for contrast in the cardiac chambers and thoracic aorta, it has been suggested that 20 minutes be permitted to elapse between each injection to allow for subsidence of hemodynamic disturbances.

Adult Dosage: Adult dose of HYPAQUE-M, 90 percent is usually 35 mL to 50 mL into either left or right chamber, outflow tracts, or aorta. The individual dose for intravenous angiocardiography ranges from 70 mL to 100 mL often injected simultaneously bilaterally by pressure injection, half of the dose into each antecubital vein.

Pediatric Dosage: The usual dose is 0.5 mL to 1 mL per kg for a subject with heart of normal size and intact valves and septum. For patients with stenotic lesions, 0.5 mL per kg is recommended. Doses up to 1.5 mL per kg may be required in cardiomegaly, large volume shunts, or where right cardiac injection is also intended to opacify left chambers.

Young Infant Dosage: The individual dose is similar to that described under Pediatric Dosage. It has been suggested, however, that the total dosage administered should be maintained below 3 mL per kg in infants under two months of age in any one procedure.

Arteriography

Coronary Arteriography
Coronary arteriography should only be used in carefully selected patients when the value of the anticipated information outweighs the risk involved.

Contraindication
Routine coronary arteriography should be deferred for four weeks in patients with clinically apparent myocardial infarction.

Precaution
Continuous EKG monitoring for early detection of arrhythmias is desirable.

Adverse Reactions
Transitory EKG changes occur almost inevitably with good filling. Transient arrhythmia may occur. (See ADVERSE REACTIONS—General.) Serum enzymes may be elevated for 24 hours.

Dosage and Administration
The usual dose for adults is 50 mL of HYPAQUE-M, 90 percent delivered into the **root of the aorta** for simultaneous bilateral angiograms. For injection at the **sinus of Valsalva**, the usual dose is 15 mL to 25 mL on either side. For **selective coronary procedures,** as by the Sones technique, the individual dose recommended is 3 mL to 5 mL into either artery. This dose may be injected alternately into the right and left coronary artery, and repeated.

Abdominal Aortography
HYPAQUE-M, brand of diatrizoate meglumine and diatrizoate sodium injection, 90 percent solution may be injected by commonly accepted techniques, such as translumbar, retrograde catheter, retrograde pressure injection (by cannula) or by antegrade (brachial) catheter for examination of the aorta and its major branches.

Warnings
During aortography by the translumbar technique, extreme care is advised to avoid inadvertent intrathecal injection since the injection of even small amounts (5 mL to 7 mL) of the contrast medium may cause convulsions, permanent sequelae, or fatality. Should the accident occur, the patient should be placed upright to confine the hyperbaric solution to a low level, anesthesia may be required to control convulsions, and if there is evidence of a large dose having been administered, a careful cerebrospinal fluid exchange-washout should be considered.

Pheochromocytoma: Administration of angiographic media to patients known or suspected to have pheochromocytoma can cause dangerous changes in blood pressure. A minimum dose should be injected. The blood pressure should be carefully monitored and measures for controlling major fluctuations should be available.

Precautions
The presence of a vigorous pulsatile flow should be established before using a catheter or pressure injection technique. A small "pilot" dose (about 2 mL) should be administered to locate the exact site of needle or catheter tip to help prevent injection of the main dose into a branch of the aorta or intramurally. In the translumbar technique, severe pain during injection may indicate intramural placement and abdominal or back pain afterwards may indicate hemorrhage from the injection site. Following catheter procedures, gentle pressure hemostasis for 5 to 10 minutes is advised, followed by observation for 30 to 60 minutes and immobilization of the limb for several hours to prevent hemorrhage from the site of arterial puncture.

Under conditions of <u>slowed</u> aortic circulation there is an increased likelihood of aortography causing muscle spasm. Occasional serious neurologic complications, including paraplegia, have also been reported in patients with aortic-iliac or even femoral artery bed obstruction, abdominal compression, hypotension, hypertension, spinal anesthesia, injection of vasopressors to increase contrast, and low injection sites (L2–3). In these patients the concentration, dose, and number of repeat injections of the medium should be maintained at a minimum with appropriate intervals between injections. The position of the patient and catheter tip should be carefully evaluated.

Adverse Reactions
The only adverse reaction expected is a mild burning sensation on injection. Unusual reactions can occur, as in angiocardiography. An abrupt hypertensive episode can occur following entry of the medium into the renal artery in patients with pheochromocytoma. Mesenteric necrosis, acute pancreatitis, and renal shutdown (usually transitory) and neurologic complications have been reported following inadvertent injection of a large part of the aortic dose into a branch of the aorta. Entry of the large aortic dose into the renal artery can cause, even in the absence of symptoms, albuminuria, cylindruria, and hematuria, and an elevated BUN. Rapid and complete return of function usually follows.

Dosage and Administration
The average adult dose range of HYPAQUE-M, 90 percent is 10 mL to 15 mL by translumbar technique and by retrograde catheter, 15 mL to 25 mL. In infants and children and thin adults, the use of a less concentrated medium for aortography, such as diatrizoate sodium 50 percent, is advised in doses of 0.5 mL per kg. For retrograde pressure injection (cannula) the usual adult dose is 35 mL to 40 mL of HYPAQUE-M, brand of diatrizoate meglumine and diatrizoate sodium injection, 90 percent solution.

Peripheral Arteriography
The use of HYPAQUE-M, 90 percent is sometimes preferred over less concentrated media in selected cases for femoral and brachio-axillary arteriography in adults.

Precautions
Pulsation should be present in the artery to be injected. In thromboangiitis obliterans, or ascending infection associated with severe ischemia, angiography should be performed with extreme caution, if at all.

Adverse Reactions
Pain or a burning sensation with some spasm may occur, and is more marked in patients with arterial insufficiency. Therefore, the procedure is more satisfactorily performed under general or, for the lower extremity, spinal anesthesia.

Arterial thrombosis, displacement of arterial plaques, and ipsilateral venous thrombosis are very rare complications.

Dosage and Administration
The usual dose of HYPAQUE-M, 90 percent is 10 mL to 25 mL, which may be repeated. Appropriate dosage in infants and children of a less concentrated medium, such as diatrizoate sodium 50 percent, will usually provide adequate contrast.

Urography

Nephrotomography And "Adequate" Or High Dose Urography
HYPAQUE-M, 90 percent solution may be used for excretory urography in selected patients. It may be used when prior urography has failed to provide diagnostic contrast and for preliminary excretory tract study to detect obstruction in azotemic patients or to avoid retrograde instrumentation. It may also be used as a high dosage medium to intensify and prolong the nephrographic effect when the prime purpose is examination of the renal parenchyma, especially with tomography. When combined with a urea "washout" technique, HYPAQUE-M, 90 percent provides the necessary increased pyelographic contrast and diuresis required for screening or special examination of patients with suspected renal hypertension.

Contraindication
Urography is contraindicated in patients with anuria.

Precautions
Although azotemia is not considered a contraindication, care is required in patients with advanced renal failure. The usual preparatory dehydration should be omitted, and urinary output should be observed for one to two days in these patients.

When HYPAQUE-M, 90 percent is used with a urea "washout" procedure, the patient should also be observed for a few hours to detect signs of undue dehydration caused by increased diuresis induced by both the medium and the urea. Ingestion of water may be required for rehydration.

In myelomatosis, urography should only be performed with caution. If a weak protein-binding agent such as a diatrizoate is used for the procedure, it is essential to omit preparatory dehydration, administer fluids, and attempt to alkalinize the urine.

Preparatory Dehydration: Preparatory dehydration is dangerous in infants, young children, the elderly, and azotemic patients (especially those with polyuria, oliguria, diabetes, advanced vascular disease, or preexisting dehydration). The undesirable dehydration in these patients may be accentuated by the osmotic diuretic action of the medium.

Adverse Reactions
Side effects following this relatively high dose urography are usually mild and transitory and do not appear to occur more frequently or severely than those induced by "standard dose" urography. Nausea, facial flushing, and emesis are not uncommon reactions. (See ADVERSE REACTIONS—General.)

Dosage and Administration
In adults, the single dose of HYPAQUE-M, 90 percent is usually 50 mL. The dose in infants and children is 0.5 mL to 1 mL per kg (not to exceed 50 mL). It is injected rapidly intravenously.

Hysterosalpingography
HYPAQUE-M, brand of diatrizoate meglumine and diatrizoate sodium injection, 90 percent may be selected when a viscous medium of high density is required. Otherwise, a less dense and less viscous medium, such as diatrizoate sodium 50 percent, may be used.

Contraindications
The procedure should not be performed during the menstrual period or when menstrual flow is imminent. It should not be performed when infection is present in any portion of the genital tract. The procedure is also contraindicated for pregnant women or for those in whom pregnancy is suspected. Its use is not advised for six months after termination of pregnancy, or for thirty days after conization or curettage.

This product information was effective as of December 3, 1984. On these and other products of Winthrop-Breon Laboratories, detailed information may be obtained on a current basis by direct inquiry to the Professional Services Department, 90 Park Avenue, New York, NY 10016 (212) 907-2525.

Continued on next page

Winthrop-Breon—Cont.

Precautions
In patients with carcinoma or in those in whom the condition is suspected, caution should be exercised to avoid possible spread of the lesion by the procedure. The effect on PBI or RAI studies is similar to that in Angiography. (See WARNINGS—General.)

Adverse Reactions
Cramping may occur during the injection and sometimes mild lower abdominal pain may be present for an hour or two afterwards. Even when the medium gains entrance into venous or lymphatic channels, systemic effects are rare. Generalized urticaria or slight transient hyperpyrexia, however, has been reported.

Dosage and Administration
Approximately 4 mL of HYPAQUE-M, 90 percent will fill the uterine cavity and an additional 3 mL to 4 mL will fill the fallopian tubes in normal subjects. A larger volume may be required in some disease states. Slow injection is advisable.

How Supplied: Vials of 50 mL, rubber stoppered, box of 25 (NDC 0024-0788-04)

HW-28-T

TELEPAQUE®
brand of iopanoic acid tablets, USP

℞

Description: TELEPAQUE, brand of iopanoic acid tablets, is a diagnostic enteral cholecystographic radiopaque agent used for radiographic visualization of the gallbladder and biliary tract. TELEPAQUE is an oral radiopaque medium for cholecystography and cholangiography. Each off-white, scored tablet contains 500 mg iopanoic acid. TELEPAQUE is a cream-colored solid which is insoluble in water. It contains 66.68 percent organically bound iodine. The molecular weight is 570.93.
TELEPAQUE is a substituted, triiodinated, benzoic acid derivative, and is chemically 3-amino-α-ethyl-2,4,6-triiodohydrocinnamic acid ($C_{11}H_{12}I_3NO_2$).

Clinical Pharmacology: The most important characteristic of contrast media is the iodine content. The relatively high atomic weight of iodine contributes sufficient radiodensity for radiographic contrast with surrounding tissues.
Diagnostic enteral radiopaque agents have few known pharmacological effects. They are moderately uricosuric. TELEPAQUE when absorbed systemically may have iodine-mediated thyrotropic effects described under PRECAUTIONS.

Pharmacokinetics
TELEPAQUE is absorbed by passive diffusion across the gastrointestinal mucosa. Absorption of the agent can be improved by increasing the gastrointestinal pH, drug solubility, and availability of bile salts.
Controversy exists regarding the effects of food on the absorption and clinical efficacy of the cholecystographic agents. In one study, the number of satisfactory cholecystograms obtained with iopanoic acid administered with a high-fat meal was greater than with a nonfat meal. However, the fat content of the meal had no significant effect on the number of satisfactory cholecystograms obtained with iopanoic acid. Therefore, recommendations regarding the size or content of the evening meal on the day prior to oral cholecystography are made at the discretion of the physician.
Once absorbed, oral cholecystographic agents enter the systemic circulation via the portal venous system. They are then transported to the liver and bound to plasma albumin. The affinity for albumin may determine the primary route of elimination, biliary or renal, with the more extensively bound agents primarily excreted by the hepatobiliary system.
In the liver, TELEPAQUE is metabolized to glucuronide esters which are then actively excreted into the hepatic ducts and concentrated by the gallbladder. The time of peak opacification of the gallbladder is approximately 14 to 19 hours for TELEPAQUE. However, diagnostically adequate visualization of gallbladder may occur within 5 to 6 hours.
TELEPAQUE is removed from the body by two pathways: excretion into the duodenum via the common bile duct and renal elimination. The ratio of renal to fecal elimination for TELEPAQUE is 75:25 respectively in normal subjects. It appears that the bulk of an administered dose is eliminated from the body within a week. However, effects on thyroid function tests may persist for longer periods.
Oral cholecystographic agents are excreted in breast milk. (See PRECAUTIONS—**Nursing Mothers.**)
Oral cholecystographic agents may produce changes in thyroid studies attributable to changes in circulating iodide. Thyroid function tests may not accurately reflect thyroid status for up to 1 year following cholecystography. Additionally, oral cholecystographic agents tend to elevate BSP (sulfobromophthalein) determinations. (See PRECAUTIONS—**Drug/Laboratory Test Interactions.**)

Indications and Usage: TELEPAQUE is indicated for use in oral cholecystography. It may also be used for oral cholangiography, although it is not considered the method of choice.

Contraindications: Administration of TELEPAQUE is contraindicated in severe impairment of renal function and particularly in advanced hepatorenal disease. It is also contraindicated in severe gastrointestinal disorders that prevent absorption, and in those patients who are allergic to iodinated compounds.

Precautions
General
Cholecystography in severely ill or debilitated patients or in those with severe hepatic or renal disease could result in partial or total renal shutdown.

Renal Effect
Acute renal insufficiency has followed the use of oral cholecystographic agents. Most reported cases were attributed to the use of large doses or multiple agents, to preexisting dehydration, or hepatic disease.
Patients with preexisting renal disease should not receive high doses of cholecystographic media. Possible renal irritation in susceptible individuals could result in reflex vascular spasm with partial or complete renal shutdown.

Liver Disease
TELEPAQUE is generally well tolerated by patients with moderately impaired liver function, and adequate gallbladder visualization can often be achieved in the presence of hepatic disease. However, severe, advanced liver disease (eg, bilirubin exceeding 5 mg per 100 mL) very frequently results in nonvisualization of the gallbladder.
Severe, advanced liver disease may interfere with metabolism of the radiopaque medium, and therefore, a greater amount of unchanged TELEPAQUE will be diverted for renal excretion, increasing the load on the kidneys. Although renal difficulty has rarely been attributed to TELEPAQUE, renal function in patients with severe, advanced liver disease should be assessed before cholecystography, and renal output and hepatic function should be observed for a few days after the procedure.

Dehydration
All patients, especially those with renal or hepatic diseases, should not be dehydrated beforehand and should drink liberal amounts of fluids after taking the tablets.

Uricosuric Effect
It has been shown that TELEPAQUE has uricosuric activity. Therefore, patients with hyperuricemia should be well hydrated to maintain adequate urinary output to prevent uric acid crystal formation.

Coronary Disease
Caution is advised in patients with coronary disorders, especially those with recent symptoms of coronary artery disease. Blood pressure should be observed after administration of cholecystographic media to these patients.

Thyroid Disease
Caution should be exercised when administering cholecystographic agents to hyperthyroid and euthyroid goiterous patients (see ADVERSE REACTIONS).

Elderly Patients
For elderly patients, see DOSAGE AND ADMINISTRATION.

Information for the Patient
Patients receiving oral cholecystographic agents should be given the following information and instructions.
This drug has been prescribed to perform an x-ray study of the gallbladder. All the medication must be taken with water following dinner the evening prior to the test. Thereafter, nothing except water should be taken until the test has been completed.
Patients should be questioned regarding medicines, including nonprescription drugs, currently being used. Allergies to iodine, any foods, or x-ray dyes should also be disclosed.
Patients should inform the physician of any liver or kidney disease or pregnancy before taking this drug.
Patients should consult the physician if, at some future date, any thyroid tests are planned. The iodine in this agent may interfere with later thyroid tests.
This drug may cause abdominal cramping, nausea, vomiting, diarrhea, skin rashes, itching, heartburn, dizziness or headache in some patients but most reactions are mild and pass quickly.

Drug Interactions
Concurrent administration of cholestyramine and iopanoic acid reportedly resulted in abnormal cholecystography. In vitro studies indicate that cholestyramine has an apparent high affinity for iopanoic acid. To avoid nonvisualization or poor visualization, oral cholecystogrphy should be performed after cholestyramine has been discontinued long enough for complete evacuation from at least the small bowel.
The administration of both oral cholecystographic agents and intravenous iodipamide meglumine within 24 hours is not recommended. The prior administration of an oral cholecystographic agent seems to block the hepatic excretion of the intravenously administered iodipamide meglumine. Renal toxicity has been reported in a few patients with liver dysfunction who were given oral cholecystographic agents followed by urographic agents. Administration of urographic agents should therefore be postponed in any patient with a known or suspected hepatic or biliary disorder who has recently taken a cholecystographic contrast agent.

Drug/Laboratory Test Interactions
Thyroid Function Tests
The results of PBI and RAI uptake studies, which depend on iodine estimations, will not reflect thyroid function for several months following administration of cholecystographic media. However, function tests not depending on iodine estimations, eg, T_3 resin uptake or free thyroxine assays, are not affected.

Liver Function Tests
Bilirubin, thymol turbidity, cephalin flocculation, and serum enzyme values are unaffected but TELEPAQUE may delay BSP clearance values for up to two days.

Urine Tests
Pseudoalbuminuria may be present for three days in response to certain chemical protein precipitation tests. Positive reactions should be verified by the heat-and-acetic acid or colorimetric dip-strip methods.

Uricosuric Effect
TELEPAQUE may increase the rate of excretion of uric acid, lowering blood levels and raising urinary excretion values for a few days.

Carcinogenesis, Mutagenesis, Impairment of Fertility
Long-term studies in animals have not been performed in order to evaluate the carcinogenic potential, mutagenesis, or whether TELEPAQUE can affect fertility in males or females.

Pregnancy Category C
Animal reproduction studies have not been conducted with TELEPAQUE. It is also not known whether TELEPAQUE can cause fetal harm when administered to a pregnant woman or can affect reproduction capacity. TELEPAQUE should be given to a pregnant woman only if clearly needed.

Nursing Mothers
TELEPAQUE is excreted in the milk of nursing mothers. Therefore, caution should be exercised when TELEPAQUE is administered.

Adverse Reactions: Most reactions following the oral administration of TELEPAQUE have been mild and transitory. Moderately severe reactions are unusual and severe reactions or morbidity is extremely rare.

Gastrointestinal: By far the most frequent adverse response to TELEPAQUE is gastrointestinal, mostly affecting the lower bowel (20%). Thus a few loose stools are common, frank diarrhea or abdominal cramps unusual and severe diarrhea with prostration is rare.

Mild nausea (10%) with vomiting (1%) is also frequent.

Allergic: (0.5%)—Skin, mucous membrane, and systemic hypersensitivity reactions are unusual and include urticaria with or without pruritus, erythema, morbilliform rash, and localized areas of edema. Rarely a systemic serum sickness-type reaction with fever, rash, and arthralgia. A few cases of transitory thrombocytopenia with petechiae have been reported.

Urinary: A mild stinging sensation during urination may occur (3%).

Hepatorenal and Cardiovascular: Very rare disturbances in function have been reported, usually occurring in patients with preexisting disease (see PRECAUTIONS—**General**).

Goiter: Cases of hyperthyroidism have been reported with the use of oral contrast media. Some of these patients reportedly had multinodular goiters which may have been responsible for the increased hormone synthesis in response to excess iodine. Thyroid storm has occurred in these patients.

Overdosage: A few cases of large overdoses of iopanoic acid have been reported, involving ingestion of 30 g, 36 g, and 75 g of the drug. Mild transient renal dysfunction was reported. All patients experienced extreme nausea, diarrhea, and vomiting, but survived without permanent adverse effects.

Based upon the clinical pharmacology of iopanoic acid, the following treatment measures are recommended. While specific recommendations for other enteral radiopaque agents are unavailable, the following measures may be beneficial:
• Lavage the stomach and administer enemas to remove remaining potentially absorbable contrast material.
• Force fluids to avoid concentration and possible precipitation or crystallization of the contrast material or uric acid in the kidneys.
• Alkalinize the urine to increase the solubility of the drug-glucuronide complex and of uric acid.
• Administer cholestyramine to chelate and reduce absorption of the drug.
• Monitor blood pressure.

The acute oral LD_{50} of iopanoic acid in the mouse is 6.6 ± 0.7 to 15.8 ± 1.1 g/kg $\pm$ Standard Error.

Dosage and Administration: The standard adult dose of 3 g (six tablets) administered individually is usually ingested with water in the evening after a fat-free dinner, about 14 hours before the cholecystography. In some instances, double doses of 6 g (12 tablets) may be ingested, eg, for duct visualization or for some repeat examinations made over 7 days later. Many radiologists prefer that the patient take a laxative (eg, castor oil) about four to six hours before ingesting TELEPAQUE. (See also Nonvisualization—Repeat Examination.) Preparatory dehydration is unnecessary and undesirable, especially in elderly patients.

The use of large or repeated doses over a number of days to force visualization of a poorly functioning gallbladder *in elderly patients* is not recommended.

DIET before Cholecystigraphy
Patients presenting for a cholecystogram are frequently on various types of diet, eg, weight reducing diet, gallbladder diet. In these diets the fat content is low or absent. The resulting gallbladder stasis often results in a viscous inspissated bile content in a distended bladder, making entry of TELEPAQUE opacified bile difficult. It is recommended, therefore, that these patients be placed on a normal (fat containing) diet for several days before TELEPAQUE cholecystography.

The Evening Meal—Fat Content
There is not a consensus as to whether or not the evening meal immediately prior to TELEPAQUE cholecystography should contain fat. This is based on the following two considerations:
• Fat is a prolonged cholecystogogue causing intermittent gallbladder emptying for up to eight hours. This renders accumulation and concentration by the healthy gallbladder difficult and may account for spurious nonvisualization on the first examination in some patients.
• A normal fat containing diet, including fat in the evening meal, promotes increased opacified bile flow facilitating gallbladder accumulation and concentration.

Both views are based on animal and clinical observation. The radiologist should choose which regimen for the patient to follow in preparation for the cholecystogram.

Fatty Meal after Cholecystography
After the gallbladder has been visualized the patient may be given a fat-containing meal or a commercially available cholecystagogue, for determining the extent and duration of gallbladder contractility (thus, the degree of function), to help identify small radiolucent stones or to visualize the bile ducts. In recent years most radiologists consider the value of the fat meal in this manner mostly unrewarding and have dispensed with its routine use.

Duct Visualization
Occasionally, the bile ducts may be visualized on the original film during cholecystography. However, in a substantial percentage of patients, administration of a fat is necessary. The more frequent the roentgenographic exposures, the greater the probability of visualization of the ducts; however, the best time intervals are usually 20 and 30 minutes after the fatty meal. Some investigators believe contrast in the ducts is enhanced by an increased dose of TELEPAQUE (up to 6 g).

Nonvisualization—Repeat Examination
Nonvisualization (or nondiagnostic faint visualization) following a primary examination can occur in up to 15% to 20% of cholecystographic examinations, irrespective of the medium used. This is only "indicative" evidence of gallbladder disease. There are, however, also a large number of extrabiliary diseases and situations which can result in nonvisualization. Following nonvisualization on the first examination, a repeat cholecystogram using a single dose is therefore indicated to exclude extrabiliary causes. The radiologic diagnosis is based on the results of the repeat examination. If nonvisualization also occurs following the second examination, gallbladder disease may be inferred with reasonable certainty (98% to 100%).

For repeat examination on the same day as the initial cholecystographic procedure, on additional 3 g (six tablets) may be given. However, if repeat cholecystography is to be performed with a double dose, a period of at least five to seven days should intervene between the first and the repeat examinations. No more than a total of 6 g (12 tablets) should be ingested during a 24-hour period.

How Supplied: Tablets of 500 mg, envelopes of 6 tablets, box of 25 (NDC 0024-1931-03)
Protect from light.

TW-27 X

This product information was effective as of December 3, 1984. On these and other products of Winthrop-Breon Laboratories, detailed information may be obtained on a current basis by direct inquiry to the Professional Services Department, 90 Park Avenue, New York, NY 10016 (212) 907-2525.

Conversion Tables

Metric Doses With Approximate Apothecary Equivalents

The approximate dose equivalents represent the quantities usually prescribed by physicians using, respectively, the metric and apothecary system of weights and measures. When prepared dosage forms such as tablets, capsules, etc. are prescribed in the metric system, the pharmacist may dispense the corresponding approximate equivalent in the apothecary system and vice versa. (Note: A milliliter [mL] is the approximate equivalent of a cubic centimeter [cc]). Exact equivalents, which appear in the United States Pharmacopeia and the National Formulary, must be used to calculate quantities in pharmaceutical formulas and prescription compounding:

LIQUID MEASURE Metric	Approximate Apothecary Equivalents	LIQUID MEASURE Metric	Approximate Apothecary Equivalents	LIQUID MEASURE Metric	Approximate Apothecary Equivalents	LIQUID MEASURE Metric	Approximate Apothecary Equivalents
1000 mL	1 quart	3 mL	45 minims	30 mL	1 fluid ounce	0.25 mL	4 minims
750 mL	1½ pints	2 mL	30 minims	15 mL	4 fluid drams	0.2 mL	3 minims
500 mL	1 pint	1 mL	15 minims	10 mL	2½ fluid drams	0.1 mL	1½ minims
250 mL	8 fluid ounces	0.75 mL	12 minims	8 mL	2 fluid drams	0.06 mL	1 minim
200 mL	7 fluid ounces	0.6 mL	10 minims	5 mL	1¼ fluid drams	0.05 mL	¾ minim
100 mL	3½ fluid ounces	0.5 mL	8 minims	4 mL	1 fluid dram	0.03 mL	½ minim
50 mL	1¾ fluid ounces	0.3 mL	5 minims				

WEIGHT Metric	Approximate Apothecary Equivalents	WEIGHT Metric	Approximate Apothecary Equivalents	WEIGHT Metric	Approximate Apothecary Equivalents	WEIGHT Metric	Approximate Apothecary Equivalents
30g	1 ounce	30mg	1/2 grain	500mg	7½ grains	1.2 mg	1/50 grain
15g	4 drams	25mg	3/8 grain	400mg	6 grains	1 mg	1/60 grain
10g	2½ drams	20mg	1/3 grain	300mg	5 grains	800 µg	1/80 grain
7.5g	2 drams	15mg	1/4 grain	250mg	4 grains	600 µg	1/100 grain
6g	90 grains	12mg	1/5 grain	200mg	3 grains	500 µg	1/120 grain
5g	75 grains	10mg	1/6 grain	150mg	2½ grains	400 µg	1/150 grain
4g	60 grains (1 dram)	8mg	1/8 grain	125mg	2 grains	300 µg	1/200 grain
3g	45 grains	6mg	1/10 grain	100mg	1½ grains	250 µg	1/250 grain
2g	30 grains (½ dram)	5mg	1/12 grain	75mg	1¼ grains	200 µg	1/300 grain
1.5g	22 grains	4mg	1/15 grain	60mg	1 grain	150 µg	1/400 grain
1g	15 grains	3mg	1/20 grain	50mg	¼ grain	120 µg	1/500 grain
750mg	12 grains	2mg	1/30 grain	40mg	⅔ grain	100 µg	1/600 grain
600mg	10 grains	1.5mg	1/40 grain				

Approximate Household Equivalents

For household purposes, an American Standard Teaspoon is defined by the American National Standards Institute as containing 4.93 ± 0.24 mL. The USP states that in view of the almost universal practice of employing teaspoons ordinarily available in the household for administration of medicine, the teaspoon may be regarded as representing 5 mL. Household units of measure often are used to inform patients of the size of a liquid dose. Because of difficulties involved in measuring liquids under normal conditions of use, household spoons are not appropriate when accurate measurement of a liquid dose is required. When accurate measurement of a liquid dose is required, the USP recommends that a calibrated oral syringe or dropper be used.

1 fluid dram = 1 teaspoonful = 5 mL
2 fluid drams = 1 dessertspoonful = 10 mL
4 fluid drams = 1 tablespoonful = 15 mL
2 fluid ounces = 1 wineglassful = 60 mL
4 fluid ounces = 1 teacupful = 120 mL
8 fluid ounces = 1 tumblerful = 240 mL

Temperature Conversion Table:

$9 \times °C = (5 \times °F) - 160$

Centigrade to Fahrenheit = $(°C \times 9/5) + 32 = °F$
Fahrenheit to Centigrade = $(°F - 32) \times 5/9 = °C$

Milliequivalents per Liter (mEq/L)

$$mEq/L = \frac{\text{weight of salt (g)} \times \text{valence of ion} \times 1000}{\text{molecular weight of salt}}$$

$$\text{weight of salt (g)} = \frac{mEq/L \times \text{molecular weight of salt}}{\text{valence of ion} \times 1000}$$

Pounds—Kilograms (kg) Conversion

1 pound = 0.453592 kg
1 kg = 2.2 pounds

GUIDE TO MANAGEMENT OF DRUG OVERDOSE

Prepared by:
Eric G. Comstock, M.D.
and
Eugene V. Boisaubin, M.D.
Department of Medicine
Baylor College of Medicine
Houston, Texas

INTRODUCTION: The following discussion is designed for use in adult patients. In the pediatric age group, general principles apply, but the volumes of fluid or suggested medication must be adjusted for body size. Symptomatic and supportive care is the basis for treatment of drug overdose. All other approaches are secondary. Procedures directed toward the offending substance, such as the performance of gastric lavage or the administration of a specific pharmacologic antagonist, should be undertaken only after adequate vital function has been assured. Procedures to facilitate excretion of toxic substances, such as peritoneal or extracorporeal dialysis and forced diuresis are required infrequently, and should never be relied upon as the primary approach to treatment. For sedative, hypnotic, and tranquilizer drugs, alone or in combination, supportive care is sufficient as outlined in the following discussion.

INITIAL ASSESSMENT: If the patient is symptomatic, determine the adequacy of respiration and cardiac function and note reflex activity, such as pupillary, corneal, gag and deep tendon. If vital function is compromised, or consciousness is impaired, proceed immediately to supportive measures.

THE ASYMPTOMATIC PATIENT: The drug overdosed patient may be asymptomatic because he has not ingested a sufficient dose of the drugs, or because a sufficient quantity has not been absorbed to produce symptoms. After the ingestion of a life threatening quantity of drugs, symptoms may be delayed as long as six hours, although ordinarily symptoms are manifested within thirty (30) minutes to two (2) hours. Ingestion of alcohol simultaneoulsy with drugs may shorten the time for symptoms to appear. Vomiting should be induced only during the asymptomatic interval. If significant central nervous system depression intervenes between the administration of emetic and the occurrence of vomiting, then the airway should be protected by insertion of a cuffed endotracheal tube. Fluids must be forced orally to obtain satisfactory results from any effort to induce vomiting. An alternate approach to the asymptomatic patient alleged to have ingested drugs, is the administration by mouth of a slurry of no less than 100 grams of activated charcoal powder (USP) in water. Gastric lavage with a large caliber tube (34 French) may be performed in the asymptomatic patient. Any patient whose consciousness is impaired to the point where a cuffed endotracheal tube will be tolerated should be intubated prior to the performance of gastric lavage.

THE SYMPTOMATIC PATIENT: If the patient is symptomatic all treatment procedures directed toward the toxic substance are secondary to the support of vital function. If the patient is in coma, attention to respiratory support and cardiac function should proceed immediately.

RESPIRATORY SUPPORT: Examine the mouth. Remove all foreign material including dentures. Position the head so that respiration is not sonorous and so that regurgitated stomach contents are not readily aspirated. If respiration is not present, provide ventilation by mouth-to-mouth, ambu bag, or positive pressure respirator until the patient is adequately oxygenated. Insert an oropharyngeal airway and suction excess secretions while preparing to insert an endotracheal tube. A cuffed endotracheal tube should be inserted and inflated. Bronchial suction should be administered to clear mucus and foreign material. Determine that the chest is being inflated symmetrically and that breath sounds are audible bilaterally. After the acute emergency, determine placement of the endotracheal tube by x-ray. Monitor adequacy of ventilation using arterial blood gases.

IV ACCESS AND CARDIAC FUNCTION: While one member of the treatment team is assuring adequate ventilation, a second member of the team should be assuring adequate IV access by insertion of an 18 gauge venous catheter and initiation of IV fluid administration such as Ringers Lactate or $\frac{1}{2}$ normal saline at a maintenance rate in adults of 150 ml. per hour. Since hypotension from sedative drug intoxication results from relative hypovolemia complicated frequently by dehydration, the rate of intravenous infusion should be increased to 10-20 cc per minute if the systolic pressure is under 80 mm of mercury. Placing the patient in the Trendelenburg position may quickly correct small to moderate degrees of hypotension. A central venous pressure catheter or a Swan-Ganz catheter is required if the continuous high rate infusion reaches one (1) liter within one hour or if the positive fluid balance exceeds two (2) liters during the first two hours. Intermittent monitoring of central venous pressure should continue throughout the period of intensive supportive care. A baseline electrocardiogram should be obtained as soon as vital functions have been supported. The appearance of conduction defects should lead to suspicion of drugs with direct cardiac effects, such as the tricyclic antidepressants. In uncomplicated sedative drug overdose, the central venous pressure will be under ten centimeters of water and will not change appreciably with high volume fluid infusion. If the central venous pressure increases abruptly in excess of five centimeters of water, or if the CVP exceeds 16 centimeters of water, high rate fluid infusion should be stopped pending evaluation of cardiac status. Adequate tissue perfusion is obtained with a systolic pressure in the range of 80 to 100 milliliters of mercury. A systolic pressure higher than this is required only in the patient with pre-existing hypertension. The formation of urine is an indication that tissue perfusion is adequate.

URINARY CATHETERIZATION: An in-dwelling urinary catheter should be inserted early in the course of treatment of any unconscious drug overdose patient. Upon insertion of the catheter, the volume of residual urine should be measured and the specimen should be saved separately for urinalysis including specific gravity, labeled for drug analysis, and sent to the laboratory to be retained for 24 hours. Recording of urine output hourly is necessary to maintain fluid balance records. Abrupt cessation of urine output most frequently is due to an obstructed catheter, but deserves immediate appraisal. Anuria for a period in excess of one hour should lead to reduction of high rate intravascular volume infusion until cardiac and renal status has been reappraised. Failure to achieve adequate urinary output after initial emptying of the bladder may reflect uncompensated dehydration and relative hypovolemia, each of which must be corrected before balanced fluid intake and output plus insensible loss can be achieved. The immediate or automatic use of diuretics at this stage only aggravates the basic defect and may result in intractable hypotension. Addition of vasopressor drugs at this stage may precipitate renal failure. Electrolyte solutions as transient volume expanders are preferred to whole